# Martindale

## The complete drug reference

**Thirty-fourth edition**

Edited by

**Sean C Sweetman**

BPharm, FRPharmS

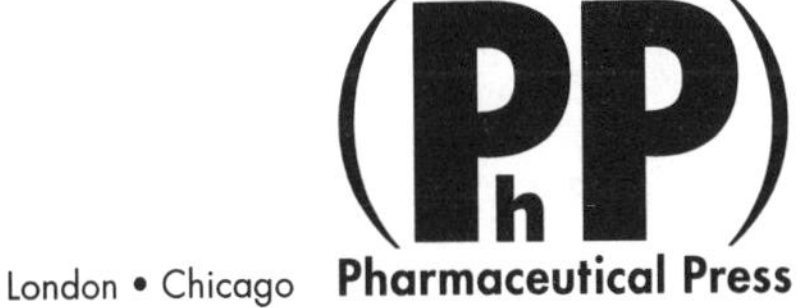


London • Chicago Pharmaceutical Press

**Published by the Pharmaceutical Press**
Publications division of the Royal Pharmaceutical Society of Great Britain

1 Lambeth High Street, London SEI 7JN, UK
100 South Atkinson Road, Suite 206, Grayslake, IL 60030-7820, USA



First edition of *Martindale: The Extra Pharmacopoeia* was published in 1883. *Squire's Companion* was incorporated in the twenty-third edition in 1952.

Thirty-fourth edition published 2005

Printed in Great Britain by William Clowes, Suffolk

ISBN 0 85369 550 4

ISSN 0263-5364



*A catalogue record for this book is available from the British Library*

# Martindale: The Complete Drug Reference

*Editor:* Sean C Sweetman, BPharm, FRPharmS

*Senior Assistant Editor:* Paul S Blake, BPharm, GradDipHealthInformatics, MRPharmS

*Assistant Editors:* Julie M McGlashan, BPharm, DipInfSc, MRPharmS
Gail C Neathercoat, BSc, MRPharmS
Anne V Parsons, BPharm, MRPharmS

*Staff Editors:* Bosede O Abe, BSc, BPharm, MRPharmS
Alison Brayfield, BPharm, MRPharmS
Catherine RM Cadart, BPharm, GradDipHospPharm, MRPharmS
Kathleen Eager, BPharm, MRPharmS
Prakash Gotecha, BSc, MRPharmS
Susan L Handy, BPharm, DipClinPharm, MRPharmS
Sue W Ho, BPharm, MRPharmS
Bryce H Kivell, BPharm, MRPharmS, MPS (NZ)
Valerie A Lee, BSc, CertPharmPractice, MRPharmS
Keith S Riley, BPharm, MRPharmS
Louise M Sheridan, BPharm, MRPharmS
Sandra Sutton, BPharm, MSc Med, Cert Proj Mngt, SAPC (SA)
Gerda W Viedge, BPharm, MRPharmS, DO

*Editorial Assistant:* Marian E Quinn, BSc, MSc

*Clerical Assistants:* Christine L Iskandar
Claire R Ryan

# Contents

Preface v

Abbreviations vii

Contracted Names for Ions and Groups ix

Atomic Weights of the Elements x

**Part 1 • Monographs on drugs and ancillary substances**

Analgesics Anti-inflammatory Drugs and Antipyretics 1

Anthelmintics 97

Antibacterials 116

Antidepressants 278

Antidiabetics 324

Antiepileptics 349

Antifungals 386

Antigout Drugs 412

Antihistamines 419

Antimalarials 444

Antimigraine Drugs 464

Antimuscarinics 475

Antineoplastics 492

Antiprotozoals 595

Antivirals 618

Anxiolytic Sedatives Hypnotics and Antipsychotics 663

Blood Products Plasma Expanders and Haemostatics 732

Bone Modulating Drugs 762

Bronchodilators and Anti-asthma Drugs 777

Cardiovascular Drugs 809

Chelators Antidotes and Antagonists 1030

Colouring Agents 1056

Contrast Media 1059

Corticosteroids 1068

Cough Suppressants Expectorants Mucolytics and Nasal Decongestants 1112

Dermatological Drugs and Sunscreens 1133

Disinfectants and Preservatives 1164

Dopaminergics 1196

Electrolytes 1217

Gases 1235

Gastrointestinal Drugs 1239

General Anaesthetics 1295

Hypothalamic and Pituitary Hormones 1312

Immunosuppressants 1344

Local Anaesthetics 1367

Muscle Relaxants 1386

Neuromuscular Blockers 1397

Nonionic Surfactants 1411

Nutritional Agents and Vitamins 1417

Organic Solvents 1471

Paraffins and Similar Bases 1479

Parasympathomimetics 1484

Pesticides and Repellents 1499

Prostaglandins 1511

Radiopharmaceuticals 1522

Sex Hormones 1527

Soaps and Other Anionic Surfactants 1574

Stabilising and Suspending Agents 1576

Stimulants and Anorectics 1583

Thyroid and Antithyroid Drugs 1594

Vaccines Immunoglobulins and Antisera 1605

**Part 2 • Supplementary drugs and other substances** 1645

**Part 3 • Preparations** 1767

**Directory of Manufacturers** 2397

**General Index** 2443

# Preface

The aim of Martindale is to provide healthcare professionals with unbiased evaluated information on drugs and medicines used throughout the world. It therefore has to develop as the body of knowledge on existing drugs grows, new drugs emerge, new preparations are launched, and old preparations are abandoned, reformulated, or redefined. It also has to reflect the changing needs of those practising pharmacy and medicine. We try to ensure that each new edition continues to meet all these needs.

Since the 31st edition, Martindale has been published every 3 years. To meet the need for more up-to-date information this edition has been produced in 2½ years. For those who require even more up-to-date information from Martindale there are various electronic versions, sections of which are updated more frequently.

All the drug monographs from the last edition have been revised, more than 110 having been deleted and more than 220 added, and organised into chapters that reflect the uses of the drugs being described. The chapter on Antineoplastics and Immunosuppressants has now been split into its two main drug types whereas the chapter on Sunscreens has been incorporated into the chapter on Dermatological Drugs.

The disease treatment reviews, 649 in all and generally located in the chapter introductions, have also been thoroughly revised in order to reflect current trends and provide key references. Cross-references to these reviews appear in the monographs of the drugs cited; the reviews can also be accessed via the general index. It is hoped that these reviews will be of use to readers who want an overview of a particular disease and its drug treatment and will provide a useful starting point for those who want to pursue particular aspects further.

The information on proprietary preparations, an important feature of Martindale, has been updated and a much wider range of countries has been covered for this edition.

Martindale is based on published information and more than 37 500 selected references are included. The amount of drug information now published electronically has increased significantly since the last printed edition of Martindale and this edition now includes nearly 1000 citations to material available on the Internet as web pages.

Our aim is to evaluate the literature, covering important studies, guidelines, and useful reviews and placing them in context. Multicentre studies, meta-analyses, and systematic reviews play an important role in the study of drug treatment, and their findings and conclusions are considered in many of our chapters. However, there is also a place for the anecdotal report and the small study, and information from such sources is included where appropriate. Acknowledgement is also given to information referenced from a number of authoritative sources including the *British National Formulary*, the *British Pharmacopoeia*, the *European Pharmacopoeia*, the *United States National Formulary*, and the *United States Pharmacopeia*.

The year 2003 saw the publication of the first Spanish edition of Martindale, the translation having been undertaken by our colleagues at Grupo Ars XXI. As a result of the close co-operation between the two teams the reader will notice that the coverage of Spanish drug synonyms has been greatly expanded.

Once again strenuous editorial efforts have been made to produce a book of manageable size without sacrificing content. The use of more headings and other changes to the typography and layout have been introduced to improve readability.

Martindale is not a book of standards. Inclusion of a substance or a preparation is not to be considered as a recommendation for use, nor does it confer any status on the substance or preparation. While considerable efforts have been made to check the material in Martindale, the publisher cannot accept any responsibility for errors and omissions. Also the reader is assumed to possess the necessary knowledge to interpret the information that Martindale provides.

## Arrangement

PART 1 (pages 1–1644) contains 4418 monographs arranged in 51 chapters. These chapters generally bring together monographs on drugs and groups of drugs that have similar uses or actions. The introductions of those chapters that describe drugs used in the management of disease may contain disease treatment reviews—descriptions of those diseases together with reviews of the choice of treatments.

PART 2 (pages 1645–1766) consists of a series of 926 monographs arranged in the alphabetical order of their main titles. It includes monographs on drugs not easily classified, on herbals, and on drugs no longer used clinically but still of interest. There are also monographs on toxic substances, the effects of which may require drug therapy.

PART 3 (pages 1767–2396) contains proprietary preparations from a range of countries. For this edition we have covered Argentina, Australia, Austria, Belgium, Brazil, Canada, Chile, Denmark, Finland, France, Germany, Greece, Hong Kong, India, Ireland, Israel, Italy, Malaysia, Mexico, the Netherlands, New Zealand, Norway, Portugal, Singapore, South Africa, Spain, Sweden, Switzerland, Thailand, the United Arab Emirates, UK, and USA. We have also included some proprietary preparations from Japan. The information provided includes the proprietary name, the manufacturer or distributor, the active ingredients with cross-references to the drug monographs, and a summary of the indications as given by the manufacturer.

## Indexes

DIRECTORY OF MANUFACTURERS. In Martindale the names of manufacturers and distributors are abbreviated. Their full names are given in this directory together with the full address if it is available. This directory contains some 9500 entries.

GENERAL INDEX. To make fullest use of the contents of Martindale the general index should always be consulted. The exhaustive index includes entries for drugs (approved names, synonyms, and chemical names), preparations, pharmacological and therapeutic groups, and clinical uses (disease treatment reviews). As in previous editions, the index is arranged alphabetically 'word-by-word' rather than 'letter-by-letter'. The index indicates the column in which the relevant entry appears as well as the page.

## Nomenclature

TITLES AND SYNONYMS. The title of each monograph is in English, with preference usually being given to International Nonproprietary Names (INN), British Approved Names (BAN), and United States Adopted Names (USAN). These 3 authorities are shown where appropriate. A European Directive (92/27/EEC) requires the use of Recommended International Nonproprietary Names (rINNs) in the labelling of medicinal products throughout member states of the European Community and where the BAN and INN differed in the past the BAN has been changed to accord with the rINN. The major exception to this convention is the retention of the names adrenaline and noradrenaline, these being the terms used as the titles of the monographs in the European Pharmacopoeia and therefore the official names in the member states. In some approved names it is now general policy to use 'f' for 'ph' in sulpha, 't' for 'th', and 'i' for 'y'; for this reason entries in alphabetical lists and indexes should be sought in alternative spellings if the expected spellings are not found. Inevitably there may be some inconsistencies of style with older approved names but wherever possible the names used for drugs or radicals in Martindale have been altered in accordance with the guidelines on the use of INNs for pharmaceutical substances. A table of contracted names for ions and groups used in approved names and titles is given on page ix. BAN names for substance combinations and United States Pharmacy Equivalent Names (PEN) for dosage forms containing two or more active ingredients are given in the text of the relevant mongraphs; these names start with the prefix 'Co-'.

This section also includes names given as synonyms such as commonly used abbreviated names; Latin versions of the titles in the European Pharmacopoeia; English, American, and Latin synonyms; names used in other languages when these may not be readily identifiable; manufacturers' code numbers; and chemical names. Official titles and synonyms used in the British, European, and US Pharmacopoeias are given in the section on pharmacopoeias where the relevant pharmacopoeial substance is described.

CAS REGISTRY NUMBERS. Chemical Abstracts Service (CAS) registry numbers are provided, where available, for each monograph substance to help readers refer to other information systems. Numbers for various forms of the monograph substance are listed with the variation in form given in parentheses.

ATC CODES. Codes from the Anatomical Therapeutic Chemical (ATC) classification system (see http://www.whocc.no) have been provided, where available, for each monograph substance to help readers refer to other information systems.

## Atomic and Molecular Weights

Atomic weights are based on the table of Atomic Weights as revised in 2001 by the Commission on Atomic Weights and Isotopic Abundance, International Union of Pure and Applied Chemistry (IUPAC) and based on the $^{12}C$ scale (see page x). Molecular weights are given corrected to one place of decimals or to four significant figures for relative weights of less than 100.

## Pharmacopoeias

The selected pharmacopoeias in which each substance appears are listed. A description of the substance and a summary of the pharmaceutical information (see below) that appears in the British, European, or US Pharmacopoeias is also included. Current copies of the pharmacopoeias and their addenda should be consulted for confirmation and for details of standards.

The pharmacopoeias covered include: *British, British Veterinary, Chinese, European, French, German, International, Italian, Japanese, Polish, Spanish, Swiss, United States* (including the *National Formulary*), and *Vietnamese*. They either appeared as new editions or were revised by supplements since the last edition of Martindale, and have been examined for this 34th edition.

The abbreviations for these pharmacopoeias are included in the list of abbreviations used in Martindale, see page vii, which also includes details of the edition and/or supplement(s) consulted.

Several countries are parties to the Convention on the Elaboration of a European Pharmacopoeia. This means that they must adopt the standards of the European Pharmacopoeia. These countries are currently Austria, Belgium, Bosnia and Herzegovina, Croatia, Cyprus, the Czech Republic, Denmark, Estonia, Finland, France, Germany, Greece, Hungary, Iceland, Ireland, Italy, Latvia, Luxembourg, the Netherlands, Norway, Portugal, Romania, Serbia and Montenegro, Slovak Republic, Slovenia, Spain, Sweden, Switzerland, Turkey, the United Kingdom, and the Former Yugoslav Republic of Macedonia. Hence the European Pharmacopoeia is cited in the drug monograph lists of pharmacopoeias rather than these individual national pharmacopoeias.

Official preparations, mainly from the current British, European, and US Pharmacopoeias, are listed at the end of drug monographs.

## Pharmaceutical Information

Information on the chemical and physical properties of each substance is given when it is likely to be of use or interest, but only when it is certain that it applies to the form of substance being described in the monograph.

PERCENTAGE STRENGTHS. Unless otherwise stated, solutions of solids in liquids are expressed as percentage w/v, of liquids in liquids as percentage v/v, and of gases in liquids as percentage w/w.

SOLUBILITY. The figures given for solubility in each monograph have generally been obtained from the major pharmacopoeias in which the substance is described, but should not be considered absolute. Unless otherwise indicated in the text, the figures are for solubility at temperatures between 15° and 25°. The information usually relates to w/v solubilities but in some cases is v/v if the monograph substance itself is a liquid. Where solubilities are given in words, the following terms describe the indicated solubility ranges:

| **solubility** | |
|---|---|
| very soluble | 1 in less than 1 |
| freely soluble | 1 in 1 to 1 in 10 |
| soluble | 1 in 10 to 1 in 30 |
| sparingly soluble | 1 in 30 to 1 in 100 |
| slightly soluble | 1 in 100 to 1 in 1000 |
| very slightly soluble | 1 in 1000 to 1 in 10 000 |
| practically insoluble | 1 in more than 10 000 |

STORAGE. Substances and preparations should be stored under conditions which prevent contamination and diminish deterioration, and the conditions of storage given in the text indicate the precautions recommended in specific cases. The term 'a cool place' is generally used to describe a place in which the temperature is between 8° and 15°. In general, the storage conditions apply to the monograph substance and not its solutions or preparations.

TEMPERATURE. Temperatures are expressed in degrees Celsius (centigrade) unless otherwise indicated.

## Pharmacological and Therapeutic Information

Information on adverse effects, treatment of adverse effects, precautions (including contra-indications), interactions, pharmacokinetics, and uses and administration of each substance is provided by concise statements and these may be elaborated and expanded by referenced reviews and abstracts from papers and other publications. This edition contains about 13 000 such abstracts or reviews based on information in an ever widening range of publications.

Much information has been found in sources such as World Health Organization publications, government reports and legislation, and other official and standard publications. Manufacturers' literature has been considered in the light of other available information.

The risks of administering drugs in pregnancy are well known and the general principle is to give a drug only when the benefit to the individual mother outweighs the risk to the fetus. Where there is a clear risk it is noted under the Precautions or Adverse Effects heading but safety should not be inferred from the absence of a statement for any drug.

Some drugs given to the mother are distributed into breast milk and therefore may pose a risk to a breast-fed infant. Whenever possible, information has been included to help determine the safety of continuing to breast feed while the mother is receiving a particular drug. Safety during breast feeding should not be inferred from the absence of a statement for any drug.

## Doses

Doses are described under the Uses and Administration heading with as much detail as is necessary and available. Unless otherwise stated the doses represent the average range of quantities which are generally regarded as suitable for adults when administered by mouth. More information on doses and drug administration may be given in the abstracts or reviews. Unless otherwise specified, glucose injection is 5% w/v and sodium chloride injection is 0.9% w/v.

When doses for children are expressed as a range of quantities within specified age limits, the lower dose applies at the lower age and the higher dose at the higher age.

## Acknowledgements

The Editor gratefully acknowledges the advice and assistance of the many experts who have suggested amendments to the text of Martindale. Thanks are due to G Duncan, K Galbraith, PR Jackson, PM Mason, SJ Shankie, G Vernon, and N Wilson-Baig for reading and commenting on drafts of the 34th edition. Thanks are also due to K Baxter, IH Stockley, and P St Leger for advice and comments on specific issues during revision. The Editor is grateful to the many organisations that have helped in providing information, including the World Health Organization, the British Pharmacopoeia Commission, P.R. Vademecum, and our Spanish colleagues at Grupo Ars XXI.

Martindale staff have been able to call on the expertise of other members of the Royal Pharmaceutical Society's staff. In particular the Editor is grateful to DK Mehta and the staff of the British National Formulary, and the staff of the library and information department. Thanks are due to I Baxter, M Davis, S Driver, LY Galichet, M Kouimtzi, EJ Laughton, CR Lee, R McLarney, SC Owen, and SJ Shankie for their editorial tasks. Thanks are also due to C Fry the Society's Director of Publications and to the staff of the Pharmaceutical Press for their support.

The contents of this 34th edition were planned, written, checked, indexed, keyed, proofed, and processed by the Martindale staff. The Editor is pleased to acknowledge the skills and commitment of all the Martindale staff and to record his gratitude: to Christine Iskandar and Claire Ryan for clerical assistance; to Marian Quinn for editorial assistance; to the Staff Editors Bosede Abe, Alison Brayfield, Catherine Cadart, Kathleen Eager, Prakash Gotecha, Sue Handy, Sue Ho, Bryce Kivell, Valerie Lee, Keith Riley, Louise Sheridan, Sandra Sutton, and Gerda Viedge; to the Assistant Editors Julie McGlashan, Gail Neathercoat, and Anne Parsons; and to the Senior Assistant Editor Paul Blake.

London August 2004

# Abbreviations

For abbreviations of the names of manufacturers or their distributors, see Directory of Manufacturers, p.2397.

**ACE**—angiotensin-converting enzyme.
**agg.**—aggregate (in botanical names), including 2 or more species which resemble each other closely.
**AIDS**—acquired immunodeficiency syndrome.
**a.m.**—*ante meridiem*, 'before noon'.
**ARC**—AIDS-related complex.
***Arg.***—Argentina.
**ATC**—Anatomical Therapeutic Chemical classification.
***Austral.***—Australia.
**BAN**—British Approved Name.
**BANM**—British Approved Name Modified.
***Belg.***—Belgium.
**BMA**—British Medical Association.
**b.p.**—boiling point.
**BP**—British Pharmacopoeia. Unless otherwise specified, BP references are to the 2003 edition.
**BP(Vet)**—British Pharmacopoeia (Veterinary) 2003.
**BPC**—British Pharmaceutical Codex.
***Br.***—British.
***Braz.***—Brazil.
**BUN**—Blood-urea-nitrogen.
**°C**—degrees Celsius (centigrade). Unless otherwise indicated in the text, temperatures are expressed in this thermometric scale.
***Canad.***—Canada.
**CAPD**—continuous ambulatory peritoneal dialysis.
***CAS***—Chemical Abstracts Service.
**CCPD**—continuous cycle peritoneal dialysis.
**CDC**—Centers for Disease Control (USA).
***Chin. P.***—Chinese Pharmacopoeia 2000.
**CI**—Colour Index.
**CNS**—central nervous system.
**cP**—centipoise(s).
**CPMP**—Committee on Proprietary Medicinal Products of the European Union.
**CRM**—the former Committee on the Review of Medicines (UK).
**CSF**—cerebrospinal fluid.
**CSM**—Committee on Safety of Medicines (UK).
**cSt**—centistokes.
**D & C**—designation applied in USA to dyes permitted for use in drugs and cosmetics.
**d.c.**—direct current.
***Denm.***—Denmark.
**DHSS**—the former Department of Health and Social Security (UK).
**dL**—decilitre(s).
**DNA**—deoxyribonucleic acid.
**DoH**—Department of Health (UK).
**DTF**—Drug Tariff Formulary.
**ECG**—electrocardiogram.
**ECT**—electroconvulsive therapy.
***Ecuad.***—Ecuador.
**ed.**—editor(s) *or* edited by *or* edition.
**EEC**—European Economic Community, now the European Union.
**EEG**—electro-encephalogram.
**e.g.**—*exempli gratia* 'for example'.
**ENL**—erythema nodosum leprosum.
**ESRD**—end-stage renal disease.
***et al.***—*et alii*, 'and others': for three or more co-authors or co-workers.
***et seq.***—and what follows.
**EU**—European Union.
***Eur. P.***—see Ph. Eur.
**Ext. D & C**—designation applied in USA to dyes permitted for use in external drug and cosmetic preparations.
**°F**—degrees Fahrenheit.
**FAC**—Food Additives and Contaminants Committee of the former Ministry of
Agriculture, Fisheries and Food (UK).
**FAO**—Food and Agriculture Organization of the United Nations.
**FAO/WHO**—Food and Agriculture Organization of the United Nations *and the* World Health Organization.
**FDA**—Food and Drug Administration of USA.
**FdAC**—Food Advisory Committee of the former Ministry of Agriculture, Fisheries and Food (UK).
**FD & C**—designation applied in USA to dyes permitted for use in foods, drugs, and cosmetics.
**$FEV_1$**—forced expiratory volume in 1 second.
***Fin.***—Finland.
**FIP**—Fédération Internationale Pharmaceutique.
**f.p.**—freezing point.
**FPA**—Family Planning Association (UK).
***Fr.***—France.
***Fr. P.***—French Pharmacopoeia 1982 (Pharmacopée Francaise, X$^e$ Edition) and updates up to 2003.
**g**—gram(s).
***Ger.***—Germany.
***Ger. P.***— German Pharmacopoeia (Deutsches Arzneibuch, 2003).
**GFR**—glomerular filtration rate.
***Gr.***—Greece.
**Hb**— haemoglobin.
**Hib**—*Haemophilus influenzae* type b.
**HIV**—human immunodeficiency virus.
**HLA**—human lymphocyte antigens.
**HLB**—hydrophilic-lipophilic balance.
**HRT**—hormone replacement therapy.
**HSE**—Health and Safety Executive (UK).
***Hung.***—Hungary.
**IARC**—International Agency for Research on Cancer.
***ibid.***—*ibidem*, 'in the same place (journal or book)'.
***idem***—'the same': used for the same authors and titles.
**i.e.**—*id est*, 'that is'.
**Ig**—immunoglobulin.
**INN**—International Nonproprietary Name.
**INNM**—International Nonproprietary Name Modified.
***Int. P.***—International Pharmacopoeia 3rd ed., Volume 1, 1979; Volume 2, 1981; Volume 3, 1988; Volume 4, 1994; and Volume 5, 2003.
**IPCS**—International Programme on Chemical Safety.
**IQ**—intelligence quotient.
***Irl.***—Ireland.
**ISH**—International Society of Hypertension.
***It. P.***—Italian Pharmacopoeia 11ed., 2002 (Farmacopea Ufficiale della Repubblica Italiana, XI Edizione, 2002).
***Ital.***—Italy.
**IUD**—intra-uterine device.
**IUPAC**—International Union of Pure and Applied Chemistry.
**J**—joule(s).
***Jpn***—Japan.
***Jpn P.***—The Pharmacopoeia of Japan, 14th ed., 2001 and Supplement 1.

**K**—kelvin.
**kcal**—kilocalorie(s).
**kg**—kilogram(s).
**kJ**—kilojoule(s).
**lb**—pound(s) avoirdupois.
**$LD_{50}$**—a dose lethal to 50% of the specified animals or micro-organisms.
**m**—metre(s).
**$m^2$**—square metre(s).
**$m^3$**—cubic metre(s).
**M**—molar.
**MAFF**—the former Ministry of Agriculture, Fisheries and Food (UK), now Department of Environment, Food, and Rural Affairs (DeFRA).
**MAOI**—monoamine oxidase inhibitor.
**max.**—maximum.
**MBC**—minimum bactericidal concentration.
**MCA**—Medicines Control Agency (UK).
**mEq**—milliequivalent(s).
***Mex.***—Mexico.
**mg**—milligram(s).
**MIC**—minimum inhibitory concentration.
**min**—minute.
**min.**—minimum.
**MJ**—megajoule(s).
**mL**—millilitre(s).
**mm**—millimetre(s).
**$mm^2$**—square millimetre(s).
**$mm^3$**—cubic millimetre(s).
**mmHg**—millimetre(s) of mercury.
**mmol**—millimole.
**mol**—mole.
**mol. wt**—molecular weight.
***Mon.***—Monaco.
**mosmol**—milliosmole.
**m.p.**—melting point.
**MRC**—Medical Research Council (UK).
**μg**—microgram(s).
**μm**—micrometre(s).
***Neth.***—The Netherlands.
**NIH**—National Institutes of Health (USA).
**nm**—nanometre(s).
**NMDA**—*N*-methyl-D-aspartate.
***Norw.***—Norway.
**NSAID**—nonsteroidal anti-inflammatory drug.
***NZ***—New Zealand.
**OP**—over proof.
**o/w**—oil-in-water.
***P***—probability.
**Pa**—pascal(s).
**$pCO_2$**—plasma partial pressure (concentration) of carbon dioxide.
**$p_aCO_2$**—arterial plasma partial pressure (concentration) of carbon dioxide.
**PEN**—Pharmacy Equivalent Name, see page v.
**pg**—picogram(s).
**pH**—the negative logarithm of the hydrogen ion concentration.
**Ph. Eur.**—European Pharmacopoeia, 5th ed., 2005.
***Pharm. Soc. Lab. Rep.***—Royal Pharmaceutical Society's Laboratory Report.
**PHLS**—Public Health Laboratory Service (UK).
**pINN**—Proposed International Nonproprietary Name.
**pINNM**—Proposed International Nonproprietary Name Modified.
**$pK_a$**—the negative logarithm of the dissociation constant.
**p.m.**—*post meridiem*, 'afternoon'.
**$pO_2$**—plasma partial pressure (concentration) of oxygen.
**$p_aO_2$**—arterial plasma partial pressure (concentration) of oxygen.
***Pol.***—Poland.
***Pol. P.***—Polish Pharmacopoeia 6th ed., 2002 (Farmakopea Polska VI, 2002).
***Port.***—Portugal.
**ppm**—parts per million.
**PSGB**—The Pharmaceutical Society of Great Britain. Now the Royal Pharmaceutical Society of Great Britain.
**RCGP**—Royal College of General Practitioners (UK).
**RIMA**—reversible inhibitor of monoamine oxidase type A.
**rINN**—Recommended International Nonproprietary Name.
**rINNM**—Recommended International Nonproprietary Name Modified.
**RNA**—ribonucleic acid.
**RPSGB**—The Royal Pharmaceutical Society of Great Britain.
***S. Afr.***—South Africa.
**SGOT**—serum glutamic oxaloacetic transaminase (serum aspartate aminotransferase *now preferred*).
**SGPT**—serum glutamic pyruvic transaminase (serum alanine aminotransferase *now preferred*).
**SI**—Statutory Instrument *or* Système International d'Unités (International System of Units).
***sic***—written exactly as it appears in the original.
**SLE**—systemic lupus erythematosus.
**sp.**—species (plural spp.).
**sp. gr.**—specific gravity.
***Span.***—Spanish.
***Span. P.***—Spanish Pharmacopoeia 2nd ed., 2002 (Real Farmacopoea Española, Segunda Edición, 2002) and Supplement 2.1.
**SSRI**—selective serotonin reuptake inhibitor.
**St**—stokes.
**subsp.**—subspecies.
**suppl**—supplement(s).
***Swed.***—Sweden.
***Swiss P.***—Swiss Pharmacopoeia 2003 (Pharmacopoea Helvetica, 9ᵉ édition, Edition Française) and Supplement 9.1 and 9.2.
***Switz.***—Switzerland.
***Thai.***—Thailand.
**TPN**—total parenteral nutrition.
***UAE***—United Arab Emirates.
***UK***—United Kingdom.
**UNICEF**—United Nations Children's Fund.
**UP**—under proof.
***US*** and ***USA***—United States of America.
**USAN**—United States Adopted Name.
**USNF**—The United States 'National Formulary 22', 2004, and Supplements 1 and 2.
**USP**—The United States Pharmacopeia 27, 2004, and Supplements 1 and 2.
**UV**—ultraviolet.
**var.**—variety.
***Viet.***—Vietnamese.
***Viet. P.***—Vietnamese Pharmacopoeia 2002 (Pharmacopoeia Vietnamica, Editio III).
**vol.**—volume(s).
**v/v**—volume in volume.
**v/w**—volume in weight.
**WHO**—World Health Organization.
**w/o**—water-in-oil.
**wt**—weight.
**wt per mL**—weight per millilitre.
**w/v**—weight in volume.
**w/w**—weight in weight.

# Contracted Names for Ions and Groups

| Contracted Name | Chemical Name |
|---|---|
| **acetonide** | isopropylidene ether of a dihydric alcohol |
| **aceturate** | *N*-acetylglycinate |
| **acistrate** | 2′-acetate (ester) and stearate (salt) |
| **acoxil** | acetoxymethyl |
| **amsonate** | 4,4′-diaminostilbene-2,2′-disulphonate |
| **anisatil** | 2-(4-methoxyphenyl)-2-oxoethyl |
| **axetil** | 1-acetoxyethyl |
| **besilate (besylate)** | benzenesulphonate |
| **bezomil** | (benzoyloxy)methyl |
| **buciclate** | *trans*-4-butylcyclohexanecarboxylate |
| **bunapsilate** | 3,7-di-*tert*-butylnaphthalene-1,5-disulphonate |
| **buteprate** | 17-(1-oxobutoxy) (ester) and 21-(1-oxopropoxy) (ester) |
| **camsilate (camsylate)** | camphor-10-sulphonate |
| **caproate** | hexanoate |
| **carbesilate** | 4-carboxybenzenesulphonate |
| **ciclotate (cyclotate)** | 4-methylbicyclo[2.2.2]oct-2-ene-l-carboxylate |
| **cilexetil** | (*RS*)-1-{[(cyclohexyloxy)carbonyl]oxy}ethyl |
| **cipionate (cypionate)** | 3-cyclopentylpropionate |
| **closilate (closylate)** | 4-chlorobenzenesulphonate |
| **crobefate** | (±)-(*E*)-6-hydroxy-4′-methoxy-3-(*p*-methoxybenzylidene)flavone phosphate ion (2−) |
| **cromacate** | [(6-hydroxy-4-methyl-2-oxo-2*H*-chromen-7-yl)oxy]acetate |
| **cromesilate** | 6,7-dihydroxycoumarin-4-methanesulphonate |
| **deanil** | 2-dimethylaminoethyl |
| **dibudinate** | 2,6-di-*tert*-butylnaphthalene-1,5-disulphonate |
| **dibunate** | 2,6-di-*tert*-butyl-l-naphthalenesulphonate |
| **digolil** | 2-(2-hydroxyethoxy)ethyl |
| **diolamine** | diethanolamine |
| **dofosfate** | octadecyl hydrogen phosphate |
| **edamine** | ethylenediamine |
| **edetate** | ethylenediamine-*NNN′N′*-tetra-acetate |
| **edisilate (edisylate)** | ethane-1,2-disulphonate |
| **embonate** | 4,4′-methylenebis(3-hydroxy-2-naphthoate) (=pamoate) |
| **enantate (enanthate)** | heptanoate |
| **epolamine** | 1-pyrrolidineethanol |
| **erbumine** | *tert*-butylamine |
| **esilate (esylate)** | ethanesulphonate |
| **estolate** | propionate dodecyl sulphate |
| **etabonate** | (ethoxycarbonyl)oxy (=ethyl carbonate) |
| **farnesil** | (2*E*,6*E*)-3,7,11-trimethyl-2,6,10-dodecatrienyl |
| **fendizoate** | 2-[(2′-hydroxy-4-biphenylyl)carbonyl]benzoate |
| **fostedate** | tetradecyl hydrogen phosphate |
| **gluceptate** | glucoheptonate |
| **hibenzate (hybenzate)** | 2-(4-hydroxybenzoyl)benzoate |
| **hyclate** | monohydrochloride hemi-ethanolate hemihydrate |
| **isetionate (isethionate)** | 2-hydroxyethanesulphonate |
| **laurilsulfate (lauryl sulphate)** | dodecyl sulphate |
| **megallate** | 3,4,5-trimethoxybenzoate |
| **meglumine** | *N*-methylglucamine |
| **mesilate (mesylate)** | methanesulphonate |
| **metembonate** | 4,4′-methylenebis(3-methoxy-2-naphthoate) |
| **mofetil** | 2-(morpholino)ethyl |
| **napadisilate (napadisylate)** | naphthalene-1,5-disulphonate |
| **napsilate (napsylate)** | naphthalene-2-sulphonate |
| **olamine** | ethanolamine |
| **oxoglurate** | 2-oxoglutarate |
| **pamoate** | 4,4′-methylenebis(3-hydroxy-2-naphthoate) (=embonate) |
| **pendetide** | $N^6$-{*N*-[2-({2-[bis(carboxymethyl)amino]ethyl}(carboxymethyl)amino)ethyl]-*N*-(carboxymethyl)glycyl}-$N^2$-(*N*-glycyl-L-tyrosyl)-L-lysine |
| **pentexil** | 1-hydroxyethyl pivalate |
| **phenpropionate** | 3-phenylpropionate |
| **pivalate** | trimethylacetate |
| **pivoxetil** | 1-(2-methoxy-2-methylpropionyloxy)ethyl |
| **pivoxil** | (2,2-dimethyl-1-oxopropoxy)methyl or (pivaloyloxy)methyl |
| **polistirex** | sulphonated styrene-divinylbenzene copolymer complex |
| **probutate** | 17-(1-oxobutoxy) (ester) and 21-(1-oxopropoxy) (ester) |
| **proxetil** | 1-[(isopropoxycarbonyl)oxy]ethyl |
| **soproxil** | [(isopropoxycarbonyl)oxy]methyl |
| **steaglate** | stearoyloxyacetate |
| **suleptanate** | sodium 7-[methyl(2-sulphonatomethyl)carbamoyl]heptanoyl |
| **tebutate** | *tert*-butylacetate |
| **tenoate** | 2-thiophenecarboxylate |
| **teoclate (theoclate)** | 8-chlorotheophyllinate |
| **teprosilate** | 3-(theophyllin-7-yl)propanesulphonate |
| **tofesilate** | 2-(theophyllin-7-yl)ethanesulphonate |
| **tosilate (tosylate)** | toluene-4-sulphonate |
| **triclofenate** | 2,4,5-trichlorophenolate |
| **triflutate** | trifluoroacetate |
| **trolamine** | triethanolamine |
| **troxundate** | 3,6,9-trioxaundecanoate |
| **xinafoate** | 1-hydroxy-2-naphthoate |

# Atomic Weights of the Elements— $^{12}C=12$

| Atomic Number | Name | Symbol | Atomic Weight |
|---|---|---|---|
| 89 | Actinium | Ac | * |
| 13 | Aluminium | Al | 26.981538 |
| 95 | Americium | Am | * |
| 51 | Antimony | Sb | 121.760 |
| 18 | Argon | Ar | 39.948 |
| 33 | Arsenic | As | 74.92160 |
| 85 | Astatine | At | * |
| 56 | Barium | Ba | 137.327 |
| 97 | Berkelium | Bk | * |
| 4 | Beryllium | Be | 9.012182 |
| 83 | Bismuth | Bi | 208.98038 |
| 107 | Bohrium | Bh | * |
| 5 | Boron | B | 10.811 |
| 35 | Bromine | Br | 79.904 |
| 48 | Cadmium | Cd | 112.411 |
| 55 | Caesium | Cs | 132.90545 |
| 20 | Calcium | Ca | 40.078 |
| 98 | Californium | Cf | * |
| 6 | Carbon | C | 12.0107 |
| 58 | Cerium | Ce | 140.116 |
| 17 | Chlorine | Cl | 35.453 |
| 24 | Chromium | Cr | 51.9961 |
| 27 | Cobalt | Co | 58.933200 |
| 29 | Copper | Cu | 63.546 |
| 96 | Curium | Cm | * |
| 105 | Dubnium | Db | * |
| 66 | Dysprosium | Dy | 162.500 |
| 99 | Einsteinium | Es | * |
| 68 | Erbium | Er | 167.259 |
| 63 | Europium | Eu | 151.964 |
| 100 | Fermium | Fm | * |
| 9 | Fluorine | F | 18.9984032 |
| 87 | Francium | Fr | * |
| 64 | Gadolinium | Gd | 157.25 |
| 31 | Gallium | Ga | 69.723 |
| 32 | Germanium | Ge | 72.64 |
| 79 | Gold | Au | 196.96655 |
| 72 | Hafnium | Hf | 178.49 |
| 108 | Hassium | Hs | * |
| 2 | Helium | He | 4.002602 |
| 67 | Holmium | Ho | 164.93032 |
| 1 | Hydrogen | H | 1.00794 |
| 49 | Indium | In | 114.818 |
| 53 | Iodine | I | 126.90447 |
| 77 | Iridium | Ir | 192.217 |
| 26 | Iron | Fe | 55.845 |
| 36 | Krypton | Kr | 83.798 |
| 57 | Lanthanum | La | 138.9055 |
| 103 | Lawrencium | Lr | * |
| 82 | Lead | Pb | 207.2 |
| 3 | ‡Lithium | Li | 6.941 |
| 71 | Lutetium | Lu | 174.967 |
| 12 | Magnesium | Mg | 24.3050 |
| 25 | Manganese | Mn | 54.938049 |
| 109 | Meitnerium | Mt | * |
| 101 | Mendelevium | Md | * |
| 80 | Mercury | Hg | 200.59 |
| 42 | Molybdenum | Mo | 95.94 |
| 60 | Neodymium | Nd | 144.24 |
| 10 | Neon | Ne | 20.1797 |
| 93 | Neptunium | Np | * |
| 28 | Nickel | Ni | 58.6934 |
| 41 | Niobium | Nb | 92.90638 |
| 7 | Nitrogen | N | 14.0067 |

| Atomic Number | Name | Symbol | Atomic Weight |
|---|---|---|---|
| 102 | Nobelium | No | * |
| 76 | Osmium | Os | 190.23 |
| 8 | Oxygen | O | 15.9994 |
| 46 | Palladium | Pd | 106.42 |
| 15 | Phosphorus | P | 30.973761 |
| 78 | Platinum | Pt | 195.078 |
| 94 | Plutonium | Pu | * |
| 84 | Polonium | Po | * |
| 19 | Potassium | K | 39.0983 |
| 59 | Praseodymium | Pr | 140.90765 |
| 61 | Promethium | Pm | * |
| 91 | †Protactinium | Pa | 231.03588 |
| 88 | Radium | Ra | * |
| 86 | Radon | Rn | * |
| 75 | Rhenium | Re | 186.207 |
| 45 | Rhodium | Rh | 102.90550 |
| 37 | Rubidium | Rb | 85.4678 |
| 44 | Ruthenium | Ru | 101.07 |
| 104 | Rutherfordium | Rf | * |
| 62 | Samarium | Sm | 150.36 |
| 21 | Scandium | Sc | 44.955910 |
| 106 | Seaborgium | Sg | * |
| 34 | Selenium | Se | 78.96 |
| 14 | Silicon | Si | 28.0855 |
| 47 | Silver | Ag | 107.8682 |
| 11 | Sodium | Na | 22.989770 |
| 38 | Strontium | Sr | 87.62 |
| 16 | Sulfur | S | 32.065 |
| 73 | Tantalum | Ta | 180.9479 |
| 43 | Technetium | Tc | * |
| 52 | Tellurium | Te | 127.60 |
| 65 | Terbium | Tb | 158.92534 |
| 81 | Thallium | Tl | 204.3833 |
| 90 | †Thorium | Th | 232.0381 |
| 69 | Thulium | Tm | 168.93421 |
| 50 | Tin | Sn | 118.710 |
| 22 | Titanium | Ti | 47.867 |
| 74 | Tungsten | W | 183.84 |
| 112 | Ununbium | Uub | * |
| 116 | Ununhexium | Uuh | * |
| 110 | Ununnilium | Uun | * |
| 114 | Ununquadium | Uuq | * |
| 111 | Unununium | Uuu | * |
| 92 | †Uranium | U | 238.02891 |
| 23 | Vanadium | V | 50.9415 |
| 54 | Xenon | Xe | 131.293 |
| 70 | Ytterbium | Yb | 173.04 |
| 39 | Yttrium | Y | 88.90585 |
| 30 | Zinc | Zn | 65.409 |
| 40 | Zirconium | Zr | 91.224 |

Elements marked (*) have no stable nuclides and IUPAC states "there is no general agreement on which of the isotopes of the radioactive elements is, or is likely to be judged 'important' and various criteria such as 'longest half-life', 'production in quantity', 'used commercially', etc., have been applied in the Commission's choice." However, atomic weights are given for radioactive elements marked (†) as they do have a characteristic terrestrial isotopic composition. Commercially available lithium (‡) materials have atomic weights ranging from 6.939 to 6.996; if a more accurate value is required, it must be determined for the specific material.

IUPAC Commission on Atomic Weights and Isotopic Abundances. Atomic Weights of the Elements 2001. Available at http://www.chem.qmul.ac.uk/iupac/AtWt/

# Part 1

# Monographs on Drugs and Ancillary Substances

## Analgesics Anti-inflammatory Drugs and Antipyretics


Analgesia and Pain, p.2
- Choice of analgesic, p.2
- Choice of analgesics in children, p.3
- Nerve blocks, p.3
- Patient-controlled analgesia, p.3
- Postoperative analgesia, p.4
- Rubefacients and topical analgesia, p.4
- Specific pain states, p.4
  - Biliary and renal colic, p.4
  - Cancer pain, p.5
  - Central post-stroke pain, p.5
  - Complex regional pain syndrome, p.5
  - Diabetic neuropathy, p.6
  - Dysmenorrhoea, p.6
  - Headache, p.6
  - Labour pain, p.6
  - Low back pain, p.7
  - Myocardial infarction pain, p.7
  - Neuropathic pain syndromes, p.7
  - Orofacial pain, p.7
  - Pancreatic pain, p.7
  - Phantom limb pain, p.7
  - Postherpetic neuralgia, p.7
  - Sickle-cell crisis, p.8
  - Trigeminal neuralgia, p.8

Increased Body Temperature, p.8
- Fever and hyperthermia, p.8

Musculoskeletal and Joint Disorders, p.9
- Juvenile idiopathic arthritis, p.9
- Osteoarthritis, p.9
- Rheumatoid arthritis, p.9
- Soft-tissue rheumatism, p.11
- Spondyloarthropathies, p.11
- Still's disease, p.11


The drugs described in this chapter are used mainly in the relief of pain, inflammation and, in some cases, fever. They can be grouped broadly into one of the categories briefly described below.

### Aspirin and other Salicylates

Aspirin and other salicylates have analgesic, anti-inflammatory, and antipyretic properties. Like other NSAIDs (see below) they are inhibitors of the enzyme cyclo-oxygenase; however, aspirin (though not the non-acetylated salicylates) irreversibly acetylates the enzyme whereas other NSAIDs compete with arachidonic acid for the active site. Salicylates are used for the relief of mild to moderate pain, minor febrile conditions, and for acute and chronic inflammatory disorders such as osteoarthritis, rheumatoid arthritis, juvenile idiopathic arthritis, and ankylosing spondylitis. Some salicylates are applied topically in rubefacient preparations for the relief of muscular and rheumatic pain. Aspirin also inhibits platelet aggregation and is used in cardiovascular disorders. Non-acetylated salicylates do not have antiplatelet activity.

For further discussion of the actions and uses of salicylates, see Aspirin, p.15.

Described in this chapter are


Aloxiprin, p.14
Aluminium Aspirin, p.14
Ammonium Salicylate, p.14
Amyl Salicylate, p.14
Aspirin, p.15
Bornyl Salicylate, p.21
Carbasalate Calcium, p.25
Choline Magnesium Trisalicylate, p.26
Choline Salicylate, p.26
Diethylamine Salicylate, p.34
Diflunisal, p.34
Ethenzamide, p.37
Ethyl Salicylate, p.37
Fosfosal, p.44
Glycol Salicylate, p.44
Imidazole Salicylate, p.47
Lithium Salicylate, p.54
Lysine Aspirin, p.54
Magnesium Salicylate, p.55
Methyl Butetisalicylate, p.59
Methyl Salicylate, p.59
Morpholine Salicylate, p.63
Picolamine Salicylate, p.84
Salamidacetic Acid, p.87
Salicylamide, p.87
Salix, p.87
Salol, p.88
Salsalate, p.88
Sodium Salicylate, p.90
Sodium Thiosalicylate, p.90
Thurfyl Salicylate, p.93
Trolamine Salicylate, p.95


### Disease-modifying Antirheumatic Drugs

Disease-modifying antirheumatic drugs (DMARDs) have anti-inflammatory properties thought to be mediated, in some cases, by the inhibition of the release or activity of cytokines. They are used in the treatment of rheumatoid arthritis and juvenile idiopathic arthritis; some are also of benefit in psoriatic arthritis. Many DMARDs also possess other therapeutic properties and are used in non-rheumatic conditions. The DMARD gold is referred to below; other DMARDs include the antimalarials chloroquine (p.448) and hydroxychloroquine (p.452), sulfasalazine (p.1291), penicillamine (p.1046), and the immunosuppressants azathioprine (p.1349), ciclosporin (p.1351), cyclophosphamide (p.540), and methotrexate (p.568).

Described in this chapter are


Adalimumab, p.12
Anakinra, p.14
Etanercept, p.36
Infliximab, p.50
Leflunomide, p.53


### Gold Compounds

Gold compounds are used mainly for their anti-inflammatory effect in active progressive rheumatoid arthritis and progressive juvenile idiopathic arthritis; they may also be beneficial in psoriatic arthritis. The mechanism of action of gold compounds in rheumatic disorders is as yet unknown.

For further discussion of the actions and uses of gold compounds, see Sodium Aurothiomalate, p.88.

Described in this chapter are


Auranofin, p.19
Aurothioglucose, p.19
Aurotioprol, p.20
Gold Keratinate, p.45
Sodium Aurothiomalate, p.88
Sodium Aurotiosulfate, p.90


### Nonsteroidal Anti-inflammatory Drugs

Nonsteroidal anti-inflammatory drugs (NSAIDs) are a group of unrelated organic acids that have analgesic, anti-inflammatory, and antipyretic properties (see p.67). NSAIDs are inhibitors of the enzyme cyclo-oxygenase, and so directly inhibit the biosynthesis of prostaglandins and thromboxanes from arachidonic acid (see p.1511). There are 2 forms of cyclo-oxygenase (COX), COX-1, which is the constitutive form of the enzyme, and COX-2, which is the form induced in the presence of inflammation. Inhibition of COX-2 is therefore thought to be responsible for at least some of the analgesic, anti-inflammatory, and antipyretic properties of NSAIDs whereas inhibition of COX-1 is thought to produce some of their toxic effects, particularly those on the gastrointestinal tract. Most of the NSAIDs currently available for clinical use inhibit both COX-1 and COX-2, although selective COX-2 inhibitors such as celecoxib and rofecoxib are now available.

NSAIDs are used for the relief of mild to moderate pain, minor febrile conditions, and for acute and chronic inflammatory disorders such as osteoarthritis, rheumatoid arthritis, juvenile idiopathic arthritis, and ankylosing spondylitis. Indometacin and some other NSAIDs are used to close patent ductus arteriosus in premature neonates. Some NSAIDs are applied topically for the relief of muscular and rheumatic pain, and some are used in ophthalmic preparations for ocular inflammatory disorders. Aspirin (see above) is considered to be an NSAID, although it also has other properties.

Described in this chapter are


Aceclofenac, p.11
Acemetacin, p.11
Alminoprofen, p.14
Aminophenazone, p.14
Aminopropylone, p.14
Ampiroxicam, p.14
Amtolmetin Guacil, p.14
Azapropazone, p.20
Bendazac, p.20
Benoxaprofen, p.21
Benzydamine, p.21
Beta-aminopropionitrile, p.21
Bromfenac, p.21
Bufexamac, p.21
Bumadizone, p.21
Butibufen Sodium, p.23
Carprofen, p.25
Celecoxib, p.25
Ibuproxam, p.47
Indometacin, p.47
Isonixin, p.51
Kebuzone, p.51
Ketoprofen, p.51
Ketorolac, p.52
Lonazolac, p.54
Lornoxicam, p.54
Loxoprofen, p.54
Meclofenamate, p.55
Mefenamic Acid, p.55
Meloxicam, p.56
Mofebutazone, p.60
Mofezolac, p.60
Nabumetone, p.63
Naproxen, p.65
Nifenazone, p.66
Niflumic Acid, p.67
Clofexamide, p.26
Clofezone, p.26
Clonixin, p.26
Diclofenac, p.32
Dipyrone, p.35
Droxicam, p.36
Eltenac, p.36
Epirizole, p.36
Etodolac, p.37
Etofenamate, p.38
Etoricoxib, p.38
Felbinac, p.39
Fenbufen, p.39
Fenoprofen, p.39
Fentiazac, p.43
Fepradinol, p.43
Feprazone, p.43
Floctafenine, p.43
Flufenamic Acid, p.43
Flunixin, p.43
Flunoxaprofen, p.43
Flurbiprofen, p.43
Furprofen, p.44
Glafenine, p.44
Glucametacin, p.44
Ibuprofen, p.45
Morniflumate, p.60
Nimesulide, p.67
Oxaprozin, p.75
Oxyphenbutazone, p.76
Parecoxib, p.79
Phenazone, p.82
Phenylbutazone, p.83
Piketoprofen, p.84
Piroxicam, p.84
Pranoprofen, p.85
Proglumetacin, p.85
Propyphenazone, p.85
Proquazone, p.86
Ramifenazone, p.86
Rofecoxib, p.86
Sulindac, p.91
Suprofen, p.93
Suxibuzone, p.93
Tenoxicam, p.93
Tetridamine, p.93
Tiaprofenic Acid, p.93
Tiaramide, p.94
Tolfenamic Acid, p.94
Tolmetin, p.94
Valdecoxib, p.96
Vedaprofen, p.96
Zaltoprofen, p.96


### Opioid Analgesics

Opioid analgesics include the opium alkaloids morphine and codeine and their derivatives as well as synthetic substances with agonist, partial agonist, or mixed agonist and antagonist activity at opioid receptors (see p.71). The term opiate analgesics refers only to those opioids derived from opium, or their semisynthetic congeners. The term narcotic analgesics has legal connotations and is no longer used pharmacologically or clinically.

The majority of opioids are used as analgesics, and morphine is the standard against which all other opioid analgesics are compared. Opioids such as codeine or dextropropoxyphene are used in the treatment of less severe pain, and are often combined with non-opioid analgesics such as aspirin, other NSAIDs, or paracetamol. More potent opioids such as morphine are used in severe acute and chronic pain, including cancer pain. Some opioids such as codeine, morphine, and diamorphine are also used as antitussives, although the latter two are usually reserved for use in terminal lung disease. Some opioid analgesics such as fentanyl and its congeners are used mainly as adjuncts to anaesthesia; some of these may also be used in higher doses as the sole anaesthetic drug.

Some opioids are rarely if ever used as analgesics and are described elsewhere; they include the antitussives dextromethorphan (p.1117) and pholcodine (p.1128), and the antidiarrhoeals diphenoxylate (p.1261) and loperamide (p.1271).

Opioids can produce physical dependence and withdrawal symptoms on sudden discontinuation. They are also subject to abuse.

Described in this chapter are


Alfentanil, p.12
Anileridine, p.15
Bezitramide, p.21
Ketobemidone, p.51
Levacetylmethadol, p.54
Levomethadone, p.54

Buprenorphine, p.21
Butorphanol, p.23
Carfentanil, p.25
Codeine, p.27
Dextromoramide, p.28
Dextropropoxyphene, p.28
Dezocine, p.30
Diamorphine, p.30
Dihydrocodeine, p.34
Dipipanone, p.35
Embutramide, p.36
Ethoheptazine, p.37
Ethylmorphine, p.37
Etorphine, p.38
Fentanyl, p.40
Hydrochlorides of Mixed Opium Alkaloids, p.74
Hydrocodone, p.45
Hydromorphone, p.45
Levorphanol, p.54
Meptazinol, p.56
Methadone, p.57
Morphine, p.60
Nalbuphine, p.64
Nicomorphine, p.66
Opium, p.74
Oxycodone, p.75
Oxymorphone, p.76
Papaveretum, p.74
Pentazocine, p.79
Pethidine, p.80
Phenazocine, p.82
Phenoperidine, p.83
Piritramide, p.84
Remifentanil, p.86
Sufentanil, p.90
Tilidine, p.94
Tramadol, p.94

### Paracetamol and other Para-aminophenols

Paracetamol is the principal para-aminophenol derivative in use. Acetanilide and phenacetin have generally been replaced by safer analgesics. Propacetamol is hydrolysed to paracetamol in the plasma.

Paracetamol has analgesic and antipyretic properties and weak anti-inflammatory activity. The mechanism of analgesic action remains to be fully elucidated, but may be due to inhibition of prostaglandin synthesis both centrally and peripherally. Paracetamol is used for the relief of mild to moderate pain and minor febrile conditions.

Described in this chapter are

Acetanilide, p.11
Paracetamol, p.76
Phenacetin, p.82
Propacetamol, p.85

## Analgesia and Pain

Pain is defined by the International Association for the Study of Pain as 'an unpleasant sensory and emotional experience associated with actual or potential tissue damage, or described in terms of such damage.'

Under normal circumstances pain is the result of stimulation of peripheral receptors which transmit impulses through pain pathways to the brain. Pain receptors or nociceptors are of two basic types:

- *mechanoheat receptors* have a high stimulation threshold and respond to intense or potentially damaging noxious stimuli. These receptors are associated with rapidly conducting, thinly myelinated Aδ fibres, and their stimulation produces rapid sharp localised pain that serves to activate withdrawal reflexes
- *polymodal nociceptors* respond to mechanical, thermal, or chemical insults. These receptors are also activated by cellular components that are released following tissue damage. Their impulses are transmitted slowly along unmyelinated C type fibres and produce dull, aching, and poorly localised pain with a slower onset.

Nerve fibres from nociceptors terminate in the dorsal root of the spinal cord before transmission by ascending pathways to the brain. There have been many theories on the processing of pain signals at the spinal level but the 'gate theory' proposed by Melzack and Wall is one of the best known. This theory postulates that the transmission of impulses to the brain is modulated by a gate mechanism in the substantia gelatinosa. Stimulation of small fibres opens the gate and facilitates transmission whereas stimulation of large fibres, which normally carry non-painful sensory input, can close the gate and inhibit transmission. Transmission also appears to be modulated by several other mechanisms which can influence the sensitivity of the gate.

Inflammatory mediators such as bradykinin, histamine, serotonin, and prostaglandins produced in response to tissue damage can produce peripheral sensitisation so that receptors respond to low intensity or innocuous stimuli; central sensitisation also occurs. Pain associated with tissue damage hence results in increased sensitivity of the sensory system so that the pain can occur in the absence of a clear stimulus. There may be a reduction in the pain threshold (*allodynia*) resulting in an exaggerated response (*hyperalgesia*) or a prolonged effect (*hyperpathia*).

Pain is often classified as being acute or chronic in nature.

- **Acute pain** is associated with trauma or disease and usually has a well-defined location, character, and timing. It is accompanied by symptoms of autonomic hyperactivity such as tachycardia, hypertension, sweating, and mydriasis.
- **Chronic pain** is usually regarded as pain lasting more than a few months. It may not be clearly associated with trauma or disease or may persist after the initial injury has healed; its localisation, character, and timing are more vague than with acute pain. Furthermore, as the autonomic nervous system adapts, the signs of autonomic hyperactivity associated with acute pain disappear. Some forms of pain regarded as being chronic may consist of intermittent attacks of pain followed by relatively long pain-free periods. Patients with chronic pain experience physical, psychological, social, and functional deterioration which contributes towards exacerbation of the pain.

Physiologically, pain may be divided into nociceptive pain and neuropathic pain.

- **Nociceptive pain** follows activation of nociceptors by noxious stimuli as described above but is not associated with injury to peripheral nerves or the CNS. It may be somatic or visceral, depending on which receptors or nerves are involved. *Somatic pain* is usually well localised and may be described as deeply located, sharp or dull, nagging, stabbing, throbbing, or pressure-like. *Visceral pain* is generally less localised and more diffuse than somatic pain and may be referred to remote areas of the body. Depending on the structure involved it is variously described as deeply located, aching, nagging, cramping, or pressing and may be accompanied by nausea and vomiting. Nociceptive pain usually responds to treatment with conventional analgesics.
- Pain resulting from damage or dysfunction of peripheral nerves/receptors or of the CNS is known as **neuropathic pain** (or neurogenic pain). The term covers *sympathetically maintained pain* including causalgia and reflex sympathetic dystrophy, and painful conditions such as postherpetic and trigeminal neuralgia, and diabetic neuropathy. Neuropathic pain associated with central nervous tissue, such as in central post-stroke pain (the thalamic syndrome) is referred to as *central pain*. The clinical signs of neuropathic pain can vary greatly. Some of the more common features include heightened pain sensitivity and sensations of superficial burning or stabbing (lancinating) pain. The pain may be associated with areas of sensory deficit or some form of autonomic instability. Neuropathic pain responds poorly to conventional analgesics and can be difficult to treat.

Early **treatment** of pain is important as unrelieved pain can have profound psychological effects on the patient, and acute pain that is poorly managed initially can degenerate into chronic pain, which may prove to be much more difficult to treat. It is important to assess and treat the mental and emotional aspects of the pain as well as its physical aspects. Although drug therapy is a mainstay of pain treatment (see below), physical methods such as physiotherapy (including massage and the application of heat and cold), surgery, and nervous system stimulation techniques such as acupuncture and transcutaneous electrical nerve stimulation (TENS) are also used.

◊ General references to pain and its management.

1. Melzack R, Wall PD. Pain mechanisms: a new theory. *Science* 1965; **150:** 971–9.
2. International Association for the Study of Pain. Classification of chronic pain: descriptions of chronic pain syndromes and definitions of pain terms. *Pain* 1986; (suppl 3): S1–S225.
3. Lewis KS, *et al.* Effect of analgesic treatment on the physiological consequences of acute pain. *Am J Hosp Pharm* 1994; **51:** 1539–54.
4. Justins DM. Chronic pain management. *Br J Hosp Med* 1994; **52:** 12–16.
5. Reidenberg MM, Portenoy RK. The need for an open mind about the treatment of chronic nonmalignant pain. *Clin Pharmacol Ther* 1994; **55:** 367–9.
6. American Pain Society Quality of Care Committee. Quality improvement guidelines for the treatment of acute pain and cancer pain. *JAMA* 1995; **274:** 1874–80.
7. Anonymous. Pain: under-recognized and undertreated? *WHO Drug Inf* 1996; **10:** 36–8.
8. Markenson JA. Mechanisms of chronic pain. *Am J Med* 1996; **101** (suppl 1A): 6S–18S.
9. Katz WA. Approach to the management of nonmalignant pain. *Am J Med* 1996; **101** (suppl 1A): 54S–63S.
10. McQuay H, *et al.* Treating acute pain in hospital. *BMJ* 1997; **314:** 1531–5.
11. American Academy of Pain Medicine and the American Pain Society. The use of opioids for the treatment of chronic pain: a consensus statement. *Clin J Pain* 1997; **13:** 6–8.
12. American Society of Anesthesiologists Task Force on Pain Management, Chronic Pain Section. Practice guidelines for chronic pain management. *Anesthesiology* 1997; **86:** 995–1004.
13. Barnes J, White A. Acupuncture. *Pharm J* 1998; **260:** 664–7.
14. Loeser JD, Melzack R. Pain: an overview. Available at: http://www.thelancet.com/journal/vol357/iss s1/full/llan.357.s1.pain_series.15830.1 (accessed 01/07/04)
15. Ashburn MA, Staats PS. Management of chronic pain. Available at: http://www.thelancet.com/journal/vol357/iss s1/full/llan.357.s1.pain_series.15831.1 (accessed 01/07/04)
16. Woolf CJ, Mannion RJ. Neuropathic pain: aetiology, symptoms, mechanisms, and management. Available at: http://www.thelancet.com/journal/vol357/iss s1/full/llan.357.s1.pain_series.15832.1 (accessed 01/07/04)
17. Carr DB, Goudas LC. Acute pain. Available at: http://www.thelancet.com/journal/vol357/iss s1/full/llan.357.s1.pain_series.15828.1 (accessed 01/07/04)
18. Cervero F, Laird JMA. Visceral pain. Available at: http://www.thelancet.com/journal/vol357/iss s1/full/llan.357.s1.pain_series.15834.1 (accessed 01/07/04)
19. Holdcroft A, Power I. Management of pain. *BMJ* 2003; **326:** 635–9.

### Choice of analgesic

**Paracetamol** and **NSAIDs** are the first choice analgesics for treating mild to moderate pain and are also used in moderate to severe pain to potentiate the effects of opioids. They are suitable for use in acute or chronic pain. Aspirin and paracetamol are of similar potency in most types of pain but paracetamol only has a weak anti-inflammatory effect. NSAIDs are particularly effective in bone pain of malignant origin and pain due to inflammation. The selective inhibitors of cyclo-oxygenase-2 (COX-2) are said to be as effective as the non-selective NSAIDS. Dependence and tolerance are not a problem with non-opioid analgesics but as the dose is increased, their efficacy reaches a ceiling. Aspirin and other non-selective NSAIDs inhibit blood platelet function, adversely affect the gastrointestinal tract, and can precipitate hypersensitivity reactions including asthma. The risk of serious upper gastrointestinal adverse effects is lower with the COX-2 inhibitors than the non-selective NSAIDs; however, in other respects, the COX-2 inhibitors share similar side-effect profiles to those of the non-selective NSAIDs. Paracetamol does not have the haematological or gastrointestinal adverse effects of aspirin but large doses can produce severe or sometimes fatal hepatotoxicity.

For the treatment of moderate or moderate to severe opioid-sensitive pain **codeine** is the traditional choice; alternatives include **dextropropoxyphene** and **dihydrocodeine**. They are often given together with non-opioid analgesics. Combinations of codeine with paracetamol produce a small but significant increase in analgesia compared with paracetamol alone and might be appropriate for occasional pain relief, but the incidence of adverse effects increases with repeated use. Combinations of dextropropoxyphene with paracetamol or aspirin are no more effective in acute pain than the non-opioid alone; efficacy in chronic pain is unclear and adverse effects may become troublesome.

More potent opioids such as **morphine** are mainly used in the treatment of severe acute non-malignant pain and cancer pain (see below). Their use in chronic non-malignant pain is somewhat controversial because of fears of psychological dependence and respiratory depression. However, in practice such problems rarely occur and those fears should not prevent patients being given effective analgesic therapy. Opioids may also be of value in neuropathic pain in some patients.

Morphine is the opioid of choice in severe pain. It is well absorbed when given orally and has a short half-life so that the use of immediate-release oral preparations offers a flexible means of dosage titration. Once initial pain relief has been achieved, administration of a modified-release preparation every 12 or 24 hours is more convenient for maintenance of analgesia in severe chronic pain. It may also be given parenterally (e.g. for emergency pain control or patient-controlled analgesia—see also below), or rectally or transdermally, where there would be problems with the oral route.

Occasionally **other opioids** may be useful as an alternative to morphine. Methadone or oxycodone have a longer duration of action than morphine, but it should be noted that methadone, which has a long half-life, should not be given more than twice daily when used long term because of the risk of progressive CNS depression and overdosage. A rapid onset of action is provided by pethidine, alfentanil, and fentanyl. Diamorphine or hydromorphone may be preferred to morphine when the parenteral route has to be used because they are more soluble and can be given in a smaller volume.

Adverse effects of opioids include sedation, nausea, vomiting, constipation, and, most seriously, respiratory depression. Tolerance generally develops to all of these effects except constipation, which may be prevented by regular use of laxatives.

A number of other groups of drugs have significant roles in pain management either alone or as **analgesic adjuvants**.

Subantidepressant doses of tricyclic **antidepressants** (usually amitriptyline) are considered to be useful in refractory chronic pain, including neuropathic pain of the burning, dysaesthetic type such as postherpetic neuralgia and diabetic neuropathy; shooting pain has also been reported to respond. They may be used in addition to conventional analgesics, notably in the treatment of cancer pain of mixed aetiology. There is little evidence for benefit in acute pain although musculoskeletal pain has sometimes responded. Amitriptyline has also been found to be useful for tension-type headache and for the prophylaxis of migraine. The role of other antidepressants in the treatment of neuropathic pain is less clear although venlafaxine may be useful.

**Antiepileptics** (often carbamazepine and, more recently, gabapentin) have been found useful in the relief of neuropathic pain especially when there is a stabbing (lancinating) element, as in trigeminal neuralgia; there have also been reports of efficacy in the treatment of diabetic neuropathy and for migraine prophylaxis.

**Benzodiazepines** and **other muscle relaxants** such as baclofen or dantrolene are useful for relieving painful muscle spasm in acute or chronic conditions.

**Bone modulating drugs** such as calcitonin and bisphosphonates may be useful in cancer pain arising from bone metastases (see below) but have a slow onset of action and are second choice to NSAIDs. Bisphosphonates may cause an initial transient increase in bone pain.

**Caffeine** has been used with the aim of enhancing the effects of non-opioid and opioid analgesics but is of debatable benefit. There are similar doubts about whether caffeine enhances the effect of ergotamine in the treatment of migraine (see Pharmacokinetics, p.468); it may also add to gastrointestinal adverse effects and in large doses can itself cause headache.

**Corticosteroids** have produced improvement, often substantial, in neuropathic pain. They can also relieve headache caused by raised intracranial pressure and refractory pain caused by bone metastases, and have the added benefits of increasing well-being and appetite.

Some **inhalational anaesthetics** are used in subanaesthetic doses as inhalation analgesics for acute pain. In particular, nitrous oxide is given with oxygen for pain relief in obstetrics and during dental and other procedures, and in emergency management. Isoflurane, enflurane, and in some countries methoxyflurane or trichloroethylene have been used similarly.

**Miscellaneous drugs.** Following the discovery that epidural or intrathecal injection of opioids can produce effective analgesia many other drugs have been tried by these routes, either alone or with opioids or local anaesthetics, but their role, if any, in the management of pain remains to be determined. Some of these drugs, such as clonidine and ketamine, also appear to have analgesic properties when given by other routes. Some antiarrhythmics may be effective in chronic neuropathic pain, but must be used with extreme caution. The use of antipsychotics, such as the phenothiazines, as adjuvant analgesics is controversial; levomepromazine is sometimes used as an adjunct in palliative care.

See below for discussions of the use of patient-controlled analgesia, and rubefacients and topical analgesics. Nerve blocks are discussed under Pain, on p.1369.

References.


1. Pon D, Hart LL. IV lidocaine as an analgesic. *DICP Ann Pharmacother* 1989; **23:** 602–4.
2. American Pain Society. Principles of analgesic use in the treatment of acute pain and chronic cancer pain, 2nd edition. *Clin Pharm* 1990; **9:** 601–11.
3. Bushnell TG, Justins DM. Choosing the right analgesic: a guide to selection. *Drugs* 1993; **46:** 394–408.
4. Rummans TA. Nonopioid agents for treatment of acute and subacute pain. *Mayo Clin Proc* 1994; **69:** 481–90.
5. Patt RB, *et al.* The neuroleptics as adjuvant analgesics. *J Pain Symptom Manage* 1994; **9:** 446–53.
6. Sawynok J. Pharmacological rationale for the clinical use of caffeine. *Drugs* 1995; **49:** 37–50.
7. McQuay H, *et al.* Anticonvulsant drugs for management of pain: a systematic review. *BMJ* 1995; **311:** 1047–52.
8. McQuay HJ, *et al.* A systematic review of antidepressants in neuropathic pain. *Pain* 1996; **68:** 217–27.
9. McQuay HJ, Moore RA. Antidepressants and chronic pain: effective analgesia in neuropathic pain and other syndromes. *BMJ* 1997; **314:** 763–4.
10. Tremont-Lukats IW, *et al.* Anticonvulsants for neuropathic pain syndrome: mechanisms of action and place in therapy. *Drugs* 2000; **60:** 1029–52.
11. Watson CP. The treatment of neuropathic pain: antidepressants and opioids. *Clin J Pain* 2000; **16** (suppl): S49–S55.
12. Mattia C, *et al.* New antidepressants in the treatment of neuropathic pain: a review. *Minerva Anestesiol* 2002; **68:** 105–14.
13. Curatolo M, Sveticic G. Drug combinations in pain treatment: a review of the published evidence and a method for finding the optimal combination. *Best Pract Res Clin Anaesthesiol* 2002; **16:** 507–19.
14. Backonja M. Anticonvulsants for the treatment of neuropathic pain syndromes. *Curr Pain Headache Rep* 2003; **7:** 39–42.


## Choice of analgesics in children

Pain has often been undertreated in infants and children because of fears of respiratory depression, cardiovascular collapse, depressed levels of consciousness, and addiction with potent opioid analgesics. Assessment of pain is also a problem in children of all ages and it is not that long since it was widely believed that neonates were incapable of feeling pain.

**Non-opioid analgesics** are used in ***infants and children***, either alone for minor pain or as an adjunct to opioid analgesics in severe pain. Paracetamol is frequently used but it lacks any anti-inflammatory effect. NSAIDs such as ibuprofen are useful for pain associated with inflammation. The use of aspirin is greatly restricted by its association with Reye's syndrome.

The **opioids** are still the mainstay of analgesia for moderate to severe pain in paediatric patients, and morphine is the standard against which the others are compared. Continuous intravenous infusion with or without initial loading doses has become popular for postoperative pain relief, but titration of the infusion rate is necessary to achieve a balance between analgesia and respiratory depression (particular care is needed in neonates, see below). Subcutaneous infusions of morphine have also been used, mostly for the relief of terminal cancer pain in children. Intramuscular injections can provide excellent analgesia but are painful and therefore probably only suitable for short-term use. Fentanyl has also been widely used for short-term analgesia in surgical procedures, and a variety of other opioids have been given. Patient-controlled analgesia using morphine has been tried in children (see below).

Morphine has also been given to children by the epidural route; experience with the intrathecal route is more limited. Other methods of opioid drug delivery of possible value in paediatric analgesia include transmucosal, nasal, and transdermal administration.

Cancer pain in children may be treated using the analgesic ladder scheme described under Cancer Pain (see below).

**Local anaesthetics** are especially suitable for the management of acute pain in day-care situations. Single injections given by the epidural route are often used to provide analgesia during and after surgery. Continuous epidural infusions of local anaesthetics have also been used. However, simpler techniques such as wound infiltration or peripheral nerve blocks can also provide effective analgesia for some procedures and are free of the problems of lower limb weakness or urinary retention associated with caudal blocks. Application of eutectic creams (see Surface Anaesthesia, p.1380) containing lidocaine with prilocaine to intact skin, to produce surface anaesthesia, may be sufficient for some minor painful procedures in children.

**Ketamine** is used in outpatients for brief, painful procedures such as fracture reduction and to provide immobility for repair of facial lacerations in young children. The emergence reactions that limit its use in adults are less common in children.

Most ***neonates*** requiring analgesia and receiving respiratory support can be managed with an infusion of morphine but in neonates who are breathing spontaneously there is a substantial risk of respiratory depression. Morphine has been used in such neonates but should be limited to those under intensive care, as for example after major surgery (see also Intensive Care under Sedation, p.666). Fentanyl citrate and codeine phosphate have also been used in neonates. **Sucrose** and other sweet tasting solutions have been shown to reduce physiologic and behavioural indicators of stress and pain in neonates undergoing painful procedures although there had been some doubt expressed over whether this indicates effective analgesia.

The use of **analgesic adjuncts** (see Choice of Analgesic, above) has also been advocated in some children.

References.


1. Lloyd-Thomas AR. Pain management in paediatric patients. *Br J Anaesth* 1990; **64:** 85–104.
2. Commission on the provision of surgical services. *Report of the working party on pain after surgery.* London: Royal College of Surgeons of England and College of Anaesthetists, 1990.
3. Schecter NL, *et al.* Report of the consensus conference on the management of pain in childhood cancer. *Pediatrics* 1990; **86:** 813–34.
4. Gaukroger PB. Paediatric analgesia: which drug? which dose? *Drugs* 1991; **41:** 52–9.
5. Bhatt-Mehta V, Rosen DA. Management of acute pain in children. *Clin Pharm* 1991; **10:** 667–85.
6. Selbst SM. Analgesia in children: why is it underused in emergency departments? *Drug Safety* 1992; **7:** 8–13.
7. Burrows FA, Berde CB. Optimal pain relief in infants and children. *BMJ* 1993; **307:** 815–16.
8. Anonymous. Treating moderate and severe pain in infants. *Drug Ther Bull* 1994; **32:** 21–4.
9. Anonymous. Managing acute pain in children. *Drug Ther Bull* 1995; **33:** 41–4 and 79.
10. Anonymous. Managing chronic pain in children. *Drug Ther Bull* 1995; **33:** 52–5.
11. Bhatt-Mehta V. Current guidelines for the treatment of acute pain in children. *Drugs* 1996; **51:** 760–76.
12. Ball AJ, Ferguson S. Analgesia and analgesic drugs in paediatrics. *Br J Hosp Med* 1996; **55:** 586–90.
13. Anderson BJ, *et al.* Size, myths and the clinical pharmacokinetics of analgesia in paediatric patients. *Clin Pharmacokinet* 1997; **33:** 313–27.
14. Alder Hey Royal Liverpool Children's NHS Trust. Guidelines on the management of pain in children. 1st edn, 1998. Available at: http://www.dal.ca/~painsrc/pdfs/pps55.pdf (accessed 01/07/04)
15. Morton NS. Prevention and control of pain in children. *Br J Anaesth* 1999; **83:** 118–29.
16. American Academy of Pediatrics and Canadian Paediatric Society. Prevention and management of pain and stress in the neonate. *Pediatrics* 2000; **105:** 454–61. Also available at: http://aappolicy.aappublications.org/cgi/content/full/pediatrics;105/2/454 (accessed 01/07/04)
17. Krauss B, Green SM. Sedation and analgesia for procedures in children. *N Engl J Med* 2000; **342:** 938–45.
18. American Academy of Pediatrics Committee on Psychosocial Aspects of Child and Family Health, American Pain Society Task Force on Pain in Infants, Children, and Adolescents. The assessment and management of acute pain in infants, children, and adolescents. *Pediatrics* 2001; **108:** 793–7.
19. Anand KJ; International Evidence-Based Group for Neonatal Pain. Consensus statement for the prevention and management of pain in the newborn. *Arch Pediatr Adolesc Med* 2001; **155:** 173–80.
20. Berde CB, Sethna NF. Analgesics for the treatment of pain in children. *N Engl J Med* 2002; **347:** 1094–1103.
21. Chambliss CR, *et al.* The assessment and management of chronic pain in children. *Paediatr Drugs* 2002; **4:** 737–46.


## Nerve blocks

For a discussion of the use of nerve blocks in the management of pain, see under Pain, p.1369.

## Patient-controlled analgesia

Patient-controlled analgesia involves the use of automated delivery systems that enable patients to receive doses of an analgesic on demand. Doses of **opioids** are usually given intravenously, their frequency being controlled by each patient within the safety limits of the delivery system. The technique is useful for the control of pain from a variety of causes including postoperative pain[1,2] and has been used successfully by children as young as 4 years of age and by the elderly.[3]

The safety and efficacy of patient-controlled opioid analgesia largely depends on the availability of adequately trained staff and reliable pumps designed to minimise the possibility of programming errors or tampering by patients or visitors.[3] There have been isolated reports of patients receiving very large doses through deliberate operation of the system by relatives,[4] electrical interference,[5] or incorrect use by the patient or staff.[6,7]

In the simplest type of patient-controlled analgesia the patient is able to self-administer a fixed bolus dose on demand; further doses are not then permitted until a pre-programmed lockout interval has expired. Bolus doses are adjusted to prevent overdosage but maintain analgesic blood concentrations. Variable-dose patient-controlled analgesia has also been tried in which the patient selects one of several doses, although this method may offer no advantage over fixed-dose systems.[8] Some devices allow the dose to be given as a short infusion to reduce adverse effects associated with high peak concentrations of opioids. In another commonly used method, sometimes described as patient-augmented analgesia, the patient is given a continuous background infusion which is supplemented by self-administered bolus doses. However, with this method patients may receive more opioids without any improvement in analgesia;[3,9,10] they may also experience more adverse effects such as nausea and vomiting, respiratory depression, drowsiness, and pruritus,[10,11] although this may depend on the size of the dose used for the background infusion.[12] It remains to be seen if there is any advantage with the more sophisticated devices that can be programmed to adjust the background infusion according to the frequency of the bolus demands.[3]

Morphine or pethidine are the most common opioids for patient-controlled analgesia but consideration should be given to the risks from the accumulation of the pethidine metabolite, norpethidine. Oxymorphone or hydromorphone may be useful alternatives, and the agonist-antagonist nalbuphine has been used because of its ceiling effect on respiratory depression. The use of buprenorphine and methadone is limited by their long half-lives, while the action of drugs such as fentanyl and its analogues may be too short.

Most experience has been with the intravenous route, but the intramuscular, subcutaneous, epidural, and intrathecal routes have also been used. Epidural or intrathecal use may allow the use of smaller doses but the development of respiratory depression can be delayed when using the epidural route; a greater degree of patient monitoring may be required when using either of these routes.[13] Epidural **local anaesthetic** (bupivacaine) with an opioid analgesic such as fentanyl has been tried for use in patient-controlled analgesia, and may allow reduced opioid doses, although whether this confers any clinical benefit is questionable.[14]

Other routes are also being investigated.

Inhaled **nitrous oxide** in oxygen has a long history of effective use in patient-controlled analgesia during childbirth; patient-controlled opioid analgesia may not be suitable for such pain although local anaesthetics have been used with satisfactory results.[15,16]


1. Rowbotham DJ. The development and safe use of patient-controlled analgesia. *Br J Anaesth* 1992; **68:** 331–2.
2. Walder B, *et al.* Efficacy and safety of patient-controlled opioid analgesia for acute postoperative pain: a quantitative systematic review. *Acta Anaesthesiol Scand* 2001; **45:** 795–804.
3. Macintyre PE. Safety and efficacy of patient-controlled analgesia. *Br J Anaesth* 2001; **87:** 36–46.
4. Lam FY. Patient-controlled analgesia by proxy. *Br J Anaesth* 1993; **70:** 113.
5. Notcutt WG, *et al.* Overdose of opioid from patient-controlled analgesia pumps. *Br J Anaesth* 1992; **69:** 95–7.
6. Farmer M, Harper NJN. Unexpected problems with patient controlled analgesia. *BMJ* 1992; **304:** 574.
7. Johnson T, Daugherty M. Oversedation with patient controlled analgesia. *Anaesthesia* 1992; **47:** 81–2.
8. Love DR, *et al.* A comparison of variable-dose patient-controlled analgesia with fixed-dose patient-controlled analgesia. *Anesth Analg* 1996; **83:** 1060–4.
9. Parker RK, *et al.* Patient-controlled analgesia: does a concurrent opioid infusion improve pain management after surgery? *JAMA* 1991; **266:** 1947–52.
10. Doyle E, *et al.* Comparison of patient-controlled analgesia with and without a background infusion after lower abdominal surgery in children. *Br J Anaesth* 1993; **71:** 670–3.
11. Smythe MA, *et al.* Patient-controlled analgesia versus patient-controlled analgesia plus continuous infusion after hip replacement surgery. *Ann Pharmacother* 1996; **30:** 224–7.
12. Doyle E, *et al.* Patient-controlled analgesia with low dose background infusions after lower abdominal surgery in children. *Br J Anaesth* 1993; **71:** 818–22.
13. Hill HF, Mather LE. Patient-controlled analgesia: pharmacokinetic and therapeutic considerations. *Clin Pharmacokinet* 1993; **24:** 124–40.
14. Cooper DW, *et al.* Patient-controlled extradural analgesia with bupivacaine, fentanyl, or a mixture of both, after Caesarean section. *Br J Anaesth* 1996; **76:** 611–15.
15. McIntosh DG, Rayburn WF. Patient-controlled analgesia in obstetrics and gynecology. *Obstet Gynecol* 1991; **78:** 1129–35.
16. van der Vyver M, *et al.* Patient-controlled epidural analgesia versus continuous infusion for labour analgesia: a meta-analysis. *Br J Anaesth* 2002; **89:** 459–65.


### Postoperative analgesia

Pain relief following surgery has often been inadequate and it is now recognised that pain control should be adjusted for each patient and each situation. Where it can be done safely, the pain control should be established on a preventative basis (pre-emptive analgesia), but caution is necessary since any residual respiratory depression is liable to be enhanced by injection of an opioid postoperatively.

**Opioid analgesics**, in particular morphine, are still the mainstay of the treatment of postoperative pain. Opioids can control most postoperative pain, but the desired degree of analgesia needs to be balanced against adverse effects such as nausea, vomiting, and respiratory depression. Alternatives to morphine include alfentanil, fentanyl, papaveretum, and remifentanil. Partial opioid agonists or mixed agonist-antagonists such as buprenorphine, nalbuphine, and meptazinol, although less likely to produce respiratory depression, have a weaker analgesic action than morphine and are rarely used for postoperative pain. Giving a fixed intramuscular dose of an opioid on an 'as required' basis is painful, demanding of nursing time, and can produce widely fluctuating plasma concentrations (with associated risk of sudden respiratory depression). The intravenous route is more satisfactory and is now widely used; in the immediate postoperative period a useful strategy is to give a variable rate intravenous infusion with an initial bolus dose and subsequent top-up boluses if necessary. Patient-controlled analgesia (see above) has also proved popular by the intravenous route.

Opioids injected centrally via the epidural and intrathecal routes provide effective analgesia; a catheter can be inserted during surgery to permit continuous infusion or bolus injections; however, there is a high incidence of nausea, vomiting, urinary retention, pruritus, and respiratory depression (which may be delayed, calling for close monitoring of respiratory function). Morphine is the opioid most commonly given centrally, but others such as fentanyl, which is more lipid soluble, may be preferable in the case of epidural injection. The epidural and intrathecal routes have also been used for patient-controlled analgesia. For use of opioids with local anaesthetics, see below.

Oral opioids are not suitable in the immediate postoperative period, but may be convenient later, when gastrointestinal function has recovered. Opioids have also been given by the rectal, subcutaneous, sublingual, buccal, transdermal, and intranasal routes for postoperative pain, but, because of unreliable absorption and/or slow onset of action, these routes are not usually suitable for use immediately after surgery.

The lack of sedative effects with **NSAIDs** makes them of particular value in the management of acute pain after day-case surgery, but they are usually considered to be unsuitable as sole analgesics immediately after major surgery. They can, however, be used effectively with other drugs, and use of an NSAID with an opioid enables the dose of the opioid to be reduced without loss of analgesic effect. However, the risk of gastric ulceration, impaired coagulation, and reduced renal function may limit the use of NSAIDs in some patients. Diclofenac, flurbiprofen, ketoprofen, ketorolac, and lornoxicam are among the NSAIDs used for postoperative pain; the selective inhibitors of cyclo-oxygenase-2 (COX-2) including parecoxib and rofecoxib have also been used. Diclofenac, ketoprofen, ketorolac, and parecoxib may be given by injection.

Nerve blocks with **local anaesthetics** carried out during surgery often produce profound analgesia in the immediate postoperative period. However, effects are only temporary and repeated use may be impractical. Local infiltration of anaesthetic at the site of operation is a simple method of preventing postoperative wound pain. Central nerve blocks obtained with epidural or intrathecal local anaesthetics produce excellent analgesia and use of a long-acting drug such as bupivacaine can produce prolonged pain relief. Insertion of a catheter during the operation allows subsequent infusion or bolus injection. Hypotension is a potentially serious problem with central nerve blocks and constant monitoring of blood pressure is required. Giving mixtures of opioids and local anaesthetics epidurally or intrathecally has permitted good postoperative analgesia to be obtained in some situations using relatively smaller doses of each drug. A wide range of **other drugs** such as clonidine has also been tried by these routes, either alone or with opioids or local anaesthetics, but their role, if any, remains to be determined.

References.


1. Commission on the provision of surgical services. *Report of the working party on pain after surgery.* London: Royal College of Surgeons of England and College of Anaesthetists, 1990.
2. Anonymous. Managing postoperative pain. *Drug Ther Bull* 1993; **31:** 11–12.
3. Nuutinen LS, *et al.* A risk-benefit appraisal of injectable NSAIDs in the management of postoperative pain. *Drug Safety* 1993; **9:** 380–93.
4. Howard R. Preoperative and postoperative pain control. *Arch Dis Child* 1993; **69:** 699–703.
5. Katz J. Preop analgesia for postop pain. *Lancet* 1993; **342:** 65–6.
6. Kehlet H. Postoperative pain relief—what is the issue? *Br J Anaesth* 1994; **72:** 375–8.
7. Leith S, *et al.* Extradural infusion analgesia for postoperative pain relief. *Br J Anaesth* 1994; **73:** 552–8.
8. Chrubasik S, Chrubasik J. Selection of the optimum opioid for extradural administration in the treatment of postoperative pain. *Br J Anaesth* 1995; **74:** 121–2.
9. Cashman J, McAnulty G. Nonsteroidal anti-inflammatory drugs in perisurgical pain management: mechanisms of action and rationale for optimum use. *Drugs* 1995; **49:** 51–70.
10. American Society of Anesthesiologists Task Force on Pain Management, Acute Pain Section. Practice guidelines for acute pain management in the perioperative setting. *Anesthesiology* 1995; **82:** 1071–81.
11. McQuay HJ. Pre-emptive analgesia: a systematic review of clinical studies. *Ann Med* 1995; **27:** 249–56.
12. Raja SN. Is an ounce of preoperative local anesthetic better than a pound of postoperative analgesic? *Reg Anesth* 1996; **21:** 277–80.
13. Follin SL, Charland SL. Acute pain management: operative or medical procedures and trauma. *Ann Pharmacother* 1997; **31:** 1068–76.
14. Holder KA, *et al.* Postoperative pain management. *Int Anesthesiol Clin* 1998; **36:** 71–86.
15. Kehlet H, *et al.* Balanced analgesia: what is it and what are its advantages in postoperative pain? *Drugs* 1999; **58:** 793–7.
16. Dahl V, Raeder JC. Non-opioid postoperative analgesia. *Acta Anaesthesiol Scand* 2000; **44:** 1191–1203.
17. Rawal N. Treating postoperative pain improves outcome. *Minerva Anestesiol* 2001; **67** (suppl 1): 200–5.
18. Shang AB, Gan TJ. Optimising postoperative pain management in the ambulatory patient. *Drugs* 2003; **63:** 855–67.
19. Rosenquist RW, *et al.* Postoperative pain guidelines. *Reg Anesth Pain Med* 2003; **28:** 279–88. Also available at: http://www.oqp.med.va.gov/cpg/PAIN/PAIN_base.htm (accessed 09/06/04)
20. Block BM, *et al.* Efficacy of postoperative epidural analgesia: a meta-analysis. *JAMA* 2003; **290:** 2455–63.


### Rubefacients and topical analgesia

Rubefacients or counter-irritants can relieve superficial or deep-seated pain probably by producing counter stimulation, which according to the 'gate theory' of pain (see Analgesia and Pain, above) helps to inhibit the transmission of pain signals. Their topical application produces hyperaemia or irritation of the skin and they are used alone or as an adjunct to massage in the management of a variety of painful musculoskeletal conditions.[1] Some are also traditionally used in preparations for the symptomatic relief of minor peripheral vascular disorders such as chilblains. Substances commonly used in **rubefacient** preparations include nicotinate and salicylate compounds, essential oils, capsicum, solutions of ammonia, camphor, and nonivamide. **Capsaicin**, which is one of the active ingredients of capsicum, is used alone as a topical analgesic in a range of painful conditions, including neuropathic pain and rheumatic disorders. It does not rely on vasodilatation in the skin and it is therefore not considered to be a traditional counter-irritant.

Some **NSAIDs** have been used topically in the treatment of soft-tissue injuries and inflammatory musculoskeletal conditions, although this route does not necessarily avoid the adverse effects of systemic treatment. There is some evidence[2] to suggest that topical NSAIDs might be more effective than placebo but without comparative studies against other forms of treatment their therapeutic role is considered to be unclear.[3]

**Other agents** used as topical analgesics include compounds such as ethyl chloride and the halogenated hydrocarbon propellants; their evaporation produces an intense cold that numbs the tissues. Transdermal clonidine has been used in the treatment of chronic pain.

**Local anaesthetics** are sometimes included in topical preparations used for the relief of painful skin and musculoskeletal disorders.

Application of heat to the skin can also help to relieve pain and melted hard paraffin has been used in wax baths as an adjunct to physiotherapy for painful joints and sprains. Warm kaolin poultices have also been used as a means of applying heat for pain relief.


1. Sawynok J. Topical and peripherally acting analgesics. *Pharmacol Rev* 2003; **55:** 1–20.
2. Moore RA, *et al.* Quantitative systematic review of topically applied non-steroidal anti-inflammatory drugs. *BMJ* 1998; **316:** 333–8.
3. Duerden M, *et al.* Topical NSAIDs are better than placebo. *BMJ* 1998; **317:** 280–1.


## Specific pain states

**Biliary and renal colic.** Gallstones (see Ursodeoxycholic Acid, p.1761) or other biliary disorders that result in obstruction of the bile ducts may produce **biliary colic**. Morphine may relieve the accompanying pain, but as it can also produce spasm of the sphincter of Oddi it can raise intrabiliary pressure and exacerbate the pain. It is therefore usually recommended that morphine and its derivatives should either be avoided in patients with biliary disorders or that they should be given with an antispasmodic. Pethidine, which has less smooth muscle activity than morphine, may be more suitable. Prostaglandins have also been implicated in the aetiology of biliary colic and NSAIDs such as diclofenac or ketorolac have been successfully used to relieve the pain.[1-3] Antimuscarinics have been tried for their action on biliary smooth muscle and the sphincter of Oddi.

Ureteral obstruction, such as in the formation and passage of renal calculi (see p.936), produces painful **renal** or **ureteral colic**.[4-6] The acute pain of renal or ureteral colic may be relieved using opioid analgesics such as pethidine that have a minimal effect on smooth muscle although morphine has also been used.[5,6] NSAIDs are increasingly used in the treatment of renal colic and appear to be comparable in terms of efficacy to the opioids.[4-6] They can be given by a variety of routes including intramuscularly, intravenously, orally, and rectally although oral and rectal dosage may be less reliable. Diclofenac sodium given intramuscularly is recommended as first-line treatment by some authors.[6] Parenteral ketorolac also seems to be effective.[5] The use of intranasal desmopressin is also being studied.[4,5]


1. Akriviadis EA, *et al.* Treatment of biliary colic with diclofenac: a randomized, double-blind, placebo-controlled study. *Gastroenterology* 1997; **113:** 225–31.
2. Dula DJ, *et al.* A prospective study comparing im ketorolac with im meperidine in the treatment of acute biliary colic. *J Emerg Med* 2001; **20:** 121–4.
3. Henderson SO, *et al.* Comparison of intravenous ketorolac and meperidine in the treatment of biliary colic. *J Emerg Med* 2002; **23:** 237–41.

4. Shokeir AA. Renal colic: new concepts related to pathophysiology, diagnosis and treatment. *Curr Opin Urol* 2002; **12:** 263–9.
5. Heid F, Jage J. The treatment of pain in urology. *BJU Int* 2002; **90:** 481–8.
6. Wright PJ, *et al.* Managing acute renal colic across the primary-secondary care interface: a pathway of care based on evidence and consensus. *BMJ* 2002; **325:** 1408–12.

**Cancer pain.** The pain cancer patients experience may be acute, chronic, or intermittent. It may result from tumour involvement of the viscera and extension into soft tissues, tumour-induced nerve compression and injury, raised intracranial pressure, or bone metastases. Pain may also arise as a result of side-effects of treatment, or from a concurrent disease, and may be exacerbated by emotional or mental changes. Many patients will have more than one type of pain. There may also be exacerbations due to movement (incident pain) or worsening of cancer.

Pain relief involves the treatment of the cause of the pain as well as treatment of the pain itself, together with explanation, reassurance, and supportive care to improve any mental and social complicating factors. The mainstay of cancer pain management is drug treatment with non-opioid or opioid analgesics, or both together, plus adjuvant analgesics if necessary. A small proportion of patients (about 10 to 20%) may experience pain that responds poorly or not at all to opioid analgesics given at tolerable doses, e.g. neuropathic pain resulting from nerve destruction or compression, incident bone pain, pancreatic pain, and muscle spasm.

In the management of cancer pain the aim is to achieve adequate continuous pain relief with the minimum of side-effects and this calls for regular monitoring of the treatment. Guidelines for the relief of cancer pain, published by WHO in 1986[1] and revised in 1996,[2] are widely endorsed by specialists in pain relief and the care of the terminally ill;[3-19] in the UK, guidelines[20] issued by the Scottish Intercollegiate Guidelines Network in 2000 are also widely referred to. Specific guidelines for the relief of cancer pain in children have also been published.[21] Regardless of age, patients need to be assessed individually and, wherever possible, treatment is given by mouth. It should be given regularly and should follow the accepted three-step **'analgesic ladder'**.[1,2] This approach is often described as treatment 'by mouth, by the clock, and by the ladder'. Regular dosage rather than treatment as required aims to prevent pain re-emerging and to minimise the expectation of pain. The analgesic ladder consists of 3 stages, treatment beginning at step 1 and progressing to step 3 if pain is uncontrolled or increases. The stages are as follows:

1. a non-opioid analgesic such as aspirin, other NSAIDs, or paracetamol; an adjuvant (see below) may also be given if necessary to tackle specific pain or associated symptoms
2. an opioid analgesic such as codeine, dihydrocodeine, or tramadol plus a non-opioid analgesic; an adjuvant may also be given
3. a potent opioid analgesic such as oral morphine; a non-opioid analgesic may also be given, as may an adjuvant.

Using analgesics with different pharmacological actions together can produce additive or synergistic increases in analgesia but only one analgesic from each of the 3 groups (non-opioid, less potent opioid, potent opioid) should be used at the same time.

Unmanageable adverse effects of one analgesic may be eliminated by changing to another or possibly by altering the route.[22,23] Any sedation should be assessed, for while it may be useful in the management of acute pain, it is undesirable in patients with chronic pain. Although tolerance, physical dependence, and withdrawal symptoms can occur with continued use of opioids, this does not prevent their effective use for cancer pain. Withdrawal symptoms may be avoided by gradually tapering doses on stopping a drug. Psychological dependence and addictive behaviour do not occur when opioids are used in cancer patients, so fears of their development should not restrict use of these analgesics, and opioid-sensitive pain appears to protect against respiratory depression, although it may occur if the source of opioid-sensitive pain is removed (e.g. by surgery) without adequate reduction in opioid dosage.

The opioid of choice for moderate to severe pain is morphine. It is given by mouth as a solution or tablets every 4 hours or as modified-release formulations every 12 or 24 hours. Individualisation of dosage by gradual adjustment is important; doses have ranged from 2.5 mg to more than 1 g of morphine sulfate every 4 hours, although most patients need far less than 100 mg every 4 hours. In patients receiving modified-release preparations the oral solution or standard tablets are used for breakthrough pain pending an increase in modified-release dosage (for further details see under Uses and Administration of Morphine, p.63). Patients vary in their response to opioids and sequential trials may be needed to identify the drug which yields the most favourable balance between analgesia and adverse effects. Alternatives to morphine include hydromorphone, methadone, oxycodone, and fentanyl. 'Brompton Cocktail' mixtures or elixirs, which contained diamorphine or morphine and cocaine with or without chlorpromazine, are now obsolete.

Although the oral route is generally preferred, other routes, such as the rectal route, may be necessary if, for example, there is intractable vomiting, inability to swallow, or unconsciousness. When injections become necessary a continuous subcutaneous infusion may be preferable to repeated subcutaneous or intramuscular injections. In the UK diamorphine hydrochloride is often preferred to morphine sulfate for parenteral use because it is more soluble and allows a smaller dose volume; hydromorphone hydrochloride is an alternative to diamorphine. Morphine has also been given intravenously by bolus injection or infusion.

Epidural or intrathecal opioids, either by injection or infusion, has been used when conventional routes have failed. Some advocate the use of these routes because smaller doses may produce analgesia equivalent to that of larger doses given by mouth or parenterally, although there has been little conclusive evidence for a lower incidence of side-effects or a better quality of analgesia.

The buccal, sublingual, and nebulised routes have been investigated, but these are not recommended for morphine because there is no current evidence of clinical advantage over conventional routes.[15] However, buprenorphine is given sublingually and may be a useful alternative in patients with dysphagia, although experience of long-term use in cancer pain is limited. Buprenorphine and fentanyl can be given via a transdermal system that provides continuous and controlled delivery for 72 hours. A lozenge-on-a-stick-lollipop dosage form of fentanyl is also available for the management of breakthrough cancer pain.

Automated delivery systems for self-administration of parenteral analgesics (patient-controlled analgesia) have been used to administer opioid analgesics (see above).

**Adjuvant drugs** that may be necessary at any stage include antidepressants, antiepileptics, and class I antiarrhythmics for neuropathic pain, corticosteroids for nerve compression and headache resulting from raised intracranial pressure, and muscle relaxants for muscle spasm. Radiotherapy and radioisotopes such as strontium-89 may be of use when the bone pain of metastases is unresponsive to NSAIDs alone. Bone modulating drugs such as calcitonin and bisphosphonates may be of additional benefit but have a slow onset of action and bisphosphonates may cause an initial transient increase in pain. Corticosteroids have been used as an alternative to NSAIDs in refractory bone pain but long-term use should be avoided. Nerve blocks with local anaesthetics or neurolytic solutions may benefit a few patients, in particular those with sympathetically maintained pain or specific localised pain (see under Pain, p.1369). Physiotherapy and relaxation techniques may be useful for painful muscle spasm. The addition of an NMDA antagonist such as dextromethorphan or ketamine to conventional analgesic regimens has been tried with some success in patients with refractory pain.[22,23] Adjuvant therapy should be fully explored before moving on to the next 'rung' of the treatment ladder or increasing the dosage of an opioid analgesic. For further details of analgesic adjuvants, see Choice of Analgesic, above.

1. WHO. *Cancer pain relief.* Geneva: WHO, 1986.
2. WHO. *Cancer pain relief.* 2nd ed. Geneva: WHO, 1996.
3. Hillier R. Control of pain in terminal cancer. *Br Med Bull* 1990; **46:** 279–91.
4. American Pain Society. Principles of analgesic use in the treatment of acute pain and chronic cancer pain, 2nd edition. *Clin Pharm* 1990; **9:** 601–11.
5. WHO. Cancer pain relief and palliative care: report of a WHO expert committee. *WHO Tech Rep Ser 804* 1990.
6. Schechter NL, *et al.* Report of the consensus conference on the management of pain in childhood cancer. *Pediatrics* 1990; **86:** 813–34.
7. Hanks GW, Justins DM. Cancer pain: management. *Lancet* 1992; **339:** 1031–6.
8. Davis CL, Hardy JR. Palliative care. *BMJ* 1994; **308:** 1359–62.
9. Hammack JE, Loprinzi CL. Use of orally administered opioids for cancer-related pain. *Mayo Clin Proc* 1994; **69:** 384–90.
10. Lamer TJ. Treatment of cancer-related pain: when orally administered medications fail. *Mayo Clin Proc* 1994; **69:** 473–80.
11. US Agency for Health Care Policy and Research. Management of cancer pain: adults. *Am J Hosp Pharm* 1994; **51:** 1643–56.
12. American Society of Anesthesiologists Task Force on Pain Management, Cancer Pain Section. Practice guidelines for cancer pain management. *Anesthesiology* 1996; **84:** 1243–57.
13. Marshall KA. Managing cancer pain: basic principles and invasive treatments. *Mayo Clin Proc* 1996; **71:** 472–7.
14. Levy MH. Pharmacologic treatment of cancer pain. *N Engl J Med* 1996; **335:** 1124–32.
15. Expert Working Group of the European Association for Palliative Care. Morphine in cancer pain: modes of administration. *BMJ* 1996; **312:** 823–6.
16. Thürlimann B, de Stoutz ND. Causes and treatment of bone pain of malignant origin. *Drugs* 1996; **51:** 383–98.
17. O'Neill B, Fallon M. ABC of palliative care. Principles of palliative care and pain control. *BMJ* 1997; **315:** 801–4.
18. Sykes J, *et al.* ABC of palliative care. Difficult pain problems. *BMJ* 1997; **315:** 867–9.
19. Portenoy RK, Lesage P. Management of cancer pain. *Lancet* 1999; **353:** 1695–1700. Also available at: http://www.thelancet.com/journal/vol357/iss1/full/llan.357.s1.pain_series.15835.1 (accessed 01/07/04)
20. Scottish Intercollegiate Guidelines Network. Control of pain in patients with cancer: a national clinical guideline (June 2000). Available at: http://www.sign.ac.uk/pdf/sign44.pdf (accessed 01/07/04)
21. WHO. *Cancer pain relief and palliative care in children.* Geneva: WHO, 1998.
22. Vielhaber A, *et al.* Advances in cancer pain management. *Hematol Oncol Clin North Am* 2002; **16:** 527–41.
23. Lucas LK, Lipman AG. Recent advances in pharmacotherapy for cancer pain management. *Cancer Pract* 2002; **10** (suppl 1): S14–S20.

**Central post-stroke pain.** Central pain is a neuropathic pain arising from lesions of the CNS.[1-4] Pain following a cerebrovascular accident has been referred to as thalamic syndrome but is now commonly known as central post-stroke pain and may arise not only from classical stroke but also from surgery or trauma to the head. The pain, which has been described as burning, stabbing, and aching, may be mild to intolerable and occurs spontaneously or in response to a mild stimulus.

As in other types of neuropathic pain whether opioid analgesics can be of benefit is controversial: it has been suggested that the value of conventional opioids such as high-dose morphine is modest, but that NMDA receptor antagonists such as methadone may be of more benefit.[4] Ketamine, which is also an NMDA antagonist, may also be of value. Conventional management of central post-stroke pain involves the use of antidepressants such as amitriptyline and antiepileptics including lamotrigine. Early peripheral sympathetic blockade may produce temporary relief in some cases. Mexiletine may be of use in patients with refractory pain; it has often been given with amitriptyline. Transcutaneous electrical nerve stimulation (TENS) may occasionally be of help but some advocate brain or spinal cord stimulation. Surgical treatment generally gives disappointing results.

1. Illis LS. Central pain. *BMJ* 1990; **300:** 1284–6.
2. Bowsher D. Cerebrovascular disease: sensory consequences of stroke. *Lancet* 1993; **341:** 156.
3. Bowsher D. The management of central post-stroke pain. *Postgrad Med J* 1995; **71:** 598–604.
4. Bowsher D. Central post-stroke ('thalamic syndrome') and other central pains. *Am J Hosp Palliat Care* 1999; **16:** 593–7.

**Complex regional pain syndrome.** Complex regional pain syndrome (CRPS) is a regional, post-traumatic neuropathic pain that generally affects the limbs. CRPS has also been referred to as reflex sympathetic dystrophy, post-traumatic dystrophy, causalgia, Sudeck's atrophy, and shoulder-hand syndrome. Causalgia has also been used to describe the burning pain that follows a penetrating injury. Historically, it was considered that the pain was maintained by the sympathetic nervous system and the term 'reflex sympathetic dystrophy' was commonly used to describe the syndrome; however, recent studies have shown that the sympathetic nervous system is not always involved.

CRPS may be described as type I or type II; the latter is associated with an injury to a major peripheral nerve. Clinically the two subsets are identical and typical symptoms include pain, allodynia, and hyperalgesia; as the syndrome becomes chronic, trophic changes to the muscles and skin may occur. Sympathetic dysfunction may also be present. If the pain is relieved by a sympathetic block (see below), this pain is regarded as 'sympathetically-maintained', if not it is known as 'sympathetically-independent' pain.

The treatment of CRPS is difficult especially in chronic disorders and is usually aimed at pain control and restoring limb function. The cornerstone of treatment is physiotherapy, with pain relief provided in order to allow physical exercise. Patients with mild disease may not require pain management; those with moderate pain should be tried with a tricyclic antidepressant, an antiepileptic such as gabapentin, or a less potent opioid. A sympathetic nerve block with a local anaesthetic may be useful in carefully selected patients with sympathetically-maintained pain; those who do not respond to a sympathetic nerve block may be given an epidural block. Other methods that have been tried in refractory patients include spinal cord stimulation and intrathecal baclofen or opioids. There are small studies or anecdotal reports of the use of a variety of other drugs.

References.


1. Kingery WS. A critical review of controlled clinical trials for peripheral neuropathic pain and complex regional pain syndromes. *Pain* 1997; **73:** 123–39.
2. Baron R, Wasner G. Complex regional pain syndromes. *Curr Pain Headache Rep* 2001; **5:** 114–23.
3. Schott GD. Reflex sympathetic dystrophy. *J Neurol Neurosurg Psychiatry* 2001; **71:** 291–5.
4. Rho RH, *et al.* Complex regional pain syndrome. *Mayo Clin Proc* 2002; **77:** 174–80.
5. Wasner G, *et al.* Complex regional pain syndrome—diagnostic, mechanisms, CNS involvement and therapy. *Spinal Cord* 2003; **41:** 61–75.
6. Hord ED, Oaklander AL. Complex regional pain syndrome: a review of evidence-supported treatment options. *Curr Pain Headache Rep* 2003; **7:** 188–96.


**Diabetic neuropathy.** Sensory polyneuropathy, a complication of diabetes mellitus, is the commonest of the neuropathies producing neuropathic pain. The pain is mainly experienced as a burning sensation, sometimes accompanied by shooting, or aching pain. Painful neuropathy benefits from optimal diabetic control (see p.326). Non-opioid analgesics such as aspirin or other NSAIDs, or paracetamol may be tried, although neuropathic pain is often resistant to conventional analgesics, and the treatment of painful diabetic neuropathy is generally as for postherpetic neuralgia (see below). Relief may be obtained using tricyclic antidepressants and the *British National Formulary* considers them to be the drugs of choice. SSRIs have been tried but studies suggest that they are ineffective or less effective than tricyclic antidepressants. Antiepileptics such as carbamazepine, gabapentin, and phenytoin can be used to control any shooting or stabbing components of the pain; lamotrigine and topiramate are also under investigation. Antiarrhythmics such as lidocaine given intravenously or mexiletine given orally have been shown to be effective against some components of the pain. Topical application of capsaicin may have some effect.

References.


1. Bowsher D. Neurogenic pain syndromes and their management. *Br Med Bull* 1991; **47:** 644–66.
2. Fedele D, Giugliano D. Peripheral diabetic neuropathy: current recommendations and future prospects for its prevention and management. *Drugs* 1997; **54:** 414–21.
3. Collins SL, *et al.* Antidepressants and anticonvulsants for diabetic neuropathy and postherpetic neuralgia: a quantitative systematic review. *J Pain Symptom Manage* 2000; **20:** 449–58.
4. Jensen PG, Larson JR. Management of painful diabetic neuropathy. *Drugs Aging* 2001; **18:** 737–49.
5. Boulton AJ. Treatments for diabetic neuropathy. *Curr Diab Rep* 2001; **1:** 127–32.
6. Barbano R, *et al.* Pharmacotherapy of painful diabetic neuropathy. *Curr Pain Headache Rep* 2003; **7:** 169–77.


**Dysmenorrhoea.** Dysmenorrhoea is painful menstruation. The primary form arises from uterine contractions produced by release of prostaglandins from the endometrium in the luteal phase of the menstrual cycle. For this reason, drugs that inhibit ovulation or prostaglandin production are often effective treatments.[1] NSAIDs inhibit cyclo-oxygenase (prostaglandin synthetase) and are usually the drugs of first choice. They are taken at the onset of discomfort and continued for a few days while symptoms persist. Those most commonly used have included aspirin, diflunisal, flurbiprofen, ibuprofen, indometacin, ketoprofen, mefenamic acid, naproxen, and piroxicam. Theoretically, mefenamic acid has the advantage of inhibiting both the synthesis and the peripheral action of prostaglandins, but clinical studies have not consistently shown fenamates to be more effective than other cyclo-oxygenase inhibitors. Paracetamol has also been given for pain relief. A systematic review[2] comparing several of these drugs concluded that ibuprofen appeared to have the best risk-benefit ratio in dysmenorrhoea and was the preferred analgesic; naproxen, mefenamic acid, and aspirin were also effective, but the limited data on paracetamol did not demonstrate such clear benefits. Another such review considered that there was insufficient evidence to determine which NSAID should be preferred.[3]

Patients who fail to respond to analgesics may benefit from the use of progestogens either alone for part of the cycle or more usually together with oestrogens in the form of oral contraceptive preparations.

Antispasmodic drugs such as hyoscine butylbromide are included in some preparations promoted for the relief of spasm associated with dysmenorrhoea but the *British National Formulary* considers that they do not generally provide significant relief.

Secondary dysmenorrhoea is associated with various other disorders such as endometriosis, and treatment is primarily aimed at the underlying cause.


1. Shapiro SS. Treatment of dysmenorrhoea and premenstrual syndrome with non-steroidal anti-inflammatory drugs. *Drugs* 1988; **36:** 475–90.
2. Zhang WY, Li Wan Po A. Efficacy of minor analgesics in primary dysmenorrhoea: a systematic review. *Br J Obstet Gynaecol* 1998; **105:** 780–9.
3. Marjoribanks J, *et al.* Nonsteroidal anti-inflammatory drugs for primary dysmenorrhoea. Available in The Cochrane Library; Issue 2. Chichester: John Wiley; 2004.


**Headache.** Aspirin and other NSAIDs, or paracetamol are often tried first for the symptomatic treatment of various types of headache including migraine (p.464) and tension-type headache (p.465). NSAIDs may also be effective for the prophylaxis of migraine, although they are not considered first-line options.

Opioid analgesics such as codeine are sometimes included in oral compound analgesic preparations used in the initial treatment of migraine or tension-type headache, but are best avoided, especially in patients who experience frequent attacks.

**Labour pain.** It is important to assess the adverse effects, on both the mother and the fetus, when selecting any method for the management of labour pain. Non-drug measures such as relaxation and massage, and warm baths are often advocated, but pharmacological methods of analgesia are requested by the majority of women in labour.[1,2]

The inhalational anaesthetic **nitrous oxide**, given with oxygen, is suitable for self-administration and is commonly used to relieve labour pain. It is relatively safe and can produce substantial analgesia in most patients. Other inhalational analgesics are also sometimes used (see Choice of Analgesic, above).

**Opioid analgesics** have been given systemically in the management of labour pain for many years, although they do not appear to provide adequate analgesia in most patients at a tolerable dosage.[3,4] Pethidine has been used widely for this purpose. Unfortunately, like all opioids, it can cross the placenta and produce respiratory depression in the fetus and, when given by intramuscular injection, the onset of action can be unpredictable. Intermittent intravenous doses, or continuous infusion, or patient-controlled intravenous analgesia have been tried to improve pain control, but epidural blocks (see below) seem to be more effective.

**Epidural analgesia** with a *local anaesthetic* provides the most effective pain relief during labour.[2,4-6] Medical indications may include a history of malignant hyperthermia, certain cardiovascular or respiratory disorders, or pre-eclampsia, but the primary indication is the patient's desire for pain relief.[4,5]

Epidural block has few contra-indications and serious adverse events are rare. Nonetheless, it has been associated with an increased risk of prolonged labour, forceps delivery, and caesarean section[4-7] (although meta-analysis[3] and a systematic review[6] refute the latter), and it may not improve maternal experience of childbirth. Profound hypotension can occur as a result of sympathetic block.[8] Other effects may include diminished patient awareness of uterine contractions and of giving birth, sensations of weakness, numbness and paraesthesia of the lower limbs, impaired mobility, bladder distension, and pyrexia or uncontrollable shivering.[1,9] Many of these effects are associated with motor block and can be reduced by using doses of local anaesthetic lower than those required for surgery. Epidural analgesia can also prolong the second stage of labour and the use of oxytocin may be required.[9] However, since a request for epidural analgesia is most likely from women experiencing a slow, complicated, painful labour it is difficult to quantify the effect of the epidural itself.[10,11] Further details of the adverse effects of and precautions for epidural block can be found under Central Block on p.1367 and p.1368, respectively. Occasionally epidural local anaesthetic does not produce adequate analgesia due to patchy or incomplete block.[8]

Bupivacaine is one of the local anaesthetics most often used in epidural analgesia.

*Opioid analgesics* have been given epidurally but are not particularly effective for labour pain when used alone.[8,12] Adequate analgesia is usually only obtained with doses that are associated with nausea, sedation, and disorientation.[1] Severe pruritus can also be a problem with some opioids such as morphine. Delayed respiratory depression is also a potential hazard, but may be less of a problem with drugs such as pethidine or fentanyl.[1,8] Epidural opioids are considered to be most useful when given with epidural local anaesthetics. The addition of small doses of opioid analgesics to bupivacaine provides additional pain relief and reduces the amount of local anaesthetic required as well as the degree of motor block.[2,4,8,12] The addition of an opioid can also control epidural-induced shivering.[12] Several opioids have been tried epidurally with bupivacaine but it has not yet been determined which is the most suitable for pain relief during labour; favourable results have been obtained with drugs such as fentanyl or sufentanil. The use of drugs such as clonidine with local anaesthetics or opioids is also being studied.

Once the initial block is established additional analgesia can be provided through a catheter by intermittent 'top-up' doses or by a continuous epidural infusion;[1,13] a combination of the two methods forms the basis of some types of patient-controlled epidural analgesia.[13-15]

A spinal block given before the epidural block reduces the degree of motor block associated with epidural analgesia and allows the patient to be ambulatory during labour.[14,16-19] Combined **spinal-epidural analgesia** provides the rapid onset of spinal block and the flexibility of continuous epidural block,[4,5,10,13,20] and may have advantages when analgesia is requested late in labour, where maternal distress is severe, and in situations where epidural analgesia has proved unsatisfactory.[15]

Although there is renewed interest in the use of **spinal blocks** in labour[14] they do not appear to have been widely used alone for the relief of labour pain and it is considered[10] that no single drug or combination of drugs by this route reliably provides adequate analgesia for the duration of labour. The use of spinal blocks in obstetrics has been more commonly associated with anaesthesia and management of postoperative pain in caesarean section.[1,2] Spinal blocks with local anaesthetics have a greater tendency to produce hypotension and headache than epidural blocks, and this appears to be particularly so in pregnant patients.[21] Although spinal block using opioids may control labour pain, some consider that they are unsuitable for use alone because they also produce a greater incidence of adverse effects in pregnant patients.[21] Further details of the adverse effects of and precautions for spinal block can be found under Central Block on p.1367 and p.1368, respectively.

Pudendal nerve blocks with lidocaine followed by administration of a local anaesthetic into the perineum provides pain relief during labour.[2] However, the technique of paracervical local anaesthetic block has been largely abandoned in labour pain[1] because of the high incidence of fetal arrhythmias, acidosis, and asphyxia and isolated reports of fetal death.


1. Brownridge P. Treatment options for the relief of pain during childbirth. *Drugs* 1991; **41:** 69–80.
2. Findley I, Chamberlain G. ABC of labour care. Relief of pain. *BMJ* 1999; **318:** 927–30.
3. Halpern SH, *et al.* Effect of epidural vs parenteral opioid analgesia in the progress of labor. *JAMA* 1998; **280:** 2105–10.
4. Goetzl LM, *et al.* ACOG Practice Bulletin. Clinical management guidelines for obstetrician-gynecologists number 36, July 2002: obstetric analgesia and anesthesia. *Obstet Gynecol* 2002; **100:** 177–91.
5. Eltzschig HK, *et al.* Regional anesthesia and analgesia for labor and delivery. *N Engl J Med* 2003; **348:** 319–32.
6. Howell CJ. Epidural versus non-epidural analgesia for pain relief in labour. Available in The Cochrane Library; Issue 2. Chichester: John Wiley; 2004.
7. Thorp JA, *et al.* The effect of intrapartum epidural analgesia on nulliparous labor: a randomized, controlled, prospective trial. *Am J Obstet Gynecol* 1993; **169:** 851–8.
8. Anonymous. Pain relief in labour: old drugs, new route. *Lancet* 1991; **337:** 1446–7.
9. Reynolds F. Epidural analgesia in obstetrics. *BMJ* 1989; **299:** 751–2.
10. Eberle RL, Norris MC. Labour analgesia: a risk-benefit analysis. *Drug Safety* 1996; **14:** 239–51.
11. McGrady EM. Extradural analgesia: does it affect progress and outcome in labour? *Br J Anaesth* 1997; **78:** 115–17.
12. Reynolds F. Extradural opioids in labour. *Br J Anaesth* 1989; **63:** 251–3.
13. Collis RE. Regional analgesia in labour: a new look. *Hosp Med* 1998; **59:** 388–92.
14. Kan RE, Hughes SC. Recent developments in analgesia during labour. *Drugs* 1995; **50:** 417–22.
15. Paech M. New epidural techniques for labour analgesia: patient-controlled epidural analgesia and combined spinal-epidural analgesia. *Baillieres Clin Obstet Gynaecol* 1998; **12:** 377–95.
16. Collis RE, *et al.* Combined spinal epidural analgesia with ability to walk throughout labour. *Lancet* 1993; **341:** 767–8. Correction *ibid.*; 1038.
17. Camann W, Abouleish A. Spinal epidural analgesia and walking throughout labour. *Lancet* 1993; **341:** 1095.
18. Collis RE, *et al.* Randomised comparison of combined spinal-epidural and standard epidural analgesia in labour. *Lancet* 1995; **345:** 1413–16.
19. Nageotte MP, *et al.* Epidural analgesia compared with combined spinal-epidural analgesia during labor in nulliparous women. *N Engl J Med* 1997; **337:** 1715–19.
20. Hughes D, *et al.* Combined spinal-epidural versus epidural analgesia in labour. Available in The Cochrane Library; Issue 2. Chichester: John Wiley; 2004.
21. Kestin IG. Spinal anaesthesia in obstetrics. *Br J Anaesth* 1991; **66:** 596–607.

**Low back pain.** Low back pain (sometimes referred to as lumbago), is a common complaint but only a small percentage of patients suffer from a recognised organic disease, most frequently disc disease. In patients with a herniated or prolapsed disc, the rupture of one of the fibrocartilagenous intervertebral discs can exert pressure on spinal nerves and produce a condition characterised by severe and often acute pain radiating from the back along the distribution of the nerves affected. In lumbar disc herniation the sciatic nerve may be involved and patients experience pain (sciatica), usually in one leg along the typical distribution of the nerve.

Treatment for **acute back pain** should be given early to prevent the condition becoming chronic. For simple back pain (in the absence of nerve root symptoms or signs of serious spinal pathology) paracetamol is tried, and if this fails to give relief an NSAID is substituted. If neither of these drugs controls the pain adequately, paracetamol may be combined with an opioid such as codeine; more potent opioid analgesics such as morphine should be avoided if possible. Analgesics should be given regularly rather than when required. A short course of a muscle relaxant such as diazepam or baclofen may also be considered. Unless patients are in severe pain or unable to stand or walk, bed rest is no longer recommended; if it is necessary, bed rest should be limited to up to 3 days. Early physical activity, even if it causes some discomfort, improves the rate of recovery. Specific exercises do not appear to be useful for acute back pain but manipulation may be considered during the first weeks after onset.

Bed rest was often advocated in the treatment of **sciatica** but it has subsequently been found to be no more useful than watchful waiting. Epidural injections of corticosteroids with or without local anaesthetics, using either the caudal or lumbar route, may facilitate recovery. Manipulation should not be used for patients with evidence of nerve root entrapment as it may exacerbate the lesion. Surgery is indicated in patients with herniated disc if conservative treatment fails or if there is severe nerve compression. Dissolution of the disc by injection of enzymes (chemonucleolysis) such as chymopapain or collagenase appears to be an effective alternative to surgery, but anaphylactic reactions may occur.

The prevalence of **chronic or recurrent back problems** is high, and in the majority of cases, the source of the pain cannot be identified. Chronic pain is not necessarily the same as prolonged acute back pain and treatment is difficult. Surgery may be indicated for disc disease (see above) or spondylosis, and local injections of corticosteroids, sclerosant injections into ligaments, or cryotherapy to facet joints have all been tried, but the success rate of these procedures is low. Rehabilitation programmes combining physical and psychological approaches to managing back pain, transcutaneous electrical nerve stimulation (TENS), acupuncture, and neurolytic nerve blocks are other methods that have been tried for intractable chronic back pain.

References.


1. Bush K. Lower back pain and sciatica: how best to manage them. *Br J Hosp Med* 1994; **51:** 216–22.
2. Royal College of General Practitioners. *Clinical guidelines for the management of acute low back pain: low back pain evidence review.* London: Royal College of General Practitioners, 1996.
3. Jayson MIV. Back pain. *BMJ* 1996; **313:** 355–8.
4. Deyo RA. Acute low back pain: a new paradigm for management. *BMJ* 1996; **313:** 1343–4.
5. Jayson MIV. Why does acute back pain become chronic? *BMJ* 1997; **314:** 1639–40.
6. van Tulder MW, *et al.* Conservative treatment of acute and chronic nonspecific low back pain: a systematic review of randomized controlled trials of the most common interventions. *Spine* 1997; **22:** 2128–56.
7. Anonymous. Managing acute low back pain. *Drug Ther Bull* 1998; **12:** 93–5.
8. Vroomen PCAJ, *et al.* Lack of effectiveness of bed rest for sciatica. *N Engl J Med* 1999; **340:** 418–23.
9. Malanga GA, Nadler SF. Nonoperative treatment of low back pain. *Mayo Clin Proc* 1999; **74:** 1135–48.
10. Deyo RA, Weinstein JN. Low back pain. *N Engl J Med* 2001; **344:** 363–70.
11. Priest TD, Hoggart B. Chronic pain: mechanisms and treatment. *Curr Opin Pharmacol* 2002; **2:** 310–15.
12. Ehrlich GE. Low back pain. *Bull WHO* 2003; **81:** 671–6.
13. Bogduk N. Management of chronic low back pain. *Med J Aust* 2004; **180:** 79–83.
14. Speed C. Low back pain. In: Snaith ML, ed. *ABC of rheumatology.* 3rd ed. London: BMJ Publishing Group, 2004: 15–18.


**Myocardial infarction pain.** The severe pain of acute myocardial infarction is located in the retrosternal area with radiation to the arms, neck, jaw, and epigastrium. Pain relief is of benefit not only in its own right but also because pain may cause adverse haemodynamic effects such as increases in blood pressure, heart rate, and stroke volume. Although early treatment of the myocardial infarction (p.828) may relieve pain dramatically, opioid analgesics are the first-line treatment for pain and should be given intravenously as soon as possible, that is before hospital admission, to patients with suspected infarction.[1-4] Opioids can also help to reduce anxiety. An inhaled mixture of nitrous oxide and oxygen has sometimes been used to provide pain relief before arrival in hospital; sublingual glyceryl trinitrate or an alternative fast-acting nitrate may also be given.

Diamorphine or morphine given by slow intravenous injection have generally been the opioids of choice, partly because of a more advantageous haemodynamic profile, but pethidine has also been used. An antiemetic such as metoclopramide or, if left ventricular function is not compromised, cyclizine, by intravenous injection should also be given. The intramuscular route should only be used if venous access is unobtainable since it is relatively ineffective in shocked patients, complicates the enzymatic assessment of the infarction, and may result in large haematomas when patients are given thrombolytics. Alternative analgesics include nalbuphine or buprenorphine, although the latter may not produce pain relief as quickly as diamorphine. The cardiovascular effects of pentazocine make it unsuitable for use during or after myocardial infarction.


1. Wyllie HR, Dunn FG. Pre-hospital opiate and aspirin administration in patients with suspected myocardial infarction. *BMJ* 1994; **308:** 760–1.
2. Weston CFM, *et al.* Guidelines for the early management of patients with myocardial infarction. *BMJ* 1994; **308:** 767–71.
3. Ryan TJ, *et al.* 1999 update: ACC/AHA guidelines for the management of patients with acute myocardial infarction: a report of the American College of Cardiology/American Heart Association Task Force on Practice Guidelines (Committee on Management of Acute Myocardial Infarction). *J Am Coll Cardiol* 1999; **34:** 890–911.
4. Gershlick AH. The acute management of myocardial infarction. *Br Med Bull* 2001; **59:** 89–112.


**Neuropathic pain syndromes.** The definition and characteristics of neuropathic pain are described under Analgesia and Pain, above. Treatment can be difficult and is best undertaken in specialist pain clinics, since neuropathic pain often responds poorly to conventional analgesics.[1-3] The painful disorders characterised by neuropathic pain (either as the predominant form of pain or as one component of the overall pain) discussed in this section are Central Post-stroke Pain, Diabetic Neuropathy, Phantom Limb Pain, Postherpetic Neuralgia, Sympathetic Pain Syndromes such as reflex sympathetic dystrophy and causalgia, and Trigeminal Neuralgia.


1. Anonymous. Drug treatment of neuropathic pain. *Drug Ther Bull* 2000; **38:** 89–93.
2. Attal N. Pharmacologic treatment of neuropathic pain. *Acta Neurol Belg* 2001; **101:** 53–64.
3. Hempenstall K, Rice ASC. Current treatment options in neuropathic pain. *Curr Opin Investig Drugs* 2002; **3:** 441–8.


**Orofacial pain.** Orofacial pain may arise from a wide range of disorders so its effective management depends very much on the correct identification and treatment of any underlying cause, which may include dental disease, cluster headache (p.464), migraine (p.464), trigeminal neuralgia (see below), sinusitis (p.146), ear disease such as otitis media (p.138), giant cell arteritis (p.1080), aneurysms, and neoplasms. In the treatment of dental pain, analgesics are used judiciously as a temporary measure until the underlying cause has been effectively managed. Paracetamol or aspirin or other NSAIDs are adequate for most purposes. Opioid analgesics are relatively ineffective and are rarely needed.

In addition, a large number of patients have a type of facial pain of unknown cause which is typically exacerbated by stress and can develop into a chronic debilitating disorder. Many patients with such idiopathic facial pain respond to non-opioid analgesics, explanation, and reassurance. Antidepressants such as the tricyclics are often of value. Antiepileptics, including carbamazepine and sodium valproate, and the oral lidocaine analogue mexiletine have been used as adjuncts to the tricyclics. Topical treatment with capsaicin has also been tried. Treatment needs to be continued for several months to avoid pain recurrence on withdrawal. Psychological treatments can also be helpful. Botulinum A toxin has been tried for the relief of facial pain associated with some disorders of the orofacial muscles.

References.


1. Hunter S. The management of "psychogenic" orofacial pain. *BMJ* 1992; **304:** 329–30.
2. Feinmann C, Peatfield R. Orofacial neuralgia: diagnosis and treatment guidelines. *Drugs* 1993; **46:** 263–8.
3. Vickers ER, Cousins MJ. Neuropathic orofacial pain part 2–diagnostic procedures, treatment guidelines and case reports. *Aust Endod J* 2000; **26:** 53–63.
4. List T, *et al.* Pharmacologic interventions in the treatment of temporomandibular disorders, atypical facial pain, and burning mouth syndrome: a qualitative systematic review. *J Orofac Pain* 2003; **17:** 301–10.


**Pancreatic pain.** Pain in pancreatitis (p.1726) can be severe and may require opioid analgesics. Concerns over the long-term use of opioids in non-malignant pain should not prevent the patient being given effective analgesia which may be achieved by following the general principles recommended by the WHO for treatment of cancer pain (see above):

- mild attacks of pain may be treated using non-opioid analgesics including NSAIDs, with or without antispasmodics such as antimuscarinics
- patients experiencing inadequate pain relief may progress to opioids such as codeine
- if necessary, more potent opioids including morphine are given. Morphine and its derivatives can produce spasm of the sphincter of Oddi, and should be given with an antispasmodic. Pethidine has a minimal effect on smooth muscle and may be given intravenously for pain relief in acute pancreatitis

Analgesics are given before meals to help to alleviate the postprandial exacerbation of pain. Administration should be on a regular basis and doses titrated for each patient. Pancreatic extracts may ease the pain but are otherwise reserved for those with symptomatic malabsorption. Coeliac plexus block has been used for the relief of severe intractable pain in some patients with chronic pancreatitis; it has also been used similarly in patients with cancer of the pancreas. However, the benefits of such a block are unclear.

References.


1. Trewby PN. Chronic pancreatitis. *Prescribers' J* 1991; **31:** 111–17.
2. Caraceni A, Portenoy RK. Pain management in patients with pancreatic carcinoma. *Cancer* 1996; **78:** 639–53.
3. Mergener K, Baillie J. Chronic pancreatitis. *Lancet* 1997; **350:** 1379–85.
4. Ischia S, *et al.* Celiac block for the treatment of pancreatic pain. *Curr Rev Pain* 2000; **4:** 127–33.
5. Khalid A, Whitcomb DC. Conservative treatment of chronic pancreatitis. *Eur J Gastroenterol Hepatol* 2002; **14:** 943–9.
6. El Kamar FG, *et al.* Metastatic pancreatic cancer: emerging strategies in chemotherapy and palliative care. *Oncologist* 2003; **8:** 18–34.


**Phantom limb pain.** Phantom limb pain is associated with an amputated limb and is more common when there has been severe pre-amputation pain. It is frequently a mixture of neuropathic and other types of pain. Management may be difficult[1-5] but in a survey of war veteran amputees, for those who took any form of treatment for phantom limb pain, conventional analgesics such as NSAIDs or paracetamol with or without opioid analgesics were reported as being satisfactory.[2] Transcutaneous electrical nerve stimulation (TENS) was another method used by some and considered to be at least as effective as other therapies.[2] Tricyclic antidepressants and antiepileptics may be of help for the neuropathic components of the pain[1,3,5,6] and some relief may be obtained with sympathetic blocks.[1] Intravenous ketamine may also be of use.[4,5] From a review[7] of studies investigating the effect of regional anaesthesia in preventing phantom limb pain in patients undergoing lower-limb amputation it appeared that epidural blockade started before and continuing for the duration of surgery or for several days after amputation conferred more protection from long-term pain than blockade commenced late intra-operatively or postoperatively. However, a randomised, double-blind, controlled trial[8] failed to demonstrate any beneficial effect of pre-emptive analgesia using epidural blockade in such patients. A more recent review[4] which included this trial concluded that the pre-emptive use of epidural block was of limited success.


1. Stannard CF. Phantom limb pain. *Br J Hosp Med* 1993; **50:** 583–7.
2. Wartan SW, *et al.* Phantom pain and sensation among British veteran amputees. *Br J Anaesth* 1997; **78:** 652–9.
3. Flor H. Phantom-limb pain: characteristics, causes, and treatment. *Lancet Neurol* 2002; **1:** 182–9.
4. Halbert J, *et al.* Evidence for the optimal management of acute and chronic phantom pain: a systemic review. *Clin J Pain* 2002; **18:** 84–92.
5. Nikolajsen L, Jensen TS. Phantom limb pain. *Br J Anaesth* 2001; **87:** 107–16.
6. Ward A, *et al.* Phantom limb pain—a pain beyond reach? *Hosp Pharm* 1998; **5:** 241–6.
7. Katz J. Prevention of phantom limb pain by regional anaesthesia. *Lancet* 1997; **349:** 519–20.
8. Nikolajsen L, *et al.* Randomised trial of epidural bupivacaine and morphine in prevention of stump and phantom pain in lower-limb amputation. *Lancet* 1997; **350:** 1353–7.


**Postherpetic neuralgia.** About 10% of patients who have had acute herpes zoster still experience neuropathic pain resulting from peripheral nerve injury one month or more after the rash has healed. The elderly are the most susceptible. The affected area (commonly head, neck, and limbs) is extremely sensitive to any stimuli; even the pressure of clothing can produce unbearable pain. Spontaneous remission occurs in many patients within a few months. However, in a small percentage of patients the pain can last for several years.

Attempts have been made to **prevent** the development of postherpetic neuralgia. A meta-analysis[1] concluded that, if started within 72 hours of the onset of rash, aciclovir might reduce the incidence of residual pain at 6 months in some patients. A more recent analysis[2] considered that there was only marginal evidence of a decreased incidence of postherpetic neuralgia with aciclovir treatment and that there was no reduction in incidence with either famciclovir or valaciclovir treatments. It is, however, generally agreed that antiviral treatment does reduce the duration of postherpetic neuralgia.[2-5] Other drugs such as corticosteroids and local and regional anaesthesia have also been tried but without noted success in the prevention of postherpetic neuralgia,[6] although corticosteroids may reduce its duration.

Various **treatments** have been tried once neuralgia develops.[2-13] The value of conventional analgesics is limited because of the neuropathic character of the pain although opioid analgesics have been used in refractory cases (see below). Tricyclic antidepressants appear to help some patients and the early use of low-dose amitriptyline during the acute phase of the disease may also reduce the duration of the neuralgia. Nortriptyline has also been tried and may be better tolerated in elderly patients. Where amitriptyline fails to control the pain an antiepileptic such as gabapentin (alone or with a tricyclic) may be helpful. Opioids, including methadone, morphine, and oxycodone, are also effective but they are usually reserved for patients who fail to respond to tricyclics or gabapentin.[12] Topical application of capsaicin or lidocaine may produce some benefit. Nerve blocks and surgical techniques may provide temporary pain relief, but results have generally been disappointing. The use of intrathecal methylprednisolone is controversial.[12] Transcutaneous electrical nerve stimulation (TENS) has also been tried. Topical preparations of aspirin or indometacin, have shown some promise.


1. Jackson JL, *et al.* The effect of treating herpes zoster with oral acyclovir in preventing postherpetic neuralgia: a meta-analysis. *Arch Intern Med* 1997; **157:** 909–12.
2. Alper BS, Lewis PR. Does treatment of acute herpes zoster prevent or shorten postherpetic neuralgia? *J Fam Pract* 2000; **49:** 255–64.
3. Lee JJ, Gauci CAG. Postherpetic neuralgia: current concepts and management. *Br J Hosp Med* 1994; **52:** 565–70.
4. Kost RG, Straus SE. Postherpetic neuralgia—pathogenesis, treatment, and prevention. *N Engl J Med* 1996; **335:** 32–42.
5. Panlilio LM, *et al.* Current management of postherpetic neuralgia. *Neurolog* 2002; **8:** 339–50.
6. Robertson DRC, George CF. Treatment of post herpetic neuralgia in the elderly. *Br Med Bull* 1990; **46:** 113–123.
7. Anonymous. Postherpetic neuralgia. *Lancet* 1990; **336:** 537–8.
8. Bowsher D. Neurogenic pain syndromes and their management. *Br Med Bull* 1991; **47:** 644–66.
9. Bowsher D. The management of postherpetic neuralgia. *Postgrad Med J* 1997; **73:** 623–9.
10. Collins SL, *et al.* Antidepressants and anticonvulsants for diabetic neuropathy and postherpetic neuralgia: a quantitative systematic review. *J Pain Symptom Manage* 2000; **20:** 449–58.
11. Kanazi GE, *et al.* Treatment of postherpetic neuralgia: an update. *Drugs* 2000; **59:** 1113–26.
12. Johnson RW, Dworkin RH. Treatment of herpes zoster and postherpetic neuralgia. *BMJ* 2003; **326:** 748–50.
13. Dworkin RH, Schmader KE. Treatment and prevention of postherpetic neuralgia. *Clin Infect Dis* 2003; **36:** 877–82.


**Sickle-cell crisis.** The management of pain of sickle-cell crisis (p.734) is similar to that of other forms of acute pain. The pain of mild crises may be controlled using oral analgesics such as paracetamol, an NSAID, codeine, or dihydrocodeine. Partial agonist and antagonist opioids such as buprenorphine are not recommended to treat acute pain before transfer to hospital.[1] Crises severe enough to necessitate hospital admission usually require the use of more potent parenteral opioid analgesics but NSAIDs may be useful as an adjunct for bone pain. In most centres, morphine is the opioid of choice for moderate to severe pain. Some patients appear to prefer pethidine but many clinicians[2-7] avoid its use if possible as control of pain may be inadequate and doses of pethidine needed to manage crises may lead to accumulation of its neuroexcitatory metabolite norpethidine and precipitate seizures (see also Effects on the Nervous System, p.80). UK guidelines[8] recommend that pethidine should only be used in exceptional circumstances such as in patients hypersensitive to other opioids. Diamorphine, fentanyl, hydromorphone, and methadone have been used as alternatives to morphine. As the dose of opioid required to control the pain can vary considerably, not only during each episode but also from one episode to another and between individual patients, patient-controlled analgesia (see above) may be of help to manage the pain once initial pain relief has been obtained with loading doses of parenteral opioids;[4,9] opioids used have included morphine and fentanyl. The use of continuous epidural analgesia with local anaesthetics alone or with opioids has been tried. However, a randomised trial[10] of morphine for the management of severe painful sickle-cell crises in children showed that oral modified-release morphine was a safe and effective alternative to continuous intravenous morphine. Inhalation of a mixture of nitrous oxide and oxygen may be a useful analgesic during transfer to hospital.[1,8]


1. Report of a working party of the Standing Medical Advisory Committee on sickle cell, thalassaemia and other haemoglobinopathies. London: HMSO, 1993.
2. Pryle BJ, *et al.* Toxicity of norpethidine in sickle cell crisis. *BMJ* 1992; **304:** 1478–9.
3. Davies SC, Oni L. Management of patients with sickle cell disease. *BMJ* 1997; **315:** 656–60.
4. Vijay V, *et al.* The anaesthetist's role in acute sickle cell crisis. *Br J Anaesth* 1998; **80:** 820–8.
5. Marlowe KF, Chicella MF. Treatment of sickle cell pain. *Pharmacotherapy* 2002; **22:** 484–91.
6. Stinson J, Naser B. Pain management in children with sickle cell disease. *Paediatr Drugs* 2003; **5:** 229–41.
7. Yaster M, *et al.* The management of pain in sickle cell disease. *Pediatr Clin North Am* 2000; **47:** 699–710.
8. Rees DC, *et al.* Guidelines for the management of the acute painful crisis in sickle cell disease. *Br J Haematol* 2003; **120:** 744–52.
9. Grundy R, *et al.* Practical management of pain in sickling disorders. *Arch Dis Child* 1993; **69:** 256–9.
10. Jacobson SJ, *et al.* Randomised trial of oral morphine for painful episodes of sickle-cell disease in children. *Lancet* 1997; **350:** 1358–61.


**Trigeminal neuralgia.** Trigeminal neuralgia (tic douloureux) is a neuropathic pain characterised by sudden, brief, sharp, agonising, episodic pain in the distribution of one or more branches of the fifth cranial nerve. There may be several episodes (lasting several seconds or minutes) a day over a number of weeks, followed by a pain-free interval which may last for weeks or years. Trigeminal neuralgia generally has a 'trigger zone' in which even a very light stimulus such as a draught of air produces pain. In some cases firm pressure applied around but not to the zone itself may help to relieve pain. Trigeminal neuralgia may be idiopathic or may be secondary to nerve compression (such as that caused by a tumour), facial injury, or multiple sclerosis.

Carbamazepine is the drug of choice for the management of trigeminal neuralgia and initially may produce satisfactory pain relief in 70% or more of patients, although increasingly large doses may be required.[1-6] If pain relief is inadequate phenytoin or baclofen may be added to carbamazepine therapy; these drugs may also be used alone in patients intolerant of carbamazepine.[5] Other antiepileptics such as gabapentin, lamotrigine, oxcarbazepine, valproate, and clonazepam have also been used in patients intolerant of, or resistant to, carbamazepine.[1-6]

In some patients drug therapy eventually fails to control the pain or produces unacceptable side-effects and invasive procedures become necessary. These may include the selective destruction of pain bearing nerve fibres with radiofrequency thermocoagulation, instillation of glycerol (although the efficacy and safety of the procedure is debatable), and microvascular decompression of the trigeminal nerve root.[3,4]


1. Green MW, Selman JE. Review article: the medical management of trigeminal neuralgia. *Headache* 1991; **31:** 588–92.
2. Zakrzewska JM. Trigeminal neuralgia. *Prim Dent Care* 1997; **4:** 17–19.
3. Joffroy A, *et al.* Trigeminal neuralgia: pathophysiology and treatment. *Acta Neurol Belg* 2001; **101:** 20–5.
4. Nurmikko TJ, Eldridge PR. Trigeminal neuralgia—pathophysiology, diagnosis and current treatments. *Br J Anaesth* 2001; **87:** 117–32.
5. Rozen TD. Antiepileptic drugs in the management of cluster headache and trigeminal neuralgia. *Headache* 2001; **41** (suppl 1): S25–S32.
6. Sindrup SH, Jensen TS. Pharmacotherapy of trigeminal neuralgia. *Clin J Pain* 2002; **18:** 22–7.


## Increased Body Temperature

The hypothalamus is the centre of the thermoregulatory system and is responsible for maintaining the body temperature at a set point (known as the set-point temperature) which is normally 37°. Mechanisms which produce or conserve body heat include passive heat absorption from the environment, peripheral vasoconstriction, and thermogenic processes such as metabolic reactions and shivering. Heat loss is achieved mainly through sweating and peripheral vasodilatation. Various states may lead to an abnormal increase in body temperature.

### Fever and hyperthermia

Fever (pyrexia) is an increase in body temperature due to an elevated set-point temperature. Common causes of fever include infections, inflammatory disorders, neoplastic disease, and some drug treatment. Hyperthermia (hyperpyrexia) implies a disturbance of thermoregulatory control. This may be caused by injury to the hypothalamus, or heat stroke following defective heat loss as occurs in dehydration or excessive heat production following strenuous activities; it may also be caused by excessive dosage of some drugs or a reaction to certain drugs such as anaesthetics (malignant hyperthermia, p.1394) or antipsychotics (neuroleptic malignant syndrome, p.677). Underlying thermoregulatory defects may be a particular problem in sedentary elderly subjects.

Whenever possible the underlying cause of **fever** should be identified and treated.[1] Apart from pregnant women or patients who are already dehydrated or malnourished or those with cardiac, respiratory, or neurological diseases, body temperatures up to 41° are relatively harmless.[1] It is not clear if there is any value in treating fever at lower temperatures.

Both physical means and antipyretics may be used to reduce body temperature in fever. Maintaining an adequate fluid intake is important. Fanning and tepid sponging are often employed,[1-5] but cold baths should not be used as they may actually increase body temperature by inducing vasoconstriction, and the risks of a cold-induced pressor response should be borne in mind. Antipyretics appear mostly to help return the set-point temperature to normal by inhibiting central synthesis and release of prostaglandin $E_2$, which mediates the effect of endogenous pyrogens in the hypothalamus.[6] Antipyretics cannot lower the body temperature below normal, and are ineffective against raised body temperature not associated with fever.

Paracetamol is usually the antipyretic of choice in children. However, in a systematic review[7] there was inconsistent evidence to support any advantage of using paracetamol to reduce fever in children, since the number of reliable studies was too low to be sure that it was effective. Another review[8] considered that treatment with paracetamol should only be given to those children in obvious discomfort. Salicylates (including aspirin) are generally contra-indicated because of the possible link between their use and the development of Reye's syndrome. Ibuprofen appears to be at least as effective as paracetamol.[6,9,10]

However, antipyretic treatment of febrile children does not necessarily improve their comfort[11] and might even prolong any infection.[2] It has also been suggested[12] that in severe infection the use of antipyretics might increase mortality: the WHO recommend that in developing countries antipyretics should not be given routinely to children with fever but should be reserved for those with severe discomfort or high fever. In the UK, the Joint Committee on Vaccination and Immunisation recommends antipyretic therapy to treat post-immunisation fever developing after some vaccines. However, if the fever persists after the second dose of antipyretic medical advice should be sought.

Antipyretics have also been given as *prophylaxis* against febrile convulsions, especially in those with a previous history of such seizures or in those with epilepsy. However, antipyretic therapy does not appear to prevent recurrence of febrile convulsions (p.353).[1,3,13] There is also little to support the use of antipyretics for prophylaxis of post-immunisation fever although some suggest offering it to infants at higher risk of seizures receiving diphtheria-tetanus-pertussis or polio immunisation.[14]

**Hyperthermia** may produce body temperatures greater than 41°. These high temperatures are life-threatening and need to be lowered immediately. Antipyretics are ineffective since the high temperatures are a result of thermoregulatory failure. One of the most rapid and effective means of cooling is to immerse the patient in very cold water but core temperature should be monitored to avoid inducing hypothermia.[15] Evaporative cooling methods may be more efficient.[16] Intravenous or intraperitoneal administration of cool fluids, gastric lavage or enemas with ice water have also been used.[15,17]

When hyperthermia is associated with muscle rigidity and fulminant hypermetabolism of skeletal muscle, as in the neuroleptic malignant syndrome and malignant hyperthermia, temperature reductions may be obtained using the muscle relaxant dantrolene. There is also anecdotal evidence that dantrolene may produce beneficial effects for the treatment of similar symptoms resulting from poisoning with various agents. However, dantrolene is not an effective treatment for all types of hyperthermia and rigidity accompanying poisoning. Although dantrolene has been tried in patients with heat stroke, there is no evidence that it affects outcome.[18] In severe cases of hyperthermia when neuromuscular hyperactivity may also impair ventilation, a neuromuscular blocker has been used, although suxamethonium is best avoided as it can itself precipitate malignant hyperthermia.


1. Drwal-Klein LA, Phelps SJ. Antipyretic therapy in the febrile child. *Clin Pharm* 1992; **11:** 1005–21.
2. Plaisance KI, Mackowiak PA. Antipyretic therapy: physiologic rationale, diagnostic implications, and clinical consequences. *Arch Intern Med* 2000; **160:** 449–56.
3. Joint Working Group of the Research Unit of the Royal College of Physicians and the British Paediatric Association. Guidelines for the management of convulsions with fever. *BMJ* 1991; **303:** 634–6.
4. Kinmonth A-L, *et al.* Management of feverish children at home. *BMJ* 1992; **305:** 1134–6.
5. Meremikwu M, Oyo-Ita A. Physical methods for treating fever in children. Available in The Cochrane Library; Issue 2. Chichester: John Wiley; 2004.
6. Aronoff DM, Nielson EG. Antipyretics: mechanism of action and clinical use in fever suppression. *Am J Med* 2001; **111:** 304–15.
7. Meremikwu M, Oyo-Ita A. Paracetamol for treating fever in children. Available in The Cochrane Library; Issue 2. Chichester: John Wiley; 2004.
8. Russell FM, *et al.* Evidence on the use of paracetamol in febrile children. *Bull WHO* 2003; **81:** 367–72.
9. McIntyre J, Hull D. Comparing efficacy and tolerability of ibuprofen and paracetamol in fever. *Arch Dis Child* 1996; **74:** 164–7.
10. Anonymous. Junifen suspension—ibuprofen for febrile children. *Drug Ther Bull* 1991; **29:** 11–12.
11. Kramer MS, *et al.* Risks and benefits of paracetamol antipyresis in young children with fever of presumed viral origin. *Lancet* 1991; **337:** 591–4.
12. Shann F. Antipyretics in severe sepsis. *Lancet* 1995; **345:** 338.
13. Uhari M, *et al.* Effect of acetaminophen and of low intermittent doses of diazepam on prevention of recurrences of febrile seizures. *J Pediatr* 1995; **126:** 991–5.
14. Anonymous. Prophylactic paracetamol with childhood immunisation? *Drug Ther Bull* 1990; **28:** 73–4.
15. Simon HB. Hyperthermia. *N Engl J Med* 1993; **329:** 483–7.
16. Slovis CM. Hyperthermia. *N Engl J Med* 1994; **330:** 218–19.
17. Duthie DJR. Heat-related illness. *Lancet* 1998; **352:** 1329–30.
18. Bouchama A, Knochel JP. Heat stroke. *N Engl J Med* 2002; **346:** 1978–88.


## Musculoskeletal and Joint Disorders

The **rheumatic disorders** are a wide range of painful disorders affecting primarily the joints and related structures of the musculoskeletal system, but there may also be widespread involvement of other systems. The term arthritis is used when the disease is largely confined to the joints. Some of the most common forms of arthritis are discussed in this section and these include rheumatoid arthritis, osteoarthritis, juvenile idiopathic arthritis, and the spondyloarthropathies such as ankylosing spondylitis. Other conditions that are associated with arthritis and which are discussed elsewhere include gout (p.412) and systemic lupus erythematosus (p.1088).

The names **soft-tissue rheumatism** (see below) and **non-articular rheumatism** have been used to describe a number of painful conditions associated with disease of the structures that surround a joint. For a discussion of the management of **low back pain**, see above.

### Juvenile idiopathic arthritis

Juvenile idiopathic arthritis (juvenile chronic arthritis) is a term used to describe a clinically heterogeneous group of idiopathic arthritides occurring in children under 16 years of age.

Treatment depends on the number of joints affected, but is generally similar to that for rheumatoid arthritis in adults (see below), although for some drugs there is limited evidence for their use in children. NSAIDs, corticosteroids (particularly by intra-articular injection), and methotrexate or sulfasalazine are mainstays of treatment. Juvenile idiopathic arthritis is one of the limited number of indications for the use of aspirin in children, although other NSAIDs are preferred. Etanercept may be used in patients who fail to respond to methotrexate. Autologous stem cell transplantation has been investigated as a treatment of last resort.

References.


1. Malleson PN. Management of childhood arthritis. Part 2: chronic arthritis. *Arch Dis Child* 1997; **76:** 541–4.
2. Schaller JG. Juvenile rheumatoid arthritis. *Pediatr Rev* 1997; **18:** 337–49.
3. Woo P, Wedderburn LR. Juvenile chronic arthritis. *Lancet* 1998; **351:** 969–73. Correction. *ibid.*; 1292.
4. Cassidy JT. Medical management of children with juvenile rheumatoid arthritis. *Drugs* 1999; **58:** 831–50.
5. Hull RG, *et al.* Guidelines for management of childhood arthritis. *Rheumatology (Oxford)* 2001; **40:** 1309–12.
6. Ilowite NT. Current treatment of juvenile rheumatoid arthritis. *Pediatrics* 2002; **109:** 109–15.
7. Cron RQ. Current treatment for chronic arthritis in childhood. *Curr Opin Pediatr* 2002; **14:** 684–7.
8. Wilkinson N, *et al.* Biologic therapies for juvenile arthritis. *Arch Dis Child* 2003; **88:** 186–91.
9. Cleary AG, *et al.* Intra-articular corticosteroid injections in juvenile idiopathic arthritis. *Arch Dis Child* 2003; **88:** 192–6.
10. Ramanan AV, *et al.* Use of methotrexate in juvenile idiopathic arthritis. *Arch Dis Child* 2003; **88:** 197–200.
11. Wedderburn LR, *et al.* Autologous haematopoietic stem cell transplantation in juvenile idiopathic arthritis. *Arch Dis Child* 2003; **88:** 201–5.
12. Friswell M, Southwood TR. Juvenile idiopathic arthritis. In: Snaith ML, ed. *ABC of rheumatology.* 3rd ed. London: BMJ Publishing Group, 2004: 68–74.


### Osteoarthritis

Osteoarthritis is a diverse collection of diseases also known as osteoarthrosis, degenerative joint disease, or joint failure. It is characterised by progressive disintegration of articular cartilage, usually accompanied by new bone formation at joint margins and beneath the involved cartilage. There may be synovial inflammation, particularly in advanced disease, but it is different in nature from that seen with rheumatoid arthritis and is usually only a minor component of the disease. Osteoarthritis may be a sequel to trauma, inflammation, or metabolic disorders, but usually the underlying origin is not apparent.

Despite claims based largely on *animal* studies, there is no evidence from controlled studies in humans that any treatment affects disease progression. Management is therefore aimed at relief of pain and maintenance of joint function.

Physical methods of treatment include physiotherapy, heat and cold therapy, exercises, splinting, and weight reduction in the obese. Acupuncture and transcutaneous electrical nerve stimulation (TENS) may also be tried.

For pain relief, paracetamol is often sufficient and should be used first. A low-dose NSAID may be tried when paracetamol is ineffective or when there is a significant inflammatory component but there is the risk of adverse effects with prolonged use of NSAIDs, especially in the elderly. There has also been concern that NSAIDs such as indometacin may accelerate osteoarthritis. UK and US guidelines recommend that treatment with NSAIDs such as celecoxib and rofecoxib that are selective inhibitors of cyclo-oxygenase-2 is limited to those patients considered to be at high risk of developing serious gastrointestinal problems if given a non-selective NSAID (see p.68). If pain relief is inadequate, paracetamol may be combined with an NSAID; opioids such as codeine or dihydrocodeine are sometimes also used with paracetamol. Tramadol may also be given. Dietary supplements such as glucosamine and chondroitin may have some benefit.

Topical analgesics such as NSAIDs, or capsaicin or rubefacients, may provide some relief of pain.

Systemic corticosteroids have no place in the management of osteoarthritis. Intra-articular or peri-articular injections of corticosteroids are somewhat controversial but may be of help in some patients with localised inflammation, although if used they should only be given infrequently and as adjunctive therapy. Intra-articular injections of hyaluronic acid may improve the viscosity and elasticity of the synovial fluid; they may be useful in osteoarthritis of the knee.

Surgery, including joint replacement, is of great benefit to patients with severe osteoarthritis that cannot be effectively managed by physical or medical therapy.

References.


1. Ghosh P. Nonsteroidal anti-inflammatory drugs and chondroprotection: a review of the evidence. *Drugs* 1993; **46:** 834–46.
2. Puett DW, Griffin MR. Published trials of nonmedicinal and noninvasive therapies for hip and knee osteoarthritis. *Ann Intern Med* 1994; **121:** 133–40.
3. Brandt KD. Toward pharmacologic modification of joint damage in osteoarthritis. *Ann Intern Med* 1995; **122:** 874–5.
4. Wollheim FA. Current pharmacological treatment of osteoarthritis. *Drugs* 1996; **52** (suppl 3): 27–38.
5. Anonymous. What can be done about osteoarthritis? *Drug Ther Bull* 1996; **34:** 33–5.
6. Creamer P, Hochberg MC. Osteoarthritis. *Lancet* 1997; **350:** 503–9.
7. Eccles M, *et al.* North of England evidence based guideline development project: summary guideline for non-steroidal anti-inflammatory drugs versus basic analgesia in treating the pain of degenerative arthritis. *BMJ* 1998; **317:** 526–30.
8. LaPrade RF, Swiontkowski MF. New horizons in the treatment of osteoarthritis of the knee. *JAMA* 1999; **281:** 876–8.
9. American College of Rheumatology Subcommittee on Osteoarthritis Guidelines. Recommendations for the medical management of osteoarthritis of the hip and knee: 2000 update. *Arthritis Rheum* 2000; **43:** 1905–15. Also available at: http://www.rheumatology.org/publications/guidelines/oa-mgmt/oa-mgmt.asp (accessed 01/07/04)
10. Walker-Bone K, *et al.* Medical management of osteoarthritis. *BMJ* 2000; **321:** 936–40.
11. Felson DT, *et al.* Osteoarthritis: new insights. Part 1: the disease and its risk factors. *Ann Intern Med* 2000; **133:** 635–46.
12. Felson DT, *et al.* Osteoarthritis: new insights. Part 2: treatment approaches. *Ann Intern Med* 2000; **133:** 726–37.
13. Manek NJ. Medical management of osteoarthritis. *Mayo Clin Proc* 2001; **76:** 533–9.
14. National Institute for Clinical Excellence. Guidance on the use of cyclo-oxygenase (Cox) II selective inhibitors, celecoxib, rofecoxib, meloxicam and etodolac for osteoarthritis and rheumatoid arthritis (issued July 2001). Available at: http://www.nice.org.uk/pdf/coxiifullguidance.pdf (accessed 01/07/04)
15. March LM, Stenmark J. Non-pharmacological approaches to managing arthritis. *Med J Aust* 2001; **175** (suppl): S102–S107.
16. McColl GJ. Pharmacological therapies for the treatment of osteoarthritis. *Med J Aust* 2001; **175** (suppl): S108–S111.
17. Hogue JH, Mersfelder TL. Pathophysiology and first-line treatment of osteoarthritis. *Ann Pharmacother* 2002; **36:** 679–86.
18. Schnitzer TJ, *et al.* Update of ACR guidelines for osteoarthritis: role of the coxibs. *J Pain Symptom Manage* 2002; **23** (suppl): S24–S30.
19. Chard J, Dieppe P. Update: treatment of osteoarthritis. *Arthritis Rheum* 2002; **47:** 686–90.
20. Raj N, Jones A. Osteoarthritis. In: Snaith ML, ed. *ABC of rheumatology.* 3rd ed. London: BMJ Publishing Group, 2004: 34–8.


### Rheumatoid arthritis

Rheumatoid arthritis is a common chronic systemic inflammatory disease that results in progressive disability and increased mortality. Early disease is characterised primarily by inflammation of the synovium (the inner membrane of the capsule of synovial joints); as the disease progresses the patient suffers destruction of cartilage and bone. Extra-articular features commonly include general malaise, fatigue, weight loss, fever, and anaemia. More severe disease may be associated with vasculitis, pericarditis, pleurisy, pleural effusion, pulmonary interstitial fibrosis, peripheral neuropathies, subcutaneous and pulmonary nodules, scleritis, and Sjögren's syndrome. Palindromic rheumatism is characterised by repeated episodes of arthritis and periarthritis without fever; the joints appear normal between attacks.

The severity and course of rheumatoid arthritis varies greatly between patients. Some experience brief attacks with little or no disease progression, but the majority will have slowly progressive joint destruction and deformity despite intermittent relapses and remissions; a few patients may have very severe and rapidly progressive disease.

Since there is no cure, management is aimed at relieving pain and improving or maintaining joint function, using physiotherapy as well as drugs. In some cases surgery may be required.

The choice of **drugs for relief of pain** depends upon the severity of symptoms. In mild cases an analgesic such as paracetamol may be all that is required but most patients need the additional anti-inflammatory effect provided by an NSAID. Although there is little apparent difference between the various NSAIDs in terms of anti-inflammatory activity, patient responses vary widely. When starting an NSAID the dose is gradually increased to the recommended maximum over 1 to 2 weeks; if the response is inadequate after a total of about 4 weeks, or if adverse effects are intolerable, other NSAIDs are tried. Treatment with NSAIDs such as celecoxib and rofecoxib that are selective inhibitors of cyclo-oxygenase-2 is limited to those patients considered to be at high risk of developing serious gastrointestinal problems if given a non-selective NSAID[1] (see p.68). Topical analgesics such as NSAIDs or capsaicin, or rubefacients may provide slight relief of pain but their role, if any, is unclear.

Although NSAIDs provide symptomatic relief they do not affect the course of the disease or prevent joint destruction. Consequently, they should not be used alone in the treatment of rheumatoid arthritis.[2] The use of **disease-modifying antirheumatic drugs** (DMARDs) (also referred to as second-line drugs) had conventionally been delayed until there was overt evidence of progressive disease but it is now clear that irreversible joint damage commonly occurs early in the disease and rheumatologists now generally add a DMARD shortly after rheumatoid arthritis has been diagnosed.[2,3] US guidelines recommend that a DMARD is started within 3 months of diagnosis for patients not controlled by NSAIDs, although immediate treatment is recommended for those who present with persistent synovitis and joint damage.[2] The *British National Formulary* states that DMARDs should be started as soon as diagnosis, progression, and severity of the disease has been confirmed. It is unclear whether early use of DMARDs will reduce long-term disability[3] but data from 2888 patients with rheumatoid arthritis followed up for an average of 9 years indicated that consistent use of DMARDs was associated with an improvement in long-term functional outcomes.[4]

DMARDs include antimalarials (chloroquine, hydroxychloroquine), sulfasalazine, gold compounds (auranofin, sodium aurothiomalate), penicillamine, and immunosuppressants (methotrexate, adalimumab, anakinra, azathioprine, ciclosporin, cyclophosphamide, etanercept, infliximab, and leflunomide). It is thought that most DMARDs inhibit the release or activity of cytokines involved in maintaining the inflammatory process, although other actions may also contribute.[5] Any therapeutic effect may not be apparent for 4 to 6 months.

- Intramuscular *gold* has long been used for the treatment of rheumatoid arthritis, but although it is still prescribed, its toxicity and poor long-term efficacy have led to debate over its place in antirheumatic therapy.[6,7] Oral gold is less toxic but is also much less effective.
- Early enthusiasm for *penicillamine* has also been curtailed by a high incidence of adverse effects although better tolerability than gold or antimalarials has been reported if the dose is limited to 500 mg daily or less.[8]
- The antimalarials are less effective than most other DMARDs but as they are generally less toxic and better tolerated they may be preferred in patients with milder forms of disease. *Hydroxychloroquine* is generally preferred to *chloroquine*.
- *Sulfasalazine* is often one of the DMARDs of first choice[3,9] especially in milder forms of rheumatoid arthritis.[2] About 60% of patients given the drug are still taking it after 3 years.[10]
- Immunosuppressants are also used in rheumatoid arthritis. *Methotrexate* can improve disease activity when given once weekly in doses too small to produce systemic immunosuppression, and when used in this manner adverse effects are usually mild. In a recent long-term study[11] almost two-thirds of patients were still taking methotrexate after 5 years. Folic acid or folinic acid can reduce the toxicity of methotrexate without reducing efficacy,[12,13] but the timing of the dose may be important. The risk of hepatotoxicity remains a concern, but many rheumatologists[2,3,14] nevertheless consider methotrexate to be a first choice DMARD. Improvement generally begins earlier with methotrexate than with other DMARDs. The use of other immunosuppressants is more debatable but *azathioprine* and *cyclophosphamide* are used in some patients with severe disease who have failed to respond to other drugs. *Ciclosporin* is effective but, because of concern over nephrotoxicity, it is reserved for refractory disease; the use of low-dose regimens may help to minimise adverse effects.[15,16]
- The immunosuppressant *leflunomide*, and the cytokine modulators *adalimumab*, *anakinra*, *etanercept*, and *infliximab* have recently been introduced for the treatment of rheumatoid arthritis.[2,10,17-19] Leflunomide is said to be equivalent in efficacy to sulfasalazine; comparative data with methotrexate is, however, conflicting. Adverse effects, particularly the increased risk of serious infection, may be a problem with these newer drugs. Long-term data is also lacking and they are usually reserved for second-line DMARD therapy.

At present, data from comparative studies are insufficient to allow more than a crude ranking of DMARDs with regard to efficacy and toxicity, but a number of reviews and analyses have been published to aid rational selection.[3,9,10,14,20-26] Some meta-analyses[20,22] of generally short-term comparative studies suggest that methotrexate, intramuscular gold (sodium aurothiomalate), sulfasalazine, and penicillamine are more or less equivalent in efficacy, while the antimalarials and oral gold (auranofin) appear to be somewhat less effective. Intramuscular gold exhibited the highest toxicity while the antimalarials and oral gold had relatively low toxicity rates.[20] Another meta-analysis[21] considered that antimalarials and methotrexate had the best ratio of toxicity to efficacy. However, as adverse reactions with any DMARDs may be life threatening, all patients require careful monitoring.[27,28]

The long-term use of DMARDs is limited by toxicity and loss of efficacy and many patients do not continue to take a particular drug for more than 1 or 2 years. Stopping therapy in a patient who has shown improvement may cause a relapse, but drug withdrawal may be considered on an empirical basis by some clinicians for patients in complete remission.[29] In a randomised, placebo-controlled study[30] of stopping DMARDs in rheumatoid arthritis, the risk of synovitis was doubled in patients who stopped active therapy but 62% of the placebo group went for a full year without experiencing a rheumatoid flare. In a further study[31] in patients who had stopped DMARDs, restarting therapy with the same antirheumatic drug when the disease flared up again was effective in most cases.

As the effects of a DMARD are not immediate, treatment may need to be continued for 6 months (or 3 months if at maximum treatment) before any objective benefit is seen. If there is no benefit after this time another DMARD should be tried. Patients who relapse during treatment with one DMARD may also benefit from substitution. Combining DMARDs is being tried in refractory cases and some rheumatologists are increasingly using combination therapy.[2,10] A meta-analysis[32] of 5 different combinations of DMARDs found that although efficacy might be greater, toxicity was also increased. Nonetheless, some combinations, particularly methotrexate with the newer immunosuppressants, have produced favourable results.[2,17,33] Combination of 2 or 3 DMARDs has also been tried in early disease to maximise control; once achieved, the number of DMARDs is reduced or 'stepped-down'.[2]

The use of **corticosteroids** in rheumatoid arthritis is controversial. Although systemic corticosteroids can suppress the symptoms of the disease, their value is limited by adverse effects. They are usually reserved for patients with severe rapidly progressing disease that has failed to respond to other antirheumatics, or when there are severe extra-articular effects, or to control disease activity temporarily during initiation of DMARDs. However, it has been suggested that, in line with current thinking on the earlier use of more aggressive therapy, early use of short-term corticosteroids might also be appropriate.[34] Although corticosteroids are associated with bone loss,[35] this appears to be dose-related[36] and, at low doses, the benefits of corticosteroid therapy on inflammation and mobility might result in a reduced loss of bone in patients with rheumatoid arthritis. The rate of joint destruction may be substantially reduced by corticosteroids in low doses (such as prednisolone 7.5 mg daily) in patients with moderate to severe rheumatoid arthritis of less than 2 years duration;[37] the corticosteroid should be gradually discontinued after 2 to 4 years to avoid long-term adverse effects. Reduction in joint destruction should be distinguished from symptomatic improvement, which, at low corticosteroid doses, lasts only for 6 to 12 months. Such symptomatic benefits have been confirmed by two recent meta-analyses.[38,39] The authors considered that the short-term, intermittent use of low-dose corticosteroids (not exceeding the equivalent of 15 mg of prednisolone per day) may be justified, particularly in patients not controlled by other means,[38] and that benefit persisted in moderate-term use (at least 3 months).[39] Intra-articular injections of corticosteroids may be used when there are acute flares affecting one or a few individual joints[40] but they should be used with care.

There is little good evidence to support most **other drugs** tried in rheumatoid arthritis.[2,23,26,41,42] Studies[43,44] indicate that minocycline can produce modest beneficial effects in patients with advanced rheumatoid arthritis, but the clinical significance of these improvements has been questioned.[45] Greater symptomatic improvements have been obtained in early disease;[46] continued treatment with minocycline may also reduce the need for DMARDs.[47] Testosterone has produced clinical improvement in male and postmenopausal female patients. Much research has been conducted into immunomodulators and immunotherapy. Interferons have produced results similar to conventional DMARDs but the need for repeated injections is a drawback. Other drugs that have been tried[48-50] include amiprilose, mycophenolate mofetil, zileuton, oral desensitisation with collagen, and immunoglobulins. Tumour necrosis factor (TNF) is involved in the inflammatory process and inhibitors of TNF-α under investigation include tumour necrosis factor receptor fusion protein, as well as interleukin antagonists.[51,52] (The TNF-α inhibitors etanercept and infliximab and the interleukin-1 inhibitor anakinra are now licensed for use in rheumatoid arthritis, see above). A CD4 antibody (IDEC-CE9.1) and matrix metalloprotease inhibitors have also been studied. Other methods of treatment that are under investigation include gene therapy and autologous bone marrow transplantation. A rheumatoid arthritis vaccine is also in clinical trials. Some studies suggest that addition of fish oils[53] and/or evening primrose oil to standard antirheumatic therapy might help to reduce pain and joint swelling.

Findings that significant skeletal bone loss occurs early in the disease have raised the question of the need for general measures to prevent osteoporosis in patients with rheumatoid arthritis.[34] Some[34] consider the use of oestrogen therapy in postmenopausal women with rheumatoid arthritis to be appropriate but it appears to have little effect on disease activity.[54] The use of bisphosphonates is being studied.[55]

The treatment of rheumatoid arthritis during **pregnancy** presents its own problems; the rational selection of suitable drugs has been discussed in a number of reviews.[56,57]


1. National Institute for Clinical Excellence. Guidance on the use of cyclo-oxygenase (Cox) II selective inhibitors, celecoxib, rofecoxib, meloxicam and etodolac for osteoarthritis and rheumatoid arthritis (issued July 2001). Available at: http://www.nice.org.uk/pdf/coxiifullguidance.pdf (accessed 01/07/04)
2. American College of Rheumatology Subcommittee on Rheumatoid Arthritis. Guidelines for the management of rheumatoid arthritis. *Arthritis Rheum* 2002; **46:** 328–46.
3. Anonymous. Modifying disease in rheumatoid arthritis. *Drug Ther Bull* 1998; **36:** 3–6.
4. Fries JF, *et al.* Reduction in long-term disability in patients with rheumatoid arthritis by disease-modifying antirheumatic drug-based treatment strategies. *Arthritis Rheum* 1996; **39:** 616–22.
5. Choy E, Kingsley G. How do second-line agents work? *Br Med Bull* 1995; **51:** 472–92.
6. Anonymous. Gold therapy in rheumatoid arthritis. *Lancet* 1991; **338:** 19–20.
7. Pincus T, Wolfe F. Treatment of rheumatoid arthritis: challenges to traditional paradigms. *Ann Intern Med* 1991; **115:** 825–7.
8. Jessop JD, *et al.* A long-term five-year randomized controlled trial of hydroxychloroquine, sodium aurothiomalate, auranofin and penicillamine in the treatment of patients with rheumatoid arthritis. *Br J Rheumatol* 1998; **37:** 992–1002.
9. Jackson CG, Williams HJ. Disease-modifying antirheumatic drugs: using their clinical pharmacological effects as a guide to their selection. *Drugs* 1998; **56:** 337–44.
10. Akil M, Veerapen K. Rheumatoid arthritis: treatment. In: Snaith ML, ed. *ABC of rheumatology.* 3rd ed. London: BMJ Publishing Group, 2004: 56–60.
11. Weinblatt ME, *et al.* Methotrexate in rheumatoid arthritis: a five-year prospective multicenter study. *Arthritis Rheum* 1994; **37:** 1492–8.
12. Shiroky JB, *et al.* Low-dose methotrexate with leucovorin (folinic acid) in the management of rheumatoid arthritis: results of a multicenter randomized, double-blind, placebo-controlled trial. *Arthritis Rheum* 1993; **36:** 795–803.
13. Morgan SL, *et al.* Supplementation with folic acid during methotrexate therapy for rheumatoid arthritis: a double-blind, placebo-controlled trial. *Ann Intern Med* 1994; **121:** 833–41.
14. Cash JM, Klippel JH. Second-line drug therapy for rheumatoid arthritis. *N Engl J Med* 1994; **330:** 1368–75.
15. Tugwell P. International consensus recommendations on cyclosporin use in rheumatoid arthritis. *Drugs* 1995; **50:** 48–56.
16. Cush JJ, *et al.* US consensus guidelines for the use of cyclosporin A in rheumatoid arthritis. *J Rheumatol* 1999; **26:** 1176–86.
17. Kremer JM. Rational use of new and existing disease-modifying agents in rheumatoid arthritis. *Ann Intern Med* 2001; **134:** 695–706.
18. Luong BT, *et al.* Treatment options for rheumatoid arthritis: celecoxib, leflunomide, etanercept, and infliximab. *Ann Pharmacother* 2000; **34:** 743–60.
19. Drosos AA. Newer immunosuppressive drugs: their potential role in rheumatoid arthritis therapy. *Drugs* 2002; **62:** 891–907.
20. Felson DT, *et al.* The comparative efficacy and toxicity of second-line drugs in rheumatoid arthritis. *Arthritis Rheum* 1990; **33:** 1449–61.
21. Felson DT, *et al.* Use of short-term efficacy/toxicity tradeoffs to select second-line drugs in rheumatoid arthritis: a metaanalysis of published clinical trials. *Arthritis Rheum* 1992; **35:** 1117–25.
22. Capell HA, *et al.* Second line (disease modifying) treatment in rheumatoid arthritis: which drug for which patient? *Ann Rheum Dis* 1993; **52:** 423–8.
23. Brooks PM. Clinical management of rheumatoid arthritis. *Lancet* 1993; **341:** 286–90.
24. Porter DR, Sturrock RD. Medical management of rheumatoid arthritis. *BMJ* 1993; **307:** 425–8.
25. Kalla AA, *et al.* A risk-benefit assessment of slow-acting antirheumatic drugs in rheumatoid arthritis. *Drug Safety* 1994; **11:** 21–36.
26. Luqmani R, *et al.* Clinical pharmacology and modification of autoimmunity and inflammation in rheumatoid disease. *Drugs* 1994; **47:** 259–85.
27. Wijnands MJH, van Riel PLCM. Management of adverse effects of disease-modifying antirheumatic drugs. *Drug Safety* 1995; **13:** 219–27.
28. Lehmann T, *et al.* Toxicity of antirheumatic drugs. *Med J Aust* 1997; **116:** 378–83.
29. Gómez-Reino JJ. Long-term therapy for rheumatoid arthritis. *Lancet* 1996; **347:** 343–4.
30. ten Wolde S, *et al.* Randomised placebo-controlled study of stopping second-line drugs in rheumatoid arthritis. *Lancet* 1996; **347:** 347–52.
31. ten Wolde S, *et al.* Effect of resumption of second line drugs in patients with rheumatoid arthritis that flared up after treatment discontinuation. *Ann Rheum Dis* 1997; **56:** 235–9.
32. Felson DT, *et al.* The efficacy and toxicity of combination therapy in rheumatoid arthritis: a meta-analysis. *Arthritis Rheum* 1994; **37:** 1487–91.
33. Möttönen T, *et al.* FIN-RACo trial group. Comparison of combination therapy with single-drug therapy in early rheumatoid arthritis: a randomised trial. *Lancet* 1999; **353:** 1568–73.
34. Sambrook PN. Osteoporosis in rheumatoid arthritis: what is the role of antirheumatic therapy? *Lancet* 1994; **344:** 3–4.
35. Laan RFJM, *et al.* Low-dose prednisone induces rapid reversible axial bone loss in patients with rheumatoid arthritis: a randomized, controlled study. *Ann Intern Med* 1993; **119:** 963–8.
36. Saag KG, *et al.* Low dose long-term corticosteroid therapy in rheumatoid arthritis: an analysis of serious adverse events. *Am J Med* 1994; **96:** 115–23.
37. Kirwan JR. The Arthritis and Rheumatism Council Low-dose Glucocorticoid Study Group. The effect of glucocorticoids on joint destruction in rheumatoid arthritis. *N Engl J Med* 1995; **333:** 142–6.
38. Gotzsche PC, Johansen HK. Short-term low-dose corticosteroids vs placebo and nonsteroidal antiinflammatory drugs in rheumatoid arthritis. Available in The Cochrane Library; Issue 2. Chichester: John Wiley; 2004.
39. Criswell LA, *et al.* Moderate-term, low-dose corticosteroids for rheumatoid arthritis. Available in The Cochrane Library; Issue 2. Chichester: John Wiley; 2004.
40. Hunter JA, Blyth TH. A risk-benefit assessment of intra-articular corticosteroids in rheumatic disorders. *Drug Safety* 1999; **21:** 353–65.
41. Capell HA, Brzeski M. Slow drugs: slow progress? Use of slow acting antirheumatic drugs (SAARDs) in rheumatoid arthritis. *Ann Rheum Dis* 1992; **51:** 424–9.
42. Miller-Blair DJ, Robbins DL. Rheumatoid arthritis: new science, new treatment. *Geriatrics* 1993; **48:** 28–38.
43. Kloppenburg M, *et al.* Minocycline in active rheumatoid arthritis. *Arthritis Rheum* 1994; **37:** 629–36.
44. Tilley BC, *et al.* Minocycline in rheumatoid arthritis: a 48-week, double-blind, placebo-controlled trial. *Ann Intern Med* 1995; **122:** 81–9.

45. McKendry RJR. Is rheumatoid arthritis caused by an infection? *Lancet* 1995; **345:** 1319–20.
46. O'Dell JR, *et al.* Treatment of early rheumatoid arthritis with minocycline or placebo. *Arthritis Rheum* 1997; **40:** 842–8.
47. O'Dell JR, *et al.* Treatment of early seropositive rheumatoid arthritis with minocycline: four-year followup of a double-blind, placebo-controlled trial. *Arthritis Rheum* 1999; **42:** 1691–5.
48. Panush RS, Arend WP. Rheumatology. *JAMA* 1997; **277:** 1899–1900.
49. Choy EHS, Scott DL. Drug treatment of rheumatic diseases in the 1990s: achievements and future developments. *Drugs* 1997; **53:** 337–48.
50. Schiff M. Emerging treatments for rheumatoid arthritis. *Am J Med* 1997; **102** (suppl 1A): 11S–15S.
51. Buckley CD. Treatment of rheumatoid arthritis. *BMJ* 1997; **315:** 236–8.
52. Koopman WJ, Moreland LW. Rheumatoid arthritis: anticytokine therapies on the horizon. *Ann Intern Med* 1998; **128:** 231–3.
53. Cleland LG, *et al.* The role of fish oils in the treatment of rheumatoid arthritis. *Drugs* 2003; **63:** 845–53.
54. Bijlsma JW. Can we use steroid hormones to immunomodulate rheumatic diseases? Rheumatoid arthritis as an example. *Ann N Y Acad Sci* 1999; **876:** 366–7.
55. Maillefert JF, *et al.* Bisphosphonates in rheumatoid arthritis (osteoporosis excluded). *Rev Rhum Engl Ed* 1999; **66:** 442–5.
56. Witter FR. Clinical pharmacokinetics in the treatment of rheumatoid arthritis in pregnancy. *Clin Pharmacokinet* 1993; **25:** 444–9.
57. Østensen M, Ramsey-Goldman R. Treatment of inflammatory rheumatic disorders in pregnancy: what are the safest treatment options? *Drug Safety* 1998; **19:** 389–410.


### Soft-tissue rheumatism

Soft-tissue rheumatism includes a number of conditions such as fibromyalgia (fibrositis, muscular rheumatism, myofascial pain), humeral epicondylitis (e.g. tennis or golfer's elbow), frozen shoulder, Tietze's syndrome, fasciitis, tendinitis, tenosynovitis, bursitis (e.g. housemaid's knee), and sprains and strains. Inflamed or displaced tissue may also impinge on nearby nerves and produce compression neuropathies such as carpal tunnel syndrome.

Some forms of soft-tissue rheumatism will respond to selective rest of the affected region and splinting where appropriate. Gentle exercise, massage, and application of heat, cold, or rubefacients can also be of benefit. Many soft tissue lesions respond to local injection of a corticosteroid with a local anaesthetic. Short-term use of oral NSAIDs may help to relieve pain and reduce inflammation of soft-tissue trauma. The role of topical NSAIDs is unclear. Capsaicin has also been tried as a topical analgesic.

Patients with fibromyalgia have a number of other somatic symptoms including disturbed sleep and depression, in addition to their musculoskeletal pain. Pain and sleep quality may both be improved by low doses of amitriptyline with fluoxetine. If these drugs are ineffective after a trial of 4 to 6 weeks dosulepin may be tried; if there is still no response after a month, further drug treatment is probably best avoided. Exercise has also been shown to be of benefit.

References.


1. Dawson DM. Entrapment neuropathies of the upper extremities. *N Engl J Med* 1993; **329:** 2013–18.
2. Campbell P, Lawton JO. Heel pain: diagnosis and management. *BMJ* 1994; **52:** 380–5.
3. Muhammed N, *et al.* Peripheral nerve entrapment syndromes: diagnosis and management. *Br J Hosp Med* 1995; **53:** 141–6.
4. Caldwell JR. Intra-articular corticosteroids. *Drugs* 1996; **52:** 507–14.
5. Reveille JD. Soft-tissue rheumatism: diagnosis and treatment. *Am J Med* 1997; **102** (suppl 1A): 23S–29S.
6. Leventhal LJ. Management of fibromyalgia. *Ann Intern Med* 1999; **131:** 850–8.
7. Goldenberg DL. Fibromyalgia syndrome a decade later: what have we learned? *Arch Intern Med* 1999; **159:** 777–85.
8. Forseth KØ, Gran JT. Management of fibromyalgia: what are the best treatment choices? *Drugs* 2002; **62:** 577–92.
9. Shipley MA. Pain in the wrist and hand. In: Snaith ML, ed. *ABC of rheumatology*. 3rd ed. London: BMJ Publishing Group, 2004: 4–9.
10. Speed C. Pain in the neck, shoulder, and upper arm. In: Snaith ML, ed. *ABC of rheumatology*. 3rd ed. London: BMJ Publishing Group, 2004: 10–14.
11. Ryan S, Browne A. Fibromyalgia: musculoskeletal distress. In: Snaith ML, ed. *ABC of rheumatology*. 3rd ed. London: BMJ Publishing Group, 2004: 30–3.


### Spondyloarthropathies

The spondyloarthropathies are a group of seronegative arthritides which include ankylosing spondylitis, psoriatic arthritis, arthritis associated with inflammatory bowel disorders (enteropathic arthritis), and arthritis associated with infection as in reactive arthritis (aseptic arthritis).

**Ankylosing spondylitis** is characterised by arthritis of the spine and sacroiliac joints and sometimes there is also asymmetrical peripheral involvement. Males under 40 years of age are predominantly affected. The aim of management of the disease is to reduce pain and stiffness and to prevent spine and joint deformity, which is accomplished using a combination of active physical therapy and drug therapy. Exercises are used to strengthen muscles and to maintain a good posture and range of movement in joints. NSAIDs are used to relieve pain and inflammation, thus allowing the exercises to be performed; they do not influence the progression of the disease. Some patients may require concomitant treatment with other non-opioid analgesics such as paracetamol for additional pain control. Phenylbutazone is sometimes used when other drugs are unsuitable but in the UK its use is limited to hospital rheumatology departments because of the risk of serious adverse effects. Systemic corticosteroids are rarely indicated but intra-articular injections of corticosteroids may be beneficial when one or two peripheral joints are severely affected. The disease-modifying antirheumatic drug (DMARD) sulfasalazine, which has proven efficacy in ankylosing spondylitis (mainly in patients with peripheral involvement), may help to control severe or refractory disease. The tumour necrosis factor-α inhibitors, etanercept and infliximab, may also be of benefit in severe cases. The efficacy of other DMARDs used in rheumatoid arthritis (see above) remains to be demonstrated.

**Psoriatic arthritis** (or psoriatic arthropathy) is an inflammatory seronegative arthritis occurring in patients with psoriasis. In some patients the spine may be involved when the condition may be indistinguishable from ankylosing spondylitis. Less frequently some patients have a form of symmetrical arthritis resembling rheumatoid arthritis. The psoriasis (p.1137) and the arthritis usually require separate treatment. Treatment of the arthritis is initially as for ankylosing spondylitis with NSAIDs and physical therapy. If these methods fail treatment with a DMARD may be instituted, although chloroquine and hydroxychloroquine should be avoided since they may precipitate skin reactions (see Psoriatic Arthritis, p.450). Etanercept and leflunomide have recently been approved for the treatment of active arthritis in patients with psoriatic arthritis; infliximab is also effective. Systemic corticosteroids have little or no place in the management of psoriatic arthritis.

**Reactive arthritis** is characterised by sterile synovitis following 1 to 4 weeks after an infection most commonly of the gastrointestinal or genito-urinary tract. Extra-articular features involving the skin, eyes, or genito-urinary tract may or may not be present. Reactive arthritis is also a feature of Reiter's syndrome. Reactive arthritis is treated with physical therapy and NSAIDs and, if indicated, intra-articular injections of corticosteroids; the role of antibacterials is less certain (see Bone and Joint Infections, p.122).

References.


1. Svenungsson B. Reactive arthritis. *BMJ* 1994; **308:** 671–2.
2. Toussirot E, Wendling D. Current guidelines for the drug treatment of ankylosing spondylitis. *Drugs* 1998; **56:** 225–40.
3. Khan MA. Update on spondyloarthropathies. *Ann Intern Med* 2002; **136:** 896–907.
4. Lee RZ, Veale DJ. Management of spondyloarthropathy: new pharmacological treatment options. *Drugs* 2002; **62:** 2349–59.
5. Sieper J, *et al.* Ankylosing spondylitis: an overview. *Ann Rheum Dis* 2002; **61** (suppl III): iii8–iii18.
6. van der Horst-Bruinsma IE, *et al.* Treatment of ankylosing spondylitis with disease modifying antirheumatic drugs. *Clin Exp Rheumatol* 2002; **20** (suppl 28): S67–S70.
7. Brockbank J, Gladman D. Diagnosis and management of psoriatic arthritis. *Drugs* 2002; **62:** 2447–57.
8. Kingsley G, Pugh N. Spondyloarthropathies. In: Snaith ML, ed. *ABC of rheumatology*. 3rd ed. London: BMJ Publishing Group, 2004: 61–7.
9. Jones G, *et al.* Interventions for treating psoriatic arthritis. Available in The Cochrane Library; Issue 2. Chichester: John Wiley; 2004.


### Still's disease

Still's disease is characterised by a high fever, polyarthritis, and an evanescent pink macular rash that is most prominent during bouts of fever; patients are seronegative for rheumatoid factor. Onset is usually in children under 5 years of age, but can occur in adults. Treatment is usually with NSAIDs or corticosteroids.

The name Still's disease has also been used rather inconsistently to describe some types of juvenile idiopathic arthritis (above).

References.


1. Evans RH. Pyrexia of unknown origin. *BMJ* 1997; **314:** 583–6.


## Aceclofenac (BAN, rINN)

Aceclofenaco; Aceclofenacum. [*o*-(2,6-Dichloroanilino)phenyl]acetate glycolic acid ester; 2-(2,6-Dichloroanalino)phenylacetoxyacetic acid.

$C_{16}H_{13}Cl_2NO_4$ = 354.2.
*CAS — 89796-99-6.*
*ATC — M01AB16.*

**Pharmacopoeias.** In *Eur.* (see p.vi).

**Ph. Eur. 5.0** (Aceclofenac). A white or almost white, crystalline powder. Practically insoluble in water; soluble in alcohol; freely soluble in acetone. Store in airtight containers. Protect from light.

### Adverse Effects

As for NSAIDs in general, p.67.

**Hypersensitivity.** Leukocytoclastic vasculitis, a type III hypersensitivity reaction, with lung haemoptysis has been reported in a patient following therapy with aceclofenac.[1]


1. Epelde F, Boada L. Leukocytoclastic vasculitis and hemoptysis after treatment with aceclofenac. *Ann Pharmacother* 1995; **29:** 1168.


### Precautions

As for NSAIDs in general, p.69.

Aceclofenac should be avoided in patients with moderate to severe renal impairment.

### Interactions

For interactions associated with NSAIDs, see p.69.

### Pharmacokinetics

Aceclofenac is well absorbed from the gastrointestinal tract; peak plasma concentrations are reached 1 to 3 hours after an oral dose. Aceclofenac is more than 99% bound to plasma proteins. The plasma-elimination half-life is approximately 4 hours. About two-thirds of a dose is excreted in the urine, mainly as hydroxymetabolites.

### Uses and Administration

Aceclofenac, a phenylacetic acid derivative, is an NSAID (see p.70) related to diclofenac (p.33). It is used in the management of osteoarthritis, rheumatoid arthritis, and ankylosing spondylitis, in usual doses of 100 mg twice daily by mouth. Reduced doses should be used in patients with hepatic impairment, see below.

◊ Reviews.


1. Dooley M, *et al.* Aceclofenac: a reappraisal of its use in the management of pain and rheumatic disease. *Drugs* 2001; **61:** 1351–78.


**Administration in hepatic impairment.** The initial dose of aceclofenac should be reduced to 100 mg daily in patients with hepatic impairment.

### Preparations

**Proprietary Preparations** (details are given in Part 3)
***Arg.:*** Berlofen; Bristaflam; ***Austria:*** Beofenac; ***Belg.:*** Air-Tal; Biofenac; ***Braz.:*** Aceflan; Proflam; ***Chile:*** Airtal; Bristaflam; ***Denm.:*** Barcan; ***Fin.:*** Barcan; ***Ger.:*** Beofenac; ***Gr.:*** Biofenac; Sovipan; ***Irl.:*** Airtal†; ***Mex.:*** Bristaflam; ***Neth.:*** Biofenac; ***Norw.:*** Barcan; ***Port.:*** Airtal; Biofenac; ***Spain:*** Airtal; Airtal Difucrem; Falcol; Gerbin; Sanein; ***Swed.:*** Barcan; ***Switz.:*** Locomin; ***UAE:*** Aceclofar; ***UK:*** Preservex.

## Acemetacin (BAN, rINN)

Acemetacina; Bay-f-4975; TVX-1322. *O*-[(1-*p*-Chlorobenzoyl-5-methoxy-2-methylindol-3-yl)acetyl]glycolic acid.

$C_{21}H_{18}ClNO_6$ = 415.8.
*CAS — 53164-05-9.*
*ATC — M01AB11.*

### Profile

Acemetacin, a glycolic acid ester of indometacin, is an NSAID (p.67). Its pharmacological activity is due to both acemetacin and its major metabolite, indometacin (p.47). Acemetacin is used in rheumatoid arthritis, osteoarthritis, and low back pain, and for postoperative pain and inflammation. Usual daily doses are 120 to 180 mg by mouth in divided doses. Acemetacin is eliminated by both hepatic and renal routes, although pharmacokinetics are not affected by moderate renal or hepatic impairment and appear to be unchanged in the elderly.

◊ References.


1. Jones RW, *et al.* Comparative pharmacokinetics of acemetacin in young subjects and elderly patients. *Br J Clin Pharmacol* 1991; **31:** 543–5.
2. Hazleman B, Bernstein RM. Acemetacin in the long-term therapy of rheumatoid arthritis. *Curr Med Res Opin* 1993; **13:** 119–26.
3. Chou CT, Tsai YY. A double-blind, randomized, controlled parallel group study evaluating the efficacy and safety of acemetacin for the management of osteoarthritis. *Int J Clin Pharmacol Res* 2002; **22:** 1–6.


### Preparations

**Proprietary Preparations** (details are given in Part 3)
***Austria:*** Rheutrop; ***Ger.:*** Acemetadoc; Acephlogont; Peran†; Rantudil; ***Gr.:*** Gamespir; Rantudal; ***Ital.:*** Acemix; Solart; ***Mex.:*** Rantudil; ***Port.:*** Rantudil; ***Singapore:*** Rantudil†; ***Spain:*** Espledol; Oldan; ***Switz.:*** Tilur; ***UK:*** Emflex.

**Multi-ingredient:** ***Arg.:*** Rucaten Forte; Rucaten Prednisolona.

## Acetanilide

Acetanilida; Antifebrin. *N*-Phenylacetamide.

$C_8H_9NO$ = 135.2.
*CAS — 103-84-4.*

**Pharmacopoeias.** In *Fr.*

### Profile

Acetanilide, a para-aminophenol derivative related to paracetamol (p.76), has analgesic and antipyretic properties. It was replaced by safer analgesics.

## Actarit *(rINN)*

(*p*-Acetamidophenyl)acetic acid.

$C_{10}H_{11}NO_3$ = 193.2.

*CAS — 18699-02-0.*

### Profile

Actarit is reported to be a disease-modifying antirheumatic drug. It is given by mouth in the treatment of rheumatoid arthritis in a usual dose of 100 mg three times daily.

**Adverse effects.** A photosensitivity reaction developed in a 52-year-old woman one month after starting actarit and doxycycline.[1] Photopatch tests for both drugs were only positive for the patches containing actarit.

1. Kawada A, *et al.* Photosensitivity due to actarit. *Contact Dermatitis* 1997; **36:** 175–6.

**Use.** References.

1. Nobunaga M. Long term administration study of a new DMARD actarit on rheumatoid arthritis. *Rinsho Iyaku* 1994; **10:** 947–62.
2. Nakamura H, *et al.* Clinical effects of actarit in rheumatoid arthritis: improvement of early disease activity mediated by reduction of serum concentrations of nitric oxide. *Clin Exp Rheumatol* 2000; **18:** 445–50.

### Preparations

**Proprietary Preparations** (details are given in Part 3)
***Jpn:*** Mover; Orcl.

## Adalimumab *(BAN, USAN, rINN)*

D2E7; LU-200134.

*CAS — 331731-18-1.*

*ATC — L04AA17.*

### Adverse Effects and Precautions

As for Infliximab, p.50.

Injection site reactions including erythema, itching, pain, and swelling are the most common adverse reactions with adalimumab; however, most reactions are mild and do not result in drug withdrawal. Other common reactions include headache, rashes, back pain, hypertension, hypercholesterolaemia, increased alkaline phosphate levels, and haematuria.

Autoantibodies to adalimumab have been detected.

### Interactions

As for Infliximab, p.50.

Methotrexate is reported to reduce the clearance of adalimumab by up to 44% but the manufacturer of the latter considers that dosage adjustment for either drug does not appear to be necessary.

### Pharmacokinetics

Adalimumab is reported to have linear pharmacokinetics at usual dosages. Following subcutaneous injection peak concentrations are reached after about 3 to 8 days and bioavailability is estimated to be 64%. The mean terminal half-life is about 2 weeks.

### Uses and Administration

Adalimumab is a monoclonal tumour necrosis factor antibody used alone or with methotrexate or other disease-modifying antirheumatic drugs in the treatment of rheumatoid arthritis (p.9) unresponsive to the latter alone. It is given by subcutaneous injection in a dose of 40 mg every other week; some patients not receiving methotrexate may benefit from increasing the dose to 40 mg every week.

◊ References.

1. den Broeder AA, *et al.* Long-term anti-tumour necrosis factor alpha monotherapy in rheumatoid arthritis: effect on radiological course and prognostic value of markers of cartilage turnover and endothelial activation. *Ann Rheum Dis* 2002; **61:** 311–18.
2. Rau R. Adalimumab (a fully human anti-tumour necrosis factor alpha monoclonal antibody) in the treatment of active rheumatoid arthritis: the initial results of five trials. *Ann Rheum Dis* 2002; **61** (suppl 2): 70–3.
3. Weinblatt ME, *et al.* Adalimumab, a fully human anti-tumor necrosis factor alpha monoclonal antibody, for the treatment of rheumatoid arthritis in patients taking concomitant methotrexate: the ARMADA trial. *Arthritis Rheum* 2003; **48:** 35–45.
4. Furst DE, *et al.* Adalimumab, a fully human anti tumor necrosis factor-alpha monoclonal antibody, and concomitant standard antirheumatic therapy for the treatment of rheumatoid arthritis: results of STAR (Safety Trial of Adalimumab in Rheumatoid Arthritis). *J Rheumatol* 2003; **30:** 2563–71.
5. van de Putte LB, *et al.* Efficacy and safety of adalimumab as monotherapy in patients with rheumatoid arthritis for whom previous disease modifying antirheumatic drug treatment has failed. *Ann Rheum Dis* 2004; **63:** 508–16.
6. Keystone EC, *et al.* Radiographic, clinical, and functional outcomes of treatment with adalimumab (a human anti-tumor necrosis factor monoclonal antibody) in patients with active rheumatoid arthritis receiving concomitant methotrexate therapy: a randomized, placebo-controlled, 52-week trial. *Arthritis Rheum* 2004; **50:** 1400–11.

### Preparations

**Proprietary Preparations** (details are given in Part 3)
***Austral.:*** Humira; ***Fr.:*** Humira; ***UK:*** Humira; ***USA:*** Humira.

## Alfentanil Hydrochloride

*(BANM, USAN, rINNM)*

Alfentanili Hydrochloridum; Hidrocloruro de alfentanilo; R-39209. *N*-{1-[2-(4-Ethyl-5-oxo-2-tetrazolin-1-yl)ethyl]-4-(methoxymethyl)-4-piperidyl}propionanilide hydrochloride.

$C_{21}H_{32}N_6O_3,HCl$ = 453.0.

*CAS — 71195-58-9 (alfentanil); 69049-06-5 (anhydrous alfentanil hydrochloride); 70879-28-6 (alfentanil hydrochloride monohydrate).*

*ATC — N01AH02.*

**Pharmacopoeias.** In *Eur.* (see p.vi) and *US.*

**Ph. Eur. 5.0** (Alfentanil Hydrochloride). A white or almost white powder. Freely soluble in water, in alcohol, and in methyl alcohol. Protect from light.

**USP 27** (Alfentanil Hydrochloride). A white to almost white powder. Soluble in water; freely soluble in alcohol, in chloroform, and in methyl alcohol; sparingly soluble in acetone. Store in airtight containers.

### Dependence and Withdrawal

As for Opioid Analgesics, p.71.

### Adverse Effects and Treatment

As for Opioid Analgesics in general, p.72, and for Fentanyl, p.40.

**Effects on the cardiovascular system.** There have been 2 cases of sinus arrest occurring[1] during intubation following the administration of alfentanil 30 micrograms/kg.

1. Maryniak JK, Bishop VA. Sinus arrest after alfentanil. *Br J Anaesth* 1987; **59:** 390–1.

**Effects on mental function.** Like fentanyl, alfentanil 7.5 or 15 micrograms/kg intravenously had no effect on memory in healthy subjects.[1] In another study impairment of memory for new facts did occur 2 hours after operation in patients anaesthetised with alfentanil 7.5 micrograms/kg, but not in those given fentanyl;[2] methohexital might have contributed to the impairment.

1. Scamman FL, *et al.* Ventilatory and mental effects of alfentanil and fentanyl. *Acta Anaesthesiol Scand* 1984; **28:** 63–7.
2. Kennedy DJ, Ogg TW. Alfentanil and memory function: a comparison with fentanyl for day case termination of pregnancy. *Anaesthesia* 1985; **40:** 537–40.

**Effects on the respiratory system.** Alfentanil, like other opioid agonists, causes dose-related respiratory depression; it is significant with doses of more than 1 mg. Recovery has been reported to be faster after alfentanil than after fentanyl (see p.40),[1,2] possibly reflecting the shorter elimination half-life of alfentanil. Even so, accumulation of alfentanil is possible with large doses over a prolonged period. Profound analgesia is accompanied by marked respiratory depression which may persist or recur postoperatively.

After an initial rapid recovery from anaesthesia, 2 patients suffered sudden respiratory arrest about an hour after the end of alfentanil infusion;[3] both responded to treatment with naloxone. Close monitoring of respiration in the initial postoperative period was recommended and this was reinforced by the manufacturers;[4] factors such as hyperventilation and the use of opioid premedication might enhance or prolong the respiratory depressant effects of alfentanil.

1. Andrews CJH, *et al.* Ventilatory effects during and after continuous infusion of fentanyl or alfentanil. *Br J Anaesth* 1983; **55:** 211S–16S.
2. Scamman FL, *et al.* Ventilatory and mental effects of alfentanil and fentanyl. *Acta Anaesthesiol Scand* 1984; **28:** 63–7.
3. Sebel PS, *et al.* Respiratory depression after alfentanil infusion. *BMJ* 1984; **289:** 1581–2.
4. Waldron HA, Cookson RF. Respiratory depression after alfentanil infusion. *BMJ* 1985; **290:** 319.

### Precautions

As for Opioid Analgesics in general, p.72.

**Children.** Alfentanil given to preterm infants undergoing paralysis and mechanical ventilation for respiratory distress syndrome resulted in a rapid and significant fall in heart rate and blood pressure, emphasising that proper evaluation of the pharmacological and clinical effects was necessary.[1]

1. Marlow N, *et al.* Hazards of analgesia for newborn infants. *Arch Dis Child* 1988; **63:** 1293.

**The elderly.** An early study found that elderly patients had increased brain sensitivity to alfentanil as demonstrated by EEG changes,[1] and lower doses might be indicated in older patients for pharmacodynamic rather than pharmacokinetic reasons. See also under Pharmacokinetics, below.

1. Scott JC, Stanski DR. Decreased fentanyl and alfentanil dose requirements with age: a simultaneous pharmacokinetic and pharmacodynamic evaluation. *J Pharmacol Exp Ther* 1987; **240:** 159–66.

**Handling.** Avoid contact with the skin and the inhalation of particles of alfentanil hydrochloride.

**Inflammatory bowel disease.** Patients with Crohn's disease required higher doses of alfentanil than control patients[1] although there were no differences in alfentanil pharmacokinetics between the 2 groups of patients.

1. Gesink-van der Veer BJ, *et al.* Influence of Crohn's disease on the pharmacokinetics and pharmacodynamics of alfentanil. *Br J Anaesth* 1993; **71:** 827–34.

**Pregnancy.** The UK manufacturers contra-indicate the use of alfentanil in labour, or before clamping of the cord during caesarean section, because placental transfer means there is a risk of neonatal respiratory depression.

### Interactions

For interactions associated with opioid analgesics, see p.73.

Drugs that depress the heart or increase vagal tone, such as beta blockers and anaesthetic drugs, may predispose patients given alfentanil to develop bradycardia and hypotension. Use of alfentanil with non-vagolytic neuromuscular blockers may produce bradycardia and possibly asystole.

The metabolism of alfentanil via the cytochrome P450 isoenzyme CYP3A4 may be reduced by potent inhibitors of this isoenzyme, resulting in a risk of prolonged or delayed respiratory depression. Reduced doses of alfentanil may be required if given with a CYP3A4 inhibitor such as cimetidine, diltiazem, erythromycin, fluconazole, itraconazole, ketoconazole, or ritonavir.

**Antibacterials.** The elimination half-life of alfentanil was increased and clearance decreased when given after a 7-day course of *erythromycin* by mouth in healthy subjects.[1] Other hepatic enzyme inhibitors and drugs interfering with hepatic blood flow might also affect the clearance of alfentanil.

1. Bartkowski RR, *et al.* Inhibition of alfentanil metabolism by erythromycin. *Clin Pharmacol Ther* 1989; **46:** 99–102.

**Antifungals.** Azole antifungals such as *ketoconazole* or *fluconazole* can inhibit the metabolism of alfentanil. In a study, giving alfentanil 1 hour after intravenous or oral fluconazole decreased the clearance of alfentanil by 60 and 55%, respectively and increased the mean half-life of alfentanil from 1.5 hours to 2.7 and 2.5 hours, respectively.[1]

1. Palkama VJ, *et al.* The effect of intravenous and oral fluconazole on the pharmacokinetics and pharmacodynamics of intravenous alfentanil. *Anesth Analg* 1998; **87:** 190–4.

### Pharmacokinetics

After parenteral doses alfentanil hydrochloride has a rapid onset and short duration of action. Alfentanil is about 90% protein bound and has a small volume of distribution. Its terminal elimination half-life is about 1 to 2 hours. It is metabolised in the liver; oxidative *N*- and *O*-dealkylation by the cytochrome P450 isoenzyme CYP3A4 leads to inactive metabolites which are excreted in the urine. Alfentanil crosses the blood-brain barrier and the placenta and has been detected in colostrum.

◊ Alfentanil is less lipid-soluble than fentanyl, but more so than morphine. It is highly bound to plasma protein, principally to $\alpha_1$-acid glycoprotein. Decreased lipid solubility can be expected to limit penetration of the blood-brain barrier when compared with fentanyl, but the majority of unbound alfentanil is unionised and can rapidly gain access to the CNS. Alfentanil has a smaller volume of distribution than fentanyl and its elimination half-life is shorter. The manufacturers have given values for a three-compartment pharmacokinetic model with a distribution half-life of 0.4 to 3.1 minutes, a redistribution half-life of 4.6 to 21.6 minutes, and a terminal elimination half-life of 64.1 to 129.3 minutes following single bolus injections of 50 or 125 micrograms/kg. Accumulation is less likely than with fentanyl, but can occur following repeated or continuous administration especially in patients with reduced clearance. The mean elimination half-life reported is usually about 90 minutes, but this is reduced in children and increased in the elderly, in hepatic impairment, in the obese, and during cardiopulmonary bypass (see below).

◊ Reviews.

1. Hull CJ. The pharmacokinetics of alfentanil in man. *Br J Anaesth* 1983; **55:** 157S–64S.
2. Mather LE. Clinical pharmacokinetics of fentanyl and its newer derivatives. *Clin Pharmacokinet* 1983; **8:** 422–46.
3. Davis PJ, Cook DR. Clinical pharmacokinetics of the newer intravenous anaesthetic agents. *Clin Pharmacokinet* 1986; **11:** 18–35.
4. Bodenham A, Park GR. Alfentanil infusions in patients requiring intensive care. *Clin Pharmacokinet* 1988; **15:** 216–26.
5. Scholz J, *et al.* Clinical pharmacokinetics of alfentanil, fentanyl and sufentanil. *Clin Pharmacokinet* 1996; **31:** 275–92.

**Administration.** CONTINUOUS INTRAVENOUS INFUSION. Small studies of alfentanil by continuous intravenous infusion[1-3] have found pharmacokinetic parameters to be similar to those after a single bolus injection, but with some conflicting results. In 29 patients undergoing orthopaedic surgery an initial bolus intravenous injection of alfentanil 50 micrograms/kg was followed by intravenous infusion of 1 microgram/kg per minute, continued for 44 to 445 minutes; a second bolus injection of

50 micrograms/kg was given immediately before incision and an additional bolus injection of 1 mg given if necessary.[4] The time course of the plasma-alfentanil concentration fitted a two-compartmental model in 26 patients. Terminal half-lives varied widely from 56 to 226 minutes (mean 106 minutes), the highest values being mainly in patients over 60 years. There was no significant correlation between pharmacokinetic parameters and the duration of the infusion or the total dose. Plasma clearance and volumes of distribution did not correlate significantly with body-weight although steady-state volume of distribution was enlarged with increasing age. The mean estimated steady-state concentration was 293 nanograms/mL (range 147 to 636 nanograms/mL).

1. Fragen RJ, *et al.* Pharmacokinetics of the infusion of alfentanil in man. *Br J Anaesth* 1983; **55:** 1077–81.
2. Shafer A, *et al.* Pharmacokinetics and pharmacodynamics of alfentanil infusions during general anesthesia. *Anesth Analg* 1986; **65:** 1021–8.
3. Reitz JA, *et al.* The pharmacokinetics of alfentanil in gynecologic surgical patients. *J Clin Pharmacol* 1986; **26:** 60–4.
4. van Beem H, *et al.* Pharmacokinetics of alfentanil during and after a fixed rate infusion. *Br J Anaesth* 1989; **62:** 610–15.

INTRAMUSCULAR. See under The Elderly, below.

**Burns.** The volume of distribution and total clearance of alfentanil were reduced and its elimination half-life prolonged in patients with burns.[1] This was due, in part, to raised concentrations of $\alpha_1$-acid glycoprotein leading to increased protein binding.

1. Macfie AG, *et al.* Disposition of alfentanil in burns patients. *Br J Anaesth* 1992; **69:** 447–50.

**Cardiopulmonary bypass.** The elimination half-life of alfentanil increased from 72 minutes before cardiopulmonary bypass to 195 minutes afterwards in 5 patients.[1] This was attributed to an increase in volume of distribution, based in part on a dilution-induced decrease in plasma protein binding. Others[2,3] found that on starting cardiopulmonary bypass total serum concentrations of alfentanil were halved, mainly because of dilution of $\alpha_1$-acid glycoprotein and an increase in unbound alfentanil.

1. Hug CC, *et al.* Alfentanil pharmacokinetics in patients before and after cardiopulmonary bypass. *Anesth Analg* 1983; **62:** 266.
2. Kumar K, *et al.* The effect of cardiopulmonary bypass on plasma protein binding of alfentanil. *Eur J Clin Pharmacol* 1988; **35:** 47–52.
3. Hynynen M, *et al.* Plasma concentration and protein binding of alfentanil during high-dose infusion for cardiac surgery. *Br J Anaesth* 1994; **72:** 571–6.

**Children.** Alfentanil has been shown to have a shorter elimination half-life (about 40 minutes) and a smaller volume of distribution in children than in adults.[1] See also under Hepatic Impairment, below.

1. Meistelman C, *et al.* A comparison of alfentanil pharmacokinetics in children and adults. *Anesthesiology* 1987; **66:** 13–16.

**The elderly.** Plasma clearance of alfentanil following 50 micrograms/kg as a single intravenous dose was reduced in patients more than 65 years old when compared with that in healthy young adults.[1] Mean elimination half-life was 137 minutes in the elderly and 83 minutes in the young adults. Volumes of distribution were similar and it was considered that reduced clearance might be due to decreased hepatic metabolism in the elderly. In a study in male patients the terminal elimination half-life of alfentanil increased with age, although clearance was not significantly affected.[2] In patients given alfentanil 1 microgram/kg per minute by continuous intravenous infusion during orthopaedic surgery,[3] terminal half-life increased linearly with age in those older than 40 years and steady-state volume of distribution was enlarged with increasing age; clearance did not correlate significantly with age and was thought to be more variable during a continuous infusion in long-term surgery than after a single bolus injection. Others have reported[4] that the effects of age on alfentanil pharmacokinetics are dependent on gender. In this study total plasma clearance decreased and terminal half-life increased with increasing age in women, but not in men. It has been suggested that this effect in women may be more dependent on menopausal status than on age.[5]

In a study[6] in elderly patients plasma concentrations of alfentanil were greater and the maximum concentration occurred earlier when alfentanil was injected into the deltoid muscle compared with injection into the gluteal muscle.

1. Helmers H, *et al.* Alfentanil kinetics in the elderly. *Clin Pharmacol Ther* 1984; **36:** 239–43.
2. Scott JC, Stanski DR. Decreased fentanyl and alfentanil dose requirements with age: a simultaneous pharmacokinetic and pharmacodynamic evaluation. *J Pharmacol Exp Ther* 1987; **240:** 159–66.
3. van Beem H, *et al.* Pharmacokinetics of alfentanil during and after a fixed rate infusion. *Br J Anaesth* 1989; **62:** 610–15.
4. Lemmens HJM, *et al.* Influence of age on the pharmacokinetics of alfentanil: gender dependence. *Clin Pharmacokinet* 1990; **19:** 416–22.
5. Rubio A, Cox C. Sex, age and alfentanil pharmacokinetics. *Clin Pharmacokinet* 1991; **21:** 81.
6. Virkkilä M, *et al.* Pharmacokinetics and effects of im alfentanil as premedication for day-case ophthalmic surgery in elderly patients. *Br J Anaesth* 1993; **71:** 507–11.

**Hepatic impairment.** Total plasma clearance and protein binding of alfentanil were decreased in patients with alcoholic cirrhosis when compared with control subjects. Elimination half-life was prolonged from 90 to 219 minutes in the cirrhotic patients following a single intravenous dose of 50 micrograms/kg and was attributed in part to alterations in binding sites of $\alpha_1$-acid glycoprotein.[1] There might be different effects on alfentanil disposition in patients with non-alcoholic cirrhosis or other liver disorders.[2] The pharmacokinetics of alfentanil were apparently not affected in children with cholestatic hepatic disease whereas clearance was reduced postoperatively in 3 patients who had undergone liver transplantation.[3]

1. Ferrier C, *et al.* Alfentanil pharmacokinetics in patients with cirrhosis. *Anesthesiology* 1985; **62:** 480–4.
2. Bower S, *et al.* Effects of different hepatic pathologies on disposition of alfentanil in anaesthetized patients. *Br J Anaesth* 1992; **68:** 462–5.
3. Davis PJ, *et al.* Effects of cholestatic hepatic disease and chronic renal failure on alfentanil pharmacokinetics in children. *Anesth Analg* 1989; **68:** 579–83.

**Obesity.** The pharmacokinetics of alfentanil are reportedly altered in obesity.[1] Elimination half-life was 172 minutes in 6 obese patients compared with 92 minutes in 7 who were not obese. Plasma clearance of alfentanil was also decreased, although others[2] found that obesity had no effect on clearance, but it did have a direct relationship with the volume of the central compartment.

1. Bentley JB, *et al.* Obesity and alfentanil pharmacokinetics. *Anesth Analg* 1983; **62:** 251.
2. Maitre PO, *et al.* Population pharmacokinetics of alfentanil: the average dose-plasma concentration relationship and interindividual variability in patients. *Anesthesiology* 1987; **66:** 3–12.

**Renal impairment.** The pharmacokinetics of alfentanil were not affected significantly in adults[1] or children[2] with chronic renal failure. In another study[3] increased volume of distribution of alfentanil at steady state was associated with decreased plasma protein binding in patients with chronic renal failure.

1. Van Peer A, *et al.* Alfentanil kinetics in renal insufficiency. *Eur J Clin Pharmacol* 1986; **30:** 245–7.
2. Davis PJ, *et al.* Effects of cholestatic hepatic disease and chronic renal failure on alfentanil pharmacokinetics in children. *Anesth Analg* 1989; **68:** 579–83.
3. Chauvin M, *et al.* Pharmacokinetics of alfentanil in chronic renal failure. *Anesth Analg* 1987; **66:** 53–6.

## Uses and Administration

Alfentanil is a short-acting opioid analgesic (p.73) related to fentanyl (p.41).

Alfentanil is used in surgical procedures as an analgesic and adjunct to general anaesthetics or as a primary anaesthetic. It is also used as an analgesic and respiratory depressant in the management of mechanically ventilated patients under intensive care.

Alfentanil is given intravenously as the hydrochloride although doses are expressed in terms of alfentanil base. Alfentanil hydrochloride 108.8 micrograms is approximately equivalent to 100 micrograms of alfentanil. A peak effect may be seen within 1.5 to 2 minutes of an injection and analgesia can be expected to last for up to 10 minutes; dose supplements are therefore required if it is to be used for more prolonged surgical procedures. It may be given by continuous intravenous infusion in ventilated patients.

The dosage of alfentanil used depends on whether the patient has spontaneous respiration or assisted ventilation and on the expected duration of anaesthesia. Doses are adjusted according to the needs of the patient. Children may require higher or more frequent doses than adults, whereas the elderly or debilitated patients may require lower or less frequent doses. Obese patients may require doses based on their lean body mass.

When used as an adjunct in the **maintenance of general anaesthesia** the recommended initial dose in the UK is as follows:

- in adults with *spontaneous respiration*, up to 500 micrograms given slowly over about 30 seconds; supplementary doses of 250 micrograms may be given.
- *ventilated* adults and children may be given 30 to 50 micrograms/kg with supplements of 15 micrograms/kg. When given by infusion to ventilated adults and children there is an initial loading dose of 50 to 100 micrograms/kg given as a bolus or by infusion over 10 minutes, and this is followed by infusion at a rate of 0.5 to 1 microgram/kg per minute.

Typical doses that have been used in the USA are as follows:

- for procedures lasting *less than 30 minutes* in adults with spontaneous respiration or assisted ventilation, the dose is 8 to 20 micrograms/kg; this may be followed by supplementary doses of 3 to 5 micrograms/kg every 5 to 20 minutes or an infusion of 0.5 to 1 microgram/kg per minute.
- when the expected duration of anaesthesia is *longer than 30 minutes*, the initial dose for adults with assisted ventilation is 20 to 75 micrograms/kg, followed by either supplementary doses of 5 to 15 micrograms/kg or an infusion of 0.5 to 3 micrograms/kg per minute. If alfentanil has been given in anaesthetic doses (see below) for the induction of anaesthesia, infusion rates may need to be reduced by 30 to 50% during the first hour of maintenance.

Maintenance infusions of alfentanil should be discontinued 10 to 30 minutes before the anticipated end of surgery.

The dose for the **induction of anaesthesia** in patients with assisted ventilation undergoing procedures of at least 45 minutes is 130 to 245 micrograms/kg, followed by an inhalation anaesthetic or maintenance doses of alfentanil of 0.5 to 1.5 micrograms/kg per minute.

In **intensive care** ventilated adults may be given alfentanil initially at an infusion rate of 2 mg/hour or a loading dose of 5 mg may be given in divided doses over 10 minutes or more slowly if hypotension or bradycardia occur. Thereafter a suitable rate of infusion should be determined for each patient (rates of 0.5 to 10 mg/hour have been used); patients should be carefully monitored and the duration of treatment should not generally exceed 4 days. During continuous infusion additional bolus injections of 0.5 to 1 mg may be given if required to provide analgesia for short painful procedures that may be carried out in intensive care.

**Administration.** Alfentanil is usually given by intravenous injection or infusion, but has also been given intramuscularly[1,2] or epidurally (see under Pain, below).

1. Arendt-Nielsen L, *et al.* Analgesic efficacy of im alfentanil. *Br J Anaesth* 1990; **65:** 164–8.
2. Virkkilä M, *et al.* Pharmacokinetics and effects of im alfentanil as premedication for day-case ophthalmic surgery in elderly patients. *Br J Anaesth* 1993; **71:** 507–11.

**Anaesthesia.** Alfentanil, like fentanyl (p.42), appears to produce fewer circulatory changes than morphine and may be preferred for anaesthetic use, especially in cardiovascular surgery. It is generally considered to have a shorter duration of action than fentanyl. It has been used with propofol to facilitate intubation, and for total intravenous anaesthesia.

For a discussion of the drugs used to facilitate intubation and of opioids such as alfentanil used to control the pressor response and the rise of intra-ocular pressure associated with intubation, see under Anaesthesia, p.1397. For reference to a study indicating that pretreatment with alfentanil can reduce the pain associated with injection of propofol, see p.1306.

CAESAREAN SECTION. The UK manufacturers contra-indicate the use of alfentanil before clamping the cord during caesarean section because of the risk of respiratory depression in the neonate. A study of alfentanil 30 micrograms/kg in women undergoing caesarean section was abandoned after massive respiratory depression had occurred in 4 of 5 neonates.[1] However, alfentanil has been used successfully to minimise haemodynamic responses to intubation and surgery in patients with severe cardiovascular disorders undergoing caesarean section.[2,3] A baby delivered after the successful use of alfentanil 35 micrograms/kg in a mother with severe aortic stenosis[2] was apnoeic and unresponsive with poor muscle tone; the baby responded rapidly to naloxone. Alfentanil 10 micrograms/kg immediately before induction attenuated the cardiovascular response to intubation in patients with severe pregnancy-induced hypertension[3] and was considered a suitable alternative to fentanyl 2.5 micrograms/kg; no effect on neonatal mortality could be attributed to anaesthetic technique. However, it has been suggested that the use of smaller doses of alfentanil of 7.5 micrograms/kg with magnesium sulfate 30 mg/kg may provide better cardiovascular control.[4]

1. Leuwer M, *et al.* Pharmacokinetics and pharmacodynamics of an equipotent fentanyl and alfentanil dose in mother and infant during caesarean section. *Br J Anaesth* 1990; **64:** 398P–9P.
2. Redfern N, *et al.* Alfentanil for caesarean section complicated by severe aortic stenosis: a case report. *Br J Anaesth* 1987; **59:** 1309–12.
3. Rout CC, Rocke DA. Effects of alfentanil and fentanyl on induction of anaesthesia in patients with severe pregnancy-induced hypertension. *Br J Anaesth* 1990; **65:** 468–74.
4. Ashton WB, *et al.* Attenuation of the pressor response to tracheal intubation by magnesium sulphate with and without alfentanil in hypertensive proteinuric patients undergoing caesarean section. *Br J Anaesth* 1991; **67:** 741–7.

PHAEOCHROMOCYTOMA. Alfentanil does not release histamine and was of value in the anaesthetic management of patients with phaeochromocytoma.[1] It has a very rapid onset of action, good vasodilating properties, and a relatively short elimination half-life. These patients are often very somnolent for the first 48 hours after surgery and postoperative opioid dosage requirements may be less than expected. Alfentanil infusion continued into the postoperative period allows careful titration of dosage.

1. Hull CJ. Phaeochromocytoma: diagnosis, preoperative preparation and anaesthetic management. *Br J Anaesth* 1986; **58:** 1453–68.

**Pain.** POSTOPERATIVE ANALGESIA. Continuous on-demand epidural infusions of alfentanil 200 micrograms/hour or fentanyl 20 micrograms/hour provided comparable analgesia to morphine 200 micrograms/hour in the early postoperative period;[1] alfentanil (16 minutes) and fentanyl (13 minutes) had the advantage of more rapid onset of analgesia than morphine (44 minutes). However, some considered that there was no overall advantage of epidural over intravenous alfentanil either as patient-controlled analgesia[2] or by continuous infusion.[3]

1. Chrubasik J, *et al.* Relative analgesic potency of epidural fentanyl, alfentanil, and morphine in treatment of postoperative pain. *Anesthesiology* 1988; **68:** 929–33.
2. Chauvin M, *et al.* Equivalence of postoperative analgesia with patient-controlled intravenous or epidural alfentanil. *Anesth Analg* 1993; **76:** 1251–8.
3. van den Nieuwenhuyzen MCO, *et al.* Epidural vs intravenous infusion of alfentanil in the management of postoperative pain following laparotomies. *Acta Anaesthesiol Scand* 1996; **40:** 1112–18.

### Preparations

***USP 27:*** Alfentanil Injection.

**Proprietary Preparations** (details are given in Part 3)
***Arg.:*** Brevafen; ***Austral.:*** Rapifen; ***Austria:*** Rapifen; ***Belg.:*** Rapifen; ***Braz.:*** Alfast; Rapifen; ***Canad.:*** Alfenta; ***Chile:*** Rapifen; ***Denm.:*** Rapifen; ***Fin.:*** Rapifen; ***Fr.:*** Rapifen; ***Ger.:*** Rapifen; ***Gr.:*** Rapifen; ***Hong Kong:*** Rapifen; ***Irl.:*** Rapifen; ***Israel:*** Rapifen; ***Ital.:*** Fentalim; ***Malaysia:*** Rapifen; ***Mex.:*** Rapifen; ***Neth.:*** Rapifen; ***Norw.:*** Rapifen; ***NZ:*** Rapifen; ***S.Afr.:*** Rapifen; ***Spain:*** Fanaxal; Limifen; ***Swed.:*** Rapifen; ***Switz.:*** Rapifen; ***UK:*** Rapifen; ***USA:*** Alfenta.

## Alminoprofen *(rINN)*

Alminoprofeno. 4-[(2-Methylallyl)amino]hydratropic acid.

$C_{13}H_{17}NO_2$ = 219.3.
*CAS — 39718-89-3.*
*ATC — M01AE16.*

### Profile

Alminoprofen, a propionic acid derivative related to ibuprofen (p.45), is an NSAID (p.67). It has been used in inflammatory and rheumatic disorders in doses of up to 900 mg daily by mouth.

### Preparations

**Proprietary Preparations** (details are given in Part 3)
***Fr.:*** Minalfene.

## Aloxiprin *(BAN, rINN)*

Aloxiprina.
*CAS — 9014-67-9.*
*ATC — B01AC15; N02BA02.*

**Pharmacopoeias.** In *Br.*

**BP 2003** (Aloxiprin). A polymeric condensation product of aluminium oxide and aspirin. A fine, white or slightly pink powder, odourless or almost odourless. It contains not less than 7.5% and not more than 8.5% of aluminium and not less than 79.0% and not more than 87.4% of total salicylates, calculated as aspirin, $C_9H_8O_4$, both calculated with reference to the dried substance. Practically insoluble in water, in alcohol, and in ether; slightly soluble in chloroform.

### Profile

Aloxiprin, a polymeric condensation product of aluminium oxide and aspirin, has actions similar to those of aspirin (p.15); aloxiprin 600 mg is approximately equivalent to 500 mg of aspirin. Aloxiprin has been used as an analgesic and anti-inflammatory in musculoskeletal and joint disorders. It has also been used in the treatment and prevention of thromboembolic disorders.

### Preparations

***BP 2003:*** Aloxiprin Tablets.

**Proprietary Preparations** (details are given in Part 3)
***Austria:*** Palaprin†; ***Switz.:*** Thrombace†.

**Multi-ingredient:** ***UK:*** Askit.

## Aluminium Aspirin

Acetilsalicilato de aluminio; Aluminum Acetylsalicylate; Aluminum Aspirin; Aspirin Aluminium. Bis(2-acetoxybenzoato-*O*′)hydroxyaluminium.

$C_{18}H_{15}AlO_9$ = 402.3.
*CAS — 23413-80-1.*

**Pharmacopoeias.** In *Jpn.*

### Profile

Aluminium aspirin is a salicylic acid derivative (see Aspirin, p.15) that has been given by mouth in the management of fever, pain, and musculoskeletal and joint disorders.

### Preparations

**Proprietary Preparations** (details are given in Part 3)
***Ital.:*** Alupir†; ***Port.:*** Aluprim†.

**Multi-ingredient:** ***S.Afr.:*** Analgen-SA.

## Aminophenazone *(rINN)*

Amidazofen; Amidopyrine; Amidopyrine-Pyramidon; Aminofenazona; Aminopyrine; Dimethylaminoantipyrine; Dimethylaminophenazone. 4-Dimethylamino-1,5-dimethyl-2-phenyl-4-pyrazolin-3-one.

$C_{13}H_{17}N_3O$ = 231.3.
*CAS — 58-15-1.*
*ATC — N02BB03.*

**Pharmacopoeias.** In *It.*

### Profile

Aminophenazone, a pyrazolone derivative, is an NSAID (p.67), but the risk of agranulocytosis is sufficiently great to render it unsuitable for use. Onset of agranulocytosis may be sudden and unpredictable. Aminophenazone has been used in the form of a variety of salts or complexes including topically as the salicylate.

**Precautions.** CARCINOGENICITY. Some[1] consider that aminophenazone should be regarded as a potential carcinogen because it reacted readily with nitrous acid to form dimethylnitrosamine. The reaction was catalysed by thiocyanate present in the saliva particularly in smokers.

1. Boyland E, Walker SA. Catalysis of the reaction of aminopyrine and nitrite by thiocyanate. *Arzneimittelforschung* 1974; **24:** 1181–4.

PORPHYRIA. Aminophenazone has been associated with acute attacks of porphyria and is considered unsafe in porphyric patients.

### Preparations

**Proprietary Preparations** (details are given in Part 3)
***Mex.:*** Flumil.

**Multi-ingredient:** ***Braz.:*** Gineburno; ***Ital.:*** Virdex; ***Switz.:*** Thermocutan.

## Aminopropylone

Aminopropilona; Aminopropylon. *N*-(2,3-Dihydro-1,5-dimethyl-3-oxo-2-phenyl-1*H*-pyrazol-4-yl)-2-(dimethylamino)propanamide.

$C_{16}H_{22}N_4O_2$ = 302.4.
*CAS — 3690-04-8.*

### Profile

Aminopropylone is an NSAID (p.67) used in topical preparations, usually in a concentration of 5% with a heparinoid, for the local treatment of pain and inflammatory conditions. The hydrochloride has been used similarly.

### Preparations

**Proprietary Preparations** (details are given in Part 3)
**Multi-ingredient:** ***Ital.:*** Artrocur†; Vessiflex.

## Ammonium Salicylate

Salicilato de amonio.

$C_7H_9NO_3$ = 155.2.
*CAS — 528-94-9.*

### Profile

Ammonium salicylate is a salicylic acid derivative used topically in rubefacient preparations similarly to methyl salicylate (p.59) for the relief of pain in musculoskeletal and joint disorders.

### Preparations

**Proprietary Preparations** (details are given in Part 3)
**Multi-ingredient:** ***Austral.:*** Radian-B; ***Irl.:*** Radian-B; ***UK:*** Aspellin†; Radian-B.

## Ampiroxicam *(BAN, rINN)*

CP-65703. 4-[1-(Ethoxycarbonyloxy)ethoxy]-2-methyl-*N*[2]-pyridyl-2*H*-1,2-benzothiazine-3-carboxamide 1,1-dioxide.

$C_{20}H_{21}N_3O_7S$ = 447.5.
*CAS — 99464-64-9.*

### Profile

Ampiroxicam is an NSAID (p.67) that is reported to be metabolised to piroxicam (p.84). It is used for the relief of pain and inflammation particularly in musculoskeletal disorders such as rheumatoid arthritis and osteoarthritis. Ampiroxicam is given by mouth in doses of 27 mg daily as a single dose.

**Adverse effects.** Photosensitivity reactions have occurred during ampiroxicam treatment.[1-3]

1. Kurumaji Y. Ampiroxicam-induced photosensitivity. *Contact Dermatitis* 1996; **34:** 298–9.
2. Toyohara A, *et al.* Ampiroxicam-induced photosensitivity. *Contact Dermatitis* 1996; **35:** 101–2.
3. Chishiki M, *et al.* Photosensitivity due to ampiroxicam. *Dermatology* 1997; **195:** 409–10.

### Preparations

**Proprietary Preparations** (details are given in Part 3)
***Braz.:*** Artricam†; ***Jpn:*** Flucam.

## Amtolmetin Guacil *(rINN)*

Amtolmetina guacilo; MED-15; ST-679. *N*-[(1-Methyl-5-*p*-toluoylpyrrol-2-yl)acetyl]glycine.

$C_{24}H_{24}N_2O_5$ = 420.5.
*CAS — 87344-06-7.*

### Profile

Amtolmetin guacil is an NSAID (p.67). It is an ester prodrug of tolmetin (p.94) used in painful and inflammatory disorders. It is given by mouth in daily doses of 600 to 1200 mg.

### Preparations

**Proprietary Preparations** (details are given in Part 3)
***Ital.:*** Artromed; Eufans.

## Amyl Salicylate

Isoamyl Salicylate; Isopentyl Salicylate; Salicilato de isoamilo. 3-Methylbutyl 2-hydroxybenzoate.

$C_{12}H_{16}O_3$ = 208.3.
*CAS — 87-20-7.*

**Pharmacopoeias.** In *Fr.*

### Profile

Amyl salicylate is a salicylic acid derivative used topically in rubefacient preparations similarly to methyl salicylate (p.59) for its analgesic and anti-inflammatory actions. It has also been used in perfumery.

### Preparations

**Proprietary Preparations** (details are given in Part 3)
**Multi-ingredient:** ***Arg.:*** Atomo Desinflamante C; Atomo Desinflamante Familiar; Rati Salil Crema; ***Fr.:*** Baume Dalet†; Baume Saint-Bernard†; Sedartryl; ***Spain:*** Balsamo Analgesic Karmel†; Linimento Klari.

## Anakinra *(BAN, USAN, rINN)*

rhIL-1ra.
*CAS — 143090-92-0.*
*ATC — L04AA14.*

### Adverse Effects and Precautions

Mild to moderate injection site reactions with symptoms of erythema, bruising, swelling, and pain are common with anakinra particularly in the first month of treatment. Other common reactions include headache, nausea, diarrhoea, and abdominal pain. Antibodies to anakinra may develop, and rashes have been reported rarely.

Upper respiratory-tract infections and sinusitis have been reported with anakinra. Serious infections have also occurred, mainly in patients with asthma, and anakinra should be stopped if these develop. Likewise, therapy should not be begun in patients with active infections, including chronic or localised infections; caution is recommended in those with a history of recurrent infections or with underlying conditions that may predispose to infections.

Blood dyscrasias, especially neutropenia, have been reported rarely with anakinra. It should not be used in patients with a history of neutropenia; a similar effect may occur with other tumour necrosis factor antagonists.

### Interactions

Live vaccines should not be given with anakinra as its effect on vaccine efficacy or the risk of infection transmission is unknown. The risk of serious infection and neutropenia is increased when anakinra and etanercept are used together; a similar effect may occur with other tumour necrosis factor antagonists.

### Pharmacokinetics

After subcutaneous doses, peak plasma concentrations of anakinra are reached in 3 to 7 hours. Its terminal half-life is about 4 to 6 hours. Anakinra is excreted mainly in the urine.

### Uses and Administration

Anakinra is a recombinant receptor antagonist of interleukin-1 (p.1701), an inflammatory mediator found in the plasma and synovial fluid of patients with rheumatoid arthritis.

Anakinra is used for the treatment of the signs and symptoms of moderate to severely active rheumatoid arthritis in patients who have had an inadequate response to methotrexate or another disease-modifying antirheumatic drug (DMARD) alone (but see below). In the UK, it should only be given with methotrexate; however, in the USA, it may be given either alone or with another DMARD although not one which inhibits tumour necrosis factor (see Interactions, above). The usual dose is 100 mg once daily by subcutaneous injection. The dose should be given at about the same time each day.

Anakinra has been tried in septic shock and graft-versus-host disease in transplant recipients, but results were disappointing.

**Administration in renal impairment.** A study[1] in patients with varying degrees of renal function indicated that no dosage adjustment was needed for anakinra in patients with mild or moderate renal impairment but a reduction in dosage to administration on alternate days appeared advisable in those with severe renal impairment. Dialysis does not affect anakinra concentrations to any significant degree.

1. Yang B-B, *et al.* Pharmacokinetics of anakinra in subjects with different levels of renal function. *Clin Pharmacol Ther* 2003; **74:** 85–94.

**Rheumatoid arthritis.** In the UK, anakinra is licensed for the treatment of rheumatoid arthritis in patients with an inadequate response to methotrexate alone; however, the National Institute of Clinical Excellence (NICE) does not recommend its use except in the context of a controlled, long-term clinical study.

References.


1. Bresnihan B, *et al.* Treatment of rheumatoid arthritis with recombinant human interleukin-1 receptor antagonist. *Arthritis Rheum* 1998; **41:** 2196–2204.
2. Cohen S, *et al.* Treatment of rheumatoid arthritis with anakinra, a recombinant human interleukin-1 receptor antagonist, in combination with methotrexate: results of a twenty-four-week, multicenter, randomized, double-blind, placebo-controlled trial. *Arthritis Rheum* 2002; **46:** 614–24.
3. Nuki G, *et al.* Long-term safety and maintenance of clinical improvement following treatment with anakinra (recombinant human interleukin-1 receptor antagonist) in patients with rheumatoid arthritis: extension phase of a randomized, double-blind, placebo-controlled trial. *Arthritis Rheum* 2002; **46:** 2838–46.
4. Fleischmann RM, *et al.* Anakinra, a recombinant human interleukin-1 receptor antagonist (r-metHuIL-1ra), in patients with rheumatoid arthritis: a large, international, multicenter, placebo-controlled trial. *Arthritis Rheum* 2003; **48:** 927–34.
5. National Institute for Clinical Excellence. Anakinra for rheumatoid arthritis (issued November 2003). Available at: http://www.nice.org.uk/pdf/TA072guidance.pdf (accessed 25/05/04)


### Preparations

**Proprietary Preparations** (details are given in Part 3)
***Fr.:*** Kineret; ***Irl.:*** Kineret; ***Port.:*** Kineret; ***UK:*** Kineret; ***USA:*** Kineret.

---

## Anileridine *(BAN, rINN)*

Anileridina. Ethyl 1-(4-aminophenethyl)-4-phenylpiperidine-4-carboxylate.

$C_{22}H_{28}N_2O_2$ = 352.5.
*CAS — 144-14-9.*
*ATC — N01AH05.*

**Pharmacopoeias.** In *US.*

**USP 27** (Anileridine). A white to yellowish-white, odourless or practically odourless, crystalline powder. When exposed to light and air it oxidises and darkens in colour. It exhibits polymorphism, and of two crystalline forms observed, one melts at about 80° and the other at about 89°. Very slightly soluble in water; soluble 1 in 2 of alcohol and 1 in 1 of chloroform; soluble in ether but solutions may be turbid. Store in airtight containers. Protect from light.

## Anileridine Hydrochloride *(BANM, rINNM)*

Hidrocloruro de anileridina.

$C_{22}H_{28}N_2O_2,2HCl$ = 425.4.
*CAS — 126-12-5.*

**Pharmacopoeias.** In *US.*

**USP 27** (Anileridine Hydrochloride). A white or nearly white odourless crystalline powder. Soluble 1 in 5 of water and 1 in 80 of alcohol; practically insoluble in chloroform and in ether. pH of a 5% solution in water is 2.5 to 3.0. Store in airtight containers. Protect from light.

## Anileridine Phosphate *(BANM, rINNM)*

Fosfato de anileridina.

$C_{22}H_{28}N_2O_2,H_3PO_4$ = 450.5.
*CAS — 4268-37-5.*

### Profile

Anileridine, a phenylpiperidine derivative, is an opioid analgesic (p.71) chemically related to pethidine (p.80) and with similar actions. It has been used as the hydrochloride in the management of moderate to severe pain. Doses have been expressed as anileridine base; anileridine hydrochloride 30 mg is approximately equivalent to 25 mg of anileridine. The usual dose by mouth is the equivalent of 25 to 50 mg every 6 hours, as required.

Anileridine has also been given by injection as the phosphate.

### Preparations

***USP 27:*** Anileridine Hydrochloride Tablets; Anileridine Injection.

**Proprietary Preparations** (details are given in Part 3)
***Canad.:*** Leritine†.

---

# Aspirin *(BAN)*

Acetilsalicílico, ácido; Acetylsal. Acid; Acetylsalicylic Acid; Acidum Acetylsalicylicum; Polopiryna; Salicylic Acid Acetate. *O*-Acetylsalicylic acid; 2-Acetoxybenzoic acid.

$C_9H_8O_4$ = 180.2.
*CAS — 50-78-2.*
*ATC — A01AD05; B01AC06; N02BA01.*

NOTE. The use of the name Aspirin is limited; in some countries it is a trade-mark.

Compounded preparations of aspirin may be represented by the following names:

- Co-codaprin (*BAN*)—aspirin 50 parts and codeine phosphate 1 part (w/w)
- Co-codaprin (*PEN*)—aspirin and codeine phosphate.

The symbol † denotes a preparation no longer actively marketed

**Pharmacopoeias.** In *Chin., Eur.* (see p.vi), *Int., Jpn, Pol., US,* and *Viet.*

**Ph. Eur. 5.0** (Acetylsalicylic Acid; Aspirin BP 2003). White, crystalline powder or colourless crystals. Slightly soluble in water; freely soluble in alcohol. Store in airtight containers.

**USP 27** (Aspirin). White crystals, commonly tabular or needle-like, or white crystalline powder; odourless or has a faint odour. Is stable in dry air; in moist air it gradually hydrolyses to salicylic and acetic acids. Soluble 1 in 300 of water, 1 in 5 of alcohol, 1 in 17 of chloroform, and 1 in 10 to 15 of ether; sparingly soluble in absolute ether. Store in airtight containers.

## Adverse Effects and Treatment

Aspirin has many properties in common with the non-aspirin NSAIDs, the adverse effects of which are described on p.67.

The most common adverse effects of therapeutic doses of aspirin are gastrointestinal disturbances such as nausea, dyspepsia, and vomiting. Gastrointestinal symptoms may be minimised by giving aspirin with food. Irritation of the gastric mucosa with erosion, ulceration, haematemesis, and melaena may occur. Histamine $H_2$-antagonists, proton pump inhibitors, and prostaglandin analogues such as misoprostol may be used in the management of aspirin-induced mucosal damage (see under Peptic Ulcer Disease, p.1246). Slight blood loss, which is often asymptomatic, may occur in about 70% of patients; it is not usually of clinical significance but may, in a few patients, cause iron-deficiency anaemia during long-term therapy. Such occult blood loss is not affected by giving aspirin with food but may be reduced by use of enteric-coated or other modified-release tablets, $H_2$-antagonists, or high doses of antacids. Major upper gastrointestinal bleeding occurs rarely.

Some persons, especially those with asthma, chronic urticaria, or chronic rhinitis, exhibit notable hypersensitivity to aspirin (see also below), which may provoke various reactions including urticaria and other skin eruptions, angioedema, rhinitis, and severe, even fatal, paroxysmal bronchospasm and dyspnoea. Persons sensitive to aspirin often exhibit cross-sensitivity to other NSAIDs.

Aspirin increases bleeding time, decreases platelet adhesiveness, and, in large doses, may cause hypoprothrombinaemia. It may cause other blood disorders, including thrombocytopenia.

Aspirin and other salicylates may cause hepatotoxicity, particularly in patients with juvenile idiopathic arthritis or other connective tissue disorders. In children the use of aspirin has been implicated in some cases of Reye's syndrome, leading to severe restrictions on the indications for aspirin therapy in children. For further details see under Reye's Syndrome, below.

Aspirin given rectally may cause local irritation; anorectal stenosis has been reported.

Mild chronic salicylate intoxication, or salicylism, usually occurs only after repeated use of large doses. Salicylism can also occur following excessive topical application of salicylates. Symptoms include dizziness, tinnitus, deafness, sweating, nausea and vomiting, headache, and confusion, and may be controlled by reducing the dosage. Tinnitus can occur at the plasma concentrations of 150 to 300 micrograms/mL required for optimal anti-inflammatory activity; more serious adverse effects occur at concentrations above 300 micrograms/mL. Symptoms of more severe intoxication or of acute poisoning following overdosage include hyperventilation, fever, restlessness, ketosis, and respiratory alkalosis and metabolic acidosis. Depression of the CNS may lead to coma; cardiovascular collapse and respiratory failure may also occur. In children drowsiness and metabolic acidosis commonly occur; hypoglycaemia may be severe.

In acute oral salicylate overdosage repeated doses of activated charcoal may be given by mouth if the patient is suspected of ingesting more than 250 mg/kg of salicylate. Activated charcoal not only prevents the absorption of any salicylate remaining in the stomach but also aids the elimination of any that has been absorbed. Measurement of plasma-salicylate concentration should be carried out in patients who have ingested more than 120 mg/kg of salicylate, although the severity of poisoning cannot be estimated from plasma concentrations alone. Absorption of aspirin can be delayed due to reduced gastric emptying, formation of concretions in the stomach, or as a result of ingestion of enteric-coated preparations. In consequence, plasma concentrations should be measured at least 2 hours after ingestion and repeated 2 hours later. Patients who overdose with enteric preparations require continual monitoring of plasma concentrations.

Fluid and electrolyte management is essential to correct acidosis, hyperpyrexia, hypokalaemia, and dehydration. Intravenous sodium bicarbonate is given to enhance urinary salicylate excretion if plasma salicylate concentrations exceed 500 micrograms/mL (350 micrograms/mL in children). Haemodialysis or haemoperfusion are also effective methods of removing salicylate from the plasma. The *British National Formulary* considers haemodialysis the method of choice in severe poisoning; it should be seriously considered when the plasma salicylate concentration is more than 700 micrograms/mL or if there is severe metabolic acidosis. Vulnerable patients such as children or the elderly may require dialysis at an earlier stage.

◊ References to salicylate toxicity and its management.


1. Notarianni L. A reassessment of the treatment of salicylate poisoning. *Drug Safety* 1992; **7:** 292–303.
2. Woods D, *et al.* Acute toxicity of drugs: salicylates. *Pharm J* 1993; **250:** 576–8.
3. Collee GG, Hanson GC. The management of acute poisoning. *Br J Anaesth* 1993; **70:** 562–73.
4. Watson JE, Tagupa ET. Suicide attempt by means of aspirin enema. *Ann Pharmacother* 1994; **28:** 467–9.
5. Dargan PI, *et al.* An evidence based flowchart to guide the management of acute salicylate (aspirin) overdose. *Emerg Med J* 2002; **19:** 206–9.


**Effects on the blood.** In addition to its beneficial effects on platelets aspirin can cause adverse blood effects. An indication of this toxicity is given by an early reference[1] to reports submitted to the UK Committee on Safety of Medicines (CSM). There were 787 reports of adverse reactions to aspirin reported to the CSM between June 1964 and January 1973. These included 95 reports of blood disorders (17 fatal) including thrombocytopenia (26; 2 fatal), aplastic anaemia (13; 7 fatal), and agranulocytosis or pancytopenia (10; 2 fatal). Aspirin has also been associated with haemolytic anaemia in patients with G6PD deficiency.[2]


1. Cuthbert MF. Adverse reactions to non-steroidal antirheumatic drugs. *Curr Med Res Opin* 1974; **2:** 600–9.
2. Magee P, Beeley L. Drug-induced blood dyscrasias. *Pharm J* 1991; **246:** 396–7.


**Effects on the cardiovascular system.** Salicylate poisoning may result in cardiovascular collapse but details of such cases have not been widely reported. In 2 patients with salicylate intoxication asystole developed after intravenous diazepam.[1] It was suggested that diazepam-induced respiratory depression affected the acid-base balance so that the concentration of non-ionised membrane-penetrating fraction of salicylate was increased. For reference to the effects of aspirin on blood pressure compared with other NSAIDs, see Effects on the Cardiovascular System, p.67.


1. Berk WA, Andersen JC. Salicylate-associated asystole: report of two cases. *Am J Med* 1989; **86:** 505–6.


**Effects on the gastrointestinal tract.** Clinical and epidemiological evidence suggests that aspirin produces dose-related gastrointestinal toxicity[1,2] that is sometimes, but rarely, fatal.[2] Meta-analysis[3] suggests that the risk of gastrointestinal bleeding is not significantly lowered with the use of low-dose aspirin (less than 300 mg daily). A systemic review[4] of observational epidemiologic studies also concurred with this finding. Although it was suggested that very small doses of aspirin can produce prophylactic benefits in cardiovascular disease without the risk of gastrointestinal toxicity,[5] others have reported gastric injury even with doses of 10 mg daily.[6] There appears to be no convincing evidence that the risk of major gastrointestinal bleeding associated with a 75-mg dose is reduced by using enteric-coated or modified-release formulations rather than soluble aspirin,[3,4,7] although individual studies have reported a reduction in acute mucosal injury with enteric coating.[8] All known NSAIDs have the potential for causing acute damage to the gastric mucosa (see p.68), and comparative studies of acute gastric mucosal damage caused by such drugs consistently associate aspirin with the most severe lesions.[1] Gastric mucosal injury can occur even with cutaneous application.[9]


1. Graham DY, Smith JL. Aspirin and the stomach. *Ann Intern Med* 1986; **104:** 390–8.
2. Roderick PJ, *et al.* The gastrointestinal toxicity of aspirin: an overview of randomised controlled trials. *Br J Clin Pharmacol* 1993; **35:** 219–26.
3. Derry S, Loke YK. Risk of gastrointestinal haemorrhage with long term use of aspirin: meta-analysis. *BMJ* 2000; **321:** 1183–7.

4. Garcia Rodríguez LA, *et al.* Association between aspirin and upper gastrointestinal complications: systematic review of epidemiologic studies. *Br J Clin Pharmacol* 2001; **52:** 563–71.
5. Lee M, *et al.* Dose effects of aspirin on gastric prostaglandins and stomach mucosal injury. *Ann Intern Med* 1994; **120:** 184–9.
6. Cryer B, Feldman M. Effects of very low dose daily, long-term aspirin therapy on gastric, duodenal, and rectal prostaglandin levels and on mucosal injury in healthy humans. *Gastroenterology* 1999; **117:** 17–25.
7. Anonymous. Which prophylactic aspirin? *Drug Ther Bull* 1997; **35:** 7–8.
8. Cole AT, *et al.* Protection of human gastric mucosa against aspirin—enteric coating or dose reduction? *Aliment Pharmacol Ther* 1999; **13:** 187–93.
9. Cryer B, *et al.* Effects of cutaneous aspirin on the human stomach and duodenum. *Proc Assoc Am Physicians* 1999; **111:** 448–56.


**Effects on hearing.** Studies have indicated that tinnitus develops at serum-salicylate concentrations above 200 micrograms/mL.[1] However, there appears to be considerable intersubject variation in the response of the ear to salicylate;[2] tinnitus may occur at lower concentrations, whereas patients with pre-existing hearing loss may not experience tinnitus despite serum-salicylate concentrations of 311 to 677 micrograms/mL.[1] A graded increase in intensity of ototoxicity with increasing salicylate dose and plasma concentration has been demonstrated.[2] For example, at an average total plasma-salicylate concentration of 110 micrograms/mL, the hearing loss at any given frequency was about 12 decibels; such a deficit might be relevant to patients with pre-existing hearing impairment.[2]


1. Mongan E, *et al.* Tinnitus as an indication of therapeutic serum salicylate levels. *JAMA* 1973; **226:** 142–5.
2. Day RO, *et al.* Concentration-response relationships for salicylate-induced ototoxicity in normal volunteers. *Br J Clin Pharmacol* 1989; **28:** 695–702.


**Effects on the kidneys.** Although abuse of combined analgesic preparations containing aspirin has been implicated in the development of analgesic nephropathy, kidney damage associated with the therapeutic use of aspirin alone appears to be comparatively rare. Many studies have failed to find an increased risk of renal damage in patients taking aspirin.[1-8]


1. New Zealand Rheumatism Association Study. Aspirin and the kidney. *BMJ* 1974; **1:** 593–6.
2. Walker BR, *et al.* Aspirin and renal function. *N Engl J Med* 1977; **297:** 1405.
3. Akyol SM, *et al.* Renal function after prolonged consumption of aspirin. *BMJ* 1982; **284:** 631–2.
4. Bonney SL, *et al.* Renal safety of two analgesics used over the counter: ibuprofen and aspirin. *Clin Pharmacol Ther* 1986; **40:** 373–7.
5. Sandler DP, *et al.* Analgesic use and chronic renal disease. *N Engl J Med* 1989; **320:** 1238–43.
6. Pommer W, *et al.* Regular analgesic intake and the risk of end-stage renal failure. *Am J Nephrol* 1989; **9:** 403–12.
7. Dubach UC, *et al.* An epidemiologic study of abuse of analgesic drugs: effects of phenacetin and salicylate on mortality and cardiovascular morbidity (1968 to 1987). *N Engl J Med* 1991; **324:** 155–60.
8. Perneger TV, *et al.* Risk of kidney failure associated with the use of acetaminophen, aspirin, and nonsteroidal antiinflammatory drugs. *N Engl J Med* 1994; **331:** 1675–9.


**Effects on the liver.** Aspirin-induced hepatic injury is generally mild and manifests as a mild to moderate elevation in aminotransferase values; however, there is a risk of severe liver injury.[1] One review[2] reported an increase in aminotransferase values in 59 of 439 patients given aspirin; the increase was considered to be probably related to aspirin in 23. Hepatotoxicity appears to be correlated with serum-salicylate concentrations greater than 150 micrograms/mL and with active rheumatoid disease. Aspirin-induced liver injury is usually reversible on stopping the drug.[2]

See also under Reye's Syndrome, below.


1. Lewis JH. Hepatic toxicity of nonsteroidal anti-inflammatory drugs. *Clin Pharm* 1984; **3:** 128–38.
2. Freeland GR, *et al.* Hepatic safety of two analgesics used over the counter: ibuprofen and aspirin. *Clin Pharmacol Ther* 1988; **43:** 473–9.


**Effects on the mouth.** Aspirin burn (ulceration of the mucosal layer of the lips) developed in a 26-year-old woman after taking an aspirin-containing powder for a migraine.[1] The woman had swallowed the powder undissolved rather than adding to water.


1. Dellinger TM, Livingston HM. Aspirin burn of the oral cavity. *Ann Pharmacother* 1998; **32:** 1107.


**Hypersensitivity.** The main clinical features of patients who have aspirin hypersensitivity include middle-age, female sex, diagnoses of asthma or rhinitis, a personal or family history of atopy, and a history of nasal polyps.[1,2] The occurrence of aspirin sensitivity in patients with asthma and nasal polyps has been referred to in some reports as the 'aspirin triad'. Other sensitivities often found concomitantly include allergy to food dyes such as tartrazine and to other drugs such as other NSAIDs. The response to individual NSAIDs is believed to be closely linked to the extent to which they inhibit prostaglandin synthesis.[3,4] There may be a dose threshold below which no detectable symptoms occur and patients who may be tolerant of regular low-dose aspirin may develop symptoms when they take larger doses.[4] Some[4] use a formal challenge with a 300-mg dose of aspirin by mouth to confirm a diagnosis of NSAID sensitivity but others[5] consider this to be a dangerous technique and use inhalation of lysine aspirin which they consider to be a safer and more predictable alternative. Intranasal challenge with lysine aspirin has also been used.[6]


1. Kwoh CK, Feinstein AR. Rates of sensitivity reactions to aspirin: problems in interpreting the data. *Clin Pharmacol Ther* 1986; **40:** 494–505.
2. Schiavino D, *et al.* The aspirin disease. *Thorax* 2000; **55** (suppl 2): S66–S69.
3. Power I. Aspirin-induced asthma. *Br J Anaesth* 1993; **71:** 619–21.
4. Frew A. Selected side-effects: 13. non-steroidal anti-inflammatory drugs and asthma. *Prescribers' J* 1994; **34:** 74–7.
5. Davies BH. NSAIDs and asthma. *Prescribers' J* 1994; **34:** 163–4.
6. Casadevall J *et al.* Intranasal challenge with aspirin in the diagnosis of aspirin intolerant asthma: evaluation of nasal response by acoustic rhinometry. *Thorax* 2000; **55:** 921–4.


DESENSITISATION. Successful desensitisation has been achieved using various oral aspirin challenge protocols.[1,2] Incremental doses of aspirin (starting at 30 mg) are given until an allergic response is obtained; aspirin is readministered at the dose that caused the response and again incremental doses are given until finally a 650-mg dose is tolerated. After desensitisation, an interruption of continuous aspirin administration results in the reappearance of sensitivity.


1. Asad SI, *et al.* Effect of aspirin in "aspirin sensitive" patients. *BMJ* 1984; **288:** 745–8.
2. Stevenson DD. Desensitization of aspirin-sensitive asthmatics: a therapeutic alternative? *J Asthma* 1983; **20:** 31–8.


**Hypoglycaemia.** A review of the literature[1] on drug-induced hypoglycaemia highlighted the fact that overdosage with salicylates could produce hypoglycaemia in children. Although therapeutic doses of salicylates in adults can lower blood-glucose concentrations in diabetic and non-diabetic subjects alike, opinion on the clinical significance of this effect varies. Salicylates have been implicated in a few cases of hypoglycaemia in adults[1] and some[2] suggest that patients with renal impairment or those receiving large doses, such as in the treatment of rheumatoid arthritis, may be at risk. Hypoglycaemia has been reported in a patient with renal failure following excessive application of a topical preparation containing salicylic acid.[3]


1. Seltzer HS. Drug-induced hypoglycemia: a review of 1418 cases. *Endocrinol Metab Clin North Am* 1989; **18:** 163–83.
2. Pandit MK, *et al.* Drug-induced disorders of glucose tolerance. *Ann Intern Med* 1993; **118:** 529–39.
3. Raschke R, *et al.* Refractory hypoglycemia secondary to topical salicylate intoxication. *Arch Intern Med* 1991; **151:** 591–3.


**Reye's syndrome.** Reye's syndrome is a disorder characterised by acute encephalopathy and fatty degeneration of the liver. It occurs almost exclusively in children although cases have been seen[1] in patients over the age of 12. Many factors may be involved in its aetiology but it typically occurs after a viral infection such as chickenpox or influenza and may be precipitated by a chemical trigger. Several large studies, as well as individual case reports, have found an association between Reye's syndrome and the prior ingestion of aspirin.[2-5] The evidence for other salicylates could not be adequately evaluated.[4] Although the role of aspirin and possibly other salicylates in the pathogenesis of Reye's syndrome remains to be determined, the use of aspirin and other acetylated salicylates as analgesics or antipyretics is generally considered contra-indicated in children under the age of 12 years and, in some countries, in teenagers. For example, the UK Committee on Safety of Medicines has recommended that all children under 16 should not take aspirin.[6] (This advice superseded their earlier recommendations to avoid aspirin during fever or viral infection in children under 16 years; the Committee felt that this advice was too complex for products on general sale and, given the wide availability of other analgesic preparations, there was no need to expose this age group to any risk.) Some countries also extend these recommendations to non-acetylated salicylates. Most authorities consider one of the few acceptable indications remaining for the use of aspirin in children to be juvenile idiopathic arthritis. One group of workers[7] who re-examined some of the original studies suggested that there might also be a link between Reye's syndrome and the use of antiemetics, phenothiazines, and some other antihistamines, but their conclusions have been criticised.[8]


1. Hall SM, Lynn R. Reye's syndrome. *N Engl J Med* 1999; **341:** 845–6.
2. Waldman RJ, *et al.* Aspirin as a risk factor in Reye's syndrome. *JAMA* 1982; **247:** 3089–94.
3. Halpin TJ, *et al.* Reye's syndrome and medication use. *JAMA* 1982; **248:** 687–91.
4. Hurwitz ES, *et al.* Public health service study of Reye's syndrome and medications: report of the main study. *JAMA* 1987; **257:** 1905–11.
5. Hall SM, *et al.* Preadmission antipyretics in Reye's syndrome. *Arch Dis Child* 1988; **63:** 857–66.
6. Committee on Safety of Medicines/Medicines Control Agency. Medicines Control Agency statement: new advice on aspirin and under 16. Available at: http://www.mca.gov.uk/whatsnew/pressreleases/ aspirin.pdf (accessed 02/07/04)
7. Casteels-Van Daele M, Eggermont E. Reye's syndrome. *BMJ* 1994; **308:** 919–20.
8. Hall SM. Reye's syndrome. *BMJ* 1994; **309:** 411.


## Precautions

Aspirin has many properties in common with the non-aspirin NSAIDs, the precautions of which are described on p.69.

Aspirin should be used cautiously, if at all, in patients prone to dyspepsia or known to have a lesion of the gastric mucosa. It should not be given to patients with haemophilia or other haemorrhagic disorders, or to treat patients with gout since low doses increase urate concentrations.

Aspirin should be used with caution in patients with asthma or allergic disorders. It should not be given to patients with a history of sensitivity reactions to aspirin or other NSAIDs, including those in whom attacks of asthma, angioedema, urticaria, or rhinitis have been precipitated by such drugs (for further details of risk factors see Hypersensitivity under Adverse Effects, above).

Caution is necessary when renal or hepatic function is impaired; aspirin should be avoided in severe renal or hepatic impairment. Aspirin should be used cautiously in dehydrated patients and in the presence of uncontrolled hypertension.

High doses may precipitate acute haemolytic anaemia in patients with G6PD deficiency. Aspirin may interfere with insulin and glucagon control in diabetics (see Hypoglycaemia under Adverse Effects, above).

The use of aspirin in children is extremely limited because of the risk of Reye's syndrome (see under Adverse Effects, above, and under Uses and Administration, below).

Although low-dose aspirin might be used in some pregnant patients, analgesic doses of aspirin should not be used at term as they may be associated with delayed onset and prolongation of labour and with maternal and neonatal bleeding. High doses may cause closure of fetal ductus arteriosus *in utero* and possibly persistent pulmonary hypertension in the newborn (but see under Pregnancy, below); kernicterus may occur in jaundiced neonates.

Continuous prolonged use of aspirin should be avoided in the elderly because of the risk of gastrointestinal bleeding.

Aspirin should be discontinued several days before scheduled surgical procedures (see below).

Aspirin and other salicylates can interfere with thyroid function tests.

**Breast feeding.** The American Academy of Pediatrics[1] considers that salicylates should be given with caution to breast-feeding mothers, since aspirin has been associated with metabolic acidosis in the infant.[2] The *British National Formulary* also recommends that aspirin should be avoided in breast-feeding mothers because of the possible risk of Reye's syndrome in nursing infants; they also advise that infants with neonatal vitamin K deficiency may be at risk of hypoprothrombinaemia following the regular use of high doses of aspirin in breast-feeding mothers.


1. American Academy of Pediatrics. The transfer of drugs and other chemicals into human milk. *Pediatrics* 2001; **108:** 776–89. Correction. *ibid.*; 1029. Also available at: http://aappolicy.aappublications.org/cgi/content/full/pediatrics%3b108/3/776 (accessed 02/07/04)
2. Clark JH, Wilson WG. A 16-day-old breast-fed infant with metabolic acidosis caused by salicylate. *Clin Pediatr (Phila)* 1981; **20:** 53–4.


**Pregnancy.** The potential adverse effects of aspirin when used during pregnancy have been reviewed.[1] Salicylates readily cross the placenta and have been shown to be teratogenic in *animals*. Although some studies and anecdotal reports have implicated aspirin in the formation of congenital abnormalities, most large studies[2-4] have failed to find any significant risk or evidence of teratogenicity. Analysis of data collected by the Slone Epidemiology Unit Birth Defects Study suggests that use of aspirin during the early months of pregnancy, when the fetal heart is developing, is not associated with an increased risk of cardiac defects.[5] The ability of aspirin, however, to alter platelet function may be a potential risk. There have been a few reports of haemorrhagic disorders in infants whose mothers had consumed aspirin during pregnancy[6] and of salicylate-associated haemorrhagic complications in mothers.[7] However, no clinically significant adverse effects on maternal or neonatal bleeding or on fetal ductus flow were reported in 6 controlled studies which evaluated low-dose aspirin (less than 325 mg daily) in pregnancy-induced hypertension.[8] It appeared that the degree of cyclo-oxygenase inhibition produced by aspirin was unlikely to be great enough to cause premature closure of the ductus arteriosus or to affect the pulmonary blood vessels.[1] However, in some studies in patients considered to have high-risk pregnancies the risk of abruptio placentae[9] or consequent perinatal death[10] was increased by maternal administration of aspirin. For reference to a possible association between aspirin and other NSAIDs and persistent pulmonary hypertension of the newborn, see under NSAIDs, p.69.

Although aspirin has the potential to inhibit uterine contractions of labour it was considered that intermittent or low-dose aspirin was unlikely to inhibit cyclo-oxygenase for long enough to prolong pregnancy or labour.[1]

1. de Swiet M, Fryers G. The use of aspirin in pregnancy. *J Obstet Gynaecol* 1990; **10:** 467–82.
2. Slone D, *et al.* Aspirin and congenital malformations. *Lancet* 1976; **1:** 1373–5.
3. Shapiro S, *et al.* Perinatal mortality and birth-weight in relation to aspirin taken during pregnancy. *Lancet* 1976; **i:** 1375–6.
4. Winship KA, *et al.* Maternal drug histories and central nervous system anomalies. *Arch Dis Child* 1984; **59:** 1052–60.
5. Werler MM, *et al.* The relation of aspirin use during the first trimester of pregnancy to congenital cardiac defects. *N Engl J Med* 1989; **321:** 1639–42.
6. Bleyer WA, Breckenridge RT. Studies on the detection of adverse drug reactions in the newborn II: the effects of prenatal aspirin on newborn hemostasis. *JAMA* 1970; **213:** 2049–53.
7. Collins E, Turner G. Maternal effects of regular salicylate ingestion in pregnancy. *Lancet* 1975; **ii:** 335–7.
8. Imperiale TF, Petrulis AS. A meta-analysis of low-dose aspirin for the prevention of pregnancy-induced hypertensive disease. *JAMA* 1991; **266:** 261–4.
9. Sibai BM, *et al.* Prevention of preeclampsia with low-dose aspirin in healthy, nulliparous pregnant women. *N Engl J Med* 1993; **329:** 1213–18.
10. Hamid R, *et al.* Low dose aspirin in women with raised maternal serum alpha-fetoprotein and abnormal Doppler waveform patterns from the uteroplacental circulation. *Br J Obstet Gynaecol* 1994; **101:** 481–4.

**Surgical procedures.** Aspirin prolongs bleeding time, mainly by inhibiting platelet aggregation. This effect is irreversible and new platelets must be released into the circulation before bleeding time can return to normal. Therefore aspirin therapy should be stopped several days before surgical procedures. In some clinical situations, aspirin may have been given shortly before a surgical procedure. When emergency coronary bypass surgery is required for myocardial infarction, most patients would have received aspirin as part of the initial treatment for infarction. Perioperative bleeding, transfusion requirements, and surgical re-exploration rates may be increased when aspirin is given.[1] Desmopressin may reduce the risk of perioperative bleeding (see under Haemorrhagic Disorders, p.1323).

Aspirin is sometimes given during the second and third trimester for the prevention of pregnancy-induced hypertensive disease (see under Hypertension, p.825). Studies indicate that when given in a dose of 325 mg daily or less, clinically significant effects on maternal or neonatal bleeding do not occur.[2] Some have suggested that aspirin therapy may increase the risk of formation of extradural haematoma thus making epidural anaesthesia inadvisable[3] but a subsequent study[4] found that low-dose aspirin during pregnancy did not increase the risk of bleeding complications during epidural anaesthesia.

Patients on low-dose aspirin, in whom tourniquets are used for nerve blocks or other procedures, may be at increased risk of developing purpuric rash.[5]

It has been suggested that in patients undergoing dermatological surgery, aspirin need only be stopped before surgery in those patients with a prolonged bleeding time, whereas patients with a normal bleeding time could continue therapy.[6]

1. Goldman S, *et al.* Improvement in early saphenous vein graft patency after coronary artery bypass surgery with antiplatelet therapy: results of a Veterans Administration Cooperative Study. *Circulation* 1988; **77:** 1324–32.
2. Imperiale TF, Petrulis AS. A meta-analysis of low-dose aspirin for the prevention of pregnancy-induced hypertensive disease. *JAMA* 1991; **266:** 260–4.
3. Macdonald R. Aspirin and extradural blocks. *Br J Anaesth* 1991; **66:** 1–3.
4. Sibai BM, *et al.* Low-dose aspirin in nulliparous women: safety of continuous epidural block and correlation between bleeding time and maternal-neonatal bleeding complications. *Am J Obstet Gynecol* 1995; **172:** 1553–7.
5. Runcie CJ, *et al.* Aspirin and intravenous regional blocks. *Br J Hosp Med* 1990; **43:** 229–30.
6. Lawrence C, *et al.* Effect of aspirin and nonsteroidal antiinflammatory drug therapy on bleeding complications in dermatologic surgical patients. *J Am Acad Dermatol* 1994; **31:** 988–92.

## Interactions

Aspirin has many properties in common with the non-aspirin NSAIDs, the interactions of which are described on p.69.

Some of the effects of aspirin on the gastrointestinal tract are enhanced by alcohol. Use of aspirin with dipyridamole may result in an increase in plasma-salicylate concentrations. Drugs such as metoclopramide in patients with migraine headache result in earlier absorption of aspirin and higher peak plasma-salicylate concentrations. Metoprolol may increase peak plasma-salicylate concentrations. Salicylate intoxication has occurred in patients on high-dose salicylate regimens and carbonic anhydrase inhibitors. Plasma-salicylate concentrations may be reduced by corticosteroids. This interaction is likely to be important in patients receiving high-dose long-term salicylate treatment. Conversely, salicylate toxicity may occur if corticosteroids are withdrawn. Also the risk of gastrointestinal bleeding and ulceration associated with aspirin is increased when used with corticosteroids. Antacids may increase the excretion of aspirin in alkaline urine. Use of gold compounds with aspirin may exacerbate aspirin-induced liver damage. Aspirin may enhance the activity of coumarin anticoagulants, sulfonylurea hypoglycaemic drugs, zafirlukast, methotrexate, phenytoin, and valproate. Aspirin diminishes the effects of uricosurics such as probenecid and sulfinpyrazone. Use of aspirin with other NSAIDs should be avoided because of the increased risk of adverse effects; the cardioprotective effects of aspirin may be abolished by ibuprofen. Aspirin may decrease the plasma concentration of some other NSAIDs, for example, fenbufen, indometacin, and piroxicam. The manufacturer of mifepristone advises of a theoretical risk that prostaglandin synthetase inhibition by aspirin or NSAIDs may alter the efficacy of mifepristone.

◊ A review[1] of potential drug interactions related to aspirin.

1. Miners JO. Drug interactions involving aspirin (acetylsalicylic acid) and salicylic acid. *Clin Pharmacokinet* 1989; **17:** 327–44.

**ACE inhibitors.** For a discussion of aspirin and other NSAIDs reducing the activity of ACE inhibitors, see p.845.

**Antifungals.** Plasma-salicylate concentrations in an 8-year-old child receiving long-term aspirin therapy for rheumatic heart disease were markedly reduced when treatment with *griseofulvin* was started.[1] It was suggested that griseofulvin might interfere with absorption of aspirin.

1. Phillips KR, *et al.* Griseofulvin significantly decreases serum salicylate concentrations. *Pediatr Infect Dis J* 1993; **12:** 350–2.

**Calcium-channel blockers.** The antiplatelet effects of aspirin and calcium-channel blockers may be increased when they are used together; there have been isolated reports[1,2] of disturbed haemostasis including abnormal bruising, prolonged bleeding times and ecchymosis in patients taking aspirin and *verapamil* concurrently.

1. Ring ME, *et al.* Clinically significant antiplatelet effects of calcium-channel blockers. *J Clin Pharmacol* 1986; **26:** 719–20.
2. Verzino E, *et al.* Verapamil-aspirin interaction. *Ann Pharmacother* 1994; **28:** 536–7.

**General anaesthetics.** For the effect of aspirin on *thiopental* anaesthesia, see p.1309.

**NSAIDS.** It has been suggested that *ibuprofen* may reduce the cardioprotective effect of aspirin. A study involving 7107 patients prescribed low-dose aspirin for cardiovascular disease found that those also taking ibuprofen had an increased cardiovascular mortality (adjusted hazard ratio 1.73 times that of patients not taking ibuprofen).[1] In addition, a larger study[2] found that risk of myocardial infarction in patients receiving low-dose aspirin and NSAIDs (not specifically ibuprofen) was increased in those taking regular rather than intermittent NSAID treatment. However, another study in 70 316 patients found that the risk of death in patients prescribed aspirin and ibuprofen was comparable to that of patients prescribed aspirin alone or with another NSAID.[3] There are limitations to all these studies and further studies are needed before any recommendations can be made.[4,5]

1. MacDonald TM, Wei L. Effect of ibuprofen on cardioprotective effect of aspirin. *Lancet* 2003; **361:** 573–4.
2. Kurth T, *et al.* Inhibition of clinical benefits of aspirin on first myocardial infarction by nonsteroidal antiinflammatory drugs. *Circulation* 2003; **108:** 1191–5.
3. Curtis JP, *et al.* Aspirin, ibuprofen, and mortality after myocardial infarction: retrospective cohort study. *BMJ* 2003; **327:** 1322–3.
4. Etminan M, Samii A. Effect of ibuprofen on cardioprotective effect of aspirin. *Lancet* 2003; **361:** 1558–9.
5. Kimmel SE, Strom BL. Giving aspirin and ibuprofen after myocardial infarction. *BMJ* 2003; **327:** 1298–9.

**Spironolactone.** For the effect of aspirin in patients taking spironolactone, see p.1004.

## Pharmacokinetics

Aspirin and other salicylates are absorbed rapidly from the gastrointestinal tract when taken orally but absorption following rectal administration is less reliable. Aspirin and other salicylates can also be absorbed through the skin.

After oral doses, absorption of non-ionised aspirin occurs in the stomach and intestine. Some aspirin is hydrolysed to salicylate in the gut wall. Once absorbed aspirin is rapidly converted to salicylate but during the first 20 minutes after a dose by mouth, aspirin is the predominant form of the drug in the plasma. Aspirin is 80 to 90% bound to plasma proteins and is widely distributed; its volume of distribution is reported to be 170 mL/kg in adults. As plasma-drug concentrations increase, the binding sites on the proteins become saturated and the volume of distribution increases. Both aspirin and salicylate have pharmacological activity although only aspirin has an anti-platelet effect. Salicylate is extensively bound to plasma proteins and is rapidly distributed to all body parts. Salicylate appears in breast milk and crosses the placenta.

Salicylate is mainly eliminated by hepatic metabolism; the metabolites include salicyluric acid, salicyl phenolic glucuronide, salicylic acyl glucuronide, gentisic acid, and gentisuric acid. The formation of the major metabolites, salicyluric acid and salicyl phenolic glucuronide, is easily saturated and follows Michaelis-Menten kinetics; the other metabolic routes are first-order processes. As a result, steady-state plasma-salicylate concentrations increase disproportionately with dose. After a 325-mg aspirin dose, elimination is a first-order process and the plasma-salicylate half-life is about 2 to 3 hours; at high aspirin doses, the half-life increases to 15 to 30 hours. Salicylate is also excreted unchanged in the urine; the amount excreted by this route increases with increasing dose and also depends on urinary pH, about 30% of a dose being excreted in alkaline urine compared with 2% of a dose in acidic urine. Renal excretion involves glomerular filtration, active renal tubular secretion, and passive tubular reabsorption.

Salicylate is removed by haemodialysis.

◊ References.

1. Needs CJ, Brooks PM. Clinical pharmacokinetics of the salicylates. *Clin Pharmacokinet* 1985; **10:** 164–77.

## Uses and Administration

Aspirin is a salicylate NSAID and has many properties in common with non-aspirin NSAIDs (p.70). Aspirin and other salicylates have analgesic, anti-inflammatory, and antipyretic properties; they act as inhibitors of the enzyme cyclo-oxygenase, which results in the direct inhibition of the biosynthesis of prostaglandins and thromboxanes from arachidonic acid (see p.1511). Aspirin also inhibits platelet aggregation; non-acetylated salicylates do not.

Aspirin is used for the relief of mild to moderate pain such as headache, dysmenorrhoea, myalgias, and dental pain. It has also been used in the management of pain and inflammation in acute and chronic rheumatic disorders such as rheumatoid arthritis, juvenile idiopathic arthritis, osteoarthritis, and ankylosing spondylitis. In the treatment of minor febrile conditions, such as colds or influenza, aspirin can reduce temperature and relieve headache and joint and muscle pains.

Aspirin is also used for its antiplatelet activity in the initial treatment of cardiovascular disorders such as angina pectoris and myocardial infarction and for the prevention of cardiovascular events in patients at risk. Other such uses include the treatment and prevention of cerebrovascular disorders such as stroke. For further details see under Antiplatelet Therapy, below.

Aspirin is usually taken by mouth. Gastric irritation may be reduced by taking doses after food. Various dosage forms are available including plain uncoated tablets, buffered tablets, dispersible tablets, enteric-coated tablets, and modified-release tablets. In some instances aspirin may be given rectally by suppository.

The usual oral dose of aspirin as an analgesic and antipyretic is 300 to 900 mg, repeated every 4 to 6 hours according to clinical needs, to a maximum of 4 g daily. The dose as suppositories is 600 to 900 mg every 4 hours to a maximum of 3.6 g daily.

Plasma-salicylate concentrations of 150 to 300 micrograms/mL are required for optimal anti-inflammatory activity (but see also Adverse Effects, above). Doses need to be adjusted individually to achieve optimum concentrations. Generally doses of about 4 to 8 g daily in divided doses are used for acute rheumatic disorders such as rheumatoid arthritis or osteoarthritis. Doses of up to 5.4 g daily in divided doses may be sufficient in chronic conditions.

Indications for aspirin therapy in children are extremely limited because of the risk of Reye's syndrome (see under Adverse Effects, above), but include juvenile idiopathic arthritis and Still's disease. Suggested doses for children are 80 to 100 mg/kg daily in 5 or 6 divided doses; up to 130 mg/kg daily may be used for acute exacerbations if necessary.

Sodium aspirin has also been used for the treatment of pain and fever.

**Antiplatelet therapy.** Aspirin is an inhibitor of the enzyme cyclo-oxygenase, the **action** being considered to be due to an irreversible acetylation process.

- In blood platelets such enzyme inhibition prevents the synthesis of thromboxane $A_2$, a compound which is a vasoconstrictor, causes platelet aggregation, and is thus potentially thrombotic.
- In blood vessel walls the enzyme inhibition prevents the synthesis of prostacyclin, which is a vasodilator, has anti-aggregating properties, and is thus potentially anti-thrombotic.

Aspirin therefore appears to have paradoxical biological effects. The duration of these effects, however, may differ, with the *effects on the vascular tissue generally being shorter than the effects on the platelets* (although the animal species studied, the type of blood vessel employed, and the prevailing experimental conditions may alter the results). The difference may be explained by the fact that vascular cells regain the ability to regenerate prostacyclin in a few hours but platelets are unable to re-synthesise cyclo-oxygenase, which results in no new thromboxane $A_2$ being produced for about 24 hours until more platelets are released by the bone marrow; as platelet activity in bone marrow may also be affected by aspirin it is generally considered that aspirin only needs to be given once daily for inhibition of platelet aggregation to occur. The inhibitory effect on thromboxane is rapid and unrelated to serum concentrations of aspirin, probably because of the inactivation of cyclo-oxygenase in platelets in the presystemic circulation. Since the effect is unrelated to systemic bioavailability, modified-release and dermal delivery preparations which do not achieve high systemic concentrations of aspirin are being developed to limit extraplatelet effects of aspirin. Inhibition is cumulative on repeated dosage, and it has been estimated that a daily dose of 20 to 50 mg will result in virtually complete suppression of platelet thromboxane synthesis within a few days. Large doses of 150 to 300 mg can produce maximum suppression almost instantaneously.

**Uses.** Aspirin's antiplatelet activity has led to its use or investigation in a variety of disorders.[1-4]

- It is used as part of the initial **treatment** of unstable *angina* (p.813) and is given in the early treatment of *myocardial infarction* (p.828); it is also of benefit in the initial treatment of acute *ischaemic stroke* (p.836).
- Aspirin is used for its combination of anti-inflammatory, antipyretic, and antiplatelet activity in the treatment of *Kawasaki disease* (see below). It is also used to treat thrombotic symptoms associated with *antiphospholipid syndrome*, such as occurs in patients with systemic lupus erythematosus (p.1088), and has been recommended for prophylactic use in pregnant patients with antiphospholipid antibodies who are at risk of fetal loss. Aspirin has also been tried in *pregnancy-induced hypertension* (see under Hypertension, p.825) for the prevention of pre-eclampsia and intra-uterine growth retardation but it appears that its use may be justified only in women at high risk.
- It is of value for the **prevention** of cardiovascular events in patients at high risk, including those with stable or unstable angina, current or previous myocardial infarction, ischaemic stroke, or transient ischaemic attack (see Cardiovascular Risk Reduction, p.819). It has also been used in the long-term management of atrial fibrillation (see under Cardiac Arrhythmias, p.816) for the prevention of stroke in patients with contra-indications to warfarin or if there are no other risk factors for stroke.
- The value of aspirin for **primary prevention** of cardiovascular events, particularly *myocardial infarction* and *stroke* depends upon the accurate estimation of overall cardiovascular risk but is probably not justified in healthy individuals.[5-7]

  Although aspirin may prevent *venous thromboembolism* (p.839) following surgery other treatments have been preferred. However, it is recommended for use in preventing thrombotic complications associated with procedures such as angioplasty and coronary bypass grafting (see under Reperfusion and Revascularisation Procedures, p.834). Aspirin is often given as an adjunct to patients with *peripheral arterial thromboembolism* (p.830) to prevent propagation of the clot and also to prevent postoperative complications. It may have some effect in delaying disease progression and reducing vascular events in patients with *peripheral arterial disease* (p.831) but a recent analysis[8] concluded that there was insufficient evidence to support its prophylactic use in patients with intermittent claudication but no additional cardiovascular risk factors.

  The benefit of aspirin for the primary prevention of cardiovascular events in patients with *diabetes mellitus* (see under Diabetic Complications, p.326) and who have no other cardiovascular risk factors remains to be determined.[6] The value of adding aspirin to anticoagulants for the prophylaxis of thromboembolism in patients with *artificial heart valves* (see p.838) is still to be firmly established. It is usually recommended as an adjunct in patients with other risk factors. Aspirin alone may be considered in patients with bioprosthetic valves who do not require anticoagulation.

Several pharmacological studies have attempted to find a **dose** of aspirin that would inhibit synthesis of platelet thromboxane $A_2$ while sparing the effect on prostacyclin production[9-11] but it has been pointed out[4] that in patients with vascular disease accompanying or caused by endothelial dysfunction, such as in atherosclerosis, a selective sparing of vascular prostacyclin production may not be obtained at any effective antiplatelet dose. However, the clinical relevance of inhibiting the synthesis of prostacyclin may have been exaggerated.[12] Experimental evidence indicates that aspirin is thrombogenic only at extremely high doses (200 mg/kg), far exceeding the minimum dose required to inhibit prostacyclin production. Also aspirin is clinically effective as an antithrombotic drug at doses that inhibit the synthesis of prostacyclin. Further support for the lack of importance of inhibition of prostacyclin synthesis comes from epidemiological studies in patients with arthritis given large doses of aspirin and patients with congenital cyclo-oxygenase deficiency; neither of these groups of patients have experienced an excess of thrombotic episodes.

In a meta-analysis conducted by the Antithrombotic Trialists' Collaboration[6] daily doses of 75 to 325 mg appeared to be equally effective for their antiplatelet effect; doses greater than 500 mg did not appear to be superior and caused more gastrointestinal adverse effects. Whether doses less than 75 mg offer the same efficacy with reduced gastrointestinal toxicity remains to be determined (see Effects on the Gastrointestinal Tract, above). The meta-analysis concluded that for the long-term prevention of serious vascular events in high-risk patients, a daily dose of aspirin in the range of 75 to 150 mg should be effective; if an immediate effect is required as in the initial treatment of acute myocardial infarction, acute ischaemic stroke, or unstable angina, a loading dose of 150 to 300 mg may be given. Another analysis[8] has made similar dose recommendations. Aspirin should be chewed or dispersed in water; chewing a tablet of aspirin ensures that some buccal absorption occurs.


1. Patrono C. Aspirin as an antiplatelet drug. *N Engl J Med* 1994; **330:** 1287–94.
2. Lutomski DM, *et al.* Pharmacokinetic optimisation of the treatment of embolic disorders. *Clin Pharmacokinet* 1995; **28:** 67–92.
3. Catella-Lawson F, Fitzgerald GA. Long term aspirin in the prevention of cardiovascular disorders: recent developments and variations on a theme. *Drug Safety* 1995; **13:** 69–75.
4. Schrör K. Antiplatelet drugs: a comparative review. *Drugs* 1995; **50:** 7–28.
5. Sanmuganathan PS, *et al.* Aspirin for primary prevention of coronary heart disease: safety and absolute benefit related to coronary risk derived from meta-analysis of randomised trials. *Heart* 2001; **85:** 265–71.
6. Antithrombotic Trialists' Collaboration. Collaborative meta-analysis of randomised trials of antiplatelet therapy for prevention of death, myocardial infarction, and stroke in high risk patients. *BMJ* 2002; **324:** 71–86. Correction. *ibid.*; 141.
7. Collaborative Group of the Primary Prevention Project. Low-dose aspirin and vitamin E in people at cardiovascular risk: a randomised trial in general practice. *Lancet* 2001; **357:** 89–95.
8. Eccles M, *et al.* North of England evidence based guideline development project: guideline on the use of aspirin as secondary prophylaxis for vascular disease in primary care. *BMJ* 1998; **316:** 1303–9.
9. Patrignani P, *et al.* Selective cumulative inhibition of platelet thromboxane production by low-dose aspirin in healthy subjects. *J Clin Invest* 1982; **69:** 1366–72.
10. Weksler BB, *et al.* Differential inhibition by aspirin of vascular and platelet prostaglandin synthesis in atherosclerotic patients. *N Engl J Med* 1983; **308:** 800–5.
11. McLeod LJ, *et al.* The effects of different doses of some acetylsalicylic acid formulations on platelet function and bleeding times in healthy subjects. *Scand J Haematol* 1986; **36:** 379–84.
12. Hirsh J, *et al.* Aspirin and other platelet active drugs: relationship among dose, effectiveness, and side effects. *Chest* 1989; **95** (suppl 2): 12S–18S.


**Behçet's syndrome.** For reference to the use of aspirin in the management of vasculitic symptoms of Behçet's syndrome, see p.1076.

**Cataract.** Evidence to support or disprove the hypothesis that aspirin has a protective effect against cataract formation is considered inconclusive.[1,2] One study in the US in over 22 000 males concluded that low-dose aspirin (325 mg on alternate days) for 5 years was unlikely to have a major effect on cataract formation but that a slightly decreased risk for cataract extraction could not be excluded.[3] In a later study[4] in the UK ophthalmic examination of over 1800 patients who were receiving 300 mg to 1.2 g of aspirin daily for transient ischaemic attacks failed to confirm any protective effect. Re-analysis[5] of the results of the original US study identified additional cases of cataract formation or extraction although these cases did not affect the overall conclusions of the original study. However, when the study patients were followed up over 15 years, observational data[6] suggested that the use of low-dose aspirin may, in fact, increase the risk of cataract development. It was considered that further trials were needed to establish the role of long-term aspirin in cataract prevention.


1. Cheng H. Aspirin and cataract. *Br J Ophthalmol* 1992; **76:** 257–8.
2. Anonymous. Preventing cataract. *Lancet* 1992; **340:** 883–4.
3. Seddon JM, *et al.* Low dose aspirin and risks of cataract in a randomised trial of US physicians. *Arch Ophthalmol* 1991; **109:** 252–5.
4. UK-TIA Study Group. Does aspirin affect the rate of cataract formation? Cross-sectional results during a randomised double-blind placebo controlled trial to prevent serious vascular events. *Br J Ophthalmol* 1992; **76:** 259–61.
5. Christen WG, *et al.* Low-dose aspirin and risk of cataract and subtypes in a randomized trial of U.S. physicians. *Ophthalmic Epidemiol* 1998; **5:** 133–42.
6. Christen WG, *et al.* Aspirin use and risk of cataract in posttrial follow-up of Physicians' Health Study I. *Arch Ophthalmol* 2001; **119:** 405–12.


**Dysmenorrhoea.** Drugs such as aspirin and other NSAIDs that inhibit prostaglandin production through inhibition of cyclo-oxygenase are effective drugs in the treatment of dysmenorrhoea (p.6).

**Fever.** Methods for controlling fever (see p.8) include the use of antipyretics and/or physical cooling methods. Paracetamol, salicylates such as aspirin, and some other NSAIDs are the main antipyretics used. However, salicylates are generally contra-indicated for the management of fever in children because of the possible link between their use and the development of Reye's syndrome (see under Adverse Effects, above).

**Headache.** Aspirin is often used for the symptomatic treatment of various types of headache including migraine (see p.464) and tension-type headache (see p.465). Aspirin given at the onset of symptoms can successfully treat an acute attack of migraine. However, absorption may be poor due to gastric stasis which is commonly present in migraine. For this reason dispersible and effervescent preparations and compound preparations containing drugs such as metoclopramide which relieve gastric stasis have been advocated.

References.


1. Tfelt-Hansen P, Olesen J. Effervescent metoclopramide and aspirin (Migravess) versus effervescent aspirin or placebo for migraine attacks: a double-blind study. *Cephalalgia* 1984; **4:** 107–11.
2. Buring JE, *et al.* Low-dose aspirin for migraine prophylaxis. *JAMA* 1990; **264:** 1711–13.
3. The Oral Sumatriptan and Aspirin plus Metoclopramide Comparative Study Group. A study to compare oral sumatriptan with oral aspirin plus oral metoclopramide in the acute treatment of migraine. *Eur Neurol* 1992; **32:** 177–84.
4. Tfelt-Hansen P, *et al.* The effectiveness of combined oral lysine acetylsalicylate and metoclopramide compared with oral sumatriptan for migraine. *Lancet* 1995; **346:** 923–6.


**Kawasaki disease.** Aspirin has been given in regimens with normal immunoglobulins to children with Kawasaki disease (p.1629) because of its anti-inflammatory, antipyretic, and antiplatelet activity.[1,2]

The optimum dose and duration of treatment with aspirin have not yet been established but the usual practice is to use an anti-inflammatory regimen until the fever has settled and then convert to an antithrombotic regimen. Usual initial doses used have ranged from 30 to 120 mg/kg daily. Some clinicians recommend a dose of 80 to 100 mg/kg daily in 4 divided doses until the patient is afebrile or for the first 14 days after the onset of symptoms. Once fever and signs of inflammatory disease resolve, the aspirin dose is reduced to 3 to 5 mg/kg daily as a single dose for its antiplatelet effect. Aspirin may be discontinued 6 to 8 weeks after the onset of illness but is usually continued for at least one year if coronary abnormalities are present and is continued indefinitely if coronary aneurysms persist.

It has been noted[3] that aspirin has never been demonstrated in a prospective study to reduce the prevalence of coronary artery abnormalities in children with Kawasaki disease and some studies[4,5] indicate that the incidence of such abnormalities following treatment was similar for regimens using high or low doses of aspirin. In view of the potential risks and lack of obvious cardiac benefits of high-dose aspirin some[3] consider that an argument could be made for use of a low dose such as 3 to 5 mg/kg daily to prevent thrombosis, with other drugs such as paracetamol or ibuprofen being added for fever control or severe arthritis.


1. Williams RV, *et al.* Pharmacological therapy for patients with Kawasaki disease. *Paediatr Drugs* 2001; **3:** 649–60.
2. Brogan PA, *et al.* Kawasaki disease: an evidence based approach to diagnosis, treatment, and proposals for future research. *Arch Dis Child* 2002; **86:** 286–90.
3. Newburger JW. Treatment of Kawasaki disease. *Lancet* 1996; **347:** 1128.
4. Durongpisitkul K, *et al.* The prevention of coronary artery aneurysm in Kawasaki disease: a meta-analysis on the efficacy of aspirin and immunoglobulin treatment. *Pediatrics* 1995; **96:** 1057–61.
5. Terai M, Shulman ST. Prevalence of coronary artery abnormalities in Kawasaki disease is highly dependent on gamma globulin dose but independent of salicylate dose. *J Pediatr* 1997; **131:** 888–93.


**Leg ulcers.** A 4-month placebo controlled study[1] in 20 patients suggested that aspirin 300 mg daily aided healing of chronic venous leg ulcers; the mechanism of action was unclear.[2] However, the validity of the findings has been challenged.[3] The management of leg ulcers is discussed on p.1139.


1. Layton AM, *et al.* Randomised trial of oral aspirin for chronic venous leg ulcers. *Lancet* 1994; **344:** 164–5.
2. Ibbotson SH, *et al.* The effect of aspirin on haemostatic activity in the treatment of chronic venous leg ulceration. *Br J Dermatol* 1995; **132:** 422–6.
3. Ruckley CV, Prescott RJ. Treatment of chronic leg ulcers. *Lancet* 1994; **344:** 1512–13.


**Malignant neoplasms.** For references to studies suggesting that regular use of aspirin and other NSAIDs may reduce the risk of developing malignant neoplasms of the gastrointestinal tract, see under NSAIDs, p.71.

**Myeloproliferative disorders.** Aspirin in low doses may be used to provide symptomatic relief for erythromelalgia (burning pain and erythema of the hands and feet) in patients with polycythaemia vera (p.508) and primary thrombocythaemia (p.509).

**Pain.** Aspirin, along with other NSAIDs and paracetamol, may be used for treating mild or moderate pain (see Choice of Analgesic, p.2) and is also used in moderate or severe pain to potentiate the effects of opioids. It is suitable for use in acute or chronic pain. Aspirin should not be used for pain relief in children because of its association with Reye's syndrome (see under Adverse Effects, above).

Dependence and tolerance are not a problem with non-opioid analgesics such as aspirin, but there is a ceiling of efficacy, above which increasing the dose has no further therapeutic effect.

References.


1. Hersch EV, *et al.* Over-the-counter analgesics and antipyretics: a critical assessment. *Clin Ther* 2000; **22:** 500–48.
2. Edwards JE, *et al.* Single dose oral aspirin for acute pain. Available in The Cochrane Library; Issue 2. Chichester: John Wiley; 2004.


**Rheumatic disorders.** Aspirin was once widely used in the treatment of rheumatoid arthritis (p.9) but has been superseded by better tolerated NSAIDs; however, juvenile chronic arthritis (p.9) and Still's disease (p.11) are among the limited number of indications for aspirin use in children.

## Preparations

***BP 2003:*** Aspirin and Caffeine Tablets; Aspirin Tablets; Co-codaprin Tablets; Dispersible Aspirin Tablets; Dispersible Co-codaprin Tablets; Effervescent Soluble Aspirin Tablets; Enteric-coated Aspirin Tablets;
***USP 27:*** Acetaminophen and Aspirin Tablets; Acetaminophen, Aspirin, and Caffeine Tablets; Aspirin and Codeine Phosphate Tablets; Aspirin Capsules; Aspirin Delayed-release Capsules; Aspirin Delayed-release Tablets; Aspirin Effervescent Tablets for Oral Solution; Aspirin Extended-release Tablets; Aspirin Suppositories; Aspirin Tablets; Aspirin, Alumina, and Magnesia Tablets; Aspirin, Alumina, and Magnesium Oxide Tablets; Buffered Aspirin Tablets; Butalbital and Aspirin Tablets; Butalbital, Aspirin, and Caffeine Capsules; Butalbital, Aspirin, and Caffeine Tablets; Butalbital, Aspirin, Caffeine, and Codeine Phosphate Capsules; Carisoprodol and Aspirin Tablets; Carisoprodol, Aspirin, and Codeine Phosphate Tablets; Oxycodone and Aspirin Tablets; Pentazocine Hydrochloride and Aspirin Tablets; Propoxyphene Hydrochloride, Aspirin, and Caffeine Capsules; Propoxyphene Napsylate and Aspirin Tablets.

**Proprietary Preparations** (details are given in Part 3)
***Arg.:*** Adiro; Aspirinetas; Bayaspirina; Bufferin; Cardioaspirina; Desenfriolito; Geniol AP; Geniol SC sin Cafeina; Geniolito; Nuevapina; ***Austral.:*** Aspro; Astrix; Bex; Cardiprin; Cartia; Disprin; Disprin Direct; Ecotrin; Solprin; Spren; Vincent's Powders; ***Austria:*** Acekapton; Algobene†; Aspiricor; Aspro; ASS; ASSbene; Corsalbene†; Herz ASS; RheumaASS; Salimont; Thrombo ASS; Togal Mono; ***Belg.:*** Acenterine; Asaflow; Asarid; Aspirine; Aspro; Cardioaspirine; Catalgix†; Dispril†; Rhodine†; Rhonal†; Sedergine; Therasa; ***Braz.:*** AAS; Aceticil; Acetin†; Alidor†; Analgesin; Antifebrin; Aspirina; Aspisin†; Aspylin†; Bufferin; Caas; Cimaas; Doraine†; Ecasil; Endosalil†; Hipotermal; Melhoral Infantil†; Ronal†; Salicil; Somalgin; ***Canad.:*** Asaphen; Aspergum; Aspirin with Stomach Guard; Bufferin; Coryphen†; Entrophen; Headache Tablets†; Novasen; Rivasa; Tri-Buffered ASA; ***Chile:*** Aspirina; Cardioaspirina; Disgren; Ecotrin; Hassapirin Puro; Thrombo AS; ***Denm.:*** Acetard†; Albyl†; Hjertealbyl†; Hjertemagnyl; Idotyl; Iskaemyl†; Magnyl; ***Fin.:*** Aspirin Cardio; Disperin; Primaspan; ***Fr.:*** Aspirine; Aspirine pH8; Aspirisucre; Aspro; Catalgine†; Claragine; Juvepirine†; Sargepirine†; ***Ger.:*** Acesal; Acesal Calcium†; Acetylin; Aspro; ASS; Godamed; Hermes ASS†; HerzASS; Micristin†; Miniasal; Neuralgin ASS†; Romigal†; Santasal N; Spalt†; Thomapyrin akut; Togal ASS; ***Gr.:*** Salospir; Upsalgin-N; ***Hong Kong:*** Ascriptin†; Aspilets; Aspro†; Astrix; Cardiprin; Cartia; Disprin; Ecotrin; ***India:*** ASA; Aspicot; Colsprin; Ecosprin; ***Irl.:*** Ascriptin†; Aspro; Caprin; Clonteric†; Disprin; Lowasa; Nu-Seals; Resprin; ***Israel:*** Acetosal; Alka-Seltzer; Ascriptin; Cartia; Ecoprin; Godamed; Micropirin; Rhonal†; Tevapirin; ***Ital.:*** Acesal; ASA-ratio; Ascriptin; Aspiglicina; Aspirina; Aspirina 03 and 05; Aspirina 05†; Aspirinetta; Aspro; Bufferin; Cardioaspirin; Cemirit; Kilios; Upsalgina†; ***Malaysia:*** Bufferin Low Dose; Cardiprin; Casprin; Disprin; Dusil; Glyprin; ***Mex.:*** Acetin; Aciben†; Acitab; Adiro; Antacsal; ASA†; Asawin†; Ascriptin; Aspirina; Axal†; Disprina; Dolmex†; Ecotrin; Labysal†; Mejoral†; Midolen; Rhonal†; ***Neth.:*** Aspirine Protect; Aspro; ***Norw.:*** Albyl-E; Bamycor†; Dispril; Globentyl†; Globoid; Novid†; ***NZ:*** Aspec; Aspro; Cardiprin; Cartia; Disprin; Ecotrin; Pharmacare Aspec†; Solprin; ***Port.:*** AAS; ASP†; Aspirina; Aspro; Cartia; Melhoral Infantil; Migraspirina; Salycilina; Sedergine†; Toldex; ***S.Afr.:*** ASAtard†; Aspro†; Disprin; Ecotrin; Myoprin; ***Singapore:*** Aspro; Astrix; Bokey EMC; Bufferin; Cardiprin; Disprin; Dusil; ***Spain:*** AAS; Adiro; Algho†; Aspinfantil; Aspirina; Aspro†; Bioplak; Calmantina†; Helver Sal; Lafena†; Mejoral; Okal; Orravina; Rhonal; Saspryl; Sedergine; Tromalyt; Upsalgina†; ***Swed.:*** Albyl minor; Bamycor; Bamyl; Bamyl S; Dispril†; Emotpin; Magnecyl; Trombyl; ***Switz.:*** Asperivo; Aspro; ASS; Demoprin nouvelle formule†; Thrombace Neo; Tiatral 100 SR; Togal ASS; ***Thai.:*** Ascot; Aspent; Aspilets; Caparin; Cardiprin; Comoprin; Entrarin; Seferin; V-AS; ***UAE:*** Jusprin; ***UK:*** Alka; Angettes; Aspro; Beechams Lemon Tablets†; Caprin; Disprin; Disprin CV†; Disprin Direct; Enprin; Gencardia†; Micropirin; Nu-Seals; PostMI†; Pure Health; ***USA:*** Adprin-B; Arthritis Foundation Pain Reliever†; Arthritis Pain Formula; Ascriptin; Aspergum; Asprimox; Bayer Low Adult Strength; Bufferin; Buffex; Cama Arthritis Pain Reliever; Easprin; Ecotrin; Empirin; Extra Strength Bayer Plus; Genprin; Halfprin; Magnaprin; Norwich Extra Strength; Regular Strength Bayer; St. Joseph Adult Chewable; ZORprin.

**Multi-ingredient:** numerous preparations are listed in Part 3.

# Auranofin *(BAN, USAN, rINN)*

Auranofina; SKF-39162; SKF-D-39162. (1-Thio-β-D-glucopyranosato)(triethylphosphine)gold 2,3,4,6-tetra-acetate.

$C_{20}H_{34}AuO_9PS$ = 678.5.

*CAS — 34031-32-8.*

*ATC — M01CB03.*

## Adverse Effects and Treatment

The most common adverse effects of auranofin involve the gastrointestinal tract and include nausea, abdominal pain, and sometimes vomiting, but most often diarrhoea, which can affect up to 50% of patients and may be severe enough to cause patients to withdraw from treatment. Other adverse effects are similar to those experienced with sodium aurothiomalate (p.88), although they appear to be less troublesome since fewer patients stop treatment with auranofin than with injectable gold. As with other gold salts, treatment of adverse effects is generally symptomatic (see p.89). A bulking agent such as bran or modifying the diet to increase bulk or a temporary reduction in dosage may help the diarrhoea.

◊ Reviews.


1. Tozman ECS, Gottlieb NL. Adverse reactions with oral and parenteral gold preparations. *Med Toxicol* 1987; **2:** 177–89.


**Effects on the gastrointestinal tract.** Diarrhoea and abdominal pain are frequent adverse effects of auranofin. The mechanism of gastrointestinal toxicity has not been established but may be associated with a reversible defect in intestinal permeability.[1] Colitis and eosinophilia have been reported in a patient taking auranofin.[2]


1. Behrens R, *et al.* Investigation of auranofin-induced diarrhoea. *Gut* 1986; **27:** 59–65.
2. Michet CJ, *et al.* Auranofin-associated colitis and eosinophilia. *Mayo Clin Proc* 1987; **62:** 142–4.


**Effects on the kidneys.** In a retrospective review[1] of 1283 patients who had received auranofin for treatment of rheumatoid arthritis 41 (3.2%) were found to have developed proteinuria. Treatment of proteinuria in the majority of patients consisted of discontinuing auranofin therapy. Long-term follow-up of 36 patients indicated that proteinuria had resolved in 31 within 2 years and in 29 within 1 year. Seven of 8 patients later rechallenged with auranofin had no relapses. In a further review of 2 comparative double-blind studies using gold compounds in the treatment of rheumatoid arthritis, proteinuria was found to have developed in 27% (23 of 85) of patients treated with sodium aurothiomalate, in 17% (42 of 247) of those treated with auranofin, and in 17% (36 of 210) of those receiving placebo. All patients were receiving NSAIDs.


1. Katz WA, *et al.* Proteinuria in gold-treated rheumatoid arthritis. *Ann Intern Med* 1984; **101:** 176–9.


## Precautions

As for Sodium Aurothiomalate, p.89. Urine and blood tests should be carried out before starting auranofin and monthly thereafter; the UK manufacturer advises that auranofin should be withdrawn if the platelet count falls below 100 000 per $mm^3$ or if signs and symptoms suggestive of thrombocytopenia occur. Auranofin should be used with caution in patients with inflammatory bowel disease.

**Porphyria.** Auranofin has been associated with acute attacks of porphyria and is considered unsafe in porphyric patients.

## Interactions

As for Sodium Aurothiomalate, p.89.

## Pharmacokinetics

Auranofin is incompletely absorbed from the gastrointestinal tract, only about 25% of the gold being absorbed. Gold from auranofin is bound to plasma proteins as well as to red blood cells. After 2 to 3 months of treatment the steady-state concentration of gold in the blood is reported to be about 0.7 micrograms/mL. The average terminal plasma half-life of gold at steady state is about 26 days while the biological half-life is 81 days. Tissue retention and total gold accumulation in the body are less than with intramuscular gold. Gold from auranofin penetrates into synovial fluid.

Most of a dose of auranofin appears in the faeces due to its poor absorption. About 60% of the absorbed gold from auranofin is excreted in the urine and the remainder in the faeces.

◊ Reviews.


1. Blocka KLN, *et al.* Clinical pharmacokinetics of oral and injectable gold compounds. *Clin Pharmacokinet* 1986; **11:** 133–43.


## Uses and Administration

Auranofin is a gold compound with a gold content of about 29%; it has similar actions and uses to those of sodium aurothiomalate (p.89). It is given by mouth in active progressive rheumatoid arthritis (below); such oral treatment is less toxic than intramuscular gold but is also much less effective. The usual initial dose of auranofin is 6 mg daily either as a single dose or in two divided doses. Treatment should be continued for at least 6 months to assess the response; the dose may be increased after 6 months, if the response is inadequate, to 3 mg three times daily. If the response is still inadequate after 3 months at this dosage, then treatment should be discontinued.

**Asthma.** A systematic review[1] found that oral or parenteral gold compounds reduced corticosteroid requirements in the management of asthma (p.777); however, it was considered that the effect was probably of limited clinical significance and, given the adverse effects and monitoring requirements of gold compounds, their use in asthma could not be recommended.


1. Evans DJ, *et al.* Gold as an oral corticosteroid sparing agent in stable asthma. Available in The Cochrane Library; Issue 2. Chichester: John Wiley; 2004.


**Lupus.** Since the introduction of less toxic drugs gold compounds are now rarely used in the treatment of systemic lupus erythematosus, however, there have been anecdotal reports suggesting that auranofin may still be of use in patients with discoid lupus erythematosus[1] or cutaneous lupus erythematosus[2] refractory to conventional treatment.


1. Dalziel K, *et al.* Treatment of chronic discoid lupus erythematosus with an oral gold compound (auranofin). *Br J Dermatol* 1986; **115:** 211–16.
2. Farrell AM, Bunker CB. Oral gold therapy in cutaneous lupus erythematosus (revisited). *Br J Dermatol* 1996; **135** (suppl 47): 41.


**Psoriasis.** Although efficacy for topical auranofin in the treatment of plaque-type psoriasis (p.1137) has been demonstrated in a placebo-controlled study,[1] the high incidence of adverse skin reactions, such as contact dermatitis, was thought to outweigh any benefit.


1. Helm KF, *et al.* Topical auranofin ointment for the treatment of plaque psoriasis. *J Am Acad Dermatol* 1995; **33:** 517–19.


**Rheumatic disorders.** Gold compounds are among the disease-modifying antirheumatic drugs (DMARDs) that may be used in the treatment of rheumatoid arthritis (p.9) and juvenile idiopathic arthritis (p.9). There is little agreement on which of the various DMARDs should be tried first and their selection is largely based on individual experience and preference. Oral gold is less toxic than intramuscular gold but is also much less effective. Gold compounds may also be of benefit in psoriatic arthritis (see under Spondyloarthropathies, p.11).

References.


1. Suarez-Almazor ME, *et al.* Auranofin versus placebo in rheumatoid arthritis. Available in The Cochrane Library; Issue 2. Chichester: John Wiley; 2004.


## Preparations

**Proprietary Preparations** (details are given in Part 3)
***Austral.:*** Ridaura; ***Austria:*** Ridaura; ***Belg.:*** Ridaura; ***Braz.:*** Ridaura; ***Canad.:*** Ridaura; ***Denm.:*** Ridaura; ***Fin.:*** Ridaura; ***Fr.:*** Ridauran; ***Ger.:*** Ridaura; ***Gr.:*** Ridaura; ***Hong Kong:*** Ridaura; ***India:*** Goldar; ***Irl.:*** Ridaura; ***Israel:*** Ridaura; ***Ital.:*** Ridaura; ***Mex.:*** Ridaura†; ***Neth.:*** Ridaura; ***Norw.:*** Ridaura; ***NZ:*** Ridaura; ***Port.:*** Ridaura; ***S.Afr.:*** Ridaura; ***Singapore:*** Ridaura†; ***Spain:*** Ridaura; ***Swed.:*** Ridaura; ***Switz.:*** Ridaura; ***Thai.:*** Ridaura†; ***UK:*** Ridaura; ***USA:*** Ridaura.

# Aurothioglucose

1-Aurothio-D-glucopyranose; Aurotioglucosa; (D-Glucosylthio)gold; Gold Thioglucose. (1-Thio-D-glucopyranosato)gold.

$C_6H_{11}AuO_5S$ = 392.2.

*CAS — 12192-57-3.*

*ATC — M01CB04.*

**Pharmacopoeias.** In *US.*

**USP 27** (Aurothioglucose). A yellow odourless or practically odourless powder. An aqueous solution is unstable on long standing. It is stabilised by the addition of a small amount of sodium acetate. pH of a 1% solution in water is about 6.3. Freely soluble in water; practically insoluble in alcohol, in acetone, in chloroform, and in ether. Store in airtight containers. Protect from light.

## Adverse Effects, Treatment, and Precautions

As for Sodium Aurothiomalate, p.88.

## Interactions

As for Sodium Aurothiomalate, p.89.

## Pharmacokinetics

As for Sodium Aurothiomalate, p.89; absorption is slower and more irregular.

## Uses and Administration

Aurothioglucose is a gold compound with a gold content of about 50%; it has similar actions and uses to those of sodium aurothiomalate (p.89). It is used in the treatment of active rheumatoid arthritis (p.9) and juvenile idiopathic arthritis (p.9). Aurothioglucose is given intramuscularly as a suspension in oil in an initial weekly dose of 10 mg increasing gradually to up to 50 mg weekly. Therapy is continued at weekly intervals until a total dose of 0.8 to 1 g has been given; if improvement has occurred with no signs of toxicity 50 mg may then be given at intervals of 3 or 4 weeks. Children aged 6 to 12 years may be given one-quarter the adult dose, to a maximum of 25 mg per dose.

## Preparations

***USP 27:*** Aurothioglucose Injectable Suspension.

**Proprietary Preparations** (details are given in Part 3)
***Austral.:*** Gold-50†; ***Canad.:*** Solganal; ***Ger.:*** Aureotan†; ***Israel:*** nal†; ***Neth.:*** Auromyose; ***USA:*** Solganal.

## Aurotioprol

Sodium 3-aurothio-2-hydroxypropane-1-sulphonate.
$C_3H_6AuNaO_4S_2$ = 390.2.
*CAS — 27279-43-2.*
*ATC — M01CB05.*

### Profile

Aurotioprol is a gold compound with a gold content of about 50%; it has similar actions and uses to those of sodium aurothiomalate (p.88). It is given by intramuscular injection for the treatment of rheumatoid arthritis (p.9). The initial dose is 25 mg weekly, increased to 50 to 100 mg weekly, until a total dose of 1.2 to 1.5 g has been given. If improvement has occurred with no signs of toxicity, this may be followed by a dose of 50 to 100 mg intramuscularly every month.

### Preparations

**Proprietary Preparations** (details are given in Part 3)
***Belg.:*** Allochrysine; ***Fr.:*** Allochrysine.

---

## Azapropazone *(BAN, rINN)*

AHR-3018; Apazone *(USAN)*; Azapropazona; Mi85; NSC-102824. 5-Dimethylamino-9-methyl-2-propylpyrazolo[1,2-*a*][1,2,4]benzotriazine-1,3(2*H*)-dione.
$C_{16}H_{20}N_4O_2$ = 300.4.
*CAS — 13539-59-8.*
*ATC — M01AX04.*

**Pharmacopoeias.** *Br.* includes the dihydrate.

**BP 2003** (Azapropazone). The dihydrate is a white to pale yellow crystalline powder. Very slightly soluble in water and in chloroform; soluble in alcohol; dissolves in solutions of alkali hydroxides.

### Adverse Effects

As for NSAIDs in general, p.67. Some adverse effects appear to be more common with azapropazone than with other NSAIDs (see below).

◊ Analysis of spontaneous reporting of adverse reactions to the UK Committee on Safety of Medicines revealed that azapropazone had been associated with the highest risk of gastrointestinal reactions compared with 6 other NSAIDs.[1] Renal, hepatic, allergic, and haematological reactions also occur with a relatively high frequency.

1. Committee on Safety of Medicines/Medicines Control Agency. Relative safety of oral non-aspirin NSAIDs. *Current Problems* 1994; **20:** 9–11.

**Effects on the blood.** Auto-immune haemolytic anaemia, occasionally fatal, often with pulmonary infiltration, allergic alveolitis, pulmonary fibrosis, or fibrosing alveolitis, has been reported in patients receiving azapropazone.[1-3]

1. Chan-Lam D, *et al.* Red cell antibodies and autoimmune haemolysis after treatment with azapropazone. *BMJ* 1986; **293:** 1474.
2. Albazzaz MK, *et al.* Alveolitis and haemolytic anaemia induced by azapropazone. *BMJ* 1986; **293:** 1537–8.
3. Montgomery RD, Babb RG. Alveolitis and haemolytic anaemia induced by azapropazone. *BMJ* 1987; **294:** 375.

**Effects on the gastrointestinal tract.** In a review[1] of the relative safety of 7 oral NSAIDs, the UK Committee on Safety of Medicines (CSM) commented that azapropazone was associated with the highest risk of gastrointestinal reactions in both epidemiological studies and an analysis of spontaneous reporting of adverse reactions. Although it appeared that some patients over 60 years of age had received doses exceeding those recommended for this age group, it was considered that even when this was taken into account a marked difference remained between gastrointestinal reactions for azapropazone compared with other NSAIDs. *The CSM recommended that azapropazone should be restricted to use in rheumatoid arthritis, ankylosing spondylitis, and acute gout and only when other NSAIDs have been ineffective. Its use in patients with a history of peptic ulceration was contra-indicated. It was also recommended that when used in patients over 60 years of age for rheumatoid arthritis or ankylosing spondylitis the dose should be restricted to a maximum of 600 mg daily.*

1. Committee on Safety of Medicines/Medicines Control Agency. Relative safety of oral non-aspirin NSAIDs. *Current Problems* 1994; **20:** 9–11.

**Effects on the lungs.** See under Effects on the Blood, above.

**Effects on the skin.** Of 917 reports of adverse reactions associated with azapropazone forwarded to the WHO Collaborating Centre for International Drug Monitoring[1] before September 1984, 190 (21%) were of photosensitivity. Of 154 reports of photosensitivity evaluated a causal relationship to use of azapropazone was considered certain in 6, probable in 138, and possible in 10. In May 1994 the UK Committee on Safety of Medicines stated[2] that since 1976 they had received 464 reports of photosensitivity reactions associated with azapropazone and commented that, when corrected for prescription volume, reporting of this reaction was 50 times greater than with other commonly prescribed NSAIDs. They recommended that patients should be advised to avoid direct exposure to sunlight or to use sunblock preparations.

1. Olsson S, *et al.* Photosensitivity during treatment with azapropazone. *BMJ* 1985; **291:** 939.
2. Committee on Safety of Medicines/Medicines Control Agency. Photosensitivity associated with azapropazone (Rheumox). *Current Problems* 1994; **20:** 6.

### Precautions

As for NSAIDs in general, p.69. Azapropazone is also contra-indicated in patients with a history or evidence of peptic ulceration, inflammatory bowel disorders, or blood disorders. Reduced doses should be given to elderly patients and patients with renal impairment; its use should be avoided in patients with severe renal impairment.

Photosensitivity reactions may occur with azapropazone and patients should be advised to avoid direct exposure to sunlight or to use sunblock preparations.

**Breast feeding.** The American Academy of Pediatrics[1] states that there have been no reports of any clinical effect on the infant associated with the use of azapropazone by breast-feeding mothers, and that therefore it may be considered to be usually compatible with breast feeding. However, since small quantities of azapropazone are excreted into breast milk,[2] the manufacturers advise that it should not be used in breast-feeding mothers.

1. American Academy of Pediatrics. The transfer of drugs and other chemicals into human milk. *Pediatrics* 2001; **108:** 776–89. Correction. *ibid.*; 1029. Also available at: http://aappolicy.aappublications.org/cgi/content/full/pediatrics%3b108/3/776 (accessed 02/07/04)
2. Bald R, *et al.* Excretion of azapropazone in human breast milk. *Eur J Clin Pharmacol* 1990; **39:** 271–3.

**Porphyria.** Azapropazone is considered to be unsafe in patients with porphyria because it has been shown to be porphyrinogenic in *animals*.

### Interactions

For interactions associated with NSAIDs, see p.69. Like phenylbutazone, azapropazone may be particularly likely to cause interactions with oral anticoagulants such as warfarin.

### Pharmacokinetics

Azapropazone is absorbed from the gastrointestinal tract and peak plasma concentrations are reached about 4 hours after administration. It is highly protein bound. A half-life of 12 to 24 hours has been reported. Azapropazone is excreted in the urine as unchanged drug (about 65%), 8-hydroxyazapropazone, and glucuronide or sulfate metabolites. Very small amounts are distributed into breast milk.

### Uses and Administration

Azapropazone is an NSAID (see p.70), structurally related to phenylbutazone (p.84). It also has uricosuric properties. Because azapropazone appears to be associated with a higher incidence of adverse effects than with some other NSAIDs its use in the UK is restricted to the treatment of rheumatoid arthritis, ankylosing spondylitis, and acute gout in patients for whom other NSAIDs have been ineffective.

Azapropazone is used as the dihydrate and doses are expressed in terms of this hydrated form. Azapropazone dihydrate 300 mg is approximately equivalent to 268 mg of azapropazone. For the treatment of rheumatoid arthritis or ankylosing spondylitis the usual dose in the UK is 1.2 g daily in 2 or 4 divided doses by mouth. Patients *over 60 years of age* may be given 300 mg twice daily. Reduced doses are also recommended in patients with renal impairment, see below.

Usually uricosuric drugs should not be given during an acute attack of gout as they may prolong its duration, but azapropazone appears to be suitable for the treatment of acute gout. In acute gout 1.8 g of the dihydrate may be given daily in divided doses until the attack is resolving (usually by the fourth day), then reduced to 1.2 g daily until symptoms have disappeared. An adequate fluid intake should be maintained. If symptoms persist appropriate alternative treatment (see p.412) should be considered. For patients over 60 years of age, provided their renal function is normal, the dose is 1.8 g daily in divided doses for the first 24 hours only, followed by 1.2 g daily. This should be reduced as soon as possible to a maximum of 600 mg daily. Azapropazone should not be used to treat gout in elderly patients with even mild renal impairment. Patients under 60 years with renal impairment should be given reduced doses, see below.

Azapropazone has been given intravenously in some countries.

**Administration in renal impairment.** In the treatment of *rheumatoid arthritis* or *ankylosing spondylitis* in patients with reduced renal function the usual dose is 300 mg of azapropazone dihydrate twice daily; azapropazone should be avoided in patients with severe renal impairment.

In *acute gout*, patients with mildly reduced renal function (a creatinine clearance of 60 mL or more per minute) may be given 1.8 g daily in divided doses for the first 24 hours only, followed by 1.2 g daily. This should be reduced as soon as possible to a maximum of 600 mg daily. Azapropazone should be avoided altogether for gout in elderly patients with even mild renal impairment and in all patients with moderate or severe impairment.

### Preparations

***BP 2003:*** Azapropazone Capsules; Azapropazone Tablets.

**Proprietary Preparations** (details are given in Part 3)
***Arg.:*** Debelex; ***Austria:*** Prolixan; ***Ger.:*** Tolyprin†; ***Gr.:*** Prolixan; ***Irl.:*** Rheumox; ***Neth.:*** Prolixan; ***Port.:*** Prolixan; ***Swed.:*** Prolixana†; ***Switz.:*** Prolixan†; ***UK:*** Rheumox.

**Multi-ingredient:** ***Austria:*** Algo-Prolixan; ***Switz.:*** Dolo-Prolixan†.

---

## Bendazac *(BAN, USAN, rINN)*

AF-983; Bendazaco; Bindazac. (1-Benzyl-1*H*-indazol-3-yloxy)acetic acid.
$C_{16}H_{14}N_2O_3$ = 282.3.
*CAS — 20187-55-7.*
*ATC — M02AA11.*

## Bendazac Lysine *(BANM, rINNM)*

AF-1934; Bendazaco de lisina. L-Lysine-(1-benzyl-1*H*-indazol-3-yloxy)acetic acid.
$C_{22}H_{28}N_4O_5$ = 428.5.
*CAS — 81919-14-4.*
*ATC — S01BC07.*

### Profile

Bendazac is an NSAID (p.67) structurally related to indometacin (p.47). It has been used topically in preparations containing 1 or 3% for the treatment of various inflammatory skin disorders.

Bendazac lysine has been used in the management of cataract, 2 drops of a 0.5% solution being instilled three times daily.

◊ References.

1. Balfour JA, Clissold SP. Bendazac lysine: a review of its pharmacological properties and therapeutic potential in the management of cataracts. *Drugs* 1990; **39:** 575–96.

### Preparations

**Proprietary Preparations** (details are given in Part 3)
***Austria:*** Versus; ***Ital.:*** Bendalina; Versus; ***Port.:*** Bendalina; Benzum†.

---

## Benorilate *(BAN, rINN)*

Benorilato; Benorylate; FAW-76; Fenasprate; Win-11450. 4-Acetamidophenyl *O*-acetylsalicylate.
$C_{17}H_{15}NO_5$ = 313.3.
*CAS — 5003-48-5.*
*ATC — N02BA10.*

**Pharmacopoeias.** In *Br.* and *Chin.*

**BP 2003** (Benorilate). A white or almost white, odourless or almost odourless, crystalline powder. Practically insoluble in water; sparingly soluble in alcohol and in methyl alcohol; soluble in acetone and in chloroform.

### Adverse Effects, Treatment, and Precautions

As for Aspirin, p.15, and Paracetamol, p.76.

Benorilate may cause nausea, indigestion, heartburn, and constipation; drowsiness, diarrhoea, and skin rashes have also been reported. Some patients have experienced dizziness, tinnitus, and deafness associated with high blood-salicylate concentrations.

Benorilate, like aspirin (see p.16), should not generally be given to children because of the risk of Reye's syndrome.

When an overdose of benorilate is suspected, it has been suggested that plasma concentrations of both salicylate and paracetamol should be measured since a normal plasma-paracetamol concentration cannot necessarily be assumed from a normal plasma-salicylate measurement.

◊ References.

1. Aylward M. Toxicity of benorylate. *BMJ* 1973; **2:** 118.
2. Symon DNK, *et al.* Fatal paracetamol poisoning from benorylate therapy in child with cystic fibrosis. *Lancet* 1982; **ii:** 1153–4.

### Interactions

For the interactions associated with aspirin, see p.17, and for those associated with paracetamol, see p.78.

### Pharmacokinetics

Benorilate is slowly absorbed virtually unchanged from the gastrointestinal tract. Following absorption, benorilate is rapidly metabolised to salicylate and paracetamol. It is excreted mainly as metabolites of salicylic acid and paracetamol in the urine.

### Uses and Administration

Benorilate is an aspirin-paracetamol ester with analgesic, anti-inflammatory, and antipyretic properties. It is used in the treatment of mild to moderate pain (see Choice of Analgesic, p.2) and fever (p.8). It is also used in osteoarthritis (p.9), rheumatoid arthritis (p.9), and soft-tissue rheumatism (p.11). Benorilate is given by mouth, preferably after food, in doses of 2 g twice daily for mild to moderate pain and fever. Doses for osteoarthritis, quiescent rheumatoid arthritis, and soft-tissue rheumatism are up to 6 g daily in divided doses. In active rheumatoid arthritis 4 g twice daily may be required. In elderly patients reduced doses of 2 g twice daily or possibly 2 g in the morning and 4 g at night should be given; a maximum daily dose of 6 g should not be exceeded.

### Preparations

***BP 2003:*** Benorilate Oral Suspension; Benorilate Tablets.

**Proprietary Preparations** (details are given in Part 3)
***Belg.:*** Duvium; ***Fr.:*** Longalgic†; Salipran; ***Irl.:*** Benoral; ***Spain:*** Doline†; Vetedol†; ***Switz.:*** Duvium; ***UK:*** Benoral†.

## Benoxaprofen *(BAN, USAN, rINN)*

Benoxaprofeno; Compound 90459; LRCL-3794. 2-[2-(4-Chlorophenyl)benzoxazol-5-yl]propionic acid.

$C_{16}H_{12}ClNO_3$ = 301.7.

*CAS — 51234-28-7.*

*ATC — M01AE06.*

### Profile

Benoxaprofen is an NSAID (p.67) structurally related to ibuprofen (p.45). It was formerly given by mouth in rheumatoid arthritis and osteoarthritis but because of reports of adverse reactions and fatalities the manufacturers halted worldwide marketing of the preparation known as Opren in the early 1980s. Side-effects that have occurred with benoxaprofen include skin disorders, notably photosensitivity reactions but also erythema multiforme and the Stevens-Johnson syndrome, onycholysis and other nail disorders, gastrointestinal disturbances including peptic ulceration and bleeding, blood disorders such as thrombocytopenia, cholestatic jaundice and other liver or biliary disorders, and renal failure.

## Benzydamine Hydrochloride *(BANM, USAN, rINNM)*

AF-864; Benzindamine Hydrochloride; Hidrocloruro de bencidamina. 3-(1-Benzyl-1*H*-indazol-3-yloxy)-*NN*-dimethylpropylamine hydrochloride.

$C_{19}H_{23}N_3O,HCl$ = 345.9.

*CAS — 642-72-8 (benzydamine); 132-69-4 (benzydamine hydrochloride).*

**Pharmacopoeias.** In *Br.* and *Pol.*

**BP 2003** (Benzydamine Hydrochloride). A white crystalline powder. Very soluble in water; freely soluble in alcohol and in chloroform; practically insoluble in ether. A 10% solution in water has a pH of 4.0 to 5.5.

### Adverse Effects

Following topical application to the skin local reactions such as erythema or rash may occur and photosensitivity has been reported. Following use as mouth and throat preparations, numbness or stinging sensations of the oral mucosa have been reported; hypersensitivity reactions including urticaria, photosensitivity, and bronchospasm may also occur rarely.

**Effects on the kidneys.** A 57-year-old woman who had used 400 g of a topical cream containing benzydamine hydrochloride 3% over a period of 4 months was found to have raised plasma concentrations of creatinine and urea consistent with a substantial reduction in glomerular filtration rate.[1]

1. O'Callaghan CA, *et al.* Renal disease and use of topical non-steroidal anti-inflammatory drugs. *BMJ* 1994; **308:** 110–11.

**Overdose.** A 6-year old girl experienced hallucinations[1] after receiving 500 mg of benzydamine orally; it had been intended as a vaginal douche for pruritus vulvae. She recovered spontaneously.

1. Gómez-López L, *et al.* Acute overdose due to benzydamine. *Hum Exp Toxicol* 1999; **18:** 471–3.

### Uses and Administration

Benzydamine hydrochloride is an NSAID (p.70). It is used topically on the skin in concentrations of 3 to 5% in painful musculoskeletal and soft-tissue disorders. Benzydamine hydrochloride is also used as a mouthwash or spray in concentrations of 0.15% for the relief of inflammatory conditions of the mouth and throat. It has been given by mouth or rectally for the relief of painful and inflammatory conditions, and as a topical solution for vaginal irrigation.

Benzydamine salicylate (benzasal) has been used topically on the skin as a 6% cream or spray.

**Mouth disorders.** Results of a randomised placebo-controlled study in patients undergoing radiotherapy for oropharyngeal cancer indicated that benzydamine as an oral rinse was effective in reducing the area and severity of mucositis.[1] Benzydamine is also used locally for the management of mouth ulcers (p.1245) although a study[2] found it no more useful than placebo.

1. Epstein JB, *et al.* Benzydamine HCl for prophylaxis of radiation-induced oral mucositis: results from a multicenter, randomized, double-blind, placebo-controlled clinical trial. *Cancer* 2001; **92:** 875–85.
2. Matthews RW, *et al.* Clinical evaluation of benzydamine, chlorhexidine, and placebo mouthwashes in the management of recurrent aphthous stomatitis. *Oral Surg Oral Med Oral Pathol* 1987; **63:** 189–91.

### Preparations

***BP 2003:*** Benzydamine Cream; Benzydamine Mouthwash; Benzydamine Oromucosal Spray.

**Proprietary Preparations** (details are given in Part 3)

***Arg.:*** Ernex; Sandival Desleible; ***Austral.:*** Difflam; Difflam Anti-inflammatory Throat Spray; Difflam Solution; ***Austria:*** Tantum; Tantumar; ***Braz.:*** Benflogin; Benziflex†; Benzitrat; Ciclinalgin†; Ciflogex; Eridamin†; Flogin-Ped; Flogo Rosa; Flogoral; Fonergoral; Gino-Panflogin†; Neoflogin; Panflogin†; Petiflog†; Top Flog†; ***Canad.:*** Sun-Benz; Tantum; ***Denm.:*** Andolex; ***Fr.:*** Opalgyne; ***Ger.:*** Tantum Verde; ***Hong Kong:*** Difflam; Verax; ***Irl.:*** Difflam; ***Israel:*** Easy gel; ***Ital.:*** Afloben; Benzirin; Ginesal; Lagin; Multum; Saniflor Collutorio; Saniflor Vena†; Tantum; Verax; ***Malaysia:*** Difflam Anti-inflammatory Lozenges; Difflam Solution; ***Mex.:*** Lonol; Vantal; ***Neth.:*** Tantum†; ***NZ:*** Difflam; ***Port.:*** Flogoral; Rosalgin; Tantum; Tantum Verde; ***S.Afr.:*** Andolex; ***Singapore:*** Difflam; ***Spain:*** Cratimon†; Fulgium; Rosalgin; Tantum; Tantum Verde; ***Swed.:*** Andolex; ***Switz.:*** Bucco-Tantum; ***Thai.:*** Difflam; ***UK:*** Difflam.

**Multi-ingredient:** ***Arg.:*** Buchex; Dresan; Dresan Biotic; Espectocural; Pentadent; ***Austral.:*** Difflam Anti-inflammatory Cough Lozenges; Difflam Lozenges; Difflam Mouth Gel; Difflam-C; Logicin Rapid Relief; ***Braz.:*** Angino-Rub; ***Fr.:*** Hexo-Imotryl†; ***Hong Kong:*** Difflam-C; Logicin Rapid Relief; ***Ital.:*** Algolisina; Gola Action; Leucorsan†; Linea F; Mediplus; ***Malaysia:*** Difflam Anti-inflammatory Lozenges (with Antibacterial); Difflam Mouth Gel; Difflam-C; ***Mex.:*** Lonol Sport; ***NZ:*** Difflam Anti-inflammatory Antibacterial Lozenges†; Difflam Cough; Difflam Mouth Gel; Difflam-C; ***Port.:*** Tantum Rosa; Tantum Verde; ***S.Afr.:*** Andolex-C; ***Singapore:*** Difflam Mouth Gel; Difflam-C; ***Spain:*** Bristaciclina Dental; Dolosarto; Etermol Antitusivo; Mentamida; Prosturol; Tantum; Tantum Ciclina†; Vinciseptil Otico.

## Benzyl Nicotinate

Nicotinato de bencilo. Benzyl pyridine-3-carboxylate.

$C_{13}H_{11}NO_2$ = 213.2.

*CAS — 94-44-0.*

**Pharmacopoeias.** In *Ger.*

### Profile

Benzyl nicotinate is used in topical preparations as a rubefacient.

### Preparations

**Proprietary Preparations** (details are given in Part 3)

***Ger.:*** Pernionin Teil-Bad; Pykaryl T; Rheubalmin Bad Nico†; Rubriment.

**Multi-ingredient:** ***Arg.:*** Butidiona; Oxa Sport; Pergalen; ***Austria:*** Ambenat; Bayolin; Derivon; Expectal-Balsam; Igitur-antirheumatische; Igitur-Rheumafluid; Menthoneurin; Mobilisin plus; Pelvichthol†; Rheumex; Rubizon-Rheumagel; Rubriment; Thermo-Rheumon; Thrombophob; Tifen-so†; ***Belg.:*** Forapin†; ***Braz.:*** Etrat; Pergalen†; Trombofob; ***Chile:*** Bayro-Therm; ***Fin.:*** Trombosol; ***Fr.:*** Lumbalgine; ***Ger.:*** ABC Warme-Salbe; Akrotherm†; Ambene N; Arthrodestal N; Bartelin nico†; Brachont†; Camphopin; Capsamol; Caye Balsam; Contrheuma†; Cor-Select; Dolo-Menthoneurin CreSa†; Dolorgiet†; DoloVisano Salbe; Emasex-N; exrheudon OPT†; Fibraflex†; Flexocutan N†; Forapin E; Heilit†; Hot Thermo; Intradermi Fluid N†; Lomazell forte N; Marament Balsam W†; Menthoneurin-Vollbad N†; mikanil; Myalgol N†; Nitro-Praecordin N†; Ortholan mit Salicylester†; Ostochont; Pelvichthol N; Percutase N†; Pernionin Voll-Bad N; Pernionin†; Phardol Rheuma; Phlogont-Thermal; Praecordin S; Reumaless†; Rheubalmin Thermo; Rheubalmin†; Rheuma-Bad†; Rheuma-Liquidum†; Rheuma-Salbe; Rheuma-Salbe N; Rheumasalbe; Rheumasan N; Rheumasit; Rosarthron forte†; Rubriment; Rubriment-N; Salhumin Gel N†; Tachyneng Campher Herzsalbe; Tachynerg N†; Thermo Mobilisin†; thermo-loges†; Thermo-Menthoneurin; Thermo-Menthoneurin Bad†; Thermo-Rheumon; Thermosenex; Togal Mobil Rheuma-Bad†; Togal Mobil-Gel; Warme-Gel; zuk thermo; ***Hong Kong:*** Salomethyl; ***India:*** Beparine; K5 Hair Tincture; Thrombophob; ***Ital.:*** Lasoreuma†; Salonpas; Sloan; ***Mex.:*** Bayro Termo; ***Neth.:*** Menthoneurin†; Sloan's balsem; ***Port.:*** Adrinex; DM Termo†; Medalginan; ***S.Afr.:*** Thrombophob†; ***Switz.:*** Artragel†; Assan-Thermo; Demotherm Pommade contre le rhumatisme; Dolo Demotherm; Forapin; Histalgane; Incutin†; Marament-N; Roliwol S†; Thermocutan; ***UK:*** Salonair.

## Beta-aminopropionitrile

Aminopropionitrile; β-Aminopropionitrile; β-Aminopropionitrilo; BAPN. 3-Aminopropionitrile.

$C_3H_6N_2$ = 70.09.

*CAS — 151-18-8.*

### Profile

Beta-aminopropionitrile, a lysyl oxidase inhibitor, is an anti-inflammatory used as the fumarate in veterinary medicine for the treatment of tendinitis.

## Bezitramide *(BAN, rINN)*

Bezitramida; R-4845. 4-[4-(2,3-Dihydro-2-oxo-3-propionyl-1*H*-benzimidazol-1-yl)piperidino]-2,2-diphenylbutyronitrile.

$C_{31}H_{32}N_4O_2$ = 492.6.

*CAS — 15301-48-1.*

*ATC — N02AC05.*

### Profile

Bezitramide is an opioid analgesic (p.71) that has been given by mouth in the treatment of severe pain. Its action is slow in onset, but prolonged.

◊ References.

1. Meijer DKF, *et al.* Pharmacokinetics of the oral narcotic analgesic bezitramide and preliminary observations on its effect on experimentally induced pain. *Eur J Clin Pharmacol* 1984; **27:** 615–18.

### Preparations

**Proprietary Preparations** (details are given in Part 3)

***Belg.:*** Burgodin†.

## Bornyl Salicylate

Borneol Salicylate; Salicilato de bornilo. 2-Hydroxybenzoic acid 1,7,7-trimethylbicyclo[2.2.1]hept-2-yl ester.

$C_{17}H_{22}O_3$ = 274.4.

*CAS — 560-88-3.*

### Profile

Bornyl salicylate is a salicylic acid derivative that is used topically in rubefacient preparations similarly to methyl salicylate (p.59) for the relief of pain in musculoskeletal and joint disorders.

### Preparations

**Proprietary Preparations** (details are given in Part 3)

**Multi-ingredient:** ***Belg.:*** Forapin†; ***Ger.:*** Contrheuma-Gel forte N†; Forapin E; ***Switz.:*** Acidodermil†; Forapin; Hygiodermil; Sedodermil†.

## Bromfenac Sodium *(USAN, rINNM)*

AHR-10282; AHR-10282B; Bromfenaco sódico. Sodium [2-amino-3-(*p*-bromobenzoyl)phenyl]acetate sesquihydrate.

$C_{15}H_{11}BrNNaO_3,1\frac{1}{2}H_2O$ = 383.2.

*CAS — 91714-94-2 (bromfenac); 91714-93-1 (bromfenac sodium); 120638-55-3 (bromfenac sodium).*

### Profile

Bromfenac sodium, a phenylacetic acid derivative related to diclofenac (p.32), is an NSAID (p.67). It is used as 0.1% eye drops for ocular inflammation. It was formerly given by mouth in the management of acute pain but was withdrawn from the market following reports of severe and sometimes fatal hepatic failure.

### Preparations

**Proprietary Preparations** (details are given in Part 3)

***Jpn:*** Bronuck.

## Bufexamac *(BAN, rINN)*

Bufexamaco; Bufexamacum. 2-(4-Butoxyphenyl)acetohydroxamic acid.

$C_{12}H_{17}NO_3$ = 223.3.

*CAS — 2438-72-4.*

*ATC — M01AB17; M02AA09.*

**Pharmacopoeias.** In *Eur.* (see p.vi) and *Jpn.*

**Ph. Eur. 5.0** (Bufexamac). A white or almost white, crystalline powder. Practically insoluble in water; soluble in dimethylformamide; slightly soluble in ethyl acetate and in methyl alcohol. Protect from light.

### Profile

Bufexamac is an NSAID (p.67) that is applied topically in concentrations of 5% in various skin disorders. Stinging and burning may occur after application; hypersensitivity reactions have been reported.

### Preparations

**Proprietary Preparations** (details are given in Part 3)

***Arg.:*** Parfenac; ***Austral.:*** Paraderm; ***Austria:*** Bufex; Bufexan; Droxaryl; Parfenac; ***Belg.:*** Bufexine; Droxaryl; ***Canad.:*** Norfemac†; ***Fr.:*** Calmaderm†; Parfenac; ***Ger.:*** Allergipuran N†; Bufederm; duradermal; Ekzemase†; Haemo-Exhirud Bufexamac; Jomax; Malipuran; Parfenac; Windol; ***Ital.:*** Fansamac; Parfenal†; Viafen; ***Neth.:*** Parfenac; ***Port.:*** Parfenac; ***S.Afr.:*** Parfenac†; ***Switz.:*** Flogocid†; Parfenac; ***Thai.:*** Droxaryl†.

**Multi-ingredient:** ***Austral.:*** Paraderm Plus; Resolve; ***Austria:*** Droxaryl; ***Belg.:*** Flogocid†; ***Ger.:*** Bufeproct†; Faktu akut; Haemomac†; Hamo-ratiopharm N; Hamoagil plus; Mastu S; Proctoparf†; ***Hong Kong:*** Mastu S; ***NZ:*** Paraderm Plus; ***Switz.:*** Flogocid NN†; ***Thai.:*** Mastu S.

## Bumadizone Calcium *(rINNM)*

Bumadizona cálcica. Calcium 2-(1,2-diphenylhydrazinocarbonyl)hexanoate hemihydrate.

$(C_{19}H_{21}N_2O_3)_2Ca,\frac{1}{2}H_2O$ = 699.8.

*CAS — 3583-64-0 (bumadizone); 34461-73-9 (bumadizone calcium).*

### Profile

Bumadizone calcium is an NSAID (p.67) that is reported to be metabolised to phenylbutazone (p.83) and oxyphenbutazone (p.76). Its use was limited by the risk of agranulocytosis and other haematological adverse effects.

### Preparations

**Proprietary Preparations** (details are given in Part 3)

***Braz.:*** Eumotol†; ***Mex.:*** Desflam; Dibilan F†.

## Buprenorphine *(BAN, rINN)*

Buprenorfina; Buprenorphinum; RX-6029-M. (6*R*,7*R*,14*S*)-17-Cyclopropylmethyl-7,8-dihydro-7-[(1*S*)-1-hydroxy-1,2,2-trimethylpropyl]-6-*O*-methyl-6,14-ethano-17-normorphine; (2*S*)-2-[(−)-(5*R*,6*R*,7*R*,14*S*)-9a-Cyclopropylmethyl-4,5-epoxy-3-hydroxy-6-methoxy-6,14-ethanomorphinan-7-yl]-3,3-dimethylbutan-2-ol.

$C_{29}H_{41}NO_4$ = 467.6.

*CAS — 52485-79-7.*

*ATC — N02AE01; N07BC01.*

**Pharmacopoeias.** In *Eur.* (see p.vi).

**Ph. Eur. 5.0** (Buprenorphine). A white or almost white crystalline powder. Very slightly soluble in water; freely soluble in acetone; slightly soluble in cyclohexane; soluble in methyl alcohol. It dissolves in dilute solutions of acids. Protect from light.

## Buprenorphine Hydrochloride *(BANM, USAN, rINNM)*

Buprenorphini Hydrochloridum; CL-112302; Hidrocloruro de buprenorfina; NIH-8805; UM-952.

$C_{29}H_{41}NO_4,HCl$ = 504.1.

*CAS — 53152-21-9.*

**Pharmacopoeias.** In *Chin., Eur.* (see p.vi), and *US.*

**Ph. Eur. 5.0** (Buprenorphine Hydrochloride). A white or almost white crystalline powder. Sparingly soluble in water; soluble in alcohol; practically insoluble in cyclohexane; freely soluble in methyl alcohol. Protect from light.

**USP 27** (Buprenorphine Hydrochloride). pH of a 1% solution in water is between 4.0 and 6.0. Store in airtight containers. Protect from light.

## Dependence and Withdrawal

As for Opioid Analgesics, p.71.

Buprenorphine may have a lower potential for producing dependence than pure agonists such as morphine. However, it has been subject to abuse. Abrupt withdrawal of buprenorphine is said to produce only a mild abstinence syndrome.

## Adverse Effects and Treatment

As for Opioid Analgesics in general, p.72.

Local reactions such as rash, erythema, and itching have been reported with the transdermal patches. In isolated cases delayed local allergic reactions with marked signs of inflammation have occurred; the patches should be withdrawn in such cases.

Treatment of adverse effects is similar to that for other opioid analgesics (p.72). The effects of buprenorphine are only partially reversed by naloxone (see under Effects on the Respiratory System, below) but use of the latter is still recommended.

**Incidence of adverse effects.** Adverse effects reported[1] after buprenorphine injection in 8187 patients were nausea (8.8%), vomiting (7.4%), drowsiness (4.3%), sleeping (1.9%), dizziness (1.2%), sweating (0.98%), headache (0.55%), confusion (0.53%), lightheadedness (0.38%), blurred vision (0.28%), euphoria (0.27%), dry mouth (0.11%), depression (0.09%), and hallucinations (0.09%). Some studies have reported nausea, vomiting, and dizziness to be more troublesome with buprenorphine than with morphine.[2,3]

In a trial of *sublingual* buprenorphine 50 of 141 cancer patients withdrew because of side-effects, especially dizziness, nausea, vomiting, and drowsiness; constipation was not reported.[4] A woman developed a painless ulcer on the upper surface of her tongue after she had put sublingual buprenorphine tablets on rather than under her tongue.[5]

Shock occurred[6] in 2 patients 2 hours after receiving *epidural* buprenorphine 300 micrograms; treatment with naloxone was unsuccessful but symptoms disappeared spontaneously after 2 to 3 hours.


1. Harcus AW, *et al.* Methodology of monitored release of a new preparation: buprenorphine. *BMJ* 1979; **2:** 163–5.
2. Sear JW, *et al.* Buprenorphine for postoperative analgesia. *Br J Anaesth* 1979; **51:** 71.
3. Kjaer M, *et al.* A comparative study of intramuscular buprenorphine and morphine in the treatment of chronic pain of malignant origin. *Br J Clin Pharmacol* 1982; **13:** 487–92.
4. Robbie DS. A trial of sublingual buprenorphine in cancer pain. *Br J Clin Pharmacol* 1979; **7** (suppl 3): 315S–17S.
5. Lockhart SP, Baron JH. Tongue ulceration after lingual buprenorphine. *BMJ* 1984; **288:** 1346.
6. Christensen FR, Andersen LW. Adverse reaction to extradural buprenorphine. *Br J Anaesth* 1982; **54:** 476.


**Effects on the heart.** For a report of myocardial infarction associated with abuse of buprenorphine, see Abuse under Precautions, below.

**Effects on mental function.** Psychotomimetic effects have been relatively uncommon with buprenorphine. Hallucinations were reported[1] in only 7 of 8147 patients (0.09%) given buprenorphine by injection. There have been reports of hallucinations following sublingual[2] or epidural[3] administration.


1. Harcus AW, *et al.* Methodology of monitored release of a new preparation: buprenorphine. *BMJ* 1979; **2:** 163–5.
2. Paraskevaides EC. Near fatal auditory hallucinations after buprenorphine. *BMJ* 1988; **296:** 214.
3. MacEvilly M, O'Carroll C. Hallucinations after epidural buprenorphine. *BMJ* 1989; **298:** 928–9.


**Effects on the respiratory system.** There have been varying reports on the occurrence of respiratory depression with buprenorphine. It might be subject to a 'ceiling effect' as respiratory depression does not necessarily increase proportionately with dose. However, high doses of 30 or 40 micrograms/kg given as sole intravenous analgesic in balanced anaesthesia have been associated with severe respiratory depression.[1]

Respiratory depression may be delayed in onset and more prolonged than with morphine and is only partially reversed by naloxone, possibly because buprenorphine is very firmly bound to opioid receptors. A study of sublingual buprenorphine for postoperative pain relief was abandoned when 3 of the first 16 patients showed signs of late-onset respiratory depression after the second dose of buprenorphine; the respiratory depression did not respond to naloxone.[2] Successful reversal has been demonstrated in healthy subjects with buprenorphine-induced respiratory depression given large doses of naloxone 5 or 10 mg, but not with 1 mg; reversal was gradual in onset and decreased the duration of the normally prolonged respiratory depression.[3] The respiratory depressant and analgesic effects of buprenorphine were decreased by the *concomitant* administration of naloxone.[4]


1. Schmidt JF, *et al.* Postoperative pain relief with naloxone: severe respiratory depression and pain after high dose buprenorphine. *Anaesthesia* 1985; **40:** 583–6.
2. Thörn S-E, *et al.* Prolonged respiratory depression caused by sublingual buprenorphine. *Lancet* 1988; **i:** 179–80.
3. Gal TJ. Naloxone reversal of buprenorphine-induced respiratory depression. *Clin Pharmacol Ther* 1989; **45:** 66–71.
4. Lehmann KA, *et al.* Influence of naloxone on the postoperative analgesic and respiratory effects of buprenorphine. *Eur J Clin Pharmacol* 1988; **34:** 343–52.


## Precautions

As for Opioid Analgesics in general, p.72.

Buprenorphine has opioid antagonist actions and may precipitate withdrawal symptoms if given to patients physically dependent on opioids.

Respiratory depression, if it occurs, is relatively slow in onset and of prolonged duration; it may be only partially reversed by naloxone.

Absorption of buprenorphine from transdermal patches may be increased as the temperature rises and patients should therefore avoid exposing the patch to external heat; similarly, patients with fever may require monitoring because of increased absorption. It may take 30 hours for plasma concentrations of buprenorphine to decrease by 50% after removal of a patch; patients who have experienced adverse effects should be monitored during this period.

◊ There is a risk that, with opioid agonist-antagonists such as buprenorphine, their antagonistic effects might impair more effective analgesic therapy. This appeared to happen in 2 cancer patients both of whom were given sublingual buprenorphine that was later substituted by morphine.[1] Conventional doses of morphine were inadequate and in one patient raising the dose of morphine proved fatal.


1. Overweg-van Kints J, Stricker BHC. Falende pijnbestrijding tijdens sublinguaal gebruik van buprenorfine. *Ned Tijdschr Geneeskd* 1987; **131:** 1973–4.


**Abuse.** A 22-year-old man experienced chest pains on each of two occasions after he had inhaled crushed buprenorphine tablets.[1] An ECG taken after the second episode suggested that the patient had suffered a myocardial infarction. The use of adulterants in illicit preparations may also cause adverse effects: 4 patients on substitution treatment developed candida endophthalmitis after intravenously injecting sublingual buprenorphine diluted with lemon juice.[2]


1. Cracowski J-L, *et al.* Myocardial infarction associated with buprenorphine. *Ann Intern Med* 1999; **130:** 537.
2. Cassoux N, *et al.* Presumed ocular candidiasis in drug misusers after intravenous use of oral high dose buprenorphine (Subutex). *Br J Ophthalmol* 2002; **86:** 940–1.


**Breast feeding.** The *British National Formulary* considers that the amount of buprenorphine distributed into breast milk is probably too small to be harmful to a breast-fed infant. However, the manufacturers state that buprenorphine should not be used for substitution treatment in opioid-dependent mothers who are breast feeding.

From a study[1] of a breast-feeding mother who was receiving buprenorphine 4 mg daily, it was estimated that at the age of 4 weeks the total amount ingested by the infant during a 24-hour period was 3.28 micrograms for buprenorphine and 0.33 micrograms for norbuprenorphine.


1. Marquet P, *et al.* Buprenorphine withdrawal syndrome in a newborn. *Clin Pharmacol Ther* 1997; **62:** 569–71.


**Pregnancy.** An infant born to a mother who was being treated with buprenorphine 4 mg daily for diamorphine addiction suffered a minor withdrawal syndrome 2 days after birth.[1] The infant rapidly recovered without any treatment. No further signs of withdrawal occurred when breast feeding was abruptly stopped at the age of 8 weeks. In another report[2] of 15 opioid-dependent mothers who had received buprenorphine maintenance during their pregnancies, withdrawal symptoms were either absent or mild in 12 of the neonates. The remaining 3 neonates required treatment with morphine. There appeared to be no correlation between the buprenorphine dose and the degree of withdrawal symptoms.


1. Marquet P, *et al.* Buprenorphine withdrawal syndrome in a newborn. *Clin Pharmacol Ther* 1997; **62:** 569–71.
2. Fischer G, *et al.* Treatment of opioid-dependent pregnant women with buprenorphine. *Addiction* 2000; **95:** 239–44.


## Interactions

For interactions associated with opioid analgesics, see p.73. Buprenorphine is metabolised by the cytochrome P450 isoenzyme CYP3A4; consequently, use with other drugs that induce or inhibit this isoenzyme may result in changes in plasma concentrations of buprenorphine and, possibly adverse effects. The dose of buprenorphine should be halved when starting treatment with the potent CYP3A4 inhibitor, ketoconazole; a similar reduction should be considered with other CYP3A4 inhibitors.

## Pharmacokinetics

After intramuscular injection, buprenorphine rapidly reaches peak plasma concentrations. Absorption also takes place through the buccal mucosa after sublingual doses and peak plasma concentrations are achieved after 90 minutes. Transdermal application results in absorption through the skin; the minimum effective concentration is reached in 12 to 24 hours and peak plasma concentrations are achieved after about 60 hours. Buprenorphine is about 96% bound to plasma proteins. Plasma elimination half-lives have ranged from 1.2 to 7.2 hours; there is a lack of correlation between plasma concentrations and analgesic activity. Metabolism takes place in the liver by oxidation via the cytochrome P450 isoenzyme CYP3A4 to *N*-dealkylbuprenorphine (norbuprenorphine), and by conjugation to glucuronide metabolites. Buprenorphine is subject to considerable first-pass metabolism after oral doses. However, when given by the usual routes buprenorphine is excreted predominantly unchanged in the faeces; there is some evidence for enterohepatic recirculation. The terminal elimination half-life after sublingual doses is 20 to 25 hours; elimination following transdermal application is slower, with a half-life of about 30 hours. Metabolites are excreted in the urine, but very little unchanged drug is excreted in this way. Small amounts of buprenorphine are distributed into breast milk.

**Administration.** BUCCAL ROUTE. Absorption of sublingual buprenorphine is relatively slow. In a 10-hour study[1] plasma concentrations following 400 or 800 micrograms sublingually peaked at about 200 minutes (range 90 to 360 minutes) and buprenorphine was still detected in plasma at the end of the study. Systemic availability was about 55% (range 16 to 94%) and absorption was more or less complete 5 hours after a dose. However, the authors of a subsequent study[2] considered that this was an overestimation, possibly due to methodological flaws. The later study results indicated that the bioavailability of sublingual buprenorphine is about 30% and that sublingual holding times between 3 and 5 minutes are bioequivalent. Another study found that the bioavailability of sublingual buprenorphine was 50% less from a tablet than from a liquid formulation.[3]


1. Bullingham RES, *et al.* Sublingual buprenorphine used postoperatively: ten hour plasma drug concentration analysis. *Br J Clin Pharmacol* 1982; **13:** 665–73.
2. Mendelson J, *et al.* Bioavailability of sublingual buprenorphine. *J Clin Pharmacol* 1997; **37:** 31–7.
3. Nath RP, *et al.* Buprenorphine pharmacokinetics: relative bioavailability of sublingual tablet and liquid formulations. *J Clin Pharmacol* 1999; **39:** 619–23.


**Children.** The terminal elimination half-life of buprenorphine was only about 1 hour in small children aged 4 to 7 years given 3 micrograms/kg intravenously as premedication, but could not be estimated reliably because of the rapid decline in plasma-buprenorphine concentrations.[1] Clearance values did however appear higher than in adults; steady-state volume of distribution was similar. Premature neonates (gestational age 27 to 32 weeks) given a similar dose followed by an infusion of 0.72 micrograms/kg per hour had a considerably lower clearance rate and had a mean elimination half-life of 20 hours.[2] Although this dosing regimen appeared to be safe, sedation was judged to be inadequate in 4 of the 12 neonates studied. It was suggested that as buprenorphine given by infusion might not produce consistent sedation and analgesia in premature neonates, it could not be recommended for use in neonatal care.


1. Olkkola KT, *et al.* Pharmacokinetics of intravenous buprenorphine in children. *Br J Clin Pharmacol* 1989; **28:** 202–4.
2. Barrett DA, *et al.* The pharmacokinetics and physiological effect of buprenorphine infusion in premature neonates. *Br J Clin Pharmacol* 1993; **36:** 215–19.


**Renal impairment.** Buprenorphine clearance appears to occur mainly by hepatic extraction and metabolism and would not be expected to be related to renal function, whereas metabolites are excreted in urine. In a study, buprenorphine kinetics were similar in anaesthetised healthy patients to those in patients with renal impairment, with a mean elimination half-life of 398 and 239 minutes, respectively.[1] Plasma concentrations of the metabolites norbuprenorphine and buprenorphine-3-glucuronide were increased about 4 times and 15 times respectively in patients with renal impairment,[1] but significant pharmacological activity was unlikely since norbuprenorphine has little analgesic activity compared with the parent compound and buprenorphine-3-glucuronide has none.


1. Hand CW, *et al.* Buprenorphine disposition in patients with renal impairment: single and continuous dosing, with special reference to metabolites. *Br J Anaesth* 1990; **64:** 276–82.

## Uses and Administration

Buprenorphine is an opioid analgesic (p.73) classified as an opioid agonist and antagonist. It is used for the relief of moderate to severe pain and as an adjunct to anaesthesia. Buprenorphine is also used in the treatment of opioid dependence.

Buprenorphine has a relatively slow onset but prolonged duration of action. On intramuscular injection analgesia is apparent within 15 minutes and lasts up to 6 hours. A slower, more prolonged response is achieved after sublingual doses. The analgesic effects of buprenorphine after transdermal application may not be seen for at least 12 to 24 hours.

Buprenorphine is usually given by intramuscular or intravenous injection or sublingually as the hydrochloride or as transdermal patches as the base. For all routes doses are expressed in terms of the base. Buprenorphine hydrochloride 107.8 micrograms is approximately equivalent to 100 micrograms of buprenorphine.

Buprenorphine is given by all the above routes for opioid analgesia in moderate to severe **pain**.

- The dose by intramuscular or slow intravenous injection is 300 to 600 micrograms repeated every 6 to 8 hours as required. Children over 6 months may be given 3 to 6 micrograms/kg by injection every 6 to 8 hours; up to 9 micrograms/kg may be given if required in refractory cases
- By the sublingual route, doses of 200 to 400 micrograms are given every 6 to 8 hours. Suggested sublingual doses for children over 6 years are: 16 to 25 kg, 100 micrograms; 25 to 37.5 kg, 100 to 200 micrograms; and 37.5 to 50 kg, 200 to 300 micrograms
- For opioid treatment of chronic pain in adults transdermal patches delivering amounts of buprenorphine ranging from 35 to 70 micrograms/hour are available. Doses should be individually titrated for each patient according to previous opioid usage. Initial dosages should not exceed 35 micrograms/hour in *opioid-naive* patients. For *patients who have been receiving a strong opioid analgesic* the initial dose of the buprenorphine patch should be based on the previous 24-hour opioid requirement. Use of a patch providing 35 micrograms/hour of buprenorphine is roughly equivalent to 30 to 60 mg of morphine sulfate daily by mouth. During transfer to treatment with buprenorphine patches previous opioid analgesic therapy should be phased out gradually in order to allow for the gradual increase in plasma-buprenorphine concentrations. Patches should be replaced every 72 hours with the new patch being applied to a different site; use of the same area of the skin should be avoided for at least 6 days. More than one patch may be applied if required (apply at the same time to avoid confusion). Buprenorphine patches are not appropriate for acute pain

When used in balanced **anaesthesia** 300 micrograms may be given intramuscularly or 400 micrograms sublingually for premedication; 300 to 450 micrograms may be given intravenously as a perioperative analgesic supplement.

In the treatment of **opioid dependence** in adults and adolescents over 16 years, the initial dose is 0.8 to 4 mg sublingually once daily. The dose may be increased as necessary but maintenance doses should not exceed 32 mg daily. Once the patient has been stabilised, the dosage should be reduced gradually to a lower maintenance dose; treatment may eventually be discontinued if appropriate. For addicts who have not undergone opioid withdrawal before starting buprenorphine, the first dose of buprenorphine should not be given until the first signs of craving appear or until at least 4 hours after the last opioid use. In those already receiving methadone replacement, the dose of methadone should be reduced to a maximum of 30 mg daily before starting buprenorphine therapy. As a deterrent to abuse, a combined sublingual preparation of buprenorphine hydrochloride and naloxone hydrochloride is available in some countries for the treatment of opioid dependence.

**Action.** Buprenorphine is generally described as a mixed agonist-antagonist acting mainly as a partial agonist at μ opioid receptors, with some antagonist activity at κ receptors. It has also been shown to bind at μ, δ, and κ opioid binding sites and to have high affinity for the μ and δ receptors and lesser affinity for the κ receptor.[1] Buprenorphine, like fentanyl, has high lipid solubility, but has a lower intrinsic activity than fentanyl. Differences between buprenorphine and pure μ opioid agonists such as fentanyl, including relatively slow onset of action, prolonged duration of action, resistance to antagonism by naloxone, and lack of correlation between plasma concentrations and analgesic effects, have been explained by differences in the way buprenorphine binds to opioid receptors. In a study *in vitro* buprenorphine had slow rates of association and dissociation from the opioid receptor when compared with fentanyl.[2]

1. Bovill JG. Which potent opioid? Important criteria for selection. *Drugs* 1987; **33:** 520–30.
2. Boas RA, Villiger JW. Clinical actions of fentanyl and buprenorphine: the significance of receptor binding. *Br J Anaesth* 1985; **57:** 192–6.

**Anaesthesia.** In addition to its standard uses in anaesthesia (see above) buprenorphine was shown in a study[1] to antagonise the respiratory rate depression following fentanyl as effectively as naloxone.

1. Boysen K, *et al.* Buprenorphine antagonism of ventilatory depression following fentanyl anaesthesia. *Acta Anaesthesiol Scand* 1988; **32:** 490–2.

**Opioid dependence.** Buprenorphine is used in the treatment of opioid dependence (p.71). Its agonist-antagonist properties may mean that it has a lower potential for dependence and a lower risk of respiratory depression in overdose than pure agonists such as methadone. However, although it has potential in acute management of withdrawal, and is effective for maintenance, its place in clinical practice as an alternative to methadone remains to be proven. Abuse of the preparation, as with other substitution therapies, may be a problem. In patients dependent on high doses of opioids buprenorphine may precipitate withdrawal due to its partial antagonist properties; the daily opioid dose should be reduced gradually in such patients before beginning buprenorphine.

References.

1. Fudala PJ, *et al.* Use of buprenorphine in the treatment of opioid addiction: II physiologic and behavioural effects of daily and alternate-day administration and abrupt withdrawal. *Clin Pharmacol Ther* 1990; **47:** 525–34.
2. Ling W, *et al.* A controlled trial comparing buprenorphine and methadone maintenance in opioid dependence. *Arch Gen Psychiatry* 1996; **53:** 401–407.
3. O'Connor PG, *et al.* A randomized trial of buprenorphine maintenance for heroin dependence in a primary care clinic for substance users versus a methadone clinic. *Am J Med* 1998; **105:** 100–105.
4. Kakko J, *et al.* 1-year retention and social function after buprenorphine-assisted relapse prevention treatment for heroin dependence in Sweden: a randomised, placebo-controlled trial. *Lancet* 2003; **361:** 662–8.
5. Mattick RP, *et al.* Buprenorphine maintenance versus placebo or methadone maintenance for opioid dependence. Available in The Cochrane Library; Issue 2. Chichester: John Wiley; 2004.
6. Gowing L, *et al.* Buprenorphine for the management of opioid withdrawal. Available in The Cochrane Library; Issue 2. Chichester: John Wiley; 2004.

**Pain.** ACUTE PAIN. The *British National Formulary* considers that buprenorphine may antagonise the analgesic effect of previously administered opioids and is generally not to be recommended for the management of *postoperative* pain. Nonetheless, it can be given intramuscularly, intravenously, or sublingually for this purpose, although the intravenous route may be preferred for acute pain relief. The epidural route has also been used.[1] Patient-controlled analgesia with intravenous[2] and intramuscular[3] buprenorphine has been effective although its long half-life may limit such use.

Buprenorphine had no adverse cardiovascular effects when given intravenously after open-heart surgery,[4] suggesting that it was a suitable analgesic for patients with unstable circulation. Epidural analgesia with buprenorphine has also been used after cardiac surgery.[5] Buprenorphine was also considered suitable for the relief of pain in *myocardial infarction*.[6]

1. Miwa Y, *et al.* Epidural administered buprenorphine in the perioperative period. *Can J Anaesth* 1996; **43:** 907–13.
2. Dingus DJ, *et al.* Buprenorphine versus morphine for patient-controlled analgesia after cholecystectomy. *Surg Gynecol Obstet* 1993; **177:** 1–6.
3. Harmer M, *et al.* Intramuscular on demand analgesia: double blind controlled trial of pethidine, buprenorphine, morphine, and meptazinol. *BMJ* 1983; **286:** 680–2.
4. Rosenfeldt FL, *et al.* Haemodynamic effects of buprenorphine after heart surgery. *BMJ* 1978; **2:** 1602–3.
5. Mehta Y, *et al.* Lumbar versus thoracic epidural buprenorphine for postoperative analgesia following coronary artery bypass graft surgery. *Acta Anaesthesiol Scand* 1999; **43:** 388–93.
6. Hayes MJ, *et al.* Randomised trial comparing buprenorphine and diamorphine for chest pain in suspected myocardial infarction. *BMJ* 1979; **2:** 300–2.

CHRONIC PAIN. Transdermal buprenorphine is used for chronic intractable cancer pain.[1] It has also been used successfully in chronic non-cancer pain;[1,2] however, the manufacturers state that this route is not suitable for the treatment of acute pain.

1. Böhme K. Buprenorphine in a transdermal therapeutic system – a new option. *Clin Rheumatol* 2002; **21** (suppl 1): S13–S16.
2. Bálint G. Buprenorphine treatment of patients with non-malignant musculoskeletal diseases. *Clin Rheumatol* 2002; **21** (suppl 1): S17–S18.

### Preparations

**Proprietary Preparations** (details are given in Part 3)
***Arg.:*** Magnogen; Temgesic; ***Austral.:*** Subutex; Temgesic; ***Austria:*** Subutex; Temgesic; ***Belg.:*** Subutex; Temgesic; Transtec; ***Braz.:*** Temgesic; ***Denm.:*** Anorfin; Subutex; Temgesic; ***Fin.:*** Subutex; Temgesic; ***Fr.:*** Subutex; Temgesic; ***Ger.:*** Subutex; Temgesic; Transtec; ***Gr.:*** Subutex; ***Hong Kong:*** Subutex; Temgesic; ***India:*** Norphin; Pentorel; Tidigesic; ***Irl.:*** Temgesic; Transtec; ***Israel:*** Nopan; Subutex; ***Ital.:*** Subutex; Temgesic; ***Malaysia:*** Subutex; Temgesic; ***Mex.:*** Temgesic; ***Neth.:*** Temgesic; ***Norw.:*** Temgesic; ***NZ:*** Temgesic; Temgesic-nX†; ***Port.:*** Buprex; Subutex; Transtec; ***S.Afr.:*** Temgesic; ***Singapore:*** Subutex; Temgesic; ***Spain:*** Buprex; Prefin; Subutex; Transtec; ***Swed.:*** Subutex; Temgesic; ***Switz.:*** Subutex; Temgesic; Transtec; ***Thai.:*** Buprine; Temgesic; ***UK:*** Subutex; Temgesic; Transtec; ***USA:*** Buprenex; Subutex.

**Multi-ingredient:** ***USA:*** Suboxone.

## Butibufen Sodium *(rINNM)*

Butibufén sódico; FF-106 (butibufen). Sodium 2-(4-isobutylphenyl)butyrate.

$C_{14}H_{19}NaO_2$ = 242.3.

*CAS — 55837-18-8 (butibufen); 60682-24-8 (butibufen sodium).*

### Profile

Butibufen sodium is an NSAID (p.67) that has been used by mouth in inflammatory and rheumatic disorders.

### Preparations

**Proprietary Preparations** (details are given in Part 3)
***Spain:*** Mijal†.

## Butorphanol Tartrate *(BANM, USAN, rINNM)*

*levo*-BC-2627 (butorphanol); Tartrato de butorfanol. (−)-17-(Cyclobutylmethyl)morphinan-3,14-diol hydrogen tartrate.

$C_{21}H_{29}NO_2,C_4H_6O_6$ = 477.5.

*CAS — 42408-82-2 (butorphanol); 58786-99-5 (butorphanol tartrate).*

*ATC — N02AF01.*

**Pharmacopoeias.** In *US.*

**USP 27** (Butorphanol Tartrate). A white powder. Its solutions are slightly acidic. Sparingly soluble in water; insoluble in alcohol, in chloroform, in ether, in ethyl acetate, and in hexane; slightly soluble in methyl alcohol; soluble in dilute acids. Store in airtight containers at a temperature of 25°, excursions permitted between 15° and 30°.

### Dependence and Withdrawal

As for Opioid Analgesics, p.71.

Butorphanol may have a lower potential for producing dependence than pure agonists such as morphine. However, it has been subject to abuse. Abruptly stopping chronic butorphanol has produced a less severe withdrawal syndrome than with morphine.

### Adverse Effects and Treatment

As for Opioid Analgesics in general, p.72, and for Pentazocine, p.80.

Headache, and feelings of floating may also occur. Hallucinations and other psychotomimetic effects are rare and have been reported less frequently than with pentazocine. In addition insomnia and nasal congestion may occur frequently when butorphanol is given intranasally.

Because butorphanol has opioid agonist and antagonist activity, naloxone is the recommended antagonist for the treatment of overdosage.

**Effects on the respiratory system.** Butorphanol 2 mg produces a similar degree of respiratory depression to morphine 10 mg, but a ceiling effect is apparent with higher doses of butorphanol.[1] It has been reported to be a less potent respiratory depressant than fentanyl,[2] but more potent than nalbuphine.[3]

1. Nagashima H, *et al.* Respiratory and circulatory effects of intravenous butorphanol and morphine. *Clin Pharmacol Ther* 1976; **19:** 738–45.
2. Dryden GE. Voluntary respiratory effects of butorphanol and fentanyl following barbiturate induction: a double-blind study. *J Clin Pharmacol* 1986; **26:** 203–7.
3. Zucker JR, *et al.* Respiratory effects of nalbuphine and butorphanol in anesthetized patients. *Anesth Analg* 1987; **66:** 879–81.

### Precautions

As for Opioid Analgesics in general, p.72.

Although cardiovascular effects may be less than with pentazocine, butorphanol should generally be avoided after myocardial infarction.

Butorphanol may precipitate withdrawal symptoms if given to patients physically dependent on opioids. The dosage regimen of butorphanol may need to be adjusted in the elderly and in patients with hepatic or renal impairment.

**Abuse.** There has been a report of fibrous myopathy associated with chronic intramuscular abuse of butorphanol.[1]

1. Wagner JM, Cohen S. Fibrous myopathy from butorphanol injections. *J Rheumatol* 1991; **18:** 1934–5.

**Breast feeding.** No adverse effects have been observed in breast-feeding infants whose mothers were receiving butorphanol, and the American Academy of Pediatrics considers[1] that it is therefore usually compatible with breast feeding.

In a study[2] of 12 lactating women, butorphanol was detected in breast milk after both intramuscular and oral administration. However, the milk-to-plasma ratio following a 2-mg intramuscular dose (0.7) was significantly less than that following an 8-mg oral dose (1.9). Although the mothers were not breast feeding at the time of the study, the authors concluded that the potential for any adverse effects on nursing infants following maternal butorphanol use would be minimal.

1. American Academy of Pediatrics The transfer of drugs and other chemicals into human milk. *Pediatrics* 2001; **108:** 776–89. Correction. *ibid.*; 1029. Also available at: http://aappolicy.aappublications.org/cgi/content/full/pediatrics%3b108/3/776 (accessed 02/07/04)
2. Pittman KA, *et al.* Human perinatal distribution of butorphanol. *Am J Obstet Gynecol* 1980; **138:** 797–800.

**Pregnancy.** Two instances of sinusoidal fetal heart rate pattern were noted out of 188 consecutive cases of butorphanol administration in active-phase labour.[1]

1. Welt SI. Sinusoidal fetal heart rate and butorphanol administration. *Am J Obstet Gynecol* 1985; **152:** 362–3.

## Interactions

For interactions associated with opioid analgesics, see p.73.

## Pharmacokinetics

Butorphanol is absorbed from the gastrointestinal tract but it undergoes extensive first-pass metabolism. Peak plasma concentrations occur 0.5 to 1 hour after intramuscular and nasal doses and 1 to 1.5 hours after oral doses. Butorphanol has a plasma elimination half-life of about 3 hours. About 80% is bound to plasma proteins.

Butorphanol is extensively metabolised in the liver through hydroxylation, *N*-dealkylation, and conjugation, only 5% being excreted unchanged. Excretion is mainly in the urine; about 15% of a parenteral dose is excreted in the bile. It crosses the placenta and is distributed into breast milk.

◊ References.

1. Shyu WC, *et al.* Multiple-dose phase I study of transnasal butorphanol. *Clin Pharmacol Ther* 1993; **54:** 34–41.
2. Shyu WC, *et al.* The absolute bioavailability of transnasal butorphanol in patients experiencing rhinitis. *Eur J Clin Pharmacol* 1993; **45:** 559–62.
3. Shyu WC, *et al.* The effects of age and sex on the systemic availability and pharmacokinetics of transnasal butorphanol. *Eur J Clin Pharmacol* 1994; **47:** 57–60.

## Uses and Administration

Butorphanol tartrate, a phenanthrene derivative, is an opioid analgesic (p.73) with opioid agonist and antagonist properties; it is pharmacologically similar to pentazocine (p.80). Butorphanol is used for the relief of moderate to severe pain and as an adjunct to anaesthesia. Onset of analgesia occurs within 10 to 15 minutes of intramuscular injection and may last for 3 to 4 hours. With intranasal use, onset of action is also within 10 to 15 minutes but duration of action can be up to 5 hours.

For the relief of moderate to severe **pain**, butorphanol tartrate is given in doses of 1 to 4 mg by intramuscular injection or in doses of 0.5 to 2 mg by intravenous injection every 3 to 4 hours. It may also be given as a nasal spray, in usual doses of 1 mg (1 spray in 1 nostril), repeated after 60 to 90 minutes, if necessary. This sequence may be repeated after 3 to 4 hours as needed. An initial dose of 2 mg (1 spray in each nostril) may be given for severe pain, but should not be repeated until 3 to 4 hours later.

In **anaesthesia**, 2 mg may be given intramuscularly for premedication 60 to 90 minutes before surgery. For use in balanced anaesthesia a usual dose is 2 mg given intravenously shortly before induction followed by 0.5 to 1 mg intravenously in increments during anaesthesia.

**Dosage adjustment** may be needed in the elderly. When given by injection the initial dose of butorphanol for pain should be half the usual initial adult dose. Subsequent doses should be determined by the patient's response; a dosage interval of at least 6 hours has been recommended. For nasal use the initial dose should be limited to 1 mg followed by 1 mg after 90 to 120 minutes if necessary; subsequent doses if required should generally be given at intervals of not less than 6 hours. Similar recommendations have also been made for patients with hepatic or renal impairment, see below.

◊ References.

1. Atkinson BD, *et al.* Double-blind comparison of intravenous butorphanol (Stadol) and fentanyl (Sublimaze) for analgesia during labor. *Am J Obstet Gynecol* 1994; **171:** 993–8.
2. Gillis JC, *et al.* Transnasal butorphanol: a review of its pharmacodynamic and pharmacokinetic properties, and therapeutic potential in acute pain management. *Drugs* 1995; **50:** 157–75.

**Administration in hepatic or renal impairment.** The dosage of butorphanol may need to be adjusted in patients with hepatic or renal impairment. When given by injection the initial dose for pain should be half the usual initial adult dose (see above). Subsequent doses should be determined by the patient's response; a dosage interval of at least 6 hours has been recommended. For nasal use the initial dose should be limited to 1 mg followed by 1 mg after 90 to 120 minutes if necessary; subsequent doses if required should generally be given at intervals of not less than 6 hours.

**Headache.** Butorphanol has been advocated for use as a nasal spray in the treatment of migraine, but its place in therapy, if any, remains to be established.

References.

1. Freitag FG. The acute treatment of migraine with transnasal butorphanol (TNB). *Headache Q* 1993; **4** (suppl 3): 22–8.
2. Hoffert MJ, *et al.* Transnasal butorphanol in the treatment of acute migraine. *Headache* 1995; **35:** 65–9.
3. Melanson SW, *et al.* Transnasal butorphanol in the emergency department management of migraine headache. *Am J Emerg Med* 1997; **15:** 57–61.

**Pruritus.** Preliminary results from a small study[1] of 6 patients with severe opioid-induced pruritus unresponsive to diphenhydramine indicated that intranasal butorphanol 2 mg administered every 4 to 6 hours may be an effective treatment.

1. Dunteman E, *et al.* Transnasal butorphanol for the treatment of opioid-induced pruritus unresponsive to antihistamines. *J Pain Symptom Manage* 1996; **12:** 255–60.

## Preparations

***USP 27:*** Butorphanol Tartrate Injection.

**Proprietary Preparations** (details are given in Part 3)
***Canad.:*** Stadol; ***Chile:*** Stadol; ***Israel:*** Stadol†; ***Mex.:*** Stadol; ***Spain:*** Verstadol†; ***USA:*** Stadol.

---

## Capsaicin

Capsaicina. (*E*)-8-Methyl-*N*-vanillylnon-6-enamide.
$C_{18}H_{27}NO_3$ = 305.4.
*CAS — 404-86-4.*
*ATC — N01BX04.*

NOTE. Do not confuse capsaicin with capsicin (p.1667) which is capsicum oleoresin.

**Pharmacopoeias.** In *US.*

**USP 27** (Capsaicin). An off-white powder. M.p. 57° to 66°. Practically insoluble in cold water; soluble in alcohol, in chloroform, and in benzene; slightly soluble in carbon disulfide. Store in a cool place in airtight containers. Protect from light.

## Adverse Effects

A warm, stinging, or burning sensation may be experienced at the site of application; this usually disappears after a few days of use but may persist longer if applications are less frequent than recommended (see Uses and Administration, below). Coughing, sneezing, or other signs of respiratory irritation may occur if dried residue from topical preparations is inhaled.

## Precautions

Capsaicin should be handled with care. Particles should not be inhaled nor come into contact with any part of the body.

For topical application, contact with eyes and broken or irritated skin should be avoided. The hands should be washed after application of the cream, unless the hands are the treated areas, in which case, they should be washed 30 minutes after application. If bandages are used to cover treated areas they should not be wound too tightly. Heating pads should not be used with capsaicin, and patients should avoid taking a hot bath or shower immediately before or after application, as the burning sensation may be exacerbated. Thick applications of the cream should be avoided.

## Uses and Administration

Capsaicin is the active principle of the dried ripe fruits of *Capsicum* spp. It is used as a topical analgesic (p.4) in painful conditions such as postherpetic neuralgia after the lesions have healed, diabetic neuropathy, osteoarthritis, and rheumatoid arthritis. Capsaicin is usually applied sparingly 3 or 4 times daily as a 0.025% or 0.075% cream; in the UK this is only licensed for use over 12 years of age, but in the USA it may be used in children over 2 years of age. A more concentrated cream containing 0.25% capsaicin is available in some countries. Capsaicin cream should be rubbed well into the skin until little or no residue is left on the surface. Therapeutic response may not be evident for 1 to 2 weeks for arthritic disorders, or 2 to 4 weeks for neuralgias (or even longer if the head or neck are involved). The UK manufacturer recommends that for the management of painful diabetic neuropathy, capsaicin should only be used under specialist supervision and that treatment should be reviewed after the first 8 weeks and regularly re-evaluated thereafter. Although not a counter-irritant itself, capsaicin has been included in rubefacient preparations for the relief of muscular and rheumatic pain.

**Action.** The analgesic effect following topical application of capsaicin is attributed to its ability to deplete the neuropeptide substance P from local sensory C-type nerve fibres.[1-5] Its action in depleting substance P, after repeated applications, serves to reduce the transmission of pain impulses to the CNS. Since the effect of capsaicin does not rely on vasodilatation in the skin it is therefore not considered to be a traditional counter-irritant.

A vanilloid receptor, activated not only by capsaicin and related substances but also by heat and acids, has been identified.[6]

1. Rumsfield JA, West DP. Topical capsaicin in dermatologic and peripheral pain disorders. *DICP Ann Pharmacother* 1991; **25:** 381–7.
2. Cordell GA, Araujo OE. Capsaicin: identification, nomenclature, and pharmacotherapy. *Ann Pharmacother* 1993; **27:** 330–6.
3. Winter J, *et al.* Capsaicin and pain mechanisms. *Br J Anaesth* 1995; **75:** 157–68.
4. Del Bianco E, *et al.* The effects of repeated dermal application of capsaicin to the human skin on pain and vasodilatation induced by intradermal injection of acid and hypertonic solutions. *Br J Clin Pharmacol* 1996; **41:** 1–6.
5. Fusco BM, Giacovazzo M. Peppers and pain: the promise of capsaicin. *Drugs* 1997; **53:** 909–14.
6. Szallasi A, Blumberg PM. Vanilloid (capsaicin) receptors and mechanisms. *Pharmacol Rev* 1999; **51:** 159–211.

**Cluster headache.** Prevention of occurrence of attacks of cluster headache (p.464) using repeated applications of capsaicin to the nasal mucosa has been reported.[1]

1. Fusco BM, *et al.* Preventative effect of repeated nasal applications of capsaicin in cluster headache. *Pain* 1994; **59:** 321–5.

**Micturition disorders.** Intravesical capsaicin has been tried for painful bladder disorders and to treat bladder detrusor hyperreflexia.[1-5] Results have been variable, and the characteristic sensory effects of capsaicin make blinding of studies difficult, but some patients have reported benefit particularly those with neurological bladder disorders. Instillation into the ureter has also been tried in the management of the loin pain/haematuria syndrome.[6]

1. Nitti VW. Intravesical capsaicin for treatment of neurogenic bladder. *Lancet* 1994; **343:** 1448.
2. Lazzeri M, *et al.* Intravesical capsaicin for treatment of severe bladder pain: a randomized placebo controlled study. *J Urol (Baltimore)* 1996; **156:** 947–52.
3. de Sèze M, *et al.* Capsaicin and neurogenic detrusor hyperreflexia: a double-blind placebo-controlled study in 20 patients with spinal cord lesions. *Neurourol Urodyn* 1998; **17:** 513–23.
4. Petersen T, *et al.* Intravesical capsaicin in patients with detrusor hyper-reflexia: a placebo-controlled cross-over study. *Scand J Urol Nephrol* 1999; **33:** 104–10.
5. de Sèze M, *et al.* Intravesical instillation of capsaicin in urology: a review of the literature. *Eur Urol* 1999; **36:** 267–77.
6. Bultitude MI. Capsaicin in treatment of loin pain/haematuria syndrome. *Lancet* 1995; **345:** 921–2.

**Neuropathic pain.** Capsaicin has been tried topically in various types of pain that may be mediated by the neurotransmitter substance P, including neuropathic pain, which does not generally respond to conventional systemic analgesics. Topical capsaicin is used in the management of diabetic neuropathy (p.6) and postherpetic neuralgia (p.7), but while a meta-analysis[1] of randomised, double-blind, placebo-controlled studies and later studies[2] suggested that it is effective in painful diabetic neuropathy the evidence for efficacy in postherpetic neuralgia was considered[1] to be less convincing. Another meta-analysis suggested that capsaicin was of benefit in neuropathic pain,[3] but noted the difficulty of blinding in placebo-controlled trials of this substance, because of the burning sensation it produces. Other types of neuropathic pain that capsaicin has been tried in include reflex sympathetic dystrophy[4] (see Complex Regional Pain Syndrome, p.5), postmastectomy neuroma,[5,6] and stump pain.[7]

1. Zhang WY, Li Wan Po A. The effectiveness of topically applied capsaicin. *Eur J Clin Pharmacol* 1994; **46:** 517–22.
2. Biesbroeck R, *et al.* A double-blind comparison of topical capsaicin and oral amitriptyline in painful diabetic neuropathy. *Adv Therapy* 1995; **12:** 111–20.
3. Kingery WS. A critical review of controlled clinical trials for peripheral neuropathic pain and complex regional pain syndromes. *Pain* 1997; **73:** 123–39.
4. Cheshire WP, Snyder CR. Treatment of reflex sympathetic dystrophy with topical capsaicin: case report. *Pain* 1990; **42:** 307–11.
5. Watson CPN, Evans RJ. The postmastectomy pain syndrome and topical capsaicin: a randomized trial. *Pain* 1992; **51:** 375–9.
6. Dini D, *et al.* Treatment of the post-mastectomy pain syndrome with topical capsaicin. *Pain* 1993; **54:** 223–6.
7. Rayner HC, *et al.* Relief of local stump pain by capsaicin cream. *Lancet* 1989; **ii:** 1276–7.

**Pruritus.** Substance P is a possible mediator of itch sensations and capsaicin has been tried in the relief of pruritus (p.1137) associated with various diseases and haemodialysis.[1-5] It has also been used to provide relief from pruritus induced by hetastarch[6] and for the itch and pain associated with PUVA therapy.[7,8]

1. Breneman DL, *et al.* Topical capsaicin for treatment of hemodialysis-related pruritus. *J Am Acad Dermatol* 1992; **26:** 91–4.
2. Leibsohn E. Treatment of notalgia paresthetica with capsaicin. *Cutis* 1992; **49:** 335–6.
3. Fölster-Holst R, Brasch J. Effect of topically applied capsaicin on pruritus in patients with atopic dermatitis. *J Dermatol Treat* 1996; **7:** 13–15.
4. Hautmann G, *et al.* Aquagenic pruritus, PUVA and capsaicin treatments. *Br J Dermatol* 1994; **131:** 920–1.
5. Ständer S, *et al.* Treatment of prurigo nodularis with topical capsaicin. *J Am Acad Dermatol* 2001; **44:** 471–8.
6. Szeimies R-M, *et al.* Successful treatment of hydroxyethyl starch-induced pruritus with topical capsaicin. *Br J Dermatol* 1994; **131:** 380–2.
7. Burrows NP, Norris PG. Treatment of PUVA-induced skin pain with capsaicin. *Br J Dermatol* 1994; **131:** 584–5.
8. Kirby B, Rogers S. Treatment of PUVA itch with capsaicin. *Br J Dermatol* 1997; **137:** 152.

**Psoriasis.** Since substance P has been implicated in the pathophysiology of several inflammatory dermatological processes, capsaicin has been tried with some benefit in a number of skin disorders including psoriasis.[1,2]

The usual management of psoriasis is discussed on p.1137.

1. Bernstein JE, *et al.* Effects of topically applied capsaicin on moderate and severe psoriasis vulgaris. *J Am Acad Dermatol* 1986; **15:** 504–7.
2. Ellis CN, *et al.* A double-blind evaluation of topical capsaicin in pruritic psoriasis. *J Am Acad Dermatol* 1993; **29:** 438–42.

**Rheumatic disorders.** Topical capsaicin is used for the temporary relief of the pain of arthritis. From the results of a meta-analysis[1] of randomised, double-blind, placebo-controlled studies and later studies[2,3] it appears that capsaicin is effective in easing the pain of osteoarthritis (p.9) but its role, if any, is unclear; published evidence[4] for efficacy in rheumatoid arthritis (p.9) appears to be limited. Capsaicin may be a useful therapy for pain associated with primary fibromyalgia,[5] which responds poorly to conventional treatment.


1. Zhang WY, Li Wan Po A. The effectiveness of topically applied capsaicin. *Eur J Clin Pharmacol* 1994; **46:** 517–22.
2. Altman RD, *et al.* Capsaicin cream 0.025% as monotherapy for osteoarthritis: a double-blind study. *Semin Arthritis Rheum* 1994; **23** (suppl 3): 25–33.
3. McCleane G. The analgesic efficacy of topical capsaicin is enhanced by glyceryl trinitrate in painful osteoarthritis: a randomized, double blind, placebo controlled study. *Eur J Pain* 2000; **4:** 355–60.
4. Deal CL, *et al.* Treatment of arthritis with topical capsaicin: a double-blind trial. *Clin Ther* 1991; **13:** 383–95.
5. McCarty DJ, *et al.* Treatment of pain due to fibromyalgia with topical capsaicin: a pilot study. *Semin Arthritis Rheum* 1994; **23** (suppl 3): 41–7.


### Preparations

**Proprietary Preparations** (details are given in Part 3)
***Austral.:*** Zostrix; ***Braz.:*** Moment; ***Canad.:*** Antiphlogistine Rub A-535 Capsaicin; Arthricare Hand & Body; Arthritic Pain Relief†; Axsain†; Capzasin-P†; Zostrix; ***Chile:*** Presyc; ***Irl.:*** Axsain; Zacin; ***Israel:*** Zostrix; ***Mex.:*** Capsidol; ***NZ:*** Zostrix; ***Spain:*** Capsicin; Capsicum Farmaya; Capsidol; Gelcen; Katrum; Priltam†; ***Swed.:*** Capsina; ***UK:*** Axsain; Zacin; ***USA:*** Capsin; Capzasin-P; Dolorac; Doublecap; No Pain-HP; R-Gel; Rid-a-Pain HP; Theragen; Zostrix.

**Multi-ingredient:** ***Arg.:*** Atomo Desinflamante C; Rati Salil Crema; ***Austria:*** Rubizon-Rheumagel; ***Braz.:*** Infrarub†; ***Canad.:*** Arthricare Odor Free; Arthricare Ultra; Heet; Methacin; Midalgan; ***Fr.:*** Capsic†; Cliptol Sport; ***Ger.:*** Capsamol; ***Hong Kong:*** Salomethyl; ***India:*** Nimulid Nugel; ***Irl.:*** Algipan; Radian-B; ***Ital.:*** Disalgil; ***UK:*** NatraFlex; ***USA:*** Arthricare Odor Free; Heet; Menthacin; Pain Doctor; Ziks.

## Carbasalate Calcium *(BAN, rINN)*

Calcium Acetylsalicylate Carbamide; Calcium Carbaspirin; Carbasalato cálcico; Carbasalatum Calcicum; Carbasalatum Calcium; Carbaspirin Calcium *(USAN)*. Calcium bis[2-(acetoxy)benzoate]—urea.

$C_{19}H_{18}CaN_2O_9$ = 458.4.
*CAS — 5749-67-7.*
*ATC — B01AC08; N02BA15.*

**Pharmacopoeias.** In *Eur.* (see p.vi).

**Ph. Eur. 5.0** (Carbasalate Calcium). A white crystalline powder. It contains not less than 99.0% and not more than the equivalent of 101.0% of an equimolecular compound of calcium di[2-(acetyloxy)benzoate] and urea, calculated with reference to the anhydrous substance. Freely soluble in water and in dimethylformamide; practically insoluble in acetone and in anhydrous methyl alcohol. Store in airtight containers.

### Adverse Effects, Treatment, and Precautions

As for Aspirin, p.15.

Carbasalate calcium, like aspirin, should not generally be given to children because of the risk of Reye's syndrome.

### Interactions

For interactions associated with aspirin, see p.17.

### Uses and Administration

Carbasalate calcium is a 1:1 complex of calcium acetylsalicylate and urea. It is metabolised to aspirin following absorption and thus has the actions of aspirin (p.17). Carbasalate calcium is given in doses equivalent to 500 mg to 1 g of aspirin (maximum 3 g daily) for pain or fever and in doses equivalent to 0.5 to 2 g of aspirin every 4 hours (maximum 6 g daily) for rheumatic disorders. Carbasalate calcium has also been used in the management of thromboembolic disorders.

### Preparations

**Proprietary Preparations** (details are given in Part 3)
***Austria:*** Iromin; ***Belg.:*** Solupsa†; Upsalgine†; ***Fr.:*** Cardiosolupsan; Solupsan†; ***Neth.:*** Ascal; ***Spain:*** Ascal; ***Switz.:*** Alcacyl.

**Multi-ingredient:** ***Austria:*** Irocopar c C; Irocophan; Iromin-Chinin-C; ***Braz.:*** Gripefin†; ***Fr.:*** Cephalgan; ***Switz.:*** Alca-C; Calonat†.

## Carfentanil Citrate *(USAN, rINNM)*

Citrato de carfentanilo; R-33799. Methyl 1-phenethyl-4-(*N*-phenylpropionamido)isonipecotate citrate.

$C_{24}H_{30}N_2O_3,C_6H_8O_7$ = 586.6.
*CAS — 59708-52-0 (carfentanil); 61380-27-6 (carfentanil citrate).*

### Profile

Carfentanil citrate is an opioid analgesic related to fentanyl (p.40). It is used in veterinary medicine.

## Carprofen *(BAN, USAN, rINN)*

C-5720; Carprofeno; Ro-20-5720/000. (±)-2-(6-Chlorocarbazol-2-yl)propionic acid.

$C_{15}H_{12}ClNO_2$ = 273.7.
*CAS — 53716-49-7.*

### Profile

Carprofen, a propionic acid derivative, is an NSAID (p.67) that is used in veterinary medicine.

## Celecoxib *(BAN, USAN, rINN)*

SC-58635. *p*-[5-*p*-Tolyl-3-(trifluoromethyl)pyrazol-1-yl]benzenesulfonamide.

$C_{17}H_{14}F_3N_3O_2S$ = 381.4.
*CAS — 169590-42-5.*
*ATC — L01XX33; M01AH01.*

### Adverse Effects and Precautions

As for NSAIDs in general, p.67. Celecoxib should not be used in patients with severe hepatic impairment. Therapy should be withdrawn if signs or symptoms of hepatic toxicity develop. Celecoxib should not be given to patients with a history of hypersensitivity to sulfonamides. It is also contra-indicated in patients with severe heart failure, inflammatory bowel disease, and renal impairment associated with a creatinine clearance of less than 30 mL/minute.

**Effects on the cardiovascular system.** Although a large prelicensing study[1] found no increase in the risk of serious cardiovascular events such as myocardial infarction with celecoxib when compared with non-selective NSAIDs, the results are confounded as the study also permitted the use of aspirin for cardiovascular risk reduction. However, a retrospective analysis[2] of these data has also suggested that there is no increase in the risk of serious thrombotic events with celecoxib compared with non-selective NSAIDs regardless of aspirin use. Nonetheless, the UK Committee on Safety of Medicines had received a small number of reports[3] of *myocardial infarction* or *ischaemia* in association with the selective cyclo-oxygenase-2 (COX-2) inhibitors as of February 2001. COX-2 inhibitors such as celecoxib do not possess the intrinsic antiplatelet activity associated with aspirin and possibly other non-selective NSAIDs and consequently do not provide protection against ischaemic cardiac events.[3,4] There have also been 3 cases of *torsade de pointes* associated with celecoxib use.[5]

For a comparison of the *hypertensive effects* of celecoxib and rofecoxib, see p.86.


1. Silverstein FE, *et al.* Gastrointestinal toxicity with celecoxib vs nonsteroidal anti-inflammatory drugs for osteoarthritis and rheumatoid arthritis. The CLASS study: a randomized controlled trial. *JAMA* 2000; **284:** 1247–55.
2. White WB, *et al.* Comparison of thromboembolic events in patients treated with celecoxib, a cyclooxygenase-2 specific inhibitor, versus ibuprofen or diclofenac. *Am J Cardiol* 2002; **89:** 425–30.
3. Committee on Safety of Medicines/Medicines Control Agency. COX-2 selective NSAIDs lack antiplatelet activity. *Current Problems* 2001; **27:** 7. Also available at: http://www.mca.gov.uk/ourwork/monitorsafequalmed/currentproblems/cpfeb2001.pdf (accessed 02/07/04)
4. Bing RJ, Lomnicka M. Why do cyclo-oxygenase-2 inhibitors cause cardiovascular events? *J Am Coll Cardiol* 2002; **39:** 521–2.
5. Pathak A, *et al.* Celecoxib-associated torsade de pointes. *Ann Pharmacother* 2002; **36:** 1290–1.


**Effects on the gastrointestinal tract.** It is generally accepted that the inhibition of cyclo-oxygenase-1 (COX-1) results in the adverse gastrointestinal effects of the NSAIDs, and that the selective inhibition of the other isoform, COX-2, by NSAIDs such as celecoxib may cause less gastrotoxicity than that seen with the non-selective inhibition of the traditional NSAIDs.

Results from controlled trials confirm that NSAIDs selective for COX-2 are associated with a lower incidence of serious gastrointestinal effects. In a placebo-controlled trial[1] the incidence of endoscopically determined gastroduodenal ulcers in patients taking celecoxib for rheumatoid arthritis (dose range 200 to 800 mg daily) was not significantly different to that seen with the placebo group. Another study[2] in patients taking celecoxib at supratherapeutic doses (800 mg daily) concluded that there was a lower combined incidence of symptomatic gastrointestinal ulcers and ulcer complications (bleeding, perforation, and obstruction) after 6 months of treatment when compared with non-selective NSAIDS (ibuprofen 2.4 g daily or diclofenac 150 mg daily). However, the incidence of ulcer complications alone was not significantly different to that seen with other NSAIDs. A re-analysis of the study by the FDA, including both the 6 month and full term data, also found that there was no significant reduction in the rate of ulcer complications with celecoxib compared to the non-selective NSAIDs although, in subjects not taking aspirin, there was a strong trend in favour of celecoxib compared to ibuprofen.[3] The risk of ulcer complications was also significantly increased in celecoxib users taking concomitant low-dose aspirin.[2] A recent systematic review[4] of studies of patients receiving celecoxib or NSAIDs for at least 12 weeks claimed to demonstrate improved gastrointestinal safety and tolerability in those receiving celecoxib (including in patients also taking low-dose aspirin) but has been criticised on grounds of data selection.[5,6] It has been noted that the use of aspirin appears to nullify any potential protective effect of COX-2 selectivity by celecoxib.[7,8]

There have been individual case reports of gastrotoxicity with celecoxib.[9-11]


1. Simon LS, *et al.* Anti-inflammatory and upper gastrointestinal effects of celecoxib in rheumatoid arthritis: a randomized controlled trial. *JAMA* 1999; **282:** 1921–8.
2. Silverstein FE, *et al.* Gastrointestinal toxicity with celecoxib vs nonsteroidal anti-inflammatory drugs for osteoarthritis and rheumatoid arthritis. The CLASS study: a randomized controlled trial. *JAMA* 2000; **284:** 1247–55.
3. US Food and Drug Administration. Celebrex capsules (celecoxib) NDA 20-998/S009—Medical Officer Review. 2000. Available at: http://www.fda.gov/ohrms/dockets/ac/01/briefing/3677b1_03_med.pdf (accessed 02/07/04)
4. Deeks JJ, *et al.* Efficacy, tolerability, and upper gastrointestinal safety of celecoxib for treatment of osteoarthritis and rheumatoid arthritis: systematic review of randomised controlled trials. *BMJ* 2002; **325:** 619–23.
5. Jüni P, *et al.* Systematic review of celecoxib for osteoarthritis and rheumatoid arthritis: problems compromise review's validity. *BMJ* 2003; **326:** 334.
6. Metcalfe S, *et al.* Systematic review of celecoxib for osteoarthritis and rheumatoid arthritis: celecoxib's relative gastrointestinal safety is overstated. *BMJ* 2003; **326:** 334–5.
7. Lichtenstein DR, Wolfe MM. COX-2-selective NSAIDs: new and improved? *JAMA* 2000; **284:** 1297–9.
8. Bates DE, Lemaire JB. Possible celecoxib-induced gastroduodenal ulceration. *Ann Pharmacother* 2001; **35:** 782–3.
9. Mohammed S, Croom DW. Gastropathy due to celecoxib, a cyclooxygenase-2 inhibitor. *N Engl J Med* 1999; **340:** 2005–6.
10. Anonymous. Celecoxib: early Australian reporting experience. *Aust Adverse Drug React Bull* 2000; **19:** 6–7. Also available at: http://www.tga.health.gov.au/docs/html/aadrbltn/aadr0006.htm (accessed 02/07/04)
11. Anonymous. Serious gastrointestinal effects with celecoxib and rofecoxib. *Aust Adverse Drug React Bull* 2003; **22:** 15. Also available at: http://www.tga.health.gov.au/adr/aadrb/aadr0308.htm (accessed 02/07/04)


**Effects on the kidneys.** Increasing evidence of the renal toxicity of the selective cyclo-oxygenase-2 (COX-2) inhibitors such as celecoxib suggests that such NSAIDs appear to have effects on renal function similar to those of the non-selective NSAIDs (see p.68).

Some references to the adverse renal effects of celecoxib.


1. Boyd IW, *et al.* COX-2 inhibitors and renal failure: the triple whammy revisited. *Med J Aust* 2000; **173:** 274.
2. Perazella MA, Tray K. Selective cyclooxygenase-2 inhibitors: a pattern of nephrotoxicity similar to traditional nonsteroidal anti-inflammatory drugs. *Am J Med* 2001; **111:** 64–7.
3. Graham MG. Acute renal failure related to high-dose celecoxib. *Ann Intern Med* 2001; **135:** 69–70.
4. Alkhuja S, *et al.* Celecoxib-induced nonoliguric acute renal failure. *Ann Pharmacother* 2002; **36:** 52–4.
5. Ahmad SR, *et al.* Renal failure associated with the use of celecoxib and rofecoxib. *Drug Safety* 2002; **25:** 537–44.
6. Alper AB, *et al.* Nephrotic syndrome and interstitial nephritis associated with celecoxib. *Am J Kidney Dis* 2002; **40:** 1086–90.


**Effects on the liver.** Cholestatic hepatitis developed in a 54-year-old woman taking celecoxib;[1] her liver function tests improved and her symptoms resolved following drug withdrawal. Despite the temporal relationship between celecoxib treatment and the onset of hepatotoxicity, the manufacturers have stated that current evidence does not support such a relationship.[2] Another case[3] has since been reported.

For a case of acute hepatitis with pancreatitis, see Pancreatitis, below.


1. O'Beirne JP, Cairns SR. Cholestatic hepatitis in association with celecoxib. *BMJ* 2001; **323:** 23.
2. Arellano FM, *et al.* Case of cholestatic hepatitis with celecoxib did not fulfil international criteria. *BMJ* 2002; **324:** 789–90.
3. Grieco A, *et al.* Acute cholestatic hepatitis associated with celecoxib. *Ann Pharmacother* 2002; **36:** 1887–9.


**Effects on the nervous system.** Acute neuropsychiatric reactions such as confusion, somnolence, and insomnia, have occurred following celecoxib use.[1]


1. Anonymous. Acute neuropsychiatric events with celecoxib and rofecoxib. *Aust Adverse Drug React Bull* 2003; **22:** 3. Also available at: http://www.tga.health.gov.au/adr/aadrb/aadr0302.htm (accessed 02/07/04)


**Hypersensitivity.** A 52-year-old man suffered an allergic vasculitis after 8 days of treatment with celecoxib.[1] Despite intensive treatment the patient died from multiple organ failure and diffuse cutaneous necrolysis. The authors noted that potentially fatal skin reactions have occurred with other sulfa-containing drugs, although there is some evidence suggesting that the potential for cross-reactivity in patients sensitive to sulfonamides is relatively low;[2] nonetheless the manufacturers contra-indicate the use of celecoxib in such patients.


1. Schneider F, *et al.* Fatal allergic vasculitis associated with celecoxib. *Lancet* 2002; **359:** 852–3.
2. Shapiro LE, *et al.* Safety of celecoxib in individuals allergic to sulfonamide: a pilot study. *Drug Safety* 2003; **26:** 187–95.


**Pancreatitis.** Acute hepatitis and pancreatitis developed in an elderly patient with a reported history of hypersensitivity to sulfonamides who was given celecoxib.[1] Symptoms resolved on discontinuation of the drug. Pancreatitis has also been reported in a patient known to be tolerant of sulfonamides.[2]


1. Carrillo-Jimenez R, Nurnberger M. Celecoxib-induced acute pancreatitis and hepatitis: a case report. *Arch Intern Med* 2000; **160:** 553–4.
2. Baciewicz AM, *et al.* Acute pancreatitis associated with celecoxib. *Ann Intern Med* 2000; **132:** 680.

### Interactions

The metabolism of celecoxib is mediated mainly by the cytochrome P450 isoenzyme CYP2C9. Use with other drugs that inhibit or induce or are metabolised by this isoenzyme may result in changes in plasma concentration of celecoxib; fluconazole has increased plasma concentrations of celecoxib and the manufacturers recommend that the dose of celecoxib should be halved when given with fluconazole.

Celecoxib is an inhibitor of the isoenzyme CYP2D6 and the potential therefore exists for an effect on drugs metabolised by this enzyme.

For interactions associated with NSAIDs in general, see p.69.

### Pharmacokinetics

Celecoxib is absorbed from the gastrointestinal tract, peak plasma concentrations being achieved after about 3 hours. Protein binding is about 97%. Celecoxib is metabolised in the liver mainly by the cytochrome P450 isoenzyme CYP2C9; the three identified metabolites are inactive as inhibitors of COX-1 or COX-2 enzymes. It is eliminated mainly as metabolites in the faeces and urine; less than 3% is recovered as unchanged drug. The effective terminal half-life is about 11 hours. The pharmacokinetics of celecoxib may vary in different ethnic groups; it has been stated that the area under the curve is elevated in patients of Afro-Caribbean origin, although any clinical significance is unclear.

◊ References.

1. Davies NM, *et al.* Clinical pharmacokinetics and pharmacodynamics of celecoxib: a selective cyclo-oxygenase-2 inhibitor. *Clin Pharmacokinet* 2000; **38:** 225–42.

### Uses and administration

Celecoxib is an NSAID (p.70) reported to be a selective inhibitor of cyclo-oxygenase-2 (COX-2). It is used in the treatment of rheumatoid arthritis and osteoarthritis and in the adjunctive treatment of adenomatous colorectal polyps. Celecoxib is also used in the management of acute pain and dysmenorrhoea.

For osteoarthritis the recommended dose is 200 mg daily given by mouth as a single dose or in 2 divided doses. If necessary a dose of 200 mg twice daily may be used. For rheumatoid arthritis the dose is 100 to 200 mg given twice daily. In elderly patients treatment should be initiated at the lowest recommended dose.

In the treatment of pain and dysmenorrhoea, an initial dose of 400 mg followed by an additional dose of 200 mg, if necessary, is recommended on the first day; thereafter the dose is 200 mg twice daily.

Celecoxib is also used as an adjunct to standard therapy to reduce the number of adenomatous colorectal polyps in patients with familial adenomatous polyposis. For this purpose it may be given in doses of 400 mg twice daily with food.

Reduced doses are recommended in patients with hepatic impairment (see below).

◊ Reviews.

1. Clemett D, Goa KL. Celecoxib: a review of its use in osteoarthritis, rheumatoid arthritis and acute pain. *Drugs* 2000; **59:** 957–80.

**Administration in hepatic impairment.** The manufacturers recommend that doses of celecoxib should be reduced by 50% in patients with moderate hepatic impairment.

**Familial adenomatous polyposis.** Celecoxib is used in the treatment of familial adenomatous polyposis, an inherited syndrome known to predispose sufferers to the development of colonic cancer (see Malignant Neoplasms of the Gastrointestinal Tract, p.516). A randomised trial[1,2] found that treatment with celecoxib reduced the number of colonic polyps; the authors considered celecoxib to be a useful adjunct to the standard therapy of colectomy.

1. Steinbach G, *et al.* The effect of celecoxib, a cyclooxygenase-2 inhibitor, in familial adenomatous polyposis. *N Engl J Med* 2000; **342:** 1946–52.
2. Phillips RKS, *et al.* A randomised, double blind, placebo controlled study of celecoxib, a selective cyclooxygenase 2 inhibitor, on duodenal polyposis in familial adenomatous polyposis. *Gut* 2002; **50:** 857–60.

**Musculoskeletal and joint disorders.** Celecoxib is used in the treatment of osteoarthritis (p.9) and rheumatoid arthritis (p.9). However, in the UK it is recommended that the use of celecoxib and other selective cyclo-oxygenase-2 (COX-2) inhibitors be limited to those patients considered to be at high risk of developing serious gastrointestinal problems if given a non-selective NSAID. High-risk patients include the elderly, the debilitated, and those already receiving gastrotoxic drugs.

Celecoxib has also been tried in the treatment of ankylosing spondylitis.

References.

1. Bensen WG, *et al.* Treatment of osteoarthritis with celecoxib, a cyclooxygenase-2 inhibitor: a randomized controlled trial. *Mayo Clin Proc* 1999; **74:** 1095–1105.
2. Anonymous. Celecoxib for arthritis. *Med Lett Drugs Ther* 1999; **41:** 11–12.
3. Simon LS, *et al.* Anti-inflammatory and upper gastrointestinal effects of celecoxib in rheumatoid arthritis: a randomized controlled trial. *JAMA* 1999; **282:** 1921–28.
4. Emery P, *et al.* Celecoxib versus diclofenac in long-term management of rheumatoid arthritis: randomised double-blind comparison. *Lancet* 1999; **354:** 2106–11.
5. Dougados M, *et al.* Efficacy of celecoxib, a cyclooxygenase 2-specific inhibitor, in the treatment of ankylosing spondylitis: a six-week controlled study with comparison against placebo and against a conventional nonsteroidal antiinflammatory drug. *Arthritis Rheum* 2001; **44:** 180–5.
6. Tindall EA, *et al.* A 12-month, multicenter, prospective, open-label trial of radiographic analysis of disease progression in osteoarthritis of the knee or hip in patients receiving celecoxib. *Clin Ther* 2002; **24:** 2051–63.
7. Stengaard-Pedersen K, *et al.* Celecoxib 200 mg qd is efficacious in the management of osteoarthritis of the knee or hip regardless of the time of dosing. *Rheumatology (Oxford)* 2004; **43:** 592–5.

### Preparations

**Proprietary Preparations** (details are given in Part 3)
***Arg.:*** Celebrex; Celemax; Coxel; Coxtenk; Niflam; Tisorek; ***Austral.:*** Celebrex; ***Austria:*** Celebrex; Solexa; ***Belg.:*** Celebrex; ***Braz.:*** Celebra; ***Canad.:*** Celebrex; ***Chile:*** Celebra; ***Denm.:*** Celebra; ***Fin.:*** Celebra; ***Fr.:*** Celebrex; ***Ger.:*** Celebrex; ***Hong Kong:*** Celebrex; ***India:*** Celib; Zycel; ***Irl.:*** Celebrex; ***Israel:*** Celcox; Celebra; ***Ital.:*** Artilog; Celebrex; Solexa; ***Malaysia:*** Celebrex; ***Mex.:*** Celebrex; ***Neth.:*** Celebrex; Solexa; ***Norw.:*** Celebra; ***NZ:*** Celebrex; ***Port.:*** Celebrex; Solexa; ***S.Afr.:*** Celebrex; ***Singapore:*** Celebrex; ***Spain:*** Celebrex; ***Swed.:*** Celebra; ***Switz.:*** Celebrex; ***Thai.:*** Celebrex; ***UK:*** Celebrex; ***USA:*** Celebrex.

## Choline Magnesium Trisalicylate

Trisalicilato de colina y magnesio.
*CAS — 64425-90-7.*

### Adverse Effects, Treatment, and Precautions

As for Aspirin, p.15.

The use of aspirin and other acetylated salicylates is generally not recommended for children unless specifically indicated, because of the risk of Reye's syndrome. US licensing information extends this precaution to choline magnesium trisalicylate.

**Effects on the liver.** References.

1. Cersosimo RJ, Matthews SJ. Hepatotoxicity associated with choline magnesium trisalicylate: case report and review of salicylate-induced hepatotoxicity. *Drug Intell Clin Pharm* 1987; **21:** 621–5.

### Interactions

For interactions associated with salicylates, see Aspirin, p.17.

### Uses and Administration

Choline magnesium trisalicylate is a combination of the salicylic acid derivatives choline salicylate (p.26) and magnesium salicylate (p.55). It has analgesic, anti-inflammatory, and antipyretic actions similar to those of aspirin (p.17). Following oral administration, choline magnesium trisalicylate dissociates and the salicylate moiety is rapidly absorbed. Each unit dose of 500 mg of salicylate is provided by approximately 293 mg of choline salicylate with 362 mg of magnesium salicylate (anhydrous). Choline magnesium trisalicylate is used in osteoarthritis, rheumatoid arthritis, and other arthritides in doses equivalent to 1 or 1.5 g of salicylate twice daily by mouth; doses may also be given as a single daily dose if required. A dose of 750 mg given three times daily may be more suitable for elderly patients. Choline magnesium trisalicylate is also used in similar doses in the general management of other forms of pain and for fever.

### Preparations

**Proprietary Preparations** (details are given in Part 3)
***Canad.:*** Trilisate; ***USA:*** Trilisate†.

## Choline Salicylate *(BAN, USAN, rINN)*

Salicilato de colina. (2-Hydroxyethyl)trimethylammonium salicylate.
$C_{12}H_{19}NO_4$ = 241.3.
*CAS — 2016-36-6.*
*ATC — N02BA03.*

**Pharmacopoeias.** *Br.* includes a solution.

**BP 2003** (Choline Salicylate Solution). An aqueous solution containing 47.5 to 52.5% of choline salicylate. It is a clear colourless liquid. It may contain a suitable antimicrobial preservative.

### Profile

Choline salicylate is a salicylic acid derivative (see Aspirin, p.15) used in the treatment of pain and fever, and in the management of rheumatic disorders. In terms of salicylate content, choline salicylate 435 mg is approximately equivalent to 325 mg of aspirin. Choline salicylate is given by mouth in doses of 435 to 870 mg every four hours as necessary for pain and fever, and in doses of 4.8 to 7.2 g daily in divided doses for rheumatic disorders.

Choline salicylate is also used as a local analgesic. Solutions containing up to about 20% choline salicylate are used in ear disorders such as the relief of pain in otitis media and externa but are considered to be of doubtful value; they are also used to soften ear wax as an aid to removal (see p.1262). An 8.7% gel is used for lesions of the mouth (p.1245). Choline salicylate has also been applied topically in a rubefacient preparation for the relief of muscular and rheumatic pain.

Choline salicylate is also given in the form of choline magnesium trisalicylate (see above).

**Adverse effects.** A 21-month-old boy developed salicylate poisoning after his mother had rubbed the contents of 3 tubes of 'Bonjela' teething ointment (containing a total of 2.61 g of choline salicylate) on his gums over 48 hours.[1]

1. Paynter AS, Alexander FW. Salicylate intoxication caused by teething ointment. *Lancet* 1979; **ii:** 1132.

### Preparations

***BP 2003:*** Choline Salicylate Ear Drops; Choline Salicylate Oromucosal Gel.

**Proprietary Preparations** (details are given in Part 3)
***Arg.:*** Dercolina; ***Austral.:*** Applicaine; Herron Baby Teething Gel; Ora-Sed Jel; ***Belg.:*** Teejel; ***Canad.:*** Teejel; ***Ger.:*** Audax; ***Hong Kong:*** Ora-Sed; ***India:*** Gelora; Zytee; ***Irl.:*** Audax; Teejel; ***Israel:*** Teejel; ***NZ:*** Applicaine†; Ora-Sed; ***Singapore:*** Ora-Sed; ***UK:*** Audax; Dinnefords Teejel; ***USA:*** Arthropan.

**Multi-ingredient:** ***Arg.:*** Pansoral; ***Austral.:*** Bonjela; Seda-Gel; ***Austria:*** Mundisal; Tifenso†; ***Belg.:*** Givalex; ***Fr.:*** Givalex; Pansoral; ***Ger.:*** Givalex; Mundisal; ***Hong Kong:*** Bonjela; Dermojela; ***Irl.:*** Bonjela; ***Israel:*** Bonjela; ***Malaysia:*** Bonjela; ***NZ:*** Bonjela; ***Port.:*** Bucagel; ***S.Afr.:*** Bonjela; ***Singapore:*** Bonjela; ***Spain:*** Aldo Otico; ***Switz.:*** Mundisal; Pansoral†; ***Thai.:*** Bonjela; ***UK:*** Bonjela; Earex Plus.

## Clofexamide *(rINN)*

ANP-246; Clofexamida. 2-(4-Chlorophenoxy)-*N*-(2-diethylaminoethyl)acetamide.
$C_{14}H_{21}ClN_2O_2$ = 284.8.
*CAS — 1223-36-5.*

### Profile

Clofexamide has been used topically as the hydrochloride in preparations for musculoskeletal, joint, and soft-tissue disorders.

### Preparations

**Proprietary Preparations** (details are given in Part 3)
**Multi-ingredient:** ***Fr.:*** Perclusone†.

## Clofezone *(rINN)*

ANP-3260; Clofezona. An equimolar combination of clofexamide and phenylbutazone.
$C_{14}H_{21}ClN_2O_2,C_{19}H_{20}N_2O_2,2H_2O$ = 629.2.
*CAS — 60104-29-2.*
*ATC — M01AA05; M02AA03.*

### Profile

Clofezone, a combination molecule containing clofexamide (above) and phenylbutazone (p.83), has been used topically in preparations for musculoskeletal, joint, and soft-tissue disorders.

### Preparations

**Proprietary Preparations** (details are given in Part 3)
**Multi-ingredient:** ***Fr.:*** Perclusone†.

## Clonixin *(USAN, rINN)*

CBA-93626; Clonixino; Sch-10304. 2-(3-Chloro-*o*-toluidino)nicotinic acid.
$C_{13}H_{11}ClN_2O_2$ = 262.7.
*CAS — 17737-65-4.*

### Profile

Clonixin is an NSAID (p.67). It has been used as the lysine salt in doses of up to 250 mg four times daily by mouth for the relief of pain. Clonixin lysine has also been given by intramuscular or intravenous injection and as a rectal suppository.

◊ References.

1. Eberhardt R, *et al.* Analgesic efficacy and tolerability of lysine-clonixinate versus ibuprofen in patients with gonarthrosis. *Curr Ther Res* 1995; **56:** 573–80.

### Preparations

**Proprietary Preparations** (details are given in Part 3)
***Arg.:*** Clonixil; Diclen; Dolex; Dolnot; Dorixina; ***Braz.:*** Dolamin; ***Chile:*** Blonax; Clonalgin; Colmax; Dentagesic; Diminon; Dolalgial; Lafigesic; Medigesic; Nefersil; Traumicid; ***Mex.:*** Disinal; Donodol; Dorixina; Firac; Prestodol; ***Port.:*** Algimate; Clonix; ***Spain:*** Dolalgial.

**Multi-ingredient:** ***Arg.:*** Amplibenzatin Bronquial; Aseptobron Ampicilina; Dorixina B1 B6 B12; Dorixina Relax; Espasmo Dolex; Migra Dorixina; Mikesan; Nova Paratropina Compositum; Sertal Compuesto; ***Chile:*** Clonalgin Compuesto; Ergonef; Migra-Nefersil; Nefersil B; Neurocam; ***Mex.:*** Donodol Compuesto; Espacil Compuesto; Firac Plus; Plidan Compuesto.

## Codeine (BAN)

Codeína; Codeinum; Methylmorphine; Metilmorfina; Morphine Methyl Ether. 7,8-Didehydro-4,5-epoxy-3-methoxy-17-methylmorphinan-6-ol monohydrate.

$C_{18}H_{21}NO_3,H_2O$ = 317.4.

*CAS — 76-57-3 (anhydrous codeine); 6059-47-8 (codeine monohydrate).*

*ATC — R05DA04.*

**Pharmacopoeias.** In *Eur.* (see p.vi), *Int., US,* and *Viet.*

**Ph. Eur. 5.0** (Codeine). White or almost white, crystalline powder or colourless crystals. Soluble in boiling water; freely soluble in alcohol. Protect from light.

**USP 27** (Codeine). Colourless or white crystals or white crystalline powder. It effloresces slowly in dry air. Soluble 1 in 120 of water, 1 in 2 of alcohol, 1 in 0.5 of chloroform, and 1 in 50 of ether. Its saturated solution in water is alkaline to litmus. Store in airtight containers. Protect from light.

### Codeine Hydrochloride (BANM)

Codeína, hidrocloruro de; Codeini Hydrochloridum Dihydricum.

$C_{18}H_{21}NO_3,HCl,2H_2O$ = 371.9.

*CAS — 1422-07-7 (anhydrous codeine hydrochloride).*

**Pharmacopoeias.** In *Eur.* (see p.vi).

**Ph. Eur. 5.0** (Codeine Hydrochloride Dihydrate; Codeine Hydrochloride BP 2003). Small colourless crystals or a white or almost white, crystalline powder. Soluble in water; slightly soluble in dehydrated alcohol; practically insoluble in cyclohexane. Protect from light.

### Codeine Phosphate (BANM)

Codeína, fosfato de; Codeine Phosphate Hemihydrate; Codeini Phosphas; Codeini Phosphas Hemihydricus; Codeinii Phosphas; Methylmorphine Phosphate.

$C_{18}H_{21}NO_3,H_3PO_4,\frac{1}{2}H_2O$ = 406.4.

*CAS — 52-28-8 (anhydrous codeine phosphate); 41444-62-6 (codeine phosphate hemihydrate); 5913-76-8 (codeine phosphate sesquihydrate).*

NOTE. Compounded preparations of codeine phosphate may be represented by the following names:

- Co-codamol *x/y* (*BAN*)—where *x* and *y* are the strengths in milligrams of codeine phosphate and paracetamol respectively
- Co-codAPAP (*PEN*)—codeine phosphate and paracetamol
- Co-codaprin (*BAN*)—codeine phosphate 1 part and aspirin 50 parts (w/w)
- Co-codaprin (*PEN*)—codeine phosphate and aspirin.

**Pharmacopoeias.** In *Chin., Eur.* (see p.vi), *Int., Jpn, Pol., US,* and *Viet.*

Pharmacopoeias may specify the hemihydrate, sesquihydrate, or both, either under one monograph or as separate monographs.

**Ph. Eur. 5.0** (Codeine Phosphate Hemihydrate; Codeine Phosphate BP 2003). A white or almost white, crystalline powder or small, colourless crystals. Freely soluble in water; slightly soluble or very slightly soluble in alcohol. A 4% solution in water has a pH of 4.0 to 5.0. Protect from light.

**Ph. Eur. 5.0** (Codeine Phosphate Sesquihydrate; Codeini Phosphas Sesquihydricus). A white or almost white, crystalline powder or small, colourless crystals. Freely soluble in water; slightly soluble in alcohol. A 4% solution in water has a pH of 4.0 to 5.0. Protect from light.

**USP 27** (Codeine Phosphate). The hemihydrate occurs as fine, white, needle-shaped crystals or white crystalline powder; odourless. Soluble 1 in 2.5 of water, 1 in 0.5 of water at 80°, 1 in 325 of alcohol, and 1 in 125 of boiling alcohol. Its solutions are acid to litmus. Store in airtight containers at a temperature of 25°, excursions permitted between 15° and 30°. Protect from light.

**Incompatibility.** Acetylation of codeine phosphate by aspirin has occurred in solid dosage forms containing the two drugs, even at a low moisture level.[1] *Animal* work suggested that the analgesic activity of codeine was not affected by acetylation.[2]

1. Galante RN, *et al.* Solid-state acetylation of codeine phosphate by aspirin. *J Pharm Sci* 1979; **68:** 1494–8.
2. Buckett WR, *et al.* The analgesic properties of some 14-substituted derivatives of codeine and codeinone. *J Pharm Pharmacol* 1964; **16:** 174–82.

### Codeine Sulfate

Codeína, sulfato de; Codeine Sulphate (BANM).

$(C_{18}H_{21}NO_3)_2,H_2SO_4,3H_2O$ = 750.9.

*CAS — 1420-53-7 (anhydrous codeine sulfate); 6854-40-6 (codeine sulfate trihydrate).*

**Pharmacopoeias.** In *US.*

**USP 27** (Codeine Sulfate). White crystals, usually needle-like, or white crystalline powder. Soluble 1 in 30 of water, 1 in 6.5 of water at 80°, and 1 in 1300 of alcohol; insoluble in chloroform and in ether. Store in airtight containers. Protect from light.

**Stability.** Codeine sulfate solutions appear to be intrinsically more stable than codeine phosphate solutions.[1]

1. Powell MF. Enhanced stability of codeine sulfate: effect of pH, buffer, and temperature on the degradation of codeine in aqueous solution. *J Pharm Sci* 1986; **75:** 901–3.

### Dependence and Withdrawal

As for Opioid Analgesics, p.71. Codeine is subject to abuse (see under Precautions, below), but produces less euphoria and sedation than morphine.

**Neonatal abstinence syndrome.** Some of the symptoms characteristic of the neonatal abstinence syndrome were seen in a neonate whose mother had taken about 90 mg of codeine daily during the last 2 months of pregnancy.[1]

1. Khan K, Chang J. Neonatal abstinence syndrome due to codeine. *Arch Dis Child* 1997; **76:** F59–F60.

### Adverse Effects and Treatment

As for Opioid Analgesics in general, p.72.

In therapeutic doses codeine is much less liable than morphine to produce adverse effects, although constipation may be troublesome with long-term use. Following large doses of codeine, excitement and convulsions may occur.

Codeine, like morphine, has a dose-related histamine-releasing effect. Anaphylactic reactions after intravenous use have been reported rarely.

**Effects on mental function.** Central effects of codeine phosphate appeared to be limited, but dose-related, in subjects given 30, 60, or 90 mg; visuo-motor coordination was altered with doses of 60 and 90 mg and dynamic visual acuity with 90 mg.[1] Drowsiness reported by subjects receiving 90 mg of codeine phosphate could not be linked with impaired performance whereas nausea could.

1. Bradley CM, Nicholson AN. Effects of a μ-opioid receptor agonist (codeine phosphate) on visuo-motor coordination and dynamic visual acuity in man. *Br J Clin Pharmacol* 1986; **22:** 507–12.

**Effects on the pancreas.** A 26-year-old woman developed acute pancreatitis on 2 separate occasions a few hours after taking a single, 40-mg dose of codeine.[1] There was no history of alcohol consumption and her recovery was uneventful.

1. Hastier P, *et al.* Pancreatitis induced by codeine: a case report with positive rechallenge. *Gut* 1997; **41:** 705–6.

**Effects on the skin.** Pruritus and burning erythemato-vesicular plaques that developed in a patient in response to oral codeine were attributed to a fixed drug eruption.[1]

1. Gonzalo-Garijo MA, Revenga-Arranz F. Fixed drug eruption due to codeine. *Br J Dermatol* 1996; **135:** 498–9.

**Overdosage.** Acute codeine intoxication in 430 children, due to accidental ingestion of antitussive preparations, was analysed.[1] The children were nearly all between 1 and 6 years old. Symptoms in decreasing order of frequency included somnolence, rash, miosis, vomiting, itching, ataxia, and swelling of the skin. Respiratory failure occurred in 8 children and 2 died; all 8 had taken 5 mg/kg or more. Infants are at special risk and there have been fatalities[2,3] or near fatalities[4] following inappropriate treatment in infants given mixtures containing codeine.

Opioid toxicity, in addition to severe salicylate toxicity, has occurred in adults following overdoses of aspirin and codeine tablets.[5]

1. von Mühlendahl KE, *et al.* Codeine intoxication in childhood. *Lancet* 1976; **ii:** 303–5.
2. Ivey HH, Kattwinkel J. Danger of Actifed-C. *Pediatrics* 1976; **57:** 164–5.
3. Magnani B, Evans R. Codeine intoxication in the neonate. Abstract: *Pediatrics* 1999; **104:** 1379. Full version: http://pediatrics.aappublications.org/cgi/content/full/104/6/e75 (accessed 02/07/04)
4. Wilkes TCR, *et al.* Apnoea in a 3-month-old baby prescribed compound linctus containing codeine. *Lancet* 1981; **i:** 1166–7.
5. Leslie PJ, *et al.* Opiate toxicity after self poisoning with aspirin and codeine. *BMJ* 1986; **292:** 96.

### Precautions

As for Opioid Analgesics in general, p.72.

**Abuse.** Although the risk of dependence on codeine is low with normal use,[1] it is the subject of deliberate abuse. In the UK linctuses containing codeine are particularly liable to abuse. Reports in the literature include the use in New Zealand of codeine-containing preparations to produce demethylated products known as "Homebake" containing variable amounts of morphine[2] and abuse of co-codaprin tablets for their codeine content.[3-5]

1. Rowden AM, Lopez JR. Codeine addiction. *DICP Ann Pharmacother* 1989; **23:** 475–7.
2. Shaw JP. Drug misuse in New Zealand. *Pharm J* 1987; **238:** 607.
3. Sakol MS, Stark CR. Codeine abuse. *Lancet* 1989; **ii:** 1282.
4. Paterson JR, *et al.* Codeine abuse from co-codaprin. *Lancet* 1990; **335:** 224.
5. Sakol MS, Stark CR. Codeine abuse from co-codaprin. *Lancet* 1990; **335:** 224.

**Breast feeding.** No adverse effects have been observed in breast-feeding infants whose mothers were receiving codeine, and the American Academy of Pediatrics considers[1] that it is therefore usually compatible with breast feeding.

A small study[2] found very low levels of free codeine and its metabolite morphine in the plasma of breast-fed infants whose mothers had taken a 60-mg dose of codeine. It was considered that such levels were subtherapeutic and unlikely to cause respiratory depression.

1. American Academy of Pediatrics. The transfer of drugs and other chemicals into human milk. *Pediatrics* 2001; **108:** 776–89. Correction. *ibid.*; 1029. Also available at: http://aappolicy.aappublications.org/cgi/content/full/pediatrics%3b108/3/776 (accessed 02/07/04)
2. Meny RG, *et al.* Codeine and the breastfed neonate. *J Hum Lact* 1993; **9:** 237–40.

**Children.** See under Overdosage, above, and under Uses and Administration, below.

**Driving.** Codeine phosphate 50 mg alone and in combination with alcohol had a deleterious effect on driving skills in a simulated driving test.[1]

1. Linnoila M, Häkkinen S. Effects of diazepam and codeine, alone and in combination with alcohol, on simulated driving. *Clin Pharmacol Ther* 1974; **15:** 368–73.

### Interactions

For interactions associated with opioid analgesics, see p.73.

**Quinidine.** For reference to a suggestion that quinidine can inhibit the analgesic effect of codeine, see under Metabolism in Pharmacokinetics, below.

### Pharmacokinetics

Codeine and its salts are absorbed from the gastrointestinal tract. Rectal absorption of codeine phosphate has been reported. Ingestion of codeine phosphate produces peak plasma-codeine concentrations in about one hour. Codeine is metabolised by *O*- and *N*-demethylation in the liver to morphine, norcodeine, and other metabolites including normorphine and hydrocodone. Codeine and its metabolites are excreted almost entirely by the kidney, mainly as conjugates with glucuronic acid.

The plasma half-life has been reported to be between 3 and 4 hours after a dose by mouth or intramuscular injection.

◊ References.

1. Guay DR, *et al.* Pharmacokinetics of codeine after single- and multiple-oral-dose administration to normal volunteers. *J Clin Pharmacol* 1987; **27:** 983–7.
2. Persson K, *et al.* The postoperative pharmacokinetics of codeine. *Eur J Clin Pharmacol* 1992; **42:** 663–6.
3. Lafolie P, *et al.* Urine and plasma pharmacokinetics of codeine in healthy volunteers: implications for drugs-of-abuse testing. *J Anal Toxicol* 1996; **20:** 541–6.

**Administration.** In a comparative study[1] codeine had an oral/intramuscular analgesic relative potency ratio of 6:10. This was high compared with that of morphine and was attributed to protection from rapid first-pass metabolism rather than more efficient absorption after oral doses.

1. Beaver WT, *et al.* Analgesic studies of codeine and oxycodone in patients with cancer I: comparisons of oral with intramuscular codeine and of oral with intramuscular oxycodone. *J Pharmacol Exp Ther* 1978; **207:** 92–100.

**Metabolism.** The analgesic effect of codeine may be partly due to its metabolite morphine and it has been suggested that its efficacy may be impaired in patients who are poor metabolisers of codeine[1-3] or in those who are also receiving drugs, such as quinidine, that impair its metabolism.[1] However, patients unable to demethylate codeine to produce detectable plasma concentrations of morphine obtained a similar analgesic effect to patients with detectable plasma morphine concentrations.[4] A study[5] involving infants aged 6 to 10 months has indicated that children were capable of demethylating codeine to morphine at the age of 6 months although glucuronidation of the morphine appeared to be impaired when compared with older children.

1. Desmeules J, *et al.* Impact of environmental and genetic factors on codeine analgesia. *Eur J Clin Pharmacol* 1991; **41:** 23–6.
2. Chen ZR, *et al.* Disposition and metabolism of codeine after single and chronic doses in one poor and seven extensive metabolisers. *Br J Clin Pharmacol* 1991; **31:** 381–90.
3. Sindrup SH, *et al.* Codeine increases pain thresholds to copper vapor laser stimuli in extensive but not poor metabolizers of sparteine. *Clin Pharmacol Ther* 1991; **49:** 686–93.
4. Quiding H, *et al.* Analgesic effect and plasma concentrations of codeine and morphine after two dose levels of codeine following oral surgery. *Eur J Clin Pharmacol* 1993; **44:** 319–23.
5. Quiding H, *et al.* Infants and young children metabolise codeine to morphine: a study after single and repeated rectal administration. *Br J Clin Pharmacol* 1992; **33:** 45–9.

### Uses and Administration

Codeine, a phenanthrene derivative, is an opioid analgesic (p.73) obtained from opium or made by methylating morphine. It is much less potent as an analgesic than morphine and has relatively mild sedative effects.

Codeine or its salts, especially the phosphate, are given by mouth in the form of linctuses for the relief of cough, and as tablets for the relief of mild to moderate pain, often in association with a non-opioid analgesic such as aspirin or paracetamol. The phosphate is also given by intramuscular or subcutaneous injection, in doses similar to those by mouth, for the relief of pain; the intravenous route has also been used in adults.

For the relief of **pain** codeine phosphate may be given in doses of 30 to 60 mg every 4 hours to a usual maximum of 240 mg daily. Children aged 1 to 12 years may be given 500 micrograms/kg 4 to 6 times daily.

To allay unproductive **cough** codeine phosphate may be given in doses of 15 to 30 mg three or four times daily. Children aged 5 to 12 years may be given 7.5 to 15 mg three or four times daily and those aged 1 to 5 years, 3 mg three or four times daily (but see below).

Codeine phosphate is also used as tablets or in mixtures for the symptomatic relief of **acute diarrhoea** in adults in a dose of 30 mg given 3 or 4 times daily.

Other codeine salts used include the hydrochloride, sulfate, acefyllinate, camsilate, and hydrobromide. Codeine polistirex (a codeine and sulfonated diethenylbenzene-ethenylbenzene copolymer complex) is used in modified-release preparations.

**Administration in children.** Dosage recommendations for codeine in the treatment of *pain* or cough are generally restricted to those over 1 year of age. However, some have considered codeine to be an effective analgesic in neonates and children.[1] With a single dose of codeine phosphate 1 mg/kg by mouth or by intramuscular injection there was a relatively small risk of respiratory depression in neonates, but significant respiratory depression has occurred with multiple doses and patients should be observed closely.[1] Case reports of adverse reactions such as vasodilatation, severe hypotension, and apnoea in infants and children after intravenous doses of codeine have precluded its use by this route in children of all ages.[2]

Antimotility drugs such as codeine should not be used in infants and young children with acute *diarrhoea*.[3,4]

*Cough* suppressants containing codeine or similar opioids are generally not recommended for children and should be avoided in those under 1 year of age.

1. Lloyd-Thomas AR. Pain management in paediatric patients. *Br J Anaesth* 1990; **64:** 85–104.
2. Marsh DF, *et al.* Opioid systems and the newborn. *Br J Anaesth* 1997; **79:** 787–95.
3. Anonymous. Drugs in the management of acute diarrhoea in infants and young children. *Bull WHO* 1989; **67:** 94–6.
4. Cimolai N, Carter JE. Antimotility agents for paediatric use. *Lancet* 1990; **336:** 874.

**Cough.** A systematic review[1] of over-the-counter preparations for acute cough concluded that codeine appeared no more effective than placebo in reducing cough symptoms in adults or children, although the number of patients in the studies considered was small.

See also under Administration in Children, above.

1. Schroeder K, Fahey T. Over-the-counter medications for acute cough in children and adults in ambulatory settings. Available in The Cochrane Library; Issue 2. Chichester: John Wiley; 2004.

**Pain.** Systematic reviews[1,2] comparing paracetamol-codeine combinations versus paracetamol alone concluded that in single dose studies addition of codeine to paracetamol produced a comparatively small but statistically significant increase in analgesic effect; however, there was an increased incidence of side-effects with the combination.

1. de Craen AJM, *et al.* Analgesic efficacy and safety of paracetamol-codeine combinations versus paracetamol alone: a systematic review. *BMJ* 1996; **313:** 321–5.
2. Moore A, *et al.* Single dose paracetamol (acetaminophen), with and without codeine, for postoperative pain. Available in The Cochrane Library; Issue 2. Chichester: John Wiley; 2004.

## Preparations

***BP 2003:*** Co-codamol Tablets; Co-codaprin Tablets; Codeine Linctus; Codeine Phosphate Oral Solution; Codeine Phosphate Tablets; Dispersible Co-codaprin Tablets; Effervescent Co-codamol Tablets; Paediatric Codeine Linctus;
***USP 27:*** Acetaminophen and Codeine Phosphate Capsules; Acetaminophen and Codeine Phosphate Oral Solution; Acetaminophen and Codeine Phosphate Oral Suspension; Acetaminophen and Codeine Phosphate Tablets; Aspirin and Codeine Phosphate Tablets; Bromodiphenhydramine Hydrochloride and Codeine Phosphate Oral Solution; Butalbital, Aspirin, Caffeine, and Codeine Phosphate Capsules; Carisoprodol, Aspirin, and Codeine Phosphate Tablets; Codeine Phosphate Injection; Codeine Phosphate Tablets; Codeine Sulfate Tablets; Guaifenesin and Codeine Phosphate Syrup; Terpin Hydrate and Codeine Elixir.

**Proprietary Preparations** (details are given in Part 3)
***Austral.:*** Actacode; ***Austria:*** Codipertussin; Codipront Mono; Coditard; Tricodein; ***Belg.:*** Bromophar; Bronchodine†; Bronchosedal; Codocalyptol†; Eulyptan; Gloceda; Glottyl; Toularynx; ***Fr.:*** Codedrill; Codenfan; Neo-Codion; Paderyl; Pneumogenol†; ***Ger.:*** Antitussivum Burger; Bronchicum Mono Codein; codi OPT; Codicaps mono; Codicaps N; Codicompren; Codifortон†; Codipertussin; Codipront Mono; Dicton†; Makatussin Codein; Melrosum Codein Hustensirup; Neo-Codion NN; Optipect Kodein; Tricodein†; Tryasol; Tussamag Codeintropfen†; Tussoret; ***Gr.:*** Codipront N; ***Hong Kong:*** Codipront N; ***Irl.:*** Codant; ***Israel:*** Codical; Rekod; ***Malaysia:*** Setlinctus; ***Port.:*** Codeisan†; ***Spain:*** Analgiol†; Bisoltus; Codeisan; Fludan Codeina; Histaverin; Perduretas Codeina; Toseina NF; ***Switz.:*** Makatussin nouvelle formule; Tricodein; ***UK:*** Evacode†; Galcodine.

**Multi-ingredient:** numerous preparations are listed in Part 3.

## Croton Oil

Aceite de crotón; Oleum Crotonis; Oleum Tiglii.
*CAS — 8001-28-3.*

**Pharmacopoeias.** *Chin.* includes fruits of *Croton tiglium.*

### Profile

Croton oil is an oil expressed from the seeds of *Croton tiglium* (Euphorbiaceae). Externally, it is a powerful counter-irritant and vesicant. It is used in homoeopathic medicine. It has such a violent purgative action that it should not be used as a laxative. Croton oil contains phorbol esters, which are carcinogenic.

### Preparations

**Proprietary Preparations** (details are given in Part 3)
**Multi-ingredient:** ***Canad.:*** Rheumalan.

## Cymene

Cimeno; *p*-Cymene; *p*-Cymol. 4-Isopropyl-1-methylbenzene; 4-Isopropyltoluene.
$C_{10}H_{14}$ = 134.2.
*CAS — 25155-15-1; 99-87-6 (p-cymene).*

### Profile

Cymene has been used as a topical local analgesic for the relief of pain in rheumatic conditions. It is also used in perfumery.

### Preparations

**Proprietary Preparations** (details are given in Part 3)
**Multi-ingredient:** ***Fr.:*** Neuriplege†.

## Devil's Claw Root

Harpagophyti Radix; Harpagophyton; Harpagophytum; Harpagophytum Procumbens; Raíz de harpagofito; Teufelskrallenwurzel.

**Pharmacopoeias.** In *Eur.* (see p.vi).

**Ph. Eur. 5.0** (Devil's Claw Root; Devil's Claw BP 2003). The cut and dried tuberous, secondary roots of *Harpagophytum procumbens* and/or *H. zeyheri*. Greyish-brown to dark brown with a bitter taste. Contains not less than 1.2% harpagoside ($C_{24}H_{30}O_{11}$ = 494.5), calculated with reference to the dried drug. Protect from light.

### Profile

Devil's claw root is used in herbal remedies for musculoskeletal and joint disorders.

### Preparations

**Proprietary Preparations** (details are given in Part 3)
***Arg.:*** Herbaccion Flex; ***Austral.:*** Doloteffin†; ***Fr.:*** Harpadol; Harpagocid; ***Ger.:*** Ajuta; Allya; Arthrosetten H; Arthrotabs; Cefatec; Defencid†; Dolo-Arthrodynat; Dolo-Arthrosetten H; Doloteffin; flexi-loges; Harpagoforte Asmedic; HarpagoMega; Herbadon; Jucurba; Matai; Pargo; Rheuferm Phyto; Rheuma-Sern; Rheuma-Teufelskralle HarpagoMega†; Rivoltan; Salus†; Sogoon; Teltonal; Teufelskralle; ***Spain:*** Fitokey Harpagophytum; Harpagofito Orto; Hartiosen†.

**Multi-ingredient:** ***Austral.:*** Arthriforte†; Arthritic Pain Herbal Formula 1†; Bioglan Arthri Plus†; Devils Claw Plus†; Extralife Arthri-Care†; Harpagophytum Complex†; Herbal Arthritis Formula†; Lifesystem Herbal Formula 1 Arthritic Aid†; Lifesystem Herbal Formula 12 Willowbark†; Prost-1†; Willowbark Plus Herbal Formula 11†; ***Fr.:*** Actisane Douleurs Articulaires†; Arkophytum; Artrosan†; ***Ger.:*** Dr Wiemanns Rheumatonikum; ***Ital.:*** Artoxan†; Bodyguard; Nevril; Pik-Gel†; ***Spain:*** Dolosul; Natusor Harpagosinol; ***UK:*** Arthrotone†.

## Dextromoramide *(BAN, pINN)*

Dextrodiphenopyrine; Dextromoramida; *d*-Moramid; Pyrrolamidol. (+)-1-(3-Methyl-4-morpholino-2,2-diphenylbutyryl)pyrrolidine.
$C_{25}H_{32}N_2O_2$ = 392.5.
*CAS — 357-56-2.*
*ATC — N02AC01.*

### Dextromoramide Tartrate *(BANM, pINNM)*

Bitartrate de Dextromoramide; Dextromoramide Acid Tartrate; Dextromoramide Hydrogen Tartrate; Dextromoramidi Tartras; Tartrato de dextromoramida.
$C_{25}H_{32}N_2O_2,C_4H_6O_6$ = 542.6.
*CAS — 2922-44-3.*

**Pharmacopoeias.** In *Eur.* (see p.vi).

**Ph. Eur. 5.0** (Dextromoramide Tartrate). A white crystalline or amorphous powder. Soluble in water; sparingly soluble in alcohol. A 1% solution in water has a pH of 3.0 to 4.0.

### Profile

Dextromoramide is an opioid analgesic (p.73) structurally related to methadone (p.58). It has been used in the treatment of severe pain although it was not recommended for use in obstetric analgesia because of an increased risk of neonatal depression. Dextromoramide is subject to abuse.

Dextromoramide has been given as the tartrate by mouth. It has also been given rectally as suppositories and by subcutaneous or intramuscular injection; similar analgesic effects have been claimed for the same dose whether given by mouth or by injection.

### Preparations

***BP 2003:*** Dextromoramide Tablets.

**Proprietary Preparations** (details are given in Part 3)
***Austral.:*** Palfium†; ***Belg.:*** Palfium†; ***Irl.:*** Palfium; ***Neth.:*** Palfium; ***UK:*** Palfium†.

## Dextropropoxyphene *(BAN, pINN)*

Dextropropoxifeno; Propoxyphene. (+)-(1*S*,2*R*)-1-Benzyl-3-dimethylamino-2-methyl-1-phenylpropyl propionate.
$C_{22}H_{29}NO_2$ = 339.5.
*CAS — 469-62-5.*
*ATC — N02AC04.*

### Dextropropoxyphene Hydrochloride

*(BANM, pINNM)*

Dextropropoxypheni Hydrochloridum; Hidrocloruro de dextropropoxifeno; Propoxyphene Hydrochloride *(USAN).*
$C_{22}H_{29}NO_2,HCl$ = 375.9.
*CAS — 1639-60-7.*

NOTE. Compounded preparations of dextropropoxyphene hydrochloride may be represented by the following names:

- Co-proxamol *(BAN)*—dextropropoxyphene hydrochloride 1 part and paracetamol 10 parts (w/w).

**Pharmacopoeias.** In *Eur.* (see p.vi) and *US.*

**Ph. Eur. 5.0** (Dextropropoxyphene Hydrochloride). A white or almost white crystalline powder. Very soluble in water; freely soluble in alcohol. Protect from light.

**USP 27** (Propoxyphene Hydrochloride). A white odourless crystalline powder. Freely soluble in water; soluble in alcohol, in acetone, and in chloroform; practically insoluble in ether and in benzene. Store in airtight containers.

### Dextropropoxyphene Napsilate *(BANM, pINNM)*

Dextropropoxyphene Napsylate; Napsilato de dextropropoxifeno; Propoxyphene Napsylate *(USAN).* Dextropropoxyphene naphthalene-2-sulphonate monohydrate.
$C_{22}H_{29}NO_2,C_{10}H_8O_3S,H_2O$ = 565.7.
*CAS — 17140-78-2 (anhydrous dextropropoxyphene napsilate); 26570-10-5 (dextropropoxyphene napsilate monohydrate).*

NOTE. Compounded preparations of dextropropoxyphene napsilate may be represented by the following names:

- Co-proxAPAP *(PEN)*—dextropropoxyphene napsilate and paracetamol.

**Pharmacopoeias.** In *Br.* and *US.*

**BP 2003** (Dextropropoxyphene Napsilate). An odourless or almost odourless white powder. It exhibits polymorphism. Practically insoluble in water; soluble in alcohol; freely soluble in chloroform.

**USP 27** (Propoxyphene Napsylate). A white powder having essentially no odour. Very slightly soluble in water; soluble 1 in 15 of alcohol and 1 in 10 of chloroform; soluble in acetone and in methyl alcohol. Store in airtight containers.

### Dependence and Withdrawal

As for Opioid Analgesics, p.71. Dextropropoxyphene has been subject to abuse (see under Precautions, below).

◊ Reports of dextropropoxyphene dependence and its treatment.

1. Wall R, *et al.* Addiction to Distalgesic (dextropropoxyphene). *BMJ* 1980; **280:** 1213–14.
2. D'Abadie NB, Lenton JD. Propoxyphene dependence: problems in management. *South Med J* 1984; **77:** 299–301.

### Adverse Effects

As for Opioid Analgesics in general, p.72. In the recommended dosage the adverse effects of dextropropoxyphene are less marked than those of morphine. Gastrointestinal effects, dizziness, and drowsiness are the most common. Liver impairment has been reported.

There are a disturbing number of fatalities from either accidental or intentional overdosage with dextropropoxyphene. Many reports emphasise the rapidity with which death ensues; death within an hour of overdosage is not uncommon, and it can occur within 15 minutes. Overdosage is often complicated by patients also taking alcohol and using mixed preparations such as dextropropoxyphene with paracetamol or aspirin.

Symptoms of overdosage are similar to those of opioid poisoning in general, but in addition patients may experience psychotic reactions. There may be cardiac conduction abnormalities and arrhythmias.

Dextropropoxyphene injections are painful and have had a very destructive effect on soft tissues and veins when dextropropoxyphene has been abused in this way.

Anorectal reactions have followed the prolonged use of suppositories containing dextropropoxyphene; the reactions appear to be dose dependent.

**Effects on the blood.** A 12-year history of haemolysis and subsequent significant haemolytic anaemia in an elderly woman[1] was associated with chronic, periodic, and occasionally excessive intake of co-proxamol.

1. Fulton JD, McGonigal G. Steroid responsive haemolytic anaemia due to dextropropoxyphene paracetamol combination. *J R Soc Med* 1989; **82:** 228.

**Effects on the ears.** A report of complete nerve deafness associated with chronic abuse of co-proxamol was made to the UK Committee on Safety of Medicines.[1] The Committee had received 2 other reports of permanent hearing loss attributed to co-proxamol abuse; transient hearing loss had also been reported in 2 patients taking usual doses; 7 further reports described tinnitus.

1. Ramsay BC. Complete nerve deafness after abuse of co-proxamol. *Lancet* 1991; **338:** 446–7.

**Effects on the liver.** There have been occasional reports of jaundice in patients taking dextropropoxyphene without paracetamol. Many of the 49 suspected hepatic reactions with dextropropoxyphene reported to the UK Committee on Safety of Medicines by 1985[1] had involved dextropropoxyphene in association with paracetamol; clinical features including malaise, jaundice, raised serum transaminases, and sometimes fever, were however generally characteristic of dextropropoxyphene alone. Relapsing jaundice mimicking biliary disease was attributable to the dextropropoxyphene component of co-proxamol in 3 patients,[2] whereas there was no abnormality of liver function in 11 patients on long-term co-proxamol analgesia.[3] Another report of 9 cases also found that the hepatotoxic effects of dextropropoxyphene mimicked symptoms of large bile duct obstruction, and suggested that such toxicity might be misdiagnosed.[4]

1. Committee on Safety of Medicines. Hepatotoxicity with dextropropoxyphene. *Current Problems 17* 1986.
2. Bassendine MF, *et al.* Dextropropoxyphene induced hepatotoxicity mimicking biliary tract disease. *Gut* 1986; **27:** 444–9.
3. Hutchinson DR, *et al.* Liver function in patients on long-term paracetamol (co-proxamol) analgesia. *J Pharm Pharmacol* 1986; **38:** 242–3.
4. Rosenberg WMC, *et al.* Dextropropoxyphene induced hepatotoxicity: a report of nine cases. *J Hepatol* 1993; **19:** 470–4.

**Effects on the lungs.** Hypersensitivity pneumonitis and skin rash has been reported in a patient taking co-proxamol.[1] No such reaction occurred when the patient was subsequently given paracetamol alone.

1. Matusiewicz SP, *et al.* Hypersensitivity pneumonitis associated with co-proxamol (paracetamol + dextropropoxyphene) therapy. *Postgrad Med J* 1999; **75:** 475–6.

**Hypoglycaemia.** References to a hypoglycaemic effect of dextropropoxyphene.[1-3]

1. Wiederholt IC, *et al.* Recurrent episodes of hypoglycemia induced by propoxyphene. *Neurology* 1967; **17:** 703–4.
2. Almirall J, *et al.* Propoxyphene-induced hypoglycemia in a patient with chronic renal failure. *Nephron* 1989; **53:** 273–5.
3. Lowenstein W, *et al.* Hypoglycémie au dextropropoxyphène: une urgence chez le toxicomane. *Presse Med* 1993; **22:** 133.

**Overdosage.** There have been several reviews or retrospective studies of acute self-poisoning with dextropropoxyphene.[1-4] At a symposium on the safety and efficacy of dextropropoxyphene[5] many of the participants dealt with the problems of dextropropoxyphene overdosage, often in conjunction with paracetamol and sometimes with alcohol. Profound and even fatal CNS depression can develop rapidly as a result of the dextropropoxyphene content and in many cases death has occurred within an hour;[6] it was suggested that as few as 15 to 20 tablets of co-proxamol might be fatal.[7,8] Analysis of suicides involving drugs in England and Wales between 1997 and 1999 revealed that the odds of dying after overdose with co-proxamol were 2.3 times that for tricyclic antidepressant overdose, and 28.1 times greater than for paracetamol.[9] In the USA[10] the incidence of dextropropoxyphene-associated deaths reached a peak in 1977 and then fell at a rate that was not matched by a decline in prescribing. However, the number of deaths associated with dextropropoxyphene poisoning continues to be high in some countries.[4] It is not clear whether the metabolite, nordextropropoxyphene, plays an important role in fatalities.[10] However, nordextropropoxyphene, like dextropropoxyphene, is considered to have local anaesthetic activity and the membrane stabilising activity of dextropropoxyphene has been implicated as a major factor responsible for its severe cardiac depressant effect.[11]

1. Young RJ. Dextropropoxyphene overdosage: pharmacological considerations and clinical management. *Drugs* 1983; **26:** 70–9.
2. Madsen PS, *et al.* Acute propoxyphene self-poisoning in 222 consecutive patients. *Acta Anaesthesiol Scand* 1984; **28:** 661–5.
3. Segest E. Poisoning with dextropropoxyphene in Denmark. *Hum Toxicol* 1987; **6:** 203–7.
4. Jonasson U, *et al.* Correlation between prescription of various dextropropoxyphene preparations and their involvement in fatal poisonings. *Forensic Sci Int* 1999; **103:** 125–32.
5. Bowen D, *et al.* (ed). Distalgesic; safety and efficacy. *Hum Toxicol* 1984; **3** (suppl): 1S–238S.
6. Proudfoot AT. Clinical features and management of Distalgesic overdose. *Hum Toxicol* 1984; **3** (suppl): 85S–94S.
7. Whittington RM. Dextropropoxyphene deaths: coroner's report. *Hum Toxicol* 1984; **3** (suppl): 175S–85S.
8. Young RJ, Lawson AAH. Distalgesic poisoning—cause for concern. *BMJ* 1980; **280:** 1045–7.
9. Hawton K, *et al.* Co-proxamol and suicide: a study of national mortality statistics and local non-fatal self-poisonings. *BMJ* 2003; **326:** 1006–8.
10. Finkle BS. Self-poisoning with dextropropoxyphene and dextropropoxyphene compounds: the USA experience. *Hum Toxicol* 1984; **3** (suppl): 115S–34S.
11. Henry JA, Cassidy SL. Membrane stabilising activity: a major cause of fatal poisoning. *Lancet* 1986; **i:** 1414–17.

## Treatment of Adverse Effects

As for Opioid Analgesics in general, p.72.

Rapid treatment of overdosage with naloxone and assisted respiration is essential. Cardiac effects may not be reversed by naloxone. Gastric lavage and activated charcoal may be of value within 1 hour of ingestion, but dialysis is of little use.

Convulsions may require control with an anticonvulsant, bearing in mind that the CNS depressant effects of dextropropoxyphene might be exacerbated (see also under Interactions, below). Stimulants should not be used because of the risk of inducing convulsions.

Patients taking overdoses of dextropropoxyphene with paracetamol will also require treatment for paracetamol poisoning (p.76). Mixtures of dextropropoxyphene and aspirin may be involved; the treatment of aspirin poisoning is described on p.15.

## Precautions

As for Opioid Analgesics in general, p.72.

**Abuse.** There have been reports of the abuse of dextropropoxyphene,[1] and some[2] considered that the ready availability of dextropropoxyphene made it liable to abuse although it was a relatively weak opioid analgesic. However, others[3] thought there was no evidence that dextropropoxyphene was frequently associated with abuse, or concluded that, although there was abuse potential, it was of relatively low importance in terms of the community as a whole.[4]

A severe withdrawal syndrome has been reported[5] in an elderly patient who covertly consumed a daily dose of dextropropoxyphene of 1 to 3 g for at least 12 months. The patient was treated by a gradually decreasing dosage schedule of dextropropoxyphene over 9 weeks.

1. Tennant FS. Complications of propoxyphene abuse. *Arch Intern Med* 1973; **132:** 191–4.
2. Lader M. Abuse of weak opioid analgesics. *Hum Toxicol* 1984; **3** (suppl): 229S–36S.
3. Finkle BS. Self-poisoning with dextropropoxyphene and dextropropoxyphene compounds: the USA experience. *Hum Toxicol* 1984; **3** (suppl): 115S–34S.
4. Turner P. Final remarks. *Hum Toxicol* 1984; **3** (suppl): 237S–8S.
5. Hedenmalm K. A case of severe withdrawal syndrome due to dextropropoxyphene. *Ann Intern Med* 1995; **123:** 473.

**Breast feeding.** No adverse effects have been observed in breast-feeding infants whose mothers were receiving dextropropoxyphene, and the American Academy of Pediatrics considers[1] that it is therefore usually compatible with breast feeding. The *British National Formulary* also considers that the amount of dextropropoxyphene in breast milk is too small to be harmful.

1. American Academy of Pediatrics. The transfer of drugs and other chemicals into human milk. *Pediatrics* 2001; **108:** 776–89. Correction. *ibid.*; 1029. Also available at: http://aappolicy.aappublications.org/cgi/content/full/pediatrics%3b108/3/776 (accessed 05/07/04)

**Porphyria.** Dextropropoxyphene has been associated with acute attacks of porphyria and is considered unsafe in porphyric patients.

## Interactions

For interactions associated with opioid analgesics, see p.73.

Plasma concentrations of dextropropoxyphene are increased by ritonavir, with a resultant risk of toxicity; they should not be given together.

CNS depressants, including alcohol, may contribute to the hazards of dextropropoxyphene. The convulsant action of high doses of dextropropoxyphene may be enhanced by CNS stimulants.

Dextropropoxyphene interacts with several other drugs through inhibition of liver metabolism. Drugs reported to be affected include antidepressants, benzodiazepines, beta blockers, carbamazepine (see p.355), phenobarbital (see p.368), phenytoin (see p.372), and warfarin.

**Antimuscarinics.** A suggested interaction between *orphenadrine* and dextropropoxyphene has been questioned (see p.486).

## Pharmacokinetics

Dextropropoxyphene is readily absorbed from the gastrointestinal tract, the napsilate tending to be more slowly absorbed than the hydrochloride, but both are subject to considerable first-pass metabolism. Peak plasma concentrations occur about 2 to 2.5 hours after ingestion. It is rapidly distributed and concentrated in the liver, lungs, and brain. About 80% of dextropropoxyphene and its metabolites are reported to be bound to plasma proteins. Dextropropoxyphene crosses the placenta. It has been detected in breast milk.

Dextropropoxyphene is *N*-demethylated to nordextropropoxyphene (norpropoxyphene) in the liver. It is excreted in the urine mainly as metabolites. It is now recognised that dextropropoxyphene and nordextropropoxyphene have prolonged elimination half-lives; values of 6 to 12 hours and 30 to 36 hours, respectively, have been reported. Accumulation of dextropropoxyphene and its metabolites may occur with repeated doses and nordextropropoxyphene may contribute to the toxicity seen with overdosage.

◊ Reviews.

1. Pearson RM. Pharmacokinetics of propoxyphene. *Hum Toxicol* 1984; **3** (suppl): 37S–40S.

**The elderly.** The elimination half-lives of dextropropoxyphene and its metabolite nordextropropoxyphene were prolonged in healthy elderly subjects when compared with young controls.[1] After multiple dosing median half-lives of dextropropoxyphene and nordextropropoxyphene were 36.8 and 41.8 hours respectively in the elderly compared with 22.0 and 22.1 hours in the young subjects. In this study[1] there was a strong correlation between half-life of nordextropropoxyphene and estimated creatinine clearance.

1. Flanagan RJ, *et al.* Pharmacokinetics of dextropropoxyphene and nordextropropoxyphene in young and elderly volunteers after single and multiple dextropropoxyphene dosage. *Br J Clin Pharmacol* 1989; **28:** 463–9.

**Hepatic impairment.** Plasma concentrations of dextropropoxyphene were higher in patients with cirrhosis given the drug than in healthy controls whereas concentrations of nordextropropoxyphene were lower.[1]

1. Giacomini KM, *et al.* Propoxyphene and norpropoxyphene plasma concentrations after oral propoxyphene in cirrhotic patients with and without surgically constructed portacaval shunt. *Clin Pharmacol Ther* 1980; **28:** 417–24.

**Renal impairment.** Higher and more persistent plasma concentrations of dextropropoxyphene and nordextropropoxyphene in anephric patients when compared with healthy subjects[1] were attributed to decreased first-pass metabolism of dextropropoxyphene and decreased renal excretion of nordextropropoxyphene in the anephric patients.

1. Gibson TP, *et al.* Propoxyphene and norpropoxyphene plasma concentrations in the anephric patient. *Clin Pharmacol Ther* 1980; **27:** 665–70.

## Uses and Administration

Dextropropoxyphene is an opioid analgesic (p.73) structurally related to methadone (p.58). It has mild analgesic activity and is given by mouth as the hydrochloride or napsilate to alleviate mild to moderate pain. Unlike the laevo-isomer (levopropoxyphene, p.1124), dextropropoxyphene has little antitussive activity.

Dextropropoxyphene is mainly used in conjunction with other analgesics with anti-inflammatory and antipyretic effects, such as aspirin or paracetamol. In the UK the usual dose is 65 mg of the hydrochloride or 100 mg of the napsilate given three or four times daily. In the USA similar doses are given every 4 hours up to a maximum total daily dose of 390 mg of the hydrochloride and 600 mg of the napsilate.

**Pain.** A detailed review[1] of the analgesic effectiveness of dextropropoxyphene suggested that with respect to single oral doses, recommended doses of dextropropoxyphene were no more (and probably less) effective than usual doses of paracetamol, aspirin, or other NSAIDs. However, the comparative effectiveness may vary substantially depending on the cause of the pain.

When it comes to comparative studies involving combinations of dextropropoxyphene with other analgesics, findings are even less clear-cut.[2] The effectiveness of co-proxamol has long been a matter of controversy yet despite this a survey[3] conducted in 30 UK teaching hospitals found that co-proxamol was the most widely used paracetamol-containing analgesic. It was suggested that the popularity of co-proxamol was purely down to prescribing habits passed on to new medical staff, rather than hard evidence regarding efficacy. This view has been refuted by others[4] who say that a large number of studies have demonstrated clear analgesic effects for dextropropoxyphene. However, any assumption that the combination was widely used because it was more effective than paracetamol alone was not supported by a systematic overview of single-dose studies.[5] This concluded that while co-proxamol was indeed an effective analgesic it was no better than paracetamol alone. Although the evidence from this and other systematic reviews indicate that co-proxamol should be replaced by paracetamol alone for acute pain, the position for chronic use is considered to be not so clear.[6]

1. Beaver WT. Analgesic efficacy of dextropropoxyphene and dextropropoxyphene-containing combinations: a review. *Hum Toxicol* 1984; **3** (suppl): 191S–220S.
2. Collins SL, *et al.* Single dose dextropropoxyphene, alone and with paracetamol (acetaminophen), for postoperative pain. Available in The Cochrane Library; Issue 2. Chichester: John Wiley; 2004.
3. Haigh S. 12 Years on: co-proxamol revisited. *Lancet* 1996; **347:** 1840–1. Correction. *ibid.*; **348:** 346.
4. Sykes JV, *et al.* Coproxamol revisited. *Lancet* 1996; **348:** 408.
5. Li Wan Po A, Zhang WY. Systematic overview of co-proxamol to assess analgesic effects of addition of dextropropoxyphene to paracetamol. *BMJ* 1997; **315:** 1565–71. Correction *ibid.* 1998; **316:** 116 and 656.
6. Anonymous. Co-proxamol or paracetamol for acute pain? *Drug Ther Bull* 1998; **36:** 80.

## Preparations

***BP 2003:*** Co-proxamol Tablets; Dextropropoxyphene Capsules;
***USP 27:*** Propoxyphene Hydrochloride and Acetaminophen Tablets; Propoxyphene Hydrochloride Capsules; Propoxyphene Hydrochloride, Aspirin, and Caffeine Capsules; Propoxyphene Napsylate and Acetaminophen Tablets; Propoxyphene Napsylate and Aspirin Tablets; Propoxyphene Napsylate Oral Suspension; Propoxyphene Napsylate Tablets.

**Proprietary Preparations** (details are given in Part 3)
***Austral.:*** Doloxene; ***Belg.:*** Depronal; ***Canad.:*** 642; Darvon-N; Novo-Propoxyn†; ***Denm.:*** Abalgin; Doloxene; ***Fin.:*** Abalgin; ***Fr.:*** Antalvic†; ***Ger.:*** Develin†; ***Gr.:*** Romidon; Zideron; ***Hong Kong:*** Doloxene†; ***India:*** Parvodex; ***Irl.:*** Doloxene; ***Ital.:*** Liberen; ***Mex.:*** Darvon Simple; Darvon-N†; Dibagesic†; Trolibert†; ***Neth.:*** Depronal; ***NZ:*** Doloxene; ***Port.:*** Algifene; ***S.Afr.:*** Doloxene; Doxypol†; ***Spain:*** Darvon; Deprancol; ***Swed.:*** Dexofen; Dolotard†; Doloxene; ***Switz.:*** Depronal†; ***UK:*** Doloxene†; ***USA:*** Darvon; Darvon-N.

**Multi-ingredient:** ***Arg.:*** Artifene; Calmopirin; Canovex; D-P; Dextro + Dipirona; Dextrodip; Klosidol; Klosidol B1 B6 B12; Supragesic; Vicefeno; ***Austral.:*** Capadex; Di-Gesic; Paradex; ***Austria:*** Algo-Prolixan; APA; Contraforte; Sigmalin $B_6$ forte; ***Belg.:*** Algophene; Distalgic; Yamalen†; ***Braz.:*** Algafan†; Doloxene-A; ***Canad.:*** 692†; ***Fin.:*** Paraflex comp; ***Fr.:*** Algoced†; Di Dolko; Di-Antalvic; Diadupsan†; Dialgirex; Dioalgo; Propofan; Starem†; ***Hong Kong:*** Cosalgesic; Distalgesic; Dologesic†; Doloxene Compound†; Dolpocetmol; Medonol; ***India:*** Buta-Proxyvon; Ibu-Proxyvon; Parvon; Parvon Forte; Parvon-N; Parvon-Spas; Proxytab; Proxyvon; Spasmo-Proxyvon; Sudhinol; Walagesic; Wygesic; ***Irl.:*** Cosalgesic†; Distalgesic; Doloxene Compound†; ***Israel:*** Algolysin; Proxol; Rogaan; ***Mex.:*** Darvon-N Compuesto; Qual; ***Norw.:*** Aporex; ***NZ:*** Apo-Paradex†; Capadex; Di-Gesic†; Paradex; ***Port.:*** Algifene†; ***S.Afr.:*** Distalgesic; Doloxene Co; Doxyfene; Lentogesic; Synap; ***Swed.:*** Dexodon†; Distalgesic; Doleron; Paraflex comp; ***Switz.:*** Distalgesic; Dolo-Prolixan†; ***UK:*** Cosalgesic; Distalgesic; ***USA:*** Darvocet; Darvocet-N; Darvon Compound; PC-Cap; Propacet; Wygesic.

## Dezocine *(USAN, rINN)*

Dezocina; Wy-16225. (−)-13β-Amino-5,6,7,8,9,10,11α,12-octahydro-5α-methyl-5,11-methanobenzocyclodecen-3-ol.
$C_{16}H_{23}NO$ = 245.4.
*CAS — 53648-55-8.*
*ATC — N02AX03.*

### Profile

Dezocine is an opioid analgesic (p.71). It is structurally related to pentazocine (p.79) and, likewise, has mixed opioid agonist and antagonist actions. Dezocine has been given by injection for the relief of moderate to severe pain.

**Abuse.** Opioid-dependent subjects maintained on oral methadone in a daily dose of 30 mg were challenged with different doses of intramuscular dezocine ranging from 7.5 to 60 mg.[1] Dezocine produced primarily antagonist-like effects and precipitated a withdrawal syndrome which was not directly dose-related in magnitude. The greatest withdrawal effects were seen in the mid-dose range and the least with the higher doses. These results suggest that lower doses of dezocine should have a relatively low abuse liability in opioid-dependent patients. Assessment of the morphine-like subjective and miotic effects of dezocine indicated that it had the potential to be abused, but suggested that its abuse potential was less than that of morphine.[2]

1. Strain EC, *et al.* Opioid antagonist effects of dezocine in opioid-dependent humans. *Clin Pharmacol Ther* 1996; **60:** 206–17.
2. Jasinski DR, Preston KL. Assessment of dezocine for morphine-like subjective effects and miosis. *Clin Pharmacol Ther* 1985; **38:** 544–8.

### Preparations

**Proprietary Preparations** (details are given in Part 3)
***USA:*** Dalgan†.

## Diacerein *(rINN)*

Diacereína; Diacerhein; Diacetylrhein; Rhein Diacetate; SF-277. 9,10-Dihydro-4,5-dihydroxy-9,10-dioxo-2-anthroic acid diacetate.
$C_{19}H_{12}O_8$ = 368.3.
*CAS — 13739-02-1.*
*ATC — M01AX21.*

### Profile

Diacerein is an anthraquinone derivative that has been used in osteoarthritis (p.9) in doses of 50 mg twice daily by mouth. Doses should be halved in patients with creatinine clearance less than 30 mL/minute. Its active metabolite, rhein, a constituent of rhubarb (p.1287), is reported to act as an interleukin-1 inhibitor. Diarrhoea is a common side-effect with diacerein.

◊ References.

1. Debord P, *et al.* Influence of renal function on the pharmacokinetics of diacerein after a single oral dose. *Eur J Drug Metab Pharmacokinet* 1994; **19:** 13–19.
2. Spencer CM, Wilde MI. Diacerein. *Drugs* 1997; **53:** 98–106.
3. Nicolas P, *et al.* Clinical pharmacokinetics of diacerein. *Clin Pharmacokinet* 1998; **35:** 347–59.
4. Pelletier JP, *et al.* Efficacy and safety of diacerein in osteoarthritis of the knee: a double-blind, placebo-controlled trial. *Arthritis Rheum* 2000; **43:** 2339–48.
5. Falgarone G, Dougados M. Diacerein as a disease-modulating agent in osteoarthritis. *Curr Rheumatol Rep* 2001; **3:** 479–83.
6. Dougados M, *et al.* Evaluation of the structure-modifying effects of diacerein in hip osteoarthritis: ECHODIAH, a three-year, placebo-controlled trial. Evaluation of the chondromodulating effect of diacerein in OA of the hip. *Arthritis Rheum* 2001; **44:** 2539–47.

### Preparations

**Proprietary Preparations** (details are given in Part 3)
***Arg.:*** Artrodar; Artroglobina; Matrix; ***Braz.:*** Artrodar; ***Chile:*** Artrizona; ***Fr.:*** Art; Zondar; ***Gr.:*** Verboril; ***Israel:*** Art; ***Ital.:*** Artrodar†; Fisiodar; ***Port.:*** Artrolyt†; Cartivix.

## Diamorphine Hydrochloride *(BANM)*

Diacetilmorfina, hidrocloruro de; Diacetylmorphine Hydrochloride; Heroin Hydrochloride. 4,5-Epoxy-17-methylmorphinan-3,6-diyl diacetate hydrochloride monohydrate.
$C_{21}H_{23}NO_5,HCl,H_2O$ = 423.9.
*CAS — 561-27-3 (diamorphine); 1502-95-0 (diamorphine hydrochloride).*
*ATC — N02AA09.*

**Pharmacopoeias.** In *Br.* and *Swiss. Swiss* also includes the anhydrous form.

**BP 2003** (Diamorphine Hydrochloride). A white or almost white crystalline powder, odourless when freshly prepared but develops an odour characteristic of acetic acid on storage. Freely soluble in water and in chloroform; soluble in alcohol; practically insoluble in ether. Protect from light.

**Incompatibility.** Diamorphine hydrochloride is incompatible with mineral acids and alkalis and with chlorocresol.[1]

Cyclizine may precipitate from mixtures with diamorphine hydrochloride at concentrations of cyclizine greater than 10 mg/mL, or in the presence of sodium chloride, or as the concentration of diamorphine relative to cyclizine increases; mixtures of diamorphine and cyclizine are also liable to precipitate after 24 hours.

Mixtures of diamorphine and haloperidol are liable to precipitate after 24 hours if the haloperidol concentration is above 2 mg/mL. Under some conditions mixtures of metoclopramide and diamorphine may become discoloured and should be discarded.

1. McEwan JS, Macmorran GH. The compatibility of some bactericides. *Pharm J* 1947; **158:** 260–2.

**Stability.** Diamorphine is relatively unstable in aqueous solution and is hydrolysed to 6-*O*-monoacetylmorphine and then morphine to a significant extent at room temperature; 3-*O*-monoacetylmorphine is only occasionally detected. The rate of decomposition is at a minimum at about pH 4.[1,2]

In a study of the stability of aqueous solutions of diamorphine in chloroform water it was concluded that such solutions should be used within 3 weeks of preparation when stored at room temperature.[3] Another study[4] noted that the degradation products of diamorphine were not devoid of analgesic activity. Using a more sensitive analytical method it was reported that although the pH range of maximum stability of diamorphine in aqueous solution was 3.8 to 4.4, the addition of buffers reduced stability.[5] Simple unbuffered chloroform water gave maximum stability, the shelf-life of such a solution being 4 weeks at room temperature.

The BP 2003 recommends that solutions for injection be prepared immediately before use by dissolving Diamorphine Hydrochloride for Injection in Water for Injections. This may pose a problem with solutions for subcutaneous infusion when concentrated solutions may remain in infusion pump reservoirs for some time.[6] Investigation of 9 concentrations of diamorphine stored at 4 different temperatures for 8 weeks[7] revealed instability under conditions of concentration, time, and temperature prevalent during subcutaneous infusion. Degradation of diamorphine occurred at all concentrations (0.98 to 250 mg/mL) at temperatures of 4° and above; the effect of temperature was significant at 21° and 37°. The percentage fall in diamorphine concentration was directly related to initial concentration and was accompanied by a corresponding increase in 6-*O*-monoacetylmorphine and, to a lesser extent, morphine; other possible breakdown products such as 3-*O*-monoacetylmorphine were not present in detectable quantities. Diamorphine degradation was associated with a fall in pH and the development of a strong acetic acid-like odour. Precipitation and a white turbidity was seen in solutions of 15.6 mg/mL and above after incubation for 2 weeks at 21° and 37°. It has been noted that solutions for infusion are generally freshly prepared and used within 24 hours, but that signs of precipitation should be watched for, especially when using longer-term infusions and high concentrations of diamorphine.[7]

In another stability study[8] diamorphine hydrochloride in concentrations of both 1 and 20 mg/mL in sodium chloride 0.9% was stable for a minimum of 15 days at room temperature (23° to 25°) and 4° when stored in a PVC container. In one type of disposable infusion device (Infusor) similar solutions were stable for 15 days even at 31°. In another infusion device (Intermate 200) diamorphine was stable for a minimum of 15 days at both concentrations and all temperatures except for the 1 mg/mL solution kept at 31° when stability was only maintained for a minimum of 2 days. When stored in glass syringes both strengths of diamorphine hydrochloride were stable for 15 days at 4° and at room temperature the 1 mg/mL solution was stable for a minimum of 7 days and the 20 mg/mL solution was stable for a minimum of 12 days. There were no substantial changes in physical appearance or pH.

1. Davey EA, Murray JB. Hydrolysis of diamorphine in aqueous solutions. *Pharm J* 1969; **203:** 737.
2. Davey EA, Murray JB. Determination of diamorphine in the presence of its degradation products using gas liquid chromatography. *Pharm J* 1971; **207:** 167.
3. Cooper H, *et al.* Stability of diamorphine in chloroform water mixture. *Pharm J* 1981; **226:** 682–3.
4. Twycross RG. Stability of diamorphine in chloroform water. *Pharm J* 1981; **227:** 218.
5. Beaumont IM. Stability of diamorphine in chloroform water. *Pharm J* 1981; **227:** 41.
6. Jones VA, *et al.* Diamorphine stability in aqueous solution for subcutaneous infusion. *Br J Clin Pharmacol* 1987; **23:** 651P.
7. Omar OA, *et al.* Diamorphine stability in aqueous solution for subcutaneous infusion. *J Pharm Pharmacol* 1989; **41:** 275–7.
8. Kleinberg ML, *et al.* Stability of heroin hydrochloride in infusion devices and containers for intravenous administration. *Am J Hosp Pharm* 1990; **47:** 377–81.

### Dependence and Withdrawal

As for Opioid Analgesics, p.71. Diamorphine is subject to abuse (see under Adverse Effects, Treatment, and Precautions, below).

Diamorphine is used for substitution therapy in the management of opioid dependence (see under Uses and Administration, below).

### Adverse Effects, Treatment, and Precautions

As for Opioid Analgesics in general, p.72.

Pulmonary oedema after overdosage is a common cause of fatalities among diamorphine addicts. Nausea and hypotension are claimed to be less common than with morphine.

There are many reports of adverse effects associated with the abuse of diamorphine, usually obtained illicitly in an adulterated form.

**Abuse.** Most of the reports of adverse effects with diamorphine involve its abuse. In addition to the central effects, there are effects caused by the administration methods and by the adulterants.[1] Thus in many instances it is difficult to identify the factor causing the toxicity. Most body systems are involved including the immune system,[2] kidneys,[3] liver,[4] respiratory system,[5-7] and the nervous system.[8-11]

Other aspects of the illicit use of diamorphine include fatal overdose[12] and smuggling by swallowing packages of drug[13] or other methods of internal bodily concealment.

1. Hendrickse RG, *et al.* Aflatoxins and heroin. *BMJ* 1989; **299:** 492–3.
2. Husby G, *et al.* Smooth muscle antibody in heroin addicts. *Ann Intern Med* 1975; **83:** 801–5.
3. Cunningham EE, *et al.* Heroin-associated nephropathy. *JAMA* 1983; **250:** 2935–6.
4. Weller IVD, *et al.* Clinical, biochemical, serological, histological and ultrastructural features of liver disease in drug abusers. *Gut* 1984; **25:** 417–23.
5. Anderson K. Bronchospasm and intravenous street heroin. *Lancet* 1986; **i:** 1208.
6. Hughes S, Calverley PMA. Heroin inhalation and asthma. *BMJ* 1988; **297:** 1511–12.
7. Boto de los Bueis A, *et al.* Bronchial hyperreactivity in patients who inhale heroin mixed with cocaine vaporized on aluminium foil. *Chest* 2002; **121:** 1223–30.
8. Sempere AP, *et al.* Spongiform leucoencephalopathy after inhaling heroin. *Lancet* 1991; **338:** 320.
9. Roulet Perez E, *et al.* Toxic leucoencephalopathy after heroin ingestion in a 2½-year-old child. *Lancet* 1992; **340:** 729.
10. Zuckerman GB. Neurologic complications following intranasal administration of heroin in an adolescent. *Ann Pharmacother* 1996; **30:** 778–81.
11. Kriegstein AR, *et al.* Heroin inhalation and progressive spongiform leukoencephalopathy. *N Engl J Med* 1997; **336:** 589–90.
12. Kintz P, *et al.* Toxicological data after heroin overdose. *Hum Toxicol* 1989; **8:** 487–9.
13. Stewart A, *et al.* Body packing—a case report and review of the literature. *Postgrad Med J* 1990; **66:** 659–61.

**Administration.** Although generally free from complications, sterile abscess formation was reported in 2 patients with advanced cancer receiving diamorphine by continuous *subcutaneous* infusions.[1] Acute dysphoric reactions have been reported after the use of *epidural* diamorphine.[2]

1. Hoskin PJ, *et al.* Sterile abscess formation by continuous subcutaneous infusion of diamorphine. *BMJ* 1988; **296:** 1605.
2. Holder KJ, Morgan BM. Dysphoria after extradural diamorphine. *Br J Anaesth* 1994; **72:** 728.

**Breast feeding.** The American Academy of Pediatrics has stated[1] that, when used as a drug of abuse by breast-feeding mothers, diamorphine has caused adverse effects in the infant, notably tremors, restlessness, vomiting, and poor feeding.

See also under Opioid Dependence in Uses and Administration, below.


1. American Academy of Pediatrics. The transfer of drugs and other chemicals into human milk. *Pediatrics* 2001; **108:** 776–89. Correction. *ibid.*; 1029. Also available at: http://aappolicy.aappublications.org/cgi/content/full/pediatrics%3b108/3/776 (accessed 05/07/04)


**Phaeochromocytoma.** Diamorphine can liberate endogenous histamine which may in turn stimulate release of catecholamines. Its use provoked hypertension and tachycardia in a patient with phaeochromocytoma.[1]


1. Chaturvedi NC, *et al.* Diamorphine-induced attack of paroxysmal hypertension in phaeochromocytoma. *BMJ* 1974; **2:** 538.


**Pregnancy and the neonate.** Some references to diamorphine dependence in pregnant women and the effects on the fetus and neonate.


1. Fricker HS, Segal S. Narcotic addiction, pregnancy, and the newborn. *Am J Dis Child* 1978; **132:** 360–6.
2. Ostrea EM, Chavez CJ. Perinatal problems (excluding neonatal withdrawal) in maternal drug addiction: a study of 830 cases. *J Pediatr* 1979; **94:** 292–5.
3. Lifschitz MH, *et al.* Fetal and postnatal growth of children born to narcotic-dependent women. *J Pediatr* 1983; **102:** 686–91.
4. Klenka HM. Babies born in a district general hospital to mothers taking heroin. *BMJ* 1986; **293:** 745–6.
5. Gregg JEM, *et al.* Inhaling heroin during pregnancy: effects on the baby. *BMJ* 1988; **296:** 754.
6. Little BB, *et al.* Maternal and fetal effects of heroin addiction during pregnancy. *J Reprod Med* 1990; **35:** 159–62.


## Interactions

For interactions associated with opioid analgesics, see p.73.

## Pharmacokinetics

Diamorphine hydrochloride is well absorbed from the gastrointestinal tract and after subcutaneous or intramuscular injection. On injection it is rapidly converted to the active metabolite 6-*O*-monoacetylmorphine (6-acetylmorphine) in the blood and then to morphine. Oral doses are subject to extensive first-pass metabolism to morphine; neither diamorphine nor 6-acetylmorphine have been detected in the blood after giving diamorphine by this route. Both diamorphine and 6-acetylmorphine readily cross the blood-brain barrier. Morphine glucuronides are the main excretion products in the urine. A small amount is excreted in the faeces.

◊ Reviews and studies of the pharmacokinetics of diamorphine.


1. Boerner U, *et al.* The metabolism of morphine and heroin in man. *Drug Metab Rev* 1975; **4:** 39–73.
2. Inturrisi CE, *et al.* The pharmacokinetics of heroin in patients with chronic pain. *N Engl J Med* 1984; **310:** 1213–17.
3. Moore RA, *et al.* Opiate metabolism and excretion. *Baillieres Clin Anaesthesiol* 1987; **1:** 829–58.
4. Barrett DA, *et al.* Morphine kinetics after diamorphine infusion in premature neonates. *Br J Clin Pharmacol* 1991; **32:** 31–7.


**Administration.** Diamorphine is much more lipid-soluble and has a more rapid onset and shorter duration of action than morphine. Although deacetylation to morphine occurs rapidly in the blood it occurs only slowly in the CSF following intraspinal injection of diamorphine.[1] After intrathecal injection diamorphine was removed from the CSF much more rapidly than morphine.[2] Peak plasma concentrations of morphine following epidural diamorphine injection were significantly higher and were achieved significantly faster than after epidural injection of morphine.[3]


1. Morgan M. The rational use of intrathecal and extradural opioids. *Br J Anaesth* 1989; **63:** 165–88.
2. Moore A, *et al.* Spinal fluid kinetics of morphine and heroin. *Clin Pharmacol Ther* 1984; **35:** 40–5.
3. Watson J, *et al.* Plasma morphine concentrations and analgesic effects of lumbar extradural morphine and heroin. *Anesth Analg* 1984; **63:** 629–34.


**Children.** Loading doses of diamorphine of either 50 micrograms/kg or 200 micrograms/kg were given as an infusion over 30 minutes to 19 ventilated neonates followed by a continuous infusion of 15 micrograms/kg per hour, and the pharmacokinetics of the products of diamorphine metabolism (morphine, morphine-6-glucuronide, and morphine-3-glucuronide) studied.[1] Although the overall elimination of morphine was reduced compared with adults, the relative contributions of the various metabolic routes of morphine remained similar between neonates and adults. Data from this study did not indicate any advantage for the higher loading dose (see also under Uses and Administration, below).


1. Barrett DA, *et al.* Morphine, morphine-6-glucuronide and morphine-3-glucuronide pharmacokinetics in newborn infants receiving diamorphine infusions. *Br J Clin Pharmacol* 1996; **41:** 531–7.


## Uses and Administration

Diamorphine hydrochloride is an acetylated morphine derivative and is a more potent opioid analgesic (p.73) than morphine (p.62). Diamorphine is used for the relief of severe pain especially in palliative care. It is also used similarly to morphine for the relief of dyspnoea due to pulmonary oedema resulting from left ventricular failure. Diamorphine has a powerful cough suppressant effect and has been given as Diamorphine Linctus (BPC 1973) to control cough associated with terminal lung cancer although morphine is now preferred.

In the treatment of acute pain standard doses of diamorphine hydrochloride by subcutaneous or intramuscular injection are 5 to 10 mg every 4 hours. Doses equivalent to one-quarter to one-half of the corresponding intramuscular dose may be given by slow intravenous injection. For the pain of myocardial infarction diamorphine hydrochloride is given in doses of 5 mg by slow intravenous injection at a rate of 1 mg/minute with a further dose of 2.5 to 5 mg if required; doses may be reduced by one-half for elderly or frail patients. Doses of 2.5 to 5 mg may be given intravenously at the same rate for acute pulmonary oedema. For chronic pain 5 to 10 mg may be given by subcutaneous or intramuscular injection every 4 hours; the dose may be increased according to needs. Similar doses may be given by mouth, although it is converted to morphine by first-pass metabolism (see Pharmacokinetics, above). Diamorphine hydrochloride may also be given by continuous subcutaneous infusion or intraspinally.

◊ Because of its abuse potential, supply of diamorphine is carefully controlled and in many countries it is not available for clinical use; morphine can provide equivalent analgesia by dose adjustment. There has been much debate regarding the relative merits of analgesia with diamorphine or morphine. Many now regard oral morphine to be the opioid analgesic of choice although diamorphine hydrochloride may be preferred for injection because it is more soluble in water thus allowing the use of smaller dose volumes. Diamorphine hydrochloride may also be preferred to morphine salts for intraspinal use because it is more lipid-soluble.

As a guide to relative potency diamorphine hydrochloride 5 mg intramuscularly is approximately equivalent to 10 mg by mouth which in turn is approximately equivalent to morphine sulfate 15 mg by mouth.

**Administration in children.** In a study[1] of the effects of diamorphine in 34 premature infants (gestational age 26 to 40 weeks), a loading dose of 50 micrograms/kg given as an intravenous infusion over 30 minutes followed by a continuous infusion at a rate of 15 micrograms/kg per hour was considered to be safe and resulted in plasma concentrations of morphine comparable with those that usually produce adequate analgesia in children and adults; the duration of the infusion ranged from 14 to 149 hours. Small but significant reductions in heart rate and mean blood pressure were noted but these were not associated with any clinical deterioration. The fall in respiration rate reflected the desired intention to encourage synchronisation of the infants' breathing with the ventilator. The authors concluded that intravenous diamorphine could be given safely to neonates and would provide adequate analgesia. A later study[2] indicated that the use of a 200 micrograms/kg loading dose conferred no benefit over a 50 micrograms/kg dose and might produce undesirable physiological effects. In a comparative study[3] with morphine (200 micrograms/kg loading dose over 2 hours, followed by maintenance infusion of 25 micrograms/kg per hour) in ventilated preterm neonates requiring sedation, diamorphine (120 micrograms/kg over 2 hours and then 15 micrograms/kg per hour) was as effective as morphine in producing sedation and also had a faster onset of action. The small but significant drop in blood pressure noted during morphine infusions was not seen with diamorphine infusions. Continuous intravenous infusions of 7 micrograms/kg per hour have been used in neonates not requiring ventilation.[4]

The subcutaneous route appeared to be as effective and safe as the intravenous route for infusions in children for postoperative pain relief after elective abdominal surgery.[5] The dose of diamorphine used in both groups of children was 1 mg/kg given at a rate of 20 micrograms/kg per hour. Intranasal diamorphine has been investigated in adults and children, and appears to be effective and well tolerated; because it does not require a needle it may offer particular advantages in children.[6]


1. Elias-Jones AC, *et al.* Diamorphine infusion in the preterm neonate. *Arch Dis Child* 1991; **66:** 1155–7.
2. Barker DP, *et al.* Randomised, double blind trial of two loading dose regimens of diamorphine in ventilated newborn infants. *Arch Dis Child* 1995; **73:** F22–F26.
3. Wood CM, *et al.* Randomised double blind trial of morphine versus diamorphine for sedation of preterm neonates. *Arch Dis Child Fetal Neonatal Ed* 1998; **79:** F34–F39.
4. Blanchard S. Analgesic use in neonatal necrotising enterocolitis. *Pharm J* 1992; **248:** 52.
5. Semple D, *et al.* Comparison of iv and sc diamorphine infusions for the treatment of acute pain in children. *Br J Anaesth* 1996; **76:** 310–12.
6. Kendall JM, Latter VS. Intranasal diamorphine as an alternative to intramuscular morphine: pharmacokinetic and pharmacodynamic aspects. *Clin Pharmacokinet* 2003; **42:** 501–13.


**Opioid dependence.** Many opiate misusers have expressed a preference for withdrawal using diamorphine rather than methadone. In a comparative study stabilisation was achieved using either diamorphine or methadone 1 mg/mL oral solutions;[1] patients could not identify which they had been given. Whenever signs of physical withdrawal were observed 10 mL of either solution was given and the total amount over the first 24 hours taken as the patient's daily requirement. The mean dose of diamorphine required for stabilisation was 55 mg compared with 36 mg for methadone. Some centres have administered diamorphine in the form of reefers.

Breast feeding has been used to treat diamorphine dependence in the offspring of dependent mothers but this is no longer considered to be the best method and some authorities recommend that breast feeding should be stopped.


1. Ghodse AH, *et al.* Comparison of oral preparations of heroin and methadone to stabilise opiate misusers as inpatients. *BMJ* 1990; **300:** 719–20.


**Pain.** ACUTE PAIN. Rapid pain relief may be obtained with the intravenous injection of diamorphine. Other routes include the intraspinal route for which diamorphine is well suited because of its lipid solubility and pharmacokinetics. Epidural doses of diamorphine have ranged from 0.5 to 10 mg.[1] One study[2] found that diamorphine 5 mg produced rapid analgesia whether given intramuscularly (in 1 mL of 0.9% sodium chloride) or epidurally (in 10 mL of 0.9% sodium chloride) for pain following caesarean section, but analgesia was significantly more prolonged and more intense following epidural injection; itching was reported by 50% of patients undergoing epidural analgesia. Continuous epidural infusion of diamorphine 0.5 mg/hour in 15 mL of 0.125% bupivacaine provided postoperative analgesia superior to that with either drug alone in patients undergoing major abdominal gynaecological surgery.[3] Continuous epidural infusion of diamorphine 0.4 to 0.6 mg/hour in 0.15% bupivacaine produced analgesia superior to that with either epidural bolus injection of diamorphine 3.6 mg in 9 mL of 0.9% saline or patient-controlled intravenous administration of diamorphine at a maximum rate of 1 mg per 5 minutes in patients undergoing total abdominal hysterectomy.[4] However, more patients receiving the continuous epidural infusion were hypoxaemic than in the other 2 groups. Diamorphine 5 mg in 8 mL of 0.9% sodium chloride produced comparable analgesia to 8 mL of 0.375% bupivacaine when given epidurally during labour but the duration was longer with diamorphine; addition of adrenaline appeared to improve the quality and duration of analgesia with diamorphine.[5] The addition of diamorphine 5 mg to 10 mL of 0.25% bupivacaine also enhanced pain relief when given epidurally in the first stage of labour.[6] In a similar study addition of diamorphine to bupivacaine produced a high incidence of pruritus and drowsiness.[7]

Diamorphine has also been given intrathecally for postoperative analgesia and should be effective at lower doses than with the epidural route because of greater CSF concentrations. Diamorphine 0.25 or 0.5 mg administered intrathecally with bupivacaine spinal anaesthesia both provided greater postoperative analgesia than bupivacaine alone,[8] but the incidence of adverse effects, especially nausea, vomiting, and urinary retention, was still high with either dose and routine use of this technique was not recommended. Intrathecal administration of diamorphine with bupivacaine has also been used for analgesia during labour.[9]

Diamorphine has been extensively used by cardiologists in the UK for the management of pain in acute left ventricular failure, unstable angina, and myocardial infarction. It has been theorised that diamorphine may offer benefits over morphine because its stimulatory effects at opioid δ receptors on the myocardium may reduce the extent of myocardial damage.[10] Evidence to support this theory is, however, lacking.


1. Morgan M. The rational use of intrathecal and extradural opioids. *Br J Anaesth* 1989; **63:** 165–88.
2. Macrae DJ, *et al.* Double-blind comparison of the efficacy of extradural diamorphine, extradural phenoperidine and im diamorphine following caesarean section. *Br J Anaesth* 1987; **59:** 354–9.
3. Lee A, *et al.* Postoperative analgesia by continuous extradural infusion of bupivacaine and diamorphine. *Br J Anaesth* 1988; **60:** 845–50.
4. Madej TH, *et al.* Hypoxaemia and pain relief after lower abdominal surgery: comparison of extradural and patient-controlled analgesia. *Br J Anaesth* 1992; **69:** 554–7.
5. Keenan GMA, *et al.* Extradural diamorphine with adrenaline in labour: comparison with diamorphine and bupivacaine. *Br J Anaesth* 1991; **66:** 242–6.
6. McGrady EM, *et al.* Epidural diamorphine and bupivacaine in labour. *Anaesthesia* 1989; **44:** 400–3.
7. Bailey CR, *et al.* Diamorphine-bupivacaine mixture compared with plain bupivacaine for analgesia. *Br J Anaesth* 1994; **72:** 58–61.
8. Reay BA, *et al.* Low-dose intrathecal diamorphine analgesia following major orthopaedic surgery. *Br J Anaesth* 1989; **62:** 248–52.
9. Kestin IG, *et al.* Analgesia for labour and delivery using incremental diamorphine and bupivacaine via a 32-gauge intrathecal catheter. *Br J Anaesth* 1992; **68:** 244–7.
10. Poullis M. Diamorphine and British cardiology: so we are right! *Heart* 1999; **82:** 645–6.

CHRONIC PAIN. Patients with chronic opioid-sensitive pain are often treated with diamorphine given by continuous subcutaneous infusion using a small battery-operated syringe driver. The following technique has been described.[1] Diamorphine hydrochloride 1 g can be dissolved in 1.6 mL of water to give a solution with a volume of 2.4 mL (415 mg/mL), but the maximum suggested concentration is 250 mg/mL. If the analgesic requirement is not known the following protocol is recommended:

- Start injections every 4 hours of 2.5 or 5 mg diamorphine, or, if the patient has already been taking opioids, a dose that is equivalent to the last dose
- If this is unsatisfactory increase this dose in 50% increments until the patient reports even a little pain relief
- Calculate the 24-hour requirement by multiplying by six, and start the infusion at this level
- Increase the 24-hour dosage in the pump by 50% increments until the pain is controlled. Note that requirements may vary from less than 20 mg to more than 5 g per 24 hours.

When starting an infusion it is important not to allow any breakthrough pain. This may be achieved either by starting the infusion more than 2 hours before the previous oral dose wears off or by giving a loading dose injection of the 4-hourly requirement.

Although generally free from complications, sterile abscess formation was reported in 2 patients with advanced cancer receiving diamorphine by continuous subcutaneous infusions.[2]

The intraventricular route was used successfully in 2 patients with intractable cancer pain.[3]


1. Dover SB. Syringe driver in terminal care. *BMJ* 1987; **294:** 553–5.
2. Hoskin PJ, *et al.* Sterile abscess formation by continuous subcutaneous infusion of diamorphine. *BMJ* 1988; **296:** 1605.
3. Reeve WG, Todd JG. Intraventricular diamorphine via an Ommaya shunt for intractable cancer pain. *Br J Anaesth* 1990; **65:** 544–7.


## Preparations

***BP 2003:*** Diamorphine Injection;
***BPC 1973:*** Diamorphine Linctus.

**Proprietary Preparations** (details are given in Part 3)
**UK:** Diagesil†; Diamorf†.

# Diclofenac (*BAN, rINN*)

Diclofenaco. [2-(2,6-Dichloroanilino)phenyl]acetic acid.
$C_{14}H_{11}Cl_2NO_2$ = 296.1.
*CAS — 15307-86-5.*
*ATC — M01AB05; M02AA15; S01BC03.*

## Diclofenac Diethylamine (*BANM*)

Diclofenac Diethylammonium; Diclofenaco dietilamina.
$C_{18}H_{22}Cl_2N_2O_2$ = 369.3.
*CAS — 78213-16-8.*

**Pharmacopoeias.** In *Br.*

**BP 2003** (Diclofenac Diethylamine). A white to light beige, crystalline powder. Sparingly soluble in water and in acetone; freely soluble in alcohol and in methyl alcohol; practically insoluble in 1M sodium hydroxide. The pH of a 1% solution in alcohol (10%) is between 6.4 and 8.4. Store in airtight containers. Protect from light.

## Diclofenac Potassium (*BANM, USAN, rINNM*)

CGP-45840B; Diclofenaco potásico; Diclofenacum Kalicum. Potassium [o-(2,6-dichloroanilino)phenyl]acetate.
$C_{14}H_{10}Cl_2KNO_2$ = 334.2.
*CAS — 15307-81-0.*

**Pharmacopoeias.** In *Eur.* (see p.vi).

**Ph. Eur. 5.0** (Diclofenac Potassium). A white or slightly yellowish, slightly hygroscopic, crystalline powder. Sparingly soluble in water; soluble in alcohol; slightly soluble in acetone; freely soluble in methyl alcohol. Store in airtight containers. Protect from light.

## Diclofenac Sodium (*BANM, USAN, rINNM*)

Diclofenaco sódico; Diclofenacum Natricum; Diclophenac Sodium; GP-45840. Sodium [2-(2,6-dichloroanilino)phenyl]acetate.
$C_{14}H_{10}Cl_2NNaO_2$ = 318.1.
*CAS — 15307-79-6.*

NOTE. DICL is a code approved by the BP 2003 for use on single unit doses of eye drops containing diclofenac sodium where the individual container may be too small to bear all the appropriate labelling information.

**Pharmacopoeias.** In *Chin., Eur.* (see p.vi), *Jpn, US,* and *Viet.*

**Ph. Eur. 5.0** (Diclofenac Sodium). A white to slightly yellowish, slightly hygroscopic, crystalline powder. Sparingly soluble in water; soluble in alcohol; slightly soluble in acetone; freely soluble in methyl alcohol. Store in airtight containers. Protect from light.

**USP 27** (Diclofenac Sodium). A white to off-white, hygroscopic, crystalline powder. Sparingly soluble in water; soluble in alcohol; practically insoluble in chloroform and in ether; freely soluble in methyl alcohol. pH of a 1% solution in water is between 7.0 and 8.5. Store in airtight containers. Protect from light.

## Adverse Effects

As for NSAIDs in general, p.67.

There may be pain and, occasionally, tissue damage at the site of injection when diclofenac is given intramuscularly. Diclofenac suppositories may cause local irritation. Transient burning and stinging may occur with diclofenac ophthalmic solution; more serious corneal adverse effects have also occurred (see Effects on the Eyes, below).

**Incidence of adverse effects.** A review of worldwide clinical studies with diclofenac[1] has reported the incidence of drug-associated adverse effects to be about 12%; about 16% of patients who experienced adverse effects discontinued treatment (a figure corresponding to about 2% of the entire patient sample). The most frequently reported adverse effects were gastrointestinal and were reported in 7.6% of patients. CNS-related adverse effects were reported in 0.7% of patients and allergy or local reactions in 0.4%. This and other reviews[2] have shown that adverse effects associated with diclofenac are usually mild and transient and appear to be unrelated to the dose of drug given.


1. Willkens RF. Worldwide clinical safety experience with diclofenac. *Semin Arthritis Rheum* 1985; **15** (suppl 1): 105–10.
2. Small RE. Diclofenac sodium. *Clin Pharm* 1989; **8:** 545–8.


**Effects on the blood.** Results of a large survey undertaken to assess the relation between agranulocytosis, aplastic anaemia, and drug exposure indicated that diclofenac was significantly associated with aplastic anaemia, providing an estimated tenfold increase in risk.[1] There are reports of other haematological abnormalities including haemolytic anaemia,[2] thrombocytopenia,[3,4] neutropenia,[4] and agranulocytosis[5] occurring in patients given diclofenac.

Localised spontaneous bleeding,[6] bruising,[7] inhibition of platelet aggregation,[6] and prolonged bleeding time[7] have been reported.


1. The International Agranulocytosis and Aplastic Anemia Study. Risks of agranulocytosis and aplastic anemia: a first report of their relation to drug use with special reference to analgesics. *JAMA* 1986; **256:** 1749–57.
2. López A, *et al.* Autoimmune hemolytic anemia induced by diclofenac. *Ann Pharmacother* 1995; **29:** 787.
3. George S, Rahi AHS. Thrombocytopenia associated with diclofenac therapy. *Am J Health-Syst Pharm* 1995; **52:** 420–1.
4. Kim HL, Kovacs MJ. Diclofenac-associated thrombocytopenia and neutropenia. *Ann Pharmacother* 1995; **29:** 713–15.
5. Colomina P, Garcia S. Agranulocytosis caused by diclofenac. *DICP Ann Pharmacother* 1989; **23:** 507.
6. Price AJ, Obeid D. Spontaneous non-gastrointestinal bleeding associated with diclofenac. *Lancet* 1989; **ii:** 1520.
7. Khazan U, *et al.* Diclofenac sodium and bruising. *Ann Intern Med* 1990; **112:** 472–3.


**Effects on electrolytes.** Use of diclofenac has been associated with cases resembling the syndrome of inappropriate antidiuretic hormone secretion in elderly women.[1,2] Also the UK Committee on Safety of Medicines had received a report of fatal hyponatraemia in another elderly woman.[2]


1. Petersson I, *et al.* Water intoxication associated with non-steroidal anti-inflammatory drug therapy. *Acta Med Scand* 1987; **221:** 221–3.
2. Cheung NT, *et al.* Syndrome of inappropriate secretion of antidiuretic hormone induced by diclofenac. *BMJ* 1993; **306:** 186.


**Effects on the eyes.** A patient who had been taking oral diclofenac for several years and had increasingly complained of dry, gritty eyes noticed that eye irritation disappeared within 3 days when diclofenac had to be discontinued because of gastrointestinal effects.[1]

Ocular diclofenac has been implicated in reports of corneal toxicity. Ulceration of the conjunctiva or cornea, corneal or scleral melts, and perforations have been reported in patients using diclofenac eye drops, particularly after cataract surgery.[2-4] Keratitis and perforations were also reported with ketorolac eye drops,[4] although less frequently.


1. Reid ALA, Henderson R. Diclofenac and dry, irritable eyes. *Med J Aust* 1994; **160:** 308.
2. Lin JC, *et al.* Corneal melting associated with use of topical nonsteroidal anti-inflammatory drugs after ocular surgery. *Arch Ophthalmol* 2000; **118:** 1129–32.
3. Congdon NG, *et al.* Corneal complications associated with topical ophthalmic use of nonsteroidal antiinflammatory drugs. *J Cataract Refract Surg* 2001; **27:** 622–31.
4. Guidera AC, *et al.* Keratitis, ulceration, and perforation associated with topical nonsteroidal anti-inflammatory drugs. *Ophthalmology* 2001; **108:** 936–44.


**Effects on the gastrointestinal tract.** The most frequent adverse effects reported in patients given diclofenac systemically are gastrointestinal in nature. Typical reactions include epigastric pain, nausea, vomiting, and diarrhoea. Rarely peptic ulcer and gastrointestinal bleeding have occurred. Diclofenac has also been implicated as the causative agent in colonic ulceration,[1] small bowel perforation,[2] and pseudomembranous colitis.[3] Rectal administration of diclofenac suppositories may cause local reactions such as itching, burning, or exacerbation of haemorrhoids.


1. Carson J, *et al.* Colonic ulceration and bleeding during diclofenac therapy. *N Engl J Med* 1990; **323:** 135.
2. Deakin M, *et al.* Small bowel perforation associated with an excessive dose of slow release diclofenac sodium. *BMJ* 1988; **297:** 488–9.
3. Gentric A, Pennec YL. Diclofenac-induced pseudomembranous colitis. *Lancet* 1992; **340:** 126–7.


**Effects on the kidneys.** Renal papillary necrosis[1] and nephrotic syndrome[2-4] have been reported in patients taking diclofenac. See also under Effects on Electrolytes, above.


1. Scott SJ, *et al.* Renal papillary necrosis associated with diclofenac sodium. *BMJ* 1986; **292:** 1050.
2. Beun GDM, *et al.* Isolated minimal change nephropathy associated with diclofenac. *BMJ* 1987; **295:** 182–3.
3. Yinnon AM, *et al.* Nephrotic syndrome associated with diclofenac sodium. *BMJ* 1987; **295:** 556.
4. Tattersall J, *et al.* Membranous nephropathy associated with diclofenac. *Postgrad Med J* 1992; **68:** 392–3.


**Effects on the liver.** Elevations of serum aminotransferase activity and clinical hepatitis,[1-6] including fatal fulminant hepatitis[2,5] have occurred in patients taking diclofenac. There has also been a case report of hepato-renal damage attributed to diclofenac.[7] Analysis[8] of 180 of the cases of diclofenac-associated hepatic injury received by the FDA between November 1988 and June 1991 suggested an increased risk of hepatotoxicity in female patients and those taking diclofenac for osteoarthritis. Hepatotoxicity had been detected within 6 months of starting diclofenac in 85% of the patients. The biochemical pattern of injury was hepatocellular or mixed hepatocellular in 66% of patients and cholestatic injury was found in 8% of patients. Signs of hypersensitivity were uncommon and it was considered that the mechanism of hepatic injury was likely to be a metabolic idiosyncratic reaction rather than due to intrinsic toxicity of diclofenac.


1. Dunk AA, *et al.* Diclofenac hepatitis. *BMJ* 1982; **284:** 1605–6.
2. Breen EG, *et al.* Fatal hepatitis associated with diclofenac. *Gut* 1986; **27:** 1390–3.
3. Schapira D, *et al.* Diclofenac-induced hepatotoxicity. *Postgrad Med J* 1986; **62:** 63–5.
4. Ryley NG, *et al.* Diclofenac associated hepatitis. *Gut* 1989; **30:** A708.
5. Helfgott SM, *et al.* Diclofenac-associated hepatotoxicity. *JAMA* 1990; **264:** 2660–2.
6. Purcell P, *et al.* Diclofenac hepatitis. *Gut* 1991; **32:** 1381–5.
7. Diggory P, *et al.* Renal and hepatic impairment in association with diclofenac administration. *Postgrad Med J* 1989; **64:** 507–8.
8. Banks AT, *et al.* Diclofenac-associated hepatotoxicity: analysis of 180 cases reported to the Food and Drug Administration as adverse reactions. *Hepatology* 1995; **22:** 820–7.


**Effects on the skin.** Self-limiting skin reactions such as rash or pruritus may occur in patients given diclofenac. More serious skin reactions attributed to diclofenac include bullous dermatitis[1] and erythema multiforme.[2] Local irritation and necrosis has occurred on intramuscular injection of diclofenac.[3,4]


1. Gabrielsen TØ, *et al.* Drug-induced bullous dermatosis with linear IgA deposits along the basement membrane. *Acta Derm Venereol (Stockh)* 1981; **61:** 439–41.
2. Morris BAP, Remtulla SS. Erythema multiforme major following use of diclofenac. *Can Med Assoc J* 1985; **133:** 665.
3. Stricker BHC, van Kasteren BJ. Diclofenac-induced isolated myonecrosis and the Nicolau syndrome. *Ann Intern Med* 1992; **117:** 1058.
4. Pillans PI, O'Connor N. Tissue necrosis and necrotising fasciitis after intramuscular administration of diclofenac. *Ann Pharmacother* 1995; **29:** 264–6.


**Hypersensitivity.** Aspirin-sensitive asthmatic patients have developed reactions (rhinorrhoea, tightness of chest, wheezing, dyspnoea) when challenged with diclofenac in doses of 10 to 25 mg[1] and the UK Committee on Safety of Medicines has received a report of an aspirin-sensitive patient who died from acute asthma 4 hours after a single 25-mg dose of diclofenac.[2]

Anaphylactic shock has been reported.[3]


1. Szczeklik A, *et al.* Asthmatic attacks induced in aspirin-sensitive patients by diclofenac and naproxen. *BMJ* 1977; **2:** 231–2.
2. Committee on Safety of Medicines/Medicines Control Agency. Avoid all NSAIDs in aspirin-sensitive patients. *Current Problems* 1993; **19:** 8.
3. Dux S, *et al.* Anaphylactic shock induced by diclofenac. *BMJ* 1983; **286:** 1861.


## Precautions

As for NSAIDs in general, p.69.

Ophthalmic preparations containing diclofenac should not be used by patients who wear soft contact lenses.

Use of intravenous diclofenac is contra-indicated in patients with moderate or severe renal impairment, hypovolaemia, or dehydration; in addition, intravenous diclofenac should not be used in patients with a history of haemorrhagic diathesis, cerebrovascular bleeding (including suspected), or asthma nor in patients undergoing surgery with a high risk of haemorrhage.

**Breast feeding.** Diclofenac is distributed into breast milk although the *British National Formulary* and some manufacturers consider the amount to be too small to be harmful to breast-fed infants.

**Porphyria.** Diclofenac sodium has been associated with acute attacks of porphyria and is considered unsafe in porphyric patients.

## Interactions

For interactions associated with NSAIDs, see p.69.

Diclofenac should not be given intravenously to patients already receiving other NSAIDs or anticoagulants including low-dose heparin.

**Ciclosporin.** Deterioration in renal function has been attributed to the use of diclofenac with ciclosporin.[1] Increased concentrations of diclofenac were also noted with ciclosporin;[2] the manufacturer of ciclosporin recommends that the dosage of diclofenac should be reduced by about one-half when the two are given together.


1. Branthwaite JP, Nicholls A. Cyclosporin and diclofenac interaction in rheumatoid arthritis. *Lancet* 1991; **337:** 252.
2. Kovarik JM, *et al.* Cyclosporine and nonsteroidal antiinflammatory drugs: exploring potential drug interactions and their implications for the treatment of rheumatoid arthritis. *J Clin Pharmacol* 1997; **37:** 336–43.


**Diuretics.** Deterioration in renal function has been attributed to the use of diclofenac with *triamterene*.[1]


1. Härkönen M, Ekblom-Kullberg S. Reversible deterioration of renal function after diclofenac in patient receiving triamterene. *BMJ* 1986; **293:** 698–9.


**Gastrointestinal drugs.** A decrease in the plasma concentration of diclofenac has been reported[1] when given after *sucralfate*.


1. Pedrazzoli J, *et al.* Short-term sucralfate administration alters potassium diclofenac absorption in healthy male volunteers. *Br J Clin Pharmacol* 1997; **43:** 104–108.


**Lipid regulating drugs.** *Colestyramine* appears substantially to reduce the bioavailability of diclofenac when the two drugs are given together;[1] *colestipol* produces a similar but smaller effect.


1. al-Balla SR, *et al.* The effects of cholestyramine and colestipol on the absorption of diclofenac in man. *Int J Clin Pharmacol Ther* 1994; **32:** 441–5.


**Misoprostol.** The plasma concentration of diclofenac was reduced when it was given as a 100-mg dose daily in the form of a modified-release preparation to subjects receiving misoprostol 800 micrograms daily.[1] Use together was also associated with an increase in the incidence and severity of gastrointestinal effects. Studies by the manufacturer[2] had failed to find any significant pharmacokinetic interactions between diclofenac and misoprostol when given in a formulation containing diclofenac 50 mg and misoprostol 200 micrograms.


1. Dammann HG, *et al.* Differential effects of misoprostol and ranitidine on the pharmacokinetics of diclofenac and gastrointestinal symptoms. *Br J Clin Pharmacol* 1993; **36:** 345–9.
2. Karim A. Pharmacokinetics of diclofenac and misoprostol when administered alone or as a combination product. *Drugs* 1993; **45** (suppl 1): 7–14.


**Parasympathomimetics.** The manufacturer of acetylcholine chloride ophthalmic preparations has stated that there have been reports that *acetylcholine* and *carbachol* have been ineffective when used in patients treated with topical (ophthalmic) NSAIDs.

## Pharmacokinetics

Diclofenac is rapidly absorbed when given as an oral solution, sugar-coated tablets, rectal suppository, or by intramuscular injection. It is absorbed more slowly when given as enteric-coated tablets, especially when this dosage form is given with food. Although diclofenac given orally is almost completely absorbed, it is subject to first-pass metabolism so that about 50% of the drug reaches the systemic circulation in the unchanged form. Diclofenac is also absorbed percutaneously. At therapeutic concentrations it is more than 99% bound to plasma proteins. Diclofenac penetrates synovial fluid where concentrations may persist even when plasma concentrations fall; small amounts are distributed into breast milk. The terminal plasma half-life is about 1 to 2 hours. Diclofenac is metabolised to 4′-hydroxydiclofenac, 5-hydroxydiclofenac, 3′-hydroxydiclofenac and 4′,5-dihydroxydiclofenac. It is then excreted in the form of glucuronide and sulfate conjugates, mainly in the urine (about 60%) but also in the bile (about 35%); less than 1% is excreted as unchanged diclofenac.

◊ References.


1. Fowler PD, *et al.* Plasma and synovial fluid concentrations of diclofenac sodium and its major hydroxylated metabolites during long-term treatment of rheumatoid arthritis. *Eur J Clin Pharmacol* 1983; **25:** 389–94.
2. Maggi CA, *et al.* Comparative bioavailability of diclofenac hydroxyethylpyrrolidine vs diclofenac sodium in man. *Eur J Clin Pharmacol* 1990; **38:** 207–8.
3. Davies NM, Anderson KE. Clinical pharmacokinetics of diclofenac: therapeutic insights and pitfalls. *Clin Pharmacokinet* 1997; **33:** 184–213.
4. Brenner SS, *et al.* Influence of age and cytochrome P450 2C9 genotype on the steady-state disposition of diclofenac and celecoxib. *Clin Pharmacokinet* 2003; **42:** 283–92.


## Uses and Administration

Diclofenac, a phenylacetic acid derivative, is an NSAID (p.70). It is used mainly as the sodium salt for the relief of pain and inflammation in various conditions: musculoskeletal and joint disorders such as rheumatoid arthritis, osteoarthritis, and ankylosing spondylitis; peri-articular disorders such as bursitis and tendinitis; soft-tissue disorders such as sprains and strains; and other painful conditions such as renal colic, acute gout, dysmenorrhoea, migraine, and following some surgical procedures. It has also been used in some countries for the management of actinic keratoses and fever. Eye drops of diclofenac sodium are used for the prevention of intra-operative miosis during cataract extraction, for the treatment of inflammation following surgery or laser treatment of the eye, for pain in corneal epithelial defects following surgery or accidental trauma, and for the relief of ocular signs and symptoms of seasonal allergic conjunctivitis.

The usual dose of diclofenac sodium **by mouth** or **rectally** is 75 to 150 mg daily in divided doses. Modified-release preparations of diclofenac sodium are available for oral use. Diclofenac has also been given in equivalent doses by mouth as the free acid in dispersible preparations for short-term treatment up to 3 months long. Diclofenac is also given by mouth as the potassium salt. Doses of the potassium salt are similar to those for diclofenac sodium. Diclofenac potassium is also used in the treatment of migraine in an initial dose of 50 mg taken at the first signs of an attack; an additional dose of 50 mg may be taken after 2 hours if symptoms persist. If necessary further doses of 50 mg may be taken every 4 to 6 hours to a maximum daily dose of 200 mg.

Diclofenac sodium may also be given by deep intramuscular **injection** into the gluteal muscle in a dose of 75 mg once daily or, if required in severe conditions, 75 mg twice daily. Diclofenac sodium may also be given as a continuous or intermittent intravenous infusion in glucose 5% or sodium chloride 0.9% (both previously buffered with sodium bicarbonate). For the treatment of postoperative pain a dose of 75 mg may be given over 30 to 120 minutes. The dose may be repeated if necessary after 4 to 6 hours. To prevent postoperative pain, 25 to 50 mg diclofenac sodium may be given after surgery over 15 to 60 minutes followed by 5 mg/hour to a maximum of 150 mg daily. The maximum period recommended for parenteral use is 2 days. Diclofenac sodium is also used intramuscularly in renal colic in a dose of 75 mg repeated once after 30 minutes if necessary.

In children 1 to 12 years old the dose by mouth or rectally for juvenile idiopathic arthritis is 1 to 3 mg/kg daily in divided doses.

Diclofenac sodium is used as a 0.1% **ophthalmic solution** in a number of situations:

- for the prevention of intra-operative miosis during cataract surgery, it is instilled in the appropriate eye 4 times during the 2 hours before surgery
- for the treatment of postoperative inflammation following cataract surgery, it is instilled 4 times daily for up to 28 days starting 24 hours after surgery
- for the control of post-photorefractive keratectomy pain, it is instilled twice in the hour before surgery, then one drop twice at 5-minute intervals immediately after the procedure, and then every 2 to 5 hours while awake for up to 24 hours
- for pain control following accidental trauma one drop is instilled 4 times daily for up to 2 days
- in the treatment of inflammation and discomfort after strabismus surgery one drop is instilled 4 times daily for the first week; this is reduced to 3 times daily in the second week, twice daily in the third week, and as required for the fourth week
- for the control of inflammation after argon laser trabeculoplasty one drop is instilled 4 times during the 2 hours before the procedure followed by one drop 4 times daily for up to 7 days after the procedure
- for the treatment of pain and discomfort after radial keratotomy one drop is given before surgery followed by one drop immediately after surgery and then one drop 4 times daily for up to 2 days
- to relieve symptoms of seasonal allergic conjunctivitis one drop is instilled 4 times daily as necessary

Diclofenac diethylamine is used **topically** as a gel containing the equivalent of 1% of diclofenac sodium for the local symptomatic relief of pain and inflammation; it is applied to the affected site 3 or 4 times daily; treatment should be reviewed after 14 days or after 28 days if used for osteoarthritis. A topical solution of diclofenac sodium 1.6% is also available for the treatment of osteoarthritis; it is applied in small aliquots to achieve a total of 20 to 40 drops, repeated four times daily. Diclofenac is also used in the management of actinic keratoses; it is applied twice daily as diclofenac sodium gel 3% for 60 to 90 days but the optimum therapeutic effect may not be seen until 30 days after the end of treatment. Diclofenac epolamine (diclofenac hydroxyethylpyrrolidine; DHEP) is also used topically.

Diclofenac is available in combination with misoprostol (see p.1519) for patients at risk of NSAID-induced peptic ulceration.

◊ Reviews.


1. Todd PA, Sorkin EM. Diclofenac sodium: a reappraisal of its pharmacodynamic and pharmacokinetic properties, and therapeutic efficacy. *Drugs* 1988; **35:** 244–85.
2. Small RE. Diclofenac sodium. *Clin Pharm* 1989; **8:** 545–8.
3. Barden J, *et al.* Single dose oral diclofenac for postoperative pain. Available in The Cochrane Library; Issue 2. Chichester: John Wiley; 2004.


**Administration.** TOPICAL. Some references to the use of plasters providing sustained topical release of diclofenac epolamine.


1. Galeazzi M, Marcolongo R. A placebo-controlled study of the efficacy and tolerability of a nonsteroidal anti-inflammatory drug, DHEP plaster, in inflammatory peri- and extra-articular rheumatological diseases. *Drugs Exp Clin Res* 1993; **19:** 107–15.
2. Dreiser RL, Tisne-Camus M. DHEP plasters as a topical treatment of knee osteoarthritis—a double-blind placebo-controlled study. *Drugs Exp Clin Res* 1993; **19:** 117–23.


**Actinic keratoses.** Diclofenac sodium 3% in hyaluronic acid gel is used[1,2] in the treatment of actinic keratoses (see Basal Cell and Squamous Cell Carcinoma, p.522) despite previous concerns that the preparation may not be significantly more effective than hyaluronic acid gel alone.[3]


1. Rivers JK, McLean DI. An open study to assess the efficacy and safety of topical 3% diclofenac in a 2.5% hyaluronic acid gel for the treatment of actinic keratoses. *Arch Dermatol* 1997; **133:** 1239–42.
2. Rivers JK, *et al.* Topical treatment of actinic keratoses with 3.0% diclofenac in 2.5% hyaluronan gel. *Br J Dermatol* 2002; **146:** 94–100.
3. McEwan LE, Smith JG. Topical diclofenac/hyaluronic acid gel in the treatment of solar keratoses. *Australas J Dermatol* 1997; **38:** 187–9.


**Headache.** Diclofenac potassium may provide rapid relief in the treatment of acute migraine (p.464).[1]


1. McNeely W, Goa KL. Diclofenac-potassium in migraine. *Drugs* 1999; **57:** 991–1003.


## Preparations

***BP 2003:*** Diclofenac Gel; Diclofenac Tablets; Slow Diclofenac Tablets;
***USP 27:*** Diclofenac Sodium Delayed-release Tablets.

**Proprietary Preparations** (details are given in Part 3)

***Arg.:*** Ainedif; Aktiosan; Atomo Desinflamante Geldic; Banoclus; Blokium; Cataflam; Curinflam; Damixa; Desinflam; DFN; Diastone; Diclac; Dicloge-sic; Diclogrand; Diclomar; Dioxaflex; Disipan; Dolo Tomanil; Flotac; Flux-piren; Gel Antiinflamatorio; Imanol; Indofeno; Klonafenac; Lenitil; Leve-dad; Metaflex NF; Natura Fenac; Oxa; Oxaprost; Rodinac; Tomanil; Vesalion; Vimultisa; Voltaren; Voltaren Colirio; Xedenol; Xinia; ***Austral.:*** Arthrotec; Dencorub Anti-Inflammatory; Diclac; Diclohexal; Dinac; Fenac; Imflac; Voltaren; Voltaren Ophtha; ***Austria:*** Algefit; Arthrotec; Dedolor; Deflamat; Deflamm; Diclac; Diclaxol; Diclo-B; Diclobene; Di-clomelan; Diclostad; Diclosyl; Difene; Dolpasse; Fenaren; Flector; Maglu-phen; Tratul; Voltaren; Zymamed; ***Belg.:*** Arthrotec; Cataflam; Flector; Motifene; Voltaren; ***Braz.:*** Ana-Flex; Artren; Augelit; Bel-Gel; Benevran; Biofenac; Cataflam; Catalgem†; Cataren†; Cinaflan†; Clofaren; Clofen†; Clofenak; Deltaflogin; Deltaren; Desinflex; Diclac; Diclo P; Diclofen; Di-clofenax†; Diclogenom; Difenan; Dnaren; Dorflan; Dorgen; Doriflan; Dorpiren†; Fenaflan; Fenaren; Fenburil; Fisioren; Flanakin; Flanaren; Flex-amina; Flogan; Flogesic; Flogiren; Flogonac; Flotac; Gezon†; Infladoren; In-flamax; Inflaren†; Kindaren; Luparen; Neocoflan; Neotaflan; Neotaren; Olfen; Ortoflan; Probenxil; Reumadil†; Reumaren†; Reutaren†; Sin-tofenac; Still; Tricin; Vendrex; Voltaflan; Voltaflex; Voltaren; Voltaren Co-lirio; Voltrix; ***Canad.:*** Apo-Diclo; Arthrotec; Diclotec; Novo-Difenac; Nu-Diclo; Vofenal†; Voltaren; Voltaren Ophtha; ***Chile:*** 3A Ofteno; Ar-tren; Autdol; Cataflam; Deflamat; Dicogel; Dignofenac; Elitiran; Exflam; Flotac; Lertus; Merpal; Noxiflex; Oftic; Pirexyl; Piroflam; Pro Lertus; Sipirac; Turbogesic; Voltaren; ***Denm.:*** Arthrotec; Diclodan; Diclogea; Di-clon; Difenet; Modifenac; Voltaren; Vostar; ***Fin.:*** Arthrotec; Diclometin; Diclomex; Motifene; Trabona; Voltaren; ***Fr.:*** Artotec; Flector; Voldal; Voltarene; Xenid; ***Ger.:*** Allvoran; Arthotec; Arthrex Duo†; Arthrex†; Benfofen; Delphinac; Diclac; Diclo; Diclo-Divido; Diclo-Puren; Diclo-saar; Diclo-Spondyril†; Diclo-Tablinen†; Diclo†; Diclodoc; Diclofenbeta; Dic-logrun†; Diclomerck†; Diclophlogont; Diclorektal†; Dolgit-Diclo; dura-volten; Effekton; Jenafenac; Lexobene; Monoflam; Myogit; Rewodina; Si-gafenac; Solaraze; Toryxil†; Voltaren; Voltaren Ophtha; ***Gr.:*** Anthraxiton; Cataflam; Delimon; Denaclof; Diclophlogont; Evinopon; Fenoclof; Opto-bet; Rheumavek; Ruvominox; Urigon; Voltaren; Vurdon; ***Hong Kong:*** Abitren†; Almiral; Analpan; Apo-Diclo; Arthrotec; Cataflam; Clofec; Clofenac; Diclo-Denk; Diclofen; Diclogesic; Diclowal; Difenat†; Difenac; Difenol; Flector; Grofenac; Inflanac; Novo-Difenac; Olfen; Remafen; Remethan; Rhemofenax; Uniren; Voltaren; Voltaren Ophtha; ***India:*** Di-clomol; Diclonac; Dicloran; Doflex; Esgipyrin DS; Fensaide; I-Gesic; Jonac; Nac; Nacgel; Oxalgin; Relaxyl; Solunac; Tromagesic; Voveran; ***Irl.:*** Arthro-tec; Cataflam; Diclac; Diclo; Diclomel; Difene; Vologen; Voltarol; Voltarol Ophtha; ***Israel:*** Abitren; Arthrotec; Betaren; Cataflam; Dicloplast; Di-clorengel; Olfen; Voltaren; Voltaren Ophtha; ***Ital.:*** Algosenac; Artrofenac; Artrotec; Cataflam†; Dealgic; Deflamat; Diclocular; Diclodol†; Diclofan; Dicloftil; Dicloral; Dicloreum; Dolaut; Fenadol; Fender; Flector; Flogofenac; Forgenac; Lisiflen; Misofenac; Molfenac; Novapirina; Ribex Flu; Topfans; Voltaren; Voltfast; Zeroflog; **Malaysia:** Almiral; Apo-Diclo; Cataflam; Clofec; Clofenac; Difnal; Fenadium; Neo-Pyrazon; Olfen; Remafen; Remethan; Rhewlin; Taks; Voltaren; Voren; Wari-Diclowal; Zolterol; **Mex.:** 3-A; Algenac†; Alsidexten; Artrenac; Artrenac Pro; Artrotec; Cataflam; Clo-Far; Clonodifen; Deflox; Dicfafena; Dicloran; Dioxaflex; Dirret; Dofen; Dolaren; Dolflam; Dolofenac†; Ehlifena†; Evadol; Flankol; Flogoken; Flotac; Fustaren; Galedol; Lifenac; Liroken; Lodyfen; Logesic†; Mafena; Merxil; Practiser; Precifenac†; Selectofen; Vicmafen; Volfenac; Voltaren; **Neth.:** Arthrotec; Cataflam; Naclof; Voltaren; **Norw.:** Arthrotec; Cataflam; Modifenac; Otriflu; Voltaren; Voltaren Ophtha; **NZ:** Anfenax†; Apo-Diclo; Cataflam; Diclax; Flameril; Voltaren; Voltaren Ophtha; **Port.:** Arthrotec; Cataflam; Dicloftal; Diclotec; Difnan; Dorcalor; Fenil-V; Flameril; Olfen; Painex; Voltaren; **S.Afr.:** Arcanafenac†; Arthrotec; Athru-Derm; Cataflam; Dicloflam; Diclohexal; Flexagen†; Fortfen; Infla-Ban; Naclof†; Panamor; Sodiclo†; Veltex; Voltaren; Voltaren Ophtha; **Singapore:** Almiral; Arthrotec†; Biclopan†; Cataflam; Clofec; Clofenac; Diclo-Denk; Diclowal; Difenac; Difnal; Inac; Inflanac; Neo-Pyrazon; Olfen; Remafen; Remethan; Rhewlin; Ultrafen; Uniren; Voltaren; Voltaren Ophtha; Voren; Zolterol; **Spain:** Artrotec; Di Retard; Dolo Nervobion; Dolo-Voltaren; Dolotren; Liberalgium†; Luase; Normulen; Voltaren; Voltaren Emulgel; **Swed.:** Arthrotec; Modifenac; Solaraze; Voltaren; Voltaren Ophtha; Voltaren T; **Switz.:** Agofenac; Arthrotec; Athrofen; Deflamat; Diclo; diclobasan; Diclosifar; Ecofenac; Flector; Fortenac; Grofenac; Inflamac; Olfen; Primofenac; Rheufenac†; Traumasport†; Vifenac; Voltaren Emulgel; Voltaren Ophta; Voltarene; Voltarene Rapide; **Thai.:** Abitren†; Almiral; Ammi-Votara; Amminac; Arclonac; Arthrotec; Cataflam; Catanac; Chinclonac; Clofec; Clofon; Demac; Diclofen; Diclogel; Diclolan; Diclomol; Diclosian; Difelene; Difen; Difenac; Difeno; Dinac; Dinefec; Dosanac; Fenac; Fenagel; Inflanac; Lofenac; Masaren; Medaren; Myonac; Naclof; Olfen; Ostaren; Posnac; Putaren; Remethan; Rhumanol; Rumatab; Silflam; Subsyde; Taks; Tarjen; Tarjena; Uniren; Veenac; Volfenac; Volnac; Volta; Voltanac; Voltaren; Volverac; Voren†; Votamed; **UAE:** Clofen; **UK:** Acoflam; Arthrotec; Defanac; Dexomon; Dicloflex; Diclomax; Diclotard†; Diclovol; Diclozip; Econac; Fenactol; Flamatak; Flamrase; Flexotard†; Isclofen†; Lofensaid; Motifene; Pennsaid; Rheumatac; Rhumalgan; Slofenac; Solaraze; Volraman; Volsaid; Voltarol; Voltarol Ophtha; **USA:** Arthrotec; Cataflam; Solaraze; Voltaren.

**Multi-ingredient:** **Arg.:** Albesine Biotic; Algio Nervomax; Algio Nervomax Fuerte; Amixen Plus; Belmalen; Blokium B12; Blokium Flex; Blokium Gesic; Corteroid Gesic; Delta Tomanil B12; Desinflam Biotic; Diclogesic Relax; Diclomar Flex; Dioxaflex B12; Dioxaflex Forte; Dioxaflex Gesic; Dioxaflex Plus; Dolo Nervobion; Flaval; Hyanac; Lertus Biotic; Metaflex Plus NF; Meticil; Oxa B12; Oxa Forte; Oxa Sport; Oxadisten; Oxagesic; Rodinac Biotic; Rodinac Flex; Rodinac Gesic; Vesalion B12; Vesalion Flex; Vesalion Gesic; Virobron B12 NF; Voltaren Flex; Voltaren Forte; Xedenol B12; Xedenol Flex; **Austria:** Diclovit; Dolo-Neurobion; Neodolpasse; Neurofenac; Voltamicin; **Belg.:** Ocubrax; **Braz.:** Algi-Butazolon; Algi-Tanderil; Beserol; Diclofetamol; Dorpinol†; Sedilax; Tandene; Tanderalgin; Tandriflan; Tandrilax; Torsilax; Trilax; Voltamicin†; **Fr.:** Voltamicine†; **Ger.:** Combaren; **Hong Kong:** Neurofenac; Vidaclofen-Plus; **India:** Actimol; Buta-Proxyvon; Diclogenta; Diclomol; Dicloran-A; Duoflam Gel; Esgipyrin; Fenaplus; Fenaplus-MR; Fenaside-P; Flamar-MX; Myospaz Forte; Osteoflam-MR; Oxalgin-DP; Relaxyl Plus; Spasmo-Proxyvon Forte; Systaflam; **Ital.:** Voltamicin; **Malaysia:** Voren Plus; **Mex.:** Dolaren; Dolo-Neurobion; Dolo-Pangavit; Duciclon; Duoflex; Trazinac†; **Singapore:** Voltamicin; **Spain:** Ocubrax; **Switz.:** Tobrafen; Voltamicin.

## Diethylamine Salicylate

Salicilato de dietilamina.

$C_{11}H_{17}NO_3$ = 211.3.

*CAS — 4419-92-5.*

**Pharmacopoeias.** In *Br.* and *Chin.*

**BP 2003** (Diethylamine Salicylate). White or almost white, odourless or almost odourless crystals. Very soluble in water; freely soluble in alcohol and in chloroform. Protect from light. Avoid contact with iron or iron salts.

### Profile

Diethylamine salicylate is a salicylic acid derivative used topically in rubefacient preparations similarly to methyl salicylate (p.59) for rheumatic and muscular pain.

### Preparations

***BP 2003:*** Diethylamine Salicylate Cream.

**Proprietary Preparations** (details are given in Part 3)
**Belg.:** Algesal; **Canad.:** Algesal†; Physiogesic; **Fin.:** Algesal; **India:** Multigesic; **Ital.:** Algesal; Algoflex Samet†; **Neth.:** Algesal; **Norw.:** Algesal; **Port.:** Algiderma; Massagim; **Spain:** Artrogota†; **Swed.:** Algesal; **UK:** Algesal; Lloyd's Cream.

**Multi-ingredient:** **Arg.:** Algesal; Feparil; Rati Salil Flex; Salicrem; **Austral.:** Rubesal; **Austria:** Algesal; Derivon; Dolo-Menthoneurin; Dolorex; Igitur-antirheumatische; Igitur-Rheumafluid; Latesyl; Pasta rubra salicylata; Reparil; Rheugesal; Thermal; **Belg.:** Reparil; **Braz.:** Geloril†; Reparil; **Chile:** Repariven; **Fr.:** Algesal Suractive†; Reparil; Traumalgyl; **Ger.:** ABC Warme-Salbe; Algesal; Algesalona; Bartelin N†; Bartelin nico†; Contrheuma V + T Bad N†; Dolo-Menthoneurin; Doloneuro; Reparil-Gel N; Rheubalmin†; Rheuma V + T Bad N†; Rheuma-Bad†; Rheumichthol Bad†; **Hong Kong:** Reparil; Rubesal; **Ital.:** Aspercreme†; Edeven; Reparil; Sedalpan; Via Mal Traumagel; **Mex.:** Algesal; **Neth.:** Algesal Forte; **Norw.:** Thermal; **Port.:** Algesal; Latesil; Medalginan; Venoparil; **S.Afr.:** Reparil; **Spain:** Algesal; Contusin; Doctomitil; Dolmitin; Feparil; Radio Salil; **Switz.:** Algesal; Algesalona; Proctalgen; Reparil; Reparil N†; Roliwol B†; **Thai.:** Reparil; **UAE:** Rubicalm; **UK:** Fiery Jack; Transvasin Heat Spray.

## Diflunisal *(BAN, USAN, rINN)*

Diflunisalum; MK-647. 5-(2,4-Difluorophenyl)salicylic acid.

$C_{13}H_8F_2O_3$ = 250.2.

*CAS — 22494-42-4.*

*ATC — N02BA11.*

**Pharmacopoeias.** In *Eur.* (see p.vi) and *US.*

**Ph. Eur. 5.0** (Diflunisal). A white or almost white, crystalline powder. Practically insoluble in water; soluble in alcohol; dissolves in dilute solutions of alkali hydroxides. Protect from light.

**USP 27** (Diflunisal). A white to off-white, practically odourless, powder. Insoluble in water and in hexane; freely soluble in alcohol and in methyl alcohol; soluble in acetone and in ethyl acetate; slightly soluble in carbon tetrachloride, in chloroform, and in dichloromethane.

### Adverse Effects and Treatment

As for NSAIDs in general, p.67. The commonest side-effects occurring with diflunisal are gastrointestinal disturbances, headache, and rash. Peptic ulceration and gastrointestinal bleeding have been reported. Dizziness, drowsiness, insomnia, and tinnitus may also occur.

**Effects on the blood.** Haematological adverse effects associated with diflunisal appear to be infrequent. Thrombocytopenia associated with diflunisal-induced peripheral platelet destruction has been reported in a patient with rheumatoid arthritis.[1] Heinz-body haemolytic anaemia has also been reported, see under Hypersensitivity, below.

1. Bobrove AM. Diflunisal-associated thrombocytopenia in a patient with rheumatoid arthritis. *Arthritis Rheum* 1988; **31:** 148–9.

**Effects on the kidneys.** Acute interstitial nephritis, presenting as acute oliguric renal failure, erythroderma, and eosinophilia has followed the use of diflunisal.[1]

1. Chan LK, *et al.* Acute interstitial nephritis and erythroderma associated with diflunisal. *BMJ* 1980; **280:** 84–5.

**Effects on the lungs.** For reference to pneumonitis associated with diflunisal therapy, see under Hypersensitivity, below.

**Effects on the skin.** Reports of Stevens-Johnson syndrome associated with diflunisal.[1,2] See also under Hypersensitivity, below.

1. Hunter JA, *et al.* Diflunisal and Stevens-Johnson syndrome. *BMJ* 1978; **2:** 1088.
2. Grom JA, *et al.* Diflunisal-induced erythema multiforme major. *Hosp Formul* 1986; **21:** 353–4.

**Hypersensitivity.** Three cases of hypersensitivity to diflunisal in which the main clinical features were fever, elevated liver enzyme values, erythroderma, and eosinophilia, have been reported.[1] Heinz-body haemolytic anaemia occurred in one of the patients. Other hypersensitivity reactions associated with diflunisal therapy have included pneumonitis[2] and fulminant necrotising fasciitis.[3]

1. Cook DJ, *et al.* Three cases of diflunisal hypersensitivity. *Can Med Assoc J* 1988; **138:** 1029–30.
2. Rich MW, Thomas RA. A case of eosinophilic pneumonia and vasculitis induced by diflunisal. *Chest* 1997; **111:** 1767–9.
3. Krige JEJ, *et al.* Necrotising fasciitis after diflunisal for minor injury. *Lancet* 1985; **ii:** 1432–3.

**Overdosage.** Diflunisal poisoning has sometimes been fatal.[1,2] A dose of 15 g has been reported to have caused death when no other drugs were involved but a dose of 7.5 g has also been fatal when taken with other drugs.

1. Court H, Volans GN. Poisoning after overdose with non-steroidal anti-inflammatory drugs. *Adverse Drug React Acute Poisoning Rev* 1984; **3:** 1–21.
2. Levine B, *et al.* Diflunisal related fatality: a case report. *Forensic Sci Int* 1987; **35:** 45–50.

### Precautions

As for NSAIDs in general, p.69. Diflunisal may need to be given in reduced dosage in patients with significant renal impairment and should not be given when renal impairment is severe. Aspirin and other acetylated salicylates are not recommended for use in children unless specifically indicated, because of the risk of Reye's syndrome. Although this precaution has not been specifically extended to diflunisal it is not generally licensed for use in children.

### Interactions

For interactions associated with NSAIDs, see p.69.

Aspirin may produce a small decrease in the plasma concentration of diflunisal. Diflunisal has been reported to increase the plasma concentrations of indometacin and paracetamol; diflunisal with indometacin has been associated with fatal gastrointestinal haemorrhage and therefore the combination should not be used. Regular use of antacids may reduce the absorption of diflunisal.

**Benzodiazepines.** For the effect of diflunisal on plasma concentrations of *oxazepam*, see p.692.

**Probenecid.** Average steady-state plasma concentrations of diflunisal were increased by 65% when it was given with probenecid.[1] This was due mainly to reduced formation of the phenolic and acyl glucuronides. However, plasma concentrations of these glucuronides and the sulfate conjugate were also increased even more because probenecid also reduced their renal clearance.

1. Macdonald JI, *et al.* Effect of probenecid on the formation and elimination kinetics of the sulphate and glucuronide conjugates of diflunisal. *Eur J Clin Pharmacol* 1995; **47:** 519–23.

### Pharmacokinetics

Diflunisal is well absorbed from the gastrointestinal tract and peak plasma concentrations occur about 2 to 3 hours after ingestion of a single dose. It is more than 99% bound to plasma protein and has a plasma half-life of about 8 to 12 hours. Diflunisal exhibits non-linear pharmacokinetics so that doubling the dose more than doubles drug accumulation. Due to the long half-life and non-linear kinetics, several days are required to reach steady-state plasma concentrations following multiple dosing. The time to steady-state concentrations can be reduced by giving an initial loading dose. Concentrations of diflunisal in synovial fluid reach about 70% of those in plasma. Diflunisal is excreted in the urine mainly as glucuronide conjugates. Some biliary recycling may also occur. Diflunisal is distributed into breast milk with concentrations reported to be about 2 to 7% of those in plasma.

◊ References.

1. Loewen GR, *et al.* Effect of dose on the glucuronidation and sulphation kinetics of diflunisal in man: single dose studies. *Br J Clin Pharmacol* 1988; **26:** 31–9.
2. Eriksson L-O, *et al.* Influence of renal failure, rheumatoid arthritis and old age on the pharmacokinetics of diflunisal. *Eur J Clin Pharmacol* 1989; **36:** 165–74.
3. Verbeeck RK, *et al.* The effect of multiple dosage on the kinetics of glucuronidation and sulphation of diflunisal in man. *Br J Clin Pharmacol* 1990; **29:** 381–9.
4. Macdonald JI, *et al.* Sex-difference and the effects of smoking and oral contraceptive steroids on the kinetics of diflunisal. *Eur J Clin Pharmacol* 1990; **38:** 175–9.
5. Nuernberg B, *et al.* Pharmacokinetics of diflunisal in patients. *Clin Pharmacokinet* 1991; **20:** 81–9.

### Uses and Administration

Diflunisal is a salicylic acid derivative (see Aspirin, p.17) but it is not hydrolysed to salicylate and its clinical effects resemble more closely those of propionic acid derivative NSAIDs (p.70). Diflunisal is used in the acute or long-term management of mild to moderate pain, pain and inflammation associated with osteoarthritis and rheumatoid arthritis, and symptoms of primary dysmenorrhoea. The usual initial dose for pain relief is 1 g followed by a maintenance dose of 500 mg every 12 hours. In some patients 250 mg every 8 to 12 hours may be sufficient but some may require 500 mg every 8 hours. Maintenance doses greater than 1.5 g daily are not recommended. The usual dose for arthritis is 500 mg to 1 g daily given as a single dose or in 2 divided doses. Doses may need to be reduced in patients with renal impairment, see below.

Diflunisal arginine has been used similarly given by mouth or by intramuscular or intravenous injection.

**Administration in renal impairment.** Diflunisal may need to be given in reduced dosage in patients with significant renal impairment and should not be given when renal impairment is severe.

### Preparations

***BP 2003:*** Diflunisal Tablets;
***USP 27:*** Diflunisal Tablets.

**Proprietary Preparations** (details are given in Part 3)
**Austral.:** Dolobid; **Austria:** Fluniget; **Belg.:** Biartac; Diflusal; **Braz.:** Dorbid†; **Canad.:** Dolobid†; **Denm.:** Diflonid†; Donobid; **Fin.:** Donobid; **Fr.:** Dolobis; **Ger.:** Fluniget†; **Gr.:** Analeric; **Hong Kong:** Dolobid†; **Irl.:** Dolobid; **Israel:** Dolobid; **Ital.:** Aflogos†; Artrodol; Difludol†; Dolobid; Fludonil†; **Mex.:** Dolobid; **Neth.:** Dolocid; **Norw.:** Diflonid†; Donobid; **Port.:** Dolobid; Flunidor; **S.Afr.:** Dolobid†; **Spain:** Dolobid; **Swed.:** Donobid; **Switz.:** Unisal; **Thai.:** Dolobid; **UK:** Dolobid; **USA:** Dolobid.

## Dihydrocodeine Phosphate

*(BANM, rINNM)*

Fosfato de dihidrocodeína; Hydrocodeine Phosphate.

$C_{18}H_{23}NO_3,H_3PO_4$ = 399.4.

*CAS — 24204-13-5.*

*ATC — N02AA08.*

**Pharmacopoeias.** In *Jpn.*

## Dihydrocodeine Tartrate *(BANM, rINNM)*

Dihydrocodeine Acid Tartrate; Dihydrocodeine Bitartrate; Dihydrocodeine Hydrogen Tartrate; Dihydrocodeini Hydrogenotartras; Drocode Bitartrate; Hydrocodeine Bitartrate; Tartrato de dihidrocodeína. 4,5-Epoxy-3-methoxy-17-methylmorphinan-6-ol hydrogen tartrate.

$C_{18}H_{23}NO_3,C_4H_6O_6$ = 451.5.

*CAS — 125-28-0 (dihydrocodeine); 5965-13-9 (dihydrocodeine tartrate).*

NOTE. Compounded preparations of dihydrocodeine tartrate may be represented by the following names:

- Co-dydramol (*BAN*)—dihydrocodeine tartrate 1 part and paracetamol 50 parts (w/w).

**Pharmacopoeias.** In *Eur.* (see p.vi) and *US.*
*Pol.* includes the monohydrate.

**Ph. Eur. 5.0** (Dihydrocodeine Hydrogen Tartrate; Dihydrocodeine Tartrate BP 2003). A white or almost white crystalline powder. Freely soluble in water; sparingly soluble in alcohol; practically insoluble in cyclohexane. A 10% solution in water has a pH of 3.2 to 4.2. Protect from light.

**USP 27** (Dihydrocodeine Bitartrate). pH of a 10% solution in water is between 3.2 and 4.2. Store in airtight containers.

## Dependence and Withdrawal

As for Opioid Analgesics, p.71. Dihydrocodeine has been subject to abuse (see under Precautions, below).

## Adverse Effects and Treatment

As for Opioid Analgesics in general, p.72; side-effects from dihydrocodeine are less pronounced than those from morphine.

**Overdosage.** A 29-year-old man who had taken 2.1 g of dihydrocodeine had biochemical evidence of acute renal and hepatic impairment when admitted 13 hours after the overdose.[1] Severe life-threatening respiratory depression subsequently developed 36 hours after the overdose and only responded to treatment with naloxone after large doses (a total of 46.6 mg of naloxone) over a long period (106 hours). Commenting on this report some questioned the evidence for hepatic impairment and considered that the raised liver enzyme values were of muscular origin as a result of rhabdomyolysis.[2-4] Rhabdomyolysis might also have contributed to renal failure.

An anaphylactoid reaction following an overdose of an unspecified number of dihydrocodeine tablets[5] appeared to respond to intravenous naloxone.

1. Redfern N. Dihydrocodeine overdose treated with naloxone infusion. *BMJ* 1983; **287:** 751–2.
2. Buckley BM, Vale JA. Dihydrocodeine overdose treated with naloxone infusion. *BMJ* 1983; **287:** 1547.
3. Blain PG, Lane RJM. Dihydrocodeine overdose treated with naloxone infusion. *BMJ* 1983; **287:** 1547.
4. Wen P. Dihydrocodeine overdose treated with naloxone infusion. *BMJ* 1983; **287:** 1548.
5. Panos MZ, *et al.* Use of naloxone in opioid-induced anaphylactoid reaction. *Br J Anaesth* 1988; **61:** 371.

**Pain.** For reference to increased postoperative pain associated with the use of dihydrocodeine, see under Pain in Uses and Administration, below.

## Precautions

As for Opioid Analgesics in general, p.72.

**Abuse.** Dihydrocodeine has been reported to be widely abused by opiate addicts.[1-4]

1. Swadi H, *et al.* Misuse of dihydrocodeine tartrate (DF 118) among opiate addicts. *BMJ* 1990; **300:** 1313.
2. Robertson JR, *et al.* Misuse of dihydrocodeine tartrate (DF 118) among opiate addicts. *BMJ* 1990; **301:** 119.
3. Strang J, *et al.* Misuse of dihydrocodeine tartrate (DF 118) among opiate addicts. *BMJ* 1990; **301:** 119.
4. Seymour A, *et al.* The role of dihydrocodeine in causing death among drug users in the west of Scotland. *Scott Med J* 2001; **46:** 143–6.

**The elderly.** Despite some renal impairment an elderly group of patients[1] appeared to handle dihydrocodeine similarly to healthy young subjects. There was marked variability in all measurements and on the basis of this study no clear conclusions on guidelines for dosage in elderly patients could be drawn. However, the recommendation that small doses be given initially with subsequent doses according to response was endorsed.

1. Davies KN, *et al.* The effect of ageing on the pharmacokinetics of dihydrocodeine. *Eur J Clin Pharmacol* 1989; **37:** 375–9.

**Renal impairment.** Caution is necessary when giving dihydrocodeine to patients with severe renal impairment. Severe narcosis occurred in a patient with anuria and on maintenance haemodialysis after she had received dihydrocodeine by mouth for 4 days.[1] She responded to treatment with naloxone.

See also under Pharmacokinetics, below.

1. Barnes JN, Goodwin FJ. Dihydrocodeine narcosis in renal failure. *BMJ* 1983; **286:** 438–9.

## Interactions

For interactions associated with opioid analgesics, see p.73.

**Quinidine.** Dihydrocodeine is metabolised via the cytochrome P450 isoenzyme CYP2D6 to active metabolites, which it has been suggested may play a role in its analgesic activity in extensive metabolisers; quinidine impairs this metabolism, but a study in 11 healthy subjects did not demonstrate any reduced analgesic activity when dihydrocodeine and quinidine were given concomitantly, despite a three- to fourfold reduction in plasma concentrations of the metabolite dihydromorphine.[1]

1. Wilder-Smith CH, *et al.* The visceral and somatic antinociceptive effects of dihydrocodeine and its metabolite, dihydromorphine: a cross-over study with extensive and quinidine-induced poor metabolizers. *Br J Clin Pharmacol* 1998; **45:** 575–81.

## Pharmacokinetics

After oral doses peak concentrations of dihydrocodeine occur after about 1.2 to 1.8 hours; oral bioavailability is only about 20%, probably because of substantial first-pass metabolism in the gut wall or liver. Dihydrocodeine is metabolised in the liver via the cytochrome P450 isoenzyme CYP2D6, to dihydromorphine, which has potent analgesic activity, although the analgesic effect of dihydrocodeine appears to be primarily due to the parent compound; some is also converted via CYP3A4 to nordihydrocodeine. Dihydrocodeine is excreted in urine as unchanged drug and metabolites, including glucuronide conjugates. Elimination half-life is reported to range from about 3.5 to 5 hours.

◊ References.

1. Rowell FJ, *et al.* Pharmacokinetics of intravenous and oral dihydrocodeine and its acid metabolites. *Eur J Clin Pharmacol* 1983; **25:** 419–24.
2. Fromm MF, *et al.* Dihydrocodeine: a new opioid substrate for the polymorphic CYP2D6 in humans. *Clin Pharmacol Ther* 1995; **58:** 374–82.
3. Ammon S, *et al.* Pharmacokinetics of dihydrocodeine and its active metabolite after single and multiple dosing. *Br J Clin Pharmacol* 1999; **48:** 317–22.
4. Webb JA, *et al.* Contribution of dihydrocodeine and dihydromorphine to analgesia following dihydrocodeine administration in man: a PK-PD modelling analysis. *Br J Clin Pharmacol* 2001; **52:** 35–43.

**Renal impairment.** The pharmacokinetics of dihydrocodeine tartrate, given by mouth as a single 60-mg dose, were affected in 9 patients with chronic renal failure treated with haemodialysis when compared with 9 healthy subjects.[1] Time to peak plasma concentration in those with renal failure was 3 hours compared with 1 hour in healthy subjects; the area under the plasma concentration/time curve was greater in those with renal failure; and after 24 hours dihydrocodeine was still detectable in the plasma of all renal failure patients, but in only 3 of the healthy subjects.

1. Barnes JN, *et al.* Dihydrocodeine in renal failure: further evidence for an important role of the kidney in the handling of opioid drugs. *BMJ* 1985; **290:** 740–2.

## Uses and Administration

Dihydrocodeine is an opioid analgesic (p.73). It is related to codeine (p.27) and has similar analgesic activity. Dihydrocodeine is used for the relief of moderate to severe pain, often in combination with paracetamol. It has also been used as a cough suppressant.

For **analgesia** the usual dose of dihydrocodeine tartrate by mouth is 30 mg after food every 4 to 6 hours; up to 240 mg daily may be given for severe pain. Children over 4 years of age may be given 0.5 to 1 mg/kg every 4 to 6 hours. Modified-release preparations are available for twice daily administration in adults with chronic severe pain.

Dihydrocodeine tartrate may also be given by deep subcutaneous or intramuscular injection in doses of up to 50 mg every 4 to 6 hours. Doses equivalent to those used orally in children may be given parenterally to children over 4 years of age.

As a **cough suppressant** dihydrocodeine tartrate may be given by mouth in doses of 10 to 30 mg up to three times daily.

Dihydrocodeine phosphate has also been used. Other salts of dihydrocodeine used, mainly for their antitussive effects, include the hydrochloride and the thiocyanate. Dihydrocodeine polistirex has been used in modified-release preparations.

**Dyspnoea.** Dihydrocodeine has been reported[1] to have produced benefit in normocapnic patients severely disabled by breathlessness due to chronic airflow obstruction. A dose of 15 mg was taken 30 minutes before exercise up to three times a day.

1. Johnson MA, *et al.* Dihydrocodeine for breathlessness in 'pink puffers'. *BMJ* 1983; **286:** 675–7.

**Pain.** Dihydrocodeine is used in the management of moderate to severe pain. However, dose-related increase in postoperative pain has been seen[1] in patients given 25 or 50 mg dihydrocodeine tartrate intravenously following dental surgery, and it has been proposed that dihydrocodeine might act as an antagonist in situations where acute pain was accompanied by high opioid activity.[2] Systematic review of the use of single oral doses of dihydrocodeine has indicated that these are insufficient to provide adequate relief of postoperative pain, and that dihydrocodeine is less effective than ibuprofen.[3]

1. Seymour RA, *et al.* Dihydrocodeine-induced hyperalgesia in postoperative dental pain. *Lancet* 1982; **i:** 1425–6.
2. Henry JA. Dihydrocodeine increases dental pain. *Lancet* 1982; **ii:** 223.
3. Edwards JE, *et al.* Single dose dihydrocodeine for acute postoperative pain. Available in The Cochrane Library; Issue 2. Chichester: John Wiley; 2004.

## Preparations

***BP 2003:*** Co-dydramol Tablets; Dihydrocodeine Injection; Dihydrocodeine Oral Solution; Dihydrocodeine Tablets.

**Proprietary Preparations** (details are given in Part 3)

***Austral.:*** Paracodin; Rikodeine; ***Austria:*** Codidol; Paracodin; ***Belg.:*** Codicontin; Paracodine; ***Fr.:*** Dicodin; ***Ger.:*** DHC; Paracodin; Paracodin N; Remedacen; Tiamon Mono; ***Hong Kong:*** DF 118; ***Irl.:*** DF 118; DHC Continus; Hydol†; Paracodin; ***Israel:*** DHC Continus†; ***Ital.:*** Paracodina; ***Malaysia:*** Codesic; DF 118; ***NZ:*** DHC Continus; ***Port.:*** Didor; Paracodina†; ***S.Afr.:*** DF 118; Paracodin; ***Spain:*** Contugesic; Paracodina; Tosidrin; ***Switz.:*** Codicontin; Hydrocodeinon; Paracodin; ***UK:*** DF 118; DHC Continus.

**Multi-ingredient: *Austral.:*** Codox; ***Austria:*** Paracodin; ***Belg.:*** Paracodine; ***Ger.:*** Antitussivum Burger N; Makatussin Tropfen forte; Paracodin retard; ***Hong Kong:*** Codaewon; ***Irl.:*** Paramol; ***Ital.:*** Cardiazol-Paracodina; Paracodina; ***Malaysia:*** Codimol; ***Spain:*** Traquivan†; ***Switz.:*** Escotussin; Makatussin Comp; Makatussin forte†; Neo Makatussin N†; Paracodin retard; ***UK:*** Boots Dental Pain Relief†; Galake†; Paramol; Remedeine; ***USA:*** DHC Plus; DiHydro-CP; DiHydro-GP; Pancof; Pancof PD; Pancof-EXP; Panlor DC; Synalgos-DC.

---

# Dipipanone Hydrochloride *(BANM, rINNM)*

Hidrocloruro de dipipanona; Phenylpiperone Hydrochloride; Piperidyl Methadone Hydrochloride; Piperidylamidone Hydrochloride. (±)-4,4-Diphenyl-6-piperidinoheptan-3-one hydrochloride monohydrate.

$C_{24}H_{31}NO,HCl,H_2O$ = 404.0.

*CAS — 467-83-4 (dipipanone); 856-87-1 (dipipanone hydrochloride).*

**Pharmacopoeias.** In *Br.*

**BP 2003** (Dipipanone Hydrochloride). An odourless or almost odourless, white, crystalline powder. Sparingly soluble in water; freely soluble in alcohol and in acetone; practically insoluble in ether. A 2.5% solution in water has a pH of 4.0 to 6.0.

## Profile

Dipipanone hydrochloride is an opioid analgesic (p.71) structurally related to methadone (p.57). Used alone it is reported to be less sedating than morphine. It is used in the treatment of moderate to severe pain.

Dipipanone hydrochloride is usually given with cyclizine hydrochloride in order to reduce the incidence of nausea and vomiting, but the use of opioid preparations containing an antiemetic is not recommended for the management of chronic pain as an antiemetic is usually only required for the first few days of treatment. The usual oral dose of dipipanone hydrochloride is 10 mg, repeated every 6 hours. The dose may be increased if necessary in increments of 5 mg; it is seldom necessary to exceed a dose of 30 mg. After a dose by mouth the effect begins within an hour and lasts about 4 to 6 hours.

Preparations of dipipanone hydrochloride with cyclizine hydrochloride are subject to abuse.

## Preparations

***BP 2003:*** Dipipanone and Cyclizine Tablets.

**Proprietary Preparations** (details are given in Part 3)

**Multi-ingredient: *Hong Kong:*** Wellconal; ***Irl.:*** Diconal; ***S.Afr.:*** Wellconal; ***UK:*** Diconal.

---

# Diproqualone *(rINN)*

Diprocualona. 3-(2,3-Dihydroxypropyl)-2-methyl-4(3*H*)-quinazolinone.

$C_{12}H_{14}N_2O_3$ = 234.3.

*CAS — 36518-02-2.*

## Profile

Diproqualone is an analgesic that has been given as the camsilate.

## Preparations

**Proprietary Preparations** (details are given in Part 3)

**Multi-ingredient: *Switz.:*** Algopriv†.

---

# Dipyrone *(BAN, USAN)*

Metamizole Sodium *(pINN)*; Aminopyrine-sulphonate Sodium; Analginum; Metamizol sódico; Metamizolum Natricum; Methampyrone; Methylmelubrin; Natrium Novaminsulfonicum; Noramidazophenum; Novamidazofen; Novaminsulfone Sodium; NSC-73205; Sodium Noramidopyrine Methanesulphonate; Sulpyrine. Sodium *N*-(2,3-dimethyl-5-oxo-1-phenyl-3-pyrazolin-4-yl)-*N*-methylaminomethanesulphonate monohydrate.

$C_{13}H_{16}N_3NaO_4S,H_2O$ = 351.4.

*CAS — 68-89-3 (anhydrous dipyrone); 5907-38-0 (dipyrone monohydrate).*

*ATC — N02BB02.*

NOTE. Dipyrone is referred to in some countries by the colloquial name 'Mexican aspirin'. The names noraminophenazonum and novaminsulfon have apparently been applied to dipyrone, but it is not clear whether these are the sodium salt.

**Pharmacopoeias.** In *Chin., Eur.* (see p.vi), *Jpn*, and *Pol.*

**Ph. Eur. 5.0** (Metamizole Sodium; Dipyrone BP 2003). A white or almost white crystalline powder. Very soluble in water; soluble in alcohol. Protect from light.

## Adverse Effects and Precautions

Use of dipyrone is associated with an increased risk of agranulocytosis and with shock.

◊ References.

1. Levy M. Hypersensitivity to pyrazolones. *Thorax* 2000; **55** (suppl 2): S72–S74.

**Effects on the blood.** Data collected from 8 population groups in Europe and Israel by the International Agranulocytosis and Aplastic Anemia Study[1] revealed that there was a significant regional variability in the rate-ratio estimate for agranulocytosis and dipyrone (0.9 in Budapest to 33.3 in Barcelona). Although a large relative increase in risk between agranulocytosis and use of dipyrone was found, the incidence was less than some previous reports had suggested.

1. The International Agranulocytosis and Aplastic Anemia Study. Risks of agranulocytosis and aplastic anemia: a first report of their relation to drug use with special reference to analgesics. *JAMA* 1986; **256:** 1749–57.

**Effects on the skin.** Dipyrone has been considered responsible for a case of drug-induced toxic epidermal necrolysis.[1]

1. Roujeau J-C, *et al.* Sjögren-like syndrome after drug-induced toxic epidermal necrolysis. *Lancet* 1985; **i:** 609–11.

**Hypersensitivity.** Cross-sensitivity between aspirin and dipyrone occurred in a patient.[1] Dipyrone produced an exacerbation of dyspnoea, cyanosis, and respiratory arrest.

1. Bartoli E, *et al.* Drug-induced asthma. *Lancet* 1976; **i:** 1357.

**Porphyria.** Dipyrone has been associated with acute attacks of porphyria and is considered unsafe in porphyric patients.

## Pharmacokinetics

After oral doses dipyrone is rapidly hydrolysed in gastric juice to the active metabolite 4-methyl-amino-antipyrine which after absorption undergoes metabolism to 4-formyl-amino-antipyrine and other metabolites. Dipyrone is also rapidly undetectable in plasma after intravenous doses. None of the metabolites of dipyrone are extensively bound to plasma proteins. Most of a dose is excreted in the urine as metabolites. Dipyrone metabolites are also distributed into breast milk.

◊ References.

1. Heinemeyer G, *et al.* The kinetics of metamizol and its metabolites in critical-care patients with acute renal dysfunction. *Eur J Clin Pharmacol* 1993; **45:** 445–50.
2. Levy M, *et al.* Clinical pharmacokinetics of dipyrone and its metabolites. *Clin Pharmacokinet* 1995; **28:** 216–34.
3. Zylber-Katz E, *et al.* Dipyrone metabolism in liver disease. *Clin Pharmacol Ther* 1995; **58:** 198–209.

## Uses and Administration

Dipyrone is the sodium sulfonate of aminophenazone (p.14) and has similar properties. Because of the risk of serious adverse effects, in many countries its use is considered justified only in severe pain where no alternative is available or suitable. Dipyrone has been given by mouth in doses of 0.5 to 4 g daily in divided doses. It has also been given by intramuscular or intravenous injection and rectally as a suppository.

A magnesium congener of dipyrone, metamizole magnesium has been used similarly to dipyrone as has the calcium congener metamizole calcium.

## Preparations

**Proprietary Preparations** (details are given in Part 3)

***Arg.:*** Algiopiret; Dioxadol; Dipigrand; Ditral; Integrobe; Lisalgil; Novacler; Novalgina; Novemina; Unibios Simple; ***Austria:*** Inalgon Neu; Novalgin; Spasmo Inalgon Neu; ***Belg.:*** Analgine; Novalgine; ***Braz.:*** Algirona; Anador; Analgesil; Analgex; Analginat; Apiron; Baralgin M; Bioscinat; Conmel; Debelat; Dipimax; Dipirex; Dipiron; Dipironax; Dorant; Dorilan; Dornal; Dorona; Evergint; Fimdort; Findor; Magnodor; Magnopyrol; Maxiliv; Nevralginat; Nofebrin; Novalgina; Pirogina; Termonal; Termoprin; Termopriona; Toloxin; ***Chile:*** Baralgina M; Conmel; Novalgina; ***Fr.:*** Novalgine; ***Ger.:*** Analgin; Analgit†; Baralgin†; Berlosin; Metalgin; Nopain; Novalgin; Novaminsulfon; ***Hong Kong:*** Metilon; Novaminsulfon†; Sulpyrin†; ***India:*** Novalgin; ***Israel:*** Novalgin; Optalgin; Phanalgin; V-Talgin; ***Ital.:*** Novalgina; Trisalgina†; ***Mex.:*** Alnex; Anaprol; Apixol; Avafontan; Avaldrian; Ayoral Simple; Conmel; Dalmasin†; Dalsin; Dimetirol; Dipiraxil†; Dipydol; Dofisan; Dolgan; Dolofur; Domenal; Exalgin; Exodalina; Fandall; Fardolpin; Farlin†; Indigon; Mach-2†; Macodin; Magnil; Magnol; Magnopyrol; Magsons; Mayopirina†; Mecoten; Medipirol; Mermid; Metapirona; Midelin; Minoral; Mizoltec; Neo-Melubrina; Neomelin; Nesol†; Odon-Pyr†; Paleodina; Pifrol†; Piramagno; Pirandall; Pirawil†; Pirinovag; Piromebrina; Pironal†; Pirongil†; Poloren; Precidona†; Prodolina; Profelina†; Propiral†; Pyranol; Pyril†; Pyron†; Sesalgin†; Suprim; Termonil; Therma Ayoral†; Tredol†; Utidol; Vegal†; Zolidin†; ***Neth.:*** Novalgin; ***Port.:*** Conmel; Dolocalma; Nolotil; Novalgina†; ***Spain:*** Adolkin†; Afebrin†; Algi; Dolemicin†; Lasain; Neo Melubrina; Nolotil; Optalgin†; ***Swed.:*** Novalgin†; ***Switz.:*** Minalgin; Novalgine; ***Thai.:*** Acodon; Centagin; Deparon; Genergin; Invoigin; Kno-Paine; Medalgin; Mezabox; Nivagin; Nominfone†; Novalgin; Olan-Gin.

**Multi-ingredient:** ***Arg.:*** Antispasmina; Anuar; Apasmo; Apasmo Compuesto; Artifene; Bellatotal; Buscapina Compositum; Calmopirin; Canovex; Cifespasmo Compuesto; Colobolina D; Craun; Cronopen Balsamico; D-P; Dentolina Plus; Dextro + Dipirona; Dextrodip; Dioxadol; Dolo Nervobion 10000; Dresan; Dresan Biotic; Espasmo Biotenk; Espasmo Dioxadol; Febrimicina; Flexicamin A; Keptan Compuesto; Klosidol; Klosidol B1 B6 B12; Lisalgil Compuesto; Luar-G Compositum; Migra Dioxadol; Migral; Migral Compositum; Multin; Novopasmil Compuesto; Paratropina Compuesta; Pasmosedan Compuesto; Rupe-N Compuesto; Saldeva; Sumal; Tetralgin; Tetralgin Novo; Vicefeno; ***Austria:*** Buscopan Compositum; Spasmium comp; ***Belg.:*** Buscopan Compositum; Visceralgine Compositum†; ***Braz.:*** Adegrip†; Adegripan†; Algi-Ped†; Algice; Algiflex†; Aminocid; Analgex C†; Analgin C-R; Analgosedan†; Analverin; Analverin Composto; Anapirol†; Apracur†; Baldin-CE†; Banidor†; Bicavine; Binospan Composto; Bioscina Composta; Bipasmin Composto†; Bromalgina; Broncopinol; Buscopan Composto; Buscoveran Composto; Butilamin†; Cafalena†; Cefaldina; Cefaliv; Codeverin; Cortagrip D†; Cortagrip†; Cortegripan†; Dalgex; Dexalgen; Diarona†; Dilubrin†; Dimex; Dipirol; Disbuspan; Doralgina; Doralon†; Dorflex; Doricin; Doridina; Dorscopena; Dorsedin; Dorspan; Dorzone; Ductopan; Espasmobel†; Espasmocron; Espasmodid Composto; Espasmosan Composto†; Eucalliptan; Eucaliptol Composto†; Eucaliptol†; Flenalgin†; Flexdor; Gripanil; Gripefago C†; Gripion†; Gripol C Capuride†; Gripol C†; Gripol Composto Xarope†; Gripol Composto†; Gripomatine; Griponia; Gripsay; Hiospan Composto; Inatrex Balsamico†; Inib-Dor†; Itaiflex†; Killgrip; Kindpasm; Lisador; Melpaz†; Metilsedor†; Migraliv; Mionevrix; Miorrelax; Napiro†; Neocopan; Neomigran; Neosaldina; Nevralgex; Novalgrip†; Par; Pasmalgin†; Plenocedan†; Plenogripe†; Pulmodex-C†; Pulmorien†; Relaflex†; Resfrialgina†; Rielex; Sedabel; Sedalene; Sedalex; Sedalgina; Sedobion†; Sedol; Somaflex†; Spasmotropin; Sulindor†; Tebasedan†; Tensaldin; Tetrapulmo; Theopirina; Tropinal; Uzara†; Veratropan Composto; ***Chile:*** Bramedil Compuesto; Buscapina Compositum; Cefalmin; Cinabel; Dioran; Dolcopin; Dolnix; Dolo-Neurobionta; Dolonase; Fredol; Migragesic; Migranol; Migratam; Neo Butartrol; Nospasmin Compuesto; Piretanyl; Scopanil; Silartrin; Silrelax; Sistalgina; Ultrimin; Viadil Compuesto; ***Fin.:*** Litalgin; ***Fr.:*** Avafortan; Cefaline-Pyrazole; Optalidon a la Noramidopyrine†; Salgydal a la noramidopyrine; Visceralgine Forte; ***Hung.:*** Quarelin; ***Ital.:*** Soma Complex; ***Mex.:*** Algosfar; Ayoral; Bipasmin Compuesto; Buscapina Compositum; Busconet; Busepan; Busprina; Colepren; Dolnefort; Dolo-Tiaminal; Hiosinotil Compuesto; Korifen; Neobrontyl; Ortran; Pasmodil; Pirobutil; Retodol Compositum; Selpiran; Singril; ***S.Afr.:*** Buscopan Compositum; Norifortan†; Scopex Co; ***Spain:*** Buscapina Compositum; Nolotil Compositum; Vapin Complex†; ***Thai.:*** Butarion; Novapam.

---

## Droxicam (*rINN*)

5-Methyl-3-(2-pyridyl)-2*H*,5*H*-1,3-oxazino[5,6-c]-[1,2]benzothiazine-2,4(3*H*)-dione 6,6-dioxide.

$C_{16}H_{11}N_3O_5S$ = 357.3.
*CAS* — *90101-16-9.*
*ATC* — *M01AC04.*

### Profile

Droxicam is an NSAID (p.67) reported to act as a prodrug for piroxicam (p.84). It has been given by mouth for pain and inflammation associated with musculoskeletal, joint, and soft-tissue disorders but marketing was suspended in December 1994 because it was associated with adverse liver effects.

**Effects on the liver.** Up to October 1993 the Spanish National System of Pharmacovigilance had received 82 spontaneous reports of hepatic damage associated with droxicam[1] and in December 1994 the European Union Committee for Proprietary Medicinal Products recommended that marketing authorisation for droxicam should be suspended pending further studies. An industry sponsored study[1] (submitted in December 1994) of 8910 patients who had taken droxicam identified one patient whose hepatic damage was considered to be attributable to droxicam, a figure comparable with the base-line estimate observed for NSAIDs in general (see p.69).

1. García-Rodríguez LA, *et al.* Acute liver injury and droxicam use in the region of Friuli-Venezia Giulia. *Br J Clin Pharmacol* 1995; **40:** 103–6.

### Preparations

**Proprietary Preparations** (details are given in Part 3)
***Braz.:*** Ombolan†.

---

## Eltenac (*rINN*)

Eltenaco. 4-(2,6-Dichloroanilino)-3-thiopheneacetic acid.

$C_{12}H_9Cl_2NO_2S$ = 302.2.
*CAS* — *72895-88-6.*

### Profile

Eltenac is an NSAID (p.67) used in veterinary medicine.

---

## Embutramide (*BAN, USAN, rINN*)

Embutramida; Hoe-18-680. *N*-(β,β-Diethyl-*m*-methoxyphenethyl)-4-hydroxybutyramide.

$C_{17}H_{27}NO_3$ = 293.4.
*CAS* — *15687-14-6.*

### Profile

Embutramide is an opioid analgesic used in veterinary medicine for euthanasia.

---

## Enoxolone (*BAN, rINN*)

Enoxolona; Enoxolonum; Glycyrrhetic Acid; Glycyrrhetinic Acid. 3β-Hydroxy-11-oxo-olean-12-en-30-oic acid.

$C_{30}H_{46}O_4$ = 470.7.
*CAS* — *471-53-4.*

**Pharmacopoeias.** In *Eur.* (see p.vi).

**Ph. Eur. 5.0** (Enoxolone). A white or almost white, crystalline powder. It exhibits polymorphism. Practically insoluble in water; soluble in dehydrated alcohol; sparingly soluble in dichloromethane. Protect from light.

### Profile

Enoxolone is a complex triterpene prepared from glycyrrhizinic acid, a constituent of liquorice. Enoxolone is used locally in preparations for the treatment of non-infective inflammatory disorders of the skin, mouth, throat, and rectum.

Derivatives of enoxolone, including its aluminium salt (p.1264) and carbenoxolone (p.1254) are used in the treatment of benign peptic ulcer disease and other gastrointestinal disorders.

◊ Enoxolone is a potent inhibitor of the enzyme 11β-hydroxysteroid dehydrogenase which inactivates cortisol and concomitant application of enoxolone with hydrocortisone has been shown in *animal* studies to potentiate the activity of hydrocortisone in skin.[1] Whether this also increased the systemic absorption and toxicity of hydrocortisone was unclear.[2]

1. Teelucksingh S, *et al.* Potentiation of hydrocortisone activity in skin by glycyrrhetinic acid. *Lancet* 1990; **335:** 1060–3.
2. Greaves MW. Potentiation of hydrocortisone activity in skin by glycerrhetinic acid. *Lancet* 1990; **336:** 876.

### Preparations

**Proprietary Preparations** (details are given in Part 3)
***Fr.:*** Arthrodont; P.O. 12.

**Multi-ingredient:** ***Arg.:*** Anastim con RTH; ***Braz.:*** Acti Valda Diet†; ***Chile:*** Gingilacer; Suaviget; ***Fr.:*** Apaisance; Dermeol†; Fluocaril dents sensibles; Hexalyse; Lelong Irritations†; Nightpeel; Phlebocreme†; Phlebosup†; Pyreflor; Sedorrhoide†; Tiq'Aouta; Valda Septol†; Vocadys; ***Hong Kong:*** Hexalyse; ***Ital.:*** Acnesan; Biothymus DS; Eudent con Glysan; Fluocaril; Lenipasta; Lenirose; Lisomucil Gola; Neo-Stomygen; Pastiglie Valda; Valda F3†; Viderm; ***Mex.:*** Periodentyl; ***Port.:*** Despigmentante; Hyseke†; ***Spain:*** Angileptol; Anginovag; Pentalmicina†; Roberfarin; ***UK:*** Gelclair.

---

## Epirizole (*USAN, pINN*)

DA-398; Epirizol; Mepirizole. 4-Methoxy-2-(5-methoxy-3-methylpyrazol-1-yl)-6-methylpyrimidine.

$C_{11}H_{14}N_4O_2$ = 234.3.
*CAS* — *18694-40-1.*

**Pharmacopoeias.** In *Jpn.*

### Profile

Epirizole is an NSAID (p.67) that has been used by mouth in a usual dose of 150 to 450 mg daily in divided doses; larger doses of up to 600 mg daily have been used in patients with rheumatoid arthritis.

### Preparations

**Proprietary Preparations** (details are given in Part 3)
***Braz.:*** Mebron; ***Jpn:*** Mebron.

---

## Etanercept (*BAN, USAN, rINN*)

rhu-TNFR:Fc. A dimer of 1-235 tumour necrosis factor receptor (human) fusion protein with 236-467-immunoglobulin G1 (human γ1-chain Fc fragment).

*CAS* — *185243-69-0.*
*ATC* — *L04AA11.*

### Adverse Effects and Precautions

As for Infliximab, p.50.

Mild to moderate injection site reactions with symptoms of erythema, itching, pain, or swelling are common with etanercept. Other common reactions include headache, dizziness, asthenia, nausea and vomiting, abdominal pain, dyspepsia, and allergic reactions. Antibodies to etanercept may develop.

Blood dyscrasias, including pancytopenia and aplastic anaemia, have been reported rarely with etanercept treatment; in some cases the outcome was fatal. Etanercept should be used with caution in patients with a history of blood dyscrasias.

Etanercept should be used with caution in patients with heart failure.

**Effects on the skin.** Discoid lupus and necrotising vasculitis have been reported with etanercept treatment.[1,2] Urticaria has also been seen in 2 patients receiving etanercept for juvenile idiopathic arthritis.[3]

1. Brion PH, *et al.* Autoimmune skin rashes associated with etanercept for rheumatoid arthritis. *Ann Intern Med* 1999; **131:** 634.
2. Misery L, *et al.* Dermatological complications of etanercept therapy for rheumatoid arthritis. *Br J Dermatol* 2002; **146:** 334–5.
3. Skyttä E, *et al.* Etanercept and urticaria in patients with juvenile idiopathic arthritis. *Clin Exp Rheumatol* 2000; **18:** 533–4.

### Interactions

As for Infliximab, p.50.

The risk of infection is increased when anakinra and etanercept are used together.

### Pharmacokinetics

After a single subcutaneous dose of etanercept the UK manufacturer states that the mean half-life is about 70 hours, and the time to peak serum concentration 48 hours. In contrast, the US manufacturer gives the half-life as 102 hours and the time to peak concentration as about 70 hours, although with a considerable range. Repeated dosing was noted to result in a two- to sevenfold increase in serum levels of etanercept in some patients.

◊ References.

1. Korth-Bradley JM, *et al.* The pharmacokinetics of etanercept in healthy volunteers. *Ann Pharmacother* 2000; **34:** 161–4.

## Uses and Administration

Etanercept is a recombinant version of soluble human tumour necrosis factor (TNF) receptor that binds specifically to tumour necrosis factor (p.590) and blocks its interaction with endogenous cell-surface TNF receptors. This interaction prevents the important effect of TNF in the inflammatory processes of rheumatoid arthritis (p.9); elevated TNF levels are also found in the synovium of patients with psoriatic arthritis (see Spondyloarthropathies, p.11).

Etanercept is used in the treatment of moderately to severely active **rheumatoid arthritis** and active and progressive **psoriatic arthritis**. In the UK, its use is usually limited to patients who have had an inadequate response to standard disease-modifying antirheumatic drugs although, in severe rheumatoid arthritis, it may be used in patients not previously treated with methotrexate; in the USA it may be used for treating early rheumatoid arthritis or psoriatic arthritis, to reduce the signs and symptoms and delay structural damage. In both indications, it is given as a subcutaneous injection in a dose of 25 mg twice weekly at intervals of 72 to 96 hours. The equivalent weekly dose of 50 mg may also be given as two separate 25-mg injections on the same day. In the UK, the National Institute of Clinical Excellence recommends, based on guidelines from the British Society of Rheumatology, that treatment be discontinued if there is no response after 3 months. Etanercept is also indicated in the treatment of **ankylosing spondylitis** in doses similar to those used for rheumatoid arthritis.

Etanercept is also used in the treatment of unresponsive moderate to severe polyarticular **juvenile idiopathic arthritis** (p.9) in children and adolescents aged 4 years and over. It is given subcutaneously in a dose of 400 micrograms/kg (up to a maximum dose of 25 mg) twice weekly at intervals of 72 to 96 hours. The equivalent weekly dose may also be given as two separate injections on the same day. In the UK, the National Institute of Clinical Excellence recommends, based on guidelines from the British Paediatric Rheumatology Group, that treatment be discontinued in children if there is no response after 6 months, or an initial response is not maintained.

In the USA, etanercept is also used in the treatment of chronic, moderate to severe plaque **psoriasis** in patients over 18 years. The recommended initial dose is 50 mg twice weekly at intervals of 72 to 96 hours for 3 months; the dose should then be reduced to 50 mg weekly. Initial doses of 25 or 50 mg weekly have also been shown to be effective.

**Psoriasis.** Etanercept is effective in patients with moderate to severe plaque psoriasis;[1] efficacy appears to be dose-related with 25% of patients in the low-dose (25 mg once weekly) group showing at least a 75% improvement compared to 59% in the high-dose group (50 mg twice weekly) after 24 weeks of etanercept treatment.

1. Leonardi CL, *et al.* Etanercept as monotherapy in patients with psoriasis. *N Engl J Med* 2003; **349:** 2014–22.

**Psoriatic arthritis.** Etanercept may be useful in the treatment of psoriatic arthritis (see Spondyloarthropathies, p.11).

References.

1. Mease PJ, *et al.* Etanercept in the treatment of psoriatic arthritis and psoriasis: a randomised trial. *Lancet* 2000; **356:** 385–90.
2. Mease PJ. Etanercept, a TNF antagonist for treatment for psoriatic arthritis and psoriasis. *Skin Therapy Lett* 2003; **8:** 1–4.

**Rheumatoid arthritis.** Some references to the use of etanercept in rheumatoid arthritis and juvenile idiopathic arthritis.

1. Weinblatt ME, *et al.* A trial of etanercept, a recombinant tumor necrosis factor receptor: Fc fusion protein, in patients with rheumatoid arthritis receiving methotrexate. *N Engl J Med* 1999; **340:** 253–9.
2. Moreland LW, *et al.* Etanercept therapy in rheumatoid arthritis: a randomized, controlled trial. *Ann Intern Med* 1999; **130:** 478–86.
3. Jarvis B, Faulds O. Etanercept: a review of its use in rheumatoid arthritis. *Drugs* 1999; **57:** 945–66.
4. Garrison L, McDonnell ND. Etanercept: therapeutic use in patients with rheumatoid arthritis. *Ann Rheum Dis* 1999; **58** (suppl 1): 165–169.
5. Lovell DJ, *et al.* Etanercept in children with polyarticular juvenile rheumatoid arthritis. *N Engl J Med* 2000; **342:** 763–9.
6. Bathon JM, *et al.* A comparison of etanercept and methotrexate in patients with early rheumatoid arthritis. *N Engl J Med* 2000; **343:** 1586–93. Correction. *ibid.* 2001; **344:** 76.
7. Seymour HE, *et al.* Anti-TNF agents for rheumatoid arthritis. *Br J Clin Pharmacol* 2001; **51:** 201–8.
8. Johnson CJ, *et al.* Etanercept in juvenile rheumatoid arthritis. *Ann Pharmacother* 2001; **35:** 464–71.
9. Genovese MC, *et al.* Etanercept versus methotrexate in patients with early rheumatoid arthritis: two-year radiographic and clinical outcomes. *Arthritis Rheum* 2002; **46:** 1443–50.
10. Culy CR, Keating GM. Etanercept: an updated review of its use in rheumatoid arthritis, psoriatic arthritis and juvenile rheumatoid arthritis. *Drugs* 2002; **62:** 2493–2537.
11. National Institute for Clinical Excellence. Guidance on the use of etanercept for the treatment of juvenile idiopathic arthritis (March 2002). Available at: http://www.nice.org.uk/pdf/JIA-PDF.pdf (accessed 05/07/04)
12. National Institute for Clinical Excellence. Guidance on the use of etanercept and infliximab for the treatment of rheumatoid arthritis (March 2002). Available at: http://www.nice.org.uk/pdf/RA-PDF.pdf (accessed 05/07/04)
13. Klareskog L, *et al.* Therapeutic effect of the combination of etanercept and methotrexate compared with each treatment alone in patients with rheumatoid arthritis: double-blind randomised controlled trial. *Lancet* 2004; **363:** 675–81.

### Preparations

**Proprietary Preparations** (details are given in Part 3)

***Arg.:*** Enbrel; ***Austral.:*** Enbrel; ***Belg.:*** Enbrel; ***Canad.:*** Enbrel; ***Chile:*** Enbrel; ***Fin.:*** Enbrel; ***Fr.:*** Enbrel; ***Ger.:*** Enbrel; ***Israel:*** Enbrel; ***Ital.:*** Enbrel; ***Mex.:*** Enbrel; ***Norw.:*** Enbrel; ***NZ:*** Enbrel; ***Port.:*** Enbrel; ***Spain:*** Enbrel; ***Swed.:*** Enbrel; ***Switz.:*** Enbrel; ***UK:*** Enbrel; ***USA:*** Enbrel.

## Ethenzamide *(BAN, rINN)*

Aethoxybenzamidum; Etenzamida; Etenzamide; Ethoxybenzamide; Ethylsalicylamide; HP-209. 2-Ethoxybenzamide.

$C_9H_{11}NO_2$ = 165.2.

*CAS — 938-73-8.*

*ATC — N02BA07.*

**Pharmacopoeias.** In *Jpn.*

### Profile

Ethenzamide is a salicylic acid derivative (see Aspirin, p.15) given by mouth in painful and inflammatory conditions and to reduce fever.

### Preparations

**Proprietary Preparations** (details are given in Part 3)

**Multi-ingredient:** ***Austria:*** Coldadolin; Dolmix; Helopyrin; Nisicur; Seltoc; ***Braz.:*** Recilugo†; ***Ger.:*** Antifohnon-N†; Glutisal; Kolton grippale N; ***Port.:*** Cephyl; Katagrip†; ***Switz.:*** Algopriv†; Ergosanol a la cafeine†; Ergosanol special a la cafeine†; Ergosanol special†; Nicaphlogyl; Seranex sans codeine.

## Ethoheptazine Citrate *(BANM, rINNM)*

Citrato de etoheptacina; Wy-401. Ethyl 1-methyl-4-phenylperhydroazepine-4-carboxylate dihydrogen citrate.

$C_{16}H_{23}NO_2,C_6H_8O_7$ = 453.5.

*CAS — 77-15-6 (ethoheptazine); 6700-56-7 (ethoheptazine citrate); 2085-42-9 ((±)-ethoheptazine citrate).*

### Profile

Ethoheptazine citrate is an opioid analgesic (p.71) structurally related to pethidine (p.80). It has been used as an analgesic in the short-term treatment of mild to moderate pain, usually with other drugs such as aspirin and meprobamate.

### Preparations

**Proprietary Preparations** (details are given in Part 3)

**Multi-ingredient:** ***Canad.:*** Equagesic†; ***India:*** Equagesic; ***S.Afr.:*** Equagesic†; ***UK:*** Equagesic†.

## Ethyl Nicotinate

Nicotinato de etilo.

$C_8H_9NO_2$ = 151.2.

*CAS — 614-18-6.*

### Profile

Ethyl nicotinate is used in concentrations of up to 2% in topical rubefacient preparations for the relief of pain in musculoskeletal, joint, and soft-tissue disorders. It has also been used as suppositories in anorectal disorders.

### Preparations

**Proprietary Preparations** (details are given in Part 3)

***Austria:*** Mucotherm.

**Multi-ingredient:** ***Austria:*** Thermal; ***Belg.:*** Transvane†; ***Ger.:*** Striatridin†; ***Irl.:*** Transvasin; ***Norw.:*** Thermal; ***NZ:*** Transvasin†; ***Swed.:*** Transvasin†; ***Switz.:*** Baume Esco Forte; Sloan Baume†; Thermocutan; ***UK:*** PR Heat Spray; Transvasin Heat Rub.

## Ethyl Salicylate

Salicilato de etilo. Ethyl 2-hydroxybenzoate.

$C_9H_{10}O_3$ = 166.2.

*CAS — 118-61-6.*

### Profile

Ethyl salicylate is a salicylic acid derivative that is used similarly to methyl salicylate (p.59) in concentrations of up to 5% in topical rubefacient preparations for the relief of pain in musculoskeletal, joint, and soft-tissue disorders.

### Preparations

**Proprietary Preparations** (details are given in Part 3)

**Multi-ingredient:** ***Austral.:*** Deep Heat; Radian-B; ***Belg.:*** Rado-Salil; ***Ger.:*** Contrheuma-Gel forte N†; ***Israel:*** Deep Heat Spray; ***Ital.:*** Remy; ***Singapore:*** Deep Heating Spray; ***Switz.:*** Alginex; ***UK:*** Aspellin†; Deep Heat Spray; Dubam; Ralgex.

## Ethylmorphine Hydrochloride *(BANM)*

Aethylmorphinae Hydrochloridum; Aethylmorphini Hydrochloridum; Chlorhydrate de Codéthyline; Ethylmorphini Hydrochloridum; Ethylmorphinium Chloride; Etilmorfina, hidrocloruro de. 3-*O*-Ethylmorphine hydrochloride dihydrate; 7,8-Didehydro-4,5-epoxy-3-ethoxy-17-methylmorphinan-6-ol hydrochloride dihydrate.

$C_{19}H_{23}NO_3,HCl,2H_2O$ = 385.9.

*CAS — 76-58-4 (ethylmorphine); 125-30-4 (ethylmorphine hydrochloride).*

*ATC — R05DA01; S01XA06.*

**Pharmacopoeias.** In *Chin., Eur.* (see p.vi), *Jpn*, and *Pol.*

**Ph. Eur. 5.0** (Ethylmorphine Hydrochloride). A white or almost white crystalline powder. Soluble in water and in alcohol. A 2% solution in water has a pH of 4.3 to 5.7. Protect from light.

### Profile

Ethylmorphine hydrochloride is an opioid analgesic (p.71) and has properties similar to those of codeine (p.27). It is used mainly as a cough suppressant. It has also been used for its analgesic and antidiarrhoeal properties. It was formerly given in eye drops as a lymphagogue.

Ethylmorphine free base and the camphorate and camsilate have also been used.

◊ References.

1. Aasmundstad TA, *et al.* Biotransformation and pharmacokinetics of ethylmorphine after a single oral dose. *Br J Clin Pharmacol* 1995; **39:** 611–20.

### Preparations

**Proprietary Preparations** (details are given in Part 3)

***Arg.:*** Dionina; ***Belg.:*** Codethyline; ***Fin.:*** Cocillana; ***Fr.:*** Codethyline†; Dithiol; Trachyl†; ***UK:*** Collins Elixir.

**Multi-ingredient:** ***Austria:*** Modiscop; ***Belg.:*** Longbalsem; Solucamphre†; Theralene Pectoral†; Tux; ***Chile:*** Codelasa; ***Denm.:*** Cosylan†; ***Fin.:*** Indalgin; ***Fr.:*** Bronpax†; Ephydion; Humex; Marrubene Codethyline†; Peter's Sirop†; Sedophon†; Sirop Pectoral adulte†; Sirop Pectoral enfant†; Thiosedal†; Tussipax; Tussipax a l'Euquinine†; Vegetoserum; ***India:*** Bell Diono Resolvent; Bell Resolvent; ***Ital.:*** Codetilina-Eucaliptolo He†; Mindol-Merck; ***Norw.:*** Cosylan; Solvipect comp; Sterk hostesirup†; ***Port.:*** Bronquiasmol; Calmarum; Fluidin Nocturno†; Gotas Zimaia†; Xarope Antigripal; ***Spain:*** Demusin; Sedalmerck; ***Swed.:*** Cocillana-Etyfin; Cosylan†; Lepheton; ***Switz.:*** Ipeca; Phol-Tux; Saintbois; Sano Tuss.

# Etodolac *(BAN, USAN, rINN)*

AY-24236; Etodolaco; Etodolacum; Etodolic Acid. 1,8-Diethyl-1,3,4,9-tetrahydropyrano[3,4-*b*]indol-1-ylacetic acid.

$C_{17}H_{21}NO_3$ = 287.4.

*CAS — 41340-25-4.*

*ATC — M01AB08.*

**Pharmacopoeias.** In *Eur.* (see p.vi) and *US.*

**Ph. Eur. 5.0** (Etodolac). A white or almost white crystalline powder. Practically insoluble in water; freely soluble in dehydrated alcohol and in acetone.

**USP 27** (Etodolac). Store in airtight containers.

## Adverse Effects and Precautions

As for NSAIDs in general, p.67.

The presence of phenolic metabolites of etodolac in the urine may give rise to a false-positive reaction for bilirubin.

**Effects on the blood.** Agranulocytosis has been reported in a patient receiving etodolac.[1] Coombs-positive haemolytic anaemia due to sensitivity to etodolac metabolites has also been reported.[2]

1. Cramer RL, *et al.* Agranulocytosis associated with etodolac. *Ann Pharmacother* 1994; **28:** 458–60.
2. Cunha PD, *et al.* Immune hemolytic anemia caused by sensitivity to a metabolite of etodolac, a nonsteroidal anti-inflammatory drug. *Transfusion* 2000; **40:** 663–8.

**Effects on the gastrointestinal tract.** Etodolac is reported to be a preferential inhibitor of cyclo-oxygenase 2 (COX-2) and consequently it may produce less gastric toxicity than the non-selective NSAIDs such as naproxen.[1,2]

1. Taha AS, *et al.* Effect of repeated therapeutic doses of naproxen and etodolac on gastric and duodenal mucosal prostaglandins (PGs) in rheumatoid arthritis (RA). *Gut* 1989; **30:** A751.
2. Bianchi Porro G, *et al.* A double-blind gastroscopic evaluation of the effects of etodolac and naproxen on the gastrointestinal mucosa of rheumatic patients. *J Intern Med* 1991; **229:** 5–8.

## Interactions

For interactions associated with NSAIDs, see p.69.

## Pharmacokinetics

Etodolac is a chiral compound given as the racemate. Peak plasma concentrations of the active (S)-enantiomer and of the inactive (R)-enantiomer are usually obtained within about 2 hours of a dose by mouth but plasma concentrations of the (R)-enantiomer have been reported to greatly exceed those of the (S)-enantiomer. Both enantiomers are highly bound to plasma protein. Both are also distributed to the synovial fluid, although the difference in their concentrations may not be as marked as the difference in plasma concentrations. The plasma half-life of total etodolac has been reported to be about 7 hours; excretion is mainly in the urine as hydroxylated metabolites and glucuronide conjugates; some may be excreted in the bile.

◊ References.

1. Brocks DR, *et al.* Stereoselective disposition of etodolac enantiomers in synovial fluid. *J Clin Pharmacol* 1991; **31:** 741–6.
2. Brocks DR, *et al.* The stereoselective pharmacokinetics of etodolac in young and elderly subjects, and after cholecystectomy. *J Clin Pharmacol* 1992; **32:** 982–9.
3. Brocks DR, Jamali F. Etodolac clinical pharmacokinetics. *Clin Pharmacokinet* 1994; **26:** 259–74.
4. Boni J, *et al.* Pharmacokinetic and pharmacodynamic action of etodolac in patients after oral surgery. *J Clin Pharmacol* 1999; **39:** 729–37.

## Uses and Administration

Etodolac, a pyrano-indoleacetic acid derivative, is an NSAID (p.70) reported to be a preferential inhibitor of cyclo-oxygenase 2 (COX-2). It is used for rheumatoid arthritis, including juvenile idiopathic arthritis, and osteoarthritis and for the treatment of acute pain.

For the treatment of rheumatoid arthritis and osteoarthritis, the recommended dose by mouth is initially 600 to 1000 mg daily in divided doses adjusted according to response to a maximum of 1.2 g daily. Modified-release preparations are available for once daily use in these conditions. In the USA modified-release preparations may also be given for the treatment of juvenile idiopathic arthritis in children aged 6 to 16 years. Doses are given once daily and are 400 mg in those weighing 20 to 30 kg, 600 mg in those weighing 31 to 45 kg, 800 mg in those weighing 46 to 60 kg, and 1000 mg in those weighing over 60 kg.

For the treatment of acute pain, the recommended dose is 200 to 400 mg every 6 to 8 hours to a usual maximum of 1 g daily although some patients have been given up to 1.2 g daily.

## Preparations

**BP 2003:** Etodolac Capsules; Etodolac Tablets;
**USP 27:** Etodolac Capsules; Etodolac Tablets.

**Proprietary Preparations** (details are given in Part 3)
***Austria:*** Lodine; ***Braz.:*** Flancox†; ***Canad.:*** Ultradol; ***Denm.:*** Todolac; ***Fin.:*** Lodine; ***Fr.:*** Lodine; ***Gr.:*** Lonine; ***Hong Kong:*** Elderin†; Lodine; ***Israel:*** Etopan; ***Ital.:*** Lodine; ***Jpn:*** Hypen; ***Mex.:*** Lodine; ***Port.:*** Acudor; Articulan; Dualgan; Lodine; Lodot; Metazin; Sodolac; ***Switz.:*** Lodine; ***Thai.:*** Etonox; ***UK:*** Eccoxolac; Lodine; ***USA:*** Lodine.

---

## Etofenamate *(BAN, USAN, rINN)*

B-577; Bay-d-1107; Etofenamato; Etofenamatum; TV-485; TVX-485; WHR-5020. 2-(2-Hydroxyethoxy)ethyl *N*-(ααα-trifluoro-*m*-tolyl)anthranilate.

$C_{18}H_{18}F_3NO_4$ = 369.3.
*CAS — 30544-47-9.*
*ATC — M02AA06.*

**Pharmacopoeias.** In *Eur.* (see p.vi).

**Ph. Eur. 5.0** (Etofenamate). A yellowish viscous liquid. Practically insoluble in water; miscible with alcohol and with ethyl acetate.

### Profile

Etofenamate is an NSAID (p.67) that has been applied topically in a concentration of 5 or 10% for the relief of pain and inflammation associated with musculoskeletal, joint, and soft-tissue disorders. It has also been given by deep intramuscular injection in single doses of 1 g.

### Preparations

**Proprietary Preparations** (details are given in Part 3)
***Arg.:*** Bayrogel; Flogol-gel; ***Austria:*** Rheumon; Traumon; ***Belg.:*** Flexium; ***Braz.:*** Bayro; ***Chile:*** Bayro; Flogojet; Master-Gel; Valorel; ***Ger.:*** Algesalona E; Rheuma-Gel; Rheumon; Traumon; ***Gr.:*** Roiplon; ***Ital.:*** Bayro; ***Mex.:*** Bayro; Reumagel†; ***Port.:*** Fenogel; Reumon; ***Spain:*** Afrolate†; Aspitopic; Bayro†; Flogoprofen; Zenavan; ***Switz.:*** Activon; Etofen; Rheumon; Traumalix.

**Multi-ingredient:** ***Austria:*** Thermo-Rheumon; ***Chile:*** Bayro-Therm; ***Ger.:*** Thermo-Rheumon; ***Mex.:*** Bayro Termo.

---

## Etoricoxib *(BAN, USAN, rINN)*

L-791456; MK-0663. 5-Chloro-6′-methyl-3-[*p*-(methylsulfonyl)phenyl]-2,3′-bipyridine.

$C_{18}H_{15}ClN_2O_2S$ = 358.8.
*CAS — 202409-33-4.*
*ATC — M01AH05.*

### Adverse Effects and Precautions

As for NSAIDs in general, p.67. Etoricoxib should be avoided in patients with severe hepatic impairment. Therapy should be discontinued if persistently abnormal liver enzyme values are seen. Etoricoxib is also contra-indicated in patients with inflammatory bowel disease, severe heart failure, and renal impairment associated with a creatinine clearance of less than 30 mL/minute.

Caution is recommended when using etoricoxib in dehydrated patients; it may be advisable to rehydrate patients before giving etoricoxib.

**Effects on the cardiovascular system.** Cyclo-oxygenase-2 (COX-2) inhibitors such as etoricoxib do not possess the intrinsic antiplatelet activity associated with aspirin and possibly other non-selective NSAIDs and consequently do not provide protection against ischaemic cardiac events.

**Effects on the gastrointestinal tract.** It is generally accepted that the inhibition of cyclo-oxygenase-1 (COX-1) results in the adverse gastrointestinal effects of the NSAIDs, and that the selective inhibition of the other isoform, COX-2, by NSAIDs such as etoricoxib may cause less gastrotoxicity than that seen with the non-selective inhibition of the traditional NSAIDs. However, the manufacturers report that upper gastrointestinal perforation, ulceration, and bleeds have occurred with etoricoxib treatment and therefore it should be used with caution in patients with a history of such events.

**Effects on the kidneys.** Limited evidence of the renal toxicity of the selective cyclo-oxygenase-2 (COX-2) inhibitors such as etoricoxib suggests that such NSAIDs appear to have effects on renal function similar to those of the non-selective NSAIDs (see p.68).

### Interactions

The metabolism of etoricoxib is mediated by the cytochrome P450 isoenzyme CYP3A4. Use with of other drugs that inhibit or induce this isoenzyme may result in changes in plasma concentration of etoricoxib. In addition, *in vitro* studies suggest that several other isoenzymes may also mediate the main metabolic pathway of etoricoxib. Rifampicin, a potent inducer of CYP isoenzymes, has produced decreased plasma concentrations of etoricoxib.

Etoricoxib is an inhibitor of human sulfotransferase activity and has been shown to increase the plasma concentration of ethinylestradiol. Interactions with other drugs, such as oral salbutamol and minoxidil, also metabolised by this enzyme may be a possibility and the manufacturers advise care with such combinations.

For interactions associated with NSAIDs in general, see p.69.

### Pharmacokinetics

Etoricoxib is well absorbed from the gastrointestinal tract after oral doses. Peak plasma concentrations are reached in approximately 1 hour and plasma protein binding is about 92%. At steady state the half-life of etoricoxib is about 22 hours. Etoricoxib is extensively metabolised with less than 2% of a dose recovered in the urine as the parent drug. The major route of metabolism is via cytochrome P450 isoenzymes including CYP3A4 to form the 6′-hydroxymethyl derivative of etoricoxib, which is then oxidised to the 6′-carboxylic acid derivative, the major metabolite. Both are inactive or only weak cyclo-oxygenase-2 (COX-2) inhibitors. Excretion is mainly via the urine (70%) with only 20% of a dose appearing in the faeces.

◊ References.

1. Agrawal NGB, *et al.* Single- and multiple-dose pharmacokinetics of etoricoxib, a selective inhibitor of cyclooxygenase-2, in man. *J Clin Pharmacol* 2003; **43:** 268–76.

### Uses and Administration

Etoricoxib is an NSAID (p.67) reported to be a selective inhibitor of cyclo-oxygenase-2 (COX-2). It is used in the symptomatic relief of rheumatoid arthritis, osteoarthritis, and acute gouty arthritis.

In osteoarthritis, etoricoxib is given by mouth in a dose of 60 mg once daily. The recommended dose in rheumatoid arthritis is 90 mg once daily; higher doses of 120 mg once daily are used in gouty arthritis although such doses should only be used for the acute symptomatic period. For dosage recommendations in patients with hepatic impairment, see below.

◊ References.

1. Patrignani P, *et al.* Clinical pharmacology of etoricoxib: a novel selective COX2 inhibitor. *Expert Opin Pharmacother* 2003; **4:** 265–84.

**Administration in hepatic impairment.** The dose of etoricoxib in patients with mild hepatic impairment is 60 mg once daily; those with moderate impairment should be given 60 mg every other day. Etoricoxib should not be given to patients with severe hepatic impairment.

**Musculoskeletal and joint disorders.** The selective cyclo-oxygenase-2 (COX-2) inhibitor etoricoxib is used in the treatment of the musculoskeletal disorders osteoarthritis and rheumatoid arthritis (see p.9 and p.9, respectively). However, in the UK, it is recommended that the use of selective COX-2 inhibitors is limited to those patients considered to be at high risk of developing serious gastrointestinal problems if given a non-selective NSAID (see p.68).

Etoricoxib is also used in gouty arthritis (p.412).

References.

1. Cochrane DJ, *et al.* Etoricoxib. *Drugs* 2002; **62:** 2637–51.
2. Schumacher HR, *et al.* Randomised double blind trial of etoricoxib and indometacin in treatment of acute gouty arthritis. *BMJ* 2002; **324:** 1488–92.
3. Gottesdiener K, *et al.* Results of a randomized, dose-ranging trial of etoricoxib in patients with osteoarthritis. *Rheumatology (Oxford)* 2002; **41:** 1052–61.

### Preparations

**Proprietary Preparations** (details are given in Part 3)
***Irl.:*** Arcoxia; ***NZ:*** Arcoxia; ***UK:*** Arcoxia.

---

## Etorphine Hydrochloride *(BANM, rINNM)*

Hidrocloruro de etorfina; M-99; 19-Propylorvinol Hydrochloride. (6*R*,7*R*,14*R*)-7,8-Dihydro-7-(1*R*-1-hydroxy-1-methylbutyl)-6-*O*-methyl-6,14α-ethenomorphine hydrochloride; (2*R*)-2-[(−)-(5*R*,6*R*,7*R*,14*R*)-4,5-Epoxy-3-hydroxy-6-methoxy-9a-methyl-6,14-ethenomorphinan-7-yl]pentan-2-ol hydrochloride.

$C_{25}H_{33}NO_4$,HCl = 448.0.
*CAS — 14521-96-1 (etorphine); 13764-49-3 (etorphine hydrochloride).*

**Pharmacopoeias.** In *BP(Vet).*

**BP(Vet) 2003** (Etorphine Hydrochloride). A white or almost white microcrystalline powder. Sparingly soluble in water and in alcohol; very slightly soluble in chloroform; practically insoluble in ether. A 2% solution in water has a pH of 4.0 to 5.5. Protect from light.

### Dependence and Withdrawal

As for Opioid Analgesics, p.71.

### Adverse Effects and Treatment

As for Opioid Analgesics in general, p.72. Etorphine is not used therapeutically in humans.

Etorphine hydrochloride is highly potent and rapid acting; minute amounts can exert serious effects leading to coma. It may be absorbed through skin and mucous membranes. It is thus advisable to inject an antagonist *immediately* following contamination of skin or mucous membranes with preparations containing etorphine hydrochloride and to wash the affected areas copiously. Accidental injection or needle scratch should also be treated immediately by injecting an antagonist. Naloxone is preferred as the antagonist in medical treatment. However, veterinary preparations of etorphine are supplied with a preparation containing diprenorphine hydrochloride (Revivon) and this should be used for immediate first-aid antagonism if naloxone is not available.

### Uses and Administration

Etorphine hydrochloride is a highly potent opioid analgesic (p.73) used for reversible neuroleptanalgesia (see under Anaesthetic Techniques, p.1296) in veterinary medicine. It is given with acepromazine maleate or levomepromazine (Immobilon) to restrain animals and before minor veterinary surgery. The duration of action of etorphine is up to about 45 to 90 minutes depending on the species but it may be longer in man, especially if the large animal preparation is involved.

---

## Famprofazone *(BAN, rINN)*

Famprofazona. 4-Isopropyl-2-methyl-3-[methyl(α-methylphenethyl)aminomethyl]-1-phenyl-3-pyrazolin-5-one.

$C_{24}H_{31}N_3O$ = 377.5.
*CAS — 22881-35-2.*

### Profile

Famprofazone has analgesic and antipyretic properties and has been given by mouth, usually in conjunction with other analgesics.

### Preparations

**Proprietary Preparations** (details are given in Part 3)
**Multi-ingredient:** ***Ger.:*** Gewodin†.

## Felbinac (BAN, USAN, rINN)

CL-83544; Felbinaco; LJC-10141. Biphenyl-4-ylacetic acid.

$C_{14}H_{12}O_2$ = 212.2.

CAS — 5728-52-9.

ATC — M02AA08.

**Pharmacopoeias.** In *Br.*

**BP 2003** (Felbinac). A fine white, crystalline powder. Practically insoluble in water; sparingly soluble in dehydrated alcohol; freely soluble in dimethylformamide.

### Adverse Effects and Precautions

Mild local reactions such as erythema, dermatitis, and pruritus have occurred in patients using felbinac topically. More serious side-effects including bullous dermatoses such as epidermal necrolysis and erythema multiforme, photosensitivity, anaphylaxis, and bronchospasm or wheeziness have also been reported. Gastrointestinal disturbances may occur.

Felbinac preparations should be avoided in patients with a history of hypersensitivity reactions to aspirin or other NSAIDs.

◊ The UK Committee on Safety of Medicines had received 49 reports of adverse reactions associated with felbinac by October 1989, about 11 months after it was released on the UK market.[1] Bronchospasm or wheeziness was reported in 8 patients using felbinac gel. Four of these patients had a history of asthma of whom 3 were reported to have had a similar reaction to aspirin or other NSAIDs. Other reported reactions included skin rashes (17 cases), local application site reactions (7), and dyspepsia (6).

1. Committee on Safety of Medicines. Felbinac (Traxam) and bronchospasm. *Current Problems 27* 1989.

### Uses and Administration

Felbinac, an active metabolite of fenbufen (p.39), is an NSAID (p.70). It is used topically in the symptomatic treatment of musculoskeletal pain including that due to soft-tissue injuries. It is applied as a 3% gel or a 3.17% foam to unbroken skin over affected areas 2 to 4 times daily. The total daily dose of gel or foam should not exceed 25 g regardless of the size or number of affected areas. Therapy should be reviewed after 14 days.

Diisopropanolamine felbinac has been used similarly.

◊ References.

1. Hosie GAC. The topical NSAID, felbinac, versus oral ibuprofen: a comparison of efficacy in the treatment of acute lower back injury. *Br J Clin Res* 1993; **4:** 5–17.

### Preparations

***BP 2003:*** Felbinac Cutaneous Foam; Felbinac Gel.

**Proprietary Preparations** (details are given in Part 3)

***Austria:*** Target; ***Belg.:*** Flexfree†; ***Denm.:*** Dolinac†; ***Ger.:*** Dolinac†; Spalt Schmerz-Gel; Target†; ***Irl.:*** Traxam; ***Ital.:*** Dolinac; Traxam; ***Jpn:*** Seltouch; ***S.Afr.:*** Dolinac†; ***Switz.:*** Dolo Target; Target†; ***UK:*** Traxam.

## Fenbufen (BAN, USAN, rINN)

CL-82204; Fenbufén; Fenbufenum. 4-(Biphenyl-4-yl)-4-oxobutyric acid.

$C_{16}H_{14}O_3$ = 254.3.

CAS — 36330-85-5.

ATC — M01AE05.

**Pharmacopoeias.** In *Chin., Eur.* (see p.vi), and *Jpn.*

**Ph. Eur. 5.0** (Fenbufen). A white fine crystalline powder. Very slightly soluble in water; slightly soluble in alcohol, in acetone, and in dichloromethane.

### Adverse Effects and Precautions

As for NSAIDs in general, p.67, although the commonest side-effects of fenbufen are skin rashes, particularly in women and in patients with seronegative rheumatoid arthritis or psoriatic arthritis. Disorders such as erythema multiforme and Stevens-Johnson syndrome have also been reported. A small number of patients who develop rash may go on to develop a severe illness characterised by pulmonary eosinophilia or allergic alveolitis. Treatment with fenbufen should be stopped immediately if a rash appears.

**Breast feeding.** The UK manufacturer advises that fenbufen should be avoided in breast-feeding mothers, because of the presence of its metabolites in breast milk.

**Effects on the blood.** Haemolytic anaemia[1] and aplastic anaemia[2] have been reported in patients receiving fenbufen.

1. Martland T, Stone WD. Haemolytic anaemia associated with fenbufen. *BMJ* 1988; **297:** 921.
2. Andrews R, Russell N. Aplastic anaemia associated with a non-steroidal anti-inflammatory drug: relapse after exposure to another such drug. *BMJ* 1990; **301:** 38.

**Effects on the lungs.** In January 1989 the UK Committee on Safety of Medicines reported that it had received 7 reports of a suspected association between rash and an allergic interstitial lung disorder in patients receiving fenbufen.[1] In 5 patients, the lung disorder was diagnosed as pulmonary eosinophilia; in the 2 other patients the pulmonary component of the reaction was described as allergic alveolitis. Several of these reactions have been reported in the literature.[2,3]

1. Committee on Safety of Medicines. Fenbufen, rash and pulmonary eosinophilia. *Current Problems 24* 1989.
2. Swinburn CR. Alveolitis and haemolytic anaemia induced by azapropazone. *BMJ* 1987; **294:** 375.
3. Burton GH. Rash and pulmonary eosinophilia associated with fenbufen. *BMJ* 1990; **300:** 82–3.

**Effects on the skin.** In September 1988 the UK Committee on Safety of Medicines reported[1] that it was still receiving large numbers of reports of adverse reactions to fenbufen when such reports were expected to have declined. Fenbufen was the most commonly reported suspect drug in 1986 and 1987. At the time of the report more than 6000 such reports had been received, 80% concerning mucocutaneous reactions and most involving a generalised florid erythematous rash, often with pruritus. There were 178 reports of erythema multiforme, 30 of Stevens-Johnson syndrome, and 2 fatalities.

1. Committee on Safety of Medicines. Fenbufen and mucocutaneous reactions. *Current Problems 23* 1988.

**Hypersensitivity.** See under Effects on the Lungs (above).

### Interactions

For interactions associated with NSAIDs, see p.69.

Use of fenbufen with aspirin may result in decreased serum concentrations of fenbufen and its metabolites.

### Pharmacokinetics

Fenbufen is absorbed from the gastrointestinal tract and peak plasma concentrations are reached in about 70 minutes. Fenbufen is over 99% bound to plasma proteins. It is metabolised in the liver to the active metabolites, biphenylacetic acid and 4-hydroxy-biphenylbutyric acid. Fenbufen and its metabolites are reported to have plasma half-lives of about 10 to 17 hours and are mainly eliminated as conjugates in the urine. Metabolites of fenbufen have been detected in breast milk in small amounts.

### Uses and Administration

Fenbufen, a propionic acid derivative, is an NSAID (p.70). It is given for the relief of pain and inflammation associated with musculoskeletal and joint disorders such as rheumatoid arthritis, osteoarthritis, and ankylosing spondylitis in doses of 900 mg daily by mouth; the dose may be either 450 mg in the morning and evening or 300 mg in the morning with 600 mg in the evening.

### Preparations

***BP 2003:*** Fenbufen Capsules; Fenbufen Tablets.

**Proprietary Preparations** (details are given in Part 3)

***Austria:*** Lederfen; ***Denm.:*** Cinopal†; ***Fr.:*** Cinopal†; ***Irl.:*** Lederfen; ***Israel:*** Lederfen†; ***Ital.:*** Cinopal†; ***Port.:*** Reugast; ***S.Afr.:*** Cinopal†; ***Spain:*** Cinopal†; ***Thai.:*** Cepal; Cinopal; ***UK:*** Lederfen.

## Fenoprofen Calcium (BANM, USAN, rINNM)

Fenoprofeno cálcico; Lilly-69323; Lilly-53858 (fenoprofen); Lilly-61169 (fenoprofen sodium). Calcium (±)-2-(3-phenoxyphenyl)propionate dihydrate.

$(C_{15}H_{13}O_3)_2Ca,2H_2O$ = 558.6.

CAS — 31879-05-7 (fenoprofen); 34597-40-5 (anhydrous fenoprofen calcium); 53746-45-5 (fenoprofen calcium dihydrate).

ATC — M01AE04.

**Pharmacopoeias.** In *Br., Chin.,* and *US.*

**BP 2003** (Fenoprofen Calcium). A white or almost white odourless or almost odourless crystalline powder. Slightly soluble in water and in chloroform; soluble in alcohol.

**USP 27** (Fenoprofen Calcium). A white crystalline powder. Slightly soluble in water, in methyl alcohol, and in n-hexanol; practically insoluble in chloroform. Store in airtight containers.

### Adverse Effects and Precautions

As for NSAIDs in general, p.67. Dysuria, cystitis, haematuria, interstitial nephritis, and acute renal insufficiency have been reported with fenoprofen. Nephrotic syndrome, which may be preceded by fever, rash, arthralgia, oliguria, azotaemia, and anuria, has also occurred. Upper respiratory-tract infection and nasopharyngitis have been reported. There have been reports of severe hepatic reactions, including jaundice and fatal hepatitis.

**Breast feeding.** Fenoprofen is distributed into breast milk although the amount is considered by the *British National Formulary* to be too small to be harmful to a breast-fed infant. In contrast, the UK manufacturers do not recommend its use since safety has not been established.

**Effects on the blood.** Haematological adverse effects including agranulocytosis,[1] aplastic anaemia,[2] and thrombocytopenia[3,4] have been reported in patients taking fenoprofen; the UK manufacturers also report haemolytic anaemia.

1. Simon SD, Kosmin M. Fenoprofen and agranulocytosis. *N Engl J Med* 1978; **299:** 490.
2. Ashraf M, *et al.* Aplastic anaemia associated with fenoprofen. *BMJ* 1982; 284: 1301–2.
3. Simpson RE, *et al.* Acute thrombocytopenia associated with fenoprofen. *N Engl J Med* 1978; **298:** 629–30.
4. Katz ME, Wang P. Fenoprofen-associated thrombocytopenia. *Ann Intern Med* 1980; **92:** 262.

**Effects on the liver.** Cholestatic jaundice and hepatitis developed in a 68-year-old woman after receiving fenoprofen 600 mg four times daily for 7 weeks. Subsequent use of naproxen and indometacin did not result in hepatotoxicity.[1] However, there has been a report of cross-hepatotoxicity between fenoprofen and naproxen.[2]

1. Stennett DJ, *et al.* Fenoprofen-induced hepatotoxicity. *Am J Hosp Pharm* 1978; **35:** 901.
2. Andrejak M, *et al.* Cross hepatotoxicity between non-steroidal anti-inflammatory drugs. *BMJ* 1987; **295:** 180–1.

**Effects on the skin.** Toxic epidermal necrolysis was associated with fenoprofen in 2 patients.[1]

1. Stotts JS, *et al.* Fenoprofen-induced toxic epidermal necrolysis. *J Am Acad Dermatol* 1988; **18:** 755–7.

**Overdosage.** A report of coma, respiratory depression, hypotension, and metabolic acidosis in a patient who had ingested between 24 and 36 g of fenoprofen.[1] The patient responded to gastric lavage and activated charcoal and intensive supportive care.

1. Kolodzik JM, *et al.* Nonsteroidal anti-inflammatory drugs and coma: a case report of fenoprofen overdose. *Ann Emerg Med* 1990; **19:** 378–81.

### Interactions

For interactions associated with NSAIDs, see p.69.

Aspirin is reported to reduce plasma concentrations of fenoprofen.

**Antiepileptics.** *Phenobarbital* might increase the rate of metabolism of fenoprofen.[1]

1. Helleberg L, *et al.* A pharmacokinetic interaction in man between phenobarbitone and fenoprofen, a new anti-inflammatory agent. *Br J Clin Pharmacol* 1974; **1:** 371–4.

### Pharmacokinetics

Fenoprofen is readily absorbed from the gastrointestinal tract; bioavailability is about 85% but food and milk may reduce the rate and extent of absorption. Peak plasma concentrations occur 1 to 2 hours after a dose. The plasma half-life is about 3 hours. Fenoprofen is 99% bound to plasma proteins. About 90% of a dose is excreted in the urine in 24 hours, chiefly as the glucuronide and the glucuronide of hydroxylated fenoprofen. Fenoprofen is distributed into breast milk.

### Uses and Administration

Fenoprofen, a propionic acid derivative, is an NSAID (p.70) used in the management of mild to moderate pain and for the relief of pain and inflammation associated with disorders such as osteoarthritis, rheumatoid arthritis, and ankylosing spondylitis. It is given as the calcium salt although doses are expressed in terms of the base; fenoprofen calcium (dihydrate) 1.2 g is approximately equivalent to 1 g of fenoprofen. A usual dose is the equivalent of 300 to 600 mg of fenoprofen three or four times daily, adjusted thereafter according to response. It has been recommended that the total daily dose should not exceed 3 g (UK) or 3.2 g (USA). In the USA, lower doses of 200 mg every 4 to 6 hours are recommended for mild to moderate pain.

### Preparations

***BP 2003:*** Fenoprofen Tablets;
***USP 27:*** Fenoprofen Calcium Capsules; Fenoprofen Calcium Tablets.

**Proprietary Preparations** (details are given in Part 3)

***Austria:*** Nalfon†; ***Braz.:*** Trandor; ***Canad.:*** Nalfon; ***Denm.:*** Nalfon; ***Fr.:*** Nalgesic†; ***Gr.:*** Expron; ***Hong Kong:*** Fenopron†; ***Irl.:*** Fenopron†; ***Ital.:*** Fepron†; ***Mex.:*** Nalfon; ***S.Afr.:*** Fenopron; ***Spain:*** Nalfon†; ***UK:*** Fenopron; ***USA:*** Nalfon.

## Fentanyl *(BAN, rINN)*

Fentanilo; Fentanylum. *N*-(1-Phenethyl-4-piperidyl) propionanilide.

$C_{22}H_{28}N_2O$ = 336.5.
*CAS — 437-38-7.*
*ATC — N01AH01; N02AB03.*

**Pharmacopoeias.** In *Eur.* (see p.vi).

**Ph. Eur. 5.0** (Fentanyl). A white or almost white polymorphic powder. Practically insoluble in water; freely soluble in alcohol and in methyl alcohol. Protect from light.

## Fentanyl Citrate *(BANM, USAN, rINNM)*

Citrato de fentanilo; Fentanyli Citras; McN-JR-4263-49; Phentanyl Citrate; R-4263. *N*-(1-Phenethyl-4-piperidyl)propionanilide dihydrogen citrate.

$C_{22}H_{28}N_2O,C_6H_8O_7$ = 528.6.
*CAS — 990-73-8.*

**Pharmacopoeias.** In *Chin., Eur.* (see p.vi), *Jpn, Pol.,* and *US.*

**Ph. Eur. 5.0** (Fentanyl Citrate). White or almost white powder. Soluble in water; sparingly soluble in alcohol; freely soluble in methyl alcohol. Protect from light.

**USP 27** (Fentanyl Citrate). A white crystalline powder or white glistening crystals. Sparingly soluble in water; slightly soluble in chloroform; soluble in methyl alcohol. Store at a temperature of 25°, excursions permitted between 15° and 30°. Protect from light.

**Handling.** Avoid contact with skin and the inhalation of particles of fentanyl citrate.

**Incompatibility.** Fentanyl citrate is incompatible with thiopental sodium and methohexital sodium.

A thick white precipitate formed in the intravenous tubing when fentanyl citrate with droperidol was given shortly after nafcillin sodium. There was no precipitate when fentanyl citrate alone was mixed with nafcillin sodium.[1]

Fentanyl citrate underwent rapid and extensive loss when admixed with fluorouracil in PVC containers.[2] The loss was due to sorption of fentanyl to the PVC as a result of the alkaline pH of the admixture, and presumably could occur from admixture of fentanyl citrate with any sufficiently alkaline drug.

See also under Stability, below.


1. Jeglum EL, *et al.* Nafcillin sodium incompatibility with acidic solutions. *Am J Hosp Pharm* 1981; **38:** 462, 464.
2. Xu QA, *et al.* Rapid loss of fentanyl citrate admixed with fluorouracil in polyvinyl chloride containers. *Ann Pharmacother* 1997; **31:** 297–302.


**Stability.** In a 48-hour study fentanyl citrate in glucose 5% or sodium chloride 0.9% was stable when stored at room temperature under usual light conditions in glass or PVC containers;[1] the concentration of fentanyl delivered by a patient-controlled system was relatively constant throughout a 30-hour study period. Fentanyl citrate injection diluted to 20 micrograms/mL with sodium chloride 0.9% was stable for 30 days at 3° or 23° in PVC reservoirs for portable infusion pumps.[2] An admixture of fentanyl citrate and bupivacaine in sodium chloride 0.9% appeared[3] compatible and stable when stored for up to 30 days at 3° or 23° in a portable infusion pump. In another study[4] the stability of solutions containing fentanyl, bupivacaine, and adrenaline, alone and in combination was studied over a period of 56 days when stored at various temperatures in the light or in the dark in PVC bags. Both fentanyl and bupivacaine were adsorbed from solution onto the PVC for the first 3 days but thereafter concentrations of these drugs remained relatively stable; freezing appeared to slow the concentration change for bupivacaine but not for fentanyl. Solutions containing adrenaline became more acidic during the study as the adrenaline progressively deteriorated but this was greatly reduced by freezing. Autoclaving produced a further reduction in the concentration of all drugs. There was no sign of precipitation from any of the solutions studied. Fentanyl is potentially unstable in PVC containers when admixed with alkaline drugs (see under Incompatibility, above).


1. Kowalski SR, Gourlay GK. Stability of fentanyl citrate in glass and plastic containers and in a patient-controlled delivery system. *Am J Hosp Pharm* 1990; **47:** 1584–7.
2. Allen LV, *et al.* Stability of fentanyl citrate in 0.9% sodium chloride solution in portable infusion pumps. *Am J Hosp Pharm* 1990; **47:** 1572–4.
3. Tu Y-H, *et al.* Stability of fentanyl citrate and bupivacaine hydrochloride in portable pump reservoirs. *Am J Hosp Pharm* 1990; **47:** 2037–40.
4. Dawson PJ, *et al.* Stability of fentanyl, bupivacaine and adrenaline solutions for extradural infusion. *Br J Anaesth* 1992; **68:** 414–17.


## Dependence and Withdrawal

As for Opioid Analgesics, p.71. Fentanyl and illicitly manufactured analogues are subject to abuse (see under Precautions, below).

◊ Movement disorders, extreme irritability, and symptoms characteristic of opioid abstinence syndrome have been reported in children after withdrawal of prolonged fentanyl infusions.[1,2] Plasma concentrations required to produce satisfactory sedation have been reported to increase steadily in neonates receiving continuous infusions, suggesting the development of tolerance to the sedating effects of fentanyl.[3]

Acute opioid withdrawal syndrome has also been seen in cancer patients switched from modified-release oral morphine to transdermal fentanyl despite adequate analgesia being maintained.[4]


1. Lane JC, *et al.* Movement disorder after withdrawal of fentanyl infusion. *J Pediatr* 1991; **119:** 649–51.
2. Dominguez KD, *et al.* Opioid withdrawal in critically ill neonates. *Ann Pharmacother* 2003 **37:** 473–7.
3. Arnold JH, *et al.* Changes in the pharmacodynamic response to fentanyl in neonates during continuous infusion. *J Pediatr* 1991; **119:** 639–43.
4. Anonymous. Opiate withdrawal with transdermal fentanyl. *Pharm J* 1995; **255:** 680.


## Adverse Effects and Treatment

As for Opioid Analgesics in general, p.72.

Respiratory depression, which occurs especially with high doses of fentanyl, responds to naloxone (see also under Effects on the Respiratory System, below). Atropine may be used to block the vagal effects of fentanyl such as bradycardia. Unlike morphine, fentanyl is reported not to cause significant histamine release. Transient hypotension may follow intravenous administration. Muscle rigidity may occur and may require neuromuscular blockers.

Local reactions such as rash, erythema, and itching have been reported with the transdermal patches.

**Effects on the cardiovascular system.** For a reference to the effects of fentanyl on histamine release compared with some other opioids, see under Pethidine, p.80.

**Effects on mental function.** Fentanyl had some dose-related effects on mental function and motor activity in healthy subjects,[1] but immediate and delayed recall were not affected. See also under Alfentanil (p.12).

Acute toxic delirium has been reported following treatment with transdermal fentanyl.[2]


1. Scamman FL, *et al.* Ventilatory and mental effects of alfentanil and fentanyl. *Acta Anaesthesiol Scand* 1984; **28:** 63–7.
2. Kuzma PJ, *et al.* Acute toxic delirium: a uncommon reaction to transdermal fentanyl. *Anesthesiology* 1995; **83:** 869–71.


**Effects on the nervous system.** There have been reports of seizures with low and high doses of fentanyl or sufentanil.[1] There was, however, no EEG evidence of cortical seizure activity in a patient who had seizure-like muscle movements during a fentanyl infusion;[2] the muscle movements might have been due to myoclonus produced by depression of higher CNS inhibitory centres or to a pronounced form of opioid-induced muscle rigidity.

For a report of encephalopathy associated with prolonged use of fentanyl and midazolam in infants in intensive care, see under Encephalopathy in the Adverse Effects of Diazepam, p.691.


1. Zaccara G, *et al.* Clinical features, pathogenesis and management of drug-induced seizures. *Drug Safety* 1990; **5:** 109–51.
2. Scott JC, Sarnquist FH. Seizure-like movements during a fentanyl infusion with absence of seizure activity in a simultaneous EEG recording. *Anesthesiology* 1985; **62:** 812–14.


**Effects on the respiratory system.** Fentanyl, like other opioid agonists, causes dose-related respiratory depression; it is significant with *intravenous* fentanyl doses of more than 200 micrograms and may be more prolonged than analgesia. Anaesthesia with fentanyl may result in either prolonged or delayed respiratory depression postoperatively.[1] If present at the end of operation it should be reversed by an opioid antagonist such as naloxone; alternatively a respiratory stimulant such as doxapram that does not reverse analgesia has been given. Buprenorphine has also been tried for the reversal of respiratory depression induced by fentanyl (see Anaesthesia, p.23). Because of the risk of delayed respiratory depression patients should continue to be monitored postoperatively until spontaneous breathing has been re-established. Severe respiratory depression in a 14-month-old child following intravenous sedation with fentanyl and midazolam has highlighted the necessity for careful monitoring when giving respiratory depressants concurrently.[2]

Rigidity of the respiratory muscles (chest wall rigidity) may occur during fentanyl anaesthesia. The effects can be minimised by using a slow intravenous injection but a neuromuscular blocker may be required to allow artificial ventilation; rigidity has been reversed postoperatively by naloxone. Similar muscle rigidity induced by alfentanil could be attenuated by pretreatment with a benzodiazepine whereas small doses of neuromuscular blockers appeared to be ineffective.[3]

The risk of respiratory depression associated with *epidural* doses of fentanyl, a highly lipid-soluble opioid, has been considered relatively small and only slight ventilatory depression was noted[4] following a dose of 50 micrograms. However, profound delayed respiratory depression has been reported in 2 women 100 minutes[5] and 80 minutes[6] respectively after fentanyl 100 micrograms had been given epidurally for caesarean section. No adverse effects on neonatal respiration or neurobehaviour were detected in a study[7] of neonates of mothers given epidural infusions of bupivacaine and fentanyl during labour.

Respiratory depression is also a risk with *topically* applied fentanyl preparations. Severe hypoventilation with some fatalities has occurred in patients receiving fentanyl through a transdermal patch for minor painful conditions.[8]


1. Bennett MRD, Adams AP. Postoperative respiratory complications of opiates. *Clin Anaesthesiol* 1983; **1:** 41–56.
2. Yaster M, *et al.* Midazolam-fentanyl intravenous sedation in children: case report of respiratory arrest. *Pediatrics* 1990; **86:** 463–7.
3. Sanford TJ, *et al.* Pretreatment with sedative-hypnotics, but not with nondepolarizing muscle relaxants, attenuates alfentanil-induced muscle rigidity. *J Clin Anesth* 1994; **6:** 473–80.
4. Morisot P, *et al.* Ventilatory response to carbon dioxide during extradural anaesthesia with lignocaine and fentanyl. *Br J Anaesth* 1989; **63:** 97–102.
5. Brockway MS, *et al.* Profound respiratory depression after extradural fentanyl. *Br J Anaesth* 1990; **64:** 243–5.
6. Wang CY. Respiratory depression after extradural fentanyl. *Br J Anaesth* 1992; **69:** 544.
7. Porter J, *et al.* Effect of epidural fentanyl on neonatal respiration. *Anesthesiology* 1998; **89:** 79–85.
8. *FDC Reports Pink Sheet* 1994; January 24: 12.


**Effects on the skin.** A patient developed a macular rash covering the whole body, except for the face and scalp, while using transdermal fentanyl patches.[1]


1. Stoukides CA, Stegman M. Diffuse rash associated with transdermal fentanyl. *Clin Pharm* 1992; **11:** 222.


**Effects on the urinary tract.** Urinary retention developed in 2 premature infants following sedation with fentanyl infusion at a dose of 3 micrograms/kg per hour.[1] In both cases catheterisation relieved symptoms.


1. Das UG, Sasidharan P. Bladder retention of urine as a result of continuous intravenous infusion of fentanyl: 2 case reports. *Pediatrics* 2001; **108:** 1012–1015.


## Precautions

As for Opioid Analgesics in general, p.72.

Caution is advised in patients with myasthenia gravis; the effects of muscular rigidity on respiration may be particularly pronounced in these patients.

Absorption of fentanyl from transdermal patches may be increased as the temperature rises and patients should therefore avoid exposing the patch to external heat; similarly, patients with fever may require monitoring because of increased absorption. It may take 17 hours or longer for plasma concentrations of fentanyl to decrease by 50% after removal of a patch; patients who have experienced side-effects should be monitored for up to 24 hours and those requiring replacement opioid therapy should initially receive low doses increased gradually thereafter.

**Abuse.** Several synthetic analogues of fentanyl, so-called 'designer drugs', have been manufactured illicitly for recreational use, particularly in the USA. They are highly potent and respiratory depression and death may occur very rapidly.[1] The 'fentanyls' have been smoked or snorted as well as injected intravenously.

Fentanyl analogues identified by WHO[2,3] as being subject to street abuse or likely to be abused include: alpha-methylfentanyl (also known as 'China white' or 'synthetic heroin'), 3-methylfentanyl, acetyl-alpha-methylfentanyl, alpha-methylthiofentanyl, para-fluorofentanyl, beta-hydroxyfentanyl, beta-hydroxy-3-methylfentanyl, thiofentanyl, and 3-methylthiofentanyl.

Fentanyl itself is also subject to illicit use. It is chemically unrelated to morphine and does not react in screening tests for morphine-related opioids. It has therefore been recommended[4] that fentanyl should be tested for specifically in cases with suspected opioid misuse.

Used fentanyl transdermal patches may contain significant amounts of fentanyl[5] and have been subject to abuse. In some cases the contents of the patches have been injected intravenously; such abuse has resulted in death.[6] The manufacturers advise that used patches should be folded firmly in half, adhesive side inwards to conceal the release membrane, and disposed of safely.


1. Buchanan JF, Brown CR. 'Designer drugs': a problem in clinical toxicology. *Med Toxicol* 1988; **3:** 1–17.
2. WHO. WHO expert committee on drug dependence: twenty-fourth report. *WHO Tech Rep Ser 761* 1988.
3. WHO. WHO expert committee on drug dependence: twenty-sixth report. *WHO Tech Rep Ser 787* 1989.
4. Berens AIL, *et al.* Illicit fentanyl in Europe. *Lancet* 1996; **347:** 1334–5.
5. Marquardt KA, *et al.* Fentanyl remaining in a transdermal system following three days of continuous use. *Ann Pharmacother* 1995; **29:** 969–71.
6. Reeves MD, Ginifer CJ. Fatal intravenous misuse of transdermal fentanyl. *Med J Aust* 2002; **177:** 552–3.


**Administration.** Fentanyl is much more lipid-soluble than morphine and after standard single intravenous doses has a rapid onset and short duration of action. However, fentanyl is rapidly redistributed in the body and has a longer elimination half-life than morphine (see Pharmacokinetics, below). Hence with high or repeated doses fentanyl becomes a relatively long-acting drug and to avoid accumulation patients should be monitored and doses adjusted accordingly.

Repeated intra-operative doses of fentanyl should be given with care, since not only may the respiratory depression persist into the postoperative period but it may become apparent for the first time postoperatively when the patient is away from immediate nursing attention.

**Breast feeding.** The American Academy of Pediatrics[1] states that there have been no reports of any clinical effect on the infant associated with the use of fentanyl by breast-feeding mothers, and that therefore it may be considered to be usually compatible with breast feeding. However, the UK manufacturers consider that, since fentanyl is distributed into breast milk, it should be avoided in nursing mothers because of the possibility of sedation or respiratory depression in breast-fed infants.

1. American Academy of Pediatrics. The transfer of drugs and other chemicals into human milk. *Pediatrics* 2001; **108:** 776–89. Correction. *ibid.*; 1029. Also available at: http://aappolicy.aappublications.org/cgi/content/full/pediatrics%3b108/3/776 (accessed 05/07/04)

**Exercise.** Opioid toxicity requiring naloxone administration has been reported in a patient who wore a fentanyl patch whilst engaging in vigorous outdoor exercise.[1] Physicians should be aware that along with fever and external heat sources, physical activity may cause increased absorption of transdermal fentanyl.

1. Carter KA. Heat-associated increase in transdermal fentanyl absorption. *Am J Health-Syst Pharm* 2003; **60:** 191–2.

## Interactions

For interactions associated with opioid analgesics, see p.73.

**Antivirals.** *Ritonavir* might prolong fentanyl-induced respiratory depression. The plasma clearance of fentanyl was decreased, and the elimination half-life and area under the plasma concentration-time curve increased, when given with ritonavir in a study in healthy subjects.[1]

1. Olkkola KT, *et al.* Ritonavir's role in reducing fentanyl clearance and prolonging its half-life. *Anesthesiology* 1999; **91:** 681–5.

**Benzodiazepines.** For the effects of opioids such as fentanyl with benzodiazepines, see under Analgesics in the Interactions of Diazepam, p.692.

**Propofol.** For reference to the effect that fentanyl has on blood concentrations of propofol, see p.1306.

## Pharmacokinetics

After parenteral doses fentanyl citrate has a rapid onset and short duration of action. After transmucosal delivery, about 25% of the dose is rapidly absorbed from the buccal mucosa; the remaining 75% is swallowed and slowly absorbed from the gastrointestinal tract. Some first-pass metabolism occurs via this route. The absolute bioavailability of transmucosal delivery is 50% of that for intravenous fentanyl. Absorption is slow after transdermal application. Fentanyl is metabolised in the liver by *N*-dealkylation and hydroxylation via the cytochrome p450 isoenzyme CYP3A4. Metabolites and some unchanged drug are excreted mainly in the urine. The short duration of action is probably due to rapid redistribution into the tissues rather than metabolism and excretion. The relatively longer elimination half-life reflects slower release from tissue depots. About 80% has been reported to be bound to plasma proteins. Fentanyl appears in the CSF. It crosses the placenta and has been detected in breast milk.

◊ Marked differences in results of pharmacokinetic studies of fentanyl have been attributed[1] to differences in assay methods. The need for sensitive assay methods has been emphasised because the potency of fentanyl means that small doses are used. However, there are differences in pharmacokinetics between bolus doses and prolonged infusion with highly lipophilic drugs such as fentanyl.[2] Terminal half-lives ranging from 2 to 7 hours have been reported in healthy subjects and surgical patients. However, the duration of action of fentanyl after a single intravenous dose of up to 100 micrograms may be only 30 to 60 minutes as a result of rapid redistribution into the tissues. The manufacturers have given values for a three-compartment pharmacokinetic model with a distribution time of 1.7 minutes, a redistribution time of 13 minutes, and a terminal elimination half-life of 219 minutes. Giving repeated or large doses, or continuous infusions, may result in accumulation and a more prolonged action.

The clinical significance of secondary peak plasma-fentanyl concentrations and the possible role of entero-systemic recirculation[3] has been controversial, but some[4] considered that irregular decay curves were not unlikely for lipophilic compounds such as fentanyl, especially in patients undergoing operations and subject to large changes in blood flow. Unexpectedly high plasma-fentanyl concentrations in a patient following epidural use were thought to be a result of aortic clamping and might reflect the effect of changes in blood flow.[5]

The main metabolites of fentanyl, which are excreted in the urine, have been identified as 4-*N*-(*N*-propionylanilino) piperidine and 4-*N*-(*N*-hydroxypropionylanilino) piperidine; 1-(2-phenethyl)-4-*N*-(*N*-hydroxypropionylanilino) piperidine is a minor metabolite.[6] Fentanyl has no active or toxic metabolites.[4]

1. Mather LE. Clinical pharmacokinetics of fentanyl and its newer derivatives. *Clin Pharmacokinet* 1983; **8:** 422–46.
2. Scholz J, *et al.* Clinical pharmacokinetics of alfentanil, fentanyl and sufentanil: an update. *Clin Pharmacokinet* 1996; **31:** 275–92.
3. Bennett MRD, Adams AP. Postoperative respiratory complications of opiates. *Clin Anaesthesiol* 1983; **1:** 41–56.
4. Moore RA, *et al.* Opiate metabolism and excretion. *Baillieres Clin Anaesthesiol* 1987; **1:** 829–58.
5. Bullingham RES, *et al.* Unexpectedly high plasma fentanyl levels after epidural use. *Lancet* 1980; **i:** 1361–2.
6. Goromaru T, *et al.* Identification and quantitative determination of fentanyl metabolites in patients by gas chromatography-mass spectrometry. *Anesthesiology* 1984; **61:** 73–7.

**Administration.** Some references to the pharmacokinetics of fentanyl following constant rate intravenous infusion,[1] transdermal application,[2] use of the oral transmucosal route,[3] intranasal administration,[4] subcutaneous infusion,[5] and epidural administration.[6,7]

1. Duthie DJR, *et al.* Pharmacokinetics of fentanyl during constant rate iv infusion for the relief of pain after surgery. *Br J Anaesth* 1986; **58:** 950–6.
2. Grond S, *et al.* Clinical pharmacokinetics of transdermal opioids: focus on transdermal fentanyl. *Clin Pharmacokinet* 2000; **38:** 59–89.
3. Streisand JB, *et al.* Absorption and bioavailability of oral transmucosal fentanyl citrate. *Anesthesiology* 1991; **75:** 223–9.
4. Walter SH, *et al.* Pharmacokinetics of intranasal fentanyl. *Br J Anaesth* 1993; **70** (suppl 1): 108.
5. Miller RS, *et al.* Plasma concentrations of fentanyl with subcutaneous infusion in palliative care patients. *Br J Clin Pharmacol* 1995; **40:** 553–6.
6. Gourlay GK, *et al.* Pharmacokinetics of fentanyl in lumbar and cervical CSF following lumbar epidural and intravenous administration. *Pain* 1989; **38:** 253–9.
7. Bader AM, *et al.* Maternal and neonatal fentanyl and bupivacaine concentrations after epidural infusion during labor. *Anesth Analg* 1995; **81:** 829–32.

**Cardiopulmonary bypass.** In general, studies[1,2] indicate that serum concentrations of fentanyl during cardiopulmonary bypass decrease initially and then remain stable. The fall in concentrations has been attributed to haemodilution although adsorption to the bypass apparatus has also been found.

1. Buylaert WA, *et al.* Cardiopulmonary bypass and the pharmacokinetics of drugs: an update. *Clin Pharmacokinet* 1989; **17:** 10–26.
2. Gedney JA, Ghosh S. Pharmacokinetics of analgesics, sedatives and anaesthetic agents during cardiopulmonary bypass. *Br J Anaesth* 1995; **75:** 344–51.

**Children.** The disposition of intravenous fentanyl 10 to 50 micrograms/kg in 14 neonates undergoing various major surgical procedures was highly variable.[1] The mean elimination half-life of 317 minutes and other pharmacokinetic parameters including volume of distribution and total body clearance were greater than reported in adults, but both pharmacodynamic and pharmacokinetic mechanisms appeared responsible for the very prolonged respiratory depression that can occur in neonates after fentanyl anaesthesia. In 9 premature neonates given fentanyl 30 micrograms/kg intravenously for induction of anaesthesia[2] the elimination half-life ranged from 6 to 32 hours, but cautious interpretation was advised because of the method of calculation.

1. Koehntop DE, *et al.* Pharmacokinetics of fentanyl in neonates. *Anesth Analg* 1986; **65:** 227–32.
2. Collins C, *et al.* Fentanyl pharmacokinetics and hemodynamic effects in preterm infants during ligation of patent ductus arteriosus. *Anesth Analg* 1985; **64:** 1078–80.

**The elderly.** In one study the elimination half-life of fentanyl increased from 265 minutes in patients with a mean age of 36 years to 945 minutes in those with a mean age of 67 years.[1] The authors of another study were critical of the relatively short sampling time used and in contrast found that major fentanyl pharmacokinetic parameters did not correlate with age.[2] However, elderly patients had increased brain sensitivity to fentanyl, as demonstrated by EEG changes[2] and lower doses might be indicated in older patients for pharmacodynamic rather than pharmacokinetic reasons.

1. Bentley JB, *et al.* Age and fentanyl pharmacokinetics. *Anesth Analg* 1982; **61:** 968–71.
2. Scott JC, Stanski DR. Decreased fentanyl and alfentanil dose requirements with age: a simultaneous pharmacokinetic and pharmacodynamic evaluation. *J Pharmacol Exp Ther* 1987; **240:** 159–66.

**Hepatic impairment.** The pharmacokinetics of fentanyl were not affected significantly in surgical patients with cirrhosis of the liver.[1] A 1987 review[2] considered that fentanyl had not been associated with clinical problems when given to patients with liver dysfunction.

1. Haberer JP, *et al.* Fentanyl pharmacokinetics in anaesthetized patients with cirrhosis. *Br J Anaesth* 1982; **54:** 1267–70.
2. Moore RA, *et al.* Opiate metabolism and excretion. *Baillieres Clin Anaesthesiol* 1987; **1:** 829–58.

**Renal impairment.** Clearance of fentanyl from plasma was reported to be enhanced in surgical patients with end-stage renal disease,[1] although clearance was reduced and elimination half-life increased in patients with renal failure undergoing transplantation,[2] possibly because of the influence of uraemia on metabolism in the liver. Nevertheless, a 1987 review[2] noted that fentanyl had no active or toxic metabolites and had not been associated with clinical problems when given to patients with renal dysfunction.

1. Corall IM, *et al.* Plasma concentrations of fentanyl in normal surgical patients and those with severe renal and hepatic disease. *Br J Anaesth* 1980; **52:** 101P.
2. Moore RA, *et al.* Opiate metabolism and excretion. *Baillieres Clin Anaesthesiol* 1987; **1:** 829–58.

## Uses and Administration

Fentanyl, a phenylpiperidine derivative, is a potent opioid analgesic (p.73) chemically related to pethidine (p.81) and is primarily a μ-opioid agonist.

Fentanyl is used as an analgesic, an adjunct to general anaesthetics, and as an anaesthetic for induction and maintenance. It is also used as a respiratory depressant in the management of mechanically ventilated patients under intensive care. When used with an antipsychotic such as droperidol it can induce a state of neuroleptanalgesia in which the patient is calm and indifferent to his surroundings and is able to cooperate with the surgeon.

Fentanyl is usually given by intramuscular or intravenous injection as the citrate or in transdermal patches as the base. It has also been given by epidural injection or by the transmucosal route as the citrate. Fentanyl citrate 157 micrograms is approximately equivalent to 100 micrograms of fentanyl. Doses are expressed in terms of the base.

It is more lipid soluble than morphine and following an intravenous injection of 100 micrograms the effects of fentanyl begin almost immediately, although maximum analgesia and respiratory depression may not occur for several minutes; the duration of action of fentanyl depends on the dose and the intensity of the pain involved, and may vary from 10 minutes to several hours.

For **premedication** the equivalent of 50 to 100 micrograms of fentanyl may be given *intramuscularly* 30 to 60 minutes before the induction of anaesthesia.

As an **adjunct** to general anaesthesia, fentanyl is usually given by *intravenous* injection. Dosage recommendations show a wide range depending on the technique.

- *Patients with spontaneous respiration* may be given 50 to 200 micrograms of fentanyl as an initial dose with supplements of 50 micrograms. In the USA it is recommended that doses above 2 micrograms/kg be accompanied by assisted ventilation. Significant respiratory depression follows doses of more than 200 micrograms
- *Patients whose ventilation is assisted* may be given 300 micrograms to 3.5 mg (up to 50 micrograms/kg) as an initial dose, with supplements of 100 to 200 micrograms or higher depending on the patient's response. High doses have been reported to moderate or attenuate the response to surgical stress (see under Anaesthesia, below)
- Reduced doses are used in *the elderly* or debilitated patients
- In the UK recommended initial doses for use as an adjunct to general anaesthesia for *children* above 2 years of age range from 3 to 5 micrograms/kg intravenously for those with *spontaneous respiration*; supplements of 1 microgram/kg may be given. When *ventilation is assisted*, the initial recommended dose is 15 micrograms/kg, with supplements of 1 to 3 micrograms/kg. In the USA doses as low as 2 to 3 micrograms/kg are employed in children between the ages of 2 and 12 years. See also under Administration in Children, below.

Similar doses to those used for premedication may also be given by *intramuscular* injection **postoperatively**, and by *intramuscular* or *slow intravenous injection* as an adjunct to **regional anaesthesia**.

For the treatment of intractable **chronic pain** in adults when opioid analgesia is indicated *transdermal* patches delivering amounts of fentanyl ranging from 25 to 100 micrograms/hour are available.

- Doses should be individually titrated for each patient according to previous opioid usage. Initial dosages should not exceed 25 micrograms/hour in *opioid-naive* patients
- For *patients who have been receiving a strong opioid analgesic* the initial dose of the fentanyl patch should be based on the previous 24-hour opioid requirement. Use of a patch providing 25 micrograms

of fentanyl per hour is approximately equivalent to oral administration of 90 mg of morphine sulfate daily. During transfer to treatment with fentanyl patches previous opioid analgesic therapy should be phased out gradually in order to allow for the gradual increase in plasma-fentanyl concentrations

- More than one patch may be applied if doses greater than 100 micrograms/hour are required (applied at the same time to avoid confusion); additional or alternative analgesic therapy should be considered if doses greater than 300 micrograms/hour are required. Patches should be replaced every 72 hours with the new patch being applied to a different site; use of the same area of the skin should be avoided for several days. Elderly or debilitated patients should be observed carefully for signs of toxicity and the dose reduced if necessary

Fentanyl patches are not appropriate for acute or postoperative pain.

A lozenge-on-a-stick lollipop dosage form of fentanyl citrate for *transmucosal* delivery is used as a premedicant and analgesic in anaesthesia and as an analgesic in the management of breakthrough cancer pain in those already receiving and tolerant to opioid treatment. Lozenges containing the equivalent of 100 micrograms to up to 1.6 mg of fentanyl base are available.

- In *anaesthesia*, adults may receive up to a maximum of 5 micrograms/kg (2.5 to 5 micrograms/kg in the elderly); children weighing more than 10 kg may receive up to 15 micrograms/kg. The maximum dose for adults and children, regardless of weight, is 400 micrograms. Patients receiving the lozenges in this setting require constant supervision, including monitoring of respiratory function
- In *cancer* patients, an initial unit dose of 200 micrograms may be taken over 15 minutes for an episode of breakthrough pain and repeated if necessary after a further 15 minutes. Doses are subsequently titrated according to response, up to a unit dose of 1.6 mg if necessary. Once the patient has been stabilised on an effective dose, no more than 4 doses should be taken daily.

◊ References.

1. Clotz MA, Nahata MC. Clinical uses of fentanyl, sufentanil, and alfentanil. *Clin Pharm* 1991; **10:** 581–93.

**Administration.** INHALATION ROUTE. A study[1] indicating that inhaled fentanyl can provide plasma concentrations similar to those after intravenous doses and that it can be used for patient-controlled analgesia.

1. Mather LE, *et al.* Pulmonary administration of aerosolised fentanyl: pharmacokinetic analysis of systemic delivery. *Br J Clin Pharmacol* 1998; **46:** 37–43.

INTRANASAL ROUTE. Studies[1-3] indicating that intranasal fentanyl is as effective as intravenous for postoperative pain management and that it can be used in a patient-controlled analgesia system.

1. Striebel HW, *et al.* Intranasal fentanyl titration for postoperative pain management in an unselected population. *Anaesthesia* 1993; **48:** 753–7.
2. Striebel HW, *et al.* Patient-controlled intranasal analgesia: a method for noninvasive postoperative pain management. *Anesth Analg* 1996; **83:** 548–51.
3. Toussaint S, *et al.* Patient-controlled intranasal analgesia: effective alternative to intravenous PCA for postoperative pain relief. *Can J Anaesth* 2000; **47:** 299–302.

TRANSDERMAL ROUTE. Transdermal fentanyl is used for chronic intractable cancer pain in adults.[1-3] Its use in children with cancer pain is not recommended by the manufacturers although a small study[4] has shown that transdermal fentanyl is well tolerated in this group; the authors have suggested that further trials are warranted.

Transdermal fentanyl is also used in the treatment of chronic non-cancer pain;[5] however the manufacturers state that its use is contra-indicated in the management of acute or postoperative pain because the problems of dose titration in the short term increase the possibility of development of significant respiratory depression (see also under Adverse Effects, above).

Although the licensed dosage interval for transdermal patches of fentanyl is 72 hours studies have suggested that up to about 25% of cancer patients may require more frequent application with some patients requiring fresh patches every 48 hours.[6,7] Equally, in an attempt to supply lower doses than are allowed for by existing transdermal dosage forms, they have sometimes been cut, folded, or partially masked with non-porous dressings; the manufacturers do not recommend such practices as they consider the dose supplied will be unreliable, and there is potential for overdosage.

1. Jeal W, Benfield P. Transdermal fentanyl: a review of its pharmacological properties and therapeutic efficacy in pain control. *Drugs* 1997; **53:** 109–38.
2. Muijsers RBR, Wagstaff AJ. Transdermal fentanyl: an updated review of its pharmacological properties and therapeutic efficacy in chronic cancer pain control. *Drugs* 2001; **61:** 2289–2307.
3. Gourlay GK. Treatment of cancer pain with transdermal fentanyl. *Lancet Oncol* 2001; **2:** 165–72.
4. Collins JJ, *et al.* Transdermal fentanyl in children with cancer pain: feasibility, tolerability, and pharmacokinetic correlates. *J Pediatr* 1999; **134:** 319–23.
5. Allan L, *et al.* Randomised crossover trial of transdermal fentanyl and sustained release oral morphine for treating chronic non-cancer pain. *BMJ* 2001; **322:** 1154–8.
6. Radbruch L, *et al.* Transdermal fentanyl for the management of cancer pain: a survey of 1005 patients. *Palliat Med* 2001; **15:** 309–21.
7. Donner B, *et al.* Long-term treatment of cancer pain with transdermal fentanyl. *J Pain Symptom Manage* 1998; **15:** 168–75.

TRANSMUCOSAL ROUTE. References to the use of transmucosal fentanyl for sedation and analgesia before anaesthesia or painful procedures,[1-3] and for breakthrough cancer pain in opioid-tolerant patients.[4-6] It has been noted[7] that this route of administration can cause all the adverse effects of parenteral opioids; nausea and vomiting are common and potentially lethal respiratory depression can occur.

1. Nelson PS, *et al.* Comparison of oral transmucosal fentanyl citrate and an oral solution of meperidine, diazepam, and atropine for premedication in children. *Anesthesiology* 1989; **70:** 616–21.
2. Schechter NL, *et al.* The use of oral transmucosal fentanyl citrate for painful procedures in children. *Pediatrics* 1995; **95:** 335–9.
3. Macaluso AD, *et al.* Oral transmucosal fentanyl citrate for premedication in adults. *Anesth Analg* 1996; **82:** 158–61.
4. Farrar JT, *et al.* Oral transmucosal fentanyl citrate: randomized, double-blinded, placebo-controlled trial for treatment of breakthrough pain in cancer patients. *J Natl Cancer Inst* 1998; **15:** 611–16.
5. Christie JM, *et al.* Dose-titration, multicenter study of oral transmucosal fentanyl citrate for the treatment of breakthrough pain in cancer patients using transdermal fentanyl for persistent pain. *J Clin Oncol* 1998; **16:** 3238–45.
6. Coluzzi PH, *et al.* Breakthrough cancer pain: a randomized trial comparing oral transmucosal fentanyl citrate (OTFC) and morphine sulfate immediate release (MSIR). *Pain* 2001; **91:** 123–30.
7. Anonymous. Oral transmucosal fentanyl citrate. *Med Lett Drugs Ther* 1994; **36:** 24–5.

**Administration in children.** Satisfactory *anaesthesia* has been reported[1] with high-dose fentanyl citrate (30 to 50 micrograms/kg) in premature infants when used as sole anaesthetic, in conjunction with pancuronium, for ligation of patent ductus arteriosus; cardiovascular stability was maintained throughout the procedure. However, others[2] found significant hypotension in preterm infants given either fentanyl 20 micrograms/kg, isoflurane, halothane, or ketamine; systolic arterial pressure was best maintained with the ketamine technique. The surgical stress response in preterm babies was abolished by the addition of fentanyl 10 micrograms/kg intravenously to an anaesthetic regimen of nitrous oxide and tubocurarine.[3] Dose responses of fentanyl in neonatal anaesthesia have been discussed.[4]

For sedation and analgesia during *intensive care* an infusion rate of 2 to 4 micrograms/kg per hour has been useful and associated with cardiovascular stability.[5] Although the use of fentanyl for prolonged sedation of infants and children during ventilatory support is reported to be widespread there is a lack of evidence of its safety and efficacy for this use.[6] In a double-blind placebo-controlled study[7] investigating the use of a continuous fentanyl infusion for 5 days in premature neonates receiving mechanical ventilation for respiratory distress syndrome, it was noted that although fentanyl was effective in reducing physiological indicators of pain and stress, there was an increased need for ventilatory support associated with the use of fentanyl compared with placebo. Fentanyl was infused initially in a dose of 5 micrograms/kg over 20 minutes, and thereafter in a decreasing dosage schedule over 120 hours from a rate of 2 micrograms/kg per hour to 0.5 micrograms/kg per hour. The authors pointed out that the results of this study could not assess the effects of fentanyl on long-term outcome and a larger multicentre study was required. There have also been reports of possible tolerance and withdrawal symptoms associated with prolonged administration of fentanyl (see under Dependence and Withdrawal, above).

See also under Transdermal Route and Transmucosal Route, above, and Postoperative Pain, below.

1. Robinson S, Gregory GA. Fentanyl-air-oxygen anesthesia for ligation of patent ductus arteriosus in preterm infants. *Anesth Analg* 1981; **60:** 331–4.
2. Friesen RH, Henry DB. Cardiovascular changes in preterm neonates receiving isoflurane, halothane, fentanyl, and ketamine. *Anesthesiology* 1986; **64:** 238–42.
3. Anand KJS, *et al.* Randomised trial of fentanyl anaesthesia in preterm babies undergoing surgery: effects on the stress response. *Lancet* 1987; **i:** 243–8.
4. Yaster M. The dose response of fentanyl in neonatal anesthesia. *Anesthesiology* 1987; **66:** 433–5.
5. Lloyd-Thomas AR. Pain management in paediatric patients. *Br J Anaesth* 1990; **64:** 85–104.
6. Kauffman RE. Fentanyl, fads, and folly: who will adopt the therapeutic orphans? *J Pediatr* 1991; **119:** 588–9.
7. Orsini AJ, *et al.* Routine use of fentanyl infusions for pain and stress reduction in infants with respiratory distress syndrome. *J Pediatr* 1996; **129:** 140–5.

**Anaesthesia.** Fentanyl and its congeners alfentanil and sufentanil are shorter-acting than morphine and appear to produce fewer circulatory changes; they are preferred for use as supplements during anaesthesia with inhalational or intravenous drugs. Fentanyl is widely used as the analgesic component of balanced anaesthesia. It has been used to attenuate cardiovascular stress responses to intubation (see under Anaesthesia, p.1397), and may be used in higher doses in an attempt to reduce the cardiovascular, endocrine, and metabolic changes that may accompany surgery. When attenuation of surgical stress is especially important, for example in cardiac surgery, intravenous fentanyl 50 to 100 micrograms/kg in conjunction with oxygen and a neuromuscular blocker, and sometimes up to 150 micrograms/kg, may be used for general anaesthesia. Total intravenous anaesthesia with fentanyl and propofol has been successful.[1]

For the use of fentanyl for anaesthesia in neonates and children, see under Administration in Children, above.

*Neuroleptanalgesia.* An injection of short-acting fentanyl 50 micrograms/mL with the longer-acting antipsychotic droperidol 2.5 mg/mL has been used for neuroleptanalgesia, premedication, and as an adjunct to anaesthesia. However, the use of such a fixed-ratio combination cannot be recommended.

1. Jenstrup M, *et al.* Total iv anaesthesia with propofol-alfentanil or propofol-fentanyl. *Br J Anaesth* 1990; **64:** 717–22.

PHAEOCHROMOCYTOMA. Unlike morphine and some other opioids, fentanyl and alfentanil do not release histamine and may be used safely in the anaesthetic management of patients with phaeochromocytoma.[1]

1. Hull CJ. Phaeochromocytoma: diagnosis, preoperative preparation and anaesthetic management. *Br J Anaesth* 1986; **58:** 1453–68.

POSTOPERATIVE SHIVERING. As pethidine appears to be effective in the treatment of postoperative shivering a number of other opioids including fentanyl have also been tried. Not all opioids are necessarily effective but fentanyl has been reported to be so,[1] although information is scanty.[2]

1. Alfonsi P, *et al.* Fentanyl, as pethidine, inhibits post anaesthesia shivering. *Br J Anaesth* 1993; **70** (suppl 1): 38.
2. Kranke P, *et al.* Pharmacological treatment of postoperative shivering: a quantitative systematic review of randomized controlled trials. *Anesth Analg* 2002; **94:** 453–60.

**Intensive care.** Despite the short duration of action of fentanyl after single doses, rapid redistribution in the body results in an elimination half-life longer than that of morphine. Consequently fentanyl is not a short-acting drug when used for analgesia in intensive care, and may offer little advantage over morphine.[1]

See also under Administration in Children, above.

1. Aitkenhead AR. Analgesia and sedation in intensive care. *Br J Anaesth* 1989; **63:** 196–206.

**Pain.** CANCER PAIN. Transdermal fentanyl is used in the management of chronic intractable cancer pain; for references see Administration, Transdermal Route, above. For references to the use of transmucosal fentanyl in the management of breakthrough cancer pain, see Administration, Transmucosal Route, above.

LABOUR PAIN. Fentanyl has been reported to be an effective intravenous analgesic during active labour. Epidural fentanyl is unreliable when used alone,[1] although it does enhance the epidural analgesia achieved with the local anaesthetic bupivacaine. The reduction in the minimum local analgesic concentration of epidural bupivacaine for labour pain increased with increasing dose of fentanyl added to bupivacaine.[2] However, the incidence of pruritus increased significantly with fentanyl in a dose of 4 micrograms/mL and therefore the optimum dose of fentanyl may be 3 micrograms/mL for bupivacaine-sparing epidural analgesia during labour. Respiratory depression has also been reported with the combination.[3]

1. Reynolds F. Extradural opioids in labour. *Br J Anaesth* 1989; **63:** 251–3.
2. Lyons G, *et al.* Extradural pain relief in labour: bupivacaine sparing by extradural fentanyl is dose dependent. *Br J Anaesth* 1997; **78:** 493–7.
3. McClure JH, Jones G. Comparison of bupivacaine and bupivacaine with fentanyl in continuous extradural analgesia during labour. *Br J Anaesth* 1989; **63:** 637–40.

POSTOPERATIVE PAIN. Small intravenous bolus doses of opioid analgesic may be injected immediately after surgery for postoperative analgesia and faster acting opioids such as fentanyl may be preferable to morphine.[1] Fentanyl has also been given by epidural injection in doses of 100 or 200 micrograms or by continuous epidural infusion in doses of 20 to 80 micrograms/hour; patient-controlled systems have been used.[2]

Epidural fentanyl or sufentanil provided effective postoperative analgesia following caesarean section with comparable adverse effect profiles.[3] The suggested optimal dose of fentanyl was 100 micrograms. For references comparing epidural fentanyl with alfentanil, see Postoperative Analgesia in Uses and Administration of Alfentanil, p.14. In a review[4] of perioperative pain management epidural opioids were considered to provide effective analgesia at lower doses than systemic opioids. Fentanyl may be given through a lumbar epidural catheter that is often inserted immediately postoperatively. After an initial loading dose of 1 to 1.5 micrograms/kg of fentanyl, infusion at the rate of 0.7 to 2 micrograms/kg per hour is begun and continued for about 48 hours on average. Some prefer to use intermittent injection.

Combined opioid and local anaesthetic epidural infusions have also proved effective, for example fentanyl 1 microgram/mL with bupivacaine 0.1%; both could be infused at lower rates than either drug alone. Although a study[5] comparing bupivacaine-fentanyl combinations with each drug alone for epidural analgesia following caesarean section confirmed an additive analgesic effect for the combination, there was no demonstrable clinical benefit compared with fentanyl alone in this patient group who expect early mobilisation. However, the combination may be of greater benefit in patients for whom early ambulation is not routine.

Fentanyl has also been given by epidural injection to children for postoperative analgesia.[6]

Fentanyl has been tried by intrathecal injection for postoperative pain.[7]


1. Mitchell RWD, Smith G. The control of acute postoperative pain. *Br J Anaesth* 1989; **63:** 147–58.
2. Morgan M. The rational use of intrathecal and extradural opioids. *Br J Anaesth* 1989; **63:** 165–88.
3. Grass JA, *et al.* A randomized, double-blind, dose-response comparison of epidural fentanyl versus sufentanil analgesia after cesarean section. *Anesth Analg* 1997; **85:** 365–71.
4. Swarm RA, *et al.* Pain treatment in the perioperative period. *Curr Probl Surg* 2001; **38:** 835–920.
5. Cooper DW, *et al.* Patient-controlled extradural analgesia with bupivacaine, fentanyl, or a mixture of both, after caesarean section. *Br J Anaesth* 1996; **76:** 611–15.
6. Lejus C, *et al.* Postoperative extradural analgesia in children: comparison of morphine with fentanyl. *Br J Anaesth* 1994; **72:** 156–9.
7. Sudarshan G, *et al.* Intrathecal fentanyl for post-thoracotomy pain. *Br J Anaesth* 1995; **75:** 19–22.


### Preparations

***BP 2003:*** Fentanyl Injection;
***USP 27:*** Fentanyl Citrate Injection.

**Proprietary Preparations** (details are given in Part 3)
***Arg.:*** Durogesic; Fentax; Nafluvent; Sublimaze; ***Austral.:*** Actiq; Durogesic; Sublimaze; ***Austria:*** Durogesic; ***Belg.:*** Durogesic; ***Braz.:*** Durogesic; Fentabbott; Fentanest; ***Canad.:*** Duragesic; Sublimaze†; ***Chile:*** Durogesic; ***Denm.:*** Durogesic; Haldid; ***Fin.:*** Durogesic; ***Fr.:*** Actiq; Durogesic; ***Ger.:*** Actiq; Durogesic; Fenta-Hameln; ***Gr.:*** Durogesic; ***Hong Kong:*** Durogesic; ***India:*** Durogesic; Trofentyl; ***Irl.:*** Durogesic; Sublimaze; ***Israel:*** Durogesic; Tanyl; ***Ital.:*** Durogesic; Fentanest; ***Malaysia:*** Durogesic; ***Mex.:*** Durogesic; Fenodid; Fentanest; ***Neth.:*** Durogesic; ***Norw.:*** Durogesic; Leptanal; ***NZ:*** Durogesic; Sublimaze; ***Port.:*** Durogesic; ***S.Afr.:*** Durogesic; Sublimaze; Tanyl†; ***Singapore:*** Durogesic; ***Spain:*** Actiq; Durogesic; Fentanest; ***Swed.:*** Actiq; Durogesic; Leptanal; ***Switz.:*** Durogesic; Sintenyl; ***Thai.:*** Durogesic; ***UK:*** Actiq; Durogesic; Sublimaze; ***USA:*** Actiq; Duragesic; Sublimaze.

**Multi-ingredient:** ***Arg.:*** Disifelit; ***Austral.:*** Marcain with Fentanyl; Naropin with Fentanyl; ***Austria:*** Thalamonal†; ***Belg.:*** Thalamonal†; ***Braz.:*** Inoval†; Nilperidol; ***Ger.:*** Thalamonal†; ***Ital.:*** Leptofen; ***Neth.:*** Thalamonal†; ***NZ:*** Bupafen; Marcain with Fentanyl; Naropin with Fentanyl; ***USA:*** Innovar†.

## Fentiazac *(BAN, USAN, rINN)*

BR-700; Fentiazaco; Wy-21894. [4-(4-Chlorophenyl)-2-phenylthiazol-5-yl]acetic acid.

$C_{17}H_{12}ClNO_2S$ = 329.8.
*CAS — 18046-21-4.*
*ATC — M01AB10; M02AA14.*

### Profile

Fentiazac is an NSAID (p.67) that has been used for the relief of pain and inflammation associated with musculoskeletal, joint, peri-articular, and soft-tissue disorders. It has also been used in the treatment of fever. Fentiazac has been given in usual doses of 100 to 200 mg once or twice daily by mouth. Fentiazac has also been applied topically and has been given rectally as the calcium salt.

### Preparations

**Proprietary Preparations** (details are given in Part 3)
***Austria:*** Norvedan†; ***Braz.:*** Atilan†; ***Ital.:*** Flogene†; O-Flam; ***Port.:*** Donorest; IDR; Norvedan; ***Spain:*** Donorest†; Riscalon†.

## Fepradinol *(rINN)*

(±)-α-{[(2-Hydroxy-1,1-dimethylethyl)amino]methyl}benzyl alcohol.

$C_{12}H_{19}NO_2$ = 209.3.
*CAS — 63075-47-8.*

### Profile

Fepradinol is an NSAID (p.67) that has been used topically in a concentration of 6% for the relief of pain and inflammation. The hydrochloride has been used similarly.

### Preparations

**Proprietary Preparations** (details are given in Part 3)
***Chile:*** Sinalgia; ***Spain:*** Dalgen; Flexidol.

## Feprazone *(BAN, rINN)*

DA-2370; Feprazona; Phenylprenazone; Prenazone. 4-(3-Methylbut-2-enyl)-1,2-diphenylpyrazolidine-3,5-dione.

$C_{20}H_{20}N_2O_2$ = 320.4.
*CAS — 30748-29-9 (feprazone); 57148-60-4 (feprazone piperazine salt 1:1).*
*ATC — M01AX18; M02AA16.*

### Profile

Feprazone, a phenylbutazone (p.83) derivative, is an NSAID (p.67). It has been given by mouth in the treatment of mild to moderate pain, fever, and inflammation associated with musculoskeletal and joint disorders. Feprazone has also been given rectally and used topically as a 5% cream.

Pinazone, the piperazine salt of feprazone, has been used similarly.

### Preparations

**Proprietary Preparations** (details are given in Part 3)
***Austria:*** Zepelin†; ***Braz.:*** Metrazone†; Zepelan†; ***Ital.:*** Zepelin; ***Spain:*** Brotazona; Reuflodol†.

## Floctafenine *(BAN, USAN, rINN)*

Floctafenina; R-4318; RU-15750. 2,3-Dihydroxypropyl N-(8-trifluoromethyl-4-quinolyl)anthranilate.

$C_{20}H_{17}F_3N_2O_4$ = 406.4.
*CAS — 23779-99-9.*
*ATC — N02BG04.*

### Adverse Effects and Precautions

As for NSAIDs in general, p.67. Anaphylactic shock has been reported in patients given floctafenine; anaphylactic reactions may be preceded by minor allergic manifestations, therefore floctafenine should be discontinued in any patient who develops signs suggestive of allergy (such as pruritus or urticaria). Reactions may also involve the liver. Floctafenine may cross-react with glafenine (p.44) and should not be given to patients who have experienced glafenine-associated reactions.

**Porphyria.** Floctafenine is considered to be unsafe in patients with porphyria because it has been shown to be porphyrinogenic in *in-vitro* systems.

### Interactions

For interactions associated with NSAIDs, see p.69.

### Pharmacokinetics

Floctafenine is absorbed from the gastrointestinal tract; peak plasma concentrations are obtained 1 to 2 hours after ingestion. Its plasma half-life is about 8 hours. It is metabolised in the liver to floctafenic acid. It is excreted mainly as glucuronide conjugates in the urine and bile.

### Uses and Administration

Floctafenine, an anthranilic acid derivative related to glafenine (p.44), is an NSAID (p.70) used in doses of up to 1.2 g daily, in divided doses, by mouth for the short-term relief of pain.

### Preparations

**Proprietary Preparations** (details are given in Part 3)
***Braz.:*** Idarac†; ***Canad.:*** Idarac; ***Fr.:*** Idarac; ***Irl.:*** Idarac; ***Ital.:*** Idarac†; ***Neth.:*** Idalon†; ***Spain:*** Idarac†; ***Thai.:*** Idarac.

## Flufenamic Acid *(BAN, USAN, rINN)*

Ácido flufenámico; CI-440; CN-27554; INF-1837; NSC-82699. N-(ααα-Trifluoro-m-tolyl)anthranilic acid.

$C_{14}H_{10}F_3NO_2$ = 281.2.
*CAS — 530-78-9.*
*ATC — M01AG03.*

### Adverse Effects and Precautions

As for NSAIDs in general, p.67.

**Breast feeding.** No adverse effects have been observed in breast-feeding infants whose mothers were receiving flufenamic acid, and the American Academy of Pediatrics considers[1] that it is therefore usually compatible with breast feeding.

An early study[2] found that only very small amounts of flufenamic acid were excreted into breast milk after oral doses.

1. American Academy of Pediatrics. The transfer of drugs and other chemicals into human milk. *Pediatrics* 2001; **108:** 776–89. Correction. *ibid.*; 1029. Also available at: http://aappolicy.aappublications.org/cgi/content/full/pediatrics%3b108/3/776 (accessed 05/07/04)
2. Buchanan RA, *et al.* The breast milk excretion of flufenamic acid. *Curr Ther Res* 1969; **11:** 533–8.

**Effects on the gastrointestinal tract.** Acute proctocolitis associated with oral flufenamic acid in a patient.[1]

1. Ravi S, *et al.* Colitis caused by non-steroidal anti-inflammatory drugs. *Postgrad Med J* 1986; **62:** 773–6.

**Porphyria.** Flufenamic acid has been associated with acute attacks of porphyria and is considered unsafe in porphyric patients.

### Uses and Administration

Flufenamic acid, an anthranilic acid derivative related to mefenamic acid (p.56), is an NSAID (p.70). Flufenamic acid is mainly used in topical preparations in a concentration of 3 or 3.5% for the relief of pain and inflammation associated with musculoskeletal, joint, and soft-tissue disorders. It has also been given by mouth.

### Preparations

**Proprietary Preparations** (details are given in Part 3)
***Ger.:*** Dignodolin; Rheuma Lindofluid†.

**Multi-ingredient:** ***Austria:*** Mobilisin; Mobilisin plus; Rheugesal; ***Belg.:*** Mobilisin; ***Braz.:*** Mobilisin Composto; ***Ger.:*** Algesalona; Flexocutan N†; Mobilisin†; Thermo Mobilisin†; ***Hong Kong:*** Movilisin†; ***Ital.:*** Mobilisin; ***Port.:*** Latesil; Mobilisin; ***Spain:*** Movilisin; ***Switz.:*** Algesalona; Assan; Assan-Thermo; Mobilisin.

## Flunixin Meglumine *(BANM, USAN, rINNM)*

Flunixino meglumina; Sch-14714 (flunixin). 2-{[2-Methyl-3-(trifluoromethyl)phenyl]amino}-3-pyridinecarboxylic acid compounded with 1-deoxy-1-(methylamino)-D-glucitol (1:1); 2-($\alpha^3$,$\alpha^3$,$\alpha^3$-Trifluoro-2,3,-xylidino)nicotinic acid compounded with 1-deoxy-1-(methylamino)-D-glucitol (1:1).

$C_{14}H_{11}F_3N_2O_2,C_7H_{17}NO_5$ = 491.5.
*CAS — 38677-85-9 (flunixin); 42461-84-7 (flunixin meglumine).*

**Pharmacopoeias.** In *BP(Vet).* Also in *US* for veterinary use only.

**BP(Vet) 2003** (Flunixin Meglumine). A white to almost white powder. Freely soluble in water, in alcohol, and in methyl alcohol; practically insoluble in ethyl acetate. A 5% solution in water has a pH of 7.0 to 8.5. Store in airtight containers at a temperature not exceeding 25°.

**USP 27** (Flunixin Meglumine). A white to off-white crystalline powder. Soluble in water, in alcohol, and in methyl alcohol; practically insoluble in ethyl acetate. pH of a 5% solution in water is between 7.0 and 9.0. Store at a temperature of 25°, excursions permitted between 15° and 30°.

### Profile

Flunixin meglumine is an NSAID (p.67) used in veterinary medicine for relief of pain and inflammation in acute and chronic disorders and as adjunctive therapy in the treatment of endotoxic or septic shock and mastitis.

## Flunoxaprofen *(rINN)*

Flunoxaprofeno; RV-12424. (+)-2-(p-Fluorophenyl)-α-methyl-5-benzoxazoleacetic acid.

$C_{16}H_{12}FNO_3$ = 285.3.
*CAS — 66934-18-7.*
*ATC — G02CC04; M01AE15.*

### Profile

Flunoxaprofen, a propionic acid derivative, is an NSAID (p.67) that has been given for the relief of painful and inflammatory conditions.

### Preparations

**Proprietary Preparations** (details are given in Part 3)
***Ital.:*** Priaxim†.

## Flupirtine Maleate *(BANM, USAN, rINNM)*

D-9998; Maleato de flupirtina; W-2964M. Ethyl 2-amino-6-(4-fluorobenzylamino)-3-pyridylcarbamate maleate.

$C_{15}H_{17}FN_4O_2,C_4H_4O_4$ = 420.4.
*CAS — 56995-20-1 (flupirtine); 75507-68-5 (flupirtine maleate).*
*ATC — N02BG07.*

### Profile

Flupirtine maleate is an analgesic that has been given for the relief of pain (see Choice of Analgesic, p.2) in usual doses of 100 mg three or four times daily by mouth, or 150 mg three or four times daily as a rectal suppository; daily doses of up to 600 mg by mouth or 900 mg rectally have been used where necessary. Flupirtine has also been given by injection as the gluconate in the management of pain.

There has been some interest in the potential of flupirtine to treat prion diseases such as Creutzfeldt-Jakob disease.

◊ References.

1. Friedel HA, Fitton A. Flupirtine: a review of its pharmacological properties, and therapeutic efficacy in pain states. *Drugs* 1993; **45:** 548–69.

### Preparations

**Proprietary Preparations** (details are given in Part 3)
***Braz.:*** Katadolon; ***Ger.:*** Katadolon; Trancopal Dolo; ***Port.:*** Metanor.

## Flurbiprofen *(BAN, USAN, rINN)*

BTS-18322; Flurbiprofeno; Flurbiprofenum; U-27182. 2-(2-Fluorobiphenyl-4-yl)propionic acid.

$C_{15}H_{13}FO_2$ = 244.3.
*CAS — 5104-49-4.*
*ATC — M01AE09; M02AA19; S01BC04.*

**Pharmacopoeias.** In *Eur.* (see p.vi), *Jpn,* and *US.*

**Ph. Eur. 5.0** (Flurbiprofen). A white or almost white crystalline powder. Practically insoluble in water; freely soluble in alcohol and in dichloromethane; dissolves in aqueous solutions of alkali hydroxides and carbonates.

**USP 27** (Flurbiprofen). A white crystalline powder. Practically insoluble in water; freely soluble in dehydrated alcohol, in acetone, in ether, and in methyl alcohol; soluble in acetonitrile. Store in airtight containers.

### Flurbiprofen Sodium (BANM, rINNM)

Flurbiprofeno sódico. Sodium (±)-2-(2-fluoro-4-biphenylyl)propionate dihydrate.

$C_{15}H_{12}FNaO_2,2H_2O$ = 302.3.
CAS — 56767-76-1.

**Pharmacopoeias.** In *Br.* and *US.*

**BP 2003** (Flurbiprofen Sodium). A white to creamy-white, crystalline powder. Sparingly soluble in water; soluble in alcohol; practically insoluble in dichloromethane.

## Adverse Effects

As for NSAIDs in general, p.67.

Minor symptoms of ocular irritation including transient burning and stinging have been reported following the instillation of flurbiprofen sodium eye drops; there may be increased bleeding from ocular surgery and wound healing may be delayed. Local irritation may also follow rectal use, and local effects including a sensation of warming or burning in the mouth may be seen after using flurbiprofen lozenges.

◊ Reports from the manufacturers on the range and incidence of the side-effects of flurbiprofen.[1,2]

1. Sheldrake FE, *et al.* A long-term assessment of flurbiprofen. *Curr Med Res Opin* 1977; **5:** 106–16.
2. Brooks CD, *et al.* Clinical safety of flurbiprofen. *J Clin Pharmacol* 1990; **30:** 342–51.

**Effects on the CNS.** A severe symmetrical parkinsonian syndrome developed in a 52-year-old man who had taken flurbiprofen for 7 days.[1]

1. Enevoldson TP, *et al.* Acute parkinsonism associated with flurbiprofen. *BMJ* 1990; **300:** 540–1.

**Effects on the kidneys.** Renal papillary necrosis has been described in a patient who had used flurbiprofen for many years.[1] Acute flank pain and reversible renal dysfunction, similar to that seen with suprofen (see p.93) has been reported in 2 patients treated with flurbiprofen.[2,3]

1. Nafría EC, *et al.* Renal papillary necrosis induced by flurbiprofen. *DICP Ann Pharmacother* 1991; **25:** 870–1.
2. Kaufhold J, *et al.* Flurbiprofen-associated tubulointerstitial nephritis. *Am J Nephrol* 1991; **11:** 144–6.
3. McIntire SC, *et al.* Acute flank pain and reversible renal dysfunction associated with nonsteroidal anti-inflammatory drug use. *Pediatrics* 1993; **92:** 459–60.

**Effects on the liver.** A case of cholestatic jaundice probably due to flurbiprofen has been reported.[1]

1. Kotowski KE, Grayson MF. Side effects of non-steroidal anti-inflammatory drugs. *BMJ* 1982; **285:** 377.

**Effects on the skin.** Cutaneous vasculitis apparently due to flurbiprofen occurred in a 59-year-old woman with long-standing rheumatoid arthritis.[1]

1. Wei N. Flurbiprofen and cutaneous vasculitis. *Ann Intern Med* 1990; **112:** 550–1.

## Precautions

As for NSAIDs in general, p.69.

**Breast feeding.** Flurbiprofen is distributed into breast milk; however, the *British National Formulary* and some manufacturers consider the amount to be too small to be harmful to a breast-fed infant.

**Herpes simplex keratitis.** Whether flurbiprofen can exacerbate infection when used to treat ocular herpes simplex is unclear from *animal* studies,[1,2] but the manufacturer of flurbiprofen sodium eye drops recommends that they should not be used in patients with active epithelial herpes simplex keratitis. Patients with a history of herpes simplex keratitis should also be monitored closely when undergoing treatment with these eye drops.

1. Trousdale MD, *et al.* Effect of flurbiprofen on herpes simplex keratitis in rabbits. *Invest Ophthalmol Vis Sci* 1980; **19:** 267–70.
2. Hendricks RL, *et al.* The effect of flurbiprofen on herpes simplex virus type 1 stromal keratitis in mice. *Invest Ophthalmol Vis Sci* 1990; **31:** 1503–11.

## Interactions

For interactions associated with NSAIDs, see p.69.

**Parasympathomimetics.** The manufacturers of acetylcholine chloride ophthalmic preparations and of flurbiprofen sodium eye drops have both stated that there have been reports that *acetylcholine* and *carbachol* have been ineffective when used in patients treated with topical (ophthalmic) NSAIDs.

## Pharmacokinetics

Flurbiprofen is readily absorbed from the gastrointestinal tract after oral doses with peak plasma concentrations occurring about 1 to 2 hours after ingestion. Absorption after rectal doses may be more rapid. It is about 99% bound to plasma proteins and has a plasma half-life of about 3 to 6 hours. It is metabolised mainly by hydroxylation (via the cytochrome P450 isoenzyme CYP2C9) and conjugation in the liver and excreted in urine. Flurbiprofen is distributed into breast milk.

Flurbiprofen is a chiral compound given as the racemate and the above pharmacokinetic characteristics refer to the racemic mixture. Allowance may have to be made for the different activities of the enantiomers.

◊ References.

1. Aarons L, *et al.* Plasma and synovial fluid kinetics of flurbiprofen in rheumatoid arthritis. *Br J Clin Pharmacol* 1986; **21:** 155–63.
2. Smith IJ, *et al.* Flurbiprofen in post-partum women: plasma and breast milk disposition. *J Clin Pharmacol* 1989; **29:** 174–84.
3. Kean WF, *et al.* The pharmacokinetics of flurbiprofen in younger and elderly patients with rheumatoid arthritis. *J Clin Pharmacol* 1992; **32:** 41–8.
4. Davies NM. Clinical pharmacokinetics of flurbiprofen and its enantiomers. *Clin Pharmacokinet* 1995; **28:** 100–14.

## Uses and Administration

Flurbiprofen, a propionic acid derivative, is an NSAID (p.70). It is used in musculoskeletal and joint disorders such as ankylosing spondylitis, osteoarthritis, and rheumatoid arthritis, in soft-tissue disorders such as sprains and strains, for postoperative pain, and in mild to moderate pain including dysmenorrhoea and migraine. Flurbiprofen is also used as lozenges in the symptomatic relief of sore throat. Flurbiprofen sodium is used in eye drops to inhibit intra-operative miosis and to control postoperative inflammation of the anterior segment of the eye.

For **pain and inflammation**, flurbiprofen is given in usual doses of 150 to 200 mg daily by mouth in divided doses, increased to 300 mg daily in acute or severe conditions if necessary. A modified-release preparation for once daily use is also available. Patients with dysmenorrhoea may be given an initial dose of 100 mg followed by 50 to 100 mg every four to six hours to a maximum total daily dose of 300 mg. Doses given rectally as suppositories are similar to those given by mouth.

For the relief of **sore throat**, a lozenge containing 8.75 mg of flurbiprofen may be sucked or allowed to dissolve slowly in the mouth every 3 to 6 hours to a maximum daily dose of 5 lozenges. It is recommended that treatment should be limited to a maximum of 3 days.

To inhibit intra-operative miosis during **ocular surgery** one drop of flurbiprofen sodium 0.03% is instilled into the eye every 30 minutes beginning 2 hours before surgery and ending not less than 30 minutes before surgery. To control postoperative inflammation the same dosage regimen is used before ocular surgery followed 24 hours after surgery by the instillation of one drop 4 times daily for 1 to 3 weeks. Flurbiprofen sodium eye drops have also been used in the topical treatment of cystoid macular oedema.

Flurbiprofen axetil has been given in some countries by intravenous injection for severe pain.

## Preparations

***BP 2003:*** Flurbiprofen Eye Drops; Flurbiprofen Suppositories; Flurbiprofen Tablets;
***USP 27:*** Flurbiprofen Sodium Ophthalmic Solution; Flurbiprofen Tablets.

**Proprietary Preparations** (details are given in Part 3)
***Arg.:*** Clinadol; Flurbid; Luarprofeno; Tolerane; ***Austral.:*** Ocufen; Strepfen; ***Austria:*** Froben; Ocuflur; ***Belg.:*** Froben; Ocuflur; ***Braz.:*** Evril†; Ocufen; Targus; ***Canad.:*** Ansaid; Froben; Novo-Flurprofen; Ocufen; ***Chile:*** Ansaid; Distex; Ocufen; ***Denm.:*** Flurofen; Ocufen†; ***Fr.:*** Cebutid; Ocufen; ***Ger.:*** Froben†; Ocuflur; ***Gr.:*** Bonatol-R; Flurofen; Fluroptic; Ocuflur; ***Hong Kong:*** Froben†; Ocufen; ***India:*** Arflur; Froben; Ocuflur; ***Irl.:*** Fenomel†; Froben; Ocufen; ***Ital.:*** Benactiv; Froben; Ocufen; Transact Lat; ***Jpn:*** Ropion; ***Mex.:*** Ansaid; Froben†; Ocufen; ***Mon.:*** Antadys; ***Neth.:*** Froben; ***NZ:*** Froben†; Ocufen; Strepfen; ***Port.:*** Edolfene; Froben; Ocuflur; Reupax; Strepfen; Transact Lat; ***S.Afr.:*** Froben; Ocufen; Transact; ***Singapore:*** Acustop Cataplasma; Froben†; Ocufen; ***Spain:*** Froben; Neo Artrol; Ocuflur; Tulip†; ***Switz.:*** Froben; Ocuflur; ***Thai.:*** Flurozin; Ocufen†; ***UK:*** Froben; Ocufen; Strefen; Streflam†; ***USA:*** Ansaid; Ocufen.

### Fosfosal (rINN)

UR-1521. 2-Phosphono-oxybenzoic acid.

$C_7H_7O_6P$ = 218.1.
CAS — 6064-83-1.

**Profile**

Fosfosal is a salicylic acid derivative (see Aspirin, p.15). It has been given in usual doses of up to 3.6 g daily by mouth for the treatment of pain.

## Preparations

**Proprietary Preparations** (details are given in Part 3)
***Spain:*** Aydolid; Disdolen; Protalgia†.
**Multi-ingredient:** ***Spain:*** Aydolid Codeina; Disdolen Codeina.

### Furprofen

Furprofeno. 4-(2-Furanylcarbonyl)-α-methylbenzeneacetic acid.

$C_{14}H_{12}O_4$ = 244.2.
CAS — 66318-17-0.

**Profile**

Furprofen, a propionic acid derivative, is an NSAID (p.67) that has been given by mouth in doses of 200 to 400 mg daily for the relief of pain.

## Preparations

**Proprietary Preparations** (details are given in Part 3)
***Ital.:*** Dolex.

### Glafenine (rINN)

Glafenina; Glaphenine. 2,3-Dihydroxypropyl *N*-(7-chloro-4-quinolyl)anthranilate.

$C_{19}H_{17}ClN_2O_4$ = 372.8.
CAS — 3820-67-5.
ATC — N02BG03.

**Profile**

Glafenine, an anthranilic acid derivative, is an NSAID (p.67) that was used for the relief of all types of pain. However, its high incidence of anaphylactic reactions has led to its withdrawal from the market in most countries. Glafenine hydrochloride was also used.

**Adverse effects and precautions.** Glafenine is a common cause of anaphylaxis. There may be hepatotoxicity (which may be fatal), nephrotoxicity, and gastrointestinal disturbances. It should be discontinued at the first sign of any allergic reaction. Crystallisation of glafenine in the urinary tract has also occurred. Cross-reactivity with floctafenine has been reported.

### Glucametacin (rINN)

Glucametacina. 2-{2-[1-(4-Chlorobenzoyl)-5-methoxy-2-methylindol-3-yl]acetamido}-2-deoxy-D-glucose.

$C_{25}H_{27}ClN_2O_8$ = 518.9.
CAS — 52443-21-7.

**Profile**

Glucametacin, a derivative of indometacin (p.47), is an NSAID (p.67) that has been given by mouth in musculoskeletal, joint, peri-articular, and soft-tissue disorders.

## Preparations

**Proprietary Preparations** (details are given in Part 3)
***Braz.:*** Teoremin; ***Mex.:*** Teoremac.
**Multi-ingredient:** ***Chile:*** Fibrorelax.

### Glycol Salicylate

Ethylene Glycol Monosalicylate; Hydroxyethylis Salicylas; Salicilato de glicol. 2-Hydroxyethyl salicylate.

$C_9H_{10}O_4$ = 182.2.
CAS — 87-28-5.

**Pharmacopoeias.** In *Eur.* (see p.vi).

**Ph. Eur. 5.0** (Hydroxyethyl Salicylate). An oily, colourless or almost colourless liquid or colourless crystals. M.p. about 21°. Sparingly soluble in water; freely soluble in alcohol; very soluble in acetone and in dichloromethane. Protect from light.

**Profile**

Glycol salicylate is a salicylic acid derivative used similarly to methyl salicylate (p.59) in topical rubefacient preparations in usual concentrations of 5 to 15% for the relief of muscular and rheumatic pain. Dipropylene glycol salicylate has been used in similar preparations.

## Preparations

**Proprietary Preparations** (details are given in Part 3)
***Ger.:*** Auroanalin N; Dolo-Arthrosenex N; Dolo-Rubriment H; Kytta; Lumbinon; Mobilat Akut HES; Phardol mono; Phlogont; Phlogont Rheuma; Rheubalmin N; Salhumin Gel; Traumasenex; zuk Schmerzgel, zuk Schmerzsalbe.

**Multi-ingredient:** ***Arg.:*** Infrarub; Venostasin; ***Austral.:*** Deep Heat; Goanna Analgesic Ice; ***Austria:*** Ambenat; Bayolin; Dolex†; Etrat; Igitur-Rheumafluid; Menthoneurin; Mobilisin; Moviflex; Rheumex; Rubizon-Rheumagel; Rubriment; Sportino Akut; Venosin; ***Belg.:*** Algipan; Mobilisin; Percutalgine; Rado-Salil; Rado-Spray; Stilene; ***Braz.:*** Emplastro Salonpas†; Etrat; Infrarub†; Mobilisin Composto; Salonpas†; Venostasin Composto†; ***Canad.:*** Midalgan; ***Fin.:*** Moviflex; ***Fr.:*** Algipan; Cortisal; Lao-Dal†; Le Thermogene; Lumbalgine; Percutalgine; ***Ger.:*** Ambene N; Arthrodestal N; Brachont†; Caye Balsam; Contrheuma V + T Bad N†; Contrheuma†; Dolo Mobilat; Dolo-Menthoneurin CreSa†; Doloneuro; Dolorgiet†; DoloVisano Salbe; Essaven Sport; Etrat Sportgel; exrheudon OPT†; Fibraflex†; Flexocutan N†; Heparin Plus; Hot Thermo; Infrotto Ultra; Li-iL Rheuma-Bad†; Menthoneurin-Salbe; Menthoneurin-Vollbad N†; Midysalb†; mikanil; Mobilisin†; Myalgol N†; Ortholan mit Salicylester†; Ostochont; Percutase N†; Phardol Rheuma; Phlogont-Thermal; Rheubalmin Thermo; Rheuma V + T Bad N†; Rheuma-Bad†; Rheuma-Liquidum†; Rheuma-Salbe; Rheuma-Salbe N; Rheumichthol Bad†; Rubriment-N; Salhumin Gel N†; Sportino Akut; Thermo-Menthoneurin; Thermo-Menthoneurin Bad†; Thermosenex; Togal Mobil-Gel; Trauma-Puren; Venoplant AHS; Venostasin; Vertebralon N; Warme-Gel; zuk thermo; **Hong Kong:** Movilisin†; New Patecs A; Prelloran; Salomethyl; **India:** Algipan; **Irl.:** Algipan; **Israel:** Deep Heat Spray; **Ital.:** Balsamo Sifcamina; Disalgil; Lasoreumat†; Mobilisin; Salonpas; Sloan; **Malaysia:** Salonpas; **Neth.:** Menthoneurin†; Sloan's balsem; **Port.:** DM Creme; DM Gel; DM Termo†; Etrat†; Midalgan; **Singapore:** Deep Heating Spray; Saak; **Spain:** Movilisin; Percutalin†; **Switz.:** Artragel†; Assan; Assan-Thermo; Demotherm Pommade contre le rhumatisme; Dolo Demotherm; Dolo-Arthrosenex; Dolo-Arthrosenex sine Heparino; Dolo-Veniten; Dolorex Neo†; Dolorex†; Histalgane; Histalgane mite; Incutin†; Midalgan; Mobilisin; Phlebostasin compositum; Prelloran; Radalgin; Remexal; Roliwol B†; Roliwol S†; Sportusal; Sportusal Spray sine heparino; Venoplant comp; Venucreme; Venugel; **Thai.:** Percutalgine; **UK:** Algipan†; Cremalgin; Deep Heat Spray; Dubam; Fiery Jack; Ralgex; Ralgex Freeze Spray; Ralgex Heat Spray (low-odour); Salonair; Salonpas; Transvasin Heat Spray.

## Gold Keratinate

Aurothiopolypeptide.

*CAS — 9078-78-8.*

### Profile

Gold keratinate is a gold compound with a gold content of about 13%; It has similar actions and uses to those of sodium aurothiomalate (p.88). It is given by intramuscular injection as the calcium salt for the treatment of rheumatoid arthritis.

### Preparations

**Proprietary Preparations** (details are given in Part 3)
**Arg.:** Aurochobet.

## Hexyl Nicotinate

Nicotinato de hexilo. *n*-Hexyl nicotinate.

$C_{12}H_{17}NO_2$ = 207.3.

*CAS — 23597-82-2.*

### Profile

Hexyl nicotinate is used in topical preparations as a rubefacient.

### Preparations

**Proprietary Preparations** (details are given in Part 3)
**Multi-ingredient: Belg.:** Transvane†; **Irl.:** Transvasin; **NZ:** Transvasin†; **Port.:** Hipodor; **Swed.:** Transvasin†; **UK:** Transvasin Heat Rub.

## Hydrocodone Hydrochloride *(BANM, rINNM)*

Hidrocloruro de hidrocodona.

$C_{18}H_{21}NO_3,HCl,2\frac{1}{2}H_2O$ = 380.9.

*CAS — 25968-91-6 (anhydrous hydrocodone hydrochloride).*

*ATC — R05DA03.*

## Hydrocodone Tartrate *(BANM, rINNM)*

Dihydrocodeinone Acid Tartrate; Hidrocodona, tartrato de; Hydrocodone Acid Tartrate; Hydrocodone Bitartrate *(USAN)*; Hydrocodoni Bitartras; Hydrocone Bitartrate. 6-Deoxy-3-*O*-methyl-6-oxomorphine hydrogen tartrate hemipentahydrate; (−)-(5*R*)-4,5-Epoxy-3-methoxy-9a-methylmorphinan-6-one hydrogen tartrate hemipentahydrate.

$C_{18}H_{21}NO_3,C_4H_6O_6,2\frac{1}{2}H_2O$ = 494.5.

*CAS — 125-29-1 (hydrocodone); 143-71-5 (anhydrous hydrocodone tartrate); 34195-34-1 (hydrocodone tartrate hemipentahydrate).*

*ATC — R05DA03.*

NOTE. Compounded preparations of hydrocodone tartrate may be represented by the following names:

- Co-hycodAPAP *(PEN)*—hydrocodone tartrate and paracetamol.

**Pharmacopoeias.** In *Ger., Swiss,* and *US.*

**USP 27** (Hydrocodone Bitartrate). Fine, white crystals or crystalline powder. Soluble in water; slightly soluble in alcohol; insoluble in chloroform and in ether. pH of a 2% solution in water is between 3.2 and 3.8. Store in airtight containers. Protect from light.

### Profile

Hydrocodone, a phenanthrene derivative, is an opioid analgesic (p.71) related to codeine (p.27) and has similar actions, but is more potent on a weight for weight basis. Hydromorphone (below) is one of the metabolites of hydrocodone.

Hydrocodone is used chiefly as the tartrate in preparations for the relief of irritant cough, though it has no particular advantage over codeine. It is also used for the relief of moderate to moderately severe pain, usually with paracetamol.

Hydrocodone tartrate is taken by mouth in doses of 5 to 10 mg every 4 to 6 hours.

Hydrocodone hydrochloride is given by mouth and also by injection. The polistirex derivative (a hydrocodone and sulfonated diethenylbenzene-ethenylbenzene copolymer complex) is used in modified-release preparations.

Hydrocodone has also been used in the treatment of dyspnoea.

**Effects on the ears.** Sensorineural hearing loss in 12 patients has been associated with the overuse or abuse of the hydrocodone and paracetamol preparation, Vicodin.[1] Cochlear implants improved the hearing loss in some of the patients.

1. Friedman RA, *et al.* Profound hearing loss associated with hydrocodone/acetaminophen abuse. *Am J Otol* 2000; **21:** 188–91.

### Preparations

**USP 27:** Hydrocodone Bitartrate and Acetaminophen Tablets; Hydrocodone Bitartrate Tablets.

**Proprietary Preparations** (details are given in Part 3)
**Belg.:** Biocodone; **Canad.:** Hycodan; Robidone†; **Ger.:** Dicodid; **Switz.:** Dicodid.

**Multi-ingredient: Arg.:** Hidronovag Complex; **Canad.:** Caldomine-DH†; Calmydone; Coristex-DH; Coristine-DH; Dalmacol; Dimetane Expectorant DC; Hycomine; Mercodol with Decapryn†; Novahistex DH; Novahistex DH Expectorant†; Novahistine DH; Triaminic Expectorant DH†; Tussaminic DH†; Tussionex; **India:** Cardiazol-Dicodid; **USA:** Alor; Anaplex HD; Anexsia; Atuss EX; Atuss G; Atuss HD; Bancap HC; Ceta Plus; Co-Gesic; Co-Tuss V; Codal-DH; Codamine†; Codiclear DH; Codimal DH; Cophene XP; Cyndal HD; Cytuss HC; Damason-P; De-Chlor G; De-Chlor HC; De-Chlor HD; De-Chlor MR; De-Chlor NX; Deconamine CX; Dolacet; Donatussin DC; Drocon-CS; Duocet; Duratuss HD†; ED Tuss HC; ED-TLC; Endagen-HD; Endal HD; Endal-HD Plus; Endal-HD†; Entex HC; Entuss Expectorant; Entuss-D; Entuss-D Jr; H-Tuss-D; Histex HC; Histinex D; Histinex HC; Histinex PV; Histussin D; Histussin HC; Hy-KXP; Hy-Phen; HycoClear Tuss; Hycodan; Hycomine Compound; Hycomine†; Hycotuss; Hydro DP; Hydro PC; Hydro-GP; Hydro-Tussin HD; Hydrocet; Hydrocodone CP; Hydrocodone GF; Hydrocodone HD; Hydrocodone PA†; Hydrogesic; Hydromet; Hydron CP; Hydron EX; Hydron KGS; Hydron PSC; Hydropane; Hyphed; Iodal; Iotussin HC; Kwelcof; Levall; Lorcet 10/650; Lorcet Plus; Lorcet-HD; Lortab; Lortab ASA; Lortuss HC; Marcof; Margesic H; Maxi-Tuss HCG; Maxi-Tuss HCX; Maxidone; Nalex DH; Norco; Notuss PD; Oncet; P-V-Tussin; Panacet†; Panasal†; Pancof XP; Pancof-HC; Pancof-XL; Para-Hist HD; Pneumotussin; Poly-Tussin; Protuss; Protuss-D; Relacon-HC; Rolatuss with Hydrocodone†; Ru-Tuss with Hydrocodone†; S-T Forte 2; S-T Forte†; SRC Expectorant; Stagesic; Statuss Green†; Su-Tuss HD; T-Gesic; Triaminic Expectorant DH†; Tussafed HC; Tussafin Expectorant; Tussanil DH; Tussend; Tussigon; Tussionex Pennkinetic; Tyrodone; Unituss HC; Vanex Expectorant; Vanex-HD; Vetuss HC†; Vicodin; Vicodin Tuss; Vicoprofen; Vitussin; Z-Cof HC; Zydone.

## Hydromorphone Hydrochloride

*(BANM, rINNM)*

Dihydromorphinone Hydrochloride; Hidrocloruro de hidromorfona; Hydromorphoni Hydrochloridum. 6-Deoxy-7,8-dihydro-6-oxomorphine hydrochloride; (−)-(5*R*)-4,5-Epoxy-3-hydroxy-9a-methylmorphinan-6-one hydrochloride.

$C_{17}H_{19}NO_3,HCl$ = 321.8.

*CAS — 466-99-9 (hydromorphone); 71-68-1 (hydromorphone hydrochloride).*

**Pharmacopoeias.** In *Eur.* (see p.vi) and *US.*

**Ph. Eur. 5.0** (Hydromorphone Hydrochloride). A white or almost white, crystalline powder. Freely soluble in water; very slightly soluble in alcohol; practically insoluble in dichloromethane. Protect from light.

**USP 27** (Hydromorphone Hydrochloride). A fine white, or practically white, odourless, crystalline powder. Soluble 1 in 3 of water; sparingly soluble in alcohol; practically insoluble in ether. Store in airtight containers at a temperature of 25°, excursions permitted between 15° and 30°. Protect from light.

**Incompatibility.** Colour change from pale yellow to light green occurred when solutions of minocycline hydrochloride or tetracycline hydrochloride were mixed with hydromorphone hydrochloride in 5% glucose injection.[1] Mixtures of hydromorphone hydrochloride and dexamethasone sodium phosphate exhibited concentration-dependent incompatibility.[2] White cloudiness, haziness, or precipitation developed 4 hours after mixing thiopental sodium and hydromorphone hydrochloride.[3]

Stability of mixtures of fluorouracil and hydromorphone hydrochloride in 0.9% sodium chloride or 5% glucose depended on the concentration of fluorouracil present.[4] Hydromorphone hydrochloride 0.5 mg/mL with fluorouracil 1 mg/mL was stable for at least 7 days at 32° and for at least 35 days at 23°, 4°, or −20°. When the concentration of fluorouracil was increased to 16 mg/mL, hydromorphone was noted to decompose incurring unacceptable losses after 3 days at 32° or after 7 days at 23°, but was stable for at least 35 days at 4° or −20°.

1. Nieves-Cordero AL, *et al.* Compatibility of narcotic analgesic solutions with various antibiotics during simulated Y-site injection. *Am J Hosp Pharm* 1985; **42:** 1108–9.
2. Walker SE, *et al.* Compatibility of dexamethasone sodium phosphate with hydromorphone hydrochloride or diphenhydramine hydrochloride. *Am J Hosp Pharm* 1991; **48:** 2161–6.
3. Chiu MF, Schwartz ML. Visual compatibility of injectable drugs used in the intensive care unit. *Am J Health-Syst Pharm* 1997; **54:** 64–5.
4. Xu QA, *et al.* Stability and compatibility of fluorouracil with morphine sulfate and hydromorphone hydrochloride. *Ann Pharmacother* 1996; **30:** 756–61.

### Dependence and Withdrawal

As for Opioid Analgesics, p.71.

### Adverse Effects, Treatment, and Precautions

As for Opioid Analgesics in general, p.72.

### Interactions

For interactions associated with opioid analgesics, see p.73.

### Pharmacokinetics

Hydromorphone hydrochloride is rapidly but incompletely absorbed from the gastrointestinal tract after oral doses. Oral bioavailability is about 50%. A plasma elimination half-life of about 2.5 hours has been reported after oral or intravenous doses. Hydromorphone appears to be widely distributed in the tissues and it crosses the placenta. It is metabolised in the liver and excreted in the urine mainly as conjugated hydromorphone, dihydroisomorphine, and dihydromorphine.

◊ References.

1. Vallner JJ, *et al.* Pharmacokinetics and bioavailability of hydromorphone following intravenous and oral administration to human subjects. *J Clin Pharmacol* 1981; **21:** 152–6.

### Uses and Administration

Hydromorphone hydrochloride, a phenanthrene derivative, is an opioid analgesic (p.73). It is related to morphine (p.62) but with a greater analgesic potency. It is a useful alternative to morphine for subcutaneous use since its greater solubility in water allows a smaller dose volume. After injection onset of action usually occurs within 15 minutes and analgesia is reported to last for about 3 to 5 hours; after oral doses onset of analgesia is usually within 30 minutes.

Hydromorphone hydrochloride is used for the relief of moderate to severe pain. It is given by subcutaneous or intramuscular injection in initial doses of 1 to 2 mg every 4 to 6 hours as necessary. It may also be given by slow intravenous injection or by intravenous or subcutaneous infusion, with doses adjusted according to individual requirements. Higher parenteral doses may be given to opioid-tolerant patients using a highly concentrated solution containing 10 mg/mL that allows smaller dose volumes. In the UK, the initial dose of hydromorphone hydrochloride by mouth is 1.3 mg every 4 hours; thereafter the dose may be increased as necessary. In the USA doses of 2 mg may be given by mouth every 4 to 6 hours; doses may be increased to 4 mg or more for severe pain. Modified-release formulations of hydromorphone hydrochloride are available for twice-daily administration. By rectum, the usual dose is 3 mg every 6 to 8 hours.

Hydromorphone hydrochloride is given, as a syrup, in doses of 1 mg repeated every 3 to 4 hours for the relief of non-productive cough.

◊ References.

1. Searle NR, *et al.* Hydromorphone patient-controlled analgesia (PCA) after coronary artery bypass surgery. *Can J Anaesth* 1994; **41:** 198–205.
2. Hays H, *et al.* Comparative clinical efficacy and safety of immediate release and controlled release hydromorphone for chronic severe cancer pain. *Cancer* 1994; **74:** 1808–16.
3. Bruera E, *et al.* A randomized, double-blind, double-dummy, crossover trial comparing the safety and efficacy of oral sustained-release hydromorphone with immediate-release hydromorphone in patients with cancer pain. *J Clin Oncol* 1996; **14:** 1713–17.
4. Miller MG, *et al.* Continuous subcutaneous infusion of morphine vs. hydromorphone: a controlled trial. *J Pain Symptom Manage* 1999; **18:** 9–16.

### Preparations

**USP 27:** Hydromorphone Hydrochloride Injection; Hydromorphone Hydrochloride Tablets.

**Proprietary Preparations** (details are given in Part 3)
**Arg.:** Dolonovag; **Austral.:** Dilaudid; **Austria:** Dilaudid; Hydal; **Canad.:** Dilaudid; Hydromorph; **Denm.:** Opidol; **Fin.:** Opidol†; **Fr.:** Sophidone; **Ger.:** Dilaudid; Palladon; **Irl.:** Palladone; **Israel:** Palladone; **Swed.:** Opidol; **Switz.:** Opidol; **UK:** Palladone; **USA:** Dilaudid; Palladone.

**Multi-ingredient: Ger.:** Dilaudid-Atropin†; **Swed.:** Dilaudid-Atropin; **Switz.:** Dilaudid-Atropin; **USA:** Dilaudid Cough.

## Ibuprofen *(BAN, USAN, rINN)*

Ibuprofeno; Ibuprofenum; RD-13621; U-18573. 2-(4-Isobutylphenyl)propionic acid.

$C_{13}H_{18}O_2$ = 206.3.

*CAS — 15687-27-1.*

*ATC — G02CC01; M01AE01; M02AA13.*

**Pharmacopoeias.** In *Chin., Eur.* (see p.vi), *Int., Jpn, Pol., US,* and *Viet.*

**Ph. Eur. 5.0** (Ibuprofen). A white crystalline powder or colourless crystals. M.p. 75° to 78°. Practically insoluble in water; freely soluble in acetone, in dichloromethane, and in methyl alcohol; it dissolves in dilute solutions of alkali hydroxides and carbonates.

**USP 27** (Ibuprofen). A white to off-white crystalline powder having a slight characteristic odour. Practically insoluble in water; very soluble in alcohol, in acetone, in chloroform, and in methyl alcohol; slightly soluble in ethyl acetate. Store in airtight containers.

## Dexibuprofen (BAN, USAN, rINN)

S-(+)-Ibuprofen.

CAS — 51146-56-6.

ATC — M01AE14.

## Adverse Effects, Treatment, and Precautions

As for NSAIDs in general, p.67. Ibuprofen may be better tolerated than other NSAIDs.

Symptoms of nausea, vomiting, and tinnitus have been reported after ibuprofen overdosage. More serious toxicity is uncommon, but gastric emptying followed by supportive measures is recommended if the quantity ingested within the previous hour exceeds 400 mg/kg.

**Breast feeding.** No adverse effects have been observed in breast-feeding infants whose mothers were receiving ibuprofen, and the American Academy of Pediatrics considers[1] that it is therefore usually compatible with breast feeding. The *British National Formulary* also considers the amount of ibuprofen distributed into breast milk to be too small to be harmful to a breast-fed infant. A study[2] estimated that a breast-fed infant would ingest about 0.0008% of the maternal dose. However, some manufacturers recommend that breast feeding should be avoided during ibuprofen treatment, including topical application.

1. American Academy of Pediatrics. The transfer of drugs and other chemicals into human milk. *Pediatrics* 2001; **108:** 776–89. Correction. *ibid.*; 1029. Also available at: http://aappolicy.aappublications.org/cgi/content/full/pediatrics%3b108/3/776 (accessed 05/07/04)
2. Walter K, Dilger C. Ibuprofen in human milk. *Br J Clin Pharmacol* 1997; **44:** 211–12.

**Children.** An analysis[1] of the outcome of treatment of 83 915 children found that the risk of hospitalisation for gastrointestinal bleeding, renal failure, or anaphylaxis was no greater in children given ibuprofen than in those given paracetamol.

1. Lesko SM, Mitchell AA. An assessment of the safety of pediatric ibuprofen. *JAMA* 1995; **273:** 929–33.

**Effects on the blood.** Blood disorders including agranulocytosis, aplastic anaemia,[1] pure white-cell aplasia,[2] and thrombocytopenia[3] have been reported in patients taking ibuprofen. Fatal haemolytic anaemia occurred in a man taking ibuprofen and oxazepam.[4]

1. Gryfe CI, Rubenzahl S. Agranulocytosis and aplastic anemia possibly due to ibuprofen. *Can Med Assoc J* 1976; **114:** 877.
2. Mamus SW, *et al.* Ibuprofen-associated pure white-cell aplasia. *N Engl J Med* 1986; **314:** 624–5.
3. Jain S. Ibuprofen-induced thrombocytopenia. *Br J Clin Pract* 1994; **48:** 51.
4. Guidry JB, *et al.* Fatal autoimmune hemolytic anemia associated with ibuprofen. *JAMA* 1979; **242:** 68–9.

**Effects on the CNS.** Aseptic meningitis has occurred in patients taking NSAIDs. A review[1] of NSAID-related CNS adverse effects summarised 23 literature reports of NSAID-associated aseptic meningitis; 17 reports involved ibuprofen, 4 sulindac, 1 naproxen, and 1 tolmetin. Of the 23 reports, 11 involved patients with a diagnosis of systemic lupus erythematosus. Typically the reaction is seen in patients who have just restarted NSAID therapy after a gap in their treatment. Within a few hours of restarting the NSAID the patient experiences fever, headache, and a stiff neck; abdominal pain may be present. The patient may become lethargic and eventually comatose. Symptoms resolve if the NSAID is stopped. It is believed to be a hypersensitivity reaction but there does not appear to be cross-reactivity between NSAIDs. More recently, a 56-year-old man with rheumatoid arthritis developed symptoms of aseptic meningitis 2 hours after ingesting ibuprofen.[2] The authors believed this to be the first reported case of ibuprofen-induced aseptic meningitis in a patient with rheumatoid arthritis.

1. Hoppmann RA, *et al.* Central nervous system side effects of nonsteroidal anti-inflammatory drugs: aseptic meningitis, psychosis, and cognitive dysfunction. *Arch Intern Med* 1991; **151:** 1309–13.
2. Horn AC, Jarrett SW. Ibuprofen-induced aseptic meningitis in rheumatoid arthritis. *Ann Pharmacother* 1997; **31:** 1009–11.

**Effects on electrolytes.** Hyponatraemia has been described in patients receiving ibuprofen;[1-3] other risk factors such as pre-existing renal impairment or concomitant use of desmopressin were generally present.

1. Blum M, Aviram A. Ibuprofen induced hyponatraemia. *Rheumatol Rehabil* 1980; **19:** 258–9.
2. Rault RM. Case report: hyponatremia associated with nonsteroidal antiinflammatory drugs. *Am J Med Sci* 1993; **305:** 318–20.
3. García EBG, *et al.* Hyponatraemic coma induced by desmopressin and ibuprofen in a woman with von Willebrand's disease. *Haemophilia* 2003; **9:** 232–4.

**Effects on the eyes.** Reversible amblyopia has been reported in patients receiving ibuprofen.[1,2] For reference to effects on the optic nerve associated with ibuprofen, see p.68.

1. Collum LMT, Bowen DI. Ocular side-effects of ibuprofen. *Br J Ophthalmol* 1971; **55:** 472–7.
2. Palmer CAL. Toxic amblyopia from ibuprofen. *BMJ* 1972; **3:** 765.

**Effects on the gastrointestinal tract.** Ibuprofen may be associated with a lower risk of upper gastrointestinal effects than some other NSAIDs, but nonetheless it can cause dyspepsia, nausea and vomiting, gastrointestinal bleeding, and peptic ulcers and perforation. Colitis and its exacerbation have occurred.[1,2]

1. Ravi S, *et al.* Colitis caused by non-steroidal anti-inflammatory drugs. *Postgrad Med J* 1986; **62:** 773–6.
2. Clements D, *et al.* Colitis associated with ibuprofen. *BMJ* 1990; **301:** 987.

**Effects on the kidneys.** Reports of adverse renal effects with ibuprofen include an increase in serum creatinine concentration,[1] acute renal failure,[2-5] and nephrotic syndrome.[6] Cystitis, haematuria, and interstitial nephritis may occur. Acute flank pain and reversible renal dysfunction, similar to that seen with suprofen (p.93), has been reported in some patients treated with ibuprofen.[7,8] See also under Effects on Electrolytes, above.

1. Whelton A, *et al.* Renal effects of ibuprofen, piroxicam, and sulindac in patients with asymptomatic renal failure: a prospective, randomized, crossover comparison. *Ann Intern Med* 1990; **112:** 568–76.
2. Brandstetter RD, Mar DD. Reversible oliguric renal failure associated with ibuprofen treatment. *BMJ* 1978; **2:** 1194–5.
3. Kimberly RP, *et al.* Apparent acute renal failure associated with therapeutic aspirin and ibuprofen administration. *Arthritis Rheum* 1979; **22:** 281–5.
4. Spierto RJ, *et al.* Acute renal failure associated with the use of over-the-counter ibuprofen. *Ann Pharmacother* 1992; **26:** 714.
5. Fernando AHN, *et al.* Renal failure after topical use of NSAIDs. *BMJ* 1994; **308:** 533.
6. Justiniani FR. Over-the-counter ibuprofen and nephrotic syndrome. *Ann Intern Med* 1986; **105:** 303.
7. McIntire SC, *et al.* Acute flank pain and reversible renal dysfunction associated with nonsteroidal anti-inflammatory drug use. *Pediatrics* 1993; **92:** 459–60.
8. Wattad A, *et al.* A unique complication of nonsteroidal anti-inflammatory drug use. *Pediatrics* 1994; **93:** 693.

**Effects on the liver.** Raised liver transaminase levels were noted in 3 patients with chronic hepatitis C infection after taking ibuprofen.[1] Levels returned to normal on discontinuation of the drug; the effect recurred in one patient who was re-exposed.

1. Riley TR, Smith JP. Ibuprofen-induced hepatotoxicity in patients with chronic hepatitis C: a case series. *Am J Gastroenterol* 1998; **93:** 1563–5.

**Effects on the skin.** Skin rashes may occur during hypersensitivity reactions although serious dermatological effects attributed to ibuprofen are rare. Reports of more serious effects have included Stevens-Johnson syndrome (often associated with hepatotoxicity),[1,2] photosensitivity,[3] and bullous leukocytoclastic vasculitis.[4]

1. Sternlieb P, Robinson RM. Stevens-Johnson syndrome plus toxic hepatitis due to ibuprofen. *N Y State J Med* 1978; **78:** 1239–43.
2. Srivastava M, *et al.* Drug-associated acute-onset vanishing bile duct and Stevens-Johnson syndromes in a child. *Gastroenterology* 1998; **115:** 743–6.
3. Bergner T, Przybilla B. Photosensitization caused by ibuprofen. *J Am Acad Dermatol* 1992; **26:** 114–16.
4. Davidson KA, *et al.* Ibuprofen-induced bullous leukocytoclastic vasculitis. *Cutis* 2001; **67:** 303–7.

**Hypersensitivity.** A fatal asthma attack occurred in a 65-year-old-woman, with adult-onset asthma, 30 minutes after ingestion of ibuprofen 800 mg.[1]

For other hypersensitivity reactions or possible reactions see also under Effects on the CNS and under Effects on the Skin, above.

1. Ayres JG, *et al.* Asthma death due to ibuprofen. *Lancet* 1987; **i:** 1082.

**Meningitis.** For reports of aseptic meningitis following administration of ibuprofen, see under Effects on the CNS, above.

**Overdosage.** There was a substantial increase in the number of cases of ibuprofen overdose reported to the National Poisons Information Service of the UK in the 2 years following its introduction as an 'over-the-counter' medication.[1] However, no concurrent increase in severity of poisoning was demonstrated and in only 1 of 203 cases was ibuprofen thought to have caused serious problems. It was concluded that ibuprofen appeared to be much less toxic in acute overdose than either aspirin or paracetamol. Current advice is that doses below 100 mg/kg are unlikely to cause toxicity in *children*, whereas clinical features will occur in children who have ingested more than 400 mg/kg. In *adults* the dose-response effect is less clear cut, but those who have ingested less than 100 mg/kg are unlikely to require treatment.

Nonetheless, reports illustrate the complexity of major overdosage with ibuprofen. A syndrome of coma, hyperkalaemia with cardiac arrhythmias, metabolic acidosis, pyrexia, and respiratory and renal failure was reported[2] in a 17-year-old man following major overdosage with ibuprofen and minor overdosage with doxepin. Hyperkalaemia was not evident until 14 hours after hospital admission and was thought to be due to a combination of potassium replacement for initial hypokalaemia, acidosis, muscle damage, and ibuprofen-induced renal failure. A 6-year-old child developed[3] shock, coma, and metabolic acidosis after ingestion of a dose of ibuprofen equivalent to 300 mg/kg. Treatment consisting of intubation, mechanical ventilation, fluid resuscitation, gastric lavage, and activated charcoal proved successful. In another report,[4] in which a 21-month-old child had ingested the equivalent of 500 mg/kg of ibuprofen, the presenting symptoms were acute renal failure with severe metabolic acidosis. The child developed tonic-clonic seizures 46 hours after ingestion, with significant hypocalcaemia and hypomagnesaemia, which may have been exacerbated by the administration of sodium polystyrene sulfonate and furosemide. The seizures, which could not be controlled with diazepam, phenytoin, and phenobarbital, ceased following correction of electrolyte balance.

1. Perry SJ, *et al.* Ibuprofen overdose: the first two years of over–the–counter sales. *Hum Toxicol* 1987; **6:** 173–8.
2. Menzies DG, *et al.* Fulminant hyperkalaemia and multiple complications following ibuprofen overdose. *Med Toxicol Adverse Drug Exp* 1989; **4:** 468–71.
3. Zuckerman GB, Uy CC. Shock, metabolic acidosis, and coma following ibuprofen overdose in a child. *Ann Pharmacother* 1995; **29:** 869–71.
4. Al-Harbi NN, *et al.* Hypocalcemia and hypomagnesemia after ibuprofen overdose. *Ann Pharmacother* 1997; **31:** 432–4.

## Interactions

For interactions associated with NSAIDs, see p.69.

**Aspirin.** It has been suggested that ibuprofen may reduce the cardioprotective effect of aspirin but see under Interactions of Aspirin, p.17.

**Lipid regulating drugs.** For a report of rhabdomyolysis and renal failure attributed to an interaction between ibuprofen and *ciprofibrate*, see p.874.

**Muscle relaxants.** *Baclofen* toxicity may develop after starting ibuprofen; for further details, see p.1387.

## Pharmacokinetics

Ibuprofen is absorbed from the gastrointestinal tract and peak plasma concentrations occur about 1 to 2 hours after ingestion. Ibuprofen is also absorbed following rectal administration. There is some absorption following topical application to the skin. For example, some manufacturers report that percutaneous absorption from topical gel is about 5% of that obtained following administration of an oral dose form. Ibuprofen is 90 to 99% bound to plasma proteins and has a plasma half-life of about 2 hours. It is rapidly excreted in the urine mainly as metabolites and their conjugates. About 1% is excreted in urine as unchanged ibuprofen and about 14% as conjugated ibuprofen. There appears to be little if any distribution into breast milk.

The above figures refer to racemic ibuprofen. However, ibuprofen's disposition is stereoselective and there is some metabolic conversion of the inactive *R*-(−)-enantiomer to the active *S*-(+)-enantiomer (dexibuprofen).

◊ References.

1. Davies NM. Clinical pharmacokinetics of ibuprofen: the first 30 years. *Clin Pharmacokinet* 1998; **34:** 101–54.

## Uses and Administration

Ibuprofen, a propionic acid derivative, is an NSAID (p.70). Its anti-inflammatory properties may be weaker than those of some other NSAIDs.

Ibuprofen is used in the management of mild to moderate pain and inflammation in conditions such as dysmenorrhoea, headache including migraine, postoperative pain, dental pain, musculoskeletal and joint disorders such as ankylosing spondylitis, osteoarthritis, and rheumatoid arthritis including juvenile idiopathic arthritis, peri-articular disorders such as bursitis and tenosynovitis, and soft-tissue disorders such as sprains and strains. It is also used to reduce fever.

Ibuprofen has also been used as an alternative to indometacin in the treatment of patent ductus arteriosus.

The usual dose **by mouth** for painful conditions in *adults* is 1.2 to 1.8 g daily in divided doses although maintenance doses of 600 mg to 1.2 g daily may be effective in some patients. If necessary the dose may be increased; in the UK the maximum recommended dose is 2.4 g daily whereas in the USA it is 3.2 g daily. Modified-release preparations of ibuprofen are available for once- or twice daily dosing, although actual dosages vary with different preparations. Patients with rheumatoid arthritis generally require higher doses of ibuprofen than those with osteoarthritis. The recommended dose for fever reduction in adults is 200 to 400 mg every 4 to 6 hours to a maximum of 1.2 g daily.

In the UK the usual dose by mouth for the treatment of pain or fever in *children* is 20 to 30 mg/kg daily in divided doses. Alternatively, total daily doses to be given in divided doses may be expressed in terms of age and are: 6 to 12 months, 150 mg; 1 to 2 years, 150 to 200 mg; 3 to 7 years, 300 to 400 mg; and 8 to 12 years, 600 to 800 mg. Up to 40 mg/kg may be given daily in juvenile idiopathic arthritis if necessary. Ibuprofen is not generally recommended for children weighing less than 7 kg and some manufacturers suggest a maximum daily dose of 500 mg in those weighing less than 30 kg. For post-immunisation pyrexia, a dose of 50 mg has been recommended; a second dose may be given after six hours. If the pyrexia persists after the second dose, medical advice should be sought. Infants aged 2 to 3 months may also be given a 50-mg dose of ibuprofen for post-immunisation pyrexia on the advice of a doctor.

In the USA, suggested doses for children are: for fever, 5 to 10 mg/kg (depending on the severity of the fever) and for pain, 10 mg/kg; doses may be given every 6 to 8 hours up to a maximum daily dose of 40 mg/kg. A usual daily dose in the USA for juvenile idiopathic arthritis is 30 to 40 mg/kg in divided doses.

Ibuprofen is also applied **topically** as a 5% cream, foam, gel, or spray solution; a 10% gel is also available.

Ibuprofen is usually given as the base but **derivatives**, including various salts, esters, and other complexes, are also used. These include lysine and sodium salts, guaiacol and pyridoxine esters, and mabuprofen (ibuprofen aminoethanol), isobutanolammonium, and meglumine derivatives.

Ibuprofen is usually given as a racemic mixture but preparations containing only the *S*-(+)-isomer dexibuprofen are available in some countries. The usual adult dose is between 450 mg and 1.2 g daily by mouth in divided doses.

**Cachexia.** For reference to the use of ibuprofen in combination with megestrol to treat cancer cachexia, see p.1558.

**Cystic fibrosis.** In patients with cystic fibrosis (see p.123), the inflammatory response to chronic pulmonary infection with *Pseudomonas* organisms contributes to lung destruction. Ibuprofen and other NSAIDs have been studied in patients with cystic fibrosis as an alternative to corticosteroids to reduce pulmonary inflammation, but despite some evidence of benefit their place in therapy is yet to be established.[1] A study[2] in patients with cystic fibrosis and mild lung disease indicated that ibuprofen given in high doses for 4 years slowed the progression of the lung disease without serious adverse effects. Initial doses were in the region of 20 to 30 mg/kg to a maximum of 1600 mg but were then adjusted individually to achieve peak plasma concentrations of 50 to 100 micrograms/mL.

1. Dezateux C, Crighton A. Oral non-steroidal anti-inflammatory drug therapy for cystic fibrosis. Available in The Cochrane Library; Issue 2. Chichester: John Wiley; 2004.
2. Konstan MW, *et al.* Effect of high-dose ibuprofen in patients with cystic fibrosis. *N Engl J Med* 1995; **332:** 848–54.

**Patent ductus arteriosus.** For a suggestion that ibuprofen might be a better choice than indometacin for the treatment of patent ductus arteriosus, see p.49.

### Preparations

***BP 2003:*** Ibuprofen Cream; Ibuprofen Gel; Ibuprofen Oral Suspension; Ibuprofen Tablets;
***USP 27:*** Ibuprofen and Pseudoephedrine Hydrochloride Tablets; Ibuprofen Oral Suspension; Ibuprofen Tablets.

**Proprietary Preparations** (details are given in Part 3)
***Arg.:*** Algioprofen; Bistryl; Brunal; Butidiona; Copiron; Dextropirac; Dolomin; Dolorsyn; Druisel; Febratic; Ibu Evanol; Ibu-Lady; Ibu-Novalgina; Ibucler; Ibufabra; Ibufix; Ibumar; Ibupirac; Ibupiretas; Ibusi; Ibusumal; Ibutenk; Ibuzidine; Kesan; Motrax; Oxibut; Pakurat; Paraflex Crema; Ponstil Mujer; Ponstin; Sindol; ***Austral.:*** ACT-3; Actiprofen; Brufen; Bugesic; Hexal Compufen; Nurofen; Rafen; Tri-Profen; ***Austria:*** Actifen; Advil; Avallone; Brufen; Dismenol Neu; Dolgit; Dolibu; Dolofort; Duafen; Ibudol†; Ibufem; Ibugel; Ibumetin; Ibupron; Iburem; Ibutop; Imbun; Kratalgin; Movone; Nurofen; ratioDolor; Seractil; Tabcin; Urem; ***Belg.:*** Advil Mono†; Brufen; Bufedon†; Decontractyl New†; Extrapan; Ibu-Slow; Ibumed†; Ibutop; Inabrin†; Junifen; Malafene; Motrin†; Nurofen; Perviam; Siprofen; Spidifen; ***Braz.:*** Actiprofen; Advil; Algiflex; Artril; Benotrin†; Dalsy; Danilon†; Doraplax; Doretrim; Ibufran; Ibupril; Ibuprofan; Lombalgina; Motrin; Parartrin; Sanafen†; Spidufen; Uniprofen; ***Canad.:*** Actiprofen†; Advil; Motrin; Novo-Profen; ***Chile:*** Advil; Bediatil; Bladex; Deucodol; Dexelle; Dolorub; Fenpic; Fortapal; Ibu; Ibu-4; Ibu-6; Ibupirac; Ipson; Kin; Motrin; Niofen; Pediaprofen; Pironal; Pyriped; Tifen; ***Denm.:*** Apain; Brufen; Ibumetin; Ibunet†; Ibureumin; Ibutop; Ipren; Nurofen†; Seractiv; Solpaflex; ***Fin.:*** Brufen; Burana; Dexit; Ibumax; Ibumetin; Ibusal; Ibuxin; ***Fr.:*** Advil; Algifene†; Anadvil; Antarene; Brufen; Doctril†; Dolgit; Ergix; Expanfen; Gelufene; Hemagene Tailleur; Ibualgic; Ibutop; Intralgis; Nureflex; Nurofen; Oralfene†; Solufen; Syntofene†; Tiburon†; Upfen; ***Ger.:*** Aktren; Anco†; Brufen†; Contraneural; Deltaran; Dentigoa†; Dignoflex†; Dismenol N; Dolgit; Dolo neos†; Dolo Sanol; Dolo-Puren; Dolodoc; Dolormin; dura-Ibu†; duralbuprofen†; Esprenit; Eudorlin Extra; Exneural†; Fibraflex†; Gyno-Neuralgin; Gynofug; Ibu; ibu-Attritin; Ibu-ratiopharm; Ibu-Vivimed†; Ibubest†; Ibubeta; Ibudolor; Ibuflam; Ibufug†; Ibuhexal; Ibumerck; Ibuphlogont; Ibuprof; Ibutad; Ibutop; Ilvico grippal; Imbun; Jenaprofen; Kontagripp Mono; Mensoton; Migranin Ibuprofen; Mobilat†; Novogent; Nurofen; Optalidon; Opturem; Parsal; Pfeil; Phamoprofen; ratioDolor; Schmerz-Dolgit; Seclodin†; Spalt; Tabalon; Tempil; Tispol Ibu-DD; Togal Ibuprofen; Trauma-Dolgit; Urem; ***Gr.:*** Algofren; Brufen; Rozovin; ***Hong Kong:*** Advil; Bifen; Brufen; Bupogesic; Ibufac; Ibupen; Ibuslow†; Nurofen; Perofen; Rupan; ***India:*** Brufen; Emflam; Ibugesic; ***Irl.:*** Advil; Brufen; Bufigen; Cunil†; Ibugel; Melfen; Nurofen; Phorpain; Proflex; Solfen; ***Israel:*** Adex; Advil; Artofen; Ibufen; Ibuleve; Nurofen; ***Ital.:*** Aciril†; Algofen; Antalgil; Antalisin; Arfen; Asepsal†; Benfast†; Benflogin; Brufen; Brufort†; Buscofen; Calmine; Cibalgina Due Fast; Dolocyl; Dolofast; Edenil; Faspic; Ganaprofene; Gineflor; Ginenorm; Kos†; Moment; Neo-Mindol†; Nureflex; Nurofen; Zafen; ***Malaysia:*** Bifen; Brugesic; Ibufen; Nurofen; Perofen; Rupan; ***Mex.:*** Adivon†; Advil; Ainex†; Algidol†; Bestafen; Butacortelone†; Citalgan; Days; Dibufen; Dipofen†; Diprodol; Dolprin; Dolprofen; Dolval; Dolver; Eufenil†; Febratic; Flexafen; Gobrosan†; Ibuflam; Ibuflex; Ibupril†; Medifen; Mejorultra†; Micarzin†; Motrin; Natiken†; Novartril; Offeno; Proartinal; Quadrax; Realdrax; Ribufen†; Tabalon; ***Neth.:*** Advil; Brufen; Femapirin†; Nurofen; Seractil; Zafen; ***Norw.:*** Brufen; Ibumetin; Ibux; ***NZ:*** ACT-3; Anafen†; Brufen; Nurofen; Panafen; ***Port.:*** Arfen; Belep†; Brufen; Dolocyl; Ibupax; Inabrin†; Moment; Motrin; Nuprilan; Ozonol; Spidifen; Trifene; ***S.Afr.:*** Adfen†; Antiflam; Betagesic; Betaprofen; Brufen; Brugesic; Dynofen†; Iboflam; Ibopain†; Ibuleve; Ibumed; Inza; Lenafen; Norflam T; Nurofen; Painil; Ranfen; ***Singapore:*** Ampifen; Bifen; Brufen†; Ibufen; Ibuloid; Nurofen; ***Spain:*** Actimidol†; Advil; Aldospray Analgesico; Algiasdin; Algidrin; Algisan†; Alogesia; Altior; Atriscal; Babypiril; Dalsy; Diltix; Doctril; Dolorac; Dorival; Ediluna†; Espidifen; Faspic†; Femaprin†; Femidol†; Feminalin; Gelofeno; Ibenon†; Ibufen; Ibumac; Ibuprox; Ibuscent†; Inadol; Isdibudol; Isdol; Junifen; Kalma†; Leonal†; Narfen†; Neobrufen; Noalgil†; Nodolfen; Norvectan; Nureflex†; Nurofen; Pocyl; Remidol; Sadefen†; Saetil; Seractil; Solufena†; Solvium; Todalgil†; ***Swed.:*** Alindrin; Brufen; Ibumetin; Ipren; Nurofen†; Tradil; ***Switz.:*** Algifor; Artofen; Brufen; Bufeno†; DexOptifen; Dismenol N; Dolgit†; Dolo-Dismenol; Dolo-Spedifen; Dolocyl; Dologel†; Ecoprofen; Faspic†; Grefen; Ibufen-L; Ibugel†; Ibumed†; Ibusifar; Iproben; Iprogel; Irfen; Nurofen; Optifen; Panax N†; Redufen†; Seractil; Serviprofen†; Solufen†; Spedifen; ***Thai.:*** Ambufen; Anbifen; Aprofen; Babefen Sus; Borafen; Borakid; Brufen; Brumed; Bruprin; Brusil; Bumed; Cefen; Duran; Faspic; G-Fen; Greatofen; Heidi; Ibrofen; Ibu; Ibufac; Ibufen†; Ibugan; Ibulan; Iburen; Junifen; Mafen†; Nurofen; Ostofen; P-Fen; Perofen; Pippen; Probufen; Profena; Profeno; Rheumanox; Rumasian; Rumatifen; Rupan; Schufen; Serviprofen†; Skelan IB; Tofen; Trofen; ***UAE:*** Profinal; ***UK:*** Advil; Anadin Ibuprofen; Anadin Ultra; Arthrofen; Brufen; Calprofen; Cuprofen; Ebufac; Fenbid; Fenpaed; Feverfen; Galprofen; Hedex Ibuprofen; Ibrufhalal; Ibufac†; Ibufem; Ibugel; Ibular†; Ibuleve; Ibumousse; Ibuspray; Ibutop Cuprofen; Ibutop Ralgex; Inoven†; Isisfen†; Librofem; Lidifen†; Mandafen; Manorfen; Mentholatum Ibuprofen; Migrafen; Motrin; Novaprin; Nurofen; Nurofen Advance†; Nurofen Migraine; Obifen; Orbifen; Pacifene; Phensic Ibuprofen†; Phor Pain; Proflex; Radian-B Ibuprofen; Relcofen; Rimafen; ***USA:*** Advil; Bayer Select Pain Relief Formula†; Genpril; Haltran; Ibu; Ibu-Tab; Ibu-4, -6, -8; Ibuprin†; Ibuprohm†; Ibutab; Menadol; Midol Cramp & Body Aches; Motrin; Nuprin; Saleto-200.

**Multi-ingredient: *Arg.:*** Bioneural B12; Butidiona; Causalon Gesic; Deep Relief; Espasmo Ibupirac; Espasmo Motrax; Espasmofin; Ibu-Buscapina; Ibu-Tetralgin; Ibudolofrix; Ibudristan; Ibumar Migra; Ibupirac Fem; Ibupirac Flex; Ibupirac Migra; Mensalgin; Migral II; Novo Wilpan; Roveril; Supragesic; ***Austral.:*** Nurofen Cold & Flu; Nurofen Plus; Sudafed Congestion & Sinus Pain Relief; Tri-Profen Cold & Flu; ***Austria:*** Advil Cold; Ardinex; ***Belg.:*** Nurofen + Codeine†; ***Braz.:*** Algi-Danilon†; Algi-Itamanil; Algi-Reumatril†; Algifen; Fymnal; Reuplex; ***Canad.:*** Advil Cold & Sinus; Dayquil Sinus and Pain Relief; Dristan Sinus; Sudafed Sinus Advance; ***Chile:*** Adona; Butartrol; Dioran; Dolnix; Dolo-Octirona; Dolonase; Gedol; Ibupirac Compuesto; Midol; Neo Butartrol; Niofen Flu; Predual DI; Silartrin; ***Fin.:*** Ardinex; Burana-C; ***Fr.:*** Anadvil Rhume; Cliptol; Nurofen Rhume; Rhinadvil; Rhinureflex; Vicks Rhume; ***India:*** Acks; Anaflam; Combiflam; Duoflam; Duoflam Plus; Emflam Plus; Ibu-Proxyvon; Ibuflamar-P; Ibugesic Plus; Ibugesic-M; Parvon Forte; Reducin-A; Robiflam; Somaflam; ***Irl.:*** Advil Cold & Flu; Codafen Continus; Nurofen Cold & Flu; Nurofen Plus; ***Ital.:*** Solviflu; ***Mex.:*** Algitrin; Bipasmin Compuesto NF; Carbager-Plus; Dolocibal†; ***NZ:*** Nurofen Cold & Flu; Nurofen Plus; ***S.Afr.:*** Advil CS; Lotem; Mybulen; Mypaid; Myprodol; Nurofen Cold & Flu; Sinumax IB; ***Spain:*** Nurofen Complex; Nurogrip†; Salvarina; ***Swed.:*** Ardinex; ***Switz.:*** Ibufen-L; ***Thai.:*** Alaxan Pl; Brustan; Cetan†; Dologen; Rumatifen-Plus; Skelan; ***UK:*** Advil Cold & Sinus†; Codafen Continus; Cuprofen Plus; Deep Relief; Lemsip Flu 12Hr; Lemsip Pharmacy Powercaps; Non-Drowsy Sudafed Dual Relief Max; Nurofen Cold & Flu; Nurofen Plus; Nurofen Sinus; Solpaflex; Vicks Action†; ***USA:*** Advil Allergy Sinus; Advil Cold & Sinus; Childrens Advil Cold; Childrens Motrin Cold; Dimetapp Sinus; Dristan Sinus; Motrin IB Sinus; Sine-Aid IB; Vicoprofen.

---

## Ibuproxam *(rINN)*

4-Isobutylhydratropohydroxamic acid.

$C_{13}H_{19}NO_2$ = 221.3.
*CAS — 53648-05-8.*
*ATC — M01AE13.*

### Profile

Ibuproxam is an NSAID (p.67) that has been used in musculoskeletal, joint, and soft-tissue disorders.

### Preparations

**Proprietary Preparations** (details are given in Part 3)
***Ital.:*** Ibudros; ***Spain:*** Nialen.

---

## Imidazole Salicylate *(rINN)*

Salicilato de imidazol. Imidazole compounded with salicylic acid.

$C_{10}H_{10}N_2O_3$ = 206.2.
*CAS — 36364-49-5.*
*ATC — N02BA16.*

### Profile

Imidazole salicylate is a salicylic acid derivative (see Aspirin, p.15) that has been used in the treatment of fever and inflammatory respiratory-tract and otorhinolaryngeal disorders. Imidazole salicylate has been given in doses of up to 2.25 g daily in divided doses by mouth. It has also been given as a rectal suppository and has been applied topically as a 5% gel for the relief of muscular and rheumatic pain.

### Preparations

**Proprietary Preparations** (details are given in Part 3)
***Ital.:*** Flogozen†; Fluenzen†; Selezen.

---

## Indometacin *(BAN, rINN)*

Indometacina; Indometacinum; Indomethacin *(USAN)*. [1-(4-Chlorobenzoyl)-5-methoxy-2-methylindol-3-yl]acetic acid.

$C_{19}H_{16}ClNO_4$ = 357.8.
*CAS — 53-86-1.*
*ATC — C01EB03; M01AB01; M02AA23; S01BC01.*

**Pharmacopoeias.** In *Chin., Eur.* (see p.vi), *Int., Jpn, US,* and *Viet.*

**Ph. Eur. 5.0** (Indometacin). A white or yellow, crystalline powder. Practically insoluble in water; sparingly soluble in alcohol. Protect from light.

**USP 27** (Indomethacin). A pale yellow to yellow-tan, crystalline powder having not more than a slight odour. It exhibits polymorphism. Practically insoluble in water; soluble 1 in 50 of alcohol, 1 in 30 of chloroform, and 1 in 40 of ether. Protect from light.

**Stability.** Indometacin is unstable in alkaline solution.

## Indometacin Sodium *(BANM, rINNM)*

Indometacina sódica; Indometacin Sodium *(USAN)*; Indomethacin Sodium Trihydrate. Sodium 1-(4-chlorobenzoyl)-5-methoxy-2-methylindole-3-acetate, trihydrate.

$C_{19}H_{15}ClNNaO_4,3H_2O$ = 433.8.
*CAS — 74252-25-8.*

**Pharmacopoeias.** In *US.*

**USP 27** (Indomethacin Sodium). Protect from light.

**Incompatibility.** Indometacin sodium injection is reconstituted with preservative-free sodium chloride for injection 0.9% or water for injection. Preparations containing glucose should not be used; reconstitution at a pH below 6 may cause precipitation of indometacin. Visual incompatibility has been reported between indometacin sodium injection and tolazoline hydrochloride,[1] 7.5 and 10% glucose injection, calcium gluconate, dobutamine, dopamine, cimetidine,[2] gentamicin sulfate, levofloxacin,[3] and tobramycin sulfate.[4] A pH below 6 may account for the visual incompatibility of indometacin sodium and several of these drugs.

1. Marquardt ED. Visual compatibility of tolazoline hydrochloride with various medications during simulated Y-site injection. *Am J Hosp Pharm* 1990; **47:** 1802–3.
2. Ishisaka DY, *et al.* Visual compatibility of indomethacin sodium trihydrate with drugs given to neonates by continuous infusion. *Am J Hosp Pharm* 1991; **48:** 2442–3.
3. Saltsman CL, *et al.* Compatibility of levofloxacin with 34 medications during simulated Y-site administration. *Am J Health-Syst Pharm* 1999; **56:** 1458–90.
4. Thompson DF, Heflin NR. Incompatibility of injectable indomethacin with gentamicin sulfate or tobramycin sulfate. *Am J Hosp Pharm* 1992; **49:** 836–8.

**Stability.** A reconstituted solution of indometacin sodium 500 micrograms/mL was stable for 14 days when stored at 2° to 6° in either the manufacturer's original glass vial or in a polypropylene syringe.[1]

1. Walker SE, *et al.* Stability of reconstituted indomethacin sodium trihydrate in original vials and polypropylene syringes. *Am J Health-Syst Pharm* 1998; **55:** 154–8.

### Adverse Effects

As for NSAIDs in general, p.67.

Adverse effects are more frequent with indometacin than with many other NSAIDs, the most common being gastrointestinal disturbances, headache, vertigo, dizziness, and lightheadedness. Gastrointestinal perforation, ulceration, and bleeding may also occur; rarely, intestinal strictures have been reported. Other adverse effects include depression, drowsiness, tinnitus, confusion, insomnia, psychiatric disturbances, syncope, convulsions, coma, peripheral neuropathy, blurred vision, corneal deposits and other ocular effects, oedema and weight gain, hypertension, haematuria, skin rashes, pruritus, urticaria, stomatitis, alopecia, and hypersensitivity reactions. Leucopenia, purpura, thrombocytopenia, aplastic anaemia, haemolytic anaemia, agranulocytosis, epistaxis, hyperglycaemia, hypoaldosteronism and hyperkalaemia, and vaginal bleeding have been reported. There have also been reports of hepatitis, jaundice, and renal failure. Hypersensitivity reactions may also occur in aspirin-sensitive patients. Rectal irritation and bleeding has been reported occasionally in patients who have received indometacin suppositories.

Adverse effects associated with the use of indometacin in premature **neonates** also include haemorrhagic, renal, gastrointestinal, metabolic, and coagulation disorders; pulmonary hypertension, intracranial bleeding, fluid retention, and exacerbation of infection may also occur.

**Effects on the blood.** There were 1261 reports of adverse reactions to indometacin reported to the UK Committee on Safety of Medicines between June 1964 and January 1973. These included 157 reports of blood disorders (25 fatal) including thrombocytopenia (35; 5 fatal), aplastic anaemia (17; no fatalities), and agranulocytosis or leucopenia (21; 3 fatal).[1] Subsequently, the First Report from the International Agranulocytosis and Aplastic Anemia Study confirmed a significant relationship between the use of indometacin and agranulocytosis and aplastic anaemia.[2]

Although use of indometacin in 20 women being treated for premature labour did not affect maternal prothrombin or activated partial thromboplastin time, maternal bleeding time during therapy was increased.[3] However, no cases of neonatal intraventricular haemorrhage or maternal postpartum haemorrhage were seen.

1. Cuthbert MF. Adverse reactions to non-steroidal antirheumatic drugs. *Curr Med Res Opin* 1974; **2:** 600–10.
2. The International Agranulocytosis and Aplastic Anemia Study. Risks of agranulocytosis and aplastic anemia: a first report of their relation to drug use with special reference to analgesics. *JAMA* 1986; **256:** 1749–57.
3. Lunt CC, *et al.* The effect of indomethacin tocolysis on maternal coagulation status. *Obstet Gynecol* 1994; **84:** 820–2.

**Effects on cerebral blood flow.** See under Patent Ductus Arteriosus in Uses and Administration, below.

**Effects on the eyes.** Severe and irreversible retinopathy, presumably due to long-term ingestion of high doses of indometacin occurred in a 33-year-old man.[1] A summary of previous literature reports of indometacin-induced ocular effects indicated that indometacin was retinotoxic, although to what degree was uncertain. For reference to effects on the optic nerve associated with indometacin, see p.68.

1. Graham CM, Blach RK. Indomethacin retinopathy: case report and review. *Br J Ophthalmol* 1988; **72:** 434–8.

**Effects on the gastrointestinal tract.** Nausea, vomiting, dyspepsia, gastrointestinal lesions, and serious reactions including gastrointestinal bleeding, ulceration, and perforation have occurred in patients receiving indometacin. Although it is well established that NSAIDs can produce adverse effects on the upper gastrointestinal tract, indometacin and other NSAIDs can also affect the large intestines.[1] Administration of indometacin to preterm neonates increases the risk of small bowel perforation and necrotising enterocolitis.[2-4] Risk seems to be increased in very-low-birthweight or extremely premature infants.

1. Oren R, Ligumsky M. Indomethacin-induced colonic ulceration and bleeding. *Ann Pharmacother* 1994; **28:** 883–5.
2. Grosfeld JL, *et al.* Increased risk of necrotizing enterocolitis in premature infants with patent ductus arteriosus treated with indomethacin. *Ann Surg* 1996; **224:** 350–7.
3. Shorter NA, *et al.* Indomethacin-associated bowel perforations: a study of possible risk factors. *J Pediatr Surg* 1999; **34:** 442–4.
4. Fujii AM. Neonatal necrotizing enterocolitis with intestinal perforation in extremely premature infants receiving early indomethacin treatment for patent ductus arteriosus. *J Perinatol* 2002; **22:** 535–40.

**Effects on the joints.** For references to concern that NSAIDs such as indometacin may accelerate the rate of cartilage destruction in patients with osteoarthritis, see under NSAIDs, p.68.

**Effects on the kidneys.** Acute renal failure,[1] nephrotic syndrome,[2] and renal papillary necrosis[3] have been reported in patients given indometacin. There have been suggestions that misoprostol might reduce the risk of indometacin-induced renal toxicity.[4,5]

Renal impairment has also occurred in **neonates** given indometacin intravenously for patent ductus arteriosus. Although rare, and usually reversible, the effect may be serious in neonates with pre-existing renal disorders.[6] Serious or fatal renal toxicity has been reported in neonates exposed to indometacin due to maternal ingestion.[7] The renal effects of prenatal indometacin may be prolonged.[8]

1. Chan X. Fatal renal failure due to indomethacin. *Lancet* 1987; **ii:** 340.
2. Boiskin I, *et al.* Indomethacin and the nephrotic syndrome. *Ann Intern Med* 1987; **106:** 776–7.
3. Mitchell H, *et al.* Indomethacin-induced renal papillary necrosis in juvenile chronic arthritis. *Lancet* 1982; **ii:** 558–9.
4. Weir MR, *et al.* Minimization of indomethacin-induced reduction in renal function by misoprostol. *J Clin Pharmacol* 1991; **31:** 729–35.
5. Wong F, *et al.* The effect of misoprostol on indomethacin-induced renal dysfunction in well-compensated cirrhosis. *J Hepatol* 1995; **23:** 1–7.
6. Cuzzolin L, *et al.* NSAID-induced nephrotoxicity from the fetus to the child. *Drug Safety* 2001; **24:** 9–18.
7. van der Heijden BJ, *et al.* Persistent anuria, neonatal death, and renal microcystic lesions after prenatal exposure to indomethacin. *Am J Obstet Gynecol* 1994; **171:** 617–23.
8. Butler-O'Hara M, D'Angio CT. Risk of persistent renal insufficiency in premature infants following the prenatal use of indomethacin for suppression of preterm labor. *J Perinatol* 2002; **22:** 541–6.

**Effects on the liver.** Cholestasis occurred in a 52-year-old woman several days after starting indometacin;[1] liver function values returned to normal once indometacin was discontinued.

1. Cappell MS, *et al.* Indomethacin-associated cholestasis. *J Clin Gastroenterol* 1988; **10:** 445–7.

**Hypersensitivity.** Hypersensitivity reactions including acute asthma have been reported following the use of indometacin suppositories,[1] eye drops,[2] or capsules[3] by patients who were aspirin-sensitive or had a history of asthma.

1. Timperman J. A fatal asthmatic attack following administration of an indomethacin suppository. *J Forensic Med* 1971; **18:** 30–2.
2. Sheehan GJ, *et al.* Acute asthma attack due to ophthalmic indomethacin. *Ann Intern Med* 1989; **111:** 337–8.
3. Johnson NM, *et al.* Indomethacin-induced asthma in aspirin-sensitive patients. *BMJ* 1977; **2:** 1291.

## Precautions

As for NSAIDs in general, p.69.

Indometacin should be used with caution in patients with epilepsy, parkinsonism, or psychiatric disorders. Dizziness may affect the performance of skilled tasks such as driving. Patients on long-term indometacin therapy should be examined regularly for adverse effects, and the *British National Formulary* particularly recommends periodic blood and ophthalmic examinations. Rectal administration should be avoided in patients with proctitis and haemorrhoids.

In addition indometacin should not be given to **neonates** with untreated infection, with significant renal impairment, or with necrotising enterocolitis. Infants who are bleeding (especially gastrointestinal bleeding or intracranial haemorrhage) or who have thrombocytopenia or coagulation defects should not be given indometacin and those receiving indometacin should be monitored during treatment for signs of bleeding. Electrolytes and renal function should also be monitored and if anuria or marked oliguria is evident at the time of a scheduled second or third dose, it should be delayed until renal function has returned to normal.

False-negative results in the dexamethasone suppression test have been reported in patients taking indometacin.

**Breast feeding.** Convulsions in a one-week old breast-fed infant appeared to be associated with ingestion of indometacin by the mother;[1] the child had normal motor and mental development at the age of 1 year and seizures had not recurred.

Indometacin has been detected in breast milk, but some workers[2,3] consider that the amount is so small that it should not constitute a contra-indication to breast feeding. The American Academy of Pediatrics[4] also states that indometacin is usually compatible with breast feeding despite acknowledging the above case report of convulsions.

1. Eeg-Olofsson O, *et al.* Convulsions in a breast-fed infant after maternal indomethacin. *Lancet* 1978; **ii:** 215.
2. Beaulac-Baillargeon L, Allard G. Distribution of indomethacin in human milk and estimation of its milk to plasma ratio in vitro. *Br J Clin Pharmacol* 1993; **36:** 413–16.
3. Lebedevs TH, *et al.* Excretion of indomethacin in breast milk. *Br J Clin Pharmacol* 1991; **32:** 751–4.
4. American Academy of Pediatrics. The transfer of drugs and other chemicals into human milk. *Pediatrics* 2001; **108:** 776–89. Correction. *ibid.*; 1029. Also available at: http://aappolicy.aappublications.org/cgi/content/full/pediatrics%3b108/3/776 (accessed 05/07/04)

**The elderly.** Following a study[1] of the pharmacokinetics of indometacin in the elderly it was suggested that the maintenance dose of indometacin in elderly patients should be reduced by 25%. The total clearance of indometacin in elderly subjects had been reduced when compared with that in young subjects; this was thought to be due to reduced hepatic metabolism in the elderly.

1. Oberbauer R, *et al.* Pharmacokinetics of indomethacin in the elderly. *Clin Pharmacokinet* 1993; **24:** 428–34.

**Pregnancy.** See under Premature Labour in Uses and Administration, below.

## Interactions

For interactions associated with NSAIDs, see p.69.

Anti-inflammatory doses of aspirin decrease indometacin blood concentrations by about 20%. Diflunisal decreases the renal clearance and increases plasma concentrations of indometacin. Use of diflunisal with indometacin has also resulted in fatal gastrointestinal haemorrhage, and the two should not be used together. Plasma concentrations of indometacin are likely to be increased in patients receiving probenecid.

**Antibacterials.** Indometacin has been reported to increase plasma concentrations of *aminoglycoside antibiotics*.

**Antipsychotics.** A report[1] of severe drowsiness and confusion in patients given *haloperidol* with indometacin.

1. Bird HA, *et al.* Drowsiness due to haloperidol/indomethacin in combination. *Lancet* 1983; **i:** 830–1.

**Bone modulating drugs.** Indometacin has been reported to increase the bioavailability of *tiludronate*, see p.776.

**Desmopressin.** The effect of desmopressin may be enhanced by indometacin.

**Parasympathomimetics.** The manufacturer of acetylcholine chloride ophthalmic preparations has stated that there have been reports that *acetylcholine* and *carbachol* have been ineffective when used in patients treated with topical (ophthalmic) NSAIDs.

## Pharmacokinetics

Indometacin is readily absorbed from the gastrointestinal tract in adults; peak plasma concentrations are reached about 2 hours after a dose. Absorption may be slowed by food or by aluminium or magnesium containing antacids. In premature neonates, absorption of oral indometacin is poor and incomplete. The bioavailability of rectal suppositories in adults has been reported to be comparable with or slightly less than the bioavailability with oral dosage forms.

Indometacin is about 99% bound to plasma proteins. It is distributed into synovial fluid, the CNS, and placenta. Low concentrations have been distributed into breast milk. The terminal plasma half-life has been reported to range from 2.6 to 11.2 hours in adults. The terminal half-life in neonates has been reported to be between 12 and 28 hours. Indometacin is metabolised in the liver to its glucuronide conjugate and to desmethylindomethacin, desbenzoylindomethacin, desmethyl-desbenzoylindomethacin, and to their glucuronides. Some indometacin undergoes N-deacylation. Indometacin and its conjugates undergo enterohepatic circulation. Excretion of indometacin and its metabolites is mainly in the urine with lesser amounts appearing in the faeces.

◊ References.

1. Moise KJ, *et al.* Placental transfer of indomethacin in the human pregnancy. *Am J Obstet Gynecol* 1990; **162:** 549–54.
2. Wiest DB, *et al.* Population pharmacokinetics of intravenous indomethacin in neonates with symptomatic patent ductus arteriosus. *Clin Pharmacol Ther* 1991; **49:** 550–7.

## Uses and Administration

Indometacin, an indole acetic acid derivative, is an NSAID (p.70). It is used in musculoskeletal and joint disorders including ankylosing spondylitis, osteoarthritis, rheumatoid arthritis, and acute gout, and in periarticular disorders such as bursitis and tendinitis. It may also be used in inflammation, pain, and oedema following orthopaedic procedures, in mild to moderate pain in conditions such as dysmenorrhoea, and it has been used in the management of postoperative pain as an adjunct to opioids, and in the treatment of fever. Indometacin is also used as the sodium salt to close patent ductus arteriosus in premature infants (see below).

The usual initial dose by mouth in **chronic musculoskeletal and joint disorders** is 25 mg two or three times daily increased, if required, by 25 to 50 mg daily at weekly intervals to 150 to 200 mg daily. To alleviate night pain and morning stiffness, up to 100 mg of the total daily dose may be given by mouth, or rectally as a suppository, on retiring. Alternatively, the total daily dose may be given rectally as 100 mg in the morning and at night. The total daily combined dose by mouth and by rectum should not exceed 200 mg. In acute gout the daily dose is 150 to 200 mg in divided doses until all symptoms and signs subside; in dysmenorrhoea up to 75 mg daily has been suggested.

Modified-release preparations of indometacin are available for use once or twice daily.

Indometacin has been used topically as 0.5 or 1% eye drops to **prevent miosis during cataract surgery**; the usual dose is one drop instilled 4 times daily, beginning on the day before surgery, and one drop 45 minutes before surgery. The eye drops may then be instilled 4 times daily for up to 10 to 12 weeks postoperatively to prevent cystoid macular oedema.

When used to **close patent ductus arteriosus** in premature infants indometacin sodium is given as three intravenous doses at 12- to 24-hour intervals; each dose should be infused over 20 to 30 minutes. Indometacin sodium injection is reconstituted with preservative-free sodium chloride 0.9% for injection or water for injection; glucose solutions should not be used. The dose of indometacin sodium (expressed as indometacin) depends upon the age of the neonate and the following doses have been suggested based upon the age at the first dose: less than 48 hours old, 200 micrograms/kg initially followed by two further doses of 100 micrograms/kg each; 2 to 7 days old, three doses of 200 micrograms/kg each; over 7 days old, 200 micrograms/kg initially followed by two further doses of 250 micrograms/kg each. If, 48 hours after this course of therapy the ductus remains open or re-opens a second course of therapy may be used, but if this produces no response surgery may be necessary.

Meglumine indometacin and a lipid soluble ester of indometacin, indometacin farnesil ($C_{34}H_{40}ClNO_4$ = 562.1), have also been given for painful and inflammatory conditions. A complex of indometacin and L-arginine, known as indoarginine, has also been used.

**Bartter's syndrome.** The treatment of Bartter's syndrome can often be difficult (see p.1220). Blocking the kinin-prostaglandin axis with a cyclo-oxygenase inhibitor such as indometacin improves hypokalaemia and other clinical features (including growth retardation) in children with the syndrome.[1-3]

1. Littlewood JM, *et al.* Treatment of childhood Bartter's syndrome with indomethacin. *Lancet* 1976; **ii:** 795.
2. Seidel C, *et al.* Pre-pubertal growth in the hyperprostaglandin E syndrome. *Pediatr Nephrol* 1995; **9:** 723–8.
3. Craig JC, Falk MC. Indomethacin for renal impairment in neonatal Bartter's syndrome. *Lancet* 1996; **347:** 550.

**Diabetes insipidus.** Indometacin and other prostaglandin synthetase inhibitors have been reported to decrease urine volume in all types of nephrogenic diabetes insipidus (p.1314).

References.

1. Rosen GH, *et al.* Indomethacin for nephrogenic diabetes insipidus in a four-week-old infant. *Clin Pharm* 1986; **5:** 254–6.
2. Libber S, *et al.* Treatment of nephrogenic diabetes insipidus with prostaglandin synthesis inhibitors. *J Pediatr* 1986; **108:** 305–11.
3. Allen HM, *et al.* Indomethacin in the treatment of lithium-induced nephrogenic diabetes insipidus. *Arch Intern Med* 1989; **149:** 1123–6.
4. Martinez EJ, *et al.* Lithium-induced nephrogenic diabetes insipidus treated with indomethacin. *South Med J* 1993; **86:** 971–3.

**Malignant neoplasms.** In common with some other NSAIDs (see p.71) it has been suggested that indometacin might possess some antineoplastic activity.[1] Some NSAIDs such as indometacin may also be of value for the differential diagnosis and the management of neoplastic fever, as they appear to be more effective in reducing this type of fever than against fever associated with infections.[2] Indometacin has also been tried for the treatment of fever and flu-like symptoms associated with interleukin-2 therapy although there has been concern over exacerbation of renal toxicity (see NSAIDs, under Interactions, p.563).

1. Mertens WC, *et al.* Effect of indomethacin plus ranitidine in advanced melanoma patients on high-dose interleukin-2. *Lancet* 1992; **340:** 397–8.
2. Engervall P, *et al.* Antipyretic effect of indomethacin in malignant lymphoma. *Acta Med Scand* 1986; **219:** 501–5.

**Neonatal intraventricular haemorrhage.** Indometacin has been tried prophylactically to prevent the development of intraventricular haemorrhage in neonates at risk (see p.740). Several mechanisms have been proposed for its possible action including reduction of cerebral flow as a result of vasoconstriction, reduction of oxygen free-radical damage, and accelerated maturation of blood vessels around the ventricles. Early studies[1-3] of the use of indometacin for prevention of intraventricular haemorrhage produced conflicting results. A subsequent large multicentre study[4] suggested that indometacin could reduce the incidence and severity of intraventricular haemorrhage, especially for the more severe forms. Neonates who received indometacin were given a dose of 100 micrograms/kg intravenously at 6 to 12 hours after delivery and then every 24 hours for 2 additional doses. Despite concern[5] that an unusually large number of neonates with severe intraventricular haemorrhage in the control group might have biased the findings, a systematic review has also come to similar conclusions about the benefit.[6]

A concern with the use of indometacin is the possibility that it may produce cerebral ischaemia due to its vasoconstrictor action and therefore increase the risk of developmental handicaps. However, follow-up at 3 years,[7] at 4½ years,[8] and at 8 years of age[9] in the infants included in the multicentre study reported no adverse effects on cognitive or motor development. A review[6] of studies of prophylactic indometacin has also concluded that there is no evidence to suggest either harm or benefit in neurodevelopment or other longer term outcomes.

Indometacin does not appear to prevent the progression of existing haemorrhage.[10]

1. Ment LR, *et al.* Randomized indomethacin trial for prevention of intraventricular hemorrhage in very low birth weight infants. *J Pediatr* 1985; **107:** 937–43.
2. Rennie JM, *et al.* Early administration of indomethacin to preterm infants. *Arch Dis Child* 1986; **61:** 233–8.
3. Bada HS, *et al.* Indomethacin reduces the risks of severe intraventricular hemorrhage. *J Pediatr* 1989; **115:** 631–7.
4. Ment LR, *et al.* Low-dose indomethacin and prevention of intraventricular hemorrhage: a multicenter randomized trial. *Pediatrics* 1994; **93:** 543–50.
5. Volpe JJ. Brain injury caused by intraventricular hemorrhage: is indomethacin the silver bullet for prevention? *Pediatrics* 1994; **93:** 673–7.
6. Fowlie PW, Davis PG. Prophylactic intravenous indomethacin for preventing mortality and morbidity in preterm infants. Available in The Cochrane Library; Issue 2. Chichester: John Wiley; 2004.
7. Ment LR, *et al.* Neurodevelopmental outcome at 36 months' corrected age of preterm infants in the multicenter indomethacin intraventricular hemorrhage prevention trial. *Pediatrics* 1996; **98:** 714–18.
8. Ment LR, *et al.* Outcome of children in the indomethacin intraventricular hemorrhage prevention trial. *Pediatrics* 2000; **105:** 485–91.
9. Vohr BR, *et al.* School-age outcomes of very low birth weight infants in the indomethacin intraventricular hemorrhage prevention trial. Abstract: *Pediatrics* 2003; **111:** 874. Full version: http://pediatrics.aappublications.org/cgi/content/full/111/4/e340 (accessed 05/07/04)
10. Ment LR, *et al.* Low-dose indomethacin therapy and extension of intraventricular hemorrhage: a multicenter randomized trial. *J Pediatr* 1994; **124:** 951–5.

**Patent ductus arteriosus.** In the fetal circulation the ductus arteriosus connects the pulmonary artery and the descending aorta. After birth, various mechanisms, including a fall in prostaglandin concentration, trigger its closure but in some infants the ductus arteriosus fails to close, a condition known as persistent patent ductus arteriosus. This condition may be found in infants with congenital heart defects but is more commonly seen in premature neonates, especially those with respiratory distress syndrome.

- Some infants may be asymptomatic or have only slight clinical symptoms and no immediate intervention is required. In many cases spontaneous closure will occur after several months, or else surgical ligation may be performed if clinical symptoms persist.
- In some infants a patent ductus arteriosus is necessary for maintaining some oxygenation of the blood, for example in pulmonary artery atresia or transposition of the great arteries. These infants require treatment with a prostaglandin such as *alprostadil* or *dinoprostone* to maintain patency of the ductus arteriosus until surgery can be performed to correct the malformation.
- Infants with haemodynamically significant ductus arteriosus, signs of heart failure, and who require ventilation should undergo treatment to close the patent ductus arteriosus.

Initial **management** involves fluid restriction, diuretics, correction of anaemia, and support of respiration. *Chlorothiazide* and *furosemide* are common diuretics used. There has been concern that furosemide might delay closure in infants with respiratory distress syndrome.[1,2] A systematic review[3] concluded that this did not seem to be the case, and that the diuretic might reduce adverse renal effects of indometacin; however, the evidence for this was limited and it was felt that there was not enough evidence to support the administration of furosemide to infants treated with indometacin. If initial treatment fails to control symptoms after 24 to 48 hours then *indometacin* is generally given to promote closure of the ductus.[1,4-6] The benefits of treatment with indometacin as soon as symptoms become apparent, rather than delaying treatment until signs of congestive failure develop, have been debated.[7,8] Early treatment may significantly reduce the morbidities arising from a persistent patent ductus arteriosus.[7] However, delaying treatment until the end of the first week of life may result in spontaneous closure and avoid the need of exposing infants to the toxic effects of indometacin.[8]

Indometacin probably leads to closure of the ductus through inhibition of prostaglandin synthesis. It is usually given intravenously as the sodium salt. The current practice is to give 3 doses at usual intervals of 12 to 24 hours with the amount depending on the age of the neonate. Indometacin has been given by mouth where the injection is unavailable, but absorption of oral indometacin is poor and incomplete in premature neonates. A second course of injections may be given 48 hours after the first course if the ductus remains open or has re-opened. Should that fail (which may be the case in 25% of infants treated[4,9]) then surgery is required.

A decreased need for surgical closure and reduced recurrences were seen in neonates in whom standard intravenous indometacin therapy was then followed by maintenance therapy (intravenous indometacin 200 micrograms/kg per day for an additional 5 days).[10] Similar beneficial findings were reported[11] in infants given prolonged low-dose indometacin therapy (100 micrograms/kg per day for 6 days). An additional benefit was a lower incidence of adverse effects; fewer infants experienced a rise in serum creatinine or urea concentrations. However, a later study[12] has suggested that prolonged administration of low-dose indometacin (100 micrograms/kg per day for 7 days) is less effective than standard therapy and may be associated with more adverse effects.

Prophylactic administration of indometacin reduces the chance of developing symptomatic patent ductus arteriosus,[7,13] but not morbidity. A systematic review[13] found no evidence of either benefit or harm in neurological development or other longer term outcomes.

Some other NSAIDs have also been tried in the treatment of patent ductus arteriosus. Ibuprofen appears to be effective in closing a patent ductus arteriosus,[14] and it has been suggested that ibuprofen might be a better choice than indometacin as, unlike indometacin, it does not have adverse effects on renal, mesenteric, and cerebral haemodynamics. However, a recent systematic review[14] found no significant difference in the effectiveness of ibuprofen compared to indometacin and, although the risk of oliguria was reduced with ibuprofen, the risk for chronic lung disease may be increased. Ibuprofen is also effective when used prophylactically; however, there have been reports of pulmonary hypertension with such use and ibuprofen is not recommended.[15]

1. Bhatt V, Nahata MC. Pharmacologic management of patent ductus arteriosus. *Clin Pharm* 1989; **8:** 17–33.
2. Anonymous. Delayed closure of the ductus. *Lancet* 1983; **ii:** 436.
3. Brion LP, Campbell DE. Furosemide for prevention of morbidity in indomethacin-treated infants with patent ductus arteriosus. Available in The Cochrane Library; Issue 2. Chichester: John Wiley; 2004.
4. Silove ED. Pharmacological manipulation of the ductus arteriosus. *Arch Dis Child* 1986; **61:** 827–9.
5. Barst RJ, Gersony WM. The pharmacological treatment of patent ductus arteriosus: a review of the evidence. *Drugs* 1989; **38:** 249–66.
6. Archer N. Patent ductus arteriosus in the newborn. *Arch Dis Child* 1993; **69:** 529–32.
7. Clyman RI. Recommendations for the postnatal use of indomethacin: an analysis of four separate treatment strategies. *J Pediatr* 1996; **128:** 601–7.
8. Van Overmeire B, *et al.* Early versus late indomethacin treatment for patent ductus arteriosus in premature infants with respiratory distress syndrome. *J Pediatr* 2001; **138:** 205–11.
9. Gersony WM, *et al.* Effects of indomethacin in premature infants with patent ductus arteriosus: results of a national collaborative study. *J Pediatr* 1983; **102:** 895–906.
10. Hammerman C, Aramburo MJ. Prolonged indomethacin therapy for the prevention of recurrences of patent ductus arteriosus. *J Pediatr* 1990; **117:** 771–6.
11. Rennie JM, Cooke RWI. Prolonged low dose indomethacin for persistent ductus arteriosus of prematurity. *Arch Dis Child* 1991; **66:** 55–8.
12. Tammela O, *et al.* Short versus prolonged indomethacin therapy for patent ductus arteriosus in preterm infants. *J Pediatr* 1999; **134:** 552–7.
13. Fowlie PW, Davis PG. Prophylactic intravenous indomethacin for preventing mortality and morbidity in preterm infants. Available in The Cochrane Library; Issue 2. Chichester: John Wiley; 2004.
14. Ohlsson A, *et al.* Ibuprofen for the treatment of patent ductus arteriosus in preterm and/or low birth weight infants. Available in The Cochrane Library; Issue 2. Chichester: John Wiley; 2004.
15. Shah SS, Ohlsson A. Ibuprofen for the prevention of patent ductus arteriosus in preterm and/or low birth weight infants. Available in The Cochrane Library; Issue 2. Chichester: John Wiley; 2004.

**Polyhydramnios.** Reports[1-3] of the beneficial effects of indometacin in the management of polyhydramnios (an excessive accumulation of amniotic fluid).

1. Cabrol D, *et al.* Treatment of symptomatic polyhydramnios with indomethacin. *Eur J Obstet Gynecol Reprod Biol* 1996; **66:** 11–15.
2. Abhyankar S, Salvi VS. Indomethacin therapy in hydramnios. *J Postgrad Med* 2000; **46:** 176–8.
3. Kriplani A, *et al.* Indomethacin therapy in the treatment of polyhydramnios due to placental chorioangioma. *J Obstet Gynaecol Res* 2001; **27:** 245–8.

**Premature labour.** The most common approach to postponing premature labour (p.794) with drugs has historically been with a selective beta$_2$ agonist. However, as prostaglandins have a role in uterine contraction and cervical ripening and dilatation, prostaglandin synthetase inhibitors such as indometacin have also been used. Comparative studies[1,2] have demonstrated that indometacin and ritodrine are equally effective in inhibiting uterine contractions and delaying delivery in patients in preterm labour who have intact membranes and in whom the gestational age is less than or equal to 34 weeks. In one study[2] an initial oral loading dose of indometacin 50 mg was given, followed by 25 to 50 mg orally every 4 hours until contractions stopped and then by a maintenance dose of 25 mg every 4 to 6 hours. In the other comparative study[1] indometacin was given as a 100-mg rectal suppository followed by 25 mg orally every 4 hours for 48 hours; if regular uterine contractions persisted 1 to 2 hours after the initial suppository, an additional 100-mg suppository was given before beginning oral therapy. Terbutaline was given for maintenance therapy.

Unfortunately indometacin can constrict the ductus arteriosus[3,4] which may lead to pulmonary hypertension,[2] and has also been associated with bronchopulmonary dysplasia,[5] reduced volume of amniotic fluid (oligohydramnios)[2,4] and possible renal damage (see Effects on the Kidneys, above) in the fetus. Another complication is that prenatal indometacin exposure may increase both the incidence and severity of patent ductus arteriosus in premature infants,[6,7] as shown by the increased need for postnatal indometacin therapy and surgical ligation in such infants. Some consider the benefits to outweigh the potential risks,[8] but indometacin is generally reserved as a second-line tocolytic or for combination with an intravenous tocolytic when an additive effect is required.

1. Morales WJ, *et al.* Efficacy and safety of indomethacin versus ritodrine in the management of preterm labor: a randomized study. *Obstet Gynecol* 1989; **74:** 567–72.
2. Besinger RE, *et al.* Randomized comparative trial of indomethacin and ritodrine for the long-term treatment of preterm labor. *Am J Obstet Gynecol* 1991; **164:** 981–8.
3. Moise KJ, *et al.* Indomethacin in the treatment of premature labor: effects on the fetal ductus arteriosus. *N Engl J Med* 1988; **319:** 327–31.
4. Hallak M, *et al.* Indomethacin for preterm labor: fetal toxicity in a dizygotic twin gestation. *Obstet Gynecol* 1991; **78:** 911–13.
5. Eronen M, *et al.* Increased incidence of bronchopulmonary dysplasia after antenatal administration of indomethacin to prevent preterm labor. *J Pediatr* 1994; **124:** 782–8.
6. Norton ME, *et al.* Neonatal complications after the administration of indomethacin for preterm labor. *N Engl J Med* 1993; **329:** 1602–7.

7. Hammerman C, *et al.* Indomethacin tocolysis increases post-natal patent ductus arteriosus severity. Abstract: *Pediatrics* 1998; **102:** 1202–3. Full version: http://pediatrics.aappublications.org/cgi/content/full/102/5/e56 (accessed 05/07/04)
8. Macones GA, Robinson CA. Is there justification for using indomethacin in preterm labor? An analysis of neonatal risks and benefits. *Am J Obstet Gynecol* 1997; **177:** 819–24.

### Preparations

***BP 2003:*** Indometacin Capsules; Indometacin Suppositories;
***USP 27:*** Indomethacin Capsules; Indomethacin Extended-release Capsules; Indomethacin for Injection; Indomethacin Oral Suspension; Indomethacin Suppositories.

**Proprietary Preparations** (details are given in Part 3)
***Arg.:*** Agilex; IM 75; Indotex; Klonametacina; ***Austral.:*** Arthrexin; Hicin†; Indocid; Indocid PDA; Indoptol†; Indospray†; ***Austria:*** Flexidin; Indo; Indobene; Indocid; Indocollyre; Indohexal; Indomelan; Indoptol; Indostad; Liometacen; Luiflex; Ralicid; ***Belg.:*** Dolcidium; Indocid; Indoptol†; Luiflex; ***Braz.:*** Agilisin; Indocid; Indocid Colírio; Metacidil; ***Canad.:*** Indocid; Indocid PDA; Indocollyre†; Indotec; Novo-Methacin; Nu-Indo; Rhodacine; ***Chile:*** Flexono; Moviflex; ***Denm.:*** Confortid; Indocid; Indonet†; ***Fin.:*** Confortid; Indocid; Indometin; ***Fr.:*** Ainscrid†; Chrono-Indocid; Indocid; Indocollyre; ***Ger.:*** Amuno†; Chibro-Amuno 3†; Confortid; Elmetacin; Indo; Indo Top; Indo-paed; Indo-Phlogont; Indo-Tablinen†; Indocolir; Indocontin; Indomet; Indomet-ratiopharm; Indomet-ratiopharm m; Indometacinum-mp†; Indomisal; Indorektal†; Inflam; Jenatacin†; Mobilat Akut Indo; Rheubalmin Indo; Sigadoc; ***Gr.:*** Fortathrin; Indocid; Itapredin; Reumacid; ***Hong Kong:*** Imbrilon†; Indocid; Indocid PDA; Indocollyre†; Indogesic; Indomet; ***India:*** Idicin; Indocap; ***Irl.:*** Cidomel; Flexin Continus; Idomed†; Indocid; Indocid PDA; Indomod†; ***Israel:*** Indocollyre; Indomed; Indoptic; Indotard; Indovis; ***Ital.:*** Imet; Indocid; Indocollirio; Indom; Indoxen; Liometacen; Metacen; ***Jpn:*** Catlep; Infree; ***Malaysia:*** Arthrexin; Domicap; Indo; Indocid; Indomen; ***Mex.:*** Antalgin; Endacil†; Grindocin; Indocarsil; Indocid; Indoman; Indosan†; Indotrin; Italon; Labymetacyn†; Malival; Mefazil†; Reumin†; ***Neth.:*** Indocid; Indocid PDA; Indoptol; ***Norw.:*** Confortid; Indocid; ***NZ:*** Arthrexin; Elmetacin; Indocid PDA; Indocid†; Rheumacin; ***Port.:*** Autritis; Dolovin; Elmetacin; Indocid; Indocollyre; ***S.Afr.:*** Acuflex†; Adco-Indogel; Aflamin; Arthrexin; Betacin; Elmetacin; Flamaret; Flamecid; Indocid; Mediflex; Methocaps; Nisaid; Restameth-SR; ***Singapore:*** Bonidon†; Indocollyre; Indoflam†; Indomen; Methacin†; ***Spain:*** Aliviosin; Artrinovo; Flogoter; Inacid; Indo Framan†; Indocaf; Indoftol†; Indolgina; Indonilo; Mederreumol; Neo Decabutin; Reumo; Reusin; ***Swed.:*** Confortid; Indomee; ***Switz.:*** Bonidon; Elmetacin; Helvecin†; Indo-Mepha; Indocid; Indophtal; Indoptic†; ***Thai.:*** Ammi-Indocin; Bucin; Elmego; Elmetacin; Idc; Indocid; Indocollyre; Indomed; Indono; Inflamate; Inthacine; Liometacen†; Metindo; Putatone†; Servindomet†; ***UAE:*** Rothacin; ***UK:*** Flexin Continus; Indocid PDA; Indocid†; Indolar SR; Indomax; Indomod; Indotard†; Pardelprin; Rheumacin; Rimacid; Slo-Indo; ***USA:*** Indochron†; Indocin.

**Multi-ingredient:** ***Austria:*** Vonum; ***Fin.:*** Indalgin; ***Fr.:*** Indobiotic; ***Ger.:*** Inflam; ***Ital.:*** Difmetre; ***Mex.:*** Artridol; Malival Compuesto; Morlan FB 25; ***Port.:*** Indobiotic; ***Spain:*** Artri; Betartrinovo†; Fiacin; ***Switz.:*** Indobiotic; Ralur; ***Thai.:*** Sancago†.

---

## Infliximab *(BAN, rINN)*

cA2; CenTNF.
*CAS — 170277-31-3.*
*ATC — L04AA12.*

### Adverse Effects, Treatment, and Precautions

Infliximab may cause acute infusion reactions during or within 1 to 2 hours of administration, particularly with the first or second dose. Symptoms include fever, chills, pruritus, urticaria, dyspnoea, chest pain, and hypertension or hypotension. Mild reactions may respond to a reduced rate of infusion or a temporary interruption. If reactions are more severe, discontinuation of therapy should be considered. Pretreatment with paracetamol and antihistamines may be considered. Infliximab should only be given where facilities for resuscitation are available. Delayed reactions have occurred 3 to 12 days after infusion, including myalgia, arthralgia, fever, and rash (see below).

Other, common, adverse effects include nausea and vomiting, abdominal pain, diarrhoea, fatigue, dizziness, headache, and back pain. Antibodies to infliximab (human antichimeric antibodies) may develop, and are associated with an increased incidence of hypersensitivity reactions. Antinuclear antibodies and anti-double-stranded-DNA antibodies have also developed with tumour necrosis factor (TNF) inhibitor therapy. A lupus-like syndrome has occurred rarely; treatment should be discontinued if it develops.

Infections are common in patients treated with infliximab or other drugs that inhibit TNF, and most often affect the upper respiratory tract and the urinary tract. TNF inhibitors have also been associated rarely with the development of serious opportunistic infections, sepsis, and onset or re-activation of tuberculosis (see below), particularly in patients with underlying conditions predisposing them to infections; in some cases death has resulted. TNF inhibitors should not be given to patients with severe infection, including active tuberculosis and opportunistic infections, and should be discontinued if these develop. They should also be used with care in those with a history of recurrent infections or with underlying conditions that may predispose to infections. Patients should be evaluated for latent and active tuberculosis before beginning therapy; if evidence of latent tuberculosis is found the risks and benefits of treatment should be considered carefully and chemoprophylaxis should be given. Patients should be instructed to seek medical advice if symptoms suggestive of tuberculosis (such as persistent cough, weight loss, or low grade fever) occur. Patients should be monitored for signs of infection for 6 months after treatment.

Infliximab should be avoided in patients with a history of hypersensitivity to the drug or other murine proteins. Caution is required if infliximab therapy is repeated after a prolonged period of no treatment (see Delayed Reactions, below).

Infliximab has been associated in rare cases with clinical or radiological worsening of demyelinating disorders such as multiple sclerosis or optic neuritis; care is required in prescribing it to patients with such disorders or symptoms suggestive of their onset.

Infliximab is contra-indicated in patients with moderate to severe heart failure. It must be used with caution in patients with mild heart failure; such patients should be closely monitored and infliximab discontinued in those who develop new or worsening symptoms of heart failure.

**Delayed reactions.** Ten of 37 patients re-treated with infliximab after a 2 to 4 year period without treatment experienced delayed hypersensitivity reactions, of which 6 were considered serious. None of the patients had experienced infusion-related adverse effects with their original infliximab therapy. Adverse reactions developed in 9 of the 23 patients originally treated with a discontinued liquid formulation, and in 1 of the 14 patients who previously received the marketed formulation, leading to speculation that the formulation may have been a contributing factor.

**Effects on the CNS.** Aseptic meningitis developed in a 53-year-old after his fifth injection of infliximab for rheumatoid arthritis.[1] Similar symptoms also occurred after a sixth injection. Three cases of bilateral optic neuropathy associated with infliximab therapy have also been reported.[2]

1. Marotte H, *et al.* Infliximab-induced aseptic meningitis. *Lancet* 2001; **358:** 1784.
2. ten Tusscher MPM, *et al.* Bilateral anterior toxic optic neuropathy and the use of infliximab. *BMJ* 2003; **326:** 579.

**Effects on the heart.** The FDA have reported[1] on 47 patients who developed heart failure while receiving long-term therapy with tumour necrosis factor antibodies (etanercept and infliximab). Of these, 38 developed new-onset heart failure, 19 having documented risk factors for heart failure, and 9 had exacerbation of existing heart failure. The median time to new-onset heart failure occurring was 3.5 months.

1. Kwon HJ, *et al.* Case reports of heart failure after therapy with a tumor necrosis factor antagonist. *Ann Intern Med* 2003; **138:** 807–11.

**Effects on the liver.** A 44-year-old woman developed cholestatic jaundice 19 days after a single infusion of infliximab for Crohn's disease.[1] Her symptoms resolved following supportive treatment.

1. Menghini VV, Arora AS. Infliximab-associated reversible cholestatic liver disease. *Mayo Clin Proc* 2001; **76:** 84–6.

**Infection.** There have been spontaneous reports of onset or re-activation of *tuberculosis* in patients treated with infliximab, including cases of miliary tuberculosis and unusual extrapulmonary disease.[1] The UK Committee on Safety of Medicines noted in February 2001 that there had been 28 such reports worldwide. The US manufacturers subsequently reported[2] (in October 2001) that other serious opportunistic infections, including *histoplasmosis, listeriosis,* and *pneumocystosis* had occurred, and had led to some deaths; the number of reported cases of tuberculosis had risen to 84. Although the majority of patients also had a history of treatment with immunosuppressants including corticosteroids, the inhibition of tumour necrosis factor may affect normal immune responses and predispose patients to opportunistic infections.

In addition to those infections reported by the US manufacturers, there has been a case of *aspergillosis* associated with infliximab treatment.[3]

1. Committee on Safety of Medicines/Medicines Control Agency. Infliximab (Remicade) and tuberculosis. *Current Problems* 2001; **27:** 7. Also available at: http://www.mca.gov.uk/ourwork/monitorsafequalmed/currentproblems/cpfeb2001.pdf (accessed 05/07/04)
2. Schaible TF [Centocor, Inc.]. Important drug warning (issued 05/10/01). Available at: http://www.fda.gov/medwatch/safety/2001/remicadeTB_deardoc.pdf (accessed 05/07/04)
3. Warris A, *et al.* Invasive pulmonary aspergillosis associated with infliximab therapy. *N Engl J Med* 2001; **344:** 1099–1100.

**Lymphomas.** Lymphomas have been seen in patients treated with inhibitors of tumour necrosis factor for rheumatoid arthritis or Crohn's disease but further epidemiological studies are required to determine if there is a causal relationship.[1]

1. Brown SL, *et al.* Tumor necrosis factor antagonist therapy and lymphoma development: twenty-six cases reported to the Food and Drug Administration. *Arthritis Rheum* 2002; **46:** 3151–8.

### Interactions

Live vaccines should not be given with infliximab or other drugs that inhibit tumour necrosis factor (TNF) as the effect of such drugs on vaccine efficacy or the risk of infection transmission is unknown. The use of TNF inhibitors with anakinra may increase the risk of adverse effects.

### Pharmacokinetics

Infliximab shows linear pharmacokinetics. It is distributed primarily in the vascular compartment and has a terminal elimination half-life of 8 to 9.5 days. After recommended doses, infliximab has been detected in serum for at least 8 weeks.

### Uses and Administration

Infliximab is a chimeric monoclonal antibody to tumour necrosis factor α (TNF), a pro-inflammatory mediator. Elevated levels of TNF have been found in the joints of patients with rheumatoid arthritis (p.9) and in the colon of patients with Crohn's disease (see Inflammatory Bowel Disease, p.1243).

Infliximab is used in the management of rheumatoid arthritis, ankylosing spondylitis (see Spondyloarthropathies, p.11), and Crohn's disease in patients who have not responded to conventional treatments for these conditions. It is given by intravenous infusion over a period of not less than 2 hours.

In **rheumatoid arthritis**, infliximab is given in a dose of 3 mg/kg repeated at 2 and 6 weeks then every 8 weeks thereafter, in combination with methotrexate. In the USA, the dose may be increased up to 10 mg/kg or repeated as often as every 4 weeks in those with an incomplete response. In the UK the National Institute for Clinical Excellence recommends, based on guidelines from the British Society for Rheumatology, that infliximab be withdrawn if there is no response within 3 months of starting treatment.

In severe active **Crohn's disease**, a single infliximab dose of 5 mg/kg is given. In those who respond, this may be followed by a maintenance regimen of additional infusions of 5 mg/kg at 2 and 6 weeks after the initial infusion and then every 8 weeks, or the drug may be readministered when signs and symptoms of the disease recur (but see below). A similar regimen is used in patients with fistulising Crohn's disease although therapy should not be considered ineffective until after the third dose of infliximab. The US manufacturers suggest that doses of up to 10 mg/kg may be used in patients with Crohn's disease who relapse after an initial response.

If the signs and symptoms of rheumatoid arthritis or Crohn's disease recur infliximab may be readministered if within 16 weeks of the last infusion. Readministration after a drug-free interval of more than 16 weeks may be associated with an increased risk of delayed hypersensitivity (see above) and consequently is not recommended.

The initial dose in **ankylosing spondylitis** is 5 mg/kg, repeated at 2 and 6 weeks and then every 6 to 8 weeks; if there is no response after 2 doses no further treatment should be given.

◊ References.

1. Onrust SV, Lamb HM. Infliximab: a review of its use in Crohn's disease and rheumatoid arthritis. *BioDrugs* 1998; **10:** 397–422.
2. Anonymous. Infliximab (Remicade) for Crohn's disease. *Med Lett Drug Ther* 1999; **41:** 19–20.
3. Present DH, *et al.* Infliximab for the treatment of fistulas in patients with Crohn's disease. *N Engl J Med* 1999; **340:** 1398–1405.
4. Maini R, *et al.* Infliximab (chimeric anti-tumour necrosis factor α monoclonal antibody) versus placebo in rheumatoid arthritis patients receiving concomitant methotrexate: a randomised phase III trial. *Lancet* 1999; **354:** 1932–9.
5. Lipsky PE, *et al.* Infliximab and methotrexate in the treatment of rheumatoid arthritis. *N Engl J Med* 2000; **343:** 1594–1602.
6. Markham A, Lamb HM. Infliximab: a review of its use in the management of rheumatoid arthritis. *Drugs* 2000; **59:** 1341–59.

7. Anonymous. Etanercept and infliximab for rheumatoid arthritis. *Drug Ther Bull* 2001; **39:** 49–52.
8. Lamprecht P, *et al.* Effectiveness of TNF-α blockade with infliximab in refractory Wegener's granulomatosis. *Rheumatology (Oxford)* 2002; **41:** 1303–7.
9. Brandt J, *et al.* Infliximab in the treatment of active and severe ankylosing spondylitis. *Clin Exp Rheumatol* 2002; **20** (suppl 28): S106–S110.
10. Nahar IK, *et al.* Infliximab treatment of rheumatoid arthritis and Crohn's disease. *Ann Pharmacother* 2003; **37:** 1256–65.
11. Sands BE, *et al.* Infliximab maintenance therapy for fistulizing Crohn's disease. *N Engl J Med* 2004; **350:** 876–85.


**Sarcoidosis.** For a mention of possible benefit from infliximab in sarcoidosis, see p.1087.

## Preparations

**Proprietary Preparations** (details are given in Part 3)
***Arg.:*** Remicade; Revellex; ***Austral.:*** Remicade; ***Belg.:*** Remicade; ***Braz.:*** Remicade†; ***Canad.:*** Remicade; ***Chile:*** Remicade; ***Denm.:*** Remicade; ***Fin.:*** Remicade; ***Fr.:*** Remicade; ***Ger.:*** Remicade; ***Gr.:*** Remicade; ***Irl.:*** Remicade; ***Israel:*** Remicade; ***Ital.:*** Remicade; ***Mex.:*** Remicade; ***Neth.:*** Remicade; ***Norw.:*** Remicade; ***NZ:*** Remicade; ***Port.:*** Remicade†; ***S.Afr.:*** Revellex; ***Spain:*** Remicade; ***Swed.:*** Remicade; ***Switz.:*** Remicade; ***UK:*** Remicade; ***USA:*** Remicade.

---

# Isonixin *(rINN)*

Isonixino. 2-Hydroxy-*N*-(2,6-dimethylphenyl)nicotinamide.
$C_{14}H_{14}N_2O_2$ = 242.3.
*CAS — 57021-61-1.*

## Profile

Isonixin is an NSAID (p.67) that has been used in the management of pain and inflammation associated with musculoskeletal and joint disorders. Isonixin has been used in doses of 400 mg two to four times daily by mouth or by rectal suppository. It has also been applied topically as a 2.5% cream.

## Preparations

**Proprietary Preparations** (details are given in Part 3)
***Spain:*** Nixyn.
**Multi-ingredient: *Spain:*** Nixyn.

---

# Kebuzone *(rINN)*

Kebuzona; Ketophenylbutazone. 4-(3-Oxobutyl)-1,2-diphenylpyrazolidine-3,5-dione.
$C_{19}H_{18}N_2O_3$ = 322.4.
*CAS — 853-34-9.*
*ATC — M01AA06.*

## Profile

Kebuzone, a phenylbutazone derivative, is an NSAID (p.67). It has been used in musculoskeletal, joint, and soft-tissue disorders in doses of up to 1.5 g daily in divided doses by mouth. Kebuzone has also been given as the sodium salt by intramuscular injection in doses equivalent to 1 g of base.

**Porphyria.** Kebuzone is considered to be unsafe in patients with porphyria because it has been shown to be porphyrinogenic in *animals* or *in-vitro* systems.

## Preparations

**Proprietary Preparations** (details are given in Part 3)
***Austria:*** Ketazon; ***Ger.:*** Ketazon†.
**Multi-ingredient: *Austria:*** Rheumesser.

---

# Ketobemidone Hydrochloride *(BANM, rINNM)*

Cetobemidone Hydrochloride; Cetobemidoni Hydrochloridum. 1-(4-*m*-Hydroxyphenyl-1-methyl-4-piperidyl)propan-1-one hydrochloride.
$C_{15}H_{21}NO_2$,HCl = 283.8.
*CAS — 469-79-4 (ketobemidone); 5965-49-1 (ketobemidone hydrochloride).*
*ATC — N02AB01.*

**Pharmacopoeias.** In *Eur.* (see p.vi).
**Ph. Eur. 5.0** (Ketobemidone Hydrochloride). White or almost white, crystalline powder. Freely soluble in water; soluble in alcohol; very slightly soluble in dichloromethane. A 1% solution in water has a pH of 4.5 to 5.5.

## Profile

Ketobemidone is an opioid analgesic (p.71). It has been given as the hydrochloride by mouth, by injection, or rectally, sometimes with an antispasmodic.

◊ References.


1. Al-Shurbaji A, Tokics L. The pharmacokinetics of ketobemidone in critically ill patients. *Br J Clin Pharmacol* 2002 **54:** 583–6.


## Preparations

**Proprietary Preparations** (details are given in Part 3)
***Denm.:*** Ketodur; ***Norw.:*** Ketodur; Ketorax; ***Swed.:*** Ketodur; Ketogan Novum.
**Multi-ingredient: *Denm.:*** Ketogan; ***Norw.:*** Ketogan; ***Swed.:*** Ketogan.

---

# Ketoprofen *(BAN, USAN, rINN)*

Ketoprofeno; Ketoprofenum; RP-19583. (*RS*)-2-(3-Benzoylphenyl)propionic acid.
$C_{16}H_{14}O_3$ = 254.3.
*CAS — 22071-15-4 (ketoprofen); 57469-78-0 (ketoprofen lysine); 57495-14-4 (ketoprofen sodium).*
*ATC — M01AE03; M02AA10.*

**Pharmacopoeias.** In *Chin., Eur.* (see p.vi), *Jpn, Pol.,* and *US.*
**Ph. Eur. 5.0** (Ketoprofen). A white or almost white, crystalline powder. M.p. 94° to 97°. Practically insoluble in water; freely soluble in alcohol, in acetone, and in dichloromethane.
**USP 27** (Ketoprofen). Store in airtight containers.

## Dexketoprofen Trometamol *(BANM, rINNM)*

Dexketoprofeno trometamol.
*CAS — 22161-81-5 (dexketoprofen).*

## Adverse Effects and Precautions

As for NSAIDs in general, p.67.

When ketoprofen is given intramuscularly there may be pain at the injection site and occasionally tissue damage. Ketoprofen suppositories may cause local irritation. Ketoprofen should be used with caution in patients with renal or hepatic impairment; it should not be used in those with severe renal impairment. In some countries ketoprofen is also considered to be contra-indicated in patients with heart failure; however, evidence that ketoprofen is any more likely than other NSAIDs to precipitate or aggravate heart failure (see p.67) seems to be lacking.

Dexketoprofen should be avoided in patients with moderate to severe renal or severe hepatic impairment, and in those with severe heart failure.

**Hypersensitivity.** Life-threatening asthma, urticaria, and angioedema developed in 2 aspirin-sensitive patients after taking ketoprofen 50 mg by mouth.[1] Cardiac and respiratory arrest occurred in an asthmatic patient shortly after taking ketoprofen.[2] There has been a report[3] of delayed skin hypersensitivity in a patient who used a topical gel containing ketoprofen. The reaction recurred on rechallenge to ketoprofen gel but not to a similar gel containing diclofenac. The authors of the report noted that the UK Committee on Safety of Medicines had received 15 reports of skin reactions to ketoprofen gel, including two each of dermatitis and urticaria.


1. Frith P, *et al.* Life-threatening asthma, urticaria, and angiœdema after ketoprofen. *Lancet* 1978; **ii:** 847–8.
2. Schreuder G. Ketoprofen: possible idiosyncratic acute bronchospasm. *Med J Aust* 1990; **152:** 332–3.
3. Oh VMS. Ketoprofen gel and delayed hypersensitivity dermatitis. *BMJ* 1994; **309:** 512.


**Myasthenia gravis.** There has been a brief report[1] of a cholinergic crisis precipitated by a single dose of ketoprofen 50 mg by mouth in a patient with well-controlled myasthenia gravis. The patient had previously noted a similar but milder reaction with aspirin, but not with paracetamol.


1. McDowell IFW, McConnell JB. Cholinergic crisis in myasthenia gravis precipitated by ketoprofen. *BMJ* 1985; **291:** 1094.


**Pancreatitis.** A report of pancreatitis associated with ketoprofen.[1]


1. Cobb TK, Pierce JR. Acute pancreatitis associated with ketoprofen. *South Med J* 1992; **85:** 430–1.


**Photosensitivity.** Ketoprofen causes photosensitivity reactions[1,2] and cross-sensitivity to other drugs, notably the fibrates bezafibrate, ciprofibrate, and fenofibrate, has also been reported. The cross reactions were attributed to the benzoyl ketone structure that the drugs have in common.


1. Bagheri H, *et al.* Photosensitivity to ketoprofen: mechanisms and pharmacoepidemiological data. *Drug Safety* 2000; **22:** 339–49.
2. Veyrac G, *et al.* Bilan de l'enquête nationale sur les effets indésirables cutanés du kétoprofène gel enregistrés entre le 01/09/1996 et le 31/08/2000. *Therapie* 2002; **57:** 55–64.


**Renal impairment.** The elimination half-life and unbound plasma concentrations of dexketoprofen are increased in patients with renal impairment given racemic ketoprofen;[1,2] this appears to be principally attributable to impaired renal clearance of the acyl-glucuronide conjugates in a stereoselective fashion, with subsequent hydrolysis of the unstable conjugate back to the aglycone producing increased plasma-ketoprofen concentrations.[2,3] It has been suggested[3] that dosage adjustments of racemic ketoprofen are indicated only for patients with moderately severe renal failure (creatinine clearance of less than 20 mL/minute).


1. Hayball PJ, *et al.* The influence of renal function on the enantioselective pharmacokinetics and pharmacodynamics of ketoprofen in patients with rheumatoid arthritis. *Br J Clin Pharmacol* 1993; **36:** 185–93.
2. Grubb NG, *et al.* Stereoselective pharmacokinetics of ketoprofen and ketoprofen glucuronide in end-stage renal disease: evidence for a 'futile cycle' of elimination. *Br J Clin Pharmacol* 1999; **48:** 494–500.
3. Skeith KJ, *et al.* The influence of renal function on the pharmacokinetics of unchanged and acyl-glucuroconjugated ketoprofen enantiomers after 50 and 100 mg racemic ketoprofen. *Br J Clin Pharmacol* 1996; **42:** 163–9.


## Interactions

For interactions associated with NSAIDs, see p.69.

Probenecid delays the excretion of ketoprofen and decreases its extent of protein binding resulting in increased plasma-ketoprofen concentrations.

## Pharmacokinetics

Ketoprofen is readily absorbed from the gastrointestinal tract; peak plasma concentrations occur about 0.5 to 2 hours after a dose. When ketoprofen is given with food, the bioavailability is not altered but the rate of absorption is slowed. Ketoprofen is well absorbed from the intramuscular and rectal routes; only a small amount of ketoprofen is absorbed following topical application. Ketoprofen is 99% bound to plasma proteins and substantial concentrations of drug are found in the synovial fluid. The elimination half-life in plasma is about 1.5 to 4 hours. Ketoprofen is metabolised mainly by conjugation with glucuronic acid, and is excreted mainly in the urine.

Ketoprofen possesses a chiral centre. It is usually given as the racemate but its pharmacological actions appear to be due largely to the (*S*)-enantiomer, dexketoprofen. The pharmacokinetics of ketoprofen appear to exhibit little stereoselectivity (but see under Renal Impairment, above).

◊ References.


1. Debruyne D, *et al.* Clinical pharmacokinetics of ketoprofen after single intravenous administration as a bolus or infusion. *Clin Pharmacokinet* 1987; **12:** 214–21.
2. Flouvat B, *et al.* Pharmacokinetics of ketoprofen in man after repeated percutaneous administration. *Arzneimittelforschung* 1989; **39:** 812–15.
3. Jamali F, Brocks DR. Clinical pharmacokinetics of ketoprofen and its enantiomers. *Clin Pharmacokinet* 1990; **19:** 197–217.
4. Geisslinger G, *et al.* Pharmacokinetics of ketoprofen enantiomers after different doses of the racemate. *Br J Clin Pharmacol* 1995; **40:** 73–5.
5. Barbanoj MJ, *et al.* Pharmacokinetics of dexketoprofen trometamol in healthy volunteers after single and repeated oral doses. *J Clin Pharmacol* 1998; **38:** 33S–40S.
6. Kokki H, *et al.* Pharmacokinetics of ketoprofen syrup in small children. *J Clin Pharmacol* 2000; **40:** 354–9.
7. Barbanoj M-J, *et al.* Clinical pharmacokinetics of dexketoprofen. *Clin Pharmacokinet* 2001; **40:** 245–62.


## Uses and Administration

Ketoprofen, a propionic acid derivative, is an NSAID (p.70). Its anti-inflammatory properties may be weaker than those of some other NSAIDs. Ketoprofen is a racemic mixture; in *animal* studies the S-(+) enantiomer, dexketoprofen, has approximately twice the analgesic activity of ketoprofen by weight.

Ketoprofen is used in musculoskeletal and joint disorders such as ankylosing spondylitis, osteoarthritis, and rheumatoid arthritis, and in peri-articular disorders such as bursitis and tendinitis. It is also used in dysmenorrhoea, postoperative pain, in painful and inflammatory conditions such as acute gout or soft-tissue disorders, and to reduce fever. Dexketoprofen is used in the treatment of mild to moderate pain such as musculoskeletal pain, dysmenorrhoea, or dental pain.

In the treatment of rheumatic disorders a usual daily dose of *ketoprofen* by mouth is 100 to 200 mg in 2 to 4 divided doses; modified-release formulations taken once daily may also be used. In the USA some manufacturers suggest initial oral doses of 75 mg three times daily or 50 mg four times daily increased as needed to a maximum of 300 mg daily in divided doses. Ketoprofen may also be given rectally as suppositories in a usual dose of 100 mg at night. In the UK, it is recommended that the total daily combined dose by mouth and by rectum should not exceed 200 mg. The dose by mouth for the treatment of other painful conditions including dysmenorrhoea is 25 to 50 mg every 6 to 8 hours.

Ketoprofen may be given by deep intramuscular injection into the gluteal muscle for acute exacerbations of musculoskeletal, joint, peri-articular and soft-tissue disorders and in the management of pain following orthopaedic surgery. Doses of 50 to 100 mg may be given every 4 hours, up to a maximum dose of 200 mg in 24 hours for up to 3 days.

Ketoprofen may be applied as a 2.5% gel for local pain relief. Doses vary slightly between preparations: a typical regimen is application 2 or 3 times daily for up to 10 days.

*Dexketoprofen* is given by mouth as the trometamol salt. Doses are expressed in terms of the base; dexketoprofen trometamol 36.9 mg is approximately equivalent to 25 mg of dexketoprofen. Usual doses are 12.5 mg every 4 to 6 hours or 25 mg every 8 hours; the total daily dose should not exceed 75 mg. Elderly patients should be started on a total daily dose not exceeding 50 mg. Dose reductions are also necessary in patients with hepatic or renal impairment, see below.

Ketoprofen has also been used as the lysine and as the sodium salt.

◊ Reviews.


1. Mauleón D, *et al.* Preclinical and clinical development of dexketoprofen. *Drugs* 1996; **52:** 24–46.


**Administration in hepatic or renal impairment.** The manufacturers of dexketoprofen recommend a reduced initial daily dose of 50 mg in patients with mild to moderate hepatic or mild renal impairment. Dexketoprofen should not be used in patients with severe hepatic or moderate to severe renal impairment.

### Preparations

***BP 2003:*** Ketoprofen Capsules; Ketoprofen Gel.

**Proprietary Preparations** (details are given in Part 3)
***Arg.:*** Enantyum; Helenil; Orudis; Profenid; Salicrem K; ***Austral.:*** Orudis; Oruvail; ***Austria:*** Actron; Keprodol; Profenid; Prontoket; Toprek†; ***Belg.:*** Birofenid; Fastum; Rofenid; Toprek†; ***Braz.:*** Algiprofen†; Artrinid; Artrosil; Bi-Profenid; Ceprofen; Keduril†; Ketop; Profenid; ***Canad.:*** Apo-Keto; Novo-Keto; Orafen; Orudis; Oruvail†; Rhodis; Rhovail; ***Chile:*** Dolo-Ketazon; Dolofar; Fastum; Flogofin; Profenid; Relatene; Talflex; ***Denm.:*** Orofen; Orudis; ***Fin.:*** Keto; Ketofen†; Ketomex; Ketorin; Orudis; Zon; ***Fr.:*** Actroneffix†; Bi-Profenid; Ketum; Profenid; Topfena; Toprec; ***Ger.:*** Alrheumun; Gabrilen; Ketolist; Orudis; Spondylon; Sympal; ***Gr.:*** Farbovil; Nosatel; Oruvail; ***Hong Kong:*** Apo-Keto†; Fastum; Orudis; Oruvail; ***Irl.:*** Fastum; Keral; Orudis; Orugesic; Oruvail; ***Israel:*** Ketonal; Oruvail; Profenid; ***Ital.:*** Alket; Artrosilene; Desketo; Dolgosin; Enantyum; Euketos; Fastum; Flexen; Ibifen; Ketalgesic†; Ketartrium; Ketesse; Ketodol; Ketofen†; Ketoplus; Ketoselect; Meprofen; Oki; Orudis; Reuprofen; Sinketol†; Toprek; Zepelindue; ***Jpn:*** Mohrus; ***Malaysia:*** Apo-Keto; Fastum; Kenhancer; Orudis; Oruvail; Provail; ***Mex.:*** Efiken; K-Profen; Keduril; Kezer†; Orudis; Piketofen†; Profenid; ***Neth.:*** Orudis; Oscorel; ***Norw.:*** Orudis; ***NZ:*** Kefen†; Orudis; Oruvail; ***Port.:*** Artrofene; Deflogix; Fastum; Ketesse; Ketofene; Profenid; ***S.Afr.:*** Fastum; Ketoflam; Myproflam; Orucote; Oruject; Oruvail; ***Singapore:*** Apo-Keto; Fastum; Kefentech; Kenhancer; Ketotop; Oruvail; Provail; ***Spain:*** Adolquir; Arcental; Badyket; Enangel; Enantyum; Extraplus; Fastum; Ketesse; Ketosolan; Orudis; Quiralam; Quirgel; Reumoquin†; ***Swed.:*** Orudis; Prodon; Siduro; Zon; ***Switz.:*** Fastum; Ketesse; Orudis†; ***Thai.:*** Fastum; Oruvail; Profenid; Rofepain; ***UK:*** Fenoket†; Jomethid†; Keral; Ketil; Ketocid; Ketotard†; Ketovail; Ketozip; Larafen; Orudis; Oruvail; Powergel; Solpaflex†; ***USA:*** Actron†; Orudis; Oruvail.

**Multi-ingredient: *Mex.:*** Bifebral; Reumophan.

---

## Ketorolac Trometamol *(BANM, rINNM)*

Ketorolac Tromethamine *(USAN)*; Ketorolaco trometamol; RS-37619-00-31-3. (±)-5-Benzoyl-2,3-dihydro-1*H*-pyrrolizine-1-carboxylic acid compound with 2-amino-2-(hydroxymethyl)-1,3-propanediol (1 : 1).

$C_{19}H_{24}N_2O_6$ = 376.4.

*CAS — 74103-06-3 (ketorolac); 74103-07-4 (ketorolac trometamol).*

*ATC — M01AB15; S01BC05.*

**Pharmacopoeias.** In *US.*

**USP 27** (Ketorolac Tromethamine). A white to off-white, crystalline powder. Freely soluble in water and in methyl alcohol; slightly soluble in alcohol, in dehydrated alcohol, and in tetrahydrofuran; practically insoluble in acetone, in acetonitrile, in butyl alcohol, in dichloromethane, in dioxan, in ethyl acetate, in hexane, and in toluene. pH of a 1% solution in water is between 5.7 and 6.7. Store in airtight containers at a temperature of 25°, excursions permitted between 15° and 30°. Protect from light.

### Adverse Effects

As for NSAIDs in general, p.67.

Concern over the high incidence of reported adverse effects with ketorolac trometamol has led to its withdrawal in some countries while in others its permitted dosage and maximum duration of treatment have been reduced. Adverse effects reported include gastrointestinal disturbances including gastrointestinal bleeding (especially in the elderly), perforation, and peptic ulceration. Hypersensitivity reactions such as anaphylaxis, rash, bronchospasm, laryngeal oedema, and hypotension have also occurred. Other adverse effects reported include drowsiness, dizziness, headache, mental and sensory changes, psychotic reactions, sweating, dry mouth, thirst, fever, convulsions, myalgia, aseptic meningitis, hypertension, dyspnoea, pulmonary oedema, bradycardia, chest pain, palpitations, fluid retention, increases in blood urea and creatinine, acute renal failure, oedema, hyponatraemia, hyperkalaemia, urinary frequency or retention, nephrotic syndrome, flank pain with or without haematuria, purpura, thrombocytopenia, epistaxis, inhibition of platelet aggregation, increased bleeding time, postoperative wound haemorrhage, haematoma, flushing or pallor, and pancreatitis. Severe skin reactions including Stevens-Johnson syndrome and Lyell's syndrome have been reported. Liver function changes may occur; hepatitis and liver failure have been reported. There may be pain at the site of injection.

Ketorolac eye drops may produce transient stinging and other minor symptoms of ocular irritation. As with some other NSAIDs used in the eye, ketorolac has been implicated in reports of corneal toxicity (see p.32).

◊ Adverse effects reported with ketorolac are mainly those common to all NSAIDs with gastrointestinal reactions being the most frequent followed by haematological, renal, hypersensitivity, and then neurological reactions. From 1990 to 1993, 97 reactions with a fatal outcome were reported worldwide.[1] The causes of death were: gastrointestinal bleeding or perforation (47 cases); renal impairment or insufficiency (20); anaphylaxis or asthma (7); haemorrhagic reactions (4); and unexplained or miscellaneous causes (19). Concern over the safety of ketorolac has led to adverse reactions being monitored closely and to the implementation of restrictions on dose and duration of treatment (see under Uses and Administration, below). A postmarketing surveillance study[2] examined the risks of parenteral ketorolac in 9 900 patients who received 10 272 courses of ketorolac. The results indicated a dose-response relationship with average daily ketorolac dose for both gastrointestinal bleeding and operative site bleeding, the expected major risks, and an association between gastrointestinal bleeding and therapy for over 5 days. The risk of serious gastrointestinal bleeding and operative site bleeding was higher for elderly patients [the manufacturer recommends that the elderly should not receive daily parenteral doses greater than 60 mg]. Although the overall associations between ketorolac use and both gastrointestinal bleeding and operative site bleeding are small, the risk becomes clinically important as doses increase, in elderly patients, and, for gastrointestinal bleeding only, when used for longer than 5 days. The US manufacturer has consequently emphasised that ketorolac is a potent NSAID and is indicated only for the short-term management of moderate to severe pain and not for minor or chronic painful conditions; its administration carries many risks and related adverse effects can be serious especially when used inappropriately. After examining data from the above study the EU Committee for Proprietary Medicinal Products adopted the opinion that ketorolac had a narrow therapeutic margin but that it was indicated for the short-term management of moderate to severe acute postoperative pain.

Further references to ketorolac's adverse effects are given below.[3-12]


1. Committee on Safety of Medicines/Medicines Control Agency. Ketorolac: new restrictions on dose and duration of treatment. *Current Problems* 1993; **19:** 5–6.
2. Strom BL, *et al.* Parenteral ketorolac and risk of gastrointestinal and operative site bleeding: a postmarketing surveillance study. *JAMA* 1996; **275:** 376–82.
3. Rotenberg FA, Giannini VS. Hyperkalemia associated with ketorolac. *Ann Pharmacother* 1992; **26:** 778–9.
4. Boras-Uber LA, Brackett NC. Ketorolac-induced acute renal failure. *Am J Med* 1992; **92:** 450–2. Correction *ibid.*; **93:** 117.
5. Schoch PH, *et al.* Acute renal failure in an elderly woman following intramuscular ketorolac administration. *Ann Pharmacother* 1992; **26:** 1233–6.
6. Goetz CM, *et al.* Anaphylactoid reaction following ketorolac tromethamine administration. *Ann Pharmacother* 1992; **26:** 1237–8.
7. Randi ML, *et al.* Haemolytic uraemic syndrome during treatment with ketorolac trometamol. *BMJ* 1993; **306:** 186.
8. Fong J, Gora ML. Reversible renal insufficiency following ketorolac therapy. *Ann Pharmacother* 1993; **27:** 510–12.
9. Corelli RL, Gericke KR. Renal insufficiency associated with intramuscular administration of ketorolac tromethamine. *Ann Pharmacother* 1993; **27:** 1055–7.
10. Buck ML, Norwood VF. Ketorolac-induced acute renal failure in a previously healthy adolescent. *Pediatrics* 1996; **98:** 294–6.
11. Feldman HI, *et al.* Parenteral ketorolac: the risk for acute renal failure. *Ann Intern Med* 1997; **126:** 193–9.
12. Reinhart DJ, *et al.* Minimising the adverse effects of ketorolac. *Drug Safety* 2000; **22:** 487–97.


### Precautions

As for NSAIDs in general, p.69.

In light of the concern over the toxicity of ketorolac it has been recommended that it should not be used during pregnancy or labour and that it should not be given to mothers who are breast feeding.

Ketorolac is contra-indicated in patients with a history of hypersensitivity to aspirin or other NSAIDs, a history of asthma, nasal polyps, bronchospasm, or angioedema, a history of peptic ulceration or gastrointestinal bleeding, in patients with moderate or severe renal impairment, and in those with hypovolaemia or dehydration. Ketorolac should not be given to patients with coagulation or haemorrhagic disorders or those with confirmed or suspected cerebrovascular bleeding. It is contra-indicated as a prophylactic analgesic before surgery and for intraoperative use because of its inhibitory effects on platelets; it should also not be given postoperatively to those who have undergone procedures with a high risk of haemorrhage.

The dose of ketorolac should be reduced in the elderly and in patients weighing less than 50 kg. It is recommended that patients with mild renal impairment should receive a reduced dose of ketorolac and undergo close monitoring of renal function. Ketorolac should be used with caution in heart failure, hepatic impairment and conditions leading to reduction in blood volume or in renal blood flow. Ketorolac should be withdrawn if clinical symptoms of liver disease develop.

Dizziness may affect the performance of skilled tasks such as driving.

**Breast feeding.** The American Academy of Pediatrics[1] states that there have been no reports of any clinical effect on the infant associated with the use of ketorolac by breast-feeding mothers, and that therefore it may be considered to be usually compatible with breast feeding. However, the *British National Formulary* and both the UK and US manufacturers recommend that ketorolac should be avoided in mothers who are breast-feeding.

A study[2] concluded that the concentration of ketorolac distributed into breast milk was very low and the amount ingested by the infant would probably be too small to be harmful.


1. American Academy of Pediatrics. The transfer of drugs and other chemicals into human milk. *Pediatrics* 2001; **108:** 776–89. Correction. *ibid.*; 1029. Also available at: http://aappolicy.aappublications.org/cgi/content/full/pediatrics%3b108/3/776 (accessed 05/07/04)
2. Wischnik A, *et al.* The excretion of ketorolac tromethamine into breast milk after multiple oral dosing. *Eur J Clin Pharmacol* 1989; **36:** 521–4.


### Interactions

For interactions associated with NSAIDs, see p.69.

Ketorolac should not be given to patients already receiving anticoagulants or to those who will require prophylactic anticoagulant therapy, including low-dose heparin. The risk of ketorolac-associated bleeding is also increased by other NSAIDs or aspirin and by pentoxifylline and concomitant use should be avoided. Probenecid increases the half-life and plasma concentrations of ketorolac and the two drugs should not be given together.

**Parasympathomimetics.** The manufacturer of acetylcholine chloride ophthalmic preparations has stated that there have been reports that *acetylcholine* and *carbachol* have been ineffective when used in patients treated with topical (ophthalmic) NSAIDs.

### Pharmacokinetics

Ketorolac trometamol is absorbed after intramuscular or oral doses. At physiological pH ketorolac trometamol dissociates to form an anionic ketorolac molecule which is less hydrophilic than the trometamol salt. The peak plasma concentration of ketorolac is reached within about 30 to 60 minutes; absorption after intramuscular injection may be slower than that after oral doses in some individuals. Ketorolac is over 99% bound to plasma protein. It does not readily penetrate the blood-brain barrier. Ketorolac crosses the placenta and small amounts of drug are distributed into breast milk. The terminal plasma half-life is about 4 to 6 hours, but is about 6 to 7 hours in the elderly and 9 to 10 hours in patients with renal dysfunction. The major metabolic pathway is glucuronic acid conjugation; there is some *para*-hydroxylation. About 90% of a dose is excreted in urine as unchanged drug and conjugated and hydroxylated metabolites, the remainder is excreted in the faeces.

### Uses and Administration

Ketorolac, a pyrrolizine carboxylic acid derivative structurally related to indometacin (p.48), is an NSAID (p.70). It is used principally as an analgesic.

Ketorolac is used intramuscularly, intravenously, or orally as the trometamol salt in the short-term management of moderate to severe **postoperative pain**. However, it should be noted that because of concerns over the high incidence of reported adverse effects with ketorolac its dosage and maximum duration of use are restricted. The recommended maximum duration for parenteral therapy is 2 days in the UK, and patients should be transferred to oral therapy as soon as possible. In the USA it is recommended that the maximum combined duration of use of parenteral and oral ketorolac should not exceed 5 days.

- In the UK the recommended initial dose by the *parenteral* route is 10 mg of ketorolac trometamol followed by 10 to 30 mg every 4 to 6 hours as required, although ketorolac may be given as often as every 2 hours in the initial postoperative period if required. The total maximum daily dose is 90 mg (60 mg in the elderly, patients with mild renal impairment, and in those weighing less than 50 kg). Intravenous injections should be given over at least 15 seconds. During transfer from parenteral to oral therapy the combined daily dose for all forms of ketorolac trometamol should not exceed 90 mg (60 mg in the elderly, patients with mild renal impairment, and in those weighing less than 50 kg) of which no more than 40 mg should be given orally.
- Regimens in use in the USA include a single intramuscular dose of 60 mg or a single intravenous dose of 30 mg, or a multiple-dose regimen comprising 30 mg every 6 hours intramuscularly or intravenously, up to a maximum of 120 mg daily. These doses should be halved in the elderly, those with renal impairment, and those weighing less than 50 kg. Children aged between 2 to 16 years may be given a single intramuscular dose of 1 mg/kg up to a maximum of 30 mg or a single intravenous dose of 0.5 mg/kg up to a maximum of 15 mg.
- The recommended *oral* dose in the UK is 10 mg every 4 to 6 hours (every 6 to 8 hours in the elderly) to a maximum of 40 mg daily for a maximum duration of 7 days.
- In the USA the recommended oral dose is 20 mg (10 mg in the elderly, the renally impaired, and those weighing under 50 kg), followed by 10 mg every 4 to 6 hours to a maximum of 40 mg daily.

Ketorolac trometamol is used as 0.5% eye drops to relieve **ocular itching** associated with seasonal allergic conjunctivitis. Ketorolac trometamol eye drops 0.5% have also been used for the topical treatment of **cystoid macular oedema** and for the prevention and reduction of **inflammation** associated with ocular surgery. In the USA, a 0.4% eye drop is also available for postoperative ocular inflammation.

◊ Reviews.


1. Gillis JC, Brogden RN. Ketorolac: a reappraisal of its pharmacodynamic and pharmacokinetic properties and therapeutic use in pain management. *Drugs* 1997; **53:** 139–88.


**Administration in renal impairment.** Ketorolac is contra-indicated in patients with moderate to severe renal impairment; for suggested doses in less advanced renal impairment see Uses and Administration, above.

### Preparations

***USP 27:*** Ketorolac Tromethamine Injection; Ketorolac Tromethamine Tablets.

**Proprietary Preparations** (details are given in Part 3)
***Arg.:*** Acular; Dolten; Kelac; Kemanat; Kerarer; Ketopharm; Klenac; Nolarac; Poenkerat; Sinalgico; Tenkdol; ***Austral.:*** Acular; Toradol; ***Austria:*** Acular; ***Belg.:*** Aculare; Taradyl; ***Braz.:*** Acular; Cetrolac; ***Canad.:*** Acular; Toradol; ***Chile:*** Acular; Brodifac; Burten; Dilox; Dolgenal; Findedol; Netaf; Poenkerat; Syndol; ***Denm.:*** Acular; Toradol; ***Fin.:*** Acular; Toradol; ***Fr.:*** Acular; ***Ger.:*** Acular; ***Hong Kong:*** Acular; Toradol; ***India:*** Cadolac; Ketanov; Ketlur; Ketonic; Torolac; ***Irl.:*** Acular; ***Israel:*** Topadol; ***Ital.:*** Acular; Lixidol; Tora-Dol; ***Malaysia:*** Acular; Ketanov; Keto; ***Mex.:*** Acularen; Alidol; Celfax; Dolac; Dolotor; Estopein; Findol; Glicima; Onemer; Supradol; Toloran; Toral; Tromedal; ***Norw.:*** Toradol; ***NZ:*** Acular; ***Port.:*** Acular; Toradol; ***S.Afr.:*** Acular; Tora-Dol; ***Singapore:*** Acular; Keto; Toradol; ***Spain:*** Acular; Algikey; Droal; Tonum; Toradol; ***Swed.:*** Toradol; ***Switz.:*** Acular; Tora-Dol; ***Thai.:*** Acular; ***UK:*** Acular; Toradol; ***USA:*** Acular; Toradol.

## Lefetamine Hydrochloride *(rINNM)*

Hidrocloruro de lefetamina. (−)-*N*,*N*-Dimethyl-1,2-diphenylethylamine hydrochloride.
$C_{16}H_{19}N,HCl$ = 261.8.
*CAS — 7262-75-1 (lefetamine); 14148-99-3 (lefetamine hydrochloride).*

### Profile

Lefetamine hydrochloride has analgesic properties and has been given by intramuscular or subcutaneous injection.

### Preparations

**Proprietary Preparations** (details are given in Part 3)
***Ital.:*** Santenol†.

## Leflunomide *(BAN, USAN, rINN)*

HWA-486; Leflunomida; SU-101. α,α,α-Trifluoro-5-methyl-4-isoxazolecarboxy-*p*-toluidide.
$C_{12}H_9F_3N_2O_2$ = 270.2.
*CAS — 75706-12-6.*
*ATC — L04AA13.*

### Adverse Effects, Treatment and Precautions

Common adverse effects seen with leflunomide are hypertension, gastrointestinal disturbances, weight loss, headache, dizziness, asthenia, paraesthesia, joint disorders and synovitis, alopecia, eczema, and dry skin. Leucopenia may occur. Hypersensitivity reactions may occur and a few cases of Stevens-Johnson syndrome or toxic epidermal necrolysis have been reported. Hepatotoxicity has occurred. It is usually mild and reversible but rare cases of severe, sometimes fatal, liver disease, including acute hepatic necrosis, have been observed particularly in the first 6 months of therapy. There have been occasional reports of pancreatitis, interstitial lung disease, and severe infections, including fatal sepsis.

The active metabolite of leflunomide, A771726, has a half-life of about 2 weeks. Consequently the adverse effects of leflunomide may continue even after therapy has been stopped. When severe reactions occur, a drug washout procedure (see below) may be required.

Leflunomide should not be given to immunocompromised patients or to patients with severe infections, hepatic or moderate to severe renal impairment, severe hypoproteinaemia, or bone-marrow dysplasia. Patients with a history of tuberculosis should be carefully monitored because of the possibility of reactivation of the infection. Intra-uterine devices should be used with caution during immunosuppressive treatment as there is an increased risk of infection. Live vaccines should be avoided for the same reason. Blood pressure and blood counts should be monitored regularly during therapy.

In the UK liver enzyme values should be checked before beginning therapy and at fortnightly intervals during the first 6 months of treatment; the US manufacturer recommends monthly monitoring for the first 6 months. Subsequent monitoring should be carried out at 6- to 8-week intervals. Dosage should be reduced if moderate elevations of liver enzyme values occur (see below); for persistent or more severe elevations leflunomide should be stopped and washout procedures begun. Monitoring of liver enzymes should be continued after stopping therapy until they return to within the normal range. Blood counts should also be checked at the same time as liver enzyme values.

**Pregnancy.** Leflunomide is contra-indicated during pregnancy as its active metabolite has been shown to be teratogenic in *animals*. Women wishing to become pregnant should wait for 2 years after discontinuation of therapy, or if this is infeasible, a washout procedure should be performed and a waiting period of six weeks be observed from the time plasma concentrations of the metabolite fall below 20 nanograms/mL before attempting conception. A washout procedure is also recommended in men who wish to father children, and should be carried out if a patient becomes pregnant during therapy.

**Washout procedure.** If serious adverse effects occur during leflunomide therapy, the manufacturers recommend that a drug washout procedure is performed. This may also be considered if a patient becomes pregnant while taking leflunomide, or if it is necessary to swap to another disease-modifying antirheumatic drug.

For the washout procedure, either 8 g colestyramine is given by mouth 3 times daily or 50 g of activated charcoal is given by mouth 4 times daily. Therapy is normally continued for 11 days, but should be repeated until verified plasma concentrations of the primary metabolite A771726 are below 20 nanograms/mL.

### Interactions

Use of leflunomide with other hepatotoxic or haematotoxic drugs should be avoided; if a patient is to be transferred to treatment with another hepatotoxic or haematotoxic antirheumatic drug such as methotrexate a drug washout procedure (above) should be performed first. See above for precautions about use with live vaccines.

**Anticoagulants.** For reference to the effects of leflunomide on the activity of *warfarin*, see under Immunosuppressants, p.1027.

### Pharmacokinetics

After oral doses leflunomide undergoes first-pass metabolism to A771726 (teriflunomide), which is responsible for the majority of the *in vivo* activity. The bioavailability of leflunomide after oral doses ranges from 82 to 95%. Peak plasma concentrations of the active metabolite may occur from 1 to 24 hours after a dose. A771726 has an elimination half-life of approximately 2 weeks, which is thought to be mainly due to enterohepatic recycling. Colestyramine or activated charcoal are able to interrupt recycling and can therefore accelerate drug elimination.

A771726 is more than 99% bound to plasma proteins. It is metabolised in the gut wall and the liver. Approximately 43% of a dose is eliminated in the urine, mainly as glucuronides, and 48% is eliminated in the faeces via the bile.

◊ References.


1. Rozman B. Clinical pharmacokinetics of leflunomide. *Clin Pharmacokinet* 2002; **41:** 421–30.


### Uses and Administration

Leflunomide has immunosuppressant and antiproliferative properties. It is used as a disease-modifying antirheumatic drug in the treatment of active rheumatoid arthritis (p.9). It is also used in the treatment of active psoriatic arthritis (p.11) and is being investigated in the management of various solid neoplasms.

Because of the long half-life of the principal metabolite a loading dose of leflunomide is required to reach steady-state concentrations relatively rapidly. Therapy for rheumatoid arthritis should be begun with a loading dose of 100 mg once daily by mouth for 3 days. The maintenance dose is 10 to 20 mg once daily for rheumatoid arthritis and 20 mg once daily for psoriatic arthritis. Dose adjustments may be necessary in patients who develop abnormal liver enzyme values, see below. The therapeutic effect usually starts after 4 to 6 weeks of therapy and further improvements may occur for up to 6 months.

◊ References.


1. Hudes G. Signaling inhibitors in the clinic: new agents and new challenges. *J Clin Oncol* 1999; **17:** 1093–4.
2. Strand V, *et al.* Treatment of active rheumatoid arthritis with leflunomide compared with placebo and methotrexate. *Arch Intern Med* 1999; **159:** 2542–50.
3. Prakash A, Jarvis B. Leflunomide: a review of its use in active rheumatoid arthritis. *Drugs* 1999; **58:** 1137–64.
4. Emery P, *et al.* A comparison of the efficacy and safety of leflunomide and methotrexate for the treatment of rheumatoid arthritis. *Rheumatology (Oxford)* 2000; **39:** 655–65.
5. Cohen S, *et al.* Two-year, blinded, randomized, controlled trial of treatment of active rheumatoid arthritis with leflunomide compared with methotrexate. *Arthritis Rheum* 2001; **44:** 1984–92.
6. Scott DL, *et al.* Treatment of active rheumatoid arthritis with leflunomide: two year follow up of a double blind, placebo controlled trial versus sulfasalazine. *Ann Rheum Dis* 2001; **60:** 913–23.
7. Williams JW, *et al.* Experiences with leflunomide in solid organ transplantation. *Transplantation* 2002; **73:** 358–66.
8. McCarey DW, *et al.* Leflunomide in treatment of rheumatoid arthritis. *Lancet* 2002; **359:** 1158.
9. Kiely PD, Johnson DM. Infliximab and leflunomide combination therapy in rheumatoid arthritis: an open-label study. *Rheumatology (Oxford)* 2002; **41:** 631–7.
10. Kremer JM, *et al.* Concomitant leflunomide therapy in patients with active rheumatoid arthritis despite stable doses of methotrexate: a randomized, double-blind, placebo-controlled trial. *Ann Intern Med* 2002; **137:** 726–33.
11. Miceli-Richard C, Dougados M. Leflunomide for the treatment of rheumatoid arthritis. *Expert Opin Pharmacother* 2003; **4:** 987–97.


**Administration in hepatic impairment.** Leflunomide is contra-indicated in patients with hepatic impairment. Patients who develop moderate elevations of liver enzyme values while receiving leflunomide treatment should have their dose reduced to 10 mg daily; if necessary, monitoring of liver enzyme values should also be performed at weekly intervals. If moderate elevations persist or if severe elevations occur, leflunomide should be discontinued and washout procedures started (see above).

### Preparations

**Proprietary Preparations** (details are given in Part 3)
***Arg.:*** Arava; Filartros; Inmunoartro; Molagar; ***Austral.:*** Arava; ***Belg.:*** Arava; ***Braz.:*** Arava; ***Canad.:*** Arava; ***Chile:*** Arava; ***Denm.:*** Arava; ***Fin.:*** Arava; ***Fr.:*** Arava; ***Ger.:*** Arava; ***Gr.:*** Arava; ***Hong Kong:*** Arava; ***India:*** Arava; ***Irl.:*** Arava; ***Israel:*** Arava; ***Ital.:*** Arava; ***Malaysia:*** Arava; ***Mex.:*** Arava; ***Neth.:*** Arava; ***Norw.:*** Arava; ***NZ:*** Arava; ***Port.:*** Arava; ***S.Afr.:*** Ar-

ava; **Singapore:** Arava; **Spain:** Arava; **Swed.:** Arava; **Switz.:** Arava; **Thai.:** Arava; **UK:** Arava; **USA:** Arava.

## Levacetylmethadol *(rINN)*

*l*-α-Acetylmethadol; LAAM (levacetylmethadol or levacetylmethadol hydrochloride); LAM; Levacetilmetadol; Levomethadyl Acetate *(USAN)*; *l*-Methadyl Acetate. (−)-4-Dimethylamino-1-ethyl-2,2-diphenylpentyl acetate.

$C_{23}H_{31}NO_2$ = 353.5.

*CAS — 1477-40-3 (levomethadyl); 34433-66-4 (levacetylmethadol).*

*ATC — N07BC03.*

## Levacetylmethadol Hydrochloride *(rINNM)*

LAAM (levacetylmethadol or levacetylmethadol hydrochloride); Levomethadyl Acetate Hydrochloride *(USAN)*; MK-790-. (−)-(3S,6S)-6-(Dimethylamino)-4,4-diphenyl-3-heptanol acetate hydrochloride.

$C_{23}H_{31}NO_2,HCl$ = 390.0.

*CAS — 43033-72-3.*

*ATC — N07BC03.*

### Profile

Levacetylmethadol, a diphenylheptane derivative, is a long-acting opioid analgesic (p.73); it is a derivative of methadone (p.58). It was used in the management of opioid dependence. However, the proarrhythmic effects led to its withdrawal in the European Union and the USA.

◊ References.

1. Eissenberg T, *et al.* Dose-related efficacy of levomethadyl acetate for treatment of opioid dependence: a randomized clinical trial. *JAMA* 1997; **277:** 1945–51.

### Preparations

**Proprietary Preparations** (details are given in Part 3)
**Denm.:** OrLAAM†; **Irl.:** OrLAAM†; **Spain:** OrLAAM†; **UK:** OrLAAM†; **USA:** OrLAAM†.

## Levomethadone Hydrochloride *(rINNM)*

Hidrocloruro de levometadona; Levomethadoni Hydrochloridum; (−)-Methadone Hydrochloride. (−)-6-Dimethylamino-4,4-diphenylheptan-3-one hydrochloride.

$C_{21}H_{27}NO,HCl$ = 345.9.

*CAS — 125-58-6 (levomethadone); 5967-73-7 (levomethadone hydrochloride).*

**Pharmacopoeias.** In *Eur.* (see p.vi).

**Ph. Eur. 5.0** (Levomethadone Hydrochloride). A white, crystalline powder. Soluble in water; freely soluble in alcohol. Protect from light.

### Profile

Levomethadone is an opioid analgesic (p.71). It is the active isomer of racemic methadone (p.57) and is used similarly as the hydrochloride in the treatment of severe pain.

### Preparations

**Proprietary Preparations** (details are given in Part 3)
**Ger.:** L-Polamidon.

## Levorphanol Tartrate *(BANM, rINNM)*

Levorphan Tartrate; Levorphanol Bitartrate; Methorphinan Tartrate; Tartrato de levorfanol. (−)-9a-Methylmorphinan-3-ol hydrogen tartrate dihydrate.

$C_{17}H_{23}NO,C_4H_6O_6,2H_2O$ = 443.5.

*CAS — 77-07-6 (levorphanol); 125-72-4 (anhydrous levorphanol tartrate); 5985-38-6 (levorphanol tartrate dihydrate).*

**Pharmacopoeias.** In *US.*

**USP 27** (Levorphanol Tartrate). A practically white, odourless, crystalline powder. Soluble 1 in 50 of water and 1 in 120 of alcohol; insoluble in chloroform and in ether. Store at a temperature of 25°, excursions permitted between 15° and 30°.

### Profile

Levorphanol tartrate, a phenanthrene derivative, is a potent opioid analgesic (p.71) used in the management of moderate to severe pain and for premedication. The analgesic effect usually begins about 10 to 60 minutes after oral administration and lasts up to about 8 hours.

In the management of pain a usual initial dose of levorphanol tartrate by mouth is 2 mg repeated in 3 to 8 hours if necessary. The maximum initial daily dose in non-opioid tolerant patients should not exceed 16 mg.

Levorphanol tartrate may be given by intramuscular or subcutaneous injection in initial doses of 1 to 2 mg, repeated in 6 to 8 hours if necessary. Levorphanol tartrate may also be given by slow intravenous injection in an initial dose of up to 1 mg in divided doses, repeated in 3 to 6 hours if necessary. The maximum initial daily dose by the parenteral route in non-opioid tolerant patients should not exceed 8 mg.

For premedication, a usual dose is 1 to 2 mg by intramuscular or subcutaneous injection given 60 to 90 minutes before surgery. Elderly or debilitated patients may require lower doses.

### Preparations

**USP 27:** Levorphanol Tartrate Injection; Levorphanol Tartrate Tablets.

**Proprietary Preparations** (details are given in Part 3)
**USA:** Levo-Dromoran.

## Lithium Salicylate

Salicilato de litio.

$C_7H_5LiO_3$ = 144.1.

*CAS — 552-38-5.*

### Profile

Lithium salicylate is a salicylic acid derivative (see Aspirin, p.15) that has been used in rheumatic disorders, but its use cannot be recommended because of the pharmacological effect of the lithium ion.

### Preparations

**Proprietary Preparations** (details are given in Part 3)
**Multi-ingredient: Fr.:** Antigoutteux Rezall†.

## Lonazolac Calcium *(rINNM)*

Lonazolaco cálcico. Calcium 3-(4-chlorophenyl)-1-phenylpyrazol-4-ylacetate.

$C_{34}H_{24}CaCl_2N_4O_4$ = 663.6.

*CAS — 53808-88-1 (lonazolac); 75821-71-5 (lonazolac calcium).*

*ATC — M01AB09.*

### Profile

Lonazolac calcium is an NSAID (p.67). It has been used in pain, inflammation, and musculoskeletal and joint disorders in usual doses of up to 600 mg daily, in divided doses, by mouth. Suppositories have also been given in doses of 400 mg twice daily.

### Preparations

**Proprietary Preparations** (details are given in Part 3)
**Austria:** Irritren; **Ger.:** Argun; arthro akut; Irritren†; **Hong Kong:** Irritren†; **Port.:** Atrilon.

## Lornoxicam *(BAN, USAN, rINN)*

Chlorotenoxicam; Chlortenoxicam; CTX; Ro-13-9297. 6-Chloro-4-hydroxy-2-methyl-*N*-2-pyridyl-2*H*-thieno[2,3-e][1,2]-thiazine-3-carboxamide 1,1-dioxide.

$C_{13}H_{10}ClN_3O_4S_2$ = 371.8.

*CAS — 70374-39-9.*

*ATC — M01AC05.*

### Adverse Effects and Precautions

As for NSAIDs in general, p.67. Lornoxicam should not be used in patients with severe renal impairment. Intramuscular or intravenous use of lornoxicam is also contra-indicated in moderate to severe renal impairment, severe hepatic impairment, severe cardiac insufficiency, hypovolaemia, dehydration, confirmed or suspected cerebrovascular bleeding, haemorrhagic diathesis, and operations with a risk of haemorrhage or incomplete haemostasis.

### Interactions

For interactions associated with NSAIDs, see p.69. Increased plasma concentrations of lornoxicam have occurred when given with cimetidine.

### Pharmacokinetics

Lornoxicam is almost completely absorbed from the gastrointestinal tract after oral doses with peak concentrations reached in 1 to 2 hours. After intramuscular doses peak concentrations are reached in about 25 minutes. Lornoxicam is 99% bound to plasma proteins. Lornoxicam is metabolised to its inactive hydroxylated metabolite. About one-third of a dose is excreted via the urine as inactive metabolites. The mean elimination half-life is 3 to 4 hours.

### Uses and Administration

Lornoxicam, an oxicam derivative, is an NSAID (p.70). It is used in musculoskeletal and joint disorders such as osteoarthritis and rheumatoid arthritis; it is also used in the treatment of other painful conditions including postoperative pain.

In the treatment of osteoarthritis and rheumatoid arthritis lornoxicam is given by mouth in a daily dose of 12 mg in two or three divided doses.

Lornoxicam is given in doses of 8 to 16 mg daily by mouth for the treatment of pain. Doses above 8 mg should be given in divided doses. Similar doses may be given by intravenous or intramuscular injection, although in rare cases the maximum initial daily dose may be increased to 24 mg; treatment by injection should be limited to 2 days.

◊ References.

1. Balfour JA, *et al.* Lornoxicam: a review of its pharmacology and therapeutic potential in the management of painful and inflammatory conditions. *Drugs* 1996; **51:** 639–57.
2. Skjodt NM, Davies NM. Clinical pharmacokinetics of lornoxicam: a short half-life oxicam. *Clin Pharmacokinet* 1998; **34:** 421–8.
3. Staunstrup H, *et al.* Efficacy and tolerability of lornoxicam versus tramadol in postoperative pain. *J Clin Pharmacol* 1999; **39:** 834–41.

### Preparations

**Proprietary Preparations** (details are given in Part 3)
**Arg.:** Acabel; **Austria:** Artok; Lornox; Xefo; **Chile:** Acabel; **Denm.:** Xefo; **Fin.:** Xefo†; **Ger.:** Telos; **Gr.:** Xefo; **Ital.:** Taigalor; **Port.:** Acabel; **S.Afr.:** Xefo; **Spain:** Acabel; Bosporon; **Swed.:** Xefo; **Thai.:** Xefo; **UK:** Xefo†.

## Loxoprofen Sodium *(rINNM)*

CS-600 (loxoprofen); Loxoprofeno sódico. Sodium (±)-*p*-[(2-oxocyclopentyl)methyl]hydratropate dihydrate.

$C_{15}H_{17}O_3Na,2H_2O$ = 304.3.

*CAS — 68767-14-6 (loxoprofen); 80382-23-6 (loxoprofen sodium dihydrate).*

**Pharmacopoeias.** In *Jpn.*

### Profile

Loxoprofen sodium is an NSAID (p.67) given by mouth for the management of pain and inflammation associated with musculoskeletal and joint disorders or operative procedures. Loxoprofen sodium is given as the dihydrate although doses are expressed in terms of the anhydrous salt. Anhydrous loxoprofen sodium 10 mg is approximately equivalent to 11.3 mg of loxoprofen sodium dihydrate. A usual dose equivalent to 60 mg of the anhydrous form has been given by mouth three times daily.

### Preparations

**Proprietary Preparations** (details are given in Part 3)
**Arg.:** Oxeno; **Braz.:** Loxonin; **Jpn:** Lobu; Loxonin; **Thai.:** Loxonin.

## Lumiracoxib *(USAN, rINN)*

Cox-189. 2-{[(2-Chloro-6-fluorophenyl)amino]-5-methylphenyl}acetic acid.

$C_{15}H_{13}ClFNO_2$ = 293.7.

*CAS — 220991-20-8.*

*ATC — M01AH06.*

### Profile

Lumiracoxib is an NSAID (p.67) reported to be a selective inhibitor of cyclo-oxygenase-2 (COX-2). It has been approved for use in the treatment of moderate to severe acute pain and of osteoarthritis.

## Lysine Aspirin

Acetilsalicilato de lisina; Aspirin DL-Lysine; Lysine Acetylsalicylate; DL-Lysine Acetylsalicylate.

$C_{15}H_{22}N_2O_6$ = 326.3.

*CAS — 62952-06-1.*

**Pharmacopoeias.** In *Fr.*

### Adverse Effects, Treatment, and Precautions

As for Aspirin, p.15. Anaphylactic shock has been reported in patients given lysine aspirin by injection.

Lysine aspirin, like aspirin, should not generally be given to children because of the risk of Reye's syndrome.

**Hypersensitivity.** For a suggestion that lysine aspirin might be more suitable than aspirin for the diagnosis of sensitivity to NSAIDs, see under Hypersensitivity on p.16.

### Interactions

For interactions associated with aspirin, see p.17.

### Uses and Administration

Lysine aspirin has analgesic, anti-inflammatory, and antipyretic actions similar to those of aspirin (see p.17). When given, lysine aspirin dissociates into lysine and aspirin; aspirin is then hydrolysed to salicylic acid. Lysine aspirin 900 mg is approximately equivalent to 500 mg of aspirin.

Lysine aspirin is used in the treatment of pain, fever, and rheumatic disorders. It is given by mouth in doses equivalent to 0.5 to 1 g of aspirin, repeated every 4 hours as needed up to a maximum of 3 g of aspirin daily (2 g daily in the elderly) for pain and fever. The dose for rheumatic disorders is equivalent to 4 to 6 g of aspirin daily in 3 or 4 divided doses. Lysine aspirin is also given intramuscularly or intravenously in similar doses; the maximum daily parenteral dose is equivalent to 4 g of aspirin for very severe pain and to 6 g of aspirin for rheumatic disorders.

Lysine aspirin is also used with metoclopramide in the treatment of migraine.

Lysine aspirin has also been used in the management of thromboembolic disorders.

**Headache.** Some references to the use of lysine aspirin, often with metoclopramide, in the treatment of migraine.

1. Tfelt-Hansen P, *et al.* The effectiveness of combined oral lysine acetylsalicylate and metoclopramide compared with oral sumatriptan for migraine. *Lancet* 1995; **346:** 923–6.
2. Diener HC. Efficacy and safety of intravenous acetylsalicylic acid lysinate compared to subcutaneous sumatriptan and parenteral placebo in the acute treatment of migraine. A double-blind, double-dummy, randomized, multicenter, parallel group study. *Cephalalgia* 1999; **19:** 581–8.
3. Tfelt-Hansen P. The effectiveness of combined oral lysine acetylsalicylate and metoclopramide (Migpriv®) in the treatment of migraine attacks: comparison with placebo and oral sumatriptan. *Funct Neurol* 2000; **15** (suppl 3): 196–201.

### Preparations

**Proprietary Preparations** (details are given in Part 3)
***Arg.:*** Corplus; Decitriol; ***Belg.:*** Aspegic; Cardegic; ***Braz.:*** Kardegic†; ***Fr.:*** Aspegic; Kardegic; ***Ger.:*** Aspisol; ***Gr.:*** Egicalm; ***Israel:*** Lysoprin; ***Ital.:*** Aspegic; Aspidol; Cardirene; Flectadol; ***Malaysia:*** Aspegic; ***Mex.:*** Coraspir; ***Neth.:*** Aspegic; Cardegic; ***Port.:*** Aspegic; Evasprin†; Lisaspin; Tiplac; ***Spain:*** ASL; Inyesprin; Lysinotol; Solusprin; ***Switz.:*** Alcacyl instant; Aspegic; Kardegic.

**Multi-ingredient: *Belg.:*** Migpriv; ***Chile:*** Dolotol 12; ***Denm.:*** Migpriv; ***Fin.:*** Migpriv; ***Fr.:*** Migpriv; ***Ital.:*** Migpriv; Migraprim; ***Neth.:*** Migrafin; ***Norw.:*** Migpriv; ***Spain:*** Fluxal; Neurodif†; ***Swed.:*** Migpriv; ***Switz.:*** Migpriv; ***UK:*** Migramax.

## Magnesium Salicylate

Salicilato magnésico.

$C_{14}H_{10}MgO_6,4H_2O = 370.6$.

*CAS — 18917-89-0 (anhydrous magnesium salicylate); 18917-95-8 (magnesium salicylate tetrahydrate).*

**Pharmacopoeias.** In *Chin.* and *US.*

**USP 27** (Magnesium Salicylate). A white, odourless, efflorescent, crystalline powder. Soluble in water and in alcohol; slightly soluble in ether; freely soluble in methyl alcohol. Store in airtight containers.

### Adverse Effects, Treatment, and Precautions

As for Aspirin, p.15.

The use of aspirin and other acetylated salicylates is generally not recommended for children because of the risk of Reye's syndrome, unless specifically indicated. Some licensing information extends this precaution to magnesium salicylate.

There is an additional caution in renal impairment because of the risk of hypermagnesaemia.

### Interactions

For interactions associated with salicylates, see Aspirin, p.17.

### Uses and Administration

Magnesium salicylate has analgesic, anti-inflammatory, and antipyretic actions similar to those of aspirin (see p.17). Anhydrous magnesium salicylate 1 g is approximately equivalent to 1.2 g of aspirin. It is used in the treatment of pain and fever and in the management of inflammatory conditions such as osteoarthritis, rheumatoid arthritis, and other arthritides. Usual doses of magnesium salicylate, expressed in terms of anhydrous magnesium salicylate, are about 300 to 600 mg by mouth every 4 hours for pain or fever. A total daily dose of about 3.5 g should not be exceeded. A dose of 545 mg to 1.2 g given 3 or 4 times daily is used for arthritic disorders.

### Preparations

***USP 27:*** Magnesium Salicylate Tablets.

**Proprietary Preparations** (details are given in Part 3)
***Arg.:*** Rati Salil E; ***Canad.:*** Back-Ese M†; Doans Backache Pills†; Herbogesic†; ***USA:*** Backache Maximum Strength Relief; Bayer Select Maximum Strength Backache; Doans; Magan; Mobidin; Momentum Muscular Backache Formula; Novasal; Nuprin Backache.

**Multi-ingredient: *USA:*** Extra Strength Doans PM; Magsal†; Maximum Strength Arthritien†; Mobigesic; Painaid BRF Back Relief Formula; Tetra-Mag.

## Meclofenamic Acid *(BAN, USAN, rINN)*

Ácido meclofenámico; CI-583; INF-4668. N-(2,6-Dichloro-m-tolyl)anthranilic acid.

$C_{14}H_{11}Cl_2NO_2 = 296.1$.

*CAS — 644-62-2.*

*ATC — M01AG04; M02AA18.*

**Pharmacopoeias.** In *BP(Vet).*

**BP(Vet) 2003** (Meclofenamic Acid). A white or almost white, odourless or almost odourless, crystalline powder. Practically insoluble in water; slightly soluble in alcohol and in chloroform; sparingly soluble in ether; soluble in dimethylformamide and in 1M sodium hydroxide.

## Meclofenamate Sodium *(BANM, USAN, rINNM)*

Meclofenamato sódico.

$C_{14}H_{10}Cl_2NNaO_2,H_2O = 336.1$.

*CAS — 6385-02-0.*

**Pharmacopoeias.** In *US.*

**USP 27** (Meclofenamate Sodium). A white to creamy white, odourless to almost odourless, crystalline powder. Freely soluble in water, the solution sometimes being somewhat turbid due to partial hydrolysis and absorption of carbon dioxide; the solution is clear above pH 15. Slightly soluble in chloroform; practically insoluble in ether; soluble in methyl alcohol. Store in airtight containers. Protect from light.

### Adverse Effects and Precautions

As for NSAIDs in general, p.67.

**Incidence of adverse effects.** The commonest adverse effect in 2500 patients who received meclofenamate sodium was gastrointestinal disturbance.[1] Diarrhoea occurred in 11.2% of patients in double-blind studies and 32.8% of patients in long-term studies (up to 3 years). Ulcers were detected in 22 patients during therapy and skin rashes occurred in 4% of patients. Transient increases in serum aminotransferases and BUN occurred in some patients.

1. Preston SN. Safety of sodium meclofenamate (Meclomen™). *Curr Ther Res* 1978; **23** (suppl 4S): S107–12.

**Effects on the blood.** Case reports of agranulocytosis[1] and thrombocytopenia[2] associated with meclofenamate therapy.

1. Wishner AJ, Milburn PB. Meclofenamate sodium-induced agranulocytosis and suppression of erythropoiesis. *J Am Acad Dermatol* 1985; **13:** 1052–3.
2. Rodriguez J. Thrombocytopenia associated with meclofenamate. *Drug Intell Clin Pharm* 1981; **15:** 999.

### Interactions

For interactions associated with NSAIDs, see p.69.

### Pharmacokinetics

Meclofenamate sodium is readily absorbed when given by mouth. Peak plasma concentrations occur about 0.5 to 2 hours after ingestion. Meclofenamate is over 99% bound to plasma proteins. The plasma elimination half-life of meclofenamate sodium is about 2 to 4 hours. It is metabolised by oxidation, hydroxylation, dehalogenation, and conjugation with glucuronic acid and excreted in urine mainly as glucuronide conjugates of the metabolites. About 20 to 30% is recovered in the faeces. One of the metabolites, a 3-hydroxymethyl compound, is reported to be active.

◊ References.

1. Koup JR, *et al.* A single and multiple dose pharmacokinetic and metabolism study of meclofenamate sodium. *Biopharm Drug Dispos* 1990; **11:** 1–15.

### Uses and Administration

Meclofenamic acid, an anthranilic acid derivative similar to mefenamic acid (below), is an NSAID (p.70). It is given by mouth as the sodium salt in musculoskeletal and joint disorders such as osteoarthritis and rheumatoid arthritis, in mild to moderate pain, and in dysmenorrhoea and menorrhagia.

Doses of meclofenamate sodium are expressed in terms of the equivalent amount of meclofenamic acid. Meclofenamic acid 100 mg is approximately equivalent to 113.5 mg of meclofenamate sodium. In arthritic conditions it is given in doses equivalent to 200 to 400 mg daily; daily doses are usually given in 3 or 4 divided doses. For relief of mild to moderate pain doses are 50 to 100 mg every 4 to 6 hours; the daily dose should not exceed 400 mg. The dose in the treatment of dysmenorrhoea and menorrhagia is 100 mg three times daily for up to 6 days during menstruation.

Meclofenamic acid has been given as a rectal suppository and is also used in veterinary medicine.

### Preparations

***USP 27:*** Meclofenamate Sodium Capsules.

**Proprietary Preparations** (details are given in Part 3)
***Austria:*** Meclomen†; ***Chile:*** Meclomen; ***Hong Kong:*** Meclomen†; ***Ital.:*** Lenidolor; Meclodol; Movens; ***S.Afr.:*** Meclomen†; ***Spain:*** Meclomen.

## Mefenamic Acid *(BAN, USAN, rINN)*

Ácido mefenámico; Acidum Mefenamicum; CI-473; CN-35355; INF-3355. N-(2,3-Xylyl)anthranilic acid.

$C_{15}H_{15}NO_2 = 241.3$.

*CAS — 61-68-7.*

*ATC — M01AG01.*

**Pharmacopoeias.** In *Chin., Eur.* (see p.vi), *Jpn, Pol.,* and *US.*

**Ph. Eur. 5.0** (Mefenamic Acid). A white to almost white, microcrystalline powder. Practically insoluble in water; slightly soluble in alcohol and in dichloromethane; dissolves in dilute solutions of alkali hydroxides.

**USP 27** (Mefenamic Acid). A white to off-white, crystalline powder. Practically insoluble in water; slightly soluble in alcohol and in methyl alcohol; sparingly soluble in chloroform; soluble in solutions of alkali hydroxides. Store in airtight containers. Protect from light.

### Adverse Effects and Precautions

As for NSAIDs in general, p.67. Treatment should be discontinued if diarrhoea and rashes occur. Other effects reported include drowsiness, and effects on the blood including thrombocytopenia, occasionally haemolytic anaemia, and rarely aplastic anaemia. Convulsions are a prominent feature of overdosage with mefenamic acid.

Mefenamic acid is contra-indicated in patients with inflammatory bowel disease. The manufacturers recommend that blood counts and liver function should be monitored during long-term therapy. Drowsiness may affect the performance of skilled tasks.

Mefenamic acid may give a false positive in tests for the presence of bile in the urine.

**Breast feeding.** No adverse effects have been observed in breast-feeding infants whose mothers were receiving mefenamic acid, and the American Academy of Pediatrics considers[1] that it is therefore usually compatible with breast feeding. The *British National Formulary* also considers that the amount of mefenamic acid distributed into breast milk is too small to be harmful to a breast-fed infant. An early study[2] confirms that the distribution of mefenamic acid into breast milk is minimal. However, the manufacturers interpret this more cautiously and contra-indicate the use of mefenamic acid in nursing mothers.

1. American Academy of Pediatrics. The transfer of drugs and other chemicals into human milk. *Pediatrics* 2001; **108:** 776–89. Correction. *ibid.;* 1029. Also available at: http://aappolicy.aappublications.org/cgi/content/full/pediatrics%3b108/3/776 (accessed 05/07/04)
2. Buchanan RA, *et al.* The breast milk excretion of mefenamic acid. *Curr Ther Res* 1968; **10:** 592–6.

**Effects on the blood.** References to haematological reactions in patients taking mefenamic acid including haemolytic anaemia,[1] leucopenia,[2] neutropenia,[3] and agranulocytosis.[4]

1. Scott GL, *et al.* Autoimmune haemolytic anaemia and mefenamic acid therapy. *BMJ* 1968; **3:** 534–5.
2. Burns A, Young RE. Mefenamic acid induced leucopenia in the elderly. *Lancet* 1984; **ii:** 46.
3. Handa SI, Freestone S. Mefenamic acid-induced neutropenia and renal failure in elderly females with hypothyroidism. *Postgrad Med J* 1990; **66:** 557–9.
4. Muroi K, *et al.* Treatment of drug-induced agranulocytosis with granulocyte-colony stimulating factor. *Lancet* 1989; **ii:** 55.

**Effects on the gastrointestinal tract.** Reversible steatorrhoea has occurred[1] and mefenamic acid may provoke colitis in patients without a past history of this condition.[2]

1. Marks JS, Gleeson MH. Steatorrhoea complicating therapy with mefenamic acid. *BMJ* 1975; **4:** 442.
2. Ravi S, *et al.* Colitis caused by non-steroidal anti-inflammatory drugs. *Postgrad Med J* 1986; **62:** 773–6.

**Effects on the kidneys.** Nonoliguric renal failure has occurred in elderly patients who had experienced diarrhoea and vomiting while taking mefenamic acid and had continued to take the drug. It is normally recommended that mefenamic acid be discontinued in the event of diarrhoea and it was suggested that in these patients the gastrointestinal toxicity had led to fluid and electrolyte depletion, thus predisposing these patients to mefenamic acid's nephrotoxicity.[1] There has been a subsequent report[2] of nonoliguric renal failure in elderly patients given mefenamic acid for musculoskeletal pain.

1. Taha A, *et al.* Non-oliguric renal failure during treatment with mefenamic acid in elderly patients: a continuing problem. *BMJ* 1985; **291:** 661–2.
2. Grant DJ, MacConnachie AM. Mefenamic acid is more dangerous than most. *BMJ* 1995; **311:** 392.

**Effects on the skin.** Bullous pemphigoid, together with haemolytic anaemia and diarrhoea,[1] and fixed drug eruptions[2,3] have been associated with the use of mefenamic acid. Additionally, Stevens-Johnson syndrome, together with cholestatic hepatitis and haemolytic anaemia, in one patient has been attributed to mefenamic acid therapy.[4] It is generally recommended that mefenamic acid should be withdrawn if skin reactions develop.

1. Shepherd AN, *et al.* Mefenamic acid-induced bullous pemphigoid. *Postgrad Med J* 1986; **62:** 67–8.
2. Wilson CL, Otter A. Fixed drug eruption associated with mefenamic acid. *BMJ* 1986; **293:** 1243.
3. Long CC, *et al.* Fixed drug eruption to mefenamic acid: a report of three cases. *Br J Dermatol* 1992; **126:** 409–11.
4. Chan JCN, *et al.* A case of Stevens-Johnson syndrome, cholestatic hepatitis and haemolytic anaemia associated with use of mefenamic acid. *Drug Safety* 1991; **6:** 230–4.

**Overdosage.** Mefenamic acid overdose has been associated with CNS toxicity, especially with convulsions.[1] Coma[2,3] has also been reported.

1. Court H, Volans GN. Poisoning after overdose with non-steroidal anti-inflammatory drugs. *Adverse Drug React Acute Poisoning Rev* 1984; **3:** 1–21.
2. Gössinger H, *et al.* Coma in mefenamic acid poisoning. *Lancet* 1982; **ii:** 384.
3. Hendrickse MT. Mefenamic acid overdose mimicking brainstem stroke. *Lancet* 1988; **ii:** 1019.

**Pancreatitis.** A report of pancreatitis associated with mefenamic acid.[1]

1. van Walraven AA, *et al.* Pancreatitis caused by mefenamic acid. *Can Med Assoc J* 1982; **126:** 894.

**Porphyria.** Mefenamic acid is considered to be unsafe in patients with porphyria although there is conflicting experimental evidence of porphyrinogenicity.

### Interactions

For interactions associated with NSAIDs, see p.69.

### Pharmacokinetics

Mefenamic acid is absorbed from the gastrointestinal tract. Peak plasma concentrations occur about 2 to 4 hours after ingestion. The plasma elimination half-life is reported to be 2 to 4 hours. Mefenamic acid is extensively bound to plasma proteins. It is distributed into breast milk. Mefenamic acid is metabolised by the cytochrome P450 isoenzyme CYP2C9 to 3-hydroxymethyl mefenamic acid which may then be oxidised to 3-carboxymefenamic acid. Over 50% of a dose may be recovered in the urine, as unchanged drug or conjugates of mefenamic acid and its metabolites.

### Uses and Administration

Mefenamic acid, an anthranilic acid derivative, is an NSAID (p.70), although its anti-inflammatory properties are considered to be minor.

It is used in mild to moderate pain including headache, dental pain, postoperative and postpartum pain, and dysmenorrhoea, in musculoskeletal and joint disorders such as osteoarthritis and rheumatoid arthritis, in menorrhagia, and in children with fever and juvenile idiopathic arthritis. The usual dose by mouth is up to 500 mg three times daily. A suggested dose for children over 6 months of age is 25 mg/kg daily in divided doses. Alternatively, doses in children may be given according to age: 6 months to under 2 years, 50 mg; 2 years to under 5 years, 100 mg; 5 years to under 9 years, 150 mg; 9 years to 12 years, 200 mg. These doses may be repeated as necessary, up to three times daily. In the USA, where mefenamic acid is only licensed for the treatment of moderate pain in adults, it is recommended that it should not be given for longer than 7 days at a time, but in the UK this restriction is only applied to children unless they are receiving mefenamic acid for juvenile chronic arthritis.

### Preparations

***BP 2003:*** Mefenamic Acid Capsules; Mefenamic Acid Tablets;
***USP 27:*** Mefenamic Acid Capsules.

**Proprietary Preparations** (details are given in Part 3)
***Arg.:*** Ponstil; ***Austral.:*** Mefic; Ponstan; ***Austria:*** Parkemed; ***Braz.:*** Ponstan; Pontin; ***Canad.:*** Ponstan; ***Chile:*** Algifemin; Dolcin; Flipal; Sicadol; Tanston; Templadol; ***Fin.:*** Ponstan; ***Fr.:*** Ponstyl; ***Ger.:*** Parkemed; Ponalar; ***Gr.:*** Aidol; Ponstan; Vidan; ***Hong Kong:*** Dyspen; Hamitan; Hostan; Medicap; Mefacap†; Mefamic; Mefic; Napan; Ponstan; Pontacid; Sefmic; ***India:*** Dysmen-500; Ponstan; ***Irl.:*** Mefac; Pinalgesic†; Ponalgic; Ponmel; Ponstan; ***Ital.:*** Lysalgo; ***Malaysia:*** Beafemic; Mefen; Mefic; Namic; Napan; Pongesic; Ponstan; Pontalon; ***Mex.:*** Artriden; Namifen; Ponstan; ***NZ:*** Ponstan; ***Port.:*** Ponstan; ***S.Afr.:*** Fenamin; Ponac; Ponstan; Ponstel; ***Singapore:*** Beafemic; Mefacap; Mefenix; Ponstan; Pontalon; Pontyl; ***Spain:*** Coslan; ***Switz.:*** mefe-basan; Mefenacide; Melur; Mephadolor; Ponstan; Spiralgin; ***Thai.:*** Conamic; Dyspen; Femen; Fenamic; Gandin; Manic; Mednil; Mefa; Mefen; Mefenan; Mefenix†; Namic; Painnox; Panamic; Pefamic; Pondnadysmen; Ponnac†; Ponnesia; Ponstan; Pontalon†; Prostan; Pynamic; Sefmic; ***UK:*** Dysman; Ponstan; ***USA:*** Ponstel.

**Multi-ingredient:** ***India:*** Cyclo-Meff; Dysmen; Dysmen Forte; ***Thai.:*** Difemic; Mainnox; Med-Anspasmic.

---

## Meloxicam *(BAN, USAN, rINN)*

UH-AC-62; UH-AC-62XX. 4-Hydroxy-2-methyl-*N*-(5-methyl-2-thiazolyl)-2*H*-1,2-benzothiazine-3-carboxamide 1,1-dioxide.

$C_{14}H_{13}N_3O_4S_2$ = 351.4.
*CAS — 71125-38-7.*
*ATC — M01AC06.*

**Pharmacopoeias.** In *Br.*

**BP 2003** (Meloxicam). A pale yellow powder. Practically insoluble in water; very slightly soluble in alcohol and in methyl alcohol; slightly soluble in acetone; soluble in dimethylformamide.

### Adverse Effects

As for NSAIDs in general, p.67.

**Incidence of adverse effects.** Between September 1996, when meloxicam was first marketed in the UK, and mid June 1998 the UK Committee on Safety of Medicines had received a total of 773 reports of 1339 suspected adverse reactions for meloxicam.[1] Of all the reactions 41% were gastrointestinal and of these 18% involved gastrointestinal perforation, ulceration and/or bleeding; the mean age of the patients involved was 64 years. Although most patients recovered after withdrawal of meloxicam and/or treatment, 5 died. A total of 193 reactions involved the skin, the most common being pruritus, rash, and urticaria. There were also reports of angioedema (25), photosensitivity (12), and bullous dermatoses, including erythema multiforme and Stevens Johnson syndrome (5). No patients died from skin reactions and most recovered after meloxicam was withdrawn. Other frequently reported reactions were neurological (mostly headache), cardiovascular (oedema and palpitations), dizziness, flushing, and fatigue. A prescription event monitoring study has also analysed events reported with meloxicam use.[2] In a cohort of 19 087 patients who had received meloxicam some time between December 1996 and March 1997, 203 patients had experienced 252 events considered to be suspected adverse reactions. The majority of reactions were not serious or were labelled side-effects of meloxicam. Rare, serious suspected adverse reactions included 2 reports of thrombocytopenia and 1 each of interstitial nephritis and idiosyncratic liver abnormality. The most frequent gastrointestinal event was dyspepsia; other more serious gastrointestinal events occurring during meloxicam exposure included upper gastrointestinal bleeding (33 reports) and peptic ulcer (19 reports). However it was considered that the incidence of gastrointestinal disturbance was low in the absence of gastrointestinal risk factors. Adverse drug reactions reported during the first year of marketing of meloxicam to the Swedish Medical Products Agency suggested a similar safety profile to other NSAIDs.[3] Of the 15 reports, 6 were for gastrointestinal disturbances and 5 involved skin reactions.

It has been proposed that preferential inhibitors of cyclo-oxygenase-2, such as meloxicam, might produce fewer adverse effects than other NSAIDs but there has been little convincing evidence that the risk of severe gastrointestinal events is lower with meloxicam than with other NSAIDs at equi-effective doses.[4] Two recent large multicentre studies[5,6] have reported a lower incidence of gastrointestinal adverse effects with meloxicam than with non-selective cyclo-oxygenase inhibitors (diclofenac[5] or piroxicam[6]) but in one of these[5] the dose of meloxicam given also appeared to be less effective than the reference drug.


1. Committee on Safety of Medicines/Medicines Control Agency. Meloxicam (Mobic): gastrointestinal and skin reactions. *Current Problems* 1998; **24:** 13. Also available at: http://www.mca.gov.uk/ourwork/monitorsafequalmed/currentproblems/cpvol24csec4.htm (accessed 05/07/04)
2. Martin RM, *et al.* The incidence of adverse events and risk factors for upper gastrointestinal disorders associated with meloxicam use amongst 19 087 patients in general practice in England: cohort study. *Br J Clin Pharmacol* 2000; **50:** 35–42.
3. Anonymous. Meloxicam safety similar to other NSAIDs. *WHO Drug Information* 1998; **12:** 147.
4. Anonymous. Meloxicam—a safer NSAID? *Drug Ther Bull* 1998; **36:** 62–4.
5. Hawkey C, *et al.* Gastrointestinal tolerability of meloxicam compared to diclofenac in osteoarthritis patients. *Br J Rheumatol* 1998; **37:** 937–45.
6. Dequeker J, *et al.* Improvement in gastrointestinal tolerability of the selective cyclooxygenase (COX)-2 inhibitor, meloxicam, compared with piroxicam: results of the safety and efficacy large-scale evaluation of COX-inhibiting therapies (SELECT) trial in osteoarthritis. *Br J Rheumatol* 1998; **37:** 946–51.


### Precautions

As for NSAIDs in general, p.69.

Meloxicam should be avoided in severe hepatic impairment, in bleeding disorders, and in patients with renal failure unless receiving dialysis. Rectal use should be avoided in patients with a history of proctitis, haemorrhoids, or rectal bleeding.

**Renal impairment.** The pharmacokinetics of meloxicam were not substantially altered in patients with a creatinine clearance of 41 to 60 mL/minute compared with those with normal renal function.[1] In those with a creatinine clearance of 20 to 40 mL/minute, total plasma-meloxicam concentrations were lower but meloxicam free fractions were higher. Such free meloxicam concentrations were similar to the other groups. On the basis of these results, it was suggested that it was not necessary to reduce meloxicam doses in patients with a creatinine clearance greater than 20 mL/minute.


1. Boulton-Jones JM, *et al.* Meloxicam pharmacokinetics in renal impairment. *Br J Clin Pharmacol* 1997; **43:** 35–40.


### Interactions

For interactions associated with NSAIDs, see p.69.

There may be an increased risk of bleeding during concomitant use of meloxicam and pentoxifylline.

### Pharmacokinetics

Meloxicam is well absorbed after oral doses. It is 99% bound to plasma proteins. Meloxicam has a plasma-elimination half-life of about 20 hours. It is extensively metabolised mainly by oxidation and excreted in similar amounts in the urine and in the faeces; less than 3% of a dose is excreted unchanged. The volume of distribution is increased in renal failure.

◊ References.


1. Narjes H, *et al.* Pharmacokinetics and tolerability of meloxicam after i.m. administration. *Br J Clin Pharmacol* 1996; **41:** 135–9.
2. Türck D, *et al.* Clinical pharmacokinetics of meloxicam. *Arzneimittelforschung* 1997; **47:** 253–8.
3. Davies NM, Skjodt NM. Clinical pharmacokinetics of meloxicam: a cyclooxygenase-2 preferential nonsteroidal anti-inflammatory drug. *Clin Pharmacokinet* 1999; **36:** 115–26.


**Renal impairment.** For reference to the pharmacokinetics of meloxicam in renal impairment, see under Precautions, above.

### Uses and Administration

Meloxicam, an oxicam derivative, is an NSAID (p.70). It is reported to be a selective inhibitor of cyclo-oxygenase-2 (COX-2). Meloxicam is used in the management of rheumatoid arthritis, for the short-term symptomatic treatment of acute exacerbations of osteoarthritis, and for the symptomatic treatment of ankylosing spondylitis.

In the treatment of rheumatoid arthritis and ankylosing spondylitis, meloxicam is given by mouth in a usual dose of 15 mg daily as a single dose. Those with an increased risk of adverse reactions should be started on 7.5 mg daily. A dose of 7.5 mg daily is recommended for long-term treatment in the elderly. In the treatment of acute exacerbations of osteoarthritis the usual daily dose of meloxicam by mouth is 7.5 mg, increased if necessary to a maximum of 15 mg daily given as a single dose.

Meloxicam may be given by rectal suppository in doses similar to those used orally but use should be limited to the shortest time possible.

For the dose of meloxicam in patients with renal impairment, see below.

**Administration in renal impairment.** Meloxicam is normally contra-indicated in patients with severe renal impairment. However, in dialysed patients, meloxicam may be given in a dose of 7.5 mg daily by mouth or by rectal suppository.

**Musculoskeletal and joint disorders.** Meloxicam is used in the treatment of osteoarthritis (see p.9) and rheumatoid arthritis (see p.9). However, in the UK, it is recommended that the use of meloxicam and other selective cyclo-oxygenase-2 (COX-2) inhibitors is limited to those patients considered to be at high risk of developing serious gastrointestinal problems if given a non-selective NSAID (see p.68).

References.


1. Lemmel EM, *et al.* Efficacy and safety of meloxicam in patients with rheumatoid arthritis. *J Rheumatol* 1997; **24:** 282–90.
2. Yocum D, *et al.* Safety and efficacy of meloxicam in the treatment of osteoarthritis: a 12-week, double-blind, multiple-dose, placebo-controlled trial. The Meloxicam Osteoarthritis Investigators. *Arch Intern Med* 2000; **160:** 2947–54.
3. Combe B, *et al.* Comparison of intramuscular and oral meloxicam in rheumatoid arthritis patients. *Inflamm Res* 2001; **50** (suppl 1): S10–16.
4. Fleischmann R, *et al.* Meloxicam. *Expert Opin Pharmacother* 2002; **3:** 1501–12.


### Preparations

**Proprietary Preparations** (details are given in Part 3)
***Arg.:*** Flexidol; Loxitenk; Merapiran; Miogesil; Mobic; Skudal; Telaroid; Tenaron; ***Austral.:*** Mobic; ***Austria:*** Mobic; Movalis; ***Belg.:*** Mobic; ***Braz.:*** Alivian; Bioflac; Diatec†; Dormelox; Flamatec†; Flexican†; Inicox; Leutrol; Lonaflam; Loxam; Loxiflan; Melotec; Meloxigran; Meloxil; Mevamox; Movacox; Movatec; Movoxicam; ***Canad.:*** Mobicox; ***Chile:*** Anposel; Ecax; Hyflex; Isox; Melodol; Mobex; Tenaron; Zix; ***Denm.:*** Mobic; ***Fin.:*** Mobic; ***Fr.:*** Mobic; ***Ger.:*** Mobec; ***Gr.:*** Loxitan; Movatec; ***Hong Kong:*** Mobic; ***India:*** Mel-OD; ***Irl.:*** Mobic; ***Ital.:*** Leutrol; Mobic; ***Malaysia:*** Mobic; ***Mex.:*** Aflamid; Exel; Loxibest; Masflex; Melosteral; Mobicox; ***Neth.:*** Movicox; ***Norw.:*** Mobic; ***NZ:*** Mobic; ***Port.:*** Movalis; Ziloxican; ***S.Afr.:*** Coxflam; Mobic; ***Singapore:*** Mobic; ***Spain:*** Movalis; Parocin; Uticox; ***Swed.:*** Latonid; Mobic; ***Switz.:*** Mobicox; Zilutrol; ***Thai.:*** Mobic; ***UK:*** Mobic; ***USA:*** Mobic.

---

## Meptazinol Hydrochloride

*(BANM, USAN, rINNM)*

Hidrocloruro de meptazinol; IL-22811 (meptazinol); Wy-22811 (meptazinol). 3-(3-Ethyl-1-methylperhydroazepin-3-yl)phenol hydrochloride.

$C_{15}H_{23}NO,HCl$ = 269.8.
*CAS — 54340-58-8 (meptazinol); 59263-76-2 (meptazinol hydrochloride); 34154-59-1 (±-meptazinol hydrochloride).*

**Pharmacopoeias.** In *Br.*

**BP 2003** (Meptazinol Hydrochloride). A white or almost white powder. Very soluble in water and in methyl alcohol; freely soluble in alcohol; very slightly soluble in acetone; dissolves in dilute solutions of alkali hydroxides. Store at a temperature not exceeding 25°.

### Dependence and Withdrawal

As for Opioid Analgesics, p.71.

◊ In assessing the dependence potential of meptazinol, a WHO expert committee[1] noted in 1989 that abrupt discontinuation of chronic meptazinol administration precipitated only slight withdrawal signs in *animals* and that meptazinol did not suppress opioid withdrawal signs and symptoms in humans dependent on morphine. Abuse had not been reported. They considered that the likelihood of abuse was moderate and that international control was not warranted at that time.


1. WHO. WHO expert committee on drug dependence: twenty-fifth report. *WHO Tech Rep Ser 775* 1989.


### Adverse Effects, Treatment, and Precautions

As for Opioid Analgesics in general, p.72.

Meptazinol is claimed to have a low incidence of respiratory depression. There have been occasional reports of psychiatric disorders such as hallucinations, confusion, and depression. As meptazinol has both antagonist and agonist properties its effects may be only partially reversed by naloxone, but use of the latter is still recommended in overdosage.

Meptazinol has the potential to precipitate withdrawal symptoms if given to patients who are physically dependent on opioids.

**Effects on the respiratory system.** Meptazinol is said to have a relatively low potential for respiratory depression and in healthy subjects was reported to produce substantially less respiratory depression than morphine or pentazocine at usual analgesic doses.[1] However, respiratory depression does occur in anaesthetised patients given meptazinol[2] and the effects on respiration may be similar to those of morphine[3,4] or pethidine.[5,6] Compensatory mechanisms may come into play following repeated doses of meptazinol but the intravenous administration of meptazinol during anaesthesia should be viewed with as much caution as with any other opioid.[6]

Respiratory arrest occurred after an *overdose* of 50 meptazinol 200-mg tablets and a quarter of a bottle of whisky.[7] Full recovery eventually followed supportive measures although spontaneous respiration was not re-established by naloxone intravenously to a cumulative total dose of 10 mg.


1. Jordan C, *et al.* A comparison of the respiratory effects of meptazinol, pentazocine and morphine. *Br J Anaesth* 1979; **51:** 497–502.

2. Hardy PAJ. Meptazinol and respiratory depression. *Lancet* 1983; **ii:** 576.
3. Frater RAS, *et al.* Analgesia-induced respiratory depression: comparison of meptazinol and morphine in the postoperative period. *Br J Anaesth* 1989; **63:** 260–5.
4. Verborgh C, Camu F. Post-surgical pain relief with zero-order intravenous infusions of meptazinol and morphine: a double-blind placebo-controlled evaluation of their effects on ventilation. *Eur J Clin Pharmacol* 1990; **38:** 437–42.
5. Wilkinson DJ, *et al.* Meptazinol— a cause of respiratory depression in general anaesthesia. *Br J Anaesth* 1985; **57:** 1077–84.
6. Lee A, Drummond GB. Ventilatory effects of meptazinol and pethidine in anaesthetised patients. *Br J Anaesth* 1987; **59:** 1127–33.
7. Davison AG, *et al.* Meptazinol overdose producing near fatal respiratory depression. *Hum Toxicol* 1987; **6:** 331.

## Interactions

For interactions associated with opioid analgesics, see p.73.

## Pharmacokinetics

After oral doses of meptazinol peak plasma concentrations have been achieved within 0.5 to 2 hours, but bioavailability is low since it undergoes extensive first-pass metabolism. Systemic availability is improved after rectal doses. Peak plasma concentrations have been achieved 30 minutes after rectal or intramuscular use. Plasma protein binding has averaged only about 27%. Elimination half-lives of about 2 hours have been reported. Meptazinol is extensively metabolised in the liver and is excreted mainly in the urine as the glucuronide conjugate. Less than 10% of a dose has been recovered from the faeces. Meptazinol crosses the placenta.

◊ References.

1. Franklin RA, *et al.* Studies on the metabolism of meptazinol, a new analgesic drug. *Br J Clin Pharmacol* 1976; **3:** 497–502.
2. Franklin RA, *et al.* Studies on the absorption and disposition of meptazinol following rectal administration. *Br J Clin Pharmacol* 1977; **4:** 163–7.
3. Davies G, *et al.* Pharmacokinetics of meptazinol in man following repeated intramuscular administration. *Eur J Clin Pharmacol* 1982; **23:** 535–8.
4. Norbury HM, *et al.* Pharmacokinetics of the new analgesic, meptazinol, after oral and intravenous administration to volunteers. *Eur J Clin Pharmacol* 1983; **25:** 77–80.
5. Murray GR, *et al.* The systemic availability of meptazinol in man after oral and rectal doses. *Eur J Clin Pharmacol* 1989; **36:** 279–82.

**The elderly.** A lower clearance and longer elimination half-life has been reported for meptazinol in elderly patients, but dosage reduction was not considered warranted on pharmacokinetic grounds. Mean half-lives in elderly and young subjects were 3.39 and 1.94 hours respectively following single oral doses[1] and 2.93 and 2.06 hours respectively after intravenous doses.[2]

1. Norbury HM, *et al.* Pharmacokinetics of meptazinol after single and multiple oral administration to elderly patients. *Eur J Clin Pharmacol* 1984; **27:** 223–6.
2. Murray GR, *et al.* Pharmacokinetics of meptazinol after parenteral administration in the elderly. *Eur J Clin Pharmacol* 1987; **31:** 733–6.

**Hepatic impairment.** Oral bioavailability of meptazinol appeared to be enhanced in patients with liver disease. Mean peak plasma concentrations of 184 nanograms/mL, 131 nanograms/mL, and 53 nanograms/mL were measured in cirrhotic patients, patients with non-cirrhotic liver disease, and patients with normal liver function, respectively, after a single oral dose of meptazinol, although there was no evidence of accumulation after chronic dosing.[1] There were no significant differences in plasma clearance after an intravenous dose. Reduced oral doses of meptazinol might be advisable in cirrhotic patients.

1. Birnie GG, *et al.* Enhanced oral bioavailability of meptazinol in cirrhosis. *Gut* 1987; **28:** 248–54.

**Pregnancy.** In women given an intramuscular injection of 100 to 150 mg during labour, meptazinol was found to cross the placenta readily but was rapidly eliminated from the neonate.[1] This contrasted with pethidine which was known to be excreted very slowly from neonates. As in the adult, elimination of meptazinol by the neonate appeared to take place mainly by conjugation with glucuronic acid.[2] A half-life of 3.4 hours, similar to that in adults, has been reported in the neonate,[3] in contrast to 22.7 hours for pethidine in neonates.

Disposition of meptazinol appears not to be significantly affected by pregnancy. Mean half-lives of 1.36 and 1.68 hours were reported in pregnant and non-pregnant women, respectively,[4] compared with 2.06 hours in men.

1. Franklin RA, *et al.* Preliminary studies on the disposition of meptazinol in the neonate. *Br J Clin Pharmacol* 1981; **12:** 88–90.
2. Dowell PS, *et al.* Routes of meptazinol conjugation in the neonate. *Br J Clin Pharmacol* 1982; **14:** 748–9.
3. Jackson MBA, Robson PJ. Preliminary clinical and pharmacokinetic experiences in the newborn when meptazinol is compared with pethidine as an obstetric analgesic. *Postgrad Med J* 1983; **59** (suppl 1): 47–51.
4. Murray GR, *et al.* The disposition of meptazinol after single and multiple intravenous administration to pregnant and non-pregnant women. *Eur J Clin Pharmacol* 1989; **36:** 273–7.

## Uses and Administration

Meptazinol is a mixed opioid agonist and antagonist with partial opioid agonist activity at the $\mu_1$ opioid receptor (see p.73); it also has cholinergic activity. Meptazinol is used in the treatment of moderate to severe pain. It has a shorter duration of action than morphine.

Meptazinol hydrochloride is given by mouth or by intramuscular or intravenous injection; doses are expressed in terms of the base. Meptazinol hydrochloride 115.6 mg is approximately equivalent to 100 mg of meptazinol. For the short-term treatment of moderate pain meptazinol is given by mouth in a dose of 200 mg every 3 to 6 hours. The intramuscular dose is 75 to 100 mg given every 2 to 4 hours; for obstetric pain a dose of 2 mg/kg (100 to 150 mg) may be used. Meptazinol is also given by slow intravenous injection in doses of 50 to 100 mg every 2 to 4 hours.

**Administration.** EPIDURAL ROUTE. Epidural administration of meptazinol 90 mg for postoperative pain was reported to be superior to intramuscular administration of 90 mg.[1] However, in another study[2] a 30-mg dose was ineffective and associated with an unacceptable incidence of adverse effects. A 60-mg dose was also found to be ineffective because of its short duration of action.[3]

The manufacturers in the UK state that the injectable formulation is not suitable for epidural or intrathecal use.

1. Verborgh C, *et al.* Meptazinol for postoperative pain relief in man: comparison of extradural and im administration. *Br J Anaesth* 1987; **59:** 1134–9.
2. Francis RI, Lockhart AS. Epidural meptazinol. *Anaesthesia* 1986; **41:** 88–9.
3. Birks RJS, Marsh DRG. Epidural meptazinol. *Anaesthesia* 1986; **41:** 883.

**Administration in hepatic impairment.** See under Pharmacokinetics, above for a suggestion that doses may need to be reduced in patients with cirrhosis.

## Preparations

***BP 2003:*** Meptazinol Injection; Meptazinol Tablets.

**Proprietary Preparations** (details are given in Part 3)
***Austria:*** Meptidol; ***Ger.:*** Meptid; ***Irl.:*** Meptid; ***UK:*** Meptid.

# Methadone Hydrochloride

*(BANM, pINNM)*

Amidine Hydrochloride; Amidone Hydrochloride; Hidrocloruro de metadona; (±)-Methadone Hydrochloride; Methadoni Hydrochloridum; Phenadone. (±)-6-Dimethylamino-4,4-diphenylheptan-3-one hydrochloride.

$C_{21}H_{27}NO,HCl = 345.9.$

*CAS — 76-99-3 (methadone); 297-88-1 (±methadone); 1095-90-5 (methadone hydrochloride); 125-56-4 (±methadone hydrochloride).*

*ATC — N07BC02.*

**Pharmacopoeias.** In *Chin., Eur.* (see p.vi), and *US.*

**Ph. Eur. 5.0** (Methadone Hydrochloride). White crystalline powder. Soluble in water; freely soluble in alcohol. Protect from light.

**USP 27** (Methadone Hydrochloride). Odourless colourless crystals or white crystalline powder. Soluble in water; freely soluble in alcohol and in chloroform; practically insoluble in ether and in glycerol. pH of a 1% solution in water is between 4.5 and 6.5. Store in airtight containers at a temperature of 25°, excursions permitted between 15° and 30°. Protect from light.

**Incompatibility.** There appears to be adequate evidence that stable solutions containing methadone hydrochloride and hydroxybenzoate esters can be formulated but the risk of precipitation exists if syrup preserved with hydroxybenzoates is used to extemporaneously prepare a methadone mixture 1 mg/mL to the DTF formula.[1] An oral formulation of methadone hydrochloride 5 mg/mL containing methyl hydroxybenzoate 0.1% as preservative rather than chloroform has been reported stable for at least 4 months at room temperature.[2]

1. *PSGB Lab Report P/80/1* 1980.
2. Ching MS, *et al.* Stability of methadone mixture with methyl hydroxybenzoate as a preservative. *Aust J Hosp Pharm* 1989; **19:** 159–61.

## Dependence and Withdrawal

As for Opioid Analgesics, p.71. Methadone withdrawal symptoms are similar to, but more prolonged than, those produced by morphine or diamorphine. They develop more slowly and do not usually appear until 24 to 48 hours after the last dose.

Methadone is used for substitution therapy in the management of opioid dependence (see under Uses and Administration, below).

## Adverse Effects and Treatment

As for Opioid Analgesics in general, p.72.

Methadone has a more prolonged effect than morphine and readily accumulates with repeated doses. It may have a relatively greater respiratory depressant effect than morphine and, although reported to be less sedating, repeated doses of methadone may result in marked sedation. After gross overdosage symptoms are similar to those of morphine poisoning. Pulmonary oedema after overdosage is a common cause of fatalities among addicts.

Methadone causes pain at injection sites; subcutaneous injection causes local tissue irritation and induration.

◊ It has been pointed out[1] that most cases of methadone poisoning occurred in persons not on maintenance, who were often children or family members of maintenance patients. Methadone is highly toxic to anyone who is not tolerant to opioids; 50 to 100 mg can be life-threatening in non-tolerant adults and 10 mg can be fatal in a young child.

A group[2] in Australia has found that the risk of death from methadone toxicity is greatest during the first 2 weeks of maintenance therapy. This has been attributed to the difficulty in determining a safe and effective starting dose of methadone and unreliable accounts of a patient's recent drug use.

1. Harding-Pink D. Opioid toxicity: methadone: one person's maintenance dose is another's poison. *Lancet* 1993; **341:** 665–6.
2. Caplehorn JRM, Drummer OH. Mortality associated with New South Wales methadone programs in 1994: lives lost and saved. *Med J Aust* 1999; **170:** 104–9.

**Effects on the endocrine system.** Hypoadrenalism has been demonstrated in chronic methadone addicts. Findings consistent with deficient ACTH production and subsequent secondary hypoadrenalism have been reported[1] although there is also evidence[2] of methadone-induced primary adrenal cortical hypofunction.

1. Dackis CA, *et al.* Methadone induced hypoadrenalism. *Lancet* 1982; **ii:** 1167.
2. Pullan PT, *et al.* Methadone-induced hypoadrenalism. *Lancet* 1983; **i:** 714.

**Effects on the nervous system.** Choreic movements in a patient on long-term methadone maintenance treatment for diamorphine addiction disappeared when methadone was discontinued.[1]

1. Wasserman S, Yahr MD. Choreic movements induced by the use of methadone. *Arch Neurol* 1980; **37:** 727–8.

**Effects on sexual function.** Sexual performance was impaired in 29 male diamorphine addicts receiving methadone maintenance therapy.[1] The function of secondary sex organs was markedly suppressed when compared with untreated diamorphine addicts or controls and serum-testosterone concentrations were 43% lower in those on methadone.

1. Cicero TJ, *et al.* Function of the male sex organs in heroin and methadone users. *N Engl J Med* 1975; **292:** 882–7.

## Precautions

As for Opioid Analgesics in general, p.72.

**Administration.** Methadone has a long half-life and accumulation may occur with repeated doses, especially in elderly or debilitated patients.[1] An 81-year-old woman given methadone 5 mg three times daily by mouth for 2 days became deeply unconscious but awoke immediately when given naloxone 400 micrograms intravenously.[2]

Sudden death in 10 diamorphine addicts occurred between 2 and 6 days after starting a methadone maintenance programme.[3] The mean prescribed dose of methadone at the time of death had been about 60 mg. There was evidence of chronic persistent hepatitis in all cases and liver disease could have reduced methadone clearance resulting in higher than expected blood concentrations. Liver function tests and urine testing for the presence of drugs prior to entry into methadone maintenance programmes and lower starting doses might decrease the likelihood of such deaths. Like dextropropoxyphene, methadone has membrane stabilising activity and can block nerve conduction, and it was suggested[4] that the sudden deaths were mainly due to accumulation of methadone over several days resulting in complications such as cardiac arrhythmias or cardiovascular collapse. See also under Adverse Effects, above.

For the effects of hepatic and renal impairment on the disposition of methadone, see under Pharmacokinetics, below.

1. Twycross RG. A comparison of diamorphine-with-cocaine and methadone. *Br J Clin Pharmacol* 1977; **4:** 691–3.
2. Symonds P. Methadone and the elderly. *BMJ* 1977; **i:** 512.
3. Drummer OH, *et al.* Deaths of heroin addicts starting on a methadone maintenance programme. *Lancet* 1990; **335:** 108.
4. Wu C, Henry JA. Deaths of heroin addicts starting on methadone maintenance. *Lancet* 1990; **335:** 424.

**Breast feeding.** The American Academy of Pediatrics considers that the use of methadone in breast-feeding mothers is usually compatible with breast feeding.[1] The *British National Formulary* also permits breast feeding by mothers on methadone maintenance although the dose should be as low as possible and the infant monitored to avoid sedation. Others have suggested that the amount of methadone in breast milk is unlikely to have any pharmacological effect on the infant.[2-5] However, in the past, there has been a report of the death of a 5-week-old breast-fed infant whose mother was on methadone maintenance.[6]

1. American Academy of Pediatrics. The transfer of drugs and other chemicals into human milk. *Pediatrics* 2001; **108:** 776–89. Correction. *ibid.*; 1029. Also available at: http://aappolicy.aappublications.org/cgi/content/full/pediatrics%3b108/3/776 (accessed 05/07/04)
2. Blinick G, *et al.* Methadone assays in pregnant women and progeny. *Am J Obstet Gynecol* 1975; **121:** 617–21.
3. Wojnar-Horton RE, *et al.* Methadone distribution and excretion into breast milk of clients in a methadone maintenance programme. *Br J Clin Pharmacol* 1997; **44:** 543–7.
4. Geraghty B, *et al.* Methadone levels in breast milk. *J Hum Lact* 1997; **13:** 227–30.
5. McCarthy JJ, Posey BL. Methadone levels in human milk. *J Hum Lact* 2000; **16:** 115–20.
6. Smialek JE, *et al.* Methadone deaths in children. *JAMA* 1977; **238:** 2516–17.

**Pregnancy.** Methadone is not recommended for use in labour because its prolonged duration of action increases the risk of neonatal respiratory depression.

Neonatal withdrawal syndrome and low birth-weight are immediate problems in the infants born to women receiving methadone for the management of opioid addiction; increased stillbirth rates have also been noted.[1-3] In the neonatal period moderate to severe opioid abstinence syndrome occurred in 75% of infants in one study,[2] as well as reduced head circumference and raised systolic blood pressure. At follow-up over 18 months these children had a higher incidence of otitis media, of reduced head circumference, and of abnormal eye findings when compared with drug-free controls. Neurobehavioural abnormalities and lower scores on mental and motor developmental indices were thought to be possible predictors of later learning and behavioural problems. However, no specific effect of methadone or diamorphine has been noted on intra-uterine and postnatal growth.[4]

1. Blinick G, *et al.* Methadone maintenance, pregnancy, and progeny. *JAMA* 1973; **225:** 477–9.
2. Rosen TS, Johnson HL. Children of methadone-maintained mothers: follow-up to 18 months of age. *J Pediatr* 1982; **101:** 192–6.
3. Kalter H, Warkany J. Congenital malformations. *N Engl J Med* 1983; **308:** 491–7.
4. Lifschitz MH, *et al.* Fetal and postnatal growth of children born to narcotic-dependent women. *J Pediatr* 1983; **102:** 686–91.

## Interactions

For interactions associated with opioid analgesics, see p.73. Methadone is metabolised in the liver primarily via the cytochrome P450 isoenzyme CYP3A4; the cytochromes CYP2D6, CYP2C9, CYP2C19, and CYP1A2 are also thought to play minor roles. Consequently, use with other drugs that induce or inhibit these isoenzymes may result in changes in plasma concentrations of methadone and, possibly adverse effects.

◊ Drugs that *acidify* or *alkalinise* the urine may have an effect on methadone pharmacokinetics since body clearance is increased at acidic pH and decreased at alkaline pH.[1]

1. Nilsson M-I, *et al.* Effect of urinary pH on the disposition of methadone in man. *Eur J Clin Pharmacol* 1982; **22:** 337–42.

**Antibacterials.** Withdrawal symptoms have been reported in patients maintained on methadone when they were given the enzyme inducer *rifampicin*.[1-3] Conversely, the use of *ciprofloxacin*, which inhibits CYP1A2 and CYP3A4, has resulted in signs of methadone toxicity.[4]

1. Kreek MJ, *et al.* Rifampin-induced methadone withdrawal. *N Engl J Med* 1976; **294:** 1104–6.
2. Bending MR, Skacel PO. Rifampicin and methadone withdrawal. *Lancet* 1977; **i:** 1211.
3. Raistrick D, *et al.* Methadone maintenance and tuberculosis treatment. *BMJ* 1996; **313:** 925–6.
4. Herrlin K, *et al.* Methadone, ciprofloxacin, and adverse drug reactions. *Lancet* 2000; **356:** 2069–70.

**Antidepressants.** *SSRIs* such as fluoxetine[1] and fluvoxamine[1,2] may enhance the effects of some opioid analgesics; such interactions may lead to methadone toxicity.

1. Eap CB, *et al.* Fluvoxamine and fluoxetine do not interact in the same way with the metabolism of the enantiomers of methadone. *J Clin Psychopharmacol* 1997; **17:** 113–17.
2. Bertschy G, *et al.* Probable metabolic interaction between methadone and fluvoxamine in addict patients. *Ther Drug Monit* 1994; **16:** 42–5.

**Antiepileptics.** Withdrawal symptoms have been reported in patients maintained on methadone when they were given *carbamazepine*,[1,2] *phenobarbital*[3] or *phenytoin*.[4,5]

1. Bell J, *et al.* The use of serum methadone levels in patients receiving methadone maintenance. *Clin Pharmacol Ther* 1988; **43:** 623–9.
2. Saxon AJ, *et al.* Valproic acid, unlike other anticonvulsants, has no effects on methadone metabolism: two cases. *J Clin Psychiatry* 1989; **50:** 228–9.
3. Liu S-J, Wang RIH. Case report of barbiturate-induced enhancement of methadone metabolism and withdrawal syndrome. *Am J Psychiatry* 1984; **141:** 1287–8.
4. Finelli PF. Phenytoin and methadone tolerance. *N Engl J Med* 1976; **294:** 227.
5. Tong TG, *et al.* Phenytoin-induced methadone withdrawal. *Ann Intern Med* 1981; **94:** 349–51.

**Antifungals.** Use of methadone with *fluconazole* has been reported[1] to result in increased serum concentrations of methadone although the authors of the study considered that for patients being treated for opioid dependence the interaction was unlikely to require adjustment of the methadone dose.

1. Cobb MN, *et al.* The effect of fluconazole on the clinical pharmacokinetics of methadone. *Clin Pharmacol Ther* 1998; **63:** 655–62.

**Antivirals.** Methadone possibly increases plasma concentrations of *zidovudine* (see p.659). There is limited evidence[1] that *nelfinavir* or *ritonavir* may reduce plasma concentrations of methadone; *indinavir* and *saquinavir* had no effect on plasma-methadone. *Lopinavir-ritonavir* may also reduce methadone concentrations.[2] *Nevirapine* has been reported to reduce plasma-methadone concentrations and withdrawal symptoms have occurred when it was given to patients receiving methadone.[3,4] A similar interaction has occurred when *efavirenz* has been taken with methadone.[5,6]

1. Beauverie P, *et al.* Therapeutic drug monitoring in HIV-infected patients receiving protease inhibitors. *AIDS* 1998; **12:** 2510–11.
2. McCance-Katz EF, *et al.* The protease inhibitor lopinavir-ritonavir may produce opiate withdrawal in methadone-maintained patients. *Clin Infect Dis* 2003; **37:** 476–82.
3. Altice FL, *et al.* Nevirapine induced opiate withdrawal among injection drug users with HIV infection receiving methadone. *AIDS* 1999; **13:** 957–62.
4. Clarke SM, *et al.* Pharmacokinetic interactions of nevirapine and methadone and guidelines for use of nevirapine to treat injection drug users. *Clin Infect Dis* 2001: **33:** 1595–7.
5. Pinzani V, *et al.* Methadone withdrawal symptoms with nevirapine and efavirenz. *Ann Pharmacother* 2000; **34:** 405–7.
6. Clarke SM, *et al.* The pharmacokinetics of methadone in HIV-positive patients receiving the non-nucleoside reverse transcriptase inhibitor efavirenz. *Br J Clin Pharmacol* 2001; **51:** 213–17.

**Gastrointestinal drugs.** Histamine $H_2$-antagonists such as *cimetidine* (see p.73) may enhance the effects of some opioid analgesics; such interactions may lead to methadone toxicity.

## Pharmacokinetics

Methadone hydrochloride is readily absorbed from the gastrointestinal tract and following subcutaneous or intramuscular injection. It is widely distributed in the tissues, diffuses across the placenta, and is distributed into breast milk. It is extensively protein bound. Methadone is metabolised in the liver, mainly by *N*-demethylation and cyclisation, and the metabolites are excreted in the bile and urine. Metabolism is primarily catalysed by CYP3A4, although other cytochrome P450 isoenzymes also play a role (see Interactions, above). It has a prolonged half-life and is subject to accumulation.

◊ In reviews of the pharmacokinetics of methadone[1-3] particular reference has been made to its long elimination half-life, accumulation following repeated doses, and wide interindividual variations.

Methadone is rapidly absorbed after administration by mouth and has high oral bioavailability. Peak plasma concentrations have been reported 1 to 5 hours after oral administration of a single dose in tablet form. It undergoes considerable tissue distribution and protein binding is reported to be 60 to 90% with $\alpha_1$-acid glycoprotein being the main binding protein in plasma. Metabolism to the major metabolite 2-ethylidine-1,5-dimethyl-3,3-diphenylpyrrolidine and the minor metabolite 2-ethyl-3,3-diphenyl-5-methylpyrrolidine, both of them inactive, occurs in the liver. These metabolites are excreted in the faeces and urine together with unchanged methadone. Other metabolites, including methadol and normethadol, have also been described. The liver may also serve as a major storage site of unchanged methadone which is taken up, bound non-specifically by the liver, and released again mainly unchanged. Urinary excretion of methadone is pH-dependent, the lower the pH the greater the clearance.

In addition to marked interindividual variations there are differences in the pharmacokinetics of methadone following single or multiple doses. Elimination half-lives vary considerably (a range of 15 to 60 hours has been quoted) and may be much longer than the 18 hours reported following a single dose. Careful adjustment of dosage is necessary with repeated administration.

Most studies have been in addicts. Plasma concentrations have been found to vary widely during methadone maintenance therapy with large differences between patients and wide fluctuations in individual patients. Interindividual variations in kinetics have also been seen in cancer patients.

1. Säwe J. High-dose morphine and methadone in cancer patients: clinical pharmacokinetic considerations of oral treatment. *Clin Pharmacokinet* 1986; **11:** 87–106.
2. Moore RA, *et al.* Opiate metabolism and excretion. *Baillieres Clin Anaesthesiol* 1987; **1:** 829–58.
3. Eap CB, *et al.* Interindividual variability of the clinical pharmacokinetics of methadone: implications for the treatment of opioid dependence. *Clin Pharmacokinet* 2002; **41:** 1153–93.

**Administration.** Methadone is considerably more lipid-soluble than morphine. A study of plasma concentrations and analgesia following intramuscular injection indicated that more rapid and greater relief of pain might be achieved if lipid-soluble opioid analgesics were injected into the deltoid rather than the gluteal muscle; there was no significant difference in absorption of morphine from the two sites.[1]

Other routes investigated in pharmacokinetic studies include continuous intravenous infusion[2] and continuous epidural infusion.[3]

1. Grabinski PY, *et al.* Plasma levels and analgesia following deltoid and gluteal injections of methadone and morphine. *J Clin Pharmacol* 1983; **23:** 48–55.
2. Denson DD, *et al.* Pharmacokinetics of continuous intravenous infusion of methadone in the early post-burn period. *J Clin Pharmacol* 1990; **30:** 70–5.
3. Shir Y, *et al.* Plasma concentrations of methadone during postoperative patient-controlled extradural analgesia. *Br J Anaesth* 1990; **65:** 204–9.

**Hepatic impairment.** Overall hepatic dysfunction does not seem unduly to disrupt methadone metabolism[1] and it has been suggested[2] that maintenance dosage of methadone need not be changed in stable chronic liver disease, although abrupt changes in hepatic status might result in substantial alterations in methadone disposition requiring dosage adjustments.

In a study of patients on methadone maintenance therapy[2] apparent terminal half-life of methadone was prolonged from a mean of 18.8 hours in those with healthy livers to 35.5 hours in patients with severe chronic liver disease. However plasma concentrations were not increased in such patients.

1. Moore RA, *et al.* Opiate metabolism and excretion. *Baillieres Clin Anaesthesiol* 1987; **1:** 829–58.
2. Novick DM, *et al.* Methadone disposition in patients with chronic liver disease. *Clin Pharmacol Ther* 1981; **30:** 353–62.

**Pregnancy.** Plasma concentrations of methadone were reduced in methadone-maintained pregnant women, probably due to enhanced metabolism.[1] It was suggested that the dose of methadone might need to be increased in such patients.

1. Pond SM, *et al.* Altered methadone pharmacokinetics in methadone-maintained pregnant women. *J Pharmacol Exp Ther* 1985; **233:** 1–6.

**Renal impairment.** The urinary excretion of methadone was reduced in renal failure,[1] but plasma concentrations were within the usual range and faecal excretion accounted for the majority of the dose. Very little methadone was removed by peritoneal dialysis or haemodialysis.

1. Kreek MJ, *et al.* Methadone use in patients with chronic renal disease. *Drug Alcohol Depend* 1980; **5:** 197–205.

## Uses and Administration

Methadone hydrochloride, a diphenylheptane derivative, is an opioid analgesic (p.73) that is primarily a μ opioid agonist. Single doses of methadone have a less marked sedative action than single doses of morphine. Methadone is a racemic mixture and levomethadone (p.54) is the active isomer. Methadone hydrochloride is used in the treatment of severe pain; it may be of use for those patients who experience excitation or exacerbation of pain with morphine. Levomethadone is used similarly in the treatment of severe pain. Methadone is also used in the management of opioid dependence. It has a depressant action on the cough centre and has been used as a cough suppressant in terminal illness, although the *British National Formulary* discourages this use because of the risks of accumulation.

The analgesic effect of methadone begins about 10 to 20 minutes after parenteral injection and about 30 to 60 minutes after doses by mouth, the effect of a single dose usually lasting about 4 hours. As accumulation occurs with repeated doses, the effects become more prolonged.

The dose of methadone hydrochloride used for **pain relief** ranges from 2.5 to 10 mg given at intervals of 3 to 8 hours depending on the pain. A commonly used range is 5 to 10 mg every 6 to 8 hours initially, adjusted according to response. To avoid the risk of accumulation and opioid overdosage it is recommended that in prolonged use methadone should not be given more than twice daily. It may be given by mouth or by subcutaneous or intramuscular injection; if repeated injections are required the intramuscular route is preferred to the subcutaneous.

Methadone hydrochloride is used as part of the treatment of **dependence on opioids**, although prolonged use of methadone itself may result in dependence. In the treatment of opioid withdrawal, or detoxification, methadone is given initially in doses sufficient to suppress withdrawal symptoms. A mixture containing 1 mg/mL of methadone hydrochloride is used in the UK for opioid dependent persons. A daily dose of 10 to 20 mg of methadone hydrochloride by mouth may be given initially and increased as necessary by 10 to 20 mg daily until there are no signs of withdrawal or intoxication. After stabilisation, which can often be achieved with a daily dose of 40 to 60 mg, the dose of methadone is gradually decreased until total withdrawal is achieved. Similar doses may also be given by subcutaneous or intramuscular injection. Some treatment schedules for opioid dependence involve prolonged maintenance therapy with methadone where the daily dose is adjusted carefully for the individual; there have been reports of some patients receiving 120 mg or more daily.

For the control of intractable **cough** associated with terminal lung cancer, methadone hydrochloride is usually given in the form of a linctus in a dose of 1 to 2 mg every 4 to 6 hours, but reduced to twice daily on prolonged use.

**Administration.** Although duration of action after single doses of methadone is similar to that of morphine, it increases considerably with multiple dosing of methadone because of the long elimination half-life (see Pharmacokinetics, above). The minimum effective dose of methadone can be difficult to titrate for the individual patient. A fixed 10-mg oral dose with a flexible patient-controlled dosage interval has been used in patients with chronic cancer pain.[1] Dosage not more frequently than every 4 hours during the first 3 to 5 days, followed by a fixed dose every 8 to 12 hours depending on the patient's requirements, was advised.

A suggested dose for patients who need to switch from oral morphine to methadone because of poor pain control is one tenth of the total daily dose of morphine, but not greater than 100 mg given at intervals determined by the patient and not more frequently than every 3 hours.[2]

When switching from oral to parenteral use it was suggested[3] that the dose of methadone should be halved and adjusted thereafter as necessary.

Apart from subcutaneous or intramuscular injection methadone has also been given intravenously or intraspinally. Evidence of the prolonged effect of methadone was demonstrated when a single intravenous bolus dose of 20 mg resulted in postoperative analgesia lasting about 25 hours.[4] Methadone has also been tried intravenously in children to prevent postoperative pain; a dose of 200 micrograms/kg was given perioperatively followed postoperatively by 50 micrograms/kg every 10 minutes until the patient was both comfortable and adequately alert.[5] An initial 2-hour loading intravenous infusion of methadone 100 to 200 micrograms/kg per hour to provide rapid analgesia followed by infusion at a lower maintenance rate of 10 to 20 micrograms/kg per hour for continuous pain relief has been used in burn patients.[6] Epidural methadone has been used successfully in doses of up to 5 mg for analgesia in association with bupivacaine.[7,8]


1. Säwe J, *et al.* Patient-controlled dose regimen of methadone for chronic cancer pain. *BMJ* 1981; **282:** 771–3.
2. Morley JS, *et al.* Methadone in pain uncontrolled by morphine. *Lancet* 1993; **342:** 1243.
3. Säwe J. High-dose morphine and methadone in cancer patients: clinical pharmacokinetic considerations of oral treatment. *Clin Pharmacokinet* 1986; **11:** 87–106.
4. Gourlay GK, *et al.* Methadone produces prolonged postoperative analgesia. *BMJ* 1982; **284:** 630–1.
5. Berde CB, *et al.* Comparison of morphine and methadone for prevention of postoperative pain in 3- to 7-year-old children. *J Pediatr* 1991; **119:** 136–41.
6. Denson DD, *et al.* Pharmacokinetics of continuous intravenous infusion of methadone in the early post-burn period. *J Clin Pharmacol* 1990; **30:** 70–5.
7. Drenger B, *et al.* Extradural bupivacaine and methadone for extracorporeal shock-wave lithotripsy. *Br J Anaesth* 1989; **62:** 82–6.
8. Martin CS, *et al.* Extradural methadone and bupivacaine in labour. *Br J Anaesth* 1990; **65:** 330–2.


**Cancer pain.** Methadone is used as an alternative to morphine in the treatment of severe cancer pain. A better understanding of its pharmacokinetics and of equianalgesic doses may address early concerns about the risk of cumulative toxicity associated with prolonged use. However, its long terminal half-life makes it less suitable for the treatment of breakthrough pain.

Methadone has been given by the oral, rectal, and parenteral routes.

References.


1. Ayonrinde OT, Bridge DT. The rediscovery of methadone for cancer pain management. *Med J Aust* 2000; **173:** 536–40.
2. Bruera E, Sweeney C. Methadone use in cancer patients with pain: a review. *J Palliat Med* 2002; **5:** 127–38.
3. Nicholson AB. Methadone for cancer pain. Available in The Cochrane Library; Issue 2. Chichester: John Wiley; 2004.


**Opioid dependence.** The treatment of opioid dependence is discussed on p.71. In the UK, oral liquid preparations of methadone hydrochloride 1 mg/mL are widely used for this purpose. It is important to note that these preparations are 2.5 times **stronger** than Methadone Linctus (BP 2003), and although some are licensed for analgesia in severe pain, many are licensed for the treatment of opioid dependence only. Methadone Oral Solution (1 mg/mL) (BP 2003) is available as a ready-to-use solution or may be prepared from Methadone Hydrochloride Oral Concentrate. However, most commercially available preparations in the UK still follow an earlier formula formerly listed in the Drug Tariff Formulary (DTF):

**Methadone Mixture 1 mg/mL**
methadone hydrochloride 10 mg
Green S and Tartrazine Solution (BP 1980) 0.02 mL
Compound Tartrazine Solution (BP 1980) 0.08 mL
syrup, unpreserved 5 mL
chloroform water, double-strength to 10 mL.

Some commercially available forms of DTF Methadone Mixture 1 mg/mL use a preservative system based on hydroxybenzoate esters rather than chloroform; however, syrup preserved with hydroxybenzoate esters may be unsuitable for extemporaneous dispensing (see under Incompatibility, above).

References.


1. Ghodse AH, *et al.* Comparison of oral preparations of heroin and methadone to stabilise opiate misusers as inpatients. *BMJ* 1990; **300:** 719–20.
2. Wolff K, *et al.* Measuring compliance in methadone maintenance patients: use of a pharmacologic indicator to "estimate" methadone plasma levels. *Clin Pharmacol Ther* 1991; **50:** 199–207.
3. Wilson P, *et al.* Methadone maintenance in general practice: patients, workload, and outcomes. *BMJ* 1994; **309:** 641–4.
4. Farrell M, *et al.* Methadone maintenance treatment in opiate dependence: a review. *BMJ* 1994; **309:** 997–1001.
5. Henry JA. Methadone: where are we now? *Hosp Med* 1999; **60:** 161–4.
6. Amato L, *et al.* Methadone at tapered doses for the management of opioid withdrawal. Available in The Cochrane Library; Issue 2. Chichester: John Wiley; 2004.
7. Faggiano F, *et al.* Methadone maintenance at different dosages for opioid [sic] dependence. Available in The Cochrane Library; Issue 2. Chichester: John Wiley; 2004.
8. Mattick RP, *et al.* Methadone maintenance therapy versus no opioid replacement therapy for opioid dependence. Available in The Cochrane Library; Issue 2. Chichester: John Wiley; 2004.


### Preparations

***BP 2003:*** Methadone Injection; Methadone Linctus; Methadone Oral Solution (1 mg per mL); Methadone Tablets;
***USP 27:*** Methadone Hydrochloride Injection; Methadone Hydrochloride Oral Concentrate; Methadone Hydrochloride Oral Solution; Methadone Hydrochloride Tablets; Methadone Hydrochloride Tablets for Oral Suspension.

**Proprietary Preparations** (details are given in Part 3)
***Arg.:*** Gobbidona; ***Austral.:*** Biodone Forte; Physeptone; ***Austria:*** Heptadon; ***Braz.:*** Metadon; ***Canad.:*** Metadol; ***Chile:*** Amidona; ***Fin.:*** Dolmed; ***Ger.:*** L-Polamidon; Methaddict†; ***Hong Kong:*** Physeptone; ***Irl.:*** Phymet DTF; Physeptone; Pinadone DTF; ***Israel:*** Adolan; ***Ital.:*** Eptadone; ***Neth.:*** Symoron; ***NZ:*** Biodone; Methatabs; Pallidone; ***S.Afr.:*** Physeptone; ***Singapore:*** Physeptone; ***Spain:*** Metasedin; Sedo†; ***Switz.:*** Ketalgine; ***UK:*** Martindale Methadone Mixture DTF; Methadose; Methex†; Physeptone; Synastone; ***USA:*** Dolophine; Methadose.

## Methyl Butetisalicylate

Butetisalicilato de metilo; Methyl Diethylacetylsalicylate. Methyl *O*-(2-ethylbutyryl)salicylate.
$C_{14}H_{18}O_4$ = 250.3.

### Profile

Methyl butetisalicylate is a salicylic acid derivative that has been used similarly to methyl salicylate (p.59) as a rubefacient for the relief of musculoskeletal, joint, and soft-tissue pain.

### Preparations

**Proprietary Preparations** (details are given in Part 3)
***Fr.:*** Dolodermt†; ***Ital.:*** Doloderm.

## Methyl Gentisate

Gentisato de metilo. 2,5-Dihydroxybenzoic acid methyl ester.
$C_8H_8O_4$ = 168.1.
*CAS — 2150-46-1.*

### Profile

Methyl gentisate has been used topically for the relief of musculoskeletal and joint pain.

### Preparations

**Proprietary Preparations** (details are given in Part 3)
**Multi-ingredient:** ***Ital.:*** Reumacort.

## Methyl Nicotinate *(USAN)*

Nicotinato de metilo. Methyl pyridine-3-carboxylate.
$C_7H_7NO_2$ = 137.1.
*CAS — 93-60-7.*

**Pharmacopoeias.** In *Br.*

**BP 2003** (Methyl Nicotinate). White or almost white crystals or crystalline powder with a characteristic odour; m.p. 40° to 42°. Very soluble in water, in alcohol, and in chloroform; freely soluble in ether.

### Profile

Methyl nicotinate is used in topical preparations as a rubefacient.

### Preparations

**Proprietary Preparations** (details are given in Part 3)
***UK:*** Pickles Chilblain Cream.

**Multi-ingredient:** ***Arg.:*** Infrarub; Medex Rub; ***Austral.:*** Deep Heat; ***Austria:*** Berggeist; ***Belg.:*** Algipan; Decontractyl†; Percutalgine; Rado-Spray; ***Braz.:*** Ateroide†; Infrarub†; ***Canad.:*** Arthricare Odor Free; Arthricare Triple Medicated; Midalgan; ***Chile:*** Frixio; Konirub; ***Fr.:*** Algipan; Capsic†; Cliptol Sport; Decontractyl; Gel Rubefiant; Percutalgine; Sedartryl; ***Ger.:*** Contrheuma-Gel forte N†; Doloneuro; Forapin E; Kytta-Balsam f; Menthoneurin-Vollbad N†; Midysalb†; Pernionin Voll-Bad N; Pernionin†; Rheumasan N†; Spondylon; Thermo-Menthoneurin Bad†; ***India:*** Algipan; Flamar; Medicreme; Relaxyl; ***Irl.:*** Algipan; ***Israel:*** Deep Heat Spray; ***Ital.:*** Aspercreme†; Balsamo Sifcamina; Relaxar; Sedalpan; ***Port.:*** Midalgan; ***S.Afr.:*** Sportsman Rub†; ***Singapore:*** Deep Heating Spray; ***Spain:*** Balsamo Midalgan†; Doctofril Antiinflamat; Doctomitil; Percutalin†; Radio Salil; ***Switz.:*** Kytta Baume; Midalgan; Radalgin; Roliwol†; ***Thai.:*** Percutalgine; ***UK:*** Algipan†; Cremalgin; Deep Heat Spray; Dubam; Fiery Jack; Radian-B Red Oils; Ralgex; Ralgex Heat Spray (low-odour); Red Oil; Transvasin Heat Spray; ***USA:*** Arthricare Odor Free; Arthricare Triple Medicated; Musterole.

## Methyl Salicylate

Methyl Sal.; Methylis Salicylas; Salicilato de metilo. Methyl 2-hydroxybenzoate.
$C_8H_8O_3$ = 152.1.
*CAS — 119-36-8.*

NOTE. Methyl salicylate and methyl salicylate liniment have been known previously as oil of wintergreen, wintergreen, and wintergreen oil. Wintergreen oil has also been known as sweet birch oil.

**Pharmacopoeias.** In *Eur.* (see p.vi), *Jpn, Pol.,* and *Viet.* Also in *USNF.*

**Ph. Eur. 5.0** (Methyl Salicylate). A colourless or slightly yellow liquid. Very slightly soluble in water; miscible with alcohol, and with fatty and essential oils. Protect from light.

**USNF 22** (Methyl Salicylate). It is produced synthetically or is obtained from the leaves of *Gaultheria procumbens* (Ericaceae) [wintergreen] or from the bark of *Betula lenta* (Betulaceae) [sweet or black birch]. The source of the methyl salicylate must be indicated on the label.

A colourless, yellowish, or reddish liquid having the characteristic odour of wintergreen. Slightly soluble in water; soluble in alcohol and in glacial acetic acid. Store in airtight containers.

**Storage.** Certain plastic containers, such as those made from polystyrene, are unsuitable for liniments or ointments containing methyl salicylate.

### Adverse Effects, Treatment, and Precautions

Salicylate intoxication can occur following ingestion or topical application of methyl salicylate (see Adverse Effects of Aspirin, p.15).

**Overdosage.** Ingestion of methyl salicylate poses the threat of severe, rapid-onset salicylate poisoning because of its liquid concentrated form and lipid solubility.[1] It is readily absorbed from the gastrointestinal tract and most is rapidly hydrolysed to free salicylate. The symptoms, which may appear within 2 hours of ingestion, are similar to those of salicylate poisoning in general (see Adverse Effects of Aspirin, p.15), although methyl salicylate is expected to be more toxic because of its lipid solubility. There have been reports of fatalities following ingestion of as little as 4 mL in a child and 6 mL in an adult, although the adult lethal dose is estimated to be 30 mL.[1] Topical Chinese herbal medicinal oils may contain methyl salicylate in variable amounts, and salicylate poisoning has been reported in a woman who had attempted suicide by taking such a preparation, Red Flower Oil.[2] The authors also noted that some patients took small amounts of this preparation orally in an attempt to enhance its analgesic effects.


1. Chan TYK. Potential dangers from topical preparations containing methyl salicylate. *Hum Exp Toxicol* 1996; **15:** 747–50.
2. Chan TH, *et al.* Severe salicylate poisoning associated with the intake of Chinese medicinal oil ('Red Flower Oil'). *Aust N Z J Med* 1995; **25:** 57.


**Percutaneous absorption.** Like other salicylates, methyl salicylate may be absorbed through intact skin.[1] Percutaneous absorption is enhanced by exercise, heat, occlusion, or disruption of the integrity of the skin. The amount absorbed will also be increased by application to large areas of skin. Results from a study in healthy subjects demonstrated that a considerable amount of salicylic acid may be absorbed through the skin after topical application of products containing methyl salicylate.[2] Both the rate and extent of absorption increased after repeated application; the bioavailability of the ointment preparation used in the study increased from 15% after the second dose to 22% after the third to eighth dose. The authors recommend that topical analgesic preparations containing methyl salicylate or other salicylates should be used with caution in patients at increased risk of developing salicylate adverse effects (see Precautions of Aspirin, p.16). Results from another study[3] demonstrating high tissue to plasma ratios following topical application of a methyl salicylate formulation suggest that direct penetration and not recirculation in the blood is responsible for the salicylate concentrations found. The results also demonstrated that methyl salicylate is extensively metabolised to salicylic acid in the dermal and subcutaneous tissues following topical administration.


1. Chan TYK. Potential dangers from topical preparations containing methyl salicylate. *Hum Exp Toxicol* 1996; **15:** 747–50.
2. Morra P, *et al.* Serum concentrations of salicylic acid following topical applied salicylate derivatives. *Ann Pharmacother* 1996; **30:** 935–40.
3. Cross SE, *et al.* Is there tissue penetration after application of topical salicylate formulations? *Lancet* 1997; **350:** 636.


### Interactions

Absorption of methyl salicylate through the skin can occur following excessive topical application (see above), and interactions would be expected to be as for other salicylates (see Interactions of Aspirin, p.17).

**Anticoagulants.** Potentiation of warfarin anticoagulation has been reported[1-3] following topical application of methyl salicylate preparations.


1. Littleton F. Warfarin and topical salicylates. *JAMA* 1990; **263:** 2888.
2. Tam LS, *et al.* Warfarin interactions with Chinese traditional medicines: danshen and methyl salicylate medicated oil. *Aust N Z J Med* 1995; **25:** 258.
3. Joss JD, LeBlond RF. Potentiation of warfarin anticoagulation associated with topical methyl salicylate. *Ann Pharmacother* 2000; **34:** 729–33.


## Uses and Administration

Methyl salicylate is a salicylic acid derivative that is irritant to the skin and is used topically in rubefacient preparations for the relief of pain in musculoskeletal, joint, and soft-tissue disorders. It is also used for minor peripheral vascular disorders such as chilblains and as an ingredient in inhalations for the symptomatic relief of upper respiratory-tract disorders.

## Preparations

***BP 2003:*** Kaolin Poultice; Methyl Salicylate Liniment; Methyl Salicylate Ointment; Surgical Spirit.

**Proprietary Preparations** (details are given in Part 3)
***Arg.:*** Aspi-Rub; Rati Salil Gel; ***Austral.:*** Linsal; Metsal Liniment†; ***Braz.:*** Dul-X†; Gellodex†; ***Ger.:*** Hewedolor N; Rheumax†; ***Mex.:*** Tolan; ***Port.:*** Balsamo Analgesico Labesfal; ***S.Afr.:*** Thermo-Rub; ***Thai.:*** Mygesal†; ***USA:*** Argesic; Exocaine; Gordogesic.

**Multi-ingredient:** numerous preparations are listed in Part 3.

## Mofebutazone *(rINN)*

Mofebutazona; Monobutazone; Monophenylbutazone. 4-Butyl-1-phenylpyrazolidine-3,5-dione.

$C_{13}H_{16}N_2O_2$ = 232.3.
*CAS — 2210-63-1.*
*ATC — M01AA02; M02AA02.*

### Profile

Mofebutazone, a derivative of phenylbutazone (p.83), is an NSAID (p.67). It has been used in the management of musculoskeletal and joint disorders. The sodium salt has been given by intramuscular injection.

### Preparations

**Proprietary Preparations** (details are given in Part 3)
***Ger.:*** Diadin M†; Mofesal N; Mofesal†.

**Multi-ingredient: *Ger.:*** Vasotonin forte†.

## Mofezolac *(rINN)*

Mofezolaco; N-22. 3,4-Bis(*p*-methoxyphenyl)-5-isoxazoleacetic acid.

$C_{19}H_{17}NO_5$ = 339.3.
*CAS — 78967-07-4.*

### Profile

Mofezolac is an NSAID (p.67).

## Morniflumate *(USAN, rINN)*

Morniflumato; UP-164. 2-Morpholinoethyl 2-(α,α,α-trifluoro-*m*-toluidino)nicotinate.

$C_{19}H_{20}F_3N_3O_3$ = 395.4.
*CAS — 65847-85-0.*
*ATC — M01AX22.*

### Profile

Morniflumate, the morpholinoethyl ester of niflumic acid (p.67), is an NSAID (p.67). It has been used in inflammatory conditions in doses of 700 mg given twice daily by mouth or rectally as suppositories.

### Preparations

**Proprietary Preparations** (details are given in Part 3)
***Fr.:*** Nifluril; ***Ital.:*** Flomax; Morniflu; Niflam; ***Spain:*** Niflactol; ***Switz.:*** Nifluril†.

# Morphine *(BAN)*

Morfina. 7,8-Didehydro-4,5-epoxy-17-methylmorphinan-3,6-diol.

$C_{17}H_{19}NO_3$ = 285.3.
*CAS — 57-27-2 (anhydrous morphine); 6009-81-0 (morphine monohydrate).*
*ATC — N02AA01.*

## Morphine Hydrochloride *(BANM)*

Morfina, hidrocloruro de; Morphini Hydrochloridum; Morphinii Chloridum; Morphinum Chloratum.

$C_{17}H_{19}NO_3,HCl,3H_2O$ = 375.8.
*CAS — 52-26-6 (anhydrous morphine hydrochloride); 6055-06-7 (morphine hydrochloride trihydrate).*

**Pharmacopoeias.** In *Chin., Eur.* (see p.vi), *Int., Jpn, Pol.,* and *Viet.*

**Ph. Eur. 5.0** (Morphine Hydrochloride). Colourless, silky needles, cubical masses or a white or almost white, crystalline powder. It is efflorescent in a dry atmosphere. Soluble in water and in glycerol; slightly soluble in alcohol. Protect from light.

**Incompatibility.** See under Morphine Sulfate, below.

## Morphine Sulfate

Morfina, sulfato de; Morphine Sulphate *(BANM)*; Morphini Sulfas.

$(C_{17}H_{19}NO_3)_2,H_2SO_4,5H_2O$ = 758.8.
*CAS — 64-31-3 (anhydrous morphine sulfate); 6211-15-0 (morphine sulfate pentahydrate).*

**Pharmacopoeias.** In *Chin., Eur.* (see p.vi), *Int., Pol.,* and *US.*

**Ph. Eur. 5.0** (Morphine Sulphate). A white or almost white, crystalline powder. Soluble in water; very slightly soluble in alcohol; practically insoluble in toluene. Protect from light.

**USP 27** (Morphine Sulfate). White, feathery, silky crystals, cubical masses of crystals, or a white crystalline powder. Is odourless and when exposed to air it gradually loses water of hydration. It darkens on prolonged exposure to light. Soluble 1 in 16 of water and 1 in 1 of water at 80°; soluble 1 in 570 of alcohol and 1 in 240 of alcohol at 60°; insoluble in chloroform and in ether. Store in airtight containers at a temperature of 25°, excursions permitted between 15° and 30°. Protect from light.

**Incompatibility.** Morphine salts are sensitive to changes in pH and morphine is liable to be precipitated out of solution in an alkaline environment. Compounds incompatible with morphine salts include aminophylline and sodium salts of barbiturates and phenytoin. Other incompatibilities, sometimes attributed to particular formulations, have included:

- Aciclovir sodium—precipitate noted 2 hours after admixture with morphine sulfate solution[1]
- Chlorpromazine hydrochloride injection—precipitation was considered to be due to chlorocresol present in the morphine sulfate injection[2]
- Doxorubicin—addition of morphine sulfate 1 mg/mL to doxorubicin hydrochloride liposomal injection 400 micrograms/mL in dextrose 5% resulted in turbidity changes[3]
- Fluorouracil—immediate precipitate formed after admixture of fluorouracil 1 or 16 mg/mL with morphine sulfate 1 mg/mL in dextrose 5% or sodium chloride 0.9%[4]
- Furosemide—precipitate noted 1 hour after admixture with morphine sulfate solution[1]
- Heparin sodium—incompatibility has been reported from straightforward additive studies.[5] A more recent study[6] indicated that morphine sulfate and heparin sodium were only incompatible at morphine sulfate concentrations greater than 5 mg/mL and that this incompatibility could be prevented by using 0.9% sodium chloride solution as the admixture diluent rather than water
- Pethidine hydrochloride—incompatibility has been noted following admixture with morphine sulfate[5,7]
- Prochlorperazine edisilate—immediate precipitation was attributed to phenol in the morphine sulfate injection formulation[8,9]
- Promethazine hydrochloride—cloudiness was reported to develop when 12.5 mg of promethazine hydrochloride was drawn into a syringe containing morphine sulfate 8 mg.[10] Others[7] have noted no incompatibility
- Tetracyclines—colour change from pale yellow to light green occurred when solutions of minocycline hydrochloride or tetracycline hydrochloride were mixed with morphine sulfate in 5% glucose injection[11]


1. Pugh CB, *et al.* Visual compatibility of morphine sulphate and meperidine hydrochloride with other injectable drugs during simulated Y-site injection. *Am J Hosp Pharm* 1991; **48:** 123–5.
2. Crapper JB. Mixing chlorpromazine and morphine. *BMJ* 1975; **i:** 33.
3. Trissel LA, *et al.* Compatibility of doxorubicin hydrochloride liposome injection with selected other drugs during simulated Y-site administration. *Am J Health-Syst Pharm* 1997; **54:** 2708–13.
4. Xu QA, *et al.* Stability and compatibility of fluorouracil with morphine sulfate and hydromorphone hydrochloride. *Ann Pharmacother* 1996; **30:** 756–61.
5. Patel JA, Phillips GL. A guide to physical compatibility of intravenous drug admixtures. *Am J Hosp Pharm* 1966; **23:** 409–11.
6. Baker DE, *et al.* Compatibility of heparin sodium and morphine sulfate. *Am J Hosp Pharm* 1985; **42:** 1352–5.
7. Parker WA. Physical compatibilities of preanesthetic medications. *Can J Hosp Pharm* 1976; **29:** 91–2.
8. Stevenson JG, Patriarca C. Incompatibility of morphine sulfate and prochlorperazine edisylate in syringes. *Am J Hosp Pharm* 1985; **42:** 2651.
9. Zuber DEL. Compatibility of morphine sulfate injection and prochlorperazine edisylate injection. *Am J Hosp Pharm* 1987; **44:** 67.
10. Fleischer NM. Promethazine hydrochloride—morphine sulfate incompatibility. *Am J Hosp Pharm* 1973; **30:** 665.
11. Nieves-Cordero AL, *et al.* Compatibility of narcotic analgesic solutions with various antibiotics during simulated Y-site injection. *Am J Hosp Pharm* 1985; **42:** 1108–9.


**Stability.** INTRAVENOUS PREPARATIONS. Solutions of morphine sulfate for intravenous infusion appear to be relatively stable. In a study[1] solutions containing 40 micrograms/mL and 400 micrograms/mL retained more than 90% of their initial concentration of morphine sulfate when stored at 4° or 23° for 7 days, whether or not they were protected from light. Solutions prepared from commercially available injection or from powder, in 0.9% sodium chloride or 5% glucose, and stored in PVC bags or glass bottles did not differ in stability from one another. In a further study[2] 10 mg/mL or 5 mg/mL solutions of morphine sulfate in glucose or sodium chloride and stored in portable infusion pump cassettes retained more than 95% of their initial concentration when kept at 23° for 30 days. A 0.9% solution of sodium chloride containing morphine sulfate 2 mg/mL was stable for 6 weeks when stored in polypropylene syringes at ambient temperatures in the light or dark but a similar solution which also contained 0.1% sodium metabisulfite lost 15% of its potency during the same period.[3] Stability of such a solution with or without sodium metabisulfite was considered to be unacceptable when stored in glass syringes in the dark.[4]


1. Vecchio M, *et al.* The stability of morphine intravenous infusion solutions. *Can J Hosp Pharm* 1988; **41:** 5–9, 43.
2. Walker SE, *et al.* Hydromorphone and morphine stability in portable infusion pump cassettes and minibags. *Can J Hosp Pharm* 1988; **41:** 177–82.
3. Grassby PF. The stability of morphine sulphate in 0.9 per cent sodium chloride stored in plastic syringes. *Pharm J* 1991; **248:** HS24–HS25.
4. Grassby PF, Hutchings L. Factors affecting the physical and chemical stability of morphine sulphate solutions stored in syringes. *Int J Pharm Pract* 1993; **2:** 39–43.


ORAL PREPARATIONS. Studies[1,2] have shown that for optimum stability of morphine content, Kaolin and Morphine Mixture (BP) needed to be stored in well-filled glass containers.


1. Helliwell K, Game P. Stability of morphine in kaolin and morphine mixture BP. *Pharm J* 1981; **227:** 128–9.
2. Helliwell K, Jennings P. Kaolin and morphine mixture BP: effects of containers on the stability of morphine. *Pharm J* 1984; **232:** 682.


## Morphine Tartrate *(BANM)*

Morfina, tartrato de.

$(C_{17}H_{19}NO_3)_2,C_4H_6O_6,3H_2O$ = 774.8.
*CAS — 302-31-8 (anhydrous morphine tartrate); 6032-59-3 (morphine tartrate trihydrate).*

**Incompatibility.** See under Morphine Sulfate, above.

## Dependence and Withdrawal

As for Opioid Analgesics, p.71.

Dependence associated with morphine and closely related μ-agonists appears to result in more severe withdrawal symptoms than that associated with κ-receptor agonists. With morphine, withdrawal symptoms usually begin within a few hours, reach a peak within 36 to 72 hours, and then gradually subside.

## Adverse Effects and Treatment

As for Opioid Analgesics in general, p.72.

**Effects on the cardiovascular system.** For a reference to the effects of morphine on histamine release compared with some other opioids, see under Pethidine, p.80.

**Effects on the muscles.** There has been a report of severe rectovaginal spasms in a patient given intrathecal morphine.[1] The spasms were successfully controlled with midazolam.


1. Littrell RA, *et al.* Muscle spasms associated with intrathecal morphine therapy: treatment with midazolam. *Clin Pharm* 1992; **11:** 57–9.


**Effects on the nervous system.** Myoclonus has been reported in patients with advanced malignant disease receiving high doses of morphine.[1] It was unrelated to plasma-morphine concentrations and was attributed in part to the concurrent use of other drugs including antidepressants, antipsychotics, and NSAIDs. The diagnosis of myoclonus and the role of morphine in this case has been questioned;[2] others[3] also criticised the importance attached to myoclonus and considered it probably the least common and least important of all the side-effects of morphine.

Myoclonus was also reported[4] in 2 cancer patients with renal impairment on high stable doses of morphine; the metabolite normorphine, found in the plasma of both patients, might have been responsible.

It has been reported that myoclonus induced by morphine may be successfully controlled using a benzodiazepine such as midazolam.[5]


1. Potter JM, *et al.* Myoclonus associated with treatment with high doses of morphine: the role of supplemental drugs. *BMJ* 1989; **299:** 150–3.
2. Quinn N. Myoclonus associated with high doses of morphine. *BMJ* 1989; **299:** 683–4.
3. McQuay HJ, *et al.* Myoclonus associated with high doses of morphine. *BMJ* 1989; **299:** 684.
4. Glare PA, *et al.* Normorphine, a neurotoxic metabolite? *Lancet* 1990; **335:** 725–6.
5. Holdsworth MT, *et al.* Continuous midazolam infusion for the management of morphine-induced myoclonus. *Ann Pharmacother* 1995; **29:** 25–9.


## Precautions

As for Opioid Analgesics in general, p.72.

**Biliary-tract disorders.** See under Precautions of Opioid Analgesics, p.73.

**Breast feeding.** The American Academy of Pediatrics[1] states that the use of morphine is usually compatible with breast feeding; although the infant may have measurable blood concentrations of the drug, no adverse effects have been reported.[2,3]


1. American Academy of Pediatrics. The transfer of drugs and other chemicals into human milk. *Pediatrics* 2001; **108:** 776–89. Correction. *ibid.*; 1029. Also available at: http://aappolicy.aappublications.org/cgi/content/full/pediatrics%3b108/3/776 (accessed 06/07/04)
2. Robieux I, *et al.* Morphine excretion in breast milk and resultant exposure of a nursing infant. *J Toxicol Clin Toxicol* 1990; **28:** 365–70.
3. Oberlander TF, *et al.* Prenatal and breast milk morphine exposure following maternal intrathecal morphine treatment. *J Hum Lact* 2000; **16:** 137–42.


**Hepatic impairment.** In view of its hepatic metabolism, caution is generally advised when giving morphine to patients with hepatic impairment (but see under Pharmacokinetics, below). The *British National Formulary* advises that use should be avoided or the dose reduced because of the risk of precipitating a coma although it is also noted that many patients with hepatic impairment tolerate morphine well. Others have considered that severe hepatic impairment may affect morphine metabolism but less severe impairment does not.[1]

The mean elimination half-life of morphine in 12 patients with cirrhosis was almost twice that in 10 healthy subjects after administration of a modified-release oral morphine preparation (MST-Continus) and peak serum concentrations were almost three times as high.[2] Patients with cirrhosis exhibited a greater degree of sedation but none developed encephalopathy. It was recommended that the dose for modified-release preparations should be reduced and that it be given less often when patients have cirrhosis.


1. Twycross RG, Lack SA. *Oral morphine in advanced cancer.* 2nd ed. Beaconsfield: Beaconsfield Publishers, 1989.
2. Kotb HIM, *et al.* Pharmacokinetics of controlled release morphine (MST) in patients with liver cirrhosis. *Br J Anaesth* 1997; **79:** 804–6.


**Phaeochromocytoma.** Morphine and some other opioids can induce the release of endogenous histamine and thereby stimulate catecholamine release making them unsuitable for use in patients with phaeochromocytoma. For further details, see p.73.

**Renal impairment.** Severe and prolonged respiratory depression has occurred in patients with renal impairment given morphine. Toxicity in 3 such patients was attributed to the accumulation of the active metabolite morphine-6-glucuronide.[1] Plasma concentrations of this metabolite were found[2] to be ten times higher than normal in a 7-year-old girl with haemolytic uraemic syndrome given morphine intravenously although the half-life of morphine was also prolonged. Plasma concentrations of morphine-6-glucuronide were also reported[3] to be persistently increased 19 days after stopping morphine by intravenous infusion in a 17-year-old girl with normal renal function. The authors of the report suggested that alterations in bowel flora following antibiotic therapy or inhibition of morphine-3-glucuronide glucuronidation by lorazepam might be responsible. It has also been reported[4] that accumulation of morphine can occur in renal failure, although to a lesser extent than accumulation of metabolites (see also under Pharmacokinetics, below).


1. Osborne RJ, *et al.* Morphine intoxication in renal failure: the role of morphine-6-glucuronide. *BMJ* 1986; **292:** 1548–9.
2. Hasselström J, *et al.* Long lasting respiratory depression induced by morphine-6-glucuronide? *Br J Clin Pharmacol* 1989; **27:** 515–18.
3. Calleja MA, *et al.* Persistently increased morphine-6-glucuronide concentrations. *Br J Anaesth* 1990; **64:** 649.
4. Osborne R, *et al.* The pharmacokinetics of morphine and morphine glucuronides in kidney failure. *Clin Pharmacol Ther* 1993; **54:** 158–67.


## Interactions

For interactions associated with opioid analgesics, see p.73.

◊ For references to myoclonus associated with morphine and the concurrent use of other drugs, see Effects on the Nervous System under Adverse Effects, above.

**Antibacterials.** There is some evidence[1] that the potent enzyme inducer *rifampicin* can reduce the serum concentration of morphine and decrease its analgesic effect; induction of the enzymes responsible for conversion of morphine to the active glucuronide metabolite did not seem to occur.


1. Fromm MF, *et al.* Loss of analgesic effect of morphine due to coadministration of rifampin. *Pain* 1997; **72:** 261–7.


**Benzodiazepines.** An additive sedative effect is to be expected between opioid analgesics and benzodiazepines and has been reported with morphine and *midazolam*.[1]

For reference to a suggestion that *lorazepam* may inhibit morphine-3-glucuronide glucuronidation, see Renal Impairment under Precautions, above.


1. Tverskoy M, *et al.* Midazolam-morphine sedative interaction in patients. *Anesth Analg* 1989; **68:** 282–5.


**Cisapride.** Plasma concentrations of morphine have been increased by oral cisapride.[1]


1. Rowbotham DJ, *et al.* Effect of cisapride on morphine absorption after oral administration of sustained-release morphine. *Br J Anaesth* 1991; **67:** 421–5.


**Histamine $H_2$-antagonists.** See under Opioid Analgesics, p.73.

**Local anaesthetics.** Prior use of epidural *chloroprocaine* has been reported[1] to reduce the duration of epidural morphine analgesia.


1. Eisenach JC, *et al.* Effect of prior anesthetic solution on epidural morphine analgesia. *Anesth Analg* 1991; **73:** 119–23.


**Metoclopramide.** Reports on the effects of metoclopramide on morphine have included an increased rate of onset and degree of sedation when metoclopramide was given by mouth with modified-release morphine[1] and antagonism of the effects of morphine on gastric emptying by intravenous metoclopramide.[2]


1. Manara AR, *et al.* The effect of metoclopramide on the absorption of oral controlled release morphine. *Br J Clin Pharmacol* 1988; **25:** 518–21.
2. McNeill MJ, *et al.* Effect of iv metoclopramide on gastric emptying after opioid premedication. *Br J Anaesth* 1990; **64:** 450–2.


**Tricyclic antidepressants.** Both *clomipramine* and *amitriptyline* significantly increased the plasma availability of morphine when given to cancer patients taking oral morphine solution.[1] It was noted however that the potentiation of the analgesic effects of morphine by these drugs might not be confined to increased bioavailability of morphine; the dose of tricyclic to use with morphine in the treatment of cancer pain should be decided by clinical evaluation rather than by pharmacokinetic data.


1. Ventafridda V, *et al.* Antidepressants increase bioavailability of morphine in cancer patients. *Lancet* 1987; **i:** 1204.


## Pharmacokinetics

Morphine salts are well absorbed from the gastrointestinal tract but have poor oral bioavailability since they undergo extensive first-pass metabolism in the liver and gut. After subcutaneous or intramuscular injection morphine is readily absorbed into the blood. The majority of a dose of morphine is conjugated with glucuronic acid in the liver and gut to produce morphine-3-glucuronide and morphine-6-glucuronide. The latter is considered to contribute to the analgesic effect of morphine, especially when repeated doses are given by mouth. Morphine-3-glucuronide on the other hand can antagonise the analgesic action and might be responsible for the paradoxical pain observed in some patients given morphine. Other active metabolites include normorphine, codeine, and morphine ethereal sulfate. Enterohepatic circulation probably occurs. Morphine is distributed throughout the body but mainly in the kidneys, liver, lungs, and spleen, with lower concentrations in the brain and muscles. Morphine crosses the blood-brain barrier less readily than more lipid-soluble opioids such as diamorphine, but it has been detected in the CSF as have its highly polar metabolites morphine-3-glucuronide and morphine-6-glucuronide. Morphine diffuses across the placenta and traces also appear in breast milk and sweat. About 35% is protein bound. Mean plasma elimination half-lives of about 2 hours for morphine and 2.4 to 6.7 hours for morphine-3-glucuronide have been reported.

Up to 10% of a dose of morphine may eventually be excreted, as conjugates, through the bile into the faeces. The remainder is excreted in the urine, mainly as conjugates. About 90% of total morphine is excreted in 24 hours with traces in urine for 48 hours or more.

◊ Much has been published on the metabolism and disposition of morphine and its relevance to the clinical use of morphine, in particular the analgesic effect of repeated oral doses and the relative potency of oral to parenteral doses. There has been uncertainty as to the contributions in man of first-pass metabolism in the liver and gut,[1-4] the possible role of renal metabolism,[2,3,5,6] the analgesic activity and clinical importance of the metabolite morphine-6-glucuronide,[2,7-18] and enterohepatic circulation.[2,9] There has also been interest in the effects of the metabolite morphine-3-glucuronide.[19-21]


1. Hanks GW, Aherne GW. Morphine metabolism: does the renal hypothesis hold water? *Lancet* 1985; **i:** 221–2.
2. Hanks GW, *et al.* Explanation for potency of repeated oral doses of morphine? *Lancet* 1987; **ii:** 723–5.
3. Bodenham A, *et al.* Extrahepatic morphine metabolism in man during the anhepatic phase of orthotopic liver transplantation. *Br J Anaesth* 1989; **63:** 380–4.
4. Moore RA, *et al.* Opiate metabolism and excretion. *Baillieres Clin Anaesthesiol* 1987; **1:** 829–58.
5. McQuay H, Moore A. Metabolism of narcotics. *BMJ* 1984; **288:** 237.
6. Moore A, *et al.* Morphine kinetics during and after renal transplantation. *Clin Pharmacol Ther* 1984; **35:** 641–5.
7. McQuay HJ, *et al.* Potency of oral morphine. *Lancet* 1987; **ii:** 1458–9.
8. Hanks GW, *et al.* Enterohepatic circulation of morphine. *Lancet* 1988; **i:** 469.
9. Osborne R, *et al.* Analgesic activity of morphine-6-glucuronide. *Lancet* 1988; **i:** 828.
10. Hanks GW, Wand PJ. Enterohepatic circulation of opioid drugs: is it clinically relevant in the treatment of cancer patients? *Clin Pharmacokinet* 1989; **17:** 65–8.
11. Paul D, *et al.* Pharmacological characterization of morphine-6β-glucuronide, a very potent morphine metabolite. *J Pharmacol Exp Ther* 1989; **251:** 477–83.
12. Hanna MH, *et al.* Analgesic efficacy and CSF pharmacokinetics of intrathecal morphine-6-glucuronide: comparison with morphine. *Br J Anaesth* 1990; **64:** 547–50.
13. Osborne R, *et al.* Morphine and metabolite behavior after different routes of morphine administration: demonstration of the importance of the active metabolite morphine-6-glucuronide. *Clin Pharmacol Ther* 1990; **47:** 12–19.
14. McQuay HJ, *et al.* Oral morphine in cancer pain: influences on morphine and metabolite concentration. *Clin Pharmacol Ther* 1990; **48:** 236–44.
15. Hanna MH, *et al.* Disposition of morphine-6-glucuronide and morphine in healthy volunteers. *Br J Anaesth* 1991; **66:** 103–7.
16. Portenoy RK, *et al.* The metabolite morphine-6-glucuronide contributes to the analgesia produced by morphine infusion in patients with pain and normal renal function. *Clin Pharmacol Ther* 1992; **51:** 422–31.
17. Thompson PI, *et al.* Respiratory depression following morphine and morphine-6-glucuronide in normal subjects. *Br J Clin Pharmacol* 1995; **40:** 145–52.
18. Lötsch J, Geisslinger G. Morphine-6-glucuronide: an analgesic of the future? *Clin Pharmacokinet* 2001; **40:** 485–99.
19. Smith MT, *et al.* Morphine-3-glucuronide—a potent antagonist of morphine analgesia. *Life Sci* 1990; **47:** 579–85.
20. Morley JS, *et al.* Paradoxical pain. *Lancet* 1992; **340:** 1045.
21. Morley JS, *et al.* Methadone in pain uncontrolled by morphine. *Lancet* 1993; **342:** 1243.


**Administration.** There have been many studies on the pharmacokinetics of morphine after administration by various routes and methods. These include the buccal route (see below), modified-release oral preparations,[1,2] the rectal route,[3,4] the pulmonary route,[5,6] continuous subcutaneous compared with intravenous infusion,[7] and the intraspinal route.[8-12]

Slow dural transfer of morphine and its prolonged presence in the CSF appear to correlate with its slow onset and long duration of action by epidural and intrathecal injection.[13] More lipid-soluble opioids, such as diamorphine and pethidine, enter and leave the CSF more rapidly than morphine.

The pharmacokinetics of morphine given by 5 different routes—intravenous bolus injection and oral, sublingual, buccal, and modified-release buccal tablets—were studied[14] with particular reference to morphine-6-glucuronide, the active metabolite. This metabolite occurred in large quantities after intravenous doses and plasma concentrations rapidly exceeded those of morphine. After oral doses morphine-6-glucuronide and morphine-3-glucuronide were present in quantities similar to those seen after intravenous morphine; morphine concentrations in plasma were very low and the mean morphine-6-glucuronide to morphine area under the curve ratio was 9.7 to 1. There was delayed absorption with attenuation and delay of peak morphine and metabolite plasma concentrations following sublingual or buccal administration.

Compared with oral doses, concentrations of morphine were higher and those of its glucuronides lower when morphine was given rectally,[15] suggesting avoidance of first-pass metabolism.


1. Pinnock CA, *et al.* Absorption of controlled release morphine sulphate in the immediate postoperative period. *Br J Anaesth* 1986; **58:** 868–71.
2. Savarese JJ, *et al.* Steady-state pharmacokinetics of controlled release oral morphine sulphate in healthy subjects. *Clin Pharmacokinet* 1986; **11:** 505–10.
3. Moolenaar F, *et al.* Drastic improvement in the rectal absorption profile of morphine in man. *Eur J Clin Pharmacol* 1985; **29:** 119–21.
4. Cole L, *et al.* Further development of a morphine hydrogel suppository. *Br J Clin Pharmacol* 1990; **30:** 781–6.
5. Ward ME, *et al.* Morphine pharmacokinetics after pulmonary administration from a novel aerosol delivery system. *Clin Pharmacol Ther* 1997; **62:** 596–609.
6. Masood AR, Thomas SHL. Systemic absorption of nebulized morphine compared with oral morphine in healthy subjects. *Br J Clin Pharmacol* 1996; **41:** 250–2.
7. Waldmann CS, *et al.* Serum morphine levels: a comparison between continuous subcutaneous infusion and continuous intravenous infusion in postoperative patients. *Anaesthesia* 1984; **39:** 768–71.
8. Gustafsson LL, *et al.* Disposition of morphine in cerebrospinal fluid after epidural administration. *Lancet* 1982; **i:** 796.
9. Moore A, *et al.* Spinal fluid kinetics of morphine and heroin. *Clin Pharmacol Ther* 1984; **35:** 40–5.
10. Max MB, *et al.* Epidural and intrathecal opiates: cerebrospinal fluid and plasma profiles in patients with chronic cancer pain. *Clin Pharmacol Ther* 1985; **38:** 631–41.
11. Nordberg G, *et al.* Extradural morphine: influence of adrenaline admixture. *Br J Anaesth* 1986; **58:** 598–604.
12. Ionescu TI, *et al.* The pharmacokinetics of intradural morphine in major abdominal surgery. *Clin Pharmacokinet* 1988; **14:** 178–86.
13. Morgan M. The rational use of intrathecal and extradural opioids. *Br J Anaesth* 1989; **63:** 165–88.
14. Osborne R, *et al.* Morphine and metabolite behavior after different routes of morphine administration: demonstration of the importance of the active metabolite morphine-6-glucuronide. *Clin Pharmacol Ther* 1990; **47:** 12–19.
15. Babul N, Darke AC. Disposition of morphine and its glucuronide metabolites after oral and rectal administration: evidence of route specificity. *Clin Pharmacol Ther* 1993; **54:** 286–92.


BUCCAL ROUTE. Conflicting results from studies on buccal morphine may reflect differences in formulation[1] and hence absorption. Some[2] reported equivalent analgesia with buccal and intramuscular morphine although others[3] found marked inter-individual variability with mean peak serum concentrations of morphine some eight times lower after a buccal tablet than after an intramuscular injection and occurring a mean of 4 hours later. Morphine sulfate in aqueous solution has been reported to be moderately well absorbed from the buccal mucosa.[4] Absolute bioavailability for morphine was estimated to be 23.8% after an oral solution, 22.4% after a modified-release oral tablet (MST Continus), and 20.2% after a modified-release buccal tablet, with maximum plasma-morphine concentrations at 45 minutes, 2.5 hours, and 6 hours respectively; mean ratios of area under the plasma concentration-time curve for morphine-6-glucuronide to morphine in plasma were 11:1 after buccal and oral morphine compared with 2:1 for intravenous morphine.[5] There was considerable inter-subject variation in plasma concentrations of the morphine metabolites, morphine-3-glucuronide and morphine-6-glucuronide after buccal doses of morphine as a modified-release formulation,[6] and lack of pain relief was subsequently reported with this buccal formulation.[7] Poor absorption of morphine from modified-release buccal tablets when compared with intramuscular injection was also reported;[8] bitterness of the tablets, leading to their premature removal, and poor dissolution may have contributed.

1. Calvey TN, Williams NE. Pharmacokinetics of buccal morphine. *Br J Anaesth* 1990; **64:** 256.
2. Bell MDD, *et al.* Buccal morphine—a new route for analgesia? *Lancet* 1985; **i:** 71–3.
3. Fisher AP, *et al.* Serum morphine concentrations after buccal and intramuscular morphine administration. *Br J Clin Pharmacol* 1987; **24:** 685–7.
4. Al-Sayed-Omar O, *et al.* Influence of pH on the buccal absorption of morphine sulphate and its major metabolite, morphine-3-glucuronide. *J Pharm Pharmacol* 1987; **39:** 934–5.
5. Hoskin PJ, *et al.* The bioavailability and pharmacokinetics of morphine after intravenous, oral and buccal administration in healthy volunteers. *Br J Clin Pharmacol* 1989; **27:** 499–505.
6. Manara AR, *et al.* Pharmacokinetics of morphine following administration by the buccal route. *Br J Anaesth* 1989; **62:** 498–502.
7. Manara AR, *et al.* Analgesic efficacy of perioperative buccal morphine. *Br J Anaesth* 1990; **64:** 551–5.
8. Simpson KH, *et al.* An investigation of premedication with morphine given by the buccal or intramuscular route. *Br J Clin Pharmacol* 1989; **27:** 377–80.

**Children.** The pharmacokinetics of morphine in *children* are generally considered similar to those in adults;[1-3] in both an elimination half-life of about 2 hours has been reported following intravenous administration of morphine. In *neonates*, however, clearance is generally reduced[4-6] and pharmacokinetics are more variable.[7-9] Elimination half-lives of 6.7 and 10 hours have been reported in term and preterm infants, respectively following a single intravenous dose of morphine, with nearly 80% of the dose remaining unbound.[9] The reduced clearance, which is dependent on gestational age and birth weight,[10,11] is probably due to reduced metabolism in neonates as well as immature renal function: the capacity to conjugate morphine by glucuronidation is diminished in preterm infants,[6-8] and some premature neonates may lack the capacity entirely.[8]

1. Dahlström B, *et al.* Morphine kinetics in children. *Clin Pharmacol Ther* 1979; **26:** 354–65.
2. Stanski DR, *et al.* Kinetics of high-dose intravenous morphine in cardiac surgery patients. *Clin Pharmacol Ther* 1976; **19:** 752–6.
3. Olkkola KT, *et al.* Clinical pharmacokinetics and pharmacodynamics of opioid analgesics in infants and children. *Clin Pharmacokinet* 1995; **5:** 385–404.
4. Koren G, *et al.* Postoperative morphine infusion in newborn infants: assessment of disposition characteristics and safety. *J Pediatr* 1985; **107:** 963–7.
5. Lynn AM, Slattery JT. Morphine pharmacokinetics in early infancy. *Anesthesiology* 1987; **66:** 136–9.
6. Choonara IA, *et al.* Morphine metabolism in children. *Br J Clin Pharmacol* 1989; **28:** 599–604.
7. Hartley R, *et al.* Pharmacokinetics of morphine infusion in premature neonates. *Arch Dis Child* 1993; **69:** 55–8.
8. Bhat R, *et al.* Morphine metabolism in acutely ill preterm newborn infants. *J Pediatr* 1992; **120:** 795–9.
9. Bhat R, *et al.* Pharmacokinetics of a single dose of morphine in preterm infants during the first week of life. *J Pediatr* 1990; **117:** 477–81.
10. Scott CS, *et al.* Morphine pharmacokinetics and pain assessment in premature newborns. *J Pediatr* 1999; **135:** 423–9.
11. Saarenmaa E, *et al.* Morphine clearance and effects in newborn infants in relation to gestational age. *Clin Pharmacol Ther* 2000; **68:** 160–6.

**The elderly.** The pharmacokinetics of morphine were compared[1] in 7 elderly (60 to 69 years) and 13 young (24 to 28 years) subjects, all of them healthy, following a single intravenous injection of morphine sulfate 10 mg per 70 kg. Although the terminal rate of drug disappearance from plasma was faster in the elderly group, apparent volume of distribution at steady state was about half that of the young group and plasma clearance was reduced.

1. Owen JA, *et al.* Age-related morphine kinetics. *Clin Pharmacol Ther* 1983; **34:** 364–8.

**Hepatic impairment.** The liver is a major site of morphine metabolism and therefore hepatic impairment could be expected to affect elimination. There is some evidence that in cirrhosis glucuronidation might be relatively spared compared with other metabolic processes and that some extrahepatic metabolism may occur. Several studies have served to illustrate these points:

- Hepatic extraction of morphine was impaired in cirrhotic patients, but less than expected[1]
- Morphine metabolism was minimal during the anhepatic phase of liver transplantation, but increased markedly when the new liver was reperfused[2]
- Morphine metabolism was virtually complete following liver transplantation with only 4.5% unchanged morphine being excreted in the urine 24 hours after administration[3]
- Morphine elimination was reduced when hepatic blood flow was impaired[4]

1. Crotty B, *et al.* Hepatic extraction of morphine is impaired in cirrhosis. *Eur J Clin Pharmacol* 1989; **36:** 501–6.
2. Bodenham A, *et al.* Extrahepatic morphine metabolism in man during the anhepatic phase of orthotopic liver transplantation. *Br J Anaesth* 1989; **63:** 380–4.
3. Shelly MP, *et al.* Pharmacokinetics of morphine in patients following orthotopic liver transplantation. *Br J Anaesth* 1989; **63:** 375–9.
4. Manara AR, *et al.* Morphine elimination and liver blood flow: a study in patients undergoing distal splenorenal shunt. *Br J Hosp Med* 1989; **42:** 148 (abstract).

**Renal impairment.** Only a small amount of morphine is excreted unchanged in the urine. There are conflicting reports of morphine accumulation in patients with renal impairment; some for,[1,2] others against.[3-5] It does seem clear though that morphine metabolites accumulate in such patients;[5-9] the half-life of the active metabolite morphine-6-glucuronide was reported to be prolonged and its clearance reduced when morphine-6-glucuronide was administered to patients with renal impairment.[10] Opioid intoxication[11] and a prolonged opioid effect[12] in patients with renal failure has been associated with morphine-6-glucuronide (see also under Precautions, above).

1. Ball M, *et al.* Renal failure and the use of morphine in intensive care. *Lancet* 1985; **i:** 784–6.
2. Osborne R, *et al.* The pharmacokinetics of morphine and morphine glucuronides in kidney failure. *Clin Pharmacol Ther* 1993; **54:** 158–67.
3. Säwe J, *et al.* Kinetics of morphine in patients with renal failure. *Lancet* 1985; **ii:** 211.
4. Woolner DF, *et al.* Renal failure does not impair the metabolism of morphine. *Br J Clin Pharmacol* 1986; **22:** 55–9.
5. Chauvin M, *et al.* Morphine pharmacokinetics in renal failure. *Anesthesiology* 1987; **66:** 327–31.
6. Säwe J, Odar-Cederlöf I. Kinetics of morphine in patients with renal failure. *Eur J Clin Pharmacol* 1987; **32:** 377–82.
7. Wolff J, *et al.* Influence of renal function on the elimination of morphine and morphine glucuronides. *Eur J Clin Pharmacol* 1988; **34:** 353–7.
8. Sear JW, *et al.* Studies on morphine disposition: influence of renal failure on the kinetics of morphine and its metabolites. *Br J Anaesth* 1989; **62:** 28–32.
9. Peterson GM, *et al.* Plasma levels of morphine and morphine glucuronides in the treatment of cancer pain: relationship to renal function and route of administration. *Eur J Clin Pharmacol* 1990; **38:** 121–4.
10. Hanna MH, *et al.* Morphine-6-glucuronide disposition in renal impairment. *Br J Anaesth* 1993; **70:** 511–14.
11. Osborne RJ, *et al.* Morphine intoxication in renal failure: the role of morphine-6-glucuronide. *BMJ* 1986; **292:** 1548–9.
12. Bodd E, *et al.* Morphine-6-glucuronide might mediate the prolonged opioid effect of morphine in acute renal failure. *Hum Exp Toxicol* 1990; **9:** 317–21.

## Uses and Administration

Morphine, a phenanthrene derivative, is the chief alkaloid of opium (p.74). It is now commonly obtained from whole opium poppies (*Papaver somniferum*) which are harvested as poppy straw; a concentrate of poppy straw is known as CPS.

Morphine is an opioid analgesic (p.73) with agonist activity mainly at μ opioid receptors and perhaps at κ and δ receptors. It acts mainly on the CNS and smooth muscle. Although morphine is predominantly a CNS depressant it has some central stimulant actions which result in nausea and vomiting and miosis. Morphine generally increases smooth muscle tone, especially the sphincters of the gastrointestinal and biliary tracts.

Morphine may produce both physical and psychological dependence (see p.71) and should therefore be used with discrimination. Tolerance may also develop.

Morphine is used for the relief of moderate to severe pain, especially in pain associated with cancer, myocardial infarction, and surgery. In addition to relieving pain, morphine also alleviates the anxiety associated with severe pain and it is useful as a hypnotic where sleeplessness is due to pain.

Morphine reduces intestinal motility but its role, if any, in the symptomatic treatment of diarrhoea is very limited. It also relieves dyspnoea associated with various conditions, including that due to pulmonary oedema resulting from left ventricular failure. It is an effective cough suppressant, but codeine is usually preferred as there is less risk of dependence; morphine may however be necessary to control intractable cough associated with terminal lung cancer. Morphine has been used pre-operatively as an adjunct to anaesthesia for pain relief and to allay anxiety. It has also been used in high doses as a general anaesthetic in specialised procedures.

Morphine is usually **administered** as the sulfate, although the hydrochloride and the tartrate are used in similar doses. Doses are expressed as the salts. Routes of administration include the oral, subcutaneous, intramuscular, intravenous, intraspinal, and rectal routes. Subcutaneous injections are considered unsuitable for oedematous patients. Parenteral doses may be intermittent injections or continuous or intermittent infusions adjusted according to individual analgesic requirements.

Doses should generally be reduced in the elderly or debilitated or in patients with hepatic or renal impairment (see also under Precautions, above).

Doses *by mouth* for **pain** are usually in the range of 5 to 20 mg every 4 hours and may be given as an aqueous solution of the hydrochloride or sulfate, as modified-release granules or tablets, or as tablets. With modified-release preparations the 24-hour dose may be given as a single dose or in 2 divided doses (additional doses of a conventional formulation may also be needed if breakthrough pain occurs). As with the other routes, high oral doses may be required for effective analgesia in palliative care.

Morphine is sometimes given *rectally* generally as suppositories in doses of 10 to 30 mg every 4 hours. A modified-release suppository of morphine sulfate for once daily administration has also been used.

The usual dose by *subcutaneous* or *intramuscular* injection is 10 mg every 4 hours but may range from 5 to 20 mg. Children up to 1 month of age may be given 150 micrograms/kg every 4 hours; those aged 1 to 12 months, 200 micrograms/kg; 1 to 5 years, 2.5 to 5 mg; 6 to 12 years, 5 to 10 mg. See also under Administration in Children, below.

Doses of up to 15 mg have been given by slow *intravenous* injection, sometimes as a loading dose for continuous or patient-controlled infusion. For continuous intravenous administration maintenance doses have generally ranged from 0.8 to 80 mg/hour, although some patients have required and been given much higher doses. Similar doses have been given by continuous subcutaneous infusion.

For myocardial infarction 10 mg may be given by intravenous injection at a rate of 2 mg/minute followed by a further 5 to 10 mg if necessary; half this dose should be used in elderly or debilitated patients.

Intraspinal doses are in the region of 5 mg for an initial *epidural* injection; if pain relief is unsatisfactory after one hour, further doses of 1 to 2 mg may be given up to a total dose of 10 mg per 24 hours. The recommended initial dose for continuous epidural infusion is 2 to 4 mg per 24 hours increased if necessary by further 1 to 2 mg daily increments. A modified-release formulation of liposomal morphine sulfate for lumbar epidural use is also available for the treatment of pain after major surgery; doses range from 10 to 20 mg, depending on the type of surgery, and should be given before the operation, or after clamping of the umbilical cord if used during caesarean section. It is intended for single-use only and no other drugs should be administered into the epidural space for at least the next 48 hours.

*Intrathecal* use of morphine and its salts has tended to be less common than epidural. Doses of 0.2 to 1 mg have been injected intrathecally on a single occasion.

In **acute pulmonary oedema** 5 to 10 mg may be given by intravenous injection at a rate of 2 mg/minute.

For the control of intractable **cough** associated with terminal lung cancer, morphine hydrochloride oral solution is given in an initial dose of 5 mg every 4 hours.

**Administration.** CONTINUOUS INFUSION. Both acute and chronic pain have been controlled satisfactorily by continuous intravenous or subcutaneous infusions of morphine sulfate[1-3] but diamorphine hydrochloride or hydromorphone hydrochloride may be preferred for subcutaneous infusion because their greater solubility in water allows a smaller dose volume. Continuous subcutaneous infusions may be preferred to continuous intravenous infusions.[4] Continuous subcutaneous infusion may be less effective than epidural administration for relief of post-operative pain;[5] however, it was still considered to provide simple and relatively effective analgesia with a low rate of adverse effects.

See also under Patient-controlled Analgesia, below.

1. Waldmann CS, *et al.* Serum morphine levels: a comparison between continuous subcutaneous infusion and continuous intravenous infusion in postoperative patients. *Anaesthesia* 1984; **39:** 768–71.
2. Goudie TA, *et al.* Continuous subcutaneous infusion of morphine for postoperative pain relief. *Anaesthesia* 1985; **40:** 1086–92.
3. Stuart GJ, *et al.* Continuous intravenous morphine infusions for terminal pain control: a retrospective review. *Drug Intell Clin Pharm* 1986; **20:** 968–72.

4. Drexel H. Long-term continuous subcutaneous and intravenous opioid infusions. *Lancet* 1991; **337:** 979.
5. Hindsholm KB, *et al.* Continuous subcutaneous infusion of morphine—an alternative to extradural morphine for postoperative pain relief. *Br J Anaesth* 1993; **71:** 580–2.

INTRA-ARTICULAR ROUTE. Intra-articular injection of morphine into the knee at the end of arthroscopy has been reported to provide some degree of postoperative pain relief;[1,2] such pain relief may be more pronounced than that produced by the same dose given intravenously.[1] The effect appears to be due to the action of morphine on peripheral opioid receptors.[3] However, there have been conflicting results on whether addition of morphine to intra-articular bupivacaine improves analgesia.[4,5] Doses of morphine reported to have been injected intra-articularly have ranged from 1 to 5 mg.

1. Stein C, *et al.* Analgesic effect of intra-articular morphine after arthroscopic knee surgery. *N Engl J Med* 1991; **325:** 1123–6.
2. Joshi GP, *et al.* Intra-articular morphine for pain relief after anterior cruciate ligament repair. *Br J Anaesth* 1993; **70:** 87–8.
3. Stein C, *et al.* Local analgesic effect of endogenous opioid peptides. *Lancet* 1993; **342:** 321–4.
4. Laurent SC, *et al.* Addition of morphine to intra-articular bupivacaine does not improve analgesia after day-case arthroscopy. *Br J Anaesth* 1994; **72:** 170–3.
5. Heine MF, *et al.* Intra-articular morphine after arthroscopic knee operation. *Br J Anaesth* 1994; **73:** 413–15.

INTRASPINAL ROUTE. Morphine is given epidurally and intrathecally to relieve both acute and chronic pain. However, reviews on the role of spinal opioids have generally concluded that they should be reserved for pain not controlled by more conventional routes.[1-3] When converting from conventional routes it has been suggested that 1% of the total daily dose could be tried as the daily intrathecal dose and 10% as the epidural dose.[3]

Intrathecal morphine may be delivered continuously via an implanted programmable infusion pump for the long-term management of chronic non-malignant and cancer pain.

See also under Patient-controlled Analgesia, below.

1. Anonymous. Spinal opiates revisited. *Lancet* 1986; **i:** 655–6.
2. Gustafsson LL, Wiesenfeld-Hallin Z. Spinal opioid analgesia: a critical update. *Drugs* 1988; **35:** 597–603.
3. McQuay HJ. Opioids in chronic pain. *Br J Anaesth* 1989; **63:** 213–26.

PATIENT-CONTROLLED ANALGESIA. Morphine is one of the most frequently used opioid analgesics for patient-controlled analgesia (see p.3). Most experience has been with the intravenous route, but the intramuscular, subcutaneous, oral, pulmonary, and epidural[1] routes have also been used. Reasonable initial settings recommended for intravenous use have been a demand dose of 1 mg of morphine sulfate (or its equivalent) and a lockout interval of 5 to 10 minutes.[2]

1. Sjöström S, *et al.* Patient-controlled analgesia with extradural morphine or pethidine. *Br J Anaesth* 1988; **60:** 358–66.
2. Anonymous. Patient-controlled analgesia. *Med Lett Drugs Ther* 1989; **31:** 104.

PULMONARY ROUTE. For reference to the use of nebulised morphine see under Dyspnoea, below.

TOPICAL ROUTE. Morphine has been applied topically for local analgesia in cutaneous ulceration.[1-3]

1. Twillman RK, *et al.* Treatment of painful skin ulcers with topical opioids. *J Pain Symptom Manage* 1999; **17:** 288–92.
2. Krajnik M, *et al.* Potential uses of topical opioids in palliative care–report of 6 cases. *Pain* 1999; **80:** 121–5.
3. Cerchietti LC, *et al.* Effect of topical morphine for mucositis-associated pain following concomitant chemoradiotherapy for head and neck carcinoma. *Cancer* 2000; **15:** 2230–6. Correction. *ibid.* 2003; **97:** 1137.

**Administration in children.** The management of pain in children is discussed on p.3. Morphine is widely used[1] and may be given to *neonates* who require analgesia as a result of surgery, invasive procedures, or intensive care. They do however have enhanced susceptibility to the respiratory depression associated with opioids although those already receiving respiratory support are at less risk; a transient drop in blood pressure may also be noted on initiation of the infusion in preterm neonates.[2] Allowance also has to be made for morphine's altered pharmacokinetics in this group (see above). Most neonates receiving respiratory support can be managed with an infusion of morphine 10 micrograms/kg per hour; the dose should not exceed 15 micrograms/kg per hour. In neonates who are breathing spontaneously there is a substantial risk of respiratory depression with powerful opioid analgesics such as morphine, and administration should be limited to those under intensive care. Morphine 5 to 7 micrograms/kg per hour by intravenous infusion allows adequate analgesia without respiratory depression, but the infusion rate should be titrated against response. Suggested infusion rates range from 5 to 15 micrograms/kg per hour. Bolus injections should be avoided. The use of opioids for sedation and analgesia in neonates in intensive care is mentioned on p.666; morphine is considered to be a more rational choice than fentanyl in a setting where long-term infusions are required.

In *infants and children* opioids are still the mainstay of analgesia and morphine is the standard against which the others are compared. Techniques of continuous intravenous infusion have become popular for postoperative pain relief. From the age of 5 to 6 months morphine metabolism appears to conform to an adult pattern; in younger infants the regimens for neonates (see above) should be followed. Titration of infusion rate against patient response minimises the risks and most have found 10 to 30 micrograms/kg per hour to be satisfactory with minimal respiratory depression; if required a loading dose of morphine 100 to 200 micrograms/kg may be given initially with bolus top-up doses of 50 to 100 micrograms/kg every 4 hours. Subcutaneous infusions of morphine 30 to 60 micrograms/kg per hour have been used for the relief of terminal cancer pain in children, but for postoperative analgesia the dose needed should be similar to that for intravenous infusion. An intramuscular injection of morphine 100 to 200 micrograms/kg provides excellent short-term analgesia. Patient-controlled analgesia using morphine has been tried in children as young as 5 years of age.

Some spinal doses of morphine in children are as follows:

- Caudal epidural block, 100 micrograms/kg
- Thoracic or lumbar epidural block, 50 micrograms/kg
- Intrathecal doses of 20 or 30 micrograms/kg have provided satisfactory postoperative pain relief, but respiratory depression occurred in 10 and 25%, respectively

Guidelines[3] for analgesia in children in Accident and Emergency departments in the UK recommend the use of oral morphine for *moderate pain* (e.g. burns not requiring intravenous resuscitation). Suggested doses in children aged 1 to 12 years are 200 to 400 micrograms/kg, given every 4 to 6 hours, although caution is recommended before giving these doses to children less than 2 years old. For *severe pain* such as that associated with major trauma, opioid analgesics may be used even in young infants, provided that great care is taken in calculating the dose. Intravenous morphine is recommended in the following doses:

- 1 to 3 months of age, 25 micrograms/kg
- 3 to 6 months, 50 micrograms/kg (in children with major burns an initial dose of 25 micrograms/kg is advocated at all ages up to 6 months)
- 6 to 12 months, 100 micrograms/kg (half this dose in children with major burns)
- 1 to 12 years, 100 to 200 micrograms/kg

Doses should be given slowly over 10 minutes as a dilute solution (e.g. 1 mg/mL), and titrated against response. A further dose may be given after at least 5 to 10 minutes if analgesia is inadequate. In children with *major head injury* a more cautious approach is recommended: an initial dose of 25 micrograms/kg should be given by slow intravenous bolus, then repeated as necessary after 3 to 5 minutes, up to a maximum of 200 micrograms/kg in a 4-hour period.

1. Lloyd-Thomas AR. Pain management in paediatric patients. *Br J Anaesth* 1990; **64:** 85–104.
2. Wood CM, *et al.* Randomised double blind trial of morphine versus diamorphine for sedation of preterm neonates. *Arch Dis Child Fetal Neonatal Ed* 1998; **79:** F34–F39.
3. British Association for Accident and Emergency Medicine. Guidelines for analgesia in children in the Accident and Emergency department. Available at: http://www.baem.org.uk/pedangls.htm (accessed 06/07/04)

**Cancer pain.** The starting dose of morphine in cancer pain depends on the type of analgesic previously taken; 5 to 10 mg by mouth every 4 hours is enough to replace a non-opioid or a less potent opioid analgesic whereas 10 to 20 mg or more may be necessary to replace an opioid of equivalent strength to morphine. Doses should be increased gradually until the lowest effective analgesic dose is reached, taking into account any 'rescue' doses that have been administered to relieve breakthrough pain. There are no 'standard' doses; they have ranged from 2.5 to over 2500 mg of morphine sulfate every 4 hours, although most patients need far less than 100 mg every 4 hours. For patients on 4-hourly regimens, a double dose may be taken at bedtime to avoid waking up in the night.

Modified-release preparations are also used and, depending on the preparation, can be given either twice daily or as a single daily dose. The initial dose of a modified-release preparation is 10 to 20 mg every 12 hours if replacing paracetamol or no previous analgesic, but 20 to 30 mg every 12 hours if replacing a less potent opioid. The dose and not the frequency of administration should be altered if required. Some argue that dose titration should always be carried out with immediate-release preparations, only transferring to modified-release formulations once the optimum analgesic dose has been achieved. When transferring a patient, the same total 24-hour immediate-release dose is given as a modified-release preparation (divided into two equal 12-hourly doses if necessary), with the first dose given 4 hours after the last immediate-release dose. Any breakthrough pain during titration or as a result of loss of analgesic control should be managed with immediate-release formulations.

If the patient is unable to swallow, parenteral morphine may be given. The equivalent intramuscular dose of morphine is half the oral dose; if a modified-release preparation has been used, the total 24-hour dose should be halved to give the intramuscular daily dose, which is given in 6 divided doses, at 4-hourly intervals. The rectal route may also be used in patients who have difficulty swallowing.

References.

1. Expert Working Group of the European Association for Palliative Care. Morphine in cancer pain: modes of administration. *BMJ* 1996; **312:** 823–6.

**Dyspnoea.** In the treatment of dyspnoea, doses of morphine tend to be smaller than those used for pain relief. Morphine hydrochloride or sulfate may be given as an oral solution in carefully titrated doses, starting at a dose of 5 mg every 4 hours; as little as 2.5 mg every 4 hours may be sufficient for opioid-naive patients.[1] In acute pulmonary oedema, 5 to 10 mg may be given by slow intravenous injection. In incurable malignant chest disease a test dose of 5 mg by mouth should be repeated every 4 hours with 5 to 10 mg at bedtime; if necessary the dose may be increased gradually up to 15 to 20 mg every 4 hours. If the patient is already receiving morphine for pain a 50% increase in dose may be tried.[2] Patients have also obtained relief from subcutaneous injection.[3]

Although it has been reported that a low dose of nebulised morphine (mean dose 1.7 mg) improved exercise endurance in patients with dyspnoea due to advanced chronic lung disease,[4] several subsequent studies[5-7] have failed to obtain significant improvements with doses up to 40 mg. It is considered that current evidence does not support the use of nebulised morphine for breathlessness.[1,8] Furthermore, bronchospasm can be a problem, particularly at high doses, and there is no consensus on the optimal dose, schedule, or method of dose titration.

1. Davis CL. ABC of palliative care: breathlessness, cough, and other respiratory problems. *BMJ* 1997; **315:** 931–4.
2. Twycross RG, Lack SA. *Oral morphine in advanced cancer.* 2nd ed. Beaconsfield: Beaconsfield Publishers, 1989.
3. Bruera E, *et al.* Subcutaneous morphine for dyspnea in cancer patients. *Ann Intern Med* 1993; **119:** 906–7.
4. Young IH, *et al.* Effect of low dose nebulised morphine on exercise endurance in patients with chronic lung disease. *Thorax* 1989; **44:** 387–90.
5. Beauford W, *et al.* Effects of nebulized morphine sulfate on the exercise tolerance of the ventilatory limited COPD patients. *Chest* 1993; **104:** 175–8.
6. Noseda A, *et al.* Disabling dyspnoea in patients with advanced disease: lack of effect of nebulized morphine. *Eur Respir J* 1997; **10:** 1079–83.
7. Jankelson D, *et al.* Lack of effect of high doses of inhaled morphine on exercise endurance in chronic obstructive pulmonary disease. *Eur Respir J* 1997; **10:** 2270–4.
8. Polosa R, *et al.* Nebulised morphine for severe interstitial lung disease. Available in The Cochrane Library; Issue 2. Chichester: John Wiley; 2004.

**Intensive care.** When used to provide analgesia for patients in intensive care, morphine has a relatively slow onset of action, but longer term rather than rapid-onset analgesia can be achieved by a loading dose of 10 to 15 mg, in adults, followed by an infusion of 2 to 3 mg/hour; the dose must be individually titrated.

## Preparations

***BP 2003:*** Chloroform and Morphine Tincture; Morphine and Atropine Injection; Morphine Sulphate Injection; Morphine Suppositories; Morphine Tablets; Prolonged-release Morphine Tablets;
***USP 27:*** Morphine Sulfate Extended-Release Capsules; Morphine Sulfate Injection; Morphine Sulfate Suppositories.

**Proprietary Preparations** (details are given in Part 3)
***Arg.:*** Algedol; Amidiaz; Analmorph; Duramorph; GNO; MST Continus; Neocalmans; ***Austral.:*** Anamorph; Kapanol; MS Contin; MS Mono; Ordine; ***Austria:*** Compensan; Kapabloc; Kapanol; M-Dolor; M-long; Morapid; Mundidol; Oramorph; Substitol; Vendal; ***Belg.:*** Kapanol; MS Contin; MS Direct; Skenan†; Stellorphinad; Stellorphine; ***Braz.:*** Astramorph†; Dimorf; MS-Long; MST Continus; ***Canad.:*** Kadian; M-Eslon; Morphitec; MOS; MS Contin; MSIR; Oramorph; Statex; ***Chile:*** M-Eslon; ***Denm.:*** Contalgin; Depolan; Doltard; Duralgin†; Kapanol†; Malfin†; Repriadol†; ***Fin.:*** Depolan; Dolcontin; ***Fr.:*** Actiskenan; Kapanol; Moscontin; Sevredol; Skenan; ***Ger.:*** Capros; Kapanol; M-beta; M-Dolor; M-long; M-Stada; Mogetic; MSI; MSR; MST; Onkomorphin; Sevredol; ***Hong Kong:*** MST Continus; ***India:*** Morcontin; ***Irl.:*** Morstel; MST Continus; MXL; Oramorph; Sevredol; Slo-Morph; ***Israel:*** Kapanol; MCR; MIR; Morphex; MSP; ***Ital.:*** MS Contin; Oramorph; Skenan; ***Mex.:*** Analfin; Duralmor; Graten; Kapanol†; MST Continus†; ***Neth.:*** Kapanol; MS Contin; Noceptin; Sevredol; ***Norw.:*** Dolcontin; Kapanol†; ***NZ:*** Kapanol; LA Morph; MST Continus; RA Morph; RMS†; Sevredol; ***Port.:*** MST; MXL; Sevredol; Skenan; ***S.Afr.:*** MST Continus; SRM-Rhotard; ***Singapore:*** MST Continus†; SRM-Rhotard; Statex; ***Spain:*** MST Continus; MST Unicontinus; Oblioser†; Oglos; Sevredol; Skenan; Uni Mist†; ***Swed.:*** Depolan; Dolcontin; Loceptin†; Maxidon†; Oramorph†; ***Switz.:*** Kapanol; MST Continus; Sevre-Long; Sevredol; ***UK:*** Filnarine; Moraxen†; Morcap; Morphgesic; MST Continus; MXL; Oramorph; Sevredol; Zomorph; ***USA:*** Astramorph PF; Avinza; Duramorph; Infumorph; Kadian; MS Contin; MSIR; OMS Concentrate†; Oramorph; RMS; Roxanol.

**Multi-ingredient:** ***Austral.:*** Morphalgin; ***Austria:*** Modiscop; ***Belg.:*** Spasma; ***Irl.:*** Cyclimorph; ***Ital.:*** Cardiostenol; ***S.Afr.:*** Chloropect; Collodyne†; Cyclimorph; Enterodyne; Pectrolyte; ***Swed.:*** Spasmofen; ***Switz.:*** Spasmosol; ***UK:*** Collis Browne's; Cyclimorph; Diocalm Dual Action; Enterosan†; Opazimes.

---

# Morpholine Salicylate

Salicilato de morfolinio. 2-Hydroxybenzoic acid compounded with morpholine (1 : 1).

$C_{11}H_{15}NO_4$ = 225.2.
*CAS — 147-90-0.*
*ATC — N02BA08.*

## Profile

Morpholine salicylate is a salicylic acid derivative (see Aspirin, p.15) that has been used for musculoskeletal disorders.

## Preparations

**Proprietary Preparations** (details are given in Part 3)
***Israel:*** Dolical.

---

# Nabumetone *(BAN, USAN, rINN)*

BRL-14777; Nabumetona; Nabumetonum. 4-(6-Methoxy-2-naphthyl)butan-2-one.

$C_{15}H_{16}O_2$ = 228.3.
*CAS — 42924-53-8.*
*ATC — M01AX01.*

**Pharmacopoeias.** In *Eur.* (see p.vi) and *US.*

**Ph. Eur. 5.0** (Nabumetone). A white or almost white crystalline powder. Practically insoluble in water; freely soluble in acetone;

slightly soluble in methyl alcohol. Protect from light.

**USP 27** (Nabumetone). A white or almost white crystalline powder. Practically insoluble in water; sparingly soluble in alcohol and in methyl alcohol; freely soluble in acetone. Store in airtight containers. Protect from light.

## Adverse Effects and Precautions

As for NSAIDs in general, p.67.

**Effects on the gastrointestinal tract.** Like other NSAIDs nabumetone can produce adverse effects on the gastrointestinal tract, although some studies have produced favourable comparisons with ibuprofen[1] or naproxen.[2] It has been suggested[3] that nabumetone may be a preferential inhibitor of cyclo-oxygenase-2 (COX-2) but the significance of this in determining its adverse effects is uncertain.

1. Roth SH, *et al.* A controlled study comparing the effects of nabumetone, ibuprofen, and ibuprofen plus misoprostol on the upper gastrointestinal tract mucosa. *Arch Intern Med* 1993; **153:** 2565–71.
2. Roth SH, *et al.* A longterm endoscopic evaluation of patients with arthritis treated with nabumetone vs naproxen. *J Rheumatol* 1994; **21:** 1118–23.
3. Davies NM. Clinical pharmacokinetics of nabumetone: the dawn of selective cyclo-oxygenase-2 inhibition? *Clin Pharmacokinet* 1997; **33:** 403–16.

**Effects on the lungs.** Pulmonary fibrosis developed in a 68-year-old woman receiving nabumetone 1500 mg; symptoms appeared after 2 weeks of therapy and worsened during the next 6 weeks.[1] There was rapid resolution on withdrawal of nabumetone and treatment with oral corticosteroids.

1. Morice A, *et al.* Pulmonary fibrosis associated with nabumetone. *Postgrad Med J* 1991; **67:** 1021–2.

**Effects on the skin.** Pseudoporphyria characterised by blistering on the neck and hands developed in a 36-year-old woman taking nabumetone and auranofin for rheumatoid arthritis.[1] Stopping auranofin had no effect on the blistering which only resolved once nabumetone was withdrawn. The authors of the report stated that the UK Committee on Safety of Medicines had received 3 additional reports of pseudoporphyria suspected to be caused by nabumetone.

1. Varma S, Lanigan SW. Pseudoporphyria caused by nabumetone. *Br J Dermatol* 1998; **138:** 549–50. Correction. *ibid.* **139:** 759. [dose]

## Interactions

For interactions associated with NSAIDs, see p.69.

## Pharmacokinetics

Although nabumetone is well absorbed from the gastrointestinal tract, plasma concentrations after oral doses are too small to be measured as it undergoes rapid and extensive first-pass metabolism in the liver to the principal active compound 6-methoxy-2-naphthylacetic acid (6-MNA) and other inactive metabolites. 6-MNA is more than 99% bound to plasma proteins. 6-MNA diffuses into synovial fluid. It crosses the placenta and is distributed into breast milk. There is considerable interindividual variation in the plasma elimination half-life of 6-MNA, especially in the elderly; some reported mean values at steady state include 22 to about 27 hours for young adults and about 25 and 34 hours in elderly patients. 6-MNA eventually undergoes further metabolism by *O*-methylation and conjugation. About 80% of a dose is excreted in the urine as inactive or conjugated metabolites and less than 1% as unchanged 6-MNA.

◊ References.

1. Brier ME, *et al.* Population pharmacokinetics of the active metabolite of nabumetone in renal dysfunction. *Clin Pharmacol Ther* 1995; **57:** 622–7.
2. Davies NM. Clinical pharmacokinetics of nabumetone: the dawn of selective cyclo-oxygenase-2 inhibition? *Clin Pharmacokinet* 1997; **33:** 403–16.

## Uses and Administration

Nabumetone is a non-active prodrug whose major metabolite is an NSAID (p.70) structurally similar to naproxen (p.65). It is used for the relief of pain and inflammation associated with osteoarthritis and rheumatoid arthritis in a usual dose of 1 g by mouth taken as a single dose in the evening; if necessary 0.5 to 1 g may be given additionally in the morning. It has been recommended that a dose of 1 g daily should not be exceeded in elderly patients and that 500 mg daily may be satisfactory in some cases.

◊ References.

1. Anonymous. Nabumetone—a new NSAID. *Med Lett Drugs Ther* 1992; **34:** 38–40.
2. Friedel HA, *et al.* Nabumetone: a reappraisal of its pharmacology and therapeutic use in rheumatic diseases. *Drugs* 1993; **45:** 131–56.
3. Proceedings of a symposium: continuing developments with nabumetone: an investigators' update. *Am J Med* 1993; 95 (suppl 2A): 1S–45S.
4. Dahl SL. Nabumetone: a "nonacidic" nonsteroidal antiinflammatory drug. *Ann Pharmacother* 1993; **27:** 456–63.

## Preparations

***BP 2003:*** Nabumetone Oral Suspension; Nabumetone Tablets;
***USP 27:*** Nabumetone Tablets.

**Proprietary Preparations** (details are given in Part 3)

***Braz.:*** Relifex; ***Canad.:*** Relafen; ***Denm.:*** Relifex; ***Fin.:*** Relifex; ***Fr.:*** Nabucox; ***Ger.:*** Arthaxan†; ***Gr.:*** Akratol; Mevedal; Nabuton; Naditone; Relifex; ***Hong Kong:*** Relifex; ***Irl.:*** Relifex; ***Israel:*** Nabuco; Relifex; ***Ital.:*** Artaxan; Nabuser; ***Jpn:*** Relifen; ***Mex.:*** Relifex; ***Neth.:*** Mebutan; ***Norw.:*** Relifex; ***Port.:*** Balmox; Elitar; ***S.Afr.:*** Relifen; Relisan; Relitone; ***Singapore:*** Relifex†; ***Spain:*** Dolsinal†; Listran; Relif; ***Swed.:*** Relifex; ***Switz.:*** Balmox; ***Thai.:*** Nabone; Nabonet; Naflex; Nametone; Relifex; ***UK:*** Relifex; ***USA:*** Relafen.

# Nalbuphine Hydrochloride

*(BANM, USAN, rINNM)*

EN-2234A; Hidrocloruro de nalbufina; Nalbufine Hydrochloride. 17-Cyclobutylmethyl-7,8-dihydro-14-hydroxy-17-normorphine hydrochloride; (−)-(5R,6S,14S)-9a-Cyclobutylmethyl-4,5-epoxy-morphinan-3,6,14-triol hydrochloride.

$C_{21}H_{27}NO_4,HCl = 393.9.$

*CAS — 20594-83-6 (nalbuphine); 23277-43-2 (nalbuphine hydrochloride).*

*ATC — N02AF02.*

**Incompatibility.** Incompatibility has been reported between injections of nalbuphine hydrochloride and nafcillin sodium,[1] diazepam,[2] pentobarbital sodium,[2] or thiethylperazine maleate.[2]

1. Jeglum EL, *et al.* Nafcillin sodium incompatibility with acidic solutions. *Am J Hosp Pharm* 1981; **38:** 462–4.
2. Jump WG, *et al.* Compatibility of nalbuphine hydrochloride with other preoperative medications. *Am J Hosp Pharm* 1982; **39:** 841–3.

## Dependence and Withdrawal

As for Opioid Analgesics, p.71.

◊ A WHO expert committee considered in 1989 that the likelihood of nalbuphine abuse was low to moderate and was not great enough to warrant international control.[1] Abuse had been reported infrequently and the withdrawal syndrome produced when naloxone was given after continuous nalbuphine administration was less severe than that in morphine dependence. Subsequently, there have been reports of abuse among athletes.[2,3]

1. WHO. WHO expert committee on drug dependence: twenty-fifth report. *WHO Tech Rep Ser 775* 1989.
2. McBride AJ, *et al.*. Three cases of nalbuphine hydrochloride dependence associated with anabolic steroid use. *Br J Sports Med* 1996; **30:** 69–70.
3. Wines JD, *et al.*. Nalbuphine hydrochloride dependence in anabolic steroid users. *Am J Addict* 1999; **8:** 161–4.

## Adverse Effects and Treatment

As for Opioid Analgesics in general, p.72.

Headache may occur. Nausea and vomiting occur less than with other opioids. Hallucinations and other psychotomimetic effects are rare and have been reported less frequently than with pentazocine. As nalbuphine has both antagonist and agonist activity its effects may be only partially reversed by naloxone, but use of the latter is still recommended in nalbuphine overdose.

**Effects on the respiratory system.** Nalbuphine produces similar respiratory depression to morphine at equianalgesic doses, but there is a ceiling effect with nalbuphine and, unlike morphine, respiratory depression does not increase appreciably with higher doses.[1] In a cumulative-dose study[2] a plateau effect was seen with nalbuphine above a total dose of 30 mg per 70 kg intravenously. Similar ventilatory depression has been noted[3] with single intravenous doses of nalbuphine of 15, 30, or 60 mg per 70 kg; naloxone failed to reverse the depression at the highest dose.

1. Klepper ID, *et al.* Respiratory function following nalbuphine and morphine in anaesthetized man. *Br J Anaesth* 1986; **58:** 625–9.
2. Romagnoli A, Keats AS. Ceiling effect for respiratory depression by nalbuphine. *Clin Pharmacol Ther* 1980; **27:** 478–85.
3. Pugh GC, *et al.* Effect of nalbuphine hydrochloride on the ventilatory and occlusion pressure responses to carbon dioxide in volunteers. *Br J Anaesth* 1989; **62:** 601–9.

## Precautions

As for Opioid Analgesics in general, p.72.

Nalbuphine may precipitate withdrawal symptoms if given to patients physically dependent on opioids.

The dose of nalbuphine should be reduced in patients with hepatic or renal impairment.

**Abuse.** See under Dependence and Withdrawal, above.

**Pregnancy.** When nalbuphine is used for analgesia during labour there is more placental transfer and sedation in mothers and their infants than with pethidine.[1] There have also been reports of bradycardia and respiratory depression in neonates whose mothers received nalbuphine during labour.[2,3] It was considered that nalbuphine should be given with caution during labour, especially by the intravenous route. Some[2] have recommended subcutaneous administration and advised that nalbuphine should not be given around the expected time of delivery.

Further references on the transplacental transfer of nalbuphine are given under Pharmacokinetics, below.

1. Wilson CM, *et al.* Transplacental gradient of pethidine and nalbuphine in labour. *Br J Clin Pharmacol* 1986; **21:** 571P–2P.
2. Guillonneau M, *et al.* Perinatal adverse effects of nalbuphine given during parturition. *Lancet* 1990; **335:** 1588.
3. Sgro C, *et al.* Perinatal adverse effects of nalbuphine given during labour. *Lancet* 1990; **336:** 1070.

## Interactions

For interactions associated with opioid analgesics, see p.73.

## Pharmacokinetics

On intramuscular injection nalbuphine has been reported to produce peak plasma concentrations after 30 minutes. It is metabolised in the liver and is excreted in the urine and faeces as unchanged drug and conjugates.

Nalbuphine crosses the placenta.

There appears to be considerable first-pass metabolism of nalbuphine after oral doses.

◊ References.

1. Sear JW, *et al.* Disposition of nalbuphine in patients undergoing general anaesthesia. *Br J Anaesth* 1987; **59:** 572–5.
2. Kay B, *et al.* Pharmacokinetics of oral nalbuphine in postoperative patients. *Br J Anaesth* 1987; **59:** 1327P.
3. Aitkenhead AR, *et al.* The pharmacokinetics of oral and intravenous nalbuphine in healthy volunteers. *Br J Clin Pharmacol* 1988; **25:** 264–8.
4. Jaillon P, *et al.* Pharmacokinetics of nalbuphine in infants, young healthy volunteers, and elderly patients. *Clin Pharmacol Ther* 1989; **46:** 226–33.

**Pregnancy.** References.

1. Wilson CM, *et al.* Transplacental gradient of pethidine and nalbuphine in labour. *Br J Clin Pharmacol* 1986; **21:** 571P–2P.
2. Dadabhoy ZP, *et al.* Transplacental transfer of nalbuphine in patients undergoing cesarean section: a pilot study. *Acta Anaesthesiol Ital* 1988; **39:** 227–32.
3. Nicolle E, *et al.* Therapeutic monitoring of nalbuphine: transplacental transfer and estimated pharmacokinetics in the neonate. *Eur J Clin Pharmacol* 1996; **49:** 485–9.

## Uses and Administration

Nalbuphine hydrochloride, a phenanthrene derivative, is an opioid analgesic (p.73). It has mixed opioid agonist and antagonist activity. It is used for the relief of moderate to severe pain, including that associated with myocardial infarction, and as an adjunct to anaesthesia. Nalbuphine hydrochloride is reported to act within 15 minutes of subcutaneous or intramuscular injection or within 2 to 3 minutes of intravenous injection and generally to produce analgesia for 3 to 6 hours. It is given subcutaneously, intramuscularly, or intravenously; intravenous infusion as part of a patient-controlled analgesia system is also permitted.

The dose of nalbuphine hydrochloride for **pain** relief is 10 to 20 mg every 3 to 6 hours as required. Doses of 10 to 30 mg have been given by slow intravenous injection in myocardial infarction; a second dose of 20 mg may be given after 30 minutes if necessary. Children may be given up to 300 micrograms/kg initially, repeated once or twice as necessary.

**Premedication** has been carried out using doses of 100 to 200 micrograms/kg. As an adjunct to anaesthesia a usual dose is 0.3 to 1 mg/kg given intravenously over 10 to 15 minutes at induction; in the USA doses of up to 3 mg/kg have been used. Maintenance doses of 250 to 500 micrograms/kg are given at half-hourly intervals.

**Action.** Nalbuphine is generally described as a mixed agonist and antagonist acting mainly as an agonist at κ opioid receptors and as an antagonist or partial agonist at μ receptors. It has shown antagonist activity similar to that seen with naloxone in opioid-dependent subjects.[1] Nalbuphine is structurally related to naloxone and oxymorphone. Pharmacologically nalbuphine is qualitatively similar to pentazocine, but nalbuphine is a more potent antagonist at μ opioid receptors, is less likely to produce psychotomimetic effects such as hallucinations, and is reported to produce no significant cardiovascular effects in patients with ischaemic heart disease. It differs from pure μ agonists such as morphine in that its analgesic, sedative, and respiratory depressant actions are subject to a 'ceiling' effect and may not increase proportionately with dose.

1. Preston KL, *et al.* Antagonist effects of nalbuphine in opioid-dependent human volunteers. *J Pharmacol Exp Ther* 1989; **248:** 929–37.

## Preparations

**Proprietary Preparations** (details are given in Part 3)

***Arg.:*** Naltrox; Nubaina; Nubak; Onfor; ***Austria:*** Nubain; ***Braz.:*** Nubain; ***Canad.:*** Nubain; ***Fr.:*** Azerty†; Nubain; ***Ger.:*** Nubain; ***Gr.:*** Nubain; ***Hong Kong:*** Intapan; Nubain; ***Israel:*** Nubain; ***Malaysia:*** Nubain; ***Mex.:*** Bufigen; Bufilem; Nalbu†; Nalcryn; Nubain; ***NZ:*** Nubain†; ***S.Afr.:*** Nubain; ***Singapore:*** Nubain; ***Switz.:*** Nubain; ***Thai.:*** Nubain; ***UK:*** Nubain; ***USA:*** Nubain.

## Naproxen (BAN, USAN, rINN)

Naproxeno; Naproxenum; RS-3540. (+)-2-(6-Methoxy-2-naphthyl)propionic acid.

$C_{14}H_{14}O_3$ = 230.3.

*CAS — 22204-53-1.*

*ATC — G02CC02; M01AE02; M02AA12.*

**Pharmacopoeias.** In *Chin., Eur.* (see p.vi), *Jpn*, and *US.*

**Ph. Eur. 5.0** (Naproxen). A white or almost white, crystalline powder. Practically insoluble in water; soluble in alcohol and in methyl alcohol. Protect from light.

**USP 27** (Naproxen). A white to off-white, practically odourless, crystalline powder. Practically insoluble in water; soluble in alcohol; freely soluble in dehydrated alcohol and in chloroform; sparingly soluble in ether. Store in airtight containers.

## Naproxen Sodium (BANM, USAN, rINNM)

Naproxeno sódico; RS-3650.

$C_{14}H_{13}NaO_3$ = 252.2.

*CAS — 26159-34-2.*

**Pharmacopoeias.** In *Chin.* and *US.*

**USP 27** (Naproxen Sodium). A white to creamy crystalline powder. Soluble in water and in methyl alcohol; sparingly soluble in alcohol; very slightly soluble in acetone; practically insoluble in chloroform and in toluene. Store in airtight containers.

## Adverse Effects and Precautions

As for NSAIDs in general, p.67.

Administration of suppositories containing naproxen may cause rectal irritation and occasional bleeding.

◊ Reviews.

1. Bansal V, *et al.* A look at the safety profile of over-the-counter naproxen sodium: a meta-analysis. *J Clin Pharmacol* 2001; **41:** 127–38.

**Breast feeding.** The American Academy of Pediatrics[1] states that there have been no reports of any clinical effect on the infant associated with the use of naproxen by breast-feeding mothers, and that therefore it may be considered to be usually compatible with breast feeding. The *British National Formulary* also considers that the amount of naproxen distributed into breast milk is too small to be harmful to a breast-fed infant; however, some manufacturers recommend that breast feeding should be avoided during naproxen therapy.

In a study[2] of a breast-fed infant only 0.26% of the mother's dose was recovered from the infant.

1. American Academy of Pediatrics. The transfer of drugs and other chemicals into human milk. *Pediatrics* 2001; **108:** 776–89. Correction. *ibid.*; 1029. Also available at: http://aappolicy.aappublications.org/cgi/content/full/pediatrics%3b108/3/776 (accessed 06/07/04)
2. Jamali F, Stevens DRS. Naproxen excretion in milk and its uptake by the infant. *Drug Intell Clin Pharm* 1983; **17:** 910–11.

**Effects on the blood.** Haematological adverse effects reported in patients receiving naproxen include haemolytic anaemia,[1,2] aplastic anaemia,[3] and agranulocytosis.[4]

1. Hughes JA, Sudell W. Hemolytic anemia associated with naproxen. *Arthritis Rheum* 1983; **26:** 1054.
2. Lo TCN, Martin MA. Autoimmune haemolytic anaemia associated with naproxen suppositories. *BMJ* 1986; **292:** 1430.
3. McNeil P, *et al.* Naproxen-associated aplastic anaemia. *Med J Aust* 1986; **145:** 53–4.
4. Nygard N, Starkebaum G. Naproxen and agranulocytosis. *JAMA* 1987; **257:** 1732.

**Effects on the cardiovascular system.** For a discussion of the suggestion that naproxen may have a cardioprotective effect, see p.67.

**Effects on the CNS.** Aseptic meningitis has been associated with naproxen therapy;[1,2] attacks may be recurrent and cross-sensitivity with other NSAIDs has occurred.[2]

There has been a report[3] of a patient with Parkinson's disease whose symptoms had previously been well controlled but who deteriorated when she was given naproxen. She improved on withdrawal of naproxen and the effect was confirmed by rechallenge. It was noted that the UK Committee on Safety of Medicines had records of a case of parkinsonism associated with a combined preparation of naproxen and misoprostol and 12 other reports of tremor or ataxia precipitated by naproxen.

1. Weksler BB, Lehany AM. Naproxen-induced recurrent aseptic meningitis. *DICP Ann Pharmacother* 1991; **25:** 1183–4.
2. Seaton RA, France AJ. Recurrent aseptic meningitis following non-steroidal anti-inflammatory drugs – a reminder. *Postgrad Med J* 1999; **75:** 771–2.
3. Shaunak S, *et al.* Exacerbation of idiopathic Parkinson's disease by naproxen. *BMJ* 1995; **311:** 422.

**Effects on the eyes.** Keratopathy, characterised by whorl-like corneal opacities, occurred in a woman receiving naproxen; complete regression occurred after discontinuation of naproxen.[1] There has also been a report of exacerbation of glaucoma in a 65-year-old woman given naproxen.[2]

For reference to effects on the optic nerve associated with naproxen, see p.68.

1. Szmyd L, Perry HD. Keratopathy associated with the use of naproxen. *Am J Ophthalmol* 1985; **99:** 598.
2. Fincham JE. Exacerbation of glaucoma in an elderly female taking naproxen sodium: a case report. *J Geriatr Drug Ther* 1989; **3:** 139–43.

**Effects on the gastrointestinal tract.** Gastrointestinal adverse effects are among the most frequently reported during short- and long-term treatment with naproxen. Acute proctocolitis associated with the use of naproxen has been reported[1] in a patient. Oesophageal ulceration reported in 7 patients[2] may have arisen due to incorrect consumption (such as taking the dosage without fluids or lying down after administration) but other causes could not be dismissed.

1. Ravi S, *et al.* Colitis caused by non-steroidal anti-inflammatory drugs. *Postgrad Med J* 1986; **62:** 773–6.
2. Kahn LH, *et al.* Over-the-counter naproxen sodium and esophageal injury. *Ann Intern Med* 1997; **126:** 1006.

**Effects on the kidneys.** Acute renal failure,[1] renal papillary necrosis,[2] interstitial nephritis,[3] and hyperkalaemia[1] have been reported in patients receiving naproxen. As with other NSAIDs, renal adverse effects occur more frequently in patients with certain risk factors such as volume depletion, diuretic therapy, heart failure, and pre-existing renal dysfunction.[1]

1. Todd PA, Clissold SP. Naproxen: a reappraisal of its pharmacology, and therapeutic use in rheumatic diseases and pain states. *Drugs* 1990; **40:** 91–137.
2. Caruana RJ, Semble EL. Renal papillary necrosis due to naproxen. *J Rheumatol* 1984; **11:** 90–1.
3. Quigley MR, *et al.* Concurrent naproxen- and penicillamine-induced renal disease in rheumatoid arthritis. *Arthritis Rheum* 1982; **25:** 1016–19.

**Effects on the liver.** There have been a few reports[1,2] of moderate to severe jaundice attributed to naproxen including one in which the patient also had a similar reaction with fenoprofen.[2]

1. Victorino RMM, *et al.* Jaundice associated with naproxen. *Postgrad Med J* 1980; **56:** 368–70.
2. Andrejak M, *et al.* Cross hepatotoxicity between non-steroidal anti-inflammatory drugs. *BMJ* 1987; **295:** 180–1.

**Effects on the lungs.** See under Hypersensitivity, below.

**Effects on the salivary glands.** For reference to salivary gland swelling associated with naproxen therapy, see under Hypersensitivity, below.

**Effects on the skin.** Cutaneous reactions reported in patients receiving naproxen include erythema nodosum,[1] lichen planus,[2] toxic pustular skin eruption,[3] and bullous dermatosis.[4] Photodermatitis, characterised by vesicle formation or increased skin fragility on sun-exposed skin, has been reported in adults[5-7] and children.[8,9]

A relapse of subacute cutaneous lupus erythematosus was reported to be possibly associated with naproxen.[10]

For reference to facial scars of unknown origin developing in children receiving NSAIDs, and in particular naproxen, see under NSAIDs, p.69.

1. Grattan CEH, Kennedy CTC. Naproxen induced erythema nodosum. *BMJ* 1984; **288:** 114.
2. Heymann WR, *et al.* Naproxen-induced lichen planus. *J Am Acad Dermatol* 1984; **10:** 299–301.
3. Page SR, Grattan CEH. Pustular reaction to naproxen with cholestatic jaundice. *BMJ* 1986; **293:** 510.
4. Bouldin MB, *et al.* Naproxen-associated linear IgA bullous dermatosis: case report and review. *Mayo Clin Proc* 2000; **75:** 967–70.
5. Howard AM, *et al.* Pseudoporphyria due to naproxen. *Lancet* 1985; **i:** 819–20.
6. Rivers JK, Barnetson RS. Naproxen-induced bullous photodermatitis. *Med J Aust* 1989; **151:** 167–8.
7. Levy ML, *et al.* Naproxen-induced pseudoporphyria: a distinctive photodermatitis. *J Pediatr* 1990; **117:** 660–4.
8. Parodi A, *et al.* Possible naproxen-induced relapse of subacute cutaneous lupus erythematosus. *JAMA* 1992; **268:** 51–2.
9. Lang BA, Finlayson LA. Naproxen-induced pseudoporphyria in patients with juvenile rheumatoid arthritis. *J Pediatr* 1994; **124:** 639–42.
10. Cox NH, Wilkinson DS. Dermatitis artefacta as the presenting feature of auto-erythrocyte sensitization syndrome and naproxen-induced pseudoporphyria in a single patient. *Br J Dermatol* 1992; **126:** 86–9.

**Hypersensitivity.** All of 11 aspirin-sensitive asthmatic patients developed reactions (rhinorrhoea, tightness of chest, wheezing, dyspnoea) after taking naproxen in doses of 40 to 80 mg.[1] Hypersensitivity to individual NSAIDs is believed to be closely linked to the extent to which these drugs inhibit prostaglandin (see under Aspirin, p.16). There may therefore be a dose threshold below which no detectable symptoms occur. Such an effect has been reported[2] in a patient previously stabilised on naproxen for about one year who had a hypersensitivity reaction following a dosage increase.

A hypersensitivity reaction characterised by pulmonary infiltrates with eosinophilia[3,4] has been reported in patients taking naproxen. There has also been a report of a generalised hypersensitivity reaction with acute eosinophilic colitis in a 57-year-old woman treated with naproxen for osteoarthritis.[5] Bilateral swelling of the major salivary glands, a generalised rash, and eosinophilia suggestive of a hypersensitivity response was reported in another patient following use of naproxen.[6]

1. Szczeklik A, *et al.* Asthmatic attacks induced in aspirin-sensitive patients by diclofenac and naproxen. *BMJ* 1977; **2:** 231–2.
2. Briscoe-Dwyer L, Etzel JV. Dyspnea and periorbital edema following an increase in naproxen dose. *Ann Pharmacother* 1994; **28:** 1110.
3. Nader DA, Schillaci RF. Pulmonary infiltrates with eosinophilia due to naproxen. *Chest* 1983; **83:** 280–2.
4. Buscaglia AJ, *et al.* Pulmonary infiltrates associated with naproxen. *JAMA* 1984; **251:** 65–6.
5. Bridges AJ, *et al.* Acute eosinophilic colitis and hypersensitivity reaction associated with naproxen therapy. *Am J Med* 1990; **89:** 526–7.
6. Knulst AC, *et al.* Salivary gland swelling following naproxen therapy. *Br J Dermatol* 1995; **133:** 647–9.

**Parkinsonism.** For a report of a patient whose symptoms of Parkinson's disease were exacerbated by naproxen, see under Effects on the CNS, above.

## Interactions

For interactions associated with NSAIDs, see p.69.

The excretion of naproxen is delayed by probenecid resulting in raised plasma concentrations of naproxen.

**Antiepileptics.** For the effect of naproxen on the protein binding of valproic acid, see p.381.

## Pharmacokinetics

Naproxen and naproxen sodium are readily absorbed from the gastrointestinal tract. Peak plasma concentrations are attained about 1 to 2 hours after ingestion of naproxen sodium and in about 2 to 4 hours after ingestion of naproxen. Food reduces the rate but not the extent of absorption. Naproxen and naproxen sodium are also well absorbed rectally. At therapeutic concentrations naproxen is more than 99% bound to plasma proteins. Plasma concentrations of naproxen increase proportionally with dose up to about 500 mg daily; at higher doses there is an increase in clearance caused by saturation of plasma proteins. Naproxen diffuses into synovial fluid; it crosses the placenta and is distributed into breast milk in small amounts. Naproxen has a plasma elimination half-life of about 13 hours. About 95% of a dose is excreted in urine as naproxen and 6-*O*-desmethylnaproxen and their conjugates. Less than 5% of a dose appears in the faeces.

◊ References.

1. Bruno R, *et al.* Naproxen kinetics in synovial fluid of patients with osteoarthritis. *Br J Clin Pharmacol* 1988; **26:** 41–4.
2. Bertin P, *et al.* Sodium naproxen: concentration and effect on inflammatory response mediators in human rheumatoid synovial fluid. *Eur J Clin Pharmacol* 1994; **46:** 3–7.
3. Davies NM, Anderson KE. Clinical pharmacokinetics of naproxen. *Clin Pharmacokinet* 1997; **32:** 268–93.

## Uses and Administration

Naproxen, a propionic acid derivative, is an NSAID (p.70).

Naproxen is used in musculoskeletal and joint disorders such as ankylosing spondylitis, osteoarthritis, and rheumatoid arthritis including juvenile idiopathic arthritis. It is also used in dysmenorrhoea, headache including migraine, postoperative pain, soft-tissue disorders, acute gout, and to reduce fever. Naproxen is usually given by mouth as the free acid or as the sodium salt. The doses in the manufacturers product information are expressed in terms of the free acid or the sodium salt as appropriate for an individual preparation; however, the doses given below are expressed in terms of the equivalent amount of free acid only. Each 550 mg of naproxen sodium is approximately equivalent to 500 mg of naproxen.

In the treatment of rheumatic disorders, the usual dose of naproxen or naproxen sodium is the equivalent of 500 mg to 1 g of naproxen daily either as a single dose or in 2 divided doses. A dose of 10 mg/kg daily of naproxen in 2 divided doses has been used in children over 5 years of age with juvenile idiopathic arthritis.

In other painful conditions such as dysmenorrhoea and acute musculoskeletal disorders the usual initial dose is the equivalent of 500 mg of naproxen followed by 250 mg every 6 to 8 hours, up to a maximum daily dose of 1250 mg after the first day.

In acute gout an initial dose equivalent to 750 mg of naproxen followed by 250 mg every 8 hours is used.

Modified-release preparations are available in some countries for once daily use.

For the treatment of migraine, the equivalent of 750 mg of naproxen can be given at the first symptom of an impending attack and, if necessary, this may be followed after at least half an hour by further doses of 250 to 500 mg throughout the day to a total maximum daily dose of 1250 mg. See below for a suggested dose for the prophylaxis of migraine.

Naproxen is sometimes given rectally in single doses of 500 mg.

Naproxen has also been used as the piperazine, aminobutanol, and lysine salts and as naproxen cetrimonium. Naproxen is available in combination with misoprostol (p.1519) for patients at risk of NSAID-induced peptic ulceration. Alternatively, packs containing naproxen with lansoprazole capsules are available in some countries for such patients.

◊ Reviews.


1. Todd PA, Clissold SP. Naproxen: a reappraisal of its pharmacology, and therapeutic use in rheumatic diseases and pain states. *Drugs* 1990; **40:** 91–137.


**Headache.** An NSAID such as naproxen is among the drugs tried first for the symptomatic treatment of various types of headache including migraine (p.464) and tension-type headache (p.465). An NSAID given at the onset of symptoms can successfully treat an acute attack of migraine.[1] NSAIDs also appear to be effective for the prophylaxis of migraine, although propranolol or pizotifen are generally preferred. Studies have indicated that naproxen sodium 550 mg [equivalent to 500 mg of naproxen] given twice daily may be useful for reducing the number of attacks suffered.[2-5]


1. Treves TA, *et al.* Naproxen sodium versus ergotamine tartrate in the treatment of acute migraine attacks. *Headache* 1992; **32:** 280–2.
2. Sargent J, *et al.* A comparison of naproxen sodium to propranolol hydrochloride and a placebo control for the prophylaxis of migraine headache. *Headache* 1985; **25:** 320–4.
3. Welch KMA, *et al.* Successful migraine prophylaxis with naproxen sodium. *Neurology* 1985; **35:** 1304–10.
4. Sances G, *et al.* Naproxen sodium in menstrual migraine prophylaxis: a double-blind placebo controlled study. *Headache* 1990; **30:** 705–9.
5. Bellavance AJ, Meloche JP. A comparative study of naproxen sodium, pizotyline and placebo in migraine prophylaxis. *Headache* 1990; **30:** 710–15.


**Malignant neoplasms.** Some NSAIDs such as naproxen may be of value both for the differential diagnosis and the management of neoplastic fever[1,2] as they appear to be more effective in reducing this type of fever than against fever associated with infections.


1. Chang JC, Gross HM. Neoplastic fever responds to the treatment of an adequate dose of naproxen. *J Clin Oncol* 1985; **3:** 552–8.
2. Azeemuddin SK, *et al.* The effect of naproxen on fever in children with malignancies. *Cancer* 1987; **59:** 1966–8.


## Preparations

***BP 2003:*** Enteric-coated Naproxen Tablets; Naproxen Oral Suspension; Naproxen Suppositories; Naproxen Tablets;
***USP 27:*** Naproxen Oral Suspension; Naproxen Sodium Tablets; Naproxen Tablets.

**Proprietary Preparations** (details are given in Part 3)

***Arg.:*** Aleve; Algioprux; Alidase; Bumaflex N; Causalon Pro; Congex; Debril; Fabralgina; Fadalivio; Flogocefal; Melgar; Monarit; Naprofidex; Naprogen; Naprontag; Naprux; Neuralprona; Sicadentol Plus; Tundra; Veradol; Xicane; ***Austral.:*** Aleve; Anaprox; Chemists Own Period Pain Tablets; Crysanal; Inza; Naprogesic; Naprosyn; Nurolasts; Proxen; ***Austria:*** Aleve; Miranax; Naprobene; Nycopren; Proxen; ***Belg.:*** Aleve; Apra-Gel†; Apranax; Naprosyne; ***Braz.:*** Flanax†; Naprosyn†; Naprox; ***Canad.:*** Anaprox; Apo-Napro-Na; Naprosyn; Naxen; Novo-Naprox; Nu-Naprox; Rhodiaprox†; Roche†; Synflex; ***Chile:*** Deucoval; Eurogesic Gel; Inveoxel; Naprogesic; Reprost; Triox NF; ***Denm.:*** Alpoxen†; Bonyl; Daprox†; Miranax; Napronet†; Naprosyn; Nycopren†; ***Fin.:*** Alpoxen; Miranax; Naprometin; Napromex; Naprosyn; Naxopren; Nycopren†; Pronaxen; ***Fr.:*** Aleve; Apranax; Naprosyne; ***Ger.:*** Aleve; Apranax†; Dysmenalgit; Malexin†; Napro-Dorsch†; Proxen; ***Gr.:*** Anaprox; Naprosyn; Nycopren; ***Hong Kong:*** Apo-Napro-Na; Genoxen†; Inza; Naprorex; Naprosyn; Napxen; Noflam-N; Proxen; Soren; Synflex; ***India:*** Artagen; Naprosyn; Xenobid; ***Irl.:*** Gerinap; Napmel; Naprex; Naprosyn; Synflex; ***Israel:*** Aponacin†; Naprex†; Naproxi; Narocin; Naxyn; Point; ***Ital.:*** Akudol†; Aleve; Algonapril; Aperdan; Artroxen†; AS/85†; Axer; D/N PR†; Floginax; Flogogin; Floxalin; Gibinap†; Gibixen; Gynestrel; Laser; Leniartril†; Momendol; Napreben; Naprius; Naprocet; Naprodol†; Naprorex; Naprosyn; Natrioxen†; Neo Eblimon; Nitens; Numidan†; Piproxen†; Prexan; Primeral†; Proxine†; Synalgo; Synflex; Ticoflex; Xenar; ***Malaysia:*** Apo-Napro-Na; Inza; Roxyn; Seladin; Sunprox; ***Mex.:*** Actiquim; Alxen†; Anaflin†; Anapsyl; Artron; Atiflan†; Bioxan; Dafloxen; Dartrox†; Deflamox; Diferbest; Dolnaxen†; Doloatrixen†; Dolxen; Donaprox†; Faraxen†; Flanax; Flexen; Flogen; Fuxen; Genalgen; Iqfasol; Kenaprox†; Lixogan†; Lorexen; Naflapen; Naprodil; Nasocan†; Navixen†; Naxen; Naxil†; Neonaxil; Nixal; Novadex†; Novaxen; Pactens; Patxen†; Pronat; Pronax-P†; Pronaxil; Pronoxen; Proxalin; Sertrixen; Sodixen; Tandax; Tanizona; Velsay; ***Neth.:*** Aleve; Femex; Naprocoat; Naprosyne†; Naprovite; Nycopren; ***Norw.:*** Alpoxen; Ledox; Napren; Naprosyn; ***NZ:*** Naprogesic; Naprosyn; Naxen; Noflam†; Synflex; ***Port.:*** Momendol; Naprosyn; Reuxen; ***S.Afr.:*** Acusprain†; Aleve; Fibroxyn; Nafasol; Napflam; Naprel; Naproscript; Naprosyn; Pranoxen†; Synflex; Traumox†; ***Singapore:*** Anax†; Apo-Napro-Na; Bipronyl; Gesiprox; Inza; Naprosyn†; Noflam-N; Nuprafen; Seladin; Soden; Soproxen; Sunprox†; Synflex†; Zynal; ***Spain:*** Aleve; Alivi-omas; Anaprox†; Antalgin; Denaxpren; Ilagane†; Lundiran; Naprokes†; Naprosyn; Naproval; Proxen†; Tacron; ***Swed.:*** Alpoxen; Miranax†; Naprosyn; Pronaxen; ***Switz.:*** Aleve; Apranax; Naprosyn; Nycopren; Proxen; Servinaprox†; ***Thai.:*** Annoxen; Artagen†; Flexin†; Naprosian; Naproso†; Naprosyn; Napsen; Napxen; Narzen; Polyxen; Proxen; Roxen; Serviproxan; Soproxen; Synflex; Synogin†; U-Proxyn; Vinsen; ***UK:*** Arthrosin†; Arthroxen; Condrotec†; Laraflex†; Napratec; Naprosyn; Nycopren; Rimoxyn†; Synflex; Timpron†; ***USA:*** Aleve; Anaprox; Naprelan; Naprosyn; Prevacid NapraPAC.

**Multi-ingredient:** ***Arg.:*** Naprontag Flex; Papasine; ***Ital.:*** Flogogin†; ***Mex.:*** Acxen; Bifardol S; Blocacid; Dafloxen F; Decosil; Dolotandax; Farxen; Febrax; Grifed; Naxodol; Proxalin-Plus; Somalgesic; Viplus.

---

# Nefopam Hydrochloride

*(BANM, USAN, rINNM)*

Benzoxazocine; Fenazoxine; Hidrocloruro de nefopam; R-738.
3,4,5,6-Tetrahydro-5-methyl-1-phenyl-1*H*-2,5-benzoxazocine hydrochloride.
$C_{17}H_{19}NO,HCl = 289.8.$
*CAS — 13669-70-0 (nefopam); 23327-57-3 (nefopam hydrochloride).*
*ATC — N02BG06.*

**Pharmacopoeias.** In *Chin.*

## Adverse Effects and Treatment

Side-effects occurring with nefopam include gastrointestinal disturbances, such as nausea and vomiting, sweating, drowsiness, insomnia, urinary retention, dizziness, hypotension, tremor, paraesthesia, palpitations, lightheadedness, nervousness, confusion, blurred vision, headache, dry mouth, syncope, angioedema, and tachycardia. Euphoria, hallucinations, and convulsions have occasionally been reported, as has temporary pink discoloration of the urine. Symptoms of overdosage have included CNS and cardiovascular toxicity.

**Effects on the urinary tract.** In January 1989, the UK Committee on Safety of Medicines[1] reported that it had received 53 reports in which nefopam was associated with the development of urinary retention or symptoms of hesitancy, poor stream, or dribbling. In one case there was a history of prostatism.


1. Committee on Safety of Medicines. Nefopam hydrochloride (Acupan). *Current Problems 24* 1989.


**Overdosage.** There have been reports of fatal overdoses with nefopam.[1-3] One report[1] also provided details of 9 other patients who recovered with routine supportive treatment.


1. Piercy DM, *et al.* Death due to overdose of nefopam. *BMJ* 1981; **283:** 1508–9.
2. Urwin SC, Smith HS. Fatal nefopam overdose. *Br J Anaesth* 1999; **83:** 501–2.
3. Tracqui A, *et al.* Fatal overdosage with nefopam (Acupan®). *J Anal Toxicol* 2002; **26:** 239–43.


## Precautions

Nefopam is contra-indicated in patients with a history of convulsive disorders. It should be used with caution in the elderly and in patients with glaucoma, urinary retention, or impaired hepatic or renal function.

**Abuse.** A report of 3 cases of nefopam abuse.[1]


1. Villier C, Mallaret MP. Nefopam abuse. *Ann Pharmacother* 2002; **36:** 1564–6.


**Breast feeding.** No adverse effects have been observed in breast-feeding infants whose mothers were receiving nefopam, and the American Academy of Pediatrics considers[1] that it is therefore usually compatible with breast feeding.

Studies in 5 healthy nursing mothers given nefopam for post-episiotomy pain indicated that nefopam was present in human milk in an equivalent concentration to that in plasma.[2] It was calculated that on a body-weight basis a breast-fed infant would receive less than 3% of the maternal dose.


1. American Academy of Pediatrics. The transfer of drugs and other chemicals into human milk. *Pediatrics* 2001; **108:** 776–89. Correction. *ibid.*: 1029. Also available at: http://aappolicy.aappublications.org/cgi/content/full/pediatrics%3b108/3/776 (accessed 09/07/04)
2. Liu DTY, *et al.* Nefopam excretion in human milk. *Br J Clin Pharmacol* 1987; **23:** 99–101.


## Interactions

It has been recommended that nefopam should not be given to patients receiving MAOIs and should be used cautiously in those receiving tricyclic antidepressants. The adverse effects of nefopam may be additive to those of other drugs with antimuscarinic or sympathomimetic activity.

## Pharmacokinetics

Nefopam is absorbed from the gastrointestinal tract. Peak plasma concentrations occur 1 to 3 hours after a dose by mouth and about 1.5 hours after intramuscular injection. About 73% is bound to plasma proteins. Nefopam is distributed into breast milk. It has an elimination half-life of about 4 hours. It is extensively metabolised and excreted mainly in urine, in which less than 5% of a dose is excreted unchanged. About 8% of a dose is excreted via the faeces.

## Uses and Administration

Nefopam hydrochloride is a non-opioid analgesic considered to act centrally, although its mechanism of action is unclear. It also has some antimuscarinic and sympathomimetic actions. Nefopam hydrochloride is used for the relief of moderate acute and chronic pain. The usual dose range by mouth is 30 to 90 mg three times daily; the recommended initial dose is 60 mg (or 30 mg in elderly patients) three times daily. Nefopam hydrochloride may also be given in doses of 20 mg by intramuscular injection, repeated every 6 hours if necessary; it is recommended that the patient should always be lying down when receiving the injection and should remain so for 15 to 20 minutes afterwards. It has also been given by slow intravenous injection in similar doses.

**Hiccup.** In two case series[1,2] involving 10 patients in total, hiccups refractory to standard treatment stopped after treatment with intravenous nefopam. A protocol for the management of intractable hiccups may be found under Chlorpromazine, p.682.


1. Bilotta F, Rosa G. Nefopam for severe hiccups. *N Engl J Med* 2000; **343:** 1973–4.
2. Bilotta F, *et al.* Nefopam for refractory postoperative hiccups. *Anesth Analg* 2001; **93:** 1358–60.


## Preparations

**Proprietary Preparations** (details are given in Part 3)

***Belg.:*** Acupan; ***Fr.:*** Acupan; ***Ger.:*** Ajan; Silentan; ***Irl.:*** Acupan; ***Israel:*** Acupan; ***Ital.:*** Nefadol†; Nefam; Oxadol; ***NZ:*** Acupan; ***Spain:*** Acupan†; ***Switz.:*** Acupan; ***UK:*** Acupan.

---

# Nicoboxil *(rINN)*

Butoxyethyl Nicotinate; Nicoboxilo. 2-Butoxyethyl nicotinate.
$C_{12}H_{17}NO_3 = 223.3.$
*CAS — 13912-80-6.*

## Profile

Nicoboxil is a nicotinate used in topical preparations as a rubefacient. It is also included in some topical preparations used for the treatment of acne vulgaris.

## Preparations

**Proprietary Preparations** (details are given in Part 3)

**Multi-ingredient:** ***Austral.:*** Finalgon; ***Austria:*** Finalgon; ***Canad.:*** Actinac†; Finalgon; ***Ger.:*** Finalgon; ***Irl.:*** Actinac†; ***Ital.:*** Anti-Acne; ***NZ:*** Finalgon; ***Port.:*** Finalgon; ***Spain:*** Finalgon; ***UK:*** Actinac.

---

# Nicomorphine Hydrochloride *(BANM, rINNM)*

Hidrocloruro de nicomorfina. 3,6-Di-*O*-nicotinoylmorphine hydrochloride; (−)-(5*R*,6*S*)-4,5-Epoxy-9a-methylmorphin-7-en-3,6-diyl dinicotinate hydrochloride.
$C_{29}H_{25}N_3O_5,HCl = 532.0.$
*CAS — 639-48-5 (nicomorphine); 12040-41-4 (nicomorphine hydrochloride); 35055-78-8 (nicomorphine xHCl).*
*ATC — N02AA04.*

## Profile

Nicomorphine hydrochloride is an opioid analgesic (p.71) used in the treatment of moderate to severe pain. It is given by mouth in initial doses of 5 to 10 mg daily or by intramuscular, slow intravenous, or subcutaneous injection in usual doses of 10 to 20 mg; it may also be given rectally.

◊ References.


1. Koopman-Kimenai PM, *et al.* Pharmacokinetics of intramuscular nicomorphine and its metabolites in man. *Eur J Clin Pharmacol* 1991; **41:** 375–8.
2. Koopman-Kimenai PM, *et al.* Pharmacokinetics of intravenously administered nicomorphine and its metabolites in man. *Eur J Anaesthesiol* 1993; **10:** 125–32.
3. Koopman-Kimenai PM, *et al.* Rectal administration of nicomorphine in patients improves biological availability of morphine and its glucuronide conjugates. *Pharm World Sci* 1994; **16:** 248–53.


## Preparations

**Proprietary Preparations** (details are given in Part 3)

***Austria:*** Vilan; ***Denm.:*** Vilan; ***Neth.:*** Vilan; ***Switz.:*** Vilan.

---

# Nifenazone *(BAN, rINN)*

Nifenazona. *N*-(2,3-Dimethyl-5-oxo-1-phenyl-3-pyrazolin-4-yl)nicotinamide.
$C_{17}H_{16}N_4O_2 = 308.3.$
*CAS — 2139-47-1.*
*ATC — M02AA24; N02BB05.*

## Profile

Nifenazone is an NSAID (p.67) that has been used in musculoskeletal and joint disorders.

## Preparations

**Proprietary Preparations** (details are given in Part 3)

***Ital.:*** Reumatosil†.

## Niflumic Acid *(rINN)*

Ácido niflúmico; UP-83. 2-(ααα-Trifluoro-*m*-toluidino)nicotinic acid.

$C_{13}H_9F_3N_2O_2$ = 282.2.
*CAS — 4394-00-7.*
*ATC — M01AX02; M02AA17.*

**Pharmacopoeias.** In *Fr.*

### Adverse Effects and Precautions

As for NSAIDs in general, p.67. Fluoride-associated osteosis has been reported with prolonged use. Niflumic acid should be discontinued if hypersensitivity skin reactions appear.

**Effects on the skin.** From a case-control study[1] of children admitted to a hospital emergency department in Italy it was calculated that the odds-ratio of users of niflumic acid, or its derivative morniflumate, developing serious cutaneous reactions was 4.9. Given this figure and the fact that safer drugs were available the authors considered that there was no indication for which niflumic acid was required in children.

1. Menniti-Ippolito F, *et al.* Niflumic acid and cutaneous reactions in children. *Arch Dis Child* 2001; **84:** 430–1.

### Uses and Administration

Niflumic acid, a nicotinic acid derivative, is an NSAID (p.70). It has been used in inflammatory and musculoskeletal and joint disorders in usual doses of about 250 mg three or four times daily by mouth; up to 1500 mg daily has been used in severe disorders. It has also been used topically as a 3% cream or ointment or 2.5% gel. The morpholinoethyl ester, morniflumate (p.60), has similar uses.

Niflumic acid glycinamide has been used topically in inflammatory mouth disorders.

### Preparations

**Proprietary Preparations** (details are given in Part 3)
***Arg.:*** Flogovital; ***Austria:*** Actol†; ***Belg.:*** Niflugel; Nifluril; ***Fr.:*** Flunir; Niflugel; Nifluril; ***Gr.:*** Niflamol; ***Hong Kong:*** Nifluril†; ***Ital.:*** Niflam; ***Port.:*** Nifluril; ***Spain:*** Niflactol; ***Switz.:*** Niflugel†; Nifluril†.

**Multi-ingredient:** ***Arg.:*** Flogodisten; ***Fr.:*** Nifluril†; ***Port.:*** Nifluril†.

## Nimesulide *(BAN, rINN)*

Nimesulida; Nimesulidum; R-805. 4′-Nitro-2′-phenoxymethanesulphonanilide.

$C_{13}H_{12}N_2O_5S$ = 308.3.
*CAS — 51803-78-2.*
*ATC — M01AX17.*

**Pharmacopoeias.** In *Eur.* (see p.vi).

**Ph. Eur. 5.0** (Nimesulide). A yellowish crystalline powder. It exhibits polymorphism. Practically insoluble in water; slightly soluble in dehydrated alcohol; freely soluble in acetone.

### Profile

Nimesulide is an NSAID (p.67) reported to be a selective inhibitor of cyclo-oxygenase-2 (COX-2). It may be given in doses of up to 100 mg twice daily by mouth or rectally for inflammatory conditions, fever, and pain. It has also been applied topically as a 3% gel. Nimesulide betadex (nimesulide betacyclodextrin complex) has been used similarly.

◊ References.

1. Bennett A, *et al.* Nimesulide: a multifactorial therapeutic approach to the inflammatory process? a 7-year clinical experience. *Drugs* 1993; **46:** (suppl 1): 1–283.
2. Davis R, Brogden RN. Nimesulide: an update of its pharmacodynamic and pharmacokinetic properties, and therapeutic efficacy. *Drugs* 1994; **48:** 431–54.
3. Senna GE, *et al.* Nimesulide in the treatment of patients intolerant of aspirin and other NSAIDs. *Drug Safety* 1996; **14:** 94–103.
4. Vizzardi M, *et al.* Nimesulide beta cyclodextrin (nimesulide-betadex) versus nimesulide in the treatment of pain after arthroscopic surgery. *Curr Ther Res* 1998; **59:** 162–71.
5. Bernareggi A. Clinical pharmacokinetics of nimesulide. *Clin Pharmacokinet* 1998; **35:** 247–74.
6. Shah AA, *et al.* Selective inhibition of COX-2 in humans is associated with less gastrointestinal injury: a comparison of nimesulide and naproxen. *Gut* 2001; **48:** 339–46.
7. Nüing RM, *et al.* Pathogenetic role of cyclooxygenase-2 in hyperprostaglandin E syndrome/antenatal Bartter syndrome: therapeutic use of the cyclooxygenase-2 inhibitor nimesulide. *Clin Pharmacol Ther* 2001; **70:** 384–90.

**Adverse effects.** Although *thrombocytopenia* is a common feature in patients infected with HIV, a group of workers considered that thrombocytopenia in one of their patients was related to the use of nimesulide.[1]

There have been reports[2-4] of *hepatotoxicity* after treatment with nimesulide. Data from spontaneous reports has also suggested that nimesulide may be associated with a higher risk of hepatotoxicity than other NSAIDs.[4] A cohort study[5] involving about 400 000 users of NSAIDs in one region of Italy between 1997 and 2001 found that those taking nimesulide were 1.3 times more likely to develop hepatotoxicity than users of other NSAIDs and 1.9 times more likely to suffer severe liver injury.

There has been a report[6] of *toxic pustuloderma* (acute generalised exanthematous pustulosis) after receiving oral nimesulide.

An infant developed hypotension and hypothermia after inadvertently taking an *overdose* of 8 times the recommended daily dose of nimesulide.[7] The patient recovered after gastric lavage with activated charcoal and supportive therapy.

1. Pasticci MB, *et al.* Nimesulide, thrombocytopenic purpura, and human immunodeficiency virus (HIV) infection. *Ann Intern Med* 1990; **112:** 233–4.
2. McCormick PA, *et al.* COX 2 inhibitor and fulminant hepatic failure. *Lancet* 1999; **353:** 40–1.
3. Sbeit W, *et al.* Nimesulide-induced acute hepatitis. *Ann Pharmacother* 2001; **35:** 1049–52.
4. Maciá MA, *et al.* Hepatotoxicity associated with nimesulide: data from the Spanish pharmacovigilance system. *Clin Pharmacol Ther* 2002; **72:** 596–7.
5. Traversa G, *et al.* Cohort study of hepatotoxicity associated with nimesulide and other non-steroidal anti-inflammatory drugs. *BMJ* 2003; **327:** 18–22.
6. Lateo S, Boffa MJ. Localized toxic pustuloderma associated with nimesulide therapy confirmed by patch testing. *Br J Dermatol* 2002; **147:** 624–5.
7. Yapakci E, *et al.* Hypoglycaemia and hypothermia due to nimesulide overdose. *Arch Dis Child* 2001; **85:** 510.

**Pregnancy and the neonate.** Irreversible *end-stage renal failure* has been reported in a neonate born to a mother who received nimesulide as a tocolytic from the 26th to the 32nd week of pregnancy.[1] Others have reported neonatal renal failure associated with nimesulide.[2]

1. Peruzzi L, *et al.* Neonatal end-stage renal failure associated with maternal ingestion of cyclo-oxygenase-type-2 selective inhibitor nimesulide as tocolytic. *Lancet* 1999; **354:** 1615. Correction. *ibid.* 2000; **355:** 238.
2. Balasubramaniam J. Nimesulide and neonatal renal failure. *Lancet* 1999; **355:** 575.

**Premature labour.** Nimesulide has been tried as an alternative to indometacin to delay labour in patients with a history of preterm delivery. Nimesulide was given from 16 to 34 weeks of gestation and a successful delivery started 6 days after withdrawal.[1] There appeared to be no adverse effect on fetal renal function or the ductus arteriosus. The authors suggested that fetal prostaglandin synthesis might be mainly mediated through cyclo-oxygenase-1 and that a relatively selective cyclo-oxygenase-2 inhibitor such as nimesulide might produce fewer adverse effects on the fetus than other non-selective NSAIDs. However, in a small study short-term effects on the fetus were similar for nimesulide, indometacin, and sulindac.[2]

Adverse renal effects have been reported in some neonates whose mothers received nimesulide for premature labour, see above.

1. Sawdy R, *et al.* Use of a cyclo-oxygenase type-2-selective non-steroidal anti-inflammatory agent to prevent preterm delivery. *Lancet* 1997; **350:** 265–6.
2. Sawdy RJ, *et al.* A double-blind randomized study of fetal side effects during and after the short-term maternal administration of indomethacin, sulindac, and nimesulide for the treatment of preterm labor. *Am J Obstet Gynecol* 2003; **188:** 1046–51.

### Preparations

**Proprietary Preparations** (details are given in Part 3)
***Arg.:*** Aldoron; Aulin; Doloctaprin; Flogovital NF; Metaflex; Virobron; ***Austria:*** Aulin; Mesulid; ***Belg.:*** Mesulid; ***Braz.:*** Antiflogil; Cimelide; Deflogen; Deltaflan; Fasulide; Flogilid; Inflalid; Lidaflan†; Maxsulid†; Neosulida; Nimalgex; Nimeflan†; Nimesilam; Nimesulin†; Nimesulix; Nimesulon; Nisalgen; Nisuflex; Nisulid; Nodor†; Optaflan†; Scaflam; Scalid; Sintalgin; ***Chile:*** Ainex; Aulin; Doloc; Nimepast; Nimesyl; Nimesyl Gel; Nimex; Nisulid; Nisural; ***Fin.:*** Nimed; ***Fr.:*** Nexen; ***Gr.:*** Aflogen; Alencast; Amocetin; Chemisulide; Cliovyl; Discorid; Edrigyl; Elinap; Erlecit; Flogostop; G-Revm; Kartal; Lemesil; Lizepat; Melicat; Mesulid; Mesupon; Min-A-Pon; Multiformil; Myxina; Niberan; Nimelide; Nimesul; Ristolzit; Ritamine; Rolaket; Scaflam; Specilid; Tranzicalm; Ventor; Volonten; ***Hong Kong:*** Mesulid; Nidol; ***India:*** Mesulid; Nimfast; Nimulid; Nimusyp; Nimutab; Nise; ***Irl.:*** Aulin; Mesulid; ***Israel:*** Mesulid; ***Ital.:*** Algimesil; Algolider; Antalgo; Areuma; Aulin; Biosal; Delfos; Dimesul; Doleside; Doloxtren; Domes; Edemax; Efridol; Eudolene; Fansidol; Fenisal†; Flolid; Idealid; Isodol; Laidor; Ledolid; Ledoren; Lidenix; Mesid†; Mesulid; MF 110†; Nerelid; Nide; Nidol†; Nimedex; Nimenol; Nimesil; Nimesulene; Nimexan; Nims; Nisal†; Noalgos; Noxalide; Remov; Resulin; Solving; Sulidamor; Sulide; Teonim†; ***Malaysia:*** Nidol; ***Mex.:*** Apolide†; Degorflan; Eskaflam; Flamide; Lusemin; Mesulid; Redaflam; Severin; ***Port.:*** Aulin; Donulide; Gerilide; Jabasulide; Nimed; Sulidamor; ***Singapore:*** Nidol; Nise; ***Spain:*** Antifloxil†; Guaxan†; ***Switz.:*** Aulin; Nisulid; ***Thai.:*** Nidol.

**Multi-ingredient:** ***Arg.:*** Doloctaprin Plus; Metaflex Plus; Mio Aldoron; Mio-Virobron; ***India:*** Nimulid Nugel.

## Nonivamide *(rINN)*

Nonivamida; Nonylvanillamide; PAVA; Pelargonyl Vanillylamide; Pseudocapsaicin. *N*-Vanillylnonamide; *N*-[(4-Hydroxy-3-methoxyphenyl)methyl]nonanamide.

$C_{17}H_{27}NO_3$ = 293.4.
*CAS — 2444-46-4.*

NOTE. Use of the term 'synthetic capsaicin' to describe nonivamide has arisen from the use of nonivamide as an adulterant for capsaicin and capsicum oleoresin.

### Profile

Nonivamide is a synthetic analogue of capsaicin (p.24) that is used in topical preparations for the relief of muscular and rheumatic pain.

Nonivamide has also been used as a food flavour and in 'pepper sprays' for law enforcement and self defence.

### Preparations

**Proprietary Preparations** (details are given in Part 3)
***Ger.:*** ABC Warme-Pflaster Sensitive; Gothaplast Capsicum-Warmepflaster.

**Multi-ingredient:** ***Austral.:*** Finalgon; ***Austria:*** Finalgon; Rubriment; ***Belg.:*** Forapin†; ***Canad.:*** Finalgon; ***Ger.:*** ABC Warme-Salbe; Akrotherm†; Finalgon; Histajodol N†; Infrotto Ultra; Lomazell forte N; Ostochont; Rheuma-Liquidum†; Rheumasalbe; Rubriment; Vertebralon N; ***NZ:*** Finalgon; ***Port.:*** Finalgon; ***Spain:*** Finalgon; ***Switz.:*** Forapin; Histalgane; Radalgin; Roliwol S†; Thermocutan.

# Nonsteroidal Anti-inflammatory Drugs

Fármacos antiinflamatorios no esteroideos; NSAIDs.

### Adverse Effects and Treatment

The commonest side-effects of NSAIDs are generally gastrointestinal disturbances, such as gastrointestinal discomfort, nausea, and diarrhoea; these are usually mild and reversible but in some patients peptic ulceration and severe gastrointestinal bleeding may occur. It is generally agreed that the gastrointestinal effects of NSAIDs are due to inhibition of cyclo-oxygenase-1 (COX-1); the selective inhibition of COX-2 improves gastrointestinal tolerance.

CNS-related side-effects include headache, vertigo, dizziness, nervousness, tinnitus, depression, drowsiness, and insomnia. Hypersensitivity reactions may occur occasionally and include fever, angioedema, bronchospasm, and rashes. Hepatotoxicity and aseptic meningitis, which occur rarely, may also be hypersensitivity reactions. Some patients may experience visual disturbances.

Haematological adverse effects of NSAIDs include anaemias, thrombocytopenia, neutropenia, eosinophilia, and agranulocytosis. Unlike aspirin, inhibition of platelet aggregation is reversible with other NSAIDs.

Some NSAIDs have been associated with nephrotoxicity such as interstitial nephritis and nephrotic syndrome; renal failure may be provoked by NSAIDs especially in patients with pre-existing renal impairment. Haematuria has also occurred. Fluid retention may occur, rarely precipitating heart failure in elderly patients. Long-term use or abuse of analgesics, including NSAIDs, has been associated with nephropathy.

Other adverse effects include photosensitivity. Alveolitis, pulmonary eosinophilia, pancreatitis, Stevens-Johnson syndrome, and toxic epidermal necrolysis are other rare adverse effects. Induction or exacerbation of colitis has also been reported.

Further details concerning the adverse effects of the individual NSAIDs may be found under their respective monographs.

◊ The relative toxicity of NSAIDs is a continuing subject of debate.[1] Attempts have been made to rank these drugs according to their toxicity on various body systems.[2] For further details see below under individual headings.

1. Skeith KJ, *et al.* Differences in NSAID tolerability profiles: fact or fiction? *Drug Safety* 1994; **10:** 183–95.
2. Committee on Safety of Medicines/Medicines Control Agency. Relative safety of oral non-aspirin NSAIDs. *Current Problems* 1994; **20:** 9–11.

**Effects on the blood.** The UK Committee on Safety of Medicines has provided data on the reports it had received between July 1963 and January 1993 on agranulocytosis and neutropenia.[1] Several groups of drugs were commonly implicated, among them NSAIDs for which there were 133 reports of agranulocytosis (45 fatal) and 187 of neutropenia (15 fatal). The most frequently implicated NSAID was phenylbutazone with 74 reports of agranulocytosis (39 fatal) and 40 of neutropenia (4 fatal).

1. Committee on Safety of Medicines/Medicines Control Agency. Drug-induced neutropenia and agranulocytosis. *Current Problems* 1993; **19:** 10–11.

**Effects on the cardiovascular system.** A meta-analysis[1] of 50 randomised trials studying the effects of NSAIDs on *blood pressure* in a total of 771 patients found that NSAIDs had elevated mean supine blood pressure by 5 mmHg. Piroxicam, indometacin, and ibuprofen had produced the greatest increase but the effect was only found to be statistically significant for piroxicam. Aspirin, sulindac, and flurbiprofen produced the smallest elevation in blood pressure while the effect of tiaprofenic acid, diclofenac, and naproxen was intermediate. The increase was more marked in studies in which patients had received antihypertensive therapy than in those where such treatment had not been used. NSAIDs had antagonised all antihypertensive therapy but the effect had been greater against beta blockers and vasodilators than against diuretics. An earlier meta-analysis of intervention studies had produced similar results.[2] Of the 1324 patients who had received NSAIDs, increases in mean arterial pressure were greatest in hypertensive patients who had taken either indometacin, naproxen, or piroxicam, although results were only significant for indometacin and naproxen. Sulindac and aspirin had minimal effects on mean arterial pressure.

It has been suggested that the use of NSAIDs in the elderly may increase the risk of the need for antihypertensive therapy.[3] A study[3] of 9411 patients aged 65 years or older who had just started treatment with antihypertensives found that 41% had used NSAIDs in the previous year compared with 26% of 9629 control patients not being treated with antihypertensives.

The recent use of NSAIDs has also been associated with an increased risk of developing *heart failure* in elderly patients.[4] A case-control study[5] found that the use of an NSAID in the previous week doubled the odds of being admitted to hospital with heart failure; this risk was increased tenfold in those with a history of heart disease. The study also suggested an association between both high-dose and long drug plasma half-life and an increased risk of heart failure.

Although the *cardioprotective effects* of aspirin are well recognised, it is unclear whether such effects are seen with other non-aspirin NSAIDs. It has been suggested that naproxen may have a protective effect against myocardial infarction, in comparison to other non-aspirin NSAIDs.[6] However, the results of this case-control study have been criticised.[7] In addition, a recent cohort study[8] found no evidence of an increase or decrease in the risk of serious coronary heart disease and myocardial infarction in high-risk patients taking non-aspirin NSAIDs including naproxen. Another study,[9] in patients with no history of cardiovascular disease, also considered that there was no decrease in the risk of myocardial infarction in those taking non-aspirin NSAIDs. More worryingly, it has been suggested that NSAIDs may reduce the cardioprotective effect of aspirin, but see under Interactions of Aspirin, p.17.

For mention of the cardiovascular effects of the selective cyclo-oxygenase-2 inhibitors including their lack of antiplatelet activity, see under Rofecoxib, p.86.


1. Johnson AG, *et al.* Do nonsteroidal anti-inflammatory drugs affect blood pressure? *Ann Intern Med* 1994; **121:** 289–300.
2. Pope JE, *et al.* A meta-analysis of the effects of nonsteroidal anti-inflammatory drugs on blood pressure. *Arch Intern Med* 1993; **153:** 477–84.
3. Gurwitz JH, *et al.* Initiation of antihypertensive treatment during nonsteroidal anti-inflammatory drug therapy. *JAMA* 1994; **272:** 781–6.
4. Bleumink GS, *et al.* Nonsteroidal anti-inflammatory drugs and heart failure. *Drugs* 2003; **63:** 525–34.
5. Page J, Henry D. Consumption of NSAIDs and the development of congestive heart failure in elderly patients: an underrecognised public health problem. *Arch Intern Med* 2000; **160:** 777–84.
6. Rahme E, *et al.* Association between naproxen use and protection against acute myocardial infarction. *Arch Intern Med* 2002; **162:** 1111–15.
7. Mukherjee D, *et al.* Lack of cardioprotective effect of naproxen. *Arch Intern Med* 2002; **162:** 2637.
8. Ray WA, *et al.* Non-steroidal anti-inflammatory drugs and risk of serious coronary heart disease: an observational cohort study. *Lancet* 2002; **359:** 118–23.
9. Schlienger RG, *et al.* Use of nonsteroidal anti-inflammatory drugs and the risk of first-time acute myocardial infarction. *Br J Clin Pharmacol* 2002; **54:** 327–32.


**Effects on the CNS.** A literature review[1] revealed that headache, hearing loss, and tinnitus are the most frequent CNS adverse effects in patients taking NSAIDs. Aseptic meningitis had occurred rarely in patients using NSAIDs such as naproxen, sulindac, or tolmetin, but the most common reports were in patients with systemic lupus erythematosus who were receiving ibuprofen (see also p.46). Reports of psychosis appeared to be rare and have involved indometacin or sulindac, but in the reviewers' experience it was probably under-reported and was typically seen in elderly patients given indometacin.

The role of NSAIDs in the development of cognitive decline in the elderly is unclear. They have been associated with memory impairment and attention deficits in elderly patients,[1,2] especially when given in high doses;[3] however, some authors have also reported that long-term NSAID use may reduce the rate of cognitive decline[3,4] or the risk of developing Alzheimer's disease.[5,6]


1. Hoppmann RA, *et al.* Central nervous system side effects of nonsteroidal anti-inflammatory drugs: aseptic meningitis, psychosis, and cognitive dysfunction. *Arch Intern Med* 1991; **151:** 1309–13.
2. Saag KG, *et al.* Nonsteroidal antiinflammatory drugs and cognitive decline in the elderly. *J Rheumatol* 1995; **22:** 2142–7.
3. Karplus TM, Saag KG. Nonsteroidal anti-inflammatory drugs and cognitive function - do they have a beneficial or deleterious effect? *Drug Safety* 1998; **19:** 427–33.
4. Rozzini R, *et al.* Protective effect of chronic NSAID use on cognitive decline in older persons. *J Am Geriatr Soc* 1996; **44:** 1025–9.
5. Stewart WF, *et al.* Risk of Alzheimer's disease and duration of NSAID use. *Neurology* 1997; **48:** 626–32.
6. in 't Veld BA, *et al.* Nonsteroidal antiinflammatory drugs and the risk of Alzheimer's disease. *N Engl J Med* 2001; **345:** 1515–21.


**Effects on electrolytes.** See under Effects on the Kidneys, below.

**Effects on the eyes.** Ocular effects such as blurred vision occur rarely in patients taking NSAIDs. Other more serious effects on the eyes associated with NSAIDs also appear to be rare. In the USA the National Registry of Drug-Induced Ocular Side Effects analysed 144 reports they received of possible adverse optic nerve reactions associated with the use of NSAIDs.[1] Of the 24 cases of papilloedema with or without pseudotumour cerebri more than half were associated with propionic acid derivatives, but it was considered that the data indicated that, on rare occasions, most NSAIDs could cause this effect; the number of reports for individual drugs was: 7 for ibuprofen, 5 each for indometacin and naproxen, 3 for meclofenamate, and 1 each for diflunisal, ketoprofen, sulindac, and tolmetin. Almost two-thirds of the 120 cases of optic or retrobulbar neuritis were also associated with propionic acid derivatives; the number of reports for individual drugs was: ibuprofen 43, naproxen 17, indometacin 9, benoxaprofen 8, phenylbutazone 8, piroxicam 8, zomepirac 7, sulindac 6, fenoprofen 5, oxyphenbutazone 3, meclofenamate 2, tolmetin 2, diflunisal 1, and ketoprofen 1.

Ocular adverse effects have also been reported with the selective COX-2 inhibitors.[2]

There have been reports of severe corneal toxicity associated with the use of some topical NSAIDs, such as diclofenac and ketorolac, in the eye (see p.32).


1. Fraunfelder FT, *et al.* Possible optic nerve side effects associated with nonsteroidal anti-inflammatory drugs. *J Toxicol Cutan Ocul Toxicol* 1994; **13:** 311–16.
2. Coulter DM, *et al.* Celecoxib, rofecoxib, and acute temporary visual impairment. *BMJ* 2003; **327:** 1214–15.


**Effects on fertility.** There have been several reports of reversible infertility occurring in women on long-term NSAIDs.[1,2] Prostaglandins are considered to be involved in the processes of ovulation and it is thought that NSAIDs may compromise ovulation via inhibition of cyclo-oxygenase-2. Women trying to become pregnant may need to avoid treatment with NSAIDs.


1. Norman RJ. Reproductive consequences of COX-2 inhibition. *Lancet* 2001; **358:** 1287–8.
2. Stone S, *et al.* Nonsteroidal anti-inflammatory drugs and reversible female infertility: is there a link? *Drug Safety* 2002; **25:** 545–51.


**Effects on the gastrointestinal tract.** NSAIDs can cause clinically important damage of the gastrointestinal tract, increasing the incidence of bleeding in the upper gastrointestinal tract and of perforation, although serious complications are relatively infrequent. They have also been associated with damage to the distal small intestine and colon.[1-3]

The complex **mechanisms** involved are not fully understood, although it is generally accepted that the inhibition of cyclo-oxygenase-1 (COX-1) results in gastrointestinal toxicity and that the selective COX-2 inhibitors are less gastrotoxic than the traditional NSAIDs (see below).[4-8] The gastric mucosa is damaged both by local and systemic effects of NSAIDs.[5] The local effect is pH-dependent and varies between individual drugs. The systemic effect is pH-independent, can occur with any route of administration, and is less drug specific; it is this effect that is thought to involve COX-1 inhibition.

**Risk factors** continue to be studied and so far the most important patient-related factors for upper gastrointestinal toxicity are old age, a history of peptic ulcers or bleeding of the gastrointestinal tract, and concomitant use of corticosteroids.[9] A pilot study has also suggested that risk is increased in children.[10] *Helicobacter pylori* infection exacerbates the risk of ulceration, but patients remain at increased risk even if infection is eradicated.[11] Duration of therapy is not thought to influence the risk for serious events; a cohort study[12] found that the risk of gastrointestinal bleeding or perforation with NSAIDs was constant throughout treatment, and risk quickly declines following NSAID withdrawal.[13]

Several studies[14-17] have been conducted on the **relative toxicity** of oral NSAIDs on the upper gastrointestinal tract and various rankings of these drugs have been discussed.[18-20] The UK Committee on Safety of Medicines (CSM)[20] examined 10 epidemiological studies for 7 oral non-aspirin NSAIDs and also examined the spontaneous reports they had received of gastrointestinal effects associated with NSAIDs. The CSM concluded that:

- azapropazone was associated with the *highest* risk of gastrointestinal reactions
- ibuprofen carried the *lowest* risk (but this may be related to dose, see below)
- piroxicam, ketoprofen, indometacin, naproxen, and diclofenac had an *intermediate* risk; it was considered that the risk for piroxicam might be higher than for the other NSAIDs with intermediate toxicity

A recent update[21] confirms these findings. In a systematic review[22] of controlled epidemiological studies that found a relation between NSAID use and hospital admission for gastric haemorrhage or perforation, the low risk of serious gastric toxicity with ibuprofen appeared to be attributable mainly to the low doses used clinically; higher doses of ibuprofen were associated with a similar risk to indometacin and naproxen. For reference to an association between aspirin and the most severe gastric lesions compared with other NSAIDs, see p.15.

Results from controlled trials have confirmed that the **selective COX-2 inhibitors** are associated with a lower incidence of serious gastrointestinal effects, such as bleeding, perforation, and obstruction, than the traditional NSAIDs[23] (see also Celecoxib, p.25 and Rofecoxib, p.86 for further details). However, since the risk of such effects is inherently low in those with no history of peptic ulcer disease, the general prescribing of selective COX-2 inhibitors to all patients requiring an NSAID is questioned. Indeed, in the UK, the use of selective COX-2 inhibitors is limited to those at high risk of developing serious gastrointestinal problems if given a non-selective NSAID. High-risk patients include the elderly, those already receiving gastrotoxic drugs, and those with existing gastrointestinal disorders.

There has been concern that **topical** use of NSAIDs may also be associated with gastrointestinal toxicity but a case-controlled study[24] concluded that topical administration was not associated with significant upper gastrointestinal bleeding or perforation.

Apart from the selection of an NSAID with a lower risk for gastrointestinal toxicity, other methods used for the **prevention** or **treatment** of NSAID-associated ulceration are discussed under the treatment of peptic ulcer disease on p.1246.


1. Kwo PY, Tremaine WJ. Nonsteroidal anti-inflammatory drug-induced enteropathy: case discussion and review of the literature. *Mayo Clin Proc* 1995; **70:** 55–61.
2. Gleeson MH, *et al.* Non-steroidal anti-inflammatory drugs, salicylates, and colitis. *Lancet* 1996; **347:** 904–5.
3. Evans JMM, *et al.* Nonsteroidal anti-inflammatory drugs are associated with emergency admission to hospital for colitis due to inflammatory bowel disease. *Gut* 1997; **40:** 619–22.
4. Hayllar J, Bjarnason I. NSAIDs, Cox-2 inhibitors, and the gut. *Lancet* 1995; **346:** 521–2.
5. Bjorkman DJ. Nonsteroidal anti-inflammatory drug-induced gastrointestinal injury. *Am J Med* 1996; **101** (suppl 1A): 25S–32S.
6. Soll A. Pathogenesis of nonsteroidal anti-inflammatory drug-related upper gastrointestinal toxicity. *Am J Med* 1998; **105** (suppl 5A): 10S–16S.
7. Hawkey CJ. COX-2 inhibitors. *Lancet* 1999; **353:** 307–14. Correction. *ibid.* 1440. [dose]
8. Wolfe MM, *et al.* Gastrointestinal toxicity of nonsteroidal anti-inflammatory drugs. *N Engl J Med* 1999; **340:** 1888–99.
9. Seager JM, Hawkey CJ. ABC of the upper gastrointestinal tract: indigestion and non-steroidal anti-inflammatory drugs. *BMJ* 2001; **323:** 1236–9.
10. Mulberg AE, *et al.* Identification of nonsteroidal antiinflammatory drug-induced gastroduodenal injury in children with juvenile rheumatoid arthritis. *J Pediatr* 1993; **122:** 647–9.
11. Pounder RE. Helicobacter pylori and NSAIDs—the end of the debate? *Lancet* 2002; **358:** 3–4.
12. MacDonald TM, *et al.* Association of upper gastrointestinal toxicity of non-steroidal anti-inflammatory drugs with continued exposure: cohort study. *BMJ* 1997; **315:** 1333–7.
13. Mellemkjaer L, *et al.* Upper gastrointestinal bleeding among users of NSAIDs: a population-based cohort study in Denmark. *Br J Clin Pharmacol* 2002; **53:** 173–81.
14. Kaufman DW, *et al.* Nonsteroidal anti-inflammatory drug use in relation to major upper gastrointestinal bleeding. *Clin Pharmacol Ther* 1993; **53:** 485–94.
15. García Rodríguez LA, Jick H. Risk of upper gastrointestinal bleeding and perforation associated with individual non-steroidal anti-inflammatory drugs. *Lancet* 1994; **343:** 769–72.
16. Langman MJS, *et al.* Risks of bleeding peptic ulcer associated with individual non-steroidal anti-inflammatory drugs. *Lancet* 1994; **343:** 1075–8.
17. Lewis SC, *et al.* Dose–response relationships between individual nonaspirin nonsteroidal anti-inflammatory drugs (NANSAIDs) and serious upper gastrointestinal bleeding: a meta-analysis based on individual patient data. *Br J Clin Pharmacol* 2002; **54:** 320–6.
18. Bateman DN. NSAIDs: time to re-evaluate gut toxicity. *Lancet* 1994; **343:** 1051–2.
19. Smith CC, *et al.* NSAIDs and gut toxicity. *Lancet* 1994; **344:** 56–7.
20. Committee on Safety of Medicines/Medicines Control Agency. Relative safety of oral non-aspirin NSAIDs. *Current Problems* 1994; **20:** 9–11.
21. Committee on Safety of Medicines/Medicines Control Agency. Non-Steroidal Anti-Inflammatory Drugs (NSAIDs) and gastrointestinal (GI) safety. *Current Problems* 2002; **28:** 5. Also available at: http://medicines.mhra.gov.uk/ourwork/monitorsafequalmed/currentproblems/cpapril2002.pdf (accessed 06/07/04)
22. Henry D, *et al.* Variability in risk of gastrointestinal complications with individual non-steroidal anti-inflammatory drugs: results of a collaborative meta-analysis. *BMJ* 1996; **312:** 1563–6.
23. Fitzgerald GA, Patrono C. The coxibs, selective inhibitors of cyclooxygenase-2. *N Engl J Med* 2001; **345:** 433–42.
24. Evans JMM, *et al.* Topical non-steroidal anti-inflammatory drugs and admission to hospital for upper gastrointestinal bleeding and perforation: a record linkage case-control study. *BMJ* 1995; **311:** 22–6.


**Effects on the joints.** There is concern that NSAIDs such as indometacin may accelerate the rate of cartilage destruction in patients with osteoarthritis.[1,2]


1. Rashad S, *et al.* Effect of non-steroidal anti-inflammatory drugs on the course of osteoarthritis. *Lancet* 1989; **ii:** 519–22.
2. Huskisson EC, *et al.* Effects of antiinflammatory drugs on the progression of osteoarthritis of the knee. *J Rheumatol* 1995; **22:** 1941–6.


**Effects on the kidneys.** NSAIDs can produce renal disorders on systemic or topical use,[1] some of which are due to their inhibition of prostaglandin synthesis.[2,3] In the presence of renal vasoconstriction the vasodilator action of prostaglandins increases renal blood flow and thereby helps to maintain renal function.[4,5] Patients whose renal function is being maintained by prostaglandins are therefore at risk from NSAIDs. Such patients include those with impaired circulation, the elderly, those on diuretics, and those with heart failure or renal vascular disease.[2,4] Other risk factors for renal impairment with NSAIDs include dehydration, cirrhosis, surgery, sepsis,[6] and a history of gout or hyperuricaemia.[6,7] The half-life of an NSAID may be a more important determinant of the risk of developing functional renal impairment than the ingested dose.[7] Evidence of renal toxicity due to cyclo-oxygenase-2 (COX-2) selective inhibitors is less extensive; however, such NSAIDS appear to have effects on renal function similar to those of the non-selective NSAIDs.[8,9]

ACE inhibitors can also produce renal impairment and combined use with NSAIDs should be undertaken with great care. The Australian Adverse Drug Reactions Advisory Committee[10] stated in August 2003 that over 50% of cases of renal failure reported to the committee were associated with use of NSAIDs, ACE inhibitors, or diuretics (alone or together); where all these were taken together the fatality rate for reported cases of renal failure was 10%. Prostaglandin inhibition may also lead to salt and water retention particularly when there is pre-existing hypertension or sodium depletion.[4] NSAIDs, therefore, tend to counteract the action of diuretics and antihypertensives.[2,4] There have been isolated reports of severe hyponatraemia and other symptoms resembling the syndrome of inappropriate antidiuretic hormone secretion in patients taking NSAIDs.[11,12]

Potassium homoeostasis is less dependent on prostaglandins and hyperkalaemia occurs infrequently with NSAIDs.[3] It is more likely to occur in patients with specific risk factors such as those receiving potassium supplements or potassium-sparing diuretics.[3] Indometacin appears to be the main NSAID implicated.

NSAIDs may cause acute interstitial nephritis, perhaps involving an allergic response,[2,3,13] and it may progress to interstitial fibrosis or papillary necrosis.[3,14]

Analgesic abuse or prolonged excessive use can produce nephropathy, a condition characterised by renal papillary necrosis and chronic interstitial nephritis, and, eventually, renal failure.[15] Phenacetin, a para-aminophenol derivative, has long been recognised as being one of the main drugs responsible for analgesic nephropathy,[16,17] but nephropathy has also been associated with the long-term use of NSAIDs and paracetamol without phenacetin.[18]


1. O'Callaghan CA, *et al.* Renal disease and use of topical non-steroidal anti-inflammatory drugs. *BMJ* 1994; **308:** 110–11.
2. Kendall MJ, Horton RC. Clinical pharmacology and therapeutics. *Postgrad Med J* 1990; **66:** 166–85.
3. Whelton A, Hamilton CW. Nonsteroidal anti-inflammatory drugs: effects on kidney function. *J Clin Pharmacol* 1991; **31:** 588–98.
4. Harris K. The role of prostaglandins in the control of renal function. *Br J Anaesth* 1992; **69;** 233–5.
5. Kenny GNC. Potential renal, haematological and allergic adverse effects associated with nonsteroidal anti-inflammatory drugs. *Drugs* 1992; **44** (suppl 5): 31–7.
6. MacDonald TM. Selected side-effects: 14. non-steroidal anti-inflammatory drugs and renal damage. *Prescribers' J* 1994; **34:** 77–80.
7. Henry D, *et al.* Consumption of non-steroidal anti-inflammatory drugs and the development of functional renal impairment in elderly subjects: results of a case-control study. *Br J Clin Pharmacol* 1997; **44:** 85–90.
8. Perazella MA, Tray K. Selective cyclooxygenase-2 inhibitors: a pattern of nephrotoxicity similar to traditional nonsteroidal anti-inflammatory drugs. *Am J Med* 2001; **111:** 64–7.
9. Noroian G, Clive D. Cyclo-oxygenase-2 inhibitors and the kidney: a case for caution. *Drug Safety* 2002; **25:** 165–72.
10. Anonymous. ACE inhibitor, diuretic and NSAID: a dangerous combination. *Aust Adverse Drug React Bull* 2003; **22:** 14–15. Also available at: http://www.tga.health.gov.au/adr/aadrb/aadr0308.htm (accessed 06/07/04)
11. Petersson I, *et al.* Water intoxication associated with non-steroidal anti-inflammatory drug therapy. *Acta Med Scand* 1987; **221:** 221–3.
12. Cheung NT, *et al.* Syndrome of inappropriate secretion of antidiuretic hormone induced by diclofenac. *BMJ* 1993; **306:** 186.
13. Ravnskov U. Glomerular, tubular and interstitial nephritis associated with non-steroidal antiinflammatory drugs. Evidence of a common mechanism. *Br J Clin Pharmacol* 1999; **47:** 203–10.
14. Sandler DP, *et al.* Nonsteroidal anti-inflammatory drugs and the risk for chronic renal disease. *Ann Intern Med* 1991; **115:** 165–72.
15. De Broe ME, Elseviers MM. Analgesic nephropathy. *N Engl J Med* 1998; **338:** 446–52.
16. Sandler DP, *et al.* Analgesic use and chronic renal disease. *N Engl J Med* 1989; **320:** 1238–43.
17. Dubach UC, *et al.* An epidemiologic study of abuse of analgesic drugs: effects of phenacetin and salicylate on mortality and cardiovascular morbidity (1968 to 1987). *N Engl J Med* 1991; **324:** 155–60.
18. Perneger TV, *et al.* Risk of kidney failure associated with the use of acetaminophen, aspirin, and nonsteroidal antiinflammatory drugs. *N Engl J Med* 1994; **331:** 1675–9.


**Effects on the liver.** A retrospective study involving over 220 000 adults who were either using, or had used, NSAIDs identified a small excess risk of serious, acute non-infectious liver injury; in current users there was a twofold increase in risk and there was a predominance of the cholestatic type of liver injury among such patients. Nonetheless, admissions to hospital for liver injury had been rare.[1] In a review[2] of cohort and case-control studies describing an association between NSAIDs and liver disease, the strongest evidence emerged for sulindac. There were also a significant number of reports of hepatotoxicity on rechallenge with diclofenac. Evidence of hepatotoxicity for other NSAIDs was weak, although the risk appeared to be high when they were used with other hepatotoxic drugs. However, the overall incidence of liver disease with NSAIDs was very low.


1. García Rodríguez LA, *et al.* The role of non-steroidal anti-inflammatory drugs in acute liver injury. *BMJ* 1992; **305:** 865–8. Correction. *ibid.*: 920.
2. Manoukian AV, Carson JL. Nonsteroidal anti-inflammatory drug-induced hepatic disorders. *Drug Safety* 1996; **15:** 64–71.


**Effects on the lungs.** Adverse pulmonary effects such as pneumonitis, alveolitis, pulmonary infiltrates, and pulmonary fibrosis, often suggestive of an allergic or immune reaction, have been reported with a number of NSAIDs. For references, see under individual monographs.

**Effects on the pancreas.** A review[1] of drug-induced pancreatitis considered that sulindac was amongst the drugs for which a definite association with pancreatitis had been established. There had been isolated reports of pancreatitis with ketoprofen, mefenamic acid, and piroxicam but any association was considered to be questionable. For further references see under individual monographs.


1. Underwood TW, Frye CB. Drug-induced pancreatitis. *Clin Pharm* 1993; **12:** 440–8.


**Effects on the skin.** The diverse cutaneous reactions to NSAIDs have been reviewed.[1] Of 250 children attending a rheumatology clinic 34 (13.6%) were found to have 4 or more facial scars of unknown origin.[2] This number of scars was found in 22.2% of the 116 children who had received naproxen and in 9.2% of the 87 who had received other NSAIDs. Children affected were more likely to have light skin and blue or green eyes. It was not known whether this was a form of phototoxic reaction but pseudoporphyria-like eruptions associated with NSAIDs, and naproxen in particular (see p.65), have been reported.[3,4]

See also under Hypersensitivity, below.


1. Bigby M, Stern R. Cutaneous reactions to nonsteroidal anti-inflammatory drugs. *J Am Acad Dermatol* 1985; **12:** 866–76.
2. Wallace CA, *et al.* Increased risk of facial scars in children taking nonsteroidal antiinflammatory drugs. *J Pediatr* 1994; **125:** 819–22.
3. Checketts SR, *et al.* Nonsteroidal anti-inflammatory-induced pseudoporphyria: is there an alternative drug? *Cutis* 1999; **63:** 223–5.
4. Al-Khenaizan S, *et al.* Pseudoporphyria induced by propionic acid derivatives *J Cutan Med Surg* 1999; **3:** 162–6.


**Hypersensitivity.** NSAIDs have produced a wide range of hypersensitivity reactions in susceptible individuals; the most common include skin rashes, urticaria, rhinitis, angioedema, bronchoconstriction, and anaphylactic shock. Hypersensitivity to NSAIDs appears to occur more frequently in patients with asthma or allergic disorders but other risk factors have been identified (for further details see under Aspirin, p.16). The occurrence of aspirin sensitivity in patients with asthma and nasal polyps has been referred to as the 'aspirin triad'. There is considerable cross-reactivity between aspirin and other NSAIDs and it is generally recommended that patients who have had a hypersensitivity reaction to aspirin or any other NSAID should avoid all NSAIDs. For references to hypersensitivity reactions associated with NSAIDs, see under individual monographs.

**Overdosage.** In general, symptoms of NSAID poisoning are mild, and usually include nausea and vomiting, headache, drowsiness, blurred vision, and dizziness. There have been isolated case reports of more serious toxicity, including seizures, hypotension, apnoea, coma, and renal failure, although usually after ingestion of substantial quantities. Seizures are a particular problem with mefenamic acid overdosage.

Treatment of NSAID overdosage is entirely supportive. Gastric lavage and activated charcoal may be of benefit within 1 hour of ingestion. Multiple doses of activated charcoal may be useful in enhancing elimination of NSAIDs with long half-lives such as piroxicam and sulindac. Forced diuresis, haemodialysis, or haemoperfusion are unlikely to be of benefit for NSAID overdosage, although haemodialysis may be required if oliguric renal failure develops.

## Precautions

All NSAIDs are contra-indicated in patients with active peptic ulceration; in addition, the non-selective NSAIDs should be used with caution, if at all, in patients with a history of such disorders. To reduce the risk of gastrointestinal effects, NSAIDs may be taken with or after food or milk. Histamine $H_2$-antagonists, omeprazole, or misoprostol may be used for a similar purpose in high-risk patients taking non-selective NSAIDs (see under Peptic Ulcer Disease, p.1246). However, food, milk, and such measures may reduce the rate and extent of drug absorption. In the UK the Committee on Safety of Medicines recommends that NSAIDs associated with the lowest risk of gastrointestinal toxicity (see Effects on the Gastrointestinal Tract, under Adverse Effects, above) should be tried first in the lowest recommended dose, and not more than one oral NSAID should be used at a time; selective inhibitors of COX-2 should be reserved for patients at high-est risk. There is no evidence to justify the use of gastro-protective drugs with selective inhibitors of cyclo-oxygenase-2 (COX-2) to further reduce the risk of gastrointestinal effects.

NSAIDs should be used with caution in patients with infections, since symptoms such as fever and inflammation may be masked (for the suggestion that they should not be used in children with varicella see below). They should also be used with caution in patients with asthma or allergic disorders. NSAIDs (including topical NSAIDs) are contra-indicated in patients with a history of hypersensitivity reactions to such drugs, including those in whom attacks of asthma, angioedema, urticaria, or rhinitis have been precipitated by aspirin or any other NSAID.

Other general precautions to be observed include use in patients with haemorrhagic disorders, hypertension, and impaired renal, hepatic, or cardiac function. Patients undergoing therapy with some NSAIDs may need to be monitored for the development of blood, kidney, liver, or eye disorders. NSAIDs should be used with caution in the elderly and may need to be given in reduced doses.

Regular use of NSAIDs during the third trimester of pregnancy may result in closure of fetal ductus arteriosus *in utero*, and possibly in persistent pulmonary hypertension of the newborn. The onset of labour may be delayed and its duration increased.

Some NSAIDs can interfere with thyroid function tests by lowering serum-thyroid hormone concentrations.

Further details concerning the precautions of the individual NSAIDs may be found under their respective monographs.

**Pregnancy.** Results from a case-control interview study[1] suggested that prenatal ingestion of aspirin or other NSAIDs might be implicated in persistent pulmonary hypertension of the newborn. The authors suggested that these drugs may be responsible for gestational structural or functional alterations of the pulmonary vasculature. However, the primary cause might also have been the underlying disorder for which the NSAIDs or aspirin were ingested. They were unable to pinpoint in which trimester the drugs might have their proposed action, and concluded that further evaluation was necessary. A more recent study[2] has found that persistent pulmonary hypertension of the newborn is significantly associated with *in utero* NSAID exposure, particularly to aspirin, ibuprofen, and naproxen. Fetal exposure to an NSAID was confirmed by meconium analysis.

The risk of miscarriage may be increased with NSAID use;[3,4] however, this observation remains to be confirmed. One study[3] also found no association between NSAID use and congenital abnormalities, low birth weight, or preterm birth.

Most manufacturers recommend avoidance of NSAIDs during pregnancy, unless the proposed benefit outweighs the risks, but in many cases published data on use of the drugs in pregnancy is scanty or absent, making an informed decision difficult.


1. Van Marter LJ, *et al.* Persistent pulmonary hypertension of the newborn and smoking and aspirin and nonsteroidal antiinflammatory drug consumption during pregnancy. *Pediatrics* 1996; **97:** 658–63.
2. Alano MA, *et al.* Analysis of nonsteroidal antiinflammatory drugs in meconium and its relation to persistent pulmonary hypertension of the newborn. *Pediatrics* 2001; **107:** 519–23.
3. Nielsen GL, *et al.* Risk of adverse birth outcome and miscarriage in pregnant users of non-steroidal anti-inflammatory drugs: population based observational study and case-control study. *BMJ* 2001; **322:** 266–70.
4. Li D-K, *et al.* Exposure to non-steroidal anti-inflammatory drugs during pregnancy and risk of miscarriage: population based cohort study. *BMJ* 2003; **327:** 368–71.


**Renal impairment.** The *British National Formulary* recommends that NSAIDs in general should be given at the lowest effective dose in patients with mild renal impairment and that renal function should be carefully monitored; they should be avoided if possible in patients with moderate to severe renal impairment. See also under individual monographs.

**Thyroid function tests.** References[1,2] to the interference with thyroid function tests by some NSAIDs.


1. Bishnoi A, *et al.* Effect of commonly prescribed nonsteroidal anti-inflammatory drugs on thyroid hormone measurements. *Am J Med* 1994; **96:** 235–8.
2. Samuels MH, *et al.* Variable effects of nonsteroidal antiinflammatory agents on thyroid test results. *J Clin Endocrinol Metab* 2003; **88:** 5710–16.


**Varicella.** The French regulatory authorities noted in July 2004 that following the report of 3 cases of septic shock, 1 fatal, in children treated with NSAIDs for fever and pain, pharmacovigilance studies had discovered a number of other cases of severe complications relating to infection of the skin lesions of chickenpox in NSAID-treated children. Although these, and a few reports in the literature[1,2] could not establish a causal relation, it was considered prudent to avoid the use of NSAIDs in children with chickenpox, and licensed information for the relevant drugs was to be modified appropriately.[3]


1. Zerr DM, *et al.* A case-control study of necrotizing fasciitis during primary varicella. *Pediatrics* 1999; **103:** 783–90.
2. Lesko SM, *et al.* Invasive group A streptococcal infection and nonsteroidal antiinflammatory drug use among children with primary varicella. *Pediatrics* 2001; **107:** 1108–15.
3. Agence Française de Sécurité Sanitaire des Produits de Santé. L'utilisation d'anti-inflammatoires nonstéroïdiens (AINS), dans le traitement de la fièvre et/ou de la douleur, n'est pas recommandée chez l'enfant atteint de varicelle (issued 15/07/04). Available at: http://www.agmed.sante.gouv.fr/htm/10/filltrpsc/lp040701.htm (accessed 20/07/04)


## Interactions

Interactions involving NSAIDs include enhancement of the effects of oral anticoagulants (especially by azapropazone and phenylbutazone) and increased plasma concentrations of lithium, methotrexate, and cardiac glycosides. The risk of nephrotoxicity may be increased if given with ACE inhibitors, ciclosporin, tacrolimus, or diuretics. Effects on renal function may lead to reduced excretion of some drugs. There may also be an increased risk of hyperkalaemia with ACE inhibitors and potassium-sparing diuretics. The antihypertensive effects of some antihypertensives including ACE inhibitors, beta blockers, and diuretics may be reduced. Convulsions may occur due to an interaction with quinolones. NSAIDs may enhance the effects of phenytoin and sulfonylurea antidiabetics.

Use of more than one NSAID together (including aspirin) should be avoided because of the increased risk of adverse effects. The risk of gastrointestinal bleeding and ulceration associated with NSAIDs is increased when used with corticosteroids, the SSRIs, the antiplatelets clopidogrel and ticlopidine, or, possibly, alcohol, bisphosphonates, or pentoxifylline. There may be an increased risk of haematotoxicity during concomitant use of zidovudine and NSAIDs. Ritonavir may increase the plasma concentrations of NSAIDs. The manufacturer of mifepristone advises of a theoretical risk that prostaglandin synthetase inhibition by NSAIDs or aspirin may alter the efficacy of mifepristone. There have been occasional reports of increased adverse effects when NSAIDs were given with misoprostol although such combinations have sometimes been used to *decrease* the gastrointestinal toxicity of NSAIDs.

Further details concerning the interactions of the individual NSAIDs may be found under their respective monographs.

◊ References.

1. Brouwers JRBJ, de Smet PAGM. Pharmacokinetic-pharmacodynamic drug interactions with nonsteroidal anti-inflammatory drugs. *Clin Pharmacokinet* 1994; **27:** 462–85.

**Antihypertensives.** For reference to the relative effects of NSAIDs in antagonising different types of antihypertensive drugs, see Effects on the Cardiovascular System and Effects on the Kidneys under Adverse Effects, above.

**Aspirin.** It has been suggested that NSAIDS such as ibuprofen may reduce the cardioprotective effect of aspirin but see under Interactions of Aspirin, p.17.

## Pharmacokinetics

Details of the pharmacokinetics of individual NSAIDs may be found under their respective monographs.

◊ General reviews.

1. Woodhouse KW, Wynne H. The pharmacokinetics of non-steroidal anti-inflammatory drugs in the elderly. *Clin Pharmacokinet* 1987; **12:** 111–22.
2. Walson PD, Mortensen ME. Pharmacokinetics of common analgesics, anti-inflammatories and antipyretics in children. *Clin Pharmacokinet* 1989; **17** (suppl 1): 116–37.
3. Simkin PA, *et al.* Articular pharmacokinetics of protein-bound antirheumatic agents. *Clin Pharmacokinet* 1993; **25:** 342–50.
4. Lapicque F, *et al.* Protein binding and stereoselectivity of nonsteroidal anti-inflammatory drugs. *Clin Pharmacokinet* 1993; **25:** 115–25.
5. Day RO, *et al.* Pharmacokinetics of nonsteroidal anti-inflammatory drugs in synovial fluid. *Clin Pharmacokinet* 1999; **36:** 191–210.

## Uses and Administration

Given as single doses or in short-term intermittent therapy NSAIDs can relieve mild to moderate pain. However, it may take up to 3 weeks of use before their anti-inflammatory effects become evident. The combined analgesic and anti-inflammatory effects make them particularly useful for the symptomatic relief of painful and/or inflammatory conditions including rheumatic disorders such as rheumatoid arthritis, osteoarthritis, and the spondyloarthropathies, and also in peri-articular disorders, and soft-tissue rheumatism. Some NSAIDs are used in the management of postoperative pain. Some NSAIDs, but not aspirin or other salicylates, are also used to treat acute gouty arthritis.

Generally, it is felt that there are only small differences in anti-inflammatory activity between the various NSAIDs and choice is largely empirical. Responses of individual patients vary widely. Thus, if a patient fails to respond to one NSAID, another drug may be successful. However, it has been recommended that NSAIDs associated with a low risk of gastrointestinal toxicity should generally be preferred and the lowest effective dose used. Treatment with NSAIDs that are selective inhibitors of cyclo-oxygenase-2, such as celecoxib and rofecoxib, is limited in the UK to those patients with a history of serious gastrointestinal problems or considered to be at high risk of developing such problems if given a non-selective NSAID (see Effects on the Gastrointestinal Tract, above).

NSAIDs are usually given by mouth, with or after food, although some such as diclofenac, ketoprofen, ketorolac, lornoxicam, piroxicam, parecoxib, and tenoxicam can be given intramuscularly; diclofenac, ketorolac, lornoxicam, parecoxib, and tenoxicam can also be given intravenously. Some NSAIDs are applied topically or given rectally as suppositories.

Several NSAIDs are used in ophthalmic preparations for the inhibition of intra-operative miosis, control of postoperative ocular inflammation, and prevention of cystoid macular oedema.

**Action.** Cyclo-oxygenases play an important role in the biosynthesis of prostaglandins (p.1511). NSAIDs inhibit cyclo-oxygenase-1 (COX-1) and cyclo-oxygenase-2 (COX-2) and it is thought that inhibition of COX-1 is associated with adverse gastrointestinal effects while inhibition of COX-2 is associated with anti-inflammatory activity,[1-6] hence the interest[7] in preferential or selective inhibitors of COX-2. COX-2 inhibitors may also have a potential use in other diseases in which COX-2 might be implicated.[4] Meloxicam and nimesulide are preferential inhibitors of COX-2, (i.e. they have a higher selectivity for COX-2 than COX-1 but are not exclusive COX-2 inhibitors); etodolac and nabumetone are also claimed to have preference for COX-2 although there is less evidence for this. Drugs with a very high selectivity for COX-2 have also been developed. Celecoxib and rofecoxib are two examples. Although the selective inhibition of COX-2 may be associated with reduced gastrointestinal toxicity, adverse effects associated with such inhibition have been noted in other body systems, see Effects on the Cardiovascular System and Effects on the Kidneys, above.

There is evidence that NSAIDs may also have a central mechanism of action that augments the peripheral mechanism.[6]

Many NSAIDs possess centres of chirality within their molecular structure, with different chiral forms (enantiomers) having different degrees of pharmacological activity.[8,9] For example, indometacin, its analogues, and some arylpropionic acids are chiral drugs with the S(+)-enantiomer in most cases showing the dominant pharmacological activity. However, the ratio of S/R activity varies between drugs and between *animal* species. NSAIDs are generally used clinically as the racemate with only a few currently being given as the (S)-enantiomer (for example, dexketoprofen). The chirality of a drug may have subtle effects on its toxicity and interactions, and it may be more desirable to use a drug as its active enantiomer.[9]

1. Hayllar J, Bjarnason I. NSAIDs, Cox-2 inhibitors, and the gut. *Lancet* 1995; **346:** 521–2.
2. Bennett A, Tavares IA. NSAIDs, Cox-2 inhibitors, and the gut. *Lancet* 1995; **346:** 1105.
3. Vane JR. NSAIDs, Cox-2 inhibitors, and the gut. *Lancet* 1995; **346:** 1105–6.
4. Jouzeau J-Y, *et al.* Cyclo-oxygenase isoenzymes: how recent findings affect thinking about nonsteroidal anti-inflammatory drugs. *Drugs* 1997; **53:** 563–82.
5. Richardson C, Emery P. The clinical implications of inhibition of the inducible form of cyclo-oxygenase. *Drug Safety* 1996; **15:** 249–60.
6. Cashman JN. The mechanisms of action of NSAIDs in analgesia. *Drugs* 1996; **52** (suppl 5): 13–23.
7. Hawkey CJ. COX-2 inhibitors. *Lancet* 1999; **353:** 307–14. Correction. *ibid.* 1440. [dose]
8. Kean WF, *et al.* Chirality in antirheumatic drugs. *Lancet* 1991; **338:** 1565–8.
9. Hayball PJ. Chirality and nonsteroidal anti-inflammatory drugs. *Drugs* 1996; **52** (suppl 5): 47–58.

**Colic pain.** Prostaglandins have been implicated in the aetiology of biliary colic (p.4), and some NSAIDs such as diclofenac, indometacin, and ketoprofen have been used to relieve such pain.

**Dementia.** A systematic review[1] of observational studies suggested that the risk of dementia is lower in patients who are taking NSAIDs. However, a randomised trial[2] found no benefit from treatment with naproxen or rofecoxib in patients with mild to moderate Alzheimer's disease. Further randomised trials are needed to determine their role in dementia.

1. Etminan M, *et al.* Effect of non-steroidal anti-inflammatory drugs on risk of Alzheimer's disease: systematic review and meta-analysis of observational studies. *BMJ* 2003; **327:** 128–31.
2. Aisen PS, *et al.* Effects of rofecoxib or naproxen vs placebo on Alzheimer disease progression: a randomized controlled trial. *JAMA* 2003; **289:** 2819–26.

**Ectopic ossification.** NSAIDs are an effective alternative to radiotherapy for prevention of ectopic ossification (p.762) after surgery or trauma. Indometacin is widely used for this purpose.

References.

1. Pagnani MJ, *et al.* Effect of aspirin on heterotopic ossification after total hip arthroplasty in men who have osteoarthrosis. *J Bone Joint Surg Am* 1991; **73A:** 924–9.
2. Knelles D, *et al.* Prevention of heterotopic ossification after total hip replacement: a prospective, randomised study using acetylsalicylic acid, indomethacin and fractional or single-dose irradiation. *J Bone Joint Surg Br* 1997; **79B:** 596–602.
3. Moore KD, *et al.* Indomethacin versus radiation therapy for prophylaxis against heterotopic ossification in acetabular fractures: a randomised, prospective study. *J Bone Joint Surg Br* 1998; **80:** 259–63.
4. Kolbl O, *et al.* Preoperative irradiation versus the use of nonsteroidal anti-inflammatory drugs for prevention of heterotopic ossification following total hip replacement: the results of a randomized trial. *Int J Radiat Oncol Biol Phys* 1998; **42:** 397–401.
5. Sell S, *et al.* The suppression of heterotopic ossifications: radiation versus NSAID therapy–a prospective study. *J Arthroplasty* 1998; **13:** 854–9.
6. Kienapfel H, *et al.* Prevention of heterotopic bone formation after total hip arthroplasty: a prospective randomised study comparing postoperative radiation therapy with indomethacin medication. *Arch Orthop Trauma Surg* 1999; **119:** 296–302.
7. Neal B, *et al.* Non-steroidal anti-inflammatory drugs for preventing heterotopic bone formation after hip arthroplasty. Available in The Cochrane Library; Issue 2. Chichester: John Wiley; 2004.

**Eye disorders.** Miosis resistant to conventional mydriatics often develops during ocular surgery, possibly due to release of prostaglandins and other substances associated with trauma. NSAIDs, which are prostaglandin synthetase inhibitors, are therefore used prophylactically as eye drops before ocular surgery to ameliorate intra-operative miosis but there has been some doubt that the effect they produce is of clinical significance. Those commonly used include diclofenac, indometacin, and flurbiprofen. These drugs do not possess intrinsic mydriatic properties.

Some NSAIDs are used topically or systemically in a number of inflammatory ocular disorders, including inflammation and cystoid macular oedema following ocular surgery (see below). However, their role in the treatment of macular oedema associated with uveitis (p.1090) is less clear. NSAIDs are also used in the treatment of scleritis (see p.1088). Diclofenac and ketorolac have also both been used in the management of seasonal allergic conjunctivitis (see p.421).

References.

1. Flach AJ. Cyclo-oxygenase inhibitors in ophthalmology. *Surv Ophthalmol* 1992; **36:** 259–84.
2. Koay P. The emerging roles of topical non-steroidal anti-inflammatory agents in ophthalmology. *Br J Ophthalmol* 1996; **80:** 480–5.

POSTOPERATIVE INFLAMMATORY OCULAR DISORDERS. Corticosteroids are used topically for the control of **postoperative ocular inflammation** but caution is required as they can delay wound healing and mask postoperative infection. They should only be used for short periods as they can cause glaucoma in susceptible individuals. Topical NSAIDs have also been tried. Despite some doubts over efficacy several studies have found eye drops containing diclofenac sodium to be effective in controlling signs of inflammation after ocular surgery,[1-3] but there has been some concern about reports of corneal toxicity (see p.32).

**Cystoid macular oedema** may follow cataract or retinal detachment surgery due to a disturbance of the blood-retinal barrier. A number of NSAIDs,[3-6] including diclofenac, flurbiprofen, indometacin, and ketorolac are used topically with or without corticosteroids to prevent or relieve cystoid macular oedema. NSAIDs such as indometacin are also used systemically in its management.

1. Kraff MC, *et al.* Inhibition of blood-aqueous humor barrier breakdown with diclofenac: a fluorophotometric study. *Arch Ophthalmol* 1990; **108:** 380–3.
2. Wright M, *et al.* Comparison of the efficacy of diclofenac and betamethasone following strabismus surgery. *Br J Ophthalmol* 1997; **81:** 299–301.
3. Italian Diclofenac Study Group. Efficacy of diclofenac eyedrops in preventing postoperative inflammation and long-term cystoid macular edema. *J Cataract Refract Surg* 1997; **23:** 1183–9.
4. Jampol LM. Pharmacologic therapy of aphakic and pseudophakic cystoid macular edema. *Ophthalmology* 1985; **92:** 807–10.
5. Flach AJ, *et al.* Effectiveness of ketorolac tromethamine 0.5% ophthalmic solution for chronic aphakic and pseudophakic cystoid macular edema. *Am J Ophthalmol* 1987; **103:** 479–86.
6. Jampol LM, *et al.* Nonsteroidal anti-inflammatory drugs and cataract surgery. *Arch Ophthalmol* 1994; **112:** 891–4.

**Fever.** Paracetamol, salicylates and some other NSAIDs are the main antipyretics used to control fever (p.8). Paracetamol is usually the antipyretic of choice in infants and children but ibuprofen appears to be an effective alternative; salicylates are generally contra-indicated in these patients because of the possible link between their use and the development of Reye's syndrome (see under Adverse Effects of Aspirin, p.16).

**Gout.** NSAIDs are the drugs usually used first for the treatment of acute attacks of gout (p.412). Since the treatment of chronic gout can lead to the mobilisation of urate crystals from established tophi to produce acute attacks, NSAIDs may also be used for the prophylaxis of acute gout during the first few months of urate-lowering therapy.

**Headache.** An NSAID is often tried first for the symptomatic treatment of various types of headache including migraine (p.464) and tension-type headache (p.465). NSAIDs may also be effective prophylactic drugs for migraine, although propranolol or pizotifen are generally preferred. Chronic paroxysmal hemicrania, a rare variant of cluster headache (p.464), responds to indometacin.

**Kidney disorders.** Although NSAIDs can produce adverse effects on the kidney (see above) they may have a role in the management of some types of glomerular kidney disease (p.1080). They may be of use for the control of proteinuria due to nephrotic syndrome except when there is overt renal failure.

**Malignant neoplasms.** Results of a study by the American Cancer Society[1] have suggested that regular use of aspirin may reduce the risk of developing fatal cancer of the oesophagus, stomach, colon, or rectum. Death rates due to other gastrointestinal cancers did not appear to be affected. Other studies[2-10] appear to support the reduced risk of colorectal cancer (p.516) in regular users of aspirin or other NSAIDs, particularly in high-risk patients, conclusions that were cautiously endorsed by a systematic review.[11] A large case-control study,[12] using data held on the UK general practice research database, has examined information on NSAID use and the development of common cancers. This study also found that the use of NSAIDs (including aspirin) may protect against cancer of the oesophagus, stomach, colon, and rectum. However, the study failed to show any decrease in risk of non-gastrointestinal cancers. In addition, an earlier study[13] found no evidence of an association between the use of aspirin and the incidence of colorectal cancer, although the authors suggest that these results may be explained by the short treatment period and the low dose of aspirin used. Long-term use of aspirin may itself be associated with an increased risk of certain other diseases.

Treatment with sulindac (p.92) has been found to reduce the number of polyps in patients with familial adenomatous polyposis, a condition which predisposes to development of colorectal cancer. Celecoxib is now indicated for use in such patients.


1. Thun MJ, *et al.* Aspirin use and the risk of fatal cancer. *Cancer Res* 1993; **53:** 1322–7.
2. Rosenberg L, *et al.* A hypothesis: nonsteroidal anti-inflammatory drugs reduce the incidence of large-bowel cancer. *J Natl Cancer Inst* 1991; **83:** 355–8.
3. Logan RFA, *et al.* Effect of aspirin and non-steroidal anti-inflammatory drugs on colorectal adenomas: case-control study of subjects participating in the Nottingham faecal occult blood screening programme. *BMJ* 1993; **307:** 285–9.
4. Giovannucci E, *et al.* Aspirin use and the risk for colorectal cancer and adenoma in male health professionals. *Ann Intern Med* 1994; **121:** 241–6.
5. Giovannucci E, *et al.* Aspirin and the risk of colorectal cancer in women. *N Engl J Med* 1995; **333:** 609–14.
6. Sandler RS, *et al.* Aspirin and nonsteroidal anti-inflammatory agents and risk for colorectal adenomas. *Gastroenterology* 1998; **114:** 441–7.
7. Smalley W, *et al.* Use of nonsteroidal anti-inflammatory drugs and incidence of colorectal cancer: a population-based study. *Arch Intern Med* 1999; **159:** 161–6.
8. Jolly K, *et al.* NSAIDs and gastrointestinal cancer prevention. *Drugs* 2002; **62:** 945–56.
9. Sandler RS, *et al.* A randomized trial of aspirin to prevent colorectal adenomas in patients with previous colorectal cancer. *N Engl J Med* 2003; **348:** 883–90.
10. Baron JA, *et al.* A randomized trial of aspirin to prevent colorectal adenomas. *N Engl J Med* 2003; **348:** 891–9.
11. Asano TK, McLeod RS. Non steroidal anti-inflammatory drugs (NSAID) and aspirin for preventing colorectal adenomas and carcinomas. Available in The Cochrane Library; Issue 2. Chichester: John Wiley; 2004.
12. Langman MJS, *et al.* Effect of anti-inflammatory drugs on overall risk of common cancer: case-control study in general practice research database. *BMJ* 2000; **320:** 1642–6.
13. Stürmer T, *et al.* Aspirin use and colorectal cancer: post-trial follow-up data from the Physicians' Health Study. *Ann Intern Med* 1998; **128:** 713–20.


**Menstrual disorders.** Menorrhagia (p.1567) is thought to be associated with abnormalities of prostaglandin production. Treatment with NSAIDs such as ibuprofen, mefenamic acid, or naproxen during menstruation, can reduce uterine blood loss by an average of 30% in women with menorrhagia. There does not appear to be any evidence that one NSAID is more effective than another.

NSAIDs are usually the first choice for the pain of dysmenorrhoea (p.6). Mefenamic acid may have a theoretical advantage over other NSAIDs in being able to inhibit both the synthesis and the peripheral action of prostaglandins, but clinical studies have not shown fenemates to be more effective, and systematic review has suggested that ibuprofen may have the best risk/benefit ratio.

**Migraine.** See under Headache, above.

**Orthostatic hypotension.** Fludrocortisone is usually the first drug tried in the treatment of orthostatic hypotension (p.1100) when nonpharmacological treatment has failed. NSAIDs such as flurbiprofen, ibuprofen, or indometacin may be used alone or added to treatment if the response is inadequate.

**Pain.** NSAIDs have a similar analgesic effect to aspirin and paracetamol in single doses but, in regular full dosage, they have both a lasting analgesic and an anti-inflammatory effect. They are used in the management of mild to moderate pain (see Choice of Analgesic, p.2) and are of particular value in pain due to inflammation. NSAIDs may be of benefit for inflammatory pain in infants and children (p.3), although paracetamol is generally the preferred non-opioid analgesic in this age group. NSAIDs may be used in the treatment of acute low back pain (p.7) if paracetamol fails to provide adequate pain relief. NSAIDs may also be used as an adjunct to opioids in the management of severe pain such as cancer pain (p.5) and are particularly effective in bone pain of malignant origin. NSAIDs may be used for postoperative analgesia (p.4), and are of particular value following day-case surgery because of their lack of sedative effects. They are not usually considered to be strong enough as the sole analgesic following major surgery, but may be used with stronger analgesics and may allow dosage reduction of concomitant opioids. The pain of mild sickle-cell crises (p.8) may be controlled by analgesics such as NSAIDs or less potent opioids, for example codeine or dihydrocodeine; NSAIDs may be used with more potent opioids such as morphine for severe crises.

Dependence and tolerance are not a problem with non-opioid analgesics such as NSAIDs, but there is a ceiling of efficacy, above which, increasing the dose has no further therapeutic effect.

**Rheumatic disorders.** NSAIDs provide symptomatic relief for rheumatic disorders such as rheumatoid arthritis (p.9) and spondyloarthropathies (p.11), but they do not alter the course of the disease and additional antirheumatic drugs may need to be given to prevent irreversible joint damage. NSAIDs may also be used as an alternative to paracetamol for osteoarthritis (p.9). Short-term use of oral NSAIDs may help to relieve pain and reduce inflammation of soft-tissue rheumatism (p.11); topical formulations of some NSAIDs are also used but their therapeutic role, if any, is unclear.

---

# Opioid Analgesics

Analgésicos opiáceos.

## Dependence and Withdrawal

Repeated use of opioids is associated with the development of psychological and physical dependence. Although this is less of a problem with legitimate therapeutic use, dependence may develop rapidly when opioids are regularly abused for their euphoriant effects. Drug dependence of the opioid type is characterised by an overwhelming need to keep taking the drug (or one with similar properties), by a physical requirement for the drug in order to avoid withdrawal symptoms, and by a tendency to increase the dose owing to the development of tolerance.

Abrupt withdrawal of opioids from persons physically dependent on them precipitates a withdrawal syndrome, the severity of which depends on the individual, the drug used, the size and frequency of the dose, and the duration of drug use. Withdrawal symptoms may also follow the use of an opioid antagonist such as naloxone or a mixed agonist and antagonist such as pentazocine to opioid-dependent persons. Neonatal abstinence syndrome may occur in the offspring of opioid-dependent mothers and these infants can suffer withdrawal symptoms at birth.

Opioid analgesics can be classified according to the receptors at which they act (see under Uses and Administration, below) and withdrawal syndromes are characteristic for a receptor type. Cross-tolerance and cross-dependence can be expected between opioids acting at the same receptors. Dependence associated with morphine and closely related μ-agonists appears to result in more severe withdrawal symptoms than that associated with κ-receptor agonists. Onset and duration of withdrawal symptoms also vary according to the duration of action of the specific drug. With morphine and diamorphine *withdrawal symptoms* usually begin within a few hours, reach a peak within 36 to 72 hours, and then gradually subside; they develop more slowly with methadone. Withdrawal symptoms include yawning, mydriasis, lachrymation, rhinorrhoea, sneezing, muscle tremor, weakness, sweating, anxiety, irritability, disturbed sleep or insomnia, restlessness, anorexia, nausea, vomiting, loss of weight, diarrhoea, dehydration, leucocytosis, bone pain, abdominal and muscle cramps, gooseflesh, vasomotor disturbances, and increases in heart rate, respiratory rate, blood pressure, and temperature. Some physiological values may not return to normal for several months following the acute withdrawal syndrome.

Withdrawal symptoms may be terminated by a suitable dose of the original or a related opioid. Tolerance diminishes rapidly after withdrawal so that a previously tolerated dose may prove fatal.

For a discussion of the treatment of opioid dependence and neonatal abstinence syndrome, see below.

◊ Review.


1. Van Ree JM, *et al.* Opioids, reward and addiction: an encounter of biology, psychology, and medicine. *Pharmacol Rev* 1999; **51:** 341–96.


**Diagnosis.** Naloxone (p.1045) and other opioid antagonists have been used to diagnose opioid dependence.

**Treatment of opioid dependence.** The treatment of opioid dependence has been the subject of a number of reviews and discussions.[1-11]

Planned withdrawal (**detoxification**) may be effected slowly or rapidly. The usual method in many countries is to replace the drug of dependence with *methadone* (an opioid agonist) given as a liquid oral preparation, and then gradually withdraw the methadone if possible. Methadone is suitable for withdrawal therapy because it can be given orally and its long half-life allows once daily administration. Oral *diamorphine* has been used similarly to methadone; reefers containing diamorphine have also been used in some centres. *Dihydrocodeine* tablets have been used successfully. The partial opioid agonist *buprenorphine*, given sublingually, is another alternative to methadone in the treatment of opioid dependence. However, it should only be given to patients with moderate dependence; those dependent on high doses of opioids may experience withdrawal symptoms when given buprenorphine. The methadone derivative *levacetylmethadol* was a more recent introduction but its proarrhythmic effects have led to its use being suspended.

Iatrogenic opioid dependence may occur in patients receiving μ-agonists such as morphine, fentanyl, or pethidine for the management of acute pain or in an intensive care setting for more than 5 to 10 days. Methadone has been used successfully to manage opioid withdrawal in adult intensive care patients.[12] However, some[13] avoid using methadone to manage withdrawal in children because of the stigma of its associations with managing withdrawal in drug addicts. In physically dependent but non-addicted patients, gradual weaning using the same opioid that was used therapeutically is preferred where possible, although in some cases, it may be necessary to change to a different opioid because of ease of administration, duration of action, and ability to taper the dose; virtually any opioid can be used.[13]

Other drugs used in the management of opioid withdrawal include alpha$_2$-adrenoceptor agonists such as *clonidine* and opioid antagonists such as *naltrexone* and *naloxone*. Clonidine may help to suppress symptoms of opioid withdrawal, such as anxiety, insomnia, and muscle aches. It appears to be more effective when used in the control of symptoms following abrupt withdrawal than when used during gradual withdrawal of methadone. Hypotension may limit its usefulness in some patients. The clonidine analogue *lofexidine* may produce similar results to those obtained with clonidine and appears to be less sedating and hypotensive.

Naltrexone and naloxone block the euphoriant effects of opioids although their use in detoxification as monotherapy is limited by unacceptable opioid withdrawal effects. Naltrexone may be used with clonidine and in some cases withdrawal has been achieved within a few days using combined therapy.[14] Moreover, naloxone and naltrexone are being used in the relatively new technique of rapid or ultra rapid opioid detoxification,[15-17] which is achieved while the patient is heavily sedated or under *general anaesthesia* and hence unaware of any unpleasant withdrawal symptoms. However, although detoxification may be achieved within 24 hours and has a high initial success rate, the technique itself is not without risks and it does not obviate the need for maintenance treatment (see below).

Concomitant counselling and other psychosocial services have been shown to be important in the outcome of withdrawal therapy.[18] Detoxification alone does not ensure long-term abstinence.

A number of other drugs may be of use as **adjuncts** in the management of withdrawal symptoms. *Diphenoxylate* with atropine or *loperamide* may be used for the control of diarrhoea. *Promethazine* has been used for its antiemetic and sedative actions. Beta blockers such as *propranolol* may be of use for patients with pronounced somatic anxiety symptoms. *Benzodiazepines* or *clomethiazole* can be given to relieve anxiety and associated insomnia but only short courses should be used in order to minimise the risk of dependence and abuse.

Long-term **maintenance** treatment (stabilisation treatment) with an opioid is sometimes used, in conjunction with psychosocial support, to enable the patient to acquire some form of social stability. *Methadone* is most commonly used; the use of *diamorphine* although feasible[19,20] is controversial[21] and is advocated by only a few individual centres. *Buprenorphine* is another possibility.[22] The use of methadone for maintenance has been reviewed.[23-25] *Naltrexone* can be effective in maintaining abstinence in opioid addicts following detoxification, especially after rapid or ultra rapid detoxification. It is considered that naltrexone would probably be of most use in highly motivated addicts with good sociological and psychological support to discourage impulsive use of opioids.[1,26,27]

The problems associated with the management of the **pregnant** patient with opioid dependence have been discussed.[28] The aim should be to stabilise the patient first using *methadone* since acute withdrawal can result in fetal death. Drug withdrawal is best done slowly during the second trimester. It has been suggested that if patients present during the final trimester and cannot be detoxified, maintenance with *diamorphine* might be preferable to the use of methadone as it might produce less severe withdrawal symptoms in the neonate.[29] The management of neonatal abstinence syndrome is discussed below.


1. Herridge P, Gold MS. Pharmacological adjuncts in the treatment of opioid and cocaine addicts. *J Psychoactive Drugs* 1988; **20:** 233–42.
2. Guthrie SK. Pharmacologic interventions for the treatment of opioid dependence and withdrawal. *DICP Ann Pharmacother* 1990; **24:** 721–34.
3. Wodak A. Managing illicit drug use: a practical guide. *Drugs* 1994; **47:** 446–57.
4. Mattick RP, Hall W. Are detoxification programmes effective? *Lancet* 1996; **347:** 97–100.

5. Seivewright NA, Greenwood J. What is important in drug misuse treatment? *Lancet* 1996; **347:** 373–6.
6. National Concensus Development Panel on Effective Medical Treatment of Opiate Addiction. Effective medical treatment of opiate addiction. *JAMA* 1998; **280:** 1936–43.
7. DOH. *Drug misuse and dependence: guidelines on clinical management.* London: The Stationery Office, 1999. Also available at: http://www.dh.gov.uk/assetRoot/04/07/81/98/04078198.pdf (accessed 06/07/04)
8. O'Connor PG, Fiellin DA. Pharmacological treatment of heroin-dependent patients. *Ann Intern Med* 2000; **133:** 40–54.
9. Gonzalez G, *et al.* Treatment of heroin (diamorphine) addiction: current approaches and future prospects. *Drugs* 2002; **62:** 1331–43.
10. Raisch DW, *et al.* Opioid dependence treatment, including buprenorphine/naloxone. *Ann Pharmacother* 2002; **36:** 312–21.
11. Gonzalez G, *et al.* Treatment of heroin (diamorphine) addiction: current approaches and future prospects. *Drugs* 2002 **62:** 1331–43.
12. Böhrer H, *et al.* Methadone treatment of opioid withdrawal in intensive care patients. *Lancet* 1993; **341:** 636–7.
13. Yaster M, *et al.* The management of opioid and benzodiazepine dependence in infants, children, and adolescents. *Pediatrics* 1996; **98:** 135–40.
14. Gowing L, *et al.* Opioid antagonists with minimal sedation for opioid withdrawal. Available in The Cochrane Library; Issue 2. Chichester: John Wiley; 2004.
15. Justins D. Rapid opioid detoxification under anaesthesia. *Hosp Med* 1998; **59:** 180.
16. Cook TM, Collins PD. Rapid opioid detoxification under anaesthesia. *Hosp Med* 1998; **59:** 245–7.
17. Gowing L, *et al.* Opioid antagonists under heavy sedation or anaesthesia for opioid withdrawal. Available in The Cochrane Library; Issue 2. Chichester: John Wiley; 2004.
18. McLellan AT, *et al.* The effects of psychosocial services in substance abuse treatment. *JAMA* 1993; **269:** 1953–9.
19. Perneger TV, *et al.* Randomised trial of heroin maintenance programme for addicts who fail in conventional drug treatments. *BMJ* 1998; **317:** 13–18.
20. Rehm J, *et al.* Feasibility, safety, and efficacy of injectable heroin prescription for refractory opioid addicts: a follow-up study. *Lancet* 2001; **358:** 1417–20.
21. Farrell M, Hall W. The Swiss heroin trials: testing alternative approaches. *BMJ* 1998; **316:** 639.
22. Kakko J, *et al.* 1-year retention and social function after buprenorphine-assisted relapse prevention treatment for heroin dependence in Sweden: a randomised, placebo-controlled trial. *Lancet* 2003; **361:** 662–8.
23. Farrell M, *et al.* Methadone maintenance treatment in opiate dependence: a review. *BMJ* 1994; **309:** 997–1001.
24. Ward J, *et al.* Role of maintenance treatment in opioid dependence. *Lancet* 1999; **353:** 221–6.
25. Bell J, Zador D. A risk-benefit analysis of methadone maintenance treatment. *Drug Safety* 2000; **22:** 179–90.
26. Ginzburg HM, MacDonald MG. The role of naltrexone in the management of drug abuse. *Med Toxicol* 1987; **2:** 83–92.
27. Gonzalez JP, Brogden RN. Naltrexone: a review of its pharmacodynamic and pharmacokinetic properties and therapeutic efficacy in the management of opioid dependence. *Drugs* 1988; **35:** 192–213.
28. Gerada C, *et al.* Management of the pregnant opiate user. *Br J Hosp Med* 1990; **43:** 138–41.
29. Thomas CS, Osborn M. Inhaling heroin during pregnancy. *BMJ* 1988; **296:** 1672.

NEONATAL ABSTINENCE SYNDROME. Infants born to opioid-dependent mothers may suffer withdrawal, with signs including CNS hyperirritability, gastrointestinal dysfunction, respiratory distress, yawning, sneezing, mottling, and fever. Onset of symptoms is partly dependent on the drug and varies from shortly after birth to 2 weeks of age, although most symptoms appear within 72 hours. Some symptoms may persist for 3 months or more.

The American Academy of Pediatrics (AAP)[1] recommended that treatment of the neonate with abstinence syndrome should be primarily supportive and considered that many infants manifesting signs of drug withdrawal could be managed in this way. They advised adoption of abstinence scoring methods to judge the need for drug therapy, although such systems do not appear to have been validated. Drugs that have been used for opioid withdrawal include paregoric (a USP 27 preparation containing opium), diluted tincture of opium, morphine, methadone, diazepam, chlorpromazine, phenobarbital, and clonidine. Naloxone should not routinely be given to infants of opioid-dependent mothers because of the risk of seizures with abrupt opioid withdrawal. The AAP[1] made no definite recommendations but considered that, when appropriate, specific drug therapy should be used for treatment of withdrawal symptoms. Thus for opioid withdrawal, tincture of opium was the preferred drug. Others favour treatment with oral morphine solution.[2]

Practice varies widely and evidence for the efficacy of particular drugs in the management of neonatal abstinence syndrome is scanty and difficult to compare.[3,4] It has been suggested that diazepam may be less useful than phenobarbital or paregoric but the use of paregoric (which contains both camphor and alcohol) has been questioned. In the UK, chlorpromazine has also been widely used.[5]

1. American Academy of Pediatrics, Committee on Drugs. Neonatal drug withdrawal. *Pediatrics* 1998; **101:** 1079–88. Correction. *ibid.*; **102:** 660 [dosage error].
2. Gregg JEM, *et al.* Maternal narcotic abuse and the newborn. *Arch Dis Child* 1988; **63:** 684.
3. Theis JGW, *et al.* Current management of the neonatal abstinence syndrome: a critical analysis of the evidence. *Biol Neonate* 1997; **71:** 345–56.
4. Johnson K, *et al.* Treatment of neonatal abstinence syndrome. *Arch Dis Child Fetal Neonatal Ed* 2003; **88:** F2–F5.
5. Morrison CL, Siney C. A survey of the management of neonatal opiate withdrawal in England and Wales. *Eur J Pediatr* 1996; **155:** 323–6.

## Adverse Effects

In normal doses the commonest side-effects of opioid analgesics are nausea, vomiting, constipation, drowsiness, and confusion; tolerance to these (except constipation) generally develops with long-term use. Micturition may be difficult and there may be ureteric or biliary spasm; the latter may be associated with alterations in liver enzyme values. There is also an antidiuretic effect. Dry mouth, dizziness, sweating, facial flushing, headache, vertigo, bradycardia, tachycardia, palpitations, orthostatic hypotension, hypothermia, restlessness, changes of mood, decreased libido or potency, hallucinations, and miosis also occur. These effects tend to occur more commonly in ambulant patients than in those at rest in bed and in those without severe pain. Raised intracranial pressure occurs in some patients. Muscle rigidity has been reported following high doses. The euphoric activity of opioids has led to their abuse. For a discussion of opioid dependence, see above.

Larger doses of opioids produce respiratory depression and hypotension, with circulatory failure and deepening coma. Convulsions may occur, especially in infants and children. Rhabdomyolysis progressing to renal failure has been reported in overdosage. Death may occur from respiratory failure. Toxic doses of specific opioids vary considerably with the individual and regular users may tolerate large doses. The triad of coma, pinpoint pupils, and respiratory depression is considered indicative of opioid overdosage; dilatation of the pupils occurs as hypoxia develops. Pulmonary oedema after overdosage is a common cause of fatalities among opioid addicts.

Morphine and some other opioids have a dose-related histamine-releasing effect which may be responsible in part for reactions such as urticaria and pruritus as well as hypotension and flushing. Contact dermatitis has been reported and pain and irritation may occur on injection. Anaphylactic reactions following intravenous injection have been reported rarely.

◊ The adverse effects associated with individual opioid analgesics may reflect to some extent their activity at specific opioid receptors (see Uses and Administration, below) or may result from a direct toxic effect.[1,2] Some adverse effects of pure opioid agonists, such as the respiratory depressant effect of morphine, are dose-related, whereas agonist-antagonists such as buprenorphine, butorphanol, and nalbuphine exhibit a 'ceiling effect' as the dose increases.

The type and extent of side-effects experienced in practice may depend on whether or not opioid-sensitive pain is present, whether the opioid analgesic is being given for the control of chronic severe pain or acute pain, and the route of administration. In a review[3] of the use of opioids in *chronic pain* it was noted that, despite worries to the contrary, respiratory depression and dependence liability are not generally a problem when appropriate doses are used to treat opioid-sensitive pain. In fact the presence of opioid-sensitive pain appears to protect against the respiratory depressant effect, although it may occur if the source of opioid-sensitive pain is removed (e.g. by surgery) without adequate reduction in opioid dosage. The side-effects of opioid analgesics when used in advanced cancer have also been discussed.[4] Constipation was considered to be the most troublesome adverse effect; significant respiratory depression was rarely seen with recommended regimens, since pain antagonises the central depressant effects of morphine.

In the context of *acute postoperative pain* opioid-induced respiratory depression is of concern but short-term postoperative use is unlikely to cause dependence (although see under Treatment of Opioid Dependence, above for references to iatrogenic physical dependence).[5] It was hoped that administration of opioids by the *spinal route* would result in fewer side-effects, especially respiratory depression. In postoperative pain relief with spinal opioids, the incidence of side-effects is said to be low when patients are properly monitored.[6] However, some[7] have reported pruritus, nausea and vomiting, and urinary retention to be common and respiratory depression to occur; more seriously the appearance of respiratory depression could be considerably delayed. These effects were more common with morphine, but all opioid analgesics had the propensity to produce respiratory depression when given spinally.[7] Delayed respiratory depression has been attributed to the poor lipid solubility of morphine, but does occur after other opioids. Some have considered that despite earlier worries, potentially fatal late respiratory depression was as rare with the spinal route as postoperative respiratory depression with the conventional route.[8,9] Disputes regarding the frequency of respiratory depression associated with even conventional methods of administration of opioid analgesics might be due to the methods used for measuring respiratory effects.[10] The incidence of ventilatory depression has been reported to be higher following intrathecal than epidural administration of morphine.[11]

1. Duthie DJR, Nimmo WS. Adverse effects of opioid analgesic drugs. *Br J Anaesth* 1987; **59:** 61–77.
2. Schug SA, *et al.* Adverse effects of systemic opioid analgesics. *Drug Safety* 1992; **7:** 200–13.
3. McQuay HJ. Opioids in chronic pain. *Br J Anaesth* 1989; **63:** 213–26.
4. Twycross RG, Lack SA. *Oral morphine in advanced cancer.* 2nd ed. Beaconsfield: Beaconsfield Publishers, 1989.
5. Mitchell RWD, Smith G. The control of acute postoperative pain. *Br J Anaesth* 1989; **63:** 147–58.
6. Lutz LJ, Lamer TJ. Management of postoperative pain: review of current techniques and methods. *Mayo Clin Proc* 1990; **65:** 584–96.
7. Morgan M. The rational use of intrathecal and extradural opioids. *Br J Anaesth* 1989; **63:** 165–88.
8. Anonymous. Spinal opiates revisited. *Lancet* 1986; **i:** 655–6.
9. McQuay HJ. Spinal opiates. *Br J Hosp Med* 1987; **37:** 354–5.
10. Wheatley RG, *et al.* Postoperative hypoxaemia: comparison of extradural, i.m. and patient-controlled opioid analgesia. *Br J Anaesth* 1990; **64:** 267–75.
11. Gustafsson LL, *et al.* Adverse effects of extradural and intrathecal opiates: report of a nationwide survey in Sweden. *Br J Anaesth* 1982; **54:** 479–85.

**Effects on the cardiovascular system.** For reference to histamine release and cardiovascular effects following the intravenous administration of some opioids see under Pethidine, p.80.

**Effects on the endocrine system.** Endogenous opioid peptides may have a role in the regulation of endocrine function. Like endorphin and enkephalins, morphine has been found to stimulate prolactin release[1] and synthetic analogues of morphine are reported to have similar properties; long-term intrathecal opioids (morphine or hydromorphone) have been reported to produce hypogonadotrophic hypogonadism, adrenal insufficiency, and growth hormone deficiency, although tolerance to the effects on prolactin develops with long-term use.[2] Opioids such as morphine are also part of a large group of drugs implicated in causing hyperglycaemia.[3]

1. Hell K, Wernze H. Drug-induced changes in prolactin secretion: clinical implications. *Med Toxicol* 1988; **3:** 463–98.
2. Abs R, *et al.* Endocrine consequences of long-term intrathecal administration of opioids. *J Clin Endocrinol Metab* 2000; **85:** 2215–22.
3. O'Byrne S, Feely J. Effects of drugs on glucose tolerance in non-insulin-dependent diabetics (part II). *Drugs* 1990; **40:** 203–19.

## Treatment of Adverse Effects

Activated charcoal may be given by mouth in conscious patients if a substantial overdose has been ingested within 1 hour or so; it should be considered in all patients if a substantial amount of a sustained release preparation has been ingested. Gastric lavage has been used.

Intensive supportive therapy may be required to correct respiratory failure and shock. In addition, the specific antagonist naloxone is used for rapid reversal of the severe respiratory depression and coma produced by excessive doses of opioid analgesics (see p.1045). Since naloxone has a shorter duration of action than many opioids patients who have already responded should be kept under close observation for signs of relapse and repeated injections given according to the respiratory rate and depth of coma. Alternatively, in situations where one of the longer acting opioids is known or suspected to be the cause of symptoms, a continuous intravenous infusion of naloxone, adjusted according to response, may be used.

The use of opioid antagonists such as naloxone in persons physically dependent on opioids may induce withdrawal symptoms.

**Constipation.** For reference to the use of naloxone to relieve opioid-induced constipation without compromising analgesic control in patients receiving long-term therapy with opioids, see under Reversal of Opioid Effects in the Uses and Administration of Naloxone, p.1045.

## Precautions

Opioid analgesics are generally contra-indicated in acute respiratory depression and obstructive airways disease, although opioids such as morphine are used in some forms of dyspnoea (see below). They are also contra-indicated or should be used with great caution in acute alcoholism, convulsive disorders, head injuries, and conditions in which intracranial pressure is raised. They should not be given to comatose patients.

Opioid analgesics should be given with caution or in reduced doses to patients with hypothyroidism, adrenocortical insufficiency, asthma or decreased respiratory reserve, renal or hepatic impairment, prostatic hyperplasia, hypotension, shock, inflammatory or obstructive bowel disorders, or myasthenia gravis. Dosage should be reduced in elderly or debilitated patients.

Opioid analgesics should be given with great care to infants, especially neonates. Their use during labour may cause respiratory depression in the neonate. Babies born to opioid-dependent mothers may suffer withdrawal symptoms (see under Neonatal Abstinence Syndrome, above).

Discontinuation of therapy with opioid analgesics should be carried out gradually in patients who may have developed physical dependence, to avoid precipitating withdrawal symptoms (see Dependence, above). Opioid analgesics with some antagonist activity, such as buprenorphine, butorphanol, nalbuphine, or pentazocine, may precipitate withdrawal symptoms in physically dependent patients who have recently used pure agonists such as morphine.

Drowsiness may affect the ability to perform skilled tasks; those so affected should not drive or operate machinery.

**Asthma.** Opioids are usually contra-indicated in asthma.[1] However it has been suggested that they are safe in controlled asthma, but should be avoided during acute exacerbations.[2]

1. Gorchein A. Difficult asthma. *BMJ* 1989; **299:** 1031.
2. Barnes PJ, Chung KF. Difficult asthma. *BMJ* 1989; **299:** 1031–2.

**Biliary-tract disorders.** It is usually recommended that opioids such as morphine should either be avoided in patients with biliary disorders or that they should be given with an antispasmodic. Morphine can cause an increase in intrabiliary pressure as a result of effects on the sphincter of Oddi[1] and might therefore be expected to exacerbate rather than relieve pain in patients with biliary colic (p.4) or other biliary-tract disorders. Biliary-type pain has also been induced in patients given morphine after cholecystectomy.[2]

Morphine caused a more marked delay in gallbladder emptying than pethidine, pentazocine, or butorphanol in a study[3] in healthy subjects; this was considered confirmation that morphine should be avoided in biliary disorders. In another study[4] fentanyl and sufentanil did not constrict the common bile duct like morphine; they may be suitable for perioperative pain control in patients in whom spasm of the common bile duct is undesirable. The suggestion that pethidine should be preferred to morphine in patients with acute pancreatitis, because of its lesser effect on the bile duct, has been questioned.[5]

1. Helm JF, *et al.* Effects of morphine on the human sphincter of Oddi. *Gut* 1988; **29:** 1402–7.
2. Roberts-Thomson IC, *et al.* Sympathetic activation: a mechanism for morphine induced pain and rises in liver enzymes after cholecystectomy? *Gut* 1990; **31:** 217–21.
3. Hahn M, *et al.* The effect of four narcotics on cholecystokinin octapeptide stimulated gall bladder contraction. *Aliment Pharmacol Ther* 1988; **2:** 129–34.
4. Vieira ZEG, *et al.* Evaluation of fentanyl and sufentanil on the diameter of the common bile duct by ultrasonography in man: a double blind, placebo controlled study. *Int J Clin Pharmacol Ther* 1994; **32:** 274–7.
5. Thompson DR. Narcotic analgesic effects on the sphincter of Oddi: a review of the data and therapeutic implications in treating pancreatitis. *Am J Gastroenterol* 2001; **96:** 1266–72.

**Children.** There is some evidence to suggest that children under 6 months of age are more sensitive to opioids; neonates in particular may be more sensitive to respiratory depression with morphine than adults. Pharmacokinetic differences may contribute to this increased sensitivity. Nonetheless, neonates can be treated with opioids such as morphine if receiving respiratory support.

Older infants and children can be treated effectively with morphine or other opioid analgesics and from the age of 5 or 6 months morphine metabolism follows the course seen in adults.

For a discussion of the choice of analgesic in children see p.3. The use of opioids for sedation and analgesia in neonates in intensive care is mentioned on p.666.

References.

1. Choonara IA. Pain relief. *Arch Dis Child* 1989; **64:** 1101–2.
2. Lloyd-Thomas AR. Pain management in paediatric patients. *Br J Anaesth* 1990; **64:** 85–104.
3. Bhatt-Mehta V. Current guidelines for the treatment of acute pain in children. *Drugs* 1996; **51:** 760–76.
4. Marsh DF, *et al.* Opioid systems and the newborn. *Br J Anaesth* 1997; **79:** 787–95.

**Hepatic impairment.** Although some patients with hepatic dysfunction have been reported to be particularly sensitive to opioids, many patients with liver impairment have been reported to tolerate opioids normally.[1] See also under the individual monographs.

1. Hanks GW, Aherne GW. Morphine metabolism: does the renal hypothesis hold water? *Lancet* 1985; **i:** 221–2.

**Phaeochromocytoma.** Morphine and some other opioids can induce the release of endogenous histamine and thereby stimulate catecholamine release. Both diamorphine[1] and pethidine[2] have been reported to cause hypertension when given to patients with phaeochromocytoma and histamine-releasing opioids should be avoided in such patients. Alfentanil, like fentanyl, does not release histamine and may be the opioid of choice in the anaesthetic management of patients with phaeochromocytoma.[3]

1. Chaturvedi NC, *et al.* Diamorphine-induced attack of paroxysmal hypertension in phaeochromocytoma. *BMJ* 1974; **2:** 538.
2. Lawrence CA. Pethidine-induced hypertension in phaeochromocytoma. *BMJ* 1978; **1:** 149–50.
3. Hull CJ. Phaeochromocytoma: diagnosis, preoperative preparation and anaesthetic management. *Br J Anaesth* 1986; **58:** 1453–68.

## Interactions

As serious and sometimes fatal reactions have followed use of pethidine in patients receiving MAOIs (including moclobemide), pethidine and related drugs are contra-indicated in patients taking MAOIs or within 14 days of stopping such treatment; other opioid analgesics should be avoided or given with extreme caution (for further details, see p.314). Life-threatening reactions have also been reported when selegiline, a selective inhibitor of monoamine oxidase type B, has been given with pethidine. The depressant effects of opioid analgesics are enhanced by other CNS depressants such as alcohol, anaesthetics, anxiolytics, hypnotics, tricyclic antidepressants, and antipsychotics. Cyclizine may counteract the haemodynamic benefits of opioids. Cimetidine inhibits the metabolism of some opioids, especially pethidine.

The actions of opioids may in turn affect the activities of other drugs. For instance, their gastrointestinal effects may delay absorption as with mexiletine or may be counteractive as with cisapride, metoclopramide, or domperidone. Opioid premedicants such as papaveretum have been reported to reduce serum concentrations of ciprofloxacin.

**Antivirals.** Interactions between opioid analgesics and ritonavir, other *HIV-protease inhibitors*, or *reverse transcriptase inhibitors* are complex, and the results of the limited number of studies and reports *in vivo* have not always borne out predictions about the nature of potential interactions.

- Substantial **decreases** in the area under the plasma concentration-time curve (AUC) and in the plasma concentration have been reported for both methadone and for pethidine when given with *ritonavir*. In the case of pethidine, however, plasma concentrations of the toxic metabolite norpethidine are greatly **increased**, and the manufacturers of ritonavir counsel against such combined use. The HIV-protease inhibitors *amprenavir* and *nelfinavir* may also reduce methadone concentrations and provoke withdrawal symptoms in dependent patients. Patients requiring methadone may need an increase in the dose of this drug if given with amprenavir, nelfinavir, or ritonavir. Similar interactions with methadone have been noted with the non-nucleoside reverse transcriptase inhibitors *efavirenz* and *nevirapine* and the nucleoside reverse transcriptase inhibitor *abacavir*; again, a dose increase in methadone may be required. The HIV-protease inhibitors *indinavir* and *saquinavir* do not appear to interact with methadone. Ritonavir is predicted to reduce plasma concentrations of morphine.
- In contrast, an **increase** in AUC and in elimination half-life has been reported in subjects given fentanyl with *ritonavir*. The manufacturers of ritonavir also consider that increased plasma concentrations of dextropropoxyphene and tramadol, with an increased likelihood of opioid toxicity, may occur if either drug is given during ritonavir treatment.

**Histamine $H_2$-antagonists.** Histamine $H_2$-antagonists may enhance the effects of some opioid analgesics. *Cimetidine* was reported to alter the clearance and volume of distribution of pethidine[1] whereas *ranitidine* did not.[2] Morphine has been considered less likely to interact with cimetidine than pethidine because of differences in metabolism. However, although cimetidine did not affect the disposition of morphine in healthy subjects in a study[3] there have been isolated reports of possible interactions between morphine and $H_2$-antagonists; apnoea, confusion, and muscle twitching have been associated with concomitant cimetidine and morphine,[4] and confusion associated with concomitant ranitidine and morphine.[5] There has also been a report[6] of a patient receiving regular analgesia with oral methadone and subcutaneous morphine who became unresponsive 6 days after starting cimetidine for prophylaxis of peptic ulcer; treatment with naloxone was required.

1. Guay DRP, *et al.* Cimetidine alters pethidine disposition in man. *Br J Clin Pharmacol* 1984; **18:** 907–14.
2. Guay DRP, *et al.* Ranitidine does not alter pethidine disposition in man. *Br J Clin Pharmacol* 1985; **20:** 55–9.
3. Mojaverian P, *et al.* Cimetidine does not alter morphine disposition in man. *Br J Clin Pharmacol* 1982; **14:** 809–13.
4. Fine A, Churchill DN. Potentially lethal interaction of cimetidine and morphine. *Can Med Assoc J* 1981; **124:** 1434, 1436.
5. Martinez-Abad M, *et al.* Ranitidine-induced confusion with concomitant morphine. *Drug Intell Clin Pharm* 1988; **22:** 914–15.
6. Sorkin EM, Ogawa GS. Cimetidine potentiation of narcotic action. *Drug Intell Clin Pharm* 1983; **17:** 60–1.

## Uses and Administration

Opioid analgesics possess some of the properties of naturally occurring or **endogenous opioid peptides**. Endogenous opioid peptides are widely distributed in the CNS and are also found in other parts of the body. They appear to function as neurotransmitters, modulators of neurotransmission, or neurohormones. Their presence in the hypothalamus suggests a role in the regulation of endocrine function. Opioids have been shown to stimulate the release of some pituitary hormones, including prolactin and growth hormone, and to inhibit the release of others, including corticotropin.

Endogenous peptides include the enkephalins, endorphins, and dynorphins; their polypeptide precursors may also be precursors for non-opioid peptides. Proenkephalin is the precursor of met- and leu-enkephalin; pro-opiomelanocortin is the precursor of beta-endorphin, beta-lipotrophin, melanocyte-stimulating hormone, and corticotropin; and prodynorphin is the precursor of dynorphins and neoendorphins.

Pharmacologically the opioid analgesics are broadly similar; qualitative and quantitative differences may be dependent on their interaction with **opioid receptors**. There are several types of opioid receptor and they are distributed in distinct patterns through the central and peripheral nervous systems. The three main types in the CNS were originally designated μ (mu), κ (kappa), and δ (delta) although they have more recently been reclassified as $OP_3$, $OP_2$, and $OP_1$, respectively. Activities attributed to the stimulation of these receptors have been as follows:

- μ—analgesia (mainly at supraspinal sites), respiratory depression, miosis, reduced gastrointestinal motility, and euphoria; $\mu_1$ (supraspinal analgesia) and $\mu_2$ (respiratory depression and gastrointestinal activity) subtypes have been postulated;
- κ—analgesia (mainly in the spinal cord); less intense miosis and respiratory depression, dysphoria and psychotomimetic effects;
- δ—less certain in man, but probably analgesia; selective for enkephalins.
- Other receptors include σ (sigma) and ε (epsilon) receptors. The psychotomimetic effects of agonist-antagonists such as pentazocine that are poorly antagonised by naloxone have been thought by some to be mediated by σ receptors.

Opioids act at one or more of these receptors as full or partial agonists, or as antagonists. Morphine and similar opioid agonists (sometimes called μ agonists) are considered to act primarily at μ and perhaps at κ and δ receptors. Opioid agonist-antagonists such as pentazocine appear to act as κ agonists and μ antagonists whereas buprenorphine is a partial agonist at μ receptors with some antagonist activity at κ receptors. The opioid antagonist naloxone acts at μ, κ, and δ receptors.

In addition to differing affinities for particular receptors the degree of activation once bound also differs. The full agonist morphine produces maximum activation at the μ receptor and its effects increase with dose, whereas partial agonists and agonist-antagonists may demonstrate a 'ceiling effect' in that above a certain level their effects do not increase proportionately with dose.

Other differences between opioid analgesics may relate to their lipid solubility and pharmacokinetics; speed of onset and duration of action may influence the choice of analgesic.

Opioid analgesics were traditionally classified as weak opioids or strong opioids; however this classification has largely been replaced by the one used in the WHO three-step analgesic ladder (see Cancer Pain, p.5). In this system opioids are divided into those that are used for **mild to moderate pain** and those that are used for **moderate to severe pain**. Examples of opioids in the first group include codeine, dextropropoxyphene, and dihydrocodeine; such opioids are distinguished by the existence of a ceiling effect and are often used with non-opioid analgesics. The principal opioid for the treatment of moderate to severe pain is morphine. Others include: diamorphine, fentanyl, methadone, and pethidine.

In addition to the relief of pain opioids are used in **anaesthesia** for premedication, induction, or maintenance. In balanced anaesthesia they are used with an anaesthetic and a neuromuscular blocker. When used with an antipsychotic they can produce a state of mild sedation with analgesia called neuroleptanalgesia.

Some opioids are used for analgesia, sedation, and suppression of respiration in the management of mechanically ventilated patients under **intensive care** (p.666).

Codeine is used for the suppression of **cough**; for intractable cough in terminal illness morphine may be used.

Opioids may relieve some forms of **dyspnoea**; morphine and diamorphine are probably the most commonly used in the UK, but dihydrocodeine and hydrocodone have also been tried.

Methadone and buprenorphine are used in the treatment of opioid **dependence** (see above).

◊ References.

1. Cherny NI. Opioid analgesics: comparative features and prescribing guidelines. *Drugs* 1996; **51:** 713–37.
2. Upton RN, *et al.* Pharmacokinetic optimisation of opioid treatment in acute pain therapy. *Clin Pharmacokinet* 1997; **33:** 225–44.

**Action.** Some references to opioid receptors.

1. Pleuvry BJ. Opioid receptors and their ligands: natural and unnatural. *Br J Anaesth* 1991; **66:** 370–80.
2. Pleuvry BJ. Opioid receptors and awareness of the Greek alphabet. *Br J Hosp Med* 1992; **48:** 678–81.
3. Atcheson R, Lambert DG. Update on opioid receptors. *Br J Anaesth* 1994; **73:** 132–4.
4. Dhawan BN, *et al.* International Union of Pharmacology. XII. Classification of opioid receptors. *Pharmacol Rev* 1996; **48:** 567–86.
5. Lambert DG. Recent advances in opioid pharmacology. *Br J Anaesth* 1998; **81:** 1–2.

**Administration in children.** See under Precautions, above.

**Anaesthesia.** Opioid analgesics have been given intravenously as supplements during general anaesthesia with inhalational or intravenous drugs. They have also been widely used as premedication before surgery to reduce anxiety, for smooth induction of anaesthesia, to reduce overall anaesthetic requirements, and to provide postoperative pain relief. Such use of opioids is now rare and is restricted to patients already in pain or to those who will experience pain before induction of anaesthesia. Very high doses of morphine have been infused intravenously to produce anaesthesia for cardiac surgery, but shorter acting drugs such as fentanyl and related opioids are generally used now; some may prefer agonist-antagonist opioids. Sedation and respiratory depression may be prolonged necessitating assisted ventilation; reversal of these effects can be achieved by opioid antagonists such as naloxone. For a discussion of the various drugs used to achieve and maintain conditions suitable for surgery, including the use of opioids in the induction and maintenance of anaesthesia, see p.1296. Opioid analgesics, most commonly fentanyl, have been used with a neuroleptic to induce a state known as neuroleptanalgesia in which the patient is calm and indifferent to the surroundings yet is responsive to commands. For a brief discussion of neuroleptanalgesia and similar anaesthetic techniques, see p.1296.

References.

1. Sear JW. Recent advances and developments in the clinical use of i.v. opioids during the peroperative period. *Br J Anaesth* 1998; **81:** 38–50.

POSTOPERATIVE SHIVERING. Pethidine appears to be effective in the treatment of postoperative shivering (see p.1295) but not all opioids are necessarily effective.

**Cough.** Opioids are used to suppress cough (p.1112). Pholcodine (p.1128) and dextromethorphan (p.1117), which lack classical analgesic activity, are the most commonly used opioids. Of the analgesic opioids, codeine is the most widely used as a cough suppressant. However, these opioids are seldom sufficiently potent to be effective in severe cough. Morphine and diamorphine are used for the relief of intractable cough in terminal illness, although morphine is now preferred. Methadone has also been used but should be avoided as it has a long duration of action and tends to accumulate.

Cough suppressants containing codeine or similar opioids are not recommended for use in children, and should be avoided in those under 1 year of age.

**Diarrhoea.** Oral rehydration therapy, which is the treatment of choice for acute diarrhoea (p.1241), prevents dehydration, but it does not necessarily shorten the duration of the diarrhoea. Preparations containing morphine or other opioids have therefore been used for their antimotility action as adjuncts in the management of acute diarrhoea. However, the WHO considers that such antidiarrhoeal drug therapy is of limited value, may delay the expulsion of causative organisms, and should never be given to children. Furthermore opioids should not be used in conditions where inhibition of peristalsis should be avoided, where abdominal distension develops, or in diarrhoeal conditions such as severe ulcerative colitis or antibiotic-associated colitis.

**Dyspnoea.** Dyspnoea (a subjective feeling of abnormally uncomfortable, difficult, or laboured breathing) is associated with diseases that interfere with oxygenation of the blood. It is best relieved by treatment of the underlying disorder (the treatment of dyspnoea associated with asthma and chronic obstructive pulmonary disease is discussed on p.777 and p.779, respectively). Where this is impossible or ineffective, symptomatic management is required.

Oxygen may reduce dyspnoea in some patients even if dyspnoea is not related to hypoxia. A flow of air directed across the face by a fan can also be effective. Despite the hazards of using benzodiazepines in patients with any form of respiratory depression or pulmonary insufficiency (see Precautions for Diazepam, p.692), drugs such as diazepam, lorazepam, or midazolam may be helpful in patients with advanced cancer who have rapid shallow respiration, especially when this is associated with anxiety.[1,2] Levomepromazine is occasionally used as an alternative.

Opioids may relieve some forms of dyspnoea,[2,3] such as those due to acute left ventricular failure, pulmonary oedema, and malignant chest disease. The cause of dyspnoea should be established since the use of opioids is generally not advised, or only with extreme caution, in patients with obstructive airways disease whose dyspnoea may be relieved by other means. In the UK, morphine and diamorphine are probably the most commonly used opioids for dyspnoea, but dihydrocodeine, hydrocodone, and oxymorphone have also been tried.

Nebulised morphine, hydromorphone, or fentanyl have been tried for the management of dyspnoea, and there are anecdotal reports of benefit, especially in palliative care, but evidence from controlled studies to date does not support such use.[2-4]

In patients with advanced cancer and intractable dyspnoea unresponsive to the above measures, chlorpromazine may be useful to relieve air hunger and sedate dying patients who have unrelieved distress;[1] midazolam may be used as an alternative. Promethazine has also been used. High doses of a corticosteroid such as dexamethasone may help to relieve dyspnoea in patients with airways obstruction due to a tumour by reducing oedema around the tumour.

1. Walsh D. Dyspnoea in advanced cancer. *Lancet* 1993; **342:** 450–1.
2. Davis CL. ABC of palliative care: breathlessness, cough, and other respiratory problems. *BMJ* 1997; **315:** 931–4.
3. Jennings AL, *et al.* Opioids for the palliation of breathlessness in terminal illness. Available in The Cochrane Library; Issue 2. Chichester: John Wiley; 2004.
4. Chandler S. Nebulized opioids to treat dyspnea. *Am J Hosp Palliat Care* 1999; **16:** 418–22.

**Pain.** Opioid analgesics are used for the relief of acute and chronic pain (see Choice of Analgesic, p.2). Not every type of pain responds; neuropathic pain, for example, may not be alleviated by opioid therapy. For further discussion of specific pain states and the role of opioid analgesics in their treatment see p.4 onwards.

There has also been interest in the local analgesic effects of opioids themselves.[1,2]

1. Thompson DF, Pierce DR. Local analgesia with opioid drugs. *Ann Pharmacother* 1995; **29:** 189–90.
2. Stein C. The control of pain in peripheral tissue by opioids. *N Engl J Med* 1995; **332:** 1685–90.

HEADACHE. Opioid analgesics such as codeine are sometimes included in oral compound analgesic preparations used in the initial treatment of migraine (see p.464) or tension-type headache (see p.465), but are best avoided, especially in patients who experience frequent attacks.

**Restless legs syndrome.** Some opioids may be beneficial in the treatment of restless legs syndrome (see Parasomnias, p.667), although evidence is scanty.

**Sedation.** In addition to their analgesic action opioids have been used in a variety of procedures for their sedative properties. Mention of this use of opioids can be found in the discussions of anaesthesia (p.1296), endoscopy (p.666), and intensive care (p.666).

**Tetanus.** Opioid analgesics can be used to provide analgesia and additional sedation in patients undergoing treatment for tetanus (p.149 and p.1398). Morphine has also been given to control the sympathetic overactivity in such patients.[1]

1. Rocke DA, *et al.* Morphine in tetanus—the management of sympathetic nervous system overactivity. *S Afr Med J* 1986; **70:** 666–8.

---

## Opium

Gum Opium; Opio; Opium Crudum; Raw Opium.

*ATC — A07DA02; N02AA02.*

**Pharmacopoeias.** In *Chin., Eur.* (see p.vi), and *US.*

*Chin., Eur.,* and *US* also include a monograph for prepared or powdered opium. *Jpn* includes prepared opium and a diluted opium powder containing 1% of anhydrous morphine.

**Ph. Eur. 5.0** (Opium, Raw; Opium BP 2003). The air-dried latex obtained by incision from the unripe capsules of *Papaver somniferum* L. It has a characteristic odour and a blackish-brown colour. It should contain not less than 10% of anhydrous morphine, not less than 2% of anhydrous codeine, and not more than 3% of anhydrous thebaine. Protect from light.

**Ph. Eur. 5.0** (Opium, Prepared; Opii Pulvis Normatus). Raw opium powdered and dried at a temperature not exceeding 70°. It is a yellowish-brown or dark brown powder and contains 9.8 to 10.2% of morphine and not less than 1.0% of codeine, calculated with reference to the dried drug. The content may be adjusted by adding a suitable excipient or raw opium powder.

**USP 27** (Opium). The air-dried milky exudate obtained by incising the unripe capsules of *Papaver somniferum* (Papaveraceae). Externally it is pale olive-brown or olive-grey; internally it is reddish-brown. It has a very characteristic odour and a very bitter taste. It yields not less than 9.5% of anhydrous morphine.

**USP 27** (Powdered Opium). Opium dried at a temperature not exceeding 70°, and reduced to a very fine light brown or moderately yellowish-brown powder that yields not less than 10% and not more than 10.5% of anhydrous morphine. It may contain any of the permitted diluents with the exception of starch.

### Profile

Opium is the air-dried latex obtained by incision from the unripe capsules of *Papaver somniferum* (Papaveraceae). It contains morphine, codeine, and thebaine and a variable mixture of other alkaloids including noscapine and papaverine. The exuded latex is dried and manipulated to form cakes of uniform composition, variously shaped according to the country of origin, and known in commerce as Turkish, Indian, or European opium.

Opium has the properties of opioid analgesics (p.71). Its analgesic and sedative actions are due mainly to its content of morphine (p.62). It acts less rapidly than morphine since opium appears to be more slowly absorbed; the relaxing action of the papaverine and noscapine on intestinal muscle makes it more constipating than morphine.

Opium is intended only as the starting material for the manufacture of galenical preparations and is not dispensed as such. It is used as Prepared Opium (Ph. Eur. 5.0), as Powdered Opium (USP 27), as Opium Tincture (BP 2003 or USP 27), or as Camphorated Opium Tincture (BP 2003) or Paregoric (USP 27) in various oral preparations. These have included Opiate Squill Linctus (BP 2003) (Gee's linctus) for cough.

Paregoric (USP 27) has been advocated in the USA for the treatment of neonatal opioid dependence.

**Abuse.** Reports of squill-associated cardiac toxicity resulting from the abuse of opiate squill linctus (Gee's linctus).[1,2]

1. Thurston D, Taylor K. Gee's linctus. *Pharm J* 1984; **233:** 63.
2. Smith W, *et al.* Wenckebach's phenomenon induced by cough linctus. *BMJ* 1986; **292:** 868.

### Preparations

***BP 2003:*** Camphorated Opium Tincture; Concentrated Camphorated Opium Tincture; Opium Tincture;
***USP 27:*** Opium Tincture; Paregoric.

**Proprietary Preparations** (details are given in Part 3)
***Braz.:*** Elixir Paregorico.

**Multi-ingredient:** ***Braz.:*** Camomila†; Elixir de Marinheiro†; ***Canad.:*** Diban†; Donnagel-PG†; ***Denm.:*** Pectyl; ***Fin.:*** Tannopon; ***Fr.:*** Colchimax; Lamaline; Paregorique; ***Hong Kong:*** Vida Brown Mixture; ***Israel:*** Davilla; Doveri; ***Mex.:*** Reglosedyl; ***S.Afr.:*** Stilpane; ***Spain:*** Digestovital; Tanagel; ***Switz.:*** Bromocod N; Pectocalmine; ***USA:*** B & O Supprettes No. 15A; B & O Supprettes No. 16A.

---

## Hydrochlorides of Mixed Opium Alkaloids

Alkaloidosum Opii Hydrochloridum; Extractum Concentratum Opii; Mezclas de hidrocloruros de alcaloides del opio; Omnoponum; Opialum; Opium Concentratum.

**Pharmacopoeias.** Preparations of the hydrochlorides of mixed opium alkaloids are included in *Jpn.*

## Papaveretum *(BAN)*

A mixture of 253 parts of morphine hydrochloride, 23 parts of papaverine hydrochloride, and 20 parts of codeine hydrochloride.

*CAS — 8002-76-4.*
*ATC — N02AA10.*

NOTE. Do not confuse papaveretum with papaverine (p.1728).

**Pharmacopoeias.** In *Br.*

**BP 2003** (Papaveretum). It contains 80.0 to 88.4% of anhydrous morphine hydrochloride, 8.3 to 9.2% of papaverine hydrochloride, and 6.6 to 7.4% of anhydrous codeine hydrochloride. A white or almost white crystalline powder. Soluble in water, sparingly soluble in alcohol. A 1.5% solution in water has a pH of 3.7 to 4.7. Protect from light.

### Profile

The opium alkaloids are the prototypical opioid analgesics (p.71). Mixtures of opium alkaloids such as papaveretum have the analgesic and sedative properties of morphine (p.62) and are used in the treatment of moderate to severe pain and for pre-operative sedation. 15.4 mg of Papaveretum (BP 2003) contains the equivalent of approximately 10 mg of the major component, anhydrous morphine.

- In the UK, papaveretum formerly contained the hydrochlorides of morphine, codeine, noscapine, and papaverine. However, because of concern over the potential genotoxicity of noscapine (p.1125) UK preparations containing papaveretum were reformulated to exclude the noscapine component and the name papaveretum was redefined in the BP 1993 to reflect this change of formulation. It is possible that in other countries the term papaveretum is still being used to describe a mixture containing noscapine.

In adults papaveretum is generally given by subcutaneous or intramuscular injection in doses of 7.7 to 15.4 mg every 4 hours. The initial dose in the elderly or debilitated patients should not exceed 7.7 mg. Children aged 1 to 5 years may be given 1.93 to

3.85 mg and those 6 to 12 years, 3.85 to 7.7 mg. In infants, dosage is calculated by body-weight: infants aged up to 1 month may be given 115 micrograms/kg and infants aged up to 1 year, 154 micrograms/kg.

Papaveretum may also be given intravenously in doses of one-quarter to one-half the corresponding subcutaneous or intramuscular dose.

For pre-operative medication papaveretum is given intramuscularly or subcutaneously sometimes with hyoscine hydrobromide.

Papaveretum has also been given by mouth with aspirin for the management of moderate to severe pain.

◊ Papaveretum has been confused with papaverine (p.1728) and in one such case[1] a patient became unconscious after self-injection of papaveretum in mistake for papaverine.

1. Robinson LQ, Stephenson TP. Self injection treatment for impotence. *BMJ* 1989; **299:** 1568.

### Preparations

***BP 2003:*** Papaveretum Injection.

**Proprietary Preparations** (details are given in Part 3)
***S.Afr.:*** Omnopon.
**Multi-ingredient:** ***UK:*** Aspav.

## Oxaprozin *(BAN, USAN, rINN)*

Oxaprozina; Wy-21743. 3-(4,5-Diphenyloxazol-2-yl)propionic acid.

$C_{18}H_{15}NO_3$ = 293.3.
*CAS — 21256-18-8.*
*ATC — M01AE12.*

**Pharmacopoeias.** In *Chin., Jpn.,* and *US.*

**USP 27** (Oxaprozin). A white to yellowish-white, crystalline powder.

### Adverse Effects and Precautions

As for NSAIDs in general, p.67.

**Diagnosis and testing.** False-positive results for testing of benzodiazepines in urine have been reported in patients taking oxaprozin.[1] The manufacturer[2] has commented that the interaction occurs with some immunoassay tests and that thin-layer chromatography can successfully discriminate between benzodiazepines and oxaprozin. False-positive results for a fluorescence polarisation immunoassay for phenytoin have also been reported in patients receiving oxaprozin.[3]

1. Pulini M. False-positive benzodiazepine urine test due to oxaprozin. *JAMA* 1995; **273:** 1905.
2. Raphan H, Adams MH. False-positive benzodiazepine urine test due to oxaprozin. *JAMA* 1995; **273:** 1905–6.
3. Patel T, *et al.* Assay interaction between oxaprozin and phenytoin. *Ann Pharmacother* 1997; **31:** 254.

**Effects on the liver.** A report[1] of fatal fulminant hepatitis in a 56-year-old woman who had received 600 to 1200 mg of oxaprozin daily for about 6 weeks. In another patient symptomatic hepatitis developing during oxaprozin use resolved on discontinuation of the drug.[2]

1. Purdum PP, *et al.* Oxaprozin-induced fulminant hepatitis. *Ann Pharmacother* 1994; **28:** 1159–61.
2. Kethu SR, *et al.* Oxaprozin-induced symptomatic hepatotoxicity. *Ann Pharmacother* 1999; **33:** 942–4.

### Interactions

For interactions associated with NSAIDs, see p.69.

### Pharmacokinetics

Oxaprozin is slowly but extensively absorbed from the gastrointestinal tract and is highly bound to plasma proteins. Peak plasma concentrations are reached after about 2 to 4 hours. At steady state, the biological half-life is about 50 hours. Oxaprozin is metabolised mainly in the liver by microsomal oxidation and conjugation with glucuronic acid to form inactive metabolites which are excreted in the urine and faeces.

◊ References.

1. Karim A. Inverse nonlinear pharmacokinetics of total and protein unbound drug (oxaprozin): clinical and pharmacokinetic implications. *J Clin Pharmacol* 1996; **36:** 985–97.
2. Karim A, *et al.* Oxaprozin and piroxicam, nonsteroidal antiinflammatory drugs with long half-lives: effect of protein-binding differences on steady-state pharmacokinetics. *J Clin Pharmacol* 1997; **37:** 267–78.
3. Davies NM. Clinical pharmacokinetics of oxaprozin. *Clin Pharmacokinet* 1998; **35:** 425–36.

### Uses and Administration

Oxaprozin, a propionic acid derivative, is an NSAID (p.70). It is used in the treatment of osteoarthritis and rheumatoid arthritis in a usual dose of 1.2 g given once daily by mouth, although in osteoarthritis, patients with low body-weight or mild disease may respond to an initial dose of 600 mg daily. The recommended maximum daily dose is 1.8 g or 26 mg/kg, whichever is the lower.

◊ References.

1. Miller LG. Oxaprozin: a once-daily nonsteroidal anti-inflammatory drug. *Clin Pharm* 1992; **11:** 591–603.
2. Anonymous. Oxaprozin for arthritis. *Med Lett Drugs Ther* 1993; **35:** 15–16.

### Preparations

***USP 27:*** Oxaprozin Tablets.

**Proprietary Preparations** (details are given in Part 3)
***Braz.:*** Prozina†; ***Canad.:*** Daypro; ***Chile:*** Duraprox; ***Ital.:*** Walix; ***S.Afr.:*** Deflam; ***USA:*** Daypro.

## Oxycodone Hydrochloride

*(BANM, USAN, rINNM)*

7,8-Dihydro-14-hydroxycodeinone hydrochloride; Dihydrone Hydrochloride; Hidrocloruro de oxicodona; NSC-19043 (oxycodone); Oxycone Hydrochloride; Thecodine. 6-Deoxy-7,8-dihydro-14-hydroxy-3-*O*-methyl-6-oxomorphine hydrochloride; (−)-(5*R*,6*S*,14*S*)-4,5-Epoxy-14-hydroxy-3-methoxy-9a-methylmorphinan-6-one hydrochloride.

$C_{18}H_{21}NO_4,HCl$ = 351.8.
*CAS — 76-42-6 (oxycodone); 124-90-3 (oxycodone hydrochloride).*
*ATC — N02AA05.*

NOTE. Compounded preparations of oxycodone may be represented by the following names:

- Co-oxycodAPAP (*PEN*)—oxycodone and paracetamol.

**Pharmacopoeias.** In *US. Fr.* and *Jpn* include the trihydrate.

**USP 27** (Oxycodone Hydrochloride). A white to off-white, odourless, hygroscopic crystals or powder. Soluble in water; slightly soluble in alcohol. Store in airtight containers.

### Oxycodone Terephthalate

Oxicodona, tereftalato de. 4,5α-Epoxy-14-hydroxy-3-methoxy-17-methylmorphinan-6-one 1,4-benzenedicarboxylate (2:1) salt.

$(C_{18}H_{21}NO_4)_2,C_8H_6O_4$ = 796.9.
*CAS — 64336-55-6.*

**Pharmacopoeias.** In *US.*

**USP 27** (Oxycodone Terephthalate). Store in airtight containers.

### Dependence and Withdrawal

As for Opioid Analgesics in general, p.71.

### Adverse Effects, Treatment, and Precautions

As for Opioid Analgesics in general, p.72.

The UK manufacturers contra-indicate the use of oxycodone in patients with moderate to severe hepatic impairment or severe renal impairment; however, manufacturers in the USA permit its cautious use in patients with severe hepatic or severe renal impairment although they recommended that doses may need to be reduced.

**Abuse.** Oxycodone hydrochloride modified-release tablets have been subject to abuse. The crushed tablets have been inhaled or injected by addicts and in some cases this has resulted in fatalities.

**Effects on the respiratory system.** References[1,2] to respiratory depression occurring in children given oxycodone.

1. Olkkola KT, *et al.* Pharmacokinetics and ventilatory effects of intravenous oxycodone in postoperative children. *Br J Clin Pharmacol* 1994; **38:** 71–6.
2. Kalso E. Pharmacokinetics and ventilatory effects of intravenous oxycodone in postoperative children. *Br J Clin Pharmacol* 1995; **39:** 214.

**Hepatic impairment.** The clearance and elimination of oxycodone were prolonged in 6 women with end-stage liver cirrhosis awaiting liver transplantations.[1] Significant ventilatory depression also occurred. Pharmacokinetic values after successful transplantation were similar to those previously reported for healthy adults. It was recommended that, when giving oxycodone to patients with end-stage liver disease, the dosing frequency should be reduced and the dose lowered.

1. Tallgren M, *et al.* Pharmacokinetics and ventilatory effects of oxycodone before and after liver transplantation. *Clin Pharmacol Ther* 1997; **61:** 655–61.

**Porphyria.** Oxycodone is considered to be unsafe in patients with porphyria because it has been shown to be porphyrinogenic in *animals.*

### Interactions

For interactions associated with opioid analgesics, see p.73.

**Antidepressants.** For reference to a possible case of serotonin syndrome when *sertraline* was given with high doses of oxycodone, see p.296.

### Pharmacokinetics

Oxycodone is absorbed from the gastrointestinal tract. It is metabolised to noroxycodone, via cytochrome P450 isoenzymes of the CYP3A family, and, to a lesser extent, to oxymorphone (p.76) via CYP2D6. Both metabolites undergo glucuronidation and are excreted with unchanged drug in urine. The elimination half-life of oxycodone is reported to be 2 to 4 hours. Oxycodone is distributed into breast milk.

◊ References.

1. Pöyhiä R, *et al.* The pharmacokinetics of oxycodone after intravenous injection in adults. *Br J Clin Pharmacol* 1991; **32:** 516–18.
2. Leow KP, *et al.* Single-dose and steady-state pharmacokinetics and pharmacodynamics of oxycodone in patients with cancer. *Clin Pharmacol Ther* 1992; **52:** 487–95.
3. Olkkola KT, *et al.* Pharmacokinetics and ventilatory effects of intravenous oxycodone in postoperative children. *Br J Clin Pharmacol* 1994; **38:** 71–6.
4. Mandema JW, *et al.* Characterization and validation of a pharmacokinetic model for controlled-release oxycodone. *Br J Clin Pharmacol* 1996; **42:** 747–56.
5. Kaiko RF, *et al.* Pharmacokinetic-pharmacodynamic relationships of controlled-release oxycodone. *Clin Pharmacol Ther* 1996; **59:** 52–61.
6. Gammaitoni AR, Davis MW. Comparison of the pharmacokinetics of oxycodone administered in three Percocet™ formulations. *J Clin Pharmacol* 2002; **42:** 192–7.

### Uses and Administration

Oxycodone, a phenanthrene derivative, is an opioid analgesic (p.73). Oxycodone hydrochloride is given by mouth or subcutaneously or intravenously for the relief of moderate to severe pain. A usual oral starting dose for opioid naive patients in severe pain is 5 mg every 4 to 6 hours increased thereafter as necessary according to response. For patients who have been receiving a strong opioid analgesic the initial dose of oxycodone should be based on the daily opioid requirement; the UK manufacturers suggest that use of 10 mg of oral oxycodone is approximately equivalent to 20 mg of oral morphine. Most patients do not require more than 400 mg daily. Preparations containing oxycodone hydrochloride and aspirin or paracetamol are also used. Oxycodone hydrochloride may also be given orally as a modified-release preparation every 12 hours.

Intravenous doses of oxycodone hydrochloride range from 1 to 10 mg, given over 1 to 2 minutes, and repeated not more often than every 4 hours; a dose of 2 mg/hour is the recommended starting dose as an intravenous infusion. The intravenous route may also be used for patient-controlled analgesia. When given subcutaneously, the starting dose is 5 mg every 4 hours; subcutaneous infusions should be started at 7.5 mg daily in opioid naive patients. When transferring between oral and parenteral oxycodone, the UK manufacturers advise that, as a guide, 2 mg of oral oxycodone is approximately equivalent to 1 mg of parenteral oxycodone.

Oxycodone has been given rectally as suppositories containing 30 mg of oxycodone (as the pectinate) or 10 or 20 mg of oxycodone hydrochloride; the dose may be repeated every 6 to 8 hours.

For doses in patients with hepatic or renal impairment see below.

Oxycodone terephthalate is also used by mouth.

**Administration in hepatic or renal impairment.** The plasma concentrations of oxycodone may be increased in patients with hepatic or renal impairment and consequently dosage adjustment may be necessary in such patients. In the UK, the manufacturers recommend that the oral starting dose for patients with mild hepatic impairment or mild to moderate renal impairment should be 2.5 mg given every 6 hours; they contra-indicate the use of oxycodone in those with moderate to severe hepatic impairment or severe renal impairment. The US manufacturers permit the cautious use of oxycodone in patients with severe hepatic or renal impairment.

**Pain.** References.

1. Kalso E, Vainio A. Morphine and oxycodone hydrochloride in the management of cancer pain. *Clin Pharmacol Ther* 1990; **47:** 639–46.
2. Sunshine A, *et al.* Analgesic efficacy of controlled-release oxycodone in postoperative pain. *J Clin Pharmacol* 1996; **36:** 595–603.
3. Curtis GB, *et al.* Relative potency of controlled-release oxycodone and controlled-release morphine in a postoperative pain model. *Eur J Clin Pharmacol* 1999; **55:** 425–9.
4. Gimbel JS, *et al.* Controlled-release oxycodone for pain in diabetic neuropathy: a randomized controlled trial. *Neurology* 2003; **60:** 927–34.

### Preparations

***USP 27:*** Oxycodone and Acetaminophen Capsules; Oxycodone and Acetaminophen Tablets; Oxycodone and Aspirin Tablets; Oxycodone Hydrochloride Oral Solution; Oxycodone Hydrochloride Tablets.

**Proprietary Preparations** (details are given in Part 3)
***Arg.:*** Oxinovag; Oxycontin; ***Austral.:*** Endone; Oxycontin; Oxynorm; Proladone; ***Braz.:*** Oxycontin; ***Canad.:*** Oxycontin; Supeudol; ***Chile:*** Oxycontin; ***Denm.:*** Oxycontin; Oxynorm; ***Fin.:*** Oxanest; Oxycontin; Oxynorm; ***Fr.:*** Eubine; Oxycontin; ***Ger.:*** Oxygesic; ***Irl.:*** Oxycontin; Oxynorm; ***Israel:*** Oxycod; Oxycontin; ***Mex.:*** Oxycontin; ***Norw.:*** Oxycontin; Oxynorm; ***NZ:*** Proladone†; ***Swed.:*** Oxycontin; Oxynorm; ***Switz.:*** Oxycontin; ***UK:*** Oxycontin; Oxynorm; ***USA:*** Endocodone; Oxycontin; Oxyfast; OxyIR; Percolone; Roxicodone.

**Multi-ingredient:** ***Arg.:*** Oxinovag Complex; ***Canad.:*** Endocet; Endodan; Oxycocet; Oxycodan; Percocet; Percodan; Roxicet†; ***Israel:*** Percocet; Percodan; ***USA:*** Endocet; Percocet; Percodan; Roxicet; Roxilox; Roxiprin; Tylox.

## Oxymorphone Hydrochloride *(BANM, rINNM)*

7,8-Dihydro-14-hydroxymorphinone hydrochloride; Hidrocloruro de oximorfona; Oximorphone Hydrochloride. 6-Deoxy-7,8-dihydro-14-hydroxy-6-oxomorphine hydrochloride; (−)-(5*R*,6*S*,14*S*)-4,5-Epoxy-3,14-dihydroxy-9a-methylmorphinan-6-one hydrochloride.

$C_{17}H_{19}NO_4,HCl$ = 337.8.
*CAS — 76-41-5 (oxymorphone); 357-07-3 (oxymorphone hydrochloride).*

**Pharmacopoeias.** In *US.*

**USP 27** (Oxymorphone Hydrochloride). A white or slightly off-white odourless powder, darkening on exposure to light. Its aqueous solutions are slightly acidic. Soluble 1 in 4 of water, 1 in 100 of alcohol, and 1 in 25 of methyl alcohol; very slightly soluble in chloroform and in ether. Store in airtight containers at a temperature of 25°, excursions permitted between 15° and 30°. Protect from light.

### Profile

Oxymorphone hydrochloride, a phenanthrene derivative, is an opioid analgesic (p.71) with actions and uses similar to those of morphine (p.60), apart from a lack of cough suppressant activity. Oxymorphone is used in the treatment of moderate to severe pain, including pain in obstetrics, and is reported to provide analgesia for 3 to 6 hours. It may also be used as an adjunct to anaesthesia and to relieve dyspnoea due to pulmonary oedema resulting from left ventricular failure.

Oxymorphone hydrochloride is given by intramuscular or subcutaneous injection in initial doses of 1 to 1.5 mg, repeated every 4 to 6 hours as necessary; 500 micrograms may be given by intravenous injection. The usual dose for analgesia during labour is 0.5 to 1 mg intramuscularly.

Oxymorphone hydrochloride is also given rectally as a suppository in a dose of 5 mg every 4 to 6 hours.

### Preparations

***USP 27:*** Oxymorphone Hydrochloride Injection; Oxymorphone Hydrochloride Suppositories.

**Proprietary Preparations** (details are given in Part 3)
***Canad.:*** Numorphan; ***USA:*** Numorphan.

## Oxyphenbutazone *(BAN, rINN)*

G-27202; Hydroxyphenylbutazone; Oxifenbutazona; Oxyphenbutazonum. 4-Butyl-1-(4-hydroxyphenyl)-2-phenylpyrazolidine-3,5-dione monohydrate.

$C_{19}H_{20}N_2O_3,H_2O$ = 342.4.
*CAS — 129-20-4 (anhydrous oxyphenbutazone); 7081-38-1 (oxyphenbutazone monohydrate).*
*ATC — M01AA03; M02AA04; S01BC02.*

### Adverse Effects and Precautions

As for Phenylbutazone, p.83. Adverse effects on the blood may be more frequent with oxyphenbutazone than with phenylbutazone.

**Porphyria.** Oxyphenbutazone has been associated with acute attacks of porphyria and is considered unsafe in porphyric patients.

### Interactions

For interactions associated with NSAIDs, see p.69.

### Uses and Administration

Oxyphenbutazone, a metabolite of phenylbutazone (p.84), is an NSAID (p.67). It has been applied topically to the eye as an anti-inflammatory ointment in conditions such as episcleritis. Oxyphenbutazone was used systemically in disorders such as ankylosing spondylitis, osteoarthritis, and rheumatoid arthritis but such use is no longer considered justified owing to the risk of severe haematological adverse effects.

The piperazine salt has also been used.

### Preparations

**Proprietary Preparations** (details are given in Part 3)
***Austria:*** Tanderil; ***Braz.:*** Tandrex†; ***India:*** Sioril; ***Mex.:*** Butafen†; Edefen; Maderil†; Oxabenal†; Redolet; Tandorene†; ***Spain:*** Diflamil†.

**Multi-ingredient:** ***Braz.:*** Algi-Peralgin†; Algi-Reumac†; Algiflamanil†; Algizolin†; Analtrix; Febupen; Flamanan; Reumazine†; Tandrex A†.

## Paracetamol *(BAN, rINN)*

Acetaminophen; *N*-Acetyl-*p*-aminophenol; Paracetamolum. 4′-Hydroxyacetanilide; *N*-(4-Hydroxyphenyl)acetamide.

$C_8H_9NO_2$ = 151.2.
*CAS — 103-90-2.*
*ATC — N02BE01.*

NOTE. Compounded preparations of paracetamol may be represented by the following names:

- Co-bucafAPAP (*PEN*)—butalbital, paracetamol, and caffeine
- Co-codamol *x/y* (*BAN*)—where *x* and *y* are the strengths in milligrams of codeine phosphate and paracetamol respectively
- Co-codAPAP (*PEN*)—paracetamol and codeine phosphate
- Co-dydramol (*BAN*)—dihydrocodeine tartrate 1 part and paracetamol 50 parts (w/w)
- Co-hycodAPAP (*PEN*)—hydrocodone tartrate and paracetamol
- Co-methiamol *x/y* (*BAN*)—where *x* and *y* are the strengths in milligrams of DL-methionine and paracetamol respectively
- Co-oxycodAPAP (*PEN*)—oxycodone and paracetamol
- Co-proxamol (*BAN*)—dextropropoxyphene hydrochloride 1 part and paracetamol 10 parts (w/w)
- Co-proxAPAP (*PEN*)—dextropropoxyphene napsilate and paracetamol.

**Pharmacopoeias.** In *Chin., Eur.* (see p.vi), *Int., Jpn, Pol., US,* and *Viet.*

**Ph. Eur. 5.0** (Paracetamol). A white crystalline powder. Sparingly soluble in water; freely soluble in alcohol; very slightly soluble in dichloromethane. Protect from light.

**USP 27** (Acetaminophen). A white odourless crystalline powder. Soluble 1 in 20 of boiling water, 1 in 10 of alcohol, and 1 in 15 of 1*N* sodium hydroxide. Store in airtight containers. Protect from light.

### Adverse Effects and Treatment

Side-effects of paracetamol are rare and usually mild, although haematological reactions including thrombocytopenia, leucopenia, pancytopenia, neutropenia, and agranulocytosis have been reported. Skin rashes, and other hypersensitivity reactions occur occasionally.

Overdosage with paracetamol can result in severe liver damage and sometimes acute renal tubular necrosis. Prompt treatment with acetylcysteine or methionine is essential and is discussed under Overdosage, below.

**Effects on the kidneys.** For reference to evidence that abuse or prolonged excessive use of analgesics, including paracetamol, can produce nephropathy, see under NSAIDs, p.68.
See also under Overdosage, below.

**Effects on the respiratory tract.** The results of a case-control study[1] have suggested that the frequent (daily or weekly) use of paracetamol may be associated with asthma. However, the UK Committee on Safety of Medicines has commented that the results of this study do not alter any advice regarding the use of paracetamol and that it remains a safe and effective pain killer for many patients including asthmatics.

1. Shaheen SO, *et al.* Frequent paracetamol use and asthma in adults. *Thorax* 2000; **55:** 266–70.

**Hypersensitivity.** Reactions, characterised by urticaria, dyspnoea, and hypotension, have occurred following the use of paracetamol in adults[1-3] and children.[4] Angioedema has also been reported.[5] Fixed drug eruptions, confirmed by rechallenge, have been described,[6-9] and toxic epidermal necrolysis has occurred.[10]

1. Stricker BHC, *et al.* Acute hypersensitivity reactions to paracetamol. *BMJ* 1985; **291:** 938–9.
2. Van Diem L, Grilliat JP. Anaphylactic shock induced by paracetamol. *Eur J Clin Pharmacol* 1990; **38:** 389–90.
3. Kumar RK, Byard I. Paracetamol as a cause of anaphylaxis. *Hosp Med* 1999; **60:** 66–7.
4. Ellis M, *et al.* Immediate adverse reactions to acetaminophen in children: evaluation of histamine release and spirometry. *J Pediatr* 1989; **114:** 654–6.
5. Idoko JA, *et al.* Angioneurotic oedema following ingestion of paracetamol. *Trans R Soc Trop Med Hyg* 1986; **80:** 175.
6. Thomas RHM, Munro DD. Fixed drug eruption due to paracetamol. *Br J Dermatol* 1986; **115:** 357–9.
7. Cohen HA, *et al.* Fixed drug eruption caused by acetaminophen. *Ann Pharmacother* 1992; **26:** 1596–7.
8. Harris A, Burge SM. Vasculitis in a fixed drug eruption due to paracetamol. *Br J Dermatol* 1995; **133:** 790–1.
9. Hern S, *et al.* Bullous fixed drug eruption due to paracetamol with an unusual immunofluorescence pattern. *Br J Dermatol* 1998; **139:** 1129–31.
10. Halevi A, *et al.* Toxic epidermal necrolysis associated with acetaminophen ingestion. *Ann Pharmacother* 2000; **34:** 32–4.

**Overdosage.** Acute overdosage with paracetamol, whether accidental or deliberate, is relatively common and can be extremely serious because of the narrow margin between therapeutic and toxic doses. Ingestion of as little as 10 to 15 g of paracetamol by adults may cause severe hepatocellular necrosis and, less often, renal tubular necrosis. Patients should be considered at risk of severe liver damage if they have ingested more than 150 mg/kg of paracetamol or 12 g or more in total, whichever is the smaller. The risk of severe toxicity after acute paracetamol overdose appears to be less in children than in adults at comparable doses; however, chronic use of supratherapeutic doses in children has resulted in unintentional overdoses and severe hepatotoxicity.[1,2]

Early features of overdosage (very commonly nausea and vomiting although they may also include lethargy and sweating) usually settle within 24 hours. Abdominal pain may be the first indication of liver damage, which is not usually apparent for 24 to 48 hours and sometimes may be delayed for up to 4 to 6 days after ingestion. Liver damage is generally at a maximum 72 to 96 hours after ingestion. Hepatic failure, encephalopathy, coma, and death may result. Complications of hepatic failure include acidosis, cerebral oedema, haemorrhage, hypoglycaemia, hypotension, infection, and renal failure. Prothrombin time increases with deteriorating liver function and some recommend that it be measured regularly. Measurement of serum concentrations of aspartate aminotransferase and alanine aminotransferase is also of value.[3] Patients receiving enzyme-inducing drugs or those with a history of alcohol abuse are at special risk of hepatic damage, as may be patients suffering from malnutrition such as those with anorexia or AIDS. It has also been suggested that fasting may predispose to hepatotoxicity.[4]

Acute renal failure with acute tubular necrosis may develop, even in the absence of severe liver damage. Other non-hepatic symptoms that have been reported following paracetamol overdosage include myocardial abnormalities and pancreatitis.

Toxicity following overdosage with paracetamol has been attributed to the production of a minor but highly reactive metabolite, *N*-acetyl-*p*-benzoquinoneimine (NABQI) by cytochrome P450 isoenzymes (mainly CYP2E1 and CYP3A4)[2] in the liver and kidney. The amount of NABQI produced after normal doses of paracetamol is usually completely detoxified by conjugation with glutathione and excreted as mercaptopurine and cysteine conjugates. In paracetamol overdosage, tissue stores of glutathione become depleted, allowing NABQI to accumulate and bind to sulfhydryl groups within hepatocytes causing cell damage. Substances capable of replenishing depleted stores of glutathione, such as acetylcysteine or methionine, are therefore used as antidotes in paracetamol overdosage. Acetylcysteine may also be involved in the repair of damaged tissue.

**Treatment of paracetamol overdosage.** The management of paracetamol overdosage as practised in the UK and US has been the subject of numerous reviews.[3-13] Guidelines have also been issued in the UK by the Paracetamol Information Centre.[14]

*Prompt treatment is essential,* even when there are no obvious symptoms, and all patients should be admitted to hospital; full supportive measures should also be instituted.

- Activated charcoal may be used to reduce gastrointestinal absorption, if it can be given within 1 hour of the overdose, and if more than 150 mg/kg of paracetamol has been ingested. However, if acetylcysteine or methionine is to be given by mouth the charcoal is best cleared from the stomach to prevent it reducing the absorption of the antidote
- There is little evidence that gastric lavage is of benefit in those who have overdosed solely with paracetamol
- The plasma-paracetamol concentration should be determined as soon as possible, but not within 4 hours of ingestion, to ensure that peak concentrations are recorded. The risk of liver damage is determined by comparison with a nomogram reference line on a plot of plasma-paracetamol concentration against hours after ingestion. A semi-logarithmic plot or a linear plot may be used, see Figure 1 (p.77) and Figure 2 (p.77). Generally, antidote treatment is required if the patient's plasma-paracetamol concentration is higher than the appropriate line (but see below)
- Patients receiving enzyme-inducing drugs such as carbamazepine, phenytoin, phenobarbital, rifampicin, and hypericum, or those with malnutrition or a history of alcohol abuse, are considered at high risk, and should receive an antidote even if their plasma-paracetamol concentrations are up to 50% below the standard reference line
- Plasma-paracetamol concentrations measured more than 15 hours after ingestion are not reliable indicators of hepatic toxicity. Furthermore, the nomogram may not be suitable for use when patients have taken modified-release preparations of paracetamol.[15,16] Some suggestions for modified strategies for the use of the Rumack-Matthew nomogram in the face of overdosage with modified-release preparations have been made[17-19]
- Plasma-paracetamol concentrations are also of little value in patients who have taken several overdoses of paracetamol over a short period of time: such patients should be considered as at serious risk and given antidote treatment
- Deaths from liver failure have occurred in patients presenting with plasma-paracetamol concentrations below the treatment line: suggested explanations include inadequate patient histories and a need for a lower treatment threshold[20]
- If there is any doubt about timing or the need to treat, then a patient **should** be treated with an antidote. In some centres, patients who have ingested 150 mg/kg or more of paracetamol are treated regardless of plasma-paracetamol concentrations[21]
- Antidote treatment should be started as soon as possible after suspected paracetamol ingestion and should not be delayed while awaiting the results of plasma assays. Once the results become available, treatment may be stopped if the initial concentration was below the nomogram reference line. However, if the initial concentration is above the reference line, the full course of antidote must be given and should not be stopped when subsequent plasma concentrations fall below the reference line.

**Figure 1.** A semi-logarithmic plot of plasma-paracetamol concentration against hours after ingestion.

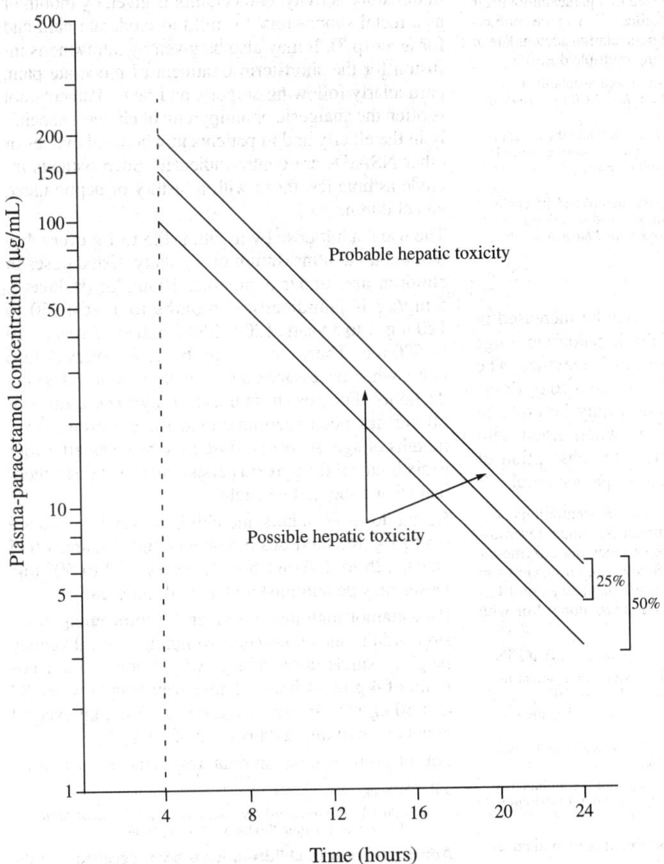


Adapted from Rumack BH, Matthew HJ. Acetaminophen poisoning and toxicity. *Pediatrics* 1975; **55:** 871–6.

Notes for the use of this chart:

1. The time coordinates refer to time after ingestion.
2. Plasma-paracetamol concentrations drawn before 4 hours may not represent peak concentrations.
3. The graph should be used only in relation to a single acute ingestion.
4. The solid line 25% below the standard nomogram is included to allow for possible errors in plasma assays and estimated time from ingestion of an overdose.
5. The solid line 50% below the standard nomogram is to assess the possible hepatic toxicity in patients receiving enzyme-inducing drugs or with malnutrition or a history of alcohol abuse.
6. The value of such charts is uncertain if the patient is first seen 15 hours or more after ingestion, or has taken modified release preparations of paracetamol.

**Figure 2.** A linear plot of plasma-paracetamol concentration against hours after ingestion.

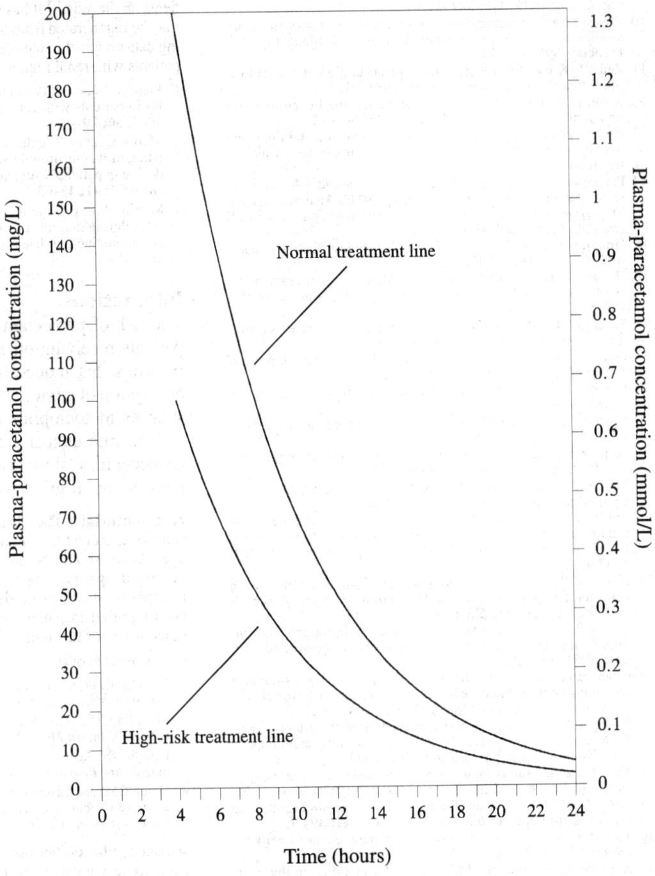


Courtesy of P A Routledge.

Notes for the use of this chart:

1. The time coordinates refer to time after ingestion.
2. Plasma-paracetamol concentrations drawn before 4 hours may not represent peak concentrations.
3. The graph should be used only in relation to a single acute ingestion.
4. Patients whose plasma-paracetamol concentrations are above the normal treatment line should be treated.
5. Patients on enzyme-inducing drugs or with malnutrition or a history of alcohol abuse should be treated if their plasma-paracetamol concentrations are above the high-risk treatment line.
6. The value of such charts is uncertain if the patient is first seen 15 hours or more after ingestion, or has taken modified release preparations of paracetamol.

*Choice of antidote.* Acetylcysteine (p.1112) is usually the antidote of choice but the route of administration varies, and the best protocol has yet to be determined.[13] Intravenous use has been associated with anaphylactic reactions but is the preferred route in the UK because of fears that oral absorption might be reduced by vomiting or activated charcoal. However, in the USA the oral route is usual, and is clearly effective. The use of methionine (p.1042) by mouth is licensed in the UK, despite the same risks of impaired absorption due to vomiting or activated charcoal. It is cheaper and easier to give than intravenous acetylcysteine and may be used in situations where a patient cannot be transferred to hospital, provided it is given within 10 to 12 hours of the overdose and the patient is not vomiting.

*Acetylcysteine* is most effective when given during the first 8 hours following ingestion of the overdose and the effect diminishes progressively thereafter. It used to be believed that starting treatment more than 15 hours after overdosage was of no benefit and might aggravate the risk of hepatic encephalopathy. However, late administration was subsequently shown to be safe,[22] and studies of patients treated up to 36 hours after ingestion suggest that benefit may be obtained up to and possibly beyond 24 hours.[23,24] Furthermore, giving intravenous acetylcysteine to patients who had already developed fulminant hepatic failure has been shown to reduce morbidity and mortality.[25]

- In the UK, an initial dose of 150 mg/kg of acetylcysteine in 200 mL of glucose 5% is given intravenously over 15 minutes, followed by an intravenous infusion of 50 mg/kg in 500 mL of glucose 5% over the next 4 hours and then 100 mg/kg in one litre over the next 16 hours. Sodium chloride 0.9% may be used where glucose 5% is unsuitable. The volume of intravenous fluids should be modified for children. If an anaphylactoid reaction develops, the infusion should be stopped and an antihistamine given; it may be possible to continue the acetylcysteine infusion at a slower rate
- In the USA, acetylcysteine is given by mouth in an initial dose of 140 mg/kg as a 5% solution followed by 70 mg/kg every 4 hours for an additional 17 doses. Some[26] have suggested increasing the loading dose of oral acetylcysteine when it is given after activated charcoal, whereas others[27] have found that the efficacy of acetylcysteine is not reduced by use of activated charcoal beforehand and consider a larger acetylcysteine dose unnecessary.

*Methionine*, like acetylcysteine, is most effective when given as early as possible following paracetamol overdosage. However, it is not as effective if treatment is delayed[5,28-30] and hepatic damage is more frequent and severe if treatment with methionine is started more than 10 hours after ingestion; it may also precipitate hepatic encephalopathy.[5]

- The usual dose of methionine in adults and children over 6 years is 2.5 g by mouth every 4 hours for 4 doses starting less than 10 to 12 hours after ingestion of the paracetamol and provided the patient is not vomiting. Children under 6 years should be given 1 g every 4 hours for 4 doses. It has also been given intravenously

The literature relating to the use of methionine in paracetamol poisoning is, in general, imprecise as to the form of methionine used. In the UK, the doses quoted above refer to DL-methionine. Preparations containing both methionine and paracetamol (co-methiamol) have been formulated for use in situations where overdosage may occur. However, the issue of whether methionine should be routinely added to paracetamol preparations is contentious for medical and ethical reasons.

*Histamine $H_2$-antagonists.* It has been suggested that since cimetidine blocks the hepatic cytochrome P450 mixed function oxidase system, it might be of use as an adjunct to acetylcysteine for patients whose production of the toxic metabolite of paracetamol is increased due to enzyme induction. Although there have been several anecdotal reports claiming benefit for cimetidine in patients with paracetamol poisoning, there is no current evidence to support these claims.[10,11,13,31]

*Liver transplantation* may be considered as a last recourse in some patients.

1. Miles FK, *et al.* Accidental paracetamol overdosing and fulminant hepatic failure in children. *Med J Aust* 1999; **171:** 472–5.
2. American Academy of Pediatrics Committee on Drugs. Acetaminophen toxicity in children. *Pediatrics* 2001; **108:** 1020–4.
3. Routledge P, *et al.* Paracetamol (acetaminophen) poisoning. *BMJ* 1998; **317:** 1609–10.
4. Whitcomb DC, *et al.* Association of acetaminophen hepatotoxicity with fasting and ethanol use. *JAMA* 1994; **272:** 1845–50.
5. Janes J, Routledge PA. Recent advances in the management of paracetamol (acetaminophen) poisoning. *Drug Safety* 1992; **7:** 170–7.
6. Bray GP. Liver failure induced by paracetamol. *BMJ* 1993; **306:** 157–8.

7. Collee GG, Hanson GC. The management of acute poisoning *Br J Anaesth* 1993; **70:** 562–73.
8. Makin AJ, *et al.* Management of severe cases of paracetamol overdosage. *Br J Hosp Med* 1994; **52:** 210–13.
9. Vale JA, Proudfoot AT. Paracetamol (acetaminophen) poisoning. *Lancet* 1995; **346:** 547–52.
10. Prescott LF. Paracetamol overdose. In: *Paracetamol (acetaminophen): a critical bibliographic review.* London: Taylor & Francis, 1996: 401–73.
11. Zed PJ, Krenzelok EP. Treatment of acetaminophen overdose. *Am J Health-Syst Pharm* 1999; **56:** 1081–91.
12. Kozer E, Koren G. Management of paracetamol overdose: current controversies. *Drug Safety* 2001; **24:** 503–12.
13. Brok J *et al.* Interventions for paracetamol (acetaminophen) overdoses. Available in The Cochrane Library, Issue 2. Chichester: John Wiley; 2004.
14. Paracetamol Information Centre. *Guidelines for the management of acute paracetamol overdosage 2003.* Also available at: http://www.pharmweb.net/pwmirror/pwy/paracetamol/chart.html (accessed 06/07/04)
15. Graudins A, *et al.* Overdose of extended-release acetaminophen. *N Engl J Med* 1995; **333:** 196.
16. Vassallo S, *et al.* Use of the Rumack-Matthew nomogram in cases of extended-release acetaminophen toxicity. *Ann Intern Med* 1996; **125:** 940.
17. Temple AR, Mrazik TJ. More on extended-release acetaminophen. *N Engl J Med* 1995; **333:** 1508.
18. Graudins A, *et al.* More on extended-release acetaminophen. *N Engl J Med* 1995; **333:** 1508–9.
19. Cetaruk EW, *et al.* Extended-release acetaminophen overdose. *JAMA* 1996; **275:** 686.
20. Bridger S, *et al.* Deaths from low dose paracetamol poisoning. *BMJ* 1998; **316:** 1724–5.
21. Aujla KS, *et al.* Nomogram does not show absolute concentration for treatment. *BMJ* 1998; **317:** 1655.
22. Parker D, *et al.* Safety of late acetylcysteine treatment in paracetamol poisoning. *Hum Exp Toxicol* 1990; **9:** 25–7.
23. Smilkstein MJ, *et al.* Efficacy of oral N-acetylcysteine in the treatment of acetaminophen overdose: analysis of the National Multicenter Study (1976 to 1985). *N Engl J Med* 1988; **319:** 1557–62.
24. Harrison PM, *et al.* Improved outcome of paracetamol-induced fulminant hepatic failure by late administration of acetylcysteine. *Lancet* 1990; **335:** 1572–3.
25. Keays R, *et al.* Intravenous acetylcysteine in paracetamol induced fulminant hepatic failure: a prospective controlled trial. *BMJ* 1991; **303:** 1026–9.
26. Chamberlain JM, *et al.* Use of activated charcoal in a simulated poisoning with acetaminophen: a new loading dose for N-acetylcysteine? *Ann Emerg Med* 1993; **22:** 1398–1402.
27. Spiller HA, *et al.* A prospective evaluation of the effect of activated charcoal before oral N-acetylcysteine in acetaminophen overdose. *Ann Emerg Med* 1994; **23:** 519–23.
28. Vale JA, *et al.* Intravenous N-acetylcysteine: the treatment of choice in paracetamol poisoning? *BMJ* 1979; **2:** 1435–6.
29. Vale JA, *et al.* Treatment of acetaminophen poisoning: the use of oral methionine. *Arch Intern Med* 1981; **141:** 394–6.
30. Tee LGB, *et al.* N-Acetylcysteine for paracetamol overdose. *Lancet* 1986; **i:** 331–2.
31. Kaufenberg AJ, Shepherd MF. Role of cimetidine in the treatment of acetaminophen poisoning. *Am J Health-Syst Pharm* 1998; **55:** 1516–19.

**Pancreatitis.** A review of drug-induced pancreatitis reported that pancreatitis associated with paracetamol had only occurred in patients taking more than recommended doses and even then it had been a rare reaction.[1]

1. Underwood TW, Frye CB. Drug-induced pancreatitis. *Clin Pharm* 1993; **12:** 440–8.

## Precautions

Paracetamol should be given with care to patients with impaired kidney or liver function. It should also be given with care to patients with alcohol dependence.

**Breast feeding.** No adverse effects have been observed in breast-feeding infants whose mothers were receiving paracetamol, and the American Academy of Pediatrics considers[1] that it is therefore usually compatible with breast feeding. The *British National Formulary* also considers that the amount of paracetamol distributed into breast milk is too small to be harmful to a breast-fed infant.

Pharmacokinetic studies in 12 nursing mothers given a single dose of paracetamol showed that peak paracetamol concentrations in breast milk of 10 to 15 micrograms/mL were achieved in 1 to 2 hours. Plasma concentrations were determined in 2 mothers; a breast milk/plasma ratio of about 1 was reported.[2] Similar findings have been reported from other studies.[3,4]

1. American Academy of Pediatrics. The transfer of drugs and other chemicals into human milk. *Pediatrics* 2001; **108:** 776–89. Correction. *ibid.*; 1029. Also available at: http://aappolicy.aappublications.org/cgi/content/full/pediatrics%3b108/3/776 (accessed 06/07/04)
2. Berlin CM, *et al.* Disposition of acetaminophen in milk, saliva, and plasma of lactating women. *Pediatr Pharmacol* 1980; **1:** 135–41.
3. Hurden EL, *et al.* Excretion of paracetamol in human breast milk. *Arch Dis Child* 1980; **55:** 969–72.
4. Bitzén P-O, *et al.* Excretion of paracetamol in human breast milk. *Eur J Clin Pharmacol* 1981; **20:** 123–5.

**Pregnancy.** Paracetamol is generally considered to be the analgesic of choice in pregnant patients. However, the frequent use of paracetamol (defined as most days or daily use) in late pregnancy may be associated with an increased risk of persistent wheezing in the infant.[1] The authors emphasised that the number of pregnant women taking frequent doses was very small and they recommended that *infrequent* paracetamol should remain the analgesic of choice in pregnancy.

1. Shaheen SO, *et al.* Paracetamol use in pregnancy and wheezing in early childhood. *Thorax* 2002; **57:** 958–63.

**Renal impairment.** Caution is recommended when giving paracetamol to patients with renal impairment. Plasma concentrations of paracetamol and its glucuronide and sulfate conjugates are increased in patients with moderate renal failure and in patients on dialysis.[1-3] It has been suggested that paracetamol itself may be regenerated from these metabolites.[1,2] There are conflicting data on whether the conjugates of paracetamol accumulate in patients with renal impairment receiving multiple doses.[2,3]

1. Prescott LF, *et al.* Paracetamol disposition and metabolite kinetics in patients with chronic renal failure. *Eur J Clin Pharmacol* 1989; **36:** 291–7.
2. Martin U, *et al.* The disposition of paracetamol and the accumulation of its glucuronide and sulphate conjugates during multiple dosing in patients with chronic renal failure. *Eur J Clin Pharmacol* 1991; **41:** 43–6.
3. Martin U, *et al.* The disposition of paracetamol and its conjugates during multiple dosing in patients with end-stage renal failure maintained on haemodialysis. *Eur J Clin Pharmacol* 1993; **45:** 141–5.

## Interactions

The risk of paracetamol toxicity may be increased in patients receiving other potentially hepatotoxic drugs or drugs that induce liver microsomal enzymes. The absorption of paracetamol may be accelerated by drugs such as metoclopramide. Excretion may be affected and plasma concentrations altered when given with probenecid. Colestyramine reduces the absorption of paracetamol if given within 1 hour of paracetamol.

**Antibacterials.** The plasma-paracetamol concentrations considered an indication for antidote treatment (see under Overdosage, above) should be halved in patients receiving enzyme-inducing drugs such as *rifampicin*. Severe hepatotoxicity at therapeutic doses or moderate overdoses of paracetamol has been reported in patients receiving *isoniazid*, alone[1-3] or with other drugs for tuberculosis.[4]

For the effects of paracetamol on chloramphenicol, see p.186.

1. Murphy R, *et al.* Severe acetaminophen toxicity in a patient receiving isoniazid. *Ann Intern Med* 1990; **113:** 799–800.
2. Moulding TS, *et al.* Acetaminophen, isoniazid, and hepatic toxicity. *Ann Intern Med* 1991; **114:** 431.
3. Crippin JS. Acetaminophen hepatotoxicity: potentiation by isoniazid. *Am J Gastroenterol* 1993; **88:** 590–2.
4. Nolan CM, *et al.* Hepatotoxicity associated with acetaminophen usage in patients receiving multiple drug therapy for tuberculosis. *Chest* 1994; **105:** 408–11.

**Anticoagulants.** For the effects of paracetamol on oral anticoagulants, see under Warfarin, p.1023.

**Antiepileptics.** The plasma-paracetamol concentrations considered an indication for antidote treatment (see under Overdosage, above) should be halved in patients receiving enzyme-inducing drugs such as *carbamazepine, phenobarbital, phenytoin,* or *primidone*.

For the effects of paracetamol on *lamotrigine*, see p.364.

**Antivirals.** For reports of adverse effects on the liver associated with concomitant use of paracetamol and antiviral drugs, see under Interferons, p.642 and Zidovudine, p.659.

**Probenecid.** Pretreatment with probenecid can decrease paracetamol clearance and increase its plasma half-life.[1] Although urinary excretion of the sulfate and glucuronide conjugates of paracetamol are reduced, that of paracetamol is unchanged.

1. Kamali F. The effect of probenecid on paracetamol metabolism and pharmacokinetics. *Eur J Clin Pharmacol* 1993; **45:** 551–3.

## Pharmacokinetics

Paracetamol is readily absorbed from the gastrointestinal tract with peak plasma concentrations occurring about 10 to 60 minutes after oral doses. Paracetamol is distributed into most body tissues. It crosses the placenta and is present in breast milk. Plasma-protein binding is negligible at usual therapeutic concentrations but increases with increasing concentrations. The elimination half-life of paracetamol varies from about 1 to 3 hours.

Paracetamol is metabolised predominantly in the liver and excreted in the urine mainly as the glucuronide and sulfate conjugates. Less than 5% is excreted as unchanged paracetamol. A minor hydroxylated metabolite (*N*-acetyl-*p*-benzoquinoneimine), is usually produced in very small amounts by cytochrome P450 isoenzymes (mainly CYP2E1 and CYP3A4) in the liver and kidney. It is usually detoxified by conjugation with glutathione but may accumulate following paracetamol overdosage and cause tissue damage.

**Absorption.** The absorption of paracetamol was slow and incomplete in vegetarian subjects compared with non-vegetarian subjects.[1]

1. Prescott LF, *et al.* Impaired absorption of paracetamol in vegetarians. *Br J Clin Pharmacol* 1993; **36:** 237–40.

## Uses and Administration

Paracetamol, a para-aminophenol derivative, has analgesic and antipyretic properties and weak anti-inflammatory activity. Paracetamol is given by mouth or as a rectal suppository for mild to moderate pain and for fever (p.8). It may also be given by intravenous infusion for the short-term treatment of moderate pain, particularly following surgery, and fever. Paracetamol is often the analgesic or antipyretic of choice, especially in the elderly and in patients in whom salicylates or other NSAIDs are contra-indicated. Such patients include asthmatics, those with a history of peptic ulcer, and children.

The usual adult dose by mouth is 0.5 to 1 g every 4 to 6 hours up to a maximum of 4 g daily. Usual doses in children are: under 3 months, 10 mg/kg (reduce to 5 mg/kg if jaundiced); 3 months to 1 year, 60 to 120 mg; 1 to 5 years, 120 to 250 mg; 6 to 12 years, 250 to 500 mg. These doses may be given every 4 to 6 hours when necessary up to a maximum of 4 doses in 24 hours. For post-immunisation pyrexia, a dose of 60 mg has been recommended for children 2 to 3 months of age. A second dose may be given after four to six hours; if the pyrexia persists after that dose, medical advice should be sought.

Rectal doses for adults and children over 12 years are 0.5 to 1 g. Rectal doses in younger children are: 1 to 5 years, 125 to 250 mg; 6 to 12 years, 250 to 500 mg. Doses may be administered up to 4 times daily.

Paracetamol may also be given by intravenous infusion. Adults and adolescents weighing over 50 kg may be given single doses of 1 g every 4 hours to a maximum of 4 g in 24 hours. Those weighing between 33 and 50 kg may be given a dose of 15 mg/kg every 4 hours to a maximum daily dose of 60 mg/kg.

For intravenous doses in renal impairment, see below.

◊ References.

1. Prescott LF. *Paracetamol (acetaminophen): a critical bibliographic review.* London: Taylor & Francis, 1996.

**Administration in children.** It has been suggested[1] that the recommended doses of paracetamol for children may result in subtherapeutic blood concentrations, and that an initial loading dose should be given, followed by regular doses up to the recommended maximum daily dose. However, the appropriate maximum daily dose remains controversial, and there is obvious concern given the risks of overdosage. For recommended doses in children see above.

1. Zacharias M, Watts D. Pain relief in children. *BMJ* 1998; **316:** 1552.

**Administration in renal impairment.** In patients with a creatinine clearance of 30 mL/minute or less it is recommended that the interval between each intravenous paracetamol dose is increased to 6 hours.

**Headache.** Non-opioid analgesics such as paracetamol, aspirin, and other NSAIDs are often tried first for the symptomatic treatment of various types of headache including migraine (see p.464) and tension-type headache (see p.465). These drugs given at the onset of symptoms can successfully treat an acute attack of migraine. However, absorption may be poor due to gastric stasis which is commonly present in migraine. For this reason dispersible and effervescent preparations and compound preparations containing drugs such as metoclopramide which relieve gastric stasis have been advocated.

**Pain.** Paracetamol is used in the management of mild to moderate pain (see Choice of Analgesic, p.2). It is of similar potency to aspirin, but with weak anti-inflammatory activity. Paracetamol may also be used as an adjunct to opioids in the management of severe pain such as cancer pain (p.5). Paracetamol is the preferred choice for pain in children (p.3) because of the association of aspirin with Reye's syndrome in this age group (see p.16). In the treatment of rheumatic disorders, a weak anti-inflammatory effect limits the role of paracetamol. However, it may be of benefit for simple pain control in rheumatoid arthritis (p.9) and ankylosing spondylitis (see under Spondyloarthropathies, p.11), although these patients usually require the additional anti-inflammatory effects provided by NSAIDs. Synovial inflammation is usually only a minor component of osteoarthritis (p.9), and paracetamol is generally recommended as first choice of treatment before NSAIDs are tried. Paracetamol is useful for the relief of acute low back pain (p.7).

Dependence and tolerance are not a problem with non-opioid analgesics such as paracetamol, but there is a ceiling of efficacy, above which increasing the dose has no further therapeutic effect.

## Preparations

**BP 2003:** Co-codamol Tablets; Co-dydramol Tablets; Co-proxamol Tablets; Dispersible Paracetamol Tablets; Effervescent Co-codamol Tablets;

Paediatric Paracetamol Oral Solution; Paracetamol Oral Suspension; Paracetamol Suppositories; Paracetamol Tablets; Soluble Paracetamol Tablets; ***USP 27:*** Acetaminophen and Aspirin Tablets; Acetaminophen and Caffeine Tablets; Acetaminophen and Codeine Phosphate Capsules; Acetaminophen and Codeine Phosphate Oral Solution; Acetaminophen and Codeine Phosphate Oral Suspension; Acetaminophen and Codeine Phosphate Tablets; Acetaminophen and Diphenhydramine Citrate Tablets; Acetaminophen and Pseudoephedrine Hydrochloride Tablets; Acetaminophen Capsules; Acetaminophen for Effervescent Oral Solution; Acetaminophen Oral Solution; Acetaminophen Oral Suspension; Acetaminophen Suppositories; Acetaminophen Tablets; Acetaminophen, Aspirin, and Caffeine Tablets; Acetaminophen, Dextromethorphan Hydrobromide, Doxylamine Succinate, and Pseudoephedrine Hydrochloride Oral Solution; Acetaminophen, Diphenhydramine Hydrochloride, and Pseudoephedrine Hydrochloride Tablets; Butalbital, Acetaminophen, and Caffeine Capsules; Butalbital, Acetaminophen, and Caffeine Tablets; Hydrocodone Bitartrate and Acetaminophen Tablets; Isometheptene Mucate, Dichloralphenazone, and Acetaminophen Capsules; Oxycodone and Acetaminophen Capsules; Oxycodone and Acetaminophen Tablets; Propoxyphene Hydrochloride and Acetaminophen Tablets; Propoxyphene Napsylate and Acetaminophen Tablets.

**Proprietary Preparations** (details are given in Part 3)

***Arg.:*** Acetolit; Apracur Antifebril; Causalon; Custodial; Dirox; Dristancito; Fiebrolito; Guemusin; Mejoral; Multifebrin; Nodipir; Nodolex; Para Z Mol; Paratral; PH 4 Plus; Plovacal; Predualito; Tafirol; Termofren; Tylenol; Vick Vitapyrena; Viclor; ***Austral.:*** Chemists Own Pain & Fever; Childrens Panadol†; Dymadon; Febridol; Lemsip Headcold†; Lemsip Max†; Lemsip†; Ordov Febrigesic†; Panadol; Panamax; Parahexal; Paralgin; Setamol; Tempra†; Tylenol; ***Austria:*** Apacet†; Becetamol; Ben-u-ron; Duaneo; Enelfa; Gewamol; Kratofin simplex; Mexalen; Momentum; Parakapton; Peinfort; Tylenol†; ***Belg.:*** Curpol; Dafalgan; Dolprone; Efferalgan†; Lemgrip†; Lonarid Mono†; Neuridon†; Panadol; Pe-Tam†; Perdolan; Sanicopyrine†; Tempra†; ***Braz.:*** Acetamol†; Acetofen; Anatyl; Baicurina†; Calpol†; Cefabrina; Cetafrin; Cetynol†; Chalena†; Contradol; Dordendril†; Dorfen; Dorib†; Dorico; Dorvan; Febralgin†; Fervex†; Gripeonil; Gripotermon; Pacemol; Parador†; Paralgen; Piramin; Pyrimel; Termo-Ped; Termol; Tilekin; Trifen†; Tylenol; Tylephen; Tylidol; Unigrip; ***Canad.:*** 222 AF†; Abenol; Acet; Acetab†; AF Anacin†; Alsiphene; Artritol; Atasol; Cephanol; Childrens Feverhalt; Multi-gesic; Novo-Gesic; Pain Aid Free; Panadol; Pediatrix; Robigesic; Rounox†; Tantaphen; Tempra; Tylenol; ***Chile:*** Acamol; Asafen Nueva Formula; Cotibin Compuesto; Cryogenine Plus; Daimeton; Fibrimol; Geniol-P; Kitadol; Panadol; Panagesic; Parox Meltab; Rapidol; Tapsin sin Cafeina; Winasorb; Zolben; ***Denm.:*** Pamol; Panodil; Pinex; ***Fin.:*** Panadol; Para-Suppo; Para-Tabs; ***Fr.:*** Aferadol†; Claradol; Compralsol†; Dafalgan; Dolflash†; Doliprane; Dolitabs; Dolko; Dolotec; Efferalgan; Efferalganodis; Expandox; Febrectol; Geluprane; Gynospasmine†; Oralgan†; Panadol; Paralyoc; Perfalgan; ***Ger.:*** Anti-Algos†; Antipanin N†; Antipanin P†; Ben-u-ron; Captin; Contac Erkaltungs-Trunk; Doloreduct; Dorocoff-Paracetamol; duracetamol†; Enelfa; Fensum; Finiweh†; Grippostad Heissgetrank; Larylin Heissgetrank gegen Schmerzen und Fieber†; Mandrogripp†; Momentum Analgetikum†; Mono Praecimed; NeoCitran†; NilnOcen†; Paedialgon; Parapaed; PCM; Pyromed; RubieMol; Sinpro N; Togal; Treupel mono†; Vivimed†; ***Gr.:*** Apotel; Dalminette; Depon; Depon Maximum; Dolal; Lonarid Aplo; Panadol; ***Hong Kong:*** Afebrin; Angenol; Apap†; Arfen; Ben-u-ron; Biogesic; Calpol; Children's Tylenol; Cortal for Children; Dhamol; Fortolin; Infant's Tylenol; Junior Strength Tylenol; Panadol; Parmol; Progesic; Setamol; Tiffy; Tylenol; Uni-Febrin; ***India:*** Calpol; Crocin; Doliprane; Malidens; Pacimol; Paracin; Pyrexon; Pyrigesic; Ultragin; ***Irl.:*** Calpol; Disprol; Hedex; Panadol; Paralief; Paralink; Parapaed; Tylenol; ***Israel:*** Abrol; Abrolet; Acamol; Acamoli; Aldolor; Dexamol; Dexamol Kid; Efferalgan; Liqiprin†; Paramolan; Rokamol; Supramol; Vimoli; ***Ital.:*** Acetamol; Efferalgan; Levadol; Neo-Fepramol†; Normaflu; Panadol; Puernol; Tachipirina; ***Malaysia:*** Acet; Arfen; Biogesic; Dhamol; Dumin; Naprex; Panadol; Partamol; Poro; Rapidol; Serimol; Setromol; Uphamol; ***Mex.:*** Acetafen; Acetif; Alpirex; Amolgen; Analmex†; Andopan; Andox; Antidol; Brontonyl†; Calinofen; Calpol†; Carofril†; Colderina†; Coriver; Datril; Dismifen; Dolotemp; Doluvital; Dolviran; Farpik; Febran; Febrim†; Febronyl†; Frilen; Icetazol; Ifutemp; Infalgina; Magnidol-Plus; Masferol; Mejoralito; Minofen†; Minomex†; Neodol; Neodolito; Notem; Panadol†; Parengesico†; Pharmacen; Piraldin†; Precifen†; Resfin†; Sedalito; Sinedol; Sons Piral; Sudis; Temperal; Tempire; Tempofin; Tempra; Temprin†; Temzzard; Termotrin; Terol†; Tylenol; Tylex; Verbalem†; Wifibrin†; Winasorb; ***Neth.:*** Daro†; Darocet†; Hedex†; Kinder Finimal; Momentum; Panadol; Sinaspril-Paracetamol; ***Norw.:*** Alvedon†; Pamol; Panodil; Paracet; Pinex; ***NZ:*** Disprol; Lemsip Cold & Flu Original, Cold & Flu Max; Pacimol; Pamol; Panadol; Paracare; Paratabs†; ***Port.:*** Atralidon; Ben-u-ron; Dafalgan; Efferalgan; Panadol; Panasorbe; Paramolan; Parsel; Supofen; Tylenol; Zaramol; ***S.Afr.:*** Antalgic; Arcanagesic†; Brunomol; Calpol; Dolorol; Doxypol†; Dynadol†; Empaped; Entalgic†; Farmacetamol†; Fevamol; Go-Pain P; Junior Disprin; Maxadol-P†; Medpramol†; Merck-Gesic; Napamol; Pacimol; Painamol; Pamol†; Panado; Prolief; Pyradol; Tylenol; Winpain; ***Singapore:*** Acet; Biogesic; Calpol; Childrens Panadol Drops for Infants; Dhamol; Fibrexin; Milidon; Napa; Naprex; Pacemol; Panadol; Poro; Rapidol; Remedol; Setamol†; Tempra†; ***Spain:*** Acertol; Actron; Akindol†; Analter†; Antidol; Apiretal; Aspac†; Asplin†; Bandol; Calmanticold; Cupanol; Dafalgan; Dolefin Paracetamol†; Dolgesic; Dolostop; Duorol; Efferalgan; Eftazid†; Febranine†; Febrectal; Gelocatil; Hedex†; Melabon Infantil; Nofedol†; Panadol; Pediapirin; Pirinasol†; Resakal; Sinmol; Stopain†; Temperal; Tempra†; Termalgin; Tylenol; Zatinol†; ***Swed.:*** Alvedon; Curadon; Lemsip†; Panodil; Reliv; ***Switz.:*** Acetalgine; Becetamol; Ben-u-ron; Comprimes analgesiques no 534†; Contre-Douleurs P; Dafalgan; Democyl; Demogripal; Dolprone; Douleurs & Fievre; Fortalidon P†; Influbene N; Nina; Ortensan†; Panadol; Rivodol; Spalt N†; Termalgin†; Treupel N†; Treuphadol; Tylenol; Zolben; ***Thai.:*** Aceta-P; Acetasil; Algogen; Biogesic; Calpol; Cemol; Daga; Detamol; Fenn; Kit-Syrup; Lotemp; Nutamol; Panadol; Paracap; Paracet; Paramol; Paramol TP; Paranal; Paranal-L; Parat; Paratol; Partamol; Pemol; Pyracon; Pyretal; Ramol; Sara; Saridon†; Temolan†; Tempra; Tumdi; Tylenol; Tymol; Unimol; Vemol; Xebramol; ***UAE:*** Adol; ***UK:*** Abdine Cold Relief; Alvedon; Anadin Paracetamol; Boots Pain Relief Suspension 6 Years Plus; Calpol; Disprol; Elkamol†; Fanalgic†; Fennings Childrens Cooling Powders; Galpamol; Hedex; Infadrops; Mandanol; Medinol; Miradol; Obimol; Pain Relief Syrup for Children†; Paldesic; Panadol; Panaleve; Paracets; Paraclear; Paramin†; Parapaed; Perfalgan; Salzone; Tixymol†; ***USA:*** Acephen; Aceta; Apacet; Apap; Apra; Arthritis Pain Formula Aspirin Free; Aspirin Free Anacin; Aspirin Free Pain Relief; Bromo Seltzer; Childrens Dynafed Jr; Childrens Mapap; Dolono; Dynafed EX; Feverall; Genapap; Genebs; Halenol; Infantaire; Liquiprin; Mapap; Maranox; Meda; Oraphen-PD; Panadol; Panitone; Redutemp; Ridenol; Silapap; Tapanol; Tempra; Tylenol; UN-Aspirin; Uni-Ace.

**Multi-ingredient:** numerous preparations are listed in Part 3.

## Parecoxib Sodium *(BANM, USAN, rINNM)*

Parecoxib sódico; SC-69124A. *N*-{[*p*-(5-Methyl-3-phenyl-4-isoxazolyl)phenyl]sulfonyl}propionamide sodium.

$C_{19}H_{17}N_2NaO_4S = 392.4$.

*CAS — 198470-84-7 (parecoxib); 197502-82-2 (parecoxib sodium).*

*ATC — M01AH04.*

**Incompatibility.** Parecoxib sodium should not be mixed with products other than those recommended by the manufacturer (see Uses and Administration, below). In particular, the use of lactated Ringer's solution with or without glucose will cause parecoxib to precipitate. Parecoxib should also not be given in the same syringe as opioids. The use of sterile water for injection is not recommended as the resulting solution is not isotonic.

### Adverse Effects and Precautions

As for NSAIDs in general, p.67. Hypersensitivity reactions, including anaphylaxis and angioedema and serious skin reactions, have been reported with valdecoxib and may therefore occur with parecoxib, a prodrug of valdecoxib. Some of these reactions occurred in patients with a history of allergic reactions to sulfonamides and the use of parecoxib is contra-indicated in such patients. Parecoxib should also be avoided in patients with severe hepatic impairment, inflammatory bowel disease, and severe heart failure.

Parecoxib should be used with caution following coronary artery bypass graft surgery as there may be an increased risk of adverse effects such as stroke, renal impairment, and wound complications, especially in obese patients or those with a history of stroke. Caution is also recommended when using parecoxib in dehydrated patients; rehydration may be advisable before giving parecoxib.

**Effects on the cardiovascular system.** The selective cyclo-oxygenase-2 (COX-2) inhibitors such as parecoxib do not possess the intrinsic antiplatelet activity associated with aspirin (and possibly other non-selective NSAIDs), and consequently do not provide protection against ischaemic cardiac events.

**Effects on the gastrointestinal tract.** It is generally accepted that the inhibition of cyclo-oxygenase-1 (COX-1) results in the adverse gastrointestinal effects of the NSAIDs, and that the selective inhibition of the other isoform, COX-2, by NSAIDs such as parecoxib may cause less gastrotoxicity than that seen with the non-selective inhibition of the traditional NSAIDs. However, the manufacturers report that upper gastrointestinal perforation, ulceration, and bleeds have occurred with parecoxib treatment and therefore it should be used with caution in patients with a history of such events.

### Interactions

For interactions associated with NSAIDs, see p.69. Parecoxib is rapidly hydrolysed to its active metabolite, valdecoxib; for interactions associated with valdecoxib, see p.96.

### Pharmacokinetics

Following intravenous or intramuscular injection, parecoxib is rapidly hydrolysed in the liver to its active metabolite, valdecoxib, and propionic acid. The plasma half-life of parecoxib is about 22 minutes. No unchanged parecoxib is found in the urine with only trace amounts in the faeces. The pharmacokinetics of valdecoxib are discussed on p.96.

◊ References.

1. Karim A, *et al.* A pharmacokinetic study of intramuscular (IM) parecoxib sodium in normal subjects. *J Clin Pharmacol* 2001; **41:** 1111–19.

### Uses and Administration

Parecoxib is an NSAID (p.70) reported to be a selective inhibitor of cyclo-oxygenase-2 (COX-2). It is a prodrug of valdecoxib (p.96) and is used in the short-term treatment of postoperative pain. Parecoxib is given as the sodium salt although doses are expressed as the base; 42.4 mg of parecoxib sodium is equivalent to 40 mg of parecoxib base. The recommended dose is 40 mg given by intravenous or slow intramuscular injection; this may be followed by 20 or 40 mg every 6 to 12 hours as required. The maximum daily dose is 80 mg. Elderly patients weighing less than 50 kg should begin treatment with half the usual dose, repeated to a maximum of 40 mg daily. Doses may need to be reduced in hepatic impairment, see below.

Parecoxib should be reconstituted with either glucose 5% or sodium chloride 0.45% with glucose 5%; no other solvents are recommended by the manufacturer. In addition the reconstituted solution may only be injected into intravenous lines delivering sodium chloride 0.9%, glucose 5%, sodium chloride 0.45% with glucose 5%, or lactated Ringer's solution. (See above for details on incompatibilities.)

◊ References.

1. Cheer SM, Goa KL. Parecoxib (parecoxib sodium). *Drugs* 2001; **61:** 1133–41.

**Administration in hepatic impairment.** The UK manufacturer states that no dosage adjustment is generally necessary for parecoxib in patients with *mild* hepatic impairment. For those with *moderate* impairment parecoxib should be given at half the usual dose (see above), repeated to a maximum dose of 40 mg daily. Use in patients with *severe* impairment is not recommended as there is no clinical experience in such patients.

### Preparations

**Proprietary Preparations** (details are given in Part 3)

***Austral.:*** Dynastat; ***Irl.:*** Dynastat; ***Norw.:*** Dynastat; ***Port.:*** Dynastat; ***UK:*** Dynastat.

## Pentazocine *(BAN, USAN, rINN)*

NIH-7958; NSC-107430; Pentazocina; Pentazocinum; Win-20228. (2*R**,6*R**,11*R**)-1,2,3,4,5,6-Hexahydro-6,11-dimethyl-3-(3-methylbut-2-enyl)-2,6-methano-3-benzazocin-8-ol.

$C_{19}H_{27}NO = 285.4$.

*CAS — 359-83-1.*

*ATC — N02AD01.*

**Pharmacopoeias.** In *Eur.* (see p.vi), *Jpn*, and *US*.

**Ph. Eur. 5.0** (Pentazocine). A white or almost white powder. It shows polymorphism. Practically insoluble in water; soluble in alcohol; freely soluble in dichloromethane. Protect from light.

**USP 27** (Pentazocine). A white or very pale, tan-coloured powder. Practically insoluble in water; soluble 1 in 11 of alcohol, 1 in 2 of chloroform, and 1 in 42 of ether; soluble in acetone; sparingly soluble in ethyl acetate and in benzene. Store in airtight containers. Protect from light.

## Pentazocine Hydrochloride *(BANM, USAN, rINNM)*

Hidrocloruro de pentazocina; Pentazocini Hydrochloridum.

$C_{19}H_{27}NO,HCl = 321.9$.

*CAS — 2276-52-0; 64024-15-3.*

**Pharmacopoeias.** In *Eur.* (see p.vi) and *US*.

**Ph. Eur. 5.0** (Pentazocine Hydrochloride). A white or almost white powder. It shows polymorphism. Sparingly soluble in water and in dichloromethane; soluble in alcohol. A 1% solution in water has a pH of 4.0 to 6.0. Protect from light.

**USP 27** (Pentazocine Hydrochloride). A white crystalline powder. It exhibits polymorphism, one form melting at about 254° and the other at about 218°. Soluble 1 in 30 of water, 1 in 20 of alcohol, and 1 in 4 of chloroform; very slightly soluble in acetone and in ether; practically insoluble in benzene. Store in airtight containers. Protect from light.

## Pentazocine Lactate *(BANM, USAN, rINNM)*

Lactato de pentazocina.

$C_{19}H_{27}NO,C_3H_6O_3 = 375.5$.

*CAS — 17146-95-1.*

**Pharmacopoeias.** In *Br. US* includes only Pentazocine Lactate Injection.

**BP 2003** (Pentazocine Lactate). A white to pale cream powder. Sparingly soluble in water, in alcohol, and in chloroform; freely soluble in methyl alcohol. A 1% solution in water has a pH of 5.5 to 6.5.

**Incompatibility.** Commercial injections of pentazocine lactate are reported to be incompatible with soluble barbiturates and other alkaline substances including sodium bicarbonate. Diazepam and chlordiazepoxide have also been reported to be incompatible, as have glycopyrronium bromide[1] and nafcillin sodium.[2]

1. Ingallinera TS, *et al.* Compatibility of glycopyrrolate injection with commonly used infusion solutions and additives. *Am J Hosp Pharm* 1979; **36:** 508–10.
2. Jeglum EL, *et al.* Nafcillin sodium incompatibility with acidic solutions. *Am J Hosp Pharm* 1981; **38:** 462, 464.

### Dependence and Withdrawal

As for Opioid Analgesics, p.71. Pentazocine is subject to abuse.

◊ Pentazocine does produce physical dependence, but withdrawal symptoms are substantially less severe than with morphine. It does not typically produce drug-seeking behaviour of the same degree or intensity as morphine or other prototypic μ agonists, nor does it substitute for morphine in dependent subjects.[1] Pentazocine injection has been abused,[2] but street abuse, especially in the USA, has more often involved the intravenous use of crushed tablets of pentazocine and tripelennamine ('T's and Blues').[3-5] A decreased incidence of pentazocine abuse in the USA appeared to coincide with the introduction of oral tablets incorporating naloxone,[1] the rationale being that naloxone antagonises the effect of pentazocine if illicitly injected, but has no effect when taken by mouth. Some continued to abuse the new pentazocine/naloxone formulation;[6] intravenous abuse in one woman, who was unaware of the reformulation, resulted in opioid withdrawal symptoms and severe hypertension.[7] A 1989 report from the WHO committee[1] rated the likelihood of abuse of pentazocine as moderate, based on its pharmacological profile, dependence potential, and actual abuse. The committee considered that it should continue to be scheduled as a psychotropic substance rather than a narcotic drug.

1. WHO. WHO expert committee on drug dependence: twenty-fifth report. *WHO Tech Rep Ser 775* 1989.
2. Hunter R, Ingram IM. Intravenous pentazocine abuse by a nurse. *Lancet* 1983; **ii:** 227.
3. Poklis A, Whyatt PL. Current trends in the abuse of pentazocine and tripelennamine: the metropolitan St. Louis experience. *J Forensic Sci* 1980; **25:** 72–8.
4. Senay EC. Clinical experience with T's and B's. *Drug Alcohol Depend* 1985; **14:** 305–11.
5. Jackson C, *et al.* Fatal intracranial hemorrhage associated with phenylpropanolamine, pentazocine, and tripelennamine overdose. *J Emerg Med* 1985; **3:** 127–32.

6. Reed DA, Schnoll SH. Abuse of pentazocine-naloxone combination. *JAMA* 1986; **256:** 2562–4.
7. Reinhart S, Barrett SM. An acute hypertensive response after intravenous use of a new pentazocine formulation. *Ann Emerg Med* 1985; **14:** 591–3.

### Adverse Effects

As for Opioid Analgesics in general, p.72.

Pentazocine may cause hallucinations and other psychotomimetic effects such as nightmares and thought disturbances. High doses may result in hypertension and tachycardia; increased aortic and pulmonary artery pressure with an increase in cardiac work has followed intravenous use in patients with myocardial infarction. Like morphine it causes respiratory depression, but pentazocine is said to have a 'ceiling' effect and the depth of respiratory depression does not increase proportionately with higher doses.

Rare adverse effects with pentazocine have included agranulocytosis and toxic epidermal necrolysis.

Pentazocine injections may be painful. Local tissue damage may occur at injection sites particularly after subcutaneous injection or multiple doses; there have been reports of muscle fibrosis associated with intramuscular injections.

**Effects on the blood.** There have been reports of agranulocytosis associated with pentazocine.[1-3]

1. Marks A, Abramson N. Pentazocine and agranulocytosis. *Ann Intern Med* 1980; **92:** 433.
2. Haibach H, *et al.* Pentazocine-induced agranulocytosis. *Can Med Assoc J* 1984; **130:** 1165–6.
3. Sheehan M, *et al.* Pentazocine-induced agranulocytosis. *Can Med Assoc J* 1985; **132:** 1401.

**Effects on the CNS.** Oculogyric crisis has been associated with the use of pentazocine.[1]

1. Burstein AH, Fullerton T. Oculogyric crisis possibly related to pentazocine. *Ann Pharmacother* 1993; **27:** 874–6.

**Effects on the skin.** Toxic epidermal necrolysis in a 62-year-old man was attributed to pentazocine;[1] he had taken 50 to 75 mg every 4 hours for 8 days. His severe uraemia was attributed to fluid loss through the skin.

1. Hunter JAA, Davison AM. Toxic epidermal necrolysis associated with pentazocine therapy and severe reversible renal failure. *Br J Dermatol* 1973; **88:** 287–90.

### Treatment of Adverse Effects

As for Opioid Analgesics in general, p.72. As pentazocine has both opioid agonist and antagonist activity its effects may not be completely reversed by naloxone, but use of the latter is still recommended in pentazocine overdosage.

### Precautions

As for Opioid Analgesics in general, p.72.

Pentazocine has weak opioid antagonist actions and may precipitate withdrawal symptoms if given to patients who are physically dependent on opioids. It should generally be avoided after myocardial infarction and in patients with heart failure or arterial or pulmonary hypertension.

When frequent injections are needed, pentazocine should be given intramuscularly rather than subcutaneously and the injection sites should be varied.

**Abuse.** See under Dependence and Withdrawal, above.

**Porphyria.** Pentazocine has been associated with acute attacks of porphyria and is considered unsafe in porphyric patients.

### Interactions

For interactions associated with opioid analgesics, see p.73.

**Tobacco smoking.** Smokers metabolised about 40% more pentazocine than non-smokers, although there was large inter-subject variation;[1] tobacco smoking might induce liver enzymes responsible for drug oxidation.[1]

1. Vaughan DP, *et al.* The influence of smoking on the inter-subject variation in pentazocine elimination. *Br J Clin Pharmacol* 1976; **3:** 279–83.

### Pharmacokinetics

Pentazocine is absorbed from the gastrointestinal tract; after a dose by mouth, peak plasma concentrations are reached in 1 to 3 hours and the half-life is reported to be about 2 to 3 hours. After intramuscular injection, peak plasma concentrations are reached in 15 minutes to 1 hour. About 60% has been reported to be bound to plasma protein. Pentazocine undergoes extensive first-pass metabolism in the liver; oral bioavailability is low with only about half of a dose reaching the systemic circulation. Metabolites and a small amount of unchanged drug are excreted in the urine. It crosses the placenta and is distributed into breast milk.

**Hepatic impairment.** Clearance of pentazocine was significantly reduced and terminal half-life and oral bioavailability increased in cirrhotic patients when compared with healthy subjects.[1]

1. Neal EA, *et al.* Enhanced bioavailability and decreased clearance of analgesics in patients with cirrhosis. *Gastroenterology* 1979; **77:** 96–102.

### Uses and Administration

Pentazocine, a benzomorphan derivative, is an opioid analgesic (p.73) that has mixed opioid agonist and antagonist actions. Agonist activity is thought to be predominantly at $\kappa$ opioid receptors (with possibly some $\sigma$ receptor activity); it acts as a weak antagonist or partial agonist at $\mu$ receptors. Pentazocine is used for the relief of moderate to severe pain. Combined preparations with paracetamol or aspirin may also be used in the treatment of moderate pain. It may also be used for pre-operative sedation and as an adjunct to anaesthesia. Its analgesic effect declines more rapidly than that of morphine.

Pentazocine is given orally as the hydrochloride; doses may be expressed as either the base or the salt. Pentazocine is also given by subcutaneous, intramuscular, and intravenous injection as the lactate; doses are expressed in terms of the base. Pentazocine 100 mg is approximately equivalent to 112.8 mg of pentazocine hydrochloride or 131.6 mg of pentazocine lactate.

A usual oral dose is the equivalent of 50 to 100 mg of pentazocine or pentazocine hydrochloride every 3 to 4 hours after food, to a maximum of 600 mg daily. Children aged 6 to 12 years may be given 25 mg every 3 to 4 hours.

The usual dose by subcutaneous, intramuscular, or intravenous injection is the equivalent of pentazocine 30 to 60 mg every 3 to 4 hours; it should not be necessary to exceed 360 mg daily. Also if frequent injections are needed, the intramuscular route should be used rather than the subcutaneous route, and the injection sites should be varied. In the USA single intravenous doses of not more than 30 mg are advised.

Children aged 1 to 12 years may be given doses of up to 1 mg/kg by subcutaneous or intramuscular injection or up to 500 micrograms/kg by intravenous injection.

Pentazocine is also given rectally as the lactate in suppositories usually in a dose equivalent to pentazocine 50 mg up to 4 times daily.

As a deterrent to abuse a combined oral preparation of pentazocine hydrochloride and naloxone hydrochloride is available in some countries.

### Preparations

***BP 2003:*** Pentazocine Capsules; Pentazocine Injection; Pentazocine Suppositories; Pentazocine Tablets;
***USP 27:*** Pentazocine and Naloxone Hydrochlorides Tablets; Pentazocine Hydrochloride and Aspirin Tablets; Pentazocine Lactate Injection.

**Proprietary Preparations** (details are given in Part 3)
***Austral.:*** Fortral; ***Austria:*** Fortral; ***Belg.:*** Fortal; ***Canad.:*** Talwin; ***Denm.:*** Fortral; ***Fr.:*** Fortal; ***Ger.:*** Fortral; ***Gr.:*** Fortal; ***India:*** Fortwin; Pentawin; ***Irl.:*** Fortral†; ***Israel:*** Rafazocine; Talwin; Talwin NX; ***Ital.:*** Pentalgina†; Talwin; ***Jpn:*** Peltazon; Pentagin; Sosegon; ***Neth.:*** Fortral; ***Norw.:*** Fortralin; ***NZ:*** Fortral; ***Port.:*** Sosegon; ***S.Afr.:*** Ospronim†; Sosenol; ***Singapore:*** Talwin†; ***Spain:*** Sosegon; ***Swed.:*** Fortalgesic†; ***Switz.:*** Fortalgesic; ***Thai.:*** Fortwin; Pangon; Sosegon; ***UK:*** Fortral; ***USA:*** Talwin; Talwin NX.

**Multi-ingredient:** ***India:*** Expergesic; Foracet; ***Irl.:*** Fortagesic; ***Israel:*** Rafazocine X†; ***USA:*** Emergent-Ez; Talacen; Talwin Compound.

---

## Pethidine Hydrochloride *(BANM, rINNM)*

Hidrocloruro de petidina; Meperidine Hydrochloride; Pethidini Hydrochloridum. Ethyl 1-methyl-4-phenylpiperidine-4-carboxylate hydrochloride.

$C_{15}H_{21}NO_2,HCl = 283.8.$

*CAS — 57-42-1 (pethidine); 50-13-5 (pethidine hydrochloride).*

*ATC — N02AB02.*

**Pharmacopoeias.** In *Chin., Eur.* (see p.vi), *Int., Jpn, Pol., US,* and *Viet.*

**Ph. Eur. 5.0** (Pethidine Hydrochloride). A white crystalline powder. Very soluble in water; freely soluble in alcohol. Store in airtight containers. Protect from light.

**USP 27** (Meperidine Hydrochloride). A fine white odourless crystalline powder. Very soluble in water; soluble in alcohol; sparingly soluble in ether. pH of a 5% solution in water is about 5. Store at a temperature of 25°, excursions permitted between 15° and 30°. Protect from light.

**Incompatibility.** Solutions of pethidine hydrochloride are acidic. They are incompatible with barbiturate salts and loss of clarity was also observed in an early additive study[1] with other drugs including aminophylline, heparin sodium, meticillin sodium, morphine sulfate, nitrofurantoin sodium, phenytoin sodium, sodium iodide, sulfadiazine sodium, and sulfafurazole diolamine. Colour change from pale yellow to light green occurred when solutions of minocycline hydrochloride or tetracycline hydrochloride were mixed with pethidine hydrochloride in 5% glucose injection.[2] In the same study an immediate precipitate occurred on admixture with cefoperazone sodium or mezlocillin sodium; with nafcillin sodium an immediate cloudy appearance cleared on agitation. Incompatibility has also been observed between pethidine hydrochloride and aciclovir sodium, imipenem, furosemide,[3] liposomal doxorubicin hydrochloride,[4] and idarubicin.[5] Solutions of cefazolin sodium[6] and pethidine hydrochloride mixed in 5% glucose injection turned light yellow after 5 days storage at 25°; the admixture was stable for at least 20 days at 4°.

1. Patel JA, Phillips GL. A guide to physical compatibility of intravenous drug admixtures. *Am J Hosp Pharm* 1966; **23:** 409–11.
2. Nieves-Cordero AL, *et al.* Compatibility of narcotic analgesic solutions with various antibiotics during simulated Y-site injection. *Am J Hosp Pharm* 1985; **42:** 1108–9.
3. Pugh CB, *et al.* Visual compatibility of morphine sulfate and meperidine hydrochloride with other injectable drugs during simulated Y-site injection. *Am J Hosp Pharm* 1991; **48:** 123–5.
4. Trissel LA, *et al.* Compatibility of doxorubicin hydrochloride liposome injection with selected other drugs during simulated Y-site administration. *Am J Health-Syst Pharm* 1997; **54:** 2708–13.
5. Turowski RC, Durthaler JM. Visual compatibility of idarubicin hydrochloride with selected drugs during simulated Y-site injection. *Am J Hosp Pharm* 1991; **48:** 2181–4.
6. Lee DKT, *et al.* Stability of cefazolin sodium and meperidine hydrochloride. *Am J Health-Syst Pharm* 1996; **53:** 1608–10.

**Stability.** Pethidine hydrochloride injection 100 mg/mL was stable[1] for at least 24 hours at room temperature when diluted to a concentration of 300 mg/litre in glucose 5% and 4% and in sodium chloride injection (0.9%) and sodium chloride injection (0.9%) diluted 1 in 5.

Accelerated stability studies using elevated temperatures and humidities to simulate tropical conditions classified pethidine hydrochloride as a 'less stable drug substance'.[2] It was suggested that during quality assurance of preparations containing pethidine hydrochloride particular attention should be paid to their stability.

1. Rudd L, Simpson P. Pethidine stability in intravenous solutions. *Med J Aust* 1978; **2:** 34.
2. WHO. WHO expert committee on specifications for pharmaceutical preparations: thirty-first report. *WHO Tech Rep Ser 790* 1990.

### Dependence and Withdrawal

As for Opioid Analgesics, p.71. Doses of pethidine as large as 3 or 4 g daily have been taken by addicts. As tolerance to the CNS stimulant and antimuscarinic effects is not complete with these very large doses, muscle twitching, tremor, mental confusion, dilated pupils, and sometimes convulsions may be present.

Withdrawal symptoms appear more rapidly than with morphine and are of shorter duration.

For the abuse of pethidine analogues, see under Precautions, below.

### Adverse Effects and Treatment

As for Opioid Analgesics in general, p.72.

The effects on smooth muscle may be relatively less intense than with morphine and constipation occurs less frequently. Local reactions often follow injection of pethidine; general hypersensitivity reactions occur rarely. Pethidine given intravenously may increase the heart rate. After overdosage, symptoms are generally similar to those of morphine poisoning. However, stimulation of the CNS and convulsions may also occur, especially in tolerant individuals or after toxic doses by mouth; these have been attributed mainly to the metabolite norpethidine.

**Incidence of adverse effects.** The incidence of adverse effects in hospitalised patients receiving pethidine was monitored by the Boston Collaborative Drug Surveillance Program.[1] Following pethidine by mouth adverse reactions were reported in 16 of 366 patients and mainly involved the gastrointestinal tract. Following pethidine by injection 102 of 3268 patients had adverse effects, the CNS being involved in 38.

1. Miller RR, Jick H. Clinical effects of meperidine in hospitalized medical patients. *J Clin Pharmacol* 1978; **18:** 180–9.

**Effects on the cardiovascular system.** Histamine release was more frequent after pethidine than after morphine, fentanyl, or sufentanil given intravenously for the induction of anaesthesia.[1] Increased plasma-histamine concentrations occurred in 5 of 16 patients given pethidine in a mean dose of 4.3 mg/kg and were generally accompanied by hypotension, tachycardia, erythema, and increased plasma-adrenaline concentrations. Only 1 of 10 given morphine and none of those receiving fentanyl or sufentanil showed evidence of histamine release. All of the histamine releasers were young women.

1. Flacke JW, *et al.* Histamine release by four narcotics: a double-blind study in humans. *Anesth Analg* 1987; **66:** 723–30.

**Effects on the nervous system.** CNS excitatory effects of pethidine such as tremors, muscle twitches, and convulsions have been associated with toxic doses and have been attributed to the metabolite norpethidine. Accumulation of norpethidine may occur if large doses of pethidine are repeated at short intervals (including for patient-controlled analgesia) and is especially likely when renal function is impaired.[1-13]

1. Kaiko RF, *et al.* Central nervous system excitatory effects of meperidine in cancer patients. *Ann Neurol* 1983; **13:** 180–5.
2. Lieberman AN, Goldstein M. Reversible parkinsonism related to meperidine. *N Engl J Med* 1985; **312:** 509.
3. Mauro VF, *et al.* Meperidine-induced seizure in a patient without renal dysfunction or sickle cell anemia. *Clin Pharm* 1986; **5:** 837–9.
4. Morisy L, Platt D. Hazards of high-dose meperidine. *JAMA* 1986; **255:** 467–8.
5. Armstrong PJ, Bersten A. Normeperidine toxicity. *Anesth Analg* 1986; **65:** 536–8.
6. Eisendrath SJ, *et al.* Meperidine-induced delirium. *Am J Psychiatry* 1987; **144:** 1062–5.
7. Kyff JV, Rice TL. Meperidine-associated seizures in a child. *Clin Pharm* 1990; **9:** 337–8.
8. Pryle BJ, *et al.* Toxicity of norpethidine in sickle cell crisis. *BMJ* 1992; **304:** 1478–9.
9. Hagmeyer KO, *et al.* Meperidine-related seizures associated with patient-controlled analgesia pumps. *Ann Pharmacother* 1993; **27:** 29–32.
10. Stone PA, *et al.* Norpethidine toxicity and patient controlled analgesia. *Br J Anaesth* 1993; **71:** 738–40.
11. Marinella MA. Meperidine-induced generalized seizures with normal renal function. *South Med J* 1997; **90:** 556–8.

12. McHugh GJ. Norpethidine accumulation and generalized seizure during pethidine patient-controlled analgesia. *Anaesth Intensive Care* 1999; **27:** 289–91.
13. Hubbard GP, Wolfe KR. Meperidine misuse in a patient with sphincter of Oddi dysfunction. *Ann Pharmacother* 2003; **37:** 534–7.

## Precautions

As for Opioid Analgesics in general, p.72. Pethidine should also be given cautiously to patients with a history of convulsive disorders.

**Abuse.** A synthetic analogue of pethidine, MPPP (1-methyl-4-phenyl-4-propionoxypiperidine), manufactured illicitly for recreational use, achieved notoriety when it was accidentally contaminated with MPTP (1-methyl-4-phenyl-1,2,3,6-tetrahydropyridine) leading to an epidemic of parkinsonism among intravenous drug abusers.[1] WHO has also identified another analogue, PEPAP (1-phenylethyl-4-phenyl-4-acetoxypiperidine) as being liable to abuse.[2]

1. Buchanan JF, Brown CR. 'Designer drugs': a problem in clinical toxicology. *Med Toxicol* 1988; **3:** 1–17.
2. WHO. WHO expert committee on drug dependence: twenty-fourth report. *WHO Tech Rep Ser 761* 1988.

**Breast feeding.** No adverse effects have been observed in breast-feeding infants whose mothers were receiving pethidine, and the American Academy of Pediatrics considers[1] that it is therefore usually compatible with breast feeding.

1. American Academy of Pediatrics. The transfer of drugs and other chemicals into human milk. *Pediatrics* 2001; **108:** 776–89. Correction. *ibid.*; 1029. Also available at: http://aappolicy.aappublications.org/cgi/content/full/pediatrics%3b108/3/776 (accessed 06/07/04)

**The elderly.** Pethidine had a slower elimination rate in elderly compared with young patients and a reduction in total daily dose might be necessary in elderly patients receiving repeated doses of pethidine.[1] Another study concluded that age-related changes in disposition were not sufficient to warrant modification of pethidine dosage regimens.[2]

1. Holmberg L, *et al.* Comparative disposition of pethidine and norpethidine in old and young patients. *Eur J Clin Pharmacol* 1982; **22:** 175–9.
2. Herman RJ, *et al.* Effects of age on meperidine disposition. *Clin Pharmacol Ther* 1985; **37:** 19–24.

**Phaeochromocytoma.** Pethidine provoked episodes of hypertension in a patient with phaeochromocytoma; the effect was suppressed by labetalol.[1] Like other histamine-releasing opioids, pethidine should be used with caution in such patients.

1. Lawrence CA. Pethidine-induced hypertension in phaeochromocytoma. *BMJ* 1978; **1:** 149–50.

**Pregnancy and the neonate.** Pethidine is widely used for analgesia during labour. It rapidly crosses the placenta and like other opioid analgesics may cause respiratory depression in the neonate although this may be less than with morphine. Respiratory depression varies according to the timing and size of the maternal dose.

Fetal depression was not apparent when delivery occurred within 1 hour of giving pethidine, but was present in 6 of 24 infants delivered 1 to 3 hours after injection and in all of 5 infants delivered 3 to 6 hours after injection.[1] However, higher blood concentrations of pethidine were seen in infants delivered within 1 hour of an intramuscular dose of pethidine compared with those delivered 1 to 4 hours after injection. The role of pethidine metabolites was uncertain. It has also been reported[2] that depressed neonatal responses persisted for the first 2 days of life; depression was dose-related being greatest with the highest dose of pethidine (75 to 150 mg within 4 hours of delivery). Neonates appear able to metabolise pethidine, although probably more slowly than adults.[3] The amounts of pethidine and norpethidine excreted by the neonate increased significantly with the maternal dose-delivery interval for intervals of up to 5 hours and most of the placentally transferred pethidine should be excreted by the third day. Elimination of pethidine took up to 6 days in the neonates in another study.[4]

Further references on the transplacental transfer of pethidine can be found under Pregnancy in Pharmacokinetics, below.

Neither psychological nor physical effects were found in 5-year-olds born to mothers who had received pethidine during labour.[5] Neonatal behaviour does not appear to have been affected significantly by pethidine, although it has been acknowledged that the relationship between maternal analgesia in labour and subsequent infant behaviour is by no means simple.[6] The results of early studies which suggested an excess of cases of cancer in children whose mothers received pethidine during labour have been refuted by a later and larger study.[7]

1. Morrison JC, *et al.* Metabolites of meperidine related to fetal depression. *Am J Obstet Gynecol* 1973; **115:** 1132–7.
2. Hodgkinson R, *et al.* Double-blind comparison of the neurobehaviour of neonates following the administration of different doses of meperidine to the mother. *Can Anaesth Soc J* 1978; **25:** 405–11.
3. Hogg MIJ, *et al.* Urinary excretion and metabolism of pethidine and norpethidine in the newborn. *Br J Anaesth* 1977; **49:** 891–9.
4. Cooper LV, *et al.* Elimination of pethidine and bupivacaine in the newborn. *Arch Dis Child* 1977; **52:** 638–41.
5. Buck C. Drugs in pregnancy. *Can Med Assoc J* 1975; **112:** 1285.
6. Anonymous. To measure life. *Lancet* 1981; **ii:** 291–2.
7. Golding J, *et al.* Childhood cancer, intramuscular vitamin K, and pethidine given during labour. *BMJ* 1992; **305:** 341–6.

**Renal impairment.** Caution is necessary when pethidine is given to patients with renal impairment; some UK manufacturers recommend that it should be avoided if impairment is severe. Evidence of CNS excitation, including seizures and twitches, in 2 patients with renal insufficiency receiving multiple doses of pethidine was attributed to accumulation of the metabolite norpethidine; both patients had high norpethidine : pethidine plasma concentration ratios.[1]

See also under Pharmacokinetics, below.

1. Szeto HH, *et al.* Accumulation of normeperidine, an active metabolite of meperidine, in patients with renal failure or cancer. *Ann Intern Med* 1977; **86:** 738–41.

## Interactions

For interactions associated with opioid analgesics, see p.73.

Very severe reactions, including coma, severe respiratory depression, cyanosis, and hypotension have occurred in patients receiving MAOIs (including moclobemide and selegiline) and given pethidine. There are also reports of hyperexcitability, convulsions, tachycardia, hyperpyrexia, and hypertension. Pethidine should not be given to patients receiving MAOIs or within 14 days of their discontinuation. Use of pethidine with phenothiazines has produced severe hypotensive episodes and may prolong the respiratory depression due to pethidine.

Plasma concentrations of norpethidine are increased by ritonavir, with a resultant risk of toxicity; use together should be avoided (see also p.73).

**Barbiturates.** Opioid analgesics and barbiturates can be expected to have additive CNS depressant effects. Prolonged sedation with pethidine in the presence of *phenobarbital* has also been attributed to induction of *N*-demethylation of pethidine, resulting in the enhanced formation of the potentially neurotoxic metabolite norpethidine.[1,2]

1. Stambaugh JE, *et al.* A potentially toxic drug interaction between pethidine (meperidine) and phenobarbitone. *Lancet* 1977; **i:** 398–9.
2. Stambaugh JE, *et al.* The effect of phenobarbital on the metabolism of meperidine in normal volunteers. *J Clin Pharmacol* 1978; **18:** 482–90.

**Histamine $H_2$-antagonists.** *Cimetidine* reduced the clearance and volume of distribution of pethidine in healthy subjects,[1] whereas ranitidine did not.[2]

1. Guay DRP, *et al.* Cimetidine alters pethidine disposition in man. *Br J Clin Pharmacol* 1984; **18:** 907–14.
2. Guay DRP, *et al.* Ranitidine does not alter pethidine disposition in man. *Br J Clin Pharmacol* 1985; **20:** 55–9.

**MAOIs.** Some of the most serious interactions involving pethidine have been with non-selective MAOIs and have been manifest as enhanced depressant effects or hyperexcitability (see above). However, a life-threatening interaction has also been reported between pethidine and *selegiline*, a selective monoamine oxidase type B inhibitor.[1] Also, symptoms suggestive of a mild serotonin syndrome developed in a 73-year-old woman taking *moclobemide* (a reversible inhibitor of monoamine oxidase type A), nortriptyline, and lithium after she was given pethidine intravenously.[2]

1. Zornberg GL, *et al.* Severe adverse interaction between pethidine and selegiline. *Lancet* 1991; **337:** 246. Correction. *ibid.*; 440.
2. Gillman PK. Possible serotonin syndrome with moclobemide and pethidine. *Med J Aust* 1995; **162:** 554.

**Phenothiazines.** *Prochlorperazine* prolonged the respiratory depressant effect of pethidine in healthy subjects.[1] Enhanced CNS depression and hypotension were reported when healthy subjects were given *chlorpromazine* in addition to pethidine; there was evidence of increased *N*-demethylation of pethidine.[2]

1. Steen SN, Yates M. Effects of benzquinamide and prochlorperazine, separately and combined with meperidine, on the human respiratory center. *Clin Pharmacol Ther* 1972; **13:** 153.
2. Stambaugh JE, Wainer IW. Drug interaction: meperidine and chlorpromazine, a toxic combination. *J Clin Pharmacol* 1981; **21:** 140–6.

**Phenytoin.** The hepatic metabolism of pethidine appears to be enhanced by phenytoin; use together resulted in reduced half-life and bioavailability in healthy subjects; blood concentrations of norpethidine were increased.[1]

1. Pond SM, Kretschzmar KM. Effect of phenytoin on meperidine clearance and normeperidine formation. *Clin Pharmacol Ther* 1981; **30:** 680–6.

## Pharmacokinetics

Pethidine hydrochloride is absorbed from the gastrointestinal tract, but only about 50% of the drug reaches the systemic circulation because of first-pass metabolism. Absorption following intramuscular injection is variable. Peak plasma concentrations have been reported 1 to 2 hours after oral doses. It is about 60 to 80% bound to plasma proteins.

Pethidine is metabolised in the liver by hydrolysis to pethidinic acid (meperidinic acid) or demethylation to norpethidine (normeperidine) and hydrolysis to norpethidinic acid (normeperidinic acid), followed by partial conjugation with glucuronic acid. Norpethidine is pharmacologically active and its accumulation may result in toxicity. Pethidine is reported to have a plasma elimination half-life of about 3 to 6 hours in healthy subjects; the metabolite norpethidine is eliminated more slowly, with a half-life reported to be up to about 20 hours. Both pethidine and norpethidine appear in the CSF. At the usual values of urinary pH or if the urine is alkaline, only a small amount of pethidine is excreted unchanged; urinary excretion of pethidine and norpethidine is enhanced by acidification of the urine. Pethidine crosses the placenta and is distributed into breast milk.

◊ Reviews.

1. Edwards DJ, *et al.* Clinical pharmacokinetics of pethidine: 1982. *Clin Pharmacokinet* 1982; **7:** 421–33.
2. Moore RA, *et al.* Opiate metabolism and excretion. *Baillieres Clin Anaesthesiol* 1987; **1:** 829–58.

**Administration.** The elimination half-life of pethidine was prolonged and plasma clearance decreased when given perioperatively compared with postoperatively.[1]

During labour the pharmacokinetics of pethidine may depend on how it is given. In a comparison of intramuscular injection at different sites, absorption of pethidine from the gluteus muscle was impaired and the deltoid muscle was preferred.[2]

No statistically significant differences were found in pharmacokinetic parameters for deltoid and gluteal intramuscular injections in elderly postoperative patients.[3] However, substantial interpatient variability was noted for both sites, and the authors suggested that more rapid and predictable routes such as intravenous injection may be more appropriate for postoperative use in the elderly.

1. Tamsen A, *et al.* Patient-controlled analgesic therapy, part 1: pharmacokinetics of pethidine in the per- and postoperative periods. *Clin Pharmacokinet* 1982; **7:** 149–63.
2. Lazebnik N, *et al.* Intravenous, deltoid, or gluteus administration of meperidine during labor? *Am J Obstet Gynecol* 1989; **160:** 1184–9.
3. Erstad BL, *et al.* Site-specific pharmacokinetics and pharmacodynamics of intramuscular meperidine in elderly postoperative patients. *Ann Pharmacother* 1997; **31:** 23–8.

**Hepatic impairment.** The terminal half-life of pethidine was prolonged to about 7 hours in cirrhotic patients compared with 3 hours in healthy subjects, which was attributed to impairment of the drug-metabolising activity of the liver.[1] Another study concluded that although impaired hepatic metabolism might confer relative protection from norpethidine toxicity in patients with cirrhosis, there might be an increased risk of cumulative toxicity because of slow elimination of the metabolite.[2]

1. Klotz U, *et al.* The effect of cirrhosis on the disposition and elimination of meperidine in man. *Clin Pharmacol Ther* 1974; **16:** 667–75.
2. Pond SM, *et al.* Presystemic metabolism of meperidine to normeperidine in normal and cirrhotic subjects. *Clin Pharmacol Ther* 1981; **30:** 183–8.

**Pregnancy.** Some references to the pharmacokinetics of pethidine during labour are given below.

1. Tomson G, *et al.* Maternal kinetics and transplacental passage of pethidine during labour. *Br J Clin Pharmacol* 1982; **13:** 653–9.
2. Kuhnert BR, *et al.* Disposition of meperidine and normeperidine following multiple doses during labor: I mother. *Am J Obstet Gynecol* 1985; **151:** 406–9.
3. Kuhnert BR, *et al.* Disposition of meperidine and normeperidine following multiple doses during labor: II fetus and neonate. *Am J Obstet Gynecol* 1985; **151:** 410–15.

**Renal impairment.** Plasma protein binding of pethidine was reported to be decreased in renal disease and ranged from 58.2% in healthy subjects to 31.8% in anuric patients.[1] The same workers also reported prolonged elimination of pethidine in patients with renal dysfunction.[2]

See also under Precautions, above.

1. Chan K, *et al.* Plasma protein binding of pethidine in patients with renal disease. *J Pharm Pharmacol* 1983; **35:** 94P.
2. Chan K, *et al.* Pharmacokinetics of low-dose intravenous pethidine in patients with renal dysfunction. *J Clin Pharmacol* 1987; **27:** 516–22.

## Uses and Administration

Pethidine, a phenylpiperidine derivative, is a synthetic opioid analgesic (p.73) that acts mainly as a μ opioid agonist. Pethidine is used for the relief of most types of moderate to severe acute pain including the pain of labour. It is more lipid soluble than morphine and has a less potent and shorter lasting analgesic effect; analgesia usually lasts for 2 to 4 hours. Its short duration of action and accumulation of its potentially neurotoxic metabolite norpethidine on repeated administration make it unsuitable for the management of chronic pain. Pethidine has a weaker action on smooth muscle than morphine and its lower potential to increase biliary pressure may make it a more suitable opioid analgesic for pain associated with biliary colic and pancreatitis (but see p.73). It is also used as pre-operative medication and as an adjunct to anaesthesia. It has been given with phenothiazines such as promethazine to achieve basal narcosis. Pethidine has little effect on cough or on diarrhoea.

For the relief of **pain**, pethidine hydrochloride is given in doses of 50 to 150 mg by mouth every 4 hours. It may also be given by intramuscular or subcutaneous injection in doses of 25 to 100 mg and by slow intravenous injection in doses of 25 to 50 mg repeated after 4 hours. For *postoperative* pain the subcutaneous or intramuscular doses may be given every 2 to 3 hours if necessary. In children, doses of 0.5 to 2 mg/kg may be given by mouth or by intramuscular injection.

In *obstetric analgesia* 50 to 100 mg may be given by intramuscular or subcutaneous injection as soon as contractions occur at regular intervals. This dose may be repeated after 1 to 3 hours if necessary up to a maximum of 400 mg in 24 hours.

For **pre-operative** medication 25 to 100 mg may be given intramuscularly or subcutaneously about 1 hour before surgery; children may be given 0.5 to 2 mg/kg. As an adjunct to nitrous oxide-oxygen anaesthesia 10 to 25 mg may be given by slow intravenous injection.

**Administration.** In addition to conventional routes of administration pethidine has been given epidurally[1-4] and intrathecally.[5,6] It has also been given via various routes as a patient-controlled system.[7-10] However, some consider that the use of pethidine should be avoided for patient-controlled analgesia because of the increased risk of norpethidine-induced seizures[11] (see also under Effects on the Nervous System, above).

1. Perriss BW. Epidural pethidine in labour: a study of dose requirements. *Anaesthesia* 1980; **35:** 380–2.
2. Husemeyer RP, *et al.* A study of pethidine kinetics and analgesia in women in labour following intravenous, intramuscular and epidural administration. *Br J Clin Pharmacol* 1982; **13:** 171–6.
3. Perriss BW, *et al.* Analgesia following extradural and im pethidine in post-caesarean section patients. *Br J Anaesth* 1990; **64:** 355–7.
4. Blythe JG, *et al.* Continuous postoperative epidural analgesia for gynecologic oncology patients. *Gynecol Oncol* 1990; **37:** 307–10.
5. Acalovschi I, *et al.* Saddle block with pethidine for perineal operations. *Br J Anaesth* 1986; **58:** 1012–16.
6. Yu SC, *et al.* Addition of meperidine to bupivacaine for spinal anaesthesia for caesarean section. *Br J Anaesth* 2002; **88:** 379–83.
7. Striebel HW, *et al.* Patient-controlled intranasal analgesia (PCINA) for the management of postoperative pain: a pilot study. *J Clin Anesth* 1996; **8:** 4–8.
8. Kee N, *et al.* Comparison of patient-controlled epidural analgesia with patient-controlled intravenous analgesia using pethidine or fentanyl. *Anaesth Intensive Care* 1997; **25:** 126–32.
9. Sharma SK, *et al.* Cesarean delivery: a randomized trial of epidural versus patient-controlled meperidine analgesia during labor. *Anesthesiology* 1997; **87:** 487–94.
10. Chen PP, *et al.* Patient-controlled pethidine after major upper abdominal surgery: comparison of the epidural and intravenous routes. *Anaesthesia* 2001; **56:** 1106–12.
11. Hagmeyer KO, *et al.* Meperidine-related seizures associated with patient-controlled analgesia pumps. *Ann Pharmacother* 1993; **27:** 29–32.

**Eclampsia and pre-eclampsia.** See Lytic Cocktails under Sedation, below.

**Pain.** Pethidine produces prompt but short-lasting analgesia, and may be preferred to morphine when rapid control of acute pain is required. It is widely used in obstetrics to control the pain of labour (although the *British National Formulary* notes that morphine or other opioids are often preferred for obstetric pain), and for postoperative pain relief following caesarean section or other surgical procedures.

In a study of patients with intractable pain the minimum effective analgesic blood concentration ranged from 100 to 820 nanograms/mL (median 250 nanograms/mL) in 15 of 16; the remaining patient failed to obtain analgesia with pethidine. Additional measures were considered necessary[1] if the minimum effective concentration exceeded 400 nanograms/mL.

Pethidine has traditionally been given by intermittent intramuscular injection in the treatment of acute pain, but inconsistent pain relief can be expected because of fluctuating blood-pethidine concentrations;[2] continuous intravenous infusion might be more effective for acute pain. For reference to various routes of administration, see Administration, above.

1. Mather LE, Glynn CJ. The minimum effective analgesic blood concentration of pethidine in patients with intractable pain. *Br J Clin Pharmacol* 1982; **14:** 385–90.
2. Edwards DJ, *et al.* Clinical pharmacokinetics of pethidine: 1982. *Clin Pharmacokinet* 1982; **7:** 421–33.

SICKLE-CELL CRISIS. Concern has been expressed over the continued use of pethidine for analgesia in painful crises in sickle-cell disease. Control of pain may be inadequate and doses commonly used to manage crises may lead to accumulation of the neuroexcitatory metabolite of pethidine and precipitate seizures.[1,2] See also under Effects on the Nervous System, above.

1. Pryle BJ, *et al.* Toxicity of norpethidine in sickle cell crisis. *BMJ* 1992; **304:** 1478–9.
2. Harrison JFM, *et al.* Pethidine in sickle cell crisis. *BMJ* 1992; **305:** 182.

**Sedation.** Some references to the use of pethidine for endoscopy are given below.

1. Bahal-O'Mara N, *et al.* Sedation with meperidine and midazolam in pediatric patients undergoing endoscopy. *Eur J Clin Pharmacol* 1994; **47:** 319–23.
2. Diab FH, *et al.* Efficacy and safety of combined meperidine and midazolam for EGD sedation compared with midazolam alone. *Am J Gastroenterol* 1996; **91:** 1120–5.
3. Laluna L, *et al.* The comparison of midazolam and topical lidocaine spray versus the combination of midazolam, meperidine, and topical lidocaine spray to sedate patients for upper endoscopy. *Gastrointest Endosc* 2001; **53:** 289–93.

LYTIC COCKTAILS. Lytic cocktails consisting of chlorpromazine, pethidine, and/or promethazine have been given intravenously in some countries for the management of pre-eclampsia and imminent eclampsia. However, the use of phenothiazines is generally not recommended late in pregnancy, and other treatments are preferred for hypertension (see Hypertension in Pregnancy, under Hypertension, p.825); the management of eclampsia, which is the convulsive phase, is discussed on p.352. Lytic cocktails have also been used for sedation and analgesia in children, by intramuscular or occasionally intravenous injection. However, there is a high rate of therapeutic failure as well as serious adverse effects with such combinations, and the American Academy of Pediatrics[1] has recommended that alternative sedatives and analgesics should be considered; guidelines have been drawn up should it be appropriate to use a lytic cocktail. Lytic cocktails are not the most appropriate means of sedation for short procedures since patients must be monitored for about 1 hour before the procedure while the drugs take effect, and for even longer during the recovery period.[2]

1. American Academy of Pediatrics Committee on Drugs. Reappraisal of Lytic cocktail/Demerol, Phenergan, and Thorazine (DPT) for the sedation of children. *Pediatrics* 1995; **95:** 598–602.
2. Barst SM, *et al.* A comparison of propofol and Demerol-Phenergan-Thorazine for brief, minor, painful procedures in a pediatric hematology-oncology clinic. *Int J Pediatr Hematol/Oncol* 1995; **1:** 587–91.

**Shivering.** For reference to the use of pethidine in the management of shivering associated with anaesthesia, see under Adverse Effects of General Anaesthetics, p.1295. Pethidine has also been used to treat amphotericin B-induced shaking chills.[1]

1. Burks LC, *et al.* Meperidine for the treatment of shaking chills and fever. *Arch Intern Med* 1980; **140:** 483–4.

## Preparations

***BP 2003:*** Pethidine Injection; Pethidine Tablets;
***USP 27:*** Meperidine Hydrochloride Injection; Meperidine Hydrochloride Syrup; Meperidine Hydrochloride Tablets.

**Proprietary Preparations** (details are given in Part 3)
***Arg.:*** Cluyer; Meperol; ***Austria:*** Alodan; ***Belg.:*** Dolantine; ***Braz.:*** Demerol†; Dolantina; Dolosal; ***Canad.:*** Demerol; ***Chile:*** Demerol; ***Fr.:*** Dolosal†; ***Ger.:*** Dolantin; ***Israel:*** Dolestine; ***Spain:*** Dolantina; ***Switz.:*** Centralgine†; ***USA:*** Demerol.

**Multi-ingredient:** ***Austral.:*** Marcain with Pethidine; ***NZ:*** Marcain with Pethidine†; ***UK:*** Pamergan P100; ***USA:*** Atropine and Demerol†; Mepergan†.

## Phenacetin *(rINN)*

Aceto-*p*-phenetidide; Acetophenetidin; Acetylphenetidin; Fenacetina; Paracetophenetidin; Phenacetinum. *p*-Acetophenetidide; 4′-Ethoxyacetanilide; *N*-(4-Ethoxyphenyl)acetamide.

$C_{10}H_{13}NO_2$ = 179.2.
*CAS — 62-44-2.*
*ATC — N02BE03.*

**Pharmacopoeias.** In *Jpn.*

### Adverse Effects and Precautions

Phenacetin may cause methaemoglobinaemia, sulfhaemoglobinaemia, and haemolytic anaemia.

Prolonged use of large doses of analgesic mixtures containing phenacetin has been associated with the development of renal papillary necrosis (see Effects on the Kidneys, p.68) and transitional-cell carcinoma of the renal pelvis.

**Porphyria.** Phenacetin is considered to be unsafe in patients with porphyria because it has been shown to be porphyrinogenic in *animals.*

### Uses and Administration

Phenacetin, a para-aminophenol derivative, has analgesic and antipyretic properties. It was usually given with aspirin, caffeine, or codeine but is now little used because of adverse haematological effects and nephrotoxicity.

## Phenazocine Hydrobromide *(BANM, rINNM)*

Hidrobromuro de fenazocina. 1,2,3,4,5,6-Hexahydro-6,11-dimethyl-3-phenethyl-2,6-methano-3-benzazocin-8-ol hydrobromide hemihydrate.

$C_{22}H_{27}NO,HBr,\frac{1}{2}H_2O$ = 411.4.
*CAS — 127-35-5 (phenazocine); 1239-04-9 (anhydrous phenazocine hydrobromide).*
*ATC — N02AD02.*

### Profile

Phenazocine hydrobromide is an opioid analgesic (p.71). It is considered to be less sedating than morphine and has a weaker action on smooth muscle. It was given by mouth or sublingually for the relief of severe pain.

### Preparations

**Proprietary Preparations** (details are given in Part 3)
***UK:*** Narphen†.

## Phenazone *(BAN, rINN)*

Analgésine; Antipyrin; Antipyrine; Azophenum; Fenazona; Phenazonum; Phenyldimethylpyrazolone. 1,5-Dimethyl-2-phenyl-4-pyrazolin-3-one.

$C_{11}H_{12}N_2O$ = 188.2.
*CAS — 60-80-0.*
*ATC — N02BB01.*

**Pharmacopoeias.** In *Eur.* (see p.vi), *Jpn,* and *US.*

**Ph. Eur. 5.0** (Phenazone). White or almost white crystalline powder or colourless crystals. Very soluble in water, in alcohol, and in dichloromethane. Protect from light.

**USP 27** (Antipyrine). Colourless crystals or white crystalline powder. Is odourless. Very soluble in water; freely soluble in alcohol and in chloroform; sparingly soluble in ether. Solutions are neutral to litmus. Store in airtight containers.

## Phenazone and Caffeine Citrate

Antipyrino-Coffeinum Citricum; Fenazona y citrato de cafeína; Migrenin; Phenzone and Caffeine Citrate.

**Description.** Phenazone and caffeine citrate is a powder usually containing phenazone 90%, caffeine 9%, and citric acid monohydrate 1%.

**Pharmacopoeias.** In *Jpn.*

## Phenazone Salicylate

Antipyrin Salicylate; Fenazona salicilato; Salipyrin.

$C_{11}H_{12}N_2O,C_7H_6O_3$ = 326.3.
*CAS — 520-07-0.*

**Pharmacopoeias.** In *Fr.*

### Adverse Effects and Precautions

Phenazone is liable to give rise to skin eruptions and in susceptible individuals even small doses may have this effect. Hypersensitivity reactions and nephrotoxicity have been reported. Large doses by mouth may cause nausea, drowsiness, coma, and convulsions.

**Effects on the blood.** Phenazone can cause haemolytic anaemia in certain individuals with a deficiency of G6PD.[1] Episodes of agranulocytosis were reported[2] in 6 women using a cream containing phenazone; all recovered on withdrawal.

1. Prankerd TAJ. Hemolytic effects of drugs and chemical agents. *Clin Pharmacol Ther* 1963; **4:** 334–50.
2. Delannoy A, Schmit J-C. Agranulocytosis after cutaneous contact with phenazone. *Eur J Haematol* 1993; **50:** 124.

**Effects on the kidneys.** Phenazone is considered nephrotoxic but only limited clinical information on phenazone is available because it has been mainly used in association with phenacetin.[1]

1. Prescott LF. Analgesic nephropathy: a reassessment of the role of phenacetin and other analgesics. *Drugs* 1982; **23:** 75–149.

**Effects on the skin.** In a summary[1] of 77 cases of fixed drug eruption phenazone derivatives were considered to be the causative agent in 9 of the 14 cases that were severe generalised reactions.

1. Stubb S, *et al.* Fixed drug eruptions: 77 cases from 1981 to 1985. *Br J Dermatol* 1989; **120:** 583.

**Hypersensitivity.** Immediate allergic reactions to phenazone have been reported.[1,2] In one patient leucopenia was detected 8 weeks later.[1]

1. Kadar D, Kalow W. Acute and latent leukopenic reaction to antipyrine. *Clin Pharmacol Ther* 1980; **28:** 820–22.
2. McCrea JB, *et al.* Allergic reaction to antipyrine, a marker of hepatic enzyme activity. *DICP Ann Pharmacother* 1989; **23:** 38–40.

**Porphyria.** Phenazone is considered to be unsafe in patients with porphyria because it has been shown to be porphyrinogenic in *animals.*

### Interactions

Phenazone affects the metabolism of some other drugs and its own metabolism is affected by other drugs that increase or reduce the activity of liver enzymes.

### Pharmacokinetics

Phenazone is absorbed from the gastrointestinal tract and peak plasma concentrations are obtained within 1 to 2 hours of ingestion. It is distributed throughout the body fluids with concentrations in the saliva and breast milk reaching about the same levels as those in plasma. Less than 10% is bound to plasma proteins and it has an elimination half-life of about 12 hours. Phenazone is metabolised in the liver to 3 major metabolites, 3-hydroxymethylphenazone, 4-hydroxyphenazone, and norphenazone. Phenazone, 3-hydroxymethylphenazone, and glucuronidated metabolites are all excreted in the urine. A small portion may be eliminated via the bile.

## Uses and Administration

Phenazone is an NSAID (p.70) and has been given by mouth; phenazone and caffeine citrate and phenazone salicylate have similarly been given by mouth as analgesics.

Solutions containing about 5% of phenazone have been used topically as ear drops in disorders such as acute otitis media (but see below).

Phenazone is used as a test for the activity of drug-metabolising enzymes in the liver.

**Diagnosis and testing.** A review[1] of normal plasma-phenazone pharmacokinetics, urinary metabolite disposition, and total body clearances of phenazone in the presence of cirrhosis, fatty liver, hepatitis, and cholestatis.

1. St Peter JV, Awni WM. Quantifying hepatic function in the presence of liver disease with phenazone (antipyrine) and its metabolites. *Clin Pharmacokinet* 1991; **20:** 50–65.

**Otitis media.** There seems to be no justification[1] for the inclusion of phenazone in topical preparations used in treating acute otitis media (p.138). It is presumably included in such preparations because it is believed to have a local anti-inflammatory and, therefore, analgesic action. It would, however, seem unlikely that phenazone would have any action on the skin of the intact tympanic membrane and, therefore, on the pain which is due primarily to the stretching and distention of the membrane.

1. Carlin WV. Is there any justification for using phenazone in a local application prescribed for the treatment of acute otitis media? *BMJ* 1987; **294:** 1333.

## Preparations

***USP 27:*** Antipyrine and Benzocaine Otic Solution; Antipyrine, Benzocaine, and Phenylephrine Hydrochloride Otic Solution.

**Proprietary Preparations** (details are given in Part 3)
***Austral.:*** Erasol†; ***Ger.:*** Aequiton-P; Eu-Med†; Migrane-Kranit mono; ***Irl.:*** Tropex; ***S.Afr.:*** Aurone; Oto-Phen; ***Swed.:*** Spalt N†.

**Multi-ingredient:** ***Arg.:*** Bajumol; Cristalomicina; Irix; Kalopsis; Leroid; Otalex G; Otoclean Gotas Oticas; Otocuril; Otonorthia; Sincerum; ***Austral.:*** Auralgan; ***Austria:*** Asthma Efeum; Coffo Selt; Otalgan; Spalt; ***Belg.:*** Otalgan†; Otipax†; Otocalmine; Ouate Hemostatique; Parmentier†; Tympalgine; ***Braz.:*** Anestesiol; Auditol†; Espasmalgon; Osmotil†; Otovix†; ***Canad.:*** Auralgan; ***Denm.:*** Koffisal; ***Fr.:*** Brulex; HEC; Otipax; Ovules Sedo-Hemostatiques du Docteur Jouve†; ***Ger.:*** Coffeemed N; Felsol Neo†; Migranin; Otalgan; Otodolor†; Titralgan; ***India:*** Tytin; ***Israel:*** Anaesthetic Ear Drops; Otidin; ***Ital.:*** Otalgan; Otomidone; Otopax; ***Norw.:*** Antineuralgica; Codalgin†; Fanalgin; ***NZ:*** Auralgan; Degest 2; ***Port.:*** Otalgan†; Otipax†; Otocalma; Profrin-A; ***S.Afr.:*** Auralgicin†; Aurasept; Aurone Forte; Covancaine; Ilvico; Otised; Oto-Phen Forte; Universal Earache Drops†; ***Singapore:*** HEC†; Tropex; ***Spain:*** AB FE; Epistaxol; Hemostatico Antisep Asen†; Otalgan; Otosedol; Pomada Heridas; Quimpedor; Tabletas Quimpe; ***Swed.:*** Doleron; Koffazon; ***Switz.:*** Otalgan; Otipax; Otosan; Otothricinol; Seranex sans codeine; Spedralgin sans codeine; Spirogel†; ***Thai.:*** Auralgan; ***USA:*** Allergen; Auralgan; Auroguard Otic; Auroto; Cy-Gesic; Otocalm; Tympagesic.

---

# Phenazopyridine Hydrochloride *(BANM, USAN, rINNM)*

Chloridrato de Fenazopiridina; Hidrocloruro de fenazopiridina; NC-150; NSC-1879; W-1655. 3-Phenylazopyridine-2,6-diyldiamine hydrochloride.

$C_{11}H_{11}N_5,HCl = 249.7$.

*CAS — 94-78-0 (phenazopyridine); 136-40-3 (phenazopyridine hydrochloride).*

*ATC — G04BX06.*

**Pharmacopoeias.** In *Pol.* and *US.*

**USP 27** (Phenazopyridine Hydrochloride). A light or dark red to dark violet crystalline powder. Is odourless or with a slight odour. Soluble 1 in 300 of cold water, 1 in 20 of boiling water, 1 in 59 of alcohol, 1 in 331 of chloroform, and 1 in 100 of glycerol; very slightly soluble in ether. Store in airtight containers.

**Removal of stains.** Phenazopyridine stains may be removed from fabric by soaking in a 0.25% solution of sodium dithionite.

## Adverse Effects

Phenazopyridine hydrochloride has caused gastrointestinal side-effects, headache, and rashes. Hepatotoxicity, haemolytic anaemia, methaemoglobinaemia, and acute renal failure have also been reported, generally associated with overdosage or with therapeutic doses in patients with renal impairment. Crystal deposits of phenazopyridine have formed in the urinary tract.

Abnormal coloration of body tissues or fluids may occur. Urine is tinged either orange or red and underclothes are apt to be stained.

**Effects on the CNS.** A case of aseptic meningitis, with distinct episodes of fever and confusion, was associated with the administration of phenazopyridine.[1]

1. Herlihy TE. Phenazopyridine and aseptic meningitis. *Ann Intern Med* 1987; **106:** 172–3.

## Precautions

Phenazopyridine hydrochloride is contra-indicated in patients with impaired renal function or severe hepatitis and should be used with caution in those with G6PD deficiency. Treatment should be discontinued if the skin or sclerae become discoloured; this may indicate accumulation as a result of impaired renal excretion. Phenazopyridine may interfere with urinalysis based on colour reactions or spectrometry.

Staining of contact lenses may occur.

## Pharmacokinetics

Phenazopyridine hydrochloride is absorbed from the gastrointestinal tract. It is excreted mainly in the urine; up to 65% may be excreted as unchanged phenazopyridine and 18% as paracetamol.

## Uses and Administration

Phenazopyridine is an azo dye that exerts an analgesic effect on the mucosa of the urinary tract and is used to provide symptomatic relief of pain and irritability in conditions such as cystitis and prostatitis (see under Urinary-tract Infections, p.153), and urethritis (p.152). Phenazopyridine hydrochloride has been given by mouth in usual doses of about 200 mg three times daily after food. It may be given with an antibacterial for the treatment of urinary-tract infections, usually for up to 2 days, although lower doses have been given as part of a combined preparation for at least a week.

**Urinary-tract infections.** There is currently no well-substantiated role for phenazopyridine in the treatment of urinary-tract infections and its adverse effects are potentially serious.[1]

1. Zelenitsky SA, Zhanel GG. Phenazopyridine in urinary tract infections. *Ann Pharmacother* 1996; **30:** 866–8.

## Preparations

***USP 27:*** Phenazopyridine Hydrochloride Tablets.

**Proprietary Preparations** (details are given in Part 3)
***Arg.:*** Cistalgina; ***Belg.:*** Uropyrine†; ***Braz.:*** Pyridium; Urologin; Urotril; ***Canad.:*** Phenazo; Pyridium; ***Chile:*** Nazamit; Nordox; Pyridium; ***Hong Kong:*** Phenazo†; Pyridium; ***India:*** Pyridium; ***Israel:*** Sedural; ***Mex.:*** Bioferina; Pirimir; Umizan†; ***S.Afr.:*** Pyridium; ***Singapore:*** Urogesic; ***Thai.:*** Amilazo; Anazo; Phendiridine; Sumedium; ***USA:*** Azo-Standard; Baridium; Prodium; Pyridiate; Pyridium; Re-Azo; Urogesic.

**Multi-ingredient:** ***Arg.:*** Bacti-Uril; Nor 2; Priper Plus; Urisept NF; Urobactrim; ***Austria:*** Gastrotest†; ***Braz.:*** Azo-Wintomylon†; Mictrex†; Mina-zol; Uretil†; Urizal†; Uro Bac Septin†; Uro Bactrim†; Uro Batrox†; Uro Duoctrim†; Uro Heractrim†; Uro Septoprin†; Uro-Bacteracin†; Uro-Baxapril; Uro-Leotrim†; Uro-Septiolan†; Uro-Teutrim†; Urobactrex†; Urobioctrin†; Urobiotic; Uroctrin; Urofar†; Urofen; Uromix†; Uroneotrim†; Uropac; Uropielon; Uropirite†; Uropol; Uroseptin†; Uroxazol†; Utrim†; ***Chile:*** Uro-Micinovo; ***Ger.:*** Urospasmon; ***India:*** Nephrogesic; ***Mex.:*** Azo-Gen; Azo-Wintomylon; Nalixone; Naxilan-Plus; Pirifur; Urovec; ***Spain:*** Micturol Sedante; ***USA:*** Pyridium Plus; Urelief Plus; Urobiotic-250.

---

# Phenicarbazide *(rINN)*

Fenicarbazida; Phenylsemicarbazide. 1-Phenylsemicarbazide.

$C_7H_9N_3O = 151.2$.

*CAS — 103-03-7.*

## Profile

Phenicarbazide has analgesic properties. It has been given by mouth and rectally.

---

# Phenoperidine Hydrochloride *(BANM, rINNM)*

Hidrocloruro de fenoperidina; R-1406. Ethyl 1-(3-hydroxy-3-phenylpropyl)-4-phenylpiperidine-4-carboxylate hydrochloride.

$C_{23}H_{29}NO_3,HCl = 403.9$.

*CAS — 562-26-5 (phenoperidine); 3627-49-4 (phenoperidine hydrochloride).*

*ATC — N01AH04.*

## Profile

Phenoperidine hydrochloride is an opioid analgesic (p.71) related to pethidine (p.80). It has been used to produce surgical analgesia and also to induce neuroleptanalgesia. It has also been given as an analgesic and respiratory depressant in patients requiring long-term assisted ventilation in intensive care.

## Preparations

**Proprietary Preparations** (details are given in Part 3)
***Swed.:*** Lealgin†.

---

# Phenylbutazone *(BAN, rINN)*

Butadione; Fenilbutazona; Phenylbutazonum. 4-Butyl-1,2-diphenylpyrazolidine-3,5-dione.

$C_{19}H_{20}N_2O_2 = 308.4$.

*CAS — 50-33-9 (phenylbutazone); 129-18-0 (phenylbutazone sodium); 4985-25-5 (phenylbutazone piperazine).*

*ATC — M01AA01; M02AA01.*

**Pharmacopoeias.** In *Eur.* (see p.vi), *Jpn, Pol.,* and *US.*

**Ph. Eur. 5.0** (Phenylbutazone). A white or almost white, crystalline powder. Practically insoluble in water; sparingly soluble in alcohol; it dissolves in alkaline solutions. Protect from light.

**USP 27** (Phenylbutazone). A white to off-white, odourless, crystalline powder. Very slightly soluble in water; soluble in alcohol; freely soluble in acetone and in ether. Store in airtight containers.

## Adverse Effects

Nausea, vomiting, epigastric distress, diarrhoea, oedema due to salt and water retention, skin rashes, dizziness, drowsiness, headache, and blurred vision may occur with phenylbutazone. More serious reactions include gastric irritation with ulceration and gastrointestinal bleeding, ulcerative stomatitis, hepatitis, jaundice, haematuria, nephritis, renal failure, pancreatitis, ocular toxicity, and goitre. Phenylbutazone may precipitate heart failure and may also cause an acute pulmonary syndrome with dyspnoea and fever. Salivary gland enlargement (parotitis), hypersensitivity reactions including asthma, and severe generalised reactions including lymphadenopathy, erythema multiforme, Stevens-Johnson syndrome, toxic epidermal necrolysis, and exfoliative dermatitis have been reported.

The most serious adverse effects of phenylbutazone are related to bone-marrow depression and include agranulocytosis and aplastic anaemia. Leucopenia, pancytopenia, haemolytic anaemia, and thrombocytopenia may also occur. These adverse haematological reactions have resulted in the indications for use of phenylbutazone being restricted (see under Uses and Administration, below). Blood disorders may develop soon after starting treatment or may occur suddenly after prolonged treatment, and regular haematological monitoring should be carried out as discussed under Precautions, below.

The adverse effects of NSAIDs in general are described on p.67.

**Effects on the blood.** Both phenylbutazone[1-3] and oxyphenbutazone[1,3] are well known for their adverse effects on the blood and especially for fatal agranulocytosis and aplastic anaemia. The UK Committee on Safety of Medicines[4] noted that between July 1963 and January 1993 it had received 74 reports of agranulocytosis (39 fatal) associated with phenylbutazone and 40 reports of neutropenia (4 fatal). Up-to-date figures were not provided on oxyphenbutazone, but it is considered to be more toxic to the bone marrow than phenylbutazone.[1]

1. Anonymous. Phenylbutazone and oxyphenbutazone: time to call a halt. *Drug Ther Bull* 1984; **22:** 5–6.
2. Böttiger LE, Westerholm B. Drug-induced blood dyscrasias in Sweden. *BMJ* 1973; **3:** 339–43.
3. The International Agranulocytosis and Aplastic Anemia Study. Risks of agranulocytosis and aplastic anemia: a first report of their relation to drug use with special reference to analgesics. *JAMA* 1986; **256:** 1749–57.
4. Committee on Safety of Medicines/Medicines Control Agency. Drug-induced neutropenia and agranulocytosis. *Current Problems* 1993; **19:** 10–11.

## Precautions

Phenylbutazone is contra-indicated in patients with blood disorders or active gastrointestinal disorders such as peptic ulcer disease or inflammatory bowel disease and in those with a history of such disorders. It is also contra-indicated in patients with cardiovascular, pulmonary, or thyroid disease, severe impairment of hepatic or renal function, or a history of hypersensitivity to aspirin or other NSAIDs. It is further contra-indicated in patients with salivary gland disorders or Sjögren's syndrome. It may aggravate systemic lupus erythematosus.

Blood-cell counts should be performed before and regularly during therapy in patients receiving the drug for more than 1 week but should not be relied upon to predict dysplasia; monitoring of hepatic and renal function is also recommended. Patients or their carers should be told to discontinue the drug at the first signs of toxic effects and to report at once the appearance of symptoms such as fever, sore throat, stomatitis, skin rashes, bruising, and weight gain or oedema. Treatment should also be withdrawn if symptoms of the acute pulmonary syndrome, including dyspnoea and fever, develop.

It should be used with caution in elderly patients who may require reduced doses.

Courses of treatment should be kept as short as possible. Dizziness or drowsiness may affect the performance of skilled tasks such as driving.

The precautions to be taken with NSAIDs in general are described on p.69.

**Breast feeding.** No adverse effects have been observed in breast-feeding infants whose mothers were receiving phenylbutazone, and the American Academy of Pediatrics considers[1] that it is therefore usually compatible with breast feeding. However, the *British National Formulary* has advised that phenylbutazone should be avoided during breast feeding as small amounts are distributed into breast milk.

1. American Academy of Pediatrics. The transfer of drugs and other chemicals into human milk. *Pediatrics* 2001; **108:** 776–89. Correction. *ibid.*; 1029. Also available at: http://aappolicy.aappublications.org/cgi/content/full/pediatrics%3b108/3/776 (accessed 06/07/04)

**Porphyria.** Phenylbutazone has been associated with acute attacks of porphyria and is considered unsafe in porphyric patients.

## Interactions

For interactions associated with NSAIDs, see p.69. Like azapropazone, phenylbutazone may be particularly likely to cause interactions with oral anticoagulants such as warfarin. The elimination half-life of phenylbutazone is reduced in patients pretreated with drugs that increase liver microsomal enzyme activity. Use of methylphenidate or anabolic steroids with phenylbutazone may increase the serum concentration of the metabolite oxyphenbutazone. Colestyramine reduces the absorption of phenylbutazone.

**Misoprostol.** A report[1] in 2 patients of side-effects including headaches, dizziness, ambulatory instability, tingles, and transient diplopia suggesting a potentiation of neurological adverse effects attributed to use of phenylbutazone with misoprostol.

1. Jacquemier JM, *et al.* Neurosensory adverse effects after phenylbutazone and misoprostol combined treatment. *Lancet* 1989; **ii:** 1283.

## Pharmacokinetics

Phenylbutazone is readily absorbed from the gastrointestinal tract with peak plasma concentrations occurring about 2 hours after oral ingestion. It is also readily absorbed when administered rectally. Phenylbutazone is widely distributed throughout body fluids and tissues; it diffuses into the synovial fluid, crosses the placenta, and small amounts enter the CNS and breast milk. It is 98% bound to plasma proteins. It is extensively metabolised in the liver by oxidation and by conjugation with glucuronic acid. Oxyphenbutazone, γ-hydroxyphenbutazone, and *p*,γ-dihydroxyphenylbutazone are formed by oxidation but only small amounts appear in urine, the remainder being further metabolised. It is mainly excreted in the urine as metabolites although about a quarter of a dose may be excreted in the faeces. The plasma elimination half-life is about 70 hours but it is subject to large inter-individual variations.

### Uses and Administration

Phenylbutazone, a pyrazolone derivative, is an NSAID (p.70). However, because of its toxicity it is not used as a general analgesic or antipyretic. Although phenylbutazone is effective in almost all musculoskeletal and joint disorders including ankylosing spondylitis, acute gout, osteoarthritis, and rheumatoid arthritis, it should only be used in acute conditions where less toxic drugs have failed. In the UK its use is restricted to the hospital treatment of ankylosing spondylitis unresponsive to other drugs, when the recommended initial dose is 200 mg given by mouth two or three times daily for 2 days. The dose is then reduced to the minimum effective amount, which is usually 200 to 300 mg daily given in divided doses. Treatment should be given for the shortest period possible. Elderly patients may require reduced doses.

In some countries phenylbutazone has also been given as a rectal suppository and applied topically for musculoskeletal pain and in soft-tissue injury. It has also been given intramuscularly as the sodium salt. Other salts of phenylbutazone that have been used in musculoskeletal, joint, and soft-tissue disorders include the calcium, megallate, and piperazine salts.

### Preparations

***USP 27:*** Phenylbutazone Tablets.

**Proprietary Preparations** (details are given in Part 3)
***Austral.:*** Butazolidin†; ***Austria:*** Butazolidin; ***Belg.:*** Butazolidin; ***Braz.:*** Butazolidina; Butazolon; Butazona; Butazonil; Neo Butazol; Peralgin†; ***Canad.:*** Novo-Butazone†; ***Fr.:*** Butazolidine; Carudol†; ***Ger.:*** Ambene; Butazolidin†; Demoplas†; exrheudon OPT; ***Ital.:*** Kadol; ***Mex.:*** Aflamina†; Bloken; Bresal; Butalen; Butazolidina; Delbulasa; Fenibent†; Fezona; Lorfenil; Rudesol†; Tisatin†; ***Neth.:*** Butazolidin; ***Port.:*** Basireuma; ***S.Afr.:*** Inflazone; ***Spain:*** Butazolidina; Carudol†; ***Switz.:*** Butadion; Butazolidine†; ***Thai.:*** Buta; ***UK:*** Butacote†; Butazone†.

**Multi-ingredient:** ***Austria:*** Ambene; Ambene N; ***Braz.:*** Alginflan†; Betazon†; Butapirin†; Butazil; Dorend; Mioflex; Reumat†; Reumix†; ***Chile:*** Balsamo Analgesico con Fenilbutazona; ***Fr.:*** Dextrarine Phenylbutazone; ***Ger.:*** Ambene Comp; ***Hong Kong:*** Trabit†; ***Mex.:*** Butayonacol; Vengesic; Zolidime; ***Spain:*** Artrodesmol Extra; Doctofril Antiinflamat; ***Switz.:*** Butaparin; Carudol†; Hepabuzone; ***Thai.:*** Alaxan; Asialax; Buta Pee Dee; Butarion; Myophen; Neo-Pyrazol; Trabit.

## Picolamine Salicylate *(rINNM)*

Salicilato de picolamina.
*CAS — 3731-52-0 (picolamine).*

### Profile

Picolamine salicylate is a salicylic acid derivative that has been used similarly to methyl salicylate (p.59) in topical rubefacient preparations for the treatment of musculoskeletal, joint, peri-articular, and soft-tissue disorders.

### Preparations

**Proprietary Preparations** (details are given in Part 3)
***Fr.:*** Reflex†.

## Piketoprofen *(rINN)*

Piketoprofeno. *m*-Benzoyl-*N*-(4-methyl-2-pyridyl)hydratropamide.
$C_{22}H_{20}N_2O_2$ = 344.4.
*CAS — 60576-13-8.*

### Profile

Piketoprofen is an NSAID (p.67) that has been used topically as the base or hydrochloride in concentrations of about 2% in musculoskeletal, joint, peri-articular, and soft-tissue disorders.

### Preparations

**Proprietary Preparations** (details are given in Part 3)
***Port.:*** Picalm; Zemalex; ***Spain:*** Calmatel; Triparsean.

## Piritramide *(BAN, rINN)*

Pirinitramide; Piritramida; R-3365. 1-(3-Cyano-3,3-diphenylpropyl)-4-piperidinopiperidine-4-carboxamide.
$C_{27}H_{34}N_4O$ = 430.6.
*CAS — 302-41-0.*
*ATC — N02AC03.*

### Profile

Piritramide is an opioid analgesic (p.71).

It is used for the management of severe pain including postoperative pain, for premedication, and to provide analgesia during anaesthesia. It is given by intramuscular, subcutaneous, or slow intravenous injection as the tartrate in doses equivalent of up to about 30 mg of the base.

◊ Reviews.

1. Kumar N, Rowbotham DJ. Piritramide. *Br J Anaesth* 1999; **82:** 3–5.

**Porphyria.** Piritramide is considered to be unsafe in patients with porphyria because it has been shown to be porphyrinogenic in *animals* or *in vitro* systems.

### Preparations

**Proprietary Preparations** (details are given in Part 3)
***Austria:*** Dipidolor; ***Belg.:*** Dipidolor; ***Ger.:*** Dipidolor; ***Neth.:*** Dipidolor.

## Piroxicam *(BAN, USAN, rINN)*

CP-16171; Piroxicamum. 4-Hydroxy-2-methyl-*N*-(2-pyridyl)-2*H*-1,2-benzothiazine-3-carboxamide 1,1-dioxide.
$C_{15}H_{13}N_3O_4S$ = 331.3.
*CAS — 36322-90-4.*
*ATC — M01AC01; M02AA07; S01BC06.*

**Pharmacopoeias.** In *Chin., Eur.* (see p.vi), *US,* and *Viet.*

**Ph. Eur. 5.0** (Piroxicam). A white or slightly yellow, crystalline powder. It shows polymorphism. Practically insoluble in water; slightly soluble in dehydrated alcohol; soluble in dichloromethane. Store in airtight containers. Protect from light.

**USP 27** (Piroxicam). An off-white to light tan or light yellow, odourless powder. It forms a monohydrate that is yellow. Very slightly soluble in water, in dilute acids, and in most organic solvents; slightly soluble in alcohol and in aqueous alkaline solutions. Store in airtight containers. Protect from light.

## Piroxicam Betadex *(USAN, rINNM)*

CHF-1194; Piroxicam Beta Cyclodextrin; Piroxicam Beta Cyclodextrin Complex.
$(C_{15}H_{13}N_3O_4S)_2,-(C_{42}H_{70}O_{35})_5$ = 6337.6.
*CAS — 96684-40-1.*

### Adverse Effects

As for NSAIDs in general, p.67.

Local irritation and occasionally bleeding may occur with piroxicam suppositories and there may be pain and occasionally tissue damage at the injection site on intramuscular administration.

Piroxicam is considered to be associated with an intermediate risk of gastrointestinal effects although there is some suggestion that the risk may be higher than for other intermediate-risk NSAIDs (p.68). There is little evidence to support the manufacturer's claim that piroxicam betadex has improved gastrointestinal tolerability.

◊ A report[1] of the adverse reactions associated with piroxicam in South Africa during 1981-86 including two reactions, paraesthesia and hair loss, not previously recorded in the literature.

1. Gerber D. Adverse reactions of piroxicam. *Drug Intell Clin Pharm* 1987; **21:** 707–10.

**Effects on the blood.** Decreases in haemoglobin and haematocrit not associated with obvious gastrointestinal bleeding, have occurred in patients taking piroxicam. Thrombocytopenia, thrombocytopenic purpura,[1] and aplastic anaemia[2] have been described in patients on piroxicam.

1. Bjørnstad H, Vik Ø. Thrombocytopenic purpura associated with piroxicam. *Br J Clin Pract* 1986; **40:** 42.
2. Lee SH, *et al.* Aplastic anaemia associated with piroxicam. *Lancet* 1982; **i:** 1186.

**Effects on electrolytes.** Reversible hyperkalaemic hyperchloraemic acidosis has been reported[1,2] in patients receiving piroxicam. Severe hyponatraemia and symptoms resembling the syndrome of inappropriate antidiuretic hormone secretion have also been associated with piroxicam.[3]

See also under Effects on the Kidneys, below.

1. Grossman LA, Moss S. Piroxicam and hyperkalemic acidosis. *Ann Intern Med* 1983; **99:** 282.
2. Miller KP, *et al.* Severe hyperkalemia during piroxicam therapy. *Arch Intern Med* 1984; **144:** 2414–15.
3. Petersson I, *et al.* Water intoxication associated with non-steroidal anti-inflammatory drug therapy. *Acta Med Scand* 1987; **221:** 221–3.

**Effects on the kidneys.** Acute nephropathy with characteristic features of Henoch-Schönlein purpura,[1] acute renal failure,[2] uraemia with hyperkalaemia, and acute interstitial nephritis[3] have been associated with systemic use of piroxicam. Nephrotic syndrome and interstitial nephritis have followed topical use of piroxicam gel.[4]

1. Goebel KM, Mueller-Brodmann W. Reversible overt nephropathy with Henoch-Schönlein purpura due to piroxicam. *BMJ* 1982; **284:** 311–12.
2. Frais MA, *et al.* Piroxicam-induced renal failure and hyperkalemia. *Ann Intern Med* 1983; **99:** 129–30.
3. Mitnick PD, Klein WJ. Piroxicam-induced renal disease. *Arch Intern Med* 1984; **144:** 63–4.
4. O'Callaghan CA, *et al.* Renal disease and use of topical non-steroidal anti-inflammatory drugs. *BMJ* 1994; **308:** 110–11.

**Effects on the liver.** Necrosis of the liver has been associated with piroxicam. Details have been supplied on 3 patients,[1,2] of whom 2 died.

1. Lee SM, *et al.* Subacute hepatic necrosis induced by piroxicam. *BMJ* 1986; **293:** 540–1.
2. Paterson D, *et al.* Piroxicam induced submassive necrosis of the liver. *Gut* 1992; **33;** 1436–8.

**Effects on the skin.** As with other NSAIDs, rash has occurred in patients taking piroxicam. Phototoxic reactions have been described.[1] Serious skin reactions attributed to piroxicam therapy include toxic epidermal necrolysis,[2] pemphigus vulgaris,[3] and Stevens-Johnson syndrome.[4]

1. Stern RS. Phototoxic reactions to piroxicam and other nonsteroidal antiinflammatory agents. *N Engl J Med* 1983; **309:** 186–7.
2. Chosidow O, *et al.* Intestinal involvement in drug-induced toxic epidermal necrolysis. *Lancet* 1991; **337:** 928.
3. Martin RL, *et al.* Fatal pemphigus vulgaris in a patient taking piroxicam. *N Engl J Med* 1983; **309:** 795–6.
4. Katoh N, *et al.* Piroxicam induced Stevens-Johnson syndrome. *J Dermatol* 1995; **22:** 677–80.

**Overdosage.** Details of 16 patients who were considered to have taken an overdosage of piroxicam alone were reported[1] to the National Poisons Information Service of the UK. Thirteen patients (including 5 children) experienced no symptoms after doses estimated to be up to 300 to 400 mg; 2 patients complained of dizziness and blurred vision after 200 to 300 mg; the last patient who claimed to have taken 600 mg presented in coma, regained consciousness within one hour, and had recovered fully within 24 hours. Severe multisystem toxicity has been reported in a 2-year-old child after ingestion of 100 mg of piroxicam.[2]

1. Court H, Volans GN. Poisoning after overdose with non-steroidal anti-inflammatory drugs. *Adverse Drug React Acute Poisoning Rev* 1984; **3:** 1–21.
2. MacDougall LG, *et al.* Piroxicam poisoning in a 2-year-old child: a case report. *S Afr Med J* 1984; **66:** 31–3.

**Pancreatitis.** A report[1] of pancreatitis associated with piroxicam.

1. Haye OL. Piroxicam and pancreatitis. *Ann Intern Med* 1986; **104:** 895.

### Precautions

As for NSAIDs in general, p.69.

**Breast feeding.** No adverse effects have been observed in breast-feeding infants whose mothers were receiving piroxicam, and the American Academy of Pediatrics considers[1] that it is therefore usually compatible with breast feeding. The *British National Formulary* also considers the amount excreted into breast milk to be too small to be harmful to a breast-fed infant.

Piroxicam appears in breast milk in concentrations of about 1% of those in the maternal plasma.[2] Similar data are also included in the manufacturer's product literature although they do not recommend piroxicam use during pregnancy as clinical safety has not been established.

1. American Academy of Pediatrics. The transfer of drugs and other chemicals into human milk. *Pediatrics* 2001; **108:** 776–89. Correction. *ibid.*; 1029. Also available at: http://aappolicy.aappublications.org/cgi/content/full/pediatrics%3b108/3/776 (accessed 06/07/04)
2. Østensen M. Piroxicam in human breast milk. *Eur J Clin Pharmacol* 1983; **25:** 829–30.

**Porphyria.** Piroxicam has been associated with acute attacks of porphyria and is considered unsafe in porphyric patients.

### Interactions

For interactions associated with NSAIDs, see p.69.

Use of aspirin with piroxicam results in decreased plasma concentrations of piroxicam to about 80% of normal. The UK manufacturer of ritonavir suggests that use of piroxicam with ritonavir may result in increased plasma concentrations of piroxicam and an increased risk of toxicity; they recommend that use together should be avoided.

### Pharmacokinetics

Piroxicam is well absorbed from the gastrointestinal tract; peak plasma concentrations are reached 3 to 5 hours after an oral dose. Piroxicam is also absorbed to some degree after topical application. Piroxicam is 99% bound to plasma proteins. It has been detected in breast milk. Piroxicam has a long plasma elimination half-life of about 50 hours. Because of this, steady-state concentrations are not reached for 7 to 12 days. It is metabolised in the liver by hydroxylation and conjugation with glucuronic acid and excreted mainly in the urine with smaller amounts in the faeces. Enterohepatic recycling occurs. Less than 5% of the dose is excreted unchanged in the urine and faeces.

Piroxicam betadex dissociates in the gastrointestinal tract to piroxicam and beta-cyclodextrin. Piroxicam absorption from piroxicam betadex is more rapid than that of unmodified piroxicam; peak plasma concentrations of piroxicam are reached 30 to 60 minutes after an oral dose. Beta-cyclodextrin is not absorbed but is metabolised in the colon to various sugars.

◊ References.


1. Richardson CJ, *et al.* Piroxicam and 5′-hydroxypiroxicam kinetics following multiple dose administration of piroxicam. *Eur J Clin Pharmacol* 1987; **32:** 89–91.
2. Mäkelä A-L, *et al.* Steady state pharmacokinetics of piroxicam in children with rheumatic diseases. *Eur J Clin Pharmacol* 1991; **41:** 79–81 (higher clearance and shorter half-life in children).
3. Rudy AC, *et al.* The pharmacokinetics of piroxicam in elderly persons with and without renal impairment. *Br J Clin Pharmacol* 1994; **37:** 1–5.
4. Deroubaix X, *et al.* Oral bioavailability of CHF1194, an inclusion complex of piroxicam and β-cyclodextrin, in healthy subjects under single dose and steady-state conditions. *Eur J Clin Pharmacol* 1995; **47:** 531–6.
5. Karim A, *et al.* Oxaprozin and piroxicam, nonsteroidal antiinflammatory drugs with long half-lives: effect of protein-binding differences on steady-state pharmacokinetics. *J Clin Pharmacol* 1997; **37:** 267–78.
6. Wang D, *et al.* Comparative population pharmacokinetic-pharmacodynamic analysis for piroxicam-β-cyclodextrin and piroxicam. *J Clin Pharmacol* 2000; **40:** 1257–66.


## Uses and Administration

Piroxicam, an oxicam derivative, and piroxicam betadex are NSAIDs (p.70). Piroxicam betadex may have a more rapid onset of therapeutic effect due to its enhanced solubility (see Pharmacokinetics above). Both are used in musculoskeletal and joint disorders such as ankylosing spondylitis, osteoarthritis, rheumatoid arthritis including juvenile idiopathic arthritis, in soft-tissue disorders, in acute gout, and in postoperative pain.

In rheumatic disorders a usual initial dose of *piroxicam* by mouth is 20 mg daily as a single dose. Daily maintenance doses may vary between 10 and 30 mg given in single or divided doses; use of doses in excess of 20 mg daily for more than a few days is associated with an increased risk of gastrointestinal adverse effects. In acute musculoskeletal conditions an initial dose of 40 mg daily may be given for 2 days followed by 20 mg daily for a total of 1 to 2 weeks. Piroxicam is also used in acute gout, the usual dose being 40 mg daily for 5 to 7 days. In the treatment of postoperative pain following dental or minor surgery, the dose of piroxicam is 20 mg daily; higher doses of 40 mg daily for the first 2 days are recommended following orthopaedic surgery. Piroxicam is given in similar doses as a rectal suppository or on a short-term basis by intramuscular injection.

Piroxicam (given as dispersible tablets) may also be used in children aged 6 years or over with juvenile idiopathic arthritis. The usual dose by mouth is:

- 5 mg once daily in those weighing less than 15 kg
- 10 mg once daily in those weighing 16 to 25 kg
- 15 mg once daily in those weighing 26 to 45 kg
- 20 mg once daily in those weighing 46 kg or over

Piroxicam is also used in the local treatment of a variety of painful or inflammatory conditions as a topical gel in a concentration of 0.5% applied three or four times daily; treatment should be reviewed after 4 weeks. A 1% gel is also available. Piroxicam has been used in some countries as a 0.5 or 1% cream and as eye drops in a concentration of 0.5%.

Doses of piroxicam betadex are expressed in terms of the equivalent amount of piroxicam. Piroxicam betadex 191.3 mg is approximately equivalent to 20 mg of piroxicam. In rheumatic and acute musculoskeletal disorders *piroxicam betadex* is given in a dose equivalent to 20 mg of piroxicam daily as a single dose. This dose may be reduced to 10 mg daily in elderly patients.

*Other salts* or compounds that have also been used include piroxicam cinnamate (cinnoxicam), piroxicam choline, and piroxicam pivalate.

◊ Reviews.


1. Lee CR, Balfour JA. Piroxicam-β-cyclodextrin: a review of its pharmacodynamic and pharmacokinetic properties, and therapeutic potential in rheumatic diseases and pain states. *Drugs* 1994; **48:** 907–29.
2. Edwards JE, *et al.* Single dose piroxicam for acute postoperative pain. Available in The Cochrane Library; Issue 2. Chichester: John Wiley; 2004.


### Preparations

***BP 2003:*** Piroxicam Capsules; Piroxicam Gel;
***USP 27:*** Piroxicam Capsules.

**Proprietary Preparations** (details are given in Part 3)
***Arg.:*** Axis; Benisan; Brionot; Calmapir; Fabopxicam; Feldene; Flogosine; Homocalmefyba; Ketazon; Micar; Nac; Nalgesic; Osteocalmine; Piroalgin; Pirofix; Roxicam; Sindrolen; Solocalm; Tirovel; Tricifa; Truxa; Truxa R; Vefren; Velaned; ***Austral.:*** Candyl; Feldene; Mobilis; Pirohexal-D; Pirox†; Rosig; ***Austria:*** Brexin; Felden; Pirocal; Pirocam; Pirorheum; Pirox; Piroxistad; Piroxityrol; Tonimed; ***Belg.:*** Brexine; Feldene; Solicam; ***Braz.:*** Anartrit; Anflene; Brexin; Cicladol; Feldene; Feldexican†; Feldox; Felnan†; Flamadene†; Flamarene†; Flamostat; Flogene; Flogoxen; Floxicam; Inflamene; Inflanan; Inflanox; Inflax; Lisedema; Piroxene; Piroxifen; Piroxiflam; Piroxil; Piroxiplus; Prodoxidil; ***Canad.:*** Brexidol; Feldene; Fexicam; Novo-Pirocam; Nu-Pirox; ***Chile:*** Fabudol; Feldene; Foldox; Notagol; Pemar; Pricam; Sinartrol; ***Denm.:*** Brexidol; Felden; Pirkam†; Pirom; Pironet†; Piroxigea; ***Fin.:*** Brexidol; Felden; Piroxal; Piroxin†; ***Fr.:*** Brexin; Cycladol; Feldene; Flexirox†; Geldene; Inflaced; Olcam†; Proxalyoc; Zofora; ***Ger.:*** Brexidol; durapirox; Fasax†; Felden; Flexase; Jenapirox; Mobilat Akut Piroxicam; Piro; Piro KD; Piro-Phlogont; Piro-Puren†; Pirobeta; Piroflam; Piroflex; Pirorheum; PirorheumA; Pirox; Pirox-Spondyril†; Piroximerck†; Pra-Brexidol; ratioMobil; Rheumitin; ***Gr.:*** Bleduran; Brexin; Feldene; Flodeneu; Neo Axedil; Pedifan; Proponol; Ruvamed; Sinartrol; Zerospam; Zitumex; ***Hong Kong:*** Brexin†; Feldene; Felxicam; Flamatrol; Hotemin; Pirox; Sefdene; Sotilen; Synoxicam; Vidapirocam; ***India:*** Brexic-DT; Dolonex; Movon; Pirox; Suganril; ***Irl.:*** Feldene; Geroxicam†; Pericam; ***Israel:*** Exipan; Feldene; ***Ital.:*** Algoxam; Antiflog; Artroxicam; Brexin; Brexivel; Bruxicam; Cicladol; Ciclafast; Clevian; Dexicam; Euroxi; Feldene; Flodol; Flogobene†; Lampoflex; Nirox†; Oxicam; Piroftal; Pivaloxicam†; Polipirox; Reucam; Reudene; Reumagil; Riacen; Roxene; Roxenil; Roxiden; Sinartrol; Zacam†; Zelis; Zen†; Zunden†; ***Jpn:*** Baxo; ***Malaysia:*** Brexin; Feldene; Focam; Roxitan; Uphaxicam; ***Mex.:*** Androxicam; Apopiran†; Arlexicam†; Artinor; Artyflam; Bioximil; Brexicam; Brexodin; Citoken T; Dixonal; Dolzycam; Facicam; Farmicam†; Feldene; Flogosan†; Glandicin; Osteral; Oxicanol; Perfarin†; Pirodax; Piromav†; Piroxan; Piroxen†; R-Tyflam; Reucam; Reufel†; Reutricam; Rogal†; Vatrem†; ***Neth.:*** Brexine; Feldene; ***Norw.:*** Brexidol; Felden; Pirox; Tetram†; ***NZ:*** Candyl-D; Feldene†; Piram-D; ***Port.:*** Brexin; Feldene; Flexar; Flogocan; Reumoxican; Roxazin; ***S.Afr.:*** Brexecam; Feldene; Pixicam; Pyrocaps; Rheugesic; Xycam; ***Singapore:*** Brexin; Capxidin; Feldene; Mobilis†; Rosiden; Sotilen†; Vitaxicam†; ***Spain:*** Artragil; Brexinil; Cycladol; Dekamega†; Doblexan; Feldegel; Feldene; Improntal; Salcacam†; Salvacam; Sasulen; Vitaxicam; ***Swed.:*** Brexidol; Felden; ***Switz.:*** Brexidol; Felden; Pirocam; Pirosol; pirox-basan; ***Thai.:*** Ammidene; Bicam; Brexin; Candyl†; Felcam; Feldene; Felrox; Finfo†; Flamic; Ifemed; Maswin; Moxicam; Neogel; Neotica; Piram; Pirax; Pirox; Piroxam; Piroxcin; Piroxen; Piroxsil; Polyxicam; Posedene; Pyroxy; Roccaxin; Roxifen; Roxium; Roxycam; Rumadene; Sotilen; Xicam; ***UK:*** Brexidol; Feldene; Flamatrol†; Larapam†; Pirozip†; ***USA:*** Feldene.

**Multi-ingredient:** ***Arg.:*** Algio-Truxa; Buta Rut B12; Calmapir-P; Flexicamin; Flexicamin A; Flexicamin B12; Flexicamin Crema; Flogiatrin; Flogiatrin B12; Ketazon Flex; Peganix; Rumisedan; Rumisedan Fuerte; Sindrolen; Sindrolen Vitaminado; Solocalm Plus; Solocalm-B; Solocalm-Flex; Vefren.

---

## Pranoprofen (rINN)

Pranoprofeno. α-Methyl-5*H*-[1]-benzopyrano[2,3-*b*]pyridine-7-acetic acid.

$C_{15}H_{13}NO_3$ = 255.3.
*CAS — 52549-17-4.*
*ATC — S01BC09.*

**Pharmacopoeias.** In *Jpn.*

### Profile

Pranoprofen, a propionic acid derivative, is an NSAID (p.67). It is used as eye drops in a concentration of 0.1% for ocular inflammation. Pranoprofen has also been given by mouth for the treatment of pain, inflammation, and fever.

◊ References.


1. Notivol R, *et al.* Treatment of chronic nonbacterial conjunctivitis with a cyclo-oxygenase inhibitor or a corticosteroid. *Am J Ophthalmol* 1994; **117:** 651–6.


### Preparations

**Proprietary Preparations** (details are given in Part 3)
***Belg.:*** Pranox; ***Braz.:*** Difen; ***Ital.:*** Oftalar; Pranoflog; ***Jpn:*** Niflan; ***Port.:*** Oftalar; ***Spain:*** Oftalar.

---

## Proglumetacin Maleate (BANM, rINNM)

CR-604; Maleato de proglumetacina; Protacine Maleate. 3-{4-[2-(1-*p*-Chlorobenzoyl-5-methoxy-2-methylindol-3-ylacetoxy)ethyl]piperazin-1-yl}propyl 4-benzamido-*N*,*N*-dipropylglutaramate dimaleate.

$C_{46}H_{58}ClN_5O_8,2C_4H_4O_4$ = 1076.6.
*CAS — 57132-53-3 (proglumetacin); 59209-40-4 (proglumetacin maleate).*
*ATC — M01AB14.*

### Profile

Proglumetacin maleate, an indoleacetic acid derivative related to indometacin (p.47), is an NSAID (p.67). It has been used in musculoskeletal and joint disorders in doses of up to 600 mg daily, in divided doses, by mouth. Similar doses have also been given as rectal suppositories.

◊ References.


1. Appelboom T, Franchimont P. Proglumetacin versus indometacin in rheumatoid arthritis: a double-blind multicenter study. *Adv Therapy* 1994; **11:** 228–34.
2. Martens M. Double-blind randomized comparison of proglumetacin and naproxen sodium in the treatment of patients with ankle sprains. *Curr Ther Res* 1995; **56:** 639–48.


### Preparations

**Proprietary Preparations** (details are given in Part 3)
***Arg.:*** Alaidol; Bruxel; ***Austria:*** Protaxon; ***Belg.:*** Tolindol; ***Chile:*** Afloxan; ***Ger.:*** Protaxon; ***Hong Kong:*** Afloxan; ***Ital.:*** Afloxan; Proxil; ***Port.:*** Protaxil; ***Spain:*** Prodamox; Protaxil†; ***Thai.:*** Afloxan.

---

## Propacetamol Hydrochloride (BANM, rINNM)

Hidrocloruro de propacetamol; Propacetamoli Hydrochloridum.
The hydrochloride of *N*,*N*-diethylglycine ester with paracetamol; 4-Acetamidophenyl diethylaminoacetate hydrochloride.

$C_{14}H_{20}N_2O_3,HCl$ = 300.8.
*CAS — 66532-85-2 (propacetamol).*
*ATC — N02BE05.*

**Pharmacopoeias.** In *Eur.* (see p.vi).

**Ph. Eur. 5.0** (Propacetamol Hydrochloride). A white or almost white crystalline powder. Freely soluble in water; slightly soluble in dehydrated alcohol; practically insoluble in acetone. Protect from moisture.

### Profile

Propacetamol hydrochloride, a para-aminophenol derivative, is hydrolysed to paracetamol (p.76) in the plasma. It has been given intramuscularly or intravenously in usual doses of 1 to 2 g for the treatment of pain (see Choice of Analgesic, p.2) and fever (p.8).

**Adverse effects.** A report[1] of occupational contact dermatitis in 3 nurses arising from the preparation of injections of propacetamol.


1. Barbaud A, *et al.* Occupational allergy to propacetamol. *Lancet* 1995; **346:** 902.


### Preparations

**Proprietary Preparations** (details are given in Part 3)
***Belg.:*** Pro-Dafalgan; ***Denm.:*** Pro-Dafalgan; ***Fin.:*** Pro-Dafalgan; ***Fr.:*** Pro-Dafalgan†; ***Ital.:*** Pro-Efferalgan; ***Mex.:*** Tempra; ***Norw.:*** Pro-Dafalgan; ***Port.:*** Pro-Dafalgan; ***Spain:*** Pro-Efferalgan; ***Swed.:*** Pro-Dafalgan; ***Switz.:*** Pro-Dafalgan.

---

## Propyl Nicotinate

Nicotinato de propilo.

$C_9H_{11}NO_2$ = 165.2.

### Profile

Propyl nicotinate is used in topical preparations as a rubefacient.

### Preparations

**Proprietary Preparations** (details are given in Part 3)
***Ger.:*** Elacur; Nicodan; Nicodan N.

---

## Propyphenazone (BAN, rINN)

Isopropylantipyrine; Isopropylantipyrinum; Isopropylphenazone; Propifenazona; Propyphenazonum. 4-Isopropyl-2,3-dimethyl-1-phenyl-3-pyrazolin-5-one.

$C_{14}H_{18}N_2O$ = 230.3.
*CAS — 479-92-5.*
*ATC — N02BB04.*

**Pharmacopoeias.** In *Eur.* (see p.vi) and *Jpn.*

**Ph. Eur. 5.0** (Propyphenazone). A white or slightly yellowish crystalline powder. Slightly soluble in water; freely soluble in alcohol and in dichloromethane. Protect from light.

### Profile

Propyphenazone, a pyrazolone derivative related to phenazone (p.82), has analgesic and antipyretic properties. It has been given by mouth and as a rectal suppository in the treatment of pain and fever. The usual adult dose by mouth is 0.5 to 1 g three times daily. There have been some reports of severe hypersensitivity reactions in patients receiving propyphenazone.

**Porphyria.** Propyphenazone has been associated with acute attacks of porphyria and is considered unsafe in porphyric patients.

### Preparations

**Proprietary Preparations** (details are given in Part 3)
***Austria:*** Dim-Antos; ***Ger.:*** Demex; Eufibron; Hewedolor propy; Isoprochin P; ***Ital.:*** Pireuma†.

**Multi-ingredient:** ***Arg.:*** Algio-Bladuril; Espasmo Cibalena; Espasmo Cibalena Fuerte; Saridon; ***Austria:*** Adolorin; Adoluron CC; APA; Asthma†; Asticol†; Avamigran; Coldagrippin; Contraforte; Contralorin; Eu-Med; Gewadal; Influvidon; Melabon; Migradon; Montamed; Neokratin; Nervan; Normensan†; Rapidol; Saridon; Spasmoplus; Tonopan; Toximer; Vivimed; ***Belg.:*** Kranit Nova; Migraine-Kranit Nova†; Neuridon Forte†; Optalidon; Saridon; Spasmo-Cibalgine†; Spasmoplus; ***Braz.:*** Optalidon†; Saridon; Tonopan; ***Chile:*** Abalgin; Droxel; Espasmo Cibalgina; Espasmo Cibalgina Compuesta; Feminosan; Gripasan Compuesto; Immediat; SAE; ***Denm.:*** Kodamid; ***Ger.:*** Avamigran N; Cibalgin Compositum N; Copyrkal N; Ergo-Kranit; Eudorlin; Fomagrippin N; Gewodin†; Ichtho-Bellol compositum S; Migrane-Kranit Duo; Migrane-Kranit Kombi†; Migrane-Kranit N; Migratan S; Milneuron Plus†; Norgesic N; Novo Petrin; Optalidon N; Optalidon special NOC; RubieNex spezial; Saridon; Schworalgan; Spasmo-Cibalgin compositum S†; Spasmo-Cibalgin S; Tispol S†; Titretta; ***Hong Kong:*** APA†; Epizon; Saridon; Tonterin; ***Ital.:*** Alfazina†; Azerodol†; Caffalgina†; Cistalgan; Flexidone†; Influrem; Influvit; Micranet; Mindol-Merck; Neo-Optalidon; Odontalgico Dr. Knapp con Vit. B1; Omniadol†; Optalidon; Ribelfan†; Saridon; Sedol; Spasmo-Cibalgina; Spasmoplus; Uniplus; Upsa Plus†; Veramon; Vitialgin†; ***Mex.:*** Espasmo Cibalgina; Tonopan; ***Neth.:*** Daro Hoofdpijnpoeders†; Sanalgin; Saridon; ***Port.:*** Avamigran; Optalidon; Saridon N; ***S.Afr.:*** Ilvico; ***Spain:*** Abdominol; Bronquimar†; Calmoplex; Dolodens; Fenalgin†; Flexagil; Hubergrip; Melabon; Meloka; Optalidon; Quimpedor; Saridon; Sedalmerck; Sulmetin Papaver; Sulmetin Papaverina; Tabletas Quimpe; Tonopan; ***Switz.:*** Angifebrine†; Barbamin; Caposan; Cerebrol; Comprimes analgesiques "S"; Dialgine forte; Dolopyrine; Dolostop; Escalgin sans codeine; Escogripp sans codeine; Febracyl†; Gewodine; Gubamine†; Kafa; Nicaphlogyl; Novidol†; Saridon; Seranex sans codeine; Sinedal; Siniphen†; Sonotryl†; Spasmo-Barbamin; Spasmo-Barbamine compositum; Spasmo-Cibalgin; Spasmo-Cibalgin comp; Spedralgin sans codeine; Tonopan.

**Proquazone** *(BAN, USAN, rINN)*

43-715; Procuazona; RU-43-715-n. 1-Isopropyl-7-methyl-4-phenylquinazolin-2(1*H*)-one.

$C_{18}H_{18}N_2O$ = 278.3.
*CAS — 22760-18-5.*
*ATC — M01AX13.*

**Profile**

Proquazone is an NSAID (p.67) that has been used in musculoskeletal and joint disorders.

---

**Ramifenazone** *(rINN)*

Isopropylaminophenazone; Isopyrin; Ramifenazona. 4-Isopropylamino-2,3-dimethyl-1-phenyl-3-pyrazolin-5-one.

$C_{14}H_{19}N_3O$ = 245.3.
*CAS — 3615-24-5.*

NOTE. The name Isopyrin has also been applied to isoniazid.

**Profile**

Ramifenazone is an NSAID (p.67) that has been used in preparations for painful and inflammatory conditions. It has also given as the hydrochloride and the salicylate.

---

## Remifentanil Hydrochloride

*(BANM, USAN, rINNM)*

GI-87084B; Hidrocloruro de remifentanilo. 4-Carboxyl-4-(*N*-phenylpropionamido)-1-piperidine propionic acid dimethyl ester monohydrate.

$C_{20}H_{28}N_2O_5,HCl$ = 412.9.
*CAS — 132539-07-2.*
*ATC — N01AH06.*

**Incompatibility.** Remifentanil hydrochloride should not be mixed in the same intravenous solution as blood products. The UK manufacturer states that it should not be mixed with lactated Ringer's injection with or without 5% glucose; however, in the USA the manufacturer's literature states that remifentanil hydrochloride is stable for 4 hours at room temperature following reconstitution and dilution to 20 to 250 micrograms/mL with lactated Ringer's injection and for 24 hours if lactated Ringer's with 5% glucose is used. Incompatibilities have been reported between chlorpromazine hydrochloride 2 mg/mL and remifentanil 25 micrograms/mL (as the hydrochloride) in 5% glucose and cefoperazone sodium 40 mg/mL or amphotericin B 0.6 mg/mL and remifentanil 250 micrograms/mL (as the hydrochloride) in 5% glucose.[1]

1. Trissel LA, *et al.* Compatibility of remifentanil hydrochloride with selected drugs during simulated Y-site administration. *Am J Health-Syst Pharm* 1997; **54:** 2192–6.

### Dependence and Withdrawal

As for Opioid Analgesics, p.71.

### Adverse Effects and Treatment

As for Opioid Analgesics in general, p.72 and for Fentanyl, p.40.

### Precautions

As for Opioid Analgesics in general, p.72.

**Administration.** Remifentanil hydrochloride injections containing glycine should not be given by the epidural or intrathecal routes.

**Hepatic impairment.** Although the pharmacokinetics of remifentanil are not changed in patients with severe hepatic impairment, such patients may be more sensitive to the respiratory depressant effects and should be monitored with doses titrated to individual requirements.

**Renal impairment.** The pharmacokinetics of remifentanil are not changed in patients with severe renal impairment (a creatinine clearance of less than 10 mL/minute) and the manufacturers have stated that the carboxylic acid metabolite is unlikely to accumulate to clinically active concentrations in such patients following remifentanil infusions of up to 2 micrograms/kg per minute for up to 12 hours. Dosage adjustment is considered to be unnecessary.

### Interactions

For interactions associated with opioid analgesics, see p.73.

### Pharmacokinetics

On parenteral use remifentanil hydrochloride has a rapid onset and short duration of action. Its effective biological half-life is about 3 to 10 minutes and is independent of dose. Remifentanil is about 70% bound to plasma proteins, principally to $\alpha_1$-acid glycoprotein. It is hydrolysed by non-specific esterases in blood and tissues to an essentially inactive carboxylic acid metabolite. Approximately 95% of a dose of remifentanil is excreted in the urine as the metabolite.

◊ The manufacturers of remifentanil have given values for a three-compartment pharmacokinetic model with a rapid distribution half-life of 1 minute, a slower distribution half-life of 6 minutes, and a terminal elimination half-life of 10 to 20 minutes.

References.

1. Egan TD. Remifentanil pharmacokinetics and pharmacodynamics: a preliminary appraisal. *Clin Pharmacokinet* 1995; **29:** 80–94.

### Uses and Administration

Remifentanil, an anilidopiperidine derivative, is an opioid analgesic (p.73) related to fentanyl (p.41). It is a short-acting μ-receptor opioid agonist used for analgesia during induction and/or maintenance of general anaesthesia. It is also used to provide analgesia into the immediate postoperative period, and may be used as the analgesic component of local or regional anaesthesia with or without benzodiazepine sedation. Remifentanil is also used to provide analgesia and sedation in ventilated adult patients under intensive care.

Remifentanil is given intravenously as the hydrochloride, usually by infusion. Its onset of action is within 1 minute and the duration of action is 5 to 10 minutes. Doses are expressed in terms of remifentanil base; remifentanil hydrochloride 1.1 mg is approximately equivalent to 1 mg of remifentanil. Initial doses for anaesthesia in elderly patients should be half the recommended adult doses and then titrated to individual requirements.

When used to provide **analgesia** during *induction* of anaesthesia an intravenous infusion is given in doses of 0.5 to 1 microgram/kg per minute. An additional initial intravenous bolus of 1 microgram/kg may be given over 30 to 60 seconds if the patient is to be intubated less than 8 minutes after the start of the infusion.

For provision of analgesia during *maintenance* of anaesthesia in ventilated patients, usual infusion doses range from 0.05 to 2 micrograms/kg per minute depending on the anaesthetic drug employed and adjusted according to patient response. Supplemental intravenous boluses of 0.5 to 1 microgram/kg may be given every 2 to 5 minutes in response to light anaesthesia or intense surgical stress. The infusion dosage in spontaneous respiration is initially 0.04 micrograms/kg per minute adjusted according to response within a usual range of 0.025 to 0.1 microgram/kg per minute. Bolus doses are not recommended during spontaneous ventilation.

For continuation of analgesia into the immediate *postoperative* period typical doses by intravenous infusion have ranged from 0.025 to 0.2 micrograms/kg per minute; supplemental intravenous bolus doses are not recommended during the postoperative period.

To provide **analgesia and sedation** in ventilated adult patients under intensive care, remifentanil is given as an intravenous infusion at an initial rate of 0.1 to 0.15 micrograms/kg per minute. Doses should then be titrated to provide adequate analgesia and sedation; a period of 5 minutes should be allowed between dose adjustments. Additional sedative drugs should be given to those patients inadequately sedated with remifentanil infusions of 0.2 micrograms/kg per minute. An increase in the rate of remifentanil infusion may be necessary if additional analgesia is required to cover stimulating or painful procedures such as wound dressing. Doses of up to 0.75 micrograms/kg per minute have been given in some patients. Bolus doses of remifentanil are not recommended in intensive care.

Remifentanil has a very rapid offset of action and no residual opioid action remains 5 to 10 minutes after stopping an infusion. When appropriate, alternative analgesics should be given before stopping remifentanil, in sufficient time to provide continuous and more prolonged pain relief.

◊ References and reviews.

1. Bacon R, *et al.* Early extubation after open-heart surgery with total intravenous anaesthetic technique. *Lancet* 1995; **345:** 133–4.
2. Duthie DJR, *et al.* Remifentanil and coronary artery surgery. *Lancet* 1995; **345:** 649–50.
3. Patel SS, Spencer CM. Remifentanil. *Drugs* 1996; **52:** 417–27.
4. Duthie DJR. Remifentanil and tramadol. *Br J Anaesth* 1998; **81:** 51–7.

### Preparations

**Proprietary Preparations** (details are given in Part 3)
***Arg.:*** Ultiva; ***Austral.:*** Ultiva; ***Austria:*** Ultiva; ***Belg.:*** Ultiva; ***Braz.:*** Ultiva; ***Canad.:*** Ultiva; ***Chile:*** Ultiva; ***Denm.:*** Ultiva; ***Fin.:*** Ultiva; ***Fr.:*** Ultiva; ***Ger.:*** Ultiva; ***Gr.:*** Ultiva; ***Hong Kong:*** Ultiva; ***Irl.:*** Ultiva; ***Israel:*** Ultiva; ***Ital.:*** Ultiva; ***Mex.:*** Ultiva†; ***Neth.:*** Ultiva; ***Norw.:*** Ultiva; ***NZ:*** Ultiva; ***Port.:*** Ultiva; ***S.Afr.:*** Ultiva; ***Singapore:*** Ultiva; ***Spain:*** Ultiva; ***Swed.:*** Ultiva; ***Switz.:*** Ultiva; ***UK:*** Ultiva; ***USA:*** Ultiva.

---

## Rofecoxib *(BAN, USAN, rINN)*

MK-0966. 4-[*p*-(Methylsulfonyl)phenyl]-3-phenyl-2(5*H*)-furanone.

$C_{17}H_{14}O_4S$ = 314.4.
*CAS — 162011-90-7.*
*ATC — M01AH02.*

### Adverse Effects and Precautions

As for NSAIDs in general, p.67. Mouth ulcers, chest pain, weight gain, atopic eczema, and muscle cramps have also been reported. Rofecoxib is contra-indicated in some patients with hepatic impairment (see Administration in Hepatic Impairment, below). Therapy should be discontinued in patients if persistently abnormal liver function tests are detected. Rofecoxib is also contra-indicated in patients with severe heart failure, inflammatory bowel disease, and renal impairment associated with a creatinine clearance of less than 30 mL/minute. It should be used with caution in those with ischaemic heart disease.

◊ References.

1. Bannwarth B, *et al.* Adverse events associated with rofecoxib therapy: results of a large study in community-derived osteoarthritis patients. *Drug Safety* 2003; **26:** 49–54.
2. Layton D, *et al.* Safety profile of rofecoxib as used in general practice in England: results of a prescription-event monitoring study. *Br J Clin Pharmacol* 2003; **55:** 166–74.

**Effects on the cardiovascular system.** As of February 2001, the UK Committee on Safety of Medicines has received a small number of reports of *myocardial infarction* or *ischaemia* in association with the selective cyclo-oxygenase-2 (COX-2) inhibitors.[1] COX-2 inhibitors such as rofecoxib do not possess the intrinsic antiplatelet activity associated with aspirin (and possibly other non-selective NSAIDs), and consequently do not provide protection against ischaemic cardiac events. Data from a large, randomised trial also showed the incidence of myocardial infarction to be greater in patients taking rofecoxib than in those taking naproxen.[2] It has been suggested[3] that this difference in incidence may be due to a cardioprotective effect of naproxen although the evidence for such an effect has been criticised, see Effects on the Cardiovascular System in NSAIDs, p.67. The cardiovascular effects of rofecoxib may also be dose-related. A recent study[4] has found that the risk of events such as acute myocardial infarction with rofecoxib was greater with doses over 25 mg daily; doses of 25 mg daily or less were associated with a risk similar to that of celecoxib, ibuprofen, or naproxen.

A review[5] of prospective studies evaluating the effect of selective COX-2 inhibitors on blood pressure was unable to determine if there was any association between the use of these drugs and blood pressure elevations. Of the studies considered, a randomised trial in elderly, hypertensive patients with osteoarthritis has suggested that the risk of developing *increased systolic blood pressure* is greater in those patients receiving rofecoxib than in those receiving celecoxib.[6] However, the manufacturers of rofecoxib have pointed out that the trial used doses of rofecoxib greater than those recommended for elderly or hypertensive patients.

1. Committee on Safety of Medicines/Medicines Control Agency. COX-2 selective NSAIDs lack antiplatelet activity. *Current Problems* 2001; **27:** 7. Also available at: http://medicines.mhra.gov.uk/ourwork/monitorsafequalmed/currentproblems/cpfeb2001.pdf (accessed 06/07/04)
2. Bombardier C, *et al.* Comparison of upper gastrointestinal toxicity of rofecoxib and naproxen in patients with rheumatoid arthritis. *N Engl J Med* 2000; **343:** 1520–8.
3. Dalen JE. Selective COX-2 inhibitors, NSAIDs, aspirin, and myocardial infarction. *Arch Intern Med* 2002; **162:** 1091–2.
4. Ray WA, *et al.* COX-2 selective non-steroidal anti-inflammatory drugs and risk of serious coronary heart disease. *Lancet* 2002; **360:** 1071–3.
5. Johnson DL, *et al.* Effect of cyclooxygenase-2 inhibitors on blood pressure. *Ann Pharmacother* 2003; **37:** 442–6.
6. Whelton A, *et al.* Cyclooxygenase-2-specific inhibitors and cardiorenal function: a randomized, controlled trial of celecoxib and rofecoxib in older hypertensive osteoarthritis patients. *Am J Ther* 2001; **8:** 85–95.

**Effects on the gastrointestinal tract.** It is generally accepted that the inhibition of cyclo-oxygenase-1 (COX-1) results in the adverse gastrointestinal effects of the NSAIDs, and that the selective inhibition of the other isoform, COX-2, by NSAIDs such as rofecoxib may cause less gastrotoxicity than that seen with the non-selective inhibition of the traditional NSAIDs.

Results from controlled trials confirm that NSAIDs selective for COX-2 are associated with a lower incidence of serious gastrointestinal effects. A combined analysis of 8 pre-licensing trials concluded that the risk of upper gastrointestinal perforation, symptomatic gastroduodenal ulcers, or upper gastrointestinal bleeding with rofecoxib was significantly less than that with ibuprofen, diclofenac, or nabumetone.[1] In a comparative study,[2] rofecoxib given in doses of 50 mg daily (twice the maximum recommended dose for osteoarthritis) was associated with a significantly lower incidence of endoscopically-detected gastroduodenal ulceration than maximum recommended doses of ibuprofen (2.4 g daily). Another comparative study[3] in patients with rheumatoid arthritis also found rofecoxib, in doses of 50 mg daily, to be associated with significantly fewer incidences of clinically serious upper gastrointestinal events than naproxen, given in doses of 1 g daily.

An observational study[4] comparing the effects of celecoxib and rofecoxib on the risk of gastrointestinal toxicity unexpectedly found that the rate of upper gastrointestinal haemorrhage was significantly higher with rofecoxib than with celecoxib. However, for both drugs, the rates were less than those seen with the non-selective NSAIDs.

There have been individual case reports of gastrotoxicity with rofecoxib.[5]


1. Langman MJ, *et al.* Adverse upper gastrointestinal effects of rofecoxib compared with NSAIDs. *JAMA* 1999; **282:** 1929–33.
2. Hawkey C, *et al.* Comparison of the effect of rofecoxib (a cyclooxygenase 2 inhibitor), ibuprofen, and placebo on the gastroduodenal mucosa of patients with osteoarthritis: a randomized, double-blind, placebo-controlled trial. *Arthritis Rheum* 2000; **43:** 370–7.
3. Bombardier C, *et al.* Comparison of upper gastrointestinal toxicity of rofecoxib and naproxen in patients with rheumatoid arthritis. *N Engl J Med* 2000; **343:** 1520–8.
4. Mamdani M, *et al.* Observational study of upper gastrointestinal haemorrhage in elderly patients given selective cyclo-oxygenase-2 inhibitors or conventional non-steroidal anti-inflammatory drugs. *BMJ* 2002; **325:** 624–7.
5. Committee on Safety of Medicines/Medicines Control Agency. Rofecoxib (Vioxx). *Current Problems* 2000; **26:** 13. Also available at: http://www.mca.gov.uk/ourwork/monitorsafequalmed/currentproblems/cpsept2000.pdf (accessed 06/07/04)


**Effects on the kidneys.** Increasing evidence of the renal toxicity of the selective cyclo-oxygenase-2 (COX-2) inhibitors such as rofecoxib suggests that such NSAIDs appear to have effects on renal function similar to those of the non-selective NSAIDs (see p.68).

Some references to the adverse renal effects of rofecoxib.


1. Swan SK, *et al.* Effect of cyclooxygenase-2 inhibition on renal function in elderly persons receiving a low-salt diet: a randomized controlled trial. *Ann Intern Med* 2000; **133:** 1–9.
2. Wolf G, *et al.* Acute renal failure associated with rofecoxib. *Ann Intern Med* 2000; **133:** 394.
3. Perazella MA, Tray K. Selective cyclooxygenase-2 inhibitors: a pattern of nephrotoxicity similar to traditional nonsteroidal anti-inflammatory drugs. *Am J Med* 2001; **111:** 64–7.
4. Rocha JL, Fernández-Alonso J. Acute tubulointerstitial nephritis associated with the selective COX-2 enzyme inhibitor, rofecoxib. *Lancet* 2001: **357:** 1946–7.
5. Ahmad SR, *et al.* Renal failure associated with the use of celecoxib and rofecoxib. *Drug Safety* 2002; **25:** 537–44.


**Effects on the nervous system.** Acute neuropsychiatric reactions such as confusion, somnolence, and insomnia, have occurred following rofecoxib use.[1] There have also been case reports of aseptic meningitis[2] and a paraesthesia-type reaction[3] with rofecoxib.


1. Anonymous. Acute neuropsychiatric events with celecoxib and rofecoxib. *Aust Adverse Drug React Bull* 2003; **22:** 3. Also available at: http://www.tga.health.gov.au/adr/aadrb/aadr0302.htm (accessed 06/07/04)
2. Bonnel RA, *et al.* Aseptic meningitis associated with rofecoxib. *Arch Intern Med* 2002; **162:** 713–15.
3. Daugherty KK, Gora-Harper ML. Idiopathic paresthesia reaction associated with rofecoxib. *Ann Pharmacother* 2002; **36:** 264–6.


**Hypersensitivity.** Although some patients with a history of hypersensitivity reactions to NSAIDs (including aspirin) have taken rofecoxib without any adverse reactions,[1,2] it may not be safe in all hypersensitive patients. There is a report[3] of a patient experiencing hypersensitivity symptoms with both diclofenac and rofecoxib.

The manufacturers of rofecoxib contra-indicate its use in patients who have experienced hypersensitivity reactions such as asthma and rhinitis with aspirin or other NSAIDs.


1. Nettis E, *et al.* Tolerability of rofecoxib in patients with cutaneous adverse reactions to nonsteroidal anti-inflammatory drugs. *Ann Allergy Asthma Immunol* 2002; **88:** 331–4.
2. Martín-García C, *et al.* Safety of a cyclooxygenase-2 inhibitor in patients with aspirin-sensitive asthma. *Chest* 2002; **121:** 1812–17.
3. Schellenberg RR, Isserow SH. Anaphylactoid reaction to a cyclooxygenase-2 inhibitor in a patient who had a reaction to a cyclooxygenase-1 inhibitor. *N Engl J Med* 2001; **345:** 1856.


## Interactions

For interactions associated with NSAIDs, see p.69. Data from *in vivo* studies suggest that rofecoxib is a modest inhibitor of the cytochrome P450 isoenzyme CYP1A2; consequently, rofecoxib should be used with caution with drugs that are metabolised by this isoenzyme, such as clozapine, olanzapine, tacrine, theophylline, and zileuton.

**Rifampicin.** Use of rifampicin with rofecoxib has resulted in a 50% decrease in rofecoxib plasma concentrations; the manufacturers recommend that the maximum dose (see below) be used when rofecoxib is given with potent inducers of hepatic metabolism.

## Pharmacokinetics

Rofecoxib is well absorbed from the gastrointestinal tract after oral doses. Peak plasma concentrations are reached in approximately 2 to 4 hours. Plasma protein binding is about 85%. Rofecoxib is extensively metabolised in the liver, mainly by reduction to *cis-* and *trans-*dihydrorofecoxib (as hydroxyl acids), which together account for 56% of a dose recovered in the urine. The 5-hydroxy glucuronide metabolite is also present. Excretion is mainly via the urine (72%) with only 14% of a dose appearing in the faeces. The elimination half-life is about 17 hours at steady state.

◊ References.


1. Davies NM, *et al.* Pharmacokinetics of rofecoxib: a specific cyclo-oxygenase-2 inhibitor. *Clin Pharmacokinet* 2003; **42:** 545–56.


## Uses and Administration

Rofecoxib is an NSAID (p.70) reported to be a selective inhibitor of cyclo-oxygenase-2 (COX-2). It is given by mouth for symptomatic relief in the treatment of osteoarthritis and rheumatoid arthritis, and is used in the management of acute pain and dysmenorrhoea. In the USA, it is also used for the acute treatment of migraine (p.464).

In **osteoarthritis**, the usual starting dose is 12.5 mg once daily, which may be increased to a maximum of 25 mg once daily. Patients with rheumatoid arthritis should receive 25 mg once daily.

An initial dose of 50 mg once daily is permitted for the short-term treatment of acute symptomatic **pain**; thereafter daily doses are 25 or 50 mg. In the USA, treatment is limited to 5 days.

In the acute treatment of **migraine**, the initial dose is 25 mg once daily, which may be increased to 50 mg daily, if necessary.

◊ References.


1. Ehrich EW, *et al.* Characterization of rofecoxib as a cyclooxygenase-2 isoform inhibitor and demonstration of analgesia in the dental pain model. *Clin Pharmacol Ther* 1999; **65:** 336–47.
2. Scott LJ, Lamb HM. Rofecoxib. *Drugs* 1999; **58:** 499–505.
3. Matheson AJ, Figgitt DP. Rofecoxib: a review of its use in the management of osteoarthritis, acute pain and rheumatoid arthritis. *Drugs* 2001; **61:** 833–65.


**Administration in hepatic impairment.** In the treatment of osteoarthritis and rheumatoid arthritis, no dose adjustment of rofecoxib is necessary for patients with mild hepatic impairment. In patients with moderate hepatic impairment the dose should not exceed 12.5 mg once daily. Rofecoxib should not be given to patients with severe impairment.

In the UK, the use of rofecoxib for acute pain is contra-indicated in all degrees of hepatic impairment.

**Bartter's syndrome.** There are reports[1,2] of benefit with rofecoxib in the treatment of Bartter's syndrome (p.1220).


1. Kleta R, *et al.* New treatment options for Bartter's syndrome. *N Engl J Med* 2000; **343:** 661–2.
2. Haas NA, *et al.* Successful management of an extreme example of neonatal hyperprostaglandin-E syndrome (Bartter's syndrome) with the new cyclooxygenase-2 inhibitor rofecoxib. *Pediatr Crit Care Med* 2003; **4:** 249–51.


**Musculoskeletal and joint disorders.** Rofecoxib is used in the treatment of the musculoskeletal disorders osteoarthritis and rheumatoid arthritis (see p.9 and p.9, respectively). However, in the UK, it is recommended that the use of rofecoxib and other selective cyclo-oxygenase-2 (COX-2) inhibitors is limited to those patients considered to be at high risk of developing serious gastrointestinal problems if given a non-selective NSAID (see p.68).

References.


1. Schnitzer TJ, *et al.* The safety profile, tolerability, and effective dose range of rofecoxib in the treatment of rheumatoid arthritis. *Clin Ther* 1999; **21:** 1688–1702.
2. Saag K, *et al.* Rofecoxib, a new cyclooxygenase 2 inhibitor, shows sustained efficacy, comparable with other nonsteroidal anti-inflammatory drugs: a 6-week and a 1-year trial in patients with osteoarthritis. *Arch Fam Med* 2000; **9:** 1124–34.
3. Schmidt H, *et al.* Benefit-risk assessment of rofecoxib in the treatment of osteoarthritis. *Drug Safety* 2004; **27:** 185–96.
4. Garner S, *et al.* Rofecoxib for rheumatoid arthritis. Available in The Cochrane Library; Issue 2. Chichester: John Wiley; 2004.


## Preparations

**Proprietary Preparations** (details are given in Part 3)
***Arg.:*** Algioxib; Antidol; Befol; Blokium Cox; Coxiro; Doxtran; Foldoxx; Silfox; Toloxane; Unicalm; Viartril; Vioxx; ***Austral.:*** Vioxx; ***Austria:*** Coxxil; Vioxx; ***Belg.:*** Vioxx; ***Braz.:*** Vioxx; ***Canad.:*** Vioxx; ***Chile:*** Ceoxx; ***Denm.:*** Vioxx; Vioxxalt; ***Fin.:*** Vioxx; ***Fr.:*** Vioxx; ***Ger.:*** Vioxx; ***Gr.:*** Vioxx; ***Hong Kong:*** Vioxx; ***India:*** Alrof; Dolib; Rofetab; Rofiz; ***Irl.:*** Ceoxx; Vioxx; ***Israel:*** Vioxx; ***Ital.:*** Arofexx; Coxxil; Dolcoxx; Miraxx; Vioxx; ***Malaysia:*** Vioxx; ***Mex.:*** Vioxx; ***Neth.:*** Vioxx; ***Norw.:*** Vioxx; ***NZ:*** Vioxx; ***Port.:*** Ceoxx; Coxxil; Vioxx; ***S.Afr.:*** Vioxx; ***Singapore:*** Vioxx; ***Spain:*** Ceoxx; Vioxx; ***Swed.:*** Vioxx; ***Switz.:*** Vioxx; ***Thai.:*** Vioxx; ***UK:*** Vioxx; ***USA:*** Vioxx.

## Salamidacetic Acid

Carbamoylphenoxyacetic acid; Salamidacético, ácido; Salicylamide *O*-acetic acid. (2-Carbamoylphenoxy)acetic acid.
$C_9H_9NO_4$ = 195.2.
*CAS — 25395-22-6 (salamidacetic acid); 3785-32-8 (sodium salamidacetate).*

### Profile

Salamidacetic acid is a salicylic acid derivative (see Aspirin, p.15) that has also been used as the sodium and diethylamine salts for the treatment of musculoskeletal and joint disorders.

### Preparations

**Proprietary Preparations** (details are given in Part 3)
***Austria:*** Akistin; ***Ger.:*** Clinit N; Hewedolor forte†.

**Multi-ingredient: *Austria:*** Ambene; Rheumesser; ***Ger.:*** Caye Balsam; Flexurat†; ***Thai.:*** Trabit.

## Salicylamide *(BAN, rINN)*

Salicilamida. 2-Hydroxybenzamide.
$C_7H_7NO_2$ = 137.1.
*CAS — 65-45-2.*
*ATC — N02BA05.*

**Pharmacopoeias.** In *Pol.* and *US.*

**USP 27** (Salicylamide). A white practically odourless crystalline powder. Slightly soluble in water and in chloroform; soluble in alcohol and in propylene glycol; freely soluble in ether and in solutions of alkalis.

### Profile

Salicylamide is a salicylic acid derivative (see Aspirin, p.15) but is not hydrolysed to salicylate; it is almost completely metabolised to inactive metabolites during absorption and on first pass through the liver. It is given in doses of 325 to 650 mg or more by mouth, usually with other analgesics, three or four times daily for pain and fever. Salicylamide has also been applied topically in rubefacient preparations in concentrations of about 5% for the relief of muscular and rheumatic pain.

### Preparations

**Proprietary Preparations** (details are given in Part 3)
***Austria:*** Isosal.

**Multi-ingredient: *Arg.:*** Finagrip; Venter; ***Austria:*** Influvidon; Isosal; Rilfit; Rubriment; Sigmalin $B_6$; Sigmalin $B_6$ forte; Sigmalin $B_6$ ohne Coffein; Spalt; ***Belg.:*** Myalgesic†; Percutalgine; ***Braz.:*** Benegrip†; Coristina R; Coristina Reforcada†; Gripin C†; Neo Sativan†; Resfry Infantil†; Resprax; Termogripe C; Vita Grip†; ***Denm.:*** Kodamid; Koffisal; ***Fr.:*** Percutalgine; ***Ger.:*** Glutisal; Salistoperm; ***Hong Kong:*** Antiflu Forte; Antiflu-N-Forte; Coryaid†; DF Multi-Symptom; Neosed†; Neozep; ***Israel:*** Novocalm; ***Ital.:*** Anticorizza; Azerodol†; ***Mex.:*** Artrilan; Butayonacol; Zolidime; ***NZ:*** Calm-U; ***S.Afr.:*** Colcaps; Flutex; Histamed Compound; Ilvico; ***Spain:*** Coricidin; Doloana†; Hubergrip; Percutalin†; Pridio; Rinomicine; Rinomicine Activada; Yendol; ***Switz.:*** Escalgin sans codeine; Escogripp sans codeine; Grippalgine N; No Grip†; Novidol†; Osa†; Siniphen†; ***Thai.:*** Apracur; Fecol; Percutalgine; ***UAE:*** Adol Compound; Flukit; ***UK:*** Intralgin†; ***USA:*** Anabar; BC; Lobac; Painaid; Saleto; Saleto-D†; Trim-Elim.

## Salix

Corteza de sauce; Salicis Cortex; Willow Bark.

**Pharmacopoeias.** In *Eur.* (see p.vi) and *Pol.*

**Ph. Eur. 5.0** (Willow Bark). The whole or fragmented dried bark of young branches or whole dried pieces of current year twigs of various species of the genus *Salix*, including *Salix purpurea*, *S. daphnoides*, and *S. fragilis*. It contains not less than 1.5% of total salicylic derivatives, expressed as salicin ($C_{13}H_{18}O_7$ = 286.3), calculated with reference to the dried drug. Protect from light.

### Profile

Salix contains variable amounts of tannin and also of salicin which has antipyretic and analgesic actions similar to those of aspirin. Salix has been used in a variety of herbal remedies for painful and inflammatory conditions and for fever. It was once used as a bitter.

◊ References.


1. Chrubasik S, *et al.* Treatment of low back pain exacerbations with willow bark extract: a randomized double-blind study. *Am J Med* 2000; **109:** 9–14.


### Preparations

**Proprietary Preparations** (details are given in Part 3)
***Austria:*** Biogelat Erkaltungs & Grippe†; ***Canad.:*** Saliton†; ***Ger.:*** Assalix; Assplant; Lintia; Rheumakaps; Rheumatab Salicis; Tamanybonsan†.

**Multi-ingredient: *Austral.:*** Arthritic Pain Herbal Formula 1†; Bioglan Arthri Plus†; Extralife Migrai-Care†; Extralife PMS-Care†; Harpagophytum Complex†; Lifesystem Herbal Formula 1 Arthritic Aid†; Lifesystem Herbal Formula 12 Willowbark†; Prost-1†; Salagesic†; Willowbark Plus Herbal Formula 11†; ***Austria:*** Apotheker Ehrmanns Grippekapseln; Curol; Digestodoron; Grippefloran; Kneipp Grippe-Tee; Krauterpfarrer Weidinger Rheumatee; Naturland Rheuma Tee; ***Braz.:*** Akhauma†; Calman; Calmiplan; Pasalix; Passi Catha†; Passicarbone†; Passiflorine; ***Canad.:*** Arthrisant†; ***Fr.:*** Arkophytum; Mediflor Tisane Circulation du Sang No 12; Santane $A_4$†; ***Ger.:*** Dr Wiemanns Rheumatonikum; Hevert-Erkaltungs-Tee†; Hevert-Gicht-Rheuma-Tee comp†; Kneipp Rheuma Tee N†; ***Ital.:*** Biothymus DS; Bodyguard; Depurativo†; Donalg; Fluend†; Influ-Zinc; Nevril; Passiflorine; Tauma†; **Mex.:** Ifupasil; **Port.:** Bio-Strath No 5†; Neurocardol; **Spain:** Dolosul; Jaqueso; Mesatil; Natusor Harpagosinol; Natusor Jaquesan; **Switz.:** Dragees antirhumatismales; Dragees contre les maux de tete†; Phytomed Rhino†; Tisane antirhumatismale; **UK:** Bio-Strath Willow Formula; Gerard House Ligvites†; Gerard House Reumalex; Herbal Pain Relief; Hofels White Willow and Burdock†; St Johns-wort Compound.

## Salol

Salicilato de fenilo. Phenyl salicylate.

$C_{13}H_{10}O_3$ = 214.2.

*CAS — 118-55-8.*

*ATC — G04BX12.*

**Pharmacopoeias.** In *Pol.*

### Profile

Salol is a salicylic acid derivative (see Aspirin, p.15). It was formerly used as an intestinal antiseptic, but effective doses were toxic owing to the liberation of phenol. It is used in oral preparations containing methenamine for the treatment of lower urinary-tract infections.

Salol has been used topically as a sunscreen.

### Preparations

**Proprietary Preparations** (details are given in Part 3)
**Austral.:** Aussie Tan Sunstick†.

**Multi-ingredient:** **Austria:** Carl Baders Divinal; **Braz.:** Malvosulfam†; Talco Alivio; **Canad.:** Franzbranns; **Chile:** Galutec; Polisep; **Fr.:** Borostyrol; Dermophil Indien; **Ger.:** Parodontal F5 med†; **Switz.:** Borostyrol N; Dermophil Indien Nouvelle formule; **USA:** Atrosept; Dolsed; MHP-A; MSP-Blu; Prosed/DS; Trac Tabs 2X; UAA; Urelle; Uretron; Uridon Modified; Urimar-T; Urimax; Urised; Uriseptic; Uritact; Uro Blue; Urogesic Blue; Utira.

## Salsalate *(BAN, USAN, rINN)*

NSC-49171; Salicyl Salicylate; Salicylosalicylic Acid; Salicylsalicylic Acid; Salsalato; Salysal; Sasapyrine. *O*-(2-Hydroxybenzoyl)salicylic acid.

$C_{14}H_{10}O_5$ = 258.2.

*CAS — 552-94-3.*

*ATC — N02BA06.*

**Pharmacopoeias.** In *Chin.* and *US.*

**USP 27** (Salsalate). Store in airtight containers.

### Adverse Effects, Treatment, and Precautions

As for Aspirin, p.15.

The use of aspirin and other acetylated salicylates is generally not recommended for children because of the risk of Reye's syndrome, unless specifically indicated. Some licensing information extends this precaution to salsalate.

**Effects on the gastrointestinal tract.** Salsalate is associated with less faecal blood loss than aspirin and has been reported to cause fewer gastric lesions than piroxicam.[1] However, small-bowel ulcerations were reported in a patient when salsalate was added to a regimen of ranitidine and metoclopramide which had been prescribed for duodenal ulcer.[2]

1. Porro GB, *et al.* Salsalate in the treatment of rheumatoid arthritis: a double-blind clinical and gastroscopic trial versus piroxicam: II—endoscopic evaluation. *J Int Med Res* 1989; **17:** 320–3.
2. Souza Lima MA. Ulcers of the small bowel associated with stomach-bypassing salicylates. *Arch Intern Med* 1985; **145:** 1139.

**Effects on the kidneys.** A case of minimal-change nephrotic syndrome associated with salsalate use.[1]

1. Vallès M, Tovar JL. Salsalate and minimal-change nephrotic syndrome. *Ann Intern Med* 1987; **107:** 116.

**Effects on the mouth.** Ulcerated lesions on the tongue of a 77-year-old man were found to be due to incorrect administration of salsalate tablets.[1] The patient had placed the tablets under his tongue rather than swallowing them whole, resulting in prolonged, direct contact with the tongue.

1. Ruscin JM, Astroth JD. Lingual lesions secondary to prolonged contact with salsalate tablets. *Ann Pharmacother* 1998; **32:** 1248.

### Interactions

For interactions associated with salicylates, see Aspirin, p.17.

### Pharmacokinetics

Salsalate is insoluble in acidic gastric fluids but is soluble in the small intestine. One molecule of salsalate is hydrolysed to 2 molecules of salicylic acid; hydrolysis occurs both in the small intestine and following absorption of the parent compound. Additional details on the pharmacokinetics of salicylic acid are provided in aspirin (see p.17). Not all of the absorbed salsalate is hydrolysed and about 13% of salsalate is excreted as glucuronide conjugates in the urine; thus, the amount of salicylic acid available from salsalate is less than that from aspirin when the two drugs are given in equimolar equivalents of salicylic acid.

### Uses and Administration

Salsalate is a salicylic acid derivative that has analgesic, anti-inflammatory, and antipyretic actions similar to those of aspirin (see p.17). It is used for pain and fever and also in inflammatory disorders such as osteoarthritis and rheumatoid arthritis. A usual dose is up to 3 g daily given by mouth in divided doses with food.

### Preparations

**USP 27:** Salsalate Capsules; Salsalate Tablets.

**Proprietary Preparations** (details are given in Part 3)
**Canad.:** Disalcid†; **Spain:** Umbradol†; **USA:** Amigesic; Argesic-SA; Artha-G; Disalcid; Marthritic; Mono-Gesic†; Salflex; Salsitab.

## Sarracenia Purpurea

Pitcher Plant; Sarracenia purpurea.

### Profile

The roots and leaves of *Sarracenia purpurea* (Sarraceniaceae) have been used in the form of an aqueous distillate, administered by local injection, for neuromuscular or neuralgic pain.

### Preparations

**Proprietary Preparations** (details are given in Part 3)
**USA:** Sarapin.

## Sodium Aurothiomalate *(rINN)*

Aurotiomalato de sodio; Gold Sodium Thiomalate; Sodium Aurothiosuccinate.

*CAS — 12244-57-4 (anhydrous xNa); 39377-38-3 (disodium monohydrate).*

*ATC — M01CB01.*

**Pharmacopoeias.** In *Br., Jpn,* and *US.*

**BP 2003** (Sodium Aurothiomalate). Fine, pale yellow, hygroscopic powder with a slight odour. It consists mainly of the disodium salt of (aurothio)succinic acid ($C_4H_3AuNa_2O_4S$ = 390.1) and has a gold content of 44.5 to 46.0% calculated on the dried material. Very soluble in water. A 10% solution in water has a pH of 6.0 to 7.0. Protect from light.

**USP 27** (Gold Sodium Thiomalate). A mixture of the monosodium and disodium salts of gold thiomalic acid [(aurothio)succinic acid] ($C_4H_4AuNaO_4S$ = 368.1 and $C_4H_3AuNa_2O_4S$ = 390.1) that has a gold content of 44.8 to 49.6%, and 49.0 to 52.5% calculated on the dried alcohol-free and glycerol-free material. pH of a 10% solution in water is between 5.8 and 6.5. Store in airtight containers at a temperature of 25°, excursions permitted between 15° and 30°. Protect from light.

### Adverse Effects

Reports show a wide range for the incidence of adverse effects of sodium aurothiomalate. However, authorities consider that with careful treatment about one-third of patients will experience adverse effects. It is also considered that about 5% of patients will experience severe adverse effects and that some of the effects will be fatal. The most common effects involve the skin and mucous membranes with pruritus (an early sign of intolerance) and stomatitis (often with a metallic taste) being the most prominent. Rashes with pruritus often occur after 2 to 6 months of intramuscular treatment and may necessitate discontinuation of therapy. Other reactions affecting the skin and mucous membranes include erythema, maculopapular eruptions, erythema multiforme, urticaria, eczema, seborrhoeic dermatitis, lichenoid eruptions, alopecia, exfoliative dermatitis, glossitis, pharyngitis, vaginitis, photosensitivity reactions, and irreversible pigmentation (chrysiasis).

Toxic effects on the blood include eosinophilia, thrombocytopenia, leucopenia, agranulocytosis, and aplastic anaemia.

Effects on the kidneys include mild transient proteinuria which may lead to heavy proteinuria, haematuria, and nephrosis.

Other effects reported include pulmonary fibrosis, toxic hepatitis, cholestatic jaundice, peripheral neuritis, encephalitis, psychoses, fever, and gastrointestinal disorders including enterocolitis. Gold deposits may occur in the eyes. Vasomotor or nitritoid reactions, with weakness, flushing, palpitations, and dyspnoea, may occur following injection of sodium aurothiomalate. Local irritation may also follow injection.

Sometimes there is an initial exacerbation of the arthritic condition.

A number of the adverse effects of gold have an immunogenic component.

◊ Reviews.

1. Tozman ECS, Gottlieb NL. Adverse reactions with oral and parenteral gold preparations. *Med Toxicol* 1987; **2:** 177–89.

**Effects on the blood.** Blood disorders such as leucopenia, granulocytopenia, and thrombocytopenia have occurred in patients receiving gold therapy. Eosinophilia has been reported to be the most frequent haematological abnormality.[1] It has been estimated that thrombocytopenia develops in 1 to 3% of patients receiving gold salts.[2]

Fatal consumption coagulopathy occurred in 4 children following the second injection of sodium aurothioglucose or sodium aurothiomalate.[3]

1. Foster RT. Eosinophilia—a marker of gold toxicity. *Can J Hosp Pharm* 1985; **85:** 150–1.
2. Coblyn JS, *et al.* Gold-induced thrombocytopenia: a clinical and immunogenetic study of twenty-three patients. *Ann Intern Med* 1981; **95:** 178–81.
3. Jacobs JC, *et al.* Consumption coagulopathy after gold therapy for JRA. *J Pediatr* 1984; **105:** 674–5.

**Effects on the cardiovascular system.** Vasomotor or nitritoid reactions associated with gold compounds are usually transient and self-limiting and although they may be mild there have been isolated reports of associated complications such as myocardial infarction, stroke, transient ischaemic attack, and transient monocular visual loss.[1] Most reactions have been associated with sodium aurothiomalate (a reported incidence of 4.7%) but they have also occurred with auranofin and sodium aurothioglucose. Tachyphylaxis usually occurs to the reactions and most patients are able to continue treatment but paradoxically in some the severity increases with repeated doses; 2.8% of patients receiving sodium aurothiomalate may require a change of treatment due to recurrent reactions. It is important to distinguish such reactions from true anaphylactic reactions to gold.[1] Patients taking ACE inhibitors may be at increased risk of nitritoid reactions. Transfer of the patient to sodium aurothioglucose or reduction of the dose by 50%, injection in the recumbent position, and observation for 20 minutes have been recommended for the next few injections following a reaction.[2]

1. Ho M, Pullar T. Vasomotor reactions with gold. *Br J Rheumatol* 1997; **36:** 154–6.
2. Arthur AB, *et al.* Nitritoid reactions: case reports, review, and recommendations for management. *J Rheumatol* 2001; **28:** 2209–12.

**Effects on the gastrointestinal tract.** A case report of enterocolitis due to sodium aurothiomalate has been published[1] and 27 other cases associated with gold therapy reviewed.

1. Jackson CW, *et al.* Gold induced enterocolitis. *Gut* 1986; **27:** 452–56.

**Effects on the immune system.** Details of a patient who developed an immune deficiency syndrome that was attributed to gold therapy with sodium aurothiomalate.[1]

1. Haskard DO, Macfarlane D. Adult acquired combined immune deficiency in a patient with rheumatoid arthritis on gold. *J R Soc Med* 1988; **81:** 548–9.

**Effects on the kidneys.** Proteinuria developed in 21 patients while receiving a standard regimen of sodium aurothiomalate.[1] The severity of the proteinuria varied greatly and in 11 it increased for 4 months after treatment was stopped. Eight patients were considered to have developed the nephrotic syndrome. The median duration of proteinuria was 11 months, resolving in all 21 patients when treatment was withdrawn; at 24 months 3 patients were still experiencing proteinuria and it was not until 39 months that all were free of the condition. Renal biopsy indicated several types of kidney damage.

See under Auranofin (p.19) for a comparative incidence of proteinuria in patients receiving sodium aurothiomalate or auranofin.

1. Hall CL, *et al.* The natural course of gold nephropathy: long term study of 21 patients. *BMJ* 1987; **295:** 745–8.

**Effects on the lungs.** 'Gold lung' is the term used to describe symptoms of dyspnoea on exertion, weakness, dry cough, and malaise developing some weeks or months after starting gold treatment. Pulmonary insufficiency may eventually develop. The pulmonary lesions usually subside on withdrawal of gold therapy, although persistent symptoms have been reported. Nonbacterial thrombotic endocarditis associated with gold-induced pulmonary disease has also been reported.[1] This was considered to be a manifestation of gold-induced immune complex deposition.

1. Kollef MH, *et al.* Nonbacterial thrombotic endocarditis associated with gold induced pulmonary disease. *Ann Intern Med* 1988; **108:** 903–4.

**Effects on the nails.** A 34-year-old woman with severe rheumatoid arthritis receiving intramuscular gold developed yellow thickened toenails and fingernails after 2 years of treatment.[1] Although there was some improvement in nail growth on stopping treatment, some light yellow discoloration in all 20 nails persisted.

1. Roest MAB, Ratnavel R. Yellow nails associated with gold therapy for rheumatoid arthritis. *Br J Dermatol* 2001; **145:** 855–6.

**Effects on the nervous system.** Neurological complications with gold salts are infrequent but may include peripheral neuropathy, Guillain-Barré syndrome, myokymia (repeated involuntary contractions of muscle fibre), and encephalopathy. Some reports[1-6] are given below.

1. Dick DJ, Raman D. The Guillain-Barre syndrome following gold therapy. *Scand J Rheumatol* 1982; **11:** 119–20.
2. Schlumpf U, *et al.* Neurologic complications induced by gold treatment. *Arthritis Rheum* 1983; **26:** 825–31.
3. Cerinic MM, *et al.* Gold polyneuropathy in juvenile rheumatoid arthritis. *BMJ* 1985; **290:** 1042.
4. Cohen M, *et al.* Acute disseminated encephalomyelitis as a complication of treatment with gold. *BMJ* 1985; **290:** 1179–80.
5. Dubowitz MN, *et al.* Gold-induced neuroencephalopathy responding to dimercaprol. *Lancet* 1991; **337:** 850–1.
6. Garrido JA, *et al.* Mioquimias inducidas por sales de oro. *Neurologia* 1995; **10:** 235–7.

**Effects on the skin.** Chrysiasis is a distinctive pigmentation that develops in light-exposed skin of patients receiving parenteral gold salts. In a study[1] of 31 patients with chrysiasis who were receiving intramuscular sodium aurothiomalate for rheumatoid arthritis, it was noted that visible changes developed above a threshold equivalent to 20 mg/kg gold content. The severity of the pigmentation depended upon cumulative dose. Focal aggregates of gold are deposited in the reticular and papillary dermis with no obvious increase in melanin. The pigmentation is permanent but benign, although the cosmetic effects may cause some patients distress. Prevention of chrysiasis is difficult but avoidance of exposure to sunlight may be helpful.

1. Smith RW, *et al.* Chrysiasis revisited: a clinical and pathological study. *Br J Dermatol* 1995; **133:** 671–8.

**Hypersensitivity.** Many adverse effects associated with gold treatment have an immunological basis. Patients with contact allergy to gold may exhibit a flare-up, associated with cytokine release, when given sodium aurothiomalate intramuscularly.[1] Small amounts of nickel have been detected in sodium aurothiomalate injection[2] and in sodium aurothioglucose injection[3] and it has been suggested that gold therapy may also exacerbate or induce hypersensitivity to nickel.[2-4]

Anaphylaxis may occur occasionally[5] but vasomotor or 'nitritoid' reactions (see Effects on the Cardiovascular System, above) may produce similar symptoms.

1. Möller H, *et al.* The flare-up reactions after systemic provocation in contact allergy to nickel and gold. *Contact Dermatitis* 1999; **40:** 200–4.
2. Choy EHS, *et al.* Nickel contamination of gold salts: link with gold-induced skin rash. *Br J Rheumatol* 1997; **36:** 1054–8.
3. Wijnands MJH, *et al.* Chrysotherapy provoking exacerbation of contact hypersensitivity to nickel. *Lancet* 1990; **335:** 867–8.
4. Fulton RA, *et al.* Another hazard of gold therapy? *Ann Rheum Dis* 1982; **41:** 100–1.
5. Neustadt DH. Another anaphylactic reaction after gold (aurothiomalate) injection. *J Rheumatol* 1995; **22:** 190.

**Pancreatitis.** It was suggested that pancreatitis reported in a woman receiving gold injections and in a woman on oral gold therapy may have been due to a hypersensitivity reaction.[1]

1. Eisemann AD, *et al.* Pancreatitis and gold treatment of rheumatoid arthritis. *Ann Intern Med* 1989; **111:** 860–1.

## Treatment of Adverse Effects

The treatment of the adverse effects of gold is usually symptomatic and most effects resolve when gold therapy is withdrawn. In severe cases a chelator such as dimercaprol (p.1037) may be used.

## Precautions

Gold therapy is contra-indicated in exfoliative dermatitis, systemic lupus erythematosus, necrotising enterocolitis, and pulmonary fibrosis. It should be used with caution in the elderly and in renal or hepatic impairment; use is contra-indicated if renal or hepatic disorders are severe. Patients with a history of haematological disorders or who have previously shown toxicity to heavy metals should not be given gold salts, nor should any severely debilitated patient.

It is recommended that diabetes mellitus and heart failure should be adequately controlled in any patient before gold is given. Patients with a history of urticaria, eczema, or colitis should be treated with caution. Patients with a poor sulfoxidation status may be more susceptible to adverse effects of sodium aurothiomalate.

Use of gold compounds with other therapy capable of inducing blood disorders should be undertaken with caution, if at all.

Due to the possibility of vasomotor reactions, patients should remain recumbent for about 10 minutes after each injection.

The urine should be tested for albumin before each injection and the blood should be examined for signs of depressed haematopoiesis. Patients receiving gold compounds either orally or parenterally should be warned to report the appearance of sore throat or tongue, metallic taste, pruritus, rash, buccal ulceration, easy bruising, purpura, epistaxis, bleeding gums, unexplained bleeding, menorrhagia, pyrexia, indigestion, diarrhoea, or unexplained malaise. The development of breathlessness or cough should also be reported. Effects such as eosinophilia, proteinuria, pruritus, and rash arising during gold treatment should be allowed to resolve before therapy is continued.

The manufacturer recommends that annual chest X-rays should be carried out.

**Breast feeding.** The American Academy of Pediatrics considers that gold compounds are usually compatible with breast feeding.[1]

Gold has been detected in breast milk[2-4] and found bound to the red blood cells of breast-fed babies.[3,4] In a report[2] of a breast-fed infant it was calculated that the weight-adjusted dose of gold received by the infant exceeded that received by the mother although the infant exhibited no ill-effects during 100 days of breast feeding and developed normally thereafter. Nonetheless, because of the relatively high exposure it was recommended that breast-fed infants should be closely monitored.

1. American Academy of Pediatrics. The transfer of drugs and other chemicals into human milk. *Pediatrics* 2001; **108:** 776–89. Correction. *ibid*; 1029. Also available at: http://aappolicy.aappublications.org/cgi/content/full/pediatrics%3b108/3/776 (accessed 06/07/04)
2. Bennett PN, *et al.* Use of sodium aurothiomalate during lactation. *Br J Clin Pharmacol* 1990; **29:** 777–9.
3. Needs CJ, Brooks PM. Antirheumatic medication during lactation. *Br J Rheumatol* 1985; **24:** 291–7.
4. Blau SP. Metabolism of gold during lactation. *Arthritis Rheum* 1973; **16:** 777–8.

**Porphyria.** Sodium aurothiomalate has been associated with acute attacks of porphyria and is considered unsafe in porphyric patients.

**Pregnancy.** Although there have been a number of healthy neonates born after *in-utero* exposure to gold compounds,[1,2] *animal* studies and a report[1] of malformation in a child born to a woman treated with sodium aurothiomalate led to a suggestion that gold might possibly have teratogenic effects. The manufacturer advises that sodium aurothiomalate should be avoided during pregnancy.

1. Rogers JG, *et al.* Possible teratogenic effects of gold. *Aust Paediatr J* 1980; **16:** 194–5.
2. Bennett PN, *et al.* Use of sodium aurothiomalate during lactation. *Br J Clin Pharmacol* 1990; **29:** 777–9.

## Interactions

There is an increased risk of toxicity when gold compounds are given with other nephrotoxic, hepatotoxic, or myelosuppressive drugs. Use of gold compounds with penicillamine may increase the risk of haematologic or renal adverse reactions.

◊ For a discussion on the effects of previous therapy with gold salts affecting *penicillamine* toxicity, see p.1048. For a possible increased risk of nitritoid reactions when gold compounds are given to patients taking *ACE inhibitors*, see Effects on the Cardiovascular System, p.88.

## Pharmacokinetics

Sodium aurothiomalate is absorbed readily after intramuscular injection and 85 to 95% becomes bound to plasma proteins. With doses of 50 mg weekly a steady-state serum concentration of gold of about 3 to 5 micrograms/mL is reached in 5 to 8 weeks. It is widely distributed to body tissues and fluids, including synovial fluid, and accumulates in the body.

The serum half-life of gold is about 5 to 6 days but this increases after successive doses and after a course of treatment, gold may be found in the urine for up to 1 year or more owing to its presence in deep body compartments. Sodium aurothiomalate is mainly excreted in the urine, with smaller amounts in the faeces.

Gold has been detected in the fetus following administration of sodium aurothiomalate to the mother. Gold is distributed into breast milk.

◊ Reviews.

1. Blocka KLN, *et al.* Clinical pharmacokinetics of oral and injectable gold compounds. *Clin Pharmacokinet* 1986; **11:** 133–43.
2. Tett SE. Clinical pharmacokinetics of slow-acting antirheumatic drugs. *Clin Pharmacokinet* 1993; **25:** 392–407.

## Uses and Administration

Sodium aurothiomalate and other gold compounds are used mainly for their anti-inflammatory effect in active progressive rheumatoid arthritis and progressive juvenile idiopathic arthritis; they may also be beneficial in psoriatic arthritis. They are generally used as disease-modifying antirheumatic drugs in patients whose symptoms are unresponsive to or inadequately controlled by NSAIDs alone.

Sodium aurothiomalate therapy should only be undertaken where facilities are available to carry out the tests specified under Precautions, above.

Sodium aurothiomalate is given by deep intramuscular injection; the area should be gently massaged and, due to the possibility of vasomotor reactions, the patient should remain recumbent for 10 minutes and kept under close observation for 30 minutes after each injection. In the UK, 10 mg is given in the first week to test the patient's tolerance. If satisfactory, this may be followed by doses of 50 mg at weekly intervals until signs of remission occur; the dosage interval is then increased to 2 weeks until full remission occurs and then increased gradually to every 4 to 6 weeks. Treatment may be continued for up to 5 years after remission.

Improvement may not be seen until a total dose of 300 to 500 mg has been given. If no major improvement has occurred after a total of 1 g has been given (excluding the test dose) therapy should be stopped; alternatively in the absence of toxicity, 100 mg may be given weekly for a further 6 weeks; should there be no response at this dose other forms of therapy should be tried. In patients who relapse while receiving maintenance therapy, the interval between doses should be reduced to one week and should not be increased again until control has been obtained but if no response is obtained within 2 months, alternative treatment should be used. It is important to avoid complete relapse since a second course of gold therapy is not usually effective.

For children with progressive juvenile idiopathic arthritis the suggested initial weekly dose is 1 mg/kg to a maximum of 50 mg weekly (one-tenth to one-fifth of the calculated initial weekly dose may be given for 2 to 3 weeks to test the patient's tolerance). With full remission, the dosage interval may be increased gradually to every 4 weeks. If no improvement has occurred after 20 weeks, the dose could be raised slightly or another antirheumatic drug tried.

NSAIDs may be continued when sodium aurothiomalate therapy is begun.

Other gold compounds that have been used include auranofin (p.19), aurothioglucose (p.19), aurotioprol (p.20), gold keratinate (p.45), and sodium aurotiosulfate (p.90).

**Asthma.** For comment on the use of parenteral gold compounds in the treatment of asthma, see p.19.

**Pemphigus and pemphigoid.** Corticosteroids are the main treatment for blistering in pemphigus and pemphigoid (p.1137). Intramuscular gold therapy has been used concomitantly to permit a reduction in corticosteroid dosage although evidence for the steroid-sparing effect is lacking;[1,2] it has been suggested that gold therapy should be reserved for patients who cannot tolerate corticosteroids or in whom they are contra-indicated.[1]

1. Bystryn J-C, Steinman NM. The adjuvant therapy of pemphigus: an update. *Arch Dermatol* 1996; **132:** 203–12.
2. Pandya AG, Dyke C. Treatment of pemphigus with gold. *Arch Dermatol* 1998; **134:** 1104–7.

**Rheumatic disorders.** Gold compounds are among the disease-modifying antirheumatic drugs (DMARDs) that may be used in the treatment of rheumatoid arthritis (p.9) and juvenile idiopathic arthritis (p.9). There is little agreement on which of the various DMARDs should be tried first and their selection is largely based on individual experience and preference. Despite its toxicity intramuscular gold has long been used for the treatment of rheumatoid arthritis and is often the standard against which the efficacy of other treatments is measured. Oral gold is less toxic but is also much less effective. Gold compounds may also be of benefit in psoriatic arthritis (see under Spondyloarthropathies, p.11).

References.

1. Epstein WV, *et al.* Effect of parenterally administered gold therapy on the course of adult rheumatoid arthritis. *Ann Intern Med* 1991; **114:** 437–44.
2. Anonymous. Gold therapy in rheumatoid arthritis. *Lancet* 1991; **338:** 19–20.
3. Klinkhoff AV, Teufel A. How low can you go? Use of very low dosage of gold in patients with mucocutaneous reactions. *J Rheumatol* 1995; **22:** 1657–9.
4. Clark P, *et al.* Injectable gold for rheumatoid arthritis. Available in The Cochrane Library; Issue 2. Chichester: John Wiley; 2004.

## Preparations

***BP 2003:*** Sodium Aurothiomalate Injection;
***USP 27:*** Gold Sodium Thiomalate Injection.

**Proprietary Preparations** (details are given in Part 3)

***Austral.:*** Myocrisin; ***Austria:*** Tauredon; ***Braz.:*** Myochrysine†; ***Canad.:*** Myochrysine; ***Denm.:*** Myocrisin; ***Fin.:*** Myocrisin; ***Ger.:*** Tauredon; ***Hong Kong:*** Myocrisin†; ***Irl.:*** Myocrisin; ***Norw.:*** Myocrisin; ***NZ:*** Myocrisin; ***Port.:*** Tauredon; ***S.Afr.:*** Myocrisin; ***Singapore:*** Miocrin; ***Spain:*** Miocrin; ***Swed.:*** Myocrisin; ***Switz.:*** Tauredon; ***Thai.:*** Myocrisin; ***UK:*** Myocrisin; ***USA:*** Aurolate; Myochrysine.

## Sodium Aurotiosulfate *(rINN)*

Aurotiosulfato de sodio; Gold Sodium Thiosulphate; Sodium Aurothiosulphate; Sodium Dithiosulfatoaurate.

$Na_3Au(S_2O_3)_2,2H_2O$ = 526.2.

*CAS — 10233-88-2 (anhydrous sodium aurotiosulfate); 10210-36-3 (sodium aurotiosulfate dihydrate).*

*ATC — M01CB02.*

### Profile

Sodium aurotiosulfate has a gold content of about 37%. It has similar actions and uses to those of sodium aurothiomalate (p.88). It has been given by intramuscular injection.

### Preparations

**Proprietary Preparations** (details are given in Part 3)
***Arg.:*** Crytion; ***Ital.:*** Fosfocrisolo.

## Sodium Gentisate *(rINN)*

Gentisato de sodio; Gentisato Sodico; Natrii Gentisas. Sodium 2,5-dihydroxybenzoate dihydrate.

$C_7H_5NaO_4,2H_2O$ = 212.1.

*CAS — 490-79-9 (gentisic acid); 4955-90-2 (anhydrous sodium gentisate).*

**Pharmacopoeias.** In *Fr.*

### Profile

Sodium gentisate has been used as an analgesic in the treatment of musculoskeletal and joint disorders. It is also used as a preservative.

## Sodium Salicylate

Natrii Salicylas; Salicilato sódico. Sodium 2-hydroxybenzoate.

$C_7H_5NaO_3$ = 160.1.

*CAS — 54-21-7.*

*ATC — N02BA04.*

**Pharmacopoeias.** In *Eur.* (see p.vi), *Int., Jpn, Pol., US,* and *Viet.*

**Ph. Eur. 5.0** (Sodium Salicylate). Colourless small crystals or shiny flakes, or white crystalline powder. Freely soluble in water; sparingly soluble in alcohol. Store in airtight containers. Protect from light.

**USP 27** (Sodium Salicylate). Amorphous or microcrystalline powder or scales. It is colourless or has not more than a faint pink tinge. It is odourless or has a faint characteristic odour. A freshly made 10% solution in water is neutral or acid to litmus. Freely (and slowly) soluble in water and in glycerol; very soluble in boiling water and in boiling alcohol; slowly soluble in alcohol. Protect from light.

### Adverse Effects, Treatment, and Precautions

As for Aspirin, p.15.

Although sodium salicylate has been used in the treatment of rheumatic fever, its high sodium content may cause problems in patients with cardiac complications.

The use of aspirin and other acetylated salicylates is generally not recommended for children because of the risk of Reye's syndrome, unless specifically indicated. Some licensing information extends this precaution to sodium salicylate.

**Effects on the eyes.** Retinal haemorrhages were reported in a 60-year-old woman taking sodium salicylate 6 g daily by mouth for 2 months and in a 10-year-old girl taking sodium salicylate, 4 g daily by mouth, for 40 days.[1] In both cases the haemorrhages gradually resolved after the treatment was stopped.

1. Mortada A, Abboud I. Retinal haemorrhages after prolonged use of salicylates. *Br J Ophthalmol* 1973; **57:** 199–200.

### Interactions

For interactions associated with salicylates, see Aspirin, p.17.

### Uses and Administration

Sodium salicylate is a salicylic acid derivative that has analgesic, anti-inflammatory, and antipyretic actions similar to those of aspirin (p.17). Sodium salicylate 1 g is approximately equivalent to 1.1 g of aspirin. It is used in the treatment of pain, fever, and in rheumatic disorders such as osteoarthritis and rheumatoid arthritis. The usual oral dose of sodium salicylate for pain or fever is 325 to 650 mg every four hours as required. The oral dose for rheumatic disorders is 3.6 to 5.4 g daily in divided doses. Sodium salicylate has also been used in the symptomatic treatment of rheumatic fever but its high sodium content may cause problems in patients with cardiac complications.

Sodium salicylate has also been given by intravenous infusion and topically.

◊ References.

1. Seymour RA, *et al.* The efficacy and pharmacokinetics of sodium salicylate in post-operative dental pain. *Br J Clin Pharmacol* 1984; **17:** 161–3.

### Preparations

***USP 27:*** Sodium Salicylate Tablets.

**Proprietary Preparations** (details are given in Part 3)
***Canad.:*** Dodds; Saljject; ***NZ:*** Hairscience Shampoo; ***UK:*** Jackson's Pain & Fever.

**Multi-ingredient:** ***Belg.:*** Baseler Haussalbe†; ***Braz.:*** A Saude da Mulher; Abacateirol†; Angi-a-Mid†; Pilulas De Witt's; ***Canad.:*** Plax; Thunas Tab for Menstrual Pain; ***Fr.:*** Aromabyl†; Brulex; Buccawalter†; ***Ger.:*** Gelonida NA; Salimar-Bad L†; ***Mon.:*** Glyco-Thymoline; ***S.Afr.:*** Colphen; Ilvico; ***UK:*** Antiseptic Mouthwash; Doans Backache Pills; TCP; ***USA:*** Cystex; Pabalate†; Scot-Tussin Original 5-Action; Tussirex.

## Sodium Thiosalicylate

Tiosalicilato sódico.

$C_7H_5O_2NaS$ = 176.2.

### Profile

Sodium thiosalicylate is a salicylic acid derivative (see Aspirin, p.15) used parenterally in the treatment of musculoskeletal disorders, osteoarthritis, rheumatic fever, and acute gout.

### Preparations

**Proprietary Preparations** (details are given in Part 3)
***USA:*** Rexolate.

# Sufentanil *(BAN, rINN)*

R-30730; Sufentanilum. *N*-{4-(Methoxymethyl)-1-[2-(2-thienyl)ethyl]-4-piperidyl}propionanilide.

$C_{22}H_{30}N_2O_2S$ = 386.6.

*CAS — 56030-54-7.*

*ATC — N01AH03.*

**Pharmacopoeias.** In *Eur.* (see p.vi).

**Ph. Eur. 5.0** (Sufentanil). A white or almost white powder. Practically insoluble in water; freely soluble in alcohol and in methyl alcohol. Protect from light.

## Sufentanil Citrate *(BANM, USAN, rINNM)*

Citrato de sufentanilo; R-33800; Sufentanili Citras. *N*-{4-(Methoxymethyl)-1-[2-(2-thienyl)ethyl]-4-piperidyl}propionanilide citrate.

$C_{22}H_{30}N_2O_2S,C_6H_8O_7$ = 578.7.

*CAS — 60561-17-3.*

*ATC — N01AH03.*

**Pharmacopoeias.** In *Eur.* (see p.vi) and *US.*

**Ph. Eur. 5.0** (Sufentanil Citrate). A white or almost white powder. Soluble in water and in alcohol; freely soluble in methyl alcohol. Protect from light.

**USP 27** (Sufentanil Citrate). A white powder. Soluble in water; sparingly soluble in alcohol, in acetone, and in chloroform; freely soluble in methyl alcohol. Store at a temperature of 25°, excursions permitted between 15° and 30°.

## Dependence and Withdrawal

As for Opioid Analgesics, p.71.

## Adverse Effects, Treatment, and Precautions

As for Opioid Analgesics in general, p.72 and Fentanyl, p.40.

**Breast feeding.** Concentrations of sufentanil were similar in colostrum and serum in 7 women given sufentanil by continuous epidural infusion during the first postoperative day following caesarean section. In the light of its poor oral availability such an amount was not considered to be a hazard to the breast-feeding infant, and a maternal dose of 5 micrograms/hour epidurally was considered to be safe for such infants.[1]

1. Ausseur A, *et al.* Continuous epidural infusion of sufentanil after caesarean section: concentration in breast milk. *Br J Anaesth* 1994; **72** (suppl 1): 106.

**Effects on the cardiovascular system.** For a reference to the effects of sufentanil on histamine release compared with some other opioids, see under Pethidine, p.80.

**Effects on the nervous system.** There have been reports of tonic-clonic movements or seizures in a few patients receiving sufentanil.[1] There was no evidence of cortical seizure activity in a patient whose EEG was recorded,[2] suggesting that the observed myoclonus was not a convulsion or seizure.

1. Zaccara G, *et al.* Clinical features, pathogenesis and management of drug-induced seizures. *Drug Safety* 1990; **5:** 109–51.
2. Bowdle TA. Myoclonus following sufentanil without EEG seizure activity. *Anesthesiology* 1987; **67:** 593–5.

**Effects on the respiratory system.** Sufentanil, like other opioid agonists, causes dose-related respiratory depression. There have been reports of significant respiratory depression associated with chest wall rigidity in the early postoperative period after anaesthesia with sufentanil.[1,2]

1. Goldberg M, *et al.* Postoperative rigidity following sufentanil administration. *Anesthesiology* 1985; **63:** 199–201.
2. Chang J, Fish KJ. Acute respiratory arrest and rigidity after anesthesia with sufentanil: a case report. *Anesthesiology* 1985; **63:** 710–11.

**Handling.** Avoid contact with skin and the inhalation of particles of sufentanil citrate.

**The elderly.** The pharmacokinetics of sufentanil in elderly patients have been variable in different studies, but a review[1] considered that there had been no evidence overall for differences between the elderly and younger adults. Nevertheless, as with fentanyl, the manufacturer advises reduced initial doses in the elderly.

1. Monk JP, *et al.* Sufentanil: a review of its pharmacological properties and therapeutic use. *Drugs* 1988; **36:** 286–313.

**Obesity.** The elimination half-life and volume of distribution of sufentanil were increased in obese subjects.[1] The manufacturers recommend that for obese patients more than 20% above ideal body-weight the dosage of sufentanil should be determined on the basis of the patients' lean body-weight.

1. Schwartz AE, *et al.* Pharmacokinetics of sufentanil in the obese. *Anesthesiology* 1986; **65** (suppl 3A): A562.

## Interactions

For interactions associated with opioid analgesics, see p.73.

**Benzodiazepines.** For the effects of using opioids such as sufentanil with benzodiazepines, see under Analgesics in the Interactions of Diazepam, p.692.

## Pharmacokinetics

After parenteral doses sufentanil citrate has a rapid onset and short duration of action. The terminal elimination half-life of sufentanil is about 2.5 hours. It is extensively bound to plasma proteins (about 90%). It is metabolised in the liver and small intestine by *N*-dealkylation and *O*-demethylation and the metabolites are excreted in the urine.

◊ The pharmacokinetics of sufentanil have been reviewed.[1,2] Sufentanil is very lipid-soluble. Like alfentanil it is highly bound to plasma protein, principally to $\alpha_1$-acid glycoprotein. The elimination half-life lies between that of alfentanil and fentanyl. The manufacturers of sufentanil have given values for a three-compartment pharmacokinetic model with a distribution half-life of 1.4 minutes, a redistribution half-life of 17.1 minutes, and an elimination half-life of 164 minutes. Accumulation may be relatively limited when compared with fentanyl. In practice the pharmacokinetics of sufentanil may vary according to the age and condition of the patient and the procedures undertaken. For example, the elimination half-life of sufentanil has been reported to be longer in patients undergoing cardiac surgery (595 minutes),[3] in hyperventilated patients (232 minutes),[4] and in those undergoing abdominal aortic surgery (more than 12 hours).[5]

1. Monk JP, *et al.* Sufentanil: a review of its pharmacological properties and therapeutic use. *Drugs* 1988; **36:** 286–313.
2. Scholz J, *et al.* Clinical pharmacokinetics of alfentanil, fentanyl and sufentanil: an update. *Clin Pharmacokinet* 1996; **31:** 275–92.
3. Howie MB, *et al.* Serum concentrations of sufentanil and fentanyl in the post-operative course in cardiac surgery patients. *Anesthesiology* 1984; **61:** A131.
4. Schwartz AE, *et al.* Pharmacokinetics of sufentanil in neurosurgical patients undergoing hyperventilation. *Br J Anaesth* 1989; **63:** 385–8.
5. Hudson RJ, *et al.* Pharmacokinetics of sufentanil in patients undergoing abdominal aortic surgery. *Anesthesiology* 1989; **70:** 426–31.

**Administration.** References to the pharmacokinetics of sufentanil given epidurally,[1] intrathecally,[1] or transdermally.[2]

1. Ionescu TI, *et al.* Pharmacokinetic study of extradural and intrathecal sufentanil anaesthesia for major surgery. *Br J Anaesth* 1991; **66:** 458–64.
2. Sebel PS, *et al.* Transdermal absorption of fentanyl and sufentanil in man. *Eur J Clin Pharmacol* 1987; **32:** 529–31.

**Children.** Neonates (up to 1 month old) had a significantly lower plasma clearance rate and greater elimination half-life than infants (1 month to 2 years), children, and adolescents.[1] Others[2] have found that infants and small children (1 month to 3 years) with cardiac disease had higher clearance rates and shorter elimination half-lives than reported for adults.

1. Greeley WJ, *et al.* Sufentanil pharmacokinetics in pediatric cardiovascular patients. *Anesth Analg* 1987; **66:** 1067–72.
2. Davis PJ, *et al.* Pharmacodynamics and pharmacokinetics of high-dose sufentanil in infants and children undergoing cardiac surgery. *Anesth Analg* 1987; **66:** 203–8.

**Hepatic impairment.** Because of the efficient hepatic extraction and clearance of sufentanil[1] liver dysfunction might be expected to affect its pharmacokinetics. However, elimination kinetics and plasma protein binding were found to be similar in cirrhotic and non-cirrhotic patients after a single dose of sufentanil.[2]

1. Schedewie H, *et al.* Sufentanil and fentanyl hepatic extraction rate and clearance in obese patients undergoing gastroplasty. *Clin Pharmacol Ther* 1988; **43:** 132.
2. Chauvin M, *et al.* Sufentanil pharmacokinetics in patients with cirrhosis. *Anesth Analg* 1989; **68:** 1–4.

**Renal impairment.** The pharmacokinetics of sufentanil were reported[1] to be unaffected in patients with chronic renal failure, although elevated plasma concentrations of sufentanil have been noted[2] in one such patient.

1. Sear JW. Sufentanil disposition in patients undergoing renal transplantation: influence of choice of kinetic model. *Br J Anaesth* 1989; **63:** 60–7.
2. Wiggum DC, *et al.* Postoperative respiratory depression and elevated sufentanil levels in a patient with chronic renal failure. *Anesthesiology* 1985; **63:** 708–10.

### Uses and Administration

Sufentanil, a phenylpiperidine derivative, is an opioid analgesic (p.73) related to fentanyl (p.41). It is highly lipid-soluble and more potent than fentanyl. Sufentanil is used as an analgesic adjunct in anaesthesia and as a primary anaesthetic drug in procedures requiring assisted ventilation. It has a rapid onset and recovery is considered to be more rapid than with fentanyl. It has also been used for the postoperative management of pain.

Sufentanil is given intravenously as the citrate either by slow injection or as an infusion. Doses are expressed as the base; sufentanil citrate 15 micrograms is equivalent to about 10 micrograms of sufentanil. Lower initial doses are advised in the elderly and debilitated patients. For obese patients more than 20% above ideal body-weight the dosage of sufentanil should be determined on the basis of the patient's lean body-weight. In all patients supplementary maintenance doses should be based on individual response and length of procedure. Doses of up to the equivalent of 8 micrograms/kg of sufentanil produce profound analgesia. Higher doses produce a deep level of anaesthesia but are associated with prolonged respiratory depression and assisted ventilation may be required in the postoperative period.

When used as an analgesic **adjunct to anaesthesia** with nitrous oxide and oxygen for surgical procedures lasting up to 8 hours, the total dosage should not exceed 1 microgram/kg per hour. It is customary to give up to 75% of the dose before intubation followed as necessary during surgery by additional injections of 10 to 50 micrograms or by a suitable continuous or intermittent infusion given so that the total hourly dose is not exceeded. Thus, for an operation lasting 1 to 2 hours the total dose would be 1 to 2 micrograms/kg with 0.75 to 1.5 micrograms/kg being given before intubation.

When used as the **primary anaesthetic** drug in major surgery doses of 8 to 30 micrograms/kg are given with 100% oxygen; doses of 25 to 30 micrograms/kg block sympathetic response including catecholamine release and are indicated in procedures such as cardiovascular surgery or neurosurgery. Anaesthesia may be maintained by additional injections of 0.5 to 10 micrograms/kg or by a suitable continuous or intermittent infusion given so that the total dosage for the procedure does not exceed 30 micrograms/kg.

All the above doses relate to the use of sufentanil in adults; experience of paediatric use is more limited. **Children** undergoing cardiovascular surgery may be given sufentanil, with 100% oxygen, in an initial dose of 10 to 25 micrograms/kg with maintenance doses of up to 25 to 50 micrograms.

For the postoperative management of **pain**, sufentanil is given in an initial dose of 30 to 60 micrograms, which should provide analgesia for 4 to 6 hours. Additional boluses of up to 25 micrograms may be given at intervals of not less than 1 hour if necessary.

Sufentanil has also been given **epidurally** for the relief of pain (see below). Recommended doses for labour and delivery are 10 to 15 micrograms given epidurally with 10 mL bupivacaine 0.125% with or without adrenaline; the dose may be repeated twice at not less than one-hour intervals until delivery. The total dose of sufentanil should not exceed 30 micrograms.

◊ General reviews of sufentanil.


1. Monk JP, *et al.* Sufentanil: a review of its pharmacological properties and therapeutic use. *Drugs* 1988; **36:** 286–313.
2. Clotz MA, Nahata MC. Clinical uses of fentanyl, sufentanil, and alfentanil. *Clin Pharm* 1991; **10:** 581–93.


**Administration.** Sufentanil is usually given intravenously, but the epidural route is also used (see below). Intranasal administration (see under Anaesthesia and under Sedation, below) or intrathecal administration (see below) have also been tried.

EPIDURAL. In a laboratory assessment of epidural sufentanil in healthy subjects,[1] a dose of 50 micrograms produced analgesia for 2 to 3 hours; analgesia was intensified and prolonged and respiratory and other side-effects, especially drowsiness, were reduced by the addition of adrenaline. Epidural sufentanil or fentanyl provided effective postoperative analgesia following caesarean section with comparable adverse effect profiles.[2] Sufentanil doses of 20 and 30 micrograms showed equivalent efficacy and provided greater analgesia for a longer duration than a dose of 10 micrograms. Addition of sufentanil to the local anaesthetic bupivacaine has improved the quality of epidural analgesia.[3]

Effective analgesia has been achieved in children with epidural sufentanil.[4]

Epidural administration of sufentanil has been tried for patient-controlled analgesia but appeared to have little advantage over patient-controlled analgesia using intravenous morphine.[5]


1. Klepper ID, *et al.* Analgesic and respiratory effects of extradural sufentanil in volunteers and the influence of adrenaline as an adjuvant. *Br J Anaesth* 1987; **59:** 1147–56.
2. Grass JA, *et al.* A randomized, double-blind, dose-response comparison of epidural fentanyl versus sufentanil analgesia after cesarean section. *Anesth Analg* 1997; **85:** 365–71.
3. Reynolds F. Extradural opioids in labour. *Br J Anaesth* 1989; **63:** 251–3.
4. Benlabed M, *et al.* Analgesia and ventilatory response to $CO_2$ following epidural sufentanil in children. *Anesthesiology* 1987; **67:** 948–51.
5. Grass JA, *et al.* Patient-controlled analgesia after cesarean delivery: epidural sufentanil versus intravenous morphine. *Reg Anesth* 1994; **19:** 90–7.


INTRATHECAL. Sufentanil has been given intrathecally for labour pain. There was no significant difference in terms of effects on fetal heart rate when intrathecal sufentanil was compared with epidural bupivacaine,[1] although it was suggested that fetal heart rate should be monitored carefully when either drug is used. A combination of sufentanil, bupivacaine, and adrenaline given intrathecally provided excellent analgesia during labour and had a more rapid onset, a longer duration of action, and reduced local anaesthetic requirements compared with epidural administration.[2] Intrathecal sufentanil and bupivacaine provided shorter duration of analgesia when given during the advanced stages of labour compared with early labour.[3]


1. Nielsen PE, *et al.* Fetal heart rate changes after intrathecal sufentanil or epidural bupivacaine for labor analgesia: incidence and clinical significance. *Anesth Analg* 1996; **83:** 742–6.
2. Kartawiadi SL, *et al.* Spinal analgesia during labor with low-dose bupivacaine, sufentanil, and epinephrine: a comparison with epidural analgesia. *Reg Anesth* 1996; **21:** 191–6.
3. Viscomi CM, *et al.* Duration of intrathecal labor analgesia: early versus advanced labor. *Anesth Analg* 1997; **84:** 1108–12.


**Anaesthesia.** Sufentanil, like fentanyl (p.42), appears to produce fewer circulatory changes than morphine, which may offer some advantages in cardiovascular surgery.

*Premedication* with sufentanil given intranasally has been tried in children[1,2] and in adults.[3]

*Neuroleptanalgesia.* Sufentanil is one of the opioids that have been used with a neuroleptic to produce neuroleptanalgesia.


1. Henderson JM, *et al.* Pre-induction of sufentanil. *Anesthesiology* 1988; **68:** 671–5.
2. Zedie N, *et al.* Comparison of intranasal midazolam and sufentanil premedication in pediatric outpatients. *Clin Pharmacol Ther* 1996; **59:** 341–8.
3. Helmers JHJH, *et al.* Comparison of intravenous and intranasal sufentanil absorption and sedation. *Can J Anaesth* 1989; **36:** 494–7.


**Pain.** For the use of sufentanil in the management of pain, see under Epidural and Intrathecal Administration, above.

**Sedation.** Some references to the use of sufentanil for sedation are given below. See also under Anaesthesia, above.


1. Bates BA, *et al.* A comparison of intranasal sufentanil and midazolam to intramuscular meperidine, promethazine, and chlorpromazine for conscious sedation in children. *Ann Emerg Med* 1994; **24:** 646–51.
2. Lefrant JY, *et al.* Sufentanil short duration infusion for postoperative sedation in critically ill patients. *Br J Anaesth* 1995; **74** (suppl 1): 114.


### Preparations

***USP 27:*** Sufentanil Citrate Injection.

**Proprietary Preparations** (details are given in Part 3)
***Arg.:*** Sufenta; ***Austria:*** Sufenta; ***Belg.:*** Sufenta; ***Braz.:*** Fastfen; Sufenta; ***Canad.:*** Sufenta; ***Chile:*** Sufenta; ***Denm.:*** Sufenta; ***Fin.:*** Sufenta; ***Fr.:*** Sufenta; ***Ger.:*** Sufenta; ***Ital.:*** Fentatienil; ***Malaysia:*** Sufenta; ***Neth.:*** Sufenta; ***Norw.:*** Sufenta; ***S.Afr.:*** Sufenta; ***Swed.:*** Sufenta; ***Switz.:*** Sufenta; ***USA:*** Sufenta.

## Sulindac *(BAN, USAN, rINN)*

MK-231; Sulindaco; Sulindacum. (*Z*)-[5-Fluoro-2-methyl-1-(4-methylsulphinylbenzylidene)inden-3-yl]acetic acid.

$C_{20}H_{17}FO_3S$ = 356.4.

*CAS — 38194-50-2.*

*ATC — M01AB02.*

**Pharmacopoeias.** In *Chin., Eur.* (see p.vi), and *US.*

**Ph. Eur. 5.0** (Sulindac). A yellow, polymorphic, crystalline powder. Very slightly soluble in water and in ether; sparingly soluble in alcohol; soluble in dichloromethane; dissolves in dilute solutions of alkali hydroxides. Protect from light.

**USP 27** (Sulindac). A yellow, odourless or practically odourless, crystalline powder. Practically insoluble in water and in hexane; slightly soluble in alcohol, in acetone, in chloroform, and in methyl alcohol; very slightly soluble in ethyl acetate and in isopropyl alcohol.

### Adverse Effects and Precautions

As for NSAIDs in general, p.67. Urine discoloration has occasionally been reported with sulindac.

Sulindac metabolites have been reported as major or minor components in renal stones. It should therefore be used with caution in patients with a history of renal stones and such patients should be kept well hydrated while receiving sulindac.

Patients with hepatic impairment should not be given sulindac. The dose of sulindac may need to be reduced in those with renal impairment.

**Effects on the blood.** Agranulocytosis,[1] thrombocytopenia,[2] haemolytic anaemia,[3] and aplastic anaemia[4] have been reported in patients taking sulindac.


1. Romeril KR, *et al.* Sulindac induced agranulocytosis and bone marrow culture. *Lancet* 1981; **ii:** 523.
2. Karachalios GN, Parigorakis JG. Thrombocytopenia and sulindac. *Ann Intern Med* 1986; **104:** 128.
3. Johnson FP, *et al.* Immune hemolytic anemia associated with sulindac. *Arch Intern Med* 1985; **145:** 1515–16.
4. Andrews R, Russell N. Aplastic anaemia associated with a non-steroidal anti-inflammatory drug: relapse after exposure to another such drug. *BMJ* 1990; **301:** 38.


**Effects on the CNS.** Acute deterioration of parkinsonism occurred in a patient after starting sulindac.[1]

See also under Hypersensitivity, below.


1. Sandyk R, Gillman MA. Acute exacerbation of Parkinson's disease with sulindac. *Ann Neurol* 1985; **17:** 104–5.


**Effects on the endocrine system.** A case of reversible gynaecomastia associated with sulindac therapy has been reported.[1] There has also been a report[2] of reversible hypothyroidism in an elderly patient taking sulindac.


1. Kapoor A. Reversible gynecomastia associated with sulindac therapy. *JAMA* 1983; **250:** 2284–5.
2. Iyer RP, Duckett GK. Reversible secondary hypothyroidism induced by sulindac. *BMJ* 1985; **290:** 1788.


**Effects on the gallbladder.** A "sludge" composed of crystalline metabolites of sulindac has been found in the common bile duct during surgery for biliary obstruction in patients who had been taking sulindac.[1]


1. Anonymous. Rare complication with sulindac. *FDA Drug Bull* 1989; **19:** 4.


**Effects on the kidneys.** Sulindac-induced renal impairment, interstitial nephritis, and nephrotic syndrome have been reported.[1] It has been suggested that sulindac, as a prodrug, may not inhibit renal prostaglandin synthesis in therapeutic doses. However, this potentially important therapeutic advantage has not been uniformly observed in short-term studies in patients with renal dysfunction.[2-4]

There have been reports of renal stones consisting of between 10 and 90% of sulindac metabolites developing in patients treated with sulindac.[5]


1. Whelton A, *et al.* Sulindac and renal impairment. *JAMA* 1983; **249:** 2892.
2. Klassen DK, *et al.* Sulindac kinetics and effects on renal function and prostaglandin excretion in renal insufficiency. *J Clin Pharmacol* 1989; **29:** 1037–42.
3. Eriksson L-O, *et al.* Effects of sulindac and naproxen on prostaglandin excretion in patients with impaired renal function and rheumatoid arthritis. *Am J Med* 1990; **89:** 313–21.
4. Whelton A, *et al.* Renal effects of ibuprofen, piroxicam, and sulindac in patients with asymptomatic renal failure. *Ann Intern Med* 1990; **112:** 568–76.
5. Anonymous. Rare complication with sulindac. *FDA Drug Bull* 1989; **19:** 4.


**Effects on the liver.** Hepatotoxicity reported in patients receiving sulindac includes hepatocellular injury and cholestatic jaundice.[1,2] Symptoms of hypersensitivity including rash, fever, or eosinophilia have been reported in 35 to 55% of patients with sulindac-induced liver damage;[2] in these patients the liver damage occurred usually within 4 to 8 weeks of beginning sulindac therapy. For reference to a report citing the strongest evidence for an association of sulindac with liver disease compared with other NSAIDs, see under NSAIDs, p.69.

See also under Effects on the Skin, below.


1. Gallanosa AG, Spyker DA. Sulindac hepatotoxicity: a case report and review. *Clin Toxicol* 1985; **23:** 205–38.
2. Tarazi EM, *et al.* Sulindac-associated hepatic injury: analysis of 91 cases reported to the Food and Drug Administration. *Gastroenterology* 1993; **104:** 569–74.


**Effects on the lungs.** For reference to pneumonitis associated with sulindac therapy, see under Hypersensitivity, below.

**Effects on the skin.** Toxic epidermal necrolysis has occurred in patients taking sulindac.[1] In a patient toxic hepatitis and the Stevens-Johnson/toxic epidermal necrolysis syndrome resulted in death.[2]

An unusual pernio-like reaction affecting the toes, which was also confirmed by rechallenge, has also been reported.[3]

Sulindac has also been reported to cause photosensitivity reactions.[4]


1. Small RE, Garnett WR. Sulindac-induced toxic epidermal necrolysis. *Clin Pharm* 1988; **7:** 766–71.
2. Klein SM, Khan MA. Hepatitis, toxic epidermal necrolysis and pancreatitis in association with sulindac therapy. *J Rheumatol* 1983; **10:** 512–13.

3. Reinertsen JL. Unusual pernio-like reaction to sulindac. *Arthritis Rheum* 1981; **24:** 1215.
4. Anonymous. Drugs that cause photosensitivity. *Med Lett Drugs Ther* 1986; **28:** 51–2.

**Hypersensitivity.** Hypersensitivity reactions to sulindac include pneumonitis,[1,2] generalised lymphadenopathy,[3] aseptic meningitis,[4] and anaphylactoid reaction.[5]

See also under Effects on the Liver and under Effects on the Skin, above.

1. Smith FE, Lindberg PJ. Life-threatening hypersensitivity to sulindac. *JAMA* 1980; **244:** 269–70.
2. Fein M. Sulindac and pneumonitis. *Ann Intern Med* 1981; **95:** 245.
3. Sprung DJ. Sulindac causing a hypersensitivity reaction with peripheral and mediastinal lymphadenopathy. *Ann Intern Med* 1982; **97:** 564.
4. Fordham von Reyn C. Recurrent aseptic meningitis due to sulindac. *Ann Intern Med* 1983; **99:** 343–4.
5. Hyson CP, Kazakoff MA. A severe multisystem reaction to sulindac. *Arch Intern Med* 1991; **151:** 387–8.

**Pancreatitis.** Reports[1-4] of pancreatitis associated with sulindac therapy.

1. Goldstein J, *et al.* Sulindac associated with pancreatitis. *Ann Intern Med* 1980; **93:** 151.
2. Siefkin AD. Sulindac and pancreatitis. *Ann Intern Med* 1980; **93:** 932–3.
3. Lilly EL. Pancreatitis after administration of sulindac. *JAMA* 1981; **246:** 2680.
4. Memon AN. Pancreatitis and sulindac. *Ann Intern Med* 1982; **97:** 139.

## Interactions

For interactions associated with NSAIDs, see p.69.

Dimethyl sulfoxide reduces plasma concentrations of the active metabolite of sulindac and use of the two drugs together has also resulted in peripheral neuropathy. Diflunisal and aspirin are reported to reduce the plasma concentration of the active metabolite of sulindac. Unlike other NSAIDs, sulindac is reported not to reduce the antihypertensive effects of drugs such as thiazide diuretics, but nevertheless the manufacturers recommend that blood pressure be closely monitored in patients taking antihypertensives and sulindac together.

## Pharmacokinetics

Sulindac is absorbed from the gastrointestinal tract. It is metabolised by reversible reduction to the sulfide metabolite, which appears to be the biologically active form, and by irreversible oxidation to the sulfone metabolite. Peak plasma concentrations of the sulfide metabolite are achieved in about 2 hours. The mean elimination half-life of sulindac is about 7.8 hours and of the sulfide metabolite about 16.4 hours. Sulindac and its metabolites are highly bound to plasma protein. About 50% is excreted in the urine mainly as the sulfone metabolite and its glucuronide conjugate, with smaller amounts of sulindac and its glucuronide conjugate; about 25% appears in the faeces, primarily as sulfone and sulfide metabolites. Sulindac and its metabolites are also excreted in bile and undergo extensive enterohepatic circulation.

◊ References.

1. Davies NM, Watson MS. Clinical pharmacokinetics of sulindac: a dynamic old drug. *Clin Pharmacokinet* 1997; **32:** 437–59.

## Uses and Administration

Sulindac is an NSAID (p.70) structurally related to indometacin (p.48); its biological activity appears to be due to its sulfide metabolite. Sulindac is used in musculoskeletal and joint disorders such as ankylosing spondylitis, osteoarthritis, and rheumatoid arthritis, and also in the short-term management of acute gout and peri-articular conditions such as bursitis and tendinitis. It is also used to reduce fever.

A usual initial dose of sulindac by mouth is 150 or 200 mg twice daily, reduced according to response. The maximum recommended daily dose is 400 mg and doses may need reduction in renal impairment. The UK manufacturers recommend that the treatment of peri-articular disorders should be limited to 7 to 10 days; for acute gout, 7 days of therapy is usually adequate.

Sulindac sodium has been given by rectal suppository.

**Administration in renal impairment.** The dose of sulindac may need to be reduced in patients with renal function impairment.

**Gastrointestinal disorders.** In placebo-controlled studies[1,2] sulindac 150 to 200 mg twice daily for 6 to 9 months has reduced the number and size of polyps in patients with familial adenomatous polyposis but the effect may be incomplete and in a study[2] only polyps less than 2 mm in size regressed. In addition, the size and number of polyps has been reported[1] to increase on discontinuation of treatment and long-term therapy is therefore being studied. However, some workers[3] have observed diminution of sulindac's effectiveness with long-term treatment although others[4] have reported that they have managed recurrences by adjustment of the maintenance dosage used; it appeared that there were individual variations in sensitivity to sulindac with respect to prevention of polyp recurrence although 200 mg daily appeared to be an average maintenance dose needed.[4] There is evidence[5] that sulindac alters the ratio of apoptosis of surface cells relative to those lying deeper in the crypt of rectal mucosa, thus altering epithelial homoeostasis. Whether sulindac prevents malignant degeneration is unknown but there has been a report[6] of a patient who developed rectal cancer during long-term therapy for familial adenomatous polyposis. A more recent, placebo-controlled trial[7] has also reported that sulindac did not reduce the development of adenomas in patients with familial adenomatous polyposis. Some[1,7] consider that sulindac is unlikely to replace surgery as primary therapy for familial adenomatous polyposis.

Sulindac has also been reported to have produced beneficial effects in a patient with duodenal polyps associated with Gardner's syndrome[8] but a placebo-controlled study has suggested that it may not be effective against sporadic type colonic polyps.[9]

For a discussion of evidence suggesting that regular use of NSAIDs may protect against various types of malignant neoplasms of the gastrointestinal tract, see under Malignant Neoplasms in NSAIDs, p.71.

1. Giardiello FM, *et al.* Treatment of colonic and rectal adenomas with sulindac in familial adenomatous polyposis. *N Engl J Med* 1993; **328:** 1313–16.
2. Debinski HS, *et al.* Effect of sulindac on small polyps in familial adenomatous polyposis. *Lancet* 1995; **345:** 855–6.
3. Tonelli F, Valanzano R. Sulindac in familial adenomatous polyposis. *Lancet* 1993; **342:** 1120.
4. Labayle D, *et al.* Sulindac in familial adenomatous polyposis. *Lancet* 1994; **343:** 417–18.
5. Keller JJ, *et al.* Rectal epithelial apoptosis in familial adenomatous polyposis patients treated with sulindac. *Gut* 1999; **45:** 822–8.
6. Thorson AG, *et al.* Rectal cancer in FAP patient after sulindac. *Lancet* 1994; **343:** 180.
7. Giardiello FM, *et al.* Primary chemoprevention of familial adenomatous polyposis with sulindac. *N Engl J Med* 2002; **346:** 1054–9.
8. Parker AL, *et al.* Disappearance of duodenal polyps in Gardner's syndrome with sulindac therapy. *Am J Gastroenterol* 1993; **88:** 93–4.
9. Ladenheim J, *et al.* Effect of sulindac on sporadic colonic polyps. *Gastroenterology* 1995; **108:** 1083–7.

**Premature labour.** The most common approach to postponing premature labour (p.794) with drugs has historically been with a selective $beta_2$ agonist. However, as prostaglandins have a role in uterine contraction and cervical ripening and dilatation, prostaglandin synthetase inhibitors such as indometacin have also been used. Sulindac has also been tried[1,2] as an alternative to indometacin as it appears to have little placental transfer and may therefore have fewer fetal side-effects.[1] However, the authors of a more recent study suggested that sulindac has many of the same adverse fetal effects as indometacin and its use can only be described as investigational.[3]

1. Carlan SJ, *et al.* Randomized comparative trial of indomethacin and sulindac for the treatment of refractory preterm labor. *Obstet Gynecol* 1992; **79:** 223–8.
2. Carlan SJ, *et al.* Outpatient oral sulindac to prevent recurrence of preterm labor. *Obstet Gynecol* 1995; **85:** 769–74.
3. Kramer WB, *et al.* A randomized double-blind study comparing the fetal effects of sulindac to terbutaline during the management of preterm labor. *Am J Obstet Gynecol* 1999; **180:** 396–401.

## Preparations

***BP 2003:*** Sulindac Tablets;
***USP 27:*** Sulindac Tablets.

**Proprietary Preparations** (details are given in Part 3)
***Austral.:*** Aclin; Clinoril; Saldac†; ***Austria:*** Clinoril; ***Belg.:*** Clinoril; ***Canad.:*** Apo-Sulin; Clinoril†; Novo-Sundac; ***Denm.:*** Clinoril; ***Fr.:*** Arthrocine; ***Hong Kong:*** Aclin; Clinoril; ***Irl.:*** Clinoril; ***Ital.:*** Aflodac†; Algocetil; Citireuma†; Clinoril; Lyndak†; Sulartrene†; Sulen; Sulinol†; ***Malaysia:*** Aclin; Apo-Sulin; Clinoril; ***Mex.:*** Bio-Dac; Clinoril; Copal; Kenalin; ***Neth.:*** Clinoril; ***Norw.:*** Clinoril; ***NZ:*** Clinoril; Daclin; Saldac†; ***Port.:*** Artribid; ***S.Afr.:*** Clinoril†; ***Spain:*** Sulindal; ***Swed.:*** Clinoril; ***Switz.:*** Clinoril; ***Thai.:*** Cenlidac; Clinoril; ***UK:*** Clinoril; ***USA:*** Clinoril.

## Superoxide Dismutase

SOD; Superóxido dismutasa.

**Description.** Superoxide dismutase represents a group of water-soluble protein congeners widely distributed in nature which catalyse the conversion of superoxide radicals to peroxide. Several different forms exist, which vary in their metal content; forms containing copper or copper and zinc are common.

## Orgotein *(BAN, USAN, rINN)*

Bovine Superoxide Dismutase; Orgoteína; Ormetein.
*CAS — 9016-01-7.*
*ATC — M01AX14.*

**Description.** Orgotein is a superoxide dismutase produced from beef liver as Cu-Zn mixed chelate. Mol. wt about 33 000 with a compact conformation maintained by about 4 gram-atoms of chelated divalent metal.

## Pegorgotein *(USAN, rINN)*

Pegorgoteína; PEG-SOD; Win-22118.
*CAS — 155773-57-2.*

**Description.** Pegorgotein is a superoxide dismutase conjugated with polyethylene glycol to prolong its duration of action.

## Sudismase *(rINN)*

Sudismasa.
*CAS — 110294-55-8.*

**Description.** Sudismase is a human *N*-acetylsuperoxide dismutase produced by recombinant DNA technology and containing a copper and zinc prosthetic group.

## Adverse Effects

Anaphylaxis and other hypersensitivity reactions, sometimes fatal, have been reported with orgotein. Local reactions and pain may occur at the site of injection of orgotein.

## Pharmacokinetics

◊ References.

1. Tsao C, *et al.* Pharmacokinetics of recombinant human superoxide dismutase in healthy volunteers. *Clin Pharmacol Ther* 1991; **50:** 713–20.
2. Uematsu T, *et al.* Pharmacokinetics and safety of intravenous recombinant human superoxide dismutase (NK341) in healthy subjects. *Int J Clin Pharmacol Ther* 1994; **32:** 638–41.
3. Jadot G, *et al.* Clinical pharmacokinetics and delivery of bovine superoxide dismutase. *Clin Pharmacokinet* 1995; **28:** 17–25.
4. Rosenfeld WN, *et al.* Safety and pharmacokinetics of recombinant human superoxide dismutase administered intrathecally to premature neonates with respiratory distress syndrome. *Pediatrics* 1996; **97:** 811–17.
5. Davis JM, *et al.* Safety and pharmacokinetics of multiple doses of recombinant human CuZn superoxide dismutase administered intrathecally to premature neonates with respiratory distress syndrome. *Pediatrics* 1997; **100:** 24–30.

## Uses and Administration

Superoxide dismutases have anti-inflammatory properties. Orgotein, a bovine derived superoxide dismutase, has been given by local injection, into the joints for degenerative joint disorders, but hypersensitivity reactions have limited its use. It has also been tried for the amelioration of side-effects from radiotherapy. Forms of human superoxide dismutase derived by recombinant DNA technology have been developed.

Superoxide dismutases are also under investigation for their free-radical scavenging properties in a variety of conditions including the prevention of bronchopulmonary dysplasia in neonates.

**Bronchopulmonary dysplasia.** Use of sudismase in premature infants treated for respiratory distress syndrome did not prevent development of bronchopulmonary dysplasia (p.1077) in the first month.[1] However, treated infants subsequently showed a lower incidence of severe respiratory disease and hospitalisations in the first year, suggesting a reduction in chronic lung injury. The antioxidant was given intratracheally in a dose of 5 mg/kg every 48 hours as long as intubation and ventilation were necessary. A systematic review[2] was unable to reach a firm conclusion about the efficacy of superoxide dismutases in preventing chronic lung disease.

1. Davis JM, *et al.* Pulmonary outcome at 1 year corrected age in premature infants treated at birth with recombinant human CuZn superoxide dismutase. *Pediatrics* 2003; **111:** 469–76.
2. Suresh GK, *et al.* Superoxide dismutase for preventing chronic lung disease in mechanically ventilated preterm infants. Available in The Cochrane Library; Issue 2. Chichester: John Wiley; 2004.

**Head injury.** Pegorgotein was found[1] to be little more effective than placebo in improving neurological outcome or reducing mortality in patients with severe head injury.

1. Young B, *et al.* Effects of pegorgotein on neurologic outcome of patients with severe head injury: a multicenter, randomized controlled trial. *JAMA* 1996; **276:** 538–43.

**Motor neurone disease.** A small percentage of patients with familial amyotrophic lateral sclerosis (see Motor Neurone Disease, p.1739) have been shown to have a mutation in the gene encoding for the enzyme copper-zinc superoxide dismutase but there has been no consensus as to whether patients with this mutation should be given superoxide dismutase supplements.[1]

1. Orrell RW, deBelleroche JS. Superoxide dismutase and ALS. *Lancet* 1994; **344:** 1651–2.

**Radiotherapy.** Although some studies[1,2] indicate that orgotein can ameliorate the side-effects of radiotherapy for bladder tumours, another study[3] was terminated prematurely because of unacceptable hypersensitivity reactions and apparent inefficacy.

1. Valencia J, *et al.* The efficacy of orgotein in the treatment of acute toxicity due to radiotherapy on head and neck tumors. *Tumori* 2002; **88:** 385–9.
2. Sanchiz F, *et al.* Prevention of radioinduced cystitis by orgotein: a randomized study. *Anticancer Res* 1996; **16:** 2025–8.
3. Nielsen OS, *et al.* Orgotein in radiation treatment of bladder cancer: a report on allergic reactions and lack of radioprotective effect. *Acta Oncol* 1987; **26:** 101–4.

### Preparations

**Proprietary Preparations** (details are given in Part 3)
***Spain:*** Ontosein.

## Suprofen *(BAN, USAN, rINN)*

R-25061; Suprofeno; Sutoprofen. 2-[4-(2-Thenoyl)phenyl]propionic acid.

$C_{14}H_{12}O_3S$ = 260.3.
*CAS — 40828-46-4.*
*ATC — M01AE07.*

**Pharmacopoeias.** In *US.*

**USP 27** (Suprofen). A white to off-white powder, odourless or having a slight odour. Sparingly soluble in water.

### Adverse Effects and Precautions

Suprofen eye drops may cause local reactions including discomfort, itching, redness, iritis, pain, chemosis, photophobia, and rarely punctate epithelial staining. Hypersensitivity may occur. They should not be used in patients with active herpes simplex keratitis.

Adverse renal reactions after oral doses have ended its use as an oral NSAID.

**Breast feeding.** No adverse effects have been observed in breast-feeding infants whose mothers were receiving oral suprofen, and the American Academy of Pediatrics considers[1] that it is therefore usually compatible with breast feeding. However, oral dosage forms have been discontinued because of renal toxicity.

1. American Academy of Pediatrics. The transfer of drugs and other chemicals into human milk. *Pediatrics* 2001; **108:** 776–89. Correction. *ibid.*; 1029. Also available at: http://aappolicy.aappublications.org/cgi/content/full/pediatrics%3b108/3/776 (accessed 06/07/04)

**Effects on the kidneys.** A clinical syndrome of flank pain and acute renal failure associated with oral suprofen has been reported;[1] the syndrome is unlike other nephrotoxic syndromes related to NSAIDs.

1. Hart D, *et al.* Suprofen-related nephrotoxicity: a distinct clinical syndrome. *Ann Intern Med* 1987; **106:** 235–8.

### Interactions

◊ The manufacturer of acetylcholine chloride ophthalmic preparations has stated that there have been reports that *acetylcholine* and *carbachol* have been ineffective when used in patients treated with topical (ophthalmic) NSAIDs.

### Uses and Administration

Suprofen is an NSAID (p.70). Suprofen is used as 1% eye drops to inhibit the miosis that may occur during ocular surgery. On the day of surgery, 2 drops are instilled into the conjunctival sac 3 hours, 2 hours, and then 1 hour before surgery. Two drops may also be instilled every 4 hours during the day before surgery.

It was formerly given by mouth in mild to moderate pain and in osteoarthritis and rheumatoid arthritis but, following reports of adverse renal reactions, marketing of the oral dose form was suspended worldwide.

### Preparations

***USP 27:*** Suprofen Ophthalmic Solution.

**Proprietary Preparations** (details are given in Part 3)
***Braz.:*** Procofen†; ***USA:*** Profenal.

## Suxibuzone *(BAN, rINN)*

Suxibuzona; Suxibuzonum. 4-Butyl-4-hydroxymethyl-1,2-diphenylpyrazolidine-3,5-dione hydrogen succinate (ester).

$C_{24}H_{26}N_2O_6$ = 438.5.
*CAS — 27470-51-5.*
*ATC — M02AA22.*

**Pharmacopoeias.** In *Eur.* (see p.vi).

**Ph. Eur. 5.0** (Suxibuzone). A white crystalline powder. Practically insoluble in water; soluble in alcohol; freely soluble in acetone; practically insoluble in cyclohexane.

### Profile

Suxibuzone, a derivative of phenylbutazone (p.83), is an NSAID (p.67) that has been applied topically at a concentration of about 7% in musculoskeletal and joint disorders. Concern over safety and toxicity following oral use has led to its withdrawal from the market in many countries.

### Preparations

**Proprietary Preparations** (details are given in Part 3)
***Spain:*** Danilon.

## Tenoxicam *(BAN, USAN, rINN)*

Ro-12-0068; Ro-12-0068/000; Tenoxicamum. 4-Hydroxy-2-methyl-*N*-(2-pyridyl)-2*H*-thieno[2,3-e][1,2]thiazine-3-carboxamide 1,1-dioxide.

$C_{13}H_{11}N_3O_4S_2$ = 337.4.
*CAS — 59804-37-4.*
*ATC — M01AC02.*

**Pharmacopoeias.** In *Eur.* (see p.vi).

**Ph. Eur. 5.0** (Tenoxicam). A yellow, polymorphic, crystalline powder. Practically insoluble in water; very slightly soluble in dehydrated alcohol; sparingly soluble in dichloromethane; it dissolves in solutions of acids and alkalis. Protect from light.

### Adverse Effects and Precautions

As for NSAIDs in general, p.67.

**Incidence of adverse effects.** Adverse effects associated with tenoxicam have been reviewed.[1] The majority of adverse effects relate to the gastrointestinal tract (11.4%), nervous system (2.8%), or skin (2.5%).

1. Todd PA, Clissold SP. Tenoxicam: an update of its pharmacology and therapeutic efficacy in rheumatic diseases. *Drugs* 1991; **41:** 625–46.

**Effects on the kidneys.** A review[1] of the effects of tenoxicam on renal function concluded that tenoxicam could be given at normal recommended doses to elderly patients or those with mild to moderate renal impairment who were not at high risk of renal failure or receiving potentially nephrotoxic therapy. Data from the manufacturer's database[1] on 67 063 patients, including 17 005 over 65 years of age, who had received tenoxicam indicated that there had been 45 adverse events relating to urinary system function, described as severe in 7. The prevalence of adverse events was similar in elderly and non-elderly patients, the most common effects being dysuria and renal pain.

1. Heintz RCA. Tenoxicam and renal function. *Drug Safety* 1995; **12:** 110–19.

**Effects on the liver.** A report[1] of acute hepatitis associated with the use of tenoxicam.

1. Sungur C, *et al.* Acute hepatitis caused by tenoxicam. *Ann Pharmacother* 1994; **28:** 1309.

**Effects on the skin.** A report of 3 cases of toxic epidermal necrolysis (Lyell's syndrome) associated with tenoxicam.[1]

For the general incidence of dermatological effects see above.

1. Chosidow O, *et al.* Toxidermies sévères au ténoxicam (Tilcotil®). *Ann Dermatol Venereol* 1991; **118:** 903–4.

### Interactions

For interactions associated with NSAIDs, see p.69.

### Pharmacokinetics

Tenoxicam is well absorbed after oral doses; peak plasma concentrations occur within about 2 hours in fasting subjects; this may be delayed to about 6 hours when tenoxicam is given with food but the extent of absorption is not affected. Tenoxicam is over 98.5% protein bound and penetrates synovial fluid. The plasma elimination half-life is about 60 to 75 hours; with daily administration, steady-state concentrations are reached within 10 to 15 days. Tenoxicam is completely metabolised to inactive metabolites which are excreted mainly in the urine; there is some biliary excretion of glucuronide conjugates of the metabolites.

◊ References.

1. Nilsen OG. Clinical pharmacokinetics of tenoxicam. *Clin Pharmacokinet* 1994; **26:** 16–43.
2. Guentert TW, *et al.* Relative bioavailability of oral dosage forms of tenoxicam. *Arzneimittelforschung* 1994; **44:** 1051–4.

### Uses and Administration

Tenoxicam, a piroxicam (p.85) analogue, is an NSAID (p.70). It is used in the symptomatic management of musculoskeletal and joint disorders such as osteoarthritis and rheumatoid arthritis, and also in the short-term management of soft-tissue injury. Tenoxicam is given by mouth as a single daily dose usually of 20 mg. In acute musculoskeletal disorders treatment for up to 7 days is usually sufficient but in severe cases it may be given for up to a maximum of 14 days. Doses similar to those given by mouth have been given by intramuscular or intravenous injection for initial treatment for 1 to 2 days. Tenoxicam has also been given by rectal suppository.

◊ References.

1. Todd PA, Clissold SP. Tenoxicam: an update of its pharmacology and therapeutic efficacy in rheumatic diseases. *Drugs* 1991; **41:** 625–46.

### Preparations

***BP 2003:*** Tenoxicam Injection; Tenoxicam Tablets.

**Proprietary Preparations** (details are given in Part 3)
***Arg.:*** Mefenix; ***Austral.:*** Tilcotil†; ***Austria:*** Liman†; Tilcotil; ***Belg.:*** Tilcotil; ***Braz.:*** Legil†; Teflan; Tenocam; Tenotec; Tenoxen; Tilatil; Tiloxican; ***Canad.:*** Mobiflex†; ***Chile:*** Avancel; Bioflam; Mitrotil; Recaflex; Texicam; Tilcotil; ***Denm.:*** Tilcotil; ***Fin.:*** Tilcotil; ***Fr.:*** Tilcotil; ***Ger.:*** Liman†; Tilcotil†; ***Gr.:*** Admiral; Algin-Vek; Amcinafal; Artroxicam; Artruic; Aspagin; Docticam; Dranat; Hobatícam; Indo-bros; Istotosal; Liaderyl; Neo-adlibamin; Neo-antiperstam; Neo-endusix; Octiveran; Oxytel; Ponsolit; Redac; Soral; Tilcitin; Toscacalm; Voir; Zibelant; ***Hong Kong:*** Nadamen; Seftil; Tilcotil; ***India:*** Tobitil; ***Irl.:*** Mobiflex; ***Ital.:*** Dolmen; Rexalgan; Tilcotil; ***Jpn:*** Tilcotil; ***Malaysia:*** Nadamen; Seftil; Sinoral; ***Mex.:*** Tilcotil; ***Neth.:*** Tilcotil; ***NZ:*** Tilcotil; ***Port.:*** Bioreucam; Calibral; Doxican; Tenalgin; Tilcotil; ***S.Afr.:*** Tilcotil; Tobitil; ***Singapore:*** Nadament†; Tilcotil†; ***Spain:*** Artriunic; Reutenox; Tilcotil; ***Swed.:*** Alganex; ***Switz.:*** Tilcotil; ***Thai.:*** Memzotil; Menzotil†; Nadamen; Seftil; Sinoral; Teconam; Tenax; Tenocam; Tenox; Tenoxil; Tilcotil; Tonox; ***UK:*** Mobiflex.

**Multi-ingredient:** ***Arg.:*** Mefenix Relax.

## Tetridamine *(rINN)*

POLI-67; Tetridamina; Tetrydamine *(USAN)*. 4,5,6,7-Tetrahydro-2-methyl-3-(methylamino)-2*H*-indazole.

$C_9H_{15}N_3$ = 165.2.
*CAS — 17289-49-5.*

### Profile

Tetridamine is an NSAID (p.67) that has been used as the maleate as a douche in the treatment of vaginitis.

### Preparations

**Proprietary Preparations** (details are given in Part 3)
***Ital.:*** Deb; ***Spain:*** Fomene; Tesos†.

## Thurfyl Salicylate

Salicilato de turfilo. Tetrahydrofurfuryl salicylate.

$C_{12}H_{14}O_4$ = 222.2.
*CAS — 2217-35-8.*

### Profile

Thurfyl salicylate is a salicylic acid derivative that has been used similarly to methyl salicylate (p.59) in topical rubefacient preparations at concentrations of up to 14% for musculoskeletal, joint, peri-articular, and soft-tissue disorders.

### Preparations

**Proprietary Preparations** (details are given in Part 3)
**Multi-ingredient:** ***Belg.:*** Transvane†; ***Irl.:*** Transvasin; ***NZ:*** Transvasin†; ***Swed.:*** Transvasin†; ***UK:*** Transvasin Heat Rub.

## Tiaprofenic Acid *(BAN, rINN)*

Ácido tiaprofénico; FC-3001; RU-15060. 2-(5-Benzoyl-2-thienyl)propionic acid.

$C_{14}H_{12}O_3S$ = 260.3.
*CAS — 33005-95-7.*
*ATC — M01AE11.*

**Pharmacopoeias.** In *Eur.* (see p.vi).

**Ph. Eur. 5.0** (Tiaprofenic Acid). A white or almost white, crystalline powder. Practically insoluble in water; freely soluble in alcohol, in acetone, and in dichloromethane. Protect from light.

### Adverse Effects and Precautions

As for NSAIDs in general, p.67.

Tiaprofenic acid may cause cystitis, bladder irritation, and other urinary-tract symptoms (see below). It should not be given to patients with active urinary-tract disorders or prostatic disease or a history of recurrent urinary-tract disorders. It should be stopped immediately if urinary-tract symptoms occur and urinalysis and urine culture performed.

**Breast feeding.** Although tiaprofenic acid is distributed into breast milk, the amount is considered by the *British National Formulary* to be too small to be harmful to a breast-fed infant.

**Effects on the urinary tract.** Cystitis and bladder irritation have been associated with the use of tiaprofenic acid.[1-6] In August 1994 the UK Committee on Safety of Medicines (CSM) stated[4] that since the introduction of tiaprofenic acid in the UK in 1982 they had received 69 reports of cystitis and 32 other reports of urinary-tract symptoms associated with tiaprofenic acid including frequency, dysuria, and haematuria whereas only 8 cases of cystitis had been reported for all other NSAIDs combined. Analysis of spontaneous reports received by WHO[7] confirmed that cystitis was more commonly associated with tiaprofenic acid than with other NSAIDs. The Australian Adverse Drug Reaction Advisory Committee had received similar reports.[3] Since the 1994 warning, the CSM[8] had received reports of a further 74 cases of cystitis, but the majority of these had occurred before the warning was issued. The duration of treatment in patients affected had varied considerably. Most patients recovered when tiaprofenic acid was withdrawn.

The CSM recommended that tiaprofenic acid should not be given to patients with urinary-tract disorders and that it should be stopped in patients who develop urinary-tract symptoms. Patients should be advised that if they develop symptoms such as urinary frequency, nocturia, urgency, or pain on urination, or have blood in their urine they should stop taking tiaprofenic acid and consult their doctor.

1. Ahmed M, Davison OW. Severe cystitis associated with tiaprofenic acid. *BMJ* 1991; **303:** 1376.
2. O'Neill GFA. Tiaprofenic acid as a cause of non-bacterial cystitis. *Med J Aust* 1994; **160:** 123–5.
3. Australian Adverse Drug Reactions Advisory Committee. Update on tiaprofenic acid and urinary symptoms. *Aust Adverse Drug React Bull* 1994; **13:** 6.
4. Committee on Safety of Medicines/Medicines Control Agency. Severe cystitis with tiaprofenic acid (Surgam). *Current Problems* 1994; **20:** 11.
5. Harrison WJ, *et al.* Adverse reactions to tiaprofenic acid mimicking interstitial cystitis. *BMJ* 1994; **309:** 574.
6. Mayall FG, *et al.* Cystitis and ureteric obstruction in patients taking tiaprofenic acid. *BMJ* 1994; **309:** 599.
7. The ADR Signals Analysis Project (ASAP) Team. How does cystitis affect a comparative risk profile of tiaprofenic acid with other non-steroidal antiinflammatory drugs? An international study based on spontaneous reports and drug usage data. *Pharmacol Toxicol* 1997; **80:** 211–17.
8. Crawford MLA, *et al.* Severe cystitis associated with tiaprofenic acid. *Br J Urol* 1997; **79:** 578–84.

### Interactions

For interactions associated with NSAIDs, see p.69.

### Pharmacokinetics

Tiaprofenic acid is absorbed from the gastrointestinal tract with peak plasma concentrations being reached within about 1.5 hours after oral doses. It has a short elimination half-life of about 2 hours and is highly bound to plasma proteins (about 98%). Excretion of tiaprofenic acid and its metabolites is mainly in the urine in the form of acyl glucuronides; some is excreted in the bile. Tiaprofenic acid is distributed into breast milk.

◊ References.

1. Davies NM. Clinical pharmacokinetics of tiaprofenic acid and its enantiomers. *Clin Pharmacokinet* 1996; **31:** 331–47.

### Uses and Administration

Tiaprofenic acid, a propionic acid derivative, is an NSAID (p.70). It is used for the relief of pain and inflammation in musculoskeletal and joint disorders such as ankylosing spondylitis, osteoarthritis, and rheumatoid arthritis, in peri-articular disorders such as fibrositis and capsulitis, and in soft-tissue disorders such as sprains and strains. The usual dose by mouth is 600 mg daily given in 2 or 3 divided doses or once daily as a modified-release preparation. Tiaprofenic acid has also been given rectally. It has been given intramuscularly as the trometamol salt in acute conditions.

◊ References.

1. Plosker GL, Wagstaff AJ. Tiaprofenic acid: a reappraisal of its pharmacological properties and use in the management of rheumatic diseases. *Drugs* 1995; **50:** 1050–75.

### Preparations

**Proprietary Preparations** (details are given in Part 3)
***Austral.:*** Surgam; ***Belg.:*** Artiflam†; Surgam†; ***Canad.:*** Albert Tiafen; Surgam; ***Denm.:*** Surgamyl; ***Fin.:*** Surgamyl; ***Fr.:*** Flamirex†; Flanid; Surgam; ***Ger.:*** Lindotab†; Surgam; ***Irl.:*** Surgam; ***Ital.:*** Artroreuma†; Suralgan; Surgamyl; Tiaprofen; Tiaprorex†; ***Mex.:*** Surdolin†; Surgam; ***Neth.:*** Surgam; ***NZ:*** Surgam; ***Port.:*** Surgam; ***S.Afr.:*** Surgam; ***Spain:*** Derilate†; Surgamic†; ***Thai.:*** Anafen†; Fengam; Gasam†; Surgam; ***UK:*** Surgam.

---

## Tiaramide Hydrochloride *(BANM, USAN, rINNM)*

Hidrocloruro de tiaramida; NTA-194; Tiaperamide Hydrochloride. 5-Chloro-3-{2-[4-(2-hydroxyethyl)piperazin-1-yl]-2-oxoethyl}benzothiazolin-2-one hydrochloride.

$C_{15}H_{18}ClN_3O_3S,HCl = 392.3.$

*CAS — 32527-55-2 (tiaramide); 35941-71-0 (tiaramide hydrochloride).*

**Pharmacopoeias.** In *Jpn.*

### Profile

Tiaramide hydrochloride is an NSAID (p.67) that has been given by mouth for the relief of pain and inflammation. Doses are expressed in terms of the base; tiaramide hydrochloride 110.3 mg is approximately equivalent to 100 mg of tiaramide. The usual dose is equivalent to 100 mg of tiaramide up to three times daily.

### Preparations

**Proprietary Preparations** (details are given in Part 3)
***Jpn:*** Solantal.

---

## Tilidine Hydrochloride *(USAN, pINNM)*

Gö 1261-C; Hidrocloruro de tilidina; Tilidate Hydrochloride *(BANM)*; Tilidini Hydrochloridum Hemihydricum; W-5759A. (±)-Ethyl *trans*-2-dimethylamino-1-phenylcyclohex-3-ene-1-carboxylate hydrochloride hemihydrate.

$C_{17}H_{23}NO_2,HCl,\frac{1}{2}H_2O = 318.8.$

*CAS — 20380-58-9 (tilidine); 27107-79-5 (anhydrous tilidine hydrochloride); 24357-97-9 (anhydrous +-trans-tilidine hydrochloride).*

*ATC — N02AX01.*

**Pharmacopoeias.** In *Eur.* (see p.vi).

**Ph. Eur. 5.0** (Tilidine Hydrochloride Hemihydrate). A white or almost white, crystalline powder. A suitable antoxidant may be added. Freely soluble in water and in alcohol; very soluble in dichloromethane. Protect from light.

### Dependence and Withdrawal

As for Opioid Analgesics in general, p.71.

### Adverse Effects, Treatment, and Precautions

As for Opioid Analgesics in general, p.72.

**Overdosage.** Cyanosis, respiratory depression, and seizures developed in a 28-year-old woman after an overdose of a combination preparation of tilidine and naloxone.[1] The authors commented that the amount of naloxone included in the preparation, in order to prevent abuse, was insufficient to prevent respiratory depression after severe overdose.

1. Regenthal R, *et al.* Poisoning with tilidine and naloxone: toxicokinetic and clinical observations. *Hum Exp Toxicol* 1998; **17:** 593–7.

**Porphyria.** Tilidine has been associated with acute attacks of porphyria and is considered unsafe in porphyric patients.

### Interactions

For interactions associated with opioid analgesics, see p.73.

### Pharmacokinetics

Tilidine is absorbed from the gastrointestinal tract. It is metabolised and excreted in the urine mainly as metabolites nortilidine (nortilidate) and bisnortilidine (bisnortilidate). Nortilidine is responsible for the analgesic activity of tilidine.

◊ References.

1. Vollmer K-O, *et al.* Pharmacokinetics of tilidine and metabolites in man. *Arzneimittelforschung* 1989; **39:** 1283–8.
2. Seiler K-U, *et al.* Pharmacokinetics of tilidine in terminal renal failure. *J Clin Pharmacol* 2001; **41:** 79–84.
3. Hajda JP, *et al.* Sequential first-pass metabolism of nortilidine: the active metabolite of the synthetic opioid drug tilidine. *J Clin Pharmacol* 2002; **42:** 1257–61.

### Uses and Administration

Tilidine hydrochloride is an opioid analgesic (p.73). It is used in the control of moderate to severe pain.

Tilidine hydrochloride may be given by intravenous, intramuscular, or subcutaneous injection in doses of up to 400 mg daily; usual doses as a suppository are 75 mg three or four times daily, or by mouth 50 mg four times daily. Tilidine has also been given as the phosphate in modified release tablets. As a deterrent to abuse combined oral preparations of tilidine hydrochloride with naloxone hydrochloride are available in some countries.

### Preparations

**Proprietary Preparations** (details are given in Part 3)
***Belg.:*** Valoron; Valtran; ***Ger.:*** Andolor; Findol N; Gruntin Tropfen; Nalidin; Tili; Tili Comp; Tili-Puren; Tilicomp; Tilidalor; Tilidin comp; Tilidin N; Tilidin plus; Tilidin-saar; Tilidura; Tiligetic; Tilimerck; tilnalox; Valoron N; ***S.Afr.:*** Valoron; ***Spain:*** Tilitrate†; ***Switz.:*** Valoron.

---

## Tolfenamic Acid *(BAN, rINN)*

Ácido tolfenámico; Acidum Tolfenamicum. *N*-(3-Chloro-o-tolyl)anthranilic acid.

$C_{14}H_{12}ClNO_2 = 261.7.$

*CAS — 13710-19-5.*

*ATC — M01AG02.*

**Pharmacopoeias.** In *Eur.* (see p.vi).

**Ph. Eur. 5.0** (Tolfenamic Acid). A white or slightly yellow crystalline powder. Practically insoluble in water; sparingly soluble in dehydrated alcohol and in dichloromethane; soluble in dimethylformamide. It dissolves in dilute solutions of alkali hydroxides. Protect from light.

### Adverse Effects and Precautions

As for NSAIDs in general, p.67. Dysuria, most commonly in males and probably due to local irritation of the urethra by a metabolite, has been reported. Tremor, euphoria, and fatigue have also occurred.

**Effects on the lungs.** Pulmonary infiltration has been associated with tolfenamic acid treatment in 6 patients.[1]

1. Strömberg C, *et al.* Pulmonary infiltrations induced by tolfenamic acid. *Lancet* 1987; **ii:** 685.

### Interactions

For interactions associated with NSAIDs, see p.69.

### Pharmacokinetics

Tolfenamic acid is readily absorbed from the gastrointestinal tract. Peak plasma concentrations are reached about 60 to 90 minutes after an oral dose. Tolfenamic acid is about 99% bound to plasma proteins. The plasma half-life is about 2 hours. Tolfenamic acid is metabolised in the liver; the metabolites and unchanged drug are conjugated with glucuronic acid. About 90% of an ingested dose is excreted in the urine and the remainder in the faeces. Tolfenamic acid is distributed into breast milk.

### Uses and Administration

Tolfenamic acid, an anthranilic acid derivative related to mefenamic acid (p.56), is an NSAID (p.70). In the treatment of acute attacks of migraine tolfenamic acid is given in a usual dose of 200 mg by mouth when the first symptoms appear; if a satisfactory response is not obtained this dose may be repeated once after 1 to 2 hours. Tolfenamic acid has also been given for the relief of mild to moderate pain in disorders such as dysmenorrhoea, rheumatoid arthritis, or osteoarthritis in doses of 100 to 200 mg three times daily.

### Preparations

**Proprietary Preparations** (details are given in Part 3)
***Arg.:*** Flocur; ***Austria:*** Clotam†; ***Braz.:*** Clotan†; Fenamic; ***Denm.:*** Clotam; Migea; ***Fin.:*** Clotam; Migea; ***Gr.:*** Clotam; Gantil; Polmonin; Purfalox; Tolfamic; Turbaund; ***Mex.:*** Bifenac; Flocur†; ***Neth.:*** Rociclyn; ***Norw.:*** Migea; ***Swed.:*** Migea; ***Switz.:*** Clotam; ***UK:*** Clotam.

---

## Tolmetin Sodium *(BANM, USAN, rINNM)*

McN-2559-21-98; McN-2559 (tolmetin); Tolmetina sódica. Sodium (1-methyl-5-*p*-toluoylpyrrol-2-yl)acetate dihydrate.

$C_{15}H_{14}NNaO_3,2H_2O = 315.3.$

*CAS — 26171-23-3 (tolmetin); 35711-34-3 (anhydrous tolmetin sodium); 64490-92-2 (tolmetin sodium dihydrate).*

*ATC — M01AB03; M02AA21.*

**Pharmacopoeias.** In *US.*

**USP 27** (Tolmetin Sodium). A light yellow to light orange crystalline powder. Freely soluble in water and in methyl alcohol; slightly soluble in alcohol; very slightly soluble in chloroform.

### Adverse Effects and Precautions

As for NSAIDs in general, p.67.

**Breast feeding.** No adverse effects have been observed in breast-feeding infants whose mothers were receiving tolmetin, and the American Academy of Pediatrics considers[1] that it is therefore usually compatible with breast feeding. However, the manufacturers recommend that tolmetin should be avoided in nursing mothers.

1. American Academy of Pediatrics. The transfer of drugs and other chemicals into human milk. *Pediatrics* 2001; **108:** 776–89. Correction. *ibid.*; 1029. Also available at: http://aappolicy.aappublications.org/cgi/content/full/pediatrics%3b108/3/776 (accessed 07/07/04)

**Effects on the blood.** Case reports of agranulocytosis[1] and thrombocytopenia[2] associated with tolmetin.

1. Sakai J, Joseph MW. Tolmetin and agranulocytosis. *N Engl J Med* 1978; **298:** 1203.
2. Lockhart JM. Tolmetin-induced thrombocytopenia. *Arthritis Rheum* 1982; **25:** 1144–5.

**Effects on the CNS.** See under Hypersensitivity, below.

**Effects on the gastrointestinal tract.** Erosive oesophagitis has been reported[1] in an 11-year-old child following ingestion of a dose of tolmetin while lying down and without drinking any water.

1. Palop V, *et al.* Tolmetin-induced esophageal ulceration. *Ann Pharmacother* 1997; **31:** 929.

**Effects on the kidneys.** Interstitial nephritis[1] and nephrotic syndrome[2,3] have been reported in patients given tolmetin.

1. Katz SM, *et al.* Tolmetin: association with reversible renal failure and acute interstitial nephritis. *JAMA* 1981; **246:** 243–5.
2. Chatterjee GP. Nephrotic syndrome induced by tolmetin. *JAMA* 1981; **246:** 1589.
3. Tietjen DP. Recurrence and specificity of nephrotic syndrome due to tolmetin. *Am J Med* 1989; **87:** 354–5.

**Hypersensitivity.** Anaphylactic shock,[1] urticaria and angioedema,[2] and aseptic meningitis[3] are among the hypersensitivity reactions reported in patients taking tolmetin.

1. Rossi AC, Knapp DE. Tolmetin-induced anaphylactoid reactions. *N Engl J Med* 1982; **307:** 499–500.
2. Ponte CD, Wisman R. Tolmetin-induced urticaria/angioedema. *Drug Intell Clin Pharm* 1985; **19:** 479–80.
3. Ruppert GB, Barth WF. Tolmetin-induced aseptic meningitis. *JAMA* 1981; **245:** 67–8.

### Interactions

For interactions associated with NSAIDs, see p.69.

### Pharmacokinetics

Tolmetin is almost completely absorbed from the gastrointestinal tract and peak plasma concentrations are attained about 30 to 60 minutes after ingestion. It is extensively bound to plasma proteins (over 99%) and has a biphasic plasma half-life of about 1 to 2 hours and 5 hours, respectively. Tolmetin penetrates synovial fluid and very small amounts are distributed into breast milk. It is excreted in the urine as an inactive dicarboxylic acid metabolite and its glucuronide and as tolmetin glucuronide with small amounts of unchanged drug.

### Uses and Administration

Tolmetin sodium is an NSAID (p.70). It is used in musculoskeletal and joint disorders such as osteoarthritis and rheumatoid arthritis, including juvenile idiopathic arthritis. It is given by mouth as the sodium salt although doses are expressed in terms of the base; tolmetin sodium dihydrate 122.5 mg is approximately equivalent to 100 mg of tolmetin base.

For the treatment of rheumatoid arthritis and osteoarthritis, the usual initial dose in adults is the equivalent of 400 mg of tolmetin three times daily by mouth; maintenance doses of 600 mg to a maximum of 1800 mg daily in divided doses have been used. For the treatment of juvenile idiopathic arthritis in children aged 2 years and over it is given in usual initial doses equivalent to 20 mg/kg of tolmetin daily in three or four divided doses; maintenance doses of 15 mg/kg to a maximum of 30 mg/kg daily have been used.

Tolmetin as the free acid has been applied as a 5% topical gel.

### Preparations

***USP 27:*** Tolmetin Sodium Capsules; Tolmetin Sodium Tablets.

**Proprietary Preparations** (details are given in Part 3)
***Austria:*** Tolectin; ***Belg.:*** Tolectin†; ***Canad.:*** Tolectin; ***Denm.:*** Tolectin†; ***Irl.:*** Tolectin†; ***Ital.:*** Tolectin†; ***Mex.:*** Tolectin; ***Neth.:*** Tolectin; ***S.Afr.:*** Tolectin†; ***Spain:*** Artrocaptin; ***Switz.:*** Tolectin; ***USA:*** Tolectin.

---

## Tramadol Hydrochloride

*(BANM, USAN, rINNM)*

CG-315; CG-315E; Hidrocloruro de tramadol; Tramadoli Hydrochloridum; U-26225A. (±)-*trans*-2-Dimethylaminomethyl-1-(3-methoxyphenyl)cyclohexanol hydrochloride.

$C_{16}H_{25}NO_2,HCl = 299.8.$

*CAS — 27203-92-5 (tramadol); 22204-88-2 (tramadol hydrochloride); 36282-47-0 (tramadol hydrochloride).*

*ATC — N02AX02.*

**Pharmacopoeias.** In *Chin.* and *Eur.* (see p.vi).

**Ph. Eur. 5.0** (Tramadol Hydrochloride). A white crystalline powder. Freely soluble in water and in methyl alcohol; very slightly soluble in acetone. Protect from light.

**Incompatibility.** The UK manufacturers state that tramadol hydrochloride injection 50 mg/mL is incompatible with injections of diazepam, diclofenac sodium, indometacin, midazolam, piroxicam, phenylbutazone, and lysine aspirin if mixed in the same syringe.

### Dependence and Withdrawal

As for Opioid Analgesics, p.71. Tramadol may have lower potential for producing dependence than morphine.

◊ The UK Committee on Safety of Medicines[1] commented in October 1996 that since June 1994 they had received reports of drug dependence in 5 patients and withdrawal symptoms associated with tramadol in 28 patients, which corresponded to a reporting rate of about 1 in 6000. Doses in excess of the recommended maximum of 400 mg daily had been taken by 5 of the patients. The duration of treatment before onset of these effects ranged from 10 to 409 days (average 3 months). Withdrawal symptoms reported were typically those of opioid withdrawal in general.

1. Committee on Safety of Medicines/Medicines Control Agency. Tramadol—(Zydol, Tramake and Zamadol). *Current Problems* 1996; **22:** 11. Also available at: http://www.mca.gov.uk/ourwork/monitorsafequalmed/currentproblems/cp11.htm (accessed 07/07/04)

## Adverse Effects and Treatment

As for Opioid Analgesics in general, p.72. Tramadol may produce fewer typical opioid adverse effects such as respiratory depression and constipation.

In addition to hypotension, hypertension has occasionally occurred.

**Effects on the CNS.** The UK Committee on Safety of Medicines (CSM)[1] commented in February 1995 that since June 1994 they had received reports of 15 patients who had experienced *confusion* and/or *hallucinations* while taking tramadol. The majority of the reactions developed 1 to 7 days after starting treatment and in most patients resolved rapidly on withdrawal. It was noted that psychiatric reactions comprised about 10% of all reactions reported with tramadol.

In a later comment[2] in October 1996, the CSM noted that 27 reports of *convulsions* and one of worsening epilepsy had been received, which corresponded to a reporting rate of about 1 in 7000. Of the 5 patients receiving intravenous tramadol, 2 had been given doses well in excess of those recommended (equivalent to 1.45 and 4 g daily). Of the patients receiving oral tramadol, the majority were taking other drugs known to cause convulsions, including tricyclic antidepressants and SSRIs. A similar pattern has been reported in the USA[3] and Australia.[4]

A debilitating CNS-mediated reaction to an initial dose of tramadol has been described in a patient.[5] Symptoms, which lasted approximately 4 hours, included ataxia, dilatation of the pupils, numbness in all limbs, tremulousness, and dysphoria. Although the exact mechanism of the reaction was not known, it was suggested that since the patient was an extensive metaboliser with very high activity of the cytochrome P450 isoenzyme CYP2D6, high concentrations of the active *O*-desmethyl metabolite were the cause. The patient recovered with no sequelae. It is possible that this represents a case of the *serotonin syndrome*, since tramadol is known to be associated with this condition, particularly at high doses or when given with other drugs that raise serotonin concentrations.[4]

1. Committee on Safety of Medicines/Medicines Control Agency. Tramadol (Zydol)—psychiatric reactions. *Current Problems* 1995; **21:** 2.
2. Committee on Safety of Medicines/Medicines Control Agency. Tramadol—(Zydol, Tramake and Zamadol). *Current Problems* 1996; **22:** 11. Also available at: http://www.mca.gov.uk/ourwork/monitorsafequalmed/currentproblems/cp11.htm (accessed 07/07/04)
3. Kahn LH, *et al.* Seizures reported with tramadol. *JAMA* 1997; **278:** 1661.
4. Adverse Drug Reactions Advisory Committee (ADRAC). Tramadol - four years experience. *Aust Adverse Drug React Bull* 2003; **22:** 1–2. Also available at: http://www.tga.health.gov.au/adr/aadrb/aadr0302.htm (accessed 07/07/04)
5. Gleason PP, *et al.* Debilitating reaction following the initial dose of tramadol. *Ann Pharmacother* 1997; **31:** 1150–2.

**Effects on the respiratory system.** Respiratory depression has been reported after tramadol infusion anaesthesia,[1] although in a postoperative study[2] tramadol had no significant respiratory depressant effect when equianalgesic doses of morphine, pentazocine, pethidine, piritramide, and tramadol were compared.

1. Paravicini D, *et al.* Tramadol-infusionsanaesthesie mit Substitution von Enfluran und differenten Lachgaskonzentrationen. *Anaesthesist* 1985; **34:** 20–7.
2. Fechner R, *et al.* Clinical investigations on the effect of morphine, pentazocine, pethidine, piritramide and tramadol on respiration. *Anasth Intensivmed* 1985; **26:** 126–32.

## Precautions

As for Opioid Analgesics in general, p.72.

Tramadol should be used with caution in patients with renal or hepatic impairment and should be avoided if renal impairment is severe. Removal by haemodialysis is reported to be very slow.

Tramadol should be used with care in patients with a history of epilepsy or those susceptible to seizures. See also Effects on the CNS under Adverse Effects, above.

**Anaesthesia.** The manufacturers warn against using tramadol during very light planes of general anaesthesia because of possible intra-operative awareness, although it may be used intra-operatively provided anaesthesia is maintained by the continuous administration of a potent volatile or intravenous anaesthetic. Intra-operative awareness was reported in 65% of a group of 20 patients when used to provide analgesia during light general anaesthesia with nitrous oxide and intermittent enflurane.[1] However, in a study[2] of 51 patients given tramadol during stable light continuous isoflurane-nitrous oxide anaesthesia there was no clinically significant lightening of anaesthesia and others have commented that during extensive use of tramadol intra-operatively over several years, there had not been any incidence of recall in any patient treated at their clinic.[3]

1. Lehmann KA, *et al.* Zur Bedeutung von Tramadol als intraoperativem Analgetikum: eine randomisierte Doppelblindstudie im Vergleich zu Placebo. *Der Anaesthetist* 1985; **34:** 11–19.
2. Coetzee JF, *et al.* Effect of tramadol on depth of anaesthesia. *Br J Anaesth* 1996; **76:** 415–18.
3. Budd K. Tramadol. *Br J Anaesth* 1995; **75:** 500.

## Interactions

For interactions associated with opioid analgesics, see p.73.

Carbamazepine is reported to diminish the analgesic activity of tramadol by reducing serum concentrations.

The risk of seizures is increased if tramadol is used with other drugs that have the potential to lower the seizure threshold. See also under Effects on the CNS under Adverse Effects, above.

Tramadol inhibits reuptake of noradrenaline and serotonin and enhances serotonin release and there is the possibility that it may interact with other drugs that enhance monoaminergic neurotransmission including lithium, tricyclic antidepressants, and SSRIs; it should not be given to patients receiving MAOIs or within 14 days of their discontinuation.

◊ Metabolism of tramadol is mediated by the cytochrome P450 isoenzyme CYP2D6. Use with specific inhibitors of this enzyme, such as *quinidine*, may increase concentrations of tramadol and lower concentrations of its active metabolite but the clinical consequences of this effect are unclear.

**Anticoagulants.** Tramadol is reported to have potentiated the anticoagulant effect of *phenprocoumon* and of *warfarin*.[1,2] However, a randomised, double-blind, placebo-controlled study[3] in 19 patients failed to find evidence of an interaction between phenprocoumon and tramadol.

1. Scher ML, *et al.* Potential interaction between tramadol and warfarin. *Ann Pharmacother* 1997; **31:** 646–7.
2. Jensen K. Interaktion mellem tramadol og orale antikoagulantia. *Ugeskr Laeger* 1997; **159:** 785–6.
3. Boeijinga JK, *et al.* Lack of interaction between tramadol and coumarins. *J Clin Pharmacol* 1998; **38:** 966–70.

**Antidepressants.** For reference to a possible case of serotonin syndrome associated with concomitant use of tramadol and *SSRIs*, see under Fluoxetine, p.296.

**5-HT$_3$-receptor antagonists.** The pre-operative use of *ondansetron* has been noted to reduce the postoperative analgesic efficacy of tramadol.[1] The cumulative dose of tramadol was up to 35% greater in those patients who also received ondansetron compared to those who received no antiemetic. In addition there was no difference in the incidence of postoperative nausea and vomiting between the two groups.

1. De Witte JL, *et al.* The analgesic efficacy of tramadol is impaired by concurrent administration of ondansetron. *Anesth Analg* 2001; **92:** 1319–21.

## Pharmacokinetics

Tramadol is readily absorbed following oral administration but is subject to first-pass metabolism. Tramadol is metabolised by *N*- and *O*-demethylation via the cytochrome P450 isoenzymes CYP3A4 and CYP2D6 and glucuronidation or sulfation in the liver. The metabolite *O*-desmethyltramadol is pharmacologically active. Tramadol is excreted mainly in the urine predominantly as metabolites. Tramadol is widely distributed, crosses the placenta, and appears in small amounts in breast milk. The elimination half-life following oral administration is about 6 hours.

**Metabolism.** Production of the active metabolite *O*-desmethyltramadol is dependent on the cytochrome P450 isoenzyme CYP2D6, which exhibits genetic polymorphism.[1] For a reference to a debilitating CNS-mediated reaction in a patient who was an extensive metaboliser with high CYP2D6 activity, see under Effects on the CNS in Adverse Effects, above.

1. Poulsen L, *et al.* The hypoalgesic effect of tramadol in relation to CYP2D6. *Clin Pharmacol Ther* 1996; **60:** 636–44.

## Uses and Administration

Tramadol hydrochloride is an opioid analgesic (p.73). It also has noradrenergic and serotonergic properties that may contribute to its analgesic activity. Tramadol is used for moderate to severe pain.

Tramadol hydrochloride is given by mouth, intravenously, or rectally as a suppository. The intramuscular route has also been used. It may also be given by infusion or as part of a patient-controlled analgesia system. Usual doses by mouth are 50 to 100 mg every 4 to 6 hours. Tramadol hydrochloride may also be given orally as a modified-release preparation once or twice daily. The total daily dosage by mouth should not exceed 400 mg.

A dose of 50 to 100 mg may be given every 4 to 6 hours by intramuscular injection or intravenous injection over 2 to 3 minutes, or by intravenous infusion. For the treatment of postoperative pain, the initial dose is 100 mg followed by 50 mg every 10 to 20 minutes if necessary to a total maximum (including the initial dose) of 250 mg in the first hour. Thereafter, doses are 50 to 100 mg every 4 to 6 hours up to a total daily dose of 600 mg.

Rectal doses by suppository are 100 mg up to 4 times daily.

For doses in patients with hepatic or renal impairment, see below.

◊ References.

1. Anonymous. Tramadol—a new analgesic. *Drug Ther Bull* 1994; **32:** 85–6. Correction. *ibid.*: 96.
2. Radbruch L, *et al.* A risk-benefit assessment of tramadol in the management of pain. *Drug Safety* 1996; **15:** 8–29.
3. Lewis KS, Han NH. Tramadol: a new centrally acting analgesic. *Am J Health-Syst Pharm* 1997; **54:** 643–52.
4. Duthie DJR. Remifentanil and tramadol. *Br J Anaesth* 1998; **81:** 51–7.
5. Budd K, Langford R. Tramadol revisited. *Br J Anaesth* 1999; **82:** 493–5.
6. Scott LJ, Perry CM. Tramadol: a review of its use in perioperative pain. *Drugs* 2000; **60:** 139–76.

**Administration in hepatic or renal impairment.** The dosage interval should be increased to 12 hours in patients with a creatinine clearance less than 30 mL/minute; in the USA the manufacturers suggest that the maximum dose by mouth should not exceed 200 mg daily in these patients. Tramadol should not be given to patients with more severe renal impairment (creatinine clearance less than 10 mL/minute). A dosage interval of 12 hours is also recommended in severe hepatic impairment.

## Preparations

**Proprietary Preparations** (details are given in Part 3)
***Arg.:*** Adamon; Calmador; Trama-Klosidol; Tramal; Tramalan; ***Austral.:*** Tramal; Zydol; ***Austria:*** Adamon; Dolol; Lanalget; Nycodol; Tradolan; Tramabene; Tramadolor; Tramal; Tramamed; Tramastad; Tramatyrol; Tramundal; ***Belg.:*** Contramal; Dolzam; Tradonal; ***Braz.:*** Dorless†; Sensitram; Sylador; Timasen; Trabilin; Tramadon; Tramal; ***Chile:*** Minidol; Timarol; Tramal; Zodol; ***Denm.:*** Dolol; Mandolgin; Nobligan; Tradolan; ***Fin.:*** Tramadin; Tramagetic; Tramal; Trambo; ***Fr.:*** Biodalgic; Contramal; Predalgic†; Takadol; Topalgic; Trasedal; Zamudol; Zumalgic; ***Ger.:*** Amadol; Tial; Tradol; Trama; Trama-Dorsch; Tramabeta; Tramadoc; Tramadol-Dolgit; Tramadolor; Tramadura; Tramagetic; Tramagit; Tramal; Tramamerck†; Tramedphano†; Tramundin; ***Hong Kong:*** Acugesic; Mabron; Sefmal; Tradonal; Tramal; Tramo; ***India:*** Contramal; Tramazac; TRD-Contin; Urgendol; ***Irl.:*** By-Madol; Tradol; Tramake; Tramapine; Tramex; Xymel; Zydol; ***Israel:*** Trabar; Tramadex; ***Ital.:*** Contramal; Fortradol; Fraxidol; Prontalgin; Tradonal; ***Malaysia:*** Mabron; Tramal; ***Mex.:*** Nobligan; Prontofort; Tradol; Tralic; Trexol; Veldrol; ***Neth.:*** Theradol; Tramagetic; Tramal; ***Norw.:*** Nobligan; Tradolan; Tramagetic; ***NZ:*** Tramal; Zytram; ***Port.:*** Paxilfar; Tramal; Travex; ***S.Afr.:*** Tramahexal; Tramal; ***Singapore:*** Mabron; Pengesic; Sefmal; Tradol; Tramal; ***Spain:*** Adolonta; Tioner; Tradonal; Tralgiol; Zytram; ***Swed.:*** Nobligan; Tiparol; Tradolan; ***Switz.:*** Ecodolor; Tramadolor†; Tramal; ***Thai.:*** Ammitram; Anadol; Analab; Mabron; Madol; Madola; Paindol; Pharmadol; Sefmal; Tamolan; Tracine; Tradolgesic; Tradonal; Tramal; Tramalan†; Tramamed; Tramax; Tramoda; Trosic; Volcidol-S; ***UK:*** Dromadol; Tramake; Zamadol; Zydol; ***USA:*** Ultram.

**Multi-ingredient:** ***Chile:*** Zaldiar; ***Fr.:*** Ixprim; Zaldiar; ***Switz.:*** Zaldiar; ***UK:*** Tramacet; ***USA:*** Ultracet.

## Trimeperidine Hydrochloride *(BANM, rINNM)*

Promedolum. 1,2,5-Trimethyl-4-phenyl-4-piperidyl propionate hydrochloride.

$C_{17}H_{25}NO_2,HCl = 311.8.$

*CAS — 64-39-1 (trimeperidine); 125-80-4 (hydrochloride).*

### Profile

Trimeperidine hydrochloride is an opioid analgesic (p.71) with actions and uses similar to those of pethidine (p.80).

## Trolamine Salicylate *(pINNM)*

Salicilato de trietanolamina; Triethanolamine Salicylate.

$C_{13}H_{21}NO_6 = 287.3.$

*CAS — 2174-16-5.*

**Pharmacopoeias.** In *US.*

**USP 27** (Trolamine Salicylate). A compounded mixture of trolamine and salicylic acid in propylene glycol. pH of a 5% solution in water is between 6.5 and 7.5. Store in airtight containers in a cool place.

### Profile

Trolamine salicylate is a salicylic acid derivative used similarly to methyl salicylate (p.59) in topical rubefacient preparations in a concentration of 10 to 20% for the relief of muscular and rheumatic pain. It has also been used as a sunscreen.

**Percutaneous absorption.** In contrast to methyl salicylate, which undergoes considerable absorption and produces high subcutaneous and dermal concentrations of salicylic acid after application to intact skin, concentrations of salicylic acid after topical application of trolamine salicylate were substantially lower in tissue[1] and undetectable in serum.[2]

1. Cross SE, *et al.* Is there tissue penetration after application of topical salicylate formulations? *Lancet* 1997; **350:** 636.
2. Morra P, *et al.* Serum concentrations of salicylic acid following topically applied salicylate derivatives. *Ann Pharmacother* 1996; **30:** 935–40.

## Preparations

**Proprietary Preparations** (details are given in Part 3)
***Arg.:*** Geniol Flex; ***Austral.:*** Dencorub Arthritis; Goanna Arthritis Cream; Metsal AR Analgesic; ***Canad.:*** Antiphlogistine Rub A-535 No Odour; Aspercreme; Ben-Gay No Odor; Miosal†; Myoflex; Royflex†; ***Mex.:*** Myoflex; ***Spain:*** Bexidermil; Topicrem†; ***USA:*** Analgesia Creme; Aspercreme; Coppertone Tan Magnifier; Flex-Power Performance Sports; Mobisyl; Myoflex; Sportscreme; Tropical Blend Tan Magnifier.

**Multi-ingredient:** ***Arg.:*** Duo Minoxi; ***Austral.:*** Metsal Analgesic†; ***Canad.:*** Ease Pain Away†; Myoflex Ice Plus.

## Valdecoxib *(BAN, USAN, rINN)*

SC-65872. *p*-(5-Methyl-3-phenyl-4-isoxazolyl)benzenesulfonamide.

$C_{16}H_{14}N_2O_3S$ = 314.4.
*CAS — 181695-72-7.*
*ATC — M01AH03.*

### Adverse Effects and Precautions

As for NSAIDs in general, p.67. Serious skin reactions such as exfoliative dermatitis, Steven-Johnson syndrome, and toxic epidermal necrolysis have been reported with valdecoxib. Other hypersensitivity reactions including anaphylaxis and angioedema have also occurred. Valdecoxib should be discontinued at the first signs of hypersensitivity. Some of these reactions have been seen in patients with a history of allergic reactions to sulfonamides and the use of valdecoxib is contra-indicated in such patients. It should also be avoided in patients with severe hepatic impairment, inflammatory bowel disease, and severe heart failure.

Valdecoxib should be used with caution following coronary artery bypass graft surgery as there may be an increased risk of adverse effects such as stroke, renal impairment, and sternal wound complications, especially in obese patients or those with a history of stroke. Caution is also recommended when using valdecoxib in dehydrated patients; rehydration may be advisable before giving valdecoxib.

**Effects on the cardiovascular system.** The selective cyclo-oxygenase-2 (COX-2) inhibitors such as valdecoxib do not possess the intrinsic antiplatelet activity associated with aspirin (and possibly other non-selective NSAIDs), and consequently do not provide protection against ischaemic cardiac events.

**Effects on the gastrointestinal tract.** It is generally accepted that the inhibition of cyclo-oxygenase-1 (COX-1) results in the adverse gastrointestinal effects of the NSAIDs, and that the selective inhibition of the other isoform, COX-2, by NSAIDs such as valdecoxib may cause less gastrotoxicity than that seen with the non-selective inhibition of the traditional NSAIDs. However, the manufacturers report that upper gastrointestinal perforation, ulceration, and bleeds have occurred with valdecoxib treatment and therefore it should be used with caution in patients with a history of such events.

Results from controlled trials confirm that NSAIDs selective for COX-2 are associated with a lower incidence of serious gastrointestinal effects. In a comparative study[1], valdecoxib (in doses of 10 or 20 mg daily) was associated with a lower incidence of endoscopically-detected gastroduodenal ulceration than diclofenac (150 mg daily) or ibuprofen (2.4 g daily). However, as with other selective COX-2 inhibitors, the concomitant use of low-dose aspirin significantly increased the risk of ulceration with valdecoxib.

1. Sikes DH, *et al.* Incidence of gastroduodenal ulcers associated with valdecoxib compared with that of ibuprofen and diclofenac in patients with osteoarthritis. *Eur J Gastroenterol Hepatol* 2002; **14:** 1101–11.

**Effects on the skin.** Toxic epidermal necrolysis developed in a patient who took valdecoxib for 8 days, despite stopping the drug at the first signs of a rash and starting treatment with oral prednisolone;[1] the patient had a history of hypersensitivity to sulfonamides. Health Canada noted[2] in January 2004 that it had received 5 reports of serious cutaneous adverse reactions associated with valdecoxib over less than 1 year from marketing of the drug in December 2002. However, none of these were erythema multiforme, Stevens-Johnson syndrome, or toxic epidermal necrolysis although these reactions had been reported to other regulatory authorities.

1. Glasser DL, Burroughs SH. Valdecoxib-induced toxic epidermal necrolysis in a patient allergic to sulfa drugs. *Pharmacotherapy* 2003; **23:** 551–3.
2. Health Canada/Santé Canada. Valdecoxib (Bextra®): severe cutaneous reactions. *Can Adverse React News* 2004; **14:** 1–2. Also available at: http://www.hc-sc.gc.ca/hpfb-dgpsa/tpd-dpt/adrv14n1_e.pdf (accessed 07/07/04)

### Interactions

For interactions associated with NSAIDs, see p.69. The metabolism of valdecoxib is mainly mediated by the cytochrome P450 isoenzymes CYP3A4 and CYP2C9 and consequently caution is recommended when using valdecoxib with inhibitors of such isoenzymes. The manufacturers have advised that valdecoxib should be started at the lowest recommended dose when given with fluconazole, a CYP2C9 inhibitor, or ketoconazole, a CYP3A4 inhibitor. Studies with the CYP3A4 inducer phenytoin did not result in a significant reduction in valdecoxib plasma concentrations and no dosage adjustment is necessary. However, there may be clinically significant interactions with other CYP3A4 inducers such as carbamazepine and dexamethasone and with potent enzyme inducers such as rifampicin.

Valdecoxib has been noted to increase the plasma levels of dextromethorphan, a CYP2D6 substrate, and therefore caution is recommended when giving valdecoxib with drugs that are metabolised via CYP2D6 and that have a narrow therapeutic index. Such drugs include flecainide, metoprolol, and propafenone. Valdecoxib may also affect the plasma levels of drugs that are metabolised via CYP2C19: an increase in the plasma levels of omeprazole was seen in patients using valdecoxib.

### Pharmacokinetics

Valdecoxib is well absorbed from the gastrointestinal tract after oral doses. Peak plasma concentrations are reached in approximately 3 hours. Plasma protein binding is about 98%. Valdecoxib is extensively metabolised in the liver; pathways involved include those via the cytochrome P450 isoenzymes CYP3A4 and CYP2C9, and glucuronidation. An active metabolite has been identified but it is not considered to contribute significantly to the activity of valdecoxib. Excretion is mainly via the urine with about 70% of a dose appearing as inactive metabolites. Less than 5% of a dose appears unchanged in the urine and faeces. The elimination half-life is about 8 to 11 hours.

### Uses and Administration

Valdecoxib is an NSAID (p.70) reported to be a selective inhibitor of cyclo-oxygenase-2 (COX-2). It is given by mouth in the treatment of osteoarthritis and rheumatoid arthritis and for the pain of dysmenorrhoea.

In **rheumatoid arthritis** and **osteoarthritis**, valdecoxib is given in a dose of 10 mg once daily increasing to a maximum of 20 mg once daily, if necessary. The lowest recommended dose should be used in elderly patients particularly those weighing less than 50 kg.

The dose in **dysmenorrhoea** is 40 mg daily, given as a single dose or in 2 divided doses; in the UK, on the first day of treatment *only*, an additional 40 mg-dose may be taken.

For dosage recommendations in patients with hepatic impairment, see below.

**Administration in hepatic impairment.** No dose adjustment of valdecoxib is necessary in patients with *mild* hepatic impairment. In those with *moderate* impairment the lowest recommended dose (10 mg once daily) should be used for osteoarthritis and rheumatoid arthritis and for dysmenorrhoea the dose should not exceed 20 mg daily. Valdecoxib is not recommended for patients with *severe* impairment as there is no clinical experience in such patients.

**Musculoskeletal and joint disorders.** Valdecoxib is used in the treatment of the musculoskeletal disorders osteoarthritis (p.9) and rheumatoid arthritis (p.9). However, in the UK it is recommended that the use of selective cyclo-oxygenase-2 (COX-2) inhibitors such as valdecoxib be limited to those patients considered to be at high risk of developing serious gastrointestinal problems if given a non-selective NSAID.

References.

1. Ormrod D, *et al.* Valdecoxib. *Drugs* 2002; **62:** 2059–71.
2. Bensen W, *et al.* Efficacy and safety of valdecoxib in treating the signs and symptoms of rheumatoid arthritis: a randomized, controlled comparison with placebo and naproxen. *Rheumatology (Oxford)* 2002; **41:** 1008–16.
3. Kivitz A, *et al.* Randomized placebo-controlled trial comparing efficacy and safety of valdecoxib with naproxen in patients with osteoarthritis. *J Fam Pract* 2002; **51:** 530–7.

**Pain.** Valdecoxib has been tried in the treatment of acute pain including postoperative pain.

References.

1. Desjardins PJ, *et al.* A single preoperative oral dose of valdecoxib, a new cyclooxygenase-2 specific inhibitor, relieves post-oral surgery or bunionectomy pain. *Anesthesiology* 2002; **97:** 565–73.

## Preparations

**Proprietary Preparations** (details are given in Part 3)
***Chile:*** Bextra; ***India:*** Valus; ***Switz.:*** Bextra; ***UK:*** Bextra; ***USA:*** Bextra.

## Vedaprofen *(BAN, USAN, rINN)*

CERM-10202; PM-150; Vedaprofeno. (±)-4-Cyclohexyl-α-methyl-1-naphthaleneacetic acid.

$C_{19}H_{22}O_2$ = 282.4.
*CAS — 71109-09-6.*

### Profile

Vedaprofen, a propionic acid derivative, is an NSAID used in veterinary medicine for the treatment of inflammation and pain.

## Viminol Hydroxybenzoate *(rINNM)*

Diviminol Hydroxybenzoate; Hidroxibenzoato de viminol; Z-424 (viminol). 1-[1-(2-Chlorobenzyl)pyrrol-2-yl]-2-(di-sec-butyl)aminoethanol 4-hydroxybenzoate.

$C_{21}H_{31}ClN_2O,C_7H_6O_3$ = 501.1.
*CAS — 21363-18-8 (viminol); 21466-60-4 (viminol hydroxybenzoate); 23784-10-3 (viminol hydroxybenzoate).*
*ATC — N02BG05.*

### Profile

Viminol hydroxybenzoate has analgesic and antipyretic properties. The equivalent of 400 mg of viminol has been given daily in divided doses by mouth.

## Preparations

**Proprietary Preparations** (details are given in Part 3)
***Ital.:*** Dividol.

## Zaltoprofen *(rINN)*

CN-100; Zaltoprofeno; ZC-102. (±)-10,11-Dihydro-α-methyl-10-oxodibenzo[*b*,*f*]thiepin-2-acetic acid.

$C_{17}H_{14}O_3S$ = 298.4.
*CAS — 89482-00-8.*

### Profile

Zaltoprofen is an NSAID (p.67) which has been given by mouth for musculoskeletal and joint disorders.

◊ References.

1. Ishizaki T, *et al.* Pharmacokinetic profile of a new nonsteroidal anti-inflammatory agent, CN-100, in humans. *Drug Invest* 1991; **3:** 1–7.
2. Hatori M, Kokubun S. The long-term efficacy and tolerability of the new anti-inflammatory agent zaltoprofen in rheumatoid arthritis. *Curr Med Res Opin* 1998; **14:** 79–87.

## Ziconotide *(USAN, rINN)*

CI-1009; SNX-111; Ziconotida. L-Cysteinyl-L-lysylglycyl-L-lysylglycl-L-alanyl-L-lysyl-L-cysteinyl-L-seryl-L-arginyl-L-leucyl-L-methionyl-L-tyrosyl-L-α-aspartyl-L-cysteinyl-L-cysteinyl-L-threonylglycyl-L-seryl-L-cysteinyl-L-arginyl-L-serylglycyl-L-lysyl-L-cysteinamide cyclic(1→16),(8→20),(15→25)-tris(disulfide).

$C_{102}H_{172}N_{36}O_{32}S_7$ = 2639.1.
*CAS — 107452-89-1.*

### Profile

Ziconotide is a peptide derived from sea snails. It is reported to be a neurone-specific calcium antagonist. Ziconotide is used intrathecally in the management of various types of pain, including neuropathic pain. It has also been tried in other conditions such as head trauma.

◊ References.

1. Verweij BH, *et al.* Mitochondrial dysfunction after experimental and human brain injury and its possible reversal with a selective N-type calcium channel antagonist (SNX-111). *Neurol Res* 1997; **19:** 334–9.
2. Penn RD, Paice JA. Adverse effects associated with the intrathecal administration of ziconotide. *Pain* 2000; **85:** 291–6.
3. Jain KK. An evaluation of intrathecal ziconotide for the treatment of chronic pain. *Expert Opin Invest Drugs* 2000; **9:** 2403–10.
4. Staats PS, *et al.* Intrathecal ziconotide in the treatment of refractory pain in patients with cancer or AIDS: a randomized controlled trial. *JAMA* 2004; **291:** 63–70.

# Anthelmintics


Ancylostomiasis, p.97
Angiostrongyliasis, p.97
Ascariasis, p.97
Capillariasis, p.98
Clonorchiasis, p.98
Cutaneous larva migrans, p.98
Cysticercosis, p.98
Diphyllobothriasis, p.98
Dracunculiasis, p.98
Echinococcosis, p.98
Enterobiasis, p.99
Fascioliasis, p.99
Fasciolopsiasis, p.99
Gnathostomiasis, p.99
Heterophyiasis, p.99
Hookworm infections, p.99
Hymenolepiasis, p.99
Intestinal fluke infections, p.99
Liver fluke infections, p.99
Loiasis, p.99
Lung fluke infections, p.99
Lymphatic filariasis, p.100
Mansonella infections, p.100
Metagonimiasis, p.100
Nanophyetiasis, p.100
Necatoriasis, p.100
Onchocerciasis, p.100
Opisthorchiasis, p.100
Paragonimiasis, p.100
Schistosomiasis, p.100
Strongyloidiasis, p.100
Syngamosis, p.101
Taeniasis, p.101
Toxocariasis, p.101
Trichinosis, p.101
Trichostrongyliasis, p.101
Trichuriasis, p.101


This chapter describes the important helminth or worm infections that occur in man (see Table 1, p.98) and the anthelmintics used to treat them.

## Choice of Anthelmintic

Helminth infections are among the most common infections in man, affecting a large proportion of the world's population, mainly in tropical regions. In developing countries they pose a large threat to public health, and contribute to the prevalence of malnutrition, anaemia, eosinophilia, and pneumonia. Helminth infections causing severe morbidity include lymphatic filariasis (a cause of elephantiasis), onchocerciasis (river blindness), and schistosomiasis. These infections can affect the majority of populations in endemic areas with major economic and social consequences. WHO is making strenuous efforts to control a number of these infections in endemic areas. Control of these infections in both individuals and populations depends not only on the use of chemotherapeutic agents but also on preventing transmission by advice on food preparation and hygiene, the provision of adequate sanitation and sewage treatment (especially where sewage is used as fertiliser), the provision of safe potable water supplies, and effective vector control.

The worms that cause infection in man generally fall either into the phylum Nematoda, which includes the nematodes or roundworms, or into the phylum Platyhelminthes, which includes the cestodes or tapeworms and the trematodes or flukes.

The **nematodes** (or roundworms) are a large group of worms, some of which are capable of producing infections in man. In many cases man is the primary (definitive) host but human infections caused by parasites for which animals are the primary hosts also occur. Nematodes do not generally multiply in man; strongyloidiasis is an exception as re-infection can occur without environmental re-exposure. Nematode infections are most common in warm, moist climates, but some species of nematode can tolerate cool or arid conditions and infective forms can persist in the environment for long periods. An understanding of the life cycle of the infective species is necessary for diagnostic tests to be made at appropriate times, usually to coincide with the infective stage of the cycle, and for the choice of appropriate control measures.

The nematode infections can be divided into filarial infections, intestinal infections, and tissue infections.

*Filarial nematodes* are endemic in large areas of the tropics and produce considerable morbidity. The adult worms may live for several years, releasing large numbers of motile embryos known as microfilariae into the blood or skin, depending on the species. Transmission is usually by biting insects which form the intermediate host. In some endemic areas multiple infections with filarial nematodes are common.

Filarial nematode infections include:

- loiasis
- lymphatic filariasis
- mansonella infections
- onchocerciasis.

*Intestinal nematode* infections (roundworms) are very common especially in developing countries in the tropics and subtropics. Children are particularly at risk and these infections contribute to morbidity through malnutrition, vitamin deficiencies, diarrhoea, anaemia, and pneumonia. Poor sanitation and sewage disposal perpetuate infections with soil-borne nematodes. Often several different worm infections are endemic in the same region, resulting in mixed infections. When this occurs, broad-spectrum anthelmintics may be used to reduce the overall infection burden in the population (see under Ascariasis, below).

Intestinal nematode infections include:

- angiostrongyliasis
- ascariasis
- capillariasis
- enterobiasis
- hookworm infections
- strongyloidiasis
- trichostrongyliasis
- trichuriasis.

The *tissue nematodes* represent a miscellaneous group causing a variety of pathological conditions in man. In cutaneous larva migrans and toxocariasis, the nematodes have a primary animal host and the human disease is caused by infection with infective larvae which do not subsequently mature in man. Trichinosis and gnathostomiasis affect a number of carnivorous animals and man is an incidental host. Syngamosis is primarily an infection of domestic fowl and wild birds although infection in man has been reported rarely. In dracunculiasis, man is the primary (definitive) host. Although these diseases are not generally fatal they cause a considerable degree of morbidity and treatment is complicated by the lack of effective, non-toxic systemic anthelmintics.

Tissue nematode infections include:

- angiostrongyliasis
- cutaneous larva migrans
- dracunculiasis
- gnathostomiasis
- syngamosis
- toxocariasis
- trichinosis.

The **cestodes** (flatworms, segmented worms, or tapeworms) cause infection in man in most parts of the world. Man may be the primary host, harbouring the adult worm in the intestine, or an intermediate host carrying the larval form. With the exception of *Hymenolepis nana* the adult worms do not usually multiply within the same host. However, larval forms may be produced and, as with infection or ingestion of these forms, systemic infection may develop.

Cestode infections include:

- cysticercosis
- diphyllobothriasis
- echinococcosis
- hymenolepiasis
- taeniasis.

**Trematode** (or fluke) infections are caused by parasitic worms of the class Trematoda. There are 4 categories of fluke which are pathogenic in man; the blood flukes *Schistosoma* spp., the intestinal flukes *Fasciolopsis, Heterophyes, Metagonimus,* and *Nanophyetus* spp., the liver flukes *Clonorchis*, *Fasciola*, and *Opisthorchis* spp., and the lung flukes *Paragonimus* spp. Symptoms are usually only seen in heavy infections and commonly include fever, pain, and eosinophilia.

Trematode infections include:

- intestinal fluke infections
- liver fluke infections
- lung fluke infections
- schistosomiasis.

### Ancylostomiasis

See under Hookworm Infections, below. Larvae of *Ancylostoma* spp. are also a cause of cutaneous larva migrans (see below).

### Angiostrongyliasis

Two forms of angiostrongyliasis are recognised and both are due to accidental infection with species of the animal nematode *Angiostrongylus*.

Infection with the larvae of the rat lungworm *A. cantonensis* causes an eosinophilic meningoencephalitis. Transmission follows ingestion of raw or undercooked snails or crustaceans, or of contaminated vegetables. The disease is generally self-limiting.

Intestinal infection with *A. costaricensis* can cause eosinophilic gastro-enteritis. It most commonly occurs in children following ingestion of vegetables contaminated by infected slugs. Surgical resection of the affected bowel may be necessary.

Mebendazole was formerly suggested for treatment of both these infections but current opinion is that there is no convincing evidence to support its use; in addition, in *A. cantonensis* infection, severe host reaction to the dying larvae may result.

### Ascariasis

Ascariasis is an infection caused by *Ascaris lumbricoides*, the common or giant roundworm. The term roundworm is also applied to nematodes in general. It is usually an infection of the small intestine but on rare occasions there may be severe ectopic infections. It is commonly found in the tropics and especially in rural areas. Eggs are excreted in the faeces and can remain viable in moist soil for several years. On ingestion of mature eggs the larvae hatch and penetrate the intestinal wall. They migrate in the bloodstream via the liver to the lungs where they enter the alveoli. The larvae then move up the bronchial tree and are swallowed. The mature adult develops in the intestines, and it has been estimated that a gravid female is produced about 2 months after infection. The life span of the adult worm is 1 to 2 years. Ascariasis may be asymptomatic. When symptoms of intestinal infection do occur they include anorexia, abdominal pain, and diarrhoea; nutritional deficiency may result. The pulmonary stage may cause pneumonitis and bronchospasm often accompanied by eosinophilia. Heavy infections can cause intestinal or biliary obstruction. Migration of the worm from the small intestine can produce ectopic infection of the genito-urinary tract, lungs, liver, or heart. Such infections are rare but serious.

Children are at greatest risk of *Ascaris* infection and a study[1] has suggested that child-targeted treatment could be more cost effective in reducing disease cases than programmes of mass chemotherapy in areas where infection is endemic.

Treatment is with a benzimidazole carbamate derivative such as albendazole or mebendazole with both drugs being equally highly effective. Pyrantel embonate is an alternative. Such broad-spectrum therapy can be useful if the patient is suffering from a mixed intestinal nematode infection. Drugs such as tiabendazole with little or no activity against *Ascaris* should be avoided for the initial treatment of mixed infections since they may stimulate the worm to migrate to a different body site. Other anthelmintics effective in ascariasis include levamisole and piperazine salts.


1. Guyatt HL, *et al.* Control of Ascaris infection by chemotherapy: which is the most cost-effective option? *Trans R Soc Trop Med Hyg* 1995; **89:** 16–20.

**Table 1.** Helminths: classification and diseases.

| Group | Helminth | Common Name | Clinical infection |
|---|---|---|---|
| **Nematodes** (filarial) | *Brugia malayi* | | lymphatic filariasis (Malayan, brugian) |
| | *Brugia timori* | | lymphatic filariasis (Timorian, brugian) |
| | *Loa loa* | eye-worm | loiasis |
| | *Mansonella* spp. | | Mansonella infections |
| | *Onchocerca volvulus* | | onchocerciasis (river blindness) |
| | *Wuchereria bancrofti* | | lymphatic filariasis (bancroftian) |
| **Nematodes** (intestinal) | *Ancylostoma duodenale* | Old World hookworm | ancylostomiasis |
| | *Angiostrongylus costaricensis* | | angiostrongyliasis |
| | *Ascaris lumbricoides** | common roundworm, giant roundworm | ascariasis |
| | *Capillaria philippinensis* | | capillariasis |
| | *Enterobius vermicularis** | threadworm, pinworm | enterobiasis |
| | *Necator americanus* | New World hookworm | necatoriasis |
| | *Strongyloides stercoralis* | sometimes called threadworm in USA | strongyloidiasis |
| | *Trichostrongylus* spp. | | trichostrongyliasis |
| | *Trichuris trichiura** | whipworm | trichuriasis |
| **Nematodes** (tissue) | *Ancylostoma* spp. | dog/cat hookworm | cutaneous larva migrans (creeping eruption) |
| | *Angiostrongylus cantonensis* | | angiostrongyliasis |
| | *Dracunculus medinensis* | guinea-worm | dracunculiasis (dracontiasis) |
| | *Gnathostoma spinigerum* | | gnathostomiasis |
| | *Syngamus* spp. | gapeworm | syngamosis |
| | *Toxocara* spp.* | | toxocariasis (visceral larva migrans, ocular larva migrans) |
| | *Trichinella spiralis** | | trichinosis (trichinellosis) |
| **Cestodes** (tapeworms) | *Diphyllobothrium latum* | broad fish tapeworm | diphyllobothriasis |
| | *Echinococcus* spp. | | echinococcosis (hydatid disease) |
| | *Hymenolepis nana* | dwarf tapeworm | hymenolepiasis |
| | *Taenia saginata** | beef tapeworm | taeniasis |
| | *Taenia solium** | pork tapeworm | cysticercosis (larval form), taeniasis (adult worm) |
| **Trematodes** (flukes) | *Clonorchis sinensis* | Chinese liver fluke | clonorchiasis |
| | *Fasciola hepatica* | liver fluke | fascioliasis |
| | *Fasciolopsis buski* | intestinal fluke | fasciolopsiasis |
| | *Heterophyes heterophyes* | intestinal fluke | heterophyiasis |
| | *Metagonimus yokogawi* | intestinal fluke | metagonimiasis |
| | *Nanophyetus salmincola* | intestinal fluke | nanophyetiasis |
| | *Opisthorchis* spp. | liver fluke | opisthorchiasis |
| | *Paragonimus* spp. | oriental lung fluke | paragonimiasis |
| | *Schistosoma* spp. | blood fluke | schistosomiasis |

NOTE: Infections due to worms marked with an asterisk may occur in temperate climates. Infections due to other worms are generally limited to tropical or localised areas, but may occur in travellers who have visited those areas.

### Capillariasis

Capillariasis is caused by infection with *Capillaria philippinensis,* a nematode endemic in the Philippines and southern Thailand. Infection in man is through eating raw or undercooked freshwater fish containing infective larvae. The larvae mature in the intestines and the adults produce both eggs and infective larvae so that auto-infection occurs and heavy infections can result. Symptoms are mostly gastrointestinal, with abdominal pain, vomiting, and severe prolonged diarrhoea leading to cachexia and muscle wasting. The infection has a mortality rate of between 20 and 30% if untreated. Prolonged treatment with mebendazole or, alternatively, albendazole, is necessary.

### Clonorchiasis

See under Liver Fluke Infections, below.

### Cutaneous larva migrans

Cutaneous larva migrans (creeping eruption) occurs when man becomes infected with the larvae of animal hookworms, usually *Ancylostoma braziliense* or *A. caninum,* hookworms of cats and dogs. Other hookworms may also be involved or may cause other infections (see Hookworm Infections, below). The larvae penetrate the skin and then migrate causing characteristic trails in the skin. This migration can persist for several months and can be a source of intense pruritus. Occasionally larvae migrate to the lungs causing eosinophilia and pulmonary symptoms. Albendazole or ivermectin may be given by mouth and may be better tolerated than oral tiabendazole; tiabendazole can also be applied topically but is of limited value for multiple lesions.

Infection with *Gnathostoma spinigerum* or *Strongyloides stercoralis* can also cause cutaneous larva migrans (see Gnathostomiasis and Strongyloidiasis, below). Ocular and visceral larva migrans are features of toxocariasis (see below).

References.

1. Caumes E. Treatment of cutaneous larva migrans. *Clin Infect Dis* 2000; **30:** 811–14.

### Cysticercosis

Cysticercosis is a systemic infection caused by the larval form (cysticercus) of *Taenia solium.* Infection is acquired through ingestion of eggs in contaminated food or water, or directly from individuals harbouring the adult worm. The eggs hatch in the intestine and the larvae spread systemically to almost any body tissue. Invasion of the brain is known as neurocysticercosis and is a common cause of epilepsy in endemic areas. The most effective treatment for neurocysticercosis has been debated.[1] In the absence of large randomised studies, opinion has been divided over whether cysticidal drugs should be given routinely in neurocysticercosis or reserved for selected patients.[1] Some have suggested that they might be associated with long-term sequelae,[2] and have reiterated that the ideal solution is prevention by ensuring adequate sanitation and sewage treatment and thorough cooking of meat that may be contaminated. A systematic review[3] has concluded that there is insufficient evidence to assess the benefit of cysticidal therapy in neurocysticercosis. When anthelmintics are considered necessary, praziquantel is used to treat neurocysticercosis and is usually given with a corticosteroid to prevent an inflammatory response to dead and dying larvae. Alternatively, some prefer albendazole; a corticosteroid or antihistamine is also given to counter any inflammatory reaction. In some cases surgical removal of cysts may be the preferred treatment.

Infection with the adult worm of *T. solium* is discussed under Taeniasis, below.

1. Anonymous. Cerebral cysticercosis: what can be expected of cysticidal drugs? *WHO Drug Inf* 1995; **9:** 135–8.
2. Carpio A, *et al.* Is the course of neurocysticercosis modified by treatment with antihelminthic agents? *Arch Intern Med* 1995; **155:** 1982–8.
3. Salinas R, Prasad K. Drugs for treating neurocysticercosis (tapeworm infection of the brain). Available in The Cochrane Library; Issue 2. Chichester: John Wiley; 2004.

### Diphyllobothriasis

Diphyllobothriasis is an intestinal infection with the fish tapeworm *Diphyllobothrium latum* and other *Diphyllobothrium* spp. and is acquired in man through ingestion of raw, infected, freshwater fish. The infection is rarely symptomatic. However, because the adult worm competes for vitamin $B_{12}$, some patients may develop megaloblastic anaemia with its associated neurological symptoms. Concentrations of other vitamins may also be reduced. Treatment is with a single dose of praziquantel. Niclosamide is an alternative. Vitamin supplements should also be given to correct any deficiencies.

### Dracunculiasis

Dracunculiasis (dracontiasis, guinea-worm infection) is caused by infection with the nematode *Dracunculus medinensis.* It has been endemic in parts of Africa and Asia but is increasingly coming under control and the hope is that it will soon be eradicated.[1] The disease is transmitted through drinking water containing larvae that develop in freshwater crustaceans. The larvae penetrate the intestinal mucosa and mature in connective tissue. The adult female migrates to the subcutaneous tissues, normally of the legs, after about 1 year. Ulceration of the overlying skin releases larvae which are ingested by the crustacean host to complete the life cycle. The first symptom is the lesion caused by the emerging worm, although a generalised hypersensitivity reaction may also occur. Secondary infection is a common complication.

The most effective method of controlling dracunculiasis is by provision of safe drinking water. The WHO eradication campaign is based on health education, and the provision of safe water by measures including water treatment with pesticides such as temefos and encouraging the use of domestic filters.

There is no effective direct drug therapy against any stage in man. The traditional treatment is removal of the adult worm by gentle traction sometimes over several weeks. Metronidazole or tiabendazole may provide symptomatic benefit in the management of dracunculiasis although they have no direct anthelmintic effect. They are thought to act by weakening the anchorage of the worms within the subcutaneous tissues, thus allowing them to be removed more quickly.

1. WHO. Dracunculiasis. Available at: http://www.who.int/ctd/dracun/index.html (accessed 01/06/04)

### Echinococcosis

Echinococcosis, or hydatid disease, in man is infection with the larval stage of the cestode *Echinococcus granulosus* or *E. multilocularis.* These two species cause distinct forms of the disease known as cystic echinococcosis and alveolar echinococcosis respectively. Various animals are involved in the transmission of the disease, man becoming infected through ingestion of eggs from contaminated faeces. The eggs hatch in the intestine and the embryos penetrate the intestinal wall and invade body organs, usually the liver. The embryo develops into a cyst which slowly increases in size and may remain intact for many years. Symptomatic infection usually only occurs when the cyst is large enough to cause obstruction or to compress adjacent structures, or if rupture occurs. Where possible, surgical removal of the intact cyst is the first line of treatment.

In **cystic echinococcosis**, drugs may be given locally or systemically before surgery to kill infective larvae within the cyst and reduce the risk of further infection. They are also given postoperatively if a cyst ruptures during surgery. Local injection of a larvicidal agent such as alcohol, cetrimide, or hypertonic saline has been used. Chemotherapy is also used as an adjunct or when surgery is not possible. The preferred drug for associated systemic treatment is albendazole. Mebendazole may be used, although some have suggested it is not as effective as albendazole. Praziquantel has also been reported to be effective. Albendazole may be a suitable alternative to surgery as initial treatment in uncomplicated cases; use with cimetidine (to inhibit its metabolism) may increase its effectiveness.

A further option when surgery is not possible is the PAIR (puncture/aspiration/injection/re-aspiration) procedure which consists of ultrasound-guided cyst puncture followed by aspiration of the cyst fluid, local injection of alcohol or hypertonic saline into the cyst, and re-aspiration of the cyst contents. Concomitant chemotherapy is recommended.

*E. multilocularis* infection (**alveolar echinococcosis**) is more invasive and is characterised by a tumour-like infiltrative growth; it usually requires both surgery and long-term treatment with a benzimidazole, such as albendazole, although some patients have improved on albendazole alone.

References.


1. Kumar A, Chattopadhyay TK. Management of hydatid disease of the liver. *Postgrad Med J* 1992; **68:** 853–6.
2. Wen H, *et al.* Diagnosis and treatment of human hydatidosis. *Br J Clin Pharmacol* 1993; **35:** 565–74.
3. WHO Informal Working Group on Echinococcosis. Guidelines for treatment of cystic and alveolar echinococcosis in humans. *Bull WHO* 1996; **74:** 231–42.
4. Reuter S, *et al.* Benzimidazoles in the treatment of alveolar echinococcosis: a comparative study and review of the literature. *J Antimicrob Chemother* 2000; **46:** 451–6.
5. Mcmanus DP, *et al.* Echinococcosis. *Lancet* 2003; **362:** 1295–1304.


### Enterobiasis

Enterobiasis is an infection with *Enterobius vermicularis* (pinworm, threadworm). It is one of the few intestinal nematodes which is common in temperate climates and is particularly common in young children. Like trichuriasis (below) it is an infection of the large intestine and transmission follows ingestion or inhalation of mature eggs. The larvae mature in the gut in about 2 months. The eggs are not released into the gut contents but the mature female migrates to the anus at night and lays its eggs on the perianal and perineal skin. The eggs become infective within 6 hours. Diagnosis is based on detecting eggs around the anus. The most common symptom is perianal itching but many infections are asymptomatic. Rarely ectopic disease such as appendicitis or salpingitis may occur. The adult worm has a life span of about 6 weeks and, if re-infection can be prevented, the infection is self-limiting. While additional hygiene measures can prevent re-infection, treatment of the whole family with an anthelmintic should remain the main therapeutic response; more than one course may be required.

Treatment is with a benzimidazole carbamate derivative, such as albendazole or mebendazole, or with pyrantel embonate. Such broad-spectrum therapy can be useful if the patient is suffering from a mixed intestinal nematode infection. Other anthelmintics used in enterobiasis include piperazine or pyrvinium embonate.

### Fascioliasis

See under Liver Fluke Infections, below.

### Fasciolopsiasis

See under Intestinal Fluke Infections, below.

### Gnathostomiasis

Gnathostomiasis is an infection with, in most cases, the larval form of the nematode *Gnathostoma spinigerum*, although other *Gnathostoma* spp. have been identified. *G. spinigerum* inhabits the stomach of cats and dogs. Eggs shed in their faeces are ingested by freshwater crustaceans and hatch into larvae which are ingested by fish or other animals; man acquires the infection by consumption of the raw or undercooked flesh of these secondary hosts. Once ingested the larva penetrates the gut wall and migrates via the liver to other tissues including skin, eyes, and CNS. Rarely, dermal infiltration may result in cutaneous larva migrans (above).

The preferred treatment of gnathostomiasis is surgical removal of the gnathostome but this is rarely possible. Albendazole or, alternatively, ivermectin, may be used.

### Heterophyiasis

See under Intestinal Fluke Infections, below.

### Hookworm infections

Infections with the hookworms *Ancylostoma duodenale* (ancylostomiasis) and *Necator americanus* (necatoriasis) are a major cause of iron-deficiency anaemia in large areas of the tropics and sub-tropics, especially in rural communities. Eggs deposited in warm moist soil hatch into larvae which develop further into the infective form. Infection is normally by penetration through the skin although it may be by ingestion. The larvae migrate to the lungs and are subsequently swallowed and mature to the adult form in the small intestine. Eggs appear in the faeces about 6 to 8 weeks after infection and the adult worm may live for several years. *A. duodenale* larvae are capable of remaining dormant in the tissues, only maturing to the adult when climatic conditions are favourable. Symptoms correspond to the stage of infection. Visitors to endemic areas may develop intense pruritus, erythema, and papulovesicular eruption at the site of infection, known as ground itch. Migration through the lungs during the first infection may cause pneumonitis and bronchospasm with accompanying eosinophilia. The main symptoms of intestinal infection are iron-deficiency anaemia and severe hypoalbuminaemia. In addition, abdominal pain, diarrhoea, and weight loss may occur.

Treatment is usually with a benzimidazole carbamate derivative such as mebendazole or albendazole, and such broad-spectrum therapy can also be useful if the patient has a mixed intestinal nematode infection. Other anthelmintics used in hookworm infections include levamisole or pyrantel embonate, but these may be less effective against *N. americanus* than against *A. duodenale*. Iron-deficiency anaemia caused by hookworm infections responds rapidly to oral iron therapy; folic acid supplements may be necessary in some patients. Mass treatment programmes may be necessary in endemic areas to reduce the overall burden of infection.[1-4]

There is some evidence to suggest[5] that human infection with animal hookworms, some of which were previously thought to cause only cutaneous larva migrans (above), may also occasionally cause enteric infections characterised by eosinophilia.


1. Nahmias J, *et al.* Evaluation of albendazole, pyrantel, bephenium, pyrantel-praziquantel, and pyrantel-bephenium for single-dose mass treatment of necatoriasis. *Ann Trop Med Parasitol* 1989; **83:** 625–9.
2. Bradley M, *et al.* The epidemiology and control of hookworm infection in the Burma Valley area of Zimbabwe. *Trans R Soc Trop Med Hyg* 1993; **87:** 145–7.
3. Krepel HP, *et al.* Treatment of mixed Oesophagostomum and hookworm infection: effect of albendazole, pyrantel pamoate, levamisole and thiabendazole. *Trans R Soc Trop Med Hyg* 1993; **87:** 87–9.
4. Idris MA, *et al.* Effective control of hookworm infection in school children from Dhofar, Sultanate of Oman: a four-year experience with albendazole mass chemotherapy. *Acta Trop* 2001; **80:** 139–43.
5. Schad GA. Hookworms: pets to humans. *Ann Intern Med* 1994; **120:** 434–5.


### Hymenolepiasis

Hymenolepiasis is an infection of the intestine with *Hymenolepis nana*, or dwarf tapeworm. Infection is acquired through ingestion of eggs in contaminated food or water or on hands and can be passed directly from person to person. It is more common in children. Clinical symptoms occur in heavy infections and include diarrhoea and abdominal pain. Treatment is with a single dose of praziquantel. Niclosamide has also been used.

### Intestinal fluke infections

The intestinal fluke infections **fasciolopsiasis, heterophyiasis, metagonimiasis**, and **nanophyetiasis** are caused by *Fasciolopsis buski, Heterophyes heterophyes* and some other *Heterophyes* spp., *Metagonimus yokogawai*, and *Nanophyetus salmincola* respectively. Fasciolopsiasis, heterophyiasis, and metagonimiasis are endemic in the Far East and Southeast Asia, and heterophyiasis is also common in the Middle East. Nanophyetiasis has occurred increasingly in the Pacific northwest of the USA. Fasciolopsiasis is caused by the ingestion of infected aquatic plants, while undercooked or raw infected fish are the sources of *H. heterophyes, M. yokogawai*, and *N. salmincola* infections.

Fasciolopsiasis is usually asymptomatic, but heavy infections can cause diarrhoea, abdominal pain, and, rarely, intestinal obstruction and an allergic oedematous reaction. Metagonimiasis is also generally asymptomatic but may cause mild diarrhoea, while pain and mucous diarrhoea are common in heterophyiasis. Similar gastrointestinal symptoms plus eosinophilia occur in nanophyetiasis. Eggs of *M. yokogawai* and *H. heterophyes* may rarely penetrate the bowel wall and enter the bloodstream to be deposited in various organs, leading to serious complications such as heart failure or fatal embolism in the heart or brain.

Treatment of intestinal fluke infections is with praziquantel.[1]


1. WHO. Control of foodborne trematode infections. *WHO Tech Rep Ser 849* 1995.


### Liver fluke infections

*Fasciola hepatica, Opisthorchis viverrini, O. felineus*, and *Clonorchis sinensis* are liver flukes transmitted by the ingestion of infected aquatic plants, grasses or water (*F. hepatica*), or raw or undercooked fish (*Opisthorchis* spp., *C. sinensis*). **Fascioliasis** is primarily a disease of sheep and cattle and human infections may occur wherever these animals are raised, whereas **clonorchiasis** and **opisthorchiasis** are seen mainly in Southeast Asia and eastern Europe.

Fascioliasis in the acute phase is usually characterised by fever, gastrointestinal symptoms, pain due to liver enlargement, and marked eosinophilia, but these symptoms decline as the worms enter their final habitat in the bile ducts. Acute symptoms occur rarely with clonorchiasis and opisthorchiasis and infections tend to be asymptomatic for many years. Adult flukes live in the bile ducts and symptoms of biliary-tract obstruction appear after repeated or heavy infections with liver flukes. Cholangiocarcinoma (bile duct cancer) is now generally accepted to be associated with liver fluke infection although its exact pathogenesis is unclear.

Praziquantel is used for the treatment of most liver fluke infections.[1] Bithionol is more effective than praziquantel in fascioliasis and has been the preferred treatment, although in the USA the CDC considers triclabendazole to be the treatment of choice; dehydroemetine has also been used.

Praziquantel remains the treatment of choice for clonorchiasis and opisthorchiasis.[1] Albendazole is a suggested alternative for clonorchiasis.


1. WHO. Control of foodborne trematode infections. *WHO Tech Rep Ser 849* 1995.


### Loiasis

Loiasis is an infection with the filarial nematode *Loa loa* which occurs in areas of Central and West Africa. It is transmitted by the biting tabanid fly *Chrysops*. The infective larvae mature to adult worms which migrate through subcutaneous tissues and occasionally the subconjunctiva. Symptoms include pruritus, swelling, and pain, with occasional subcutaneous swellings, often on the arms or legs, that are characteristic of the disease. Passage of a worm through the subconjunctiva produces intense conjunctivitis. Eosinophilia may be severe, especially in visitors from non-endemic areas. Other complications include renal disease, endomyocardial fibrosis, encephalopathy, and peripheral neuropathy.

Diethylcarbamazine is effective against the microfilariae, larval forms, and a proportion of adult worms. In some cases, treatment has been associated with acute encephalitis, particularly in patients with heavy microfilaraemia. It has been assumed that this is related to blockage of capillaries in the brain and meninges and for this reason small doses of diethylcarbamazine are given initially in combination with a corticosteroid and antihistamine, gradually increasing to full therapeutic doses over several days. However this does not eliminate the risk of encephalitis entirely and the role of the microfilariae in this syndrome has been questioned. Some consider that ivermectin could be useful but, as with diethylcarbamazine, there is concern over its potential neurotoxic effects in patients with heavy microfilaraemia.

Diethylcarbamazine is also used for prophylaxis but it has been suggested that it should be reserved for subjects at high risk of exposure. Vector control is regarded as impractical and methods aimed at reducing contact with the vector such as window screens and protective clothing are recommended.

### Lung fluke infections

The lung fluke infection **paragonimiasis** is caused by *Paragonimus* spp., commonly *P. westermani*, and occurs in Asia, Africa, and Central or South America. The disease is transmitted by the ingestion of raw infected freshwater crabs or crayfish, or from drinking infected water.

The flukes mature in the lungs where they cause local necrosis, haemorrhage, inflammation, and fibrosis. Symptoms of paragonimiasis include fever, pain, and chest complaints, but the majority of light to moderate infections are asymptomatic. The worms may also develop at other sites, particularly the brain where they can cause epilepsy, symptoms of cerebral tumours, or cerebral embolism, which may be fatal.

Treatment is with praziquantel or bithionol. Triclabendazole has been studied.

### Lymphatic filariasis

Lymphatic filariasis arises from infection with *Wuchereria bancrofti* (bancroftian filariasis), *Brugia malayi*, or *B. timori* (both known as brugian filariasis and as Malayan and Timorian filariasis respectively). It occurs in tropical and subtropical regions. Larval forms are transmitted by mosquitoes. The larvae penetrate the lymphatic system where they mature to adult worms that may live for many years. Infective microfilariae are produced within 3 to 6 months and enter the peripheral bloodstream, from where they are ingested by further mosquito vectors in which new larvae develop.

Lymphatic filariasis may be asymptomatic but both acute and chronic symptoms also occur. Inflammatory reactions to immature and adult worms in the lymphatic system produce episodic adenolymphangitis with fever. In men, bancroftian filariasis characteristically presents as epididymo-orchitis. Abscesses may occasionally occur, particularly with brugian filariasis. Chronic lymphadenopathy is frequently seen. The main clinical features in chronic bancroftian filariasis are hydrocele, lymphoedema, elephantiasis, and chyluria. Chronic brugian filariasis typically causes lymphoedema and elephantiasis in the limb below the knee or elbow. Tropical pulmonary eosinophilia is a clinical variant of filarial disease, particularly of *W. bancrofti* infection. The symptoms include cough, wheezing, and eosinophilia. If untreated the condition can progress to chronic interstitial fibrosis.

There is no entirely satisfactory treatment of lymphatic filariasis. Diethylcarbamazine kills microfilariae and a proportion of immature and adult worms and is widely used for both treatment and prophylaxis. Treatment can precipitate severe immunological reactions to the dead and dying worms. Large hydroceles and elephantiasis are generally not reversible and usually require surgical intervention.[1,2] However, treatment with coumarins may reduce the lymphoedema and so lead to improvement.[3,4] There has also been a suggestion that elephantiasis may be linked to local secondary bacterial or fungal infections, and that simple measures such as regular washing could also produce improvement.[5] Tropical pulmonary eosinophilia responds to diethylcarbamazine but about 20% of patients may relapse and require re-treatment.[1] Diethylcarbamazine (p.105) is also used in the mass control of filariasis in all subjects in endemic areas. Ivermectin (p.106), which is also effective against microfilariae, has produced promising results in several studies. Albendazole, combined with diethylcarbamazine or ivermectin, has also shown promise and these combinations (with albendazole and ivermectin being donated by *GlaxoSmithKline* and *Merck* respectively) are being used in mass treatment programmes as part of a global elimination campaign launched by WHO together with other international agencies. In areas where loiasis or onchocerciasis are co-endemic with bancroftian filariasis, albendazole and ivermectin are used together and where there is no loiasis or onchocerciasis then albendazole is given with diethylcarbamazine.

Control measures aimed at reducing the intensity of transmission include educating local communities on the use of insecticidal sprays and impregnated bed nets, and the use of mass chemotherapy treatment. Effective vector control is considered to be too expensive in most endemic areas.


1. WHO. Lymphatic filariasis: the disease and its control: fifth report of the WHO expert committee on filariasis. *WHO Tech Rep Ser 821* 1992.
2. WHO. Lymphatic filariasis. Available at: http://www.who.int/tdr/diseases/lymphfil/diseaseinfo.htm (accessed 01/06/04)
3. Casley-Smith JR, *et al.* Treatment of filarial lymphoedema and elephantiasis with 5,6-benzo-α-pyrone (coumarin). *BMJ* 1993; **307:** 1037–41.
4. Anonymous. Coumarins: symptomatic relief of filarial lymphoedema. *WHO Drug Inf* 1993; **7:** 177–8.
5. McGregor A. Washing off elephantiasis. *Lancet* 1994; **344:** 121.


### Mansonella infections

Infections with the filarial nematodes *Mansonella perstans, M. ozzardi,* and *M. streptocerca* are generally asymptomatic but a variety of symptoms including malaise, fever, joint pain, and meningeal symptoms have been described. Infection is transmitted by biting midges and flies. Treatment with diethylcarbamazine may be effective depending on the infecting species (although it has no effect in *M. ozzardi* infections). Mebendazole may be effective alone or in combination with levamisole in *M. perstans*; albendazole has also been used in this infection. Ivermectin has been suggested for *M. ozzardi* infections and may be the drug of choice for *M. streptocerca*.

### Metagonimiasis

See under Intestinal Fluke Infections, above.

### Nanophyetiasis

See under Intestinal Fluke Infections, above.

### Necatoriasis

See under Hookworm Infections, above.

### Onchocerciasis

Onchocerciasis (river blindness) is caused by infection with the filarial nematode *Onchocerca volvulus*. It is endemic in large areas of Africa and areas of Central or South America. It is particularly prevalent near fast flowing rivers, the breeding ground of the blackfly which is the vector of the parasite. Following infection, the larvae mature into adults in fibrous nodules, usually in the subcutaneous tissue. The adults release large numbers of microfilariae which have been considered responsible for the major symptoms of the disease in the skin and the eye, although there is some evidence that symbiotic *Wolbachia* bacteria within the nematodes play a role.[1] Symptoms of skin involvement range from an intensely pruritic erythematous rash to chronic skin changes and severe pendulous lymphoedema. Infection of the eye is a major cause of blindness in endemic areas.

Onchocerciasis is controlled with ivermectin.[2-6] Ivermectin rapidly eliminates microfilariae from the skin and more gradually from the eye.[3] It does not eliminate the adult worms although it suppresses release of microfilariae for several cycles. Ivermectin is donated by *Merck* through the Mectizan Expert Committee (MEC) for human use in community-wide mass treatment programmes in all countries in which onchocerciasis is endemic, where it is given to all but pregnant women, breast-feeding mothers of recently born babies, children weighing less than 15 kg, and those unable to walk or otherwise seriously ill.[7] Control of the disease in endemic areas thus relies upon the administration of ivermectin once or twice a year and this may be combined with vector control. For further details, see under Ivermectin, p.106.

Before the introduction of ivermectin, diethylcarbamazine was the usual treatment for onchocerciasis, but it is no longer recommended by WHO.[2,3] The major limitations to its use are the severe allergic reaction (the Mazzotti reaction) associated with its microfilaricidal action, aggravation of existing ocular lesions or precipitation of new ones, and the need to give repeated courses of treatment for continued suppression of the disease.[3] Suramin has also been used in the treatment of onchocerciasis and is effective against adult worms.[2,3] However, its use is restricted because of its toxicity. Amocarzine has also been evaluated in onchocerciasis.[3]

There is current interest in the use of antibacterials against *Wolbachia* as a potential approach to treatment of onchocerciasis.[8]


1. Saint André A, *et al.* The role of endosymbiotic Wolbachia bacteria in the pathogenesis of river blindness. *Science* 2002; **295:** 1892–5.
2. *WHO model prescribing information: drugs used in parasitic diseases.* 2nd ed. Geneva: WHO, 1995.
3. WHO. Onchocerciasis and its control: report of a WHO expert committee on onchocerciasis control. *WHO Tech Rep Ser 852* 1995.
4. Van Laethem Y, Lopes C. Treatment of onchocerciasis. *Drugs* 1996; **52:** 861–9.
5. Burnham G. Onchocerciasis. *Lancet* 1998; **351:** 1341–6.
6. WHO. Onchocerciasis. Available at: http://www.who.int/tdr/diseases/oncho/diseaseinfo.htm (accessed 01/06/04)
7. Pond B. Distribution of ivermectin by health workers. *Lancet* 1990; **335:** 1539.
8. Hoerauf A, *et al.* Onchocerciasis. *BMJ* 2003; **326:** 207-10.


### Opisthorchiasis

See under Liver Fluke Infections, above.

### Paragonimiasis

See under Lung Fluke Infections, above.

### Schistosomiasis

Schistosomiasis (bilharziasis) is a parasitic infection caused by *Schistosoma* spp., largely *S. mansoni, S. japonicum,* and *S. haematobium*, and to a lesser extent *S. intercalatum* and *S. mekongi*. The disease is seen mainly in Africa, Asia, South America, and the Caribbean, where it is a hazard to individuals exposed to fresh water containing the intermediate host, infected freshwater snails.

Free-swimming cercariae are released from the snail and penetrate human skin causing a pruritic papular rash in sensitised individuals (swimmer's itch). Parasites mature in the lungs and liver within about 6 weeks, then migrate to the blood vessels, the bladder, or intestines. Mature female worms produce eggs which are excreted in urine or stools, or become lodged in tissues, and immunological reaction to these eggs results in disease. The acute reaction to egg deposition has been termed Katayama fever, a self-limiting but sometimes fatal illness resembling serum sickness and most frequently seen in *S. japonicum* infection. The chronic phase of infection is often asymptomatic for many years, but usually results in granuloma formation and fibrosis in tissues where eggs are deposited, such as the liver, lungs, intestines, or urinary tract, the site depending on the infecting species.

Praziquantel is used for the treatment of chronic schistosomiasis[1-5] and is effective against all species of schistosomes. Metrifonate and oxamniquine are alternatives that may be used against *S. haematobium*[1,2] and *S. mansoni*[1,3-5] respectively. Artemisinin derivatives are also under investigation for *S. mansoni* infection.[6,7]

Niclosamide is used as a molluscicide for the treatment of water in schistosomiasis control programmes. Copper sulfate or sodium pentachlorophenate have also been used but to a lesser extent.

Schistosomiasis vaccines are in development.


1. WHO. The control of schistosomiasis: second report of the WHO expert committee. *WHO Tech Rep Ser 830* 1993.
2. Squires N. Interventions for treating schistosomiasis haematobium. Available in The Cochrane Library; Issue 2. Chichester: John Wiley; 2004.
3. Saconato H, Atallah A. Interventions for treating schistosomiasis mansoni. Available in The Cochrane Library; Issue 2. Chichester: John Wiley; 2004.
4. WHO. Schistosomiasis. Available at: http://www.who.int/tdr/diseases/schisto/diseaseinfo.htm (accessed 01/06/04)
5. Ross AGP, *et al.* Schistosomiasis. *N Engl J Med* 2002; **346:** 1212–20.
6. De Clercq D, *et al.* Efficacy of artesunate against Schistosoma mansoni infections in Richard Toll, Senegal. *Trans R Soc Trop Med Hyg* 2000; **94:** 90–1.
7. Utzinger J, *et al.* Oral artemether for prevention of Schistosoma mansoni infection: randomised controlled trial. *Lancet* 2000; **355:** 1320–5.


### Strongyloidiasis

Strongyloidiasis is an infection of the small intestine caused by *Strongyloides stercoralis*, known as threadworm in the USA. It generally occurs in the tropics and subtropics and can also occur in some areas of South and East Europe, Japan, and the USA. In contrast with other intestinal nematodes, the eggs of *S. stercoralis* hatch before leaving the gastrointestinal tract, and can cause autoinfection, particularly in immunocompromised patients. Larvae reaching the soil can either mature into free-living adults or remain in an infective larval stage. Infective larvae cause infection by penetrating the skin. The larvae migrate to the lungs, move up the bronchial tree to be swallowed, and finally penetrate the mucosa of the small intestine where they mature. Eggs are deposited about 28 days after initial infection.

Infection may be asymptomatic, but commonly patients have symptoms relating to the stages of infection. Penetration of larvae through the skin causes intense pruritus and an erythematous rash. The rash may follow the course of migration and is one of the causes of cutaneous larva migrans (above). An inflammatory response to migration through the lungs may be seen and may include pneumonitis and bronchospasm. In heavy infections, which are most common in immunocompromised patients as a result of autoinfection, massive pulmonary invasion can occur resulting in fatal alveolar haemorrhage. Abdominal symptoms include colicky pain, diarrhoea, and vomiting, leading to nutritional deficiencies and weight loss. Eosinophilia may also be present. Disseminated disease may occur in immunocompromised patients and produce severe pulmonary and abdominal symptoms, shock, encephalopathy, meningitis, and Gram-negative septicaemia. Since strongyloidiasis is commonly fatal in these patients, vulnerable patients from endemic areas should be screened regularly and treated promptly at the first sign of infection.

Ivermectin is considered to be the treatment of choice. Tiabendazole was widely used, and still is in some countries, but albendazole is more effective and better tolerated. Mebendazole has also been suggested but it must be administered for longer periods than albendazole since it has only a limited effect on migrating larvae. These broad-spectrum anthelmintics (tiabendazole excepted) are also useful if the patient is suffering from a mixed intestinal nematode infection.

### Syngamosis

Syngamosis, or gapeworm infection, is caused by *Syngamus* and *Mammomonogamus* spp. and is primarily an infection of domestic fowl and wild birds and mammals, although infection in man has been reported very rarely. Man may become infected by eating foods contaminated with infective larvae which penetrate the intestinal wall and migrate to the lungs, where they mature into adult worms. The major symptom is cough, due to irritation of the bronchi and increased mucus production. The infection may be confused with asthma. Tiabendazole and mebendazole have been used successfully to treat the infection in man.

### Taeniasis

Taeniasis is an infection of the intestine with beef tapeworm, *Taenia saginata*, or pork tapeworm, *T. solium*, acquired through ingestion of contaminated raw or undercooked meat. The larval form of *T. solium* can cause the systemic infection cysticercosis (see above).

Infection with the adult worm usually produces symptoms only when the worm reaches a size that can cause obstruction or related problems. Segments of the worm containing eggs may be excreted in the faeces so maintaining the cycle of reproduction. Treatment is with a single dose of praziquantel, which has the advantage of also being active, in higher doses, against the larval form of *T. solium*. Niclosamide is also effective but is only active against adult worms.

### Toxocariasis

Toxocariasis is infection with the larval form of *Toxocara canis* or, less commonly, *T. cati*. The adult worms live in the intestines of dogs and cats respectively, and man becomes infected when eggs excreted in animal faeces are ingested. Once ingested the eggs hatch and the larvae migrate from the intestine to other organs, most commonly the liver, lung, and eye. Most infections are asymptomatic but two clinical syndromes, ocular larva migrans and visceral larva migrans, can occur, usually in children.

Ocular larva migrans occurs when larvae invade the eye causing a granuloma which may impair vision and can cause blindness. There is no specific treatment.[1] Anthelmintics such as albendazole or tiabendazole, corticosteroids, ocular surgery, and laser photocoagulation have been used but assessment of their efficacy is difficult because of the variable natural course of the disease.

The clinical symptoms of visceral larva migrans depend upon the organs involved but commonly include cough, wheezing, fever, and hepatomegaly. Encephalitis and seizures may occur and there is usually eosinophilia. Acute infection normally resolves without treatment.[2] However, severe or prolonged infections may be treated with diethylcarbamazine. Albendazole, mebendazole, and tiabendazole have also been used.

1. Shields JA. Ocular toxocariasis: a review. *Surv Ophthalmol* 1984; **28:** 361–81.
2. Gillespie SH. Human toxocariasis. *Commun Dis Rep* 1993; **3:** R140–R143.

### Trichinosis

Trichinosis (trichinellosis) is an infection caused by *Trichinella spiralis*. Man becomes infected through ingestion of raw or undercooked meat, usually pork, containing infective larvae. The larvae mature into adult worms in the small intestine and the mature females deposit larvae which migrate in the blood to skeletal muscle and sometimes to the myocardium. Symptoms usually occur only in heavy infections. Invasion of the intestines by the maturing adult worms can cause diarrhoea, abdominal pain, and vomiting followed about a week later by hypersensitivity reactions to the migrating larvae. These may include eosinophilia, fever, muscle pain, periorbital oedema and, more rarely, encephalitis, myocarditis, or pneumonia which may be fatal.

All patients with confirmed or suspected infection should be treated to prevent the continued production of larvae. Mebendazole is considered to be the anthelmintic of choice in some countries. Albendazole, flubendazole, tiabendazole, or pyrantel embonate may also be effective. A corticosteroid should be given for severe hypersensitivity reactions.

### Trichostrongyliasis

Trichostrongyliasis is an infection of the small intestine caused by *Trichostrongylus* spp. including *T. colubriformis*. *Trichostrongylus* spp. are normally parasites of herbivores, but infections in man have been found. They have a similar life cycle to *Ancylostoma duodenale* (see Hookworm Infections, above). Pyrantel embonate, albendazole, or mebendazole are recommended for the treatment of trichostrongyliasis.

### Trichuriasis

Trichuriasis is an infection of the large intestine with *Trichuris trichiura*, sometimes known as whipworm. Distribution is worldwide, but most infections occur in the tropics and subtropics. Eggs are excreted in the faeces and can remain viable in the soil for extended periods. Under optimum conditions the eggs become infective in about 2 to 4 weeks. Following ingestion, larvae are released from the eggs and develop within the wall of the small intestine for about 3 to 10 days, before migrating to the lumen of the large intestine where they remain attached to the mucosal lining. Eggs are detectable in the faeces about 1 to 3 months after infection. Trichuriasis is often asymptomatic, but heavy infection can result in anaemia, diarrhoea, and rectal prolapse.

Treatment is with a benzimidazole carbamate derivative such as albendazole or mebendazole and such broad-spectrum therapy can be useful if the patient is suffering from a mixed intestinal nematode infection. Albendazole may be given with ivermectin.

---

## Abamectin *(USAN, rINN)*

Abamectina; MK-0936. A mixture of abamectin component $B_{1a}$ and abamectin component $B_{1b}$.

*CAS — 65195-55-3 (component $B_{1a}$); 65195-56-4 (component $B_{1b}$).*

### Profile

Abamectin is an avermectin anthelmintic used in veterinary medicine for nematode infections. It is also used as a systemic veterinary ectoparasiticide.

---

## Albendazole *(BAN, USAN, rINN)*

Albendazol; Albendazolum; SKF-62979. Methyl 5-propylthio-1*H*-benzimidazol-2-ylcarbamate.

$C_{12}H_{15}N_3O_2S$ = 265.3.

*CAS — 54965-21-8.*

*ATC — P02CA03.*

**Pharmacopoeias.** In *Chin., Eur.* (see p.vi), *Int., US,* and *Viet.*

**Ph. Eur. 5.0** (Albendazole). A white to faintly yellowish powder. Practically insoluble in water and in alcohol; very slightly soluble in dichloromethane; freely soluble in anhydrous formic acid. Protect from light.

**USP 27** (Albendazole). A white to faintly yellowish powder. Practically insoluble in water and in alcohol; very slightly soluble in ether and in dichloromethane; freely soluble in anhydrous formic acid. Store in airtight containers.

### Adverse Effects and Precautions

As for Mebendazole, p.108.

◊ Albendazole should only be used in the treatment of echinococcosis if there is constant medical supervision with regular monitoring of serum-transaminase concentrations and of leucocyte and platelet counts. Patients with liver damage should be treated with reduced doses of benzimidazole carbamates, if at all.[1]

1. Davis A, *et al.* Multicentre clinical trials of benzimidazolecarbamates in human cystic echinococcosis (phase 2). *Bull WHO* 1989; **67:** 503–8.

**Incidence of adverse effects.** Although generally well-tolerated, the following adverse reactions were reported in the first phase of WHO-coordinated studies[1] involving 30 patients given *high-dose* therapy with albendazole for the treatment of cystic echinococcosis (hydatid disease): raised serum-transaminase levels (2 patients), reduced leucocyte counts (1), gastrointestinal symptoms (1), allergic conditions (1), and loss of hair (1). Treatment was stopped in a further patient with alveolar echinococcosis because of depressed bone-marrow activity. In the second phase of these studies,[2] of 109 patients given albendazole for cystic echinococcosis, 20 experienced adverse effects; similar findings were reported with mebendazole. The range of effects with albendazole was: elevation of transaminases (5 patients), abdominal pain and other gastrointestinal symptoms (7), severe headache (4), loss of hair (2), leucopenia (2), fever and fatigue (1), thrombocytopenia (1), and urticaria and itching (1). Albendazole had to be withdrawn in 5 patients because of adverse effects, although in 3 the withdrawal was only temporary.

1. Davis A, *et al.* Multicentre clinical trials of benzimidazolecarbamates in human echinococcosis. *Bull WHO* 1986; **64:** 383–8.
2. Davis A, *et al.* Multicentre clinical trials of benzimidazolecarbamates in human cystic echinococcosis (phase 2). *Bull WHO* 1989; **67:** 503–8.

**Effects on growth.** A multiple-dose regimen of albendazole in children with asymptomatic trichuriasis has been reported to be associated with impaired growth in those with low levels of infection.[1] However it was considered that this should not prevent the use of single doses in mass treatment programmes.[2]

1. Forrester JE, *et al.* Randomised trial of albendazole and pyrantel in symptomless trichuriasis in children. *Lancet* 1998; **352:** 1103–8.
2. Winstanley P. Albendazole for mass treatment of asymptomatic trichuris infections. *Lancet* 1998; **352:** 1080–1.

**Effects on the liver.** In a series of 40 patients given albendazole for echinococcosis, 7 developed abnormalities in liver function tests during therapy.[1] Six had a hepatocellular type of abnormality attributable to albendazole; the seventh had cholestatic jaundice which was probably not due to albendazole. See also Incidence of Adverse Effects, above.

1. Morris DL, Smith PG. Albendazole in hydatid disease—hepatocellular toxicity. *Trans R Soc Trop Med Hyg* 1987; **81:** 343–4.

**Pregnancy.** Albendazole is teratogenic in some *animals* and the manufacturers note that there are no adequate and well controlled studies in human pregnancy. Albendazole is therefore usually contra-indicated during pregnancy and the manufacturers caution against becoming pregnant while taking albendazole or within one month of completing treatment.

### Interactions

**Anthelmintics.** The plasma concentration of albendazole sulfoxide has been increased by *praziquantel*,[1] although the practical consequences of this were considered uncertain.

1. Homeida M, *et al.* Pharmacokinetic interaction between praziquantel and albendazole in Sudanese men. *Ann Trop Med Parasitol* 1994; **88:** 551–9.

**Corticosteroids.** Plasma concentrations of the active metabolite of albendazole (albendazole sulfoxide) were reported to be raised by approximately 50% in a study in 8 patients receiving *dexamethasone*.[1]

1. Jung H, *et al.* Dexamethasone increases plasma levels of albendazole. *J Neurol* 1990; **237:** 279–80.

**Histamine $H_2$-antagonists.** Concentrations of albendazole sulfoxide have been found to be raised in bile and hydatid cyst fluid when albendazole was given with *cimetidine*, which may increase effectiveness in the treatment of echinococcosis.[1]

1. Wen H, *et al.* Initial observation on albendazole in combination with cimetidine for the treatment of human cystic echinococcosis. *Ann Trop Med Parasitol* 1994; **88:** 49–52.

### Pharmacokinetics

Absorption of albendazole from the gastrointestinal tract is poor but may be enhanced by a fatty meal. Albendazole rapidly undergoes extensive first-pass metabolism. Its principal metabolite albendazole sulfoxide has anthelmintic activity and a plasma half-life of about 8.5 hours. Albendazole sulfoxide is widely distributed throughout the body including into the bile and the CSF. It is about 70% bound to plasma protein. Albendazole sulfoxide is eliminated in the bile; only a small amount appears to be excreted in the urine.

◊ References.

1. Marriner SE, *et al.* Pharmacokinetics of albendazole in man. *Eur J Clin Pharmacol* 1986; **30:** 705–8.
2. Morris DL, *et al.* Penetration of albendazole sulphoxide into hydatid cysts. *Gut* 1987; **28:** 75–80.
3. Steiger U, *et al.* Albendazole treatment of echinococcosis in humans: effects on microsomal metabolism and drug tolerance. *Clin Pharmacol Ther* 1990; **47:** 347–53.
4. Jung H, *et al.* Clinical pharmacokinetics of albendazole in patients with brain cysticercosis. *J Clin Pharmacol* 1992; **32:** 28–31.
5. Jung H, *et al.* Clinical pharmacokinetics of albendazole in children with neurocysticercosis. *Am J Ther* 1997; **4:** 23–6.

### Uses and Administration

Albendazole is a benzimidazole carbamate anthelmintic structurally related to mebendazole (p.108) and with similar activity. It is used in relatively high doses in the treatment of the cestode infections cysticercosis and echinococcosis (hydatid disease). In some countries albendazole is used in the treatment of single and mixed intestinal nematode infections including ascariasis, enterobiasis, hookworm, strongyloidiasis, and trichuriasis. It may also be used in the treatment of capillariasis, gnathostomiasis, and trichostrongyliasis. Albendazole may be effective in the treatment of the tissue nematode infections cutaneous larva migrans, toxocariasis, and trichinosis and, in combination with other anthelmintics, in the management of the filarial nematode infection lymphatic filariasis. For discussions of these infections and their treatment, see under Choice of Anthelmintic (p.97), and under the individual headings below.

In the treatment of **echinococcosis**, albendazole is given by mouth with meals in a dose of 400 mg twice daily for 28 days for patients weighing over 60 kg. A dose of 15 mg/kg daily in two divided doses (to a maximum total daily dose of 800 mg) is used for patients weighing less than 60 kg. For cystic echinococcosis, the 28-day course may be repeated after 14 days without treatment to a total of 3 treatment cycles. For alveolar echinococcosis, cycles of 28 days of treatment followed by 14 days without treatment may need to continue for months or years.

In the treatment of **neurocysticercosis**, albendazole 400 mg twice daily for patients weighing over 60 kg (or 15 mg/kg daily in two divided doses to a maximum total daily dose of 800 mg in those weighing less than 60 kg) is given by mouth for 8 to 30 days.

Albendazole is given by mouth, usually as a single dose, in the treatment of single or mixed **intestinal nematode infections**. The usual dose for adults and children aged 2 years or over with ascariasis, enterobiasis, hookworm infections, or trichuriasis is 400 mg as a single dose. In enterobiasis, the dose may be repeated in 1 to 4 weeks. Some consider that children of 1 to 2 years of age may be given 200 mg for enterobiasis. In strongyloidiasis, 400 mg is given once or twice daily for 3 consecutive days; this may be repeated after 3 weeks if necessary.

Albendazole has also been used to treat **giardiasis** (p.596); suggested doses are 400 mg daily by mouth for 5 days.

**Ascariasis.** Albendazole is used as an alternative to mebendazole in the treatment of ascariasis (p.97). Both drugs are equally highly effective with a cure rate greater than 98% reported for albendazole in one study.[1]

1. Albonico M, *et al.* A randomized controlled trial comparing mebendazole and albendazole against Ascaris, Trichuris and hookworm infections. *Trans R Soc Trop Med Hyg* 1994; **88:** 585–9.

**Capillariasis.** Albendazole in a dose of 400 mg daily for 10 days has been suggested[1] as an alternative to mebendazole for the treatment of capillariasis (p.98).

1. Medical Letter on Drugs and Therapeutics. Drugs for parasitic infections (issued April 2002). Available at: http://www.medicalletter.com/freedocs/parasitic.pdf (accessed 01/06/04)

**Cutaneous larva migrans.** Albendazole has been reported[1-4] to be effective in the treatment of cutaneous larva migrans (p.98) and is an alternative to tiabendazole or ivermectin. Albendazole, generally in a dose of 400 mg daily for three[1] or five[2] days, has alleviated the discomfort of cutaneous larva migrans; treatment for seven days may be more effective and has not been associated with an increased incidence of adverse effects.[4] A single dose of 400 mg has also been effective.[3]

1. Jones SK, *et al.* Oral albendazole for the treatment of cutaneous larva migrans. *Br J Dermatol* 1990; **122:** 99–101.
2. Sanguigni S, *et al.* Albendazole in the therapy of cutaneous larva migrans. *Trans R Soc Trop Med Hyg* 1990; **84:** 831.
3. Oriheula AR, Torres JR. Single dose of albendazole in the treatment of cutaneous larva migrans. *Arch Dermatol* 1990; **126:** 398–9.
4. Veraldi S, Rizzitelli G. Effectiveness of a new therapeutic regimen with albendazole in cutaneous larva migrans. *Eur J Dermatol* 1999; **9:** 352–3.

**Cysticercosis.** Albendazole is used in the treatment of neurocysticercosis (p.98) as an alternative to praziquantel;[1,2] some consider albendazole to be preferable.[3-5] Albendazole has also been reported to be effective in extra-ocular cysticercosis.[6]

1. Sotelo J, *et al.* Short course of albendazole therapy for neurocysticercosis. *Arch Neurol* 1988; **45:** 1130–3.
2. Botero D, *et al.* Short course albendazole treatment for neurocysticercosis in Columbia. *Trans R Soc Trop Med Hyg* 1993; **87:** 576–7.
3. Cruz M, *et al.* Albendazole versus praziquantel in the treatment of cerebral cysticercosis: clinical evaluation. *Trans R Soc Trop Med Hyg* 1991; **85:** 244–7.
4. Takayanagui OM, Jardim E. Therapy for neurocysticercosis: comparison between albendazole and praziquantel. *Arch Neurol* 1992; **49:** 290–4.
5. Mehta SS, *et al.* Albendazole versus praziquantel for neurocysticercosis. *Am J Health-Syst Pharm* 1998; **55:** 598–600.
6. Sihota R, Honavar SG. Oral albendazole in the management of extraocular cysticercosis. *Br J Ophthalmol* 1994; **78:** 621–3.

**Echinococcosis.** Albendazole is used in the treatment of echinococcosis (p.98) as an adjunct to, or instead of, surgery. It is generally preferred to mebendazole.

References.

1. Teggi A, *et al.* Therapy of human hydatid disease with mebendazole and albendazole. *Antimicrob Agents Chemother* 1993; **37:** 1679–84.
2. Gil-Grande LA, *et al.* Randomised controlled trial of efficacy of albendazole in intra-abdominal hydatid disease. *Lancet* 1993; **342:** 1269–72.
3. Wen H, *et al.* Initial observation on albendazole in combination with cimetidine for the treatment of human cystic echinococcosis. *Ann Trop Med Parasitol* 1994; **88:** 49–52.
4. Wen H, *et al.* Albendazole chemotherapy for human cystic and alveolar echinococcosis in north-western China. *Trans R Soc Trop Med Hyg* 1994; **88:** 340–3.
5. Liu Y, *et al.* Continuous long-term albendazole therapy in intraabdominal cystic echinococcosis. *Chin Med J (Engl)* 2000; **113:** 827–32.
6. Keshmiri M, *et al.* Albendazole versus placebo in treatment of echinococcosis. *Trans R Soc Trop Med Hyg* 2001; **95:** 190–4.

**Gnathostomiasis.** Albendazole has been reported to be effective in the treatment of gnathostomiasis (p.99). Doses of 400 mg once or twice daily have been given for 2 or 3 weeks.[1-4]

1. Kraivichian P, *et al.* Albendazole for the treatment of human gnathostomiasis. *Trans R Soc Trop Med Hyg* 1992; **86:** 418–21.
2. Suntharasamai P, *et al.* Albendazole stimulates outward migration of Gnathostoma spinigerum to the dermis in man. *Southeast Asian J Trop Med Public Health* 1992; **23:** 716–22.
3. Nontasut P, *et al.* Comparison of ivermectin and albendazole treatment for gnathostomiasis. *Southeast Asian J Trop Med Public Health* 2000; **31:** 374–7.
4. Medical Letter on Drugs and Therapeutics. Drugs for parasitic infections (issued April 2002). Available at: http://www.medicalletter.com/freedocs/parasitic.pdf (accessed 02/06/04)

**Hookworm infections.** Hookworm infections (p.99) are commonly treated with benzimidazole carbamates such as albendazole. In 77 patients with light necatoriasis (*Necator americanus* infection) albendazole, in a single 400-mg dose, produced an 84% cure rate and an 82% reduction in egg count in those patients not cured.[1] In another study,[2] although the cure rate was only 56.8% following a single 400-mg dose of albendazole this was superior to treatment with mebendazole which had a cure rate of 22.4%. A further study[3] comparing albendazole with mebendazole and pyrantel in the treatment of necatoriasis also found albendazole to be the most effective.

Albendazole is given in mass treatment programmes to reduce the overall burden of infection.[1,4]

1. Nahmias J, *et al.* Evaluation of albendazole, pyrantel, bephenium, pyrantel-praziquantel and pyrantel-bephenium for single-dose mass treatment of necatoriasis. *Ann Trop Med Parasitol* 1989; **83:** 625–9.
2. Albonico M, *et al.* A randomized controlled trial comparing mebendazole and albendazole against Ascaris, Trichuris and hookworm infections. *Trans R Soc Trop Med Hyg* 1994; **88:** 585–9.
3. Sacko M, *et al.* Comparison of the efficacy of mebendazole, albendazole and pyrantel in treatment of human hookworm infections in the southern region of Mali, West Africa. *Trans R Soc Trop Med Hyg* 1999; **93:** 195–203.
4. Idris MA, *et al.* Effective control of hookworm infection in school children from Dhofar, Sultanate of Oman: a four-year experience with albendazole mass chemotherapy. *Acta Trop* 2001; **80:** 139–43.

**Lymphatic filariasis.** Albendazole is used in the management of lymphatic filariasis (p.100). In endemic areas where more than 5% of the population is infected, mass treatment of the entire population (excluding neonates, pregnant women, and debilitated individuals) can reduce the intensity of transmission and the incidence of disease. A global elimination campaign launched by WHO, together with other international agencies, advocates a single dose of albendazole 400 mg together with either a single dose of ivermectin 200 micrograms/kg (for bancroftian filariasis if there is co-endemic loiasis or onchocerciasis) or with a single dose of diethylcarbamazine 6 mg/kg (if there is no co-endemic loiasis or onchocerciasis); these doses are given once each year for 4 to 6 years.

**Microsporidiosis.** Albendazole has been tried[1-5] in the treatment of the protozoal infection microsporidiosis (p.598) in patients with AIDS. Albendazole has also been used empirically in the treatment of HIV-associated diarrhoea (p.623).

1. Blanshard C, *et al.* Treatment of intestinal microsporidiosis with albendazole in patients with AIDS. *AIDS* 1992; **6:** 311–13.
2. Dieterich DT, *et al.* Treatment with albendazole for intestinal disease due to Enterocytozoon bieneusi in patients with AIDS. *J Infect Dis* 1994; **169:** 178–82.
3. Franzen C, *et al.* Intestinal microsporidiosis with Septata intestinalis in a patient with AIDS—response to albendazole. *J Infect* 1995; **31:** 237–9.
4. Dore GJ, *et al.* Disseminated microsporidiosis due to Septata intestinalis in nine patients infected with the human immunodeficiency virus: response to therapy with albendazole. *Clin Infect Dis* 1995; **21:** 70–6.
5. Molina J-M, *et al.* Albendazole for treatment and prophylaxis of microsporidiosis due Encephalitozoon intestinalis in patients with AIDS: a randomized double-blind controlled trial. *J Infect Dis* 1998; **177:** 1373–7.

**Strongyloidiasis.** Albendazole is generally preferred to tiabendazole or mebendazole in the treatment of strongyloidiasis (p.100) although some authorities now consider ivermectin to be the drug of choice.

References.

1. Rossignol JF, Maisonneuve H. Albendazole: placebo-controlled study in 870 patients with intestinal helminthiasis. *Trans R Soc Trop Med Hyg* 1983; **77:** 707–11.
2. Chanthavanich P, *et al.* Repeated doses of albendazole against strongyloidiasis in Thai children. *Southeast Asian J Trop Med Public Health* 1989; **20:** 221–6.
3. Mojon M, Nielsen PB. Treatment of Strongyloides stercoralis with albendazole: a cure rate of 86 per cent. *Zentralbl Bakteriol Mikrobiol Hyg [A]* 1987; **263:** 619–24.
4. Archibald LK, *et al.* Albendazole is effective treatment for chronic strongyloidiasis. *Q J Med* 1993; **86:** 191–5.

**Toxocariasis.** Albendazole is one of the drugs that might be used for the treatment of toxocariasis (p.101) and in a small study[1] it produced improvement similar to that achieved with tiabendazole but with fewer problems.

1. Stürchler D, *et al.* Thiabendazole vs albendazole in treatment of toxocariasis: a clinical trial. *Ann Trop Med Parasitol* 1989; **83:** 473–8.

**Trichinosis.** Albendazole may be effective in the treatment of trichinosis (p.101). A retrospective study in 44 patients with trichinosis comparing albendazole treatment with tiabendazole found that, while the two drugs were of comparable efficacy, albendazole was the better tolerated.[1] Albendazole has been used to treat a patient infected with *Trichinella pseudospiralis*, an organism related to *T.spiralis*, the usual cause of trichinosis.[2]

1. Cabié A, *et al.* Albendazole versus thiabendazole as therapy for trichinosis: a retrospective study. *Clin Infect Dis* 1996; **22:** 1033–5.
2. Andrews JRH, *et al.* Trichinella pseudospiralis in humans: description of a case and its treatment. *Trans R Soc Trop Med Hyg* 1994; **88:** 200–3.

**Trichostrongyliasis.** Albendazole in a single dose of 400 mg has been suggested[1] as an alternative to pyrantel embonate or mebendazole in the treatment of trichostrongyliasis (p.101).

1. Medical Letters on Drugs and Therapeutics. Drugs for parasitic infections (issued April 2002). Available at: http://www.medicalletter.com/freedocs/parasitic.pdf (accessed 02/06/04)

**Trichuriasis.** Albendazole is used in the treatment of trichuriasis (p.101). It is normally given in a single dose and is often used in mixed intestinal nematode infections.[1] However, it has been reported[1-3] that in children with mixed intestinal worm infections single doses of albendazole are ineffective in eliminating *Trichuris trichiura* and multiple doses are required to produce worthwhile reductions in egg production. Treatment for 3 days has been suggested for heavy infection[4] (for a suggestion that such regimens may be associated with impaired growth in less heavily infected children, see Effects on Growth under Adverse Effects, above). Combined use of albendazole with ivermectin may prove useful.[5]

1. Hall A, Anwar KS. Albendazole and infections with Trichuris trichiura and Giardia intestinalis. *Southeast Asian J Trop Med Public Health* 1991; **22:** 84–7.
2. Hall A, Nahar Q. Albendazole and infections with Ascaris lumbricoides and Trichuris trichiura in children in Bangladesh. *Trans R Soc Trop Med Hyg* 1994; **88:** 110–12.
3. Albonico M, *et al.* A randomized controlled trial comparing mebendazole and albendazole against Ascaris, Trichuris and hookworm infections. *Trans R Soc Trop Med Hyg* 1994; **88:** 585–9.
4. Medical Letter on Drugs and Therapeutics. Drugs for parasitic infections (issued April 2002). Available at: http://www.medicalletter.com/freedocs/parasitic.pdf (accessed 02/06/04)
5. Ismail MM, Jayakody RL. Efficacy of albendazole and its combinations with ivermectin or diethylcarbamazine (DEC) in the treatment of Trichuris trichiura infections in Sri Lanka. *Ann Trop Med Parasitol* 1999; **93:** 501–4.

## Preparations

***USP 27:*** Albendazole Tablets.

**Proprietary Preparations** (details are given in Part 3)
***Arg.:*** Vastus; ***Austral.:*** Eskazole; Zentel; ***Austria:*** Eskazole; ***Braz.:*** Alba-3; Alben†; Albendrox; Albendy†; Albentel; Albenzonil; Alib†; Alin; Amplozol†; Bentiamin; Dazol†; Helmintal†; Imavermil; Mebenix; Monozol; Neo Bendazol; Parasin; Totelmin; Vermiclase†; Vermital; Zentel; Zolben†; ***Chile:*** Ceprazol; Zentel; ***Fr.:*** Eskazole†; Zentel; ***Ger.:*** Eskazole; ***Gr.:*** Zentel; ***India:*** Albezole; Emanthal; Nemozole; Zentel; ***Israel:*** Eskazole; ***Ital.:*** Zentel; ***Malaysia:*** Thelban; Vemizol; Zentel; Zoben; ***Mex.:*** Albensil†; Alfazol; Bendapar; Bradelmin; Dabenzol†; Dazocan†; Dazolin; Digezanol; Entoplus; Eskazole; Euralben†; Gascop; Helmisons; Loveral; Lurdex; Tenibex; Veranzol; Vermilan; Vermin-Plus; Vermisen; Zelfin†; Zenaxin; Zentel; ***Neth.:*** Eskazole; ***Port.:*** Zentel; ***S.Afr.:*** Bendex; Paranthil†; Zentel; ***Singapore:*** Alzental; Zentel; ***Spain:*** Eskazole; ***Switz.:*** Zentel; ***Thai.:*** Abentel; Albatel; Alben; Albenda; Alda; Alfuca; Alzol; Anthel; Gendazel; Labenda; Leo-400; Masaworm; Mesin; Mycotel; Vermixide; Zeben; Zentel; Zenzera; ***UAE:*** Albenda; ***UK:*** Eskazole†; ***USA:*** Albenza.

---

## Amocarzine *(rINN)*

Amocarzina; CGP-6140. 4-Methyl-4′-(*p*-nitroanilino)thio-1-piperazinecarboxanilide.

$C_{18}H_{21}N_5O_2S$ = 371.5.
*CAS — 36590-19-9.*

NOTE. Amocarzine has sometimes been referred to as thiocarbamazine.

### Profile

Amocarzine is an antifilarial anthelmintic that is active against the adult worms of *Onchocerca volvulus*. It is under investigation for the oral treatment of onchocerciasis (p.100).

◊ References.

1. Poltera AA, *et al.* Onchocercacidal effects of amocarzine (CGP 6140) in Latin America. *Lancet* 1991; **337:** 583–4.
2. Cooper PJ, *et al.* Onchocerciasis in Ecuador: evolution of chorioretinopathy after amocarzine treatment. *Br J Ophthalmol* 1996; **80:** 337–42.

## Trivalent Antimony Compounds

Compuestos de antimonio trivalente.

### Antimony Potassium Tartrate

Antim. Pot. Tart.; Antimónico potásico, tartrato; Brechweinstein; Kalii Stibyli Tartras; Potassium Antimonyltartrate; Stibii et Kalii Tartras; Tartar Emetic; Tartarus Stibiatus. Dipotassium bis{μ-[2,3-dihydroxybutanedioato(4-)-$O^1$,$O^2$:$O^3$,$O^4$]}-diantimonate(2-) trihydrate; Dipotassium bis[μ-tartrato(4-)]diantimonate(2-) trihydrate.

$C_8H_4K_2O_{12}Sb_2,3H_2O$ = 667.9.

*CAS — 11071-15-1 (anhydrous antimony potassium tartrate); 28300-74-5 (antimony potassium tartrate trihydrate).*

**Pharmacopoeias.** In *US.*

**USP 27** (Antimony Potassium Tartrate). Odourless, colourless, transparent crystals or white powder. The crystals effloresce on exposure to air and do not readily rehydrate even on exposure to high humidity. Soluble 1 in 12 of water, 1 in 3 of boiling water, and 1 in 15 of glycerol; insoluble in alcohol. Its solutions are acid to litmus.

### Antimony Sodium Tartrate

Antim. Sod. Tart.; Antimónico sódico, tartrato; Sodium Antimonyltartrate; Stibium Natrium Tartaricum. Disodium bis{μ-[2,3-dihydroxybutanedioato(4-)-$O^1$,$O^2$:$O^3$,$O^4$]}diantimonate(2-); Disodium bis{μ-[L-(+)-tartrato(4-)]}diantimonate(2-).

$C_8H_4Na_2O_{12}Sb_2$ = 581.6.

*CAS — 34521-09-0.*

**Pharmacopoeias.** In *Int.* (as $C_4H_4NaO_7Sb$ = 308.8) and *US.*

**USP 27** (Antimony Sodium Tartrate). Odourless, colourless, transparent crystals or white powder. The crystals effloresce on exposure to air. Freely soluble in water; insoluble in alcohol.

### Sodium Stibocaptate (BAN, rINN)

Antimony Sodium Dimercaptosuccinate; Estibocaptato de sodio; Ro-4-1544/6; Sb-58; Stibocaptate; TWSb/6. Antimony sodium *meso*-2,3-dimercaptosuccinate. The formula varies from $C_{12}H_{11}NaO_{12}S_6Sb_2$ = 806.1 to $C_{12}H_6Na_6O_{12}S_6Sb_2$ = 916.0.

*CAS — 3064-61-7 ($C_{12}H_6Na_6O_{12}S_6Sb_2$).*

### Stibophen

Estibofeno; Fouadin; Stibophenum. Bis[4,5-dihydroxybenzene-1,3-disulphonato(4–)-$O^4$,$O^5$]antimonate(5–) pentasodium heptahydrate.

$C_{12}H_4Na_5O_{16}S_4Sb,7H_2O$ = 895.2.

*CAS — 15489-16-4 (stibophen heptahydrate).*

*ATC — P02BX03.*

#### Adverse Effects and Treatment

Trivalent antimony compounds are more toxic than pentavalent antimonials such as sodium stibogluconate, possibly because they are excreted much more slowly. The most serious adverse effects are on the heart and liver. There are invariably ECG changes during treatment, but hypotension, bradycardia, and cardiac arrhythmias are more serious. Sudden death or cardiovascular collapse may occur at any time. Elevated liver enzyme values are common; liver damage with hepatic failure and death is more likely in patients with pre-existing hepatic disease.

Adverse effects immediately after intravenous use of trivalent antimonials, in particular the tartrates, have included coughing, chest pain, pain in the arms, vomiting, abdominal pain, fainting, and collapse, especially after rapid injection. Extravasation during injection is extremely painful because of tissue damage. An anaphylactoid reaction characterised by an urticarial rash, husky voice, and collapse has been reported after the sixth or seventh intravenous injection of a course of treatment.

Numerous less immediate adverse effects have occurred including gastrointestinal disturbances, muscular and joint pains, arthritis, pneumonia, dyspnoea, headache, dizziness, weakness, pruritus, skin rashes, facial oedema, fever, haemolytic anaemia, and kidney damage.

Large doses of antimony compounds taken by mouth have an emetic action. Continuous treatment with small doses of antimony may give rise to symptoms of subacute poisoning similar to those of chronic arsenical poisoning.

Treatment of severe poisoning with antimony compounds is similar to that for arsenic poisoning (p.1657); dimercaprol may be of benefit.

◊ References.


1. Stemmer KL. Pharmacology and toxicology of heavy metals: antimony. *Pharmacol Ther* 1976; **1:** 157–60.


#### Precautions

Trivalent antimony therapy has generally been superseded by less toxic treatment. It is contra-indicated in the presence of lung, heart, liver, or kidney disease. Intravenous injections should be given very slowly and stopped if coughing, vomiting, or substernal pain occurs; extravasation should be avoided.

Some antimony compounds such as the tartrates cause severe pain and tissue necrosis and should not be given by intramuscular or subcutaneous injection.

**Breast feeding.** The American Academy of Pediatrics[1] states that there have been no reports of any clinical effect on the infant associated with the use of antimony by breast-feeding mothers, and that therefore it may be considered to be usually compatible with breast feeding.


1. American Academy of Pediatrics. The transfer of drugs and other chemicals into human milk. *Pediatrics* 2001; **108:** 776–89. Correction. *ibid.*; 1029. Also available at: http://aappolicy.aappublications.org/cgi/content/full/pediatrics%3b108/3/776 (accessed 02/06/04)


**Glucose-6-phosphate dehydrogenase deficiency.** In the event of trivalent antimony compounds being used, patients with G6PD deficiency should be excluded. WHO lists stibophen[1] among the anthelmintics to be avoided in patients with this deficiency.


1. WHO. Glucose-6-phosphate dehydrogenase deficiency. *Bull WHO* 1989; **67:** 601–11.


#### Pharmacokinetics

Antimony compounds are poorly absorbed from the gastrointestinal tract. They are slowly excreted, mainly in the urine, after parenteral doses. Antimony accumulates in the body during treatment and persists for several months afterwards. Trivalent antimony has a greater affinity for cell proteins than for plasma proteins.

#### Uses and Administration

Trivalent antimony compounds were used in the treatment of the protozoal infection leishmaniasis until the advent of the less toxic pentavalent compounds. They continued to be used in the treatment of schistosomiasis, but have now been superseded by less toxic and more easily administered drugs such as praziquantel.

Antimony sodium tartrate was formerly used as an emetic. The sodium tartrate and potassium tartrate have also been used as expectorants.

#### Preparations

**Proprietary Preparations** (details are given in Part 3)

**Multi-ingredient:** ***Fr.:*** Montavon†; ***Hong Kong:*** Cocillana Compound; ***Thai.:*** Brown Mixture.

## Ascaridole

Ascaridol. 1-Isopropyl-4-methyl-2,3-dioxabicyclo[2.2.2]oct-5-ene.

$C_{10}H_{16}O_2$ = 168.2.

*CAS — 512-85-6.*

#### Profile

Ascaridole is the active principle of chenopodium oil (p.103) and has the same actions.

**Handling.** Ascaridole is an unstable liquid which is liable to explode when heated or when treated with organic acids.

## Bephenium Hydroxynaphthoate (BAN, rINN)

Hidroxinaftoato de befenio; Naphthammonum. Benzyldimethyl(2-phenoxyethyl)ammonium 3-hydroxy-2-naphthoate.

$C_{28}H_{29}NO_4$ = 443.5.

*CAS — 7181-73-9 (bephenium); 3818-50-6 (bephenium hydroxynaphthoate).*

*ATC — P02CX02.*

**Pharmacopoeias.** In *Int.*

#### Profile

Bephenium hydroxynaphthoate is an anthelmintic formerly used in the treatment of hookworm infections, ascariasis, and trichostrongyliasis.

#### Preparations

**Proprietary Preparations** (details are given in Part 3)

***Braz.:*** Debefenium†.

## Betanaphthol

Betanaftol; β-Naftol; Naphthol. Naphth-2-ol.

$C_{10}H_8O$ = 144.2.

*CAS — 135-19-3.*

**Pharmacopoeias.** In *Pol.* and *Swiss.*

#### Profile

Betanaphthol was formerly used as an anthelmintic in hookworm and tapeworm infections, but it has been superseded by less toxic and more efficient drugs.

Betanaphthol has a potent parasiticidal effect and has been used topically in the treatment of scabies, ringworm, and other skin diseases.

Betanaphthyl benzoate has been used in preparations for the treatment of gastrointestinal disorders.

#### Preparations

**Proprietary Preparations** (details are given in Part 3)

**Multi-ingredient:** ***Arg.:*** Hekabetol; ***Austria:*** Salvyl; ***Spain:*** Salva Infantes†.

## Bithionol (BAN, rINN)

Bitionol. 2,2′-Thiobis(4,6-dichlorophenol).

$C_{12}H_6Cl_4O_2S$ = 356.1.

*CAS — 97-18-7.*

*ATC — D10AB01; P02BX01.*

**Pharmacopoeias.** *Fr.* includes bithionol oxide for veterinary use.

#### Adverse Effects

Adverse effects in patients taking bithionol by mouth include anorexia, nausea, vomiting, abdominal discomfort, diarrhoea, salivation, dizziness, headache, and skin rashes.

Photosensitivity reactions have occurred in persons using soap containing bithionol. Cross-sensitisation with other halogenated disinfectants has also occurred.

#### Uses and Administration

Bithionol is a chlorinated bis-phenol with bactericidal and anthelmintic properties. It is active against most trematodes (flukes). Bithionol is used in preference to praziquantel in fascioliasis (p.99) and is also used in paragonimiasis (p.99) as an alternative to praziquantel. It may be given in a dose of 30 to 50 mg/kg by mouth on alternate days for 10 to 15 doses. Alternatively, for fascioliasis, WHO recommends a regimen of 30 mg/kg daily for 5 days.

Bithionol was formerly used topically as a bactericide but this use has declined because of photosensitivity reactions.

#### Preparations

**Proprietary Preparations** (details are given in Part 3)

**Multi-ingredient:** ***Arg.:*** Fonergine.

## Bromofenofos (rINN)

Bromfenofos; Bromofenofós; Bromophenophos; Bromphenphos. 3,3′,5,5′-Tetrabromo-2,2′-biphenyldiolmono(dihydrogen phosphate).

$C_{12}H_7Br_4O_5P$ = 581.8.

*CAS — 21466-07-9.*

#### Profile

Bromofenofos is an organophosphorus compound (see Organophosphorus Insecticides, p.1507) used as an anthelmintic in veterinary medicine for the treatment of fluke infections.

## Cambendazole (BAN, USAN, rINN)

MK-905. Isopropyl 2-(thiazol-4-yl)-1*H*-benzimidazol-5-ylcarbamate.

$C_{14}H_{14}N_4O_2S$ = 302.4.

*CAS — 26097-80-3.*

#### Profile

Cambendazole is a benzimidazole carbamate anthelmintic structurally related to tiabendazole (p.114). It is used in the treatment of strongyloidiasis.

#### Preparations

**Proprietary Preparations** (details are given in Part 3)

***Braz.:*** Cambem.

**Multi-ingredient:** ***Braz.:*** Exelmin.

## Chenopodium Oil

Aceite de quenopodio; Aetheroleum Chenopodii; Esencia de Quenopodio Vermifuga; Oil of American Wormseed; Wurmsamenöl.

*CAS — 8006-99-3.*

#### Profile

Chenopodium oil is distilled with steam from the fresh flowering and fruiting plants, excluding roots, of *Chenopodium ambrosioides* var. *anthelminticum.* It contains ascaridole. It was formerly used as an anthelmintic for the expulsion of roundworms (*Ascaris*) and hookworms. It is toxic and has caused numerous fatalities.

**Handling.** Chenopodium oil may explode when heated.

## Clorsulon (BAN, USAN, rINN)

Clorsulón; MK-401. 4-Amino-6-(trichlorovinyl)benzene-1,3-disulphonamide.

$C_8H_8Cl_3N_3O_4S_2$ = 380.7.

*CAS — 60200-06-8.*

**Pharmacopoeias.** In *US* for veterinary use only.

**USP 27** (Clorsulon). A white to off-white powder. Slightly soluble in water; freely soluble in acetonitrile and in methyl alcohol; very slightly soluble in dichloromethane.

#### Profile

Clorsulon is an anthelmintic used in veterinary medicine for the treatment of liver fluke infections.

## Closantel (BAN, USAN, rINN)

R-31520. 5′-Chloro-4′-(4-chloro-α-cyanobenzyl)-3,5-di-iodosalicyl-o-toluidide.

$C_{22}H_{14}Cl_2I_2N_2O_2$ = 663.1.

*CAS — 57808-65-8.*

## Closantel Sodium (BANM, rINNM)

R-34828.

$C_{22}H_{14}Cl_2I_2N_2O_2Na$ = 686.1.

**Pharmacopoeias.** In *Eur.* (see p.vi) as the dihydrate for veterinary use.

**Ph.Eur. 5.0** (Closantel Sodium Dihydrate for Veterinary Use). A yellow, slightly hygroscopic, powder. It exhibits polymorphism. Very slightly soluble in water; freely soluble in alcohol; soluble in methyl alcohol. Store in airtight containers. Protect from light.

### Profile

Closantel is an anthelmintic used in veterinary medicine for the treatment of fluke and nematode infections.

**Effects on the eyes.** Loss of eyesight was reported in 11 women who received closantel (Flukiver) in mistake for a gynaecological product.[1] Sight was restored after closantel was stopped but incapacitating eye pain remained.

1. 't Hoen E, *et al.* Harmful human use of donated veterinary drug. *Lancet* 1993; **342:** 308–9.

## Diamfenetide (BAN, rINN)

Diamfenetida; Diamfenetidum; Diamphenethide. β,β′-Oxybis(aceto-*p*-phenetidide).

$C_{20}H_{24}N_2O_5$ = 372.4.

*CAS — 36141-82-9.*

### Profile

Diamfenetide is an anthelmintic that has been used in veterinary medicine for the control of fascioliasis in sheep.

## Dichlorophen (BAN, rINN)

Diclorofeno; Di-phenthane-70; G-4. 2,2′-Methylenebis(4-chlorophenol).

$C_{13}H_{10}Cl_2O_2$ = 269.1.

*CAS — 97-23-4.*

*ATC — P02DX02.*

**Pharmacopoeias.** In *Br.* and *Fr.*

**BP 2003** (Dichlorophen). A white or slightly cream-coloured powder with a not more than slightly phenolic odour. Practically insoluble in water; freely soluble in alcohol; very soluble in ether.

### Profile

Dichlorophen is an anthelmintic that was used in the treatment of infection by tapeworms but has been superseded by praziquantel or niclosamide.

Dichlorophen also has antifungal and antibacterial activity and has been used topically in the treatment of fungal infections and as a germicide in soaps and cosmetics.

### Preparations

***BP 2003:*** Dichlorophen Tablets.

**Proprietary Preparations** (details are given in Part 3)

**Multi-ingredient:** ***S.Afr.:*** Mycota; ***UK:*** Germolene; Mycota.

# Diethylcarbamazine Citrate

(BANM, rINNM)

Citrato de dietilcarbamazina; Diethylcarbam. Cit.; Diethylcarbamazine Acid Citrate; Diethylcarbamazini Citras; Ditrazini Citras; RP-3799. *NN*-Diethyl-4-methylpiperazine-1-carboxamide dihydrogen citrate.

$C_{10}H_{21}N_3O,C_6H_8O_7$ = 391.4.

*CAS — 90-89-1 (diethylcarbamazine); 1642-54-2 (diethylcarbamazine citrate).*

*ATC — P02CB02.*

**Pharmacopoeias.** In *Chin., Eur.* (see p.vi), *Int., Jpn,* and *US.*

**Ph. Eur. 5.0** (Diethylcarbamazine Citrate). A white, crystalline, slightly hygroscopic powder. Very soluble in water; soluble in alcohol; practically insoluble in acetone. Store in airtight containers.

**USP 27** (Diethylcarbamazine Citrate). A white, crystalline, slightly hygroscopic powder, odourless or has a slight odour. Very soluble in water; sparingly soluble in alcohol; practically insoluble in acetone, in chloroform, and in ether. Store in airtight containers.

## Adverse Effects

Adverse effects directly attributable to diethylcarbamazine include nausea and vomiting. Headache, dizziness, and drowsiness may occur.

Hypersensitivity reactions arise from the death of the microfilariae. These can be serious, especially in onchocerciasis where there may also be sight-threatening ocular toxicity; fatalities have been reported. Encephalitis may be exacerbated in patients with loiasis and fatalities have occurred.

◊ Reactions occurring during diethylcarbamazine treatment of **lymphatic filariasis** are basically of 2 types: pharmacological dose-dependent responses and a response of the infected host to the destruction and death of parasites.[1]

- Reactions of the first type include weakness, dizziness, lethargy, anorexia, and nausea. They begin within 1 to 2 hours of taking diethylcarbamazine, and persist for a few hours.
- Reactions of the second type are less likely to occur and are less severe in bancroftian than in brugian filariasis. They may be systemic or local, both with or without fever.

*Systemic reactions* may occur a few hours after the first oral dose of diethylcarbamazine and generally do not last for more than 3 days. They include headache, aches in other parts of the body, joint pain, dizziness, anorexia, malaise, transient haematuria, allergic reactions, vomiting, and sometimes attacks of bronchial asthma in asthmatic patients. Fever and systemic reactions are positively associated with microfilaraemia. Systemic reactions are reduced if diethylcarbamazine is given in spaced doses or in repeated small doses. They eventually cease spontaneously and interruption of treatment is rarely necessary; symptomatic treatment with antipyretics or analgesics may be helpful.

*Local reactions* tend to occur later in the course of treatment and last longer; they also disappear spontaneously and interruption of treatment is not necessary. Local reactions include lymphadenitis, abscess, ulceration, and transient lymphoedema; funiculitis and epididymitis may also occur in bancroftian filariasis.

It has been suggested that the release of interleukin-6 may be implicated in diethylcarbamazine's adverse effects in patients with lymphatic filariasis.[2]

In most patients with **onchocerciasis**, the microfilaricidal activity of diethylcarbamazine leads to a series of events with dermal, ocular, and systemic components, known as the *Mazzotti reaction*, within minutes to hours after its use.[3]

- Clinical manifestations can be severe, dangerous, and debilitating. Systemic reactions include increased itching, rash, headache, aching muscles, joint pain, painful swollen and tender lymph nodes, fever, tachycardia and hypotension, and vertigo. Most patients experience eye discomfort in the first few hours after diethylcarbamazine treatment. Punctate keratitis can develop as can optic neuritis and visual field loss.

WHO no longer recommends the use of diethylcarbamazine in onchocerciasis as safer alternatives exist.

1. WHO. Lymphatic filariasis: the disease and its control: fifth report of the WHO expert committee on filariasis. *WHO Tech Rep Ser 821* 1992.
2. Yazdanbakhsh M, *et al.* Serum interleukin-6 levels and adverse reactions to diethylcarbamazine in lymphatic filariasis. *J Infect Dis* 1992; **166:** 453–4.
3. WHO. WHO expert committee on onchocerciasis: third report. *WHO Tech Rep Ser 752* 1987.

## Precautions

Treatment with diethylcarbamazine should be closely supervised since hypersensitivity reactions are common and may be severe, especially in patients with onchocerciasis or loiasis. Patients with onchocerciasis should be monitored for eye changes. (The use of diethylcarbamazine to treat onchocerciasis is no longer recommended.) In patients with heavy *Loa loa* infection there is a small risk of encephalopathy and diethylcarbamazine should be stopped at the first sign of cerebral involvement.

Infants, pregnant women, the elderly, and the debilitated, especially those with cardiac or renal disease, are normally excluded when diethylcarbamazine is used in mass treatment schedules.

**Pregnancy.** Pregnant women are normally excluded when diethylcarbamazine is used in mass treatment schedules.

*Animal* studies[1] suggest that the uterine hypermotility induced by diethylcarbamazine is mediated via prostaglandin synthesis; this might explain the mechanism of the abortifacient action previously reported.[2]

1. Joseph CA, Dixon PAF. Possible prostaglandin-mediated effect of diethylcarbamazine on rat uterine contractility. *J Pharm Pharmacol* 1984; **36:** 281–2.
2. Subbu VSV, Biswas AR. Ecbolic effect of diethyl carbamazine. *Indian J Med Res* 1971; **59:** 646–7.

**Renal impairment.** For a study on the effects of renal impairment on the pharmacokinetics of diethylcarbamazine, see under Pharmacokinetics, below.

## Pharmacokinetics

Diethylcarbamazine is readily absorbed from the gastrointestinal tract and also through the skin and conjunctiva. It is widely distributed in tissues and is mainly excreted in the urine unchanged and as the *N*-oxide metabolite. Urinary excretion and hence plasma half-life is dependent on urinary pH. Approximately 5% of a dose is eliminated in the faeces.

**Disposition.** A pharmacokinetic study in 6 patients with onchocerciasis[1] indicated that diethylcarbamazine is absorbed quickly and almost completely from the gastrointestinal tract, and is eliminated largely as unchanged drug in urine, with relatively small amounts being excreted as the *N*-oxide metabolite. Following a single radioactively labelled dose of diethylcarbamazine citrate 0.5 mg/kg by mouth as an aqueous solution, peak plasma concentrations of 100 to 150 nanograms/mL were achieved in 1 to 2 hours, followed by a sharp decline, then a marked secondary rise 3 to 6 hours after dosing, followed by a steady decline. The half-life ranged from 9 to 13 hours. Urinary excretion of diethylcarbamazine and diethylcarbamazine *N*-oxide was complete within 96 hours; between 4 and 5% of the dose was recovered in the faeces. Disposition was similar in 5 healthy subjects given a single 50-mg tablet of diethylcarbamazine citrate. Peak plasma concentrations were initially 80 to 200 nanograms/mL, with a secondary rise 3 to 9 hours after dosing, the terminal half-life ranged from 5 to 13 hours, and urinary excretion of unchanged diethylcarbamazine and the *N*-oxide was complete within 48 hours.

When an alkaline urinary pH was maintained, the elimination half-life of diethylcarbamazine and the area under the plasma concentration versus time curve were significantly increased compared with when an acidic urinary pH was maintained.[2]

1. Edwards G, *et al.* Diethylcarbamazine disposition in patients with onchocerciasis. *Clin Pharmacol Ther* 1981; **30:** 551–7.
2. Edwards G, *et al.* The effect of variations in urinary pH on the pharmacokinetics of diethylcarbamazine. *Br J Clin Pharmacol* 1981; **12:** 807–12.

**Renal impairment.** Results in patients with chronic renal impairment and in healthy subjects, given a single 50-mg dose of diethylcarbamazine citrate by mouth, indicated that the plasma half-life of diethylcarbamazine is prolonged and its 24-hour urinary excretion considerably reduced in those with moderate and severe degrees of renal impairment.[1] Mean plasma half-lives in 7 patients with severe renal impairment (creatinine clearance less than 25 mL/minute), in 5 patients with moderate renal impairment (creatinine clearance between 25 and 60 mL/minute), and in 4 healthy subjects, were 15.1, 7.7, and 2.7 hours, respectively. The patient with the longest plasma half-life of 32 hours did not have the poorest renal function, but it was considered likely that the abnormally slow elimination of diethylcarbamazine was due to the high urinary pH (7) resulting from sodium bicarbonate therapy. A further patient with a half-life longer than expected also had a less acidic urine.

1. Adjepon-Yamoah KK, *et al.* The effect of renal disease on the pharmacokinetics of diethylcarbamazine in man. *Br J Clin Pharmacol* 1982; **13:** 829–34.

## Uses and Administration

Diethylcarbamazine is an anthelmintic used in the treatment of lymphatic filariasis due to *Wuchereria bancrofti* (bancroftian filariasis), *Brugia malayi*, or *B. timori* (both known as brugian filariasis and as Malayan and Timorian filariasis respectively). It is also used in loiasis due to *Loa loa*. It was used in onchocerciasis due to *Onchocerca volvulus* before ivermectin became available. Diethylcarbamazine is active against both the microfilariae and adult worms of *W. bancrofti, B. malayi*, and *Loa loa*, but only against the microfilariae of *O. volvulus*. It has been tried in *Mansonella* infections and may be most effective against *M. streptocerca*. Diethylcarbamazine is also used in the treatment of toxocariasis (visceral larva migrans). For discussions of these infections and their treatment, see under Choice of Anthelmintic, p.97, and under the individual headings below.

Diethylcarbamazine is usually given by mouth as the citrate.

In the treatment of filarial infections due to *W. bancrofti, B. malayi, B. timori*, and *Loa loa*, the recommended dose of diethylcarbamazine citrate is 6 mg/kg daily in 3 divided doses for 3 weeks, given in an initial dosage of 1 mg/kg daily, gradually increased to 6 mg/kg daily over 3 days then maintained for 3 weeks, to reduce the incidence and severity of hypersensitivity reactions due to the destruction of microfilariae. However, in bancroftian filariasis, WHO recommends 6 mg/kg daily in divided doses for 12 days and, in brugian filariasis, WHO recommends a dose of 3 to 6 mg/kg daily in divided doses for 6 to 12 days. In the treatment of loiasis, WHO recommends a dose of 1 mg/kg as a single dose initially, doubled on two successive days and then adjusted to 2 to 3 mg/kg three times daily for a further 18 days. A corticosteroid may be given concurrently in the treatment of filarial infections. Similar doses are given for 3 weeks in the treatment of toxocariasis.

In the prophylaxis of loiasis, a dose of 300 mg weekly is recommended by WHO.

In areas where lymphatic filariasis is endemic, mass treatment campaigns can reduce the intensity of transmission and incidence of disease. Diethylcarbamazine may also be used in the form of medicated salt to control lymphatic filariasis. For further details, see below.

**Administration.** Diethylcarbamazine was first used as the chloride, but is now produced as the dihydrogen citrate which contains only half its weight as base. In reporting doses it is therefore important to indicate whether they refer to a specific salt or to the base; unless otherwise stated, it can generally be assumed that the dose refers to the citrate.[1]

1. WHO. Lymphatic filariasis: fourth report of the WHO expert committee on filariasis. *WHO Tech Rep Ser 702* 1984.

**Loiasis.** Diethylcarbamazine is the main drug used in the management of loiasis (p.99).

References.

1. Nutman TB, *et al.* Loa loa infection in temporary residents of endemic regions: recognition of a hyperresponsive syndrome with characteristic clinical manifestations. *J Infect Dis* 1986; **154:** 10–18.
2. Nutman TB, *et al.* Diethylcarbamazine prophylaxis for human loiasis: results of a double-blind study. *N Engl J Med* 1988; **319:** 752–6.
3. Nutman TB, Ottesen EA. Diethylcarbamazine and human loiasis. *N Engl J Med* 1989; **320:** 320.
4. Klion AD, *et al.* Effectiveness of diethylcarbamazine in treating loiasis acquired by expatriate visitors to endemic regions: long-term follow-up. *J Infect Dis* 1994; **169:** 604–10.

**Lymphatic filariasis.** Diethylcarbamazine is used in the management of lymphatic filariasis (p.100). In endemic areas where more than 5% of the population is infected, mass treatment of the entire population (excluding neonates, pregnant women, and debilitated individuals) can reduce the intensity of transmission and the incidence of disease. In countries where there is no co-endemic loiasis or onchocerciasis, a global elimination campaign launched by WHO together with other international agencies advocates a single dose of diethylcarbamazine 6 mg/kg together with a single dose of albendazole 400 mg, given once each year for 4 to 6 years. If diethylcarbamazine-medicated salt is to be employed then intake of salt needs to be on a daily basis for 6 to 12 months.

## Preparations

**USP 27:** Diethylcarbamazine Citrate Tablets.

**Proprietary Preparations** (details are given in Part 3)

***Canad.:*** Hetrazan†; ***Fr.:*** Notezine; ***Gr.:*** Hetrazan; ***India:*** Banocide; Hetrazan; ***Thai.:*** Diethizine; ***UK:*** Hetrazan†.

**Multi-ingredient:** ***India:*** Helmazan; Unicarbazan.

## Disophenol

Disofenol. 2,6-Diiodo-4-nitrophenol.

$C_6H_3I_2NO_3$ = 390.9.

*CAS — 305-85-1.*

### Profile

Disophenol is an anthelmintic used in veterinary medicine.

## Doramectin *(BAN, USAN, rINN)*

Doramectina; UK-67994.

*CAS — 117704-25-3.*

### Profile

Doramectin is an avermectin anthelmintic used in veterinary medicine for nematode infections. It is also used as a systemic veterinary ectoparasiticide.

## Embelia

Vidang.

*CAS — 550-24-3 (embelic acid).*

### Profile

Embelia consists of the dried fruits of *Embelia ribes* and *E. robusta* ( = *E. tsjeriamcottam*) (Myrsinaceae), containing about 2.5% of embelic acid (embelin). It has been used in India and other Asian countries for the expulsion of tapeworms.

## Eprinomectin *(USAN, rINN)*

Eprinomectina; MK-397. A mixture of eprinomectin component $B_{1a}$ and eprinomectin component $B_{1b}$.

*CAS — 159628-36-1 (eprinomectin); 123997-26-2 (eprinomectin); 133305-88-1 (component $B_{1a}$); 133305-89-2 (component $B_{1b}$).*

### Profile

Eprinomectin is an avermectin anthelmintic used in veterinary medicine for nematode infections. It is also used as a systemic veterinary ectoparasiticide.

## Epsiprantel *(BAN, rINN)*

BRL-38705. 2-Cyclohexylcarbonyl-1,2,3,4,6,7,8,12b-octahydropyrazino[2,1-*a*][2]benzazepin-4-one.

$C_{20}H_{26}N_2O_2$ = 326.4.

*CAS — 98123-83-2.*

### Profile

Epsiprantel is an anthelmintic closely related to praziquantel. It is used in veterinary medicine.

## Febantel *(BAN, USAN, rINN)*

Bay-h-5757; Bay-Vh-5757. 2′-[2,3-Bis(methoxycarbonyl)guanidino]-5′-phenylthio-2-methoxyacetanilide; Dimethyl {2-[2-(2-methoxyacetamido)-4-(phenylthio)phenyl]imidocarbonyl}dicarbamate.

$C_{20}H_{22}N_4O_6S$ = 446.5.

*CAS — 58306-30-2.*

### Profile

Febantel is an anthelmintic used in veterinary medicine for the treatment of nematode infections of the gastrointestinal tract and lungs and in tapeworm infections.

## Fenbendazole *(BAN, USAN, rINN)*

Fenbendazol; Hoe-881V. Methyl 5-phenylthio-1*H*-benzimidazol-2-ylcarbamate.

$C_{15}H_{13}N_3O_2S$ = 299.3.

*CAS — 43210-67-9.*

*ATC — P02CA06.*

**Pharmacopoeias.** In *Eur.* (see p.vi) for veterinary use only.

**Ph. Eur. 5.0** (Fenbendazole for Veterinary Use). A white or almost white powder. Practically insoluble in water; sparingly soluble in dimethylformamide; very slightly soluble in methyl alcohol. Protect from light.

### Profile

Fenbendazole is a benzimidazole carbamate anthelmintic structurally related to mebendazole (p.108). It is used in veterinary medicine.

## Flubendazole *(BAN, USAN, rINN)*

Flubendazol; Flubendazolum; Fluoromebendazole; R-17889. Methyl 5-(4-fluorobenzoyl)-1*H*-benzimidazol-2-ylcarbamate.

$C_{16}H_{12}FN_3O_3$ = 313.3.

*CAS — 31430-15-6.*

*ATC — P02CA05.*

**Pharmacopoeias.** In *Eur.* (see p.vi).

**Ph. Eur. 5.0** (Flubendazole). A white or almost white powder. It exhibits polymorphism. Practically insoluble in water, in alcohol, and in dichloromethane. Protect from light.

### Profile

Flubendazole, a benzimidazole carbamate anthelmintic, is an analogue of mebendazole (p.108) and has similar actions and uses.

For the treatment of enterobiasis in adults and children, flubendazole 100 mg is given by mouth as a single dose, repeated after 2 to 3 weeks. For ascariasis, hookworm infections, and trichuriasis 100 mg is given twice daily for 3 days. For discussions of these infections and their treatment, see under Choice of Anthelmintic, p.97.

### Preparations

**Proprietary Preparations** (details are given in Part 3)

***Arg.:*** Flumoxal; ***Fr.:*** Fluvermal; ***Port.:*** Fluvermal; Teniverme; ***Spain:*** Flicum.

## Haloxon *(BAN, rINN)*

Haloxón. Bis(2-chloroethyl) 3-chloro-4-methylcoumarin-7-yl phosphate.

$C_{14}H_{14}Cl_3O_6P$ = 415.6.

*CAS — 321-55-1.*

### Profile

Haloxon is an organophosphorus compound (see Organophosphorus Insecticides, p.1507) used as an anthelmintic in veterinary medicine.

## Hycanthone Mesilate *(rINNM)*

Hycanthone Mesylate; Hydroxylucanthone Methanesulphonate; Mesilato de hicantona; NSC-134434 (hycanthone); Win-24933 (hycanthone). 1-(2-Diethylaminoethylamino)-4-hydroxymethylthioxanthen-9-one methanesulphonate.

$C_{20}H_{24}N_2O_2S,CH_3SO_3H$ = 452.6.

*CAS — 3105-97-3 (hycanthone); 23255-93-8 (hycanthone mesilate).*

NOTE. Hycanthone is *USAN.*

### Profile

Hycanthone has been used as a schistosomicide in the individual or mass treatment of infection with *Schistosoma haematobium* and *S. mansoni.*

Owing to its toxicity and concern about possible carcinogenicity, mutagenicity, and teratogenicity, hycanthone has been replaced by other drugs such as praziquantel.

## Hygromycin B

Higromicina B. *O*-6-Amino-6-deoxy-L-glycero-D-galacto-heptopyranosylidene-(1→2-3)-*O*-β-D-talopyranosyl-(1→5)-2-deoxy-$N^3$-methyl-D-streptamine.

$C_{20}H_{37}N_3O_{13}$ = 527.5.

### Profile

Hygromycin B is an anthelmintic used in veterinary medicine for nematode infections.

## Ivermectin *(BAN, USAN, rINN)*

Ivermectina.

*CAS — 70288-86-7 (ivermectin); 70161-11-4 (component $B_{1a}$); 70209-81-3 (component $B_{1b}$).*

*ATC — P02CF01.*

**Pharmacopoeias.** In *Eur.* (see p.vi) and *US.*

**Ph. Eur. 5.0** (Ivermectin). A mixture of ivermectin component $H_2B_{1a}$ (5-*O*-demethyl-22,23-dihydroavermectin $A_{1a}$; $C_{48}H_{74}O_{14}$ = 875.1) and ivermectin component $H_2B_{1b}$ (5-*O*-demethyl-25-de(1-methylpropyl)-25-(1-methylethyl)-22,23-dihydroavermectin $A_{1a}$; $C_{47}H_{72}O_{14}$ = 861.1).

A white or yellowish-white, slightly hygroscopic, crystalline powder. Practically insoluble in water; soluble in alcohol; freely soluble in dichloromethane. Store in airtight containers.

**USP 27** (Ivermectin). A mixture of component $H_2B_{1a}$ (5-*O*-demethyl-22,23-dihydro-avermectin $A_{1a}$; $C_{48}H_{74}O_{14}$ = 875.1) and component $H_2B_{1b}$ (5-*O*-demethyl-25-de(1-methylpropyl)-22,23-dihydro-25-(1-methylethyl)-avermectin $A_{1a}$; $C_{47}H_{72}O_{14}$ = 861.1). It contains not less than 90% of component $H_2B_{1a}$, calculated on the anhydrous and alcohol- and formamide-free basis. It may contain small amounts of suitable antoxidant and chelating agents.

A white to yellowish-white, slightly hygroscopic, crystalline powder. Practically insoluble in water and in petroleum spirit; soluble in acetone and in acetonitrile; freely soluble in dichloromethane and in methyl alcohol.

### Adverse Effects and Precautions

The adverse effects reported with ivermectin are generally consistent with a mild Mazzotti reaction arising from its effect on the microfilariae. They include fever, pruritus, skin rashes, arthralgia, myalgia, asthenia, postural hypotension, tachycardia, oedema, lymphadenopathy, gastrointestinal symptoms, sore throat, cough, and headache. The effects tend to be transient and if treatment is required they respond to analgesics and antihistamines.

Ivermectin may cause mild ocular irritation. Somnolence, transient eosinophilia, and raised liver enzyme values have also been reported.

Ivermectin is not recommended during pregnancy. Mass treatment is generally withheld from pregnant women (see Pregnancy, below), children under 15 kg, and the seriously ill.

**Incidence of adverse effects.** Some studies have shown quite a high incidence of adverse effects with ivermectin and have associated the effects with the severity of infection.[1-3] However, in none of these studies were the reactions considered to be life-threatening and only symptomatic treatment was required. The severity, incidence, and duration of adverse reactions was reported to be reduced after repeated annual administration.[4] When larger groups of patients were considered in the Onchocerciasis Control Programme (OCP) in West Africa, a much lower incidence of adverse reactions was observed in patients given ivermectin for the first time[5] and when treatment was repeated a year later that incidence was reduced even further. The results from several trials in this programme[6] showed 93 severe reactions in 50 929 patients (1.83%), most of the reactions being postural hypotension or dizziness (53). A more recent study[7] found 22 severe reactions in 17 877 patients treated for onchocerciasis in an area also endemic for *Loa loa* infection, and demonstrated a relationship to heavy *L. loa* microfilaraemia. It was suggested that ivermectin should be used with caution for mass onchocerciasis treatment programmes in areas where loiasis and onchocerciasis co-exist.

Some supervision is considered necessary after administration of ivermectin;[2,6] the OCP recommendation[6] is for resident nurses to monitor patients for a period of 36 hours after treatment, whatever the level of endemicity. However, the incidence of adverse reactions reported after repeated doses appears to be lower than after the first dose and the need for supervision on re-treatment has been questioned.[8]

Neurotoxicity observed in some breeds of *dogs* has not been seen in *cattle* or *horses*[9] and nor was it reported in man in the above studies. Another potential concern was the prolongation of prothrombin times observed in 28 patients given ivermectin,[10] but others have not confirmed this effect[11] or observed any bleeding disorders.[12]

There has been some concern over the use of ivermectin to treat scabies in elderly patients following a report suggesting a possible link to an increased incidence of death among a cohort of 47 patients.[13] It has, however, been argued that no such association has been seen in other populations of elderly patients and that the statistical methods used by the original authors were deficient.[14-16] There was no evidence of an increase in death rate associated with ivermectin in a community-based trial in Papua New Guinea of diethylcarbamazine with or without ivermectin for lymphatic filariasis.[17]


1. Kumaraswami V, *et al.* Ivermectin for the treatment of Wuchereria bancrofti filariasis: efficacy and adverse reactions. *JAMA* 1988; **259:** 3150–3.
2. Rothova A, *et al.* Side-effects of ivermectin in treatment of onchocerciasis. *Lancet* 1989; **i:** 1439–41.
3. Zea-Flores R, *et al.* Adverse reactions after community treatment of onchocerciasis with ivermectin in Guatemala. *Trans R Soc Trop Med Hyg* 1992; **86:** 663–6.
4. Burnham GM. Adverse reactions to ivermectin treatment for onchocerciasis: results of a placebo-controlled, double-blind trial in Malawi. *Trans R Soc Trop Med Hyg* 1993; **87:** 313–17.
5. De Sole G, *et al.* Lack of adverse reactions in ivermectin treatment of onchocerciasis. *Lancet* 1990; **335:** 1106–7.
6. De Sole G, *et al.* Adverse reactions after large-scale treatment of onchocerciasis with ivermectin: combined results from eight community trials. *Bull WHO* 1989; **67:** 707–19.
7. Gardon J, *et al.* Serious reactions after mass treatment of onchocerciasis with ivermectin in an area endemic for Loa loa infection. *Lancet* 1997; **350:** 18–22.
8. Whitworth JAG, *et al.* A community trial of ivermectin for onchocerciasis in Sierra Leone: adverse reactions after the first five treatment rounds. *Trans R Soc Trop Med Hyg* 1991; **85:** 501–5.
9. WHO. WHO expert committee on onchocerciasis: third report. *WHO Tech Rep Ser 752* 1987.
10. Homeida MMA, *et al.* Prolongation of prothrombin time with ivermectin. *Lancet* 1988; **i:** 1346–7.
11. Richards FO, *et al.* Ivermectin and prothrombin time. *Lancet* 1989; **i;** 1139–40.
12. Pacque MC, *et al.* Ivermectin and prothrombin time. *Lancet* 1989; **i:** 1140.
13. Barkwell R, Shields S. Deaths associated with ivermectin treatment of scabies. *Lancet* 1997; **349:** 1144–5.
14. Diazgranados JA, Costa JL. Deaths after ivermectin treatment. *Lancet* 1997; **349:** 1698.
15. Reintjes R, Hoek C. Deaths associated with ivermectin for scabies. *Lancet* 1997; **350:** 215.
16. Coyne PE, Addiss DG. Deaths associated with ivermectin for scabies. *Lancet* 1997; **350:** 215–16.
17. Alexander NDE, *et al.* Absence of ivermectin-associated excess deaths. *Trans R Soc Trop Med Hyg* 1998; **92:** 342.


**Breast feeding.** Mean ivermectin concentrations in the breast milk of 4 healthy lactating women who had been given a standard dose of ivermectin were 14.13 nanograms/mL.[1] It was felt that in view of this low concentration the precaution of excluding lactating mothers from ivermectin mass treatment programmes should be reconsidered. Some authorities have recommended that ivermectin should not be given to mothers who are breast feeding until the infant is at least one week old. The American Academy of Pediatrics states that, since no adverse effects have been observed in breast-fed infants whose mothers were receiving ivermectin, it may be considered to be usually compatible with breast feeding.[2]


1. Ogbuokiri JE, *et al.* Ivermectin levels in human breast milk. *Eur J Clin Pharmacol* 1994; **46:** 89–90.
2. American Academy of Pediatrics. The transfer of drugs and other chemicals into human milk. *Pediatrics* 2001; **108:** 776–89. Correction. *ibid.*; 1029. Also available at: http://aappolicy.aappublications.org/cgi/content/full/pediatrics%3b108/3/776 (accessed 02/06/04)


**Pregnancy.** Ivermectin is teratogenic in *animals* and the manufacturers note that there are no adequate and well controlled studies in human pregnancy. Ivermectin treatment is therefore usually contra-indicated during pregnancy and pregnant women should be excluded from mass treatment schedules with ivermectin. However, women not yet diagnosed as pregnant or unwilling to admit their pregnancy have been treated. An assessment[1] of 203 pregnancy outcomes to women who had received ivermectin during pregnancy, mostly during the first 12 weeks, found that the rates of major congenital malformation, miscarriage, and still-birth associated with ivermectin were similar to those in untreated mothers. In another study, 110 women also inadvertently given ivermectin during pregnancy experienced a similar lack of adverse effect on pregnancy outcome;[2] it was considered that the precaution of avoiding the use of ivermectin in women notifying a pregnancy should be adequate.


1. Pacqué M, *et al.* Pregnancy outcome after inadvertent ivermectin treatment during community-based distribution. *Lancet* 1990; **336:** 1486–9.
2. Chippaux J-P, *et al.* Absence of any adverse effect of inadvertent ivermectin treatment during pregnancy. *Trans R Soc Trop Med Hyg* 1993; **87:** 318.


## Pharmacokinetics

Ivermectin is absorbed following oral administration with peak plasma concentrations being obtained after about 4 hours. Ivermectin is reported to be about 93% bound to plasma proteins and has a plasma elimination half-life of about 12 hours. It undergoes metabolism and is excreted largely as metabolites over a period of about 2 weeks, chiefly in the faeces, with less than 1% appearing in the urine and less than 2% in breast milk (see also Breast Feeding, above).

## Uses and Administration

Ivermectin is a semisynthetic derivative of one of the avermectins, a group of macrocyclic lactones produced by *Streptomyces avermitilis*.

It has a microfilaricidal action in onchocerciasis and reduces the microfilarial load without the toxicity seen with diethylcarbamazine. Ivermectin also has a microfilaricidal action in lymphatic filariasis and is used in its management. Ivermectin is active in some other worm infections. It is used in the treatment of strongyloidiasis and has been tried in some *Mansonella* infections. For details of these infections and their treatment, see under Choice of Anthelmintic, p.97, and under the individual headings below.

In the treatment of onchocerciasis, a single dose of 3 to 12 mg of ivermectin, based roughly on 150 micrograms/kg by mouth for patients weighing more than 15 kg and over 5 years of age, is given annually or every 6 months. This schedule has been adopted for mass treatment in infected areas. No food should be taken for 2 hours before or after the dose.

Ivermectin 200 micrograms/kg as a single dose, or daily on two consecutive days, is used for the treatment of strongyloidiasis.

◊ Reviews.


1. Ottesen EA, Campbell WC. Ivermectin in human medicine. *J Antimicrob Chemother* 1994; **34:** 195–203.


**Cutaneous larva migrans.** There are some reports[1,2] of ivermectin being effective in the treatment of cutaneous larva migrans (p.98).


1. Caumes E, *et al.* Efficacy of ivermectin in the therapy of cutaneous larva migrans. *Arch Dermatol* 1992; **128:** 994–5.
2. Caumes E, *et al.* A randomized trial of ivermectin versus albendazole for the treatment of cutaneous larva migrans. *Am J Trop Med Hyg* 1993; **49:** 641–4.


**Intestinal nematode infections.** Ivermectin activity has been observed in man against *Ascaris lumbricoides*, *Strongyloides stercoralis*, and *Trichuris trichiura*;[1] although some have failed to detect activity against *Trichuris*,[2] ivermectin given with albendazole has been studied for the treatment of trichuriasis (p.101) and may prove useful. Roundworm expulsion has been reported as a 'side-effect' of ivermectin when used in community-based treatment of onchocerciasis.[3] In a controlled study,[4] single doses of ivermectin 150 or 200 micrograms/kg produced cure rates of 94% in strongyloidiasis (see below) and above 67% in ascariasis, trichuriasis, and enterobiasis. Although some activity has been observed against *Necator americanus*,[1] cure rates for hookworm were considered unsatisfactory.[4]


1. Freedman DO, *et al.* The efficacy of ivermectin in the chemotherapy of gastrointestinal helminthiasis in humans. *J Infect Dis* 1989; **159:** 1151–3.
2. Whitworth JAG, *et al.* A field study of the effect of ivermectin on intestinal helminths in man. *Trans R Soc Trop Med Hyg* 1991; **85:** 232–4.
3. Whitworth JAG, *et al.* Community-based treatment with ivermectin. *Lancet* 1988; **ii:** 97–8.
4. Naquira C, *et al.* Ivermectin for human strongyloidiasis and other intestinal helminths. *Am J Trop Med Hyg* 1989; **40:** 304–9.


**Loiasis.** There is evidence of reduced microfilaraemia following ivermectin treatment[1-5] in patients with loiasis (p.99), but concern over its potential for neurotoxicity in patients with a high microfilarial burden.[6,7]


1. Martin-Prevel Y, *et al.* Reduction of microfilaraemia with single high-dose of ivermectin in loiasis. *Lancet* 1993; 342: 442.
2. Ranque S, *et al.* Decreased prevalence and intensity of Loa loa infection in a community treated with ivermectin every three months for two years. *Trans R Soc Trop Med Hyg* 1996; **90:** 429–30.
3. Duong TH, *et al.* Reduced Loa loa microfilaria count ten to twelve months after a single dose of ivermectin. *Trans R Soc Trop Med Hyg* 1997; **91:** 592–3.
4. Gardon J, *et al.* Marked decrease in Loa loa microfilaraemia six and twelve months after a single dose of ivermectin. *Trans R Soc Trop Med Hyg* 1997; **91:** 593–4.
5. Chippaux J-P, *et al.* Impact of repeated large scale ivermectin treatments on the transmission of Loa loa. *Trans R Soc Trop Med Hyg* 1998; **92:** 454–8.
6. Anonymous. Encephalitis following treatment of loiasis. *WHO Drug Inf* 1991; **5:** 113–14.
7. Gardon J, *et al.* Serious reactions after mass treatment of onchocerciasis with ivermectin in an area endemic for Loa loa infection. *Lancet* 1997; **350:** 18–22.


**Lymphatic filariasis.** Ivermectin is used in the management of lymphatic filariasis (p.100). In endemic areas where more than 5% of the population is infected, mass treatment of the entire population (excluding neonates, pregnant women, and debilitated individuals) can reduce the intensity of transmission and the incidence of disease. For bancroftian filariasis in countries where there is co-endemic loiasis or onchocerciasis, a global elimination campaign launched by WHO, together with other international agencies, advocates a single dose of ivermectin 200 micrograms/kg together with a single dose of albendazole 400 mg given once each year for 4 to 6 years.

**Mansonella infections.** The response of *Mansonella* infections (p.100) to ivermectin depends on the species. It may be effective against *Mansonella ozzardi*, but studies in *M. perstans* infection have not shown ivermectin to produce a substantial reduction in microfilaraemia.[1,2] A good response to ivermectin has been reported in infections with *M. streptocerca*.[3,4]


1. Van den Enden E, *et al.* Treatment failure of a single high dose of ivermectin for Mansonella perstans filariasis. *Trans R Soc Trop Med Hyg* 1993; **87:** 90.
2. Schulz-Key H, *et al.* Efficacy of ivermectin in the treatment of concomitant Mansonella perstans infections in onchocerciasis patients. *Trans R Soc Trop Med Hyg* 1993; **87:** 227–9.
3. Fischer P, *et al.* Treatment of human Mansonella streptocerca infection with ivermectin. *Trop Med Int Health* 1997; **2:** 191–9.
4. Fischer P, *et al.* Long-term suppression of Mansonella streptocerca microfilariae after treatment with ivermectin. *J Infect Dis* 1999; **180:** 1403–5.


**Onchocerciasis.** Ivermectin has a microfilaricidal action against *Onchocerca volvulus* and is the main drug used in the control of onchocerciasis (p.100). A single dose rapidly eliminates microfilariae from the skin and gradually eliminates them from the cornea and anterior chamber of the eye.[1] Ivermectin does not eliminate the adult worms but does suppress the release of microfilariae from the adult worm for several cycles which accounts for its prolonged activity. Its action against *O. volvulus* has been attributed to a GABA-agonist effect. Studies have also indicated that ivermectin inhibits the transmission of microfilariae by reducing their uptake from man by the insect vector.[2-5]

Ivermectin is donated by *Merck* through the Mectizan Expert Committee (MEC) for human use in community-wide mass treatment programmes in all countries in which onchocerciasis is endemic, where it is given once or twice a year to all but pregnant women, breast-feeding mothers of recently born babies, children weighing less than 15 kg, and those unable to walk or otherwise seriously ill.[6] Several studies have confirmed the long-term safety and efficacy of such programmes.[7-11]

The ocular microfilarial load can be safely reduced by ivermectin[1,12] and early lesions of the anterior segment of the eye have improved.[12] A reduction in the incidence[13] and progression[14] of optic nerve damage has also been reported, but the effect on posterior segment disease is less certain.[15] Improvements in skin lesions have been reported.[16] Giving it every 6 months produces a more rapid reduction of microfilariae than dosage once a year,[17] but it is difficult to tell whether any long-term advantages outweigh the disadvantages of more frequent doses. In non-endemic areas, repeated doses may be necessary to reduce recurrence; a study in the UK found that patients given three doses at monthly intervals had fewer relapses at 6 months than patients who received a single dose, but relapses were nevertheless seen in 50% of patients at 12 months.[18] Others have suggested that treatment may need to be repeated every 4 to 6 months.[19]


1. Newland HS, *et al.* Effect of single-dose ivermectin therapy on human Onchocerca volvulus infection with onchocercal ocular involvement. *Br J Ophthalmol* 1988; **72:** 561–9.
2. Taylor HR, *et al.* Impact of mass treatment of onchocerciasis with ivermectin on the transmission of infection. *Science* 1990; **250:** 116–18.
3. Trpis M, *et al.* Effect of mass treatment of a human population with ivermectin on transmission of Onchocerca volvulus by Simulium yahense in Liberia, West Africa. *Am J Trop Med Hyg* 1990; **42:** 148–56.
4. Chavasse DC, *et al.* Low level ivermectin coverage and the transmission of onchocerciasis. *Trans R Soc Trop Med Hyg* 1995; **89:** 534–7.
5. Boussinesq M, *et al.* Onchocerca volvulus: striking decrease in transmission in the Vina valley (Cameroon) after eight annual large scale ivermectin treatments. *Trans R Soc Trop Med Hyg* 1997; **91:** 82–6.
6. Pond B. Distribution of ivermectin by health workers. *Lancet* 1990; **335:** 1539.
7. De Sole G, *et al.* Adverse reactions after large-scale treatment of onchocerciasis with ivermectin: combined results from eight community trials. *Bull WHO* 1989; **67:** 707–19.
8. Pacqué M, *et al.* Safety of and compliance with community-based ivermectin therapy. *Lancet* 1990; **335:** 1377–80.
9. Pacqué M, *et al.* Community-based treatment of onchocerciasis with ivermectin: safety, efficacy, and acceptability of yearly treatment. *J Infect Dis* 1991; **163:** 381–5.
10. Steel C, *et al.* Immunologic responses to repeated ivermectin treatment in patients with onchocerciasis. *J Infect Dis* 1991; **164:** 581–7.

11. Whitworth JAG, *et al.* A community trial of ivermectin for onchocerciasis in Sierra Leone: clinical and parasitological responses to four doses given at six-monthly interval. *Trans R Soc Trop Med Hyg* 1992; **86:** 277–80.
12. Dadzie KY, *et al.* Changes in ocular onchocerciasis after two rounds of community-based ivermectin treatment in a holo-endemic onchocerciasis focus. *Trans R Soc Trop Med Hyg* 1991; **85:** 267–71.
13. Abiose A, *et al.* Reduction in incidence of optic nerve disease with annual ivermectin to control onchocerciasis. *Lancet* 1993; **341:** 130–4.
14. Cousens SN, *et al.* Impact of annual dosing with ivermectin on progression of onchocercal visual field loss. *Bull WHO* 1997; **75:** 229–36.
15. Whitworth JAG, *et al.* Effects of repeated doses of ivermectin on ocular onchocerciasis: community-based trial in Sierra Lione. *Lancet* 1991; **338:** 1100–1103.
16. Pacqué M, *et al.* Improvements in severe onchocercal skin disease after a single dose of ivermectin. *Am J Med* 1991; **90:** 590–4.
17. Greene BM, *et al.* A comparison of 6-, 12-, and 24-monthly dosing with ivermectin for treatment of onchocerciasis. *J Infect Dis* 1991; **163:** 376–80.
18. Churchill DR, *et al.* A trial of a three-dose regimen of ivermectin for the treatment of patients with onchocerciasis in the UK. *Trans R Soc Trop Med Hyg* 1994; **88:** 242.
19. Greene BM. Modern medicine versus an ancient scourge: progress toward control of onchocerciasis. *J Infect Dis* 1992; **166:** 15–21.

**Scabies and pediculosis.** Scabies (p.1499) is usually treated with a topically applied acaricide. However, a single oral dose of ivermectin has been reported to be effective.[1,2] In a study of 11 patients with uncomplicated scabies, a single oral dose of ivermectin 200 micrograms/kg was effective in curing infection after 4 weeks. In a group of 11 patients, also infected with HIV, scabies was cured in 8 after 2 weeks.[1] Two of the remaining 3 patients received a second dose of ivermectin which cured the scabies infection by the fourth week. A single oral dose of ivermectin 150 micrograms/kg was partially effective in an outbreak of scabies in 1153 Tanzanian patients.[3] Crusted (Norwegian) scabies has also been reported to be effectively treated by a single oral dose of 12 mg of ivermectin in addition to topical application of 3% salicylic acid ointment in 2 patients; the treatment was effective in under one week.[2] A single oral dose of ivermectin 200 micrograms/kg was effective for crusted scabies in a 2-year-old infant who had contracted the disease following long-term corticosteroid use.[4]

Ivermectin has also been investigated as a possible treatment for pediculosis (p.1499) although, again, topically applied insecticides are the usual method of control. A study *in vitro* and in *animals* showed that ivermectin killed nymphs and females of the human body louse (*Pediculus humanus humanus*). Ivermectin was known to be effective against other louse species that infect a range of *animals*.[5]

1. Meinking TL, *et al.* The treatment of scabies with ivermectin. *N Engl J Med* 1995; **333:** 26–30.
2. Aubin F, Humbert P. Ivermectin for crusted (Norwegian) scabies. *N Engl J Med* 1995; **332:** 612.
3. Leppard B, Naburi AE. The use of ivermectin in controlling an outbreak of scabies in a prison. *Br J Dermatol* 2000; **143:** 520–3.
4. Marlière V, *et al.* Crusted (Norwegian) scabies induced by use of topical corticosteroids and treated successfully with ivermectin. *J Pediatr* 1999; **135:** 122–4.
5. Mumcuoglu KY, *et al.* Systemic activity of ivermectin on the human body louse (Anoplura: Pediculidae). *J Med Entomol* 1990; **27:** 72–5.

**Strongyloidiasis.** Ivermectin is effective in the treatment of strongyloidiasis (p.100) and is considered by some authorities to be the drug of choice.

References.

1. Naquira C, *et al.* Ivermectin for human strongyloidiasis and other intestinal helminths. *Am J Trop Med Hyg* 1989; **40:** 304–9.
2. Wijesundera M de S, Sanmuganathan PS. Ivermectin therapy in chronic strongyloidiasis. *Trans R Soc Trop Med Hyg* 1992; **86:** 291.
3. Lyagoubi M, *et al.* Chronic persistent strongyloidiasis cured by ivermectin. *Trans R Soc Trop Med Hyg* 1992; **86:** 541.
4. Datry A, *et al.* Treatment of Strongyloides stercoralis infection with ivermectin compared with albendazole: results of an open study of 60 cases. *Trans R Soc Trop Med Hyg* 1994; **88:** 344–5.
5. Gann PH, *et al.* A randomized trial of single- and two-dose ivermectin versus thiabendazole for treatment of strongyloidiasis. *J Infect Dis* 1994; **169:** 1076–9.
6. Marti H, *et al.* A comparative trial of a single-dose ivermectin versus three days of albendazole for treatment of Strongyloides stercoralis and other soil-transmitted helminth infections in children. *Am J Trop Med Hyg* 1996; **55:** 477–81.

## Preparations

**Proprietary Preparations** (details are given in Part 3)
***Arg.:*** Securo; ***Austral.:*** Stromectol; ***Braz.:*** Revectina; ***Fr.:*** Mectizan; Stromectol; ***USA:*** Mectizan; Stromectol.

# Levamisole *(BAN, rINN)*

(S)-2,3,5,6-Tetrahydro-6-phenylimidazo[2,1-*b*][1,3]thiazole.
$C_{11}H_{12}N_2S$ = 204.3.
*CAS — 14769-73-4.*
*ATC — P02CE01.*

**Pharmacopoeias.** In *Eur.* (see p.vi) for veterinary use only.

**Ph. Eur. 5.0** (Levamisole for Veterinary Use). A white or almost white powder. It exhibits polymorphism. Slightly soluble in water; freely soluble in alcohol and in methyl alcohol. Store in airtight containers. Protect from light.

## Levamisole Hydrochloride *(BANM, USAN, rINNM)*

Cloridrato de Levamizol; Hidrocloruro de levamisol; ICI-59623; Levamisoli Hydrochloridum; NSC-177023; R-12564; RP-20605; *l*-Tetramisole Hydrochloride; *l*-Tetramisole Hydrochloride.
$C_{11}H_{12}N_2S,HCl$ = 240.8.
*CAS — 16595-80-5.*
*ATC — P02CE01.*

**Pharmacopoeias.** In *Chin., Eur.* (see p.vi), *Int., Pol., US,* and *Viet.*

**Ph. Eur. 5.0** (Levamisole Hydrochloride). A white to almost white crystalline powder. Freely soluble in water; soluble in alcohol; slightly soluble in dichloromethane. A 5% solution in water has a pH of 3.0 to 4.5. Protect from light.

**USP 27** (Levamisole Hydrochloride). A white or almost white crystalline powder. Freely soluble in water; soluble in alcohol; slightly soluble in dichloromethane; practically insoluble in ether. pH of a 5% solution in water is between 3.0 and 4.5. Protect from light.

## Adverse Effects

When given in single doses for the treatment of ascariasis or other worm infections, levamisole is generally well tolerated and side-effects are usually limited to nausea, vomiting, diarrhoea, abdominal pain, dizziness, and headache.

When levamisole is used as an immunostimulant and given for longer periods, adverse effects are more frequent and diverse and, in common with other immunomodulators, may sometimes result from exacerbation of the primary underlying disease. Adverse effects associated especially with the more prolonged use of levamisole have included: hypersensitivity reactions such as fever, a flu-like syndrome, arthralgia, muscle pain, skin rashes, and cutaneous vasculitis; CNS effects including headache, insomnia, dizziness, and convulsions; haematological abnormalities such as agranulocytosis, leucopenia, and thrombocytopenia; and gastrointestinal disturbances, including an abnormal taste in the mouth.

**Incidence of adverse effects.** In a review[1] (by the manufacturers) of 46 controlled studies in which 2635 cancer patients received adjuvant levamisole treatment, most patients received levamisole on 3 consecutive days every 2 weeks (1102 patients) or on 2 consecutive days every week (1156 patients), usually in a daily dose of 150 mg. Levamisole caused several side-effects, such as skin rash, nausea, vomiting, and a metallic or bitter taste in the mouth, which although troublesome were relatively trivial and often regressed during therapy or disappeared on cessation of therapy. A total of 38 patients developed agranulocytosis and of these 36 had received weekly treatment. Several contracted possible life-threatening infections and 2 died of septic shock.

1. Amery WK, Butterworth BS. Review/commentary: the dosage regimen of levamisole in cancer: is it related to efficacy and safety? *Int J Immunopharmacol* 1983; **5:** 1–9.

**Effects on the endocrine system.** Rechallenge confirmed that levamisole was responsible for inappropriate antidiuretic hormone syndrome in a patient receiving levamisole with fluorouracil.[1]

1. Tweedy CR, *et al.* Levamisole-induced syndrome of inappropriate antidiuretic hormone. *N Engl J Med* 1992; **326:** 1164.

**Effects on the liver.** Elevated aspartate aminotransferase concentrations in 2 of 11 patients given levamisole for recurrent pyoderma suggested liver toxicity, a very rarely occurring side-effect.[1] More recently, liver enzyme concentrations were reported to be raised in a 14-year-old boy treated with levamisole for minimal change nephrotic syndrome.[2]

1. Papageorgiou P, *et al.* Levamisole in chronic pyoderma. *J Clin Lab Immunol* 1982; **8:** 121–7.
2. Bulugahapitiya DTD. Liver toxicity in a nephrotic patient treated with levamisole. *Arch Dis Child* 1997; **76:** 289.

**Effects on the nervous system.** Reports[1,2] of inflammatory leukoencephalopathy were associated with the use of fluorouracil and levamisole in 4 patients being treated for adenocarcinoma of the colon. Active demyelination was demonstrated in 2 patients.[1] Clinical improvement occurred when chemotherapy was stopped; 3 patients were treated with corticosteroids.[1] A similar syndrome has been reported in a patient with a history of hepatitis C who received levamisole alone.[3]

1. Hook CC, *et al.* Multifocal inflammatory leukoencephalopathy with 5-fluorouracil and levamisole. *Ann Neurol* 1992; **31:** 262–7.
2. Kimmel DW, Schutt AJ. Multifocal leukoencephalopathy: occurrence during 5-fluorouracil and levamisole therapy and resolution after discontinuation of chemotherapy. *Mayo Clin Proc* 1993; **68:** 363–5.
3. Lucia P, *et al.* Multifocal leucoencephalopathy induced by levamisole. *Lancet* 1996; **348:** 1450.

## Precautions

The use of levamisole should be avoided in patients with pre-existing blood disorders. Patients receiving levamisole with fluorouracil should undergo appropriate monitoring of haematological and hepatic function.

**Rheumatoid arthritis.** The presence of HLA B27 in seropositive rheumatoid arthritis is an important predisposing factor to the development of agranulocytosis with levamisole; it is recommended that the use of levamisole in this group should be avoided.[1]

1. Mielants H, Veys EM. A study of the hematological side effects of levamisole in rheumatoid arthritis with recommendations. *J Rheumatol* 1978; **5** (suppl 4): 77–83.

**Sjögren's syndrome.** The appearance of side-effects in 9 of 10 patients with rheumatoid arthritis and Sjögren's syndrome while being treated with levamisole led to abandonment of the study.[1] Levamisole should be given with caution, if at all, to patients with Sjögren's syndrome.

1. Balint G, *et al.* Sjögren's syndrome: a contraindication to levamisole treatment? *BMJ* 1977; **2:** 1386–7.

## Interactions

**Alcohol.** The US manufacturer reports that levamisole can produce a disulfiram-like reaction with *alcohol.*

**Anticoagulants.** For an increase in the activity of *warfarin* when given with levamisole and fluorouracil, see Interactions, Levamisole, under Warfarin, p.1027.

**Antiepileptics.** For increased *phenytoin* concentrations when given with levamisole and fluorouracil, see Interactions, Antineoplastics, under Phenytoin, p.373.

## Pharmacokinetics

Levamisole is rapidly absorbed from the gastrointestinal tract. Maximum plasma concentrations are attained within 1.5 to 2 hours. It is extensively metabolised in the liver. The plasma half-life for levamisole is 3 to 4 hours and for the metabolites is 16 hours. It is excreted mainly in the urine as metabolites and a small proportion in the faeces. About 70% of a dose is excreted in the urine over 3 days, with about 5% as unchanged levamisole.

◊ References.

1. Luyckx M, *et al.* Pharmacokinetics of levamisole in healthy subjects and cancer patients. *Eur J Drug Metab Pharmacokinet* 1982; **7:** 247–54.
2. Kouassi E, *et al.* Novel assay and pharmacokinetics of levamisole and p-hydroxylevamisole in human plasma and urine. *Biopharm Drug Dispos* 1986; **7:** 71–89.

## Uses and Administration

Levamisole hydrochloride is the active laevo-isomer of tetramisole hydrochloride. It is used as an anthelmintic and as an adjuvant in malignant disease. It has also been tried in several conditions where its stimulant effect on the depressed immune response might be useful.

Levamisole is active against intestinal nematode worms and appears to act by paralysing susceptible worms which are subsequently eliminated from the intestines. In particular, levamisole is effective in the treatment of ascariasis (p.97). It is also used in hookworm infections (p.99).

Doses of levamisole hydrochloride are expressed in terms of the equivalent amount of levamisole. Levamisole hydrochloride 1.18 g is approximately equivalent to 1 g of levamisole. The usual adult dose in ascariasis is 150 mg of levamisole by mouth as a single dose; children have been given 3 mg/kg as a single dose. For the hookworm infection ancylostomiasis or for mixed ascariasis-hookworm infections, both adults and children may be given 2.5 mg/kg as a single dose, repeated after 7 days in cases of severe hookworm infection. Levamisole influences host defences by modulating cell-mediated immune responses; it restores depressed T-cell functions and has been described as an immunostimulant, although stimulation above normal levels does not seem to occur. It has been tried in many disorders, including bacterial and viral infections and rheumatic disorders, although in these conditions results have not been encouraging.

Levamisole has also been used as an adjunct in patients with malignant disease, although it is not clear that any response is due to its action on the immune system. Adjuvant treatment with levamisole and fluorouracil has been given to reduce recurrence following resection of adenocarcinoma of the colon with regional lymph node involvement (but see Malignant Neoplasms, below).

◊ Reviews.

1. Janssen PAJ. The levamisole story. *Prog Drug Res* 1976; **20:** 347–83.
2. Renoux G. The general immunopharmacology of levamisole. *Drugs* 1980; **20:** 89–99.
3. Amery WKP, Bruynseels JPJM. Levamisole, the story and the lessons. *Int J Immunopharmacol* 1992; **14:** 481–6.

**Malignant neoplasms.** Levamisole has been tried in the adjuvant treatment of various malignant neoplasms[1,2] with conflicting results. Based on the results of early adjuvant trials,[3-5] levamisole was used as standard therapy to modulate fluorouracil in patients with colorectal cancer (p.516), particularly in the USA. However, whether levamisole actually added to the beneficial effect of adjuvant fluorouracil was unclear. Adjuvant levamisole alone was no more effective than placebo in 1 study,[6] and more recent trials have indicated that levamisole is no more effective than placebo when added to fluorouracil,[7] or to fluorouracil plus folinic acid.[8]

1. Spreafico F. Use of levamisole in cancer patients. *Drugs* 1980; **20:** 105–16.
2. Amery WK, Butterworth BS. Review/commentary: the dosage regimen of levamisole in cancer: is it related to efficacy and safety? *Int J Immunopharmacol* 1983; **5:** 1–9.
3. Laurie JA, *et al.* Surgical adjuvant therapy of large-bowel carcinoma: an evaluation of levamisole and the combination of levamisole and fluorouracil: the North Central Cancer Treatment Group and the Mayo Clinic. *J Clin Oncol* 1989; **7:** 1447–56.
4. Moertel CG, *et al.* Levamisole and fluorouracil for adjuvant therapy of resected colon carcinoma. *N Engl J Med* 1990; **322:** 352–8.
5. Moertel CG, *et al.* Fluorouracil plus levamisole as effective adjuvant therapy after resection of stage III colon carcinoma: a final report. *Ann Intern Med* 1995; **122:** 321–6.
6. Chlebowski RT, *et al.* Long-term survival following levamisole or placebo adjuvant treatment of colorectal cancer: a Western Cancer Study Group trial. *Oncology* 1988; **45:** 141–3.
7. QUASAR Collaborative Group. Comparison of fluorouracil with additional levamisole, higher-dose folinic acid, or both, as adjuvant chemotherapy for colorectal cancer: a randomised trial. *Lancet* 2000; **355:** 1588–96.
8. Wolmark N, *et al.* Clinical trial to assess the relative efficacy of fluorouracil and leucovorin, fluorouracil and levamisole, and fluorouracil, leucovorin, and levamisole in patients with Dukes' B and C carcinoma of the colon: results from National Surgical Adjuvant Breast and Bowel Project C-04. *J Clin Oncol* 1999; **17:** 3553–9.

**Mansonella infections.** Levamisole is one of the drugs that has been suggested for the treatment of *Mansonella* infections (p.100). There have been reports[1,2] of response when given with mebendazole.

1. Maertens K, Wery M. Effect of mebendazole and levamisole on Onchocerca volvulus and Dipetalonema perstans. *Trans R Soc Trop Med Hyg* 1975; **69:** 359–60.
2. Bernberg HC, *et al.* The combined treatment with levamisole and mebendazole for a perstans-like filarial infection in Rhodesia. *Trans R Soc Trop Med Hyg* 1979; **73:** 233–4.

**Mouth ulceration.** Levamisole might be beneficial in severe mouth ulceration (p.1245) but is limited by its adverse effects. A review[1] of its use in recurrent aphthous stomatitis indicated that beneficial results have been reported with levamisole in open studies, but results of double-blind studies have been conflicting. Nevertheless, there have been patients with severe recurrent aphthous stomatitis refractory to all other modes of treatment who have responded to levamisole. Dosage has been with 150 mg daily in divided doses given for 3 days at the first sign of ulceration, followed by 11 days without treatment, repeated as necessary.

1. Miller MF. Use of levamisole in recurrent aphthous stomatitis. *Drugs* 1980; **20:** 131–6.

**Renal disorders.** In a randomised double-blind study, children with frequently relapsing corticosteroid-sensitive and corticosteroid-dependent nephrotic syndrome were given placebo or levamisole 2.5 mg/kg on alternate days and steroid therapy was gradually withdrawn.[1] Of 31 children being treated with levamisole, 14 were still in remission 112 days after the start of the study compared with 4 of 30 receiving placebo. For a discussion of the treatment of glomerular kidney disorders, including the nephrotic syndrome, see p.1080.

1. British Association for Paediatric Nephrology. Levamisole for corticosteroid-dependent nephrotic syndrome in childhood. *Lancet* 1991; **337:** 1555–7.

**Vitiligo.** In a study[1] involving 36 patients with limited slow-spreading vitiligo, response to levamisole treatment occurred in 34 within 2 to 4 months. Patients received 150 mg of oral levamisole daily on 2 consecutive days each week. Patients who were additionally treated with topical fluocinolone or clobetasol had higher rates of repigmentation.

The usual treatment of vitiligo is discussed under Pigmentation Disorders, p.1137.

1. Pasricha JS, Khera V. Effect of prolonged treatment with levamisole on vitiligo with limited and slow-spreading disease. *Int J Dermatol* 1994; **33:** 584–7.

## Preparations

***USP 27:*** Levamisole Hydrochloride Tablets.

**Proprietary Preparations** (details are given in Part 3)

***Arg.:*** Meglum; ***Austral.:*** Ergamisol; ***Belg.:*** Ergamisol; ***Braz.:*** Ascaridil; ***Canad.:*** Ergamisol; ***Ger.:*** Ergamisol; ***Hong Kong:*** Decaris; ***India:*** Vermisol; Vizole; ***Irl.:*** Ketrax; ***Israel:*** Ergamisol; ***Ital.:*** Ergamisol†; ***Mex.:*** Decaris; ***Neth.:*** Ergamisol; ***S.Afr.:*** Ergamisol; ***UK:*** Ketrax; ***USA:*** Ergamisol.

## Male Fern

Aspidium; Farnwurzel; Felce Maschio; Feto Macho; Filix Mas; Fougère Mâle; Helecho Macho; Helecho macho; Rhizoma Filicis Maris.

**Pharmacopoeias.** In *Chin.*

### Profile

Male fern consists of the rhizome, frond-bases, and apical bud of *Dryopteris filix-mas* agg. (Polypodiaceae), collected late in the autumn, divested of the roots and dead portions and carefully dried, retaining the internal green colour. It contains not less than 1.5% of filicin. During storage the green colour of the interior gradually disappears, often after a lapse of 6 months, and such material is unfit for medicinal use.

Filicin is the mixture of ether-soluble substances obtained from male fern. Its activity is chiefly due to flavaspidic acid, a phloroglucinol derivative.

Male fern has anthelmintic properties and was formerly administered as male fern extract (aspidium oleoresin) for the expulsion of tapeworms. However, male fern is highly toxic and has been superseded by other drugs.

Adverse effects include headache, nausea and vomiting, severe abdominal cramp, diarrhoea, dyspnoea, albuminuria, hyperbilirubinaemia, dizziness, tremors, convulsions, visual disturbances including blindness (possibly permanent), stimulation of uterine muscle, coma, respiratory failure, bradycardia, and cardiac failure. Fatalities have occurred.

### Preparations

**Proprietary Preparations** (details are given in Part 3)

**Multi-ingredient:** ***Austria:*** Digestodoron; ***Ger.:*** Discmigon†.

## Mebendazole *(BAN, USAN, rINN)*

Mebendazol; Mebendazolum; R-17635. Methyl 5-benzoyl-1*H*-benzimidazol-2-ylcarbamate.

$C_{16}H_{13}N_3O_3$ = 295.3.

*CAS — 31431-39-7.*

*ATC — P02CA01.*

**Pharmacopoeias.** In *Chin., Eur.* (see p.vi), *Int., Pol., US,* and *Viet.*

**Ph. Eur. 5.0** (Mebendazole). A white or almost white powder. It shows polymorphism. Practically insoluble in water, in alcohol, and in dichloromethane. Protect from light.

**USP 27** (Mebendazole). A white to slightly yellow, almost odourless, powder. Practically insoluble in water, in alcohol, in chloroform, in ether, and in dilute mineral acids; freely soluble in formic acid.

### Adverse Effects

Since mebendazole is poorly absorbed from the gastrointestinal tract at the usual therapeutic doses, adverse effects have generally been restricted to gastrointestinal disturbances, such as transient abdominal pain and diarrhoea, and have tended to occur in patients being treated for heavy intestinal infection. Headache and dizziness have been reported. Adverse effects have been reported more frequently with the high doses tried in echinococcosis and have included allergic reactions, raised liver enzyme values, alopecia, and bone marrow depression.

**Incidence of adverse effects.** In the first phase[1] of WHO-coordinated multicentre studies on the treatment of echinococcosis (hydatid disease) involving *Echinococcus granulosus* or *E. multilocularis*, the most frequent adverse effects in the 139 patients given *high-dose* mebendazole, generally for 3 months, were reduced leucocyte count (25 patients), gastrointestinal symptoms (22), and raised serum-transaminase values (22). Other adverse effects were allergic conditions such as fever and skin reactions (4), CNS symptoms including headache (6), and loss of hair (7). Seven patients stopped treatment because of side-effects.

The second phase of studies[2] compared albendazole with mebendazole in more prolonged high-dosage schedules for cystic *E. granulosus* infection. Adverse effects were similar to those reported with the first phase. However, in the first phase the allergic consequences of the 14 ruptured lung cysts and the 4 ruptured liver cysts that occurred with mebendazole were not reported. In the second phase, 2 patients suffered anaphylactic shock as a result of rupture of a lung cyst and a cyst in the abdominal cavity. These 2 patients were withdrawn from mebendazole treatment, as were another 4 patients as a consequence of their adverse reactions, although in 3 the withdrawal was only temporary.

Although albendazole is preferred to mebendazole in the treatment of echinococcosis, if either drug is used there should be constant medical supervision with regular monitoring of serum-transaminase concentrations and of leucocyte and platelet counts. Patients with liver damage should be treated with reduced doses of benzimidazole carbamates, if at all.[2]

1. Davis A, *et al.* Multicentre clinical trials of benzimidazolecarbamates in human echinococcosis. *Bull WHO* 1986; **64:** 383–8.
2. Davis A, *et al.* Multicentre clinical trials of benzimidazolecarbamates in human cystic echinococcosis (phase 2). *Bull WHO* 1989; **67:** 503–8.

**Overdosage.** Respiratory arrest and tachyarrhythmia associated with continuous convulsions were reported[1] in an 8-week-old infant following accidental poisoning with mebendazole. Treatment by exchange transfusion and anticonvulsants was successful.

1. el Kalla S, Menon NS. Mebendazole poisoning in infancy. *Ann Trop Paediatr* 1990; **10:** 313–14.

### Precautions

Patients receiving high doses of mebendazole, such as those with echinococcosis, should be supervised closely with blood counts and liver function being monitored; such high-dose therapy may be inappropriate in those with hepatic impairment (see under Incidence of Adverse Effects, above).

**Monitoring drug concentrations.** In a retrospective analysis of patients who had received high doses of mebendazole for echinococcosis,[1] no relationship was found between dose and plasma concentration of mebendazole and considerable intra- and interindividual variation in plasma concentrations was observed, emphasising the need for repeated monitoring. Several patients appeared to have what were considered to be subtherapeutic plasma concentrations.

1. Luder PJ, *et al.* Treatment of hydatid disease with high oral doses of mebendazole: long-term follow-up of plasma mebendazole levels and drug interactions. *Eur J Clin Pharmacol* 1986; **31:** 443–8.

**Pregnancy.** Mebendazole is teratogenic in *rats* and the manufacturers note that there are no adequate and well controlled studies in human pregnancy. Mebendazole is therefore usually contra-indicated during pregnancy. However, it was noted that in a survey of a limited number of pregnant women who had inadvertently taken mebendazole during the first trimester, the incidence of malformation and spontaneous abortion was no greater than that observed in the general population.

### Interactions

**Antiepileptics.** *Phenytoin* or *carbamazepine* have been reported to lower plasma-mebendazole concentrations in patients receiving high doses for echinococcosis, presumably as a result of enzyme induction; *valproate* had no such effect.[1]

1. Luder PJ, *et al.* Treatment of hydatid disease with high oral doses of mebendazole: long-term follow-up of plasma mebendazole levels and drug interactions. *Eur J Clin Pharmacol* 1986; **31:** 443–8.

**Histamine $H_2$-antagonists.** Plasma concentrations of mebendazole have been raised when the enzyme inhibitor *cimetidine* was also given, and this has resulted in the resolution of previously unresponsive hepatic hydatid cysts.[1]

1. Bekhti A, Pirotte J. Cimetidine increases serum mebendazole concentrations: implications for treatment of hepatic hydatid cysts. *Br J Clin Pharmacol* 1987; **24:** 390–2.

### Pharmacokinetics

Mebendazole is poorly absorbed from the gastrointestinal tract and undergoes extensive first-pass elimination, being metabolised in the liver, eliminated in the bile as unchanged drug and metabolites, and excreted in the faeces. Only about 2% of a dose is excreted unchanged or as metabolites in the urine.

Mebendazole is highly protein bound.

### Uses and Administration

Mebendazole, a benzimidazole carbamate derivative, is an anthelmintic with activity against most nematodes and some other worms; activity against some larval stages and ova has also been demonstrated. It inhibits or destroys cytoplasmic microtubules in the worm's intestinal or absorptive cells. Inhibition of glucose uptake and depletion of glycogen stores follow as do other inhibitory effects leading to death of the worm within several days.

Mebendazole, being poorly absorbed from the gastrointestinal tract, is used principally in the treatment of the intestinal nematode infections ascariasis (roundworm infection), enterobiasis (pinworm or threadworm infections), hookworm (ancylostomiasis and necatoriasis), and trichuriasis (whipworm infection); it is useful in mixed infections. During treatment with mebendazole, migration of worms with expulsion through the mouth and nose has occurred in some patients heavily infected with *Ascaris*. Mebendazole is also used in the treatment of capillariasis and trichostrongyliasis and has been used in strongyloidiasis. Other nematode infections which may respond to mebendazole are infection with the filarial nematode *Mansonel-*

*la perstans*, and the tissue infections toxocariasis and trichinosis. Mebendazole has also been tried in high doses in the treatment of echinococcosis (hydatid disease). For discussions of these infections and their treatment, see under Choice of Anthelmintic, p.97, and under the individual headings below.

Mebendazole is given by mouth. The usual dose for adults and children aged over 2 years with enterobiasis is 100 mg as a single dose, repeated if necessary after 2 to 3 weeks; for ascariasis, hookworm infections, and trichuriasis the usual dose is 100 mg twice daily for 3 days, although a single dose of 500 mg may be effective.

**Angiostrongyliasis.** Mebendazole was formerly used for the treatment of angiostrongyliasis (p.97) but current opinion is that there is no convincing evidence to support its use.

**Capillariasis.** Mebendazole in a dose of 200 mg twice daily for 20 days has been used[1] for the treatment of capillariasis (p.98).

1. Medical Letter on Drugs and Therapeutics. Drugs for parasitic infections (issued April 2002). Available at: http://www.medicalletter.com/freedocs/parasitic.pdf (accessed 02/06/04)

**Echinococcosis.** Mebendazole has been used[1-7] in echinococcosis (p.98), but albendazole is generally preferred. The usual dose of mebendazole in cystic echinococcosis is 40 to 50 mg/kg daily for at least 3 to 6 months.[8] A similar dose is used as an adjuvant to surgery. For alveolar echinococcosis, the dose is adjusted after 4 weeks to produce a plasma concentration of at least 250 nanomoles/litre (74 nanograms/mL), although adults should not receive more than 6 g daily. Treatment is continued for at least 2 years following radical surgery, or indefinitely in inoperable cases.

1. Ammann RW, *et al.* Recurrence rate after discontinuation of long-term mebendazole therapy in alveolar echinococcosis (preliminary results). *Am J Trop Med Hyg* 1990; **43:** 506–15.
2. Messaritakis J, *et al.* High mebendazole doses in pulmonary and hepatic hydatid disease. *Arch Dis Child* 1991; **66:** 532–3.
3. Teggi A, *et al.* Therapy of human hydatid disease with mebendazole and albendazole. *Antimicrob Agents Chemother* 1993; **37:** 1679–84.
4. Göçmen A, *et al.* Treatment of hydatid disease in childhood with mebendazole. *Eur Respir J* 1993; **6:** 253–7.
5. Ammann RW, *et al.* Effect of chemotherapy on the larval mass and the long-term course of alveolar echinococcosis. *Hepatology* 1994; **19:** 735–42.
6. Erdinçler P, *et al.* The role of mebendazole in the surgical treatment of central nervous system hydatid disease. *Br J Neurosurg* 1997; **11:** 116–20.
7. Vutova K, *et al.* Effect of mebendazole on human cystic echinococcosis: the role of dosage and treatment duration. *Ann Trop Med Parasitol* 1999; **93:** 357–65.
8. WHO Informal Working Group on Echinococcosis. Guidelines for treatment of cystic and alveolar echinococcosis in humans. *Bull WHO* 1996; **74:** 231–42.

**Giardiasis.** For mention of the use of mebendazole for the treatment of giardiasis, see p.596.

**Mansonella infections.** Mebendazole is one of the drugs that has been suggested for the treatment of infections with *Mansonella perstans* (p.100). Some patients have responded to mebendazole with levamisole[1,2] or to mebendazole alone.[3]

1. Maertens K, Wery M. Effect of mebendazole and levamisole on Onchocerca volvulus and Dipetalonema perstans. *Trans R Soc Trop Med Hyg* 1975; **69:** 359–60.
2. Bernberg HC, *et al.* The combined treatment with levamisole and mebendazole for a perstans-like filarial infection in Rhodesia. *Trans R Soc Trop Med Hyg* 1979; **73:** 233–4.
3. Wahlgren M, Frolov I. Treatment of Dipetalonema perstans infections with mebendazole. *Trans R Soc Trop Med Hyg* 1983; **77:** 422–3.

**Strongyloidiasis.** Mebendazole has been used for the treatment of strongyloidiasis (p.100), but needs to be given for longer periods than albendazole to control auto-infection, so that, of the two, albendazole is preferred.[1-3]

1. Wilson KH, Kauffman CA. Persistent Strongyloides stercoralis in a blind loop of the bowel: successful treatment with mebendazole. *Arch Intern Med* 1983; **143:** 357–8.
2. Mravak S, *et al.* Treatment of strongyloidiasis with mebendazole. *Acta Trop (Basel)* 1983; **40:** 93–4.
3. Pelletier LL, Baker CB. Treatment failures following mebendazole therapy for chronic strongyloidiasis. *J Infect Dis* 1987; **156:** 532–3.

**Syngamosis.** Mebendazole has been used successfully[1] to treat syngamosis (p.101).

1. Timmons RF, *et al.* Infection of the respiratory tract with Mammomanogamus (Syngamus) laryngeus: a new case in Largo, Florida, and a summary of previously reported cases. *Am Rev Respir Dis* 1983; **128:** 566–9.

**Toxocariasis.** Mebendazole has been used in the treatment of toxocariasis (p.101). In comparative studies, mebendazole has been reported to produce similar improvements to those obtained with tiabendazole[1] and with diethylcarbamazine,[2] in each case with a lower incidence of adverse effects.

1. Magnaval JF, Charlet JP. Efficacité comparée du thiabendazole et du mébendazole dans le traitement de la toxocarose. *Therapie* 1987; **42:** 541–4.
2. Magnaval J-F. Comparative efficacy of diethylcarbamazine and mebendazole for the treatment of human toxocariasis. *Parasitology* 1995; **110:** 529–33.

**Trichinosis.** Mebendazole is used for the treatment of trichinosis (p.101) in some countries.

References.

1. Levin ML. Treatment of trichinosis with mebendazole. *Am J Trop Med Hyg* 1983; **32:** 980–3.

## Preparations

***USP 27:*** Mebendazole Tablets.

**Proprietary Preparations** (details are given in Part 3)
***Arg.:*** Mebutar; Nemasole; Tesical; ***Austral.:*** Chemists Own De Worm; Combantrin-1 with Mebendazole; Vermox; ***Austria:*** Pantelmin; ***Belg.:*** Vermox; ***Braz.:*** Ascariobel; Ascaritor†; Ascarobex†; Athelmin†; Averpan†; Belmirax†; Bendrax; Bivalem†; Certovermil†; Cessaverm†; Crisdazol; Divermil; Ductelmin; Eraverm; Feller†; Geophagol; Gran-Verm†; Helmizil†; Ibdazol†; Kindelmin; Meben†; Mebendazotil†; Mebendil†; Mebental; Moben; Multielmin; Necamin; Neo Mebend; Novelmin; Panfugan; Pantelmin; Panverm; Paraverm†; Parelmin†; Pentazole†; Pluriverm; Pluriverm†; Politelmin†; Quintelmin; Sirben; Tetrahelmin; Vermepen†; Vermionon; Vermirax; Vermonon†; Vermoplex; Vermoral; Verzol; Zol-Triq†; ***Canad.:*** Vermox; ***Chile:*** Diacor; ***Denm.:*** Vermox; ***Ger.:*** Surfont; Vermox; ***Gr.:*** Vermox; ***Hong Kong:*** Elmetin; Vermox; ***India:*** Mebex; Wormin; ***Irl.:*** Vermox; ***Israel:*** Vermox; ***Ital.:*** Vermox; ***Malaysia:*** Quemox; Thelmox; Vermox; ***Mex.:*** Amycil†; Benedaxol†; Bensolmin†; Bestelar; Carbatil; Daben; Diazolen; Exaverm†; Exbenzol; Exteny; Fanciadazol; Hedazol†; Helminzole†; Lumbicid; M-Bentabs; Marben†; Meb-Overoid; Meban†; Mebandozer†; Mebelmin†; Mebensole; Mebentiasis†; Mebentine†; Mebentral; Mizolmex†; Nemapres†; Oxizole†; Panvermin; Paranzol; Prodazol†; Profenzol; Revapol; Soltric; Vermicol; Vermidil; Vermin-Dazol; Vermox; Vertex; Vertizole; ***Neth.:*** Madicure; Vermox; ***Norw.:*** Vermox; ***NZ:*** Combantrin-1; Mindol; Vermox; ***Port.:*** Pantelmin; Toloxim; ***S.Afr.:*** Anthex; Cipex; D-Worm; Vermox; Wormgo; Wormstop; ***Spain:*** Bantenol; Lomper; Mebendan; Oxitover; Sufil; ***Swed.:*** Vermox; ***Switz.:*** Vermox; ***Thai.:*** Benda; Drivermide; Elmetin†; Fugacar; Masaworm-1; Meba†; Meben; Mebenda-P; Mebenlax†; Medazole; Noxworm; Vagaka; Warca; ***UAE:*** Mebzol; ***UK:*** Boots Threadworm Tablets 2 Years Plus; Ovex; Pripsen; Vermox; ***USA:*** Vermox.

**Multi-ingredient:** ***Arg.:*** Aduar; Mebutar Compuesto; Tru Compuesto; ***Braz.:*** Exelmin; Flenverme†; Forverm; Helmi-Ped; Helmib†; Helmiben; Helmidrax; Neovermin; Octelmin; Poliben; Profium; Prohelmin; Vermol; Zoles; ***Mex.:*** Mebeciclol.

---

## Melarsomine *(rINN)*

Melarsomina. Bis(2-aminoethyl) *p*-[(4,6-diamino-s-triazin-2-yl)amino]dithiobenzenearsonite.

$C_{13}H_{21}AsN_8S_2$ = 428.4.
*CAS* — *128470-15-5.*

### Profile

Melarsomine is a trivalent arsenical derivative used in veterinary practice for the control of canine heartworm (dirofilariasis).

---

## Metrifonate *(BAN, rINN)*

Bayer-L-1359; DETF; Metrifonato; Metrifonatum; Metriphonate; Trichlorfon *(USAN)*; Trichlorphon. Dimethyl 2,2,2-trichloro-1-hydroxyethylphosphonate.

$C_4H_8Cl_3O_4P$ = 257.4.
*CAS* — *52-68-6.*
*ATC* — *P02BB01.*

**Pharmacopoeias.** In *Eur.* (see p.vi), *Int.*, and *US.*

**Ph. Eur. 5.0** (Metrifonate). A white crystalline powder. M.p. is between 76° and 81°. Freely soluble in water, in alcohol, and in acetone; very soluble in dichloromethane. Protect from light.

**USP 27** (Metrifonate). A white crystalline powder. M.p. about 78° with decomposition. Freely soluble in water, in alcohol, in acetone, in chloroform, in ether, and in benzene; very soluble in dichloromethane; very slightly soluble in hexane and in pentane. Decomposed by alkali. Store at a temperature not exceeding 25°.

## Adverse Effects, Treatment, and Precautions

Metrifonate is generally well tolerated, but may cause nausea, vomiting, abdominal pain, diarrhoea, headache, dizziness, and weakness.

It is an organophosphorus compound and because of its anticholinesterase properties depresses plasma-cholinesterase concentrations. For a description of the toxic effects of organophosphorus compounds and the treatment of acute poisoning, see Organophosphorus Insecticides, p.1507. Atropine has been used to relieve cholinergic side-effects without affecting metrifonate's activity against *Schistosoma haematobium.*

**Anticholinesterase effects.** Metrifonate depresses cholinesterase activity and there has been the occasional report of severe cholinergic adverse effects.[1] However, it does not usually give rise to troublesome effects at doses normally used, even though there may temporarily be almost complete inhibition of plasma cholinesterase and considerable inhibition of erythrocyte cholinesterase[2] (but see also under Alzheimer's Disease, below).

The environmental aspects of metrifonate usage have been considered by WHO.[3]

1. Jamnadas VP, Thomas JEP. Metriphonate and organophosphate poisoning. *Cent Afr J Med* 1979; **25:** 130.
2. Pleština R, *et al.* Effect of metrifonate on blood cholinesterases in children during the treatment of schistosomiasis. *Bull WHO* 1972; **46:** 747–59.
3. Trichlorfon. *Environmental Health Criteria 132.* Geneva: WHO, 1992.

**Handling.** Metrifonate is very toxic when inhaled, swallowed, or spilled on the skin. It can be removed from the skin by washing with soap and water. Contaminated material should be immersed in a 2% aqueous solution of sodium hydroxide for several hours.

**Pregnancy.** WHO reported[1] that metrifonate had not shown embryotoxicity or teratogenicity, but did not recommend the use of metrifonate in pregnant patients unless immediate intervention was essential. There has been a report of an infant born with massive hydrocephalus and a large meningomyelocele whose mother had been treated twice with metrifonate during the second month of pregnancy.[2] A possible link between congenital abnormalities and the use of metrifonate to eradicate fish parasites has also been postulated.[3]

1. WHO. The control of schistosomiasis: second report of the WHO expert committee. *WHO Tech Rep Ser 830* 1993.
2. Monson MH, Alexander K. Metrifonate in pregnancy. *Trans R Soc Trop Med Hyg* 1984; **78:** 565.
3. Czeizel AE, *et al.* Environmental trichlorfon and cluster of congenital abnormalities. *Lancet* 1993; **341:** 539–42.

## Interactions

Patients treated with metrifonate should not be given depolarising neuromuscular blockers such as suxamethonium for at least 48 hours.The use of metrifonate should be avoided in those recently exposed to insecticides or other agricultural chemicals with anticholinesterase activity.

## Pharmacokinetics

Metrifonate is absorbed after oral doses and some is converted to dichlorvos which is considered to be the active moiety. Plasma concentrations of dichlorvos are about 1% of those of metrifonate with peak concentrations of both substances occurring within 2 hours. Excretion is via the kidney, mainly as glucuronides.

◊ References.

1. Nordgren I, *et al.* Plasma levels of metrifonate and dichlorvos during treatment of schistosomiasis with Bilarcil. *Am J Trop Med Hyg* 1980; **29:** 426–30.
2. Nordgren I, *et al.* Levels of metrifonate and dichlorvos in plasma and erythrocytes during treatment of schistosomiasis with Bilarcil. *Acta Pharmacol Toxicol (Copenh)* 1981; **49** (suppl V): 79–86.
3. Pettigrew LC, *et al.* Pharmacokinetics, pharmacodynamics, and safety of metrifonate in patients with Alzheimer's disease. *J Clin Pharmacol* 1998; **38:** 236–45.

## Uses and Administration

Metrifonate is an organophosphorus compound and is converted in the body to the active metabolite dichlorvos (p.1503), an anticholinesterase.

Metrifonate has anthelmintic activity against *Schistosoma haematobium* and is given by mouth as an alternative to praziquantel in the treatment of schistosomiasis due to *S. haematobium.* It is usually given in three doses of 7.5 to 10 mg/kg at intervals of 2 weeks.

Metrifonate has also been used as an insecticide and as a parasiticide in fish and domestic animals.

**Alzheimer's disease.** Metrifonate, like a number of other cholinesterase inhibitors, has been tried in the treatment of Alzheimer's disease (see Dementia, p.1484). Clinical studies[1,2] produced modest benefits but research was discontinued following reports of muscle weakness, sometimes requiring respiratory support.

1. Becker RE, *et al.* Effects of metrifonate on cognitive decline in Alzheimer disease: a double-blind, placebo-controlled, 6-month study. *Alzheimer Dis Assoc Disord* 1998; **12:** 54–7.
2. Morris JC, *et al.* Metrifonate benefits cognitive, behavioral, and global function in patients with Alzheimer's disease. *Neurology* 1998; **50:** 1222–30.

**Schistosomiasis.** While praziquantel is now the main treatment for schistosomiasis (p.100), metrifonate is an alternative for infection due to *Schistosoma haematobium.*

Metrifonate owes its activity against *S. haematobium* to its metabolite dichlorvos which is a cholinesterase inhibitor; it is not active against other *Schistosoma* spp. The standard dose in the treatment of *S. haematobium* infection is 7.5 to 10 mg/kg given on 3 occasions at intervals of 2 weeks.[1] Cure rates with this schedule in schistosomiasis control programmes range from 40 to more than 80%, with a reduction of more than 80% in egg counts among those not cured. A comparison with praziquantel has shown praziquantel to be the more effective drug.[2] In addition, metrifonate's dosage schedule of 3 doses at intervals of 2 weeks has caused problems of patient compliance.[3] Other dosage schedules have been tried. In one group of trials, the cure rate at 6 months following treatment with 1, 2, or 3 doses was 28, 65, and 84% respectively. Another study showed that 5 mg/kg given three times in one day produced similar results to a standard dosage schedule.[4]

1. WHO. WHO model prescribing information: drugs used in parasitic diseases. Geneva: WHO, 1995.

2. Squires N. Interventions for treating schistosomiasis haematobium. Available in The Cochrane Library; Issue 2. Chichester: John Wiley; 2004.
3. Aden Abdi Y, Gustafsson LL. Poor patient compliance reduces the efficacy of metrifonate treatment of Schistosoma haematobium in Somalia. *Eur J Clin Pharmacol* 1989; **36:** 161–4.
4. Aden Abdi Y, Gustafsson LL. Field trial of the efficacy of a simplified and standard metrifonate treatments of Schistosoma haematobium. *Eur J Clin Pharmacol* 1989; **37:** 371–4.

## Milbemycin Oxime

CGA-179246; Milbemicina oxima. A mixture of milbemycin $A_4$ 5-oxime and milbemycin $A_3$ 5-oxime.
*CAS — 129496-10-2.*

### Profile

Milbemycin oxime is an anthelmintic used in veterinary medicine.

## Morantel Citrate *(BANM, pINNM)*

Citrato de morantel. (*E*)-1,4,5,6-Tetrahydro-1-methyl-2-[2-(3-methyl-2-thienyl)vinyl]pyrimidine citrate monohydrate.
$C_{12}H_{16}N_2S,C_6H_8O_7,H_2O = 430.5.$
*CAS — 20574-50-9 (morantel); 69525-81-1 (morantel citrate).*

## Morantel Tartrate *(BANM, USAN, pINNM)*

CP-12009-18; Moranteli Hydrogenotartras; Tartrato de morantel; UK-2964-18.
$C_{12}H_{16}N_2S,C_4H_6O_6 = 370.4.$
*CAS — 20574-50-9 (morantel); 26155-31-7 (morantel tartrate).*

**Pharmacopoeias.** In *Eur.* (see p.vi) for veterinary use only.

**Ph. Eur. 5.0** (Morantel Hydrogen Tartrate for Veterinary Use). A white or pale yellow, crystalline powder. Very soluble in water and in alcohol; practically insoluble in ethyl acetate. A 1% solution in water has a pH of 2.8 to 3.2. Protect from light.

### Profile

Morantel is an analogue of pyrantel. The citrate and the tartrate are used as anthelmintics in veterinary medicine for the treatment of gastrointestinal roundworms.

## Moxidectin *(BAN, USAN, rINN)*

CL-301423; Moxidectina. (6*R*,15*S*)-5-*O*-Demethyl-28-deoxy-25-[(*E*)-1,3-dimethylbut-1-enyl]-6,28-epoxy-23-oxomilbemycin B (*E*)-23-*O*-methyloxime.
$C_{37}H_{53}NO_8 = 639.8.$
*CAS — 113507-06-5.*

### Profile

Moxidectin is an anthelmintic used in veterinary medicine. It is also used as a systemic veterinary ectoparasiticide.

## Naftalofos *(BAN, USAN, rINN)*

Bay-9002; E-9002; ENT-25567; Naftalofós; Naphthalophos; Phthalophos; S-940. Diethyl naphthalimido-oxyphosphonate.
$C_{16}H_{16}NO_6P = 349.3.$
*CAS — 1491-41-4.*

### Profile

Naftalofos is an organophosphorus compound (see Organophosphorus Insecticides, p.1507) used as an anthelmintic in veterinary medicine.

## Netobimin *(BAN, USAN, rINN)*

Netobimina; Sch-32481. 2-{3-Methoxycarbonyl-2-[2-nitro-5-(propylthio)phenyl]guanidino}ethanesulphonic acid.
$C_{14}H_{20}N_4O_7S_2 = 420.5.$
*CAS — 88255-01-0.*

### Profile

Netobimin is an anthelmintic used in veterinary medicine.

# Niclosamide *(BAN, USAN, rINN)*

Anhydrous Niclosamide; Bay-2353; Niclosamida; Niclosamida Anidra; Niclosamidum Anhydricum; Phenasale. 2′,5-Dichloro-4′-nitrosalicylanilide; 5-Chloro-*N*-(2-chloro-4-nitrophenyl)-2-hydroxybenzamide.
$C_{13}H_8Cl_2N_2O_4 = 327.1.$
*CAS — 50-65-7.*
*ATC — P02DA01.*

**Pharmacopoeias.** In *Chin., Eur.* (see p.vi), and *Pol.*
*Int.* permits the anhydrous substance or the monohydrate under the title Niclosamide.

**Ph. Eur. 5.0** (Niclosamide, Anhydrous). Yellowish-white to yellowish, fine crystals. Practically insoluble in water; slightly soluble in dehydrated alcohol; sparingly soluble in acetone. Store in airtight containers. Protect from light.

## Niclosamide Monohydrate *(BANM)*

Niclosamida Mono-hidratada; Niclosamida monohidrato; Niclosamidum Monohydricum.
$C_{13}H_8Cl_2N_2O_4,H_2O = 345.1.$
*ATC — P02DA01.*

**Pharmacopoeias.** In *Eur.* (see p.vi).
*Int.* permits the monohydrate or the anhydrous substance under the title Niclosamide.

**Ph. Eur. 5.0** (Niclosamide Monohydrate). Yellowish, fine crystals. Practically insoluble in water; slightly soluble in dehydrated alcohol; sparingly soluble in acetone. Protect from light.

### Adverse Effects

Gastrointestinal disturbances may occur occasionally with niclosamide. Lightheadedness and pruritus have been reported less frequently.

### Pharmacokinetics

Niclosamide is not significantly absorbed from the gastrointestinal tract.

### Uses and Administration

Niclosamide is an anthelmintic which is active against most tapeworms, including the beef tapeworm (*Taenia saginata*), the pork tapeworm (*T. solium*), the fish tapeworm (*Diphyllobothrium latum*), the dwarf tapeworm (*Hymenolepis nana*), and the dog tapeworm (*Dipylidium caninum*). For discussions of the treatment of tapeworm infections, see Diphyllobothriasis, p.98, Hymenolepiasis, p.99, and Taeniasis, p.101. The activity of niclosamide against these worms appears to be due to inhibition of mitochondrial oxidative phosphorylation; anaerobic ATP production is also affected.

Niclosamide is given as tablets, which must be chewed thoroughly before swallowing and washed down with water.

For infections with pork tapeworm a single 2-g dose is given after a light breakfast. Niclosamide is not active against the larval form (cysticerci) and, although the risk of inducing cysticercosis appears to be theoretical, a laxative is given about 2 hours after the dose to expel the killed worms and minimise the possibility of the migration of ova of *T. solium* into the stomach; an antiemetic may also be given before treatment.

For infections with beef or fish tapeworms the 2-g dose of niclosamide may be divided, with 1 g taken after breakfast and 1 g an hour later.

In dwarf-tapeworm infections an initial dose of 2 g is given on the first day followed by 1 g daily for 6 days.

Children aged 2 to 6 years are given half the above doses and those under 2 years of age are given one-quarter the above doses.

Unless expulsion of the worm is aided by a laxative, portions are voided in a partially digested form after treatment with niclosamide; the scolex is rarely identifiable.

Niclosamide is used as a molluscicide for the treatment of water in schistosomiasis control programmes (p.100).

### Preparations

***BP 2003:*** Niclosamide Tablets.

**Proprietary Preparations** (details are given in Part 3)
***Belg.:*** Yomesan; ***Braz.:*** Atenase; ***Denm.:*** Yomesan; ***Fin.:*** Kontal; ***Fr.:*** Tredemine; ***Ger.:*** Yomesan; ***Gr.:*** Tredemine; ***India:*** Niclosan; ***Israel:*** Yomesan; ***Ital.:*** Yomesan; ***Mex.:*** Overoid; ***Neth.:*** Yomesan; ***S.Afr.:*** Yomesan; ***Swed.:*** Yomesan; ***Thai.:*** Niclosan; Telmitin; Unicide; Yomesan; ***UK:*** Yomesan.

**Multi-ingredient:** ***Thai.:*** Zenda.

## Nitroscanate *(BAN, USAN, rINN)*

CGA-23654; Nitroscanato. 4-(4-Nitrophenoxy)phenyl isothiocyanate.
$C_{13}H_8N_2O_3S = 272.3.$
*CAS — 19881-18-6.*

### Profile

Nitroscanate is an isothiocyanate anthelmintic used in veterinary medicine.

## Nitroxinil *(BAN, rINN)*

Nitroxinilo; Nitroxynil. 4-Hydroxy-3-iodo-5-nitrobenzonitrile.
$C_7H_3IN_2O_3 = 290.0.$
*CAS — 1689-89-0 (nitroxinil); 27917-82-4 (nitroxinil eglumine).*

**Pharmacopoeias.** In *BP(Vet).* Also in *Fr.* for veterinary use only.

**BP(Vet) 2003** (Nitroxynil). A yellow to yellowish brown powder. Practically insoluble in water; slightly soluble in alcohol; sparingly soluble in ether; it dissolves in solutions of alkali hydroxides. Protect from light.

### Profile

Nitroxinil is an anthelmintic used in veterinary medicine for the treatment of fascioliasis and some gastrointestinal roundworms in cattle and sheep.

# Oxamniquine *(BAN, USAN, rINN)*

Oxamniquina; UK-4271. 1,2,3,4-Tetrahydro-2-isopropylaminomethyl-7-nitro-6-quinolylmethanol.
$C_{14}H_{21}N_3O_3 = 279.3.$
*CAS — 21738-42-1.*
*ATC — P02BA02.*

**Pharmacopoeias.** In *Fr.* and *Int.*

### Adverse Effects

Oxamniquine causes severe pain at the injection site when given intramuscularly and is no longer given by this route.

It is generally well tolerated following doses by mouth, although dizziness with or without drowsiness occurs in at least a third of patients, beginning up to 3 hours after a dose and usually lasting for up to 6 hours. Headache and gastrointestinal effects such as nausea, vomiting, and diarrhoea are also common.

Allergic-type reactions including urticaria, pruritic skin rashes, and fever may occur. Liver enzyme values have been raised transiently in some patients. Epileptiform convulsions have been reported, especially in patients with a history of convulsive disorders. Hallucinations and excitement have occurred rarely.

A reddish discoloration of urine, probably due to a metabolite of oxamniquine, has been reported.

**Effects on body temperature.** A review[1] in 1987 noted that although a modest post-treatment rise in temperature had been reported occasionally, fever was not a common side-effect of oxamniquine, except in Egypt where it appeared to be characteristic. The cause was not known. Increased immune complexes and excretion of antigens occurred in only half the cases, there was no evidence that Egyptian patients metabolised the drug differently to produce a pyrogenic metabolite, and the effect had not been seen in other areas where a similar high-dose regimen was used.[1]

1. Foster R. A review of clinical experience with oxamniquine. *Trans R Soc Trop Med Hyg* 1987; **81:** 55–9.

**Effects on the nervous system.** In 37 patients with *Schistosoma mansoni* infection treated successfully with oxamniquine,[1] dizziness and drowsiness were most common, but the most significant adverse effect was the development of EEG abnormalities in 6 of 34 patients whose pre-treatment EEG was normal. Of the 3 patients with pre-existing EEG abnormalities, 1 suffered a tonic-clonic seizure during therapy as previously reported,[2] 1 did not suffer seizures, and the third received phenytoin prophylaxis during oxamniquine therapy. It was considered prudent to give antiepileptics before starting oxamniquine in patients with a history of seizure disorder. After completion of this study, a patient with no history of seizures suffered a tonic-clonic seizure 2 hours after each of the second and third doses of oxamniquine.

The main neuropsychiatric side-effects seen in 180 Brazilian patients with *Schistosoma mansoni* infection treated with single oral doses of oxamniquine were: drowsiness (50.6%), dizziness (41.1%), headache (16.1%), temporary amnesia (2.2%), behavioural disturbances (1.7%), chills (1.1%), and seizures (1.1%).[3] An EEG was performed before and after treatment in 20 patients; there were alterations in 3 but they were not associated with neuropsychiatric changes.

1. Krajden S, *et al.* Safety and toxicity of oxamniquine in the treatment of Schistosoma mansoni infections, with particular reference to electroencephalographic abnormalities. *Am J Trop Med Hyg* 1983; **32:** 1344–6.
2. Keystone JS. Seizures and electroencephalograph changes associated with oxamniquine therapy. *Am J Trop Med Hyg* 1978; **27:** 360–2.
3. de Carvalho SA, *et al.* Neurotoxicidade do oxamniquine no tratamento da infeçåo humana pelo Schistosoma mansoni. *Rev Inst Med Trop Sao Paulo* 1985; **27:** 132–42.

### Precautions

Oxamniquine should be used with caution in patients with epilepsy or a history of convulsive disorders. Patients should be warned that oxamniquine can cause dizziness or drowsiness and if affected they should not drive or operate machinery.

### Pharmacokinetics

Oxamniquine is readily absorbed after oral doses. Peak plasma concentrations are achieved 1 to 3 hours after a dose and the plasma half-life is 1 to 2.5 hours.

It is extensively metabolised to inactive metabolites, principally the 6-carboxy derivative, which are excreted in the urine. About 70% of a dose of oxamniquine is excreted as the 6-carboxy metabolite within 12 hours of a dose; traces of the 2-carboxy metabolite have also been detected in the urine.

### Uses and Administration

Oxamniquine is an anthelmintic used in the treatment of schistosomiasis caused by *Schistosoma mansoni*, but not by other *Schistosoma* spp. It causes worms to shift from the mesenteric veins to the liver where the male worms are retained; the female worms return to the mesentery, but can no longer release eggs. Resistance may occur.

Oxamniquine is given by mouth, preferably after food. Dosage depends on the geographical origin of the infection and total doses range from 15 mg/kg as a single dose to 60 mg/kg given over 2 to 3 days. A single dose should not exceed 20 mg/kg.

**Schistosomiasis.** Oxamniquine is an alternative to praziquantel for the treatment of schistosomiasis (p.100) due to *Schistosoma mansoni*, although resistance has occurred, particularly in South America.[1]

The dose ranges between a single dose of 15 mg/kg and 60 mg/kg given over 2 or 3 days.[1,2] Doses in the low range have been used effectively in South America, the Caribbean, and West Africa while patients in Egypt, South Africa, and Zimbabwe require doses at the top end of the range; intermediate doses may be effective in other parts of Africa.[2]

After the appropriate therapeutic dose of oxamniquine, cure rates of at least 60%, and often more than 90%, can be expected. Egg excretion in those not cured will be reduced by over 80%, and usually by over 90%, one year after treatment.[2]

1. WHO. The control of schistosomiasis: second report of the WHO expert committee. *WHO Tech Rep Ser 830* 1993.
2. WHO. The control of schistosomiasis: report of a WHO expert committee. *WHO Tech Rep Ser 728* 1985.

### Preparations

**Proprietary Preparations** (details are given in Part 3)
***Braz.:*** Mansil; ***Gr.:*** Vansil; ***USA:*** Vansil†.

---

## Oxantel Embonate *(BANM, rINNM)*

CP-14445-16; Embonato de oxantel; Oxantel Pamoate *(USAN)*. (*E*)-3-[2-(1,4,5,6-Tetrahydro-1-methylpyrimidin-2-yl)vinyl]phenol 4,4′-methylenebis(3-hydroxy-2-naphthoate).

$C_{13}H_{16}N_2O,C_{23}H_{16}O_6$ = 604.6.
*CAS — 36531-26-7 (oxantel); 68813-55-8 (oxantel embonate); 42408-84-4 (oxantel embonate).*
*ATC — P02CC02.*

### Profile

Oxantel is an analogue of pyrantel that has been used as the embonate in the treatment of trichuriasis. It is used in combination with pyrantel for various intestinal nematode infections.

---

## Oxfendazole *(BAN, USAN, rINN)*

Oxfendazol; Oxfendazolum; RS-8858. Methyl 5-phenylsulphinyl-1*H*-benzimidazol-2-ylcarbamate.

$C_{15}H_{13}N_3O_3S$ = 315.3.
*CAS — 53716-50-0.*

**Pharmacopoeias.** In *Eur.* (see p.vi) and *US* for veterinary use only.

**Ph. Eur. 5.0** (Oxfendazole for Veterinary Use). A white or almost white powder. It shows polymorphism. Practically insoluble in water; slightly soluble in alcohol and in dichloromethane. Protect from light.

**USP 27** (Oxfendazole). A white or almost white powder. Practically insoluble in water; slightly soluble in alcohol and in dichloromethane. Protect from light.

### Profile

Oxfendazole is a benzimidazole carbamate anthelmintic structurally related to mebendazole (p.108). It is used in veterinary medicine.

---

## Oxibendazole *(BAN, USAN, rINN)*

Oxibendazol; SKF-30310. Methyl 5-propoxy-1*H*-benzimidazol-2-ylcarbamate.

$C_{12}H_{15}N_3O_3$ = 249.3.
*CAS — 20559-55-1.*

### Profile

Oxibendazole is a benzimidazole carbamate anthelmintic structurally related to mebendazole (p.108). It is used in veterinary medicine.

---

## Oxyclozanide *(BAN, rINN)*

ICI-46683; Oxiclozanida. 3,3′,5,5′,6-Pentachloro-2′-hydroxysalicylanilide.

$C_{13}H_6Cl_5NO_3$ = 401.5.
*CAS — 2277-92-1.*

**Pharmacopoeias.** In *BP(Vet).*

**BP(Vet) 2003** (Oxyclozanide). A pale cream or cream-coloured, odourless or almost odourless powder. Very slightly soluble in water; soluble in alcohol; freely soluble in acetone; slightly soluble in chloroform.

### Profile

Oxyclozanide is an anthelmintic used in veterinary medicine for the control of fascioliasis in cattle and sheep.

---

# Piperazine

Piperazina.

$C_4H_{10}N_2$ = 86.14.
*CAS — 110-85-0.*
*ATC — P02CB01.*

**Pharmacopoeias.** In *US.*

**USP 27** (Piperazine). White to off-white lumps or flakes having an ammoniacal odour. Soluble in water and in alcohol; insoluble in ether. Store in airtight containers. Protect from light.

## Piperazine Adipate

Piperaz. Adip.; Piperazina, adipato de; Piperazini Adipas; Piperazinum Adipicum.

$C_4H_{10}N_2,C_6H_{10}O_4$ = 232.3.
*CAS — 142-88-1.*
*ATC — P02CB01.*

**Pharmacopoeias.** In *Eur.* (see p.vi), *Int., Jpn,* and *Viet.*

**Ph. Eur. 5.0** (Piperazine Adipate). A white crystalline powder. Soluble in water; practically insoluble in alcohol.

## Piperazine Citrate

Hydrous Tripiperazine Dicitrate; Piperazina, citrato de; Piperazini Citras.

$(C_4H_{10}N_2)_3,2C_6H_8O_7,xH_2O$ = 642.7 (anhydrous substance).
*CAS — 144-29-6 (anhydrous piperazine citrate); 41372-10-5 (piperazine citrate hydrate).*
*ATC — P02CB01.*

**Pharmacopoeias.** In *Chin., Eur.* (see p.vi), *Int., US,* and *Viet.*

**Ph. Eur. 5.0** (Piperazine Citrate). A white granular powder. It contains a variable amount of water. Freely soluble in water; practically insoluble in alcohol.

**USP 27** (Piperazine Citrate). A white, crystalline powder having not more than a slight odour. Soluble in water; insoluble in alcohol and in ether. pH of a 10% solution in water is about 5.

**Stability.** A decrease in the content of piperazine [as citrate] in syrups on storage was attributed to interaction with fructose and glucose formed by hydrolysis of sucrose.[1] A syrup prepared with sorbitol lost no potency when stored at 25° for 14 months.

1. Nielsen A, Reimer P. The stability of piperazine in syrup. *Arch Pharm Chemi (Sci)* 1975; **3:** 73–8.

## Piperazine Hydrate

Piperazina hexahidrato; Piperazini Hydras; Piperazinum Hydricum. Piperazine Hexahydrate.

$C_4H_{10}N_2,6H_2O$ = 194.2.
*CAS — 142-63-2.*
*ATC — P02CB01.*

**Pharmacopoeias.** In *Eur.* (see p.vi) and *Viet.*

**Ph. Eur. 5.0** (Piperazine Hydrate). Colourless deliquescent crystals. M.p. about 43°. Freely soluble in water and in alcohol. A 5% solution in water has a pH of 10.5 to 12.0. Store in airtight containers. Protect from light.

## Piperazine Phosphate

Piperazina, fosfato de; Piperazini Phosphas.

$C_4H_{10}N_2,H_3PO_4,H_2O$ = 202.1.
*CAS — 14538-56-8 (anhydrous piperazine phosphate); 18534-18-4 (piperazine phosphate monohydrate).*
*ATC — P02CB01.*

**Pharmacopoeias.** In *Br., Chin., Jpn,* and *Viet.*

**BP 2003** (Piperazine Phosphate). A white odourless or almost odourless crystalline powder. Sparingly soluble in water; practically insoluble in alcohol. A 1% solution in water has a pH of 6.0 to 6.5.

### Adverse Effects

Serious adverse effects are rare with piperazine and generally indicate overdosage or impaired excretion. Nausea, vomiting, diarrhoea, abdominal pain, headache, skin rashes, and urticaria occasionally occur. Severe neurotoxicity and EEG abnormalities have been reported with symptoms including somnolence, dizziness, nystagmus, muscular incoordination and weakness, ataxia, paraesthesia, myoclonic contractions, choreiform movements, tremor, convulsions, and loss of reflexes.

Transient visual disturbances such as blurred vision have occurred occasionally and there were reports of cataract formation after treatment with piperazine although they do not appear to have been substantiated.

Hypersensitivity reactions such as bronchospasm, Stevens-Johnson syndrome, and angioedema have occurred in some individuals.

◊ Piperazine has been taken off the market in some European countries because of general concern about its safety.[1] A study carried out in Sweden on 2 healthy subjects had indicated that mononitrosation of piperazine can occur in the stomach to produce the potential carcinogen *N*-mononitrosopiperazine; the more potent *N,N*-dinitrosopiperazine was not found.[2] However, the disease risk to man from such *N*-nitroso compounds has been questioned[3] and certainly reports of tumours associated with the use of piperazine have not been traced. Also, in the UK the Committee on Review of Medicines concluded that the incidence of serious adverse effects associated with piperazine was low and that, with appropriate pack warnings, piperazine products could remain as medicines available to the public through pharmacies.[1]

1. Anonymous. Data sheet changes for piperazine in pregnancy. *Pharm J* 1988; **240:** 367.
2. Bellander BTD, *et al.* Nitrosation of piperazine in the stomach. *Lancet* 1981; **ii:** 372.
3. Tannenbaum SR. N-nitroso compounds: a perspective on human exposure. *Lancet* 1983; **i:** 629–32.

**Effects on the blood.** A 4-year-old African boy with G6PD deficiency developed haemolytic anaemia; no cause for the haemolysis was found except that 2 days previously he had taken Pripsen (piperazine and senna).[1] Severe thrombocytopenia with epistaxis and haemoptysis, which developed in a 61-year-old man after piperazine self-medication, was probably the result of sensitisation to piperazine 15 years earlier.[2]

1. Buchanan N, *et al.* G-6-PD deficiency and piperazine. *BMJ* 1971; **2:** 110.
2. Cork MJ, *et al.* Pruritus ani, piperazine, and thrombocytopenia. *BMJ* 1990; **301:** 1398.

**Effects on the liver.** A reaction resembling viral hepatitis occurred on 2 occasions in a 25-year-old woman after use of piperazine; it appeared to be a hypersensitivity reaction.[1]

1. Hamlyn AN, *et al.* Piperazine hepatitis. *Gastroenterology* 1976; **70:** 1144–7.

**Hypersensitivity.** There has been a report[1] of a patient experiencing a serum-sickness-like illness associated with piperazine, which was followed by a delayed hypersensitivity vasculitis.

See also Effects on the Blood and Effects on the Liver, above.

1. Balzan M, Cacciottolo JM. Hypersensitivity vasculitis associated with piperazine therapy. *Br J Dermatol* 1994; **131:** 133–4.

### Precautions

Piperazine is contra-indicated in patients with epilepsy or severe renal impairment and should be given with care to patients with neurological disturbances or mild to moderate renal impairment. It should also be avoided or given with extreme caution in patients with hepatic impairment.

**Breast feeding.** The UK manufacturers of Pripsen (piperazine and senna) report that piperazine is distributed into breast milk. Mothers should be advised to take a dose after breast feeding then not to breast feed for 8 hours during which period milk should be expressed and discarded at the regular feeding times.

**Pregnancy.** It has been reported that piperazine is teratogenic in *rabbits* and that there have been isolated reports of fetal malformations following clinical use, though no causal relationship has been established. Two infants with malformations have been described briefly:[1] one had bilateral hare lip, cleft palate, and anophthalmia; the other had an abnormality of one foot. Both mothers had taken Pripsen (piperazine and senna). The UK manufacturers of Pripsen advise against use in pregnancy, especially during the first trimester, unless immediate treatment with piperazine is essential.

1. Leach FN. Management of threadworm infestation during pregnancy. *Arch Dis Child* 1990; **65:** 399–400.

## Interactions

The anthelmintic effects of piperazine and pyrantel may be antagonised when the two compounds are used together. The possibility that piperazine may enhance the adverse effects of phenothiazines such as chlorpromazine is discussed on p.680.

## Pharmacokinetics

Piperazine is readily absorbed from the gastrointestinal tract and is excreted in the urine within 24 hours, partly as metabolites. The rate at which different individuals excrete piperazine has been reported to vary widely. It is distributed into breast milk.

## Uses and Administration

Piperazine is an anthelmintic effective against the intestinal nematodes *Ascaris lumbricoides* (roundworm) and *Enterobius vermicularis* (pinworm, threadworm), although other anthelmintics are usually preferred (see the discussions on the treatment of ascariasis and enterobiasis on p.97 and p.99). In roundworms piperazine produces a neuromuscular block leading to a flaccid muscle paralysis in susceptible worms, which are then easily dislodged by the movement of the gut and expelled in the faeces.

Piperazine is usually given as the citrate or phosphate, but the adipate may also be used. The dosage of the salts of piperazine is usually expressed in terms of piperazine hydrate; 100 mg of piperazine hydrate is equivalent to about 44.4 mg of piperazine, 120 mg of piperazine adipate, 125 mg of piperazine citrate (110 mg of anhydrous piperazine citrate), and to 104 mg of piperazine phosphate.

For the treatment of ascariasis, a single dose, repeated once after 14 days, has been used. In adults and children over 12 years of age, a dose equivalent to 4.5 g of piperazine hydrate is given by mouth. Children aged 9 to 12 years may be given the equivalent of 3.75 g, those aged 6 to 8 years the equivalent of 3 g, those aged 4 to 5 years the equivalent of 2.25 g, and those aged 1 to 3 years the equivalent of 1.5 g. Children under 1 year should receive piperazine on medical advice only; a dose equivalent to 120 mg/kg has been suggested.

For enterobiasis, piperazine has been given for 7 days. A second course after a 7-day interval may be required. Adults and children over 12 years of age are given the equivalent of 2.25 g of the hydrate once daily, children aged 7 to 12 years the equivalent of 1.5 g daily, those aged 4 to 6 years the equivalent of 1.125 g daily, and those aged 1 to 3 years the equivalent of 750 mg daily. Children under 1 year should receive piperazine on medical advice only; a dose equivalent to 45 to 75 mg/kg has been suggested.

Piperazine is also used as a preparation with senna in a single dose of 4 g of the phosphate for adults and children over 6 years of age, repeated after 14 days for enterobiasis, or repeated monthly if necessary for up to 3 months to treat and prevent ascariasis.

## Preparations

***BP 2003:*** Piperazine Citrate Elixir; Piperazine Phosphate Tablets;
***USP 27:*** Piperazine Citrate Syrup; Piperazine Citrate Tablets.

**Proprietary Preparations** (details are given in Part 3)
***Braz.:*** Ascarin†; Ascarinase†; Ortovermim†; Oxiurazina†; Pipercream†; Pipervermin†; Trivermon†; Vermifran; Vermilen; ***Canad.:*** Entacyl; Verigat; Verimex†; ***Fr.:*** Antelmina†; Solucamphre†; Vermifuge; ***Ital.:*** Citropiperazina; ***Mex.:*** Desparasil; Helmifar; Lu-Peracina†; Overpon; Pipemed†; Piperawitt DS; Piperazil; Pipermed; Pirzinol; Verfid†; Vermin; ***Port.:*** Lombrimade; Pipermel; Pipertox; ***S.Afr.:*** Pipralen†; Piprine; ***Spain:*** Mimedran; Vermi; ***Thai.:*** Antepar†; Vermex; ***UK:*** Ectodyne†; Pripsen; Worm†; Wormex†.

**Multi-ingredient:** ***Belg.:*** Solucamphre†; ***Braz.:*** Licor de Cacau†; Lumbriquil†; Vermilen Composto; ***India:*** Helmazan; ***Irl.:*** Pripsen; ***Port.:*** Urocrasina†; ***Switz.:*** Carudol†; ***UK:*** Pripsen.

---

# Pomegranate Bark

Granado; Granati Cortex; Granatrinde; Granatum; Grenadier; Melograno; Pomegranate; Pomegranate Root Bark; Romeira.

## Profile

Pomegranate bark, the dried bark of the stem and root of *Punica granatum* (Punicaceae) containing about 0.4 to 0.9% of alkaloids,, has been used for the expulsion of tapeworms.

---

# Praziquantel *(BAN, USAN, rINN)*

EMBAY-8440; Prazicuantel; Praziquantelum. 2-Cyclohexylcarbonyl-1,2,3,6,7,11b-hexahydropyrazino[2,1-*a*]isoquinolin-4-one.
$C_{19}H_{24}N_2O_2$ = 312.4.
*CAS — 55268-74-1.*
*ATC — P02BA01.*

**Pharmacopoeias.** In *Chin., Eur.* (see p.vi), *Int.,* and *US.*

**Ph. Eur. 5.0** (Praziquantel). White or almost white crystalline powder. It exhibits polymorphism. Very slightly soluble in water; freely soluble in alcohol and in dichloromethane. Protect from light.

**USP 27** (Praziquantel). A white or practically white crystalline powder; odourless or with a faint characteristic odour. Very slightly soluble in water; freely soluble in alcohol and in chloroform. Protect from light.

## Adverse Effects

Adverse effects with praziquantel may be common but are usually mild and transient. Headache, diarrhoea, dizziness, drowsiness, malaise, abdominal discomfort, nausea, and vomiting have been reported most frequently. Hypersensitivity reactions such as fever, urticaria, pruritic skin rashes, and eosinophilia can occur; they may be due to death of the infecting parasites. Raised liver enzyme values have been reported rarely.

Most patients with neurocysticercosis who are given praziquantel suffer CNS effects, including headache, hyperthermia, seizures, and intracranial hypertension, which are thought to result from an inflammatory response to dead and dying parasites in the CNS. Use with corticosteroids is advised in such patients.

**Effects on the gastrointestinal tract.** Colicky abdominal pain and bloody diarrhoea occurred in a small community in Zaire shortly after treatment for *Schistosoma mansoni* infection with single doses of praziquantel 40 mg/kg by mouth.[1] A similar syndrome has been reported in some patients with *Schistosoma japonicum* infection given praziquantel.[2] The abdominal pain occurring in these patients was very different from the mild abdominal discomfort much more commonly reported with praziquantel therapy.

1. Polderman AM, *et al.* Side effects of praziquantel in the treatment of Schistosoma mansoni in Maniema, Zaire. *Trans R Soc Trop Med Hyg* 1984; **78:** 752–4.
2. Watt G, *et al.* Bloody diarrhoea after praziquantel therapy. *Trans R Soc Trop Med Hyg* 1986; **80:** 345–6.

**Effects on the nervous system.** Adverse nervous system effects are common in patients with neurocysticercosis given praziquantel. Neurological symptoms have also been reported[1] with the much lower doses of praziquantel used in the treatment of taeniasis in a patient with undiagnosed neurocysticercosis.

1. Flisser A, *et al.* Neurological symptoms in occult neurocysticercosis after single taenicidal dose of praziquantel. *Lancet* 1993; **342:** 748.

## Precautions

Praziquantel should not be used in patients with ocular cysticercosis because of the risk of severe eye damage resulting from destruction of the parasite.

Patients should be warned that praziquantel may cause dizziness or drowsiness and if affected they should not drive or operate machinery during or for 24 hours after treatment.

**Breast feeding.** Praziquantel is distributed into breast milk and mothers should not breast feed during treatment or for 72 hours thereafter.

## Interactions

**Anthelmintics.** For reference to plasma concentrations of the active metabolite of *albendazole* being increased by praziquantel, see p.101.

**Antiepileptics.** *Carbamazepine* and *phenytoin* have been reported to reduce the bioavailability of praziquantel.[1]

1. Quinn DI, Day RO. Drug interactions of clinical importance: an updated guide. *Drug Safety* 1995; **12:** 393–452.

**Antimalarials.** *Chloroquine* has been reported to reduce the bioavailability of praziquantel.[1]

1. Masimirembwa CM, *et al.* The effect of chloroquine on the pharmacokinetics and metabolism of praziquantel in rats and in humans. *Biopharm Drug Dispos* 1994; **15:** 33–43.

**Corticosteroids.** Some workers have proposed the use of *dexamethasone* to prevent the inflammatory response due to destroyed cysticerci in praziquantel treatment of cysticercosis. However, since dexamethasone roughly halves plasma concentrations of praziquantel,[1] it has been suggested that it be reserved for the short-term treatment of praziquantel-induced intracranial hypertension.

1. Vazquez ML, *et al.* Plasma levels of praziquantel decrease when dexamethasone is given simultaneously. *Neurology* 1987; **37:** 1561–2.

**Histamine $H_2$-antagonists.** *Cimetidine* has been reported to increase praziquantel bioavailability.[1,2]

1. Metwally A, *et al.* Effect of cimetidine, bicarbonate and glucose on the bioavailability of different formulations of praziquantel. *Arzneimittelforschung* 1995; **45:** 516–18.
2. Jung H, *et al.* Pharmacokinetic study of praziquantel administered alone and in combination with cimetidine in a single-day therapeutic regimen. *Antimicrob Agents Chemother* 1997; **41:** 1256–9.

## Pharmacokinetics

Praziquantel is rapidly absorbed after oral doses; more than 80% of a dose is reported to be absorbed. Peak plasma concentrations occur 1 to 3 hours after a dose, but there is a pronounced first-pass effect and praziquantel undergoes rapid and extensive metabolism in the liver, being hydroxylated to metabolites that are thought to be inactive. It is distributed into the CSF. The plasma elimination half-life of praziquantel is about 1 to 1.5 hours and that of the metabolites about 4 hours.

It is excreted in the urine, mainly as metabolites, about 80% of the dose being eliminated within 4 days and more than 90% of this in the first 24 hours.

Praziquantel is distributed into breast milk (see Breast Feeding under Precautions, above).

◊ References.

1. Leopold G, *et al.* Clinical pharmacology in normal volunteers of praziquantel, a new drug against schistosomes and cestodes: an example of a complex study covering both tolerance and pharmacokinetics. *Eur J Clin Pharmacol* 1978; **14:** 281–91.
2. Bühring KU, *et al.* Metabolism of praziquantel in man. *Eur J Drug Metab Pharmacokinet* 1978; **3:** 179–90.
3. Patzschke K, *et al.* Serum concentrations and renal excretion in humans after oral administration of praziquantel—results of three determination methods. *Eur J Drug Metab Pharmacokinet* 1979; **3:** 149–56.
4. Mandour M El M, *et al.* Pharmacokinetics of praziquantel in healthy volunteers and patients with schistosomiasis. *Trans R Soc Trop Med Hyg* 1990; **84:** 389–93.

## Uses and Administration

Praziquantel is an anthelmintic with a broad spectrum of activity against trematodes (flukes) including all species of *Schistosoma* pathogenic to man, and against cestodes (tapeworms). It is used in the treatment of cysticercosis, diphyllobothriasis, hymenolepiasis, schistosomiasis, taeniasis, and intestinal, liver, and lung fluke infections. For discussions of these infections and their treatment, see under Choice of Anthelmintic, p.97, and under the individual headings below.

Praziquantel is given by mouth with food.

In the treatment of schistosomiasis in adults and children it is given on one day as three doses of 20 mg/kg at intervals of 4 to 6 hours or it is given as a single dose of 40 mg/kg (but see below).

Doses in adults and children in the liver fluke infections clonorchiasis and opisthorchiasis are 25 mg/kg three times daily for one or two days or a single dose of 40 mg/kg. Similar doses may be used in intestinal fluke and lung fluke infections (see below).

Single doses of 5 to 25 mg/kg are used in adults and children in tapeworm infections.

Praziquantel is used in the treatment of neurocysticercosis in a dose of 50 mg/kg daily in 3 divided doses for 14 days. A corticosteroid should be given to reduce the severity of adverse effects.

◊ Reviews.

1. Pearson RD, Guerrant RL. Praziquantel: a major advance in anthelmintic therapy. *Ann Intern Med* 1983; **99:** 195–8. Correction. *ibid.*; 574.
2. King CH, Mahmoud AAF. Drugs five years later: praziquantel. *Ann Intern Med* 1989; **110:** 290–6.

**Cysticercosis.** Praziquantel is used in the treatment of neurocysticercosis (p.98) although albendazole may be more effective. References.

1. Sotelo J, *et al.* Therapy of parenchymal brain cysticercosis with praziquantel. *N Engl J Med* 1984; **310:** 1001–7.
2. Sotelo J, *et al.* Praziquantel for cysticercosis of the brain parenchyma. *N Engl J Med* 1984; **311:** 734.
3. Del Brutto OH, Sotelo J. Neurocysticercosis: an update. *Rev Infect Dis* 1988; **10:** 1075–87.
4. Ciferri F. Delayed CSF reaction to praziquantel. *Lancet* 1988; **i:** 642–3.
5. Moodley M, Moosa A. Treatment of neurocysticercosis: is praziquantel the new hope? *Lancet* 1989; **i:** 262–3.
6. Sotelo J. Praziquantel for neurocysticercosis. *Lancet* 1989; **i:** 897.
7. Crimmins D, *et al.* Neurocysticercosis: an under-recognized cause of neurological problems. *Med J Aust* 1990; **152:** 434–8.

8. Takayanagui JM, Jardim E. Therapy for neurocysticercosis: comparison between albendazole and praziquantel. *Arch Neurol* 1992; **49:** 290–4.
9. Mehta SS, *et al.* Albendazole versus praziquantel for neurocysticercosis. *Am J Health-Syst Pharm* 1998; **55:** 598–600.
10. Del Brutto OH, *et al.* Single-day praziquantel versus 1-week albendazole for neurocysticercosis. *Neurology* 1999; **52:** 1079–81.

**Echinococcosis.** Praziquantel may be used as an adjunct to surgery in echinococcosis (p.98). Praziquantel has been reported to possess a scolicidal effect *in vitro* against *Echinococcus granulosus*[1] and there has been a report of the successful treatment of disseminated peritoneal hydatid disease with praziquantel and surgery.[2] In this case praziquantel was effective against the small cysts; 2 large cysts were removed surgically, one before praziquantel was started. However, activity in 9 other patients given praziquantel was disappointing.[3]

1. Morris DL, *et al.* Protoscolicidal effect of praziquantel— in vitro and electron microscopical studies on Echinococcus granulosus. *J Antimicrob Chemother* 1986; **18:** 687–91.
2. Henriksen T-H, *et al.* Treatment of disseminated peritoneal hydatid disease with praziquantel. *Lancet* 1989; **i:** 272.
3. Piens MA, *et al.* Praziquantel dans l'hydatidose humaine: évaluation par traitement médical pré-opératoire. *Bull Soc Pathol Exot Filiales* 1989; **82:** 503–12.

**Intestinal fluke infections.** Praziquantel is used in the treatment of intestinal fluke infections (see p.99). In the treatment of fasciolopsiasis, heterophyiasis, and metagonimiasis, the usual recommended dose is 25 mg/kg three times daily for one day.[1] However, a single dose of 25 mg/kg has also been recommended.[2] Single doses of 15 mg/kg, 25 mg/kg, or 40 mg/kg all yielded a cure rate of 100% in a study in 72 primary-school children in Thailand who were harbouring *Fasciolopsis buski*, suggesting that a single dose of 15 mg/kg at bedtime might be tried.[3] In another study, 9 patients infected with the trematode *Nanophyetus salmincola* were treated with praziquantel 20 mg/kg three times daily for one day and were negative for eggs in their stools 2 to 12 weeks later,[4] and this has become the usual recommended dose.[1]

1. Medical Letter on Drugs and Therapeutics. Drugs for parasitic infections (issued April 2002). Available at: http://www.medicalletter.com/freedocs/parasitic.pdf (accessed 02/06/04)
2. WHO. *WHO model prescribing information: drugs used in parasitic diseases.* Geneva: WHO, 1995.
3. Harinasuta T, *et al.* Efficacy of praziquantel on fasciolopsiasis. *Arzneimittelforschung* 1984; **34:** 1214–15.
4. Fritsche TR, *et al.* Praziquantel for treatment of human Nanophyetus salmincola (Troglotrema salmincola) infection. *J Infect Dis* 1989; **160:** 896–9.

**Liver fluke infections.** Praziquantel is used in the treatment of clonorchiasis and opisthorchiasis, and has also been used in the treatment of fascioliasis (p.99) although in this latter infection bithionol or triclabendazole are preferred.

Various studies have shown praziquantel to be effective in clonorchiasis[1-4] and opisthorchiasis,[5,6] although one study in opisthorchiasis[7] showed that re-infection was common despite praziquantel therapy, particularly in those with heavy initial infection. A study in Thailand[8] confirmed that mass treatment for opisthorchiasis with a single dose of praziquantel was beneficial, although it was suggested that ideally treatment should be given twice a year.

While praziquantel is not the drug of choice for fascioliasis, there has been a report[9] of successful treatment of a patient with severe infection. Subsequent studies[10-12] have, however, shown praziquantel to be of little benefit.

1. Soh C-J. Clonorchis sinensis: experimental and clinical studies with praziquantel in Korea. *Arzneimittelforschung* 1984; **34:** 1156–9.
2. Chen C-Y, Hsieh W-C. Clonorchis sinensis: epidemiology in Taiwan and clinical experience with praziquantel. *Arzneimittelforschung* 1984; **34:** 1160–2.
3. Kuang Q-H, *et al.* Clonorchiasis: treatment with praziquantel in 50 cases. *Arzneimittelforschung* 1984; **34:** 1162–3.
4. Lee S-H. Large scale treatment of clonorchis sinensis infections with praziquantel under field conditions. *Arzneimittelforschung* 1984; **34:** 1227–8.
5. Bunnag D, *et al.* Opisthorchis viverrini: clinical experience with praziquantel in hospital for tropical diseases. *Arzneimittelforschung* 1984; **34:** 1173–4.
6. Ambroise-Thomas P, *et al.* Therapeutic results in opisthorchiasis with praziquantel in a reinfection-free environment in France. *Arzneimittelforschung* 1984; **34:** 1177–9.
7. Upatham ES, *et al.* Rate of re-infection by Opisthorchis viverrini in an endemic northeast Thai community after chemotherapy. *Int J Parasitol* 1988; **18:** 643–9.
8. Pungpak S, *et al.* Opisthorchis viverrini infection in Thailand: studies on the morbidity of the infection and resolution following praziquantel treatment. *Am J Trop Med Hyg* 1997; **56:** 311–14.
9. Schiappacasse RH, *et al.* Successful treatment of severe infection with Fasciola hepatica with praziquantel. *J Infect Dis* 1985; **152:** 1339–40.
10. Farag HF, *et al.* A short note on praziquantel in human fascioliasis. *J Trop Med Hyg* 1986; **89:** 79–80.
11. Farid Z, *et al.* Unsuccessful use of praziquantel to treat acute fascioliasis in children. *J Infect Dis* 1986; **154:** 920–1.
12. Farid Z, *et al.* Treatment of acute toxaemic fascioliasis. *Trans R Soc Trop Med Hyg* 1988; **82:** 299.

**Lung fluke infections.** Praziquantel is used in the treatment of the lung fluke infection paragonimiasis (p.99).

References.

1. Vanijanonta S, *et al.* Paragonimus heterotremus and other Paragonimus spp. in Thailand: pathogenesis clinic and treatment. *Arzneimittelforschung* 1984; **34:** 1186–8.
2. Pachucki CT, *et al.* American paragonimiasis treated with praziquantel. *N Engl J Med* 1984; **311:** 582–3.

**Schistosomiasis.** Praziquantel is the main drug used in the treatment of schistosomiasis (p.100). It is effective against all species of schistosomes.[1] The manufacturers recommend a dose of 20 mg/kg given three times in one day for all schistosomal infections. WHO[1] recommends a single dose of 40 mg/kg. WHO considers[1] that in the field such treatment will produce a cure rate of 60 to 90% with a reduction in egg count in those not cured of 90 to 95%. Good as such results are, a single dose or one day's sole treatment should not be considered to be all that is required to achieve a permanent cure or prevent re-infection, and any treatment plan should be reassessed after 6 or 12 months.[2,3] Such an approach with annual screening and targeted chemotherapy can provide, at least in some endemic areas, successful protection for children against intense infection and consequent hepatic disease.[3]

Several studies indicate that doses lower than those recommended above might be effective and in some control programmes 20 mg/kg might be enough for *S. haematobium*[4-6] or 30 mg/kg for *S. mansoni.*[4] The extent to which low doses contribute to resistance, as has been suggested with oxamniquine,[7] is unclear, but refractory infections have been reported. A 4-day treatment course was needed to produce a complete cure in a patient who relapsed twice following standard one-day treatment regimens.[8] Hepatic impairment, specifically hepatic fibrosis, is a feature of some schistosomal infections and patients with such liver involvement have benefited from treatment with praziquantel.[3,9]

1. WHO. The control of schistosomiasis: second report of the WHO expert committee. *WHO Tech Rep Ser 830* 1993.
2. Anonymous. The chemotherapy of schistosomiasis control. *Bull WHO* 1986; **64:** 23–5.
3. Anonymous. Mass treatment of schistosomiasis with praziquantel. *WHO Drug Inf* 1988; **2:** 184–5.
4. Taylor P, *et al.* Efficacy of low doses of praziquantel for Schistosoma mansoni and S. haematobium. *J Trop Med Hyg* 1988; **91:** 13–17.
5. King CH, *et al.* Dose-finding study for praziquantel therapy of Schistosoma haematobium in Coast Province, Kenya. *Am J Trop Med Hyg* 1989; **40:** 507–13.
6. Hatz C, *et al.* Ultrasound scanning for detecting morbidity due to Schistosoma haematobium and its resolution following treatment with different doses of praziquantel. *Trans R Soc Trop Med Hyg* 1990; **84:** 84–8.
7. Coles GC, *et al.* Tolerance of Kenyan Schistosoma mansoni to oxamniquine. *Trans R Soc Trop Med Hyg* 1987; **81:** 782–5.
8. Murray-Smith SQ, *et al.* A case of refractory schistosomiasis. *Med J Aust* 1996; **165:** 458.
9. Zwingenberger K, *et al.* Praziquantel in the treatment of hepatosplenic schistosomiasis: biochemical disease markers indicate deceleration of fibrogenesis and diminution of portal flow obstruction. *Trans R Soc Trop Med Hyg* 1990; **84:** 252–6.

**Taeniasis.** Praziquantel is used in the treatment of taeniasis (p.101). It has been studied in the mass control of taeniasis when a single dose of 5 mg/kg was used.[1]

Praziquantel is also effective against the larval form of *Taenia solium* and is used to treat neurocysticercosis (see above).

1. Cruz M, *et al.* Operational studies on the control of Taenia solium taeniasis/cysticercosis in Ecuador. *Bull WHO* 1989; **67:** 401–7.

## Preparations

**USP 27:** Praziquantel Tablets.

**Proprietary Preparations** (details are given in Part 3)
***Austral.:*** Biltricide; ***Braz.:*** Cestox; Cisticid; ***Canad.:*** Biltricide; ***Chile:*** Cesol; Cisticid; ***Fr.:*** Biltricide; ***Ger.:*** Biltricide; Cesol; Cysticide; ***Gr.:*** Biltricide; ***Hong Kong:*** Biltricide; ***Israel:*** Biltricide; ***Mex.:*** Bio-Cest; Cercon†; Cesol; Cisticid; Ehliten†; Extiser Q; Prozitel; Sincerck†; Teniken†; Waycital†; Zifartel†; ***Neth.:*** Biltricide; ***S.Afr.:*** Biltricide; Cysticide; ***Thai.:*** Biltricide†; Mycotricide; Opticide; Praquantel; Prasikon; Prazite; ***USA:*** Biltricide.

# Pyrantel Embonate *(BANM, rINNM)*

CP-10423-16; Embonato de pirantel; Pirantel Pamoate; Pyrantel Pamoate *(USAN)*; Pyranteli Embonas. 1,4,5,6-Tetrahydro-1-methyl-2-[(E)-2-(2-thienyl)vinyl]pyrimidine 4,4′-methylenebis(3-hydroxy-2-naphthoate).

$C_{11}H_{14}N_2S,C_{23}H_{16}O_6$ = 594.7.

*CAS — 15686-83-6 (pyrantel); 22204-24-6 (pyrantel embonate).*

*ATC — P02CC01.*

**Pharmacopoeias.** In *Chin., Eur.* (see p.vi), *Int., Jpn, Pol.,* and *US.*

**Ph. Eur. 5.0** (Pyrantel Embonate). A pale yellow or yellow powder. Practically insoluble in water and in methyl alcohol; soluble in dimethyl sulfoxide. Protect from light.

**USP 27** (Pyrantel Pamoate). A yellow to tan solid. Practically insoluble in water and in methyl alcohol; soluble in dimethyl sulfoxide; slightly soluble in dimethylformamide. Protect from light.

## Adverse Effects and Precautions

The adverse effects of pyrantel embonate are generally mild and transient. The most frequent are gastrointestinal effects such as nausea and vomiting, anorexia, abdominal pain, and diarrhoea. Other adverse effects reported include headache, dizziness, drowsiness, insomnia, skin rashes, and raised liver enzyme values. Pyrantel embonate should be used with caution in patients with hepatic impairment.

## Interactions

The anthelmintic effects of both pyrantel and piperazine may be antagonised when the two drugs are used together.

## Pharmacokinetics

Only a small proportion of a dose of pyrantel embonate is absorbed from the gastrointestinal tract. Up to about 7% is excreted as unchanged drug and metabolites in the urine but over half of the dose is excreted unchanged in the faeces.

## Uses and Administration

Pyrantel embonate is an anthelmintic effective against intestinal nematodes including roundworms (*Ascaris lumbricoides*), threadworms (*Enterobius vermicularis*), and *Trichostrongylus* spp., the tissue nematode *Trichinella spiralis*, and hookworms, although it is possibly less effective against *Necator americanus* hookworms than against *Ancylostoma duodenale*. Pyrantel embonate is one of the anthelmintics that may be used in the treatment of infections with these worms, as discussed under Choice of Anthelmintic, p.97. It appears to act by paralysing susceptible worms which are then dislodged by peristaltic activity.

Pyrantel is given by mouth as the embonate, but doses are described in terms of the base. Pyrantel embonate 2.9 g is approximately equivalent to 1 g of pyrantel.

Single or mixed infections due to susceptible worms in adults and children may be treated with the equivalent of pyrantel 10 mg/kg as a single oral dose. Ascariasis occurring alone may only require 5 mg/kg; a single dose of 2.5 mg/kg given three or four times a year has been used in mass treatment programmes. In necatoriasis, 10 mg/kg daily for 3 days or 20 mg/kg daily for 2 days may be necessary. The response in enterobiasis may be improved by repeating the 10 mg/kg dose after 2 to 4 weeks. In trichinosis, a dose of 10 mg/kg daily for 5 days has been used.

## Preparations

**USP 27:** Pyrantel Pamoate Oral Suspension.

**Proprietary Preparations** (details are given in Part 3)
***Arg.:*** Aut; ***Austral.:*** Anthel; Combantrin; Early Bird; ***Austria:*** Combantrin; ***Braz.:*** Ascarical; ***Canad.:*** Combantrin; Jaa Pyral; ***Fr.:*** Combantrin; Helmintox; ***Ger.:*** Helmex; ***Gr.:*** Combantrin; ***Hong Kong:*** Combantrin; Pyrantin; Pyrantrin; ***India:*** Nemocid; ***Israel:*** Combantrin; ***Ital.:*** Combantrin; ***Mex.:*** Combantrin; Pirantrim†; ***NZ:*** Combantrin; ***Port.:*** Combantrin; Vertel; ***S.Afr.:*** Combantrin; ***Spain:*** Lombriareu; Trilombrin; ***Switz.:*** Cobantril; ***Thai.:*** Bantel; Combantrin†; Pyrapam; ***USA:*** Antiminth; Pin-Rid; Pin-X; Reese's Pinworm.

# Pyrvinium Embonate *(rINNM)*

Embonato de pirvinio; Pyrvinium Pamoate *(BAN)*; Viprynium Embonate; Viprynium Pamoate. Bis{6-dimethylamino-2-[2-(2,5-dimethyl-1-phenylpyrrol-3-yl)vinyl]-1-methylquinolinium} 4,4′-methylenebis(3-hydroxy-2-naphthoate).

$C_{52}H_{56}N_6,C_{23}H_{14}O_6$ = 1151.4.

*CAS — 3546-41-6.*

*ATC — P02CX01.*

**Pharmacopoeias.** In *US.*

**USP 27** (Pyrvinium Pamoate). A bright orange or orange-red to practically black crystalline powder. Practically insoluble in water and in ether; slightly soluble in chloroform and in methoxyethanol; freely soluble in glacial acetic acid; very slightly soluble in methyl alcohol. Store in airtight containers. Protect from light.

## Adverse Effects

Pyrvinium occasionally causes nausea, vomiting, abdominal pain, and diarrhoea. Hypersensitivity reactions and photosensitivity have been reported. Headache may occur.

Pyrvinium stains the stools bright red and may stain clothing if vomiting occurs.

## Pharmacokinetics

Pyrvinium embonate is not significantly absorbed from the gastrointestinal tract.

## Uses and Administration

Pyrvinium embonate is an effective anthelmintic in the treatment of enterobiasis (p.99), but has generally been superseded by other drugs.

Pyrvinium is given as the embonate but doses are described in terms of the base. Pyrvinium embonate 7.5 mg is approximately equivalent to 5 mg of pyrvinium.

It has been administered by mouth in a single dose equivalent to pyrvinium 5 mg/kg, repeated after 2 to 3 weeks.

### Preparations

**USP 27:** Pyrvinium Pamoate Oral Suspension; Pyrvinium Pamoate Tablets.

**Proprietary Preparations** (details are given in Part 3)
***Arg.:*** Tru; ***Austria:*** Molevac; ***Braz.:*** Enterocid; Pyr-Pam; Pyvermt†; ***Canad.:*** Vanquin; ***Denm.:*** Vanquin; ***Fin.:*** Pyrvin; ***Fr.:*** Povanyl; ***Ger.:*** Molevac; Pyrcon; ***Norw.:*** Vanquin; ***Spain:*** Pamoxan; ***Swed.:*** Vanquin; ***Switz.:*** Molevac†.

**Multi-ingredient:** ***Braz.:*** Contrelmin†; Vermizol†.

## Rafoxanide *(BAN, USAN, rINN)*

MK-990; Rafoxanida. 3′-Chloro-4′-(4-chlorophenoxy)-3,5-di-iodosalicylanilide.

$C_{19}H_{11}Cl_2I_2NO_3$ = 626.0.
*CAS — 22662-39-1.*

### Profile

Rafoxanide is an anthelmintic used in veterinary medicine for the treatment of fascioliasis in cattle and sheep.

## Santonin

Santonina; Santoninum. (3S,3aS,5aS,9bS)-3a,5,5a,9b-Tetrahydro-3,5a,9-trimethylnaphtho[1,2-*b*]furan-2,8(3*H*,4*H*)-dione.

$C_{15}H_{18}O_3$ = 246.3.
*CAS — 481-06-1.*

**Pharmacopoeias.** In *Jpn.*

### Profile

Santonin is a crystalline lactone obtained from the dried unexpanded flowerheads of *Artemisia cina* (santonica, wormwood) and other species of *Artemisia* (Compositae). It was formerly used as an anthelmintic in the treatment of roundworm (*Ascaris*) infection, but has been superseded by other less toxic anthelmintics.

It is used as a flavour in food.

## Selamectin *(USAN, rINN)*

Selamectina; UK-124114. (2aE,4E,5′S,6S,6′S,7S,8E,11R,13R,15S,17aR,20aR,20bS)-6′-Cyclohexyl-7-[(2,6-dideoxy-3-*O*-methyl-α-L-*arabino*-hexopyranosyl)oxy]-3′,4′,5′,6,6′,7,10,11,14,15,20a,20b-dodecahydro-20b-hydroxy-5′,6,8,19-tetramethylspiro(11,15-methano-2*H*,13*H*,17*H*-furo[4,3,2-*p*,*q*][2,6]benzodioxacyclooctadecin-13,2′-[2*H*]pyran)-17,20(17a*H*)-dione 20-oxime.

$C_{43}H_{63}NO_{11}$ = 770.0.
*CAS — 165108-07-6.*

### Profile

Selamectin is an avermectin anthelmintic and ectoparasiticide used in veterinary medicine.

## Tetramisole Hydrochloride *(BANM, USAN, rINNM)*

Hidrocloruro de tetramisol; ICI-50627; McN-JR-8299-11; R8299. (±)-2,3,5,6-Tetrahydro-6-phenylimidazo[2,1-*b*]thiazole hydrochloride.

$C_{11}H_{12}N_2S,HCl$ = 240.8.
*CAS — 5036-02-2 (tetramisole); 5086-74-8 (tetramisole hydrochloride).*

**Pharmacopoeias.** In *Fr.* for veterinary use only.

### Profile

Tetramisole hydrochloride is an anthelmintic used in veterinary medicine for the control of nematode infections. It is a racemic mixture and the laevo-isomer, levamisole hydrochloride (p.107), accounts for most of its activity.

### Preparations

**Proprietary Preparations** (details are given in Part 3)
***Braz.:*** Ascarotrat†; Ascaverm†; Cofasol†; Tetramizotil.

**Multi-ingredient:** ***Braz.:*** Tetramizol Composto†; Vermizol†; ***India:*** Jetomisol-P.

## Thiacetarsamide

Tiacetarsamida. *p*-[Bis(carboxymethylmercapto)arsino]benzamide; 4-Carbamylphenyl bis[carboxymethylthio]arsenite.

$C_{11}H_{12}AsNO_5S_2$ = 377.3.
*CAS — 531-72-6.*

### Profile

Thiacetarsamide is an anthelmintic used in veterinary medicine.

## Thiophanate *(BAN)*

Tiofanato. 4,4′-*o*-Phenylenebis(ethyl 3-thioallophanate).

$C_{14}H_{18}N_4O_4S_2$ = 370.4.
*CAS — 23564-06-9.*

### Profile

Thiophanate is an anthelmintic used in veterinary medicine for the control of nematode infections.

## Tiabendazole *(BAN, rINN)*

E233; MK-360; Thiabendazole *(USAN)*; Tiabendazol; Tiabendazolum. 2-(Thiazol-4-yl)-1*H*-benzimidazole.

$C_{10}H_7N_3S$ = 201.2.
*CAS — 148-79-8.*
*ATC — D01AC06; P02CA02.*

**Pharmacopoeias.** In *Chin., Eur.* (see p.vi), *Int.*, and *US.*

**Ph. Eur. 5.0** (Tiabendazole). A white or almost white crystalline powder. Practically insoluble in water; slightly soluble in alcohol and in dichloromethane; it dissolves in dilute mineral acids. Protect from light.

**USP 27** (Thiabendazole ). A white to practically white, odourless or practically odourless, powder. Practically insoluble in water; slightly soluble in alcohol and in acetone; very slightly soluble in chloroform and in ether.

### Adverse Effects

Dizziness and gastrointestinal disturbances, especially anorexia, nausea and vomiting, diarrhoea, and abdominal pain are common during treatment with tiabendazole. Other adverse effects occurring occasionally include pruritus, skin rashes, headache, fatigue, drowsiness, drying of mucous membranes, hyperglycaemia, disturbance of vision including colour vision, leucopenia, tinnitus, effects on the liver including cholestasis and parenchymal damage (in some cases severe and irreversible), enuresis, crystalluria, and bradycardia and hypotension. There have also been reports of erythema multiforme, fatal Stevens-Johnson syndrome, toxic epidermal necrolysis, convulsions, and effects on mental state.

Fever, chills, angioedema, and lymphadenopathy have been reported, but may represent allergic response to dead parasites rather than to tiabendazole.

The urine of some patients taking tiabendazole may have a characteristic odour similar to that following the ingestion of asparagus; it is attributed to the presence of a tiabendazole metabolite.

**Effects on the salivary glands.** Dry mouth with swollen parotid and salivary glands suggestive of the sicca complex preceded the development of cholestatic jaundice in a 17-year-old boy given tiabendazole.[1]

1. Davidson RN, *et al.* Intrahepatic cholestasis after thiabendazole. *Trans R Soc Trop Med Hyg* 1988; **82:** 620.

**Hypersensitivity.** Severe erythema multiforme developed in a patient 16 days after a course of tiabendazole.[1] Many of the lesions encircled pre-existing melanocytic naevi.

1. Humphreys F, Cox NH. Thiabendazole-induced erythema multiforme with lesions around melanocytic naevi. *Br J Dermatol* 1988; **118:** 855–6.

### Precautions

Tiabendazole should be used with caution in patients with hepatic or renal impairment. Tiabendazole causes drowsiness in some patients and those affected should not drive or operate machinery.

Tiabendazole should not be used in mixed worm infections involving *Ascaris lumbricoides* as it can cause these roundworms to migrate; live roundworms have emerged through the mouth or nose.

**Pregnancy.** Tiabendazole is teratogenic in *mice* although the manufacturers note that there are no adequate and well controlled studies in human pregnancy.

**Renal impairment.** Tiabendazole and its 5-hydroxy metabolite did not accumulate in an anephric patient on haemodialysis and haemoperfusion who was receiving treatment for severe strongyloidiasis.[1] However, the potentially toxic conjugated glucuronide and sulfate metabolites did accumulate. The clearance of all 3 metabolites was poor by haemodialysis; haemoperfusion was much more efficient, although for rapid removal the haemoperfusion columns should be changed every hour.

1. Bauer L, *et al.* The pharmacokinetics of thiabendazole and its metabolites in an anephric patient undergoing hemodialysis and hemoperfusion. *J Clin Pharmacol* 1982; **22:** 276–80.

### Interactions

**Xanthines.** For the effect of tiabendazole on serum concentrations of *theophylline*, see p.803.

### Pharmacokinetics

Tiabendazole is readily absorbed from the gastrointestinal tract and reaches peak concentrations in the plasma after 1 to 2 hours. It is metabolised to 5-hydroxythiabendazole and excreted principally in the urine as glucuronide or sulfate conjugates; about 90% is recovered in the urine within 48 hours of ingestion, but only 5% in the faeces. Absorption may occur from preparations applied to the skin or eyes.

◊ References.

1. Tocco DJ, *et al.* Absorption, metabolism, and excretion of thiabendazole in man and laboratory animals. *Toxicol Appl Pharmacol* 1966; **9:** 31–9.

### Uses and Administration

Tiabendazole, a benzimidazole derivative, is an anthelmintic with activity against most nematode worms; activity against some larval stages and ova has also been demonstrated. The mode of action is not certain, but tiabendazole may inhibit the fumarate-reductase system of worms thereby interfering with their source of energy.

Tiabendazole is used in the treatment of cutaneous larva migrans, dracunculiasis (guinea worm infection), and toxocariasis. It may also be used in the treatment of strongyloidiasis, and can provide symptomatic relief during the larval invasion stage of trichinosis. Tiabendazole is also active against some intestinal nematodes, but should not be used as primary therapy; the treatment of mixed infections including ascariasis is not recommended since tiabendazole may cause the worms to migrate to other body organs causing serious complications. For discussions of the treatment of the above infections see under Choice of Anthelmintic, p.97, and under the individual headings below.

Tiabendazole is given by mouth, with meals, usually in a dose of 25 mg/kg twice daily for 2 or more days, the duration depending on the type of infection; the daily dose should not exceed 3 g. For those unable to tolerate 2 doses daily, 25 mg/kg may be given after the largest meal on day 1 and repeated 24 hours later after a similar meal on day 2. For mass treatment, a single dose of 50 mg/kg after the evening meal is suggested although the incidence of adverse effects may be higher than with 2 doses of 25 mg/kg.

In cutaneous larva migrans, 25 mg/kg may be given twice daily for 2 days, repeated after 2 days if necessary; topical treatment with a 10 to 15% suspension intended for oral use has also been advocated as an alternative or adjunct to oral treatment.

In dracunculiasis, 25 to 50 mg/kg may be given twice daily for one day; in massive infection a further 50 mg/kg may be given after 5 to 8 days.

In strongyloidiasis, 25 mg/kg may be given twice daily for 2 or 3 days or 50 mg/kg as a single dose; when the infection is disseminated treatment for at least 5 days may be necessary.

In trichinosis, 25 mg/kg may be given twice daily for 2 to 4 successive days.

In toxocariasis, 25 mg/kg may be given twice daily for 7 days.

Tiabendazole also has some antifungal activity. It is used as a fungicidal preservative for certain foods.

**Dracunculiasis.** Tiabendazole[1,2] may be used for symptomatic treatment of dracunculiasis (p.98), although it has no direct anthelmintic effect. It is used to facilitate removal of the worm from subcutaneous tissues.

1. Muller R. Guinea worm disease: epidemiology, control, and treatment. *Bull WHO* 1979; **57:** 683–9.
2. Kale OO, *et al.* Controlled comparative trial of thiabendazole and metronidazole in the treatment of dracontiasis. *Ann Trop Med Parasitol* 1983; **77:** 151–7.

**Strongyloidiasis.** Tiabendazole may be used in the treatment of strongyloidiasis (p.100), but albendazole or ivermectin are generally preferred.

References.

1. Grove DI. Treatment of strongyloidiasis with thiabendazole: an analysis of toxicity and effectiveness. *Trans R Soc Trop Med Hyg* 1982; **76:** 114–18.

2. Barnish G, Barker J. An intervention study using thiabendazole suspension against strongyloides fuelleborni-like infections in Papua New Guinea. *Trans R Soc Trop Med Hyg* 1987; **81:** 60–3.
3. Boken DJ, *et al.* Treatment of Strongyloides stercoralis hyperinfection syndrome with thiabendazole administered per rectum. *Clin Infect Dis* 1993; **16:** 123–6.
4. Gann PH, *et al.* A randomized trial of single- and two-dose ivermectin versus thiabendazole for treatment of strongyloidiasis. *J Infect Dis* 1994; **169:** 1076–9.
5. Pitisuttithum P, *et al.* A randomized comparative study of albendazole and thiabendazole in chronic strongyloidiasis. *Southeast Asian J Trop Med Public Health* 1995; **26:** 735–8.
6. Schaffel R, *et al.* Thiabendazole for the treatment of strongyloidiasis in patients with hematologic malignancies. *Clin Infect Dis* 2000; **31:** 821–2.


**Syngamosis.** Tiabendazole has been used successfully[1,2] to treat syngamosis (p.101) when it has occurred in man.


1. Grell GAC, *et al.* Syngamus in a West Indian. *BMJ* 1978; **2:** 1464.
2. Leers W-D, *et al.* Syngamosis, an unusual case of asthma: the first reported case in Canada. *Can Med Assoc J* 1985; **132:** 269–70.


## Preparations

***BP 2003:*** Tiabendazole Tablets;
***USP 27:*** Thiabendazole Oral Suspension; Thiabendazole Tablets.

**Proprietary Preparations** (details are given in Part 3)

***Arg.:*** Foldan; ***Austral.:*** Mintezol; ***Braz.:*** Benzol; Foldan; Folderm†; Thiaben; Thianax; Tiabenzol; Tiabiose†; Tiaplex; Tutiverm†; ***Canad.:*** Mintezol†; ***Chile:*** Soldrin; ***Gr.:*** Mintezol; ***Irl.:*** Mintezol†; ***Mex.:*** Eprofil†; ***Spain:*** Triasox; ***UK:*** Mintezol†; ***USA:*** Mintezol.

**Multi-ingredient:** ***Braz.:*** Contrelmin†; Derms; Flenverme†; Folderm Pomada; Forverm; Helmi-Ped; Helmib†; Helmiben; Helmidrax; Micoplex; Neovermin; Octelmin; Poliben; Profium; Prohelmin; Tetramizol Composto†; Thiabena; Travogyn; Vermilen Composto; Vermol; Zoles.

## Triclabendazole *(BAN, rINN)*

Triclabendazol. 5-Chloro-6-(2,3-dichlorophenoxy)-2-(methylthio)benzimidazole.

$C_{14}H_9Cl_3N_2OS$ = 359.7.

*CAS — 68786-66-3.*

*ATC — P02BX04.*

### Profile

Triclabendazole is a benzimidazole anthelmintic used in veterinary medicine for the treatment of fascioliasis. It is also increasingly being used in the treatment of human fascioliasis, and is under investigation for the treatment of human paragonimiasis.

**Liver fluke infections.** Although bithionol or praziquantel are used to treat fascioliasis (p.99), some consider triclabendazole to be the drug of choice.[1] A suggested dose is 10 mg/kg, given as a single dose after food.[1] Several studies[2-5] have demonstrated the efficacy of triclabendazole in fascioliasis.


1. Medical Letter on Drugs and Therapeutics. Drugs for parasitic infections (issued April 2002). Available at: http://www.medicalletter.com/freedocs/parasitic.pdf (accessed 02/06/04)
2. Apt W, *et al.* Treatment of human chronic fascioliasis with triclabendazole: drug efficacy and serologic response. *Am J Trop Med Hyg* 1995; **52:** 532–5.
3. El-Karaksy H, *et al.* Human fascioliasis in Egyptian children: successful treatment with triclabendazole. *J Trop Pediatr* 1999; **45:** 135–8.
4. Millán JC, *et al.* The efficacy and tolerability of triclabendazole in Cuban patients with latent and chronic Fasciola hepatica infection. *Am J Trop Med Hyg* 2000; **63:** 264–9.
5. Graham CS, *et al.* Imported Fasciola hepatica infection in the United States and treatment with triclabendazole. *Clin Infect Dis* 2001; **33:** 1–5.


**Lung fluke infections.** Encouraging results were reported from a pilot study of triclabendazole[1] in the treatment of paragonimiasis (p.99). In an open comparative study[2] in 62 patients, a more rapid parasitological response was obtained with triclabendazole in doses of 5 mg/kg once daily for 3 days, 10 mg/kg twice on one day, or 10 mg/kg as a single dose, than with praziquantel. Clinical symptoms resolved at a comparable rate in all groups.


1. Ripert C, *et al.* Therapeutic effect of triclabendazole in patients with paragonimiasis in Cameroon: a pilot study. *Trans R Soc Trop Med Hyg* 1992; **86:** 417.
2. Calvopiña M, *et al.* Treatment of human pulmonary paragonimiasis with triclabendazole: clinical tolerance and drug efficacy. *Trans R Soc Trop Med Hyg* 1998; **92:** 566–9.

# Antibacterials

Drug Groups, p.116
- Aminoglycosides, p.116
- Antimycobacterials, p.117
- Cephalosporins and related Beta Lactams, p.117
- Chloramphenicols, p.117
- Glycopeptides, p.118
- Lincosamides, p.118
- Macrolides, p.118
- Penicillins, p.118
- Quinolones, p.119
- Sulfonamides and Diaminopyrimidines, p.119
- Tetracyclines, p.119
- Miscellaneous Antibacterials, p.120

Choice of Antibacterial, p.120
- Abscess, abdominal, p.120
- Abscess, brain, p.120
- Abscess, liver, p.120
- Abscess, lung, p.120
- Actinomycosis, p.120
- Anaerobic bacterial infections, p.121
- Anthrax, p.121
- Antibiotic-associated colitis, p.121
- Arthritis, bacterial, p.121
- Bacillary angiomatosis, p.121
- Bacterial vaginosis, p.121
- Biliary-tract infections, p.121
- Bites and stings, p.121
- Bone and joint infections, p.122
- Botulism, p.122
- Bronchitis, p.122
- Brucellosis, p.122
- Campylobacter enteritis, p.123
- Cat scratch disease, p.123
- Cellulitis, p.123
- Cervicitis, p.123
- Chancroid, p.123
- Chlamydial infections, p.123
- Cholera and other vibrio infections, p.123
- Cystic fibrosis, p.123
- Diarrhoea, infective, p.125
- Diphtheria, p.125
- Ear infections, p.125
- Ehrlichiosis, p.125
- Endocarditis, p.125
- Endometritis, p.126
- Enterococcal infections, p.126
- Epididymitis, p.127
- Epiglottitis, p.127
- Escherichia coli enteritis, p.127
- Eye infections, p.127
- Gas gangrene, p.127
- Gastro-enteritis, p.127
  - Antibiotic-associated colitis, p.128
  - Campylobacter enteritis, p.128
  - Cholera and other vibrio infections, p.128
  - Escherichia coli enteritis, p.129
  - Necrotising enterocolitis, p.129
  - Salmonella enteritis, p.129
  - Shigellosis, p.130
  - Yersinia enteritis, p.130
- Gonorrhoea, p.130
- Granuloma inguinale, p.131
- Haemophilus influenzae infections, p.131
- Helicobacter pylori infections, p.131
- Infections in immunocompromised patients, p.131
- Intensive care, p.132
- Legionnaires' disease, p.133
- Leprosy, p.133
- Leptospirosis, p.133
- Listeriosis, p.134
- Lyme disease, p.134
- Lymphogranuloma venereum, p.134
- Melioidosis, p.134
- Meningitis, p.134
- Meningococcal infections, p.135
- Mouth infections, p.136
- Mycetoma, p.136
- Necrotising enterocolitis, p.136
- Necrotising fasciitis, p.136
- Neonatal conjunctivitis, p.136
- Nocardiosis, p.137
- Obstetric disorders, p.137
- Opportunistic mycobacterial infections, p.137
- Osteomyelitis, p.138
- Otitis externa, p.138
- Otitis media, p.138
- Pancreatitis, p.139
- Pelvic inflammatory disease, p.139
- Peptic ulcer disease, p.139
- Perinatal streptococcal infections, p.139
- Peritonitis, p.140
- Pertussis, p.140
- Pharyngitis, p.140
- Pinta, p.141
- Plague, p.141
- Pneumonia, p.141
- Pregnancy and the neonate, p.143
- Premature labour, p.143
- Proctitis, p.143
- Prostatitis, p.143
- Psittacosis, p.143
- Q fever, p.143
- Relapsing fever, p.143
- Respiratory-tract infections, p.144
- Rheumatic fever, p.144
- Rickettsial infections, p.144
- Salmonella enteritis, p.144
- Salpingitis, p.144
- Septicaemia, p.144
- Sexually transmitted diseases, p.145
- Shigellosis, p.145
- Sickle-cell disease, p.146
- Sinusitis, p.146
- Skin infections, p.146
- Spleen disorders, p.146
- Spotted fevers, p.147
- Staphylococcal infections, p.147
- Surgical infection, p.147
- Syphilis, p.148
- Tetanus, p.149
- Tonsillitis, p.149
- Toxic shock syndrome, p.149
- Trachoma, p.149
- Trench fever, p.150
- Tuberculosis, p.150
- Tularaemia, p.152
- Typhoid and paratyphoid fever, p.152
- Typhus, p.152
- Urethritis, p.152
- Urinary-tract infections, p.153
  - Catheter-related, p.153
  - The elderly, p.153
  - Infants and children, p.153
  - Men, p.153
  - Pregnancy, p.153
  - Women, p.153
- Whipple's disease, p.153
- Yaws, p.153
- Yersinia enteritis, p.153

This chapter includes antimicrobial drugs that are used principally in the treatment and prophylaxis of bacterial infections. In practice the term 'antibiotics' is often, and in some instances erroneously, used to encompass all of these drugs. In *Martindale* the term antibacterial is generally used in this chapter. The various groups into which these drugs may be categorised are described below. Antibacterials described elsewhere in *Martindale* include metronidazole (p.607) which, as well as being an antiprotozoal, is used in the treatment of anaerobic bacterial infections.

Immunological approaches to the treatment and prophylaxis of bacterial infections are discussed under Vaccines Immunoglobulins and Antisera, p.1605.

In addition, disinfectants and preservatives (p.1164) are used to kill or inhibit the growth of micro-organisms.

## Drug Groups

Although antibacterials are a very diverse class of compounds they are often classified and discussed in groups. They may be classified according to their mode of action or spectrum of antimicrobial activity, but generally those with similar chemical structures are grouped together.

### Aminoglycosides

The aminoglycosides are a closely related group of bactericidal antibacterials derived from bacteria of the order Actinomycetales or, more specifically, the genus *Streptomyces* (framycetin, kanamycin, neomycin, paromomycin, streptomycin, and tobramycin) and the genus *Micromonospora* (gentamicin and sisomicin). They are polycationic compounds that contain an aminocyclitol, usually 2-deoxystreptamine, or streptidine in streptomycin and related compounds, with cyclic amino-sugars attached by glycosidic linkages. Therefore, they have also been termed aminoglycosidic aminocyclitols. The sulfate salts are generally used.

The aminoglycosides have broadly similar toxicological features. Ototoxicity is a major limitation to their use; streptomycin and gentamicin are generally considered to be more toxic to the vestibular branch of the eighth cranial nerve and neomycin and kanamycin to be more toxic to the auditory branch. Other adverse effects common to the group include nephrotoxicity, neuromuscular blockade, and allergy, including cross-reactivity.

The pharmacokinetics of the aminoglycosides are very similar. Little is absorbed from the gastrointestinal tract but they are generally well distributed in the body after parenteral administration although penetration into the CSF is poor. They are excreted unchanged in the urine by glomerular filtration.

The aminoglycosides have a similar antimicrobial spectrum and appear to act by interfering with bacterial protein synthesis, possibly by binding irreversibly to the 30S and to some extent the 50S portions of the bacterial ribosome. The manner in which they bring about cell death is not fully understood. They are most active against Gram-negative rods. *Staphylococcus aureus* is susceptible to the aminoglycosides but otherwise most Gram-positive bacteria, and also anaerobic bacteria, are naturally resistant. Aminoglycosides show enhanced activity with penicillins against some enterococci and streptococci. Bacterial resistance to streptomycin may occur by mutation, whereas with the other aminoglycosides it is usually associated with the plasmid-mediated production of inactivating enzymes which are capable of phosphorylation, acetylation, or adenylation. The aminoglycosides have a postantibiotic effect, that is antibacterial activity persisting after concentrations have dropped below minimum inhibitory concentrations.

*Streptomycin* was the first aminoglycoside to become available commercially and was isolated from a strain of *Streptomyces griseus* in 1944. Its use is now restricted mainly to the treatment of tuberculosis when it is always given with other antituberculous drugs because of the rapid development of resistance. *Dihydrostreptomycin*, a reduction product of streptomycin, is only rarely used because of its toxicity. The *neomycin* complex of antibacterials were the next to be isolated; neomycin itself is mainly a mixture of the B and C isomers and neomycin B is considered to be identical with *framycetin*. Because of their toxicity they are not given systemically. The related compound *paromomycin* (p.612) also has antiprotozoal and anthelmintic properties and may be used in the treatment of intestinal amoebiasis, cestode infections, cryptosporidiosis, and leishmaniasis. *Kanamycin* is less toxic than neomycin and can be used systemically. Although it has been used in penicillin-resistant gonorrhoea, it is not active against *Pseudomonas aeruginosa* and has generally been replaced by gentamicin and other newer aminoglycosides.

*Gentamicin* was isolated from *Micromonospora purpurea* in 1963 and, being active against *Ps. aeruginosa* and *Serratia marcescens*, is widely used in the treatment of life-threatening infections. *Tobramycin* is one of several components of the nebramycin complex of aminoglycosides produced by *Streptomyces tenebrarius*. It has an antimicrobial spectrum very similar to that of gentamicin and is reported to be more active against *Ps. aeruginosa*. *Amikacin*, a semisynthetic derivative of kanamycin, has a side-chain rendering it less susceptible to inactivating enzymes. It has a spectrum of activity like that of gentamicin but Gram-negative bacteria resistant to gentamicin, tobramycin, and kanamycin are often sensitive. *Sisomicin* is closely related structurally to gentamicin. *Netilmicin*, the

*N*-ethyl derivative of sisomicin, may be active against some gentamicin-resistant strains of bacteria although not to the same extent as amikacin. Other aminoglycosides include *apramycin, arbekacin, astromicin, bekanamycin, dibekacin, isepamicin, and micronomicin*.

Aminoglycosides should in general only be used for the treatment of serious infections because of their potential toxicity and antimicrobial spectrum. Doses must be carefully regulated to maintain plasma concentrations within the therapeutic range but avoid accumulation, especially in patients with renal impairment. Neomycin and framycetin, which are considered too toxic to be given parenterally, have been given by mouth to suppress the intestinal flora. The topical use of neomycin and gentamicin has been associated with allergic reactions and the emergence of resistant bacteria. Gentamicin or tobramycin are the drugs of choice in the treatment of life-threatening infections due to aminoglycoside-sensitive organisms and are often used with other antibacterials. With the continuing emergence of resistant strains, amikacin and netilmicin should be reserved for severe infections resistant to gentamicin and the other aminoglycosides.

Described in this chapter are


Amikacin, p.154
Apramycin, p.158
Arbekacin, p.158
Astromicin, p.158
Bekanamycin, p.162
Dibekacin, p.205
Dihydrostreptomycin, p.205
Framycetin, p.215
Gentamicin, p.217
Isepamicin, p.222
Kanamycin, p.224
Micronomicin, p.231
Neomycin, p.235
Netilmicin, p.236
Sisomicin, p.254
Streptomycin, p.256
Tobramycin, p.271


## Antimycobacterials

The antimycobacterials are a miscellaneous group of antibacterials whose spectrum of activity includes *Mycobacterium* spp. and which are used in the treatment of tuberculosis, leprosy, and other mycobacterial infections. They include the rifamycins, also known as ansamycins or rifomycins, a group of antibacterials isolated from a strain of *Amycolatopsis mediterranei* (*Nocardia mediterranei*; *Streptomyces mediterranei*). The main antibacterial in this group, *rifampicin*, is a mainstay of regimens for the treatment of tuberculosis and leprosy, and is increasingly being used for other infections. The related drug *rifabutin* is also used in mycobacterial disease, especially opportunistic mycobacterial infections due to *Mycobacterium avium* complex (MAC). Other rifamycins described in this chapter include *rifapentine, rifaximin* which is poorly absorbed and is mainly used for a local effect on the gastrointestinal tract, and *rifamycin sodium*, a rifamycin rarely used as it has been superseded by more effective drugs.

Another drug widely used for tuberculosis is *isoniazid*, a derivative of isonicotinic acid; it is invariably used with other drugs to avoid or delay emergence of resistance. *Pyrazinamide*, a nicotinamide derivative, is also an important component of regimens for tuberculosis, while *ethambutol* and the aminoglycoside *streptomycin* are added when resistance to first-line drugs is likely. The thiosemicarbazone derivative *thioacetazone* is now less widely used in tuberculosis because of its toxicity and because more effective drugs are available, but is sometimes used in developing countries. Other drugs that have been used to treat tuberculosis including *aminosalicylic acid* and its salts, *capreomycin, cycloserine, ethionamide, protionamide*, and *kanamycin* are regarded as secondary drugs and are reserved for patients in whom resistance or toxicity to first-line drugs is a problem.

The sulfones have been used since the 1940s in the treatment of leprosy, but the only one widely used now is *dapsone*, an important component of multidrug regimens. Its action is thought to involve inhibition of folate metabolism, similarly to the sulfonamides, and dapsone is also used for the prophylaxis of malaria and for prophylaxis and treatment of *Pneumocystis carinii* pneumonia. Also important in the treatment of leprosy is the phenazine dye *clofazimine*. Additionally, it has a role in the treatment of type 2 lepra reactions and has been used in other mycobacterial infections. The thioamides *ethionamide* and *protionamide* have been used in the treatment of leprosy and tuberculosis, but have generally been replaced by less toxic drugs, for example *clarithromycin, ofloxacin, minocycline*, or *pefloxacin*, in alternative antileprotic regimens.

Described in this chapter are


Aminosalicylic Acid, p.154
Capreomycin, p.166
Clofazimine, p.197
Cycloserine, p.202
Dapsone, p.202
Methaniazide, p.230
Morinamide, p.233
Protionamide, p.246
Pyrazinamide, p.246
Rifabutin, p.249
Rifampicin, p.250
Ethambutol, p.211
Ethionamide, p.212
Ftivazide, p.215
Isoniazid, p.222
Rifamycin, p.253
Rifapentine, p.253
Rifaximin, p.254
Thioacetazone, p.269


## Cephalosporins and related Beta Lactams

The cephalosporins or cephem antibacterials are semisynthetic antibacterials derived from cephalosporin C a natural antibacterial produced by the mould *Cephalosporium acremonium*. The active nucleus, 7-aminocephalosporanic acid, is very closely related to the penicillin nucleus, 6-aminopenicillanic acid, and consists of a beta-lactam ring fused with a 6-membered dihydrothiazine ring and having an acetoxymethyl group at position 3. Cephalosporin C has a side-chain at position 7 derived from D-α-aminoadipic acid. Chemical modification of positions 3 and 7 has resulted in a series of drugs with different characteristics. Substitution at the 7-amino group tends to affect antibacterial action whereas at position 3 it may have more of an effect on pharmacokinetic properties.

The cephalosporins are bactericidal and, similarly to the penicillins, they act by inhibiting synthesis of the bacterial cell wall. The most widely used system of classification of cephalosporins is by generations and is based on the general features of their antibacterial activity, but may depend to some extent on when they were introduced. Succeeding generations generally have increasing activity against Gram-negative bacteria. *Cefalotin* was one of the first cephalosporins to become available and is representative of the **first-generation** cephalosporins. It has good activity against a wide spectrum of Gram-positive bacteria including penicillinase-producing, but not meticillin-resistant, staphylococci; enterococci are, however, resistant. Its activity against Gram-negative bacteria is modest. Cefalotin is not absorbed from the gastrointestinal tract and must be given parenterally although intramuscular administration is painful. Cefalotin has generally been replaced by *cefazolin* or *cefradine*. *Cefaloridine* is now rarely used because of its nephrotoxicity. Cefradine is absorbed from the gastrointestinal tract and can be administered both by mouth and by injection. *Cefadroxil, cefatrizine*, and *cefalexin* are all given orally. All of these drugs have a very similar spectrum of antimicrobial activity to cefalotin. *Cefaclor* is also given by mouth. It has similar activity to cefalotin against Gram-positive cocci, but because of its greater activity against Gram-negative bacteria, particularly *Haemophilus influenzae*, it is often classified as a second-generation drug. *Cefprozil* is an oral cephalosporin with a longer half-life than cefaclor.

*Cefamandole* was the first available **second-generation** cephalosporin. It has similar or slightly less activity than cefalotin against Gram-positive bacteria, but greater stability to hydrolysis by beta lactamases produced by Gram-negative bacteria and enhanced activity against many of the Enterobacteriaceae and *Haemophilus influenzae*. It is given parenterally. *Cefuroxime* has a similar spectrum of activity to cefamandole although it is even more resistant to hydrolysis by beta lactamases. It is given parenterally but, *cefuroxime axetil*, the acetoxyethyl ester of cefuroxime, is given orally. Other drugs classified as second-generation cephalosporins and administered parenterally include *cefonicid, ceforanide*, and *cefotiam*; these all have spectra of activity similar to cefamandole. Cephamycins (see below) are also classified with second-generation cephalosporins.

The **third-generation** cephalosporins, sometimes referred to as **extended-spectrum** cephalosporins, are even more stable to hydrolysis by beta lactamases than cefamandole and cefuroxime. Compared with the earlier generations of cephalosporins they have a wider spectrum and greater potency of activity against Gram-negative organisms, including most clinically important Enterobacteriaceae. Their activity against Gram-positive organisms is said to be less than that of the first-generation drugs, but they are very active against streptococci. *Cefotaxime* was the first of this group to become available and it has relatively modest activity against *Pseudomonas aeruginosa*. *Cefmenoxime, cefodizime, ceftizoxime*, and *ceftriaxone* are all very similar to cefotaxime in their antimicrobial activity. These drugs are all given parenterally and differ mainly in their pharmacokinetic characteristics. *Cefixime* is a third-generation cephalosporin given by mouth; others include *cefdinir, cefetamet pivoxil, cefpodoxime proxetil*, and *ceftibuten*. *Ceftazidime* is typical of a group of parenteral third-generation cephalosporins with enhanced activity against *Ps. aeruginosa*. *Cefoperazone* is similar in its activity to ceftazidime. *Cefpiramide* is structurally related to cefoperazone and has comparable activity. Although *cefsulodin* is classified as a third-generation cephalosporin its activity against Gram-negative bacteria is confined to *Ps. aeruginosa*. *Latamoxef* is an **oxacephalosporin** which differs from the true cephalosporins in that the sulfur atom of the 7-aminocephalosporanic acid nucleus is replaced by an oxygen atom. It differs from cefotaxime mainly in its enhanced activity against *Bacteroides fragilis*.

The newer cephalosporins *cefepime* and *cefpirome* are generally considered to be **fourth-generation** because of their broad spectrum of activity.

The semisynthetic **cephamycins** are chemical modifications of cephamycin C, a beta-lactam antibacterial produced naturally by *Streptomyces* spp. They differ from the cephalosporins by the addition of a 7-α-methoxy group to the 7-aminocephalosporanic acid nucleus. Steric hindrance by this methoxy group is considered to be responsible for their greater stability to beta lactamases. For practical purposes they are generally classified with the second-generation cephalosporins, but are more active against anaerobic bacteria, especially *Bacteroides fragilis*. *Cefoxitin* was one of the first cephamycins available; *cefmetazole* and *cefotetan* have been introduced more recently. Another is *cefminox*. All these cephamycins must be given parenterally.

*Imipenem* was the first of the **carbapenem** group of antibacterials to become available; it is the *N*-formimidoyl derivative of thienamycin which is produced by *Streptomyces cattleya*. It is bactericidal, and, similarly to the cephalosporins, acts by inhibiting synthesis of the bacterial cell wall. It has a very broad spectrum of antimicrobial activity including Gram-positive and Gram-negative aerobic and anaerobic organisms; it has good activity against both *Ps. aeruginosa* and *B. fragilis*. Imipenem is given parenterally with cilastatin, a dehydropeptidase I inhibitor that inhibits the renal metabolism of imipenem. Similarly, the carbapenem panipenem is given with the renal protectant betamipron. Two other carbapenems, *ertapenem* and *meropenem*, are relatively stable to renal dehydropeptidase and can be used without such an inhibitor. Ertapenem has a narrower spectrum of activity than other carbapenems, including no activity against *Ps. aeruginosa*.

The **monobactams** were first identified as monocyclic beta lactams isolated from bacteria; they are now produced synthetically. *Aztreonam* was the first commercially available monobactam. It is bactericidal with a similar action on bacterial cell-wall synthesis to the cephalosporins. Its antimicrobial activity, however, differs from imipenem and the newer cephalosporins in that it is restricted to Gram-negative aerobic organisms. It has good activity against *Ps. aeruginosa*. Aztreonam is given parenterally. Other monobactams include *carumonam*.

**Carbacephems** are structurally related to the cephalosporins, but the sulfur atom of the 7-aminocephalosporanic acid nucleus is replaced by a methylene group. *Loracarbef* is an oral carbacephem.

Described in this chapter are


Aztreonam, p.160
Betamipron, p.165
Biapenem, p.165
Carumonam, p.166
Cefaclor, p.167
Cefadroxil, p.167
Cefalexin, p.168
Cefalonium, p.168
Cefaloridine, p.168
Cefalotin, p.168
Cefamandole, p.169
Cefapirin, p.170
Cefatrizine, p.170
Cefazolin, p.170
Cefcapene, p.171
Cefdinir, p.171
Cefditoren, p.172
Cefepime, p.172
Cefetamet, p.172
Cefixime, p.172
Cefluprenam, p.173
Cefmenoxime, p.173
Cefmetazole, p.173
Cefminox, p.174
Cefodizime, p.174
Cefonicid, p.174
Cefoperazone, p.174
Ceforanide, p.175
Cefoselis, p.175
Cefotaxime, p.175
Cefotetan, p.177
Cefotiam, p.177
Cefoxitin, p.177
Cefozopran, p.178
Cefpiramide, p.178
Cefpirome, p.178
Cefpodoxime, p.178
Cefprozil, p.179
Cefquinome, p.179
Cefradine, p.179
Cefsulodin, p.180
Ceftazidime, p.180
Cefteram, p.181
Ceftezole, p.182
Ceftibuten, p.182
Ceftiofur, p.182
Ceftizoxime, p.182
Ceftriaxone, p.182
Cefuroxime, p.184
Cilastatin, p.188
Ertapenem, p.207
Faropenem, p.213
Flomoxef, p.213
Imipenem, p.221
Latamoxef, p.225
Loracarbef, p.228
Meropenem, p.229
Panipenem, p.241


## Chloramphenicols

*Chloramphenicol* is an antibacterial which was first isolated from cultures of *Streptomyces venezuelae* in 1947 but is now produced synthetically. It has a relatively simple structure and is a derivative of dichloroacetic acid with a nitrobenzene moiety. Chloramphenicol was the first broad-spectrum antibacterial to be discovered; it acts by interfering with bacterial protein synthesis and is mainly bacteriostatic. Its range of activity is similar to that of tetracycline and includes Gram-positive and Gram-negative bacteria, Rickettsia spp., and Chlamydiaceae. The sensitivities of *Salmonella typhi, Haemophilus influenzae*, and *Bacteroides fragilis* to chloramphenicol have dictated the principal indications for its use.

Shortly after its introduction chloramphenicol was found to have a serious and sometimes fatal depressant effect on the bone marrow. The 'grey syndrome', another potentially fatal adverse effect, was reported later in neonates. As a result of this toxicity the systemic use of chloramphenicol has been restricted in many countries; it should only be given when there is no suitable alternative and never for minor infections.

Chloramphenicol is active when given orally and, unlike most other antibacterials, it diffuses into the CSF even when the meninges are not inflamed. The majority of a dose is inactivated in the liver, only a small proportion appearing unchanged in the urine.

Chloramphenicol is widely used for typhoid fever, although resistance is a problem in some countries. For *Haemophilus influenzae* infections, especially meningitis, the emergence of ampicillin-resistant strains led to a reappraisal of the use of chloramphenicol, and suggestions that ampicillin and chloramphenicol should both be given empirically to patients with meningitis until the sensitivity of the infecting organisms was known, but the newer third-generation cephalosporins are increasingly preferred because of resistance. For proven *H. influenzae* meningitis, chloramphenicol is used as an alternative to the third-generation cephalosporins, which are now regarded as treatment of choice. Chloramphenicol is also effective against many anaerobic bacteria and may be valuable in such conditions as cerebral abscess where anaerobes such as *Bacteroides fragilis* are often involved, although metronidazole may be preferred.

Chloramphenicol sodium succinate is used parenterally and the palmitate is given orally. Ophthalmic and other topical preparations of chloramphenicol are used widely in some countries for a variety of infections.

*Thiamphenicol* is a semisynthetic derivative of chloramphenicol in which the nitro group on the benzene ring has been replaced by a methylsulfonyl group, resulting, in general, in a loss of activity *in vitro*. It has been claimed that thiamphenicol is less toxic than chloramphenicol and there have been fewer reports of aplastic anaemia but reversible bone-marrow depression may occur more frequently. It is also less likely to cause the 'grey syndrome'. Unlike chloramphenicol, thiamphenicol is not metabolised in the liver to any extent and is excreted largely unchanged in the urine. It has been used similarly to chloramphenicol in some countries.

*Azidamfenicol* is another analogue of chloramphenicol that has been used topically in the treatment of eye infections.

Described in this chapter are

Azidamfenicol, p.159
Chloramphenicol, p.185
Florfenicol, p.213
Thiamphenicol, p.269

## Glycopeptides

*Vancomycin* has a glycopeptide structure; it acts by interfering with bacterial cell wall synthesis and is very active against Gram-positive cocci. Intravenous vancomycin is reserved for the treatment of severe staphylococcal infections and for the treatment and prophylaxis of endocarditis when other antibacterials cannot be used, either because of patient sensitivity or bacterial resistance. It is the treatment of choice for infections caused by meticillin-resistant staphylococci. Vancomycin hydrochloride is poorly absorbed when taken orally; it is used in the treatment of pseudomembranous colitis. *Teicoplanin* is a glycopeptide with similar properties to vancomycin, but a longer duration of action. It can be given intramuscularly as well as intravenously. *Ramoplanin* is under investigation, especially for the prevention of infection due to vancomycin-resistant enterococci.

Described in this chapter are

Avoparcin, p.159
Norvancomycin, p.239
Oritavancin, p.240
Ramoplanin, p.249
Teicoplanin, p.264
Vancomycin, p.275

## Lincosamides

*Lincomycin* is an antibacterial produced by a strain of *Streptomyces lincolnensis* and was first described in 1962; *clindamycin* is the 7-chloro-7-deoxy derivative of lincomycin.

Although not related structurally to erythromycin and the other macrolide antibacterials, the lincosamides have similar antimicrobial activity and act at the same site on the bacterial ribosome to suppress protein synthesis.

The lincosamides are bacteriostatic or bactericidal, depending on the concentration, and are active mainly against Gram-positive bacteria, and against *Bacteroides* spp. They also appear to have some antiprotozoal activity. Clindamycin and lincomycin have qualitatively similar activity but clindamycin is more active than lincomycin *in vitro*. Cross-resistance occurs between the lincosamides, macrolides, and streptogramins.

The lincosamides have been used, like erythromycin, as an alternative to penicillin, but reports of severe and sometimes fatal pseudomembranous colitis in association with lincomycin and clindamycin have led to the recommendation that they should only be used when there is no suitable alternative.

Both lincomycin and clindamycin can be given orally and parenterally, but clindamycin is much better absorbed from the gastrointestinal tract and less affected by the presence of food in the stomach. They both penetrate well into bone and have been used successfully in osteomyelitis. They have also been used topically in the treatment of acne vulgaris.

The main indication for the use of lincosamides is now in the treatment of severe anaerobic infections, although metronidazole (p.609) or some beta lactams may be a more suitable choice in such infections. Clindamycin also has a role in the prophylaxis of endocarditis in penicillin-allergic patients and has been used, usually with other antiprotozoals, in babesiosis, chloroquine-resistant malaria, toxoplasmosis, and *Pneumocystis carinii* pneumonia.

Described in this chapter are

Clindamycin, p.194
Lincomycin, p.226
Pirlimycin, p.244

## Macrolides

The macrolides are a large group of antibacterials mainly derived from *Streptomyces* spp. and having a common macrocyclic lactone ring to which one or more sugars are attached. They are all weak bases and only slightly soluble in water. Their properties are very similar and in general they have low toxicity and a similar spectrum of antimicrobial activity with cross-resistance between individual members of the group. The macrolides are bacteriostatic or bactericidal, depending on the concentration and the type of micro-organism, and are thought to interfere with bacterial protein synthesis. Their antimicrobial spectrum is similar to that of benzylpenicillin but they are also active against such organisms as *Legionella pneumophila, Mycoplasma pneumoniae*, and some rickettsias, chlamydias, and chlamydophilas. Macrolides and related drugs have a postantibiotic effect: that is, antibacterial activity persists after concentrations have dropped below the minimum inhibitory concentration.

*Erythromycin* was discovered in 1952 and is the macrolide used most widely. It is destroyed by gastric acid and must therefore be given as enteric-coated formulations or as one of its more stable salts or esters such as the stearate or ethyl succinate. Hepatotoxicity has been reported after the use of erythromycin, most commonly as the estolate. Erythromycin lactobionate or gluceptate may be given intravenously. Cardiac arrhythmias have been reported occasionally after intravenous administration. Erythromycin is used as an alternative to penicillin in many infections, especially in patients who are allergic to penicillin. It has similar uses to tetracycline in the treatment of infections due to *Mycoplasma pneumoniae* and *Chlamydia trachomatis*, and in acne vulgaris. It is also used in the treatment of infections caused by *Legionella pneumophila*.

More recently developed macrolides include *azithromycin, clarithromycin, dirithromycin*, and *roxithromycin*. These drugs all appear to have essentially similar properties to erythromycin although they may differ in their pharmacokinetics. Clarithromycin and, to a lesser extent, azithromycin are more active than erythromycin against opportunistic mycobacteria such as *Mycobacterium avium* complex. Clarithromycin is also used in the treatment of leprosy and in regimens for the eradication of *Helicobacter pylori* in peptic ulcer disease. Both azithromycin and clarithromycin have activity against protozoa including *Toxoplasma gondii*.

*Flurithromycin* is another newer macrolide in use.

Other macrolides include *spiramycin*, which has been used extensively in Europe and has also been used in the treatment and prophylaxis of toxoplasmosis. It may be useful in the treatment of cryptosporidiosis.

*Oleandomycin* has been used orally and parenterally as the phosphate. Its ester, *troleandomycin*, is better absorbed from the gastrointestinal tract but, like erythromycin estolate, has proved hepatotoxic. *Josamycin, kitasamycin, midecamycin*, and *rokitamycin* have been used in Europe and/or Japan.

The **streptogramin** group of antibacterials are also derived from *Streptomyces* spp. and include *pristinamycin* and *virginiamycin*. They consist of two components that act synergistically and are therefore also known as synergistins. One of the components is structurally related to the macrolides, and they have a similar spectrum of antimicrobial activity to erythromycin. Semisynthetic derivatives such as *quinupristin/dalfopristin* may be useful in the treatment of infections with multidrug-resistant organisms including meticillin-resistant *Staphylococcus aureus* and vancomycin-resistant enterococci.

Cross-resistance is often observed between the macrolides, lincosamides, and streptogramins. The **ketolide** antibacterials *telithromycin* and *cethromycin* are semi-synthetic derivatives of erythromycin A that have been developed to overcome macrolide resistance in respiratory tract pathogens.

Described in this chapter are

Azithromycin, p.159
Cethromycin, p.185
Clarithromycin, p.192
Dirithromycin, p.206
Erythromycin, p.208
Flurithromycin, p.214
Josamycin, p.224
Kitasamycin, p.225
Midecamycin, p.231
Oleandomycin, p.240
Pristinamycin, p.246
Quinupristin/Dalfopristin, p.248
Rokitamycin, p.254
Roxithromycin, p.254
Spiramycin, p.255
Telithromycin, p.265
Tilmicosin, p.271
Troleandomycin, p.274
Tylosin, p.274
Virginiamycin, p.277

## Penicillins

Penicillin was the first antibacterial to be used therapeutically and was originally obtained, as a mixture of penicillins known as F, G, X, and K, from the mould *Penicillium notatum*. Better yields were achieved using *P. chrysogenum* and benzylpenicillin (penicillin G) was selectively produced by adding the precursor phenylacetic acid to the fermentation medium. The term 'penicillin' is now used generically for the entire group of natural and semisynthetic penicillins. Penicillins are still widely used; they are generally well tolerated, apart from hypersensitivity reactions, and are usually bactericidal by virtue of their inhibitory action on the synthesis of the bacterial cell wall.

Penicillins all have the same ring structure and are monobasic acids which readily form salts and esters; 6-aminopenicillanic acid, the penicillin nucleus, consists of a fused thiazolidine ring and a beta-lactam ring with an amino group at the 6-position.

The earlier or so-called 'natural' penicillins were produced by adding different side-chain precursors to fermentations of the *Penicillium* mould; *benzylpenicillin*, with a phenylacetamido side-chain at the 6-position, and *phenoxymethylpenicillin* (penicillin V), with a phenoxyacetamido side-chain, were 2 of the first and are still widely used. Benzylpenicillin can be considered the parent compound of the penicillins and is active mainly against Gram-positive bacteria and *Neisseria* spp. It is inactivated by penicillinase-producing bacteria and because of its instability in gastric acid it is usually injected. Long-acting preparations include *procaine benzylpenicillin* and *benzathine benzylpenicillin*, which slowly release benzylpenicillin after injection. Phenoxymethylpenicillin is acid-stable and is therefore given orally but it is also inactivated by penicillinase. It is generally used for relatively mild infections.

When no side-chain precursor is added to the fermentation medium, 6-aminopenicillanic acid itself is obtained. A range of penicillins has been synthesised from 6-aminopenicillanic acid by substitution at the 6-amino position in an effort to improve on the instability of benzylpenicillin to gastric acid and penicillinases, to widen its antimicrobial spectrum, and to reduce its rapid rate of renal excretion. Two phenoxypenicillins in which the side-chain is α-phenoxypropionamido (*pheneticillin*) or α-phenoxybutyramido (*propicillin*) are more stable to acid than benzylpenicillin but offer no advantage over phenoxymethylpenicillin.

*Meticillin* has a 2,6-dimethoxybenzamido group at the 6-position and was the first penicillin found to be resistant to destruction by staphylococcal penicillinase. However, it is not acid-resistant and has to be injected. The isoxazolyl penicillins, *cloxacillin, dicloxacillin, flucloxacillin,* and *oxacillin,* are resistant to penicillinase and gastric acid. They have very similar chemical structures and differ mainly in their absorption characteristics. *Nafcillin* is a similar penicillinase-resistant antibacterial but is irregularly absorbed when taken orally.

*Ampicillin* has a D(−)-α-aminophenylacetamido side-chain and a broader spectrum of activity than benzylpenicillin; although generally less active against Gram-positive bacteria, some Gram-negative organisms including *Escherichia coli, Haemophilus influenzae,* and *Salmonella* spp. are sensitive although resistance is being reported increasingly. *Pseudomonas* spp. are not sensitive. Ampicillin is acid-stable and can be given orally but is destroyed by penicillinase. A number of prodrugs including *bacampicillin, metampicillin,* and *pivampicillin* are also said to be better absorbed and are hydrolysed to ampicillin *in vivo*. *Amoxicillin,* with a D(−)-α-aminohydroxyphenylacetamido side-chain, only differs from ampicillin by the addition of a hydroxyl group, but is better absorbed from the gastrointestinal tract.

*Carbenicillin,* with an α-carboxyphenylacetamido side-chain, has marked activity against *Pseudomonas aeruginosa* and some *Proteus* spp. but otherwise is generally less active than ampicillin. It has to be given by injection and large doses are required. *Carfecillin* and *carindacillin* are the phenyl and indanyl esters of carbenicillin respectively and are hydrolysed to carbenicillin *in vivo* when taken by mouth. *Sulbenicillin* has an α-phenylsulfoacetamido side-chain and *ticarcillin* an α-carboxythienylacetamido side-chain and both have similar activity to carbenicillin; ticarcillin is more active against *Ps. aeruginosa*. The ureidopenicillins *azlocillin* and *mezlocillin*, and the closely related drug *piperacillin* are more active than carbenicillin against *Ps. aeruginosa* and have a wider range of activity against Gram-negative bacteria.

*Temocillin,* a 6-α-methoxy derivative of ticarcillin, is resistant to many beta lactamases and is active against most Gram-negative aerobic bacteria, but not *Ps. aeruginosa*.

*Mecillinam* is a penicillanic acid derivative with a substituted amidino group in the 6-position. Unlike the 6-aminopenicillanic acid derivatives it is active mainly against Gram-negative bacteria, although *Ps. aeruginosa,* and *Bacteroides* spp. are considered resistant. Mecillinam is not active orally and is given by mouth as *pivmecillinam,* which is hydrolysed to mecillinam on absorption.

The beta-lactamase inhibitors *clavulanic acid, sulbactam,* and *tazobactam* are used to extend the antimicrobial range of certain beta-lactam antibacterials.

Described in this chapter are


Amoxicillin, p.155
Ampicillin, p.157
Aspoxicillin, p.158
Azidocillin, p.159
Azlocillin, p.160
Bacampicillin, p.161
Benethamine Penicillin, p.162
Benzathine Benzylpenicillin, p.162
Benzathine Phenoxymethylpenicillin, p.163
Benzylpenicillin, p.163
Carbenicillin, p.166
Carfecillin, p.166
Carindacillin, p.166
Ciclacillin, p.188
Clavulanic Acid, p.193
Clemizole Penicillin, p.194
Clometocillin, p.198
Cloxacillin, p.198
Dicloxacillin, p.205
Flucloxacillin, p.213
Mecillinam, p.228
Metampicillin, p.229
Meticillin, p.230
Mezlocillin, p.231
Nafcillin, p.233
Oxacillin, p.240
Penethamate, p.242
Pheneticillin, p.242
Phenoxymethylpenicillin, p.242
Piperacillin, p.243
Pivampicillin, p.244
Pivmecillinam, p.244
Procaine Benzylpenicillin, p.246
Propicillin, p.246
Sulbactam, p.257
Sulbenicillin, p.257
Sultamicillin, p.264
Tazobactam, p.264
Temocillin, p.266
Ticarcillin, p.270


## Quinolones

The quinolonecarboxylic acids, carboxyquinolones, or 4-quinolones are a group of synthetic antibacterials structurally related to nalidixic acid. The term 4-quinolone has been used as a generic name for the common 4-oxo-1,4-dihydroquinoline skeleton. Under this system nalidixic acid, a naphthyridene derivative, is an 8-aza-4-quinolone, cinoxacin, a cinnoline derivative, is a 2-aza-4-quinolone, and pipemidic and piromidic acids, pyrido-pyrimidine derivatives, are 6,8-diaza-4-quinolones.

*Nalidixic acid* is active against Gram-negative bacteria but has little activity against *Pseudomonas* and Gram-positive organisms. Because bactericidal concentrations can only be achieved in urine its use has generally been limited to the treatment of urinary-tract infections.

Modification of the structure of nalidixic acid has produced related antibacterials such as *oxolinic acid, cinoxacin,* and *rosoxacin*. Although some of these have a greater activity *in vitro* against Gram-negative organisms and activity against some Gram-positive organisms, none has been considered to represent a significant clinical advance over nalidixic acid; rosoxacin is only used in the treatment of gonorrhoea. Addition of a piperazinyl radical at position 7, as in *pipemidic acid,* appears to confer some activity against *Pseudomonas*. *Flumequine* was the first fluorinated 4-quinolone to be synthesised, but has no piperazinyl group. Addition of the 7-piperazinyl group and a fluorine atom at position 6 has produced a group of fluorinated piperazinyl quinolones or fluoroquinolones with a broader spectrum of activity than nalidixic acid and pharmacokinetic properties more suitable for the treatment of systemic infections. They include *ciprofloxacin, enoxacin, fleroxacin, gatifloxacin, gemifloxacin, levofloxacin, lomefloxacin, moxifloxacin, nadifloxacin, norfloxacin, ofloxacin, pazufloxacin, pefloxacin, rufloxacin, sparfloxacin,* and *trovafloxacin*. Marketing of trovafloxacin and its prodrug, alatrofloxacin, has been suspended in some countries following reports of unpredictable hepatotoxicity, including some fatalities. *Danofloxacin, enrofloxacin, marbofloxacin, orbifloxacin,* and *sarafloxacin* are used in veterinary practice. Development of *difloxacin* for human use was suspended because of the high incidence of adverse effects, but it is used in veterinary practice. *Temafloxacin* and, more recently, *grepafloxacin* were withdrawn worldwide because of toxicity.

The fluoroquinolones are very active against aerobic Gram-negative bacilli and cocci including the Enterobacteriaceae, *Haemophilus influenzae, Moraxella catarrhalis* (*Branhamella catarrhalis*), and *Neisseria gonorrhoeae* and are also active against *Pseudomonas aeruginosa*. They are generally less active against Gram-positive organisms such as staphylococci and much less active against streptococci such as *Streptococcus pneumoniae,* although some fluoroquinolones now developed have increased activity against these organisms. They also have activity against mycobacteria, mycoplasmas, rickettsias, and *Plasmodium falciparum*. Some, for example ofloxacin, have useful activity against *Chlamydia trachomatis*. Activity against anaerobic bacteria is generally poor. There is concern that the emergence of resistant strains of organisms may limit the usefulness of fluoroquinolones in future.

One disadvantage of the quinolone antibacterials is that they are generally not recommended for use in children, adolescents, and pregnant and breast-feeding women because of their propensity to cause joint erosions in immature *animals*.

Described in this chapter are


Alatrofloxacin, p.154
Balofloxacin, p.162
Cinoxacin, p.188
Ciprofloxacin, p.188
Clinafloxacin, p.194
Danofloxacin, p.202
Difloxacin, p.205
Enoxacin, p.207
Enrofloxacin, p.207
Fleroxacin, p.213
Flumequine, p.214
Gatifloxacin, p.216
Gemifloxacin, p.216
Grepafloxacin, p.220
Levofloxacin, p.225
Lomefloxacin, p.227
Marbofloxacin, p.228
Moxifloxacin, p.233
Nadifloxacin, p.233
Nalidixic Acid, p.234
Norfloxacin, p.238
Ofloxacin, p.239
Orbifloxacin, p.240
Oxolinic Acid, p.240
Pazufloxacin, p.241
Pefloxacin, p.241
Pipemidic Acid, p.243
Piromidic Acid, p.244
Prulifloxacin, p.246
Rosoxacin, p.254
Rufloxacin, p.254
Sarafloxacin, p.254
Sparfloxacin, p.255
Temafloxacin, p.266
Tosufloxacin, p.272
Trovafloxacin, p.274


## Sulfonamides and Diaminopyrimidines

The sulfonamides are analogues of *p*-aminobenzoic acid. The first sulfonamide of clinical importance was *Prontosil,* an azo dye that is metabolised *in vivo* to *sulfanilamide*. It was synthesised in Germany in 1932. Many sulfonamides have since been synthesised; they differ only slightly in their antimicrobial activity, but vary in their pharmacokinetic properties. The sulfonamides have been classified according to their rate of excretion as short-, medium- or intermediate-, long-, and ultra-long-acting. The **short-acting** sulfonamides are excreted in the urine in high concentrations and have therefore been of particular use in the treatment of urinary-tract infections. The solubility in urine of earlier short-acting sulfonamides, such as *sulfapyridine,* and their acetyl metabolites is low and hence crystalluria has been reported frequently. Of the short-acting sulfonamides most commonly used, *sulfadiazine* also has low solubility in urine whereas *sulfadimidine* and *sulfafurazole* and their acetyl conjugates are very soluble. Three short-acting sulfonamides (triple sulfonamides) have been given together to reduce the risk of crystalluria, as the constituent sulfonamides can co-exist in solution in urine without affecting each other's solubility. Preparations of mixed sulfonamides have, however, generally been replaced by the more soluble sulfonamides. The **medium-acting** sulfonamides such as *sulfamethoxazole,* the **long-acting** sulfonamides such as *sulfadimethoxine, sulfamethoxypyridazine,* and *sulfametoxydiazine,* and the **ultra-long-acting** sulfonamides such as *sulfadoxine* and *sulfametopyrazine* do not attain such high concentrations in the urine and rarely cause crystalluria. Sulfonamides that are slowly excreted from the body do appear, however, to have been more commonly implicated in the development of reactions such as the Stevens-Johnson syndrome.

The sulfonamides are usually bacteriostatic, and interfere with folic acid synthesis of susceptible organisms; their broad spectrum of antimicrobial activity has, however, been limited by the development of resistance. The clinical use of sulfonamides has therefore been greatly reduced; in general they are indicated only in the treatment of urinary-tract infections and a few other disorders such as nocardiosis. Sulfonamides such as *sulfaguanidine, succinylsulfathiazole,* and *phthalylsulfathiazole* are poorly absorbed from the gastrointestinal tract and have been used for the treatment of gastrointestinal infections although they are now rarely indicated. *Sulfadiazine silver* and *mafenide* are applied topically for their antibacterial action in patients with burns. *Sulfasalazine* (p.1291), a conjugate of 5-aminosalicylic acid (mesalazine) and sulfapyridine, is used in the treatment of inflammatory bowel diseases and in rheumatoid arthritis.

*Trimethoprim* is a diaminopyrimidine that also inhibits folic acid synthesis but at a different stage in the metabolic pathway to that inhibited by the sulfonamides. It has a similar spectrum of antimicrobial activity to sulfonamides and often shows synergy *in vitro* with these drugs. Trimethoprim was initially available only in combination with sulfonamides, most commonly with sulfamethoxazole as co-trimoxazole. It is now used alone particularly in the treatment of infections of the urinary and respiratory tracts. Analogues of trimethoprim include *baquiloprim, brodimoprim, ormetoprim,* and *tetroxoprim*.

*Co-trimoxazole* generally replaced use of sulfonamides alone in the treatment of systemic infections, although its use has also been restricted in some countries and trimethoprim may be preferred. Co-trimoxazole is however indicated for *Pneumocystis carinii* pneumonia and nocardiosis and may be useful in protozoal infections such as toxoplasmosis. Other sulfonamides which have been used in combination with trimethoprim include sulfadiazine (see *co-trimazine*), sulfamethoxypyridazine, sulfametopyrazine, sulfametrole, and sulfamoxole (see *co-trifamole*). Sulfadiazine has been used in combination with tetroxoprim (see *co-tetroxazine*).

Sulfonamides have also been used with the diaminopyrimidine, pyrimethamine (p.458) in the treatment or prophylaxis of some protozoal infections. Commonly used combinations are sulfadoxine and pyrimethamine for malaria, and sulfadiazine and pyrimethamine for the treatment of toxoplasmosis.

Described in this chapter are


Baquiloprim, p.162
Brodimoprim, p.165
Co-tetroxazine, p.199
Co-trifamole p.199
Co-trimazine, p.199
Co-trimoxazole, p.199
Formosulfathiazole, p.214
Mafenide, p.228
Ormetoprim, p.240
Phthalylsulfathiazole, p.242
Succinylsulfathiazole, p.257
Sulfabenzamide, p.257
Sulfacarbamide, p.257
Sulfacetamide, p.257
Sulfachlorpyridazine, p.258
Sulfachrysoidine, p.258
Sulfaclozine, p.258
Sulfadiazine, p.258
Sulfadiazine Silver, p.259
Sulfadicramide, p.259
Sulfadimethoxine, p.259
Sulfadimidine, p.259
Sulfadoxine, p.259
Sulfafurazole, p.260
Sulfaguanidine, p.260
Sulfamerazine, p.260
Sulfamethizole, p.260
Sulfamethoxazole, p.261
Sulfamethoxypyridazine, p.263
Sulfamethylthiazole, p.263
Sulfametopyrazine, p.263
Sulfametrole, p.263
Sulfamonomethoxine, p.263
Sulfamoxole, p.263
Sulfanilamide, p.263
Sulfapyridine, p.263
Sulfaquinoxaline, p.263
Sulfasuccinamide, p.264
Sulfathiazole, p.264
Sulfatroxazole, p.264
Sulfisomidine, p.264
Tetroxoprim, p.269
Trimethoprim, p.272


## Tetracyclines

The tetracyclines are a group of antibacterials, originally derived from certain *Streptomyces* spp., having the same tetracyclic nucleus, naphthacene, and similar properties. Unlike the penicillins and aminoglycosides they are usually bacteriostatic at the concentrations achieved in the body but act similarly to the aminoglycosides by interfering with protein synthesis in susceptible organisms.

Tetracyclines all have a broad spectrum of activity which includes Gram-positive and Gram-negative bacteria, chlamydias and chlamydophilas, rickettsias, mycoplasmas, spirochaetes, some mycobacteria, and some protozoa, but the emergence of resistant strains and the development of other antimicrobials has often reduced their value. Adverse effects have also restricted their usefulness. Gastrointestinal disturbances are common and other important toxic effects include deposition in bones and teeth, precluding their use in pregnancy and young children; anti-anabolic effects, especially in patients with renal impairment; fatty changes in the liver; and photosensitivity, especially with demeclocycline. Allergic reactions are relatively uncommon. Because of these adverse effects tetracyclines should be avoided in pregnant women, children, and, apart from doxycycline and minocycline, patients with renal impairment.

The first tetracycline to be introduced was *chlortetracycline* in 1948 and, like chloramphenicol which was discovered at about the same time, it was found to have a broad spectrum of activity and to be active by mouth unlike benzylpenicillin or streptomycin, the only other antibacterials then in use. The discovery of chlortetracycline was followed closely by that of *oxytetracycline* and then *tetracycline*, a reduction product of chlortetracycline which may be produced semisynthetically. All three have very similar properties, although chlortetracycline is less well absorbed and oxytetracycline may cause less staining of teeth. *Demeclocycline*, demethylated chlortetracycline, has a longer half-life than tetracycline. However, phototoxic reactions have been reported most frequently with demeclocycline. It has been used with some success in patients with the syndrome of inappropriate secretion of antidiuretic hormone.

These four tetracyclines are all natural products that have been isolated from *Streptomyces* spp. The more recent tetracyclines, namely methacycline, doxycycline, and minocycline, are semisynthetic derivatives. *Methacycline*, like demeclocycline, has a longer half-life than tetracycline and has been given twice daily. *Doxycycline* and *minocycline* are both more active *in vitro* than tetracycline against many species. More importantly, minocycline is active against some tetracycline-resistant bacteria, including strains of staphylococci. Both are well absorbed and, unlike the other tetracyclines, absorption is not significantly affected by the presence of food. They can be given in lower doses than the older members of the group and, having long half-lives, doxycycline is usually given once daily and minocycline twice daily. Also, they do not accumulate significantly in patients with renal impairment and can, therefore, be given to such patients. Both doxycycline and minocycline are more lipid-soluble than the other tetracyclines and they penetrate well into tissues. The use of minocycline may, however, be limited by its vestibular adverse effects.

Tetracyclines are not generally the antibacterials of choice in Gram-positive or Gram-negative infections because of the emergence of resistant organisms and the discovery of drugs with narrower antimicrobial spectra. However, they have a place in the treatment of chlamydial infections, rickettsial infections such as typhus and the spotted fevers, mycoplasmal infections such as atypical pneumonia, pelvic inflammatory disease, Lyme disease, brucellosis, tularaemia, plague, cholera, periodontal disease, and acne. The tetracyclines have also been useful in the treatment of penicillin-allergic patients suffering from venereal diseases, anthrax, actinomycosis, bronchitis, and leptospirosis. Minocycline may sometimes be used in multidrug regimens for leprosy.

Described in this chapter are


Chlortetracycline, p.187
Demeclocycline, p.204
Doxycycline, p.206
Lymecycline, p.228
Meclocycline, p.229
Methacycline, p.230
Minocycline, p.231
Oxytetracycline, p.241
Rolitetracycline, p.254
Tetracycline, p.266


## Miscellaneous Antibacterials

*Spectinomycin* is an aminocyclitol antibacterial with some similarities to streptomycin although it is not an aminoglycoside. Spectinomycin is active against a wide range of bacteria but its clinical use is restricted to the treatment of chancroid and gonorrhoea. Trospectomycin, a water-soluble derivative, has been investigated.

*Mupirocin* is an antibacterial produced by *Pseudomonas fluorescens* with activity against most strains of staphylococci and streptococci and also some Gram-negative bacteria. It is applied topically.

*Fosfomycin* is a derivative of phosphonic acid; it is active against a range of Gram-positive and Gram-negative bacteria and is administered by mouth or parenterally.

The fusidane antibacterial *fusidic acid* is derived from *Fusidium coccineum* and has a narrow spectrum of antibacterial activity, but it is very active against *Staphylococcus aureus* and has been used both topically and systemically in the treatment of staphylococcal infections. Resistance develops readily and it is often used with other antibacterials.

The polymyxins are basic antibacterials produced by the growth of different strains of *Bacillus polymyxa* (*B. aerosporus*). *Polymyxin B* and *colistin* have been used clinically, but their systemic use has been more or less abandoned because of their toxicity, notably to the kidneys and nervous system. They are not absorbed when taken orally and have therefore been given in gastrointestinal infections for their bactericidal activity against Gram-negative bacteria. They continue to be widely used as components of topical preparations.

*Bacitracin*, *gramicidin*, and *tyrothricin* are polypeptide antibacterials also produced by certain strains of *Bacillus* spp. but they are active against Gram-positive bacteria. Like the polymyxins, they are toxic when used systemically and are therefore mainly used topically.

The halogenated hydroxyquinoline *clioquinol* has antibacterial, antifungal, and antiprotozoal activity. It was formerly used in gastrointestinal infections including amoebiasis but is of little value and can produce severe neurotoxicity. It is now mainly used locally for superficial infections of the skin and external ear. *Chlorquinaldol* and *halquinol* are used similarly.

Urinary antimicrobials such as *nitrofurantoin*, and also *methenamine* which has generally been given as the hippurate or mandelate, may be used in the treatment and prophylaxis of infections of the lower urinary tract. They are concentrated in the urine, but do not usually achieve antimicrobial concentrations in the blood.

The oxazolidinone *linezolid* has activity against Gram-positive organisms including vancomycin-resistant enterococci and meticillin-resistant *Staphylococcus aureus*. It is used in infections of the skin and respiratory tract due to these organisms.

Described in this chapter are


Acediasulfone, p.153
Arsanilic Acid, p.158
Avilamycin, p.159
Bacitracin, p.161
Bambermycin, p.162
Carbadox, p.166
Chlorquinaldol, p.187
Clioquinol, p.196
Clofoctol, p.198
Colistin, p.198
Daptomycin, p.204
Fosfomycin, p.214
Furaltadone, p.215
Furazidin, p.215
Fusafungine, p.215
Fusidic Acid, p.215
Gramicidin, p.220
Halquinol, p.220
Linezolid, p.226
Magainins, p.228
Mandelic Acid, p.228
Methenamine, p.230
Mupirocin, p.233
Nifuroxazide, p.237
Nifurtoinol, p.237
Nifurzide, p.237
Nisin, p.237
Nitrofurantoin, p.237
Nitrofurazone, p.238
Nitroxoline, p.238
Novobiocin, p.239
Polymyxin B, p.245
Spectinomycin, p.255
Sulfamazone, p.260
Taurolidine, p.264
Terizidone, p.266
Thenoic Acid, p.269
Thiostrepton, p.270
Tiamulin, p.270
Trospectomycin, p.274
Tyrothricin, p.275
Valnemulin, p.275
Xibornol, p.277


## Choice of Antibacterial

Ideally, antibacterial treatment of infections should be chosen after the infecting organisms have been identified and the results of sensitivity tests are known. In practice, empirical treatment is often necessary initially, bearing in mind local patterns of infection and resistance. Other factors such as site of infection and tissue penetration are also important in deciding which antibacterial to give.

The prophylactic use of antibacterials is restricted mainly to patients undergoing some types of surgery. Other groups requiring infection prophylaxis include patients at special risk of developing endocarditis and those who have had rheumatic fever, who are splenectomised, or who are immunocompromised.

### Abscess, abdominal

See under Abscess, Liver, below, and under Peritonitis, p.140.

### Abscess, brain

Brain abscesses can result from otitis media, sinusitis, trauma, or dental sepsis, or they may be metastatic secondary to, for example, lung abscesses. Opportunistic infections in immunocompromised patients may present as brain abscesses.

Treatment of brain abscesses entails removal of pus or excision and use of high doses of antibacterials. Ideally the choice of antibacterial depends on the infecting organisms and penetration by the antibacterial into brain tissue and abscess pus. Until organisms can be cultured empirical treatment should be given.

There is very little good quality published information on the treatment of brain abscess. For many years, combined treatment with benzylpenicillin and chloramphenicol was the mainstay of empirical therapy, but a report by the British Society for Antimicrobial Chemotherapy,[1] based on published information and the authors' expertise, has recommended the following regimens for first-line empirical treatment, according to the site of the abscess and origin of the infection:

- for frontal lobe abscesses originating from infection of the paranasal sinuses or teeth, a combination of metronidazole with one of cefuroxime, cefotaxime, or ceftriaxone
- for temporal lobe or cerebellar abscesses originating from infection of the middle ear or sphenoidal sinuses, ampicillin and metronidazole with either ceftazidime or gentamicin
- for abscesses associated with penetrating trauma, flucloxacillin, cefuroxime, cefotaxime, or ceftriaxone
- for metastatic abscesses, usually in the area supplied by the middle cerebral artery, one of cefuroxime, cefotaxime, or ceftriaxone, with or without metronidazole, or, if associated with endocarditis or cyanotic congenital heart disease, benzylpenicillin


1. Infection in Neurosurgery Working Party of the British Society for Antimicrobial Chemotherapy. The rational use of antibiotics in the treatment of brain abscess. *Br J Neurosurg* 2000; **14:** 525–30.


### Abscess, liver

Bacteria commonly responsible for pyogenic liver abscesses include Enterobacteriaceae, especially *Escherichia coli*; anaerobes, especially *Bacteroides fragilis*; and *Streptococcus milleri* (these can be microaerophilic). As elsewhere in the abdomen (see under Peritonitis, p.140), infections are often mixed. Treatment involves removal of pus and the use of high doses of antibacterials. Broad-spectrum empirical therapy should be started immediately; more specific therapy may be possible when the results of cultures following diagnostic percutaneous aspiration of the abscess are known. Gentamicin with clindamycin has been commonly used[1,2] but various combinations of other antibacterials, including cefoxitin, chloramphenicol, carboxypenicillins, third-generation cephalosporins, and metronidazole, might be appropriate.[2] Antibacterial therapy has been successful without surgical intervention, but may not be consistently so,[3] although this might be due to inadequate treatment against enteric anaerobes, especially *B. fragilis*.[2]

For the treatment of amoebic liver abscess, see under Amoebiasis in Antiprotozoals, p.595.


1. Herbert DA, *et al.* Pyogenic liver abscesses: successful non-surgical therapy. *Lancet* 1982; **i:** 134–6.
2. Herbert DA, *et al.* Medical management of pyogenic liver abscesses. *Lancet* 1985; **i:** 1384.
3. McCorkell SJ, Niles NL. Pyogenic liver abscesses: another look at medical management. *Lancet* 1985; **i:** 803–6.


### Abscess, lung

Lung abscesses are often secondary to aspiration pneumonia and are discussed under Pneumonia, p.141. The organisms involved are commonly anaerobic bacteria.

### Actinomycosis

Actinomycosis is mainly caused by the oral commensal *Actinomyces israelii*, a Gram-positive anaerobic or microaerophilic bacterium. Other species sometimes responsible include *A. meyeri*, *A. naeslundii*, and *A. viscosus*. One of the commonest forms has been cervicofacial actinomycosis, generally associated with poor oral hygiene and dental procedures.[1] Other forms include abdominal,[2] pulmonary, and disseminated actinomycosis; pelvic actinomycosis is associated with the use of intra-uterine contraceptive devices.

The antibacterial of choice is benzylpenicillin given intravenously in high doses for several weeks, followed by oral penicillin (e.g. phenoxymethylpenicillin) for several months.[1,2] Strains relatively resistant to benzylpenicillin have proved sensitive to amoxicillin.[3] Tetracycline is an alternative in patients allergic to penicillin. Other alternatives include erythromycin or clindamycin. In one patient, actinomycosis resistant to conventional treatment responded to a prolonged course of ciprofloxacin.[4]


1. Anonymous. Essential drugs: systemic mycoses. *WHO Drug Inf* 1991; **5:** 129–36.
2. Stringer MD, Cameron AEP. Abdominal actinomycosis: a forgotten disease? *Br J Hosp Med* 1987; **38:** 125–7.
3. Martin MV. The use of oral amoxycillin for the treatment of actinomycosis: a clinical and in vitro study. *Br Dent J* 1984; **156:** 252–4.
4. Macfarlane DJ, *et al.* Treatment of recalcitrant actinomycosis with ciprofloxacin. *J Infect* 1993; **27:** 177–80.


### Anaerobic bacterial infections

Anaerobic bacteria predominate in the normal microbial flora of man and are a common cause of infections, especially those arising from the gastrointestinal tract, upper respiratory tract, skin, or vagina. Common anaerobic pathogens are *Bacteroides*, *Prevotella* (formerly non-fragilis *Bacteroides*), *Fusobacterium*, *Clostridium*, *Peptostreptococcus*, and *Actinomyces* spp. Apart from single species infections such as tetanus, gas gangrene, pseudomembranous colitis, and actinomycosis, most anaerobic infections are of mixed aetiology. Abscesses are often a feature. Infections include: brain abscess; acute necrotising gingivitis and other periodontal infections; chronic otitis media and chronic sinusitis; aspiration pneumonia and lung abscess; peritonitis and intra-abdominal abscess; bacterial vaginosis and pelvic inflammatory disease; cellulitis, ulcers, bites, and other wound infections.[1]

Sensitivity testing *in vitro* is often impractical and treatment is usually empirical.[1-4] Benzylpenicillin was traditionally considered the antibacterial of choice when *B. fragilis* was unlikely (infections above the diaphragm) although resistance is increasingly a problem. Antibacterials with activity against the *B. fragilis* group and other anaerobic pathogens include metronidazole and other 5-nitroimidazole derivatives, chloramphenicol, clindamycin, cefoxitin, antipseudomonal penicillins, imipenem-cilastatin, and combinations of a beta lactam and a beta-lactamase inhibitor.[2]

Surveys of susceptibility patterns in clinical isolates of anaerobic bacteria have shown increasing resistance of the *B. fragilis* group (including *B. distasonis*, *B. fragilis*, *B. ovatus*, *B. thetaiotaomicron*, and *B. vulgatus*) to clindamycin, continuing penicillin resistance in non-fragilis *Bacteroides* spp. (now reclassified as *Prevotella* spp. and including the type species *P. melaninogenica*), and rare beta-lactamase-mediated resistance of *Fusobacterium* to penicillin. Resistance of some *Clostridium* spp. to penicillin and clindamycin had declined, but no changes were noted for *Cl. perfringens*.

The *B. fragilis* group are the most frequently isolated anaerobic bacteria in clinical infections and all members of the group may be pathogenic.[5] Most strains produce beta lactamase and thus are resistant to penicillins and cephalosporins although there is varied susceptibility within the group.[6] In a survey of susceptibility patterns[7] the most active drugs *in vitro* against *B. fragilis* group strains were imipenem, metronidazole, and chloramphenicol; resistance to cefoxitin, clindamycin, and piperacillin was not widespread and combinations of beta-lactamase inhibitors with penicillins or cephalosporins (e.g. ampicillin or cefoperazone with sulbactam; ticarcillin with clavulanate) were also very active. Others have reported similar results.[6] On the basis of activity *in vitro* in another study[8] metronidazole, imipenem, ticarcillin with clavulanate, cefoxitin, and amoxicillin with clavulanate were considered suitable for the treatment of *B. fragilis* group infections. A clinical isolate of *B. fragilis*, simultaneously resistant to metronidazole, amoxicillin with clavulanate, and imipenem, was reported in the UK;[9] treatment with clindamycin was successful on this occasion.


1. Styrt B, Gorbach SL. Recent developments in the understanding of the pathogenesis and treatment of anaerobic infections (first of two parts). *N Engl J Med* 1989; **321:** 240–6.
2. Styrt B, Gorbach SL. Recent developments in the understanding of the pathogenesis and treatment of anaerobic infections (second of two parts). *N Engl J Med* 1989; **321:** 298–302.
3. Finegold SM, Wexler HM. Present status of therapy for anaerobic infections. *Clin Infect Dis* 1996; **23** (suppl 1): S9–S14.
4. Brook I. Anaerobic infections. *Rev Med Microbiol* 1999; **10:** 137–53.
5. Brook I. The clinical importance of all members of the Bacteroides fragilis group. *J Antimicrob Chemother* 1990; **25:** 473–4.
6. Cuchural GJ, *et al.* Comparative activities of newer β-lactam agents against members of the Bacteroides fragilis group. *Antimicrob Agents Chemother* 1990; **34:** 479–80.
7. Cornick NA, *et al.* The antimicrobial susceptibility patterns of the Bacteroides fragilis group in the United States, 1987. *J Antimicrob Chemother* 1990; **25:** 1011–19.
8. Jacobs MR, *et al.* β-Lactamase production, β-lactam sensitivity and resistance to synergy with clavulanate of 737 Bacteroides fragilis group organisms from thirty-three US centres. *J Antimicrob Chemother* 1990; **26:** 361–70.
9. Turner P, *et al.* Simultaneous resistance to metronidazole, co-amoxiclav, and imipenem in clinical isolate of Bacteroides fragilis. *Lancet* 1995; **345:** 1275–7.


### Anthrax

Anthrax is a zoonotic disease caused by *Bacillus anthracis*, a spore-forming Gram-positive aerobe.[1] It is rare in western countries. The commonest type is cutaneous anthrax; pulmonary, gastrointestinal, and meningeal anthrax can also occur and in these types the prognosis is poor.

Benzylpenicillin has traditionally been the antibacterial of choice,[2] but resistant strains of *B. anthracis* have been reported and ciprofloxacin or doxycycline or other tetracycline may now be preferred, with benzylpenicillin or erythromycin recommended as alternatives.[3] Once septicaemia has developed a fatal outcome is likely due to toxin release; the use of anthrax antitoxin, if available, in conjunction with antibacterials has been advised.[2] Benzylpenicillin 10 mg/kg intramuscularly every 12 hours for 5 to 7 days has been used prophylactically if contaminated meat has been ingested or if *B. anthracis* has been inadvertently injected beneath the skin. Vaccine is available for active immunisation against anthrax. Combined penicillin and vaccine prophylaxis has been used for pulmonary anthrax prophylaxis.[2]

Guidelines[4-6] for the treatment of clinically evident infection following the use of *B. anthracis* for biological warfare or terrorism also recommend the initial use of ciprofloxacin or doxycycline.


1. Dixon TC, *et al.* Anthrax. *N Engl J Med* 1999; **341:** 815–26.
2. Knudson GB. Treatment of anthrax in man: history and current concepts. *Mil Med* 1986; **151:** 71–7.
3. Anonymous. The choice of antibacterial drugs. In: *Handbook of antimicrobial therapy.* 16th ed. New York: The Medical Letter, 2002: 34–52.
4. Centers for Disease Control. Update: investigation of bioterrorism-related anthrax and interim guidelines for exposure management and antimicrobial therapy, October 2001. *MMWR* 2001; **50:** 909–19. Also available at: http://www.cdc.gov/mmwr/preview/mmwrhtml/mm5042a1.htm (accessed 17/05/04) Correction. *ibid.*; 962.
5. Inglesby TV, *et al.* Anthrax as a biological weapon, 2002: updated recommendations for management. *JAMA* 2002; **287:** 2236–52.
6. Health Protection Agency. *Anthrax: interim guidelines for action in the event of a deliberate release.* Version 5.2; issued 12/08/03. Available at: http://www.hpa.org.uk/infections/topics_az/deliberate_release/Anthrax/PDFs/anthrax_guidelines.pdf (accessed 17/05/04)


### Antibiotic-associated colitis

See under Gastro-enteritis, p.128.

### Arthritis, bacterial

See under Bone and Joint Infections, p.122.

### Bacillary angiomatosis

See under Cat Scratch Disease, p.123.

### Bacterial vaginosis

Bacterial vaginosis (anaerobic vaginosis; non-specific vaginitis) is a common and often distressing vaginal condition that may or may not be sexually transmitted and is associated with a fishy-smelling vaginal discharge and an abnormal vaginal flora. The abnormal flora comprises *Gardnerella vaginalis*, *Mycoplasma hominis*, or *Mobiluncus* or *Prevotella* spp.

Guidelines produced by WHO[1] and in the UK[2] and USA[3] for the treatment of bacterial vaginosis are as follows, although relapse is common following any regimen:

- **WHO:** metronidazole 400 or 500 mg twice daily orally for 7 days; alternatives are metronidazole 2 g orally as a single dose, or metronidazole 5 g of a 0.75% gel twice daily intravaginally for 5 days, or clindamycin either 300 mg twice daily orally or 5 g of a 2% cream at bedtime intravaginally for 7 days
- **UK:** metronidazole 400 or 500 mg twice daily orally for 5 to 7 days or as a single 2-g dose; alternatives are metronidazole 0.75% gel once daily intravaginally for 5 days, or clindamycin either 300 mg twice daily orally or as a 2% cream once daily intravaginally for 7 days
- **USA:** metronidazole 500 mg twice daily orally for 7 days or 5 g of a 0.75% gel once daily intravaginally for 5 days, or clindamycin 5 g of a 2% cream at bedtime intravaginally for 7 days; alternatives are metronidazole 2 g orally as a single dose, or clindamycin either 300 mg twice daily orally for 7 days or 100 mg at bedtime intravaginally for 3 days.

An association has been reported between bacterial vaginosis and premature births of low-weight infants, and some have advised treatment early in the second trimester of pregnancy.[4,5] A systematic review[6] of randomised studies has concluded that the current evidence does not support screening and treatment of all pregnant women for bacterial vaginosis to prevent premature birth and its consequences, and that there is little suggestion that detection and treatment of bacterial vaginosis is effective in preventing premature birth in women with a history of a previous premature birth, although it may reduce the risk of low birth-weight and of preterm rupture of membranes.


1. WHO. Guidelines for the management of sexually transmitted infections. Geneva: WHO, 2003. Also available at: http://whqlibdoc.who.int/publications/2003/9241546263.pdf (accessed 22/06/04)
2. Clinical Effectiveness Group (Association for Genitourinary Medicine and the Medical Society for the Study of Venereal Diseases). 2001 National guideline for the management of bacterial vaginosis. Available at: http://www.bashh.org/guidelines/2002/BV_06_01.pdf (accessed 22/06/04)
3. Centers for Disease Control. Sexually transmitted diseases treatment guidelines 2002. *MMWR* 2002; **51**(RR-6): 1–80. Also available at: http://www.cdc.gov/mmwr/PDF/rr/rr5106.pdf (accessed 17/05/04)
4. Hay PE. Therapy of bacterial vaginosis. *J Antimicrob Chemother* 1998; **41:** 6–9.
5. Anonymous. Management of bacterial vaginosis. *Drug Ther Bull* 1998; **36:** 33–5.
6. McDonald H, *et al.* Antibiotics for treating bacterial vaginosis in pregnancy. Available in The Cochrane Library; Issue 2. Chichester: John Wiley; 2004.


### Biliary-tract infections

Infections of the biliary tract are usually associated with obstructive and inflammatory conditions such as cholecystitis and cholangitis. Complications can include gangrene, hepatic or intraperitoneal abscesses, peritonitis, and septicaemia. The organisms involved are typically gut flora, including Gram-negative aerobes such as *Escherichia coli* and *Klebsiella* spp., and anaerobes including *Bacteroides fragilis*.

Treatment of uncomplicated acute cholecystitis is usually conservative. Antibacterials including cephalosporins, tetracyclines, or broad-spectrum penicillins are commonly given, although some have questioned their use.[1] For more severe infections including suppurative cholangitis, prompt treatment with appropriate antibacterial drugs is necessary. Since biliary obstruction prevents adequate concentrations of many antibacterials being achieved in the bile, the main aim of treatment is to control bacteraemia. Antibacterials used, often in combination, include cephalosporins, aminoglycosides, ampicillin (or amoxicillin), piperacillin, fluoroquinolones, metronidazole, clindamycin, and imipenem.[2-4] In most cases of obstruction, definitive treatment depends on restoring drainage of bile by surgical or medical treatment of gallstones (p.1761).

Antibacterial prophylaxis is commonly used in biliary surgery (see Surgical Infection, p.147) to prevent acute cholangitis and wound infections. Cephalosporins are often used for this purpose.[2]

Antibacterials may also have a role as maintenance therapy in recurrent cholangitis.


1. Bouchier IAD. Gallstones. *BMJ* 1990; **300:** 592–7.
2. van den Hazel SJ, *et al.* Role of antibiotics in the treatment and prevention of acute and recurrent cholangitis. *Clin Infect Dis* 1994; **19:** 279–86.
3. Peña C, Gudiol F. Cholecystitis and cholangitis: spectrum of bacteria and role of antibiotics. *Dig Surg* 1996; **13:** 317–20.
4. Westphal J-F, Brogard J-M. Biliary tract infections: a guide to drug treatment. *Drugs* 1999; **57:** 81–91.


### Bites and stings

Wound infections following cat or dog bites may be due to a mixture of organisms,[1] often including the Gram-negative aerobe *Pasteurella multocida*. The treatment of choice for *P. multocida* is benzylpenicillin[2] and it should be given for infections evident within 24 hours of a bite;[3] alternatives are amoxicillin-clavulanic acid, ampicillin-sulbactam, or a cephalosporin.[2] Tetracycline is a further alternative in patients allergic to penicillin. The fluoroquinolone ciprofloxacin has been used successfully to treat *P. multocida* cellulitis associated with a cat bite.[4]

In addition to *P. multocida*, other bacteria involved in cat or dog bite wound infections include *Staphylococcus, Streptococcus, Bacteroides,* and *Fusobacterium* spp. and their presence will influence the choice of treatment. For example, a penicillinase-resistant penicillin may be necessary if *Staph. aureus* is present. Also, combinations of antibacterials may be necessary in patients allergic to penicillin since tetracycline, the alternative suggested against *P. multocida* infection, has only limited activity against aerobic Gram-positive cocci.

More unusual organisms include *Capnocytophaga canimorsus* (formerly called dysgonic fermenter type 2 or DF-2) which has been associated in particular with dog bites,[5,6] but also with cat bites. It is an opportunistic pathogen especially hazardous to immunocompromised patients including splenectomised patients; the best treatment is benzylpenicillin,[7] amoxicillin-clavulanic acid, or erythromycin.[8] Infection with *C. canimorsus* following dog bites may be severe and has led to fatal septicaemia, disseminated intravascular coagulation, meningitis, or endocarditis,[5] highlighting the importance of early antibacterial treatment and debridement.

See also under Cat Scratch Disease (p.123).

A systematic review[9] has concluded that there is no evidence that the use of prophylactic antibacterials is effective for cat or dog bites, though, if necessary, prophylaxis or treatment for rabies (p.1636) should be instituted.

Among the more unusual infections acquired from animals is seal finger, caused by an as yet unidentified organism and treated with tetracycline.[10] The Gram-negative bacilli *Spirillum minus* (or *minor*) and *Streptobacillus moniliformis* are both causes of rat-bite fever. In each case the treatment of choice is benzylpenicillin;[2] a tetracycline or streptomycin are alternatives.

Envenomation following bites and stings by snakes, scorpions, spiders, and some marine animals is usually treated symptomatically and with specific antivenoms and antisera (see Box Jellyfish Sting, p.1621, Scorpion Stings, p.1638, Snake Bites, p.1639, Spider Bites, p.1640, and Stone Fish Venom Antisera, p.1640).


1. Talan DA, *et al.* Bacteriologic analysis of infected dog and cat bites. *N Engl J Med* 1999; **340:** 85–92.
2. Anonymous. The choice of antibacterial drugs. In: *Handbook of antimicrobial therapy.* 16th ed. New York: The Medical Letter, 2002: 34–52.
3. Elliot DL, *et al.* Pet-associated illness. *N Engl J Med* 1985; **313:** 985–95.
4. Richards CAL, Emmanuel FXS. Treatment of Pasteurella multocida cellulitis with ciprofloxacin. *J Infect* 1992; **24:** 216–17.
5. Pers C, *et al.* Capnocytophaga canimorsus septicemia in Denmark, 1982-1995: review of 39 cases. *Clin Infect Dis* 1996; **23:** 71–5.
6. Le Moal G, *et al.* Meningitis due to Capnocytophaga canimorsus after receipt of a dog bite: case report and review of the literature. *Clin Infect Dis* 2003; **36:** e42–e46.
7. McCarthy M, Zumla A. DF-2 infection. *BMJ* 1988; **297:** 1355–6.
8. Morgan MS, Cruickshank JG. Prevention of postsplenectomy sepsis. *Lancet* 1993; **341:** 700–1.
9. Medeiros I, Saconato H. Antibiotic prophylaxis for mammalian bites. Available in The Cochrane Library; Issue 2. Chichester: John Wiley; 2004.
10. Hartley JW, Pitcher D. Seal finger—tetracycline is first line. *J Infect* 2002; **45:** 71–5.


## Bone and joint infections

In *bacterial arthritis* (septic arthritis) joints may be infected via the blood with a variety of organisms, including staphylococci, streptococci, enterococci, Enterobacteriaceae, *Pseudomonas aeruginosa*, and anaerobes, although the commonest is probably *Staphylococcus aureus*. *Haemophilus influenzae* is a common cause in young children, as is *Neisseria gonorrhoeae* in sexually active young adults. In addition to gonococcal arthritis, other specific types of bacterial arthritis include Lyme disease and meningococcal, salmonellal, and tuberculous arthritis (see under the appropriate disease for further details).

With the exception of *N. gonorrhoeae*, infecting organisms in *osteomyelitis* (infection of bone) are similar to those in bacterial arthritis.[1-3]

In *reactive arthritis* (aseptic arthritis) joint inflammation follows infection elsewhere in the body. It is generally secondary to sexually transmitted, especially chlamydial, infections, or to enteric infections. Reactive arthritis in association with urethritis or cervicitis, or both, is termed Reiter's syndrome.

Empirical treatment regimens for bacterial arthritis or osteomyelitis usually include antistaphylococcal antibacterials such as flucloxacillin, nafcillin, clindamycin, and fusidic acid; vancomycin is used to combat possible meticillin-resistant *Staph aureus*. Children under 5 years may be given amoxicillin or cefuroxime because of the likelihood of *H. influenzae* infection. Treatment is generally initiated with high doses given intravenously and may need to continue for 6 weeks in acute bacterial arthritis or osteomyelitis. Chronic disease may require longer term treatment although the oral route may be used after initial parenteral therapy.

A systematic review and meta-analysis[4] of antibacterial treatment of bone and joint infections concluded that most studies were methodologically flawed and that there was little high-quality evidence regarding treatment. Oral ciprofloxacin[5,6] or other fluoroquinolones[7,8] have been used successfully in the treatment of osteomyelitis due to susceptible organisms, but the value of fluoroquinolones against Gram-positive bacteria has been questioned and there is increasing resistance to them among meticillin-resistant *Staph. aureus* and coagulase-negative staphylococci.[9] Rifampicin has also been used, sometimes with other drugs; in one study[10] use of rifampicin with ciprofloxacin improved control of staphylococcal bone infections related to orthopaedic devices in comparison with ciprofloxacin alone.

For reference to infection prophylaxis in orthopaedic patients, see under Surgical Infection, below.

Reactive arthritis is treated with anti-inflammatories; the role of antibacterials is less certain.[11] Results in arthritis associated with chlamydial infections have been more promising than in that triggered by enteric infections.[12] Long-term treatment with a tetracycline in addition to an NSAID has been reported to shorten the duration of reactive arthritis resulting from *Chlamydia trachomatis* infection.[13]

For mention of the use of tetracyclines, usually minocycline, in the treatment of *rheumatoid arthritis*, see under Rheumatic Disorders, p.268.


1. Lew DP, Waldvogel FA. Osteomyelitis. *N Engl J Med* 1997; **336:** 999–1007.
2. Mader JT, *et al.* A practical guide to the diagnosis and management of bone and joint infections. *Drugs* 1997; **54:** 253–64.
3. Goldenberg DL. Septic arthritis. *Lancet* 1998; **351:** 197–202.
4. Stengel D, *et al.* Systematic review and meta-analysis of antibiotic therapy for bone and joint infections. *Lancet Infect Dis* 2001; **1:** 175–88. Correction. *ibid.* 2002; **2:** 125.
5. Gentry LO, Rodriguez GG. Oral ciprofloxacin compared with parenteral antibiotics in the treatment of osteomyelitis. *Antimicrob Agents Chemother* 1990; **34:** 40–3.
6. Dan M, *et al.* Oral ciprofloxacin treatment of Pseudomonas aeruginosa osteomyelitis. *Antimicrob Agents Chemother* 1990; **34:** 849–52.
7. Gentry LO, Rodriguez-Gomez G. Ofloxacin versus parenteral therapy for chronic osteomyelitis. *Antimicrob Agents Chemother* 1991; **35:** 538–41.
8. Greenberg RN, *et al.* Ciprofloxacin, lomefloxacin, or levofloxacin as treatment for chronic osteomyelitis. *Antimicrob Agents Chemother* 2000; **44:** 164–6.
9. Cruciani M, Bassetti D. The fluoroquinolones as treatment for infections caused by Gram-positive bacteria. *J Antimicrob Chemother* 1994; **33:** 403–17.
10. Zimmerli W, *et al.* Role of rifampin for treatment of orthopedic implant-related staphylococcal infections: a randomized controlled trial. *JAMA* 1998; **279:** 1537–41.
11. Toivanen A. Bacteria-triggered reactive arthritis: implications for antibacterial treatment. *Drugs* 2001; **61:** 343–51.
12. Svenungsson B. Reactive arthritis. *BMJ* 1994; **308:** 671–2.
13. Lauhio A. Reactive arthritis: consider combination treatment. *BMJ* 1994; **308:** 1302–3.


## Botulism

For a discussion of botulism and its management, see p.1611.

## Bronchitis

Bronchitis may be defined as inflammation of the bronchi and is associated with excessive sputum production and cough. The bronchi of healthy people are said to be nearly always sterile whereas the upper respiratory tract is often colonised with commensal bacteria including *Streptococcus pneumoniae* and *Haemophilus influenzae*.

*Acute bronchitis* in previously healthy subjects is commonly associated with viral respiratory infections such as colds and influenza. There may sometimes be secondary bacterial infection that responds to antibacterial therapy as for acute exacerbations of chronic bronchitis (see below). *Acute bronchiolitis* occurs in infants as a result mainly of viral infection and antibacterials are not given routinely (see Respiratory Syncytial Virus Infection, p.625).

*Chronic bronchitis* and emphysema often occur together and have been termed chronic obstructive pulmonary disease (p.779). Acute exacerbations of chronic bronchitis may be viral in origin, but bacteria are often present in purulent sputum, the commonest being *Str. pneumoniae* and *H. influenzae*; *Moraxella catarrhalis* (*Branhamella catarrhalis*) is increasingly reported.

The value of antibacterial treatment in both acute bronchitis and acute exacerbation of chronic disease has been controversial and difficult to assess.[1-5] Following a comparison of a broad-spectrum antibacterial (amoxicillin, co-trimoxazole, or doxycycline) with placebo,[6] it was considered that antibacterials were justified in exacerbations of chronic obstructive pulmonary disease characterised by increased dyspnoea, sputum production, and sputum purulence. Also, a meta-analysis of randomised studies indicated a small improvement due to therapy in patients with exacerbations of disease.[7] However, a further meta-analysis[8] assessing the use of antibacterials for acute bronchitis concluded that, although there was some benefit to be obtained this did not outweigh the risks of adverse effects and increased resistance and that the use of antibacterials could therefore not be advocated in otherwise healthy patients with no evidence of chronic disease. A systematic review[9] also concluded that the modest benefit associated with antibacterial use in acute disease was of similar magnitude to the detriment from potential adverse effects. If antibacterials are given it is common practice to give a 7- to 10-day oral course of a broad-spectrum drug such as amoxicillin (alone or with clavulanic acid), ampicillin, an oral cephalosporin such as cefaclor or cefuroxime axetil, co-trimoxazole, erythromycin or a newer macrolide such as azithromycin or clarithromycin, tetracycline, or trimethoprim (preferred to co-trimoxazole in the UK), the choice depending on local patterns of resistance.

Long-term prophylaxis in patients with frequent exacerbations of bronchitis is controversial. A systematic review[10] of the value of antibacterial prophylaxis in chronic bronchitis concluded that it did have a small but significant effect in reducing the number of days of illness, but that it had no place in routine therapy because of concerns over adverse effects and the development of resistance.

Bronchitis associated with *Chlamydophila pneumoniae* (*Chlamydia pneumoniae*) and responding to tetracycline or erythromycin has also been reported.[11]


1. Anonymous. Antibiotics for exacerbations of chronic bronchitis? *Lancet* 1987; **ii:** 23–4.
2. Staley H, *et al.* Is an objective assessment of antibiotic therapy in exacerbations of chronic bronchitis possible? *J Antimicrob Chemother* 1993; **31:** 193–7.
3. Gonzales R, Sande M. What will it take to stop physicians from prescribing antibiotics in acute bronchitis? *Lancet* 1995; **345:** 665–6.
4. Hahn DL. Antibiotics in acute bronchitis. *Lancet* 1995; **345:** 1244–5.
5. O'Brien KL, *et al.* Cough illness/bronchitis—principles of judicious use of antimicrobial agents. *Pediatrics* 1998; **101** (suppl): 178–81.
6. Anthonisen NR, *et al.* Antibiotic therapy in exacerbations of chronic obstructive pulmonary disease. *Ann Intern Med* 1987; **106:** 196–204.
7. Saint S, *et al.* Antibiotics in chronic obstructive pulmonary disease exacerbations: a meta-analysis. *JAMA* 1995; **273:** 957–60.
8. Bent S, *et al.* Antibiotics in acute bronchitis: a meta-analysis. *Am J Med* 1999; **107:** 62–7.
9. Smucny J, *et al.* Antibiotics for acute bronchitis. Available in The Cochrane Library; Issue 2. Chichester: John Wiley; 2004.
10. Staykova T, *et al.* Prophylactic antibiotic therapy for chronic bronchitis. Available in The Cochrane Library; Issue 2. Chichester: John Wiley; 2004.
11. Grayston JT, *et al.* A new respiratory tract pathogen: Chlamydia pneumoniae strain TWAR. *J Infect Dis* 1990; **161:** 618–25.


## Brucellosis

Brucellosis (formerly known as undulant fever) is caused by *Brucella* spp., aerobic Gram-negative bacteria found primarily in animals and transmitted to humans. The principal species affecting man are *Brucella abortus*, from cattle; *B. melitensis*, from sheep, goats, camels, and sometimes cattle; and *B. suis* from pigs. Brucellosis has often been associated with consumption of unpasteurised milk or its products and although rare or controlled in countries such as the UK it remains a problem in many areas, including the Mediterranean region and Middle East. Rarely, human infection can result from exposure to live veterinary vaccines.[1]

Treatment of brucellosis has been with rifampicin plus doxycycline, but some now prefer doxycycline plus streptomycin. The regimen recommended by WHO is rifampicin 600 to 900 mg with doxycycline 200 mg, both given daily in the morning as a single dose for at least 6 weeks.[2] Use of doxycycline and rifampicin for 30 days was found by some workers[3] to result in higher relapse rates than those for the regimen of tetracycline and streptomycin previously recommended by WHO. However, in a multinational comparative study of 143 patients with acute brucellosis,[4] a 45-day regimen of rifampicin and doxycycline was comparable with a regimen of doxycycline 200 mg daily with a meal for 45 days and streptomycin 1 g intramuscularly daily for 21 days; a third regimen of tetracycline 500 mg 4 times daily for 21 days and streptomycin 1 g intramuscularly daily for 14 days was associated with a 41% failure rate and could not be recommended. Doxycycline for 6 weeks and streptomycin for the first 2 weeks also proved effective in a Spanish study,[5] and was considered preferable to doxycycline and rifampicin. An overview of studies also indicated that doxycycline plus streptomycin was associated with lower relapse rates than rifampicin plus doxycycline, and recommended the former as the preferred combination.[6] An interaction between rifampicin and doxycycline, in which concentrations of doxycycline were reduced when the two were given together,[7] might explain the reduced efficacy of this combination. A suggested regimen in non-pregnant adults is thus doxycycline 200 mg daily for 6 weeks together with streptomycin 1 g daily for 2 to 3 weeks.[8]

Resistance to rifampicin has emerged following therapy despite administration with doxycycline.[9]

Although treatment usually uses combinations of drugs, co-trimoxazole has been used alone but relapse was common.[2]

Rifampicin with co-trimoxazole was effective in the treatment of **children**,[10] although the authors of a multicentre study in Kuwaiti children[11] considered that rifampicin should be reserved for complicated brucellosis because of the risk of serious adverse effects and development of resistance in areas endemic for tuberculosis. They recommended oxytetracycline or doxycycline for 3 weeks with gentamicin intramuscularly for the first 5 days in children over 8 years old, co-trimoxazole being given instead of a tetracycline in younger children.

For the treatment of brucellosis during **pregnancy**, WHO recommends rifampicin as the drug of choice and that co-trimoxazole or tetracycline should only be given if rifampicin is unavailable; streptomycin is contra-indicated.[2]

In the treatment of **neurobrucellosis**, the length of therapy appears to be of critical importance; relapses may occur after treatment lasting only 2 to 3 weeks and a regimen of tetracycline 2 g daily and rifampicin 600 to 900 mg daily given for 8 to 12 weeks supplemented with streptomycin 1 g daily for 6 weeks has consequently been recommended.[12] There have also been reports of the successful use of similar triple therapy in the treatment of endocarditis due to *Brucella melitensis*.[13]

A vaccine is available in some countries for active immunisation of individuals at high risk of contracting brucellosis.


1. Blasco JM, Díaz R. Brucella melitensis Rev-1 vaccine as a cause of human brucellosis. *Lancet* 1993; **342:** 805.
2. FAO/WHO. Joint FAO/WHO expert committee on brucellosis: sixth report. *WHO Tech Rep Ser 740* 1986.
3. Ariza J, *et al.* Comparative trial of rifampin-doxycycline versus tetracycline-streptomycin in the therapy of human brucellosis. *Antimicrob Agents Chemother* 1985; **28:** 548–51.
4. Acocella G, *et al.* Comparison of three different regimens in the treatment of acute brucellosis: a multicenter multinational study. *J Antimicrob Chemother* 1989; **23:** 433–9. Correction *ibid.*; **24:** 629.
5. Cisneros JM, *et al.* Multicenter prospective study of treatment of Brucella melitensis brucellosis with doxycycline for 6 weeks plus streptomycin for 2 weeks. *Antimicrob Agents Chemother* 1990; **34:** 881–3.
6. Solera J, *et al.* Recognition and optimum treatment of brucellosis. *Drugs* 1997; **53:** 245–56.
7. Colmenero JD, *et al.* Possible implications of doxycycline-rifampin interaction for treatment of brucellosis. *Antimicrob Agents Chemother* 1994; **38:** 2798–2802.
8. Friedland JS. Brucellosis. *Prescribers' J* 1993; **33:** 24–8.
9. De Rautlin de la Roy YM, *et al.* Rifampicin resistance in a strain of Brucella melitensis after treatment with doxycycline and rifampicin. *J Antimicrob Chemother* 1986; **18:** 648–9.
10. Llorens-Terol J, Busquets RM. Brucellosis treated with rifampicin. *Arch Dis Child* 1980; **55:** 486–8.
11. Lubani MM, *et al.* A multicenter therapeutic study of 1100 children with brucellosis. *Pediatr Infect Dis* 1989; **8:** 75–8.
12. Shakir RA. Neurobrucellosis. *Postgrad Med J* 1986; **62:** 1077–9.
13. Farid Z, Trabolsi B. Successful treatment of two cases of brucella endocarditis with rifampicin. *BMJ* 1985; **291:** 110.


## Campylobacter enteritis

See under Gastro-enteritis, p.128.

## Cat scratch disease

Cat scratch disease usually occurs after a cat scratch or bite. The condition is characterised by regional lymphadenopathy and is often self-limiting, but may be disseminated in immunocompromised patients.

In the 1980s a Gram-negative bacillus presumed to be responsible for cat scratch disease was isolated[1,2] and subsequently named *Afipia felis*.[3] However, it now appears that *Bartonella henselae* (formerly *Rochalimaea henselae*) is the main cause of cat scratch disease[3-5] and that *A. felis* causes few, if any, cases, although there is some evidence that both organisms might have a joint role.[6] With uncertainty over aetiology there has been no specific antibacterial therapy, but there are reports of successful treatment with gentamicin[7] or co-trimoxazole[8] in children and with ciprofloxacin[9] in adults. Azithromycin has also been found to be of benefit in adults[10] and may now be the treatment of choice. Bacillary angiomatosis, in which both *B. henselae* and *B. quintana*[11] (the causative organism of trench fever) have been implicated, may represent a disseminated form of cat scratch disease occurring predominantly in HIV-infected patients. In contrast, the disseminated disease in immunocompromised patients has not responded to ciprofloxacin,[12,13] but has responded to treatment with doxycycline[12-15] or erythromycin[12] or azithromycin. Care is required in patients with AIDS since the lesions of bacillary angiomatosis closely resemble those of Kaposi's sarcoma, and if the diagnosis is missed, life-saving antibacterial therapy may not be given.[16]


1. Wear DJ, *et al.* Cat scratch disease: a bacterial infection. *Science* 1983; **221:** 1403–5.
2. English CK, *et al.* Cat-scratch disease: isolation and culture of the bacterial agent. *JAMA* 1988; **259:** 1347–52.
3. Birtles RJ, *et al.* Cat scratch disease and bacillary angiomatosis: aetiological agents and the link with AIDS. *Commun Dis Rep* 1993; **3:** R107–R110.
4. Relman DA, *et al.* The agent of bacillary angiomatosis: an approach to the identification of uncultured pathogens. *N Engl J Med* 1990; **323:** 1573–80.
5. Flexman JP, *et al.* Bartonella henselae is a causative agent of cat scratch disease in Australia. *J Infect* 1995; **31:** 241–5.
6. Alkan S, *et al.* Dual role for Afipia felis and Rochalimaea henselae in cat-scratch disease. *Lancet* 1995; **345:** 385.
7. Bogue CW, *et al.* Antibiotic therapy for cat-scratch disease? *JAMA* 1989; **262:** 813–16.
8. Collipp PJ. Cat-scratch disease therapy. *Am J Dis Child* 1989; **143:** 1261.
9. Holley HP. Successful treatment of cat-scratch disease with ciprofloxacin. *JAMA* 1991; **265:** 1563–5.
10. Bass JW, *et al.* Prospective randomized double blind placebo-controlled evaluation of azithromycin for treatment of cat-scratch disease. *Pediatr Infect Dis J* 1998; **17:** 447–52.
11. Koehler JE, *et al.* Isolation of Rochalimaea species from cutaneous and osseous lesions of bacillary angiomatosis. *N Engl J Med* 1992; **327:** 1625–31.
12. Tappero JW, Koehler JE. Cat-scratch disease and bacillary angiomatosis. *JAMA* 1991; **266:** 1938–9.
13. Tucker RM, *et al.* Cat-scratch disease and bacillary angiomatosis. *JAMA* 1991; **266:** 1939.
14. Kemper CA, *et al.* Visceral bacillary epithelioid angiomatosis: possible manifestations of disseminated cat scratch disease in the immunocompromised host: a report of two cases. *Am J Med* 1990; **89:** 216–22.
15. Mui BSK, *et al.* Response of HIV-associated disseminated cat scratch disease to treatment with doxycycline. *Am J Med* 1990; **89:** 229–31.
16. Taylor AG, *et al.* Cat-scratch, Kaposi's sarcoma, and bacillary angiomatosis. *Lancet* 1993; **342:** 686.


## Cellulitis

See under Skin Infections, p.146.

## Cervicitis

Gonorrhoea in women occurs mainly as cervicitis, but mucopurulent cervicitis is frequently caused by sexually transmitted *Chlamydia trachomatis*. The two infections often occur together and should be treated concurrently. Guidelines for treatment are given under Gonorrhoea, p.130, and Chlamydial Infections, below.

## Chancroid

Chancroid is a sexually transmitted disease caused by the Gram-negative bacterium *Haemophilus ducreyi*. It occurs worldwide, but is endemic in parts of Africa and South East Asia, where it is a frequent cause of genital ulceration and a risk factor in the transmission of HIV. Chancroid has also become an important sexually transmitted disease in the USA.[1]

Specific treatment guidelines have been provided in the UK,[2] the USA,[1] and by WHO.[3] Treatment failure may be more common in patients also infected with HIV, especially with single-dose regimens,[1] although, in other patients, single-dose treatment regimens might be preferable if compliance is a problem. Recommendations in the UK and USA are azithromycin 1 g by mouth as a single dose, or ceftriaxone 250 mg intramuscularly as a single dose, or ciprofloxacin 500 mg twice daily by mouth for 3 days.[1,2] A further alternative is erythromycin 500 mg, recommended either four times daily by mouth for 7 days in the UK[2] or three times daily by mouth for 7 days in the USA.[1] Also recommended in the UK are ciprofloxacin 500 mg as a single dose by mouth, or single oral doses of other fluoroquinolones such as fleroxacin 400 mg or norfloxacin 800 mg, or a single intramuscular injection of spectinomycin 2 g.[2] WHO recommends[3] ciprofloxacin 500 mg twice daily by mouth for 3 days, or erythromycin 500 mg four times daily by mouth for 7 days, or azithromycin 1 g as a single oral dose; an alternative is a single intramuscular injection of ceftriaxone 250 mg.

Sexual partners of patients with chancroid should also be treated.


1. Centers for Disease Control. Sexually transmitted diseases treatment guidelines 2002. *MMWR* 2002; **51**(RR-6): 1–80. Also available at: http://www.cdc.gov/mmwr/PDF/rr/rr5106.pdf (accessed 17/05/04)
2. Clinical Effectiveness Group (Association for Genitourinary Medicine and the Medical Society for the Study of Venereal Diseases). 2001 National guideline for the management of chancroid. Available at: http://www.bashh.org/guidelines/2002/chancroid%2009%2001b.pdf (accessed 17/05/04)
3. WHO. Guidelines for the management of sexually transmitted infections. Geneva: WHO, 2003. Also available at: http://whqlibdoc.who.int/publications/2003/9241546263.pdf (accessed 22/06/04)


## Chlamydial infections

The family Chlamydiaceae is divided into two genera, *Chlamydia* and *Chlamydophila*. Species that are pathogenic in man are *Chlamydophila pneumoniae*, *Chlamydophila psittaci*, and *Chlamydia trachomatis* and are generally sensitive to tetracyclines or erythromycin. *C. pneumoniae* (formerly TWAR strain of *C. psittaci*) is a respiratory pathogen. It was first described as a cause of community-acquired pneumonia (see Pneumonia, p.141), but has since been associated with a wide variety of clinical presentations including pharyngitis (see p.140) and has been implicated in the pathogenesis of ischaemic heart disease (see Atherosclerosis, p.815). *C. psittaci* is transmitted to man from birds and causes psittacosis which also affects the lungs (see Psittacosis, p.143).

*C. trachomatis* causes a wide range of diseases. Many are sexually transmitted and the spectrum is similar to that with *Neisseria gonorrhoeae* (see Gonorrhoea, p.130); infections with the two organisms often occur concurrently. Pregnant women infected with *C. trachomatis* may be at risk of premature rupture of membranes and preterm labour (see Premature Labour, p.143). They may also infect their offspring to cause ophthalmia neonatorum (see Neonatal Conjunctivitis, p.136) or pneumonia (p.141).

Treatment is with oral antibacterials. Guidelines for the treatment of uncomplicated anogenital infection with *C. trachomatis* have been published by WHO,[1] as well as in the UK[2] and USA.[3] All recommend doxycycline 100 mg twice daily by mouth for 7 days or a single dose of azithromycin 1 g by mouth. Alternatives, which are broadly similar, are: WHO, oral amoxicillin, erythromycin, ofloxacin, or tetracycline; UK, oral erythromycin, ofloxacin, or other tetracyclines; USA, oral levofloxacin, ofloxacin, or erythromycin. Sexual partners of those infected with *C. trachomatis* should be tested and treated.[1-3] Pregnant women should be given erythromycin or amoxicillin[1-3] to eradicate *C. trachomatis* infection and prevent perinatal transmission. Azithromycin[3] or clindamycin[4] are further alternatives.

In the USA, the US Preventive Services Task Force has recommended routine screening for *C. trachomatis* infection in all sexually active women aged 25 years or less, whether or not they are pregnant, and in women aged over 25 years if they are considered to be at increased risk of infection.[5]

For further reference to sexually transmitted *C. trachomatis* infections, see under Epididymitis (p.127), Pelvic Inflammatory Disease (p.139), and Urethritis (p.152)

Specific serotypes of *C. trachomatis* are responsible for another sexually transmitted disease, lymphogranuloma venereum (p.134).

Reactive arthritis (see Bone and Joint Infections, p.122) may be secondary to chlamydial infections.

Other *C. trachomatis* infections that are not sexually transmitted include trachoma and inclusion conjunctivitis in adults (see Trachoma, p.149).


1. WHO. Guidelines for the management of sexually transmitted infections. Geneva: WHO, 2003. Also available at: http://whqlibdoc.who.int/publications/2003/9241546263.pdf (accessed 22/06/04)
2. Clinical Effectiveness Group (Association for Genitourinary Medicine and the Medical Society for the Study of Venereal Diseases). Clinical effectiveness guideline for the management of Chlamydia trachomatis genital tract infection. Available at: http://www.bashh.org/guidelines/2002/C4A%2009%2001c.pdf (accessed 17/05/04)
3. Centers for Disease Control. Sexually transmitted diseases treatment guidelines 2002. *MMWR* 2002; **51**(RR-6): 1–80. Also available at: http://www.cdc.gov/mmwr/PDF/rr/rr5106.pdf (accessed 17/05/04)
4. Brocklehurst P, Rooney G. Interventions for treating genital Chlamydia trachomatis infection in pregnancy. Available in The Cochrane Library; Issue 2. Chichester: John Wiley; 2004.
5. US Preventive Services Task Force. Chlamydia trachomatis screening recommendations. *MMWR* 2002; **51** (RR-15): 37. Also available at: http://www.ahcpr.gov/clinic/uspstf/uspschlm.htm (accessed 17/05/04)


## Cholera and other vibrio infections

See under Gastro-enteritis, p.128.

## Cystic fibrosis

Cystic fibrosis is a genetic disorder associated with the production of abnormally viscous mucus. The underlying defect is mutation in the gene which codes for cystic fibrosis transmembrane conductance regulator (CFTR), a protein which functions as a chloride channel. Mutations result in defective ion transport with reduced chloride ion secretion and accelerated sodium ion absorption, and related changes in the composition and properties of mucin secreted. Now that patients with cystic fibrosis usually survive into adulthood, it is increasingly seen to be a multisystem disease. However, the main clinical manifestations are still pulmonary disease, with recurrent bacterial infections and the production of copious viscous sputum, and malabsorption due to pancreatic insufficiency. Other complications include male infertility and hepatobiliary disease. There is increased salt loss in sweat.

Various diagnostic methods are available[1-3] and clinical diagnosis of cystic fibrosis may be confirmed by establishing that chloride concentrations in sweat are raised. This may be done by using the pilocarpine sweat test (see Pilocarpine, p.1495, and for further details, see *Martindale*, 29th ed. p.1335). Identification of gene mutation is possible and may be used for further confirmation of the diagnosis and identification of carrier status.[4]

The reduced morbidity and improved survival in patients with cystic fibrosis are largely due to the management of pulmonary disease with antibacterials and physiotherapy and to nutritional management. Several reviews have discussed both established and experimental therapy.[5-7]

**Pulmonary disease** is the major cause of mortality. Cystic fibrosis is an underlying cause of bronchiectasis (chronic dilatation of the bronchi) as a result of excessive secretion of mucus and recurrent infections. Cough and excessive production of sputum are characteristic of cystic fibrosis and the lungs are generally colonised with bacterial pathogens, especially mucoid strains of *Pseudomonas aeruginosa*. Pseudomonal pulmonary infection is the major cause of morbidity and mortality in cystic fibrosis. Monitoring of bacterial pathogens in the sputum, including their sensitivity, is necessary for rational treatment. Apart from *Ps. aeruginosa*, *Staphylococcus aureus* is often present and may be the predominant pathogen in infants. *Burkholderia cepacia* (*Pseudomonas cepacia*) has been recognised as a cause of serious lung infection in cystic fibrosis. In a proportion who acquire it, *B. cepacia* has been associated with rapid deterioration and death.[8] Other bacteria isolated include *Haemophilus influenzae* and atypical *Mycobacteria* spp.

The approach to managing lung infections varies and the development of a consensus view has been hampered by the lack of clinical trials of sufficient power. Staphylococcal infections commonly develop during the first decade of life, and some clinicians start antistaphylococcal antibacterials on diagnosis of cystic fibrosis. Others wait until the first clinical infection occurs before starting treatment. Once started, antistaphylococcal therapy is continued indefinitely in some centres, while others only treat when symptomatic exacerbations or positive sputum cultures occur. Systematic reviews confirmed that antistaphylococcal treatment is effective and also concluded that prophylaxis is likely to be beneficial in young children with cystic fibrosis.[9,10] There was, however, insufficient evidence to determine whether intermittent or continuous therapy produces the best clinical outcome. In an accompanying editorial, concerns were expressed about the basis for even these conclusions.[11] Other potential disadvantages to prophylaxis are the possible early acquisition of *P. aeruginosa* infection[12] and an increased incidence of drug-resistant staphylococci with continuous therapy.[11]

Once present, eradication of *Ps. aeruginosa* is difficult and not permanent. Acute exacerbations of pulmonary infection are treated with antipseudomonal antibacterials intravenously, usually an aminoglycoside (e.g. tobramycin) with either a penicillin (e.g. ticarcillin) or a third-generation cephalosporin (e.g. ceftazidime); monotherapy, usually with ceftazidime, has also been given, but has been implicated in the emergence of resistant organisms.[13] High doses are necessary because of the poor penetration of these antipseudomonal antibacterials into the site of infection and their increased renal clearance in patients with cystic fibrosis.[14,15]

There is no consensus over the best strategy for managing chronic infection.[13] Some treat acute exacerbations as they occur whereas others give regular intermittent courses of intravenous antipseudomonal antibacterials. In one study,[16] chronic colonisation was prevented by giving oral ciprofloxacin and inhalations of colistin for 3 weeks whenever *Ps. aeruginosa* was isolated from routine sputum cultures. Intermittent elective intravenous therapy has become more practical with the development of regimens that enable patients to be treated at home.[13,17] Inhaled antibacterials, particularly tobramycin (either alone[18,19] or with ticarcillin[20]), have become increasingly popular.[21,22] Studies have shown that nebulised tobramycin given twice daily every alternate month produces clinical benefits[23] and is not associated with increased resistance or bacterial superinfections.[24] Gentamicin with carbenicillin,[25] and colistin[26] have also been used by inhalation. Active immunisation with a *Pseudomonas aeruginosa* vaccine or passive immunisation with antibodies against *Ps. aeruginosa* are under investigation.

Infection with *B. cepacia* is difficult to treat because the majority of antipseudomonal antibacterials are not effective. Co-trimoxazole has been suggested for *B. cepacia* infections.[27] Results of a pilot study indicating that nebulised taurolidine may be beneficial have not been supported by a double-blind placebo-controlled crossover clinical trial.[28] Transmission of *B. cepacia* in cystic fibrosis patients appears to be mainly by social contact,[29,30] although some have reported otherwise.[31]

The effects of cystic fibrosis in the lungs are complex and treatment of infections may not halt the progression of lung destruction. Many other interventions have been tried.[32,33] Dornase alfa[34] is given by aerosol inhalation and reduces the viscosity of the sputum by breaking down the large quantities of DNA released by degenerating inflammatory cells. The use of dornase alfa has been associated with some improvement in lung function and it might be a useful adjunct to bronchial drainage, although it is unclear whether it prevents the development of progressive lung damage (see p.1119). However, a randomised, multicentre, placebo-controlled study in children showed that dornase alfa maintained lung function and reduced the risk of exacerbations over a period of 96 weeks.[35] Mucolytics such as acetylcysteine are generally not considered to be effective in cystic fibrosis.[36]

Bronchodilators including both beta agonists and antimuscarinics may be useful in selected patients although there are few meaningful clinical trial results.[32,33,37] A therapeutic trial is often justified in individual patients since it is difficult to predict which patients will respond.[32] While administration by nebuliser is regarded as most effective, inhalers may be more practical where compatibility with other nebulised drugs could be a problem.[33]

Other interventions tried with some evidence of benefit include management of the inflammatory response in the lungs with corticosteroids[38] (by mouth[39] or more usually by inhalation,[32] although a systematic review[40] of randomised studies concluded that there was insufficient evidence to establish whether there was a beneficial or harmful effect of inhaled corticosteroids in cystic fibrosis patients), or, less commonly, with the NSAID ibuprofen.[41] Azithromycin may also have a potential role in the management of cystic fibrosis but more studies are needed;[42-44] its beneficial effects are thought to be due more to its anti-inflammatory properties than to its antibacterial action. Alpha$_1$-proteinase inhibitor, the main inhibitor of neutrophil elastase in the lung has also been investigated[45] as has pentoxifylline,[46] a drug with anticytokine activity.

Experimental treatment aimed at modifying the pulmonary disease process has included ion transport therapy. This involves the use of aerosolised drugs that either inhibit sodium ion absorption across airway epithelia (for example the sodium channel blocker amiloride[47]) or induce chloride ion secretion. However, nebulised amiloride was not found to be a useful adjunct in patients on optimal treatment.[48,49]

In patients with severe lung disease, oxygen therapy may give some relief of symptoms but its effect on mortality and morbidity is uncertain.[50,51] At present the only available treatment for patients with end stage pulmonary disease is lung transplantation.

**Nutritional management** of cystic fibrosis should ensure adequate calorie intake from a balanced diet in order to counteract malabsorption due to pancreatic insufficiency and the increased metabolic requirements of patients with cystic fibrosis.[52,53] Supplements of the fat-soluble vitamins A, D, and E, and sometimes vitamin K, may be necessary. Investigation of bone mineral density[54] and direct assessment of vitamin status[55] suggest that current supplements may be inadequate. Pancreatic enzymes, as pancreatin or pancrelipase, are taken before or with each meal or snack.

Somatic **gene therapy** represents the nearest approach to a cure for cystic fibrosis.[56] It aims to introduce the normal CFTR gene sequence into cells of affected tissue. Most effort has been directed at gene delivery to the lungs using adenovirus vectors or liposomes, but results have been variable.[57-60] Difficulties encountered include inefficient gene transfer, immunity to viral vectors, and a systemic inflammatory reaction provoked by plasmid DNA.[4] For a discussion of the general principles of gene therapy, see p.1691.


1. Stern RC. The diagnosis of cystic fibrosis. *N Engl J Med* 1997; **336:** 487–91.
2. Wallis C. Diagnosing cystic fibrosis: blood, sweat, and tears. *Arch Dis Child* 1997; **76:** 85–91.
3. Rosenstein BJ, *et al.* The diagnosis of cystic fibrosis: a consensus statement. *J Pediatr* 1998; **132:** 589–95.
4. Geddes DM, Alton EWFW. The CF gene: 10 years on. *Thorax* 1999; **54:** 1052–3.
5. Doull IJM. Recent advances in cystic fibrosis. *Arch Dis Child* 2001; **85:** 62–6.
6. Tonelli MR, Aitken ML. New and emerging therapies for pulmonary complications of cystic fibrosis. *Drugs* 2001; **61:** 1379–85.
7. Ratjen F, Döring G. Cystic fibrosis. *Lancet* 2003; **361:** 681–9.
8. Walters S, Smith EG. Pseudomonas cepacia in cystic fibrosis: transmissibility and its implications. *Lancet* 1993; **342:** 3–4.
9. McCaffery K, *et al.* Systematic review of antistaphylococcal antibiotic therapy in cystic fibrosis. *Thorax* 1999; **54:** 380–3.
10. Smyth A, Walters S. Prophylactic antibiotics for cystic fibrosis. Available in The Cochrane Library; Issue 2. Chichester: John Wiley; 2004.
11. Elborn JS. Treatment of Staphylococcus aureus in cystic fibrosis. *Thorax* 1999; **54:** 377–8.
12. Stutman HR, *et al.* Antibiotic prophylaxis in infants and young children with cystic fibrosis: a randomized controlled trial. *J Pediatr* 2002; **140:** 299–305.
13. Banerjee D, Stableforth D. The treatment of respiratory Pseudomonas infection in cystic fibrosis: what drug and which way? *Drugs* 2000; **60:** 1053–64.
14. Rey E, *et al.* Drug disposition in cystic fibrosis. *Clin Pharmacokinet* 1998; **35:** 313–29.
15. Touw DJ, *et al.* Pharmacokinetic optimisation of antibacterial treatment in patients with cystic fibrosis: current practice and suggestions for future directions. *Clin Pharmacokinet* 1998; **35:** 437–59.
16. Valerius NH, *et al.* Prevention of chronic Pseudomonas aeruginosa colonisation in cystic fibrosis by early treatment. *Lancet* 1991; **338:** 725–6.
17. Wolter JM, *et al.* Home intravenous therapy in cystic fibrosis: a prospective randomized trial examining clinical, quality of life and cost aspects. *Eur Respir J* 1997; **10:** 896–900.
18. Pai VB, Nahata MC. Efficacy and safety of aerosolized tobramycin in cystic fibrosis. *Pediatr Pulmonol* 2001; **32:** 314–27.
19. Moss RB. Long-term benefits of inhaled tobramycin in adolescent patients with cystic fibrosis. *Chest* 2002; **121:** 55–63.
20. Wall MA, *et al.* Inhaled antibiotics in cystic fibrosis. *Lancet* 1983; **i:** 1325.
21. Conway SP. Evidence for using nebulised antibiotics in cystic fibrosis. *Arch Dis Child* 1999; **80:** 307–9.
22. Campbell PW, Saiman L. Use of aerosolized antibiotics in patients with cystic fibrosis. *Chest* 1999; **116:** 775–88.
23. Ramsey BW, *et al.* Intermittent administration of inhaled tobramycin in patients with cystic fibrosis. *N Engl J Med* 1999; **340:** 23–30.
24. Burns JL, *et al.* Effect of chronic intermittent administration of inhaled tobramycin on respiratory microbial flora in patients with cystic fibrosis. *J Infect Dis* 1999; **179:** 1190–6.
25. Hodson ME, *et al.* Aerosol carbenicillin and gentamicin treatment of Pseudomonas aeruginosa infection in patients with cystic fibrosis. *Lancet* 1981; **ii:** 1137–9.
26. Beringer P. The clinical use of colistin in patients with cystic fibrosis. *Curr Opin Pulm Med* 2001; **7:** 434–40.
27. Anonymous. The choice of antibacterial drugs. In: *Handbook of antimicrobial therapy.* 16th ed. New York: The Medical Letter, 2002: 34–52.
28. Ledson MJ, *et al.* Nebulised taurolidine and B cepacia bronchiectasis. *Thorax* 2000; **55:** 91–2.
29. Govan JRW, *et al.* Evidence for transmission of Pseudomonas cepacia by social contact in cystic fibrosis. *Lancet* 1993; **342:** 15–19.
30. Mahenthiralingam E, *et al.* Burkholderia cepacia in cystic fibrosis. *N Engl J Med* 1995; **332:** 819.
31. Steinbach S, *et al.* Transmissibility of Pseudomonas cepacia infection in clinic patients and lung-transplant recipients with cystic fibrosis. *N Engl J Med* 1994; **331:** 981–7.
32. Conway SP, Watson A. Nebulised bronchodilators, corticosteroids, and rhDNase in adult patients with cystic fibrosis. *Thorax* 1997; **52** (suppl 2): S64–8.
33. Spencer DA. Nebulised bronchodilators, antibiotics and rhDNase for children with cystic fibrosis. *Thorax* 1997; **52** (suppl 2): S89–S91.
34. Jones AP, *et al.* Recombinant human deoxyribonuclease for cystic fibrosis. Available in The Cochrane Library; Issue 2. Chichester: John Wiley; 2004.
35. Quan JM, *et al.* A two-year randomized, placebo-controlled trial of dornase alfa in young patients with cystic fibrosis with mild lung function abnormalities. *J Pediatr* 2001; **139:** 813–20.
36. Duijvestijn YCM, Brand PLP. Systematic review of N-acetylcysteine in cystic fibrosis. *Acta Paediatr* 1999; **88:** 38–41.
37. Ziebach R, *et al.* Bronchodilatory effects of salbutamol, ipratropium bromide, and their combination: double-blind, placebo-controlled crossover study in cystic fibrosis. *Pediatr Pulmonol* 2001; **31:** 431–5.
38. Konstan MW. Therapies aimed at airway inflammation in cystic fibrosis. *Clin Chest Med* 1998; **19:** 505–13.
39. Cheng K, *et al.* Oral steroids for cystic fibrosis. Available in The Cochrane Library; Issue 2. Chichester: John Wiley; 2004.
40. Balfour-Lynn I, *et al.* Inhaled corticosteroids for cystic fibrosis. Available in The Cochrane Library; Issue 2. Chichester: John Wiley; 2004.
41. Konstan MW, *et al.* Effect of high-dose ibuprofen in patients with cystic fibrosis. *N Engl J Med* 1995; **332:** 848–54.
42. Wolter J, *et al.* Effect of long term treatment with azithromycin on disease parameters in cystic fibrosis: a randomised trial. *Thorax* 2002; **57:** 212–16.
43. Equi A, *et al.* Long term azithromycin in children with cystic fibrosis: a randomised, placebo-controlled crossover trial. *Lancet* 2002; **360:** 978–84.
44. Saiman L, *et al.* Azithromycin in patients with cystic fibrosis chronically infected with Pseudomonas aeruginosa: a randomized controlled trial. *JAMA* 2003; **290:** 1749–56.
45. McElvaney NG, *et al.* Aerosol α-1-antitrypsin treatment for cystic fibrosis. *Lancet* 1991; **337:** 392–4.
46. Aronoff SC, *et al.* Effects of pentoxifylline on sputum neutrophil elastase and pulmonary function in patients with cystic fibrosis: preliminary observations. *J Pediatr* 1994; **125:** 992–7.
47. Knowles MR, *et al.* A pilot study of aerosolized amiloride for the treatment of lung disease in cystic fibrosis. *N Engl J Med* 1990; **322:** 1189–94.
48. Bowler IM, *et al.* Nebulised amiloride in respiratory exacerbations of cystic fibrosis: a randomised controlled trial. *Arch Dis Child* 1995; **73:** 427–30.
49. Graham A, *et al.* No added benefit from nebulized amiloride in patients with cystic fibrosis. *Eur Respir J* 1993; **6:** 1243–8.

50. Zinman R, *et al.* Nocturnal home oxygen in the treatment of hypoxemic cystic fibrosis patients. *J Pediatr* 1989; **114:** 368–77.
51. Dinwiddie R, *et al.* Oxygen therapy for cystic fibrosis. *J R Soc Med* 1999; **92** (suppl 37): 19–22.
52. Bowler IM, *et al.* Resting energy expenditure and substrate oxidation rates in cystic fibrosis. *Arch Dis Child* 1993; **68:** 754–9.
53. Green MR, *et al.* Nutritional management of the infant with cystic fibrosis. *Arch Dis Child* 1995; **72:** 452–6.
54. Haworth CS, *et al.* Low bone mineral density in adults with cystic fibrosis. *Thorax* 1999; **54:** 961–7.
55. Feranchak AP, *et al.* Prospective, long-term study of fat-soluble vitamin status in children with cystic fibrosis identified by newborn screen. *J Pediatr* 1999; **135:** 601–10.
56. Jaffé A, *et al.* Prospects for gene therapy in cystic fibrosis. *Arch Dis Child* 1999; **80:** 286–9.
57. Colledge WH, Evans MJ. Cystic fibrosis gene therapy. *Br Med Bull* 1995; **51:** 82–90.
58. Coutelle C. Gene therapy approaches for cystic fibrosis. *Biologicals* 1995; **23:** 21–5.
59. Southern KW. Gene therapy for cystic fibrosis: current issues. *Br J Hosp Med* 1996; **55:** 495–9.
60. Flotte TR, Laube BL. Gene therapy in cystic fibrosis. *Chest* 2001; **120:** 124S–131S.

## Diarrhoea, infective

See under Gastro-enteritis, p.127.

## Diphtheria

Diphtheria is caused by infection, usually of the upper respiratory tract or the skin, with the Gram-positive aerobe *Corynebacterium diphtheriae*. It occurs worldwide and, despite the effectiveness of immunisation (see Diphtheria Vaccines, p.1612), is still common in parts of the world, including the tropics. Although the risk to travellers is said to be low, diphtheria should be considered in patients returning from tropical countries with a sore throat. Russia and other republics of the former USSR have experienced an epidemic.

The most serious manifestations of infection are due to exotoxin produced by toxigenic strains and thus treatment is primarily with diphtheria antitoxin. Erythromycin or benzylpenicillin are also given to eliminate *C. diphtheriae*, thereby terminating toxin production and preventing the spread of infection to contacts. Close contacts of primary cases of diphtheria may be given a 7-day prophylactic course of erythromycin orally or a single intramuscular dose of benzylpenicillin,[1] in addition to boosters or primary immunisation with diphtheria vaccine. Non-toxigenic *C. diphtheriae* is the most common isolate in clinical cases in the UK[1,2] and generally causes a less severe form of the disease; it does, however, have the potential to cause invasive disease in some patients.[3]

Asymptomatic carriers may harbour non-toxigenic strains of *C. diphtheriae* that can be converted to toxigenic strains. A single intramuscular injection of benzathine benzylpenicillin has been less effective than oral erythromycin, but may be used if compliance is uncertain;[4] clindamycin for 7 days by mouth has also eliminated the carrier state,[4] but erythromycin remains the drug of choice. Bacteriological follow-up should be carried out 2 weeks after completing treatment to be certain *C. diphtheriae* has been eradicated from carriers.[5]

1. Bonnet JM, Begg NT. Control of diphtheria: guidance for consultants in communicable disease control. *Commun Dis Public Health* 1999; **2:** 242–9.
2. Begg N, Balraj V. Diphtheria: are we ready for it? *Arch Dis Child* 1995; **73:** 568–72.
3. Efstratiou A, *et al.* Non-toxigenic Corynebacterium diphtheriae var gravis in England. *Lancet* 1993; **341:** 1592–3.
4. McCloskey RV, *et al.* Treatment of diphtheria carriers: benzathine penicillin, erythromycin, and clindamycin. *Ann Intern Med* 1974; **81:** 788–91.
5. Miller LW, *et al.* Diphtheria carriers and the effect of erythromycin therapy. *Antimicrob Agents Chemother* 1974; **6:** 166–9.

## Ear infections

See under Otitis Externa, and Otitis Media, p.138.

## Ehrlichiosis

Infections with rickettsia-like bacteria of the *Ehrlichia* genus are rare and at one time the only species isolated from humans was *E. sennetsu*, the cause of Sennetsu fever in Japan. *E. canis* is responsible for a tick-borne disease in *dogs* and a closely related species, *E. chaffeensis*, causes human monocytic ehrlichiosis.[1] *Anaplasma phagocytophilum* (*E. phagocytophila*; *E. equi*) is responsible for cases of human granulocytic ehrlichiosis reported in parts of the USA[1-3] and Europe.[4,5] *E. ewingii* has also been identified as a human pathogen.[6] A large proportion of infections occur after a tick bite (*Ixodes* spp.). As with other rickettsial infections, treatment is with a tetracycline, commonly doxycycline;[1,2,7] chloramphenicol has been used as an alternative.[7] Antibacterial susceptibility testing has suggested that rifamycins and fluoroquinolones are promising alternatives in the granulocytic form of infections.[8] Successful treatment with rifampicin has been reported in 2 patients.[9]

1. Dumler JS, Bakken JS. Ehrlichial diseases of humans: emerging tick-borne infections. *Clin Infect Dis* 1995; **20:** 1102–10.
2. Bakken JS, *et al.* Clinical and laboratory characteristics of human granulocytic ehrlichiosis. *JAMA* 1996; **275:** 199–205.
3. IJdo JW, *et al.* The emergence of another tickborne infection in the 12-town area around Lyme, Connecticut: human granulocytic ehrlichiosis. *J Infect Dis* 2000; **181:** 1388–93.
4. Brouqui P, *et al.* Human granulocytic ehrlichiosis in Europe. *Lancet* 1995; **346:** 782–3.
5. Blanco JR, Oteo JA. Human granulocytic ehrlichiosis in Europe. *Clin Microbiol Infect* 2002; **8:** 763–72.
6. Buller RS, *et al.* Ehrlichia ewingii, a newly recognized agent of human ehrlichiosis. *N Engl J Med* 1999; **341:** 148–55.
7. Schaffner W, Standaert SM. Ehrlichiosis—in pursuit of an emerging infection. *N Engl J Med* 1996; **334:** 262–3.
8. Klein MB, *et al.* Antibiotic susceptibility of the newly cultivated agent of human granulocytic ehrlichiosis: promising activity of quinolones and rifamycins. *Antimicrob Agents Chemother* 1997; **41:** 76–9.
9. Buitrago MI, *et al.* Human granulocytic ehrlichiosis during pregnancy treated successfully with rifampin. *Clin Infect Dis* 1998; **27:** 213–15.

## Endocarditis

Infective endocarditis is caused by infection of the endocardium following invasion of the bloodstream by bacteria or fungi and particularly affects the heart valves. Infection may follow an acute or subacute course depending in part on the organisms responsible. Virtually any organism can cause endocarditis but streptococci, enterococci, and staphylococci continue to be major culprits. The commonest bacteria responsible are the alpha-haemolytic streptococci originating mainly from the mouth and throat; they have been called viridans streptococci or even '*Streptococcus viridans*' (although this is not a true species) and include *Str. mitis*, *Str. mutans*, *Str. oralis*, *Str. salivarius*, and *Str. sanguis*. Other streptococci originate in the gut and include *Str. bovis*. Enterococci (faecal streptococci) also originate in the gut and include *Enterococcus faecalis* and, to a lesser extent, *E. faecium*. Endocarditis due to any of these bacteria is commonly subacute or insidious. Acute endocarditis is often due to *Staphylococcus aureus*, a common cause in intravenous drug abusers, but may also be caused by coagulase-negative staphylococci, particularly *Staph. lugdunensis*. Prosthetic valve infection is often caused by *Staph. epidermidis*. Less common causes of endocarditis are: Gram-negative bacteria such as the Enterobacteriaceae, *Pseudomonas* spp., and the HACEK group of slow-growing organisms (*Haemophilus*, *Actinobacillus*, *Cardiobacterium*, *Eikenella*, *Kingella*); the rickettsia *Coxiella burnetii* (the cause of Q fever, p.143); and fungi such as *Candida* and *Aspergillus*.

There are consensus recommendations for the treatment and prophylaxis of endocarditis.

**Endocarditis treatment**. Guidelines for the treatment of streptococcal, enterococcal, and staphylococcal endocarditis were produced by the British Society for Antimicrobial Chemotherapy in 1998[1] and, with the addition of HACEK endocarditis, by the American Heart Association in 1995.[2] Although these guidelines are broadly accepted there may be differing views on detail including choice of antibacterial, route of administration, and duration of treatment. Treatment depends on identification of the infecting organisms and their sensitivity to antibacterials. Blood should therefore be taken for culture before treatment is started; MICs should be measured. *Empirical treatment* with benzylpenicillin plus gentamicin should then be given until the laboratory results are known; vancomycin should be given instead of benzylpenicillin if staphylococcal infection is likely.[1] There is synergy between penicillin and aminoglycosides against streptococci. Viridans streptococci are generally much more sensitive to penicillin than enterococci and gentamicin may sometimes be stopped once the laboratory results are known.

Briefly, the 1998 **UK** guidelines[1] are as follows.

- STREPTOCOCCAL ENDOCARDITIS

  For *penicillin-sensitive streptococci* (viridans streptococci and *Str. bovis* with a benzylpenicillin MIC of 0.1 microgram or less per mL): intravenous bolus injections of benzylpenicillin 1.2 g every 4 hours and gentamicin 80 mg twice daily both given for 2 weeks.

  For *streptococci less sensitive to penicillin* (viridans streptococci and *Str. bovis* with a benzylpenicillin MIC of more than 0.1 microgram/mL): benzylpenicillin and gentamicin as above, but both given for 4 weeks.

  For *streptococci in penicillin-allergic patients*: initially either vancomycin 1 g intravenously twice daily or teicoplanin 400 mg intravenously every 12 hours for three doses and then a maintenance dose of 400 mg daily; either drug should be given for 4 weeks, together with gentamicin as above for the first 2 weeks.

- ENTEROCOCCAL ENDOCARDITIS

  For *gentamicin-sensitive or low-level resistant enterococci* (MIC less than 100 micrograms/mL): intravenous bolus injections of ampicillin or amoxicillin 2 g every 4 hours and gentamicin 80 mg twice daily, both given for 4 weeks.

  For *gentamicin highly-resistant enterococci* (MIC at least 2000 micrograms/mL): ampicillin or amoxicillin as above, but for a minimum of 6 weeks; streptomycin may also be given if sensitivity can be demonstrated.

  For *enterococci in penicillin-allergic patients*: as for streptococci in penicillin-allergic patients above, except that gentamicin should be given for all 4 weeks of treatment.

- STAPHYLOCOCCAL ENDOCARDITIS

  For *penicillin-sensitive staphylococci*: intravenous bolus injections of benzylpenicillin 1.2 g every 4 hours for 4 weeks plus gentamicin 80 to 120 mg every 8 hours for the first week.

  For *staphylococci resistant to penicillins generally but sensitive to meticillin/flucloxacillin*: intravenous bolus injections of flucloxacillin 2 g every 4 hours for 4 weeks plus gentamicin as for penicillin-sensitive staphylococci.

  For *staphylococci resistant to meticillin/flucloxacillin* and in *penicillin-allergic patients*: vancomycin 1 g intravenously twice daily for 4 weeks plus gentamicin as for penicillin-sensitive staphylococci.

  In difficult cases of endocarditis due to coagulase-negative staphylococci or *Staph. aureus*, rifampicin may occasionally be added to therapy, usually with vancomycin.

The 1995 **USA** guidelines[2] are as follows.

- STREPTOCOCCAL AND ENTEROCOCCAL ENDOCARDITIS

  For *penicillin-sensitive streptococci* (viridans streptococci and *Str. bovis* with a benzylpenicillin MIC of 0.1 microgram or less per mL): there are 3 alternative regimens, namely benzylpenicillin alone for 4 weeks; or ceftriaxone alone for 4 weeks; or benzylpenicillin with gentamicin, each for 2 weeks only. Streptomycin has been used as an alternative to gentamicin but gentamicin is now preferred. Doses are: intravenous benzylpenicillin 7.2 to 10.8 g daily by continuous infusion or in 6 divided doses; intravenous or intramuscular ceftriaxone 2 g once daily; intramuscular or intravenous gentamicin 1 mg/kg every 8 hours.

  For *relatively resistant streptococci* (viridans streptococci and *Str. bovis* with a benzylpenicillin MIC greater than 0.1 microgram/mL but less than 0.5 micrograms/mL): intravenous benzylpenicillin 10.8 g daily by continuous infusion or in 6 divided doses for 4 weeks with gentamicin as above for 2 weeks.

  For *more resistant bacteria* (enterococci or viridans streptococci with a benzylpenicillin MIC of 0.5 micrograms or more per mL): there are 3 alternative regimens, namely intravenous benzylpenicillin 10.8 to 18 g daily by continuous infusion or in 6 divided doses with gentamicin as above; or intravenous ampicillin 12 g daily by continuous infusion or in 6 divided doses again with gentamicin as above; or intravenous vancomycin 30 mg/kg daily in 2 divided doses, the total daily dose not exceeding 2 g, again with gentamicin as above. Both drugs in each regimen should be given for 4 to 6 weeks. Streptomycin has again been used as an alternative to gentamicin but gentamicin is now preferred. Resistance is, however, emerging among enterococcal strains to vancomycin and to gentamicin and streptomycin as well as to the penicillins. Where resistance to vancomycin is modest, teicoplanin is suggested as an alternative. Some patients with multiply-resistant enterococcal infection whose treatment fails may need to be considered for surgical intervention.

  For *streptococci and enterococci in penicillin-allergic patients or those allergic to other beta lactams*: intravenous vancomycin 30 mg/kg daily in 2 divided doses for 4 weeks, the total daily dose not exceeding 2 g. For more resistant bacteria, vancomycin should be given with gentamicin as above, both for 4 to 6 weeks.

- STAPHYLOCOCCAL ENDOCARDITIS

  For *meticillin-susceptible staphylococci in the absence of prosthetic material*: intravenous nafcillin or oxacillin 2 g every 4 hours for 4 to 6 weeks with or without gentamicin 1 mg/kg intramuscularly or intravenously every 8 hours for 3 to 5 days.

  For *meticillin-resistant staphylococci in the absence of prosthetic material*, intravenous vancomycin 30 mg/kg daily in 2 divided doses for 4 to 6 weeks, the total daily dose not exceeding 2 g.

For *meticillin-susceptible staphylococci in the presence of prosthetic material*: intravenous nafcillin or oxacillin 2 g every 4 hours with oral rifampicin 300 mg every 8 hours for 6 weeks or more and gentamicin as above for the initial 2 weeks.

For *meticillin-resistant staphylococci in the presence of prosthetic material*, nafcillin or oxacillin are replaced by intravenous vancomycin 30 mg/kg daily in 2 or 4 divided doses for 6 weeks or more, the total daily dose not exceeding 2 g.

For *meticillin-susceptible staphylococci in penicillin-allergic patients or those allergic to other beta lactams in the absence of prosthetic material*, intravenous cefazolin 2 g every 8 hours for 4 to 6 weeks or other first-generation cephalosporin (except in immediate-type hypersensitivity) with or without gentamicin as above for 3 to 5 days. Alternatively, intravenous vancomycin 30 mg/kg daily in 2 divided doses is given for 4 to 6 weeks, the total daily dose not exceeding 2 g.

For *meticillin-susceptible staphylococci in penicillin-allergic patients or those allergic to other beta lactams in the presence of prosthetic material*, as above but with nafcillin or oxacillin replaced by vancomycin or a first-generation cephalosporin.

- HACEK ENDOCARDITIS

Traditionally the HACEK group of organisms have been susceptible to ampicillin, but recently resistant strains have been identified and monotherapy with ampicillin is no longer recommended. Preferred treatment is therefore with intramuscular or intravenous ceftriaxone 2 g once daily for 4 weeks, although cefotaxime or other third-generation cephalosporin may be substituted. Alternatively, intravenous ampicillin 12 g daily by continuous infusion or in 6 divided doses with intramuscular or intravenous gentamicin 1 mg/kg every 8 hours may be given, both for 4 weeks. Therapy should be extended to 6 weeks for prosthetic valve endocarditis.

**Endocarditis prophylaxis**. Patients at risk of developing endocarditis, including those with valvular heart disease, prosthetic valves, or other cardiac abnormalities and those with a history of endocarditis or rheumatic fever, should be given antibacterials prophylactically when about to undergo dental operations, tonsillectomy, or other procedures liable to lead to bacteraemia. Antibacterials should be administered so that adequate blood and tissue concentrations are achieved throughout the procedure. They are generally given as a single dose before the procedure, sometimes repeated about 6 hours later; the oral route is used if possible. A penicillin such as amoxicillin, with or without an aminoglycoside such as gentamicin, is used, reflecting the bacteria usually responsible (see above). Clindamycin, vancomycin, or teicoplanin are used in penicillin-allergic patients. UK and USA guidelines for prophylaxis are similar. Recommendations from the British Society for Antimicrobial Chemotherapy were published in 1982[3] and amended in 1986,[4] 1990,[5] 1992,[6] and 1997.[7] Updated recommendations from the American Heart Association were also published in 1997.[8]

**UK** guidelines are as follows.

- DENTAL PROCEDURES

Prior application of chlorhexidine or other suitable antiseptic to the gingival margins may reduce the severity of any bacteraemia.

*Under local or no anaesthesia* (including patients with a prosthetic valve, but not in those who have had endocarditis): amoxicillin or clindamycin by mouth. Amoxicillin is preferred provided that patients are not penicillin-allergic and have not received penicillin more than once in the previous month. Doses are: amoxicillin 3 g or clindamycin 600 mg as a single oral dose 1 hour before the procedure.

*Under general anaesthesia*: amoxicillin in one of 3 regimens, namely: amoxicillin 1 g intravenously just before induction then 500 mg by mouth 6 hours later; or 3 g by mouth 4 hours before anaesthesia and repeated once as soon as possible after the procedure; or amoxicillin 3 g with probenecid 1 g both by mouth 4 hours before the procedure. Those who are allergic to penicillin or have received it more than once in the previous month should be referred to hospital.

*In special-risk patients referred to hospital* (i.e. those who are to have a general anaesthetic and have prosthetic heart valves or are unable to receive penicillin because of allergy or receipt of penicillin more than once in the previous month; those who have previously had endocarditis): amoxicillin plus gentamicin or vancomycin plus gentamicin. When penicillin *can* be given: amoxicillin 1 g and gentamicin 120 mg both intravenously just before induction and amoxicillin 500 mg by mouth 6 hours later. When penicillin *cannot* be used: vancomycin 1 g by slow intravenous infusion over at least 100 minutes followed by gentamicin 120 mg intravenously just before induction or 15 minutes before the procedure. Intravenous teicoplanin 400 mg just before induction or 15 minutes before the procedure may be substituted for vancomycin. A second alternative is clindamycin 300 mg intravenously over at least 10 minutes just before induction or 15 minutes before the procedure followed 6 hours later by 150 mg by mouth or by intravenous infusion over at least 10 minutes.

- UPPER RESPIRATORY-TRACT PROCEDURES

As for dental procedures (above), but the postoperative antibacterial may need to be given parenterally if swallowing is painful.

- GENITO-URINARY PROCEDURES

As for dental procedures in special-risk patients (above), but not clindamycin. If there is urinary infection prophylaxis should also be effective against these infecting organisms.

- GASTROINTESTINAL, OBSTETRIC, AND GYNAECOLOGICAL PROCEDURES

Prophylaxis is only necessary in patients with prosthetic valves or those who have previously had endocarditis and then as for dental procedures in special-risk patients (above), but not clindamycin.

**USA** guidelines[8] are as follows.

- DENTAL, ORAL, RESPIRATORY-TRACT, OR OESOPHAGEAL PROCEDURES

*Standard oral regimen*: amoxicillin 2 g given 1 hour beforehand.

*Patients unable to take oral antibacterials*: ampicillin 2 g intravenously or intramuscularly up to 30 minutes before the procedure.

*Penicillin-allergic patients*: clindamycin 600 mg by mouth an hour beforehand, or cefalexin or cefadroxil 2 g by mouth 1 hour beforehand, or azithromycin or clarithromycin 500 mg by mouth 1 hour beforehand.

*Penicillin-allergic patients unable to take oral antibacterials*: clindamycin 600 mg intravenously or cefazolin 1 g intravenously or intramuscularly up to 30 minutes before the procedure.

- GENITO-URINARY AND GASTROINTESTINAL (EXCLUDING OESOPHAGEAL) PROCEDURES

*Moderate-risk patients*: amoxicillin 2 g by mouth 1 hour beforehand, or ampicillin 2 g intravenously or intramuscularly up to 30 minutes before the procedure.

*Moderate-risk patients who are penicillin-allergic*: vancomycin 1 g intravenously over 1 to 2 hours, with completion of the infusion up to 30 minutes before the procedure.

*High-risk patients*: ampicillin 2 g plus gentamicin 1.5 mg/kg (up to a maximum total of 120 mg) intravenously or intramuscularly up to 30 minutes before the procedure, followed 6 hours later by ampicillin 1 g intravenously or intramuscularly or by amoxicillin 1 g by mouth.

*High-risk patients who are penicillin-allergic*: vancomycin 1 g intravenously over 1 to 2 hours plus gentamicin 1.5 mg/kg (up to 120 mg) intravenously or intramuscularly, with completion of the infusion and injection up to 30 minutes before the procedure.

1. Working Party of the British Society for Antimicrobial Chemotherapy. Antibiotic treatment of streptococcal, enterococcal, and staphylococcal endocarditis. *Heart* 1998; **79:** 207–10.
2. Wilson WR, *et al.* Antibiotic treatment of adults with infective endocarditis due to streptococci, enterococci, staphylococci, and HACEK microorganisms. *JAMA* 1995; **274:** 1706–13.
3. Working Party of the British Society for Antimicrobial Chemotherapy. The antibiotic prophylaxis of infective endocarditis. *Lancet* 1982; **ii:** 1323–6.
4. Simmons NA, *et al.* Prophylaxis of infective endocarditis. *Lancet* 1986; **i:** 1267.
5. Endocarditis Working Party of the British Society for Antimicrobial Chemotherapy. Antibiotic prophylaxis of infective endocarditis. *Lancet* 1990; **335:** 88–9.
6. Simmons NA, *et al.* Antibiotic prophylaxis and infective endocarditis. *Lancet* 1992; **339:** 1292–3.
7. Littler WA, *et al.* Changes in recommendations about amoxycillin prophylaxis for prevention of endocarditis. *Lancet* 1997; **350:** 1100.
8. Dajani AS, *et al.* Prevention of bacterial endocarditis: recommendations by the American Heart Association. *JAMA* 1997; **277:** 1794–1801.

## Endometritis

Endometritis (or endomyometritis) is a uterine infection that may be a part of pelvic inflammatory disease (p.139) or may be a postoperative complication of caesarean section.

Antibacterial prophylaxis may be given at caesarean section after cord clamping to prevent postpartum endometritis as well as wound infection. While the use of antimicrobial prophylaxis in patients at high risk of infection is well established, prophylaxis in low-risk patients remains controversial. A systematic literature review[1] has shown prophylaxis to be beneficial following both elective and non-elective caesarean section, but USA surgical guidelines do not recommend routine prophylaxis in low-risk patients.[2] A penicillin or first-generation cephalosporin such as cefazolin is commonly used.[2,3]

Early postpartum endometritis has a polymicrobial aetiology. In one study the most common organisms isolated included *Gardnerella vaginalis*, *Peptococcus* spp., *Bacteroides* spp., *Staphylococcus epidermidis*, group B streptococci, and *Ureaplasma urealyticum*.[4] *Chlamydia trachomatis* has been implicated more often in late postpartum endometritis, but a wide variety of micro-organisms may also be responsible including genital mycoplasmas and, to a lesser extent, facultative and anaerobic bacteria.[5]

In the USA, standard empirical therapy for postpartum endometritis has been a short course of intravenous antibacterials, often clindamycin with gentamicin, given until the patient has been afebrile and asymptomatic for 24 to 48 hours and sometimes followed by a course of oral treatment, often amoxicillin. A systematic review[6] has confirmed the suitability of clindamycin with gentamicin and indicated that oral therapy is not necessary after successful intravenous therapy. It may, however, be recommended in patients with staphylococcal bacteraemia.[2]

1. Smaill F, Hofmeyr GJ. Antibiotic prophylaxis for cesarean section. Available in The Cochrane Library; Issue 2. Chichester: John Wiley; 2004.
2. ACOG. Antimicrobial therapy for obstetric patients. *Int J Gynecol Obstet* 1998; **61:** 299–308.
3. Hopkins L, Smaill F. Antibiotic prophylaxis regimens and drugs for cesarean section. Available in The Cochrane Library; Issue 2. Chichester: John Wiley; 2004.
4. Rosene K, *et al.* Polymicrobial early postpartum endometritis with facultative and anaerobic bacteria, genital mycoplasmas, and Chlamydia trachomatis: treatment with piperacillin or cefoxitin. *J Infect Dis* 1986; **153:** 1028–37.
5. Hoyme UB, *et al.* Microbiology and treatment of late postpartum endometritis. *Obstet Gynecol* 1986; **68:** 226–32.
6. French LM, Smaill FM. Antibiotic regimens for endometritis after delivery. Available in The Cochrane Library; Issue 2. Chichester: John Wiley; 2004.

## Enterococcal infections

Enterococcal infections are causing increasing concern, particularly with the emergence of drug-resistant strains.[1-6] Enterococci, principally *Enterococcus faecalis* (formerly *Streptococcus faecalis*) but also *E. faecium* and *E. avium*, can cause a variety of infections including those of the biliary tract and urinary tract, endocarditis, and peritonitis. Since they are frequently present in the gut flora they are a common cause of nosocomial infections. Enterococci are resistant to cephalosporins, tetracyclines, macrolides, and chloramphenicol. The emergence of resistance to gentamicin, penicillins, and the glycopeptide antimicrobials vancomycin and teicoplanin has compromised the previously standard treatment for enterococcal infections of a penicillin or glycopeptide with gentamicin. Two further therapeutic options have more recently emerged with the development of linezolid and quinupristin/dalfopristin for the treatment of vancomycin-resistant enterococcal infections,[7,8] although the latter is active against *E. faecium* but not against *E. faecalis.* There has, however, been a report of enterococcal resistance to linezolid.[9] In general, there can be no recommendations for treatment at present and the choice of antibacterial should be made according to local patterns of resistance and antibacterial sensitivity tests. The lack of effective antibacterials has placed emphasis on measures to prevent the spread of vancomycin-resistant enterococci. Guidelines were published in 1995 by the USA Hospital Infection Control Practices Advisory Committee,[10] and it has been suggested that they could be adapted for use in other countries.[11]

1. Landman D, Quale JM. Management of infections due to resistant enterococci: a review of therapeutic options. *J Antimicrob Chemother* 1997; **40:** 161–70.
2. Murray BE. Vancomycin-resistant enterococci. *Am J Med* 1997; **102:** 284–93.
3. Antony SJ. Multidrug-resistant enterococci: the dawn of a new era in resistant pathogens. *J Natl Med Assoc* 1998; **90:** 537–40.
4. Moellering RC. Vancomycin-resistant enterococci. *Clin Infect Dis* 1998; **26:** 1196–9.

5. Linden PK, Miller CB. Vancomycin-resistant enterococci: the clinical effect of a common nosocomial pathogen. *Diagn Microbiol Infect Dis* 1999; **33:** 113–20.
6. Murray BE. Vancomycin-resistant enterococcal infections. *N Engl J Med* 2000; **342:** 710–21.
7. Gold HS. Vancomycin-resistant enterococci: mechanisms and clinical observations. *Clin Infect Dis* 2001; **33:** 210–19.
8. Linden PK. Treatment options for vancomycin-resistant enterococcal infections. *Drugs* 2002; **62:** 425–41.
9. Auckland C, *et al.* Linezolid-resistant enterococci: report of the first isolates in the United Kingdom. *J Antimicrob Chemother* 2002; **50:** 743–6.
10. Hospital Infection Control Practices Advisory Committee (HICPAC). Recommendations for preventing the spread of vancomycin resistance. *MMWR* 1995; **44** (RR-12): 1–13. Also available at: http://www.cdc.gov/mmwr/PDF/rr/rr4412.pdf (accessed 18/05/04)
11. Fraise AP. The treatment and control of vancomycin resistant enterococci. *J Antimicrob Chemother* 1996; **38:** 753–6.

## Epididymitis

Epididymitis is often associated with urethritis and in young men occurs most commonly as a complication of sexually transmitted infection with *Neisseria gonorrhoeae* and especially *Chlamydia trachomatis*, but may occur in homosexual males as a result of infection with enteric organisms, particularly *Escherichia coli*.

In men over 35 years and in children epididymitis is usually secondary to urinary-tract infection with *Pseudomonas aeruginosa* and other Gram-negative bacilli and is not sexually transmitted.

For chlamydial epididymitis, WHO[1] recommends a 7-day oral course of doxycycline 100 mg twice daily or azithromycin 1 g as a single dose. Alternatives are 7-day courses of amoxicillin 500 mg three times daily, or erythromycin 500 mg four times daily, or ofloxacin 300 mg twice daily, or tetracycline 500 mg four times daily. Unless it can be excluded, patients should also be treated concurrently for gonorrhoea (p.130).

In the UK, the recommended treatment[2] for disease most probably due to gonococcal infection is a single intramuscular dose of ceftriaxone 250 mg or a single oral dose of ciprofloxacin 500 mg plus doxycycline 100 mg by mouth twice daily for 10 to 14 days. For probable chlamydial infections or infections with other non-gonococcal, non-enteric organisms, doxycycline 100 mg by mouth twice daily for 10 to 14 days is recommended, and for infections with enteric organisms, ofloxacin 200 mg by mouth twice daily for 14 days, or ciprofloxacin 500 mg by mouth twice daily for 10 days, is recommended. In patients allergic to cephalosporins and/or tetracyclines, ofloxacin 200 mg by mouth twice daily for 14 days may be used for infections of all causes.

In the USA, the Centers for Disease Control[3] recommends empirical treatment for epididymitis likely to have been caused by gonococcal or chlamydial infection with a single intramuscular dose of ceftriaxone 250 mg together with doxycycline 100 mg twice daily by mouth for 10 days; if the cause is thought to be an enteric organism, ofloxacin 300 mg twice daily by mouth or levofloxacin 500 mg once daily by mouth, in each case for 10 days, is recommended.

1. WHO. Guidelines for the management of sexually transmitted infections. Geneva: WHO, 2003. Also available at: http://whqlibdoc.who.int/publications/2003/9241546263.pdf (accessed 22/06/04)
2. Clinical Effectiveness Group (Association for Genitourinary Medicine and the Medical Society for the Study of Venereal Diseases). 2001 National guideline for the management of epididymo-orchitis. Available at: http://www.bashh.org/guidelines/2002/epididymoorchitis%200601.pdf (accessed 18/05/04)
3. Centers for Disease Control. Sexually transmitted diseases treatment guidelines 2002. *MMWR* 2002; **51**(RR-6): 1–80. Also available at: http://www.cdc.gov/mmwr/PDF/rr/rr5106.pdf (accessed 18/05/04)

## Epiglottitis

In acute epiglottitis rapid swelling of the epiglottis and surrounding soft tissues results in sudden airway obstruction which can be fatal. It is often due to bacteraemic infection with *Haemophilus influenzae* type b (see p.131) and has occurred primarily in young children. However, the incidence has decreased in this age group since the introduction of Haemophilus influenzae vaccine.[1] Acute epiglottitis also occurs in adults.[1]

Treatment and prophylaxis is similar to that for Haemophilus influenzae meningitis (see under Meningitis, p.134). Immediate management includes the maintenance of an adequate airway and the intravenous use of antibacterials active against *H. influenzae* type b. Chloramphenicol has been the drug of choice, but third-generation cephalosporins such as cefotaxime and ceftriaxone are increasingly used.[2] Prophylaxis with rifampicin may be given to index cases and contacts.

1. Frantz TD, *et al.* Acute epiglottitis in adults: analysis of 129 cases. *JAMA* 1994; **272:** 1358–60.
2. Sawyer SM, *et al.* Successful treatment of epiglottitis with two doses of ceftriaxone. *Arch Dis Child* 1994; **70:** 129–32.

## Escherichia coli enteritis

See under Gastro-enteritis, p.129.

## Eye infections

**Conjunctivitis** is a common superficial eye disorder and may be caused by infection with a wide range of bacteria, viruses, and, less frequently, fungi. Acute bacterial conjunctivitis is commonly caused by staphylococci or streptococci in adults, and *Haemophilus influenzae* and *Moraxella catarrhalis* (*Branhamella catarrhalis*) particularly in children. Other causes of bacterial conjunctivitis include gonococci (see Gonorrhoea, p.130) and *Chlamydia trachomatis* (see Trachoma, p.149). Neonatal chlamydial and gonococcal conjunctivitis are discussed under Neonatal Conjunctivitis, p.136. Uncomplicated bacterial conjunctivitis may be self-limiting but empirical treatment with topical antibacterials is often given. In the UK, topical chloramphenicol remains the treatment of choice despite concerns over the potential risk of aplastic anaemia (see Ocular Use under Precautions of Chloramphenicol, p.185). Alternatives include gentamicin, tobramycin, erythromycin (especially when infection with Gram-positive organisms is suspected), fluoroquinolones including ciprofloxacin and ofloxacin, framycetin, fusidic acid (especially for staphylococcal infections), and polymyxin B in combination with bacitracin, trimethoprim, or neomycin.

**Blepharitis** is an infection of the lid margins. It usually presents as a chronic condition and may require prolonged treatment, typically involving local hygiene to remove encrustations and topical application of a broad-spectrum antibacterial ointment.

**Keratitis** may be caused by infection of the cornea by bacteria, fungi, viruses, or protozoa usually following trauma to the surface of the eye, including that due to contact lens wear (see Contact Lens Care, p.1164). Common bacterial pathogens include staphylococci, streptococci, *Pseudomonas* spp., and Enterobacteriaceae. Bacterial keratitis is potentially sight-threatening and requires prompt aggressive treatment with broad-spectrum antibacterials. It is customary to obtain material for sensitivity testing, but increasingly, empirical treatment is then instituted without delay. Frequent or continuous topical application of drops or the use of local drug delivery devices have been used to ensure prolonged elevated drug concentrations. Subconjunctival or systemic therapy may occasionally be necessary. Topical treatment with cefazolin and either gentamicin or tobramycin has traditionally been used when *Pseudomonas* is not suspected. More recently, fluoroquinolones or ceftazidime have been used, and semisynthetic penicillins or vancomycin are other alternatives. For the treatment of Acanthamoeba keratitis, see p.595.

**Endophthalmitis** is a devastating ocular disease resulting from infection of the ocular cavity, usually following penetrating trauma or surgery. Depending on the route of infection, causative organisms commonly include staphylococci, streptococci, *H. influenzae*, *Bacillus cereus*, and *Propionibacterium acnes*. Fungal infections occur less commonly. Bacterial endophthalmitis requires immediate aggressive treatment with antibacterials, usually given intravitreally. The value of concurrent parenteral antibacterials is unclear. The choice of antibacterial for intravitreal use depends on the most likely pathogen. Third-generation cephalosporins or vancomycin are used, but aminoglycosides may produce retinal toxicity. Clindamycin may be effective if *B. cereus* is suspected. Adjunctive treatment includes vitrectomy, surgical removal of infected lens structures, and corticosteroids to control inflammatory and immune responses.

For a discussion of fungal infections of the eye, see p.388; for cytomegalovirus retinitis and ocular herpes simplex infections, see under Cytomegalovirus Infections, p.619, and Herpes Simplex Infections, p.620, respectively.

Some general references are given below.

1. Baum J. Infections of the eye. *Clin Infect Dis* 1995; **21:** 479–88.
2. Leeming JP. Treatment of ocular infections with topical antibacterials. *Clin Pharmacokinet* 1999; **37:** 351–60.
3. Robert P-Y, Adenis J-P. Comparative review of topical ophthalmic antibacterial preparations. *Drugs* 2001; **61:** 175–85.
4. Sheikh A, *et al.* Antibiotics versus placebo for acute bacterial conjunctivitis. Available in The Cochrane Library; Issue 2. Chichester: John Wiley; 2004.

## Gas gangrene

*Clostridium* spp. are anaerobic Gram-positive bacteria some of which cause gas gangrene with muscle necrosis and systemic toxicity as a result of toxin formation. *Cl. perfringens* is the species most frequently responsible. Gas gangrene is usually associated with traumatic or surgical wounds. Treatment is primarily by surgical debridement of all necrotic muscle and large doses of benzylpenicillin. Alternative antibacterials have included clindamycin, metronidazole, imipenem, a tetracycline, or chloramphenicol. Hyperbaric oxygen is used as an adjunct to surgical debridement. Gas-gangrene antitoxins are rarely used nowadays.

Benzylpenicillin is also recommended as prophylaxis against gas gangrene in patients undergoing high amputations of lower limbs or following major trauma; metronidazole is an alternative in patients allergic to penicillin.

## Gastro-enteritis

Diarrhoea is a symptom of simple gastro-enteritis and of most intestinal infections. It is a major problem in developing countries, but is common worldwide. Although viruses are often responsible, the severest forms of infectious diarrhoea are generally those due to bacteria. Common bacterial pathogens include *Campylobacter jejuni, Escherichia coli, Salmonella enteritidis, Shigella* spp., *Vibrio cholerae*, and *Yersinia enterocolitica*. Intestinal protozoa also cause diarrhoea and are of increasing importance in AIDS-associated diarrhoea. For discussions of viral and protozoal gastro-enteritis and their treatment, see p.618 and p.596, respectively. In acute diarrhoea of any aetiology the priority is to maintain hydration by prevention or treatment of fluid and electrolyte depletion, especially in infants and the elderly. Rehydration therapy is discussed under Diarrhoea on p.1241.

Acute, watery diarrhoea caused by non-invasive pathogens is usually self-limiting and may be treated conservatively. Inflammatory diarrhoea, predominantly caused by invasive pathogens and affecting the colon, often requires treatment with antibacterials. Guidelines published in the UK[1] recommended that empirical treatment of acute diarrhoea with antibacterials should be reserved for patients with symptoms suggesting infection with invasive pathogens and those at high risk of complications. Similarly antibacterial treatment was considered appropriate in tropical regions for diarrhoea due to invasive but not non-invasive organisms.[2] Nevertheless, some clinicians consider such an approach to be unnecessarily conservative in adults with severe acute diarrhoea in developed countries[3] in whom empirical treatment with fluoroquinolones can relieve symptoms and shorten the illness without significant adverse effects. In the USA, empirical therapy is considered for any patients in whom a bacterial cause is suspected; stool samples should be obtained for identification of the causative organism.[4]

In **infants and children** oral rehydration therapy is universally recognised as initial treatment of acute diarrhoea, but has been underutilised in both developed and developing countries.[2,5,6] Nutritional support and management of secondary complications, including systemic infections, is also particularly important in this age group.[2] Antibacterials have little place in management in most cases and their inappropriate use has contributed to a high prevalence of resistance in commensal bacteria.[5] WHO[6,7] has stipulated that antibacterials should only be used in children with acute diarrhoea when there is dysentery or suspected cholera; *Shigella* is the most important cause of dysentery in young children. Giardiasis and amoebiasis should also be treated. WHO emphasised[6] that oral preparations containing streptomycin or dihydrostreptomycin, neomycin, halogenated hydroxyquinolines, or nonabsorbable sulfonamides (sulfaguanidine, succinylsulfathiazole, phthalylsulfathiazole) should not be used.

Persistent or prolonged diarrhoea may not have an infective cause and antibacterial treatment should not be started unless a pathogen can be identified. **Tropical sprue**, a syndrome characterised by malabsorption often presenting as chronic diarrhoea, is believed to have an infective component and may respond to tetracycline, although this may be less effective in indigenous populations than in expatriates.[2]

**HIV-associated diarrhoea**. As discussed on p.623, diarrhoea is common in HIV infection and AIDS and causative organisms may be bacterial, protozoal, or viral. The most common bacterial cause is the *Mycobacterium avium* complex (see Opportunistic Mycobacterial Infections, p.137); others include *Campylobacter*, *Salmonella*, and

*Shigella* spp. Supportive care and appropriate conventional antibacterial therapy may be adequate, as described under the specific infections, below.

**'Food poisoning'** is generally a self-limiting form of gastro-enteritis, although serious outbreaks of foodborne illness have been associated with bacteria such as *Salmonella enteritidis*. Other common food-poisoning organisms include *Listeria monocytogenes*, *Campylobacter* spp., *Yersinia enterocolitica*, *Vibrio parahaemolyticus*, and *E. coli*. An enterotoxin is responsible for food poisoning associated with *Staphylococcus aureus*, *Clostridium* spp., and *Bacillus* spp.[8,9]

**Travellers' diarrhoea.** Acute diarrhoea associated with travel occurs worldwide. The most common bacterial pathogen is enterotoxigenic *E. coli*, although enteroadherent *E. coli* is also sometimes involved. Other bacteria include *Campylobacter jejuni*, *Salmonella* and *Shigella* spp., *Vibrio cholerae*, and non-cholera vibrios such as *V. parahaemolyticus*. Viruses and the protozoa *Giardia intestinalis*, *Entamoeba histolytica*, and *Cryptosporidium* may also be responsible. Recommendations for the management of travellers' diarrhoea are published by national and international bodies including WHO, the Department of Health in the UK, and the Centers for Disease Control in the USA. Clinical features depend on the pathogen responsible and treatment varies according to severity and duration of diarrhoea. Onset of diarrhoea is generally delayed with *Giardia* and *Entamoeba* because of the incubation period. Diarrhoea is often mild and self-limiting and increased fluid intake or oral rehydration therapy is usually all that will be required. Symptomatic treatment with antimotility drugs such as loperamide may be of benefit in mild to moderate diarrhoea. Bismuth salicylate may be used to reduce the frequency of diarrhoea. Although antimicrobial therapy is not indicated in most cases of infective diarrhoea, empirical treatment with a fluoroquinolone has been effective for moderate to severe attacks. Co-trimoxazole has also been used, but its use is restricted by its toxicity and increasingly widespread bacterial resistance is of concern. When the infecting bacteria are known, specific therapy may be necessary, as described below.

The risk of developing travellers' diarrhoea can be reduced by avoiding possibly contaminated foods as embodied in the advice to '***cook it, boil it, peel it, or forget it***'. A number of prophylactic drug regimens have been suggested, including various antibacterials, usually a fluoroquinolone or co-trimoxazole, in addition to bismuth salicylate. However, routine antimicrobial prophylaxis is not generally recommended because of the danger of drug reactions, supra-infections, and increasing bacterial resistance and should be reserved for those at special risk.[10] Many authorities prefer early treatment, including self-medication, with clear instructions on when medical help should be sought.


1. Farthing M, *et al.* The management of infective gastroenteritis in adults: a consensus statement by an expert panel convened by the British Society for the Study of Infection. *J Infect* 1996; **33:** 143–52.
2. Mathan VI. Diarrhoeal diseases. *Br Med Bull* 1998; **54:** 407–19.
3. Gorbach SL. Treating diarrhoea. *BMJ* 1997; **314:** 1776–7.
4. Guerrant RL, *et al.* Infectious Diseases Society of America. Practice guidelines for the management of infectious diarrhea. *Clin Infect Dis* 2001; **32:** 331–50. Also available at: http://www.journals.uchicago.edu/CID/journal/issues/v32n3/001387/001387.web.pdf (accessed 18/05/04)
5. Walker-Smith JA. Underutilisation of oral rehydration in the treatment of gastroenteritis. *Drugs* 1988; **36** (suppl 4): 61–4.
6. WHO. *The rational use of drugs in the management of acute diarrhoea in children.* Geneva: WHO, 1990.
7. WHO. *The management and prevention of diarrhoea: practical guidelines.* 3rd ed. Geneva: WHO, 1993.
8. Waites WM, Arbuthnott JP. Foodborne illness: an overview. *Lancet* 1990; **336:** 722–5.
9. Roberts D. Sources of infection: food. *Lancet* 1990; **336:** 859–61.
10. Rendi-Wagner P, Kollaritsch H. Drug prophylaxis for travelers' diarrhea. *Clin Infect Dis* 2002; **34:** 628–33.


**Antibiotic-associated colitis.** Although other organisms, including *Candida* spp.,[1] have been implicated in antibiotic-associated diarrhoea, colonisation of the colon with *Clostridium difficile*, a toxin-producing Gram-positive anaerobe, is the most common identifiable cause of antibiotic-associated colitis and pseudomembranous colitis. Restrictive antibacterial policies have decreased the incidence of *Cl. difficile*-associated diarrhoea in some hospitals[2] but it remains a major hazard of antibacterial use. Antibiotic-associated colitis has been associated with the use of most antibacterials, but particularly with clindamycin, lincomycin, ampicillin, amoxicillin, and cephalosporins and, less frequently, with fluoroquinolones, tetracycline, carbapenems, and trimethoprim. The diarrhoea may be mild and self-limiting or debilitating and persistent and can be life-threatening. Although the diarrhoea generally resolves within a few days of stopping the offending drug, together with fluid and electrolyte replacement, early specific antibacterial therapy should be given to patients with severe illness characterised by high fever, marked abdominal pain, and marked leucocytosis and to elderly, toxic, or debilitated patients, or those unresponsive to supportive therapy.[3,4] Antidiarrhoeal drugs should be avoided since they may aggravate the condition and may occasionally increase the possibility of toxic megacolon.[3]

Vancomycin or metronidazole are widely used when antibacterial treatment is necessary.[3-5] Metronidazole tends to be the drug of first choice and vancomycin is reserved for those who do not respond to, or who cannot tolerate, metronidazole, for those who are severely immunocompromised, and for those with severe illness.[3-6] This view is also endorsed by expert bodies in the USA whose aim is to provide guidelines for preventing the spread of vancomycin resistance.[7] Metronidazole can be given orally or intravenously as appropriate. Vancomycin is only given orally; it should not be given intravenously since it does not give rise to adequate concentrations of the drug in the bowel lumen.[3] The severity of the diarrhoea often decreases within 48 to 72 hours, but may not stop for a week or more. Treatment is usually continued for 10 days.[5] Relapses are quite common,[6] but usually respond to re-treatment with vancomycin or metronidazole.[3,6]

Other drugs that have been investigated in the treatment of antibiotic-associated colitis include teicoplanin,[8-10] fusidic acid,[10,11] and bacitracin,[12] although experience with their use remains limited.

The anion-exchange resins colestyramine and colestipol hydrochloride have been shown to bind the *Cl. difficile* toxin *in vitro*, and colestyramine has been used to treat pseudomembranous colitis.[13] The use of vancomycin together with colestyramine has been suggested,[14] but the value of the combination is uncertain. In general, the use of colestyramine is not recommended.[5]

Oral immunoglobulin A, used with vancomycin, was effective in controlling severe diarrhoea in a child who had not responded to other therapies.[15] Normal immunoglobulin given intravenously was also effective when added to vancomycin and metronidazole therapy in 2 elderly patients unresponsive to antibacterials alone.[16]

Treatment and prevention strategies aimed at colonising the gut with non-pathogenic organisms have included use of lactic-acid-producing organisms such as *Lactobacillus*,[4,17] and the yeasts *Saccharomyces boulardii*,[4] and *S. cerevisiae*.[18]


1. Danna PL, *et al.* Role of candida in pathogenesis of antibiotic-associated diarrhoea in elderly inpatients. *Lancet* 1991; **337:** 511–14.
2. Gorbach SL. Antibiotics and Clostridium difficile. *N Engl J Med* 1999; **341:** 1690–1.
3. Tabaqchali S, Jumaa P. Diagnosis and management of Clostridium difficile infection. *BMJ* 1995; **310:** 1375–80.
4. Malnick SDH, Zimhony O. Treatment of Clostridium difficile-associated diarrhea. *Ann Pharmacother* 2002; **36:** 1767–75. **269:** 71–5.
5. ASHP. ASHP therapeutic position statement on the preferential use of metronidazole for the treatment of Clostridium difficile-associated disease. *Am J Health-Syst Pharm* 1998; **55:** 1407–11.
6. Fekety R. Guidelines for the diagnosis and management of Clostridium difficile-associated diarrhea and colitis. *Am J Gastroenterol* 1997; **92:** 739–50.
7. Hospital Infection Control Practices Advisory Committee (HICPAC). Recommendations for preventing the spread of vancomycin resistance. *MMWR* 1995; **44** (RR-12): 1–13. Also available at: http://www.cdc.gov/mmwr/PDF/rr/rr4412.pdf (accessed 18/05/04)
8. de Lalla F, *et al.* Treatment of Clostridium difficile-associated disease with teicoplanin. *Antimicrob Agents Chemother* 1989; **33:** 1125–7.
9. de Lalla F, *et al.* Prospective study of oral teicoplanin versus oral vancomycin for therapy of pseudomembranous colitis and Clostridium difficile-associated diarrhea. *Antimicrob Agents Chemother* 1992; **36:** 2192–6.
10. Wenisch C, *et al.* Comparison of vancomycin, teicoplanin, metronidazole, and fusidic acid for the treatment of Clostridium difficile-associated diarrhea. *Clin Infect Dis* 1996; **22:** 813–18.
11. Cronberg S, *et al.* Fusidic acid for the treatment of antibiotic-associated colitis induced by Clostridium difficile. *Infection* 1984; **12:** 276–9.
12. Dudley MN, *et al.* Oral bacitracin vs vancomycin therapy for Clostridium difficile-induced diarrhea: a randomized double-blind trial. *Arch Intern Med* 1986; **146:** 1101–4.
13. Pruksananonda P, Powell KR. Multiple relapses of Clostridium difficile-associated diarrhea responding to an extended course of cholestyramine. *Pediatr Infect Dis J* 1989; **8:** 175–8.
14. Shwed JA, Rodvold KA. Anion-exchange resins and oral vancomycin in pseudomembranous colitis. *DICP Ann Pharmacother* 1989; **23:** 70–1.
15. Tjellström B, *et al.* Oral immunoglobulin A supplement in treatment of Clostridium difficile enteritis. *Lancet* 1993; **341:** 701–2.
16. Salcedo J, *et al.* Intravenous immunoglobulin therapy for severe Clostridium difficile colitis. *Gut* 1997; **41:** 366–70.
17. Vanderhoof JA, *et al.* Lactobacillus GG in the prevention of antibiotic-associated diarrhea in children. *J Pediatr* 1999; **135:** 564–8.
18. Schellenberg D, *et al.* Treatment of Clostridium difficile diarrhoea with brewer's yeast. *Lancet* 1994; **343:** 171–2.


**Campylobacter enteritis.** *Campylobacter jejuni* is a major cause of acute diarrhoea. *C. coli* is less common and *C. upsaliensis* has more recently been identified as an enteropathogen.[1,2] Food is a common source of infection.[3,4] In the UK, several sources are responsible[5] including contaminated food and water and one important source is from doorstep deliveries of foil-topped bottled milk that have been pecked by birds.[5-7]

The macrolides erythromycin or azithromycin, or a fluoroquinolone are of benefit[8] in severely affected patients, but the infection is usually self-limiting and fluid and electrolyte replacement is generally sufficient. A tetracycline or gentamicin may be alternative antimicrobials.[8] Treatment with erythromycin can eradicate the organism from the faeces,[9-11] but may not reduce the duration of symptoms unless treatment is started early in the course of the disease.[9-11] Some strains of *Campylobacter* are resistant to erythromycin,[12] and resistance is also an increasing problem with ciprofloxacin.[13,14] Multiple drug resistance has been reported.[15,16]

Severe systemic infections with *C. fetus* require parenteral therapy with a carbapenem or gentamicin,[8] depending on susceptibility.

There is some evidence of an association between *C. jejuni* infection and the Guillain-Barré syndrome.[17,18]


1. Bourke B, *et al.* Campylobacter upsaliensis: waiting in the wings. *Clin Microbiol Rev* 1998; **11:** 440–9.
2. Jenkin GA, Tee W. Campylobacter upsaliensis-associated diarrhea in human immunodeficiency virus-infected patients. *Clin Infect Dis* 1998; **27:** 816–21.
3. Skirrow MB. Foodborne illness: Campylobacter. *Lancet* 1990; **336:** 921–3.
4. Allos BM. Campylobacter jejuni infections: update on emerging issues and trends. *Clin Infect Dis* 2001; **32:** 1201–6.
5. Pebody RG, *et al.* Outbreaks of campylobacter infection: rare events for a common pathogen. *Commun Dis Rep* 1997; **7:** R33–R37.
6. Phillips CA. Bird attacks on milk bottles and campylobacter infection. *Lancet* 1995; **346:** 386.
7. Stuart J, *et al.* Outbreak of campylobacter enteritis in a residential school associated with bird pecked bottle tops. *Commun Dis Rep* 1997; **7:** R38–R40.
8. Anonymous. The choice of antibacterial drugs. In: *Handbook of antimicrobial therapy.* 16th ed. New York: The Medical Letter, 2002: 34–52.
9. Anders BJ, *et al.* Double-blind placebo controlled trial of erythromycin for treatment of campylobacter enteritis. *Lancet* 1982; **i:** 131–2.
10. Mandal BK, *et al.* Double-blind placebo-controlled trial of erythromycin in the treatment of clinical campylobacter infection. *J Antimicrob Chemother* 1984; **13:** 619–23.
11. Williams D, *et al.* Early treatment of Campylobacter jejuni enteritis. *Antimicrob Agents Chemother* 1989; **33:** 248–50.
12. Taylor DN, *et al.* Erythromycin-resistant campylobacter infections in Thailand. *Antimicrob Agents Chemother* 1987; **31:** 438–42.
13. Piddock LJV. Quinolone resistance and Campylobacter spp. *J Antimicrob Chemother* 1995; **36:** 891–8.
14. Campylobacter Sentinel Surveillance Scheme Collaborators. Ciprofloxacin resistance in Campylobacter jejuni: case-case analysis as a tool for elucidating risks at home and abroad. *J Antimicrob Chemother* 2002; **50:** 561–8.
15. Winstanley TG, *et al.* Multiple antibiotic resistance in a strain of Campylobacter jejuni acquired in Jordan. *J Antimicrob Chemother* 1993; **31:** 178–9.
16. Gaudreau C, Michaud S. Cluster of erythromycin- and ciprofloxacin-resistant Campylobacter jejuni subsp jejuni from 1999 to 2001 in men who have sex with men, Quebec, Canada. *Clin Infect Dis* 2003; **37:** 131–6.
17. Rees JH, *et al.* Campylobacter jejuni infection and Guillain-Barré syndrome. *N Engl J Med* 1995; **333:** 1374–9.
18. Allos BM. Association between Campylobacter infection and Guillain-Barré syndrome. *J Infect Dis* 1997; **176** (suppl 2): S125–S128.


**Cholera and other vibrio infections.** Cholera results from infection with the enterotoxin-producing Gram-negative bacillus *Vibrio cholerae* which causes acute secretory diarrhoea. It can be associated with two serogroups of *V. cholerae*, O1 and O139. Serogroup O1 can then be divided into two biotypes (classical and El Tor) and each of these has three serotypes (Inaba, Ogawa, and Hikojima). The seventh pandemic[1-6] began in 1961 in South East Asia, reached South America in January 1991, and still shows no sign of abating. This pandemic is caused by *V. cholerae* O1 biotype El Tor. In late 1992 and 1993 epidemic cholera caused by *V. cholerae* O139 was reported in India and Bangladesh and subsequently identified in Thailand and other Asian countries. *V. cholerae* O139 became the dominant strain in India in less than 2 months and some workers declared it responsible for the eighth cholera pandemic.[2] However, there was some evidence that by 1994 it was abating and that by 1996 O1 was again the prevalent type in India and Bangladesh. There appears to be no cross-immunity between O1 and the O139 serogroup.

Individuals can reduce the risk of contracting cholera by avoiding possibly contaminated foodstuffs, good personal hygiene, and boiling or otherwise disinfecting drinking water. Methods of preventing or containing cholera epidemics include ensuring a safe water supply, providing good sanitation, and promoting safe handling and preparation of foods. Mass chemoprophylaxis, vaccination, and travel and trade restrictions are not effective[7] although oral vaccines show more promise.

The majority of cases of vibrio gastro-enteritis are mild to moderate and generally require no therapy other than fluid and electrolyte replacement with an appropriate oral rehydration solution (see Diarrhoea, p.1241). Patients with severe gastro-enteritis, dehydration, and shock should receive vigorous fluid replacement, preferably intravenously.[8] Antimicrobial therapy has been shown to decrease the duration and volume of diarrhoea in cholera and may also decrease the duration of other vibrio diarrhoeas.[9] WHO recommends a single dose of doxycycline as the treatment of choice for adults except pregnant women. Tetracycline, ciprofloxacin, co-trimoxazole, furazolidone, erythromycin, and chloramphenicol are alternatives, with furazolidone being preferred for pregnant women and erythromycin for children. Recommendations from the USA for adults specify a tetracycline as the first choice with co-trimoxazole or a fluoroquinolone such as ciprofloxacin as alternatives.[10] One study has suggested that single-dose ciprofloxacin might be preferred to doxycycline, particularly in areas of tetracycline resistance,[11] and in Bangladesh, ampicillin has been found to be as effective as either erythromycin or tetracycline[12] and may be a useful alternative in children. The O139 strain is reported to be sensitive to ciprofloxacin,[13] erythromycin,[13] and tetracyclines,[2] but resistant to co-trimoxazole.[2] There has also been some resistance to furazolidone.[2] Multiple drug resistance may be a problem; differing sensitivity and resistance patterns have been reported for the 2 biotypes classical and El Tor *V. cholerae*.[14] The outbreak strain in Rwandan refugees was resistant to tetracycline, doxycycline, co-trimoxazole, chloramphenicol, and ampicillin.[2]

Mass chemoprophylaxis is not recommended but may be justified for household contacts,[1,15] especially those at high risk because of age or pregnancy.[1] The type of cholera vaccines traditionally available are not very effective although promising results have been reported with the use of oral vaccines in areas where cholera is endemic.

Marine or halophilic *Vibrio* spp. known to cause gastro-enteritis include *V. parahaemolyticus* which is responsible for food poisoning from raw or undercooked seafood, especially in Japan.[16,17] Another halophilic sp., *V. vulnificus*, is increasingly associated with wound infection and septicaemia.[16] On the basis of *in-vitro* sensitivity testing[18] and anecdotal clinical experience, empirical therapy with aminoglycosides, ceftazidime, imipenem, or ciprofloxacin should all be effective.[19]


1. Anonymous. Cholera. *Commun Dis Rep* 1991; **1:** R48–50.
2. Crowcroft NS. Cholera: current epidemiology. *Commun Dis Rep* 1994; **4:** R157–64.
3. Swerdlow SL, Ries AA. Vibrio cholerae non-O1—the eighth pandemic? *Lancet* 1993; **342:** 382–3.
4. Mahon BE, *et al.* Reported cholera in the United States, 1992-1994: a reflection of global changes in cholera epidemiology. *JAMA* 1996; **276:** 307–12.
5. Seas C, Gotuzzo E. Cholera: overview of epidemiologic, therapeutic, and preventive issues learned from recent epidemics. *Int J Infect Dis* 1996; **1:** 37–46.
6. Sánchez JL, Taylor DN. Cholera. *Lancet* 1997; **349:** 1825–30.
7. WHO. *Guidelines for cholera control.* Geneva: WHO, 1993.
8. Morris JG, Black RE. Cholera and other vibrioses in the United States. *N Engl J Med* 1985; **312:** 343–50.
9. Blake PA. Vibrios on the half shell: what the walrus and the carpenter didn't know. *Ann Intern Med* 1983; **99:** 558–9.
10. Anonymous. The choice of antibacterial drugs. In: *Handbook of antimicrobial therapy.* 16th ed. New York: The Medical Letter, 2002: 34–52.
11. Khan WA, *et al.* Randomised controlled comparison of single-dose ciprofloxacin and doxycycline for cholera caused by Vibrio cholerae O1 or O139. *Lancet* 1996; **348:** 296–300.
12. Roy SK, *et al.* A randomized clinical trial to compare the efficacy of erythromycin, ampicillin and tetracycline for the treatment of cholera in children. *Trans R Soc Trop Med Hyg* 1998; **92:** 460–2.
13. Dhar U, *et al.* Clinical features, antimicrobial susceptibility and toxin production in Vibrio cholerae O139 infection: comparison with V. cholerae O1 infection. *Trans R Soc Trop Med Hyg* 1996; **90:** 402–5.
14. Siddique AK, *et al.* Simultaneous outbreaks of contrasting drug resistant classic and El Tor Vibrio cholerae O1 in Bangladesh. *Lancet* 1989; **ii:** 396.
15. WHO. WHO expert committee on cholera: second report. *WHO Tech Rep Ser 352* 1967.
16. Anonymous. Shuck your oysters with care. *Lancet* 1990; **336:** 215–16.
17. Doyle MP. Foodborne illness: pathogenic Escherichia coli, Yersinia enterocolitica, and Vibrio parahaemolyticus. *Lancet* 1990; **336:** 1111–15.
18. French GL, *et al.* Antimicrobial susceptibilities of halophilic vibrios. *J Antimicrob Chemother* 1989; **24:** 183–94.
19. French GL. Antibiotics for marine vibrios. *Lancet* 1990; **336:** 568–9.


**Escherichia coli enteritis.** *Escherichia coli* is a normal intestinal commensal and member of the Gram-negative family of bacteria the Enterobacteriaceae. Pathogenic strains causing distinct syndromes of diarrhoeal disease and also associated with foodborne illness include: enteropathogenic *E. coli* (EPEC)—an important cause of infantile diarrhoea in many developing countries; enteroinvasive *E. coli* (EIEC)—producing an invasive type of diarrhoea resembling that of *Shigella* dysentery; enterotoxigenic *E. coli* (ETEC)—an important cause of travellers' diarrhoea (see Gastro-enteritis, above); and enterohaemorrhagic *E. coli* (EHEC)—associated with haemorrhagic colitis, haemolytic-uraemic syndrome, and thrombotic thrombocytopenic purpura.[1] Enteroadherent *E. coli* (EAEC) is a cause of chronic diarrhoea in young children.[2]

Although these organisms are generally sensitive to a wide range of antibacterials only special categories of *E. coli* diarrhoea should be treated.[2]

Neonates with severe EPEC diarrhoea have been given oral non-absorbable antibacterials such as neomycin or gentamicin although in older children or adults this diarrhoea is said by some to be self-limiting.[2] Evidence for the efficacy of neomycin is largely limited to uncontrolled studies.[3] However, improvement with antibacterials has been noted beyond the neonatal period;[4] EPEC infection has been reported to be a common treatable cause of life-threatening *chronic* diarrhoea in infancy, possibly associated with travel to a developing country.[5] Symptoms could become persistent and life-threatening in previously healthy infants, requiring intravenous rehydration and parenteral antibacterials such as gentamicin and penicillin.[5]

Vero cytotoxin-producing strains of EHEC (VTEC; Shiga toxin producing *E. coli*; STEC), in particular serotype O157, have been associated with bloody diarrhoea, haemorrhagic colitis, and haemolytic-uraemic syndrome.[6,7] Children and the elderly are regarded to be at high risk of severe disease,[6] but the illness is usually self-limiting.[7] Cases have generally been linked with the consumption of foods derived from cattle, especially undercooked beef and unpasteurised milk, although there have been outbreaks associated with the consumption of fresh vegetables and unpasteurised juices, probably as a result of faecal contamination. Person-to-person spread is also common, and direct spread from infected animals may occur. *E. coli* O157 has also been reported as a cause of epidemic haemorrhagic colitis in Africa, where it may be difficult to distinguish from shigellosis.[8,9] Treatment is generally supportive, including correcting and maintaining the fluid and electrolyte balance.[7] Antibacterial treatment is controversial and there is uncertainty as to whether it influences the course of enterohaemorrhagic *E. coli* infection and the development of haemolytic-uraemic syndrome[10] or thrombotic thrombocytopenic purpura;[6,7,11] the non-antibacterial treatment of these two latter complications is discussed in Plasma, under Thrombotic Microangiopathies, p.758. Oral preparations of Vero cytotoxin-binding resins are under investigation.


1. Doyle MP. Pathogenic Escherichia coli, Yersinia enterocolitica, and Vibrio parahaemolyticus. *Lancet* 1990; **336:** 1111–15.
2. Gorbach SL. Bacterial diarrhoea and its treatment. *Lancet* 1987; **ii:** 1378–82.
3. WHO. *The rational use of drugs in the management of acute diarrhoea in children.* Geneva: WHO, 1990.
4. Hill SM, *et al.* Antibiotics for Escherichia coli gastroenteritis. *Lancet* 1988; **i:** 771–2.
5. Hill SM, *et al.* Enteropathogenic Escherichia coli and life threatening chronic diarrhoea. *Gut* 1991; **32:** 154–8.
6. Mead PS, Griffin PM. Escherichia coli O157:H7. *Lancet* 1998; **352:** 1207–12.
7. Subcommittee of the PHLS Advisory Committee on Gastrointestinal Infections. Guidelines for the control of infection with Vero cytotoxin producing Escherichia coli (VTEC). *Commun Dis Public Health* 2000; **3:** 14–23.
8. Isaäcson M, *et al.* Haemorrhagic colitis epidemic in Africa. *Lancet* 1993; **341:** 961.
9. Paquet C, *et al.* Aetiology of haemorrhagic colitis epidemic in Africa. *Lancet* 1993; **342:** 175.
10. Safdar N, *et al.* Risk of hemolytic uremic syndrome after antibiotic treatment of Escherichia coli O157:H7 enteritis: a meta-analysis. *JAMA* 2002; **288:** 996–1001.
11. Farthing M, *et al.* The management of infective gastroenteritis in adults: a consensus statement by an expert panel convened by the British Society for the Study of Infection. *J Infect* 1996; **33:** 143–52.


**Necrotising enterocolitis.** Necrotising enterocolitis in the newborn is thought to result from hypoxia or ischaemic injury to the intestinal mucosa with subsequent infection. Bacteria implicated in the disease include *Pseudomonas*, *Escherichia coli*, *Klebsiella*, *Salmonella* spp., and *Clostridium* spp. Treatment involves suspension of oral feeding, intravenous fluid therapy, and surgical excision of the affected gut. References to the use of oral vancomycin for the treatment[1] of neonatal necrotising enterocolitis indicate that it may be of benefit. In a comparison of intravenous regimens to treat the condition it was reported that ampicillin with gentamicin appeared as effective as vancomycin with cefotaxime in neonates over 2.2 kg birth-weight, but in smaller neonates results were better with vancomycin and cefotaxime.[2] A systematic review has concluded that prophylactic oral antibacterials might well reduce the incidence of necrotising enterocolitis in low birth-weight or preterm infants in a high-risk environment,[3] but there are concerns about adverse outcomes, and prophylactic use (particularly of vancomycin) is not generally recommended because of the risk of inducing resistance. It has been suggested[4] that oral immunoglobulins may prevent necrotising enterocolitis in low-birth-weight infants; however, a systematic review[5] concluded that the available evidence did not support this claim.

Necrotising enteritis in older children and adults, known as pigbel, has been attributed to toxins produced by *Clostridium perfringens*. Both sporadic and epidemic forms are predominantly seen in the highlands of Papua New Guinea, but sporadic cases have been reported elsewhere. Treatment is supportive with surgical intervention where necessary. A vaccine is available for prophylaxis.


1. Han VKM. An outbreak of Clostridium difficile necrotizing enterocolitis: a case for oral vancomycin therapy? *Pediatrics* 1983; **71:** 935–41.
2. Scheifele DW, *et al.* Comparison of two antibiotic regimens for neonatal necrotizing enterocolitis. *J Antimicrob Chemother* 1987; **20:** 421–9.
3. Bury RG, Tudehope D. Enteral antibiotics for preventing necrotizing enterocolitis in low birthweight or preterm infants. Available in The Cochrane Library; Issue 2. Chichester: John Wiley; 2004.
4. Eibl MM, *et al.* Prevention of necrotizing enterocolitis in low-birth-weight infants by IgA-IgG feeding. *N Engl J Med* 1988; **319:** 1–7.
5. Foster J, Cole M. Oral immunoglobulin for preventing necrotizing enterocolitis in preterm and low birth-weight neonates. Available in The Cochrane Library; Issue 2. Chichester: John Wiley; 2004.


**Salmonella enteritis.** *Salmonella* spp. are Gram-negative bacteria belonging to the Enterobacteriaceae family. They can be divided into those causing enteric fever, namely *S. typhi* and *S. paratyphi*, where infection is systemic although affecting the gastrointestinal tract (see under Typhoid and Paratyphoid Fever, p.152) and non-typhoid *Salmonella*, including *S. enteritidis* and *S. typhimurium* which cause acute gastro-enteritis, usually through food poisoning. There are numerous *Salmonella* serotypes identified with food poisoning and they have often been named according to the place where they were first isolated. The increase in salmonellosis in Great Britain has been almost entirely due to *S. enteritidis*[1] and this reflects an increase internationally.[2] Non-typhoid *Salmonella* spp. can cause invasive salmonellosis which may present as septicaemia or localised infections such as meningitis or osteomyelitis.

Uncomplicated non-typhoid *Salmonella* enteritis is usually managed by fluid and electrolyte replacement. Antibacterial therapy produces no clinical benefit in uncomplicated *Salmonella* enteritis[3] and may prolong *Salmonella* detection in stools.[3] Attempts to eradicate the carrier state with antibacterial therapy (for example fluoroquinolones) appear to have been unsuccessful so far[4] and routine use is not recommended.[5] Patients with underlying debility or evidence of invasive salmonellosis should be given antibacterial therapy. Amoxicillin, ampicillin, or co-trimoxazole have been suggested[6,7] as have trimethoprim, cefotaxime,[7] ceftriaxone,[7] a fluoroquinolone[7] such as ciprofloxacin,[8] or chloramphenicol.[7] However, there is concern over the emergence of resistant strains, particularly to the fluoroquinolones.[9,10] Resistance to cephalosporins has also been recognised.[11,12] Multiresistant R-type strains of *S. typhimurium* DT 104 (another common cause of *Salmonella* enteritis in the UK) have severely limited the treatment options for infections with this organism.[13-16]


1. Baird-Parker AC. Foodborne salmonellosis. *Lancet* 1990; **336:** 1231–5.
2. Rodrigue DC, *et al.* International increase in Salmonella enteritidis: a new pandemic? *Epidemiol Infect* 1990; **105:** 21–7.
3. Sirinavin S, Garner P. Antibiotics for treating salmonella gut infections. Available in The Cochrane Library; Issue 2. Chichester: John Wiley; 2004.
4. Nagler JM, *et al.* Salmonella gastroenteritis: longterm follow-up of an outbreak after treatment with norfloxacin or co-trimoxazole. *J Antimicrob Chemother* 1994; **34:** 291–4.
5. Farthing M. The management of infective gastroenteritis in adults: a consensus statement by an expert panel convened by the British Society for the Study of Infection. *J Infect* 1996; **33:** 143–52.
6. Gorbach SL. Bacterial diarrhoea and its treatment. *Lancet* 1987; **ii:** 1378–82.
7. Anonymous. The choice of antibacterial drugs. In: *Handbook of antimicrobial therapy.* 16th ed. New York: The Medical Letter, 2002: 34–52.
8. Leigh DA. The treatment of a large outbreak of acute bacterial gastroenteritis with ciprofloxacin. *J Antimicrob Chemother* 1992; **30:** 733–5.
9. Wilcox MH, Spencer RC. Quinolones and salmonella gastroenteritis. *J Antimicrob Chemother* 1992; **30:** 221–8.
10. Frost JA, *et al.* Increasing ciprofloxacin resistance in salmonellas in England and Wales 1991-1994. *J Antimicrob Chemother* 1996; **37:** 85–91.

11. Tzouvelekis LS, *et al.* Emergence of resistance to third-generation cephalosporins amongst Salmonella typhimurium isolates in Greece: report of the first three cases. *J Antimicrob Chemother* 1998; **42:** 273–5.
12. Dunne EF, *et al.* Emergence of domestically acquired ceftriaxone-resistant Salmonella infections associated with AmpC beta-lactamase. *JAMA* 2000; **284:** 3151–6.
13. Threlfall EJ, *et al.* Increasing spectrum of resistance in multiresistant Salmonella typhimurium. *Lancet* 1996; **347:** 1053–4.
14. Anonymous. Multidrug-resistant Salmonella serotype typhimurium—United States, 1996. *JAMA* 1996; **277:** 1513.
15. Anonymous. Emergence of multidrug-resistant salmonella. *WHO Drug Inf* 1997; **11:** 21.
16. Threlfall EJ, *et al.* Multiresistant Salmonella typhimurium DT 104 and salmonella bacteraemia. *Lancet* 1998; **352:** 287–8.

**Shigellosis.** Shigellosis (bacillary dysentery) is an enteric infection caused by the *Shigella* spp. *S. dysenteriae*, *S. flexneri*, *S. boydii*, or *S. sonnei*. They are Gram-negative bacteria belonging to the Enterobacteriaceae family and are able to invade the colon. Depending on the species involved, the disease ranges from mild self-limiting secretory diarrhoea to severe colitis and dysentery with blood and mucus in the stools. *S. dysenteriae* is the most common in the developing world and causes the most severe disease. In developed countries *S. flexneri* and *S. sonnei* are more common. Some *S. flexneri* can cause severe colitis and toxic dilatation of the colon has been reported in travellers.[1] *S. sonnei* is the least pathogenic of the species.

As with any form of diarrhoea, rehydration is the key to treatment. Antibacterial therapy may be with ampicillin (amoxicillin appears to be less effective), co-trimoxazole (or trimethoprim), nalidixic acid, or fluoroquinolones such as ciprofloxacin, but will depend on the prevailing resistance patterns (see below) and the severity of the disease. Bacterial resistance is common and some consider that antibacterials should be restricted to the most severe cases, particularly those due to *S. dysenteriae*;[2] in the UK, the Public Health Laboratory Services (PHLS) Working Group has concluded that therapy is seldom indicated for *S. sonnei* infections.[3] WHO[4] has advised that children with *Shigella* dysentery should be given antimicrobial therapy and recommended co-trimoxazole as treatment of choice with nalidixic acid or ampicillin as alternatives; it was noted that resistance to ampicillin is frequent.[5]

The rapid development of resistance and the emergence of multiresistant strains of *Shigella*, particularly in developing countries, has led to some changes in treatment recommendations.[5] In 1992, nalidixic acid had become the preferred drug in developing countries unless ampicillin or co-trimoxazole were known to be effective in the region.[6] For *S. dysenteriae* it might be necessary to use pivmecillinam. It was concluded that the fluoroquinolones should continue to be reserved for infections resistant to nalidixic acid or pivmecillinam.[6] Reduced susceptibility to fluoroquinolones of some strains of *S. sonnei* has been reported from Japan.[7] Fluoroquinolones are generally not used in children, although a study[8] in Bangladesh has used ciprofloxacin in children with shigellosis and found it to be of similar efficacy to pivmecillinam. In studies from Israel, the third-generation cephalosporins ceftriaxone[9] or cefixime[10] were more effective than ampicillin or co-trimoxazole, respectively, in children with shigellosis. Other studies in adults in Bangladesh found cefixime to be ineffective compared with pivmecillinam[11] and azithromycin to be effective, although slightly less so, than ciprofloxacin.[12]

Vitamin A may be a useful adjunct to treatment, especially in children in developing countries (see Vitamin A, p.1454).

Oral shigella vaccines are being studied for prophylaxis.

1. Wilson APR, *et al.* Toxic dilatation of the colon in shigellosis. *BMJ* 1990; **301:** 1325–6.
2. Kaya IS, *et al.* Danger of antibiotic resistance in shigellosis. *Lancet* 1990; **336:** 186.
3. PHLS Working Group on the control of Shigella sonnei infection. Revised guidelines for the control of Shigella sonnei infection and other infective diarrhoeas. *Commun Dis Rep* 1993; **3:** R69–70.
4. WHO. *The rational use of drugs in the management of acute diarrhoea in children.* Geneva: WHO, 1990.
5. WHO. *The management and prevention of diarrhoea: practical guidelines.* 3rd ed. Geneva: WHO, 1993.
6. Bennish ML, Salam MA. Rethinking options for the treatment of shigellosis. *J Antimicrob Chemother* 1992; **30:** 243–7.
7. Horiuchi S, *et al.* Reduced susceptibilities of Shigella sonnei strains isolated from patients with dysentery to fluoroquinolones. *Antimicrob Agents Chemother* 1993; **37:** 2486–9.
8. Salam MA, *et al.* Randomised comparison of ciprofloxacin suspension and pivmecillinam for childhood shigellosis. *Lancet* 1998; **352:** 522–7.
9. Varsano I, *et al.* Comparative efficacy of ceftriaxone and ampicillin for treatment of severe shigellosis in children. *J Pediatr* 1991; **118:** 627–32.
10. Ashkenazi S, *et al.* A randomized, double-blind study comparing cefixime and trimethoprim-sulfamethoxazole in the treatment of childhood shigellosis. *J Pediatr* 1993; **123:** 817–21.
11. Salam MA, *et al.* Treatment of shigellosis: IV. Cefixime is ineffective in shigellosis in adults. *Ann Intern Med* 1995; **123:** 505–8.
12. Khan WA, *et al.* Treatment of shigellosis: V. Comparison of azithromycin and ciprofloxacin. *Ann Intern Med* 1997; **126:** 697–703.

**Yersinia enteritis.** *Yersinia enterocolitica* is a Gram-negative bacteria of the Enterobacteriaceae family and the species most commonly responsible for yersiniosis. The predominant form of infection is an enteric illness with or without mesenteric adenitis[1] although clinical manifestations can range from self-limited enterocolitis to potentially fatal systemic infection, and post-infection complications can include erythema nodosum and reactive arthritis.[2] *Y. enterocolitica* is a recognised foodborne pathogen[3] and in some temperate countries rivals *Salmonella* and exceeds *Shigella* as a cause of acute gastro-enteritis; pigs are a major reservoir. Increased susceptibility to *Yersinia* infection has occurred in patients with iron overload treated with desferrioxamine (see p.1034).

Isolates of *Y. enterocolitica* are reported to be susceptible to co-trimoxazole, aminoglycosides, chloramphenicol, tetracycline, third-generation cephalosporins, and quinolones *in vitro*.[1,2] As with any form of diarrhoea, rehydration is the key to treatment and most forms of mild uncomplicated enteritis do not require antibacterial treatment. There has been no general consensus concerning the antibacterial of choice when treatment becomes necessary: as with many other enteric infections there is a lack of good clinical evidence. Drugs with good intracellular activity such as trimethoprim, co-trimoxazole, tetracycline, chloramphenicol, or fluoroquinolones may be preferred.[1] Doxycycline or co-trimoxazole have been recommended[2] for complicated gastrointestinal and focal extra-intestinal infections or doxycycline and an aminoglycoside empirically in bacteraemia. Co-trimoxazole as first choice or alternatively a fluoroquinolone, an aminoglycoside, cefotaxime, or ceftizoxime have also been recommended.[4] A patient with chronic *Yersinia* infection who responded well to tetracycline or co-trimoxazole, but relapsed on withdrawal, was treated successfully with ciprofloxacin.[5]

1. Hoogkamp-Korstanje JAA. Antibiotics in Yersinia enterocolitica infections. *J Antimicrob Chemother* 1987; **20:** 123–31.
2. Cover TL, Aber RC. Yersinia enterocolitica. *N Engl J Med* 1989; **321:** 16–24.
3. Doyle MP. Pathogenic Escherichia coli, Yersinia enterocolitica, and Vibrio parahaemolyticus. *Lancet* 1990; **336:** 1111–15.
4. Anonymous. The choice of antibacterial drugs. In: *Handbook of antimicrobial therapy.* 16th ed. New York: The Medical Letter, 2002: 34–52.
5. Read RC, Barry RE. Relapsing yersinia infection. *BMJ* 1990; **300:** 1694.

## Gonorrhoea

Gonorrhoea is a sexually transmitted disease caused by infection of mucosa with *Neisseria gonorrhoeae* (gonococcus), a Gram-negative bacterium. It occurs mainly as urethritis in men and cervicitis in women, but also as pharyngitis, proctitis, or conjunctivitis. Complications of gonococcal infections include pelvic inflammatory disease (p.139) in women and epididymitis (p.127) in men. Disseminated gonococcal infection results from gonococcal bacteraemia and may lead to septic arthritis, an arthritis-dermatitis syndrome (not to be confused with Reiter's disease which has been associated with non-gonococcal or non-specific urethritis), and more rarely with conditions such as endocarditis or meningitis. Gonorrhoea in pregnant women may cause neonatal gonococcal conjunctivitis (ophthalmia neonatorum).

Infection with *Chlamydia trachomatis* (see under Chlamydial Infections, p.123) often occurs along with gonorrhoea and should be tested for or treated presumptively.

*N. gonorrhoeae* used to be sensitive to penicillins and tetracyclines but in some areas, including the USA, this is no longer the case. Gonococcal resistance includes plasmid-mediated penicillin resistance due to penicillinase-producing *N. gonorrhoeae* (PPNG), high-level plasmid-mediated tetracycline resistance (TRNG), and chromosomally mediated resistance (CMRNG) to penicillin, tetracycline, cefoxitin, or spectinomycin that is not due to beta-lactamase production.[1]

Although resistant strains of *N. gonorrhoeae* have generally been slower to emerge in the UK than in some other parts of the world, increasing world travel and population mixing means that clinicians in the UK have to be aware of the possibility of antibacterial resistant infections. Increasing resistance of gonococci is now monitored in England and Wales via the Gonococcal Resistance to Antimicrobials Surveillance Programme (GRASP).[2] Although GRASP has reported increasing resistance to fluoroquinolones, current UK guidelines[3] for treatment of gonorrhoea still recommend single doses of ciprofloxacin or ofloxacin for uncomplicated infections unless the organism can be demonstrated to be fully sensitive to penicillins, in which case ampicillin plus probenecid may be used.[3] Infections acquired outside the UK are presumed to be resistant to penicillins, tetracycline, and possibly fluoroquinolones, and treatment with an alternative regimen comprising a single intramuscular dose of ceftriaxone, cefotaxime, or spectinomycin should be considered.[3]

In the USA, the wide distribution of antimicrobial-resistant *N. gonorrhoeae*, as documented by the Gonococcal Isolate Surveillance Project,[1] has necessitated revised treatment guidelines. The Centers for Disease Control (CDC)[4] recommends single-dose cephalosporins or fluoroquinolones as the treatment of choice for uncomplicated gonorrhoea, rather than penicillin or tetracycline, plus treatment for chlamydial infection (see below for details).

Of concern are the increasing number of reports worldwide of resistance to newer antigonococcal drugs such as the fluoroquinolones.

Recommended treatment regimens from WHO[5] in 2003 and CDC[4] in 2002 are as follows. Where possible, sexual partners should be tested and treated.

- UNCOMPLICATED GONOCOCCAL INFECTIONS IN ADULTS.

  **WHO** (for anogenital infections): a single oral dose of ciprofloxacin 500 mg or cefixime 400 mg, or a single intramuscular dose of ceftriaxone 125 mg or spectinomycin 2 g.

  **CDC** (for uncomplicated infections in general): a single oral dose of cefixime 400 mg, or ciprofloxacin 500 mg, or ofloxacin 400 mg, or levofloxacin 250 mg, or a single intramuscular dose of ceftriaxone 125 mg. Other cephalosporins or fluoroquinolones may be substituted. Spectinomycin 2 g as a single intramuscular dose is an alternative in patients who cannot tolerate cephalosporins or fluoroquinolones. For pharyngeal infections a single oral dose of ciprofloxacin 500 mg, or a single intramuscular dose of ceftriaxone 125 mg is recommended. (In the UK,[3] these drugs are also recommended for pharyngeal infections, although the recommended dose for ceftriaxone is 250 mg; a further recommended alternative is ofloxacin 400 mg orally as a single dose.) In each case CDC advocates concomitant treatment for presumptive chlamydial infections with either azithromycin 1 g orally as a single dose or doxycycline 100 mg twice daily for 7 days.[4]

  **CDC** recommends a cephalosporin or spectinomycin for pregnant women with gonorrhoea, and erythromycin or amoxicillin for chlamydial infection.[4]

- GONOCOCCAL EYE INFECTIONS IN ADULTS.

  **WHO**[5] recommends a single dose of ceftriaxone 125 mg intramuscularly, or spectinomycin 2 g intramuscularly, or ciprofloxacin 500 mg by mouth, together with frequent irrigation of the infected eye with saline. Kanamycin 2 g intramuscularly is another alternative.

  **CDC**[4] recommends a single dose of ceftriaxone 1 g intramuscularly together with irrigation of the infected eye with saline.

- DISSEMINATED GONOCOCCAL INFECTIONS IN ADULTS.

  **WHO**[5] recommends ceftriaxone 1 g intramuscularly or intravenously once daily for 7 days or spectinomycin 2 g intramuscularly twice daily for 7 days. Another third-generation cephalosporin may be substituted if neither of these drugs is available.

  **CDC**[4] recommends the following regimens: initially ceftriaxone 1 g intramuscularly or intravenously every 24 hours; alternatives are ceftizoxime 1 g intravenously every 8 hours or cefotaxime 1 g intravenously every 8 hours. Ciprofloxacin 400 mg intravenously every 12 hours, or ofloxacin 400 mg intravenously every 12 hours, or levofloxacin 250 mg intravenously once daily, or spectinomycin 2 g intramuscularly every 12 hours may be substituted in patients allergic to beta lactams. Once improvement has been established for 24 to 48 hours, oral therapy with cefixime 400 mg twice daily, or ciprofloxacin 500 mg twice daily, or ofloxacin 400 mg twice daily, or levofloxacin 500 mg once daily may be substituted until at least a 1-week treatment period is complete. For gonococcal *meningitis* and *endocarditis*, CDC advises ceftriaxone 1 to 2 g intravenously every 12 hours; treatment for meningitis should continue for 10 to 14 days and for endocarditis for at least 4 weeks.

- GONOCOCCAL INFECTIONS IN NEONATES AND CHILDREN.

  *Neonates* born to mothers with gonorrhoea are at high risk of infection and require prophylaxis.

  **WHO**[5] recommends a single intramuscular injection of ceftriaxone 50 mg/kg (maximum 125 mg) or, if ceftriaxone is not available, spectinomycin 25 mg/kg (maximum 75 mg) or kanamycin 25 mg/kg (maximum 75 mg).

**CDC**[4] recommends a single intramuscular or intravenous injection of ceftriaxone 25 to 50 mg/kg (maximum 125 mg). For those neonates with disseminated gonococcal infection (sepsis, arthritis, meningitis), ceftriaxone 25 to 50 mg/kg intramuscularly or intravenously once daily for 7 days or cefotaxime 25 mg/kg intramuscularly or intravenously every 12 hours for 7 days is recommended, in each case extended to 10 to 14 days if meningitis is present. The prevention and treatment of neonatal gonococcal conjunctivitis is discussed under Neonatal Conjunctivitis, p.136.

The treatment recommended by CDC[4] for *children* with gonococcal infections, most commonly due to sexual abuse in pre-adolescents, is as for adults in those weighing 45 kg or more. For those weighing less than 45 kg, CDC recommends a single intramuscular dose of ceftriaxone 125 mg or spectinomycin 40 mg/kg (maximum 2 g) for those with uncomplicated infections. For disseminated infection in all children they recommend an intramuscular or intravenous dose of ceftriaxone 50 mg/kg once daily for 7 days, up to a maximum dose of 1 g in those weighing less than 45 kg.

1. Centers for Disease Control. Sexually transmitted disease surveillance 2001 supplement: Gonococcal Isolate Surveillance Project (GISP) annual report—2001. Available at: http://www.cdc.gov/std/GISP2001/GISP2001Text&Fig.pdf (accessed 18/05/04)
2. Health Protection Agency. GRASP The Gonococcal Resistance to Antimicrobials Surveillance Programme: annual report, year 2002 collection. Available at: http://www.hpa.org.uk/infections/topics_az/hiv_and_sti/sti-gonorrhoea/publications/grasp_report_2002.pdf (accessed 18/05/04)
3. Clinical Effectiveness Group (Association for Genitourinary Medicine and the Medical Society for the Study of Venereal Diseases). 2001 National guideline on the management of gonorrhoea in adults. Available at: http://www.bashh.org/guidelines/2002/gc%200601.pdf (accessed 18/05/04)
4. Centers for Disease Control. Sexually transmitted diseases treatment guidelines 2002. *MMWR* 2002; **51**(RR-6): 1–80. Also available at: http://www.cdc.gov/mmwr/PDF/rr/rr5106.pdf (accessed 18/05/04)
5. WHO. Guidelines for the management of sexually transmitted infections. Geneva: WHO, 2003. Also available at: http://whqlibdoc.who.int/publications/2003/9241546263.pdf (accessed 22/06/04)

## Granuloma inguinale

Granuloma inguinale or donovanosis is caused by the Gram-negative bacterium *Calymmatobacterium granulomatis* and occurs most commonly in the tropics and subtropics, especially Papua New Guinea and India. It is characterised by genital ulcers and is generally considered to be a sexually transmitted disease.

WHO[1] recommends azithromycin 1 g by mouth on the first day then 500 mg by mouth once daily, or doxycycline 100 mg orally twice daily. Alternative drugs include erythromycin, tetracycline, or co-trimoxazole. The addition of parenteral gentamicin should be considered for HIV-infected patients. All treatment should be continued until all lesions have completely resolved. Streptomycin is no longer recommended because of its toxicity and the need to reserve it for tuberculosis.

In the USA, the Centers for Disease Control[2] recommend treatment with doxycycline 100 mg twice daily or co-trimoxazole 960 mg twice daily, both for a minimum of 3 weeks; alternatives are ciprofloxacin 750 mg twice daily, or erythromycin 500 mg four times daily, or azithromycin 1 g once weekly by mouth, all also for 3 weeks. The addition of an aminoglycoside may be considered if lesions do not respond during the first few days of treatment.

Other drugs shown to be effective include ceftriaxone and norfloxacin.[3]

1. WHO. Guidelines for the management of sexually transmitted infections. Geneva: WHO, 2003. Also available at: http://whqlibdoc.who.int/publications/2003/9241546263.pdf (accessed 22/06/04)
2. Centers for Disease Control. Sexually transmitted diseases treatment guidelines 2002. *MMWR* 2002; **51**(RR-6): 1–80. Also available at: http://www.cdc.gov/mmwr/PDF/rr/rr5106.pdf (accessed 18/05/04)
3. Clinical Effectiveness Group (Association for Genitourinary Medicine and the Medical Society for the Study of Venereal Diseases). 2001 National guideline for the management of donovanosis (granuloma inguinale). Available at: http://www.bashh.org/guidelines/2002/donovanosis%2009%2001b.pdf (accessed 18/05/04)

## Haemophilus influenzae infections

*Haemophilus influenzae* is a Gram-negative bacterium that colonises the upper respiratory tract in the majority of healthy people. Most are carriers of non-encapsulated strains, but a small proportion carry *H. influenzae* type b, the commonest encapsulated strain. Serious invasive infections have usually been caused by type b strains and have occurred mainly in young children. They include the bacteraemic diseases meningitis, pneumonia, epiglottitis, cellulitis, and arthritis. Non-encapsulated strains commonly cause otitis media, sinusitis, and conjunctivitis and infect patients with chronic bronchitis. However, they too can cause invasive infections such as pneumonia, septicaemia, and meningitis and, with the introduction of *H. influenzae* type b vaccines, non-encapsulated strains may be responsible for a greater proportion of invasive *H. influenzae* disease.

For further details of these infections and their management, see under the specific disease side-headings.

Ampicillin and chloramphenicol have been the antibacterials of choice against *H. influenzae*, but increasing resistance, especially to ampicillin, should be borne in mind; there have been several reports of multiresistant strains.[1-4] Injectable cephalosporins are popular alternatives for multiresistant type b organisms although there is controversy over their effectiveness against fully sensitive strains when compared with ampicillin or chloramphenicol or both; experience has been favourable with cefotaxime and ceftriaxone, but there have been treatment failures in *H. influenzae* meningitis with cefuroxime and there is argument over its efficacy.[5] Meropenem is a further alternative.[6]

For serious *H. influenzae* infections cefotaxime or ceftriaxone are currently preferred. For less serious infections, co-trimoxazole (or trimethoprim in the UK) is preferred; ampicillin, amoxicillin (with or without clavulanic acid), oral second- or third-generation cephalosporins, a tetracycline, a fluoroquinolone, or the macrolides azithromycin or clarithromycin are suggested alternatives.[6]

In the UK, secondary prophylaxis with rifampicin is given following *H. influenzae* type b meningitis (see p.134). A vaccine against *H. influenzae* type b is available and vaccination is included in the infant immunisation schedules in some countries including the UK and USA.

1. Sturm AW, *et al.* Outbreak of multiresistant non-encapsulated Haemophilus influenzae infections in a pulmonary rehabilitation centre. *Lancet* 1990; **335:** 214–16.
2. Brightman CAJ, *et al.* Family outbreak of chloramphenicol-ampicillin resistant Haemophilus influenzae type b disease. *Lancet* 1990; **335:** 351–2.
3. Barclay K, *et al.* Multiresistant Haemophilus influenzae. *Lancet* 1990; **335:** 549.
4. Scott GM, *et al.* Outbreaks of multiresistant Haemophilus influenzae infection. *Lancet* 1990; **335:** 925.
5. Powell M. Chemotherapy for infections caused by Haemophilus influenzae: current problems and future prospects. *J Antimicrob Chemother* 1991; **27:** 3–7.
6. Anonymous. The choice of antibacterial drugs. In: *Handbook of antimicrobial therapy.* 16th ed. New York: The Medical Letter, 2002: 34–52.

## Helicobacter pylori infections

Antibacterial therapy is used to eradicate *Helicobacter pylori* infection in peptic ulcer disease (p.1246) and MALT lymphoma of the stomach (p.511). The role of *H. pylori* and the value of its eradication in dyspepsia (p.1242) and gastro-oesophageal reflux disease (p.1242) is less clear.

## Infections in immunocompromised patients

Patients with a defective immune system are at special risk of infection. Primary immune deficiency is rare, whereas secondary deficiency is more common: immunosuppressive therapy, cancer and its treatment, HIV infection, and splenectomy may all cause neutropenia and impaired humoral and cellular immunity in varying degrees. The risk and severity of infections depends upon the duration of compromised immunity, the degree to which immune function is compromised, whether cellular or humoral functions are affected, and upon breaches in physical barriers, for example by severe mucositis or prolonged vascular access. Thus patients with profound neutropenia or a history of splenectomy are prone to rapidly progressive and potentially life-threatening infections; those with neutropenia induced by cytotoxic chemotherapy or by preparation for transplantation are particularly vulnerable to acute infections whereas those in whom immunosuppression results from viral infections or congenital defects are at lower risk of acute infections.[1] Patients in whom neutropenia persists for more than 10 days are not only at risk of opportunistic bacterial infections but also susceptible to viral, fungal, and parasitic infections.

Infectious diseases are a major cause of morbidity and mortality in patients with AIDS (see HIV-associated Infections, p.623). Some are due to common pathogens, but others are opportunistic and are caused by normally avirulent commensals. Children with HIV infection appear to be at special risk of serious bacterial infections with common encapsulated bacteria. For further reference to some bacterial infections associated with AIDS, see under Gastro-enteritis (p.127), Opportunistic Mycobacterial Infections (p.137), and Tuberculosis (p.150). Fungal, protozoal, and viral infections which can affect immunocompromised patients are discussed in the relevant chapters under Infections in Immunocompromised Patients, p.388, p.597, and p.624, respectively.

Common causative organisms of unexplained fever in neutropenic patients include the Gram-negative bacteria *Pseudomonas aeruginosa, Escherichia coli*, and *Klebsiella* spp. and Gram-positive organisms particularly staphylococci, streptococci, enterococci, and *Corynebacterium* spp. Gram-negative organisms have historically been responsible for most immediate life-threatening infections, but Gram-positive infections are increasing in importance and now predominate in many areas.[1,2] Factors influencing this change include the wider use of selective gut decontamination and of central venous catheters,[3] and possibly the prophylactic use of quinolones.

TREATMENT. Onset of fever in neutropenic patients is indicative of potentially serious infection which may progress to septicaemia and death. The severity of infections depends on numerous factors (see above) and it is therefore difficult to produce a standard drug regimen; in addition, the choice of empirical therapy must be adapted according to prevailing local antibacterial susceptibility patterns. Nevertheless, guidelines have been produced by the Infectious Diseases Society of America[4] for both the initial and subsequent management of febrile neutropenic patients. Initial assessment should be performed to determine whether the patient is at low or high risk of life-threatening infection. If the risk is considered high, empirical intravenous antibacterial therapy should be started immediately. Secondly, consideration should be given to whether the patient requires vancomycin therapy. If so, treatment should begin with vancomycin plus cefepime, ceftazidime, or a carbapenem, with or without an aminoglycoside. If vancomycin is not indicated, intravenous monotherapy should be given with either a cephalosporin (cefepime or ceftazidime) or a carbapenem (imipenem-cilastatin or meropenem) for uncomplicated cases; in more complicated cases, or where resistance is a problem, combined treatment should be given with an aminoglycoside and one of cefepime, ceftazidime, a carbapenem, or an antipseudomonal penicillin such as ticarcillin with clavulanic acid or piperacillin with tazobactam. Low-risk patients may be treated empirically either orally with ciprofloxacin and amoxicillin with clavulanic acid, or intravenously as for uncomplicated cases above. Initial treatment with oral antibacterials alone is, however, not recommended for children.[4]

The initial regimen usually needs to be given for 3 to 5 days in order to determine its efficacy. In patients in whom fever resolves and in whom a causative organism is identified, antibacterial treatment should be modified for the specific organisms and broad-spectrum antibacterials continued for at least 7 days or until culture results are negative and the patient has clinically recovered.[4] In afebrile patients in whom no causative organism is found but who were considered at high risk at the onset of treatment, the same antibacterials should be continued intravenously; those considered at low risk initially may be switched to oral therapy with ciprofloxacin plus either amoxicillin-clavulanic acid (adults) or cefixime (children).[4]

Patients in whom fever persists throughout the first 3 to 5 days but for whom no aetiology is determined may have a non-bacterial infection, a bacterial infection that is refractory to treatment, the emergence of a second infection, or drug fever.[4] Such patients should be reassessed and then one of three options followed. If the patient's condition is clinically stable, the same antibacterial treatment may be continued; if there is still no change in the patient's condition, consideration should be given to stopping vancomycin if it has been given. Alternatively, if there is evidence of progressive disease or drug toxicity, the antibacterials given may be changed; if vancomycin has not been given, it may be added to the regimen. The third option is to add an antifungal drug (amphotericin B) with or without a change to the antibacterial regimen if the patient is febrile through days 5 to 7 and resolution of neutropenia is not imminent.[4]

The optimum duration of therapy is governed by the clinical situation. The most important determinant of successful discontinuation of antibacterials is the neutrophil count.[4] If no infection is identified after day 3, the neutrophil count exceeds 500 cells/mm$^3$ for 2 consecutive days, and the patient has been afebrile for at least 48 hours, then antibacterial treatment may be stopped. If neutropenia persists in the absence of fever, it is reasonable to stop antibacterial treatment after 5 to 7 days in patients who were initially considered at low risk and who are clinically well, though such patients should be closely monitored and intravenous antibacterials reinstigated immediately on recurrence of fever or evidence of infection.[4] In afebrile patients with profound neutropenia (less than 100 cells/mm$^3$), or in those with mucositis or other risk factors, continuous antibacterial treatment should be considered throughout the entire neutropenic period. In patients with persistent fever and prolonged neutropenia in whom haematological recovery cannot be anticipated, consideration may be given to stopping antibacterials after 2 weeks if no infection has been identified and careful observation is possible.[4] Clinically well patients with persistent fever may have their antibacterials stopped after 4 to 5 days if the neutrophil count remains at least 500 cells/mm$^3$ throughout this period and there is no sign of infection and no response to therapy; such patients should be closely monitored for subsequent infections which are usually easily treatable, and empirical amphotericin B should be considered despite cessation of antibacterials if fever persists for 5 to 7 days after the start of initial therapy.[4] Patients who remain febrile after recovery from neutropenia and despite broad-spectrum antibacterials should be reassessed for undiagnosed infection which may be fungal, mycobacterial, or viral.

The routine use of colony-stimulating factors as an adjunct to antibacterial treatment is not generally recommended[4] but may be indicated in neutropenic patients at high risk of serious infections or infection-related complications; examples include some patients with malignant neoplasms[5] and those with persistent severe neutropenia and infections that are not responsive to antibacterials alone.[4] A systematic review[6] of the use of colony-stimulating factors in patients with febrile neutropenia due to cancer chemotherapy concluded that their use did not affect overall mortality but did reduce time spent in hospital and the neutrophil recovery time.

**PROPHYLAXIS.** Most infections in immunocompromised patients are caused by organisms from their own alimentary tract and in cancer patients, for example, may follow chemotherapy-induced mucosal damage to the tract. Although antibacterial prophylaxis may be effective in afebrile patients likely to be neutropenic, the efficacy of empirical treatment means that prophylaxis is less widely used[7] and the Infectious Diseases Society of America[4] discourages routine use; reasons include toxicity of the antibacterial, potential fungal overgrowth, and problems of bacterial resistance (see below). Most experience with prophylaxis has been in patients with leukaemia. Possible prophylactic regimens have included selective decontamination of the alimentary tract using oral nonabsorbable antibacterials (see also under Intensive Care, below). Co-trimoxazole has also been widely used.[7] More recently, prophylaxis with fluoroquinolones has been commonly used although, generally, prophylaxis with these drugs has resulted in reduction in Gram-negative but not in Gram-positive infections in immunocompromised patients,[8] and improved morbidity and mortality has not been observed.[9] Combination prophylaxis with fluoroquinolones and phenoxymethylpenicillin[10] or rifampicin[11] has been tried to improve cover against Gram-positive organisms. Nevertheless, concern about the emergence of resistant organisms has led to the recommendation that routine prophylaxis should be avoided.[4]

Immunocompromised patients may benefit from appropriate immunisation against common infections, although precautions relating to the use of live vaccines in such patients should be observed (p.1606).

The duration and severity of neutropenia can be reduced by the use granulocyte or granulocyte-macrophage colony-stimulating factors, and this may be a useful adjunct in infection control in selected patients.[5] Bone marrow protective agents such as amifostine are also being studied.

For further reference to prophylaxis in high-risk patients, see under Intensive Care, below.


1. Pizzo PA. Fever in immunocompromised patients. *N Engl J Med* 1999; **341:** 893–900.
2. Plunkett T, *et al.* Complications of chemotherapy 1: the management of neutropenia and febrile neutropenia. *CME Oncol* 1998; **1:** 40–4.
3. Oppenheim BA. The changing pattern of infection in neutropenic patients. *J Antimicrob Chemother* 1998; **41** (suppl D): 7–11.
4. Infectious Diseases Society of America. 2002 Guidelines for the use of antimicrobial agents in neutropenic patients with cancer. *Clin Infect Dis* 2002; **34:** 730–51.
5. American Society of Clinical Oncology. 2000 Update of recommendations for the use of hematopoietic colony-stimulating factors: evidence-based, clinical practice guidelines. *J Clin Oncol* 2000; **18:** 3558–85.
6. Clark OAC, *et al.* Colony stimulating factors for chemotherapy induced febrile neutropenia. Available in The Cochrane Library; Issue 2. Chichester: John Wiley; 2004.
7. Kerr KG. The prophylaxis of bacterial infections in neutropenic patients. *J Antimicrob Chemother* 1999; **44:** 587–91.
8. Engels EA, *et al.* Efficacy of quinolone prophylaxis in neutropenic cancer patients: a meta-analysis. *J Clin Oncol* 1998; **16:** 1179–87.
9. Cruciani M, *et al.* Prophylaxis with fluoroquinolones for bacterial infections in neutropenic patients: a meta-analysis. *Clin Infect Dis* 1996; **23:** 795–805.
10. International Antimicrobial Therapy Cooperative Group of the European Organization for Research and Treatment of Cancer (EORTC). Reduction of fever and streptococcal bacteremia in granulocytopenic patients with cancer: a trial of oral penicillin V or placebo combined with pefloxacin. *JAMA* 1994; **272:** 1183–9.
11. Bow EJ, *et al.* Quinolone-based antibacterial chemoprophylaxis in neutropenic patients: effect of augmented gram-positive activity on infectious morbidity. *Ann Intern Med* 1996; **125:** 183–90.


## Intensive care

Similarly to immunocompromised patients (above), those in intensive care units are often very susceptible to endogenous infections, especially respiratory and urinary-tract infections, arising from gastrointestinal colonisation by aerobic Gram-negative bacilli acquired in hospital. Selective digestive tract decontamination (SDD), using oral non-absorbable antibacterial regimens, and selective parenteral and enteral antisepsis regimens (SPEAR), incorporating selective decontamination together with systemic antibacterial prophylaxis, have been used in an attempt to prevent colonisation and infection in these high-risk patients, although their effectiveness is debated. SDD has generally not been widely adopted in the USA[1] particularly in relation to prevention of nosocomial pneumonia.[2,3] It may be more effective in surgical patients.[4]

Selective decontamination is achieved by elimination of aerobic, potentially pathogenic, organisms from the throat and intestines while preserving the indigenous, mostly anaerobic, flora.[5,6] Regimens commonly include two or three non-absorbable or poorly absorbed antibacterial drugs, for example colistin, neomycin, norfloxacin, or polymyxin, in combination with an antifungal, usually amphotericin B. The drugs are usually applied topically to the oropharyngeal mucosa in addition to oral or intragastric administration, although local application to the oropharynx alone is also reported to be effective.[7,8] A parenteral third-generation cephalosporin, usually cefotaxime, may be given for a few days until oral medication takes effect.[9,10] Strict adherence to the protocol is reported to be necessary for maximum efficacy[11] and constant monitoring for the emergence of antimicrobial resistance is considered essential[10,11] although so far this has rarely been seen in practice.[11,12] However, most regimens have little or no activity against potential Gram-positive pathogens such as *Enterococcus* spp., and so their use may increase the risk for colonisation and infection with these organisms.[13] There is particular concern over the emergence of vancomycin-resistant strains.

Despite numerous clinical studies, many of which have shown a reduction in potential Gram-negative pathogens[9,10,14] and in the incidence of respiratory-tract infections,[7,8] it has been difficult to demonstrate that SDD or SPEAR reduces mortality.[15-18] Although meta-analyses[19,20] of randomised controlled trials concluded that a combination of a systemic and topical antibacterial could be beneficial it has been argued that the effect was largely due to the systemic component of the treatment.[21] It has been suggested[22] that equivalent infection control could be achieved more economically by emphasis on high standards of hygiene and avoidance of histamine $H_2$-receptor antagonists, which could allow overgrowth of potentially pathogenic bacteria as a result of the change in gastric pH.

Another potential source of infection in intensive care is from the use of **intravascular catheters**. The organisms implicated most frequently have been coagulase-negative staphylococci.[23] Prevention and control of infection depend on good aseptic technique and care of the insertion site, and also catheter design;[23,24] guidelines have been produced in the USA for the prevention of infection.[25] Catheters should be removed as soon as possible (often after 48 to 72 hours for peripheral lines) and any infections treated promptly with antibacterials; vancomycin or teicoplanin are appropriate for empirical treatment provided resistance is not a problem.[23] There have been some favourable results with antibacterial prophylaxis, but their use is discouraged because of concern over the emergence of resistant organisms.[26] Topical antiseptics and antibacterials have produced promising results.[23] Antibacterials could also prove useful in reducing or eliminating colonisation of the catheter lumen[27] and catheters coated with antibacterials[28] or heparin[29] are under investigation. Randomised clinical studies have shown that the use of catheters coated with minocycline and rifampicin[30] or with antiseptics (p.1165) can reduce the risk of systemic infections. Current evidence suggests that catheters impregnated with minocycline and rifampicin are more effective in minimising risk of infection than those coated with chlorhexidine or sulfadiazine silver.[31]

The importance of maintaining high standards of infection control, including handwashing, in intensive care units has been reinforced by the increasing incidence of nosocomial infections that are difficult to treat such as those due to vancomycin-resistant enterococci and *Acinetobacter.* In one such outbreak due to *A. baumannii* some strains were resistant to imipenem and all other antibacterials except polymyxin B and sulbactam.[32] Intensive infection control measures and irrigation of all open wounds with polymyxin B solution were used to eliminate infection and colonisation.


1. Kollef MH. The prevention of ventilator-associated pneumonia. *N Engl J Med* 1999; **340:** 627–34. Correction. *ibid.*; **341:** 294.
2. American Thoracic Society. Hospital-acquired pneumonia in adults: diagnosis, assessment of severity, initial antimicrobial therapy, and preventative strategies: a consensus statement. *Am J Respir Crit Care Med* 1996; **153:** 1711–25. Also available at: http://www.thoracic.org/adobe/statements/hosp1-15.pdf (accessed 19/05/04)
3. Centers for Disease Control. Guidelines for prevention of nosocomial pneumonia. *MMWR* 1997; **46** (RR-1): 1–79. Also available at: http://www.cdc.gov/mmwr/PDF/rr/rr4601.pdf (accessed 19/05/04)
4. Nathens AB, Marshall JC. Selective decontamination of the digestive tract in surgical patients: a systematic review of the evidence. *Arch Surg* 1999; **134:** 170–6.
5. van Saene HKF, Stoutenbeek CP. Selective decontamination. *J Antimicrob Chemother* 1987; **20:** 462–5.
6. Krueger WA, Unertl KE. Selective decontamination of the digestive tract. *Curr Opin Crit Care* 2002; **8:** 139–44.
7. Rodriguez-Roldan JM, *et al.* Prevention of nosocomial lung infection in ventilated patients: use of an antimicrobial pharyngeal nonabsorbable paste. *Crit Care Med* 1990; **18:** 1239–42.
8. Pugin J, *et al.* Oropharyngeal decontamination decreases incidence of ventilator-associated pneumonia: a randomized, placebo-controlled, double-blind clinical trial. *JAMA* 1991; **265:** 2704–10.
9. Ledingham IM, *et al.* Triple regimen of selective decontamination of the digestive tract, systemic cefotaxime, and microbiological surveillance for prevention of acquired infection in intensive care. *Lancet* 1988; **i:** 785–90.
10. Tetteroo GWM, *et al.* Selective decontamination to reduce gram-negative colonisation and infections after oesophageal resection. *Lancet* 1990; **335:** 704–7.
11. Tetteroo GWM, *et al.* Bacteriology of selective decontamination: efficacy and rebound colonisation. *J Antimicrob Chemother* 1994; **34:** 139–48.
12. van Saene HKF, *et al.* Cefotaxime combined with selective decontamination in long term intensive care unit patients: virtual absence of emergence of resistance. *Drugs* 1988; **35** (suppl 2): 29–34.
13. Bonten MJM, *et al.* Colonization and infection with Enterococcus faecalis in intensive care units: the role of antimicrobial agents. *Antimicrob Agents Chemother* 1995; **39:** 2783–6.
14. Aerdts SJA, *et al.* Prevention of bacterial colonization of the respiratory tract and stomach of mechanically ventilated patients by a novel regimen of selective decontamination in combination with initial systemic cefotaxime. *J Antimicrob Chemother* 1990; **26** (suppl A): 59–76.
15. Loirat P, *et al.* Selective digestive decontamination in intensive care unit patients. *Intensive Care Med* 1992; **18:** 182–8.
16. Vandenbroucke-Grauls CMJE, Vandenbroucke JP. Effect of selective decontamination of the digestive tract on respiratory tract infections and mortality in the intensive care unit. *Lancet* 1991; **338:** 859–62.
17. van Saene HKF, *et al.* Selective decontamination of the digestive tract in the intensive care unit: current status and future prospects. *Crit Care Med* 1992; **20:** 691–703.
18. Selective Decontamination of the Digestive Tract Trialists' Collaborative Group. Meta-analysis of randomised controlled trials of selective decontamination of the digestive tract. *BMJ* 1993; **307:** 525–32.
19. Liberati A, *et al.* Antibiotic prophylaxis to reduce respiratory tract infections and mortality in adults receiving intensive care. Available in The Cochrane Library; Issue 2. Chichester: John Wiley; 2004.
20. D'Amico R, *et al.* Effectiveness of antibiotic prophylaxis in critically ill adult patients: systematic review of randomised controlled trials. *BMJ* 1998; **316:** 1275–85.
21. Kollef MH. The prevention of ventilator-associated pneumonia. *N Engl J Med* 1999; **341:** 294.
22. Atkinson SW, Bihari DJ. Selective decontamination of the gut. *BMJ* 1993; **306:** 286–7.
23. Elliott TSJ. Line-associated bacteraemias. *Commun Dis Rep* 1993; **3:** R91–R96.
24. Raad I. Intravascular-catheter-related infections. *Lancet* 1998; **351:** 893–8.
25. O'Grady NP, *et al.* Guidelines for the prevention of intravascular catheter-related infections. *MMWR* 2002; **51**(RR-10): 1–29. Correction. *ibid.*; **51:** 711. Also available at: http://www.cdc.gov/mmwr/PDF/rr/rr5110.pdf (accessed 12/07/04)
26. McGee DC, Gould MK. Preventing complications of central venous catheterization. *N Engl J Med* 2003; **348:** 1123–33.
27. Yassien M, *et al.* Modulation of biofilms of Pseudomonas aeruginosa by quinolones. *Antimicrob Agents Chemother* 1995; **39:** 2262–8.
28. Raad I, *et al.* Antibiotics and prevention of microbial colonization of catheters. *Antimicrob Agents Chemother* 1995; **39:** 2397–2400.
29. Appelgren P, *et al.* Does surface heparinisation reduce bacterial colonisation of central venous catheters? *Lancet* 1995; **345:** 130.

30. Raad I, *et al.* Central venous catheters coated with minocycline and rifampin for the prevention of catheter-related colonization and bloodstream infections: a randomized, double-blind trial. *Ann Intern Med* 1997; **127:** 267–74.
31. Darouiche RO, *et al.* A comparison of two antimicrobial-impregnated central venous catheters. *N Engl J Med* 1999; **340:** 1–8.
32. Go ES, *et al.* Clinical and molecular epidemiology of acinetobacter infections sensitive only to polymyxin B and sulbactam. *Lancet* 1994; **344:** 1329–32.

## Legionnaires' disease

Legionnaires' disease is a legionella pneumonia caused by the Gram-negative bacterium *Legionella pneumophila*. Serious outbreaks have been associated with infected air-conditioning systems or water supplies. Pontiac fever is a milder, usually self-limiting, flu-like illness also caused by *L. pneumophila* as well as by other *Legionella* spp. Legionellosis has been suggested as a broad term to cover pneumonic and non-pneumonic clinical syndromes caused by any *Legionella* spp., which may include *L. bozemanii, L. micdadei* (Pittsburgh pneumonia agent), and *L. wadsworthii.*

The usual treatment for *Legionella* infections is with a macrolide, with azithromycin now increasingly used in preference to erythromycin;[1-3] clarithromycin may be a further acceptable alternative macrolide.[3,4] Fluoroquinolones are also increasingly recommended as alternatives to the macrolides.[1-4] Doxycycline or co-trimoxazole are further alternatives.[5] Rifampicin has been given in addition to fluoroquinolones or doxycycline, especially in severe or deteriorating illness or in immunocompromised patients,[4] although some consider this to be of little further benefit.[1]

1. Edelstein PH. Antimicrobial chemotherapy for Legionnaires disease: time for a change. *Ann Intern Med* 1998; **129:** 328–30.
2. Dedicoat M, Venkatesan P. The treatment of Legionnaires' disease. *J Antimicrob Chemother* 1999; **43:** 747–52.
3. Roig J, Rello J. Legionnaires' disease: a rational approach to therapy. *J Antimicrob Chemother* 2003; **51:** 1119–29.
4. Stout JE, Yu VL. Legionellosis. *N Engl J Med* 1997; **337:** 682–7.
5. Anonymous. The choice of antibacterial drugs. In: *Handbook of antimicrobial therapy.* 16th ed. New York: The Medical Letter, 2002: 34–52.

## Leprosy

Leprosy (Hansen's disease) is a chronic disease caused by *Mycobacterium leprae*; it affects the peripheral nervous system, the skin, and some other tissues. It is transmitted from person to person when bacilli are shed from the nose and skin lesions of infected patients, but most individuals are naturally immune, and symptoms are suppressed. Clinical leprosy may be regarded as a consequence of deficient cell-mediated immunity in susceptible individuals. For the purpose of grouping patients for chemotherapy, leprosy may be classified as multibacillary or paucibacillary.

- **Multibacillary** leprosy occurs when cellular immunity is largely deficient, and includes the sub-groups lepromatous (LL), borderline lepromatous (BL), and midborderline leprosy (BB), as well as any other types giving a positive skin smear for acid-fast bacilli. Generally the lepromin test (p.1706) is negative.
- **Paucibacillary** leprosy results when cellular immunity is only partially deficient, and includes the sub-groups borderline tuberculoid (BT), tuberculoid (TT), and indeterminate leprosy (I) when the skin smear is negative. Generally the lepromin test is positive.

For the purpose of treatment, WHO classifies patients with more than 5 skin lesions as multibacillary, and those with 1 to 5 skin lesions as paucibacillary. The use of this clinical classification avoids the necessity to provide facilities for bacteriological examination of skin smears.

Reactive episodes may be seen in leprosy patients undergoing treatment; they are known as **lepra reactions** and unless treated may lead to deformity and disability. Most reactions belong to one of two main types.

- **Type 1** lepra reactions, or reversal reactions, are delayed hypersensitivity reactions (type IV hypersensitivity). Prompt treatment with corticosteroids is necessary to prevent permanent nerve damage.[1-3]
- **Type 2** lepra reactions, also known as erythema nodosum leprosum (ENL), represent a humoral antibody response (type III hypersensitivity) to dead bacteria. Mild type 2 reactions may be treated with anti-inflammatories but moderate or severe reactions should be treated with corticosteroids or thalidomide.[1-4] The incidence of neuritis has decreased since the inclusion of clofazimine in multidrug regimens, probably owing to the drug's anti-inflammatory action; a further reduction in high-risk patients has been achieved by the use of an initial loading dose.[5] Clofazimine does not act as rapidly as either corticosteroids or thalidomide, nor is it as effective, but it may be used in chronic type 2 reactions in doses of up to 300 mg daily.[1,2,4,6] Antileprotic drug therapy is generally continued during lepra reactions.

Dapsone given on its own was for a long time the mainstay of leprosy treatment. However, the emergence of resistance to dapsone and to other antileprotics led to the use of multidrug therapy regimens consisting of 2 or 3 drugs with dapsone, rifampicin, and clofazimine being the standard ones. Newer alternatives include clarithromycin, minocycline, and fluoroquinolones such as ofloxacin. Ethionamide or protionamide have been used in place of clofazimine in light-skinned patients, but are no longer recommended because of their severe hepatotoxicity.

The most widely used multidrug regimens are those recommended by WHO[2] and in these the choice of drugs and length of treatment are based on the clinical classification outlined above.

- MULTIBACILLARY LEPROSY

The standard regimen recommended by WHO for multibacillary leprosy[2,3] is rifampicin 600 mg and clofazimine 300 mg both given once a month, together with clofazimine 50 mg and dapsone 100 mg both daily. Treatment is continued for 12 months.[3] When multidrug therapy was introduced patient compliance was considered essential for successful treatment. Ideally, the monthly rifampicin and clofazimine doses were given under supervision and dapsone ingestion could be verified by a urine spot test. Subsequent demonstration of the high efficacy of the regimen has allowed WHO to take a pragmatic approach, recommending flexible delivery systems to ensure that patients have access to treatment even when supervision of the monthly dose is impractical.[2,3] A 2-year treatment duration was chosen originally because it is highly effective in the majority of cases and avoids the need to assess response with skin smears. However, such a long treatment duration is an obstacle to implementing treatment programmes in areas where healthcare is inaccessible or infrastructure poor. Ongoing clinical studies and experience with patients defaulting from treatment have encouraged WHO to now recommend that treatment for 12 months is adequate.[3] Nevertheless, there has been concern that prolonged treatment (beyond 2 years) may be necessary in patients with high pretreatment bacterial loads.[7-10] Early hopes that reducing duration of treatment to as little as one month would be possible have not been supported by a study using daily rifampicin and ofloxacin.[11]

In patients for whom rifampicin is unsuitable because of resistance or intolerance, WHO recommends[2] daily treatment with clofazimine 50 mg, ofloxacin 400 mg, and minocycline 100 mg for the first 6 months; treatment is then continued for at least a further 18 months with clofazimine together with either minocycline or ofloxacin. When clofazimine cannot be given because of unacceptable skin pigmentation, ofloxacin 400 mg daily or minocycline 100 mg daily may be substituted in the standard regimen.[12] Alternatively, rifampicin 600 mg, ofloxacin 400 mg, and minocycline 100 mg could be administered once a month for 24 months.[2]

- PAUCIBACILLARY LEPROSY

The WHO recommended regimen[2,3] for paucibacillary leprosy is rifampicin 600 mg monthly and dapsone 100 mg daily. Treatment is continued for 6 months. If there are severe toxic effects with dapsone it should be substituted with clofazimine.[12] On the basis of a clinical study[13] showing that a single dose each of rifampicin 600 mg, ofloxacin 400 mg, and minocycline 100 mg given in combination is only slightly less effective than standard multidrug treatment, WHO has suggested that this is a suitable alternative for patients with single-lesion paucibacillary leprosy.[2] However, reservations have been expressed about the study including concerns regarding the short follow-up[14] and poor microbiological rationale.[15]

- RELAPSE

Relapse following a recommended course of multidrug therapy for multibacillary or paucibacillary leprosy can occur and WHO recommends re-treatment with the appropriate regimen.[2,3] Although the relapse rate following multidrug therapy for multibacillary leprosy generally appears to be low,[2,16] there is concern that further reduction of treatment duration could be detrimental (see above).

- PREGNANCY

Leprosy patients who are pregnant or breast feeding experience clinical deterioration and, in general, antileprotic therapy is continued in such patients.

- PROPHYLAXIS

Leprosy is spread from person to person, so household contacts may be at risk. A systematic review and meta-analysis[17] has concluded that prophylaxis, usually with dapsone, in some household contacts may prevent disease in this high-risk group. WHO[2] suggests that contacts of newly diagnosed cases should be examined for evidence of leprosy and then advised how to watch for early signs of the disease; prophylaxis with rifampicin or other antileprotics is not recommended in leprosy control programmes. BCG vaccine appears to be protective. Vaccines specifically against leprosy are under investigation.

- ELIMINATION

The multidrug therapy regimens recommended by WHO have been widely implemented in recent years. Their success led to the World Health Assembly setting a goal in 1991 of elimination of leprosy as a public health problem by the year 2000: that is, reducing the prevalence to less than 1 case per 10 000 population in endemic areas. Considerable progress towards this target was made, and it was announced in 2001 that the global level of leprosy had decreased by over 90%, and that global elimination had been achieved. Full control of leprosy, however, had still not been attained in several countries and continued efforts were necessary. WHO has now set a goal for elimination of leprosy at a national level by the year 2005.

1. Britton WJ, Lockwood DNJ. Leprosy reactions: current and future approaches to management. *Baillieres Clin Infect Dis* 1997; **4:** 1–23.
2. WHO. WHO expert committee on leprosy. *WHO Tech Rep Ser 874* 1998.
3. WHO. *Guide to eliminate leprosy as a public health problem.* 1st ed. Geneva: WHO, 2000. Also available at: http://www.who.int/lep/disease/Eliminate_Leprosy_V8.pdf (accessed 19/05/04)
4. Lockwood DNJ. The management of erythema nodosum leprosum: current and future options. *Lepr Rev* 1996; **67:** 253–9.
5. Arunthathi S, Satheesh KK. Does clofazimine have a prophylactic role against neuritis? *Lepr Rev* 1997; **68:** 233–41.
6. Jacobson RR, Krahenbuhl JL. Leprosy. *Lancet* 1999; **353:** 655–60.
7. Waters MFR. Relapse following various types of multidrug therapy in multibacillary leprosy. *Lepr Rev* 1995; **66:** 1–9. Correction. *ibid.;* 192.
8. Jamet P, *et al.* Relapse after long-term follow-up of multibacillary patients treated by WHO multidrug regimen. *Int J Lepr* 1995; **63:** 195–201.
9. Waters MFR. Is it safe to shorten multidrug therapy for lepromatous (LL and BL) leprosy to 12 months? *Lepr Rev* 1998; **69:** 110–11.
10. Girdhar BK, *et al.* Relapses in multibacillary leprosy patients: effect of length of therapy. *Lepr Rev* 2000; **71:** 144–53.
11. Ji B, *et al.* High relapse rate among lepromatous leprosy patients treated with rifampin plus ofloxacin daily for 4 weeks. *Antimicrob Agents Chemother* 1997; **41:** 1953–6.
12. WHO. Chemotherapy of leprosy. *WHO Tech Rep Ser 847* 1994.
13. Single-lesion Multicentre Trial Group. Efficacy of single-dose multidrug therapy for the treatment of single-lesion paucibacillary leprosy. *Lepr Rev* 1997; **68:** 341–9.
14. Lockwood DNJ. Rifampicin/minocycline and ofloxacin (ROM) for single lesions—what is the evidence? *Lepr Rev.* 1997; **68:** 299–300.
15. Katoch VM. Is there a microbiological rationale for single-dose treatment of leprosy? *Lepr Rev* 1998; **69:** 2–5.
16. World Health Organisation Leprosy Unit. Risk of relapse in leprosy. *Indian J Lepr* 1995; **67:** 13–26.
17. Smith CM, Smith WCS. Chemoprophylaxis is effective in the prevention of leprosy in endemic countries: a systematic review and meta-analysis. *J Infect* 2000; **41:** 137–42.

## Leptospirosis

Leptospirosis[1] is an infectious disease caused by serovars of the spirochaete *Leptospira interrogans*, the commonest in the UK being *L. hardjo* and *L. icterohaemorrhagiae*.[2] *Leptospira* are widely distributed in wild and domestic animals, including cattle. Rats are a common source of infection in man and transmission is often by contact with water or soil contaminated with infected urine. The main occupational group at risk in the UK has been farmers and agricultural workers, although there have been outbreaks elsewhere among recreational water users such as canoeists.[3] The majority of symptomatic patients have no more than a mild flu-like illness, although a small proportion develop Weil's disease with haemorrhagic complications and severe hepatic and renal impairment.

The use of antibacterials is controversial since many patients recover without treatment. There is insufficient evidence to conclude whether treatment with antibacterials is worthwhile.[4] However, treatment for suspected leptospirosis within 4 to 7 days has been recommended to prevent complications.[5,6] The intravenous use of either benzylpenicillin 900 mg, ampicillin 1 g, or erythromycin 500 mg every 6 hours, or the oral use of amoxicillin 500 mg every 8 hours or doxycycline 100 mg twice daily has been suggested;[6] treatment is continued for 7 days. Benzylpenicillin has been given intravenously in higher doses for severe leptospirosis; 7.2 to 9.6 g daily for 5 days followed by 1.44 g daily for a further 5 days has been advocated.[7] However, intravenous doses of 900 mg every 6 hours for 7 days have proved successful even when given late in the course of illness.[8] In severe infections, supportive therapy with analgesics and antiemetics may be required. Renal function should be monitored and dialysis instigated if necessary, and blood products may be necessary to control haemorrhagic complications.[5]

The incidence of leptospirosis in USA soldiers in Panama was reduced when they were given doxycycline prophylactically.[9] Leptospirosis vaccines are available in some countries.


1. WHO, International Leptospirosis Society. *Human leptospirosis: guidance for diagnosis, surveillance and control.* Geneva: WHO, 2003.
2. Ferguson IR. Leptospirosis update. *BMJ* 1991; **302** 128–9.
3. Centers for Disease Control. Outbreak of leptospirosis among white-water rafters—Costa Rica, 1996. *MMWR* 1997; **46:** 577–9.
4. Guidugli F, *et al.* Antibiotics for leptospirosis. Available in The Cochrane Library; Issue 2. Chichester: John Wiley; 2004.
5. Ferguson I. Uncommon infections I: leptospirosis. *Prescribers' J* 1991; **31:** 185–9.
6. Ferguson IR. Leptospirosis surveillance: 1990-1992. *Commun Dis Rep* 1993; **3:** R47–R48.
7. Anonymous. Leptospira outbreak in cattle and man. *J R Coll Gen Pract* 1985; **35:** 36.
8. Watt G, *et al.* Placebo-controlled trial of intravenous penicillin for severe and late leptospirosis. *Lancet* 1988; **i:** 433–5.
9. Takafuji ET, *et al.* An efficacy trial of doxycycline chemoprophylaxis against leptospirosis. *N Engl J Med* 1984; **310:** 497–500.


### Listeriosis

Listeriosis is caused by *Listeria monocytogenes*, a Gram-positive bacterium widespread in the environment and capable of growing at low temperatures. Increased awareness of *L. monocytogenes* as a human pathogen has followed epidemics of listeriosis associated with the consumption of contaminated food products including soft cheeses, coleslaw, and milk. *L. monocytogenes* has since been detected in many types of food, especially uncooked hot dogs, undercooked chicken, and pâté. It has been acknowledged[1,2] that it is a relatively rare infection and that despite epidemics associated with identified food products it typically occurs sporadically and the source is usually not certain. Infection occurs primarily in pregnant women, neonates, the elderly, and immunocompromised patients. Clinical manifestations vary. Pregnant women may have relatively mild flu-like symptoms, but infection may result in spontaneous abortion, fetal death, or perinatal sepsis or meningitis in the neonate. Non-perinatal listeriosis may cause sepsis but commonly presents as meningitis. Endocarditis has occurred in patients with cardiac lesions. Focal infections following initial bacteraemia occur mainly in immunocompromised patients.

The treatment of choice is generally ampicillin with gentamicin,[1-4] although some have advocated ampicillin alone;[5] synergy has been reported *in vitro*. Ampicillin or amoxicillin alone may be used in pregnant women.[6] In penicillin-allergic patients co-trimoxazole, erythromycin, and tetracycline are alternatives,[1] but the choice of treatment in these patients is more difficult. Gentamicin with chloramphenicol or with vancomycin has been used[3] as has erythromycin plus gentamicin.[7] According to some,[3] tetracycline should not be used to treat listeriosis in the UK because of bacterial resistance.

Further details specifically concerning neonatal listerial meningitis and its treatment can be found under Meningitis, p.134.


1. Gellin BG, Broome CV. Listeriosis. *JAMA* 1989; **261:** 1313–20.
2. Schlech WF. Foodborne listeriosis. *Clin Infect Dis* 2000; **31:** 770–5. Correction. *ibid.* 2001; **32:** 1518–19.
3. MacGowan AP. Listeriosis—the therapeutic options. *J Antimicrob Chemother* 1990; **26:** 721–2.
4. Temple ME, Nahata MC. Treatment of listeriosis. *Ann Pharmacother* 2000; **34:** 656–61.
5. Kessler SL, Dajani AS. Listeria meningitis in infants and children. *Pediatr Infect Dis J* 1990; **9:** 61–3.
6. Wilkinson P. Uncommon infections 2: listeriosis. *Prescribers' J* 1992; **32:** 26–31.
7. MacGowan AP, *et al.* Maternal listeriosis in pregnancy without fetal or neonatal infection. *J Infect* 1991; **22:** 53–7.


### Lyme disease

Lyme disease is a seasonal infectious disease caused by the spirochaete *Borrelia burgdorferi* and transmitted primarily by *Ixodes* ticks. It was first recognised in the 1970s in Lyme, Connecticut, but when the spirochaete responsible was later identified, Lyme disease was found to occur worldwide with regional variations. Lyme disease is a multisystem disease that principally affects the skin, nervous system, heart, and joints, and can be divided into 3 stages. In the early stage a characteristic skin lesion, erythema migrans, may be accompanied by flu-like or meningitis-like symptoms. This may be followed weeks or months later by signs of disseminated infection, including neurological and cardiac abnormalities, and even years later by chronic arthritis and the late skin manifestation acrodermatitis chronica atrophicans, both signs of persistent infection.

Appropriate treatment should prove curative, especially in the early stages. Current recommendations for treatment[1-3] give oral doxycycline (or tetracycline) or amoxicillin as the antibacterials of choice for **early stage** Lyme disease and mild neurological and cardiac symptoms. Alternatives include oral cephalosporins such as cefuroxime or the macrolides azithromycin or clarithromycin. In pregnant women or young children amoxicillin (or phenoxymethylpenicillin) may be used or erythromycin in those allergic to penicillin, although erythromycin has been associated with a high failure rate. In general duration of treatment ranges from 14 to 21 days, but depends on individual response. One study[4] has suggested, however, that 10 days' therapy with doxycycline may be sufficient in some patients.

Intravenous ceftriaxone, cefotaxime, or benzylpenicillin are recommended for early stage Lyme disease with acute neurological symptoms of meningitis or radiculopathy, or for **late stage** Lyme disease including meningitis, serious cardiac symptoms, and arthritis; doxycycline or amoxicillin by mouth for 28 days may also be used in Lyme arthritis without clinically evident neurological disease.

A small percentage of patients continue to experience non-specific symptoms after appropriate treatment of Lyme disease; there is some controversy over whether prolonged treatment is effective in these patients and one placebo-controlled study has suggested otherwise.[5]

**Preventive** measures against Lyme disease include the use of tick repellents and physical protection.[2,6,7] Some consider that empirical treatment with doxycycline may be warranted following tick bites in endemic areas where the probability of infection is high,[8] but generally the risk of infection is low,[9] particularly if the tick is removed promptly. The risk of infection may be greater if the tick has fed to repletion.[10] Most guidelines[2,6] do not support the use of empirical antibacterial therapy following tick bites, and the cost effectiveness of parenteral therapy in those with positive serological test results and non-specific symptoms has been questioned.[11,12] Lyme disease vaccines are available in some countries.


1. Loewen PS, *et al.* Systematic review of the treatment of early Lyme disease. *Drugs* 1999; **57:** 157–73.
2. Infectious Diseases Society of America. Practice guidelines for the treatment of Lyme disease. *Clin Infect Dis* 2000; **31** (suppl 1): S1–S14. Also available at: http://www.journals.uchicago.edu/CID/journal/issues/v31nS1/000342/000342.web.pdf (accessed 19/05/04)
3. Steere AC. Lyme disease. *N Engl J Med* 2001; **345:** 115–25.
4. Wormser GP, *et al.* Duration of antibiotic therapy for early Lyme disease: a randomized, double-blind, placebo-controlled trial. *Ann Intern Med* 2003; **138:** 697–704.
5. Klempner MS, *et al.* Two controlled trials of antibiotic treatment in patients with persistent symptoms and a history of Lyme disease. *N Engl J Med* 2001; **345:** 85–92.
6. American Academy of Pediatrics Committee on Infectious Diseases. Prevention of Lyme disease. *Pediatrics* 2000; **105:** 142–7.
7. Hayes EB, Piesman J. How can we prevent Lyme disease? *N Engl J Med* 2003; **348:** 2424–30.
8. Nadelman RB, *et al.* Prophylaxis with single-dose doxycycline for the prevention of Lyme disease after an Ixodes scapularis tick bite. *N Engl J Med* 2001; **345:** 79–84.
9. Shapiro ED, *et al.* A controlled trial of antimicrobial prophylaxis for Lyme disease after deer-tick bites. *N Engl J Med* 1992; **327:** 1769–73.
10. Matuschka F-R, Spielman A. Risk of infection from and treatment of tick bite. *Lancet* 1993; **342:** 529–30.
11. Lightfoot RW, *et al.* Empiric parenteral antibiotic treatment of patients with fibromyalgia and fatigue and a positive serologic result for lyme disease: a cost-effectiveness analysis. *Ann Intern Med* 1993; **119:** 503–9.
12. Luft BJ, *et al.* Appropriateness of parenteral antibiotic treatment for patients with presumed Lyme disease: a joint statement of the American College of Rheumatology and the Council of the Infectious Diseases Society of America. *Ann Intern Med* 1993; **119:** 518.


### Lymphogranuloma venereum

Lymphogranuloma venereum or chlamydial lymphogranuloma is caused by infection with certain serotypes of *Chlamydia trachomatis* and is endemic in tropical areas, but may also occur in the developed world. It is a sexually transmitted disease and in the early phase may cause genital ulceration although the commonest clinical manifestation is inguinal lymphadenopathy. There is multisystem involvement and late complications, including those related to fibrosis and abnormal lymphatic drainage, may require surgery.

WHO[1] recommends treatment with doxycycline 100 mg twice daily, erythromycin 500 mg four times daily, or tetracycline 500 mg four times daily, in each case given by mouth for 2 weeks. UK[2] and US[3] guidelines recommend treatment for 3 weeks with doxycycline 100 mg twice daily or alternatively with erythromycin 500 mg four times daily.


1. WHO. Guidelines for the management of sexually transmitted infections. Geneva: WHO, 2003. Also available at: http://whqlibdoc.who.int/publications/2003/9241546263.pdf (accessed 22/06/04)
2. Clinical Effectiveness Group (Association for Genitourinary Medicine and the Medical Society for the Study of Venereal Diseases). 2001 National guideline for the management of lymphogranuloma venereum (LGV). Available at: http://www.bashh.org/guidelines/2002/LGV%2006%2001.pdf (accessed 19/05/04)
3. Centers for Disease Control. Sexually transmitted diseases treatment guidelines 2002. *MMWR* 2002; **51**(RR-6): 1–80. Also available at: http://www.cdc.gov/mmwr/PDF/rr/rr5106.pdf (accessed 19/05/04)


### Melioidosis

Melioidosis is caused by the Gram-negative aerobic bacterium *Burkholderia pseudomallei* (*Pseudomonas pseudomallei*), and has been found mainly in south-east Asia and northern Australia.[1] Its true incidence and distribution may be much wider than originally thought;[2] diagnosis is difficult because of the broad spectrum of clinical manifestations. Pulmonary melioidosis is probably the commonest form and has been treated with doxycycline for 3 to 6 months.[3] Chronic or subacute non-bacteraemic melioidosis has also been treated long term with tetracycline or co-trimoxazole.[3]

Septicaemic melioidosis is an important cause of death in Thailand. Because *B. pseudomallei* is intrinsically resistant to many antibacterials, including aminoglycosides and the early beta lactams, it has been unresponsive to many empirical regimens for septicaemia.[2] Treatment was based on anecdotal regimens until, in a study from Thailand,[4] intravenous ceftazidime halved the mortality of severe melioidosis when compared with conventional parenteral treatment with high doses of chloramphenicol intravenously, doxycycline, and co-trimoxazole. As a result ceftazidime came to be considered the treatment of choice for septicaemic melioidosis.[2] A systematic review[5] of treatment of acute melioidosis has also concluded that regimens should contain ceftazidime or imipenem parenterally. Parenteral treatment for a minimum of 7 days is followed by oral maintenance therapy with amoxicillin-clavulanic acid or the conventional regimen (chloramphenicol, doxycycline, and co-trimoxazole);[1,4] amoxicillin-clavulanic acid has shown promise[4] and appears to be a safe alternative to the conventional regimen for the oral treatment of melioidosis.[6] However, resistance to ceftazidime and amoxicillin-clavulanic acid has been reported,[7] emphasising the importance of careful monitoring for the emergence of resistance during treatment. Ceftazidime plus co-trimoxazole, both given intravenously, has been advocated by some for severe melioidosis, especially in patients with septicaemia.[8]

*B. pseudomallei* has the potential for prolonged latency as demonstrated by a Vietnam war veteran who presented with melioidosis of the bone 18 years after exposure to the organism.[9] He was treated with ceftriaxone intravenously for 8 weeks followed by oral ciprofloxacin.


1. White NJ. Melioidosis. *Lancet* 2003; **361:** 1715–22.
2. Dance DAB. Pseudomonas pseudomallei: danger in the paddy fields. *Trans R Soc Trop Med Hyg* 1991; **85:** 1–3.
3. Guard RW, *et al.* Melioidosis in far north Queensland: a clinical and epidemiological review of twenty cases. *Am J Trop Med Hyg* 1984; **33:** 467–73.
4. White NJ, *et al.* Halving of mortality of severe melioidosis by ceftazidime. *Lancet* 1989; **ii:** 697–701.
5. Samuel M, Ti TY. Interventions for treating melioidosis. Available in The Cochrane Library; Issue 2. Chichester: John Wiley; 2004.
6. Rajchanuvong A, *et al.* A prospective comparison of co-amoxiclav and the combination of chloramphenicol, doxycycline, and co-trimoxazole for the oral maintenance treatment of melioidosis. *Trans R Soc Trop Med Hyg* 1995; **89:** 546–9.
7. Dance DAB, *et al.* Development of resistance to ceftazidime and co-amoxiclav in Pseudomonas pseudomallei. *J Antimicrob Chemother* 1991; **28:** 321–4.
8. Sookpranee M, *et al.* Multicenter prospective randomized trial comparing ceftazidime plus co-trimoxazole with chloramphenicol plus doxycycline and co-trimoxazole for treatment of severe melioidosis. *Antimicrob Agents Chemother* 1992; **36:** 158–62.
9. Koponen MA, *et al.* Melioidosis: forgotten but not gone. *Arch Intern Med* 1991; **151:** 605–8.


### Meningitis

Initiation of bacterial meningitis involves colonisation of the nasopharynx by the bacterial pathogen, invasion into the bloodstream (bacteraemia), survival in the bloodstream (enhanced in encapsulated bacteria), invasion of the meninges, bacterial replication, and subarachnoid-space inflammation. The bacteria most often responsible for meningitis are *Streptococcus pneumoniae* (pneumococci), *Haemophilus influenzae*, and *Neisseria meningitidis* (meningococci). Other causes include *Listeria mono-*

*cytogenes*, *Pseudomonas aeruginosa*, and Gram-negative enteric bacilli. *H. influenzae* is more common in infants and young children, whereas in neonates *Escherichia coli* and group B streptococci are the most frequent causes. Overall *H. influenzae* meningitis has appeared to be more common in the USA than in the UK but, as elsewhere, its incidence has decreased following the introduction of immunisation with *H. influenzae* type b vaccine.

**Choice of treatment**. Doctors in the UK are advised[1] to give emergency treatment with parenteral benzylpenicillin to all suspected cases of meningitis before transfer to hospital (see also under Meningococcal Meningitis, below). Subsequent treatment depends on identification of the infecting organism and its susceptibility to antibacterials. Other factors affecting choice of antibacterial include penetration into the CSF and bactericidal activity once there. Once in hospital, cefotaxime or ceftriaxone may be given **empirically** until the results of culture and susceptibility tests are known.[2-4] Ampicillin should be added in patients less than 3 months of age[2,3] or in older patients (50 to 55 years of age)[2-4] in whom Listeria meningitis is more prevalent. Vancomycin is also recommended in addition to any empirical regimen when highly penicillin-resistant or cephalosporin-resistant pneumococcal meningitis is suspected.[2-4] Vancomycin with ceftazidime is recommended in patients with recent head trauma, neurosurgery or CSF shunts.[3] Immunocompromised patients should receive ampicillin with ceftazidime.[3] Penicillin-allergic patients can be given chloramphenicol but it may not be effective against Gram-negative enteric bacilli or resistant pneumococci. Encouraging results have been obtained with meropenem as an alternative to cephalosporins for empirical treatment.[5,6]

The chosen antibacterials are generally given intravenously in relatively high doses. Treatment regimens should be reconsidered as soon as microbiological information is available. Management of the commonest forms of bacterial meningitis is discussed below.

**Neonatal meningitis** is uncommon but remains a life-threatening emergency often associated with bacteraemia and shock. Group B streptococci and *E. coli* are the commonest pathogens; other Gram-negative rods, *L. monocytogenes* and *Str. pneumoniae* are also responsible. USA authors[2] have advised that, for neonates up to 4 weeks of age, ampicillin plus cefotaxime or ampicillin plus an aminoglycoside should be given; vancomycin should also be added when highly penicillin-resistant or cephalosporin-resistant pneumococcal meningitis is suspected. In preterm, low-birth-weight neonates, vancomycin should be given with ceftazidime because of the higher risk of nosocomial infection with staphylococci or Gram-negative bacilli.[3] A committee of the American Academy of Pediatrics[7] has recommended that, once the infecting organism is known, benzylpenicillin or ampicillin be given for group B streptococci and ampicillin for *L. monocytogenes*, both for 14 days; treatment of Gram-negative enteric infection should be based on susceptibility tests and continued for at least 3 weeks. A later update[8] suggested that vancomycin should be considered as additional therapy for suspected pneumococcal meningitis.

In the UK[9] an aggressive approach to the treatment of neonatal meningitis is advocated. Lumbar puncture should be performed in all neonates with suspected meningitis, with suspected or proven late-onset sepsis, and should be considered if there are any signs of sepsis. Initial empirical treatment should consist of ampicillin with cefotaxime and gentamicin. Once the infecting organisms are known, high-dose penicillin should be given in the case of group B streptococci, or cefotaxime, with an aminoglycoside for the first 2 weeks, for Gram-negative enteric organisms.

In **infants** immediately beyond the neonatal period (1 to 3 months of age) infecting organisms may be as for neonates or children older than 3 months (*N. meningitidis*, *Str. pneumoniae*, or *H. influenzae*) and initial treatment with ampicillin together with cefotaxime or ceftriaxone has been recommended in the UK.[10] Authors from the USA,[2,3] have advised ampicillin with either cefotaxime or ceftriaxone for infants aged 4 to 12 weeks; vancomycin should also be added when highly penicillin-resistant or cephalosporin-resistant pneumococcal meningitis is suspected.[2] A committee of the American Academy of Pediatrics has recommended[8] vancomycin plus cefotaxime or ceftriaxone for the initial treatment of all children older than 1 month with definite or probable meningitis. For **older infants and children** the UK authors[10] have recommended cefotaxime or ceftriaxone in preference to benzylpenicillin or ampicillin. Opinion in the USA[2] is that ampicillin may or may not be given with the cephalosporin.

**Adjunctive treatment**. Mortality and morbidity, including deafness in children, remain high in meningitis despite increasingly effective antibacterials. As well as microbial virulence the host response to infection is important. Endotoxins and other microbial products, resulting from bacterial lysis following antibacterial treatment, are able to provoke an inflammatory response by triggering the release of cytokines including interleukin-1 and tumour necrosis factor. There is thus a possible role for anti-inflammatory drugs in the treatment of bacterial meningitis. The role of corticosteroids has been the subject of considerable debate in the past. However, a systematic review[11] of trials in both children and adults showed that, in childhood bacterial meningitis, the use of adjuvant corticosteroids reduces the risk of severe hearing loss, and that in adults mortality is reduced. Thus, adjuvant treatment is now generally advocated.

- GRAM-NEGATIVE ENTERIC AND PSEUDOMONAL MENINGITIS

Meningitis due to Gram-negative enteric bacteria occurs especially in neonates (see above), the elderly, and the immunocompromised and as a complication of neurosurgery. Treatment is generally with a third-generation cephalosporin such as cefotaxime; gentamicin or another suitable aminoglycoside may sometimes be given as well. For meningitis caused by *Pseudomonas aeruginosa* ceftazidime plus an aminoglycoside is used.[2,3] Intraventricular administration of an aminoglycoside has sometimes been judged necessary, but see under Neonatal Meningitis, above.

- HAEMOPHILUS INFLUENZAE MENINGITIS

This is mainly a disease of pre-school children and was nearly always caused by encapsulated type b strains of *H. influenzae* acquired from close contact, but the incidence has decreased as a result of immunisation. A third-generation cephalosporin such as cefotaxime or ceftriaxone is the treatment of choice.[2,3] Chloramphenicol is an alternative. Ampicillin is less useful now because of resistance, but can be given for beta-lactamase-negative strains. Treatment for a minimum of 7 to 10 days after fever has subsided may be necessary. For a discussion of the treatment of *H. influenzae* infections in general, see p.131.

*Prophylaxis*. Since treatment does not eliminate nasopharyngeal carriage of *H. influenzae* type b, rifampicin should be given to index cases in the usual prophylactic dose for 4 days before discharge from hospital. Secondary cases should be prevented by giving rifampicin for 4 days to household and classroom contacts.

For active immunisation of children against *H. influenzae* type b, see under Haemophilus Influenzae Vaccines, p.1616.

- LISTERIA MENINGITIS

See above under Neonatal Meningitis. See also under Listeriosis, p.134.

- MENINGOCOCCAL MENINGITIS

Benzylpenicillin is the treatment of choice for meningitis caused by *N. meningitidis*,[2,3] probably the commonest form of meningococcal infection (see under Meningococcal Infections, below), although reduced sensitivity has been reported in some strains and has resulted in treatment failure; high doses of benzylpenicillin are recommended. Alternatives are third-generation cephalosporins such as cefotaxime or ceftriaxone.[2,3] Parenteral benzylpenicillin is given, preferably intravenously, before transfer to hospital if meningococcal infection seems likely.[1] Duration of treatment is empirical but since *N. meningitidis* is rapidly cleared from the CSF and relapse is uncommon, treatment is generally continued for 5 days after resolution of fever and signs of meningitis; a 7-day course is generally effective. A single intramuscular dose of oily chloramphenicol may be a possibility in developing countries.[12]

*Prophylaxis*. Penicillin may not eliminate the carrier state and therefore rifampicin should be given for 2 days prior to hospital discharge, in the usual prophylactic dose. Secondary cases of meningococcal infection should be prevented by giving prophylactic treatment to close contacts of the index case, especially members of the same household who have had close prolonged contact with the case.[1,13] Rifampicin given for 2 days is the prophylactic of choice for the prevention of secondary cases.[1,13] Alternatives to rifampicin include a single oral dose of ciprofloxacin or an intramuscular dose of ceftriaxone.[1,13]

Where possible, vaccination should be performed in those contacts who have received prophylaxis.[1,13] Vaccines are available against group A and C meningococci or against groups A, C, Y, and W135 meningococci, and are under investigation against group B.

- PNEUMOCOCCAL MENINGITIS

Meningitis due to *Str. pneumoniae* is most common in adults and infants, but can occur at any age. It is said to be the most serious form of meningitis with mortality exceeding 20%. Benzylpenicillin or phenoxymethylpenicillin have been treatments of choice although strains with reduced sensitivity to penicillins are increasingly reported (see under Pneumonia, p.141) and a third-generation cephalosporin such as cefotaxime or ceftriaxone is often the initial treatment of choice; benzylpenicillin may be substituted if the organism is subsequently shown to be sensitive to it. Treatment should generally continue for 7 to 10 days after fever subsides, with some clinicians preferring treatment for 10 to 14 days. Pneumococcal strains resistant to cephalosporins have recently emerged and vancomycin is recommended with or without rifampicin in addition to cefotaxime or ceftriaxone where such pneumococci are prevalent.[2,3] However, one difficulty is that third-generation cephalosporins may not be available in developing countries; chloramphenicol may still prove useful in those countries with a high incidence of bacterial meningitis,[14,15] but treatment failures have been reported with chloramphenicol in penicillin-resistant pneumococcal meningitis.[16]

*Prophylaxis*. A pneumococcal vaccine is available, but its effectiveness in preventing meningitis has not been established.


1. PHLS, Public Health Medicine Environmental Group, Scottish Centre for Infection and Environmental Health. Guidelines for public health management of meningococcal disease in the UK. *Commun Dis Public Health* 2002; **5:** 187–204. Also available at: http://www.hpa.org.uk/cdph/issues/CDPHvol5/no3/Meningococcal_Guidelines.pdf (accessed 19/05/04)
2. Tunkel AR, Scheld WM. Acute bacterial meningitis. *Lancet* 1995; **346:** 1675–80.
3. Quagliarello VJ, Scheld WM. Treatment of bacterial meningitis. *N Engl J Med* 1997; **336:** 708–16.
4. British Infection Society. Early management of suspected bacterial meningitis and meningococcal septicaemia in adults. Available at: http://www.britishinfectionsociety.org/meningitis.html (accessed 19/05/04)
5. Schmutzhard E, *et al.* A randomised comparison of meropenem with cefotaxime or ceftriaxone for the treatment of bacterial meningitis in adults. *J Antimicrob Chemother* 1995; **36** (suppl A): 85–97.
6. Odio CM, *et al.* Prospective, randomized, investigator-blinded study of the efficacy and safety of meropenem vs cefotaxime therapy in bacterial meningitis in children: Meropenem Meningitis Study Group. *Pediatr Infect Dis J* 1999; **18:** 581–90.
7. American Academy of Pediatrics Committee on Infectious Diseases. Treatment of bacterial meningitis. *Pediatrics* 1988; **81:** 904–7. [See also Savarino SJ, *et al. Pediatrics* 1989; **83:** 632–3 and McCracken GH, *ibid.*, 633 (correction; cefotaxime should *not* be used for pseudomonal meningitis).]
8. American Academy of Pediatrics. Therapy for children with invasive pneumococcal infections. *Pediatrics* 1997; **99:** 289–99.
9. Heath PT, *et al.* Neonatal meningitis. *Arch Dis Child Fetal Neonatal Ed* 2003; **88:** F173–F178.
10. El Bashir H, *et al.* Diagnosis and treatment of bacterial meningitis. *Arch Dis Child* 2003; **88:** 615–20.
11. van de Beek D, *et al.* Corticosteroids in acute bacterial meningitis. Available in The Cochrane Library; Issue 2. Chichester: John Wiley; 2004.
12. Lewis RF, *et al.* Long-acting oily chloramphenicol for meningococcal meningitis. *Lancet* 1998; **352:** 823.
13. American Academy of Pediatrics, Canadian Paediatric Society. Meningococcal disease prevention and control strategies for practice-based physicians. *Pediatrics* 1996; **97:** 404–11.
14. Pécoul B, *et al.* Long-acting chloramphenicol versus intravenous ampicillin for treatment of bacterial meningitis. *Lancet* 1991; **338:** 862–6.
15. Kumar P, Verma IC. Antibiotic therapy for bacterial meningitis in children in developing countries. *Bull WHO* 1993; **71:** 183–8.
16. Friedland IR, Klugman KP. Failure of chloramphenicol therapy in penicillin-resistant pneumococcal meningitis. *Lancet* 1992; **339:** 405–8.


## Meningococcal infections

The meningococcus *Neisseria meningitidis* is a Gram-negative bacterium classified into several serotypes including groups A, B, and C. It occurs worldwide and can cause endemic and epidemic infection. Group A is mainly responsible for epidemics in the developing world. In the USA, most infections have been caused by group B or group C meningococci; the relative importance of group C has been increasing in North America. Group B has been the most prevalent in the UK and Europe, although there has been some increase in group C infections. Infections have occurred predominantly in young children under 5 years, but there has been an increased incidence in teenagers and young adults in recent UK outbreaks. Meningococcal disease has traditionally been associated with poverty and overcrowding; the only established risk factor is close contact with an index case, hence the importance of prophylaxis. Clinical infection is preceded by asymptomatic nasopharyngeal carriage of meningococci and spread of infection is usually via respiratory droplets from asymptomatic carriers. Bacteraemia is probably the primary event in all forms of meningococcal disease; clinical manifestations range from mild sore throat or transient fever to fulminant disease. A vasculitic rash (petechiae or purpura) is often associated with meningococcal infection. Meningococcal infection most commonly manifests as septicaemia, which can be rapidly fatal, particularly if fulminating, with mortality ranging from 15% up to 80% in severe forms, or as meningococcal meningitis, in which the infection is confined to the CNS and is associated with mortality rates of 5% or less. Meningococcal meningitis may also occur in conjunction with meningococcal septicaemia. Less usual forms of metastatic meningococcal infection include polyarthritis, pericarditis, pneumonitis, and genito-urinary-tract infections.

Despite some uncertainty as to whether patients with suspected meningococcal septicaemia rather than meningitis would benefit from early penicillin treatment, it is still generally recommended for all patients with suspected meningococcal disease. Thus, when meningococcal infection seems likely benzylpenicillin should be given parenterally, preferably intravenously, before transfer to hospital. For details of the treatment and prophylaxis of meningococcal infections, see Meningococcal Meningitis, under Meningitis, above.

References.


1. American Academy of Pediatrics and Canadian Paediatric Society. Meningococcal disease prevention and control strategies for practice-based physicians. *Pediatrics* 1996; **97:** 404–11.
2. Pollard AJ, *et al.* Emergency management of meningococcal disease. *Arch Dis Child* 1999; **80:** 290–6.
3. American Academy of Pediatrics, Committee on Infectious Diseases. Meningococcal disease prevention and control strategies for practice-based physicians (Addendum: recommendations for college students). *Pediatrics* 2000; **106:** 1500–4.
4. Rosenstein NE, *et al.* Meningococcal disease. *N Engl J Med* 2001; **344:** 1378–88.
5. PHLS, Public Health Medicine Environmental Group, Scottish Centre for Infection and Environmental Health. Guidelines for public health management of meningococcal disease in the UK. *Commun Dis Public Health* 2002; **5:** 187–204. Also available at: http://www.hpa.org.uk/cdph/issues/CDPHvol5/no3/Meningococcal_Guidelines.pdf (accessed 19/05/04)
6. British Infection Society. Early management of suspected bacterial meningitis and meningococcal septicaemia in adults. Available at: http://www.britishinfectionsociety.org/meningitis.html (accessed 19/05/04)


## Mouth infections

Infections of the mouth include those of dental origin such as dental caries, abscesses, gingivitis, and periodontal infections, and those without a dental origin. Infections arising in the nasal cavity, middle ear, oropharynx, and paranasal sinuses can also affect the oral cavity. Emphasis has shifted from treatment to prevention of oral diseases.[1] This discussion deals mainly with infections of dental origin.

The organisms most often encountered in oral infections are viridans streptococci, a variety of anaerobes, and facultative streptococci.[2]

**Dental caries** is caused by the erosion of tooth enamel due to acid produced by bacteria (usually *Streptococcus mutans*) in plaque. Fluoride in various forms is used in dental caries prophylaxis, where it may promote remineralisation or reduce acid production by plaque bacteria.[1] Sugar-free chewing gum can help prevent caries by stimulating the production of saliva.[3] Dental caries vaccines have also been investigated.

The term **periodontal disease** encompasses specific conditions affecting the gingiva and the supporting connective tissue and alveolar bone. **Gingivitis** is thought to be caused by a non-specific bacterial plaque flora that gradually changes from predominantly Gram-positive to more Gram-negative. Gingivitis may or may not develop into periodontitis, but periodontitis is always preceded by gingivitis. **Periodontitis** is associated with a Gram-negative anaerobic microflora. Most gingivitis and periodontitis can be prevented and treated by adequate oral hygiene and plaque removal using mechanical means such as toothbrushing. Mechanical removal of calculus is necessary where the build up is significant. Antiseptics may also help to reduce plaque accumulation and several, but most notably chlorhexidine, have been used.[4,5]

Penicillin has continued to be an effective drug in combating oral pathogens, and erythromycin or metronidazole are alternatives. Fusiform bacteria and spirochaetes have been linked with acute necrotising ulcerative gingivitis (also called Vincent's infection or trench mouth);[6] systemic metronidazole is often the treatment of choice. Tinidazole has also been used. Tetracyclines or metronidazole have been used for chronic periodontal disease.[7] Antibacterials and antiseptics delivered locally to the periodontal pocket may be of value.[5]


1. WHO. Recent advances in oral health: report of a WHO expert committee. *WHO Tech Rep Ser 826* 1992.
2. Guralnick W. Odontogenic infections. *Br Dent J* 1984; **156:** 440–7.
3. Edgar WM. Sugar substitutes, chewing gum and dental caries—a review. *Br Dent J* 1998; **184:** 29–32.
4. Eley BM. Antibacterial agents in the control of supragingival plaque—a review. *Br Dent J* 1999; **186:** 286–96.
5. Greenwell H, Bissada NF. Emerging concepts in periodontal therapy. *Drugs* 2002; **62:** 2581–7.
6. Johnson BD, Engel D. Acute necrotizing ulcerative gingivitis: a review of diagnosis, etiology and treatment. *J Periodontol* 1986; **57:** 141–50.
7. Watts TLP. Periodontitis for medical practitioners. *BMJ* 1998; **316:** 993–6.


## Mycetoma

Mycetoma is a localised chronic infection seen especially in the tropics and subtropics and involving subcutaneous tissue, bone, and skin. It has been termed Madura foot when affecting the sole of the foot. Mycetomas caused by fungi (p.388) such as *Madurella mycetomatis* are called eumycetomas and those caused by the filamentous bacteria, actinomycetes, are called actinomycetomas. *Nocardia brasiliensis* is the commonest actinomycete responsible; others include *Actinomadura madurae*, *A. pelletieri*, and *Streptomyces somaliensis*. For details of systemic infections caused by *Nocardia* spp., see under Nocardiosis, p.137.

Various treatment regimens for actinomycetomas have been tried. Co-trimoxazole with streptomycin or dapsone with streptomycin have been found[1] to be the most effective although *S. somaliensis* infection did not always respond. Two further regimens, sulfadoxine with pyrimethamine and streptomycin, or rifampicin with streptomycin, were suitable for second-line therapy.[1] Cures were achieved after treatment for 4 to 24 months.[1] In a study of antibacterial activity *in vitro* against strains of *S. somaliensis* isolated from mycetoma patients, rifampicin was the most effective followed in decreasing order of activity by erythromycin, tobramycin, fusidic acid, and streptomycin; all strains were resistant to trimethoprim.[2] The successful use of hyperbaric oxygen in addition to co-trimoxazole[3] or of amoxicillin-clavulanic acid[4] in the treatment of *N. brasiliensis* actinomycetoma previously resistant to conventional therapy has been described.


1. Mahgoub ES. Medical management of mycetoma. *Bull WHO* 1976; **54:** 303–10.
2. Nasher MA, *et al.* In vitro studies of antibiotic sensitivities of Streptomyces somaliensis—a cause of human actinomycetoma. *Trans R Soc Trop Med Hyg* 1989; **83:** 265–8.
3. Walker RM, *et al.* Beneficial effects of hyperbaric oxygen therapy in Nocardia brasiliensis soft-tissue infection. *Med J Aust* 1991; **155:** 122–3.
4. Gomez A, *et al.* Amoxicillin and clavulanic acid in the treatment of actinomycetoma. *Int J Dermatol* 1993; **32:** 218–20.


## Necrotising enterocolitis

See under Gastro-enteritis, p.129.

## Necrotising fasciitis

Necrotising fasciitis is a severe soft-tissue infection resulting in necrosis of the subcutaneous tissue and adjacent fascia, together with severe systemic illness. It may be caused by a mixture of aerobic and anaerobic organisms, but can be due to group A streptococci or staphylococci alone and may be associated with a toxic shock syndrome (p.149).

Treatment involving radical surgical excision of the affected tissues may be avoided in some patients treated with large doses of appropriate antibacterials.[1] For streptococcal necrotising fasciitis, high-dose benzylpenicillin should be used; clindamycin may be added in severe cases.[2] Erythromycin should be avoided because of the risk of resistance.[2] Staphylococcal infections are treated with a penicillinase-resistant penicillin, cefazolin, or vancomycin (for resistant strains).[1] Since diagnosis can be difficult, it may be advisable initially to treat as for a mixed infection with antibacterials active against anaerobes (e.g. clindamycin) and also an aminoglycoside or third-generation cephalosporin active against Gram-negative rods, in addition to benzylpenicillin.[3] A broad-spectrum penicillin-beta-lactamase-inhibitor combination or imipenem-cilastatin may also be used.[1] Hyperbaric oxygen therapy has also been beneficial although prospective controlled studies are lacking.[4]


1. Gorbach SL. IDCP guidelines: necrotizing skin and soft tissue infections. Part I: necrotizing fasciitis. *Infect Dis Clin Pract* 1996; **5:** 406–11.
2. Anonymous. Invasive group A streptococcal infections in Gloucestershire. *Commun Dis Rep* 1994; **4:** 97.
3. Chelsom J, *et al.* Necrotising fasciitis due to group A streptococci in western Norway: incidence and clinical features. *Lancet* 1994; **344:** 1111–15.
4. Leach RM, *et al.* Hyperbaric oxygen therapy. *BMJ* 1998; **317:** 1140–3.


## Neonatal conjunctivitis

Conjunctivitis of the newborn, also known as ophthalmia neonatorum, is defined as any conjunctivitis with discharge occurring during the first 28 days of life.[1] That due to *Neisseria gonorrhoeae* is the most serious; it usually appears by the third day after birth and can rapidly result in blindness; systemic infections, especially severe septicaemia, may occur. *Chlamydia trachomatis* is another major cause of neonatal conjunctivitis; it characteristically occurs 5 to 14 days after birth and is less threatening to sight than gonococcal infection, but may also infect the nasopharynx and may cause pneumonia. Chlamydial conjunctivitis is more common than gonococcal conjunctivitis in developed countries. Both organisms are sexually transmitted and the infants of mothers with such genital-tract infections are infected during their passage through the birth canal. Other less serious bacterial causes of neonatal conjunctivitis include *Staphylococcus aureus*, *Streptococcus pneumoniae*, *Haemophilus* spp., and *Pseudomonas* spp.; they are often hospital-acquired.[1]

The management of gonococcal and chlamydial neonatal conjunctivitis varies from country to country depending on the prevalence of gonorrhoea and *C. trachomatis* infection and on bacterial resistance.

• PROPHYLAXIS

The ideal method of prophylaxis is to treat the infected mother during pregnancy, but this is not always possible. Where the risk of *gonococcal infection* is high, ocular prophylaxis at birth is particularly important because of the rapid onset of conjunctivitis and its potential seriousness and is preferable to early diagnosis and treatment of the neonate.[2] Cleansing of the neonate's eyes immediately after birth followed by the topical application of either tetracycline 1% eye ointment, erythromycin 0.5% eye ointment, or silver nitrate 1% eye drops is advised[3,4] and is sometimes required by law.[3] Silver nitrate[1] is active against all strains of *N. gonorrhoeae* regardless of their susceptibility to antibacterials; it is inexpensive and widely available, but may cause chemical conjunctivitis and has been ineffective in preventing chlamydial conjunctivitis (see below). Tetracycline has been reported to be as effective as silver nitrate in protecting against gonococcal conjunctivitis caused by multiresistant strains[5] and WHO now lists both drugs as the drugs of choice.[4]

The value of prophylaxis against *chlamydial neonatal conjunctivitis* is less certain. Tetracycline ointment has been reported to be less effective in preventing chlamydial infection than gonococcal infection[5] and erythromycin ointment has also been unreliable.[6] Silver nitrate is generally considered ineffective,[1] despite an unexpected reduction in the incidence of chlamydial conjunctivitis in one study.[5] Screening and treatment of pregnant women for *C. trachomatis* infection may be a more effective method of control than ocular prophylaxis.[5,7] This approach also tackles the more serious problem of pneumonia.[8]

Neonatal conjunctivitis continues to cause blindness, especially in developing countries. Povidone-iodine is less expensive and perhaps more readily available in such countries than silver nitrate or erythromycin. In a study in Kenya involving more than 3000 infants[9] a 2.5% ophthalmic solution of povidone-iodine appeared to be a more effective prophylactic than either a 1% ophthalmic solution of silver nitrate or erythromycin 0.5% eye ointment. In particular, there were fewer cases of chlamydial conjunctivitis with povidone-iodine.

• TREATMENT

All cases of neonatal conjunctivitis should be treated for both *N. gonorrhoeae* and *C. trachomatis* because of the possibility of mixed infection.[4] *Gonococcal neonatal conjunctivitis* must be treated systemically. WHO[4] recommends ceftriaxone 50 mg/kg by intramuscular injection as a single dose (to a maximum of 125 mg) or, if ceftriaxone is not available, spectinomycin 25 mg/kg (to a maximum of 75 mg) or kanamycin 25 mg/kg (to a maximum of 75 mg) by intramuscular injection as a single dose.

In the USA, CDC[3] recommends a single intravenous or intramuscular injection of ceftriaxone 25 to 50 mg/kg (up to 125 mg) when there is no evidence of disseminated infection.

See also under Gonorrhoea (p.130) for the treatment of infants exposed to gonorrhoea at birth or with established gonococcal infection at any site.

For *nongonococcal neonatal conjunctivitis* WHO[4] and CDC[3] recommend erythromycin 50 mg/kg daily in 4 divided doses by mouth for 14 days; WHO[4] recommend co-trimoxazole 240 mg twice daily for 14 days as an alternative. There is no indication that topical therapy is of additional benefit.[3,4]


1. WHO. *Conjunctivitis of the newborn: prevention and treatment at the primary health care level.* Geneva: WHO, 1986.
2. Laga M, *et al.* Epidemiology and control of gonococcal ophthalmia neonatorum. *Bull WHO* 1989; **67:** 471–8.
3. Centers for Disease Control. Sexually transmitted diseases treatment guidelines 2002. *MMWR* 2002; **51**(RR-6): 1–80. Also available at: http://www.cdc.gov/mmwr/PDF/rr/rr5106.pdf (accessed 19/05/04)
4. WHO. Guidelines for the management of sexually transmitted infections. Geneva: WHO, 2003. Also available at: http://whqlibdoc.who.int/publications/2003/9241546263.pdf (accessed 22/06/04)
5. Laga M, *et al.* Prophylaxis of gonococcal and chlamydial ophthalmia neonatorum: a comparison of silver nitrate and tetracycline. *N Engl J Med* 1988; **318:** 653–7.
6. Black-Payne C, *et al.* Failure of erythromycin ointment for post natal ocular prophylaxis of chlamydial conjunctivitis. *Pediatr Infect Dis J* 1989; **8:** 491–5.
7. Hammerschlag MR, *et al.* Efficacy of neonatal ocular prophylaxis for the prevention of chlamydial and gonococcal conjunctivitis. *N Engl J Med* 1989; **320:** 769–72.
8. Schachter J. Why we need a program for the control of Chlamydia trachomatis. *N Engl J Med* 1989; **320:** 802–4.
9. Isenberg SJ, *et al.* A controlled trial of povidone-iodine as prophylaxis against ophthalmia neonatorum. *N Engl J Med* 1995; **332:** 562–6.


## Nocardiosis

*Nocardia* spp. are Gram-positive aerobic branching bacteria that cause systemic or localised infection. The principal pathogenic species in man is *N. asteroides*; others include *N. brasiliensis, N. pseudobrasiliensis,* and *N. caviae*. Localised chronic infection or actinomycetoma is described under Mycetoma (p.136). Systemic nocardiosis is primarily a lung infection and often involves abscess formation; it occurs especially in immunocompromised patients and may be disseminated with abscesses in the brain and subcutaneous tissues.

The treatment of choice has been a sulfonamide such as sulfadiazine or co-trimoxazole,[1-4] although a study *in vitro* indicated that the fixed ratio of trimethoprim:sulfamethoxazole in co-trimoxazole might contain too little trimethoprim for optimal activity.[5] Sulfafurazole[6] has been used successfully. There have been reports of the effective treatment of nocardiosis with amikacin,[7,8] linezolid,[9] minocycline,[10,11] or ciprofloxacin with doxycycline.[12] Other suggested alternatives include imipenem or meropenem.[13] Treatment needs to be prolonged and may continue for 6 to 12 months.


1. Abdi EA, *et al.* Nocardia infection in splenectomized patients: case reports and a review of the literature. *Postgrad Med J* 1987; **63:** 455–8.
2. Smego RA, *et al.* Treatment of systemic nocardiosis. *Lancet* 1987; **i:** 456.
3. Filice GA. Treatment of nocardiosis. *Lancet* 1987; **i:** 1261–2.
4. Varghese GK, *et al.* Nocardia brasiliensis meningitis. *Postgrad Med J* 1992; **68:** 986.
5. Bennett JE, Jennings AE. Factors influencing susceptibility of Nocardia species to trimethoprim-sulfamethoxazole. *Antimicrob Agents Chemother* 1978; **13:** 624–7.
6. Poland GA, *et al.* Nocardia asteroides pericarditis: report of a case and review of the literature. *Mayo Clin Proc* 1990; **65:** 819–24.
7. Goldstein FW, *et al.* Amikacin-containing regimens for treatment of nocardiosis in immunocompromized patients. *Eur J Clin Microbiol* 1987; **6:** 198–200.
8. Meier B, *et al.* Successful treatment of a pancreatic Nocardia asteroides abscess with amikacin and surgical drainage. *Antimicrob Agents Chemother* 1986; **29:** 150–1.
9. Moylett EH, *et al.* Clinical experience with linezolid for the treatment of Nocardia infection. *Clin Infect Dis* 2003; **36:** 313–18.
10. Petersen EA, *et al.* Minocycline treatment of pulmonary nocardiosis. *JAMA* 1983; **250:** 930–2.
11. Naka W, *et al.* Unusually located lymphocutaneous nocardiosis caused by Nocardia brasiliensis. *Br J Dermatol* 1995; **132:** 609–13.
12. Bath PMW, *et al.* Treatment of multiple subcutaneous Nocardia asteroides abscesses with ciprofloxacin and doxycycline. *Postgrad Med J* 1989; **65:** 190–1.
13. Anonymous. The choice of antibacterial drugs. In: *Handbook of antimicrobial therapy.* 16th ed. New York: The Medical Letter, 2002: 34–52.


## Obstetric disorders

See under: Endometritis (the prophylaxis and treatment of postpartum endometritis), p.126; Premature Labour, p.143; and Urinary-Tract Infections in Pregnancy, p.153. See also Neonatal Conjunctivitis, p.136, and Perinatal Streptococcal Infections, p.139.

## Opportunistic mycobacterial infections

Environmental mycobacteria are widespread, and a number of species other than those responsible for leprosy and tuberculosis are facultative parasites capable of producing disease in man. These organisms, which have been referred to as atypical, nontuberculous, tuberculoid, opportunistic, or MOTT mycobacteria (mycobacteria other than tuberculous), are rarely, if ever, transmitted from person to person but are acquired from the environment. The diseases produced include localised skin and soft tissue lesions, pulmonary infections, and lymphadenitis, but disseminated infections may develop rapidly in immunocompromised patients such as those with AIDS and now represent some of the most common opportunistic bacterial infections in patients with advanced AIDS.

Localised lesions, invariably following inoculation, are most commonly due to the slow-growing species *Mycobacterium marinum* ('swimming pool' or 'fish-tank' granuloma), *M. ulcerans* (Buruli ulcer), and the fast-growing species *M. chelonae* (*M. chelonei*), *M. abscessus* (formerly *M. chelonae* subspecies), and *M. fortuitum*. Ulcerated lesions due to *M. haemophilum* have been described mainly in immunocompromised patients.

Pulmonary disease, which is clinically indistinguishable from pulmonary tuberculosis, has most frequently been attributed to the *M. avium* complex (MAC; *M. avium-intracellulare* complex; MAIC), *M. kansasii*, and to a lesser extent *M. xenopi*; less common causes include *M. abscessus, M. asiaticum, M. celatum, M. chelonae, M. fortuitum, M. malmoense, M. scrofulaceum, M. simiae*, and *M. szulgai*.

Lymphadenitis, which is usually self-limiting and occurs particularly in children under 5 years of age, may be caused by many species but the great majority of cases are due to the related *M. avium* complex, *M. genavense, M. malmoense*, and *M. scrofulaceum* (sometimes collectively known as the MAIS complex).

Dissemination of opportunistic mycobacterial infections may occur rapidly in patients with depressed cellular immunity. The majority of cases have been attributed to the *M. avium* complex; species implicated more recently include *M. abscessus, M. celatum, M. chelonae, M. genavense, M. haemophilum, M. kansasii, M. malmoense, M. scrofulaceum*, and *M. simiae*.

The course of treatment depends on the site and nature of infection. Response to chemotherapy is often difficult to predict as the response obtained *in vivo* may not reflect *in-vitro* sensitivity of the organisms.

Both HIV-negative and HIV-positive patients may be affected and the British Thoracic Society has published guidelines[1] on the management of opportunistic mycobacterial infections. It is noted that, on the whole, the evidence is not derived from controlled clinical trials as very few have been reported. In patients receiving antiretroviral therapy, the possibility of drug interactions should be borne in mind.

- MYCOBACTERIUM AVIUM COMPLEX (MAC)

In HIV-negative patients with MAC pulmonary disease, treatment should be with rifampicin and ethambutol for 24 months; isoniazid may also be given if necessary. In extrapulmonary disease affecting lymph nodes, surgical excision of the nodes should be undertaken; chemotherapy with rifampicin, ethambutol, and clarithromycin for up to 2 years should be considered if disease recurs or where the excision is incomplete or impossible. In sites other than lymph nodes, chemotherapy should be given for 18 to 24 months.[1]

Treatment for HIV-positive patients with MAC pulmonary disease should consist of rifampicin (or rifabutin), ethambutol, and clarithromycin (or azithromycin). A quinolone such as ciprofloxacin, or even amikacin, may be added for patients who are intolerant of these drugs or who fail to respond. Treatment should be lifelong. In disseminated disease, the same treatment should be given and continued indefinitely.[1]

*Chemoprophylaxis* is used to reduce the incidence of disseminated MAC disease in patients with HIV infection. There appears to be a tendency to delay starting prophylaxis until later in the disease process; the guidelines[2] from the US Public Health Service and the Infectious Diseases Society of America (USPHS/IDSA) recommend starting prophylaxis at a CD4+ count of less than 50 cells/microlitre.

In the UK, the British Thoracic Society note there is no general agreement about when prophylaxis should be used. If prophylaxis is to be given to patients with a CD4+ count below 50 cells/microlitre the first drug of choice would be azithromycin; clarithromycin is an alternative and azithromycin with rifabutin would be a third choice.[1] The UK guidelines recommend that prophylaxis be continued indefinitely.[1] The US guidelines,[2] however, state that prophylaxis need not be lifelong in patients responding to highly active antiretroviral therapy (HAART); specifically, primary prophylaxis should be discontinued in patients whose CD4+ count has increased to more than 100 cells/microlitre for 3 months or more, but should be restarted if the CD4+ count falls to below 50 to 100 cells/microlitre again. The US guidelines[2] also state that it may be possible to discontinue secondary prophylaxis (chronic maintenance therapy) in HIV-infected patients who have completed at least 12 months' treatment for MAC, who remain asymptomatic with respect to MAC, and who have a sustained response to HAART (CD4+ count greater than 100 cells/microlitre). Secondary prophylaxis should be restarted if CD4+ count falls below 100 cells/microlitre.

- MYCOBACTERIUM KANSASII INFECTION

Infections with *M. kansasii* may be treated with rifampicin (or rifabutin) and ethambutol.[1] For pulmonary disease, HIV-negative patients usually need only 9 months of therapy whereas HIV-positive patients should receive therapy for 2 years or until the sputum has been negative for 12 months. For disseminated infection in HIV-positive patients, clarithromycin should be added and possibly also isoniazid. The place of macrolides and fluoroquinolones in pulmonary or disseminated *M. kansasii* infection remain to be established. In extrapulmonary disease in HIV-negative patients, chemotherapy with rifampicin and ethambutol may be used prior to excision of an infected lymph node. In other extrapulmonary disease the data is rather insufficient to make recommendations, but rifampicin and ethambutol for 9 months appears sensible with the addition of protionamide and streptomycin and/or a macrolide if the condition is not responding.[1]

- OTHER OPPORTUNISTIC MYCOBACTERIA

In *M. malmoense* and *M. xenopi* pulmonary disease, rifampicin and ethambutol should be given for 2 years in HIV-negative states. Extrapulmonary *M. malmoense* infections should be treated in the same manner as extrapulmonary MAC or *M. kansasii* infections. *M. malmoense* infection rarely occurs in AIDS patients, but if necessary, treatment with rifampicin, ethambutol, and clarithromycin, and possibly isoniazid should be used. For *M. xenopi* in HIV-positive patients there is no evidence on which to base recommendations; treatment as for pulmonary or disseminated MAC infection is suggested.[1]

For pulmonary disease due to rapidly growing bacteria (*M. abcessus, M. chelonae, M. fortuitum*, and *M. gordonae*) and other species (*M. genavense, M. haemophilum, M. simiae, M. szulgai*, and *M. ulcerans*) surgery should be used if possible. Drug therapy should probably include rifampicin, ethambutol, and clarithromycin. Amikacin, cefoxitin, imipenem, quinolones, and sulfonamides may have a place in treatment. For extrapulmonary disease due to these organisms, there have been several anecdotal reports outlining treatment but there is no evidence from controlled clinical trials.[1] For *M. marinum* infections (swimming-pool granuloma or fish-tank granuloma) numerous antibacterial regimens have been used,[3] including rifampicin with ethambutol[4] or isoniazid, rifabutin with ciprofloxacin,[5] minocycline with co-trimoxazole,[6] clarithromycin with rifabutin[7] or ciprofloxacin[5] or ethambutol,[5] and monotherapy with clarithromycin, minocycline, doxycycline, or co-trimoxazole[8] have each been used, mainly in small series of patients. Surgical treatment and intensive antibacterial regimens have been used for *M. scrofulaceum* infections,[9] while Buruli ulcer, due to *M. ulcerans*, is difficult to treat and often requires surgery; responses to antimycobacterials have been disappointing.[10,11] Phenytoin, applied locally, was reported to induce healing in 3 patients with Buruli ulcer.[12] *M. haemophilum* infection in a patient with rheumatoid arthritis and ulcerated nodules on his legs responded to treatment with rifampicin, ciprofloxacin, and clarithromycin.[13] Symptomatic improvement was achieved in an AIDS patient with *M. celatum* infection with a regimen of isoniazid, rifampicin, and ethambutol.[14] Successful treatment of *M. simiae* infection in patients with AIDS was reported with clarithromycin, ethambutol, and ciprofloxacin.[15]


1. Subcommittee of the Joint Tuberculosis Committee of the British Thoracic Society. Management of opportunist mycobacterial infections: Joint Tuberculosis Committee guidelines 1999. *Thorax* 2000; **55:** 210–18. Also available at: http://www.brit-thoracic.org.uk/docs/OppMyco.pdf (accessed 19/05/04)

2. Centers for Disease Control and Prevention. Guidelines for preventing opportunistic infections among HIV-infected persons—2002: recommendations of the US Public Health Service and the Infectious Diseases Society of America. *MMWR* 2002; **51** (RR-8): 1–52. Also available at: http://www.cdc.gov/mmwr/PDF/rr/rr5108.pdf (accessed 19/05/04)
3. Aubry A, *et al.* Sixty-three cases of Mycobacterium marinum infection: clinical features, treatment, and antibiotic susceptibility of causative isolates. *Arch Intern Med* 2002; **162:** 1746–52.
4. Donta ST, *et al.* Therapy of Mycobacterium marinum infections: use of tetracyclines vs rifampin. *Arch Intern Med* 1986; **146:** 902–4.
5. Laing RBS, *et al.* Antimicrobial treatment of fish tank granuloma. *J Hand Surg* 1997; **22B:** 135–7.
6. Gray SF, *et al.* Fish tank granuloma. *BMJ* 1990; **300:** 1069–70.
7. Laing RBS, *et al.* New antimicrobials against Mycobacterium marinum infection. *Br J Dermatol* 1994; **131:** 914.
8. American Thoracic Society. Diagnosis and treatment of disease caused by nontuberculous mycobacteria. *Am J Respir Crit Care Med* 1997; **156:** S1–S25.
9. Bailey WC. Treatment of atypical mycobacterial disease. *Chest* 1983; **84:** 625–8.
10. van der Werf TS, *et al.* Mycobacterium ulcerans infection. *Lancet* 1999; **354:** 1013–18.
11. Thangaraj HS, *et al.* Mycobacterium ulcerans disease; Buruli ulcer. *Trans R Soc Trop Med Hyg* 1999; **93:** 337–40.
12. Adjei O, *et al.* Phenytoin in the treatment of Buruli ulcer. *Trans R Soc Trop Med Hyg* 1998; **92:** 108–9.
13. Darling TN, *et al.* Treatment of Mycobacterium haemophilum infection with an antibiotic regimen including clarithromycin. *Br J Dermatol* 1994; **131:** 376–9.
14. Piersimoni C, *et al.* Disseminated infection due to Mycobacterium celatum in patient with AIDS. *Lancet* 1994; **344:** 332.
15. Barzilai A, *et al.* Successful treatment of disseminated Mycobacterium simiae infection in AIDS patients. *Scand J Infect Dis* 1998; **30:** 143–6.

### Osteomyelitis

See under Bone and Joint Infections, p.122.

### Otitis externa

Otitis externa or inflammation of the skin of the external auditory canal may be due to infection with bacteria, viruses, or fungi or secondary to skin disorders such as eczema, although more than one factor is often responsible for chronic disease. Treatment includes thorough cleansing and the use of appropriate antibacterial ear drops, often containing a corticosteroid as well, even though some have doubted the value of topical antibacterials. (Note that the UK Committee on Safety of Medicines has warned[1] that ear drops containing aminoglycosides, such as gentamicin, neomycin, or framycetin, or polymyxins should not be used when the ear drum is perforated because of the risk of ototoxicity.) Systemic antibacterials may be necessary in severe cases of otitis externa.

The various types of otitis externa and their management have been described.[2,3] Briefly, for *acute localised otitis externa (furunculosis)*, commonly due to *Staphylococcus aureus*, local heat application and systemic treatment with a penicillinase-resistant penicillin such as flucloxacillin or a first-generation cephalosporin such as cefalexin may be used.[2] In *acute diffuse otitis externa* (*swimmer's ear*), *Staphylococcus aureus* and *Pseudomonas* spp. are often present. Treatment includes thorough cleansing of the ear canal and instillation of ear drops including antibacterials such as aminoglycosides, fluoroquinolones, chloramphenicol, or polymyxin B, with or without corticosteroids such as dexamethasone. Antifungals may sometimes be required. A wick may be used if administration proves difficult.[2] Topical gentamicin has generally been successful and oral fluoroquinolones effective in most cases not responding to topical treatment.[4] *Necrotising (malignant) otitis externa*, due to fulminating infection, especially with *Pseudomonas*, is uncommon but can occur in, for example, elderly diabetics. Topical antibacterials are not effective and systemic treatment with antipseudomonal drugs such as gentamicin or ceftazidime or a fluoroquinolone is needed.[2] However, resistance to ciprofloxacin has been reported.[5] In *eczematous otitis externa* gentamicin with hydrocortisone ear drops can be used if infection is suspected.

1. Committee on Safety of Medicines. Preparations used in the topical treatment of otitis externa. *Current Problems 5* 1981.
2. Brook I. Treatment of otitis externa in children. *Paediatr Drugs* 1999; **1:** 283–9.
3. Hughes E, Lee JH. Otitis externa. *Pediatr Rev* 2001; **22:** 191–7.
4. Elies W. Local chemotherapy of selected bacterial infections of the ear. *J Antimicrob Chemother* 1990; **26:** 303–5.
5. Cooper MA, *et al.* Ciprofloxacin resistance developing during treatment of malignant otitis externa. *J Antimicrob Chemother* 1993; **32:** 163–4.

### Otitis media

Otitis media or inflammation of the middle ear is one of the most frequent childhood illnesses seen in general practice. Despite this, there has been much confusion over terminology and differences in management. Diagnosis can be difficult and some consider that it can only be achieved by viewing the tympanic membrane (ear drum) or by the presence of a discharge.[1,2] The following classification has been applied[1] to otitis media:

- *acute serous otitis media*, secondary to Eustachian tube dysfunction and characterised by discomfort
- *acute suppurative otitis media*, due to bacterial or viral infection, with pain ranging from mild earache to severe pain and a red ear drum bulging from an acute purulent effusion that may rupture with purulent discharge
- *chronic serous otitis media*, or the 'glue ear' syndrome, characterised by deafness
- *chronic suppurative otitis media*, associated with perforation and/or cholesteatoma and characterised by discharge and deafness.

There may be some overlap in the use of these terms. It has been stated[3] that *serous otitis media* (also termed secretory or non-suppurative otitis media, otitis media with effusion, and 'glue ear') is the commonest middle ear disorder in children; the fluid present may be serous, mucoid, mucopurulent, or of mixed variety; there are no acute symptoms and signs of inflammation; and the fluid is often sterile. Some[4] consider terms such as 'acute suppurative' or 'acute serous' otitis media to be unhelpful since the diagnosis cannot be made in practice, and prefer the use of acute otitis media.

**Acute otitis media** is seen especially in young children and is often due to bacterial or viral infection (frequently both), although infecting organisms are not always identified. It is sometimes associated with upper respiratory-tract infection. The commonest bacterial pathogens are *Streptococcus pneumoniae*, followed by *Haemophilus influenzae*, with *Moraxella catarrhalis* (*Branhamella catarrhalis*)[5] an increasingly important cause. Treatment aims to relieve symptoms, avoid complications, and prevent relapse, recurrence, and progression to the chronic state.[1] Sometimes an analgesic such as paracetamol may be all that is required as long as frequent inspection is possible. However, it is common practice to prescribe a systemic antibacterial as well as an analgesic,[2,6] although the need for routine antibacterial treatment is questionable.[4,7-9] Ear drops containing antibacterials, corticosteroids, or local anaesthetics are not effective, neither are topical and systemic decongestants, antihistamines, and mucolytics.[10] Systemic antibacterial treatment aims to speed resolution and prevent complications. However, while clinical studies have shown only modest benefits from routine use of antibacterials[11-13] and experience from countries where antibacterials are not given routinely for acute otitis media suggests that there is no consequent increase in complications,[8,13] some clinicians argue that the routine use of antibacterials is clinically justifiable[14-17] and a systematic review[18] has concluded that it does provide a small benefit in children. Another suggested approach has been to delay the start of antibacterials for 72 hours and to then only administer them if the patient remains unwell.[19] Amoxicillin is often the drug of choice; alternatives include erythromycin with or without a sulfonamide such as sulfafurazole, or an oral cephalosporin. Co-trimoxazole is used in some countries but it is not recommended in the UK for acute otitis media unless there is good reason to prefer it. Amoxicillin with clavulanic acid may be given when beta-lactamase-resistant strains of *H. influenzae* or *M. catarrhalis* are prevalent. Penicillin-resistant strains of *Str. pneumoniae* have been reported in children with otitis media[20] and are reported to be increasingly prevalent.[21] However, many penicillin-resistant strains remain sensitive to amoxicillin, although the situation will need continued evaluation.[21,22] The American Academy of Pediatrics has produced guidelines[23] for the diagnosis and management of acute otitis media, in which high-dose amoxicillin is recommended for most children. In children with severe illness, amoxicillin with clavulanic acid should be given.[23] Alternatively, in children allergic to penicillin but in whom the allergic reaction is not a type I hypersensitivity reaction, cefdinir, cefpodoxime, or cefuroxime can be given. If the reaction is a type I hypersensitivity reaction, azithromycin or clarithromycin may be tried; other possibilities include erythromycin with sulfafurazole, or co-trimoxazole.[23] Penicillin-allergic children with acute otitis media known or suspected to be caused by penicillin-resistant *Str. pneumoniae* may alternatively be given clindamycin.[23] Parenteral ceftriaxone may be given to children unable to tolerate oral medication.[23] Duration of therapy for acute otitis media has varied from 5 to 10 or more days; some have claimed that the shorter courses of 5 days are as effective as 7 days or more[24,25] and, in one study,[26] amoxicillin for 3 days appeared to be as effective as for 10 days. However, a further study[27] has found a 10-day course of amoxicillin with clavulanic acid to be more effective than a 5-day course in children aged up to 30 months who were assessed 12 to 14 days after initiation of treatment, and it is considered by some that short courses should probably not be used in children under 2 years of age[17,24] or in others at high risk of treatment failure.[24] Longer treatment for 20 days has not been found to be more efficacious than for 10 days.[28]

Antibacterial prophylaxis has been tried in children at high risk including those with *recurrent acute otitis media*,[29] but it remains controversial.[1,2] In the UK, it is suggested that prophylaxis with amoxicillin may be tried during the winter. The use of xylitol, which inhibits the growth of *Str. pneumoniae*, as chewing gum[30] or as syrup[31] has been reported to reduce the incidence of acute otitis media, although a randomised trial[32] found xylitol to be ineffective when it was used only during an acute respiratory-tract infection. There is also the prospect of vaccination against acute otitis media with pneumococcal vaccines, and one study has found such a vaccine to be safe and efficacious;[33] the results of this study were, however, questioned. Vaccination may also have a role in reducing incidence and in preventing the development of antibacterial resistance.[34]

**Serous otitis media** (otitis media with effusion) is common in children and may be associated with recurrent upper respiratory-tract infection. Many are asymptomatic, the fluid is usually sterile, and the condition can resolve spontaneously.[3] Optimal treatment is controversial. Careful assessment and follow-up without medication is the conservative approach, but some have advocated a broad-spectrum antibacterial such as amoxicillin for 5 to 10 days in young children with serous otitis media following an infection. However, a meta-analysis[35] failed to find any evidence to justify the use of antibacterials. Those at special risk such as children with cleft palate should be referred to a specialist.

**Chronic otitis media** can include recurrent episodes of acute infection, chronic suppurative otitis media, and prolonged serous otitis media. There have been various definitions of *chronic suppurative otitis media*. One classification[1] has divided it into 2 types associated with deafness and/or discharge. In one (tubo-tympanic disease) there is typically perforation of the ear drum, deafness, and a profuse mucoid discharge associated with upper respiratory-tract infection, the commonest infecting organisms being *Str. pneumoniae*, *Staph. aureus*, and *H. influenzae*. In the other (attico-antral disease) there may be cholesteatoma with bone involvement and the commonest infecting organisms are *Pseudomonas aeruginosa* and *Proteus* spp. Treatment of chronic suppurative otitis media is controversial. Although the value of systemic antibacterials has been debated,[1] in the UK they are recommended for use during acute exacerbations. The mainstay of treatment is thorough cleansing. Local treatment with corticosteroids or astringents as in otitis externa (above) may be beneficial, particularly with infections of mastoid cavities. Antibacterial ear drops are suggested when perforation of the ear drum is present. The UK Committee on Safety of Medicines has warned[36] of the dangers of ototoxicity when ear drops containing aminoglycosides or polymyxins are used in the presence of a perforated ear drum in patients with otitis externa, but specialists consider that untreated chronic suppurative otitis media is more likely to result in deafness than is the use of these ear drops.[1] In *Pseudomonas* infection ear drops containing gentamicin and hydrocortisone are frequently used.[1] Local application of the fluoroquinolones ciprofloxacin or ofloxacin[15] has shown promise and may prove a safer alternative than these ear drops.[37] A systematic review[38] has concluded that aural toilet procedures and topical antibacterials, particularly quinolones, are effective in resolving otorrhoea and eradicating bacteria from the middle ear.

In the USA, initial oral therapy with amoxicillin with clavulanic acid, cefaclor, or erythromycin-sulfafurazole has been advocated for chronic suppurative otitis media,[39] but despite this ear drops continue to be popular. In a study from Israel[40] intravenous mezlocillin or ceftazidime together with daily suction and debridement, but no topical antibacterial therapy, was reported to be successful in treating children with chronic suppurative otitis media without cholesteatoma; *Ps. aeruginosa* had been present in most cultures and other organisms included Gram-negative enteric bacilli, *Staph. aureus*, and *H. influenzae*. Anaerobic organisms have also been implicated frequently.[41]

1. Glover GW. Otitis media. *Prescribers' J* 1990; **30:** 218–24.
2. Hendley JO. Otitis media. *N Engl J Med* 2002; **347:** 1169–74.
3. Shah NS. Serous otitis media. *Prescribers' J* 1990; **30:** 225–8.
4. Bollag U, Bollag-Albrecht E. Recommendations derived from practice audit for the treatment of acute otitis media. *Lancet* 1991; **338:** 96–9.

5. Marchant CD. Spectrum of disease due to Branhamella catarrhalis in children with particular reference to acute otitis media. *Am J Med* 1990; **88** (suppl 5A): 15S–19S.
6. Anonymous. Management of acute otitis media and glue ear. *Drug Ther Bull* 1995; **33:** 12–15.
7. Browning GG. Childhood otalgia: acute otitis media 1. *BMJ* 1990; **300:** 1005–6.
8. Majeed A, Harris T. Acute otitis media in children. *BMJ* 1997; **315:** 321–2.
9. Damoiseaux RAMJ, *et al.* Primary care based randomised, double blind trial of amoxicillin versus placebo for acute otitis media in children aged under 2 years. *BMJ* 2000; **320:** 350–4.
10. Flynn CA, *et al.* Decongestants and antihistamines for acute otitis media in children. Available in The Cochrane Library; Issue 2. Chichester: John Wiley; 2004.
11. Rosenfeld RM, *et al.* Clinical efficacy of antimicrobial drugs for acute otitis media: metaanalysis of 5400 children from thirty-three randomized trials. *J Pediatr* 1994; **124:** 355–67.
12. Del Mar C, *et al.* Are antibiotics indicated as initial treatment for children with acute otitis media? A meta-analysis. *BMJ* 1997; **314:** 1526–9.
13. Froom J, *et al.* Antimicrobials for acute otitis media? A review from the International Primary Care Network. *BMJ* 1997; **315:** 98–102.
14. Carlin SA, *et al.* Host factors and the early therapeutic response in acute otitis media. *J Pediatr* 1991; **118:** 178–83.
15. Burke P, *et al.* Acute red ear in children: controlled trial of non-antibiotic treatment in general practice. *BMJ* 1991; **303:** 558–62.
16. Dowell SF, *et al.* Otitis media—principles of judicious use of antimicrobial agents. *Pediatrics* 1998; **101** (suppl): 165–71.
17. Paradise JL. Short-course antimicrobial treatment for acute otitis media: not best for infants and young children. *JAMA* 1997; **278:** 1640–2.
18. Glasziou PP, *et al.* Antibiotics for acute otitis media in children. Available in The Cochrane Library; Issue 2. Chichester: John Wiley; 2004.
19. Little P, *et al.* Pragmatic randomised controlled trial of two prescribing strategies for childhood acute otitis media. *BMJ* 2001; **322:** 336–42.
20. Klugman KP. Management of antibiotic-resistant pneumococcal infections. *J Antimicrob Chemother* 1994; **34:** 191–3.
21. Klugman KP. Epidemiology, control and treatment of multiresistant pneumococci. *Drugs* 1996; **52** (suppl 2): 42–6.
22. Pelton SI. New concepts in the pathophysiology and management of middle ear disease in childhood. *Drugs* 1996; **52** (suppl 2): 62–7.
23. American Academy of Pediatrics. Clinical practice guideline: diagnosis and management of acute otitis media. *Pediatrics* 2004; **113:** 1451–65. Also available at: http://www.aap.org/policy/aomfinal.pdf (accessed 11/06/04)
24. Pichichero ME. Changing the treatment paradigm for acute otitis media in children. *JAMA* 1998; **279:** 1748–50.
25. Kozyrskyj AL, *et al.* Short course antibiotics for acute otitis media. Available in The Cochrane Library; Issue 2. Chichester: John Wiley; 2004.
26. Chaput de Saintonge DM, *et al.* Trial of three-day and ten-day courses of amoxycillin in otitis media. *BMJ* 1982; **284:** 1078–81.
27. Cohen R, *et al.* A multicenter, randomized, double-blind trial of 5 versus 10 days of antibiotic therapy for acute otitis media in young children. *J Pediatr* 1998; **133:** 634–9.
28. Mandel EM, *et al.* Efficacy of 20- versus 10-day antimicrobial treatment for acute otitis media. *Pediatrics* 1995; **96:** 5–13.
29. Paradise JL. Antimicrobial drugs and surgical procedures in the prevention of otitis media. *Pediatr Infect Dis J* 1989; **8** (suppl 1): S35–7.
30. Uhari M, *et al.* Xylitol chewing gum in prevention of acute otitis media: double blind randomised trial. *BMJ* 1996; **313:** 1180–4.
31. Uhari M, *et al.* Xylitol in preventing acute otitis media. *Vaccine* 2001; **19:** S144–S147.
32. Tapiainen T, *et al.* Xylitol administered only during respiratory infections failed to prevent acute otitis media. Abstract: *Pediatrics* 2002; **109:** 302. Full version: http://pediatrics.aappublications.org/cgi/content/full/109/2/e19 (accessed 19/05/04)
33. Eskola J, *et al.* Efficacy of a pneumococcal conjugate vaccine against acute otitis media. *N Engl J Med* 2001; **344:** 403–9.
34. Jacobs MR. Prevention of otitis media: role of pneumococcal conjugate vaccines in reducing incidence and antibiotic resistance. *J Pediatr* 2002; **141:** 287–93.
35. Cantekin EI, McGuire TW. Antibiotics are not effective for otitis media with effusion: reanalysis of meta-analyses. *Otorhinolaryngol Nova* 1998; **8:** 214–22.
36. Committee on Safety of Medicines. Preparations used in the topical treatment of otitis externa. *Current Problems 5*; 1981.
37. Elies W. Local chemotherapy of selected bacterial infections of the ear. *J Antimicrob Chemother* 1990; **26:** 303–5.
38. Acuin J, *et al.* Interventions for chronic suppurative otitis media. Available in The Cochrane Library; Issue 2. Chichester: John Wiley; 2004.
39. Nelson JD. Chronic suppurative otitis media. *Pediatr Infect Dis J* 1988; **7:** 446–8.
40. Fliss DM, *et al.* Medical management of chronic suppurative otitis media without cholesteatoma in children. *J Pediatr* 1990; **116:** 991–6.
41. Wintermeyer SM, Nahata MC. Chronic suppurative otitis media. *Ann Pharmacother* 1994; **28:** 1089–99.


## Pancreatitis

The overall management of pancreatitis is discussed on p.1726. Although there has been some uncertainty about the value of prophylactic antibacterials in acute pancreatitis, early treatment with cefuroxime markedly reduced mortality in a study of patients with acute necrotising pancreatitis[1] and a retrospective study[2] reported a reduction in the incidence, but not in the time of onset, of infection in those receiving prophylactic therapy. A meta-analysis[3] of 8 studies showed a positive benefit for prophylactic antibacterials in reducing mortality in patients with acute pancreatitis. The advantage was limited to patients with severe pancreatitis who received broad-spectrum drugs that achieved therapeutic levels in pancreatic tissue, such as imipenem or a fluoroquinolone.


1. Sainio V, *et al.* Early antibiotic treatment in acute necrotising pancreatitis. *Lancet* 1995; **346:** 663–7.
2. Ho HS, Frey CF. The role of antibiotic prophylaxis in severe acute pancreatitis. *Arch Surg* 1997; **132:** 487–93.
3. Golub R, *et al.* Role of antibiotics in acute pancreatitis: a meta-analysis. *J Gastrointest Surg* 1998; **2:** 496–503.


## Pelvic inflammatory disease

Pelvic inflammatory disease is a broad term for infectious disorders of the upper genital tract in women and may include endometritis, salpingitis, tubo-ovarian abscess, and pelvic peritonitis. It is generally due to ascending infection through the cervix and uterus to the fallopian tubes, resulting in salpingitis, and from there may extend to the ovaries and peritoneum. Long-term complications include infertility and ectopic pregnancy. Pelvic inflammatory disease has become more common and has been the subject of several reviews.[1-3] The use of intra-uterine contraceptive devices might increase the likelihood of pelvic inflammatory disease although the risk may have been overstated;[1] it appears to be greatest during the first 20 days after insertion of the device.[4]

The majority of these infections are probably sexually transmitted and at one time were mainly due to *Neisseria gonorrhoeae*, but *Chlamydia trachomatis* is increasingly responsible and may be the commonest cause of pelvic inflammatory disease in some areas. Other organisms that have been isolated include *Mycoplasma hominis*; *Ureaplasma urealyticum*; anaerobes such as *Bacteroides*, *Peptococcus*, and *Peptostreptococcus* spp.; Gram-negative enteric aerobes such as *Escherichia coli*; and Gram-positive aerobes such as group B streptococci. Some of these organisms occur in the abnormal vaginal flora associated with bacterial vaginosis (p.121). Thus, the aetiology of pelvic inflammatory disease appears to be polymicrobial; some think that primary infection with *N. gonorrhoeae* or *C. trachomatis*, or both, allows opportunistic infection with aerobic and anaerobic bacteria.[1]

Treatment regimens are of necessity broad spectrum and empirical and should include antibacterials active against the major pathogens. Many consider that treatment should be started in hospital so that drugs can be given parenterally.

**WHO** recommends three possible treatment regimens for inpatients:[5]

- intramuscular ceftriaxone, plus oral or intravenous doxycycline or oral tetracycline, plus oral or intravenous metronidazole or chloramphenicol
- intravenous clindamycin plus intravenous gentamicin
- oral ciprofloxacin or intramuscular spectinomycin, plus oral or intravenous doxycycline or oral tetracycline, plus oral or intravenous metronidazole or chloramphenicol.

Therapy should be continued for at least 48 hours after clinical improvement, and then followed by doxycycline or tetracycline orally for 14 days. For outpatients a single-dose treatment for uncomplicated gonorrhoea such as ceftriaxone intramuscularly is recommended[5] (see Gonorrhoea, p.130) together with metronidazole and either doxycycline or tetracycline orally for 14 days.

In the **UK**, recommended regimens[6] are:

- cefoxitin intravenously plus doxycycline intravenously (or orally if tolerated) then doxycycline plus metronidazole orally for a total of 14 days
- clindamycin plus gentamicin both intravenously followed by either clindamycin orally or doxycycline plus metronidazole both orally for a total of 14 days
- ofloxacin plus metronidazole both orally for 14 days
- single intramuscular doses of ceftriaxone or cefoxitin with probenecid orally followed by doxycycline plus metronidazole both orally for 14 days.

Intravenous therapies should be continued until 24 hours after clinical improvement is noted and then oral therapy should be substituted.[6] Alternative regimens[6] are:

- ofloxacin plus metronidazole both intravenously
- ciprofloxacin plus metronidazole both intravenously, plus doxycycline intravenously or orally.

Further examples of suitable treatment regimens have been provided by the CDC in the **USA**.[7] For parenteral administration:

- cefoxitin or cefotetan intravenously together with doxycycline orally or intravenously (regimen A)
- clindamycin intravenously together with gentamicin intramuscularly or intravenously (regimen B)

In each case treatment is continued for 24 hours after substantial clinical improvement has occurred and then followed by doxycycline by mouth to complete a total of 14 days' treatment.[7] In regimen A, clindamycin or metronidazole may be added to doxycycline for continued therapy in patients with tubo-ovarian abscesses. In regimen B, continuation may be with oral clindamycin rather than doxycycline.[7]

For oral treatment:

- ofloxacin or levofloxacin, with or without metronidazole orally, for 14 days (regimen A)
- cefoxitin as a single intramuscular dose plus probenecid orally, or a single intramuscular dose of ceftriaxone or equivalent cephalosporin, together with doxycycline orally, with or without oral metronidazole, for 14 days (regimen B).


1. Pearce JM. Pelvic inflammatory disease. *BMJ* 1990; **300:** 1090–1.
2. Dodson MG. Optimum therapy for acute pelvic inflammatory disease. *Drugs* 1990; **39:** 511–22.
3. McCormack WM. Pelvic inflammatory disease. *N Engl J Med* 1994; **330:** 115–19.
4. Farley TMM, *et al.* Intrauterine devices and pelvic inflammatory disease: an international perspective. *Lancet* 1992; **339:** 785–8.
5. WHO. Guidelines for the management of sexually transmitted infections. Geneva: WHO, 2003. Also available at: http://whqlibdoc.who.int/publications/2003/9241546263.pdf (accessed 22/06/04)
6. Clinical Effectiveness Group (Association for Genitourinary Medicine and the Medical Society for the Study of Venereal Diseases). 2001 Guidelines for the management of pelvic infection and perihepatitis. Available at: http://www.bashh.org/guidelines/2002/Pid%2006%2001.pdf (accessed 19/05/04)
7. Centers for Disease Control. Sexually transmitted diseases treatment guidelines 2002. *MMWR* 2002; **51** (RR-6): 1–80. Also available at: http://www.cdc.gov/mmwr/PDF/rr/rr5106.pdf (accessed 19/05/04)


## Peptic ulcer disease

The Gram-negative bacterium *Helicobacter pylori* is involved in the aetiology of gastritis and peptic ulceration, and treatment regimens to eradicate the organism are recommended in peptic ulcer disease (p.1246).

## Perinatal streptococcal infections

Group B streptococci are a major cause of perinatal infections, often leading to neonatal pneumonia or septicaemia, sometimes with meningitis, although the incidence varies in different parts of the world. Infections are acquired through maternal genital carriage during pregnancy. *Prevention* of group B streptococcal infection in infants may be achieved by giving appropriate antibacterials to the mother during labour.[1] Ideally maternal carriers of group B streptococci would be identified during pregnancy, but this may not be practical. Factors that increase the risk of acquiring neonatal infection include premature labour, prolonged rupture of membranes, maternal fever, a previous child with neonatal group B streptococcal infection, and multiple pregnancy and they will influence the decision of whether or not to give intrapartum antibacterial prophylaxis to the mother. A penicillin is the preferred drug.

Guidelines from the USA[1] recommend prophylaxis based on universal prenatal screening. Where required, they recommend benzylpenicillin or, alternatively, ampicillin, given intravenously during labour. In women allergic to penicillin but who are not considered to be at high risk of anaphylaxis, intravenous cefazolin is recommended as an alternative; those considered to be at high risk of anaphylaxis should be given clindamycin or erythromycin intravenously or, where there is resistance to clindamycin and erythromycin or susceptibility is unknown, intravenous vancomycin.

In other parts of the world, including Europe, the incidence of neonatal streptococcal infections is much lower and the US model for prophylaxis may not be appropriate.[2,3]

Another strategy suggested for areas with a high incidence of neonatal group B streptococcal disease (above 1.5 per 1000 live births) is administration of a single dose of penicillin to all neonates at birth.[4]

As mentioned under Premature Labour, p.143, the elimination of group B streptococci in pregnant women might also reduce the risk of premature labour.

Streptococcus group B vaccines are under investigation for administration to pregnant women to prevent neonatal infection.


1. Centers for Disease Control. Prevention of perinatal group B streptococcal disease: revised guidelines from CDC. *MMWR* 2002; **51** (RR-11): 1–22. Also available at: http://www.cdc.gov/mmwr/PDF/rr/rr5111.pdf (accessed 20/05/04)

2. Simpson AJA, Heard SR. Group B Streptococcus. *Lancet* 1995; **346:** 700.
3. Jakobi P, *et al.* New CDC guidelines for prevention of perinatal group B streptococcal disease. *Lancet* 2003; **361:** 351.
4. Siegel JD, Cushion NB. Prevention of early-onset group B streptococcal disease: another look at single-dose penicillin at birth. *Obstet Gynecol* 1996; **87:** 692–8.

### Peritonitis

Intra-abdominal infections include peritonitis, which may be complicated by intraperitoneal abscesses, and abscesses of the intra-abdominal viscera such as those of the liver (see under Abscess, Liver, p.120), pancreas, and spleen. Infective peritonitis may be primary or secondary or may be a complication of continuous ambulatory peritoneal dialysis (CAPD).

**Primary peritonitis.** In primary or spontaneous bacterial peritonitis there is no specific focus of infection and it occurs most often as a complication of ascites. Infecting bacteria include *Escherichia coli*, other Enterobacteriaceae, and streptococci. Initial empirical treatment has been with broad-spectrum chemotherapy such as ampicillin plus an aminoglycoside, but third-generation cephalosporins such as cefotaxime are considered by some to be the treatment of choice.[1-3] Other alternatives include other broad-spectrum penicillins, carbapenems, and combinations of penicillins with beta-lactamase inhibitors.[2,3] Oral ofloxacin has been reported to be as effective as intravenous cefotaxime in uncomplicated infections.[4] If infection with anaerobic organisms is suspected, metronidazole or clindamycin may be added to the chosen regimen.[2] In cirrhotic patients with low levels of ascitic fluid protein[5] the use of oral norfloxacin for selective intestinal decontamination appeared to prevent spontaneous bacterial peritonitis and prophylaxis with norfloxacin has been recommended to decrease the recurrence of spontaneous bacterial peritonitis.[1] However, prophylaxis with norfloxacin will not prevent infection by Gram-positive bacteria including *Staphylococcus aureus* or quinolone-resistant Gram-negative bacteria.[2] Co-trimoxazole has also been reported to be an effective prophylactic.[6]

**Secondary peritonitis.** Secondary peritonitis is associated with perforation of the gastrointestinal tract, conditions such as appendicitis and diverticulitis, and contamination at surgery. Infections are generally mixed and originate from the gastrointestinal tract. Bacteria responsible include *E. coli* and other Enterobacteriaceae, anaerobes (especially *Bacteroides fragilis*), enterococci, and sometimes *Pseudomonas aeruginosa*. Broad-spectrum antibacterial therapy is therefore usually used, at least until the infecting organisms are known, and a combination of two or three drugs is often given. The intravenous route is generally preferred. Nevertheless, it is difficult to assess the relative merits of surgical therapy against medical management that includes antibacterial therapy.[2] An aminoglycoside such as gentamicin or a cephalosporin, plus metronidazole or clindamycin, have often been used, but many other regimens have been tried. Patterns of resistance further complicate the choice of antibacterial: resistance to beta lactams may emerge among some Gram-negative organisms, which are most likely to infect patients with prolonged hospital stays, previous antibacterial treatment, postoperative peritonitis, or recurrent peritonitis. Such patients are best treated with a regimen that includes a carbapenem, cefepime, a fluoroquinolone, or an aminoglycoside.[2] Resistant isolates of *B. fragilis* and *Clostridium difficile* (with associated diarrhoea) are more common after clindamycin than after metronidazole.[2] Microaerophilic Gram-positive cocci are resistant to metronidazole but not to clindamycin,[2] so metronidazole should be used with a beta lactam other than aztreonam.[2]

For reference to the prevention of postoperative infection, see under Surgical Infection, p.147.

**CAPD peritonitis.** Peritonitis is the main complication of CAPD, a technique widely used in end-stage renal failure. Unlike secondary peritonitis, above, a single infecting organism is often responsible. The most common infections have usually been due to Gram-positive organisms, especially staphylococci, but infections with Gram-negative bacteria (typically Enterobacteriaceae) are becoming more common,[7] and fungi are an increasingly important cause of peritonitis in CAPD.[2] The empirical treatment of CAPD peritonitis has changed in recent years because of the emergence of vancomycin-resistant organisms. While vancomycin in combination with an aminoglycoside has been recommended,[8] in order to avoid unnecessary exposure to vancomycin the International Society for Peritoneal Dialysis now recommends the use of a first-generation cephalosporin with ceftazidime, given intraperitoneally by mixing the antibacterials with the dialysate.[7] Alternatives to ceftazidime in this regimen are cefazolin or cefalotin in combination with an aminoglycoside, or clindamycin, or vancomycin, in that order of preference. Once-daily dosing regimens for aminoglycosides are considered appropriate for CAPD patients.[7] Once the infecting organism is identified, an appropriate narrow-spectrum antibacterial can be substituted. Treatment is generally continued for 14 days in patients who have a clinical response.[7] Treatment should be extended to 21 days in patients with *Staph. aureus* infections, and also in those with pseudomonal infections.[7]

Exit-site infections can be treated with an oral penicillinase-resistant penicillin, cefalexin, or co-trimoxazole for Gram-positive infections, or an oral fluoroquinolone such as ciprofloxacin for Gram-negative infections.[7] Intraperitoneal ceftazidime may be added in cases of pseudomonal infection where resolution of infection is slow or where there is recurrence.

Long-term antibacterial prophylaxis is not generally effective, but *Staph. aureus* nasal carriage is associated with increased risk of exit-site infections and intranasal or exit-site mupirocin or oral rifampicin have been used to reduce them.[7] Dramatic reductions in peritonitis rates have been achieved with programmes based on stringent aseptic wound care and on minimising contact of the CAPD system with domestic water.[9]

1. Gilbert JA, Kamath PS. Spontaneous bacterial peritonitis: an update. *Mayo Clin Proc* 1995; **70:** 365–70.
2. Johnson CC, *et al.* Peritonitis: update on pathophysiology, clinical manifestations, and management. *Clin Infect Dis* 1997; **24:** 1035–47.
3. Rimola A, *et al.* Diagnosis, treatment and prophylaxis of spontaneous bacterial peritonitis: a consensus document. *J Hepatol* 2000; **32:** 142–53.
4. Navasa M *et al.* Randomized comparative study of oral ofloxacin versus intravenous cefotaxime in spontaneous bacterial peritonitis. *Gastroenterology* 1996; **111:** 1011–17.
5. Soriano G, *et al.* Selective intestinal decontamination prevents spontaneous bacterial peritonitis. *Gastroenterology* 1991; **100:** 477–81.
6. Singh N, *et al.* Trimethoprim-sulfamethoxazole for the prevention of spontaneous bacterial peritonitis in cirrhosis: a randomized trial. *Ann Intern Med* 1995; **122:** 595–8.
7. Keane WF, *et al.* Adult peritoneal dialysis-related peritonitis treatment recommendations: 2000 update. *Perit Dial Int* 2000; **20:** 396–411. Correction. *ibid.*; 828–9. Also available at: http://www.ispd.org/2000_treatment_recommendations.html (accessed 20/05/04)
8. Working Party of the British Society for Antimicrobial Chemotherapy. Diagnosis and management of peritonitis in continuous ambulatory peritoneal dialysis. *Lancet* 1987; **i:** 845–9.
9. Ludlam H, *et al.* Prevention of peritonitis in continuous ambulatory peritoneal dialysis. *Lancet* 1990; **335:** 1161.

### Pertussis

Pertussis or whooping cough is caused by infection with the respiratory pathogen *Bordetella pertussis*, a Gram-negative aerobic bacterium. The related species *B. parapertussis* causes a similar but generally milder illness. Pertussis is very infectious and occurs most frequently in children, but may be more common in adults than once thought.[1-3] The incidence of pertussis has been greatly reduced by the active immunisation of infants (see under Pertussis Vaccines, p.1632) and effective prevention by the adequate uptake of vaccine remains the ultimate objective. In addition to an accelerated schedule of vaccination, prompt use of erythromycin for treatment and prophylaxis may help to contain epidemics.[4]

Erythromycin is the antibacterial of choice at any stage of the disease.[5] Once infection has occurred erythromycin is thought to render the patient non-infectious by eliminating nasopharyngeal carriage of *B. pertussis*. Such treatment is unlikely to affect the clinical course of pertussis because diagnosis is difficult until the paroxysmal stage, by which time the bacteria have already damaged the respiratory tract and released their toxins.[6] Erythromycin is also given prophylactically to close contacts. Erythromycin 50 mg/kg daily for 14 days, whether for treatment or prophylaxis, has been recommended,[7] and the estolate ester was favoured in order to achieve maximum blood concentrations. However, a 7-day course of erythromycin was reported to be as effective as a 14-day course for treatment.[8] Courses of azithromycin for 3 or 5 days or clarithromycin for 7 days are also effective.[9-11] Decreased transmission and severity of the disease has been seen in adults and adolescents in a confined setting, when erythromycin was used for treatment, and prophylaxis in those exposed, and especially when started within 14 days of the first case being identified.[12] Erythromycin prophylaxis was also effective in a family setting, especially if started before the occurrence of the first secondary case.[13]

Strains of *B. pertussis* resistant to erythromycin have been reported in the USA, but do not appear to be widespread.[14] Co-trimoxazole has been suggested as an alternative to erythromycin for both treatment and prophylaxis.[14]

1. Mortimer EA. Pertussis and its prevention: a family affair. *J Infect Dis* 1990; **161:** 473–9.
2. Wright SW, *et al.* Pertussis infection in adults with persistent cough. *JAMA* 1995; **273:** 1044–6.
3. Cherry JD. Pertussis in adults. *Ann Intern Med* 1998; **128:** 64–6.
4. Christie CDC, *et al.* The 1993 epidemic of pertussis in Cincinnati: resurgence of disease in a highly immunized population of children. *N Engl J Med* 1994; **331:** 16–21.
5. Kerr JR, Preston NW. Current pharmacotherapy of pertussis. *Expert Opin Pharmacother* 2001; **2:** 1275–82.
6. Moxon ER, Rappuoli R. Modern vaccines: Haemophilus influenzae infections and whooping cough. *Lancet* 1990; **335:** 1324–9.
7. Bass JW. Pertussis: current status of prevention and treatment. *Pediatr Infect Dis* 1985; **4:** 614–19.
8. Halperin SA, *et al.* Seven days of erythromycin estolate is as effective as fourteen days for the treatment of Bordetella pertussis infections. *Pediatrics* 1997; **100:** 65–71.
9. Aoyama T, *et al.* Efficacy of short-term treatment of pertussis with clarithromycin and azithromycin. *J Pediatr* 1996; **129:** 761–4.
10. Baće A, *et al.* Short-term treatment of pertussis with azithromycin in infants and young children. *Eur J Clin Microbiol Infect Dis* 1999; **18:** 296–8.
11. Lebel MH, Mehra S. Efficacy and safety of clarithromycin versus erythromycin for the treatment of pertussis: a prospective, randomized, single blind trial. *Pediatr Infect Dis J* 2001; **20:** 1149–54.
12. Steketee RW, *et al.* Evidence for a high attack rate and efficacy of erythromycin prophylaxis in a pertussis outbreak in a facility for the developmentally disabled. *J Infect Dis* 1988; **157:** 434–40.
13. De Serres G, *et al.* Field effectiveness of erythromycin prophylaxis to prevent pertussis within families. *Pediatr Infect Dis J* 1995; **14:** 969–75.
14. Centers for Disease Control. Erythromycin-resistant Bordetella pertussis—Yuma County, Arizona, May-October 1994. *MMWR* 1994; **43:** 807–10.

### Pharyngitis

Pharyngitis and tonsillitis are upper respiratory-tract infections with similar causes and occur especially in children. Acute pharyngitis is an inflammatory syndrome of the oropharynx that may include the tonsils whereas tonsillitis is, strictly speaking, a more localised infection. The commonest causes are viral and a sore throat is often a symptom of the common cold as well as influenza and infectious mononucleosis. For further details of these viral infections, see under Choice of Antiviral, p.618.

The most important bacterial cause of acute pharyngitis and tonsillitis is the group A beta-haemolytic streptococcus, *Streptococcus pyogenes*. An erythrogenic toxin-producing strain causes pharyngitis and tonsillitis in scarlet fever.

In view of the prevalence of a viral cause, opinions have differed over whether and when to treat pharyngitis with antimicrobial drugs. Some have advocated waiting until a definite diagnosis of *Str. pyogenes* infection is made, but others treat immediately if streptococcal pharyngitis is suspected because of the risk of longer term complications such as rheumatic fever and the need to eradicate *Str. pyogenes* from the throat.[1-3] The incidence of rheumatic fever has been low for many years in developed countries, but there was evidence of a resurgence in parts of the USA in the mid-1980s. Thus, in addition to shortening the illness and interrupting transmission, the antibacterial treatment of streptococcal pharyngitis also serves as primary prevention of rheumatic fever (see below). However, in countries in which the incidence of rheumatic fever remains low the routine use of antibacterials for the management of sore throats is discouraged.[4,5]

Penicillin is the standard treatment for streptococcal pharyngitis or tonsillitis,[6-8] generally as phenoxymethylpenicillin by mouth for 10 days; benzylpenicillin may be given by injection initially. A single intramuscular injection of benzathine benzylpenicillin is perhaps the treatment of choice, especially if compliance with a 10-day course of oral penicillin is unlikely, and is advocated by WHO and the American Heart Association for the primary prevention of rheumatic fever (see under Rheumatic Fever, p.144), but the injection may not be available in some countries. Ampicillin should probably be avoided because of the risk of maculopapular rash if the patient proves to have infectious mononucleosis.[9] Erythromycin or another macrolide may be given to penicillin-allergic patients, except where there is evidence of significant resistance, as in some parts of Europe,[6] the USA,[10] Japan,[11] and Finland;[12] it may also be a better choice than penicillin if there is a likelihood of infection with *Arcanobacterium haemolyticum* (*Corynebacterium haemolyticum*) (see below). Oral cephalosporins are another alternative.

Despite the general effectiveness of penicillin a trend of increasing numbers of relapses and recurrent infections has been noted.[13] Some treatment failures have been attributed to poor patient compliance with a 10-day course of penicillin and attempts to overcome this have included giving fewer daily doses or shortening the length of treatment. Meta-analysis of studies supports the use of twice-daily dosing of phenoxymethylpenicillin which appears to be as effective as doses three or four times daily,[14] but a single daily dose is less effective. Courses of phenoxymethylpenicillin shorter than 10 days have not proved effective.[15,16] There is some evidence that shorter courses may be possible with some alternative antibacterials. Studies have shown that courses of 5 days or less of erythromycin,[17] cefotiam hexetil,[18] azithromycin,[19,20] clarithromycin,[21] or cefuroxime axetil[22,23] may be as effective as a 10-day course of phenoxymethylpenicillin. However, definitive studies have not been done, and the broader spectrum and higher cost of these regimens are drawbacks.[6,7]

Penicillin resistance in *Str. pyogenes* remains rare. In addition to poor compliance, treatment failures with penicillin, leading to recurrent infection, might be explained by the presence of beta-lactamase-producing oropharyngeal bacteria that are able to protect *Str. pyogenes* against penicillin,[24] although this theory was not supported by a study in 462 children.[25] Antibacterials less susceptible to beta lactamase have been effective, sometimes more so than phenoxymethylpenicillin. They include the oral cephalosporins cefaclor,[26] cefuroxime axetil,[27] cefixime,[28] cefprozil,[29] and cefadroxil[30] and the combined preparation amoxicillin with clavulanic acid[31,32] (like ampicillin, amoxicillin should perhaps be avoided because of the risk of maculopapular rash if the patient proves to have infectious mononucleosis). Clindamycin has eradicated *Str. pyogenes* and beta-lactamase-producing bacteria in children of 12 years and under with recurrent tonsillitis, but might be less effective in older patients.[33] It was also effective where penicillin and erythromycin had failed in an outbreak of streptococcal pharyngitis.[34]

Pharyngeal carriage of *Str. pyogenes* is common, especially in primary-school children and thus its presence does not necessarily reflect acute infection. Eradication may be beneficial in selected cases and has been achieved by a single intramuscular injection of benzathine benzylpenicillin together with a 4-day course of oral rifampicin;[35] a 10-day course of oral clindamycin has also been effective.[36] In order to ensure that outbreaks of *Str. pyogenes* are prevented in closely confined populations, some have recommended prophylactic antibacterials for *all* members of these populations, without exception.[37]

Other bacterial causes of pharyngitis include *Arcanobacterium haemolyticum* (*Corynebacterium haemolyticum*), *Chlamydophila pneumoniae* (*Chlamydia pneumoniae*), *Corynebacterium diphtheriae* (see under Diphtheria, p.125), *Neisseria gonorrhoeae* (see under Gonorrhoea, p.130), group C beta-haemolytic streptococci, and anaerobic bacteria.

*A. haemolyticum* is thought to be an important cause of pharyngitis in adolescents and young adults; there is often an accompanying scarlatiniform rash. It has been reported to respond to a single injection of benzathine benzylpenicillin or a 10-day course of oral erythromycin, but not to phenoxymethylpenicillin.[7]

Pharyngitis is often associated with *Chlamydophila pneumoniae* infection and tetracycline or erythromycin are effective antibacterials.[38]


1. Anonymous. Bacterial pharyngitis. *Lancet* 1987; **i:** 1241–2.
2. Marcovitch H. Sore throats. *Arch Dis Child* 1990; **65:** 249–50.
3. Lang SDR, Singh K. The sore throat: when to investigate and when to prescribe. *Drugs* 1990; **40:** 854–62.
4. Little P, *et al.* Reattendance and complications in a randomised trial of prescribing strategies for sore throat: the medicalising effect of prescribing antibiotics. *BMJ* 1997; **315:** 350–2.
5. Del Mar CB, *et al.* Antibiotics for sore throat. Available in The Cochrane Library; Issue 2. Chichester: John Wiley; 2004.
6. WHO. *WHO model prescribing information: drugs used in the treatment of streptococcal pharyngitis and prevention of rheumatic fever.* Geneva: WHO, 1999.
7. Bisno AL. Acute pharyngitis. *N Engl J Med* 2001; **344:** 205–11.
8. Bisno AL, *et al.* Practice guidelines for the diagnosis and management of group A streptococcal pharyngitis. *Clin Infect Dis* 2002; **35:** 113–25.
9. Green AD. Treatment of choice for childhood tonsillitis. *BMJ* 1986; **293:** 1030.
10. Martin JM, *et al.* Erythromycin-resistant group A streptococci in schoolchildren in Pittsburgh. *N Engl J Med* 2002; **346:** 1200–6.
11. Maruyama S, *et al.* Sensitivity of group A streptococci to antibiotics: prevalence of resistance to erythromycin in Japan. *Am J Dis Child* 1979; **133:** 1143–5.
12. Seppälä H, *et al.* Resistance to erythromycin in group A streptococci. *N Engl J Med* 1992; **326:** 292–7.
13. Dillon HC. Streptococcal pharyngitis in the 1980s. *Pediatr Infect Dis J* 1987; **6:** 123–30.
14. Lan AJ, *et al.* The impact of dosing frequency on the efficacy of 10-day penicillin or amoxicillin therapy for streptococcal tonsillopharyngitis: a meta-analysis. Abstract: *Pediatrics* 2000; **105:** 414. Full version: http://pediatrics.aappublications.org/cgi/content/full/105/2/e19 (accessed 20/05/04)
15. Gerber MA, *et al.* Five vs ten days of penicillin V therapy for streptococcal pharyngitis. *Am J Dis Child* 1987; **141:** 224–7.
16. Strömberg A, *et al.* Five versus ten days treatment of group A streptococcal pharyngotonsillitis: a randomized controlled clinical trial with phenoxymethylpenicillin and cefadroxil. *Scand J Infect Dis* 1988; **20:** 37–46.
17. Adam D, *et al.* Five days of erythromycin estolate versus ten days of penicillin V in the treatment of group A streptococcal tonsillopharyngitis in children. *Eur J Clin Microbiol Infect Dis* 1996; **15:** 712–17.
18. Carbon C, *et al.* A double-blind randomized trial comparing the efficacy and safety of a 5-day course of cefotiam hexetil with that of a 10-day course of penicillin V in adult patients with pharyngitis caused by group A β-haemolytic streptococci. *J Antimicrob Chemother* 1995; **35:** 843–54.
19. O'Doherty B, *et al.* Azithromycin versus penicillin V in the treatment of paediatric patients with acute streptococcal pharyngitis/tonsillitis. *Eur J Clin Microbiol Infect Dis* 1996; **15:** 718–24.
20. Hooton TM. A comparison of azithromycin and penicillin V for the treatment of streptococcal pharyngitis. *Am J Med* 1991; **91**(3A): 23S–26S.
21. Portier H, *et al.* Five day clarithromycin modified release versus 10 day penicillin V for group A streptococcal pharyngitis: a multi-centre, open-label, randomized study. *J Antimicrob Chemother* 2002; **49:** 337–44.
22. Aujard Y, *et al.* Comparative efficacy and safety of four-day cefuroxime axetil and ten-day penicillin treatment of group A beta-hemolytic streptococcal pharyngitis in children. *Pediatr Infect Dis J* 1995; **14:** 295–300.
23. Adam D, *et al.* Comparison of short-course (5 day) cefuroxime axetil with a standard 10 day oral penicillin V regimen in the treatment of tonsillopharyngitis. *J Antimicrob Chemother* 2000; **45** (suppl): 23–30.
24. Brook I. The role of β-lactamase-producing bacteria in the persistence of streptococcal tonsillar infection. *Rev Infect Dis* 1984; **6:** 601–7.
25. Gerber MA, *et al.* Potential mechanisms for failure to eradicate group A streptococci from the pharynx. *Pediatrics* 1999; **104:** 911–17.
26. Stillerman M. Comparison of oral cephalosporins with penicillin therapy for group A streptococcal pharyngitis. *Pediatr Infect Dis* 1986; **5:** 649–54.
27. Gooch WM, *et al.* Efficacy of cefuroxime axetil suspension compared with that of penicillin V suspension in children with group A streptococcal pharyngitis. *Antimicrob Agents Chemother* 1993; **37:** 159–63.
28. Kiani R, *et al.* Comparative, multicenter studies of cefixime and amoxicillin in the treatment of respiratory tract infections. *Am J Med* 1988; **85** (suppl 3A): 6–13.
29. Milatovic D, *et al.* Cefprozil versus penicillin V in treatment of streptococcal tonsillopharyngitis. *Antimicrob Agents Chemother* 1993; **37:** 1620–3.
30. Milatovic D, Knauer J. Cefadroxil versus penicillin in the treatment of streptococcal tonsillopharyngitis. *Eur J Clin Microbiol Infect Dis* 1989; **8:** 282–8.
31. Brook I. Treatment of patients with acute recurrent tonsillitis due to group A β-haemolytic streptococci: a prospective randomized study comparing penicillin and amoxycillin/clavulanate potassium. *J Antimicrob Chemother* 1989; **24:** 227–33.
32. Dykhuizen RS, *et al.* Phenoxymethyl penicillin versus co-amoxiclav in the treatment of acute streptococcal pharyngitis, and the role of β-lactamase activity in saliva. *J Antimicrob Chemother* 1996; **37:** 133–8.
33. Foote PA, Brook I. Penicillin and clindamycin therapy in recurrent tonsillitis: effect of microbial flora. *Arch Otolaryngol Head Neck Surg* 1989; **115:** 856–9.
34. Raz R, *et al.* Clindamycin in the treatment of an outbreak of streptococcal pharyngitis in a kibbutz due to beta-lactamase producing organisms. *J Chemother* 1990; **2:** 182–4.
35. Tanz RR, *et al.* Penicillin plus rifampin eradicates pharyngeal carriage of group A streptococci. *J Pediatr* 1985; **106:** 876–80.
36. Tanz RR, *et al.* Clindamycin treatment of chronic pharyngeal carriage of group A streptococci. *J Pediatr* 1991; **119:** 123–8.
37. Gray GC, *et al.* Hyperendemic Streptococcus pyogenes infection despite prophylaxis with penicillin G benzathine. *N Engl J Med* 1991; **325:** 92–7.
38. Grayston JT, *et al.* A new respiratory tract pathogen: Chlamydia pneumoniae strain TWAR. *J Infect Dis* 1990; **161:** 618–25.


### Pinta

See under Syphilis, p.148.

### Plague

Plague is caused by the Gram-negative bacillus *Yersinia pestis* (*Yersinia pseudotuberculosis* subsp. *pestis*) and is usually transmitted to man via rodents and their infected fleas. It has occurred as worldwide pandemics, for example, the Black Death in Europe in the Middle Ages. In the 1980s the largest numbers of cases reported were in Tanzania, Vietnam, Brazil, and Peru.[1] More recently there has been a re-emergence in Madagascar.[2] Plague may take several forms of which bubonic plague is the most common; others include pneumonic, septicaemic, and meningitic plague. Treatment with streptomycin, tetracycline, or chloramphenicol is highly effective in all forms if recognised early.[3] Many consider streptomycin to be the antibacterial of choice,[1] but the possibility of a Jarisch-Herxheimer reaction resulting from the bactericidal effect of streptomycin has prompted some to prefer tetracycline or to use lower doses of streptomycin together with tetracycline. Doxycycline, chloramphenicol, gentamicin, or streptomycin are recommended by WHO.[4] Chloramphenicol has been preferred in meningitic plague because it crosses the blood-brain barrier.

Commenting on the plague epidemic that occurred in India in 1994, workers from the US Centers for Disease Control[5] also noted that streptomycin continues to be the drug of choice for treating plague, that tetracycline and gentamicin are alternatives, and that chloramphenicol is preferred for plague meningitis. They considered that prophylaxis should be given to those who have had face-to-face contact or who have occupied a closed space with someone who has pneumonic plague. For prophylaxis, tetracycline can be given to adults and older children or sulfonamides to children of 8 years or less; chloramphenicol is also effective.[5]

Infection with a strain of *Y. pestis* resistant to all the drugs usually effective against plague identified in a patient from Madagascar[6] responded to treatment with co-trimoxazole and streptomycin.

A consensus statement[7] produced in the USA by the Working Group on Civilian Biodefense has mentioned that, in addition to standard treatment, studies *in vitro* and in *animals* indicate that fluoroquinolones such as ciprofloxacin may be an effective alternative in the event of the use of plague for the purposes of biological warfare.

A vaccine is available for active immunisation.


1. Butler T. The black death past and present 1: plague in the 1980s. *Trans R Soc Trop Med Hyg* 1989; **83:** 458–60.
2. Chanteau S, *et al.* Plague, a reemerging disease in Madagascar. *Emerg Infect Dis* 1998; **4:** 101–4.
3. Public Health Laboratory Service Communicable Disease Surveillance Centre. Plague. *BMJ* 1983; **287:** 118–19.
4. WHO. *WHO model prescribing information: drugs used in bacterial infections.* Geneva: WHO, 2001.
5. Campbell GL, Hughes JM. Plague in India: a new warning from an old nemesis. *Ann Intern Med* 1995; **122:** 151–3.
6. Galimand M, *et al.* Multidrug resistance in Yersinia pestis mediated by a transferable plasmid. *N Engl J Med* 1997; **337:** 677–80.
7. Inglesby TV, *et al.* Plague as a biological weapon: medical and public health management. *JAMA* 2000; **283:** 2281–90.


### Pneumonia

Pneumonia, or inflammation of the lungs with consolidation, is mostly due to bacterial or viral infection, but may be caused by fungi in immunocompromised patients or by the aspiration of chemical irritants. Interstitial pneumonitis is a common complication in cancer patients and has also been associated with certain drugs, for example amiodarone, bleomycin, and nitrofurantoin; sometimes a hypersensitivity reaction has been suspected.

The aetiology of infective pneumonia, and therefore the choice of treatment, differs according to whether it is community-acquired or hospital-acquired (nosocomial) and whether the patient was previously healthy, has chronic lung disease or other debilitating condition, is very young or very old, is immunocompromised, or has pneumonia as a result of aspiration.

**Community-acquired pneumonia.** In community-acquired pneumonia[1-3] the commonest pathogen in previously healthy subjects is *Streptococcus pneumoniae* (pneumococcus). Onset of pneumococcal pneumonia can be very rapid and treatment should be started promptly. *Str. pneumoniae* has usually been considered to be sensitive to penicillins (benzylpenicillin, amoxicillin, or ampicillin), cephalosporins, erythromycin, or co-trimoxazole, but there is increasing prevalence of global resistance although there are marked geographical differences.[4-7] A survey[7] which, during 1999 to 2000, collected data from 69 centres in 25 countries found 22.1% resistance overall to benzylpenicillin (but 71.5% in South Korea, 46.2% in France, 42.1% in Spain, 32.6% in the USA, 15.3% in Latin America, 5.5% in the UK, 4.4% in Australia, and 0% in the Netherlands); resistance overall to erythromycin was 31.0% (87.6% in South Korea, 57.6% in France, 28.6% in Spain, 30.9% in the USA, 15.3% in Latin America, 13.2% in the UK, 12.3% in Australia, and 7.8% in the Netherlands). Fluoroquinolone resistance was low overall (1%) although 14.3% of isolates were resistant in Hong Kong. However, the routine use of penicillin for community-acquired pneumonia may still be reasonable in many countries; indeed, one study in Spain[8] noted that, although there were increased levels of resistance to penicillins and to cephalosporins, this had not been associated with increased mortality so that these antibacterials remained the drugs of choice.

*Mycoplasma pneumoniae* is also an important cause of community-acquired pneumonia. Epidemics occur about every 4 years and the one underway in Europe in 1991 would probably have been responsible for up to 20% of all community-acquired pneumonia during 1992.[9]

Other bacteria that may be responsible for community-acquired pneumonia include *Staphylococcus aureus*, which usually occurs as a secondary bacterial infection following influenza and is associated with high mortality; *Haemophilus influenzae* and *Moraxella catarrhalis* (*Branhamella catarrhalis*), especially in patients with chronic lung disease; *Legionella pneumophila* (see Legionnaires' Disease, p.133); Gram-negative enteric bacilli; *Pseudomonas aeruginosa*; *Chlamydophila psittaci* (*Chlamydia *psittaci*) (see Psittacosis, p.143); *Chlamydophila pneumoniae* (*Chlamydia pneumoniae*); and *Coxiella burnetii* (see Q Fever, p.143). Gram-negative bacilli rarely cause pneumonia in the community, especially in previously healthy patients, although the frequency of such infections is increasing.[10] Anaerobic bacteria are associated with aspiration pneumonia. Viruses are the commonest pathogens in young children.

Guidelines for the management of community-acquired pneumonia in the UK and in the USA have been published by the British[10] and the American[11] Thoracic Societies (BTS and ATS) and the Infectious Diseases Society of America (IDSA).[12] In the UK,[10] preferred initial *empirical* treatment in the community is usually with amoxicillin. Erythromycin is an alternative in penicillin-allergic patients and should also be given during epidemics of mycoplasmal pneumonia and when *Legionella* is suspected; clarithromycin may be given if there is gastrointestinal intolerance to erythromycin.

In those patients hospitalised with non-severe community-acquired pneumonia there is an increased likelihood of infection with atypical pathogens, or with *Legionella* spp.; consequently, combined empirical treatment orally with amoxicillin plus either erythromycin or clarithromycin is preferred.[10] When oral therapy is inappropriate, intravenous ampicillin or benzylpenicillin is given, together with intravenous erythromycin or, preferably, clarithromycin. For those intolerant of beta lactams and macrolides or when there are local concerns over *Clostridium difficile*-associated diarrhoea, levofloxacin, a fluoroquinolone with enhanced activity against pneumococci, may be given orally or intravenously as an alternative.[10] In practice, however, many patients with non-severe community-acquired pneumonia are admitted to hospital for non-clinical reasons such as old age, family preference, inadequate home care, or adverse social circumstances, and in these patients it is considered appropriate to treat with monotherapy as for patients treated in the community (see above).[10]

Patients hospitalised with severe community-acquired pneumonia should receive parenteral empirical treatment regardless of their ability to take oral medication. Since community-acquired pneumonia caused by *Legionella* spp. is more likely to result in severe disease, the initial empirical regimen should include appropriate therapy. Current recommendations[10] are for combined intravenous treatment with a broad-spectrum beta-lactamase-stable antibacterial such as amoxicillin with clavulanic acid or a second- or third-generation cephalosporin such as cefuroxime, cefotaxime, or ceftriaxone, together with a macrolide (clarithromycin or erythromycin). For life-threatening infection where *Legionella* is suspected, the further addition of rifampicin is recommended;[10] although rifampicin may result in reduced serum concentrations of macrolides, this is not known to be of clinical significance when treating community-acquired pneumonia. As in non-severe infection, in patients who are intolerant of beta lactams and macrolides or when there are local concerns over *C. difficile*-associated diarrhoea, levofloxacin may be given as an alternative, but with the addition of benzylpenicillin for severe infection.[10]

The following treatments are recommended in the UK,[10] in conjunction with local microbiological advice, for the minority of patients with community-acquired pneumonia in whom the causative organism has been identified, usually in hospital:

- *Str. pneumoniae*: preferred treatment, oral amoxicillin or intravenous benzylpenicillin; alternatives, oral erythromycin or clarithromycin, or intravenous cefuroxime, cefotaxime, or ceftriaxone
- *M. pneumoniae* or *C. pneumoniae*: preferred treatment, oral or intravenous erythromycin or clarithromycin; alternatives, oral tetracycline or oral or intravenous fluoroquinolone
- *C. psittaci* or *C. burnetii*: preferred treatment, oral or intravenous tetracycline; alternatives, oral or intravenous erythromycin or clarithromycin
- *Legionella* spp.: preferred treatment, oral or intravenous clarithromycin with or without oral or intravenous rifampicin; alternative, oral or intravenous fluoroquinolone
- *H. influenzae* (non-beta-lactamase-producing): preferred treatment, oral amoxicillin or intravenous ampicillin; alternatives, intravenous cefuroxime, cefotaxime, or ceftriaxone, or oral or intravenous fluoroquinolone
- *H. influenzae* (beta-lactamase-producing): preferred treatment, oral or intravenous amoxicillin with clavulanic acid; alternatives, intravenous cefuroxime, cefotaxime, or ceftriaxone, or oral or intravenous fluoroquinolone
- Gram-negative enteric bacilli: preferred treatment, intravenous cefuroxime, cefotaxime, or ceftriaxone; alternatives, intravenous fluoroquinolone, imipenem, or meropenem
- *Ps. aeruginosa*: preferred treatment, intravenous ceftazidime plus either gentamicin or tobramycin; alternatives, intravenous ciprofloxacin or piperacillin plus either gentamicin or tobramycin
- *Staph. aureus* (non-meticillin-resistant): preferred treatment, intravenous flucloxacillin with or without oral or intravenous rifampicin; alternative, intravenous teicoplanin with or without oral or intravenous rifampicin
- *Staph. aureus* (meticillin-resistant): preferred treatment, intravenous vancomycin; alternative, intravenous teicoplanin with or without oral or intravenous rifampicin

In the USA, guidelines for the management of community-acquired pneumonia in adults have been produced by the ATS[11] and by the IDSA.[12] For outpatients with uncomplicated disease, the ATS recommends azithromycin or clarithromycin, or doxycycline if patients are intolerant of macrolides.[11] The IDSA similarly recommends one of erythromycin, azithromycin, clarithromycin, or doxycycline.[12] In those who have received antibacterial therapy within the previous 3 months, the IDSA recommends a respiratory fluoroquinolone (moxifloxacin, gatifloxacin, levofloxacin, or gemifloxacin) alone, or azithromycin or clarithromycin plus high-dose amoxicillin with or without clavulanic acid.[12] In outpatients who have co-existing cardiopulmonary disease and/or other complicating factors, the ATS recommends a beta lactam such as oral cefpodoxime, cefuroxime, high-dose amoxicillin with or without clavulanic acid, or parenteral ceftriaxone followed by oral cefpodoxime, in addition to a macrolide or doxycycline; alternatively such patients may be given monotherapy with an antipneumococcal fluoroquinolone.[11] Similarly the IDSA recommends that such patients receive a respiratory fluoroquinolone alone or azithromycin or clarithromycin, with the addition of a beta lactam (high-dose amoxicillin with or without clavulanic acid, or cefpodoxime, cefprozil, or cefuroxime) to the macrolide if the patient has also received antibacterial therapy within the previous 3 months.[12] Clindamycin or amoxicillin with clavulanic acid should be given to patients with suspected aspiration.[12] Patients with influenza and bacterial superinfection should be given high-dose amoxicillin with or without clavulanic acid, cefpodoxime, cefprozil, cefuroxime, or a respiratory fluoroquinolone.[12] In hospitalised patients who are not in intensive care and who have uncomplicated disease, the ATS recommends intravenous azithromycin alone or, if there is macrolide intolerance, doxycycline with a beta lactam; alternatively such patients may be given monotherapy with an antipneumococcal fluoroquinolone.[11] Inpatients not in intensive care, but who have co-existing cardiopulmonary disease and/or other complicating factors, should receive an intravenous beta lactam (cefotaxime, ceftriaxone, or ampicillin with or without sulbactam) together with an intravenous or oral macrolide or doxycycline; alternatively they may be given an intravenous antipneumococcal fluoroquinolone alone.[11] The IDSA recommends a respiratory fluoroquinolone alone, or azithromycin or clarithromycin plus a beta lactam (cefotaxime, ceftriaxone, ampicillin-sulbactam, or ertapenem) for inpatients not in intensive care.[12] Inpatients who are in intensive care but in whom there is no risk of *Pseudomonas aeruginosa* infection, should receive an intravenous beta lactam such as cefotaxime, ceftriaxone, ampicillin-sulbactam, or ertapenem, together with either intravenous azithromycin or an intravenous fluoroquinolone.[11,12] Alternatively, patients in intensive care not at risk of *Ps. aeruginosa* but who are allergic to beta lactams may be given a respiratory fluoroquinolone with or without clindamycin.[12] Where there is a risk of *Ps. aeruginosa*, an intravenous antipseudomonal beta lactam (such as cefepime, imipenem, meropenem, or piperacillin with or without tazobactam) should be given with either an intravenous antipseudomonal quinolone such as ciprofloxacin, or an intravenous aminoglycoside and either intravenous azithromycin or an intravenous respiratory fluoroquinolone.[11,12] In patients at risk of *Ps. aeruginosa* who are allergic to beta lactams, the ATS states that aztreonam may be given in their place;[11] the IDSA recommends either aztreonam plus levofloxacin, or aztreonam plus one of moxifloxacin or gatifloxacin with or without an aminoglycoside for such patients.[12] For patients receiving treatment while resident in nursing homes, the IDSA recommends a respiratory fluoroquinolone alone or amoxicillin with clavulanic acid plus either azithromycin or clarithromycin.[12]

In **children** pneumonia is caused by a wider spectrum of organisms than in adults. Viruses, especially respiratory syncytial virus, are very common pathogens in infants and children up to 4 years of age and, as in adults, pneumococci are very common bacterial pathogens. Guidelines for the management of community-acquired pneumonia in children have been produced by the BTS.[13] Amoxicillin is considered the antibacterial of first choice for empirical oral therapy in children under 5 years of age because it is effective against the majority of causative organisms. Alternatives are amoxicillin with clavulanic acid, cefaclor, erythromycin, clarithromycin, or azithromycin. Macrolides should be given as first-line empirical therapy in children over 5 years since *M. pneumoniae* pneumonia is more prevalent in older children. Macrolides should also be used in children of any age if either *M. pneumoniae* or *C. pneumoniae* are suspected. Amoxicillin should be used as first line treatment at any age if *Str. pneumoniae* is thought to be the likely pathogen. If *Staph. aureus* is suspected then a macrolide or a combination of flucloxacillin with amoxicillin is appropriate. Intravenous therapy should be given in severe infection or when the child is unable to absorb oral antibacterials, for example due to vomiting; appropriate intravenous drugs for severe pneumonia include amoxicillin with clavulanic acid, cefuroxime, or cefotaxime. If the causative organism is known to be *Str. pneumoniae* a penicillin may be used alone. *Chlamydia trachomatis* is another common cause in infants up to 3 months of age for which erythromycin may be used or, alternatively, sulfafurazole.

Pneumonia in neonates is usually due to organisms acquired from the mother's genital tract, especially group B streptococci, *Escherichia coli*, and *Klebsiella pneumoniae*; initial treatment with gentamicin and benzylpenicillin or ampicillin has been suggested. For prophylaxis against group B streptococci in neonates, see under Perinatal Streptococcal Infections, p.139.

**Hospital-acquired pneumonia**. Most reports on hospital-acquired or nosocomial pneumonia have been from the USA. The organisms most commonly responsible for hospital-acquired pneumonia are Gram-negative enteric bacilli, *Staph. aureus*, *Str. pneumoniae*, and *H. influenzae*; others that may need to be considered, particularly in the presence of specific risk factors, are *Legionella* spp., *Ps. aeruginosa*, anaerobes and, in severe infection, *Acinetobacter* spp.

Broad spectrum antibacterial therapy is essential for hospital-acquired pneumonia. Guidelines[14] produced by the ATS recommend the following treatments: core treatment, given to patients without unusual risk factors who present either with mild to moderate hospital-acquired pneumonia, or with severe infection of early onset, may usually consist of monotherapy using a second-generation cephalosporin such as cefuroxime, a nonpseudomonal third-generation cephalosporin such as cefotaxime or ceftriaxone, or a beta lactam with a beta-lactamase inhibitor such as ampicillin-sulbactam, ticarcillin-clavulanic acid, or piperacillin-tazobactam. A third-generation cephalosporin should be combined with another drug where *Enterobacter* infection is suspected. A fluoroquinolone or, alternatively, clindamycin plus aztreonam, may be used in penicillin-allergic patients.[14]

Patients with specific risk factors presenting with mild to moderate hospital-acquired pneumonia should receive core treatment as above, with additional drugs given according to the likely pathogen.[14] Clindamycin or metronidazole are active against anaerobes and can be given in cases of known or suspected aspiration (see also below under Aspiration Pneumonia), although a beta lactam with a beta-lactamase inhibitor may be sufficient. Patients with suspected meticillin-resistant *Staph. aureus* infection should be given vancomycin until it is excluded. Where there is suspected *Legionella* infection a macrolide should be given.[14]

Patients with severe hospital-acquired pneumonia of early onset but who have specific risk factors, or those with severe infection of late onset, should receive core treatment with the addition of an aminoglycoside or a fluoroquinolone such as ciprofloxacin, plus one of an antipseudomonal penicillin, a beta lactam with a beta-lactamase inhibitor, ceftazidime or cefoperazone, imipenem, or, when appropriate, aztreonam. Where meticillin-resistant *Staph. aureus* is a concern, vancomycin should also be considered.[14]

Nosocomial pneumonia is especially likely in immunocompromised or neutropenic patients. Prophylactic measures in ventilated patients are those mentioned under Intensive Care, p.132.

**Immunocompromised patients.** Immunosuppressed patients are at special risk of pneumonia. In addition to the bacteria mentioned above they are susceptible to opportunistic infections with *Mycobacterium tuberculosis* (see under Tuberculosis, p.150); viruses such as *Cytomegalovirus* and fungi, in particular *Pneumocystis carinii* (see p.389), are also causes of pneumonia in these patients.

Interstitial pneumonitis is a common complication in cancer patients. It may sometimes be drug-related, but diagnosis of the cause is difficult. Early empirical treatment with erythromycin and co-trimoxazole, active against *Legionella*, *Mycoplasma*, and *Pneumocystis carinii*, has been advocated,[15] although individualised patient-directed care may be preferable.[16]

**Aspiration pneumonia.** Aspiration of organisms present in the upper respiratory tract into the lungs, often as a result of loss of consciousness or difficulty in swallowing, can cause aspiration pneumonia.[17] When community acquired the organisms responsible are predominantly anaerobes, but in hospital-acquired aspiration pneumonia Gram-negative bacilli and *Staph. aureus* are also found. Confusion has arisen over the term 'aspiration pneumonia' because it has also been applied more generally to aspiration, for example, of gastric acid (Mendelson's syndrome), resulting in chemical pneumonitis and not associated with bacterial infection. *Lung abscess* generally characterises late-stage aspiration pneumonia involving anaerobic bacteria. The aetiology is rarely established, but specific anaerobic bacteria involved include *Peptostreptococcus*, *Prevotella melaninogenica* (*Bacteroides melaninogenicus*), and *Fusobacterium nucleatum*. Nearly all patients with anaerobic pulmonary infections are treated empirically. Some[17] have expressed the view that penicillin and clindamycin are inadequate and that antibacterials with activity against Gram-negative organisms, such as third-generation cephalosporins, fluoroquinolones, and piperacillin are usually required even in community-acquired aspiration pneumonia. Most patients with lung abscess receive parenteral therapy until they become afebrile and show clinical improvement; oral therapy may then continue for weeks or months if necessary.


1. Bartlett JG, Mundy LM. Community-acquired pneumonia. *N Engl J Med* 1995; **333:** 1618–24.
2. Brown PD, Lerner SA. Community-acquired pneumonia. *Lancet* 1998; **352:** 1295–1302.
3. File TM. Community-acquired pneumonia. *Lancet* 2003; **362:** 1991–2001.
4. Friedland IR, McCracken GH. Management of infections caused by antibiotic-resistant Streptococcus pneumoniae. *N Engl J Med* 1994; **331:** 377–82.
5. Goldsmith CE, *et al.* Pneumococcal resistance in the UK. *J Antimicrob Chemother* 1997; **40** (suppl A): 11–18.
6. Garau J. Treatment of drug-resistant pneumococcal pneumonia. *Lancet Infect Dis* 2002; **2:** 404–15.
7. Felmingham D, *et al.* Increasing prevalence of antimicrobial resistance among isolates of Streptococcus pneumoniae from the PROTEKT surveillance study, and comparative in vitro activity of the ketolide, telithromycin. *J Antimicrob Chemother* 2002; **50** (suppl S1): 25–37.
8. Pallares R, *et al.* Resistance to penicillin and cephalosporin and mortality from severe pneumococcal pneumonia in Barcelona, Spain. *N Engl J Med* 1995; **333:** 474–80. Correction. *ibid.*; 1655.
9. Anonymous. Mycoplasma pneumoniae. *Lancet* 1991; **337:** 651–2.
10. British Thoracic Society. BTS Guidelines for the management of community acquired pneumonia in adults. *Thorax* 2001; **56** (suppl IV): iv1–iv64. Also available at: http://www.brit-thoracic.org.uk/docs/cap.pdf (accessed 20/05/04)
11. American Thoracic Society. Guidelines for the management of adults with community-acquired pneumonia: diagnosis, assessment of severity, antimicrobial therapy, and prevention. *Am J Respir Crit Care Med* 2001; **163:** 1730–54. Also available at: http://www.thoracic.org/adobe/statements/commacq1-25.pdf (accessed 20/05/04)
12. Infectious Diseases Society of America. Update of practice guidelines for the management of community-acquired pneumonia in immunocompetent adults. *Clin Infect Dis* 2003; **37:** 1405–33. Also available at: http://www.journals.uchicago.edu/CID/journal/issues/v37n11/32441/32441.web.pdf (accessed 20/05/04)
13. British Thoracic Society. BTS Guidelines for the management of community acquired pneumonia in childhood. *Thorax* 2002; **57** (suppl 1): i1–i24. Also available at: http://www.brit-thoracic.org.uk/docs/paediatriccap.pdf (accessed 20/05/04)
14. American Thoracic Society. Hospital-acquired pneumonia in adults: diagnosis, assessment of severity, initial antimicrobial therapy, and preventative strategies: a consensus statement. *Am J Respir Crit Care Med* 1996; **153:** 1711–25. Also available at: http://www.thoracic.org/adobe/statements/hosp1-15.pdf (accessed 20/05/04)
15. Browne MJ, *et al.* A randomized trial of open lung biopsy versus empiric antimicrobial therapy in cancer patients with diffuse pulmonary infiltrates. *J Clin Oncol* 1990; **8:** 222–9.
16. Bustamante CI, Wade JC. Treatment of interstitial pneumonia in cancer patients: is empiric antibiotic therapy the answer? *J Clin Oncol* 1990; **8:** 200–2.
17. Marik PE. Aspiration pneumonitis and aspiration pneumonia. *N Engl J Med* 2001; **344:** 665–71.


## Pregnancy and the neonate

For infections associated specifically with pregnancy, see under Endometritis (p.126), Perinatal Streptococcal Infections (p.139), and Premature Labour (below).

## Premature labour

There is evidence of an association between premature rupture of membranes, maternal genito-urinary infection, and preterm labour. Various bacteria have been implicated, including group B streptococci, *Chlamydia trachomatis*, and those associated with bacterial vaginosis, and adjunctive antibacterial treatment has been evaluated. However, concerns have been expressed that delaying delivery in the presence of a subclinical infection may not produce the best outcome for the neonate.[1]

A meta-analysis[2] and a systematic review[3] of studies of the routine use of antibacterials as adjuncts in the management of premature labour in women with intact membranes have failed to demonstrate an overall improvement in neonatal morbidity; indeed, an increase in neonatal mortality was actually noted.[2]

In women with preterm premature rupture of membranes, meta-analyses[4,5] and a systematic review[6] have shown that antibacterials could delay delivery, and reduce both maternal morbidity (chorioamnionitis and postpartum infections) and some aspects of neonatal morbidity (sepsis, pneumonia, and intraventricular haemorrhage). No effects on neonatal mortality or gestational age-related morbidity were noted.[5,6] An increased incidence of neonatal necrotising enterocolitis has been found following maternal use of amoxicillin with clavulanic acid and it is considered best avoided in women at risk of premature delivery; erythromycin may be the antibacterial of choice.[6]

Clinical infections of the genito-urinary tract during pregnancy are a cause of significant morbidity in the neonate and intrapartum antimicrobial treatment is necessary (see Bacterial Vaginosis, p.121, Chlamydial Infections, p.123, and Perinatal Streptococcal Infections, p.139).


1. Brocklehurst P. Infection and preterm delivery. *BMJ* 1999; **318:** 548–9.
2. Egarter C, *et al.* Adjunctive antibiotic treatment in preterm labor and neonatal morbidity: a meta-analysis. *Obstet Gynecol* 1996; **88:** 303–9.
3. King J, Flenady V. Prophylactic antibiotics for inhibiting preterm labour with intact membranes. Available in The Cochrane Library; Issue 2. Chichester: John Wiley; 2004.
4. Mercer BM, Arheart KL. Antimicrobial therapy in expectant management of preterm premature rupture of the membranes. *Lancet* 1995; **346:** 1271–9. Correction. *ibid.* 1996; **347:** 410.
5. Egarter C, *et al.* Antibiotic treatment in preterm premature rupture of membranes and neonatal morbidity: a metaanalysis. *Am J Obstet Gynecol* 1996; **174:** 589–97.
6. Kenyon S, *et al.* Antibiotics for preterm rupture of membranes. Available in The Cochrane Library; Issue 2. Chichester: John Wiley; 2004.


## Proctitis

The treatment of rectal infections caused by *Chlamydia trachomatis* and *Neisseria gonorrhoeae* is discussed under Chlamydial Infections and Gonorrhoea, p.123 and p.130, respectively.

Ceftriaxone 125 mg intramuscularly with doxycycline 100 mg twice daily by mouth for 7 days is recommended by the Centers for Disease Control in the USA[1] for empirical treatment of sexually transmitted proctitis and should be effective against *C. trachomatis* and *N. gonorrhoeae*.

Proctitis may also be associated with herpes simplex infections (p.620).


1. Centers for Disease Control. Sexually transmitted diseases treatment guidelines 2002. *MMWR* 2002; **51**(RR-6): 1–80. Also available at: http://www.cdc.gov/mmwr/PDF/rr/rr5106.pdf (accessed 20/05/04)


## Prostatitis

See under Urinary-tract Infections, p.153.

## Psittacosis

The causative organism of psittacosis (ornithosis) is *Chlamydophila psittaci* (*Chlamydia psittaci*). It is usually transmitted to humans by direct or indirect contact with infected birds and the primary site of infection is the lung.[1] The clinical presentation of psittacosis can vary widely from a mild 'flu-like' illness to a fulminating toxic state with multiple organ involvement.[1] Most patients will have a cough, although this is not always prominent. Tetracyclines are the treatment of choice[1,2] and early therapy may be life-saving; a 21-day course has been recommended since relapses have occurred after shorter periods.[1] An alternative is chloramphenicol.[2] Erythromycin or a similar macrolide have also been used successfully.[3,4]


1. Macfarlane JT, Macrae AD. Psittacosis. *Br Med Bull* 1983; **39:** 163–7.
2. Anonymous. The choice of antibacterial drugs. In: *Handbook of antimicrobial therapy.* 16th ed. New York: The Medical Letter, 2002: 34–52.
3. Morrison WM, *et al.* An outbreak of psittacosis. *J Infect* 1991; **22:** 71–5.
4. Chang KP, Veitch PC. Fever, haematuria, proteinuria, and a parrot. *Lancet* 1997; **350:** 1674.


## Q fever

Q fever (or query fever) is a rickettsial infection (p.144) caused by *Coxiella burnetii*. It is a zoonosis occurring worldwide and is transmitted to humans from domestic animals such as cattle and sheep, mainly by inhalation of infected dust. Acute infection generally presents as a febrile flu-like illness that may progress to pneumonia. Endocarditis is the most frequent manifestation of chronic infection and the most serious form of Q fever; infection may be difficult to eradicate and prolonged treatment is generally required. There is also evidence of long-term sequelae including lethargy and fatigue in patients who have not experienced cardiac involvement.

A tetracycline such as doxycycline has been the treatment of choice for Q fever; alternatively chloramphenicol has been used. Erythromycin may be adequate for Q fever pneumonia,[1] at least in mild cases;[2] results with erythromycin were favourable in a retrospective review.[3] However, Q fever pneumonia may often resolve without treatment and the role of antibacterial therapy is not clear.[4]

Q fever endocarditis is more difficult to treat. Tetracycline has been described as the mainstay of treatment,[5] although it fails to eradicate *C. burnetii* when used alone and various combinations of antibacterials have been tried. A study *in vitro*[6] showed that isolates of *C. burnetii* associated with chronic infection were less sensitive to antibacterials than those from acute Q fever, but that fluoroquinolones alone or with rifampicin might be of value. Long-term treatment with doxycycline plus rifampicin[7] or with ciprofloxacin alone[8] has been successful in individual patients with endocarditis, whereas pefloxacin alone[9] was not. Following a retrospective comparison of doxycycline alone or with rifampicin, fluoroquinolones (ofloxacin or pefloxacin), or co-trimoxazole, treatment for at least 3 years with doxycycline plus a fluoroquinolone was recommended;[10] doxycycline plus rifampicin also appeared effective, but in most cases rifampicin had been stopped after a few months because of interactions with anticoagulants often prescribed at the same time. Different authors have also concluded[5] that no current treatment eradicated Q fever endocarditis within 2 years and similarly recommended[5] that it be treated with doxycycline together with a fluoroquinolone for a minimum of 3 years. Other regimens that have been investigated have included doxycycline with chloroquine[5,11] or with hydroxychloroquine.[12]

A vaccine is available in some countries for use in occupational groups who regularly handle potentially infected animal tissues.


1. D'Angelo LJ, Hetherington R. Q fever treated with erythromycin. *BMJ* 1979; **2:** 305–6.
2. Marrie TJ, *et al.* Q fever pneumonia associated with exposure to wild rabbits. *Lancet* 1986; **i:** 427–9.
3. Pérez-del-Molino A, *et al.* Erythromycin and the treatment of Coxiella burnetii pneumonia. *J Antimicrob Chemother* 1991; **28:** 455–9.
4. Lieberman D, *et al.* Q-fever pneumonia in the Negev region of Israel: a review of 20 patients hospitalised over a period of one year. *J Infect* 1995; **30:** 135–40.
5. Raoult D. Treatment of Q fever. *Antimicrob Agents Chemother* 1993; **37:** 1733–6.
6. Yeaman MR, *et al.* Antibiotic susceptibilities of two Coxiella burnetii isolates implicated in distinct clinical syndromes. *Antimicrob Agents Chemother* 1989; **33:** 1052–7.
7. Brecker SJD, Eykyn SJ. Q-fever endocarditis twenty-five years on. *Lancet* 1989; **ii:** 684–5.
8. Yebra M, *et al.* Ciprofloxacin in a case of Q fever endocarditis. *N Engl J Med* 1990; **323:** 614.
9. Cacoub P, *et al.* Q-fever endocarditis and treatment with the fluoroquinolones. *Arch Intern Med* 1991; **151:** 816, 818.
10. Levy PY, *et al.* Comparison of different antibiotic regimens for therapy of 32 cases of Q fever endocarditis. *Antimicrob Agents Chemother* 1991; **35:** 533–7.
11. Calza L, *et al.* Doxycycline and chloroquine as treatment for chronic Q fever endocarditis. *J Infect* 2002; **45:** 127–9.
12. Raoult D, *et al.* Treatment of Q fever endocarditis: comparison of 2 regimens containing doxycycline and ofloxacin or hydroxychloroquine. *Arch Intern Med* 1999; **159:** 167–73.


## Relapsing fever

Relapsing fever is caused by spirochaetes of the *Borrelia* genus that are transmitted to humans by body lice or *Ornithodoros* ticks. *B. recurrentis* causes louse-borne relapsing fever and can occur widely, but is endemic especially in Ethiopia. Many species of *Borrelia* may cause tick-borne relapsing fever.

The treatment of choice for infection due to *B. recurrentis* is a tetracycline; benzylpenicillin is an alternative.[1] Therapy with single oral doses of tetracycline,[2,3] erythromycin,[2,3] or chloramphenicol[3] has been effective. Antibacterial treatment often causes a Jarisch-Herxheimer reaction characterised by rigor, fever and hypotension, which may be fatal.[2,4] Therapies used in an attempt to prevent this reaction include paracetamol and corticosteroids;[2,4] the use of antibodies against tumour necrosis factor α has shown promise.[5]

Tick-borne relapsing fever is milder than the louse-borne variety, but has been treated similarly.


1. Anonymous. The choice of antibacterial drugs. In: *Handbook of antimicrobial therapy.* 16th ed. New York: The Medical Letter, 2002: 34–52.
2. Butler T, *et al.* Borrelia recurrentis infection: single-dose antibiotic regimens and management of the Jarisch-Herxheimer reaction. *J Infect Dis* 1978; **137:** 573–7.
3. Perine PL, Teklu B. Antibiotic treatment of louse-borne relapsing fever in Ethiopia: a report of 377 cases. *Am J Trop Med Hyg* 1983; **32:** 1096–1100.
4. Butler T. Relapsing fever: new lessons about antibiotic action. *Ann Intern Med* 1985; **102:** 397–9.
5. Fekade D, *et al.* Prevention of Jarisch-Herxheimer reactions by treatment with antibodies against tumor necrosis factor α. *N Engl J Med* 1996; **335:** 311–15.


## Respiratory-tract infections

Principal community-acquired bacterial pathogens in the respiratory tract are *Streptococcus pneumoniae* and *Haemophilus influenzae*, although *Moraxella catarrhalis* (*Branhamella catarrhalis*)[1] is increasingly important in some areas. Other respiratory pathogens include *Chlamydophila pneumoniae* (*Chlamydia pneumoniae*), *Legionella pneumophila*, and *Mycoplasma pneumoniae*. *Streptococcus pyogenes* is the predominant cause of pharyngitis. *Staphylococcus aureus* and aerobic Gram-negative bacilli such as *Pseudomonas aeruginosa* and *Klebsiella* spp. may be responsible for hospital-acquired (nosocomial) infections.

Community-acquired lower respiratory-tract infections are very common and are traditionally considered to be viral in origin, but bacterial pathogens similar to those causing pneumonia are commonly isolated from patients with these milder respiratory infections;[2] even so, about one-quarter of patients fail to respond satisfactorily to empirical antibacterial treatment. For previously healthy adults with non-specific upper respiratory-tract infection, US guidelines[3] recommend that antibacterials are not given.

Broad-spectrum antibacterials such as a penicillin or erythromycin may be necessary in some cases of uncomplicated upper or lower respiratory-tract infection. First line empirical treatment with a fluoroquinolone has been avoided in the past because of poor activity against streptococci,[4,5] although some newer fluoroquinolones have much greater activity against streptococci.[6]

In respiratory-tract infections complicating chronic obstructive pulmonary disease, amoxicillin has been recommended for first-line treatment.[7] If a further course is necessary, drugs with activity against penicillin-resistant *H. influenzae* and *M. catarrhalis* should probably be given, such as amoxicillin with clavulanic acid, a fluoroquinolone (bearing in mind that some are not very active against *Str. pneumoniae*), or a second-generation cephalosporin. Ofloxacin has been reported to be beneficial in patients with chronic obstructive pulmonary disease who require mechanical ventilation.[8]

For details on infections of the upper respiratory tract, see under Epiglottitis (p.127), Pharyngitis (p.140), and Sinusitis (p.146); see also Otitis Media (p.138). For infections of the lower respiratory tract, see under Bronchitis (p.122), Cystic Fibrosis (p.123), and Pneumonia (p.141); those with a specific cause include Legionnaires' Disease (p.133), Nocardiosis (p.137), Pertussis (p.140), and Tuberculosis (p.150).


1. Murphy TF. Branhamella catarrhalis: epidemiological and clinical aspects of a human respiratory tract pathogen. *Thorax* 1998; **53:** 124–8.
2. Macfarlane JT, *et al.* Prospective study of aetiology and outcome of adult lower-respiratory-tract infections in the community. *Lancet* 1993; **341:** 511–14.
3. Snow V, *et al.* Principles of appropriate antibiotic use for treatment of nonspecific upper respiratory tract infections in adults. *Ann Intern Med* 2001; **134:** 487–9.
4. Körner RJ, *et al.* Dangers of oral fluoroquinolone treatment in community acquired upper respiratory tract infections. *BMJ* 1994; **308:** 191–2.
5. Hosker HSR, *et al.* Management of community acquired lower respiratory tract infection. *BMJ* 1994; **308:** 701–5.
6. Guthrie R. Community-acquired lower respiratory tract infections: etiology and treatment. *Chest* 2001; **120:** 2021–34.
7. Hosker H, *et al.* Antibiotics in chronic obstructive pulmonary disease. *BMJ* 1994; **308:** 871–2.
8. Nouira S, *et al.* Once daily oral ofloxacin in chronic obstructive pulmonary disease exacerbation requiring mechanical ventilation: a randomised placebo-controlled trial. *Lancet* 2001; **358:** 2020–5.


## Rheumatic fever

Acute rheumatic fever occurs especially in children aged 6 to 15 years as a consequence of upper respiratory-tract infections, such as pharyngitis or tonsillitis, with rheumatogenic strains of the group A beta-haemolytic streptococcus, *Streptococcus pyogenes*. The pathogenesis of rheumatic fever is not known, but an immune mechanism may be involved. There may be a latent period of 1 to 5 weeks after the initial infection, before clinical manifestations of rheumatic fever appear. The major ones are arthritis, carditis, chorea, erythema marginatum, and subcutaneous nodules. Those affecting the heart are the most serious and are a major cause of cardiovascular death in children and young adults in developing countries. Rheumatic fever has been associated with poverty and overcrowding and has declined dramatically in developed countries, but is still a major problem in the developing world. However, in the 1980s there was evidence of a resurgence in the USA with outbreaks of rheumatic fever reported in middle-class children[1] and military recruits.[2] Increased pathogenicity of *Str. pyogenes* serotypes might have contributed to this resurgence.[3]

Similar guidelines for the primary and secondary prevention of rheumatic fever have been published in 1999 by WHO[4] and in 1995 by the American Heart Association (AHA).[5] Rheumatic fever can usually be prevented by *primary prophylaxis*, that is, by the prompt treatment of streptococcal upper respiratory-tract infection with eradication of group A streptococci from the throat. Penicillin is the drug of choice, either as a single intramuscular injection of benzathine benzylpenicillin or as a course of phenoxymethylpenicillin by mouth for 10 days. An injection containing benzathine benzylpenicillin and procaine benzylpenicillin has been used in children.[5] Erythromycin may be given to patients allergic to penicillin. Other macrolides or oral cephalosporins may also be used. For further details on the treatment of streptococcal sore throat, see under Pharyngitis, p.140. Treatment failure is more common after oral antibacterials and in the USA most of these patients are streptococcal carriers.[5] Treatment of chronic carriers is not usually necessary, but eradication of pharyngeal carriage has been achieved by an injection of benzathine benzylpenicillin plus rifampicin by mouth for 4 days;[6] a 10-day course of oral clindamycin has also been effective.[7] Broad-based primary prophylaxis in communities rather than individuals is controversial and requires careful planning, but, for example, penicillin prophylaxis did control an epidemic of acute tonsillitis associated with *Str. pyogenes* in a junior detention centre.[8] However, a study in military recruits demonstrated that *Str. pyogenes* infection could not be prevented in closely confined communities unless all individuals in the population received prophylaxis.[9]

If acute rheumatic fever occurs, a full therapeutic course of penicillin should be given initially, as for primary prevention, to eradicate group A streptococci.[5] Treatment then comprises bed rest and anti-inflammatory drugs, usually corticosteroids or salicylates, in an attempt to prevent valvular scarring. However, it is unclear whether anti-inflammatory treatment has any influence on such long-term sequelae.[10] *Secondary prevention* is then continued with prolonged antibacterial prophylaxis because of the high risk of recurrent attacks of rheumatic fever following subsequent streptococcal upper respiratory-tract infections. Again, penicillin is the preferred antibacterial, the usual recommendation being an intramuscular injection of benzathine benzylpenicillin every 4 weeks, although injections every 3 weeks may be warranted where the risk of recurrence is high.[4,5] This advice has been influenced by reports of high recurrence rates with the monthly regimen in such situations.[11] A 12-year study in Taiwan[12] confirmed that prophylaxis with benzathine benzylpenicillin injections every 3 weeks is more effective than injections every 4 weeks and it was recommended that the 3-week regimen should be used in adults and children with a recent episode of rheumatic fever, especially in developing countries where exposure to streptococci is still intense. In addition, pharmacokinetic studies have indicated relatively low serum concentrations of penicillin in the fourth week after an intramuscular injection of benzathine benzylpenicillin,[13,14] despite the successful use of monthly injections in most patients. Alternatively, oral prophylaxis with phenoxymethylpenicillin or sulfadiazine may be given; erythromycin is suggested for the rare patient who is allergic to penicillin and sulfonamides. Sulfonamides should *not* be used for primary prevention because they do not eradicate the streptococci. The duration of secondary prophylaxis depends on the individual patient, but in those who have not had rheumatic carditis it should generally continue for a minimum of 5 years after the last attack of rheumatic fever,[4,5] and at least until the age of 18 or early 20s. A study from Chile supported this view.[15] Those who have had rheumatic carditis but without residual valvular disease should perhaps receive prophylaxis for 10 years[5] or at least until the age of 25 years.[4] For those with carditis and persistent valvular disease, prophylaxis should continue at least until the age of 40 years, or sometimes for life.[5] Fears of serious allergic reactions associated with long-term benzathine benzylpenicillin prophylaxis appear to be unfounded.[16]

Household contacts of rheumatic fever patients who themselves have positive streptococcal cultures should be treated.[5]

Patients with rheumatic valvular heart disease as a result of rheumatic fever are at risk of developing infective endocarditis and should receive additional appropriate short-term antibacterial prophylaxis when undergoing dental and some surgical procedures (see Endocarditis, p.125).


1. Veasy LG, *et al.* Resurgence of acute rheumatic fever in the intermountain area of the United States. *N Engl J Med* 1987; **316:** 421–7.
2. Wallace MR, *et al.* The return of acute rheumatic fever in young adults. *JAMA* 1989; **262:** 2557–61.
3. Schwartz B, *et al.* Changing epidemiology of group A streptococcal infection in the USA. *Lancet* 1990; **336:** 1167–71.
4. WHO. *WHO model prescribing information: drugs used in the treatment of streptococcal pharyngitis and prevention of rheumatic fever.* Geneva: WHO, 1999.
5. Dajani A, *et al.* Treatment of acute streptococcal pharyngitis and prevention of rheumatic fever: a statement for health professionals. *Pediatrics* 1995; **96:** 758–64.
6. Tanz RR, *et al.* Penicillin plus rifampin eradicates pharyngeal carriage of group A streptococci. *J Pediatr* 1985; **106:** 876–80.
7. Tanz RR, *et al.* Clindamycin treatment of chronic pharyngeal carriage of group A streptococci. *J Pediatr* 1991; **119:** 123–8.
8. Colling A, *et al.* Minimum amount of penicillin prophylaxis required to control Streptococcus pyogenes epidemic in closed community. *BMJ* 1982; **285:** 95–6.
9. Gray GC, *et al.* Hyperendemic Streptococcus pyogenes infection despite prophylaxis with penicillin G benzathine. *N Engl J Med* 1991; **325:** 92–7.
10. Stollerman GH. Rheumatic fever. *Lancet* 1997; **349:** 935–42.
11. Ayoub EM. Prophylaxis in patients with rheumatic fever: every three or every four weeks? *J Pediatr* 1989; **115:** 89–91.
12. Lue H-C, *et al.* Long-term outcome of patients with rheumatic fever receiving benzathine penicillin G prophylaxis every three weeks versus every four weeks. *J Pediatr* 1994; **125:** 812–16.
13. Kaplan EL, *et al.* Pharmacokinetics of benzathine penicillin G: serum levels during the 28 days after intramuscular injection of 1,200,000 units. *J Pediatr* 1989; **115:** 146–50.
14. Meira ZMA, *et al.* Evaluation of secondary prophylactic schemes, based on benzathine penicillin G, for rheumatic fever in children. *J Pediatr* 1993; **123:** 156–8.
15. Berrios X, *et al.* Discontinuing rheumatic fever prophylaxis in selected adolescents and young adults: a prospective study. *Ann Intern Med* 1993; **118:** 401–6. Correction. *ibid.*; **119:** 173.
16. International Rheumatic Fever Study Group. Allergic reactions to long-term benzathine penicillin prophylaxis for rheumatic fever. *Lancet* 1991; **337:** 1308–10.


## Rickettsial infections

Bacteria of the Rickettsiaceae family that infect man include *Rickettsia* spp. (see under Spotted Fevers, p.147 and under Typhus, p.152) and *Coxiella burnetii* (see under Q fever, p.143). *Ehrlichia* spp. (see under Ehrlichiosis, p.125), are rickettsia-like bacteria. *Bartonella quintana* (*Rochalimaea quintana*) (see under Trench Fever, p.150) is no longer classified as a rickettsia. The treatment of choice for rickettsial infections is usually a tetracycline or chloramphenicol;[1,2] a fluoroquinolone such as ciprofloxacin has also been used.[2]


1. WHO Working Group on Rickettsial Diseases. Rickettsioses: a continuing disease problem. *Bull WHO* 1982; **60:** 157–64.
2. Raoult D, Drancourt M. Antimicrobial therapy of rickettsial diseases. *Antimicrob Agents Chemother* 1991; **35:** 2457–62.


## Salmonella enteritis

See under Gastro-enteritis, p.129.

## Salpingitis

See under Pelvic Inflammatory Disease, p.139.

## Septicaemia

Traditionally, transient bacteraemia (the presence of bacteria in the blood) has been regarded as a fairly common condition which does not usually cause complications, whereas uncontrolled bacteraemia leads to septicaemia with serious symptoms such as fever and shock. This distinction has not always been adhered to in published sources and the terms have sometimes been used interchangeably. Added to this, the identification of the cascade of inflammatory mediators involved and the realisation that what had been called 'sepsis' could arise in the absence of infection have prompted reassessment of the terminology used both in the UK and in the USA.[1] In the UK, some authorities[2] considered that the term 'septicaemia' should no longer be used since it does not distinguish between mild and severe disease. The term 'sepsis syndrome' was preferred for patients with a generalised systemic response together with evidence of organ dysfunction and 'septic shock' to describe patients who also have hypotension not due to hypovolaemia or cardiac causes. The American College of Chest Physicians and Society of Critical Care Medicine proposed the following series of definitions to cover the spectrum of syndromes resulting from this inflammatory response:[1,3]

- **systemic inflammatory response syndrome** (SIRS), the systemic inflammatory response to infection or various other severe clinical insults including pancreatitis, ischaemia, trauma, and haemorrhagic shock
- **sepsis**, the SIRS caused specifically by infection
- **severe sepsis**, sepsis associated with organ dysfunction, perfusion abnormalities (such as lactic acidosis, oliguria, or an acute alteration in mental status), or hypotension
- **septic shock**, sepsis with hypotension, despite adequate fluid resuscitation, together with perfusion abnormalities
- **multiple organ dysfunction syndrome** (MODS), the presence of altered organ function in an acutely ill patient such that homoeostasis cannot be maintained without intervention; it may be a cause as well as a consequence of SIRS.

Septicaemia can be caused by a wide range of bacteria.[4] **Community-acquired** primary septicaemia is often associated with a specific infectious disease, such as meningococcal septicaemia with meningococcal meningitis (p.134) or streptococcal septicaemia with pneumonia (p.141). *Streptococcus pneumoniae* and *Haemophilus influenzae* are common causes of primary septicaemia in children (although this pattern is changing in countries where immunisation against *H. influenzae* type b is routine); Gram-negative rods and group B streptococci are commonest in neonates. **Hospital-acquired** septicaemia is often iatrogenic and may occur as a complication of surgery or indwelling catheters[5] or may be associated with neutropenia in immunocompromised patients (see under Infections in Immunocompromised Patients, p.131). Gram-positive organisms have been reported to be responsible for the majority of infections.[6] Hospital-acquired septicaemia is often associated with acute respiratory distress syndrome (p.1075).

Whatever the cause, septicaemia requires prompt treatment without waiting for the results of laboratory tests. Choice of antibacterial depends on the probable source of infection. For example, urinary-tract infection is likely to be associated with Gram-negative septicaemia due to *Escherichia coli*; abdominal sepsis with Gram-negative septicaemia due to mixed infection with *E. coli*, enterococci, and anaerobic bacteria; and skin sepsis, bacterial arthritis, acute osteomyelitis, and cardiovascular shunts with Gram-positive septicaemia due to staphylococci. The antibacterials used should also reflect current patterns of bacterial resistance in the community or hospital. *Empirical treatment* has often been initiated with a penicillin and an aminoglycoside, metronidazole being added if anaerobic infection is suspected. In the UK, recommended initial empirical treatment for community-acquired septicaemia is with either a broad-spectrum penicillin plus an aminoglycoside, or a third-generation cephalosporin (such as cefotaxime) alone; for hospital-acquired septicaemia an aminoglycoside plus either a broad-spectrum antipseudomonal penicillin or ceftazidime is recommended, or meropenem alone, or imipenem-cilastatin alone. Metronidazole may be added if anaerobic organisms are suspected, and flucloxacillin or vancomycin if Gram-positive organisms are suspected. US guidelines[7] recommend a third- or fourth-generation cephalosporin (cefotaxime, ceftriaxone, or cefepime), or ticarcillin-clavulanic acid, or piperacillin-tazobactam, or imipenem-cilastatin, or meropenem, in each case with an aminoglycoside (gentamicin, tobramycin, or amikacin) for the initial treatment of life-threatening sepsis in adults. When there is some information on which to base choice of treatment, but before the infecting organisms are definitely known, the following treatment is suggested:

- suspected bacterial endocarditis—gentamicin with vancomycin
- suspected meticillin-resistant staphylococci—vancomycin, with or without gentamicin and/or rifampicin
- intra-abdominal or pelvic infections likely to involve anaerobes—ticarcillin-clavulanic acid, ampicillin-sulbactam, piperacillin-tazobactam, imipenem-cilastatin, cefoxitin, or cefotetan, each with or without an aminoglycoside
- suspected biliary-tract infection—piperacillin plus metronidazole, piperacillin-tazobactam, or ampicillin-sulbactam, each with or without an aminoglycoside.

Once the infecting organisms have been identified, choice of treatment will again depend on their sensitivity and current patterns of resistance in the community or hospital. For comments on the consequences of emerging multi-drug-resistant strains of enterococci and staphylococci, see Enterococcal Infections, p.126, and Staphylococcal Infections, p.147.

In addition to antimicrobial therapy, patients with sepsis or septic shock[8,9] require rigorous supportive measures (p.835).

Septicaemia is generally most lethal in the very old and the very young.

**Neonatal septicaemia** may be divided into **early-onset**, which is acquired from the mother's genital tract and manifests itself during the first few days after birth, and **late-onset** which may be nosocomially acquired. Bacteria commonly causing early-onset sepsis include enterococci, *E. coli, H. influenzae, Listeria monocytogenes,* and streptococci. Some of these organisms may also produce meningitis in the neonate (p.134). Empirical treatment for both early- and late-onset sepsis is based on similar principles to those in other patients, giving consideration to local patterns of infection and resistance and to the suitability of individual antibacterials for this age group. However, early-onset sepsis is usually best controlled by prenatal treatment of the mother or by perinatal prophylaxis. Prophylaxis for group B streptococcal infections is discussed under Perinatal Streptococcal Infections, p.139. While vancomycin has been shown to prevent infections with coagulase-negative staphylococci and to reduce the incidence of neonatal sepsis, widespread prophylactic use of this drug is not recommended.[10] Intravenous administration of normal immunoglobulin (p.1630) and of filgrastim (p.754) have been tried for the prevention of septicaemia in preterm neonates with variable results.

Treatment failure in patients with sepsis or septic shock, occurring despite apparently adequate anti-infective therapy, might be due in part to a continuing inflammatory process and attempts to modify this are under investigation.[9,11] Endotoxin, a lipopolysaccharide associated with the cell membrane of Gram-negative bacteria, is an important mediator in the septic syndrome. Endotoxin release may occur spontaneously or during antibacterial therapy.[12] When in the circulation it stimulates the release of endogenous mediators such as interleukin-1, interleukin-6, tumour necrosis factor alpha, and other cytokines.[13] These in turn induce a cascade of secondary inflammatory mediators resulting eventually in endothelial damage and severe haemodynamic and metabolic derangements. It is now understood that a similar inflammatory response also occurs following non-infective insults. However, adjunctive therapy with endotoxin antibodies, anticytokines such as anakinra and tumour necrosis factor antibodies, soluble tumour necrosis factor receptor, bactericidal permeability increasing protein, nitric oxide synthase inhibitors, guanylate cyclase inhibitors such as methylthioninium chloride, and platelet-activating factor antagonists have generally produced disappointing results.[11,14,15] A systematic review[16] of the use of intravenous polyclonal immunoglobulin has concluded that it has a promising role as adjuvant therapy in sepsis and septic shock. Specific monoclonal immunoglobulins were not effective.[16] Recent theories suggest that a more complex interplay of pro- and anti-inflammatory responses may be involved in the pathophysiology of SIRS and MODS and this may explain the failure of many of these predominantly anti-inflammatory treatment modalities.[17] Reduced mortality has been reported[18] following the treatment of patients with severe sepsis with recombinant activated protein C (drotrecogin alfa) which has antithrombotic, anti-inflammatory, and pro-fibrinolytic properties. However, trials with other physiological anticoagulants such as antithrombin III[19] and tissue factor pathway inhibitor (tifacogin)[20] have not been as successful.


1. Bone RC. Why new definitions of sepsis and organ failure are needed. *Am J Med* 1993; **95:** 348–50.
2. Lynn WA, Cohen J. Management of septic shock. *J Infect* 1995; **30:** 207–12.
3. American College of Chest Physicians/Society of Critical Care Medicine Consensus Conference Committee. Definitions for sepsis and organ failure and guidelines for the use of innovative therapies in sepsis. *Crit Care Med* 1992; **20:** 864–74.
4. Eykyn SJ, *et al.* The causative organisms of septicaemia and their epidemiology. *J Antimicrob Chemother* 1990; **25** (suppl C): 41–58.
5. Mermel LA, *et al.* Guidelines for the management of intravascular catheter-related infections. *Clin Infect Dis* 2001; **32:** 1249–72.
6. Edmond MB, *et al.* Nosocomial bloodstream infections in United States hospitals: a three-year analysis. *Clin Infect Dis* 1999; **29:** 239–44.
7. Anonymous. The choice of antibacterial drugs. In: *Handbook of antimicrobial therapy.* 16th ed. New York: The Medical Letter, 2002: 34–52.
8. Astiz ME, Rackow EC. Septic shock. *Lancet* 1998; **351:** 1501–5.
9. Wheeler AP, Bernard GR. Treating patients with severe sepsis. *N Engl J Med* 1999; **340:** 207–14.
10. Craft AP, *et al.* Vancomycin for prophylaxis against sepsis in preterm neonates. Available in The Cochrane Library; Issue 2. Chichester: John Wiley; 2004.
11. Baumgartner J-D, Calandra T. Treatment of sepsis: past and future avenues. *Drugs* 1999; **57:** 127–32.
12. Prins JM. Clinical relevance of antibiotic-induced endotoxin release. *Antimicrob Agents Chemother* 1994; **38:** 1211–18.
13. Blackwell TS, Christman JW. Sepsis and cytokines: current status. *Br J Anaesth* 1996; **77:** 110–17.
14. Verhoef J, *et al.* Issues in the adjunct therapy of severe sepsis. *J Antimicrob Chemother* 1996; **38:** 167–82.
15. Opal SM, Yu RL. Antiendotoxin strategies for the prevention and treatment of septic shock: new approaches and future directions. *Drugs* 1998; **55:** 497–508.
16. Alejandria MM, *et al.* Intravenous immunoglobulin for treating sepsis and septic shock. Available in The Cochrane Library; Issue 2. Chichester: John Wiley; 2004.
17. Bone RC. Immunologic dissonance: a continuing evolution in our understanding of the systemic inflammatory response syndrome (SIRS) and the multiple organ dysfunction syndrome (MODS). *Ann Intern Med* 1996; **125:** 680–7.
18. Bernard GR, *et al.* Efficacy and safety of recombinant human activated protein C for severe sepsis. *N Engl J Med* 2001; **344:** 699–709.
19. Warren BL, *et al.* High-dose antithrombin III in severe sepsis: a randomized controlled trial. *JAMA* 2001; **286:** 1869–78. Correction. *ibid.* 2002; **287:** 192.
20. Abraham E, *et al.* Efficacy and safety of tifacogin (recombinant tissue factor pathway inhibitor) in severe sepsis: a randomized controlled trial. *JAMA* 2003; **290:** 238–47.


## Sexually transmitted diseases

The sexually transmitted diseases, formerly termed venereal diseases, are defined as a group of communicable diseases that are transferred mainly by sexual contact. More than 20 pathogens are known to be transmitted sexually. They include the bacteria *Calymmatobacterium granulomatis* (see Granuloma Inguinale, p.131), *Chlamydia trachomatis* (see Lymphogranuloma Venereum, p.134 and Chlamydial Infections, p.123), *Haemophilus ducreyi* (see Chancroid, p.123), *Neisseria gonorrhoeae* (see Gonorrhoea, p.130), *Treponema pallidum* (see Syphilis, p.148), and mycoplasmas including *Ureaplasma urealyticum.*

Clinical syndromes associated with sexually transmitted diseases include urethritis (p.152) and epididymitis (p.127) in men; cervicitis (p.123), pelvic inflammatory disease (p.139), and bacterial vaginosis (p.121) in women; and proctitis (p.143). Perinatal transmission of sexually transmitted pathogens from the mother can result in neonatal conjunctivitis (p.136) or pneumonia (p.141).

For discussions of some viral sexually transmitted diseases, see under HIV Infection and AIDS (p.621), Hepatitis (p.618), and Herpesvirus Infections (p.619) in Antivirals. Trichomoniasis is discussed in Antiprotozoals, p.599.

The suggestion that spermicidal contraceptives may provide some protection against sexually transmitted diseases is discussed under Nonoxinols, p.1413.

General guidelines for the management of sexually transmitted diseases have been published.[1-3]


1. Centers for Disease Control. Sexually transmitted diseases treatment guidelines 2002. *MMWR* 2002; **51** (RR-6): 1–80. Also available at: http://www.cdc.gov/mmwr/PDF/rr/rr5106.pdf (accessed 21/05/04)
2. Clinical Effectiveness Group (Association for Genitourinary Medicine and the Medical Society for the Study of Venereal Diseases). UK national guidelines on sexually transmitted infections and closely related conditions. Available at: http://www.bashh.org/guidelines/ceguidelines.htm (accessed 21/05/04)
3. WHO. Guidelines for the management of sexually transmitted infections. Geneva: WHO, 2003. Also available at: http://whqlibdoc.who.int/publications/2003/9241546263.pdf (accessed 22/06/04)


## Shigellosis

See under Gastro-enteritis, p.130.

### Sickle-cell disease

For prophylaxis against pneumococcal infection in sickle-cell disease, see under Spleen Disorders, p.146.

### Sinusitis

Sinusitis or inflammation of the paranasal sinuses can be caused by viral, bacterial, or fungal infection or may be secondary to other disorders such as allergy. Serious complications include bacterial meningitis and brain abscess.

Acute sinusitis often results from viral upper respiratory-tract infections. Similarly to acute otitis media the most frequent bacterial pathogens are *Streptococcus pneumoniae* and unencapsulated *Haemophilus influenzae*, with *Moraxella catarrhalis* (*Branhamella catarrhalis*) increasingly important in children. Other bacterial causes, especially in adults, include mixed anaerobic bacteria (usually associated with dental disease and more frequent in chronic sinusitis), *Staphylococcus aureus*, *Streptococcus pyogenes*, and Gram-negative bacteria including Enterobacteriaceae and *Pseudomonas aeruginosa* (in nosocomial sinusitis). About 5% of primary sinusitis in young adults has been associated with *Chlamydophila pneumoniae* (*Chlamydia pneumoniae*).

Acute sinusitis may resolve spontaneously. In an evidence-based report on the diagnosis and treatment of rhinosinusitis,[1] the Agency for Health Care Policy and Research in the USA has stated that most patients with the acute condition will recover without antibacterial therapy, although they will recover faster if antibacterials are given. It was considered[1] that the use of new antibacterials for treating uncomplicated community-acquired acute bacterial rhinosinusitis was not justified and that amoxicillin or folate inhibitors were sufficiently effective. This view was supported by a meta-analysis.[2] Guidelines from the American Academy of Pediatrics for the management of sinusitis in children[3] recommend antibacterials be given to children clinically diagnosed with persistent or severe acute bacterial sinusitis in order to achieve a more rapid clinical cure. Similarly, US guidelines for the management of sinusitis in adults[4] state that most cases will resolve without antibacterial treatment and recommend that antibacterials should be reserved for those patients with persistent moderate or severe symptoms. A systematic review[5] has supported the use of amoxicillin in confirmed acute sinusitis. If antibacterials are considered necessary, treatment should be given for an adequate length of time, usually 2 weeks.[3,6,7] Topical decongestants may also be used to promote drainage and ventilation.[6,7] The choice of antibacterial is similar to that for acute otitis media (p.138). Effective antibacterials include amoxicillin with or without clavulanic acid, cefuroxime, clarithromycin, clindamycin and azithromycin;[3] the emergence of penicillin-resistant strains of *H. influenzae*, *M. catarrhalis*, and *Str. pneumoniae* is of concern.[8] Co-trimoxazole or erythromycin with sulfafurazole have also been used although pneumococcal resistance has been reported to be substantial.[3] Patients with evidence of severe infections may require intravenous therapy with vancomycin and ceftriaxone or cefotaxime initially.[8] Tetracycline or erythromycin are the most effective antibacterials against *Chlamydophila pneumoniae*.[9]

Failure to treat acute sinusitis that does not resolve spontaneously can result in chronic sinusitis or occasionally in complications such as brain abscess or meningitis. Exacerbations of chronic sinusitis are treated as for acute infection. Management of chronic sinusitis is based on reducing obstruction of the sinus cavity using antihistamines, decongestants, anti-inflammatory drugs (including corticosteroids), and saline washes as appropriate.[6,10,11] The usefulness of antibacterials is more contentious,[10] although some clinicians advocate prolonged courses as part of initial treatment.[6,11] Surgical intervention may be necessary if medical treatment fails.

1. Agency for Health Care Policy and Research. *Diagnosis and treatment of acute bacterial rhinosinusitis*. Evidence Report/Technology Assessment: Number 9, March 1999. Available at: http://www.ahrq.gov/clinic/tp/sinustp.htm (accessed 21/05/04)
2. de Ferranti SD, *et al*. Are amoxycillin and folate inhibitors as effective as other antibiotics for acute sinusitis? A meta-analysis. *BMJ* 1998; **317:** 632–7.
3. American Academy of Pediatrics: Subcommittee on Management of Sinusitis and Committee on Quality Improvement. Clinical practice guideline: management of sinusitis. *Pediatrics* 2001; **108:** 798–808. Corrections. *ibid.* **108** (5): A24 and *ibid.* 2002; **109** (5): A40. Also available at: http://www.aap.org/policy/0106.html (accessed 21/05/04)
4. Snow V, *et al*. Principles of appropriate antibiotic use for acute sinusitis in adults. *Ann Intern Med* 2001; **134:** 495–7.
5. Williams JW, *et al*. Antibiotics for acute maxillary sinusitis. Available in The Cochrane Library; Issue 2. Chichester: John Wiley; 2004.
6. Evans KL. Diagnosis and management of sinusitis. *BMJ* 1994; **309:** 1415–22.
7. Evans KL. Recognition and management of sinusitis. *Drugs* 1998. **56:** 59–71.
8. Gwaltney JM. Acute community-acquired sinusitis. *Clin Infect Dis* 1996; **23:** 1209–25.
9. Grayston JT, *et al*. A new respiratory tract pathogen: Chlamydia pneumoniae strain TWAR. *J Infect Dis* 1990; **161:** 618–25.
10. Rowe-Jones J, Mackay I. Management of sinusitis: sinusitis and rhinitis, or rhinosinusitis? *BMJ* 1995; **310:** 670.
11. Wald ER. Chronic sinusitis in children. *J Pediatr* 1995; **127:** 339–47.

### Skin infections

Bacterial infections of the skin may result from invasion of skin structures by endogenous skin flora or by exogenous pathogenic organisms. They include the primary pyodermas (for example, impetigo, folliculitis, furunculosis, erysipelas, cellulitis, and ecthyma) and secondary infections complicating pre-existing skin lesions, for example diabetic or other chronic superficial skin ulcers, burns, bites and stings (p.121), eczema, or may occur as opportunistic infections following skin trauma in immunocompromised patients.

The pyodermas are commonly caused by *Staphylococcus aureus* or, less commonly, by beta-haemolytic streptococci. Skin ulcers and burns may typically be colonised by *Staph. aureus* or *Pseudomonas aeruginosa*; chronic ulcers and fungating tumours may also be colonised by anaerobes which can cause an offensive odour.

Skin disorders of uncertain or mixed aetiology that are treated with antibacterials include acne (p.1133) and rosacea (p.1138). Systemic infections with cutaneous involvement include anthrax (p.121), diphtheria (p.125), and mycetoma (p.136).

Topical antibacterials and antiseptics may be useful for superficial skin infections, but antibacterials should only be used short term because of the risks of inducing bacterial resistance and contact allergy. Topical use of antibacterials that are of value systemically, such as gentamicin, is best avoided, although fusidic acid is used topically in the UK. Application of topical antibacterials to extensive areas of damaged skin can result in systemic toxicity.

Serious infections are treated systemically. Treatment of skin infections is increasingly based on knowledge of the likely infecting organisms and patterns of resistance; empirical treatment with broad-spectrum antibacterials is now discouraged in an attempt to minimise the emergence of resistant organisms.[1] For burns, however, control of infection is important to reduce the risk of sepsis. Topical application of sulfadiazine silver or mafenide acetate has been used in addition to aggressive systemic antibacterial therapy.

Gram-positive pathogens, especially staphylococci and beta-haemolytic streptococci, are commonly associated with primary pyodermas. *Staphylococcus aureus* is implicated in impetigo, cellulitis, folliculitis, furunculosis, and occasionally erysipelas and necrotising fasciitis (p.136), and may colonise burns. Staphylococcal scalded skin syndrome is a severe manifestation of bullous impetigo caused by infection with strains of *Staph. aureus* producing exfoliative exotoxins. The term toxic epidermal necrolysis is used to cover both this syndrome and a morphologically identical syndrome due to various aetiologies. A syndrome resembling scarlet fever may also occur. Staphylococcal infections are usually treated systemically with a penicillinase-resistant penicillin. Erythromycin is an alternative for patients unable to tolerate penicillin. Multidrug-resistant staphylococci are becoming increasingly common, particularly in hospitals, and treatment alternatives for infections with these organisms are discussed under Staphylococcal Infections, p.147. Less severe infections in folliculitis or furunculosis may respond to the application of moist heat without the need for antibacterials. In patients at risk of recurrent staphylococcal infections, nasal application of chlorhexidine plus neomycin or mupirocin alone is used to eliminate nasal carriage of staphylococci.

Beta-haemolytic streptococci are also implicated in pyodermas including impetigo, erysipelas, and cellulitis. Necrotising fasciitis (p.136) may be caused by group A streptococci. Streptococcal infections continue to respond to phenoxymethylpenicillin or benzylpenicillin. Erythromycin is an alternative in patients unable to tolerate penicillins, but increasing resistance may be a problem;[1] clindamycin may be effective in patients with aggressive infections not responding to penicillin.[2]

Resistance is also emerging in *Propionibacterium acnes*; strains resistant to erythromycin, clindamycin, and tetracycline are reported to be common in patients following treatment for acne.[1]

Gram-negative bacteria are less frequently implicated in skin infections, but *Pseudomonas aeruginosa* and *Proteus* spp. can cause infections, especially if the skin is subjected to damp conditions. These organisms produce proteolytic enzymes that cause the resulting skin damage. *Ps. aeruginosa* may colonise burns and skin ulcers. Pseudomonal infections are treated with aminoglycosides and the antipseudomonal penicillins.

Anaerobic organisms may colonise wounds, particularly chronic ulcers and fungating tumours. Topical metronidazole has been used to control the offensive odour caused by these infections.

1. Espersen F. Resistance to antibiotics used in dermatological practice. *Br J Dermatol* 1998; **139** (suppl 53): 4–8.
2. Bisno AL, Stevens DL. Streptococcal infections of skin and soft tissues. *N Engl J Med* 1996; **334:** 240–5.

### Spleen disorders

Splenectomised patients and those with hyposplenism associated with, for example, sickle-cell disease have impaired immunity and, like other immunocompromised patients (p.131), are at increased risk of infection. Children are at special risk. *Streptococcus pneumoniae* is the commonest infecting bacterium and may cause severe overwhelming infection that is rapid in onset and sometimes fatal. Hence, prophylaxis with an oral penicillin such as phenoxymethylpenicillin is advocated. Pneumococcal vaccine is also used; the newer ones may be more effective than earlier vaccines. Other organisms implicated include *Neisseria meningitidis*, *Haemophilus influenzae*, and *Escherichia coli* in splenectomised patients and *Salmonella* in children with sickle-cell disease. More unusual organisms include *Capnocytophaga canimorsus* (formerly called DF-2) which may cause opportunistic infections in splenectomised patients following animal bites. There may also be an increased risk of falciparum malaria and babesiosis.

- SPLENECTOMISED PATIENTS

Guidelines for prophylaxis based on published evidence and expert opinion have been published in the UK.[1] Immunisation with polyvalent pneumococcal vaccine is recommended for all asplenic patients and those with functional hyposplenism. *Haemophilus influenzae* (Hib) vaccine is recommended for all patients who have not previously received this vaccine. Influenza vaccination should be given. Meningococcal group C conjugate vaccine is recommended; however, the vaccine currently available does not protect against the group B strain of *N. meningitidis* causing the majority of infections in the UK. In addition, patients travelling abroad should receive a meningococcal vaccine which protects against Group A infections. Lifelong prophylaxis with a suitable antibacterial should be offered. Phenoxymethylpenicillin is usually given, but amoxicillin may be preferred, particularly in adults, as it is better absorbed following oral administration and has a broader spectrum of activity. Erythromycin is a suitable alternative in those unable to tolerate penicillins. On a practical level, compliance with lifelong prophylaxis is difficult, but is particularly important in patients with underlying immunodeficiency, in children up to the age of 16 years, and for the first 2 years after splenectomy. Patients should keep a supply of a suitable antibacterial for immediate administration should symptoms of infection occur, and be instructed to seek medical advice urgently.

- SICKLE-CELL DISEASE

Children with sickle-cell disease are particularly susceptible to severe pneumococcal infection which may present as septicaemia, meningitis, or pneumonia.

Penicillin prophylaxis is usually combined with early administration of a polyvalent pneumococcal vaccine. However, despite the introduction of the 23-valent vaccine, there is little evidence that it produces substantial protection in children under 2 years of age. Phenoxymethylpenicillin 125 mg twice daily is effective in young children but amoxicillin may be preferred in adults since it is better absorbed and has a broader spectrum. There is evidence to suggest that, in children who have received pneumococcal immunisation, there is no benefit in continuing penicillin prophylaxis beyond the age of 5 years,[2] although indefinite prophylaxis has been recommended for those who have had a previous pneumococcal septic event.[3] Fears that prolonged prophylaxis could encourage the emergence of resistant pneumococci have not been substantiated,[4] although the prevalence of beta-lactam-resistant pneumococci continues to increase. Neonatal screening for sickle-cell disease is advocated, but compliance with regular penicillin prophylaxis may be poor and effective follow-up is necessary if the full benefit of such screening is to be achieved.[5,6] Nevertheless, availability of penicillin in the home, even if not taken regularly, means that it can be readily used if febrile illness occurs.[5] If children with sickle-cell disease develop a febrile illness they are generally treated in hospital with intravenous antibacterials, although outpatient management may often be possible.[7]


1. British Committee for Standards in Haematology Working Party of the Haemato-Oncology Task Force. Update of guidelines for the prevention and treatment of infection in patients with an absent or dysfunctional spleen. *Clin Med* 2002; **2:** 440–3. Also available at: http://www.bcshguidelines.com/pdf/SPLEEN21.pdf (accessed 21/05/04)
2. Falletta JM, *et al.* Discontinuing penicillin prophylaxis in children with sickle cell anemia. *J Pediatr* 1995; **127:** 685–90.
3. Hongeng S, *et al.* Recurrent Streptococcus pneumoniae sepsis in children with sickle cell disease. *J Pediatr* 1997; **130:** 814–16. Correction. *ibid.*; **131:** 232.
4. Norris CF, *et al.* Pneumococcal colonization in children with sickle cell disease. *J Pediatr* 1996; **129:** 821–7.
5. Milne RIG. Assessment of care of children with sickle cell disease: implications for neonatal screening programmes. *BMJ* 1990; **300:** 371–4.
6. Cummins D, *et al.* Penicillin prophylaxis in children with sickle cell disease in Brent. *BMJ* 1991; **302:** 989–90.
7. Wilimas JA, *et al.* A randomized study of outpatient treatment with ceftriaxone for selected febrile children with sickle cell disease. *N Engl J Med* 1993; **329:** 472–6.


## Spotted fevers

Rickettsial infections of the spotted fever group are transmitted to man by ticks and have also been called tick typhus. They include Rocky Mountain spotted fever, due to *Rickettsia rickettsii* and occurring especially in the USA; boutonneuse or Mediterranean spotted fever, due to *R. conorii* and occurring in Mediterranean countries including the Middle East, Africa, and India; Queensland tick typhus, due to *R. australis* and occurring in Australia; north Asian tick typhus, due to *R. sibirica* and occurring in Siberia and Mongolia; and oriental spotted fever, due to *R. japonica* and occurring in Japan. Rickettsialpox, due to *R. akari* is transmitted from mice by mites and occurs in the USA, Russia, and Africa.

Spotted fevers are recognised increasingly as a cause of febrile illness associated usually, but not always, with a purpuric rash and are becoming an important cause of imported fevers in non-endemic areas.[1] Rocky Mountain spotted fever has been one of the most severe of these fevers, but others are potentially serious. A tetracycline, often doxycycline, or chloramphenicol is the treatment of choice for all the spotted fevers. In Rocky Mountain spotted fever, tetracycline 25 to 50 mg/kg daily or chloramphenicol 50 to 75 mg/kg daily for 7 to 10 days markedly reduced mortality.[1] Because tetracyclines are generally contra-indicated in young children, chloramphenicol has been recommended for children with Rocky Mountain spotted fever under the age of 9, but some prefer to use a tetracycline;[2,3] as demonstrated in Mediterranean spotted fever, shorter courses of tetracycline might be effective.[4] Relapses have occurred in patients with Mediterranean spotted fever treated with chloramphenicol.[5] Other alternatives to tetracycline used in Mediterranean spotted fever have included the macrolides azithromycin,[6] clarithromycin,[6] and erythromycin,[7] or ciprofloxacin[8] or rifampicin. Erythromycin was effective, but less so than tetracycline, in children with Mediterranean spotted fever.[7] Short 2-day courses of ciprofloxacin or doxycycline were curative in adults whose disease was not severe, although there was a more rapid response to doxycycline.[8] A 5-day course of ciprofloxacin has also been used successfully to treat infection with *R. australis*.[9]

Rickettsialpox can be mistaken for chickenpox. However, it will respond to tetracycline although patients have generally recovered without treatment.[10]


1. Anonymous. Bitten, hot, and mostly spotty. *Lancet* 1991; **337:** 143–4.
2. Abramson JS, Givner LB. Should tetracycline be contraindicated for therapy of presumed Rocky Mountain spotted fever in children less than 9 years of age? *Pediatrics* 1990; **86:** 123–4.
3. Cale DF, McCarthy MW. Treatment of Rocky Mountain spotted fever in children. *Ann Pharmacother* 1997; **31:** 492–4.
4. Yagupsky P. Tetracycline for Rocky Mountain spotted fever. *Pediatrics* 1991; **87:** 124.
5. Shaked Y, *et al.* Relapse of rickettsial Mediterranean spotted fever and murine typhus after treatment with chloramphenicol. *J Infect* 1989; **18:** 35–7.
6. Cascio A, *et al.* Clarithromycin versus azithromycin in the treatment of Mediterranean spotted fever in children: a randomized controlled trial. *Clin Infect Dis* 2002; **34:** 154–8.
7. Muñoz-Espin T, *et al.* Erythromycin versus tetracycline for treatment of Mediterranean spotted fever. *Arch Dis Child* 1986; **61:** 1027–9.
8. Gudiol F, *et al.* Randomized double-blind evaluation of ciprofloxacin and doxycycline for Mediterranean spotted fever. *Antimicrob Agents Chemother* 1989; **33:** 987–8.
9. Hudson BJ, *et al.* Ciprofloxacin treatment for Australian spotted fever. *Med J Aust* 1996; **165:** 588.
10. Kass EM, *et al.* Rickettsialpox in a New York City hospital, 1980 to 1989. *N Engl J Med* 1994; **331:** 1612–17.


## Staphylococcal infections

Staphylococci are Gram-positive bacteria pathogenic to man. Species may be differentiated by various methods, including the coagulase test. Those species of clinical importance are *Staphylococcus aureus*, which is usually coagulase-positive, and *Staph. epidermidis* and *Staph. saprophyticus*, which are coagulase-negative.

*Staph. aureus* colonises the skin and mucous membranes naturally and many people, including neonates, may be staphylococcal carriers from time to time. Localised *Staph. aureus* infections may follow surgery or trauma and commonly result in abscess formation. Staphylococcal skin infections include impetigo and furunculosis. Conditions associated with staphylococcal extracellular toxin production include staphylococcal scalded skin syndrome, toxic shock syndrome, and staphylococcal food poisoning. Staphylococcal septicaemia is usually a consequence of local infection and may sometimes be associated with intravascular or intraperitoneal catheters or with intravenous drug abuse. Septicaemia often results in staphylococcal endocarditis. Other possible complications of septicaemia are pneumonia and bone and joint infections, although in these cases aspiration or local trauma, respectively, may be the cause.

*Staph. epidermidis* is also a natural inhabitant of skin and mucous membranes and an increasingly important nosocomial pathogen. Many infections are hospital-acquired and are often associated with indwelling catheters. There has been an increased incidence of bacteraemia due to *Staph. epidermidis* in neonatal units.

*Staph. saprophyticus* is a common cause of urinary-tract infections in young women.

Staphylococci were sensitive to benzylpenicillin when it was first introduced, but the majority of strains are now resistant as a result of penicillinase production. Meticillin and other penicillinase-resistant penicillins such as flucloxacillin were developed because of their activity against these resistant staphylococci. However, meticillin-resistant staphylococci soon emerged. Both coagulase-negative staphylococci and *Staph. aureus* resistant to meticillin are generally resistant to all beta lactams and often exhibit multiple resistance to other antibacterials (see Meticillin, p.230). More studies have been published on meticillin-resistant *Staph. aureus* (MRSA) than meticillin-resistant coagulase-negative staphylococci, but both types are a serious problem in hospitals around the world. Resistant strains may be endemic to a single hospital or may be epidemic causing outbreaks of infection at more than one hospital. Colonisation of hospital staff and patients with meticillin-resistant staphylococci is an important factor in the spread of these infections. Current trends are towards health care at home rather than in hospital and there are reports suggesting that MRSA is becoming more prevalent in the community.[1-5]

Revised guidelines[6] for the control of MRSA in hospital were produced by a combined working party of the British Society for Antimicrobial Chemotherapy, the Hospital Infection Society, and the Infection Control Nurses Association in 1998. They advise prompt isolation of infected or colonised patients, screening of patients and staff in contact with such patients, the use of protective clothing, handwashing with an antiseptic detergent or alcoholic rub, and the use by all patients of an antiseptic detergent for washing and bathing. For eradication of nasal carriage they recommend mupirocin nasal ointment or, if the strain is mupirocin-resistant, chlorhexidine and neomycin cream. Eradication at other colonised sites is more difficult: antiseptic detergents may be used for skin and hair washing; mupirocin in a macrogol basis for small infected skin lesions, but not for burns or large raw areas; hexachlorophene dusting powder for axillae and groins; and systemic rifampicin with fusidic acid or ciprofloxacin for throat or sputum colonisation if absolutely necessary.[6] However, a systematic review[7] has concluded that there is insufficient evidence to support the use of topical or systemic antimicrobial therapy for eradicating nasal or extra-nasal MRSA. For the treatment of severe infections due to MRSA the UK guidelines[6] recommend vancomycin or teicoplanin, possibly combined with rifampicin, as the treatment of choice.

Although ciprofloxacin may be used the emergence of widespread resistance in meticillin-sensitive and meticillin-resistant *Staph. aureus* limits its usefulness (see p.190). Combination therapy may be helpful. Rifampicin is highly active against MRSA, but it must always be used in combination with another drug to prevent the emergence of resistance. Combinations of rifampicin with gentamicin, vancomycin, co-trimoxazole, fusidic acid, quinolones, or novobiocin have been tried. Newer antibacterials such as linezolid or quinupristin/dalfopristin may be effective and may assume increasing importance.

Isolated reports from around the world of MRSA with intermediate resistance or reduced susceptibility to vancomycin initially emerged in the late 1990s,[8-10] and in response the CDC produced interim[11] and later[12] guidelines for preventing the spread of vancomycin-intermediate *Staph. aureus* (VISA) and vancomycin-resistant *Staph. aureus* (VRSA).

Staphylococcal vaccines have been used for the prophylaxis and treatment of staphylococcal infections.

For the management of staphylococcal infections in general, see under the specific disease headings.


1. Rosenberg J. Methicillin-resistant Staphylococcus aureus (MRSA) in the community: who's watching? *Lancet* 1995; **346:** 132–3.
2. Herold BC, *et al.* Community-acquired methicillin-resistant Staphylococcus aureus in children with no identified predisposing risk. *JAMA* 1998; **279:** 593–8.
3. Collignon P, *et al.* Community-acquired meticillin-resistant Staphylococcus aureus in Australia. *Lancet* 1998; **352:** 145–6.
4. Lowy FD. Staphylococcus aureus infections. *N Engl J Med* 1998; **339:** 520–32.
5. Salgado CD, *et al.* Community-acquired methicillin-resistant Staphylococcus aureus: a meta-analysis of prevalence and risk factors. *Clin Infect Dis* 2003; **36:** 131–9.
6. Combined Working Party of the British Society for Antimicrobial Chemotherapy, the Hospital Infection Society and the Infection Control Nurses Association. Revised guidelines for the control of methicillin-resistant Staphylococcus aureus infection in hospitals. *J Hosp Infect* 1998; **39:** 253–90. Correction. *ibid.* 1999; **42:** 83.
7. Loeb M, *et al.* Antimicrobial drugs for treating methicillin-resistant Staphylococcus aureus colonization. Available in The Cochrane Library; Issue 2. Chichester: John Wiley; 2004.
8. CDC. Update: Staphylococcus aureus with reduced susceptibility to vancomycin—United States, 1997. *MMWR* 1997; **46:** 813–15.
9. Smith TL, *et al.* Emergence of vancomycin resistance in Staphylococcus aureus. *N Engl J Med* 1999; **340:** 493–501.
10. Rybak MJ, Akins RL. Emergence of methicillin-resistant Staphylococcus aureus with intermediate glycopeptide resistance: clinical significance and treatment options. *Drugs* 2001; **61:** 1–7.
11. CDC. Interim guidelines for prevention and control of staphylococcal infection associated with reduced susceptibility to vancomycin. *MMWR* 1997; **46:** 626–8, 635. Also available at: http://www.cdc.gov/mmwr//preview/mmwrhtml/00048384.htm (accessed 21/05/04)
12. CDC. Investigation and control of vancomycin-intermediate and resistant Staphylococcus aureus (VISA/VRSA): a guide for health departments and infection control personnel. Available at: http://www.cdc.gov/ncidod/hip/ARESIST/visa_vrsa_guide.pdf (accessed 21/05/04)


## Surgical infection

Infection is an important cause of postoperative surgical morbidity and mortality and *antimicrobial prophylaxis* is one of several strategies used to reduce the risk of infection. The value of infection prophylaxis is well established in certain types of surgery, especially abdominal surgery and where prostheses are implanted, although recommendations as to the choice of antibacterial and the route, timing, and duration of administration may vary. Surgical wounds are classified as clean, clean-contaminated (potentially contaminated), contaminated, and those following 'dirty operations'. Clean operations exclude those involving the gastrointestinal, genital, urinary, or respiratory tracts. Clean-contaminated operations include those where the gastrointestinal, genital, urinary, or respiratory tracts are opened, but without unusual contamination. Contaminated operations include those where there is acute inflammation or spillage from a hollow viscus. Dirty operations include those where there is pus, gangrene, or perforated viscera. In addition, surgery to repair compound fractures and lacerations due to animal or human bites is considered dirty. The use of antibacterials for the management of contaminated or dirty surgery is considered to be therapeutic rather than prophylactic[1,2] and should continue for several days postoperatively.[3]

Guidelines for the *treatment* of intra-abdominal infections have been produced in the USA by the Surgical Infection Society.[4]

ANTIMICROBIAL PROPHYLAXIS. Strictly speaking the term 'prophylaxis' should be confined to elective procedures with no evidence of sepsis at the time of operation. If possible any pre-existing infections should be treated before admission for surgery. For prophylaxis it is customary to give antibacterials systemically as a single pre-operative dose whereas more prolonged administration is necessary when they are given therapeutically. Antimicrobial prophylaxis is used in clean-contaminated operations and in clean operations that involve the insertion of prosthetic materials or when an infection, however unlikely, would be catastrophic.[1]

**Contaminating organisms**. The choice of prophylactic antibacterial will be influenced by the likely contaminants for a particular surgical procedure. The most frequently isolated pathogens include *Staphylococcus aureus*, coagulase-negative staphylococci, *Enterococcus* spp., and *Escherichia coli*. Infections with antimicrobial-resistant pathogens including *Candida albicans* and meticillin-resistant *Staph. aureus* (MRSA) are increasing in some hospitals.[1] The most common source of infection is the endogenous flora of the patient's skin, mucous membranes, or viscera. Thus, aerobic Gram-positive organisms (for example staphylococci) are common infecting organisms when the source is the skin and mucous membranes, while infections with enterococci, Gram-negative aerobes (for example *E. coli*), and anaerobic bacteria (for example *Bacteroides fragilis*) can arise from the gastrointestinal tract.

**Route of administration**. Systemic administration, usually by the intravenous route, is generally preferred. The chosen antibacterial is usually given as a single dose intravenously just before operation at the induction of anaesthesia. The pharmacokinetic properties should be such that adequate serum concentrations are maintained throughout the surgical procedure.[1] Additional doses may be necessary when surgery is prolonged, when there is massive blood loss, or when an antibacterial with a short half-life is used.[3] More controversial routes have included topical or intra-incisional administration and peritoneal lavage. Oral administration of non-absorbable antibacterials to suppress the intestinal flora was traditionally used before large bowel surgery and neomycin with erythromycin is still given for this purpose in the USA. For reference to selective digestive tract decontamination (SDD), see under Intensive Care, p.132. Other means of administration include bone cement and chains of beads for implantation, both containing gentamicin and used prophylactically in orthopaedic surgery,[5,6] and topical and sometimes subconjunctival antibacterials for ophthalmic surgery.[3]

**Choice of antibacterial.** The most commonly used antibacterials are cephalosporins, aminoglycosides, and metronidazole. In the UK, gentamicin or cefuroxime is given before abdominal surgery; before colorectal surgery or hysterectomy metronidazole is given in addition, or amoxicillin with clavulanic acid may be given alone; before endoscopic retrograde cholangiopancreatography gentamicin or ciprofloxacin may be given; and before joint replacements, including the hip and knee, cefuroxime or flucloxacillin. In the USA, cefazolin is commonly given before surgery, except that involving the lower gastrointestinal tract, for which cefoxitin or cefotetan are used to provide activity against anaerobes.[1-3,7] Alternatively, cefazolin may be given with metronidazole in colorectal surgery.[3] The choice of prophylaxis for patients unable to tolerate cephalosporins is less well established. Aztreonam has been suggested as an alternative to cefazolin with the addition of clindamycin or metronidazole if activity against anaerobes is necessary.[1] However, the use of aztreonam plus metronidazole may provide inadequate activity against Gram-positive cocci.[7] Another suggested alternative to cefazolin is vancomycin,[3] but the routine use of vancomycin should be avoided because of the risk of inducing resistance.[8] Vancomycin may be indicated for high-risk procedures if MRSA infections are prevalent,[8] and combination with aztreonam or an aminoglycoside has been suggested to provide activity against Gram-negative organisms.[7] If vancomycin is used for prophylaxis, no more than two doses should be given.[8] Other alternatives for colorectal procedures include an aminoglycoside with either clindamycin or metronidazole.[7]

The necessity for antibacterial prophylaxis in minimally invasive procedures such as laparoscopy and endoscopy is often not clear.[9] US guidelines[1,7] suggest that standard prophylaxis should be used pending further evidence.

Certain categories of patient continue to be at long-term risk of infection after surgery and include splenectomised patients who have impaired immunity and are at risk of pneumococcal and other infections (see under Spleen Disorders, p.146). Patients at special risk of endocarditis require prophylaxis when undergoing dental and some surgical procedures (see Endocarditis, p.125). Some have advocated similar prophylaxis in patients with joint prostheses undergoing dental treatment,[10] but a working party for the British Society for Antimicrobial Chemotherapy considers such prophylaxis to be unjustified.[11]

1. Mangram AJ, *et al.* Guideline for prevention of surgical site infection, 1999. *Infect Control Hosp Epidemiol* 1999; **20:** 250–78.
2. American Society of Health-System Pharmacists. ASHP therapeutic guidelines on antimicrobial prophylaxis in surgery. *Am J Health-Syst Pharm* 1999; **56:** 1839–88.
3. Anonymous. Antimicrobial prophylaxis in surgery. In: *Handbook of antimicrobial therapy.* 16th ed. New York: The Medical Letter, 2002: 55–63.
4. Mazuski JE, *et al.* The Surgical Infection Society guidelines on antimicrobial therapy for intra-abdominal infections: an executive summary. *Surg Infect (Larchmt)* 2002; **3:** 161–73.
5. Henry SL, Galloway KP. Local antibacterial therapy for the management of orthopaedic infections: pharmacokinetic considerations. *Clin Pharmacokinet* 1995; **29:** 36–45.
6. Wininger DA, Fass RJ. Antibiotic-impregnated cement and beads for orthopedic infections. *Antimicrob Agents Chemother* 1996; **40:** 2675–9.
7. Dellinger EP, *et al.* Quality standard for antimicrobial prophylaxis in surgical procedures. *Clin Infect Dis* 1994; **18:** 422–7.
8. CDC. Recommendations for preventing the spread of vancomycin resistance: recommendations of the Hospital Infection Control Practices Advisory Committee (HICPAC). *MMWR* 1995; **44** (RR-12): 1–13. Also available at: http://www.cdc.gov/mmwr//PDF/rr/rr4412.pdf (accessed 21/05/04)
9. Wilson APR. Antibiotic prophylaxis and infection control measures in minimally invasive surgery. *J Antimicrob Chemother* 1995; **36:** 1–5.
10. Grant A, Hoddinott C. Joint replacement, dental surgery, and antibiotic prophylaxis. *BMJ* 1992; **304:** 959.
11. Simmons NA, *et al.* Case against antibiotic prophylaxis for dental treatment of patients with joint prostheses. *Lancet* 1992; **339:** 301.

## Syphilis

Syphilis is a sexually transmitted disease caused by the spirochaete *Treponema pallidum* and occurs worldwide. Non-venereal treponematoses, occurring principally in the tropics, include endemic syphilis or bejel, also caused by *T. pallidum*; pinta, caused by *T. carateum*; and yaws, caused by *T. pertenue*.

Syphilis may be acquired or congenital and in each case has early and late stages. Syphilis may be described as latent, when serological and CSF tests are positive but the patient is asymptomatic. In acquired sexually transmitted disease the *early* stage includes primary and secondary syphilis and early latent infection; early latent infection is defined as of not more than 2 years' duration in the UK[1] and by WHO,[2,3] or of less than 1 year's duration by the Centers for Disease Control (CDC) in the USA.[4] *Late* stage disease includes late latent infection and all late clinical stages. The late clinical stages fall broadly into three types: *neurosyphilis* manifesting as neurological symptoms, commonly including dorsal column loss (tabes dorsalis), dementia, or meningovascular involvement; *cardiovascular* syphilis, characterised by aortitis which may manifest as aortic regurgitation, aortic aneurysm, or angina; and *gummata*, inflammatory fibrous nodules or plaques which may be locally destructive and which commonly affect the bone and skin but may occur in any organ. Some term all these late clinical stages tertiary syphilis whereas others use tertiary for benign gummatous syphilis and quaternary for the more serious complications of cardiovascular syphilis and neurosyphilis. The term neurosyphilis has generally been applied to late-stage symptomatic neurological disease, although it is recognised that CNS invasion by *T. pallidum* is common in early syphilis and that CNS involvement may occur at any stage.

The incidence of syphilis fell dramatically after the introduction of penicillin and *T. pallidum* remains sensitive to it. There has, however, been a resurgence of syphilis, linked in part with HIV infection. In HIV-infected patients syphilis appears more virulent and neurosyphilis occurs more quickly. Like other diseases causing genital ulcers, syphilis is a risk factor for HIV infection.

The **treatment** of choice for both early and late syphilis is still penicillin and long-acting injections are generally used. WHO guidelines[3] recommend either benzathine benzylpenicillin or procaine benzylpenicillin. The preferred penicillin in the UK is procaine benzylpenicillin[1,5] although it is no longer commercially available. Benzathine benzylpenicillin is preferred in the USA.[4] Treatment for late syphilis is less well-established than that for early disease and is usually for longer. Benzylpenicillin may be preferred for neurosyphilis and congenital syphilis. For a summary of WHO, UK, and US treatment guidelines, see below.

CSF involvement is common in early syphilis and in the USA neurosyphilis has become more prevalent, especially among HIV-infected patients. In the UK, CSF abnormalities are uncommon after treatment for early syphilis and the prevalence of late syphilis, including neurosyphilis, remains low. The lower incidence of neurosyphilis throughout Europe may have been attributable to the use of more intensive treatment courses for early syphilis than is customary in the USA, and to the choice of penicillin. In addition, since neither benzathine benzylpenicillin nor procaine benzylpenicillin achieve treponemicidal concentrations in the CNS during standard regimens, host immune responses may play an essential part. The use of multidose or augmented treatment regimens in the USA has not generally been associated with improved clinical response.[6-8] In the UK, treatment of all cases of syphilis in HIV-infected patients as for neurosyphilis is advised;[1] in the USA, standard treatment is considered sufficient (see below for details).[4]

Patients *allergic to penicillin* have been given a tetracycline or erythromycin or azithromycin although their efficacy is less well established.

A Jarisch-Herxheimer reaction may occur after the first dose of antibacterial, especially in patients with early syphilis, and corticosteroid cover may be beneficial, especially in patients with cardiovascular or neurological involvement.

*Congenital syphilis* may result from transplacental infection at any stage of pregnancy and any stage of maternal syphilis. There has been a dramatic increase in its incidence in the USA and renewed concern about the efficacy of treatment with benzathine benzylpenicillin.[9] Benzylpenicillin or procaine benzylpenicillin are preferred to benzathine benzylpenicillin for infants with congenital syphilis.[1-4]

Recommended **treatment regimens** from WHO,[3] UK,[1,5] and USA[4] for acquired and congenital syphilis are as follows. Sexual partners should be examined and treated.

- EARLY SYPHILIS

**WHO**: benzathine benzylpenicillin 1.8 g (2.4 million units) intramuscularly in a single session, usually given as 2 injections at separate sites, or procaine benzylpenicillin 1.2 g (1.2 million units) intramuscularly daily for 10 days. Alternatives for non-pregnant penicillin-allergic patients: doxycycline 100 mg orally twice daily for 14 days or tetracycline hydrochloride 500 mg by mouth four times daily for 14 days. Pregnant women allergic to penicillin may be given erythromycin 500 mg orally four times daily for 14 days (but see below).

**UK**: procaine benzylpenicillin 750 mg (750 000 units) intramuscularly daily for 10 days, or benzathine benzylpenicillin 1.8 g (2.4 million units) intramuscularly as a single dose or repeated after 7 days. Procaine benzylpenicillin may be given as a multi-ingredient preparation also containing benzylpenicillin. Additional alternative if parenteral therapy is refused: amoxicillin 500 mg plus probenecid 500 mg each four times daily orally for 14 days. Alternatives for penicillin-allergic patients: oral doxycycline 100 mg twice daily for 14 days, or oral erythromycin 500 mg four times daily for 14 days. Further options for penicillin-allergic patients are azithromycin 500 mg daily orally or, in the absence of anaphylaxis to penicillin, intramuscular ceftriaxone 500 mg daily, each for 10 days.

**USA**: benzathine benzylpenicillin 1.8 g (2.4 million units) intramuscularly in a single dose. Alternatives for penicillin-allergic patients: doxycycline 100 mg twice daily, or tetracycline 500 mg four times daily, each by mouth for 14 days; preliminary data suggest that azithromycin 2 g orally as a single dose may also be effective; as a further option ceftriaxone may also be considered.

- LATE SYPHILIS

**WHO**: benzathine benzylpenicillin 1.8 g (2.4 million units) intramuscularly once weekly for 3 consecutive weeks or procaine benzylpenicillin 1.2 g (1.2 million units) intramuscularly daily for 20 consecutive days. Alternatives for non-pregnant penicillin-allergic patients are doxycycline 100 mg twice daily, or tetracycline 500 mg four times daily, each orally for 30 days. Pregnant women allergic to penicillin may be given erythromycin 500 mg four times daily for 30 days. For those with neurosyphilis: benzylpenicillin 1.2 to 2.4 g (2 to 4 million units) intravenously every 4 hours for 14 days, or, if compliance can be ensured, procaine benzylpenicillin 1.2 g (1.2 million units) intramuscularly daily plus probenecid 500 mg orally four times daily for 10 to 14 days; non-pregnant penicillin-allergic patients may be given doxycycline 200 mg twice daily, or tetracycline 500 mg four times daily, each orally for 30 days.

**UK**: first-line therapy: procaine benzylpenicillin 750 mg (750 000 units) intramuscularly daily for 17 days. Alternative: benzathine benzylpenicillin 2.4 g (3.2 million units) intramuscularly weekly for 3 doses. Second-line therapy for patients allergic to penicillin and those declining parenteral therapy: doxycycline 200 mg orally twice daily for 28 days. Alternative if penicillin can be tolerated: amoxicillin 2 g orally three times daily plus probenecid 500 mg four times daily, both for 28 days. For neurosyphilis: procaine benzylpenicillin 2 g (2 million units) intramuscularly once daily plus probenecid 500 mg orally four times daily for 17 days. Alternative: benzylpenicillin 1.8 to 2.4 g (3 to 4 million units) intravenously every 4 hours for 17 days. Second-line therapies for neurosyphilis: doxycycline 200 mg orally twice daily for 28 days, or amoxicillin 2 g three times daily plus probenecid 500 mg four times daily, both orally, for 28 days.

**USA**: benzathine benzylpenicillin 1.8 g (2.4 million units) intramuscularly weekly for 3 consecutive weeks. Alternatives in penicillin-allergic patients: doxycycline 100 mg twice daily or tetracycline 500 mg four times daily, each orally for 28 days. For those with neurosyphilis: benzylpenicillin 1.8 to 2.4 g (3 to 4 million units) intravenously every 4 hours for 10 to 14 days (or the total daily dose may be given by continuous infusion). Alternative for neurosyphilis if outpatient compliance can be ensured: procaine benzylpenicillin 2.4 g (2.4 million units) intramuscularly daily plus probenecid 500 mg orally four times daily, both for 10 to 14 days. Since the duration of treatment for neurosyphilis is shorter than that for late syphilis in the absence of neurosyphilis, some clinicians give benzathine benzylpenicillin 1.8 g (2.4 million units) once weekly for up to 3 weeks after completion of neurosyphilis treatment to provide a comparable total duration of treatment.

• SYPHILIS IN PREGNANCY

All guidelines recommend penicillin as under early and late syphilis, together with close surveillance. In the USA, CDC[4] note that some recommend a second dose of benzathine benzylpenicillin a week after the initial dose for patients with early syphilis. According to CDC,[4] pregnant patients who are allergic to penicillin should be given penicillin, after desensitisation if necessary, since the alternatives, tetracyclines, are contra-indicated during pregnancy and erythromycin cannot be relied upon to cure an infected fetus. WHO,[3] on the other hand, advise against desensitisation in a primary care setting and suggest that erythromycin, although inferior, should be given in these circumstances; consideration should probably be given to use of a third-generation cephalosporin in the absence of anaphylaxis. Following treatment, the mother should be re-treated if there is serological evidence of re-infection or relapse, and the infant treated.[3] Similar advice to that of WHO is given in the UK.

• CONGENITAL SYPHILIS

**WHO**: for early congenital syphilis in infants up to 2 years of age and having abnormal CSF: benzylpenicillin 30 mg/kg (50 000 units/kg) intravenously twice daily for the first 7 days of life and three times daily thereafter for a total of 10 days, or procaine benzylpenicillin 50 mg/kg (50 000 units/kg) intramuscularly once daily for 10 days. For infants with normal CSF: benzathine benzylpenicillin 37.5 mg/kg (50 000 units/kg) intramuscularly as a single-session treatment (although some treat all infants as if the CSF were abnormal). Children older than 2 years: benzylpenicillin 120 to 180 mg/kg (200 000 to 300 000 units/kg) intramuscularly or intravenously daily in 4 or 6 divided doses for 10 to 14 days. An alternative regimen for penicillin-allergic infants aged over 1 month is erythromycin 7.5 to 12.5 mg/kg by mouth four times daily for 30 days.

**UK**: as for infants up to 2 years with abnormal CSF in WHO guidelines, above. Procaine benzylpenicillin may be given as a multi-ingredient preparation also containing benzylpenicillin.

**USA**: as for infants up to 2 years with abnormal and with normal CSF in WHO guidelines, above. Older infants and children thought to have congenital syphilis or neurological involvement should be given benzylpenicillin 30 mg/kg (50 000 units/kg) every 4 to 6 hours for 10 days.

• NON-VENEREAL TREPONEMATOSES

When the prevalence of endemic syphilis (bejel), pinta, or yaws is 10% or more WHO[2] recommend mass treatment of the entire population with a single intramuscular injection of benzathine benzylpenicillin 900 mg (1.2 million units) or half this dose in children under 10 years.

1. Clinical Effectiveness Group (Association for Genitourinary Medicine and the Medical Society for the Study of Venereal Diseases). UK national guidelines on the management of early syphilis. Available at: http://www.bashh.org/guidelines/2002/early$final0502.pdf (accessed 21/05/04)
2. WHO. WHO expert committee on venereal diseases and treponematoses: sixth report. *WHO Tech Rep Ser 736* 1986: 126–39.
3. WHO. Guidelines for the management of sexually transmitted infections. Geneva: WHO, 2003. Also available at: http://whqlibdoc.who.int/publications/2003/9241546263.pdf (accessed 22/06/04)
4. Centers for Disease Control. Sexually transmitted diseases treatment guidelines 2002. *MMWR* 2002; **51**(RR-6): 1–80. Also available at: http://www.cdc.gov/mmwr/PDF/rr/rr5106.pdf (accessed 21/05/04)
5. Clinical Effectiveness Group (Association for Genitourinary Medicine and the Medical Society for the Study of Venereal Diseases). UK national guideline for the management of late syphilis. Available at: http://www.bashh.org/guidelines/2002/late%20$%20final%20b%2031%2012%2002.pdf (accessed 21/05/04)
6. Malone JL, *et al.* Syphilis and neurosyphilis in a human immunodeficiency virus type-1 seropositive population: evidence for frequent serologic relapse after therapy. *Am J Med* 1995; **99:** 55–63.
7. Gordon SM, *et al.* The response of symptomatic neurosyphilis to high-dose intravenous penicillin G in patients with human immunodeficiency virus infection. *N Engl J Med* 1994; **331:** 1469–73.
8. Rolfs RT, *et al.* A randomized trial of enhanced therapy for early syphilis in patients with and without human immunodeficiency virus infection. *N Engl J Med* 1997; **337:** 307–14.
9. Ikeda MK, Janson HB. Evaluation and treatment of congenital syphilis. *J Pediatr* 1990; **117:** 843–52.

## Tetanus

*Clostridium tetani* is a Gram-positive anaerobic spore-forming bacillus present in soil and faeces. The toxin it produces, tetanospasmin, causes tetanus or lockjaw, with uncontrolled muscle spasm. Tetanus can be prevented by active immunisation with tetanus vaccine or passive immunisation with tetanus immunoglobulin. Nowadays it occurs predominantly in developing countries and especially in neonates. In developed countries immunity may be relatively low in the elderly.

In addition to the control of muscle spasm with drugs such as diazepam (see p.1398 for the symptomatic treatment of tetanus), treatment includes the use of tetanus immunoglobulin to neutralise any circulating toxin and the administration of antibacterials. Benzylpenicillin has traditionally been used, with a tetracycline or metronidazole as possible alternatives, but some now consider metronidazole to be preferable to benzylpenicillin.[1-3]

In rural developing countries where tetanus is common and active immunisation little practised, pre-operative metronidazole or penicillin might be used for patients undergoing emergency operations who have not been immunised against tetanus; the duration of antibacterial cover depends on the contamination risk.[4]

1. Ahmadsyah I, Salim A. Treatment of tetanus: an open study to compare the efficacy of procaine penicillin and metronidazole. *BMJ* 1985; **291:** 648–50.
2. Sanford JP. Tetanus—forgotten but not gone. *N Engl J Med* 1995; **332:** 812–13.
3. Anonymous. The choice of antibacterial drugs. In: *Handbook of antimicrobial therapy.* 16th ed. New York: The Medical Letter, 2002: 34–52.
4. Anonymous. Postoperative tetanus. *Lancet* 1984; **ii:** 964–5.

## Tonsillitis

See under Pharyngitis, p.140.

## Toxic shock syndrome

Toxic shock syndrome is an acute febrile illness associated with multisystem failure and caused by a toxin, usually toxic shock syndrome toxin-1 (TSST-1), produced by *Staphylococcus aureus*.[1,2] Bacteraemia has been reported to be absent in most cases.[3] In the early 1980s, toxic shock syndrome was reported predominantly in menstruating women using high-absorbency tampons, but it is now appreciated that foci of staphylococcal infection such as surgical wounds, burns, abscesses, and sinuses are often responsible.[1,2] Treatment of the acute phase requires prevention of further production or absorption of toxin by local measures such as removal of tampons or packing, wound debridement, or drainage of abscesses; elimination of the toxin-producing bacteria by antistaphylococcal antibacterials given intravenously initially; fluid replacement; and sometimes corticosteroids.[1,2] Continuing antibacterial treatment for 10 days during the convalescent phase to reduce the risk of recurrence has been recommended.[1]

Group A beta-haemolytic streptococci (*Streptococcus pyogenes*) have been associated with a similar toxin-related syndrome.[4,5] Benzylpenicillin is the treatment of choice[6] but, since it may be difficult to exclude staphylococcal toxic shock syndrome, an antistaphylococcal drug such as flucloxacillin should also be given.[6] Clinical improvement has been reported after administration of intravenous normal immunoglobulins.[7,8]

Toxic shock syndromes may be associated with necrotising fasciitis (see p.136).

1. Todd JK. Therapy of toxic shock syndrome. *Drugs* 1990; **39:** 856–61.
2. Williams GR. The toxic shock syndrome. *BMJ* 1990; **300:** 960.
3. Eykyn SJ. Staphylococcal sepsis: the changing pattern of disease and therapy. *Lancet* 1988; **i:** 100–4.
4. Cone LA, *et al.* Clinical and bacteriologic observations of a toxic shock-like syndrome due to Streptococcus pyogenes. *N Engl J Med* 1987; **317:** 146–9.
5. Stevens DL, *et al.* Severe group A streptococcal infections associated with a toxic shock-like syndrome and scarlet fever toxin A. *N Engl J Med* 1989; **321:** 1–7.
6. Sanderson P. Do streptococci cause toxic shock? *BMJ* 1990; **301:** 1006–7.
7. Barry W, *et al.* Intravenous immunoglobulin therapy for toxic shock syndrome. *JAMA* 1992; **267:** 3315–16.
8. Kaul R, *et al.* Intravenous immunoglobulin therapy for streptococcal toxic shock syndrome—a comparative observational study. *Clin Infect Dis* 1999; **28:** 800–7.

## Trachoma

Trachoma[1] results from chronic eye infection with certain *Chlamydia trachomatis* serotypes and is endemic in parts of Africa, the Middle East, and India where it is an important cause of blindness. It is not a sexually transmitted disease, but is associated with poverty, poor sanitation, and poor personal hygiene. The reservoir is chronic eye infection and transmission may be via fingers, fomites, and flies. Inclusion conjunctivitis in infants (see under Neonatal Conjunctivitis, p.136) and in adults is associated with sexually transmitted genital *C. trachomatis* infection and can progress to trachoma when there is persistent or recurrent eye infection.

Guidelines for trachoma control published by WHO in 1981 outlined topical or oral treatment with a tetracycline or alternatively with erythromycin or a sulfonamide.[2] Topical chemotherapy for trachoma must be intensive and prolonged, 6 weeks being the minimum recommended duration for continuous intensive treatment with tetracycline 1% ophthalmic ointment. With less frequent applications, the duration of treatment must be prolonged and may need to be extended to months or even years. The recommended intermittent treatment schedule consists of applications of tetracycline twice daily for 5 consecutive days or once daily for 10 days each month for 6 months each year, to be repeated as necessary. Short courses with topical tetracyclines can be used for the control of bacterial infections during seasonal epidemics of conjunctivitis and may have to be repeated annually. Oral therapy with tetracycline or doxycycline for 3 to 4 weeks has also been effective for selective treatment in well monitored programmes. Erythromycin and related macrolides administered by mouth or topically to the eye have been of benefit in trachoma, but have been less widely used. Topical therapy with sulfonamides appears only partially effective; adequate treatment with oral sulfonamides requires full therapeutic doses for about 2 to 3 weeks and may be associated with adverse reactions.

A single oral dose of azithromycin produces a similar rate of resolution to conventional treatment with topical tetracycline for 6 weeks.[3] Mass treatment of African village communities with oral azithromycin once weekly for 3 weeks has resulted in a lower incidence of trachoma at follow-up after one year than a standard course of topical tetracycline.[4,5] Many[6] now recommend azithromycin as the treatment of choice for trachoma, with combined oral and topical treatment with either a tetracycline or a sulfonamide as an alternative.

WHO[7,8] has developed the International Trachoma Initiative of which the SAFE strategy (surgery, azithromycin, facial cleanliness, and environmental improvements) is the cornerstone. The aim is to eliminate trachoma by 2020. Tetracycline is still, however, the antibacterial treatment of choice in those countries that are not yet part of the initiative program and for patients in whom azithromycin is contra-indicated.

A vaccine against *C. trachomatis* is also under investigation.[9]

1. Mabey DCW, *et al.* Trachoma. *Lancet* 2003; **362:** 223–9.
2. Dawson CR, *et al. Guide to trachoma control.* Geneva: WHO, 1981.
3. Bailey RL, *et al.* Randomised controlled trial of single-dose azithromycin in treatment of trachoma. *Lancet* 1993; **342:** 453–6.
4. Schachter J, *et al.* Azithromycin in control of trachoma. *Lancet* 1999; **354:** 630–5.
5. Fraser-Hurt N, *et al.* Efficacy of oral azithromycin versus topical tetracycline in mass treatment of endemic trachoma. *Bull WHO* 2001; **79:** 632–40.
6. Anonymous. The choice of antibacterial drugs. In: *Handbook of antimicrobial therapy.* 16th ed. New York: The Medical Letter, 2002: 34–52.
7. Bailey R, Lietman T. The SAFE strategy for the elimination of trachoma by 2020: will it work? *Bull WHO* 2001; **79:** 233–6.

8. WHO. International Trachoma Initiative. Available at: http://www.trachoma.org/home.asp (accessed 21/05/04)
9. Coghlan A. Shapely vaccine targets chlamydia. *New Scientist* 1996; **152:** 18.

### Trench fever

Trench fever is a louse-borne bacterial infection so named because of its prevalence among soldiers in the First World War. It is caused by *Bartonella quintana* (formerly *Rochalimaea quintana*) which was until recently classified as a rickettsia. *B. quintana* and *B. henselae* have also been implicated in bacillary angiomatosis, especially in immunocompromised patients, and *B. henselae* is considered to be a cause of cat scratch disease (p.123).

Reports from France[1,2] and the USA[3] of *B. quintana* bacteraemia, sometimes with endocarditis, in the urban poor prompted the suggestion that trench fever has returned.[4,5] Cases of trench fever in Marseilles have been reported[2] and might herald an increasing incidence as a result of migration from endemic areas, poverty, and louse infestation.

Treatment of trench fever has usually been with a tetracycline such as doxycycline or with a macrolide such as erythromycin. Other antibacterials, for example ceftriaxone, were also used in cases of bacteraemia,[3] but there was limited follow-up and clear recommendations could not be given. Similarly, optimal therapy for *Bartonella* endocarditis has not been identified; however, it has been suggested that the usual treatment for blood culture-negative endocarditis (a penicillin plus an aminoglycoside) should be effective.[6]

1. Drancourt M, *et al.* Bartonella (Rochalimaea) quintana endocarditis in three homeless men. *N Engl J Med* 1995; **332:** 419–23.
2. Brouqui P, *et al.* Chronic Bartonella quintana bacteremia in homeless patients. *N Engl J Med* 1999; **340:** 184–9.
3. Spach DH, *et al.* Bartonella (Rochalimaea) quintana bacteremia in inner-city patients with chronic alcoholism. *N Engl J Med* 1995; **332:** 424–8.
4. Relman DA. Has trench fever returned? *N Engl J Med* 1995; **332:** 463–4.
5. Ohl ME, Spach DH. Bartonella quintana and urban trench fever. *Clin Infect Dis* 2000; **31:** 131–5.
6. Raoult D, *et al.* Diagnosis of 22 new cases of Bartonella endocarditis. *Ann Intern Med* 1996; **125:** 646–52. Correction. *ibid.* 1997; **127:** 249.

### Tuberculosis

Tuberculosis is a chronic infectious disease caused primarily by *Mycobacterium tuberculosis* or sometimes *M. bovis*; the closely related form *M. africanum* has occasionally been implicated as a cause of human tuberculosis. Infection is usually due to inhalation of infected droplet nuclei and the lung is generally the first organ affected. The primary infection is usually asymptomatic.

In the majority of subjects infection and concomitant inflammatory reactions resolve once acquired immunity develops and any surviving organisms become dormant, but in some patients, particularly in young children or immunocompromised patients, there may be a progression to active primary disease. Dormant organisms may also become reactivated in some patients to produce disease, particularly following changes in immune status. Hypersensitivity reactions to mycobacterial proteins may cause extensive tissue damage, and virtually any organ of the body can be involved.

During recent years there has been an increase in the incidence of tuberculosis, particularly among the urban poor, and also in association with the spread of HIV infection. WHO declared tuberculosis a global emergency in 1993. Particularly worrying is the increase in multidrug-resistant strains (see below) and poor compliance with drug treatment is seen as a contributory factor. In the USA, there has been emphasis on improving compliance with drug therapy and monitoring responses to limit the further spread of multidrug-resistant disease. Direct supervision of treatment has been shown to be effective in both urban and rural settings, and generally a higher proportion of patients complete treatment under direct observation than with unsupervised treatment. However, directly observed treatment has not been successful in all settings, and cultural and social attitudes are influential. Attempts have been made to simplify drug regimens, including the use of intermittent therapy and combination preparations, and fixed dose combination tablets are recommended by WHO to aid compliance.[1] The feasibility of implantable dosage forms has also been investigated.[2]

WHO applies the term DOTS to its tuberculosis control strategy which includes standards for diagnosis, ensuring secure drug supplies, and evaluating implementation in addition to the use of directly observed short course treatment regimens; it is also used as an acronym for directly observed treatment, short-course. A survey has shown that countries adopting the WHO strategy achieve higher cure rates than those that do not.[3]

**Treatment**. The introduction of rifampicin, with its rapid bactericidal activity, in the 1970s allowed the development of short-course therapy for tuberculosis. Treatment regimens formerly relied on oral daily isoniazid and thioacetazone for periods of 12 to 18 months supplemented by parenteral streptomycin for the first 2 months. Reasons for the high failure rate commonly encountered with such regimens included poor compliance, failure of streptomycin to suppress active disease during the initial treatment phase, and toxicity of the drugs used. Modern short-course therapy involves an initial phase (2 months) using a combination of drugs to produce rapid killing of the bacilli, and a continuation phase of 4 to 6 months using fewer drugs with the aim of eliminating any remaining organisms and thus preventing recurrence. The majority of patients have no organisms detectable in sputum after 2 months with this regimen.

• FIRST-LINE DRUGS

First-choice **antituberculous drugs**, often referred to as primary or 'first-line' drugs include isoniazid, rifampicin, pyrazinamide, ethambutol, and streptomycin. Thioacetazone has also been regarded as a first-line drug in developing countries, but WHO recommends that ethambutol be substituted in patients with HIV infection whenever possible, since this patient group is at high risk of severe and sometimes fatal skin reactions with thioacetazone.[4] However, the suggestion that thioacetazone should be dropped for routine treatment[5,6] in general has proved controversial.[7,8]

The short-course regimens recommended by WHO combine drugs to ensure elimination of both metabolically active and dormant organisms: rifampicin and isoniazid are potent bactericides and one or both are used throughout the treatment course; pyrazinamide is bactericidal against intracellular organisms; and streptomycin and ethambutol are used to prevent the emergence of resistant strains. All first-line drugs except thioacetazone can be given intermittently as an alternative to daily administration.

WHO categorises patients according to the site and severity of the disease, results of the sputum smear, and whether or not the patient has received treatment previously; treatment is then recommended accordingly.[4,9] To ensure compliance, WHO considers direct observation of therapy to be essential during the initial phase and desirable in patients receiving rifampicin during the continuation phase.[4,9]

For **newly diagnosed patients** with active pulmonary tuberculosis and patients with severe tuberculosis at any site the following regimens are recommended: for the initial phase, isoniazid, rifampicin, and pyrazinamide plus either streptomycin or ethambutol daily for 2 months; then for the continuation phase either isoniazid plus rifampicin daily (or 3 times each week for both drugs for intermittent therapy) for a further 4 months or isoniazid plus ethambutol or thioacetazone daily for a further 6 months. (Ethambutol and streptomycin are omitted from the initial phase in some national guidelines for patient groups in whom the risk of drug resistance is small.)

For **re-treatment after relapse**, treatment failure, or default, patients should receive isoniazid, rifampicin, pyrazinamide, and ethambutol daily for 3 months, supplemented with streptomycin daily for the first 2 months as directly observed therapy (initial phase) then, if the sputum is smear-negative, isoniazid, rifampicin, and ethambutol daily (or 3 times each week for all drugs) for a further 5 months (continuation phase).

For patients with smear-negative pulmonary tuberculosis and patients with **less severe infections** at other sites the preferred regimen is isoniazid, rifamycin, and pyrazinamide daily for 2 months (initial phase) then either isoniazid and ethambutol daily for 6 months or isoniazid and rifampicin daily (or 3 times each week for both drugs) for 4 months (continuation phase).

Short-course therapy is unsuitable for patients who **remain smear-positive** despite supervised re-treatment. These patients usually require treatment with second-line drugs (see below).

The choice of regimen depends on local patterns of drug resistance and the availability of drugs and medical supervision, and are embodied in national and regional treatment protocols in many countries including Europe,[10] the UK,[11] and USA.[12,13] Recently there has been increased awareness of the potential hepatotoxicity of first-line drugs such as isoniazid, rifampicin, and particularly pyrazinamide. Pyrazinamide is generally regarded as being the most hepatotoxic of the three, and further details covering this and special precautions for its use in patients with liver disorders are given in the drug monograph (p.247). WHO and UK guidelines recommend interrupting drug therapy if liver dysfunction occurs, and cautiously re-introducing the same drugs (including pyrazinamide) on resolution.[4,14] Patients in whom complete cessation of therapy is hazardous may be given streptomycin and ethambutol until hepatic function recovers.

• SECOND-LINE DRUGS

Other drugs used in the treatment of tuberculosis, such as the aminosalicylates, capreomycin, cycloserine, ethionamide, protionamide, and kanamycin are considered to be secondary drugs and have been used if resistance or toxicity to first-line drugs develops during therapy, but are generally less effective and/or more toxic. The increasing problem of tuberculosis resistant to conventional first-line drugs has also led to increased interest in the development of new drugs, and use of existing drugs such as the fluoroquinolones, amoxicillin-clavulanic acid, and the rifamycin derivative rifabutin.

• RESISTANCE

The incidence of drug-resistant strains of *Mycobacterium tuberculosis* has increased steadily over recent years in many countries.[15,16] Isoniazid resistance is most common but multidrug-resistant strains have also occurred, often in HIV-infected individuals, resulting in disease which is very difficult to treat and often fatal. Such resistance is considered to result from poor management of tuberculosis control.

The key to controlling the development of multidrug-resistant tuberculosis is the adoption of the WHO DOTS programme,[17] but different strategies are necessary in areas where multidrug-resistance is established. In areas with a high rate of initial drug resistance, ethambutol or streptomycin is added during the initial phase;[4,9] drug selection may be re-evaluated once sensitivity results are available. As discussed above, patients who relapse after an initial treatment course are generally given a second prolonged and directly observed treatment course with first-line drugs. Patients who relapse following the WHO standard re-treatment regimen or who are otherwise suspected of having multidrug-resistant tuberculosis should receive at least three drugs, preferably four or five, which they have not already received and which do not share cross-resistance to drugs received previously; these should be given under direct observation for at least 3 months followed by a continuation phase of at least 18 months with at least 2 of the drugs. WHO recommends inclusion of an injectable aminoglycoside (amikacin, capreomycin, or kanamycin) and pyrazinamide, even if the patient has previously received it, in the initial phase.[18] Cross-resistance exists between fluoroquinolones, between cycloserine and terizidone, and between thioacetazone and protionamide or ethionamide.[18] Cross-resistance between rifampicin and rifabutin is also commonly observed. There appears to be no cross-resistance between fluoroquinolones and other antituberculous drugs, but fluoroquinolone-resistant tuberculosis can emerge rapidly as a result of inadequate or inappropriate treatment.[19] Cross-resistance patterns among aminoglycosides are complex.[18]

• CHILDREN

Children and infants can be treated with similar regimens to adults.[11-13] Ethambutol is not usually given to young children because of the perceived difficulty in detecting ocular toxicity in this age group although some clinicians have not found this to be a problem.[20]

• PREGNANCY AND THE NEONATE

Tuberculosis during pregnancy poses a serious risk to the mother, fetus, and neonate if not detected early and treated properly.[21] Pregnant patients with clinical tuberculosis are treated similarly to non-pregnant patients, although streptomycin, other aminoglycosides, and capreomycin should be avoided because they can cause ototoxicity in the fetus. Ethionamide and protionamide are also best avoided.[11] The importance of monitoring of liver enzymes and for symptoms of drug-induced hepatotoxicity should not be forgotten. Pregnant women who react positively to a tuberculin skin test, but who have a normal chest X-ray, may be offered immediate prophylaxis with isoniazid (see Preventive Therapy, below) if they have risk factors for tuberculosis; those without risk factors are referred for prophylaxis after delivery.[21]

Neonates of mothers with current tuberculosis should receive isoniazid for 6 weeks (UK)[22] or 6 months (USA)[13] after which time the infant should be re-evaluated. BCG vaccination is recommended by WHO and in the UK when isoniazid is stopped.[4,22]

• HIV INFECTION

Patients with HIV infection are particularly prone to active tubercular disease, both pulmonary and extrapulmonary, and mortality is higher than in HIV-negative patients.[4,23] Studies suggest that such patients respond well to conventional regimens.[24,25] However, low drug concentrations can occur[26] possibly due to malabsorption of antimycobacterials[27,28] (although it has not invariably been found[29]); malabsorption has been associated with acquired drug resistance.[30] Paradoxical worsening of symptoms has been reported in patients receiving concurrent treatment with antimycobacterials and antiretrovirals.[31] Also, there may be an increased incidence of adverse reactions to antimycobacterials in HIV-positive individuals,[24] particularly to thioacetazone.[32] WHO recommend that ethambutol should be used in place of both thioacetazone and streptomycin in patients with HIV infection.[4] Most regimens suggested for treating tuberculosis in patients with HIV infection are versions of standard short-course therapy with rifampicin, isoniazid, ethambutol, and pyrazinamide (see above), and most commentators emphasise the importance of directly observed therapy to ensure compliance.[33] It has been suggested that regimens omitting thioacetazone should be adopted for treatment of all patients regardless of HIV status, thus avoiding the necessity to test for HIV before starting treatment,[5,6] but this may not be practical in some developing countries.[7,8]

Drug interactions between rifamycins and antiretrovirals can complicate the choice of treatment.[34,35] In particular, rifamycins can reduce plasma concentrations of HIV-protease inhibitors to potentially subtherapeutic levels, and conversely, rifabutin concentrations may be increased to toxic levels (rifampicin is metabolised by a different mechanism and is not affected).

In patients who have not yet started antiretroviral therapy, it may be possible to delay it until treatment of tuberculosis is complete, but antiretroviral therapy, once started, should not be interrupted.[35] Alternatively, a regimen that does not contain a rifamycin may be used, although it is recommended that such regimens should continue for at least 9 months.[36] In addition, they typically include streptomycin and thus commit the patient to regular injections for 9 months which may jeopardize compliance. The non-rifamycin regimen recommended by the CDC consists of an initial phase of isoniazid, ethambutol, streptomycin, and pyrazinamide daily or daily then intermittently for 2 months, and a continuation phase of isoniazid, streptomycin, and pyrazinamide given 2 or 3 times weekly for 7 months.

CDC recommends that the duration of therapy (regardless of the regimen used) should be increased by a further 3 months in patients with a delayed response to treatment during the primary phase.[35]

Drug-resistant tuberculosis is a problem,[16] with up to 90% of cases of drug-resistant disease in the USA occurring in HIV-infected persons;[37] regimens must be modified as in non-HIV-infected patients. Multiple drug-resistant tuberculosis can be rapidly fatal in patients with HIV infection and early, effective treatment is essential, and should continue for 18 to 24 months after smears become negative.[38]

Prolonged or lifetime prophylaxis with isoniazid has been given to patients with HIV infection following the completion of tuberculosis treatment in the UK,[39] and has been shown to reduce the rate of recurrence in other countries.[40] Preventive therapy is also used in some countries to prevent first episodes of active disease (see below).

• ADJUNCTIVE THERAPY

Some, but not all, studies have suggested that injection of suspensions of killed *Mycobacterium vaccae* improved immune responsiveness in patients with pulmonary tuberculosis, and a systematic review[41] concluded that *M. vaccae* immunotherapy did not benefit patients with tuberculosis. Several other forms of **immunotherapy** have also been tried as adjuncts to conventional chemotherapy.

The use of **corticosteroids** in uncomplicated pulmonary tuberculosis should be avoided but they have a role in selected patients with severe pulmonary and severe extrapulmonary disease, and for patients with severe hypersensitivity reactions to antituberculous drugs.[4,42] They should never be given to patients with active disease without protective chemotherapy cover and they must be used with caution in patients with dormant disease, in whom they may reactivate disease. For further details on the possible role of corticosteroids as an adjunct to antituberculous therapy, see p.1089.

Interferons have also been tried (see p.648).

**Preventive therapy** or **chemoprophylaxis** is intended to prevent the occurrence of acute tuberculosis in patients with asymptomatic tuberculous infection (that is, those with a positive tuberculin skin test but no evidence of active disease), and in susceptible contacts, and to curb its spread through the community.

Chemoprophylaxis is not recommended routinely in developing countries and the primary objective, as elsewhere, should be to treat active tuberculosis.[4] Chemoprophylaxis is more widely used in the USA than in the UK and other countries where vaccination with BCG vaccine (p.1610) is routinely used.

The American Thoracic Society and the CDC have issued detailed recommendations for chemoprophylaxis (treatment of latent tuberculosis infection).[43] Isoniazid given for 9 months is the preferred regimen, although treatment for 6 months may be adequate. Rifampicin, alone for 4 months, or with pyrazinamide for 2 months, were considered to be alternatives, but reports of severe and fatal liver damage associated with rifampicin and pyrazinamide administration have led to revised recommendations for the use of this combination[44] and the American Thoracic Society and CDC now recommend that it should not generally be offered to persons with latent tuberculosis.[45] Prophylaxis is generally recommended for patients at high risk of developing tuberculosis and who exhibit a positive tuberculin skin test, including:

- Household members and other close associates of newly diagnosed potentially infectious tuberculosis patients
- Persons with an abnormal chest X-ray consistent with prior tuberculosis
- Recent immigrants from countries with a high prevalence of tuberculosis
- Patients in special clinical situations such as those with diabetes mellitus, lymphomas, leukaemia, carcinoma of the head or neck and lung, end-stage renal failure, or those receiving prolonged corticosteroid or immunosuppressive therapy, or intravenous drug abusers, or those with substantial rapid weight loss or chronic undernutrition

In addition, chemoprophylaxis may be offered to persons with negative skin tests in certain high-risk situations.

Prophylaxis is also recommended for persons infected with HIV who react positively to tuberculin but have no evidence of disease. HIV-positive patients should not receive BCG vaccine because of the risk of disseminated infection.[46]

For reference to prophylaxis in pregnant women and the neonate, see above.

The British Thoracic Society's Joint Tuberculosis Committee advises that chemoprophylaxis may be given to some contacts with strongly positive tuberculin Heaf test reactions, but without clinical or radiological evidence of tuberculous disease.[22] They recommend that chemoprophylaxis should be given to contacts under 16 years old who have not had BCG vaccination and have positive tuberculin reactions and should be considered in children who have received BCG vaccination and who have a strongly positive tuberculin reaction. Also, children under 2 years old who are close contacts of cases with positive sputum smears and who have not had BCG vaccination should be given chemoprophylaxis whatever their tuberculin status.[11,22] Chemoprophylaxis is also recommended for patients in whom recent tuberculin conversion has been documented.[22]

The resurgence of tuberculosis has increased the risk of nosocomial infection in patients and health care workers and has prompted guidance on preventing its transmission in health care settings.[22,47] Guidance is also given on the management of bovine tuberculosis, and the risks of tuberculosis transmission during air travel and in schools.[22]

• HIV INFECTION

Since HIV infection increases both the individual's susceptibility to primary infection with *M. tuberculosis* and to progression to active tuberculosis in individuals with existing *M. tuberculosis* infection, effective tuberculosis control is particularly important in this population. BCG immunisation is not recommended in individuals with HIV infection since there is a risk of disseminated infection. Chemoprophylaxis has been shown to reduce the incidence of tuberculosis when given to persons with HIV infection, particularly in those with a positive tuberculin reaction.[48] Current practice is to give chemoprophylaxis to individuals identified as being at greatest risk of tuberculosis, including close contacts of patients with infectious disease. In 1994, the IUATLD (International Union Against Tuberculosis and Lung Disease) and WHO[49] supported prophylaxis with isoniazid for 6 to 12 months in HIV-infected individuals with a positive tuberculin test, once active tuberculosis had been excluded. In the USA, chemoprophylaxis is also offered to HIV-infected persons who are considered to be at high risk of contracting the infection regardless of tuberculin test results.[35,46] Chemoprophylaxis may be with isoniazid for 9 months, or with rifampicin or rifabutin for 4 months, or with rifampicin or rifabutin with pyrazinamide for 2 months,[35,46,50-52] although the combination of rifampicin with pyrazinamide has been associated with fatal liver injury[44,45] (see also above). Also, as mentioned above, rifamycins may interact with antiretroviral drugs.

In developing countries with a high prevalence of tuberculosis, the difficulties in providing preventive chemotherapy to all HIV-infected individuals at risk may be overwhelming.[53] WHO has suggested that preventive chemotherapy may be restricted to selected at-risk groups such as healthcare workers and selected individuals.[4]

Inactivated *Mycobacterium vaccae* is under investigation.[54]


1. Blomberg B, Fourie B. Fixed-dose combination drugs for tuberculosis: application in standardised treatment regimens. *Drugs* 2003; **63:** 535–553.
2. Gangadharam PRJ, *et al.* Experimental chemotherapy of tuberculosis using single dose treatment with isoniazid in biodegradable polymers. *J Antimicrob Chemother* 1994; **33:** 265–71.
3. Raviglione MC, *et al.* Assessment of worldwide tuberculosis control. *Lancet* 1997; **350:** 624–9.
4. WHO. *TB/HIV: A clinical manual.* Geneva: WHO, 1996.
5. Nunn P. Thiacetazone should not be used routinely—or primum non nocere. *Tubercle Lung Dis* 1995; **76** (suppl 2): 3.
6. Elliott AM, Foster SD. Thiacetazone: time to call a halt? *Tubercle Lung Dis* 1996; **77:** 27–9.
7. Rieder HL. Controversies in tuberculosis control: thioacetazone may be used routinely—pro. *Tubercle Lung Dis* 1995; **76** (suppl 2): 3.
8. van Gorkom J, Kibuga DK. Cost-effectiveness and total costs of three alternative strategies for the prevention and management of severe skin reactions attributable to thiacetazone in the treatment of human immunodeficiency virus positive patients with tuberculosis in Kenya. *Tubercle Lung Dis* 1996; **77:** 30–6.
9. WHO. *Treatment of tuberculosis: guidelines for national programmes.* Geneva: WHO, 1997.
10. Task Force of ERS, WHO and the Europe Region of IUATLD. Tuberculosis management in Europe: recommendations of a task force of the European Respiratory Society (ERS), the World Health Organisation (WHO) and the International Union Against Tuberculosis and Lung Disease (IUATLD) Europe region. *Eur Respir J* 1999; **14:** 978–92.
11. Joint Tuberculosis Committee of the British Thoracic Society. Chemotherapy and management of tuberculosis in the United Kingdom: recommendations 1998. *Thorax* 1998; **53:** 536–48. Also available at: http://www.brit-thoracic.org.uk/docs/Chemotherapy.pdf (accessed 24/05/04)
12. Centers for Disease Control. Initial therapy for tuberculosis in the era of multidrug resistance: recommendations of the Advisory Council for the Elimination of Tuberculosis. *MMWR* 1993; **42** (RR-7): 1–8. Also available at: http://www.cdc.gov/mmwr/PDF/rr/rr4207.pdf (accessed 24/05/04)
13. American Thoracic Society, Centers for Disease Control, and the Infectious Diseases Society of America. Treatment of tuberculosis. *MMWR* 2003; **52** (RR-11): 1–77. Also available at: http://www.cdc.gov/mmwr/PDF/rr/rr5211.pdf (accessed 24/05/04)
14. Ormerod LP, *et al.* Hepatotoxicity of antituberculosis drugs. *Thorax* 1996; **51:** 111–13.
15. Espinal MA, *et al.* Global trends in resistance to antituberculosis drugs. *N Engl J Med* 2001; **344:** 1294–1303.
16. WHO. Anti-tuberculosis drug resistance in the world: report no 2: prevalence and trends. Available at: http://www.who.int/emc-documents/antimicrobial_resistance/whocdstb2000278c.html (accessed 24/05/04)
17. Farmer P, Kim JY. Community based approaches to the control of multidrug resistant tuberculosis: introducing "DOTS-plus". *BMJ* 1998; **317:** 671–4.
18. WHO. *Guidelines for the management of drug-resistant tuberculosis.* Geneva: WHO, 1997.
19. Sullivan EA, *et al.* Emergence of fluoroquinolone-resistant tuberculosis in New York City. *Lancet* 1995; **345:** 1148–50.
20. Trébucq A. Should ethambutol be recommended for routine treatment of tuberculosis in children? A review of the literature. *Int J Tuberc Lung Dis* 1997; **1:** 12–15.
21. Bothamley G. Drug treatment for tuberculosis during pregnancy: safety considerations. *Drug Safety* 2001; **24:** 553–65.
22. Joint Tuberculosis Committee of the British Thoracic Society. Control and prevention of tuberculosis in the United Kingdom: code of practice 2000. *Thorax* 2000; **55:** 887–901. Also available at: http://www.brit-thoracic.org.uk/docs/TB.pdf (accessed 24/05/04)
23. Havlir DV, Barnes PF. Tuberculosis in patients with human immunodeficiency virus infection. *N Engl J Med* 1999; **340:** 367–73.
24. Small PM, *et al.* Treatment of tuberculosis in patients with advanced human immunodeficiency virus infection. *N Engl J Med* 1991; **324:** 289–94.
25. Sterling TR, *et al.* Relapse rates after short-course (6-month) treatment of tuberculosis in HIV-infected and uninfected persons. *AIDS* 1999; **13:** 1899–1904.
26. Peloquin CA, *et al.* Low antituberculosis drug concentrations in patients with AIDS. *Ann Pharmacother* 1996; **30:** 919–25.

27. Peloquin CA, *et al.* Malabsorption of antimycobacterial medications. *N Engl J Med* 1993; **329:** 1122–3.
28. Sahai J, *et al.* Reduced plasma concentrations of antituberculosis drugs in patients with HIV infection. *Ann Intern Med* 1997; **127:** 289–93.
29. Choudhri SH, *et al.* Pharmacokinetics of antimycobacterial drugs in patients with tuberculosis, AIDS, and diarrhea. *Clin Infect Dis* 1997; **25:** 104–11.
30. Patel KB, *et al.* Drug malabsorption and resistant tuberculosis in HIV-infected patients. *N Engl J Med* 1995; **332:** 336–7.
31. Narita M, *et al.* Paradoxical worsening of tuberculosis following antiretroviral therapy in patients with AIDS. *Am J Respir Crit Care Med* 1998; **158:** 157–61.
32. Nunn P, *et al.* Cutaneous hypersensitivity reactions due to thiacetazone in HIV-1 seropositive patients treated for tuberculosis. *Lancet* 1991; **337:** 627–30.
33. De Cock KM, Wilkinson D. Tuberculosis control in resource-poor countries: alternative approaches in the era of HIV. *Lancet* 1995; **346:** 675–7.
34. Burman WJ, *et al.* Therapeutic implications of drug interactions in the treatment of human immunodeficiency virus-related tuberculosis. *Clin Infect Dis* 1999; **28:** 419–30.
35. Centers for Disease Control. Prevention and treatment of tuberculosis among patients infected with human immunodeficiency virus: principles of therapy and revised recommendations. *MMWR* 1998; **47** (RR-20): 1–58. Also available at: http://www.cdc.gov/mmwr//PDF/rr/rr4720.pdf (accessed 24/05/04)
36. Schluger NW. Issues in the treatment of active tuberculosis in human immunodeficiency virus-infected patients. *Clin Infect Dis* 1999; **28:** 130–5.
37. Snider DE, Roper WL. The new tuberculosis. *N Engl J Med* 1992; **326:** 703–5.
38. Drobniewski F. Is death inevitable with multiresistant TB plus HIV infection? *Lancet* 1997; **349:** 71–2.
39. Subcommittee of the Joint Tuberculosis Committee of the British Thoracic Society. Guidelines on the management of tuberculosis and HIV infection in the United Kingdom. *BMJ* 1992; **304:** 1231–3.
40. Fitzgerald DW, *et al.* Effect of post-treatment isoniazid on prevention of recurrent tuberculosis in HIV-1-infected individuals: a randomised trial. *Lancet* 2000; **356:** 1470–4.
41. de Bruyn G, Garner P. Mycobacterium vaccae immunotherapy for treating tuberculosis. Available in the Cochrane Library; Issue 2. Chichester: John Wiley; 2004.
42. Alzeer AH, FitzGerald JM. Corticosteroids and tuberculosis: risks and use as adjunct therapy. *Tubercle Lung Dis* 1993; **74:** 6–11.
43. American Thoracic Society and the Centers for Disease Control. Targeted tuberculin testing and treatment of latent tuberculosis infection. *Am J Respir Crit Care Med* 2000; **161** (suppl): S221–S247.
44. Centers for Disease Control. Update: fatal and severe liver injuries associated with rifampin and pyrazinamide for latent tuberculosis infection, and revisions in American Thoracic Society/CDC recommendations—United States, 2001. *MMWR* 2001; **50:** 733–5. Also available at: http://www.cdc.gov/mmwr/PDF/wk/mm5034.pdf (accessed 24/05/04)
45. Centers for Disease Control. Update: adverse event data and revised American Thoracic Society/CDC recommendations against the use of rifampin and pyrazinamide for treatment of latent tuberculosis infection—United States, 2003. *MMWR* 2003; **52:** 735–9. Also available at: http://www.cdc.gov/mmwr/preview/mmwrhtml/mm5231a4.htm (accessed 24/05/04)
46. Centers for Disease Control and Prevention. Guidelines for preventing opportunistic infections among HIV-infected persons—2002: recommendations of the US Public Health Service and the Infectious Diseases Society of America. *MMWR* 2002; **51** (RR-8): 1–52. Also available at: http://www.cdc.gov/mmwr/PDF/rr/rr5108.pdf (accessed 24/05/04)
47. ACOEM. ACOEM guidelines for protecting health care workers against tuberculosis. *J Occup Environ Med* 1998; **40:** 765–7.
48. Wilkinson D, *et al.* Effect of preventive treatment for tuberculosis in adults infected with HIV: systematic review of randomised placebo controlled trials. *BMJ* 1998; **317:** 625–9.
49. International Union Against Tuberculosis and Lung Disease (IUATLD) and the Global Programme on AIDS and the Tuberculosis Programme of the World Health Organization (WHO). Tuberculosis preventive therapy in HIV-infected individuals: a joint statement. *Tubercle Lung Dis* 1994; **75:** 96–8.
50. Halsey NA, *et al.* Randomised trial of isoniazid versus rifampicin and pyrazinamide for prevention of tuberculosis in HIV-1 infection. *Lancet* 1998; **351:** 786–92.
51. Rose DN. Short-course prophylaxis against tuberculosis in HIV-infected persons. *Ann Intern Med* 1998; **129:** 779–86.
52. Gordin F, *et al.* Rifampin and pyrazinamide vs isoniazid for prevention of tuberculosis in HIV-infected persons: an international randomized trial. *JAMA* 2000; **283:** 1445–50.
53. De Cock KM, *et al.* Preventive therapy for tuberculosis in HIV-infected persons: international recommendations, research, and practice. *Lancet* 1995; **345:** 833–6.
54. Fordham von Reyn C, *et al.* Cellular immune responses to mycobacteria in healthy and human immunodeficiency virus-positive subjects in the United States after a five-dose schedule of Mycobacterium vaccae vaccine. *Clin Infect Dis* 1998; **27:** 1517–20.

## Tularaemia

Tularaemia is caused by the Gram-negative bacillus *Francisella tularensis*, an organism that primarily affects rodents and rabbits but may be transmitted to man, usually by handling infected animals or carcasses, or by the bites of insect vectors. It may take several forms, the most common of which is the ulceroglandular form, characterised by rash and ulceration at the site of inoculation accompanied by fever and lymphadenopathy; other forms include the typhoidal and pneumonic forms, which have a higher mortality rate.

Streptomycin is still considered the antibacterial of choice in severe disease,[1,2] although gentamicin may be an alternative in patients who cannot tolerate streptomycin.[2] Tetracycline or chloramphenicol may be given orally; clinical relapses are more frequent than with the aminoglycosides,[2,3] although relapsed disease will respond to a further course. Some patients have also responded to high-dose intravenous erythromycin.[4]

Streptomycin is difficult to obtain in the USA but a review[5] of alternative drugs for the treatment of tularaemia concluded that:

- gentamicin is an acceptable alternative to streptomycin and should be considered the alternative antibacterial of choice for serious cases of nonmeningitic tularaemia
- tetracycline might be a reasonable alternative to gentamicin and could be given orally in less severely ill patients, but there is a relatively high relapse rate with tetracycline
- chloramphenicol should be considered when tularaemic meningitis is suspected—like tetracycline it is associated with a relatively high relapse rate, but has the advantage over both aminoglycosides and tetracycline of good penetration of the CNS
- imipenem-cilastatin and the fluoroquinolones ciprofloxacin and norfloxacin have shown promise in a small number of patients, but further studies were needed before they could be recommended.

A tularaemia vaccine is available in some countries for active immunisation against the disease.

1. Corwin WC, Stubbs SP. Further studies on tularemia in the Ozarks: review of forty-four cases during a three-year period. *JAMA* 1952; **149:** 343–5.
2. Evans ME, *et al.* Tularemia: a 30-year experience with 88 cases. *Medicine (Baltimore)* 1985; **64:** 251–69.
3. Ford-Jones L, *et al.* "Muskrat fever": two outbreaks of tularemia near Montreal. *Can Med Assoc J* 1982; **127:** 298–9.
4. Westerman EL, McDonald J. Tularemia pneumonia mimicking Legionnaires' disease: isolation of organism on CYE agar and successful treatment with erythromycin. *South Med J* 1983; **76:** 1169–70.
5. Enderlin G, *et al.* Streptomycin and alternative agents for the treatment of tularemia: review of the literature. *Clin Infect Dis* 1994; **19:** 42–7.

## Typhoid and paratyphoid fever

Typhoid and paratyphoid fever are systemic infections caused respectively by *Salmonella typhi* and *S. paratyphi* A, B, or C, Gram-negative bacteria belonging to the Enterobacteriaceae family. They are sometimes termed collectively 'enteric fever' but, although initial infection is intestinal, dissemination in the blood leads to more widespread systemic effects. Typhoid and paratyphoid are endemic in many countries and, in most, typhoid is more common. Most cases occurring in the UK are contracted abroad.

Treatment of typhoid fever has generally been with chloramphenicol or alternatively amoxicillin, ampicillin, or co-trimoxazole.[1] However, there has been a spread of strains of *S. typhi* resistant to chloramphenicol, ampicillin, amoxicillin, trimethoprim, and co-trimoxazole,[2] especially in the Indian subcontinent, in the Middle East, and possibly in South and South-East Asia. Fluoroquinolones such as ciprofloxacin or third-generation cephalosporins such as cefotaxime, ceftriaxone, and cefoperazone are effective for typhoid fever due to multiresistant strains. Fluoroquinolones have been the preferred alternative to chloramphenicol for patients returning to the UK from the Indian subcontinent or other regions where multidrug-resistant strains are endemic.[3,4] However, the increasing incidence of ciprofloxacin resistance in multiresistant *S. typhi* has been noted, mainly in cases originating in the Indian subcontinent,[5,6] and strains with decreased susceptibility to fluoroquinolones may now be endemic in this region.[7] There is also some concern that resistance to ceftriaxone may be emerging in the Indian subcontinent, but ciprofloxacin-resistant strains isolated in the UK have generally retained their sensitivity to cephalosporins.[7] A further alternative is azithromycin.[8-11]

Fluoroquinolones are generally contra-indicated in children and in pregnant women because of potential toxicity, but there is evidence of the successful use of ciprofloxacin or ofloxacin in multiresistant infection in children.[12-14] Similarly, ciprofloxacin was effective in the second and third trimester of pregnancy[15,16] and some have suggested that it could be used in pregnancy if the organism was resistant to amoxicillin or ampicillin.[15]

On recovery, typhoid patients may continue to excrete *S. typhi* in the faeces or urine for several weeks. Unlike these convalescent carriers, chronic carriers may excrete *S. typhi* for years without any symptoms; eradication is difficult and prolonged treatment is necessary. An increased risk of biliary-tract and bile-related cancers has been associated with chronic carriage of *S. typhi*, and the importance of eradication has been emphasised.[17]

Typhoid vaccines are used for the prevention of typhoid fever.

Paratyphoid fever is less common and generally milder than typhoid fever. Treatment is similar.

1. Parry CM, *et al.* Typhoid fever. *N Engl J Med* 2002; **347:** 1770–82.
2. Rowe B, *et al.* Multidrug-resistant Salmonella typhi: a worldwide epidemic. *Clin Infect Dis* 1997; **24** (suppl 1): S106–S109.
3. Rowe B, *et al.* Spread of multiresistant Salmonella typhi. *Lancet* 1990; **336:** 1065.
4. Rowe B, *et al.* Treatment of multiresistant typhoid fever. *Lancet* 1991; **337:** 1422.
5. Rowe B, *et al.* Ciprofloxacin-resistant Salmonella typhi in the UK. *Lancet* 1995; **346:** 1302.
6. Mitchell DH. Ciprofloxacin-resistant Salmonella typhi: an emerging problem. *Med J Aust* 1997; **167:** 172.
7. Threlfall EJ, *et al.* Ciprofloxacin-resistant Salmonella typhi and treatment failure. *Lancet* 1999; **353:** 1590–1.
8. Girgis NI, *et al.* Azithromycin versus ciprofloxacin for treatment of uncomplicated typhoid fever in a randomized trial in Egypt that included patients with multidrug resistance. *Antimicrob Agents Chemother* 1999; **43:** 1441–4.
9. Butler T, *et al.* Treatment of typhoid fever with azithromycin versus chloramphenicol in a randomized multicentre trial in India. *J Antimicrob Chemother* 1999; **44:** 243–50.
10. Chinh NT, *et al.* A randomized controlled comparison of azithromycin and ofloxacin for treatment of multidrug-resistant or nalidixic acid-resistant enteric fever. *Antimicrob Agents Chemother* 2000; **44:** 1855–9.
11. Frenck RW, *et al.* Azithromycin versus ceftriaxone for the treatment of uncomplicated typhoid fever in children. *Clin Infect Dis* 2000; **31:** 1134–8.
12. Cheesbrough JS, *et al.* Quinolones in children with invasive salmonellosis. *Lancet* 1991; **338:** 127.
13. Dutta P, *et al.* Ciprofloxacin for treatment of severe typhoid fever in children. *Antimicrob Agents Chemother* 1993; **37:** 1197–9.
14. Vinh H, *et al.* Two or three days of ofloxacin treatment for uncomplicated multidrug-resistant typhoid fever in children. *Antimicrob Agents Chemother* 1996; **40:** 958–61.
15. Leung D, *et al.* Treatment of typhoid in pregnancy. *Lancet* 1995; **346:** 648.
16. Koul PA, *et al.* Ciprofloxacin for multiresistant enteric fever in pregnancy. *Lancet* 1995; **346:** 307–8.
17. Caygill CPJ, *et al.* Cancer mortality in chronic typhoid and paratyphoid carriers. *Lancet* 1994; **343:** 83–4.

## Typhus

Rickettsial infections or fevers of the typhus group are transmitted to man by various insect vectors. Louse-borne or epidemic typhus, due to *Rickettsia prowazekii*, and flea-borne or murine typhus, due to the closely related *R. typhi* (*R. mooseri*), have occurred worldwide. Scrub typhus is due to *Orientia tsutsugamushi* (*R. tsutsugamushi*), transmitted by mites, and occurs mainly in Asia, Australia, and the Pacific Islands.

A tetracycline, often doxycycline, or chloramphenicol is the treatment of choice for these infections although strains of *O. tsutsugamushi* resistant to doxycycline and chloramphenicol have been reported in Thailand.[1,2] Ciprofloxacin may be an effective alternative,[3] and rifampicin has been shown to be more effective against scrub typhus than doxycycline.[4] Prophylaxis for scrub typhus with doxycycline has shown promise when started before exposure to infection.[5] Typhus vaccines are available for active immunisation against louse-borne typhus.

1. Watt G, *et al.* Scrub typhus infections poorly responsive to antibiotics in northern Thailand. *Lancet* 1996; **348:** 86–9.
2. Panpanich R, Garner P. Antibiotics for treating scrub typhus. Available in The Cochrane Library; Issue 2. Chichester: John Wiley; 2004.
3. Eaton M, *et al.* Ciprofloxacin treatment of typhus. *JAMA* 1989; **262:** 772–3.
4. Watt G, *et al.* Doxycycline and rifampicin for mild scrub-typhus infections in northern Thailand: a randomised trial. *Lancet* 2000; **356:** 1057–61.
5. Twartz JC, *et al.* Doxycycline prophylaxis for human scrub typhus. *J Infect Dis* 1982; **146:** 811–18.

## Urethritis

Infective urethritis is a sexually transmitted disease seen most frequently in men. One of the commonest causes is *Neisseria gonorrhoeae*. Nongonococcal urethritis or non-specific urethritis may be due to *Chlamydia trachomatis* in up to 50% of cases and *Ureaplasma urealyticum* (formerly T-strain mycoplasma) in up to 40%, but often the cause is unknown. Other organisms implicated have included *Mycoplasma genitalium*. Gonococcal and chlamydial infections frequently occur together and, since specific therapy for gonorrhoea is often not effective against *C. trachomatis*, treatment for the two infections should be given concomitantly otherwise postgonococcal urethritis due to *C. trachomatis* may follow the cure of gonorrhoea. The treatment of chlamydial urethritis is discussed under Chlamydial Infections (p.123) and that for gonococcal urethritis under Gonorrhoea (p.130).

For nongonococcal urethritis, the UK guidelines[1] recommend a single 1-g dose of azithromycin by mouth or a 7-day course of oral doxycycline 100 mg twice daily. Alternative regimens are oral erythromycin 500 mg twice daily for 14 days, or ofloxacin 400 mg daily in one single or two divided doses for 7 days. In the USA,[2] the recommended first-choice therapy is the same as that in the UK. Alternative regimens listed in the USA are oral erythromycin 500 mg four times daily, or erythromycin ethylsuccinate 800 mg four times daily, or ofloxacin 300 mg twice daily, or levofloxacin 500 mg once daily, in each case for 7 days.[2] Persistent or recurrent nongonococcal urethritis should be treated with a single oral 2-g dose of metronidazole plus oral erythromycin 500 mg four times daily, or erythromycin ethylsuccinate 800 mg four times daily, in each case for 7 days.[2]

1. Clinical Effectiveness Group (Association for Genitourinary Medicine and the Medical Society for the Study of Venereal Diseases). National guideline on the management of non-gonococcal urethritis. Available at: http://www.bashh.org/guidelines/2002/NGU%2009%2001c.pdf (accessed 24/05/04)
2. Centers for Disease Control. Sexually transmitted diseases treatment guidelines 2002. *MMWR* 2002; **51**(RR-6): 1–80. Also available at: http://www.cdc.gov/mmwr/PDF/rr/rr5106.pdf (accessed 24/05/04)

## Urinary-tract infections

Infections of the urinary tract are especially common in women. They are frequently due to enteric bacteria, in particular *Escherichia coli*, although a common cause in young women is *Staphylococcus saprophyticus*, a coagulase-negative staphylococcus. Other urinary pathogens include *Staph. epidermidis*, enterococci, and *Pseudomonas* spp. An arbitrary definition of urinary-tract infection has been significant bacteriuria with $10^5$ or more colony forming units/mL of a midstream urine specimen; some also consider lower counts to be indicative of infection. Most urinary-tract infections are isolated uncomplicated infections of the lower urinary tract. Recurrent infections may be due to relapse, or more often, re-infection, and are more serious. Patients with complicated urinary-tract infections associated with urinary-tract abnormalities or diseases such as diabetes mellitus may be at risk of kidney damage.

Infections of the lower urinary tract in *women* generally present as cystitis (inflammation of the bladder) and symptoms include dysuria, frequency, and urgency together with pyuria and significant bacteriuria; the urethral syndrome is similar, but there is no significant bacteriuria. In the upper urinary tract, acute pyelonephritis may occur as a complication of cystitis or, more rarely, may result from septicaemia. Asymptomatic bacteriuria may progress to acute pyelonephritis in *pregnant women* and should therefore be treated.

Urinary-tract infections in *men* are less common and are often associated with abnormalities of the genito-urinary tract such as prostatic hyperplasia. Acute bacterial prostatitis is usually caused by organisms similar to those responsible for cystitis in women. Chronic bacterial prostatitis is difficult to treat; the antibacterials used must be able to penetrate into the prostatic fluid. For other genito-urinary infections in men, see under Epididymitis, p.127, and under Urethritis, above.

In preschool *children*, especially girls, asymptomatic bacteriuria together with vesicoureteric reflux can result in renal scarring and should be treated; the use of prophylactic antibacterials is complex and controversial. Long-term follow-up of girls who have had asymptomatic bacteriuria suggests that new kidney damage does not occur after 4 years of age, but highlights the importance of diagnosis and treatment in younger children.

The significance of asymptomatic bacteriuria in *old age* is disputed, but most consider treatment to be unnecessary.

Infections associated with *indwelling bladder catheters* occur in both men and women and probably account for the majority of hospital-acquired urinary-tract infections.

**Treatment**. Antibacterials used to treat urinary-tract infections need to be excreted in adequate concentrations in the urine. For *acute uncomplicated infections* oral amoxicillin, ampicillin, co-trimoxazole, nalidixic acid, nitrofurantoin, or trimethoprim (preferred to co-trimoxazole in the UK) have been given, although the choice will depend on local patterns of bacterial resistance; *E. coli* resistant to ampicillin and amoxicillin is widespread. Alternatives when resistance is prevalent include amoxicillin with clavulanic acid, oral cephalosporins, fluoroquinolones, or fosfomycin. In pregnant women, nitrofurantoin or a beta lactam can be used. Standard treatment schedules have been for 5 to 7 days; 3-day or single-dose regimens can also be effective and may be preferred in women. Single-dose treatment may be associated with reduced efficacy compared with 3-day regimens. Urinary alkalinising agents such as potassium citrate and sodium citrate have been given by mouth to relieve the pain of cystitis caused by lower urinary-tract infections. Recurrent infections may require long-term low-dose antibacterial prophylaxis.

*Acute pyelonephritis* may require broad-spectrum parenteral treatment initially with, for example, aztreonam, ceftazidime, cefuroxime, ciprofloxacin, or gentamicin.

*Chronic bacterial prostatitis* may require treatment for several weeks with trimethoprim, erythromycin, or a fluoroquinolone.

*Catheter-related bladder infections* may sometimes respond to localised treatment with bladder washouts containing chlorhexidine.

GENERAL. References.

1. Kunin CM. Chemoprophylaxis and suppressive therapy in the management of urinary tract infections. *J Antimicrob Chemother* 1994; **33** (suppl A): 51–62.
2. Reeves DS. A perspective on the safety of antibacterials used to treat urinary tract infections. *J Antimicrob Chemother* 1994; **33** (suppl A): 111–20.
3. Brumfitt W, Hamilton-Miller JMT. Consensus viewpoint on management of urinary infections. *J Antimicrob Chemother* 1994; **33** (suppl A): 147–53.
4. Maskell R. Management of recurrent urinary tract infections in adults. *Prescribers' J* 1995; **35**: 1–11.
5. Ronald A, Sanche SE. Antimicrobial management of urinary tract infections. *Curr Opin Infect Dis* 1995; **8**: 420–3.
6. Nicolle LE. A practical guide to the management of complicated urinary tract infection. *Drugs* 1997; **53**: 583–92.
7. Preston SL, *et al.* Empiric treatment of uncomplicated urinary tract infections. *Ann Pharmacother* 1998; **32**: 1231–3.
8. Nicolle LE. Urinary tract infection: traditional pharmacologic therapies. *Am J Med* 2002; **113** (suppl 1A): 35S–44S.
9. Nicolle L. Best pharmacological practice: urinary tract infections. *Expert Opin Pharmacother* 2003; **4**: 693–704.

CATHETER-RELATED. References.

1. Tambyah PA, Maki DG. The relationship between pyuria and infection in patients with indwelling urinary catheters: a prospective study of 761 patients. *Arch Intern Med* 2000; **160**: 673–7.
2. Tambyah PA, Maki DG. Catheter-associated urinary tract infection is rarely symptomatic: a prospective study of 1497 catheterized patients. *Arch Intern Med* 2000; **160**: 678–82.

THE ELDERLY. References.

1. Abrutyn E, *et al.* Does asymptomatic bacteriuria predict mortality and does antimicrobial treatment reduce mortality in elderly ambulatory women? *Ann Intern Med* 1994; **120**: 827–33. Correction. *ibid.*; **121**: 901.
2. Nicolle LE. Urinary tract infection in the elderly. *J Antimicrob Chemother* 1994; **33** (suppl A): 99–109.
3. Ouslander JG, *et al.* Does eradicating bacteriuria affect the severity of chronic urinary incontinence in nursing home residents? *Ann Intern Med* 1995; **122**: 749–54.
4. Abrutyn E, *et al.* Does treatment of asymptomatic bacteriuria in older ambulatory women reduce subsequent symptoms of urinary tract infection? *J Am Geriatr Soc* 1996; **44**: 293–5.
5. Shortliffe LMD, McCue JD. Urinary tract infection at the age extremes: pediatrics and geriatrics. *Am J Med* 2002; **113** (suppl 1A): 55S–66S.
6. Lutters M, Vogt N. Antibiotic duration for treating uncomplicated, symptomatic lower urinary tract infections in elderly women. Available in The Cochrane Library; Issue 2. Chichester: John Wiley; 2004.

INFANTS AND CHILDREN. References.

1. Working Group of the Research Unit, Royal College of Physicians. Guidelines for the management of acute urinary tract infection in childhood. *J R Coll Physicians Lond* 1991; **25**: 36–42.
2. Smellie JM, *et al.* Retrospective study of children with renal scarring associated with reflux and urinary infection. *BMJ* 1994; **308**: 1193–6.
3. Ansari BM, *et al.* Urinary tract infection in children: part 1: epidemiology, natural history, diagnosis and management. *J Infect* 1995; **30**: 3–6.
4. Watson AR. Urinary tract infection in early childhood. *J Antimicrob Chemother* 1994; **34** (suppl A): 53–60. Correction. *ibid.* 1995; **35**: 561.
5. Gordon I. Vesico-ureteric reflux, urinary-tract infection, and renal damage in children. *Lancet* 1995; **346**: 489–90.
6. Anonymous. The management of urinary tract infection in children. *Drug Ther Bull* 1997; **35**: 65–9.
7. American Academy of Pediatrics Committee on Quality Improvement, Subcommittee on Urinary Tract Infection. Practice parameter: the diagnosis, treatment, and evaluation of the initial urinary tract infection in febrile infants and young children. *Pediatrics* 1999; **103**: 843–52. Corrections. *ibid.*: 1052. *ibid.* 2000; **105**: 141.
8. Williams G, *et al.* Antibiotics for the prevention of urinary tract infection in children: a systematic review of randomized controlled trials. *J Pediatr* 2001; **138**: 868–74.
9. Tran D, *et al.* Short-course versus conventional length antimicrobial therapy for uncomplicated lower urinary tract infections in children: a meta-analysis of 1279 patients. *J Pediatr* 2001; **139**: 93–9.
10. Shortliffe LMD, McCue JD. Urinary tract infection at the age extremes: pediatrics and geriatrics. *Am J Med* 2002; **113** (suppl 1A): 55S–66S.
11. Michael M, *et al.* Short versus standard duration oral antibiotic therapy for acute urinary tract infection in children. Available in The Cochrane Library; Issue 2. Chichester: John Wiley; 2004.
12. Bloomfield P, *et al.* Antibiotics for acute pyelonephritis in children. Available in The Cochrane Library; Issue 2. Chichester: John Wiley; 2004.

MEN. References.

1. Lipsky BA. Prostatitis and urinary tract infection in men: what's new; what's true? *Am J Med* 1999; **106**: 327–34.
2. Joly-Guillou M-L, Lasry S. Practical recommendations for the drug treatment of bacterial infections of the male genital tract including urethritis, epididymitis and prostatitis. *Drugs* 1999; **57**: 743–50.

PREGNANCY. References.

1. Vercaigne LM, Zhanel GG. Recommended treatment for urinary tract infection in pregnancy. *Ann Pharmacother* 1994; **28**: 248–51.
2. Bint AJ, Hill D. Bacteriuria of pregnancy—an update on significance, diagnosis and management. *J Antimicrob Chemother* 1994; **33** (suppl A): 93–7.
3. Maclean AB. Urinary tract infection in pregnancy. *Int J Antimicrob Agents* 2001; **17**: 273–6.
4. Krcmery S, *et al.* Treatment of lower urinary tract infection in pregnancy. *Int J Antimicrob Agents* 2001; **17**: 279–82.
5. Wing DA. Pyelonephritis in pregnancy: treatment options for optimal outcomes. *Drugs* 2001; **61**: 2087–96.
6. Smaill F. Antibiotics for asymptomatic bacteriuria in pregnancy. Available in The Cochrane Library; Issue 2. Chichester: John Wiley; 2004.
7. Vazquez JC, Villar J. Treatments for symptomatic urinary tract infections during pregnancy. Available in The Cochrane Library; Issue 2. Chichester: John Wiley; 2004.

WOMEN. References.

1. Hamilton-Miller JMT. The urethral syndrome and its management. *J Antimicrob Chemother* 1994; **33** (suppl A): 63–73.
2. Kunin CM. Urinary tract infections in females. *Clin Infect Dis* 1994; **18**: 1–12.
3. Anonymous. Managing urinary tract infection in women. *Drug Ther Bull* 1998; **36**: 30–2.
4. Warren JW, *et al.* Guidelines for antimicrobial treatment of uncomplicated acute bacterial cystitis and acute pyelonephritis in women. *Clin Infect Dis* 1999; **29**: 745–58.
5. Hooton TM. Recurrent urinary tract infection in women. *Int J Antimicrob Agents* 2001; **17**: 259–68.
6. Fihn SD. Acute uncomplicated urinary tract infection in women. *N Engl J Med* 2003; **349**: 259–66.

## Whipple's disease

Whipple's disease is a rare chronic systemic condition associated with infection with *Tropheryma whippelii*.[1] It was once considered to be a disease predominantly involving the small intestine and resulting in malabsorption, but may affect virtually all organs. There is probably CNS involvement in all patients with Whipple's disease, although it may only be evident in 10 to 20%. Before the use of antibacterial therapy the disease was invariably fatal. The treatment generally recommended is either benzylpenicillin (sometimes given as procaine benzylpenicillin) and streptomycin, or ceftriaxone, parenterally for two weeks, followed by co-trimoxazole orally for at least one year.[2-4] Such long-term treatment with co-trimoxazole, a drug that crosses the blood-brain barrier, is advisable because of the relatively high frequency and seriousness of CNS relapse. These relapses respond less well to antibacterial treatment; chloramphenicol has been used in those not responding to the above regimen and a patient with CNS relapse improved on ceftriaxone given intravenously.[5] Further alternatives may be a tetracycline[6] or cefixime.[3] A patient intolerant of co-trimoxazole was given phenoxymethylpenicillin and probenecid after the initial 14-day course of benzylpenicillin and streptomycin.[7] There has also been a report of benefit in a penicillin-allergic patient treated with erythromycin.[8]

1. Relman DA, *et al.* Identification of the uncultured bacillus of Whipple's disease. *N Engl J Med* 1992; **327**: 293–301.
2. Singer R. Diagnosis and treatment of Whipple's disease. *Drugs* 1998; **55**: 699–704.
3. Maiwald M, Relman DA. Whipple's disease and Tropheryma whippelii: secrets slowly revealed. *Clin Infect Dis* 2001; **32**: 457–63.
4. Marth T, Raoult D. Whipple's disease. *Lancet* 2003; **361**: 239–46.
5. Adler CH, Galetta SL. Oculo-facial-skeletal myorhythmia in Whipple disease: treatment with ceftriaxone. *Ann Intern Med* 1990; **112**: 467–9.
6. Anonymous. The choice of antibacterial drugs. In: *Handbook of antimicrobial therapy.* 16th ed. New York: The Medical Letter, 2002: 34–52.
7. Rickman LS, *et al.* Brief report: uveitis caused by Tropheryma whippelii (Whipple's bacillus). *N Engl J Med* 1995; **332**: 363–6.
8. Bowles KM, *et al.* A 35-year-old with swollen knees who had recurrent fever and pericarditis, then diarrhoea before getting better. *Lancet* 1996; **348**: 1356.

## Yaws

See under Syphilis, p.148.

## Yersinia enteritis

See under Gastro-enteritis, p.130.

---

## Acediasulfone Sodium (rINN)

Acediasulfona sódica; Sodium Diaphenylsulphonacetate. *N*-*p*-Sulphanilylphenylglycine sodium.

$C_{14}H_{13}N_2NaO_4S$ = 328.3.

*CAS — 127-60-6.*

### Profile

Acediasulfone sodium is reported to have antibacterial properties and is an ingredient of preparations used topically in the treatment of local infections of the ear.

### Preparations

**Proprietary Preparations** (details are given in Part 3)

**Multi-ingredient: *Austria:*** Ciloprin cum Anaesthetico; ***Denm.:*** Ciloprin†; ***Fin.:*** Ciloprin cum Anaesthetico; ***Swed.:*** Ciloprin†; ***Switz.:*** Ciloprine ca.

---

**Alatrofloxacin Mesilate** *(rINNM)*

Alatrofloxacin Mesylate *(USAN)*; CP-116517-27; Mesilato de alatrofloxacino. 7-{(1R,5S,6s)-6-[(S)-2-((S)-2-Aminopropionamido)propionamido]-3-azabicyclo[3.1.0]hex-3-yl}-1-(2,4-difluorophenyl)-6-fluoro-1,4-dihydro-4-oxo-1,8-naphthyridine-3-carboxylic acid monomethanesulphonate.

$C_{26}H_{25}F_3N_6O_5,CH_3SO_3H = 654.6.$

*CAS — 157182-32-6 (alatrofloxacin); 157605-25-9 (alatrofloxacin mesilate).*

**Profile**

Alatrofloxacin is a prodrug of the fluoroquinolone antibacterial trovafloxacin (p.274) and is used intravenously as the mesilate in the treatment of susceptible infections. Details of doses are given under trovafloxacin.

Alatrofloxacin and trovafloxacin preparations have been withdrawn in many countries following reports of unpredictable severe hepatic adverse effects, including some fatalities.

**Preparations**

**Proprietary Preparations** (details are given in Part 3)
***Austral.:*** Trovan†; ***Canad.:*** Trovan; ***Israel:*** Trova†; ***USA:*** Trovan.

## Amikacin *(BAN, rINN)*

Amicacina; Amikacina; Amikacinum. 6-*O*-(3-Amino-3-deoxy-α-D-glucopyranosyl)-4-*O*-(6-amino-6-deoxy-α-D-glucopyranosyl)-$N^1$-[(2S)-4-amino-2-hydroxybutyryl]-2-deoxystreptamine.

$C_{22}H_{43}N_5O_{13} = 585.6.$

*CAS — 37517-28-5.*

*ATC — D06AX12; J01GB06; S01AA21.*

**Pharmacopoeias.** In *Chin., Eur.* (see p.vi), *Int., Pol.,* and *US.*

**Ph. Eur. 5.0** (Amikacin). An antimicrobial substance obtained from kanamycin A. A white or almost white powder. Sparingly soluble in water; practically insoluble in alcohol and in acetone; slightly soluble in methyl alcohol. A 1% solution in water has a pH of 9.5 to 11.5.

**USP 27** (Amikacin). A white crystalline powder. Sparingly soluble in water. pH of a 1% solution in water is between 9.5 and 11.5. Store in airtight containers.

### Amikacin Sulfate *(USAN, rINNM)*

Amikacin Sulphate *(BANM)*; Amikacini Sulfas; BB-K8; Sulfato de amikacina.

$C_{22}H_{43}N_5O_{13},2H_2SO_4 = 781.8.$

*CAS — 39831-55-5.*

*ATC — D06AX12; J01GB06; S01AA21.*

**Pharmacopoeias.** In *Chin., Eur.* (see p.vi), *Int., Jpn, Pol.,* and *US.*

**Ph. Eur. 5.0** (Amikacin Sulphate). A white or almost white powder. It loses not more than 13.0% of its weight on drying. Freely soluble in water; practically insoluble in alcohol and in acetone. The pH of a 1% solution in water is between 2.0 and 4.0. Store in airtight containers.

**USP 27** (Amikacin Sulfate). Amikacin sulfate having a molar ratio of amikacin to $H_2SO_4$ of 1:2 contains the equivalent of not less than 674 micrograms and not more than 786 micrograms of amikacin per mg, calculated on the dried basis. Amikacin sulfate having a molar ratio of amikacin to $H_2SO_4$ of 1:1.8 contains the equivalent of not less than 691 micrograms and not more than 806 micrograms of amikacin per mg, calculated on the dried basis.

A white crystalline powder. Freely soluble in water. pH of a 1% solution in water is between 2.0 and 4.0 (1:2 salt) and 6.0 to 7.3 (1:1.8 salt). Store in airtight containers.

**Incompatibility.** For discussion of the incompatibility of aminoglycosides, including amikacin, with beta lactams, see under Gentamicin Sulfate, p.217. Amikacin is also reported to be incompatible with various other drugs. However, reports are contradictory in many cases, and other factors, such as the strength and composition of the vehicles used, may play a role.

**Stability.** Solutions may darken from colourless to pale yellow but this does not indicate a loss of potency.

### Adverse Effects, Treatment, and Precautions

As for Gentamicin Sulfate, p.217. Peak plasma concentrations of amikacin greater than 30 to 35 micrograms/mL or trough concentrations greater than 5 to 10 micrograms/mL should be avoided. Amikacin affects auditory (cochlear) function to a greater extent than gentamicin.

**Effects on the eyes.** A report of retinal damage following intravitreal injection of amikacin.[1]

1. Jackson TL, Williamson TH. Amikacin retinal toxicity. *Br J Ophthalmol* 1999; **83:** 1199–1200.

### Interactions

As for Gentamicin Sulfate, p.218.

### Antimicrobial Action

As for Gentamicin Sulfate, p.218. Amikacin is active against a similar range of organisms although it is also reported to have some activity against *Nocardia asteroides, Mycobacterium tuberculosis,* and some atypical mycobacterial strains. Amikacin is not degraded by many of the common enzymes often responsible for acquired aminoglycoside resistance. In consequence, cross-resistance with gentamicin and other aminoglycosides is infrequent and amikacin may be effective against strains resistant to other aminoglycosides. However, resistant strains of Gram-negative bacteria and staphylococci have been reported, and some authorities feel that its use should be restricted to infections resistant to other aminoglycosides, although reports differ as to the extent and speed of the development of amikacin resistance where it has been widely used.

◊ References.

1. Ho YII, *et al.* In-vitro activities of aminoglycoside-aminocyclitols against mycobacteria. *J Antimicrob Chemother* 1997; **40:** 27–32.

### Pharmacokinetics

As for Gentamicin Sulfate, p.218.

After intramuscular injection, peak plasma-amikacin concentrations of about 20 micrograms/mL are achieved 1 hour after a 500-mg dose, reducing to about 2 micrograms/mL 10 hours after injection. A plasma concentration of 38 micrograms/mL has been reported after the intravenous infusion of 500 mg over 30 minutes, reducing to 18 micrograms/mL 1 hour later. Amikacin has been detected in body tissues and fluids after injection; it crosses the placenta but does not readily penetrate into the CSF, although substantial penetration of the blood-brain barrier has been reported in children with meningitis.

A plasma half-life of about 2 to 3 hours has been reported in patients with normal renal function. Most of a dose is excreted by glomerular filtration in the urine within 24 hours.

◊ References.

1. Vanhaeverbeek M, *et al.* Pharmacokinetics of once-daily amikacin in elderly patients. *J Antimicrob Chemother* 1993; **31:** 185–7.
2. Gaillard J-L, *et al.* Cerebrospinal fluid penetration of amikacin in children with community-acquired bacterial meningitis. *Antimicrob Agents Chemother* 1995; **39:** 253–5.
3. Bressolle F, *et al.* Population pharmacokinetics of amikacin in critically ill patients. *Antimicrob Agents Chemother* 1996; **40:** 1682–9.
4. Canis F, *et al.* Pharmacokinetics and bronchial diffusion of single daily dose amikacin in cystic fibrosis patients. *J Antimicrob Chemother* 1997; **39:** 431–3.
5. Tod M, *et al.* Population pharmacokinetic study of amikacin administered once or twice daily to febrile, severely neutropenic adults. *Antimicrob Agents Chemother* 1998; **42:** 849–56.
6. Tréluyer JM, *et al.* Nonparametric population pharmacokinetic analysis of amikacin in neonates, infants, and children. *Antimicrob Agents Chemother* 2002; **46:** 1381–7.

### Uses and Administration

Amikacin is a semisynthetic aminoglycoside antibiotic derived from kanamycin and is used similarly to gentamicin (p.219) in the treatment of severe Gram-negative and other infections. It is given as the sulfate, and is generally reserved for the treatment of severe infections caused by susceptible bacteria that are resistant to gentamicin and tobramycin. Amikacin has also been given with antimycobacterials in the treatment of opportunistic mycobacterial infections (p.137). As with gentamicin, amikacin may be used with penicillins and with cephalosporins; the injections should be given at separate sites.

Doses of amikacin sulfate are expressed in terms of amikacin base. 1.3 g of amikacin sulfate is approximately equivalent to 1 g of amikacin. Adults and children may be given 15 mg/kg daily in equally divided doses every 8 or 12 hours by intramuscular injection. In life-threatening infections, the dose may be increased in adults up to a maximum of 500 mg every 8 hours. A dose of 7.5 mg/kg daily in two divided doses (equivalent to 250 mg twice daily in adults) may be given for the treatment of uncomplicated urinary-tract infections. The same doses may be given by slow intravenous injection over 2 to 3 minutes, or by intravenous infusion. In adults, 500 mg in 100 to 200 mL of diluent has been infused over 30 to 60 minutes; proportionately less fluid should be given to children.

Neonates may be given 10 mg/kg as a loading dose, followed by 15 mg/kg daily in two divided doses. If given by intravenous infusion, an infusion period of 1 to 2 hours is recommended. It has been suggested that doses may need to be adjusted in preterm neonates.

Treatment should preferably not continue for longer than 7 to 10 days, and the total dose given to adults should not exceed 15 g. Peak plasma concentrations greater than 30 to 35 micrograms/mL or trough plasma concentrations greater than 5 to 10 micrograms/mL should be avoided. Dosage should be adjusted in all patients according to plasma-amikacin concentrations, and this is particularly important where factors such as age, renal impairment, or prolonged therapy may predispose to toxicity, or where there is a risk of subtherapeutic concentrations. For discussion of the methods of calculating aminoglycoside dosage requirements, see p.219. As with some other aminoglycosides, there are preliminary results suggesting that equivalent efficacy can be obtained from once-daily dosage with amikacin without increasing toxicity, but such dosage regimens are not yet established.

A 0.25% solution has been instilled into body cavities in adults.

A liposomal formulation of amikacin is under investigation.

**Opportunistic mycobacterial infections.** Amikacin has been included in multidrug regimens for the treatment of *Mycobacterium avium* complex infections (p.137). Treatment with amikacin in combination with parenteral ethambutol and ciprofloxacin together with an oral macrolide produced negative blood cultures in 13 of 15 patients,[1] but the addition of amikacin to oral treatment with rifampicin, ciprofloxacin, clofazimine, and ethambutol did not influence the clinical response in an open study of 74 patients.[2]

1. Roger P-M, *et al.* Efficacy and safety of an intravenous induction therapy for treatment of disseminated Mycobacterium avium complex infection in AIDS patients: a pilot study. *J Antimicrob Chemother* 1999; **44:** 129–31.
2. Parenti DM, *et al.* A phase II/III trial of antimicrobial therapy with or without amikacin in the treatment of disseminated Mycobacterium avium infection in HIV-infected individuals. *AIDS* 1998; **12:** 2439–46.

### Preparations

***USP 27:*** Amikacin Sulfate Injection.

**Proprietary Preparations** (details are given in Part 3)
***Arg.:*** Biklin; Greini; Riklinak; ***Austral.:*** Amikin; ***Austria:*** Biklin; ***Belg.:*** Amukin; ***Braz.:*** Amicacil; Amicalin; Amicilon; Amikin†; Aminocina; Bactomicin; Novamin; ***Canad.:*** Amikin; ***Denm.:*** Biklin†; ***Fin.:*** Biklin; ***Fr.:*** Amiklin; ***Ger.:*** Biklin; ***Gr.:*** Amicasil; Amikan; Briklin; Farcyclin; Flexelite; Fromentyl; Kancin-Gap; Lanomycin; Lifermycin; Micalpha; Orlobin; Remikin; Roviericlin; Selaxa; Uzix; ***Hong Kong:*** Amikin; Apalin; Selemycin; ***India:*** Amicin; ***Irl.:*** Amikin; ***Israel:*** Amikin; Likacin; ***Ital.:*** Amicasil; Amikan; BB-K8; Chemacin; Dramigel; Likacin; Lukadin; Mediamik; Migracin; Mikan; Mikavir; Nekacin; Pierami; Sifamic†; ***Malaysia:*** Amikin; Selemycin; ***Mex.:*** Akacin; Amikafur; Amikalem; Amikasons; Amikavi; Amikayect; Amikin; Amiyec; AMK; Baxi-K; Beramikin; Biclin; Biokacin; Cramigen†; Gamikal; Georkacina†; Mikazul†; Oprad; Yectamid; ***Neth.:*** Amukin; ***NZ:*** Amikin; ***Port.:*** Biclin; Kamina; ***S.Afr.:*** Amikin; Kacinth†; ***Singapore:*** Amikin; Selemycin†; ***Spain:*** Biclin; Kanbine; ***Swed.:*** Biklin; ***Switz.:*** Amikine; ***Thai.:*** Akacin; Akicin; Amikasol; Amikin; Anbikin; Siamik; Tipkin; Tybikin; ***UAE:*** Mikacin; ***UK:*** Amikin; ***USA:*** Amikin.

## Aminosalicylic Acid

Aminosalicílico, ácido; 4-Aminosalicylic Acid; Aminosalylum; Para-aminosalicylic Acid; PAS; Pasalicylum. 4-Amino-2-hydroxybenzoic acid.

$C_7H_7NO_3 = 153.1.$

*CAS — 65-49-6.*

*ATC — J04AA01.*

NOTE. Distinguish from 5-aminosalicylic acid (Mesalazine, p.1273).

**Pharmacopoeias.** In *US.*

**USP 27** (Aminosalicylic Acid). A white or practically white, bulky powder that darkens on exposure to light and air; it is odourless or has a slight acetous odour. Slightly soluble in water and in ether; soluble in alcohol; practically insoluble in benzene. Under no circumstances should a solution be used if its colour is darker than that of a freshly prepared solution. pH of a saturated solution in water is between 3.0 to 3.7. Store in airtight containers at a temperature not exceeding 30°. Protect from light.

## Calcium Aminosalicylate

Aminosalicilato cálcico; Aminosalicylate calcium; Calcii Para-aminosalicylas; Calcium PAS. Calcium 4-amino-2-hydroxybenzoate trihydrate.

$(C_7H_6NO_3)_2Ca,3H_2O$ = 398.4.

*CAS — 133-15-3 (anhydrous calcium aminosalicylate).*

*ATC — J04AA03.*

**Pharmacopoeias.** *Jpn* includes the heptahydrate.

## Sodium Aminosalicylate

Aminosalicilato sódico; Aminosalicylate Sodium; Aminosalylnatrium; Monosodium 4-Aminosalicylate Dihydrate; Natrii Aminosalicylas Dihydricus; Natrii Para-aminosalicylas; Pasalicylum Solubile; Sodium Para-aminosalicylate; Sodium PAS. Sodium 4-amino-2-hydroxybenzoate dihydrate.

$C_7H_6NNaO_3,2H_2O$ = 211.1.

*CAS — 133-10-8 (anhydrous sodium aminosalicylate); 6018-19-5 (sodium aminosalicylate dihydrate).*

*ATC — J04AA02.*

**Pharmacopoeias.** In *Chin., Eur.* (see p.vi), *Pol.*, and *US.*

**Ph. Eur. 5.0** (Sodium Aminosalicylate Dihydrate). A slightly hygroscopic, white, crystalline powder, or white or almost white crystals. Freely soluble in water; sparingly soluble in alcohol, practically insoluble in dichloromethane. A 2% solution in water has a pH of 6.5 to 8.5. Store in airtight containers. Protect from light.

**USP 27** (Aminosalicylate Sodium). A white to cream-coloured, practically odourless crystalline powder. Soluble 1 in 2 of water; sparingly soluble in alcohol; very slightly soluble in chloroform and in ether. Its solutions decompose slowly and darken in colour. Prepare solutions within 24 hours of administration. Under no circumstances should a solution be used if its colour is darker than that of a freshly prepared solution. pH of a 2% solution in water is between 6.5 and 8.5. Store in airtight containers at a temperature not exceeding 40°. Protect from light.

**Stability.** Aqueous solutions of aminosalicylates are unstable and should be freshly prepared.

Solutions of sodium aminosalicylate in sorbitol or syrup degraded more quickly to *m*-aminophenol than those in glycerol or propylene glycol.[1] Colour developed in all solutions but was not found to be an accurate indicator of decomposition of sodium aminosalicylate as it reflected only oxidation of *m*-aminophenol.

1. Blake MI, *et al.* Effect of vehicle on the stability of sodium aminosalicylate in liquid dosage forms. *Am J Hosp Pharm* 1973; **30:** 441–3.

### Adverse Effects and Treatment

Aminosalicylic acid and its salts may cause the adverse effects of salicylates (see Aspirin, p.15).

Gastrointestinal effects are common and include nausea, vomiting, and diarrhoea; they may be reduced by giving doses with food or with an antacid but occasionally may be severe enough that therapy has to be withdrawn. Alteration of gastrointestinal function may lead to malabsorption of vitamin $B_{12}$, folate, and lipids. Salts of aminosalicylic acid may be better tolerated than the acid. Tolerance in children may be better than in adults.

Hypersensitivity reactions have been reported in 5 to 10% of adults, usually during the first few weeks of treatment, and include fever, skin rashes; less commonly, arthralgia, lymphadenopathy, and hepatosplenomegaly may occur and, rarely, a syndrome resembling infectious mononucleosis. Other adverse effects which have been attributed to a hypersensitivity reaction to aminosalicylate include jaundice and encephalitis. Blood disorders reported include haemolytic anaemia in patients with G6PD deficiency, agranulocytosis, eosinophilia, leucopenia, and thrombocytopenia. Psychosis may occasionally occur. Prolonged treatment may induce goitre and hypothyroidism. Crystalluria may occur.

**Effects on the liver.** Drug-induced hepatitis occurred in 0.32% of 7492 patients receiving antituberculous drugs; aminosalicylic acid was the most common cause.[1]

1. Rossouw JE, Saunders SJ. Hepatic complications of antituberculous therapy. *Q J Med* 1975; **44:** 1–16.

### Precautions

Aminosalicylic acid and its salts should be used with great care in patients with hepatic or renal impairment and in patients with gastric ulcer. They should be given with caution to patients with G6PD deficiency. The sodium salt should be used with caution in patients with heart failure.

Aminosalicylates interfere with tests for glycosuria using copper reagents and for urobilinogen using Ehrlich's reagent.

**Breast feeding.** Small amounts of aminosalicylic acid are present in breast milk. A maximum concentration of 1.1 microgram/mL has been reported in the breast milk of a lactating woman 3 hours after administration of a 4 g dose of aminosalicylic acid.[1]

1. Holdiness MR. Antituberculosis drugs and breast feeding. *Arch Intern Med* 1984; **144:** 1888.

**Pregnancy.** The use of aminosalicylic acid or its salts is not recommended in pregnant patients due to gastrointestinal intolerance.[1] In addition, one study suggested that first-trimester exposure may be associated with congenital defects although other studies had not found similar effects.[2]

1. Snider D. Pregnancy and tuberculosis. *Chest* 1984; **86:** 10S–13S.
2. Briggs GG, *et al. Drugs in pregnancy and lactation.* 6th ed. Philadelphia: Lippincott Williams and Wilkins, 2002: 51a.

### Interactions

The adverse effects of aminosalicylates and salicylates may be additive. Probenecid may also increase toxicity by delaying renal excretion and enhancing plasma concentrations of aminosalicylate. The activity of aminosalicylic acid may be antagonised by ester-type local anaesthetics such as procaine.

### Antimicrobial Action

Aminosalicylic acid is bacteriostatic and is active against *M. tuberculosis*. Other mycobacteria are usually resistant. It has a relatively weak action compared with other antituberculous drugs. Resistance develops quickly if aminosalicylic acid is used alone.

### Pharmacokinetics

When given by mouth, aminosalicylic acid and its salts are readily absorbed, and peak plasma concentrations occur after about 1 to 4 hours.

Aminosalicylate diffuses widely through body tissues and fluids, although diffusion into the CSF occurs only if the meninges are inflamed. About 15% of the sodium salt, and 50 to 70% of the acid, is bound to plasma proteins.

Aminosalicylate is metabolised in the intestine and liver primarily by acetylation. Urinary excretion is rapid, and 80% or more of a dose is excreted within 24 hours; 50% or more of the dose is excreted as the acetylated metabolite. The half-life of aminosalicylic acid is approximately 1 hour.

Aminosalicylate is distributed into breast milk (see under Precautions, above, for more details).

### Uses and Administration

Aminosalicylic acid and its salts are second-line antimycobacterials given by mouth in the treatment of tuberculosis (p.150) when other more potent drugs cannot be used. They should always be given with other antituberculous drugs.

Aminosalicylic acid may be given as the acid or as the sodium salt. Sodium aminosalicylate 1.38 g is approximately equivalent to 1 g of aminosalicylic acid. However, a usual adult daily dose is 12 g in 3 divided doses by mouth and has been recommended for products containing the acid as well as for those containing the sodium salt.

Aminosalicylate sodium is also given rectally in the treatment of ulcerative colitis in a usual dose of 2 g once daily.

A wide range of dosage forms has been used in an attempt to overcome the bulk and exceedingly unpleasant taste of the aminosalicylates. The salts appear to be better tolerated than the free acid and solutions in iced water prepared immediately before use may be less unpleasant to take.

**Administration in renal impairment.** It has been recommended that aminosalicylic acid should be avoided in patients with renal impairment.[1] An increase in plasma clearance of aminosalicylic acid (attributed to increased hepatic metabolism) has been noted in patients with renal impairment, hence attempting to give aminosalicylate in reduced doses to such patients may lead to subtherapeutic serum concentrations.[2]

1. Appel GB, Neu HC. The nephrotoxicity of antimicrobial agents (first of three parts). *N Engl J Med* 1977; **296:** 663–70.
2. Holdiness MR. Clinical pharmacokinetics of the antituberculosis drugs. *Clin Pharmacokinet* 1984; **9:** 511–44.

**Inflammatory bowel disease.** Together with corticosteroids, derivatives of 5-aminosalicylic acid are one of the mainstays of the treatment of inflammatory bowel disease (p.1243). However, aminosalicylic acid (4-aminosalicylic acid) has also been investigated, and beneficial results have been reported with enemas[1-4] and with oral administration[5] in ulcerative colitis.

1. Campieri M, *et al.* 4-Aminosalicylic acid (4-ASA) and 5-aminosalicylic acid (5-ASA) in topical treatment of ulcerative colitis patients. *Gastroenterology* 1984; **86:** 1039.
2. Ginsberg AL, *et al.* Treatment of left-sided ulcerative colitis with 4-aminosalicylic acid enemas: a double-blind, placebo-controlled trial. *Ann Intern Med* 1988; **108:** 195–9.
3. Sharma MP, Duphare HV. 4-Aminosalicylic acid enemas for ulcerative colitis. *Lancet* 1989; **i:** 450.
4. O'Donnell LJD, *et al.* Double blind, controlled trial of 4-aminosalicylic acid and prednisolone enemas in distal ulcerative colitis. *Gut* 1992; **33:** 947–9.
5. Beeken W, *et al.* Controlled trial of 4-ASA in ulcerative colitis. *Dig Dis Sci* 1997; **42:** 354–8.

### Preparations

***USP 27:*** Aminosalicylate Sodium Tablets; Aminosalicylic Acid Tablets.

**Proprietary Preparations** (details are given in Part 3)

***Canad.:*** Nemasol; ***Chile:*** Aflogol; ***Fr.:*** Quadrasa; ***Ger.:*** Pas-Fatol N; ***Ital.:*** Quadrasa; Salf-Pas; ***Switz.:*** Perfusion de PAS; ***USA:*** Paser.

***Multi-ingredient:*** ***India:*** Inapas.

## Amoxicillin *(BAN, rINN)*

Amoxicilina; Amoxycillin. (6*R*)-6-[α-D-(4-Hydroxyphenyl)glycylamino]penicillanic acid.

$C_{16}H_{19}N_3O_5S$ = 365.4.

*CAS — 26787-78-0.*

*ATC — J01CA04.*

## Amoxicillin Sodium *(BANM, USAN, rINNM)*

Amoxicilina sódica; Amoxicillinum Natricum; Amoxycillin Sodium; BRL-2333AB-B.

$C_{16}H_{18}N_3NaO_5S$ = 387.4.

*CAS — 34642-77-8.*

*ATC — J01CA04.*

**Pharmacopoeias.** In *Chin., Eur.* (see p.vi), and *Pol.*

**Ph. Eur. 5.0** (Amoxicillin Sodium). A white or almost white, very hygroscopic powder. Very soluble in water; sparingly soluble in dehydrated alcohol; very slightly soluble in acetone. A 10% solution in water has a pH of 8.0 to 10.0. Store in airtight containers.

## Amoxicillin Trihydrate *(BANM, rINNM)*

Amoxicilina trihidrato; Amoxicillin *(USAN)*; Amoxicillinum Trihydricum; Amoxycillin Trihydrate; BRL-2333.

$C_{16}H_{19}N_3O_5S,3H_2O$ = 419.4.

*CAS — 61336-70-7.*

*ATC — J01CA04.*

NOTE. Compounded preparations of amoxicillin may be represented by the following names:

- Co-amoxiclav *x/y* (*BAN*)—amoxicillin (as the trihydrate or the sodium salt) and potassium clavulanate; *x* and *y* are the strengths in milligrams of amoxicillin and clavulanic acid respectively
- Co-amoxiclav (*PEN*)—amoxicillin trihydrate and potassium clavulanate.

**Pharmacopoeias.** In *Chin., Eur.* (see p.vi), *Int., Jpn, Pol., US,* and *Viet.*

**Ph. Eur. 5.0** (Amoxicillin Trihydrate). A white or almost white, crystalline powder. Slightly soluble in water; very slightly soluble in alcohol; practically insoluble in fatty oils. It dissolves in dilute acids and in dilute solutions of alkali hydroxides. A 0.2% solution in water has a pH of 3.5 to 5.5. Store in airtight containers

**USP 27** (Amoxicillin). A white, practically odourless crystalline powder. Slightly soluble in water and in methyl alcohol; insoluble in carbon tetrachloride, in chloroform, and in benzene. pH of a 0.2% solution in water is between 3.5 and 6.0. Store in airtight containers.

### Adverse Effects and Precautions

As for Ampicillin, p.157.

The incidence of diarrhoea is less with amoxicillin than ampicillin.

Hepatitis and cholestatic jaundice have been reported with the combination amoxicillin with clavulanic acid; the clavulanic acid component has been implicated. Erythema multiforme, Stevens-Johnson syndrome, toxic epidermal necrolysis, and exfoliative dermatitis have also been attributed occasionally to the use of amoxicillin with clavulanic acid.

**Breast feeding.** Although amoxicillin is excreted in breast milk in small amounts,[1] the American Academy of Pediatrics considers that it is usually compatible with breast feeding.[2]

1. Kafetzis DA, *et al.* Passage of cephalosporins and amoxicillin into the breast milk. *Acta Paediatr Scand* 1981; **70:** 285–8.
2. American Academy of Pediatrics. The transfer of drugs and other chemicals into human milk. *Pediatrics* 2001; **108:** 776–89. Correction. *ibid.*; 1029. Also available at: http://aappolicy.aappublications.org/cgi/content/full/pediatrics%3b108/3/776 (accessed 24/05/04)

**Effects on the liver.** Hepatitis and cholestatic jaundice associated with the combination amoxicillin with clavulanic acid (co-amoxiclav) have been reported[1-4] and by 1993 the UK Committee on Safety of Medicines (CSM) had received 138 reports of hepatobiliary disorders, 3 of which were fatal.[5] It warned that, although usually reversible, the reaction often occurred after stopping therapy with a delay of up to 6 weeks. It appeared that the clavulanic acid was probably responsible. Retrospective analysis of cases reported in Australia[6] and a cohort study in the UK[7] found increasing age and prolonged treatment to be major risk factors for jaundice following co-amoxiclav; male sex is also a risk factor. By 1997 the CSM considered that cholestatic jaundice occurred with a frequency of about 1 in 6000 adult patients and that the risk of acute liver injury was about six times greater with co-amoxiclav than with amoxicillin alone. Therefore it now recommends that co-amoxiclav should be reserved for bacterial infections likely to be caused by amoxicillin-resistant strains, and that treatment should not usually exceed 14 days.[8]

1. Stricker BHC, *et al.* Cholestatic hepatitis due to antibacterial combination of amoxicillin and clavulanic acid (Augmentin). *Dig Dis Sci* 1989; **34:** 1576–80.
2. Wong FS, *et al.* Augmentin-induced jaundice. *Med J Aust* 1991; **154:** 698–701.

3. Larrey D, *et al.* Hepatitis associated with amoxycillin-clavulanic acid combination report of 15 cases. *Gut* 1992; **33:** 368–71.
4. Hebbard GS, *et al.* Augmentin-induced jaundice with a fatal outcome. *Med J Aust* 1992; **156:** 285–6.
5. Committee on Safety of Medicines/Medicines Control Agency. Cholestatic jaundice with co-amoxiclav. *Current Problems* 1993; **19:** 2.
6. Thomson JA, *et al.* Risk factors for the development of amoxycillin-clavulanic acid associated jaundice. *Med J Aust* 1995; **162:** 638–40.
7. Rodríguez LAG, *et al.* Risk of acute liver injury associated with the combination of amoxicillin and clavulanic acid. *Arch Intern Med* 1996; **156:** 1327–32.
8. Committee on Safety of Medicines/Medicines Control Agency. Revised indications for co-amoxiclav (Augmentin). *Current Problems* 1997; **23:** 8. Also available at: http://medicines.mhra.gov.uk/ourwork/monitorsafequalmed/currentproblems/volume24.htm (accessed 24/05/04)

**Effects on the teeth.** A report of tooth discoloration in 3 children associated with the use of amoxicillin with clavulanic acid.[1]

1. Garcia-López M, *et al.* Amoxycillin-clavulanic acid-related tooth discoloration in children. *Pediatrics* 2001; **108:** 819–20.

**Sodium content.** Each g of amoxicillin sodium contains about 2.6 mmol of sodium.

## Interactions

As for Ampicillin, p.157.

## Antimicrobial Action

As for Ampicillin, p.157.

Amoxicillin has been reported to be more active *in vitro* than ampicillin against *Enterococcus faecalis, Helicobacter pylori,* and *Salmonella* spp., but less active against *Shigella* spp.

Amoxicillin is inactivated by beta lactamases and complete cross-resistance has been reported between amoxicillin and ampicillin. The spectrum of activity of amoxicillin may be extended by use with a beta-lactamase inhibitor such as clavulanic acid (p.193). As well as reversing resistance to amoxicillin in beta-lactamase-producing strains of species otherwise sensitive, clavulanic acid has also been reported to enhance the activity of amoxicillin against several species not generally considered sensitive. These have included *Bacteroides, Legionella,* and *Nocardia* spp., *Haemophilus influenzae, Moraxella catarrhalis* (*Branhamella catarrhalis*), and *Burkholderia pseudomallei* (*Pseudomonas pseudomallei*). However, *Ps. aeruginosa, Serratia marcescens,* and many other Gram-negative bacteria remain resistant. Transferable resistance has been reported in *H. pylori.*

## Pharmacokinetics

Amoxicillin is resistant to inactivation by gastric acid. It is more rapidly and more completely absorbed than ampicillin when given by mouth. Peak plasma-amoxicillin concentrations of about 5 micrograms/mL have been observed 1 to 2 hours after a dose of 250 mg, with detectable amounts present for up to 8 hours. Doubling the dose can double the concentration. The presence of food in the stomach does not appear to diminish the total amount absorbed.

Concentrations of amoxicillin after intramuscular injection are similar to those achieved with oral administration.

About 20% is bound to plasma proteins and plasma half-lives of 1 to 1.5 hours have been reported. The half-life may be prolonged in neonates, the elderly, and patients with renal impairment; in severe renal impairment the half-life may be 7 to 20 hours. Amoxicillin is widely distributed at varying concentrations in body tissues and fluids. It crosses the placenta; small amounts are distributed into breast milk. Little amoxicillin passes into the CSF unless the meninges are inflamed.

Amoxicillin is metabolised to a limited extent to penicilloic acid which is excreted in the urine. About 60% of an oral dose of amoxicillin is excreted unchanged in the urine in 6 hours by glomerular filtration and tubular secretion. Urinary concentrations above 300 micrograms/mL have been reported after a dose of 250 mg. Probenecid reduces renal excretion. Amoxicillin is removed by haemodialysis. High concentrations have been reported in bile; some may be excreted in the faeces.

*Amoxicillin with clavulanic acid.* The pharmacokinetics of amoxicillin and clavulanic acid are broadly similar and neither appears to affect the other to any great extent.

## Uses and Administration

Amoxicillin is the 4-hydroxy analogue of ampicillin (p.158) and is used in a similar variety of susceptible infections. These include actinomycosis, biliary-tract infections, bronchitis, endocarditis (particularly for prophylaxis), gastro-enteritis (including salmonella enteritis, but not shigellosis), gonorrhoea, Lyme disease, mouth infections, otitis media, pneumonia, spleen disorders (pneumococcal infection prophylaxis), typhoid and paratyphoid fever, and urinary-tract infections. The beta-lactamase inhibitor clavulanic acid (p.193) widens amoxicillin's antimicrobial spectrum and a combined preparation (co-amoxiclav) can be used when resistance to amoxicillin is prevalent, for example in respiratory-tract infections due to *Haemophilus influenzae* or *Moraxella catarrhalis* (*Branhamella catarrhalis*), in the empirical treatment of animal bites, or in melioidosis. For details of these infections and their treatment, see under Choice of Antibacterial, p.120.

Amoxicillin is also given as part of treatment regimens to eradicate *Helicobacter pylori* infection in patients with peptic ulcer disease (p.1246).

*Administration and dosage.* Amoxicillin is given by mouth as the trihydrate and by injection as the sodium salt. Doses are expressed in terms of the equivalent amount of amoxicillin. 1.06 g of amoxicillin sodium and 1.15 g of amoxicillin trihydrate are each approximately equivalent to 1 g of amoxicillin.

The usual oral dose is 250 to 500 mg every 8 hours, or 500 to 875 mg every 12 hours. Children up to 10 years of age may be given 125 to 250 mg every 8 hours; for those under 40 kg, a dose of 20 to 40 mg/kg daily in divided doses every 8 hours, or 25 to 45 mg/kg daily in divided doses every 12 hours, may be used; in infants less than 3 months old, the maximum dose should be 30 mg/kg daily in divided doses every 12 hours.

Higher oral doses of amoxicillin, either as a single dose or in short courses, are used in some conditions. For example, a dose of 3 g repeated once after 8 hours may be used for dental abscesses. A 3-g dose may be given for uncomplicated acute urinary-tract infections, and repeated once after 10 to 12 hours.

A high-dose regimen of 3 g twice daily may be used in patients with severe or recurrent infections of the respiratory tract. If necessary, children aged 3 to 10 years with otitis media may be given 750 mg twice daily for 2 days. Amoxicillin has also been given as a single dose of 3 g, with probenecid 1 g, in the treatment of uncomplicated gonorrhoea in areas where gonococci remain sensitive.

For the prophylaxis of endocarditis in patients at risk, amoxicillin 2 or 3 g is given about 1 hour before dental procedures.

For the eradication of *H. pylori,* amoxicillin is given with either metronidazole or clarithromycin and a proton pump inhibitor or ranitidine bismuth citrate; usual doses of amoxicillin are 0.75 or 1 g twice daily or 500 mg three times daily.

Amoxicillin is administered by intramuscular or slow intravenous injection in doses of 500 mg every 8 hours. In severe infections, 1 g of amoxicillin may be given every 6 hours by slow intravenous injection over 3 to 4 minutes or by infusion over 30 to 60 minutes. Children up to 10 years of age may be given 50 to 100 mg/kg daily by injection in divided doses.

Doses may need to be reduced in moderate to severe renal impairment (see below).

*Amoxicillin with clavulanic acid.* Amoxicillin in combination with clavulanic acid (co-amoxiclav) is given by mouth in a ratio of amoxicillin (as the trihydrate) 2, 4, or 7 parts to 1 part of clavulanic acid (as the potassium salt), or intravenously in a ratio of 5 parts of amoxicillin (as the sodium salt) to 1 part of clavulanic acid (as the potassium salt). Doses of the combination, calculated on amoxicillin content, are similar to those for amoxicillin used alone.

◊ References.

1. Speller DCE, *et al.*, eds. Clavulanate/β-lactam antibiotics: further experience. *J Antimicrob Chemother* 1989; **24** (suppl B): 1–226.
2. Todd PA, Benfield P. Amoxicillin/clavulanic acid: an update of its antibacterial activity, pharmacokinetic properties and therapeutic use. *Drugs* 1990; **39**: 264–307.
3. Easton J, *et al.* Amoxicillin/clavulanic acid: a review of its use in the management of paediatric patients with acute otitis media. *Drugs* 2003; **63**: 311–40.

**Administration in renal impairment.** Doses of amoxicillin should be reduced in patients with moderate to severe renal impairment according to creatinine clearance (CC):

- CC 10 to 30 mL/minute: 250 to 500 mg every 12 hours
- CC less than 10 mL/minute: 250 to 500 mg every 24 hours
- haemodialysis patients: 250 to 500 mg every 24 hours and an additional dose both during and after the dialysis session.

## Preparations

***BP 2003:*** Amoxicillin Capsules; Amoxicillin Injection; Amoxicillin Oral Suspension; Co-amoxiclav Tablets;
***USP 27:*** Amoxicillin and Clavulanate Potassium for Oral Suspension; Amoxicillin and Clavulanate Potassium Tablets; Amoxicillin Capsules; Amoxicillin for Oral Suspension; Amoxicillin Tablets; Amoxicillin Tablets for Oral Suspension.

**Proprietary Preparations** (details are given in Part 3)
***Arg.:*** Abiotyl; Almorsan; Amixen; Amox-G; Amoxi; Amoxibiot; Amoxicina; Amoxicler; Amoxidal; Amoxidal Duo; Amoxigrand; Amoxipenil; Amoxipoten; Amoxitenk; Antibiocilina; Antiobiocilina; Apracur Biotic; Ardine; Atrival; Biotamoxal; Bioxilina; Darzitil; Dunox; Flemoxon; Fullcilina; Fullcilina Duo; Grinsil; Grinsil Duo; Moxitral; Nobactam; Optamox; Oximar; Trifamox; Trifamox Duo; ***Austral.:*** Alphamox; Amohexal; Amoxil; Bgramin; Cilamox; Fisamox; Maxamox; Moxacin; ***Austria:*** Amoxal; Amoxid†; Amoxihexal; Amoxilan; Amoxistad; Clamoxyl; Eramox; Gonoform; Ospamox; Supramox; ***Belg.:*** Amoxi; Clamoxyl; Flemoxin; Hiconcil; Moxaline; Novabritine; ***Braz.:*** Amox; Amoxi-Ped; Amoxidil†; Amoxifar; Amoxil; Amoxina; Amoxipen; Amoxitan; Amplal†; Amplamox; Camoxin; Cibramicina†; Farmoxil; Flemoxon; Hiconcil; Hincomox; Ibamoxil†; Licilon; Moxiplus†; Neo Moxicilin; Novacil; Novocilin; Novoxil; Penvicilin; Polibac; Polimoxil; Prodoxil; Respicilin; Trimox; Ultramox; Uni Amox; Velamox; ***Canad.:*** Amoxil†; Apo-Amoxi; Lin-Amox; Novamoxin; Nu-Amoxi; ***Chile:*** Abiolex; Amobiotic; Amoval; Amoval Duo; Amoxipenil; Optamox; ***Denm.:*** Flemoxin; Imacillin; Imadrax; ***Fin.:*** Amorion; Amoxin; Clamox; Flemoxin; Penalta; ***Fr.:*** A-Gram; Amodex; Amophar†; Bactox; Bristamox; Clamoxyl; Flemoxine; Gramidil; Hiconcil; Zamocilline†; ***Ger.:*** Amagesan; Amc-Puren; Amoxi; Amoxi-Diolan; Amoxi-Hefa; Amoxi-Puren; Amoxi-Tablinen; Amoxi-Wolff; Amoxibeta; Amoxibiocin†; Amoxidoc; Amoxihexal; Amoxillat; Amoximerck; Amoxypen; Clamoxyl; dura AX†; espa-moxin; Flui-Amoxicillin; InfectoMox; Jephoxin†; Phamoxi; Sigamopen; Ulcolind Amoxi†; ***Gr.:*** Amoxil; Aproxal; Flemoxin; Paradroxil; Stevencillin; Triodanin; ***Hong Kong:*** Amoxa; Amoxapen; Amoxil†; Apo-Amoxi; Aroxin; Betamox; Edamox; Hamoxillin; Moxilen; Moxlin; Ospamox; Unimox; ***India:*** Amoxil; Amoxivan; Biomoxil; Damoxy; Flemoxin; Hipen; Imox; Loxyn; Mox; Novamox; Ronemox; Symoxyl; ***Irl.:*** Amoxil; Clonamox; Galenamox; Geramox; Oramox; Pinamox; Roxillin†; ***Israel:*** Amoxi; Apomoxyn†; Hiconcil; Moxypen; Moxyvit; ***Ital.:*** Alfamox; Amoflux; Amosol; Amox; Amoxillin; Amoxina; Amoxipen†; Bradimox; Dodemox; Erremox; Genimox; Helimox†; Hydramox; Ibiamox; Isimoxin; Majorpen; Mopen; Moxiren; Neo-Ampiplus; Neotetranase; Oralmox; Pamocil; Progemox; Simoxil; Simplamox; Sintopen; Velamox; Zimox; ***Malaysia:*** Beamoxy; Moxacil; Moxilen; Moxipen; Ospamox; Setmoxil; ***Mex.:*** Acimox; Acroxil; Ameclina; Amobay; Amoxifur; Amoxil; Amoxinovag; Amoxisol; Amoxivet; Ampliron; AMX; Ardine; Axcil†; Brenoxil; Deniren†; Doxamil; Examolin; Flemoxon; Gimalxina; Grunicina; Hidramox; Limoxin; Lumox; Moxicel†; Moxlin†; Penamox; Penticlox; Polymox; Servamox; Servamox-F; Solciclina; Xalyn-Or; Xiprocan†; ***Neth.:*** Clamoxyl; Flemoxin; ***Norw.:*** Amimox†; Amoxillin; Imacillin; ***NZ:*** Amoxil; Apo-Amoxi†; Ibiamox; Moxlin†; Ospamox; Penamox†; ***Port.:*** Amplamox; Bodisan; Cipamox; Clamoxyl; Flemoxin; Moxadent; Moxipen; Oraminax; Ospamox; Penamox; ***S.Afr.:*** Acucil†; Amocillin; Amoxil; Amoxyfizz†; Betamox; C-Mox†; Ipcamox; Maxcil; Moxan; Moxymax†; Moxypen; Penmox; Promoxil; Ranmoxy; Saltermox†; Spectramox; Ultramox†; Xeracil†; Zoxil; ***Singapore:*** Amoxa; Amoxapen; Amoxicap; Amoxigran†; Amoxil; Amoxitab†; Apo-Amoxi; Aroxin; Moxilen†; Moxipen; Ospamox; Ranoxyl†; Unimox; ***Spain:*** Actimoxi; Agerpen; Amitron; Amoflamisan†; Amox†; Amoxaren; Amoxi Gobens; Amoxibacter; Amoxidel†; Amoximedical; Apamox; Ardine; Blenox; Bolchipen; Borbalan; Britamox; Brondix; Clamoxyl; Co Amoxin; Combitora†; Damoxicil†; Dobriciclin; Edoxil; Eupen; Flubiotic NF; Hosboral; Inexbron†; Mediamox†; Metifarma†; Morgenxil; Novagcilina†; Precopen†; Raudopen†; Reloxyl; Remisan; Riotapen†; Salvapen; Suamoxil†; Superpeni†; Tolodina; ***Swed.:*** Amimox; Bristamox†; Flemoxin†; Imacillin; ***Switz.:*** amoxi-basan; Amoxi-Cophar; Amoxi-Mepha; Amoximex; Antiotic; Azilline; Clamoxyl; Flemoxin; Helvamox†; Penimox; Rivoxicillin†; Servamox†; Spectroxyl; Supramox; ***Thai.:*** Acticillin; Amacin; Amox; Amoxa; Amoxcillin; Amoxil; Amoxy; Amoxylin; Asiamox; Biomox†; Coamox; Ibiamox; Kamoxin; Kenya-Mox; Manmox; Meixil; Milamox; Moxapen; Moxcil; Moxcin; Moxilcap; Moxilen†; Moxilin; Moximed; Moxipan; Pondnoxcill; Posmox†; Rancil; Samox; Samoxin; Servamox; Sia-Mox; Sil-A-Mox; Unimox; ***UAE:*** Julphamox; ***UK:*** Almodan†; Amix; Amopen†; Amoram; Amoxident; Amoxil; Galenamox; Rimoxallin; ***USA:*** Amoxil; DisperMox; Trimox; Wymox†.

**Multi-ingredient:** ***Arg.:*** Aclav; Albesine Biotic; Amixen Plus; Amox-G Bronquial; Amoxi Respiratorio; Amoxidal Respiratorio; Amoxidal Respiratorio Duo; Amoxigrand Bronquial; Amoxigrand Compuesto; Amoxipenil Bronquial; Amoxitenk Plus; Amoxitenk Respiratorio; Aseptobron Respiratorio; Bioxilina Plus; Clavulox; Clavulox Duo; Cloximar Duo; Darzitil Plus; Darzitil SB; Desinflam Biotic; Dibional; Fluimucil Biotic; Fullcilina Plus; Grinsil Clavulanico; Grinsil Respiratorio; Heliklar; Klonalmox; Lertus Biotic; Muco Dosodos Biotic; No-Tos Biotic; Nobactam Bronquial; Oximar Respiratorio; Rodinac Biotic; Trexirol NF; Trifamox Bronquial; Trifamox IBL; ***Austral.:*** Augmentin; Ausclav; Clamoxyl; Clavulin; Klacid HP 7; Losec Helicopak†; Losec Hp 7; Pylorid-KA; Somac-MA†; ***Austria:*** Amoclan; Amoclax; Amoxiplus; Augmentin; Clavamox; Curam; Helicocin; Lanoclav; Xiclav; ***Belg.:*** Augmentin; Clavucid; ***Braz.:*** Amoxifar Balsamico†; Anzopac; Augmentin†; Bronco Cilimox†; Bronco-Amoxil; Bronco-Polimoxil; Clavoxil; Clavulin; Erradic; Helicopac; Heliklar; Novamox; Novocilin Balsamico†; Pyloripac; Trifamox; ***Canad.:*** Clavulin; Hp-Pac; Losec 1-2-3 A; ***Chile:*** Ambilan; Ambilan Bid; Amolex; Augmentin; Augmentin Bid; Clavinex; Clavinex Duo; Clavoxilina Bid; Sulbamox; ***Denm.:*** Bioclavid; Spektramox; **Fin.:** Amoxin Comp; Augmentin; Bioclavid; Clavurion; Helipak A; Helipak K; Losec Helira; Spektramox; **Fr.:** Augmentin; Ciblor; **Ger.:** Amoclav; Amoxi-Clavulan; Amoxiclav; Amoxidura Plus; Amoxillat-Clav; Amuclan; Augmentan; Flanamox; ZacPac; **Gr.:** Augmentin; Bioclavid; Fugentin; **Hong Kong:** Amoksiklav; Augmentin; Curam; Moxiclav; **India:** Amclo; Augmentin; Bicidal Plus; Carbomox; Hipenox; Imox-Clo; Moxycarb; Novaclox; Nuclav; Respimox; Suprimox; **Irl.:** Augmentin; Clavamel; Germentin; Pinaclav; **Israel:** Amoxiclav; Augmentin; Clavamox; **Ital.:** Augmentin; Clavulin; Neoduplamox; **Malaysia:** Amoxiclav; Augmentin; Curam; Enhancin; Klacid HP 7; Moxiclav; Vestaclav; **Mex.:** Acimox-Ex; Ambrexin; Amoxibron; Amoxiclav; Augmentin; Bromixen; Cibronal; Clamoxin; Clavulin; Esteclin Bac; Eumetinex†; Gimabrol; Hidramox-M; Penamox M; Pentibroxil; Sekretovit Amoxi; Septacin Amoxi; Servamox CLV; Trifamox IBL; **Neth.:** Augmentin; PantoPAC; **Norw.:** Bremide; **NZ:** Alpha-Amoxyclav†; Augmentin; Helicosec†; Klacid HP 7; Losec Hp 7; Synermox; **Port.:** Amoclavam; Augmentin; Betamox; Clavamox; Clavepen; Penilan; **S.Afr.:** Adco-Amoclav; Amoclav; Augmaxil; Augmentin; Bio-Amoksiclav; Clamentin; Clavumox; Hiconcil-NS†; Losec 20 Triple; Macropen; Megapen; Moxyclav; Ranclav; Suprapen; **Singapore:** Amocla; Augmentin; Clamonex; Curam; Enhancin; Fugentin; Moxiclav; **Spain:** Agerpen Mucolitico†; Amo Resan; Amoclave; Amoxi Gobens Mucol; Amoxidel Bronquial†; Amoxtiol†; Amoxyplus; Ardine Bronquial; Ardineclav; Augmentine; Bigpen; Bisolvon Amoxycilina†; Bronco Tonic; Bronconovag†; Bronquium Amoxicilina†; Burmicin; Clamoxyl Mucolitico; Clavepen; Clavucid; Clavumox; Combitorax†; Damoxicil Mucolitico†; Duonasa; Edoxil Mucolitico; Eupeclanic; Eupen Bronquial; Halitol Mucolitico†; Hosboral Bronquial†; Inexbron Mucolitico†; Inmupen†; Kelsopen; Metifarma Mucolit†; Pangamox†; Precopen Mucolitico†; Pulmo Borbalan; Reloxyl Mucolitico; Remisan Mucolitico; Salvapen Mucolitico; **Swed.:** Nexium Hp; Spektramox; **Switz.:** Augmentin; Aziclav; Clavamox; Co-Amoxi; **Thai.:** Amoksiklav; Augmentin; Cavumox; Curam; Ranclav; **UAE:** Julmentin; **UK:** Amiclav; Augmentin; Augmentin-Duo; Heliclear; **USA:** Augmentin; Prevpac.

# Ampicillin *(BAN, USAN, rINN)*

Aminobenzylpenicillin; Ampicilina; Ampicillinum; Ampicillinum Anhydricum; Anhydrous Ampicillin; AY-6108; BRL-1341; NSC-528986; P-50. (6*R*)-6-(α-D-Phenylglycylamino)penicillanic acid.

$C_{16}H_{19}N_3O_4S$ = 349.4.

*CAS — 69-53-4.*

*ATC — J01CA01; S01AA19.*

NOTE. Compounded preparations of ampicillin may be represented by the following names:

- Co-fluampicil (*BAN*)—flucloxacillin 1 part and ampicillin 1 part (w/w).

**Pharmacopoeias.** In *Eur.* (see p.vi), *Jpn, Pol.,* and *Viet.* *Int.* and *US* permit anhydrous or the trihydrate.

**Ph. Eur. 5.0** (Ampicillin, Anhydrous; Ampicillin BP 2003). A white, crystalline powder. It exhibits polymorphism. Sparingly soluble in water; practically insoluble in alcohol, in acetone, and in fatty oils. It dissolves in dilute solutions of acids and of alkali hydroxides. A 0.25% solution in water has a pH of 3.5 to 5.5. Store at a temperature not exceeding 30° in airtight containers.

**USP 27** (Ampicillin). It is anhydrous or contains three molecules of water of hydration. A white, practically odourless crystalline powder. Slightly soluble in water and in methyl alcohol; insoluble in carbon tetrachloride, in chloroform, and in benzene. pH of a 1% solution in water is between 3.5 and 6.0. Store in airtight containers.

## Ampicillin Sodium *(BANM, USAN, rINNM)*

Aminobenzylpenicillin Sodium; Ampicilina sódica; Ampicillinnatrium; Ampicillinum Natricum.

$C_{16}H_{18}N_3NaO_4S$ = 371.4.

*CAS — 69-52-3.*

*ATC — J01CA01; S01AA19.*

**Pharmacopoeias.** In *Chin., Eur.* (see p.vi), *Int., Jpn, Pol.,* and *US.*

**Ph. Eur. 5.0** (Ampicillin Sodium). A white or almost white hygroscopic powder. Freely soluble in water; sparingly soluble in acetone; practically insoluble in liquid paraffin and in fatty oils. A 10% solution in water has a pH of 8.0 to 10.0. Store in airtight containers.

**USP 27** (Ampicillin Sodium). A white to off-white, odourless or practically odourless, hygroscopic, crystalline powder. Very soluble in water and in isotonic sodium chloride and glucose solutions. pH of a solution in water containing the equivalent of ampicillin 1% is between 8.0 and 10.0. Store in airtight containers.

**Incompatibility.** The incompatibility of ampicillin sodium and aminoglycosides is well established. Incompatibilities have also been reported with a wide range of other drugs, including other antibacterials, and appear to be more pronounced at higher concentrations and in solutions also containing glucose.

**Stability.** The stability of solutions of ampicillin sodium is dependent on many factors including concentration, pH, temperature, and the nature of the vehicle. Stability decreases in the presence of glucose, fructose, invert sugar, dextrans, hetastarch, sodium bicarbonate, and lactate. It is recommended that reconstituted solutions of ampicillin sodium for injection should be administered within 24 hours of preparation, and should be stored at 2° to 8° but should not be frozen. Solutions for infusion are stable for varying periods and details are given in the manufacturers' literature.

References.

1. Lynn B. The stability and administration of intravenous penicillins. *Br J Intraven Ther* 1981; **2**(Mar): 22–39.

## Ampicillin Trihydrate *(BANM, rINNM)*

Ampicilina trihidrato; Ampicillin; Ampicillinum Trihydricum.

$C_{16}H_{19}N_3O_4S,3H_2O$ = 403.5.

*CAS — 7177-48-2.*

*ATC — J01CA01; S01AA19.*

**Pharmacopoeias.** In *Eur.* (see p.vi), *Pol.,* and *Viet.* In *Chin.* and *Jpn* under the title Ampicillin. *Int.* and *US* permit anhydrous or the trihydrate under the title Ampicillin.

**Ph. Eur. 5.0** (Ampicillin Trihydrate). A white crystalline powder. Slightly soluble in water; practically insoluble in alcohol and in fatty oils. It dissolves in dilute solutions of acids and of alkali hydroxides. A 0.25% solution in water has a pH of 3.5 to 5.5. Store at a temperature not exceeding 30° in airtight containers.

**USP 27** (Ampicillin). It is anhydrous or contains three molecules of water of hydration. A white, practically odourless crystalline powder. Slightly soluble in water and in methyl alcohol; insoluble in carbon tetrachloride, in chloroform, and in benzene. pH of a 1% solution in water is between 3.5 and 6.0. Store in airtight containers.

## Adverse Effects

As for Benzylpenicillin p.163.

Skin rashes are among the most common adverse effects and are generally either urticarial or maculopapular; the urticarial reactions are typical of penicillin hypersensitivity, while the erythematous maculopapular eruptions are characteristic of ampicillin and amoxicillin and often appear more than 7 days after commencing treatment. Such rashes may be due to hypersensitivity to the beta-lactam moiety or to the amino group in the side-chain, or to a toxic reaction. The occurrence of a maculopapular rash during ampicillin use does not necessarily preclude the subsequent use of other penicillins. However, since it may be difficult in practice to distinguish between hypersensitive and toxic responses, skin testing for hypersensitivity may be advisable before another penicillin is used in patients who have had ampicillin rashes. Most patients with infectious mononucleosis develop a maculopapular rash when treated with ampicillin, and patients with other lymphoid disorders such as lymphatic leukaemia and possibly HIV infection also appear to be at higher risk. More serious skin reactions may occur and erythema multiforme associated with ampicillin has occasionally been reported.

Gastrointestinal adverse effects, particularly diarrhoea and nausea and vomiting, occur quite frequently, usually following oral use. Pseudomembranous colitis has also been reported.

## Precautions

As for Benzylpenicillin p.164.

Ampicillin should be discontinued if a skin rash occurs. It should preferably not be given to patients with infectious mononucleosis since they are especially susceptible to ampicillin-induced skin rashes; patients with lymphatic leukaemia or possibly HIV infection may also be at increased risk of developing skin rashes.

**Myasthenia gravis.** The symptoms of a woman with myasthenia gravis were exacerbated when she was given ampicillin.[1]

1. Argov Z, *et al.* Ampicillin may aggravate clinical and experimental myasthenia gravis. *Arch Neurol* 1986; **43:** 255–6.

**Sodium content.** Each g of ampicillin sodium contains about 2.7 mmol of sodium.

## Interactions

As for Benzylpenicillin, p.164.

**Allopurinol.** An increased frequency of skin rashes has been reported in patients receiving ampicillin or amoxicillin, together with allopurinol, compared with those receiving the antibacterial alone,[1] but this could not be confirmed in a subsequent study.[2]

1. Jick H, Porter JB. Potentiation of ampicillin skin reactions by allopurinol or hyperuricemia. *J Clin Pharmacol* 1981; **21:** 456–8.
2. Hoigné R, *et al.* Occurrence of exanthems in relation to aminopenicillin preparations and allopurinol. *N Engl J Med* 1987; **316:** 1217.

**Chloroquine.** The absorption of ampicillin has been reduced in healthy subjects taking chloroquine.[1]

1. Ali HM. Reduced ampicillin bioavailability following oral coadministration with chloroquine. *J Antimicrob Chemother* 1985; **15:** 781–4.

## Antimicrobial Action

Ampicillin is a beta-lactam antibiotic. It is bactericidal and has a similar mode of action to that of benzylpenicillin (p.164), but as an aminopenicillin with an amino group side-chain attached to the basic penicillin structure, ampicillin is better able to penetrate the outer membrane of some Gram-negative bacteria and has a broader spectrum of activity.

*Spectrum of activity.* Ampicillin resembles benzylpenicillin in its action against Gram-positive organisms, including *Streptococcus pneumoniae* and other streptococci, but, with the possible exception of activity against *Enterococcus faecalis,* it is slightly less potent than benzylpenicillin. *Listeria monocytogenes* is highly sensitive. The Gram-negative cocci *Moraxella catarrhalis* (*Branhamella catarrhalis*), *Neisseria gonorrhoeae,* and *N. meningitidis* are sensitive. Ampicillin is more active than benzylpenicillin against some Gram-negative bacilli, including *Haemophilus influenzae* and Enterobacteriaceae such as *Escherichia coli, Proteus mirabilis, Salmonella* and *Shigella* spp. It is inactive against *Pseudomonas aeruginosa.* Ampicillin also has activity similar to benzylpenicillin against other organisms including many anaerobes and *Actinomyces* spp.

*Activity with other antimicrobials.* There is synergy against some beta-lactamase-producing organisms between ampicillin and beta-lactamase inhibitors such as clavulanic acid or sulbactam, and also penicillinase-stable drugs such as cloxacillin or flucloxacillin. Synergy has also been demonstrated between ampicillin and aminoglycosides against a range of organisms, including enterococci. Variable effects ranging from synergy to antagonism have been reported between ampicillin and other beta lactams, bacteriostatic drugs such as chloramphenicol, and rifampicin.

*Resistance.* Like benzylpenicillin, ampicillin is inactivated by beta lactamases, although other mechanisms may be responsible for resistance in some species. There are geographical variations in the incidence of resistance, but most staphylococci and many strains of *E. coli, H. influenzae, M. catarrhalis, N. gonorrhoeae,* and *Salmonella* and *Shigella* spp. are resistant.

## Pharmacokinetics

Ampicillin is relatively resistant to inactivation by gastric acid and is moderately well absorbed from the gastrointestinal tract after oral administration. Food can interfere with the absorption of ampicillin so doses should preferably be taken at least 30 minutes before meals. Peak concentrations in plasma are attained in about 1 to 2 hours and after a 500-mg oral dose are reported to range from 3 to 6 micrograms/mL.

Peak plasma concentrations of ampicillin after a 500-mg intramuscular dose given as the sodium salt occur within about 1 hour and are reported to range from 7 to 14 micrograms/mL.

Ampicillin is widely distributed and therapeutic concentrations can be achieved in ascitic, pleural, and joint fluids. It crosses the placenta and small amounts are distributed into breast milk. There is little diffusion into the CSF except when the meninges are inflamed. About 20% is bound to plasma proteins and the plasma half-life is about 1 to 1.5 hours, but this may be increased in neonates, the elderly, and patients with renal impairment; in severe renal impairment half-lives of 7 to 20 hours have been reported.

Ampicillin is metabolised to some extent to penicilloic acid which is excreted in the urine.

Renal clearance of ampicillin occurs partly by glomerular filtration and partly by tubular secretion; it is reduced by probenecid. About 20 to 40% of an oral dose may be excreted unchanged in the urine in 6 hours; urinary concentrations have ranged from 0.25 to 1 mg/mL following a dose of 500 mg. Following parenteral administration about 60 to 80% is excreted in the urine within 6 hours. Ampicillin is removed by haemodialysis. High concentrations are reached in bile; it undergoes enterohepatic recycling and some is excreted in the faeces.

*Ampicillin with sulbactam.* The pharmacokinetics of ampicillin and sulbactam are broadly similar and neither appears to affect the other to any great extent.

## Uses and Administration

Ampicillin is used in the treatment of a variety of infections due to susceptible organisms (see Antimicrobial Action, above). They include biliary-tract infections, bronchitis, endocarditis, gastro-enteritis (including salmonella enteritis and shigellosis), gonorrhoea, listeriosis, meningitis, perinatal streptococcal infections (intrapartum prophylaxis against group B streptococci), peritonitis, pneumonia, septicaemia, typhoid and paratyphoid fever, and urinary-tract infections. Resistance to ampicillin is increasingly a problem in some infections, for example, gonorrhoea, pneumococcal infections, respiratory-tract infections due to *Haemophilus influenzae* or *Moraxella catarrhalis* (*Branhamella catarrhalis*), *Salmonella* infections, shigellosis, and infections due to *Escherichia coli*. For details of these infections and their treatment, see under Choice of Antibacterial, p.120. If beta-lactamase-producing organisms are present, ampicillin can be given with a beta-lactamase inhibitor such as sulbactam (see below) or a penicillinase-resistant drug such as cloxacillin, dicloxacillin, or flucloxacillin (known as co-fluampicil). It may also be used with an aminoglycoside to increase the spectrum of organisms covered; it is advisable to administer the injections separately.

*Administration and dosage.* The dosage of ampicillin will depend on the severity of the disease, the age of the patient, and renal function. Ampicillin is usually given by mouth as the trihydrate and by injection as the sodium salt. Doses are expressed in terms of the equivalent amount of ampicillin. 1.06 g of ampicillin sodium and 1.15 g of ampicillin trihydrate are each approximately equivalent to 1 g of ampicillin.

The usual adult dose by mouth is 0.25 to 1 g every 6 hours taken at least 30 minutes before or 2 hours after food. Children may be given half the adult dose. The usual adult dose by injection is 500 mg every 4 to 6 hours intramuscularly or by slow intravenous injection over 3 to 5 minutes or by infusion. Again, children may be given half the adult dose.

For urinary-tract infections, ampicillin 500 mg is given by mouth every 8 hours.

For typhoid and paratyphoid fever where *Salmonella typhi* strains remain sensitive to ampicillin, an oral dose of 1 to 2 g may be given every 6 hours for 2 weeks for acute infections, and for 4 to 12 weeks in carriers. An intramuscular dose of 10 mg/kg (maximum dose 250 mg) every 6 hours for 4 to 6 weeks has been suggested for children who are chronic carriers.

Ampicillin 2 g given with probenecid 1 g, as a single oral dose, has been used in the treatment of uncomplicated gonorrhoea in areas where gonococci remain sensitive; repeated doses are recommended in females.

In meningitis, higher parenteral doses of 2 to 3 g given intravenously every 4 or 6 hours have been suggested. For infants and children with meningitis, an intravenous dose of 150 mg/kg daily in divided doses may be given; a dose of 50 mg/kg (maximum 3 g) every 4 to 6 hours has also been suggested. Neonates may be given a dose of 50 mg/kg every 12 hours for those under 1 week of age, or every 8 hours for older neonates.

For intrapartum prophylaxis against group B streptococcal infection in the neonate, a maternal dose of 2 g by intravenous injection initially then 1 g every 4 hours until delivery has been suggested.

Ampicillin may also be administered by other routes, usually as a supplement to systemic therapy. Intraperitoneal or intrapleural injections are given in a dose of 500 mg daily dissolved in 5 to 10 mL of water. For intra-articular injection, ampicillin 500 mg daily is given dissolved in up to 5 mL of water or a solution of procaine hydrochloride 0.5%.

Ampicillin benzathine has also been administered by intramuscular injection.

*Ampicillin with sulbactam.* The sodium salts of ampicillin and sulbactam (p.257) may be given intramuscularly or intravenously in the treatment of infections due to beta-lactamase-producing organisms. Doses are expressed in terms of the equivalent amounts of ampicillin and sulbactam; available injections contain ampicillin and sulbactam in the ratio 2:1, respectively. The usual dose is ampicillin 1 g with sulbactam 500 mg every 6 hours; doses may be doubled in severe infections.

For oral administration sultamicillin (p.264), a mutual prodrug of ampicillin and sulbactam, may be used.

**Administration in renal impairment.** The dose of ampicillin should be reduced, or the dose interval increased, in severe renal impairment (creatinine clearance less than 10 mL/minute). Patients undergoing dialysis should receive an additional dose after the session.

## Preparations

***BP 2003:*** Ampicillin Capsules; Ampicillin Injection; Ampicillin Oral Suspension; Co-fluampicil Capsules; Co-fluampicil Oral Suspension;
***USP 27:*** Ampicillin and Probenecid for Oral Suspension; Ampicillin and Sulbactam for Injection; Ampicillin Capsules; Ampicillin for Injectable Suspension; Ampicillin for Injection; Ampicillin for Oral Suspension; Ampicillin Tablets.

**Proprietary Preparations** (details are given in Part 3)

***Arg.:*** Alpovex; Aminoxidin; Ampi; Ampi-Bis; Ampicler; Ampigen; Ampigrand; Ampitenk; Ampixen; Bactilina; Decilina; Galciclina; Grampenil; Histopen; Poenbiotico; Trifacilina; Trimicro; Welticilina; ***Austral.:*** Alphacin; Ampicyn; Austrapen; ***Austria:*** Standacillin; ***Belg.:*** Penbritin†; Pentrexyl; ***Braz.:*** Ampiciflan; Ampicil; Ampicilase; Ampicilib†; Ampicilon; Ampicimax; Ampicler com Probenecide†; Ampicler†; Ampicrom†; Ampifar; Ampigran; Ampilong†; Ampispectrin†; Ampitotal†; Ampival; Amplacilina; Amplimed†; Amplitor†; Amplofen; Bacterinil; Bacterion†; Binopen†; Binotal; Binotine†; Bipencil; Cilinon; Cilipen; Degona†; Emicilin; Expectocilin; Gonocilin†; Gonol; Gonorrels†; Gramcilina; Makrocilin†; Natuscilin†; Notacilin†; Probenzima†; Tandrexin; Totapen†; ***Canad.:*** Ampicin†; Apo-Ampi; Nu-Ampi; Penbritin†; ***Denm.:*** Anhypen†; Doktacillin; Pentrexyl; ***Fin.:*** A-Pen; ***Fr.:*** Totapen; ***Ger.:*** Ampi†; Binotal; duraampicillin†; Jenampin†; ***Gr.:*** Copercilex; Isticilline; Pentrexyl; ***Hong Kong:*** Ampilin†; Amprexyl; Dhacillin; Pamecil; Penbritin; Pentrexyl; ***India:*** Ampilin; Ampipen; Biocilin; Campicilin; Roscillin; Synthocilin; ***Irl.:*** Amfipen†; Clonamp; Novapen; Penbritin; ***Israel:*** Penibrin; Pentrexyl†; Vitapen; ***Ital.:*** Ampilisa; Ampilux; Ampiplus Simplex; Amplital; Amplizer; Citicil†; Ibimicyn; Lampocillina†; Pentrexyl; Platocillina†; ***Malaysia:*** Ampilin; Biocil; Pamecil; Setcillin; Standacillin; ***Mex.:*** Acimpil†; Alvedrin; Am-An; Ambidrin; Ambiosol; Ampex; Ampi-Quim; Ampi-Tecno; Ampibal; Ampicidar; Ampidrat; Ampigrin; Ampilon; Ampimex†; Ampiset; Ampisuspen†; Amsapen; Anglopen; Bacticil†; Binotal; Bremicina; Dibacilina; Diferin; Expicin; Fenipencil†; Flamicina; Ifecin†; Iqfacilina; Lampicin†; Linapen†; Marovilina; Meprizina; Omnipen; Penbritin; Pentiver; Pentrexyl; Prodifer; Promecilina†; Rayepen†; Riganpil†; Sinaplin; Totipen†; Tronex†; Unicilin†; Yapamicin; ***Neth.:*** Pentrexyl; ***Norw.:*** Doktacillin†; Pentrexyl; ***Port.:*** Amplifar; Britacil†; Hiperbiotico; Hiperbiotico Retard; ***S.Afr.:*** Ampimax†; Ampipen; Be-Ampicil; Co-Cillin†; Dyna-Ampcil†; Excillin†; Penbritin; Penrite†; Petercillin; Ranamp; Spectracil; ***Singapore:*** Ampicap†; Ampilin; Ampitab†; Dhacillin; Pamecil†; Penbritin†; Pricillin; Standacillin; ***Spain:*** Ampilevel; Ampiplus; Antibiopen; Bactosone Retard†; Britapen; Ciarbiot†; Electopen†; Gobemicina; Nuvapen; ***Swed.:*** Doktacillin; Pentrexyl†; ***Thai.:*** Amcillin; Amilin; Ampat†; Ampexin†; Ampicyn; Ampilin; Ampillin; Ampra; Amprexyl; Ampro; Eracillin; Penbritin; Pencotrex; Pentrexyl; Servicillin†; Siampicil; Sumapen; Vacillin; Viccillin; ***UAE:*** Julphapen; ***UK:*** Amfipen†; Flu-Amp†; Magnapen; Penbritin; Rimacillin; ***USA:*** Marcillin†; Omnipen-N†; Omnipen†; Principen; Totacillin†.

**Multi-ingredient: *Arg.:*** Aminoxidin Sulbactam; Ampi-Bis Plus; Ampigen SB; Amplibenzatin Bronquial; Aseptobron Ampicilina; Cronopen Balsamico; Grampenil Bronquial; Meticil; Prixin; Unsayna; ***Austria:*** Unasyn; ***Braz.:*** Ambezetal; Ampifar Balsamico†; Ampizan†; Amplotal; Benzotal Balsamico†; Benzotal†; Binotine Balsamico†; Dibendril†; Durapen; Durapen Balsamico†; Expectocilin Balsamico†; Genitopen†; Labfcilina†; Optacilin; Optacilin Balsamico†; Parenzyme Ampicilina; Probenzima Ampicilina†; Soma Balsamico†; Soma†; Urobiotic; Uropielon; ***Chile:*** Unasyn; ***Fr.:*** Unacim; ***Ger.:*** Unacid; ***Gr.:*** Begalin-P; ***Hong Kong:*** Ampiclox; APT-Ampicloxa; Pamedox; Unasyn; ***India:*** Adilox; Ampilox; Amplus; Ampoxin; Ampoxin-LB; Sulbacin; ***Irl.:*** Ampiclox; ***Israel:*** Unasyn; ***Ital.:*** Ampiplus; Amplium; Bethacil; Diamplicil; Duplexcillina†; Duplexil†; Infectrin†; Loricin; Unasyn; ***Jpn:*** Sulperazon; Unasyn-S; ***Malaysia:*** Unasyn; ***Mex.:*** Ampiclox-D; Mucolin A; Panac; Panac K; Pentibrom; Pentidix; Pentrexyl Expec; Unasyna; ***S.Afr.:*** Ampiclox; Apen; Cloxam; Megamox; Ranclosil; ***Singapore:*** Unasyn; ***Spain:*** Alongamicina Balsa†; Bacimex†; Bio Espectrum†; Bronco Pensusan†; Electopen Balsam Retard†; Electopen Retard†; Espectral; Espectral Balsamico†; Espectrosira; Etro Balsamico†; Etro†; Gobemicina Retard; Hispamicina Retard†; Maxicilina; Miliken Mucol Med Retard†; Miliken Mucol Retard†; Miliken Mucolitico†; Mucorex Ampicilina†; Pectosan Ampicilina†; Pectox Ampicilina†; Penisintex Bronquial; Pulminflamatoria; Pulmospin†; Pulmosterin Retard; Resan Mucolitico†; Resan Retard†; Resisten Retard†; Retarpen; Retarpen Balsamico; Retarpen Mucolitico; Sulquibron†; Ultrabion Balsamico†; Ultrabion†; Ultrapenil; Unasyn; ***Thai.:*** Ampiclox; Polyclox†; Unasyn; Viccillin-S; ***UK:*** Flu-Amp†; Magnapen; ***USA:*** Unasyn.

---

## Apramycin (BAN, USAN, rINN)

47657; EL-857; EL-857/820; Nebramycin Factor 2. 4-*O*-[(2*R*,3*R*,4a*S*,6*R*,7*S*,8*R*,8a*R*)-3-Amino-6-(4-amino-4-deoxy-α-D-glucopyranosyloxy)-8-hydroxy-7-methylaminoperhydropyrano[3,2-*b*]pyran-2-yl]-2-deoxystreptamine.

$C_{21}H_{41}N_5O_{11}$ = 539.6.
*CAS — 37321-09-8.*

## Apramycin Sulfate (rINNM)

Apramycin Sulphate (BANM); Sulfato de apramicina.

$C_{21}H_{41}N_5O_{11}.2\frac{1}{2}H_2SO_4$ = 784.8.
*CAS — 41194-16-5.*

**Pharmacopoeias.** In *BP(Vet)*.

**BP(Vet) 2003** (Apramycin Sulphate). The sulfate of an antibiotic produced by certain strains of *Streptomyces tenebrarius* or by other means. A light brown hygroscopic powder or granules. Freely soluble in water; practically insoluble in alcohol, in acetone, in ether, and in methyl alcohol. Store at a temperature not exceeding 25°.

### Profile

Apramycin is an aminoglycoside antibiotic used as the sulfate in veterinary practice for the treatment of susceptible infections.

---

## Arbekacin Sulfate (rINNM)

ABK (arbekacin); AHB-DBK (arbekacin); Arbekacin Sulphate; HABA-Dibekacin (arbekacin); Sulfato de arbekacina. *O*-3-Amino-3-deoxy-α-D-glucopyranosyl-(1→4)-*O*-[2,6-diamino-2,3,4,6-tetradeoxy-α-D-*erythro*-hexopyranosyl-(1→6)]-*N*′-[(2*S*)-4-amino-2-hydroxybutyryl]-2-deoxy-L-streptamine sulphate.

$C_{22}H_{44}N_6O_{10},xH_2SO_4$.
*CAS — 51025-85-5 (arbekacin).*

**Pharmacopoeias.** In *Jpn*.

### Profile

Arbekacin is an aminoglycoside derived from dibekacin and has general properties similar to those of gentamicin (p.217). It has been used as the sulfate in the treatment of serious infections due to meticillin-resistant *Staphylococcus aureus*.

---

## Arsanilic Acid (BAN, rINN)

Ácido arsanílico; Aminarsonic Acid; AS-101. *p*-Aminobenzenearsonic acid; 4-Aminophenylarsonic acid.

$C_6H_8AsNO_3$ = 217.1.
*CAS — 98-50-0.*

NOTE. The code AS-101 has also been used for an immunomodulator investigated as an antineoplastic and antiviral.

**Pharmacopoeias.** In *US* for veterinary use only.

**USP 27** (Arsanilic Acid). A white to off-white crystalline powder. Soluble in hot water, in amyl alcohol, and in solutions of alkali carbonates; slightly soluble in cold water, in alcohol, and in acetic acid; insoluble in acetone, in chloroform, in ether, in benzene, and in dilute mineral acids; sparingly soluble in concentrated mineral acids.

## Sodium Arsanilate (BANM, rINNM)

Arsanilato sódico; Sodium Aminarsonate; Sodium Anilarsonate. Sodium 4-aminophenylarsonate.

$C_6H_7AsNNaO_3$ = 239.0.
*CAS — 127-85-5.*

**Pharmacopoeias.** *Fr.* includes the anhydrous substance and the trihydrate.

### Profile

Arsanilic acid and sodium arsanilate have been used in veterinary medicine for the prophylaxis and treatment of enteric infections in pigs and also as growth-promoting agents.

---

## Aspoxicillin (rINN)

Aspoxicilina; TA-058. (2*S*,5*R*,6*R*)-6-{(2*R*)-2-[(2*R*)-2-Amino-3-(methylcarbamoyl)propionamido]-2-(*p*-hydroxyphenyl)acetamido}-3,3-dimethyl-7-oxo-4-thia-1-azabicyclo[3.2.0]-heptane-2-carboxylic acid.

$C_{21}H_{27}N_5O_7S$ = 493.5.
*CAS — 63358-49-6.*

**Pharmacopoeias.** *Jpn* includes the trihydrate.

### Profile

Aspoxicillin is a ureidopenicillin that has been given intravenously in the treatment of susceptible infections.

---

## Astromicin Sulfate (USAN, pINNM)

Abbott-44747; Astromicin Sulphate; Fortimicin A Sulphate; KW-1070; Sulfato de astromicina. 4-Amino-1-(2-amino-*N*-methylacetamido)-1,4-dideoxy-3-*O*-(2,6-diamino-2,3,4,6,7-pentadeoxy-β-L-*lyxo*-heptopyranosyl)-6-*O*-methyl-L-*chiro*-inositol sulphate.

$C_{17}H_{35}N_5O_6,2H_2SO_4$ = 601.6.
*CAS — 55779-06-1 (astromicin); 72275-67-3 (astromicin sulfate); 66768-12-5 ($xH_2SO_4$).*

**Pharmacopoeias.** In *Jpn*.

### Profile

Astromicin is an aminoglycoside antibiotic produced by *Micromonospora* spp. and with actions and uses similar those of gentamicin (p.217). It is used as the sulfate and doses are expressed in terms of astromicin. 594 mg of astromicin sulfate is approximately equivalent to 400 mg astromicin. It is administered intramuscularly or by intravenous infusion over 30 minutes to 1 hour in a usual dosage of 400 mg daily in 2 divided doses. Dosage should be adjusted based on serum-astromicin concentration monitoring.

### Preparations

**Proprietary Preparations** (details are given in Part 3)
***Jpn:*** Fortimicin.

## Avilamycin (BAN, USAN)

Avilamicina; LY-048740 (avilamycin or avilamycin A).

$C_{61}H_{88}Cl_2O_{32}$ (avilamycin A) = 1404.2.

*CAS — 11051-71-1 (avilamycin); 69787-79-7 (avilamycin A); 69787-80-0 (avilamycin C).*

### Profile

Avilamycin is an antibacterial used in veterinary medicine as a growth promotor.

## Avoparcin (BAN, USAN, rINN)

Avoparcina; Compound 254.

*CAS — 37332-99-3.*

### Profile

Avoparcin is a glycopeptide antibiotic usually produced by *Amycolatopsis coloradensis* (*Streptomyces candidus*). It has been incorporated into animal feedstuffs to promote growth.

◊ There is evidence of cross-resistance between avoparcin and vancomycin.[1] Suggestions that vancomycin-resistant organisms could enter the human population from the food chain as a result of the use of avoparcin as a growth promotor in animals[2,3] were disputed by the manufacturers of avoparcin.[4,5] Following a ban in the European Union on the use of avoparcin as a growth promotor in animals there has been some evidence[6] of a decrease in the occurrence of vancomycin-resistant enterococci in poultry meat.


1. Klare I, *et al.* vanA-mediated high-level glycopeptide resistance in Enterococcus faecium from animal husbandry. *FEMS Microbiol Lett* 1995; **125:** 165–72.
2. Howarth F, Poulter D. Vancomycin resistance: time to ban avoparcin? *Lancet* 1996; **347:** 1047.
3. Wise R. Avoparcin and animal feedstuff. *Lancet* 1996; **347:** 1835.
4. Mudd A. Vancomycin resistance and avoparcin. *Lancet* 1996; **347:** 1412.
5. Mudd AJ. Is it time to ban all antibiotics as animal growth-promoting agents? *Lancet* 1996; **348:** 1454–5.
6. Pantosti A, *et al.* Decrease of vancomycin-resistant enterococci in poultry meat after avoparcin ban. *Lancet* 1999; **354:** 741–2.


## Azidamfenicol (BAN, rINN)

Azidamphenicol; Azidanfenicol; Azidoamphenicol; Bayer 52910. 2-Azido-N-[(αR,βR)-β-hydroxy-α-hydroxymethyl-4-nitrophenethyl]acetamide.

$C_{11}H_{13}N_5O_5$ = 295.3.

*CAS — 13838-08-9.*

*ATC — S01AA25.*

### Profile

Azidamfenicol is an antibiotic that is related structurally to chloramphenicol (p.185). It is used as 1% eye drops or eye ointment in the treatment of bacterial eye infections.

### Preparations

**Proprietary Preparations** (details are given in Part 3)
***Ger.:*** Berlicetin; Posifenicol; Thilocanfol.

## Azidocillin Sodium (BANM, rINNM)

Azidobenzylpenicillin Sodium. Sodium (6R)-6-(D-2-azido-2-phenylacetamido)penicillanate.

$C_{16}H_{16}N_5NaO_4S$ = 397.4.

*CAS — 17243-38-8 (azidocillin); 35334-12-4 (azidocillin sodium).*

### Profile

Azidocillin is a semisynthetic penicillin with actions and uses similar to those of phenoxymethylpenicillin (p.242). It is given by mouth as the sodium salt in doses of 750 mg twice daily in the treatment of susceptible infections. The potassium salt has also been used.

### Preparations

**Proprietary Preparations** (details are given in Part 3)
***Austria:*** Longatren; ***Ger.:*** InfectoBicillin H; Syncillin†.

## Azithromycin (BAN, USAN, rINN)

Azithromycinum; Azitromicina; CP-62993; XZ-450. (2R,3S,4R,5R,8R,10R,11R,12S,13S,14R)-13-(2,6-Dideoxy-3-C-3-O-dimethyl-α-L-*ribo*-hexopyranosyloxy)-2-ethyl-3,4,10-trihydroxy-3,5,6,8,10,12,14-heptamethyl-11-(3,4,6-trideoxy-3-dimethylamino-β-D-*xylo*-hexopyranosyloxy)-1-oxa-6-azacyclopentadecan-15-one dihydrate; 9-Deoxo-9a-aza-9a-methyl-9a-homoerythromycin A dihydrate.

$C_{38}H_{72}N_2O_{12}.2H_2O$ = 785.0.

*CAS — 83905-01-5 (anhydrous azithromycin); 117772-70-0 (azithromycin dihydrate).*

*ATC — J01FA10.*

**Pharmacopoeias.** In *Chin.* and *US. Eur.* (see p.vi) includes the anhydrous form.

**Ph. Eur. 5.0** (Azithromycin). A white or almost white powder. Practically insoluble in water; freely soluble in dehydrated alcohol and in dichloromethane. A 0.2% solution in a mixture of methyl alcohol and water (1:1) has a pH of 9.0 to 11.0. Store in airtight containers.

**USP 27** (Azithromycin). pH of a 0.2% solution in a mixture of methyl alcohol and water (1:1) is between 9.0 and 11.0. Store in airtight containers.

### Adverse Effects and Precautions

As for Erythromycin, p.208. Gastrointestinal disturbances are the most frequent adverse effect but are usually mild and less frequent than with erythromycin. Headache may occur and taste disturbances have been reported rarely. Severe hypersensitivity reactions occur rarely but may be prolonged. Transient reductions in neutrophil counts have been seen in patients receiving azithromycin. Pain and inflammation may occur at the site of intravenous infusions. The UK manufacturers state that azithromycin should not be used in patients with hepatic impairment.

**Incidence of adverse effects.** In patients receiving azithromycin daily long-term for mycobacterial infections,[1] gastrointestinal disorders occurred in 32 of 39 patients (82%), hearing impairment in 10 patients (26%), tinnitus in 18 patients (46%), and poor balance or dizziness in 11 patients (28%). In general, adverse effects were associated with higher serum-azithromycin concentrations.


1. Brown BA, *et al.* Relationship of adverse events to serum drug levels in patients receiving high-dose azithromycin for mycobacterial lung disease. *Clin Infect Dis* 1997; **24:** 958–64.


**Effects on the ears.** Reversible sensorineural hearing loss was reported in 3 patients who received oral azithromycin 500 mg daily with clofazimine and ethambutol for the treatment of disseminated *Mycobacterium avium* complex infection.[1] Irreversible hearing loss has also been reported in a patient following low-dose exposure to oral azithromycin for a urinary-tract infection.[2] A patient who had received 8 days' treatment with intravenous azithromycin 500 mg daily for pneumonia reported complete deafness, which had resolved 20 days after discontinuation of the drug.[3]

See also above.


1. Wallace MR, *et al.* Ototoxicity with azithromycin. *Lancet* 1994; **343:** 241.
2. Ress BD, Gross EM. Irreversible sensorineural hearing loss as a result of azithromycin ototoxicity: a case report. *Ann Otol Rhinol Laryngol* 2000; **109:** 435–7.
3. Bizjak ED, *et al.* Intravenous azithromycin-induced ototoxicity. *Pharmacotherapy* 1999; **19:** 245–8.


**Effects on fluid and electrolyte homoeostasis.** The syndrome of inappropriate antidiuretic hormone secretion was associated with azithromycin treatment in a patient.[1,2]


1. Cadle RM, *et al.* Symptomatic syndrome of inappropriate antidiuretic hormone secretion associated with azithromycin. *Ann Pharmacother* 1997; **31:** 1308–10.
2. Kintzel PE. Correction: symptomatic syndrome of inappropriate antidiuretic hormone secretion associated with azithromycin. *Ann Pharmacother* 1998; **32:** 388.


**Effects on the kidneys.** Acute interstitial nephritis leading to irreversible renal failure has been reported in a patient who received azithromycin for 9 days.[1]


1. Mansoor GA, *et al.* Azithromycin-induced acute interstitial nephritis. *Ann Intern Med* 1993; **119:** 636–7.


**Eosinophilia.** A syndrome characterised by eosinophilia, arthralgia, fever, and rash was associated with administration of azithromycin or roxithromycin to a patient on separate occasions.[1] The original authors believed the condition represented the Churg-Strauss syndrome, although this was disputed in correspondence[2] and attributed to the eosinophilia-myalgia syndrome.


1. Hübner C, *et al.* Macrolide-induced Churg-Strauss syndrome in a patient with atopy. *Lancet* 1997; **350:** 563.
2. Kränke B, Aberer W. Macrolide-induced Churg-Strauss syndrome in patient with atopy. *Lancet* 1997; **350:** 1551–2.


### Interactions

For a discussion of drug interactions of macrolide antibacterials, see Erythromycin, p.209. Concurrent administration of antacids containing aluminium or magnesium salts can reduce the rate, but not the extent, of absorption of azithromycin; azithromycin should be given at least 1 hour before or 2 hours after the antacid.

**Nelfinavir.** Azithromycin serum levels are markedly increased when it is given with nelfinavir,[1] but the clinical significance of this is uncertain. The US manufacturer of azithromycin states that dosage adjustment is not required although the patient should be closely monitored for adverse effects.


1. Amsden GW, *et al.* A study of the pharmacokinetics of azithromycin and nelfinavir when coadministered in healthy volunteers. *J Clin Pharmacol* 2000; **40:** 1522–7.


### Antimicrobial Action

As for Erythromycin, p.209. Azithromycin is less active than erythromycin against streptococci and staphylococci, but has greater activity than erythromycin *in vitro* against some Gram-negative pathogens such as *Haemophilus influenzae* and *Moraxella catarrhalis* (*Branhamella catarrhalis*), as well as having activity against some of the Enterobacteriaceae such as *Escherichia coli* and *Salmonella* and *Shigella* spp. Azithromycin is also more active than erythromycin against *Chlamydia trachomatis* and some opportunistic mycobacteria, including *Mycobacterium avium* complex. It has activity against the protozoa *Toxoplasma gondii* and *Plasmodium falciparum*.

**Resistance.** The pattern of resistance to azithromycin is similar to that seen with clarithromycin (p.193).

### Pharmacokinetics

Azithromycin given orally is about 40% bioavailable. Absorption from capsules, but not tablets, is reduced by food. Peak plasma concentrations are achieved 2 to 3 hours after a dose, but azithromycin is extensively distributed to the tissues, and tissue concentrations subsequently remain much higher than those in the blood; in contrast to most other antibacterials, plasma concentrations are therefore of little value as a guide to efficacy. High concentrations are taken up into white blood cells. There is little diffusion into the CSF when the meninges are not inflamed. Small amounts of azithromycin are demethylated in the liver, and it is excreted in bile as unchanged drug and metabolites. About 6% of an oral dose (representing about 20% of the amount in the systemic circulation) is excreted in the urine. The terminal elimination half-life is about 68 hours.

◊ Reviews and references.


1. Lalak NJ, Morris DL. Azithromycin clinical pharmacokinetics. *Clin Pharmacokinet* 1993; **25:** 370–4.
2. Nahata MC, *et al.* Pharmacokinetics of azithromycin in pediatric patients after oral administration of multiple doses of suspension. *Antimicrob Agents Chemother* 1993; **37:** 314–16.
3. Luke DR, *et al.* Safety, toleration, and pharmacokinetics of intravenous azithromycin. *Antimicrob Agents Chemother* 1996; **40:** 2577–81.
4. Rapp RP. Pharmacokinetics and pharmacodynamics of intravenous and oral azithromycin: enhanced tissue activity and minimal drug interactions. *Ann Pharmacother* 1998; **32:** 785–93.
5. Amsden GW, *et al.* Pharmacokinetics in serum and leukocyte exposures of oral azithromycin, 1,500 milligrams, given over a 3- or 5-day period in healthy subjects. *Antimicrob Agents Chemother* 1999; **43:** 163–5.
6. Amsden GW, Gray CL. Serum and WBC pharmacokinetics of 1500 mg of azithromycin when given either as a single dose or over a 3 day period in healthy volunteers. *J Antimicrob Chemother* 2001; **47:** 61–6.
7. Blandizzi C, *et al.* Distribution of azithromycin in plasma and tonsil tissue after repeated oral administration of 10 or 20 milligrams per kilogram in pediatric patients. *Antimicrob Agents Chemother* 2002; **46:** 1594–6.


### Uses and Administration

Azithromycin is a nitrogen-containing macrolide or azalide with actions and uses similar to those of erythromycin (p.210).

Azithromycin may also be used as a component of regimens in the treatment of *Mycobacterium avium* complex (MAC) infections (see under Opportunistic Mycobacterial Infections, p.137) and may be used for prophylaxis. It is used in some countries for the prophylaxis of endocarditis in at-risk patients unable to take penicillin. It is used in the management of trachoma (p.149) and has been tried in protozoal infections such as toxoplasmosis (p.598).

It is given by mouth as the dihydrate; doses are expressed in terms of the anhydrous substance. 524 mg of azithromycin dihydrate is approximately equivalent to 500 mg of anhydrous azithromycin. The capsule formulation should be given at least 1 hour before, or 2 hours after, meals.

The usual adult dose of azithromycin is 500 mg as a single dose daily for 3 days. Alternatively, an initial dose of 500 mg may be followed by 250 mg daily for a further 4 days. For the treatment of granuloma inguinale, an initial dose of 1 g followed by 500 mg daily may be given. For uncomplicated genital infections due to *Chlamydia trachomatis*, 1 g of azithromycin is given as a single dose. A single dose of 2 g has been given for uncomplicated gonorrhoea. For prophylaxis of disseminated MAC infections, azithromycin 1.2 g may be given once weekly. In children over 6 months of age, the dose in the UK is 10 mg/kg once daily for 3 days. In the USA, the dose for children over 6 months of age for pneumonia or otitis media is 10 mg/kg on the first day, then 5 mg/kg daily for a further 4 days (alternatively, 30 mg/kg as a single dose, or 10 mg/kg daily for 3 days may be given for acute otitis media), and the dose for pharyngitis or tonsillitis in children aged over 2 years is 12 mg/kg once daily for 5 days.

Azithromycin dihydrate may also be given initially by intravenous infusion in doses equivalent to 500 mg of azithromycin as a single daily dose in the treatment of community-acquired pneumonia and pelvic inflammatory disease. It may be administered either in a solution containing 1 mg/mL over 3 hours or in a solution containing 2 mg/mL over 1 hour.

◊ Reviews.

1. Peters DH, *et al.* Azithromycin: a review of its antimicrobial activity, pharmacokinetic properties and clinical efficacy. *Drugs* 1992; **44:** 750–99.
2. Langtry HD, Balfour JA. Azithromycin: a review of its use in paediatric infectious disease. *Drugs* 1998; **56:** 273–97.
3. Alvarez-Elcoro S, Enzler MJ. The macrolides: erythromycin, clarithromycin, and azithromycin. *Mayo Clin Proc* 1999; **74:** 613–34.
4. Garey KW, Amsden GW. Intravenous azithromycin. *Ann Pharmacother* 1999; **33:** 218–28.
5. Ioannidis JPA, *et al.* Meta-analysis of randomized controlled trials on the comparative efficacy and safety of azithromycin against other antibiotics for upper respiratory tract infections. *J Antimicrob Chemother* 2001; **48:** 677–89.
6. Contopoulos-Ioannidis DG, *et al.* Meta-analysis of randomized controlled trials on the comparative efficacy and safety of azithromycin against other antibiotics for lower respiratory tract infections. *J Antimicrob Chemother* 2001; **48:** 691–703.

**Ischaemic heart disease.** Azithromycin has been investigated in the prevention of ischaemic heart disease, based on a suggested link between atherosclerosis and infection with *Chlamydophila pneumoniae* (*Chlamydia pneumoniae*) (see p.123). Pilot studies and preliminary results of prospective studies[1] demonstrated that treatment with azithromycin was tolerable. A subsequent larger study, in which 1439 patients presenting with acute myocardial infarction or unstable angina were randomised to receive a 5-day course of either azithromycin or placebo and were followed up for 6 months, it was found that short-term treatment with azithromycin did not decrease the incidence of ischaemic events compared with placebo.[2] Subsequently a larger study,[3] in which 7747 adults with previous myocardial infarction and evidence of *C. pneumoniae* infection were randomised to receive azithromycin over 12 weeks or placebo, found that azithromycin had no significant effect in reducing clinical sequelae of ischaemic heart disease.

1. Anderson JL, *et al.* Randomized secondary prevention trial of azithromycin in patients with coronary artery disease and serological evidence for Chlamydia pneumoniae infection: the Azithromycin in Coronary Artery Disease: Elimination of Myocardial Infection with Chlamydia (ACADEMIC) study. *Circulation* 1999; **99:** 1540–7.
2. Cercek B, *et al.* Effect of short-term treatment with azithromycin on recurrent ischaemic events in patients with acute coronary syndrome in the Azithromycin in Acute Coronary Syndrome (AZACS) trial: a randomised controlled trial. *Lancet* 2003; **361:** 809–13.
3. O'Connor CM, *et al.* Azithromycin for the secondary prevention of coronary heart disease events: the WIZARD study: a randomized controlled trial. *JAMA* 2003; **290:** 1459–66.

**Malaria.** Azithromycin has been studied in the management of malaria.

1. Taylor WR, *et al.* Malaria prophylaxis using azithromycin: a double-blind, placebo-controlled trial in Irian Jaya, Indonesia. *Clin Infect Dis* 1999; **28:** 74–81.
2. Krudsood S, *et al.* A randomized clinical trial of combinations of artesunate and azithromycin for treatment of uncomplicated Plasmodium falciparum malaria in Thailand. *Southeast Asian J Trop Med Public Health* 2000; **31:** 801–7.

**Typhoid fever.** Azithromycin has been tried in the treatment of typhoid fever (p.152). A suggested dose in the *British National Formulary* is 500 mg given once daily for 7 days.

## Preparations

*USP 27:* Azithromycin Capsules.

**Proprietary Preparations** (details are given in Part 3)

***Arg.:*** Arzomicin; Azitronal; Clearsing; Cronopen; Doyle; Fabramicina; Macromax; Misultina; Naxocina; Neblic; Nifostin; Novozitron; Orobiotic; Sumir; Tanezox; Triamid; Tritab; Zitromax; ***Austral.:*** Zithromax; ***Austria:*** Zithromax; ***Belg.:*** Zitromax; ***Braz.:*** Atromicin; Azi; Azimax†; Azimix; Azitrax; Azitrocin†; Azitromin; Aziton†; Azitroxil; Clindal; Clindaz†; Mazitrom; Novatrex; Selimax; Trozyman; Zimicina; Zitromax; Zitroneo; ***Canad.:*** Z-Pak; Zithromax; ***Chile:*** Abacten; Asipral; Atizor; Azitrom; Ricilina; Trex; Zithromax; ***Denm.:*** Zitromax; ***Fin.:*** Zithromax; ***Fr.:*** Azadose; Zithromax; ***Ger.:*** Ultreon; Zithromax; ***Gr.:*** Zithromax; ***Hong Kong:*** Zithromax; ***India:*** Azithral; Aziwok; ***Irl.:*** Zithromax; ***Israel:*** Azenil; Zeto; Zithromax; ***Ital.:*** Azitrocin; Ribotrex; Trozocina; Zitromax; ***Malaysia:*** Zithromax; ***Mex.:*** Azitrocin; ***Neth.:*** Zithromax; ***Norw.:*** Azitromax; ***NZ:*** Zithromax; ***Port.:*** Arzomicina; Azitrix; Farmiz; Gigatrom; Unizitro; Zithromax; ***S.Afr.:*** Zithromax; ***Singapore:*** Zithromax; ***Spain:*** Goxil; Toraseptol; Vinzam; Zentavion; Zitromax; ***Swed.:*** Azitromax; ***Switz.:*** Zithromax; ***Thai.:*** Zithromax; ***UAE:*** Azomycin; ***UK:*** Zithromax; ***USA:*** Zithromax.

## Azlocillin *(BAN, USAN)*

6-[*N*-(2-Oxoimidazolidin-1-ylcarbonyl)-D-phenylglycylamino]penicillanic acid.

$C_{20}H_{23}N_5O_6S$ = 461.5.

*CAS — 37091-66-0.*

## Azlocillin Sodium *(BANM, rINNM)*

Azlocilina sódica; Bay-e-6905. Sodium (6*R*)-6-[D-2-(2-oxoimidazolidine-1-carboxamido)-2-phenylacetamido]penicillanate.

$C_{20}H_{22}N_5NaO_6S$ = 483.5.

*CAS — 37091-65-9.*

*ATC — J01CA09.*

**Pharmacopoeias.** In *Pol.*

**Incompatibility.** Azlocillin sodium has been reported to be incompatible with aminoglycosides, ciprofloxacin, metronidazole, and tetracyclines.

### Adverse Effects and Precautions

As for Carbenicillin Sodium, p.166.

Prolongation of bleeding time has been less frequent and less severe with azlocillin than with carbenicillin.

**Hypouricaemia.** Reports of transient asymptomatic decreases in serum-uric acid concentrations during treatment with azlocillin.[1,2]

1. Faris HM, Potts DW. Azlocillin and serum uric acid. *Ann Intern Med* 1983; **98:** 414.
2. Ernst JA, Sy ER. Effect of azlocillin on uric acid levels in serum. *Antimicrob Agents Chemother* 1983; **24:** 609–10.

**Sodium content.** Each g of azlocillin sodium contains about 2.1 mmol of sodium. As azlocillin sodium has a lower sodium content than carbenicillin sodium, hypernatraemia and hypokalaemia are less likely to occur.

### Interactions

As for Benzylpenicillin, p.164.

**Antibacterials.** For the effect of azlocillin on the clearance of *cefotaxime*, and a report of neurotoxicity, see p.175. For reference to azlocillin affecting the disposition of *ciprofloxacin*, see p.190.

### Antimicrobial Action

Azlocillin has an antimicrobial action similar to that of piperacillin (p.243). Its activity *in vitro* against Enterobacteriaceae is generally less than that of mezlocillin or piperacillin, but it has comparable activity to piperacillin against *Pseudomonas aeruginosa*.

### Pharmacokinetics

Azlocillin is not absorbed from the gastrointestinal tract to any significant extent. It has nonlinear dose-dependent pharmacokinetics. Doubling of an intravenous dose results in more than double the plasma concentration. Between 20 and 46% of azlocillin in the circulation is bound to plasma proteins. The plasma half-life is usually about 1 hour, but is longer in neonates; in patients with renal impairment half-lives of 2 to 6 hours have been reported.

Azlocillin is widely distributed in body tissues and fluids. It crosses the placenta into the fetal circulation and small amounts are distributed into breast milk. There is little diffusion into the CSF except when the meninges are inflamed.

Azlocillin is metabolised to a limited extent. About 50 to 70% of a dose is excreted unchanged in the urine by glomerular filtration and tubular secretion within 24 hours of administration, so that high urinary concentrations are achieved. Azlocillin is partly excreted in the bile where it is also found in high concentrations.

Plasma concentrations are enhanced if probenecid is administered concomitantly.

Azlocillin is removed by haemodialysis.

### Uses and Administration

Azlocillin is a ureidopenicillin and, like piperacillin (p.243), is used mainly for the treatment of infections caused by *Pseudomonas aeruginosa*. It has been used particularly for septicaemia, and infections of the respiratory and urinary tracts, and also for peritonitis; for details of these infections, see under Choice of Antibacterial, p.120.

Azlocillin is commonly used with an aminoglycoside; however, they should be administered separately as they have been shown to be incompatible (see Incompatibility, above).

*Administration and dosage.* Azlocillin is administered intravenously as the sodium salt. Doses are expressed in terms of the equivalent amount of azlocillin. 1.05 g of azlocillin sodium is approximately equivalent to 1 g of azlocillin. A 10% solution in a suitable diluent is given by slow injection for doses of 2 g or less; higher doses should be infused over 20 to 30 minutes.

The usual adult dose is 5 g every 8 hours for life-threatening infections, or 2 g every 8 hours for less severe infections and urinary-tract infections.

The following doses may be used for children: premature infants, 50 mg/kg twice daily; neonates less than 7 days old, 100 mg/kg twice daily; infants between 7 days and 1 year, 100 mg/kg three times daily; children up to 14 years, 75 mg/kg three times daily.

Dosage of azlocillin may need to be adjusted in patients with hepatic or renal impairment (see below).

**Administration in hepatic or renal impairment.** The interval between doses of azlocillin may need to be increased to every 12 hours in moderate to severe renal impairment (creatinine clearance less than 30 mL/minute); additional dosage reductions may be needed in patients with both severe renal and hepatic impairment.

### Preparations

**Proprietary Preparations** (details are given in Part 3)

***Austria:*** Securopen†; ***Ger.:*** Securopen†; ***Irl.:*** Securopen†; ***Ital.:*** Securopen†; ***Norw.:*** Securopen†.

## Aztreonam *(BAN, USAN, rINN)*

Azthreonam; SQ-26776. (*Z*)-2-{2-Aminothiazol-4-yl-[(2*S*,3*S*)-2-methyl-4-oxo-1-sulphoazetidin-3-ylcarbamoyl]methyleneamino-oxy}-2-methylpropionic acid.

$C_{13}H_{17}N_5O_8S_2$ = 435.4.

*CAS — 78110-38-0.*

*ATC — J01DF01.*

**Pharmacopoeias.** In *Jpn* and *US*.

**USP 27** (Aztreonam). A white, odourless crystalline powder. Very slightly soluble in dehydrated alcohol; practically insoluble in chloroform, in ethyl acetate, and in toluene; soluble in dimethylformamide and in dimethyl sulfoxide; slightly soluble in methyl alcohol. Store in airtight containers.

**Incompatibility and stability.** Aztreonam has been reported to be incompatible with cefradine, metronidazole, nafcillin, and vancomycin.

References.

1. Bell RG, *et al.* Stability of intravenous admixtures of aztreonam and cefoxitin, gentamicin, metronidazole, or tobramycin. *Am J Hosp Pharm* 1986; **43:** 1444–53.
2. Riley CM, Lipford LC. Interaction of aztreonam with nafcillin in intravenous admixtures. *Am J Hosp Pharm* 1986; **43:** 2221–4.
3. Belliveau PP, *et al.* Stability of aztreonam and ampicillin sodium-sulbactam sodium in 0.9% sodium chloride injection. *Am J Hosp Pharm* 1994; **51:** 901–4.
4. Trissel LA, Martinez JF. Compatibility of aztreonam with selected drugs during simulated Y-site administration. *Am J Health-Syst Pharm* 1995; **52:** 1086–90.
5. Trissel LA, *et al.* Compatibility and stability of aztreonam and vancomycin hydrochloride. *Am J Health-Syst Pharm* 1995; **52:** 2560–4.

### Adverse Effects

The adverse effects of aztreonam are similar to those of other beta lactams (see Benzylpenicillin, p.163, and Cefalotin, p.168). Hypersensitivity reactions, including skin rashes, urticaria, exfoliative dermatitis, eosinophilia, and rarely anaphylaxis, may occur in patients receiving aztreonam, although it has been reported to be only weakly immunogenic (see also under Precautions, below). Gastrointestinal effects include diarrhoea, nausea, vomiting, and an abnormal taste.

Phlebitis or thrombophlebitis has been reported after the intravenous administration of aztreonam, and pain or swelling after intramuscular injection.

Use of aztreonam may result in the overgrowth of non-susceptible organisms, including Gram-positive cocci. Pseudomembranous colitis may develop.

Other adverse effects that have been reported with aztreonam include jaundice and hepatitis, increases in liver enzymes, and prolongation of prothrombin and partial thromboplastin times.

**Effects on the skin.** References.

1. McDonald BJ, *et al.* Toxic epidermal necrolysis possibly linked to aztreonam in bone marrow transplant patients. *Ann Pharmacother* 1992; **26:** 34–5.

### Precautions

Aztreonam should not be given to patients who are hypersensitive to it and should be used with caution in those known to be hypersensitive to other beta lactams, although the incidence of cross-sensitivity appears to be low (but see below).

Aztreonam should be used with caution in patients with renal or hepatic impairment.

**Breast feeding.** In a study in 12 lactating healthy women given aztreonam, peak concentrations in breast milk were found to be less than 1% of those in serum and this was considered suggestive of a low risk of adverse effects in breast-fed infants.[1] The American Academy of Pediatrics states that no adverse effects have been observed in breast-fed infants whose mothers received aztreonam and considers it to be usually compatible with breast feeding,[2] although the UK manufacturers recommend that lactating mothers should refrain from breast feeding while receiving aztreonam.

1. Fleiss PM, *et al.* Aztreonam in human serum and breast milk. *Br J Clin Pharmacol* 1985; **19:** 509–11.
2. American Academy of Pediatrics. The transfer of drugs and other chemicals into human milk. *Pediatrics* 2001; **108:** 776–89. Correction. *ibid.*; 1029. Also available at: http://aappolicy.aappublications.org/cgi/content/full/pediatrics%3b108/3/776 (accessed 25/05/04)

**Hypersensitivity.** Aztreonam is said to show little cross-reactivity with other beta lactams,[1,2] but there have been isolated reports of immediate hypersensitivity to aztreonam in patients with a history of hypersensitivity to penicillin.[3,4]

1. Saxon A, *et al.* Lack of cross-reactivity between aztreonam, a monobactam antibiotic, and penicillin in penicillin-allergic subjects. *J Infect Dis* 1984; **149:** 16–22.
2. Adkinson NF. Immunogenicity and cross-allergenicity of aztreonam. *Am J Med* 1990; **88** (suppl 3C): 12S–15S.
3. Alvarez JS, *et al.* Immediate hypersensitivity to aztreonam. *Lancet* 1990; **335:** 1094.
4. Hantson P, *et al.* Immediate hypersensitivity to aztreonam and imipenem. *BMJ* 1991; **302:** 294–5.

## Interactions

Caution is recommended in patients receiving aztreonam and oral anticoagulants because of the possibility of increased prothrombin time.

## Antimicrobial Action

Aztreonam is bactericidal and acts similarly to the penicillins by inhibiting synthesis of the bacterial cell wall; it has a high affinity for the penicillin-binding protein 3 (PBP-3) of Gram-negative bacteria. The activity of aztreonam is restricted to Gram-negative aerobic organisms, including beta-lactamase-producing strains, with poor or no activity against Gram-positive aerobes or anaerobic organisms. It is active against most Enterobacteriaceae including *Escherichia coli*, *Klebsiella*, *Proteus*, *Providencia*, *Salmonella*, *Serratia*, *Shigella*, and *Yersinia* spp. Some strains of *Enterobacter* and *Citrobacter* spp. are resistant. Aztreonam has some activity against *Pseudomonas aeruginosa*, although most strains of other *Pseudomonas* spp. are insensitive. Aztreonam has good activity against *Haemophilus influenzae* and *Neisseria* spp.

Synergy has been reported *in vitro* between aztreonam and aminoglycosides against *Ps. aeruginosa* and some *Enterobacteriaceae*.

Aztreonam is stable to hydrolysis by many beta-lactamases and appears to be a poor inducer of beta-lactamase production. Acquired resistance has occasionally been reported.

## Pharmacokinetics

Aztreonam is poorly absorbed from the gastrointestinal tract and is therefore given parenterally. Absorption after intramuscular injection is good; peak plasma concentrations of about 46 micrograms/mL have been achieved within 1 hour of a 1-g dose. Aztreonam has a plasma half-life of about 1.7 hours. The half-life may be prolonged in neonates, in the elderly, in patients with renal impairment, and to some extent in those with hepatic impairment. Aztreonam is about 56% bound to plasma proteins. It is widely distributed in body tissues and fluids, including bile. Diffusion into the CSF is poor unless the meninges are inflamed. It crosses the placenta and enters the fetal circulation; small amounts are distributed into breast milk.

Aztreonam is not extensively metabolised. The principal metabolite, SQ-26992, is inactive and is formed by opening of the beta-lactam ring; it has a much longer half-life than the parent compound. Aztreonam is excreted mainly in the urine, by renal tubular secretion and glomerular filtration; about 60 to 70% of a dose appears within 8 hours as unchanged drug with only small quantities of metabolites. Only small amounts of unchanged drug and metabolites are excreted in the faeces.

Aztreonam is removed by haemodialysis and to a lesser extent by peritoneal dialysis.

◊ Reviews.

1. Mattie H. Clinical pharmacokinetics of aztreonam: an update. *Clin Pharmacokinet* 1994; **26:** 99–106.

## Uses and Administration

Aztreonam is a monobactam or monocyclic beta-lactam antibacterial used parenterally as an alternative to aminoglycosides or third-generation cephalosporins for the treatment of infections caused by susceptible Gram-negative aerobic organisms. These have included bone and joint infections, gonorrhoea, intra-abdominal and pelvic infections, lower respiratory-tract infections including pseudomonal infections in patients with cystic fibrosis, meningitis, septicaemia, skin and soft tissue infections, and urinary-tract infections. For details of these infections and their treatment, see under Choice of Antibacterial, p.120. To broaden the spectrum of activity for empirical treatment of infections, aztreonam should be used with other antibacterials. Use with an aminoglycoside may be of benefit in serious *Pseudomonas aeruginosa* infections.

Aztreonam is usually administered parenterally by deep intramuscular injection, by slow intravenous injection over 3 to 5 minutes, or by intravenous infusion over 20 to 60 minutes. It is given to adults, in doses ranging from 1 to 8 g daily, in divided doses every 6 to 12 hours, according to the severity of the infection. Single doses over 1 g should be given by the intravenous route.

Infants older than one week and children may be given aztreonam 30 mg/kg every 6 or 8 hours. For severe infections, children of 2 years or older may be given 50 mg/kg every 6 or 8 hours up to a maximum total daily dose of 8 g.

For details of dosage in patients with renal impairment, see below.

A single intramuscular dose of 1 g has been recommended for the treatment of gonorrhoea or cystitis.

◊ General references.

1. Brogden RN, Heel RC. Aztreonam: a review of its antibacterial activity, pharmacokinetic properties and therapeutic use. *Drugs* 1986; **31:** 96–130.
2. Neu HC. ed. Aztreonam's role in the treatment of Gram-negative infections. *Am J Med* 1990; **88** (suppl 3C): 1S–43S.
3. Hellinger WC, Brewer NS. Carbapenems and monobactams: imipenem, meropenem, and aztreonam. *Mayo Clin Proc* 1999; **74:** 420–34.

**Administration in renal impairment.** Dosage of aztreonam should be reduced in moderate to severe renal impairment. Patients with renal impairment may be given a usual initial dose followed by a maintenance dose adjusted according to their creatinine clearance (CC):

- CC 10 to 30 mL/minute: half the initial dose
- CC less than 10 mL/minute: one-quarter of the initial dose
- haemodialysis patients: a supplementary dose of one-eighth of the initial dose may be given after each dialysis session

## Preparations

*USP 27:* Aztreonam for Injection; Aztreonam Injection.

**Proprietary Preparations** (details are given in Part 3)
***Arg.:*** Azactam; ***Austral.:*** Azactam; ***Austria:*** Azactam; ***Belg.:*** Azactam; ***Braz.:*** Azactam; ***Chile:*** Azactam; ***Denm.:*** Azactam; ***Fin.:*** Azactam; ***Fr.:*** Azactam; ***Ger.:*** Azactam; ***Gr.:*** Azactam; ***Hong Kong:*** Azactam; ***Irl.:*** Azactam; ***Israel:*** Azactam; ***Ital.:*** Azactam; Primbactam; ***Mex.:*** Monobac; ***Neth.:*** Azactam†; ***Norw.:*** Azactam; ***NZ:*** Azactam; ***Port.:*** Azactam; ***S.Afr.:*** Azactam; ***Singapore:*** Azactam; ***Spain:*** Azactam; Urobactam; ***Swed.:*** Azactam; ***Switz.:*** Azactam; ***Thai.:*** Azactam†; ***UK:*** Azactam; ***USA:*** Azactam.

---

# Bacampicillin Hydrochloride *(BANM, USAN, rINNM)*

Ampicillin Ethoxycarbonyloxyethyl Hydrochloride; Bacampicillini Hydrochloridum; Carampicillin; EPC-272; Hidrocloruro de bacampicilina. 1-(Ethoxycarbonyloxy)ethyl (6*R*)-6-(α-D-phenylglycylamino)penicillanate hydrochloride.

$C_{21}H_{27}N_3O_7S,HCl = 502.0.$
*CAS — 50972-17-3 (bacampicillin); 37661-08-8 (bacampicillin hydrochloride).*

**Pharmacopoeias.** In *Eur.* (see p.vi), *Jpn*, and *US.*

**Ph. Eur. 5.0** (Bacampicillin Hydrochloride). A white or almost white hygroscopic powder or granules. Soluble in water and in dichloromethane; freely soluble in alcohol. A 2% solution in water has a pH of 3.0 to 4.5. Store in airtight containers.

**USP 27** (Bacampicillin Hydrochloride). A white or practically white, hygroscopic, powder. Soluble in water and in dichloromethane; freely soluble in alcohol and in chloroform; very slightly soluble in ether. pH of a 2% solution in water is between 3.0 and 4.5. Store in airtight containers.

## Adverse Effects and Precautions

As for Ampicillin, p.157. Diarrhoea has been reported to occur less frequently with bacampicillin.

## Interactions

As for Benzylpenicillin, p.164.

## Antimicrobial Action

Bacampicillin has the antimicrobial action of ampicillin *in vivo* (p.157). It possesses no intrinsic activity and needs to be hydrolysed to ampicillin.

## Pharmacokinetics

Bacampicillin is more rapidly and completely absorbed from the gastrointestinal tract than ampicillin, to which it is hydrolysed in the intestinal wall and plasma. Peak plasma-ampicillin concentrations occur about 30 to 60 minutes after administration by mouth, and are about 2 to 3 times those after an equivalent dose of ampicillin. The absorption of bacampicillin from tablets does not appear to be affected by the presence of food in the stomach. About 75% of a dose is excreted in the urine as ampicillin within 8 hours.

## Uses and Administration

Bacampicillin has actions and uses similar to those of ampicillin (p.158) to which it is rapidly hydrolysed after administration. It is given by mouth as the hydrochloride in adult doses of 0.8 to 2.4 g daily, in 2 or 3 divided doses; children over 5 years of age have been given 25 to 50 mg/kg daily in 2 or 3 divided doses.

In uncomplicated gonorrhoea a single dose of bacampicillin hydrochloride 1.6 g together with probenecid 1 g may be given in areas where gonococci remain sensitive.

## Preparations

*USP 27:* Bacampicillin Hydrochloride for Oral Suspension; Bacampicillin Hydrochloride Tablets.

**Proprietary Preparations** (details are given in Part 3)
***Austria:*** Penglobe; ***Belg.:*** Bacampicin; Bacocil†; Penglobe†; ***Canad.:*** Penglobe; ***Denm.:*** Penglobe†; ***Fr.:*** Bacampicine; Penglobe; ***Ger.:*** Ambacamp; Penglobe†; ***Hong Kong:*** Penglobe; ***India:*** Penglobe; ***Ital.:*** Ampibac; Bacacil; Bacagen; Bacasint; Bacattiv; Bacillin; Bakam; Penglobe; Polibiotic; Rebacil; ***Malaysia:*** Penbaccin; Penglobe; ***Mex.:*** Penglobe; ***Port.:*** Bacampicin; ***Singapore:*** Penglobe†; ***Spain:*** Ambaxino; Penglobe; Velbacil†; ***Swed.:*** Penglobe; ***Switz.:*** Bacampicin†; ***Thai.:*** Penglobe; ***USA:*** Spectrobid†.

---

# Bacitracin *(BAN, rINN)*

Bacitracina; Bacitracinum.
*CAS — 1405-87-4.*
*ATC — D06AX05; R02AB04.*

**Pharmacopoeias.** In *Chin., Eur.* (see p.vi), *Int., Jpn, Pol.,* and *US.*

**Ph. Eur. 5.0** (Bacitracin). Mixture of antimicrobial polypeptides produced by certain strains of *Bacillus licheniformis* or *B. subtilis*. The potency is not less than 60 units/mg, calculated with reference to the dried substance. A white or almost white hygroscopic powder. Freely soluble in water and in alcohol. A 1% solution in water has a pH of 6.0 to 7.0. Store at a temperature of 8° to 15° in airtight containers.

**USP 27** (Bacitracin). A polypeptide produced by the growth of an organism of the *licheniformis* group of *Bacillus subtilis* (Bacillaceae). It has a potency of not less than 40 units/mg. It is a white to pale buff, hygroscopic powder, odourless or having a slight odour. Freely soluble in water; soluble in alcohol, in glacial acetic acid, and in methyl alcohol, the solution in the organic solvents usually showing some insoluble residue; insoluble in acetone, in chloroform, and in ether. Its solutions deteriorate rapidly at room temperature. It is precipitated from its solutions and is inactivated by salts of many of the heavy metals. pH of a solution in water containing 10 000 units/mL is between 5.5 and 7.5. Store in airtight containers at a temperature of 8° to 15°.

## Bacitracin Zinc *(BANM, rINNM)*

Bacitracina zinc; Bacitracins Zinc Complex; Bacitracinum Zincum; Zinc Bacitracin.
*CAS — 1405-89-6.*
*ATC — D06AX05; R02AB04.*

**Pharmacopoeias.** In *Eur.* (see p.vi), *Int., Pol.,* and *US.*

**Ph. Eur. 5.0** (Bacitracin Zinc). The zinc complex of bacitracin. The potency is not less than 60 units/mg, calculated with reference to the dried substance. A white or light-yellowish-grey hygroscopic powder. Slightly soluble in water and in alcohol. The filtrate of a saturated solution has a pH of 6.0 to 7.5. Store in airtight containers.

**USP 27** (Bacitracin Zinc). The zinc salt of a kind of bacitracin or a mixture of two or more such salts. It has a potency of not less than 40 units/mg. A white or pale tan, hygroscopic powder, odourless or having a slight odour. Sparingly soluble in water. pH of a saturated solution in water is between 6.0 and 7.5. Store in airtight containers at a temperature of 8° to 15°.

**Incompatibility.** Bacitracin was slowly inactivated in bases containing stearyl alcohol, cholesterol, polyoxyethylene derivatives, and sodium laurilsulfate, and was rapidly inactivated in bases containing water, macrogols, propylene glycol, glycerol, cetylpyridinium chloride, benzalkonium chloride, ichthammol, phenol, and tannic acid.[1]

1. Plaxco JM, Husa WJ. The effect of various substances on the antibacterial activity of bacitracin in ointments. *J Am Pharm Assoc (Sci)* 1956; **45:** 141–5.

**Stability.** Bacitracin zinc was more stable than bacitracin and could be stored for 18 months at temperatures up to 40° without appreciable loss. Lozenges of bacitracin zinc and ointments and tablets containing bacitracin zinc with neomycin were more stable than the corresponding bacitracin preparations. Bacitracin zinc was less bitter than bacitracin and the taste was more readily disguised.[1]

1. Gross HM, *et al.* Zinc bacitracin in pharmaceutical preparations. *Drug Cosmet Ind* 1954; **75:** 612–13.

## Units

The second International Standard Preparation (1964) of bacitracin zinc contains 74 units/mg.

### Adverse Effects

Bacitracin may produce severe nephrotoxicity when given systemically. Nausea and vomiting may occur, as well as pain at the site of injection. Hypersensitivity reactions, including rashes and anaphylaxis, have occurred with both systemic, and more rarely with topical, use.

### Interactions

Additive nephrotoxicity would be anticipated if bacitracin is given systemically with other nephrotoxic drugs. Bacitracin is reported to enhance the neuromuscular blocking action of other drugs.

### Antimicrobial Action

Bacitracin interferes with bacterial cell wall synthesis by blocking the function of the lipid carrier molecule that transfers cell wall subunits across the cell membrane. It is active against many Gram-positive bacteria including staphylococci, streptococci (particularly group A streptococci), and clostridia. It is also active against *Actinomyces*, *Treponema pallidum*, and some Gram-negative species such as *Neisseria* and *Haemophilus influenzae*, although most Gram-negative organisms are resistant.

Acquired bacterial resistance to bacitracin rarely occurs, but resistant strains of staphylococci have been detected.

### Pharmacokinetics

Bacitracin is not appreciably absorbed from the gastrointestinal tract. It is rapidly absorbed when given by intramuscular injection. About 10 to 40% of a single injected dose is excreted in the urine within 24 hours. Bacitracin readily diffuses into pleural and ascitic fluids but little passes into the CSF. Absorption is reported to be negligible following topical application but may occur after peritoneal lavage.

### Uses and Administration

Bacitracin and bacitracin zinc are applied topically, often with other antibacterials such as neomycin and polymyxin B, and sometimes with corticosteroids, in the treatment of local infections due to susceptible organisms. Absorption from open wounds and from the bladder or peritoneal cavity may lead to adverse effects, although the dose-limiting toxicity of combined preparations is considered to be due to neomycin.

Parenteral administration of bacitracin is usually avoided because of toxicity but it may be given intramuscularly for the treatment of infants with staphylococcal pneumonia and empyema due to susceptible organisms. Infants weighing less than 2.5 kg may be given a dose of 900 units/kg daily in 2 or 3 divided doses; those weighing more than 2.5 kg may be given 1000 units/kg daily in 2 or 3 divided doses. Bacitracin has been given by mouth in the treatment of antibiotic-associated colitis due to *Clostridium difficile*.

### Preparations

***BP 2003:*** Polymyxin and Bacitracin Eye Ointment;
***USP 27:*** Bacitracin and Polymyxin B Sulfate Topical Aerosol; Bacitracin for Injection; Bacitracin Ointment; Bacitracin Ophthalmic Ointment; Bacitracin Zinc and Polymyxin B Sulfate Ointment; Bacitracin Zinc and Polymyxin B Sulfate Ophthalmic Ointment; Bacitracin Zinc Ointment; Neomycin and Polymyxin B Sulfates and Bacitracin Ointment; Neomycin and Polymyxin B Sulfates and Bacitracin Ophthalmic Ointment; Neomycin and Polymyxin B Sulfates and Bacitracin Zinc Ointment; Neomycin and Polymyxin B Sulfates and Bacitracin Zinc Ophthalmic Ointment; Neomycin and Polymyxin B Sulfates, Bacitracin Zinc, and Hydrocortisone Acetate Ophthalmic Ointment; Neomycin and Polymyxin B Sulfates, Bacitracin Zinc, and Hydrocortisone Ointment; Neomycin and Polymyxin B Sulfates, Bacitracin Zinc, and Hydrocortisone Ophthalmic Ointment; Neomycin and Polymyxin B Sulfates, Bacitracin Zinc, and Lidocaine Ointment; Neomycin and Polymyxin B Sulfates, Bacitracin, and Hydrocortisone Acetate Ointment; Neomycin and Polymyxin B Sulfates, Bacitracin, and Hydrocortisone Acetate Ophthalmic Ointment; Neomycin and Polymyxin B Sulfates, Bacitracin, and Lidocaine Ointment; Neomycin Sulfate and Bacitracin Ointment; Neomycin Sulfate and Bacitracin Zinc Ointment; Polymyxin B Sulfate and Bacitracin in Zinc Topical Aerosol; Polymyxin B Sulfate and Bacitracin Zinc Topical Powder.

**Proprietary Preparations** (details are given in Part 3)
***Austria:*** Rhinocillin B†; ***Canad.:*** Baciguent; Bacitin; ***Hong Kong:*** Bacitin†; ***USA:*** Ak-Tracin; Baci-IM; Baciguent†.

**Multi-ingredient:** ***Arg.:*** Biotaer; Biotaer Gamma; Biotaer Nebulizable; Biotaer Ultrason Nebulizable; Butimerin; Carnot Colutorio; Cicatrex; Nebapol B; ***Austral.:*** Cicatrin; Nemdyn; Neosporin; ***Austria:*** Baneocin; Cicatrex; Eucillin; Nebacetin; ***Belg.:*** Neobacitracine; ***Braz.:*** Anaseptil; Antiseptin†; Bacigen; Bacineo; Belcetin; Cicatrene; Cicatrizan; Cutiderm; Dermacetin-Ped; Dermase; Duplocitrin†; Infectracina†; Kindcetin; Nebacetin; Nebacina†; Nebacitrin; Nebalon†; Neobacina; Neobacipan; Neobacitracina†; Neocetrin; Neotop; Neotricin; Rinogerol†; Teutomicina; ***Canad.:*** Antibiotic Ointment; Antibiotique Onguent; Baciguent Plus Pain Reliever†; Bacimyxin; Band-Aid Antibiotic; Bioderm; Cicatrin; Cortisporin; Emercreme No 4†; Johnson & Johnson First Aid Ointment; Lanabiotic†; Lid-Pack†; Neo Bace†; Neosporin; Neotopic; Optimyxin; Ozonol Antibiotic Plus; Polycidin; Polyderm; Polysporin; Polysporin Triple Antibiotic; Polytopic; Polytracin†; ***Chile:*** Bacitopic; Bacitopic Compuesto; Banedif; Banedif Oftalmico; Banedif Oftalmico con Prednisolona; Biodexin; Dermabiotico; Grifoftal; Monticina; Nasomin; Oftabiotico; Pensulan; Polvos Antibioticos; Rinobanedif; Unguento Dermico Antibiotico; ***Fin.:*** Bacibact; ***Fr.:*** Baciocoline; Collunovar; Lysopaine; Maxilase-Bacitracine†; Oropivalone Bacitracine; ***Ger.:*** Anginomycin; Batrax†; Bivacyn; Cicatrex; Nebacetin; Neobac; Neotracin†; Polyspectran; Polyspectran HC; Prednitracin†; ***Hong Kong:*** Bacimycin; Bivacyn; Nebacetin; Neosporin; Neotopic†; PMS-Baximycin; Polyfax; Polyspectran†; Prednitracin; ***India:*** Nebasulf; Neosporin; Neosporin-H; ***Irl.:*** Cicatrin; Polybactrin†; Polyfax; ***Israel:*** Bamyxin; ***Ital.:*** Bimixin; Cicatrene; Enterostop; Orobicin; ***Malaysia:*** Baneocin; ***Mex.:*** Nebacetina; Neosporin; Polixin; Tribiot; ***Neth.:*** Bacicoline-B; ***Norw.:*** Bacimycin; ***Port.:*** Baciderma; Bacitracina-Neo; Cicatrin†; Davimicina; Dermimade Bacitracina; Dermobiotico; Dimicina; Oralbiotico; Polisulfade; Tri-Sinerge†; ***S.Afr.:*** Cicatrin; Neosporin; Polysporin†; ***Singapore:*** Baneocin; Batramycin; Fast Powder†; Polybamycin; ***Spain:*** Alantomicina Complex†; Bacisporin; Banedif; Dermisone Tri Antibiotic; Dermo Hubber; Edifaringen; Linitul Antibiotico†; Lizipaina; Neo Bacitrin; Neo Bacitrin Hidrocortis†; Oxidermiol Enzima; Phonal; Pomada Antibiotica; Rinobanedif; Tulgrasum Antibiotico; Tyroneomicin†; ***Switz.:*** Bacimycin; Baneopol; Batramycine; Cicatrex; Lysopaine; Nebacetin; Neotracin; Oro-Pivalone; Prednitracin; ***Thai.:*** Banocin; Biochin; Genquin; Izac; Lobacin†; Mybacin; Mybacin Dermic; ***UK:*** Cicatrin; Polyfax; ***USA:*** Ak-Poly-Bac; Ak-Spore; Bactine First Aid Antibiotic Plus Anesthetic†; Betadine First Aid Antibiotics + Moisturizer†; Betadine Plus First Aid Antibiotics & Pain Reliever; Campho-Phenique Antibiotic Plus Pain Reliever Ointment†; Clomycin†; Cortimycin; Cortisporin; Lanabiotic; Mycitracin; Mycitracin Plus†; Neocin; Neomixin†; Neosporin; Neosporin + Pain Relief; Neosporin Plus†; Neotricin HC; Ocu-Spor-B; Ocutricin; Polycin-B; Polymycin; Polysporin; Polytracin; Septa†; Spectrocin Plus; Tri-Biozene; Tribiotic Plus†; Triple Antibiotic†.

---

## Balofloxacin *(rINN)*

Balofloxacino; Q-35. (±)-1-Cyclopropyl-6-fluoro-1,4-dihydro-8-methoxy-7-[3-(methylamino)piperidino]-4-oxo-3-quinolinecarboxylic acid.

$C_{20}H_{24}FN_3O_4$ = 389.4.
*CAS — 127294-70-6.*

### Profile

Balofloxacin is a fluoroquinolone antibacterial.

---

## Bambermycin *(BAN, pINN)*

Bambermicina; Bambermycins *(USAN)*; Flavophospholipol.
*CAS — 11015-37-5.*

### Profile

Bambermycin is an antibacterial complex containing mainly moenomycin A and moenomycin C and which may be obtained from cultures of *Streptomyces bambergiensis* or by other means. It is used as a growth promotor in veterinary practice.

---

## Baquiloprim *(BAN, rINN)*

Baquiloprima; 1380U. 5-(8-Dimethylamino-7-methyl-5-quinolylmethyl)pyrimidin-2,4-diyldiamine.

$C_{17}H_{20}N_6$ = 308.4.
*CAS — 102280-35-3.*

### Profile

Baquiloprim is a diaminopyrimidine antibacterial used in veterinary medicine with sulfadimethoxine or sulfadimidine.

---

## Bekanamycin Sulfate *(rINNM)*

Aminodeoxykanamycin Sulphate; Bekanamycin Sulphate; Bekanamycini Sulfas; Kanamycin B Sulphate; KDM; NK-1006; Sulfato de bekanamicina. 6-*O*-(3-Amino-3-deoxy-α-D-glucopyranosyl)-2-deoxy-4-*O*-(2,6-diamino-2,6-dideoxy-α-D-glucopyranosyl)-D-streptamine sulphate.

$C_{18}H_{37}N_5O_{10},2\frac{1}{2}H_2SO_4$ = 728.7.
*CAS — 4696-76-8 (bekanamycin); 70550-99-1 (bekanamycin sulfate).*

**Pharmacopoeias.** In *Jpn.*

### Profile

Bekanamycin is an aminoglycoside and is a congener of kanamycin. It has properties similar to those of gentamicin (p.217). It is given topically as the sulfate for the treatment of eye infections. It has also been given intramuscularly and by mouth. It is reported to be more toxic than kanamycin.

### Preparations

**Proprietary Preparations** (details are given in Part 3)
***Ital.:*** Kanendos†; ***Port.:*** Kanacyl.

**Multi-ingredient:** ***Ital.:*** Visucloben Antibiotico; Visumetazone Antibiotico; Visumicina†.

---

## Benethamine Penicillin *(BAN, rINN)*

Penicilina-benetamina. Benzyl(phenethyl)ammonium (6*R*)-6-(2-phenylacetamido)penicillanate.

$C_{15}H_{17}N,C_{16}H_{18}N_2O_4S$ = 545.7.
*CAS — 751-84-8.*

### Profile

Benethamine penicillin is a poorly soluble derivative of benzylpenicillin (p.163) with similar actions and uses, although it is not recommended for chronic, severe, or deep-seated infections. After deep intramuscular injection it forms a depot from which it is slowly absorbed and hydrolysed to benzylpenicillin. Benethamine penicillin is usually given with benzylpenicillin sodium and also sometimes procaine benzylpenicillin to produce both an immediate and a prolonged effect; overall, the effect lasts for 2 to 3 days.

### Preparations

**Proprietary Preparations** (details are given in Part 3)
**Multi-ingredient:** ***Fr.:*** Biclinocilline; ***Port.:*** Atralmicina.

---

## Benzathine Benzylpenicillin *(BAN, rINN)*

Benzathine Penicillin; Benzathini Benzylpenicillinum; Benzatina bencilpenicilina; Benzethacil; Benzilpenicillina Benzatinica; Benzylpenicillinum Benzathinum; Penicillin G Benzathine; Penzaethinum G. *NN'*-Dibenzylethylenediammonium bis[(6*R*)-6-(2-phenylacetamido)penicillanate].

$C_{16}H_{20}N_2(C_{16}H_{18}N_2O_4S)_2$ = 909.1.
*CAS — 1538-09-6 (anhydrous benzathine benzylpenicillin); 5928-83-6 (benzathine benzylpenicillin monohydrate); 41372-02-5 (benzathine benzylpenicillin tetrahydrate).*
*ATC — J01CE08.*

**Pharmacopoeias.** In *Chin., Eur.* (see p.vi), *Int.*, and *Pol.*
*Jpn* and *US* include the tetrahydrate.

**Ph. Eur. 5.0** (Benzylpenicillin, Benzathine). It contains a variable quantity of water. A white powder. Very slightly soluble in water; slightly soluble in alcohol; freely soluble in dimethylformamide and in formamide. Store in airtight containers.

**USP 27** (Penicillin G Benzathine). The tetrahydrate is a white, odourless, crystalline powder. Soluble 1 in 5000 of water and 1 in 65 of alcohol. pH in a solution prepared by dissolving 50 mg in 50 mL of dehydrated alcohol, and adding 50 mL of water is between 4.0 and 6.5. Store in airtight containers.

### Adverse Effects and Precautions

As for Benzylpenicillin, p.163.

Non-allergic (embolic-toxic) reactions similar to those associated with procaine benzylpenicillin, p.246, have been reported rarely with benzathine benzylpenicillin.

Benzathine benzylpenicillin should not be injected intravascularly since ischaemic reactions may occur.

### Interactions

As for Benzylpenicillin, p.164.

### Pharmacokinetics

When benzathine benzylpenicillin is given by intramuscular injection, it forms a depot from which it is slowly released and hydrolysed to benzylpenicillin. Peak plasma concentrations are produced in about 24 hours and are lower than those following an equivalent dose of benzylpenicillin potassium or sodium. However, depending on the dose, benzylpenicillin is usually detectable in plasma for up to 4 weeks (but see below). Distribution into the CSF is reported to be poor.

Due to the slow absorption from the site of injection, benzylpenicillin has been detected in the urine for up to 12 weeks after a single dose.

Benzathine benzylpenicillin is relatively stable in the presence of gastric juice, but absorption from the gastrointestinal tract is variable. Plasma concentrations of benzylpenicillin after an oral dose are lower than those from the same dose of a soluble penicillin; peak concentrations are also produced less rapidly, but may persist for longer.

**Plasma concentrations.** Benzathine benzylpenicillin has been given every 4 weeks for secondary prophylaxis against rheumatic fever, although some advocate administration every 3 weeks to ensure adequate plasma concentrations of benzylpenicillin. Typical concentrations achieved after a single intramuscular injection of benzathine benzylpenicillin 900 mg have been cited as about 100, 20, and 2 nanograms/mL on days 1, 14, and 32 respectively. In one study[1] adequate concentrations (defined as 20 nanograms or more per mL) were seen in more than 80% of serum samples at 3 weeks, but in only 36% at 4 weeks. In a further study,[2] in which single doses of 900 mg, 1.35 g and 1.8 g were compared, it appeared that doses higher than the 900-mg dose of benzathine benzylpenicillin usually recommended might prolong the duration of protective plasma concentrations of benzylpenicillin (defined as above 25 nanograms/mL) and improve the efficacy of dosing every 4 weeks for prophylaxis against rheumatic fever.

1. Kaplan EL, *et al.* Pharmacokinetics of benzathine penicillin G: serum levels during the 28 days after intramuscular injection of 1 200 000 units. *J Pediatr* 1989; **115:** 146–50.
2. Currie BJ, *et al.* Penicillin concentrations after increased doses of benzathine penicillin G for prevention of secondary rheumatic fever. *Antimicrob Agents Chemother* 1994; **38:** 1203–4.

**Pregnancy.** The pharmacokinetics of benzathine benzylpenicillin appear to be altered in late pregnancy. Of 10 healthy pregnant women given benzathine benzylpenicillin 1.8 g intramuscularly before caesarean section, only 4 achieved adequate serum concentrations of benzylpenicillin (for syphilis, at least 18 nanograms/mL) for 7 days.[1]

1. Nathan L, *et al.* Penicillin levels following the administration of benzathine penicillin G in pregnancy. *Obstet Gynecol* 1993; **82:** 338–42.

## Uses and Administration

Benzathine benzylpenicillin has the same antimicrobial action as benzylpenicillin (p.164), to which it is hydrolysed gradually following deep intramuscular injection. This results in a prolonged effect, but because of the relatively low blood concentrations of benzylpenicillin produced, its use should be restricted to micro-organisms that are highly susceptible to benzylpenicillin. In acute infections, and when bacteraemia is present, the initial treatment should be with benzylpenicillin by injection.

Infections treated with benzathine benzylpenicillin include diphtheria (asymptomatic carriers), pharyngitis (*Streptococcus pyogenes; Arcanobacterium haemolyticum* (*Corynebacterium haemolyticum*)), and syphilis (including non-venereal treponematoses). It is also used for primary and secondary prophylaxis of rheumatic fever. For details of these infections and their treatment, see under Choice of Antibacterial, p.120.

*Administration and dosage.* Benzathine benzylpenicillin is administered by deep intramuscular injection, sometimes with procaine benzylpenicillin and benzylpenicillin itself. It has been given by mouth for mild infections, although phenoxymethylpenicillin is usually preferred. Benzathine benzylpenicillin 900 mg is approximately equivalent to 720 mg of benzylpenicillin (1.2 million units).

For early syphilis, a single dose of benzathine benzylpenicillin 1.8 g by deep intramuscular injection is given, usually as 2 injections at separate sites. In late syphilis, 1.8 g is given at weekly intervals for 3 consecutive weeks. Benzathine benzylpenicillin is not usually recommended for the treatment of neurosyphilis because of reports of inadequate penetration into the CSF. Infants up to 2 years of age may be given a single intramuscular dose of 37.5 mg/kg for the treatment of congenital syphilis, provided there is no evidence of infection in the CSF.

For the treatment of other treponemal infections, such as yaws, pinta, and endemic syphilis (bejel), a single intramuscular dose of benzathine benzylpenicillin 900 mg is given; a dose of 450 mg may be used in children.

For streptococcal pharyngitis and the primary prevention of rheumatic fever, the adult dose is a single intramuscular injection of 900 mg; children under 30 kg may be given 225 to 675 mg. To prevent recurrences of acute rheumatic fever, 900 mg is given intramuscularly every 3 or 4 weeks to adults; a dose of 450 mg has been used for children under 30 kg.

## Preparations

***USP 27:*** Penicillin G Benzathine and Penicillin G Procaine Injectable Suspension; Penicillin G Benzathine Injectable Suspension; Penicillin G Benzathine Oral Suspension; Penicillin G Benzathine Tablets.

**Proprietary Preparations** (details are given in Part 3)
***Arg.:*** Benzetacil; Galtamicina; Pen di Ben; ***Austral.:*** Bicillin L-A; ***Austria:*** Retarpen; ***Belg.:*** Penadur; ***Braz.:*** Ampiretard†; Benzatron; Benzetacil; Bepeben; Longacilin; Neo Benzil; Normabenzil†; ***Canad.:*** Bicillin L-A†; Megacillin†; ***Fr.:*** Extencilline; ***Ger.:*** Pendysin; ***Gr.:*** Penadur; ***India:*** Pencom; Penidure; ***Israel:*** Durabiotic; ***Ital.:*** Diaminocillina; Wycillina; ***Malaysia:*** Retarpen; ***Mex.:*** Bencelin; Benzanil Simple; Benzetacil; Lentopenil; ***Neth.:*** Penidural; ***NZ:*** Bicillin L-A; ***Port.:*** Lentocilin-S; Penadur; ***S.Afr.:*** Bicillin L-A†; Penilente LA; ***Singapore:*** Penadur†; Retarpen; ***Spain:*** Benzetacil; Cepacilina; ***Thai.:*** Penadur; ***USA:*** Bicillin L-A; Permapen.

**Multi-ingredient:** ***Austria:*** Retarpen compositum; ***Braz.:*** Kitapen†; ***Canad.:*** Bicillin A-P†; ***Chile:*** Karbasilin; ***Ger.:*** Retacillin compositum; Tardocillin; ***Ital.:*** Tri-Wycillina; ***Mex.:*** Bencelin Combinado; Benzanil Compuesto; Benzetacil Combinado; Pendiben Compuesto; ***Neth.:*** Penidural D/F; ***Port.:*** Penadur 6.3.3; ***S.Afr.:*** Penilente Forte; Ultracillin; ***Spain:*** Benzetacil Compuesta; Cepacilina 633; Neocepacilina†; Penilevel Retard; ***USA:*** Bicillin C-R.

## Benzathine Phenoxymethylpenicillin

Benzatina fenoximetilpenicilina; Penicillin V Benzathine *(USAN)*; Phenoxymethylpenicillini Dibenzylaethylendiaminum. *N,N'*-Dibenzylethylenediammonium bis[(6*R*)-6-(2-phenoxyacetamido)penicillanate].

$(C_{16}H_{18}N_2O_5S)_2,C_{16}H_{20}N_2 = 941.1.$

*CAS — 5928-84-7 (anhydrous benzathine phenoxymethylpenicillin); 63690-57-3 (benzathine phenoxymethylpenicillin tetrahydrate).*

*ATC — J01CE10.*

**Pharmacopoeias.** In *US.*

**USP 27** (Penicillin V Benzathine). A practically white powder having a characteristic odour. Soluble 1 in 3200 of water, 1 in 330 of alcohol, 1 in 37 of acetone, 1 in 42 of chloroform, and 1 in 910 of ether. pH of a 3% suspension in water is between 4.0 and 6.5. Store in airtight containers.

### Profile

Benzathine phenoxymethylpenicillin has actions and uses similar to those of phenoxymethylpenicillin (p.242) and is given orally in the treatment of susceptible mild to moderate infections. Doses are expressed in terms of phenoxymethylpenicillin.

### Preparations

***USP 27:*** Penicillin V Benzathine Oral Suspension.

**Proprietary Preparations** (details are given in Part 3)
***Austral.:*** Abbocillin-V; Cilicaine V; ***Austria:*** Ospen; Pen-Os; Star-Pen; ***Belg.:*** Oracilline†; ***Canad.:*** Pen-Vee; PVF†; ***Fr.:*** Oracilline; ***Ger.:*** Infectobicillin; ***Gr.:*** Ospen; ***Spain:*** Benoral; ***Switz.:*** Ospen; Phenocillin.

# Benzylpenicillin *(BAN, rINN)*

Bencilpenicilina; Crystalline Penicillin G; Penicillin; Penicillin G. (2*S*,5*R*,6*R*)-3,3-Dimethyl-7-oxo-6-(2-phenylacetamido)-4-thia-1-azabicyclo[3.2.0]heptane-2-carboxylic acid; (6*R*)-6-(2-Phenylacetamido)penicillanic acid.

$C_{16}H_{18}N_2O_4S = 334.4.$

*CAS — 61-33-6.*

*ATC — J01CE01; S01AA14.*

**Description.** The name benzylpenicillin is commonly used to describe either benzylpenicillin potassium or benzylpenicillin sodium as these are the forms in which benzylpenicillin is used. In *Martindale*, benzylpenicillin means either the potassium or sodium salt.

## Benzylpenicillin Potassium *(BANM, rINNM)*

Bencilpenicilina potásica; Benzylpenicillinum Kalicum; Penicillin G Potassium.

$C_{16}H_{17}KN_2O_4S = 372.5.$

*CAS — 113-98-4.*

*ATC — J01CE01; S01AA14.*

**Pharmacopoeias.** In *Chin., Eur.* (see p.vi), *Int., Jpn, Pol., US,* and *Viet.*

**Ph. Eur. 5.0** (Benzylpenicillin Potassium). The potassium salt of a substance produced by growing certain strains of *Penicillium notatum* or related organisms or obtained by any other means. A white or almost white crystalline powder. Very soluble in water; practically insoluble in fatty oils and in liquid paraffin. A 10% solution in water has a pH of 5.5 to 7.5. Store in airtight containers.

**USP 27** (Penicillin G Potassium). Colourless or white crystals, or white crystalline powder. It is odourless or practically so, and is moderately hygroscopic. Very soluble in water, in sodium chloride 0.9%, and in glucose solutions; sparingly soluble in alcohol. Its solutions retain substantially full potency for several days at temperatures below 15°, but are rapidly inactivated by acids, by alkali hydroxides, by glycerol, and by oxidising agents. pH of a 6% solution in water is between 5.0 and 7.5. Store in airtight containers.

**Incompatibility and stability.** As for Benzylpenicillin Sodium, below.

## Benzylpenicillin Sodium *(BANM, rINNM)*

Bencilpenicilina sódica; Benzylpenicillinum Natricum; Penicillin G Sodium.

$C_{16}H_{17}N_2NaO_4S = 356.4.$

*CAS — 69-57-8.*

*ATC — J01CE01; S01AA14.*

**Pharmacopoeias.** In *Chin., Eur.* (see p.vi), *Int., Pol., US,* and *Viet.*

**Ph. Eur. 5.0** (Benzylpenicillin Sodium). The sodium salt of a substance produced by growing certain strains of *Penicillium notatum* or related organisms or obtained by any other means. A white or almost white crystalline powder. Very soluble in water; practically insoluble in fatty oils and in liquid paraffin. A 10% solution in water has a pH of 5.5 to 7.5. Store in airtight containers.

**USP 27** (Penicillin G Sodium). Colourless or white crystals, or white to slightly yellow crystalline powder. It is odourless or practically so, and is moderately hygroscopic. Its solutions lose potency fairly rapidly at room temperature, but retain substantially full potency for several days at temperatures below 15°. Its solutions are rapidly inactivated by acids, by alkali hydroxides, by oxidising agents, and by penicillinase. pH of a 6% solution in water is between 5.0 and 7.5. Store in airtight containers.

**Incompatibility.** Benzylpenicillin has been reported to be incompatible with metal ions and some rubber products. Its stability may be affected by ionic and nonionic surfactants, oxidising and reducing agents, alcohols, glycerol, glycols, macrogols and other hydroxy compounds, some paraffins and bases, some preservatives such as chlorocresol or thiomersal, carbohydrate solutions in an alkaline pH, fat emulsions, blood and blood products, and viscosity modifiers. Benzylpenicillin is incompatible with a wide range of acidic and basic drugs (see Stability, below) and with a number of other antimicrobials, including amphotericin B, some cephalosporins, and vancomycin. Benzylpenicillin and aminoglycosides are mutually incompatible and injections should be given at separate sites.

**Stability.** Benzylpenicillin is hydrolysed in aqueous solutions by degradation of the beta-lactam ring and hydrolysis is accelerated by increased temperature or alkaline conditions; inactivation also occurs under acid conditions. Degradation products include penillic, penicillenic, and penicilloic acids which lower the pH and cause a progressive increase in the rate of deterioration; *N*-formylpenicillamine and very small amounts of penicillamine have also been detected. Degradation is minimal at about pH 6.8 and deterioration of benzylpenicillin in solution may be retarded by using a citrate buffer. Dilute solutions are more stable than concentrated ones.

References.

1. Lynn B. The stability and administration of intravenous penicillins. *Br J Intraven Ther* 1981; **2** (Mar): 22–39.
2. Bird AE, *et al.* N-Formylpenicillamine and penicillamine as degradation products of penicillins in solution. *J Pharm Pharmacol* 1986; **38:** 913–17.

## Units

The second International Standard Preparation (1952) of benzylpenicillin sodium contained 1670 units of penicillin per mg but was discontinued in 1968 since penicillin can now be characterised completely by chemical tests. Despite this, doses of benzylpenicillin are still expressed in units in some countries.

Benzylpenicillin potassium 600 mg or benzylpenicillin sodium 600 mg have generally been considered to be approximately equivalent to 1 million units (1 mega unit).

## Adverse Effects

The most common adverse effects of benzylpenicillin are hypersensitivity reactions, especially skin rashes; anaphylaxis occasionally occurs and has sometimes been fatal.

Gastrointestinal effects such as diarrhoea and nausea are the most common adverse effects following oral use of benzylpenicillin; a sore mouth or tongue or a black hairy tongue have occasionally been reported. Pseudomembranous colitis has been associated with the use of most antibiotics and, of the penicillins, ampicillin or amoxicillin have been implicated most frequently (see Antibiotic-associated Colitis, p.128).

Other adverse effects have generally been associated with large intravenous doses of benzylpenicillin; patients with renal impairment are also at increased risk. These adverse effects include haemolytic anaemia and neutropenia, both of which might have some immunological basis; prolongation of bleeding time and defective platelet function; convulsions and other signs of CNS toxicity (encephalopathy has followed intrathecal administration and can be fatal); and electrolyte disturbances because of the large amounts of potassium or sodium given when benzylpenicillin potassium or sodium, respectively, are used.

Hepatitis and cholestatic jaundice have been reported rarely with some penicillins, notably penicillinase-resistant penicillins such as flucloxacillin and oxacillin, and also combinations of amoxicillin or ticarcillin with clavulanic acid.

Nephropathy and interstitial nephritis, which may have some immunological basis, have been especially associated with meticillin, but may be produced by other penicillins.

Some patients with syphilis and other spirochaete infections may experience a Jarisch-Herxheimer reaction shortly after starting treatment with penicillin, which is probably due to the release of endotoxins from the killed treponemes and should not be mistaken for a hypersensitivity reaction. Symptoms include fever, chills, headache, and reactions at the site of the lesions. The reaction can be dangerous in cardiovascular syphilis, or where there is a serious risk of increased local damage, such as with optic atrophy.

**Hypersensitivity**. The overall incidence of allergic reactions to penicillin has been reported to vary from about 1 to 10% although some patients may have been incorrectly labelled 'allergic to penicillin'. Anaphylactic reactions occur in about 0.05% of patients, usually after parenteral use, but they have also been reported after taking penicillin by mouth.

Hypersensitivity to penicillin gives rise to a wide variety of clinical syndromes. Immediate reactions include anaphylaxis, angioedema, urticaria, and some maculopapular rashes. Late reactions may include serum sickness-like reactions and haemolytic anaemia. Reactions are considered to be due mainly to breakdown products produced *in vitro* before administration or to metabolites of penicillin, and possibly penicillin itself. These act as haptens which, when combined with proteins and other macromolecules, produce potential antigens. As the hypersensitivity is related to the basic penicillin structure, patients who are genuinely allergic to benzylpenicillin must be assumed to be allergic to all penicillins; sensitised patients may also react to the cephalosporins and other beta-lactam antibiotics.

*Tests for hypersensitivity* may be used to determine those patients most likely to develop serious allergic reactions to penicillins. Skin tests are used to evaluate the current risk of immediate or accelerated IgE-mediated reactions, the most serious being anaphylaxis. Both the major and minor determinants of penicillin hypersensitivity should be used; the major determinant is available as penicilloyl-polylysine (p.1729) and a minor-determinant mixture consisting of benzylpenicillin and its derivatives, including penicilloic acid and benzylpenicilloylamine, can be used, although if this is not available a solution of benzylpenicillin may be substituted. Adrenaline should be available in case an anaphylactic reaction develops. The results of skin tests are unreliable if a significant time has elapsed before beginning therapy. A number of *in-vitro* tests including the radioallergosorbent test (RAST) have been developed.

*Desensitisation* may be attempted in patients allergic to penicillin when treatment with penicillin is considered essential. It involves very small doses of penicillin given at relatively short intervals of 15 minutes or more, and gradually increased to therapeutic concentrations. However, desensitisation may be hazardous and should only be carried out if the patient can be monitored continuously and adrenaline and resuscitation equipment are immediately available. Desensitisation should be regarded as temporary, and allergic reactions may recur during the next exposure to penicillin.

**Neutropenia**. Neutropenia has been widely reported in patients receiving high doses of beta lactams and an incidence of from 5 to more than 15% has been reported in patients treated for 10 days or more. Warning signs include fever, rash, and eosinophilia. Monitoring of the leucocyte count is recommended during long-term treatment with high doses. Some have proposed a direct toxic effect whereas others have postulated an immune mechanism.

**Effects on the blood.** References to neutropenia associated with penicillins.


1. Anonymous. Antibiotic-induced neutropenia. *Lancet* 1985; **ii:** 814.
2. Neftel KA, *et al.* Inhibition of granulopoiesis in vivo and in vitro by β-lactam antibiotics. *J Infect Dis* 1985; **152:** 90–8.
3. Olaison L, Alestig K. A prospective study of neutropenia induced by high doses of β-lactam antibiotics. *J Antimicrob Chemother* 1990; **25:** 449–53.


**Effects on the nervous system.** References to CNS effects associated with penicillins.


1. Schliamser SE, *et al.* Neurotoxicity of β-lactam antibiotics: predisposing factors and pathogenesis. *J Antimicrob Chemother* 1991; **27:** 405–25.


**Hypersensitivity.** References to hypersensitivity reactions associated with penicillins.


1. Sullivan TJ, *et al.* Skin testing to detect penicillin allergy. *J Allergy Clin Immunol* 1981; **68:** 171–80.
2. Beeley L. Allergy to penicillin. *BMJ* 1984; **288:** 511–12.
3. Holgate ST. Penicillin allergy: how to diagnose and when to treat. *BMJ* 1988; **296:** 1213–14.
4. Anonymous. Penicillin allergy in childhood. *Lancet* 1989; **i:** 420.
5. Surtees SJ, *et al.* Allergy to penicillin: fable or fact? *BMJ* 1991; **302:** 1051–2. Correspondence. *ibid.*: 1462–3.
6. Anonymous. Penicillin allergy. *Drug Ther Bull* 1996; **34:** 87–8.
7. Salkind AR, *et al.* Is this patient allergic to penicillin? An evidence-based analysis of the likelihood of penicillin allergy. *JAMA* 2001; **285:** 2498–2505.


## Precautions

Patients known to be hypersensitive to penicillins should be given an antibacterial of another class. However, sensitised patients may also react to the cephalosporins and other beta lactams. Desensitisation may be attempted if treatment with a penicillin is considered essential (see Adverse Effects, above). Penicillins should be given with caution to patients with a history of allergy, especially to drugs.

Care is necessary if very high doses of penicillins are given, especially if renal function is poor, because of the risk of neurotoxicity. The intrathecal route should be avoided. Renal, hepatic, and haematological status should be monitored during prolonged and high-dose therapy. Because of the Jarisch-Herxheimer reaction, care is also necessary when treating patients with spirochaete infections, particularly syphilis.

Skin contact with penicillins should be avoided since sensitisation may occur.

Penicillin therapy changes the normal bacterial flora and can lead to supra-infection with penicillin-resistant organisms including *Clostridium difficile* or *Candida*, particularly with prolonged use.

Penicillins may interfere with some diagnostic tests such as those for urinary glucose using copper sulfate, direct antiglobulin (Coombs') tests, and some tests for urinary or serum proteins. Penicillins may interfere with tests that use bacteria, for example the Guthrie test for phenylketonuria using *Bacillus subtilis* organisms.

**Potassium and sodium content.** Each g of benzylpenicillin potassium contains about 2.7 mmol of potassium and each g of benzylpenicillin sodium contains about 2.8 mmol of sodium. Care is necessary if large doses of the potassium or sodium salts are given to patients with renal impairment or heart failure. High doses of benzylpenicillin potassium should also be used with caution in patients receiving potassium-containing drugs or potassium-sparing diuretics.

## Interactions

Probenecid prolongs the half-life of benzylpenicillin by competing with it for renal tubular secretion and may be used therapeutically for this purpose. Benzylpenicillin may also interact with bacteriostatic antibacterials such as chloramphenicol and tetracyclines (see Antimicrobial Action, below), and may be incompatible *in vitro* with other drugs, including a number of other antibacterials (see above).

The possibility of a prolonged bleeding time following oral treatment with a broad-spectrum drug like ampicillin should be borne in mind in patients receiving anticoagulants.

**Hormonal contraceptives.** For the effect of penicillins on oral contraceptives, see p.1534.

**Methotrexate.** For the effect of penicillins on methotrexate, see p.570.

## Antimicrobial Action

Benzylpenicillin is a beta-lactam antibiotic and has a bactericidal action against Gram-positive bacteria, Gram-negative cocci, some other Gram-negative bacteria, spirochaetes, and actinomycetes.

*Mechanism of action.* It exerts its killing action on growing and dividing bacteria by inhibiting bacterial cell-wall synthesis, although the mechanisms involved are still not precisely understood. Bacterial cell walls are held rigid and protected against osmotic rupture by peptidoglycan. Benzylpenicillin inhibits the final cross-linking stage of peptidoglycan production by binding to and inactivating transpeptidases, penicillin-binding proteins on the inner surface of the bacterial cell membrane. However, it is now realised that other earlier stages in cell-wall synthesis can also be inhibited. Other mechanisms involved include bacterial lysis by the inactivation of endogenous inhibitors of bacterial autolysins.

Its action is inhibited by penicillinase and other beta-lactamases that are produced during the growth of certain micro-organisms.

Many Gram-negative organisms are intrinsically resistant by virtue of the inability of benzylpenicillin to penetrate their outer membranes. Intrinsic resistance can also be due to structural differences in the target penicillin-binding proteins. See under Resistance, below, for reference to acquired resistance.

*Spectrum of activity.* The following pathogenic organisms are usually sensitive to benzylpenicillin:

- Gram-positive aerobes and anaerobes including *Bacillus anthracis*, *Clostridium perfringens*, *Cl. tetani*, *Corynebacterium diphtheriae*, *Erysipelothrix rhusiopathiae*, *Listeria monocytogenes*, *Peptostreptococcus* spp., non-beta-lactamase-producing staphylococci, and streptococci including *Streptococcus agalactiae* (group B), *Str. pneumoniae* (pneumococci), *Str. pyogenes* (group A), and some viridans streptococci; enterococci are relatively insensitive.
- Gram-negative cocci including *Neisseria meningitidis* (meningococci) and *Neisseria gonorrhoeae* (gonococci), although beta-lactamase-producing strains are common.
- Gram-negative bacilli including *Pasteurella multocida*, *Streptobacillus moniliformis*, and *Spirillum minus* (or *minor*); most Gram-negative bacilli, including *Pseudomonas* spp. and Enterobacteriaceae, are insensitive although some strains of *Proteus mirabilis* and *Escherichia coli* may be inhibited by high concentrations of benzylpenicillin.
- Gram-negative anaerobes including *Prevotella* (non-fragilis *Bacteroides*) and *Fusobacterium* spp.
- Other organisms including *Actinomyces* and the spirochaetes, *Borrelia*, *Leptospira*, and *Treponema* spp.
- Mycobacteria, fungi, mycoplasmas, and rickettsias are not sensitive.

*Activity with other antimicrobials.* Benzylpenicillin may exhibit synergy with other antimicrobials, particularly the aminoglycosides, and such combinations have been used against enterococci and other relatively insensitive bacteria. Its activity may be enhanced by clavulanic acid and other beta-lactamase inhibitors, and both enhancement and antagonism have been demonstrated for beta-lactam combinations. Antagonism has been reported to occur with some bacteriostatic drugs, such as chloramphenicol or tetracyclines, that interfere with active bacterial growth necessary for benzylpenicillin to achieve its effect.

*Resistance.* Susceptible Gram-positive bacteria acquire resistance to beta lactams mainly through the induction of beta-lactamases, including penicillinases. These enzymes are liberated extracellularly and hydrolyse the beta-lactam ring. This resistance is usually plasmid-mediated and can be transferred from one bacterium to another. Gram-negative bacteria produce beta-lactamases within their cell membranes which may be chromosomally or plasmid-mediated; all Gram-negative species probably contain small amounts of beta-lactamases. Resistance in Gram-negative species may also be due to changes in their outer membrane resulting in the failure of beta lactams to reach their target penicillin-binding proteins. Changes in the binding characteristics of penicillin-binding proteins may also result in resistance in Gram-positive and Gram-negative bacteria.

Most strains of *Staphylococcus aureus* are now resistant to benzylpenicillin. *Streptococcus pneumoniae* with reduced susceptibility or complete resistance to benzylpenicillin have increasingly been reported. Strains of *Neisseria meningitidis* with reduced sensitivity to benzylpenicillin have been identified. Penicillinase-producing *Neisseria gonorrhoeae* are widespread; reduced sensitivity of gonococci to benzylpenicillin may also result from alterations in penicillin-binding proteins. Most strains of *Haemophilus influenzae* and *Moraxella catarrhalis* (*Branhamella catarrhalis*) are now resistant.

Some organisms, usually Gram-positive cocci such as staphylococci or streptococci, may develop tolerance and are inhibited but not killed by benzylpenicillin; in such cases the minimum bactericidal concentration is much greater than the minimum inhibitory concentration.

## Pharmacokinetics

Benzylpenicillin rapidly appears in the blood following intramuscular injection of water-soluble salts, and maximum concentrations are usually reached in 15 to 30 minutes; peak plasma concentrations of about 12 micrograms/mL have been reported after single doses of 600 mg.

When given by mouth, benzylpenicillin is inactivated fairly rapidly by gastric acid and only up to about 30% is absorbed, mainly from the duodenum; maximum plasma-penicillin concentrations usually occur in about 1 hour. In order to attain plasma-penicillin concentrations after oral use similar to those following intramuscular injection, up to 5 times as much benzylpenicillin may be necessary. Absorption varies greatly in different individuals and is better in patients with reduced gastric acid production, including neonates and the elderly. Food decreases the absorption of benzylpenicillin and oral doses are best given at least half an hour before or 2 to 3 hours after a meal.

Benzylpenicillin is widely distributed at varying concentrations in body tissues and fluids. It appears in pleural, pericardial, peritoneal, and synovial fluids, but in the absence of inflammation diffuses only to a small extent into abscess cavities, avascular areas, the eye, the middle ear, and the CSF. Inflamed tissue is, however, more readily penetrated and, for example, in meningitis higher concentrations of benzylpenicillin are achieved in the CSF. Active transport out of the CSF is reduced by probenecid. In patients with uraemia, other organic acids may accumulate in the CSF and compete with benzylpenicillin for active transport; toxic concentrations of benzylpenicillin sufficient to cause convulsions can result.

Benzylpenicillin diffuses across the placenta into the fetal circulation, and small amounts appear in breast milk.

The plasma half-life is about 30 minutes, although it may be longer in neonates and the elderly because of incomplete renal function. In renal impairment the half-life may be increased to about 10 hours. Approximately 60% is reported to be bound to plasma protein.

Benzylpenicillin is metabolised to a limited extent and the penicilloic acid derivative has been recovered in the urine. Benzylpenicillin is rapidly excreted in the urine, principally by tubular secretion and about 20% of a dose given by mouth appears unchanged in the urine; about 60 to 90% of a dose of aqueous benzylpenicillin given intramuscularly appears in the urine, mainly within the first hour. Significant concentrations are achieved in bile, but in patients with normal renal function only small amounts are excreted via the bile. Benzylpenicillin is removed by haemodialysis.

Renal tubular secretion is inhibited by probenecid (p.417), which is sometimes given to increase plasma-penicillin concentrations.

## Uses and Administration

Benzylpenicillin is used in the treatment of a variety of infections due to susceptible organisms (see Antimicrobial Action, above). They include abscess, actinomycosis, anthrax, bites and stings, diphtheria, endocarditis, gas gangrene, leptospirosis, Lyme disease, meningitis, meningococcal infections, necrotising enterocolitis, necrotising fasciitis, neonatal conjunctivitis (if gonococci are sensitive), perinatal streptococcal infections (intrapartum prophylaxis against group B streptococci), pharyngitis (or tonsillitis), pneumonia, skin infections, syphilis (neurosyphilis and congenital syphilis), tetanus, toxic shock syndrome, and Whipple's disease. It is also used for surgical infection prophylaxis in first trimester abortion in women at high risk of pelvic infection. For details of these infections and their treatment, see under Choice of Antibacterial, p.120.

*Administration and dosage.* Benzylpenicillin is usually given intramuscularly or intravenously. For some indications benzathine benzylpenicillin (p.162) or procaine benzylpenicillin (p.246), which provide a prolonged effect, are preferred; they are given intramuscularly. Benzylpenicillin is sometimes given by mouth for infections of moderate severity, but one of the acid-resistant penicillins such as phenoxymethylpenicillin (p.242) is preferable.

Benzylpenicillin is available as the potassium or sodium salt. The dose of benzylpenicillin should be sufficient to achieve an optimum bactericidal concentration in the blood as rapidly as possible; concentrations may be increased by concurrent administration of probenecid (p.417). In some countries, doses are still expressed in units. Benzylpenicillin potassium 600 mg or benzylpenicillin sodium 600 mg have generally been considered to be approximately equivalent to 1 million units (1 mega unit).

For some infections, adult doses of 0.6 to 4.8 g of benzylpenicillin daily in 2 to 4 divided doses by intramuscular or slow intravenous injection or intravenous infusion may be adequate, but higher doses given intravenously, often by infusion, are more usual for severe infections. For example, in endocarditis, benzylpenicillin 7.2 g daily (1.2 g every 4 hours) intravenously, usually with an aminoglycoside, is recommended; doses of up to 18 g daily are not unusual for less sensitive streptococci and enterococci. In meningococcal and pneumococcal meningitis, benzylpenicillin 14.4 g daily (2.4 g every 4 hours) intravenously is recommended; up to 18 g daily has been recommended for meningococcal meningitis. High doses should be given slowly to avoid irritation of the CNS and electrolyte imbalance, and a rate of not more than 300 mg/minute is recommended for intravenous doses above 1.2 g. High doses may need to be reduced in patients with renal impairment.

Infants and children from 1 month to 12 years may be given 100 mg/kg daily in 4 divided doses; infants aged 1 to 4 weeks, 75 mg/kg daily in 3 divided doses; and neonates 50 mg/kg daily in 2 divided doses.

As in adults, higher paediatric doses may be necessary in severe infections. A dose of 180 to 300 mg/kg daily given intravenously in 4 to 6 divided doses is recommended for meningococcal meningitis in infants and children from 1 month to 12 years of age; infants aged 1 to 4 weeks may be given 150 mg/kg daily in 3 divided doses; neonates up to 7 days old may be given 100 mg/kg daily in 2 divided doses.

In patients with suspected meningococcal infection, an intravenous or intramuscular injection of benzylpenicillin should be given before transfer to hospital. Doses are: adults and children aged 10 years or more, 1.2 g; children aged 1 to 9 years, 600 mg; children under 1 year, 300 mg.

A dose for intrapartum prophylaxis against group B streptococcal infection is benzylpenicillin 3 g intravenously initially, then 1.5 g every 4 hours until delivery.

*Other routes.* Benzylpenicillin eye drops and eye ointment are used in the treatment of susceptible eye infections. For subconjunctival injection, 300 or 600 mg of benzylpenicillin has been dissolved in 0.5 to 1.0 mL of water, or another suitable solvent such as lidocaine 2% with or without adrenaline 1 in 100 000.

Benzylpenicillin has also been given by mouth on an empty stomach in adult doses of 125 to 312 mg every 4 to 6 hours.

Intrathecal injections are no longer recommended.

### Preparations

***BP 2003:*** Benzylpenicillin Injection;
***USP 27:*** Penicillin G Potassium Capsules; Penicillin G Potassium for Injection; Penicillin G Potassium for Oral Solution; Penicillin G Potassium Injection; Penicillin G Potassium Tablets; Penicillin G Sodium for Injection.

**Proprietary Preparations** (details are given in Part 3)
***Arg.:*** Penilfedrin P; ***Austral.:*** Benpen; ***Braz.:*** Benzecilin; Cristalpen; Isacilin†; Megapen; Penkaron; ***Canad.:*** Crystapen; Megacillin†; Novo-Pen-G†; ***Fin.:*** Geepenil; ***India:*** Pentids; ***Irl.:*** Crystapen; ***Mex.:*** Benacilina; Pengesod; Penisol; Sodipen; Xozacil; ***NZ:*** Benpen; ***S.Afr.:*** Benzatec; Novopen; ***Spain:*** Coliriocilina; Pekamin†; Penibiot; Penibiot Lidocaina†; Penilevel; Peniroger; Sodiopen; Unicilina; ***UK:*** Crystapen; ***USA:*** Pfizerpen.

**Multi-ingredient: *Austria:*** Fortepen; Ophcillin N; Retarpen compositum; ***Braz.:*** Benapen; Benzapen G; Cibramicina†; Climacilin†; Despacilina; Drenovac; Expectovac; Ginurovac; Linfocilin; Odontovac; Ortocilin†; Pulmocilin†; Wycillin R; ***Canad.:*** Bicillin A-P†; ***Chile:*** Prevepen Forte; ***Fr.:*** Biclinocilline; Gomenol-Syner-Penicilline†; ***Ger.:*** Bipensaar; Hydracillin†; Jenacillin A; Retacillin compositum; ***India:*** Bistrepen; ***Israel:*** Duplo-Penicillin; Penicillin Fortified; ***Ital.:*** Tri-Wycillina; ***Mex.:*** Anapenil; Bencelin Combinado; Benzanil Compuesto; Benzetacil Combinado; Hidrocilina; Megapenil Forte; Pendiben Compuesto; Penicil; Penipot; Penisodina; Penprocilina; Procilin; Suipen; ***Neth.:*** Penidural D/F; ***Port.:*** Atralcilina†; Atralmicina; Penadur 6.3.3; Prevecilina; ***S.Afr.:*** Penilente Forte; Ultracillin; ***Spain:*** Anapen†; Aqucilina D A; Benzetacil Compuesta; Cepacilina 633; Neocepacilina†; Neopenyl; Penilevel Retard; ***UK:*** Bicillin†.

---

## Betamipron *(rINN)*

*N*-Benzoyl-β-alanine; CS-443. 3-Benzamidopropionic acid.

$C_{10}H_{11}NO_3$ = 193.2.
*CAS — 3440-28-6.*

### Profile

Betamipron is a renal protectant used with the carbapenem antibacterial panipenem to reduce its adverse renal effects.

### Preparations

**Proprietary Preparations** (details are given in Part 3)
**Multi-ingredient: *Jpn:*** Carbenin.

---

## Biapenem *(USAN, rINN)*

CL-186815; L-627; LJC-10627. 6-{[(4*R*,5*S*,6*S*)-2-Carboxy-6-[(1*R*)-1-hydroxyethyl]-4-methyl-7-oxo-1-azabicyclo[3.2.0]hept-2-en-3-yl]thio}-6,7-dihydro-5*H*-pyrazolo[1,2-*a*]-s-triazol-4-ium hydroxide, inner salt.

$C_{15}H_{18}N_4O_4S$ = 350.4.
*CAS — 120410-24-4.*

### Profile

Biapenem is a carbapenem beta-lactam antibacterial similar to imipenem (p.221), although it is reported to be more stable to renal dehydropeptidase I than imipenem.

◊ Reviews.

1. Perry CM, Ibbotson T. Biapenem. *Drugs* 2002; **62:** 2221–34.

---

## Brodimoprim *(rINN)*

Brodimoprima. 2,4-Diamino-5-(4-bromo-3,5-dimethoxybenzyl)pyrimidine.

$C_{13}H_{15}BrN_4O_2$ = 339.2.
*CAS — 56518-41-3.*
*ATC — J01EA02.*

### Profile

Brodimoprim is closely related structurally to trimethoprim (p.272) and has been used in the treatment of infections of the respiratory tract and ear.

◊ References.

1. Braunsteiner AR, Finsinger F. Brodimoprim: therapeutic efficacy and safety in the treatment of bacterial infections. *J Chemother* 1993; **5:** 507–11.

### Preparations

**Proprietary Preparations** (details are given in Part 3)
***Ital.:*** Unitrim†; ***Mex.:*** Novatrim.

---

## Broxyquinoline *(rINN)*

Broxichinolinum. 5,7-Dibromoquinolin-8-ol.

$C_9H_5Br_2NO$ = 303.0.
*CAS — 521-74-4.*
*ATC — A07AX01; G01AC06; P01AA01.*

### Profile

Broxyquinoline is a halogenated hydroxyquinoline used topically in vaginal infections. It was formerly given by mouth, in conjunction with broxaldine, in the treatment of intestinal protozoal infections, including amoebiasis, but less toxic drugs are preferred.

### Preparations

**Proprietary Preparations** (details are given in Part 3)
***Fin.:*** Starogyn.

**Multi-ingredient: *Braz.:*** Enterovit†; ***Fin.:*** Senikolp.

---

## Capreomycin Sulfate *(USAN, rINNM)*

34977; Capreomycin Sulphate *(BANM)*; Capromycin Sulphate; Sulfato de capreomicina.

*CAS — 11003-38-6 (capreomycin); 1405-37-4 (capreomycin sulfate).*

*ATC — J04AB30.*

**Description.** Capreomycin I consists of capreomycin IA ($C_{25}H_{44}N_{14}O_8$ = 668.7) and capreomycin IB ($C_{25}H_{44}N_{14}O_7$ = 652.7), which predominates. Capreomycin II, which makes up about 10% of the mixture, consists of capreomycin IIA and capreomycin IIB.

**Pharmacopoeias.** In *Chin.* and *US.*

**USP 27** (Capreomycin Sulfate). The disulfate of capreomycin, a polypeptide mixture produced by the growth of *Streptomyces capreolus*. It contains not less than 90% of capreomycin I. A white to practically white amorphous powder. Freely soluble in water; practically insoluble in most organic solvents. pH of a 3% solution in water is between 4.5 and 7.5. Store in airtight containers.

### Adverse Effects and Treatment

The effects of capreomycin on the kidney and eighth cranial nerve are similar to those of aminoglycosides such as gentamicin (p.217). Nitrogen retention, renal tubular dysfunction, and progressive renal damage may occur. Hypokalaemia and other electrolyte abnormalities have been reported. Vertigo, tinnitus, and hearing loss may also occur and are sometimes irreversible. Abnormalities in liver function have been reported when capreomycin has been used with other antituberculous drugs. Hypersensitivity reactions including urticaria, maculopapular rashes, and sometimes fever have been reported. Leucocytosis and leucopenia have also been observed. Thrombocytopenia has been reported rarely. Eosinophilia commonly occurs with capreomycin. Capreomycin also has a neuromuscular blocking action. There may be pain, induration, and excessive bleeding at the site of intramuscular injection; sterile abscesses may also form.

Teratogenicity has been observed following high doses in *rodents*.

Treatment of overdose is generally supportive. Patients with normal renal function should be hydrated to maintain adequate urine output. Capreomycin is removed by haemodialysis.

### Precautions

Capreomycin should be given with care and in reduced dosage to patients with renal impairment. Care is also essential in patients with signs of eighth cranial nerve damage. It is advisable to monitor renal and auditory function and serum-potassium concentrations in patients before and during therapy. Periodic assessment of hepatic function is also recommended.

### Interactions

Care should be taken when capreomycin is used with other drugs that have neuromuscular blocking activity. It should not be given with other drugs that are ototoxic or nephrotoxic.

### Antimicrobial Action

Capreomycin has activity against various mycobacteria. Resistance develops readily if capreomycin is used alone. It shows cross-resistance with kanamycin and neomycin.

◊ References.

1. Ho YII, *et al.* In-vitro activities of aminoglycoside-aminocyclitols against mycobacteria. *J Antimicrob Chemother* 1997; **40:** 27–32.

### Pharmacokinetics

Capreomycin is poorly absorbed from the gastrointestinal tract. An intramuscular dose of 1 g has been reported to give a peak serum concentration of about 30 micrograms/mL after 1 or 2 hours. About 50% of a dose is excreted unchanged in the urine by glomerular filtration within 12 hours. Capreomycin is removed by haemodialysis.

### Uses and Administration

Capreomycin is a second-line antimycobacterial that may be used in the treatment of tuberculosis (p.150) as part of a multidrug regimen when resistance to, or toxicity from, primary drugs has developed.

Capreomycin is given as the sulfate by deep intramuscular injection or by intravenous infusion. The usual adult dose is the equivalent of 1 g of capreomycin base (maximum 20 mg/kg) given daily for 2 to 4 months, then 2 or 3 times weekly for the remainder of therapy.

**Administration in renal impairment.** As with aminoglycosides, the dose of capreomycin in patients with renal impairment must be adjusted based on creatinine clearance; the desired steady-state serum capreomycin level is 10 micrograms/mL.

### Preparations

***USP 27:*** Capreomycin for Injection.

**Proprietary Preparations** (details are given in Part 3)
***Austral.:*** Capastat; ***Austria:*** Capastat; ***Canad.:*** Capastat†; ***Gr.:*** Capastat; ***Spain:*** Capastat; ***UK:*** Capastat; ***USA:*** Capastat.

---

## Carbadox *(BAN, USAN, pINN)*

GS-6244. Methyl 3-quinoxalin-2-ylmethylenecarbazate 1,4-dioxide.

$C_{11}H_{10}N_4O_4$ = 262.2.

*CAS — 6804-07-5.*

### Profile

Carbadox is an antibacterial that has been used in veterinary practice for treating swine dysentery and enteritis and for promoting growth. However, its use has been prohibited in the European Union and some other countries following reports of carcinogenicity.

---

## Carbenicillin Sodium *(BANM, rINNM)*

BRL-2064; Carbenicilina sódica; Carbenicillin Disodium *(USAN)*; Carbenicillinum Natricum; α-Carboxybenzylpenicillin Sodium; CP-15-639-2; GS-3159 (carbenicillin potassium); NSC-111071. The disodium salt of (6R)-6-(2-carboxy-2-phenylacetamido)penicillanic acid .

$C_{17}H_{16}N_2Na_2O_6S$ = 422.4.

*CAS — 4697-36-3 (carbenicillin); 4800-94-6 (carbenicillin disodium); 17230-86-3 (carbenicillin potassium).*

*ATC — J01CA03.*

**Pharmacopoeias.** In *Br., Pol.,* and *US.*

**BP 2003** (Carbenicillin Sodium). A white or slightly yellowish, hygroscopic powder. Freely soluble in water; soluble in alcohol and in methyl alcohol. A 5% solution in water has a pH of 5.5 to 7.5. Store at a temperature between 2° and 8° in airtight containers. Protect from light.

**USP 27** (Carbenicillin Disodium). A white to off-white crystalline powder. Freely soluble in water; soluble in alcohol; practically insoluble in chloroform and in ether. pH of a solution in water containing the equivalent of carbenicillin 1% is between 6.5 and 8.0. Store in airtight containers.

**Incompatibility.** Carbenicillin sodium has been reported to be incompatible with aminoglycosides, tetracyclines, and a number of other drugs including other antimicrobials and these drugs should therefore be given separately.

### Adverse Effects

As for Benzylpenicillin, p.163.

Hypersensitivity reactions have been reported to be less frequent and less severe with carbenicillin than with benzylpenicillin. Pain at the injection site and phlebitis may occur. Electrolyte disturbances, particularly hypokalaemia or hypernatraemia, may follow large doses of carbenicillin sodium.

A dose-dependent coagulation defect has been reported, especially in patients with renal impairment. Carbenicillin appears to interfere with platelet function thereby prolonging bleeding time; purpura and haemorrhage from mucous membranes and elsewhere may result.

### Precautions

As for Benzylpenicillin, p.164.

**Sodium content.** Each g of carbenicillin sodium contains about 4.7 mmol of sodium. Carbenicillin sodium should therefore be given with caution to patients on a restricted sodium diet.

### Interactions

As for Benzylpenicillin, p.164.

### Antimicrobial Action

Carbenicillin has a bactericidal mode of action similar to that of benzylpenicillin, but with an extended spectrum of activity against Gram-negative bacteria. The most important feature of carbenicillin is its activity against *Pseudomonas aeruginosa*, although high concentrations are generally necessary. Activity against *Ps. aeruginosa* and some other organisms can be enhanced by gentamicin and other aminoglycosides. Carbenicillin is also active against *Proteus*, including indole-positive spp. such as *Pr. vulgaris*. It is comparable with ampicillin against other Gram-negative bacteria. Sensitive organisms include some Enterobacteriaceae, for example *Escherichia coli* and *Enterobacter* spp.; *Haemophilus influenzae*; and *Neisseria* spp. *Klebsiella* spp. are usually not susceptible. Its activity against Gram-positive bacteria is less than that of benzylpenicillin. Anaerobic organisms are generally susceptible to carbenicillin, but high concentrations are required for *Bacteroides fragilis*.

*Resistance.* Carbenicillin is inactivated by penicillinases and some other beta-lactamases, although it is more stable to the chromosomally mediated beta-lactamases produced by some Gram-negative organisms, including *Ps. aeruginosa* and some *Proteus* spp. Resistance to carbenicillin may develop in *Ps. aeruginosa* during treatment with carbenicillin or other beta lactams. This resistance may be intrinsic where there are changes in cell wall permeability or penicillin-binding proteins, or it may be due to plasmid-mediated beta-lactamase production that may be transferred to and from certain strains of Enterobacteriaceae.

There may be cross-resistance between carbenicillin and other antipseudomonal penicillins.

Outbreaks of pseudomonal resistance to carbenicillin have been associated with extensive use in, for example, hospital burns units.

### Pharmacokinetics

Carbenicillin is not absorbed from the gastrointestinal tract and has therefore been given either intramuscularly or intravenously.

The half-life of carbenicillin is reported to be about 1 to 1.5 hours; it is increased in patients with renal impairment, especially if there is also hepatic impairment, and also in neonates. Half-lives of 10 to 18 hours have been reported in renal impairment. Clearance is enhanced in patients with cystic fibrosis. Carbenicillin is about 50% bound to plasma proteins. Distribution of carbenicillin in the body is similar to that of other penicillins. Small amounts have been detected in breast milk. There is little diffusion into the CSF except when the meninges are inflamed. Relatively high concentrations have been reported in bile, but carbenicillin is excreted principally by renal tubular secretion and glomerular filtration.

Probenecid increases and prolongs plasma concentrations of carbenicillin.

Carbenicillin is removed by haemodialysis and, to some extent, by peritoneal dialysis.

### Uses and Administration

Carbenicillin is a carboxypenicillin that has been given by injection as the disodium salt, often with gentamicin, in the treatment of infections due to *Pseudomonas aeruginosa*; however, other antipseudomonal penicillins such as ticarcillin (p.270) or piperacillin (p.243) are now preferred. It has also been given to treat serious infections due to non-penicillinase-producing strains of *Proteus* spp.

Esters of carbenicillin, such as carfecillin (p.166) and carindacillin (p.166), have been given by mouth in the treatment of urinary-tract infections.

### Preparations

***USP 27:*** Carbenicillin for Injection.

**Proprietary Preparations** (details are given in Part 3)
***Ital.:*** Geopen†; ***Mex.:*** Carbecin; Myciclid†; ***Spain:*** Geopen†.

---

## Carfecillin Sodium *(BANM, pINNM)*

BRL-3475; Carbenicillin Phenyl Sodium *(USAN)*; Carfecilina sódica. Sodium (6R)-6-(2-phenoxycarbonyl-2-phenylacetamido)penicillanate.

$C_{23}H_{21}N_2NaO_6S$ = 476.5.

*CAS — 27025-49-6 (carfecillin); 21649-57-0 (carfecillin sodium).*

*ATC — G01AA08.*

### Profile

Carfecillin is the phenyl ester of carbenicillin (p.166) to which it is hydrolysed following absorption from the gastrointestinal tract. Its use has been restricted to the treatment of urinary-tract infections due to *Pseudomonas* spp. and other sensitive bacteria including *Proteus* spp.

### Preparations

**Proprietary Preparations** (details are given in Part 3)
***Ital.:*** Urocarf†.

---

## Carindacillin Sodium *(BANM, pINNM)*

Carbenicillin Indanyl Sodium *(USAN)*; Carindacilina sódica; CP-15464-2. Sodium (6R)-6-[2-(indan-5-yloxycarbonyl)-2-phenylacetamido]penicillanate.

$C_{26}H_{25}N_2NaO_6S$ = 516.5.

*CAS — 35531-88-5 (carindacillin); 26605-69-6 (carindacillin sodium).*

*ATC — J01CA05.*

**Pharmacopoeias.** In *US.*

**USP 27** (Carbenicillin Indanyl Sodium). A white to off-white powder. Soluble in water and in alcohol. pH of a 10% solution in water is between 5.0 and 8.0. Store in airtight containers.

### Profile

Carindacillin is the indanyl ester of carbenicillin (p.166) to which it is hydrolysed following absorption from the gastrointestinal tract. Its use is restricted to the treatment of urinary-tract infections due to *Pseudomonas* spp. and other sensitive bacteria including *Proteus* spp.

Carindacillin is given by mouth as the sodium salt. 535 mg of carindacillin sodium is approximately equivalent to 382 mg of carbenicillin. Usual doses, expressed in terms of carbenicillin, are 382 to 764 mg four times daily.

**Sodium content.** Each g of carindacillin sodium contains about 1.9 mmol of sodium.

### Preparations

***USP 27:*** Carbenicillin Indanyl Sodium Tablets.

**Proprietary Preparations** (details are given in Part 3)
***Hong Kong:*** Geopen†; ***USA:*** Geocillin.

---

## Carumonam Sodium *(BANM, USAN, rINNM)*

AMA-1080 (carumonam); Carumonam sódico; Ro-17-2301 (carumonam); Ro-17-2301/006 (carumonam sodium). (Z)-(2-Aminothiazol-4-yl){[(2S,3S)-2-carbamoyloxymethyl-4-oxo-1-sulphoazetidin-3-yl]carbamoyl}methyleneamino-oxyacetic acid, disodium salt.

$C_{12}H_{12}N_6Na_2O_{10}S_2$ = 510.4.

*CAS — 87638-04-8 (carumonam); 86832-68-0 (carumonam sodium).*

**Pharmacopoeias.** In *Jpn.*

### Profile

Carumonam is a monobactam antibacterial with a spectrum of antimicrobial action *in vitro* similar to that of aztreonam (p.161). It is given by intramuscular or intravenous injection as the sodium salt and doses are expressed in terms of carumonam. 1.09 g of carumonam sodium is approximately equivalent to 1 g of carumonam. The usual dose is 1 to 2 g daily in two divided doses.

**Sodium content.** Each g of carumonam sodium contains about 3.92 mmol of sodium.

### Preparations

**Proprietary Preparations** (details are given in Part 3)
***Jpn:*** Amasulin.

## Cefaclor *(BAN, USAN, pINN)*

Cefaclorum; Compound 99638. (7R)-3-Chloro-7-(α-D-phenylglycylamino)-3-cephem-4-carboxylic acid monohydrate.

$C_{15}H_{14}ClN_3O_4S,H_2O$ = 385.8.

*CAS — 53994-73-3 (anhydrous cefaclor); 70356-03-5 (cefaclor monohydrate).*

*ATC — J01DA08.*

**Pharmacopoeias.** In *Chin., Eur.* (see p.vi), and *US. Jpn* includes the anhydrous substance.

**Ph. Eur. 5.0** (Cefaclor). A white or slightly yellow powder. Slightly soluble in water; practically insoluble in dichloromethane and in methyl alcohol. A 2.5% suspension in water has a pH of 3.0 to 4.5.

**USP 27** (Cefaclor). A white to off-white crystalline powder. Slightly soluble in water; practically insoluble in chloroform, in methyl alcohol, and in benzene. pH of a 2.5% suspension in water is between 3.0 and 4.5. Store in airtight containers.

### Adverse Effects and Precautions

As for Cefalexin, p.168.

**Hypersensitivity.** Serum-sickness-like reactions may be more common with cefaclor than several other oral antibacterials[1] especially in young children who have received a number of courses of cefaclor;[2] typical features include skin reactions and arthralgia. A relatively high incidence of anaphylactic reactions has been reported from Japan.[3]

There has been a report of myocarditis that developed as a hypersensitivity reaction to cefaclor in a 12-year-old child.[4]

1. McCue JD. Delayed detection of serum sickness caused by oral antimicrobials. *Adv Therapy* 1990; **7:** 22–7.
2. Vial T, *et al.* Cefaclor-associated serum sickness-like disease: eight cases and review of the literature. *Ann Pharmacother* 1992; **26:** 910–14.
3. Hama R, Mori K. High incidence of anaphylactic reactions to cefaclor. *Lancet* 1988; **i:** 1331.
4. Beghetti M, *et al.* Hypersensitivity myocarditis caused by an allergic reaction to cefaclor. *J Pediatr* 1998; **132:** 172–3.

### Interactions

As for Cefalexin, p.168.

**Anticoagulants.** The UK manufacturer recommends that monitoring of prothrombin time should be considered in patients receiving cefaclor and *warfarin* following rare reports of increased prothrombin times. It is not known whether this interaction is related to the vitamin K-related hypoprothrombinaemia observed with some cephalosporins (see Cefamandole, p.169), but cefaclor does not contain the side-chain usually implicated in this reaction.

### Antimicrobial Action

Cefaclor is bactericidal and has antimicrobial activity similar to that of cefalexin (p.168) but is reported to be more active against Gram-negative bacteria including *Escherichia coli, Klebsiella pneumoniae, Neisseria gonorrhoeae,* and *Proteus mirabilis,* and especially against *Haemophilus influenzae*. It is active against some beta-lactamase-producing strains of *H. influenzae*. It may be less resistant to staphylococcal penicillinase than cefalexin or cefradine and a marked inoculum effect has been reported *in vitro*.

### Pharmacokinetics

Cefaclor is well absorbed from the gastrointestinal tract. Doses of 250 mg, 500 mg, and 1 g by mouth produce peak plasma concentrations of about 7, 13, and 23 micrograms/mL respectively after 0.5 to 1 hour. The presence of food may delay the absorption of cefaclor, but the total amount absorbed is unchanged. A plasma half-life of 0.5 to 1 hour has been reported; it may be slightly prolonged in patients with renal impairment. About 25% is bound to plasma proteins.

Cefaclor appears to be widely distributed in the body; it crosses the placenta and low concentrations have been detected in breast milk. It is rapidly excreted by the kidneys; up to 85% of a dose appears unchanged in the urine within 8 hours, the greater part within 2 hours. High concentrations of cefaclor are achieved in the urine within 8 hours of a dose; peak concentrations of 600, 900, and 1900 micrograms/mL have been reported after doses of 0.25, 0.5, and 1 g respectively. Probenecid delays excretion. Some cefaclor is removed by haemodialysis.

◊ References.

1. Wise R. The pharmacokinetics of the oral cephalosporins—a review. *J Antimicrob Chemother* 1990; **26** (suppl E): 13–20.
2. Sourgens H, *et al.* Pharmacokinetic profile of cefaclor. *Int J Clin Pharmacol Ther* 1997; **35:** 374–80.

### Uses and Administration

Cefaclor is a cephalosporin antibacterial given by mouth similarly to cefalexin in the treatment of susceptible infections including upper and lower respiratory-tract infections, skin infections, and urinary-tract infections. Some classify cefaclor as a second-generation cephalosporin and its greater activity against *Haemophilus influenzae* makes it more suitable than cefalexin for the treatment of infections such as otitis media. For details of these infections and their treatment, see under Choice of Antibacterial, p.120.

Cefaclor is given as the monohydrate. Doses are expressed in terms of the equivalent amount of anhydrous cefaclor. 1.05 g of cefaclor monohydrate is approximately equivalent to 1 g of anhydrous cefaclor. The usual adult dose is 250 to 500 mg every 8 hours; up to 4 g daily has been given. A suggested dose for children over 1 month of age is 20 mg/kg daily in three divided doses, increased if necessary to 40 mg/kg daily, but not exceeding a total daily dose of 1 g. A common dosage regimen is: children over 5 years, 250 mg three times daily; 1 to 5 years, 125 mg three times daily; under 1 year, 62.5 mg three times daily.

Modified-release formulations of cefaclor are available in some countries.

### Preparations

***BP 2003:*** Cefaclor Capsules; Cefaclor Oral Suspension; Slow Cefaclor Tablets;
***USP 27:*** Cefaclor Capsules; Cefaclor Extended-Release Tablets; Cefaclor for Oral Suspension.

**Proprietary Preparations** (details are given in Part 3)
***Arg.:*** Cec; Cefral; Kwicap; ***Austral.:*** Ceclor; Cefkor; Keflor; Verceft†; ***Austria:*** Cec; Ceclor; Cefastad; Cefax; Lanacef; ***Belg.:*** Ceclor; ***Braz.:*** Ceclor; Clorcin-Ped; Faclor; Plecor; Reflax; ***Canad.:*** Ceclor; ***Chile:*** Keflor; ***Fin.:*** Kefolor; ***Fr.:*** Alfatil; Alphexine; ***Ger.:*** Cec; Ceclorbeta; Cef-Diolan; Cefa-Wolff; Cefallone†; Ceph-Biocin†; Cephalodoc; Hefaclor; InfectoCef; Kefspor†; Panoral; Sigacefal; ***Gr.:*** Afecton; Ceclor; Hetaclox; Makovan; Panclor; Phacotrex; ***Hong Kong:*** Ceclor; Cefalor; Medoclor; Soficlor; ***India:*** Keflor; ***Irl.:*** Cefager; Distaclor; Keftid; Pinaclor; ***Israel:*** Ceclor; Cefalor; ***Ital.:*** Bacticef; Cefulton; Citiclor; Clorad; Dorf; Erreclor; Eurocefix; Fuclode; Kliacef; Lafarclor; Necloral; Oralcef; Panacef; Performer; Selanir; Takecef; Tibifor; ***Malaysia:*** Distaclor; Soficlor; Vercef; ***Mex.:*** Ceclor; Cefalan; Ceflacid; Serviclor; Teraclox; ***Neth.:*** Ceclor; ***NZ:*** Ceclor†; Clorotir; ***Port.:*** Ceclor; ***S.Afr.:*** Cec; Ceclor; CloraCEF; Kloclor†; Vercef; ***Singapore:*** Cleancef; Distaclor; Soficlor; Vercef; ***Spain:*** Ceclor; ***Swed.:*** Kefolor†; ***Switz.:*** Ceclor; ***Thai.:*** Celco; Distaclor; Kefaclor; Sifaclor; Tefaclor; Vercef; ***UAE:*** Recocef; ***UK:*** Bacticlor; Distaclor; Keftid; ***USA:*** Ceclor.

**Multi-ingredient:** ***Ger.:*** Muco Panoral†.

## Cefadroxil *(BAN, USAN, pINN)*

BL-S578; Cefadroxilo; Cefadroxilum Monohydricum; Cephadroxil; MJF-11567-3. (7R)-7-(α-D-4-Hydroxyphenylglycylamino)-3-methyl-3-cephem-4-carboxylic acid monohydrate.

$C_{16}H_{17}N_3O_5S,H_2O$ = 381.4.

*CAS — 50370-12-2 (anhydrous cefadroxil); 119922-85-9 (cefadroxil hemihydrate); 66592-87-8 (cefadroxil monohydrate).*

*ATC — J01DA09.*

**Pharmacopoeias.** In *Chin., Eur.* (see p.vi), and *US. Jpn* includes the anhydrous substance.

**Ph. Eur. 5.0** (Cefadroxil Monohydrate). A white or almost white powder. Slightly soluble in water; very slightly soluble in alcohol. A 5% suspension in water has a pH of 4.0 to 6.0. Protect from light.

**USP 27** (Cefadroxil). A white to off-white crystalline powder. Slightly soluble in water; practically insoluble in alcohol, in chloroform, and in ether. pH of a 5% suspension in water is between 4.0 and 6.0. Store in airtight containers.

### Adverse Effects and Precautions

As for Cefalexin, p.168.

**Breast feeding.** Although higher concentrations of cefadroxil were reported in breast milk compared with cefalexin, cefalotin, cefapirin, and cefotaxime,[1] no detectable cefadroxil would be expected in breast-fed infants and no adverse effects have been observed in infants whose mothers were receiving cefadroxil. Accordingly, the American Academy of Pediatrics considers[2] that cefadroxil is usually compatible with breast feeding.

1. Kafetzis DA, *et al.* Passage of cephalosporins and amoxicillin into the breast milk. *Acta Paediatr Scand* 1981; **70:** 285–8.
2. American Academy of Pediatrics. The transfer of drugs and other chemicals into human milk. *Pediatrics* 2001; **108:** 776–89. Correction. *ibid.*; 1029. Also available at: http://aappolicy.aappublications.org/cgi/content/full/pediatrics%3b108/3/776 (accessed 25/05/04)

### Interactions

As for Cefalexin, p.168.

### Antimicrobial Action

As for Cefalexin, p.168.

### Pharmacokinetics

Cefadroxil is almost completely absorbed from the gastrointestinal tract. After doses of 500 mg and 1 g by mouth, peak plasma concentrations of about 16 and 30 micrograms/mL respectively are obtained after 1.5 to 2 hours. Although peak concentrations are similar to those of cefalexin, plasma concentrations are more sustained. Administration with food does not appear to affect the absorption of cefadroxil. About 20% of cefadroxil is reported to be bound to plasma proteins. The plasma half-life of cefadroxil is about 1.5 hours and is prolonged in patients with renal impairment.

Cefadroxil is widely distributed to body tissues and fluids. It crosses the placenta and appears in breast milk.

More than 90% of a dose of cefadroxil may be excreted unchanged in the urine within 24 hours by glomerular filtration and tubular secretion; peak urinary concentrations of 1.8 mg/mL have been reported after a dose of 500 mg. Cefadroxil is removed by haemodialysis.

◊ References.

1. Tanrisever B, Santella PJ. Cefadroxil: a review of its antibacterial, pharmacokinetic and therapeutic properties in comparison with cephalexin and cephradine. *Drugs* 1986; **32** (suppl 3): 1–16.
2. Wise R. The pharmacokinetics of the oral cephalosporins—a review. *J Antimicrob Chemother* 1990; **26** (suppl E): 13–20.
3. Garrigues TM, *et al.* Dose-dependent absorption and elimination of cefadroxil in man. *Eur J Clin Pharmacol* 1991; **41:** 179–83.

### Uses and Administration

Cefadroxil is a first-generation cephalosporin antibacterial that is the para-hydroxy derivative of cefalexin (p.168), and is used similarly in the treatment of mild to moderate susceptible infections. It is given by mouth, and doses are expressed in terms of the anhydrous substance. 1.04 g of cefadroxil monohydrate is approximately equivalent to 1 g of anhydrous cefadroxil. The usual adult dose is 1 to 2 g daily as a single dose or in two divided doses. The following doses are used in children: 500 mg twice daily for those over 6 years of age, 250 mg twice daily for those aged 1 to 6 years, and 25 mg/kg daily in divided doses for infants under 1 year. For details of reduced doses of cefadroxil to be used in patients with renal impairment, see below.

**Administration in renal impairment.** Following an initial loading dose of 0.5 to 1 g, dosage of cefadroxil should be adjusted in patients with renal impairment according to creatinine clearance (CC) as follows:

- CC 26 to 50 mL/minute: 0.5 to 1 g twice daily
- CC 11 to 25 mL/minute: 0.5 to 1 g once daily
- CC 10 mL/minute or less: 0.5 to 1 g every 36 hours.

### Preparations

***BP 2003:*** Cefadroxil Capsules; Cefadroxil Oral Suspension;
***USP 27:*** Cefadroxil Capsules; Cefadroxil for Oral Suspension; Cefadroxil Tablets.

**Proprietary Preparations** (details are given in Part 3)
***Arg.:*** Cefabiot; Cefacar; Cefacilina; Cefamar; Cefasin; Cefatenk; Droxil; Kandicin; Klonadroxil; Versatic; ***Austria:*** Biodroxil; Duracef; ***Belg.:*** Duracef; Moxacef; ***Braz.:*** Cefadroxon; Cefamox; Drocef†; Drofaxil; Neo Cefadril; ***Canad.:*** Duricef; ***Chile:*** Adroxef; Biodroxil; Cefamox; ***Fin.:*** Duracef; ***Fr.:*** Oracefal; ***Ger.:*** Cedrox; Gruncef; ***Gr.:*** Cefalom; Kleotrat; Moxacef; ***Hong Kong:*** Amben; Androxyl; Biodroxil; Duracef; Sofidrox; ***India:*** Lydroxil; Odoxil; Vepan; ***Irl.:*** Ultracef; ***Israel:*** Biodroxil; Duracef; ***Ital.:*** Cefadril; Ceoxil; Cephos; Crenodyn†; Foxil; Oradroxil; ***Malaysia:*** Sofidrox; ***Mex.:*** Cefamox; Duracef; ***Port.:*** Biofaxil; Cefacile; Ceforal; Cefra; ***S.Afr.:*** Cefadrox†; Cipadur; Dacef; Duracef†; ***Singapore:*** Biodroxil†; Duricef; Sofidrox; ***Spain:*** Duracef; ***Swed.:*** Cefamox; ***Switz.:*** Duracef†; ***Thai.:*** Cefadril; Duricef†; ***UK:*** Baxan; ***USA:*** Duricef.

**Multi-ingredient:** ***Arg.:*** Cefacar Mucolitico; Cefacilina Bronquial.

## Cefalexin *(BAN, pINN)*

66873; Cefalexina; Cefalexinum Monohydricum; Cephalexin *(USAN)*. (7*R*)-3-Methyl-7-(α-D-phenylglycylamino)-3-cephem-4-carboxylic acid monohydrate.

$C_{16}H_{17}N_3O_4S,H_2O$ = 365.4.

*CAS — 15686-71-2 (anhydrous cefalexin); 23325-78-2 (cefalexin monohydrate).*

*ATC — J01DA01.*

**Pharmacopoeias.** In *Chin., Eur.* (see p.vi), *Jpn, Pol., US,* and *Viet.*

**Ph. Eur. 5.0** (Cefalexin Monohydrate). A white or almost white crystalline powder. Sparingly soluble in water; practically insoluble in alcohol. A 0.5% solution in water has a pH of 4.0 to 5.5. Protect from light.

**USP 27** (Cephalexin). A white to off-white crystalline powder. Slightly soluble in water; practically insoluble in alcohol, in chloroform, and in ether. pH of a 5% suspension in water is between 3.0 and 5.5. Store in airtight containers.

### Cefalexin Hydrochloride *(BANM, pINNM)*

Cephalexin Hydrochloride *(USAN)*; Hidrocloruro de cefalexina; LY-061188.

$C_{16}H_{17}N_3O_4S,HCl,H_2O$ = 401.9.

*CAS — 105879-42-3.*

*ATC — J01DA01.*

**Pharmacopoeias.** In *US.*

**USP 27** (Cephalexin Hydrochloride). A white to off-white crystalline powder. Soluble 1 in 100 in water, in acetone, in acetonitrile, in alcohol, in dimethylformamide, and in methyl alcohol; practically insoluble in chloroform, in ether, in ethyl acetate, and in isopropyl alcohol. pH of a 1% solution in water is between 1.5 and 3.0. Store in airtight containers.

### Adverse Effects and Precautions

As for Cefalotin Sodium, p.168.

The most common adverse effects of cefalexin and other oral cephalosporins are generally gastrointestinal disturbances and hypersensitivity reactions. Pseudomembranous colitis has been reported.

◊ References.

1. Dave J, *et al.* Cephalexin induced toxic epidermal necrolysis. *J Antimicrob Chemother* 1991; **28:** 477–8.
2. Baran R, Perrin C. Fixed-drug eruption presenting as an acute paronychia. *Br J Dermatol* 1991; **125:** 592–5.
3. Clark RF. Crystalluria following cephalexin overdose. *Pediatrics* 1992; **89:** 672–4.
4. Murray KM, Camp MS. Cephalexin-induced Stevens-Johnson syndrome. *Ann Pharmacother* 1992; **26:** 1230–3.
5. Czechowicz RT, *et al.* Bullous pemphigoid induced by cephalexin. *Australas J Dermatol* 2001; **42:** 132–5.

**Porphyria.** Cefalexin is considered to be unsafe in patients with porphyria although there is conflicting experimental evidence of porphyrinogenicity.

### Interactions

The renal excretion of cefalexin, and many other cephalosporins, is delayed by probenecid.

**Hormonal contraceptives.** There have been isolated reports of cefalexin decreasing the efficacy of oestrogen-containing oral contraceptives.[1] For a discussion of decreased efficacy of oral contraceptives and the need for additional contraceptive methods in patients taking broad-spectrum antibacterials, see under Hormonal Contraceptives, p.1534.

1. Friedman M, *et al.* Cephalexin and Microgynon-30 do not go well together. *J Obstet Gynaecol* 1982; **2:** 195–6.

### Antimicrobial Action

As for Cefalotin Sodium, p.169, although cefalexin is generally less potent. Some strains of Gram-negative bacteria may be inhibited only by the high concentrations achievable in the urinary tract. *Haemophilus influenzae* is moderately resistant to cefalexin.

### Pharmacokinetics

Cefalexin is almost completely absorbed from the gastrointestinal tract and produces a peak plasma concentration of about 18 micrograms/mL 1 hour after a 500-mg oral dose. If cefalexin is taken with food, absorption may be delayed, but the total amount absorbed is not appreciably altered. Up to 15% of a dose is bound to plasma proteins. The plasma half-life is about 1 hour; it increases with reduced renal function.

Cefalexin is widely distributed in the body but does not enter the CSF in significant quantities. It crosses the placenta and small quantities are found in breast milk. Cefalexin is not metabolised. About 80% or more of a dose is excreted unchanged in the urine in the first 6 hours by glomerular filtration and tubular secretion; urinary concentrations greater than 1 mg/mL have been achieved after a dose of 500 mg. Probenecid delays urinary excretion. Therapeutically effective concentrations may be found in the bile and some may be excreted by this route.

Cefalexin is removed by haemodialysis and peritoneal dialysis.

◊ References.

1. Wise R. The pharmacokinetics of the oral cephalosporins—a review. *J Antimicrob Chemother* 1990; **26** (suppl E): 13–20.

### Uses and Administration

Cefalexin is a first-generation cephalosporin antibacterial. It is given by mouth for the treatment of susceptible infections including those of the respiratory and urinary tracts and of the skin (see under Choice of Antibacterial, p.120). For severe infections, treatment with parenteral cephalosporins is to be preferred.

Cefalexin is usually given as the monohydrate although the hydrochloride is sometimes used. Doses are expressed in terms of the equivalent amount of anhydrous cefalexin. 1.05 g of cefalexin monohydrate and 1.16 g of cefalexin hydrochloride are each approximately equivalent to 1 g of anhydrous cefalexin.

The usual dose for adults is 1 to 2 g daily given in divided doses at 6-, 8-, or 12-hourly intervals; in severe or deep-seated infections the dose can be increased to up to 6 g daily but when high doses are required the use of a parenteral cephalosporin should be considered. Children may be given 25 to 100 mg/kg daily in divided doses to a maximum of 4 g daily.

For the prophylaxis of recurrent urinary-tract infection, cefalexin may be given in a dose of 125 mg at night.

Cefalexin sodium or cefalexin lysine have been used parenterally.

**Administration in renal impairment.** Doses of cefalexin may need to be reduced in patients with renal impairment. The *British National Formulary* recommends the following maximum daily doses according to creatinine clearance (CC):

- CC 40 to 50 mL/minute: maximum 3 g daily
- CC 10 to 40 mL/minute: maximum 1.5 g daily
- CC less than 10 mL/minute: maximum 750 mg daily

### Preparations

***BP 2003:*** Cefalexin Capsules; Cefalexin Oral Suspension; Cefalexin Tablets;

***USP 27:*** Cephalexin Capsules; Cephalexin for Oral Suspension; Cephalexin Tablets; Cephalexin Tablets for Oral Suspension.

**Proprietary Preparations** (details are given in Part 3)

***Arg.:*** Beliam; Cefalexi; Cefapoten; Cefasporina; Cefosporen; Ceporexin; Keforal; Lars; Lexin; Novalexin; Pectorina; Septilisin; Velexina; ***Austral.:*** Ceflin†; Cilex; Ibilex; Keflex; Sporahexal; ***Austria:*** Cepexin; Cephalobene; Keflex; Ospexin; Sanaxin; ***Belg.:*** Ceporex; Keforal; ***Braz.:*** Betacef; Cefaben; Cefagon†; Cefagran; Cefalen†; Cefalexan; Cefanal; Cefaporex†; Cefaxon; Ceflexin; Celen; Celexin; Ceporexin; Kefalexin; Keflaxina; Keflex; Lexin; Neo Ceflex; Neoceflex; Valflex; ***Canad.:*** Apo-Cephalex; Keflex†; Novo-Lexin; Nu-Cephalex; ***Denm.:*** Keflex; ***Fin.:*** Kefalex; Kefexin; Orakef; ***Fr.:*** Cefacet; Ceporexine; Keforal; ***Ger.:*** Cephalex; Ceporexin; Oracef; ***Hong Kong:*** Anxer; Apo-Cepalex†; Cefacin-M; Cefacure; Ceporex; Felexin; Keflex; Medolexin; Ospexin; Sofilex; Solulexin; ***India:*** Alexin; Cephaxin; Nufex; Phexin; Rofex; Sepexin; Sporidex; ***Irl.:*** Ceporex; Kefexin; Keflex; ***Israel:*** Cefalin; Ceforal; Cefovit; Keflex; ***Ital.:*** Ceporex; Keforal; Lafarin; ***Malaysia:*** Cefax; Celexin; Ceporex; Felexin; Kefexin; Medolexin; Ospexin; Refex; Sofilex; Sporidex; Uphalexin; ***Mex.:*** Acacin; Cefalver; Ceporex; Facelit; Falexol†; Keflex; Meta-K†; Nafacil; Paferxin; Quimosporina; Servicef; ***Neth.:*** Keforal; ***Norw.:*** Keflex; ***NZ:*** Keflex; ***Port.:*** Ceflax; Ceporex; Keflex; ***S.Afr.:*** Betacef†; Cerexin†; Fexin; Keflex; Lenocef; Ranceph; ***Singapore:*** Celexin; Cephalen; Cephanmycin; Ceporex; Felexin; Ospexin; Sofilex; Sporidex; ***Spain:*** Bioscefal; Cefalexgobens; Cefamiso†; Defaxina; Efemida†; Karilexina†; Kefloridina; Lexibiotico†; Lexincef; Sulquipen; Torlasporin; ***Swed.:*** Keflex; ***Switz.:*** Keflex†; Servispor†; ***Thai.:*** Anxer; Cefexin; Cefxin; Celex; Celexin; Cephalexyl; Cephin; Ceporex; Farmalex; Felexin; Ibilex; Keflex; Pondnacef; Sefasin; Servispor†; Sialexin; Sporicef; Sporidex; Toflex; Zeplex; ***UAE:*** Cefrin; ***UK:*** Ceporex; Keflex; ***USA:*** Biocef; Cefanex; Keflex; Keftab.

**Multi-ingredient: *India:*** Caceff; ***Mex.:*** Mucocef; Rombox; ***Spain:*** Kefloridina Mucolitico†.

---

## Cefalonium *(BAN, pINN)*

41071; Carbamoylcefaloridine; Cefalonio; Cephalonium. (7*R*)-3-(4-Carbamoyl-1-pyridiniomethyl)-7-[2-(2-thienyl)acetamido]-3-cephem-4-carboxylate.

$C_{20}H_{18}N_4O_5S_2$ = 458.5.

*CAS — 5575-21-3.*

**Pharmacopoeias.** *BP(Vet)* includes the dihydrate.

**BP(Vet) 2003** (Cefalonium). The dihydrate is a white or almost white crystalline powder. Very slightly soluble in water and in methyl alcohol; insoluble in alcohol, in dichloromethane, and in ether; soluble in dimethyl sulfoxide. It dissolves in dilute acids and in alkaline solutions. Store at temperature not exceeding 30°. Protect from light.

### Profile

Cefalonium is a cephalosporin antibacterial used in veterinary practice.

---

## Cefaloridine *(BAN, pINN)*

40602; Cefaloridina; Cefaloridinum; Cephaloridine *(USAN)*. (7*R*)-3-(1-Pyridiniomethyl)-7-[(2-thienyl)acetamido]-3-cephem-4-carboxylate.

$C_{19}H_{17}N_3O_4S_2$ = 415.5.

*CAS — 50-59-9.*

*ATC — J01DA02.*

**Pharmacopoeias.** In *Jpn.*

### Profile

Cefaloridine was one of the first cephalosporin antibacterials to be available clinically. It has properties similar to those of cefalotin (below), but is more nephrotoxic and is seldom used now.

### Preparations

**Proprietary Preparations** (details are given in Part 3)

***Mex.:*** Ceporan†.

---

## Cefalotin Sodium *(BANM, pINNM)*

38253; Cefalotina sódica; Cefalotinum Natricum; Cephalothin Sodium *(USAN)*; Sodium Cephalothin. Sodium (7*R*)-7-[2-(2-thienyl)acetamido]cephalosporanate; Sodium (7*R*)-3-acetoxymethyl-7-[2-(2-thienyl)acetamido]-3-cephem-4-carboxylate.

$C_{16}H_{15}N_2NaO_6S_2$ = 418.4.

*CAS — 153-61-7 (cefalotin); 58-71-9 (cefalotin sodium).*

*ATC — J01DA03.*

**Pharmacopoeias.** In *Chin., Eur.* (see p.vi), *Jpn, Pol.,* and *US.*

**Ph. Eur. 5.0** (Cefalotin Sodium). A white or almost white powder. Freely soluble in water; slightly soluble in dehydrated alcohol. A 10% solution in water has a pH of 4.5 to 7.0. Store in airtight containers. Protect from light.

**USP 27** (Cephalothin Sodium). A white to off-white, practically odourless, crystalline powder. Freely soluble in water, in sodium chloride 0.9%, and in glucose solutions; insoluble in most organic solvents. pH of a 25% solution in water is between 4.5 and 7.0. Store in airtight containers.

**Incompatibility and stability.** Cefalotin sodium has been reported to be incompatible with aminoglycosides and with many other drugs. Precipitation may occur in solutions with a pH of less than 5.

### Adverse Effects

The adverse effects associated with cefalotin and other cephalosporins are broadly similar to those described for penicillins (see Benzylpenicillin, p.163). The most common are hypersensitivity reactions, including skin rashes, urticaria, eosinophilia, fever, reactions resembling serum sickness, and anaphylaxis.

There may be a positive response to the Coombs' test although haemolytic anaemia rarely occurs. Neutropenia and thrombocytopenia have occasionally been reported. Agranulocytosis has been associated rarely with some cephalosporins. Bleeding complications related to hypoprothrombinaemia and/or platelet dysfunction have occurred especially with cephalosporins and cephamycins having an *N*-methylthiotetrazole side-chain, including cefamandole, cefbuperazone, cefmenoxime, cefmetazole, cefonicid, cefoperazone, ceforanide, cefotetan, cefpiramide, and latamoxef. The presence of a methylthiadiazolethiol side-chain, as in cefazolin, or an *N*-methylthiotriazine ring, as in ceftriaxone, might also be associated with such bleeding disorders.

Nephrotoxicity has been reported with cefalotin although it is less toxic than cefaloridine. Acute renal tubular necrosis has followed excessive dosage and has also been associated with its use in older patients or those with pre-existing renal impairment, or when used with nephrotoxic drugs such as aminoglycosides. Acute interstitial nephritis is also a possibility as a manifestation of hypersensitivity.

Transient increases in liver enzyme values have been reported. Hepatitis and cholestatic jaundice have occurred rarely with some cephalosporins.

Convulsions and other signs of CNS toxicity have been associated with high doses, especially in patients with severe renal impairment.

Gastrointestinal adverse effects such as nausea, vomiting, and diarrhoea have been reported rarely. Prolonged use may result in overgrowth of non-susceptible organisms and, as with other broad-spectrum antibiotics, pseudomembranous colitis may develop (see also below).

There may be pain at the injection site following intramuscular use, and thrombophlebitis has occurred following intravenous infusion of cephalosporins. Cefalotin appears to be more likely to cause such local reactions than other cephalosporins.

**Antibiotic-associated colitis.** Pseudomembranous colitis has occurred with many antibacterials, including the cephalosporins. The newer broad-spectrum cephalosporins have also been implicated[1-3] and the UK Committee on Safety of Medicines (CSM) has warned[4] of the dangers of pseudomembranous colitis with the newer, as well as the older, oral cephalosporins. In addition to 33 reports of pseudomembranous colitis associated with cefalexin, cefradine, cefadroxil, and cefaclor, 6 of which proved fatal, they had received 12 reports of probable or confirmed cases with cefuroxime axetil and 15 with cefixime, one of them fatal. In clinical trials of cefuroxime axetil and cefixime, diarrhoea and pseudomembranous colitis appeared to be dose-related and therefore the CSM recommended that higher doses should be reserved for severe infections. In any event they advised that treatment should be discontinued if symptoms suggestive of pseudomembranous colitis arise.

For further discussion of the management of this condition, see p.128.

1. de Lalla F, *et al.* Third generation cephalosporins as a risk factor for Clostridium difficile-associated disease: a four-year survey in a general hospital. *J Antimicrob Chemother* 1989; **23:** 623–31.
2. Golledge CL, *et al.* Extended spectrum cephalosporins and Clostridium difficile. *J Antimicrob Chemother* 1989; **23:** 929–31.
3. Freiman JP, *et al.* Pseudomembranous colitis associated with single-dose cephalosporin prophylaxis. *JAMA* 1989; **262:** 902.
4. Committee on Safety of Medicines. Pseudomembranous (antibiotic-associated) colitis and diarrhoea with cephalosporins. *Current Problems 32* 1991.

**Effects on the kidneys.** References.

1. Zhanel GG. Cephalosporin-induced nephrotoxicity: does it exist? *DICP Ann Pharmacother* 1990; **24:** 262–5.

## Precautions

Cefalotin should not be given to patients who are hypersensitive to it or to other cephalosporins. Immunological studies have suggested that up to 20% of penicillin-sensitive patients may also be allergic to cephalosporins although clinical studies indicate a lower frequency and the true incidence is uncertain; great care should be taken if cefalotin is to be given to such patients. Care is also necessary in patients with a history of allergy.

Cefalotin should be given with caution to patients with renal impairment; dosage reduction may be necessary. Renal and haematological status should be monitored especially during prolonged and high-dose therapy. Cefalotin and some other cephalosporins and cephamycins (ceforanide, cefotetan, cefoxitin, and cefpirome) may interfere with the Jaffé method of measuring creatinine concentrations and may produce falsely high values; this should be borne in mind when measuring renal function. Positive results to the direct Coombs' test have been found during treatment with cefalotin and these can interfere with blood cross-matching. The urine of patients being treated with cefalotin may give false-positive reactions for glucose using copper-reduction reactions.

**Porphyria.** Cephalosporins are considered to be unsafe in patients with porphyria although there is conflicting experimental evidence of porphyrinogenicity.

**Sodium content.** Each g of cefalotin sodium contains about 2.39 mmol of sodium.

## Interactions

The use of nephrotoxic drugs such as the aminoglycosides gentamicin and tobramycin may increase the risk of kidney damage with cefalotin. There is also some evidence for enhanced nephrotoxicity with the loop diuretic furosemide, but this is less certain than for furosemide with cefaloridine. Similarly to the penicillins, the renal excretion of cefalotin and many other cephalosporins is inhibited by probenecid. There may be antagonism between cefalotin and bacteriostatic antibacterials.

## Antimicrobial Action

Cefalotin is a beta-lactam antibacterial. It is bactericidal and acts similarly to benzylpenicillin (p.164) by inhibiting synthesis of the bacterial cell wall. It is most active against Gram-positive cocci, and has moderate activity against some Gram-negative bacilli.

Sensitive Gram-positive cocci include both penicillinase- and non-penicillinase-producing staphylococci, although meticillin-resistant staphylococci are resistant; most streptococci are also sensitive, but not penicillin-resistant *Streptococcus pneumoniae;* enterococci are usually resistant. Some Gram-positive anaerobes are also susceptible. Cefalotin is usually inactive against *Listeria monocytogenes*.

Among Gram-negative bacteria cefalotin has activity against some Enterobacteriaceae including strains of *Escherichia coli*, *Klebsiella pneumoniae*, *Proteus mirabilis*, *Salmonella*, and *Shigella* spp., but not against *Enterobacter*, indole-positive *Proteus*, or *Serratia* spp. It is also active against *Moraxella catarrhalis* (*Branhamella catarrhalis*) and *Neisseria* spp., though *Haemophilus influenzae* is moderately resistant. *Bacteroides fragilis* and *Pseudomonas aeruginosa* are not sensitive and neither are mycobacteria, mycoplasma, and fungi.

*Resistance* of bacteria to cefalotin may be due to several mechanisms: the drug may be prevented from reaching its site of action, for example in some Gram-negative organisms the cell wall may be a potential barrier; the target penicillin-binding proteins may be altered so that cefalotin cannot bind with these proteins; or, most importantly, the organism may produce beta-lactamases (cephalosporinases). Cefalotin is relatively resistant to hydrolysis by staphylococcal beta-lactamase, but is inactivated by a variety of beta-lactamases produced by Gram-negative organisms; resistance of Gram-negative organisms often depends on more than one factor. Resistance can be chromosomally or plasmid-mediated and may sometimes be inducible by cephalosporins.

Certain strains of bacteria may be inhibited but not killed by cephalosporins or penicillins and in such cases the minimum bactericidal concentration is much greater than the minimum inhibitory concentration; this is known as tolerance.

As well as with other cephalosporins, some cross-resistance may occur between cefalotin and the penicillinase-resistant penicillins.

## Pharmacokinetics

Cefalotin is poorly absorbed from the gastrointestinal tract. After intramuscular injection peak plasma concentrations of about 10 and 20 micrograms/mL are achieved within 30 minutes of doses of 0.5 and 1 g, respectively. A concentration of 30 micrograms/mL has been reported 15 minutes after the intravenous injection of a 1-g dose; a range of 14 to 20 micrograms/mL has been achieved by the continuous intravenous infusion of 500 mg/hour.

Cefalotin is widely distributed in body tissues and fluids except the brain and CSF where the concentrations achieved are low and unpredictable. It crosses the placenta and low concentrations have been detected in breast milk. The plasma half-life varies from about 30 to 50 minutes, but may be longer in patients with renal impairment, especially that of the metabolite. About 70% of cefalotin is bound to plasma proteins.

Approximately 20 to 30% of cefalotin is rapidly deacetylated in the liver and about 60 to 70% of a dose is excreted in the urine by the renal tubules within 6 hours as cefalotin and the less active metabolite, desacetylcefalotin. High urine concentrations of 0.8 and 2.5 mg/mL have been observed following intramuscular doses of 0.5 and 1 g, respectively. Probenecid blocks the renal excretion of cefalotin. A very small amount is excreted in bile.

## Uses and Administration

Cefalotin is a first-generation cephalosporin antibacterial that has been used in the treatment of infections due to susceptible bacteria, particularly staphylococci, but has generally been replaced by newer cephalosporins.

Cefalotin is given as the sodium salt by slow intravenous injection over 3 to 5 minutes or by intermittent or continuous infusion. It may be given intramuscularly but this route is painful. Doses are expressed in terms of the equivalent amount of cefalotin. 1.06 g of cefalotin sodium is approximately equivalent to 1 g of cefalotin. The usual dose is 0.5 to 1 g of cefalotin every 4 to 6 hours; up to 12 g daily has been given in severe infections.

**Administration in renal impairment.** Reduced doses are recommended if cefalotin is given to patients with renal impairment. After an intravenous loading dose of 1 to 2 g patients may be given the following maximum doses according to their creatinine clearance (CC):

- CC 50 to 80 mL/minute: 2 g every 6 hours
- CC 25 to 50 mL/minute: 1.5 g every 6 hours
- CC 10 to 25 mL/minute: 1 g every 6 hours
- CC 2 to 10 mL/minute: 500 mg every 6 hours
- CC less than 2 mL/minute: 500 mg every 8 hours

## Preparations

***USP 27:*** Cephalothin for Injection; Cephalothin Injection.

**Proprietary Preparations** (details are given in Part 3)
***Arg.:*** Arecamin; Cefade; Dasuglor; Keflin; Rupecef; ***Austral.:*** Keflin Neutral; ***Austria:*** Keflin†; ***Braz.:*** Cefalot; Cefariston; Kefalotin; Keflin; ***Canad.:*** Ceporacin; Keflin†; ***Denm.:*** Keflin; ***Fin.:*** Keflin; ***Fr.:*** Keflin†; ***Israel:*** Keflin; ***Ital.:*** Keflin; ***Mex.:*** Ceftina; Falot; Keflin; Lotin; ***Neth.:*** Keflin; ***Norw.:*** Keflin; ***NZ:*** Keflin†; ***S.Afr.:*** Keflin; ***Singapore:*** Cefadin; ***Spain:*** Keflin†; ***Swed.:*** Keflin†; ***Thai.:*** Cefadin; Keflin.

# Cefamandole *(BAN, USAN, rINN)*

83405; Cefamandol; Cephamandole; Compound 83405. (7*R*)-7-D-Mandelamido-3-(1-methyl-1*H*-tetrazol-5-ylthiomethyl)-3-cephem-4-carboxylic acid; {6*R*-[6α,7β(*R**)]}-7-[(hydroxyphenylacetyl)amino]-3-{[(1-methyl-1*H*-tetrazol-5-yl)thio]methyl}-8-oxo-5-thia-1-azabicyclo[4.2.0]oct-2-ene-2-carboxylic acid.

$C_{18}H_{18}N_6O_5S_2$ = 462.5.
*CAS — 34444-01-4.*
*ATC — J01DA07.*

## Cefamandole Nafate *(BAN, USAN, rINNM)*

106223; Cefamandole Formate Sodium; Cefmandoli Nafas; Cephamandole Nafate; Nafato de cefamandol. Sodium (7*R*)-7-[(2*R*)-2-formyloxy-2-phenylacetamido]-3-(1-methyl-1*H*-tetrazol-5-ylthiomethyl)-3-cephem-4-carboxylate.

$C_{19}H_{17}N_6NaO_6S_2$ = 512.5.
*CAS — 42540-40-9.*
*ATC — J01DA07.*

**Pharmacopoeias.** In *Eur.* (see p.vi), *Pol.*, and *US*.

**Ph. Eur. 5.0** (Cefamandole Nafate). A white, or almost white powder. Freely soluble in water; sparingly soluble in methyl alcohol. A 10% solution in water has a pH, measured after 30 minutes, of 6.0 to 8.0. Store in airtight containers. Protect from light

**USP 27** (Cefamandole Nafate). A white, odourless, crystalline solid. Soluble in water and in methyl alcohol; practically insoluble in chloroform, in cyclohexane, in ether, and in benzene. pH of a 10% solution in water is between 3.5 and 7.0. Store in airtight containers.

**Incompatibility and stability.** Cefamandole nafate has been reported to be incompatible with aminoglycosides and with metronidazole. Formulations of cefamandole nafate available for injection contain sodium carbonate and are incompatible with solutions containing calcium or magnesium salts. When reconstituted with water the sodium carbonate rapidly hydrolyses about 30% of the ester to cefamandole sodium; during storage of the reconstituted solution at room temperature carbon dioxide is produced.

References.

1. Frable RA, *et al.* Stability of cefamandole nafate injection with parenteral solutions and additives. *Am J Hosp Pharm* 1982; **39:** 622–7. Correction. *ibid.*; 1479.

## Cefamandole Sodium *(BANM, rINNM)*

Cefamandol sódico; Cephamandole Sodium.

$C_{18}H_{17}N_6NaO_5S_2$ = 484.5.
*CAS — 30034-03-8.*
*ATC — J01DA07.*

**Pharmacopoeias.** In *Jpn*.

## Adverse Effects and Precautions

As for Cefalotin Sodium, p.168.

Cefamandole has an *N*-methylthiotetrazole side-chain and may cause bleeding as a result of hypoprothrombinaemia which is usually reversible with administration of vitamin K. An alteration in intestinal flora was once thought responsible for this vitamin K-associated hypoprothrombinaemia, but interference with prothrombin synthesis now seems more likely.

**Effects on the blood.** References.

1. Lipsky JJ. Antibiotic-associated hypoprothrombinaemia. *J Antimicrob Chemother* 1988; **21:** 281–300.
2. Shearer MJ, *et al.* Mechanism of cephalosporin-induced hypoprothrombinemia: relation to cephalosporin side chain, vitamin K metabolism, and vitamin K status. *J Clin Pharmacol* 1988; **28:** 88–95.
3. Welage LS, *et al.* Comparative evaluation of the pharmacokinetics of N-methylthiotetrazole following administration of cefoperazone, cefotetan, and cefmetazole. *Antimicrob Agents Chemother* 1990; **34:** 2369–74.

**Sodium content.** 1.05 g of cefamandole sodium and 1.11g of cefamandole nafate each contain about 2.2 mmol of sodium.

## Interactions

A disulfiram-like interaction with alcohol may occur and has been attributed to the *N*-methylthiotetrazole side-chain of cefamandole. Patients receiving cefamandole should therefore avoid alcohol during, and for at least several days after, treatment. Interactions are also possible with preparations containing significant amounts of alcohol.

Cefamandole, and other cephalosporins containing an *N*-methylthiotetrazole side-chain, may enhance the hypoprothrombinaemic response to anticoagulants as discussed under Warfarin (p.1024).

Probenecid reduces the renal clearance of cefamandole and many other cephalosporins.

◊ References.

1. Portier H, *et al.* Interaction between cephalosporins and alcohol. *Lancet* 1980; **ii:** 263.
2. Drummer S, *et al.* Antabuse-like effect of β-lactam antibiotics. *N Engl J Med* 1980; **303:** 1417–18.

## Antimicrobial Action

Cefamandole is bactericidal and acts similarly to cefalotin, but has a broader spectrum of activity. It generally has similar or less activity against Gram-positive staphylococci and streptococci, but is resistant to some beta-lactamases produced by Gram-negative bacteria. It is more active than cefalotin against many of the Enterobacteriaceae including some strains of *Enterobacter, Escherichia coli, Klebsiella, Salmonella,* and some *Proteus* spp. However, resistance to cefamandole and other beta lactams has emerged in some species, notably *Enterobacter,* during treatment with cefamandole. Cefamandole is very active *in vitro* against *Haemophilus influenzae* although an inoculum effect has been reported for beta-lactamase-producing strains. Like cefalotin, most strains of *Bacteroides fragilis* are resistant to cefamandole, as are *Pseudomonas* spp.

◊ References.

1. Sabath LD. Reappraisal of the antistaphylococcal activities of first-generation (narrow-spectrum) and second-generation (expanded-spectrum) cephalosporins. *Antimicrob Agents Chemother* 1989; **33:** 407–11.

## Pharmacokinetics

Cefamandole is poorly absorbed from the gastrointestinal tract. It is given intramuscularly or intravenously, usually as the nafate which is rapidly hydrolysed to release cefamandole *in vivo*. Peak plasma concentrations for cefamandole of about 13 and 25 micrograms/mL have been achieved 0.5 to 2 hours after intramuscular doses of 0.5 and 1 g respectively; concentrations are very low after 6 hours. About 70% is bound to plasma proteins. The plasma half-life varies from about 0.5 to 1.2 hours depending on the route of injection; it is prolonged in patients with renal impairment.

Cefamandole is widely distributed in body tissues and fluids including bone, joint fluid, and pleural fluid; it diffuses into the CSF when the meninges are inflamed, but concentrations are unpredictable. Cefamandole has also been detected in breast milk. It is rapidly excreted unchanged by glomerular filtration and renal tubular secretion; about 80% of a dose is excreted within 6 hours and high urinary concentrations are achieved. Probenecid competes for renal tubular secretion with cefamandole resulting in higher and prolonged plasma concentrations of cefamandole. Therapeutic concentrations of cefamandole are achieved in bile.

Cefamandole is removed by haemodialysis to some extent.

## Uses and Administration

Cefamandole is a second-generation cephalosporin antibacterial used in the treatment of infections due to susceptible bacteria and for surgical infection prophylaxis.

It is given principally as cefamandole nafate (the sodium salt of cefamandole formyl ester). Doses are expressed in terms of the equivalent amount of cefamandole. 1.05 g of cefamandole sodium and 1.11 g of cefamandole nafate are each approximately equivalent to 1 g of cefamandole. It is given by deep intramuscular injection, by slow intravenous injection over 3 to 5 minutes, or by intermittent or continuous infusion in doses of 0.5 to 2 g every 4 to 8 hours for adults depending on the severity of the infection. Children over 1 month of age may be given 50 to 100 mg/kg daily in equally divided doses; 150 mg/kg daily may be given in severe infections, but this dose should not be exceeded. For details of reduced doses to be used in patients with renal impairment, see below. If cefamandole is used with an aminoglycoside, the drugs should be administered separately.

For surgical infection prophylaxis, a dose of 1 or 2 g intravenously or intramuscularly 30 to 60 minutes before surgical incision, followed by 1 or 2 g every 6 hours for 24 to 48 hours, is recommended. For patients undergoing procedures involving implantation of prosthetic devices, cefamandole should be continued for up to 72 hours. Children over 3 months of age may be treated similarly to adults and given 50 to 100 mg/kg daily in equally divided doses.

**Administration in renal impairment.** Doses of cefamandole should be reduced for patients with renal impairment. After an initial dose of 1 to 2 g the following maintenance doses have been recommended based on creatinine clearance (CC):

- CC 50 to 80 mL/minute: 0.75 to 2 g every 6 hours
- CC 25 to 50 mL/minute: 0.75 to 2 g every 8 hours
- CC 10 to 25 mL/minute: 0.5 to 1.25 g every 8 hours
- CC 2 to 10 mL/minute: 0.5 to 1 g every 12 hours
- CC less than 2 mL/minute: 0.25 to 0.75 g every 12 hours

## Preparations

***USP 27:*** Cefamandole Nafate for Injection.

**Proprietary Preparations** (details are given in Part 3)
***Austral.:*** Mandol; ***Austria:*** Mandokef; ***Belg.:*** Mandol; ***Canad.:*** Mandol†; ***Fr.:*** Kefandol†; ***Ger.:*** Mandokef†; ***Gr.:*** Acemycin; Mandokef; ***Hong Kong:*** Mandol; ***Irl.:*** Kefadol; ***Ital.:*** Cedol†; Cefam; Cefiran†; Cemado; Lampomandol; Mancef; Mandokef; Mandolsan; Neocefal†; Septomandolo; ***Neth.:*** Mandol; ***NZ:*** Mandol; ***Port.:*** Mandokef; ***S.Afr.:*** Kefdole; Mandokef; ***Spain:*** Mandokef†; ***Switz.:*** Mandokef; ***Thai.:*** Cefadol; Cefmandol; Mandol; ***UK:*** Kefadol†; ***USA:*** Mandol†.

# Cefapirin Sodium *(BANM, pINNM)*

BL-P-1322; Cefapirina sódica; Cefapirinum Natricum; Cephapirin Sodium *(USAN)*. Sodium (7*R*)-7-[2-(4-pyridylthio)acetamido]cephalosporanate; Sodium (7*R*)-3-acetoxymethyl-7-[2-(4-pyridylthio)acetamido]-3-cephem-4-carboxylate.

$C_{17}H_{16}N_3NaO_6S_2$ = 445.4.
*CAS — 21593-23-7 (cefapirin); 24356-60-3 (cefapirin sodium).*
*ATC — J01DA30.*

**Pharmacopoeias.** In *Eur.* (see p.vi), *Jpn,* and *US.*
*US* also includes Cephapirin Benzathine for veterinary use.

**Ph. Eur. 5.0** (Cefapirin Sodium). A white or pale yellow powder. Soluble in water; practically insoluble in dichloromethane. A 1% solution in water has a pH of 6.5 to 8.5. Protect from light.

**USP 27** (Cephapirin Sodium). A white to off-white crystalline powder, odourless or having a slight odour. Very soluble in water; insoluble in most organic solvents. pH of a solution in water containing the equivalent of cefapirin 1% is between 6.5 and 8.5. Store in airtight containers.

## Profile

Cefapirin is a first-generation cephalosporin antibacterial with actions and uses very similar to those of cefalotin (p.168). It is used as the sodium salt but doses are expressed in terms of cefapirin base. 1.05 g of cefapirin sodium is approximately equivalent to 1 g of cefapirin. The usual adult dose is the equivalent of 0.5 to 1 g of cefapirin every 4 to 6 hours by intramuscular injection or intravenously. In severe infections up to 12 g daily may be given, preferably intravenously.

**Administration in renal impairment.** Reduced doses of cefapirin sodium may be necessary in patients with renal impairment. One regimen, based on creatinine clearance (CC), that has been suggested is:

- CC 5 to 20 mL/minute: 1 g every 12 hours
- CC less than 5 mL/minute: 1 g every 24 hours

Patients undergoing haemodialysis may receive 7.5 to 15 mg/kg after each dialysis.

**Sodium content.** Each g of cefapirin sodium contains about 2.2 mmol of sodium.

## Preparations

***USP 27:*** Cephapirin for Injection.

**Proprietary Preparations** (details are given in Part 3)
***Fr.:*** Cefaloject; ***Gr.:*** Cefatrex; ***Hong Kong:*** Lopitrex†; ***Spain:*** Brisfirina.
**Multi-ingredient:** ***Spain:*** Brisfirina Balsamica†.

# Cefatrizine *(BAN, USAN, pINN)*

BL-S640; Cefatrizina; SKF-60771; S-640P. (7*R*)-7-(α-D-4-Hydroxyphenylglycylamino)-3-(1*H*-1,2,3-triazol-4-ylthiomethyl)-3-cephem-4-carboxylic acid.

$C_{18}H_{18}N_6O_5S_2$ = 462.5.
*CAS — 51627-14-6.*
*ATC — J01DA21.*

# Cefatrizine Propylene Glycol *(BANM, pINNM)*

(7*R*)-7-(α-D-4-Hydroxyphenylglycylamino)-3-(1*H*-1,2,3-triazol-4-ylthiomethyl)-3-cephem-4-carboxylate propylene glycol.

$C_{18}H_{18}N_6O_5S_2, (C_3H_8O_2)_n$.
*CAS — 64217-62-5.*
*ATC — J01DA21.*

**Pharmacopoeias.** In *Eur.* (see p.vi) and *Jpn.*

**Ph. Eur. 5.0** (Cefatrizine Propylene Glycol ). A white or almost white powder. Slightly soluble in water; practically insoluble in alcohol and in dichloromethane.

## Profile

Cefatrizine is a cephalosporin antibacterial with actions and uses similar to those of cefalexin (p.168), although it might be more active *in vitro*. It is given by mouth as the base or, more commonly, as a compound with propylene glycol, in usual adult doses equivalent to 500 mg twice daily of cefatrizine.

## Preparations

**Proprietary Preparations** (details are given in Part 3)
***Belg.:*** Cefaperos; ***Fr.:*** Cefaperos; ***Gr.:*** Anfagladin; Axelorax; Banadroxin; Ceftazin; Cetrizin; Gertemycin; Izerin; Kentacef; Klevasin; Liamycin; Liferost; Lingopen; Mekan; Nibocin; Northiron; Phacobiotic; Relyovix; Specic-ef-N; ***Ital.:*** Biotrixina; Cefatrix; Cefotrizin†; Cetrazil; Cetrinox; Faretrizin; Ipatrizina; Kefoxina†; Ketrizin; Miracef; Novacef; Orotrix†; Tamyl; Tricef; Trixidine†; Trixilan†; Trizina; Zinaf†; Zitrix†; ***Port.:*** Macropen.

# Cefazolin *(BAN, pINN)*

Cefazolina; Cephazolin. 3-[(5-Methyl-1,3,4-thiadiazol-2-yl)thiomethyl]-7-(tetrazol-1-ylacetamido)-3-cephem-4-carboxylic acid.

$C_{14}H_{14}N_8O_4S_3$ = 454.5.
*CAS — 25953-19-9.*
*ATC — J01DA04.*

**Pharmacopoeias.** In *US.*

**USP 27** (Cefazolin). A white to slightly off-white, odourless crystalline powder. Slightly soluble in water, in alcohol, and in methyl alcohol; sparingly soluble in acetone; practically insoluble in chloroform, in dichloromethane, in ether, and in benzene; soluble in dimethylformamide and in pyridine; very slightly soluble in ethyl acetate, in isopropyl alcohol, and in methyl isobutyl ketone. Store in airtight containers.

# Cefazolin Sodium *(BANM, USAN, pINNM)*

46083; Cefazolina sódica; Cefazolinum Natricum; Cephazolin Sodium; SKF-41558.

$C_{14}H_{13}N_8NaO_4S_3$ = 476.5.
*CAS — 27164-46-1.*
*ATC — J01DA04.*

**Pharmacopoeias.** In *Chin., Eur.* (see p.vi), *Jpn,* and *US.*
*Jpn* also includes the pentahydrate.

**Ph. Eur. 5.0** (Cefazolin Sodium). A white or almost white, very hygroscopic powder. It exhibits polymorphism. Freely soluble in water; very slightly soluble in alcohol. A 10% solution in water has a pH of 4.0 to 6.0. Store in airtight containers. Protect from light.

**USP 27** (Cefazolin Sodium). A white to off-white, practically odourless, crystalline powder, or a white to off-white solid. Freely soluble in water, in sodium chloride 0.9%, and in glucose solutions; very slightly soluble in alcohol; practically insoluble in chloroform and in ether. pH of a solution in water containing the equivalent of cefazolin 10% is between 4.0 and 6.0. Store in airtight containers.

**Incompatibility and stability.** Cefazolin sodium has been reported to be incompatible with aminoglycosides and many other drugs. When the pH of a solution exceeds 8.5 there may be hydrolysis and when it is below 4.5 insoluble cefazolin may be precipitated.

References.

1. Nahata MC, Ahalt PA. Stability of cefazolin sodium in peritoneal dialysis solutions. *Am J Hosp Pharm* 1991; **48:** 291–2.

2. Wu C-C, *et al.* Stability of cefazolin in heparinized and non-heparinized peritoneal dialysis solutions. *Am J Health-Syst Pharm* 2002; **59:** 1537–8.
3. Lin Y-F, *et al.* Stability of cefazolin sodium in icodextrin-containing peritoneal dialysis solution. *Am J Health-Syst Pharm* 2002; **59:** 2362, 2364.

## Adverse Effects and Precautions

As for Cefalotin Sodium, p.168. Stevens-Johnson syndrome has occurred.

Similarly to cephalosporins with a *N*-methylthiotetrazole side-chain, cefazolin has been associated with hypoprothrombinaemia (see Cefamandole, p.169).

**Breast feeding.** In a study[1] of 20 lactating women receiving cefazolin, the amount of cefazolin in breast milk was found to be extremely small (equivalent to less than 0.075% of the dose). No adverse effects have been observed in breast-fed infants whose mothers were receiving cefazolin, and the American Academy of Pediatrics considers[2] that it is therefore usually compatible with breast feeding.

1. Yoshioka H, *et al.* Transfer of cefazolin into human milk. *J Pediatr* 1979; **94:** 151–2.
2. American Academy of Pediatrics. The transfer of drugs and other chemicals into human milk. *Pediatrics* 2001; **108:** 776–89. Correction. *ibid.*; 1029. Also available at: http://aappolicy.aappublications.org/cgi/content/full/pediatrics%3b108/3/776 (accessed 25/05/04)

**Effects on the nervous system.** References.

1. Manzella JP, *et al.* CNS toxicity associated with intraventricular injection of cefazolin: report of three cases. *J Neurosurg* 1988; **68:** 970–1.
2. Martin ES, *et al.* Seizures after intraventricular cefazolin administration. *Clin Pharm* 1992; **11:** 104–5.

**Sodium content.** Each g of cefazolin sodium contains about 2.1 mmol of sodium.

## Interactions

Cefazolin contains a methylthiadiazolethiol side-chain and, similarly to cephalosporins containing the related *N*-methylthiotetrazole side-chain (see Cefamandole, p.170), may have the potential to cause a disulfiram-like reaction with alcohol, and may possibly enhance the effects of warfarin.

The renal excretion of cefazolin and many other cephalosporins is delayed by probenecid.

## Antimicrobial Action

As for Cefalotin Sodium, p.169, although cefazolin is more sensitive to staphylococcal beta-lactamase.

## Pharmacokinetics

Cefazolin is poorly absorbed from the gastrointestinal tract and is given by the intramuscular or intravenous routes. Following a 500-mg dose given intramuscularly, peak plasma concentrations of 30 micrograms or more per mL are obtained after 1 hour. About 85% of cefazolin is bound to plasma proteins. The plasma half-life of cefazolin is about 1.8 hours, and is increased in patients with renal impairment. Cefazolin diffuses into bone and into ascitic, pleural, and synovial fluid but not appreciably into the CSF. It crosses the placenta; only low concentrations are detected in breast milk.

Cefazolin is excreted unchanged in the urine, mainly by glomerular filtration with some renal tubular secretion, at least 80% of a dose given intramuscularly being excreted within 24 hours. Peak urine concentrations of more than 2 and 4 mg/mL have been reported after intramuscular doses of 0.5 and 1 g respectively. Probenecid delays excretion. Cefazolin is removed to some extent by haemodialysis.

High biliary concentrations have been reported, although the amount excreted by this route is small.

## Uses and Administration

Cefazolin is a first-generation cephalosporin antibacterial used in the treatment of a variety of infections due to susceptible organisms, including biliary-tract infections, endocarditis (staphylococcal), and peritonitis (associated with continuous ambulatory peritoneal dialysis). It is also used for surgical infection prophylaxis, including prophylaxis of endometritis at caesarean section. For details of these infections and their treatment, see under Choice of Antibacterial, p.120.

*Administration and dosage.* Cefazolin is given as the sodium salt by deep intramuscular injection, by slow intravenous injection over 3 to 5 minutes, or by intravenous infusion. Doses are expressed in terms of the equivalent amount of cefazolin. 1.05 g of cefazolin sodium is approximately equivalent to 1 g of cefazolin. The usual adult dose is the equivalent of 0.5 to 1 g of cefazolin every 6 to 12 hours. The usual maximum daily dose is 6 g, although up to 12 g has been used in severe life-threatening infections. Children over 1 month may be given 25 to 50 mg/kg daily in 3 or 4 divided doses, increased in severe infections to a maximum of 100 mg/kg daily.

For the prophylaxis of infection during surgery, a 1-g dose is given half to one hour before the operation, followed by 0.5 to 1 g during surgery for lengthy procedures. A dose of 0.5 to 1 g is given every 6 to 8 hours postoperatively for 24 hours, or up to 5 days in certain cases.

For details of reduced doses of cefazolin for use in patients with renal impairment, see below.

Other routes of administration used for cefazolin sodium include intraperitoneal administration in peritoneal dialysis solutions and intra-ocular injections.

In some countries a modified-release intramuscular formulation of cefazolin sodium together with the less soluble dibenzylamine salt of cefazolin, in the ratio of 1:4, has been used.

**Administration in renal impairment.** Dosage of cefazolin should be reduced in patients with renal impairment and various modifications have been recommended. After a loading dose the manufacturers suggest the following doses for adults based on creatinine clearance (CC):

Adults

- CC 55 mL or more per minute: usual doses
- CC 35 to 54 mL/minute: usual doses but at intervals of at least 8 hours
- CC 11 to 34 mL/minute: half the usual dose every 12 hours
- CC 10 mL or less per minute: half the usual dose every 18 to 24 hours

Children

- CC 40 to 70 mL/minute: 60% of the normal daily dose in 2 divided doses
- CC 20 to 40 mL/minute: 25% of the normal daily dose in 2 divided doses
- CC 5 to 20 mL/minute: 10% of the normal daily dose every 24 hours.

One group of workers[1] found that, for patients receiving long-term haemodialysis, a dose of 20 mg/kg given postdialysis 3 times weekly maintained therapeutic cefazolin concentrations.

1. Ahern JW, *et al.* Cefazolin dosing protocol for patients receiving long-term hemodialysis. *Am J Health-Syst Pharm* 2003; **60:** 178–81.

## Preparations

***BP 2003:*** Cefazolin Injection;
***USP 27:*** Cefazolin for Injection; Cefazolin Injection; Cefazolin Ophthalmic Solution.

**Proprietary Preparations** (details are given in Part 3)
***Arg.:*** Cefalomicina; Cefamezin; ***Austral.:*** Cefamezin†; Kefzol; ***Austria:*** Gramaxin†; Kefzol; Servazolin; Zolicef; ***Belg.:*** Cefacidal; Kefzol; ***Braz.:*** Cefamezin†; Ceftrat†; Cezolin; Kefazol; ***Canad.:*** Ancef†; Kefzol; ***Chile:*** Kefzol; ***Fr.:*** Cefacidal; ***Ger.:*** Basocef; Elzogram; Gramaxin†; ***Gr.:*** Biozolin; Vifazolin; ***Hong Kong:*** Cefamezin; ***India:*** Azolin; Reflin; ***Israel:*** Cefamezin; Kefazin; Kefzol; Totacef; ***Ital.:*** Acef; Biazolina†; Cefabiozim; Cefamezin; Cefazil; Cromezin; Firmacef†; Nefazol; Recef; Sicef; Silzolin; Totacef; Zolin†; Zolisint†; ***Jpn:*** Cefamezin; ***Mex.:*** Cefacidal†; ***Neth.:*** Cefacidal; Kefzol; ***NZ:*** Kefzol; ***Port.:*** Cefamezin; Kurgan; ***S.Afr.:*** Cefacidal; Izacef†; Kefzol; Ranzol; ***Spain:*** Areuzolin; Brizolina; Camil; Caricef; Cefa Resan; Cefacene; Cefadrex; Cefakes†; Cefamezin†; Cefamusel†; Dacovo; Fazoplex; Filoklin; Gencefal; Intrazolina; Karidina†; Kefol; Kurgan; Neofazol; Tasep; Tecfazolina; Zolival; ***Switz.:*** Kefzol; Servicef†; ***Thai.:*** Cefacidal†; Cefalin; Cefamezin; Cefazillin; Cefazol; Fazolin; Kefzol†; Zefa; Zepilen; ***UK:*** Kefzol†; ***USA:*** Ancef; Kefzol†; Zolicef.

---

## Cefbuperazone *(USAN, rINN)*

BMY-25182; T-1982. 7-[(2*R*,3*S*)-2-(4-ethyl-2,3-dioxopiperazin-1-ylcarboxamido)-3-hydroxybutyramido]-7-methoxy-3-(1-methyl-1*H*-tetrazol-5-ylthiomethyl)-3-cephem-4-carboxylic acid.

$C_{22}H_{29}N_9O_9S_2$ = 627.7.
*CAS — 76610-84-9.*

## Cefbuperazone Sodium *(rINNM)*

BMY-25182; T-1982 (both cefbuperazone).
$C_{22}H_{28}N_9NaO_9S_2$ = 649.6.

**Pharmacopoeias.** In *Jpn.*

### Profile

Cefbuperazone is a cephamycin antibiotic similar to cefoxitin (p.178) and is given by injection as the sodium salt. Its spectrum of activity includes Enterobacteriaceae, but more especially anaerobic bacteria such as *Bacteroides fragilis*. Cefbuperazone does not appear to be active against cefoxitin-resistant strains of *B. fragilis*.

Cefbuperazone has an *N*-methylthiotetrazole side-chain. For adverse effects and drug interactions associated with the presence of this side-chain, see under Cephamandole, p.169.

### Preparations

**Proprietary Preparations** (details are given in Part 3)
***Jpn:*** Tomiporan.

---

## Cefcapene Pivoxil Hydrochloride *(rINNM)*

Pivaloyloxymethyl (+)-(6*R*,7*R*)-7-[(*Z*)-2-(2-amino-4-thiazolyl)-2-pentenamido]-3-(hydroxymethyl)-8-oxo-5-thia-1-azabicyclo[4.2.0]oct-2-ene-2-carboxylic acid carbamate monohydrochloride monohydrate.

$C_{23}H_{29}N_5O_8S_2,HCl,H_2O$ = 622.1.
*CAS — 135889-00-8 (cefcapene); 105889-45-0 (cefcapene pivoxil); 147816-23-7 (anhydrous cefcapene pivoxil hydrochloride); 147816-24-8 (cefcapene pivoxil hydrochloride);.*

**Pharmacopoeias.** In *Jpn.*

### Profile

Cefcapene is an oral cephalosporin antibacterial given by mouth as the pivaloyloxymethyl ester, cefcapene pivoxil hydrochloride.

For reference to carnitine deficiency occurring after the administration of some pivaloyloxymethyl esters, see Pivampicillin, p.244.

### Preparations

**Proprietary Preparations** (details are given in Part 3)
***Jpn:*** Flomox.

---

## Cefdinir *(BAN, USAN, rINN)*

CI-983; FK-482. (−)-(6*R*,7*R*)-7-[2-(2-Amino-4-thiazolyl)glyoxylamido]-8-oxo-3-vinyl-5-thia-1-azabicyclo[4.2.0]oct-2-ene-2-carboxylic acid, $7^2$-(*Z*)-oxime; 7-{(2-Amino-1,3-thiazol-4-yl)-2-[(*Z*)-hydroxyimino]acetamido}-3-vinylcephem-4-carboxylic acid.

$C_{14}H_{13}N_5O_5S_2$ = 395.4.
*CAS — 91832-40-5.*
*ATC — J01DA42.*

**Pharmacopoeias.** In *Jpn.*

### Adverse Effects and Precautions

As for Cefalotin Sodium, p.168. There have been reports of reddish stools in patients who have received cefdinir with iron supplements (see also Interactions, below).

### Interactions

Absorption of cefdinir is decreased by antacids or iron supplements and administration should be separated by an interval of at least 2 hours. Probenecid reduces the renal excretion of cefdinir.

### Antimicrobial Action

As for Cefixime, p.173. However, cefdinir is reported to be much more active *in vitro* than cefixime against *Staphylococcus aureus*, but not meticillin-resistant strains, and it is less active against some Enterobacteriaceae.

### Pharmacokinetics

Cefdinir is absorbed from the gastrointestinal tract following oral administration, peak plasma concentrations occurring 2 to 4 hours after a dose. Bioavailability following administration by mouth has been estimated to range from 16 to 25%. It is widely distributed into tissues and is 60 to 70% bound to plasma proteins. Cefdinir is not appreciably metabolised and is excreted in the urine with an elimination half-life of 1.7 hours.

Cefdinir is removed by dialysis.

### Uses and Administration

Cefdinir is a third-generation oral cephalosporin antibacterial with actions and uses similar to those of cefixime (p.172). It is given by mouth in a usual adult dose of 600 mg daily as a single dose or in two divided doses. Children may be given 14 mg/kg daily up to a maximum of 600 mg daily. Doses may need to be reduced in patients with renal impairment (see below).

◊ Reviews.

1. Guay DRP. Cefdinir: an expanded-spectrum oral cephalosporin. *Ann Pharmacother* 2000; **34:** 1469–77.
2. Guay DR, *et al.* Cefdinir: an advanced-generation, broad-spectrum oral cephalosporin. *Clin Ther* 2002; **24:** 473–89.

**Administration in renal impairment.** Doses of cefdinir should be reduced to 300 mg once daily in patients with renal impairment whose creatinine clearance is less than 30 mL/minute.

### Preparations

**Proprietary Preparations** (details are given in Part 3)
***Austria:*** Omnicef; ***India:*** Sefdin; ***Jpn:*** Cefzon; ***Thai.:*** Omnicef; ***USA:*** Omnicef.

---

**Cefditoren Pivoxil** *(rINNM)*

ME-1207; ME-1206 (cefditoren). Pivaloyloxymethyl (+)-(6R,7R)-7-[2-(2-Amino-4-thiazolyl)glyoxylamido]-3-[(Z)-2-(4-methyl-5-thiazolyl)vinyl]-8-oxo-5-thia-1-azabicyclo[4.2.0]oct-2-ene-2-carboxylic acid $7^2$-(Z)-(O-methyloxime).

$C_{25}H_{28}N_6O_7S_3$ = 620.7.

*CAS — 104145-95-1 (cefditoren); 117467-28-4 (cefditoren pivoxil).*

**Pharmacopoeias.** In *Jpn.*

### Adverse Effects and Precautions

As for Cefalotin, p.168.

The most frequently reported adverse effects of cefditoren are gastrointestinal disturbances, especially diarrhoea.

For reference to carnitine deficiency occurring after some pivaloyloxymethyl esters, see Pivampicillin, p.244.

### Interactions

Absorption of cefditoren following oral doses is decreased by antacids or histamine $H_2$-receptor antagonists. Probenecid reduces the renal excretion of cefditoren.

### Antimicrobial Action

As for Cefixime, p.173. Cefditoren also has activity against *Staphylococcus aureus.*

### Pharmacokinetics

Cefditoren pivoxil is absorbed from the gastrointestinal tract and is hydrolysed to cefditoren by esterases to release active cefditoren in the bloodstream. Peak plasma concentrations average 1.8 micrograms/mL in fasting subjects 1.5 to 3 hours after a 200-mg dose. Bioavailability is about 14% in fasting subjects and is increased when cefditoren pivoxil is given with a high fat meal. Plasma protein binding is reported to be 88%. The plasma half-life is about 1.6 hours and is prolonged in patients with renal impairment.

Cefditoren is not appreciably metabolised and is excreted mainly in the urine by glomerular filtration and tubular secretion. It is removed by haemodialysis.

### Uses and Administration

Cefditoren is a cephalosporin antibacterial with a broad spectrum of activity used in the treatment of susceptible infections, particularly of the respiratory tract and skin. It is given by mouth as the pivaloyloxymethyl ester, cefditoren pivoxil, but doses are expressed in terms of cefditoren. 245 mg of cefditoren pivoxil is approximately equivalent to 200 mg of cefditoren. A usual dose is 200 to 400 mg given twice daily.

For details of reduced doses to be used in patients with moderate to severe renal impairment, see below.

◊ Reviews.

1. Darkes MJM, Plosker GL. Cefditoren pivoxil. *Drugs* 2002; **62:** 319–36.

**Administration in renal impairment.** Doses of cefditoren pivoxil should be reduced in patients with moderate to severe renal impairment according to creatinine clearance (CC):

- CC 30 to 49 mL/minute: the dose should not exceed 200 mg twice daily
- CC less than 30 mL/minute: the dose should be 200 mg once daily.

### Preparations

**Proprietary Preparations** (details are given in Part 3)
***Jpn:*** Meiact; ***USA:*** Spectracef.

## Cefepime Hydrochloride

*(BANM, USAN, rINNM)*

BMY-28142 (cefepime); Hidrocloruro de cefepima. {6R-[6α,7β(Z)]}-1-[(7-{[(2-Amino-4-thiazolyl)-(methoxyimino)acetyl]amino}-2-carboxy-8-oxo-5-thia-1-azabicyclo[4.2.0]oct-2-en-3-yl)methyl]-1-methylpyrrolidinium chloride monohydrochloride monohydrate; 7-{(2-Amino-1,3-thiazol-4-yl)-2-[(Z)-methoxyimino]acetamido}-3-(1-methylpyrrolidiniomethyl)-3-cephem-4-carboxylate hydrochloride.

$C_{19}H_{25}ClN_6O_5S_2,HCl,H_2O$ = 571.5.

*CAS — 88040-23-7 (cefepime); 123171-59-5 (cefepime hydrochloride monohydrate).*

*ATC — J01DA24.*

**Pharmacopoeias.** In *Jpn* and *US.*

**USP 27** (Cefepime Hydrochloride). A white to off-white, non-hygroscopic, crystalline powder. Freely soluble in water. Store in airtight containers. Protect from light.

**Incompatibility and stability.** References.

1. Stewart JT, *et al.* Stability of cefepime hydrochloride injection in polypropylene syringes at −20°C, 4°C, and 22-24°C. *Am J Health-Syst Pharm* 1999; **56:** 457–9.
2. Stewart JT, *et al.* Stability of cefepime hydrochloride in polypropylene syringes. *Am J Health-Syst Pharm* 1999; **56:** 1134.
3. Williamson JC, *et al.* Stability of cefepime in peritoneal dialysis solution. *Ann Pharmacother* 1999; **33:** 906–9.
4. Baririan N, *et al.* Stability and compatibility study of cefepime in comparison with ceftazidime for potential administration by continuous infusion under conditions pertinent to ambulatory treatment of cystic fibrosis patients and to administration in intensive care units. *J Antimicrob Chemother* 2003; **51:** 651–8.
5. Trissel LA, Xu QA. Stability of cefepime hydrochloride in AutoDose infusion system bags. *Ann Pharmacother* 2003; **37:** 804–7.

### Adverse Effects and Precautions

As for Cefalotin Sodium, p.168.

◊ References.

1. Neu HC. Safety of cefepime: a new extended-spectrum parenteral cephalosporin. *Am J Med* 1996; **100** (suppl 6A): 68S–75S.

### Antimicrobial Action

Cefepime is a fourth-generation cephalosporin and is active against a wide range of Gram-positive and Gram-negative aerobic organisms. Against Gram-positive cocci, its activity is similar to that of cefotaxime (p.176) and includes staphylococci (but not meticillin-resistant *Staphylococcus aureus*) and streptococci. Against Enterobacteriaceae, it has a broader spectrum of activity than other cephalosporins, including activity against organisms producing chromosomally mediated beta-lactamases such as *Enterobacter* spp. and *Proteus vulgaris.* Against *Pseudomonas aeruginosa,* it has similar or slightly less activity than ceftazidime (p.181), although it may be active against some strains resistant to ceftazidime.

### Pharmacokinetics

Cefepime is given by injection as the hydrochloride. It is rapidly and almost completely absorbed following intramuscular injection and mean peak plasma concentrations of about 14 and 30 micrograms/mL have been reported about 1.5 hours after doses of 500 mg and 1 g respectively. Within 30 minutes of intravenous administration of similar doses, peak plasma concentrations of about 40 and 80 micrograms/mL are achieved. The plasma half-life of cefepime is approximately 2 hours and is prolonged in patients with renal impairment. About 20% of cefepime is bound to plasma proteins.

Cefepime is widely distributed in body tissues and fluids. High concentrations are achieved in bile. Low concentrations have been detected in breast milk.

Cefepime is eliminated principally by the kidneys and about 85% of a dose is recovered unchanged in the urine. Cefepime is substantially removed by haemodialysis.

◊ References.

1. Okamoto MP, *et al.* Cefepime clinical pharmacokinetics. *Clin Pharmacokinet* 1993; **25:** 88–102.
2. Rybak M. The pharmacokinetic profile of a new generation of parenteral cephalosporin. *Am J Med* 1996; **100** (suppl 6A): 39S–44S.
3. Reed MD, *et al.* Pharmacokinetics of intravenously and intramuscularly administered cefepime in infants and children. *Antimicrob Agents Chemother* 1997; **41:** 1783–7.
4. Allaouchiche B, *et al.* Pharmacokinetics of cefepime during continuous venovenous hemodiafiltration. *Antimicrob Agents Chemother* 1997; **41:** 2424–7.
5. Blumer JL, *et al.* Review of the pharmacokinetics of cefepime in children. *Pediatr Infect Dis J* 2001; **20:** 337–42.

### Uses and Administration

Cefepime is a fourth-generation cephalosporin antibacterial used in the treatment of infections due to susceptible organisms. They include infections of the urinary tract, respiratory tract, and skin. For details of these infections and their treatment, see under Choice of Antibacterial, p.120.

Cefepime is given as the hydrochloride by deep intramuscular injection, or intravenously by infusion over at least 30 minutes. Doses are expressed in terms of the equivalent amount of cefepime. 1.19 g of cefepime hydrochloride is approximately equivalent to 1 g of cefepime. The usual adult dose is 1 to 2 g daily in 2 divided doses for mild to moderate infections, increased to 4 g daily in 2 divided doses in severe infections, although up to 6 g daily in 3 divided doses has been given for febrile neutropenia. Children aged over 2 months and weighing up to 40 kg may be given 50 mg/kg twice daily; this dose may be given 3 times daily for febrile neutropenia.

For details of reduced doses to be used in renal impairment, see below.

◊ Reviews.

1. Various. Cefepime: a β-lactamase-stable extended-spectrum cephalosporin. *J Antimicrob Chemother* 1993; **32** (suppl B): 1–214.
2. Barradell LB, Bryson HM. Cefepime: a review of its antibacterial activity, pharmacokinetic properties and therapeutic use. *Drugs* 1994; **47:** 471–505.
3. Okamoto MP, *et al.* Cefepime: a new fourth-generation cephalosporin. *Am J Hosp Pharm* 1994; **51:** 463–77.
4. Wynd MA, Paladino JA. Cefepime: a fourth-generation parenteral cephalosporin. *Ann Pharmacother* 1996; **30:** 1414–24.

**Administration in renal impairment.** Dosage of cefepime should be modified in renal impairment; after a normal initial loading dose the maintenance dosage should be adjusted according to the patient's creatinine clearance (CC) and the severity of the infection:

- CC 30 to 60 mL/minute: 0.5 to 2 g every 24 hours
- CC 11 to 29 mL/minute: 0.5 to 1 g every 24 hours
- CC 10 mL/minute or less: 250 to 500 mg every 24 hours

Patients undergoing haemodialysis should be given a repeat dose (equivalent to the initial dose) after each dialysis session, while those undergoing continuous ambulatory peritoneal dialysis should receive normal recommended doses at intervals of 48 hours.

### Preparations

***USP 27:*** Cefepime for Injection.

**Proprietary Preparations** (details are given in Part 3)
***Arg.:*** Maxcef; ***Austral.:*** Maxipime; ***Austria:*** Maxipime; ***Belg.:*** Maxipime; ***Braz.:*** Maxcef; ***Canad.:*** Maxipime; ***Chile:*** Maxipime; ***Denm.:*** Maxipime; ***Fin.:*** Maxipime; ***Fr.:*** Axepim; ***Ger.:*** Maxipime; ***Gr.:*** Maxipime; ***Hong Kong:*** Maxipime; ***Irl.:*** Maxipime; ***Israel:*** Maxcef; ***Ital.:*** Cepim; Cepimex; Maxipime; ***Malaysia:*** Maxipime; ***Mex.:*** Maxipime; ***Neth.:*** Maxipime†; ***NZ:*** Maxipime; ***Port.:*** Maxipime; ***S.Afr.:*** Maxipime; ***Singapore:*** Maxipime; ***Spain:*** Maxipime; ***Swed.:*** Maxipime; ***Switz.:*** Maxipime; ***Thai.:*** Maxipime; ***USA:*** Maxipime.

**Cefetamet** *(USAN, rINN)*

LY-097964; Ro-15-8074. (Z)-7-[2-(2-Aminothiazol-4-yl)-2-methoxyiminoacetamido]-3-methyl-3-cephem-4-carboxylic acid.

$C_{14}H_{15}N_5O_5S_2$ = 397.4.

*CAS — 65052-63-3 (cefetamet).*

*ATC — J01DA26.*

**Cefetamet Pivoxil Hydrochloride** *(rINN)*

Ro-15-8075 (cefetamet pivoxil). Cefetamet pivaloyloxymethyl hydrochloride.

$C_{20}H_{25}N_5O_7S_2,HCl$ = 548.0.

*CAS — 65243-33-6 (cefetamet pivoxil); 111696-23-2 (cefetamet pivoxil hydrochloride).*

*ATC — J01DA26.*

**Pharmacopoeias.** In *Jpn.*

### Profile

Cefetamet is a third-generation cephalosporin antibacterial similar to cefixime (below). It is given by mouth as the hydrochloride of the pivaloyloxymethyl ester, cefetamet pivoxil hydrochloride, which is hydrolysed to cefetamet *in vivo.* The usual dose is 500 mg twice daily.

For reference to carnitine deficiency occurring after the administration of some pivaloyloxymethyl esters, see Pivampicillin, p.244.

◊ Reviews.

1. Bryson HM, Brogden RN. Cefetamet pivoxil: a review of its antibacterial activity, pharmacokinetic properties and therapeutic use. *Drugs* 1993; **45:** 589–621.
2. Blouin RA, Stoeckel K. Cefetamet pivoxil clinical pharmacokinetics. *Clin Pharmacokinet* 1993; **25:** 172–88.

### Preparations

**Proprietary Preparations** (details are given in Part 3)
***Braz.:*** Globocef; ***Ger.:*** Globocef; ***Hong Kong:*** Globocef; ***Ital.:*** Globocef; ***Mex.:*** Globocef†; ***Port.:*** Cefec; Globocef; ***Switz.:*** Globocef.

## Cefixime *(BAN, USAN, rINN)*

Cefixima; Cefiximum; CL-284635; FK-027; FR-17027. (Z)-7-[2-(2-Aminothiazol-4-yl)-2-(carboxymethoxyimino)acetamido]-3-vinyl-3-cephem-4-carboxylic acid trihydrate.

$C_{16}H_{15}N_5O_7S_2,3H_2O$ = 507.5.

*CAS — 79350-37-1.*

*ATC — J01DA23.*

**Pharmacopoeias.** In *Eur.* (see p.vi) and *US. Jpn* includes the anhydrous substance.

**Ph. Eur. 5.0** (Cefixime). A white or almost white, slightly hygroscopic, powder. Slightly soluble in water; sparingly soluble in dehydrated alcohol; practically insoluble in ethyl acetate; freely soluble in methyl alcohol. A 5% suspension in water has a pH of 2.6 to 4.1. Store in airtight containers. Protect from light.

**USP 27** (Cefixime). A white to light yellow crystalline powder. Practically insoluble in water, in ether, in ethyl acetate, and in hexane; slightly soluble in alcohol, in acetone, and in glycerol; soluble in methyl alcohol and in propylene glycol; very slightly soluble in 70% sorbitol and in octanol. pH of a solution in water containing the equivalent of cefixime 0.07% is between 2.6 and 4.1. Store in airtight containers.

### Adverse Effects and Precautions

As for Cefalotin Sodium, p.168.

The most frequently reported adverse effects of cefixime are gastrointestinal disturbances, especially diarrhoea. Cefixime should be discontinued if diarrhoea is severe.

Although cefixime does not have the *N*-methylthiotetrazole side-chain usually associated with hypoprothrombinaemia (see Cefamandole, p.169), increases in prothrombin times have occurred in a few patients.

**Antibiotic-associated colitis.** For reports of diarrhoea and pseudomembranous colitis associated with cefixime, see Cefalotin, p.169.

### Interactions

Care should be exercised in patients receiving anticoagulants and cefixime due to the possibility that cefixime may increase prothrombin times (see above).

### Antimicrobial Action

Cefixime is bactericidal and is stable to hydrolysis by many beta-lactamases. It has a mode of action and spectrum of activity similar to those of the third-generation cephalosporin cefotaxime (p.176), but some Enterobacteriaceae are less susceptible to cefixime. *Haemophilus influenzae*, *Moraxella catarrhalis* (*Branhamella catarrhalis*), and *Neisseria gonorrhoeae* are sensitive, including penicillinase-producing strains. Of the Gram-positive bacteria, streptococci are sensitive to cefixime but most strains of staphylococci, enterococci, and *Listeria* spp. are not.

*Enterobacter* spp., *Pseudomonas aeruginosa*, and *Bacteroides* spp. are resistant to cefixime.

### Pharmacokinetics

Only 40 to 50% of an oral dose of cefixime is absorbed from the gastrointestinal tract, whether taken before or after meals, although the rate of absorption may be decreased in the presence of food. Cefixime is better absorbed from oral suspension than from tablets. Absorption is fairly slow; peak plasma concentrations of 2 to 3 micrograms/mL and 3.7 to 4.6 micrograms/mL have been reported between 2 and 6 hours after single doses of 200 and 400 mg, respectively. The plasma half-life is usually about 3 to 4 hours and may be prolonged when there is renal impairment. About 65% of cefixime is bound to plasma proteins.

Information on the distribution of cefixime in body tissues and fluids is limited. It crosses the placenta. Relatively high concentrations may be achieved in bile and urine. About 20% of an oral dose (or 50% of an absorbed dose) is excreted unchanged in the urine within 24 hours. Up to 60% may be eliminated by nonrenal mechanisms; there is no evidence of metabolism but some is probably excreted into the faeces from bile. It is not substantially removed by dialysis.

◊ References.

1. Brittain DC, *et al.* The pharmacokinetic and bactericidal characteristics of oral cefixime. *Clin Pharmacol Ther* 1985; **38:** 590–4.
2. Guay DRP, *et al.* Pharmacokinetics of cefixime (CL-284,635; FK027) in healthy subjects and patients with renal insufficiency. *Antimicrob Agents Chemother* 1986; **30:** 485–90.
3. Faulkner RD, *et al.* Pharmacokinetics of cefixime in the young and elderly. *J Antimicrob Chemother* 1988; **21:** 787–94.
4. Stone JW, *et al.* Cefixime, in-vitro activity, pharmacokinetics and tissue penetration. *J Antimicrob Chemother* 1989; **23:** 221–8.
5. Westphal JF, *et al.* Biliary excretion of cefixime: assessment in patients provided with T-tube drainage. *Antimicrob Agents Chemother* 1993; **37:** 1488–91.
6. Somekh E, *et al.* Penetration and bactericidal activity of cefixime in synovial fluid. *Antimicrob Agents Chemother* 1996; **40:** 1198–1200.

### Uses and Administration

Cefixime is generally classified as a third-generation cephalosporin antibacterial and is given by mouth in the treatment of susceptible infections including gonorrhoea, otitis media, pharyngitis, lower respiratory-tract infections such as bronchitis, and urinary-tract infections. For details of these infections and their treatment, see under Choice of Antibacterial, p.120.

Cefixime is available as the trihydrate and doses are expressed in terms of anhydrous cefixime. It is given by mouth in adult doses of 200 to 400 mg daily as a single dose or in two divided doses. Children over 6 months and under 50 kg may be given 8 mg/kg daily as an oral suspension, again as a single dose or in two divided doses. For details of reduced dosage of cefixime in patients with moderate to severe renal impairment, see below.

For uncomplicated gonorrhoea, a single oral dose of 400 mg is given.

◊ General references.

1. Leggett NJ, *et al.* Cefixime. *DICP Ann Pharmacother* 1990; **24:** 489–95.
2. Adam D, Wallace RJ, eds. Symposium on cefixime. *Drugs* 1991; **42** (suppl 4): 1–32.
3. Markham A, Brogden RN. Cefixime: a review of its therapeutic efficacy in lower respiratory tract infections. *Drugs* 1995; **49:** 1007–22.

**Administration in renal impairment.** Doses of cefixime should be reduced in patients with moderate to severe renal impairment. A dose of 200 mg daily should not be exceeded in patients with a creatinine clearance of less than 20 mL/minute.

### Preparations

***USP 27:*** Cefixime for Oral Suspension; Cefixime Tablets.

**Proprietary Preparations** (details are given in Part 3)
***Arg.:*** Cetaxim; Novacef; Vixcef; ***Austria:*** Aerocef; Tricef; ***Braz.:*** Cefnax; Neo Cefix; Plenax; ***Canad.:*** Suprax; ***Chile:*** Cefspan; Tricef; Urotricef; ***Fin.:*** Supracef†; ***Fr.:*** Oroken; ***Ger.:*** Cephoral; Suprax; Uro-Cephoral; ***Gr.:*** Ceftoral; ***India:*** Fixx; ***Irl.:*** Suprax; ***Israel:*** Supran; ***Ital.:*** Cefixoral; Suprax; Unixime; ***Jpn:*** Cefspan; ***Mex.:*** Denvar; Novacef; ***Neth.:*** Fixim; ***Port.:*** Bonocef; Cefimix; Cefiton; Neocef; Tricef; ***S.Afr.:*** Fixime; ***Spain:*** Denvar; Necopen; ***Swed.:*** Tricef; ***Switz.:*** Cephoral; ***Thai.:*** Cefspan; ***UK:*** Suprax; ***USA:*** Suprax.

---

## Cefluprenam (*rINN*)

Cefprenam; E-1077. (–)-{(*E*)-3-[(6*R*,7*R*)-7-[2-(5-Amino-1,2,4-thiadiazol-3-yl)glyoxylamido]-2-carboxy-8-oxo-5-thia-1-azabicyclo[4.2.0]oct-2-en-3-yl]allyl}(carbamoylmethyl)ethylmethylammonium hydroxide, inner salt, 7²-(*Z*)-[*O*-(fluoromethyl)oxime].

$C_{20}H_{25}FN_8O_6S_2$ = 556.6.
*CAS — 116853-25-9.*

### Profile

Cefluprenam is a cephalosporin antibacterial. It has been investigated in the treatment of susceptible infections.

---

## Cefmenoxime Hydrochloride (*USAN, rINNM*)

Abbott-50192; Cefmenoxime Hemihydrochloride; Hidrocloruro de cefmenoxima; SCE-1365 (cefmenoxime). (*Z*)-(7*R*)-7-[2-(2-Aminothiazol-4-yl)-2-methoxyiminoacetamido]-3-[(1-methyl-1*H*-tetrazol-5-yl)thiomethyl]-3-cephem-4-carboxylic acid hydrochloride.

$(C_{16}H_{17}N_9O_5S_3)_2$,HCl = 1059.6.
*CAS — 65085-01-0 (cefmenoxime); 75738-58-8 (cefmenoxime hydrochloride).*
*ATC — J01DA16.*

**Pharmacopoeias.** In *Jpn* and *US.*

**USP 27** (Cefmenoxime Hydrochloride). White to light orange-yellow crystals or crystalline powder. Very slightly soluble in water; practically insoluble in dehydrated alcohol and in ether; freely soluble in formamide; slightly soluble in methyl alcohol. Store in airtight containers.

### Profile

Cefmenoxime is a third-generation cephalosporin antibacterial with actions and uses similar to those of cefotaxime (p.175). It is given as the hydrochloride by intramuscular injection, or intravenously by injection or infusion in the treatment of susceptible infections. Doses are expressed in terms of the equivalent amount of cefmenoxime. 1.04 g of cefmenoxime hydrochloride is approximately equivalent to 1 g of cefmenoxime. The usual adult dose is 1 to 4 g daily in 2 to 4 divided doses, although up to 9 g daily has been given in severe infections. Children have been given 40 to 80 mg/kg daily in 2 to 4 divided doses; higher doses have been used in severe infections. Neonates have been given 40 to 60 mg/kg in 2 or 3 divided doses.

Like cefamandole (p.169), cefmenoxime has an *N*-methylthiotetrazole side-chain and coagulopathy and a disulfiram-like interaction with alcohol have been reported rarely.

Cefmenoxime hydrochloride is also given as eye drops for the treatment of eye infections.

◊ Reviews.

1. Campoli-Richards DM, Todd PA. Cefmenoxime: a review of its antibacterial activity, pharmacokinetic properties and therapeutic use. *Drugs* 1987; **34:** 188–221.

### Preparations

***USP 27:*** Cefmenoxime for Injection.

**Proprietary Preparations** (details are given in Part 3)
***Austria:*** Tacef; ***Ger.:*** Tacef†; ***Jpn:*** Bestcall; Bestron.

---

## Cefmetazole (*USAN, rINN*)

Cefmetazol; U-72791. (6*R*,7*S*)-7-{2-[(Cyanomethyl)thio]acetamido}-7-methoxy-3-{[(1-methyl-1*H*-tetrazol-5-yl)thio]methyl}-8-oxo-5-thia-1-azabicyclo-[4.2.0]oct-2-ene-2-carboxylic acid.

$C_{15}H_{17}N_7O_5S_3$ = 471.5.
*CAS — 56796-20-4.*
*ATC — J01DA40.*

**Pharmacopoeias.** In *US.*

**USP 27** (Cefmetazole). Store in airtight containers.

## Cefmetazole Sodium (*USAN, rINNM*)

Cefmetazol sódico; CS-1170; SKF-83088; U-72791A.

$C_{15}H_{16}N_7NaO_5S_3$ = 493.5.
*CAS — 56796-39-5.*
*ATC — J01DA40.*

**Pharmacopoeias.** In *Jpn* and *US.*

**USP 27** (Cefmetazole Sodium). A white solid. Very soluble in water and in methyl alcohol; soluble in acetone; practically insoluble in chloroform. pH of a 10% solution in water is between 4.2 and 6.2. Store in airtight containers.

### Adverse Effects and Precautions

As for Cefalotin Sodium, p.168.

Cefmetazole contains an *N*-methylthiotetrazole side-chain and like cefamandole (p.169) has the potential to cause hypoprothrombinaemia and bleeding.

**Effects on the blood.** References.

1. Breen GA, St Peter WL. Hypoprothrombinemia associated with cefmetazole. *Ann Pharmacother* 1997; **31:** 180–4.

**Sodium content.** Each g of cefmetazole sodium contains about 2 mmol of sodium.

### Interactions

As for Cefamandole, p.170.

### Antimicrobial Action

Cefmetazole is a cephamycin antibacterial with a similar spectrum of antibacterial activity to that of cefoxitin (p.177), including the anaerobe *Bacteroides fragilis*.

◊ References.

1. Cornick NA, *et al.* Activity of cefmetazole against anaerobic bacteria. *Antimicrob Agents Chemother* 1987; **31:** 2010–12.

### Pharmacokinetics

Following cefmetazole sodium 2 g intravenously every 6 hours, peak and trough plasma concentrations of 138 and 6 micrograms/mL have been achieved. Cefmetazole is 65 to 85% bound to plasma proteins, depending on the plasma concentration. A plasma half-life of about 1.1 to 1.5 hours has been reported; it is prolonged in patients with renal impairment. Small amounts have been detected in breast milk. Relatively high concentrations have been achieved in bile.

The majority of a dose is excreted unchanged in the urine resulting in high concentrations; up to 85% of a dose has been recovered within 12 hours. Cefmetazole is partly excreted by renal tubular secretion and probenecid prolongs elimination.

Cefmetazole is removed to some extent by haemodialysis.

### Uses and Administration

Cefmetazole is a cephamycin antibacterial generally classified with the second-generation cephalosporins and used similarly to cefoxitin (p.178) in the treatment and prophylaxis of anaerobic and mixed bacterial infections, especially intra-abdominal and pelvic infections. It may also be used in the treatment of gonorrhoea. For details of these infections and their treatment, see under Choice of Antibacterial, p.120.

Cefmetazole is given intravenously as the sodium salt by infusion over 10 to 60 minutes or by slow injection over 3 to 5 minutes. Cefmetazole sodium is also used intramuscularly in some countries. Doses are expressed in terms of the equivalent amount of cefmetazole. 1.05 g of cefmetazole sodium is approximately equivalent to 1 g of cefmetazole.

The usual adult dose is 2 g intravenously every 6 to 12 hours.

For details of reduced dosage of cefmetazole to be used in patients with renal impairment, see below.

For uncomplicated gonorrhoea the usual dose is 1 g as a single intramuscular injection, together with probenecid 1 g by mouth.

For surgical infection prophylaxis, a single dose of 1 or 2 g may be given intravenously 30 to 90 minutes before surgery and repeated if necessary after 8 and 16 hours. At caesarean section a single 2-g dose may be given intravenously to the mother after the umbilical cord is clamped; alternatively a 1-g dose may be given and repeated after 8 and 16 hours.

◊ References.

1. Finch R, *et al.* eds. Cefmetazole: a clinical appraisal. *J Antimicrob Chemother* 1989; **23** (suppl D): 1–142.

**Administration in renal impairment.** Doses of cefmetazole should be reduced in patients with renal impairment. The interval between doses should be 12, 16, or 24 hours in patients with mild, moderate, or severe renal impairment, respectively; patients with virtually no renal function may be given cefmetazole every 48 hours, after haemodialysis.

### Preparations

**USP 27:** Cefmetazole for Injection; Cefmetazole Injection.

**Proprietary Preparations** (details are given in Part 3)
***Hong Kong:*** Cefmetazon; ***Ital.:*** Cefadel†; Decacef†; Metacaf; Metafar; Metasal; Metazol; ***Jpn:*** Cefmetazon; ***Spain:*** Cemetol†; ***Thai.:*** Cefmetazon†; ***USA:*** Zefazone.

## Cefminox Sodium *(pINNM)*

Cefminox sódico; MT-141. Sodium 7-{2-[(S)-2-amino-2-carboxyethyl]thioacetamido}-7-methoxy-3-(1-methyl-1*H*-tetrazol-5-ylthiomethyl)-3-cephem-4-carboxylate.

$C_{16}H_{20}N_7NaO_7S_3$ = 541.6.

*CAS — 75481-73-1 (cefminox).*

**Pharmacopoeias.** *Jpn* includes the heptahydrate.

### Profile

Cefminox sodium is a cephamycin antibacterial with properties similar to those of cefoxitin (p.177). It is given intravenously as the sodium salt but doses are expressed in terms of cefminox. 1.04 g of cefminox sodium is approximately equivalent to 1 g of cefminox. A usual adult dose is 2 to 4 g daily given in divided doses.

Cefminox has an *N*-methylthiotetrazole side-chain. For adverse effects and drug interactions associated with this side-chain, see under Cefamandole, p.169.

◊ References.

1. Watanabe S, Omoto S. Pharmacology of cefminox, a new bactericidal cephamycin. *Drugs Exp Clin Res* 1990; **16:** 461–7.
2. Soriano F, *et al.* Comparative susceptibility of cefminox and cefoxitin to β-lactamases of Bacteroides spp. *J Antimicrob Chemother* 1991; **28:** 55–60.
3. Aguilar L, *et al.* Cefminox: correlation between in-vitro susceptibility and pharmacokinetics and serum bactericidal activity in healthy volunteers. *J Antimicrob Chemother* 1994; **33:** 91–101.
4. Mayama T, *et al.* Postmarketing surveillance on side-effects of cefminox sodium (Meicelin). *Int J Clin Pharmacol Ther* 1995; **33:** 149–55.
5. Hoellman DB, *et al.* In vitro activities of cefminox against anaerobic bacteria compared with those of nine other compounds. *Antimicrob Agents Chemother* 1998; **42:** 495–501.
6. Torres AJ, *et al.* Cefminox versus metronidazole plus gentamicin in intra-abdominal infections: a prospective randomized controlled clinical trial. *Infection* 2000; **28:** 318–22.

**Sodium content.** Each g of cefminox sodium contains about 1.84 mmol of sodium.

### Preparations

**Proprietary Preparations** (details are given in Part 3)
***Jpn:*** Meicelin; ***Spain:*** Alteporina†; Tencef; ***Thai.:*** Meicelin.

## Cefodizime Sodium *(BANM, rINNM)*

Cefodizima sódica; HR-221; S-771221B; THR-221; TRH-221. (Z)-7-[2-(2-Aminothiazol-4-yl)-2-methoxyiminoacetamido]-3-(5-carboxymethyl-4-methylthiazol-2-ylthiomethyl)-3-cephem-4-carboxylic acid, disodium salt.

$C_{20}H_{18}N_6Na_2O_7S_4$ = 628.6.

*CAS — 69739-16-8 (cefodizime); 86329-79-5 (cefodizime sodium).*

*ATC — J01DA25.*

**Pharmacopoeias.** In *Jpn.*

### Adverse Effects and Precautions

As for Cefotaxime, p.175.

**Sodium content.** Each g of cefodizime sodium contains about 3.2 mmol of sodium.

### Interactions

Probenecid reduces the renal clearance of cefodizime.

### Antimicrobial Action

Cefodizime has similar antimicrobial activity to that of cefotaxime (p.176) although cefodizime has no active metabolite. It has variable activity against *Citrobacter* spp., and *Pseudomonas aeruginosa* and *Bacteroides fragilis* are generally resistant.

### Pharmacokinetics

Cefodizime is given by injection as the sodium salt. Intramuscular administration of 1 g cefodizime produces peak plasma concentrations of about 60 to 75 micrograms/mL at about 1 to 1.5 hours. Immediately after intravenous administration of 1 or 2 g cefodizime mean peak plasma concentrations of 215 and 394 micrograms/mL, respectively, have been achieved. Cefodizime is about 80% bound to plasma proteins and is widely distributed into body tissues and fluids. It crosses the placenta and small amounts have been detected in breast milk. Plasma elimination is reported to be triphasic with a terminal elimination half-life of about 4 hours. The half-life is prolonged by renal impairment.

The majority of a dose is excreted unchanged in the urine; up to 80% of a dose has been recovered within 24 hours. Cefodizime is mainly excreted by glomerular filtration with some tubular secretion. Probenecid delays excretion. Cefodizime is removed by dialysis.

### Uses and Administration

Cefodizime is a third-generation cephalosporin antibacterial with uses similar to those of cefotaxime (p.176).

Cefodizime is given as the disodium salt by intramuscular injection or intravenously by injection or infusion in the treatment of susceptible infections. Doses are expressed in terms of the equivalent amount of cefodizime. 1.08 g of cefodizime sodium is approximately equivalent to 1 g of cefodizime. Adults have usually been given 1 g every 12 hours for urinary-tract infections and lower respiratory-tract infections; alternatively, a single daily dose of 2 g has been given in urinary-tract infections. Single doses over 1 g should be given intravenously. Doses may need to be reduced in patients with renal impairment (see below).

◊ References.

1. Finch RG, *et al.*, eds. Cefodizime: a third generation cephalosporin with immunomodulating properties. *J Antimicrob Chemother* 1990; **26** (suppl C): 1–134.
2. Barradell LB, Brogden RN. Cefodizime: a review of its antibacterial activity, pharmacokinetic properties and therapeutic use. *Drugs* 1992; **44:** 800–834.

**Administration in renal impairment.** Doses of cefodizime should be reduced to one-half the usual dose in renal impairment when the creatinine clearance is less than 30 mL/minute.

### Preparations

**Proprietary Preparations** (details are given in Part 3)
***Austria:*** Timecef; ***Braz.:*** Timecef†; ***Ger.:*** Opticef†; ***Irl.:*** Modivid†; ***Ital.:*** Diezime; Modivid; Timecef; ***Mex.:*** Modivid; ***Port.:*** Modivid; ***Thai.:*** Modivid†.

## Cefonicid Sodium *(BANM, USAN, rINNM)*

Cefonicid sódico; SKF-D-75073-$Z_2$; SKF-D-75073-Z (cefonicid monosodium). 7-[(R)-Mandelamido]-3-(1-sulphomethyl-1*H*-tetrazol-5-ylthiomethyl)-3-cephem-4-carboxylic acid, disodium salt.

$C_{18}H_{16}N_6Na_2O_8S_3$ = 586.5.

*CAS — 61270-58-4 (cefonicid); 61270-78-8 (cefonicid disodium); 71420-79-6 (cefonicid monosodium).*

*ATC — J01DA17.*

**Pharmacopoeias.** In *US.*

**USP 27** (Cefonicid Sodium). A white to off-white solid. Freely soluble in water, in sodium chloride 0.9%, and in glucose 5%; very slightly soluble in dehydrated alcohol; soluble in methyl alcohol. pH of a 5% solution in water is between 3.5 and 6.5. Store in airtight containers.

### Adverse Effects and Precautions

As for Cefalotin Sodium, p.168.

Cefonicid contains a substituted *N*-methylthiotetrazole side-chain, a structure associated with hypoprothrombinaemia (see Cefamandole, p.169).

**Effects on the blood.** References.

1. Riancho JA, *et al.* Life-threatening bleeding in a patient treated with cefonicid. *Ann Intern Med* 1995; **123:** 472–3.

**Effects on the liver.** References.

1. Famularo G, *et al.* Eosinophilic hepatitis associated with cefonicid therapy. *Ann Pharmacother* 2001; **35:** 1669–71.

**Sodium content.** Each g of cefonicid sodium contains about 3.4 mmol of sodium.

### Interactions

As for Cefamandole, p.170.

### Antimicrobial Action

Cefonicid sodium has an antimicrobial action and pattern of resistance similar to those of cefamandole (p.170), although it is generally less active against Gram-positive cocci.

### Pharmacokinetics

Cefonicid is given parenterally as the sodium salt. Peak plasma concentrations ranging from 67 to 126 micrograms/mL have been achieved 1 to 2 hours after a 1-g intramuscular dose. Cefonicid is more than 90% bound to plasma proteins. It has a plasma half-life of about 4.5 hours, which is prolonged in patients with renal impairment.

Therapeutic concentrations of cefonicid have been reported in a wide range of body tissues and fluids.

Up to 99% of a dose of cefonicid is excreted unchanged in the urine within 24 hours. Probenecid reduces excretion of cefonicid.

### Uses and Administration

Cefonicid is a second-generation cephalosporin antibacterial used similarly to cefamandole (p.170) in the treatment of susceptible infections and for surgical infection prophylaxis.

It is given as the sodium salt by deep intramuscular injection, or intravenously by slow injection over 3 to 5 minutes or by infusion. Doses are expressed in terms of the equivalent amount of cefonicid. 1.08 g of cefonicid sodium is approximately equivalent to 1 g of cefonicid. The usual dose is cefonicid 1 g once daily. For uncomplicated urinary-tract infections, a dose of 500 mg once daily is recommended; up to 2 g once daily has been given in severe infections. More than 1 g should not be injected intramuscularly into a single site.

For surgical infection prophylaxis, a single dose of 1 g given 1 hour before surgical incision is usually sufficient, but may be given daily for a further 2 days in prosthetic arthroplasty or open-heart surgery.

◊ References.

1. Saltiel E, Brogden RN. Cefonicid: a review of its antibacterial activity, pharmacological properties and therapeutic use. *Drugs* 1986; **32:** 222–59.

**Administration in renal impairment.** For patients with renal impairment a loading dose equivalent to cefonicid 7.5 mg/kg is recommended, followed by reduced maintenance doses according to the creatinine clearance and the severity of the infection. A dose supplement is not required after dialysis.

### Preparations

**USP 27:** Cefonicid for Injection.

**Proprietary Preparations** (details are given in Part 3)
***Belg.:*** Monocid; ***Hong Kong:*** Monocid†; ***Israel:*** Lisa; Monocef; ***Ital.:*** Abiocef; Auricid; Bacid; Biocil; Bioticic; Cefobacter; Cefodie; Cefoger; Cefok; Cefoplus; Cefosporin; Cefovis†; Chefir; Clastidin; Daycef; Delsacid; Diespor; Emidoxin; Epicef; Fonexel; Fonicef; Fonicid; Fonisal; Framecef; Ipacid; Krucef; Lampocef; Lisa; Maxid; Microcid; Modicef; Modiem; Monobios; Monobiotic; Monocid; Necid; Nokid; Pantacid; Parecid; Praticef; Raikocef; Renbiocid; Rocid; Silvercef; Sintocef; Sofarcid; Unicef†; Unicid; Valecid; ***Port.:*** Monocid; ***Spain:*** Monocid; Unidie; ***USA:*** Monocid†.

## Cefoperazone Sodium

*(BANM, USAN, rINNM)*

Cefoperazona sódica; Cefoperazonum Natricum; CP-52640-2; CP-52640 (anhydrous cefoperazone); CP-52640-3 (cefoperazone dihydrate); T-1551 (cefoperazone or cefoperazone sodium). Sodium (7R)-7-[(R)-2-(4-ethyl-2,3-dioxopiperazin-1-ylcarboxamido)-2-(4-hydroxyphenyl)acetamido]-3-[(1-methyl-1*H*-tetrazol-5-yl)thiomethyl]-3-cephem-4-carboxylate.

$C_{25}H_{26}N_9NaO_8S_2$ = 667.6.

*CAS — 62893-19-0 (cefoperazone); 62893-20-3 (cefoperazone sodium).*

*ATC — J01DA32.*

**Pharmacopoeias.** In *Chin., Eur.* (see p.vi), *Jpn, Pol.,* and *US.*

**Ph. Eur. 5.0** (Cefoperazone Sodium). A white or slightly yellow, hygroscopic, powder. If crystalline it exhibits polymorphism. Freely soluble in water; slightly soluble in alcohol; soluble in methyl alcohol. A 25% solution in water has a pH of 4.5 to 6.5. Store in airtight containers at a temperature of 2° to 8°. Protect from light.

**USP 27** (Cefoperazone Sodium). A white to pale buff crystalline powder. Freely soluble in water and in methyl alcohol; slightly soluble in dehydrated alcohol; insoluble in acetone, in ether, and in ethyl acetate. pH of a 25% solution in water is between 4.5 and 6.5. Store in airtight containers.

**Incompatibility.** As with most beta lactams, admixture of cefoperazone sodium with aminoglycosides is not recommended because of the potential for inactivation of either drug.

There have been reports of incompatibility with other drugs including diltiazem,[1] doxorubicin,[2] pentamidine,[3] perphenazine,[4] pethidine,[5] promethazine,[6] and remifentanil.[7]

1. Gayed AA, *et al.* Visual compatibility of diltiazem injection with various diluents and medications during simulated Y-site injection. *Am J Health-Syst Pharm* 1995; **52:** 516–20.
2. Trissel LA, *et al.* Compatibility of doxorubicin hydrochloride liposome injection with selected other drugs during simulated Y-site administration. *Am J Health-Syst Pharm* 1997; **54:** 2708–13.
3. Lewis JD, El-Gendy A. Cephalosporin-pentamidine isethionate incompatibilities. *Am J Health-Syst Pharm* 1996; **53:** 1461–2.
4. Gasca M, *et al.* Visual compatibility of perphenazine with various antimicrobials during simulated Y-site injection. *Am J Hosp Pharm* 1987; **44:** 574–5.
5. Nieves-Cordero AL, *et al.* Compatibility of narcotic analgesic solutions with various antibiotics during simulated Y-site injection. *Am J Hosp Pharm* 1985; **42:** 1108–9.
6. Scott SM. Incompatibility of cefoperazone and promethazine. *Am J Hosp Pharm* 1990; **47:** 519.
7. Trissel LA, *et al.* Compatibility of remifentanil hydrochloride with selected drugs during simulated Y-site administration. *Am J Health-Syst Pharm* 1997; **54:** 2192–6.

### Adverse Effects and Precautions

As for Cefalotin Sodium, p.168.

Like cefotaxime (p.175), cefoperazone has the potential for colonisation and superinfection with resistant organisms. Changes in bowel flora may be more marked than with cefotaxime because of the greater biliary excretion of cefoperazone; diarrhoea may occur more often.

Cefoperazone contains an *N*-methylthiotetrazole side-chain, a structure associated with hypoprothrombinaemia (see Cefamandole, p.169). Hypoprothrombinaemia has been reported in patients treated with cefoperazone and has rarely been associated with bleeding episodes. Prothrombin time should be monitored in patients at risk of hypoprothrombinaemia and vitamin K used if necessary.

**Sodium content.** Each g of cefoperazone sodium contains about 1.5 mmol of sodium.

## Interactions

As for Cefamandole, p.170.

Unlike many other cephalosporins, probenecid has no effect on the renal clearance of cefoperazone.

## Antimicrobial Action

Cefoperazone has antimicrobial activity similar to that of ceftazidime (p.181), although it is slightly less active against some Enterobacteriaceae. It has good activity against *Pseudomonas aeruginosa*, but is less active than ceftazidime.

Cefoperazone is more susceptible than cefotaxime to hydrolysis by certain beta-lactamases.

Activity, particularly against Enterobacteriaceae and *Bacteroides* spp. has been enhanced in the presence of the beta-lactamase inhibitor sulbactam; resistant *Ps. aeruginosa* are not sensitive to the combination.

◊ References.

1. Fass RJ, *et al.* In vitro activities of cefoperazone and sulbactam singly and in combination against cefoperazone-resistant members of the family Enterobacteriaceae and nonfermenters. *Antimicrob Agents Chemother* 1990; **34:** 2256–9.
2. Clark RB, *et al.* Multicentre study on antibiotic susceptibilities of anaerobic bacteria to cefoperazone-sulbactam and other antimicrobial agents. *J Antimicrob Chemother* 1992; **29:** 57–67.

## Pharmacokinetics

Cefoperazone is given parenterally as the sodium salt. After intramuscular doses equivalent to cefoperazone 1 or 2 g, peak plasma concentrations of 65 and 97 micrograms/mL have been reported after 1 to 2 hours. The plasma half-life of cefoperazone is about 2 hours, but may be prolonged in neonates and in patients with hepatic or biliary-tract disease. Cefoperazone is 82 to 93% bound to plasma proteins, depending on the concentration.

Cefoperazone is widely distributed in body tissues and fluids, although penetration into the CSF is generally poor. It crosses the placenta, and low concentrations have been detected in breast milk.

Cefoperazone is excreted mainly in the bile where it rapidly achieves high concentrations. Urinary excretion is primarily by glomerular filtration. Up to 30% of a dose is excreted unchanged in the urine within 12 to 24 hours; this proportion may be increased in patients with hepatic or biliary disease. Cefoperazone A, a degradation product less active than cefoperazone, has been found only rarely *in vivo*.

## Uses and Administration

Cefoperazone is a third-generation cephalosporin antibiotic used similarly to ceftazidime (p.181) in the treatment of susceptible infections, especially those due to *Pseudomonas* spp. It is not recommended for the treatment of meningitis because of poor penetration into the CSF.

Cefoperazone is given as the sodium salt by deep intramuscular injection or intravenously by intermittent or continuous infusion. Doses are expressed in terms of the equivalent amount of cefoperazone. 1.03 g of cefoperazone sodium is approximately equivalent to 1 g of cefoperazone. The usual dose for adults is 2 to 4 g daily in 2 divided doses. In severe infections, up to 12 g daily in 2 to 4 divided doses may be given.

For details of dosage in patients with hepatic and renal impairment, see below.

If cefoperazone is used with an aminoglycoside, the drugs should be administered separately.

Cefoperazone has also been given with the beta-lactamase inhibitor sulbactam.

**Administration in hepatic and renal impairment.** In general, the dose of cefoperazone should not exceed 4 g daily in patients with liver disease or biliary obstruction or 1 to 2 g daily in those with both hepatic and renal impairment; if higher doses are used plasma concentrations of cefoperazone should be monitored.

## Preparations

***USP 27:*** Cefoperazone for Injection; Cefoperazone Injection.

**Proprietary Preparations** (details are given in Part 3)
***Arg.:*** Cefobid; ***Austria:*** Cefobid; ***Braz.:*** Cefazone; Cefobid†; Neoperazona; ***Fr.:*** Cefobis†; ***Ger.:*** Cefobis†; ***Hong Kong:*** Cefobid; Cefozone†; ***India:*** Cefomycin; Magnamycin; ***Ital.:*** Bioperazone; Cefazone†; Cefogram†; Cefoneg; Cefoper; Cefosint†; Dardum; Farecef; Ipazone; Kefazon†; Novobiocyl; Perocef†; Prontokef†; Tomabef; Zoncef; ***Jpn:*** Cefobid; ***Malaysia:*** Cefobid; Shinfomycin; ***Singapore:*** Cefobid; Cefozone; Dardum; Medocef†; ***Spain:*** Cefobid; ***Thai.:*** Cefobid; Cefozone; Medocef; ***USA:*** Cefobid.

**Multi-ingredient:** ***Arg.:*** Sulperazon; ***Chile:*** Sulperazon; ***Hong Kong:*** Sulperazon; ***Malaysia:*** Sulperazon; ***Thai.:*** Sulperazon.

---

## Ceforanide *(BAN, USAN, rINN)*

BL-S786; Ceforanida. 7-[2-(α-Amino-*o*-tolyl)acetamido]-3-(1-carboxymethyl-1*H*-tetrazol-5-ylthiomethyl)-3-cephem-4-carboxylic acid.

$C_{20}H_{21}N_7O_6S_2$ = 519.6.
*CAS — 60925-61-3.*

**Pharmacopoeias.** In *US*.

**USP 27** (Ceforanide). A white to off-white powder. Practically insoluble in water, in chloroform, in ether, and in methyl alcohol; very soluble in 1N sodium hydroxide. pH of a 5% suspension in water is between 2.5 and 4.5. Store in airtight containers.

### Profile

Ceforanide is a second-generation cephalosporin antibacterial with actions and uses similar to those of cefamandole (p.169), although it is reported to be less active *in vitro* against some bacteria, including staphylococci and *Haemophilus influenzae*. It is used in the treatment of susceptible infections and for surgical infection prophylaxis.

It is given as the lysine salt ($C_{26}H_{35}N_9O_8S_2$ = 665.7) but doses are expressed in terms of the equivalent amount of ceforanide. 1.28 g of ceforanide lysine is approximately equivalent to 1 g of ceforanide. It is given by deep intramuscular injection, or intravenously by slow injection over 3 to 5 minutes or by infusion. The usual adult dose is 1 to 2 g every 12 hours. Children may be given 20 mg/kg daily in 2 divided doses. For surgical infection prophylaxis, a dose of 1 to 2 g intravenously 1 hour before surgical incision is used in adults.

Ceforanide contains a substituted *N*-methylthiotetrazole side-chain, a structure associated with hypoprothrombinaemia and alcohol intolerance (see Cefamandole, p.169). Probenecid does not affect the renal excretion of ceforanide.

◊ References.

1. Campoli-Richards DM, *et al.* Ceforanide: a review of its antibacterial activity, pharmacokinetic properties and clinical efficacy. *Drugs* 1987; **34:** 411–37.

### Preparations

***USP 27:*** Ceforanide for Injection.

**Proprietary Preparations** (details are given in Part 3)
***Belg.:*** Precef; ***Gr.:*** Radacef.

---

## Cefoselis Sulfate *(rINNM)*

Cefoselis Sulphate; FK-037. (−)-5-Amino-2-({(6*R*,7*R*)-7-[2-(2-amino-4-thiazolyl)glyoxylamido]-2-carboxy-8-oxo-5-thia-1-azabicyclo[4.2.0]oct-2-en-3-yl}methyl)-1-(2-hydroxyethyl)pyrazolium hydroxide, inner salt, $7^2$-(*Z*)-(*O*-methyloxime) sulfate.

$C_{19}H_{22}N_8O_6S_2, H_2SO_4$ = 620.6.
*CAS — 122841-10-5 (cefoselis); 122841-12-7 (cefoselis sulfate).*

**Pharmacopoeias.** In *Jpn*.

### Profile

Cefoselis is a cephalosporin antibacterial used in the treatment of susceptible bacterial infections. It is given as the sulfate and doses are expressed in terms of cefoselis. 1.19 g of cefoselis sulfate is approximately equivalent to 1 g of cefoselis. It is given by intravenous infusion in a usual dose of 1 to 2 g daily in 2 divided doses. For severe infections, up to 4 g daily may be given.

### Preparations

**Proprietary Preparations** (details are given in Part 3)
***Jpn:*** Wincef.

---

## Cefotaxime Sodium *(BANM, USAN, rINNM)*

Cefotaxima sódica; Cefotaximum Natricum; CTX; HR-756; RU-24756. Sodium (7*R*)-7-[(*Z*)-2-(2-aminothiazol-4-yl)-2-(methoxyimino)acetamido]cephalosporanate; Sodium (7*R*)-3-acetoxymethyl-7-[(*Z*)-2-(2-aminothiazol-4-yl)-2-(methoxyimino)acetamido]-3-cephem-4-carboxylate.

$C_{16}H_{16}N_5NaO_7S_2$ = 477.4.
*CAS — 63527-52-6 (cefotaxime); 64485-93-4 (cefotaxime sodium).*
*ATC — J01DA10.*

**Pharmacopoeias.** In *Chin.*, *Eur.* (see p.vi), *Jpn*, *Pol.*, and *US*.

**Ph. Eur. 5.0** (Cefotaxime Sodium). A white or slightly yellow, hygroscopic, powder. Freely soluble in water; sparingly soluble in methyl alcohol. A 10% solution in water has a pH of between 4.5 and 6.5. Store in airtight containers at a temperature not exceeding 30°. Protect from light.

**USP 27** (Cefotaxime Sodium). An off-white to pale yellow crystalline powder. Freely soluble in water; practically insoluble in organic solvents. pH of a 10% solution in water is between 4.5 and 6.5. Store in airtight containers.

**Incompatibility.** Cefotaxime sodium has been reported to be incompatible with alkaline solutions such as sodium bicarbonate. The manufacturers recommend that it should be administered separately from aminoglycosides.

### Adverse Effects and Precautions

As for Cefalotin Sodium, p.168. Arrhythmias have been associated with rapid bolus administration through a central venous catheter in a few cases.

The broad-spectrum third-generation cephalosporins have the potential for colonisation and superinfection with resistant organisms such as *Pseudomonas aeruginosa*, *Enterobacter* spp., *Candida*, and enterococci, at various sites in the body, although the incidence has generally been low with cefotaxime. Changes in bowel flora are a predisposing factor and have been more marked with cefoperazone and ceftriaxone, possibly because of their greater biliary excretion. Pseudomembranous colitis, associated with *Clostridium difficile* infection, may occasionally be seen with any of the third-generation cephalosporins.

◊ Reviews on adverse effects associated with third-generation cephalosporins.

1. Neu HC. Third generation cephalosporins: safety profiles after 10 years of clinical use. *J Clin Pharmacol* 1990; **30:** 396–403.
2. Fekety FR. Safety of parenteral third-generation cephalosporins. *Am J Med* 1990; **88** (suppl 4A): 38S–44S.

**Antibiotic-associated colitis.** It has been suggested[1] that cefotaxime is associated with an increased risk of *Clostridium difficile* diarrhoea in elderly patients; however, the manufacturer[2] has disputed this, arguing that cefotaxime compares favourably with alternative third-generation cephalosporins.

1. Impallomeni M, *et al.* Increased risk of diarrhoea caused by Clostridium difficile in elderly patients receiving cefotaxime. *BMJ* 1995; **311:** 1345–6.
2. Rothschild E, *et al.* Risk of diarrhoea due to Clostridium difficile during cefotaxime treatment. *BMJ* 1996; **312:** 778.

**Breast feeding.** Although cefotaxime is excreted in breast milk in small amounts,[1] no adverse effects have been observed in breast-fed infants whose mothers were receiving cefotaxime, and the American Academy of Pediatrics considers[2] that it is therefore usually compatible with breast feeding.

1. Kafetzis DA, *et al.* Passage of cephalosporins and amoxicillin into the breast milk. *Acta Paediatr Scand* 1981; **70:** 285–8.
2. American Academy of Pediatrics. The transfer of drugs and other chemicals into human milk. *Pediatrics* 2001; **108:** 776–89. Correction. *ibid.*; 1029. Also available at: http://aappolicy.aappublications.org/cgi/content/full/pediatrics%3b108/3/776 (accessed 25/05/04)

**Sodium content.** Each g of cefotaxime sodium contains about 2.09 mmol of sodium.

### Interactions

As for many cephalosporins, probenecid reduces the renal clearance of cefotaxime, resulting in higher and prolonged plasma concentrations of cefotaxime and its desacetyl metabolite.

**Antibacterials.** The total body clearance of cefotaxime has been reduced in patients with normal and reduced renal function by the ureidopenicillins *azlocillin*[1] or *mezlocillin*.[2] Doses of cefotaxime may need to be reduced if either of these penicillins is being given. Encephalopathy with focal motor status and generalised convulsions have been reported in a patient with renal failure given cefotaxime and high doses of azlocillin.[3]

1. Kampf D, *et al.* Kinetic interactions between azlocillin, cefotaxime, and cefotaxime metabolites in normal and impaired renal function. *Clin Pharmacol Ther* 1984; **35:** 214–20.

2. Rodondi LC, *et al.* Influence of coadministration on the pharmacokinetics of mezlocillin and cefotaxime in healthy volunteers and in patients with renal failure. *Clin Pharmacol Ther* 1989; **45:** 527–34.

3. Wroe SJ, *et al.* Focal motor status epilepticus following treatment with azlocillin and cefotaxime. *Med Toxicol* 1987; **2:** 233–4.

## Antimicrobial Action

Cefotaxime is a third-generation cephalosporin. It has a bactericidal action similar to cefamandole, but a broader spectrum of activity. It is highly stable to hydrolysis by most beta-lactamases and has greater activity than first- or second-generation cephalosporins against Gram-negative bacteria. Although cefotaxime is generally considered to have slightly less activity than first-generation cephalosporins against Gram-positive bacteria, many streptococci are very sensitive to it.

Desacetylcefotaxime is an active metabolite of cefotaxime and there may be additive or synergistic effects against some species.

*Spectrum of activity.* Among Gram-negative bacteria, cefotaxime is active *in vitro* against many Enterobacteriaceae including *Citrobacter* and *Enterobacter* spp., *Escherichia coli*, *Klebsiella* spp., both indole-positive and indole-negative *Proteus*, *Providencia*, *Salmonella*, *Serratia*, *Shigella*, and *Yersinia* spp. Other susceptible Gram-negative bacteria, including penicillin-resistant strains, are *Haemophilus influenzae*, *Moraxella catarrhalis* (*Branhamella catarrhalis*), *Neisseria gonorrhoeae*, and *N. meningitidis*. *Brucella melitensis* is also reported to be moderately sensitive. Some strains of *Pseudomonas* spp. are moderately susceptible to cefotaxime, but most are resistant. Desacetylcefotaxime is active against many of these Gram-negative bacteria, but not against *Pseudomonas* spp.

Among Gram-positive bacteria, cefotaxime is active against staphylococci and streptococci. *Staphylococcus aureus*, including penicillinase-producing strains but not meticillin-resistant *Staph. aureus*, is sensitive. *Staph. epidermidis* is also sensitive but penicillinase-producing strains are resistant. *Streptococcus agalactiae* (group B streptococci), *Str. pneumoniae*, and *Str. pyogenes* (group A streptococci) are all very sensitive although truly penicillin-resistant pneumococci are apparently not sensitive. Enterococci and *Listeria monocytogenes* are resistant.

Cefotaxime is active against some anaerobic bacteria. *Bacteroides fragilis* may be moderately sensitive, but many strains are resistant; synergy has been demonstrated with desacetylcefotaxime *in vitro*. *Clostridium perfringens* is sensitive, but most *Cl. difficile* are resistant.

Other organisms sensitive to cefotaxime include the spirochaete *Borrelia burgdorferi* and *Haemophilus ducreyi*.

*Activity with other antimicrobials.* In addition to possible synergy or additive effects with desacetylcefotaxime, the activity of cefotaxime may be enhanced by aminoglycosides such as gentamicin; synergy has been demonstrated *in vitro* against Gram-negative bacteria including *Pseudomonas aeruginosa*. There have also been reports of enhanced activity *in vitro* with other antibacterials including fosfomycin and ciprofloxacin and variable results with penicillins.

*Resistance* may develop during treatment with cefotaxime due to derepression of chromosomally mediated beta-lactamases, and has been reported particularly in *Enterobacter* spp., with multiresistant strains emerging during treatment. This type of resistance has also developed in other bacteria including *Citrobacter*, *Serratia*, and *Pseudomonas* spp. Another mechanism of cefotaxime resistance is the development of plasma-mediated, extended-spectrum beta-lactamases, and this has occurred in *Klebsiella* spp. and also other Enterobacteriaceae. Resistance in *Str. pneumoniae* is due to the production of altered penicillin-binding proteins.

◊ References to the antimicrobial activity of cefotaxime and other third-generation cephalosporins, including the problem of bacterial resistance.

1. Neu HC. Pathophysiologic basis for the use of third-generation cephalosporins. *Am J Med* 1990; **88** (suppl 4A): 3S–11S.
2. Chow JW, *et al.* Enterobacter bacteremia: clinical features and emergence of antibiotic resistance during therapy. *Ann Intern Med* 1991; **115:** 585–90.
3. Sanders CC. New β-lactams: new problems for the internist. *Ann Intern Med* 1991; **115:** 650–1.
4. Thomson KS, *et al.* High-level resistance to cefotaxime and ceftazidime in Klebsiella pneumoniae isolates from Cleveland, Ohio. *Antimicrob Agents Chemother* 1991; **35:** 1001–3.
5. Piddock LJV, *et al.* Prevalence and mechanism of resistance to 'third-generation' cephalosporins in clinically relevant isolates of Enterobacteriaceae from 43 hospitals in the UK, 1990-1991. *J Antimicrob Chemother* 1997; **39:** 177–87.

## Pharmacokinetics

Cefotaxime is given by injection as the sodium salt. It is rapidly absorbed after intramuscular injection and mean peak plasma concentrations of about 12 and 20 micrograms/mL have been reported 30 minutes after doses of 0.5 and 1 g of cefotaxime, respectively. Immediately after intravenous injection of 0.5, 1, or 2 g of cefotaxime, mean peak plasma concentrations of 38, 102, and 215 micrograms/mL, respectively, have been achieved with concentrations ranging from about 1 to 3 micrograms/mL after 4 hours. The plasma half-life of cefotaxime is about 1 hour and that of the active metabolite desacetylcefotaxime about 1.5 hours; half-lives are increased in neonates and in patients with severe renal impairment, especially those of the metabolite, and a reduction in dosage may be necessary. The effects of liver disease on clearance of cefotaxime and its metabolite have been variable, but in general dosage adjustment has not been considered necessary. About 40% of cefotaxime is reported to be bound to plasma proteins.

Cefotaxime and desacetylcefotaxime are widely distributed in body tissues and fluids; therapeutic concentrations are achieved in the CSF particularly when the meninges are inflamed. Cefotaxime crosses the placenta and low concentrations have been detected in breast milk.

Following partial metabolism in the liver to desacetylcefotaxime and inactive metabolites, elimination is mainly by the kidneys and about 40 to 60% of a dose has been recovered unchanged in the urine within 24 hours; a further 20% is excreted as the desacetyl metabolite. Relatively high concentrations of cefotaxime and desacetylcefotaxime are achieved in bile and about 20% of a dose has been recovered in the faeces.

Probenecid competes for renal tubular secretion with cefotaxime resulting in higher and prolonged plasma concentrations of cefotaxime and its desacetyl metabolite. Cefotaxime and its metabolites are removed by haemodialysis.

When microbiological assays have been used, reported pharmacokinetic values may relate to cefotaxime plus its active metabolite, desacetylcefotaxime.

**Hepatic impairment.** References.

1. Höffken G, *et al.* Pharmacokinetics of cefotaxime and desacetyl-cefotaxime in cirrhosis of the liver. *Chemotherapy* 1984; **30:** 7–17.
2. Graninger W, *et al.* Cefotaxime and desacetyl-cefotaxime blood levels in hepatic dysfunction. *J Antimicrob Chemother* 1984; **14** (suppl B): 143–6.
3. Hary L, *et al.* The pharmacokinetics of ceftriaxone and cefotaxime in cirrhotic patients with ascites. *Eur J Clin Pharmacol* 1989; **36:** 613–16.
4. Ko RJ, *et al.* Pharmacokinetics of cefotaxime and desacetylcefotaxime in patients with liver disease. *Antimicrob Agents Chemother* 1991; **35:** 1376–80.

**Renal impairment.** References.

1. Matzke GR, *et al.* Cefotaxime and desacetyl cefotaxime kinetics in renal impairment. *Clin Pharmacol Ther* 1985; **38:** 31–6.
2. Paap CM, *et al.* Pharmacokinetics of cefotaxime and its active metabolite in children with renal dysfunction. *Antimicrob Agents Chemother* 1991; **35:** 1879–83.
3. Paap CM, *et al.* Cefotaxime and metabolite disposition in two pediatric continuous ambulatory peritoneal dialysis patients. *Ann Pharmacother* 1992; **26:** 341–3.
4. Paap CM, Nahata MC. The relation between type of renal disease and renal drug clearance in children. *Eur J Clin Pharmacol* 1993; **44:** 195–7.

## Uses and Administration

Cefotaxime is a third-generation cephalosporin antibacterial used in the treatment of infections due to susceptible organisms, especially serious and life-threatening infections. They include brain abscess, endocarditis, gonorrhoea, intensive care (selective parenteral and enteral antisepsis regimens), Lyme disease, meningitis, peritonitis (primary or spontaneous), pneumonia, septicaemia, and typhoid fever. It is also used for surgical infection prophylaxis. For details of these infections and their treatment, see under Choice of Antibacterial, p.120.

*Administration and dosage.* Cefotaxime is given as the sodium salt by deep intramuscular injection or intravenously by slow injection over 3 to 5 minutes or by infusion over 20 to 60 minutes. Doses are expressed in terms of the equivalent amount of cefotaxime. 1.05 g of cefotaxime sodium is approximately equivalent to 1 g of cefotaxime. It is usually given in doses of 2 to 6 g daily in 2 to 4 divided doses to adults. In severe infections up to 12 g may be given daily by the intravenous route in up to 6 divided doses; pseudomonal infections usually require more than 6 g daily, but a cephalosporin with greater antipseudomonal activity, such as ceftazidime, is preferable. Children may be given 100 to 150 mg/kg (50 mg/kg for neonates) daily in 2 to 4 divided doses, increased in severe infections to 200 mg/kg (150 to 200 mg/kg for neonates) daily if necessary.

For details of reduced doses to be used in patients with severe renal impairment, see below.

In the treatment of gonorrhoea, a single dose of 0.5 or 1 g of cefotaxime is given.

For surgical infection prophylaxis, 1 g is given 30 to 90 minutes before surgery. At caesarean section, 1 g is given intravenously to the mother as soon as the umbilical cord is clamped and two further doses intramuscularly or intravenously 6 and 12 hours later.

Cefotaxime may be used with an aminoglycoside as synergy may occur against some Gram-negative organisms, but the drugs should be administered separately. It has sometimes been used with another beta lactam to broaden the spectrum of activity. Cefotaxime has also been used with metronidazole in the treatment of mixed aerobic-anaerobic infections.

◊ General references to third-generation cephalosporins.

1. Neu HC, *et al.*, eds. Third-generation cephalosporins: a decade of progress in the treatment of severe infections. *Am J Med* 1990; **88** (suppl 4A): 1S–45S.

◊ General references to cefotaxime.

1. Todd PA, Brogden RN. Cefotaxime: an update of its pharmacology and therapeutic use. *Drugs* 1990; **40:** 608–51.
2. Gentry LO. Cefotaxime and prophylaxis: new approaches with a proven agent. *Am J Med* 1990; **88** (suppl 4A): 32S–37S.
3. Davies A, Speller DCE, eds. Cefotaxime—recent clinical investigations. *J Antimicrob Chemother* 1990; **26** (suppl A): 1–83.
4. Brogden RN, Spencer CM. Cefotaxime: a reappraisal of its antibacterial activity and pharmacokinetic properties, and a review of its therapeutic efficacy when administered twice daily for the treatment of mild to moderate infections. *Drugs* 1997; **53:** 483–510.

**Administration in renal impairment.** Doses of cefotaxime should be reduced in severe renal impairment; after an initial loading dose of 1 g for adults, halving the dose while maintaining the usual frequency of dosing has been suggested.

## Preparations

***BP 2003:*** Cefotaxime Injection;
***USP 27:*** Cefotaxime for Injection; Cefotaxime Injection.

**Proprietary Preparations** (details are given in Part 3)

***Arg.:*** Cefacolin; Terasep; Tizoxim; ***Austral.:*** Claforan; ***Austria:*** Claforan; ***Belg.:*** Claforan; ***Braz.:*** Ceforan; Cefotax†; Claforan†; Clafordil; Kefoxin; ***Canad.:*** Claforan; ***Chile:*** Grifotaxima; ***Denm.:*** Claforan; ***Fin.:*** Claforan; ***Fr.:*** Claforan; ***Ger.:*** Claforan; ***Gr.:*** Claforan; Letynol; Molelant; Naspor; Phacocef; Spirosine; Stoparen; ***Hong Kong:*** Claforan; Valoran; ***India:*** Biotax; Claforan; Lyforan; Omnatax; Zetaxim; ***Irl.:*** Claforan; ***Israel:*** Claforan; ***Ital.:*** Aximad; Batixim; Claforan; Refotax; Spectrocef; Zariviz; Zimanel; ***Malaysia:*** Claforan; ***Mex.:*** Benaxima; Biosint; Cefaxim†; Cefoclin†; Cefotex†; Cefradil†; Claforan; Fotexina; Sepsilem; Taporin; Tirotax; Viken; ***Neth.:*** Claforan; ***Norw.:*** Claforan; ***NZ:*** Claforan; ***Port.:*** Ralopar; Totam; ***S.Afr.:*** Claforan; Klafotaxim; Oritaxim†; Reftax; Totam; ***Singapore:*** Clacef; Claforan; ***Spain:*** Claforan; Primafen†; ***Swed.:*** Claforan; ***Switz.:*** Claforan; ***Thai.:*** Biotaxime; Cefomic; Ceforan; Cefotax; Ceftaran; Claforan; Claraxim; Fortax; Fotax; Oritaxime; Valoran; ***UAE:*** Primocef; ***UK:*** Claforan; ***USA:*** Claforan.

## Cefotetan (BAN)

ICI-156834; YM-09330. (7S)-7-[(4-Carbamoylcarboxymethylene-1,3-dithietan-2-yl)carboxamido]-7-methoxy-3-[(1-methyl-1H-tetrazol-5-yl)thiomethyl]-3-cephem-4-carboxylic acid.

$C_{17}H_{17}N_7O_8S_4$ = 575.6.
*CAS — 69712-56-7.*
*ATC — J01DA14.*

**Pharmacopoeias.** In *Jpn* and *US.*

**USP 27** (Cefotetan). Store in airtight containers.

## Cefotetan Disodium (BANM, USAN, rINNM)

Cefotetán disódico; ICI-156834; YM-09330 (both cefotetan or disodium salt). (7S)-7-[(4-Carbamoylcarboxymethylene-1,3-dithietan-2-yl)carboxamido]-7-methoxy-3-[(1-methyl-1H-tetrazol-5-yl)thiomethyl]-3-cephem-4-carboxylic acid, disodium salt.

$C_{17}H_{15}N_7Na_2O_8S_4$ = 619.6.
*CAS — 74356-00-6.*
*ATC — J01DA14.*

**Pharmacopoeias.** In *US.*

**USP 27** (Cefotetan Disodium). pH of a 10% solution in water is between 4.0 and 6.5. Store in airtight containers.

**Incompatibility and stability.** There may be incompatibility with aminoglycosides. Precipitation has been reported with promethazine hydrochloride.

References.

1. Das Gupta V, *et al.* Chemical stability of cefotetan disodium in 5% dextrose and 0.9% sodium chloride injections. *J Clin Pharm Ther* 1990; **15:** 109–14.
2. Erickson SH, Ulici D. Incompatibility of cefotetan disodium and promethazine hydrochloride. *Am J Health-Syst Pharm* 1995; **52:** 1347.

### Adverse Effects and Precautions

As for Cefalotin Sodium, p.168.

Cefotetan contains an *N*-methylthiotetrazole side-chain and like cefamandole (p.169) has the potential to cause hypoprothrombinaemia and bleeding.

Cefotetan, especially at high doses, may interfere with the Jaffé method of measuring creatinine concentrations to produce falsely elevated values; this should be borne in mind when measuring renal function.

**Effects on the blood.** Reviews of haemolytic anaemia associated with cefotetan.

1. Moes GS, MacPherson BR. Cefotetan-induced hemolytic anemia: a case report and review of the literature. *Arch Pathol Lab Med* 2000; **124:** 1344–6.
2. Viraraghavan R, *et al.* Cefotetan-induced haemolytic anaemia: a review of 85 cases. *Adverse Drug React Toxicol Rev* 2002; **21:** 101–7.

**Sodium content.** Each g of cefotetan disodium contains about 3.2 mmol of sodium.

### Interactions

As for Cefamandole, p.170.

### Antimicrobial Action

Cefotetan is a cephamycin antibiotic with a mode of action and spectrum of activity similar to those of cefoxitin (p.177). It is generally much more active *in vitro* than cefoxitin against the Gram-negative Enterobacteriaceae, but has similar activity against *Bacteroides fragilis* and may be less active against some other *Bacteroides* spp.

### Pharmacokinetics

After intramuscular injection of cefotetan, peak plasma concentrations of about 70 micrograms/mL at 1 hour and 90 micrograms/mL at 3 hours have been reported after doses of 1 and 2 g, respectively. The plasma half-life of cefotetan is usually in the range of 3.0 to 4.6 hours and is prolonged in patients with renal impairment. About 88% of cefotetan may be bound to plasma proteins, depending on the plasma concentration.

Cefotetan is widely distributed in body tissues and fluids. It crosses the placenta and low concentrations have been detected in breast milk. High concentrations are achieved in bile.

Cefotetan is excreted in the urine, primarily by glomerular filtration, as unchanged drug; 50 to 80% of a dose has been recovered in the urine in 24 hours and high concentrations are achieved. Small amounts of the tautomeric form of cefotetan have been detected in both plasma and urine.

Biliary excretion of cefotetan probably accounts for nonrenal clearance.

Some cefotetan is removed by dialysis.

◊ References.

1. Martin C, *et al.* Clinical pharmacokinetics of cefotetan. *Clin Pharmacokinet* 1994; **26:** 248–58.

### Uses and Administration

Cefotetan is a cephamycin antibacterial generally classified with the second-generation cephalosporins and used similarly to cefoxitin (p.178) in the treatment and prophylaxis of anaerobic and mixed bacterial infections, especially intra-abdominal and pelvic infections.

It is given as the disodium salt by deep intramuscular injection or intravenously by slow injection over 3 to 5 minutes or by infusion. Doses are expressed in terms of the equivalent amount of cefotetan. 1.08 g of cefotetan disodium is approximately equivalent to 1 g of cefotetan. The usual dose for adults is 1 or 2 g every 12 hours. For the treatment of life-threatening infections, 3 g every 12 hours may be given intravenously. Doses of cefotetan should be reduced in patients with moderate to severe renal impairment (see below).

For infection prophylaxis during surgical procedures, an intravenous dose of 1 or 2 g is given 30 to 60 minutes before surgery or, in caesarean section, as soon as the umbilical cord is clamped.

**Administration in renal impairment.** Dosage of cefotetan should be reduced in patients with moderate to severe renal impairment. The US manufacturer gives the following dosing guidelines based on the patient's creatinine clearance (CC):

- CC 10 to 30 mL/minute: the usual dose every 24 hours or one-half the usual dose every 12 hours
- CC less than 10 mL/minute: the usual dose every 48 hours or one-quarter the usual dose every 12 hours

In patients undergoing haemodialysis, one-quarter the usual dose may be given every 24 hours on days between dialysis and one-half the usual dose on the day of dialysis.

### Preparations

***USP 27:*** Cefotetan for Injection; Cefotetan Injection.

**Proprietary Preparations** (details are given in Part 3)
***Austral.:*** Apatef; ***Belg.:*** Apacef; ***Canad.:*** Cefotan; ***Fr.:*** Apacef; ***Ital.:*** Apatef; ***Jpn:*** Yamatetan; ***NZ:*** Apatef; ***Port.:*** Apatef; ***USA:*** Cefotan.

## Cefotiam Hydrochloride (BANM, USAN, rINNM)

Abbott-48999; CGP-14221E (cefotiam or hydrochloride); Hidrocloruro de cefotiam; SCE-963. 7-[2-(2-Amino-1,3-thiazol-4-yl)acetamido]-3-[1-(2-dimethylaminoethyl)-1H-tetrazol-5-ylthiomethyl]-3-cephem-4-carboxylic acid dihydrochloride.

$C_{18}H_{23}N_9O_4S_3,2HCl$ = 598.6.
*CAS — 61622-34-2 (cefotiam); 66309-69-1 (cefotiam hydrochloride).*
*ATC — J01DA19.*

**Pharmacopoeias.** In *Jpn* and *US. Jpn* also includes cefotiam hexetil hydrochloride.

**USP 27** (Cefotiam Hydrochloride). Store in airtight containers.

### Profile

Cefotiam is a third-generation cephalosporin antibacterial with actions and uses similar to those of cefamandole (p.169). It is given intravenously or intramuscularly as the hydrochloride but doses are expressed in terms of the base. 1.14 g of cefotiam hydrochloride is approximately equivalent to 1 g of cefotiam. The usual dose is the equivalent of up to 6 g of cefotiam daily in divided doses, according to the severity of the infection.

Cefotiam hexetil hydrochloride, a prodrug of cefotiam, is given by mouth in doses equivalent to 200 to 400 mg of cefotiam twice daily.

◊ References.

1. Brogard JM, *et al.* Clinical pharmacokinetics of cefotiam. *Clin Pharmacokinet* 1989; **17:** 163–74.

### Preparations

***USP 27:*** Cefotiam for Injection.

**Proprietary Preparations** (details are given in Part 3)
***Austria:*** Spizef; ***Fr.:*** Taketiam; Texodil; ***Ger.:*** Spizef; ***Hong Kong:*** Ceradolan†; ***Jpn:*** Pansporin; ***Singapore:*** Ceradolan; ***Thai.:*** Ceradolan.

# Cefoxitin Sodium (BANM, USAN, rINNM)

Cefoxitina sódica; Cefoxitinum Natricum; L-620388; MK-306. Sodium 3-carbamoyloxymethyl-7-methoxy-7-[2-(2-thienyl)acetamido]-3-cephem-4-carboxylate.

$C_{16}H_{16}N_3NaO_7S_2$ = 449.4.
*CAS — 35607-66-0 (cefoxitin); 33564-30-6 (cefoxitin sodium).*
*ATC — J01DA05.*

**Pharmacopoeias.** In *Eur.* (see p.vi), *Jpn, Pol.,* and *US.*

**Ph. Eur. 5.0** (Cefoxitin Sodium). A white or almost white, very hygroscopic, powder. Very soluble in water; sparingly soluble in alcohol. A 1% solution in water has a pH between 4.2 and 7.0. Store in airtight containers.

**USP 27** (Cefoxitin Sodium). White to off-white, somewhat hygroscopic, granules or powder, having a slight characteristic odour. Very soluble in water; slightly soluble in acetone; insoluble in chloroform and in ether; sparingly soluble in dimethylformamide; soluble in methyl alcohol. pH of a 10% solution in water is between 4.2 and 7.0. Store in airtight containers at a temperature not exceeding 8°.

## Adverse Effects and Precautions

As for Cefalotin Sodium, p.168.

Cefoxitin may interfere with the Jaffé method of measuring creatinine concentrations to produce falsely high values; this should be borne in mind when measuring renal function.

**Breast feeding.** Cefoxitin is distributed into breast milk but is detectable only in low concentrations. In a study[1] in which cefoxitin was given prophylactically in doses of 2 to 4 g to 18 women undergoing caesarean section, only one sample of breast milk contained measurable concentrations of cefoxitin, 19 hours after the last dose. No adverse effects have been observed in breast-fed infants whose mothers were receiving cefoxitin, and the American Academy of Pediatrics considers[2] that it is therefore usually compatible with breast feeding.

1. Roex AJM, *et al.* Secretion of cefoxitin in breast milk following short-term prophylactic administration in caesarean section. *Eur J Obstet Gynecol Reprod Biol* 1987; **25:** 299–302.
2. American Academy of Pediatrics. The transfer of drugs and other chemicals into human milk. *Pediatrics* 2001; **108:** 776–89. Correction. *ibid.*; 1029. Also available at: http://aappolicy.aappublications.org/cgi/content/full/pediatrics%3b108/3/776 (accessed 25/05/04)

**Effects on the gastrointestinal tract.** Marked changes in anaerobic, facultative, and aerobic faecal flora have been noted with cefoxitin.[1]

1. Mulligan ME, *et al.* Alterations in human fecal flora, including ingrowth of Clostridium difficile, related to cefoxitin therapy. *Antimicrob Agents Chemother* 1984; **26:** 343–6.

**Sodium content.** Each g of cefoxitin sodium contains about 2.2 mmol of sodium.

## Interactions

Probenecid reduces the renal clearance of cefoxitin.

## Antimicrobial Action

Cefoxitin is a cephamycin antibacterial which, like the other beta lactams, is bactericidal and is considered to act through the inhibition of bacterial cell wall synthesis.

It has a similar spectrum of activity to cefamandole (p.170) but is more active against anaerobic bacteria, especially *Bacteroides fragilis.*

Cefoxitin can induce the production of beta-lactamases by some bacteria, and use of cefoxitin with other beta lactams have been shown to be antagonistic *in vitro.*

Cefoxitin itself is considered to be resistant to a wide range of beta-lactamases, including those produced by *Bacteroides* spp. However, acquired resistance to cefoxitin has been reported in *B. fragilis* (see Anaerobic Bacterial Infections, p.121) and has been attributed to beta-lactamase as well as to alterations in penicillin-binding proteins or to outer membrane proteins; there may be cross-resistance to other antibacterials.

◊ References.

1. Cuchural GJ, *et al.* Transfer of β-lactamase-associated cefoxitin resistance in Bacteroides fragilis. *Antimicrob Agents Chemother* 1986; **29:** 918–20.
2. Piddock LJV, Wise R. Cefoxitin resistance in Bacteroides species: evidence indicating two mechanisms causing decreased susceptibility. *J Antimicrob Chemother* 1987; **19:** 161–70.
3. Brogan O, *et al.* Bacteroides fragilis resistant to metronidazole, clindamycin and cefoxitin. *J Antimicrob Chemother* 1989; **23:** 660–2.
4. Wexler HM, Halebian S. Alterations to the penicillin-binding proteins in the Bacteroides fragilis group: a mechanism for non-β-lactamase mediated cefoxitin resistance. *J Antimicrob Chemother* 1990; **26:** 7–20.
5. Cherubin CE, Appleman MD. Susceptibility of cefoxitin-resistant isolates of bacteroides to other agents including β-lactamase inhibitor/β-lactam combinations. *J Antimicrob Chemother* 1993; **32:** 168–70.

## Pharmacokinetics

Cefoxitin is not absorbed from the gastrointestinal tract; it is given parenterally as the sodium salt. After 1 g by intramuscular injection a peak plasma concentration of up to 30 micrograms/mL at 20 to 30 minutes has been reported whereas concentrations of 125, 72, and 25 micrograms/mL have been achieved after the intravenous administration of 1 g over 3, 30, and 120 minutes respectively. Cefoxitin is about 70% bound to plasma proteins. It has a plasma half-life of 45 to 60 minutes which is prolonged in renal impairment. Cefoxitin is widely distributed in the body but there is normally little penetration into the CSF, even when the meninges are inflamed. It crosses the placenta and has been detected in breast milk. Relatively high concentrations are achieved in bile.

The majority of a dose is excreted unchanged by the kidneys, up to about 2% being metabolised to descarbamylcefoxitin which is virtually inactive. Cefoxitin is excreted in the urine by glomerular filtration and tubular secretion and about 85% of a dose is recovered within 6 hours; probenecid slows this excretion. After an intramuscular dose of 1 g, peak concentrations in the urine are usually greater than 3 mg/mL.

Cefoxitin is removed to some extent by haemodialysis.

### Uses and Administration

Cefoxitin is a cephamycin antibacterial that differs structurally from the cephalosporins by the addition of a 7-α-methoxy group to the 7-β-aminocephalosporanic acid nucleus.

It is generally classified with the second-generation cephalosporins and can be used similarly to cefamandole (p.170) for the treatment of susceptible infections. However, because of its activity against *Bacteroides fragilis* and other anaerobic bacteria, it is used principally in the treatment and prophylaxis of anaerobic and mixed bacterial infections, especially intra-abdominal and pelvic infections. Indications include endometritis (prophylaxis at caesarean section), pelvic inflammatory disease, and surgical infection (prophylaxis). It may also be used in the treatment of gonorrhoea and urinary-tract infections. For details of these infections and their treatment, see under Choice of Antibacterial, p.120.

*Administration and dosage.* Cefoxitin is given as the sodium salt by deep intramuscular injection, by slow intravenous injection over 3 to 5 minutes, or by intermittent or continuous intravenous infusion.

Doses are expressed in terms of the equivalent amount of cefoxitin. 1.05 g of cefoxitin sodium is approximately equivalent to 1 g of cefoxitin. The usual adult dose is 1 or 2 g every 8 hours although it may be given more frequently (every 4 or 6 hours). In severe infections up to 12 g daily has been recommended. Children and neonates may be given 20 to 40 mg/kg, every 12 hours for neonates up to 1 week old, every 8 hours for those aged 1 to 4 weeks, and every 6 to 8 hours for older infants and children; in severe infections, up to 200 mg/kg daily may be given, to a maximum of 12 g daily.

For the treatment of uncomplicated urinary-tract infections, cefoxitin 1 g twice daily has been given intramuscularly.

For details of reduced doses of cefoxitin to be used in patients with renal impairment, see below.

For the treatment of uncomplicated gonorrhoea, a single dose of 2 g intramuscularly has been given with probenecid 1 g by mouth.

For surgical infection prophylaxis, the usual adult dose is cefoxitin 2 g intramuscularly or intravenously 30 to 60 minutes prior to the procedure and then every 6 hours, not usually for more than 24 hours. Infants and children undergoing surgical procedures can be given doses of 30 to 40 mg/kg, at the same time intervals as adults; neonates may be given 30 to 40 mg/kg, but at intervals of 8 to 12 hours.

At caesarean section a single 2-g dose may be given intravenously to the mother as soon as the umbilical cord is clamped. If necessary, a 3-dose regimen, with further 2-g doses 4 and 8 hours after the initial dose, may be used.

◊ Reviews.

1. DiPiro JT, May JR. Use of cephalosporins with enhanced antianaerobic activity for treatment and prevention of anaerobic and mixed infections. *Clin Pharm* 1988; **7:** 285–302.
2. Goodwin CS. Cefoxitin 20 years on: is it still useful? *Rev Med Microbiol* 1995; **6:** 146–53.

**Administration in renal impairment.** In renal impairment, dosage of cefoxitin should be reduced according to creatinine clearance (CC). In adults, after an initial loading dose of 1 to 2 g, maintenance doses are:

- CC 30 to 50 mL/minute: 1 to 2 g every 8 to 12 hours
- CC 10 to 29 mL/minute: 1 to 2 g every 12 to 24 hours
- CC 5 to 9 mL/minute: 0.5 to 1 g every 12 to 24 hours
- CC below 5 mL/minute: 0.5 to 1 g every 24 to 48 hours

In patients undergoing haemodialysis, the loading dose should be repeated after each dialysis session.

### Preparations

***BP 2003:*** Cefoxitin Injection;
***USP 27:*** Cefoxitin for Injection; Cefoxitin Injection.

**Proprietary Preparations** (details are given in Part 3)
***Arg.:*** Mefoxin; Pluricefo; ***Austral.:*** Mefoxin; ***Austria:*** Mefoxitin; ***Belg.:*** Mefoxin; ***Braz.:*** Cefoxan; Cefoxin; Cefton; Foxtil; Mefoxin; Propoten; ***Canad.:*** Mefoxin; ***Fin.:*** Mefoxin; ***Fr.:*** Mefoxin; ***Ger.:*** Mefoxitin; ***Gr.:*** Mefoxil; ***Hong Kong:*** Mefoxin; ***Irl.:*** Mefoxin†; ***Ital.:*** Betaceft†; Cefociclin; Mefoxin; Tifox; ***Neth.:*** Mefoxin; ***Norw.:*** Mefoxitin; ***NZ:*** Mefoxin; ***Port.:*** Mefoxin; ***S.Afr.:*** Mefoxin; ***Spain:*** Cefaxicina†; Mefoxitin; ***Swed.:*** Mefoxitin; ***Switz.:*** Mefoxitin; ***Thai.:*** Cefoxin; Cefxitin; ***UK:*** Mefoxin; ***USA:*** Mefoxin.

## Cefozopran Hydrochloride *(rINNM)*

(−)-1-{[(6R,7R)-7-[2-(5-Amino-1,2,4-thiadiazol-3-yl)glyoxylamido]-2-carboxy-8-oxo-5-thia-1-azabicyclo[4.2.0]oct-2-en-3-yl]methyl}-1*H*-imidazo[1,2-b]pyridazin-4-ium hydroxide inner salt, $7^2$-(*Z*)-(*O*-methyloxime), hydrochloride.

$C_{19}H_{17}N_9O_5S_2,HCl = 552.0.$

*CAS — 113359-04-9 (cefozopran); 113981-44-5 (cefozopran hydrochloride).*

**Pharmacopoeias.** In *Jpn.*

### Profile

Cefozopran is a cephalosporin antibacterial used parenterally as the hydrochloride.

◊ References.

1. Iwahi T, *et al.* In vitro and in vivo activities of SCE-2787, a new parenteral cephalosporin with a broad antibacterial spectrum. *Antimicrob Agents Chemother* 1992; **36:** 1358–66.
2. Paulfeuerborn W, *et al.* Comparative pharmacokinetics and serum bactericidal activities of SCE-2787 and ceftazidime. *Antimicrob Agents Chemother* 1993; **37:** 1835–41.
3. Fujii R, *et al.* Pharmacokinetics and clinical effects of cefozopran in pediatric patients. *Jpn J Antibiot* 1996; **49:** 17–33.

## Cefpiramide *(USAN, rINN)*

Cefpiramida; SM-1652; Wy-44635. (7R)-7-[(R)-2-(4-Hydroxy-6-methylnicotinamido)-2-(4-hydroxyphenyl)acetamido]-3-(1-methyl-1*H*-tetrazol-5-ylthiomethyl)-3-cephem-4-carboxylic acid.

$C_{25}H_{24}N_8O_7S_2 = 612.6.$

*CAS — 70797-11-4.*

*ATC — J01DA27.*

**Pharmacopoeias.** In *US.*

**USP 27** (Cefpiramide). Store in airtight containers. pH of a 0.5% suspension in water is between 3.0 and 5.0.

## Cefpiramide Sodium *(USAN, rINNM)*

Cefpiramida sódica.

$C_{25}H_{23}N_8NaO_7S_2 = 634.6.$

*CAS — 74849-93-7.*

*ATC — J01DA27.*

**Pharmacopoeias.** In *Jpn.*

### Profile

Cefpiramide is a third-generation cephalosporin antibacterial related to cefoperazone (p.174) and with similar activity against *Pseudomonas aeruginosa*, but possibly less active against Enterobacteriaceae. Cefpiramide is also active against staphylococci and streptococci and marginal activity against enterococci *in vitro* has been reported. Cefpiramide contains an *N*-methylthiotetrazole side-chain, a structure associated with hypoprothrombinaemia (see Cefamandole, p.169), alcohol intolerance, and potentiation of anticoagulants.

Cefpiramide is given by intravenous injection or infusion as the sodium salt in the treatment of susceptible infections but doses are expressed in terms of cefpiramide. 1.04 g of cefpiramide sodium is approximately equivalent to 1 g of cefpiramide. The usual adult dose is 1 to 2 g daily in 2 divided doses.

◊ References.

1. Wang H, *et al.* In-vitro antibacterial activities of cefpiramide and other broad-spectrum antibiotics against 440 clinical isolates in China. *J Infect Chemother* 2000; **6:** 81–5.

**Sodium content.** Each g of cefpiramide sodium contains about 1.6 mmol of sodium.

### Preparations

***USP 27:*** Cefpiramide for Injection.

**Proprietary Preparations** (details are given in Part 3)
***Jpn:*** Sepatren.

## Cefpirome Sulfate *(USAN, rINNM)*

Cefpirome Sulphate *(BANM)*; HR-810 (cefpirome or cefpirome sulfate); Sulfato de cefpiroma. (Z)-7-[2-(2-Aminothiazol-4-yl)-2-methoxyiminoacetamido]-3-(1-pyrindiniomethyl)-3-cephem-4-carboxylate sulphate.

$C_{22}H_{22}N_6O_5S_2,H_2SO_4 = 612.7.$

*CAS — 84957-29-9 (cefpirome); 98753-19-6 (cefpirome sulfate).*

*ATC — J01DA37.*

**Pharmacopoeias.** In *Jpn.*

### Adverse Effects and Precautions

As for Cefalotin, p.168.

Cefpirome is reported to interfere with the Jaffé method of measuring creatinine concentrations to determine renal function.

◊ References.

1. Rubinstein E, *et al.* A review of the adverse events profile of cefpirome. *Drug Safety* 1993; **9:** 340–5.

### Interactions

Probenecid reduces the renal clearance of cefpirome.

### Antimicrobial Action

Cefpirome is a fourth-generation cephalosporin that is stable to a wide range of beta-lactamases. It has a spectrum of activity similar to that of the third-generation cephalosporin cefotaxime (p.176), but it appears to be more active *in vitro* against staphylococci, some enterococci, some Enterobacteriaceae, and *Pseudomonas aeruginosa*. Cefpirome may be less active than ceftazidime (p.181) against *Ps. aeruginosa*.

### Pharmacokinetics

Cefpirome is given by injection as the sulfate. Mean peak serum concentrations of 80 to 90 micrograms/mL are attained after a single intravenous 1-g dose. The elimination half-life is about 2 hours and is prolonged in patients with renal impairment. Cefpirome is less than 10% bound to plasma proteins.

Cefpirome is widely distributed into body tissues and fluids and appears in breast milk. It is mainly excreted by the kidneys and 80 to 90% of a dose is recovered unchanged in the urine. Significant amounts are removed by haemodialysis.

### Uses and Administration

Cefpirome is a fourth-generation cephalosporin antibacterial used in the treatment of infections due to susceptible organisms. They include infections of the urinary tract, respiratory tract, and skin, and also septicaemia and infections in immunocompromised patients. For details of these infections and their treatment, see under Choice of Antibacterial, p.120.

Cefpirome is given by intravenous injection over 3 to 5 minutes or infusion over 20 to 30 minutes as the sulfate, but doses are expressed in terms of the base. 1.19 g of cefpirome sulfate is approximately equivalent to 1 g of cefpirome. The usual dose is the equivalent of 1 or 2 g of cefpirome every 12 hours. For details of reduced doses to be used in renal impairment, see below.

◊ References.

1. Brown EM, *et al.* eds. Cefpirome: a novel extended spectrum cephalosporin. *J Antimicrob Chemother* 1992; **29** (suppl A): 1–104.
2. Wiseman LR, Lamb HM. Cefpirome: a review of its antibacterial activity, pharmacokinetic properties and clinical efficacy in the treatment of severe nosocomial infections and febrile neutropenia. *Drugs* 1997; **54:** 117–40.

**Administration in renal impairment.** Dosage of cefpirome should be modified in renal impairment; after a loading dose of 1 or 2 g depending on the severity of infection, the maintenance dosage should be adjusted according to the patient's creatinine clearance (CC) and the severity of infection:

- CC 20 to 50 mL/minute: 0.5 or 1 g twice daily
- CC 5 to 20 mL/minute: 0.5 or 1 g once daily
- CC 5 mL/minute or less (in haemodialysis patients): 0.5 or 1 g once daily plus a half-dose after each dialysis session.

### Preparations

**Proprietary Preparations** (details are given in Part 3)
***Austral.:*** Cefrom; ***Austria:*** Cedixen; Cefrom; ***Belg.:*** Cefrom; ***Braz.:*** Cefron†; ***Denm.:*** Cefrom†; ***Fin.:*** Cefrom†; ***Fr.:*** Cefrom; ***Hong Kong:*** Cefrom†; ***India:*** Cefrom; ***Irl.:*** Cefrom; ***Mex.:*** Cefrom; ***Neth.:*** Cefrom; ***NZ:*** Cefrom; ***S.Afr.:*** Cefrom; ***Singapore:*** Cefrom†; ***Spain:*** Metran†; ***Swed.:*** Cefrom†; ***Switz.:*** Cefrom†; ***Thai.:*** Cefrom; ***UK:*** Cefrom.

## Cefpodoxime Proxetil *(BANM, USAN, rINNM)*

Cefpodoxima proxetilo; CS-807; R-3763(cefpodoxime); U-76252; U-76253(cefpodoxime). The 1-[(isopropoxycarbonyl)oxy]ethyl ester of (Z)-7-[2-(2-amino-1,3-thiazol-4-yl)-2-methoxyiminoacetamido]-3-methoxymethyl-3-cephem-4-carboxylic acid.

$C_{21}H_{27}N_5O_9S_2 = 557.6.$

*CAS — 80210-62-4 (cefpodoxime); 87239-81-4 (cefpodoxime proxetil).*

*ATC — J01DA33.*

**Pharmacopoeias.** In *Jpn* and *US.*

**USP 27** (Cefpodoxime Proxetil). A white to light brownish-white powder, odourless or having a faint odour. Very slightly soluble in water; freely soluble in dehydrated alcohol; soluble in acetonitrile and in methyl alcohol; slightly soluble in ether. Store in airtight containers at a temperature not exceeding 25°.

### Adverse Effects and Precautions

As for Cefalotin Sodium, p.168.

The most frequently reported adverse effects of cefpodoxime are gastrointestinal disturbances, especially diarrhoea.

### Interactions

Absorption of cefpodoxime is decreased by antacids or histamine $H_2$-receptor antagonists. Probenecid reduces the renal excretion of cefpodoxime.

### Antimicrobial Action

As for Cefixime, p.173, but cefpodoxime has greater activity against *Staphylococcus aureus*.

◊ References.

1. Valentini S, *et al.* In-vitro evaluation of cefpodoxime. *J Antimicrob Chemother* 1994; **33:** 495–508.

### Pharmacokinetics

Cefpodoxime proxetil is de-esterified in the intestinal epithelium following oral administration, to release active cefpodoxime in the bloodstream. Bioavailability is about 50% in fasting subjects and may be increased in the presence of food. Absorption is decreased in conditions of low gastric acidity. Peak plasma concentrations of about 1.5, 2.5, and 4.0 micrograms/mL have been achieved 2 to 3 hours after oral doses of 100, 200, and 400 mg cefpodoxime respectively. About 20 to 30% of cefpodoxime is bound to plasma proteins. The plasma half-life is about 2 to 3 hours and is prolonged in patients with renal impairment.

Cefpodoxime reaches therapeutic concentrations in the respiratory and genito-urinary tracts and bile. It has been detected in low concentrations in breast milk.

Cefpodoxime is excreted unchanged in the urine. Some is removed by dialysis.

### Uses and Administration

Cefpodoxime is a third-generation cephalosporin antibiotic used similarly to cefixime (p.173) in the treatment of susceptible infections. It is given by mouth as the proxetil ester, which is hydrolysed on absorption to cefpodoxime. Doses are expressed in terms of the equivalent amount of cefpodoxime. 130 mg of cefpodoxime proxetil is approximately equivalent to 100 mg of cefpodoxime. Absorption may be enhanced if cefpodoxime proxetil is given with food. The usual adult dose is 100 to 200 mg every 12 hours for respiratory-tract and urinary-tract infections. A dose of 200 or 400 mg every 12 hours may be used for skin infections. In children doses of 8 to 10 mg/kg daily may be given in 2 divided doses, up to a maximum of 200 mg daily for respiratory-tract infections or 400 mg daily for otitis media or sinusitis.

The interval between doses of cefpodoxime may need to be extended in patients with renal impairment (see below).

For uncomplicated gonorrhoea, a single dose of 200 mg may be given.

◊ References.

1. Moore EP, *et al.*, eds. Cefpodoxime proxetil: a third-generation oral cephalosporin. *J Antimicrob Chemother* 1990; **26** (suppl E): 1–101.
2. Adam D, *et al.*, eds. Cefpodoxime proxetil: a new third generation oral cephalosporin. *Drugs* 1991; **42** (suppl 3): 1–66.
3. Frampton JE, *et al.* Cefpodoxime proxetil: a review of its antibacterial activity, pharmacokinetic properties and therapeutic potential. *Drugs* 1992; **44:** 889–917.
4. Chocas EC, *et al.* Cefpodoxime proxetil: a new, broad-spectrum, oral cephalosporin. *Ann Pharmacother* 1993; **27:** 1369–77.
5. Fulton B, Perry CM. Cefpodoxime proxetil: a review of its use in the management of bacterial infections in paediatric patients. *Paediatr Drugs* 2001; **3:** 137–58.

**Administration in renal impairment.** The interval between doses of cefpodoxime should be extended in patients with renal impairment to every 24 hours in those with creatinine clearance 10 to 39 mL/minute, and to every 48 hours when the creatinine clearance is less than 10 mL/minute.

### Preparations

*USP 27:* Cefpodoxime Proxetil for Oral Suspension; Cefpodoxime Proxetil Tablets.

**Proprietary Preparations** (details are given in Part 3)
***Austral.:*** Orelox†; ***Austria:*** Biocef; Otreon; ***Braz.:*** Orelox; ***Denm.:*** Orelox†; ***Fr.:*** Orelox; ***Ger.:*** Orelox; Podomexef; ***Hong Kong:*** Banan; ***India:*** Cepodem; ***Irl.:*** Cefodox; ***Ital.:*** Cefodox; Orelox; Otreon; ***Jpn:*** Banan; ***Mex.:*** Orelox; ***Neth.:*** Orelox; ***S.Afr.:*** Orelox; ***Spain:*** Garia; Instana; Kelbium†; Orelox†; Otreon; ***Swed.:*** Orelox; ***Switz.:*** Orelox; Podomexef; ***Thai.:*** Banan; ***UK:*** Orelox; ***USA:*** Vantin.

The symbol † denotes a preparation no longer actively marketed

## Cefprozil *(BAN, USAN, rINN)*

BMY-28100-03-800; BMY-28100 (*cis*-isomer); BMY-28167 (*trans*-isomer); Cefprozilo. (6*R*,7*R*)-7-[(*R*)-2-Amino-2-(*p*-hydroxyphenyl)acetamido]-8-oxo-3-(1-propenyl)-5-thia-1-azabicyclo[4.2.0]oct-2-ene-2-carboxylic acid monohydrate; 7-(D-4-Hydroxyphenylglycylamino)-3-[(*E*)prop-1-enyl]cephem-4-carboxylic acid monohydrate.

$C_{18}H_{19}N_3O_5S,H_2O$ = 407.4.

*CAS — 92665-29-7 (anhydrous cefprozil); 121123-17-9 (cefprozil monohydrate).*

*ATC — J01DA41.*

**Pharmacopoeias.** In *US.*

**USP 27** (Cefprozil). pH of a 0.5% solution in water is between 3.5 and 6.5. Store in airtight containers.

### Adverse Effects and Precautions

As for Cefalexin, p.168.

**Breast feeding.** A study[1] in 9 healthy, lactating women found that concentrations of cefprozil in breast milk corresponded to no more than 0.3% of a dose and concluded that cefprozil could be given safely during breast feeding. The American Academy of Pediatrics[2] states that there have been no reports of any clinical effect on the infant associated with the use of cefprozil in breast-feeding mothers, and that it may be considered to be usually compatible with breast feeding.

1. Shyu WC, *et al.* Excretion of cefprozil into human breast milk. *Antimicrob Agents Chemother* 1992; **36:** 938–41.
2. American Academy of Pediatrics. The transfer of drugs and other chemicals into human milk. *Pediatrics* 2001; **108:** 776–89. Correction. *ibid.*; 1029. Also available at: http://aappolicy.aappublications.org/cgi/content/full/pediatrics%3b108/3/776 (accessed 25/05/04)

**Hypersensitivity.** Serum sickness-like reactions were reported in 4 patients, 3 of them children, given cefprozil.[1] Such reactions have been associated with cefaclor (p.167), but whether they represent a class-related hypersensitivity reaction is not clear.

1. Lowery N, *et al.* Serum sickness-like reactions associated with cefprozil therapy. *J Pediatr* 1994; **125:** 325–8.

### Interactions

As for Cefalexin, p.168.

### Antimicrobial Action

Cefprozil is bactericidal and has a similar but wider range of antimicrobial activity than cefaclor (p.167).

### Pharmacokinetics

Cefprozil is well absorbed from the gastrointestinal tract with a reported bioavailability of 90 to 95%. Doses of 0.25, 0.5, and 1 g by mouth produce peak plasma concentrations of about 6, 10, and 18 micrograms/mL respectively at 1 to 2 hours. The presence of food is reported to have little or no effect on the absorption of cefprozil. A plasma half-life of 1 to 1.4 hours has been reported; it is increased in patients with renal impairment, up to about 6 hours in those with end-stage renal failure. Approximately 35 to 45% of cefprozil is bound to plasma proteins.

Cefprozil is widely distributed in the body tissues. Concentrations of cefprozil in tonsillar and adenoidal tissue are reported to be about 40 to 50% of those in plasma, and less than 0.3% of a 1-g dose has been recovered in breast milk in 24 hours. About 60% of a dose is excreted unchanged in the urine in the first 8 hours by glomerular filtration and tubular secretion. High concentrations of cefprozil are achieved in the urine; concentrations of 700, 1000, and 2900 micrograms/mL have been reported within 4 hours of doses of 0.25, 0.5, and 1 g respectively. Some cefprozil is removed by haemodialysis.

### Uses and Administration

Cefprozil is a cephalosporin antibacterial consisting of *cis*- and *trans*- isomers in a ratio of about 90:10. It is used similarly to cefaclor (p.167) in the treatment of susceptible infections, including upper and lower respiratory-tract infections and skin and soft tissue infections, and should probably be classified as a second-generation cephalosporin.

Cefprozil is given by mouth as the monohydrate. Doses are expressed in terms of the equivalent amount of anhydrous cefprozil. 523 mg of cefprozil monohydrate is approximately equivalent to 500 mg of anhydrous cefprozil. The usual adult dose is 500 mg daily (as a single dose or in two divided doses), increased to 500 mg twice daily if necessary. Children may be given up to 20 mg/kg once or twice daily (to a maximum of 500 mg once daily, or twice daily if necessary for otitis media).

For details of reduced dosage of cefprozil in patients with renal impairment, see below.

◊ Reviews.

1. Wiseman LR, Benfield P. Cefprozil: a review of its antibacterial activity, pharmacokinetic properties, and therapeutic potential. *Drugs* 1993; **45:** 295–317.
2. Barriere SL. Review of in vitro activity, pharmacokinetic characteristics, safety, and clinical efficacy of cefprozil, a new oral cephalosporin. *Ann Pharmacother* 1993; **27:** 1082–9.

**Administration in renal impairment.** Doses of cefprozil should be reduced in patients with renal impairment; half the standard dose should be given to patients with a creatinine clearance of less than 30 mL/minute.

### Preparations

*USP 27:* Cefprozil for Oral Suspension; Cefprozil Tablets.

**Proprietary Preparations** (details are given in Part 3)
***Austria:*** Procef; ***Braz.:*** Cefzil; ***Canad.:*** Cefzil; ***Chile:*** Procef; ***Fin.:*** Procef†; ***Gr.:*** Procef; ***Hong Kong:*** Procef; ***Ital.:*** Cronocef; Procef; Rozicel; ***Malaysia:*** Procef; ***Mex.:*** Procef; ***Port.:*** Procef; ***S.Afr.:*** Prozef; ***Singapore:*** Procef; ***Spain:*** Arzimol; Brisoral; ***Switz.:*** Procef; ***Thai.:*** Procef; ***UK:*** Cefzil; ***USA:*** Cefzil.

## Cefquinome Sulfate *(USAN, rINNM)*

Cefquinome Sulphate *(BANM)*; HR-111V. {6*R*-[6α,7β(*Z*)]}-1-[(7-{[(2-amino-4-thiazolyl)-(methoxyimino)acetyl]amino}-2-carboxy-8-oxo-5-thia-1-azabicyclo[4.2.0]oct-2-en-3-yl)methyl]-5,6,7,8,-tetrahydroquinolinium sulfate (1:1).

$C_{23}H_{24}N_6O_5S_2,H_2SO_4$ = 626.7.

*CAS — 84957-30-2 (cefquinome); 118443-89-3 (cefquinome sulfate); 123766-80-3 (cefquinome sulfate).*

### Profile

Cefquinome is a fourth-generation cephalosporin antibacterial used as the sulfate in veterinary medicine.

## Cefradine *(BAN, rINN)*

Cefradina; Cefradinum; Cephradine *(USAN)*; SKF-D-39304; SQ-11436; SQ-22022 (cefradine dihydrate). (7*R*)-7-(α-D-Cyclohexa-1,4-dienylglycylamino)-3-methyl-3-cephem-4-carboxylic acid.

$C_{16}H_{19}N_3O_4S$ = 349.4.

*CAS — 38821-53-3 (anhydrous cefradine); 31828-50-9 (non-stoichiometric cefradine hydrate); 58456-86-3 (cefradine dihydrate).*

*ATC — J01DA31.*

**Pharmacopoeias.** In *Chin., Eur.* (see p.vi), *Jpn, Pol.,* and *US* (which allows the anhydrous form, the monohydrate, or the dihydrate).

**Ph. Eur. 5.0** (Cefradine). A white or slightly yellow, hygroscopic powder. Sparingly soluble in water; practically insoluble in alcohol. A 1% solution in water has a pH of 3.5 to 6.0. Store at 2° to 8° in airtight containers. Protect from light.

**USP 27** (Cephradine). A white to off-white crystalline powder. Sparingly soluble in water; very slightly soluble in alcohol and in chloroform; practically insoluble in ether. pH of a 1% solution in water is between 3.5 and 6.0. Store in airtight containers.

**Incompatibility and stability.** Commercially available injections contain sodium carbonate or arginine as neutralisers. Injections containing sodium carbonate are incompatible with solutions such as compound sodium lactate injection that contain calcium salts.

References.

1. Wang Y-C J, Monkhouse DC. Solution stability of cephradine neutralized with arginine or sodium bicarbonate. *Am J Hosp Pharm* 1983; **40:** 432.
2. Mehta AC, *et al.* Chemical stability of cephradine injection solutions. *Intensive Therapy Clin Monit* 1988; **9:** 195–6.

### Adverse Effects and Precautions

As for Cefalexin, p.168. Intramuscular injections of cefradine can be painful and thrombophlebitis has occurred following intravenous injection.

**Porphyria.** Cefradine is considered to be unsafe in patients with porphyria although there is conflicting experimental evidence of porphyrinogenicity.

### Interactions

As for Cefalexin, p.168.

### Antimicrobial Action

As for Cefalexin, p.168.

### Pharmacokinetics

Cefradine is rapidly and almost completely absorbed from the gastrointestinal tract following oral administration. Doses of 0.25, 0.5, and 1 g given by mouth have produced peak plasma concentrations of about 9, 17, and 24 micrograms/mL respectively at 1 hour and are similar to those achieved with cefalexin. Absorption is delayed by the presence of food although the total amount absorbed is not appreciably altered. Following intramuscular injection peak plasma concentrations of about 6 and 14 micrograms/mL have been obtained within 1 to 2 hours of doses of 0.5 and 1 g respectively.

Only about 8 to 12% is reported to be bound to plasma proteins. A plasma half-life of about 1 hour has been reported; this is prolonged in patients with renal impairment. Cefradine is widely distributed to body tissues and fluids, but does not enter the CSF in significant quantities. Therapeutic concentrations may be found in the bile. It crosses the placenta into the fetal circulation and is distributed in small amounts into breast milk.

Cefradine is excreted unchanged in the urine by glomerular filtration and tubular secretion, over 90% of an oral dose or 60 to 80% of an intramuscular dose being recovered within 6 hours. Peak urinary concentrations of about 3 mg/mL have been achieved after a 500-mg dose by mouth. Probenecid delays excretion.

Cefradine is removed by haemodialysis and peritoneal dialysis.

◊ References.


1. Wise R. The pharmacokinetics of the oral cephalosporins—a review. *J Antimicrob Chemother* 1990; **26** (suppl E): 13–20.
2. Schwinghammer TL, *et al.* Pharmacokinetics of cephradine administered intravenously and orally to young and elderly subjects. *J Clin Pharmacol* 1990; **30:** 893–9.


## Uses and Administration

Cefradine is a first-generation cephalosporin antibacterial given by mouth similarly to cefalexin (p.168) and by the parenteral route similarly to cefazolin (p.171) in the treatment of susceptible infections and in the prophylaxis of infections during surgical procedures.

Cefradine is given by mouth in doses of 1 to 2 g daily in 2 to 4 divided doses to adults; up to 4 g daily may be given by this route. In severe infections it should be given parenterally, by deep intramuscular injection or intravenously by slow injection over 3 to 5 minutes or by infusion, in doses of 2 to 4 g daily in 4 divided doses; up to 8 g daily may be given parenterally.

In children, the usual daily dose by mouth is 25 to 50 mg/kg in 2 to 4 divided doses, although 75 to 100 mg/kg daily may be given for otitis media. By injection, 50 to 100 mg/kg daily may be given in 4 divided doses, increasing to 300 mg/kg daily in severe infections.

For surgical infection prophylaxis, 1 to 2 g may be given pre-operatively by intramuscular or intravenous injection; subsequent parenteral or oral doses are given as appropriate.

For details of reduced doses of cefradine to be used in patients with severe renal impairment, see below.

**Administration in renal impairment.** Doses of cefradine should be reduced in patients with severe renal impairment. The following oral and parenteral doses are recommended by the UK manufacturers according to creatinine clearance (CC):

- CC more than 20 mL/minute: 500 mg every 6 hours
- CC 5 to 20 mL/minute: 250 mg every 6 hours
- CC less than 5 mL/minute: 250 mg every 50 to 70 hours

Patients undergoing chronic intermittent haemodialysis may be given a 250-mg dose at the start of the session, repeated after 6 to 12 hours, then again 36 to 48 hours after the initial dose, and again at the start of the next haemodialysis if more than 30 hours have elapsed since the previous dose.

Further dosage modification may be required in children with renal impairment.

## Preparations

***BP 2003:*** Cefradine Capsules; Cefradine Oral Suspension;
***USP 27:*** Cephradine Capsules; Cephradine for Injection; Cephradine for Oral Suspension; Cephradine Tablets.

**Proprietary Preparations** (details are given in Part 3)
***Belg.:*** Velosef; ***Chile:*** Velosef; ***Fr.:*** Cefirex†; Dexef; Doncef†; Kelsef; Zadyl†; Zeefra; ***Gr.:*** Tracilarin; Vethisel; ***Hong Kong:*** Velosef; Zeefra; ***Irl.:*** Velosef; ***Israel:*** Velosef†; ***Ital.:*** Cefrabiotic; Citicef†; Ecosporina; Lisacef; Planocid; ***Malaysia:*** Sephros; ***Mex.:*** Veracef; ***Neth.:*** Maxisporin; Velosef; ***NZ:*** Velosef; ***Port.:*** Cefradur; Novacefrex†; Velosef; ***S.Afr.:*** Bactocef†; Cefril; Ranfradin; ***Spain:*** Septacef; Velocef; ***UAE:*** Julphacef; ***UK:*** Nicef; Velosef; ***USA:*** Velosef.

## Cefsulodin Sodium *(BANM, USAN, rINNM)*

Abbott-46811; Cefsulodina sódica; CGP-7174E; SCE-129; Sulcephalosporin Sodium. Sodium 3-(4-carbamoylpyridiniomethyl)-7-[(2R)-2-phenyl-2-sulphoacetamido]-3-cephem-4-carboxylate.
$C_{22}H_{19}N_4NaO_8S_2$ = 554.5.
*CAS — 62587-73-9 (cefsulodin); 52152-93-9 (cefsulodin sodium).*
*ATC — J01DA12.*

**Pharmacopoeias.** In *Jpn.*

### Adverse Effects and Precautions

As for Cefalotin Sodium, p.168.

**Sodium content.** Each g of cefsulodin sodium contains about 1.8 mmol of sodium.

### Antimicrobial Action

Cefsulodin is a bactericidal antibiotic with activity against *Pseudomonas aeruginosa* as great as that of ceftazidime (p.181), but no significant activity against other Gram-negative bacteria. Gram-positive bacteria and anaerobes are not very susceptible. Its activity against *Ps. aeruginosa* may be enhanced by aminoglycosides.

Cefsulodin is stable to hydrolysis by many beta-lactamases, but emergence of resistant *Ps. aeruginosa* has been reported.

### Pharmacokinetics

Cefsulodin is given parenterally as the sodium salt. It has a plasma half-life of about 1.6 hours, which is prolonged in renal impairment. Up to 30% of cefsulodin in the circulation is bound to plasma proteins. Therapeutic concentrations have been reported in a wide range of body tissues and fluids. The major route of excretion of cefsulodin is via the urine, mainly by glomerular filtration. Clearance may be enhanced in cystic fibrosis, although there have been conflicting reports.

◊ References.


1. Granneman GR, *et al.* Cefsulodin kinetics in healthy subjects after intramuscular and intravenous injection. *Clin Pharmacol Ther* 1982; **31:** 95–103.
2. Reed MD, *et al.* Single-dose pharmacokinetics of cefsulodin in patients with cystic fibrosis. *Antimicrob Agents Chemother* 1984; **25:** 579–81.
3. Hedman A, *et al.* Increased renal clearance of cefsulodin due to higher glomerular filtration rate in cystic fibrosis. *Clin Pharmacokinet* 1990; **18:** 168–75.


### Uses and Administration

Cefsulodin is a third-generation cephalosporin antibiotic with a narrow spectrum of activity that has been used similarly to ceftazidime (p.181) for the treatment of infections caused by susceptible strains of *Pseudomonas aeruginosa*.

It is given as the sodium salt by intramuscular injection, or intravenously by slow injection or by infusion. Doses are expressed in terms of the equivalent amount of cefsulodin. 1.04 g of cefsulodin sodium is approximately equivalent to 1 g of cefsulodin. The usual adult dose is 1 to 4 g daily in 2 to 4 divided doses; in severe infections daily doses of 6 g or more may be required. Children may be given doses of 20 to 50 mg/kg daily; up to 100 mg/kg daily has been given in severe infections.

◊ References.


1. Smith BR. Cefsulodin and ceftazidime, two antipseudomonal cephalosporins. *Clin Pharm* 1984; **3:** 373–85.
2. Wright DB. Cefsulodin. *Drug Intell Clin Pharm* 1986; **20:** 845–9.


**Administration in renal impairment.** Patients with renal impairment should be given the usual loading dose of cefsulodin sodium; subsequent doses should be reduced or the dosage interval prolonged.

### Preparations

**Proprietary Preparations** (details are given in Part 3)
***Austria:*** Monaspor†; Pseudocef†; ***Fr.:*** Pyocefal†; ***Ger.:*** Pseudocef†; ***Jpn:*** Takesulin.

## Ceftazidime *(BAN, USAN, rINN)*

Ceftazidima; Ceftazidimum; GR-20263; LY-139381. (Z)-(7R)-7-[2-(2-Aminothiazol-4-yl)-2-(1-carboxy-1-methylethoxyimino)acetamido]-3-(1-pyridiniomethyl)-3-cephem-4-carboxylate pentahydrate.
$C_{22}H_{22}N_6O_7S_2,5H_2O$ = 636.7.
*CAS — 72558-82-8 (anhydrous ceftazidime); 78439-06-2 (ceftazidime pentahydrate).*
*ATC — J01DA11.*

**Pharmacopoeias.** In *Chin., Eur.* (see p.vi), *Jpn, Pol.,* and *US.*

**Ph. Eur. 5.0** (Ceftazidime). A white or almost white crystalline powder. Slightly soluble in water and in methyl alcohol; practically insoluble in alcohol and in acetone; it dissolves in acid and alkali solutions. A 0.5% solution in water has a pH of 3.0 to 4.0. Store in airtight containers.

**USP 27** (Ceftazidime). A white to cream-coloured crystalline powder. Slightly soluble in water, in dimethylformamide, and in methyl alcohol; insoluble in alcohol, in acetone, in chloroform, in dioxan, in ether, in ethyl acetate, and in toluene; soluble in alkali and in dimethyl sulfoxide. pH of a 0.5% solution in water is between 3.0 and 4.0. Store in airtight containers.

**Formulation.** Ceftazidime for injection is available as a dry powder containing ceftazidime together with sodium carbonate. When reconstituted ceftazidime sodium is formed with the evolution of carbon dioxide. An alternative formulation, ceftazidime with arginine, appears to overcome the problems associated with effervescence.[1] In some countries a frozen injection containing ceftazidime sodium is also used.


1. Stiles ML, *et al.* Gas production of three brands of ceftazidime. *Am J Hosp Pharm* 1991; **48:** 1727–9.


**Incompatibility.** It has been reported that ceftazidime does not cause decreased activity when incubated in solution with *gentamicin*[1] or *tobramycin*[2] at 37°, or when mixed with tobramycin in serum.[3] Ceftazidime and tobramycin[4] were also stable for up to 16 hours at room temperature when combined in a glucose-containing dialysis solution, and for a further 8 hours at 37°. However, the manufacturers recommend that ceftazidime, like most other beta lactams, should not be mixed with an aminoglycoside in the same giving set or syringe because of the potential for inactivation of either drug.

Ceftazidime is generally considered to be compatible with *metronidazole*, but degradation of ceftazidime has been reported.[5] Precipitation has occurred with *vancomycin*[6] and therefore the manufacturers consider it prudent to flush giving sets and intravenous lines between administration of the two drugs. However, in one study[7] ceftazidime and/or vancomycin were stable in a glucose-containing peritoneal dialysis solution when kept for 6 days in a refrigerator or 48 to 72 hours at room temperature, and in a further study[8] the two drugs were stable when combined in similar solutions containing 1.5% or 4.25% glucose for up to 12 hours when stored at 37° and for 24 hours when stored at 4° and 24°. Ceftazidime and *teicoplanin*[9] were stable in combination in a peritoneal dialysis solution at 37° for 8 hours when it had been previously stored at 4°, but not when previously stored at 25°. Ceftazidime was not stable when mixed in solution with *aminophylline*.[10] There was some evidence of possible incompatibility with *pentamidine*.[11]


1. Elliott TSJ, *et al.* Stability of gentamicin in combination with selected new β-lactam antibiotics. *J Antimicrob Chemother* 1984; **14:** 668–9.
2. Elliott TSJ, *et al.* Stability of tobramycin in combination with selected new β-lactam antibiotics. *J Antimicrob Chemother* 1986; **17:** 680–1.
3. Pennell AT, *et al.* Effect of ceftazidime, cefotaxime, and cefoperazone on serum tobramycin concentrations. *Am J Hosp Pharm* 1991; **48:** 520–2.
4. Mason NA, *et al.* Stability of ceftazidime and tobramycin sulfate in peritoneal dialysis solution. *Am J Hosp Pharm* 1992; **49:** 1139–42.
5. Messerschmidt W. Pharmazeutische kompatibilität von ceftazidim und metronidazol. *Pharm Ztg* 1990; **135:** 36–8.
6. Cairns CJ, Robertson J. Incompatibility of ceftazidime and vancomycin. *Pharm J* 1987; **238:** 577.
7. Vaughan LM, Poon CY. Stability of ceftazidime and vancomycin alone and in combination in heparinized and nonheparinized peritoneal dialysis solution. *Ann Pharmacother* 1994; **28:** 572–6.
8. Stamatakis MK, *et al.* Stability of high-dose vancomycin and ceftazidime in peritoneal dialysis solutions. *Am J Health-Syst Pharm* 1999; **56:** 246–8.
9. Manduru M. *et al.* Stability of ceftazidime sodium and teicoplanin sodium in a peritoneal dialysis solution. *Am J Health-Syst Pharm* 1996; **53:** 2731–4.
10. Pleasants RA, *et al.* Compatibility of ceftazidime and aminophylline admixtures for different methods of intravenous infusion. *Ann Pharmacother* 1992; **26:** 1221–6.
11. Lewis JD. El-Gendy A. Cephalosporin-pentamidine isethionate incompatibilities. *Am J Health-Syst Pharm* 1996; **53:** 1462–3.


**Stability.** References.


1. Richardson BL, *et al.* The pharmacy of ceftazidime. *J Antimicrob Chemother* 1981; **8** (suppl B): 233–6.
2. Brown AF, *et al.* Freeze thaw stability of ceftazidime. *Br J Parenter Ther* 1985; **6:** 43, 45, 50.
3. Walker SE, Dranitsaris G. Ceftazidime stability in normal saline and dextrose in water. *Can J Hosp Pharm* 1988; **41:** 65–6, 69–71.
4. Wade CS, *et al.* Stability of ceftazidime and amino acids in parenteral nutrient solutions. *Am J Hosp Pharm* 1991; **48:** 1515–19.
5. Stiles ML, *et al.* Stability of ceftazidime (with arginine) and of cefuroxime sodium in infusion-pump reservoirs. *Am J Hosp Pharm* 1992; **49:** 2761–4.
6. Stewart JT, *et al.* Stability of ceftazidime in plastic syringes and glass vials under various storage conditions. *Am J Hosp Pharm* 1992; **49:** 2765–8.
7. Nahata MC, *et al.* Stability of ceftazidime (with arginine) stored in plastic syringes at three temperatures. *Am J Hosp Pharm* 1992; **49:** 2954–6.
8. Bednar DA, *et al.* Stability of ceftazidime (with arginine) in an elastomeric infusion device. *Am J Health-Syst Pharm* 1995; **52:** 1912–14.
9. van Doorne H, *et al.* Ceftazidime degradation rates for predicting stability in a portable infusion-pump reservoir. *Am J Health-Syst Pharm* 1996; **53:** 1302–5.
10. Stendal TL, *et al.* Drug stability and pyridine generation in ceftazidime injection stored in an elastomeric infusion device. *Am J Health-Syst Pharm* 1998; **55:** 683–5.
11. Servais H, Tulkens PM. Stability and compatibility of ceftazidime administered by continuous infusion to intensive care patients. *Antimicrob Agents Chemother* 2001; **45:** 2643–7.


### Adverse Effects and Precautions

As for Cefalotin Sodium, p.168.

Like cefotaxime (p.175), ceftazidime has the potential for colonisation and superinfection with resistant organisms. The risk of superinfection with, for example, *Staphylococcus aureus* may be higher than with cefotaxime, since ceftazidime is less active against staphylococci.

**Breast feeding.** No adverse effects have been observed in breast-fed infants whose mothers were receiving ceftazidime, and the American Academy of Pediatrics considers[1] that it is therefore usually compatible with breast feeding.

1. American Academy of Pediatrics. The transfer of drugs and other chemicals into human milk. *Pediatrics* 2001; **108:** 776–89. Correction. *ibid.*; 1029. Also available at: http://aappolicy.aappublications.org/cgi/content/full/pediatrics%3b108/3/776 (accessed 25/05/04)

**Effects on the blood.** References.

1. Hui CH, Chan LC. Agranulocytosis associated with cephalosporin. *BMJ* 1993; **307:** 484.

**Effects on the nervous system.** References.

1. Al-Zahawi MF, *et al.* Hallucinations in association with ceftazidime. *BMJ* 1988; **297:** 858.
2. Jackson GD, Berkovic SF. Ceftazidime encephalopathy: absence status and toxic hallucinations. *J Neurol Neurosurg Psychiatry* 1992; **55:** 333–4.

**Effects on the skin.** References.

1. Vinks SATMM, *et al.* Photosensitivity due to ambulatory intravenous ceftazidime in cystic fibrosis patient. *Lancet* 1993; **341:** 1221–2.

## Interactions

Unlike many other cephalosporins, probenecid has little effect on the renal clearance of ceftazidime.

◊ References.

1. Verhagen CA, *et al.* The renal clearance of cefuroxime and ceftazidime and the effect of probenecid on their tubular excretion. *Br J Clin Pharmacol* 1994; **37:** 193–7.

## Antimicrobial Action

Ceftazidime has a bactericidal action and broad spectrum of activity similar to that of cefotaxime (p.176), but increased activity against *Pseudomonas* spp.; it is less active against staphylococci and streptococci. Unlike cefotaxime it has no active metabolite.

Ceftazidime is highly stable to hydrolysis by most beta-lactamases. It is active *in vitro* against many Gram-negative bacteria including *Pseudomonas aeruginosa*, *Burkholderia pseudomallei* (*Pseudomonas pseudomallei*), and Enterobacteriaceae including *Citrobacter* and *Enterobacter* spp., *Escherichia coli*, *Klebsiella* spp., both indole-positive and indole-negative *Proteus*, *Providencia*, *Salmonella*, *Serratia*, and *Shigella* spp. and *Yersinia enterocolitica*. Other susceptible Gram-negative bacteria include *Haemophilus influenzae*, *Moraxella catarrhalis* (*Branhamella catarrhalis*), and *Neisseria* spp. Among Gram-positive bacteria it is active against some staphylococci and streptococci, but meticillin-resistant staphylococci, enterococci, and *Listeria monocytogenes* are generally resistant. Ceftazidime is active against some anaerobes, although most strains of *Bacteroides fragilis* and *Clostridium difficile* are resistant.

The activity of ceftazidime against *Pseudomonas aeruginosa* and some Enterobacteriaceae may be enhanced by aminoglycosides. Antagonism has been reported *in vitro* between ceftazidime and chloramphenicol.

*Resistance.* As with cefotaxime, resistance may develop during treatment due to the derepression of chromosomally mediated beta-lactamases. It has been noted particularly in *Pseudomonas* spp. and in Enterobacteriaceae including *Citrobacter*, *Enterobacter* spp. and *Proteus vulgaris*. Resistance may also occur due to the production of plasmid-mediated extended-spectrum beta-lactamases, particularly in *Klebsiella* spp. and *E. coli*.

## Pharmacokinetics

Ceftazidime is given by injection as the sodium salt or in solution with arginine. Mean peak plasma concentrations of 17 and 39 micrograms/mL have been reported about 1 hour after intramuscular administration of 0.5 and 1 g of ceftazidime, respectively. Five minutes after intravenous bolus injections of 0.5, 1, and 2 g of ceftazidime, mean plasma concentrations of 45, 90, and 170 micrograms/mL, respectively, have been reported. The plasma half-life of ceftazidime is about 2 hours, but this is prolonged in patients with renal impairment and in neonates. Clearance may be enhanced in patients with cystic fibrosis. It is about 10% bound to plasma proteins.

Ceftazidime is widely distributed in body tissues and fluids; therapeutic concentrations are achieved in the CSF when the meninges are inflamed. It crosses the placenta and is distributed into breast milk.

Ceftazidime is passively excreted in bile, although only a small proportion is eliminated by this route. It is mainly excreted by the kidneys, almost exclusively by glomerular filtration; probenecid has little effect on the excretion. About 80 to 90% of a dose appears unchanged in the urine within 24 hours. It is removed by haemodialysis and peritoneal dialysis.

**Cystic fibrosis.** References.

1. Leeder JS, *et al.* Ceftazidime disposition in acute and stable cystic fibrosis. *Clin Pharmacol Ther* 1984; **36:** 355–62.
2. Hedman A, *et al.* Influence of the glomerular filtration rate on renal clearance of ceftazidime in cystic fibrosis. *Clin Pharmacokinet* 1988; **15:** 57–65.
3. Vinks AATMM, *et al.* Continuous infusion of ceftazidime in cystic fibrosis patients during home treatment: clinical outcome, microbiology and pharmacokinetics. *J Antimicrob Chemother* 1997; **40:** 125–33.

**The elderly.** References.

1. LeBel M, *et al.* Pharmacokinetics of ceftazidime in elderly volunteers. *Antimicrob Agents Chemother* 1985; **28:** 713–15.
2. Higbee MD, *et al.* Pharmacokinetics of ceftazidime in elderly patients. *Clin Pharm* 1989; **8:** 59–62.
3. Sirgo MA, Norris S. Ceftazidime in the elderly: appropriateness of twice-daily dosing. *DICP Ann Pharmacother* 1991; **25:** 284–8.

**Hepatic impairment.** References.

1. El Touny M, *et al.* Pharmacokinetics of ceftazidime in patients with liver cirrhosis and ascites. *J Antimicrob Chemother* 1991; **28:** 95–100.

**Neonates.** References.

1. van den Anker JN, *et al.* Ceftazidime pharmacokinetics in preterm infants: effects of renal function and gestational age. *Clin Pharmacol Ther* 1995; **58:** 650–9.
2. van den Anker JN, *et al.* Ceftazidime pharmacokinetics in preterm infants: effect of postnatal age and postnatal exposure to indomethacin. *Br J Clin Pharmacol* 1995; **40:** 439–43.
3. van den Anker JN, *et al.* Once-daily versus twice-daily administration of ceftazidime in the preterm infant. *Antimicrob Agents Chemother* 1995; **39:** 2048–50.

**Renal impairment.** References.

1. Welage LS, *et al.* Pharmacokinetics of ceftazidime in patients with renal insufficiency. *Antimicrob Agents Chemother* 1984; **25:** 201–4.
2. Leroy A, *et al.* Pharmacokinetics of ceftazidime in normal and uremic subjects. *Antimicrob Agents Chemother* 1984; **25:** 638–42.
3. Ackerman BH, *et al.* Effect of decreased renal function on the pharmacokinetics of ceftazidime. *Antimicrob Agents Chemother* 1984; **25:** 785–6.
4. Lin N-S, *et al.* Single- and multiple-dose pharmacokinetics of ceftazidime in infected patients with varying degrees of renal function. *J Clin Pharmacol* 1989; **29:** 331–7.
5. Kinowski J-M, *et al.* Multiple-dose pharmacokinetics of amikacin and ceftazidime in critically ill patients with septic multiple-organ failure during intermittent hemofiltration. *Antimicrob Agents Chemother* 1993; **37:** 464–73.
6. Demotes-Mainard F, *et al.* Pharmacokinetics of intravenous and intraperitoneal ceftazidime in chronic ambulatory peritoneal dialysis. *J Clin Pharmacol* 1993; **33:** 475–9.

## Uses and Administration

Ceftazidime is a third-generation cephalosporin antibacterial with enhanced activity against *Pseudomonas aeruginosa*. It is used in the treatment of susceptible infections especially those due to *Pseudomonas* spp. They include biliary-tract infections, bone and joint infections, cystic fibrosis (respiratory-tract infections), endophthalmitis, infections in immunocompromised patients (neutropenic patients), melioidosis, meningitis, peritonitis, pneumonia, upper respiratory-tract infections, septicaemia, skin infections (including burns, ecthyma gangrenosum, and ulceration), and urinary-tract infections. It is also used for surgical infection prophylaxis. For details of these infections and their treatment, see under Choice of Antibacterial, p.120.

*Administration and dosage.* Ceftazidime is available as the pentahydrate but it is formulated with sodium carbonate, to form the sodium salt in solution, or with arginine. Doses are expressed in terms of anhydrous ceftazidime. Ceftazidime pentahydrate 1.16 g is approximately equivalent to 1 g of anhydrous ceftazidime. It is given by deep intramuscular injection, slow intravenous injection over 3 to 5 minutes, or intravenous infusion over up to 30 minutes. The usual dose for adults ranges from 1 to 6 g daily in divided doses every 8 or 12 hours. The higher doses are used in severe infections especially in immunocompromised patients. In adults with cystic fibrosis who have pseudomonal lung infections, high doses of 90 to 150 mg/kg daily in 3 divided doses are used; up to 9 g daily has been given to adults with normal renal function. Single doses of more than 1 g should be given intravenously.

Children are usually given ceftazidime 30 to 100 mg/kg daily in 2 or 3 divided doses, but in severely ill children up to 150 mg/kg daily to a maximum of 6 g daily may be given in 3 divided doses. Neonates and infants up to 2 months have been given 25 to 60 mg/kg daily in 2 divided doses.

In the elderly the dose should generally not exceed 3 g daily.

For details of reduced doses to be used in patients with renal impairment, see below.

For surgical infection prophylaxis in patients undergoing prostatic surgery, a dose of 1 g may be given at induction of anaesthesia and repeated if necessary when the catheter is removed.

Ceftazidime can be used with an aminoglycoside, another beta lactam such as piperacillin, or vancomycin in patients with severe neutropenia, or, if infection with *Bacteroides fragilis* is suspected, with an antimicrobial such as clindamycin or metronidazole. The drugs should generally be administered separately (see also Incompatibility, above).

◊ References.

1. Rains CP, *et al.* Ceftazidime: an update of its antibacterial activity, pharmacokinetic properties and therapeutic efficacy. *Drugs* 1995; **49:** 577–617.

**Administration in renal impairment.** In patients with renal impairment the dosage of ceftazidime may need to be reduced. Following a loading dose of 1 g, maintenance doses are based on the creatinine clearance (CC):

- CC 31 to 50 mL/minute: 1 g every 12 hours
- CC 16 to 30 mL/minute: 1 g every 24 hours
- CC 6 to 15 mL/minute: 500 mg every 24 hours
- CC less than 5 mL/minute: 500 mg every 48 hours

In severe infections these doses may need to be increased by 50%. In these patients ceftazidime trough serum concentrations should not exceed 40 micrograms/mL. In patients undergoing peritoneal dialysis a loading dose of 1 g may be given followed by 500 mg every 24 hours; ceftazidime sodium may also be added to the dialysis fluid, usually 125 to 250 mg of ceftazidime for 2 litres of dialysis fluid. In patients undergoing haemodialysis a loading dose of 1 g is given and then 0.5 to 1 g after each dialysis period.

## Preparations

***USP 27:*** Ceftazidime for Injection; Ceftazidime Injection.

**Proprietary Preparations** (details are given in Part 3)

***Arg.:*** Crima; Fortum; Tinacef; ***Austral.:*** Fortum; ***Austria:*** Fortum; Kefazim; ***Belg.:*** Glazidim; Kefadim; ***Braz.:*** Cefazima; Ceftazidon; Ceften; Cetaz; Fortaz; Kefadim†; Roycefax; Tazidem†; ***Canad.:*** Ceptaz; Fortaz; Tazidime; ***Chile:*** Fortum; Kefzim; ***Denm.:*** Fortum; ***Fin.:*** Glazidim; ***Fr.:*** Fortum; Fortumset; ***Ger.:*** Fortum; ***Gr.:*** Ftazidime; Lemoxol; Solvetan; ***Hong Kong:*** Fortum; ***India:*** Ceftidin; Fortum; Zytaz; ***Irl.:*** Fortum; ***Israel:*** Fortum; ***Ital.:*** Ceftim; Glazidim; Panzid; Spectrum; Starcef; ***Malaysia:*** Fortum; ***Mex.:*** Bac-Zidim†; Fortum; Izadima; Lezidim; Tagal; Taloken; Taxifur; Waytrax†; Zadolina; Zidicef†; ***Neth.:*** Fortum; ***Norw.:*** Fortum; ***NZ:*** Fortum; ***Port.:*** Cefortam; ***S.Afr.:*** Fortum†; Kefzim; ***Singapore:*** Fortum; ***Spain:*** Fortam; Kefamin; Potendal†; ***Swed.:*** Fortum; ***Switz.:*** Fortam; ***Thai.:*** CEF-4; Cefodime; Fortum; Forzid; Fournox; Kefadim†; Zeftam; ***UAE:*** Negacef; ***UK:*** Fortum; Kefadim; ***USA:*** Ceptaz; Fortaz; Tazicef; Tazidime.

---

## Cefteram Pivoxil *(rINNM)*

T-2588. Pivaloyloxymethyl (*Z*)-7-[2-(2-aminothiazol-4-yl)-2-methoxyiminoacetamido]-3-(5-methyl-2*H*-tetrazol-2-ylmethyl)-3-cephem-4-carboxylic acid.

$C_{22}H_{27}N_9O_7S_2$ = 593.6.

*CAS — 82547-58-8 (cefteram); 82547-81-7 (cefteram pivoxil).*

**Pharmacopoeias.** In *Jpn.*

### Profile

Cefteram is a cephalosporin antibacterial used for the treatment of susceptible infections. It is given by mouth as the pivaloyloxymethyl ester, cefteram pivoxil, and doses are expressed in terms of cefteram. 186 mg of cefteram pivoxil is approximately equivalent to 150 mg of cefteram. The usual adult dose is 150 to 300 mg daily in 3 divided doses after meals. For severe infections, up to 600 mg daily may be given.

### Preparations

**Proprietary Preparations** (details are given in Part 3)

***Jpn:*** Tomiron.

---

### Ceftezole Sodium *(rINNM)*

Ceftezol sódico. Sodium (7R)-7-[2-(1H-tetrazol-1-yl)acetamido]-3-(1,3,4-thiadiazol-2-ylthiomethyl)-3-cephem-4-carboxylate.

$C_{13}H_{11}N_8NaO_4S_3$ = 462.5.

*CAS — 26973-24-0 (ceftezole); 41136-22-5 (ceftezole sodium).*

*ATC — J01DA36.*

#### Profile

Ceftezole is a cephalosporin antibacterial with properties similar to those of cefalotin (p.168). It is given as the sodium salt but doses are expressed in terms of the base. 1.05 g of ceftezole sodium is approximately equivalent to 1 g of ceftezole. The usual adult dose is 2 to 4 g daily by intramuscular injection in 2 or 3 divided doses.

**Sodium content.** Each g of ceftezole sodium contains about 2.16 mmol of sodium.

#### Preparations

**Proprietary Preparations** (details are given in Part 3)
***Ital.:*** Alomen.

## Ceftibuten *(BAN, USAN, rINN)*

Ceftibuteno; 7432-S; Sch-39720. 7-[2-(2-Amino-1,3-thiazol-4-yl)-4-carboxyisocrotonamide]-3-cephem-4-carboxylic acid.

$C_{15}H_{14}N_4O_6S_2$ = 410.4.

*CAS — 97519-39-6.*

*ATC — J01DA39.*

**Pharmacopoeias.** In *Jpn.*

#### Adverse Effects and Precautions

As for Cefalotin Sodium, p.168.

The most frequently reported adverse effects of ceftibuten are gastrointestinal disturbances, especially diarrhoea, and headache.

#### Antimicrobial Action

As for Cefixime, p.173. It is less active *in vitro* against *Streptococcus pneumoniae*.

◊ References.


1. Shawar R, *et al.* Comparative in vitro activity of ceftibuten (Sch-39720) against bacterial enteropathogens. *Antimicrob Agents Chemother* 1989; **33:** 781–4.
2. Bragman SGL, Casewell MW. The in-vitro activity of ceftibuten against 475 clinical isolates of Gram-negative bacilli, compared with cefuroxime and cefadroxil. *J Antimicrob Chemother* 1990; **25:** 221–6.
3. Wise R, *et al.* Ceftibuten—in-vitro activity against respiratory pathogens, β-lactamase stability and mechanism of action. *J Antimicrob Chemother* 1990; **26:** 209–13.


#### Pharmacokinetics

Ceftibuten is rapidly absorbed from the gastrointestinal tract, although the rate and extent of absorption are somewhat decreased by the presence of food. Peak plasma concentrations of about 17 micrograms/mL are attained about 2 hours after a 400-mg dose. The plasma half-life of ceftibuten is about 2.0 to 2.3 hours and is prolonged in patients with renal impairment. Ceftibuten is 65 to 77% bound to plasma proteins.

Ceftibuten distributes into middle-ear fluid and bronchial secretions. About 10% of a dose is converted to the *trans*-isomer, which has about one-eighth of the activity of the *cis*-isomer. Ceftibuten is excreted mainly in the urine and also in the faeces. Significant amounts are removed by haemodialysis.

#### Uses and Administration

Ceftibuten is an oral third-generation cephalosporin antibacterial used similarly to cefixime (p.173) in the treatment of urinary-tract and respiratory-tract infections. It is given by mouth as the dihydrate, but doses are expressed in terms of anhydrous ceftibuten. 435 mg of ceftibuten dihydrate is approximately equivalent to 400 mg of anhydrous ceftibuten. The usual adult dose is 400 mg once daily on an empty stomach. Children over 6 months of age and weighing 45 kg or less may be given 9 mg/kg daily as a single dose. For reduced doses to be used in patients with moderate to severe renal impairment, see below.

◊ Reviews.


1. Wiseman LR, Balfour JA. Ceftibuten: review of its antibacterial activity, pharmacokinetic properties and clinical efficacy. *Drugs* 1994; **47:** 784–808.
2. Nelson JD, McCracken GH (eds). Ceftibuten: a new orally active cephalosporin for pediatric infections. *Pediatr Infect Dis J* 1995; **14** (suppl): S76–S133.
3. Guay DRP. Ceftibuten: a new expanded-spectrum oral cephalosporin. *Ann Pharmacother* 1997; **31:** 1022–33.
4. Owens RC, *et al.* Ceftibuten: an overview. *Pharmacotherapy* 1997; **17:** 707–20.


**Administration in renal impairment.** Doses of ceftibuten should be reduced in patients with moderate to severe renal impairment. The following doses based on creatinine clearance (CC) may be used:

- CC 30 to 49 mL/minute: 200 mg once daily
- CC 5 to 29 mL/minute: 100 mg once daily

Patients undergoing haemodialysis 2 or 3 times weekly may be given a dose of 400 mg after each dialysis session.

#### Preparations

**Proprietary Preparations** (details are given in Part 3)
***Arg.:*** Cedax; Sepex; ***Austria:*** Caedax; ***Fin.:*** Cedax†; ***Ger.:*** Keimax; ***Gr.:*** Caedax; ***Hong Kong:*** Cedax; ***India:*** Procadax; ***Irl.:*** Cedax†; ***Israel:*** Cedax†; ***Ital.:*** Cedax; Isocef; ***Jpn:*** Seftem; ***Malaysia:*** Cedax; ***Mex.:*** Cedax; ***Neth.:*** Cedax; ***Port.:*** Caedax; ***S.Afr.:*** Cedax; Sepexin; ***Singapore:*** Cedax; ***Spain:*** Biocef; Cedax; Cepifran; ***Swed.:*** Cedax; ***Switz.:*** Cedax; ***Thai.:*** Cedax; ***USA:*** Cedax.

### Ceftiofur Hydrochloride *(BANM, USAN)*

U-64279A. (6R,7R)-7-[2-(2-Amino-4-thiazolyl)-glyoxylamido]-3-mercaptomethyl-8-oxo-5-thia-1-azabicyclo[4.2.0]oct-2-ene-2-carboxylate, $7^2$-(Z)-(O-methyloxime), 2-furoate (ester), monohydrochloride.

$C_{19}H_{17}N_5O_7S_3$.HCl = 560.0.

*CAS — 80370-57-6 (ceftiofur); 103980-44-5 (ceftiofur hydrochloride).*

### Ceftiofur Sodium *(BANM, USAN)*

Ceftiofur sódico; CM-31-916; U-64279E.

$C_{19}H_{16}N_5NaO_7S_3$ = 545.5.

*CAS — 104010-37-9.*

#### Profile

Ceftiofur is a cephalosporin antibacterial used as the hydrochloride and sodium salts in veterinary practice.

## Ceftizoxime Sodium *(BANM, USAN, rINNM)*

Ceftizoxima sódica; FK-749; FR-13749; SKF-88373-Z. Sodium (Z)-7-[2-(2-aminothiazol-4-yl)-2-methoxyiminoacetamido]-3-cephem-4-carboxylate.

$C_{13}H_{12}N_5NaO_5S_2$ = 405.4.

*CAS — 68401-81-0 (ceftizoxime); 68401-82-1 (ceftizoxime sodium).*

*ATC — J01DA22.*

**Pharmacopoeias.** In *Jpn* and *US.*

**USP 27** (Ceftizoxime Sodium). A white to pale yellow crystalline powder. Freely soluble in water. pH of a 10% solution in water is between 6.0 and 8.0. Store in airtight containers.

**Stability.** References.


1. Lesko AB, *et al.* Ceftizoxime stability in iv solutions. *DICP Ann Pharmacother* 1989; **23:** 615–18.


#### Adverse Effects and Precautions

As for Cefotaxime Sodium, p.175.

**Sodium content.** Each g of ceftizoxime sodium contains about 2.5 mmol of sodium.

#### Interactions

Probenecid reduces the renal clearance of ceftizoxime.

#### Antimicrobial Action

As for Cefotaxime Sodium, p.176, although ceftizoxime has no active metabolite.

#### Pharmacokinetics

After intramuscular injection of 0.5 and 1 g of ceftizoxime, mean peak plasma concentrations of about 14 and 39 micrograms/mL respectively have been reported after 1 hour. The plasma half-life of ceftizoxime is about 1.7 hours and is prolonged in neonates and in renal impairment. Ceftizoxime is 30% bound to plasma proteins.

Ceftizoxime is widely distributed in body tissues and fluids; therapeutic concentrations are achieved in the CSF when the meninges are inflamed. It crosses the placenta and low concentrations have been detected in breast milk.

Nearly all of a dose is excreted unchanged in the urine within 24 hours of administration, thus achieving high urinary concentrations. Ceftizoxime is excreted by tubular secretion as well as glomerular filtration and the concomitant administration of probenecid results in higher and more prolonged plasma concentrations. Some ceftizoxime is removed by haemodialysis.

**Neonates.** References.


1. Fujii R. Investigation of half-life and clinical effects of ceftizoxime in premature and newborn infants. *Drug Invest* 1990; **2:** 143–9.
2. Reed MD, *et al.* Ceftizoxime disposition in neonates and infants during the first six months of life. *DICP Ann Pharmacother* 1991; **25:** 344–7.


#### Uses and Administration

Ceftizoxime is a third-generation cephalosporin antibacterial used similarly to cefotaxime (p.176) for the treatment of susceptible infections.

It is given as the sodium salt by deep intramuscular injection, or intravenously as a slow injection over 3 to 5 minutes or as a continuous or intermittent infusion. If 2 g of ceftizoxime is injected intramuscularly the dose should be divided between sites.

Doses are expressed in terms of the equivalent amount of ceftizoxime. 1.06 g of ceftizoxime sodium is approximately equivalent to 1 g of ceftizoxime. It is usually given in an adult dose of 1 to 2 g every 8 to 12 hours. In severe infections 2 to 4 g may be given intravenously every 8 hours; doses up to 2 g every 4 hours have been given in life-threatening infections.

Children over 6 months of age may be given 50 mg/kg every 6 to 8 hours.

For the treatment of uncomplicated urinary-tract infections, a dose of 500 mg every 12 hours is used.

For details of reduced doses to be used in patients with renal impairment, see below.

A single intramuscular dose of 1 g has been given in uncomplicated gonorrhoea.

◊ References.


1. Richards DM, Heel RC. Ceftizoxime: a review of its antibacterial activity, pharmacokinetic properties and therapeutic use. *Drugs* 1985; **29:** 281–329.


**Administration in renal impairment.** Doses of ceftizoxime should be modified in renal impairment; after a loading dose of 0.5 to 1 g, the maintenance dosage should be adjusted according to the patient's creatinine clearance (CC) and the severity of the infection:

- CC 50 to 79 mL/minute: 0.5 to 1.5 g every 8 hours
- CC 5 to 49 mL/minute: 0.25 to 1 g every 12 hours
- CC less than 5 mL/minute: 250 to 500 mg every 24 hours or 0.5 to 1 g every 48 hours, after dialysis.

#### Preparations

***USP 27:*** Ceftizoxime for Injection; Ceftizoxime Injection.

**Proprietary Preparations** (details are given in Part 3)
***Arg.:*** Ceftix; Ceftizon; ***Austria:*** Cefizox†; ***Canad.:*** Cefizox; ***Fin.:*** Epocelin†; ***Fr.:*** Cefizox; ***Ger.:*** Ceftix†; ***India:*** Cefizox; ***Irl.:*** Cefizox†; ***Israel:*** Tefizox†; ***Ital.:*** Eposerin; ***Jpn:*** Epocelin; ***Mex.:*** Cefizox; Ultraceff†; ***Neth.:*** Cefizox; ***Port.:*** Cefizox; ***Spain:*** Cefizox†; Epocelin†; ***Thai.:*** Epocelin†; ***USA:*** Cefizox.

## Ceftriaxone Sodium *(BANM, USAN, rINNM)*

Ceftriaxona sódica; Ceftriaxonum Natricum; Ro-13-9904; Ro-13-9904/000 (ceftriaxone). (Z)-7-[2-(2-Aminothiazol-4-yl)-2-methoxyiminoacetamido]-3-[(2,5-dihydro-6-hydroxy-2-methyl-5-oxo-1,2,4-triazin-3-yl)thiomethyl]-3-cephem-4-carboxylic acid, disodium salt, sesquaterhydrate.

$C_{18}H_{16}N_8Na_2O_7S_3,3\frac{1}{2}H_2O$ = 661.6.

*CAS — 73384-59-5 (ceftriaxone); 74578-69-1 (anhydrous ceftriaxone sodium); 104376-79-6 (ceftriaxone sodium sesquaterhydrate).*

*ATC — J01DA13.*

**Pharmacopoeias.** In *Chin., Eur.* (see p.vi), *Jpn, Pol.,* and *US.*

**Ph. Eur. 5.0** (Ceftriaxone Sodium). An almost white to yellowish, slightly hygroscopic, crystalline powder. Freely soluble in water; very slightly soluble in dehydrated alcohol; sparingly soluble in methyl alcohol. A 12% solution in water has a pH of 6.0 to 8.0. Store in airtight containers. Protect from light.

**USP 27** (Ceftriaxone Sodium). A white to yellowish-orange crystalline powder. Freely soluble in water; very slightly soluble in alcohol; sparingly soluble in methyl alcohol. pH of a 10% solution in water is between 6.0 and 8.0. Store in airtight containers.

**Incompatibility.** The UK manufacturer warns of incompatibility if ceftriaxone sodium is mixed with calcium-containing solutions or with aminoglycosides, amsacrine, fluconazole, labetalol, or vancomycin. Published reports of incompatibility have included that between ceftriaxone and vancomycin[1] or pentamidine.[2]


1. Pritts D, Hancock D. Incompatibility of ceftriaxone with vancomycin. *Am J Hosp Pharm* 1991; **48:** 77.
2. Lewis JD, El-Gendy A. Cephalosporin-pentamidine isethionate incompatibilities. *Am J Health-Syst Pharm* 1996; **53:** 1461–2.


**Stability.** References.


1. Nahata MC. Stability of ceftriaxone sodium in peritoneal dialysis solutions. *DICP Ann Pharmacother* 1991; **25:** 741–2.
2. Canton E, Esteban MJ. Stability of ceftriaxone solution. *J Antimicrob Chemother* 1992; **30:** 397–8.
3. Bailey LC, *et al.* Stability of ceftriaxone sodium in injectable solutions stored frozen in syringes. *Am J Hosp Pharm* 1994; **51:** 2159–61.
4. Plumridge RJ, *et al.* Stability of ceftriaxone sodium in polypropylene syringes at −20, 4, and 20°C. *Am J Health-Syst Pharm* 1996; **53:** 2320–3.


## Adverse Effects and Precautions

As for Cefotaxime Sodium, p.175.

Changes in bowel flora may be more marked than with cefotaxime because of the greater biliary excretion of ceftriaxone; diarrhoea may occur more often, especially in children. Biliary sludge or pseudolithiasis due to a precipitate of calcium ceftriaxone has been seen occasionally in patients receiving ceftriaxone. Similarly, deposition of the calcium salt has occurred rarely in the urine. Ceftriaxone is highly protein bound and is able to displace bilirubin from albumin binding sites, causing hyperbilirubinaemia; its use should be avoided in jaundiced neonates.

Neutropenia has been reported with most cephalosporins; a complex mechanism has been attributed to that associated with ceftriaxone. There have been rare reports of fatal haemolysis associated with ceftriaxone.

Although ceftriaxone has an *N*-methylthiotriazine ring rather than the *N*-methylthiotetrazole side-chain seen in cephalosporins such as cefamandole (p.169), it might still have the potential to cause hypoprothrombinaemia.

**Breast feeding.** A study of drug distribution and protein binding between maternal blood and breast milk post partum in a 26-year-old woman receiving ceftriaxone 2 g daily by intravenous infusion for 10 days found that penetration of ceftriaxone into breast milk became greater at such high doses as protein binding capacity was saturated, although no adverse effects occurred in the infant.[1] The authors advised caution in breast-feeding mothers receiving acidic drugs which also have high protein binding such as ceftriaxone[1] although, on the basis that no adverse effects have been observed in breast-fed infants whose mothers were receiving ceftriaxone, the American Academy of Pediatrics considers[2] that it is therefore usually compatible with breast feeding.


1. Bourget P, *et al.* Ceftriaxone distribution and protein binding between maternal blood and milk postpartum. *Ann Pharmacother* 1993; **27:** 294–7.
2. American Academy of Pediatrics. The transfer of drugs and other chemicals into human milk. *Pediatrics* 2001; **108:** 776–89. Correction. *ibid.*; 1029. Also available at: http://aappolicy.aappublications.org/cgi/content/full/pediatrics%3b108/3/776 (accessed 25/05/04)


**Effects on the biliary tract.** Using abdominal ultrasonography, biliary sludge or pseudolithiasis was found in about 40% of severely ill children being treated with high doses of ceftriaxone[1] and was later reported in adults.[2,3] The sludge has been identified as a calcium salt of ceftriaxone.[4] Patients are often asymptomatic and the sludge usually dissolves once ceftriaxone is discontinued. Gallstones with ceftriaxone as a major component have been identified in a patient given long-term high-dose treatment.[5] Similarly, a bile-duct stone composed of ceftriaxone occurred with high-dose ceftriaxone in a child.[6] In another report, intractable hiccups were associated with ceftriaxone-related pseudolithiasis in a 10-year-old boy.[7]


1. Schaad UB, *et al.* Reversible ceftriaxone-associated biliary pseudolithiasis in children. *Lancet* 1988; **ii:** 1411–13.
2. Pigrau C, *et al.* Ceftriaxone-associated biliary pseudolithiasis in adults. *Lancet* 1989; **ii:** 165.
3. Heim-Duthoy KL, *et al.* Apparent biliary pseudolithiasis during ceftriaxone therapy. *Antimicrob Agents Chemother* 1990; **34:** 1146–9.
4. Park HZ, *et al.* Ceftriaxone-associated gallbladder sludge: identification of calcium-ceftriaxone salt as a major component of gallbladder precipitate. *Gastroenterology* 1991; **100:** 1665–70.
5. Lopez AJ, *et al.* Ceftriaxone-induced cholelithiasis. *Ann Intern Med* 1991; **115:** 712–14.
6. Robertson FM, *et al.* Ceftriaxone choledocholithiasis. *Pediatrics* 1996; **98:** 133–5.
7. Bonioli E, *et al.* Pseudolithiasis and intractable hiccups in a boy receiving ceftriaxone. *N Engl J Med* 1994; **331:** 1532.


**Effects on the blood.** References.


1. Haubenstock A, *et al.* Hypoprothrombinaemic bleeding associated with ceftriaxone. *Lancet* 1983; **i:** 1215–16.
2. Rey D, *et al.* Ceftriaxone-induced granulopenia related to a peculiar mechanism of granulopoiesis inhibition. *Am J Med* 1989; **87:** 591–2.
3. Bernini JC, *et al.* Fatal hemolysis induced by ceftriaxone in a child with sickle cell anemia. *J Pediatr* 1995; **126:** 813–15.
4. Lascari AD, Amyot K. Fatal hemolysis caused by ceftriaxone. *J Pediatr* 1995; **126:** 816–17.
5. Scimeca PG, *et al.* Hemolysis after treatment with ceftriaxone. *J Pediatr* 1996; **128:** 163.
6. Moallem HJ, *et al.* Ceftriaxone-related fatal hemolysis in an adolescent with perinatally acquired human immunodeficiency virus infection. *J Pediatr* 1998; **133:** 279–81.
7. Meyer O, *et al.* Fatal immune haemolysis due to a degradation product of ceftriaxone. *Br J Haematol* 1999; **105:** 1084–5.
8. Viner Y, *et al.* Severe hemolysis induced by ceftriaxone in a child with sickle-cell anemia. *Pediatr Infect Dis J* 2000; **19:** 83–5.
9. Seltsam A, Salama A. Ceftriaxone-induced immune haemolysis: two case reports and a concise review of the literature. *Intensive Care Med* 2000; **26:** 1390–4.
10. Citak A, *et al.* Ceftriaxone-induced haemolytic anaemia in a child with no immune deficiency or haematological disease. *J Paediatr Child Health* 2002; **38:** 209–10.


**Effects on the pancreas.** References.


1. Zimmermann AE, *et al.* Ceftriaxone-induced acute pancreatitis. *Ann Pharmacother* 1993; **27:** 36–7.
2. Maranan MC, *et al.* Gallstone pancreatitis caused by ceftriaxone. *Pediatr Infect Dis J* 1998; **17:** 662–3.


**Neonates.** References to the displacement of bilirubin by ceftriaxone in neonates.


1. Gulian J-M, *et al.* Bilirubin displacement by ceftriaxone in neonates: evaluation by determination of 'free' bilirubin and erythrocyte-bound bilirubin. *J Antimicrob Chemother* 1987; **19:** 823–9.
2. Fink S, *et al.* Ceftriaxone effect on bilirubin-albumin binding. *Pediatrics* 1987; **80:** 873–5.


**Sodium content.** Each g of ceftriaxone sodium contains about 3.0 mmol of sodium.

## Interactions

Ceftriaxone has an *N*-methylthiotriazine side-chain and may have the potential to increase the effects of anticoagulants and to cause a disulfiram-like reaction with alcohol.

Unlike many cephalosporins, probenecid does not affect the renal excretion of ceftriaxone.

## Antimicrobial Action

As for Cefotaxime Sodium, p.176, although ceftriaxone has no active metabolite.

◊ References.


1. Goldstein FW, *et al.* Resistance to ceftriaxone and other β-lactams in bacteria isolated in the community. *Antimicrob Agents Chemother* 1995; **39:** 2516–19.


## Pharmacokinetics

Ceftriaxone demonstrates nonlinear dose-dependent pharmacokinetics because of its protein binding; about 85 to 95% is bound to plasma protein depending on the concentration of ceftriaxone.

Mean peak plasma concentrations of about 40 and 80 micrograms/mL have been reported 2 hours after intramuscular injection of 0.5 and 1 g of ceftriaxone respectively. The plasma half-life of ceftriaxone is not dependent on the dose and varies between 6 and 9 hours; it may be prolonged in neonates. The half-life does not change appreciably in patients with moderate renal impairment, but it may be prolonged in severe renal impairment especially when there is also hepatic impairment.

Ceftriaxone is widely distributed in body tissues and fluids. It crosses both inflamed and non-inflamed meninges, generally achieving therapeutic concentrations in the CSF. It crosses the placenta and low concentrations have been detected in breast milk. High concentrations are achieved in bile.

About 40 to 65% of a dose of ceftriaxone is excreted unchanged in the urine, principally by glomerular filtration; the remainder is excreted in the bile and is ultimately found in the faeces as unchanged drug and microbiologically inactive compounds.

◊ Reviews.


1. Hayton WL, Stoeckel K. Age-associated changes in ceftriaxone pharmacokinetics. *Clin Pharmacokinet* 1986; **11:** 76–86.
2. Yuk JH, *et al.* Clinical pharmacokinetics of ceftriaxone. *Clin Pharmacokinet* 1989; **17:** 223–35.
3. Perry TR, Schentag JJ. Clinical use of ceftriaxone: a pharmacokinetic-pharmacodynamic perspective on the impact of minimum inhibitory concentration and serum protein binding. *Clin Pharmacokinet* 2001; **40:** 685–94.


**Hepatic impairment.** References.


1. Stoeckel K, *et al.* Single-dose ceftriaxone kinetics in liver insufficiency. *Clin Pharmacol Ther* 1984; **36:** 500–9.
2. Hary L, *et al.* The pharmacokinetics of ceftriaxone and cefotaxime in cirrhotic patients with ascites. *Eur J Clin Pharmacol* 1989; **36:** 613–16.
3. Toth A, *et al.* Pharmacokinetics of ceftriaxone in liver-transplant recipients. *J Clin Pharmacol* 1991; **31:** 722–8.


**Pregnancy.** References.


1. Bourget P, *et al.* Pharmacokinetics and protein binding of ceftriaxone during pregnancy. *Antimicrob Agents Chemother* 1993; **37:** 54–9.


**Renal impairment.** The pharmacokinetics of ceftriaxone are not markedly altered in mild to moderate renal impairment,[1] but the half-life can be prolonged in severe or end-stage renal disease.[1-4] Ceftriaxone is generally not removed by peritoneal dialysis[4] or by haemodialysis[1-3] although a decrease in half-life has been reported during haemodialysis.[5] In many patients no alteration in dosage is necessary, but some individuals have reduced non-renal clearance despite apparently normal hepatic function.[2,3] It is advisable to monitor plasma ceftriaxone in patients with severe renal impairment and unknown non-renal clearance.


1. Patel IH, *et al.* Ceftriaxone pharmacokinetics in patients with various degrees of renal impairment. *Antimicrob Agents Chemother* 1984; **25:** 438–42.
2. Stoeckel K, *et al.* Single-dose ceftriaxone kinetics in functionally anephric patients. *Clin Pharmacol Ther* 1983; **33:** 633–41.
3. Cohen D, *et al.* Pharmacokinetics of ceftriaxone in patients with renal failure and in those undergoing hemodialysis. *Antimicrob Agents Chemother* 1983; **24:** 529–32.
4. Ti T-Y, *et al.* Kinetic disposition of intravenous ceftriaxone in normal subjects and patients with renal failure on hemodialysis or peritoneal dialysis. *Antimicrob Agents Chemother* 1984; **25:** 83–7.
5. Garcia RL, *et al.* Single-dose pharmacokinetics of ceftriaxone in patients with end-stage renal disease and hemodialysis. *Chemotherapy* 1988; **34:** 261–6.


## Uses and Administration

Ceftriaxone is a third-generation cephalosporin antibacterial used similarly to cefotaxime for the treatment of susceptible infections. They include chancroid, endocarditis, gastro-enteritis (invasive salmonellosis; shigellosis), gonorrhoea, Lyme disease, meningitis (including meningococcal meningitis prophylaxis), pneumonia, septicaemia, syphilis, typhoid fever, and Whipple's disease. It is also used for surgical infection prophylaxis. For details of these infections and their treatment, see under Choice of Antibacterial, p.120.

*Administration and dosage.* Ceftriaxone is given as the sodium salt by slow intravenous injection over at least 2 to 4 minutes, by intermittent intravenous infusion over at least 30 minutes, or by deep intramuscular injection. If more than 1 g is to be injected intramuscularly then the dose should be divided between more than one site. Doses are expressed in terms of the equivalent amount of ceftriaxone. 1.19 g of ceftriaxone sodium is approximately equivalent to 1 g of ceftriaxone. The usual adult dose is 1 to 2 g daily as a single dose or in two divided doses; in severe infections up to 4 g daily may be given. Doses for infants and children (under 50 kg) are 20 to 50 mg/kg once daily; for severe infections up to 80 mg/kg daily may be given. In neonates, the maximum dose should not exceed 50 mg/kg daily; intravenous doses in neonates should be given over 60 minutes. Doses above 50 mg/kg should be given by intravenous infusion only.

A single intramuscular dose of 250 mg is recommended for the treatment of uncomplicated gonorrhoea in adults.

For surgical infection prophylaxis in adults, a single dose of 1 g may be given 0.5 to 2 hours before surgery; a 2-g dose is suggested before colorectal surgery.

For the prevention of secondary cases of meningococcal meningitis, a single intramuscular dose of 250 mg may be used for adults and 125 mg for children.

◊ References.


1. Brogden RN, Ward A. Ceftriaxone: a reappraisal of its antibacterial activity and pharmacokinetic properties, and an update on its therapeutic use with particular reference to once-daily administration. *Drugs* 1988; **35:** 604–45.
2. Lamb HM, *et al.* Ceftriaxone: an update of its use in the management of community-acquired and nosocomial infections. *Drugs* 2002; **62:** 1041–89.


**Administration in hepatic and renal impairment.** A reduction in dosage of ceftriaxone may be necessary in patients with severe renal impairment, in whom the daily dose should not exceed 2 g, and in those with both renal and hepatic impairment; plasma concentrations should be monitored in such patients.

## Preparations

***BP 2003:*** Ceftriaxone Injection;
***USP 27:*** Ceftriaxone for Injection; Ceftriaxone Injection.

**Proprietary Preparations** (details are given in Part 3)
***Arg.:*** Acantex; Bioteral; Ceftriaz; Exempla; Rivacefin; Soltrimox; ***Austral.:*** Rocephin; ***Austria:*** Rocephin; ***Belg.:*** Rocephine; ***Braz.:*** Amplospec; Ceft; Ceftriax; Mesporan; Neocefriona; Prodoxin; Rocefin; Rofoxin; Triaxin†; Triaxton; Trioxina; ***Canad.:*** Rocephin; ***Chile:*** Acantex; Curocef; Grifotriaxona; ***Denm.:*** Rocephalin; ***Fin.:*** Rocephalin; ***Fr.:*** Rocephine; ***Ger.:*** Rocephin; ***Gr.:*** Antibacin; Azatyl; Bresec; Farcef; Gladius; Glorixone; Labilex;

Rocephin; Travilan; Veracol; **Hong Kong:** Mesporin; Rocephin; **India:** Lyceft; Monocef; Oframax; Powercef; **Irl.:** Rocephin; **Israel:** Keftriaxon; Rocephin; **Ital.:** Rocefin; **Jpn:** Rocephin; **Malaysia:** Ceftrex; **Mex.:** Bac-Xolid†; Benaxona; Cefaxona; Cefraden†; Ceftrex; Ceftrilem; Rocephin; Tacex; Terbac; Triaken; Waysul†; Xonatil†; **Neth.:** Rocephin; **Norw.:** Rocephalin; **NZ:** Rocephin; **Port.:** Mesporin; Rocephin; **S.Afr.:** Rocephin; **Singapore:** Cefaxone; Cefin; Oframax; Rocephin; Trexofin; Tricefin; **Spain:** Rocefalin; **Swed.:** Rocephalin; **Switz.:** Rocephine; **Thai.:** CEF-3; Cefine; Ceftrex; Ceftriphin; Lephin; Oframax; Rocephin; Sedalin; Tricephin; Trixone; Zefaxone; **UAE:** Triaxone; **UK:** Rocephin; **USA:** Rocephin.

## Cefuroxime *(BAN, USAN, rINN)*

640/359; Cefuroxima. (Z)-3-Carbamoyloxymethyl-7-[2-(2-furyl)-2-methoxyiminoacetamido]-3-cephem-4-carboxylic acid.

$C_{16}H_{16}N_4O_8S$ = 424.4.

*CAS — 55268-75-2.*

*ATC — J01DA06.*

### Cefuroxime Axetil *(BANM, USAN, rINNM)*

CCI-15641; Cefuroxima axetilo; Cefuroximum Axetili.

$C_{20}H_{22}N_4O_{10}S$ = 510.5.

*CAS — 64544-07-6.*

*ATC — J01DA06.*

**Pharmacopoeias.** In *Chin., Eur.* (see p.vi), *Jpn, Pol.,* and *US.*

**Ph. Eur. 5.0** (Cefuroxime Axetil). A white or almost white powder. Slightly soluble in water and in alcohol; soluble in acetone, in ethyl acetate, and in methyl alcohol. Store in airtight containers. Protect from light.

**USP 27** (Cefuroxime Axetil). A mixture of the diasterioisomers of cefuroxime axetil. A white or almost white powder. The amorphous form is insoluble in water and in ether; slightly soluble in dehydrated alcohol; freely soluble in acetone; soluble in chloroform, in ethyl acetate, and in methyl alcohol. The crystalline form is insoluble in water and in ether; slightly soluble in dehydrated alcohol; freely soluble in acetone; sparingly soluble in chloroform, in ethyl acetate, and in methyl alcohol. Store in airtight containers.

### Cefuroxime Sodium *(BANM, rINNM)*

Cefuroxima sódica; Cefuroximum Natricum.

$C_{16}H_{15}N_4NaO_8S$ = 446.4.

*CAS — 56238-63-2.*

*ATC — J01DA06.*

**Pharmacopoeias.** In *Chin., Eur.* (see p.vi), *Jpn, Pol.,* and *US.*

**Ph. Eur. 5.0** (Cefuroxime Sodium). A white or almost white slightly hygroscopic powder. Freely soluble in water; very slightly soluble in alcohol. A 1% solution in water has a pH of 5.5 to 8.5. Store in airtight containers.

**USP 27** (Cefuroxime Sodium). A white or faintly yellow powder. Freely soluble in water; very slightly soluble in alcohol, in chloroform, in ether, and in ethyl acetate; soluble in methyl alcohol. pH of a 10% solution in water is between 6.0 and 8.5. Store in airtight containers.

**Incompatibility and stability.** Cefuroxime sodium may be incompatible with aminoglycosides.

References.

1. Barnes AR. Chemical stabilities of cefuroxime sodium and metronidazole in an admixture for intravenous infusion. *J Clin Pharm Ther* 1990; **15:** 187–96.
2. Stiles ML, *et al.* Stability of ceftazidime (with arginine) and of cefuroxime sodium in infusion-pump reservoirs. *Am J Hosp Pharm* 1992; **49:** 2761–4.
3. Hebron B, Scott H. Shelf life of cefuroxime eye-drops when dispensed in artificial tear preparations. *Int J Pharm Pract* 1993; **2:** 163–7.

## Adverse Effects and Precautions

As for Cefalotin Sodium, p.168.

Gastrointestinal disturbances, including diarrhoea, nausea, and vomiting, have occurred in some patients receiving cefuroxime axetil. There have been rare reports of erythema multiforme, Stevens-Johnson syndrome, and toxic epidermal necrolysis. Mild to moderate hearing loss has been reported in some children given cefuroxime for the treatment of meningitis.

**Antibiotic-associated colitis.** For reports of pseudomembranous colitis associated with cefuroxime axetil, see Cefalotin, p.169.

**Porphyria.** Cefuroxime is considered to be unsafe in patients with porphyria although there is conflicting experimental evidence of porphyrinogenicity.

**Sodium content.** Each g of cefuroxime sodium contains about 2.2 mmol of sodium.

## Interactions

Probenecid reduces the renal clearance of cefuroxime.

## Antimicrobial Action

Cefuroxime is bactericidal and has a similar spectrum of antimicrobial action and pattern of resistance to those of cefamandole (p.170). It is more resistant to hydrolysis by beta-lactamases than cefamandole, and therefore may be more active against beta-lactamase-producing strains of, for example, *Haemophilus influenzae* and *Neisseria gonorrhoeae*. However, treatment failures have occurred in patients with *H. influenzae* meningitis given cefuroxime and might be associated with a relatively high minimum bactericidal concentration when compared with the minimum inhibitory concentration or with a significant inoculum effect. Reduced affinity of penicillin-binding proteins for cefuroxime has also been reported to be responsible for resistance in a beta-lactamase-negative strain of *H. influenzae*.

◊ References.

1. Arditi M, *et al.* Cefuroxime treatment failure and Haemophilus influenzae meningitis: case report and review of literature. *Pediatrics* 1989; **84:** 132–5.
2. Mendelman PM, *et al.* Cefuroxime treatment failure of nontypable Haemophilus influenzae meningitis associated with alteration of penicillin-binding proteins. *J Infect Dis* 1990; **162:** 1118–23.
3. Brown NM, *et al.* Cefuroxime resistance in Haemophilus influenzae. *Lancet* 1992; **340:** 552.

## Pharmacokinetics

Cefuroxime axetil is absorbed from the gastrointestinal tract and is rapidly hydrolysed in the intestinal mucosa and blood to cefuroxime; absorption is enhanced in the presence of food. Peak plasma concentrations are reported about 2 to 3 hours after an oral dose. The sodium salt is given by intramuscular or intravenous injection. Peak plasma concentrations of about 27 micrograms/mL have been achieved 45 minutes after an intramuscular dose of 750 mg with measurable amounts present 8 hours after a dose. Up to 50% of cefuroxime in the circulation is bound to plasma proteins. The plasma half-life is about 70 minutes and is prolonged in patients with renal impairment and in neonates.

Cefuroxime is widely distributed in the body including pleural fluid, sputum, bone, synovial fluid, and aqueous humour, but only achieves therapeutic concentrations in the CSF when the meninges are inflamed. It crosses the placenta and has been detected in breast milk.

Cefuroxime is excreted unchanged, by glomerular filtration and renal tubular secretion, and high concentrations are achieved in the urine. Following injection, most of a dose of cefuroxime is excreted within 24 hours, the majority within 6 hours. Probenecid competes for renal tubular secretion with cefuroxime resulting in higher and more prolonged plasma concentrations of cefuroxime. Small amounts of cefuroxime are excreted in bile.

Plasma concentrations are reduced by dialysis.

## Uses and Administration

Cefuroxime is a second-generation cephalosporin antibacterial used in the treatment of susceptible infections. These have included bone and joint infections, bronchitis (and other lower respiratory-tract infections), gonorrhoea, meningitis (although treatment failures have been reported in *H. influenzae* meningitis), otitis media, peritonitis, pharyngitis, sinusitis, skin infections (including soft-tissue infections), and urinary-tract infections. It is also used for surgical infection prophylaxis. For details of these infections and their treatment, see under Choice of Antibacterial, p.120.

*Administration and dosage.* Cefuroxime is given by mouth as the acetoxyethyl ester, cefuroxime axetil, in the form of tablets or suspension with or after food, or by injection as the sodium salt. Cefuroxime sodium may be given by deep intramuscular injection, by slow intravenous injection over 3 to 5 minutes, or by intravenous infusion. Doses of cefuroxime axetil and cefuroxime sodium are expressed in terms of the equivalent amount of cefuroxime. 1.20 g of cefuroxime axetil and 1.05 g of cefuroxime sodium are each approximately equivalent to 1 g of cefuroxime.

Usual oral doses for adults are 125 mg twice daily for uncomplicated urinary-tract infections and 250 to 500 mg twice daily for respiratory-tract infections. A dose for children more than 3 months of age is 125 mg twice daily or 10 mg/kg twice daily to a maximum of 250 mg daily. Children over 2 years of age with otitis media may be given 250 mg twice daily or 15 mg/kg twice daily to a maximum of 500 mg daily.

By injection the usual adult dose is 750 mg of cefuroxime every 8 hours but in more severe infections 1.5 g may be given intravenously every 8, or in some cases every 6, hours. Infants and children can be given 30 to 60 mg/kg daily, increased to 100 mg/kg daily if necessary, given in 3 or 4 divided doses. Neonates may be given similar total daily doses but in 2 or 3 divided doses.

Adults with pneumonia or with acute exacerbations of chronic bronchitis may respond to sequential therapy with parenteral cefuroxime sodium 1.5 g twice daily or 750 mg twice daily respectively, followed by oral cefuroxime axetil 500 mg twice daily in each case.

For Lyme disease in adults, a dose of 500 mg is given twice daily for 20 days.

For details of reduced dosage of cefuroxime to be used in patients with renal impairment, see below.

For the treatment of meningitis due to sensitive strains of bacteria, cefuroxime is given intravenously in adult doses of 3 g every 8 hours. Infants and children are given 200 to 240 mg/kg daily intravenously in 3 or 4 divided doses, which may be decreased to 100 mg/kg daily after 3 days or when there is clinical improvement. For neonates, a dose of 100 mg/kg daily, decreased to 50 mg/kg daily when indicated, may be used.

In the treatment of gonorrhoea, a single dose of 1.5 g by intramuscular injection, divided between 2 injection sites, has been used. A single 1-g oral dose of cefuroxime has been given for uncomplicated gonorrhoea. In each case an oral dose of probenecid 1 g may be given with cefuroxime.

For surgical infection prophylaxis, the usual dose is 1.5 g of cefuroxime intravenously before the procedure; this may be supplemented by 750 mg intramuscularly every 8 hours for up to 24 to 48 hours depending upon the procedure. For total joint replacement, 1.5 g of cefuroxime powder may be mixed with the methylmethacrylate cement.

◊ Reviews.

1. Perry CM, Brogden RN. Cefuroxime axetil: a review of its antibacterial activity, pharmacokinetic properties and therapeutic efficacy. *Drugs* 1996; **52:** 125–58.
2. Scott LJ, *et al.* Cefuroxime axetil: an updated review of its use in the management of bacterial infections. *Drugs* 2001; **61:** 1455–1500.

**Administration in renal impairment.** Parenteral doses of cefuroxime may need to be reduced in renal impairment. The manufacturers suggest the following adult doses based on creatinine clearance (CC):

- CC 10 to 20 mL/minute: 750 mg twice daily
- CC less than 10 mL/minute: 750 mg once daily

Patients undergoing haemodialysis should receive an additional 750-mg dose following each dialysis; those undergoing continuous peritoneal dialysis may be given 750 mg twice daily.

## Preparations

**BP 2003:** Cefuroxime Axetil Tablets; Cefuroxime Injection;
**USP 27:** Cefuroxime Axetil for Oral Suspension; Cefuroxime Axetil Tablets; Cefuroxime for Injection; Cefuroxime Injection.

**Proprietary Preparations** (details are given in Part 3)
**Arg.:** Ceflux; Cefogram; Cefurox; Deltrox; Ligramex; **Austral.:** Zinnat; **Austria:** Curocef; Furoxim; Zinnat; **Belg.:** Kefurox; Zinacef; Zinnat; **Braz.:** Zinacef; Zinnat; **Canad.:** Ceftin; Kefurox; Zinacef; **Chile:** Curocef; Zinnat; **Denm.:** Axacef†; Lifurox†; Zinacef; Zinnat; **Fin.:** Kefurion†; Lifurox†; Zinacef; Zinnat; **Fr.:** Cepazine; Zinnat; **Ger.:** Cefudura; Cefuhexal; Cefurax; Cefuro-Puren; Cefurox-Reu†; Cefurox-Wolff; Elobact; Zinacef; Zinnat; **Gr.:** Anaptivan; Cerofene; Ceruxim; Fredyr; Galemin; Gonif; Interbion; Medoxem; Mosalan; Nipogalin; Normafenac; Receant; Vekfazolin; Yokel; Zetagal; Zilisten; Zinacef; Zinadol; **Hong Kong:** Anikef; Axetine; Zinacef; Zinnat; **India:** Supacef; **Irl.:** Zinacef; Zinnat; **Israel:** Kefurim; Zinacef; Zinnat; **Ital.:** Biociclin; Biofurex; Bioxima†; Cefamar†; Cefoprim; Cefumax; Cefur; Cefurex; Cefurin; Colifossim; Curoxim; Deltacef; Duxima; Gibicef†; Ipacef; Itorex; Kefox; Kesint; Lafurex; Medoxim†; Oraxim; Polixima†; Supero; Tilexim; Zinnat; Zinocep; Zoref; **Malaysia:** Ceflour; Zinacef; Zinnat; **Mex.:** Cefuracet; Cetoxil; Froxal; Fucerox; Lemoxin; Novador; Ximaken; Zinnat; **Neth.:** Zinacef; Zinnat; **Norw.:** Lifurox†; Zinacef; **NZ:** Zinacef; Zinnat; **Port.:** Cefofix; Curoxime; Zipos; Zoref; **S.Afr.:** Cipofix; Intracef; Lifurom; Zinacef; Zinnat; **Singapore:** Shincef; Zinacef; Zinnat; **Spain:** Curoxima; Lifurox; Nivador; Selan; Zinnat; **Swed.:** Axacef†; Lifurox†; Zinacef; Zinnat; **Switz.:** Zinacef; Zinat; **Thai.:** Axetine; Cefamar; Cefogen; Cefurim; Furoxime; Magnaspor; Zinacef; Zinnat; **UAE:** Cefuzime; **UK:** Zinacef; Zinnat; **USA:** Ceftin; Kefurox†; Zinacef.

### Cethromycin (USAN, rINN)

A-195773; Abbott-195773; ABT-773. (3aS,4R,7R,9R,10R,11R,13R,15R,15aR)-4-Ethyl-3a,7,9,11,13,15-hexamethyl-11-{[3-(quinolin-3-yl)prop-2-enyl]oxy}-10-{[3,4,6-trideoxy-3-(dimethylamino)-β-D-*xylo*-hexopyranosyl]oxy}octahydro-2*H*-oxacyclotetradecino[4,3-*d*]oxazole-2,6,8,14(1*H*,7*H*,9*H*)-tetrone.

$C_{42}H_{59}N_3O_{10}$ = 765.9.

*CAS — 205110-48-1.*

#### Profile

Cethromycin is a ketolide antibacterial under investigation for the treatment of susceptible respiratory-tract infections.

◊ References.

1. Dougherty TJ, Barrett JF. ABT-773: a new ketolide antibiotic. *Expert Opin Invest Drugs* 2001; **10:** 343–51.
2. Zhanel GC, *et al.* The ketolides: a critical review. *Drugs* 2002; **62:** 1771–1804.

## Chloramphenicol (BAN, rINN)

Chloramphenicolum; Chloranfenicol; Cloranfenicol; Kloramfenikol; Laevomycetinum. 2,2-Dichloro-*N*-[(αR,βR)-β-hydroxy-α-hydroxymethyl-4-nitrophenethyl]acetamide.

$C_{11}H_{12}Cl_2N_2O_5$ = 323.1.

*CAS — 56-75-7.*

*ATC — D06AX02; D10AF03; G01AA05; J01BA01; S01AA01; S02AA01; S03AA08.*

NOTE. CPL is a code approved by the BP 2003 for use on single unit doses of eye drops containing chloramphenicol where the individual container may be too small to bear all the appropriate labelling information.

**Pharmacopoeias.** In *Chin., Eur.* (see p.vi), *Int., Jpn, Pol., US,* and *Viet.*

**Ph. Eur. 5.0** (Chloramphenicol). A substance produced by the growth of certain strains of *Streptomyces venezuelae*, but now mainly prepared synthetically. A white, greyish-white or yellowish-white, fine crystalline powder or fine crystals, needles, or elongated plates. Slightly soluble in water; freely soluble in alcohol and in propylene glycol. Protect from light.

**USP 27** (Chloramphenicol). Fine, white to greyish-white or yellowish-white, needle-like crystals or elongated plates. Soluble 1 in 400 of water; freely soluble in alcohol, in acetone, in ethyl acetate, and in propylene glycol. pH of a 2.5% suspension in water is between 4.5 and 7.5. Its solutions are practically neutral to litmus. It is reasonably stable in neutral or moderately acid solutions. Store in airtight containers.

### Chloramphenicol Palmitate (BANM, rINNM)

Chloramphenicol α-Palmitate; Chloramphenicoli Palmitas; Palmitato de cloranfenicol; Palmitylchloramphenicol.

$C_{27}H_{42}Cl_2N_2O_6$ = 561.5.

*CAS — 530-43-8.*

*ATC — D06AX02; D10AF03; G01AA05; J01BA01; S01AA01; S02AA01; S03AA08.*

**Pharmacopoeias.** In *Chin., Eur.* (see p.vi), *Int., Jpn, US,* and *Viet.*

**Ph. Eur. 5.0** (Chloramphenicol Palmitate). A fine, white or almost white, unctuous, powder. M.p. 87° to 95°. Chloramphenicol palmitate shows polymorphism and the thermodynamically stable form has low bioavailability following oral administration. Practically insoluble in water; sparingly soluble in alcohol; freely soluble in acetone; very slightly soluble in hexane. Protect from light.

**USP 27** (Chloramphenicol Palmitate). A fine, white, unctuous, crystalline powder, having a faint odour. M.p. 87° to 95°. Insoluble in water; sparingly soluble in alcohol; freely soluble in acetone and in chloroform; soluble in ether; very slightly soluble in hexane. Store in airtight containers.

### Chloramphenicol Sodium Succinate (BANM, rINNM)

Chloramphenicol α-Sodium Succinate; Chloramphenicoli Natrii Succinas; Succinato sódico de cloranfenicol.

$C_{15}H_{15}Cl_2N_2NaO_8$ = 445.2.

*CAS — 982-57-0.*

*ATC — D06AX02; D10AF03; G01AA05; J01BA01; S01AA01; S02AA01; S03AA08.*

**Pharmacopoeias.** In *Eur.* (see p.vi), *Int., Jpn, US,* and *Viet.* *Chin.* includes Chloramphenicol Hydrogen Succinate.

**Ph. Eur. 5.0** (Chloramphenicol Sodium Succinate). A white or yellowish-white hygroscopic powder. Very soluble in water; freely soluble in alcohol. A 25% solution in water has a pH of 6.4 to 7.0. Store in airtight containers. Protect from light.

**USP 27** (Chloramphenicol Sodium Succinate). A light yellow powder. Freely soluble in water and in alcohol. pH of a solution in water containing the equivalent of chloramphenicol 25% is between 6.4 and 7.0. Store in airtight containers.

**Incompatibility.** Incompatibility or loss of activity has been reported between chloramphenicol and a wide variety of other substances. Other factors, especially drug concentration, may play a part and many incompatibilities are chiefly seen with concentrated solutions.

### Adverse Effects and Treatment

Chloramphenicol may cause serious and sometimes fatal adverse effects. Some of its toxicity is thought to be due to effects on mitochondrial protein synthesis. The most serious adverse effect of chloramphenicol is bone-marrow depression, which can take two different forms. The first is a fairly common dose-related reversible depression occurring usually when plasma-chloramphenicol concentrations exceed 25 micrograms/mL and is characterised by morphological changes in the bone marrow, decreased iron utilisation, reticulocytopenia, anaemia, leucopenia, and thrombocytopenia. This effect may be due to inhibition of protein synthesis in the mitochondria of bone marrow cells.

The second and apparently unrelated form of bone-marrow toxicity is severe irreversible aplastic anaemia. This is fairly rare, with a suggested incidence of about 1:20 000 to 1:50 000, although the incidence varies throughout the world, and is not considered to be dose-related. The aplasia usually develops after a latent period of weeks or even months and has been suggested to be the result of a nitrated benzene radical produced *in vivo*. It is considered that there may be some genetic or biochemical predisposition, but there is no way of identifying susceptible patients. Although the majority of cases have followed oral use, aplasia has also occurred after intravenous and topical (eye drops) use of chloramphenicol. Survival is most likely in those with early onset aplasia, but they may subsequently develop acute myeloid leukaemia.

A toxic manifestation—the 'grey syndrome'—characterised by abdominal distension, vomiting, ashen colour, hypothermia, progressive pallid cyanosis, irregular respiration, and circulatory collapse followed by death in a few hours or days, has occurred in premature and other newborn infants receiving large doses of chloramphenicol. The syndrome is associated with high plasma concentrations of chloramphenicol, due to reduced capacity for glucuronidation and decreased glomerular filtration in children of this age, leading to drug accumulation. Recovery is usually complete if the drug is withdrawn early enough after onset, but up to 40% of infants with the full-blown syndrome may die. The syndrome has also been reported in infants born to mothers given chloramphenicol in late pregnancy. A similar syndrome has been reported in adults and older children given very high doses.

Prolonged oral use of chloramphenicol may induce bleeding, either by bone-marrow depression or by reducing the intestinal flora with consequent inhibition of vitamin K synthesis. Haemolytic anaemia has occurred in some patients with the Mediterranean form of glucose 6-phosphate dehydrogenase deficiency, but is rare in patients with milder forms of the deficiency.

Peripheral as well as optic neuritis has been reported in patients receiving chloramphenicol, usually over prolonged periods. Although ocular symptoms are often reversible if treatment is withdrawn early, permanent visual impairment or blindness has occurred.

Other neurological symptoms have included encephalopathy with confusion and delirium, mental depression, and headache. Ototoxicity has also occurred, especially after the use of ear drops.

Hypersensitivity reactions including rashes, fever, and angioedema may occur especially after topical use; anaphylaxis has occurred but is rare. Jarisch-Herxheimer reactions may also occur. Gastrointestinal symptoms including nausea, vomiting, and diarrhoea can follow oral use. Disturbances of the oral and intestinal flora may cause stomatitis, glossitis, and rectal irritation. Patients may experience an intensely bitter taste following rapid intravenous use of chloramphenicol sodium succinate.

**Aplastic anaemia.** A review[1] of the toxicity of chloramphenicol and related drugs, including the potential role of the *p*-nitro group in producing aplastic anaemia, indicated that derivatives such as thiamphenicol, which lack this grouping, are not associated with increased incidence of aplastic anaemia.

1. Yunis AA. Chloramphenicol: relation of structure to activity and toxicity. *Ann Rev Pharmacol Toxicol* 1988; **28:** 83–100.

**Overdosage.** Charcoal haemoperfusion was found to be far superior to exchange transfusion in the removal of chloramphenicol from blood, although it did not prevent death in a 7-week-old infant with the 'grey syndrome' following a dosage error.[1]

1. Freundlich M, *et al.* Management of chloramphenicol intoxication in infancy by charcoal hemoperfusion. *J Pediatr* 1983; **103:** 485–7.

### Precautions

Chloramphenicol is contra-indicated in patients with a history of hypersensitivity or toxic reaction to the drug. It should never be given systemically for minor infections or for prophylaxis. Repeated courses and prolonged treatment should be avoided and it should not be used in patients with pre-existing bone-marrow depression or blood dyscrasias. Routine periodic blood examinations are advisable in all patients, but will not warn of aplastic anaemia.

Use of chloramphenicol with other drugs liable to depress bone-marrow function should be avoided.

Reduced doses should be given to patients with hepatic impairment. Excessive blood concentrations may also occur following usual doses in patients with severe renal impairment and in premature and full-term neonates who have immature metabolic processes. Monitoring of plasma-chloramphenicol concentrations may be desirable in patients with risk factors. A suggested range for peak plasma concentrations is 10 to 25 micrograms/mL and for trough concentrations 5 to 15 micrograms/mL.

Neonates should never be given chloramphenicol systemically, unless it may be life-saving and there is no alternative treatment, because of the risk of the 'grey syndrome'. The use of chloramphenicol is probably best avoided during pregnancy.

Chloramphenicol may interfere with the development of immunity and it should not be given during active immunisation.

**Breast feeding.** Chloramphenicol is distributed into breast milk[1] and the American Academy of Pediatrics[2] considers that its use by mothers during breast feeding may be of concern, since there have been reports of possible idiosyncratic bone-marrow suppression in the infant.

1. Havelka J, *et al.* Excretion of chloramphenicol in human milk. *Chemotherapy* 1968; **13:** 204–11.
2. American Academy of Pediatrics. The transfer of drugs and other chemicals into human milk. *Pediatrics* 2001; **108:** 776–89. Correction. *ibid.*; 1029. Also available at: http://aappolicy.aappublications.org/cgi/content/full/pediatrics%3b108/3/776 (accessed 25/05/04)

**Ocular use.** Ocular chloramphenicol is widely used in the UK for the treatment of superficial eye infections. In view of the potential for serious toxicity, such as aplastic anaemia, following systemic absorption some, particularly in the USA, have advised that its ocular use should be restricted to situations where there is no alternative treatment.[1] However, apart from patients with a personal or family history of blood dyscrasias, the use, particularly of short courses, was defended by several specialists in the UK,[2-4] and the arguments have been the subject of several reviews.[5-7] Prospective case-control studies were considered necessary to clarify the risk.[8] One such study,[9] involving 145 patients with aplastic anaemia and 1226 controls, found that only 3 of the patients had been exposed to ocular chloramphenicol, and calculated that the absolute risk was no more than 0.5 cases per million treatment courses. Similarly, data[10] from 2 other studies revealed that none of 426 patients with aplastic anaemia and 7 of 3118 controls had used chloramphenicol eye drops. In a survey[11] of patients who received prescriptions for chloramphenicol eye drops the risk of serious haematological toxicity was 3 per 442 543 patients or 3 per 674 148 prescriptions.

1. Doona M, Walsh JB. Use of chloramphenicol as topical eye medication: time to cry halt? *BMJ* 1995; **310:** 1217–18.
2. Mulla RJ, *et al.* Is it time to stop using chloramphenicol on the eye: fears are based on only six cases. *BMJ* 1995; **311:** 450.
3. Buckley RJK, *et al.* Is it time to stop using chloramphenicol on the eye: safe in patients with no history of blood dyscrasia. *BMJ* 1995; **311:** 450.
4. Hall AV, *et al.* Is it time to stop using chloramphenicol on the eye: risk is low in short courses. *BMJ* 1995; **311:** 450–1.
5. McGhee CNJ, Anastas CN. Widespread ocular use of topical chloramphenicol: is there justifiable concern regarding idiosyncratic aplastic anaemia? *Br J Ophthalmol* 1996; **80:** 182–4.
6. Rayner SA, Buckley RJ. Ocular chloramphenicol and aplastic anaemia: is there a link? *Drug Safety* 1996; **14:** 273–6.
7. Titcomb L. Ophthalmic chloramphenicol and blood dyscrasias: a review. *Pharm J* 1997; **258:** 28–35.
8. Gordon-Smith EC, *et al.* Is it time to stop using chloramphenicol on the eye: prospective study of aplastic anaemia should give definitive answer. *BMJ* 1995; **311:** 451.
9. Laporte J-R, *et al.* Possible association between ocular chloramphenicol and aplastic anaemia—the absolute risk is very low. *Br J Clin Pharmacol* 1998; **46:** 181–4.

10. Wiholm B-E, *et al.* Relation of aplastic anaemia to use of chloramphenicol eye drops in two international case-control studies. *BMJ* 1998; **316:** 666.
11. Lancaster T, *et al.* Risk of serious haematological toxicity with use of chloramphenicol eye drops in a British general practice database. *BMJ* 1998; **316:** 667.

**Porphyria.** Chloramphenicol has been associated with acute attacks of porphyria and is considered unsafe in porphyric patients.

**Sodium content.** Each g of chloramphenicol sodium succinate represents about 2.2 mmol of sodium.

## Interactions

Chloramphenicol is inactivated in the liver and may, therefore, interact with drugs that are metabolised by hepatic microsomal enzymes. For example, chloramphenicol enhances the effects of coumarin anticoagulants, such as dicoumarol and warfarin, some hypoglycaemics such as chlorpropamide and tolbutamide, and antiepileptics such as phenytoin. Conversely, the metabolism of chloramphenicol may be increased by inducers of hepatic enzymes such as phenobarbital or rifampicin. Some other interactions affecting the activity of chloramphenicol are discussed below.

Chloramphenicol may decrease the effects of iron and vitamin $B_{12}$ in anaemic patients and has occasionally impaired the action of oral contraceptives.

For the effects of chloramphenicol on the activity of other antibacterials, see under Antimicrobial Action, below.

**Antiepileptics.** Serum concentrations of chloramphenicol are usually reduced by the hepatic enzyme induction that occurs with *phenobarbital*,[1,2] and similar reductions have been reported in a case study during *phenytoin* use.[3] Conversely, elevated and potentially toxic serum-chloramphenicol concentrations have resulted during phenytoin use,[2] apparently due to competition for binding sites, although increased metabolism may alternatively lead to decreased serum-chloramphenicol concentrations.

For reference to the effects of chloramphenicol on phenobarbital and phenytoin, see p.368 and p.372, respectively.

1. Bloxham RA, *et al.* Chloramphenicol and phenobarbitone—a drug interaction. *Arch Dis Child* 1979; **54:** 76–7.
2. Krasinski K, *et al.* Pharmacologic interactions among chloramphenicol, phenytoin and phenobarbital. *Pediatr Infect Dis* 1982; **1:** 232–5.
3. Powell DA, *et al.* Interactions among chloramphenicol, phenytoin, and phenobarbital in a pediatric patient. *J Pediatr* 1981; **98:** 1001–3.

**Ciclosporin.** For the effect of chloramphenicol on ciclosporin, see p.1354.

**Cimetidine.** Fatal aplastic anaemia of rapid onset has occurred in 2 patients who received intravenous chloramphenicol and cimetidine.[1,2] As there is usually a latent period of 2 weeks to 12 months before aplastic anaemia develops following chloramphenicol therapy it is plausible that an additive or synergistic effect may have occurred between the 2 drugs to cause bone-marrow toxicity.

1. Farber BF, Brody JP. Rapid development of aplastic anemia after intravenous chloramphenicol and cimetidine therapy. *South Med J* 1981; **74:** 1257–8.
2. West BC, *et al.* Aplastic anemia associated with parenteral chloramphenicol: review of 10 cases, including the second case of possible increased risk with cimetidine. *Rev Infect Dis* 1988; **10:** 1048–51.

**Cyclophosphamide.** For the effect of chloramphenicol on cyclophosphamide, see p.541.

**Oral contraceptives.** For the effect of chloramphenicol on oral contraceptives, see Hormonal Contraceptives, p.1534.

**Paracetamol.** A report of an increase in chloramphenicol half-life from 3.25 to 15 hours when intravenous paracetamol was given to 6 patients in intensive care 2 hours after intravenous chloramphenicol[1] has not been confirmed by subsequent studies in patients receiving oral paracetamol. A study in 5 children found that the half-life of intravenous chloramphenicol was reduced from 3 to 1.2 hours, concomitant with an increase in clearance, when oral paracetamol was given 30 minutes beforehand.[2] Furthermore, a study in 26 children found no evidence of altered disposition when oral paracetamol was given to patients receiving intravenous chloramphenicol,[3] and no significant change in chloramphenicol pharmacokinetics was found in 5 patients given oral chloramphenicol and paracetamol.[4]

1. Buchanan N, Moodley GP. Interaction between chloramphenicol and paracetamol. *BMJ* 1979; **2:** 307–8.
2. Spika JS, *et al.* Interaction between chloramphenicol and acetaminophen. *Arch Dis Child* 1986; **61:** 1121–4.
3. Kearns GL, *et al.* Absence of a pharmacokinetic interaction between chloramphenicol and acetaminophen in children. *J Pediatr* 1985; **107:** 134–9.
4. Stein CM, *et al.* Lack of effect of paracetamol on the pharmacokinetics of chloramphenicol. *Br J Clin Pharmacol* 1989; **27:** 262–4.

**Tacrolimus.** For the effect of chloramphenicol on tacrolimus, see p.1364.

## Antimicrobial Action

Chloramphenicol is a bacteriostatic antibiotic with a broad spectrum of action against both Gram-positive and Gram-negative bacteria, as well as some other organisms.

*Mechanism of action.* Chloramphenicol is thought to enter sensitive cells by an active transport process. Within the cell it binds to the 50S subunit of the bacterial ribosome at a site adjacent to the site of action of the macrolides and clindamycin, and inhibits bacterial protein synthesis by preventing attachment of aminoacyl transfer RNA to its acceptor site on the ribosome, thus preventing peptide bond formation by peptidyl transferase. The block in protein synthesis results in a primarily bacteriostatic action, although it may be bactericidal to some organisms, including *Haemophilus influenzae, Neisseria meningitidis,* and *Streptococcus pneumoniae*, at higher concentrations.

*Spectrum of activity.* Chloramphenicol has activity against many types of bacteria, although in most cases there are less toxic alternatives available. The following pathogens are usually susceptible (but see also Resistance, below).

Gram-positive cocci including staphylococci such as *Staph. epidermidis* and some strains of *Staph. aureus*, and streptococci such as *Str., pneumoniae, Str. pyogenes*, and the viridans streptococci. Meticillin-resistant staphylococci and *Enterococcus faecalis* are commonly found to be resistant.

Other Gram-positive species including *Bacillus anthracis, Corynebacterium diphtheriae*, and anaerobes such as *Peptococcus* and *Peptostreptococcus* spp. are usually susceptible.

Gram-negative cocci such as *Neisseria meningitidis* and *N. gonorrhoeae* are usually highly sensitive, as are *Haemophilus influenzae* and a variety of other Gram-negative bacteria including *Bordetella pertussis, Brucella abortus, Campylobacter* spp., *Legionella pneumophila, Pasteurella*, and *Vibrio* spp. The Enterobacteriaceae vary in their susceptibility, and many strains have shown acquired resistance, but *Escherichia coli*, and strains of *Klebsiella* spp., *Proteus mirabilis, Salmonella, Shigella*, and *Yersinia* spp. have been reported to be susceptible. Many strains of *Enterobacter*, indole-positive *Proteus*, and *Serratia* spp. are resistant, or at best moderately susceptible. *Pseudomonas aeruginosa* is invariably resistant, although *Burkholderia* (formerly *Pseudomonas*) spp. may be susceptible.

Some Gram-negative anaerobes are susceptible, or moderately so, including *Bacteroides fragilis, Veillonella*, and *Fusobacterium* spp.

Other susceptible organisms include *Actinomyces* spp., *Leptospira* spp., spirochaetes such as *Treponema pallidum*, Chlamydiaceae, Mycoplasma spp., and Rickettsia spp. *Nocardia* spp. are resistant. Chloramphenicol is ineffective against fungi, protozoa, and viruses.

*Activity with other antimicrobials.* As with other bacteriostatic antimicrobials, the possibility exists of an antagonistic effect if chloramphenicol is given with a bactericidal drug, and some antagonism has been demonstrated *in vitro* between chloramphenicol and various beta lactams and aminoglycosides, but the clinical significance of most of these interactions is usually held to be doubtful. Chloramphenicol may competitively inhibit the effects of macrolides or lincosamides such as clindamycin because of the adjacency of their binding sites on the ribosome.

*Resistance.* Acquired resistance has been widely reported, although the prevalence of resistance has tended to decline where use of the drug has become less frequent. The most commonly seen form of resistance has been the production of an acetyltransferase that inactivates the drug. Such resistance is usually plasmid-mediated and may be associated with resistance to other drugs such as the tetracyclines. Other mechanisms that may reduce sensitivity to chloramphenicol include reduced permeability or uptake, and ribosomal mutation.

The actual incidence of resistance varies considerably in different countries and different centres. Epidemics of chloramphenicol-resistant *Salmonella* and *Shigella* spp. have occurred in the past, and although the prevalence of resistance in *Salmonella* spp. has been reported to be negligible except in parts of South or South-east Asia, resistant salmonellal infections acquired in these regions are increasingly being seen elsewhere. Resistance among *Haemophilus* and *Neisseria* spp. occurs, and the latter may be problematic in developing countries, although it does not yet seem to be widespread. However, resistant strains of enterococci and pneumococci are reported to be relatively common in some areas, and over 50% of staphylococcal strains have been reported to show resistance in some hospitals.

## Pharmacokinetics

Chloramphenicol is readily absorbed when given by mouth. Blood concentrations of 10 micrograms/mL or more may be reached about 1 or 2 hours after a single dose of 1 g by mouth, and blood concentrations of about 18.5 micrograms/mL have been reported after multiple 1-g doses. Chloramphenicol palmitate is hydrolysed to chloramphenicol in the gastrointestinal tract prior to absorption, and the sodium succinate, which is given parenterally, is probably hydrolysed to free drug mainly in the liver, lungs, kidneys, and plasma; such hydrolysis may be incomplete in infants and neonates, contributing to the variable pharmacokinetics in this age group. Chloramphenicol sodium succinate is, even in adults, only partially and variably hydrolysed, so that blood concentrations of chloramphenicol obtained after the sodium succinate parenterally are often lower than those obtained after chloramphenicol by mouth, with up to 30% of a dose excreted unchanged in the urine before hydrolysis can take place (but see under Administration, below).

Chloramphenicol is widely distributed in body tissues and fluids; it enters the CSF, giving concentrations of about 50% of those existing in the blood even in the absence of inflamed meninges; it diffuses across the placenta into the fetal circulation, into breast milk, and into the aqueous and vitreous humours of the eye. It also enters the aqueous humour following topical application. Up to about 60% in the circulation is bound to plasma protein. The half-life of chloramphenicol has been reported to range from 1.5 to 4 hours; the half-life is prolonged in patients with severe hepatic impairment and is also much longer in neonates. Renal impairment has relatively little effect on the half-life of the active drug, due to its extensive metabolism, but may lead to accumulation of the inactive metabolites.

Chloramphenicol is excreted mainly in the urine but only 5 to 10% of an oral dose appears unchanged; the remainder is inactivated in the liver, mostly by conjugation with glucuronic acid. About 3% is excreted in the bile. However, most is reabsorbed and only about 1%, mainly in the inactive form, is excreted in the faeces.

The absorption, metabolism, and excretion of chloramphenicol are subject to considerable interindividual variation, especially in infants and children, making monitoring of plasma concentrations necessary to determine pharmacokinetics in a given patient.

## Uses and Administration

The risk of life-threatening adverse effects, particularly bone-marrow aplasia, has severely limited the clinical usefulness of chloramphenicol, although it is still widely used in some countries. It should never be given systemically for minor infections and regular blood counts are usually advisable during treatment. The third-generation cephalosporins replaced chloramphenicol for many of its former indications. There are consequently few unambiguous indications for the use of chloramphenicol. It has been used in severe typhoid and other salmonellal infections, although it does not eliminate the carrier state. Chloramphenicol is an alternative to a third-generation cephalosporin in the treatment of bacterial meningitis, both empirically and against sensitive organisms such as *Haemophilus influenzae*. It has been used in the treatment of severe anaerobic infections, particularly in brain abscesses, and in infections below the diaphragm where *Bacteroides fragilis* is often implicated; however, other drugs are usually preferred. Although the tetracyclines remain the treatment of choice in rickettsial infections such as typhus and the spotted fevers, chloramphenicol is also used as an alternative where the tetracyclines cannot be given.

Other bacterial infections in which chloramphenicol may be used as an alternative to other drugs include anthrax, ehrlichiosis, severe gastro-enteritis (including *Salmonella* enteritis, cholera, and *Yersinia* enteritis), gas gangrene, granuloma inguinale, severe *Haemophilus influenzae* infections (for example in epiglottitis), listeriosis, severe melioidosis, plague (especially if meningitis develops), pneumonia, psittacosis, Q fever, tularaemia (especially when meningitis is suspected), and Whipple's disease. For details of these infections and their treatment, see under Choice of Antibacterial, p.120.

Chloramphenicol is extensively used in the topical treatment of ear and, in particular, eye infections, despite the fact that many of these are mild and self-limiting. It is also used topically in the treatment of skin infections.

When given by mouth, chloramphenicol is usually used as capsules or as a suspension of chloramphenicol palmitate. When oral use is not feasible, water-soluble chloramphenicol sodium succinate may be given intravenously, but oral therapy should be substituted as soon as possible; an intravenous dose should be injected over at least 1 minute. Intramuscular injection is controversial because of doubts whether absorption is adequate. In some countries chloramphenicol has been given rectally.

Doses are expressed in terms of chloramphenicol base and are similar whether given by mouth or intravenously. Chloramphenicol palmitate 1.7 g and chloramphenicol sodium succinate 1.4 g are each approximately equivalent to 1 g of chloramphenicol base.

For adults and children the usual dose is 50 mg/kg daily in divided doses every 6 hours; up to 100 mg/kg daily may be given in meningitis or severe infections due to moderately resistant organisms, although these higher doses should be reduced as soon as possible. It has been recommended that treatment should be continued after the patient's temperature has returned to normal for a further 4 days in rickettsial diseases, and for 8 to 10 days in typhoid fever, to minimise the risk of relapse.

Where there is no alternative to the use of chloramphenicol, premature and full-term neonates may be given daily doses of 25 mg/kg, in 4 divided doses, and full-term infants over the age of 2 weeks may be given up to 50 mg/kg daily, in 4 divided doses. Monitoring of plasma concentrations is essential to avoid toxicity.

In patients with hepatic impairment or severe renal impairment, the dose of chloramphenicol may need to be reduced because of decreased metabolism or excretion.

In the treatment of eye infections, chloramphenicol is usually applied as a 0.5% solution or as a 1% ointment.

For bacterial infections in otitis externa, chloramphenicol has been given as ear drops in a strength of 5 or 10%.

Chloramphenicol has also been used in the form of various other derivatives including the arginine succinate, the cinnamate, the glycinate, the glycinate sulfate, the palmitoylglycolate, the pantothenate, the steaglate, the stearate, and the hydrogen succinate.

**Administration.** When parenteral use of chloramphenicol is necessary the intravenous route is generally preferred, although the intramuscular route has been advocated. Adequate serum concentrations after intramuscular injection have been reported,[1,2] although this is contrary to the widely held belief that chloramphenicol sodium succinate is poorly absorbed by this route. Pain on injection was also claimed to be minimal.[1] Following a study in children with bacterial meningitis,[3] treatment with intramuscular chloramphenicol for 2 or 3 days followed by oral therapy has been suggested, although a later study[2] found that the intramuscular route produced therapeutic concentrations when the oral route did not. However, it has been said[4] that children describe intramuscular chloramphenicol as amongst the worst treatments they ever receive, and certainly much worse than the insertion of intravenous cannulae.


1. Shann F, *et al.* Absorption of chloramphenicol sodium succinate after intramuscular administration in children. *N Engl J Med* 1985; **313:** 410–14.
2. Weber MW, *et al.* Chloramphenicol pharmacokinetics in infants less than three months of age in the Philippines and The Gambia. *Pediatr Infect Dis J* 1999; **18:** 896–901.
3. Shann F, *et al.* Chloramphenicol alone versus chloramphenicol plus penicillin for bacterial meningitis in children. *Lancet* 1985; **ii** 681–3.
4. Coulthard MG, Lamb WH. Antibiotics: intramuscular or intravenous? *Lancet* 1985; **ii:** 1015.


**Enterococcal infections.** Chloramphenicol has been reported to be effective against vancomycin-resistant *Enterococcus faecium*.[1-3] Although no significant effect of chloramphenicol on mortality was found in one small study,[4] a retrospective analysis[5] of the outcomes of 6 patients with bacteraemia due to vancomycin-resistant *Enterococcus faecium* concluded that chloramphenicol was effective and should be considered as a treatment option.


1. Norris AH, *et al.* Chloramphenicol for the treatment of vancomycin-resistant enterococcal infections. *Clin Infect Dis* 1995; **20:** 1137–44.
2. Papanicolaou GA, *et al.* Nosocomial infections with vancomycin-resistant Enterococcus faecium in liver transplant recipients: risk factors for acquisition and mortality. *Clin Infect Dis* 1996; **23:** 760–6.
3. Mato SP, *et al.* Vancomycin-resistant Enterococcus faecium meningitis successfully treated with chloramphenicol. *Pediatr Infect Dis J* 1999; **18:** 483–4.
4. Lautenbach E, *et al.* The role of chloramphenicol in the treatment of bloodstream infection due to vancomycin-resistant Enterococcus. *Clin Infect Dis* 1998; **27:** 1259–65.
5. Ricaurte JC, *et al.* Chloramphenicol treatment for vancomycin-resistant Enterococcus faecium bacteremia. *Clin Microbiol Infect* 2001; **7:** 17–21.


## Preparations

***BP 2003:*** Chloramphenicol Capsules; Chloramphenicol Ear Drops; Chloramphenicol Eye Drops; Chloramphenicol Eye Ointment; Chloramphenicol Sodium Succinate Injection;
***USP 27:*** Chloramphenicol and Hydrocortisone Acetate for Ophthalmic Suspension; Chloramphenicol and Polymyxin B Sulfate Ophthalmic Ointment; Chloramphenicol and Prednisolone Ophthalmic Ointment; Chloramphenicol Capsules; Chloramphenicol Cream; Chloramphenicol for Ophthalmic Solution; Chloramphenicol Ophthalmic Ointment; Chloramphenicol Ophthalmic Solution; Chloramphenicol Otic Solution; Chloramphenicol Palmitate Oral Suspension; Chloramphenicol Sodium Succinate for Injection; Chloramphenicol, Polymyxin B Sulfate, and Hydrocortisone Acetate Ophthalmic Ointment.

**Proprietary Preparations** (details are given in Part 3)
***Arg.:*** A-Solmicina-C; Bio Gelin; Bioticaps; Chloromycetin; Farmicetina; Isopto Fenicol; Klonalfenicol; Pluscloran; Poenfenicol; Quemicetina; Quotal NF; ***Austral.:*** Chloromycetin; Chlorsig; ***Austria:*** Halomycetin; Kemicetin; Oleomycetin; ***Belg.:*** Kemicetina; ***Braz.:*** Arifenicol; Auridonal; Clorafenil; Cloranfenil; Clorfenil†; Farmicetina; Feniclor; Neo Fenicol; Quemicetina; Sintomicetina; Visalmin; Vixmicina; ***Canad.:*** Chloromycetin; Chloroptic†; Diochloram; Novo-Chlorocap†; Ophtho-Chloram†; Pentamycetin; ***Chile:*** Clorampast; Gemitin; Quemicetina; ***Fin.:*** Chloromycetin; Oftan Akvakol; Oftan Chlora; ***Fr.:*** Cebenicol; ***Ger.:*** Aquamycetin-N; Chloramsaar N; Oleomycetin; Paraxin; Posifenicol C; Thilocanfol C; ***Gr.:*** Chloranic; Thilocof; ***Hong Kong:*** Chloment; Chloroph; Chlorsig; Isopto Fenicol†; Kemicetine; Spersanicol; Vanafen-S†; Vista-Phenicol; Xepanicol; ***India:*** Chloromycetin; Kemicetine; Kemicetine Otological; Paraxin; Reclor; Vanmycetin; Vitamycetin; ***Irl.:*** Chloromycetin; Chloroptic†; ***Israel:*** Chloroptic; Phenicol; Synthomycine; Tarophenicol†; ***Ital.:*** Chemicetina; Chloromycetin†; Cloramfen; Mycetin; Optafen†; Sificetina; Vitamfenicolo; ***Malaysia:*** Beaphenicol; Nicol; Spersanicol; Xepanicol; ***Mex.:*** Alcan; Brocil; Cetina†; Chloromycetin; Clorafen; Cloramed; Cloramfeni; Cloramfenil†; Cloran; Clorazin; Clordil; Clorfenil; Diarman; Dilclor; Domicetina†; Exacol; Fenicol; Fenisol†; Fenizzard; Furocloran†; Italmicin†; K-Biofen†; Lebrocetin; Leclor A; Naxo; Oftadil; Omycet; Palcol†; Palmiclor†; Palmiffer†; Palmisol; Procloril; Pronicol; Quemicetina; Solufen†; Spersanicol†; Uniclor; Vixin; Wilyfenicol†; ***Neth.:*** Globenicol; ***NZ:*** Chloromycetin; Chloroptic†; Chlorsig; Isopto Fenicol; ***Port.:*** Clorocil; Dermimade Cloranfenicol; Fenoptic; Micetinoftalmina; ***S.Afr.:*** Chloramex; Chlorcol; Chlornicol†; Chloromycetin; Chloroptic; Chlorphen; Spersanicol; ***Singapore:*** Beaphenicol†; Isopto Fenicol; Kemicetine; Spersanicol; Vanafen-S; Xepanicol†; ***Spain:*** Chemicetina; Chloromycetin; Cloranfe†; Cloranfenic; Isopto Fenicol†; Normofenicol; ***Swed.:*** Chloromycetin; Isopto Fenicol†; ***Switz.:*** Chloromycetin†; Septicol; Spersanicol; ***Thai.:*** Antibi-Otic; Archifen; Chloracil; Chloram-D†; Chloramno; Chloroph; Chlorosin; Cogenate; Cogetine; Fenicol; Genercin; Kemicetine; Koro; Levomycetin; Mycochlorin; Nicolmycetin; Opsaram; Pharmacetin; Servicol†; Silmycetin; Succi Pharmacetin†; Synchlolim; Unison Ointment; Vanafen; ***UK:*** Chloromycetin; Kemicetine; Sno Phenicol†; ***USA:*** Ak-Chlor; Chloromycetin; Chloroptic.

**Multi-ingredient:** ***Arg.:*** Acnoxin; Antiflogol; Anuar; Clorfibrase; Esodar; Eubetal Biotic; Fluoropoen; Iruxol; Neocortizul; Oftal; Oftalmoflogol; Poenbioptal; Quemicetina con Hidrocortisona; Vistacloran; ***Austral.:*** Chlorocort†; ***Austria:*** Cortison Kemicetin; Oleomycetin-Prednison; ***Belg.:*** De Icol; Viscocort†; ***Braz.:*** Adermykon-C†; Dermofibrin C; Dexaclor; Dexacloran†; Dexafenicol; Epitezan; Fenidex; Fibrase; Fluo-Fenicol†; Gino-Fibrase; Gyno Iruxol; Hipoglos Oftalmico†; Iruxol; Kollagenase com cloranfenicol; Lisofenicol†; Naxogin Composto; Oto-Biotic; Otofenicol-D; Otoflogin†; Otomicina; Otopen†; Ouvidonal; Procutan; Regenom; Sulnil; ***Canad.:*** Actinac†; Elase-Chloromycetin†; Ophthocort†; Pentamycetin-HC; ***Chile:*** Cortifenol H; Gemitin con Prednisolona; Naxogin Compositum; Otandrol; Sintoftona; Spersadex Comp; ***Denm.:*** Spersadex Comp; ***Fin.:*** Iruxol; Oftan C-C; Oftan Dexa-Chlora; ***Fr.:*** Cebedexacol; ***Ger.:*** Aquapred; Berlicetin; Corti-Flexiole†; Ichthoseptal; Oleomycetin-Prednison; Spersadex Comp; Spersadexolin; ***Gr.:*** Sulfachloramphenicol; Sulfanicole; ***Hong Kong:*** Chlomy-P; Chloram-D; Cortiphenol H; Cortison Kemicetine†; Ginetris; Neo-Dex (Improved); Oftalmolosa Cusi de Icol†; Spersacet C†; Spersadex Comp; Spersadexoline; ***India:*** Chlormixin; Chloromycetin Ear Drops; Cortison Kemicetine; Dexosyn-C; Kemicetine Antiozena; Kemicetine Otological; Ocupol; Ocupol-D; Otek-AC; Paraxin Ear; Perfocyn; Pyrimon; ***Irl.:*** Actinac†; ***Israel:*** Phenimixin; Tarocidin; Tarocidin D; Threolone; ***Ital.:*** Antibioptal; Betabioptal; Cloradex; Colbiocin; Cortison Chemicetina; Cosmiciclina; Dexoline; Eubetal Antibiotico; Fluorobioptal†; Idracemi; Iruxol; Otomicetina†; Vasofen; Vitecaf; Xantervit Antibiotico; ***Malaysia:*** De Icol; Spersadex Comp; Spersadexoline; ***Mex.:*** Cloran Otico; Fibrase; Levodexan; Levofenil; Otolone; Pre Clor; Soldrin; Solfranicol; Sulfa Cloran; Trecloran; Ulcoderma; ***Norw.:*** Spersadex med kloramfenikol; ***Port.:*** Blefarida†; Cloranpectina; Clorcorticil; Medrivas Antibiotico; Predniftalmina; ***S.Afr.:*** Covomycin; Covomycin-D; Covotop; Spersacet C; Spersadex Comp; Spersadexoline; ***Singapore:*** Neo-Dex (Improved)†; Spersadex Comp; Spersadexoline; ***Spain:*** Blefarida; Clo Zinc†; Cloram Hemidexa; Cloram Zinc; Cortison Chemicet Topica; Dermisone Epitelizante; Dexa Fenic†; Dexafenicol†; Dexam Constric; Fluo Fenic; Hidroc Cloranf†; Icol; Icolamida†; Medricol†; Medrivas Antib; Otosedol Biotico; Parkelase Chloromycetin†; Predni Azuleno; ***Switz.:*** Septicortin†; Spersacet C; Spersadex Comp; Spersadexoline; ***Thai.:*** Archifen; Chlorotracin; Dermasol; Levoptin; Otosil†; Spersacet C†; Spersadexoline; Vagicin; ***UK:*** Actinac.

---

## Chlorquinaldol *(BAN, rINN)*

Clorquinaldol. 5,7-Dichloro-2-methylquinolin-8-ol.
$C_{10}H_7Cl_2NO = 228.1$.
*CAS — 72-80-0.*
*ATC — D08AH02; G01AC03; P01AA04; R02AA11.*

**Pharmacopoeias.** In *Pol.*

### Profile

Chlorquinaldol is a halogenated hydroxyquinoline with properties similar to those of clioquinol (p.196). It is mainly applied topically in infected skin conditions and in vaginal infections.

### Preparations

**Proprietary Preparations** (details are given in Part 3)
**Multi-ingredient:** ***Arg.:*** Nerisona C; ***Austria:*** Neriquinol†; ***Braz.:*** Bi-Nerisona; ***Chile:*** Bi-Nerisona; ***Denm.:*** Locoidol; ***Fin.:*** Locoidol; ***Fr.:*** Nerisone C; ***Ger.:*** Nerisona C; Proctospre; ***Hong Kong:*** Colposeptine; Nerisone C; ***Irl.:*** Locoid C; ***Israel:*** Multiderm; ***Ital.:*** Impetex; Nerisona C; ***Mex.:*** Bi-Nerisona; ***Mon.:*** Colposeptine; ***Norw.:*** Locoidol; ***NZ:*** Locoid C; Nerisone C; ***Port.:*** Locoid C; Nerisona C; Trophoseptine†; ***Singapore:*** Nerisone C; ***Spain:*** Amplidermis; Claral Plus; Quinortar; ***Switz.:*** Anginazol; Proctospre†; ***UK:*** Locoid C.

---

## Chlortetracycline *(BAN, rINN)*

Clortetraciclina. (4*S*,4a*S*,5a*S*,6*S*,12a*S*)-7-Chloro-4-dimethylamino-1,4,4a,5,5a,6,11,12a-octahydro-3,6,10,12,12a-pentahydroxy-6-methyl-1,11-dioxonaphthacene-2-carboxamide; 7-Chlorotetracycline.
$C_{22}H_{23}ClN_2O_8 = 478.9$.
*CAS — 57-62-5.*
*ATC — A01AB21; D06AA02; J01AA03; S01AA02.*

## Chlortetracycline Bisulfate *(rINNM)*

Chlortetracycline Bisulphate *(BANM)*.

**Pharmacopoeias.** In *US* for veterinary use only.
**USP 27** (Chlortetracycline Bisulfate). Store in airtight containers. Protect from light.

## Chlortetracycline Hydrochloride *(BANM, rINNM)*

Chlortetracyclini Hydrochloridum; Hidrocloruro de clortetraciclina.
$C_{22}H_{23}ClN_2O_8,HCl = 515.3$.
*CAS — 64-72-2.*
*ATC — A01AB21; D06AA02; J01AA03; S01AA02.*

**Pharmacopoeias.** In *Chin.*, *Eur.* (see p.vi), *Int.*, *Pol.*, and *US.*
**Ph. Eur. 5.0** (Chlortetracycline Hydrochloride). The hydrochloride of a substance produced by the growth of certain strains of *Streptomyces aureofaciens* or by any other means. A yellow powder. Slightly soluble in water and in alcohol; it dissolves in solutions of alkali hydroxides and carbonates. A 1% solution in water has a pH of 2.3 to 3.3. Protect from light.
**USP 27** (Chlortetracycline Hydrochloride). A yellow, odourless crystalline powder. Soluble 1 in 75 of water and 1 in 560 of alcohol; practically insoluble in acetone, in chloroform, in dioxan, and in ether; soluble in solutions of alkali hydroxides and carbonates. pH of a 1% solution in water is between 2.3 and 3.3. Store in airtight containers. Protect from light.

**Incompatibility.** Preparations of chlortetracycline have an acid pH and incompatibility may reasonably be expected with alkaline preparations or drugs unstable at low pH.

### Adverse Effects and Precautions

As for Tetracycline Hydrochloride, p.266.

### Interactions

As for Tetracycline Hydrochloride, p.267.

### Antimicrobial Action

As for Tetracycline Hydrochloride, p.267. It is somewhat less active against many Gram-negative organisms.

### Pharmacokinetics

As for Tetracycline Hydrochloride, p.268.

Chlortetracycline is poorly absorbed from the gastrointestinal tract compared with other tetracyclines. It is reported to be rapidly inactivated in the body with a half-life of about 5 to 6 hours, and is largely eliminated by biliary excretion. About 45% of a dose is protein bound. Only a small amount is excreted in the urine but chlortetracycline is not recommended in patients with renal impairment, since accumulation may occur due to an increase in half-life to 7 to 11 hours.

### Uses and Administration

Chlortetracycline is a tetracycline derivative with uses similar to those of tetracycline (p.268). It is used as the hydrochloride and is administered as a 1% ophthalmic ointment and as a 3% ointment for application to the skin. It is also sometimes given by mouth as the hydrochloride in combination with other tetracycline derivatives.

### Preparations

**BP 2003:** Chlortetracycline Eye Ointment; Chlortetracycline Ointment; **USP 27:** Chlortetracycline Hydrochloride Ointment; Chlortetracycline Hydrochloride Ophthalmic Ointment.

**Proprietary Preparations** (details are given in Part 3)
**Austral.:** Aureomycin†; **Austria:** Aureomycin; **Belg.:** Aureomycin; Aureomycine; **Canad.:** Aureomycin†; **Denm.:** Aureomycin†; **Fin.:** Aureomycin†; **Fr.:** Aureomycine; **Ger.:** Aureomycin; **Hong Kong:** Aureomycin; Chlortralim; **Irl.:** Aureomycin†; **Israel:** Aureomycin†; **Ital.:** Aureomicina; **Malaysia:** Chlortralim; **Mex.:** Aureomicina†; **Neth.:** Aureomycin†; **Norw.:** Aureomycin; **NZ:** Aureomycin†; **Port.:** Aurecil; Aureodermil; Aureomicina†; **S.Afr.:** Aureomycin†; **Singapore:** Chlortralim; **Spain:** Aureomicina; Dermosa Aureomicina; **Swed.:** Aureomycin†; **Switz.:** Aureomycine†; **Thai.:** Aureomycin; Chlortralim; **UK:** Aureomycin†.

**Multi-ingredient: Austria:** Aureocort; **Braz.:** Corciclen; **Fin.:** Aureocort†; **Ger.:** Aureodelf; Aureomycin N; **Irl.:** Aureocort†; Deteclo†; **Ital.:** Aureocort; Aureomix; **S.Afr.:** Tritet†; **Spain:** Antiblefarica†; Poliantib†; **UK:** Aureocort; Deteclo.

## Ciclacillin *(BAN, rINN)*

Ciclacilina; Cyclacillin *(USAN)*; Wy-4508. (6R)-6-(1-Aminocyclohexanecarboxamido)penicillanic acid.

$C_{15}H_{23}N_3O_4S$ = 341.4.
*CAS — 3485-14-1.*

**Pharmacopoeias.** In *Jpn.*

### Profile

Ciclacillin is an aminopenicillin with properties similar to those of ampicillin (p.157), although it is generally less active *in vitro*.

### Preparations

**Proprietary Preparations** (details are given in Part 3)
**Braz.:** Cilinase.

## Cilastatin Sodium *(BANM, USAN, rINNM)*

Cilastatina sódica; Cilastatinum Natricum; L-642957; MK-791. (Z)-(S)-6-Carboxy-6-[(S)-2,2-dimethylcyclopropanecarboxamido]hex-5-enyl-L-cysteine, monosodium salt.

$C_{16}H_{25}N_2NaO_5S$ = 380.4.
*CAS — 82009-34-5 (cilastatin); 81129-83-1 (cilastatin sodium).*

**Pharmacopoeias.** In *Eur.* (see p.vi) and *US.*

**Ph. Eur. 5.0** (Cilastatin Sodium). A white or light yellow, hygroscopic, amorphous powder. Very soluble in water and in methyl alcohol; slightly soluble in dehydrated alcohol; practically insoluble in acetone and in dichloromethane; soluble in dimethyl sulfoxide. A 1% solution in water has a pH of 6.5 to 7.5. Store at a temperature not exceeding 8° in airtight containers.

**USP 27** (Cilastatin Sodium). A white to tan-coloured powder. Soluble in water and in methyl alcohol. pH of a 1% solution in water is between 6.5 and 7.5. Store at a temperature less than 8°.

### Profile

Cilastatin is an inhibitor of dehydropeptidase I, an enzyme found in the brush border of the renal tubules. It is given as the sodium salt with the antibacterial imipenem (p.221) to prevent its renal metabolism to microbiologically inactive and potentially nephrotoxic products. This increases the concentrations of imipenem achieved in the urine and protects against any nephrotoxic effects, which were seen with high doses of imipenem given experimentally to *animals*.

Cilastatin has no antibacterial activity itself, and does not affect the antibacterial activity of imipenem.

### Preparations

**USP 27:** Imipenem and Cilastatin for Injectable Suspension; Imipenem and Cilastatin for Injection.

**Proprietary Preparations** (details are given in Part 3)
**Multi-ingredient: Arg.:** Klonam; Zienam; **Austral.:** Primaxin; **Austria:** Zienam; **Belg.:** Tienam; **Braz.:** Tienam; **Canad.:** Primaxin; **Chile:** Tienam; **Denm.:** Tienam; **Fin.:** Tienam; **Fr.:** Tienam; **Ger.:** Zienam; **Gr.:** Primaxin; **Hong Kong:** Tienam; **Israel:** Tienam; **Ital.:** Imipem; Tenacid; Tienam; **Malaysia:** Tienam; **Mex.:** Tienam; **Neth.:** Tienam; **Norw.:** Tienam; **NZ:** Primaxin; **Port.:** Tienam; **S.Afr.:** Tienam; **Singapore:** Tienam; **Spain:** Tienam; **Swed.:** Tienam; **Switz.:** Tienam; **Thai.:** Tienam; **UK:** Primaxin; **USA:** Primaxin.

## Cinoxacin *(BAN, USAN, rINN)*

64716; Azolinic Acid; Cinoxacino; Compound 64716. 1-Ethyl-1,4-dihydro-4-oxo-1,3-dioxolo[4,5-g]cinnoline-3-carboxylic acid.

$C_{12}H_{10}N_2O_5$ = 262.2.
*CAS — 28657-80-9.*
*ATC — J01MB06.*

**Pharmacopoeias.** In *US.*

**USP 27** (Cinoxacin). A white to yellowish-white, odourless crystalline solid. Insoluble in water and in most common organic solvents; soluble in alkaline solution. Store in airtight containers.

### Adverse Effects and Precautions

As for Nalidixic Acid, p.234.

Cinoxacin is not recommended in patients with severe renal impairment, and the dosage should be reduced in those with mild to moderate renal impairment.

◊ References.

1. Stricker BHC, *et al.* Anaphylactic reactions to cinoxacin. *BMJ* 1988; **297:** 1434–5.

### Interactions

As for Nalidixic Acid, p.234.

### Antimicrobial Action

As for Nalidixic Acid, p.234. Cross-resistance with nalidixic acid has been shown.

### Pharmacokinetics

Cinoxacin is rapidly and almost completely absorbed following administration by mouth. Peak serum concentrations of about 15 micrograms/mL have been obtained 2 to 3 hours after a 500-mg dose. The plasma half-life is about 1 to 2 hours. Cinoxacin has been reported to be more than 60% bound to plasma proteins.

Cinoxacin appears to be metabolised in the liver and is excreted via the kidney. Over 95% of a dose appears in the urine within 24 hours, over half as unaltered drug and the remainder as inactive metabolites. Mean urinary concentrations of about 300 micrograms/mL have been achieved during the first 4 hours after administration of a 500-mg dose by mouth. Urinary excretion is reduced by probenecid and in patients with renal impairment.

### Uses and Administration

Cinoxacin is a 4-quinolone antibacterial with actions and uses similar to those of nalidixic acid (p.234). In the treatment of urinary-tract infections the usual adult dose is 250 mg four times daily or 500 mg twice daily by mouth; for prophylaxis a single dose of 250 mg daily is given at bedtime.

For details of reduced doses to be used in renal impairment, see below.

◊ References.

1. Sisca TS, *et al.* Cinoxacin: a review of its pharmacological properties and therapeutic efficacy in the treatment of urinary tract infections. *Drugs* 1983; **25:** 544–69.

**Administration in renal impairment.** Dosage of cinoxacin should be reduced in mild to moderate renal impairment. The following doses are recommended, depending on the degree of impairment: creatinine clearance of 50 to 80 mL/minute, 250 mg three times daily; 20 to 50 mL/minute, 250 mg once or twice daily; less than 20 mL/minute, 250 mg once daily. Cinoxacin should not be given to anuric patients.

### Preparations

**USP 27:** Cinoxacin Capsules.

**Proprietary Preparations** (details are given in Part 3)
**Belg.:** Cinobac†; **Ger.:** Cinobactin†; **Gr.:** Cinobactin; **Ital.:** Cinobac; Cinocil; Cinoxen; Nossacin; Noxigram; Uroc; Uronorm; Uroxacin; **Mex.:** Gugecin; **S.Afr.:** Cinobactin†; **UK:** Cinobac†; **USA:** Cinobac.

## Ciprofloxacin *(BAN, USAN, rINN)*

Bay-q-3939; Ciprofloxacino; Ciprofloxacinum. 1-Cyclopropyl-6-fluoro-1,4-dihydro-4-oxo-7-piperazin-1-ylquinoline-3-carboxylic acid.

$C_{17}H_{18}FN_3O_3$ = 331.3.
*CAS — 85721-33-1.*
*ATC — J01MA02; S01AX13; S03AA07.*

**Pharmacopoeias.** In *Eur.* (see p.vi), *Int.*, and *US.*

**Ph. Eur. 5.0** (Ciprofloxacin). An almost white or pale yellow, slightly hygroscopic, crystalline powder. Practically insoluble in water; very slightly soluble in dehydrated alcohol and in dichloromethane. Store in airtight containers. Protect from light.

**USP 27** (Ciprofloxacin). Store in airtight containers at a temperature of 25°, excursions permitted between 15° and 30°. Avoid temperatures above 40°. Protect from light.

## Ciprofloxacin Hydrochloride *(BANM, USAN, rINNM)*

Bay-o-9867; Ciprofloxacini Hydrochloridum; Hidrocloruro de ciprofloxacino. Ciprofloxacin hydrochloride monohydrate.

$C_{17}H_{18}FN_3O_3,HCl,H_2O$ = 385.8.
*CAS — 86483-48-9 (anhydrous ciprofloxacin hydrochloride); 86393-32-0 (ciprofloxacin hydrochloride monohydrate).*

**Pharmacopoeias.** In *Chin., Eur.* (see p.vi), *Int., Pol., US,* and *Viet.*

**Ph. Eur. 5.0** (Ciprofloxacin Hydrochloride). A pale yellow, slightly hygroscopic, crystalline powder. Soluble in water; very slightly soluble in dehydrated alcohol; practically insoluble in acetone, in dichloromethane, and in ethyl acetate; slightly soluble in methyl alcohol. A 2.5% solution in water has a pH of 3.5 to 4.5. Store in airtight containers. Protect from light.

**USP 27** (Ciprofloxacin Hydrochloride). Faintly yellowish to light yellow crystals. Sparingly soluble in water; very slightly soluble in dehydrated alcohol; slightly soluble in acetic acid and in methyl alcohol; practically insoluble in acetone, in acetonitrile, in dichloromethane, in ethyl acetate, and in hexane. pH of a 2.5% solution in water is between 3.0 and 4.5. Store in airtight containers at a temperature of 25°, excursions permitted between 15° and 30°. Protect from light.

## Ciprofloxacin Lactate *(BANM, rINNM)*

Lactato de ciprofloxacino.

$C_{17}H_{18}FN_3O_3,C_3H_6O_3$ = 421.4.
*CAS — 97867-33-9.*

**Pharmacopoeias.** In *Chin.*

**Incompatibility.** Ciprofloxacin infusion is stated by the manufacturers to have a pH of 3.9 to 4.5 and to be incompatible with injections chemically or physically unstable at this pH range. Incompatibility has been reported between ciprofloxacin and a range of drugs including some other antibacterials.[1-5]

1. Lyall D, Blythe J. Ciprofloxacin lactate infusion. *Pharm J* 1987; **238:** 290.
2. Janknegt R, *et al.* Quinolones and penicillins incompatibility. *DICP Ann Pharmacother* 1989; **23:** 91–2.
3. Goodwin SD, *et al.* Compatibility of ciprofloxacin injection with selected drugs and solutions. *Am J Hosp Pharm* 1991; **48:** 2166–71.
4. Jim LK. Physical and chemical compatibility of intravenous ciprofloxacin with other drugs. *Ann Pharmacother* 1993; **27:** 704–7.
5. Elmore RL, *et al.* Stability and compatibility of admixtures of intravenous ciprofloxacin and selected drugs. *Clin Ther* 1996; **18:** 246–55.

**Stability.** For mention of loss of activity in ciprofloxacin solutions exposed to ultraviolet light see under Precautions, below.

### Adverse Effects

Ciprofloxacin is generally well tolerated. The range of adverse effects associated with ciprofloxacin and the other fluoroquinolone antibacterials is broadly similar to that with earlier quinolones such as nalidixic acid (p.234). They most often involve the gastrointestinal tract, CNS, or skin.

Gastrointestinal disturbances include nausea, vomiting, diarrhoea, abdominal pain, and dyspepsia and are the most frequent adverse effects. Pseudomembranous colitis has been reported rarely.

Headache, dizziness, and restlessness are among the commonest effects on the CNS. Others include tremor, drowsiness, insomnia, nightmares, and visual and other sensory disturbances and, more rarely, hallucinations, psychotic reactions, depression, and convulsions. Paraesthesia and peripheral neuropathy have occurred occasionally.

In addition to rash and pruritus, hypersensitivity-type reactions affecting the skin have included, rarely, vasculitis, erythema multiforme, Stevens-Johnson syndrome, and toxic epidermal necrolysis. Photosensitivity has occurred, although it may be more frequent with some newer fluoroquinolones such as lomefloxacin and sparfloxacin. Anaphylaxis has been associated with ciprofloxacin and some other quinolone antibacterials. As with other quinolone antibacterials, reversible arthralgia has sometimes occurred and joint erosions have been documented in immature *animals*. Tendon damage has been reported.

Other adverse effects reported with ciprofloxacin include transient increases in serum creatinine or blood urea nitrogen and, occasionally, acute renal failure secondary to interstitial nephritis; crystalluria; elevated liver enzyme values, jaundice, and hepatitis; haematological disturbances including eosinophilia, leucopenia, thrombocytopenia and, very rarely, pancytopenia, haemolytic anaemia or agranulocytosis; myalgia; gynaecomastia; and cardiovascular effects including tachycardia, oedema, syncope, hot flushes, and sweating.

As with other antibacterials, superinfection with organisms not very susceptible to ciprofloxacin is possible. Such organisms include *Candida, Clostridium difficile,* and *Streptococcus pneumoniae.* There is some evidence that ciprofloxacin use may be associated with an increased risk of colonisation by meticillin-resistant *Staphylococcus aureus* and vancomycin-resistant enterococci.

Pain and irritation may occur at the site of injection accompanied rarely by phlebitis or thrombophlebitis.

◊ General reviews of the adverse effects of fluoroquinolone antibacterials.


1. Stahlmann R. Safety profile of the quinolones. *J Antimicrob Chemother* 1990; **26** (suppl D): 31–44.
2. Paton JH, Reeves DS. Adverse reactions to the fluoroquinolones. *Adverse Drug React Bull* 1992; (April): 575–8.
3. Domagala JM. Structure-activity and structure-side-effect relationships for the quinolone antibacterials. *J Antimicrob Chemother* 1994; **33:** 685–706.
4. Rubinstein E, *et al.* The use of fluoroquinolones in neutropenic patients—analysis of adverse effects. *J Antimicrob Chemother* 1994; **34:** 7–19.
5. Ball P, Tillotson G. Tolerability of fluoroquinolone antibiotics: past, present and future. *Drug Safety* 1995; **13:** 343–58.
6. Lipsky BA, Baker CA. Fluoroquinolone toxicity profiles: a review focusing on newer agents. *Clin Infect Dis* 1999; **28:** 352–64.
7. Ball P, *et al.* Comparative tolerability of the newer fluoroquinolone antibacterials. *Drug Safety* 1999; **21:** 407–21.


◊ Reviews and surveys of the adverse effects of ciprofloxacin.


1. Arcieri GM, *et al.* Safety of intravenous ciprofloxacin: a review. *Am J Med* 1989; **87** (suppl 5A): 92S–97S.
2. Schacht P, *et al.* Safety of oral ciprofloxacin: an update based on clinical trial results. *Am J Med* 1989; **87** (suppl 5A): 98S–102S.
3. Kennedy N, *et al.* Safety profile of ciprofloxacin during long-term therapy for pulmonary tuberculosis. *J Antimicrob Chemother* 1993; **32:** 897–902.
4. Segev S, *et al.* Safety of long-term therapy with ciprofloxacin: data analysis of controlled clinical trials and review. *Clin Infect Dis* 1999; **28:** 299–308.


**Effects on the blood.** Haematological disturbances including eosinophilia, leucopenia, thrombocytopenia, and, very rarely, pancytopenia, haemolytic anaemia, or agranulocytosis have been reported with ciprofloxacin. In addition, transient reductions in factor VIII and von Willebrand's factor leading to bleeding in 2 patients receiving ciprofloxacin has been reported.[1]


1. Castaman G, Rodeghiero F. Acquired transitory von Willebrand syndrome with ciprofloxacin. *Lancet* 1994; **343:** 492.


**Effects on the gastrointestinal tract.** Reports of pseudomembranous colitis or superinfection with *Clostridium difficile* associated with ciprofloxacin and other fluoroquinolones.


1. Dan M, Samra Z. Clostridium difficile colitis associated with ofloxacin therapy. *Am J Med* 1989; **87:** 479.
2. Cain DB, O'Connor ME. Pseudomembranous colitis associated with ciprofloxacin. *Lancet* 1990; **336:** 946.
3. Bates CJ, *et al.* Ciprofloxacin and Clostridium difficile infection. *Lancet* 1990; **336:** 1193.
4. Low N, Harries A. Ciprofloxacin and pseudomembranous colitis. *Lancet* 1990; **336:** 1510.
5. Hillman RJ, *et al.* Ciprofloxacin as a cause of Clostridium difficile-associated diarrhoea in an HIV antibody-positive patient. *J Infect* 1990; **21:** 205–7.
6. Golledge CL, *et al.* Ciprofloxacin and Clostridium difficile-associated diarrhoea. *J Antimicrob Chemother* 1992; **30:** 141–7.
7. McFarland LV, *et al.* Ciprofloxacin-associated Clostridium difficile disease. *Lancet* 1995; **346:** 977–8.


**Effects on the kidneys.** References to renal toxicity associated with ciprofloxacin and other fluoroquinolones.


1. Rippelmeyer DJ, Synhavsky A. Ciprofloxacin and allergic interstitial nephritis. *Ann Intern Med* 1988; **109:** 170.
2. Ying LS, Johnson CA. Ciprofloxacin-induced interstitial nephritis. *Clin Pharm* 1989; **8:** 518–21.
3. Rastogi S, *et al.* Allergic nephropathy associated with ciprofloxacin. *Mayo Clin Proc* 1990; **65:** 987–9.
4. Allon M, *et al.* Acute renal failure due to ciprofloxacin. *Arch Intern Med* 1990; **150:** 2187–9.
5. George MJ, *et al.* Acute renal failure after an overdose of ciprofloxacin. *Arch Intern Med* 1991; **151:** 620.
6. Simpson J, *et al.* Typhoid fever, ciprofloxacin, and renal failure. *Arch Dis Child* 1991; **66:** 1083–4.
7. Yew WW, *et al.* Ciprofloxacin-induced renal dysfunction in patients with mycobacterial lung infections. *Tubercle Lung Dis* 1995; **76:** 173–5.
8. Hestin D, *et al.* Norfloxacin-induced nephrotic syndrome. *Lancet* 1995; **345:** 732–3.
9. Lomaestro BM. Fluoroquinolone-induced renal failure. *Drug Safety* 2000; **22:** 479–85.
10. Famularo G, De Simone C. Nephrotoxicity and purpura associated with levofloxacin. *Ann Pharmacother* 2002; **36:** 1380–2.


**Effects on the liver.** References to hepatotoxicity associated with ciprofloxacin and other fluoroquinolones.


1. Grassmick BK, *et al.* Fulminant hepatic failure possibly related to ciprofloxacin. *Ann Pharmacother* 1992; **26:** 636–9.
2. Sherman O, Beizer JL. Possible ciprofloxacin-induced acute cholestatic jaundice. *Ann Pharmacother* 1994; **28:** 1162–4.
3. Villeneuve J-P, *et al.* Suspected ciprofloxacin-induced hepatotoxicity. *Ann Pharmacother* 1995; **29:** 257–9.
4. Jones SE, Smith RH. Quinolones may induce hepatitis. *BMJ* 1997; **314:** 869.


**Effects on the musculoskeletal system.** Reversible arthralgia has sometimes occurred with the fluoroquinolone antibacterials;[1] joint erosions have been documented in immature *animals*. In one report, treatment with pefloxacin might have contributed to the destructive arthropathy that occurred in a 17-year-old youth.[2]

More recently there have been reports of tendinitis and tendon rupture associated with fluoroquinolones.[3-6] By July 1995, the UK Committee on Safety of Medicines (CSM) had received 21 reports of tendon damage, often of the Achilles tendon, associated with these antibacterials—11 with ciprofloxacin and 10 with ofloxacin.[5] In a later case-control study[7] of a cohort of 46 776 users of fluoroquinolones, 704 had Achilles tendinitis and 38 had Achilles tendon rupture; the adjusted relative risk of Achilles tendon disorders with current use was 1.9. The risk of tendon damage is increased by the concomitant use of corticosteroids and is more common with increasing age:[5] the case-control study[7] found that the relative risk for current users rose to 3.2 among those aged 60 and over, and to 6.2 in those in this age group using corticosteroids concurrently. Onset may be rapid: rupture has occurred within 48 hours of starting therapy.[8] The CSM warned that at the first sign of pain or inflammation the quinolone should be discontinued and the affected limb rested until the tendon symptoms had resolved.[5] Similar warnings have been issued in other countries.


1. Alfaham M, *et al.* Arthropathy in a patient with cystic fibrosis taking ciprofloxacin. *BMJ* 1987; **295:** 699.
2. Chevalier X, *et al.* A case of destructive polyarthropathy in a 17-year-old youth following pefloxacin treatment. *Drug Safety* 1992; **7:** 310–14.
3. Huston KA. Achilles tendinitis and tendon rupture due to fluoroquinolone antibiotics. *N Engl J Med* 1994; **331:** 748.
4. Szarfman A, *et al.* More on fluoroquinolone antibiotics and tendon rupture. *N Engl J Med* 1995; **332:** 193.
5. Committee on Safety of Medicines/Medicines Control Agency. Tendon damage associated with quinolone antibiotics. *Current Problems* 1995; **21:** 8.
6. Carrasco JM, *et al.* Tendinitis associated with ciprofloxacin. *Ann Pharmacother* 1997; **31:** 120.
7. van der Linden PD, *et al.* Fluoroquinolones and risk of Achilles tendon disorders: case-control study. *BMJ* 2002; **324:** 1306–7.
8. Committee on Safety of Medicines/Medicines Control Agency. Reminder: fluoroquinolone antibiotics and tendon disorders. *Current Problems* 2002; **28:** 3–4. Also available at: http://www.mca.gov.uk/ourwork/monitorsafequalmed/currentproblems/cpapril2002.pdf (accessed 25/05/04)


**Effects on the nervous system.** By 1991 the UK Committee on Safety of Medicines had received 26 reports of convulsions associated with ciprofloxacin, 1 with norfloxacin, and 1 with ofloxacin.[1] It was noted that convulsions could occur both in patients with epilepsy and in those with no previous history of convulsions.

Other recent reports of CNS toxicity associated with ciprofloxacin have included eosinophilic meningitis,[2] delirium,[3] and acute psychoses.[4,5] Peripheral neuropathy,[6] dysaesthesia,[7] catatonia,[8] hemiparesis,[9] and tinnitus[10] have also been reported.

There have also been reports of sleep disturbances[11] and of a Tourette-like syndrome[12] associated with ofloxacin.


1. Committee on Safety of Medicines. Convulsions due to quinolone antimicrobial agents. *Current Problems 32* 1991.
2. Asperilla MO, *et al.* Eosinophilic meningitis associated with ciprofloxacin. *Am J Med* 1989; **87:** 589–90.
3. Jay GT, Fitzgerald JM. Ciprofloxacin-induced delirium. *Ann Pharmacother* 1997; **31:** 252.
4. McCue JD, Zandt JR. Acute psychoses associated with the use of ciprofloxacin and trimethoprim-sulfamethoxazole. *Am J Med* 1991; **90:** 528–9.
5. Reeves RR. Ciprofloxacin-induced psychosis. *Ann Pharmacother* 1992; **26:** 930–1.
6. Aoun M, *et al.* Peripheral neuropathy associated with fluoroquinolones. *Lancet* 1992; **340:** 127.
7. Zehnder D, *et al.* Painful dysaesthesia with ciprofloxacin. *BMJ* 1995; **311:** 1204.
8. Akhtar S, Ahmad H. Ciprofloxacin-induced catatonia. *J Clin Psychiatry* 1993; **54:** 115–16.
9. Rosolen A, *et al.* Acute hemiparesis associated with ciprofloxacin. *BMJ* 1994; **309:** 1411.
10. Paul J, Brown NM. Tinnitus and ciprofloxacin. *BMJ* 1995; **311:** 232.
11. Upton C. Sleep disturbance in children treated with ofloxacin. *BMJ* 1994; **309:** 1411.
12. Thomas RJ, Reagan DR. Association of a Tourette-like syndrome with ofloxacin. *Ann Pharmacother* 1996; **30:** 138–41.


**Hypersensitivity.** Hypersensitivity and skin reactions have been associated with ciprofloxacin and other fluoroquinolones. Reports have included anaphylaxis (which has sometimes been fatal),[1-5] serum sickness,[6] toxic epidermal necrolysis,[7-11] laryngeal oedema,[12] and vasculitis.[13-15] Fatal vasculitis has been reported with ofloxacin.[16]


1. Davis H, *et al.* Anaphylactoid reactions reported after treatment with ciprofloxacin. *Ann Intern Med* 1989; **111:** 1041–3.
2. Peters B, Pinching AJ. Fatal anaphylaxis associated with ciprofloxacin in a patient with AIDS related complex. *BMJ* 1989; **298:** 605.
3. Wurtz RM, *et al.* Anaphylactoid drug reactions to ciprofloxacin and rifampicin in HIV-infected patients. *Lancet* 1989; **i:** 955–6.
4. Assouad M, *et al.* Anaphylactoid reactions to ciprofloxacin. *Ann Intern Med* 1995; **122:** 396–7.
5. Smythe MA, Cappelletty DM. Anaphylactoid reaction to levofloxacin. *Pharmacotherapy* 2000; **20:** 1520–3.
6. Slama TG. Serum sickness-like illness associated with ciprofloxacin. *Antimicrob Agents Chemother* 1990; **34:** 904–5.
7. Tham TCK, *et al.* Possible association between toxic epidermal necrolysis and ciprofloxacin. *Lancet* 1991; **338:** 522.
8. Moshfeghi M, Mandler HD. Ciprofloxacin-induced toxic epidermal necrolysis. *Ann Pharmacother* 1993; **27:** 1467–9.
9. Yerasi AB, Oertel MD. Ciprofloxacin-induced toxic epidermal necrolysis. *Ann Pharmacother* 1996; **30:** 297.
10. Livasy CA, Kaplan AM. Ciprofloxacin-induced toxic epidermal necrolysis: a case report. *Dermatology* 1997; **195:** 173–5.
11. Melde SL. Ofloxacin: a probable cause of toxic epidermal necrolysis. *Ann Pharmacother* 2001; **35:** 1388–90.
12. Baciewicz AM, *et al.* Laryngeal edema related to ciprofloxacin therapy. *Ann Pharmacother* 1992; **26:** 1456.
13. Choe U, *et al.* Ciprofloxacin-induced vasculitis. *N Engl J Med* 1989; **320:** 257–8.
14. Stubbings J, *et al.* Cutaneous vasculitis due to ciprofloxacin. *BMJ* 1992; **305:** 29.
15. Drago F, *et al.* Henoch-Schönlein purpura induced by fluoroquinolones. *Br J Dermatol* 1994; **131:** 448.
16. Pace JL, Gatt P. Fatal vasculitis associated with ofloxacin. *BMJ* 1989; **299:** 658.


**Superinfection.** Reports of superinfection with *Streptococcus pneumoniae* in patients receiving ciprofloxacin.[1-3] For references to superinfection with *Clostridium difficile* and associated pseudomembranous colitis, see under Effects on the Gastrointestinal Tract, above.


1. Righter J. Pneumococcal meningitis during intravenous ciprofloxacin therapy. *Am J Med* 1990; **88:** 548.
2. Gordon JJ, Kauffman CA. Superinfection with Streptococcus pneumoniae during therapy with ciprofloxacin. *Am J Med* 1990; **89:** 383–4.
3. Lee BL, *et al.* Infectious complications with respiratory pathogens despite ciprofloxacin therapy. *N Engl J Med* 1991; **325:** 520–1.


## Precautions

Ciprofloxacin should be used with caution in patients with epilepsy or a history of CNS disorders. Since ciprofloxacin and related fluoroquinolones have, like nalidixic acid, been shown to cause degenerative changes in weight-bearing joints of young *animals*, licensing information in the UK states that these drugs should not be used in children, adolescents, pregnant women, or breast-feeding mothers (but see also under Breast Feeding, below). Tendon damage may occur rarely with fluoroquinolones (see Effects on the Musculoskeletal System, above) and treatment should be discontinued if patients experience tendon pain, inflammation, or rupture; subsequent use of fluoroquinolones is contra-indicated in these patients.

Care is necessary in patients with impaired hepatic or renal function, G6PD deficiency, or myasthenia gravis. An adequate fluid intake should be maintained during treatment with ciprofloxacin and excessive alkalinity of the urine avoided because of the risk of crystalluria. Exposure to strong sunlight or sunlamps should also be avoided. The ability to drive or operate machinery may be impaired by ciprofloxacin, especially when alcohol is also taken.

Ciprofloxacin and other quinolones should be avoided in meticillin-resistant *Staphylococcus aureus* infections because of the high level of resistance.

**Administration in children.** Since ciprofloxacin and other fluoroquinolones can cause degenerative changes in weight-bearing joints of young *animals* they should only be used in children and adolescents where their use may be justified if the benefits outweigh the risks.[1,2]


1. Schaad UB, *et al.* Use of fluoroquinolones in pediatrics: consensus report of an International Society of Chemotherapy commission. *Pediatr Infect Dis J* 1995; **14:** 1–9.
2. Green SDR. Indications and restrictions of fluoroquinolone use in children. *Br J Hosp Med* 1996; **56:** 420–3.


**Breast feeding.** Ciprofloxacin was found to be undetectable in the serum of a breast-fed infant whose mother received ciprofloxacin 500 mg daily for 10 days.[1] In another study[2] involving 30 women who underwent termination of pregnancy, 10 each received ciprofloxacin, ofloxacin, or pefloxacin respectively, and all three drugs were found to be highly concentrated in breast milk with ratios exceeding 75% of the simultaneous serum concentrations 2 hours after administration; it was concluded that, because quinolones had been demonstrated to cause arthropathy in young *animals*, their potential benefits should be weighed against the risk to the infant before they were considered for use in breast-feeding women. For the same reasons, UK licensing information states that the use of ciprofloxacin should be avoided in breast-feeding mothers, although the view of the American Academy of Pediatrics is that ciprofloxacin may be considered usually compatible with breast feeding.[3]


1. Gardner DK, *et al.* Simultaneous concentrations of ciprofloxacin in breast milk and in serum in mother and breast-fed infant. *Clin Pharm* 1992; **11:** 352–4.
2. Giamarellou H, *et al.* Pharmacokinetics of three newer quinolones in pregnant and lactating women. *Am J Med* 1989; **87** (suppl 5A): 49S–51S.
3. American Academy of Pediatrics. The transfer of drugs and other chemicals into human milk. *Pediatrics* 2001; **108:** 776–89. Correction. *ibid.*; 1029. Also available at: http://aappolicy.aappublications.org/cgi/content/full/pediatrics%3b108/3/776 (accessed 25/05/04)


**Exposure to ultraviolet light.** Loss of antibacterial activity has been reported following irradiation of ciprofloxacin solutions by ultraviolet light.[1] In addition to the possible hazard of photosensitivity reactions, a reduction in both cutaneous and circulating levels of ciprofloxacin was predicted in patients exposed to sunlight through window glass or longer wavelength ultraviolet (UVA) radiation from sunbeds.[1]


1. Phillips G, *et al.* The loss of antibiotic activity of ciprofloxacin by photodegradation. *J Antimicrob Chemother* 1990; **26:** 783–9.


**Interference with diagnostic tests.** Ciprofloxacin did not interfere with determination of urinary-glucose concentrations carried out with Clinitest, Diastix, or Tes-Tape,[1] but pseudoglycosuria, a false-positive reaction for glucose in urine, has been reported with BM-Test-7 in elderly patients given ciprofloxacin for urinary-tract infections.[2]

1. Tartaglione TA, Flint NB. Effect of imipenem-cilastatin and ciprofloxacin on tests for glycosuria. *Am J Hosp Pharm* 1985; **42:** 602–5.
2. Drysdale L, *et al.* Pseudoglycosuria and ciprofloxacin. *Lancet* 1988; **ii:** 961.

**Myasthenia gravis.** Caution is advised in patients with myasthenia gravis given fluoroquinolones following reports of the possible exacerbation of symptoms in a patient,[1] and unmasking of subclinical myasthenia gravis in another,[2] by ciprofloxacin. Exacerbation of myasthenia gravis has also been reported with norfloxacin,[3] ofloxacin,[4] and pefloxacin.[5]

1. Moore B, *et al.* Possible exacerbation of myasthenia gravis by ciprofloxacin. *Lancet* 1988; **i:** 882.
2. Mumford CJ, Ginsberg L. Ciprofloxacin and myasthenia gravis. *BMJ* 1990; **301:** 818.
3. Rauser EH, *et al.* Exacerbation of myasthenia gravis by norfloxacin. *DICP Ann Pharmacother* 1990; **24:** 207–8.
4. Azevedo E, *et al.* Probable exacerbation of myasthenia gravis by ofloxacin. *J Neurol* 1993; **240:** 508.
5. Vial T, *et al.* Aggravation d'une myasthénie sous péfloxacine. *Rev Neurol (Paris)* 1995; **151:** 286–7.

## Interactions

Fluoroquinolones are known to inhibit hepatic drug metabolism and may interfere with the clearance of drugs, such as theophylline, that are metabolised by the liver. Cations such as aluminium, magnesium, or iron reduce the absorption of ciprofloxacin and related drugs when given concomitantly. Changes in the pharmacokinetics of fluoroquinolones have been reported when given with histamine $H_2$ antagonists, possibly due to changes in gastric pH, but do not seem to be of much clinical significance.

For physical or chemical incompatibilities with ciprofloxacin, see above.

**Analgesics.** Use of *fenbufen* with quinolones may increase the incidence of quinolone CNS adverse effects. Reviews[1,2] have noted cases of convulsions associated with the use of fenbufen and enoxacin reported to the Japanese regulatory authorities. The UK Committee on Safety of Medicines has recognised that convulsions may occur due to an interaction between the quinolones and NSAIDs; by 1991, 3 such interactions had been reported to them.[3] Adverse neurological effects have also been reported in a patient receiving *naproxen* and chloroquine when ciprofloxacin was given, which abated when the antirheumatic drugs were withdrawn.[4]

Ciprofloxacin also interacts with *opioid analgesics*; peak serum concentrations of ciprofloxacin given by mouth pre-operatively were significantly reduced when intramuscular *papaveretum* was injected.[5] In the UK, product information for ciprofloxacin recommends that opioid premedication should not be used if ciprofloxacin is given for surgical infection prophylaxis.

1. Janknegt R. Drug interactions with quinolones. *J Antimicrob Chemother* 1990; **26** (suppl D): 7–29.
2. Christ W. Central nervous system toxicity of quinolones: human and animal findings. *J Antimicrob Chemother* 1990; **26** (suppl B): 219–25.
3. Committee on Safety of Medicines. Convulsions due to quinolone antimicrobial agents. *Current Problems 32* 1991.
4. Rollof J, Vinge E. Neurologic adverse effects during concomitant treatment with ciprofloxacin, NSAIDs, and chloroquine: possible drug interaction. *Ann Pharmacother* 1993; **27:** 1058–9.
5. Morran C, *et al.* Brief report: pharmacokinetics of orally administered ciprofloxacin in abdominal surgery. *Am J Med* 1989; **87** (suppl 5A): 86S–88S.

**Antacids and metal ions.** The absorption of ciprofloxacin and other fluoroquinolones is reduced by *antacids* containing *aluminium* or *magnesium* and also by *calcium*, *iron*, and *zinc* salts.[1] *Sucralfate* releases aluminium ions in the stomach and thereby reduces the absorption of ciprofloxacin[2,3] and other fluoroquinolones, including norfloxacin,[4] ofloxacin, and sparfloxacin.[5] In addition, antacids or oral iron preparations might antagonise the antibacterial activity of fluoroquinolones within the gut lumen.[6] *Dairy products* with a high calcium content might also interfere with the absorption of some fluoroquinolones.[7-9] *Enteral feeds*, which contain cations, have also been found to reduce absorption of ciprofloxacin.[10] A reduction in ciprofloxacin bioavailability has also been reported after *chewable tablets* of didanosine which contain aluminium and magnesium ion buffering agents.[11]

1. Lomaestro BM, Bailie GR. Absorption interactions with fluoroquinolones: 1995 update. *Drug Safety* 1995; **12:** 314–33.
2. Garrelts JC, *et al.* Sucralfate significantly reduces ciprofloxacin concentrations in serum. *Antimicrob Agents Chemother* 1990; **34:** 931–3.
3. Van Slooten AD, *et al.* Combined use of ciprofloxacin and sucralfate. *DICP Ann Pharmacother* 1991; **25:** 578–82.
4. Parpia SH, *et al.* Sucralfate reduces the gastrointestinal absorption of norfloxacin. *Antimicrob Agents Chemother* 1989; **33:** 99–102.
5. Kamberi M, *et al.* The effect of staggered dosing of sucralfate on oral bioavailability of sparfloxacin. *Br J Clin Pharmacol* 2000; **49:** 98–103.
6. Lewin CS, Smith JT. 4-Quinolones and multivalent ions. *J Antimicrob Chemother* 1990; **26:** 149.
7. Neuvonen PJ, *et al.* Interference of dairy products with the absorption of ciprofloxacin. *Clin Pharmacol Ther* 1991; **50:** 498–502.
8. Kivistö KT, *et al.* Inhibition of norfloxacin absorption by dairy products. *Antimicrob Agents Chemother* 1992; **36:** 489–91.
9. Neuvonen PJ, Kivistö KT. Milk and yoghurt do not impair the absorption of ofloxacin. *Br J Clin Pharmacol* 1992; **33:** 346–8.
10. Healy DP, *et al.* Ciprofloxacin absorption is impaired in patients given enteral feedings orally and via gastrostomy and jejunostomy tubes. *Antimicrob Agents Chemother* 1996; **40:** 6–10.
11. Sahai J, *et al.* Cations in the didanosine tablet reduce ciprofloxacin bioavailability. *Clin Pharmacol Ther* 1993; **53:** 292–7.

**Antibacterials.** The simultaneous use of parenteral ciprofloxacin and *azlocillin* has resulted in higher and more prolonged serum concentrations of ciprofloxacin.[1]

1. Barriere SL, *et al.* Alteration in the pharmacokinetic disposition of ciprofloxacin by simultaneous administration of azlocillin. *Antimicrob Agents Chemother* 1990; **34:** 823–6.

**Anticoagulants.** For reports of ciprofloxacin and other quinolones enhancing the effect of oral anticoagulants, see under *Warfarin*, p.1024.

**Antidiabetics.** For reference to elevated glibenclamide concentrations in patients who were also given ciprofloxacin, see p.347.

**Antiepileptics.** For conflicting reports of the effect of ciprofloxacin on serum-*phenytoin* concentrations, see p.372.

**Antimigraine drugs.** For a recommendation to reduce the dosage of *zolmitriptan* when given with ciprofloxacin, see p.473.

**Antineoplastics.** Absorption of oral ciprofloxacin appears to be reduced after cytotoxic chemotherapy.[1]

1. Johnson EJ, *et al.* Reduced absorption of oral ciprofloxacin after chemotherapy for haematological malignancy. *J Antimicrob Chemother* 1990; **25:** 837–42.

**Antivirals.** Both ciprofloxacin and *foscarnet* can cause convulsions and 2 patients developed generalised tonic-clonic seizures while receiving the drugs together.[1]

For reference to reduction of ciprofloxacin bioavailability due to the antacid content of chewable *didanosine* tablets, see under Antacids and Metal Ions, above.

1. Fan-Havard P, *et al.* Concurrent use of foscarnet and ciprofloxacin may increase the propensity for seizures. *Ann Pharmacother* 1994; **28:** 869–72.

**Anxiolytics.** For an isolated report of increased blood concentrations of *midazolam* associated with the use of ciprofloxacin, see under Diazepam, p.693.

**Immunosuppressants.** For reference to possible interaction between quinolones and *ciclosporin*, see p.1354.

**Probenecid.** The urinary excretion of ciprofloxacin and some other fluoroquinolones is reduced by probenecid; plasma concentrations are not necessarily increased.

**Xanthines.** Ciprofloxacin and other fluoroquinolones (to a greater or lesser extent) decrease the clearance of *theophylline* (p.801) and *caffeine* (p.782) from the body. Seizures have occurred in patients given ciprofloxacin and theophylline and in one such report[1] serum-theophylline concentrations were normal.

1. Bader MB. Role of ciprofloxacin in fatal seizures. *Chest* 1992; **101:** 883–4.

## Antimicrobial Action

Ciprofloxacin is bactericidal and acts by inhibiting the A subunit of DNA gyrase (topoisomerase) which is essential in the reproduction of bacterial DNA. It has a broader spectrum of activity and is more potent *in vitro* than the non-fluorinated quinolone nalidixic acid. Activity may be reduced in acid media.

*Spectrum of activity.* Among Gram-negative aerobic bacteria, ciprofloxacin is active *in vitro* against Enterobacteriaceae, including *Escherichia coli* and *Citrobacter, Enterobacter, Klebsiella, Proteus, Providencia, Salmonella, Serratia, Shigella*, and *Yersinia* spp. It is also active against *Pseudomonas aeruginosa*, but less so against other *Pseudomonas* spp. *Haemophilus ducreyi, H. influenzae, Moraxella catarrhalis* (*Branhamella catarrhalis*), and *Neisseria gonorrhoeae* are all very sensitive, including beta-lactamase-producing strains; *N. meningitidis* is also susceptible. Other Gram-negative aerobic bacteria reported to be sensitive to ciprofloxacin have included *Acinetobacter* spp., *Campylobacter* spp., *Gardnerella vaginalis, Helicobacter pylori, Legionella* spp., *Pasteurella multocida*, and *Vibrio* spp. Variable activity has been reported against *Brucella melitensis*.

Among Gram-positive aerobic bacteria, ciprofloxacin is active against staphylococci, including penicillinase-producing and penicillinase-nonproducing strains, and against some meticillin-resistant strains. Streptococci, in particular *Streptococcus pneumoniae* and enterococci, are less susceptible. Other Gram-positive bacteria sensitive to ciprofloxacin *in vitro* are *Bacillus anthracis* and *Corynebacterium* spp.

Most anaerobic bacteria, including *Bacteroides fragilis* and *Clostridium difficile*, are resistant to ciprofloxacin, although some other *Clostridium* spp. may be susceptible.

Ciprofloxacin has some activity against mycobacteria, mycoplasmas, rickettsias, and the protozoan *Plasmodium falciparum*. *Chlamydia trachomatis* is moderately susceptible, and *Nocardia asteroides* and *Ureaplasma urealyticum* are usually considered to be resistant. The spirochaete *Treponema pallidum* and fungi are also resistant.

*Activity with other antimicrobials.* There have been some reports of enhanced activity *in vitro* when ciprofloxacin has been used with other antimicrobials, such as aminoglycosides or azlocillin against *Staphylococcus aureus* and *Pseudomonas aeruginosa*, imipenem against *Ps. aeruginosa*, and cefotaxime or clindamycin against anaerobic bacteria.

*Acquired resistance.* Resistant strains, particularly of *Staph. aureus* (including meticillin-resistant strains) and *Ps. aeruginosa* have emerged during treatment with ciprofloxacin (see below for reports of other resistant bacteria). There is complete cross-resistance between ciprofloxacin and the other fluoroquinolones, but not between ciprofloxacin and nalidixic acid. Like nalidixic acid, resistance to ciprofloxacin appears, so far, to be chromosomally rather than plasmid-mediated.

**Resistance.** Acquired resistance to ciprofloxacin and other fluoroquinolones has occurred most frequently in staphylococci[1-3] and *Pseudomonas aeruginosa*;[4] cross-resistance to unrelated antibacterials has been described in *Ps. aeruginosa*.[5] Resistance has also been reported in *Campylobacter* spp., initially linked with the widespread veterinary use of quinolones[6,7] and subsequently becoming more clinically important,[8,9] including isolated reports of possible resistance in *C. fetus* infections in immunocompromised patients.[10] Similarly there have been reports of increasing quinolone resistance in both non-typhoid *Salmonella* spp.,[11] as well as *S. typhi*[12-15] and *S. paratyphi*.[16] Resistance to fluoroquinolones has also been reported in other Enterobacteriaceae, including *Escherichia coli*,[17,18] *Serratia marcescens*,[19] *Shigella sonnei*,[20] and *Haemophilus influenzae*.[21,22] Decreased susceptibility of *Neisseria gonorrhoeae* has been described[23,24] and resistant strains have now been reported.[25-27] Mutational resistance has developed in mycobacteria following monotherapy with ciprofloxacin.[28] Fluoroquinolone-resistant strains of *Mycobacterium tuberculosis* have been isolated from patients with tuberculosis.[29]

Excretion of ciprofloxacin in sweat has been suggested to be a contributory factor in the development of resistance in *Staphylococcus epidermidis* and possibly other skin-dwelling bacteria.[30]

1. Oppenheim BA, *et al.* Outbreak of coagulase negative staphylococcus highly resistant to ciprofloxacin in a leukaemia unit. *BMJ* 1989; **299:** 294–7.
2. Blumberg HM, *et al.* Rapid development of ciprofloxacin resistance in methicillin-susceptible and -resistant Staphylococcus aureus. *J Infect Dis* 1991; **163:** 1279–85.
3. Trucksis M, *et al.* Emerging resistance to fluoroquinolones in staphylococci: an alert. *Ann Intern Med* 1991; **114:** 424–6.
4. Acar JF, Francoual S. The clinical problems of bacterial resistance to the new quinolones. *J Antimicrob Chemother* 1990; **26** (suppl B): 207–13.
5. Aubert G, *et al.* Emergence of quinolone-imipenem cross-resistance in Pseudomonas aeruginosa after fluoroquinolone therapy. *J Antimicrob Chemother* 1992; **29:** 307–12.
6. Endtz HP, *et al.* Quinolone resistance in campylobacter isolated from man and poultry following the introduction of fluoroquinolones in veterinary medicine. *J Antimicrob Chemother* 1991; **27:** 199–208.
7. Bowler I, Day D. Emerging quinolone resistance in campylobacters. *Lancet* 1992; **340:** 245.
8. Segreti J, *et al.* High-level quinolone resistance in clinical isolates of Campylobacter jejuni. *J Infect Dis* 1992; **165:** 667–70.
9. McIntyre M, Lyons M. Resistance to ciprofloxacin in Campylobacter spp. *Lancet* 1993; **341:** 188.
10. Meier PA, *et al.* Development of quinolone-resistant Campylobacter fetus bacteremia in human immunodeficiency virus-infected patients. *J Infect Dis* 1998; **177:** 951–4.
11. Frost JA, *et al.* Increasing ciprofloxacin resistance in salmonellas in England and Wales 1991-1994. *J Antimicrob Chemother* 1996; **37:** 85–91.
12. Rowe B, *et al.* Ciprofloxacin-resistant Salmonella typhi in the UK. *Lancet* 1995; **346:** 1302.
13. Mitchell DH. Ciprofloxacin-resistant Salmonella typhi: an emerging problem. *Med J Aust* 1997; **167:** 172.
14. Murdoch DA, *et al.* Epidemic ciprofloxacin-resistant Salmonella typhi in Tajikistan. *Lancet* 1998; **351:** 339.
15. Threlfall EJ, *et al.* Ciprofloxacin-resistant Salmonella typhi and treatment failure. *Lancet* 1999; **353:** 1590–1.
16. Bhutta ZA. Quinolone-resistant Salmonella paratyphi B meningitis in a newborn: a case report. *J Infect* 1997; **35:** 308–10.
17. Aguiar JM, *et al.* The emergence of highly fluoroquinolone-resistant Escherichia coli in community-acquired urinary tract infections. *J Antimicrob Chemother* 1992; **29:** 349–50.
18. Threlfall EJ, *et al.* High-level resistance to ciprofloxacin in Escherichia coli. *Lancet* 1997; **349:** 403.
19. Fujimaki K, *et al.* Quinolone resistance in clinical isolate of Serratia marcescens. *Antimicrob Agents Chemother* 1989; **33:** 785–7.

20. Horiuchi S, *et al.* Reduced susceptibilities of Shigella sonnei strains isolated from patients with dysentery to fluoroquinolones. *Antimicrob Agents Chemother* 1993; **37:** 2486–9.
21. Barriere SL, Hindler JA. Ciprofloxacin-resistant Haemophilus influenzae infection in a patient with chronic lung disease. *Ann Pharmacother* 1993; **27:** 309–10.
22. Gould IM, *et al.* Quinolone resistant Haemophilus influenzae. *J Antimicrob Chemother* 1994; **33:** 187–8.
23. Jephcott AE, Turner A. Ciprofloxacin resistance in gonococci. *Lancet* 1990; **335:** 165.
24. Gordon SM, *et al.* The emergence of Neisseria gonorrhoeae with decreased susceptibility to ciprofloxacin in Cleveland, Ohio: epidemiology and risk factors. *Ann Intern Med* 1996; **125:** 465–70.
25. Kam K, *et al.* Quinolone-resistant Neisseria gonorrhoeae in Hong Kong. *Sex Transm Dis* 1996; **23:** 103–8.
26. Ison CA, *et al.* Drift in susceptibility of Neisseria gonorrhoeae to ciprofloxacin and emergence of therapeutic failure. *Antimicrob Agents Chemother* 1998; **42:** 2919–22.
27. Health Protection Agency. GRASP The Gonococcal Resistance to Antimicrobials Surveillance Programme: annual report, year 2002 collection. Available at: http://www.hpa.org.uk/infections/topics_az/hiv_and_sti/sti-gonorrhoea/publications/grasp_report_2002.pdf (accessed 25/05/04)
28. Wallace RJ, *et al.* Activities of ciprofloxacin and ofloxacin against rapidly growing mycobacterial with demonstration of acquired resistance following single-drug therapy. *Antimicrob Agents Chemother* 1990; **34:** 65–70.
29. Sullivan EA, *et al.* Emergence of fluoroquinolone-resistant tuberculosis in New York City. *Lancet* 1995; **345:** 1148–50.
30. Høiby N, *et al.* Excretion of ciprofloxacin in sweat and multiresistant Staphylococcus epidermidis. *Lancet* 1997; **349:** 167–9.

## Pharmacokinetics

Ciprofloxacin is rapidly and well absorbed from the gastrointestinal tract. Oral bioavailability is approximately 70% and a peak plasma concentration of about 2.5 micrograms/mL is achieved 1 to 2 hours after a dose of 500 mg by mouth. Absorption may be delayed by the presence of food, but is not substantially affected overall. The plasma half-life is about 3.5 to 4.5 hours and there is evidence of modest accumulation. Half-life may be prolonged in renal impairment—a value of 8 hours has been reported in end-stage renal disease—and to some extent in the elderly. There is limited information on the effect of hepatic impairment; the half-life of ciprofloxacin has been reported to be slightly prolonged in patients with severe cirrhosis of the liver. With one or two exceptions, most studies have shown the pharmacokinetics of ciprofloxacin to be not markedly affected by cystic fibrosis.

Plasma protein binding ranges from 20 to 40%. Ciprofloxacin is widely distributed in the body and tissue penetration is generally good. It appears in the CSF, but concentrations are only about 10% of those in plasma when the meninges are not inflamed. Ciprofloxacin crosses the placenta and is also distributed into breast milk. High concentrations are achieved in bile.

Ciprofloxacin is eliminated principally by urinary excretion, but non-renal clearance may account for about a third of elimination and includes hepatic metabolism, biliary excretion, and possibly transluminal secretion across the intestinal mucosa. At least 4 active metabolites have been identified. Oxociprofloxacin appears to be the major urinary metabolite and sulfociprofloxacin the primary faecal metabolite. Urinary excretion is by active tubular secretion as well as glomerular filtration and is reduced by probenecid; it is virtually complete within 24 hours. About 40 to 50% of an oral dose is excreted unchanged in the urine and about 15% as metabolites. Up to 70% of a parenteral dose may be excreted unchanged within 24 hours and 10% as metabolites. Faecal excretion over 5 days has accounted for 20 to 35% of an oral dose and 15% of an intravenous dose.

Only small amounts of ciprofloxacin are removed by haemodialysis or peritoneal dialysis.

◊ Reviews of the pharmacokinetics of ciprofloxacin[1] and of the comparative pharmacokinetics of fluoroquinolones.[2]

1. Vance-Bryan K, *et al.* Clinical pharmacokinetics of ciprofloxacin. *Clin Pharmacokinet* 1990; **19:** 434–61.
2. Aminimanizani A, *et al.* Comparative pharmacokinetics and pharmacodynamics of the newer fluoroquinolone antibacterials. *Clin Pharmacokinet* 2001; **40:** 169–187.

**Distribution.** Studies on the distribution of ciprofloxacin.

1. Sweeney G, *et al.* Penetration of ciprofloxacin into the aqueous humour of the uninflamed human eye after oral administration. *J Antimicrob Chemother* 1990; **26:** 99–105.
2. Cover DL, Mueller BA. Ciprofloxacin penetration into human breast milk: a case report. *DICP Ann Pharmacother* 1990; **24:** 703–4.
3. Nau R, *et al.* Penetration of ciprofloxacin into the cerebrospinal fluid of patients with uninflamed meninges. *J Antimicrob Chemother* 1990; **25:** 965–73.
4. Trautmann M, *et al.* Penetration of ciprofloxacin into the spinal fluid in patients with viral and bacterial meningitis. *Arzneimittelforschung* 1990; **40:** 611–13.
5. Mertes PM, *et al.* Penetration of ciprofloxacin into heart valves, myocardium, mediastinal fat, and sternal bone marrow in humans. *Antimicrob Agents Chemother* 1990; **34:** 398–401.
6. Darouiche R, *et al.* Levels of rifampin and ciprofloxacin in nasal secretions: correlation with $MIC_{90}$ and eradication of nasopharyngeal carriage of bacteria. *J Infect Dis* 1990; **162:** 1124–7.
7. Jacobs F, *et al.* Penetration of ciprofloxacin into human pleural fluid. *Antimicrob Agents Chemother* 1990; **34:** 934–6.
8. Fabre D, *et al.* Steady-state pharmacokinetics of ciprofloxacin in plasma from patients with nosocomial pneumonia: penetration of the bronchial mucosa. *Antimicrob Agents Chemother* 1991; **35:** 2521–5.
9. Dan M, *et al.* Distribution of ciprofloxacin in ascitic fluid following administration of a single oral dose of 750 milligrams. *Antimicrob Agents Chemother* 1992; **36:** 677–8.
10. Dan M, *et al.* The penetration of ciprofloxacin into bronchial mucosa, lung parenchyma, and pleural tissue after intravenous administration. *Eur J Clin Pharmacol* 1993; **44:** 101–2.
11. Decré D, Bergogne-Bérézin E. Pharmacokinetics of quinolones with special reference to the respiratory tree. *J Antimicrob Chemother* 1993; **31:** 331–43.
12. Catchpole C, *et al.* The comparative pharmacokinetics and tissue penetration of single-dose ciprofloxacin 400 mg iv and 750 mg po. *J Antimicrob Chemother* 1994; **33:** 103–10.
13. Leeming JP, *et al.* Ocular penetration of topical ciprofloxacin and norfloxacin drops and their effect upon eyelid flora. *Br J Ophthalmol* 1994; **78:** 546–8.
14. Edmiston CE, *et al.* Penetration of ciprofloxacin and fleroxacin into biliary tract. *Antimicrob Agents Chemother* 1996; **40:** 787–8.

**In cystic fibrosis.** References to the pharmacokinetics of ciprofloxacin in patients with cystic fibrosis.

1. LeBel M, *et al.* Pharmacokinetics and pharmacodynamics of ciprofloxacin in cystic fibrosis patients. *Antimicrob Agents Chemother* 1986; **30:** 260–6.
2. Davis RL, *et al.* Pharmacokinetics of ciprofloxacin in cystic fibrosis. *Antimicrob Agents Chemother* 1987; **31:** 915–19.
3. Steen HJ, *et al.* Clinical and pharmacokinetic aspects of ciprofloxacin in the treatment of acute exacerbations of pseudomonas infection in cystic fibrosis patients. *J Antimicrob Chemother* 1989; **24:** 787–95.
4. Christensson BA, *et al.* Increased oral bioavailability of ciprofloxacin in cystic fibrosis patients. *Antimicrob Agents Chemother* 1992; **36:** 2512–17.
5. Schaefer HG, *et al.* Pharmacokinetics of ciprofloxacin in pediatric cystic fibrosis patients. *Antimicrob Agents Chemother* 1996; **40:** 29–34.
6. Rubio TT, *et al.* Pharmacokinetic disposition of sequential intravenous/oral ciprofloxacin in pediatric cystic fibrosis patients with acute pulmonary exacerbation. *Pediatr Infect Dis J* 1997; **16:** 112–17.
7. Odoul F, *et al.* Ciprofloxacin pharmacokinetics in young cystic fibrosis patients after repeated oral doses. *Therapie* 2001; **56:** 519–24.

**In the elderly.** References to the pharmacokinetics of ciprofloxacin in elderly patients.

1. LeBel M, *et al.* Pharmacokinetics of ciprofloxacin in elderly subjects. *Pharmacotherapy* 1986; **6:** 87–91.
2. Kees F, *et al.* Pharmacokinetics of ciprofloxacin in elderly patients. *Arzneimittelforschung* 1989; **39:** 524–7.
3. Ljungberg B, Nilsson-Ehle I. Pharmacokinetics of ciprofloxacin in the elderly: increased oral bioavailability and reduced renal clearance. *Eur J Clin Microbiol Infect Dis* 1989; **8:** 515–20.
4. Shah A, *et al.* Pharmacokinetics of high-dose intravenous ciprofloxacin in young and elderly and in male and female subjects. *Antimicrob Agents Chemother* 1995; **39:** 1003–6.

**In hepatic impairment.** References to the pharmacokinetics of ciprofloxacin in hepatic impairment.

1. Esposito S, *et al.* Pharmacokinetics of ciprofloxacin in impaired liver function. *Int J Clin Pharmacol Res* 1989; **9:** 37–41.

**In renal impairment.** References to the pharmacokinetics of ciprofloxacin in renal impairment.

1. Roberts DE, Williams JD. Ciprofloxacin in renal failure. *J Antimicrob Chemother* 1989; **23:** 820–3.
2. Dharmasena D, *et al.* Pharmacokinetics of intraperitoneal ciprofloxacin in patients on CAPD. *J Antimicrob Chemother* 1989; **23:** 253–9.
3. Plaisance KI, *et al.* Effect of renal function on the bioavailability of ciprofloxacin. *Antimicrob Agents Chemother* 1990; **34:** 1031–4.
4. MacGowan AP, *et al.* Serum ciprofloxacin concentrations in patients with severe sepsis being treated with ciprofloxacin 200 mg iv bd irrespective of renal function. *J Antimicrob Chemother* 1994; **33:** 1051–4.
5. Shah A, *et al.* Pharmacokinetics of intravenous ciprofloxacin in normal and renally impaired subjects. *J Antimicrob Chemother* 1996; **38:** 103–16.

**In the seriously ill.** References to the pharmacokinetics of ciprofloxacin in seriously ill patients.

1. Forrest A, *et al.* Development of a population pharmacokinetic model and optimal sampling strategies for intravenous ciprofloxacin. *Antimicrob Agents Chemother* 1993; **37:** 1065–72.
2. Forrest A, *et al.* Pharmacodynamics of intravenous ciprofloxacin in seriously ill patients. *Antimicrob Agents Chemother* 1993; **37:** 1073–81.
3. Cohn SM, *et al.* Enteric absorption of ciprofloxacin during the immediate postoperative period. *J Antimicrob Chemother* 1995; **36:** 717–21.
4. Garrelts JC, *et al.* Ciprofloxacin pharmacokinetics in burn patients. *Antimicrob Agents Chemother* 1996; **40:** 1153–6.
5. Owens RC, *et al.* Oral bioavailability and pharmacokinetics of ciprofloxacin in patients with AIDS. *Antimicrob Agents Chemother* 1997; **41:** 1508–11.
6. Lipman J, *et al.* Pharmacokinetic profiles of high-dose intravenous ciprofloxacin in severe sepsis. *Antimicrob Agents Chemother* 1998; **42:** 2235–9.
7. Lesne-Hulin A, *et al.* Clinical pharmacokinetics of ciprofloxacin in patients with major burns. *Eur J Clin Pharmacol* 1999; **55:** 515–19.
8. Varela JE, *et al.* Pharmacokinetics and burn eschar penetration of intravenous ciprofloxacin in patients with major thermal injuries. *J Antimicrob Chemother* 2000; **45:** 337–42.
9. Lipman J, *et al.* Ciprofloxacin pharmacokinetic profiles in paediatric sepsis: how much ciprofloxacin is enough? *Intensive Care Med* 2002; **28:** 493–500.

## Uses and Administration

Ciprofloxacin is a fluorinated 4-quinolone or fluoroquinolone antibacterial with a wider spectrum of activity than nalidixic acid (see Antimicrobial Action, above) and more favourable pharmacokinetics allowing its use in systemic infections. It has been used in the treatment of a wide range of infections including anthrax, biliary-tract infections, infected bites and stings, bone and joint infections, cat scratch disease, chancroid, exacerbations of cystic fibrosis, gastro-enteritis (including travellers' diarrhoea and campylobacter enteritis, cholera, salmonella enteritis, and shigellosis), gonorrhoea, infections in immunocompromised patients (neutropenia), legionnaires' disease, otitis externa, otitis media, peritonitis, Q fever, lower respiratory-tract infections (including pseudomonal infections in cystic fibrosis, but excluding infections due to *Streptococcus pneumoniae* such as pneumococcal pneumonia), septicaemia, skin infections (including soft-tissue infections), spotted fevers, typhoid and paratyphoid fever, typhus, and urinary-tract infections. Ciprofloxacin is used for meningococcal meningitis prophylaxis. It is also used for surgical infection prophylaxis. Fluoroquinolones such as ciprofloxacin and ofloxacin have been tried in the treatment of opportunistic mycobacterial infections and tuberculosis; ofloxacin may be used in the treatment of leprosy. Fluoroquinolones such as ciprofloxacin and ofloxacin are used topically in the treatment of eye infections. For details of all these infections and their treatment, see under Choice of Antibacterial, p.120.

*Administration and dosage.* Ciprofloxacin is given by mouth as the hydrochloride or base, by intravenous infusion as the lactate, and in eye drops or eye ointment as the hydrochloride. Doses and strengths are expressed in terms of the equivalent amount of ciprofloxacin base. 291.1 mg of ciprofloxacin hydrochloride is approximately equivalent to 250 mg of ciprofloxacin. 127 mg of ciprofloxacin lactate is approximately equivalent to 100 mg of ciprofloxacin.

The usual adult oral dose of ciprofloxacin ranges from 250 to 750 mg twice daily depending on the severity and nature of the infection. The usual adult intravenous dose is 100 to 400 mg twice daily, given over 30 to 60 minutes as a solution containing the equivalent of 1 to 2 mg/mL (but see also under Administration, below). A dose of 100 mg twice daily by mouth is suitable in women with acute uncomplicated cystitis.

For acute exacerbations of cystic fibrosis associated with *Pseudomonas aeruginosa* infection, ciprofloxacin may be given to adolescents and children aged 5 years or more in a dose of 20 mg/kg by mouth twice daily, up to a maximum of 750 mg twice daily. Alternatively, a dose of 10 mg/kg may be given by intravenous infusion over 60 minutes three times daily, to a maximum of 400 mg three times daily.

For inhalation anthrax, ciprofloxacin may be given to children and adolescents for 60 days in a dose of 15 mg/kg twice daily by mouth, up to a maximum of 500 mg twice daily. Alternatively, a dose of 10 mg/kg twice daily may be given by intravenous infusion, up to a maximum of 400 mg twice daily.

Ciprofloxacin is not generally recommended for other uses in children and adolescents (see Precautions, above) but, if considered essential, doses of 5 to 15 mg/kg twice daily by mouth or 4 to 8 mg/kg twice daily intravenously have been suggested.

Doses should be reduced in patients with severe renal impairment (see Administration in Renal Impairment, below).

Single oral doses of 250 or 500 mg are used for the treatment of gonorrhoea, depending upon patterns of resistance. A single oral dose of 500 mg is suggested for meningococcal meningitis prophylaxis. A single oral dose of 750 mg is suggested for surgical infection prophylaxis, given 60 to 90 minutes before the procedure.

For corneal ulcers and superficial ocular infections caused by susceptible strains of bacteria ciprofloxacin is given as the hydrochloride in eye drops and eye ointment containing the equivalent of 0.3% of ciprofloxacin base.

◊ General references to fluoroquinolone antibacterials.

1. Hooper DC, Wolfson JS. Fluoroquinolone antimicrobial agents. *N Engl J Med* 1991; **324:** 384–94.
2. von Rosenstiel N, Adam D. Quinolone antibacterials: an update of their pharmacology and therapeutic use. *Drugs* 1994; **47:** 872–901.
3. Balfour JA, Goa KL, eds. Proceedings of the 5th International symposium on new quinolones. *Drugs* 1995; **49** (suppl 2): 1–505.
4. Walker RC. The fluoroquinolones. *Mayo Clin Proc* 1999; **74:** 1030–7.
5. Smith A, *et al.* Fluoroquinolones: place in ocular therapy. *Drugs* 2001; **61:** 747–61.
6. Schaeffer AJ. The expanding role of fluoroquinolones. *Am J Med* 2002; **113** (suppl 1A): 45S–54S.
7. Zhanel GG, *et al.* A critical review of the fluoroquinolones: focus on respiratory infections. *Drugs* 2002; **62:** 13–59.

◊ General references to ciprofloxacin.

1. Campoli-Richards DM, *et al.* Ciprofloxacin: a review of its antibacterial activity, pharmacokinetic properties and therapeutic use. *Drugs* 1988; **35:** 373–447.
2. Neu HC, ed. Ciprofloxacin: major advances in intravenous and oral quinolone therapy. *Am J Med* 1989; **87** (suppl 5A): 1S–287S.
3. Brown EM, *et al.*, eds. Ciprofloxacin—defining its role today. *J Antimicrob Chemother* 1990; **26** (suppl F): 1–193.
4. Davis R, *et al.* Ciprofloxacin: an updated review of its pharmacology, therapeutic efficacy and tolerability. *Drugs* 1996; **51:** 1019–74.
5. Gould FK, *et al.*, eds. Ten years of ciprofloxacin: the past, present and future. *J Antimicrob Chemother* 1999; **43** (suppl A): 1–134.

**Administration.** Although the usual maximum doses of ciprofloxacin are 750 mg twice daily orally or 400 mg twice daily intravenously, higher doses have been used. Notably, the US manufacturers recommend an intravenous dose of 400 mg three times daily in severe or complicated infections of the lower respiratory tract, skin, and bones and joints. They also recommend this dose for nosocomial pneumonia, and for empirical treatment of febrile neutropenic patients in combination with piperacillin.

In a study in patients with suspected shigellosis,[1] a single oral dose of ciprofloxacin 1 g, or 1 g daily for 2 days, was as effective as the conventional dose of 500 mg twice daily for 5 days, except in patients infected with *Shigella dysenteriae* type 1. A single oral dose of ciprofloxacin 500 mg appeared to be effective when given early for the empirical treatment of travellers' diarrhoea.[2] A patient with a renal cyst infection unresponsive to conventional antibacterial therapy improved on ciprofloxacin 600 mg intravenously twice daily for 7 days, followed by oral therapy, without evidence of toxicity.[3] Long-term therapy with a single 1-g daily dose was also found to be probably more effective than 500 mg twice daily in a study in patients with pulmonary tuberculosis.[4]

1. Bennish ML, *et al.* Treatment of shigellosis III: comparison of one- or two-dose ciprofloxacin with standard 5-day therapy: a randomized, blinded trial. *Ann Intern Med* 1992; **117:** 727–34.
2. Salam I, *et al.* Randomised trial of single-dose ciprofloxacin for travellers' diarrhoea. *Lancet* 1994; **344:** 1537–9.
3. Rossi SJ, *et al.* High-dose ciprofloxacin in the treatment of a renal cyst infection. *Ann Pharmacother* 1993; **27:** 38–9.
4. Bergstermann H, Rüchardt A. Ciprofloxacin once daily versus twice daily for the treatment of pulmonary tuberculosis. *Infection* 1997; **25:** 227–32.

**Administration in renal impairment.** Doses of ciprofloxacin should be reduced in patients with severe renal impairment. Halving the dose has been suggested when the creatinine clearance is less than 20 mL/minute or alternatively the dosage interval may be increased; ideally plasma concentrations of ciprofloxacin should be monitored.

**Inflammatory bowel disease.** Ciprofloxacin has been given, sometimes in combination with metronidazole, to treat active Crohn's disease[1] (see Inflammatory Bowel Disease, p.1243).

1. Prantera C, *et al.* An antibiotic regimen for the treatment of active Crohn's disease: a randomized, controlled clinical trial of metronidazole plus ciprofloxacin. *Am J Gastroenterol* 1996; **91:** 328–32.

## Preparations

***BP 2003:*** Ciprofloxacin Intravenous Infusion; Ciprofloxacin Tablets;
***USP 27:*** Ciprofloxacin Injection; Ciprofloxacin Ophthalmic Ointment; Ciprofloxacin Ophthalmic Solution; Ciprofloxacin Tablets.

**Proprietary Preparations** (details are given in Part 3)
***Arg.:*** Argeflox; Biotic; Blader; Ciloxan; Cipro; Cipro-Otico; Ciprotenk; Cirflox-G; Ciriax; Crisacide; Exertial; Floraxina; Microsulf; Novidat; Ocefax; Omaflaxina; Plusgin; Septicide; ***Austral.:*** C-Flox; Ciloquin; Ciloxan; Ciprol; Ciproxin; Profloxin; Proquin; ***Austria:*** Agyr; Ciloxan; Ciproxin; ***Belg.:*** Ciloxan; Ciproxine; ***Braz.:*** Bactoflox; Biamotil; Ciflox; Cifloxtron; Ciloxan; Cinoflax; Ciprex†; Cipro; Ciprobiot; Ciprocin†; Ciprocina; Ciprodine; Ciprofar; Ciproflox; Cipronal; Ciproxan; Ciproxil; Flobac†; Floxan; Nixin; Ofoxin; Procin; Proflox; Proxacin; Quiflox; Quinoflox; ***Canad.:*** Ciloxan; Cipro; ***Chile:*** Baycip; Cifloxin; Ciloxacin; Ciproval; Ciproxino; Grificiprox; Oflono; Oftaciprox; ***Denm.:*** Ciloxan; Ciproxin; Sancipro; ***Fin.:*** Ciproxin; ***Fr.:*** Ciflox; Ciloxan; Uniflox; ***Ger.:*** Ciloxan; Cipro-Lich; Cipro-Wolff; Ciprobay; Ciprobeta; Ciprodura; Ciproflox; Ciprogamma; Ciprohexal; Keciflox; ***Gr.:*** Afenoxin; Aristin-C; Balepton; Bivorilan; Ciloxan; Cipromycin; Ciprospes; Ciproxin; Citrovenot; Flociprin; Forterra; Ginorectol; Glossyfin; Grenis-cipro; Labentrol; Ladinin; Nafloxin; Ravalton; Remena; Revion; Ufexil; ***Hong Kong:*** Ciloxan; Cipide; Ciproxin; ***India:*** Cifran; Cipro-Cent; Ciprobid; Ciprowin; Ificipro; Quinobact; Strox; ***Irl.:*** Ciproxin; Truoxin; ***Israel:*** Ciloxan; Ciprogis; Ciproxin; ***Ital.:*** Ciproxin; Flociprin; Oftacilox; ***Jpn:*** Ciproxan; ***Malaysia:*** Ciloxan; Ciprobay; ***Mex.:*** Arfloxina†; Bioflox; Ciloxan; Cimogal; Ciprain; Ciprobac; Ciprobiotic; Ciproflox; Ciprofur; Ciproser; Ciproxina; Ciqfadin; Ehlixacin†; Eni; Floxager; Floxakin†; Floxantina; Floxelena; Infloxa; Italnik; Kenzoflex; Lemyflox; Liferxina; Microrgan; Mitroken; Nivoflox; Novoquin; Oftaquin; Opthaflox; Pharcina; Proxitec; Quifloxona; Sophixin; Suiflox; Trigen; Zipra; ***Neth.:*** Ciproxin; ***Norw.:*** Cilox; Ciproxin; ***NZ:*** Ciloxan; Ciproxin; ***Port.:*** Carmicina; Ciflan; Ciplox; Ciproquinol; Ciproxina; Estecina; Floxacipron; Giroflox; Keefloxin; Megaflox; Nivoflox; Nixin; Oftacilox; Quinox; Xorpic; ***S.Afr.:*** Adco-Ciprin; Cifloc; Cifran; Ciloxan; Ciprobay; ***Singapore:*** Ciloxan; Ciprobay; Cycin; Neofloxin; Uroxin; ***Spain:*** Aceoto; Baycip; Belmacina; Catex; Ceprimax; Cetraxal; Cipobacter; Ciprenit Otico; Ciprok†; Cunesin; Doriman; Estecina; Felixene; Globuce; Huberdoxina; Inkamil†; Oftacilox; Piprol; Plenolyt; Quipro; Rigoran; Sepcen; Septocipro; Tam; Ultramicina; Velmonit; ***Swed.:*** Ciloxan; Ciproxin; ***Switz.:*** Ciloxan; Ciprin; Ciproxine; ***Thai.:*** C-Floxacin; Ciflolan; Cifloxin; Cifran; Cilab; Ciloxan; Cinfloxine; Cipflocin; Ciprobay; Ciprobid; Ciprocep; Ciprofin; Ciprogen; Ciproglen; Ciprolet; Cipròm-H; Ciprosun; Ciproxan; Ciproxyl; Cyflox; Forexin; Medociprin†; Poli-Cifloxin; Proflox; Serviflox; Uroxin; ***UAE:*** Sarf; ***UK:*** Ciloxan; Ciproxin; ***USA:*** Ciloxan; Cipro.

**Multi-ingredient:** ***Arg.:*** Cipro HC; Ciriax Otic; Otex HC; Otocipro; ***Austral.:*** Ciproxin HC; ***Austria:*** Ciproxin HC; ***Braz.:*** Biamotil-D; Ciloxadex; Cipro HC; ***Canad.:*** Cipro HC; ***Chile:*** Ciprodex; ***Denm.:*** Ciflox; ***Fin.:*** Ciproxin-Hydrocortison; ***Hong Kong:*** Cipro HC; ***India:*** Ciplox; ***Israel:*** Ciproxin HC; ***Mex.:*** Quinoflox; ***NZ:*** Ciproxin HC; ***S.Afr.:*** Ciprobay HC; ***Singapore:*** Ciprobay HC; ***Spain:*** Aceoto Plus; Cetraxal Plus; Cexidal Otico; Ciproxina; Ultramicina Plus; ***Switz.:*** Ciproxin HC; ***USA:*** Cipro HC; Ciprodex.

# Clarithromycin *(BAN, USAN, rINN)*

A-56268; Abbott-56268; Clarithromycinum; Claritromicina; TE-031. (2*R*,3*S*,4*S*,5*R*,6*R*,8*R*,10*R*,11*R*,12*S*,13*R*)-3-(2,6-Dideoxy-3-*C*,3*O*-dimethyl-α-L-*ribo*-hexopyranosyloxy)-11,12-dihydroxy-6-methoxy-2,4,6,8,10,12-hexamethyl-9-oxo-5-(3,4,6-trideoxy-3-dimethylamino-β-D-*xylo*-hexopyranosyloxy)pentadecan-13-olide; 6-*O*-Methylerythromycin.

$C_{38}H_{69}NO_{13}$ = 748.0.

*CAS — 81103-11-9.*

*ATC — J01FA09.*

**Pharmacopoeias.** In *Chin., Eur.* (see p.vi), *Jpn,* and *US.*

**Ph. Eur. 5.0** (Clarithromycin). A white or almost white, crystalline powder. Practically insoluble in water; soluble in acetone and in dichloromethane; slightly soluble in methyl alcohol.

**USP 27** (Clarithromycin). A white to off-white crystalline powder. Practically insoluble in water; slightly soluble in dehydrated alcohol, in methyl alcohol, and in acetonitrile; soluble in acetone; slightly soluble in phosphate buffer at pH values of 2 to 5. pH of a 0.2% suspension in a mixture of water and methyl alcohol (19:1) is between 7.5 and 10.0. Store in airtight containers.

## Adverse Effects and Precautions

As for Erythromycin, p.208. Gastrointestinal disturbances are the most frequent adverse effect but are usually mild and less frequent with clarithromycin than with erythromycin. Taste disturbances, stomatitis, glossitis, tooth discoloration, and headache have occurred. There have also been reports of transient CNS effects such as anxiety, dizziness, insomnia, hallucinations, and confusion; convulsions have also occurred. Other adverse effects include hypoglycaemia, leucopenia, and thrombocytopenia. Interstitial nephritis and renal failure have been reported rarely.

Intravenous administration may cause phlebitis and pain at the injection site.

Caution is required in patients with hepatic or renal impairment and doses should be reduced in those with severe renal impairment. It should not be used during pregnancy if possible as high doses have been associated with embryotoxicity in *animal* studies.

**Effects on the blood.** Single cases of thrombocytopenia[1] and thrombocytopenic purpura[2,3] associated with clarithromycin have been reported. A case of thrombocytopenia accompanied by interstitial nephritis, hepatitis, and elevated serum amylase levels was attributed to an allergic reaction to clarithromycin.[4]

1. Price TA, Tuazon CU. Clarithromycin-induced thrombocytopenia. *Clin Infect Dis* 1992; **15:** 563–4.
2. Oteo JA, *et al.* Clarithromycin-induced thrombocytopenic purpura. *Clin Infect Dis* 1994; **19:** 1170–1.
3. Alexopoulou A, *et al.* Thrombotic thrombocytopenic purpura in a patient treated with clarithromycin. *Eur J Haematol* 2002; **69:** 191–2.
4. Baylor P, Williams K. Interstitial nephritis, thrombocytopenia, hepatitis, and elevated serum amylase levels in a patient receiving clarithromycin therapy. *Clin Infect Dis* 1999; **29:** 1350–1.

**Effects on the eyes.** Corneal opacities, reversible on discontinuation of treatment, were reported in a patient receiving oral clarithromycin as part of a regimen for disseminated *Mycobacterium avium* complex infection.[1] Corneal subepithelial deposits have also been reported in a patient following prolonged use of clarithromycin eye drops for *Mycobacterium avium* complex keratitis. The deposits did not cause any ocular discomfort and resolved on discontinuation of therapy.[2]

1. Dorrell L, *et al.* Toxicity of clarithromycin in the treatment of Mycobacterium avium complex infection in a patient with AIDS. *J Antimicrob Chemother* 1994; **34:** 605–6.
2. Tyagi AK, *et al.* An unreported side effect of topical clarithromycin when used successfully to treat Mycobacterium avium-intracellulare keratitis. *Cornea* 1999; **18:** 606–7.

**Effects on the gastrointestinal tract.** Pseudomembranous colitis associated with *Clostridium difficile* developed in a child receiving clarithromycin.[1]

1. Braegger CP, Nadal D. Clarithromycin and pseudomembranous enterocolitis. *Lancet* 1994; **343:** 241–2.

**Effects on the heart.** QT prolongation and torsade de pointes were associated with use of clarithromycin in 2 patients.[1] Renal impairment in 1 of the patients and hepatic impairment and organic heart disease in both could have increased their susceptibility to these effects.

1. Lee KL, *et al.* QT prolongation and torsades de pointes associated with clarithromycin. *Am J Med* 1998; **104:** 395–6.

**Effects on the liver.** Progressive cholestatic jaundice, which subsequently proved fatal, developed in a 59-year-old woman after 3 days of clarithromycin therapy for acute maxillary sinusitis.[1] Fulminant hepatic failure in another patient, which developed during clarithromycin therapy, resolved once the drug was withdrawn.[2] Clarithromycin itself was considered responsible although there was the possibility that it had increased concentrations of isradipine, another known hepatotoxic drug that the patient was also receiving.

1. Fox JC, *et al.* Progressive cholestatic liver disease associated with clarithromycin treatment. *J Clin Pharmacol* 2002; **42:** 676–80.
2. Tietz A, *et al.* Fulminant liver failure associated with clarithromycin. *Ann Pharmacother* 2003; **37:** 57–60.

**Effects on the lungs.** On 2 occasions fever and pulmonary infiltration with eosinophilia occurred in a patient given clarithromycin.[1]

1. Terzano C, Petroianni A. Clarithromycin and pulmonary infiltration with eosinophilia. *BMJ* 2003; **326:** 1377–8.

**Effects on mental state.** Acute psychoses occurred in 2 patients receiving clarithromycin as part of prophylactic treatment for *Helicobacter pylori* infection and were similar to 3 previously reported cases in either AIDS patients or elderly subjects.[1]

1. Gómez-Gil E, *et al.* Clarithromycin-induced acute psychoses in peptic ulcer disease. *Eur J Clin Microbiol Infect Dis* 1999; **18:** 70–1.

**Effects on the pancreas.** A case of pancreatitis was reported in a patient receiving clarithromycin.[1]

1. Liviu L, *et al.* Pancreatitis induced by clarithromycin. *Ann Intern Med* 1996; **125:** 701.

**Effects on the skin.** In addition to skin rashes and other hypersensitivity reactions which occasionally occur in patients receiving macrolides, leukocytoclastic vasculitis has been reported in a patient receiving clarithromycin.[1]

1. Gavura SR, Nusinowitz S. Leukocytoclastic vasculitis associated with clarithromycin. *Ann Pharmacother* 1998; **32:** 543–5.

## Interactions

For a discussion of drug interactions of macrolide antibacterials, see Erythromycin, p.209.

**Antidiabetics.** For reference to hypoglycaemia resulting from the addition of clarithromycin to glibenclamide or glipizide, see p.347.

**Antiretroviral drugs.** In studies in healthy subjects,[1,2] the HIV-protease inhibitor *ritonavir* inhibited the metabolism of clarithromycin, producing elevated plasma concentrations and a prolonged half-life. The metabolism of ritonavir was not affected significantly. The two drugs may be given together in usual doses to those with normal renal function but the manufacturer recommends that the dose of clarithromycin should be reduced in patients with renal impairment receiving ritonavir and it should be noted that this is an extra reduction over and above that which may be needed for the renal impairment alone. It has been suggested that other HIV-protease inhibitors and non-nucleoside reverse transcriptase inhibitors may have a similar effect on clarithromycin. Use of *efavirenz* with clarithromycin has resulted in decreases in the plasma concentration of clarithromycin and increases in its hydroxy metabolite. The combination has been associated with a high incidence of skin rashes.

Decreased concentrations of *zidovudine* (p.659) have been reported in patients also taking clarithromycin and the manufacturer recommends that doses of the two drugs should be separated by 1 to 2 hours.

1. Ouellet D, *et al.* Assessment of the pharmacokinetic interaction between ritonavir and clarithromycin. *Clin Pharmacol Ther* 1996; **59:** 143.
2. Ouellet D, *et al.* Pharmacokinetic interaction between ritonavir and clarithromycin. *Clin Pharmacol Ther* 1998; **64:** 355–62.

**Cimetidine.** Although a study in healthy subjects suggested that some pharmacokinetic parameters of clarithromycin are altered by cimetidine,[1] the clinical significance of such changes are unknown.

1. Amsden GW, *et al.* Oral cimetidine prolongs clarithromycin absorption. *Antimicrob Agents Chemother* 1998; **42:** 1578–80.

**Colchicine.** For mention of fatal colchicine toxicity associated with concomitant use of clarithromycin, see p.415.

**Disulfiram.** For a report of an interaction between clarithromycin and *disulfiram*, see p.1682.

**Fluoxetine.** There has been a report of delirium following use of clarithromycin with fluoxetine (see p.295).

**Omeprazole.** In a study in healthy subjects, concentrations of clarithromycin and its active metabolite were increased in gastric tissue and mucus and, to a lesser extent, in plasma during use of omeprazole.[1] In addition, use of clarithromycin with omeprazole resulted in higher and more prolonged plasma concentrations of omeprazole. The investigators suggest that this interaction could account for the synergistic action observed with this combination when used for eradication of *Helicobacter pylori*. However, the manufacturers of clarithromycin state that no dosage alteration to either drug is necessary.

1. Gustavson LE, *et al.* Effect of omeprazole on concentrations of clarithromycin in plasma and gastric tissue at steady state. *Antimicrob Agents Chemother* 1995; **39:** 2078–83.

## Antimicrobial Action

As for Erythromycin, p.209. Clarithromycin is reported to be more active than erythromycin against susceptible streptococci and staphylococci *in vitro*, as well as against some other species including *Moraxella catarrhalis* (*Branhamella catarrhalis*), *Legionella* spp., *Chlamydia trachomatis*, and *Ureaplasma urealyticum*. Clarithromycin is reported to be more active than erythromycin or azithromycin against some mycobacteria, including *Mycobacterium avium* complex, and against *M. leprae*. It is reported to have some *in-vitro* activity against the protozoan *Toxoplasma gondii*, and may have some activity against cryptosporidia. The major metabolite, 14-hydroxyclarithromycin, is also active, and may enhance the activity of clarithromycin *in vivo*, notably against *Haemophilus influenzae*.

**Activity with other antimicrobials.** Clarithromycin has been reported to enhance the activity of a number of antimycobacterials including ethambutol, isoniazid, pyrazinamide, and rifampicin against *Mycobacterium tuberculosis*.[1,2]

1. Cavalieri SJ, *et al.* Synergistic activities of clarithromycin and antituberculous drugs against multi drug-resistant Mycobacterium tuberculosis. *Antimicrob Agents Chemother* 1995; **39:** 1542–5.
2. Mor N, Esfandiari A. Synergistic activities of clarithromycin and pyrazinamide against Mycobacterium tuberculosis in human macrophages. *Antimicrob Agents Chemother* 1997; **41:** 2035–6.

**Resistance.** Erythromycin-resistant isolates of *Streptococcus pneumoniae* are commonly cross-resistant to clarithromycin.[1] The incidence of resistance to clarithromycin and other macrolides is higher among penicillin-resistant strains than among penicillin-sensitive strains.[2] Clarithromycin-resistant isolates of *Helicobacter pylori* have also emerged.[3-6] Genetic mutations responsible for clarithromycin resistance have been identified in *H. pylori*[7] and in *Mycobacterium* spp.[8,9] Since resistance develops rapidly in *Mycobacterium avium* during clarithromycin monotherapy, combination therapy is usually recommended. However, resistance to clarithromycin in an AIDS patient with systemic *Mycobacterium avium* complex infection, despite combined treatment with clofazimine, has been described.[10]

1. Lonks JR, Medeiros AA. High rate of erythromycin and clarithromycin resistance among Streptococcus pneumoniae isolates from blood cultures from Providence, RI. *Antimicrob Agents Chemother* 1993; **37:** 1742–5.
2. Barry AL, *et al.* Macrolide resistance among Streptococcus pneumoniae and Streptococcus pyogenes isolates from outpatients in the USA. *J Antimicrob Chemother* 1997; **40:** 139–40.
3. López-Brea M, *et al.* Evolution of resistance to metronidazole and clarithromycin in Helicobacter pylori clinical isolates from Spain. *J Antimicrob Chemother* 1997; **40:** 279–81.
4. Hultén K, *et al.* Macrolide resistance in Helicobacter pylori: mechanism and stability in strains from clarithromycin-treated patients. *Antimicrob Agents Chemother* 1997; **41:** 2550–3.
5. Kalach N, *et al.* High levels of resistance to metronidazole and clarithromycin in Helicobacter pylori strains in children. *J Clin Microbiol* 2001; **39:** 394–7.
6. Grove DI, Koutsouridis G. Increasing resistance of Helicobacter pylori to clarithromycin: is the horse bolting? *Pathology* 2002; **34:** 71–3.
7. Versalovic J, *et al.* Mutations in 23S rRNA are associated with clarithromycin resistance in Helicobacter pylori. *Antimicrob Agents Chemother* 1996; **40:** 477–80.
8. Nash KA, Inderlied CB. Genetic basis of macrolide resistance in Mycobacterium avium isolated from patients with disseminated disease. *Antimicrob Agents Chemother* 1995; **39:** 2625–30.
9. Wallace RJ, *et al.* Genetic basis for clarithromycin resistance among isolates of Mycobacterium chelonae and Mycobacterium abscessus. *Antimicrob Agents Chemother* 1996; **40:** 1676–81.
10. De Wit S, *et al.* Acquired resistance to clarithromycin as combined therapy in Mycobacterium avium intracellulare infection. *Lancet* 1993; **341:** 53–4.

## Pharmacokinetics

Clarithromycin is rapidly absorbed from the gastrointestinal tract, and undergoes first-pass metabolism; the bioavailability of the parent drug is about 55%. The extent of absorption is relatively unaffected by the presence of food. Peak concentrations of clarithromycin and its principal active metabolite, 14-hydroxyclarithromycin, are reported to be about 900 and 600 nanograms/mL respectively following a single 250-mg dose by mouth; at steady state the same dose given every 12 hours as tablets produces peak concentrations of clarithromycin of about 1 microgram/mL. The same dose given as a suspension to fasting subjects produces a steady-state plasma concentration of about 2 micrograms/mL.

The pharmacokinetics of clarithromycin are non-linear and dose dependent; high doses may produce disproportionate increases in peak concentrations of the parent drug, due to saturation of the metabolic pathways.

Clarithromycin and its principal metabolite are widely distributed, and tissue concentrations exceed those in serum, in part because of intracellular uptake. Clarithromycin has been detected in breast milk. It is extensively metabolised in the liver, and excreted in faeces via the bile. At steady state about 20% and 30% of a 250-mg or 500-mg dose as tablets, respectively, and about 40% of a 250-mg dose as suspension, is excreted in the urine as unchanged drug. 14-Hydroxyclarithromycin as well as other metabolites are also excreted in the urine accounting for 10 to 15% of the dose. The terminal half-life of clarithromycin is reportedly about 3 to 4 hours in patients receiving 250-mg doses twice daily, and about 5 to 7 hours in those receiving 500 mg twice daily. The half-life is prolonged in renal impairment.

◊ Reviews.

1. Rodvold KA. Clinical pharmacokinetics of clarithromycin. *Clin Pharmacokinet* 1999; **37:** 385–98.

## Uses and Administration

Clarithromycin is a macrolide derived from erythromycin with similar actions and uses (p.210). It is given in the treatment of respiratory-tract infections (including otitis media) and in skin and soft-tissue infections. Clarithromycin is also used for the prophylaxis and treatment of opportunistic mycobacterial infections and has been used in the treatment of leprosy. It is used in some countries as an alternative to penicillins for prophylaxis of endocarditis. For details of all these infections and their treatment, see under Choice of Antibacterial, p.120.

Clarithromycin may be given to eradicate *Helicobacter pylori* in treatment regimens for peptic ulcer disease (p.1246). It has been tried in protozoal infections, including toxoplasmosis (p.598).

Clarithromycin is given by mouth or by intravenous infusion. Usual doses in adults are 250 mg twice daily by mouth, increased to 500 mg twice daily if necessary in severe infection. Modified-release tablets allowing once-daily use are available in some countries. A course is usually for 7 to 14 days. Children may be given 7.5 mg/kg twice daily for 5 to 10 days.

The usual intravenous dose is 500 mg twice daily, given as an intravenous infusion over 60 minutes using a solution containing about 0.2% of clarithromycin. Intravenous treatment may continue for 2 to 5 days, but should be changed to clarithromycin by mouth when possible.

For treatment and prophylaxis of disseminated infection due to *Mycobacterium avium* complex, clarithromycin may be given in a dose of 500 mg twice daily by mouth; for treatment, it should be given with other antimycobacterials. For leprosy, clarithromycin 500 mg daily by mouth has been given as part of an alternative multidrug therapy regimen (p.133).

For the eradication of *H. pylori* associated with peptic ulcer disease, clarithromycin, usually in a dose of 500 mg twice daily, is given with another antibacterial and either a proton pump inhibitor or a histamine $H_2$-receptor antagonist, for 7 to 14 days.

Doses may need to be reduced in patients with severe renal impairment (see below).

◊ Reviews.

1. Peters DH, Clissold SP. Clarithromycin: a review of its antimicrobial activity, pharmacokinetic properties and therapeutic potential. *Drugs* 1992; **44:** 117–64.
2. Barradell LB, *et al.* Clarithromycin: a review of its pharmacological properties and therapeutic use in Mycobacterium avium-intracellulare complex infection in patients with acquired immune deficiency syndrome. *Drugs* 1993; **46:** 289–312.
3. Markham A, McTavish D. Clarithromycin and omeprazole: as Helicobacter pylori eradication therapy in patients with H. pylori-associated gastric disorders. *Drugs* 1996; **51:** 161–78.
4. Alvarez-Elcoro S, Enzler MJ. The macrolides: erythromycin, clarithromycin, and azithromycin. *Mayo Clin Proc* 1999; **74:** 613–34.

**Administration in renal impairment.** In patients with severe renal impairment (creatinine clearance of less than 30 mL/minute) dosage of clarithromycin may need to be halved.

**Ischaemic heart disease.** Macrolide antibacterials, including clarithromycin,[1] have been investigated in the prevention of ischaemic heart disease, based on a suggested link between infection and the inflammation associated with myocardial infarction and unstable angina (see also Ischaemic Heart Disease, under Azithromycin, p.160).

1. Sinisalo J, *et al.* Effect of 3 months of antimicrobial treatment with clarithromycin in acute non-Q-wave coronary syndrome. *Circulation* 2002; **105:** 1555–60.

## Preparations

***USP 27:*** Clarithromycin for Oral Suspension; Clarithromycin Tablets.

**Proprietary Preparations** (details are given in Part 3)

***Arg.:*** Aeroxina; Centromicina; Clarimid; Clatromicin; Finasept; Iset; Klaricid; Klonacid; Macromicina; Orabiot UD; ***Austral.:*** Klacid; ***Austria:*** Klacid; Maclar; Monocid; ***Belg.:*** Biclar; Heliclar; Maclar; Monaxin; ***Braz.:*** Clamicin; Clarimax†; Clarineo; Claritab†; Helicocid†; Klaricid; Lagur†; ***Canad.:*** Biaxin; ***Chile:*** Clarimax; Euromicina; Infex; Klaricid; Mus; Pre-Clar; ***Denm.:*** Klacid; ***Fin.:*** Klacid; Zeclar; ***Fr.:*** Naxy; Zeclar; ***Ger.:*** Biaxin; Cyllind; Klacid; Mavid; ***Gr.:*** Klaricid; Oklaricid; Zeclaren OD; ***Hong Kong:*** Klacid; ***India:*** Claribid; Clarimac; ***Irl.:*** Klacid; ***Israel:*** Karin; Klacid; Klaridex; ***Ital.:*** Klacid; Macladin; Veclam; ***Malaysia:*** Klacid; ***Mex.:*** Adel; Gervaken; Klaricid; Mabicrol; ***Neth.:*** Klacid; ***Norw.:*** Klacid; ***NZ:*** Klacid; ***Port.:*** Klacid; Maclar†; ***S.Afr.:*** Klacid; ***Singapore:*** Klacid; ***Spain:*** Bremon; Klacid; Kofron; ***Swed.:*** Klacid; ***Switz.:*** Klacid; Klaciped; ***Thai.:*** Klacid; ***UAE:*** Clamycin; ***UK:*** Klaricid; ***USA:*** Biaxin.

**Multi-ingredient:** ***Arg.:*** Heliklar; ***Austral.:*** Klacid HP 7; Losec Hp 7; Pylorid-KA; ***Braz.:*** Anzopac; Erradic; Helicopac; Heliklar; Pyloripac; ***Canad.:*** Hp-Pac; Losec 1-2-3 A; Losec 1-2-3 M; ***Fin.:*** Helipak K; ***Ger.:*** ZacPac; ***Malaysia:*** Klacid HP 7; ***Neth.:*** PantoPAC; ***NZ:*** Klacid HP 7; Losec Hp 7; ***S.Afr.:*** Losec 20 Triple; ***Swed.:*** Nexium Hp; ***UK:*** Heliclear; HeliMet; ***USA:*** Prevpac.

---

## Clavulanic Acid *(BAN, rINN)*

Ácido clavulánico; BRL-14151; MM-14151. (*Z*)-(2*R*,5*R*)-3-(2-Hydroxyethylidene)-7-oxo-4-oxa-1-azabicyclo[3.2.0]heptane-2-carboxylic acid.

$C_8H_9NO_5$ = 199.2.

*CAS — 58001-44-8 (clavulanic acid); 57943-81-4 (sodium clavulanate).*

## Potassium Clavulanate *(BANM, rINNM)*

BRL-14151K; Clavulanate Potassium *(USAN)*; Clavulanato potásico; Kalii Clavulanas.

$C_8H_8KNO_5$ = 237.3.

*CAS — 61177-45-5.*

NOTE. Compounded preparations of potassium clavulanate may be represented by the following names:

- Co-amoxiclav *x/y* (*BAN*)—amoxicillin (as the trihydrate or the sodium salt) and potassium clavulanate; *x* and *y* are the strengths in milligrams of amoxicillin and clavulanic acid respectively
- Co-amoxiclav (*PEN*)—amoxicillin trihydrate and potassium clavulanate.

**Pharmacopoeias.** In *Chin.*, *Eur.* (see p.vi), *Jpn*, *Pol.*, and *US*.
*Eur.* also includes Diluted Potassium Clavulanate.

**Ph. Eur. 5.0** (Potassium Clavulanate). The potassium salt of a substance produced by the growth of certain strains of *Streptomyces clavuligerus* or by any other means. A white or almost white, hygroscopic, crystalline powder. Freely soluble in water; slightly soluble in alcohol; very slightly soluble in acetone. A 1% solution in water has a pH of 5.5 to 8.0. Store in airtight containers at a temperature of 2° to 8°.

**Ph. Eur. 5.0** (Potassium Clavulanate, Diluted; Kalii Clavulanas Dilutus). A dry mixture of potassium clavulanate and microcrystalline cellulose or anhydrous or hydrated colloidal silicon dioxide. A white or almost white, hygroscopic, powder. A suspension corresponding to 1% of potassium clavulanate in water has a pH of 4.8 to 8.0. Store in airtight containers.

**USP 27** (Clavulanate Potassium). A white to off-white powder. Freely soluble in water; soluble in methyl alcohol with decomposition. Stability in aqueous solutions is not good, optimum stability at a pH of 6.0 to 6.3. pH of a 1% solution in water is between 5.5 and 8.0. Store in airtight containers.

## Profile

Clavulanic acid is produced by cultures of *Streptomyces clavuligerus*. It has a beta-lactam structure resembling that of the penicillin nucleus, except that the fused thiazolidine ring of the penicillins is replaced by an oxazolidine ring. In general, clavulanic acid has only weak antibacterial activity. It is a potent progressive inhibitor of plasmid-mediated and some chromosomal beta-lactamases produced by Gram-negative bacteria including *Haemophilus ducreyi*, *H. influenzae*, *Neisseria gonorrhoeae*, *Moraxella catarrhalis* (*Branhamella catarrhalis*), *Bacteroides fragilis*, and some Enterobacteriaceae. It is also an inhibitor of the beta-lactamases produced by *Staphylococcus aureus*. Clavulanic acid can permeate bacterial cell walls and can therefore inactivate both extracellular enzymes and those that are bound to the cell. Its mode of action depends on the particular enzyme inhibited, but it generally acts as a competitive, and often irreversible, inhibitor. Clavulanic acid consequently enhances the activity of penicillin and cephalosporin antibacterials against many resistant strains of bacteria. However, it is generally less effective against chromosomally mediated type 1 beta-lactamases; therefore, many *Citrobacter, Enterobacter, Morganella*, and *Serratia* spp., and *Pseudomonas aeruginosa* remain resistant. Some plasmid-mediated extended-spectrum beta-lactamases in *Klebsiella pneumoniae*, some other Enterobacteriaceae, and *Ps. aeruginosa* are also not inhibited by beta-lactamase inhibitors.

Clavulanic acid is given as potassium clavulanate by mouth and injection in combination with amoxicillin (co-amoxiclav) (p.155), and by injection in combination with ticarcillin (p.270).

Use of clavulanate with penicillins has been associated with the development of cholestatic jaundice and hepatitis (see Amoxicillin, Adverse Effects, p.155) and therefore the use of co-amoxiclav has declined (see below).

◊ Because of the risk of cholestatic jaundice co-amoxiclav is not a treatment of choice for common bacterial infections. The UK Committee on Safety of Medicines[1] recommends that it should be reserved for bacterial infections likely to be caused by amoxicillin-resistant beta-lactamase-producing strains and that treatment should not usually exceed 14 days. It may be considered for the following main indications:

- sinusitis, otitis media, recurrent tonsillitis
- acute exacerbations of chronic bronchitis
- bronchopneumonia
- urinary-tract infections, especially when recurrent or complicated, but not prostatitis
- septic abortion, pelvic or puerperal sepsis, and intra-abdominal sepsis
- cellulitis, animal bites, and severe dental abscess with spreading cellulitis.

1. Committee on Safety of Medicines/Medicines Control Agency. Revised indications for co-amoxiclav (Augmentin). *Current Problems* 1997; **23:** 8. Also available at: http://www.mca.gov.uk/ourwork/monitorsafequalmed/currentproblems/volume24.htm (accessed 25/05/04)

### Preparations

***BP 2003:*** Co-amoxiclav Tablets;
***USP 27:*** Amoxicillin and Clavulanate Potassium for Oral Suspension; Amoxicillin and Clavulanate Potassium Tablets; Ticarcillin and Clavulanic Acid for Injection; Ticarcillin and Clavulanic Acid Injection.

**Proprietary Preparations** (details are given in Part 3)
***Arg.:*** Optamox.

**Multi-ingredient:** ***Arg.:*** Aclav; Amoxigrand Compuesto; Amoxitenk Plus; Bioxilina Plus; Clavulox; Clavulox Duo; Cloximar Duo; Darzitil Plus; Dibional; Fullcilina Plus; Grinsil Clavulanico; Klonalmox; ***Austral.:*** Augmentin; Ausclav; Clamoxyl; Clavulin; Timentin; ***Austria:*** Amoclan; Amoclax; Amoxiplus; Augmentin; Clavamox; Curam; Lanoclav; Xiclav; ***Belg.:*** Augmentin; Clavucid; Timentin; ***Braz.:*** Augmentin†; Clavoxil; Clavulin; Novamox; Timentin; ***Canad.:*** Clavulin; Timentin; ***Chile:*** Ambilan; Ambilan Bid; Amolex; Augmentin; Augmentin Bid; Clavinex; Clavinex Duo; Clavoxilina Bid; ***Denm.:*** Bioclavid; Spektramox; ***Fin.:*** Amoxin Comp; Augmentin; Bioclavid; Clavurion; Spektramox; ***Fr.:*** Augmentin; Ciblor; Claventin; ***Ger.:*** Amoclav; Amoxi-Clavulan; Amoxiclav; Amoxidura Plus; Amoxillat-Clav; Amuclan; Augmentan; Betabactyl†; ***Gr.:*** Augmentin; Bioclavid; Fugentin; Timentin; ***Hong Kong:*** Amoksiklav; Augmentin; Curam; Moxiclav; Timentin; ***India:*** Augmentin; Nuclav; Timentin; ***Irl.:*** Augmentin; Clavamel; Germentin; Pinaclav; Timentin; ***Israel:*** Amoxiclav; Augmentin; Clavamox; Timentin; ***Ital.:*** Augmentin; Clavucar; Clavulin; Neoduplamox; Timentin; ***Malaysia:*** Amoxiclav; Augmentin; Curam; Enhancin; Moxiclav; Vestaclav; ***Mex.:*** Amoxiclav; Augmentin; Clamoxin; Clavulin; Eumetinex†; Servamox CLV; Timentin; ***Neth.:*** Augmentin; Timentin; ***Norw.:*** Bremide; ***NZ:*** Alpha-Amoxyclav†; Augmentin; Synermox; Timentin; ***Port.:*** Amoclavam; Augmentin; Betamox; Clavamox; Clavepen; Penilan; ***S.Afr.:*** Adco-Amoclav; Amoclav; Augmaxil; Augmentin; Bio-Amoksiclav; Clamentin; Clavumox; Moxyclav; Ranclav; ***Singapore:*** Amocla; Augmentin; Clamonex; Curam; Enhancin; Fugentin; Moxiclav; ***Spain:*** Amoclave; Amoxyplus; Ardineclav; Augmentine; Bigpen; Burmicin; Clavepen; Clavucid; Clavumox; Duonasa; Eupeclanic; Inmupen†; Kelsopen; Pangamox†; ***Swed.:*** Spektramox; ***Switz.:*** Augmentin; Aziclav; Clavamox; Co-Amoxi; Timenten; ***Thai.:*** Amoksiklav; Augmentin; Cavumox; Curam; Ranclav; ***UAE:*** Julmentin; ***UK:*** Amiclav; Augmentin; Augmentin-Duo; Timentin; ***USA:*** Augmentin; Timentin.

## Clemizole Penicillin *(BAN, rINN)*

Clemizol penicilina; Clemizole Benzylpenicillin; Penicillin G Clemizole. 1-[1-(4-Chlorobenzyl)benzimidazol-2-ylmethyl]pyrrolidinium (6*R*)-6-(2-phenylacetamido)penicillanate.

$C_{16}H_{18}N_2O_4S,C_{19}H_{20}ClN_3$ = 660.2.
*CAS — 6011-39-8.*

### Profile

Clemizole penicillin is a long-acting preparation of benzylpenicillin (p.163) with similar properties and uses.

### Preparations

**Proprietary Preparations** (details are given in Part 3)
***Chile:*** Prevepen; ***Mex.:*** Megapenil; ***Switz.:*** Megacilline.

**Multi-ingredient:** ***Chile:*** Prevepen Forte; ***Mex.:*** Anapenil; Megapenil Forte; ***Port.:*** Prevecilina; ***Spain:*** Anapen†; Neopenyl.

## Clinafloxacin Hydrochloride *(USAN, rINNM)*

CI-960 (clinafloxacin); Hidrocloruro de clinafloxacino; PD-127391. (±)-7-(3-Amino-1-pyrrolidinyl)-8-chloro-1-cyclopropyl-6-fluoro-1,4-dihydro-4-oxo-3-quinolinecarboxylic acid hydrochloride.

$C_{17}H_{17}ClFN_3O_3,HCl$ = 402.2.
*CAS — 105956-97-6 (clinafloxacin); 105956-99-8 (clinafloxacin hydrochloride).*

### Profile

Clinafloxacin is a fluoroquinolone antibacterial.

◊ References.

1. Solomkin JS, *et al.* Results of a clinical trial of clinafloxacin versus imipenem/cilastatin for intraabdominal infections. *Ann Surg* 2001; **233:** 79–87.
2. Siami G, *et al.* Clinafloxacin versus piperacillin-tazobactam in treatment of patients with severe skin and soft tissue infections. *Antimicrob Agents Chemother* 2001; **45:** 525–31.
3. Winston DJ, *et al.* Randomized, double-blind, multicenter trial comparing clinafloxacin with imipenem as empirical monotherapy for febrile granulocytopenic patients. *Clin Infect Dis* 2001; **32:** 381–90.
4. Petermann W, *et al.* A prospective, randomized, multicenter comparative study of clinafloxacin versus a ceftriaxone-based regimen in the treatment of hospitalized patients with community-acquired pneumonia. *Scand J Infect Dis* 2001; **33:** 832–7.
5. Glauser MP, *et al.* Clinafloxacin monotherapy (CI-960) versus ceftazidime plus amikacin for empirical treatment of febrile neutropenic cancer patients. *Clin Microbiol Infect* 2002; **8:** 14–25.
6. Shah P, *et al.* Open-label, multicentre, emergency-use study of clinafloxacin (CI-960) in the treatment of patients with serious life-threatening infections. *Int J Antimicrob Agents* 2002; **19:** 245–8.

# Clindamycin *(BAN, USAN, rINN)*

U-21251. Methyl 6-amino-7-chloro-6,7,8-trideoxy-*N*-[(2*S*,4*R*)-1-methyl-4-propylprolyl]-1-thio-L-*threo*-D-*galacto*-octopyranoside.

$C_{18}H_{33}ClN_2O_5S$ = 425.0.
*CAS — 18323-44-9.*
*ATC — D10AF01; G01AA10; J01FF01.*

NOTE. The name Clinimycin, which was formerly used for clindamycin, has also been used for a preparation of oxytetracycline.

## Clindamycin Hydrochloride *(BANM, rINNM)*

Chlorodeoxylincomycin Hydrochloride; (7*S*)-Chloro-7-deoxylincomycin Hydrochloride; Clindamycini Hydrochloridum; Hidrocloruro de clindamicina.

$C_{18}H_{33}ClN_2O_5S,HCl$ = 461.4.
*CAS — 21462-39-5 (anhydrous clindamycin hydrochloride); 58207-19-5 (clindamycin hydrochloride monohydrate).*
*ATC — D10AF01; G01AA10; J01FF01.*

**Pharmacopoeias.** In *Chin., Eur.* (see p.vi), *Jpn, Pol.*, and *US.*

**Ph. Eur. 5.0** (Clindamycin Hydrochloride). A white or almost white, crystalline powder. It contains a variable quantity of water. Very soluble in water; slightly soluble in alcohol. A 10% solution in water has a pH of 3.0 to 5.0. Store in airtight containers.

**USP 27** (Clindamycin Hydrochloride). A white or practically white crystalline powder, odourless or has a faint mercaptan-like odour. Freely soluble in water, in dimethylformamide, and in methyl alcohol; soluble in alcohol; practically insoluble in acetone. pH of a 10% solution in water is between 3.0 and 5.5. Store in airtight containers.

## Clindamycin Palmitate Hydrochloride
*(BANM, USAN, rINNM)*

Hidrocloruro del palmitato de clindamicina; U-25179E. Clindamycin 2-palmitate hydrochloride.

$C_{34}H_{63}ClN_2O_6S,HCl$ = 699.9.
*CAS — 36688-78-5 (clindamycin palmitate); 25507-04-4 (clindamycin palmitate hydrochloride).*
*ATC — D10AF01; G01AA10; J01FF01.*

**Pharmacopoeias.** In *US.*

**USP 27** (Clindamycin Palmitate Hydrochloride). A white to off-white amorphous powder having a characteristic odour. Freely soluble in water, in chloroform, in ether, and in benzene; soluble 1 in 3 of alcohol and 1 in 9 of ethyl acetate; very soluble in dimethylformamide. pH of a 1% solution in water is between 2.8 and 3.8. Store in airtight containers.

## Clindamycin Phosphate *(BANM, USAN, rINNM)*

Clindamycini Phosphas; Fosfato de clindamicina; U-28508. Clindamycin 2-(dihydrogen phosphate).

$C_{18}H_{34}ClN_2O_8PS$ = 505.0.
*CAS — 24729-96-2.*
*ATC — D10AF01; G01AA10; J01FF01.*

**Pharmacopoeias.** In *Eur.* (see p.vi), *Int., Jpn*, and *US.*

**Ph. Eur. 5.0** (Clindamycin Phosphate). A white or almost white, slightly hygroscopic powder. It exhibits polymorphism. Freely soluble in water; very slightly soluble in alcohol; practically insoluble in dichloromethane. A 1% solution in water has a pH of 3.5 to 4.5. Store at a temperature not exceeding 30° in airtight containers.

**USP 27** (Clindamycin Phosphate). A white to off-white, odourless or practically odourless, hygroscopic, crystalline powder. Soluble 1 in 2.5 of water; slightly soluble in dehydrated alcohol; very slightly soluble in acetone; practically insoluble in chloroform, in ether, and in benzene. pH of a 1% solution in water is between 3.5 and 4.5. Store in airtight containers.

**Incompatibility.** Solutions of clindamycin salts have an acid pH and incompatibility may reasonably be expected with alkaline preparations, or with drugs unstable at low pH. The UK manufacturers of the injectable solution of clindamycin state that incompatibility has been reported between clindamycin and the following drugs: ampicillin, aminophylline, barbiturates, calcium gluconate, ceftriaxone, idarubicin, magnesium sulfate, phenytoin, and ranitidine.

Clindamycin phosphate is incompatible with natural rubber closures.

## Adverse Effects

Clindamycin is reported to produce diarrhoea in up to 20% of patients after systemic use; in some patients severe antibiotic-associated or pseudomembranous colitis may develop, and has proved fatal. The syndrome, which may develop during therapy or several weeks later, appears to be due to toxins produced by *Clostridium* spp., most notably *C. difficile*. It has been reported to be more frequent in women and in elderly patients, and may also occur rarely after topical use. Other gastrointestinal effects reported with clindamycin include nausea, vomiting, abdominal pain or cramps, and unpleasant or metallic taste after high intravenous doses.

Hypersensitivity reactions, including skin rashes in up to 10% of patents, urticaria, and very rarely anaphylaxis, have occurred. Other adverse effects include transient leucopenia or occasionally agranulocytosis, eosinophilia, thrombocytopenia, erythema multiforme, exfoliative and vesiculobullous dermatitis, polyarthritis, and abnormalities of liver function tests; in some cases overt jaundice and hepatic damage have been reported. Although local irritation is stated to be rare, intramuscular injection has led to sterile abscess, and thrombophlebitis may occur after intravenous use. Some parenteral formulations contain benzyl alcohol which may cause fatal 'gasping syndrome' in neonates (see p.1170).

Topical application may be associated with local irritation and contact dermatitis; sufficient clindamycin may be absorbed to produce systemic effects. Cervicitis, vaginitis, or vulvovaginal irritation has been reported with intravaginal use; a small amount of systemic absorption also occurs.

**Effects on the cardiovascular system.** Cardiac arrest occurred in a 50-year-old woman after rapid injection of 600 mg of undiluted clindamycin phosphate into a central intravenous line. Further injections were given over 30 minutes without cardiovascular complications.[1]

1. Aucoin P, *et al.* Clindamycin-induced cardiac arrest. *South Med J* 1982; **75:** 768.

**Effects on the gastrointestinal tract.** References to antibiotic-associated colitis and the role of clindamycin.

1. Tedesco FJ, *et al.* Clindamycin-associated colitis: a prospective study. *Ann Intern Med* 1974; **81:** 429–33.
2. Robertson MB, *et al.* Incidence of antibiotic-related diarrhoea and pseudomembranous colitis: a prospective study of lincomycin, clindamycin and ampicillin. *Med J Aust* 1977; **1:** 243–6.
3. Committee on Safety of Medicines. Antibiotic induced colitis. *Adverse Reactions Series 17* 1979.
4. Borriello SP, Larson HE. Antibiotic and pseudomembranous colitis. *J Antimicrob Chemother* 1981; **7** (suppl A): 53–62.
5. Milstone EB, *et al.* Pseudomembranous colitis after topical application of clindamycin. *Arch Dermatol* 1981; **117:** 154–5.
6. Parry MF, Rha C-K. Pseudomembranous colitis caused by topical clindamycin phosphate. *Arch Dermatol* 1986; **122:** 583–4.
7. Young GP, *et al.* Antibiotic-associated colitis caused by Clostridium difficile: relapse and risk factors. *Med J Aust* 1986; **144:** 303–6.
8. Meadowcroft AM, *et al.* Clostridium difficile toxin-induced colitis after use of clindamycin phosphate vaginal cream. *Ann Pharmacother* 1998; **32:** 309–11.

**Effects on the lymphatic system.** A report of lymphadenitis associated with clindamycin.[1]

1. Southern PM. Lymphadenitis associated with the administration of clindamycin. *Am J Med* 1997; **103:** 164–5.

**Effects on the skin.** A report of toxic epidermal necrolysis associated with clindamycin.[1]

1. Paquet P, *et al.* Toxic epidermal necrolysis following clindamycin treatment. *Br J Dermatol* 1995; **132:** 665–6.

## Treatment of Adverse Effects

Clindamycin should be withdrawn immediately if significant diarrhoea or colitis occurs. Metronidazole or vancomycin may be used to treat antibiotic-associated pseudomembranous colitis. For further details, see Antibiotic-associated Colitis, p.128.

## Precautions

Clindamycin should not be given to patients hypersensitive to it or to the closely related drug lincomycin. It should be used with caution in patients with gastrointestinal disease, particularly those with a history of colitis. Clindamycin should be withdrawn immediately if significant diarrhoea or colitis occurs. Elderly and female patients may be more likely to experience severe diarrhoea or pseudomembranous colitis. Caution has also been advised in atopic patients. Patients with hepatic or renal impairment may require dosage adjustment. Periodic tests of liver and kidney function and blood counts have been recommended in patients receiving prolonged therapy, and in infants. Caution is required during parenteral use in neonates, since some parenteral formulations contain benzyl alcohol which may cause fatal 'gasping syndrome' (see p.1170).

**AIDS.** Clindamycin was poorly tolerated by patients with AIDS in a study of its use for *prophylaxis* of toxoplasmic encephalitis.[1] Despite the use of relatively low doses of clindamycin (300 mg twice daily), 23 of 52 patients reported adverse effects that necessitated temporary or permanent withdrawal of the drug, the most frequent adverse reactions being diarrhoea and skin rash. The clindamycin arm of the study had to be terminated prematurely. Nevertheless, clindamycin has been used successfully in patients with AIDS for the *treatment* of both toxoplasmic encephalitis (below) and *Pneumocystis carinii* pneumonia (below).

1. Jacobson MA, *et al.* Toxicity of clindamycin as prophylaxis for AIDS-associated toxoplasmic encephalitis. *Lancet* 1992; **339:** 333–4.

**Breast feeding.** No adverse effects have been observed in breast-fed infants whose mothers were receiving clindamycin, and the American Academy of Pediatrics considers[1] that it is therefore usually compatible with breast feeding. The UK manufacturers, however, state that, although it is unlikely that a breast-fed infant could absorb a significant amount of clindamycin from its gastrointestinal tract, caution should be exercised when clindamycin is given during breast feeding.

1. American Academy of Pediatrics. The transfer of drugs and other chemicals into human milk. *Pediatrics* 2001; **108:** 776–89. Correction. *ibid.*; 1029. Also available at: http://aappolicy.aappublications.org/cgi/content/full/pediatrics%3b108/3/776 (accessed 25/05/04)

## Interactions

Clindamycin has neuromuscular blocking activity in high doses and may enhance the effect of other drugs with this action (see Atracurium, p.1400), with a potential danger of respiratory depression. Clindamycin may antagonise the activity of parasympathomimetics. For reports of synergistic and antagonistic antimicrobial activity with other antibacterials, see Antimicrobial Action, below.

**Adsorbents.** In 16 healthy subjects given clindamycin alone and with a kaolin-pectin suspension it was found that the suspension had no effect on the extent of clindamycin absorption but did markedly reduce the absorption rate.[1]

1. Albert KS, *et al.* Pharmacokinetic evaluation of a drug interaction between kaolin-pectin and clindamycin. *J Pharm Sci* 1978; **67:** 1579–82.

## Antimicrobial Action

Clindamycin is a lincosamide antibiotic with a primarily bacteriostatic action against Gram-positive aerobes and a wide range of anaerobic bacteria.

*Mechanism of action.* Lincosamides such as clindamycin bind to the 50S subunit of the bacterial ribosome, similarly to macrolides such as erythromycin (p.209), and inhibit the early stages of protein synthesis. The action of clindamycin is predominantly bacteriostatic, although high concentrations may be slowly bactericidal against sensitive strains.

*Spectrum of activity.* Clindamycin is active against most aerobic Gram-positive bacteria including streptococci, staphylococci, *Bacillus anthracis*, and *Corynebacterium diphtheriae*; enterococci, however, are generally resistant.

Clindamycin has good activity against a wide range of anaerobic bacteria. Susceptible Gram-positive anaerobes include *Eubacterium*, *Propionibacterium*, *Peptococcus*, and *Peptostreptococcus* spp., and many strains of *Clostridium perfringens* and *Cl. tetani*. Among Gram-negative anaerobes susceptible to clindamycin are *Fusobacterium* spp. (although *F. varium* is usually resistant), *Prevotella* spp., and *Bacteroides* spp., including the *B. fragilis* group.

Several *Actinomyces* spp. and *Nocardia asteroides* are reported to be susceptible. *Mycoplasma* spp. are generally resistant.

Most Gram-negative aerobic bacteria, including the Enterobacteriaceae, are resistant to clindamycin; unlike erythromycin, *Neisseria gonorrhoeae*, *N. meningitidis*, and *Haemophilus influenzae* are generally resistant to clindamycin.

Fungi, yeasts, and viruses are also resistant; however, clindamycin has been reported to have some antiprotozoal activity against *Toxoplasma gondii* and *Plasmodium* spp.

*Activity with other antimicrobials.* Synergistic activity has been reported between clindamycin and ceftazidime or metronidazole, and also with ciprofloxacin against some anaerobes. However, there is some evidence that clindamycin inhibits the bactericidal activity of the aminoglycosides, although conflicting reports have suggested variable degrees of synergy against anaerobic organisms. Because of the adjacency of their binding sites on the ribosome, clindamycin may competitively inhibit the effects of macrolides or chloramphenicol. Clindamycin has been reported to diminish the activity of ampicillin *in vitro* against *Staph. aureus*. It is reported to enhance the activity of primaquine against *Pneumocystis carinii*.

*Resistance.* Most Gram-negative aerobes, such as the Enterobacteriaceae, are intrinsically resistant to clindamycin, but acquired resistance also occurs in normally sensitive strains. The mechanisms of resistance are the same as those for erythromycin, namely methylation of the ribosomal binding site, chromosomal mutation of the ribosomal protein, and, in a few staphylococcal isolates, enzymic inactivation by a plasmid-mediated adenyltransferase. Methylation of the ribosome leads to cross-resistance between the lincosamides and macrolides and streptogramins (the $MLS_B$ phenotype); this type of resistance is usually plasmid-mediated and inducible. Complete cross-resistance exists between clindamycin and lincomycin.

The incidence of resistance varies with the organism and the geographical location; it is more frequent in organisms that are also erythromycin-resistant, and some strains of meticillin-resistant *Staphylococcus aureus* are also resistant to clindamycin. In some countries and institutions there is evidence of an increase in resistance amongst the *Bacteroides fragilis* group to 25% of strains or more.

**Action.** References suggesting that clindamycin may reduce microbial adherence and enhance phagocytosis by its effects on bacterial slime (glycocalyx)[1-3] and that its antibacterial effects may be independent of plasma concentrations.[4,5]

1. Veringa EM, *et al.* Enhancement of opsonophagocytosis of Bacteroides spp by clindamycin in subinhibitory concentrations. *J Antimicrob Chemother* 1981; **23:** 577–87.
2. Veringa EM, *et al.* The role of glycocalyx in surface phagocytosis of Bacteroides spp, in the presence and absence of clindamycin. *J Antimicrob Chemother* 1989; **23:** 711–20.
3. Khardori N, *et al.* Effect of subinhibitory concentrations of clindamycin and trospectomycin on the adherence of Staphylococcus epidermidis in an in vitro model of vascular catheter colonization. *J Infect Dis* 1991; **164:** 108–13.
4. Xue IB, *et al.* Variation in postantibiotic effect of clindamycin against clinical isolates of Staphylococcus aureus and implications for dosing of patients with osteomyelitis. *Antimicrob Agents Chemother* 1996; **40:** 1403–7.
5. Klepser ME, *et al.* Bactericidal activity of low-dose clindamycin administered at 8- and 12-hour intervals against Staphylococcus aureus, Streptococcus pneumoniae, and Bacteroides fragilis. *Antimicrob Agents Chemother* 1997; **41:** 630–5.

**Resistance.** Although there is usually cross-resistance between clindamycin and macrolides (above), a resistance pattern has recently been identified that results in streptococcal resistance to macrolides while retaining susceptibility to clindamycin.[1]

1. Sutcliffe J, *et al.* Streptococcus pneumoniae and Streptococcus pyogenes resistant to macrolides but sensitive to clindamycin: a common resistance pattern mediated by an efflux system. *Antimicrob Agents Chemother* 1996; **40:** 1817–24.

## Pharmacokinetics

About 90% of a dose of clindamycin hydrochloride is absorbed from the gastrointestinal tract; concentrations of 2 to 3 micrograms/mL occur within 1 hour after a 150-mg oral dose of clindamycin, with average concentrations of about 700 nanograms/mL after 6 hours. After doses of 300 and 600 mg, peak plasma concentrations of 4 and 8 micrograms/mL, respectively, have been reported. Absorption is not significantly diminished by food in the stomach but the rate of absorption may be reduced. Clindamycin palmitate hydrochloride is rapidly hydrolysed following oral use to provide free clindamycin.

Following parenteral use, the biologically inactive clindamycin phosphate is also hydrolysed to clindamycin. When the equivalent of 300 mg of clindamycin is injected intramuscularly, a mean peak plasma concentration of 6 micrograms/mL is achieved within 3 hours; 600 mg gives a peak concentration of 9 micrograms/mL. In children, peak concentrations may be reached within 1 hour. When the same doses are infused intravenously, peak concentrations of 7 and 10 micrograms/mL are achieved by the end of infusion.

Small amounts of clindamycin may be absorbed after topical application to the skin; bioavailability from topical preparations of the hydrochloride and phosphate (the former in an extemporaneous formulation) has been reported to be about 7.5% and 2% respectively.

About 5% of an intravaginal dose may be absorbed systemically.

Clindamycin is widely distributed in body fluids and tissues, including bone, but it does not reach the CSF in significant concentrations. It diffuses across the placenta into the fetal circulation and has been reported to appear in breast milk. High concentrations occur in bile. It accumulates in leucocytes and macrophages. Over 90% of clindamycin in the circulation is bound to plasma proteins. The half-life is 2 to 3 hours, although this may be prolonged in preterm neonates and in patients with severe renal impairment.

Clindamycin undergoes metabolism, presumably in the liver, to the active *N*-demethyl and sulfoxide metabolites, and also to some inactive metabolites. About 10% of a dose is excreted in the urine as active drug or metabolites and about 4% in the faeces; the remainder is excreted as inactive metabolites. Excretion is slow, and takes place over several days. It is not effectively removed from the blood by dialysis.

**AIDS patients.** Clindamycin was reported to have higher bioavailability, lower plasma clearance, and a lower volume of distribution in patients with AIDS than in healthy volunteers.[1] This may partly be explained by increased binding to plasma proteins.[2]

Although it is generally considered that penetration of clindamycin into the CSF is insignificant, parasiticidal CSF concentrations against *Toxoplasma gondii* were achieved following clindamycin intravenously in patients with AIDS.[3]

1. Gatti G, *et al.* Comparative study of bioavailabilities and pharmacokinetics of clindamycin in healthy volunteers and patients with AIDS. *Antimicrob Agents Chemother* 1993; **37:** 1137–43.
2. Flaherty JF, *et al.* Protein binding of clindamycin in sera of patients with AIDS. *Antimicrob Agents Chemother* 1996; **40:** 1134–8.
3. Gatti G, *et al.* Penetration of clindamycin and its metabolite N-demethylclindamycin into cerebrospinal fluid following intravenous infusion of clindamycin phosphate in patients with AIDS. *Antimicrob Agents Chemother* 1998; **42:** 3014–17.

## Uses and Administration

Clindamycin is a lincosamide antibiotic that is a chlorinated derivative of lincomycin. It is a primarily bacteriostatic antibacterial used chiefly in the treatment of serious anaerobic infections, notably due to *Bacteroides fragilis*, and in some staphylococcal and streptococcal infections. However, because of its potential for causing pseudomembranous colitis (see Adverse Effects, above) it is usually used only when alternative drugs are unsuitable. Amongst the conditions that it may be used to treat are liver abscess, actinomycosis, biliary-tract infections, staphylococcal bone and joint infections, the carrier state of diphtheria, gas gangrene, various gynaecological infections including bacterial vaginosis, endometritis, and pelvic inflammatory disease (the latter two in combination with an aminoglycoside), necrotising fasciitis, secondary peritonitis, streptococcal pharyngitis (usually to treat the carrier state), pneumonia (especially lung abscess), septicaemia, and skin infections involving heavy colonisation with streptococci or anaerobes. It is used in the prophylaxis of endocarditis in penicillin-allergic patients, in the prevention of perinatal streptococcal infections, and in combination with other drugs for the prophylaxis of surgical infection. For details of these bacterial infections and their treatment, see under Choice of Antibacterial, p.120.

Clindamycin is also applied topically in the treatment of acne (p.1133).

Clindamycin has some antiprotozoal actions, and has been used, usually with other antiprotozoals, in various infections (see below) including babesiosis, malaria, and toxoplasmosis; it may also be used with primaquine in the treatment of *Pneumocystis carinii* pneumonia (below).

Clindamycin is given **by mouth** as capsules containing the hydrochloride or as oral liquid preparations containing the palmitate hydrochloride. The capsules should be taken with a glass of water. Doses are expressed in terms of the equivalent amount of clindamycin base. 1.13 g of clindamycin hydrochloride and 1.6 g of clindamycin palmitate hydrochloride are each approximately equivalent to 1 g of clindamycin.

The usual adult dose by mouth is the equivalent of 150 to 300 mg of clindamycin every 6 hours; in severe infections the dose may be increased to 450 mg every 6 hours. Children may be given 3 to 6 mg/kg every 6 hours; those weighing 10 kg or less should receive at least 37.5 mg every 8 hours.

Clindamycin is given **parenterally** as the phosphate by intramuscular injection or by intermittent or continuous intravenous infusion over 10 minutes to 1 hour. Doses are again expressed in terms of the equivalent amount of clindamycin base. 1.2 g of clindamycin phosphate is approximately equivalent to 1 g of clindamycin. For intravenous use, a solution containing the equivalent of 6 mg of clindamycin per mL is used in the UK, although solutions containing up to 18 mg/mL are allowed in the USA; the rate of infusion should be not more than 30 mg/minute. Not more than 1.2 g should be given as a single one-hour infusion, and not more than 600 mg should be given as a single intramuscular injection.

The usual parenteral dose is the equivalent of 0.6 to 2.7 g of clindamycin daily in divided doses; up to 4.8 g daily has been given intravenously in very severe infections. Children over the age of 1 month may be given the equivalent of 15 to 40 mg/kg daily in divided doses; in severe infections they should receive a total dose of not less than 300 mg of clindamycin daily. Neonates have been given 15 to 20 mg/kg daily.

For *prophylaxis* in patients at risk of developing endocarditis and who cannot be given a penicillin, an oral dose of clindamycin 600 mg, given 1 hour before procedures such as dental extractions under local or no anaesthesia, has been suggested. For patients at special risk undergoing dental procedures involving general anaesthesia and who cannot be given a penicillin, a suggested regimen is clindamycin 300 mg given intravenously over at least 10 minutes, at induction or 15 minutes before the procedure, followed 6 hours later by oral or intravenous clindamycin 150 mg.

**Topical** formulations containing clindamycin phosphate equivalent to 1% of clindamycin are used for the treatment of acne. The hydrochloride may be applied similarly, but systemic absorption may be greater (see Pharmacokinetics, above).

Clindamycin phosphate may be given **intravaginally** as pessaries or as a 2% cream for the treatment of bacterial vaginosis; the equivalent of about 100 mg clindamycin is given at night for 3 to 7 days.

**Administration.** A number of studies have suggested that a parenteral regimen of clindamycin 600 mg three times daily is as effective as giving the same dose four times daily,[1] or as giving 900 mg three times daily.[2,3]


1. Buchwald D, *et al.* Effect of hospitalwide change in clindamycin dosing schedule on clinical outcome. *Rev Infect Dis* 1989; **11:** 619–24.
2. Chin A, *et al.* Cost analysis of two clindamycin dosing regimens. *DICP Ann Pharmacother* 1989; **23:** 980–3.
3. Chatwani A, *et al.* Clindamycin dosage scheduling for acute pelvic infection. *Am J Obstet Gynecol* 1990; **163:** 240.


**Babesiosis.** Clindamycin 1.2 g twice daily intravenously or 600 mg three times daily by mouth, for 7 to 10 days, in association with quinine 650 mg three times daily by mouth for 7 days, has been recommended in the USA for the treatment of babesiosis (p.595) caused by *Babesia microti*.[1] Children could be given clindamycin 20 to 40 mg/kg daily and quinine 25 mg/kg daily, both by mouth in 3 divided doses for 7 days.[1] However, WHO had earlier noted that although the combination was reported to be successful in the few patients requiring specific treatment, further confirmation of its effectiveness was required.[2]


1. Medical Letter on Drugs and Therapeutics. Drugs for parasitic infections (issued April 2002). Available at: http://www.medicalletter.com/freedocs/parasitic.pdf (accessed 25/05/04)
2. WHO. *WHO model prescribing information: drugs used in parasitic diseases.* 2nd ed. Geneva: WHO, 1995.


**Malaria.** Clindamycin 900 mg three times daily for 5 days in a regimen with quinine sulfate 650 mg three times daily for 3 to 7 days, both given by mouth, has been suggested in the USA for the treatment[1] of chloroquine-resistant falciparum malaria (p.444). Parenteral clindamycin plus quinine has also been tried in severe falciparum malaria.[2]

When treatment with quinine plus doxycycline would otherwise be indicated for quinine-resistant falciparum malaria clindamycin is a suitable alternative to doxycycline; in children the *British National Formulary* states that a dose of 20 to 40 mg/kg every 8 hours for 5 days may be used.


1. Medical Letter on Drugs and Therapeutics. Drugs for parasitic infections (issued April 2002). Available at: http://www.medicalletter.com/freedocs/parasitic.pdf (accessed 25/05/04)
2. Kremsner PG, *et al.* Quinine plus clindamycin improves chemotherapy of severe malaria in children. *Antimicrob Agents Chemother* 1995; **39:** 1603–5.


**Pneumocystis carinii pneumonia.** Clindamycin may be used with primaquine as an alternative to co-trimoxazole for the **treatment** of *Pneumocystis carinii* pneumonia in patients with AIDS (p.389). A suggested dose[1] is clindamycin 600 mg intravenously, or 300 to 450 mg by mouth, every 6 hours with primaquine 30 mg by mouth daily, for 21 days.

A randomised multicentre study[2] compared the use of a combination of primaquine (30 mg daily) and clindamycin (600 mg three times daily) with co-trimoxazole and with a combination of dapsone and trimethoprim in 181 AIDS patients who had confirmed mild to moderate *Pneumocystis carinii* pneumonia. Primaquine/clindamycin was as effective as the other two regimens, although the authors suggested that the combination might be best avoided in patients with severe myelosuppression.

Clindamycin with primaquine is not normally recommended for **prophylaxis** although there are reports of it being tried.[3] A retrospective examination[4] of the records of patients who had received prophylaxis found that clindamycin with primaquine was less effective than co-trimoxazole or dapsone, although this could have been due in part to underdosing.


1. Medical Letter on Drugs and Therapeutics. Drugs for parasitic infections (issued April 2002). Available at: http://www.medicalletter.com/freedocs/parasitic.pdf (accessed 25/05/04)
2. Safrin S, *et al.* Comparison of three regimens for treatment of mild to moderate Pneumocystis carinii pneumonia in patients with AIDS: a double-blind, randomized trial of oral trimethoprim-sulfamethoxazole, dapsone-trimethoprim, and clindamycin-primaquine. *Ann Intern Med* 1996; **124:** 792–802.
3. Kay R, DuBois RE. Clindamycin/primaquine therapy and secondary prophylaxis against Pneumocystis carinii pneumonia in patients with AIDS. *South Med J* 1990; **83:** 403–4.
4. Barber BA, *et al.* Clindamycin/primaquine as prophylaxis for Pneumocystis carinii pneumonia. *Clin Infect Dis* 1996; **23:** 718–22.


**Rosacea.** Topical clindamycin[1] has improved the inflammatory episodes of rosacea (p.1138), although other features of the skin disorder may not respond.


1. Wilkin JK, DeWitt S. Treatment of rosacea: topical clindamycin versus oral tetracycline. *Int J Dermatol* 1993; **32:** 65–7.


**Toxoplasmosis.** Clindamycin with pyrimethamine has been used for the treatment of toxoplasmosis (p.598) instead of the more usual treatment with pyrimethamine plus sulfadiazine, in patients unable to tolerate sulfonamides. In patients with AIDS and toxoplasmic encephalitis, a suggested dose has been clindamycin 600 mg by mouth every 6 hours for at least 3 weeks, then maintenance therapy with at least 1200 mg daily;[1] patients also received pyrimethamine. Another schedule[2] has been oral clindamycin 600 mg four times daily together with pyrimethamine 75 mg daily for 6 weeks. Other studies found acute therapy with pyrimethamine and clindamycin, 600 mg four times daily by mouth[3] or 1200 mg every 6 hours intravenously,[4] to be as effective as pyrimethamine and sulfadiazine, but maintenance therapy with pyrimethamine and clindamycin 300 mg four times daily by mouth was less effective than pyrimethamine and sulfadiazine at preventing relapses in a population followed for 3 years or more.[3] Clindamycin with fluorouracil produced beneficial responses in a study involving 16 patients.[5]

In contrast, another study, comparing clindamycin alone (in lower doses—300 mg twice daily by mouth) with pyrimethamine alone for prophylaxis of toxoplasmic encephalitis, reported an unacceptably high incidence of adverse effects with clindamycin, which forced premature termination of the clindamycin arm—see AIDS under Precautions, above.


1. Remington JS, Vildé JL. Clindamycin for toxoplasma encephalitis in AIDS. *Lancet* 1991; **338:** 1142–3.
2. Luft BJ, *et al.* Toxoplasmic encephalitis in patients with the acquired immunodeficiency syndrome. *N Engl J Med* 1993; **329:** 995–1000.
3. Katlama C, *et al.* Pyrimethamine-clindamycin vs pyrimethamine-sulphadiazine as acute and long-term therapy for toxoplasmic encephalitis in patients with AIDS. *Clin Infect Dis* 1996; **22:** 268–75.
4. Dannemann B, *et al.* Treatment of toxoplasmic encephalitis in patients with AIDS: a randomized trial comparing pyrimethamine plus clindamycin to pyrimethamine plus sulfadiazine. *Ann Intern Med* 1992; **116:** 33–43.
5. Dhiver C, *et al.* 5-Fluoro-uracil-clindamycin for treatment of cerebral toxoplasmosis. *AIDS* 1993; **7:** 143–4.


## Preparations

**BP 2003:** Clindamycin Capsules; Clindamycin Injection;
**USP 27:** Clindamycin for Injection; Clindamycin Hydrochloride Capsules; Clindamycin Hydrochloride Oral Solution; Clindamycin Injection; Clindamycin Palmitate Hydrochloride for Oral Solution; Clindamycin Phosphate Gel; Clindamycin Phosphate Topical Solution; Clindamycin Phosphate Topical Suspension; Clindamycin Phosphate Vaginal Cream; Clindamycin Phosphate Vaginal Inserts.

**Proprietary Preparations** (details are given in Part 3)
***Arg.:*** Acnestop; Clindacin; Clindopax; Clintopic; Dalacin; Dalacin C; Dalacin ST; Naxoclinda; Torgyn; ***Austral.:*** Cleocin; Clindatech; Dalacin C; Dalacin T; Dalacin V; ***Austria:*** Cleocin; Clindac; Clindal; Dalacin; Lanacine; ***Belg.:*** Dalacin C; Dalacin Topical; Dalacin Vaginal; ***Braz.:*** Clinagel; Clindacne†; Clindamin C; Clindarix; Dalacin C; Dalacin T; Dalacin V; ***Canad.:*** Dalacin C; Dalacin T; Dalacin Vaginal; ***Chile:*** Clidets; Daclin; Dalacin; Dalacin C; Dalacin T; Dalacin V; Dermabel; Divanon; Lexis; ***Denm.:*** Dalacin; ***Fin.:*** Dalacin; ***Fr.:*** Dalacine; Dalacine T; Zindacline; ***Ger.:*** Aclinda; Basocin; Clin-Sanorania; Clinda; Clinda-saar; Clindabeta; Clindahexal; Clindastad; Dentomycin; Sobelin; Turimycin; ***Gr.:*** Arfarel; Botamycin-N; Dalacin C; Dalacin-C; Edason; Lindasol; Sotomycin; Toliken; Upderm; ***Hong Kong:*** Clinac; Dalacin C; Dalacin T; Dalacin V†; Fleminosan; Topicil; ***India:*** Dalacin; Dalcap; ***Irl.:*** Dalacin; Dalacin C; Dalacin T; ***Israel:*** Dalacin C; Dalacin Vaginal; Dalagis T; ***Ital.:*** Cleocin; Dalacin C; Dalacin T; ***Malaysia:*** C-Mycin; Dalacin C; Dalacin T; Tidact; Topicil; ***Mex.:*** Clindazyn; Cutaclin; Dalacin C; Dalacin T; Dalacin V; Damiclin; Galecin; Klyndaken; Lisiken; Trexen; ***Neth.:*** Dalacin C; Dalacin T; Dalacin V; ***Norw.:*** Dalacin; ***NZ:*** Clinac; Dalacin; Dalacin T; Dalacin V†; Topicil; ***Port.:*** Dalacin C; Dalacin T; Dalacin V; ***S.Afr.:*** Clindac†; Clindahexal; Dalacin C; Dalacin T; Dalacin VC; ***Singapore:*** Climadan; Clindatech; Dalacin C; Dalacin T; Tidact; ***Spain:*** Clinwas; Dalacin; ***Swed.:*** Dalacin; ***Switz.:*** Dalacin C; Dalacin T; Dalacin V; ***Thai.:*** Chinacin-T; Dacin-F; Dalacin C; Dalacin T; Klimicin; Klinna; Lacin; ***UK:*** Dalacin; Dalacin C; Dalacin T; Zindaclin; ***USA:*** C/T/S†; Cleocin; Cleocin T; Clinda-Derm†; Clindagel; ClindaMax; Clindets.

**Multi-ingredient:** ***Ger.:*** Copal; ***Mex.:*** Femisan; ***UK:*** Duac Once Daily; ***USA:*** BenzaClin; Duac.

## Clioquinol *(BAN, rINN)*

Chinoform; Chloroiodoquine; Cliochinolum; Clioquinolum; Iodochlorhydroxyquin; Iodochlorhydroxyquinoline; Quiniodochlor. 5-Chloro-7-iodoquinolin-8-ol.

$C_9H_5ClINO$ = 305.5.
*CAS — 130-26-7.*
*ATC — D08AH30; D09AA10; G01AC02; P01AA02; S02AA05.*

**Pharmacopoeias.** In *Chin., Eur.* (see p.vi), and *US.*

**Ph. Eur. 5.0** (Clioquinol). An almost white, light yellow, brownish-yellow, or yellowish-grey powder. Practically insoluble in water; very slightly soluble or slightly soluble in alcohol; sparingly soluble in dichloromethane. Protect from light.

**USP 27** (Clioquinol). A voluminous, spongy, yellowish-white to brownish-yellow powder having a slight characteristic odour. It darkens on exposure to light. Practically insoluble in water; soluble 1 in 3500 of alcohol, 1 in 120 of chloroform, and 1 in 4500 of ether; soluble in hot ethyl acetate and in hot glacial acetic acid. Store in airtight containers. Protect from light.

### Adverse Effects and Precautions

Clioquinol may rarely cause iodism in sensitive patients. Local application of clioquinol in ointments or creams may occasionally cause severe irritation or hypersensitivity and there may be cross-sensitivity with other halogenated hydroxyquinolines.

Clioquinol stains clothing and linen yellow on contact and may stain the skin and discolour fair hair.

Clioquinol given by mouth has been associated with severe neurotoxicity. In Japan, the epidemic development of subacute myelo-opticoneuropathy (SMON) in the 1960s was associated with the ingestion of normal or high doses of clioquinol for prolonged periods, and the sale of clioquinol and related hydroxyquinolines was subsequently banned there. Symptoms of subacute myelo-opticoneuropathy are principally those of peripheral neuropathy, including optic atrophy, and myelopathy. Abdominal pain and diarrhoea often precede neurological symptoms, such as paraesthesias in the legs progressing to paraplegia in some patients, and loss of visual acuity sometimes leading to blindness. A characteristic green pigment, a chelate of clioquinol with iron, is often seen on the tongue and in the urine and faeces. Cerebral disturbances, including confusion and retrograde amnesia, have also been reported. Although many patients improved when clioquinol was withdrawn, others had residual disablement.

It was suggested that the Japanese epidemic might be due to genetic susceptibility, but a few similar cases of subacute myelo-opticoneuropathy associated with clioquinol or related hydroxyquinoline derivatives, such as broxyquinoline or diiodohydroxyquinoline have been reported from several other countries. Oral preparations of clioquinol have now been banned in most countries.

◊ Absorption of clioquinol through the skin has been noted following topical application.[1,2] The Committee on Drugs of the American Academy of Pediatrics[3] considered that there was a potential risk of toxicity to infants and children from clioquinol and diiodohydroxyquinoline applied topically. Since alternative effective preparations are available for dermatitis, the Committee recommended that products containing either of these compounds should not be used.

1. Fischer T, Hartvig P. Skin absorption of 8-hydroxyquinolines. *Lancet* 1977; **i:** 603.
2. Stohs SJ, *et al.* Percutaneous absorption of iodochlorhydroxyquin in humans. *J Invest Dermatol* 1984; **82:** 195–8.
3. Kauffman RE, *et al.* Clioquinol (iodochlorhydroxyquin, Vioform) and iodoquinol (diiodohydroxyquin): blindness and neuropathy. *Pediatrics* 1990; **86:** 797–8.

**Hypersensitivity.** Clioquinol is classified as a contact allergen which can commonly cause sensitisation, especially when applied to eczematous skin; chlorquinaldol can also cause sensitisation, although less frequently.[1] It is important to include clioquinol and chlorquinaldol in routine patch testing since the clinical reaction may be relatively mild and sensitivity easily missed, particularly in the presence of a corticosteroid which suppresses or attenuates the reaction.

1. Anonymous. Skin sensitisers in topical corticosteroids. *Drug Ther Bull* 1986; **24:** 57–9.

## Uses and Administration

Clioquinol is a halogenated hydroxyquinoline with antibacterial and antifungal activity and is used in creams and ointments, usually containing 3%, in the treatment of skin infections. It is applied together with a corticosteroid in inflammatory skin conditions complicated by bacterial or fungal infections. It is also used in ear drops for otitis externa. The treatment of bacterial and of fungal skin infections is described on p.146 and p.390 respectively.

For a discussion of the risks from topical application of clioquinol, see Adverse Effects and Precautions, above.

Clioquinol was formerly given by mouth in the treatment of intestinal amoebiasis. It was also formerly used for the prophylaxis and treatment of traveller's diarrhoea and similar infections but was of doubtful value. Oral preparations have now been withdrawn because of neurotoxicity (see Adverse Effects and Precautions, above). However, clioquinol by mouth is being investigated for its action as a chelator of copper and zinc in the treatment of Alzheimer's disease.

## Preparations

***BP 2003:*** Betamethasone and Clioquinol Cream; Betamethasone and Clioquinol Ointment; Hydrocortisone and Clioquinol Cream; Hydrocortisone and Clioquinol Ointment;
***USP 27:*** Clioquinol and Hydrocortisone Cream; Clioquinol and Hydrocortisone Ointment; Clioquinol Cream; Clioquinol Ointment; Compound Clioquinol Topical Powder.

**Proprietary Preparations** (details are given in Part 3)
***Ger.:*** Linola-sept; ***India:*** Dermoquinol; Entero-Quinol; Entrozyme Plain; ***Irl.:*** Oralcer†; ***Mex.:*** Lasalar-Y Simple; Luzolona Simple; Nolil; Quindoleina†; Vioformo; Yoquin†; ***Port.:*** Quinodermil; ***S.Afr.:*** Bioform†; ***Switz.:*** Vioform†; ***USA:*** Vioform†.

**Multi-ingredient:** ***Arg.:*** Betnovate-C; Locorten Vioformo; Quadriderm; ***Austral.:*** Hydroform; Locacorten Vioform; Quinaband; ***Austria:*** Betnovate-C; Locacorten Vioform; ***Belg.:*** Betnelan-VC; Locacortene Vioformet; ***Braz.:*** Atacoly†; Betnovate-Q; Cremederme; Dreniformio; Hidrocorte; Kaostase†; Locorten Vioformio; Poliderms; Predmicin; Quadriderm; Quadrikin; Quadrilon; Quadriplus; Tetraderm; Vioformio-Hidrocortisona; ***Canad.:*** Locacorten Vioform; Phenoris; Vioform-Hydrocortisone; ***Denm.:*** Betnovat med Chinoform; Celeston med Chinoform; Diproform†; Locacorten Vioform; Synalar med Chinoform; ***Fin.:*** Betnovat-C; Celestoderm cum Chinoform; Locacorten Vioform; ***Fr.:*** DipTosept; Locacortene Vioforme†; ***Ger.:*** Locacorten Vioform; Millicorten-Vioform†; ***Hong Kong:*** Betnovate-C; Quadriderm; Triaformo†; ***India:*** Beclate-C; Betnovate-C; Cortoquinol; Millicorten-Vioform; Polyderm; Quiss; ***Irl.:*** Betnovate-C; Synalar C; Vioform-Hydrocortisone; ***Israel:*** Betnovate-C; Topicorten V; ***Ital.:*** Diproform; Locorten; Locorten Vioformio; Viobeta†; Viocidina†; ***Mex.:*** Cetoquina Y; Clio-Betnovate; Contefur; Cortilona Compuesta; Dealan; Diprosone Y; Ditayod†; Flamin 400†; Flunal; Lasalar-Y; Luzolona Y; Sebryl; Sebryl Plus; Solfurol; Sultroquin; Synalar C; Topsyn-Y; Trilor; Ultracortin; Vioformo-Cort; Yodozona; ***Neth.:*** Celestoform; Locacorten Vioform; ***Norw.:*** Betnovat med Chinoform; Locacorten Vioform†; Synalar med Chinoform; ***NZ:*** Betnovate-C; Locorten Vioform; ***Port.:*** Betnovate-C; Dexaval V; Locorten Vioformio; Quinodermil-AS; ***S.Afr.:*** Betnovate-C; Locacorten Vioform; Quadriderm; Synalar C†; ***Singapore:*** Betnovate-C†; Quadriderm; Synalar C†; ***Spain:*** Antiblef Eczem†; Cuatroderm; Locortene Vioformo†; Menaderm Clio; Menaderm Otologico; Recto Menaderm†; Synobel; ***Swed.:*** Betnovat med Chinoform; Celeston valerat med chinoform; Locacorten Vioform; ***Switz.:*** Betnovate-C; Quadriderm; ***Thai.:*** Banocin; Beta-C; Betnovate-C; Betosone-CE; Chlorotracin; Genquin; Quadriderm†; ***UK:*** Betnovate-C; Locorten Vioform; Oralcer†; Quinaband; Synalar C; Vioform-Hydrocortisone; ***USA:*** I + I-F; Corque; Hysone; Pedi-Cort V†.

# Clofazimine *(BAN, USAN, rINN)*

B-663; Clofazimina; Clofaziminum; G-30320; NSC-141046. 3-(4-Chloroanilino)-10-(4-chlorophenyl)-2,10-dihydro-2-phenazin-2-ylideneisopropylamine.

$C_{27}H_{22}Cl_2N_4$ = 473.4.
*CAS — 2030-63-9.*
*ATC — J04BA01.*

**Pharmacopoeias.** In *Chin., Eur.* (see p.vi), *Int.*, and *US.*

**Ph. Eur. 5.0** (Clofazimine). A fine reddish-brown powder. It exhibits polymorphism. Practically insoluble in water; very slightly soluble in alcohol; soluble in dichloromethane.

**USP 27** (Clofazimine). Dark red crystals. Practically insoluble in water; sparingly soluble in alcohol, in acetone, and in ethyl acetate; soluble in chloroform and in benzene. Store in airtight containers. Protect from light.

## Adverse Effects

Adverse effects to clofazimine are dose-related, the most common being red to brown discoloration of the skin especially on areas exposed to sunlight; leprotic lesions may become mauve to black. These changes are more noticeable in light-skinned people and may limit its acceptance. The conjunctiva and cornea may also show some signs of red to brown pigmentation. The generalised discoloration may take months to years to disappear after stopping therapy with clofazimine. Discoloration of hair, tears, sweat, sputum, breast milk, urine, and faeces may occur, as may nail discoloration with high doses of 300 mg daily. Severe depression related to skin discoloration has been reported rarely.

Gastrointestinal effects are uncommon for doses of clofazimine less than 100 mg daily and usually are not severe. Symptoms of nausea, vomiting, and abdominal pain experienced shortly after the start of treatment may be due to direct irritation of the gastrointestinal tract and such symptoms usually disappear on dose reduction. Use of doses of 300 mg daily or more for several months sometimes produces abdominal pain, diarrhoea, weight loss, gastrointestinal bleeding, and in severe cases the small bowel may become oedematous and symptoms of bowel obstruction may develop. This may be due to deposition of crystals of clofazimine in the wall of the small bowel and in the mesenteric lymph nodes. Crystal deposition may also occur in other organs including the liver and spleen and cause adverse effects. Symptoms usually regress on withdrawal of treatment.

Clofazimine may produce a dryness of the skin and ichthyosis as well as decreased sweat production and rashes. Pruritus, acneiform eruptions, and photosensitivity reactions have also been reported.

Eye irritation and decreased tear production may occur.

Headache, drowsiness, dizziness, taste disorders, and elevation of blood glucose levels have been reported rarely.

**Incidence of adverse effects.** The incidence of adverse effects experienced with clofazimine was reviewed in 65 patients who were receiving, or had received, clofazimine in weekly doses of either 700 mg or less as antimycobacterial therapy, or more than 700 mg as anti-inflammatory therapy.[1] Length of treatment ranged from 1 to 83 months. Adverse effects on the skin included discoloration (20% of patients), pigmentation (64.6%), dry skin (35.4%), and pruritus (5%). Ocular adverse effects experienced were conjunctival pigmentation (49.2% of patients), subjective dimness of vision (12.3%), and dry eyes, burning, and other ocular irritation (24.6%). Gastrointestinal adverse effects included abdominal pain (33.8% of patients), nausea (9.2%), diarrhoea (9.2%), and weight loss, vomiting, or loss of appetite (13.8%). The different dose regimens for antimycobacterial therapy or anti-inflammatory effect had similar incidences of adverse effects. Skin pigmentation in 8 patients disappeared on average 8.5 months after stopping therapy with clofazimine, the maximum time required being one year. Adverse effects of clofazimine were considered to be well tolerated.

In another report covering 540 patients receiving clofazimine 100 mg on alternate days or 300 mg daily, the most common adverse effect was skin pigmentation which occurred in 77.8% of the patients. Ichthyotic changes were reported in 66.7% and pruritus in 20.2%. Gastrointestinal symptoms occurred in 20 patients (about 4%); other effects such as discoloration of sweat, urine, and tears were minor.[2]

1. Moore VJ. A review of side-effects experienced by patients taking clofazimine. *Lepr Rev* 1983; **54:** 327–35.
2. Kumar B, *et al.* More about clofazimine—3 years experience and review of the literature. *Indian J Lepr* 1987; **59:** 63–74.

**Effects on the eyes.** Accumulation of clofazimine crystals in the eye can lead to pigmentation of the cornea and conjunctiva. Degeneration of the retinal pigment epithelium has also been attributed to clofazimine therapy in a patient.[1] Slight repigmentation was observed following withdrawal of clofazimine.

1. Forster DJ, *et al.* Bull's eye retinopathy and clofazimine. *Ann Intern Med* 1992; **116:** 876–7.

**Effects on the heart.** Ventricular tachycardia, thought to be probably torsade de pointes, was reported to be associated with clofazimine.[1]

1. Choudhri SH, *et al.* Clofazimine induced cardiotoxicity—a case report. *Lepr Rev* 1995; **66:** 63–8.

**Splenic infarction.** A case report[1] of splenic infarction associated with clofazimine.

1. McDougall AC, *et al.* Splenic infarction and tissue accumulation of crystals associated with the use of clofazimine (Lamprene; B663) in the treatment of pyoderma gangrenosum. *Br J Dermatol* 1980; **102:** 227–30.

## Precautions

Clofazimine should be used with caution in patients with gastrointestinal symptoms such as abdominal pain and diarrhoea. If gastrointestinal symptoms develop during treatment, the dose should be reduced and, if necessary, the interval between doses increased, or the drug should be discontinued. Daily doses of more than 100 mg should not be used for more than 3 months because of dose-related adverse effects on the gastrointestinal tract; patients receiving doses greater than 100 mg daily should be under medical supervision.

Patients should be warned that clofazimine may cause a reddish-brown discoloration of breast milk, hair, skin, conjunctiva, tears, sputum, sweat, urine, and faeces. Nails may be discoloured at higher doses.

As clofazimine crosses the placental barrier, neonates of women receiving clofazimine may have skin discoloration at birth.

**Breast feeding.** The American Academy of Pediatrics[1] considers that the use of clofazimine by mothers during breast feeding may be of concern, since there is the possibility of transfer of a high percentage of the maternal dose and a possible increase in skin pigmentation in the infant. A small study in 8 women calculated that up to 30% of a maternal dose may be ingested by a breast-fed infant.[2]

1. American Academy of Pediatrics. The transfer of drugs and other chemicals into human milk. *Pediatrics* 2001; **108:** 776–89. Correction. *ibid.*; 1029. Also available at: http://aappolicy.aappublications.org/cgi/content/full/pediatrics%3b108/3/776 (accessed 25/05/04)
2. Venkatesan K, *et al.* Excretion of clofazimine in human milk in leprosy patients. *Lepr Rev* 1997; **68:** 242–6.

**Pregnancy.** Two successful pregnancies in women who received clofazimine throughout pregnancy have been reported[1] but a literature review revealed 3 neonatal deaths in 13 pregnancies, although the deaths could not be directly attributed to clofazimine. However, WHO[2] states that its recommended multiple drug therapy regimens, which may include clofazimine, are safe during pregnancy.

1. Farb H, *et al.* Clofazimine in pregnancy complicated by leprosy. *Obstet Gynecol* 1982; **59:** 122–3.
2. WHO. *Guide to eliminate leprosy as a public health problem.* 1st ed. Geneva: WHO, 2000.

## Interactions

Some preliminary data has suggested that the anti-inflammatory action of clofazimine in Type 2 lepra reactions may be reduced by dapsone, although the manufacturers have stated that these findings have not been confirmed; the antimycobacterial effect was not affected.

In patients receiving high doses of clofazimine and also receiving isoniazid, elevated plasma and urine concentrations of clofazimine have been detected, although skin concentrations were found to be lower.

For a report of the effect of clofazimine on rifampicin absorption, see p.251.

## Antimicrobial Action

Clofazimine is bacteriostatic and weakly bactericidal against *Mycobacterium leprae.* Tissue antimicrobial activity in humans cannot be demonstrated until after about 50 days of therapy. Clofazimine is active *in vitro* against various other species of *Mycobacterium.* Resistance has been reported rarely.

## Pharmacokinetics

Clofazimine is absorbed from the gastrointestinal tract in amounts varying from 45 to 70%. Absorption is greatest when clofazimine is given in microcrystalline formulations and when it is taken immediately after food. The time to steady-state plasma concentrations has not been determined but exceeds 42 days.

Average plasma concentrations in leprosy patients receiving 100 or 300 mg daily are reported as 0.7 micrograms/mL and 1.0 microgram/mL, respectively.

Because of its lipophilic nature, clofazimine is mainly distributed to fatty tissue and reticuloendothelial cells, including macrophages. Clofazimine is distributed to most organs and tissues and into breast milk; it crosses the placenta but not the blood-brain barrier.

The tissue half-life following a single dose has been reported to be about 10 days; that following multiple oral doses has been variously estimated to be between 25 and 90 days. Clofazimine accumulates in the body and is largely excreted unchanged in the faeces, both as unabsorbed drug and via biliary excretion. About 1% of the dose is excreted in 24 hours in the urine as unchanged clofazimine and metabolites. A small amount of clofazimine is also excreted through sebaceous and sweat glands, and in sputum.

◊ References.

1. Holdiness MR. Clinical pharmacokinetics of clofazimine: a review. *Clin Pharmacokinet* 1989; **16:** 74–85.

### Uses and Administration

Clofazimine is an antimycobacterial and is one of the main drugs used in regimens for the treatment of multibacillary leprosy (p.133), although, because of its adverse effect on skin colour, other drugs may be preferred in light-skinned patients. It has anti-inflammatory properties and has been given in chronic Type 2 lepra reactions and in a variety of skin disorders.

Clofazimine is given orally with, or immediately after, food or milk for optimum absorption.

For multibacillary leprosy the most common regimen is that recommended by WHO, in which rifampicin 600 mg and clofazimine 300 mg are both given once a month together with clofazimine 50 mg daily [or 100 mg every other day depending on what preparations are available] and dapsone 100 mg daily; this treatment continues for 12 months. Children aged 10 to 14 years may be given clofazimine 150 mg once a month and 50 mg on alternate days.

Clofazimine 50 mg daily is given with ofloxacin and minocycline in patients unable to take rifampicin. Clofazimine is not usually given in paucibacillary leprosy. However, it may be used with rifampicin instead of dapsone when the latter has caused severe toxicity.

Clofazimine has been used in the treatment of chronic Type 2 lepra reactions, although the effect may not be evident for 4 to 6 weeks. A dose of up to 300 mg daily has been suggested but it should not be given for longer than 3 months. Corticosteroids may be given with clofazimine, and standard antileprosy treatment should be continued. Clofazimine is not used in Type 1 lepra reactions.

### Preparations

***BP 2003:*** Clofazimine Capsules;
***USP 27:*** Clofazimine Capsules.

**Proprietary Preparations** (details are given in Part 3)
***Austral.:*** Lamprene; ***Braz.:*** Neozimina; ***Fr.:*** Lamprene; ***Gr.:*** Lamprene; ***Hong Kong:*** Lamprene; ***India:*** Clofozine; Hansepran; ***Jpn:*** Lampren; ***Malaysia:*** Lamprene; ***Neth.:*** Lampren; ***NZ:*** Lamprene; ***S.Afr.:*** Lamprene; ***Spain:*** Lampren; ***Switz.:*** Lamprene; ***Thai.:*** Lamcoin; ***UK:*** Lamprene†; ***USA:*** Lamprene.

## Clofoctol *(rINN)*

2-(2,4-Dichlorobenzyl)-4-(1,1,3,3-tetramethylbutyl)phenol.
$C_{21}H_{26}Cl_2O$ = 365.3.
*CAS — 37693-01-9.*
*ATC — J01XX03.*

### Profile

Clofoctol has bacteriostatic or bactericidal activity against Gram-positive organisms such as staphylococci and streptococci. It is given in doses of 20 to 40 mg/kg daily rectally in the treatment of respiratory-tract infections.

### Preparations

**Proprietary Preparations** (details are given in Part 3)
***Fr.:*** Octofene; ***Ital.:*** Gramplus; Octofene; ***Port.:*** Octofene.

## Clometocillin Potassium *(rINNM)*

Clometocilina potásica; 3,4-Dichloro-α-methoxybenzylpenicillin Potassium; Penicillin 356 (clometocillin). Potassium (6*R*)-6-[2-(3,4-dichlorophenyl)-2-methoxyacetamido]penicillanate.
$C_{17}H_{17}Cl_2KN_2O_5S$ = 471.4.
*CAS — 1926-49-4 (clometocillin); 15433-28-0 (clometocillin potassium).*
*ATC — J01CE07.*

### Profile

Clometocillin is a penicillin given by mouth as the potassium salt in the treatment of susceptible bacterial infections. Doses are expressed in terms of the base. The usual adult dose is 500 mg two or three times daily.

### Preparations

**Proprietary Preparations** (details are given in Part 3)
***Belg.:*** Rixapen.

## Cloxacillin *(BAN, rINN)*

Cloxacilina. (6*R*)-6-[3-(2-Chlorophenyl)-5-methylisoxazole-4-carboxamido]penicillanic acid.
$C_{19}H_{18}ClN_3O_5S$ = 435.9.
*CAS — 61-72-3.*
*ATC — J01CF02.*

### Cloxacillin Benzathine *(BANM)*

Cloxacilina benzatina. The *N,N'*-dibenzylethylenediamine salt of cloxacillin.
$C_{16}H_{20}N_2,(C_{19}H_{18}ClN_3O_5S)_2$ = 1112.1.
*CAS — 23736-58-5; 32222-55-2.*
*ATC — J01CF02.*

**Pharmacopoeias.** In *US* for veterinary use only. Also in *BP(Vet).*

**BP(Vet) 2003** (Cloxacillin Benzathine). A white or almost white powder. Slightly soluble in water, in alcohol, and in isopropyl alcohol; soluble in chloroform; freely soluble in methyl alcohol. Store at a temperature not exceeding 25° in airtight containers.

**USP 27** (Cloxacillin Benzathine). White or almost white, almost odourless, crystals or crystalline powder. Slightly soluble in water, in alcohol, and in isopropyl alcohol; sparingly soluble in acetone; soluble in chloroform and in methyl alcohol. pH of a 1% suspension in water is between 3.0 and 6.5. Store in airtight containers.

### Cloxacillin Sodium *(BANM, USAN, rINNM)*

BRL-1621; Cloxacilina sódica; Cloxacillinum Natricum; P-25.
$C_{19}H_{17}ClN_3NaO_5S,H_2O$ = 475.9.
*CAS — 642-78-4 (anhydrous cloxacillin sodium); 7081-44-9 (cloxacillin sodium monohydrate).*
*ATC — J01CF02.*

**Pharmacopoeias.** In *Chin., Eur.* (see p.vi), *Int., Jpn, Pol., US,* and *Viet.*

**Ph. Eur. 5.0** (Cloxacillin Sodium). A white or almost white, hygroscopic, crystalline powder. Freely soluble in water and in methyl alcohol; soluble in alcohol. A 10% solution in water has a pH of 5.0 to 7.0. Store at a temperature not exceeding 25° in airtight containers.

**USP 27** (Cloxacillin Sodium). A white, odourless, crystalline powder. Freely soluble in water; soluble in alcohol; slightly soluble in chloroform. pH of a 1% solution in water is between 4.5 and 7.5. Store in airtight containers at a temperature not exceeding 25°.

**Incompatibility.** Cloxacillin sodium has been reported to be incompatible with aminoglycosides and a number of other antimicrobials.

### Adverse Effects and Precautions

As for Flucloxacillin, p.213.

**Effects on the kidneys.** References.

1. García-Ortiz R, *et al.* Cloxacillin-induced acute tubulo interstitial nephritis. *Ann Pharmacother* 1992; **26:** 1241–2.

**Effects on the liver.** References.

1. Enat R, *et al.* Cholestatic jaundice caused by cloxacillin: macrophage inhibition factor test in preventing rechallenge with hepatotoxic drugs. *BMJ* 1980; **280:** 982–3.
2. Konikoff F, *et al.* Cloxacillin-induced cholestatic jaundice. *Am J Gastroenterol* 1986; **81:** 1082–3.
3. Goland S, *et al.* Severe cholestatic hepatitis following cloxacillin treatment. *Postgrad Med J* 1998; **74:** 59–60.

**Sodium content.** Each g of cloxacillin sodium contains about 2.1 mmol of sodium.

### Interactions

As for Benzylpenicillin, p.164.

### Antimicrobial Action

As for Flucloxacillin, p.213.

### Pharmacokinetics

Cloxacillin is incompletely absorbed from the gastrointestinal tract, and absorption is reduced by the presence of food in the stomach. After an oral dose of 500 mg, a peak plasma concentration of 7 to 15 micrograms/mL is attained in fasting subjects in 1 to 2 hours. Absorption is more complete when given by intramuscular injection and peak plasma concentrations of about 15 micrograms/mL have been observed 30 minutes after a dose of 500 mg. Doubling the dose can double the plasma concentration. About 94% of cloxacillin in the circulation is bound to plasma proteins. Cloxacillin has been reported to have a plasma half-life of 0.5 to 1 hour. The half-life is prolonged in neonates.

Cloxacillin crosses the placenta and is distributed into breast milk. There is little diffusion into the CSF except when the meninges are inflamed. Therapeutic concentrations can be achieved in pleural and synovial fluids and in bone.

Cloxacillin is metabolised to a limited extent, and the unchanged drug and metabolites are excreted in the urine by glomerular filtration and renal tubular secretion. About 35% of an oral dose is excreted in the urine and up to 10% in the bile. Cloxacillin is not removed by haemodialysis.

Plasma concentrations are enhanced by probenecid. Reduced concentrations in patients with cystic fibrosis have been attributed to both enhanced tubular secretion and enhanced nonrenal clearance of cloxacillin.

### Uses and Administration

Cloxacillin is an isoxazolyl penicillin used similarly to flucloxacillin (p.214) in the treatment of infections due to staphylococci resistant to benzylpenicillin.

Cloxacillin is given by mouth as the sodium salt and doses are expressed in terms of the equivalent amount of cloxacillin. 1.09 g of cloxacillin sodium is approximately equivalent to 1 g of cloxacillin. It should be given at least 30 minutes before meals as the presence of food in the stomach reduces absorption.

Usual oral doses are 250 to 500 mg four times daily. Children may be given 50 to 100 mg/kg daily in divided doses every 6 hours.

Cloxacillin sodium has also been given by intramuscular or slow intravenous injection or infusion. Other routes of administration have included intra-articular or intrapleural injection, and inhalation.

Cloxacillin may be used with other antibacterials, including ampicillin, to produce a wider spectrum of activity.

Cloxacillin benzathine is used in veterinary medicine.

### Preparations

***USP 27:*** Cloxacillin Sodium Capsules; Cloxacillin Sodium for Oral Solution.

**Proprietary Preparations** (details are given in Part 3)
***Belg.:*** Orbenin†; Penstaphon; ***Canad.:*** Apo-Cloxi; Novo-Cloxin; Nu-Cloxi; Tegopen†; ***Chile:*** Cloxapen; ***Denm.:*** Ekvacillin†; ***Fin.:*** Ekvacillin; Staflocil; ***Fr.:*** Orbenine; ***Gr.:*** Anaclosil; Orbenin; Staphyclox; ***Hong Kong:*** Apo-Cloxi; Cloxil; Lidoxin; Monoclox; Orbenin†; ***India:*** Bioclox; ***Irl.:*** Orbenin†; ***Israel:*** Loxavit; Orbenil; Prostaphlin-A†; ***Malaysia:*** Monoclox; Oxacil; Proxin; ***Neth.:*** Orbenin; ***Norw.:*** Ekvacillin; ***S.Afr.:*** Cloxin; Orbenin; ***Singapore:*** Axocillin; Cloxacap; Lidoxin; Monoclox†; Orbenin†; ***Spain:*** Anaclosil; Orbenin; ***Swed.:*** Ekvacillin; ***Thai.:*** Cloxa; Cloxalin; Cloxam; Cloxanbin; Cloxapan†; Cloxasian; Cloxgen; Cloxil; Cloxillin; Corbin; Greater-Gloxa; K-Cil; Lidoxin; Meiclox; Monoclox†; Orbenin; Serviclox; Socloxin; Syntoclox; Theraclox; Vaclox; ***USA:*** Cloxapen†.

**Multi-ingredient:** ***Hong Kong:*** Ampiclox; APT-Ampicloxa; Pamedox; ***India:*** Adilox; Amclo; Ampilox; Amplus; Ampoxin; Ampoxin-LB; Bicidal Plus; Hipenox; Imox-Clo; Novaclox; Suprimox; ***Irl.:*** Ampiclox; ***Ital.:*** Amplium; ***S.Afr.:*** Ampiclox; Apen; Cloxam; Megamox; Ranclosil; ***Thai.:*** Ampiclox; Polyclox†; Viccillin-S.

## Colistin Sulfate *(pINNM)*

Colistin Sulphate *(BANM)*; Colistini Sulfas; Polymyxin E Sulphate; Sulfato de colistina.
*CAS — 1066-17-7 (colistin); 1264-72-8 (colistin sulfate).*
*ATC — A07AA10; J01XB01.*

**Pharmacopoeias.** In *Chin., Eur.* (see p.vi), *Jpn, Pol.,* and *US.*

**Ph. Eur. 5.0** (Colistin Sulphate). A mixture of the sulfates of polypeptides produced by certain strains of *Bacillus polymyxa* var. *colistinus* or obtained by any other means. A white or almost white, hygroscopic powder. Freely soluble in water; slightly soluble in alcohol; practically insoluble in acetone. A 1% solution in water has a pH of 4.0 to 6.0. Store in airtight containers. Protect from light.

**USP 27** (Colistin Sulfate). The sulfate salt of an antibacterial substance produced by the growth of *Bacillus polymyxa* var. *colistinus*. It has a potency of not less than 500 micrograms of colistin per mg. A white to slightly yellow, odourless, fine powder. Freely soluble in water; insoluble in acetone and in ether; slightly soluble in methyl alcohol. pH of a 1% solution in water is between 4.0 and 7.0. Store in airtight containers.

**Stability.** Colistin base is precipitated from aqueous solution above pH 7.5.

### Colistimethate Sodium (BANM, USAN, rINN)

Colistimetato de sodio; Colistimetato de Sódio; Colistimethatum Natrium; Colistin Sulphomethate Sodium; Colistineméthanesulfonate Sodique; Pentasodium Colistinmethanesulfonate; Sodium Colistimethate; Sodium Colistinmethanesulphonate; W-1929.
*CAS — 30387-39-4 (colistimethate); 8068-28-8 (colistimethate sodium).*
*ATC — A07AA10; J01XB01.*

**Pharmacopoeias.** In *Eur.* (see p.vi), *Jpn, Pol.,* and *US.*
**Ph. Eur. 5.0** (Colistimethate Sodium). It is prepared from colistin by the action of formaldehyde and sodium bisulfite. The potency is not less than 11 500 units/mg, calculated with reference to the dried substance. A white or almost white, hygroscopic powder. Very soluble in water; slightly soluble in alcohol; practically insoluble in acetone. A 1% solution in water has a pH of 6.5 to 8.5. Store in airtight containers. Protect from light.
**USP 27** (Colistimethate Sodium). A white to slightly yellow, odourless, fine powder. It has a potency equivalent to not less than 390 micrograms of colistin per mg. Freely soluble in water; insoluble in acetone and in ether; soluble in methyl alcohol. pH of a 1% solution in water is between 6.5 and 8.5.

**Incompatibility.** Incompatibility has been reported with various drugs including other antibacterials.

## Units

The first International Standard Preparation (1968) for colistin contains 20 500 units/mg of colistin sulfate and the first International Reference Preparation (1966) for colistimethate contains 12 700 units/mg of colistimethate.

## Adverse Effects, Treatment, and Precautions

As for Polymyxin B Sulfate, p.245.

Colistin sulfate is poorly absorbed from the gastrointestinal tract and adverse effects do not normally occur with usual oral doses. Cough and bronchospasm may occur during inhalation. Overgrowth of non-susceptible organisms, particularly *Proteus* spp., may occur after prolonged use. Pain and local irritation are reported to be less troublesome after intramuscular injection of colistimethate sodium than with colistin sulfate or polymyxin B.

Plasma-concentration monitoring during systemic treatment is recommended in neonates, patients with renal impairment, and those with cystic fibrosis. Peak plasma-colistin concentrations of 10 to 15 mg/L (about 125 to 200 units/mL) are recommended.

**Cystic fibrosis.** Colistin sulfate was reported to be associated with a lower rate of severe nephrotoxicity among 19 patients with cystic fibrosis than has been previously reported in other patient populations.[1]

1. Bosso JA, *et al.* Toxicity of colistin in cystic fibrosis patients. *DICP Ann Pharmacother* 1991; **25:** 1168–70.

**Porphyria.** Colistin has been associated with acute attacks of porphyria and is considered unsafe in porphyric patients.

## Interactions

As for Polymyxin B Sulfate, p.245.

## Antimicrobial Action

The antimicrobial spectrum and mode of action of colistin is similar to that of polymyxin B (p.245) but colistin sulfate is slightly, and colistimethate significantly, less active.

## Pharmacokinetics

Colistin sulfate and colistimethate sodium are poorly absorbed from the gastrointestinal tract. They are not absorbed through intact skin. Peak plasma concentrations usually occur 2 to 3 hours after an intramuscular injection of colistimethate sodium. Some colistimethate sodium may be hydrolysed to colistin *in vivo*. The serum half-life of colistimethate sodium is 2 to 3 hours but is prolonged in renal impairment. It may initially be prolonged in neonates but has been reported to fall to 2 to 3 hours after 3 or 4 days. Colistin is reversibly bound to body tissues, but binding does not occur with colistimethate.

Colistimethate is mainly excreted by glomerular filtration as changed and unchanged drug and up to 80% of a parenteral dose may be recovered in the urine within 24 hours. Excretion is more rapid in children than in adults; it is diminished in patients with renal impairment. Colistin diffuses across the placenta but diffusion into the CSF is negligible. It is distributed into breast milk.

**Cystic fibrosis.** References.

1. Reed MD, *et al.* The pharmacokinetics of colistin in patients with cystic fibrosis. *J Clin Pharmacol* 2001; **41:** 645–54.

## Uses and Administration

Colistin is a polymyxin antibacterial that has been used in the treatment of severe Gram-negative infections, especially those due to *Pseudomonas aeruginosa*, although other drugs are usually preferred. Colistimethate sodium is used by inhalation in the management of respiratory infections, especially in patients with cystic fibrosis (p.123). Colistin has been used by mouth as the sulfate for the treatment of gastrointestinal infections and with other drugs for the selective decontamination of the gastrointestinal tract in patients at high risk of endogenous infections (see under Intensive Care, p.132).

The usual dose of colistin sulfate by mouth is 1.5 to 3 million units 3 times daily; children weighing up to 15 kg may be given 0.25 to 0.5 million units 3 times daily, and those weighing 15 to 30 kg may be given 0.75 to 1.5 million units 3 times daily.

Colistin is given parenterally, as colistimethate sodium, by intramuscular injection or slow intravenous injection or infusion. In the UK, usual doses are 1 to 2 million units 3 times daily for adults weighing more than 60 kg; children weighing up to 60 kg may be given 50 000 units/kg daily in 3 divided doses. In the USA, the usual dose is equivalent to colistin base 2.5 to 5 mg/kg daily in 2 to 4 divided doses. Monitoring of plasma concentrations is required in some patients (see Adverse Effects and Precautions, above). Doses and dosage intervals should be adjusted in patients with renal impairment (see below).

Colistimethate sodium may be given by inhalation in respiratory infections as an adjunct to systemic antibacterial therapy. The UK manufacturers recommend that children under 2 years are given 0.5 to 1 million units twice daily by inhalation and adults and children over 2 years are given 1 to 2 million units twice daily, up to a maximum of 2 million units three times daily for frequent recurrent infections.

Colistimethate sodium has also been given by subconjunctival injection and as a bladder instillation. Both colistin sulfate and colistimethate sodium have been applied topically, often with other antibacterials, in the management of ear, eye, and skin infections.

◊ Reviews.

1. Evans ME, *et al.* Polymyxin B sulfate and colistin: old antibiotics for emerging multiresistant Gram-negative bacteria. *Ann Pharmacother* 1999; **33:** 960–7.

**Administration in renal impairment.** Dosage of parenteral colistimethate sodium must be adjusted in renal impairment; both reduction in dose and decreased frequency of dosing may be required.

In the UK, the following intravenous doses have been suggested for adults based on creatinine clearance (CC):

- CC 20 to 72 mL/minute: 1 to 2 million units every 8 hours
- CC 10 to 20 mL/minute: 1 million units every 12 to 18 hours
- CC less than 10 mL/minute: 1 million units every 18 to 24 hours

The US manufacturers have also suggested dosage modifications in renal impairment.

## Preparations

**BP 2003:** Colistimethate Injection; Colistin Tablets;
**USP 27:** Colistimethate for Injection; Colistin and Neomycin Sulfates and Hydrocortisone Acetate Otic Suspension; Colistin Sulfate for Oral Suspension.

**Proprietary Preparations** (details are given in Part 3)
***Arg.:*** Alficetin; ***Austral.:*** Coly-Mycin M; ***Belg.:*** Colimycine†; ***Canad.:*** Coly-Mycin M; ***Denm.:*** Colimycin; ***Fr.:*** Colimycine; ***Ger.:*** Diaront mono; ***India:*** Walamycin; ***Irl.:*** Colomycin; ***Israel:*** Coliracin; ***Ital.:*** Colimicina; ***Neth.:*** Belcomycine; Colimycine; ***Norw.:*** Colimycin; ***NZ:*** Coly-Mycin M; ***Spain:*** Colimicina; ***UK:*** Colomycin; Promixin; ***USA:*** Coly-Mycin M.

**Multi-ingredient:** ***Arg.:*** Anuar; Eubetal Biotic; ***Austria:*** AKZ†; ***Denm.:*** Antibiotic Simplex†; ***Fr.:*** Bacicoline; Colicort†; ***Ger.:*** Ecolicin; ***Ital.:*** Colbiocin; Eubetal Antibiotico; Iducol†; ***Mex.:*** Colfur; ***Neth.:*** Bacicoline-B; ***NZ:*** Coly-Mycin S Otic†; ***Switz.:*** AKZ†; ***USA:*** Coly-Mycin S Otic; Cortisporin-TC.

---

### Co-tetroxazine (BAN)

Tetroxoprima y sulfadiazina.
*CAS — 73173-12-3.*

**Profile**

Co-tetroxazine, a mixture of tetroxoprim and sulfadiazine in the proportion of 2:5, has properties similar to those of co-trimoxazole (below) and is used similarly, mainly in the treatment of infections of the urinary and respiratory tracts, including *Pneumocystis carinii* pneumonia. It is given by mouth in an initial dose of 700 mg (tetroxoprim 200 mg or its equivalent as the embonate and sulfadiazine 500 mg), followed by 350 mg twice daily.

**Preparations**

**Proprietary Preparations** (details are given in Part 3)
***Ger.:*** Sterinor; ***Ital.:*** Oxosint†; Sterinor†.

---

### Co-trifamole (BAN)

CN-3123; Cotrifamol.
*ATC — J01EE04.*

**Profile**

Co-trifamole, a mixture of 5 parts of sulfamoxole and 1 part of trimethoprim, has properties similar to those of co-trimoxazole (below) and has been used similarly.

---

### Co-trimazine (BAN)

Trimetoprima y sulfadiazina.
*CAS — 39474-58-3.*
*ATC — J01EE02.*

**Profile**

Co-trimazine, a mixture of 5 parts of sulfadiazine and 1 part of trimethoprim, has properties similar to those of co-trimoxazole (below) and has been used similarly.

Preparations are available in some countries which contain trimethoprim and sulfadiazine in proportions different to co-trimazine.

**Preparations**

**Proprietary Preparations** (details are given in Part 3)
***Fr.:*** Trimadiaz Antrima†.

---

# Co-trimoxazole (BAN)

Cotrimoxazol.
*CAS — 8064-90-2.*
*ATC — J01EE01.*

**Description.** Co-trimoxazole is defined as a mixture of 5 parts of sulfamethoxazole and 1 part of trimethoprim.

**Stability.** Diluted infusion solutions of co-trimoxazole have a limited stability and eventually form a precipitate: this happens more rapidly at higher concentrations. The manufacturers recommend a dilution of 480 mg in 130 mL, which is usually stable for up to 6 hours, but more concentrated solutions should be used within shorter periods of time, and a dilution of 480 mg in 80 mL should be used within 1 hour. The usual diluent is glucose 5%, although other solutions, including sodium chloride 0.9%, have been stated to be compatible for adequate periods.

## Adverse Effects and Treatment

The adverse effects of co-trimoxazole are those of its components (see Sulfamethoxazole, p.261, and Trimethoprim, p.272). Gastrointestinal disturbances (mainly nausea and vomiting) and skin reactions are the most common adverse effects. There have been occasional deaths, especially in elderly patients, mainly due to blood disorders, hepatic necrosis, or severe skin reactions.

A high incidence of adverse effects has been reported in AIDS patients; desensitisation may sometimes be considered (see Immunocompromised Patients under Precautions, below).

◊ There has been concern over the safety of co-trimoxazole. In 1985, reporting on 85 deaths associated with the use of co-trimoxazole,[1] predominantly due to blood dyscrasias (50 reports) and skin reactions (14 reports), the UK Committee on Safety of Medicines (CSM) found that fatalities showed a marked increase with age: below 40 years, there were 0.25 reported deaths per million prescriptions, but for patients over 65 years of age the number of reported deaths per million prescriptions was more than 15-fold greater. However, at that time the CSM felt that it would be unwise to assume that trimethoprim was substantially less liable than co-trimoxazole to cause fatal adverse reactions.[1] Others suggested[2] that most of the deaths associated with the use of co-trimoxazole were typical of sulfonamide toxicity and that the indications for the use of co-trimoxazole should be reduced; this included the suggestion that it should be contra-indicated in the elderly. The CSM stated that their main message was that the risks of treatment with co-trimoxazole were more apparent in the elderly, but that there was no significant difference between the numbers of reports received for serious adverse reactions to trimethoprim and co-trimoxazole when corrected for prescription volumes.[3] In practice, despite further occasional reports of fatalities in elderly patients,[4] there did not appear to have been a marked reduction in the prescribing of this drug in the UK.[5] A similar warning of increased risk from co-trimoxazole in elderly patients was issued by the Adverse Drug Reactions Advisory Committee in Australia.[6]

More recently, a large population-based follow-up study in the UK[7] indicated that the risks of serious liver, blood, skin, and kidney disorders with either co-trimoxazole, trimethoprim, or cefalexin were small and were similar to those with many other antibacterials. Although in 1995 the CSM did restrict the use of co-trimoxazole on the grounds that its place in therapy had changed[8] (see under Uses and Administration, below), they also noted that co-trimoxazole continued to show a similar pattern of serious suspected adverse reactions to that reported 10 years earlier and that adverse drug reactions with trimethoprim were similar; blood dyscrasias and generalised skin disorders were the most serious reactions in each case and remained predominantly in elderly patients.

1. Committee on Safety of Medicines. Deaths associated with co-trimoxazole, ampicillin and trimethoprim. *Current Problems 15* 1985.
2. Lacey RW, *et al.* Co-trimoxazole toxicity. *BMJ* 1985; **291:** 481.
3. Goldberg A. Co-trimoxazole toxicity. *BMJ* 1985; **291:** 673.
4. Whittington RM. Toxic epidermal necrolysis and co-trimoxazole. *Lancet* 1989; **ii:** 574.
5. Carmichael AJ, Tan CY. Fatal toxic epidermal necrolysis associated with co-trimoxazole. *Lancet* 1989; **ii:** 808–9.
6. Adverse Drug Reactions Advisory Committee. Trimethoprim-sulphamethoxazole warning on elderly. *Aust Adverse Drug React Bull* February 1990.
7. Jick H, Derby LE. Is co-trimoxazole safe? *Lancet* 1995; **345:** 1118–19.
8. Committee on Safety of Medicines. Revised indications for co-trimoxazole (Septrin, Bactrim, various generic preparations). *Current Problems* 1995; **21:** 6.

## Precautions

As for Sulfamethoxazole, p.261 and Trimethoprim, p.272.

Co-trimoxazole should not be given to patients with a history of hypersensitivity to it or to the sulfonamides or trimethoprim. It should be discontinued at the first appearance of skin rash, or if blood disorders develop. It should be avoided in patients with severe hepatic impairment and used with caution in patients with lesser degrees of impairment. Like its components, co-trimoxazole should be used with caution in renal impairment, and dosage adjustment may be necessary; it should not be used in severe renal impairment without monitoring of plasma drug concentrations. An adequate fluid intake should be maintained to reduce the risk of crystalluria, but alkalinisation of the urine, although it increases urinary excretion of the sulfamethoxazole component, decreases urinary trimethoprim excretion. Regular blood counts and urinalyses and renal-function tests should be carried out in patients receiving prolonged treatment with co-trimoxazole. Elderly patients may be more susceptible to adverse effects (see above). Folate supplementation may be necessary in patients predisposed to folate deficiency, such as elderly patients and when high doses of co-trimoxazole are given for a prolonged period. Co-trimoxazole is contra-indicated in patients with megaloblastic anaemia due to folate deficiency.

**Breast feeding.** No adverse effects have been observed in breast-fed infants whose mothers were receiving co-trimoxazole, and the American Academy of Pediatrics considers[1] that it is therefore usually compatible with breast feeding. Studies have shown that significant concentrations of trimethoprim and sulfamethoxazole are present in breast milk following maternal administration;[2,3] however, the calculated dose to the infant was deemed unlikely to lead to clinical effects.

1. American Academy of Pediatrics. The transfer of drugs and other chemicals into human milk. *Pediatrics* 2001; **108:** 776–89. Correction. *ibid.*; 1029. Also available at: http://aappolicy.aappublications.org/cgi/content/full/pediatrics%3b108/3/776 (accessed 26/05/04)
2. Arnauld R, *et al.* Étude du passage de la triméthoprime dans le lait maternel. *Ouest Med* 1972; **25:** 959–64.
3. Miller RD, Salter AJ. The passage of trimethoprim/sulphamethoxazole into breast milk and its significance. *Hell Soc Chemother* 1974; **1:** 687–91.

**G6PD deficiency.** Some have expressed the opinion that co-trimoxazole should be avoided by people with G6PD deficiency.[1]

1. WHO. Glucose-6-phosphate dehydrogenase deficiency. *Bull WHO* 1989; **67:** 601–11.

**Immunocompromised patients.** An extraordinarily high frequency of adverse reactions to co-trimoxazole has been reported in **patients with AIDS** being treated for *Pneumocystis carinii* pneumonia. The comment has been made that, when therapeutic doses of co-trimoxazole are used, hypersensitivity rashes and leucopenia each develop in 30% of patients, compared with less than 5% for each complication in patients without AIDS.[1] Other studies have reported an even higher incidence of toxicity, and the overall incidence of adverse effects, including fever, malaise, and hepatitis, may be 80% or more.[2-4] Adverse reactions also appear to be unusually frequent when prophylactic doses are used.[4] A lower frequency of cutaneous reactions has been reported among African, Haitian, and American black AIDS patients compared with white AIDS patients, suggesting a genetic susceptibility to such reactions.[5]

The occurrence of high serum concentrations of trimethoprim and sulfamethoxazole in patients has been proposed as a contributing factor to the high incidence of adverse effects,[6,7] and it was noted[6] that adverse effects, and in particular myelosuppression, were kept to tolerable levels in a group of patients in whom the **dose** of co-trimoxazole was adjusted to maintain serum-trimethoprim concentrations at 5 to 8 micrograms/mL. In a study in HIV-infected patients given co-trimoxazole for the prophylaxis of *Pneumocystis carinii* pneumonia,[8] gradual initiation of therapy (increased over 2 weeks to the full therapeutic dose) was found to improve the tolerability of co-trimoxazole, when compared with patients initiated on full therapeutic doses. However, others[9] demonstrated no difference in the frequency of adverse effects when the sulfamethoxazole dose was modified.

It was suggested[10] that it was the reactive hydroxylamine **metabolites** of sulfamethoxazole which produced the adverse effects in HIV-infected individuals, but later work by the same authors[11] cast some doubt on this hypothesis.

Some workers have used diphenhydramine alone or with adrenaline to manage hypersensitivity reactions associated with co-trimoxazole therapy, thus allowing continuation of treatment,[12,13] while other workers have tried **desensitisation** to co-trimoxazole in patients with AIDS.[14-19] For mention of desensitisation to sulfonamides in patients with AIDS, see under Sulfamethoxazole, p.261.

An increased incidence of myelosuppression, although not, apparently, of other adverse effects, has been reported in **patients with leukaemia** receiving maintenance chemotherapy.[20,21]

1. Masur H. Treatment of infections and immune defects. In: Fauci AS, moderator. Acquired immunodeficiency syndrome: epidemiologic, clinical, immunologic, and therapeutic considerations. *Ann Intern Med* 1984; **100:** 92–106.
2. Gordin FM, *et al.* Adverse reactions to trimethoprim-sulfamethoxazole in patients with the acquired immunodeficiency syndrome. *Ann Intern Med* 1984; **100:** 495–9.
3. Jaffe HS, *et al.* Complications of co-trimoxazole in treatment of AIDS-associated Pneumocystis carinii pneumonia in homosexual men. *Lancet* 1983; **ii:** 1109–11.
4. Mitsuyasu R, *et al.* Cutaneous reaction to trimethoprim-sulfamethoxazole in patients with AIDS and Kaposi's sarcoma. *N Engl J Med* 1983; **308:** 1535.
5. Colebunders R, *et al.* Cutaneous reactions to trimethoprim-sulfamethoxazole in African patients with the acquired immunodeficiency syndrome. *Ann Intern Med* 1987; **107:** 599–600.
6. Sattler FR, *et al.* Trimethoprim-sulfamethoxazole compared with pentamidine for treatment of Pneumocystis carinii pneumonia in the acquired immunodeficiency syndrome. *Ann Intern Med* 1988; **109:** 280–7.
7. Stevens RC, *et al.* Pharmacokinetics and adverse effects of 20-mg/kg/day trimethoprim and 100-mg/kg/day sulfamethoxazole in healthy adult subjects. *Antimicrob Agents Chemother* 1991; **35:** 1884–90.
8. Para MF, *et al.* Reduced toxicity with gradual initiation of trimethoprim-sulfamethoxazole as primary prophylaxis for Pneumocystis carinii pneumonia: AIDS Clinical Trials Group 268. *J Acquir Immune Defic Syndr* 2000; **24:** 337–43.
9. McLean I, *et al.* Modified trimethoprim-sulphamethoxazole doses in Pneumocystis carinii pneumonia. *Lancet* 1987; **ii:** 857–8.
10. van der Ven AJAM, *et al.* Adverse reactions to co-trimoxazole in HIV infection. *Lancet* 1991; **338:** 431–3.
11. ter Hofstede HJM, *et al.* Drug reactions to cotrimoxazole in HIV infection: possibly not due to the hydroxylamine metabolites of sulphamethoxazole. *Br J Clin Pharmacol* 1999; **47:** 571–3.
12. Gibbons RB, Lindauer JA. Successful treatment of Pneumocystis carinii pneumonia with trimethoprim-sulfamethoxazole in hypersensitive AIDS patients. *JAMA* 1985; **253:** 1259–60.
13. Toma E, Fournier S. Adverse reactions to co-trimoxazole in HIV infection. *Lancet* 1991; **338:** 954.
14. Kreuz W, *et al.* "Treating through" hypersensitivity to co-trimoxazole in children with HIV infection. *Lancet* 1990; **336:** 508–9.
15. Carr A, *et al.* Efficacy and safety of rechallenge with low-dose trimethoprim-sulphamethoxazole in previously hypersensitive HIV-infected patients. *AIDS* 1993; **7:** 65–71.
16. Absar N, *et al.* Desensitization to trimethoprim/sulfamethoxazole in HIV-infected patients. *J Allergy Clin Immunol* 1994; **93:** 1001–5.
17. Cortese LM, *et al.* Trimethoprim/sulfamethoxazole desensitization. *Ann Pharmacother* 1996; **30:** 184–6.
18. Caumes E, *et al.* Efficacy and safety of desensitization with sulfamethoxazole and trimethoprim in 48 previously hypersensitive patients infected with human immunodeficiency virus. *Arch Dermatol* 1997; **133:** 465–9.
19. Demoly P, *et al.* Six-hour trimethoprim-sulfamethoxazole-graded challenge in HIV-infected patients. *J Allergy Clin Immunol* 1998; **102:** 1033–6.
20. Woods WG, *et al.* Myelosuppression associated with co-trimoxazole as a prophylactic antibiotic in the maintenance phase of childhood acute lymphocytic leukemia. *J Pediatr* 1984; **105:** 639–44.
21. Drysdale HC, Jones LF. Co-trimoxazole prophylaxis in leukaemia. *Lancet* 1982; **i:** 448.

**Interference with diagnostic tests.** Co-trimoxazole has been reported[1,2] to cause a small reduction in serum-thyroxine and tri-iodothyronine concentrations, probably due to the sulfonamide component.[2] Although co-trimoxazole had not been shown to be a cause of hypothyroidism (since all concentrations remained within the normal range), tests of thyroid function might need to be interpreted with care in patients on such treatment.

1. Cohen HN, *et al.* Effects on human thyroid function of sulphonamide and trimethoprim combination drugs. *BMJ* 1980; **281:** 646–7.
2. Cohen HN, *et al.* Trimethoprim and thyroid function. *Lancet* 1981; **i:** 676–7.

**Porphyria.** See under Sulfamethoxazole, p.261, and Trimethoprim, p.273.

## Interactions

Any of the drug interactions reported with sulfamethoxazole (p.262) or trimethoprim (p.273) may occur with co-trimoxazole.

**Rifampicin.** For reference to potential interaction between co-trimoxazole and rifampicin, see p.251.

## Antimicrobial Action

The actions and spectrum of activity of co-trimoxazole are essentially those of its components, sulfamethoxazole (p.262) and trimethoprim (p.273).

Because they act at different points of the folate metabolic pathway a potent synergy exists between its components *in vitro* with an increase of up to about 10-fold in antibacterial activity, and a frequently bactericidal action where the components individually are generally bacteriostatic. The optimum effect against most organisms is seen at a ratio of 1 part trimethoprim to 20 of sulfamethoxazole; although co-trimoxazole is formulated as a 1 to 5 ratio, differences in the pharmacokinetics of the two drugs mean that the ratio of the peak concentrations is approximately 1:20. However, it is not clear that the optimum ratio is achieved at all sites and, given that both drugs are present in therapeutic concentrations, the contribution of synergy to the effects of co-trimoxazole *in vivo* is uncertain.

Resistance to co-trimoxazole develops more slowly *in vitro* than to either component alone. Resistance has increased, and although initially slow, a more rapid increase was seen in many countries during the 1980s, occurring in both Gram-positive and Gram-negative organisms. Resistance has occurred notably among Enterobacteriaceae. Resistant strains of *Brucella melitensis*, *Haemophilus influenzae*, streptococci, and *Vibrio cholerae* have been reported rarely. Although resistant organisms are usually resistant to both components of the mixture, strains resistant to either the sulfonamide or trimethoprim, and with a reduced sensitivity to co-trimoxazole, have been reported.

◊ References.

1. Martin JN, *et al.* Emergence of trimethoprim-sulfamethoxazole resistance in the AIDS era. *J Infect Dis* 1999; **180:** 1809–18.
2. Huovinen P. Resistance to trimethoprim-sulfamethoxazole. *Clin Infect Dis* 2001; **32:** 1608–14.

## Pharmacokinetics

As for sulfamethoxazole (p.262) and trimethoprim (p.273). When co-trimoxazole is administered by mouth, plasma concentrations of trimethoprim and sulfamethoxazole are generally around the optimal ratio of 1:20, although they may vary from 1:2 to 1:30 or more. The ratio of the two drugs is usually much lower in the tissues (often around 1:2 to 1:5) since trimethoprim, the more lipophilic drug, penetrates many tissues better than sulfamethoxazole and has a much larger volume of distribution. In urine the ratio may vary from 1:1 to 1:5 depending on the pH.

## Uses and Administration

Co-trimoxazole is a mixture of the sulfonamide, sulfamethoxazole, and the diaminopyrimidine, trimethoprim, in the proportion of 5 parts of sulfamethoxazole to 1 part of trimethoprim. It has been used in a wide variety of infections due to susceptible organisms, particularly those of the urinary, respiratory, and gastrointestinal tracts, although the indications for its use are restricted in the UK (see below). Its main uses now are in *Pneumocystis carinii* pneumonia, toxoplasmosis, and nocardiosis.

Its other uses have included the treatment of acne, biliary-tract infections, brucellosis (generally in combination with other drugs), cat scratch disease, chancroid,

*Burkholderia cepacia* (*Pseudomonas cepacia*) infections in cystic fibrosis, some forms of AIDS-associated diarrhoea such as the protozoal infection isosporiasis, gonorrhoea, granuloma inguinale, listeriosis, melioidosis, mycetoma, otitis media, pertussis, typhoid and paratyphoid fever, and Whipple's disease. It has also been used for the prophylaxis of infections in immunocompromised patients. For details of the bacterial infections listed above and their treatment, see under Choice of Antibacterial, p.120.

Co-trimoxazole is usually given by mouth in an adult dose of 960 mg (trimethoprim 160 mg and sulfamethoxazole 800 mg) twice daily; in severe infections 2.88 g daily in 2 divided doses has been given. Lower doses are given for long-term treatment and in patients with renal impairment (see Administration in Renal Impairment, below).

Doses of co-trimoxazole to be given twice daily to children are: from 6 weeks to 5 months of age, 120 mg; 6 months to 5 years, 240 mg; 6 to 12 years, 480 mg. Alternatively, children may be given a dose of 24 mg/kg twice daily. Co-trimoxazole should not generally be given to infants below 6 weeks of age because of the risk of kernicterus from the sulfonamide component (see Breast Feeding, p.261, and Pregnancy, p.261, under Precautions of Sulfamethoxazole), although it may be used in infants from 4 weeks of age for the treatment or prophylaxis of *Pneumocystis carinii* pneumonia.

Higher doses of co-trimoxazole of up to 120 mg/kg daily given in 2 to 4 divided doses for 14 to 21 days are used in the treatment of *Pneumocystis carinii* pneumonia in adults and children over 4 weeks of age; serum concentrations should be monitored and folate supplementation possibly considered (but see Pneumocystis carinii Pneumonia, below). For prophylaxis in adults with AIDS, the standard dose of co-trimoxazole (960 mg twice daily) may be given, but has been associated with a high incidence of adverse effects (see under Precautions, above). Alternatively the following dose regimens may be used: 960 mg daily (7 days each week); 960 mg daily on alternate days (3 days each week); or 960 mg twice daily on alternate days (3 days each week). Children may be given standard doses (see above) for prophylaxis; doses are given on 3 consecutive days per week or for 7 days per week.

For serious infections, if oral use is not possible, co-trimoxazole may be given initially by intravenous infusion diluted immediately before use in a suitable diluent. The contents of each ampoule containing 480 mg of co-trimoxazole in 5 mL are added to 125 mL of diluent and infused over 60 to 90 minutes, unless fluid restriction is required, in which case only 75 mL of diluent may be used. Dosage is similar to that by mouth.

◊ The current place of co-trimoxazole in therapy was reviewed by the UK Committee on Safety of Medicines in 1995 (see also under Adverse Effects and Treatment, above).[1] As a result they recommended that its use should be limited to: *Pneumocystis carinii* pneumonia, toxoplasmosis, and nocardiosis; urinary-tract infections and acute exacerbations of chronic bronchitis, but only when there is bacteriological evidence of sensitivity to co-trimoxazole and good reason to prefer it to a single antibacterial; and acute otitis media in children, but again only when there is good reason to prefer it.

1. Committee on Safety of Medicines. Revised indications for co-trimoxazole (Septrin, Bactrim, various generic preparations). *Current Problems* 1995; **21:** 6.

**Administration in renal impairment.** Doses of co-trimoxazole, both orally and intravenously, should be reduced in patients with renal impairment. The following recommendations for adults and children over 12 years of age are based on creatinine clearance (CC):

- CC above 30 mL/minute: the standard dose
- CC 15 to 30 mL/minute: half the standard dose
- CC below 15 mL/minute: not recommended.

**Blastocystis infection.** For a mention of the use of co-trimoxazole in the treatment of *Blastocystis hominis* infection, see p.596.

**Cyclosporiasis.** Patients with *Cyclospora* infection (p.596) have responded to treatment with co-trimoxazole.[1-3]

1. Pape JW, *et al.* Cyclospora infection in adults infected with HIV: clinical manifestations, treatment and prophylaxis. *Ann Intern Med* 1994; **121:** 654–7.
2. Hoge CW, *et al.* Placebo-controlled trial of co-trimoxazole for cyclospora infections among travellers and foreign residents in Nepal. *Lancet* 1995; **345:** 691–3. Correction. *ibid.*: 1060.
3. Verdier R-I, *et al.* Trimethoprim-sulfamethoxazole compared with ciprofloxacin for treatment and prophylaxis of Isospora belli and Cyclospora cayetanensis infection in HIV-infected patients: a randomized, controlled trial. *Ann Intern Med* 2000; **132:** 885–8.

**Granulomatous diseases.** Although co-trimoxazole appears to be effective in reducing the incidence of bacterial infection in patients with chronic granulomatous disease,[1-3] a disorder of leucocyte function associated with recurrent life-threatening infection and granuloma formation, its use in systemic vasculitis is much more controversial. There have been a number of reports of benefit from co-trimoxazole in patients with Wegener's granulomatosis (p.1090),[4-7] but even where benefit has been reported relapse appears to be common,[6] and an analysis[8] of the experience of the USA National Institutes of Health in 158 patients, was sceptical of its value: only 1 of 9 patients given 960 mg twice daily by mouth had any prolonged improvement.

Some evidence later emerged that addition of co-trimoxazole to maintenance regimens in patients already in remission reduces the incidence of relapse,[9] although another study suggested that it might actually increase the risk of relapse.[10]

1. Mouy R, *et al.* Incidence, severity, and prevention of infections in chronic granulomatous disease. *J Pediatr* 1989; **114:** 555–60.
2. Margolis DM, *et al.* Trimethoprim-sulfamethoxazole prophylaxis in the management of chronic granulomatous disease. *J Infect Dis* 1990; **162:** 723–6.
3. Gallin JI, Malech HL. Update on chronic granulomatous diseases of childhood: immunotherapy and potential for gene therapy. *JAMA* 1990; **263:** 1533–7.
4. DeRemee RA, *et al.* Wegener's granulomatosis: observations on treatment with antimicrobial agents. *Mayo Clin Proc* 1985; **60:** 27–32.
5. Bowden FJ, Griffiths H. Co-trimoxazole in the treatment of Wegener's granulomatosis. *Med J Aust* 1989; **151:** 303–4.
6. Valeriano-Marcet J, Spiera H. Treatment of Wegener's granulomatosis with sulfamethoxazole-trimethoprim. *Arch Intern Med* 1991; **151:** 1649–52.
7. Ohtake T, *et al.* Generalized Wegener's granulomatosis responding to sulfamethoxazole-trimethoprim monotherapy. *Intern Med* 2001; **40:** 666–70.
8. Hoffman GS, *et al.* Wegener granulomatosis: an analysis of 158 patients. *Ann Intern Med* 1992; **116:** 488–98.
9. Stegeman CA, *et al.* Trimethoprim-sulfamethoxazole (co-trimoxazole) for the prevention of relapses of Wegener's granulomatosis. *N Engl J Med* 1996; **335:** 16–20.
10. de Groot K, *et al.* Therapy for the maintenance of remission in sixty-five patients with generalized Wegener's granulomatosis: methotrexate versus trimethoprim/sulfamethoxazole. *Arthritis Rheum* 1996; **39:** 2052–61.

**Isosporiasis.** For the treatment of isosporiasis (p.597), WHO recommends co-trimoxazole 960 mg four times daily for 10 days by mouth;[1] this regimen followed by 960 mg twice daily for 3 weeks was reported to be initially effective in patients with AIDS suffering from isosporiasis, and produced resolution of diarrhoea within 2 days of beginning treatment, but was associated with a high rate of recurrence.[2] A shorter initial regimen followed by indefinite prophylaxis may be preferable in persons with AIDS; in a small randomised controlled trial, co-trimoxazole 960 mg twice daily for 7 days, followed by 10 weeks' prophylaxis, was effective in HIV-infected patients with isosporiasis.[3]

1. WHO. *WHO model prescribing information: drugs used in parasitic diseases.* Geneva: WHO, 1995.
2. DeHovitz JA, *et al.* Clinical manifestations and therapy of Isospora belli infection in patients with the acquired immunodeficiency syndrome. *N Engl J Med* 1986; **315:** 87–90.
3. Verdier R-I, *et al.* Trimethoprim-sulfamethoxazole compared with ciprofloxacin for treatment and prophylaxis of Isospora belli and Cyclospora cayetanensis infection in HIV-infected patients: a randomized, controlled trial. *Ann Intern Med* 2000; **132:** 885–8.

**Nocardiosis.** Co-trimoxazole is used in the treatment of nocardiosis (p.137). There is no consensus on the optimum dosage; doses of 2.88 to 3.84 g daily in divided doses for up to 3 months have been used.

**Pneumocystis carinii pneumonia.** Co-trimoxazole is the preferred drug for both the treatment and prophylaxis of *Pneumocystis carinii* pneumonia (p.389). A single daily dose of 480 mg on every day each week may be effective and better tolerated for prophylaxis than a daily dose of 960 mg.[1] However, some still prefer the latter dose schedule[2] which is also the one preferred by the CDC in the USA[3] and is a licensed dose for prophylaxis in both the UK and USA. Various studies[1,2,4-8] have shown intermittent dosing is also effective for the prophylaxis of pneumonia and is better tolerated than daily dosing; the dose has usually been 960 mg three times each week on alternate days[1,2,4-7] although 960 mg twice daily three times each week has also been given.[8] The addition of folinic acid has no effect on tolerability and may be associated with a higher rate of therapeutic failure (see HIV Infection and AIDS, p.1431).

1. Ioannidis JPA, *et al.* A meta-analysis of the relative efficacy and toxicity of Pneumocystis carinii prophylactic regimens. *Arch Intern Med* 1996; **156:** 177–88.
2. El-Sadr WM, *et al.* A randomized trial of daily and thrice-weekly trimethoprim-sulfamethoxazole for the prevention of Pneumocystis carinii pneumonia in human immunodeficiency virus-infected persons. *Clin Infect Dis* 1999; **29:** 775–83.
3. Centers for Disease Control and Prevention. Guidelines for preventing opportunistic infections among HIV-infected persons—2002: recommendations of the US Public Health Service and the Infectious Diseases Society of America. *MMWR* 2002; **51** (RR-8): 1–52.
4. Wormser GP, *et al.* Low-dose intermittent trimethoprim-sulfamethoxazole for prevention of Pneumocystis carinii pneumonia in patients with human immunodeficiency virus infection. *Arch Intern Med* 1991; **151:** 688–92.
5. Stein DS, *et al.* Use of low-dose trimethoprim-sulfamethoxazole thrice weekly for primary and secondary prophylaxis of Pneumocystis carinii pneumonia in human immunodeficiency virus-infected patients. *Antimicrob Agents Chemother* 1991; **35:** 1705–9.
6. Ruskin J, LaRiviere M. Low-dose co-trimoxazole for prevention of Pneumocystis carinii pneumonia in human immunodeficiency virus disease. *Lancet* 1991; **337:** 468–71.
7. Bozzette SA, *et al.* The tolerance for zidovudine plus thrice weekly or daily trimethoprim-sulfamethoxazole with and without leucovorin for primary prophylaxis in advanced HIV disease. *Am J Med* 1995; **98:** 177–82.
8. Podzamczer D, *et al.* Intermittent trimethoprim-sulfamethoxazole compared with dapsone-pyrimethamine for the simultaneous primary prophylaxis of Pneumocystis pneumonia and toxoplasmosis in patients infected with HIV. *Ann Intern Med* 1995; **122:** 755–61.

**Toxoplasmosis.** There is some evidence that administration of co-trimoxazole for prophylaxis of *Pneumocystis carinii* pneumonia produces an additional benefit in acting prophylactically against toxoplasmic encephalitis in persons with HIV infection or AIDS,[1-5] but the evidence (as for other drugs) has been largely anecdotal or from small retrospective studies. In the USA, the CDC recommends[1] that co-trimoxazole 960 mg daily (as for *Pneumocystis carinii* pneumonia prophylaxis, above) be given to HIV-infected patients who are seropositive for *Toxoplasma* and have a CD4+ count below 100 cells/microlitre.

Co-trimoxazole has also produced promising results in preliminary studies for the treatment of toxoplasmic encephalitis in patients with AIDS.[6]

For a discussion of toxoplasmosis and its management, see p.598.

1. Centers for Disease Control and Prevention. Guidelines for preventing opportunistic infections among HIV-infected persons—2002: recommendations of the US Public Health Service and the Infectious Diseases Society of America. *MMWR* 2002; **51** (RR-8): 1–52.
2. Zangerle R, Allerberger F. Effect of prophylaxis against Pneumocystis carinii on toxoplasma encephalitis. *Lancet* 1991; **337:** 1232.
3. Carr A, *et al.* Low-dose trimethoprim-sulfamethoxazole prophylaxis for toxoplasmic encephalitis in patients with AIDS. *Ann Intern Med* 1992; **117:** 106–11.
4. Beaman MH, *et al.* Prophylaxis for toxoplasmosis in AIDS. *Ann Intern Med* 1992: **117:** 163–4.
5. Podzamczer D, *et al.* Intermittent trimethoprim-sulfamethoxazole compared with dapsone-pyrimethamine for the simultaneous primary prophylaxis of pneumocystis pneumonia and toxoplasmosis in patients infected with HIV. *Ann Intern Med* 1995; **122:** 755–61.
6. Torre D, *et al.* Randomized trial of trimethoprim-sulfamethoxazole versus pyrimethamine-sulfadiazine for therapy of toxoplasmic encephalitis in patients with AIDS. *Antimicrob Agents Chemother* 1998; **42:** 1346–9.

## Preparations

***BP 2003:*** Co-trimoxazole Intravenous Infusion; Co-trimoxazole Oral Suspension; Co-trimoxazole Tablets; Dispersible Co-trimoxazole Tablets; Paediatric Co-trimoxazole Oral Suspension; Paediatric Co-trimoxazole Tablets;
***USP 27:*** Sulfamethoxazole and Trimethoprim Injection; Sulfamethoxazole and Trimethoprim Oral Suspension; Sulfamethoxazole and Trimethoprim Tablets.

**Proprietary Preparations** (details are given in Part 3)
***Arg.:*** Adrenol; Bacticel; Bactrim; Cotrizol-G; Danferane; Diocla; Netocur; Novidrine; Sulfagrand; Tritenk; ***Austral.:*** Bactrim; Cosig; Resprim; Septrin; Trimoxazole; ***Austria:*** Bactrim; Cotribene; Cotristad; Eusaprim; Oecotrim; Supracombin; Trimetho comp; ***Belg.:*** Bactrim; Eusaprim; Steroprim; ***Braz.:*** Assepium; Bac Septin†; Bac-Sulfitrin; Bacfar; Bacgen†; Bacprotin; Bacris; Bacteracin; Bactox†; Bactren†; Bactricin†; Bactrim; Bactrisan; Bactrizol; Bactropin; Baklinger†; Balsandin†; Baxapril†; Becaltrin†; Belfactrin†; Benectrin; Binoctrin; Dientrin; Duoctrin; Ectrin; Enterone†; Espectrin; Gamactrin; Ibtrim†; Imuneprim; Infecteracin†; Infectrin; Katrim†; Leotrim†; Linurin; Lupectrim; Metoprin; Neotrin; Pulkrin; Qiftrin; Quimio-Ped; Roytrin; Sedactrim†; Selectrim†; Septiolan; Septoprin†; Silpin†; Sulf+Trim†; Sulfa+Trim†; Suss†; Teutrin; Trimexazol; ***Canad.:*** Apo-Sulfatrim; Bactrim†; Novo-Trimel; Nu-Cotrimox; Roubac†; Septra; ***Chile:*** Bacterol; Bactrimel; Introcin; Septrin; Trelibec; ***Denm.:*** Bactrim†; Sulfotrim; ***Fin.:*** Cotrim; ***Fr.:*** Bactrim; Cotrimazol†; Eusaprim; ***Ger.:*** Bactoreduct; Bactrim†; Berlocid; Co-trim-Tablinen†; Cotrim; Cotrim-Diolan; Cotrimhexal; Cotrimox-Wolff; Cotrimstada; Drylin; Eusaprim; Jenamoxazol†; Kepinol; Linaris†; Microtrim; Sigaprim; Supracombin; TMS; ***Gr.:*** Bactrimel; Bioprim; Septrin; ***Hong Kong:*** Apo-Sulfatrim†; Bacin†; BS†; Chemitrim; Chemoprim; Dhatrin; Letus; Septrin; ***India:*** Bactrim; Ciplin; Colizole; Oriprim; Sepmax; Septran; Trisulfose; ***Irl.:*** Bactrim†; Cotrimel†; Duobact; Septrin; Tricomox†; ***Israel:*** Diseptyl; Resprim; Septrin; Sulfatrim; ***Ital.:*** Abacin; Bacterial†; Bactrim; Chemitrim; Eusaprim; Gantrim; Isotrim†; Medixin†; Strepto-Plus†; ***Malaysia:*** Bacin; Baserin; Chemix; Cotrim; Resprim; Trimexazole; Virin; ***Mex.:*** Andoprim; Anitrim; Bacpiryl; Bactelan; Bactide; Bactilen; Bactiver; Bactrim; Bactropin; Bateral; Batrizol; Bioprim; Dertrin; Dibaprim; Ectaprim; Enterobacticel†; Esteprim; Fectri; Isobac†; Kaltrim; Lidaprim†; Maxtrim; Metoxiprim; Microbactim; Octiban; Pisatrina; Polibatrin; Protaxol; Septrin; Servitrim; Sulfawal; Sulfoid Trimetho; Sulfort†; Sulprim; Sultiprim; Supristol†; Syraprim; Thriazol; Tribakin; Trim-Vit†; Trimesul†; Trimesuxol†; Trimetoger; Trimetox; Trimexazol; Trimexole; Trimzol†; Trinelax†; Trisufin; Zaprin†; ***Neth.:*** Bactrimel; Eusaprim; Trimoxol; ***Norw.:*** Bactrim; Trimetoprim-Sulfa; ***NZ:*** Apo-Sulfatrim; Bactrim†; Trimel†; Trisul; ***Port.:*** Bactrim; Cotrim; Metomide; Septrin; ***S.Afr.:*** Acuco†; Arcanaprim†; Bactrim; Bencole; Cocydal†; Cozole; Doctrim†; Durobac; Dynazole†; Fabubac; Lagatrim; Mezenol; Purbac; Septran; Spectrim; Tri-Co†; Trimethox; Trimoks†; Trimzol†; Ultrasept†; Xerazole; Xeroprim; ***Singapore:*** Apo-Sulfatrim; Bacin; Bactrim†; BS; Chemix; Chemoprim; Dhatrin; Septrin; Suprim; Trimezole; ***Spain:*** Abactrim†; Bactifor†; Bridotrim†; Broncomega; Brongenit†; Eduprim; Gobens Trim; Momentol; Salvatrim†; Septrin; Toose†; ***Swed.:*** Bactrim; Eusaprim; ***Switz.:*** Agoprim; Bactrim; Cotrim; Escoprim; Eusaprim†; Groprim; Helveprim†; Imexim†; Lagatrim; Mediprim; Nopil; Sigaprim; Supracombin; ***Thai.:*** Actin; Bacin; Bacta; Bactrim; Baczole; Chemoprim; Co-Tasian; Co-Trimed; Conprim; Cotamox; Ko-Cap; Ko-Kure; Lastrim; Le-

tus; M-Trim; Med-Sultrim; Mega-Prim; Metrim; Metxaprim; Mycosamthong; Po-Trim; Pulvicin; Septrin; Servitrim†; Sulbacta; Sulfometh; Tampo; Toprim; Trimexazole; Trimox†; Trimoxzol†; Triprim; Trixzol; Zoleprim; **UAE:** Trimol; **UK:** Chemotrim†; Fectrim; Laratrim†; Septrin; **USA:** Bactrim; Cotrim; Septra; SMZ-TMP; Sulfatrim.

**Multi-ingredient: Arg.:** Bacti-Uril; Bactrim Balsamico; Dosulfin Bronquial; Dosulfin Fuerte; Enterobacticel; Netocur Balsamico; Neumobacticel; Urisept NF; Uro-Bactrim; **Braz.:** Assepium Balsamico; Bac Septin Balsamico†; Bacfar Balsamico†; Bacgen Balsamico†; Bacteracin Balsamico†; Bactox Balsamico†; Bactrex†; Bactricin Balsamico†; Bactrisan Balsamico†; Bactropin Balsamico†; Balsiprin†; Benectrin Balsamico; Diazol; Dispeptrin†; Diteutrin†; Duoctrin Balsamico†; Duoctrin Enterico†; Ectrin Balsamico; Entercal†; Entero Heractrin†; Heractrin†; Infectrin Balsamico†; Katrim Balsamico†; Lupectrim Balsamico†; Metoprin Balsamico†; Mictrex†; Neotrin Balsamico†; Quimio-Ped Balsamico†; Sedactrim Balsamico†; Septiolan Balsamico†; Sulfatrex†; Suss Balsamico†; Teutrin Balsamico†; Trimetoprim Balsamico†; Trimexazol Balsamico†; Trizol Balsamico†; Urizal†; Uro Bac Septin†; Uro Bactrim†; Uro Batrox†; Uro Duoctrim†; Uro Heractrim†; Uro Septoprin†; Uro-Bacteracin†; Uro-Baxapril; Uro-Leotrim†; Uro-Septiolan†; Uro-Teutrim†; Urobactrex†; Urobioctrin†; Uroctrin; Urofar†; Uroneotrim†; Uropol; Uroxazol†; Utrim†; **Chile:** Entero Micinovo; Uro-Micinovo; **Mex.:** Bactrim Compositum; Octex; Trimexole Compositum; **Spain:** Bactopumon; Balsoprim; Bronco Aseptilex Fuerte; Bronco Bactifor†; Bronco Sergot†; Broncorema†; Broncovir; Bronquicisteina; Bronquidiazina CR; Bronquimar; Bronquimucil; Bronquium†; Cotrazol; Eduprim Mucolitico; Lotusix†; Mucorama TS†; Neumopectolina; Pulmo Menal; Pulmosterin Duo; Tosdetan†; Traquivan†; Tresium†.

## Cycloserine *(BAN, rINN)*

Cicloserina; D-Cycloserin; Cycloserinum; SC-49088. (+)-(*R*)-4-Aminoisoxazolidin-3-one.

$C_3H_6N_2O_2$ = 102.1.

*CAS — 68-41-7.*

*ATC — J04AB01.*

**Description.** Cycloserine is an antimicrobial substance produced by the growth of certain strains of *Streptomyces orchidaceus* or *S. garyphalus*, or obtained by synthesis.

**Pharmacopoeias.** In *Jpn* and *US.*

**USP 27** (Cycloserine). A white to pale yellow, crystalline powder, odourless or has a faint odour. It is hygroscopic and deteriorates upon absorbing water. Freely soluble in water. pH of a 10% solution in water is between 5.5 and 6.5. Store in airtight containers.

### Adverse Effects and Treatment

The most frequent adverse effects with cycloserine involve the CNS and include anxiety, confusion, disorientation, depression, psychoses possibly with suicidal tendencies, aggression, irritability, and paranoia. Vertigo, headache, drowsiness, speech difficulties, tremor, paresis, hyperreflexia, dysarthria, paraesthesia, coma, and convulsions may also occur. Neurological reactions are dose related and may be reduced by keeping plasma concentrations below 30 micrograms/mL. It has been reported that up to 30% of patients have experienced adverse effects. These reactions usually subside when cycloserine is discontinued or the dosage is reduced. Pyridoxine has been used in an attempt to treat or prevent neurological reactions but its value is unproven.

Hypersensitivity reactions including skin reactions and photosensitivity occur rarely. Serum aminotransferase values may be raised, especially in patients with a history of liver disease. Folate and vitamin $B_{12}$ deficiency, megaloblastic anaemia, and sideroblastic anaemia have been reported occasionally when cycloserine has been used with other antituberculous drugs. Heart failure has occurred in patients receiving daily doses of 1 g or more.

### Precautions

Cycloserine is contra-indicated in patients with epilepsy, depression, psychosis, severe anxiety, severe renal impairment, or in those who misuse alcohol. Cycloserine should be discontinued, or the dose reduced, if skin reactions or symptoms of CNS toxicity develop.

Cycloserine has a low therapeutic index, and dosage should be adjusted according to plasma concentrations, which should be monitored at least weekly in patients with renal impairment, in those taking doses greater than 500 mg daily, and in patients showing signs of neurotoxicity. Plasma concentrations should be maintained below 30 micrograms/mL. Haematological, renal, and hepatic function should be monitored. Patients with mild to moderate renal impairment require lower doses.

**Breast feeding.** No adverse effects have been observed in breast-fed infants whose mothers were receiving cycloserine,[1] and the American Academy of Pediatrics considers[2] that it is therefore usually compatible with breast feeding.


1. Morton RF, *et al.* Studies on the absorption, diffusion, and excretion of cycloserine. *Antibiot Annu* 1955-56; **3:** 169–72.
2. American Academy of Pediatrics. The transfer of drugs and other chemicals into human milk. *Pediatrics* 2001; **108:** 776–89. Correction. *ibid.*; 1029. Also available at: http://aappolicy.aappublications.org/cgi/content/full/pediatrics%3b108/3/776 (accessed 26/05/04)


**Porphyria.** Cycloserine has been associated with acute attacks of porphyria and is considered unsafe in porphyric patients.

### Interactions

Patients receiving cycloserine with alcohol are at increased risk of convulsions and for a mention of increased blood-alcohol concentrations in patients receiving cycloserine, see p.1167.

Neurotoxic effects may be potentiated by use of cycloserine with ethionamide, and increased CNS toxicity, such as dizziness and drowsiness, may occur in patients receiving cycloserine and isoniazid.

### Antimicrobial Action

Cycloserine interferes with bacterial cell wall synthesis by competing with D-alanine for incorporation into the cell wall. It has variable activity against Gram-positive and Gram-negative bacteria including *Escherichia coli* and *Staphylococcus aureus*.

Cycloserine is active against *Mycobacterium tuberculosis* and some other mycobacteria. Resistance develops if cycloserine is used alone.

### Pharmacokinetics

Cycloserine is readily and almost completely absorbed from the gastrointestinal tract. Peak plasma concentrations of 10 micrograms/mL have been obtained 3 to 4 hours after a dose of 250 mg, rising to 20 to 30 micrograms/mL on repeating the dose every 12 hours. The plasma half-life is about 10 hours and is prolonged in patients with renal impairment.

Cycloserine is widely distributed into body tissues and fluids, including the CSF and breast milk. It crosses the placenta producing fetal blood concentrations approaching those in maternal serum.

Cycloserine is excreted largely unchanged by glomerular filtration. About 50% of a single 250-mg dose is excreted unchanged in the urine within 12 hours and about 70% is excreted within 72 hours. As negligible amounts of cycloserine appear in the faeces, it is assumed that the remainder of a dose is metabolised to unidentified metabolites. It is removed by haemodialysis.

**Pregnancy and breast feeding.** Cycloserine has been shown to pass to the fetus, amniotic fluid,[1] and into breast milk.[2] Concentrations in breast milk after 250 mg four times daily have been reported to range from 6 to 19 micrograms/mL.[2]


1. Holdiness MR. Transplacental pharmacokinetics of the antituberculosis drugs. *Clin Pharmacokinet* 1987; **13:** 125–9.
2. Morton RF, *et al.* Studies on the absorption, diffusion, and excretion of cycloserine. *Antibiot Annu* 1955-56; **3:** 169–72.


### Uses and Administration

Cycloserine is a second-line antimycobacterial that may be used in the treatment of tuberculosis (p.150) as part of a multidrug regimen when resistance to, or toxicity from, primary drugs has developed. It has been used in urinary-tract infections, although less toxic drugs are preferred.

The usual adult dose in tuberculosis is 250 mg twice daily by mouth for 2 weeks, followed by 0.5 to 1 g daily in divided doses. Experience in children is limited; an initial paediatric dose of 10 mg/kg daily has been suggested. Dosage in patients with mild to moderate renal impairment should be reduced and doses for all patients should be adjusted by monitoring plasma concentrations (see Precautions, above).

Cycloserine is under investigation for the adjunctive treatment of schizophrenia. L-Cycloserine has been investigated for the treatment of Gaucher disease (p.1649).

### Preparations

*USP 27:* Cycloserine Capsules.

**Proprietary Preparations** (details are given in Part 3)
**Austral.:** Closina; **Canad.:** Seromycin†; **Hong Kong:** Seromycin; **India:** Cyclorine; **UK:** Cycloserine; **USA:** Seromycin.

## Danofloxacin Mesilate *(BANM, rINNM)*

CP-76136 (danofloxacin); CP-76136-27 (danofloxacin mesilate); Danofloxacin Mesylate *(USAN)*; Mesilato de danofloxacino. 1-Cyclopropyl-6-fluoro-1,4-dihydro-7-[(1*S*,4*S*)-5-methyl-2,5-diazabicyclo[2.2.1]hept-2-yl]-4-oxo-3-quinolinecarboxylic acid monomethanesulphonate.

$C_{19}H_{20}FN_3O_3,CH_4O_3S$ = 453.5.

*CAS — 112398-08-0 (danofloxacin); 119478-55-6 (danofloxacin mesilate).*

### Profile

Danofloxacin is a fluoroquinolone antibacterial used as the mesilate in veterinary medicine.

## Dapsone *(BAN, USAN, rINN)*

DADPS; Dapsona; Dapsonum; DDS; Diaminodiphenylsulfone; Diaphenylsulfone; Disulone; NSC-6091; 4,4′-Sulfonylbis-benzenamine; Sulphonyldianiline. Bis(4-aminophenyl) sulphone.

$C_{12}H_{12}N_2O_2S$ = 248.3.

*CAS — 80-08-0.*

*ATC — J04BA02.*

**Pharmacopoeias.** In *Chin., Eur.* (see p.vi), *Int., US,* and *Viet.*

**Ph. Eur. 5.0** (Dapsone). A white or slightly yellowish-white, crystalline powder. Very slightly soluble in water; sparingly soluble in alcohol; freely soluble in acetone. It dissolves freely in dilute mineral acids. Protect from light.

**USP 27** (Dapsone). A white or creamy-white, odourless crystalline powder. Very slightly soluble in water, freely soluble in alcohol; soluble in acetone and in dilute mineral acids. Protect from light.

**Stability.** A study[1] of the stability of two extemporaneous oral suspensions of dapsone prepared from commercially available tablets found them to be stable for 3 months when stored at 4° and at 25°.


1. Nahata MC, *et al.* Stability of dapsone in two oral liquid dosage forms. *Ann Pharmacother* 2000; **34:** 848–50.


### Adverse Effects

Varying degrees of dose-related haemolysis and methaemoglobinaemia are the most frequently reported adverse effects of dapsone, and occur in most patients given more than 200 mg daily; doses of up to 100 mg daily do not cause significant haemolysis, but patients with G6PD deficiency are affected by doses above about 50 mg daily.

Although agranulocytosis has been reported rarely with dapsone when used alone, reports have been more common when it has been used with other drugs in the prophylaxis of malaria.

Rash and pruritus may develop. Serious cutaneous hypersensitivity reactions occur rarely and include maculopapular rash, exfoliative dermatitis, toxic epidermal necrolysis, and Stevens-Johnson syndrome. Fixed drug eruptions have occurred.

A 'dapsone syndrome' may occur and resembles mononucleosis in its presentation (see Hypersensitivity Reactions, below).

Peripheral neuropathy with motor loss has been reported in patients on dapsone for dermatological conditions. Peripheral neuropathy may occur as part of leprosy reaction states and is not an indication to discontinue dapsone.

Other adverse effects occur infrequently and include nausea, vomiting, anorexia, headache, hepatitis, insomnia, psychosis, and tachycardia.

**Carcinogenicity.** A survey of 1678 leprosy patients admitted for treatment to the National Hansen's Disease Center in the USA between 1939 and 1977 indicated that, although dapsone has been implicated as a carcinogen in *animals*, the use of dapsone did not appear to affect significantly the risk of cancer in these patients.[1]


1. Brinton LA, *et al.* Cancer mortality among patients with Hansen's disease. *J Natl Cancer Inst* 1984; **72:** 109–14.


**Effects on the blood.** *Haemolysis* is the most frequent serious adverse effect of dapsone and may occur at doses of 200 mg or higher daily.[1] Red blood cells may contain Heinz bodies and there is a reduction in their life span. Well-known risk factors include G6PD deficiency, methaemoglobin reductase deficiency, and haemoglobin M trait; haemoglobin E trait may also increase susceptibility to haemolytic reactions.[2] Haemolytic anaemia has been reported in a neonate following ingestion of dapsone in breast milk.[3]

*Methaemoglobinaemia*, although common, is rarely symptomatic.[1] However, severe cyanosis was associated with methaemoglobinaemia in an HIV-positive patient with suspected *Pneumocystis carinii* pneumonia following inadvertent overdosing with dapsone.[4] Methaemoglobinaemia has also been reported in an HIV-negative patient with severe renal impairment, who had previously undergone liver and kidney transplantations and who was receiving dapsone for prophylaxis of *Pneumocystis carinii* pneumonia.[5] The metabolite dapsone hydroxylamine is probably responsible for the methaemoglobinaemia and haemolysis associated with dapsone. Studies have shown[6,7] that use of dapsone with cimetidine, which inhibits production of the *N*-hydroxy metabolite, has resulted in a decrease in methaemoglobin levels, at least in the short term.

*Agranulocytosis* has occurred rarely following dapsone use in leprosy and skin disease. More cases have been observed when used for malaria prophylaxis[8] (see also under Pyrimethamine, p.458) and dermatitis herpetiformis.[9] The reaction is usually self-limiting once the drug is withdrawn, but fatalities have occurred.[9,10]

*Aplastic anaemia* has been reported.[11,12] Of 11 fatalities attributed to dapsone reported to the British and Swedish adverse reaction registers[13] between 1968 and 1988, seven were due to white blood cell dyscrasias; none were attributed to red cell dyscrasias, although such reactions formed almost half of all serious reactions reported for dapsone.

*Thrombocytosis* was reported in a patient with AIDS receiving dapsone prophylactically.[14]

See also Hypoalbuminaemia, below.


1. Jopling WH. Side-effects of antileprosy drugs in common use. *Lepr Rev* 1983; **54:** 261–70.
2. Lachant NA, Tanaka KR. Case report: dapsone-associated Heinz body hemolytic anemia in a Cambodian woman with hemoglobin E trait. *Am J Med Sci* 1987; **294:** 364–8.
3. Sanders SW, *et al.* Hemolytic anemia induced by dapsone transmitted through breast milk. *Ann Intern Med* 1982; **96:** 465–6.
4. Seaton RA, *et al.* Blue and breathless. *Hosp Med* 1999; **60:** 530.
5. Ward KE, McCarthy MW. Dapsone-induced methemoglobinemia. *Ann Pharmacother* 1998; **32:** 549–53.

6. Coleman MD, *et al.* The use of cimetidine as a selective inhibitor of dapsone N-hydroxylation in man. *Br J Clin Pharmacol* 1990; **30:** 761–7.
7. Rhodes LE, *et al.* Cimetidine improves the therapeutic/toxic ratio of dapsone in patients on chronic dapsone therapy. *Br J Dermatol* 1995; **132:** 257–62.
8. Firkin FC, Mariani AF. Agranulocytosis due to dapsone. *Med J Aust* 1977; **2:** 247–51.
9. Cockburn EM, *et al.* Dapsone-induced agranulocytosis: spontaneous reporting data. *Br J Dermatol* 1993; **128:** 702–3.
10. Barss P. Fatal dapsone agranulocytosis in a Melanesian. *Lepr Rev* 1986; **57:** 63–6.
11. Foucauld J, *et al.* Dapsone and aplastic anemia. *Ann Intern Med* 1985; **102:** 139.
12. Meyerson MA, Cohen PR. Dapsone-induced aplastic anaemia in a woman with bullous systemic lupus erythematosus. *Mayo Clin Proc* 1994; **69:** 1159–62.
13. Björkman A, Phillips-Howard PA. Adverse reactions to sulfa drugs: implications for malaria chemotherapy. *Bull WHO* 1991; **69:** 297–304.
14. Wynn RF, *et al.* Case report of dapsone-related thrombocytosis in an AIDS patient. *Am J Med* 1995; **98:** 602.

**Effects on the eyes.** References to eye damage associated with dapsone poisoning.[1-3]

1. Daneshmend TK. The neurotoxicity of dapsone. *Adverse Drug React Acute Poisoning Rev* 1984; **3:** 43–58.
2. Alexander TA, *et al.* Presumed DDS ocular toxicity. *Indian J Ophthalmol* 1989; **37:** 150–1.
3. Seo M-S, *et al.* Dapsone maculopathy. *Korean J Ophthalmol* 1997; **11:** 70–3.

**Effects on the liver.** Toxic hepatitis and cholestatic jaundice have been reported by the manufacturer to occur early in dapsone therapy. Jaundice may also form part of the dapsone reaction (see Hypersensitivity Reactions, below). Deterioration in liver function tests during dapsone treatment has been noted in a patient with dermatitis herpetiformis and primary sclerosing cholangitis.[1]

1. Kirby B, *et al.* Abnormal liver function tests induced by dapsone in a patient with dermatitis herpetiformis and primary sclerosing cholangitis. *Br J Dermatol* 1999; **141:** 172–3.

**Effects on the lungs.** Pulmonary eosinophilia occurred on 2 occasions in a woman receiving dapsone for urticaria.[1] On each occasion symptoms resolved when dapsone was stopped.

1. Jaffuel D, *et al.* Eosinophilic pneumonia induced by dapsone. *BMJ* 1998; **317:** 181.

**Effects on mental state.** Psychosis has been reported in leprosy patients receiving dapsone, but the role of dapsone in this effect is poorly defined.[1] Manic-depressive reactions have been reported in 2 patients with skin disorders. These reactions appeared to be idiosyncratic reactions to dapsone.[2,3]

1. Daneshmend T. Idiosyncratic dapsone induced manic depression. *BMJ* 1989; **299:** 324.
2. Carmichael AJ, Paul CJ. Idiosyncratic dapsone induced manic depression. *BMJ* 1989; **298:** 1524. Correction. *ibid.*; **299:** 56.
3. Gawkrodger D. Manic depression induced by dapsone in patient with dermatitis herpetiformis. *BMJ* 1989; **299:** 860.

**Effects on the nervous system.** Clinical details of 13 patients who experienced dapsone-induced neuropathy. Patients received a mean dose of 115 g (range 6 to 380 g) over 19 months for various dermatological conditions.[1] All patients had motor weakness and some experienced sensory impairment. Most recovered within several months of discontinuing dapsone.

1. Daneshmend TK. The neurotoxicity of dapsone. *Adverse Drug React Acute Poisoning Rev* 1984; **3:** 43–58.

**Effects on the pancreas.** A report[1] of acute pancreatitis associated with the use of dapsone to treat dermatitis herpetiformis in an 87-year-old man. Symptoms resolved upon discontinuation of dapsone but recurred upon rechallenge.

1. Jha SH, *et al.* Dapsone-induced acute pancreatitis. *Ann Pharmacother* 2003; **37:** 1438–40.

**Effects on taste.** A persistent sweet taste and tingling of the face and lips was described in a patient receiving dapsone for ocular cicatricial pemphigoid.[1] The symptoms resolved when dapsone was stopped.

1. Stafanous SN, Morgan SJ. A previously unrecognised side effect of dapsone. *Br J Ophthalmol* 1997; **81:** 1113–14.

**Hyperpigmentation.** Hyperpigmented macules were reported in 32 of about 800 children who received dapsone with pyrimethamine for 3 months or more for malaria prophylaxis.[1] The reaction was attributed to dapsone.

1. David KP, *et al.* Hyperpigmented dermal macules in children following the administration of Maloprim for malaria chemoprophylaxis. *Trans R Soc Trop Med Hyg* 1997; **91:** 204–8.

**Hypersensitivity reactions.** Dapsone syndrome is a rare hypersensitivity reaction, although it has been suggested[1-3] that the incidence has increased since the introduction of multidrug therapy for leprosy. It occurs in the first 6 weeks of therapy and symptoms include rash, which is always present, fever, jaundice, and eosinophilia. The syndrome has occurred in leprosy patients,[4-6] in patients with skin disorders,[7,8] and in patients taking weekly dapsone (in association with pyrimethamine) for malaria prophylaxis.[9] Fatalities have occurred.[5,10] Desensitisation has been successfully carried out in several patients with AIDS who exhibited hypersensitivity to dapsone.[11,12]

1. Richardus JH, Smith TC. Increased incidence in leprosy of hypersensitivity reactions to dapsone after introduction of multidrug therapy. *Lepr Rev* 1989; **60:** 267–73.
2. Kumar RH, *et al.* Dapsone syndrome—a five year retrospective analysis. *Indian J Lepr* 1998; **70:** 271–6.
3. Rao PN, Lakshmi TSS. Increase in the incidence of dapsone hypersensitivity syndrome—an appraisal. *Lepr Rev* 2001; **72:** 57–62.



4. Joseph MS. Hypersensitivity reaction to dapsone. *Lepr Rev* 1985; **56:** 315–20.
5. Jamrozik K. Dapsone syndrome occurring in two brothers. *Lepr Rev* 1986; **57:** 57–62.
6. Hortaleza AR, *et al.* Dapsone syndrome in a Filipino man. *Lepr Rev* 1995; **66:** 307–13.
7. Tomecki KJ, Catalano CJ. Dapsone hypersensitivity: the sulfone syndrome revisited. *Arch Dermatol* 1981; **117:** 38–9.
8. Kromann NP, *et al.* The dapsone syndrome. *Arch Dermatol* 1982; **118:** 531–2.
9. Grayson ML, *et al.* Severe dapsone syndrome due to weekly Maloprim. *Lancet* 1988; **i:** 531.
10. Frey HM, *et al.* Fatal reaction to dapsone during treatment of leprosy. *Ann Intern Med* 1981; **94:** 777–9.
11. Metroka CE, *et al.* Desensitization to dapsone in HIV-positive patients. *JAMA* 1992; **267:** 512.
12. Cook DE, Kossey JL. Successful desensitization to dapsone for Pneumocystis carinii prophylaxis in an HIV-positive patient. *Ann Pharmacother* 1998; **32:** 1302–5.

**Hypoalbuminaemia.** Severe and often life-threatening hypoalbuminaemia has been reported rarely in patients taking dapsone for extended periods for dermatitis herpetiformis.[1-3] Hypoalbuminaemia usually resolves rapidly once dapsone is withdrawn.

1. Kingham JGC, *et al.* Dapsone and severe hypoalbuminaemia. *Lancet* 1979; **ii:** 662–4 and 1018.
2. Foster PN, Swan CHJ. Dapsone and fatal hypoalbuminaemia. *Lancet* 1981; **ii:** 806–7.
3. Sinclair SA, *et al.* Life threatening hypoalbuminaemia associated with dapsone therapy. *Br J Dermatol* 1996; **135** (suppl 47): 45.

**Photosensitivity.** A report of photosensitivity in 6 patients who had taken dapsone.[1]

1. Dhanapaul S. DDS-induced photosensitivity with reference to six case reports. *Lepr Rev* 1989; **60:** 147–50.

## Treatment of Adverse Effects

In severe overdosage, repeated doses of activated charcoal should be given by mouth with the aim of preventing absorption of dapsone but also to aid the elimination of dapsone and its monoacetyl metabolite. Methaemoglobinaemia has been treated with slow intravenous injections of methylthioninium chloride 1 to 2 mg/kg repeated after 1 hour if necessary. Methylthioninium chloride should not be given to patients with G6PD deficiency since it will not be effective. Haemolysis has been treated by infusion of concentrated human red blood cells to replace the damaged cells. Supportive therapy includes administration of oxygen and fluids.

Patients who develop dapsone syndrome (see Hypersensitivity Reactions, above) may require several weeks of corticosteroid therapy.

**Overdosage.** References.

1. Dawson AH, Whyte IM. Management of dapsone poisoning complicated by methaemoglobinaemia. *Med Toxicol Adverse Drug Exp* 1989; **4:** 387–92.
2. Endre ZH, *et al.* Successful treatment of acute dapsone intoxication using charcoal hemoperfusion. *Aust N Z J Med* 1983; **13:** 509–12.
3. Hoetelmans RMW, *et al.* Combined dapsone and clofazimine intoxication. *Hum Exp Toxicol* 1996; **15:** 625–8.
4. Ferguson AJ, Lavery GG. Deliberate self-poisoning with dapsone: a case report and summary of relevant pharmacology and treatment. *Anaesthesia* 1997; **52:** 359–63.

## Precautions

Dapsone should not be used in patients with severe anaemia. It is recommended that regular blood counts be performed during treatment. Patients deficient in G6PD or methaemoglobin reductase, or with haemoglobin M are more susceptible to the haemolytic effects of dapsone.

Where possible, liver function should be monitored during treatment.

It is now generally considered that the benefits of dapsone in the treatment of leprosy during pregnancy outweigh any potential risk to the pregnant patient or fetus. Some practitioners recommend folic acid 5 mg daily for leprosy patients receiving dapsone during pregnancy.

**Breast feeding.** Dapsone is distributed into breast milk and the American Academy of Pediatrics[1] states that, although usually compatible with breast feeding, use of dapsone in a breast-feeding mother has resulted in sulfonamide detected in the infant's urine.[2] There has also been a report of haemolytic anaemia in a breast-fed infant (see Effects on the Blood, under Adverse Effects, above). A study in 3 lactating women who were given a single dose of dapsone 100 mg plus pyrimethamine and chloroquine estimated that if their infants were breast fed they would receive 4.6, 10, or 14.3%, respectively, of the maternal dose in the 9-day period following administration.[3]

1. American Academy of Pediatrics. The transfer of drugs and other chemicals into human milk. *Pediatrics* 2001; **108:** 776–89. Correction. *ibid.*; 1029. Also available at: http://aappolicy.aappublications.org/cgi/content/full/pediatrics%3b108/3/776 (accessed 26/05/04)
2. Dreisbach JA. Sulphone levels in breast milk of mothers on sulphone therapy. *Lepr Rev* 1952; **23:** 101–6.
3. Edstein MD, *et al.* Excretion of chloroquine, dapsone and pyrimethamine in human milk. *Br J Clin Pharmacol* 1986; **22:** 733–5.

**Porphyria.** Dapsone has been associated with acute attacks of porphyria and is considered unsafe in porphyric patients.

## Interactions

Serum concentrations of dapsone are increased, with a consequent increased risk of adverse effects, when given with probenecid, probably as a result of reduced renal excretion of dapsone. Increased dapsone and trimethoprim concentrations have also been reported in patients receiving both drugs, and such patients may be at increased risk of dapsone toxicity. Rifampicin reduces serum concentrations of dapsone to a level that may compromise efficacy in infections other than leprosy. Rifampicin concentrations are generally unaffected. Dapsone may antagonise the anti-inflammatory properties of clofazimine (p.197).

**Cimetidine.** Cimetidine has been reported to increase the area under the curve for dapsone, but to decrease the area under the curve for the metabolite dapsone hydroxylamine. Haematotoxicity is thought to be related to production of this metabolite (see Effects on the Blood, above).

**Pyrimethamine.** Although some manufacturers warn that dapsone-induced haematotoxicity could be potentiated by folic acid antagonists such as pyrimethamine, the tolerability of dapsone plus pyrimethamine was similar to dapsone alone when each treatment was given on a once-weekly basis to patients with HIV infection.[1] Dapsone concentrations were not significantly higher in patients receiving dapsone plus pyrimethamine than in those receiving dapsone alone.

1. Falloon J, *et al.* Pharmacokinetics and safety of weekly dapsone and dapsone plus pyrimethamine for prevention of pneumocystis pneumonia. *Antimicrob Agents Chemother* 1994; **38:** 1580–7.

**Trimethoprim.** In a study of AIDS patients with *Pneumocystis carinii* pneumonia, the mean peak serum concentrations of dapsone after 7 days were 1.5 micrograms/mL following 100 mg daily and 2.1 micrograms/mL following dapsone 100 mg daily in combination with trimethoprim 20 mg/kg daily; concentrations of trimethoprim were also increased.[1] Elevated dapsone concentrations may contribute to the toxicity and the efficacy of this combination.

1. Lee BL, *et al.* Dapsone, trimethoprim, and sulfamethoxazole plasma levels during treatment of Pneumocystis pneumonia in patients with the acquired immunodeficiency syndrome (AIDS). *Ann Intern Med* 1989; **110:** 606–11.

## Antimicrobial Action

Dapsone is a sulfone active against a wide range of bacteria, but it is mainly used for its action against *Mycobacterium leprae*. Its mechanism of action is probably similar to that of the sulfonamides, which involves inhibition of folic acid synthesis in susceptible organisms. It is usually considered to be bacteriostatic against *M. leprae*, although it may also possess weak bactericidal activity. It is also active against *Plasmodium* and *Pneumocystis carinii*. As with the sulfonamides, antibacterial activity is inhibited by *p*-aminobenzoic acid.

Secondary (acquired) dapsone resistance of *Mycobacterium leprae* is mainly associated with dapsone being used on its own. Primary dapsone resistance has also been reported with increasing frequency in areas with secondary resistance. Resistance of *M. leprae* to dapsone should be suspected whenever a patient relapses clinically and bacteriologically.

**Multidrug resistance.** Strains of *Mycobacterium leprae* with multiple resistance to rifampicin, ofloxacin, and dapsone have been isolated from patients who have previously received dapsone monotherapy followed by treatment with rifampicin in combination with ofloxacin.[1]

1. Cambau E, *et al.* Multidrug-resistance to dapsone, rifampicin, and ofloxacin in Mycobacterium leprae. *Lancet* 1997; **349:** 103–4.

## Pharmacokinetics

Dapsone is almost completely absorbed from the gastrointestinal tract with peak plasma concentrations occurring 2 to 8 hours after a dose. Steady-state concentrations are not attained until after at least 8 days of daily administration; doses of 100 mg daily provide trough concentrations of 500 nanograms/mL, which are well in excess of the MIC for *M. leprae*. About 50 to 80% of dapsone in the circulation is bound to plasma proteins and nearly 100% of its monoacetylated metabolite is bound.

Dapsone undergoes enterohepatic recycling. It is widely distributed; it is present in saliva and breast milk and crosses the placenta. The half-life ranges from 10 to 80 hours.

Dapsone is acetylated to monoacetyldapsone, the major metabolite, and other mono and diacetyl derivatives. Acetylation exhibits genetic polymorphism. Hydroxylation is the other major metabolic pathway resulting in hydroxylamine dapsone, which may be responsible for dapsone-associated methaemoglobinaemia and haemolysis.

Dapsone is mainly excreted in the urine, only 20% of a dose as unchanged drug.

◊ References.

1. Zuidema J, *et al.* Clinical pharmacokinetics of dapsone. *Clin Pharmacokinet* 1986; **11:** 299–315.
2. May DG, *et al.* The disposition of dapsone in cirrhosis. *Clin Pharmacol Ther* 1992; **51:** 689–700.
3. Mirochnick M, *et al.* Pharmacokinetics of dapsone in children. *J Pediatr* 1993; **122:** 806–9.
4. Opravil M, *et al.* Levels of dapsone and pyrimethamine in serum during once-weekly dosing for prophylaxis of Pneumocystis carinii pneumonia and toxoplasmic encephalitis. *Antimicrob Agents Chemother* 1994; **38:** 1197–9.
5. Gatti G, *et al.* Penetration of dapsone into cerebrospinal fluid of patients with AIDS. *J Antimicrob Chemother* 1997; **40:** 113–15.
6. Mirochnick M, *et al.* Pharmacokinetics of dapsone administered daily and weekly in human immunodeficiency virus-infected children. *Antimicrob Agents Chemother* 1999; **43:** 2586–91.
7. Mirochnick M, *et al.* Population pharmacokinetics of dapsone in children with human immunodeficiency virus infection. *Clin Pharmacol Ther* 2001; **70:** 24–32.

**Metabolism.** Measurement of the relative activity of the two main routes of dapsone metabolism (acetylation and hydroxylation) suggests that the risk of adverse effects is greater in individuals in whom the *N*-hydroxylation route predominates.[1] This is consistent with the hypothesis that the toxicity of dapsone is related to production of an active metabolite. See also Effects on the Blood, above.

1. Bluhm RE, *et al.* Development of dapsone toxicity in patients with inflammatory dermatoses: activity of acetylation and hydroxylation of dapsone as risk factors. *Clin Pharmacol Ther* 1999; **65:** 598–605.

## Uses and Administration

Dapsone is used as part of multidrug regimens in the treatment of all forms of leprosy (p.133). It has also been used in the prophylaxis of leprosy and in the management of household contacts of leprosy patients. Dapsone is used as an alternative to co-trimoxazole or pentamidine for the treatment and prophylaxis of *Pneumocystis carinii* pneumonia (below), and with pyrimethamine for the prophylaxis of malaria (see under Pyrimethamine, p.459). It is also used in dermatitis herpetiformis and other dermatoses (see Skin Disorders, below). It has been tried for the prophylaxis of toxoplasmosis (p.598) and for the treatment of cutaneous leishmaniasis (p.597) and actinomycetoma (p.136).

Dapsone is usually given by mouth. There are some reports of it being given by intramuscular injection, but such injections can be painful and cause abscess formation.

The most common regimens for leprosy are those recommended by WHO. For multibacillary leprosy, rifampicin 600 mg and clofazimine 300 mg are both given once a month together with dapsone 100 mg and clofazimine 50 mg both daily for 12 months. Doses of all 3 drugs are reduced in children and, in those aged 10 to 14 years, daily doses of dapsone 50 mg, or 1 to 2 mg/kg if their body-weight is low, are given. Adults weighing less than 35 kg also receive reduced doses of rifampicin and dapsone, and in such patients the dapsone dose is 50 mg or 1 to 2 mg/kg daily.

The WHO regimen for paucibacillary leprosy consists of rifampicin 600 mg once a month and dapsone 100 mg daily; both are given for 6 months. Doses are reduced in children and low-weight patients as for multibacillary leprosy.

The doses of dapsone used for the prophylaxis of *Pneumocystis carinii* pneumonia are discussed in more detail under Pneumocystis carinii Pneumonia, below. Dapsone has also been given with trimethoprim for treatment.

The adult dose of dapsone for malaria prophylaxis is 100 mg weekly with pyrimethamine 12.5 mg weekly.

The dose required for the treatment of dermatitis herpetiformis has to be titrated for individual patients, but it is usual to start with 50 mg daily by mouth, gradually increased to 300 mg daily or more if required. This dose should be reduced to a minimum as soon as possible. Maintenance dosage can often be reduced in patients receiving a gluten-free diet.

**Connective tissue disorders.** Dapsone has been used in a number of inflammatory disorders. Relapsing polychondritis (p.1086) has responded to dapsone, as has Behçet's syndrome (p.1076) and systemic lupus erythematosus. Vasculitic syndromes such as hypersensitivity vasculitis (p.1081) have also improved following dapsone.

**Pneumocystis carinii pneumonia.** Dapsone is used alone or with pyrimethamine[1] for primary prophylaxis of *Pneumocystis carinii* pneumonia (p.389) in patients unable to tolerate co-trimoxazole. A dose of dapsone 100 mg daily in one or two doses is commonly used and has been reported to have similar efficacy to co-trimoxazole.[2] Dapsone has also been given with pyrimethamine in various regimens including dapsone 50 mg daily with pyrimethamine 50 mg once weekly,[3] dapsone 100 mg plus pyrimethamine 50 mg both given twice weekly,[4] and dapsone 200 mg plus pyrimethamine 75 mg both given once weekly.[5]

For treatment, dapsone 100 mg daily with trimethoprim 5 mg/kg every 6 or 8 hours for 21 days has been suggested.

1. Centers for Disease Control and Prevention. Guidelines for preventing opportunistic infections among HIV-infected persons—2002: recommendations of the US Public Health Service and the Infectious Diseases Society of America. *MMWR* 2002; **51** (RR-8): 1–52.
2. Bozzette SA, *et al.* A randomized trial of three antipneumocystic agents in patients with advanced human immunodeficiency virus infection. *N Engl J Med* 1995; **332:** 693–9.
3. Girard P-M, *et al.* Dapsone-pyrimethamine compared with aerosolized pentamidine as primary prophylaxis against Pneumocystis carinii pneumonia and toxoplasmosis in HIV infection. *N Engl J Med* 1993; **328:** 1514–20.
4. Podzamczer D, *et al.* Intermittent trimethoprim-sulfamethoxazole compared with dapsone-pyrimethamine for the simultaneous primary prophylaxis of pneumocystis pneumonia and toxoplasmosis in patients infected with HIV. *Ann Intern Med* 1995; **122:** 755–61.
5. Opravil M, *et al.* Once-weekly administration of dapsone/pyrimethamine vs. aerosolized pentamidine as combined prophylaxis for Pneumocystis carinii pneumonia and toxoplasmic encephalitis in human immunodeficiency virus-infected patients. *Clin Infect Dis* 1995; **20:** 531–41.

**Skin disorders.** Dapsone is used in a variety of skin disorders including the suppression of skin lesions in dermatitis herpetiformis (p.1134). The mechanism of action is unknown but is unrelated to its antimicrobial activity. Reports, generally involving small numbers of patients, suggest that dapsone may also be beneficial for bullous or cicatricial pemphigoid (p.1137), pyoderma gangrenosum (p.1138), recurrent erythema multiforme (p.1135), and urticaria (p.1138). Topical administration of dapsone is under investigation for the treatment of acne.

**Spider bites.** As discussed on p.1640, necrotic araneism resulting from the bite of spiders of the genus *Loxosceles* is usually treated conservatively with surgical repair of any persistent defect. A prospective clinical study[1] of 31 patients with brown recluse spider bites indicated that treatment with dapsone 100 mg daily for 14 days followed by delayed surgical intervention if necessary reduced the incidence of wound complications and residual scarring compared with treatment by immediate surgical excision. A dose of 100 mg twice daily has also been given for 14 days.[2]

1. Rees RS, *et al.* Brown recluse spider bites: a comparison of early surgical excision versus dapsone and delayed surgical excision. *Ann Surg* 1985; **202:** 659–63.
2. King LE, Rees RS. Dapsone treatment of a brown recluse bite. *JAMA* 1983; **250:** 648.

## Preparations

***BP 2003:*** Dapsone Tablets;
***USP 27:*** Dapsone Tablets.

**Proprietary Preparations** (details are given in Part 3)
***Arg.:*** Daps; ***Canad.:*** Avlosulfon†; ***Israel:*** Avlosulfon; ***Mex.:*** Dapsoderm-X; Novasulfon; ***Port.:*** Sulfona; ***Spain:*** Sulfona; ***Thai.:*** Dopsan; Servidapsone.

**Multi-ingredient:** ***Austria:*** Isoprodian; ***Fr.:*** Disulone; ***Ger.:*** Isoprodian; ***Irl.:*** Maloprim; ***S.Afr.:*** Maloprim; ***UK:*** Maloprim†.

## Daptomycin *(BAN, USAN, rINN)*

Daptomicina; LY-146032. *N*-Decanoyl-L-tryptophyl-L-asparaginyl-L-aspartyl-L-threonylglycyl-L-ornithyl-L-aspartyl-D-alanyl-L-aspartylglycyl-D-seryl-*threo*-3-methyl-L-glutamyl-3-anthraniloyl-L-alanine 1.13-3.4-lactone.

$C_{72}H_{101}N_{17}O_{26}$ = 1620.7.
*CAS — 103060-53-3.*

### Adverse Effects and Precautions

The most common adverse effects associated with daptomycin are gastrointestinal effects including nausea and vomiting, constipation, diarrhoea, and dyspepsia. Headache, insomnia, dizziness, and fever may occur. Injection site reactions have occurred. Effects on the skin have included rash and pruritus. Abnormal liver function tests have been reported. Creatine phosphokinase concentrations may be elevated and should be monitored weekly. There may be hypertension or hypotension and renal failure has occurred. Other reported adverse effects include anaemia, dyspnoea, and musculoskeletal disorders including arthralgia and limb pain; patients should be monitored for the development of muscle pain, weakness, or neuropathy, particularly of the extremities.

### Uses and Administration

Daptomycin is a lipopeptide antibacterial that is reported to have a spectrum of antibacterial activity similar to that of vancomycin (p.276) and greater potency against many bacterial strains *in vitro*. It is reported to show antimicrobial synergy *in vitro* with the aminoglycosides against enterococci and *Staphylococcus aureus*. It is given by intravenous infusion over 30 minutes in a dose of 4 mg/kg once daily for 7 to 14 days for the intravenous treatment of susceptible infections, including complicated Gram-positive infections of the skin and soft tissues. For details of dosage modification in patients with renal impairment, see below. It has also been investigated for the treatment of vancomycin-resistant enterococcal infections, complicated urinary-tract infections, endocarditis, bacteraemia, and community-acquired pneumonia.

◊ References.

1. Pryka RD, *et al.* Clinical pharmacokinetics of daptomycin. *DICP Ann Pharmacother* 1990; **24:** 255–6.
2. Kreft B, *et al.* Experimental studies on nephrotoxicity and pharmacokinetics of LY 146032 (daptomycin) in rats. *J Antimicrob Chemother* 1990; **25:** 635–43.
3. Woodworth JR, *et al.* Single-dose pharmacokinetics and antibacterial activity of daptomycin, a new lipopeptide antibiotic, in healthy volunteers. *Antimicrob Agents Chemother* 1992; **36:** 318–25.
4. Woodworth JR, *et al.* Tobramycin and daptomycin disposition when co-administered to healthy volunteers. *J Antimicrob Chemother* 1994; **33:** 655–9.
5. Tally FP, DeBruin MF. Development of daptomycin for gram-positive infections. *J Antimicrob Chemother* 2000; **46:** 523–6.
6. Snydman DR, *et al.* Comparative in vitro activities of daptomycin and vancomycin against resistant Gram-positive pathogens. *Antimicrob Agents Chemother* 2000; **44:** 3447–50.

**Administration in renal impairment.** Doses of daptomycin should be modified to 4 mg/kg every 48 hours in patients with a creatinine clearance of less than 30 mL/minute, including those receiving dialysis.

### Preparations

**Proprietary Preparations** (details are given in Part 3)
***USA:*** Cubicin.

## Demeclocycline *(BAN, rINN)*

Demeclociclina; Demethylchlortetracycline. (4*S*,4a*S*,5a*S*,6*S*,12a*S*)-7-Chloro-4-dimethylamino-1,4,4a,5,5a,6,11,12a-octahydro-3,6,10,12,12a-pentahydroxy-1,11-dioxonaphthacene-2-carboxamide; 7-Chloro-6-demethyltetracycline.

$C_{21}H_{21}ClN_2O_8$ = 464.9.
*CAS — 127-33-3 (demeclocycline); 13215-10-6 (demeclocycline sesquihydrate).*
*ATC — D06AA01; J01AA01.*

**Pharmacopoeias.** In *US.*

**USP 27** (Demeclocycline). A yellow, odourless crystalline powder. Sparingly soluble in water; soluble 1 in 200 of alcohol and 1 in 40 of methyl alcohol; dissolves readily in 3N hydrochloric acid and in alkaline solutions. pH of a 1% solution in water is between 4.0 and 5.5. Store in airtight containers. Protect from light.

## Demeclocycline Hydrochloride *(BANM, rINNM)*

Demeclocyclini Hydrochloridum; Hidrocloruro de demeclociclina.

$C_{21}H_{21}ClN_2O_8$,HCl = 501.3.
*CAS — 64-73-3.*
*ATC — D06AA01; J01AA01.*

**Pharmacopoeias.** In *Eur.* (see p.vi), *Jpn*, and *US.*

**Ph. Eur. 5.0** (Demeclocycline Hydrochloride). The hydrochloride of a substance produced by certain strains of *Streptomyces aureofaciens* or by any other means. A yellow powder. Soluble or sparingly soluble in water; slightly soluble in alcohol; very slightly soluble in acetone. It dissolves in solutions of alkali hydroxides and carbonates. A 1% solution in water has a pH of 2.0 to 3.0. Protect from light.

**USP 27** (Demeclocycline Hydrochloride). A yellow, odourless, crystalline powder. Soluble 1 in 60 of water and 1 in 50 of methyl alcohol; slightly soluble in alcohol; practically insoluble in acetone and in chloroform; sparingly soluble in solutions of alkali hydroxides and carbonates. pH of a 1% solution in water is between 2.0 and 3.0. Store in airtight containers. Protect from light.

### Adverse Effects and Precautions

As for Tetracycline Hydrochloride, p.266.

Phototoxic reactions occur more frequently with demeclocycline than with other tetracyclines and patients should avoid direct exposure to sunlight or artificial ultraviolet light.

Reversible nephrogenic diabetes insipidus with polyuria, polydipsia, and weakness may occur in patients treated with demeclocycline. Plasma creatinine should be monitored in patients receiving demeclocycline for long periods for the treatment of inappropriate secretion of antidiuretic hormone, since tetracycline-induced renal impairment may not otherwise be apparent in the absence of oliguria. For a comment that the usefulness of demeclocycline for this indication may be limited by nephrotoxicity in patients with cardiac or hepatic disease, see Syndrome of Inappropriate ADH Secretion under Uses and Administration, below.

### Interactions

As for Tetracycline Hydrochloride, p.267.

### Antimicrobial Action

As for Tetracycline Hydrochloride, p.267. Demeclocycline is stated to be somewhat more active against certain strains of some organisms including *Neisseria gonorrhoeae* and *Haemophilus influenzae*, as well as to being the most active of the tetracyclines *in vitro* against *Brucella* spp.

### Pharmacokinetics

As for Tetracycline Hydrochloride, p.268.

About 60 to 80% of a dose of demeclocycline is absorbed from the gastrointestinal tract. Peak plasma concentrations of about 1.5 to 1.7 micrograms/mL have been reported 3 to 4 hours after a single oral dose of 300 mg, but higher plasma concentrations may be achieved with repeated dosage. Its plasma elimination half-life is about 12 hours. The renal clearance of demeclocycline is about half that of tetracycline.

### Uses and Administration

Demeclocycline is a tetracycline derivative with uses similar to those of tetracycline (p.268). It is excreted more slowly and effective blood concentrations are maintained for a longer period.

Demeclocycline is given by mouth as the hydrochloride. The usual adult dose of demeclocycline hydrochloride is 600 mg daily in 2 or 4 divided doses, preferably 1 hour before or 2 hours after meals; 900 mg daily in 3 divided doses may be given for atypical pneumonia. Older children (over 8 years) have been given approximately 6 to 12 mg/kg daily in divided doses, but the effect of tetracyclines on teeth and bones should be considered.

Demeclocycline may be given to adults in the treatment of chronic hyponatraemia associated with the syndrome of inappropriate antidiuretic hormone secretion, when water restriction has proved ineffective. Initially demeclocycline hydrochloride 900 to 1200 mg is given daily in divided doses, reduced to maintenance doses of 600 to 900 mg daily.

For dosage recommendations in patients with hepatic impairment, see below.

The calcium and magnesium salts of demeclocycline have also been used.

**Administration in hepatic impairment.** The manufacturers state that the dosage of demeclocycline should not exceed 1 g daily in patients with known liver disease.

**Syndrome of inappropriate ADH secretion.** Demeclocycline may be given in the treatment of the syndrome of inappropriate ADH (antidiuretic hormone) secretion (SIADH—p.1318) to antagonise the effect of ADH on the renal tubules; lithium has been given as an alternative. Both lithium and demeclocycline act by interfering with the cellular action of ADH to produce nephrogenic diabetes insipidus. Demeclocycline was reported to be superior to lithium[1] and became the preferred treatment for chronic SIADH if water restriction was unsuccessful,[2] although fluid restriction is probably still the treatment of choice. However, since nephrotoxicity has been reported in patients with cardiac or hepatic disease, the usefulness of demeclocycline in the treatment of hyponatraemic states might be limited; this view was supported by studies in patients with heart failure[3] and cirrhosis.[4]


1. Forrest JN, *et al.* Superiority of demeclocycline over lithium in the treatment of chronic syndrome of inappropriate secretion of antidiuretic hormone. *N Engl J Med* 1978; **298:** 173–7.
2. Schrier RW. Treatment of hyponatremia. *N Engl J Med* 1985; **312:** 1121–2.
3. Zegers de Beyl D, *et al.* Demeclocycline treatment of water retention in congestive heart failure. *BMJ* 1978; **1:** 760.
4. Miller PD, *et al.* Plasma demeclocycline levels and nephrotoxicity: correlation in hyponatremic cirrhotic patients. *JAMA* 1980; **243:** 2513–15.


### Preparations

***BP 2003:*** Demeclocycline Capsules;
***USP 27:*** Demeclocycline Hydrochloride Capsules; Demeclocycline Hydrochloride Tablets; Demeclocycline Oral Suspension.

**Proprietary Preparations** (details are given in Part 3)
***Austral.:*** Ledermycin; ***Austria:*** Ledermycin†; ***Canad.:*** Declomycin; ***India:*** Ledermycin; ***Irl.:*** Ledermycin†; ***Ital.:*** Ledermicina†; ***Neth.:*** Ledermycin; ***NZ:*** Ledermycin†; ***UK:*** Ledermycin; ***USA:*** Declomycin.

**Multi-ingredient:** ***Austria:*** Ledermix; ***Denm.:*** Ledermix; ***Irl.:*** Deteclo†; Ledermix†; ***Israel:*** Ledermix; ***Ital.:*** Rubrociclina; ***S.Afr.:*** Ledermix†; Tritet†; ***Spain:*** Varibiotic†; ***Switz.:*** Ledermix; ***UK:*** Deteclo; Ledermix.

## Dibekacin Sulfate *(rINNM)*

Dibekacin Sulphate *(BANM)*; 3′,4′-Dideoxykanamycin B; Sulfato de dibekacina. 6-*O*-(3-Amino-3-deoxy-α-D-glucopyranosyl)-2-deoxy-4-*O*-(2,6-diamino-2,3,4,6-tetradeoxy-α-D-*erythro*-hexopyranosyl)-streptamine sulphate.

$C_{18}H_{37}N_5O_8,xH_2SO_4$.

*CAS — 34493-98-6 (dibekacin); 58580-55-5 (dibekacin sulfate).*

*ATC — J01GB09.*

**Pharmacopoeias.** In *Jpn.*

### Profile

Dibekacin is an aminoglycoside derived from kanamycin with actions and uses similar to those of gentamicin (p.217). It is given intramuscularly as the sulfate in doses equivalent to dibekacin 1 to 3 mg/kg daily in divided doses; doses in the upper half of this range are mostly recommended in Europe, while those in the lower half have been preferred in the Far East. It may be given in similar doses by slow intravenous infusion and has also been given subcutaneously. Dosage should be adjusted based on serum-dibekacin concentration monitoring. It has also been used topically for eye infections.

### Preparations

**Proprietary Preparations** (details are given in Part 3)
***Belg.:*** Dikacine; ***Fr.:*** Debekacyl†; ***Jpn:*** Panimycin.

## Dicloxacillin *(BAN, USAN, rINN)*

BRL-1702; Dicloxacilina; R-13423. (6*R*)-6-[3-(2,6-Dichlorophenyl)-5-methylisoxazole-4-carboxamido]penicillanic acid.

$C_{19}H_{17}Cl_2N_3O_5S$ = 470.3.

*CAS — 3116-76-5.*

*ATC — J01CF01.*

## Dicloxacillin Sodium *(BANM, USAN, rINNM)*

Dicloxacilina sódica; Dicloxacillinum Natricum; P-1011. Sodium dicloxacillin monohydrate.

$C_{19}H_{16}Cl_2N_3NaO_5S,H_2O$ = 510.3.

*CAS — 343-55-5 (anhydrous dicloxacillin sodium); 13412-64-1 (dicloxacillin sodium monohydrate).*

*ATC — J01CF01.*

**Pharmacopoeias.** In *Eur.* (see p.vi), *Int.*, *Jpn*, and *US.*

**Ph. Eur. 5.0** (Dicloxacillin Sodium). A white or almost white, hygroscopic, crystalline powder. Freely soluble in water; soluble in alcohol and in methyl alcohol. A 10% solution in water has a pH of 5.0 to 7.0. Store at a temperature not exceeding 25° in airtight containers.

**USP 27** (Dicloxacillin Sodium). A white to off-white crystalline powder. Freely soluble in water. pH of a 1% solution in water is between 4.5 and 7.5. Store in airtight containers.

### Adverse Effects and Precautions

As for Flucloxacillin, p.213.

**Effects on the liver.** References.


1. Kleinman MS, Presberg JE. Cholestatic hepatitis after dicloxacillin-sodium therapy. *J Clin Gastroenterol* 1986; **8:** 77–8.


**Sodium content.** Each g of dicloxacillin sodium contains about 2 mmol of sodium.

### Interactions

As for Benzylpenicillin, p.164.

### Antimicrobial Action

As for Flucloxacillin, p.213.

### Pharmacokinetics

Dicloxacillin is better absorbed from the gastrointestinal tract than cloxacillin but absorption is reduced by the presence of food in the stomach. After an oral dose of 500 mg, peak plasma concentrations of 10 to 18 micrograms/mL in about 1 hour have been reported in fasting subjects. Doubling the dose can double the plasma concentration. About 97% of dicloxacillin in the circulation is bound to plasma proteins. Dicloxacillin has been reported to have a plasma half-life of 0.5 to 1 hour. The half-life is prolonged in neonates.

The distribution of dicloxacillin in body tissues and fluids is similar to that of cloxacillin (p.198).

Dicloxacillin is metabolised to a limited extent and the unchanged drug and metabolites are excreted in the urine by glomerular filtration and renal tubular secretion. About 60% of an oral dose is excreted in the urine. Only small amounts are excreted in the bile. Dicloxacillin is not removed by haemodialysis.

Plasma concentrations are enhanced by probenecid. Reduced concentrations have been reported in patients with cystic fibrosis.

### Uses and Administration

Dicloxacillin is an isoxazolyl penicillin used similarly to flucloxacillin (p.214) in the treatment of infections due to staphylococci resistant to benzylpenicillin.

Dicloxacillin is given intravenously and by mouth as the sodium salt. All doses are expressed in terms of the equivalent amount of dicloxacillin. 1.09 g of dicloxacillin sodium is approximately equivalent to 1 g of dicloxacillin. Oral doses should be taken at least 1 hour before, or 2 hours after, meals since the presence of food in the stomach reduces absorption. The usual adult dose by mouth is 250 mg every 6 hours. Similar doses may be given by slow intravenous injection or, preferably, by intravenous infusion. Doses may be doubled in severe infections.

### Preparations

***USP 27:*** Dicloxacillin Sodium Capsules; Dicloxacillin Sodium for Oral Suspension.

**Proprietary Preparations** (details are given in Part 3)
***Austral.:*** Diclocil; Dicloxsig; Distaph; ***Denm.:*** Dicillin; Diclocil; ***Fin.:*** Diclocil; ***Ger.:*** Dichlor-Stapenor†; InfectoStaph; ***Gr.:*** Diclocil; ***Hong Kong:*** Diclocil†; ***Ital.:*** Diclo†; ***Mex.:*** Brispen; Cilpen; Clomicin; Cloxil†; Cloxipen†; Diclo-Tecno; Dipxapen; Ditterolina; Dixen; Penclox; Posipen; ***Norw.:*** Diclocil; ***NZ:*** Diclocil; ***Port.:*** Diclocil; ***Swed.:*** Diclocil; ***Thai.:*** Amcidil; Cloxydin; Diclex; Diclocil; Diclocillin; Dicloson; Diclox; Dicloxia; Dicloxin; Dicloxman; Dicloxno; Diloxin; Ditum; Dixocillin; Dorox; Servidiclox; ***USA:*** Dycill†; Dynapen†; Pathocil†.

**Multi-ingredient:** ***Ital.:*** Ampiplus; Diamplicil; Duplexcillina†; Duplexil†; ***Mex.:*** Ampiclox-D; Panac; Panac K; Pentidix.

## Difloxacin Hydrochloride *(USAN, rINNM)*

A-56619; Abbott-56619; Hidrocloruro de difloxacino. 6-Fluoro-1-(*p*-fluorophenyl)-1,4-dihydro-7-(4-methyl-1-piperazinyl)-4-oxo-3-quinolinecarboxylic acid hydrochloride.

$C_{21}H_{19}F_2N_3O_3,HCl$ = 435.9.

*CAS — 98106-17-3 (difloxacin); 91296-86-5 (difloxacin hydrochloride).*

### Profile

Difloxacin is a fluoroquinolone antibacterial used as the hydrochloride in veterinary medicine. It was formerly used in humans but was associated with an unacceptably high incidence of adverse CNS effects.

## Dihydrostreptomycin Sulfate *(rINNM)*

Dihydrostreptomycin Sulphate *(BANM)*; Dihydrostreptomycini Sulfas; Sulfato de dihidroestreptomicina. *O*-2-Deoxy-2-methylamino-α-L-glucopyranosyl-(1→2)-*O*-5-deoxy-3-*C*-hydroxymethyl-α-L-lyxofuranosyl-(1→4)-$N^1$,$N^3$-diamidino-D-streptamine sulphate.

$(C_{21}H_{41}N_7O_{12})_2,3H_2SO_4$ = 1461.4.

*CAS — 128-46-1 (dihydrostreptomycin); 5490-27-7 (dihydrostreptomycin sulfate).*

*ATC — S01AA15.*

**Pharmacopoeias.** In *Eur.* (see p.vi) and *US*, both for veterinary use only.

**Ph. Eur. 5.0** (Dihydrostreptomycin Sulphate for Veterinary Use). The sulfate of a substance obtained by catalytic hydrogenation of streptomycin or by any other means. Stabilisers may be added. The potency is not less than 730 units/mg, calculated with reference to the dried substance. A white or almost white powder; it may be hygroscopic. Freely soluble in water; practically insoluble in alcohol, in acetone, and in methyl alcohol. A 25% solution in water has a pH of 5.0 to 7.0. Store in airtight containers. Protect from light.

**USP 27** (Dihydrostreptomycin Sulfate). A white or almost white amorphous or crystalline powder; the amorphous form is hygroscopic. Freely soluble in water; practically insoluble in acetone, in chloroform, and in methyl alcohol. pH of a solution in water containing the equivalent of dihydrostreptomycin 20% is between 4.5 and 7.0, except that if it is labelled as being solely for oral use, the pH is between 3.0 and 7.0. Store in airtight containers.

### Profile

Dihydrostreptomycin is an aminoglycoside antibacterial with actions similar to those of streptomycin (p.256). As it is not absorbed following oral administration, it has been given by this route for gastrointestinal infections. Since it is more likely than streptomycin to cause partial or complete loss of hearing it is not used parenterally in humans, although it is used as the sulfate in veterinary medicine.

### Preparations

**Proprietary Preparations** (details are given in Part 3)

**Multi-ingredient:** ***Arg.:*** Gemipasmol; Vagisan; Vagisan Compuesto; ***Braz.:*** Fluocal com Pectina†; ***Mex.:*** Estrefen; ***Spain:*** Cilinafosal DHD Estrep; Citrocil; Estreptoenterol; Salitanol Estreptomicina; Sulfintestin Neomicina.

## Dirithromycin *(BAN, USAN, rINN)*

ASE-136BS; Dirithromycinum; Diritromicina; LY-237216. (1R,2R,3R,6R,7S,8S,9R,10R,12R,13S,15R,17S)-7-(2,6-Dideoxy-3-C,3-O-dimethyl-α-L-*ribo*-hexopyranosyloxy)-3-ethyl-2,10-dihydroxy-15-(2-methoxyethoxymethyl)-2,6,8,10,12,17-hexamethyl-9-(3,4,6-trideoxy-3-dimethylamino-β-L-*xylo*-hexopyranosyloxy)-4,16-dioxa-14-azabicyclo[11.3.1]heptadecan-5-one; (9S)-9-Deoxo-11-deoxy-9,11-{imino[(1R)-2-(2-methoxyethoxy)-ethylidene]oxy}erythromycin.

$C_{42}H_{78}N_2O_{14}$ = 835.1.
*CAS — 62013-04-1.*
*ATC — J01FA13.*

**Pharmacopoeias.** In *Eur.* (see p.vi) and *US.*

**Ph. Eur. 5.0** (Dirithromycin). A white or almost white powder. It exhibits polymorphism. Very slightly soluble in water; very soluble in dichloromethane and in methyl alcohol.

**USP 27** (Dirithromycin). A white or practically white powder. Very slightly soluble in water; very soluble in dichloromethane and in methyl alcohol.

**Stability.** Dirithromycin is hydrolysed to erythromycylamine in acidic aqueous solutions.

### Adverse Effects and Precautions

As for Erythromycin, p.208. Dirithromycin should be used with caution in patients with moderate to severe hepatic impairment since its metabolite erythromycylamine is primarily eliminated in the bile.

### Interactions

For a discussion of drug interactions of macrolide antibacterials, see Erythromycin, p.209.

### Antimicrobial Action

As for Erythromycin, p.209.

It is reported to be generally less active than erythromycin *in vitro*, but may show greater activity *in vivo* than is indicated by *in-vitro* studies and may exert a postantibiotic effect.

### Pharmacokinetics

Dirithromycin is readily absorbed following oral doses and undergoes rapid non-enzymatic hydrolysis to erythromycylamine. Absorption is enhanced by food. Bioavailability is about 10%. Daily administration of dirithromycin 500 mg produces peak plasma concentrations of erythromycylamine of about 400 nanograms/mL.

Erythromycylamine is widely distributed and tissue concentrations exceed those in plasma. Protein binding is 15 to 30%. Erythromycylamine is mainly excreted unchanged in the bile with only about 2% in the urine. The mean plasma half-life is about 8 hours and the mean urinary terminal elimination half-life is about 44 hours.

◊ References.

1. Sides GD, *et al.* Pharmacokinetics of dirithromycin. *J Antimicrob Chemother* 1993; **31** (suppl C): 65–75.
2. LaBreque D, *et al.* Pharmacokinetics of dirithromycin in patients with impaired hepatic function. *J Antimicrob Chemother* 1993; **32:** 741–50.
3. Mazzei T, *et al.* Pharmacokinetics of dirithromycin in patients with mild or moderate cirrhosis. *Antimicrob Agents Chemother* 1999; **43:** 1556–9.

### Uses and Administration

Dirithromycin is a prodrug of the macrolide antibacterial erythromycylamine, which has similar properties to those of erythromycin (p.208) and is used in respiratory-tract, skin, and soft tissue infections caused by susceptible organisms.

Dirithromycin is given by mouth as enteric-coated tablets in a usual dose of 500 mg once daily.

◊ References.

1. Various. Dirithromycin: a new once-daily macrolide. *J Antimicrob Chemother* 1993; **31** (suppl C): 1–185.
2. Brogden RN, Peters DH. Dirithromycin: a review of its antimicrobial activity, pharmacokinetic properties and therapeutic efficacy. *Drugs* 1994; **48:** 599–616.
3. Wintermeyer SM, *et al.* Dirithromycin: a new macrolide. *Ann Pharmacother* 1996; **30:** 1141–9.
4. McConnell SA, Amsden GW. Review and comparison of advanced-generation macrolides clarithromycin and dirithromycin. *Pharmacotherapy* 1999; **19:** 404–15.

### Preparations

***USP 27:*** Dirithromycin Delayed-Release Tablets.

**Proprietary Preparations** (details are given in Part 3)

***Austria:*** Dimac†; ***Belg.:*** Unibac; ***Braz.:*** Dynabac†; ***Chile:*** Dynabac; ***Fr.:*** Dynabac; ***Gr.:*** Dynabac; ***Hong Kong:*** Dynabac†; ***Ital.:*** Dinabac†; ***Malaysia:*** Dynabac; ***Spain:*** Balodin†; Noriclan†; Nortron†; ***USA:*** Dynabac.

## Doxycycline *(BAN, USAN, rINN)*

Doxiciclina; Doxycycline Monohydrate; Doxycyclinum; GS-3065. (4S,4aR,5S,5aR,6S,12aS)-4-Dimethylamino-1,4,4a,5,5a,6,11,12a-octahydro-3,5,10,12,12a-pentahydroxy-6-methyl-1,11-dioxonaphthacene-2-carboxamide monohydrate; 6-Deoxy-5β-hydroxytetracycline monohydrate.

$C_{22}H_{24}N_2O_8,H_2O$ = 462.4.
*CAS — 564-25-0 (anhydrous doxycycline); 17086-28-1 (doxycycline monohydrate).*
*ATC — A01AB22; J01AA02.*

**Pharmacopoeias.** In *Eur.* (see p.vi) and *US.*

**Ph. Eur. 5.0** (Doxycycline Monohydrate). A yellow crystalline powder. Very slightly soluble in water and in alcohol. It dissolves in dilute solutions of mineral acids and in solutions of alkali hydroxides and carbonates. A 1% suspension in water has a pH of 5.0 to 6.5. Store in airtight containers. Protect from light.

**USP 27** (Doxycycline). A yellow crystalline powder. Very slightly soluble in water; sparingly soluble in alcohol; practically insoluble in chloroform and in ether; freely soluble in dilute acid and in alkali hydroxide solutions. pH of a 1% suspension in water is between 5.0 and 6.5. Store in airtight containers. Protect from light.

### Doxycycline Calcium *(BANM, rINNM)*

Doxiciclina cálcica.
*ATC — A01AB22; J01AA02.*

### Doxycycline Fosfatex *(BAN, USAN)*

AB-08; DMSC; Doxiciclina fosfatex. 6-Deoxy-5β-hydroxytetracycline—metaphosphoric acid—sodium metaphosphate in the ratio 3:3:1.

$(C_{22}H_{24}N_2O_8)_3(HPO_3)_3NaPO_3$ = 1675.2.
*CAS — 83038-87-3.*
*ATC — A01AB22; J01AA02.*

### Doxycycline Hyclate *(BANM, rINNM)*

Dossiciclina Iclato; Doxycycline Hydrochloride; Doxycyclini Hyclas; Hiclato de doxiciclina. Doxycycline hydrochloride hemiethanolate hemihydrate.

$C_{22}H_{24}N_2O_8,HCl,\frac{1}{2}C_2H_5OH,\frac{1}{2}H_2O$ = 512.9.
*CAS — 10592-13-9 (doxycycline hydrochloride); 24390-14-5 (doxycycline hyclate).*
*ATC — A01AB22; J01AA02.*

**Pharmacopoeias.** In *Chin., Eur.* (see p.vi), *Int., Jpn, Pol., US,* and *Viet.*

**Ph. Eur. 5.0** (Doxycycline Hyclate). A yellow hygroscopic crystalline powder. Freely soluble in water and in methyl alcohol; sparingly soluble in alcohol. It dissolves in solutions of alkali hydroxides and of carbonates. A 1% solution in water has a pH of 2.0 to 3.0. Store in airtight containers. Protect from light.

**USP 27** (Doxycycline Hyclate). A yellow crystalline powder. Soluble in water; slightly soluble in alcohol; practically insoluble in chloroform and in ether; soluble in solutions of alkali hydroxides and carbonates. pH of a solution in water containing the equivalent of doxycycline 1% is between 2.0 and 3.0. Store in airtight containers. Protect from light.

**Incompatibility.** Preparations of doxycycline hyclate have an acid pH and incompatibility may reasonably be expected with alkaline preparations or with drugs unstable at low pH. Reduced antimicrobial activity has been reported *in vitro* when doxycycline hyclate was mixed with riboflavin.

### Adverse Effects and Precautions

As for Tetracycline Hydrochloride, p.266.

Gastrointestinal disturbances with doxycycline are reported to be less frequent than with tetracycline and doxycycline may also cause less tooth discoloration.

Oesophageal ulceration may be a particular problem if capsules or tablets are taken with insufficient fluid or in a recumbent posture: doxycycline should be taken with at least half a glass of water, in an upright position, and well before retiring to bed. There is some evidence from studies in *animals* that preparations of the base, which have a higher pH, cause less oesophageal damage than those of the more acid hyclate. Dispersible tablets or liquid formulations should be used in elderly patients, who may be at greater risk of oesophageal injury.

Unlike many tetracyclines, doxycycline does not appear to accumulate in patients with impaired renal function, and aggravation of renal impairment may be less likely.

**Anosmia.** Anosmia or dysosmia (absent or impaired sense of smell) have occasionally been reported in patients receiving doxycycline, although the association has not been definitely established.[1]

1. Bleasel AF, *et al.* Anosmia after doxycycline use. *Med J Aust* 1990; **152:** 440.

**Porphyria.** Doxycycline has been associated with acute attacks of porphyria and is considered unsafe in porphyric patients.

### Interactions

As for Tetracycline Hydrochloride, p.267.

Doxycycline has a lower affinity for binding with calcium than many tetracyclines. In consequence its absorption is less likely to be affected by milk or food, although it is still affected by antacids and iron preparations.

The metabolism of doxycycline may be accelerated by drugs that induce hepatic enzymes such as alcohol (chronic use), rifampicin, and antiepileptics including carbamazepine, phenobarbital, phenytoin, and primidone. It has been suggested that doxycycline could increase ciclosporin concentrations, but evidence for this seems to be scant.

### Antimicrobial Action

As for Tetracycline Hydrochloride, p.267. Doxycycline is more active than tetracycline against many bacterial species including *Streptococcus pyogenes*, enterococci, *Nocardia* spp., and various anaerobes. Cross-resistance is common although some tetracycline-resistant *Staphylococcus aureus* respond to doxycycline. Doxycycline is also more active against protozoa, particularly *Plasmodium* spp.

### Pharmacokinetics

For the general pharmacokinetics of the tetracyclines, see Tetracycline Hydrochloride, p.268.

Doxycycline is readily and almost completely absorbed from the gastrointestinal tract and absorption is not significantly affected by the presence of food in the stomach or duodenum. Mean peak plasma concentrations of 2.6 micrograms/mL have been reported 2 hours after a 200-mg dose by mouth, falling to 1.45 micrograms/mL at 24 hours. After intravenous infusion of the same dose peak plasma concentrations are briefly somewhat higher, but become very similar to those after oral administration following equilibration into the tissues.

From 80 to 95% of doxycycline in the circulation is reported to be bound to plasma proteins. Its biological half-life varies from about 12 to 24 hours. Doxycycline is more lipid-soluble than tetracycline. It is widely distributed in body tissues and fluids.

In patients with normal renal function about 40% of a dose is slowly excreted in the urine, although more is excreted by this route if the urine is made alkaline. However, the majority of a dose of doxycycline is excreted in the faeces following chelation in the intestines. Although doxycycline has been reported to undergo some inactivation in the liver, some sources consider this doubtful; however, the kinetics of doxycycline have been reportedly altered in patients receiving drugs which induce hepatic metabolism.

Doxycycline is stated not to accumulate significantly in patients with renal impairment, although excretion in the urine is reduced; increased amounts of doxycycline are excreted in the faeces in these patients. Nevertheless, there have been reports of some accumulation in renal failure. Removal of doxycycline by haemodialysis is insignificant.

◊ Reviews.

1. Saivin S, Houin G. Clinical pharmacokinetics of doxycycline and minocycline. *Clin Pharmacokinet* 1988; **15:** 355–66.

### Uses and Administration

Doxycycline is a tetracycline derivative with uses similar to those of tetracycline (p.268). It may sometimes be preferred to other tetracyclines in the treatment of sensitive infections because of its fairly reliable absorption and its long half-life which permits less frequent (often once daily) dosage. It also has the advantage that it can be given (with care) to patients with renal impairment. However, relatively high doses may need to be given for urinary-tract infections because of its low renal excretion. Doxycycline has antiprotozoal actions and may be given in conjunction with quinine in the management of falciparum malaria resistant to chloroquine (below).

Doxycycline is normally given by mouth as doxycycline or its various derivatives, usually the hyclate. Doses are expressed in terms of doxycycline; doxycycline hyclate 115 mg is approximately equivalent to 100 mg of anhydrous doxycycline. The usual dose is 200 mg of doxycycline on the first day (as a single dose or in divided doses), followed by 100 mg daily. Older children (over 8 years) weighing 45 kg or less have been given approximately 4 mg/kg in two divided doses initially and thereafter approximately 2 mg/kg daily, but the effect of tetracyclines on teeth and bones should be considered. In severe infections the initial dosage is maintained throughout the course of treatment. In patients with sensitive gonococcal infections, doxycycline 100 mg twice daily for 7 days is given, although it has occasionally been given in a single dose of 300 mg, sometimes followed by a second similar dose 1 hour later. For syphilis, doxycycline 200 or 300 mg is given daily in divided doses for at least 14 or 10 days, respectively. In the treatment of acne, a dose of 50 mg daily may be adequate, although the *British National Formulary* advocates a dose of 100 mg daily. For relapsing fever and louse-borne typhus, doxycycline 100 or 200 mg may be given as a single dose. For prophylaxis of scrub typhus, 200 mg may be taken as a single dose.

Doxycycline capsules and tablets should be given with plenty of fluid, with the patient in an upright position, and well before retiring to bed. It may be given with food or milk if gastric irritation occurs. Dispersible tablets or liquid formulations are advisable in elderly patients.

In patients in whom oral therapy is not feasible, doxycycline may be given as the hyclate by slow intravenous infusion of a solution containing 0.1 to 1 mg/mL, in doses equivalent to those by mouth. Infusions should be given over 1 to 4 hours.

Solutions of doxycycline are also used for malignant effusions (p.512).

Doxycycline is also used as a subgingival gel for the treatment of periodontal disease. Alternatively, it may be given by mouth in low doses of 20 mg twice daily for 3 months as an adjunct to supragingival and subgingival scaling and root planing.

**Malaria.** Doxycycline is used in some areas for the treatment of chloroquine-resistant falciparum malaria (p.444) in a dose of 200 mg daily for at least 7 days following treatment with quinine. Doxycycline 100 mg daily has been used for prophylaxis in areas of high risk where other drugs are likely to be ineffective, but it is not suitable for extended prophylactic use.

## Preparations

***BP 2003:*** Dispersible Doxycycline Tablets; Doxycycline Capsules;
***USP 27:*** Doxycycline Calcium Oral Suspension; Doxycycline Capsules; Doxycycline for Injection; Doxycycline for Oral Suspension; Doxycycline Hyclate Capsules; Doxycycline Hyclate Delayed-release Capsules; Doxycycline Hyclate Tablets.

**Proprietary Preparations** (details are given in Part 3)

***Arg.:*** Doxibiot; Verboril; Vibramicina; ***Austral.:*** Doryx; Doxsig; Doxy; Doxyhexal; Doxylin; Vibra-Tabs; Vibramycin; ***Austria:*** Aliudox; Biocyclin; Dotur; Doxal; Doxybene; Doxyderm; Doxydyn; Doxyhexal; Doxylan; Doxystad; Gewacyclin; Sigadoxin†; Supracyclin; Vibramycin; Vibravenos; ***Belg.:*** Clifordin†; Dagramycine†; Doxyfim†; Doxylets; Unidox†; Vibramycine; Vibratab; ***Braz.:*** Ciclisan; Clordox; Doxina†; Protectina; Uni Doxiciclin; Vibramicina; ***Canad.:*** Apo-Doxy; Doryx†; Doxycin; Doxytec; Novo-Doxylin; Vibra-Tabs; Vibramycin†; ***Chile:*** Doxithal; Sigadoxin; Vibramicina; ***Denm.:*** Dumoxin†; Vibradox; Vibramycin; ***Fin.:*** Apodoxin; Atridox; Dosyklin; Doximed; Doximycin; Doxitin; ***Fr.:*** Doxy; Doxygram†; Doxylets†; Doxypalu; Granudoxy; Monocline†; Spanor; Tolexine; Vibramycine N; Vibraveineuse†; ***Ger.:*** Azudoxat; Bactidox†; Clinofug D; Doxakne; Doxy Komb; Doxy M; Doxy-Diolan; Doxy-HP; Doxy-N-Tablinen; Doxy-P†; Doxy-Puren; Doxy-Tablinen†; Doxy-Wolff; Doxybiocin†; Doxyderma; Doxydoc; Doxyhexal; Doxymerck; Doxymono; Doxytem†; duradoxal†; Jenacyclin; Mespafin; Neodox; Sigadoxin; Supracyclin; Vibramycin; Vibravenos; ***Gr.:*** Impalamycin; Microvibrate; Novimax; Otosal; Relyomycin; Smilitene; Vibramycin; ***Hong Kong:*** Doxy; Medomycin; Remycin; Servidoxyne†; Tolexine†; Vibramycin; Wanmycin; Zadorin; ***India:*** Biodoxi; Doxy-1; Doxypal-DR; Vibazine; ***Irl.:*** By-Mycin; Vibramycin; ***Israel:*** Apodoxy†; Doxibiotic; Doxy; Doxylin; Doxytrim; Vibramycin; Vibravenos†; ***Ital.:*** Bassado; Doxina†; Gram-Val†; Miraclin; Monodoxin†; Ribociclina†; Unacil†; ***Malaysia:*** Bronmycin; Doline; Doxacyne; Doxy; Doxycillin; Doxymycin; Medomycin; Vibramycin; Wanmycin; Zadorin; ***Mex.:*** Apociclina†; Bioximicina; Domiken; Kenciclen†; Vibramicina; Vivradoxil; ***Neth.:*** Dagracycline; Doxy-Dagra; Neo-Dagracycline; Unidox; Vibra-S; Vibramycin; ***Norw.:*** Doryx; Doxylin; Doxysol; Dumoxin; Vibramycin; ***NZ:*** Doryx†; Doxine; Doxy; ***Port.:*** Actidox; Biocin; Doxytrex; Pluridoxina; Sigadoxin; Vibramicina; ***S.Afr.:*** Cyclidox; Doryx†; Doximal; Doxitab; Doxycyl; Doxyhexal; Dumoxin; Noritet†; Randoclin; Thedox†; Viacin†; Vibramycin; ***Singapore:*** Apo-Doxy; Bronmycin; Doryx; Doxilin; Doxine; Doxycap; Doxyline; Doxymycin; Medomycin†; Remycin; Servidoxyne†; Tetradox; Vibramycin; Wanmycin; ***Spain:*** Cildox†; Clisemina†; Docostyl; Dosil; Doxi Crisol; Doxi Sergo†; Doxiclat; Doxinate; Doxiten Bio; Doxiten†; Duo Gobens†; Novelciclina†; Peledox; Proderma; Retens; Rexilen; Solupen†; Tetrasan†; Vibracina; Vibravenosa; ***Swed.:*** Atridox; Doryx; Doxyferm; Vibramycin; ***Switz.:*** Diocimex; Doxy-basan; Doxycline; Doxylag; Doxysol; Helvedoclyn†; Rudocycline; Sigadoxin; Supracycline; Vibramycine; Vibraveineuse; Zadorin; ***Thai.:*** Amermycin; Bronmycin; Docline; Doxin; Doxy; Doxy-100†; Doxy-P; Doxycline; Doxylin; Doxymycin†; Dumoxin; Ibimycin†; Madoxy; Medomycin; Medoxin; Policycline; Servidoxyne; Siadocin; Tetradox; Torymycin; Veemycin; Vibramycin; ***UAE:*** Duradox; ***UK:*** Atridox†; Cyclodox†; Demix; Doxylar; Periostat; Ramysis†; Vibramycin; ***USA:*** Adoxa; Atridox; Bio-Tab†; Doryx; Doxy†; Doxychel†; Monodox; Periostat; Vibra-Tabs; Vibramycin.

**Multi-ingredient:** ***Austria:*** Mucotectan†; ***Ger.:*** Ambrodoxy; Ambroxol AL comp; Ambroxol comp; Amdox-Puren; Azudoxat comp; Doxam; Doximucol; Doxy Comp; Doxy Lindoxyl; Doxy Plus; Doxy-duramucal†; Doxy-Wolff Mucolyt; Doxysolvat; Jenabroxol comp; Mucotectan†; Sagittamuc†; Sigamuc; Terelit; ***Spain:*** Dosil Enzimatico; Doxiten Enzimatico; Pulmotropic; Solupen Enzimatico†; Sorciclina†.

## Enoxacin *(BAN, USAN, rINN)*

AT-2266; CI-919; Enoxacino; PD-107779. 1-Ethyl-6-fluoro-1,4-dihydro-4-oxo-7-(1-piperazinyl)-1,8-naphthyridine-3-carboxylic acid.

$C_{15}H_{17}FN_4O_3$ = 320.3.
*CAS — 74011-58-8.*
*ATC — J01MA04.*

**Pharmacopoeias.** In *Jpn. Chin.* includes the sesquihydrate.

### Adverse Effects and Precautions

As for Ciprofloxacin, p.188.

### Interactions

As for Ciprofloxacin, p.190.

Of the fluoroquinolones, enoxacin has been reported to cause the strongest interaction with theophylline (p.801) and with caffeine (p.782).

### Antimicrobial Action

As for Ciprofloxacin, p.190, although enoxacin is generally less potent *in vitro*.

### Pharmacokinetics

Peak plasma concentrations of 2 to 3 micrograms/mL are achieved 1 to 2 hours after a 400-mg dose of enoxacin by mouth. A plasma half-life of about 3 to 6 hours has been reported. Plasma protein binding has ranged from 18 to 67%. Enoxacin appears to be widely distributed in the body and concentrations higher than those in plasma have been reported in tissues such as lung, kidney, and prostate. High concentrations are achieved in bile, but the extent of biliary excretion is not completely clear.

Enoxacin is eliminated from the body mainly by urinary excretion, but also by metabolism. The major metabolite, 3-oxo-enoxacin, has some antibacterial activity. Urinary excretion of enoxacin is by both tubular secretion and glomerular filtration and may be reduced by probenecid. High concentrations are achieved in the urine since about 60% of an oral dose of enoxacin appears unchanged in the urine within 24 hours; about 10% is recovered as 3-oxo-enoxacin. In renal impairment the half-life of enoxacin may be prolonged and the oxometabolite may accumulate.

### Uses and Administration

Enoxacin is a fluoroquinolone antibacterial with actions and uses similar to those of ciprofloxacin (p.191). It is used mainly in the treatment of urinary-tract infections (p.153) and gonorrhoea (p.130).

For urinary-tract infections, enoxacin is given by mouth in doses of 200 to 400 mg twice daily. A single 400-mg dose is given for uncomplicated gonorrhoea.

For details of reduced doses to be used in renal impairment, see below.

◊ References.

1. Patel SS, Spencer CM. Enoxacin: a reappraisal of its clinical efficacy in the treatment of genitourinary tract infections. *Drugs* 1996; **51:** 137–60.

**Administration in renal impairment.** Half the usual dose of enoxacin is recommended in renal impairment when the creatinine clearance is below 30 mL/minute.

### Preparations

**Proprietary Preparations** (details are given in Part 3)

***Austral.:*** Enoxin†; ***Austria:*** Enoxor; ***Fr.:*** Enoxor; ***Ger.:*** Enoxor; ***Ital.:*** Bactidan; Enoxen; ***Jpn:*** Flumark; ***Mex.:*** Comprecin†; ***Port.:*** Vinone; ***S.Afr.:*** Bactidron; ***Spain:*** Almitil†; ***USA:*** Penetrex.

## Enrofloxacin *(BAN, USAN, rINN)*

Bay-Vp-2674; Enrofloxacino. 1-Cyclopropyl-7-(4-ethylpiperazin-1-yl)-6-fluoro-1,4-dihydro-4-oxoquinoline-3-carboxylic acid.

$C_{19}H_{22}FN_3O_3$ = 359.4.
*CAS — 93106-60-6.*

### Profile

Enrofloxacin is a fluoroquinolone antibacterial that is used in veterinary practice.

## Ertapenem Sodium *(BANM, USAN, rINNM)*

L-749345; MK-826; MK-0826; ZD-4433. Sodium (4R,5S,6S)-3-({(3S,5S)-5-[(m-Carboxyphenyl)carbamoyl]-3-pyrrolidinyl}thio)-6-[(1R)-1-hydroxyethyl]-4-methyl-7-oxo-1-azabicyclo[3.2.0]hept-2-ene-2-carboxylate.

$C_{22}H_{24}N_3NaO_7S$ = 497.5.
*CAS — 153832-46-3 (ertapenem); 153832-38-3 (ertapenem disodium); 153773-82-1 (ertapenem sodium).*
*ATC — J01DH03.*

**Incompatibility and stability.** References.

1. McQuade MS, *et al.* Stability and compatibility of reconstituted ertapenem with commonly used iv infusion and coinfusion solutions. *Am J Health-Syst Pharm* 2004; **61:** 38–45.

### Adverse Effects and Precautions

As for Imipenem, p.221.

Ertapenem is more stable to renal dehydropeptidase I than imipenem and administration with cilastatin, which inhibits the enzyme, is not required.

### Interactions

Probenecid inhibits the renal excretion of ertapenem thereby increasing its plasma concentrations and prolonging its elimination half-life.

### Antimicrobial Action

As for Imipenem, p.221,

Ertapenem is reported to be slightly more active *in vitro* than imipenem but has a narrower spectrum of activity and is not active against *Acinetobacter* or *Pseudomonas aeruginosa*.

### Pharmacokinetics

Following intravenous infusion of ertapenem 1 g over 30 minutes, a mean plasma concentration of 155 micrograms/mL is attained, falling to 9 micrograms/mL after 12 hours and 1 microgram/mL after 24 hours. After the same dose intramuscularly, a plasma concentration of 67 micrograms/mL is achieved after 2 hours. Bioavailability following intramuscular injection is about 90%.

Ertapenem is more than 90% bound to plasma proteins. It is distributed into breast milk. The plasma half-life is about 4 hours and may be prolonged in patients with renal impairment.

Ertapenem is partially metabolised via hydrolysis of its beta-lactam ring by dehydropeptidase I to an open-ringed metabolite. About 80% of a dose is excreted in the urine as both unchanged drug and metabolite. Approximately 10% is excreted in faeces.

Ertapenem is removed by haemodialysis.

### Uses and Administration

Ertapenem is a carbapenem beta-lactam antibacterial with actions and uses similar to those of imipenem (p.221). It is more stable to renal dehydropeptidase I than imipenem and need not be given with an enzyme inhibitor such as cilastatin. It is used in the treatment of susceptible infections including intra-abdominal infections, pneumonia, and infections of the skin and of the urinary tract. For details of these infections and their treatment, see under Choice of Antibacterial, p.120.

Ertapenem is administered as the sodium salt, but doses are expressed in terms of the base. 1.04 g of ertapenem sodium is approximately equivalent to 1 g of ertapenem. It is given by intravenous infusion over 30 minutes or by intramuscular injection, in a usual dose of 1 g once daily.

For details of reduced doses to be used in patients with renal impairment, see below.

◊ Reviews.

1. Curran MP, *et al.* Ertapenem: a review of its use in the management of bacterial infections. *Drugs* 2003; **63:** 1855–78.

**Administration in renal impairment.** Doses of ertapenem should be reduced in patients with renal impairment whose creatinine clearance is less than 30 mL/minute. A dose of 500 mg daily should be given to these patients, including those with end-stage renal disease. Patients undergoing haemodialysis who have received the 500-mg dose within the previous 6 hours should receive an additional 150 mg following each session.

## Preparations

**Proprietary Preparations** (details are given in Part 3)
***Austral.:*** Invanz; ***Fr.:*** Invanz; ***Ger.:*** Invanz; ***Irl.:*** Invanz; ***NZ:*** Invanz; ***Singapore:*** Invanz; ***UK:*** Invanz; ***USA:*** Invanz.

---

# Erythromycin *(BAN, rINN)*

Eritromicina; Erythromycinum. Erythromycin A is (2R,3S,4S,5R,6R,8R,10R,11R,12S,13R)-5-(3-amino-3,4,6-trideoxy-N,N-dimethyl-β-D-*xylo*-hexopyranosyloxy)-3-(2,6-dideoxy-3-C,3-O-dimethyl-α-L-*ribo*-hexopyranosyloxy)-13-ethyl-6,11,12-trihydroxy-2,4,6,8,10,12-hexamethyl-9-oxotridecan-13-olide.
$C_{37}H_{67}NO_{13}$ = 733.9.
*CAS — 114-07-8.*
*ATC — D10AF02; J01FA01; S01AA17.*

**Pharmacopoeias.** In *Chin., Eur.* (see p.vi), *Int., Jpn, Pol.,* and *US.*

**Ph. Eur. 5.0** (Erythromycin). It is produced by the growth of a strain of *Streptomyces erythreus* and is a mixture of macrolide antibiotics consisting largely of erythromycin A. It occurs as a white or slightly yellow powder or colourless or slightly yellow crystals; slightly hygroscopic. Slightly soluble in water but less soluble at higher temperatures; freely soluble in alcohol; soluble in methyl alcohol. Protect from light.

**USP 27** (Erythromycin). It consists primarily of erythromycin A. A white or slightly yellow, odourless or practically odourless, crystalline powder. Soluble 1 in 1000 of water; soluble in alcohol, in chloroform, and in ether. Store in airtight containers.

## Erythromycin Acistrate *(USAN, rINN)*

Acetylerythromycin Stearate; Acistrato de eritromicina. Erythromycin 2′-acetate stearate.
$C_{39}H_{69}NO_{14},C_{18}H_{36}O_2$ = 1060.4.
*CAS — 96128-89-1.*
*ATC — D10AF02; J01FA01; S01AA17.*

## Erythromycin Estolate *(BAN, USAN, rINNM)*

Erythromycin Propionate Lauryl Sulfate; Erythromycin Propionate Lauryl Sulphate; Erythromycini Estolas; Estolato de eritromicina; Propionylerythromycin Lauryl Sulphate. Erythromycin 2′-propionate dodecyl sulphate.
$C_{40}H_{71}NO_{14},C_{12}H_{26}O_4S$ = 1056.4.
*CAS — 3521-62-8.*
*ATC — D10AF02; J01FA01; S01AA17.*

**Pharmacopoeias.** In *Chin., Eur.* (see p.vi), *Pol.,* and *US.*

**Ph. Eur. 5.0** (Erythromycin Estolate). A white, crystalline powder. The potency is not less than 610 units/mg calculated on the anhydrous basis. Practically insoluble in water; freely soluble in alcohol; soluble in acetone; practically insoluble in dilute hydrochloric acid. A saturated solution in water has a pH of 5.5 to 7.0. Store in airtight containers at a temperature not exceeding 30°. Protect from light.

**USP 27** (Erythromycin Estolate). A white, odourless or practically odourless, crystalline powder. It has a potency equivalent to not less than 600 micrograms of erythromycin per mg, calculated on the anhydrous basis. Practically insoluble in water; soluble 1 in 20 of alcohol, 1 in 15 of acetone, and 1 in 10 of chloroform. Store in airtight containers.

## Erythromycin Ethyl Succinate *(BANM)*

Eritromicina, etilsuccinato de; Erythromycin Ethylsuccinate; Erythromycini Ethylsuccinas. Erythromycin 2′-(ethylsuccinate).
$C_{43}H_{75}NO_{16}$ = 862.1.
*CAS — 41342-53-4.*
*ATC — D10AF02; J01FA01; S01AA17.*

NOTE. Compounded preparations of erythromycin ethyl succinate may be represented by the following names:

- Co-erynsulfisox *(PEN)*—erythromycin ethyl succinate and acetyl sulfafurazole.

**Pharmacopoeias.** In *Chin., Eur.* (see p.vi), *Int., Jpn, Pol.,* and *US.*

**Ph. Eur. 5.0** (Erythromycin Ethylsuccinate; Erythromycin Ethyl Succinate BP 2003). A white hygroscopic crystalline powder. Practically insoluble in water; freely soluble in dehydrated alcohol, in acetone, and in methyl alcohol. Store in airtight containers. Protect from light.

**USP 27** (Erythromycin Ethylsuccinate). A white or slightly yellow, odourless or practically odourless, crystalline powder. It has a potency equivalent to not less than 765 micrograms of erythromycin per mg, calculated on the anhydrous basis. Very slightly soluble in water; freely soluble in alcohol, in chloroform, and in macrogol 400. Store in airtight containers.

## Erythromycin Gluceptate *(BANM, rINNM)*

Gluceptato de eritromicina. Erythromycin glucoheptonate.
$C_{37}H_{67}NO_{13},C_7H_{14}O_8$ = 960.1.
*CAS — 304-63-2; 23067-13-2.*
*ATC — D10AF02; J01FA01; S01AA17.*

**Pharmacopoeias.** In *US.*

**USP 27** (Sterile Erythromycin Gluceptate). It is erythromycin gluceptate suitable for parenteral use. It has a potency equivalent to not less than 600 micrograms of erythromycin per mg, calculated on the anhydrous basis. pH of a 2.5% solution in water is between 6.0 and 8.0.

## Erythromycin Lactobionate *(BANM, rINNM)*

Erythromycini Lactobionas; Lactobionato de eritromicina. Erythromycin mono(4-O-β-D-galactopyranosyl-D-gluconate).
$C_{37}H_{67}NO_{13},C_{12}H_{22}O_{12}$ = 1092.2.
*CAS — 3847-29-8.*
*ATC — D10AF02; J01FA01; S01AA17.*

**Pharmacopoeias.** In *Chin., Eur.* (see p.vi), *Int., Jpn, Pol.,* and *US.*

**Ph. Eur. 5.0** (Erythromycin Lactobionate). White or slightly yellow, hygroscopic powder. Soluble in water; freely soluble in dehydrated alcohol and in methyl alcohol; very slightly soluble in acetone and in dichloromethane. A 2% solution in water has a pH of 6.5 to 7.5. Store in airtight containers at a temperature not exceeding 25°.

**USP 27** (Sterile Erythromycin Lactobionate). It has a potency equivalent to not less than 525 micrograms of erythromycin per mg, calculated on the anhydrous basis. pH of a solution in water containing the equivalent of erythromycin 5% is between 6.5 and 7.5.

## Erythromycin Propionate *(BANM, USAN, rINNM)*

Erythromycin Propanoate; Propionato de eritromicina; Propionylerythromycin. Erythromycin 2′-propionate.
$C_{40}H_{71}NO_{14}$ = 790.0.
*CAS — 134-36-1.*
*ATC — D10AF02; J01FA01; S01AA17.*

**Pharmacopoeias.** In *Fr.*

## Erythromycin Stearate *(BANM, rINNM)*

Erythromycini Stearas; Estearato de eritromicina. Erythromycin octadecanoate.
$C_{37}H_{67}NO_{13},C_{18}H_{36}O_2$ = 1018.4.
*CAS — 643-22-1.*
*ATC — D10AF02; J01FA01; S01AA17.*

**Pharmacopoeias.** In *Eur.* (see p.vi), *Int., Jpn, Pol., US,* and *Viet.*

**Ph. Eur. 5.0** (Erythromycin Stearate). A mixture of the stearates of erythromycin and stearic acid. A white crystalline powder. Practically insoluble in water; soluble in acetone and in methyl alcohol. Solutions may be opalescent.

**USP 27** (Erythromycin Stearate). The stearic acid salt of erythromycin with an excess of stearic acid. White or slightly yellow crystals or powder, odourless or may have a slight, earthy odour. Practically insoluble in water; soluble in alcohol, in chloroform, in ether, and in methyl alcohol. Store in airtight containers.

**Incompatibility and stability.** The stability of erythromycin derivatives is dependent upon pH, with particularly rapid degradation occurring at a pH greater than 10 or less than 5.5. Incompatibility might reasonably be expected, therefore, when erythromycin preparations are mixed with drugs or preparations that have a highly acidic or alkaline pH. In practice, reports of incompatibility are not always consistent, and other factors such as the temperature and concentration of solutions, and the diluents used, may play a role.

## Adverse Effects

Erythromycin and its salts and esters are generally well tolerated and serious adverse effects are rare. Gastrointestinal disturbances such as abdominal discomfort and cramp, nausea, vomiting, and diarrhoea are fairly common after both oral and parenteral use, probably because of the stimulant activity of erythromycin on the gut. Gastrointestinal effects are dose-related and appear to be more common in young than in older subjects. Supra-infection with resistant organisms may occur and pseudomembranous colitis has been reported. Hypersensitivity reactions appear to be uncommon, having been reported in about 0.5% of patients, and include pruritus, urticaria and skin rash as well as occasional cases of anaphylaxis. Hypersensitivity or irritation may occur following topical application of erythromycin.

A hypersensitivity reaction may also be responsible for the hepatotoxicity sometimes reported in patients receiving erythromycin or its derivatives. Symptoms indicative of cholestasis, including upper abdominal pain (sometimes very severe), nausea and vomiting, abnormal liver function values, raised serum bilirubin and usually jaundice, may be accompanied by rash, fever, and eosinophilia. Symptoms usually occur initially in patients who have been receiving the drug for more than 10 days, although they may develop more quickly in patients given the drug previously. Erythromycin may interfere with tests for serum aspartate aminotransferase, which might make diagnosis of hepatotoxicity more difficult.

The majority of reports of liver dysfunction have been in patients receiving the estolate, and it has been suggested that the propionyl ester linkage is particularly associated with hepatotoxicity, but symptoms have been reported in patients receiving the base and most of the other derivatives, both by mouth and parenterally. Hepatic dysfunction seems to be rare in children. The effects of erythromycin on the liver are generally reversible on discontinuing treatment.

A generally reversible sensorineural deafness, sometimes with tinnitus, has been reported in patients receiving erythromycin and appears to be related to serum concentration, with an increased likelihood of such effects in patients given doses of 4 g or more daily of base or its equivalent, in those given intravenous therapy, and in those with renal or hepatic impairment.

Other adverse effects that have been reported in patients receiving erythromycin include agranulocytosis, prolongation of the QT interval and other arrhythmias, central neurotoxicity including psychotic reactions and nightmares, a myasthenia-like syndrome, and pancreatitis. Parenteral formulations of erythromycin are irritant and intravenous administration may produce thrombophlebitis, particularly at high doses. Intramuscular injection is generally avoided as it may produce severe pain.

◊ General reviews.

1. Periti P, *et al.* Adverse effects of macrolide antibacterials. *Drug Safety* 1993; **9:** 346–64.
2. Principi N, Esposito S. Comparative tolerability of erythromycin and newer macrolide antibacterials in paediatric patients. *Drug Safety* 1999; **20:** 25–41.
3. Rubinstein E. Comparative safety of the different macrolides. *Int J Antimicrob Agents* 2001; **18** (suppl 1): S71–S76.

**Effects on body temperature.** A report of hypothermia associated with oral erythromycin in 2 children.[1] Symptoms resolved on withdrawal of the medication. The children were cousins, perhaps indicating a genetic predisposition to the effect.

1. Hassel B. Hypothermia from erythromycin. *Ann Intern Med* 1991; **115:** 69–70.

**Effects on the gastrointestinal tract.** Comparison in patients with upper respiratory-tract infections has suggested that erythromycin ethyl succinate may be associated with less abdominal pain than an equivalent dosage of erythromycin base; in a similar study the ethyl succinate and acistrate did not differ in their gastrointestinal tolerability.[1] Another study has indicated that there was no significant difference in gastrointestinal symptoms between plain and enteric-coated formulations of erythromycin base.[2] Severe nausea and vomiting following rapid intravenous infusion of erythromycin lactobionate ceased in 2 patients who transferred to erythromycin base or ethyl succinate by mouth.[3] However, the adverse effects may have been due to the rate of administration, since in 2 further patients symptoms resolved when the lactobionate was given more slowly as a more dilute solution.[3]

There have been a number of studies suggesting an association between erythromycin and infantile hypertrophic pyloric stenosis.[4-6] A retrospective cohort study of 469 infants who had received erythromycin found that 43 were diagnosed with the condition including 36 male infants, although erythromycin had been prescribed almost equally for males and females.[5] All the infants in whom stenosis developed were given erythromycin in the first 2 weeks of life. In another study,[6] involving 7138 infants who received erythromycin between 3 and 90 days of life, use of the drug between 3 and 13 days of life was associated with an almost 8-fold increased risk of infantile hypertrophic pyloric stenosis. However, current evidence does not support a generalisation of this association to the whole class of macrolides.[7]

For reference to the stimulant effects of erythromycin on the gastrointestinal tract, see Decreased Gastrointestinal Motility under Uses and Administration, below.

1. Saloranta P, *et al.* Erythromycin ethylsuccinate, base and acistrate in the treatment of upper respiratory tract infection: two comparative studies of tolerability. *J Antimicrob Chemother* 1989; **24:** 455–62.
2. Ellsworth AJ, *et al.* Prospective comparison of patient tolerance to enteric-coated vs non-enteric-coated erythromycin. *J Fam Pract* 1990; **31:** 265–70.

3. Seifert CF, *et al.* Intravenous erythromycin lactobionate-induced severe nausea and vomiting. *DICP Ann Pharmacother* 1989; **23:** 40–4.
4. Honein MA, *et al.* Infantile hypertrophic pyloric stenosis after pertussis prophylaxis with erythromycin: a case review and cohort study. *Lancet* 1999; **354:** 2101–5. Correction. *ibid.* 2000; **355:** 758.
5. Mahon BE, *et al.* Maternal and infant use of erythromycin and other macrolide antibiotics as risk factors for infantile hypertrophic pyloric stenosis. *J Pediatr* 2001; **139:** 380–4.
6. Cooper WO, *et al.* Very early exposure to erythromycin and infantile hypertrophic pyloric stenosis. *Arch Pediatr Adolesc Med* 2002; **156:** 647–50.
7. Hauben M, Amsden GW. The association of erythromycin and infantile hypertrophic pyloric stenosis: causal or coincidental? *Drug Safety* 2002; **25:** 929–42.

**Effects on the heart.** There have been several reports[1-6] of QT prolongation or torsade de pointes associated with erythromycin, particularly with intravenous use.

A review[7] of reports of torsade de pointes received by the FDA Adverse Event Reporting System between 1987 and December 2000 identified 156 cases associated with use of the macrolides azithromycin, clarithromycin, dirithromycin, or erythromycin. Of these reports, half involved the use of other drugs known to prolong the QT interval; co-morbid diseases and physiological abnormalities, including cardiac abnormalities, were also commonly reported.

1. McComb JM, *et al.* Recurrent ventricular tachycardia associated with QT prolongation after mitral valve replacement and its association with intravenous administration of erythromycin. *Am J Cardiol* 1984; **54:** 922–3.
2. Schoenenberger RA, *et al.* Association of intravenous erythromycin and potentially fatal ventricular tachycardia with Q-T prolongation (torsades de pointes). *BMJ* 1990; **330:** 1375–6.
3. Nattel S, *et al.* Erythromycin-induced long QT syndrome: concordance with quinidine and underlying cellular electrophysiologic mechanism. *Am J Med* 1990; **89:** 235–8.
4. Gitler B, *et al.* Torsades de pointes induced by erythromycin. *Chest* 1994; **105:** 368–72.
5. Gouyon JB, *et al.* Cardiac toxicity of intravenous erythromycin lactobionate in preterm infants. *Pediatr Infect Dis J* 1994; **13:** 840–1.
6. Drici M-D, *et al.* Cardiac actions of erythromycin: influence of female sex. *JAMA* 1998; **280:** 1774–6.
7. Shaffer D, *et al.* Concomitant risk factors in reports of torsades de pointes associated with macrolide use: review of the United States Food and Drug Administration Adverse Event Reporting System. *Clin Infect Dis* 2002; **35:** 197–200.

**Effects on the neonate.** For a suggestion that erythromycin might be associated with an increased risk of infantile hypertrophic pyloric stenosis in neonates, see under Effects on the Gastrointestinal Tract, above.

**Effects on the skin.** Skin reactions ranging from mild eruptions to erythema multiforme, Stevens-Johnson syndrome, and toxic epidermal necrolysis have rarely been reported with macrolides.

References.

1. Lestico MR, Smith AD. Stevens-Johnson syndrome following erythromycin administration. *Am J Health-Syst Pharm* 1995; **52:** 1805–7.
2. Sullivan S, *et al.* Stevens-Johnson syndrome secondary to erythromycin. *Ann Pharmacother* 1999; **33:** 1369.

**Overdosage.** Acute pancreatitis was reported in a 12-year-old girl after ingestion of about 5 g of erythromycin base.[1]

1. Berger TM, *et al.* Acute pancreatitis in a 12-year-old girl after an erythromycin overdose. *Pediatrics* 1992; **90:** 624–6.

## Precautions

Erythromycin and its derivatives should be avoided in those known to be hypersensitive to it, or in those who have previously developed jaundice. All forms of erythromycin should be used with care in patients with existing liver disease or hepatic impairment, and the estolate is best avoided in such patients. Repeated courses of the estolate or use for longer than 10 days increases the risk of hepatotoxicity. Erythromycin may aggravate muscle weakness in patients with myasthenia gravis. Erythromycin should be used with care in patients with a history of arrhythmias or a prolonged QT interval.

Erythromycin may interfere with some diagnostic tests including measurements of urinary catecholamines and 17-hydroxycorticosteroids. It has also been associated with falsely-elevated serum aspartate aminotransferase values when measured colorimetrically, although genuine elevations of this enzyme, due to hepatotoxicity, also occur, particularly with the estolate.

Erythromycin is irritant; solutions for parenteral use should be suitably diluted and given by intravenous infusion over 20 to 60 minutes to reduce the incidence of thrombophlebitis. Rapid infusion is also more likely to be associated with arrhythmias or hypotension.

**Breast feeding.** There has been a report of a breast-fed infant who developed pyloric stenosis thought to be associated with use of erythromycin by the mother.[1] (See also Effects on the Gastrointestinal Tract, above.) However, the American Academy of Pediatrics state that, although erythromycin is concentrated in human breast milk, no adverse effects have been observed in breast-fed infants whose mothers were receiving erythromycin and it is therefore usually compatible with breast feeding.[2]

1. Stang H. Pyloric stenosis associated with erythromycin ingested through breastmilk. *Minn Med* 1986; **69:** 669–70, 682.
2. American Academy of Pediatrics. The transfer of drugs and other chemicals into human milk. *Pediatrics* 2001; **108:** 776–89. Correction. *ibid.*; 1029. Also available at: http://aappolicy.aappublications.org/cgi/content/full/pediatrics%3b108/3/776 (accessed 26/05/04)

**Porphyria.** Erythromycin has been associated with acute attacks of porphyria and is considered unsafe in porphyric patients.

**Pregnancy.** Of 298 pregnant women who took erythromycin estolate, clindamycin, or placebo for 3 weeks or longer, about 14, 4, and 3% respectively had abnormally high serum aspartate aminotransferase values.[1] Erythromycin estolate should probably not be given to pregnant women.

1. McCormack WM, *et al.* Hepatotoxicity of erythromycin estolate during pregnancy. *Antimicrob Agents Chemother* 1977; **12:** 630–5.

## Interactions

Erythromycin and other macrolides have the potential to interact with a large number of drugs through their action on hepatic cytochrome P450 isoenzymes, particularly CYP1A2 and CYP3A4. Macrolides inhibit drug metabolism by microsomal cytochromes by competitive inhibition and by the formation of inactive complexes. Such interactions can result in severe adverse effects, including ventricular arrhythmias with astemizole, cisapride, and terfenadine. Enzyme inhibition is reported to be particularly pronounced with macrolides such as erythromycin and troleandomycin. Clarithromycin is less likely to inhibit the hepatic metabolism of other drugs, although those undergoing first-pass metabolism may still be affected. Other macrolides such as azithromycin and dirithromycin are reported to have little or no effect on hepatic cytochromes, and consequently may produce fewer interactions.

Macrolides themselves have been reported rarely to prolong the QT interval and should be used with care with other drugs known to also have this effect.

Other mechanisms by which macrolides cause interactions include suppression of the gastrointestinal flora responsible for the intraluminal metabolism of digoxin and possibly oral contraceptives, and the stimulant effect of macrolides on gastrointestinal motility which is believed to be responsible for the interaction between spiramycin and levodopa.

Cimetidine is one of the few drugs reported to affect erythromycin (see below).

The effect on antimicrobial action when erythromycin is given with other antimicrobials is discussed under Antimicrobial Action, below.

◊ General references to interactions associated with macrolide antibacterials.

1. von Rosenstiel N-A, Adam D. Macrolide antibacterials: drug interactions of clinical significance. *Drug Safety* 1995; **13:** 105–22.
2. Westphal JF. Macrolide-induced clinically relevant drug interactions with cytochrome P-450A (CYP) 3A4: an update focused on clarithromycin, azithromycin and dirithromycin. *Br J Clin Pharmacol* 2000; **50:** 285–95.
3. Pai MP, *et al.* Macrolide drug interactions: an update. *Ann Pharmacother* 2000; **34:** 495–513.

◊ For reference to the effects of erythromycin and other macrolides on other drugs, see

- alfentanil (p.12)
- bromocriptine (p.1202)
- buspirone (p.672)
- carbamazepine (p.355)
- ciclosporin (p.1354)
- clozapine (p.687)
- colchicine (p.415)
- digoxin (p.897)
- dihydroergotamine and ergotamine (p.468)
- disopyramide (p.904)
- levodopa (p.1208)
- midazolam and triazolam (p.693)
- phenytoin (p.372)
- pimozide (p.679 and p.715)
- quetiapine (p.718)
- quinidine (p.992)
- repaglinide (p.344)
- rifabutin (p.249)
- sildenafil (p.1744)
- simvastatin and other statins (p.998)
- tacrolimus (p.1364)
- terfenadine (p.441)
- theophylline (p.801)
- valproate (p.381)
- vinblastine (p.591)
- warfarin (p.1024)
- zopiclone (p.730)

In the case of astemizole, cisapride, and terfenadine the UK Committee on Safety of Medicines (CSM) has warned that there is a risk of inducing ventricular arrhythmias if erythromycin, or possibly other macrolides, are also given,[1,2] and that, in particular, cisapride should not be used with macrolides.[3]

1. Committee on Safety of Medicines. Ventricular arrhythmias due to terfenadine and astemizole. *Current Problems 35* 1992.
2. Committee on Safety of Medicines/Medicines Control Agency. Cisapride (Prepulsid, Alimax): interactions with antifungals and antibiotics can lead to ventricular arrhythmias. *Current Problems* 1996; **22:** 1.
3. Committee on Safety of Medicines/Medicines Control Agency. Cisapride (Prepulsid): risk of arrhythmias. *Current Problems* 1998; **24:** 11. Also available at: http://medicines.mhra.gov.uk/ourwork/monitorsafequalmed/currentproblems/volume24aug.htm (accessed 26/05/04)

**Cimetidine.** Cimetidine may increase plasma concentrations of erythromycin and deafness occurred in a patient taking both drugs.[1]

1. Mogford N, *et al.* Erythromycin deafness and cimetidine treatment. *BMJ* 1994; **309:** 1620.

**Mechanism.** In *rats* and humans, troleandomycin, and erythromycin and some of its derivatives, induce microsomal enzymes; the nitrosoalkane metabolites so formed produce stable inactive complexes with the iron of cytochrome P450. Eventually the oxidative metabolism of other drugs may be decreased. These effects are marked after troleandomycin, moderate after erythromycin, small after oleandomycin, and absent or negligible after josamycin, midecamycin, or spiramycin.[1,2]

1. Pessayre D, *et al.* Drug interactions and hepatitis produced by some macrolide antibiotics. *J Antimicrob Chemother* 1985; **16** (suppl A): 181–94.
2. Periti P, *et al.* Pharmacokinetic drug interactions of macrolides. *Clin Pharmacokinet* 1992; **23:** 106–31.

## Antimicrobial Action

Erythromycin is a macrolide antibacterial with a broad and essentially bacteriostatic action against many Gram-positive and to a lesser extent some Gram-negative bacteria, as well as other organisms including some *Mycoplasma* spp., Chlamydiaceae, *Rickettsia* spp., and spirochaetes.

*Mechanism of action.* Erythromycin and other macrolides bind reversibly to the 50S subunit of the ribosome, resulting in blockage of the transpeptidation or translocation reactions, inhibition of protein synthesis, and hence inhibition of cell growth. Its action is predominantly bacteriostatic, but high concentrations are slowly bactericidal against the more sensitive strains. Because macrolides penetrate readily into white blood cells and macrophages there has been some interest in their potential synergy with host defence mechanisms *in vivo*. The actions of erythromycin are increased at moderately alkaline pH (up to about 8.5), particularly in Gram-negative species, probably because of the improved cellular penetration of the nonionised form of the drug.

*Spectrum of activity.* Erythromycin has a broad spectrum of activity. The following pathogenic organisms are usually sensitive to erythromycin (but see also Resistance, below).

Gram-positive cocci, particularly streptococci such as *Streptococcus pneumoniae* and *Str. pyogenes* are sensitive. Most strains of *Staphylococcus aureus* remain susceptible, although resistance can emerge rapidly, and some enterococcal strains are also susceptible.

Many other Gram-positive organisms respond to erythromycin, including *Bacillus anthracis*, *Corynebacterium diphtheriae*, *Erysipelothrix rhusiopathiae*, and *Listeria monocytogenes*. Anaerobic *Clostridium* spp. are also usually susceptible, as is *Propionibacterium acnes*. *Nocardia* spp. vary in their susceptibility.

Gram-negative cocci including *Neisseria meningitidis* and *N. gonorrhoeae*, and *Moraxella catarrhalis* (*Branhamella catarrhalis*) are usually sensitive.

Other Gram-negative organisms vary in their susceptibility, but *Bordetella* spp., some *Brucella* strains, *Flavobacterium*, and *Legionella* spp. are usually susceptible. *Haemophilus ducreyi* is reportedly susceptible, but

*H. influenzae* is somewhat less so. The Enterobacteriaceae are usually resistant, although some strains may respond at alkaline pH. *Helicobacter pylori* and most strains of *Campylobacter jejuni* are sensitive (about 10% of the latter are reported to be resistant).

Among the Gram-negative anaerobes most strains of *Bacteroides fragilis* and many *Fusobacterium* strains are resistant.

Other organisms usually sensitive to erythromycin include *Actinomyces*, Chlamydiaceae, rickettsias, spirochaetes such as *Treponema pallidum* and *Borrelia burgdorferi*, some mycoplasmas (notably *Mycoplasma pneumoniae*), and some of the opportunistic mycobacteria: *Mycobacterium scrofulaceum* and *M. kansasii* are usually susceptible, but *M. intracellulare* is often resistant and *M. fortuitum* usually so.

Fungi, yeasts, and viruses are not susceptible to erythromycin.

*Activity with other antimicrobials.* As with other bacteriostatic antimicrobials, the possibility of an antagonistic effect if erythromycin is given with a bactericide exists, and some antagonism has been shown *in vitro* between erythromycin and various penicillins and cephalosporins or gentamicin. However, in practice the results of such concurrent use are complex, and depend on the organism; in some cases synergy has been seen. Because of the adjacency of their binding sites on the ribosome, erythromycin may competitively inhibit the effects of chloramphenicol or lincosamides such as clindamycin. A synergistic effect has been seen when erythromycin was combined with a sulfonamide, notably against *Haemophilus influenzae.* Erythromycin has also been reported to enhance the antiplasmodial actions of chloroquine.

*Resistance.* Several mechanisms of acquired resistance to erythromycin have been reported of which the most common is a plasmid-mediated ability to methylate ribosomal RNA, resulting in decreased binding of the antimicrobial drug. This can result in cross-resistance between erythromycin, other macrolides, lincosamides, and streptogramin B, because they share a common binding site on the ribosome and this pattern of resistance is referred to as the $MLS_B$ phenotype. It is seen in staphylococci, and to a somewhat lesser extent in streptococci, as well as in a variety of other species including *Bacteroides fragilis, Clostridium perfringens, Corynebacterium diphtheriae, Listeria,* and *Legionella* spp.

Decreased binding of antimicrobial to the ribosome may also occur as a result of a chromosomal mutation, resulting in an alteration of the ribosomal proteins in the 50S subunit, which conveys one-step high-level erythromycin resistance. This form of resistance has been demonstrated in *Escherichia coli* and some strains of *Str. pyogenes*, and probably occurs in *Staphylococcus aureus.*

Other forms of erythromycin resistance may be due to the production of a plasmid-determined erythromycin esterase which can inactivate the drug, or to decreased drug penetration. The latter may be partly responsible for the intrinsic resistance of Gram-negative bacteria like the Enterobacteriaceae, but has also been shown to be acquired as a plasmid-mediated determinant in some organisms; production of a protein which increases drug efflux from the cell is thought to explain the MS form of resistance, in which organisms are resistant to 14-carbon ring macrolides and streptogramins, but retain sensitivity to 16-carbon ring macrolides and lincosamides.

The incidence of resistance varies greatly with the area and the organism concerned and, although the emergence of resistance is rarely a problem in the short-term treatment of infection, it is quite common in conditions requiring prolonged treatment such as endocarditis due to *Staph. aureus.* The incidence of resistance in streptococci is generally lower than in *Staph. aureus* but shows geographical variation and may be increasing in some countries, including the UK. In addition, localised outbreaks of resistant strains may occur and produce a much higher incidence of resistance.

**Antipseudomonal activity.** Although macrolides have limited direct antibacterial activity against *Pseudomonas aeruginosa*, prolonged exposure has produced antipseudomonal effects *in vitro*[1,2] and synergy has been demonstrated with other antipseudomonals.[3] Erythromycin and clarithromycin appear to have the greatest activity. This action has been attributed to the ability of macrolides to reduce the protective biofilm produced by some strains of *P. aeruginosa.*[4]

1. Tateda K, *et al.* Effects of sub-MICs of erythromycin and other macrolide antibiotics on serum sensitivity of Pseudomonas aeruginosa. *Antimicrob Agents Chemother* 1993; **37:** 675–80.
2. Tateda K, *et al.* Direct evidence of antipseudomonal activity of macrolides: exposure-dependent bactericidal activity and inhibition of protein synthesis by erythromycin, clarithromycin, and azithromycin. *Antimicrob Agents Chemother* 1996; **40:** 2271–5.
3. Bui KQ, *et al.* In vitro and in vivo influence of adjunct clarithromycin on the treatment of mucoid Pseudomonas aeruginosa. *J Antimicrob Chemother* 2000; **45:** 57–62.
4. Yasuda H, *et al.* Interaction between biofilms formed by Pseudomonas aeruginosa and clarithromycin. *Antimicrob Agents Chemother* 1993; **37:** 1749–55.

**Resistance.** References to macrolide resistance.

1. Barry AL, *et al.* Macrolide resistance among Streptococcus pneumoniae and Streptococcus pyogenes isolated from outpatients in the USA. *J Antimicrob Chemother* 1997; **40:** 139–40.
2. Bingen E, *et al.* Resistance to macrolides in Streptococcus pyogenes in France in pediatric patients. *Antimicrob Agents Chemother* 2000; **44:** 1453–7.
3. Coates P, *et al.* Prevalence of antibiotic-resistant propionibacteria on the skin of acne patients: 10-year surveillance data and snapshot distribution study. *Br J Dermatol* 2002; **146:** 840–8.
4. Leclercq R. Mechanisms of resistance to macrolides and lincosamides: nature of the resistance elements and their clinical implications. *Clin Infect Dis* 2002; **34:** 482–92.

## Pharmacokinetics

Erythromycin base is unstable in gastric acid, and absorption is therefore variable and unreliable. In consequence, the base is usually given in film- or enteric-coated preparations, or one of the more acid-stable salts or esters is used. Food may reduce absorption of the base or the stearate, although this depends to some extent on the formulation; the esters are generally more reliably and quickly absorbed and their absorption is little affected by food, obviating any need to take them before food.

Peak plasma concentrations generally occur between 1 and 4 hours after a dose and have been reported to range between about 0.3 and 1.0 micrograms/mL after 250 mg of erythromycin base, and from 0.3 to 1.9 micrograms/mL after 500 mg. Similar concentrations have been seen after equivalent doses of the stearate. Somewhat higher peak concentrations may be achieved on repeated use 4 times daily. Higher total concentrations are achieved after oral doses of the estolate or ethyl succinate, but only about 20 to 30% of estolate or 55% of ethyl succinate is present as the active base, the rest being present as the inactive ester (in the case of the estolate as the propionate). Peak concentrations of about 500 nanograms/mL of erythromycin base have been reported following 250 mg of the estolate or 500 mg of the ethyl succinate. A peak of 3 to 4 micrograms/mL can be achieved after 200 mg of gluceptate or lactobionate intravenously.

Erythromycin is widely distributed throughout body tissues and fluids, although it does not cross the blood-brain barrier well and concentrations in CSF are low. Relatively high concentrations are found in the liver and spleen, and some is taken up into polymorphonuclear lymphocytes and macrophages. Around 70 to 75% of the base is protein bound, but after administration as the estolate the propionate ester is stated to be about 95% protein bound. Erythromycin crosses the placenta: fetal plasma concentrations are variously stated to be 5 to 20% of those in the mother. It is distributed into breast milk.

Erythromycin is excreted in high concentrations in the bile and 2 to 5% of an oral dose is excreted unchanged in the urine. As much as 12 to 15% of an intravenous dose may be excreted by the urinary route. Some erythromycin is demethylated in the liver but its metabolic fate has not been completely determined. The half-life of erythromycin is usually reported to be about 1.5 to 2.5 hours, although this may be slightly longer in patients with renal impairment.

## Uses and Administration

Erythromycin is a macrolide antibacterial with a wide spectrum of activity, that has been used in the treatment of a wide variety of infections caused by susceptible organisms.

Its uses have included bronchitis, severe campylobacter enteritis, chancroid, diphtheria, legionnaires' disease and other *Legionella* infections, neonatal conjunctivitis, pertussis, pneumonia (mycoplasmal and other atypical pneumonias as well as streptococcal), sinusitis, and trench fever, and, combined with neomycin, for the prophylaxis of surgical infection in patients undergoing bowel surgery.

Erythromycin is used as an alternative to penicillin in penicillin-allergic patients with various conditions including anthrax, actinomycosis, leptospirosis, listeriosis, mouth infections, otitis media (usually with a sulfonamide such as sulfafurazole), pelvic inflammatory disease caused by *Neisseria gonorrhoeae*, pharyngitis, the prevention of perinatal streptococcal infections, rheumatic fever, and infections in splenectomised patients, and staphylococcal and streptococcal skin infections. It has also been used in the treatment of penicillin-allergic patients with syphilis, but there are doubts about its efficacy. In penicillin-allergic patients in the early stages of Lyme disease, erythromycin may be used as an alternative to a tetracycline; this use is generally restricted to pregnant women and young children, since it is less effective than other drugs. It is also used as an alternative to the tetracyclines in patients with *Chlamydia* or *Chlamydophila* infections (such as epididymitis, lymphogranuloma venereum, nongonococcal urethritis, pneumonia, psittacosis, and trachoma), in Q fever, and in spotted fevers.

For details of these infections and their treatment, see under Choice of Antibacterial, p.120.

Both oral and topical erythromycin may be used in acne (see Skin Disorders, below).

*Administration and dosage.* Erythromycin may be given as the base or its salts or esters; doses are expressed in terms of the base. Each 1 g of erythromycin is approximately equivalent to the following amounts of each salt or ester:

- erythromycin estolate 1.44 g
- erythromycin ethyl succinate 1.17 g
- erythromycin gluceptate 1.3 g
- erythromycin lactobionate 1.5 g
- erythromycin propionate 1.08 g
- erythromycin stearate 1.39 g

The usual oral adult dose is the equivalent of erythromycin 1 to 2 g daily in 2 to 4 divided doses; for severe infections this may be increased to up to 4 g daily in divided doses. Daily doses higher than 1 g should be given in more than 2 divided doses. Doses may need to be reduced in patients with renal impairment (see below). For children the dose is usually about 30 to 50 mg/kg daily in divided doses although it may be doubled in severe infections; based on age, children of 2 to 8 years may be given 1 g daily in divided doses and infants and children up to 2 years of age may be given 500 mg daily in divided doses.

For the prevention of streptococcal infections in patients with evidence of rheumatic fever or heart disease, who are unable to take penicillin or sulfonamides, a dose of 250 mg twice daily may be given.

For the management of acne, maintenance doses as low as 250 mg daily have been used in adults but resistant strains of propionibacteria are widespread; the *British National Formulary* recommends a dose of 500 mg twice daily.

In patients who are unable to take erythromycin by mouth and in those who are severely ill, in whom it is necessary to attain an immediate high blood concentration, erythromycin may be given intravenously in the form of one of its more soluble salts such as the gluceptate or the lactobionate, in doses equivalent to those by mouth.

To reduce the risk of venous irritation it should be administered only by continuous or intermittent intravenous infusion of a solution containing not more than 0.5% of erythromycin. Intermittent infusions should be given every 6 hours over 20 to 60 minutes.

For the preparation of solutions of erythromycin gluceptate or lactobionate for infusion, a primary solution containing not more than 5% of erythromycin should be prepared first; only water for injection should be used in preparing the primary solution. It should be further diluted before intravenous administration with sodium chloride 0.9% or other suitable intravenous fluid. Acidic solutions, such as glucose, should only be used if neutralised with sodium bicarbonate.

*Other routes.* Erythromycin was formerly given by intramuscular injection, but such injections are painful and are no longer generally recommended. Erythromycin has been used as a 0.5 to 1% ophthalmic ointment for the treatment and prophylaxis of infections of the eye, particularly of neonatal conjunctivitis. It may also be applied topically as a 2 to 4% gel or solution for the treatment of acne vulgaris.

Propionyl erythromycin mercaptosuccinate has also been used. Erythromycin salnacedin, a prodrug of erythromycin, acetylcysteine, and salicylic acid, has been investigated for the treatment of acne. Erythromycin thiocyanate and erythromycin phosphate are used in veterinary medicine.

◊ Reviews.


1. Zhanel GG, *et al.* Review of macrolides and ketolides: focus on respiratory tract infections. *Drugs* 2001; **61:** 443–98.


**Administration.** A discussion of the significance of different formulations and salts used for oral preparations of erythromycin concluded that there was no clear evidence that any was superior in terms of clinical effect.[1]


1. Anonymous. Giving erythromycin by mouth. *Drug Ther Bull* 1995; **33:** 77–9.


**Administration in renal impairment.** A maximum dose of erythromycin 1.5 g daily has been suggested for patients with severe renal impairment.

**Decreased gastrointestinal motility.** Erythromycin stimulates gut motility, apparently by acting as a motilin receptor agonist, although it has been suggested that it may have other actions as well.[1] It has been tried, with some success, for its prokinetic action in a small number of patients with decreased gastrointestinal motility (p.1241) including those with gastroparesis,[2] reflux ileus,[3] acute colonic pseudo-obstruction (Ogilvie's syndrome),[3,4] delayed gastric emptying following pancreatic-duodenal surgery,[5] and neonatal postoperative intestinal dysmotility.[6] It has also been used to increase gastrointestinal motility in critically ill, mechanically ventilated patients[7] and in preterm very low birthweight infants.[8] However, the prophylactic or routine use of erythromycin in preterm infants has been cautioned against,[8] and adverse effects associated with the long-term use of erythromycin that is necessary in, for example, diabetic gastroparesis, may be problematic.[9]


1. Catnach SM, Fairclough PD. Erythromycin and the gut. *Gut* 1992; **33:** 397–401.
2. Maganti K, *et al.* Oral erythromycin and symptomatic relief of gastroparesis: a systematic review. *Am J Gastroenterol* 2003; **98:** 259–63.
3. Armstrong DN, *et al.* Erythromycin for reflux ileus in Ogilvie's syndrome. *Lancet* 1991; **337:** 378.
4. Bonacini M, *et al.* Erythromycin as therapy for acute colonic pseudo-obstruction (Ogilvie's syndrome). *J Clin Gastroenterol* 1991; **13:** 475–6.
5. Yeo CJ, *et al.* Erythromycin accelerates gastric emptying after pancreaticoduodenectomy: a prospective, randomized, placebo-controlled trial. *Ann Surg* 1993; **218:** 229–38.
6. Simkiss DE, *et al.* Erythromycin in neonatal postoperative intestinal dysmotility. *Arch Dis Child* 1994; **71:** F128–9.
7. Chapman MJ, *et al.* Erythromycin improves gastric emptying in critically ill patients intolerant of nasogastric feeding. *Crit Care Med* 2000; **28:** 2334–7.
8. Ng PC, *et al.* Randomised controlled study of oral erythromycin for treatment of gastrointestinal dysmotility in preterm infants. *Arch Dis Child Fetal Neonatal Ed* 2001; **84:** F177–F182.
9. Tanis AA, *et al.* Side-effects of oral erythromycin for treatment of diabetic gastroparesis. *Lancet* 1993; **342:** 1431.


**Skin disorders.** ACNE. Erythromycin may be used topically or orally in the treatment of acne (p.1133). Topical erythromycin may be used for mild inflammatory acne if benzoyl peroxide is ineffective or poorly tolerated. It is also used as adjunctive treatment in more severe acne. Erythromycin is also available as a complex with zinc acetate that has been reported to be more effective than topical erythromycin alone[1] or oral minocycline.[2] However, development of antibiotic resistance by the skin flora is an increasing problem. Combination therapy with benzoyl peroxide and erythromycin has been reported to be helpful in preventing the selection of antibiotic-resistant mutants[3,4] and to be more effective than topical clindamycin alone.[5] Alternatively, short intervening courses of benzoyl peroxide during antibacterial therapy may help to eliminate any resistant bacteria that have been selected.[6] It has also been recommended that courses of topical antibiotics be continued for no longer than necessary (although treatment should be used for at least 6 months), that the same drug be used if further treatment is required, and that concomitant treatment with different oral and topical antibiotics or antibiotic rotation be avoided.[6]

Oral erythromycin may be used as an alternative to a tetracycline in moderate acne. However, resistance to erythromycin is increasing so it is usually reserved for those patients in whom other antibacterials are unsuitable.


1. Habbema L, *et al.* A 4% erythromycin and zinc combination (Zineryt®) versus 2% erythromycin (Eryderm®) in acne vulgaris: a randomized, double-blind comparative study. *Br J Dermatol* 1989; **121:** 497–502.
2. Stainforth J, *et al.* A single-blind comparison of topical erythromycin/zinc lotion and oral minocycline in the treatment of acne vulgaris. *J Dermatol Treat* 1993; **4:** 119–22.
3. Eady EA, *et al.* Effects of benzoyl peroxide and erythromycin alone and in combination against antibiotic-sensitive and -resistant skin bacteria from acne patients. *Br J Dermatol* 1994; **131:** 331–6.
4. Eady EA, *et al.* The effects of acne treatment with a combination of benzoyl peroxide and erythromycin on skin carriage of erythromycin-resistant propionibacteria. *Br J Dermatol* 1996; **134:** 107–13.
5. Packman AM, *et al.* Treatment of acne vulgaris: combination of 3% erythromycin and 5% benzoyl peroxide in a gel compared to clindamycin phosphate lotion. *Int J Dermatol* 1996; **35:** 209–11.
6. Eady EA, *et al.* Antibiotic resistant propionibacteria in acne: need for policies to modify antibiotic usage. *BMJ* 1993; **306:** 555–6.


## Preparations

***BP 2003:*** Erythromycin Estolate Capsules; Erythromycin Ethyl Succinate Oral Suspension; Erythromycin Ethyl Succinate Tablets; Erythromycin Lactobionate Intravenous Infusion; Erythromycin Stearate Tablets; Erythromycin Tablets;

***USP 27:*** Erythromycin and Benzoyl Peroxide Topical Gel; Erythromycin Delayed-release Capsules; Erythromycin Delayed-release Tablets; Erythromycin Estolate and Sulfisoxazole Acetyl Oral Suspension; Erythromycin Estolate Capsules; Erythromycin Estolate for Oral Suspension; Erythromycin Estolate Oral Suspension; Erythromycin Estolate Tablets; Erythromycin Ethylsuccinate and Sulfisoxazole Acetyl for Oral Suspension; Erythromycin Ethylsuccinate for Oral Suspension; Erythromycin Ethylsuccinate Injection; Erythromycin Ethylsuccinate Oral Suspension; Erythromycin Ethylsuccinate Tablets; Erythromycin Lactobionate for Injection; Erythromycin Ointment; Erythromycin Ophthalmic Ointment; Erythromycin Pledgets; Erythromycin Stearate Tablets; Erythromycin Tablets; Erythromycin Topical Gel; Erythromycin Topical Solution; Sterile Erythromycin Ethylsuccinate; Sterile Erythromycin Gluceptate; Sterile Erythromycin Lactobionate.

**Proprietary Preparations** (details are given in Part 3)

***Arg.:*** Algiderm; Ambamida; Erigrand; Erisol; Eritroderm; Eritrofarm; Eritromed; Eryacne; Eryfluid; Ilosone; Iloticina; Kitacne; Lederpax; Oftalmolets; Pantomicina; Pentoclave; Stiemycin; Toperit; Trixne; Wemid; ***Austral.:*** E-Mycin; EES; Emu-V†; Eryacne; Eryc; Eryhexal; Erythrocin; Ilosone†; ***Austria:*** Akne; Aknemycin†; Eryaknen; Erybesan; Eryhexal; Erysolvan†; Erystad; Erythrocin; Ilosone†; Meromycin; Monomycin; Stiemycine; ***Belg.:*** Acneryne; Aknemycin; Eryderm; Erythrocine; Erythroforte; Inderm; ***Braz.:*** Eribiotic; Eriflogin; Eritrax; Eritrex; Eritril†; Eritrin; Eritrocin†; Eritrofar†; Eryacnen; Ilocin; Ilosone; Ilotrex†; Infectoss†; Kanazima; Lisotran; Lisotrex†; Ortociclina†; Pantomicina; Plenomicina†; Stiemycin; Valmicin; ***Canad.:*** Apo-Erythro; Diomycin; E-Mycin†; EES; Erybid; Eryc; Erysol; Erythrocin; Erythromid†; Ilosone†; Ilotycin†; Novo-Rythro†; PCE; Staticin; T-Stat; ***Chile:*** Cinactiv; Eryacnen; Gelerit; Labocne; Mercina; Pantomicina; ***Denm.:*** Abboticin; Erycin; Erystrat†; Escumycin; Hexabotin; ***Fin.:*** Abboticin; Erasis†; Ermysin; ***Fr.:*** Abboticine; Egery; Ery; Eryacne; Erycocci†; Eryfluid; Erythrocine; Erythrogel; Erythrogram; Logecine†; Propiocine†; Stimycine; ***Ger.:*** Akne Cordes; Aknederm Ery; Aknefug-EL; aknemago†; Aknemycin; Aknin†; Bisolvonat Mono†; Clinofug Gel†; duraerythromycin†; durapaediat†; Ery; Ery-Diolan; Ery-Reu†; Eryaknen; Erybeta; Erycinum; Erydermec; Eryhexal; Erysec; Erythro; Erythro-Hefa; Erythrocin; Erythrocin Neo; Erythrogenat; Erytop†; Eupragin†; Hydrodermed; Inderm; InfectoMycin; Karex; Lederpaediat†; Medismon†; Monomycin; Paediathrocin; Sanasepton; Semibiocin†; Skid E†; Stiemycine; Udima Ery†; ***Gr.:*** Acne Hermal; Erythrocin; Roug-mycin; ***Hong Kong:*** Aknemycin; Apo-Erythro; E-Mycin; EES; Eryacne; Eryc†; Eryped†; Erysol†; Erythro; Erythrocin; Ilosone†; PCE; Porphyrocin; Servitrocin†; Stiemycin; ***India:*** Acnesol; Althrocin; E-Mycin; Eltocin; Erysafe; Erythrocin; ***Irl.:*** Erymax; Erythrocin; Erythromid†; Erythroped; Ilosone†; Primacine; Stiemycin; Tiprocin†; ***Israel:*** Acnetrim; E-Mycin†; Eryc; Eryderm; Erytab†; Erythro-Teva; Erythrocin; Erythroderm†; Erythrol; Erythroped; ***Ital.:*** Eritrocina; Eritrocist†; Eryacne; Erytrociclin; Ilosone†; Lauromicina; Stellamicina†; Zalig†; ***Malaysia:*** Aknemycin; EES; Erogran; Erotab; Eryderm; Eryped; Eryson; Erythrocin; Etrogran; Etrotab; Sethro; Stiemycin; ***Mex.:*** Bestocin; Biotril; Colitromin; E-Trocima-P; Eribec; Eriber; Eribus†; Erimicina†; Erisuspen†; Eritolat†; Eritrerba†; Eritrofarmin; Eritrolat; Eritroquim; Eritrosol; Eritrovier; Eritrowel†; Eryacnen; Eryderm; Erylar†; Esteromicin†; Examicyn†; Galentromicina†; Iliocin; Ilosin; Ilosone; Iqfamicina; Latotryd; Lauricin; Laurimicina; Lauritran; Lederpax; Mexcyn†; Optomicin; Pantomicina; Procephal; Quimolauril; Sansacne; Stiemycin; T-Stat; Totatrom†; Tromigal†; Verytracin; Witromin; ***Neth.:*** Aknemycin; Eryacne; Eryc; Eryderm; Erythrocine; Inderm; Stiemycin; ***Norw.:*** Abboticin; Ery-Max; ***NZ:*** E-Mycin; EES†; Era; Eromycin†; Eryacne; Eryc†; Stiemycin; ***Port.:*** Akne-Mycin; Clinac; Eritina; Eritrocina; Eritromicina†; Eryc; Eryfluid; ESE; ***S.Afr.:*** Acu-Erylate S†; Arcanamycin†; Betamycin; E-Mycin†; Emsyn; Emu-V†; Eromel; Eromel-S†; Erycette; Eryderm; Erymax†; Erymycin; Erystat†; Erythrocin; Erythromid†; Erythroped; Estomycin†; Ilosone; Ilotycin TS; Purmycin; Ryped†; Spectrasone; Stiemycin; Succilate†; Succin†; Xeramel; ***Singapore:*** Acnetrim†; Aknemycin; E-Mycin†; EES; Ermycin; Erotab; Eryacne; Eryderm; Eryped; Erysol; Eryson; Erytab-S†; Erythrocin; Etocin†; Ranthrocin; Servitrocin†; Stiemycin; T-Stat; ***Spain:*** Bronsema; Deripil; Eridosis; Eritrogobens; Eritroveinte; Ery-Max†; Euskin; Lagarmicin; Lederpax; Loderm; Neo Iloticina; Pantodrin; Pantomicina; ***Swed.:*** Abboticin; Ery-Max; ***Switz.:*** Aknemycin; Aknilox; Cimetrin†; Ericosol†; Erios; Ery†; Eryaknen; Eryderm; Erythrocine; Erytran†; Helvemycin†; Ilotycin†; Inderm; Karex; Monomycine†; Servitrocin†; Staticine†; Stiemycine; ***Thai.:*** Elocin; Erathrom; Ericin; Erimit; Erimycin; Ery-Tab; Eryacne; Erycin; Erymin; Erysil; Eryth-mycin; Erythrocin; Etrolate; Ilosone; Malocin; Pocin†; Redrocin; Rythocin†; Servitrocin; Stacin; Stiemycin; Tomcin; ***UAE:*** Eromycin; ***UK:*** Arpimycin†; Eryacne†; Erymax; Erythrocin; Erythromid†; Erythroped; Ilosone†; Retcin†; Rommix; Ronmix†; Stiemycin; Tiloryth; ***USA:*** Akne-Mycin; ATS; Del-Mycin; E-Base; E-Mycin; EES; Emgel; Eramycin; Ery-Ped; Ery-Tab; Eryc; Erycette; Eryderm; Erygel; Erymax; Erythra-Derm†; Erythrocin; Ilosone; Ilotycin; PCE; Robimycin Robitabs; Staticin; T-Stat; Theramycin Z†.

**Multi-ingredient: *Arg.:*** Benzamycin; Ecnagel E; Erimicin; Eritrobron; Kitacne AR; Kitacne PB; Pantomucol; Pediazole; Peroximicina; Tratacne; ***Austria:*** Aknemycin compositum; AKZ†; Isotrexin; ***Belg.:*** Benzamycin; Zineryt; ***Braz.:*** Baknyl†; Benzac Eritromicina; Cifrantil†; Eritrex A; Eritrosima†; Isotrexin; ***Canad.:*** Benzamycin; Pediazole; Sans-Acne; Stievamycin; ***Chile:*** Abboderm; Benzamycin; Bioquin; Pediazole; Stievamycin; ***Denm.:*** Antibiotic Simplex†; ***Fr.:*** Antibio-Aberel†; Antibiotrex; Erylik; Pediazole; ***Ger.:*** Aknemycin; Aknemycin Plus; Bisolvonat†; Clinesfar; Ecolicin; Isotrexin; Synergomycin; Zineryt; ***Gr.:*** Pediazole; ***Hong Kong:*** Benzamycin; Dermabaz; Erylik; Pediazole; ***Irl.:*** Benzamycin; Isotrexin; Zineryt; ***Israel:*** Aknemycin; Aknemycin Plus; Benzamycin; Pediazole; ***Ital.:*** Isotrexin; Lauromicina; Rubrociclina; Zineryt; ***Malaysia:*** Aknemycin Plus; ***Mex.:*** Benzamycin; Pantobron; Pediazole†; Quimobrom; Stievamycin; ***Neth.:*** Zineryt; ***Port.:*** Isotrexin; Zineryt; ***S.Afr.:*** Benzamycine; Pediazole†; ***Singapore:*** Aknemycin Plus; Benzamycin; ***Spain:*** Bronsema Expectorante; Erifoscin†; Isotrex Eritromicina; Tosdiazina; Zineryt; ***Switz.:*** Aknemycin; AKZ†; ***UK:*** Aknemycin Plus; Benzamycin; Isotrexin; Zineryt; ***USA:*** Benzamycin; Eryzole; Pediazole.

---

# Ethambutol Hydrochloride

*(BANM, USAN, rINNM)*

CL-40881; Ethambutoli Hydrochloridum; Hidrocloruro de etambutol. (S,S)-N,N′-Ethylenebis(2-aminobutan-1-ol) dihydrochloride.

$C_{10}H_{24}N_2O_2,2HCl = 277.2.$

*CAS — 74-55-5 (ethambutol); 1070-11-7 (ethambutol hydrochloride).*

*ATC — J04AK02.*

**Pharmacopoeias.** In *Chin., Eur.* (see p.vi), *Int., Jpn, Pol., US,* and *Viet.*

**Ph. Eur. 5.0** (Ethambutol Hydrochloride). A white, crystalline powder. Freely soluble in water; soluble in alcohol. A 2% solution in water has a pH of 3.7 to 4.0. Store in airtight containers.

**USP 27** (Ethambutol Hydrochloride). A white crystalline powder. Freely soluble in water; soluble in alcohol and in methyl alcohol; slightly soluble in chloroform and in ether.

## Adverse Effects and Treatment

The most important adverse effect of ethambutol is retrobulbar neuritis with a reduction in visual acuity, constriction of visual field, central or peripheral scotoma, and green-red colour blindness. One or both eyes may be affected. The degree of visual impairment appears to depend on the dose and duration of therapy; toxicity is observed most frequently at daily doses of 25 mg/kg or more and after at least 2 months of therapy. Recovery of vision usually takes place over a period of a few weeks or months, but in rare cases it may take up to a year or more or the effect may be permanent. Retinal haemorrhage has occurred rarely.

Renal clearance of urate may be reduced and acute gout has been precipitated rarely.

Hypersensitivity reactions including skin rashes, pruritus, leucopenia, fever, and joint pains have occurred but appear to be rare with ethambutol. Other adverse effects which have been reported include confusion, disorientation, hallucinations, headache, dizziness, malaise, jaundice or transient liver dysfunction, peripheral neuritis, thrombocytopenia, pulmonary infiltrates, eosinophilia, and gastrointestinal disturbances such as nausea, vomiting, anorexia, and abdominal pain.

Teratogenicity has been observed in *animals.*

Blood concentrations of ethambutol following overdosage may be reduced by haemodialysis or peritoneal dialysis.

**Effects on the blood.** Neutropenia has been reported in a patient on ethambutol, isoniazid, and rifampicin.[1] Each drug induced neutropenia individually on rechallenge. In another patient also receiving mixed antituberculous therapy, eosinophilia and neutropenia were associated with ethambutol, although the effects recurred only on rechallenge with this drug.[2] Thrombocytopenia attributable to ethambutol has been reported in 2 patients.[3,4]


1. Jenkins PF, *et al.* Neutropenia with each standard antituberculosis drug in the same patients. *BMJ* 1980; **280:** 1069–70.
2. Wong CF, Yew WW. Ethambutol-induced neutropenia and eosinophilia. *Chest* 1994; **106:** 1638–9.
3. Rabinovitz M, *et al.* Ethambutol-induced thrombocytopenia. *Chest* 1982; **81:** 765–6.
4. Prasad R, Mukerji PK. Ethambutol-induced thrombocytopaenia. *Tubercle* 1989; **70:** 211–12.


**Effects on the eyes.** Ophthalmic effects have been found in 10 of 2184 patients receiving ethambutol in doses of 25 mg/kg or less daily, although few of the 10 patients complained of symptoms.[1] In 9 of the 10 patients, ocular changes occurred after the second month of treatment. In the 928 patients who only received 2 months of ethambutol therapy, ocular toxicity was not reported. While short-term use of ethambutol is usually safe, deterioration of vision leading to long-term blindness has been reported after only a few doses of ethambutol;[2] it was suspected that this was an idiosyncratic reaction. Rapid onset reversible ocular toxicity has also occurred.[3] Visual defects occurring with ethambutol generally resolve when the drug is discontinued; for treatment of long-term visual loss hydroxocobalamin or cyanocobalamin[2,4,5] have been used with varying success.

1. Citron KM, Thomas GO. Ocular toxicity from ethambutol. *Thorax* 1986; **41:** 737–9.
2. Karnik AM, *et al.* A case of ocular toxicity to ethambutol—an idiosyncratic reaction? *Postgrad Med J* 1985; **61:** 811–13.
3. Schild HS, Fox BC. Rapid-onset reversible ocular toxicity from ethambutol therapy. *Am J Med* 1991; **90:** 404–6.
4. Harada T, *et al.* Ocular toxicity with ethambutol. *Jpn J Clin Ophthalmol* 1979; **33:** 1345–55.
5. Guerra R, Casu L. Hydroxycobalamin for ethambutol-induced optic neuropathy. *Lancet* 1981; **ii:** 1176.

**Effects on the kidneys.** Interstitial nephritis has been reported[1,2] in 5 patients receiving ethambutol and isoniazid; 3 were also receiving additional antimycobacterials. In another patient, acute renal failure occurred secondary to interstitial nephritis which was thought to have been induced by ethambutol.[3]

1. Collier J, *et al.* Two cases of ethambutol nephrotoxicity. *BMJ* 1976; **2:** 1105–6.
2. Stone WJ, *et al.* Acute diffuse interstitial nephritis related to chemotherapy of tuberculosis. *Antimicrob Agents Chemother* 1976; **10:** 164–72.
3. García-Martín F, *et al.* Acute interstitial nephritis induced by ethambutol. *Nephron* 1991; **59:** 679–80.

**Effects on the liver.** Although transient abnormalities in liver function commonly occur during the early stages of antituberculosis treatment, drugs other than ethambutol are generally considered responsible. Ethambutol has generated fewer reports of hepatotoxicity to the UK Committee on Safety of Medicines than rifampicin, isoniazid, or pyrazinamide,[1] and the use of regimens containing ethambutol has been recommended for patients unable to tolerate standard regimens due to hepatotoxicity.[1-3]

1. Ormerod LP, *et al.* Hepatotoxicity of antituberculosis drugs. *Thorax* 1996; **51:** 111–13.
2. Ormerod LP. Chemotherapy and management of tuberculosis in the United Kingdom: recommendations of the Joint Tuberculosis Committee of the British Thoracic Society. *Thorax* 1990; **45:** 403–8.
3. WHO. *TB/HIV: a clinical manual.* Geneva: WHO, 1996.

**Effects on the skin.** Details of a patient in whom toxic epidermal necrolysis was associated with the use of ethambutol.[1] The manufacturer noted that isolated cases of photosensitive lichenoid eruptions, Stevens-Johnson syndrome, and bullous dermatitis had also occurred.

1. Pegram PS, *et al.* Ethambutol-induced toxic epidermal necrolysis. *Arch Intern Med* 1981; **141:** 1677–8.

**Hyperuricaemia.** In a controlled study of 71 patients receiving ethambutol 20 mg/kg daily by mouth with other antimycobacterials, serum-uric acid concentrations increased in 66, mainly in the first 2 weeks of treatment.[1] One patient experienced arthralgia and another acute gouty arthritis. Serum-uric acid concentrations did not change in 60 control patients receiving other antimycobacterials.

1. Khanna BK, Gupta VP. Ethambutol-induced hyperuricaemia. *Tubercle* 1984; **65:** 195–9.

## Precautions

Ethambutol is generally contra-indicated in patients with optic neuritis. It should be used with great care in patients with visual defects, the elderly, and in children in whom evaluation of changes in visual acuity may be difficult (see also Children, below). Ocular examination is recommended before treatment with ethambutol and some consider that regular examinations are necessary during treatment, especially in children. Patients should be advised to report visual disturbances immediately and to discontinue ethambutol pending visual evaluation.

Ethambutol should be given in reduced dosage to patients with renal impairment and dosage adjustments may need to be made according to serum concentrations. The *British National Formulary* recommends peak concentrations of 2 to 6 mg/L and trough concentrations of less than 1 mg/L.

Ethambutol may precipitate attacks of gout.

Although ethambutol crosses the placenta and may be teratogenic in *animals*, problems in humans have not been documented. It is generally considered that the benefits of ethambutol in the treatment of tuberculosis outweigh any potential risks in pregnancy.

**Breast feeding.** Ethambutol diffuses into breast milk to produce concentrations similar to those in plasma.[1] However, no adverse effects have been observed in breast-fed infants whose mothers were receiving ethambutol, and the American Academy of Pediatrics considers[2] that it is therefore usually compatible with breast feeding.

1. Snider DE, Powell KE. Should women taking antituberculosis drugs breast-feed? *Arch Intern Med* 1984; **144:** 589–90.
2. American Academy of Pediatrics. The transfer of drugs and other chemicals into human milk. *Pediatrics* 2001; **108:** 776–89. Correction. *ibid.*; 1029. Also available at: http://aappolicy.aappublications.org/cgi/content/full/pediatrics%3b108/3/776 (accessed 26/05/04)

**Children.** Due to the possible difficulty of evaluating changes in visual acuity that may be induced in children receiving ethambutol, the *British National Formulary* advises that it should be used with caution in children under 5 years of age whereas in the USA the manufacturers advise against use in those under 13 years of age.

The authors of a review of the use of ethambutol in children concluded that no extra precautions were necessary in children aged 5 years or more, and that it could also be used in younger children without undue fear of adverse effects.[1] Another review suggested that visual toxicity is not a particular problem except perhaps when CNS infection is involved.[2]

1. Trébucq A. Should ethambutol be recommended for routine treatment of tuberculosis in children? A review of the literature. *Int J Tuberc Lung Dis* 1997; **1:** 12–15.
2. Graham SM, *et al.* Ethambutol in tuberculosis: time to reconsider? *Arch Dis Child* 1998; **78:** 274–8.

## Antimicrobial Action

Ethambutol is active against *Mycobacterium tuberculosis* and some other mycobacteria. Resistant strains of *M. tuberculosis* are readily produced if ethambutol is used alone.

## Pharmacokinetics

About 80% of an oral dose of ethambutol is absorbed from the gastrointestinal tract. Absorption is not significantly impaired by food (but see also Bioavailability, below). After a single dose of 25 mg/kg peak plasma concentrations of up to 5 mg/L appear within 4 hours, and are less than 1 mg/L by 24 hours.

Ethambutol is distributed to most tissues, including the lungs, kidneys, and erythrocytes. About 10 to 50% may diffuse into the CSF when the meninges are inflamed. It has been reported to cross the placenta and is distributed into breast milk. The elimination half-life following oral administration is about 3 to 4 hours.

Ethambutol is partially metabolised in the liver to the aldehyde and dicarboxylic acid derivatives which are inactive and then excreted in the urine. Most of a dose appears in the urine within 24 hours as unchanged drug and 8 to 15% as the inactive metabolites. About 20% of the dose is excreted unchanged in the faeces.

**Bioavailability.** Although the absorption of ethambutol is not generally regarded as being impaired by food, a study in 14 healthy subjects[1] suggested that administration with a high fat meal or an antacid could delay absorption and reduce the maximum plasma concentration.

1. Peloquin CA, *et al.* Pharmacokinetics of ethambutol under fasting conditions, with food, and with antacids. *Antimicrob Agents Chemother* 1999; **43:** 568–72.

**Pregnancy and breast feeding.** Ethambutol crosses the placenta and is present in fetal tissue in amounts of at least 74.5% of the maternal serum concentration.[1] Ethambutol diffuses into breast milk to produce concentrations similar to those in plasma.[2]

1. Holdiness MR. Transplacental pharmacokinetics of the antituberculosis drugs. *Clin Pharmacokinet* 1987; **13:** 125–9.
2. Snider DE, Powell KE. Should women taking antituberculosis drugs breast-feed? *Arch Intern Med* 1984; **144:** 589–90.

## Uses and Administration

Ethambutol is used with other antituberculous drugs in the primary treatment of pulmonary and extrapulmonary tuberculosis (p.150) to suppress emergence of resistance to the other drugs used in the regimens. It is also used as a component of regimens for the treatment of opportunistic mycobacterial infections (p.137).

In the treatment of tuberculosis, ethambutol is given, as the hydrochloride, usually with isoniazid, rifampicin, and pyrazinamide in the initial 8-week phase and sometimes in combinations with isoniazid and rifampicin in the continuation phase. It is given by mouth in a single daily dose of 15 mg/kg, or 30 mg/kg three times weekly, or 45 mg/kg twice weekly. Initial doses of ethambutol 25 mg/kg daily for 60 days may be given to patients who have previously received antimycobacterial therapy, reduced to 15 mg/kg daily thereafter. Ethambutol has also been used occasionally with other drugs for prophylaxis if the likelihood of resistance to isoniazid is high, when daily doses of 15 mg/kg have been employed, for 6 months or more. If it is used in patients with renal impairment (see Precautions, above), then doses should be adjusted according to serum concentrations.

## Preparations

**BP 2003:** Ethambutol Tablets;
**USP 27:** Ethambutol Hydrochloride Tablets; Rifampin, Isoniazid, Pyrazinamide, and Ethambutol Hydrochloride Tablets.

**Proprietary Preparations** (details are given in Part 3)
***Austral.:*** Myambutol; ***Austria:*** Etibi; Myambutol; ***Belg.:*** Myambutol; ***Canad.:*** Etibi; Myambutol†; ***Denm.:*** Myambutol; ***Fin.:*** Oributol; ***Fr.:*** Myambutol; ***Ger.:*** EMB; Myambutol; ***Gr.:*** Myambutol; ***Hong Kong:*** Etibi†; Lambutol†; Myambutol; ***India:*** Combutol; Myambutol; Mycobutol; Rifacom E-Z; Themibutol; Tibitol; ***Irl.:*** Myambutol†; ***Israel:*** Myambutol; ***Ital.:*** Etapiam; Miambutol; ***Mex.:*** Myambutol; Tambutec; Tubetam†; ***Mon.:*** Dexambutol; ***Neth.:*** Myambutol; ***NZ:*** Myambutol; ***Port.:*** Turresis; ***S.Afr.:*** Myambutol†; ***Spain:*** Myambutol; ***Swed.:*** Myambutol; ***Switz.:*** Myambutol; ***Thai.:*** Conbutol; Etham; Ethbutol; Lambutol; Myambutol; Myrin; Myrin-P; Servambutol; Tobutol; ***USA:*** Myambutol.

**Multi-ingredient:** ***Austria:*** Myambutol-INH; ***Ger.:*** EMB-INH; Myambutol-INH; ***India:*** Akt-3; Akt-4; Combunex; Cx-4; Cx-5; Inabutol Forte; Myconex; Rifa E; Wokex-3; Wokex-4; ***Ital.:*** Etanicozid B6; Miazide B6; Miazide†; ***Mex.:*** Myambutol-INH; ***Mon.:*** Dexambutol-INH; ***S.Afr.:*** Mynah†; Myrin Plus; Myrin†; Rifafour; ***Spain:*** Isoetam†; ***Switz.:*** Myambutol-INH.

# Ethionamide *(BAN, USAN, rINN)*

Ethionamidum; 2-Ethylthioisonicotinamide; Etionamida; Etionamide; 1314-TH. 2-Ethylpyridine-4-carbothioamide.

$C_8H_{10}N_2S$ = 166.2.
*CAS — 536-33-4.*
*ATC — J04AD03.*

**Pharmacopoeias.** In *Eur.* (see p.vi), *Int., Jpn, Pol.,* and *US.*

**Ph. Eur. 5.0** (Ethionamide). Small yellow crystals or a yellow crystalline powder. Practically insoluble in water; sparingly soluble in alcohol; soluble in methyl alcohol.

**USP 27** (Ethionamide). A bright yellow powder having a faint to moderate sulfide-like odour. Slightly soluble in water, in chloroform, and in ether; sparingly soluble in alcohol and in propylene glycol; soluble in methyl alcohol. pH of a 1% slurry in water is between 6.0 and 7.0. Store in airtight containers.

## Adverse Effects and Treatment

Many patients cannot tolerate therapeutic doses of ethionamide and have to discontinue treatment. The most common adverse effects are dose-related gastrointestinal disturbances, including nausea, vomiting, diarrhoea, anorexia, excessive salivation, a metallic taste, and abdominal pain. Tolerance may be improved by reducing the dose, adjusting the timing of administration, or giving an antiemetic.

Mental disturbances including depression, anxiety, and psychosis have been provoked. Dizziness, drowsiness, headache, orthostatic hypotension, and asthenia may also occur occasionally. Peripheral and optic neuropathy, diplopia and blurred vision, and a pellagra-like syndrome have occurred. Pyridoxine or nicotinamide have been suggested for the treatment or prevention of neurotoxic effects. Hepatitis may occur occasionally, with or without jaundice. The incidence of hepatotoxicity is increased when ethionamide is given in association with rifampicin.

Other adverse effects reported include hypersensitivity reactions, thrombocytopenia and purpura, alopecia, dermatitis (including photodermatitis), endocrine disturbances, hypoglycaemia, and hypothyroidism with or without goitre.

Teratogenic effects have been reported in *animals.*

**Effects on the liver.** Use of ethionamide or protionamide with rifampicin for the treatment of multibacillary leprosy has been associated with a high incidence of hepatotoxicity. A hepatitis incidence of 4.5 to 5% has been reported for patients on ethionamide or protionamide, rifampicin, and either dapsone or clofazimine.[1,2] In these studies, diagnosis of hepatitis was based on clinical assessment. When laboratory monitoring was used, an incidence of 13% was reported with a regimen of ethionamide or protionamide with rifampicin and dapsone.[3] A regimen of protionamide, dapsone, rifampicin, and clofazimine has been associated with a 22% incidence based on laboratory monitoring.[4] Use of ethionamide with pyrazinamide has also resulted in a high incidence of abnormal liver function tests.[5]

In the above studies rifampicin was given daily during part or all of the regimens. The incidence of hepatotoxicity when ethionamide or protionamide is used with once-monthly rifampicin may be lower; hepatotoxicity was not reported in patients receiving monthly rifampicin and daily protionamide, isoniazid, and dapsone.[6]

1. Pattyn SR, *et al.* Hepatotoxicity of the combination of rifampin-ethionamide in the treatment of multibacillary leprosy. *Int J Lepr* 1984; **52:** 1–6.
2. Pattyn SR, *et al.* Combined regimens of one year duration in the treatment of multibacillary leprosy—II: combined regimens with rifampicin administered during 6 months. *Lepr Rev* 1989; **60:** 118–23.
3. Cartel J-L, *et al.* Hepatitis in leprosy patients treated by a daily combination of dapsone, rifampin, and a thioamide. *Int J Lepr* 1983; **51:** 461–5.
4. Ji B, *et al.* Hepatotoxicity of combined therapy with rifampicin and daily prothionamide for leprosy. *Lepr Rev* 1984; **55:** 283–9.
5. Schless JM, *et al.* The use of ethionamide in combined drug regimens in the re-treatment of isoniazid-resistant pulmonary tuberculosis. *Am Rev Respir Dis* 1965; **91:** 728–37.
6. Ellard GA, *et al.* Long-term prothionamide compliance: a study carried out in India using a combined formulation containing prothionamide, dapsone and isoniazid. *Lepr Rev* 1988; **59:** 163–75.

### Precautions

Ethionamide should not be used in severe hepatic impairment. Liver function tests should be carried out before and during treatment with ethionamide.

Caution is necessary in patients with depression or other psychiatric illness. Difficulty may be experienced in the management of diabetes mellitus. Periodic monitoring of blood glucose, thyroid function, and visual function is desirable.

Ethionamide is teratogenic in *animals*.

**Porphyria.** Ethionamide is considered to be unsafe in patients with porphyria because it has been shown to be porphyrinogenic in *animals* or *in-vitro* systems.

### Interactions

The adverse effects of other antimycobacterials may be increased when ethionamide is used (see Effects on the Liver, above, and under Cycloserine, Interactions, p.202).

**Alcohol.** A psychotic reaction has been reported in a patient receiving ethionamide following excessive intake of alcohol.[1]

1. Lansdown FS, *et al.* Psychotoxic reaction during ethionamide therapy. *Am Rev Respir Dis* 1967; **95:** 1053–5.

### Antimicrobial Action

Ethionamide is active only against mycobacteria including *Mycobacterium tuberculosis, M. kansasii, M. leprae*, and some strains of *M. avium* complex.

Resistance develops rapidly if used alone and there is complete cross-resistance between ethionamide and protionamide. Cross-resistance has been reported *in vitro* and in *animals* with isoniazid or with thioacetazone.

### Pharmacokinetics

Ethionamide is readily absorbed from the gastrointestinal tract, and peak plasma concentrations of about 2 micrograms/mL occur 2 hours after an oral dose of 250 mg. It is widely distributed throughout body tissues and fluids. It crosses the placenta and penetrates the uninflamed meninges, appearing in the CSF in concentrations equivalent to those in serum. It is about 30% bound to plasma proteins. The half-life is reported to be 2 to 3 hours. Ethionamide is extensively metabolised, probably in the liver, to the active sulfoxide and other inactive metabolites and less than 1% of a dose appears in the urine as unchanged drug.

**Distribution.** Following single oral doses of ethionamide 15 or 20 mg/kg in children with tuberculous meningitis, the peak spinal fluid concentration was reached in 1½ to 2½ hours.[1] A wide range of concentrations was reported but doses of 20 mg/kg were more likely to produce spinal fluid concentrations above 2.5 micrograms/mL, the concentration considered by the authors to be essential for therapeutic success.

1. Donald PR, Seifart HI. Cerebrospinal fluid concentrations of ethionamide in children with tuberculous meningitis. *J Pediatr* 1989; **115:** 483–6.

### Uses and Administration

Ethionamide is a thioamide derivative considered to be interchangeable with protionamide. It has been used with other antituberculous drugs for the treatment of tuberculosis (p.150) when resistance to, or toxicity from, primary drugs has developed. It has also been used, as a substitute for clofazimine, in regimens for the treatment of leprosy (p.133) but less toxic alternatives are now preferred.

In the treatment of resistant tuberculosis, adults may be given 15 to 20 mg/kg daily (maximum 1 g daily) by mouth. Children have been given 10 to 20 mg/kg daily (maximum 750 mg daily). Ethionamide may be given in divided doses with meals, or as a single daily dose after the evening meal, or at bedtime, to minimise gastrointestinal adverse effects. Similar doses were used for the treatment of leprosy.

Ethionamide has also been used as rectal suppositories; the hydrochloride has been given intravenously.

### Preparations

**USP 27:** Ethionamide Tablets.

**Proprietary Preparations** (details are given in Part 3)
***Gr.:*** Trecator; ***India:*** Myobid; ***S.Afr.:*** Ethatyl; ***USA:*** Trecator.

## Faropenem Sodium *(rINNM)*

ALP-201; Faropenem sódico; Fropenem Sodium; Furopenem; SUN-5555; SY-5555; Wy-49605; YM-044. Sodium (+)-(5R,6S)-6-[(1R)-1-hydroxyethyl]-7-oxo-3-[(2R)-tetrahydro-2-furyl]-4-thia-1-azabicyclo[3.2.0]hept-2-ene-2-carboxylate.

$C_{12}H_{15}NaNO_5S$ = 308.3.

*CAS — 106560-14-9 (faropenem); 122547-49-3 (faropenem sodium).*

**Pharmacopoeias.** In *Jpn*.

### Profile

Faropenem is a penem antibacterial that is given by mouth as the sodium salt for the treatment of susceptible infections.

Faropenem daloxate (Bay-56-6854) is being investigated for the treatment of respiratory-tract infections.

◊ References.

1. Critchley IA, *et al.* Activities of faropenem, an oral β-lactam, against recent US isolates of Streptococcus pneumoniae, Haemophilus influenzae, and Moraxella catarrhalis. *Antimicrob Agents Chemother* 2002; **46:** 550–5.
2. von Eiff C, *et al.* Comparative in vitro activity of faropenem against staphylococci. *J Antimicrob Chemother* 2002; **50:** 277–80.
3. Milatovic D, *et al.* In vitro activity of faropenem against 5460 clinical bacterial isolates from Europe. *J Antimicrob Chemother* 2002; **50:** 293–9.
4. Wexler HM, *et al.* In vitro activities of faropenem against 579 strains of anaerobic bacteria. *Antimicrob Agents Chemother* 2002; **46:** 3669–75.
5. Jones ME, *et al.* Activity of faropenem, a new furanem, against European respiratory pathogens collected during 2000-2001: a comparison with other beta-lactam agents. *J Antimicrob Chemother* 2003; **51:** 196–9.

### Preparations

**Proprietary Preparations** (details are given in Part 3)
***Jpn:*** Farom.

## Fleroxacin *(BAN, USAN, rINN)*

AM-833; Fleroxacino; Ro-23-6240; Ro-23-6240/000. 6,8-Difluoro-1-(2-fluoroethyl)-1,4-dihydro-7-(4-methyl-1-piperazinyl)-4-oxo-3-quinolinecarboxylic acid.

$C_{17}H_{18}F_3N_3O_3$ = 369.3.

*CAS — 79660-72-3.*

*ATC — J01MA08.*

### Profile

Fleroxacin is a fluoroquinolone antibacterial with actions and uses similar to those of ciprofloxacin (p.188), but is reported to have greater systemic bioavailability and a longer half-life. It is given by mouth or by intravenous infusion for the treatment of susceptible infections in usual doses of 200 to 400 mg once daily.

The incidence of adverse effects associated with fleroxacin has been relatively high.

◊ General references.

1. Leigh D, *et al.* eds. Fleroxacin, a long acting fluoroquinolone with broad spectrum activity. *J Antimicrob Chemother* 1988; **22** (suppl D): 1–234.
2. Balfour JA, *et al.* Fleroxacin: a review of its pharmacology and therapeutic efficacy in various infections. *Drugs* 1995; **49:** 794–850.

**Adverse effects.** References to adverse effects associated with fleroxacin.

1. Bowie WR, *et al.* Adverse reactions in a dose-ranging study with a new long-acting fluoroquinolone, fleroxacin. *Antimicrob Agents Chemother* 1989; **33:** 1778–82.
2. Geddes AM. Safety of fleroxacin in clinical trials. *Am J Med* 1993; **94** (suppl 3A): 201S–203S.
3. Kimura M, *et al.* Photosensitivity induced by fleroxacin. *Clin Exp Dermatol* 1996; **21:** 46–7.

**Breast feeding.** The American Academy of Pediatrics[1] states that fleroxacin is usually compatible with breast feeding. However, in one study,[2] in which women were given a single 400-mg dose and breast feeding was withheld for 48 hours, it was concluded that although a breast-fed infant would only receive a moderate amount (maximum 10 mg daily), fleroxacin should not be used in breast-feeding mothers due to the potential for adverse effects such as arthropathy in the infant.

1. American Academy of Pediatrics. The transfer of drugs and other chemicals into human milk. *Pediatrics* 2001; **108:** 776–89. Correction. *ibid.*; 1029. Also available at: http://aappolicy.aappublications.org/cgi/content/full/pediatrics%3b108/3/776 (accessed 26/05/04)
2. Dan M, *et al.* Penetration of fleroxacin into breast milk and pharmacokinetics in lactating women. *Antimicrob Agents Chemother* 1993; **37:** 293–6.

### Preparations

**Proprietary Preparations** (details are given in Part 3)
***Austria:*** Quinodis; ***Belg.:*** Quinodis†; ***Denm.:*** Quinodis†; ***Ger.:*** Quinodis; ***Jpn:*** Megalocin; ***Switz.:*** Quinodis†.

## Flomoxef Sodium *(rINNM)*

6315-S. 7R-7-[2-(Difluoromethylthio)acetamido]-3-[1-(2-hydroxyethyl)-1H-tetrazol-5-ylthiomethyl]-7-methoxy-1-oxa-3-cephem-4-carboxylic acid sodium.

$C_{15}H_{17}F_2N_6NaO_7S_2$ = 518.4.

*CAS — 99665-00-6 (flomoxef); 92823-03-5 (flomoxef sodium).*

**Pharmacopoeias.** In *Jpn*.

### Profile

Flomoxef is an oxacephalosporin or oxacephem antibacterial with properties similar to latamoxef (p.225). It is given intravenously as the sodium salt and doses are expressed in terms of flomoxef. 1.04 g of flomoxef sodium is approximately equivalent to 1 g of flomoxef. The usual adult dose is 1 to 2 g daily in two divided doses.

### Preparations

**Proprietary Preparations** (details are given in Part 3)
***Jpn:*** Flumarin.

## Florfenicol *(BAN, USAN, rINN)*

Sch-25298. 2,2-Dichloro-N-[(αS,βR)-α-(fluoromethyl)-β-hydroxy-4-methanesulfonylphenethyl]acetamide.

$C_{12}H_{14}Cl_2FNO_4S$ = 358.2.

*CAS — 76639-94-6.*

### Profile

Florfenicol, a fluorinated analogue of chloramphenicol, is an antibacterial used in veterinary medicine.

# Flucloxacillin *(BAN, rINN)*

BRL-2039; Floxacillin *(USAN)*; Flucloxacilina. (6R)-6-[3-(2-Chloro-6-fluorophenyl)-5-methylisoxazole-4-carboxamido]penicillanic acid.

$C_{19}H_{17}ClFN_3O_5S$ = 453.9.

*CAS — 5250-39-5.*

*ATC — J01CF05.*

NOTE. Compounded preparations of flucloxacillin may be represented by the following names:

- Co-fluampicil *(BAN)*—flucloxacillin 1 part and ampicillin 1 part (w/w).

## Flucloxacillin Magnesium *(BANM, rINNM)*

Flucloxacilina magnésica.

$(C_{19}H_{16}ClFN_3O_5S)_2Mg,8H_2O$ = 1074.2.

*CAS — 58486-36-5.*

*ATC — J01CF05.*

**Pharmacopoeias.** In *Br.*

**BP 2003** (Flucloxacillin Magnesium). A white or almost white powder. Slightly soluble in water and in chloroform; freely soluble in methyl alcohol. A 0.5% solution in water has a pH of 4.5 to 6.5. Store at a temperature not exceeding 25°. Protect from moisture.

## Flucloxacillin Sodium *(BANM, rINNM)*

Flucloxacilina sódica; Flucloxacillinum Natricum.

$C_{19}H_{16}ClFN_3NaO_5S,H_2O$ = 493.9.

*CAS — 1847-24-1.*

*ATC — J01CF05.*

**Pharmacopoeias.** In *Eur.* (see p.vi).

**Ph. Eur. 5.0** (Flucloxacillin Sodium). A white or almost white, crystalline hygroscopic, powder. Freely soluble in water and in methyl alcohol; soluble in alcohol. A 10% solution in water has a pH of 5.0 to 7.0. Store at a temperature not exceeding 25° in airtight containers.

**Incompatibility.** As with other penicillins, flucloxacillin sodium is incompatible with aminoglycosides.

### Adverse Effects and Precautions

As for Benzylpenicillin p.163.

Hepatitis and cholestatic jaundice have been reported occasionally with flucloxacillin and may be delayed in onset for up to several weeks after treatment has been stopped; older patients and those receiving flucloxacillin for more than 2 weeks are at greater risk. Agranulocytosis and neutropenia have been associated rarely with isoxazolyl penicillins such as flucloxacillin. Phlebitis has followed intravenous infusion.

**Effects on the liver.** References.

1. Fairley CK, *et al.* Flucloxacillin jaundice. *Lancet* 1992; **339:** 679.
2. Committee on Safety of Medicines. Flucloxacillin-induced cholestatic jaundice. *Current Problems 35* 1992.
3. Fairley CK, *et al.* Risk factors for development of flucloxacillin associated jaundice. *BMJ* 1993; **306:** 233–5. Correction. *ibid.*; **307:** 1179.
4. Devereaux BM, *et al.* Flucloxacillin associated cholestatic hepatitis: an Australian and Swedish epidemic? *Eur J Clin Pharmacol* 1995; **49:** 81–5.

**Porphyria.** Flucloxacillin has been associated with acute attacks of porphyria and is considered unsafe in porphyric patients.

**Sodium content.** Each g of flucloxacillin sodium contains about 2 mmol of sodium.

### Interactions

As for Benzylpenicillin, p.164.

### Antimicrobial Action

Flucloxacillin is bactericidal with a mode of action similar to that of benzylpenicillin, but is resistant to staphylococcal penicillinase. It is active therefore against penicillinase-producing and non-penicillinase-producing staphylococci. Its activity against streptococci such as *Streptococcus pneumoniae* and *Str. pyogenes* is less than that of benzylpenicillin, but sufficient to be useful when these organisms are present with penicillin-resistant staphylococci. Flucloxacillin is virtually ineffective against *Enterococcus faecalis*.

*Resistance.* The resistance of staphylococci to flucloxacillin and other penicillinase-resistant penicillins is described under meticillin (p.230).

## Pharmacokinetics

Flucloxacillin is better absorbed from the gastrointestinal tract than cloxacillin, but absorption is reduced by the presence of food in the stomach. After an oral dose of 0.25 to 1 g, in fasting subjects, peak plasma concentrations in about 1 hour are usually in the range of 5 to 15 micrograms/mL. Plasma concentrations following the intramuscular injection of flucloxacillin sodium are similar, but peak concentrations are achieved in about 30 minutes. Doubling the dose can double the plasma concentration. About 95% of flucloxacillin in the circulation is bound to plasma proteins. Flucloxacillin has been reported to have a plasma half-life of approximately 1 hour. The half-life is prolonged in neonates.

The distribution of flucloxacillin into body tissues and fluids is similar to that of cloxacillin (p.198).

Flucloxacillin is metabolised to a limited extent and the unchanged drug and metabolites are excreted in the urine by glomerular filtration and renal tubular secretion. About 66% of a dose by mouth and 76% of a parenteral dose is excreted in the urine within 8 hours. Only small amounts are excreted in the bile. Flucloxacillin is not removed by haemodialysis or peritoneal dialysis.

Plasma concentrations are enhanced by probenecid.

## Uses and Administration

Flucloxacillin is an isoxazolyl penicillin used primarily for the treatment of infections due to staphylococci resistant to benzylpenicillin. These include bone and joint infections, endocarditis, pneumonia, skin infections (including soft-tissue infections), and toxic shock syndrome. For discussions of these infections and their treatment, see under Choice of Antibacterial, p.120.

*Administration and dosage.* Flucloxacillin is given parenterally and by mouth as the sodium or magnesium salt. All doses are expressed as flucloxacillin. 2.4 g of flucloxacillin magnesium and 1.09 g of flucloxacillin sodium are each approximately equivalent to 1 g of flucloxacillin. Oral doses should be taken at least 30 minutes before meals as the presence of food in the stomach reduces absorption. In severe renal impairment a reduction in dosage may be necessary.

The usual adult dose by mouth or by intramuscular injection is 250 mg four times daily. It is given intravenously in a dose of 0.25 to 1 g four times daily by slow injection over 3 to 4 minutes or by intravenous infusion. All systemic doses may be doubled in severe infections; up to 8 g daily in 3 or 4 divided doses may be given for osteomyelitis and up to 12 g in 6 divided doses for endocarditis.

Flucloxacillin has been given by other routes in conjunction with systemic therapy. It has been given in a dose of 250 to 500 mg daily by intra-articular injection, dissolved if necessary in a 0.5% solution of lidocaine hydrochloride, or by intrapleural injection in a dose of 250 mg daily. Using powder for injection, 125 to 250 mg has been dissolved in 3 mL of sterile water and inhaled by nebuliser 4 times daily.

Children up to 2 years of age may be given one-quarter the adult dose and those aged 2 to 10 years one-half the adult dose.

Flucloxacillin may be used with other antibacterials, including ampicillin (known as co-fluampicil), to produce a wider spectrum of activity. If flucloxacillin is given with an aminoglycoside the two drugs should not be mixed.

## Preparations

**BP 2003:** Co-fluampicil Capsules; Co-fluampicil Oral Suspension; Flucloxacillin Capsules; Flucloxacillin Injection; Flucloxacillin Oral Solution; Flucloxacillin Oral Suspension.

**Proprietary Preparations** (details are given in Part 3)
**Austral.:** Flopen; Floxapen; Floxsig; Flucil; Staphylex; **Austria:** Floxapen; **Belg.:** Floxapen; Staphycid; **Chile:** Fluxacina; Vitalpen; **Denm.:** Heracillin; **Ger.:** Fluclox-Reu†; Flucloxa; Staphylex; **Hong Kong:** Flucloxil; **Irl.:** Floxapen; Flucillin; Fluclon†; Geriflox; Stafoxil†; **Ital.:** Betabiotic; Cloxillin; Evercid; Faifloc; Fareclox; Flucacid; Flucef; Flucinal; Fluclox; Fluxacil; Fluzerit; Liderclox; Nepenic; Pantaflux; **Malaysia:** Staphlex; **Mex.:** Floxapen; **Neth.:** Floxapen; Stafoxil; **NZ:** Floxapen; Flucloxin; Staphlex; **Port.:** Floxapen; Floxil; **S.Afr.:** Floxapen; **Singapore:** Fluocloxt†; Staphlex; **Swed.:** Heracillin; **Switz.:** Floxapen; Flucloxin†; **UK:** Floxapen; Fluclomix; Galfloxin†; Ladropen.

**Multi-ingredient:** **Austria:** Fluxapril†; **Ger.:** Flanamox; Fluxapril†; **Ital.:** Infectrin†; **S.Afr.:** Macropen; Megapen; Suprapen; **UK:** Flu-Amp†; Magnapen.

---

## Flumequine *(BAN, USAN, rINN)*

Flumequina; Flumequinum; R-802. 9-Fluoro-6,7-dihydro-5-methyl-1-oxo-1*H*,5*H*-pyrido[3,2,1-*ij*]quinoline-2-carboxylic acid.
$C_{14}H_{12}FNO_3$ = 261.2.
*CAS — 42835-25-6.*
*ATC — J01MB07.*

**Pharmacopoeias.** In *Eur.* (see p.vi).

**Ph. Eur. 5.0** (Flumequine). A microcrystalline white powder. Practically insoluble in water; sparingly soluble in dichloromethane; very slightly soluble in methyl alcohol; freely soluble in dilute solutions of alkali hydroxides.

### Profile

Flumequine is a 4-quinolone antibacterial with actions and uses similar to those of nalidixic acid (p.234). It may be more active *in vitro* against some Enterobacteriaceae. In the treatment of urinary-tract infections doses of 400 mg are given 3 times daily by mouth.

**Porphyria.** Flumequine is considered to be unsafe in patients with porphyria because it has been shown to be porphyrinogenic in *in-vitro* systems.

### Preparations

**Proprietary Preparations** (details are given in Part 3)
**Belg.:** Apurone†; **Fr.:** Apurone; **Ital.:** Flumural†.

---

## Flurithromycin Ethyl Succinate *(rINNM)*

(8*S*)-8-Fluoroerythromycin mono(ethyl butanedioate) ester.
$C_{43}H_{74}FNO_{16}$ = 880.0.
*CAS — 82664-20-8 (flurithromycin); 82730-23-2 (flurithromycin ethyl succinate).*

### Profile

Flurithromycin is a fluorinated macrolide antibacterial derived from erythromycin (p.208). It is given by mouth as the ethyl succinate in the treatment of susceptible infections.

◊ References.

1. Saverino D, *et al.* Antibacterial profile of flurithromycin, a new macrolide. *J Antimicrob Chemother* 1992; **30:** 261–72.

### Preparations

**Proprietary Preparations** (details are given in Part 3)
**Ital.:** Flurizic; Mizar; Ritro.

---

## Formosulfathiazole

Formaldehyde-sulphathiazole; Formosulfatiazol; Formosulphathiazole; Methylenesulfathiazole.
*CAS — 13968-86-0.*

### Profile

Formosulfathiazole, a condensation product of sulfathiazole with formaldehyde, has properties similar to those of sulfamethoxazole (p.261). It is poorly absorbed and has been given for its antibacterial action in the gastrointestinal tract, often with other antibacterials.

### Preparations

**Proprietary Preparations** (details are given in Part 3)
**Multi-ingredient:** **Spain:** Sulfintestin Neom†; Sulfintestin Neomicina.

---

## Fosfomycin *(BAN, USAN, rINN)*

Fosfomicina; MK-955; Phosphomycin; Phosphonomycin. (1*R*,2*S*)-1,2-Epoxypropylphosphonic acid.
$C_3H_7O_4P$ = 138.1.
*CAS — 23155-02-4.*
*ATC — J01XX01.*

**Description.** Fosfomycin is an antibacterial isolated from *Streptomyces fradiae* and other *Streptomyces* spp. or produced synthetically.

## Fosfomycin Calcium *(BANM, rINNM)*

Fosfomycinum Calcicum. Calcium (1*R*,2*S*)-1,2-epoxypropylphosphonate monohydrate.
$C_3H_5CaO_4P,H_2O$ = 194.1.
*CAS — 26016-98-8.*
*ATC — J01XX01.*

**Pharmacopoeias.** In *Eur.* (see p.vi) and *Jpn.*

**Ph. Eur. 5.0** (Fosfomycin Calcium). A white or almost white powder. Slightly soluble in water; practically insoluble in acetone, in dichloromethane, and in methyl alcohol. A 0.1% solution in water has a pH of 8.1 to 9.6. Store in airtight containers. Protect from light.

## Fosfomycin Sodium *(BANM, rINNM)*

Fosfomycinum Natricum. Disodium (1*R*,2*S*)-1,2-epoxypropylphosphonate.
$C_3H_5Na_2O_4P$ = 182.0.
*CAS — 26016-99-9.*
*ATC — J01XX01.*

**Pharmacopoeias.** In *Chin.*, *Eur.* (see p.vi), and *Jpn.*

**Ph. Eur. 5.0** (Fosfomycin Sodium). A white or almost white, very hygroscopic powder. Very soluble in water; practically insoluble in dehydrated alcohol and in dichloromethane; sparingly soluble in methyl alcohol. A 5% solution in water has a pH of 9.0 to 10.5. Store in airtight containers. Protect from light.

## Fosfomycin Trometamol *(BANM, rINNM)*

Fosfomycin Tromethamine *(USAN)*; Fosfomycinum Trometamol; FZ-588; Z-1282. (1*R*,2*S*)-1,2-Epoxypropylphosphonic acid, compound with 2-amino-2-(hydroxymethyl)-1,3-propanediol.
$C_3H_7O_4P,C_4H_{11}NO_3$ = 259.2.
*CAS — 78964-85-9.*
*ATC — J01XX01.*

**Pharmacopoeias.** In *Eur.* (see p.vi).

**Ph. Eur. 5.0** (Fosfomycin Trometamol). A white or almost white, hygroscopic powder. Very soluble in water; slightly soluble in alcohol and in methyl alcohol; practically insoluble in acetone. A 5% solution in water has a pH of 3.5 to 5.5. Store in airtight containers.

### Adverse Effects and Precautions

Gastrointestinal disturbances including nausea and diarrhoea, transient increases in serum concentrations of aminotransferases, headache, visual disturbances, and skin rashes have been reported following the use of fosfomycin. Eosinophilia and, rarely, angioedema, aplastic anaemia, exacerbation of asthma, cholestatic jaundice, hepatic necrosis, and toxic megacolon, have also occurred.

### Antimicrobial Action

Fosfomycin is a bactericidal antibacterial. Following active uptake into the cell it is reported to interfere with the first step in the synthesis of bacterial cell walls. It is active *in vitro* against a range of Gram-positive and Gram-negative bacteria including *Staphylococcus aureus*, some streptococci, most Enterobacteriaceae, ***Haemophilus influenzae***, ***Neisseria*** spp., and some strains of *Pseudomonas aeruginosa* although some are resistant. *Bacteroides* spp. are not sensitive.

Bacterial resistance to fosfomycin has been reported and can be chromosomal or, in some organisms, transferred by plasmids encoding multiple resistance (for example in *Serratia marcescens*). However, there appears to be little cross-resistance with other antibacterials.

Fosfomycin has been reported to demonstrate antimicrobial synergy with a wide range of antibacterials against organisms such as enterococci, meticillin-resistant *Staph. aureus*, and the enterobacteria. Such synergistic effects have been reported particularly with the beta lactams, but also with aminoglycosides, macrolides, tetracyclines, chloramphenicol, rifamycin, and lincomycin. Antimicrobial antagonism with a beta lactam has also been reported.

There is some suggestion that use of fosfomycin with an aminoglycoside may also reduce the nephrotoxicity of the latter *in vivo*.

◊ References.

1. Barry AL, Brown SD. Antibacterial spectrum of fosfomycin trometamol. *J Antimicrob Chemother* 1995; **35:** 228–30.

### Pharmacokinetics

Fosfomycin or fosfomycin calcium are poorly absorbed from the gastrointestinal tract. Peak plasma concentrations about 4 hours after a 1-g dose of fosfomycin calcium are around 7 micrograms/mL, and bioavailability has been calculated at about 30 to 40%. Similar bioavailability has been reported for the trometamol salt, and plasma concentrations of about 22 to 32 micrograms/mL have been reported 2 hours after a dose of 50 mg/kg (about 3 g fosfomycin). Fosfomycin disodium is given intramuscularly or intravenously: intravenous infusion of a 3-g dose results in peak serum concentrations of around 220 micrograms/mL. The plasma half-life is about 2 hours. Fosfomycin does not appear to be bound to plasma proteins. It crosses the placenta and is widely distributed in body fluids including the CSF; small amounts have been found in breast milk and bile. The majority of a parenteral dose is excreted unchanged in the urine, by glomerular filtration, within 24 hours.

Following fosfomycin trometamol orally, urinary concentrations of 3 mg/mL have been reported within 2 to 4 hours of a 3-g dose; therapeutic concentrations are maintained for about 36 hours following a single oral dose.

◊ References.

1. Bergan T, *et al.* Pharmacokinetic profile of fosfomycin trometamol. *Chemotherapy* 1993; **39:** 297–301.

### Uses and Administration

Fosfomycin is a phosphonic acid antibacterial given by mouth as the trometamol or calcium salt and intramuscularly or intravenously as the disodium salt in the treatment of a variety of bacterial infections due to susceptible organisms. Doses are expressed in terms of the base; fosfomycin calcium 1.4 g, fosfomycin sodium 1.3 g, and fosfomycin trometamol 1.9 g are each approximately equivalent to 1 g of fosfomycin.

In the treatment of acute uncomplicated infections of the urinary tract (p.153), fosfomycin trometamol is given as a single dose equivalent to 3 g of fosfomycin. Fosfomycin trometamol has also been used for the prophylaxis of infection in transurethral surgical procedures. For a discussion of surgical infections and their prophylaxis and treatment, see p.147.

The usual adult dose of fosfomycin calcium by mouth is the equivalent of 1 g of fosfomycin every 6 to 8 hours. Higher doses have been given parenterally as the sodium salt, with up to 20 g daily having been given intravenously in severe infection.

Fosfomycin has also been used with beta lactam antibacterials.

◊ Reviews.

1. Reeves DS. Fosfomycin trometamol. *J Antimicrob Chemother* 1994; **34:** 853–8.
2. Patel SS, *et al.* Fosfomycin tromethamine: a review of its antibacterial activity, pharmacokinetic properties and therapeutic efficacy as a single-dose oral treatment for acute uncomplicated lower urinary tract infections. *Drugs* 1997; **53:** 637–56.

### Preparations

**Proprietary Preparations** (details are given in Part 3)
***Arg.:*** Veramina; ***Austria:*** Monuril; ***Belg.:*** Monuril; ***Braz.:*** Monuril; ***Canad.:*** Monurol; ***Chile:*** Monurol; ***Fin.:*** Monurol; ***Fr.:*** Fosfocine; Monuril; Uridoz; ***Ger.:*** Fosfocin†; InfectoFos; Monuril; ***Gr.:*** Monurol; ***Hong Kong:*** Monurol; ***Irl.:*** Monuril†; ***Israel:*** Monurol; ***Ital.:*** Afos; Biocin†; Faremicin; Fonofos†; Fosfocin; Fosforal†; Foximin†; Francital; Ipamicina; Lofoxin†; Monuril; Ultramicina; ***Jpn:*** Fosmicin-S; ***Mex.:*** Fosfocil; Monurol; ***Neth.:*** Monuril; ***Port.:*** Monuril; ***S.Afr.:*** Urizone; ***Spain:*** Fosfocina; Monofoscin†; Monurol; Solufos; ***Swed.:*** Monurol; ***Switz.:*** Fosfocin†; Monuril; ***Thai.:*** Fosmicin; ***USA:*** Monurol.

**Multi-ingredient:** ***Spain:*** Erifoscin†.

## Framycetin Sulfate *(rINNM)*

Framycetin Sulphate *(BANM)*; Framycetini Sulfas; Neomycin B Sulphate; Sulfato de framicetina. 2-Deoxy-4-*O*-(2,6-diamino-2,6-dideoxy-α-D-glucopyranosyl)-5-*O*-[3-*O*-(2,6-diamino-2,6-dideoxy-β-L-idopyranosyl)-β-D-ribofuranosyl]streptamine sulphate.

$C_{23}H_{46}N_6O_{13},xH_2SO_4$.

*CAS — 119-04-0 (framycetin); 4146-30-9 (framycetin sulfate).*

*ATC — D09AA01; R01AX08; S01AA07.*

**Pharmacopoeias.** In *Eur.* (see p.vi).

**Ph. Eur. 5.0** (Framycetin Sulphate). A substance produced by growth of selected strains of *Streptomyces fradiae* or *S. decaris* or obtained by any other means. It contains not more than 3% of neomycin C (p.235) and loses not more than 8% of its weight on drying. A white or yellowish-white, hygroscopic powder. The potency is not less than 630 units of neomycin B per mg, calculated with reference to the dried substance. Freely soluble in water; very slightly soluble in alcohol; practically insoluble in acetone. A 1% solution in water has a pH of 6.0 to 7.0. Store in airtight containers. Protect from light.

### Profile

Framycetin is an aminoglycoside antibiotic which forms the major component of neomycin (p.235) and has similar actions and uses. It is used as the sulfate topically in usual concentrations of 1% for the treatment of infections of the skin, and in concentrations of 0.5% for infections of the eye and ear. It is often used with other antibacterials and corticosteroids in topical preparations.

Framycetin sulfate is poorly absorbed from the gastrointestinal tract and has been given by mouth for the treatment of gastrointestinal infections and pre-operatively for bowel preparation. It has sometimes been given prophylactically as part of regimens for the selective decontamination of the digestive tract in patients in intensive care.

### Preparations

**Proprietary Preparations** (details are given in Part 3)
***Austral.:*** Sofra-Tulle; Soframycin; ***Austria:*** Sofra-Tull; ***Belg.:*** Soframycine; ***Canad.:*** Sofra-Tulle; Soframycin; ***Denm.:*** Sofra-Tulle†; ***Fin.:*** Sofra-Tulle; ***Fr.:*** Framybiotal†; Isofra†; Rhinobiotal†; Soframycine†; ***Ger.:*** Leukase N; Sofra-Tull; ***Hong Kong:*** Sofra-Tulle; ***India:*** Sofra-Tulle; Soframycin; ***Irl.:*** Sofra-Tulle†; Soframycin; ***Israel:*** Sofra-Tulle; ***Malaysia:*** Sofra-Tulle; ***Neth.:*** Sofra-Tulle; Soframycin†; ***Norw.:*** Sofra-Tulle; ***NZ:*** Sofra-Tulle†; Soframycin; ***S.Afr.:*** Sofra-Tulle; Soframycin†; ***Singapore:*** Sofra-Tulle; Soframycin†; ***Swed.:*** Sofra-Tulle†; ***Switz.:*** Frakitacine; Sofra-Tulle; Soframycin; ***Thai.:*** Sofra-Tulle; ***UK:*** Sofra-Tulle; Soframycin.

**Multi-ingredient:** ***Arg.:*** Biotaer Nasal; ***Austral.:*** Otodex; Sofradex; Soframycin; ***Austria:*** Leukase; Leukase-Kegel; ***Belg.:*** Sofraline; Sofrasolone; ***Braz.:*** Fonergin; Oftcort†; Oftrim†; ***Canad.:*** Proctomyxin; Proctosedyl; Proctosone; Sofracort; Soframycin; ***Denm.:*** Proctosedyl; Sofradex; ***Fin.:*** Proctosedyl; Sofradex; ***Fr.:*** Cortibiotique†; Corticetine; Dermocalm†; Frakidex; Framyxone; Frazoline†; Neoparyl Framycetine†; Novomyxine; Polyfra; Rhinyl†; Soframycine Hydrocortisone†; Soframycine Naphazoline†; Topifram†; ***Ger.:*** Leukase N; ***Hong Kong:*** Frakidex; Proctosedyl; Sofradex; ***India:*** Proctosedyl; Sofracort; Sofradex; Sofradex-F; ***Irl.:*** Proctosedyl; Sofradex; Soframycin; ***Malaysia:*** Proctosedyl; Sofradex; ***Neth.:*** Proctosedyl; Sofradex; ***Norw.:*** Proctosedyl; Sofradex; ***NZ:*** Sofradex; Soframycin; ***Port.:*** Frakidex; ***S.Afr.:*** Proctosedyl; Sofradex; ***Singapore:*** Frakidex; Proctosedyl; Sofradex; Topifram†; ***Spain:*** Abrasone; Aldo Otico; Aldoderma; Nesfare; Otomidrin; ***Swed.:*** Proctosedyl; Sofradex†; ***Switz.:*** Corticetine; Dexalocal-F; Frakidex; Pulpomixine†; Septomixine; Sofradex; ***Thai.:*** Proctosedyl; Sofradex; Topifram; ***UK:*** Sofradex.

## Ftivazide *(rINN)*

Ftivazidum; Phthivazid; Phthivazidum. 2′-Vanillylideneisonicotinohydrazide monohydrate.

$C_{14}H_{13}N_3O_3,H_2O = 289.3$.

*CAS — 149-17-7 (anhydrous ftivazide).*

**Pharmacopoeias.** In *Chin.* and *Int.*

### Profile

Ftivazide is an antimycobacterial used in the treatment of tuberculosis. It is a derivative of isoniazid.

## Furaltadone Hydrochloride *(BANM, rINNM)*

Hidrocloruro de furaltadona. (±)-5-Morpholinomethyl-3-(5-nitrofurfurylideneamino)oxazolidin-2-one hydrochloride.

$C_{13}H_{16}N_4O_6,HCl = 360.8$.

*CAS — 139-91-3 (furaltadone); 59302-14-6 (±-furaltadone).*

**Pharmacopoeias.** *Fr.* includes Furaltadone for veterinary use.

### Profile

Furaltadone was formerly given orally as an antibacterial but was later withdrawn owing to its toxic effects. Furaltadone hydrochloride is still used topically in preparations for ear disorders.

Furaltadone has been used in veterinary medicine.

### Preparations

**Proprietary Preparations** (details are given in Part 3)
**Multi-ingredient:** ***Spain:*** Panotile; ***Thai.:*** Otosamthong.

## Furazidin

Furazidine. 1-{[3-(5-Nitro-2-furyl)allylidene]amino}hydantoin.

$C_{10}H_8N_4O_5 = 264.2$.

*CAS — 1672-88-4.*

### Profile

Furazidin is a nitrofuran antibacterial with properties similar to those of nitrofurantoin and is used in the treatment of urinary-tract infections.

## Fusafungine *(BAN, rINN)*

Fusafungina.

*CAS — 1393-87-9.*

*ATC — R02AB03.*

### Profile

Fusafungine is a depsipeptide antibacterial produced by *Fusarium lateritium* strain 437. It is active against some Gram-positive and Gram-negative organisms, *Candida albicans*, and *Mycoplasma pneumoniae*. It has also been stated to possess anti-inflammatory activity.

It is used in the form of an aerosol spray in the treatment of infections of the upper respiratory tract, inhaled in usual adult doses of 500 micrograms every 4 hours into each nostril or via the mouth. These routes may be used simultaneously if necessary.

### Preparations

**Proprietary Preparations** (details are given in Part 3)
***Austria:*** Locabiosol; ***Belg.:*** Locabiotal; ***Braz.:*** Locabiotal; ***Chile:*** Locabiosol; ***Fr.:*** Locabiotal; ***Ger.:*** Locabiosol; ***Hong Kong:*** Locabiotal; ***Irl.:*** Locabiotal; ***Ital.:*** Locabiotal; ***Malaysia:*** Locabiotal; ***Mex.:*** Locabiotal†; ***Port.:*** Locabiosol; ***S.Afr.:*** Locabiotal; ***Spain:*** Fusaloyos; ***Switz.:*** Locabiotal; ***UK:*** Locabiotal.

# Fusidic Acid *(BAN, USAN, rINN)*

Ácido fusídico; Acidum Fusidicum; SQ-16603. *ent*-16α-Acetoxy-3β-dihydroxy-4β,8β,14α-trimethyl-18-nor-5β,10α-cholesta-(17Z)-17(20),24-dien-21-oic acid hemihydrate.

$C_{31}H_{48}O_6,\frac{1}{2}H_2O = 525.7$.

*CAS — 6990-06-3 (anhydrous fusidic acid).*

*ATC — D06AX01; D09AA02; J01XC01; S01AA13.*

**Pharmacopoeias.** In *Eur.* (see p.vi).

**Ph. Eur. 5.0** (Fusidic Acid). An antimicrobial substance produced by the growth of certain strains of *Fusidium coccineum* or by any other means. A white or almost white crystalline powder. Practically insoluble in water; freely soluble in alcohol. Store at a temperature of 2° to 8°. Protect from light.

## Sodium Fusidate *(BANM, rINNM)*

Fusidate Sodium *(USAN)*; Fusidato sódico; Natrii Fusidas; SQ-16360.

$C_{31}H_{47}NaO_6 = 538.7$.

*CAS — 751-94-0.*

*ATC — D06AX01; D09AA02; J01XC01; S01AA13.*

**Pharmacopoeias.** In *Eur.* (see p.vi) and *Jpn.*

**Ph. Eur. 5.0** (Sodium Fusidate). A white or almost white, slightly hygroscopic, crystalline powder. Freely soluble in water and in alcohol. A 1.25% solution in water has a pH of 7.5 to 9.0. Store in airtight containers at a temperature of 2° to 8°. Protect from light.

**Incompatibility.** The UK manufacturers state that the reconstituted sodium fusidate injection is incompatible with infusion solutions containing glucose 20% or more, and that precipitation may occur in solutions with a pH of less than 7.4.

## Adverse Effects and Precautions

Apart from mild gastrointestinal upsets, fusidic acid or sodium fusidate appear to be well tolerated when given orally. Treatment with fusidates, by mouth or especially by the intravenous route, has been associated with jaundice and changes in liver function; normal liver function is usually restored when treatment is discontinued. Therefore, fusidates should be given with caution to patients with hepatic impairment, and periodic monitoring of hepatic function is recommended in these patients and in those receiving high or prolonged oral doses. Caution is also required in biliary disease or biliary obstruction.

Venospasm, thrombophlebitis, and haemolysis have occurred in patients given fusidates intravenously. To reduce this it is recommended that solutions be buffered and that the solution should be given as a slow infusion into a large vein where there is a good blood flow. Hypocalcaemia has occurred after use of intravenous doses above those recommended, and has been attributed to the phosphate-citrate buffer in the preparation. Intramuscular or subcutaneous use may lead to tissue necrosis and is contra-indicated.

Hypersensitivity reactions in the form of rashes and irritation may occur after fusidates topically; rash is rare after systemic use.

Fusidic acid competes with bilirubin for binding to albumin *in vitro* and caution has been advised if it is given to premature, jaundiced, acidotic, or seriously-ill neonates because of the risk of kernicterus.

**Effects on the blood.** There have been occasional reports of granulocytopenia[1-3] and one case of thrombocytopenia[3] following the use of fusidic acid systemically. Sideroblastic anaemia has also been reported.[4] The UK manufacturers also state that there have been isolated cases of neutropenia, agranulocytosis, and pancytopenia.

1. Revell P, *et al.* Granulocytopenia due to fusidic acid. *Lancet* 1988; **ii:** 454–5.
2. Evans DIK. Granulocytopenia due to fusidic acid. *Lancet* 1988; **ii:** 851.
3. Leibowitz G, *et al.* Leukopenia and thrombocytopenia due to fusidic acid. *Postgrad Med J* 1991; **67:** 591–2.
4. Anonymous. Sideroblastic anaemia and fusidic acid. *Prescrire Int* 2003; **12:** 19.

## Interactions

Although the exact metabolic pathways of fusidic acid are not known, an interaction with drugs metabolised by hepatic cytochrome P450 isoenzymes may be suspected and the UK manufacturers suggest avoiding their use with fusidic acid.

**Antivirals.** An HIV-infected patient had fusidic acid toxicity after taking fusidic acid orally for one week with his usual antiretroviral treatment of ritonavir, saquinavir, and stavudine.[1] The plasma-fusidic acid concentration was about twice that expected and the ritonavir and saquinavir concentrations were also elevated. Fusidic acid was stopped and the patient initially improved. However, 4 days later he presented with jaundice, nausea, weakness, and further increases in liver function tests and hence all medications were stopped. The fusidic acid concentration, as well as those of ritonavir and saquinavir, were found to be still significantly elevated 6 days after fusidic acid had been stopped. The patient was able to restart his antiretroviral therapy later with no problems. The authors suggested that this interaction may be due to mutual inhibition of metabolism between the protease inhibitors and fusidic acid, and recommended that use of fusidic acid with either saquinavir or ritonavir should be avoided.

1. Khaliq Y, *et al.* A drug interaction between fusidic acid and a combination of ritonavir and saquinavir. *Br J Clin Pharmacol* 2000; **50:** 82–3.

## Antimicrobial Action

Fusidic acid is a steroidal antibacterial with a bacteriostatic or bactericidal activity, mainly against Gram-positive bacteria.

*Mechanism of action.* Fusidic acid inhibits bacterial protein synthesis although, in contrast to drugs such as the macrolides or tetracyclines, it does not bind to the bacterial ribosome, but inhibits a factor necessary for translocation of peptide subunits and elongation of the peptide chain. It is capable of inhibiting protein synthesis in mammalian cells but exerts a selective action against susceptible infecting organisms because of poor penetration into the host cell.

*Spectrum of activity.* Fusidic acid is very active against staphylococci, notably *Staph. aureus* and *Staph. epidermidis* (including meticillin-resistant strains). *Nocardia asteroides* and many clostridial strains are also highly susceptible. The streptococci and enterococci are less susceptible.

Most Gram-negative bacteria are intrinsically resistant but fusidic acid is active against *Neisseria* spp. and *Bacteroides fragilis*. It has some activity against strains of *Mycobacterium tuberculosis* and is highly active against *M. leprae*.

Fungi are resistant, but fusidic acid has some activity against a range of protozoa including *Giardia lamblia* and *Plasmodium falciparum*. High concentrations of fusidate are reported to inhibit viral growth *in vitro*, including that of HIV, although it is unclear whether this represents a surfactant effect, a general cytotoxic effect, or a genuine antiviral action.

*Activity with other antimicrobials.* No synergy has been demonstrated *in vitro* in most studies between fusidic acid and rifampicin or vancomycin, and antagonism of the effects of ciprofloxacin has been reported. Interactions with the penicillins are complex, with either antagonism of the effect of one or both drugs, or no interaction. However, use of an antistaphylococcal penicillin with fusidic acid may prevent the emergence of fusidic acid-resistant staphylococcal mutants, and such combinations may be clinically effective.

*Resistance.* Resistant strains of staphylococci are readily selected *in vitro*, and occasionally during therapy, but the number of clinical isolates that are initially resistant remains relatively low at about 1 to 2% overall, despite widespread topical use. Resistance may be chromosomally mediated, representing altered protein synthesis, or plasmid-mediated, which appears to be due to reduced penetration of active drug into the cell.

## Pharmacokinetics

Sodium fusidate is well absorbed from the gastrointestinal tract, and a single 500-mg dose is reported to produce mean plasma concentrations of about 30 micrograms/mL 2 to 4 hours after administration, although there is considerable interindividual variation. Oral suspensions of fusidic acid are less well absorbed, and a 500-mg dose of such a suspension is reported to produce peak plasma concentrations of about 23 micrograms/mL. Absorption may be delayed by food and may be more rapid in children than adults. Some accumulation occurs with repeated administration and plasma concentrations of 100 micrograms/mL or more have been reported following 500 mg of sodium fusidate three times daily for 4 days.

Fusidate is widely distributed into tissues and body fluids, including bone, pus, and synovial fluid; it penetrates cerebral abscesses but does not enter CSF in appreciable amounts. It has been found in the fetal circulation and in breast milk. About 95% or more of fusidate in the circulation is bound to plasma protein.

Fusidate has a plasma half-life that has been variously reported as 5 to 6 and 10 to 15 hours. It is excreted in the bile, almost entirely as metabolites, some of which have weak antimicrobial activity. About 2% appears unchanged in the faeces. Little is excreted in the urine or removed by haemodialysis.

◊ References.


1. Reeves DS. The pharmacokinetics of fusidic acid. *J Antimicrob Chemother* 1987; **20:** 467–76.
2. Peter J-D, *et al.* Pharmacokinetics of intravenous fusidic acid in patients with cholestasis. *Antimicrob Agents Chemother* 1993; **37:** 501–6.
3. Brown NM, *et al.* The pharmacokinetics and protein-binding of fusidic acid in patients with severe renal failure requiring either haemodialysis or continuous ambulatory peritoneal dialysis. *J Antimicrob Chemother* 1997; **39:** 803–9.
4. Turnidge J. Fusidic acid pharmacology, pharmacokinetics and pharmacodynamics. *Int J Antimicrob Agents* 1999; **12** (suppl 2): S23–S34.


## Uses and Administration

Fusidic acid and its salts are antibacterials used mainly in the treatment of staphylococcal infections, often with other drugs. They have been used in the treatment of abscess, including brain abscess, in bone and joint infections, in staphylococcal infections in patients with cystic fibrosis, in the treatment of staphylococcal endocarditis, and topically in eye infections and infections of the skin. For details of these infections and their treatment, see under Choice of Antibacterial, p.120.

*Administration and dosage.* The fusidates are given by mouth or topically as fusidic acid or sodium fusidate, or intravenously as sodium fusidate. 1 g of sodium fusidate is approximately equivalent to 0.98 g of fusidic acid. Because of differences in absorption (see Pharmacokinetics, above) 250 mg of fusidic acid is therapeutically equivalent to only 175 mg of the sodium salt, so doses of fusidic acid suspension (commonly used in children) appear relatively higher. The diolamine salt was formerly used intravenously.

Sodium fusidate is given as tablets in a usual adult dose of 500 mg by mouth every 8 hours, although this dose may be doubled in severe infection. For cutaneous staphylococcal infections, a dose of 250 mg twice daily is suitable. Doses of fusidic acid suspension in children are: up to 1 year, 50 mg/kg daily in 3 divided doses; 1 to 5 years, 250 mg three times daily; 5 to 12 years, 500 mg three times daily; over 12 years and adults, 750 mg three times daily.

In severe infections in adults weighing over 50 kg, sodium fusidate 500 mg is given three times daily by slow intravenous infusion. Each 500-mg dose is usually administered as a buffered solution (pH 7.4 to 7.6) diluted to 500 mL with sodium chloride or other suitable intravenous solution. For children and adults weighing less than 50 kg, a dose of 6 to 7 mg/kg three times daily is used.

Sodium fusidate as a 2% ointment or medicated dressing, or fusidic acid as a 2% cream or gel, are used in the local treatment of skin infections. Eye drops containing fusidic acid 1% are used in eye infections. Topical use may lead to problems of resistance.

## Preparations

**BP 2003:** Fusidic Acid Cream; Fusidic Acid Eye Drops; Fusidic Acid Oral Suspension; Sodium Fusidate Ointment.

**Proprietary Preparations** (details are given in Part 3)
***Arg.:*** Fucidin; Fucithalmic; Fusimed; Fusitop; Gelbiotic; ***Austral.:*** Fucidin; ***Austria:*** Fucidin; Fucithalmic; ***Belg.:*** Fucidin; Fucithalmic; ***Braz.:*** Verutex; ***Canad.:*** Fucidin; Fucithalmic; ***Chile:*** Fucidin; Fucithalmic; ***Denm.:*** Fucidin; Fucithalmic; ***Fin.:*** Fucidin; Fucithalmic; ***Fr.:*** Fucidine; Fucithalmic; ***Ger.:*** Fucidine; Fucithalmic; ***Gr.:*** Fucidin; ***Hong Kong:*** Fucidin; Fucithalmic; ***India:*** Fusiwal; ***Irl.:*** Fucidin; Fucithalmic; ***Israel:*** Fucidin; Fucithalmic; ***Ital.:*** Dermomycin; Fucidin; Fucithalmic; ***Malaysia:*** Foban; Fucidin; Fucithalmic; Germacid; ***Mex.:*** Fucidin; ***Neth.:*** Fucidin; Fucithalmic; ***Norw.:*** Fucidin; Fucithalmic; ***NZ:*** Fucidin; Fucithalmic; ***Port.:*** Fucidine; Fucithalmic; ***S.Afr.:*** Fucidin; Fucithalmic; ***Singapore:*** Balad; Foban; Fucidin; Fucithalmic; ***Spain:*** Fucidine; Fucithalmic; ***Swed.:*** Fucidin; Fucithalmic; ***Switz.:*** Fucidine; Fucithalmic; ***Thai.:*** Fucidin; Fucithalmic; Fusid; ***UAE:*** Futasole; ***UK:*** Fucidin; Fucithalmic.

**Multi-ingredient:** ***Arg.:*** Fucicort; Fusimed B; Gelbiotic Plus; ***Belg.:*** Fucicort; Fucidin Hydrocortisone†; ***Canad.:*** Fucidin H; ***Chile:*** Fucicort; Fucidin H; ***Denm.:*** Fucicort; Fucidin-Hydrocortison; ***Fin.:*** Fucicort; Fucidin-Hydrocortison; ***Ger.:*** Fucicort; Fucidine plus; ***Gr.:*** Fucicort; Fucidin H; ***Hong Kong:*** Fucicort; Fucidin H; ***Irl.:*** Fucibet; Fucidin H; ***Israel:*** Fucicort; Fucidin H; ***Ital.:*** Fucicort; Fucidin H; Piodermina; ***Malaysia:*** Fobancort; Fucicort; Fucidin H; Germacort; ***Mex.:*** Fucicort; ***Norw.:*** Fucidin-Hydrocortison; ***NZ:*** Fucicort; ***Port.:*** Fucicort; Fucidine H; ***S.Afr.:*** Fucidin H; ***Singapore:*** Fobancort; Fucicort; Fucidin H; ***Spain:*** Fucibet; Fucidine H†; ***Swed.:*** Fucidin-Hydrocortison; ***Switz.:*** Fucicort; Fucidin H; ***Thai.:*** Fucicort; Fucidin H; ***UAE:*** Futasone; ***UK:*** Fucibet; Fucidin H.

# Gatifloxacin *(USAN, rINN)*

AM-1155; BMS-206584-01; CG-5501; Gatifloxacino. (±)-1-Cyclopropyl-6-fluoro-1,4-dihydro-8-methoxy-7-(3-methyl-1-piperazinyl)-4-oxo-3-quinolinecarboxylic acid sesquihydrate.

$C_{19}H_{22}FN_3O_4,1\frac{1}{2}H_2O = 402.4.$

*CAS — 160738-57-8 (anhydrous gatifloxacin); 180200-66-2 (gatifloxacin sesquihydrate).*

*ATC — J01MA16.*

## Adverse Effects and Precautions

As for Ciprofloxacin, p.188.

Gatifloxacin may have the potential to prolong the QT interval and should be avoided in patients with existing QT prolongation or uncorrected hypokalaemia.

## Interactions

As for Ciprofloxacin, p.190.

As gatifloxacin may have the potential to prolong the QT interval, it should not be given to patients receiving class Ia antiarrhythmic drugs (such as quinidine and procainamide) or class III antiarrhythmics (such as amiodarone and sotalol). In addition, caution should be exercised when gatifloxacin is used with other drugs known to have this effect (such as the antihistamines astemizole and terfenadine, cisapride, erythromycin, pentamidine, phenothiazines, or tricyclic antidepressants).

**Antidiabetics.** Severe and persistent hypoglycaemia occurred in 3 patients receiving oral hypoglycaemics (*repaglinide, glibenclamide* and *pioglitazone*, and *glimepiride*) when gatifloxacin was added to their therapy.[1]


1. Menzies DJ, *et al.* Severe and persistent hypoglycemia due to gatifloxacin interaction with oral hypoglycemic agents. *Am J Med* 2002; **113:** 232–4.


## Antimicrobial Action

As for Ciprofloxacin, p.190.

Gatifloxacin is reported to have greater activity against Gram-positive bacteria, including pneumococci, than ciprofloxacin.

## Pharmacokinetics

Gatifloxacin is readily absorbed from the gastrointestinal tract with an absolute bioavailability of 96%. Peak plasma concentrations are achieved within 1 to 2 hours of a dose. Gatifloxacin is widely distributed into body tissues and is approximately 20% bound to plasma proteins. It undergoes limited metabolism and has an elimination half-life of 7 to 14 hours. It is excreted primarily unchanged in the urine with less than 1% as metabolites. A small amount (5%) is also excreted unchanged in the faeces.

## Uses and Administration

Gatifloxacin is a fluoroquinolone antibacterial with actions and uses similar to those of ciprofloxacin (p.191). It is given by mouth, or by intravenous infusion as a 2 mg/mL solution over 60 minutes, for the treatment of susceptible infections, including respiratory- and urinary-tract infections. The usual adult dose is 400 mg once daily. A single dose of 400 mg or a dose of 200 mg daily for 3 days may be adequate for uncomplicated urinary-tract infections. A single dose of 400 mg may also be given for the treatment of uncomplicated gonorrhoea.

Gatifloxacin is also given as 0.3% eye drops for the treatment of bacterial conjunctivitis.

For details of reduced doses to be used in renal impairment, see below.

◊ Reviews.


1. Perry CM, *et al.* Gatifloxacin: a review of its use in the management of bacterial infections. *Drugs* 2002; **62:** 169–207.


**Administration in renal impairment.** Doses of gatifloxacin should be reduced in patients with renal impairment; the initial dose of 400 mg should be followed by maintenance doses of 200 mg daily in those with a creatinine clearance less than 40 mL/minute.

## Preparations

**Proprietary Preparations** (details are given in Part 3)
***Arg.:*** Tequin; ***Austral.:*** Tequin; ***Braz.:*** Tequin; ***Canad.:*** Tequin; ***Chile:*** Starox; ***India:*** Zyquin; ***Jpn:*** Gatiflo; ***Malaysia:*** Tequin; ***Mex.:*** Tequin; ***S.Afr.:*** Tequin; ***Singapore:*** Tequin; ***Thai.:*** Tequin; ***USA:*** Tequin; Zymar.

# Gemifloxacin Mesilate *(rINNM)*

Gemifloxacin Mesylate *(USAN)*; LB-20304 (gemifloxacin); LB-20304a; Mesilato de gemifloxacino; SB-265805 (gemifloxacin); SB-265805S. (±)-7-[3-(Aminomethyl)-4-oxo-1-pyrrolidinyl]-1-cyclopropyl-6-fluoro-1,4-dihydro-4-oxo-1,8-naphthyridine-3-carboxylic acid $7^4$-(Z)-(O-methyloxime) methanesulfonate.

$C_{18}H_{20}FN_5O_4,CH_4O_3S = 485.5.$

*CAS — 204519-64-2 (gemifloxacin); 204519-65-3 (gemifloxacin mesilate).*

*ATC — J01MA15.*

## Adverse Effects and Precautions

As for Ciprofloxacin, p.188.

Skin rashes may be more common with gemifloxacin and treatment should be discontinued if they occur.

## Uses and Administration

Gemifloxacin is a fluoroquinolone antibacterial given as the mesilate for the treatment of community-acquired pneumonia and acute bacterial exacerbations of chronic bronchitis. Doses are expressed in terms of the base. It is given by mouth in a dose of 320 mg once daily for 5 days in patients with bronchitis or for 7 days in those with pneumonia.

For details of dosage modification in patients with renal impairment, see below.

◊ Reviews.

1. Lowe MN, Lamb HM. Gemifloxacin. *Drugs* 2000; **59:** 1137–47.

**Administration in renal impairment.** Doses of gemifloxacin should be halved in patients with a creatinine clearance of 40 mL/minute or less, including patients receiving haemodialysis.

### Preparations

**Proprietary Preparations** (details are given in Part 3)
***USA:*** Factive.

## Gentamicin Sulfate *(USAN, pINNM)*

Gentamicin Sulphate *(BANM)*; Gentamicini Sulfas; NSC-82261; Sch-9724; Sulfato de gentamicina.

*CAS — 1403-66-3 (gentamicin); 1405-41-0 (gentamicin sulfate).*

*ATC — D06AX07; J01GB03; S01AA11; S02AA14; S03AA06.*

NOTE. GNT is a code approved by the BP 2003 for use on single unit doses of eye drops containing gentamicin sulfate where the individual container may be too small to bear all the appropriate labelling information.

**Pharmacopoeias.** In *Chin., Eur.* (see p.vi), *Int., Jpn, Pol., US,* and *Viet.*

**Ph. Eur. 5.0** (Gentamicin Sulphate). A mixture of the sulfates of antimicrobial substances produced by *Micromonospora purpurea*, the main components being gentamicins C1, C1a, C2, C2a, and C2b. It contains 20 to 40% of gentamicin C1, 10 to 30% of gentamicin C1a; the sum of gentamicins C2, C2a, and C2b is 40 to 60%. The potency is not less than 590 units/mg, calculated with reference to the anhydrous substance. A white or almost white hygroscopic powder. Freely soluble in water; practically insoluble in alcohol. A 4% solution in water has a pH of 3.5 to 5.5. Store in airtight containers.

**USP 27** (Gentamicin Sulfate). The sulfate salt, or a mixture of such salts, of antibiotic substances produced by the growth of *Micromonospora purpurea*. The content of gentamicin C1 is between 25 and 50%, the content of gentamicin C1a is between 10 and 35%, and the sum of the contents of gentamicin C2a and gentamicin C2 is between 25 and 55%. It has a potency equivalent to not less than 590 micrograms of gentamicin per mg, calculated on the dried basis. A white to buff powder. Freely soluble in water; insoluble in alcohol, in acetone, in chloroform, in ether, and in benzene. pH of a 4% solution in water is between 3.5 and 5.5. Store in airtight containers.

**Incompatibility.** The aminoglycosides are inactivated *in vitro* by various penicillins and cephalosporins via an interaction with the beta-lactam ring, the extent of inactivation depending on temperature, concentration, and duration of contact. The different aminoglycosides vary in their stability, with amikacin apparently the most resistant and tobramycin the most susceptible to inactivation; gentamicin and netilmicin are of intermediate stability. The beta lactams also vary in their ability to produce inactivation, with ampicillin, benzylpenicillin, and antipseudomonal penicillins such as carbenicillin and ticarcillin producing marked inactivation. Inactivation has also been reported with clavulanic acid.

Gentamicin is also incompatible with furosemide, heparin, sodium bicarbonate (the acid pH of gentamicin solutions may liberate carbon dioxide), and some solutions for parenteral nutrition. Interactions with preparations having an alkaline pH (for example sulfadiazine sodium), or drugs unstable at acid pH (for example erythromycin salts), might reasonably be expected.

Given their potential for incompatibility, gentamicin and other aminoglycosides should not generally be mixed with other drugs in syringes or infusion solutions nor given through the same intravenous line. When aminoglycosides are given with a beta lactam, administration should generally be at separate sites.

General references.

1. Henderson JL, *et al.* In vitro inactivation of gentamicin, tobramycin, and netilmicin by carbenicillin, azlocillin, or mezlocillin. *Am J Hosp Pharm* 1981; **38:** 1167–70.
2. Tindula RJ, *et al.* Aminoglycoside inactivation by penicillins and cephalosporins and its impact on drug-level monitoring. *Drug Intell Clin Pharm* 1983; **17:** 906–8.
3. Navarro AS, *et al.* In-vitro interaction between dibekacin and penicillins. *J Antimicrob Chemother* 1986; **17:** 83–9.
4. Courcol RJ, Martin GR. Comparative aminoglycoside inactivation by potassium clavulanate. *J Antimicrob Chemother* 1986; **17:** 682–4.

**Stability.** There was an average 16% potency loss of gentamicin sulfate from solutions containing 10 and 40 mg/mL when stored at 4° or 25° in plastic disposable syringes for 30 days, and a brown precipitate formed in several. Storage in glass disposable syringes for 30 days produced an average 7% potency loss, which was considered acceptable, but storage for longer resulted in precipitate formation in some cases and was not recommended.[1]

1. Weiner B, *et al.* Stability of gentamicin sulfate injection following unit dose repackaging. *Am J Hosp Pharm* 1976; **33:** 1254–9.

### Adverse Effects

The aminoglycosides can produce irreversible, cumulative ototoxicity affecting both the cochlea (manifest as hearing loss, initially of higher tones, and which, because speech recognition relies greatly on lower frequencies, may not be at first apparent) and the vestibular system (manifest as dizziness or vertigo). The incidence and relative toxicity with different aminoglycosides is a matter of some dispute, but netilmicin is probably less cochleotoxic than gentamicin or tobramycin, and amikacin more so. Netilmicin also exhibits less vestibular toxicity than gentamicin, tobramycin, or amikacin, while streptomycin produces a high incidence of vestibular damage. Vestibular damage is more common than hearing loss in patients receiving gentamicin.

Reversible nephrotoxicity may occur and acute renal failure has been reported, often in association with the use of other nephrotoxic drugs. Renal impairment is usually mild, although acute tubular necrosis and interstitial nephritis have occurred. Decreased glomerular filtration rate is usually seen only after several days, and may even occur after therapy has been discontinued. Electrolyte disturbances (notably hypomagnesaemia, but also hypocalcaemia and hypokalaemia) have occurred. The nephrotoxicity of gentamicin is reported to be largely due to the gentamicin $C_2$ component.

Although particularly associated with high plasma concentrations, many risk factors have been suggested for ototoxicity and nephrotoxicity in patients receiving aminoglycosides—see Precautions below.

Aminoglycosides possess a neuromuscular-blocking action and respiratory depression and muscular paralysis have been reported, notably after absorption from serous surfaces. Neomycin has the most potent action and several deaths have been associated with its use.

Hypersensitivity reactions have occurred, especially after local use, and cross-sensitivity between aminoglycosides may occur. Very rarely, anaphylactic reactions to gentamicin have occurred. Some hypersensitivity reactions have been attributed to the presence of sulfites in parenteral formulations, and endotoxic shock has also been reported.

Infrequent effects reported for gentamicin include blood dyscrasias, purpura, nausea and vomiting, stomatitis, and signs of liver dysfunction such as increased serum-aminotransferase values and increased serum-bilirubin concentrations. Neurotoxicity has occurred, with both peripheral neuropathies and central symptoms being reported including encephalopathy, confusion, lethargy, hallucinations, convulsions, and mental depression.

Atrophy or fat necrosis has been reported at injection sites. There have been isolated reports of meningeal irritation, arachnoiditis, polyradiculitis, and ventriculitis following the intrathecal, intracisternal, or intraventricular use of aminoglycosides. Subconjunctival injection of gentamicin may lead to pain, hyperaemia, and conjunctival oedema, while severe retinal ischaemia has followed intra-ocular injection.

**Effects on the ears.** Reviews and references to aminoglycoside-induced ototoxicity.

1. Cone LA. A survey of prospective, controlled clinical trials of gentamicin, tobramycin, amikacin, and netilmicin. *Clin Ther* 1982; **5:** 155–62.
2. Kahlmeter G, Dahlager JI. Aminoglycoside toxicity—a review of clinical studies published between 1975 and 1982. *J Antimicrob Chemother* 1984; **13** (suppl A): 9–22.
3. Brummett RE, Fox KE. Aminoglycoside-induced hearing loss in humans. *Antimicrob Agents Chemother* 1989; **33:** 797–800.
4. Mattie H, *et al.* Determinants of efficacy and toxicity of aminoglycosides. *J Antimicrob Chemother* 1989; **24:** 281–93.
5. Schacht J. Aminoglycoside ototoxicity: prevention in sight? *Otolaryngol Head Neck Surg* 1998; **118:** 674–7.

**Effects on the kidneys.** Reviews and references to aminoglycoside-induced nephrotoxicity.

1. Cone LA. A survey of prospective, controlled clinical trials of gentamicin, tobramycin, amikacin, and netilmicin. *Clin Ther* 1982; **5:** 155–62.
2. Lietman PS, Smith CR. Aminoglycoside nephrotoxicity in humans. *Rev Infect Dis* 1983; **5** (suppl 2): S284–93.
3. Kahlmeter G, Dahlager JI. Aminoglycoside toxicity—a review of clinical studies published between 1975 and 1982. *J Antimicrob Chemother* 1984; **13** (suppl A): 9–22.
4. Kohlhepp SJ, *et al.* Nephrotoxicity of the constituents of the gentamicin complex. *J Infect Dis* 1984; **149:** 605–14.
5. Mattie H, *et al.* Determinants of efficacy and toxicity of aminoglycosides. *J Antimicrob Chemother* 1989; **24:** 281–93.
6. Appel GB. Aminoglycoside nephrotoxicity. *Am J Med* 1990; **88** (suppl 3C): 16S–20S.
7. Bertino JS, *et al.* Incidence of and significant risk factors for aminoglycoside-associated nephrotoxicity in patients dosed by using individualized pharmacokinetic monitoring. *J Infect Dis* 1993; **167:** 173–9.

**Endotoxin reactions.** Reports of endotoxin reactions associated with intravenous gentamicin have been received by the CDC and the FDA in the USA.[1] Although endotoxin concentrations in the injections used were within USP limits, administration as a single daily dose rather than in divided doses was thought to have resulted in toxic serum concentrations of endotoxins.[1,2]

1. Centers for Disease Control. Endotoxin-like reactions associated with intravenous gentamicin—California, 1998. *MMWR* 1998; **47:** 877–80.
2. Krieger JA, Duncan L. Gentamicin contaminated with endotoxin. *N Engl J Med* 1999; **340:** 1122.

### Treatment of Adverse Effects

Aminoglycosides may be removed by haemodialysis or to a much lesser extent by peritoneal dialysis. Calcium salts given intravenously have been used to counter neuromuscular blockade; the effectiveness of neostigmine has been variable.

◊ For reference to the potential for calcium-channel blockers to reduce aminoglycoside-related nephrotoxicity, see Kidney Disorders, under Uses of Verapamil, p.1021.

### Precautions

Gentamicin is contra-indicated in patients with a known history of hypersensitivity to it, and probably in those hypersensitive to other aminoglycosides. It should be avoided in patients with myasthenia gravis, and great care is required in patients with parkinsonism and other conditions characterised by muscular weakness.

The risk of ototoxicity and nephrotoxicity from aminoglycosides is increased at high plasma concentrations and it is therefore generally desirable to determine dosage requirements by individual monitoring. In patients receiving standard multiple-dose regimens of gentamicin, dosage should be adjusted to avoid peak plasma concentrations above 10 micrograms/mL, or trough concentrations (immediately before next dose) exceeding 2 micrograms/mL. Monitoring is particularly important in patients receiving high doses or prolonged courses, in infants and the elderly, and in patients with renal impairment, who generally require reduced doses. The *British National Formulary* also considers monitoring to be important in patients with cystic fibrosis or significant obesity; again, altered doses may be required. See Pharmacokinetics below for other patient groups in whom pharmacokinetics may be altered. Impaired hepatic function or auditory function, bacteraemia, fever, and perhaps exposure to loud noises have also been reported to increase the risk of ototoxicity, while volume depletion or hypotension, liver disease, or female sex have been reported as additional risk factors for nephrotoxicity. Regular assessment of auditory and renal function is particularly necessary in patients with additional risk factors.

Topical application of gentamicin into the ear is contra-indicated in patients with known or suspected perforation of the ear drum.

Use of aminoglycosides during pregnancy may damage the eighth cranial nerve of the fetus.

**Breast feeding.** A study[1] involving 10 mothers given gentamicin and their breast-fed infants found measurable gentamicin concentrations in the serum of 5 of the 10 neonates, indicating that appreciable gastrointestinal absorption had occurred. It was, however, considered that these low concentrations would not cause clinical effects and the American Academy of Pediatrics[2] also considers that the use of gentamicin is usually compatible with breast feeding.


1. Celiloglu M, *et al.* Gentamicin excretion and uptake from breast milk by nursing infants. *Obstet Gynecol* 1994; **84:** 263–5.
2. American Academy of Pediatrics. The transfer of drugs and other chemicals into human milk. *Pediatrics* 2001; **108:** 776–89. Correction. *ibid.*; 1029. Also available at: http://aappolicy.aappublications.org/cgi/content/full/pediatrics%3b108/3/776 (accessed 27/05/04)


**Interference with assay procedures.** The implications of drug interference with assays for aminoglycosides have been reviewed.[1] A number of other antimicrobials and antineoplastics may alter the results of microbiological assays but this might be overcome by selection of an appropriate assay organism.

Microbiological assays for aminoglycosides in samples also containing *imipenem* could be accomplished by using cysteine hydrochloride to inactivate imipenem, since it is stable to most beta-lactamases and resistant strains are extremely rare.[2] Because aminoglycosides may be inactivated by *penicillins* and *cephalosporins*, it has been recommended that aminoglycoside sampling times should be chosen to coincide with a trough plasma concentration for the beta lactam. Samples should be frozen if there is to be a delay before they are assayed[3] or a penicillinase added. However, one group of workers have reported loss of gentamicin activity after storage at −60° before assay.[4] Furthermore, there have been reports that concentrations of aminoglycosides in patients also receiving beta lactams have been overestimated using a homogeneous enzyme immunoassay, probably because of an inability to differentiate between active drug and inactivated products.[5,6]

The radionuclide *gallium-67* interferes with radio-enzymatic assays, and it has been suggested that an agar diffusion method should be used in patients who have received a gallium scan.[7,8]

*Heparin* has been shown to produce underestimation of aminoglycoside concentrations when using microbiological, enzymatic, or immunoassays.[9-11] It has been recommended that either serum should be used or that blood samples should not be collected in heparinised tubes or from indwelling catheter lines. Some consider that concentrations of heparin reached in the blood of patients receiving heparin are too low to affect gentamicin.[12]

Falsely low concentrations have also been reported in microbiological assays in the presence of *zinc* salts.[13]

Heat treatment of whole *blood* to inactivate human immunodeficiency virus leads to an increase in the concentration of gentamicin subsequently found on assay.[14]


1. Yosselson-Superstine S. Drug interferences with plasma assays in therapeutic drug monitoring. *Clin Pharmacokinet* 1984; **9:** 67–87.
2. McLeod KM, *et al.* Gentamicin assay in the presence of imipenem. *J Antimicrob Chemother* 1986; **17:** 828–9.
3. Tindula RJ, *et al.* Aminoglycoside inactivation by penicillins and cephalosporins and its impact on drug-level monitoring. *Drug Intell Clin Pharm* 1983; **17:** 906–8.
4. Carlson LG, *et al.* Potential liabilities of gentamicin homogeneous enzyme immunoassay. *Antimicrob Agents Chemother* 1982; **21:** 192–4.
5. Ebert SC, Clementi WA. In vitro inactivation of gentamicin by carbenicillin, compared by Emit and microbiological assays. *Drug Intell Clin Pharm* 1983; **17:** 451.
6. Dalmady-Israel C, *et al.* Ticarcillin and assay of tobramycin. *Ann Intern Med* 1984; **100:** 460.
7. Bhattacharya I, *et al.* Effects of radiopharmaceuticals on radioenzymatic assays of aminoglycoside antibiotics: interference by gallium-67 and its elimination. *Antimicrob Agents Chemother* 1978; **14:** 448–53.
8. Shannon K, *et al.* Interference with gentamicin assays by gallium-67. *J Antimicrob Chemother* 1980; **6:** 285–300.
9. Nilsson L. Factors affecting gentamicin assay. *Antimicrob Agents Chemother* 1980; **17:** 918–21. Correction. *ibid.*; **18:** 839.
10. Nilsson L, *et al.* Inhibition of aminoglycoside activity by heparin. *Antimicrob Agents Chemother* 1981: **20:** 155–8.
11. O'Connell MB, *et al.* Heparin interference with tobramycin, netilmicin, and gentamicin concentrations determined by Emit. *Drug Intell Clin Pharm* 1984; **18:** 503–4.
12. Regamey C, *et al.* Inhibitory effect of heparin on gentamicin concentrations in blood. *Antimicrob Agents Chemother* 1972; **1:** 329–32.
13. George RH, Healing DE. The effect of zinc on aminoglycoside assay. *J Antimicrob Chemother* 1978; **4:** 186.
14. Eley A, *et al.* Effect of heat on gentamicin assays. *Lancet* 1987; **ii:** 335–6.


## Interactions

Use of other nephrotoxic drugs, including other aminoglycosides, vancomycin, some cephalosporins, ciclosporin, cisplatin, and fludarabine, or of potentially ototoxic drugs such as etacrynic acid and perhaps furosemide, may increase the risk of aminoglycoside toxicity. It has been suggested that use of an antiemetic such as dimenhydrinate may mask the early symptoms of vestibular ototoxicity. Care is also required if other drugs with a neuromuscular-blocking action are used (see Atracurium, p.1400). The neuromuscular-blocking properties of aminoglycosides may be sufficient to provoke severe respiratory depression in patients receiving general anaesthetics or opioids.

There is a theoretical possibility that the antibacterial effects of aminoglycosides could be reduced by bacteriostatic antibacterials, but such combinations have been used successfully in practice.

Since aminoglycosides have been shown to be incompatible with some beta lactams *in vitro* (see Incompatibility, above), these antibacterials should be administered separately if both are required; antagonism *in vivo* has been reported only in a few patients with severe renal impairment, in whom aminoglycoside activity was diminished. Aminoglycosides exhibit synergistic activity with a number of beta lactams *in vivo* (see Antimicrobial Action, below).

Renal excretion of zalcitabine may be reduced by aminoglycosides.

For a report of severe hypocalcaemia in a patient receiving aminoglycosides and bisphosphonates, see p.767.

Gentamicin may inhibit α-galactosidase activity and should not be used with agalsidase alfa or beta.

## Antimicrobial Action

Gentamicin is an aminoglycoside antibiotic and has a bactericidal action against many Gram-negative aerobes and against some strains of staphylococci.

*Mechanism of action.* Aminoglycosides are taken up into sensitive bacterial cells by an active transport process which is inhibited in anaerobic, acidic, or hyperosmolar environments. Within the cell they bind to the 30S, and to some extent to the 50S, subunits of the bacterial ribosome, inhibiting protein synthesis and generating errors in the transcription of the genetic code. The manner in which cell death is brought about is imperfectly understood, and other mechanisms may contribute, including effects on membrane permeability.

*Spectrum of activity.* The following pathogenic organisms are usually sensitive to gentamicin (but see also Resistance, below).

Many strains of Gram-negative bacteria including species of *Brucella, Calymmatobacterium, Campylobacter, Citrobacter, Escherichia, Enterobacter, Francisella, Klebsiella, Proteus, Providencia, Pseudomonas, Serratia, Vibrio*, and *Yersinia.* Some activity has been reported against isolates of *Neisseria*, although aminoglycosides are rarely used clinically in neisserial infections.

Among the Gram-positive organisms many strains of *Staphylococcus aureus* are highly sensitive to gentamicin. *Listeria monocytogenes* and some strains of *Staph. epidermidis* may also be sensitive to gentamicin, but enterococci and streptococci are usually insensitive to gentamicin.

Some actinomycetes and mycoplasmas have been reported to be sensitive to gentamicin, but mycobacteria are insensitive at clinically achievable concentrations; anaerobic organisms, yeasts, and fungi are resistant.

*Activity with other antimicrobials.* Gentamicin exhibits synergy with beta lactams, probably because the effects of the latter on bacterial cell walls enhance aminoglycoside penetration. Enhanced activity has been demonstrated with a penicillin (such as ampicillin or benzylpenicillin) and gentamicin against the enterococci, and gentamicin has been combined with an antipseudomonal penicillin such as ticarcillin for enhanced activity against *Pseudomonas* spp., and with vancomycin for enhanced activity against staphylococci and streptococci.

*Resistance* to the aminoglycosides may be acquired by three main mechanisms. The first is by mutation of ribosomal target sites leading to reduced affinity for binding; this type of resistance is generally only relevant for streptomycin and, even then, it appears to be rare in Gram-negative bacteria. Secondly, penetration of aminoglycosides into bacterial cells is by an oxygen-dependent active transport process and resistance may occur because of elimination or reduction of this uptake; when it occurs this generally results in cross-resistance to all aminoglycosides. Thirdly, and by far the most important cause of resistance to the aminoglycosides, is inactivation by enzymatic modification. Three main classes of enzyme conferring resistance have been found, operating by phosphorylation, acetylation, or addition of a nucleotide group, usually adenyl. Enzyme production is usually plasmid-determined and resistance can therefore be transferred between bacteria, even of different species. Resistance to other antibacterials may be transferred at the same time. In *Staph. aureus* such transfer of resistance is reportedly facilitated when these drugs are used topically. Each type of enzyme produces characteristic patterns of resistance, but their overlapping and variable affinities for their substrates result in a wide range of permutations of cross-resistance to the different aminoglycosides. The different enzymes vary in their distribution and prevalence in different locations, and at different times, presumably with variations in antibacterial usage, but relationships to the use of specific aminoglycosides are difficult to establish. These variations in drug sensitivity require local testing to determine resistance and establish susceptibility of bacteria to the aminoglycoside being used, but such local variations mean that estimates of the incidence of resistance are of limited value. In general, the occurrence of resistant pathogens seems to have been greater in southern than in northern Europe, and perhaps greater in the USA than in Europe. There has been particular concern over the increasing incidence of high-level gentamicin resistance among enterococci (in up to 50% of isolates from some centres), since they already possess inherent or acquired resistance to many drugs, including vancomycin in some cases. A similar problem exists with gentamicin resistance in meticillin-resistant strains of *Staph. aureus.* Such multiply-resistant strains pose a major therapeutic problem in those centres where they occur, since the usual synergistic combinations with other antibacterials are ineffective. However, results from some centres indicate that rational use of a wider range of aminoglycosides (including amikacin which is not affected by most of the aminoglycoside-degrading enzymes) has resulted in a modest decline in overall aminoglycoside resistance.

◊ References.


1. Mingeot-Leclercq M-P, *et al.* Aminoglycosides: activity and resistance. *Antimicrob Agents Chemother* 1999; **43:** 727–37.
2. Kotra LP, *et al.* Aminoglycosides: perspectives on mechanisms of action and resistance and strategies to counter resistance. *Antimicrob Agents Chemother* 2000; **44:** 3249–56.
3. Barclay ML, Begg EJ. Aminoglycoside adaptive resistance: importance for effective dosage regimens. *Drugs* 2001; **61:** 713–21.


## Pharmacokinetics

Gentamicin and other aminoglycosides are poorly absorbed from the gastrointestinal tract but are rapidly absorbed after intramuscular injection. Average peak plasma concentrations of about 4 micrograms/mL have been attained in patients with normal renal function 30 to 60 minutes after an intramuscular dose equivalent to gentamicin 1 mg/kg, which is similar to concentrations achieved after intravenous infusion. There may be considerable individual variation. Several doses are required before plasma equilibrium concentrations occur and this may represent the saturation of binding sites in body tissues such as the kidney. Binding of gentamicin to plasma proteins is usually low.

Following parenteral use, gentamicin and other aminoglycosides diffuse mainly into extracellular fluids. However, there is little diffusion into the CSF and even when the meninges are inflamed effective concentrations may not be achieved; diffusion into the eye is also poor. Aminoglycosides diffuse readily into the perilymph of the inner ear. They cross the placenta but only small amounts have been reported in breast milk.

Systemic absorption of gentamicin and other aminoglycosides has been reported after topical use on denuded skin and burns and following instillation into, and irrigation of, wounds, body-cavities (except the urinary bladder), and joints.

The plasma elimination half-life for gentamicin has been reported to be 2 to 3 hours though it may be considerably longer in neonates and patients with renal impairment. Gentamicin and other aminoglycosides do not appear to be metabolised and are excreted virtually unchanged in the urine by glomerular filtration. At steady state at least 70% of a dose may be recovered in the urine in 24 hours and urine concentrations in excess of 100 micrograms/mL may be achieved. However, gentamicin and the other aminoglycosides appear to accumulate in body tissues to some extent, mainly in the kidney, although the relative degree to which this occurs may vary with different aminoglycosides. Release from these sites is slow and small amounts of aminoglycosides may be detected in the urine for up to 20 days or more after administration ceases. Small amounts of gentamicin appear in the bile.

The pharmacokinetics of the aminoglycosides are affected by many factors, which may become significant because of the relatively small difference between therapeutic and toxic concentrations, reinforcing the need for monitoring.

- Absorption from intramuscular sites may be reduced in critically ill patients, especially in conditions that reduce perfusion such as shock, resulting in **reduced plasma concentrations**. Plasma concentrations may also be reduced in patients with conditions which expand extracellular fluid volume or increase renal clearance including ascites, cirrhosis, heart failure, malnutrition, spinal cord injury, burns, cystic fibrosis, and possibly leukaemia. Clearance is also reportedly increased in intravenous drug abusers, and in patients who are febrile.
- In contrast, renal impairment or reduced renal clearance for any reason (for example in neonates with immature renal function, or in the elderly in whom glomerular function tends to decline with age) can result in markedly **increased plasma concentrations** and/or prolonged half-lives. However, in neonates initial plasma concentrations may actually be reduced, due to a larger volume of distribution. Plasma concentrations may also be higher than expected for a given dose in obese patients (in whom extracellular volume is low relative to weight), and in patients with anaemia.

Renal clearance, and hence plasma concentrations, of aminoglycosides may vary according to a circadian cycle, and it has been suggested that this should be taken into account when determining and comparing plasma aminoglycoside concentrations.

## Uses and Administration

Gentamicin is an aminoglycoside antibiotic used, often with other antibacterials, to treat severe systemic infections due to sensitive Gram-negative and other organisms (see Antimicrobial Action, above). Such infections include biliary-tract infections (acute cholecystitis or cholangitis), brucellosis, cat scratch disease, cystic fibrosis, endocarditis (in the treatment and prophylaxis of endocarditis due to streptococci, enterococci, or staphylococci), endometritis, gastroenteritis, granuloma inguinale, listeriosis, meningitis, otitis externa, otitis media, pelvic inflammatory disease, peritonitis, plague, pneumonia, septicaemia, skin infections such as in burns or ulcers (given systemically for pseudomonal and other Gram-negative infections), tularaemia, and urinary-tract infections (acute pyelonephritis), as well as in the prophylaxis of surgical infection and the treatment of immunocompromised patients and those in intensive care. Gentamicin is also applied topically for localised infections. For details of these infections and their treatment, see under Choice of Antibacterial, p.120.

Gentamicin is often used with other antibacterials to extend its spectrum of activity or increase its efficacy, e.g. with a penicillin for enterococcal and streptococcal infections, or an antipseudomonal beta lactam for pseudomonal infections, or with metronidazole or clindamycin for mixed aerobic-anaerobic infections.

*Administration and dosage.* Gentamicin is used as the sulfate but doses are expressed in terms of gentamicin base. In the management of many of the infections above it is commonly given intramuscularly every 8 hours to provide a total daily dose of 3 to 5 mg/kg. Slightly lower doses have been suggested in the prophylaxis and treatment of streptococcal and enterococcal endocarditis: in the UK a dose of 80 mg twice daily in association with a penicillin or vancomycin has been suggested for treatment; a suggested dose for prophylaxis in high-risk patients is 120 mg before induction of anaesthesia, with a penicillin or vancomycin or teicoplanin. For urinary-tract infections, if renal function is not impaired, 160 mg once daily may be used.

Gentamicin sulfate may also be given intravenously in similar doses to those used intramuscularly, but there is some disagreement as to the appropriate method, since intravenous infusion has been associated with both subtherapeutic and excessive trough concentrations of gentamicin, while bolus intravenous injection may increase the risk of neuromuscular blockade. In the USA, intravenous infusion over 30 minutes to 2 hours is favoured, but sources in the UK differ, with some manufacturers recommending infusion over no more than 20 minutes, in a limited fluid volume, while others suggest that it should not be given by slow infusion, recommending bolus injection over at least 2 to 3 minutes, and yet others allow administration in a similar way to the USA.

The course of treatment should generally be limited to 7 to 10 days. As gentamicin is poorly distributed into fatty tissue it has been suggested that dosage calculations should be based on an estimate of lean body weight.

*Doses in infants and children* are usually somewhat higher than those in adults but exact dosage recommendations vary. One regimen is gentamicin 3 mg/kg every 12 hours in premature infants and those up to 2 weeks of age, with older neonates and children receiving 2 mg/kg every 8 hours. Alternatively, 2.5 mg/kg every 12 hours in the first week of life, 2.5 mg/kg every 8 hours or 3 mg/kg every 12 hours in infants and neonates, and 1.5 to 2 mg/kg every 8 hours in children has been given.

*Dose adjustment and monitoring.* Dosage should be adjusted in all patients according to plasma-gentamicin concentrations, and this is discussed in more detail under Administration and Dosage, below.

*Once-daily dosage.* Some sources consider, in contrast to what has been the accepted view, that there may be advantages to administering the total daily requirement as a single dose (see Once-daily Dosage, below). However, it is not yet clear whether once-daily dosage is as effective as conventional dosage regimens in all cases, particularly in children, or in patients with endocarditis or renal impairment. With once-daily dosage, traditional methods of monitoring peak and trough plasma concentrations may not be applicable and advice on dosage and plasma concentrations should be sought.

*Other routes.* Gentamicin has sometimes been given by mouth for enteric infections and to suppress intestinal flora and has occasionally been given by inhalation in cystic fibrosis. In meningitis it has been given intrathecally or intraventricularly usually in doses of 1 to 5 mg daily together with intramuscular therapy. Gentamicin has also been given by subconjunctival injection.

A bone cement impregnated with gentamicin is used in orthopaedic surgery. Acrylic beads containing gentamicin and threaded on to surgical wire are implanted in the management of bone infections.

Gentamicin has also been applied topically for skin infections in concentrations of 0.1%, but such use may lead to the emergence of resistance and is considered inadvisable. Concentrations of 0.3% are used in preparations for topical application to the eyes and ears.

A liposomal formulation of gentamicin is under investigation.

◊ Reviews.


1. Edson RS, Terrell CL. The aminoglycosides. *Mayo Clin Proc* 1999; **74:** 519–28.


**Administration and dosage.** CONCENTRATION MONITORING. Measurements of aminoglycoside plasma concentrations are routinely performed to individualize dosage regimens, both in terms of dose per administration and dosing interval, in order to attain the desired therapeutic range as quickly as possible.[1] This entails measurement of both peak concentrations to monitor efficacy and trough concentrations to avoid accumulation and thereby prevent toxicity. Dosage should be adjusted in all patients according to these concentrations, but this is of particular importance where factors such as age, renal impairment, or high dosage may predispose to toxicity. Although there has been some dispute about the relationship between plasma concentrations and toxicity it is generally recommended that, for multiple daily dosing with gentamicin, trough plasma concentrations (measured just before the next dose) should be less than 2 micrograms/mL, and peak concentrations should reach at least 4 micrograms/mL but not exceed 10 micrograms/mL. In the UK, peak concentrations are generally measured 1 hour after intramuscular and intravenous doses, but practice has varied between centres and countries and this may lead to difficulties when comparing figures.

Various methods exist for calculating aminoglycoside dosage requirements, though none has been universally accepted. Simple pharmacokinetic methods involve linear dosage adjustment based on peak or trough concentrations or area under the concentration-time curve, or the use of predictive nomograms.[1] For most patients receiving once daily administration (see below), the nomogram is the method of choice, primarily because of its simplicity. However, it has not been validated for children and does not work in patients with either a very high clearance of aminoglycosides or a high volume of distribution, such as those with ascites, burns, or cystic fibrosis, or in other conditions such as pregnancy where the fixed dose assumed in the construction of the nomogram is irrelevant. When a nomogram cannot be applied, a more sophisticated pharmacokinetic method is required, using either Bayesian statistics or non-Bayesian methods such as that of Sawchuk and Zaske.[2,3] Bayesian methods are favoured when the patient population's pharmacokinetic parameters are well known because of their good predictive performance. Otherwise, the Sawchuk and Zaske method is the method of choice because of its robustness and the lack of requirement for prior information about the distribution of parameters within the population.[1]


1. Tod MM, *et al.* Individualising aminoglycoside dosage regimens after therapeutic drug monitoring: simple or complex pharmacokinetic methods? *Clin Pharmacokinet* 2001; **40:** 803–14.
2. Sawchuk RJ, Zaske DE. Pharmacokinetics of dosing regimens which utilize multiple intravenous infusions: gentamicin in burn patients. *J Pharmacokinet Biopharm* 1976; **4:** 183–95.
3. Sawchuk RJ, *et al.* Kinetic model for gentamicin dosing with the use of individual patient parameters. *Clin Pharmacol Ther* 1977; **21:** 362–9.


IN NEONATES AND INFANTS. References.


1. Isemann BT, *et al.* Optimal gentamicin therapy in preterm neonates includes loading doses and early monitoring. *Ther Drug Monit* 1996; **18:** 549–55.
2. Logsdon BA, Phelps SJ. Routine monitoring of gentamicin serum concentrations in pediatric patients with normal renal function is unnecessary. *Ann Pharmacother* 1997; **31:** 1514–18.
3. Murphy JE, *et al.* Evaluation of gentamicin pharmacokinetics and dosing protocols in 195 neonates. *Am J Health-Syst Pharm* 1998; **55:** 2280–9.
4. Yeung MY, Smyth JP. Targeting gentamicin concentrations in babies: the younger the baby, the larger the loading dose and the longer the dose interval. *Aust J Hosp Pharm* 2000; **30:** 98–101.
5. Stickland MD, *et al.* An extended interval dosing method for gentamicin in neonates. *J Antimicrob Chemother* 2001; **48:** 887–93.
6. Rastogi A, *et al.* Comparison of two gentamicin dosing schedules in very low birth weight infants. *Pediatr Infect Dis J* 2002; **21:** 234–40.
7. Chattopadhyay B. Newborns and gentamicin—how much and how often? *J Antimicrob Chemother* 2002; **49:** 13–16.


IN PATIENTS WITH NON-IDEAL BODY WEIGHT. References.


1. Traynor AM, *et al.* Aminoglycoside dosing weight correction factors for patients of various body sizes. *Antimicrob Agents Chemother* 1995; **39:** 545–8.


IN RENAL IMPAIRMENT. Although a number of nomograms, schedules, and rules have been devised for the calculation of aminoglycoside dosage in renal impairment, where possible dosage modification should be based on the monitoring of individual pharmacokinetic parameters. Standard dosage calculation methods should not be used for patients undergoing dialysis as they may require supplementary post-dialysis doses.

ONCE DAILY DOSAGE. The concept of giving aminoglycosides once daily rather than in divided doses is attractive on the grounds of convenience and economy. The rationale cited by proponents of single daily doses for preferring high intermittent plasma concentrations includes the prolonged postantibiotic effect of aminoglycosides (persistent antibacterial activity after plasma concentrations have fallen below the MIC), potentially higher antibacterial concentrations at the site of infection, and theoretical reductions in the incidence of adaptive resistance, with no apparent increase in nephrotoxicity. There have been numerous clinical studies but these have generally included small numbers of patients with uncomplicated infections and have excluded patients with altered pharmacokinetic profiles. Despite the deficiencies of these studies, several meta-analyses have been published which have concluded that once-daily administration appears to be at least as effective as, and no more toxic than, multiple daily dosing in such patient populations.[1-7] Some have questioned the validity of these conclusions[8] while others take a more optimistic view.[9] Despite the reports of good tolerability, an increase in endotoxin reactions has recently been associated with the use of single daily doses (see under Adverse Effects, above).

Several methods for calculating doses and monitoring treatment have been proposed[10-12] but consensus is still needed on appropriate treatment regimens and suitable target serum concentrations.[12-14] There is currently insufficient information for pregnant or breast-feeding women, or patients with burns or impaired renal or hepatic function.[12-14] However, preliminary reports suggest that once-daily use may be practical in trauma patients,[15] neonates and children,[16-18] including those with neutropenia,[19] and patients with cystic fibrosis.[20,21] Once daily dosage may, though, be inappropriate for elderly patients[22] (due to an increased incidence of nephrotoxicity), patients in whom the volume of drug distribution or clearance is difficult to predict or markedly abnormal,[23] and in the treatment of enterococcal endocarditis.[12]


1. Barza M, *et al.* Single or multiple daily doses of aminoglycosides: a meta-analysis. *BMJ* 1996; **312:** 338–45.
2. Hatala R, *et al.* Once-daily aminoglycoside dosing in immunocompetent adults: a meta-analysis. *Ann Intern Med* 1996; **124:** 717–25.
3. Ferriols-Lisart R, Alos-Almiñana M. Effectiveness and safety of once-daily aminoglycosides: a meta-analysis. *Am J Health-Syst Pharm* 1996; **53:** 1141–50.
4. Munckhof WJ, *et al.* A meta-analysis of studies on the safety and efficacy of aminoglycosides given either once daily or as divided doses. *J Antimicrob Chemother* 1996; **37:** 645–63.
5. Bailey TC, *et al.* A meta-analysis of extended-interval dosing versus multiple daily dosing of aminoglycosides. *Clin Infect Dis* 1997; **24:** 786–95.
6. Ali MZ, Goetz MB. A meta-analysis of the relative efficacy and toxicity of single daily dosing versus multiple daily dosing of aminoglycosides. *Clin Infect Dis* 1997; **24:** 796–809.
7. Hatala R, *et al.* Single daily dosing of aminoglycosides in immunocompromised adults: a systematic review. *Clin Infect Dis* 1997; **24:** 810–15.
8. Bertino JS, *et al.* Single daily dosing of aminoglycosides—a concept whose time has not yet come. *Clin Infect Dis* 1997; **24:** 820–3.
9. Gilbert DN. Meta-analyses are no longer required for determining the efficacy of single daily dosing of aminoglycosides. *Clin Infect Dis* 1997; **24:** 816–19.
10. Begg EJ, *et al.* A suggested approach to once-daily aminoglycoside dosing. *Br J Clin Pharmacol* 1995; **39:** 605–9.
11. Prins JM, *et al.* Validation and nephrotoxicity of a simplified once-daily aminoglycoside dosing schedule and guidelines for monitoring therapy. *Antimicrob Agents Chemother* 1996; **40:** 2494–9.
12. Freeman CD, *et al.* Once-daily dosing of aminoglycosides: review and recommendations for clinical practice. *J Antimicrob Chemother* 1997; **39:** 677–86.
13. Rodvold KA, *et al.* Single daily doses of aminoglycosides. *Lancet* 1997; **350:** 1412.
14. Anonymous. Aminoglycosides once daily? *Drug Ther Bull* 1997; **35:** 36–7.
15. Finnell DL, *et al.* Validation of the Hartford nomogram in trauma surgery patients. *Ann Pharmacother* 1998; **32:** 417–21.
16. Langlass TM, Mickle TR. Standard gentamicin dosage regimen in neonates. *Am J Health-Syst Pharm* 1999; **56:** 440–3.
17. Thureen PJ, *et al.* Once- versus twice-daily gentamicin dosing in neonates ≥34 weeks' gestation: cost-effectiveness analyses. *Pediatrics* 1999; **103:** 594–8.
18. Lundergan FS, *et al.* Once-daily gentamicin dosing in newborn infants. *Pediatrics* 1999; **103:** 1228–34.
19. Tomlinson RJ, *et al.* Once daily ceftriaxone and gentamicin for the treatment of febrile neutropenia. *Arch Dis Child* 1999; **80:** 125–31.
20. Bragonier R, Brown NM. The pharmacokinetics and toxicity of once-daily tobramycin therapy in children with cystic fibrosis. *J Antimicrob Chemother* 1998; **42:** 103–6.
21. Vic P, *et al.* Efficacy, tolerance, and pharmacokinetics of once daily tobramycin for pseudomonas exacerbations in cystic fibrosis. *Arch Dis Child* 1998; **78:** 536–9.
22. Koo J, *et al.* Comparison of once-daily versus pharmacokinetic dosing of aminoglycosides in elderly patients. *Am J Med* 1996; **101:** 177–83.
23. Gerberding JL. Aminoglycoside dosing: timing is of the essence. *Am J Med* 1998; **105:** 256–8.


**Ménière's disease.** Gentamicin and streptomycin have been used for medical ablation in advanced Ménière's disease (p.422). Although gentamicin given systemically is considered to be more ototoxic than streptomycin, evidence from *animal* studies suggests that intratympanic use may be less ototoxic. This, and a higher incidence of adverse effects with streptomycin, has meant that intratympanic gentamicin is now preferred. Intratympanic gentamicin has been reported to control vertigo symptoms in the majority of patients, although some experience a worsening of their hearing loss immediately after treatment.[1-6] However, the ideal regimen for intratympanic gentamicin has yet to be defined.


1. Nedzelski JM, *et al.* Chemical labyrinthectomy: local application of gentamicin for the treatment of unilateral Meniere's disease. *Am J Otol* 1992; **13:** 18–22.
2. Pyykkö I, *et al.* Intratympanic gentamicin in bilateral Meniere's disease. *Otolaryngol Head Neck Surg* 1994; **110:** 162–7.
3. Quaranta A, *et al.* Intratympanic therapy for Ménière's disease: high-concentration gentamicin with round-window protection. *Ann N Y Acad Sci* 1999; **884:** 410–24.
4. Longridge NS, Mallinson AI. Low-dose intratympanic gentamicin treatment for dizziness in Meniere's disease. *J Otolaryngol* 2000; **29:** 35–9.
5. Quaranta A, *et al.* Intratympanic therapy for Ménière's disease: effect of administration of low concentration of gentamicin. *Acta Otolaryngol* 2001; **121:** 387–92.
6. Marzo SJ, Leonetti JP. Intratympanic gentamicin therapy for persistent vertigo after endolymphatic sac surgery. *Otolaryngol Head Neck Surg* 2002; **126:** 31–3.


## Preparations

***BP 2003:*** Gentamicin Cream; Gentamicin Eye Drops; Gentamicin Injection; Gentamicin Ointment;
***USP 27:*** Gentamicin and Prednisolone Acetate Ophthalmic Ointment; Gentamicin Injection; Gentamicin Sulfate Cream; Gentamicin Sulfate Ointment; Gentamicin Sulfate Ophthalmic Ointment; Gentamicin Sulfate Ophthalmic Solution.

**Proprietary Preparations** (details are given in Part 3)
***Arg.:*** Gentamina; Gentapharma; Gentatenk; Genticol; Gentoler; Glevomicina; Plurisemina; Provisual; Rupegen; Sintepul; Ultradermis; ***Austral.:*** Genoptic; ***Austria:*** Garamycin; Gentax; Refobacin; Sulmycin; ***Belg.:*** Gentamytrex†; Geomycine; ***Braz.:*** Ampligen†; Amplomicina†; Garacin; Garamicina; Gentac; Gentagran; Gentamil; Gentaplus†; Gentaron; Gentax; Gentaxil†; ***Canad.:*** Alcomicin; Cidomycin†; Diogent; Garamycin; Garatec; Gentacidin†; Ocugram†; ***Chile:*** Gentalyn; Oftagen; ***Denm.:*** Garamycin; Gensumycin†; Gentacoll; Hexamycin; ***Fin.:*** Gensumycin; Gentacoll; ***Fr.:*** Collatamp G; Gentabilles†; Gentalline; Ophtagram†; ***Ger.:*** Dispagent†; duragentamicin†; Gencin; Gent-Ophtal; Genta; Gentamytrex; Ophtagram; Refobacin; Sulmycin; Terramycin N; ***Gr.:*** Dabroson; Garamycin; ***Hong Kong:*** Garamycin; Genoptic; Miramycin; Optigen; ***India:*** Andregen; Biogaracin; Garamycin; Gentasporin; Genticyn; Genticyn Eye/Ear; ***Irl.:*** Cidomycin; Genticin; ***Israel:*** Cidomycin; Garamycin†; Gentatrim; Lacromycin; Opti-Genta; ***Ital.:*** Gentalyn; Gentamen; Gentibioptal; Genticol; Gentomil; Ribomicin; ***Malaysia:*** Beagenta; Garamycin; Gentamed; Gentamytrex; Miramycin; ***Mex.:*** Barmicil; Beramicina; Fustermicina; Garacoll; Garalen; Garamicina; Genemicin; Genexal†; Genkova; Genrex; Genta; Gentabac†; Gentacarnot†; Gentacin†; Gentanacin; Gentapat; Gentarim; Gentavivant†; Gentazaf Z; Gentialoquin; Geracin†; Gl; Gy-Sol†; Ikatin; Migent†; Nozolon†; Oftagen†; Quilagen†; Servigenta; Tamigen; Tondex; Yectamicina; ***Neth.:*** Garacol; Garamycin; Gentamytrex; ***Norw.:*** Garamycin; Gensumycin; ***NZ:*** Genoptic; ***Port.:*** Cronocol†; Garalone; Genta Gobens; Genticol; Ophtagram; ***S.Afr.:*** Cidomycin†; Fermentmycin†; Garacoll; Garamycin; Genoptic; Sabax Gentamix; ***Singapore:*** Garamycin; Genoptic; Gentamytrex; Miramycin; Ophtagram†; ***Spain:*** Coliriocilina Gentam; Genta Gobens; Gentalodina†; Gentamedical; Gentamival; Genticina; Gentralay†; Gevramycin; Gevramycin Topica; Lantogent†; Rexgenta; ***Swed.:*** Garamycin; Gensumycin; ***Switz.:*** Garamycin; Ophtagram; Servigenta†; Yedoc†; ***Thai.:*** Garamycin; Genta; Genta-Oph; Gentac; Gentacin; Gental; Grammicin; Grammixin; Miramycin; Servigenta†; Skinfect; Versigen; ***UAE:*** Gental; ***UK:*** Cidomycin; Garamycin†; Genticin; ***USA:*** G-Myticin†; Garamycin; Genoptic; Gentacidin; Gentak; Gentasol; Ocu-Mycin.

**Multi-ingredient:** ***Arg.:*** Adenil; Aeromicrosona C; Anginotrat; Bacticort; Bacticort Complex; Becortin; Cevaderm; Ciprocort; Denvercrem; Dermizol G; Dermizol Trio; Dermoperative; Dermosona; Dermovit; Diprogenta; Factor Dermico; Filoderma; Filoderma Plus; Gentasol; Gentocelina; Griseocrem; Hifamonil Crema; Lisoderma; Macril; Micozol Compuesto; Microsona C; Miklogen; Novo Bacticort; Novo Bacticort Complex; Otalex G; Otonorthia; Pancutan; Provisual Compuesto; Prurisedan Biotic; Quadriderm; Quadriderm CD; Quiacort G; Quiacort G Plus; Septopal; Sirotamicin BG; Start NP; Tridermal; Triefect; Triplex; Vitacortil; ***Austral.:*** Celestone VG; Palacos E with Garamycin; Palacos R with Garamycin; Septopal; ***Austria:*** Decoderm compositum; Decoderm trivalent; Dexagenta; Diprogenta; Refobacin-Palacos R†; Septopal; Voltamicin; ***Belg.:*** Decoderm Comp; Duracoll; Garasone; Palacos LV avec Gentamicine; Palacos R avec Gentamicine; Septopal†; ***Braz.:*** Cauterex; Cremederme; Dexamytrex; Diprogenta; Emecort; Garasone; Gentacort; Gino-Cauterex; Ginometrim†; Infectoflam†; Microbiogen†; Otigent†; Pan-Emecort; Poliderms; Quadriderm; Quadrikin; Quadrilon; Quadriplus; Septopal; Tetraderm; Voltamicin†; ***Canad.:*** Diprogen; Garasone; Valisone-G; ***Chile:*** Diprospan G; Gentasone; Labosona G; Mixgen; Oftagen Compuesto; Palacos R con Gentamicina; Perlas de PMMA con Gentamicina; Pred G; Vilterm; ***Denm.:*** Palacos cum Gentamicin†; Septopal; ***Fin.:*** Celestoderm cum Garamycin; Palacos R cum Gentamicin; Septopal; ***Fr.:*** Gentasone†; Indobiotic; Palacos LV avec Gentamicine; Palacos R avec Gentamicine; Voltamicine†; ***Ger.:*** Betagentam; Cibaflam; CMW mit Gentamicin; Copal; Decoderm Comp; Dexa-Gentamicin; Dexamytrex; Diprogenta; Inflanegent; Palamed G; Refobacin-Palacos R; Septocoll; Septopal; Sulmycin mit Celestan-V; Terracortril N; ***Gr.:*** Palacos-R with Gentamycin; Septopal; ***Hong Kong:*** Celestoderm-V with Garamycin; Colircusi Gentadexa†; Diprogenta; Garasone; Infectoflam†; Novoter Gentamicin†; Quadriderm; Septopal; Triderm; Triditol-G; ***India:*** Betnovate-GM; Cloben-G; Clomycin; Diclogenta; Ecodax; Genticyn B Eye/Ear; Genticyn HC; Lobate-G; Lobate-GM; Quiss; Septopal; Tenovate G; ***Irl.:*** Gentisone HC; Palacos R with Gentamicin†; Septopal†; ***Israel:*** Aflumycin; Betacorten-G; Celestoderm-V with Garamycin†; Cicloderm-C; Diprogenta; Triderm; ***Ital.:*** Citrizan Antibiotico; Diprogenta†; Formomicin; Genalfa; Genatrop; Gentacort; Gentalyn Beta; Vasosterone Oto; Voltamicin; ***Malaysia:*** Beprogent; Betagen; Celestoderm-V with Garamycin; Dermal G; Dexa-Gentamicin; Dexamytrex Ophtiole; Diprogenta; Garasone; Gentadexa; Infectoflam; Joysun; Septopal; ***Mex.:*** Diprosone G; Garamicina-V; Garasone; Genrex-B†; Miclobet; Quadriderm NF; Triderm; ***Neth.:*** Dexagenta-POS†; Dexamytrex; Palacos met gentamicine; Septopal; ***Norw.:*** Palacos cum Gentamicin†; Septopal; ***NZ:*** Palacos with Garamycin; ***Port.:*** Dexamytrex; Diprogenta; Epione; Gentadexa; Indobiotic; Palacos R com Gentamicina†; Quadriderme; ***S.Afr.:*** Celestoderm-V with Garamycin; Diprogenta; Garasone; Palacos R with Garamycin; Pred G†; Quadriderm; Septopal; ***Singapore:*** B-Tasone-G; Beprogent; Betnovate-GM†; Celestoderm-V with Garamycin; Combiderm; Conazole; Dexamytrex; Diprogenta; Garasone; Gentrisone; Infectoflam; Neoderm; Quadriderm; Refobacin-Palacos R; Septopal; Tri-Micon; Triderm; Voltamicin; ***Spain:*** Celestoderm Gentamicina; Cuatroderm; Diprogenta; Epitelizante; Flugen; Flutenal Gentamicina; Gentadexa; Gentavasor†; Interderm; Novoter Gentamicina; ***Swed.:*** Celeston valerat med gentamicin; Palacos cum Gentamicin†; Septopal; ***Switz.:*** Diprogenta; Indobiotic; Infectoflam; Ophtasone; Palacos avec Garamycin†; Pred G†; Quadriderm; Septopal; Triderm; Voltamicin; ***Thai.:*** Beprogenta; Dexamytrex; Diprogenta; Genquin; Gental-F; Infectoflam; Pred Oph; Quadriderm†; Refobacin-Palacos R; Septopal; ***UK:*** Gentisone HC; Palacos LV with Gentamicin; Palacos R with Gentamicin; Septopal; Vipsogal†; ***USA:*** Pred G.

## Gramicidin *(BAN, rINN)*

Gramicidin D; Gramicidin (Dubos); Gramicidina; Gramicidinum.
*CAS — 1405-97-6 (gramicidin); 113-73-5 (gramicidin S).*
*ATC — R02AB30.*

NOTE. The name gramicidin was formerly applied to tyrothricin.

**Pharmacopoeias.** In *Eur.* (see p.vi), *Jpn*, and *US.*

**Ph. Eur. 5.0** (Gramicidin). It consists of a family of antimicrobial linear polypeptides usually obtained by extraction from tyrothricin, the complex isolated from the fermentation broth of *Bacillus brevis.* The main component is gramicidin A1, together with gramicidins A2, B1, C1, and C2 in particular. The potency is not less than 900 units/mg calculated with reference to the dried substance. A white or almost white, slightly hygroscopic, crystalline powder. Practically insoluble in water; sparingly soluble in alcohol; soluble in methyl alcohol. Store in airtight containers. Protect from light.

**USP 27** (Gramicidin). An antibacterial substance produced by the growth of *Bacillus brevis* (Bacillaceae); it may be obtained from tyrothricin. It has a potency of not less than 900 micrograms of gramicidin per mg, calculated on the dried basis. A white or practically white, odourless, crystalline, powder. Insoluble in water; soluble in alcohol. Store in airtight containers.

## Profile

Gramicidin has properties similar to those of tyrothricin (p.275) and is too toxic to be given systemically. It is used topically for the local treatment of susceptible infections usually with other antibacterials such as neomycin and polymyxin B, and often with a corticosteroid as well.

Gramicidin S or 'Soviet gramicidin' ($C_{60}H_{92}N_{12}O_{10}$ = 1141.4) has been used.

**Porphyria.** Gramicidin is considered to be unsafe in patients with porphyria because it has been shown to be porphyrinogenic in *animals* or *in-vitro* systems.

## Preparations

***USP 27:*** Neomycin and Polymyxin B Sulfates and Gramicidin Cream; Neomycin and Polymyxin B Sulfates and Gramicidin Ophthalmic Solution; Neomycin and Polymyxin B Sulfates, Gramicidin, and Hydrocortisone Acetate Cream; Neomycin Sulfate and Gramicidin Ointment; Nystatin, Neomycin Sulfate, Gramicidin, and Triamcinolone Acetonide Cream; Nystatin, Neomycin Sulfate, Gramicidin, and Triamcinolone Acetonide Ointment.

**Proprietary Preparations** (details are given in Part 3)
***Fr.:*** Argicilline†; Pharmacilline†.

**Multi-ingredient:** ***Arg.:*** Antibiocort; Aseptobron N; Biotaer Nasal; Caext; Carnot Colutorio; Desenfriol Caramelos; Gargaletas; Gramibiotic; Graneodin; Graneodin N; Kenacomb; Nasomicina; Neo Coltirot; Neo Pelvicillin; Pantometil; Proetztotal; ***Austral.:*** Kenacomb; Neosporin; Otocomb Otic; Otodex; Sofradex; Soframycin; ***Austria:*** Mycostatin V; Topsym polyvalent; Trilon; Volon A antibiotikahaltig; ***Belg.:*** Mycolog; ***Braz.:*** Fonergin; Londerm-N; Neolon-D; Oftrim†; Omcilon A M; Onciplus; ***Canad.:*** Antibiotic Cream; Diosporin†; Kenacomb; Lidosporin†; Neosporin; Optimyxin; Optimyxin Plus; Polycidin; Polysporin; Polysporin Plus Pain Relief; Polysporin Triple Antibiotic; Polytopic; Sofracort; Soframycin; Triacomb; Viaderm-KC; ***Chile:*** Grifoftal; Oftabiotico; ***Denm.:*** Kenalog Comp med Mycostatin; Kenalog Comp†; Sofradex; ***Fin.:*** Bafucin; Polysporin; Sofradex; ***Fr.:*** Topifram†; ***Ger.:*** Polyspectran; Ultexiv†; ***Hong Kong:*** Dexa-Polyspectran†; Kenacomb; Neosporin; Polyoph; Polyspectran†; Sofradex; Triacomb; ***India:*** Kenacomb; Kenalog-S; Neosporin; Sofracort; ***Irl.:*** Graneodin; Kenacomb; Neosporin; Sofradex; Soframycin; ***Israel:*** Dermacombin; Kenacomb; ***Ital.:*** Eta Biocortilen VC; Neogram†; Vasosterone Antibiotico; ***Malaysia:*** Kenacomb; Pocin G; Sofradex; ***Mex.:*** Biotarson N; Biotarson O; Kenacomb; Neosporin; Nicobio; Polixin; Septilisin; ***Neth.:*** Mycolog; Sofradex; ***Norw.:*** Sofradex; ***NZ:*** Kenacomb; Sofradex; Soframycin; ***Port.:*** Dropcina; Gramixina†; Kenacomb; Polysporina†; ***S.Afr.:*** Kenacomb; Neosporin; Sofradex; ***Singapore:*** Kenacomb; Neosporin†; Sofradex; Topifram†; ***Spain:*** Flodermol; Fludronef; Intradermo Cort Ant Fung; Midacina; Oftalmowell; Poxider†; Spectrocin; Tivitis; Trigon Topico; ***Swed.:*** Bafucin; Sofradex†; ***Switz.:*** Angidine; Korticoid polyvalent†; Mycolog; Neosporin; Sofradex; Topsym polyvalent; Tyrothricine + Gramicidine; ***Thai.:*** Dermacombin; Kenacomb; Neosporin; Opsacin; Polyoph; Sofradex; Topifram; Xanalin; ***UAE:*** Panderm; ***UK:*** Adcortyl with Graneodin†; Graneodin; Neosporin; Sofradex; Tri-Adcortyl; ***USA:*** Ak-Spore†; Neosporin; Ocu-Spor-G; Ocutricin; Polymycin.

## Grepafloxacin Hydrochloride *(BANM, USAN, rINNM)*

Hidrocloruro de grepafloxacino; OPC-17116. (±)-1-Cyclopropyl-6-fluoro-1,4-dihydro-5-methyl-7-(3-methyl-1-piperazinyl)-4-oxo-3-quinolinecarboxylic acid monohydrochloride.
$C_{19}H_{22}FN_3O_3,HCl$ = 395.9.
*CAS — 119914-60-2 (grepafloxacin); 161967-81-3 (grepafloxacin hydrochloride).*

## Profile

Grepafloxacin is a fluoroquinolone antibacterial with properties similar to those of ciprofloxacin (p.188). It was formerly used as the hydrochloride but was withdrawn worldwide in October 1999 following reports of cardiovascular toxicity; prolongation of the QT interval was associated with the drug.

## Halquinol *(BAN)*

Chlorhydroxyquinoline; Chlorquinol; Halquinols *(USAN)*; SQ-16401. A mixture of the chlorinated products of quinolin-8-ol containing 57 to 74% of 5,7-dichloroquinolin-8-ol (chloroxine), 23 to 40% of 5-chloroquinolin-8-ol (cloxyquin), and not more than 4% of 7-chloroquinolin-8-ol.
*CAS — 8067-69-4 (halquinol); 773-76-2 (5,7-dichloroquinolin-8-ol).*

## Profile

Halquinol is a halogenated hydroxyquinoline with properties similar to those of clioquinol (p.196). It is used topically in infected skin conditions and one of its constituents, 5,7-dichloroquinolin-8-ol (chloroxine), has been applied as a 2% shampoo in the treatment of dandruff and seborrhoeic dermatitis of the scalp.

## Preparations

**Proprietary Preparations** (details are given in Part 3)
***UK:*** Valpeda; ***USA:*** Capitrol.

**Multi-ingredient:** ***Austria:*** Decoderm trivalent; ***Denm.:*** Kenacutan; ***Israel:*** Antiseptic Foot Balm†; ***Ital.:*** Beben Clorossina; ***Norw.:*** Kenacutan; ***Spain:*** Decoderm Trivalente†; ***Swed.:*** Kenacutan; ***Thai.:*** Supracortin 3; ***UK:*** Antiseptic Foot Balm†.

## Imipenem (BAN, USAN, rINN)

N-Formimidoyl Thienamycin; Imipemide; Imipenemum; MK-787; MK-0787. (5R,6S)-6-[(R)-1-Hydroxyethyl]-3-(2-iminomethylaminoethylthio)-7-oxo-1-azabicyclo[3.2.0]hept-2-ene-2-carboxylic acid monohydrate.

$C_{12}H_{17}N_3O_4S,H_2O$ = 317.4.

*CAS — 64221-86-9 (anhydrous imipenem); 74431-23-5 (imipenem monohydrate).*

**Description.** Imipenem is the *N*-formimidoyl derivative of thienamycin, an antibiotic produced by *Streptomyces cattleya.*

**Pharmacopoeias.** In *Eur.* (see p.vi), *Jpn*, and *US.*

**Ph. Eur. 5.0** (Imipenem). A white, almost white, or pale yellow powder. Sparingly soluble in water; slightly soluble in methyl alcohol. A 0.5% solution in water has a pH of 4.5 to 7.0. Store in airtight containers at a temperature of 2° to 8°.

**USP 27** (Imipenem). A white to tan-coloured crystalline powder. Sparingly soluble in water; slightly soluble in methyl alcohol. Store at a temperature not exceeding 8°.

**Incompatibility and stability.** Imipenem is unstable at alkaline or acidic pH and the commercially available injection of imipenem with cilastatin sodium for intravenous use is buffered to provide, when reconstituted, a solution with pH 6.5 to 7.5. The manufacturers advise against mixing with other antibacterials.

References.

1. Bigley FP, *et al.* Compatibility of imipenem-cilastatin sodium with commonly used intravenous solutions. *Am J Hosp Pharm* 1986; **43:** 2803–9.
2. Smith GB, *et al.* Stability and kinetics of degradation of imipenem in aqueous solution. *J Pharm Sci* 1990; **79:** 732–40.

### Adverse Effects

Imipenem is always given with the enzyme inhibitor cilastatin and thus clinical experience relates to the combination.

Adverse effects with imipenem-cilastatin are similar in general to those with other beta lactams (see Benzylpenicillin, p.163, and Cefalotin, p.168). Hypersensitivity reactions such as skin rashes, urticaria, eosinophilia, fever, and, rarely, anaphylaxis may occur. Gastrointestinal effects include nausea, vomiting, diarrhoea, tooth or tongue discoloration, and altered taste. Superinfection with non-susceptible organisms such as *Enterococcus faecium*, strains of *Pseudomonas aeruginosa* with acquired resistance, and *Candida* may also occur. Pseudomembranous colitis may develop. Erythema multiforme, exfoliative dermatitis, Stevens-Johnson syndrome, and toxic epidermal necrolysis have been reported rarely. Increases in liver enzymes and abnormalities in haematological parameters, including a positive Coombs' test, have been noted.

Local reactions such as pain or thrombophlebitis may occur following injection.

Seizures or convulsions have been reported with imipenem-cilastatin, particularly in patients with a history of CNS lesions and/or poor renal function, but sometimes in those without predisposing factors for seizures given recommended doses. Mental disturbances and confusion have also been reported.

Cilastatin has protected against the nephrotoxicity seen with high doses of imipenem given experimentally to *animals.* A harmless reddish coloration of urine has been observed in children.

**Effects on the nervous system.** References.

1. Eng RH, *et al.* Seizure propensity with imipenem. *Arch Intern Med* 1989; **149:** 1881–3.
2. Brown RB, *et al.* Seizure propensity with imipenem. *Arch Intern Med* 1990; **150:** 1551.
3. Job ML, Dretler RH. Seizure activity with imipenem therapy: incidence and risk factors. *DICP Ann Pharmacother* 1990; **24:** 467–9.
4. Leo RJ, Ballow CH. Seizure activity associated with imipenem use: clinical case reports and review of the literature. *DICP Ann Pharmacother* 1991; **25:** 351–4.
5. Duque A, *et al.* Vertigo caused by intravenous imipenem/cilastatin. *DICP Ann Pharmacother* 1991; **25:** 1009.
6. Lucena M, *et al.* Imipenem/cilastatin-associated hiccups. *Ann Pharmacother* 1992; **26:** 1459.
7. Norrby SR. Neurotoxicity of carbapenem antibacterials. *Drug Safety* 1996; **15:** 87–90.

**Superinfection.** References.

1. Gray JW, *et al.* Enterococcal superinfection in paediatric oncology patients treated with imipenem. *Lancet* 1992; **339:** 1487–8.

### Precautions

Imipenem-cilastatin should not be given to patients known to be hypersensitive to it, and should be given with caution to patients known to be hypersensitive to penicillins, cephalosporins, or other beta lactams because of the possibility of cross-sensitivity.

It should be given with caution to patients with renal impairment, and the dose reduced appropriately. Particular care is necessary in patients with CNS disorders such as epilepsy.

### Interactions

Seizures have been reported in patients given ganciclovir with imipenem-cilastatin.

### Antimicrobial Action

Imipenem is bactericidal and acts similarly to the penicillins by inhibiting synthesis of the bacterial cell wall. It has a very broad spectrum of activity *in vitro*, including activity against Gram-positive and Gram-negative aerobic and anaerobic organisms, and is stable to hydrolysis by beta-lactamases produced by most bacterial species. Cilastatin, the enzyme inhibitor given in association with imipenem, appears to have no antibacterial activity.

Most Gram-positive cocci are sensitive to imipenem including most streptococci, and both penicillinase- and non-penicillinase-producing staphylococci, although its activity against meticillin-resistant *Staphylococcus aureus* is variable. Imipenem has good to moderate activity against *Enterococcus faecalis*, but most *E. faecium* are resistant. *Nocardia, Rhodococcus,* and *Listeria* spp. are also sensitive.

Among Gram-negative bacteria, imipenem is active against many of the Enterobacteriaceae including *Citrobacter* and *Enterobacter* spp., *Escherichia coli, Klebsiella, Proteus, Providencia, Salmonella, Serratia, Shigella,* and *Yersinia* spp. Its activity against *Pseudomonas aeruginosa* is similar to that of ceftazidime. Imipenem is also active against *Acinetobacter* spp. and *Campylobacter jejuni*, and also against *Haemophilus influenzae* and *Neisseria* spp., including beta-lactamase-producing strains.

Many anaerobic bacteria, including *Bacteroides* spp., are sensitive to imipenem, but *Clostridium difficile* is only moderately susceptible.

Imipenem is not active against *Chlamydia trachomatis, Mycoplasma* spp., fungi, or viruses.

There have been reports of antagonism between imipenem and other beta lactams *in vitro.* Imipenem and aminoglycosides often act synergistically against some isolates of *Ps. aeruginosa.*

Imipenem is a potent inducer of beta-lactamases of some Gram-negative bacteria, but generally remains stable to them. Acquired resistance has been reported in *Ps. aeruginosa* during therapy with imipenem.

**Resistance.** References.

1. Ballestero S, *et al.* Carbapenem resistance in Pseudomonas aeruginosa from cystic fibrosis patients. *J Antimicrob Chemother* 1996; **38:** 39–45.
2. Rasmussen BA, Bush K. Carbapenem-hydrolyzing β-lactamases. *Antimicrob Agents Chemother* 1997; **41:** 223–32.
3. Livermore DM. Acquired carbapenemases. *J Antimicrob Chemother* 1997; **39:** 673–6.
4. MacKenzie FM, *et al.* Emergence of a carbapenem-resistant Klebsiella pneumoniae. *Lancet* 1997; **350:** 783.
5. Pikis A, *et al.* Decreased susceptibility to imipenem among penicillin-resistant Streptococcus pneumoniae. *J Antimicrob Chemother* 1997; **40:** 105–8.
6. Mainardi J-L, *et al.* Carbapenem resistance in a clinical isolate of Citrobacter freundii. *Antimicrob Agents Chemother* 1997; **41:** 2352–4.
7. Modakkas EM, Sanyal SC. Imipenem resistance in aerobic gram-negative bacteria. *J Chemother* 1998; **10:** 97–101.
8. Tsakris A, *et al.* Outbreak of infections caused by Pseudomonas aeruginosa producing VIM-1 carbapenemase in Greece. *J Clin Microbiol* 2000; **38:** 1290–2.
9. Fierobe L, *et al.* An outbreak of imipenem-resistant Acinetobacter baumannii in critically ill surgical patients. *Infect Control Hosp Epidemiol* 2001; **22:** 35–40.
10. Nagy E, *et al.* Occurrence of metronidazole and imipenem resistance among Bacteroides fragilis group clinical isolates in Hungary. *Acta Biol Hung* 2001; **52:** 271–80.
11. Gulay Z, *et al.* Clonal spread of imipenem-resistant Pseudomonas aeruginosa in the intensive care unit of a Turkish hospital. *J Chemother* 2001; **13:** 546–54.

### Pharmacokinetics

Imipenem is not appreciably absorbed from the gastrointestinal tract and is given parenterally.

Imipenem is excreted primarily in the urine by glomerular filtration and tubular secretion and undergoes partial metabolism in the kidneys by dehydropeptidase I, an enzyme in the brush border of the renal tubules, to inactive, nephrotoxic metabolites, with only 5 to 45% of a dose excreted in the urine as unchanged active drug. Imipenem is given with cilastatin sodium (p.188), a dehydropeptidase inhibitor, resulting in increased urinary-imipenem concentrations. Cilastatin does not affect serum concentrations of imipenem.

The pharmacokinetics of imipenem and cilastatin are similar and both have plasma half-lives of approximately 1 hour; half-lives, especially those of cilastatin, may be prolonged in neonates and in patients with renal impairment. Following imipenem with cilastatin, in doses of 500 or 750 mg intramuscularly, peak plasma-imipenem concentrations of 10 and 12 micrograms/mL respectively are achieved at about 2 hours and prolonged absorption results in plasma-imipenem concentrations of above 2 micrograms/mL for 6 to 8 hours. The bioavailability of imipenem after intramuscular injection is about 75%. Up to 20% of imipenem and 40% of cilastatin is bound to plasma proteins. Imipenem is widely distributed in body tissues and fluids and crosses the placenta. Information on penetration into the CSF is limited, but concentrations appear to be relatively low.

When given with cilastatin about 70% of an intravenous dose of imipenem is recovered unchanged in the urine within 10 hours. A total of 50% of an intramuscular dose is recovered in the urine and urinary concentrations above 10 micrograms/mL are maintained for 12 hours following a dose of 500 or 750 mg. Cilastatin is also excreted mainly in the urine, the majority as unchanged drug and about 12% as *N*-acetyl cilastatin. Both imipenem and cilastatin are removed by haemodialysis.

About 1% of imipenem is excreted via the bile in the faeces.

◊ Reviews.

1. Drusano GL. An overview of the pharmacology of imipenem/cilastatin. *J Antimicrob Chemother* 1986; **18** (suppl E): 79–92.
2. Watson ID, *et al.* Clinical pharmacokinetics of enzyme inhibitors in antimicrobial chemotherapy. *Clin Pharmacokinet* 1988; **15:** 133–64.
3. Mouton JW, *et al.* Comparative pharmacokinetics of the carbapenems: clinical implications. *Clin Pharmacokinet* 2000; **39:** 185–201.

**The elderly.** References.

1. Finch RG, *et al.* Pharmacokinetic studies of imipenem/cilastatin in elderly patients. *J Antimicrob Chemother* 1986; **18** (suppl E): 103–7.

**Hepatic impairment.** References.

1. Rolando N, *et al.* The penetration of imipenem/cilastatin into ascitic fluid in patients with chronic liver disease. *J Antimicrob Chemother* 1994; **33:** 163–7.

**Pregnancy and the neonate.** References.

1. Reed MD, *et al.* Clinical pharmacology of imipenem and cilastatin in premature infants during the first week of life. *Antimicrob Agents Chemother* 1990; **34:** 1172–7.
2. Heikkilä A, *et al.* Pharmacokinetics and transplacental passage of imipenem during pregnancy. *Antimicrob Agents Chemother* 1992; **36:** 2652–5.

**Renal impairment.** References.

1. Verbist L, *et al.* Pharmacokinetics and tolerance after repeated doses of imipenem/cilastatin in patients with severe renal failure. *J Antimicrob Chemother* 1986; **18** (suppl E): 115–20.
2. Alarabi AA, *et al.* Pharmacokinetics of intravenous imipenem/cilastatin during intermittent haemofiltration. *J Antimicrob Chemother* 1990; **26:** 91–8.
3. Pietroski NA, *et al.* Steady-state pharmacokinetics of intramuscular imipenem-cilastatin in elderly patients with various degrees of renal function. *Antimicrob Agents Chemother* 1991; **35:** 972–5.
4. Konishi K, *et al.* Removal of imipenem and cilastatin by hemodialysis in patients with end-stage renal failure. *Antimicrob Agents Chemother* 1991; **35:** 1616–20.
5. Chan CY, *et al.* Pharmacokinetics of parenteral imipenem/cilastatin in patients on continuous ambulatory peritoneal dialysis. *J Antimicrob Chemother* 1991; **27:** 225–32.
6. Tegeder I, *et al.* Pharmacokinetics of imipenem-cilastatin in critically ill patients undergoing continuous venovenous hemofiltration. *Antimicrob Agents Chemother* 1997; **41:** 2640–5.

### Uses and Administration

Imipenem is a carbapenem beta-lactam antibacterial, differing from the penicillins in that the 5-membered ring is unsaturated and contains a carbon rather than a sulfur atom. Since imipenem is metabolised in the kidney by the enzyme dehydropeptidase I it is always given with cilastatin (p.188), an inhibitor of the enzyme; this enhances urinary concentrations of active drug and was found to protect against the nephrotoxicity of high doses of imipenem seen in *animal* studies.

Imipenem is used for the treatment of infections caused by susceptible organisms. They include infections in immunocompromised patients (with neutropenia), intra-abdominal infections, bone and joint infections, skin and soft-tissue infections, urinary-tract infections, biliary-tract infections, hospital-acquired pneumonia, and septicaemia. It may also be used for the treatment of gonorrhoea and for surgical infection prophylaxis. For details of these infections and their treatment, see under Choice of Antibacterial, p.120. It is not indicated for CNS infections.

*Administration and dosage.* Commercial preparations contain imipenem and cilastatin, as the sodium salt, in a ratio of 1 to 1. Doses of the combination are expressed in terms of the amount of anhydrous imipenem. Imipenem is given by intravenous infusion or deep intramuscular injection. When administered intravenously, doses of 250 or 500 mg are infused over 20 to 30 minutes, and doses of 750 mg or 1 g over 40 to 60 minutes. The usual intravenous dose in adults and children weighing more than 40 kg is 1 to 2 g daily in divided doses every 6 or 8 hours, depending on the severity of the infection, although up to a maximum daily dose of 4 g or 50 mg/kg has been given in life-threatening infections.

Children of 3 months or more and weighing less than 40 kg may be given 15 to 25 mg/kg every 6 hours by intravenous infusion; the total daily dose should not usually exceed 2 g. Higher doses of up to 4 g daily have been given to children with moderately susceptible *Pseudomonas aeruginosa* infection; up to 90 mg/kg daily has been given to older children with cystic fibrosis. Neonates and infants up to 3 months of age may be given the following doses: 4 weeks to 3 months of age, 25 mg/kg every 6 hours; 1 to 4 weeks of age, 25 mg/kg every 8 hours; up to 1 week of age, 25 mg/kg every 12 hours.

For details of reduced doses to be used in renal impairment, see below.

For surgical infection prophylaxis in adults, imipenem 1 g may be given intravenously on induction of anaesthesia, followed by a further 1 g three hours later, with additional doses of 500 mg at 8 and 16 hours after induction if necessary.

Imipenem may be administered intramuscularly in adults with mild to moderate infections in doses of 500 or 750 mg every 12 hours. A single 500-mg intramuscular dose may be given in uncomplicated gonorrhoea.

◊ General reviews.


1. Balfour JA, *et al.* Imipenem/cilastatin: an update of its antibacterial activity, pharmacokinetics and therapeutic efficacy in the treatment of serious infections. *Drugs* 1996; **51:** 99–136.
2. Hellinger WC, Brewer NS. Carbapenems and monobactams: imipenem, meropenem, and aztreonam. *Mayo Clin Proc* 1999; **74:** 420–34.
3. Norrby SR. Carbapenems in serious infections: a risk-benefit assessment. *Drug Safety* 2000; **22:** 191–4.


**Administration in renal impairment.** Doses of imipenem should be reduced in patients with renal impairment; in the UK, the following are the recommended maximum *intravenous* doses based on creatinine clearance (CC):

- CC 31 to 70 mL/minute: 500 mg every 6 to 8 hours
- CC 21 to 30 mL/minute: 500 mg every 8 to 12 hours
- CC 6 to 20 mL/minute: 250 mg (or 3.5 mg/kg, whichever is the lower) every 12 hours or occasionally 500 mg every 12 hours
- CC 5 mL/minute or less: should only be given imipenem if haemodialysis is started within 48 hours

Imipenem and cilastatin are cleared from the body by haemodialysis and doses should be given after a dialysis session and then every 12 hours.

Information is lacking on the safety or effectiveness of the *intramuscular route* in patients with renal impairment.

## Preparations

***USP 27:*** Imipenem and Cilastatin for Injectable Suspension; Imipenem and Cilastatin for Injection.

**Proprietary Preparations** (details are given in Part 3)

**Multi-ingredient:** ***Arg.:*** Klonam; Zienam; ***Austral.:*** Primaxin; ***Austria:*** Zienam; ***Belg.:*** Tienam; ***Braz.:*** Tienam; ***Canad.:*** Primaxin; ***Chile:*** Tienam; ***Denm.:*** Tienam; ***Fin.:*** Tienam; ***Fr.:*** Tienam; ***Ger.:*** Zienam; ***Gr.:*** Primaxin; ***Hong Kong:*** Tienam; ***Israel:*** Tienam; ***Ital.:*** Imipem; Tenacid; Tienam; ***Malaysia:*** Tienam; ***Mex.:*** Tienam; ***Neth.:*** Tienam; ***Norw.:*** Tienam; ***NZ:*** Primaxin; ***Port.:*** Tienam; ***S.Afr.:*** Tienam; ***Singapore:*** Tienam; ***Spain:*** Tienam; ***Swed.:*** Tienam; ***Switz.:*** Tienam; ***Thai.:*** Tienam; ***UK:*** Primaxin; ***USA:*** Primaxin.

## Isepamicin *(BAN, USAN, rINN)*

HAPA-B; Isepamicina; Sch-21420; Sch-21420. 4-*O*-(6-Amino-6-deoxy-α-D-glucopyranosyl)-1-*N*-(3-amino-L-lactoyl)-2-deoxy-6-*O*-(3-deoxy-4-*C*-methyl-3-methylamino-β-L-arabinopyranosyl)streptamine; 1*N*-(*S*-3-Amino-2-hydroxypropionyl)-gentamicin B.

$C_{22}H_{43}N_5O_{12}$ = 569.6.
*CAS — 58152-03-7; 67479-40-7.*
*ATC — J01GB11.*

## Isepamicin Sulfate *(rINNM)*

Isepamicin Sulphate *(BANM)*; Sulfato de isepamicina.

$C_{22}H_{43}N_5O_{12},2H_2SO_4$ = 765.8.
*CAS — 68000-78-2.*
*ATC — J01GB11.*

**Pharmacopoeias.** In *Jpn*, which specifies a variable amount of $H_2SO_4$.

### Profile

Isepamicin is a semisynthetic aminoglycoside with actions and uses similar to those of gentamicin (p.217). It is reported not to be degraded by many of the enzymes responsible for aminoglycoside resistance. Isepamicin sulfate is given by intramuscular injection or intravenous infusion in a dose of up to 15 mg/kg daily in 2 divided doses. Once-daily dosage may be possible in selected patients. Dosage should be adjusted based on serum-isepamicin concentration monitoring. In adults, the total daily dose should not exceed 1.5 g.

◊ References.


1. Tod M, *et al.* Clinical pharmacokinetics and pharmacodynamics of isepamicin. *Clin Pharmacokinet* 2000; **38:** 205–23.


### Preparations

**Proprietary Preparations** (details are given in Part 3)

***Austria:*** Isepacin; ***Belg.:*** Isepacine; ***Fr.:*** Isepalline; ***Ital.:*** Isepacin; Vizax†; ***Mex.:*** Isepacin; ***Port.:*** Isepacin†.

## Isoniazid *(BAN, pINN)*

INAH; INH; Isoniazida; Isoniazidum; Isonicotinic Acid Hydrazide; Isonicotinylhydrazide; Isonicotinylhydrazine; Tubazid. Isonicotinohydrazide.

$C_6H_7N_3O$ = 137.1.
*CAS — 54-85-3.*
*ATC — J04AC01.*

NOTE. The name Isopyrin, which has been applied to isoniazid, has also been applied to ramifenazone.

**Pharmacopoeias.** In *Chin., Eur.* (see p.vi), *Int., Jpn, Pol., US,* and *Viet.*

**Ph. Eur. 5.0** (Isoniazid). A white, crystalline powder or colourless crystals. Freely soluble in water; sparingly soluble in alcohol. A 5% solution in water has a pH of 6.0 to 8.0.

**USP 27** (Isoniazid). Colourless, or white, odourless crystals, or white crystalline powder. Soluble 1 in 8 of water and 1 in 50 of alcohol; slightly soluble in chloroform; very slightly soluble in ether. pH of a 10% solution in water is between 6.0 and 7.5. Store in airtight containers at a temperature of 25°, excursions permitted between 15° and 30°. Protect from light.

**Incompatibility.** It has been recommended that sugars such as glucose, fructose, and sucrose should not be used in isoniazid syrup preparations because the absorption of the drug was impaired by the formation of a condensation product.[1] Sorbitol may be a suitable substitute if necessary.


1. Rao KVN, *et al.* Inactivation of isoniazid by condensation in a syrup preparation. *Bull WHO* 1971; **45:** 625–32.


**Sterilisation.** Solutions of isoniazid should be sterilised by autoclaving.

### Adverse Effects

Isoniazid is generally well tolerated at currently recommended doses. However, patients who are slow acetylators of isoniazid appear to have a higher incidence of some adverse effects. Also patients whose nutrition is poor are at risk of peripheral neuritis which is one of the commonest adverse effects of isoniazid. Other neurological adverse effects include psychotic reactions and convulsions. Pyridoxine may be given to prevent or treat these adverse effects. Optic neuritis has also been reported.

Transient increases in liver enzymes occur in 10 to 20% of patients during the first few months and usually return to normal despite continued treatment. Elevated liver enzymes associated with clinical signs of hepatitis such as nausea and vomiting, or fatigue may indicate hepatic damage; in these circumstances, isoniazid should be stopped pending evaluation and should only be reintroduced cautiously once hepatic function has recovered. The incidence of liver damage increases with age. The influence of acetylator status is uncertain. Fatalities have occurred following liver necrosis.

Haematological effects reported following use of isoniazid include various anaemias, agranulocytosis, thrombocytopenia, and eosinophilia.

Hypersensitivity reactions occur infrequently and include skin eruptions (including erythema multiforme), fever, and vasculitis.

Other adverse effects include nausea, vomiting, dry mouth, constipation, pellagra, purpura, hyperglycaemia, lupus-like syndrome, vertigo, hyperreflexia, urinary retention, and gynaecomastia.

Symptoms of overdosage include slurred speech, metabolic acidosis, hallucinations, hyperglycaemia, respiratory distress or tachypnoea, convulsions, and coma; fatalities can occur.

**Carcinogenicity.** Concern about the carcinogenicity of isoniazid arose in the 1970s when an increased risk of bladder cancer in patients treated with isoniazid was reported.[1-3] However, no evidence to support a carcinogenic effect of isoniazid was found in more than 25 000 patients followed up for 9 to 14 years in studies organised by the US Public Health Service[4] and in 3842 patients followed up for 16 to 24 years in the UK.[5]


1. Miller CT. Isoniazid and cancer risks. *JAMA* 1974; **230:** 1254.
2. Kerr WK, Chipman ML. The incidence of cancer of bladder and other sites after INH therapy. *Am J Epidemiol* 1976; **104:** 335–6.
3. Miller CT, *et al.* Relative importance of risk factors in bladder carcinogenesis. *J Chron Dis* 1978; **31:** 51–6.
4. Glassroth JL, *et al.* An assessment of the possible association of isoniazid with human cancer deaths. *Am Rev Respir Dis* 1977; **116:** 1065–74.
5. Stott H, *et al.* An assessment of the carcinogenicity of isoniazid in patients with pulmonary tuberculosis. *Tubercle* 1976; **57:** 1–15.


**Effects on the blood.** In addition to the effects mentioned above, rare reports of adverse effects of isoniazid on the blood include bleeding associated with acquired inhibition of fibrin stabilisation[1] or of factor XIII[2] and red cell aplasia.[3-5]

For a reference to neutropenia, see Effects on the Blood under Ethambutol Hydrochloride, p.211.


1. Otis PT, *et al.* An acquired inhibitor of fibrin stabilization associated with isoniazid therapy: clinical and biochemical observations. *Blood* 1974; **44:** 771–81.
2. Krumdieck R, *et al.* Hemorrhagic disorder due to an isoniazid-associated acquired factor XIII inhibitor in a patient with Waldenström's macroglobulinemia. *Am J Med* 1991; **90:** 639–45.
3. Claiborne RA, Dutt AK. Isoniazid-induced pure red cell aplasia. *Am Rev Respir Dis* 1985; **131:** 947–9.
4. Lewis CR, Manoharan A. Pure red cell hypoplasia secondary to isoniazid. *Postgrad Med J* 1987; **63:** 309–10.
5. Veale KS, *et al.* Pure red cell aplasia and hepatitis in a child receiving isoniazid therapy. *J Pediatr* 1992; **120:** 146–8.


**Effects on the CNS.** References.


1. Blumberg EA, Gil RA. Cerebellar syndrome caused by isoniazid. *DICP Ann Pharmacother* 1990; **24:** 829–31.
2. Pallone KA, *et al.* Isoniazid-associated psychosis: case report and review of the literature. *Ann Pharmacother* 1993; **27:** 167–70.
3. Cheung WC, *et al.* Isoniazid induced encephalopathy in dialysis patients. *Tubercle Lung Dis* 1993; **74:** 136–9.
4. Shah BR, *et al.* Acute isoniazid neurotoxicity in an urban hospital. *Pediatrics* 1995; **95:** 700–4.
5. Alao AO, Yolles JC. Isoniazid-induced psychosis. *Ann Pharmacother* 1998; **32:** 889–91.


**Effects on the liver.** In a review[1] of hepatotoxicity of antituberculous regimens containing isoniazid, it was stressed that hepatitis occurring during chemotherapy may be due to the disease itself, alcoholism, cirrhosis, or other infections. When treatment is implicated, it may not be possible to identify which drug or drugs are responsible.

A multicentre study[2] considered the incidence of hepatotoxicity from a short-term regimen of daily isoniazid, rifampicin, and pyrazinamide for 8 weeks in the initial phase followed by daily isoniazid and rifampicin for 16 weeks in the continuing phase. Analysis from 617 patients showed an incidence of hepatotoxic reactions of 1.6%; the incidence of elevated aspartate aminotransferase was 23.2%. In the same study, 445 patients on a nine-month regimen of daily isoniazid and rifampicin had a 1.2% incidence of hepatotoxicity and 27.1% incidence of elevated liver enzymes. A similar incidence of hepatitis of 1.4% among 350 patients on a 9-month regimen of rifampicin and isoniazid has also been reported.[3] A retrospective analysis[4] of 430 children on isoniazid and rifampicin revealed hepatotoxic reactions in 3.3%, the highest incidence being in children with severe disease. The incidence of hepatotoxicity is lower in patients receiving isoniazid for prophylaxis than in those receiving treatment for active disease. During a 7-year period[5] an incidence of 0.15% was recorded in 11 141 patients who started prophylactic therapy, whereas it was 1.25% amongst 1427 patients receiving treatment.

While increasing age,[6-9] high isoniazid doses, and pre-existing hepatic disease appear to increase the risk of isoniazid-induced hepatotoxicity, the influence of other factors is less certain. Speculation that fast acetylators of isoniazid could be at increased risk of hepatotoxicity due to production of a hepatotoxic hydrazine metabolite has not been supported;[10] in fact, slow acetylators have generally been found to have a higher risk than fast.[7,11] This could reflect a reduced rate of subsequent metabolism to non-toxic compounds. In addition, concentrations of hydrazine in the blood have not been found to correlate with acetylator status.[12,13]

The Joint Tuberculosis Committee of the British Thoracic Society is anxious that fears over the safety of treatment regimens should not compromise adequate therapy of the disease itself. They make recommendations[14] for initial measurement of liver function in all patients and regular monitoring in patients with known chronic liver disease. Tests should be repeated if symptoms of liver dysfunction occur, and details are given concerning the response to deteriorating liver function depending on the clinical situation, and include guidelines for prompt re-introduction of appropriate antituberculosis therapy once normal liver function is restored.


1. Girling DJ. The hepatic toxicity of antituberculosis regimens containing isoniazid, rifampicin and pyrazinamide. *Tubercle* 1978; **59:** 13–32.
2. Combs DL, *et al.* USPHS tuberculosis short-course chemotherapy trial 21: effectiveness, toxicity, and acceptability: the report of final results. *Ann Intern Med* 1990; **112:** 397–406.
3. Dutt AK, *et al.* Short-course chemotherapy for extrapulmonary tuberculosis: nine years' experience. *Ann Intern Med* 1986; **104:** 7–12.
4. O'Brien RJ, *et al.* Hepatotoxicity from isoniazid and rifampin among children treated for tuberculosis. *Pediatrics* 1983; **72:** 491–9.
5. Nolan CM, *et al.* Hepatotoxicity associated with isoniazid preventive therapy: a 7-year survey from a public health tuberculosis clinic. *JAMA* 1999; **281:** 1014–18.
6. Black M, *et al.* Isoniazid-associated hepatitis in 114 patients. *Gastroenterology* 1975; **69:** 289–302.
7. Dickinson DS, *et al.* Risk factors for isoniazid (INH)-induced liver dysfunction. *J Clin Gastroenterol* 1981; **3:** 271–9.
8. Stead WW, *et al.* Benefit-risk considerations in preventive treatment for tuberculosis in elderly persons. *Ann Intern Med* 1987; **107:** 843–5.
9. Døssing M, *et al.* Liver injury during antituberculosis treatment: an 11-year study. *Tubercle Lung Dis* 1996; **77:** 335–40.
10. Gurumurthy P, *et al.* Lack of relationship between hepatic toxicity and acetylator phenotype in three thousand South Indian patients during treatment with isoniazid for tuberculosis. *Am Rev Respir Dis* 1984; **129:** 58–61.
11. Pande JN, *et al.* Risk factors for hepatotoxicity from antituberculosis drugs: a case-control study. *Thorax* 1996; **51:** 132–6.
12. Gent WL, *et al.* Factors in hydrazine formation from isoniazid by paediatric and adult tuberculosis patients. *Eur J Clin Pharmacol* 1992; **43:** 131–6.
13. Donald PR, *et al.* Hydrazine production in children receiving isoniazid for the treatment of tuberculous meningitis. *Ann Pharmacother* 1994; **28:** 1340–3.
14. Ormerod LP, *et al.* Hepatotoxicity of antituberculosis drugs. *Thorax* 1996; **51:** 111–13.


**Effects on the pancreas.** Pancreatitis was associated with isoniazid therapy in 2 patients.[1,2] Chronic pancreatic insufficiency was reported in a patient following use of isoniazid, rifampicin, ethambutol, and pyrazinamide.[3]


1. Chan KL, *et al.* Recurrent acute pancreatitis induced by isoniazid. *Tubercle Lung Dis* 1994; **75:** 383–5.
2. Rabassa AA, *et al.* Isoniazid-induced acute pancreatitis. *Ann Intern Med* 1994; **121:** 433–4.
3. Liu BA, *et al.* Pancreatic insufficiency due to antituberculous therapy. *Ann Pharmacother* 1997; **31:** 724–6.


**Effects on the skin and hair.** Isoniazid causes cutaneous drug reactions in less than 1% of patients.[1,2] These reactions include urticaria, purpura, acneform syndrome,[3] a lupus erythematosus-like syndrome[4] (see below), and exfoliative dermatitis.[5] Pellagra is also associated with isoniazid.[6] Isoniazid was considered the most likely cause of alopecia in 5 patients receiving antituberculosis regimens which also included rifampicin, ethambutol, and pyrazinamide.[7]


1. Arndt KA, Jick H. Rates of cutaneous reactions to drugs: a report from the Boston Collaborative Drug Surveillance Program. *JAMA* 1976; **235:** 918–23.
2. Bigby M, *et al.* Drug-induced cutaneous reactions: a report from the Boston Collaborative Drug Surveillance Program on 15 438 consecutive inpatients, 1975 to 1982. *JAMA* 1986; **256:** 3358–63.
3. Thorne N. Skin reactions to systemic drug therapy. *Practitioner* 1973; **211:** 606–13.
4. Smith AG. Drug-induced photosensitivity. *Adverse Drug React Bull* 1989; **136:** 508–11.
5. Rosin MA, King LE. Isoniazid-induced exfoliative dermatitis. *South Med J* 1982; **75:** 81.
6. Ishii N, Nishihara Y. Pellagra encephalopathy among tuberculous patients: its relation to isoniazid therapy. *J Neurol Neurosurg Psychiatry* 1985; **48:** 628–34.
7. FitzGerald JM, *et al.* Alopecia side-effect of antituberculosis drugs. *Lancet* 1996; **347:** 472–3.


**Lupus.** Antinuclear antibodies have been reported to occur in up to 22% of patients receiving isoniazid; however, patients are usually asymptomatic and overt lupoid syndrome is rare.[1,2] The incidence of antibody induction has been reported to be higher in slow acetylators than in fast acetylators,[3] but the difference was not statistically significant and acetylator phenotype is not considered an important determinant of the risk of isoniazid-induced lupus.[1,4] The syndrome appeared to be due to isoniazid itself rather than its metabolite acetylisoniazid.[5]


1. Hughes GRV. Recent developments in drug-associated systemic lupus erythematosus. *Adverse Drug React Bull* 1987; **123:** 460–3.
2. Siddiqui MA, Khan IA. Isoniazid-induced lupus erythematosus presenting with cardiac tamponade. *Am J Ther* 2002; **9:** 163–5.
3. Alarcon-Segovia D, *et al.* Isoniazid acetylation rate and development of antinuclear antibodies upon isoniazid treatment. *Arthritis Rheum* 1971; **14:** 748–52.
4. Clark DWJ. Genetically determined variability in acetylation and oxidation: therapeutic implications. *Drugs* 1985; **29:** 342–75.
5. Sim E, *et al.* Drugs that induce systemic lupus erythematosus inhibit complement component C4. *Lancet* 1984; **ii:** 422–4.


## Treatment of Adverse Effects

Pyridoxine hydrochloride 10 mg daily is usually recommended for prophylaxis of peripheral neuritis associated with isoniazid although up to 50 mg daily may be used. A dose of 50 mg three times daily may be given for treatment of peripheral neuritis if it develops.

Nicotinamide has been given, usually with pyridoxine, to patients who develop pellagra.

Treatment of overdosage is symptomatic and supportive and consists of activated charcoal, control of convulsions, and correction of metabolic acidosis. Large doses of pyridoxine may be needed intravenously for control of convulsions and may be given in conjunction with diazepam. Isoniazid is removed by haemodialysis.

**Overdosage.** Isoniazid doses of 2 to 3 g or more are potentially toxic and doses of 10 to 15 g may be fatal without appropriate treatment. Symptoms may not occur until 2 hours after ingestion. Treatment includes early removal of the drug from the stomach, supportive treatment, and pyridoxine intravenously in a dose at least equal to the amount of isoniazid ingested. Diazepam may be given intravenously to assist seizure control and sodium bicarbonate for metabolic acidosis. Dialysis has been used but may not be necessary. An initial intravenous dose of pyridoxine hydrochloride equivalent to the estimated amount of isoniazid ingested (or, if the amount ingested is unknown, pyridoxine hydrochloride 5 g) has been recommended. If required, this dose is repeated at 5 to 30 minute intervals until the dose greatly exceeds that of ingested isoniazid, seizures cease, or consciousness is regained. Other routes for pyridoxine have been proposed, including giving the total amount of pyridoxine as a single intravenous infusion in glucose 5% over 30 to 60 minutes.[1] A maximum dose of pyridoxine has not been set; doses in the range of 70 to 357 mg/kg over 1 hour[1] and 52 g intravenously[2] have been used in isoniazid overdosage without pyridoxine toxicity.


1. Wason S, *et al.* Single high-dose pyridoxine treatment for isoniazid overdose. *JAMA* 1981; **246:** 1102–4.
2. Sievers ML, Herrier RN. Treatment of acute isoniazid toxicity. *Am J Hosp Pharm* 1975; **32:** 202–6.


**Pyridoxine deficiency.** Pyridoxine deficiency associated with isoniazid in doses of 5 mg/kg daily is uncommon. Patients at risk of developing pyridoxine deficiency include those with diabetes, uraemia, alcoholism, HIV infection, and malnutrition.[1,2] Supplementation with pyridoxine should be considered for these at-risk groups as well as for pregnant women and patients with seizure disorders.[1] For the prophylaxis of peripheral neuritis it is common practice to give pyridoxine 10 mg daily, although 6 mg daily might be sufficient.[3] However, in one patient a dose of pyridoxine 10 mg daily failed to prevent psychosis, the symptoms of which only resolved after stopping isoniazid and increasing the pyridoxine dosage to 100 mg daily.[4]


1. American Thoracic Society, Centers for Disease Control, and the Infectious Diseases Society of America. Treatment of tuberculosis. *MMWR* 2003; **52** (RR-11): 1–77. Also available at: http://www.cdc.gov/mmwr/PDF/rr/rr5211.pdf (accessed 24/05/04)
2. Joint Tuberculosis Committee of the British Thoracic Society. Chemotherapy and management of tuberculosis in the United Kingdom: recommendations 1998. *Thorax* 1998; **53:** 536–48. Also available at: http://www.brit-thoracic.org.uk/docs/Chemotherapy.pdf (accessed 24/05/04)
3. Snider DE. Pyridoxine supplementation during isoniazid therapy. *Tubercle* 1980; **61:** 191–6.
4. Chan TYK. Pyridoxine ineffective in isoniazid-induced psychosis. *Ann Pharmacother* 1999; **33:** 1123–4.


## Precautions

Isoniazid should be used with caution in patients with convulsive disorders, a history of psychosis, or hepatic or renal impairment. Patients who are at risk of neuropathy or pyridoxine deficiency, including those who are diabetic, alcoholic, malnourished, uraemic, pregnant, or infected with HIV, should receive pyridoxine usually in a dose of 10 mg daily, although up to 50 mg daily may be used. If symptoms of hepatitis such as malaise, fatigue, anorexia, and nausea develop isoniazid should be discontinued pending evaluation.

Liver function should be checked before treatment with isoniazid and special care should be taken in alcoholic patients or those with pre-existing liver disease. Regular monitoring of liver function is recommended in patients with pre-existing liver disease, and isoniazid treatment should be suspended if serum aspartate aminotransferase concentrations are elevated to more than 3 times the normal upper limit or the bilirubin concentration rises. Careful monitoring should be considered for black and Hispanic women, in whom there may be an increased risk of fatal hepatitis.

When visual symptoms occur during isoniazid treatment periodic eye examinations have been suggested.

**Breast feeding.** Peak concentrations of isoniazid in breast milk were 6 micrograms/mL following a dose of 5 mg/kg and were 16.6 micrograms/mL following a 300-mg dose.[1] Adverse effects on breast-fed infants have not been reported and the American Academy of Pediatrics thus considers isoniazid to be usually compatible with breast feeding,[2] although such infants should be monitored for toxic reactions.[1]


1. Snider D, Powell KE. Should women taking antituberculosis drugs breast-feed? *Arch Intern Med* 1984; **144:** 589–90.
2. American Academy of Pediatrics. The transfer of drugs and other chemicals into human milk. *Pediatrics* 2001; **108:** 776–89. Correction. *ibid.*; 1029. Also available at: http://aappolicy.aappublications.org/cgi/content/full/pediatrics%3b108/3/776 (accessed 27/05/04)


**Porphyria.** Isoniazid is considered to be unsafe in patients with porphyria although there is conflicting experimental evidence of porphyrinogenicity.

**Pregnancy and the neonate.** In a review[1] of antituberculous treatment in pregnant patients it was reported that over 95% of 1480 pregnancies in which isoniazid had been given resulted in a normal term infant. Slightly more than 1% of the infants/fetuses were abnormal and many of these abnormalities were CNS related. Isoniazid is therefore recognised as being suitable for use in regimens for the **treatment** of tuberculosis in **pregnant** patients.[2,3] Pyridoxine supplementation is recommended[2] (see Treatment of Adverse Effects, above). **Preventive therapy** with isoniazid is generally delayed until after delivery unless other risk factors are present.


1. Snider DE, *et al.* Treatment of tuberculosis during pregnancy. *Am Rev Respir Dis* 1980; **122:** 65–79.
2. American Thoracic Society, Centers for Disease Control, and the Infectious Diseases Society of America. Treatment of tuberculosis. *MMWR* 2003; **52** (RR-11): 1–77. Also available at: http://www.cdc.gov/mmwr/PDF/rr/rr5211.pdf (accessed 24/05/04)
3. Joint Tuberculosis Committee of the British Thoracic Society. Chemotherapy and management of tuberculosis in the United Kingdom: recommendations 1998. *Thorax* 1998; **53:** 536–48. Also available at: http://www.brit-thoracic.org.uk/docs/Chemotherapy.pdf (accessed 24/05/04)


## Interactions

The risk of hepatotoxicity may be increased in patients receiving isoniazid with rifampicin or other potentially hepatotoxic drugs.

Isoniazid can inhibit the hepatic metabolism of a number of drugs, in some cases leading to increased toxicity. These include the antiepileptics carbamazepine (p.355), ethosuximide (p.360), and phenytoin (p.372), the benzodiazepines diazepam and triazolam (p.693), chlorzoxazone (p.1393), and theophylline (p.801). The metabolism of enflurane (p.1298) may be increased in patients receiving isoniazid, resulting in potentially nephrotoxic levels of fluoride. Isoniazid has been associated with increased concentrations or toxicity of clofazimine (p.197), cycloserine (p.202), and warfarin (p.1024).

For interactions affecting isoniazid, see below.

**Alcohol.** The metabolism of isoniazid may be increased in chronic alcoholics: this may lead to reduced isoniazid effectiveness.[1] These patients may also be at increased risk of developing isoniazid-induced peripheral neuropathies and hepatic damage (see Precautions, above).


1. Anonymous. Interaction of drugs with alcohol. *Med Lett Drugs Ther* 1981; **23:** 33–4.


**Antacids.** Oral absorption of isoniazid is reduced by aluminium-containing antacids; isoniazid should be given at least 1 hour before the antacid.[1]


1. Hurwitz A, Schluzman DL. Effects of antacids on gastrointestinal absorption of isoniazid in rat and man. *Am Rev Respir Dis* 1974; **109:** 41–7.


**Antifungals.** Serum concentrations of isoniazid were below the limits of detection in a patient also receiving rifampicin and *ketoconazole*.[1] For the effect of isoniazid on ketoconazole, see p.404.


1. Abadie-Kemmerly S, *et al.* Failure of ketoconazole treatment of Blastomyces dermatitidis due to interaction of isoniazid and rifampin. *Ann Intern Med* 1988; **109:** 844–5. Correction. *ibid.* 1989; **111:** 96.


**Antivirals.** The clearance of isoniazid was approximately doubled when *zalcitabine* was given to 12 HIV-positive patients.[1] In addition, care is needed since *stavudine* and zalcitabine may also cause peripheral neuropathy; use of isoniazid with stavudine has been reported to increase its incidence.[2]


1. Lee BL, *et al.* The effect of zalcitabine on the pharmacokinetics of isoniazid in HIV-infected patients. *Intersci Conf Antimicrob Agents Chemother* 1994; **34:** 3(A4).
2. Breen RAM, *et al.* Increased incidence of peripheral neuropathy with co-administration of stavudine and isoniazid in HIV-infected individuals. *AIDS* 2000; **14:** 615.


**Corticosteroids.** Administration of *prednisolone* 20 mg to 13 slow acetylators and 13 fast acetylators receiving isoniazid 10 mg/kg reduced plasma concentrations of isoniazid by 25 and 40% respectively.[1] Renal clearance of isoniazid was also enhanced in both acetylator phenotypes and the rate of acetylation increased in slow acetylators only.[1]

The clinical significance of this effect is not established.

1. Sarma GR, *et al.* Effect of prednisolone and rifampin on isoniazid metabolism in slow and rapid inactivators of isoniazid. *Antimicrob Agents Chemother* 1980; **18:** 661–6.

**Food.** Palpitations, headache, conjunctival irritation, severe flushing, tachycardia, tachypnoea, and sweating have been reported in patients taking isoniazid following ingestion of *cheese, red wine*,[1] and some *fish*.[2,3] Accumulation of tyramine[1] or histamine[2] has been proposed as the cause of these food-related reactions, and they could be mistaken for anaphylaxis.[3]

1. Toutoungi M, *et al.* Cheese, wine, and isoniazid. *Lancet* 1985; **ii:** 671.
2. Kottegoda SR. Cheese, wine and isoniazid. *Lancet* 1985; **ii:** 1074.
3. O'Sullivan TL. Drug-food interaction with isoniazid resembling anaphylaxis. *Ann Pharmacother* 1997; **31:** 928.

## Antimicrobial Action

Isoniazid is highly active against *Mycobacterium tuberculosis* and may have activity against some strains of other mycobacteria including *M. kansasii*.

Although it is rapidly bactericidal against actively dividing *M. tuberculosis*, it is considered to be only bacteriostatic against semi-dormant organisms and has less sterilising activity than rifampicin or pyrazinamide.

Resistance of *M. tuberculosis* to isoniazid develops rapidly if it is used alone in the *treatment* of clinical infection, and may be due in some strains to loss of the gene for catalase production. Resistance is delayed or prevented by the combination of isoniazid with other antimycobacterials which appears to be highly effective in preventing emergence of resistance to other antituberculous drugs. Resistance does not appear to be a problem when isoniazid is used alone in *prophylaxis*, probably because the bacillary load is low.

**Mycobacterium avium complex.** Synergistic activity of isoniazid plus streptomycin and, to a lesser degree, isoniazid plus clofazimine, against *Mycobacterium avium* complex (MAC) has been demonstrated *in vitro* and *in vivo*.[1]

1. Reddy MV, *et al.* In vitro and in vivo synergistic effect of isoniazid with streptomycin and clofazimine against Mycobacterium avium complex (MAC). *Tubercle Lung Dis* 1994; **75:** 208–12.

## Pharmacokinetics

Isoniazid is readily absorbed from the gastrointestinal tract and following intramuscular injection. Peak concentrations of about 3 to 7 micrograms/mL appear in blood 1 to 2 hours after a fasting dose of 300 mg by mouth. The rate and extent of absorption of isoniazid is reduced by food. Isoniazid is not considered to be bound appreciably to plasma proteins and diffuses into all body tissues and fluids, including the CSF. It appears in fetal blood if given during pregnancy (see below), and is distributed into breast milk (see under Precautions, above).

The plasma half-life for isoniazid ranges from about 1 to 6 hours, those who are fast acetylators having shorter half-lives. The primary metabolic route is the acetylation of isoniazid to acetylisoniazid by *N*-acetyltransferase found in the liver and small intestine. Acetylisoniazid is then hydrolysed to isonicotinic acid and monoacetylhydrazine; isonicotinic acid is conjugated with glycine to isonicotinyl glycine (isonicotinuric acid) and monoacetylhydrazine is further acetylated to diacetylhydrazine. Some unmetabolised isoniazid is conjugated to hydrazones. The metabolites of isoniazid have no tuberculostatic activity and, apart from possibly monoacetylhydrazine, they are also less toxic. The rate of acetylation of isoniazid and monoacetylhydrazine is genetically determined and there is a bimodal distribution of persons who acetylate them either slowly or rapidly. Various ethnic groups contain differing proportions of genetic phenotypes. When isoniazid is given daily or 2 or 3 times weekly, clinical effectiveness is not influenced by acetylator status.

In patients with normal renal function, over 75% of a dose appears in the urine in 24 hours, mainly as metabolites. Small amounts of drug are also excreted in the faeces. Isoniazid is removed by dialysis.

**Distribution.** Therapeutic concentrations of isoniazid have been detected in CSF[1,2] and synovial fluid[3] several hours after an oral dose. Diffusion into saliva is good and it has been suggested that salivary concentrations could be used in place of serum concentrations in pharmacokinetic studies.[4]

1. Forgan-Smith R, *et al.* Pyrazinamide and other drugs in tuberculous meningitis. *Lancet* 1973; **ii:** 374.
2. Miceli JN, *et al.* Isoniazid (INH) kinetics in children. *Fedn Proc* 1983; **42:** 1140.
3. Mouries D, *et al.* Passage articulaire de l'isoniazide et de l'éthambutol: deux observations de synovite tuberculeuse du genou. *Nouv Presse Med* 1975; **4:** 2734.
4. Gurumurthy P, *et al.* Salivary levels of isoniazid and rifampicin in tuberculous patients. *Tubercle* 1990; **71:** 29–33.

**HIV-infected patients.** Malabsorption of isoniazid may occur in patients with HIV infection. However, it is not clear whether this is related to the infection itself or associated diarrhoea. In a report of treatment failure during antituberculosis therapy in 2 patients with HIV infection, serum concentrations of isoniazid in 1 patient were low or undetectable for up to 12 hours after a dose.[1] However, in another study, serum concentrations of isoniazid in 26 HIV-positive patients undergoing intermittent antituberculosis treatment were generally regarded as adequate in a single sample taken 2 hours after a dose.[2] A pharmacokinetic study in subjects without tuberculosis indicated that the presence of diarrhoea had a greater influence on absorption than either the presence or severity of HIV infection.[3]

1. Patel KB, *et al.* Drug malabsorption and resistant tuberculosis in HIV-infected patients. *N Engl J Med* 1995; **332:** 336–7.
2. Peloquin CA, *et al.* Low antituberculosis drug concentrations in patients with AIDS. *Ann Pharmacother* 1996; **30:** 919–25.
3. Sahai J, *et al.* Reduced plasma concentrations of antituberculosis drugs in patients with HIV infection. *Ann Intern Med* 1997; **127:** 289–93.

**Pregnancy.** Isoniazid crosses the placenta and average fetal concentrations of 61.5 and 72.8% of maternal serum or plasma concentration have been reported.[1] The half-life of isoniazid may be prolonged in neonates.[1]

1. Holdiness MR. Transplacental pharmacokinetics of the antituberculosis drugs. *Clin Pharmacokinet* 1987; **13:** 125–9.

## Uses and Administration

Isoniazid is a hydrazide derivative that is the mainstay of the primary treatment of pulmonary and extrapulmonary tuberculosis (p.150). It is used with other antituberculous drugs usually in regimens including rifampicin and pyrazinamide. Isoniazid is also used in high risk subjects for the prophylaxis of tuberculosis.

Isoniazid is given in the initial and continuation phases of short-course tuberculosis regimens. The usual adult dose is 300 mg daily by mouth on an empty stomach. Children's doses vary from 5 mg/kg daily (WHO), to 5 to 10 mg/kg daily (UK) to 10 to 15 mg/kg daily (USA), all with a maximum of 300 mg daily. For intermittent therapy, WHO recommend 10 mg/kg three times a week or 15 mg/kg twice a week, while the recommended dose in the UK is 15 mg/kg three times a week. In the USA 15 mg/kg two or three times a week is recommended for adults and 20 to 30 mg/kg (maximum 900 mg) twice a week for children. Caution is required in patients with hepatic impairment and doses may need to be reduced in those with severe renal impairment.

Similar doses to those used orally may be given by intramuscular injection when isoniazid cannot be taken by mouth; it may also be given by intravenous injection. Isoniazid has also been given intrathecally and intrapleurally.

In tuberculosis prophylaxis, daily doses of 300 mg are given for 6 months. Alternatively it may be given with rifampicin for 3 months. Doses of 5 to 10 mg/kg isoniazid daily to a maximum of 300 mg daily have been suggested for prophylaxis in children in the UK.

Isoniazid aminosalicylate (pasiniazid) and isoniazid sodium glucuronate have also been used in the treatment of tuberculosis.

## Preparations

***BP 2003:*** Isoniazid Injection; Isoniazid Tablets;
***USP 27:*** Isoniazid Injection; Isoniazid Syrup; Isoniazid Tablets; Rifampin and Isoniazid Capsules; Rifampin, Isoniazid, and Pyrazinamide Tablets; Rifampin, Isoniazid, Pyrazinamide, and Ethambutol Hydrochloride Tablets.

**Proprietary Preparations** (details are given in Part 3)
***Arg.:*** Isoniac; ***Belg.:*** Nicotibine; ***Canad.:*** Isotamine; ***Fin.:*** Tubilysin; ***Fr.:*** Rimifon; ***Ger.:*** Isozid; Isozid comp N; tebesium; tebesium-s; ***Gr.:*** Dianicotyl; Nicozid; ***Hong Kong:*** Trisofort†; ***India:*** Isokin; Isonex; Rifacom E-Z; ***Israel:*** Inazid; ***Ital.:*** Nicizina; Nicozid; ***Jpn:*** Hydra; Hydrazide; ***Mex.:*** Dipasic†; Erbazid†; Hidrasix; Pas Hain†; Valifol; ***Port.:*** Hidrazida; ***Spain:*** Cemidon; Cemidon B6; Pyreazid†; Rimifon†; ***Swed.:*** Tibinide; ***Switz.:*** Rimifon; ***Thai.:*** Myrin; Myrin-P; ***USA:*** Laniazid; Nydrazid.

**Multi-ingredient:** ***Arg.:*** Bacifim; Rifinah; Risoniac; ***Austria:*** Isoprodian; Myambutol-INH; Rifater; Rifoldin INH; Rimactan + INH; ***Braz.:*** Fluodrazin F†; ***Canad.:*** Rifater; ***Fr.:*** Rifater; Rifinah; ***Ger.:*** EMB-INH; Iso-Eremfat; Isoprodian; Myambutol-INH; Rifater; Rifinah; ***Gr.:*** Oboliz; Rifinah; Rimactazid; ***Hong Kong:*** Ricinis†; Rifater; Rifinah; ***India:*** Akt-3; Akt-4; Arzide; Combunex; Cx-3; Cx-4; Cx-5; Gocox Compound; Gocox-3; Inabutol Forte; Inapas; Ipcacin Kid; Ipcazide; Isokin-300; Isokin-T Forte; Isorifam; Myconex; R-Cinex; R-Cinex Z; Rifa; Rifa E; Rimactazid + Z; Rimpazid; Siticox-INH; Tibirim INH; Tricox; Wokex-2; Wokex-3; Wokex-4; ***Irl.:*** Rifater; Rifinah; Rimactazid; ***Ital.:*** Etanicozid B6; Miazide B6; Miazide†; Rifanicozid†; Rifater; Rifinah; ***Malaysia:*** Rimactazid; ***Mex.:*** Finater; Myambutol-INH; Rifater; Rifinah; ***Mon.:*** Dexambutol-INH; ***Neth.:*** Rifinah; ***NZ:*** Rifinah; ***Port.:*** Rifater; Rifinah; Tuberen†; ***S.Afr.:*** Mynah†; Myrin Plus; Myrin†; Pyrifin†; Rifafour; Rifater†; Rifinah; Rimactazid; Rimcure; ***Singapore:*** Rifater†; Rifinah†; Rimactazid; ***Spain:*** Amiopia; Duplicalcio 150†; Duplicalcio B12; Duplicalcio Hidraz†; Duplicalcio†; Isoetam†; Rifater; Rifazida; Rifinah; Rimactazid; Tisobrif; ***Switz.:*** Myambutol-INH; Rifater; Rifinah; Rimactazide + Z†; Rimactazide†; ***Thai.:*** Ricinis†; Rifamiso†; Rifampyzid; Rifater; Rifinah; Rimactazid; Rimcure 3-FDC; ***UK:*** Rifater; Rifinah; Rimactazid; ***USA:*** Rifamate; Rifater.

---

## Josamycin *(BAN, USAN, rINN)*

EN-141; Josamicina; Josamycinum; Leucomycin $A_3$. A stereoisomer of 7-(formylmethyl)-4,10-dihydroxy-5-methoxy-9,16-dimethyl-2-oxo-oxacyclohexadeca-11,13-dien-6-yl 3,6-dideoxy-4-*O*-(2,6-dideoxy-3-*C*-methyl-α-L-*ribo*-hexopyranosyl)-3-(dimethylamino)-β-D-glucopyranoside 4′-acetate 4″-isovalerate.

$C_{42}H_{69}NO_{15}$ = 828.0.
*CAS — 16846-24-5; 56689-45-3.*
*ATC — J01FA07.*

**Pharmacopoeias.** In *Eur.* (see p.vi) and *Jpn.*

**Ph. Eur. 5.0** (Josamycin). A macrolide antibiotic produced by certain strains of *Streptomyces narbonensis* var. *josamyceticus* var. *nova*, or obtained by any other means. A white or slightly yellowish, slightly hygroscopic powder. It contains a minimum of 900 units/mg calculated with reference to the dried substance. Very slightly soluble in water; soluble in acetone; freely soluble in dichloromethane and in methyl alcohol. Store in airtight containers.

## Josamycin Propionate *(BANM, rINNM)*

Josamycini Propionas; Propionato de josamicina; YS-20P. Josamycin 10-propionate.

$C_{45}H_{73}NO_{16}$ = 884.1.
*CAS — 56111-35-4; 40922-77-8.*
*ATC — J01FA07.*

**Pharmacopoeias.** In *Eur.* (see p.vi) and *Jpn.*

**Ph. Eur. 5.0** (Josamycin Propionate). It is derived from a macrolide antibiotic produced by certain strains of *Streptomyces narbonensis* var. *josamyceticus* var. *nova*, or obtained by any other means. A white or slightly yellowish, slightly hygroscopic, crystalline powder. It contains a minimum of 843 units/mg, calculated with reference to the dried substance. Practically insoluble in water; soluble in acetone; freely soluble in dichloromethane and in methyl alcohol. Store in airtight containers.

### Adverse Effects and Precautions

As for Erythromycin, p.208. Josamycin is reported to produce less gastrointestinal disturbance than erythromycin.

**Oedema.** A report of josamycin-induced oedema of the foot.[1]

1. Bosch X, *et al.* Josamycin-induced pedal oedema. *BMJ* 1993; **307:** 26.

### Interactions

For a discussion of drug interactions of macrolide antibacterials, see Erythromycin, p.209.

**Cytochrome P450 isoenzymes.** Josamycin is reported to have little or no effect on hepatic cytochrome P450 and may therefore interact less than erythromycin with other drugs metabolised by this enzyme system (see under Interactions of Erythromycin, Mechanism, p.209). The lack of interaction between josamycin and theophylline (p.801) would appear to support this.

### Antimicrobial Action

As for Erythromycin, p.209. Some reports suggest that josamycin may be more active against some strains of anaerobic species such as *Bacteroides fragilis*.

### Uses and Administration

Josamycin is a macrolide antibacterial with actions and uses similar to those of erythromycin (p.210). It is given by mouth as the base or the propionate but doses are calculated in terms of the base. 1.07 mg of josamycin propionate is approximately equivalent to 1 mg of josamycin base. Usual doses are 1 to 2 g daily in 2 or more divided doses.

### Preparations

**Proprietary Preparations** (details are given in Part 3)
***Austria:*** Josalid; ***Fr.:*** Josacine; ***Ger.:*** Wilprafen; ***Ital.:*** Iosalide; Josaxin; ***Jpn:*** Josamy; ***Spain:*** Josamina; Josaxin†; ***Switz.:*** Josacine†.

**Multi-ingredient:** ***Ital.:*** Corti-Fluoral.

---

# Kanamycin Acid Sulfate

Kanamicina, sulfato ácido de; Kanamycin Acid Sulphate *(BANM)*; Kanamycini Sulfas Acidus.

*ATC — A07AA08; J01GB04; S01AA24.*

**Pharmacopoeias.** In *Chin.* and *Eur.* (see p.vi).

**Ph. Eur. 5.0** (Kanamycin Acid Sulphate). A form of kanamycin sulfate prepared by adding sulfuric acid to a solution of kanamycin sulfate and drying by a suitable method. A white or almost white, hygroscopic powder containing not less than 670 units/mg and 23 to 26% of sulfate, calculated with reference to the dried material. Soluble 1 in about 1 of water; practically insoluble in alcohol and in acetone. A 1% solution in water has a pH of 5.5 to 7.5.

## Kanamycin Sulfate *(rINNM)*

Kanamycin A Sulphate; Kanamycin Monosulphate; Kanamycin Sulphate *(BANM)*; Kanamycini Monosulfas; Sulfato de kanamicina. 6-*O*-(3-Amino-3-deoxy-α-D-glucopyranosyl)-4-*O*-(6-amino-6-deoxy-α-D-glucopyranosyl)-2-deoxystreptamine sulphate monohydrate.

$C_{18}H_{36}N_4O_{11},H_2SO_4,H_2O$ = 600.6.

*CAS — 59-01-8 (kanamycin); 25389-94-0 (anhydrous kanamycin sulfate).*

*ATC — A07AA08; J01GB04; S01AA24.*

**Pharmacopoeias.** In *Eur.* (see p.vi) and *US.*

*Chin., Jpn,* and *Pol.* include the anhydrous substance.

**Ph. Eur. 5.0** (Kanamycin Monosulphate; Kanamycin Sulphate BP 2003). The sulfate of an antimicrobial substance produced by the growth of certain strains of *Streptomyces kanamyceticus.* A white or almost white, crystalline powder containing not less than 750 units/mg and 15.0 to 17.0% of sulfate, calculated with reference to the dried material. Soluble 1 in about 8 of water; practically insoluble in alcohol and in acetone. A 1% solution in water has a pH of 6.5 to 8.5.

**USP 27** (Kanamycin Sulfate). A white, odourless crystalline powder. It has a potency equivalent to not less than 750 micrograms of kanamycin per mg, calculated on the dried basis. Freely soluble in water; insoluble in acetone, in ethyl acetate, and in benzene. pH of a 1% solution in water is between 6.5 and 8.5. Store in airtight containers.

**Incompatibility.** For discussion of the incompatibility of aminoglycosides such as kanamycin with beta lactams, see under Gentamicin Sulfate, p.217. Kanamycin is also reported to be incompatible with various other drugs including some other antimicrobials as well as with some electrolytes.

### Adverse Effects, Treatment, and Precautions

As for Gentamicin Sulfate, p.217.

Peak plasma concentrations of kanamycin greater than 30 micrograms/mL, and trough concentrations greater than 10 micrograms/mL, should be avoided. Auditory (cochlear) toxicity is more frequent than vestibular toxicity.

Local pain and inflammation, as well as bruising and haematoma, have been reported at the site of intramuscular injections.

Gastrointestinal disturbances and a malabsorption syndrome, similar to that seen with oral neomycin (p.235), have occurred after oral kanamycin. Oral kanamycin should be avoided in patients with gastrointestinal ulceration.

**Breast feeding.** Although kanamycin is distributed into breast milk[1] the American Academy of Pediatrics states that no adverse effects have been observed in breast-fed infants whose mothers were receiving kanamycin, and therefore considers[2] that its use is usually compatible with breast feeding.


1. Chyo N, *et al.* Clinical studies of kanamycin applied in the field of obstetrics and gynecology. *Asian Med J* 1962; **5:** 265–75.
2. American Academy of Pediatrics. The transfer of drugs and other chemicals into human milk. *Pediatrics* 2001; **108:** 776–89. Correction. *ibid.*; 1029. Also available at: http://aappolicy.aappublications.org/cgi/content/full/pediatrics%3b108/3/776 (accessed 27/05/04)


### Interactions

As for Gentamicin Sulfate, p.218.

### Antimicrobial Action

As for Gentamicin Sulfate, p.218. It is active against a similar range of organisms although it is not active against *Pseudomonas* spp. Some strains of *Mycobacterium tuberculosis* are sensitive.

Resistance has been reported in strains of many of the organisms normally sensitive to kanamycin, and at one time was widespread, but a decline in the use of kanamycin has meant that resistance has become somewhat less prevalent. Cross-resistance occurs between kanamycin and neomycin, framycetin, and paromomycin, and partial cross-resistance has been reported between kanamycin and streptomycin.

◊ References.


1. Ho YII, *et al.* In-vitro activities of aminoglycoside-aminocyclitols against mycobacteria. *J Antimicrob Chemother* 1997; **40:** 27–32.


### Pharmacokinetics

As for Gentamicin Sulfate, p.218.

Less than 1% of an oral dose is absorbed, although this may be significantly increased if the gastrointestinal mucosa is inflamed or ulcerated.

After intramuscular injection peak plasma concentrations of kanamycin of about 20 and 30 micrograms/mL are attained in about 1 hour following doses of 0.5 and 1 g respectively. A plasma half-life of about 3 hours has been reported. Absorption after intraperitoneal instillation is similar to that from intramuscular administration.

Kanamycin is rapidly excreted by glomerular filtration and most of a parenteral dose appears unchanged in the urine within 24 hours. It has been detected in cord blood and in breast milk.

### Uses and Administration

Kanamycin is an aminoglycoside antibacterial with actions similar to those of gentamicin (p.219). It has been used in the treatment of susceptible Gram-negative and staphylococcal infections, including gonorrhoea (p.130) and neonatal gonococcal eye infections (p.136), although its use has declined in many centres because of the development of resistance. As with gentamicin it may be used with penicillins and with cephalosporins; the injections should be given at separate sites. Kanamycin has also been used as a second-line drug in tuberculosis (p.150), but other, safer drugs are usually preferred.

The sulfate or acid sulfate salts are often used: in the USA, preparations containing the bisulfate ($C_{18}H_{36}N_4O_{11},2H_2SO_4$), but referred to as the sulfate, are available. Doses are expressed in terms of kanamycin base. 1.2 g of kanamycin sulfate, and 1.34 g of kanamycin acid sulfate, are each approximately equivalent to 1 g of kanamycin. Administration is usually by intramuscular injection, and in acute infections adults may be given 15 mg/kg daily, to a maximum of 1.5 g daily, in 2 to 4 divided doses. The same doses may be given by intravenous infusion of a 0.25 to 0.5% solution over 30 to 60 minutes; in the UK, up to 30 mg/kg daily has been given in 2 or 3 divided doses by this route. Similar doses are used in children. Treatment of acute infections should preferably not continue for longer than 7 to 10 days or exceed a cumulative dose of 10 g kanamycin. A dose of 3 to 4 g weekly, given as 1 g on alternate days or as 1 g twice daily on 2 days each week, has been suggested in the UK for chronic bacterial infections, up to a maximum cumulative dose of 50 g, but prolonged use increases the risk of nephrotoxicity and is not generally recommended.

A single intramuscular dose of 2 g of kanamycin has been used in the treatment of penicillin-resistant gonorrhoea. In the treatment and prophylaxis of neonatal gonococcal infections in infants born to mothers with gonorrhoea, 25 mg/kg, up to a maximum of 75 mg, may be given as a single intramuscular dose.

Peak plasma concentrations greater than 30 micrograms/mL and trough concentrations greater than 10 micrograms/mL should be avoided. It is recommended that dosage should be adjusted in all patients according to plasma-kanamycin concentrations, and this is particularly important where factors such as age, renal impairment, or prolonged therapy may predispose to toxicity, or where there is a risk of subtherapeutic concentrations. For discussion of the methods of calculating aminoglycoside dosage requirements, see p.219.

Kanamycin has been used by mouth similarly to neomycin (p.235), for the suppression of intestinal flora. For pre-operative use, 1 g may be given every hour for 4 hours, then 1 g every 6 hours for 36 to 72 hours. In the management of hepatic encephalopathy, 8 to 12 g daily in divided doses may be given.

Kanamycin has also been administered in doses of 250 mg as a nebulised inhalation, 2 to 4 times daily. Solutions of kanamycin 0.25% have been used for the irrigation of body cavities.

Kanamycin tannate has also been used.

### Preparations

**USP 27:** Kanamycin Injection; Kanamycin Sulfate Capsules.

**Proprietary Preparations** (details are given in Part 3)
**Arg.:** Cristalomicina; **Fr.:** Kamycine†; **Ger.:** Kan-Ophtal; Kana-Stulln; Kanamytrex; **India:** Kancin; **Ital.:** Keimicina; **Malaysia:** Kancin; **Mex.:** Kanacil; Kanadrex; Kanapat; Kanibel†; Reukamicin†; Solkan; Sulmyn; **Singapore:** Kancin; Kancin-L; **Spain:** Kanacolirio†; Kanescin†; Kantrex; **Thai.:** Anbikan; Kan-Mycin; Kancin; Kangen; KMH; **USA:** Kantrex.

**Multi-ingredient: Arg.:** Cristalomicina; **Fr.:** Sterimycine; **Ital.:** Dermaflogil; Kanazone†; **S.Afr.:** Kantrexil; **Spain:** Kanafosal; Kanafosal Predni; Kanapomada†; Naso Pekamin; **Thai.:** KA-Cilone.

## Kitasamycin *(BAN, USAN, rINN)*

Kitasamicina; Leucomycin.

*CAS — 1392-21-8.*

**Pharmacopoeias.** In *Jpn* which also includes Acetylkitasamycin and Kitasamycin Tartrate.

### Profile

Kitasamycin is a macrolide antibacterial produced by *Streptomyces kitasatoensis,* consisting mainly of kitasamycins $A_4$ and $A_5$. It has actions and uses similar to those of erythromycin (p.208) and has been given by mouth as kitasamycin base or intravenously as the tartrate. Acetylkitasamycin has also been given by mouth.

## Latamoxef Disodium *(BANM, rINNM)*

Latamoxef disódico; LY-127935; Moxalactam Disodium *(USAN)*; 6059-S. (7*R*)-7-[2-Carboxy-2-(4-hydroxyphenyl)acetamido]-7-methoxy-3-(1-methyl-1*H*-tetrazol-5-ylthiomethyl)-1-oxa-3-cephem-4-carboxylic acid, disodium salt.

$C_{20}H_{18}N_6Na_2O_9S$ = 564.4.

*CAS — 64952-97-2 (latamoxef); 64953-12-4 (latamoxef disodium).*

*ATC — J01DA18.*

**Pharmacopoeias.** In *Jpn.*

### Profile

Latamoxef is an oxacephalosporin antibacterial that has been given intramuscularly or intravenously as the disodium salt in the treatment of susceptible infections. It differs from the cephalosporins in that the sulfur atom of the 7-aminocephalosporanic acid nucleus is replaced by oxygen. Like cefamandole, it has an *N*-methylthiotetrazole side-chain and may cause hypoprothrombinaemia. Serious bleeding episodes have been reported with latamoxef and prophylaxis with vitamin K and monitoring of bleeding time have been recommended during treatment. In addition to hypoprothrombinaemia, inhibition of platelet function and more rarely immune-mediated thrombocytopenia may be responsible for interference with haemostasis. As with the methylthiotetrazole-containing cephalosporins, a disulfiram-like reaction with alcohol may occur.

Latamoxef has antimicrobial activity similar to that of the third-generation cephalosporin cefotaxime (p.176), although it is generally less active against Gram-positive bacteria and more active against *Bacteroides fragilis.*

**Breast feeding.** Following a pharmacokinetic study[1] in 8 lactating women given latamoxef, the authors cautioned that there was a possibility of colonisation of the infant's bowel with Gram-positive bacteria and in consequence a risk of enterocolitis. They therefore advised against breast feeding during maternal use of the drug. However, no adverse effects have been observed in breast-fed infants whose mothers were receiving latamoxef, and the American Academy of Pediatrics considers[2] that it is therefore usually compatible with breast feeding.


1. Miller RD, *et al.* Human breast milk concentration of moxalactam. *Am J Obstet Gynecol* 1984; **148:** 348–9.
2. American Academy of Pediatrics. The transfer of drugs and other chemicals into human milk. *Pediatrics* 2001; **108:** 776–89. Correction. *ibid.*; 1029. Also available at: http://aappolicy.aappublications.org/cgi/content/full/pediatrics%3b108/3/776 (accessed 27/05/04)


### Preparations

**Proprietary Preparations** (details are given in Part 3)
**Ital.:** Mactam†; Sectam†; **Jpn:** Shiomarin.

## Levofloxacin *(BAN, USAN, rINN)*

DR-3355; HR-355; Levofloxacino; S-(−)-Ofloxacin; RWJ-25213. (−)-(*S*)-9-Fluoro-2,3-dihydro-3-methyl-10-(4-methyl-1-piperazinyl)-7-oxo-7*H*-pyrido[1,2,3-*de*]-1,4-benzoxazine-6-carboxylic acid.

$C_{18}H_{20}FN_3O_4$ = 361.4.

*CAS — 100986-85-4 (levofloxacin); 138199-71-0 (levofloxacin hemihydrate).*

*ATC — J01MA12; S01AX19.*

### Adverse Effects and Precautions

As for Ciprofloxacin, p.188.

Levofloxacin has been found in isolated cases to prolong the QT interval, particularly in overdosage.

### Interactions

For the interactions of the fluoroquinolones in general, see under Ciprofloxacin, p.190.

◊ References.

1. Gisclon LG, *et al.* Absence of a pharmacokinetic interaction between intravenous theophylline and orally administered levofloxacin. *J Clin Pharmacol* 1997; **37:** 744–50.
2. Doose DR, *et al.* Levofloxacin does not alter cyclosporine disposition. *J Clin Pharmacol* 1998; **38:** 90–3.

### Antimicrobial Action

As for Ciprofloxacin, p.190.

Levofloxacin is generally considered to be about twice as active as its isomer, ofloxacin (p.239). It has a broad spectrum of activity which includes Gram-positive bacteria.

◊ References.

1. Brown DFJ, *et al.*, eds. Levofloxacin: an extended spectrum 4-quinolone agent. *J Antimicrob Chemother* 1999; **43** (suppl C): 1–90.

### Pharmacokinetics

Levofloxacin is rapidly and almost completely absorbed following oral use with peak plasma concentrations achieved within 1 hour of a dose. It is distributed into body tissues including the bronchial mucosa and lungs, but penetration into CSF is relatively poor. Levofloxacin is approximately 30 to 40% bound to plasma proteins. It is only metabolised to a small degree to inactive metabolites. The elimination half-life of levofloxacin is 6 to 8 hours, although this may be prolonged in patients with renal impairment. Levofloxacin is excreted largely unchanged, primarily in the urine. It is not removed by haemodialysis or peritoneal dialysis.

◊ References.

1. Fish DN, Chow AT. The clinical pharmacokinetics of levofloxacin. *Clin Pharmacokinet* 1997; **32:** 101–19.
2. Chien S-C, *et al.* Pharmacokinetic profile of levofloxacin following once-daily 500-milligram oral or intravenous doses. *Antimicrob Agents Chemother* 1997; **41:** 2256–60.
3. Preston SL, *et al.* Pharmacodynamics of levofloxacin: a new paradigm for early clinical trials. *JAMA* 1998; **279:** 125–9.
4. Chien S-C, *et al.* Double-blind evaluation of the safety and pharmacokinetics of multiple oral once-daily 750-milligram and 1-gram doses of levofloxacin in healthy volunteers. *Antimicrob Agents Chemother* 1998; **42:** 885–8.
5. Piscitelli SC, *et al.* Pharmacokinetics and safety of high-dose and extended-interval regimens of levofloxacin in human immunodeficiency virus-infected patients. *Antimicrob Agents Chemother* 1999; **43:** 2323–7.
6. Chow AT, *et al.* Safety and pharmacokinetics of multiple 750-milligram doses of intravenous levofloxacin in healthy volunteers. *Antimicrob Agents Chemother* 2001; **45:** 2122–5.

### Uses and Administration

Levofloxacin is the *S*-(−)-isomer of the fluoroquinolone antibacterial ofloxacin (p.239). It is given by mouth or intravenously for the treatment of susceptible infections in a usual dose of 250 or 500 mg once or twice daily. A regimen of 750 mg once daily is recommended in the USA for complicated skin infections and for hospital-acquired pneumonia. Doses should be reduced in patients with renal impairment (see below).

Levofloxacin is also used topically as 0.5% eye drops for the treatment of bacterial conjunctivitis.

◊ Reviews.

1. Davis R, Bryson HM. Levofloxacin: a review of its antibacterial activity, pharmacokinetics and therapeutic efficacy. *Drugs* 1994; **4:** 677–700.
2. Martin SJ, *et al.* Levofloxacin and sparfloxacin: new quinolone antibiotics. *Ann Pharmacother* 1998; **32:** 320–36.
3. Martin SJ, *et al.* A risk-benefit assessment of levofloxacin in respiratory, skin and skin structure, and urinary tract infections. *Drugs* 2001; **24:** 199–222.
4. Croom KF, Goa KL. Levofloxacin: a review of its use in the treatment of bacterial infections in the United States. *Drugs* 2003; **63:** 2769–2802.

**Administration in renal impairment.** Although initial doses (see above) remain unchanged in patients with renal impairment, subsequent doses of levofloxacin should be reduced according to creatinine clearance (CC):

- CC 20 to 50 mL/minute: subsequent doses are halved
- CC 10 to 19 mL/minute: subsequent doses are reduced to one-quarter of the standard dose (a regimen of 250 mg daily should be reduced to 125 mg every other day)
- CC less than 10 mL/minute: standard doses of 250 mg or 500 mg daily are reduced to 125 mg every 48 or 24 hours respectively; a regimen of 500 mg twice daily is reduced to 125 mg every 24 hours

### Preparations

**Proprietary Preparations** (details are given in Part 3)
***Arg.:*** Floxlevo; Levaquin; Tavanic; ***Austria:*** Tavanic; ***Belg.:*** Tavanic; ***Braz.:*** Levaquin; Tavanic; ***Canad.:*** Levaquin; ***Chile:*** Auxxil; Novacilina; Quinobiot; Recamicina; Tavanic; ***Fin.:*** Tavanic; ***Fr.:*** Tavanic; ***Ger.:*** Tavanic; ***Gr.:*** Tavanic; ***Hong Kong:*** Cravit; ***India:*** Tavanic; ***Irl.:*** Tavanic; ***Israel:*** Tavanic; ***Ital.:*** Levoxacin; Prixar; Tavanic; ***Jpn:*** Cravit; ***Malaysia:*** Cravit; ***Mex.:*** Elequine; Tavanic; ***Neth.:*** Tavanic; ***Port.:*** Tavanic; ***S.Afr.:*** Tavanic; ***Singapore:*** Cravit; ***Spain:*** Tavanic; ***Swed.:*** Oftaquix; Tavanic; ***Switz.:*** Tavanic; ***Thai.:*** Cravit; ***UAE:*** Jenoquine; ***UK:*** Tavanic; ***USA:*** Levaquin; Quixin.

## Lincomycin *(BAN, USAN, rINN)*

U-10149. Methyl 6-amino-6,8-dideoxy-*N*-[(2*S*,4*R*)-1-methyl-4-propylprolyl]-1-thio-α-D-*erythro*-D-*galacto*-octopyranoside.
$C_{18}H_{34}N_2O_6S$ = 406.5.
*CAS — 154-21-2.*
*ATC — J01FF02.*

### Lincomycin Hydrochloride *(BANM, rINNM)*

Hidrocloruro de lincomicina; Lincomycini Hydrochloridum; NSC-70731. Lincomycin hydrochloride monohydrate.
$C_{18}H_{34}N_2O_6S,HCl,H_2O$ = 461.0.
*CAS — 859-18-7 (anhydrous lincomycin hydrochloride); 7179-49-9 (lincomycin hydrochloride, monohydrate).*
*ATC — J01FF02.*

**Pharmacopoeias.** In *Chin., Eur.* (see p.vi), *Jpn, Pol., US,* and *Viet.*

**Ph. Eur. 5.0** (Lincomycin Hydrochloride). An antimicrobial substance produced by *Streptomyces lincolnensis* var. *lincolnensis* or by any other means. A white or almost white crystalline powder. It contains not more than 5% of lincomycin B. Very soluble in water; slightly soluble in alcohol; very slightly soluble in acetone. A 10% solution in water has a pH of 3.5 to 5.5. Store at a temperature not exceeding 30° in airtight containers.

**USP 27** (Lincomycin Hydrochloride). A white or practically white crystalline powder, odourless or with a faint odour. Freely soluble in water; very slightly soluble in acetone; soluble in dimethylformamide. pH of a 10% solution in water is between 3.0 and 5.5. Store in airtight containers.

**Incompatibility.** Solutions of lincomycin hydrochloride have an acid pH and incompatibility may be expected with alkaline preparations, or with drugs unstable at low pH.

### Adverse Effects, Treatment, and Precautions

As for Clindamycin, p.194.

Hypotension, ECG changes, and on rare occasions cardiac arrest, have followed rapid intravenous injections. Other adverse reactions reported rarely with lincomycin include aplastic anaemia, pancytopenia, and tinnitus.

### Interactions

As for Clindamycin, p.195.

Absorption of lincomycin is reduced by adsorbent antidiarrhoeals and cyclamate sweeteners.

### Antimicrobial Action

As for Clindamycin, p.195, but it is less potent. There is complete cross-resistance between clindamycin and lincomycin.

### Pharmacokinetics

About 20 to 30% of a dose of lincomycin given by mouth is absorbed from the gastrointestinal tract and following a 500-mg dose, peak plasma concentrations of about 3 micrograms/mL are reached within 2 to 4 hours. Food markedly reduces the rate and extent of absorption. The intramuscular injection of 600 mg produces peak plasma concentrations of 9 to 18 micrograms/mL usually within 30 minutes.

The biological half-life of lincomycin is about 5 hours. Lincomycin is widely distributed in the tissues including bone and body fluids but diffusion into the CSF is poor, although it may be slightly better when the meninges are inflamed. It diffuses across the placenta and is distributed into breast milk. Lincomycin is partially inactivated in the liver; unchanged drug and metabolites are excreted in the urine, bile, and faeces. Lincomycin is not effectively removed from the blood by dialysis.

### Uses and Administration

Lincomycin is a lincosamide antibiotic with actions and uses similar to those of its chlorinated derivative, clindamycin (p.195). Clindamycin is usually preferred to lincomycin because of its greater activity and better absorption. However, the usefulness of both drugs is limited by their potential to cause pseudomembranous colitis.

Lincomycin is given by mouth as the hydrochloride but doses are expressed in terms of the base. 1.13 g of lincomycin hydrochloride is approximately equivalent to 1 g of lincomycin. The usual adult dose is the equivalent of 500 mg of lincomycin 3 or 4 times daily, taken at least 1 hour before food. It is also given parenterally by intramuscular injection in a dose of 600 mg once or twice daily, or by slow intravenous infusion in a dose of 600 mg to 1 g two or three times daily. Higher doses have been given in very severe infections, up to a total daily dose of about 8 g. For doses in renal impairment, see below. Children over the age of 1 month may be given 30 to 60 mg/kg daily in divided doses by mouth, or 10 to 20 mg/kg daily in divided doses by intramuscular injection or intravenous infusion.

Lincomycin hydrochloride may be given by subconjunctival injection in a dose equivalent to 75 mg of lincomycin.

**Administration in renal impairment.** Doses of lincomycin may need to be reduced in patients with severe renal impairment; a reduction down to 25 to 30% of the usual dose may be appropriate.

### Preparations

***BP 2003:*** Lincomycin Capsules; Lincomycin Injection;
***USP 27:*** Lincomycin Hydrochloride Capsules; Lincomycin Hydrochloride Syrup; Lincomycin Injection.

**Proprietary Preparations** (details are given in Part 3)
***Arg.:*** Frademicina; ***Austral.:*** Lincocin; ***Belg.:*** Lincocin; ***Braz.:*** Frademicina; Fredcina†; Linco-Ped†; Linco-Plus†; Lincoflan; Lincomiral; Lincomyn; Lincoplax; Lincotax; Macrolin†; Neo Linco; Teclind†; ***Canad.:*** Lincocin; ***Chile:*** Lincocin; ***Fr.:*** Lincocine; ***Ger.:*** Albiotic; ***Gr.:*** Lincocin; Pecasolin; ***Hong Kong:*** Lincocin; Medoglycin; ***India:*** Lynx; ***Ital.:*** Lincocin; ***Malaysia:*** Linco; Medoglycin; ***Mex.:*** Libiocid; Lincocin; Princol; Rimsalin; ***Neth.:*** Lincocin; ***Port.:*** Lincocina; ***S.Afr.:*** Lincocin; ***Singapore:*** Lincocin; ***Spain:*** Cillimicina; Lincocin; ***Swed.:*** Lincocin†; ***Switz.:*** Lincocin†; ***Thai.:*** Anbycin†; Linco; Lincocin; Lincogin; Lincolan; Lincomy; Lincono; Lingo; Linmycin; Utolincomycin; ***USA:*** Lincocin; Lincorex.

**Multi-ingredient:** ***Arg.:*** Nicozinc.

## Linezolid *(BAN, USAN, rINN)*

PNU-100766; U-100766. *N*-{[(*S*)-3-(3-Fluoro-4-morpholinophenyl)-2-oxo-5-oxazolidinyl]methyl}acetamide.
$C_{16}H_{20}FN_3O_4$ = 337.3.
*CAS — 165800-03-3.*
*ATC — J01XX08.*

**Incompatibility and stability.** References.

1. Zhang Y, *et al.* Compatibility and stability of linezolid injection admixed with three quinolone antibiotics. *Ann Pharmacother* 2000; **34:** 996–1001.

### Adverse Effects and Precautions

The adverse effects most frequently reported in patients receiving linezolid include diarrhoea, nausea and vomiting, metallic taste, headache, insomnia, constipation, rashes, dizziness, and abnormal liver function tests. Reversible myelosuppression including anaemia, leucopenia, pancytopenia and, in particular, thrombocytopenia has been reported and blood counts should be monitored weekly in patients receiving linezolid. Patients particularly at risk are those who have received linezolid for more than 10 to 14 days or who have pre-existing myelosuppression or severe renal impairment.

◊ References.

1. Rubinstein E, *et al.* Worldwide assessment of linezolid's clinical safety and tolerability: comparator-controlled phase III studies. *Antimicrob Agents Chemother* 2003; **47:** 1824–31.

**Effects on the blood.** Reversible myelosuppression with red cell hypoplasia occurred in 3 patients treated with linezolid.[1] Features of the myelosuppression were considered by some[1,2] to be similar to those associated with chloramphenicol, although this was disputed by the manufacturers.[3]

There have been reports of thrombocytopenia occurring at a higher incidence than that reported by the manufacturers; in one study,[4] 6 of 19 patients who had been treated with linezolid developed thrombocytopenia, while another[5] found that it occurred in 23 of 48 patients who had received the drug for more than 5 days.

During the initial 8 months of licensed use in the UK 12 reports of haematopoietic disorders (including thrombocytopenia, anaemia, leucopenia, and pancytopenia) were received by the UK Committee on Safety of Medicines.[6]

1. Green SL, *et al.* Linezolid and reversible myelosuppression. *JAMA* 2001; **285:** 1291.
2. Lawyer MC, Lawyer EZ. Linezolid and reversible myelosuppression. *JAMA* 2001; **286:** 1974.

3. Arellano FM. Linezolid and reversible myelosuppression. *JAMA* 2001; **286:** 1973–4.
4. Attassi K, *et al.* Thrombocytopenia associated with linezolid therapy. *Clin Infect Dis* 2002; **34:** 695–8.
5. Orrick JJ, *et al.* Thrombocytopenia secondary to linezolid administration: what is the risk? *Clin Infect Dis* 2002; **35:** 348–9.
6. Committee on Safety of Medicines/Medicines Control Agency. Reminder: linezolid (Zyvox) and myelosuppression. *Current Problems* 2001; **27:** 14. Also available at: http://www.mca.gov.uk/ourwork/monitorsafequalmed/currentproblems/cpaug2001.pdf (accessed 27/05/04)

**Effects on the nervous system.** Peripheral and optic neuropathy occurred in a 76-year-old man who had received linezolid for about 6 months for the treatment of meticillin-resistant *Staphylococcus aureus* infection.[1] The Australian Adverse Drug Reactions Advisory Committee[2] stated in February 2003 that it had received 4 reports of peripheral neuropathy in patients who had taken linezolid for 6 to 9 months; none of these cases had resolved at the time of the report. They suggested that the risk of peripheral neuropathy should be considered when treatment is extended beyond 28 days.

1. Corallo CE, Paull AE. Linezolid-induced neuropathy. *Med J Aust* 2002; **177:** 332.
2. Adverse Drug Reactions Advisory Committee. Linezolid and peripheral neuropathy. *Aust Adverse Drug React Bull* 2003; **22:** 3. Also available at: http://www.tga.gov.au/adr/aadrb/aadr0302.htm (accessed 27/05/04)

## Interactions

Linezolid is a reversible, nonselective MAOI and therefore has the potential to interact with adrenergic and serotonergic drugs. Enhanced pressor activity has been reported in patients receiving linezolid with phenylpropanolamine or pseudoephedrine. The interactions of conventional MAOIs, both with other drugs and with foods, are described under Phenelzine, p.314.

◊ References.

1. Wigen CL, Goetz MB. Serotonin syndrome and linezolid. *Clin Infect Dis* 2002; **34:** 1651–2.

## Antimicrobial Action

Linezolid is a oxazolidinone antibacterial with activity against a range of aerobic Gram-positive bacteria including vancomycin-resistant enterococci and meticillin-resistant *Staphylococcus aureus*. It is less active against Gram-negative bacteria, but has some *in vitro* activity against *Haemophilus influenzae, Legionella* spp., *Moraxella catarrhalis* (*Branhamella catarrhalis*), *Neisseria gonorrhoeae*, and *Pasteurella* spp. It is not active against *Acinetobacter* spp., Enterobacteriaceae, or *Pseudomonas* spp.

Oxazolidinone antibacterials are bacteriostatic and act by inhibition of ribosomal protein synthesis. Cross-resistance between oxazolidinones and other classes of antibacterial is considered unlikely.

Resistant strains of *Enterococcus faecium* have been reported.

◊ References.

1. Noskin GA, *et al.* In vitro activities of linezolid against important Gram-positive bacterial pathogens including vancomycin-resistant enterococci. *Antimicrob Agents Chemother* 1999; **43:** 2059–62.
2. Cercenado E, *et al.* In vitro activity of linezolid against multiply resistant Gram-positive clinical isolates. *J Antimicrob Chemother* 2001; **47:** 77–81.
3. Gemmell CG. Susceptibility of a variety of clinical isolates to linezolid: a European inter-country comparison. *J Antimicrob Chemother* 2001; **48:** 47–52.
4. Livermore DM. Linezolid in vitro: mechanism and antibacterial spectrum. *J Antimicrob Chemother* 2003; **51** (suppl S2): ii9–ii16.

**Resistance.** There have been reports of linezolid resistance in enterococci, involving both *Enterococcus faecium*[1-3] and *E. faecalis*.[2] There is also concern over the emergence of linezolid resistance in meticillin-resistant *Staphylococcus aureus* following reports of such resistance in 2 patients.[4,5] A survey[6] of reported resistance to linezolid in the USA found that it was still rare but was no longer limited to enterococci having also occurred in *Staph. epidermidis* and *Streptococcus oralis*.

1. Gonzales RD, *et al.* Infections due to vancomycin-resistant Enterococcus faecium resistant to linezolid. *Lancet* 2001; **357:** 1179.
2. Auckland C, *et al.* Linezolid-resistant enterococci: report of the first isolates in the United Kingdom. *J Antimicrob Chemother* 2002; **50:** 743–6.
3. Herrero IA, *et al.* Nosocomial spread of linezolid-resistant, vancomycin-resistant Enterococcus faecium. *N Engl J Med* 2002; **346:** 867–9.
4. Tsiodras S, *et al.* Linezolid resistance in a clinical isolate of Staphylococcus aureus. *Lancet* 2001; **358:** 207–8.
5. Wilson P, *et al.* Linezolid resistance in clinical isolates of Staphylococcus aureus. *J Antimicrob Chemother* 2003; **51:** 186–8.
6. Mutnick AH, *et al.* Linezolid resistance since 2001: SENTRY Antimicrobial Surveillance Program. *Ann Pharmacother* 2003; **37:** 769–74.

## Pharmacokinetics

Linezolid is rapidly and completely absorbed following oral administration and maximum plasma concentrations are achieved after 1 to 2 hours. It is about 31% bound to plasma proteins. Linezolid is reported to be distributed into bone, fat, lungs, muscle, skin blister fluids, and into the CSF. It is metabolised mainly by oxidation to 2 main inactive metabolites, the hydroxyethyl glycine metabolite (PNU-142586) and the aminoethoxyacetic acid metabolite (PNU-142300); other minor inactive metabolites have also been identified. About 40% of a dose is excreted in the urine as PNU-142586, 30% as linezolid, and 10% as PNU-142300. Small amounts of metabolites are excreted in the faeces. The elimination half-life is 4.8 hours following intravenous use and 4.6 to 5.4 hours following oral doses.

◊ References.

1. MacGowan AP. Pharmacokinetic and pharmacodynamic profile of linezolid in healthy volunteers and patients with Gram-positive infections. *J Antimicrob Chemother* 2003; **51** (suppl S2): ii17–ii25.
2. Stalker DJ, Jungbluth GL. Clinical pharmacokinetics of linezolid, a novel oxazolidinone antibacterial. *Clin Pharmacokinet* 2003; **42:** 1129–40.

## Uses and Administration

Linezolid is an oxazolidinone antibacterial used for the treatment of Gram-positive infections of the skin and respiratory tract, including those due to vancomycin-resistant enterococci and meticillin-resistant *Staphylococcus aureus*. It is given in a dose of 600 mg by mouth or by intravenous infusion every 12 hours for 10 to 28 days. In uncomplicated skin and skin structure infections the dose is 400 mg by mouth every 12 hours for 10 to 14 days.

◊ Reviews.

1. Diekema DJ, Jones RN. Oxazolidinones: a review. *Drugs* 2000; **59:** 7–16.
2. Plouffe JF. Emerging therapies for serious gram-positive bacterial infections: a focus on linezolid. *Clin Infect Dis* 2000; **31**(suppl 4): S144–S149.
3. Perry CM, Jarvis B. Linezolid: a review of its use in the management of serious gram-positive infections. *Drugs* 2001; **61:** 525–51.
4. Bain KT, Wittbrodt ET. Linezolid for the treatment of resistant gram-positive cocci. *Ann Pharmacother* 2001; **35:** 566–75.
5. Diekema DJ, Jones RN. Oxazolidinone antibiotics. *Lancet* 2001; **358:** 1975–82.
6. Paladino JA. Linezolid: an oxazolidinone antimicrobial agent. *Am J Health-Syst Pharm* 2002; **59:** 2413–25.
7. Birmingham MC, *et al.* Linezolid for the treatment of multidrug-resistant, Gram-positive infections: experience from a compassionate-use program. *Clin Infect Dis* 2003; **36:** 159–68.
8. Wilcox MH. Efficacy of linezolid versus comparator therapies in Gram-positive infections. *J Antimicrob Chemother* 2003; **51** (suppl S2): ii27–ii35.

**Administration in renal impairment.** Linezolid should be used with caution in patients with severe renal impairment. Although no dosage adjustment is required the manufacturers have reported that peak plasma concentrations of linezolid's two major metabolites were about tenfold higher in such patients after several days of treatment. As about 30% of a dose is removed during 3 hours of haemodialysis it is recommended that linezolid should be given after dialysis.

## Preparations

**Proprietary Preparations** (details are given in Part 3)
***Arg.:*** Zyvox; ***Austral.:*** Zyvox; ***Braz.:*** Zyvox; ***Canad.:*** Zyvoxam; ***Chile:*** Zyvox; ***Denm.:*** Zyvoxid; ***Fin.:*** Zyvoxid; ***Fr.:*** Zyvoxid; ***Hong Kong:*** Zyvox; ***India:*** Linox; ***Irl.:*** Zyvox; ***Israel:*** Zyvox; ***Ital.:*** Zyvoxid; ***Mex.:*** Zyvoxam; ***Neth.:*** Zyvoxid; ***Norw.:*** Zyvoxid; ***NZ:*** Zyvox; ***Port.:*** Zyvoxid; ***Singapore:*** Zyvox; ***Spain:*** Zyvoxid; ***Swed.:*** Zyvoxid; ***Switz.:*** Zyvoxid; ***UK:*** Zyvox; ***USA:*** Zyvox.

# Lomefloxacin Hydrochloride

*(BANM, USAN, rINNM)*

Hidrocloruro de lomefloxacino; NY-198; SC-47111; SC-47111A (lomefloxacin). (*RS*)-1-Ethyl-6,8-difluoro-1,4-dihydro-7-(3-methylpiperazin-1-yl)-4-oxoquinoline-3-carboxylic acid hydrochloride.

$C_{17}H_{19}F_2N_3O_3,HCl = 387.8.$

*CAS — 98079-51-7 (lomefloxacin); 98079-52-8 (lomefloxacin hydrochloride).*

*ATC — J01MA07; S01AX17.*

### Lomefloxacin Mesilate *(BANM, rINNM)*

Lomefloxacin Mesylate *(USAN)*; SC-47111B.

$C_{17}H_{19}F_2\text{-}N_3O_3, CH_4O_3S = 447.5.$

*CAS — 114394-67-1.*

## Adverse Effects and Precautions

As for Ciprofloxacin, p.188.

Concern has been expressed over the relatively high incidence of phototoxicity reactions in patients receiving lomefloxacin. Patients should be advised to avoid exposure to sunlight during, and for a few days after, lomefloxacin therapy, and to discontinue the drug immediately if phototoxicity occurs.

◊ References.

1. Arata J, *et al.* Photosensitivity reactions caused by lomefloxacin hydrochloride: a multicenter survey. *Antimicrob Agents Chemother* 1998; **42:** 3141–5.

## Interactions

As for Ciprofloxacin, p.190. Lomefloxacin does not appear to interact significantly with theophylline or caffeine.

## Antimicrobial Action

As for Ciprofloxacin, p.190. Most streptococci, including *Streptococcus pneumoniae*, are relatively resistant to lomefloxacin. Cross-resistance between lomefloxacin and other quinolones has been reported.

## Pharmacokinetics

Lomefloxacin is rapidly and almost completely absorbed following oral administration, peak plasma concentrations of about 3 micrograms/mL being attained about 1 to 1.5 hours after a 400-mg dose. Lomefloxacin is approximately 10% bound to plasma proteins. It is widely distributed into body tissues including the lungs and prostate.

The elimination half-life of lomefloxacin is about 7 to 8 hours, and is prolonged in patients with renal impairment. Lomefloxacin is excreted in the urine, mainly as unchanged drug but also in small amounts as the glucuronide and other metabolites. Small amounts are also eliminated unchanged in the faeces. Lomefloxacin is only removed in negligible amounts by haemodialysis.

◊ References.

1. Freeman CD, *et al.* Lomefloxacin clinical pharmacokinetics. *Clin Pharmacokinet* 1993; **25:** 6–19.

## Uses and Administration

Lomefloxacin is a fluoroquinolone antibacterial with actions and uses similar to those of ciprofloxacin (p.191).

It is given by mouth, as the hydrochloride, for the treatment of susceptible infections, including bronchitis due to *Haemophilus influenzae* or *Moraxella catarrhalis* (*Branhamella catarrhalis*), and urinary-tract infections. Doses are expressed in terms of lomefloxacin base. The usual dose is the equivalent of 400 mg of lomefloxacin once daily. Evening administration may minimise the risk of phototoxicity reactions.

For details of reduced doses to be used in renal impairment, see below.

Lomefloxacin is also used topically as the hydrochloride as 0.3% eye drops for the treatment of bacterial conjunctivitis and as 0.3% ear drops for the treatment of otitis externa and otitis media.

◊ General references.

1. Wadworth AN, Goa KL. Lomefloxacin: a review of its antibacterial activity, pharmacokinetic properties and therapeutic use. *Drugs* 1991; **42:** 1018–60.
2. Neu HC, ed. Lomefloxacin: development of a once-a-day quinolone. *Am J Med* 1992; **92** (suppl 4A): 1S–137S.

**Administration in renal impairment.** Dosage of lomefloxacin should be reduced in patients with moderate to severe renal impairment; the initial dose of 400 mg should be followed by maintenance doses of 200 mg daily in those with a creatinine clearance of 10 to 40 mL/minute and in those on haemodialysis.

## Preparations

**Proprietary Preparations** (details are given in Part 3)
***Arg.:*** Okacin; ***Austria:*** Okacin; Uniquin; ***Braz.:*** Maxaquin; Meflox; Okacin; ***Chile:*** Okacin; ***Denm.:*** Okacin; ***Fin.:*** Okacin; ***Fr.:*** Decalogiflox; Logiflox; ***Ger.:*** Okacin; ***Hong Kong:*** Maxaquin; Okacin; ***India:*** Lomef; Lomflox; Ontop; ***Israel:*** Maxaquin†; Okacin; ***Ital.:*** Chimono; Maxaquin; Okacin; Uniquin; ***Jpn:*** Lomeflon; ***Malaysia:*** Okacin; ***Mex.:*** Lomacin; Maxaquin; ***Port.:*** Basab; Floxaquil; Loxina; Maxaquin; Monoquin; Okacin; Uniquin; ***S.Afr.:*** Maxaquin; Okacyn; Uniquin; ***Singapore:*** Lomflox; Okacyn; ***Spain:*** Ocacin; ***Switz.:*** Maxaquin; Okacin; ***Thai.:*** Maxaquin; Okacin; ***UAE:*** Lomax; ***UK:*** Okacyn†; ***USA:*** Maxaquin.

## Loracarbef *(BAN, USAN, rINN)*

KT-3777; LY-163892. (6R,7S)-3-Chloro-8-oxo-7-D-phenylglycylamino-1-azabicyclo[4.2.0]oct-2-ene-2-carboxylic acid monohydrate.

$C_{16}H_{16}ClN_3O_4,H_2O$ = 367.8.

*CAS — 76470-66-1 (anhydrous loracarbef); 121961-22-6 (loracarbef monohydrate).*

*ATC — J01DA38.*

**Pharmacopoeias.** In *US.*

**USP 27** (Loracarbef). pH of a 10% suspension in water is between 3.0 and 5.5. Store in airtight containers.

### Adverse Effects and Precautions

Adverse effects of loracarbef are generally similar to those of other beta lactams (see Benzylpenicillin, p.163, and Cefalotin, p.168). They include gastrointestinal disturbances, particularly diarrhoea, and hypersensitivity reactions such as skin rashes. Increases in liver enzymes and abnormalities in haematological parameters have been reported.

Loracarbef should not be given to patients known to be hypersensitive to it or to other beta lactams because of the possibility of cross-sensitivity. It should be given with caution, with appropriate dosage reduction, in patients with renal impairment.

**Effects on the kidneys.** References.

1. Thieme RE, *et al.* Acute interstitial nephritis associated with loracarbef therapy. *J Pediatr* 1995; **127:** 997–1000.

### Interactions

Probenecid decreases the renal excretion of loracarbef thereby increasing its plasma concentrations.

### Antimicrobial Action

Loracarbef is bactericidal with antibacterial activity similar to that of cefaclor (p.167).

### Pharmacokinetics

Loracarbef is well absorbed from the gastrointestinal tract with a bioavailability of 90%. Peak plasma concentrations following 200- and 400-mg doses as capsules are about 8 and 14 micrograms/mL respectively at 1.2 hours. Peak concentrations are achieved more rapidly following an oral suspension and a paediatric dose of 15 mg/kg produces a concentration of approximately 19 micrograms/mL within 40 to 60 minutes. Absorption is delayed by the presence of food. A plasma half-life of about 1 hour has been reported which is prolonged in renal impairment. About 25% is bound to plasma proteins.

Loracarbef is excreted largely unchanged in the urine, and therapeutic concentrations are maintained in the urine for up to 12 hours. Probenecid delays excretion. Loracarbef is removed by haemodialysis.

### Uses and Administration

Loracarbef is an oral carbacephem antibiotic. The carbacephems are closely related to the cephalosporins, but replacement of the sulfur atom in the 7-aminocephalosporanic acid nucleus by a methylene group is said to enhance stability. It is used similarly to cefaclor in the treatment of susceptible infections of the respiratory and urinary tracts and of skin and soft tissue. For details of these infections and their treatment, see under Choice of Antibacterial, p.120.

Loracarbef should be given 1 hour before food or on an empty stomach. Loracarbef is given as the monohydrate. Doses are expressed in terms of the equivalent amount of anhydrous loracarbef. The usual adult dose is 200 to 400 mg every 12 hours. In uncomplicated urinary-tract infections, a dose of 200 mg daily may be adequate. A dose for children is 7.5 mg/kg every 12 hours for uncomplicated infections or 15 mg/kg every 12 hours for acute otitis media or acute maxillary sinusitis.

For details of reduced doses of loracarbef to be used in patients with renal impairment, see below.

◊ General references.


1. Moellering RC, Jacobs NF. Advances in outpatient antimicrobial therapy: loracarbef. *Am J Med* 1992; **92** (suppl 6A): 1S–103S.
2. Brogden RN, McTavish D. Loracarbef: a review of its antimicrobial activity, pharmacokinetic properties and therapeutic efficacy. *Drugs* 1993; **45:** 716–36.


**Administration in renal impairment.** Doses of loracarbef should be reduced in patients with renal impairment; patients with a creatinine clearance of 10 to 49 mL/minute may be given half the usual dose at the usual dosage interval or the full usual dose at twice the usual interval; patients with a creatinine clearance of less than 10 mL/minute may be treated with the usual dose given every 3 to 5 days. Patients on haemodialysis should receive another dose following dialysis.

### Preparations

***USP 27:*** Loracarbef Capsules; Loracarbef for Oral Suspension.

**Proprietary Preparations** (details are given in Part 3)
***Austria:*** Lorabid†; Lorax†; ***Ger.:*** Lorafem; ***Gr.:*** Lorbef; ***Hong Kong:*** Lorabid†; ***Ital.:*** Carbem†; ***Mex.:*** Carbac; Lorabid; ***Neth.:*** Lorax; ***S.Afr.:*** Lorabid; ***Swed.:*** Lorabid; ***USA:*** Lorabid.

---

## Lymecycline *(BAN, rINN)*

Limeciclina; Tetracyclinemethylene lysine.

$C_{29}H_{38}N_4O_{10}$ = 602.6.

*CAS — 992-21-2.*

*ATC — J01AA04.*

**Pharmacopoeias.** In *Br.*

**BP 2003** (Lymecycline). A water-soluble combination of tetracycline, lysine, and formaldehyde. The potency is not less than 900 international units/mg, calculated with reference to the anhydrous substance. A yellow, very hygroscopic, powder. Very soluble in water; slightly soluble in alcohol; practically insoluble in acetone, in chloroform, and in ether. It contains not more than 5% by weight of water. A 1% solution in water has a pH of 7.8 to 8.1. Store at a temperature not exceeding 25°. Protect from light.

### Profile

Lymecycline is a tetracycline derivative with general properties similar to those of tetracycline (p.266).

Doses of lymecycline are expressed in terms of the equivalent amount of tetracycline base. Lymecycline 407 mg is approximately equivalent to 300 mg of tetracycline and to 325 mg of tetracycline hydrochloride. The usual adult dose is the equivalent of 300 mg of tetracycline base twice daily by mouth; in severe infections total daily doses of up to the equivalent of 1.2 g may be given. In the treatment of acne, the equivalent of 300 mg of tetracycline is given daily.

### Preparations

***BP 2003:*** Lymecycline Capsules.

**Proprietary Preparations** (details are given in Part 3)
***Arg.:*** Tetralysal; ***Austria:*** Tetralysal; ***Belg.:*** Tetralysal; ***Braz.:*** Tetralysal; ***Denm.:*** Tetralysal; ***Fin.:*** Tetralysal; ***Fr.:*** Tetralysal; ***Irl.:*** Tetralysal; ***Ital.:*** Tetralysal; ***Mex.:*** Tetralisal; ***Norw.:*** Tetralysal; ***S.Afr.:*** Tetralysal; ***Swed.:*** Tetralysal; ***UK:*** Tetralysal.

---

## Mafenide *(BAN, USAN, rINN)*

NSC-34632. α-Aminotoluene-*p*-sulphonamide.

*CAS — 138-39-6.*

*ATC — D06BA03.*

## Mafenide Acetate *(BANM, rINNM)*

Acetato de mafenida.

$C_7H_{10}N_2O_2S,C_2H_4O_2$ = 246.3.

*CAS — 13009-99-9.*

*ATC — D06BA03.*

**Pharmacopoeias.** In *Chin.* and *US.*

**USP 27** (Mafenide Acetate). A white to pale yellow crystalline powder. Freely soluble in water. pH of a 10% solution in water is between 6.4 and 6.8. Store in airtight containers. Protect from light.

### Adverse Effects, Treatment, and Precautions

Mafenide is absorbed to some extent following topical application and may produce systemic effects similar to those of other sulfonamides (see Sulfamethoxazole, p.261). Fatal haemolytic anaemia with disseminated intravascular coagulation, related to G6PD deficiency, has been reported.

Mafenide cream may cause pain or a burning sensation on application to the burnt area, with occasional bleeding or excoriation. The separation of the eschar may be delayed and fungal invasion of the wound has been reported. By its action in inhibiting carbonic anhydrase, mafenide may cause metabolic acidosis and hyperventilation; acid-base balance should therefore be monitored, particularly in patients with extensive burns, or with pulmonary or renal impairment. If persistent acidosis occurs, mafenide treatment should be temporarily suspended and fluid therapy continued.

### Pharmacokinetics

Mafenide is absorbed from wounds into the circulation and is metabolised to *p*-carboxybenzenesulfonamide, which is excreted in the urine. The metabolite has no antibacterial action but retains the ability to inhibit carbonic anhydrase.

### Uses and Administration

Mafenide is a sulfonamide that is not inactivated by *p*-aminobenzoic acid or by pus and serum. The acetate is used as a cream, containing the equivalent of mafenide 8.5%, in conjunction with debridement, for the prevention and treatment of infection, including *Pseudomonas aeruginosa,* in second- and third-degree burns (p.1134). A solution containing mafenide acetate 5% is also available for use under moist dressings in burns. Mafenide hydrochloride and mafenide propionate have also been used.

### Preparations

***USP 27:*** Mafenide Acetate Cream; Mafenide Acetate for Topical Solution.

**Proprietary Preparations** (details are given in Part 3)
***USA:*** Sulfamylon.

**Multi-ingredient:** ***Braz.:*** Otosulf†; ***Spain:*** Pental Forte; Pentalmicina†.

---

## Magainins

Magaininas.

### Profile

The magainins are a group of antimicrobial peptides derived from amphibians. A number of semisynthetic derivatives including pexiganan acetate (MSI-78), MSI-93, and MSI-94 have been investigated as topical anti-infectives.

◊ References.


1. Lamb HM, Wiseman LR. Pexiganan acetate. *Drugs* 1998; **56:** 1047–52.


---

## Mandelic Acid

Amygdalic Acid; Mandélico, ácido; Phenylglycolic Acid; Racemic Mandelic Acid. 2-Hydroxy-2-phenylacetic acid.

$C_8H_8O_3$ = 152.1.

*CAS — 90-64-2; 17199-29-0 ((+)-mandelic acid); 611-71-2 ((−)-mandelic acid); 611-72-3 ((±)-mandelic acid).*

*ATC — B05CA06; J01XX06.*

### Profile

Mandelic acid has bacteriostatic properties and is used as a 1% flushing solution for the maintenance of indwelling urinary catheters. Mandelic acid and acetyl mandelic acid are used topically in preparations for the treatment of acne. It was formerly given by mouth in the treatment of urinary-tract infections, usually as the ammonium or calcium salt.

Mandelic acid is a component of methenamine mandelate (p.230).

### Preparations

**Proprietary Preparations** (details are given in Part 3)
***Fr.:*** Rolip.

**Multi-ingredient:** ***Chile:*** Neostrata; ***Fr.:*** Sphingogel; Zeniac; Zeniac LP; Zeniac LP Fort; ***Ital.:*** NeoCeuticals Clear Skin; NeoCeuticals Spot Treatment; ***Port.:*** Mandelip.

---

## Marbofloxacin *(BAN, rINN)*

Marbofloxacino. 9-Fluoro-2,3-dihydro-3-methyl-10-(4-methyl-1-piperazinyl)-7-oxo-7H-pyrido[3,2,1-*ij*][4,1,2]benzoxadiazine-6-carboxylic acid.

$C_{17}H_{19}FN_4O_4$ = 362.4.

*CAS — 115550-35-1.*

### Profile

Marbofloxacin is a fluoroquinolone antibacterial used in veterinary medicine.

---

## Mecillinam *(BAN, rINN)*

Amdinocillin *(USAN)*; FL-1060; Mecilinam; Ro-10-9070. (6R)-6-(Perhydroazepin-1-ylmethyleneamino)penicillanic acid.

$C_{15}H_{23}N_3O_3S$ = 325.4.

*CAS — 32887-01-7.*

*ATC — J01CA11.*

### Adverse Effects and Precautions

As for Benzylpenicillin, p.163.

**Porphyria.** Mecillinam has been associated with acute attacks of porphyria and is considered unsafe in porphyric patients.

### Interactions

As for Benzylpenicillin, p.164.

### Antimicrobial Action

Mecillinam is a derivative of amidinopenicillanic acid. Unlike benzylpenicillin and related antibiotics, it is active against many Gram-negative bacteria, in particular Enterobacteriaceae including *Escherichia coli, Enterobacter, Klebsiella, Salmonella,* and *Shigella* spp. The susceptibility of *Proteus* spp. varies; *Serratia marcescens* is generally resistant. It is less active against *Neisseria* spp. and *Haemophilus influenzae. Pseudomonas aeruginosa* and *Bacteroides* spp. are considered to be resistant. It is much less active against Gram-positive bacteria; enterococci including *Enterococcus faecalis* are resistant.

Mecillinam interferes with the synthesis of the bacterial cell wall by binding with a different penicillin-binding protein from benzylpenicillin. This difference in mode of action may explain the synergism against many Gram-negative organisms that has been reported *in vitro* between mecillinam and various penicillins or cephalosporins.

Mecillinam is inactivated by beta-lactamases, but is more stable than ampicillin.

### Pharmacokinetics

Mecillinam is poorly absorbed from the gastrointestinal tract. Peak plasma concentrations of about 6 and 12 micrograms/mL have been achieved half an hour after intramuscular doses of 200 and 400 mg, respectively. The usual plasma half-life of about 1 hour has been reported to be prolonged to 3 to 5 hours or more in severe renal impairment. Between 5 and 10% of mecillinam is bound to plasma proteins. Mecillinam is widely distributed into body tissues and fluids; little passes into the CSF unless the meninges are inflamed. It crosses the placenta into the fetal circulation; little appears to be distributed into breast milk.

Mecillinam is metabolised to only a limited extent. From 50 to 70% of a parenteral dose may be excreted in the urine within 6 hours by glomerular filtration and tubular secretion. Renal tubular secretion can be reduced by probenecid. Some mecillinam is excreted in bile where high concentrations are achieved.

Mecillinam is removed by haemodialysis.

### Uses and Administration

Mecillinam is a semisynthetic penicillin with a substituted amidino group at the 6-position of the penicillanic acid nucleus. It is given by slow intravenous injection, by intravenous infusion, or intramuscularly, in the treatment of susceptible Gram-negative infections (see under Antimicrobial Action, above).

For urinary-tract infections a dose of 800 mg is given every 6 to 8 hours. A total dose of up to 60 mg/kg daily may be used in very severe infections.

Mecillinam has been used with other beta lactams to extend the spectrum of antimicrobial activity to Gram-positive organisms and because of reported synergism against Gram-negative bacteria *in vitro*.

The pivaloyloxymethyl ester of mecillinam, pivmecillinam, is used orally (see p.244).

### Preparations

**Proprietary Preparations** (details are given in Part 3)
***Denm.:*** Selexid; ***Gr.:*** Selexid N; ***Norw.:*** Selexid; ***Swed.:*** Selexid.

---

## Meclocycline *(BAN, USAN, rINN)*

GS-2989; NSC-78502. (4S,4aR,5S,5aR,6S,12aS)-7-Chloro-4-dimethylamino-1,4,4a,5,5a,6,11,12a-octahydro-3,5,10,12,12a-pentahydroxy-6-methylene-1,11-dioxonaphthacene-2-carboxamide; 7-Chloro-6-demethyl-6-deoxy-5β-hydroxy-6-methylenetetracycline.

$C_{22}H_{21}ClN_2O_8$ = 476.9.
*CAS — 2013-58-3.*
*ATC — D10AF04.*

## Meclocycline Sulfosalicylate *(USAN)*

Meclociclina, sulfosalicilato de; Meclocycline Sulphosalicylate. Meclocycline 5-sulphosalicylate.

$C_{22}H_{21}ClN_2O_8,C_7H_6O_6S$ = 695.0.
*CAS — 73816-42-9.*
*ATC — D10AF04.*

**Pharmacopoeias.** In *US.*

**USP 27** (Meclocycline Sulfosalicylate). pH of a 1% solution in water is between 2.5 and 3.5. Store in airtight containers. Protect from light.

### Profile

Meclocycline is a tetracycline antibiotic derived from oxytetracycline (p.241). It is applied topically as the sulfosalicylate for the treatment of acne vulgaris and superficial skin infections. Potency is expressed in terms of meclocycline. Preparations containing the equivalent of 1 or 2% are available. Meclocycline sulfosalicylate has also been given as a pessary in the treatment of vulvovaginal infections.

### Preparations

***USP 27:*** Meclocycline Sulfosalicylate Cream.

**Proprietary Preparations** (details are given in Part 3)
***Ger.:*** Meclosorb; ***Ital.:*** Mecloderm; Mecloderm Antiacne; Mecloderm Ovuli; Mecloderm Polvere Aspersoria; Meclutin Semplice; Novacnyl†; Traumatociclina†; ***Spain:*** Quoderm†; ***USA:*** Meclan†.

**Multi-ingredient:** ***Ital.:*** Anti-Acne; Mecloderm F; Meclutin.

---

# Meropenem *(BAN, USAN, rINN)*

ICI-194660; SM-7338. (4R,5S,6S)-3-[(3S,5S)-5-Dimethylcarbamoylpyrrolidin-3-ylthio]-6-[(R)-1-hydroxyethyl]-4-methyl-7-oxo-1-azabicyclo[3.2.0]hept-2-ene-2-carboxylic acid trihydrate.

$C_{17}H_{25}N_3O_5S,3H_2O$ = 437.5.
*CAS — 96036-03-2 (meropenem); 119478-56-7 (meropenem trihydrate).*
*ATC — J01DH02.*

**Pharmacopoeias.** In *Jpn* and *US.*

**USP 27** (Meropenem). Colourless to white crystals. Sparingly soluble in water; very slightly soluble in alcohol; practically insoluble in acetone and in ether; soluble in dimethylformamide and in 5% monobasic potassium phosphate solution. pH of a 1% solution in water is between 4.0 and 6.0. Store in airtight containers.

### Adverse Effects and Precautions

As for Imipenem, p.221.

Meropenem is more stable to renal dehydropeptidase I than imipenem and administration with cilastatin, which inhibits this enzyme, is not required. Meropenem may have less potential to induce seizures than imipenem (see also below).

**Effects on the nervous system.** *Animal* studies have indicated that meropenem induces fewer seizures than imipenem-cilastatin and clinical data from the manufacturer have substantiated this.[1] Comparison of data[2] from 4872 patients with a variety of infections (including meningitis) treated with meropenem with that from 4752 patients who received other antibacterials, principally cephalosporin-based regimens or imipenem-cilastatin, showed that meropenem was not associated with any greater risk of seizures than the other antibacterials and was likely to have less neurotoxic potential than imipenem-cilastatin, making it a suitable drug to use in the treatment of meningitis.

1. Norrby SR, *et al.* Safety profile of meropenem: international clinical experience based on the first 3125 patients treated with meropenem. *J Antimicrob Chemother* 1995; **36** (suppl A): 207–23.
2. Norrby SR, Gildon KM. Safety profile of meropenem: a review of nearly 5,000 patients treated with meropenem. *Scand J Infect Dis* 1999; **31:** 3–10.

### Interactions

Probenecid inhibits the renal excretion of meropenem thereby increasing its plasma concentrations and prolonging its elimination half-life.

**Antiepileptics.** For a report of decreased plasma-*valproate* concentrations associated with antibacterial therapy containing meropenem, see p.381.

### Antimicrobial Action

As for Imipenem, p.221.

Meropenem is slightly more active than imipenem against Enterobacteriaceae and slightly less active against Gram-positive organisms.

### Pharmacokinetics

Following intravenous injection of meropenem 0.5 and 1 g over 5 minutes, peak plasma concentrations of about 50 and 112 micrograms/mL respectively are attained. The same doses infused over 30 minutes produce peak plasma concentrations of 23 and 49 micrograms/mL, respectively.

Meropenem has a plasma elimination half-life of about 1 hour; this may be prolonged in patients with renal impairment and is also slightly prolonged in children. Meropenem is widely distributed into body tissues and fluids including the CSF and bile. It is approximately 2% bound to plasma proteins. It is more stable to renal dehydropeptidase I than imipenem and is mainly excreted in the urine by tubular secretion and glomerular filtration. About 70% of a dose is recovered unchanged in the urine over a 12-hour period and urinary concentrations above 10 micrograms/mL are maintained for up to 5 hours after a 500-mg dose. Meropenem is reported to have one metabolite (ICI-213689), which is inactive and is excreted in the urine.

Meropenem is removed by haemodialysis.

◊ References.

1. Chimata M, *et al.* Pharmacokinetics of meropenem in patients with various degrees of renal function, including patients with end-stage renal disease. *Antimicrob Agents Chemother* 1993; **37:** 229–33.
2. Dagan R, *et al.* Penetration of meropenem into the cerebrospinal fluid of patients with inflamed meninges. *J Antimicrob Chemother* 1994; **34:** 175–9.
3. Mouton JW, Van den Anker JN. Meropenem clinical pharmacokinetics. *Clin Pharmacokinet* 1995; **28:** 275–86.
4. Blumer JL, *et al.* Sequential, single-dose pharmacokinetic evaluation of meropenem in hospitalized infants and children. *Antimicrob Agents Chemother* 1995; **39:** 1721–5.
5. Novelli A, *et al.* Clinical pharmacokinetics of meropenem after the first and tenth intramuscular administration. *J Antimicrob Chemother* 1996; **37:** 775–81.
6. Thalhammer F, *et al.* Continuous infusion versus intermittent administration of meropenem in critically ill patients. *J Antimicrob Chemother* 1999; **43:** 523–7.
7. Giles LJ, *et al.* Pharmacokinetics of meropenem in intensive care unit patients receiving continuous veno-venous hemofiltration or hemodiafiltration. *Crit Care Med* 2000; **28:** 632–7.
8. Thalhammer F, Horl WH. Pharmacokinetics of meropenem in patients with renal failure and patients receiving renal replacement therapy. *Clin Pharmacokinet* 2000; **39:** 271–9.
9. Ververs TF, *et al.* Pharmacokinetics and dosing regimen of meropenem in critically ill patients receiving continuous venovenous hemofiltration. *Crit Care Med* 2000; **28:** 3412–16.
10. van Enk JG, *et al.* Pharmacokinetics of meropenem in preterm neonates. *Ther Drug Monit* 2001; **23:** 198–201.
11. Goldstein SL, *et al.* Meropenem pharmacokinetics in children and adolescents receiving hemodialysis. *Pediatr Nephrol* 2001; **16:** 1015–18.

### Uses and Administration

Meropenem is a carbapenem beta-lactam antibacterial with actions and uses similar to those of imipenem (p.221). It is more stable to renal dehydropeptidase I than imipenem and need not be given in association with an enzyme inhibitor such as cilastatin. It is used in the treatment of susceptible infections including intra-abdominal infections, meningitis, respiratory-tract infections (including in cystic fibrosis patients), septicaemia, skin infections, urinary-tract infections, and infections in immunocompromised patients. For details of these infections and their treatment, see under Choice of Antibacterial, p.120.

Meropenem is given intravenously as the trihydrate, but doses are expressed in terms of the amount of anhydrous meropenem. 1.14 g of meropenem trihydrate is approximately equivalent to 1 g of anhydrous meropenem. It is given by slow injection over 3 to 5 minutes or by infusion over 15 to 30 minutes in a usual adult dose of 0.5 to 1 g every 8 hours, increased to 2 g every 8 hours for meningitis; doses of up to 2 g every 8 hours have also been used in cystic fibrosis.

For details of reduced doses to be used in renal impairment, see below.

Children over 3 months of age and weighing less than 50 kg may be given 10 to 20 mg/kg every 8 hours, increased to 40 mg/kg every 8 hours for meningitis. Doses of 25 to 40 mg/kg every 8 hours have been used in children with cystic fibrosis.

◊ Reviews.

1. Wiseman LR, *et al.* Meropenem: a review of its antibacterial activity, pharmacokinetic properties and clinical efficacy. *Drugs* 1995; **50:** 73–101.
2. Finch RG, *et al.* eds. Meropenem: focus on clinical performance. *J Antimicrob Chemother* 1995; **36** (suppl A): 1–223.
3. Hellinger WC, Brewer NS. Carbapenems and monobactams: imipenem, meropenem, and aztreonam. *Mayo Clin Proc* 1999; **74:** 420–34.
4. Hurst M, Lamb HM. Meropenem: a review of its use in patients in intensive care. *Drugs* 2000; **59:** 653–80.
5. Lowe MN, Lamb HM. Meropenem: an updated review of its use in the management of intra-abdominal infections. *Drugs* 2000; **60:** 619–46.

**Administration in renal impairment.** Doses of meropenem should be reduced in patients with renal impairment. The following doses may be given based on creatinine clearance (CC):

- CC 26 to 50 mL/minute: the usual dose given every 12 hours
- CC 10 to 25 mL/minute: one-half the usual dose every 12 hours
- CC less than 10 mL/minute: one-half the usual dose every 24 hours

### Preparations

***USP 27:*** Meropenem for Injection.

**Proprietary Preparations** (details are given in Part 3)
***Arg.:*** Merozen; Zeropenem; ***Austral.:*** Merrem; ***Austria:*** Optinem; ***Belg.:*** Meronem; ***Braz.:*** Meronem; ***Canad.:*** Merrem; ***Chile:*** Meronem; ***Denm.:*** Meronem; ***Fin.:*** Meronem; ***Ger.:*** Meronem; ***Gr.:*** Meronem; ***Hong Kong:*** Meronem; ***Irl.:*** Meronem; ***Israel:*** Meronem; ***Ital.:*** Merrem; ***Jpn:*** Meropen; ***Malaysia:*** Meronem; ***Mex.:*** Merrem; ***Neth.:*** Meronem; ***Norw.:*** Meronem; ***NZ:*** Merrem; ***Port.:*** Meronem; ***S.Afr.:*** Meronem; ***Singapore:*** Meronem; ***Spain:*** Meronem; ***Swed.:*** Meronem; ***Switz.:*** Meronem; ***Thai.:*** Meronem; ***UK:*** Meronem; ***USA:*** Merrem.

---

## Metampicillin Sodium *(rINNM)*

Metampicilina sódica. Sodium (6R)-6-(D-2-methyleneamino-2-phenylacetamido)penicillanate.

$C_{17}H_{18}N_3NaO_4S$ = 383.4.
*CAS — 6489-97-0 (metampicillin); 6489-61-8 (metampicillin sodium).*
*ATC — J01CA14.*

### Profile

Metampicillin has actions and uses similar to those of ampicillin (p.157).

After oral doses it is almost completely hydrolysed to ampicillin. When given parenterally, however, a proportion of the dose exists in the circulation as unchanged metampicillin which has some antibacterial activity of its own.

Metampicillin has been given by mouth as the sodium salt in usual doses of 1 to 2 g daily in 4 divided doses. It has also been given by intramuscular or intravenous injection.

### Preparations

**Proprietary Preparations** (details are given in Part 3)
***Braz.:*** Pravacilin†; ***Fr.:*** Suvipen†; ***Spain:*** Dompil†; Meta Framan†; Metakes†; Serfabiotic†.

**Multi-ingredient: *Arg.:*** Gentocelina.

---

## Methacycline *(BAN, USAN)*

Metacycline *(pINN)*; GS-2876. (4S,4aR,5S,5aR,6S,12aS)-4-Dimethylamino-1,4,4a,5,5a,6,11,12a-octahydro-3,5,10,12,12a-pentahydroxy-6-methylene-1,11-dioxonaphthacene-2-carboxamide; 6-Demethyl-6-deoxy-5β-hydroxy-6-methylenetetracycline.
$C_{22}H_{22}N_2O_8$ = 442.4.
*CAS — 914-00-1.*
*ATC — J01AA05.*

## Methacycline Hydrochloride *(BANM)*

Metacycline Hydrochloride *(pINNM)*; Hidrocloruro de metaciclina; Metacyclini Chloridum; Méthylènecycline Chlorhydrate; 6-Methyleneoxytetracycline Hydrochloride.
$C_{22}H_{22}N_2O_8$,HCl = 478.9.
*CAS — 3963-95-9.*
*ATC — J01AA05.*

**Pharmacopoeias.** In *Chin., Pol.,* and *US.*
**USP 27** (Methacycline Hydrochloride). A yellow to dark yellow crystalline powder. Soluble 1 in 100 of water, 1 in 300 of alcohol, and 1 in 25 of 0.1N sodium hydroxide; very slightly soluble in chloroform and in ether. pH of a solution in water containing the equivalent of methacycline 1% is between 2.0 and 3.0. Store in airtight containers. Protect from light.

### Adverse Effects and Precautions

As for Tetracycline Hydrochloride, p.266.

### Interactions

As for Tetracycline Hydrochloride, p.267.

### Antimicrobial Action

As for Tetracycline Hydrochloride, p.267.

### Pharmacokinetics

As for Tetracycline Hydrochloride, p.268.

Around 60% of an oral dose is absorbed from the gastrointestinal tract. About 80 to 95% of methacycline in the circulation is bound to plasma proteins. Plasma concentrations of 2 to 6 micrograms/mL have been reported 4 hours after a 300-mg dose of methacycline. Its plasma elimination half-life is about 14 to 15 hours. About a third of a dose is slowly excreted unchanged in the urine.

### Uses and Administration

Methacycline is a tetracycline derivative with uses similar to those of tetracycline (p.268). Like demeclocycline, it is excreted more slowly than tetracycline and effective blood concentrations are maintained for longer periods.

Methacycline hydrochloride is given by mouth in a usual dose of 600 mg daily in 2 divided doses, preferably 1 hour before or 2 hours after meals.

### Preparations

***USP 27:*** Methacycline Hydrochloride Capsules; Methacycline Hydrochloride Oral Suspension.

**Proprietary Preparations** (details are given in Part 3)
***Fr.:*** Lysocline; Physiomycine; ***Ital.:*** Esarondil; Rotilen; Stafilon.

---

## Methaniazide *(rINN)*

Isoniazid Mesylate; Isoniazid Methanesulfonate; Metaniazida. 2-Isonicotinoylhydrazinomethanesulphonic acid.
$C_7H_9N_3O_4S$ = 231.2.
*CAS — 13447-95-5 (methaniazide); 6059-26-3 (methaniazide calcium); 3804-89-5 (methaniazide sodium).*

### Profile

Methaniazide is a derivative of isoniazid (p.222). It has been used as the calcium and sodium salts in the treatment of tuberculosis.

### Preparations

**Proprietary Preparations** (details are given in Part 3)
***Austria:*** Neo-Tizide; ***India:*** Erbazide.

---

## Methenamine *(rINN)*

Aminoform; E239; Esametilentetrammina; Esammina; Formine; Hexamethylenamine; Hexamine; Metenamina; Metenammina; Methenaminum; Urotropine. Hexamethylenetetramine; 1,3,5,7-Tetraazatricyclo[3.3.1.1$^{3,7}$]decane.
$C_6H_{12}N_4$ = 140.2.
*CAS — 100-97-0.*
*ATC — J01XX05.*

**Pharmacopoeias.** In *Chin., Eur.* (see p.vi), *Pol.,* and *US.*
**Ph. Eur. 5.0** (Methenamine). A white crystalline powder or colourless crystals. Freely soluble in water; soluble in alcohol and in dichloromethane. Protect from light.

**USP 27** (Methenamine). Colourless, practically odourless, lustrous crystals or white crystalline powder. Soluble 1 in 1.5 of water, 1 in 12.5 of alcohol, 1 in 10 of chloroform, and 1 in 320 of ether. Its solutions are alkaline to litmus.

## Methenamine Hippurate *(BAN, USAN, rINNM)*

Hexamine Hippurate; Hipurato de metenamina. Hexamethylenetetramine hippurate.
$C_6H_{12}N_4,C_9H_9NO_3$ = 319.4.
*CAS — 5714-73-8.*
*ATC — J01XX05.*

**Pharmacopoeias.** In *US.*

## Methenamine Mandelate *(rINNM)*

Hexamine Amygdalate; Hexamine Mandelate; Mandelato de metenamina. Hexamethylenetetramine mandelate.
$C_6H_{12}N_4,C_8H_8O_3$ = 292.3.
*CAS — 587-23-5.*
*ATC — J01XX05.*

**Pharmacopoeias.** In *US.*
**USP 27** (Methenamine Mandelate). A white, practically odourless crystalline powder. Very soluble in water; soluble 1 in 10 of alcohol, 1 in 20 of chloroform, and 1 in 350 of ether. Its solutions have a pH of about 4.

### Adverse Effects and Precautions

Methenamine and its salts are generally well tolerated but may cause gastrointestinal disturbances such as nausea, vomiting, and diarrhoea. Skin rashes, and occasionally other hypersensitivity reactions, may occur.

Comparatively large amounts of formaldehyde may be formed during prolonged use or when large doses are given. This may produce irritation and inflammation of the urinary tract, especially the bladder, as well as painful and frequent micturition, haematuria, and proteinuria. The effect of the formaldehyde may be reduced by alkalinising drugs, such as sodium bicarbonate, or large quantities of water, but it is then less effective.

Methenamine and its salts are contra-indicated in patients with hepatic impairment because of the liberation of ammonia in the gastrointestinal tract. Although methenamine itself is not contra-indicated in renal impairment, the salts should be avoided in severe impairment because of the risk of mandelate or hippurate crystalluria. They should also be avoided in patients with severe dehydration, metabolic acidosis, or gout.

Interference with laboratory estimations for catecholamines, 17-hydroxycorticosteroids, and oestrogens in the urine has been reported.

### Interactions

The use of drugs that alkalinise the urine, including some antacids, potassium citrate, and diuretics such as acetazolamide or the thiazides, should be avoided because the activation of methenamine to formaldehyde may be inhibited (but see above).

Use of methenamine with sulfonamides may increase the risk of crystalluria since methenamine requires low urinary pH for its effect, at which sulfonamides and their metabolites are poorly soluble; methenamine may also form poorly soluble compounds with some sulfonamides.

### Antimicrobial Action

Methenamine owes its antibacterial properties to formaldehyde, a non-specific bactericide, which is slowly liberated by hydrolysis at acid pH. Most Gram-positive and Gram-negative organisms and fungi are susceptible. Hippuric and mandelic acids have some antibacterial activity *in vitro*, but their contribution to the antibacterial action of the salts *in vivo*, beyond assisting the maintenance of low urinary pH, is uncertain. Urea-splitting organisms such as *Proteus* and some *Pseudomonas* spp. tend to increase urinary pH and inhibit the release of formaldehyde, thereby decreasing the effectiveness of methenamine. The concomitant use of acetohydroxamic acid, a potent inhibitor of bacterial urease, has been suggested for urinary infections due to these organisms. True resistance to formaldehyde does not appear to be a problem in clinical use.

### Pharmacokinetics

Methenamine is readily absorbed from the gastrointestinal tract and widely distributed in the body. Under acid conditions methenamine is slowly hydrolysed to formaldehyde and ammonia: about 10 to 30% of a dose may be converted in the stomach unless it is given as an enteric-coated preparation. Almost no hydrolysis of methenamine takes place at physiological pH, and it is therefore virtually inactive in the body. The half-life is reported to be about 4 hours. Methenamine is rapidly and almost completely eliminated in the urine, and provided this is acidic (preferably below pH 5.5) bactericidal concentrations of formaldehyde are achieved. Because of the time taken for hydrolysis, however, these are not achieved until the urine reaches the bladder, with peak concentrations occurring up to 2 hours after a dose. Absorption, and hence excretion, may be somewhat delayed in patients given enteric-coated formulations.

Methenamine crosses the placenta and small amounts may be distributed into breast milk.

The mandelate and hippurate moieties are also rapidly absorbed and are excreted in urine by tubular secretion as well as glomerular filtration.

### Uses and Administration

Methenamine is used, usually as the hippurate or mandelate, in the prophylaxis and treatment of chronic or recurrent, uncomplicated, lower urinary-tract infections and asymptomatic bacteriuria. It has been considered suitable for long-term use because acquired resistance does not appear to develop.

Methenamine and its salts should not be used in upper urinary-tract infections because it is eliminated too rapidly to exert an effect, nor in acute urinary infections. It is only active in acidic urine, when formaldehyde is released, and although hippuric or mandelic acid helps to acidify the urine, ammonium chloride or ascorbic acid may be tried. If urea-splitting bacteria such as *Proteus* or some *Pseudomonas* spp. are present they may produce so much ammonia that the urine cannot be acidified (see also Antimicrobial Action, above).

The usual adult dose of methenamine or methenamine mandelate is 1 g by mouth four times daily; a dose of about 18 mg/kg four times daily has been suggested in children up to 6 years of age and 500 mg four times daily in those aged 6 to 12 years. Methenamine hippurate is given in a usual adult dose of 1 g twice daily, or 500 mg twice daily in children 6 to 12 years of age.

Methenamine has been used topically in deodorant preparations, since in the presence of acid sweat it liberates formaldehyde. Methenamine calcium thiocyanate has been used in combination preparations for upper respiratory-tract disorders.

### Preparations

***USP 27:*** Methenamine Elixir; Methenamine Hippurate Tablets; Methenamine Mandelate Delayed-release Tablets; Methenamine Mandelate for Oral Solution; Methenamine Mandelate Oral Suspension; Methenamine Mandelate Tablets; Methenamine Tablets.

**Proprietary Preparations** (details are given in Part 3)
***Austral.:*** Hiprex; ***Austria:*** Antihydral†; Hiprex; ***Belg.:*** Hiprex; ***Braz.:*** Neohexal†; ***Canad.:*** Dehydral; Hiprex; Mandelamine; Urasal; ***Denm.:*** Geasalol; Haiprex; ***Fin.:*** Hipeksal; Hiprex; ***Ger.:*** Antihydral; Mandelamine†; Urotractan; ***Irl.:*** Hiprex; ***Israel:*** Hiprex; ***Mex.:*** Bioran; Mandelan†; Mandepiril†; ***Neth.:*** Reflux†; ***Norw.:*** Hiprex; ***NZ:*** Hiprex; ***S.Afr.:*** Hippramine; Mandelamine; ***Swed.:*** Hiprex; ***Switz.:*** Antihydral; ***UK:*** Hiprex; ***USA:*** Hiprex; Mandelamine; Urex.

**Multi-ingredient: *Arg.:*** Calculina; ***Austria:*** Antihydral M†; ***Belg.:*** Carbobel; Mictasol; ***Braz.:*** Abacateirol†; Acridin; Cezane†; Colagolen†; Cystex; Metenan†; Mictarin†; Pyelodion†; Sepurin; Urodonal†; Uropirite†; Urosalin†; Uroseptin†; ***Chile:*** Uroknop; ***Fr.:*** Mictasol; ***Ger.:*** Antihydral M; ***Hong Kong:*** Antihydral M; ***Mex.:*** Furanton†; ***Port.:*** Urocrasina†; ***Switz.:*** Antihydral M†; ***USA:*** Atrosept; Cystex; Dolsed; MHP-A; MSP-Blu; Prosed/DS; Trac Tabs 2X; UAA; Urelle; Uretron; Uridon Modified; Urimar-T; Urimax; Urised; Uriseptic; Uritact; Uro Blue; Uro-Phosphate†; Urogesic Blue; Uroqid-Acid†; Utira.

---

## Meticillin Sodium *(rINNM)*

BRL-1241; Dimethoxyphenecillin Sodium; Dimethoxyphenyl Penicillin Sodium; Methicillin Sodium *(BANM, USAN)*; Meticilina sódica; Meticillinum Natricum; SQ-16123; X-1497. Sodium (6R)-6-(2,6-dimethoxybenzamido)penicillanate monohydrate.
$C_{17}H_{19}N_2NaO_6S,H_2O$ = 420.4.
*CAS — 61-32-5 (meticillin); 132-92-3 (anhydrous meticillin sodium); 7246-14-2 (meticillin sodium monohydrate).*
*ATC — J01CF03.*

**Incompatibility.** Meticillin sodium has been reported to be incompatible with aminoglycosides and a number of other antimicrobials. It has also been reported to be incompatible with acidic and alkaline drugs.

### Adverse Effects and Precautions

As for Benzylpenicillin, p.163.

Meticillin is the penicillin most commonly associated with acute interstitial nephritis.

**Effects on the kidneys.** References.

1. Sanjad SA, *et al.* Nephropathy, an underestimated complication of methicillin therapy. *J Pediatr* 1974; **84:** 873–7.
2. Galpin JE, *et al.* Acute interstitial nephritis due to methicillin. *Am J Med* 1978; **65:** 756–65.

**Sodium content.** Each g of meticillin sodium contains about 2.4 mmol of sodium.

### Interactions

As for Benzylpenicillin, p.164.

### Antimicrobial Action

Meticillin has a mode of action similar to that of benzylpenicillin (p.164) but it is resistant to staphylococcal penicillinase. There is evidence that meticillin is more stable to staphylococcal penicillinase than the other penicillinase-resistant penicillins.

Meticillin is active against both penicillinase-producing and non-penicillinase-producing staphylococci, and also against *Streptococcus pyogenes* (group A beta-haemolytic streptococci), *Str. pneumoniae*, and some viridans streptococci. Its activity against penicillin-sensitive staphylococci and streptococci is less than that of benzylpenicillin. It is virtually ineffective against *Enterococcus faecalis*.

*Resistance* of staphylococci to meticillin is due to the expression of an altered penicillin-binding protein and is not dependent on penicillinase production. There is cross-resistance with other penicillins, including the penicillinase-resistant penicillins cloxacillin, dicloxacillin, flucloxacillin, nafcillin, and oxacillin, and with the cephalosporins. Meticillin-resistant staphylococci are also frequently resistant to other antibacterials, including aminoglycosides, chloramphenicol, ciprofloxacin, clindamycin, erythromycin, and tetracycline. The incidence of such resistance has varied considerably. However, both endemic (restricted to one hospital) and epidemic (affecting more than one hospital) strains of meticillin-resistant *Staphylococcus aureus* (MRSA) are now recognised and infections are a problem in many hospitals.

There have been fewer studies on coagulase-negative staphylococci, but patterns of meticillin resistance in *Staph. epidermidis* are similar to those for MRSA and the frequency of resistance may be higher.

For further details on meticillin-resistant staphylococci and the management of infections, see under Staphylococcal Infections, p.147.

**Resistance.** References to meticillin-resistant staphylococci.

1. Hackbarth CJ, Chambers HF. Methicillin-resistant staphylococci: genetics and mechanisms of resistance. *Antimicrob Agents Chemother* 1989; **33:** 991–4.
2. Maple PAC, *et al.* World-wide antibiotic resistance in methicillin-resistant Staphylococcus aureus. *Lancet* 1989; **i:** 537–40.
3. Mouton RP, *et al.* Correlations between consumption of antibiotics and methicillin resistance in coagulase negative staphylococci. *J Antimicrob Chemother* 1990; **26:** 573–83.
4. Marples RR, Reith S. Methicillin-resistant Staphylococcus aureus in England and Wales. *Commun Dis Rep* 1992; **2:** R25–R29.
5. de Lencastre H, *et al.* Molecular aspects of methicillin resistance in Staphylococcus aureus. *J Antimicrob Chemother* 1994; **33:** 7–24.
6. Fluckiger U, Widmer AF. Epidemiology of methicillin-resistant Staphylococcus aureus. *Chemotherapy* 1999; **45:** 121–34.
7. Livermore DM. Antibiotic resistance in staphylococci. *Int J Antimicrob Agents* 2000; **16** (suppl 1): S3–S10.
8. Turnidge JD, Bell JM. Methicillin-resistant Staphylococcal aureus evolution in Australia over 35 years. *Microb Drug Resist* 2000; **6:** 223–9.

### Pharmacokinetics

Meticillin is inactivated by gastric acid and must be given by injection. Peak plasma concentrations are attained within 0.5 to 1 hour of an intramuscular injection; concentrations of up to 18 micrograms/mL have been achieved after a dose of 1 g. A half-life of 0.5 to 1 hour has been reported, although this may be increased to 3 to 6 hours in renal impairment. About 40% of the meticillin in the circulation is bound to plasma proteins. It is widely distributed in body fluids and in tissues, but there is little diffusion into the CSF unless the meninges are inflamed. Meticillin also crosses the placenta and appears in breast milk. Relatively high concentrations are achieved in bile compared with plasma, although only small amounts are excreted in bile. The majority is rapidly excreted by tubular secretion and glomerular filtration; up to 80% of an injected dose has been detected unchanged in the urine.

Plasma concentrations are enhanced by probenecid. They may be reduced in patients with cystic fibrosis.

### Uses and Administration

Meticillin is a penicillinase-resistant penicillin and has been used similarly to flucloxacillin (p.214) in the treatment of staphylococcal infections resistant to benzylpenicillin. It is not active by mouth and has been given by injection as the sodium salt.

### Preparations

**Proprietary Preparations** (details are given in Part 3)
***Denm.:*** Lucopenin†; ***Ital.:*** Staficyn†.

---

## Mezlocillin *(BAN, USAN)*

6-[*N*-(3-Methylsulfonyl-2-oxoimidazolidin-1-ylcarbonyl)-D-phenylglycylamino]penicillanic acid.

$C_{21}H_{25}N_5O_8S_2$ = 539.6.
*CAS — 51481-65-3.*
*ATC — J01CA10.*

### Mezlocillin Sodium *(BANM, rINNM)*

Bay-f-1353; Mezlocilina sódica. Sodium (6*R*)-6-[D-2-(3-mesyl-2-oxoimidazolidine-1-carboxamido)-2-phenylacetamido]penicillanate monohydrate.

$C_{21}H_{24}N_5NaO_8S_2,H_2O$ = 579.6.
*CAS — 42057-22-7 (anhydrous mezlocillin sodium); 80495-46-1 (mezlocillin sodium monohydrate).*
*ATC — J01CA10.*

**Pharmacopoeias.** In *US.*

**USP 27** (Mezlocillin Sodium). A white to pale yellow crystalline powder. Freely soluble in water. pH of a 10% solution in water is between 4.5 and 8.0. Store in airtight containers.

**Incompatibility.** Mezlocillin sodium has been reported to be incompatible with aminoglycosides, ciprofloxacin, metronidazole, and tetracyclines.

### Adverse Effects and Precautions

As for Carbenicillin Sodium, p.166.

Prolongation of bleeding time has been less frequent and less severe with mezlocillin than with carbenicillin.

**Sodium content.** Each g of mezlocillin sodium contains about 1.7 mmol of sodium. As mezlocillin sodium has a lower sodium content than carbenicillin sodium, hypernatraemia and hypokalaemia are less likely to occur.

### Interactions

As for Benzylpenicillin, p.164.

**Cefotaxime.** For the effect of mezlocillin on the clearance of cefotaxime, see p.175.

### Antimicrobial Action

Mezlocillin has a similar antimicrobial action to piperacillin (p.243). Its activity against *Pseudomonas aeruginosa* is less than that of azlocillin or piperacillin.

### Pharmacokinetics

Mezlocillin is not absorbed from the gastrointestinal tract to any significant extent. It is well absorbed after intramuscular injection, peak plasma concentrations of 15 to 25 micrograms/mL having been observed 45 to 90 minutes after a single dose of 1 g. It is reported to have nonlinear dose-dependent pharmacokinetics. Between 16 and 42% of mezlocillin in the circulation is bound to plasma proteins. Mezlocillin is reported to have a plasma half-life of about 1 hour; this is slightly prolonged in neonates, and in patients with renal impairment half-lives of up to about 6 hours have been reported.

Mezlocillin is widely distributed in body tissues and fluids. It crosses the placenta into the fetal circulation and small amounts are distributed into breast milk. There is little diffusion into CSF except when the meninges are inflamed.

Mezlocillin is reported to be metabolised to a limited extent. About 55% of a dose is excreted unchanged in the urine by glomerular filtration and tubular secretion within 6 hours of administration, hence achieving high urinary concentrations. High concentrations are also found in the bile; up to 30% of a dose has been reported to be excreted by this route.

Plasma concentrations are enhanced by probenecid.

Mezlocillin is removed by haemodialysis, and to some extent by peritoneal dialysis.

### Uses and Administration

Mezlocillin is a ureidopenicillin with uses similar to those of piperacillin (p.243). It is commonly used with an aminoglycoside; however they should be given separately as they have been shown to be incompatible.

*Administration and dosage.* Mezlocillin is given by injection as the sodium salt. Doses are expressed in terms of the equivalent amount of mezlocillin. 1.07 g of mezlocillin sodium is approximately equivalent to 1 g of mezlocillin. Dosage may need to be reduced in renal impairment. It may be given by slow intravenous injection over 3 to 5 minutes, by intravenous infusion over 30 minutes, or by deep intramuscular injection. Single intramuscular doses should not exceed 2 g.

For the treatment of serious infections, 200 to 300 mg/kg daily in divided doses may be given intravenously. For life-threatening infections, up to 350 mg/kg daily may be used, but the total daily dose should not normally exceed 24 g. For uncomplicated urinary-tract infections, a dose of 1.5 to 2 g may be given intramuscularly or intravenously every 6 hours.

Uncomplicated gonorrhoea may be treated by a single intramuscular or intravenous dose of mezlocillin 1 to 2 g. Probenecid 1 g by mouth may be given at the same time or up to 30 minutes before the injection.

For the prophylaxis of infection during surgery, an intravenous pre-operative dose of mezlocillin 4 g, repeated at 6-hourly intervals for 2 further doses, may be given.

### Preparations

***USP 27:*** Mezlocillin for Injection.

**Proprietary Preparations** (details are given in Part 3)
***Austria:*** Baypen; ***Fr.:*** Baypen; ***Ger.:*** Baypen; Melocin†; ***Israel:*** Baypen; ***Ital.:*** Baypen; ***Spain:*** Baypen†; ***USA:*** Mezlin†.

**Multi-ingredient:** ***Austria:*** Optocillin†; ***Ger.:*** Optocillin.

---

### Micronomicin Sulfate *(pINNM)*

Gentamicin $C_{2B}$ Sulphate; KW-1062 (micronomicin); 6′*N*-Methylgentamicin $C_{1A}$ Sulphate; Micronomicin Sulphate; Sagamicin Sulphate; Sulfato de micronomicina. *O*-2-Amino-2,3,4,6-tetradeoxy-6-(methylamino)-α-D-*erythro*-hexopyranosyl-(1→4)-*O*-[3-deoxy-4-*C*-methyl-3-(methylamino)-β-L-arabinopyranosyl-(1→6)]-2-deoxy-D-streptamine hemipentasulphate.

$(C_{20}H_{41}N_5O_7)_2,5H_2SO_4$ = 1417.5.
*CAS — 52093-21-7 (micronomicin).*
*ATC — S01AA22.*

**Pharmacopoeias.** In *Jpn.*

### Profile

Micronomicin is an aminoglycoside with general properties similar to those of gentamicin (p.217). It is given as the sulfate and doses are expressed in terms of micronomicin. 183 mg of micronomicin sulfate is approximately equivalent to 120 mg of micronomicin. It is given by intramuscular injection or by intravenous infusion over 30 minutes to 1 hour in doses of 120 to 240 mg daily in 2 or 3 divided doses. Dosage should be adjusted based on serum-micronomicin concentration monitoring. It is also used topically as eye drops or ointment in a concentration of 0.3% for infections of the eye.

### Preparations

**Proprietary Preparations** (details are given in Part 3)
***Ital.:*** Luxomicina; Sagamicina†; ***Jpn:*** Sagamicin; ***Mon.:*** Microphta; ***Singapore:*** Sagamicin.

---

## Midecamycin *(rINN)*

Midecamicina; Midecamycin $A_1$; Mydecamycin. 7-(Formylmethyl)-4,10-dihydroxy-5-methoxy-9,16,-dimethyl-2-oxo-oxacyclohexadeca-11,13-dien-6-yl 3,6-dideoxy-4-*O*-(2,6-dideoxy-3-*C*-methyl-α-L-*ribo*-hexopyranosyl)-3-(dimethylamino)-β-D-glucopyranoside 4′,4″-dipropionate.

$C_{41}H_{67}NO_{15}$ = 814.0.
*CAS — 35457-80-8.*
*ATC — J01FA03.*

**Pharmacopoeias.** In *Jpn.*

### Midecamycin Acetate *(rINNM)*

Acecamycin; Midecamycin Diacetate; Miocamycin; Miokamycin; MOM; Ponsinomycin; 1532-RB. 9,3″-Diacetylmidecamycin; Leucomycin V $3^B$, 9-diacetate $3,4^B$-dipropanoate.

$C_{45}H_{71}NO_{17}$ = 898.0.
*CAS — 55881-07-7.*

**Pharmacopoeias.** In *Jpn.*

### Profile

Midecamycin is a macrolide antibacterial produced by the growth of *Streptomyces mycarofaciens* with actions and uses similar to those of erythromycin (p.208) but it is somewhat less active. It is given by mouth as the acetate in doses of 1.2 to 1.8 g daily in 2 or 3 divided doses. It has also been given as the base.

### Preparations

**Proprietary Preparations** (details are given in Part 3)
***Arg.:*** Myoxam; ***Belg.:*** Merced; ***Braz.:*** Midecamin†; ***Fr.:*** Mosil; ***Gr.:*** Miocacin; Miocamen; ***Ital.:*** Macroral; Midecin; Miocamen; Miokacin; ***Jpn:*** Medemycin; Miocamycin; ***Mex.:*** Midecamin; ***Port.:*** Miocacin; ***Spain:*** Momicine; Myoxam; Normicina; ***Thai.:*** Miotin.

---

## Minocycline *(BAN, USAN, rINN)*

(4*S*,4a*S*,5a*R*,12a*S*)4,7-Bis(dimethylamino)-1,4,4a,5,5a,6,11,12a-octahydro-3,10,12,12a-tetrahydroxy-1,11-dioxonaphthacene-2-carboxamide; 6-Demethyl-6-deoxy-7-dimethylaminotetracycline.

$C_{23}H_{27}N_3O_7$ = 457.5.
*CAS — 10118-90-8;.*
*ATC — A01AB23; J01AA08.*

### Minocycline Hydrochloride *(BANM, rINNM)*

Hidrocloruro de minociclina; Minocyclini Hydrochloridum.

$C_{23}H_{27}N_3O_7,HCl$ = 493.9.
*CAS — 13614-98-7.*
*ATC — A01AB23; J01AA08.*

**Pharmacopoeias.** In *Eur.* (see p.vi), *Jpn*, and *US.*

**Ph. Eur. 5.0** (Minocycline Hydrochloride). A yellow, hygroscopic, crystalline powder. Sparingly soluble in water; slightly soluble in alcohol. It dissolves in solutions of alkali hydroxides and carbonates. A 1% solution in water has a pH of 3.5 to 4.5. Store in airtight containers. Protect from light.

**USP 27** (Minocycline Hydrochloride). A yellow crystalline powder. Sparingly soluble in water; slightly soluble in alcohol; practically insoluble in chloroform and in ether; soluble in solutions of alkali hydroxides and carbonates. pH of a solution in water containing the equivalent of minocycline 1% is between 3.5 and 4.5. Store in airtight containers. Protect from light.

**Incompatibility.** Preparations of minocycline hydrochloride have an acid pH and incompatibility may reasonably be expected with alkaline preparations or with drugs unstable at low pH.

## Adverse Effects and Precautions

As for Tetracycline Hydrochloride, p.266.

Vestibular adverse effects including dizziness or vertigo may occur with minocycline, particularly in women. Patients should be advised not to drive or operate machinery if affected.

Oesophageal ulceration has occurred and may be a particular problem if capsules or tablets are taken with insufficient fluid or in a recumbent posture: minocycline should be taken with at least half a glass of water, in an upright position, and well before retiring to bed.

Severe adverse effects including erythema nodosum, hepatitis, and systemic lupus erythematosus have been reported, often in patients taking the drug long-term for acne. Hypersensitivity reactions may include arthralgia, myalgia, pulmonary infiltration, and anaphylaxis. Other adverse effects include alopecia, myocarditis, and vasculitis. Decreased hearing has been reported rarely.

Minocycline has also been associated with pigmentation of the skin and other tissues. Three patterns of skin pigmentation have been described: blue-black macules occurring in areas of inflammation and scarring and possibly due to an iron chelate of minocycline within macrophages; blue-grey macules or hyperpigmentation affecting normal skin and which may be due to a breakdown product of minocycline; or a greyish-brown discoloration occurring particularly in sun-exposed areas of skin ('muddy skin syndrome'), apparently due to melanin deposition. Skin pigmentation appears to resolve slowly on discontinuing the drug although recovery may be incomplete.

Unlike many tetracyclines, minocycline does not appear to accumulate in patients with impaired renal function, and aggravation of renal impairment may be less likely.

◊ There have been several reports of severe complications in patients receiving minocycline for acne including serum-sickness-like disease,[1,2] lupus erythematosus,[3] and hepatitis.[3,4] The number of cases reported probably reflects the widespread use of this drug and the true incidence of such adverse effects is difficult to assess.[5] A study of 700 patients receiving minocycline for acne revealed adverse effects in 13.6%, mostly benign.[6] Gastrointestinal disturbances and vestibular disturbances were the most common, each occurring in about 2% of patients, and pigmentation in up to 4% of patients. Another problem is that of assessing the incidence of severe adverse effects relative to other antibacterials commonly used in acne such as tetracycline and erythromycin. Nevertheless, minocycline should probably be regarded as a second-line oral antibacterial for the treatment of acne until further evidence is available.[7]

1. Knowles SR, *et al.* Serious adverse reactions induced by minocycline: report of 13 patients and review of the literature. *Arch Dermatol* 1996; **132:** 934–9.
2. Harel L, *et al.* Serum-sickness-like reaction associated with minocycline therapy in adolescents. *Ann Pharmacother* 1996; **30:** 481–3.
3. Gough A, *et al.* Minocycline induced autoimmune hepatitis and systemic lupus erythematosus-like syndrome. *BMJ* 1996; **312:** 169–72.
4. Australian Adverse Drug Reactions Advisory Committee. Minocycline and the liver, the CNS, the skin. *Aust Adverse Drug React Bull* 1996; **15:** 14.
5. Seukeran DC, *et al.* Benefit-risk assessment of acne therapies. *Lancet* 1997; **349:** 1251–2.
6. Goulden V, *et al.* Safety of long-term high-dose minocycline in the treatment of acne. *Br J Dermatol* 1996; **134:** 693–5.
7. Garner SE, *et al.* Minocycline for acne vulgaris: efficacy and safety. Available in The Cochrane Library; Issue 2. Chichester: John Wiley; 2004.

**Effects on the liver.** A systematic review[1] considered 65 published case reports of hepatitis or liver damage associated with the use of minocycline for acne, including 4 fatalities, and also data held by WHO concerning 493 reactions involving the liver in 393 patients in whom the indication for the use of minocycline was largely unspecified.

Of the 65 published cases, 38 occurred in females and 61 in patients under 40 years of age. These cases appeared to be of two types:

- 16 cases appeared to be attributable to a hypersensitivity reaction, with a rapid onset usually within 1 month of starting treatment and sometimes associated with eosinophilia and exfoliative dermatitis.
- a further 29 cases of hepatitis (of which 20 were in females) appeared to be of an auto-immune nature, occurring after 1 year or more of therapy and sometimes associated with lupus-like symptoms.

The remaining 20 cases could not be definitively classified into either group.

The 393 patients described by the WHO data experienced 22 different types of hepatic reaction which could be broadly grouped into 4 categories. These were: hepatic dysfunction (32% of patients); hepatitis (26%); abnormal liver function tests (24%); and hyperbilirubinaemia or jaundice (14%). There were, in addition, several other reactions, including hepatic damage or necrosis in 11 patients and fatty liver in 7. Gender distribution was almost even. Of the 393 patients, 14 also experienced lupus-like symptoms. The outcome of the hepatic reactions was reported in less than half of the patients, although it was apparent that there had been at least 3 fatalities.

Despite these findings, the reviewers concluded[1] that there was no clear information regarding the absolute or relative risks of hepatitis in patients given minocycline, and that it was inappropriate to comment as to whether monitoring would be worthwhile. A study of the comparative rates of hepatitis in people exposed to minocycline compared with those who were not was required.

1. Lawrenson RA, *et al.* Liver damage associated with minocycline use in acne: a systematic review of the published literature and pharmacovigilance data. *Drug Safety* 2000; **23:** 333–49.

**Effects on the lungs.** References to minocycline-induced pneumonitis.

1. Guillon J-M, *et al.* Minocycline-induced cell-mediated hypersensitivity pneumonitis. *Ann Intern Med* 1992; **117:** 476–81.
2. Bridges AJ. Minocycline-induced pneumonia. *Ann Intern Med* 1993; **118:** 749–50.
3. Sigmann P. Minocycline-induced pneumonia. *Ann Intern Med* 1993; **118:** 750.
4. Sitbon O, *et al.* Minocycline pneumonitis and eosinophilia: a report on 8 patients. *Arch Intern Med* 1994; **154:** 1633–40.
5. Dykhuizen RS, *et al.* Minocycline and pulmonary eosinophilia. *BMJ* 1995; **310:** 1520–1.

**Effects on the nervous system.** References to the vestibular adverse effects of minocycline.

1. Williams DN, *et al.* Minocycline: possible vestibular side-effects. *Lancet* 1974; **ii:** 744–6.
2. Nicol CS, Oriel JD. Minocycline: possible vestibular side-effects. *Lancet* 1974; **ii:** 1260.
3. Yeadon A. Chemoprophylaxis of meningococcal infection. *Lancet* 1975; **i:** 109.
4. Fanning WL, *et al.* Side effects of minocycline: a double-blind study. *Antimicrob Agents Chemother* 1977; **11:** 712–17.
5. Gump DW, *et al.* Side effects of minocycline: different dosage regimens. *Antimicrob Agents Chemother* 1977; **12:** 642–6.
6. Greco TP, *et al.* Minocycline toxicity: experience with an altered dosage regimen. *Curr Ther Res* 1979; **25:** 193–201.

**Hyperpigmentation.** References to skin and tissue pigmentation in patients receiving minocycline.

1. Ridgway HA, *et al.* Hyperpigmentation associated with oral minocycline. *Br J Dermatol* 1982; **107:** 95–102.
2. Zijdenbos AM, Balmus KJ. Pigmentation secondary to minocycline therapy. *Br J Dermatol* 1984; **110:** 117–18.
3. Noble JG, *et al.* The black thyroid: an unusual finding during neck exploration. *Postgrad Med J* 1989; **65:** 34–5.
4. Eisen D, Hakim MD. Minocycline-induced pigmentation: incidence, prevention and management. *Drug Safety* 1998; **18:** 431–40.

## Interactions

As for Tetracycline Hydrochloride, p.267.

Minocycline has a lower affinity for binding with calcium than tetracycline. In consequence its absorption is less affected by milk and food, although it is still affected by iron salts and antacids.

## Antimicrobial Action

Minocycline has a spectrum of activity and mode of action similar to that of tetracycline (p.267) but it is more active against many species including *Staphylococcus aureus*, streptococci, *Neisseria meningitidis*, various enterobacteria, *Acinetobacter*, *Bacteroides*, *Haemophilus*, *Nocardia*, and some mycobacteria, including *M. leprae*.

Partial cross-resistance exists between minocycline and other tetracyclines but some strains resistant to other drugs of the group remain sensitive to minocycline, perhaps because of better cell-wall penetration.

## Pharmacokinetics

For the general pharmacokinetics of the tetracyclines, see Tetracycline Hydrochloride, p.268.

Minocycline is readily absorbed from the gastrointestinal tract and is not significantly affected by the presence of food or moderate amounts of milk. Oral doses of 200 mg followed by 100 mg every 12 hours are reported to produce plasma concentrations of 2 to 4 micrograms/mL. It is more lipid-soluble than doxycycline and the other tetracyclines and is widely distributed in body tissues and fluids with high concentrations being achieved in the hepatobiliary tract, lungs, sinuses and tonsils, as well as in tears, saliva, and sputum. Penetration into the CSF is relatively poor, although a higher ratio of CSF to blood concentrations has been reported with minocycline than with doxycycline. It crosses the placenta and is distributed into breast milk. About 75% of minocycline in the circulation is bound to plasma proteins. It has a low renal clearance: only about 5 to 10% of a dose is excreted in the urine and up to about 34% is excreted in the faeces. However, in contrast to most tetracyclines it appears to undergo some metabolism in the liver, mainly to 9-hydroxyminocycline. Sources differ as to whether the normal plasma half-life of 11 to 26 hours is prolonged in patients with renal impairment, with a consequent risk of accumulation; hepatic impairment does not appear to lead to accumulation. Little minocycline is removed by dialysis.

◊ Reviews.

1. Saivin S, Houin G. Clinical pharmacokinetics of doxycycline and minocycline. *Clin Pharmacokinet* 1988; **15:** 355–66.

## Uses and Administration

Minocycline is a tetracycline derivative with uses similar to those of tetracycline (p.268). It is also a component of multidrug regimens for the treatment of leprosy (p.133) and has been used in the prophylaxis of meningococcal infection to eliminate the carrier state, but the high incidence of vestibular disturbances means that it is not the drug of choice for the latter. Despite some conflicting pharmacokinetic data, patients with impaired renal function do not usually require adjustment of minocycline dosage, although this may be considered if renal impairment is severe.

Minocycline is normally given by mouth as the hydrochloride. Doses are expressed in terms of minocycline base. Minocycline hydrochloride 108 mg is approximately equivalent to 100 mg of minocycline. The usual adult dose is 200 mg of minocycline daily in divided doses, usually every 12 hours. An initial loading dose of 200 mg may be given. A dose of 50 mg twice daily or 100 mg once daily by mouth is used for the treatment of acne. For leprosy, minocycline 100 mg daily or intermittently has been recommended (by WHO) as part of alternative multidrug regimens. In asymptomatic meningococcal carriers, 100 mg may be given twice daily for 5 days, usually followed by a course of rifampicin.

Older children (over 8 years) have been given 4 mg/kg initially followed by 2 mg/kg every 12 hours, but the effect of tetracyclines on teeth and bones should be considered. Minocycline capsules and tablets should be taken with plenty of fluid, with the patient in an upright position, and well before retiring to bed.

In patients in whom oral therapy is not feasible, minocycline may be given as the hydrochloride, by slow intravenous infusion, in doses equivalent to those by mouth. In some countries it has also been given by intramuscular injection.

Minocycline is applied as a 2% gel for periodontal infections.

**Rheumatic disorders.** For reference to the use of minocycline in the treatment of rheumatoid arthritis, see under Tetracycline Hydrochloride, p.268.

### Preparations

***BP 2003:*** Minocycline Tablets;
***USP 27:*** Minocycline for Injection; Minocycline Hydrochloride Capsules; Minocycline Hydrochloride Oral Suspension; Minocycline Hydrochloride Tablets.

**Proprietary Preparations** (details are given in Part 3)
***Arg.:*** Acneclin; Asolmicina; Meibi; Minocin; ***Austral.:*** Akamin; Minomycin; ***Austria:*** Auramin; Klinoc; Minocin; Minostad; Minotyrol; Oracyclin; ***Belg.:*** Klinotab; Mino-50; Minocin; Minotab; ***Braz.:*** Minoderm; Minomax; ***Canad.:*** Minocin; ***Chile:*** Bagomicina; Minocin; Pracne; ***Fr.:*** Dermirex†; Logryx†; Mestacine; Minolis; Mynocine; Spicline†; Yelnac; Zacnan; ***Ger.:*** Akne-Puren; Aknereduct†; Aknin-Mino; Aknosan; durakne†; Icht-Oral†; Klinomycin; Lederderm; Minakne; Mino-Wolff; Minoclir; Minogalen†; Minoplus; Skid; Skinocyclin; Udima; ***Gr.:*** Minocin; ***Hong Kong:*** Minaxen; Minocin; ***India:*** Cynomycin; ***Irl.:*** Dentomycin†; Minocin; Minox; ***Israel:*** Apominolin†; Minocin; Minoclin; ***Ital.:*** Minocin; ***Jpn:*** Periocline; ***Malaysia:*** Borymycin; Minocin; ***Mex.:*** Micromycin; Minocin; ***Neth.:*** Aknemin†; Minocin; Minotab†; ***NZ:*** Minomycin; Minotabs; ***Port.:*** Minocin; Minotrex; ***S.Afr.:*** Cyclimycin; Mino T†; Minomycin†; Minotabs; Triomin; ***Singapore:*** Borymycin; Minocin; ***Spain:*** Minocin; ***Switz.:*** Aknin-N; Aknoral; Minac 50; Minocin; ***Thai.:*** Minocin; ***UK:*** Aknemin; Blemix; Dentomycin; Minocin; Minogal†; Sebomin; ***USA:*** Arestin; Dynacin; Minocin; Vectrin†.

## Morinamide (pINN)

Morinamida; Morphazinamide. N-Morpholinomethylpyrazine-2-carboxamide.

$C_{10}H_{14}N_4O_2$ = 222.2.
*CAS — 952-54-5.*
*ATC — J04AK04.*

### Profile

Morinamide is an antimycobacterial that has been given by mouth as the hydrochloride in the treatment of tuberculosis.

### Preparations

**Proprietary Preparations** (details are given in Part 3)
***Ital.:*** Piazofolina†.

## Moxifloxacin Hydrochloride (BANM, USAN, rINNM)

Bay-12-8039; Hidrocloruro de moxifloxacino. 1-Cyclopropyl-6-fluoro-1,4-dihydro-8-methoxy-7-[(4aS,7aS)-octahydro-6H-pyrrolo[3,4-b]pyridin-6-yl]-4-oxo-3-quinolinecarboxylic acid hydrochloride.

$C_{21}H_{24}FN_3O_4,HCl$ = 437.9.
*CAS — 151096-09-2 (moxifloxacin); 186826-86-8 (moxifloxacin hydrochloride).*
*ATC — J01MA14.*

### Adverse Effects and Precautions

As for Ciprofloxacin, p.188.

Moxifloxacin has been shown to prolong the QT interval and should be avoided in patients with existing QT prolongation or uncorrected hypokalaemia.

### Interactions

As for Ciprofloxacin, p.190.

As moxifloxacin has been shown to prolong the QT interval, it should not be given to patients receiving class Ia antiarrhythmic drugs (such as quinidine and procainamide) or class III antiarrhythmics (such as amiodarone and sotalol). In addition, caution should be exercised when moxifloxacin is used with other drugs known to have this effect (such as the antihistamines astemizole and terfenadine, cisapride, erythromycin, pentamidine, phenothiazines, or tricyclic antidepressants).

### Antimicrobial Action

As for Ciprofloxacin, p.190.

Moxifloxacin is reported to have greater activity against Gram-positive bacteria, including pneumococci, than ciprofloxacin.

### Pharmacokinetics

Moxifloxacin is readily absorbed from the gastrointestinal tract with an absolute bioavailability of about 90%. It is widely distributed throughout the body tissues and is approximately 50% bound to plasma proteins. Moxifloxacin has an elimination half-life of approximately 12 hours, allowing once-daily dosing. It is metabolised principally via sulfate and glucuronide conjugation, and is excreted in the urine and the faeces as unchanged drug and as metabolites, the sulfate conjugate primarily in the faeces and the glucuronide exclusively in the urine.

### Uses and Administration

Moxifloxacin is a fluoroquinolone antibacterial given by mouth or by intravenous infusion over 60 minutes as the hydrochloride in the treatment of susceptible infections. Doses are expressed in terms of the base; the usual adult dose is 400 mg once daily.

Moxifloxacin hydrochloride is also given as 0.5% eye drops for the treatment of bacterial conjunctivitis.

◊ Reviews.


1. Barman Balfour JA, Wiseman LR. Moxifloxacin. *Drugs* 1999; **57:** 363–73.
2. Barman Balfour JA, Lamb HM. Moxifloxacin: a review of its clinical potential in the management of community-acquired respiratory tract infections. *Drugs* 2000; **59:** 115–39.
3. Culley CM, *et al.* Moxifloxacin: clinical efficacy and safety. *Am J Health-Syst Pharm* 2001; **58:** 379–88.
4. Muijsers RBR, Jarvis B. Moxifloxacin in uncomplicated skin and skin structure infections. *Drugs* 2002; **62:** 967–73.


### Preparations

**Proprietary Preparations** (details are given in Part 3)
***Arg.:*** Avelox; Octegra; ***Austral.:*** Avelox; ***Austria:*** Actira; Avelox; Octegra; ***Belg.:*** Avelox; Proflox; ***Braz.:*** Avalox; ***Canad.:*** Avelox; ***Chile:*** Avelox; Octegra; ***Denm.:*** Avelox; ***Fin.:*** Avelox; ***Fr.:*** Izilox; ***Ger.:*** Avalox; ***Gr.:*** Avelox; Octegra; ***Hong Kong:*** Avelox; ***India:*** Moxif; ***Irl.:*** Avelox; ***Israel:*** Megaxin; ***Ital.:*** Avalox; Octegra; ***Malaysia:*** Avelox; ***Mex.:*** Avelox; ***NZ:*** Avelox; ***Port.:*** Avelox; Proflox; ***S.Afr.:*** Avelon; ***Singapore:*** Avelox; ***Spain:*** Actira; Octegra; Proflox; ***Swed.:*** Avelox; ***Switz.:*** Avalox; ***Thai.:*** Avelox; ***UK:*** Avelox; ***USA:*** Avelox; Vigamox.

## Mupirocin (BAN, USAN, rINN)

BRL-4910A; Mupirocina; Mupirocinum; Pseudomonic Acid. 9-[(2E)-4-[(2S,3R,4R,5S)-5-[(2S,3S,4S,5S)-2,3-Epoxy-5-hydroxy-4-methylhexyl]tetrahydro-3,4-dihydroxypyran-2-yl]-3-methylbut-2-enoyloxy]nonanoic acid; (2S-{2α(E),3β,4β,5α[2R*,3R*(1R*,2R*)]})-9-{[3-Methyl-1-oxo-4-(tetrahydro-3,4-dihydroxy-5-{[3-(2-hydroxy-1-methyl-propyl)oxiranyl]methyl}-2H-pyran-2-yl)-2-butenyl]oxy}nonanoic acid.

$C_{26}H_{44}O_9$ = 500.6.
*CAS — 12650-69-0.*
*ATC — D06AX09; R01AX06.*

The symbol † denotes a preparation no longer actively marketed

**Pharmacopoeias.** In *Eur.* (see p.vi) and *US.*

**Ph. Eur. 5.0** (Mupirocin). A white or almost white powder. It shows polymorphism. Slightly soluble in water; freely soluble in dehydrated alcohol, in acetone, and in dichloromethane. The pH of a freshly prepared saturated solution in water is 3.5 to 4.0. Protect from light.

**USP 27** (Mupirocin). A white to off-white crystalline solid. Very slightly soluble in water; freely soluble in dehydrated alcohol, in acetone, in chloroform, and in methyl alcohol; slightly soluble in ether. pH of a saturated solution in water is between 3.5 and 4.5. Store in airtight containers.

## Mupirocin Calcium (BANM, USAN, rINNM)

BRL-4910F; Mupirocinum Calcicum.

$C_{52}H_{86}O_{18}Ca,2H_2O$ = 1075.3.
*CAS — 104486-81-9 (anhydrous mupirocin calcium); 115074-43-6 (mupirocin calcium dihydrate).*
*ATC — D06AX09; R01AX06.*

**Pharmacopoeias.** In *Eur.* (see p.vi) and *Jpn.*

**Ph. Eur. 5.0** (Mupirocin Calcium). A white or almost white powder. Very slightly soluble in water; sparingly soluble in dehydrated alcohol and in dichloromethane.

### Adverse Effects and Precautions

Mupirocin is usually well tolerated but local reactions such as burning, stinging, and itching may occur after the application of mupirocin to the skin.

Some mupirocin products are formulated in a macrogol base: such formulations are not suitable for application to mucous membranes and should be used with caution in patients with extensive burns or wounds because of the possibility of macrogol toxicity. Care is also required in patients with renal impairment.

### Antimicrobial Action

Mupirocin is an antibacterial that inhibits bacterial protein synthesis by binding to isoleucyl transfer RNA synthetase. It is primarily bacteriostatic at low concentrations, although it is usually bactericidal in the high concentrations achieved by topical application to the skin. At these concentrations it may have some activity against organisms reported to be relatively resistant to mupirocin *in vitro.*

It is mainly active against Gram-positive aerobes. Most strains of staphylococci (including meticillin-resistant and multiply-resistant *Staph. aureus*) and streptococci are susceptible *in vitro*, although the enterococci are relatively resistant. Mupirocin is also active against *Listeria monocytogenes* and *Erysipelothrix rhusiopathiae*. The Gram-negative organisms are generally insensitive, but *Haemophilus influenzae*, *Neisseria* spp. and a few others are sensitive. Anaerobic organisms, both Gram-positive and Gram-negative, are generally resistant, and activity against fungi is low. Mupirocin is more active *in vitro* at acid pH than in alkaline conditions.

Naturally resistant strains of *Staph. aureus* occur rarely but resistance, including high-level plasmid-mediated transferable resistance, has emerged, particularly during long-term use. There has been some concern that inappropriate prescribing of mupirocin has led to this steadily increasing resistance.

**Activity against fungi.** Activity of mupirocin 2% *in vitro* against *Candida albicans* was comparable to that of other commonly used topical antifungals. Although MICs were considerably in excess of those reported for susceptible bacteria, clinical responses in 10 patients suggested that adequate concentrations of mupirocin were achieved following topical application.[1]


1. Rode H, *et al.* Efficacy of mupirocin in cutaneous candidiasis. *Lancet* 1991; **338:** 578.


**Resistance.** References.


1. Cookson BD. The emergence of mupirocin resistance: a challenge to infection control and antibiotic prescribing practice. *J Antimicrob Chemother* 1998; **41:** 11–18.
2. Schmitz F-J, *et al.* The prevalence of low- and high-level mupirocin resistance in staphylococci from 19 European hospitals. *J Antimicrob Chemother* 1998; **42:** 489–95.
3. Upton A, *et al.* Mupirocin and Staphylococcus aureus: a recent paradigm of emerging antibiotic resistance. *J Antimicrob Chemother* 2003; **51:** 613–17.


### Pharmacokinetics

Only very small amounts of topically applied mupirocin are absorbed into the systemic circulation where it is rapidly metabolised to monic acid.

### Uses and Administration

Mupirocin is an antibacterial produced by *Pseudomonas fluorescens*. It is applied topically as a 2% ointment in a macrogol basis, or as a cream containing mupirocin calcium equivalent to 2% mupirocin, in the treatment of various bacterial skin infections. These preparations should be applied up to 3 times daily for up to 10 days; treatment should be re-evaluated if there is no response after 3 to 5 days. They are not suitable for application to mucous membranes, and therefore mupirocin calcium is used as a 2% nasal ointment in a paraffin basis for eradication of the nasal carriage of *Staphylococcus aureus*, particularly epidemic meticillin-resistant strains.

For further details of skin infections and staphylococcal infections and their treatment, see under Choice of Antibacterial, p.146.

### Preparations

***USP 27:*** Mupirocin Ointment.

**Proprietary Preparations** (details are given in Part 3)
***Arg.:*** Bactroban; Mupax; Mupirox; Paldar; Vidox; ***Austral.:*** Bactroban; ***Austria:*** Bactroban; ***Belg.:*** Bactroban; ***Braz.:*** Bacrocin; Bactroban; Bactroneo; ***Canad.:*** Bactroban; ***Chile:*** Bactroban; Ultrabiotic; Underan; ***Denm.:*** Bactroban; ***Fin.:*** Bactroban; ***Fr.:*** Bactroban; Mupiderm; ***Ger.:*** Turixin; ***Gr.:*** Bactroban; Micoban; ***Hong Kong:*** Bactroban; ***India:*** Bactroban; ***Irl.:*** Bactroban; ***Israel:*** Bactoderm; Bactroban; ***Ital.:*** Bactroban; ***Jpn:*** Bactroban; ***Malaysia:*** Bactroban; ***Mex.:*** Bactroban; ***Neth.:*** Bactroban; ***NZ:*** Bactroban; ***Port.:*** Bactroban; ***S.Afr.:*** Bactroban; ***Singapore:*** Bactroban; ***Spain:*** Bactroban; Plasimine; ***Swed.:*** Bactroban; ***Switz.:*** Bactroban; ***Thai.:*** Bactroban; Muporin; ***UK:*** Bactroban; ***USA:*** Bactroban; Centany.

## Nadifloxacin (BAN, rINN)

Jinofloxacin; Nadifloxacino; OPC-7251. (±)-9-Fluoro-6,7-dihydro-8-(4-hydroxypiperidino)-5-methyl-1-oxo-1H,5H-benzo[ij]quinolizine-2-carboxylic acid.

$C_{19}H_{21}FN_2O_4$ = 360.4.
*CAS — 124858-35-1.*

### Profile

Nadifloxacin is a fluoroquinolone antibacterial. It is applied topically in the treatment of acne.

### Preparations

**Proprietary Preparations** (details are given in Part 3)
***Braz.:*** Nadixa†; ***Jpn:*** Acuatim; ***Mex.:*** Nadixa.

## Nafcillin Sodium (BANM, USAN, rINNM)

Nafcilina sódica; Nafcillinum Natricum; Wy-3277. Sodium (6R)-6-(2-ethoxy-1-naphthamido)penicillanate monohydrate.

$C_{21}H_{21}N_2NaO_5S,H_2O$ = 454.5.
*CAS — 147-52-4 (nafcillin); 985-16-0 (anhydrous nafcillin sodium); 7177-50-6 (nafcillin sodium monohydrate).*

**Pharmacopoeias.** In *US.*

**USP 27** (Nafcillin Sodium). A white to yellowish-white powder having not more than a slight characteristic odour. Freely soluble in water and in chloroform; soluble in alcohol. pH of a 3% solution in water is between 5.0 and 7.0. Store in airtight containers.

**Incompatibility.** Nafcillin sodium has been reported to be incompatible with aminoglycosides and a number of other antibacterials. It has also been reported to be incompatible with acidic and alkaline drugs.

### Adverse Effects and Precautions

As for Benzylpenicillin, p.163.

Thrombophlebitis may occur when nafcillin is given by intravenous injection, and tissue damage has been reported on extravasation.

**Effects on the kidneys.** References.


1. Lestico MR, *et al.* Hepatic and renal dysfunction following nafcillin administration. *Ann Pharmacother* 1992; **26:** 985–90.
2. Guharoy SR, *et al.* Suspected nafcillin-induced interstitial nephritis. *Ann Pharmacother* 1993; **27:** 170–3.


**Effects on the liver.** References.


1. Lestico MR, *et al.* Hepatic and renal dysfunction following nafcillin administration. *Ann Pharmacother* 1992; **26:** 985–90.


**Sodium content.** Each g of nafcillin sodium contains about 2.2 mmol of sodium.

### Interactions

As for Benzylpenicillin, p.164.

**Ciclosporin.** For the effect of nafcillin on ciclosporin, see p.1354.

**Warfarin.** For the effect of nafcillin on warfarin, see p.1024.

### Antimicrobial Action

As for Flucloxacillin, p.213.

### Pharmacokinetics

Nafcillin is incompletely and irregularly absorbed from the gastrointestinal tract, especially when given after food. After intramuscular injection it is absorbed more reliably, an injection of 0.5 to 1 g producing peak plasma concentrations of 5 to 8 micrograms/mL within about 0.5 to 1 hour. Up to 90% of nafcillin in the circulation is bound to plasma proteins. Nafcillin has been reported to have a plasma half-life of about 0.5 to 1.5 hours. The half-life is prolonged in neonates.

Nafcillin crosses the placenta into the fetal circulation and is distributed into breast milk. There is little diffusion into the CSF except when the meninges are inflamed. Nafcillin is distributed into pleural and synovial fluids and into bone.

Nafcillin differs from most other penicillins in that it is largely inactivated by hepatic metabolism. It is excreted via the bile although some reabsorption takes place in the small intestine. Only about 10% of a dose given by mouth before food, and about 30% of a dose given intramuscularly, is excreted in the urine.

Plasma concentrations are enhanced by probenecid.

### Uses and Administration

Nafcillin is a penicillinase-resistant penicillin used similarly to flucloxacillin (p.214) in the treatment of infections due to staphylococci resistant to benzylpenicillin.

It is given by injection as the sodium salt. Doses are expressed in terms of the equivalent amount of nafcillin. 1.1 g of nafcillin sodium is approximately equivalent to 1 g of nafcillin. Nafcillin sodium may be given intravenously by slow injection over 5 to 10 minutes or by slow infusion over at least 30 to 60 minutes; usual adult doses are 0.5 to 1 g of nafcillin every 4 hours, although it is usually recommended that it be used for not more than 24 to 48 hours because of the risk of thrombophlebitis. It has also been given by intramuscular injection in a dose of 500 mg of nafcillin every 4 to 6 hours.

Nafcillin sodium has also been given by mouth but other penicillinase-resistant penicillins are preferred.

### Preparations

***USP 27:*** Nafcillin for Injection; Nafcillin Injection; Nafcillin Sodium Capsules; Nafcillin Sodium for Oral Solution; Nafcillin Sodium Tablets.

**Proprietary Preparations** (details are given in Part 3)
***USA:*** Nallpen†; Unipen†.

## Nalidixic Acid *(BAN, USAN, rINN)*

Ácido nalidíxico; Acidum Nalidixicum; Nalidixinic Acid; NSC-82174; Win-18320. 1-Ethyl-1,4-dihydro-7-methyl-4-oxo-1,8-naphthyridine-3-carboxylic acid.

$C_{12}H_{12}N_2O_3$ = 232.2.

*CAS — 389-08-2.*

*ATC — J01MB02.*

**Pharmacopoeias.** In *Eur.* (see p.vi), *Jpn, Pol.*, and *US.*

**Ph. Eur. 5.0** (Nalidixic Acid). An almost white or pale yellow, crystalline powder. Practically insoluble in water; slightly soluble in alcohol and in acetone; soluble in dichloromethane. It dissolves in dilute solutions of alkali hydroxides. Store in airtight containers. Protect from light.

**USP 27** (Nalidixic Acid). A white to very pale yellow, odourless crystalline powder. Very slightly soluble in water and in ether; soluble 1 in 910 of alcohol and 1 in 29 of chloroform; slightly soluble in acetone, in methyl alcohol, and in toluene; soluble in dichloromethane and in solutions of fixed alkali hydroxides and carbonates. Store in airtight containers.

### Adverse Effects

The most frequent adverse reactions to nalidixic acid involve the gastrointestinal tract, skin, and CNS. Gastrointestinal effects have been reported in about 8% of patients and include nausea, vomiting, diarrhoea, and abdominal pain.

Neurological effects include visual disturbances, headache, dizziness or vertigo, drowsiness, and sometimes confusion, depression, excitement, and hallucinations. Toxic psychoses or convulsions have occurred, especially after large doses; convulsions are most likely in patients with predisposing factors such as cerebrovascular insufficiency, parkinsonism, or epilepsy. There have been reports of intracranial hypertension, especially in infants and young children, and also of metabolic acidosis. Peripheral neuropathies, muscular weakness, and myalgia are occasional adverse effects. Sixth cranial nerve palsy has been reported rarely.

Adverse effects on the skin include photosensitivity reactions with erythema and bullous eruptions, allergic rashes, urticaria, and pruritus. Erythema multiforme and Stevens-Johnson syndrome have been reported rarely. Eosinophilia, fever, angioedema, and, rarely, anaphylactoid reactions have occurred. Arthralgia has been reported (degenerative changes in weight-bearing joints of young *animals* are documented). Tendon damage has occasionally been associated with related compounds, the fluoroquinolones (see under Ciprofloxacin: Effects on the Musculoskeletal System, p.189).

Cholestatic jaundice, thrombocytopenia, and leucopenia have occurred rarely, as has haemolytic anaemia in patients who may or may not have G6PD deficiency. There have been isolated reports of fatal auto-immune haemolytic anaemia in elderly patients.

### Precautions

Nalidixic acid should be avoided in patients subject to convulsions. It should be given with care to patients with renal or hepatic impairment, severe cerebral arteriosclerosis, or G6PD deficiency. Blood counts and renal and hepatic function should be monitored if treatment continues for more than 2 weeks.

It should be avoided in infants less than 3 months old. Since nalidixic acid and related antimicrobials have been shown to cause degenerative changes in weight-bearing joints of young *animals*, it has been suggested that these compounds should not be used in children, adolescents, pregnant women, or during breast feeding (but see also below). Treatment should be discontinued if symptoms of arthralgia occur.

Exposure to strong sunlight or sunlamps should be avoided during treatment with nalidixic acid.

Nalidixic acid may cause false-positive reactions in urine tests for glucose using copper reduction methods.

**Breast feeding.** The American Academy of Pediatrics[1] states that nalidixic acid is usually compatible with breast feeding, although haemolytic anaemia has been reported[2] in a breast-fed infant, with no evidence of G6PD deficiency, whose mother had received nalidixic acid.

1. American Academy of Pediatrics. The transfer of drugs and other chemicals into human milk. *Pediatrics* 2001; **108:** 776–89. Correction. *ibid.*; 1029. Also available at: http://aappolicy.aappublications.org/cgi/content/full/pediatrics%3b108/3/776 (accessed 27/05/04)
2. Belton EM, Jones RV. Haemolytic anaemia due to nalidixic acid. *Lancet* 1965; **ii:** 691.

**Porphyria.** Nalidixic acid has been associated with acute attacks of porphyria and is considered unsafe in porphyric patients.

### Interactions

The excretion of nalidixic acid is reduced and plasma concentrations increased by probenecid. Nitrofurantoin and nalidixic acid are antagonistic *in vitro* and should not be used together. Fatal haemorrhagic enterocolitis has been associated with the use of nalidixic acid and high-dose intravenous melphalan in children. There is a possible risk of increased nephrotoxicity when nalidixic acid is given with ciclosporin.

Nalidixic acid is reported to enhance the effect of oral anticoagulants such as warfarin (p.1024); this may be due in part to displacement of anticoagulant from its plasma binding sites. The dose of anticoagulant may need to be reduced.

The effect of some quinolone antibacterials on xanthines is discussed under Caffeine, p.782, and Theophylline, p.801.

Convulsions may be precipitated by the use of some quinolones with NSAIDs (see Analgesics, under Interactions of Ciprofloxacin, p.190), although this has not been reported with nalidixic acid.

### Antimicrobial Action

Nalidixic acid is considered to act by interfering with the replication of bacterial DNA, probably by inhibiting DNA gyrase (topoisomerase) activity. It is active against Gram-negative bacteria including *Escherichia coli, Klebsiella* spp., *Proteus* spp., *Enterobacter* spp., *Salmonella* spp., and *Shigella* spp., and is usually bactericidal. *Pseudomonas aeruginosa*, Gram-positive bacteria, and anaerobes are not generally susceptible.

Bacterial resistance may develop rapidly, sometimes within a few days of commencing treatment, but it does not appear to be transferable or R-plasmid mediated (see also below). Cross-resistance occurs with oxolinic acid and cinoxacin.

The antibacterial activity of nalidixic acid is not significantly affected by differences in urinary pH. Antagonism between nitrofurantoin and nalidixic acid has been demonstrated *in vitro*.

**Resistance.** Bacterial plasmid-mediated resistance to quinolones had not been seen by the late 1980s.[1] A report[2] of such resistance to nalidixic acid in *Shigella dysenteriae* responsible for an epidemic of shigellosis in Bangladesh in 1987, was questioned at the time.[3] On reinspection of the data, chromosomal mutation rather than plasmid-mediated resistance was confirmed as the mechanism responsible so far for resistance to quinolones.[1] More recent data[4] in an isolate of *Klebsiella pneumoniae* has, however, suggested that plasma-mediated resistance to quinolones may be possible.

1. Courvalin P. Plasmid-mediated 4-quinolone resistance: a real or apparent absence? *Antimicrob Agents Chemother* 1990; **34:** 681–4.
2. Munshi MH, *et al.* Plasmid-mediated resistance to nalidixic acid in Shigella dysenteriae type 1. *Lancet* 1987; **ii:** 419–21.
3. Crumplin GC. Plasmid-mediated resistance to nalidixic acid and new 4-quinolones? *Lancet* 1987; **ii:** 854–5.
4. Martínez-Martínez L, *et al.* Quinolone resistance from a transferable plasmid. *Lancet* 1998; **351:** 797–9.

### Pharmacokinetics

Nalidixic acid is rapidly and almost completely absorbed from the gastrointestinal tract, and peak plasma concentrations of 20 to 40 micrograms/mL have been reported 2 hours after a 1-g dose by mouth. Plasma half-lives of about 1 to 2.5 hours have been reported (but see below).

Nalidixic acid is partially metabolised to hydroxynalidixic acid, which has antibacterial activity similar to that of nalidixic acid and accounts for about 30% of active drug in the blood. About 93% of nalidixic acid and 63% of hydroxynalidixic acid are bound to plasma proteins. Both nalidixic acid and hydroxynalidixic acid are rapidly metabolised to inactive glucuronide and dicarboxylic acid derivatives; the major inactive metabolite carboxynalidixic acid is usually only detected in urine.

Nalidixic acid and its metabolites are excreted rapidly in the urine, nearly all of a dose being eliminated within 24 hours. About 80 to 90% of the drug excreted in the urine is as inactive metabolites, but urinary concentrations of unchanged drug and active metabolite ranging from 25 to 250 micrograms/mL are achieved after a single 1-g dose. Hydroxynalidixic acid accounts for about 80 to 85% of activity in the urine. Urinary excretion is reduced by probenecid.

Traces of nalidixic acid are distributed into breast milk and appear to cross the placenta. About 4% of a dose is excreted in the faeces.

◊ Although a plasma half-life of 1 to 2.5 hours is generally cited for nalidixic acid, values of 6 to 7 hours have been reported for active drug (nalidixic acid and hydroxynalidixic acid) after using more specific and sensitive assay techniques and longer sampling periods than previously.[1]

The elimination rate of nalidixic acid appears to be not markedly altered by renal impairment, but the elimination of hydroxynalidixic acid is significantly reduced. 7-Carboxynalidixic acid has appeared in the plasma of patients with renal impairment.[2] Plasma concentrations of active drug were higher and the half-life prolonged in elderly subjects.[3]

1. Ferry N, *et al.* Nalidixic acid kinetics after single and repeated oral doses. *Clin Pharmacol Ther* 1981; **29:** 695–8.
2. Cuisinaud G, *et al.* Nalidixic acid kinetics in renal insufficiency. *Br J Clin Pharmacol* 1982; **14:** 489–93.
3. Barbeau G, Belanger P-M. Pharmacokinetics of nalidixic acid in old and young volunteers. *J Clin Pharmacol* 1982; **22:** 490–6.

### Uses and Administration

Nalidixic acid is a 4-quinolone antibacterial used in the treatment of uncomplicated lower urinary-tract infections due to Gram-negative bacteria other than *Pseu-*

domonas spp. (p.153). It has also been used to treat shigellosis (bacillary dysentery) (p.130).

The usual adult dose is 4 g daily by mouth in 4 divided doses for at least 7 days in acute infections, reducing to half this dose in chronic infections. Since bacterial resistance may develop rapidly it has been suggested that if treatment with nalidixic acid has not resulted in a negative urine culture within 48 hours another antimicrobial should be used. Children over 3 months have been given 50 to 55 mg/kg daily in 4 divided doses reduced to 30 to 33 mg/kg daily for prolonged treatment (but see Precautions, above).

For details of reduced doses to be used in renal impairment, see below.

Although the antibacterial activity of nalidixic acid does not appear to be influenced by urinary pH, the use of sodium bicarbonate or sodium citrate does increase the concentration of active drug in the urine. The adult dose of nalidixic acid, in conjunction with sodium citrate, is 660 mg three times daily for 3 days.

**Administration in renal impairment.** In the UK, some products of nalidixic acid are licensed for use at half the standard dose in patients with a creatinine clearance below 20 mL/minute. However, licensed data for other products does not contain this information and suggests that they should not be used in patients with severe renal impairment.

### Preparations

***BP 2003:*** Nalidixic Acid Oral Suspension; Nalidixic Acid Tablets;
***USP 27:*** Nalidixic Acid Oral Suspension; Nalidixic Acid Tablets.

**Proprietary Preparations** (details are given in Part 3)
***Arg.:*** Nalidix; Wintomylon; ***Austral.:*** Negram†; ***Braz.:*** Naluril; Wintomylon; ***Canad.:*** NegGram; ***Chile:*** Wintomylon; ***Denm.:*** Negram†; ***Fr.:*** Negram; ***Hong Kong:*** Wintomylon; ***India:*** Diarlop; Gramoneg; Negadix; ***Irl.:*** Negram; ***Israel:*** NegGram; Urigram†; ***Ital.:*** Betaxina; Nalidixin; Naligram; Nalissina†; NegGram; Uralgin†; Uri-Flor; Urogram†; ***Mex.:*** Acidix; Acinal†; Fardixon; Kamilon; Labydon†; Lidinal†; Lidixin†; Nadiwil†; Nalidixant†; Nalidoid†; Nalix†; Neo-Uridixico†; Seltomylon; Unidixina†; Urlix†; Uronalin†; Wintomylon; ***Norw.:*** Negram†; ***NZ:*** Negram†; ***Port.:*** Wintomilon; ***S.Afr.:*** Puromylon; Winlomylon; ***UK:*** Negram; Uriben; ***USA:*** NegGram.

**Multi-ingredient:** ***Braz.:*** Azo-Wintomylon†; ***Irl.:*** Mictral; ***Mex.:*** Azo-Gen; Azo-Wintomylon; Nalixone; Naxilan-Plus; Pirifur; ***UK:*** Mictral†.

---

## Neomycin *(BAN, rINN)*

Neomicina.

*CAS — 1404-04-2 (neomycin); 3947-65-7 (neomycin A); 119-04-0 (neomycin B); 66-86-4 (neomycin C).*

*ATC — A01AB08; A07AA01; B05CA09; D06AX04; J01GB05; R02AB01; S01AA03; S02AA07; S03AA01.*

**Description.** A mixture of 2 isomers, neomycin B ($C_{23}H_{46}N_6O_{13}$ = 614.6) and neomycin C ($C_{23}H_{46}N_6O_{13}$ = 614.6) with neomycin A (neamine, $C_{12}H_{26}N_4O_6$ = 322.4); neomycins B and C are glycoside esters of neamine and neobiosamines B and C. Framycetin (p.215) consists of neomycin B.

### Neomycin Sulfate *(rINNM)*

Fradiomycin Sulfate; Neomycin Sulphate *(BANM)*; Neomycini Sulfas; Sulfato de neomicina.

*CAS — 1405-10-3.*

*ATC — A01AB08; A07AA01; B05CA09; D06AX04; J01GB05; R02AB01; S01AA03; S02AA07; S03AA01.*

NOTE. NEO is a code approved by the BP 2003 for use on single unit doses of eye drops containing neomycin sulfate where the individual container may be too small to bear all the appropriate labelling information.

**Pharmacopoeias.** In *Chin., Eur.* (see p.vi), *Int., Jpn, Pol.,* and *US.*

**Ph. Eur. 5.0** (Neomycin Sulphate). A mixture of the sulfates of substances produced by the growth of certain selected strains of *Streptomyces fradiae*, the main component being the sulfate of neomycin B. The potency is not less than 680 units/mg, calculated with reference to the dried substance. A white or yellowish-white, hygroscopic powder. Very soluble in water; very slightly soluble in alcohol; practically insoluble in acetone. A 1% solution in water has a pH of 5.0 to 7.5. Store in airtight containers. Protect from light.

**USP 27** (Neomycin Sulfate). The sulfate salt of a kind of neomycin, an antibacterial substance produced by the growth of *Streptomyces fradiae* (Streptomycetaceae), or a mixture of two or more such salts. It has a potency equivalent to not less than 600 micrograms of neomycin per mg, calculated on the dried basis. A white to slightly yellow powder, or cryodesiccated solid. It is odourless or practically so, and is hygroscopic. Soluble 1 in 1 of water; very slightly soluble in alcohol; insoluble in acetone, in chloroform, and in ether. pH of a solution in water containing the equivalent of neomycin 3.3% is between 5.0 and 7.5. Store in airtight containers. Protect from light.

### Neomycin Undecenoate *(BANM, rINNM)*

Neomycin Undecylenate *(USAN)*; Undecilenato de neomicina.
The 10-undecenoate salt of neomycin.

*CAS — 1406-04-8.*

*ATC — A01AB08; A07AA01; B05CA09; D06AX04; J01GB05; R02AB01; S01AA03; S02AA07; S03AA01.*

### Adverse Effects and Treatment

As for Gentamicin Sulfate, p.217.

Neomycin has particularly potent nephrotoxic and ototoxic properties and so is generally no longer given parenterally. However, sufficient may be absorbed following administration by other routes (e.g. orally, instillation into cavities or open wounds, or topical administration to damaged skin), to produce irreversible partial or total deafness. The effect is dose-related and is enhanced by renal impairment. Nephrotoxic effects may also occur.

When given orally in large doses, neomycin causes nausea, vomiting, and diarrhoea. Prolonged oral use may cause a malabsorption syndrome with steatorrhoea and diarrhoea which can be very severe. Suprainfection may occur, especially with prolonged treatment.

Neomycin has a neuromuscular-blocking action similar to, but stronger than, that of other aminoglycosides, and respiratory depression and arrest has followed the intraperitoneal instillation of neomycin. Fatalities have occurred.

Hypersensitivity reactions, such as rashes, pruritus, and sometimes drug fever or even anaphylaxis, occur frequently during local treatment with neomycin and may be masked by the combined use of a corticosteroid. Cross-sensitivity with other aminoglycosides may occur.

### Precautions

As for Gentamicin Sulfate, p.217. Parenteral use of neomycin, or its use for irrigation of wounds or serous cavities such as the peritoneum, is no longer recommended.

Neomycin is contra-indicated for intestinal disinfection when an obstruction is present, in patients with a known history of allergy to aminoglycosides, and in infants under 1 year. It should be used with great care in patients with renal or hepatic impairment, or with neuromuscular disorders, and in those with impaired hearing. The topical use of neomycin in patients with extensive skin damage or perforated tympanic membranes may result in deafness. Neomycin sulfate should not be used topically or for urological purposes in doses greater than 1 g daily; it should not be used urologically for longer than 10 days.

Prolonged local use should be avoided as it may lead to skin sensitisation and possible cross-sensitivity to other aminoglycosides.

**Hypersensitivity and vaccination.** Neomycin was thought to be responsible for a hypersensitivity reaction[1] in a child given measles, mumps, and rubella vaccine containing neomycin 25 micrograms. However, there is also a report of successful vaccination with measles, mumps, and rubella vaccine in a neomycin-sensitive child.[2] Although the vaccine may contain small amounts of neomycin or kanamycin, and sensitivity to either is considered a contra-indication to its use, it is only rarely necessary to withhold it once appropriate expert advice has been taken. There is little logic to intradermal testing since test solutions contain 4 to 40 times as much neomycin as the vaccine.[2]

1. Kwittken PL, *et al.* MMR vaccine and neomycin allergy. *Am J Dis Child* 1993; **147:** 128–9.
2. Elliman D, Dhanraj B. Safe MMR vaccination despite neomycin allergy. *Lancet* 1991; **337:** 365.

### Interactions

As for Gentamicin Sulfate, p.218. Absorption following oral or local use may be sufficient to produce interactions with other drugs given systemically.

Neomycin orally has been reported to impair the absorption of other drugs including phenoxymethylpenicillin, digoxin, and methotrexate; the efficacy of oral contraceptives might be reduced. The effects of acarbose may be enhanced by oral neomycin.

### Antimicrobial Action

Neomycin has a mode of action and spectrum of activity similar to that of gentamicin (p.218) but it lacks activity against *Pseudomonas aeruginosa.* It is reported to be active against *Mycobacterium tuberculosis.*

Because of its extensive topical use resistance has been reported to be relatively widespread, notably among staphylococci, and some *Salmonella, Shigella,* and *Escherichia coli* strains. Cross-resistance with kanamycin, framycetin, and paromomycin occurs.

### Pharmacokinetics

Neomycin is poorly absorbed from the gastrointestinal tract, about 97% of an oral dose being excreted unchanged in the faeces. Doses of 3 g by mouth produce peak plasma concentrations of up to 4 micrograms/mL and absorption is similar after an enema. Absorption may be increased in conditions which damage or inflame the mucosa. Absorption has also been reported to occur from the peritoneum, respiratory tract, bladder, wounds, and inflamed skin.

Once neomycin is absorbed it is rapidly excreted by the kidneys in active form. It has been reported to have a half-life of 2 to 3 hours.

### Uses and Administration

Neomycin is an aminoglycoside antibiotic used topically in the treatment of infections of the skin, ear, and eye due to susceptible staphylococci and other organisms. Most preparations contain the sulfate, but neomycin undecenoate is also used. Neomycin is often used with another antibacterial such as bacitracin, colistin, gramicidin, or polymyxin B. Such combinations have been used topically in the eye before ophthalmic surgery for infection prophylaxis and, in conjunction with propamidine isetionate, in the treatment of acanthamoeba keratitis (p.595). A cream containing neomycin sulfate and chlorhexidine hydrochloride has been used for application to the nostrils in the treatment of staphylococcal nasal carriers (p.147) but, as with other topical antibacterial preparations, development of resistance may be a problem. Neomycin is often used with topical corticosteroids, but such preparations should be used with caution because of the risk that signs of resistant infection may be suppressed. Care must also be taken where there is skin trauma because of the risk of increased absorption and toxicity (see Adverse Effects, above). For details of bacterial skin infections and their treatment, see p.146.

Because neomycin sulfate is poorly absorbed from the gastrointestinal tract, it has been given by mouth for bowel preparation before abdominal surgery, often with erythromycin (p.147). Neomycin sulfate is also used with other antibacterials and antifungals in the selective decontamination of the digestive tract in patients in intensive care (p.132).

Neomycin is rarely used in the treatment of existing gastrointestinal infections. Although it has been used in the treatment of diarrhoea due to infection with enteropathogenic *Escherichia coli* (EPEC) (p.129), the use of neomycin in children with acute diarrhoea is generally not recommended.

Neomycin sulfate may be given by mouth to patients with incipient hepatic encephalopathy (p.1243) to reduce the flora of the gastrointestinal tract.

Neomycin has lipid regulating properties and has occasionally been given by mouth in the treatment of hyperlipidaemias (see below). It has also been used for the irrigation of wounds and body cavities but such use is no longer recommended because of the risk of toxicity.

*Administration and dosage.* For pre-operative use, 1 g of neomycin sulfate has been given hourly for 4 hours and then every 4 hours for 2 or 3 days before surgery; suggested doses in children, given every 4 hours, are 1 g in those aged over 12 years and 250 to 500 mg in those aged 6 to 12 years.

As an adjunct in the management of hepatic encephalopathy, 4 to 12 g may be given daily in divided doses, usually for 5 to 7 days; children may be given 50 to 100 mg/kg daily in divided doses. Prolonged administration may cause malabsorption.

Topical preparations typically contain the equivalent of 0.35% neomycin base.

Neomycin hydrochloride has also been used.

**Hyperlipidaemias.** Neomycin has been given in doses of up to 2 g daily by mouth in the treatment of hypercholesterolaemia (p.823). It is thought to reduce intestinal absorption of cholesterol through its action on microbial flora, resulting in greater catabolism of low-density lipoproteins in the body.[1] However, more effective and safer drugs are preferred.

1. Illingworth DR. Lipid-lowering drugs: an overview of indications and optimum use. *Drugs* 1987, **33:** 259–79.

## Preparations

**BP 2003:** Hydrocortisone Acetate and Neomycin Ear Drops; Hydrocortisone Acetate and Neomycin Eye Drops; Hydrocortisone Acetate and Neomycin Eye Ointment; Hydrocortisone and Neomycin Cream; Neomycin Eye Drops; Neomycin Eye Ointment; Neomycin Oral Solution; Neomycin Tablets;
**USP 27:** Colistin and Neomycin Sulfates and Hydrocortisone Acetate Otic Suspension; Neomycin and Polymyxin B Sulfates and Bacitracin Ointment; Neomycin and Polymyxin B Sulfates and Bacitracin Ophthalmic Ointment; Neomycin and Polymyxin B Sulfates and Bacitracin Zinc Ointment; Neomycin and Polymyxin B Sulfates and Bacitracin Zinc Ophthalmic Ointment; Neomycin and Polymyxin B Sulfates and Dexamethasone Ophthalmic Ointment; Neomycin and Polymyxin B Sulfates and Dexamethasone Ophthalmic Suspension; Neomycin and Polymyxin B Sulfates and Gramicidin Cream; Neomycin and Polymyxin B Sulfates and Gramicidin Ophthalmic Solution; Neomycin and Polymyxin B Sulfates and Hydrocortisone Acetate Cream; Neomycin and Polymyxin B Sulfates and Hydrocortisone Acetate Ophthalmic Suspension; Neomycin and Polymyxin B Sulfates and Hydrocortisone Ophthalmic Suspension; Neomycin and Polymyxin B Sulfates and Hydrocortisone Otic Solution; Neomycin and Polymyxin B Sulfates and Hydrocortisone Otic Suspension; Neomycin and Polymyxin B Sulfates and Lidocaine Cream; Neomycin and Polymyxin B Sulfates and Pramoxine Hydrochloride Cream; Neomycin and Polymyxin B Sulfates and Prednisolone Acetate Ophthalmic Suspension; Neomycin and Polymyxin B Sulfates Cream; Neomycin and Polymyxin B Sulfates Ophthalmic Ointment; Neomycin and Polymyxin B Sulfates Ophthalmic Solution; Neomycin and Polymyxin B Sulfates Solution for Irrigation; Neomycin and Polymyxin B Sulfates, Bacitracin Zinc, and Hydrocortisone Acetate Ophthalmic Ointment; Neomycin and Polymyxin B Sulfates, Bacitracin Zinc, and Hydrocortisone Ointment; Neomycin and Polymyxin B Sulfates, Bacitracin Zinc, and Hydrocortisone Ophthalmic Ointment; Neomycin and Polymyxin B Sulfates, Bacitracin Zinc, and Lidocaine Ointment; Neomycin and Polymyxin B Sulfates, Bacitracin, and Hydrocortisone Acetate Ointment; Neomycin and Polymyxin B Sulfates, Bacitracin, and Hydrocortisone Acetate Ophthalmic Ointment; Neomycin and Polymyxin B Sulfates, Bacitracin, and Lidocaine Ointment; Neomycin and Polymyxin B Sulfates, Gramicidin, and Hydrocortisone Acetate Cream; Neomycin for Injection; Neomycin Sulfate and Bacitracin Ointment; Neomycin Sulfate and Bacitracin Zinc Ointment; Neomycin Sulfate and Dexamethasone Sodium Phosphate Cream; Neomycin Sulfate and Dexamethasone Sodium Phosphate Ophthalmic Ointment; Neomycin Sulfate and Dexamethasone Sodium Phosphate Ophthalmic Solution; Neomycin Sulfate and Fluocinolone Acetonide Cream; Neomycin Sulfate and Fluorometholone Ointment; Neomycin Sulfate and Flurandrenolide Cream; Neomycin Sulfate and Flurandrenolide Lotion; Neomycin Sulfate and Flurandrenolide Ointment; Neomycin Sulfate and Gramicidin Ointment; Neomycin Sulfate and Hydrocortisone Acetate Cream; Neomycin Sulfate and Hydrocortisone Acetate Lotion; Neomycin Sulfate and Hydrocortisone Acetate Ointment; Neomycin Sulfate and Hydrocortisone Acetate Ophthalmic Ointment; Neomycin Sulfate and Hydrocortisone Acetate Ophthalmic Suspension; Neomycin Sulfate and Hydrocortisone Cream; Neomycin Sulfate and Hydrocortisone Ointment; Neomycin Sulfate and Hydrocortisone Otic Suspension; Neomycin Sulfate and Methylprednisolone Acetate Cream; Neomycin Sulfate and Prednisolone Acetate Ointment; Neomycin Sulfate and Prednisolone Acetate Ophthalmic Ointment; Neomycin Sulfate and Prednisolone Acetate Ophthalmic Suspension; Neomycin Sulfate and Prednisolone Sodium Phosphate Ophthalmic Ointment; Neomycin Sulfate and Triamcinolone Acetonide Cream; Neomycin Sulfate and Triamcinolone Acetonide Ophthalmic Ointment; Neomycin Sulfate Cream; Neomycin Sulfate Ointment; Neomycin Sulfate Ophthalmic Ointment; Neomycin Sulfate Oral Solution; Neomycin Sulfate Tablets; Neomycin Sulfate, Sulfacetamide Sodium, and Prednisolone Acetate Ophthalmic Ointment; Nystatin, Neomycin Sulfate, Gramicidin, and Triamcinolone Acetonide Cream; Nystatin, Neomycin Sulfate, Gramicidin, and Triamcinolone Acetonide Ointment.

**Proprietary Preparations** (details are given in Part 3)
***Arg.:*** Concatag; Neomas; ***Austral.:*** Neosulf; Siguent Neomycin; ***Austria:*** Bykomycin; ***Braz.:*** Nemicina; Neo POM; Neocina; Neogecim; Neomed; ***Canad.:*** Mycifradin†; Myciguent†; ***Fr.:*** Bacteomycine; ***Ger.:*** Bykomycin; Cysto-Myacyne N; Myacyne; Nebacetin N; Uro-Nebacetin N; Vagicillin; ***Gr.:*** Nivemycin; ***Hong Kong:*** Mycifradin†; ***Irl.:*** Mycifradin†; ***Israel:*** Neocin; ***Mex.:*** Gemicina†; Neomixen; ***NZ:*** Neosulf; ***Port.:*** Enteromicina; ***S.Afr.:*** Mycifradin†; ***UK:*** Mycifradin†; Nivemycin; ***USA:*** Mycifradin; Myciguent†; Neo-fradin.

**Multi-ingredient:** ***Arg.:*** Admericina; Antibiocort; Aseptobron N; Belbar; Betnovate-N; Biocortin; Biotaer; Biotaer Gamma; Biotaer Nebulizable; Biotaer Ultrason Nebulizable; Butimerin; Caext; Caramelos Antibioticos Bucoangin; Cicatrex; Clevosan; Cloptison-N; Decadron con Neomicina; Derivoco; Dermadex NN; Dexafurazon; Dexalergin; Endomicina; Factioneye; Farm-X Ginecologico; FML Neo; Gargaletas; Ginal Cent; Ginkan; Gramibiotic; Gramicortil; Graneodin; Graneodin N; Griseoplus; Hidrocortin; Irigal; Isoptomax; Kenacomb; Ledercort con Neomicina; Lefaenteril; Linfol; Min O; Nasojol; Nasomicina; Naxo TV; Nebapol B; Neo Coltirot; Neo Kef; Neo Pelvicillin; Neo-Currino; Neo-Mudapenil; Neobitiol Compuesto; Neodexa Plus; Neomas L; Neosona; Nexadron Compuesto; O-Biol; O-Biol P; Oftal; Opocarbon; Oto Biotaer; Otoclean Gotas Oticas; Otoseptil; Otosporin; Otosporin L; Palan; Pantometil; Plastenan con Neomicina; Poenbioptal; Polygynax; Proetztotal; Provacsin Nasal; Rezamid; Rinoflax AG M; Scheriderm; Sincerum; Sincerum Biotic; Sincerum Biotic L; Suavisan N; Tri-Emcortina; Vagicural; Vagicural Plus; ***Austral.:*** Cicatrin; Kenacomb; Nemdyn; Neo-Medrol; Neosporin; Otocomb Otic; ***Austria:*** Baneocin; Betnesol-N; Betnovate-N; Cicatrex; Dorithricin; Hydoftal; Hydrocortimycin; Locacorten mit Neomycin; Mycostatin V; Nebacetin; Neo-Delphicort; Neocones; Otosporin; Synalar N; Topsym polyvalent; Trilon; Tropoderm; Tyrothricin comp; Tyrothricin compositum; Ulcurilen; Volon A antibiotikahaltig; ***Belg.:*** Betnelan-VN†; De Icin; Decadron avec Neomycine†; Flogocid†; Maxitrol; Mycolog; Neobacitracine; Neodexon†; Otosporin; Panotile; Pimafucort†; Polydexa; Polygynax; Predmycin P; Pulvo Neomycine†; Rhinovalon Neomycine; Spitalen; Statrol; Synalar Bi-Otic; ***Braz.:*** Amigdagen; Amigdamicin; Anaseptil; Anfomicin†; Angi-a-Mid†; Angino Tricin; Antiseptin†; Atacoly†; Bacigen; Bacineo; Belcetin; Belglos†; Betazol Cort; Betnovate-N; Bismu-Jet; Cetobeta; Cicatrene; Cicatrizan; Colpagex N; Colpolase; Colutoide; Conjuntin†; Cutiderm; Decadron Nasal; Decadron Oftalmico; Dermacetin-Ped; Dermase; Dermazon†; Dermobel; Dermogen†; Dermoxin; Derms; Dexacort; Dexanil; Dexavison; Dexazona; Dimicin†; Drenison N; Duploctrin†; Elotin; Enterocler†; Enterodina†; Enteroftal†; Enterovit†; Enterozol†; Esperson N; Flumex N; Fluo-Vaso; Fluocal com Pectina†; Folderm Pomada; Gargosedans†; Ginec; Gingilone; Gotas Ototilan†; Gynax-N; Halcicomb†; Hidrocin; Hidroneo; Hipodex; Histalerg†; Infectracina†; Infepan†; Kindcetin; Larintil†; Locorten Neomicina; Londerm-N; Maxitrol; Mentodrin†; Metcort; Micoplex; Nazobel; Nebacetin; Nebacina†; Nebacitrin; Nebalon†; Neobacina; Neobacipan; Neobacitracina†; Neocetrin; Neocina; Neocinolon; Neocortin; Neodex; Neolon-D; Neomicina Composta†; Neotop; Neotricin; Novacort; Novaderm; Omcilon A M; Onciplus; Otauril†; Oto Xilodase; Oto-Ped†; Otocort; Otodol; Otolin†; Otolone†; Otomixyn; Otosporin; Otosynalar; Panotil; Parenterin; Penetran†; Poliginax; Polipred; Prenefrin†; Providex†; Rhinosept; Rinogerol†; Rinosite; Sinus†; Solemil†; Testinfex†; Teutomicina; Thiabena; Trivagel N; Trofodermin; Vagitrin-N; Xilodase; ***Canad.:*** Cicatrin; Cortimyxin; Cortisporin; Dioptrol; Diospor HC†; Diosporin†; Kenacomb; Maxitrol; Neo-Cortef; Neo-Medrol Acne; Neo-Medrol Veriderm; NeoDecadron†; Neosporin; Neotopic; Optimyxin Plus; Triacomb; Viaderm-KC; ***Chile:*** Bacitopic; Bacitopic Compuesto; Banedif; Banedif Oftalmico; Banedif Oftalmico con Prednisolona; Betnovate-N; Biodexin; Celulase Con Neomicina; Escar T-Neomicina; Fluforte N; Gotalgic; Grifoftal; Grifoftal-D; Labosona N; Madecassol Neomicina; Maxitrol; Monticina; Nasomin; Oftabiotico; Oftasona N; Otazol; Oticum; Otolisan; Otoseptil; Pensulan; Polvos Antibioticos; Rinobanedif; Trofodermin Neomicina; Unguento Dermico Antibiotico; ***Denm.:*** Decadron med Neomycin; Kenalog Comp med Mycostatin; Kenalog Comp†; ***Fin.:*** Bacibact; Maxitrol; Neo-Medrol comp; Otomize†; Pimafucort; Polysporin; ***Fr.:*** Antibio-Synalar; Antibiotulle Lumiere; Atebemyxine; Betneval-Neomycine; Cebemyxine; Chibro-Cadron; Cidermex; Corticotulle Lumiere; Dexagrane; Diprosone Neomycine; Halog Neomycine†; Locacortene†; Locoide N†; Madecassol Neomycine Hydrocortisone; Maxidrol; Myco-Ultralan†; Mycolog; Panotile; Penticort Neomycine†; Pivalone Neomycine†; Polydexa; Polydexa a la Phenylephrine†; Polygynax; Polygynax Virgo; Pulvo 47 Neomycine; Synalar Neomycine†; Tergynan†; Topsyne Neomycine†; Trofoseptine; ***Ger.:*** Antibiotulle Lumiere; Batrax†; Bivacyn; Chibro-Cadron†; Cicatrex; Corticotulle Lumiere; Cortidexason comp; Dexa Polyspectran; Dispadex comp; Efflumycin; Farco-Uromycin; Halog Tri; Isopto Max; Jellin polyvalent; Jellin-Neomycin; Jellisoft-Neomycin†; Kombi-Stulln N; Linola-H-compositum N; Lokalison-antimikrobiell Creme N; Myacyne†; Nebacetin; Neobac; Neotracin†; Otosporin†; Pimafucort†; Polygynax; Polyspectran; Prednitracin†; Pulvo Neomycin; Topoderm N†; Topsym polyvalent; Ulcurilen N; Ultexiv†; Volon A antibiotikahaltig N; ***Gr.:*** Fotocollyre; Statrol; ***Hong Kong:*** Aplosyn-Otic; Bacimycin; Betnovate-N; Bivacyn; Cebemyxine; Celestoderm-V with Neomycin†; Chlomy-P; Corticin; Decadron with Neomycin†; Dexa-Polyspectran†; Dexoph; Dextracin; Drenison N†; Flunolone; Fluonid-N; Kenacomb; Lozopin; Maxitrol; Nebacetin; Neo-Medrol Acne; Neosporin; Neotopic†; Otosporin; Polygynax; Polyoph; Polyspectran†; Prednitracin; Proctosone; Protozone†; Spersapolymyxin†; Synalar N; Synco-CFN; Triacomb; ***India:*** Beclate-N; Betnesol-N; Betnesol-N Nasal; Betnor; Betnovate-N; Candizole-T; Decdan-N; Dexona Eye/Ear; Dexosyn-N; Flucort-N; Flucreme NM; Kenacomb; Kenalog-S; Ledercort-N; Mycidex; Nebasulf; Neosporin; Neosporin-H; Stecort-NM; Surfaz-SN; Topicasone with Neomycin; Valbet; Wycort c Neomycin; ***Irl.:*** Audicort; Betnesol-N; Betnovate-N; Cicatrin; Dexa-Rhinaspray†; Graneodin; Kenacomb; Maxitrol; Naseptin; Neo-Cortef†; Neo-Medrone†; Neosporin; Otomize; Otosporin; Polybactrin†; Synalar N; Vista-Methasone N†; ***Israel:*** Bamyxin; Betnesol-N; Betnovate-N; Dermacombin; Desoren; Dethamycin; Dethaphrine; Dex-Otic; Dexamycin; Dexefrin; FML Neo†; Hycocin; Hycomycin; Kenacomb; Locacorten with Neomycin; Maxitrol; Nazodin; Neo-Medrol; Nodryl; Otomize; Otomycin; Otosporin†; Polycutan; Tevacutan; ***Ital.:*** Abiostil; Anauran; Antibioptal; Bimixin; Bio-Delta Cortilen; Cicatrene; Desalfa; Desamix-Neomicina; Doricum; Ecoval con Neomicina; Enterostop; Eta Biocortilen; Eta Biocortilen VC; Halciderm Combi; Idracemi; Idrocet; Idroneomicil; Idustatin†; Kataval; Localyn; Localyn-Neomicina; Locorten; Menaderm; Mixotone; Nefluan; Neo Cortofen; Neo-Audiocort†; Neo-Medrol Veriderm; Neogram†; Nevacort; Orobicin; Otomicetina†; Otosporin; Rinojet SF; Solprene; Streptosil con Neomicina-Fher; Trofodermin; Vasosterone Antibiotico; Vasosterone Collirio; ***Malaysia:*** Baneocin; Beavate N; Besone-N; Betacin; Betnesol-N; Betnovate-N; Dermasole N; Dextracin; Fluonid-N; Kenacomb; Maxitrol; Neo-Deca; Neo-Hydro; Neo-Medrol; Pocin G; Pocin H; Synalar N; Uniflex-N; ***Mex.:*** Alin Nasal; Alin Oftalmico; Alosol; Baycuten N; Biodexan; Biotarson N; Biotarson O; Cortisporin; Decadron con Neomicina; Dermalog-C; Dexamicin; Dexne; Dexsul; Fluforte N; Flunal-Neo; Fluo Grin; Gotadex; Hidromagma; Hidropolicin; Kaomycin; Kenacomb; Kodakon; Maxitrol; Nebacetina; Neobacigrin; Neosporin; Neoxil; Nicobio; Otilin; Polixin; Recoveron N; Recoveron NC; Scheriderm; Septilisin; Soldrin; Synalar N; Synalar Neo; Synalar O; Synalar Oftalmico; Tapzol con Neomicina; Treda; Tribiot; ***Neth.:*** Celestoderm met Neomycine; Decadron met neomycine; Mycolog; Otosporin; Panotile; Synalar Bi-Otic; ***Norw.:*** Maxitrol; ***NZ:*** Betnesol-N†; Coly-Mycin S Otic†; Kenacomb; Maxitrol; Pimafucort; Ultrazon N†; ***Port.:*** Baciderma; Bacitracina-Neo; Betnovate-N; Bienterico; Cicatrin†; Conjunctilone; Conjunctilone-S; Davimicina; Decadron com Neomicina; Dermimade Bacitracina; Dermobiotico; Dermovate-NN; Dexaval N; Dexaval O; Dimicina; FML Neo; Kenacomb; Leuco Hubber; Meocil; Neo-Davisolona; Neo-Preocil; Otolys†; Otosporin†; Pimafucort; Plastenan Neomicina; Polydexa; Polygynax†; Polysporina†; Predniderma; Tri-Sinerge†; Zotinar-N; ***S.Afr.:*** Betanoid N; Betnesol-N; Betnovate-N; Cicatrin; Covomycin; Covomycin-D; FML Neo; Kenacomb; Maxitrol; Naseptin†; Nasomixin; Neo-Medrol; Neoderm; Neopan; Neosporin; Otosporin; Synalar N†; Trialone; Vibrocil; ***Singapore:*** Baneocin; Batramycin; Besone-N; Betnovate-N†; Celestoderm-V with Neomycin; Dextracin; Fast Powder†; Flunolone; Kenacomb; Maxitrol; Neo-Deca†; Neo-Medrol; Neosporin†; Otosporin†; Pivalone Neomycin; Polybamycin; Polydexa; Polygynax; Predmycin-P; Synalar N†; Uniflex-N†; ***Spain:*** Alantomicina Complex†; Anasilpiel; Antihemorroidal; Bacisporin; Banedif; Betamatil con Neomicina†; Bexicortil; Blastoestimulina; Cilinafosal Hidrocort; Cilinafosal Neomicina†; Cilinavagin Neomicina†; Coliriocilina Espectro†; Coliriocilina Prednisona; Creanolona; Decadran Neomicina; Decoderm Trivalente†; Deltacina†; Dermisone Tri Antibiotic; Dermo Hubber; Dermomycose Talco; Drenison Neomicina†; Edifaringen; Flodermol; Fludronef; Fluo Vasoc†; FML Neo†; Gingilone; Grietalgen Hidrocort; Hidroc Neomic†; Intradermo Cort Ant Fung; Iruxol Neo; Leuco Hubber; Linitul Antibiotico†; Liquipom Dexa Antib; Maxitrol; Menaderm Neomicina; Midacina; Mirantal†; Nasotic Oto†; Neo Analsona; Neo Bacitrin; Neo Bacitrin Hidrocortis†; Neo Hubber; Neo Moderin†; Neo-Synalar†; Neocones; Neodexa; Oftalmo†; Oftalmowell; Oto Difusor†; Oto Neomicin Calm†; Oto Vitna; Otonina; Otosporin; Oxidermiol Enzima; Panotile; Pentalmicina†; Phonal; Plaskine Neomicina; Poly Pred; Pomada Antibiotica; Positon; Poxider†; Prednis Neomic; Rino Dexa; Rinobanedif; Rinoblanco Dexa Antibio†; Rinovel; Spectrocin; Statrol†; Sulfintestin Neom†; Sulfintestin Neomicina; Synalar Nasal; Synalar Neomicina; Synalar Otico; Tisuderma; Tivitis; Trigon Topico; Tulgrasum Antibiotico; Tyroneomicin†; Vasocon Ant†; Vinciseptil Otico; ***Swed.:*** Betnovat med Neomycin; Celeston valerat comp; Decadron cum neomycin; Isopto Biotic; ***Switz.:*** Bacimycin; Baneopol; Batramycine; Betnovate-N; Cicatrex; Cloptison-N†; Cortifluid N; Cortimycine; Dermovate-NN; Flogocid NN†; FML Neo; Korticoid polyvalent†; Maxitrol; Mycinopred; Mycolog; Nebacetin; Neo-Hydro; Neocones; Neosporin; Neotracin; Otosporin; Otospray; Panotile; Pivalone compositum; Polydexa; Prednitracin; Riccomycine†; Spersapolymyxin; Synalar N; Topsym polyvalent; Tyrocombine; ***Thai.:*** Archidex; Banocin; Benn†; Besone-N; Beta-Dipo; Beta-N; Betama-EN; Betameth-N; Bethasone-N; Betnovate-N; Biochin; Cadexcin-N; Celestoderm-V with Neomycin†; Coccila; Decadron with Neomycin; Dermacombin; Dex-Otic†; Dexacin; Dexasil; Dexoph; Dexylin; Disento; Eyedex; Farakil; Fluciderm-N; Flunolone; Fluonid-N; FML Neo; Izac; Kaopectal-N†; Kenacomb; Lobacin†; Maxitrol; Mybacin; Mybacin Dermic; Mysolone-N; Neo-Hytisone†; Neo-Medrol; Neo-Optal; Neodex; Neopred; Neosporin; Neozolone; Opsacin; Opsardex; Otosamthong; Otosporin; Polyoph; Predex; Predmycin; Prednisil; Prednisil-N; Spersapolymyxin; Statrol†; Supracortin 3; Supralan-N; Synalar N; Topaben-N; Trilosil N†; Trofodermin; Unipred; Valbet-N; Xanalin; ***UAE:*** Panderm; ***UK:*** Adcortyl with Graneodin†; Audicort; Betnesol-N; Betnovate-N; Cicatrin; Dermovate-NN; FML Neo Liquifilm†; Graneodin; Gregoderm; Maxitrol; Naseptin; Neo-Cortef†; Neosporin; Otomize; Otosporin; Predsol-N; Synalar N; Tri-Adcortyl; Vista-Methasone N; ***USA:*** Ak-Neo-Dex; Ak-Spore; Ak-Spore HC†; Ak-Spore†; Ak-Trol; AntibiOtic†; Bactine First Aid Antibiotic Plus Anesthetic†; Campho-Phenique Antibiotic Plus Pain Reliever Ointment†; Clomycin†; Coly-Mycin S Otic; Cortatrigen; Cortimycin; Cortisporin; Cortisporin-TC; Dexacidin; Dexacine; Dexasporin; Ear-Eze; Lanabiotic; LazerSporin-C; Maxitrol; Mycitracin; Mycitracin Plus†; Neo-Dexameth; Neocin; NeoDecadron; Neodexasone; Neomixin†; Neopolydex; Neosporin; Neosporin + Pain Relief; Neosporin GU; Neosporin Plus†; Neosporin†; Neotricin HC; Octicair; Ocu-Spor-B; Ocu-Spor-G; Ocu-Trol; Ocutricin; Otic-Care; OtiTricin; Otocort; Otomycin-HPN; Otosporin; Pediotic; Poly-Dex; Poly-Pred; Polymycin; Septa†; Spectrocin Plus; Tri-Biozene; Tribiotic Plus†; Triple Antibiotic†; UAD-Otic.

# Netilmicin Sulfate *(USAN, rINNM)*

*N*[1]-Ethylsissomicin; Netilmicin Sulphate *(BANM)*; Netilmicini Sulfas; Sch-20569; Sulfato de netilmicina. 4-*O*-[(2*R*,3*R*)-*cis*-3-Amino-6-aminomethyl-3,4-dihydro-2*H*-pyran-2-yl]-2-deoxy-6-*O*-(3-deoxy-4-*C*-methyl-3-methylamino-β-L-arabinopyranosyl)-1-*N*-ethylstreptamine sulphate.

$(C_{21}H_{41}N_5O_7)_2,5H_2SO_4 = 1441.6.$

*CAS — 56391-56-1 (netilmicin); 56391-57-2 (netilmicin sulfate).*

*ATC — J01GB07; S01AA23.*

**Pharmacopoeias.** In *Chin.*, *Eur.* (see p.vi), *Jpn*, *Pol.*, and *US*.

**Ph. Eur. 5.0** (Netilmicin Sulphate). A substance obtained by synthesis from sisomicin. The potency is not less than 650 units/mg, calculated with reference to the dried substance. A white or yellowish-white, very hygroscopic, powder. Very soluble in water; practically insoluble in alcohol and in acetone. A 4% solution in water has a pH of 3.5 to 5.5. Store in airtight containers. Protect from light.

**USP 27** (Netilmicin Sulfate). A white to pale yellowish-white powder. Freely soluble in water; practically insoluble in dehydrated alcohol and in ether. pH of a solution in water containing the equivalent of netilmicin 4% is between 3.5 and 5.5. Store in airtight containers.

**Incompatibility.** For discussion of the incompatibility of aminoglycosides, including netilmicin, with beta lactams, see under Gentamicin Sulfate, p.217. Netilmicin is also reported to be incompatible with furosemide, heparin, and vitamin B complex.

## Adverse Effects, Treatment, and Precautions

As for Gentamicin Sulfate, p.217. Some studies suggest that netilmicin is less nephrotoxic and ototoxic than gentamicin or tobramycin, although others have not found any significant differences in their toxicity.

Prolonged peak plasma concentrations of netilmicin greater than 16 micrograms/mL, and trough concentrations greater than 4 micrograms/mL, should be avoided, and the *British National Formulary* suggests that peaks should not exceed 12 micrograms/mL and troughs should be below 2 micrograms/mL.

**Effects on the cardiovascular system.** Severe hypotension was associated with netilmicin in a patient undergoing artificial ventilation.[1] Hypotensive episodes were of short duration and coincided with netilmicin injection. They almost disappeared when sedation was stopped.

1. Rygnestad T. Severe hypotension associated with netilmicin treatment. *BMJ* 1997; **315:** 31.

## Interactions

As for Gentamicin Sulfate, p.218.

## Antimicrobial Action

As for Gentamicin Sulfate, p.218. It is active against a similar range of organisms although it is also reported to have some activity against *Nocardia*. It may be somewhat less effective against *Pseudomonas aeruginosa*. It is not degraded by all of the enzymes responsible for aminoglycoside resistance, and may be active against some strains resistant to gentamicin or tobramycin, but this is less marked than with amikacin: for example, gentamicin-resistant *Providencia*, *Pseudomonas*, and *Serratia* are usually also netilmicin-resistant. Between about 5 and 20% of Gram-negative isolates are reported to be resistant to netilmicin.

## Pharmacokinetics

As for Gentamicin Sulfate, p.218.

Following intramuscular injection of netilmicin, peak plasma concentrations are achieved within 0.5 to 1 hour, and concentrations of about 7 micrograms/mL have been reported following doses of 2 mg/kg; similar concentrations are obtained after intravenous infusion of the same dose over 1 hour. Peak concentrations following rapid intravenous injection may transiently be 2 or 3 times higher than those following infusion. Standard, once-daily doses may produce transient peak concentrations of 20 to 30 micrograms/mL. In multiple dosing studies, netilmicin in usual doses every 12 hours produced steady-state concentrations on the second day which were less than 20% higher than those seen after the first dose.

The half-life of netilmicin is usually 2.0 to 2.5 hours. About 80% of a dose is excreted in the urine within 24 hours.

## Uses and Administration

Netilmicin is a semisynthetic aminoglycoside antibiotic with actions and uses similar to those of gentamicin (p.219). It may be used as an alternative to amikacin (p.154) in the treatment of infections caused by susceptible bacteria that are resistant to gentamicin and tobramycin. As with gentamicin, netilmicin may be used with penicillins and with cephalosporins; the injections should be given separately.

Netilmicin is given as the sulfate but doses are expressed in terms of the equivalent amount of base. 1.5 g of netilmicin sulfate is approximately equivalent to 1 g of netilmicin. It is usually given intramuscularly in doses of 4 to 6 mg/kg daily as a single dose; alternatively, it may be given in equally divided doses every 8 or 12 hours; for the control of life-threatening infections, up to 7.5 mg/kg may be given daily in divided doses every 8 hours for short periods. In the management of urinary-tract infections, a single daily dose of 150 mg for 5 days may be given; for complicated urinary-tract infections, 3 to 4 mg/kg daily in divided doses every 12 hours has been given. A single dose of 300 mg has been licensed for gonorrhoea (p.130).

The same doses may be given by slow intravenous injection over 3 to 5 minutes or infused intravenously over 0.5 to 2 hours in 50 to 200 mL of infusion fluid; proportionately less fluid should be given to children.

Treatment with netilmicin is usually given for 7 to 14 days. Prolonged peak plasma concentrations greater than 16 micrograms/mL and trough plasma concentrations greater than 4 micrograms/mL should be avoided. The *British National Formulary* recommends peaks below 12 micrograms/mL and troughs below 2 micrograms/mL for divided daily dose regimens.

Dosage recommendations in infants and children vary somewhat. One regimen is 7.5 to 9 mg/kg daily in infants and neonates older than 1 week, and 6 to 7.5 mg/kg daily in older children, both given in divided doses every 8 hours. Premature infants and neonates less than 1 week old may be given 6 mg/kg daily in divided doses every 12 hours. An alternative regimen is 4 to 6.5 mg/kg daily in neonates less than 6 weeks of age, in divided doses every 12 hours, and 5.5 to 8 mg/kg daily in divided doses every 8 or 12 hours in older infants and children.

Dosage should be adjusted in all patients according to plasma-netilmicin concentrations, and this is particularly important where factors such as age, renal impairment, or prolonged therapy may predispose to toxicity, or where there is a risk of subtherapeutic concentrations. For discussion of the methods of calculating aminoglycoside dosage requirements, see p.219.

## Preparations

**USP 27:** Netilmicin Sulfate Injection.

**Proprietary Preparations** (details are given in Part 3)
***Arg.:*** Netira; ***Austral.:*** Netromycin; ***Austria:*** Certomycin; ***Belg.:*** Netromycine; ***Braz.:*** Netromicina; ***Canad.:*** Netromycin; ***Denm.:*** Netilyn; ***Fin.:*** Netilyn; ***Fr.:*** Netromicine; ***Ger.:*** Certomycin; ***Gr.:*** Netromycin; ***Hong Kong:*** Netromycin; ***India:*** Netromycin; ***Irl.:*** Netillin; ***Ital.:*** Nettacin; Zetamicin; ***Mex.:*** Neticin; Netromicina; ***Neth.:*** Netromycine; ***Norw.:*** Netilyn; ***NZ:*** Netromycin; ***Port.:*** Netromicina; ***S.Afr.:*** Netromycin; ***Spain:*** Dilinar†; Netrocin; ***Swed.:*** Netilyn; ***Switz.:*** Netromycine; ***Thai.:*** Nelin; Netromycin; ***UK:*** Netillin; ***USA:*** Netromycin†.

# Nifuroxazide (rINN)

Nifuroxazida; Nifuroxazidum. 2′-(5-Nitrofurfurylidene)-4-hydroxybenzohydrazide.

$C_{12}H_9N_3O_5$ = 275.2.
*CAS — 965-52-6.*
*ATC — A07AX03.*

**Pharmacopoeias.** In *Eur.* (see p.vi).

**Ph. Eur. 5.0** (Nifuroxazide). A bright yellow crystalline powder. Practically insoluble in water; slightly soluble in alcohol; practically insoluble in dichloromethane. Protect from light.

## Profile

Nifuroxazide is an antibacterial that is poorly absorbed from the gastrointestinal tract. It is given by mouth in a dose of 800 mg daily in divided doses in the treatment of colitis and diarrhoea.

## Preparations

**Proprietary Preparations** (details are given in Part 3)
***Belg.:*** Bacifurane; Ercefuryl; ***Braz.:*** Passifuril; ***Fr.:*** Ambatrol†; Bacterix; Bifix; Ediston; Ercefuryl; Erceryl; Lumifurex; Nifur†; Panfurex; Septidiaryl; ***Hong Kong:*** Antidia†; Ercefuryl; ***Ital.:*** Diarret; Ercefuryl†; ***Mex.:*** Akabar; Diarim; Eskapar†; Topron; ***Singapore:*** Ercefuryl†; Niraben; ***Thai.:*** Ercefuryl.

**Multi-ingredient: *Chile:*** Diaren; Diarfin; Enterol Con Nifuroxacida; Imecol; Liracol; Nifurat; Testisan.

# Nifurtoinol (rINN)

Hydroxymethylnitrofurantoin. 3-Hydroxymethyl-1-(5-nitrofurfurylideneamino)hydantoin.

$C_9H_8N_4O_6$ = 268.2.
*CAS — 1088-92-2.*
*ATC — J01XE02.*

## Profile

Nifurtoinol is a nitrofuran antibacterial with properties similar to those of nitrofurantoin (p.237) and is used in the treatment of urinary-tract infections. It is given by mouth in doses of up to 300 mg daily in divided doses.

## Preparations

**Proprietary Preparations** (details are given in Part 3)
***Belg.:*** Urfadyn PL; ***Switz.:*** Urfadyne†.

# Nifurzide (rINN)

Nifurzida. 5-Nitro-2-thiophenecarboxylic acid [3-(5-nitro-2-furyl)allylidene]hydrazide.

$C_{12}H_8N_4O_6S$ = 336.3.
*CAS — 39978-42-2.*
*ATC — A07AX04.*

## Profile

Nifurzide is an antibacterial that is poorly absorbed from the gastrointestinal tract. It has been given by mouth in a dose of 450 mg daily in divided doses in the treatment of diarrhoea.

## Preparations

**Proprietary Preparations** (details are given in Part 3)
***Fr.:*** Ricridene; ***Mex.:*** Normodiar†.

# Nisin

E234; Nisina.
*CAS — 1414-45-5.*

## Profile

Nisin is a polypeptide antibacterial produced by *Streptococcus lactis*. It is used as a food preservative.

It has been investigated for the treatment of various infections, including those caused by *Helicobacter pylori* and *Clostridium difficile*.

# Nitrofurantoin (BAN, rINN)

Furadoninum; Nitrofurantoína; Nitrofurantoinum. 1-(5-Nitrofurfurylideneamino)hydantoin; 1-(5-Nitrofurfurylideneamino)imidazolidine-2,4-dione.

$C_8H_6N_4O_5$ = 238.2.
*CAS — 67-20-9 (anhydrous nitrofurantoin); 17140-81-7 (nitrofurantoin monohydrate).*
*ATC — J01XE01.*

**Pharmacopoeias.** In *Chin.* and *Eur.* (see p.vi). *Int.* and *US* specify anhydrous or monohydrate.

**Ph. Eur. 5.0** (Nitrofurantoin). A yellow, odourless or almost odourless, crystalline powder or crystals. Very slightly soluble in water and in alcohol; soluble in dimethylformamide. Store at a temperature not exceeding 25°. Protect from light.

**USP 27** (Nitrofurantoin). It is anhydrous or contains one molecule of water of hydration. Lemon-yellow, odourless crystals or fine powder. Nitrofurantoin and its solutions are discoloured by alkalis and by exposure to light, and are decomposed on contact with metals other than stainless steel or aluminium. Very slightly soluble in water and in alcohol; soluble in dimethylformamide. Store in airtight containers. Protect from light.

## Adverse Effects

The estimated incidence of adverse effects with nitrofurantoin has varied enormously, but may be around 10% overall; an incidence of serious reactions of about 0.001% for pulmonary, and 0.0007% for neurological reactions has been suggested. The most common adverse effects of nitrofurantoin involve the gastrointestinal tract. They are dose-related and generally include nausea, vomiting, and anorexia; abdominal pain and diarrhoea occur less frequently. It has been reported that adverse effects on the gastrointestinal tract are less common when nitrofurantoin is given in a macrocrystalline form or with food.

Neurological adverse effects include headache, drowsiness, vertigo, dizziness, nystagmus, and benign intracranial hypertension. Severe and sometimes irreversible peripheral polyneuropathy has developed, particularly in patients with renal impairment and in those given prolonged therapy.

Hypersensitivity reactions such as skin rashes, urticaria, pruritus, fever, sialadenitis, and angioedema may occur. Anaphylaxis, erythema multiforme, Stevens-Johnson syndrome, exfoliative dermatitis, pancreatitis, a lupus-like syndrome, myalgia, and arthralgia have also been reported. Patients with a history of asthma may experience acute asthmatic attacks.

Acute pulmonary sensitivity reactions characterised by sudden onset of fever, chills, eosinophilia, cough, chest pain, dyspnoea, pulmonary infiltration or consolidation, and pleural effusion may occur within hours to a few days of beginning therapy, but they usually resolve on discontinuation.

Subacute or chronic pulmonary symptoms including interstitial pneumonitis and pulmonary fibrosis may develop more insidiously in patients on long-term therapy and the latter are not always reversible, particularly if therapy is continued after onset of symptoms.

Hepatotoxicity including cholestatic jaundice, hepatitis, and hepatic necrosis may develop rarely, particularly in women, and may represent a hypersensitivity reaction. Other adverse effects include megaloblastic anaemia, leucopenia, granulocytopenia or agranulocytosis, thrombocytopenia, aplastic anaemia, and haemolytic anaemia in persons with a genetic G6PD deficiency. Transient alopecia has been reported.

Nitrofurantoin may cause a brownish discoloration of the urine.

There is limited evidence from *animal* studies that nitrofurantoin may be carcinogenic, although this has not been demonstrated conclusively in humans.

◊ References.


1. Koch-Weser J, *et al.* Adverse reactions to sulfisoxazole, sulfamethoxazole, and nitrofurantoin: manifestations and specific reaction rates during 2118 courses of therapy. *Arch Intern Med* 1971; **128:** 399–404.
2. Holmberg L, *et al.* Adverse reactions to nitrofurantoin: analysis of 921 reports. *Am J Med* 1980; **69:** 733–8.
3. Penn RG, Griffin JP. Adverse reactions to nitrofurantoin in the United Kingdom, Sweden, and Holland. *BMJ* 1982; **284:** 1440–2.
4. D'Arcy PF. Nitrofurantoin. *Drug Intell Clin Pharm* 1985; **19:** 540–7.


## Precautions

Nitrofurantoin should not be given to patients with renal impairment since antibacterial concentrations in the urine may not be attained and toxic concentrations in the plasma can occur. Nitrofurantoin is also contra-indicated in patients known to be hypersensitive to nitrofurans, in those with G6PD deficiency, and in infants less than 3 months old. It has been suggested that nitrofurantoin should not be used in pregnant patients at term because of the possibility of producing haemolytic anaemia in the neonate, and that it should be avoided, or used with caution, in mothers who are breast feeding infants who have G6PD deficiency, since traces are found in breast milk.

Nitrofurantoin should be used with care in the elderly, who may be at increased risk of toxicity, particularly acute pulmonary reactions. All patients undergoing prolonged therapy should be monitored for changes in pulmonary function, and the drug withdrawn at the first signs of pulmonary damage. Care is required in patients with pre-existing pulmonary, hepatic, neurological or allergic disorders, and in those with conditions (such as anaemia, diabetes mellitus, electrolyte imbalance, debility, or vitamin B deficiency) which may predispose to peripheral neuropathy. Nitrofurantoin should be withdrawn if signs of peripheral neuropathy develop.

Nitrofurantoin may cause false positive reactions in urine tests for glucose using copper reduction methods.

**Breast feeding.** The American Academy of Pediatrics considers that, although nitrofurantoin is excreted into breast milk, it is usually compatible with breast feeding, but caution is necessary in breast-fed infants with G6PD deficiency.[1]

1. American Academy of Pediatrics. The transfer of drugs and other chemicals into human milk. *Pediatrics* 2001; **108:** 776–89. Correction. *ibid.*; 1029. Also available at: http://aappolicy.aappublications.org/cgi/content/full/pediatrics%3b108/3/776 (accessed 27/05/04)

**Porphyria.** Nitrofurantoin has been associated with acute attacks of porphyria and is considered to be unsafe in porphyric patients.

## Interactions

Nitrofurantoin and the quinolone antibacterials are antagonistic *in vitro* and should not be used together. The antibacterial activity of nitrofurantoin may be decreased in the presence of carbonic anhydrase inhibitors and other drugs that alkalinise the urine.

Probenecid or sulfinpyrazone should not be given with nitrofurantoin as they may reduce its excretion. Magnesium trisilicate may reduce the absorption of nitrofurantoin but it is not clear whether this applies to other antacids.

**Antiepileptics.** For reference to the effect of nitrofurantoin on *phenytoin*, see p.372.

**Hormonal contraceptives.** For mention of a possible decrease in contraceptive efficacy when nitrofurantoin was used with oral contraceptives, see under Hormonal Contraceptives, p.1534.

## Antimicrobial Action

Nitrofurantoin is bactericidal *in vitro* to most Gram-positive and Gram-negative urinary-tract pathogens. The mode of action is uncertain but appears to depend on the formation of reactive intermediates by reduction; this process occurs more efficiently in bacterial than in mammalian cells.

It is effective against the enterococci *in vitro*, as well as various other Gram-positive species including staphylococci, streptococci, and corynebacteria, although this is of little clinical significance. Most strains of *Escherichia coli* are particularly sensitive to nitrofurantoin but *Enterobacter* and *Klebsiella* spp. are less susceptible and some may be resistant. *Pseudomonas aeruginosa* is resistant as are most strains of *Proteus* spp.

Nitrofurantoin is most active in acid urine, and if the pH exceeds 8 most of the antibacterial activity is lost. Resistance rarely develops during nitrofurantoin treatment but may occur during prolonged treatment. Plasmid-encoded resistance has been reported in *E. coli*. Resistance may be due to the loss of nitrofuran reductases which generate the active intermediates.

## Pharmacokinetics

Nitrofurantoin is readily absorbed from the gastrointestinal tract. The absorption rate is dependent on crystal size. The macrocrystalline form has slower dissolution and absorption rates, produces lower serum concentrations than the microcrystalline form, and takes longer to achieve peak concentrations in the urine. The presence of food in the gastrointestinal tract may increase the bioavailability of nitrofurantoin and prolong the duration of therapeutic urinary concentrations. Preparations of nitrofurantoin from different sources may not be bioequivalent, and care may be necessary if changing from one brand to another.

Following absorption, concentrations in blood and body tissues are low because of rapid elimination, and antibacterial concentrations are not achieved. Nitrofurantoin crosses the placenta and the blood-brain barrier and traces have been detected in breast milk. There is some disagreement about the degree of protein binding, and although figures of up to about 60% are quoted by some sources, others suggest that the figure should be as much as 90%. The plasma half-life is reported to range from 0.3 to 1 hour.

Nitrofurantoin is metabolised in the liver and most body tissues while about 30 to 40% of a dose is excreted rapidly in the urine as unchanged nitrofurantoin. Some tubular reabsorption may occur in acid urine. Average doses give a concentration of 50 to 200 micrograms/mL in the urine in patients with normal renal function.

## Uses and Administration

Nitrofurantoin is a nitrofuran derivative that is used in the treatment of uncomplicated lower urinary-tract infections (p.153), including for prophylaxis or long-term suppressive therapy in recurrent infection.

It is given by mouth, usually in a dose of 50 to 100 mg four times daily, with food or milk. Treatment is usually continued for 7 days. A dual-release formulation, consisting of macrocrystalline nitrofurantoin and nitrofurantoin monohydrate, is available in some countries and is given in a dose of 100 mg twice daily. A usual long-term prophylactic dose is 50 to 100 mg at bedtime.

Infants over 3 months of age and older children may be given 3 mg/kg daily in 4 divided doses by mouth. For long-term prophylactic therapy 1 mg/kg once daily may be adequate.

◊ Reviews.

1. Guay DR. An update on the role of nitrofurans in the management of urinary tract infections. *Drugs* 2001; **61:** 353–64.

## Preparations

***BP 2003:*** Nitrofurantoin Oral Suspension; Nitrofurantoin Tablets;
***USP 27:*** Nitrofurantoin Capsules; Nitrofurantoin Oral Suspension; Nitrofurantoin Tablets.

**Proprietary Preparations** (details are given in Part 3)
***Arg.:*** Furadantina; ***Austral.:*** Furadantin; Macrodantin; Ralodantin; ***Austria:*** Furadantin; ***Belg.:*** Furadantine†; ***Braz.:*** Hantina; Macrodantina; Nitrobid†; Uro Furan†; Urogem; ***Canad.:*** Macrobid; Macrodantin; Novo-Furantoin; ***Chile:*** Macrodantina; Macrosan; Matidan; ***Fin.:*** Nitrofur-C; ***Fr.:*** Furadantine; Furadoine; Microdoine; ***Ger.:*** Cystit†; Furadantin; Nifurantin; Nifuretten; Uro-Tablinen; ***Gr.:*** Furolin; ***India:*** Furadantin; ***Irl.:*** Furadantin; Macrobid; Macrodantin; ***Israel:*** Macrodantin; Urantoin†; Uvamin; ***Ital.:*** Cistofuran†; Furadantin; Furedan; Furil; Macrodantin; Neo-Furadantin; ***Mex.:*** Biofurin; Furadantina; Futroken†; Macrodantina; Macrofurin†; Promac†; Suronit; Teguran†; Urobac†; ***Neth.:*** Furabid; Furadantine MC; ***Norw.:*** Furadantin; ***NZ:*** Furadantin; Nifuran; ***Port.:*** Furadantina; ***S.Afr.:*** Furadantin; Macrodantin; Urantin†; ***Spain:*** Chemiofurin†; Furantoina; Furobactina; ***Swed.:*** Furadantin; ***Switz.:*** Furadantine; Urodin; Uvamine retard; ***UK:*** Furadantin; Macrobid; Macrodantin; Urantoin†; ***USA:*** Furadantin; Macrobid; Macrodantin.

**Multi-ingredient:** ***Arg.:*** Bagociletas con Anestesia; Bagociletas sin Anestesia; ***Braz.:*** Nipactrin†; Urofen; Uropac; ***Ger.:*** Nifurantin B 6; Urospasmon; Urospasmon sine; ***India:*** Nephrogesic; ***Mex.:*** Furanton†.

---

# Nitrofurazone *(BAN)*

Nitrofural *(pINN)*; Furacilinum; Nitrofuralum. 5-Nitro-2-furaldehyde semicarbazone.

$C_6H_6N_4O_4$ = 198.1.
*CAS — 59-87-0.*
*ATC — B05CA03; D08AF01; D09AA03; P01CC02; S01AX04; S02AA02.*

**Pharmacopoeias.** In *Eur.* (see p.vi), *Pol.*, and *US.*

**Ph. Eur. 5.0** (Nitrofural; Nitrofurazone BP 2003). A yellow or brownish-yellow, crystalline powder. Very slightly soluble in water; slightly soluble in alcohol. The filtrate from a 1% suspension in water has a pH of 5.0 to 7.0. Protect from light.

**USP 27** (Nitrofurazone). A lemon-yellow, odourless crystalline powder. It darkens slowly on exposure to light. Soluble 1 in 4200 of water, 1 in 590 of alcohol, and 1 in 350 of propylene glycol; practically insoluble in chloroform and in ether; soluble in dimethylformamide; slightly soluble in polyethylene glycol mixtures. The filtrate from a 1% suspension in water has a pH of 5.0 to 7.5. Store in airtight containers at a temperature not exceeding 40°. Protect from light.

**Sterilisation.** Autoclaving gauze dressings impregnated with nitrofurazone, as recommended by the US manufacturer, resulted in a greater than 10% loss of the drug.[1] Since the spectroscopic assay used may not distinguish between nitrofurazone and some of its degradation products, the degree of degradation may have been greater than this.

1. Phillips C, Fisher E. Effect of autoclaving on stability of nitrofurazone soluble dressing. *Am J Health-Syst Pharm* 1996; **53:** 1169–71.

## Adverse Effects

Sensitisation and generalised allergic skin reactions may be produced by the topical application of nitrofurazone.

Nitrofurazone is a toxic drug when given by mouth and serious adverse effects include severe peripheral neuropathy; haemolysis may occur in patients with G6PD deficiency. Nitrofurazone in high oral doses is carcinogenic in *rats*.

## Precautions

Nitrofurazone is contra-indicated in patients with known hypersensitivity. Preparations containing macrogols should be used with caution in patients with renal impairment since macrogols can be absorbed and their accumulation in such patients may result in symptoms of further impairment.

Nitrofurazone by mouth should be used with caution in patients with G6PD deficiency because of the risk of haemolysis.

## Antimicrobial Action

Nitrofurazone is a nitrofuran derivative with a broad spectrum of antibacterial activity, but with little activity against *Pseudomonas* spp. It also has antitrypanosomal activity.

## Uses and Administration

Nitrofurazone is a nitrofuran derivative which is used as a local application for wounds, burns, ulcers, and skin infections, and for the preparation of surfaces before skin grafting. It is usually applied in a concentration of 0.2% in a water-soluble or water-miscible basis. A solution of nitrofurazone is used for bladder irrigation.

## Preparations

***USP 27:*** Nitrofurazone Ointment; Nitrofurazone Topical Solution.

**Proprietary Preparations** (details are given in Part 3)
***Arg.:*** Furacin; Ivoran Pilot; Nitromed; ***Belg.:*** Furacine; ***Braz.:*** Alivioderm; Caziderm; Furacin; Sensiderme; ***Chile:*** Demodek; Furacin; ***Ger.:*** Furacin-Sol; Nifucin†; ***India:*** Furacin; ***Israel:*** Rafuzone†; ***Mex.:*** Furacin; Nifurol†; ***Neth.:*** Furacine; ***S.Afr.:*** Furacin; Furasept†; Furex; ***Spain:*** Furacin; ***Thai.:*** Bactacin; Polycin; ***USA:*** Furacin.

**Multi-ingredient:** ***Arg.:*** Fadanasal; Neo Pelvicillin; O-Biol; Vagicural; Vagisan; Vagisan Compuesto; ***Braz.:*** Colpacid†; Dermilan†; Elocort†; Furazolon†; Infladerm†; Nitrileno; Nitrolerg; Nitronasal†; Oto-Ped†; Otodol; Otolin†; Rinocron†; Solucao Nasal de Nafazolina†; ***Ger.:*** Nifucin†; ***India:*** Furacin-S; ***Ital.:*** Furanvit†; Furotricina; ***Mex.:*** Madecassol C; Madecassol N; ***Spain:*** Dertrase; ***Thai.:*** Denson.

---

# Nitroxoline *(BAN, pINN)*

Nitroxolina. 5-Nitroquinolin-8-ol.

$C_9H_6N_2O_3$ = 190.2.
*CAS — 4008-48-4.*
*ATC — J01XX07.*

## Profile

Nitroxoline has antibacterial and antifungal properties and is used in the treatment of urinary-tract infections in usual doses of 600 or 750 mg daily by mouth in divided doses before food. It has also been given with sulfamethizole.

## Preparations

**Proprietary Preparations** (details are given in Part 3)
***Fr.:*** Nibiol; ***Ger.:*** Cysto-Saar; ***Mex.:*** Noxigur†; ***S.Afr.:*** Nicene N.

**Multi-ingredient:** ***Braz.:*** Minazol; ***S.Afr.:*** Nicene†.

---

# Norfloxacin *(BAN, USAN, rINN)*

AM-715; MK-366; Norfloxacino; Norfloxacinum. 1-Ethyl-6-fluoro-1,4-dihydro-4-oxo-7-(piperazin-1-yl)quinoline-3-carboxylic acid.

$C_{16}H_{18}FN_3O_3$ = 319.3.
*CAS — 70458-96-7.*
*ATC — J01MA06; S01AX12.*

**Pharmacopoeias.** In *Chin., Eur.* (see p.vi), *Jpn, Pol.*, and *US.*

**Ph. Eur. 5.0** (Norfloxacin). A white or pale yellow, hygroscopic, photosensitive, crystalline powder. Very slightly soluble in water; slightly soluble in alcohol and in acetone. Store in airtight containers. Protect from light.

**USP 27** (Norfloxacin). A white to pale yellow crystalline powder. Slightly soluble in water, in alcohol, and in acetone; freely soluble in acetic acid; sparingly soluble in chloroform; practically insoluble in ether; very slightly soluble in ethyl acetate and in methyl alcohol. Store in airtight containers. Protect from light.

## Adverse Effects and Precautions

As for Ciprofloxacin, p.188.

**Effects on the kidneys.** References.

1. Hestin D, *et al.* Norfloxacin-induced nephrotic syndrome. *Lancet* 1995; **345:** 732–3.

## Interactions

As for Ciprofloxacin, p.190.

## Antimicrobial Action

As for Ciprofloxacin, p.190, although norfloxacin is less potent *in vitro*. Norfloxacin is not active against Chlamydiaceae, mycoplasmas, or mycobacteria.

## Pharmacokinetics

About 30 to 40% of an oral dose of norfloxacin is absorbed. Peak plasma concentrations of about 1.5 micrograms/mL have been achieved 1 to 2 hours after a 400-mg oral dose; the presence of food can delay absorption. The plasma half-life is 3 to 4 hours and may be prolonged in renal impairment; a value of 6.5 hours or more has been reported when creatinine clearance is below 30 mL/minute. Norfloxacin has been reported to be 14% bound to plasma proteins. It is probably widely distributed, but information is limited. Norfloxacin penetrates well into tissues of the genitourinary tract. It crosses the placenta. Relatively high concentrations are achieved in bile.

About 30% of a dose is excreted unchanged in the urine within 24 hours, producing high urinary concentrations; norfloxacin is least soluble at a urinary pH of 7.5. Urinary excretion is by tubular secretion and glomerular filtration and is reduced by probenecid, although plasma concentrations of norfloxacin are not generally affected. Some metabolism occurs, possibly in the liver, and several metabolites have been identified in urine, some with antibacterial activity. About 30% of an oral dose is recovered from the faeces.

## Uses and Administration

Norfloxacin is a fluoroquinolone antibacterial with properties similar to those of ciprofloxacin, but it is generally less potent *in vitro*.

Norfloxacin is used mainly in the treatment of urinary-tract infections (p.153). It is also used for the treatment of gonorrhoea (p.130).

Norfloxacin is given by mouth. In urinary-tract infections the usual dose is 400 mg twice daily for 3 to 10 days. Treatment may need to be continued for up to 12 weeks in chronic relapsing urinary-tract infections; it may be possible to reduce the dose to 400 mg once daily if there is an adequate response within the first 4 weeks.

For details of reduced doses to be used in renal impairment, see below.

A single oral dose of 800 mg is given in the treatment of uncomplicated gonorrhoea.

Eye drops containing 0.3% of norfloxacin are used to treat eye infections.

The pivaloyloxymethyl salt of norfloxacin, norfloxacin pivoxil, is also used in some countries.

**Administration in renal impairment.** Doses of norfloxacin may need to be reduced in renal impairment; for urinary-tract infections, 400 mg once daily may be given to patients with a creatinine clearance of 30 mL/minute or less.

## Preparations

***BP 2003:*** Norfloxacin Eye Drops; Norfloxacin Tablets;
***USP 27:*** Norfloxacin Ophthalmic Solution; Norfloxacin Tablets.

**Proprietary Preparations** (details are given in Part 3)

***Arg.:*** Bio Tarbun; Chibroxin; Floxamicin; Floxatral; Memento NF; Norflol; Noroxin; Norsol; Ritromine; Uro-Linfol; Urofos; Uronovag; Uroseptal; Urotem; Uroxacin; Yanurax; ***Austral.:*** Insensye; Norflohexal; Noroxin; Roxin; ***Austria:*** Floxacin; Urobacid; Zoroxin; ***Belg.:*** Chibroxol; Zoroxin; ***Braz.:*** Chibroxin; Flox; Floxacin; Floxanor; Floxatrat; Floxinol; Genitoflox; Neofloxin; Noracin†; Norflamin; Norfloxasan; Norxin; Quinoform; Respexil; Uritrat; Uroflox; Uroplex; Uroseptal; Uroxazol-N; ***Canad.:*** Apo-Norflox; Noroxin; ***Chile:*** Chibroxin; Fulgram 400; Noroxin; Urekolin; ***Denm.:*** Zoroxin; ***Fin.:*** Lexinor; Noroxin; ***Fr.:*** Chibroxine; Noroxine; ***Ger.:*** Bactracid; Barazan; Chibroxin; Firin; Norflohexal; Norflosal; Norflox; Norflox-Azu; Norflox-Puren; Norfloxbeta; ***Gr.:*** Alenbit; Constilax; Fluseminal; Grenis; Norocin; Ovinol; Pistofil; Sinobid; Sofasin; Steinaclox; Vetamol; ***Hong Kong:*** Chibroxin†; Janacin; Lexiflox; Lexinor; Rexacin; Uroctal; ***India:*** Biofloxin; Norbactin; Norflox; Normax; ***Israel:*** Apirol; Chibroxin; ***Ital.:*** Diperflox; Flossac; Fulgram; Norflox; Noroxin; Sebercim; Utinor; ***Jpn:*** Baccidal; ***Malaysia:*** Chibroxin; Floxen; Janacin; Lexinor; Norbactin; Norfloxinor; Trizolin; Urobacid; ***Mex.:*** Difoxacil; Floxacin; Microxin; Noroxin; Oranor; ***Neth.:*** Chibroxol; Noroxin; ***NZ:*** Noroxin; ***Port.:*** Chibroxol†; Noroxin; Quinoflex; Taflox; Uroflox; ***S.Afr.:*** Noroxin; Utin; ***Singapore:*** Bexinor; Chibroxin; Effectsal; Gyrablock†; Lexinor†; Norbactin; Sefnor; Trizolin; Urobacid; ***Spain:*** Amicrobin; Baccidal; Chibroxin; Esclebin; Espeden; Nalion; Norflok; Noroxin; Senro; Uroctal; Vicnas†; Xasmun; ***Swed.:*** Lexinor; ***Switz.:*** Chibroxol; Norflocine; Noroxin; Norsol; ***Thai.:*** BGB Norflox; Floxenor†; Foxin; Foxinon; Gonorcin; Gyrablock†; Janacin; Lexfor; Lexinor; Manoflox; Noracin; Noraxin†; Norbactin; Norcin; Norfcin; Norflo; Norflocin; Norfloxin; Norsa; Norxacin; Norxia; Noxine; Noxinor; Proxinor; Rexacin; Snoffocin; Trizolin; Urinox; Uritracin; Xacin; ***UAE:*** Uroxin; ***UK:*** Utinor; ***USA:*** Chibroxin†; Noroxin.

**Multi-ingredient: *Arg.:*** Nor 2.

---

# Norvancomycin Hydrochloride

*N*-Demethylvancomycin; 56-Demethylvancomycin. ($S_a$)-(3*S*,6*R*,7*R*,22*R*,23*S*,26*S*,36*R*,38a*R*)-44-{[2-*O*-(3-Amino-2,3,6-trideoxy-3-*C*-methyl-α-L-*lyxo*-hexopyranosyl)-β-D-glucopyranosyl]oxy}-3-(carbamoylmethyl)-10,19-dichloro-2,3,4,5,6,7,23,24,25,26,36,37,38,38a-tetradecahydro-7,22,28,30,32-pentahydroxy-6-[(2*R*)-4-methyl-2-(amino)valeramido]-2,5,24,38,39-pentaoxo-22*H*-8,11:18,21-dietheno-23,36-(iminomethano)-13,16:31,35-dimetheno-1*H*,16*H*-[1,6,9]oxadiazacyclohexadecino[4,5-*m*][10,2,16]-benzoxadiazacyclotetracosine-26-carboxylic acid, monohydrochloride.

$C_{65}H_{73}Cl_2N_9O_{24}$, HCl = 1471.7.
*CAS — 91700-98-0 (norvancomycin).*

**Pharmacopoeias.** In *Chin.*

## Profile

Norvancomycin is a glycopeptide antibacterial with properties similar to those of vancomycin (p.275).

---

# Novobiocin *(BAN, rINN)*

Crystallinic Acid; Novobiocina; PA-93; Streptonivicin; U-6591. 4-Hydroxy-3-[4-hydroxy-3-(3-methylbut-2-enyl)benzamido]-8-methylcoumarin-7-yl 3-*O*-carbamoyl-5,5-di-*C*-methyl-α-L-lyxo-furanoside.

$C_{31}H_{36}N_2O_{11}$ = 612.6.
*CAS — 303-81-1.*

**Description.** Novobiocin is an antimicrobial substance produced by the growth of *Streptomyces niveus* and *S. spheroides* or related organisms.

## Novobiocin Calcium *(BANM, rINNM)*

Calcium Novobiocin; Novobiocina cálcica; Novobiocinum Calcium.

$(C_{31}H_{35}N_2O_{11})_2Ca$ = 1263.3.
*CAS — 4309-70-0.*

## Novobiocin Sodium *(BANM, rINNM)*

Novobiocina sódica; Novobiocinum Natricum; Sodium Novobiocin.

$C_{31}H_{35}N_2NaO_{11}$ = 634.6.
*CAS — 1476-53-5.*

**Pharmacopoeias.** In *Fr., Int.,* and *US.*

**USP 27** (Novobiocin Sodium). A white or yellowish-white, odourless, hygroscopic crystalline powder. Freely soluble in water, in alcohol, in methyl alcohol, in glycerol, and in propylene glycol; practically insoluble in acetone, in chloroform, and in ether; slightly soluble in butyl acetate. pH of a 2.5% solution in water is between 6.5 and 8.5. Store in airtight containers.

## Profile

Novobiocin is an antimicrobial which is structurally related to coumarin. It is active against Gram-positive bacteria such as *Staphylococcus aureus* (including meticillin-resistant strains) and other staphylococci; *Enterococcus faecalis* is usually resistant but *E. faecium* may be sensitive. Some Gram-negative organisms including *Haemophilus influenzae* and *Neisseria* spp. are also susceptible, as are some strains of *Proteus*, but most of the Enterobacteriaceae are resistant. Its action is primarily bacteriostatic, although it may be bactericidal against more sensitive species at high concentrations. It is an inhibitor of DNA gyrase and is effective in eliminating plasmids, but resistance to novobiocin develops readily *in vitro* and during therapy.

Although novobiocin has been used alone or with other drugs such as rifampicin or sodium fusidate in the treatment of infections due to staphylococci and other susceptible organisms, it has been largely superseded by other drugs because of the problems of resistance and toxicity.

Novobiocin is a potent sensitiser and hypersensitivity reactions are relatively common; they include rashes, fever, and pruritus, and more serious reactions such as Stevens-Johnson syndrome and pneumonitis. Jaundice and liver damage have occurred, although apparent jaundice may be due to a yellow metabolite of the drug rather than hyperbilirubinaemia. Other adverse effects include eosinophilia, leucopenia, thrombocytopenia, agranulocytosis, and haemolytic anaemia; gastrointestinal disturbances are common.

**Porphyria.** Novobiocin has been associated with acute attacks of porphyria and is considered unsafe in porphyric patients.

## Preparations

**Proprietary Preparations** (details are given in Part 3)
***USA:*** Albamycin†.

**Multi-ingredient: *Spain:*** Tetra Tripsin†.

---

# Ofloxacin *(BAN, USAN, rINN)*

DL-8280; Hoe-280; Ofloxacino; Ofloxacinum. (±)-9-Fluoro-2,3-dihydro-3-methyl-10-(4-methyl-1-piperazinyl)-7-oxo-7*H*-pyrido[1,2,3-*de*]-1,4-benzoxazine-6-carboxylic acid.

$C_{18}H_{20}FN_3O_4$ = 361.4.
*CAS — 82419-36-1; 83380-47-6.*
*ATC — J01MA01; S01AX11.*

**Pharmacopoeias.** In *Chin., Eur.* (see p.vi), *Jpn,* and *US.*

**Ph. Eur. 5.0** (Ofloxacin). A pale yellow or bright yellow crystalline powder. Slightly soluble in water and in methyl alcohol; slightly soluble to soluble in dichloromethane; soluble in glacial acetic acid. Store in airtight containers. Protect from light.

**USP 27** (Ofloxacin). Pale yellowish-white to light yellowish-white crystals or crystalline powder. Slightly soluble in water, in alcohol, and in methyl alcohol; sparingly soluble in chloroform. Store at a temperature of 25°, excursions permitted between 15° and 30°. Protect from light.

## Adverse Effects and Precautions

As for Ciprofloxacin, p.188.

**Breast feeding.** The American Academy of Pediatrics has stated that no adverse effects have been observed in breast-fed infants whose mothers were receiving ofloxacin and that it is therefore usually compatible with breast feeding.[1] However, in a study of 10 women who received ofloxacin following termination of pregnancy, drug concentrations in breast milk were sufficiently high that it was considered that the use of ofloxacin in lactating women should be avoided.[2]

1. American Academy of Pediatrics. The transfer of drugs and other chemicals into human milk. *Pediatrics* 2001; **108:** 776–89. Correction. *ibid.*; 1029. Also available at: http://aappolicy.aappublications.org/cgi/content/full/pediatrics%3b108/3/776 (accessed 27/05/04)
2. Giamarellou H, *et al.* Pharmacokinetics of three newer quinolones in pregnant and lactating women. *Am J Med* 1989; **87** (suppl 5A): 49S–51S.

## Interactions

As for Ciprofloxacin, p.190.

## Antimicrobial Action

As for Ciprofloxacin, p.190.

Ofloxacin is more active than ciprofloxacin against *Chlamydia trachomatis*. It is also active against *Mycobacterium leprae* as well as *M. tuberculosis* and some other *Mycobacterium* spp. Synergistic activity against *M. leprae* has been reported between ofloxacin and rifabutin.

The optically active *S*-(−)-isomer levofloxacin (p.225) has twice the activity of the racemate ofloxacin.

Resistance has been reported in some strains of *Neisseria gonorrhoeae*.

◊ References.

1. Dhople AM, *et al.* In vitro synergistic activity between ofloxacin and ansamycins against Mycobacterium leprae. *Arzneimittelforschung* 1993; **43:** 384–6.
2. Kam K-M, *et al.* Ofloxacin susceptibilities of 5667 Neisseria gonorrhoea strains isolated in Hong Kong. *Antimicrob Agents Chemother* 1993; **37:** 2007–8.
3. Kam KM, *et al.* Quinolone-resistant Neisseria gonorrhoeae in Hong Kong. *Sex Transm Dis* 1996; **23:** 103–8.
4. Cambau E, *et al.* Multidrug-resistance to dapsone, rifampicin, and ofloxacin in Mycobacterium leprae. *Lancet* 1997; **349:** 103–4.

## Pharmacokinetics

Ofloxacin is rapidly and well absorbed from the gastrointestinal tract. Oral bioavailability is almost 100% and a peak plasma concentration of 3 to 5 micrograms/mL is achieved 1 to 2 hours after a dose of 400 mg by mouth. Absorption may be delayed by the presence of food, but the extent of absorption is not substantially affected. The plasma half-life ranges from 4 to 7 hours; in renal impairment values of 15 to 60 hours have been reported.

About 25% is bound to plasma proteins. Ofloxacin is widely distributed in body fluids, including the CSF, and tissue penetration is good. It crosses the placenta and is distributed into breast milk. It also appears in the bile.

There is limited metabolism to desmethyl and *N*-oxide metabolites; desmethylofloxacin has moderate antibacterial activity. Ofloxacin is eliminated mainly by the kidneys. Excretion is by tubular secretion and glomerular filtration and 65 to 80% of a dose is excreted unchanged in the urine over 24 to 48 hours, resulting in high urinary concentrations. Less than 5% is excreted in the urine as metabolites. From 4 to 8% of a dose may be excreted in the faeces.

Only small amounts of ofloxacin are removed by haemodialysis.

◊ References.

1. Lamp KC, *et al.* Ofloxacin clinical pharmacokinetics. *Clin Pharmacokinet* 1992; **22:** 32–46.
2. Flor SC, *et al.* Bioequivalence of oral and intravenous ofloxacin after multiple-dose administration to healthy male volunteers. *Antimicrob Agents Chemother* 1993; **37:** 1468–72.
3. Nau R, *et al.* Kinetics of ofloxacin and its metabolites in cerebrospinal fluid after a single intravenous infusion of 400 milligrams of ofloxacin. *Antimicrob Agents Chemother* 1994; **38:** 1849–53.
4. Tang-Liu DD-S, *et al.* Comparative tear concentrations over time of ofloxacin and tobramycin in human eyes. *Clin Pharmacol Ther* 1994; **55:** 284–92.
5. Bethell DB, *et al.* Pharmacokinetics of oral and intravenous ofloxacin in children with multidrug-resistant typhoid fever. *Antimicrob Agents Chemother* 1996; **40:** 2167–72.
6. Durmaz B, *et al.* Aqueous humor penetration of topically applied ciprofloxacin, ofloxacin and tobramycin. *Arzneimittelforschung* 1997; **47:** 413–15.
7. McMullin CM, *et al.* The pharmacokinetics of once-daily oral 400 mg ofloxacin in patients with peritonitis complicating continuous ambulatory peritoneal dialysis. *J Antimicrob Chemother* 1997; **39:** 829–31.

## Uses and Administration

Ofloxacin is a fluoroquinolone antibacterial used similarly to ciprofloxacin (p.191). It is also used in *Chlamydia* or *Chlamydophila* infections including nongonococcal urethritis (p.123 and p.152) and in the treatment of mycobacterial infections such as leprosy (p.133).

Ofloxacin is given by mouth as the base or intravenously as the hydrochloride. All doses are expressed in terms of the base.

The adult oral or intravenous dose ranges from 200 mg daily to 400 mg twice daily depending on the severity and the nature of the infection. Oral doses up to 400 mg may be given as a single dose, preferably in the morning. For intravenous use a 0.2% solution is infused over 30 minutes or a 0.4% solution over 60 minutes. A dose of 400 mg daily or intermittently by mouth has been recommended by WHO as part of alternative multidrug therapy regimens for leprosy.

For details of reduced doses to be used in renal impairment, see below.

A single 400-mg dose of ofloxacin may be given by mouth for uncomplicated gonorrhoea.

Ofloxacin is also employed as 0.3% eye drops and 0.3% ear drops.

◊ Reviews.

1. Todd PA, Faulds D. Ofloxacin: a reappraisal of its antimicrobial activity, pharmacology and therapeutic use. *Drugs* 1991; **42:** 825–76.
2. Onrust SV, *et al.* Ofloxacin: a reappraisal of its use in the management of genitourinary tract infections. *Drugs* 1998; **56:** 895–928.
3. Simpson KL, Markham A. Ofloxacin otic solution: a review of its use in the management of ear infections. *Drugs* 1999; **58:** 509–31.
4. Wai TKH, Tong MCF. A benefit-risk assessment of ofloxacin otic solution in ear infection. *Drug Safety* 2003; **26:** 405–20.

**Administration in renal impairment.** Lower doses of ofloxacin may be necessary in patients with renal impairment. Following a normal initial dose subsequent doses are modified according to creatinine clearance (CC):

- CC 20 to 50 mL/minute: doses halved to 100 to 200 mg daily or the usual dose is given every 24 hours
- CC less than 20 mL/minute: dose reduced to 100 mg every 24 hours
- patients on dialysis: 100 mg every 24 hours

## Preparations

***USP 27:*** Ofloxacin Ophthalmic Solution.

**Proprietary Preparations** (details are given in Part 3)
***Arg.:*** Floxil; Oflox; Otoflox; Quinomed; Rafocilina; ***Austral.:*** Ocuflox; Ofloceт†; ***Austria:*** Floxal; Tarivid; ***Belg.:*** Tarivid; Trafloxal; ***Braz.:*** Floxstat; Oflox; Ofloxan; Ofloxin; Quinoxan; ***Canad.:*** Apo-Oflox; Floxin; Ocuflox; ***Chile:*** Ifos; Oflox; Poenflox; ***Denm.:*** Exocin; Tarivid; ***Fin.:*** Exocin; Tarivid; ***Fr.:*** Exocine; Monoflocet; Oflocet; ***Ger.:*** Floxal; Oflodura; Oflohexal; Oflox; Tarivid; Uro-Tarivid; ***Gr.:*** Ermofan; Exocin; Hetacloxacin; Tabrin; ***Hong Kong:*** Tarivid; ***India:*** Floxur; Oflin; Tarivid; Zanocin; ***Irl.:*** Exocin; Tarivid; ***Israel:*** Oflodex; Oflox; Tarivid; Uro-Tarivid; ***Ital.:*** Exocin; Flobacin; Oflocin; ***Jpn:*** Tarivid; ***Malaysia:*** Apo-Oflox; Inoflox; Medofloxine; Ofcin; Tarivid; Zanocin; ***Mex.:*** Bactocin; Floxil; Floxstat; Ocuflox; ***Neth.:*** Tarivid; Trafloxal; ***Norw.:*** Tarivid; ***NZ:*** Oflocet†; ***Port.:*** Bactoflox; Bioquil; Exocin; Floxedol; Megacina†; Megasin; Oflocet; Tarivid; ***S.Afr.:*** Exocin; Tafloc; Tarivid; ***Singapore:*** Inoflox; Ofcin; Tarivid; ***Spain:*** Exocin; Oflovir; Surnox; Tarivid†; ***Swed.:*** Tarivid; ***Switz.:*** Floxal; Tarivid; ***Thai.:*** Konovid; O-Flox; Occidal; Oflocee; Ofloxa; Ofloxcin; Qinolon; Seracin; Tarivid; Viotisone; ***UK:*** Exocin; Tarivid; ***USA:*** Floxin; Ocuflox.

---

## Oleandomycin Phosphate *(BANM, rINNM)*

Fosfato de oleandomicina; PA-105 (oleandomycin). (2*R*,3*S*,4*R*,5*S*,6*S*,8*R*,10*R*,11*S*,12*R*,13*R*)-3-(2,6-Dideoxy-3-*O*-methyl-α-L-*arabino*-hexopyranosyloxy)-8,8-epoxymethano-11-hydroxy-2,4,6,10,12,13-hexamethyl-9-oxo-5-(3,4,6-trideoxy-3-dimethylamino-β-D-*xylo*-hexopyranosyloxy)tridecan-13-olide phosphate.

$C_{35}H_{61}NO_{12},H_3PO_4$ = 785.9.
*CAS — 3922-90-5 (oleandomycin); 7060-74-4 (oleandomycin phosphate).*
*ATC — J01FA05.*

### Profile

Oleandomycin is a macrolide antibacterial produced by the growth of certain strains of *Streptomyces antibioticus* with actions and uses similar to those of erythromycin (p.208). It has antimicrobial activity weaker than that of erythromycin. It has been given by mouth or intravenously as the phosphate.

Troleandomycin (p.274) is the triacetyl ester.

---

## Orbifloxacin *(rINN)*

Orbifloxacino. 1-Cyclopropyl-7-(*cis*-3,5-dimethyl-1-piperazinyl)-5,6,8-trifluoro-1,4-dihydro-4-oxo-3-quinolinecarboxylic acid.

$C_{19}H_{20}F_3N_3O_3$ = 395.4.
*CAS — 113617-63-3.*

### Profile

Orbifloxacin is a fluoroquinolone antibacterial used in veterinary medicine.

---

## Oritavancin *(rINN)*

LY-333328. (4″R)-22-*O*-(3-Amino-2,3,6-trideoxy-3-*C*-methyl-α-L-*arabino*-hexopyranosyl)-$N^{3''}$-[*p*-(*p*-chlorophenyl)benzyl]vancomycin.

$C_{86}H_{97}Cl_3N_{10}O_{26}$ = 1793.1.
*CAS — 171099-57-3 (oritavancin); 192564-14-0 (oritavancin phosphate).*

NOTE. Oritavancin phosphate is *USAN*.

### Profile

Oritavancin is a glycopeptide antibacterial under investigation for the treatment of complicated infections of the skin and soft tissues due to Gram-positive bacteria.

---

## Ormetoprim *(USAN, rINN)*

NSC-95072; Ormetoprima; Ro-5-9754. 5-(4,5-Dimethoxy-2-methylphenyl)methyl-2,4-pyrimidinediamine.

$C_{14}H_{18}N_4O_2$ = 274.3.
*CAS — 6981-18-6.*

### Profile

Ormetoprim is a diaminopyrimidine antibacterial used in veterinary medicine in combination with sulfadimethoxine.

---

# Oxacillin Sodium *(BANM, USAN, rINNM)*

(5-Methyl-3-phenyl-4-isoxazolyl)penicillin Sodium; Oxacilina sódica; Oxacillinum Natricum; Oxacillinum Natrium; P-12; SQ-16423. Sodium (6*R*)-6-(5-methyl-3-phenylisoxazole-4-carboxamido)penicillanate monohydrate.

$C_{19}H_{18}N_3NaO_5S,H_2O$ = 441.4.
*CAS — 66-79-5 (oxacillin); 1173-88-2 (anhydrous oxacillin sodium); 7240-38-2 (oxacillin sodium monohydrate).*
*ATC — J01CF04.*

**Pharmacopoeias.** In *Chin.* and *US.*

**USP 27** (Oxacillin Sodium). A fine white crystalline powder, odourless or having a slight odour. Freely soluble in water, in dimethyl sulfoxide, and in methyl alcohol; slightly soluble in dehydrated alcohol, in chloroform, in methyl acetate, and in pyridine; insoluble in ether, in ethyl acetate, in ethylene chloride, and in benzene. pH of a 3% solution in water is between 4.5 and 7.5. Store in airtight containers at a mean temperature not exceeding 25°.

**Incompatibility.** Oxacillin sodium has been reported to be incompatible with aminoglycosides and tetracyclines.

## Adverse Effects and Precautions

As for Flucloxacillin, p.213.

**Effects on the liver.** References.

1. Onorato IM, Axelrod JL. Hepatitis from intravenous high-dose oxacillin therapy: findings in an adult inpatient population. *Ann Intern Med* 1978; **89:** 497–500.
2. Saliba B, Herbert PN. Oxacillin hepatotoxicity in HIV-infected patients. *Ann Intern Med* 1994; **120:** 1048.
3. Maraqa NF, *et al.* Higher occurrence of hepatotoxicity and rash in patients treated with oxacillin, compared with those treated with nafcillin and other commonly used antimicrobials. *Clin Infect Dis* 2002; **34:** 50–4.

**Sodium content.** Each g of oxacillin sodium contains about 2.3 mmol of sodium.

## Interactions

As for Benzylpenicillin, p.164.

## Antimicrobial Action

As for Flucloxacillin, p.213.

**Resistance.** The isolation of pneumococci resistant to oxacillin but sensitive to benzylpenicillin has been reported.[1,2] The resistance was due to acquisition of a low-affinity penicillin-binding protein and conferred cross-resistance to meticillin and cloxacillin, and, to a lesser degree, to cefotaxime.

1. Johnson AP, *et al.* Oxacillin-resistant pneumococci sensitive to penicillin. *Lancet* 1993; **341:** 1222.
2. Dowson CG, *et al.* Genetics of oxacillin resistance in clinical isolates of Streptococcus pneumoniae that are oxacillin resistant and penicillin susceptible. *Antimicrob Agents Chemother* 1994; **38:** 49–53.

## Pharmacokinetics

Oxacillin is incompletely absorbed from the gastrointestinal tract. Absorption is reduced by the presence of food in the stomach and is less than with cloxacillin. Peak plasma concentrations of 3 to 6 micrograms/mL have been achieved 1 hour after a dose of 500 mg given by mouth to fasting subjects. Following the intramuscular injection of 500 mg, peak plasma concentrations of up to 15 micrograms/mL have been achieved after 30 minutes. Doubling the dose can double the plasma concentration. About 93% of the oxacillin in the circulation is bound to plasma proteins. Oxacillin has been reported to have a plasma half-life of about 0.5 hours. The half-life is prolonged in neonates.

The distribution of oxacillin into body tissues and fluids is similar to that of cloxacillin (p.198).

Oxacillin undergoes some metabolism, and the unchanged drug and metabolites are excreted in the urine by glomerular filtration and renal tubular secretion.

About 20 to 30% of an oral dose, and more than 40% of an intramuscular dose, is rapidly excreted in the urine. Oxacillin is also excreted in the bile.

Plasma concentrations are enhanced by probenecid.

## Uses and Administration

Oxacillin is an isoxazolyl penicillin used similarly to flucloxacillin (p.214) in the treatment of infections due to staphylococci resistant to benzylpenicillin.

Oxacillin is given by mouth or by injection as the sodium salt. Doses are expressed in terms of the equivalent amount of oxacillin. 1.1 g of oxacillin sodium is approximately equivalent to 1 g of oxacillin. Oral doses should preferably be given at least 1 hour before, or 2 hours after, meals. Usual adult oral doses are 0.5 to 1 g of oxacillin every 4 to 6 hours. Similar doses may be given by intramuscular injection, by slow intravenous injection over about 10 minutes, or by intravenous infusion.

Children weighing less than 40 kg may be given 50 to 100 mg/kg daily in divided doses by mouth or parenterally.

Doses may be increased in severe infections.

## Preparations

***USP 27:*** Oxacillin for Injection; Oxacillin Injection; Oxacillin Sodium Capsules; Oxacillin Sodium for Oral Solution.

**Proprietary Preparations** (details are given in Part 3)
***Austria:*** Stapenor; ***Belg.:*** Penstapho; ***Braz.:*** Oxacil; Oxapen; Roxacilin; Staficilin N; Teutocilin; ***Fr.:*** Bristopen; ***Ger.:*** InfectoStaph; Stapenor†; ***Ital.:*** Penstapho; ***USA:*** Bactocill†.

**Multi-ingredient:** ***Austria:*** Optocillin†; ***Ger.:*** Optocillin.

---

## Oxolinic Acid *(BAN, USAN, rINN)*

Ácido oxolínico; Acidum Oxolinicum; NSC-110364; W-4565. 5-Ethyl-5,8-dihydro-8-oxo-1,3-dioxolo[4,5-*g*]quinoline-7-carboxylic acid.

$C_{13}H_{11}NO_5$ = 261.2.
*CAS — 14698-29-4.*
*ATC — J01MB05.*

**Pharmacopoeias.** In *Eur.* (see p.vi).

**Ph. Eur. 5.0** (Oxolinic Acid). An almost white or pale yellow crystalline powder. Practically insoluble in water and in alcohol; very slightly soluble in dichloromethane; dissolves in dilute solutions of alkali hydroxides. Protect from light.

### Profile

Oxolinic acid is a 4-quinolone antibacterial with properties similar to those of nalidixic acid (p.234), although adverse effects on the CNS may be more frequent. It is given in the treatment of urinary-tract infections in a usual dose of 750 mg by mouth every 12 hours, preferably after food.

### Preparations

**Proprietary Preparations** (details are given in Part 3)
***Belg.:*** Uritrate†; ***Braz.:*** Urilin; ***Fr.:*** Urotrate†; ***Port.:*** Cistopax; ***Spain:*** Oribiox†; Oxoinex.

## Oxytetracycline *(BAN, rINN)*

Glomycin; Hydroxytetracycline; Oxitetraciclina; Oxytetracyclinum; Riomitsin; Terrafungine. 4S,4aR,5S,5aR,6S,12aS-4-Dimethylamino-1,4,4a,5,5a,6,11,12a-octahydro-3,5,6,10,12,12a-hexahydroxy-6-methylene-1,11-dioxonaphthacene-2-carboxamide; 5β-Hydroxytetracycline.

$C_{22}H_{24}N_2O_9$ = 460.4.
*CAS — 79-57-2 (anhydrous oxytetracycline); 6153-64-6 (oxytetracycline dihydrate).*
*ATC — D06AA03; G01AA07; J01AA06; S01AA04.*

**Pharmacopoeias.** In *Eur.* (see p.vi) and *Int.*, which specify the dihydrate ($C_{22}H_{24}N_2O_9,2H_2O$ = 496.5); *Pol.* and *US* allow the anhydrous substance or the dihydrate.

**Ph. Eur. 5.0** (Oxytetracycline Dihydrate). A substance produced by the growth of certain strains of *Streptomyces rimosus* or obtained by any other means. A yellow, crystalline powder. Very slightly soluble in water; dissolves in dilute acid and alkaline solutions. A 1% suspension in water has a pH of 4.5 to 7.5. Store in airtight containers. Protect from light.

**USP 27** (Oxytetracycline). A pale yellow to tan, odourless crystalline powder, that darkens on exposure to strong sunlight. Soluble 1 in 4150 of water, 1 in 66 of dehydrated alcohol, and 1 in 6250 of ether; sparingly soluble in alcohol; practically insoluble in chloroform; freely soluble in 3N hydrochloric acid and in alkaline solutions. pH of a 1% suspension in water is between 4.5 and 7.0. It loses potency in solutions of pH below 2 and is rapidly destroyed by alkali hydroxide solutions. Store in airtight containers. Protect from light.

### Oxytetracycline Calcium *(BANM, rINNM)*

Oxitetraciclina cálcica.

$C_{44}H_{46}CaN_4O_{18}$ = 958.9.
*CAS — 15251-48-6 (xCa).*
*ATC — D06AA03; G01AA07; J01AA06; S01AA04.*

**Pharmacopoeias.** In *Br.* and *US.*

**BP 2003** (Oxytetracycline Calcium). A pale yellow to greenish-fawn, crystalline powder. Practically insoluble in water; soluble in dilute acids; dissolves slowly in dilute ammonia solution. A 2.5% suspension in water has a pH of 6.0 to 7.5. Store at a temperature of 2° to 8°. Protect from light.

**USP 27** (Oxytetracycline Calcium). A yellow to light brown crystalline powder. Insoluble in water; soluble 1 in more than 1000 of alcohol, of chloroform, and of ether, and 1 in 15 of 0.1N sodium hydroxide. pH of a 2.5% suspension in water is between 6.0 and 8.0. Store in airtight containers at a temperature between 8° and 15°. Protect from light.

### Oxytetracycline Hydrochloride *(BANM, rINNM)*

Hidrocloruro de oxitetraciclina; Oxytetracyclini Hydrochloridum.

$C_{22}H_{24}N_2O_9$,HCl = 496.9.
*CAS — 2058-46-0.*
*ATC — D06AA03; G01AA07; J01AA06; S01AA04.*

**Pharmacopoeias.** In *Chin., Eur.* (see p.vi), *Int., Jpn, Pol.*, and *US.*

**Ph. Eur. 5.0** (Oxytetracycline Hydrochloride). A yellow, hygroscopic, crystalline powder. Freely soluble in water; sparingly soluble in alcohol. Solutions in water become turbid on standing owing to the precipitation of oxytetracycline. A 1% solution in water has a pH of 2.3 to 2.9. Store in airtight containers. Protect from light.

**USP 27** (Oxytetracycline Hydrochloride). A yellow, odourless, hygroscopic, crystalline powder. It decomposes at temperatures exceeding 180°, and exposure to strong sunlight or temperatures exceeding 90° in moist air causes it to darken. Its potency is diminished in solutions having a pH below 2, and it is rapidly destroyed by alkali hydroxide solutions. Freely soluble in water, but crystals of oxytetracycline separate as a result of partial hydrolysis of the hydrochloride; sparingly soluble in alcohol and in methyl alcohol, and even less soluble in dehydrated alcohol; insoluble in chloroform and in ether. pH of a 1% solution in water is between 2.0 and 3.0. Store in airtight containers. Protect from light.

**Incompatibility.** Oxytetracycline injections have an acid pH and incompatibility may reasonably be expected with alkaline preparations, or with drugs unstable at low pH. Tetracyclines can chelate metal cations to produce insoluble complexes, and incompatibility has been reported with solutions containing metallic salts.

Reports of incompatibility are not always consistent, and other factors, such as the strength and composition of the vehicles used, may play a role.

### Adverse Effects and Precautions

As for Tetracycline Hydrochloride, p.266.

Oxytetracycline may produce less tooth discoloration than some other tetracyclines but gastrointestinal symptoms tend to be more severe.

**Porphyria.** For the suggestion that oxytetracycline might be porphyrinogenic, see under Tetracycline Hydrochloride, p.267.

### Interactions

As for Tetracycline Hydrochloride, p.267.

### Antimicrobial Action

As for Tetracycline Hydrochloride, p.267. It is somewhat less active against many organisms.

### Pharmacokinetics

As for Tetracycline Hydrochloride, p.268. A dose of 500 mg every 6 hours by mouth is reported to produce steady-state plasma concentrations of 3 to 4 micrograms/mL. Plasma protein binding is reported to be about 20 to 40% and the half-life to be approximately 9 hours.

### Uses and Administration

Oxytetracycline is a tetracycline derivative with actions and uses similar to those of tetracycline (p.268).

Oxytetracycline dihydrate or hydrochloride are usually used in tablets, capsules, and injections, and the calcium salt in aqueous oral suspensions; all three are also used in topical preparations. Doses have been expressed as anhydrous oxytetracycline, the dihydrate, or the hydrochloride but in practice this appears to make little difference. Oxytetracycline dihydrate and oxytetracycline hydrochloride 1.08 g, and oxytetracycline calcium 1.04 g, are each approximately equivalent to 1 g of oxytetracycline.

Oxytetracycline is usually given in adult doses of 250 to 500 mg four times daily by mouth, usually 1 hour before food or 2 hours after food. Older children (over 8 years) have been given 25 to 50 mg/kg daily by mouth, in 4 divided doses, but the effect of tetracyclines on teeth and bones should be considered.

Doses of oxytetracycline 250 to 500 mg daily have been used in acne, although the *British National Formulary* advocates a dose of 1 g daily.

Oxytetracycline is sometimes given intramuscularly, in doses of 250 to 300 mg daily, but this route may be painful and produces lower blood concentrations than oral administration in the recommended doses. It has also been given intravenously.

Oxytetracycline and its salts have been applied topically, often with other agents, as a variety of eye and ear drops, ointments, creams, and sprays.

### Preparations

***BP 2003:*** Oxytetracycline Capsules; Oxytetracycline Tablets;
***USP 27:*** Oxytetracycline and Nystatin Capsules; Oxytetracycline and Nystatin for Oral Suspension; Oxytetracycline Calcium Oral Suspension; Oxytetracycline for Injection; Oxytetracycline Hydrochloride and Hydrocortisone Acetate Ophthalmic Suspension; Oxytetracycline Hydrochloride and Hydrocortisone Ointment; Oxytetracycline Hydrochloride and Polymyxin B Sulfate Ointment; Oxytetracycline Hydrochloride and Polymyxin B Sulfate Ophthalmic Ointment; Oxytetracycline Hydrochloride and Polymyxin B Sulfate Topical Powder; Oxytetracycline Hydrochloride and Polymyxin B Sulfate Vaginal Tablets; Oxytetracycline Hydrochloride Capsules; Oxytetracycline Injection; Oxytetracycline Tablets.

**Proprietary Preparations** (details are given in Part 3)
***Arg.:*** Terramicina; ***Braz.:*** Terramicina; ***Denm.:*** Oxytetral†; ***Fr.:*** Posycycline; Terramycine Solu-Retard†; Tetranase†; ***Ger.:*** Tetra-Tablinen†; ***Gr.:*** Terramycin; ***Hong Kong:*** Oxylim; Terramycin†; ***India:*** Terramycin; ***Irl.:*** Clinimycin; ***Malaysia:*** Oxylim; ***Mex.:*** Metrecina; Oxitraklin; Terrados; Terramicina; Tracin†; ***Norw.:*** Oxytetral; ***Port.:*** Geomicina; Terricil; ***S.Afr.:*** Acu-Oxytet†; Be-Oxytet; Cotet; Dynoxytet†; O-4 Cycline; O-Tet†; Oxyt†; Oxypan; Roxy; Spectratet†; Tetracem; Tetramel; ***Singapore:*** Oxylim; Terramycin; ***Spain:*** Terramicina; ***Swed.:*** Oxytetral; ***Thai.:*** Oxycline; Oxylim; Servicyclin†; Terramycin†; ***UK:*** Oxymycin; Oxytetramix; Terramycin†; ***USA:*** Terramycin.

**Multi-ingredient:** ***Arg.:*** Terra-Cortril; Terra-Cortril Nistatina; Terramicina con Polimixina B; ***Austria:*** Tetra-Gelomyrtol; ***Belg.:*** Eoline; Terra-Cortril; Terramycine; ***Braz.:*** Asseptobron†; Terra-Cortril; Terra-Cortril com Polimixina B†; Terramicina Pomada; ***Denm.:*** Terramycin Polymyxin B; ***Fin.:*** Terra-Cortril; Terra-Cortril P; ***Fr.:*** Auricularum; Primyxine; Ster-Dex; ***Ger.:*** Bisolvomycin†; Corti Biciron N; Farco-Tril; Oxy Biciron; Terracortril; Terramycin; Tetra-Gelomyrtol; ***Gr.:*** Oxacycle-P; Terra-Cortil; Terramycin with Polymyxin; ***Hong Kong:*** Terramycin with Polymyxin B; ***India:*** Terramycin SF; ***Irl.:*** Terra-Cortril Nystatin†; Terra-Cortril†; ***Israel:*** Auricularum; Tarocyn†; Terramycin; ***Ital.:*** Cosmiciclina; ***Malaysia:*** Terramycin; ***Mex.:*** Andociclina Balsamica; Terramicina; ***Neth.:*** Terra-Cortril Gel Steraject met polymyxine-B; Terra-Cortril met polymyxine-B; Terramycin met polymyxine-B†; ***Norw.:*** Terra-Cortril; Terra-Cortril Polymyxin B; Terramycin Polymyxin B; ***Port.:*** Corticil T; ***S.Afr.:*** Bisolvomycin†; Terra-Cortril; Terramycin; ***Singapore:*** Terramycin; ***Spain:*** Coliriocilina Espectro†; Pulmonilo Synergium†; Terra-Cortril; Terramicina; ***Swed.:*** Terracortril; Terracortril med polymyxin B; Terramycin Polymyxin B; ***Switz.:*** Terracortril; Terramycine†; ***Thai.:*** Terramycin; Terrasil; ***UK:*** Terra-Cortril; Terra-Cortril Nystatin†; Trimovate; ***USA:*** Terak; Terra-Cortril; Terramycin with Polymyxin B; Urobiotic-250.

## Panipenem *(rINN)*

(+)-(5R,6S)-3-[[(S)-1-Acetimidoyl-3-pyrrolidinyl]thio]-6-[(R)-1-hydroxyethyl]-7-oxo-1-azabicyclo[3.2.0]hept-2-ene-2-carboxylic acid.

$C_{15}H_{21}N_3O_4S$ = 339.4.
*CAS — 87726-17-8.*

**Pharmacopoeias.** In *Jpn.*

### Profile

Panipenem is a carbapenem beta-lactam antibacterial similar to imipenem (p.221). It is given with betamipron (p.165), which reduces its adverse renal effects, by intravenous infusion. The usual adult dose is 500 mg twice daily.

◊ References.

1. Goa KL, Noble S. Panipenem/betamipron. *Drugs* 2003; **63:** 913–25.

### Preparations

**Proprietary Preparations** (details are given in Part 3)
**Multi-ingredient:** ***Jpn:*** Carbenin.

## Pazufloxacin Mesilate

Pazufloxacin mesilate *(rINNM)*; T-3762; T-3761 (pazufloxacin). (−)-(3S)-10-(1-Aminocyclopropyl)-9-fluoro-2,3-dihydro-3-methyl-7-oxo-7H-pyrido[1,2,3-de]-1,4-benzoxazine-6-carboxylic acid methanesulfonate.

$C_{16}H_{15}FN_2O_4$, $CH_3SO_3H$ = 414.4.
*CAS — 127045-41-4 (pazufloxacin); 163680-77-1 (pazufloxacin mesilate).*

### Profile

Pazufloxacin is a fluoroquinolone antibacterial given by intravenous infusion as the mesilate in the treatment of susceptible infections in a usual adult dose of 1 g daily in 2 divided doses.

### Preparations

**Proprietary Preparations** (details are given in Part 3)
***Jpn:*** Pasil; Pazucross.

## Pefloxacin Mesilate *(BANM, rINNM)*

EU-5306 (pefloxacin); Mesilato de pefloxacino; Pefloxacin Mesylate *(USAN)*; Pefloxacini Mesilas Dihydricus; 1589-RB (pefloxacin); 41982-RP. 1-Ethyl-6-fluoro-1,4-dihydro-7-(4-methyl-1-piperazinyl)-4-oxo-3-quinolinecarboxylic acid methanesulphonate dihydrate.

$C_{17}H_{20}FN_3O_3,CH_4O_3S,2H_2O$ = 465.5.
*CAS — 70458-92-3 (pefloxacin); 70458-95-6 (pefloxacin mesilate).*
*ATC — J01MA03.*

**Pharmacopoeias.** In *Eur.* (see p.vi) and *Pol.*

**Ph. Eur. 5.0** (Pefloxacin Mesilate Dihydrate). A fine, white or almost white powder. Freely soluble in water; slightly soluble in alcohol; very slightly soluble in dichloromethane. A 1% solution in water has a pH of 3.5 to 4.5. Store in airtight containers. Protect from light.

### Profile

Pefloxacin is a fluoroquinolone antibacterial with actions and uses similar to those of ciprofloxacin (p.188). It also has bactericidal activity against *Mycobacterium leprae* and has been tried in the treatment of leprosy (p.133).

Pefloxacin has a longer plasma half-life than ciprofloxacin (about 8 to 13 hours) and is also extensively metabolised, the principal metabolite being *N*-desmethylpefloxacin which is otherwise known as norfloxacin (p.238).

Pefloxacin is given by mouth or by intravenous infusion as the mesilate in the treatment of susceptible infections. Doses are expressed in terms of the equivalent amount of pefloxacin and are usually 400 mg twice daily by mouth or by intravenous infusion.

Fluoroquinolones have caused adverse effects on the musculoskeletal system (see under Ciprofloxacin, p.189) and in the case of pefloxacin this has led to certain restrictions in some countries.

**Adverse effects.** References to adverse effects with pefloxacin.

1. Chevalier X, *et al.* A case of destructive polyarthropathy in a 17-year-old youth following pefloxacin treatment. *Drug Safety* 1992; **7:** 310–14.
2. Al-Hedaithy MA, Noreddin AM. Hypersensitivity anaphylactoid reaction to pefloxacin in a patient with AIDS. *Ann Pharmacother* 1996; **30:** 612–14.
3. Chang H, *et al.* Pefloxacin-induced arthropathy in an adolescent with brain abscess. *Scand J Infect Dis* 1996; **28:** 641–3.

**Pharmacokinetics.** References to the pharmacokinetics of pefloxacin.

1. Bressolle F, *et al.* Pefloxacin clinical pharmacokinetics. *Clin Pharmacokinet* 1994; **27:** 418–46.

2. Moreau JL, *et al*. Penetration of pefloxacin and its desmethyl metabolite into the uroepithelium after a 800-mg single oral dose in human patients. *Eur J Clin Pharmacol* 1996; **49:** 401–5.
3. Jacoberger B, *et al*. Concentrations of pefloxacin in plasma and tissue after administration as surgical prophylaxis. *Antimicrob Agents Chemother* 1998; **42:** 425–7.
4. Giannopoulos A, *et al*. Pharmacokinetics of intravenously administered pefloxacin in the prostate; perspectives for its application in surgical prophylaxis. *Int J Antimicrob Agents* 2001; **17:** 221–4.

### Preparations

**Proprietary Preparations** (details are given in Part 3)
***Austria:*** Peflacine†; ***Belg.:*** Peflacine†; ***Braz.:*** Floxinon; Peflacin; Pefloxidina; ***Fr.:*** Peflacine; ***Ger.:*** Peflacin†; ***Gr.:*** Idrostamin; Labocton; Peflacine; ***Hong Kong:*** Abaktal†; Peflacine†; ***India:*** Ifipef; Pefbid; Pelox; Proflox; ***Israel:*** Peflacine†; ***Ital.:*** Peflacin; Peflox; ***Malaysia:*** Peflacine; ***Mex.:*** Nopriken; Peflacina; Uroquina†; ***Port.:*** Peflacine; ***Spain:*** Azuben; Peflacine; ***Thai.:*** Abaktal; Peflacine.

## Penethamate Hydriodide *(BAN)*

Diethylaminoethyl Penicillin G Hydroiodide; Penetamato, hidroioduro de. 2-Diethylaminoethyl (6*R*)-6-(2-phenylacetamido)penicillanate hydriodide.

$C_{22}H_{31}N_3O_4S,HI$ = 561.5.

*CAS — 3689-73-4 (penethamate); 808-71-9 (penethamate hydriodide).*

### Profile

Penethamate is a penicillin antibacterial used as the hydriodide in veterinary medicine.

## Pheneticillin Potassium *(BANM, rINNM)*

Feneticilina potásica; Penicillin B; Phenethicillin Potassium; Pheneticillinum Kalicum; Potassium α-Phenoxyethylpenicillin. A mixture of the D(+)- and L(−)-isomers of potassium (6*R*)-6-(2-phenoxypropionamido)penicillanate.

$C_{17}H_{19}KN_2O_5S$ = 402.5.

*CAS — 147-55-7 (pheneticillin); 132-93-4 (pheneticillin potassium).*

*ATC — J01CE05.*

**Pharmacopoeias.** In *Jpn*.

### Profile

Pheneticillin is a phenoxypenicillin with actions and uses similar to those of phenoxymethylpenicillin (below). It has been given by mouth, as the potassium salt, for the treatment of susceptible mild to moderate infections. Pheneticillin sodium has also been used.

### Preparations

**Proprietary Preparations** (details are given in Part 3)
***Neth.:*** Broxil.

## Phenoxymethylpenicillin *(BAN, rINN)*

Fenoximetilpenicilina; Penicillin, Phenoxymethyl; Penicillin V *(USAN)*; Phénomycilline; Phenoxymethyl Penicillin; Phenoxymethylpenicillinum. (6*R*)-6-(2-Phenoxyacetamido)penicillanic acid.

$C_{16}H_{18}N_2O_5S$ = 350.4.

*CAS — 87-08-1.*

*ATC — J01CE02.*

**Pharmacopoeias.** In *Eur.* (see p.vi), *Int., Pol., US,* and *Viet.*

**Ph. Eur. 5.0** (Phenoxymethylpenicillin). A substance produced by the growth of certain strains of *Penicillium notatum* or related organisms on a culture medium containing an appropriate precursor, or obtained by any other means. A white or almost white, slightly hygroscopic, crystalline powder. Very slightly soluble in water; soluble in alcohol. A 0.5% suspension in water has a pH of 2.4 to 4.0. Store protected from moisture.

**USP 27** (Penicillin V). A white, odourless crystalline powder. Very slightly soluble in water; freely soluble in alcohol and in acetone; insoluble in fixed oils. pH of a 3% suspension in water is between 2.5 and 4.0. Store in airtight containers.

## Phenoxymethylpenicillin Calcium *(BANM, rINNM)*

Fenoximetilpenicilina cálcica; Penicillin V Calcium; Phenoxymethylpenicillinum Calcicum.

$(C_{16}H_{17}N_2O_5S)_2Ca,2H_2O$ = 774.9.

*CAS — 147-48-8 (anhydrous phenoxymethylpenicillin calcium); 73368-74-8 (phenoxymethylpenicillin calcium dihydrate).*

*ATC — J01CE02.*

**Pharmacopoeias.** In *Int.*

## Phenoxymethylpenicillin Potassium *(BANM, rINNM)*

Fenoximetilpenicilina potásica; Fenoximetilpenicilina Potássica; Penicillin V Potassium *(USAN)*; Phenoxymethylpenicillinum Kalicum.

$C_{16}H_{17}KN_2O_5S$ = 388.5.

*CAS — 132-98-9.*

*ATC — J01CE02.*

**Pharmacopoeias.** In *Chin., Eur.* (see p.vi), *Int., Pol., US,* and *Viet.*

**Ph. Eur. 5.0** (Phenoxymethylpenicillin Potassium). A white or almost white, crystalline powder. Freely soluble in water; practically insoluble in alcohol. A 0.5% solution in water has a pH of 5.5 to 7.5.

**USP 27** (Penicillin V Potassium). A white, odourless crystalline powder. Very soluble in water; soluble 1 in 150 of alcohol; insoluble in acetone. pH of a 3% solution in water is between 4.0 and 7.5. Store in airtight containers.

### Units

The first International Standard Preparation (1957) of phenoxymethylpenicillin contained 1695 units/mg but was discontinued in 1968. Despite this, doses of phenoxymethylpenicillin are still expressed in units in some countries.

Phenoxymethylpenicillin 250 mg is approximately equivalent to 400 000 units.

### Adverse Effects and Precautions

As for Benzylpenicillin, p.163.

Phenoxymethylpenicillin is usually well tolerated but may occasionally cause transient nausea and diarrhoea.

**Potassium content.** Each g of phenoxymethylpenicillin potassium contains about 2.6 mmol of potassium.

### Interactions

As for Benzylpenicillin, p.164.

**Antibacterials.** Reduced absorption was reported when phenoxymethylpenicillin was given following a course of *neomycin* by mouth.[1]

1. Cheng SH, White A. Effect of orally administered neomycin on the absorption of penicillin V. *N Engl J Med* 1962; **267:** 1296–7.

**Beta blockers.** Beta blockers might have potentiated anaphylactic reactions in 2 patients on *nadolol* and *propranolol*, respectively, who died following a dose of phenoxymethylpenicillin.[1]

1. Berkelman RL, *et al*. Beta-adrenergic antagonists and fatal anaphylactic reactions to oral penicillin. *Ann Intern Med* 1986; **104:** 134.

### Antimicrobial Action

Phenoxymethylpenicillin has a range of antimicrobial activity similar to that of benzylpenicillin (p.164) and a similar mode of action. It may be less active against some susceptible organisms, particularly Gram-negative bacteria.

The mechanisms and patterns of resistance to phenoxymethylpenicillin are similar to those of benzylpenicillin.

### Pharmacokinetics

Phenoxymethylpenicillin is more resistant to inactivation by gastric acid and is more completely absorbed than benzylpenicillin from the gastrointestinal tract. Absorption is usually rapid, although variable, with about 60% of an oral dose being absorbed. The calcium and potassium salts are better absorbed than the free acid. Peak plasma concentrations of 3 to 5 micrograms/mL have been observed 30 to 60 minutes after a dose of 500 mg. The effect of food on absorption appears to be slight. The plasma half-life of phenoxymethylpenicillin is about 30 to 60 minutes and may be increased to about 4 hours in severe renal impairment. About 80% is reported to be protein bound. The distribution and elimination of phenoxymethylpenicillin is similar to that of benzylpenicillin (p.165). It is metabolised in the liver to a greater extent than benzylpenicillin; several metabolites have been identified including penicilloic acid. The unchanged drug and metabolites are excreted rapidly in the urine. Only small amounts are excreted in the bile.

### Uses and Administration

Phenoxymethylpenicillin is used similarly to benzylpenicillin (p.165) in the treatment or prophylaxis of infections caused by susceptible organisms, especially streptococci. It is used only for the treatment of mild to moderate infections, and not for chronic, severe, or deep-seated infections since absorption can be unpredictable. Patients treated initially with parenteral benzylpenicillin may continue treatment with phenoxymethylpenicillin by mouth once a satisfactory clinical response has been obtained. Specific indications for phenoxymethylpenicillin include anthrax (mild uncomplicated infections), Lyme disease (early stage in pregnant women or young children), pharyngitis or tonsillitis, rheumatic fever (primary and secondary prophylaxis), streptococcal skin infections, and spleen disorders (pneumococcal infection prophylaxis). For details of these infections and their treatment, see under Choice of Antibacterial, p.120.

*Administration and dosage.* Phenoxymethylpenicillin is given by mouth, usually as the potassium or calcium salt, preferably at least 30 minutes before, or 2 hours after, food. Benzathine phenoxymethylpenicillin (p.163) is also used.

Doses are expressed in terms of the equivalent amount of phenoxymethylpenicillin. 1.1 g of phenoxymethylpenicillin calcium and 1.1 g of phenoxymethylpenicillin potassium are each approximately equivalent to 1 g of phenoxymethylpenicillin.

Usual adult doses have been 250 to 500 mg every 6 hours, but the *British National Formulary* recommends up to 1 g every 6 hours in severe infections. Children may be given the following doses every 6 hours: up to 1 year, 62.5 mg; 1 to 5 years, 125 mg; and 6 to 12 years, 250 mg. Dosage may need to be modified in severe renal impairment.

To prevent recurrences of rheumatic fever, WHO and the *British National Formulary* recommend 250 mg twice daily.

### Preparations

***BP 2003:*** Phenoxymethylpenicillin Oral Solution; Phenoxymethylpenicillin Tablets;
***USP 27:*** Penicillin V for Oral Suspension; Penicillin V Potassium for Oral Solution; Penicillin V Potassium Tablets; Penicillin V Tablets.

**Proprietary Preparations** (details are given in Part 3)
***Arg.:*** Pen Oral; Penagrand; Penfantil; Penicina; ***Austral.:*** Abbocillin-VK; Cilicaine VK; Cilopen VK; LPV; Penhexal VK; PVK†; ***Austria:*** Aliucillin; Cliacil; Megacillin; Ospen; Pen-V; Penbene; Penstad; Star-Pen; ***Belg.:*** Peni-Oral†; ***Braz.:*** Meracilina; Oracilin; Pen-Ve-Oral; Penicigran; ***Canad.:*** Apo-Pen-VK; Ledercillin VK†; Nadopen-V; Novo-Pen-VK; Nu-Pen-VK; Pen-Vee; PVFK; V-Cillin K†; ***Denm.:*** Calcipen; Fenoxcillin†; Pancillin; Primcillin; Rocilin; Vepicombin; ***Fin.:*** Medicillin; Milcopen; V-Pen; ***Fr.:*** Oracilline; Ospen; ***Ger.:*** Antibiocin†; Arcasin; durapenicillin; InfectoCillin; Isocillin; Ispenoral; Jenacillin V; Megacillin oral; P-Mega-Tablinen; Pen; Pen Mega; Pen-BASF†; Pen-V-Merck†; Penbeta; Penhexal; Penicillat; V-Tablopen; ***Gr.:*** Ospen; ***Hong Kong:*** Ospen; Pen-V†; ***Irl.:*** Calvepen; Kopen; ***Israel:*** Rafapen Mega; Rafapen V-K; V-Pen; ***Ital.:*** Fenospen†; ***Malaysia:*** Beapen; Ospen KV; Penoxil V; ***Mex.:*** Anapenil; Kavipen; Megapenil; Pen-Vi-K; Pota-Vi-Kin; ***Neth.:*** Acipen; Acipen-V; ***Norw.:*** Apocillin; Calcipen; Femepen†; Kavepenin; Rocilin; Weifapenin; ***NZ:*** Cilicaine VK; Compocillin†; ***S.Afr.:*** Betapen; Darocillin†; Dynapen†; Len V.K.; Novo V-K; V-Cil-K†; ***Singapore:*** Ospen; ***Spain:*** Penilevel; ***Swed.:*** Calciopen†; Kavepenin; Tikacillin; ***Switz.:*** Arcasin†; Brunocillin; Fenoxypen†; Megacilline; Ospen; pen-V-basan; Penisol; Phenocillin; Rivopen-V†; Stabicilline; ***Thai.:*** Pen-V; Pener; Penveno; Servipen-V; ***UK:*** Distaquaine V-K†; Rimapen†; ***USA:*** Beepen-VK†; Pen-Vee K; Veetids.

**Multi-ingredient:** ***Spain:*** Penilevel Retard.

## Phthalylsulfathiazole *(BAN, rINN)*

Ftalilsulfatiazol; Phthalazolum; Phthalylsulfathiazolum; Phthalylsulphathiazole; Sulfaphtalylthiazol. 4′-(1,3-Thiazol-2-ylsulphamoyl)phthalanilic acid.

$C_{17}H_{13}N_3O_5S_2$ = 403.4.

*CAS — 85-73-4.*

*ATC — A07AB02.*

**Pharmacopoeias.** In *Eur.* (see p.vi) and *Viet.*

**Ph. Eur. 5.0** (Phthalylsulfathiazole). A white or yellowish-white crystalline powder. Practically insoluble in water; slightly soluble in alcohol and in acetone; freely soluble in dimethylformamide. Protect from light.

### Profile

Phthalylsulfathiazole is a sulfonamide with properties similar to those of sulfamethoxazole (p.261). It is poorly absorbed, about 95% remaining in the intestine and only about 5% being slowly hydrolysed to sulfathiazole and absorbed.

It is given, with other antibacterials, for its antibacterial action in the gastrointestinal tract in the treatment of infections and for bowel decontamination before surgery.

### Preparations

**Proprietary Preparations** (details are given in Part 3)
***Mex.:*** Kaotalil†.

**Multi-ingredient:** ***Arg.:*** Antidiar; Carbon Tabs; Colistop; Colistoral; Diarrocalmol; Estreptocarbocaftiazol; Gemipasmol; Lefaenteril; Opocarbon; Opocler; ***Austria:*** Hylakombun†; ***Braz.:*** Enterodina†; Enteroftal†; Enteromicina†; Enterovit†; Furazolin†; Parenterin; Sanadiar†; Tratocoli†; ***Chile:*** Imecol; Liracol; Testisan; ***Mex.:*** Ditayod†; Sultroquin; ***Port.:*** Cloranpectina; ***Spain:*** Estreptoenterol; ***Thai.:*** Chlorotracin; Coccila; Disento; Mediocin.

### Pipemidic Acid (BAN, rINN)

Ácido pipemídico; Acidum Pipemidicum Trihydricum; Piperamic Acid; 1489-RB. 8-Ethyl-5,8-dihydro-5-oxo-2-(piperazin-1-yl)pyrido[2,3-*d*]pyrimidine-6-carboxylic acid.

$C_{14}H_{17}N_5O_3$ = 303.3.

*CAS — 51940-44-4 (anhydrous pipemidic acid); 72571-82-5 (pipemidic acid trihydrate).*

*ATC — J01MB04.*

**Pharmacopoeias.** In *Chin., Eur.* (see p.vi), and *Jpn* (all as the trihydrate).

**Ph. Eur. 5.0** (Pipemidic Acid Trihydrate). A pale yellow or yellow crystalline powder. Very slightly soluble in water. It dissolves in dilute solutions of acids and of alkali hydroxides. Protect from light.

#### Profile

Pipemidic acid is a 4-quinolone antibacterial with properties similar to those of nalidixic acid (p.234), but is more active *in vitro* against some bacteria, including *Pseudomonas aeruginosa*. It is used (as the trihydrate) in the treatment of urinary-tract infections in doses equivalent to 400 mg of the anhydrous substance twice daily by mouth.

**Interactions.** For the effect of pipemidic acid on the clearance of xanthines, see under Caffeine, p.782, and Theophylline, p.801.

**Porphyria.** Pipemidic acid is considered to be unsafe in patients with porphyria because it has been shown to be porphyrinogenic in *in-vitro* systems.

#### Preparations

**Proprietary Preparations** (details are given in Part 3)
***Arg.:*** Finuret; Memento; Priper; ***Austria:*** Deblaston; ***Belg.:*** Pipram†; ***Braz.:*** Balurol; Elofuran; Pipram; Pipurol; Uroxina; ***Chile:*** Nupra; Purid; Uropimide; ***Fr.:*** Pipram; ***Ger.:*** Deblaston; ***Hong Kong:*** Urotractin; ***Ital.:*** Acipem; Biopim†; Biosoviran; Cistomid; Diperpen; Faremid; Filtrax; Pipeacid; Pipedac; Pipefort; Pipemid; Pipram; Pipurin; Pro-Uro†; Tractur†; Urodene; Uropimid; Urosan; Urosetic; Urotractin; Uroval†; ***Jpn:*** Dolcol; ***Malaysia:*** Urotractin; ***Mex.:*** Anurin†; Dicofarm†; Fustermid†; Pipemidol†; Uribac†; Uriken†; Uripiser; Urmidin†; Urogal†; Uronovag; Uropipemid; Urotal†; ***Neth.:*** Pipram; ***S.Afr.:*** Deblaston; Septidron; ***Singapore:*** Urotractin; ***Spain:*** Galusan; Nuril; Urisan; Uropipedil; ***Switz.:*** Deblaston†; ***Thai.:*** Pipedic; Urotractin.

**Multi-ingredient:** ***Arg.:*** Priper Plus.

---

## Piperacillin (BAN, rINN)

Piperacilina; Piperacillinum. (6*R*)-6-[*R*-2-(4-Ethyl-2,3-dioxopiperazine-1-carboxamido)-2-phenylacetamido]penicillanic acid monohydrate; 3-Dimethyl-7-oxo-4-thia-1-azabicyclo[3.2.0]heptane-2-carboxylic acid monohydrate.

$C_{23}H_{27}N_5O_7S,H_2O$ = 535.6.

*CAS — 61477-96-1 (anhydrous piperacillin); 66258-76-2 (piperacillin monohydrate).*

*ATC — J01CA12.*

**Pharmacopoeias.** In *Chin., Eur.* (see p.vi), and *US.*

**Ph. Eur. 5.0** (Piperacillin). A white or almost white powder. Slightly soluble in water and in ethyl acetate; freely soluble in methyl alcohol.

**USP 27** (Piperacillin). A white to off-white crystalline powder. Very slightly soluble in water; slightly soluble in ethyl acetate; sparingly soluble in isopropyl alcohol; very soluble in methyl alcohol.

### Piperacillin Sodium (BANM, USAN, rINNM)

CL-227193; Piperacilina sódica; Piperacillinum Natricum; T-1220.

$C_{23}H_{26}N_5NaO_7S$ = 539.5.

*CAS — 59703-84-3.*

*ATC — J01CA12.*

**Pharmacopoeias.** In *Chin., Eur.* (see p.vi), *Jpn, Pol.,* and *US.*

**Ph. Eur. 5.0** (Piperacillin Sodium). A white or almost white, hygroscopic powder. Freely soluble in water and in methyl alcohol; practically insoluble in ethyl acetate. A 10% solution in water has a pH of 5.0 to 7.0. Store in airtight containers.

**USP 27** (Piperacillin Sodium). A white to off-white solid. Freely soluble in water and in alcohol. pH of a 40% solution in water is between 5.5 and 7.5. Store in airtight containers.

**Incompatibility.** Piperacillin sodium has been reported to be incompatible with aminoglycosides and sodium bicarbonate.

**Stability.** References.

1. Zhang Y, Trissel LA. Stability of piperacillin and ticarcillin in AutoDose Infusion System bags. *Ann Pharmacother* 2001; **35:** 1360–3.

### Adverse Effects and Precautions

As for Carbenicillin Sodium, p.166.

Prolongation of bleeding time has been less frequent and less severe with piperacillin than with carbenicillin.

**Hypersensitivity.** In the mid 1980s there were reports of a relatively high incidence of adverse reactions to piperacillin, especially fever, in patients with cystic fibrosis.[1-3] However, the manufacturers[4] considered such patients to be particularly prone to allergy and cited reactions with other semisynthetic penicillins including carbenicillin and azlocillin.

Similar apparent hypersensitivity reactions have been reported in patients taking high doses of piperacillin and other ureidopenicillins, over long periods for other indications,[5] and with other penicillins in patients with cystic fibrosis,[6] although piperacillin does appear to be most frequently implicated.[6]

1. Stead RJ, *et al.* Adverse reactions to piperacillin in cystic fibrosis. *Lancet* 1984; **i:** 857–8.
2. Strandvik B. Adverse reactions to piperacillin in patients with cystic fibrosis. *Lancet* 1984; **i:** 1362.
3. Stead RJ, *et al.* Adverse reactions to piperacillin in adults with cystic fibrosis. *Thorax* 1985; **40:** 184–6.
4. Brock PG, Roach M. Adverse reactions to piperacillin in cystic fibrosis. *Lancet* 1984; **i:** 1070–1.
5. Lang R, *et al.* Adverse reactions to prolonged treatment with high doses of carbenicillin and ureidopenicillins. *Rev Infect Dis* 1991; **13:** 68–72.
6. Pleasants RA, *et al.* Allergic reactions to parenteral beta-lactam antibiotics in patients with cystic fibrosis. *Chest* 1994; **106:** 1124–8.

**Sodium content.** Each g of piperacillin sodium contains about 1.85 mmol of sodium. As piperacillin sodium has a lower sodium content than carbenicillin sodium, hypernatraemia and hypokalaemia are less likely to occur.

### Interactions

As for Benzylpenicillin, p.164.

**Neuromuscular blockers.** Piperacillin and other ureidopenicillins are reported to prolong the action of competitive muscle relaxants such as *vecuronium* (see Atracurium, p.1400).

### Antimicrobial Action

Piperacillin has a similar antimicrobial action to carbenicillin (p.166) and ticarcillin (p.270), but is active against a wider range of Gram-negative organisms, including *Klebsiella pneumoniae*. It is also generally more active *in vitro*, especially against *Pseudomonas aeruginosa* and the Enterobacteriaceae, against Gram-positive *Enterococcus faecalis*, and possibly against *Bacteroides fragilis*. There is, however, an inoculum effect, i.e. minimum inhibitory concentrations of piperacillin increase with the size of the inoculum.

Combinations of piperacillin and aminoglycosides have been shown to be synergistic *in vitro* against *Ps. aeruginosa* and Enterobacteriaceae. The effect of using piperacillin with other beta lactams has been less predictable. The activity of piperacillin against some organisms, resistant because of the production of beta-lactamases, may be restored by tazobactam, a beta-lactamase inhibitor. Such organisms include beta-lactamase-producing strains of staphylococci, *Escherichia coli, Haemophilus influenzae*, and *Bacteroides* spp.; the activity of piperacillin against *Ps. aeruginosa* is not enhanced by tazobactam.

Resistance has developed in *Ps. aeruginosa* during treatment with piperacillin, especially when used alone. There may be some cross-resistance with other antipseudomonal penicillins.

◊ References.

1. Higashitani F, *et al.* Inhibition of β-lactamases by tazobactam and in-vitro antibacterial activity of tazobactam combined with piperacillin. *J Antimicrob Chemother* 1990; **25:** 567–74.
2. Mehtar S, *et al.* The in-vitro activity of piperacillin/tazobactam, ciprofloxacin, ceftazidime and imipenem against multiple resistant Gram-negative bacteria. *J Antimicrob Chemother* 1990; **25:** 915–19.
3. Kempers J, MacLaren DM. Piperacillin/tazobactam and ticarcillin/clavulanic acid against resistant Enterobacteriaceae. *J Antimicrob Chemother* 1990; **26:** 598–9.
4. Kadima TA, Weiner JH. Mechanism of suppression of piperacillin resistance in enterobacteria by tazobactam. *Antimicrob Agents Chemother* 1997; **41:** 2177–83.
5. Klepser ME, *et al.* Comparison of the bactericidal activities of piperacillin-tazobactam, ticarcillin-clavulanate, and ampicillin-sulbactam against clinical isolates of Bacteroides fragilis, Enterococcus faecalis, Escherichia coli, and Pseudomonas aeruginosa. *Antimicrob Agents Chemother* 1997; **41:** 435–9.

### Pharmacokinetics

Piperacillin is not absorbed from the gastrointestinal tract. It is well absorbed after intramuscular use, peak plasma concentrations of 30 to 40 micrograms/mL being observed 30 to 50 minutes after a dose of 2 g. The pharmacokinetics of piperacillin are reported to be nonlinear and dose-dependent. The plasma half-life is about 1 hour, but is prolonged in neonates. In patients with severe renal impairment there may be a threefold increase in half-life; in those with end-stage renal failure half-lives of 4 to 6 hours have been reported, and in those with both renal and hepatic impairment much longer half-lives may result. About 20% of piperacillin in the circulation is bound to plasma proteins.

Piperacillin is widely distributed in body tissues and fluids. It crosses the placenta into the fetal circulation and small amounts are distributed into breast milk. There is little diffusion into the CSF except when the meninges are inflamed.

About 60 to 80% of a dose is excreted unchanged in the urine by glomerular filtration and tubular secretion within 24 hours, achieving high concentrations. High concentrations are also found in the bile and up to 20% of a dose may be excreted by this route.

Plasma concentrations are enhanced by probenecid.

Piperacillin is removed by haemodialysis.

*Piperacillin with tazobactam.* The pharmacokinetics of piperacillin do not appear to be altered by tazobactam, but piperacillin reduces the renal clearance of tazobactam.

◊ References.

1. Heikkilä A, Erkkola R. Pharmacokinetics of piperacillin during pregnancy. *J Antimicrob Chemother* 1991; **28:** 419–23.
2. Wise R, *et al.* Pharmacokinetics and tissue penetration of tazobactam administered alone and with piperacillin. *Antimicrob Agents Chemother* 1991; **35:** 1081–4.
3. Johnson CA, *et al.* Single-dose pharmacokinetics of piperacillin and tazobactam in patients with renal disease. *Clin Pharmacol Ther* 1992; **51:** 32–41.
4. Dupon M, *et al.* Plasma levels of piperacillin and vancomycin used as prophylaxis in liver transplant patients. *Eur J Clin Pharmacol* 1993; **45:** 529–34.
5. Sörgel F, Kinzig M. The chemistry, pharmacokinetics and tissue distribution of piperacillin/tazobactam. *J Antimicrob Chemother* 1993; **31** (suppl A): 39–60.
6. Reed MD, *et al.* Single-dose pharmacokinetics of piperacillin and tazobactam in infants and children. *Antimicrob Agents Chemother* 1994; **38:** 2817–26.
7. Bourget P, *et al.* Clinical pharmacokinetics of piperacillin-tazobactam combination in patients with major burns and signs of infection. *Antimicrob Agents Chemother* 1996; **40:** 139–45.
8. Occhipinti DJ, *et al.* Pharmacokinetics and pharmacodynamics of two multiple-dose piperacillin-tazobactam regimens. *Antimicrob Agents Chemother* 1997; **41:** 2511–17.

### Uses and Administration

Piperacillin is a ureidopenicillin that is used similarly to ticarcillin (p.271) for the treatment of infections caused by *Pseudomonas aeruginosa*, and also infections due to other susceptible bacteria. It has been used particularly in immunocompromised patients (neutropenic patients) and for biliary-tract infections (cholangitis). Other indications have included uncomplicated gonorrhoea due to penicillin-sensitive gonococci, and urinary-tract infections. It has also been used for surgical infection prophylaxis. For details of these infections and their treatment, see under Choice of Antibacterial, p.120. For the treatment of serious infections piperacillin is commonly used with an aminoglycoside, but they should be given separately because of possible incompatibility.

*Administration and dosage.* Piperacillin is given by injection as the sodium salt. Doses are expressed in terms of the equivalent amount of piperacillin. 1.04 g of piperacillin sodium is approximately equivalent to 1 g of piperacillin. Doses should generally be reduced in moderate to severe renal impairment.

Piperacillin may be given by slow intravenous injection over 3 to 5 minutes, by intravenous infusion over 20 to 30 minutes, or by deep intramuscular injection. Single doses of more than 2 g for adults or 500 mg for children should not be given by the intramuscular route.

For the treatment of serious or complicated infections, adults may be given piperacillin 200 to 300 mg/kg daily in divided doses intravenously; the usual dose is 3 to 4 g every 4 or 6 hours. In life-threatening infections, particularly those caused by *Pseudomonas* or *Klebsiella* spp., it should be given in a dose of not less than 16 g daily. The usual maximum daily dose is 24 g, although this has been exceeded.

For mild or uncomplicated infections, 100 to 125 mg/kg daily may be given to adults; usual doses are 2 g every 6 or 8 hours, or 4 g every 12 hours, intravenously, or 2 g every 8 or 12 hours intramuscularly.

Uncomplicated gonorrhoea may be treated by a single intramuscular dose of 2 g. Probenecid 1 g by mouth may be given 30 minutes before the injection.

For the prophylaxis of infection during surgery, 2 g just before the procedure, or when the umbilical cord is clamped in caesarean section, followed by at least 2 doses of 2 g at intervals of 4 or 6 hours within 24 hours of the procedure, may be given.

The intravenous route is preferred for infants and children. Those aged 1 month to 12 years may be given 100 to 300 mg/kg daily in 3 or 4 divided doses. Neonates less than 7 days old or weighing less than 2 kg may be given 150 mg/kg daily in 3 divided doses. Those more than 7 days old and weighing more than 2 kg may be given 300 mg/kg daily in 3 or 4 divided doses.

*Piperacillin with tazobactam.* Piperacillin has also been used with tazobactam (p.264), a beta-lactamase inhibitor, to widen its antibacterial spectrum to organisms usually resistant because of the production of beta-lactamases. The combination is given intravenously in a ratio of piperacillin (as the sodium salt) 8 parts to 1 part of tazobactam (as the sodium salt). Doses, calculated on piperacillin content, are similar to those of piperacillin alone.

◊ References.

1. Greenwood D, Finch RG, eds. Piperacillin/tazobactam: a new β-lactam/β-lactamase inhibitor combination. *J Antimicrob Chemother* 1993; **31** (suppl A): 1–124.
2. Schoonover LL, *et al.* Piperacillin/tazobactam: a new beta-lactam/beta-lactamase inhibitor combination. *Ann Pharmacother* 1995; **29:** 501–14.
3. Perry CM, Markham A. Piperacillin/tazobactam: an updated review of its use in the treatment of bacterial infections. *Drugs* 1999; **57:** 805–43.

### Preparations

***BP 2003:*** Piperacillin Intravenous Infusion;
***USP 27:*** Piperacillin for Injection.

**Proprietary Preparations** (details are given in Part 3)
***Arg.:*** Algiseptico; Piperac; ***Austral.:*** Pipril; ***Austria:*** Pipril; ***Belg.:*** Pipcil; ***Canad.:*** Pipracil; ***Denm.:*** Ivacin; ***Fr.:*** Piperilline†; ***Ger.:*** Pipera; Pipril; ***Gr.:*** Pipril; ***Hong Kong:*** Pipracil; ***India:*** Pipracil; ***Irl.:*** Pipril; ***Israel:*** Picillin; Pipril; ***Ital.:*** Avocin; Biopiper; Cilpier; Diperil; Ecosette; Eril; Farecillin; Peracil; Picillin; Piperital; Pipersal; Pipertex; Pipracin†; Reparcillin; Semipenil; Sintoplus; Viracillina; ***Jpn:*** Pentcillin; ***Malaysia:*** Pipracil; ***Mex.:*** Tazocin; ***Neth.:*** Pipcil†; ***NZ:*** Pipril; ***S.Afr.:*** Pipril†; ***Spain:*** Pipril†; ***Swed.:*** Ivacin†; ***Switz.:*** Pipril; ***Thai.:*** Pipracil; ***UK:*** Pipril†; ***USA:*** Pipracil†.

**Multi-ingredient:** ***Arg.:*** Pipetexina; Tazonam; ***Austral.:*** Tazocin; ***Austria:*** Fluxapril†; Tazonam; ***Belg.:*** Tazocin; ***Braz.:*** Tazocin; ***Canad.:*** Tazocin; ***Chile:*** Tazonam; ***Denm.:*** Tazocin; ***Fin.:*** Tazocin; ***Fr.:*** Tazocilline; ***Ger.:*** Fluxapril†; Tazobac; ***Gr.:*** Tazocin; ***Hong Kong:*** Tazocin; ***India:*** Zosyn; ***Irl.:*** Tazocin; ***Israel:*** Tazocin; ***Ital.:*** Tazobac†; Tazocin; ***Malaysia:*** Tazocin; ***Neth.:*** Tazocin; ***Norw.:*** Tazocin; ***NZ:*** Tazocin; ***Port.:*** Tazobac; ***S.Afr.:*** Tazocin; ***Singapore:*** Tazocin; ***Spain:*** Tazocel; ***Swed.:*** Tazocin; ***Switz.:*** Tazobac; ***Thai.:*** Tazocin; ***UK:*** Tazocin; ***USA:*** Zosyn.

## Pirlimycin Hydrochloride *(USAN, rINNM)*

Hidrocloruro de pirlimicina; U-57930E. Methyl 7-chloro-6,7,8-trideoxy-6-(*cis*-4-ethyl-L-pipecolamido)-1-thio-L-*threo*-α-D-*galacto*-octopyranoside monohydrochloride monohydrate.

$C_{17}H_{31}ClN_2O_5S,HCl,H_2O$ = 465.4.
*CAS — 79548-73-5 (pirlimycin); 77495-92-2 (pirlimycin hydrochloride).*

### Profile

Pirlimycin is a lincosamide antibacterial used in veterinary medicine.

## Piromidic Acid *(rINN)*

Ácido piromídico; PD-93. 8-Ethyl-5,8-dihydro-5-oxo-2-(pyrrolidin-1-yl)pyrido[2,3-*d*]pyrimidine-6-carboxylic acid.

$C_{14}H_{16}N_4O_3$ = 288.3.
*CAS — 19562-30-2.*
*ATC — J01MB03.*

### Profile

Piromidic acid is a 4-quinolone antibacterial with properties similar to those of nalidixic acid (p.234). It is used in the treatment of susceptible infections in doses of up to 3 g daily by mouth in divided doses. There have been a number of reports of acute renal failure associated with piromidic acid.

### Preparations

**Proprietary Preparations** (details are given in Part 3)
***Ital.:*** Enteromix.

## Pivampicillin *(BAN, rINN)*

MK-191; Pivampicilina; Pivampicillinum. Pivaloyloxymethyl (6*R*)-6-(α-D-phenylglycylamino)penicillanate.

$C_{22}H_{29}N_3O_6S$ = 463.5.
*CAS — 33817-20-8.*
*ATC — J01CA02.*

**Pharmacopoeias.** In *Eur.* (see p.vi).

**Ph. Eur. 5.0** (Pivampicillin). A white or almost white crystalline powder. Practically insoluble in water; soluble in dehydrated alcohol; freely soluble in methyl alcohol. It dissolves in dilute acids. Store in airtight containers.

## Pivampicillin Hydrochloride *(BANM, USAN, rINNM)*

Hidrocloruro de pivampicilina.

$C_{22}H_{29}N_3O_6S,HCl$ = 500.0.
*CAS — 26309-95-5.*
*ATC — J01CA02.*

### Adverse Effects and Precautions

As for Ampicillin, p.157. Pivampicillin is reported to cause a lower incidence of diarrhoea than ampicillin. Upper gastrointestinal discomfort may be more frequent when pivampicillin is taken on an empty stomach.

Pivaloyloxymethyl esters such as pivampicillin have been associated with the induction of carnitine deficiency (see below).

**Carnitine deficiency.** Carnitine deficiency (see under Levocarnitine, p.1424) has been reported following the use of pivampicillin and pivmecillinam.[1] It is thought that the pivalic acid liberated on hydrolysis of these pivaloyloxymethyl esters *in vivo* is excreted as pivaloyl-carnitine with a consequent depletion in plasma and muscle concentrations of carnitine.[2] Low plasma-carnitine concentrations persisted in a patient after discontinuing pivampicillin, despite 6 weeks of replacement therapy with carnitine 1g daily by mouth. She had originally presented with skeletal myopathy after receiving pivampicillin for 3 months. A more intensive carnitine replacement regimen might be necessary in such patients.[3]

1. Holme E, *et al.* Carnitine deficiency induced by pivampicillin and pivmecillinam therapy. *Lancet* 1989; **ii:** 469–73.
2. Anonymous. Carnitine deficiency. *Lancet* 1990; **335:** 631–3.
3. Rose SJ, *et al.* Carnitine deficiency associated with long-term pivampicillin treatment: the effect of a replacement therapy regime. *Postgrad Med J* 1992; **68:** 932–4.

**Porphyria.** Pivampicillin has been associated with acute attacks of porphyria and is considered unsafe in porphyric patients.

### Interactions

As for Benzylpenicillin, p.164.

There is a theoretical possibility that carnitine deficiency may be increased in patients receiving pivampicillin and valproate.

### Antimicrobial Action

Pivampicillin has the antimicrobial activity of ampicillin to which it is hydrolysed *in vivo* (p.157).

### Pharmacokinetics

Pivampicillin is acid-stable and is readily absorbed from the gastrointestinal tract. On absorption it is rapidly and almost completely hydrolysed to ampicillin, pivalic acid, and formaldehyde. Plasma-ampicillin concentrations 1 hour after administration are 2 to 3 times those attained after an equivalent dose of ampicillin. The absorption of pivampicillin is generally not significantly affected by food. About 70% of a dose is excreted in the urine as ampicillin within 6 hours.

### Uses and Administration

Pivampicillin is the pivaloyloxymethyl ester of ampicillin (p.158) and has similar uses. 1.3 g of pivampicillin and 1.43 g of pivampicillin hydrochloride are each approximately equivalent to 1 g of ampicillin.

Pivampicillin is given by mouth to adults in doses of 500 mg twice daily with food. Doses in children are: 3 months to 1 year of age, 20 to 30 mg/kg twice daily; 1 to 3 years, 175 mg twice daily; 4 to 6 years, 262.5 mg twice daily; 7 to 10 years, 350 mg twice daily. Doses may be doubled in severe infections. In gonorrhoea a single dose of 1.5 g is given, with probenecid 1 g, in areas where gonococci remain sensitive.

Pivampicillin hydrochloride is used in some countries.

Pivampicillin has also been given with pivmecillinam (p.244).

### Preparations

**Proprietary Preparations** (details are given in Part 3)
***Canad.:*** Pondocillin; ***Denm.:*** Pondocillin; ***Fr.:*** Proampi; ***Norw.:*** Pondocillin; ***S.Afr.:*** Pondocillin†; ***Spain:*** Lervipan†; Pivamiser†; ***Swed.:*** Pondocillin.
**Multi-ingredient:** ***Austria:*** Miraxid†.

# Pivmecillinam *(BAN, rINN)*

Amdinocillin Pivoxil *(USAN)*; FL-1039; Pivamdinocillin; Pivmecillinam; Ro-10-9071. Pivaloyloxymethyl (6*R*)-6-(perhydroazepin-1-ylmethyleneamino)penicillanate.

$C_{21}H_{33}N_3O_5S$ = 439.6.
*CAS — 32886-97-8.*
*ATC — J01CA08.*

## Pivmecillinam Hydrochloride *(BANM, rINNM)*

Hidrocloruro de pivmecilinam; Pivmecillinami Hydrochloridum.

$C_{21}H_{33}N_3O_5S,HCl$ = 476.0.
*CAS — 32887-03-9.*
*ATC — J01CA08.*

**Pharmacopoeias.** In *Eur.* (see p.vi) and *Jpn.*

**Ph. Eur. 5.0** (Pivmecillinam Hydrochloride). A white or almost white crystalline powder. Freely soluble in water, in dehydrated alcohol, and in methyl alcohol; slightly soluble in acetone. A 10% solution in water has a pH of 2.8 to 3.8. Store at a temperature of 2° to 8°. Protect from light.

### Adverse Effects and Precautions

As for Benzylpenicillin, p.163.

Pivaloyloxymethyl esters such as pivmecillinam have been associated with the induction of carnitine deficiency (see Pivampicillin, above).

**Administration.** Oesophageal injury has been associated rarely with pivmecillinam tablets.[1,2] Patients are advised to take them during a meal, while sitting or standing, and with at least half a glass of water.[3]

1. Committee on Safety of Medicines. Pivmecillinam and oesophageal injury. *Current Problems 19* 1987.
2. Mortimer Ö, Wiholm B-E. Oesophageal injury associated with pivmecillinam tablets. *Eur J Clin Pharmacol* 1989; **37:** 605–7.
3. Anonymous. CSM warning on pivmecillinam. *Pharm J* 1987; **238:** 443.

**Porphyria.** Pivmecillinam has been associated with acute attacks of porphyria and is considered unsafe in porphyric patients.

### Interactions

As for Benzylpenicillin, p.164.

### Antimicrobial Action

Pivmecillinam has the antimicrobial activity of mecillinam (p.228) to which it is hydrolysed *in vivo*.

### Pharmacokinetics

Pivmecillinam is well absorbed from the gastrointestinal tract and is rapidly hydrolysed to the active drug mecillinam (p.229), pivalic acid, and formaldehyde. The presence of food in the stomach does not appear to have a significant effect on absorption. Peak plasma concentrations of mecillinam of 5 micrograms/mL have been achieved 1 to 2 hours after a 400-mg dose of pivmecillinam.

About 45% of a dose may be excreted in the urine as mecillinam, mainly within the first 6 hours.

◊ References.

1. Heikkilä A, *et al.* The pharmacokinetics of mecillinam and pivmecillinam in pregnant and non-pregnant women. *Br J Clin Pharmacol* 1992; **33;** 629–33.

### Uses and Administration

Pivmecillinam is the pivaloyloxymethyl ester of mecillinam (p.229), to which it is hydrolysed after oral administration. It is used in the treatment of urinary-tract infections (p.153).

Doses of pivmecillinam have often been expressed in a confusing manner since no differentiation has been made between the hydrochloride, used in tablets, and the base, used in suspensions for oral use. Pivmecillinam 1.35 g and pivmecillinam hydrochloride 1.46 g are each approximately equivalent to 1 g of mecillinam.

Pivmecillinam should preferably be taken with food (see also under Adverse Effects and Precautions, above).

In acute uncomplicated cystitis, the initial adult dose is 400 mg by mouth followed by 200 mg three times daily for 8 doses. In chronic or recurrent bacteriuria, 400 mg may be given 3 or 4 times daily. The dose for children (body-weight less than 40 kg) with urinary-tract infections is 20 to 40 mg/kg daily in 3 or 4 divided doses.

Pivmecillinam has been given with other beta lactams, particularly pivampicillin (p.244), to extend the spectrum of antimicrobial activity to Gram-positive organisms and because of reported synergism against Gram-negative bacteria *in vitro*.

For parenteral administration, mecillinam is used.

◊ References.

1. Nicolle LE. Pivmecillinam in the treatment of urinary tract infections. *J Antimicrob Chemother* 2000; **46** (suppl S1): 35–9.

### Preparations

**Proprietary Preparations** (details are given in Part 3)
***Austria:*** Selexid; ***Belg.:*** Selexid; ***Canad.:*** Selexid; ***Denm.:*** Selexid; ***Fin.:*** Selexid; ***Fr.:*** Selexid; ***Norw.:*** Selexid; ***NZ:*** Selexid; ***Port.:*** Selecid; ***Swed.:*** Selexid; ***UK:*** Selexid.
**Multi-ingredient:** ***Austria:*** Miraxid†.

## Polymyxin B Sulfate *(rINNM)*

Polymyxin B Sulphate *(BANM)*; Polymyxini B Sulfas; Sulfato de polimixina B.

*CAS — 1404-26-8 (polymyxin B); 1405-20-5 (polymyxin B sulfate).*

*ATC — A07AA05; J01XB02; S01AA18; S02AA11; S03AA03.*

**Pharmacopoeias.** In *Eur.* (see p.vi), *Jpn, Pol.,* and *US.*

**Ph. Eur. 5.0** (Polymyxin B Sulphate). A mixture of the sulfates of polypeptides produced by the growth of certain strains of *Bacillus polymyxa* or obtained by any other means. A white or almost white, hygroscopic powder. Soluble in water; slightly soluble in alcohol. A 2% solution in water has a pH of 5.0 to 7.0. Store in airtight containers. Protect from light.

**USP 27** (Polymyxin B Sulfate). The sulfate salt of a kind of polymyxin, a substance produced by the growth of *Bacillus polymyxa* (Bacillaceae), or a mixture of two or more such salts. A white to buff-coloured, powder, odourless or has a faint odour. It has a potency of not less than 6000 Polymyxin B units/mg, calculated on the dried substance. Freely soluble in water; slightly soluble in alcohol. pH of a 0.5% solution in water is between 5.0 and 7.5. Store in airtight containers. Protect from light.

**Incompatibility.** Incompatibility has been reported with many other drugs including antimicrobials. Polymyxin B sulfate is rapidly inactivated by strong acids and alkalis.

### Units

The second International Standard Preparation (1969) of polymyxin B sulfate contains 8403 units/mg.

NOTE. The available forms of polymyxin B sulfate are generally less pure than the International Standard Preparation and doses are sometimes stated in terms of pure polymyxin base; 100 mg of pure polymyxin B is considered to be equivalent to 1 million units (1 mega unit).

### Adverse Effects, Treatment, and Precautions

When given parenterally, the major adverse effects of the polymyxins are dose-related neurotoxicity and nephrotoxicity. Hypersensitivity reactions are rare, although rashes and fever have been reported, and polymyxins cause histamine release which may lead to bronchoconstriction and other anaphylactoid symptoms.

Neurotoxic reactions include peripheral effects such as circumoral and 'stocking-glove' pattern paraesthesias, visual disturbances, and dizziness, ataxia, confusion, drowsiness, and other central effects. The polymyxins are potent neuromuscular blockers, and respiratory paralysis and apnoea may result, especially in patients with renal impairment or pre-existing disorders of neuromuscular transmission such as myasthenia gravis, in whom particular care is needed. Neostigmine or calcium salts are usually of little value in reversing neuromuscular blockade and artificial ventilation may be required if it develops.

Nephrotoxicity may occur in up to 20% of patients following parenteral use and may be marked by nitrogen retention, haematuria, proteinuria, and tubular necrosis. Electrolyte disturbances frequently occur. Patients with pre-existing renal impairment are at particular risk and require dosage reduction. Renal function should be monitored. Signs of increasing nitrogen retention are an indication for dosage reduction in all patients and the drugs should be withdrawn if oliguria occurs. Although polymyxin B has been stated to be more nephrotoxic than colistin on a weight-for-weight basis their effects on the kidney seem to be similar at therapeutically equivalent doses.

Polymyxin B is irritant and pain following intramuscular injection may be severe. Meningeal irritation may follow intrathecal doses.

Polymyxins should be avoided in patients with a history of hypersensitivity to any of the group. Serum concentrations of polymyxins should be monitored in patients receiving parenteral therapy.

Ear drops containing polymyxins should not be used in patients with perforated ear drums, and topical application to large areas of broken skin should be avoided, because of the risk of systemic absorption.

### Interactions

Polymyxins may enhance the action of neuromuscular blockers (p.1400). Additive nephrotoxicity may occur if polymyxins are given with other potentially nephrotoxic drugs including aminoglycosides and cefalotin.

### Antimicrobial Action

Polymyxin B and the other polymyxin antibacterials act primarily by binding to membrane phospholipids and disrupting the bacterial cytoplasmic membrane. Polymyxin B has a bactericidal action on most Gram-negative bacilli except *Proteus* spp. It is particularly effective against *Pseudomonas aeruginosa*. Of the other Gram-negative organisms, *Acinetobacter* spp., *Escherichia coli, Enterobacter* and *Klebsiella* spp., *Haemophilus influenzae, Bordetella pertussis, Salmonella,* and *Shigella* spp. are sensitive. Classical *Vibrio cholerae* 01 is sensitive but the El Tor and O139 biotypes are resistant. *Serratia marcescens, Providencia* spp., and *Bacteroides fragilis* are usually resistant. It is not active against *Neisseria* spp., obligate anaerobes, and Gram-positive bacteria. Some fungi such as *Coccidioides immitis* are susceptible but most are resistant.

Polymyxins have been reported to demonstrate antimicrobial synergy with a variety of other drugs, including chloramphenicol, tetracyclines, and the sulfonamides and trimethoprim.

The action of polymyxin B is reduced by divalent cations such as calcium and magnesium, and so activity *in vivo* is less marked than *in vitro*.

Acquired resistance to polymyxin B is uncommon, although adaptive resistance may develop in enterobacteria exposed to sublethal concentrations. There is complete cross-resistance between polymyxin B and colistin.

### Pharmacokinetics

Polymyxin B sulfate is not absorbed from the gastrointestinal tract, except in the newborn. It is not absorbed through the intact skin.

Peak plasma concentrations after intramuscular use are usually obtained within 2 hours, but are variable and polymyxin B sulfate is partially inactivated by serum. It is widely distributed and extensively bound to cell membranes in the tissues. Accumulation may occur after repeated doses. Polymyxin B is reported to have a half-life of about 6 hours. There is no diffusion into the CSF.

Polymyxin B sulfate is excreted mainly by the kidneys, up to 60% being recovered in the urine, but there is a time lag of 12 to 24 hours before polymyxin B is recovered in the urine.

### Uses and Administration

Polymyxin B sulfate is used topically, often with other drugs, in the treatment of skin, ear, and eye infections due to susceptible organisms. Eye drops of polymyxin B with neomycin and gramicidin have been used for the prophylaxis of infection in patients undergoing ocular surgery and, with propamidine isetionate, for the treatment of acanthamoeba keratitis (p.595). Polymyxin B has been given orally for oropharyngeal decontamination or the suppression of intestinal flora in patients at high risk of endogenous infections (see under Intensive Care, p.132). Polymyxin B has also been used parenterally for the treatment of infections due to susceptible Gram-negative bacteria, especially *Pseudomonas aeruginosa,* but other drugs are generally preferred.

For topical application polymyxin B is usually available as a 0.1% solution or ointment, in combination with other drugs. Parenteral doses have ranged from 15 000 to 25 000 units/kg (about 1.5 to 2.5 mg/kg) daily, preferably by intravenous infusion, although the intramuscular route has been used despite the severe pain which may be associated with it. Higher doses have been given to neonates, but dosage must be reduced in patients with renal impairment.

Polymyxin B has also been given intrathecally in meningeal infection, and by subconjunctival injection for eye infections.

◊ References.

1. Evans ME, *et al.* Polymyxin B sulfate and colistin: old antibiotics for emerging multiresistant Gram-negative bacteria. *Ann Pharmacother* 1999; **33:** 960–7.

### Preparations

***BP 2003:*** Polymyxin and Bacitracin Eye Ointment;
***USP 27:*** Bacitracin and Polymyxin B Sulfate Topical Aerosol; Bacitracin Zinc and Polymyxin B Sulfate Ointment; Bacitracin Zinc and Polymyxin B Sulfate Ophthalmic Ointment; Chloramphenicol and Polymyxin B Sulfate Ophthalmic Ointment; Chloramphenicol, Polymyxin B Sulfate, and Hydrocortisone Acetate Ophthalmic Ointment; Neomycin and Polymyxin B Sulfates and Bacitracin Ointment; Neomycin and Polymyxin B Sulfates and Bacitracin Ophthalmic Ointment; Neomycin and Polymyxin B Sulfates and Bacitracin Zinc Ointment; Neomycin and Polymyxin B Sulfates and Bacitracin Zinc Ophthalmic Ointment; Neomycin and Polymyxin B Sulfates and Dexamethasone Ophthalmic Ointment; Neomycin and Polymyxin B Sulfates and Dexamethasone Ophthalmic Suspension; Neomycin and Polymyxin B Sulfates and Gramicidin Cream; Neomycin and Polymyxin B Sulfates and Gramicidin Ophthalmic Solution; Neomycin and Polymyxin B Sulfates and Hydrocortisone Acetate Cream; Neomycin and Polymyxin B Sulfates and Hydrocortisone Acetate Ophthalmic Suspension; Neomycin and Polymyxin B Sulfates and Hydrocortisone Ophthalmic Suspension; Neomycin and Polymyxin B Sulfates and Hydrocortisone Otic Solution; Neomycin and Polymyxin B Sulfates and Hydrocortisone Otic Suspension; Neomycin and Polymyxin B Sulfates and Lidocaine Cream; Neomycin and Polymyxin B Sulfates and Pramoxine Hydrochloride Cream; Neomycin and Polymyxin B Sulfates and Prednisolone Acetate Ophthalmic Suspension; Neomycin and Polymyxin B Sulfates Cream; Neomycin and Polymyxin B Sulfates Ophthalmic Ointment; Neomycin and Polymyxin B Sulfates Ophthalmic Solution; Neomycin and Polymyxin B Sulfates Solution for Irrigation; Neomycin and Polymyxin B Sulfates, Bacitracin Zinc, and Hydrocortisone Acetate Ophthalmic Ointment; Neomycin and Polymyxin B Sulfates, Bacitracin Zinc, and Hydrocortisone Ointment; Neomycin and Polymyxin B Sulfates, Bacitracin Zinc, and Hydrocortisone Ophthalmic Ointment; Neomycin and Polymyxin B Sulfates, Bacitracin Zinc, and Lidocaine Ointment; Neomycin and Polymyxin B Sulfates, Bacitracin, and Hydrocortisone Acetate Ointment; Neomycin and Polymyxin B Sulfates, Bacitracin, and Hydrocortisone Acetate Ophthalmic Ointment; Neomycin and Polymyxin B Sulfates, Bacitracin, and Lidocaine Ointment; Neomycin and Polymyxin B Sulfates, Gramicidin, and Hydrocortisone Acetate Cream; Oxytetracycline Hydrochloride and Polymyxin B Sulfate Ointment; Oxytetracycline Hydrochloride and Polymyxin B Sulfate Ophthalmic Ointment; Oxytetracycline Hydrochloride and Polymyxin B Sulfate Topical Powder; Oxytetracycline Hydrochloride and Polymyxin B Sulfate Vaginal Tablets; Polymyxin B for Injection; Polymyxin B Sulfate and Bacitracin Zinc Topical Aerosol; Polymyxin B Sulfate and Bacitracin Zinc Topical Powder; Polymyxin B Sulfate and Hydrocortisone Otic Solution; Polymyxin B Sulfate and Trimethoprim Ophthalmic Solution.

**Proprietary Preparations** (details are given in Part 3)
***Canad.:*** Aerosporin†.

**Multi-ingredient: *Arg.:*** Belbar; Ginal Cent; Ginkan; Isoptomax; Min O; Nebapol B; Neoftalm; Neoftalm Dexa; O-Biol P; Oto Biotaer; Otosporin; Otosporin L; Pantometil; Polygynax; Sincerum Biotic L; Terramicina con Polimixina B; Vagicural Plus; ***Austral.:*** Neosporin; ***Austria:*** Neocones; Otosporin; Polytrim; ***Belg.:*** De Icin; Maxitrol; Ophtalmotrim; Otosporin; Panotile; Polydexa; Polygynax; Polytrim; Predmycin P; Statrol; Synalar Bi-Otic; Terra-Cortril; Terramycine; ***Braz.:*** Anaseptil; Colpolase; Conjuntin†; Dermicin†; Elotin; Ginec; Lidosporin; Maxitrol; Oftcor†; Oftrim†; Otauril†; Oto-Ped†; Otocort; Otolone†; Otomixyn; Otosporin; Otosynalar; Panotil; Pertrim†; Poliginax; Polimixina B Composto†; Polipred; Predmicin; Terra-Cortril com Polimixina B†; Terramicina Pomada; ***Canad.:*** Antibiotic Cold Sore Ointment; Antibiotic Cream; Antibiotic Ointment; Antibiotique Onguent; Bacimyxin; Band-Aid Antibiotic; Bioderm; Cortimyxin; Cortisporin; Dioptrol; Diospor HC†; Diosporin†; Johnson & Johnson First Aid Ointment; Lanabiotic†; Lid-Pack†; Lidomyxin; Lidosporin; Maxitrol; Neo Bace†; Neosporin; Neotopic; Ophthocort†; Optimyxin; Optimyxin Plus; Ozonol Antibiotic Plus; PMS-Polytrimethoprim; Polycidin; Polyderm; Polysporin; Polysporin Plus Pain Relief; Polysporin Triple Antibiotic; Polytopic; Polytracin†; Polytrim; ***Chile:*** Dermabiotico; Gotalgic; Grifoftal; Grifoftal-D; Maxitrol; Oftabiotico; Otazol; Oticum; Otolisan; Otoseptil; Unguento Dermico Antibiotico; ***Denm.:*** Terramycin Polymyxin B; ***Fin.:*** Maxitrol; Polysporin; Terra-Cortril P; ***Fr.:*** Antibio-Synalar; Antibiotulle Lumiere; Atebemyxine; Auricularum; Cebemyxine; Corticotulle Lumiere; Framyxone; Maxidrol; Novomyxine; Panotile; Polydexa; Polydexa a la Phenylephrine†; Polyfra; Polygynax; Polygynax Virgo; Primyxine; Sterimycine; ***Ger.:*** Antibiotulle Lumiere; Corticotulle Lumiere; Dexa Polyspectran; Farco-Tril; Isopto Max; Kombi-Stulln N; Otosporin†; Panotile N; Polygynax; Polyspectran; Polyspectran HC; Terracortril; Terramycin; ***Gr.:*** Fotocollyre; Oxacycle-P; Statrol; Terramycin with Polymyxin; ***Hong Kong:*** Aplosyn-Otic; Cebemyxine; Dexa-Polyspectran†; Maxitrol; Neosporin; Neotopic†; Oftalmotrim†; Otosporin; PMS-Baximycin; Polyfax; Polygynax; Polyoph; Polyspectran†; Spersapolymyxin†; Terramycin with Polymyxin B; ***India:*** Chlormixin; Neosporin; Neosporin-H; Ocupol; Ocupol-D; ***Irl.:*** Maxitrol; Neosporin; Otosporin; Polybactrin†; Polyfax; ***Israel:*** Auricularum; Bamyxin; Desoren; Dex-Otic; Maxitrol; Otosporin†; Phenimixin; Tarocidin; Tarocidin D; Tarocyn†; Terramycin; ***Ital.:*** Anauran; Cicatrene; Dermobios†; Mixotone; Otosporin; Rinojet SF; ***Malaysia:*** Maxitrol; Oftalmotrim; Pocin G; Pocin H; Terramycin; ***Mex.:*** Alosol; Biodexan; Cortisporin; Dexsul; Hidropolicin; Maxitrol; Neobacigrin; Neosporin; Nicobio; Polixin; Septilisin; Synalar N; Synalar O; Synalar Oftalmico; Terramicina; Tribiot; ***Neth.:*** Otosporin; Panotile; Polytrim; Synalar Bi-Otic; Terra-Cortril Gel Steraject met polymyxine-B; Terra-Cortril met polymyxine-B; Terramycin met polymyxine-B†; ***Norw.:*** Maxitrol; Terra-Cortril Polymyxin B; Terramycin Polymyxin B; ***NZ:*** Maxitrol; ***Port.:*** Conjunctilone; Conjunctilone-S; Gramixina†; Oftalmotrim; Otolys†; Otosporin†; Polisulfade; Polydexa; Polygynax†; Polysporina†; ***S.Afr.:*** Maxitrol; Neosporin; Otosporin; Polysporin†; Polytrim; Terra-Cortril; Terramycin; ***Singapore:*** Lignosporin†; Maxitrol; Neosporin†; Oftalmotrim†; Otosporin†; Polybamycin; Polydexa; Polygynax; Predmycin-P; Terramycin; ***Spain:*** Bacisporin; Blastoestimulina; Creanolona; Dermisone Tri Antibiotic; Linitul Antibiotico†; Liquipom Dexa Antib; Maxitrol; Nasotic Oto†; Neocones; Oftalmotrim; Oftalmotrim Dexa; Oftalmowell; Otix; Otosporin; Panotile; Phonal; Poliantib†; Poly Pred; Pomada Antibiotica; Statrol†; Synalar Nasal; Synalar Otico; Terra-Cortril; Terramicina; Tivitis; Tulgrasum Antibiotico; Vinciseptil Otico; ***Swed.:*** Isopto Biotic; Terracortril med polymyxin B; Terramycin Polymyxin B; ***Switz.:*** Baneopol; Maxitrol; Mycinopred; Neosporin; Otosporin; Panotile; Polydexa; Pulpomixine†; Spersapolymyxin; Terracortril; Terramycine†; ***Thai.:*** Banocin; Dex-Otic†; Maxitrol; Neosporin; Opsacin; Otosamthong; Otosporin; Polyoph; Predmycin; Spersapolymyxin; Statrol†; Terramycin;

Terrasil; Xanalin; **UK:** Gregoderm; Maxitrol; Neosporin; Otosporin; Polyfax; Polytrim; **USA:** Ak-Poly-Bac; Ak-Spore; Ak-Spore HC†; Ak-Spore†; Ak-Trol; AntibiOtic†; Bactine First Aid Antibiotic Plus Anesthetic†; Betadine First Aid Antibiotics + Moisturizer†; Betadine Plus First Aid Antibiotics & Pain Reliever; Campho-Phenique Antibiotic Plus Pain Reliever Ointment†; Clomycin†; Cortatrigen; Cortimycin; Cortisporin; Dexacidin; Dexacine; Dexasporin; Ear-Eze; Lanabiotic; LazerSporin-C; Maxitrol; Mycitracin; Mycitracin Plus†; Neocin; Neomixin†; Neopolydex; Neosporin; Neosporin + Pain Relief; Neosporin GU; Neosporin Plus†; Neosporin†; Neotricin HC; Octicair; Ocu-Spor-B; Ocu-Spor-G; Ocu-Trol; Ocutricin; Otic-Care; OtiTricin; Otobiotic; Otocort; Otomycin-HPN; Otosporin; Pediotic; Poly-Dex; Poly-Pred; Polycin-B; Polymycin; Polysporin; Polytracin; Polytrim; Septa†; Spectrocin Plus; Terak; Terramycin with Polymyxin B; Tri-Biozene; Tribiotic Plus†; Triple Antibiotic†; UAD-Otic.

## Pristinamycin *(BAN, rINN)*

Pristinamicina; RP-7293.

*CAS — 11006-76-1.*

*ATC — J01FG01.*

### Profile

Pristinamycin is a streptogramin antibacterial produced by the growth of *Streptomyces pristina spiralis*, with actions and uses similar to those of virginiamycin (p.277). It is given by mouth in the treatment of susceptible infections, particularly staphylococcal infections, in a dose of 2 to 4 g daily in divided doses. Children have been given 50 to 100 mg/kg daily.

◊ Pristinamycin is a naturally occurring mixture of two synergistic components, pristinamycin I which is a macrolide, and pristinamycin II which is a depsipeptide.[1] It has been available for many years as an oral antistaphylococcal drug, and also acts against streptococci. It is effective against strains showing resistance to erythromycin; resistance to pristinamycin is rare,[2,3] although resistance in staphylococci has been reported in the past.[4,5] It is effective against meticillin-resistant *Staphylococcus aureus* (MRSA) but its usefulness in severe infection is limited by its poor solubility, which prevents development of an intravenous formulation. Oral pristinamycin has been shown to be as effective as standard therapy with intravenous then oral penicillin in the treatment of erysipelas.[6]

Mixtures of water-soluble derivatives of pristinamycins I and II, including quinupristin/dalfopristin (p.248), are in clinical use or under investigation.


1. Hamilton-Miller JMT. From foreign pharmacopoeias: 'new' antibiotics from old? *J Antimicrob Chemother* 1991; **27:** 702–5.
2. Weber P. Streptococcus pneumoniae: absence d'émergence de résistance à la pristinamycine. *Pathol Biol (Paris)* 2001; **49:** 840–5.
3. Leclercq R, *et al.* Activité in vitro de la pristinamycine vis-à-vis des staphylocoques isolés dans les hôpitaux français en 1999-2000 *Pathol Biol (Paris)* 2003; **51:** 400–4.
4. Loncle V, *et al.* Analysis of pristinamycin-resistant Staphylococcus epidermidis isolates responsible for an outbreak in a Parisian hospital. *Antimicrob Agents Chemother* 1993; **37:** 2159–65.
5. Allignet J, *et al.* Distribution of genes encoding resistance to streptogramin A and related compounds among staphylococci resistant to these antibiotics. *Antimicrob Agents Chemother* 1996; **40:** 2523–8.
6. Bernard P, *et al.* Oral pristinamycin versus standard penicillin regimen to treat erysipelas in adults: randomised, non-inferiority, open trial. *BMJ* 2002; **325:** 864–6.


### Preparations

**Proprietary Preparations** (details are given in Part 3)
**Belg.:** Pyostacine†; **Fr.:** Pyostacine; **Israel:** Pyostacine.

# Procaine Benzylpenicillin *(BAN, rINNM)*

Benzylpenicillin Novocaine; Benzylpenicillinum Procainum; Penicillin G Procaine; Procaína penicilina; Procaine Penicillin G; Procaini Benzylpenicillinum. 2-(4-Aminobenzoyloxy)ethyldiethylammonium (6*R*)-6-(2-phenylacetamido)penicillanate monohydrate.

$C_{13}H_{20}N_2O_2,C_{16}H_{18}N_2O_4S,H_2O$ = 588.7.

*CAS — 54-35-3 (anhydrous procaine benzylpenicillin); 6130-64-9 (procaine benzylpenicillin monohydrate).*

*ATC — J01CE09.*

**Pharmacopoeias.** In *Chin., Eur.* (see p.vi), *Int., Pol.,* and *US.*

**Ph. Eur. 5.0** (Benzylpenicillin, Procaine). A white, crystalline powder. Slightly soluble in water; sparingly soluble in alcohol. A 0.33% solution in water has a pH of 5.0 to 7.5. Store in airtight containers.

**USP 27** (Penicillin G Procaine). White crystals or white, very fine, microcrystalline powder, odourless or practically odourless. Slightly soluble in water; soluble in alcohol and in chloroform. It is rapidly inactivated by acids, by alkali hydroxides, and by oxidising agents. pH of a saturated solution in water is between 5.0 and 7.5.

## Adverse Effects and Precautions

As for Benzylpenicillin, p.163.

Procaine benzylpenicillin should not be given to patients known to be hypersensitive to either of its components. Procaine benzylpenicillin should not be injected intravascularly since ischaemic reactions may occur.

Severe, usually transient, reactions with symptoms of severe anxiety and agitation, confusion, psychotic reactions including visual and auditory hallucinations, seizures, tachycardia and hypertension, cyanosis, and a sensation of impending death have occasionally been reported with procaine benzylpenicillin and may be due to accidental intravascular injection. Since similar reactions have also occurred with other depot penicillin preparations that do not contain procaine, its presence is unlikely to be the major cause of such reactions, but may be a contributory factor, especially after injection of high doses. These reactions have been termed non-allergic, pseudoallergic, pseudoanaphylactic, or Hoigné's syndrome; the term 'embolic-toxic reaction' has also been proposed.

## Interactions

As for Benzylpenicillin, p.164.

## Pharmacokinetics

When procaine benzylpenicillin is given by intramuscular injection, it forms a depot from which it is slowly released and hydrolysed to benzylpenicillin. Peak plasma concentrations are produced in 1 to 4 hours, and effective concentrations of benzylpenicillin are usually maintained for 12 to 24 hours. However, plasma concentrations are lower than those following an equivalent dose of benzylpenicillin potassium or sodium.

Distribution into the CSF is reported to be poor.

## Uses and Administration

Procaine benzylpenicillin has the same antimicrobial action as benzylpenicillin (p.164) to which it is hydrolysed gradually following deep intramuscular injection. This results in a prolonged effect, but because of the relatively low blood concentrations produced, its use should be restricted to infections caused by micro-organisms that are highly sensitive to penicillin. Procaine benzylpenicillin should not be used as the sole treatment for severe acute infections, or when bacteraemia is present.

Procaine benzylpenicillin is used mainly in the treatment of syphilis; other indications have included anthrax, pneumonia (in children in developing countries), and Whipple's disease. For details of these infections and their treatment, see under Choice of Antibacterial, p.120.

*Administration and dosage.* Doses of procaine benzylpenicillin may sometimes be expressed in terms of equivalent units of benzylpenicillin. Procaine benzylpenicillin 600 mg is approximately equivalent to 360 mg of benzylpenicillin (600 000 units). Procaine benzylpenicillin is administered by deep intramuscular injection in usual doses of 0.6 to 1.2 g daily.

Patients with syphilis are given procaine benzylpenicillin 1.2 g daily for 10 to 14 days; infants up to 2 years of age with congenital syphilis may be given 50 mg/kg daily. Treatment may be continued for 3 weeks in patients with late syphilis.

Procaine benzylpenicillin is also used in combined preparations with other penicillins, including benzylpenicillin and benzathine benzylpenicillin.

## Preparations

**USP 27:** Penicillin G Benzathine and Penicillin G Procaine Injectable Suspension; Penicillin G Procaine for Injectable Suspension; Penicillin G Procaine Injectable Suspension.

**Proprietary Preparations** (details are given in Part 3)
**Arg.:** Mudapenil; Penicil Dermol; **Austral.:** Cilicaine Syringe; **Braz.:** Penkaron; Probecilin†; **Canad.:** Ayercillin†; **Ger.:** Jenacillin O; **Mex.:** Sodilin; **NZ:** Cilicaine; **S.Afr.:** Novocillin; Procillin; **Spain:** Aquicilina; Farmaproina; **USA:** Crysticillin; Wycillin†.

**Multi-ingredient: Austria:** Fortepen; Retarpen compositum; **Braz.:** Benapen; Benzapen G; Cibramicina†; Climacilin†; Despacilina; Drenovac; Expectovac; Ginurovac; Linfocilin; Odontovac; Ortocilin†; Pulmocilin†; Wycillin R; **Canad.:** Bicillin A-P†; **Chile:** Karbasalin; **Ger.:** Bipensaar; Hydracillin†; Jenacillin A; Retacillin compositum; **India:** Bistrepen; **Israel:** Duplo-Penicillin; Penicillin Fortified; **Ital.:** Tri-Wycillina; **Mex.:** Bencelin Combinado; Benzanil Compuesto; Benzetacil Combinado; Hidrocilina; Pendiben Compuesto; Penicil; Penipot; Penisodina; Penprocilina; Procilin; Suipen; **Neth.:** Penidural D/F; **Port.:** Atralcilina†; Penadur 6.3.3; **S.Afr.:** Penilente Forte; Ultracillin; **Spain:** Aquicilina D A; Benzetacil Compuesta; Cepacilina 633; Neocepacilina†; **UK:** Bicillin†; **USA:** Bicillin C-R.

## Propicillin Potassium *(BANM, pINNM)*

Potassium α-Phenoxypropylpenicillin; Propicilina potásica; Propicillinum Kalicum. A mixture of the D(+)- and L(−)-isomers of potassium (6*R*)-6-(2-phenoxybutyramido)penicillanate.

$C_{18}H_{21}KN_2O_5S$ = 416.5.

*CAS — 551-27-9 (propicillin); 1245-44-9 (propicillin potassium).*

*ATC — J01CE03.*

### Profile

Propicillin is a phenoxypenicillin with actions and uses similar to those of phenoxymethylpenicillin (p.242). It is given by mouth, as the potassium salt, for the treatment of susceptible mild to moderate infections in a usual dose of 700 mg three times daily.

### Preparations

**Proprietary Preparations** (details are given in Part 3)
**Ger.:** Baycillin; **Mex.:** Propibay†.

## Protionamide *(BAN, rINN)*

Prothionamide; Protionamida; RP-9778; TH-1321. 2-Propylpyridine-4-carbothioamide.

$C_9H_{12}N_2S$ = 180.3.

*CAS — 14222-60-7.*

*ATC — J04AD01.*

**Pharmacopoeias.** In *Chin., Int.,* and *Jpn.*

### Adverse Effects, Precautions, and Antimicrobial Action

As for Ethionamide, p.212; it may be better tolerated than ethionamide.

### Pharmacokinetics

Protionamide is readily absorbed from the gastrointestinal tract and produces peak plasma concentrations about 2 hours after a dose by mouth. It is widely distributed throughout body tissues and fluids, including the CSF. Protionamide is metabolised to the active sulfoxide and other inactive metabolites and less than 1% of a dose appears in the urine as unchanged drug.

### Uses and Administration

Protionamide is a thioamide derivative considered to be interchangeable with ethionamide (p.213) and has been used as a second-line drug in the treatment of tuberculosis. Complete cross-resistance occurs between the two drugs. Protionamide has been given by mouth in doses similar to those used for ethionamide. It has also been given as rectal suppositories; protionamide hydrochloride has been given intravenously. Like ethionamide, it has generally been replaced by less toxic antimycobacterials.

### Preparations

**Proprietary Preparations** (details are given in Part 3)
**Ger.:** ektebin; Peteha; **Hong Kong:** Peteha; **India:** Prothicid.

**Multi-ingredient: Austria:** Isoprodian; **Ger.:** Isoprodian; Peteha.

## Prulifloxacin *(rINN)*

NM-441; Prulifloxacino. (±)-7-{4-[(*Z*)-2,3-Dihydroxy-2-butenyl]-1-piperazinyl}-6-fluoro-1-methyl-4-oxo-1*H*,4*H*-[1,3]thiazeto[3,2-*a*]quinoline-3-carboxylic acid cyclic carbonate.

$C_{21}H_{20}FN_3O_6S$ = 461.5.

*CAS — 123447-62-1.*

### Profile

Prulifloxacin is a fluoroquinolone antibacterial.

◊ References.


1. Grassi C, *et al.* Randomized, double-blind study of prulifloxacin versus ciprofloxacin in patients with acute exacerbations of chronic bronchitis. *Respiration* 2002; **69:** 217–22.


# Pyrazinamide *(BAN, rINN)*

Pirazinamida; Pyrazinamidum; Pyrazinoic Acid Amide. Pyrazine-2-carboxamide.

$C_5H_5N_3O$ = 123.1.

*CAS — 98-96-4.*

*ATC — J04AK01.*

**Pharmacopoeias.** In *Chin., Eur.* (see p.vi), *Int., Jpn, Pol., US,* and *Viet.*

**Ph. Eur. 5.0** (Pyrazinamide). A white, crystalline powder. Sparingly soluble in water, slightly soluble in alcohol and in dichloromethane.

**USP 27** (Pyrazinamide). A white to practically white, odourless or practically odourless, crystalline powder. Soluble 1 in 67 of water, 1 in 175 of dehydrated alcohol, 1 in 135 of chloroform, 1 in 1000 of ether, and 1 in 72 of methyl alcohol; slightly soluble in alcohol.

## Adverse Effects and Treatment

Hepatotoxicity is the most serious adverse effect of pyrazinamide therapy and its frequency appears to be dose-related. However, in currently recommended doses, when given with isoniazid and rifampicin, the incidence of hepatitis has been reported to be less than 3%. Patients may experience a transient increase in liver enzyme values; more seriously hepatomegaly, splenomegaly, and jaundice may develop and on rare occasions death has occurred.

Hyperuricaemia commonly occurs and may lead to attacks of gout.

Other adverse effects are anorexia, nausea, vomiting, arthralgia, malaise, fever, sideroblastic anaemia, and dysuria. Photosensitivity and skin rashes have been reported on rare occasions.

**Effects on blood pressure.** Acute hypertension was associated with pyrazinamide in a previously normotensive woman.[1]

1. Goldberg J, *et al.* Acute hypertension as an adverse effect of pyrazinamide *JAMA* 1997; **277:** 1356.

**Effects on the liver.** The risk of hepatitis with antituberculous regimens containing pyrazinamide may be lower than suggested by early studies, in which large doses were used, often for long periods. The incidence of hepatitis in studies of short-course regimens containing pyrazinamide has ranged from 0.2% in Africa, to 0.6% in Hong Kong, to 2.8% in Singapore.[1] These and later studies[2-4] have shown that hepatotoxicity is not increased when pyrazinamide is added to the initial phase of short-term chemotherapy containing rifampicin and isoniazid. Nevertheless, a report[5] of 4 cases of fulminant hepatic failure in patients given triple therapy with the potentially hepatotoxic drugs rifampicin, isoniazid, and pyrazinamide (1 patient also received ethambutol) highlighted the importance of strict liver function monitoring and this was reinforced by others. However, the Joint Tuberculosis Committee of the British Thoracic Society is anxious that fears over the safety of treatment regimens do not compromise adequate therapy of the disease itself. They recommend[6] initial measurement of liver function in all patients and regular monitoring in patients with known chronic liver disease. Tests should be repeated if symptoms of liver dysfunction occur, and details are given concerning the response to deteriorating liver function and include guidelines for prompt re-introduction of appropriate antituberculous therapy once normal liver function is restored. In the USA, the CDC and the American Thoracic Society now recommend that the combination of pyrazinamide with rifampicin should not generally be offered to persons with latent tuberculosis.[7]

1. Girling DJ. The role of pyrazinamide in primary chemotherapy for pulmonary tuberculosis. *Tubercle* 1984; **65:** 1–4.
2. Parthasarathy R, *et al.* Hepatic toxicity in South Indian patients during treatment of tuberculosis with short-course regimens containing isoniazid, rifampicin and pyrazinamide. *Tubercle* 1986; **67:** 99–108.
3. Combs DL, *et al.* USPHS tuberculosis short-course chemotherapy trial 21: effectiveness, toxicity, and acceptability: the report of final results. *Ann Intern Med* 1990; **112:** 397–406.
4. le Bourgeois M, *et al.* Good tolerance of pyrazinamide in children with pulmonary tuberculosis. *Arch Dis Child* 1989; **64:** 177–8.
5. Mitchell I, *et al.* Anti-tuberculous therapy and acute liver failure. *Lancet* 1995; **345:** 555–6.
6. Ormerod LP, *et al.* Hepatotoxicity of antituberculosis drugs. *Thorax* 1996; **51:** 111–13.
7. Centers for Disease Control. Update: adverse event data and revised American Thoracic Society/CDC recommendations against the use of rifampin and pyrazinamide for treatment of latent tuberculosis infection—United States, 2003. *MMWR* 2003; **52:** 735–9. Also available at: http://www.cdc.gov/mmwr/preview/mmwrhtml/mm5231a4.htm (accessed 24/05/04)

**Effects on the nervous system.** Convulsions that developed in a 2-year-old child receiving antituberculous therapy appeared to be due to pyrazinamide, given in a dose of 250 mg daily.[1]

1. Herlevsen P, *et al.* Convulsions after treatment with pyrazinamide. *Tubercle* 1987; **68:** 145–6.

**Hyperuricaemia.** Hyperuricaemia during therapy with pyrazinamide may be due to inhibition of uric acid excretion by pyrazinoic acid, the main metabolite of pyrazinamide.[1]

In a large multicentre study,[2] the incidence of elevated serum concentrations of uric acid for patients receiving rifampicin, isoniazid, and pyrazinamide was 52.2% at 8 weeks while the incidence for patients receiving rifampicin and isoniazid was 5.4%. Arthralgia was reported in 6 of 617 patients receiving rifampicin, isoniazid, and pyrazinamide, but in none of 445 patients receiving rifampicin and isoniazid.

Slight increases in plasma concentrations of uric acid occurred in 9 of 43 children after one month's treatment with rifampicin, isoniazid, ethambutol, and pyrazinamide. Arthralgias and gout did not occur. Uric acid concentrations were normal on completion of treatment with pyrazinamide.[3] Some studies have suggested a relationship between elevated serum uric acid levels and arthralgia,[4] but this has not been confirmed.[5]

1. Ellard GA, Haslam RM. Observations on the reduction of the renal elimination of urate in man caused by the administration of pyrazinamide. *Tubercle* 1976; **57:** 97–103.
2. Combs DL, *et al.* USPHS tuberculosis short-course chemotherapy trial 21: effectiveness, toxicity, and acceptability: the report of final results. *Ann Intern Med* 1990; **112:** 397–406.
3. le Bourgeois M, *et al.* Good tolerance of pyrazinamide in children with pulmonary tuberculosis. *Arch Dis Child* 1989; **64:** 177–8.
4. Hong Kong Tuberculosis Treatment Services/British MRC. Adverse reactions to short-course regimens containing streptomycin, isoniazid, pyrazinamide and rifampicin in Hong Kong. *Tubercle* 1976; **57:** 81–95.
5. Jenner PJ, *et al.* Serum uric acid concentrations and arthralgia among patients treated with pyrazinamide-containing regimens in Hong Kong and Singapore. *Tubercle* 1981; **62:** 175–9.

**Pellagra.** Pellagra, probably due to pyrazinamide, developed in a 26-year-old woman receiving antituberculous therapy.[1] Symptoms regressed, without stopping therapy, on administration of nicotinamide.

1. Jørgensen J. Pellagra probably due to pyrazinamide: development during combined chemotherapy of tuberculosis. *Int J Dermatol* 1983; **22:** 44–5.

## Precautions

Pyrazinamide is contra-indicated in patients with liver damage, although the US manufacturers consider that it can be used with care when the liver damage is not severe. Liver function should be assessed before and regularly during treatment. The British Thoracic Society recommends that, in patients with chronic liver disease, pyrazinamide treatment should be suspended if serum aminotransferase concentrations are elevated to 5 times the normal upper limit or the bilirubin concentration rises. Although both the UK and US manufacturers recommend that pyrazinamide should not be restarted in patients with evidence of hepatocellular damage, the UK guidelines allow cautious re-introduction of antimycobacterial drugs, including pyrazinamide, once liver function has returned to normal.

Pyrazinamide should not be given to patients with acute gout or hyperuricaemia and should be used with caution in patients with a history of gout. Caution should also be observed in patients with renal impairment. Increased difficulty has been reported in controlling diabetes mellitus when diabetics are given pyrazinamide.

**Porphyria.** Pyrazinamide has been associated with acute attacks of porphyria and is considered unsafe in porphyric patients.

**Pregnancy.** Although detailed teratogenicity data are not available, WHO,[1] the IUATLD,[2] and the British Thoracic Society[3] do not contra-indicate pyrazinamide in pregnant patients.

1. WHO. *Treatment of tuberculosis: guidelines for national programmes.* Geneva: WHO, 1997.
2. Anonymous. Antituberculosis regimens of chemotherapy: recommendations from the Committee on Treatment of the International Union Against Tuberculosis and Lung Disease. *Bull Int Union Tuberc Lung Dis* 1988; **63:** 60–4.
3. Joint Tuberculosis Committee of the British Thoracic Society. Chemotherapy and management of tuberculosis in the United Kingdom: recommendations 1998. *Thorax* 1998; **53:** 536–48. Also available at: http://www.brit-thoracic.org.uk/docs/Chemotherapy.pdf (accessed 24/05/04)

## Interactions

**Probenecid.** A study of the complex interactions occurring when pyrazinamide and probenecid are given to patients with gout.[1] Urinary excretion of urate depends on the relative size and timing of doses of the two drugs. Probenecid is known to block the excretion of pyrazinamide.

1. Yü TF, *et al.* The effect of the interaction of pyrazinamide and probenecid on urinary uric acid excretion in man. *Am J Med* 1977; **63:** 723–8.

**Zidovudine.** Low or undetectable concentrations of pyrazinamide occurred in 4 patients also taking zidovudine.[1] In the same study, 6 of 7 patients with HIV infection taking pyrazinamide without zidovudine had normal serum pyrazinamide concentrations.

1. Peloquin CA, *et al.* Low antituberculosis drug concentrations in patients with AIDS. *Ann Pharmacother* 1996; **30:** 919–25.

## Antimicrobial Action

Pyrazinamide has a bactericidal effect on *Mycobacterium tuberculosis* but appears to have no activity against other mycobacteria or micro-organisms *in vitro.* It is almost completely inactive at a neutral pH, but is effective against persisting tubercle bacilli within the acidic intracellular environment of the macrophages. The initial inflammatory response to chemotherapy increases the number of organisms in the acidic environment. As inflammation subsides and pH increases, the sterilising activity of pyrazinamide decreases. This pH-dependent activity explains the clinical effectiveness of pyrazinamide as part of the initial 8-week phase in short-course treatment regimens.

Resistance to pyrazinamide rapidly develops when it is used alone.

**Action.** Although the antimicrobial activity of pyrazinamide has been recognised since the 1950s, the mode of action is still unclear. One proposal is that pyrazinoic acid is the active moiety. Pyrazinamidase produced by the tubercle bacilli is known to convert pyrazinamide to pyrazinoic acid. A further proposal[1] is that the pyrazinoic acid formed within the macrophage would be trapped, thereby lowering intracellular pH to levels toxic to tubercle bacilli.

1. Salfinger M, *et al.* Pyrazinamide and pyrazinoic acid activity against tubercle bacilli in cultured human macrophages and in the BACTEC system. *J Infect Dis* 1990; **162:** 201–7.

**Activity with other antimicrobials.** Pyrazinamide exhibited synergistic activity against *Mycobacterium tuberculosis* with clarithromycin.[1]

1. Mor N, Esfandiari A. Synergistic activities of clarithromycin and pyrazinamide against Mycobacterium tuberculosis in human macrophages. *Antimicrob Agents Chemother* 1997; **41:** 2035–6.

## Pharmacokinetics

Pyrazinamide is readily absorbed from the gastrointestinal tract. Peak serum concentrations occur about 2 hours after a dose by mouth and have been reported to be about 33 micrograms/mL after 1.5 g, and 59 micrograms/mL after 3 g. Pyrazinamide is widely distributed in body fluids and tissues and diffuses into the CSF. The half-life has been reported to be about 9 to 10 hours. It is metabolised primarily in the liver by hydrolysis to the major active metabolite pyrazinoic acid, which is subsequently hydroxylated to the major excretory product 5-hydroxypyrazinoic acid. It is excreted through the kidney mainly by glomerular filtration. About 70% of a dose appears in the urine within 24 hours mainly as metabolites and about 4% as unchanged drug. Pyrazinamide is removed by dialysis. Pyrazinamide is distributed into breast milk.

◊ A short distribution phase and an elimination phase of 9.6 hours in healthy subjects following a single oral dose of pyrazinamide 27 mg/kg has been reported;[1] the half-life for the major metabolite pyrazinoic acid was 11.8 hours.

In the major metabolic pathway, pyrazinamide was deaminated to pyrazinoic acid which was hydroxylated to hydroxypyrazinoic acid; in the minor pathway, pyrazinamide was hydroxylated to hydroxypyrazinamide which was then deaminated to hydroxypyrazinoic acid. The limiting step was deamination; oxidation by xanthine oxidase occurred very quickly.

1. Lacroix C, *et al.* Pharmacokinetics of pyrazinamide and its metabolites in healthy subjects. *Eur J Clin Pharmacol* 1989; **36:** 395–400.

**Bioavailability.** The oral bioavailability of rifampicin and isoniazid, but not of pyrazinamide, was decreased by food in one study.[1] However, another report[2] showed slightly reduced peak serum concentrations when pyrazinamide was given with a high-fat meal, and the authors suggested that pyrazinamide should preferably be given on an empty stomach.

1. Zent C, Smith P. Study of the effect of concomitant food on the bioavailability of rifampicin, isoniazid and pyrazinamide. *Tubercle Lung Dis* 1995; **76:** 109–13.
2. Peloquin CA, *et al.* Pharmacokinetics of pyrazinamide under fasting conditions, with food, and with antacids. *Pharmacotherapy* 1998; **18:** 1205–11.

**Breast feeding.** The peak concentration of pyrazinamide in breast milk of a 29-year-old woman was 1.5 micrograms/mL 3 hours after a 1-g dose.[1] The peak plasma concentration was 42 micrograms/mL after 2 hours.

1. Holdiness MR. Antituberculosis drugs and breast-feeding. *Arch Intern Med* 1984; **144:** 1888.

**Distribution.** Pyrazinamide was given to 28 patients with suspected tuberculous meningitis in doses of 34 to 41 mg/kg. The mean concentration of pyrazinamide in the CSF after 2 hours was 38.6 micrograms/mL and represented about 75% of that in serum; concentrations at 5 and 8 hours were 44.5 and 31.0 micrograms/mL respectively and were about 10% higher than those in serum.[1] The use of corticosteroids appeared to have no influence on penetration of pyrazinamide into the CSF of patients with tuberculous meningitis.[2]

1. Ellard GA, *et al.* Penetration of pyrazinamide into the cerebrospinal fluid in tuberculous meningitis. *BMJ* 1987; **294:** 284–5.
2. Woo J, *et al.* Cerebrospinal fluid and serum levels of pyrazinamide and rifampicin in patients with tuberculous meningitis. *Curr Ther Res* 1987; **42:** 235–42.

**Hepatic impairment.** A study of the pharmacokinetics of pyrazinamide was carried out in 10 patients with cirrhosis of the liver.[1] Following a dose of 19.3 mg/kg, the elimination phase was about 15 hours for pyrazinamide and 24 hours for the major metabolite pyrazinoic acid.

1. Lacroix C, *et al.* Pharmacokinetics of pyrazinamide and its metabolites in patients with hepatic cirrhotic insufficiency. *Arzneimittelforschung* 1990; **40:** 76–9.

## Uses and Administration

Pyrazinamide is used as part of multidrug regimens for the treatment of tuberculosis (p.150), primarily in the initial 8-week phase of short-course treatment. Pyrazinamide is usually given daily or 2 or 3 times weekly. In the UK, recommended doses by mouth for adults are up to 35 mg/kg daily (maximum daily dose is 3 g); children may be given 35 mg/kg daily or, for intermittent treatment, 50 mg/kg three times weekly or up to 75 mg/kg twice weekly. To standardise administration, the usual dose for patients under 50 kg is 1.5 g daily, 2 g three times weekly, or 3 g twice weekly. For patients 50 kg or greater, the usual dose is 2 g daily, 2.5 g three times weekly, or 3.5 g twice weekly. The recommended doses in the USA are 20 to 25 mg/kg daily (maximum 2 g) or 1.5 to 3 g three times weekly or 2 to 4 g twice weekly. WHO recommends 25 mg/kg daily or 35 mg/kg three times weekly or 50 mg/kg twice weekly.

Pyrazinamide is also used in the chemoprophylaxis of tuberculosis (see below).

**Administration in hepatic impairment.** See Precautions, above.

**Administration in renal impairment.** The UK manufacturer recommends dosage reduction in patients with renal impairment, although the Joint Tuberculosis Committee of the British Thoracic Society states that standard dosage may be used in such patients.[1]

In a study of 6 patients on haemodialysis,[2] the average amount of pyrazinamide and its metabolites removed during a dialysis session was 926 mg after an oral dose of 1700 mg. It was recommended that the usual pyrazinamide dose be given to patients on dialysis as the risk of accumulation was negligible, and that the dose on dialysis days be given after the procedure.

1. Joint Tuberculosis Committee of the British Thoracic Society. Chemotherapy and management of tuberculosis in the United Kingdom: recommendations 1998. *Thorax* 1998; **53:** 536–48. Also available at: http://www.brit-thoracic.org.uk/docs/Chemotherapy.pdf (accessed 24/05/04)
2. Lacroix C, *et al.* Haemodialysis of pyrazinamide in uraemic patients. *Eur J Clin Pharmacol* 1989; **37:** 309–11.

**Tuberculosis chemoprophylaxis.** In the USA, the American Thoracic Society and the CDC recommended a dose of pyrazinamide 15 to 20 mg/kg daily (maximum 2 g daily) with rifampicin 600 mg daily as an alternative to the preferred isoniazid regimen for the treatment of latent tuberculosis infection.[1] (In those unable to take rifampicin, it was substituted with rifabutin 300 mg daily.) However, owing to the risk of liver injury (see Effects on the Liver, under Adverse Effects, above) the CDC and the American Thoracic Society now recommend that the combination of pyrazinamide with rifampicin should not generally be offered to persons with latent tuberculosis.[2].

1. American Thoracic Society and the Centers for Disease Control. Targeted tuberculin testing and treatment of latent tuberculosis infection. *Am J Respir Crit Care Med* 2000; **161** (suppl): S221–S247.
2. Centers for Disease Control. Update: adverse event data and revised American Thoracic Society/CDC recommendations against the use of rifampin and pyrazinamide for treatment of latent tuberculosis infection—United States, 2003. *MMWR* 2003; **52:** 735–9. Also available at: http://www.cdc.gov/mmwr/preview/mmwrhtml/mm5231a4.htm (accessed 24/05/04)

## Preparations

***BP 2003:*** Pyrazinamide Tablets;
***USP 27:*** Pyrazinamide Tablets; Rifampin, Isoniazid, and Pyrazinamide Tablets; Rifampin, Isoniazid, Pyrazinamide, and Ethambutol Hydrochloride Tablets.

**Proprietary Preparations** (details are given in Part 3)
***Austral.:*** Zinamide; ***Austria:*** Pyrafat; ***Belg.:*** Tebrazid; ***Braz.:*** Pirazinon; ***Canad.:*** Tebrazid; ***Fin.:*** Tisamid; ***Fr.:*** Pirilene; ***Ger.:*** Pyrafat; PZA; ***Hong Kong:*** Pyrafat; ***India:*** P-Zide; Pyzin; PZA-Ciba; Rifacom E-Z; ***Irl.:*** Zinamide; ***Ital.:*** Piraldina; ***Malaysia:*** PZA; ***Mex.:*** Braccopiral†; Pirafoid†; Pirazer†; Premox†; ***NZ:*** Zinamide; ***Port.:*** Piraside; Pramide; ***S.Afr.:*** Pyrazide; Tebezide†; ***Singapore:*** PZA†; ***Thai.:*** Myrin-P; Pyratab; PZA; ***UK:*** Zinamide†.

**Multi-ingredient:** ***Austria:*** Rifater; ***Canad.:*** Rifater; ***Fr.:*** Rifater; ***Ger.:*** Rifater; ***Hong Kong:*** Rifater; ***India:*** Akt-4; Cx-5; Gocox-3; R-Cinex Z; Rimactazid + Z; Tricox; Wokex-4; ***Irl.:*** Rifater; ***Ital.:*** Rifater; ***Mex.:*** Rifater; ***Port.:*** Rifater; Tuberen†; ***S.Afr.:*** Myrin Plus; Pyrifin†; Rifafour; Rifater†; Rimcure; ***Singapore:*** Rifater†; ***Spain:*** Rifater; ***Switz.:*** Rifater; Rimactazide + Z†; ***Thai.:*** Rifampyzid; Rifater; Rimcure 3-FDC; ***UK:*** Rifater; ***USA:*** Rifater.

# Quinupristin/Dalfopristin

Quinupristin *(BAN, USAN, rINN)*; Dalfopristin *(BAN, USAN, rINN)*; Quinupristina/dalfopristina; RP-59500.

*CAS — 126602-89-9 (quinupristin/dalfopristin); 176861-85-1 (quinupristin/dalfopristin).*
*ATC — J01FG02.*

### Dalfopristin Mesilate *(BANM, rINNM)*

Dalfopristin Mesylate; Mesilato de dalfopristina; RP-54476 (dalfopristin). (3*R*,4*R*,5*E*,10*E*,12*E*,14*S*,26*R*,26a*S*)-26-{[2-(Diethylamino)ethyl]sulfonyl}-8,9,14,15,24,25,26,26a-octahydro-14-hydroxy-3-isopropyl-4,12-dimethyl-3*H*-21,18-nitrilo-1*H*,22*H*-pyrrolo[2.1-c][1,8,4,19]dioxadiazacyclotetracosine-1,7,16,22(4*H*,17*H*)-tetrone methanesulphonate; (26*R*,27*S*)-26-{[2-(Diethylamino)-ethyl]sulfonyl}-26,27-dihydrovirginiamycin $M_1$ methanesulphonate.

$C_{34}H_{50}N_4O_9S,CH_4O_3S = 787.0.$
*CAS — 112362-50-2 (dalfopristin).*

### Quinupristin Mesilate *(BANM, rINNM)*

Mesilato de quinupristina; Quinupristin Mesylate; RP-57669 (quinupristin). *N*-{(6*R*,9*S*,10*R*,13*S*,15a*S*,18*R*,22*S*,24a*S*)-22-[*p*-(Dimethylamino)benzyl]-6-ethyldocosahydro-10,23-dimethyl-5,8,12,15,17,21,24-heptaoxo-13-phenyl-18-{[(3*S*)-3-quinuclidinylthio]methyl}-12*H*-pyrido[2,1-*f*]pyrrolo[2,1-*l*][1,4,7,10,13,16]-oxapentaazacyclononadecin-9-yl}-3-hydroxy-picolinamide methanesulphonate; 4-[4-(Dimethylamino)-*N*-methyl-L-phenylalamine]-5-(*cis*-5-{[(*S*)-1-azabicyclo[2.2.2]oct-3-ylthio]methyl}-4-oxo-L-2-piperidinecarboxylic acid)-virginiamycin $S_1$ methanesulphonate.

$C_{53}H_{67}N_9O_{10}S,CH_4O_3S = 1118.3.$
*CAS — 120138-50-3 (quinupristin).*

## Adverse Effects and Treatment

The adverse effects most frequently reported in patients receiving quinupristin/dalfopristin include nausea and vomiting, diarrhoea, skin rash, pruritus, headache, and pain. Myalgia and arthralgia have occurred and may be severe; symptoms may be improved by decreasing the dose frequency. Eosinophilia, anaemia, leucopenia, and neutropenia are also common. Pseudomembranous colitis has been reported. Hyperbilirubinaemia and raised liver enzyme values may occur. Individual cases of severe thrombocytopenia and pancytopenia have been reported.

Pain and inflammation at the injection site is common, and thrombophlebitis has occurred.

Quinupristin/dalfopristin is not removed by peritoneal dialysis, and removal by haemodialysis is considered unlikely.

**Effects on the musculoskeletal system.** References.

1. Olsen KM, *et al.* Arthralgias and myalgias related to quinupristin-dalfopristin administration. Abstract: *Clin Infect Dis* 2001; **32:** 674. Full version: http://www.journals.uchicago.edu/CID/journal/issues/v32n4/000218/000218.html (accessed 28/05/04)

## Precautions

Quinupristin/dalfopristin should be used with caution in patients with hepatic impairment and is contra-indicated in severe impairment, as elevated plasma concentrations of quinupristin and dalfopristin and their metabolites have been found in patients with hepatic dysfunction, and elevated concentrations of quinupristin metabolites have occurred in patients with hyperbilirubinaemia. The combination is contra-indicated in patients who have plasma-bilirubin concentrations greater than 3 times the normal upper limit.

The UK manufacturers state that prolongation of the QT interval has been seen in *animal* studies and therefore recommend that quinupristin/dalfopristin should be used with caution in patients at risk of cardiac arrhythmias.

## Interactions

Quinupristin/dalfopristin inhibits the cytochrome P450 isoenzyme CYP3A4 and it may therefore inhibit the metabolism of a number of drugs. In particular, there is a theoretical possibility of serious ventricular arrhythmias with astemizole, cisapride, and terfenadine. Quinupristin/dalfopristin has been shown to increase plasma concentrations of ciclosporin, midazolam, nifedipine, and tacrolimus. The UK manufacturers suggest that the use of ergot alkaloids with quinupristin/dalfopristin should be avoided, and advise caution if drugs that prolong the QT interval are to be given with quinupristin/dalfopristin.

## Antimicrobial Action

Quinupristin/dalfopristin is a semisynthetic streptogramin antibacterial. Quinupristin and dalfopristin each have bacteriostatic activity and in combination usually act synergistically to produce bactericidal activity. The streptogramins act on the ribosome to block protein synthesis.

Quinupristin/dalfopristin is active against a range of Gram-positive bacteria including meticillin- and multi-drug-resistant strains of *Staphylococcus aureus*, *S. epidermidis*, vancomycin-resistant *Enterococcus faecium* (but not *E. faecalis*), and penicillin- and macrolide-resistant *Streptococcus pneumoniae*. It is also active against the anaerobe *Clostridium perfringens*, and Gram-negative bacteria *Legionella pneumophila*, *Moraxella catarrhalis* (*Branhamella catarrhalis*), *Mycoplasma pneumoniae*, and *Neisseria meningitidis*.

◊ References.

1. Schouten MA, Hoogkamp-Korstanje JAA. Comparative in-vitro activities of quinupristin-dalfopristin against Gram-positive bloodstream isolates. *J Antimicrob Chemother* 1997; **40:** 213–19.
2. Pankuch GA, *et al.* Postantibiotic effect and postantibiotic sub-MIC effect of quinupristin-dalfopristin against Gram-positive and negative organisms. *Antimicrob Agents Chemother* 1998; **42:** 3028–31.
3. Johnson AP, *et al.* Susceptibility to quinupristin/dalfopristin and other antibiotics of vancomycin-resistant enterococci from the UK, 1997 to mid-1999. *J Antimicrob Chemother* 2000; **46:** 125–8.
4. Ling TK, *et al.* In vitro activity and post-antibiotic effect of quinupristin/dalfopristin (Synercid). *Chemotherapy* 2001; **47:** 243–9.
5. Eliopoulos GM, Wennersten CB. Antimicrobial activity of quinupristin-dalfopristin combined with other antibiotics against vancomycin-resistant enterococci. *Antimicrob Agents Chemother* 2002; **46:** 1319–24.

**Resistance.** Although uncommon, isolated reports of *E. faecium* resistant to quinupristin/dalfopristin have emerged,[1-3] and have included a link to the use of the streptogramin virginiamycin as an animal food additive.[3]

1. Eliopoulos GM, *et al.* Characterization of vancomycin-resistant Enterococcus faecium isolates from the United States and their susceptibility in vitro to dalfopristin-quinupristin. *Antimicrob Agents Chemother* 1998; **42:** 1088–92.
2. Bozdogan B, *et al.* Plasmid-mediated coresistance to streptogramins and vancomycin in Enterococcus faecium HM1032. *Antimicrob Agents Chemother* 1999; **43:** 2097–8.
3. Werner G, *et al.* Association between quinupristin/dalfopristin resistance in glycopeptide-resistant Enterococcus faecium and the use of additives in animal feed. *Eur J Clin Microbiol Infect Dis* 1998; **17:** 401–2.

## Pharmacokinetics

Following parenteral administration, quinupristin and dalfopristin are rapidly metabolised. At steady state, the half-life of quinupristin and its metabolites is about 3 hours and that of dalfopristin and its metabolites about 1 hour. Elimination half-lives of unchanged quinupristin and dalfopristin are 0.9 and 0.75 hours respectively. Protein binding is 55 to 78% for quinupristin and 11 to 26% for dalfopristin. The main route of excretion is biliary, with 75 to 77% of a dose detectable in the faeces. Urinary excretion accounts for 15% of the quinupristin and 19% of the dalfopristin dose. Negligible amounts are removed by peritoneal dialysis and probably also by haemodialysis.

## Uses and Administration

Quinupristin/dalfopristin is a streptogramin antibacterial related to pristinamycin. Quinupristin and dalfopristin are semisynthetic derivatives of pristinamycin I and pristinamycin IIA respectively, and are used in the ratio 3:7. Quinupristin/dalfopristin is active against a range of Gram-positive and some Gram-negative organisms, but it is reserved for the treatment of serious infections with multidrug-resistant Gram-positive bacteria, specifically multidrug-resistant *Staphylococcus aureus* and pneumococci and vancomycin-resistant *Enterococcus faecium*.

Quinupristin/dalfopristin is given by intravenous infusion in glucose 5% over 60 minutes through a central venous catheter. The vein should be flushed following each infusion to minimise venous irritation. The injection should not be diluted with saline solutions since it is incompatible with sodium chloride. Quinupristin/dalfopristin is given as the mesilate salts in a dose of 7.5 mg/kg (equivalent to quinupristin 2.25 mg/kg and dalfopristin 5.25 mg/kg) every 8 or 12 hours for 7 to 10 days.

◊ References.

1. Bayston R, *et al.*, eds. Quinupristin/dalfopristin—update on the first injectable streptogramin. *J Antimicrob Chemother* 1997; **39** (suppl A): 1–151.
2. Wood MJ (ed). Quinupristin/dalfopristin–a novel approach for the treatment of serious Gram-positive infections. *J Antimicrob Chemother* 1999; **44** (suppl A): 1–46.
3. Lamb HM, *et al.* Quinupristin/dalfopristin: a review of its use in the management of serious Gram-positive infections. *Drugs* 1999; **58:** 1061–97.
4. Drew RH, *et al.* Treatment of methicillin-resistant Staphylococcus aureus infections with quinupristin-dalfopristin in patients intolerant of or failing prior therapy: for the Synercid Emergency-Use Study Group. *J Antimicrob Chemother* 2000; **46:** 775–84.
5. Allington DR, Rivey MP. Quinupristin/dalfopristin: a therapeutic review. *Clin Ther* 2001; **23:** 24–44.

6. Linden PK, *et al.* Treatment of vancomycin-resistant Enterococcus faecium infections with quinupristin/dalfopristin. *Clin Infect Dis* 2001; **33:** 1816–23.
7. Goff DA, Sierawski SJ. Clinical experience of quinupristin-dalfopristin for the treatment of antimicrobial-resistant gram-positive infections. *Pharmacotherapy* 2002; 748–58.

**Administration in hepatic impairment.** Quinupristin/dalfopristin is contra-indicated in patients with severe hepatic impairment. For patients with moderate impairment the UK manufacturers recommend that a dose reduction to 5 mg/kg (equivalent to quinupristin 1.5 mg/kg and dalfopristin 3.5 mg/kg) should be considered.

## Preparations

**Proprietary Preparations** (details are given in Part 3)

**Multi-ingredient:** ***Arg.:*** Synercid; ***Austral.:*** Synercid; ***Austria:*** Synercid; ***Braz.:*** Synercid; ***Canad.:*** Synercid; ***Fin.:*** Synercid; ***Fr.:*** Synercid; ***Ger.:*** Synercid; ***Irl.:*** Synercid; ***Israel:*** Synercid; ***Ital.:*** Synercid; ***Mex.:*** Synercid; ***Neth.:*** Synercid; ***S.Afr.:*** Synercid; ***Spain:*** Synercid; ***Swed.:*** Synercid; ***Switz.:*** Synercid; ***UK:*** Synercid; ***USA:*** Synercid.

## Ramoplanin *(USAN, rINN)*

A-16686; MDL-62198; Ramoplanina.

*CAS — 76168-82-6.*

### Profile

Ramoplanin is a glycopeptide antibiotic with a spectrum of activity *in vitro* similar to that of vancomycin (p.276) but considerably more potent. It is also active against *Bacteroides* spp. It is under investigation, notably in the prevention of infection due to vancomycin-resistant enterococci, and the reduction of nasal carriage of staphylococci.

◊ References.

1. Wong MT, *et al.* Effective suppression of vancomycin-resistant Enterococcus species in asymptomatic gastrointestinal carriers by a novel glycolipodepsipeptide, ramoplanin. *Clin Infect Dis* 2001; **33:** 1476–82.
2. Montecalvo MA. Ramoplanin: a novel antimicrobial agent with the potential to prevent vancomycin-resistant enterococcal infection in high-risk patients. *J Antimicrob Chemother* 2003; **51** (suppl S3): iii31 iii35.

## Rifabutin *(BAN, USAN, rINN)*

Ansamicin; Ansamycin; LM-427; Rifabutina; Rifabutine; Rifabutinum. (9*S*,12*E*,14*S*,15*R*,16*S*,17*R*,18*R*,19*R*,20*S*,21*S*,22*E*,24*Z*)-6,16,18,20-Tetrahydroxy-1′-isobutyl-14-methoxy-7,9,15,17,19,21,25-heptamethylspiro[9,4-(epoxypentadeca[1,11,13]trienimino)-2*H*-furo-[2′,3′:7,8]naphth[1,2-*d*]imidazole-2,4′-piperidine]-5,10,26-(3*H*,9*H*)-trione-16-acetate.

$C_{46}H_{62}N_4O_{11}$ = 847.0.

*CAS — 72559-06-9.*

*ATC — J04AB04.*

**Pharmacopoeias.** In *Eur.* (see p.vi) and *US.*

**Ph. Eur. 5.0** (Rifabutin). A reddish-violet amorphous powder. Slightly soluble in water and in alcohol; soluble in methyl alcohol.

**USP 27** (Rifabutin). An amorphous red-violet powder. Very slightly soluble in water; sparingly soluble in alcohol; soluble in chloroform and in methyl alcohol. Store at a temperature not exceeding 40°. Protect from light.

**Stability.** Study of the stability of two extemporaneous oral liquid preparations of rifabutin.[1]

1. Haslam JL, *et al.* Stability of rifabutin in two extemporaneously compounded oral liquids. *Am J Health-Syst Pharm* 1999; **56:** 333–6.

### Adverse Effects and Precautions

As for Rifampicin, p.250. It produces a syndrome of polyarthralgia-arthritis at doses greater than 1 g daily. Uveitis has been reported, especially in patients also receiving clarithromycin or fluconazole. Asymptomatic corneal opacities have been reported following long-term use.

◊ A polyarthralgia-arthritis syndrome has been reported[1] in 9 of 10 patients receiving a daily dose of rifabutin greater than 1 g. The syndrome did not occur in patients receiving less than 1 g daily and disappeared on drug withdrawal. Two patients with polyarthralgia-arthritis symptoms developed uveitis (see also under Effects on the Eyes, below) and aphthous stomatitis at doses of approximately 1.8 g daily.

An orange-tan skin pigmentation has been reported to occur in most patients receiving rifabutin.[1] Urine may be discoloured.[2] A flu-like syndrome has been reported in 2 of 12 patients given 300 mg daily for Crohn's disease,[3] in 1 of 16 HIV-infected patients on continuous rifabutin,[1] and in 8 of 15 HIV-infected patients receiving increasing doses of rifabutin.[2]

Other reported adverse effects include hepatitis,[1] leucopenia[2] (including neutropenia[4]), epigastric pain,[3] rash,[3] erythema,[2] and ageusia.[5] Rash, fever, and vomiting occurred in 1 of 2 children receiving 6.5 mg/kg daily.[6]

1. Siegal FP, *et al.* Dose-limiting toxicity of rifabutin in AIDS-related complex: syndrome of arthralgia/arthritis. *AIDS* 1990; **4:** 433–41.
2. Torseth J, *et al.* Evaluation of the antiviral effect of rifabutin in AIDS-related complex. *J Infect Dis* 1989; **159:** 1115–18.
3. Basilisco G, *et al.* Controlled trial of rifabutin in Crohn's disease. *Curr Ther Res* 1989; **46:** 245–50.
4. Apseloff G, *et al.* Severe neutropenia caused by recommended prophylactic doses of rifabutin. *Lancet* 1996; **348:** 685.
5. Morris JT, Kelly JW. Rifabutin-induced ageusia. *Ann Intern Med* 1993; **119:** 171–2.
6. Levin RH, Bolinger AM. Treatment of nontuberculous mycobacterial infections in pediatric patients. *Clin Pharm* 1988; **7:** 545–51.

**Effects on the eyes.** Uveitis may occur a few weeks or months after starting rifabutin, and generally necessitates withdrawal of the drug and treatment with topical or systemic corticosteroids and cycloplegics.[1] The UK Committee on Safety of Medicines was aware of 48 reports of uveitis in patients taking rifabutin.[2] Most patients were also receiving clarithromycin for treatment of AIDS-related *Mycobacterium avium* complex (MAC) infection and many were also receiving fluconazole (see Interactions, below). A dosage reduction to 300 mg rifabutin daily is now recommended in patients also receiving macrolides or triazole antifungals[2,3] and is reported to produce a satisfactory response in MAC infections.[4]

1. Tseng AL, Walmsley SL. Rifabutin-associated uveitis. *Ann Pharmacother* 1995; **29:** 1149–55.
2. Committee on Safety of Medicines. Rifabutin (Mycobutin)—uveitis. *Current Problems 20* 1994.
3. Committee on Safety of Medicines. Revised indications and drug interactions of rifabutin. *Current Problems* 1997; **23:** 14. Also available at: http://www.mca.gov.uk/ourwork/monitorsafequalmed/currentproblems/first.htm (accessed 28/05/04)
4. Shafran SD, *et al.* A comparison of two regimens for the treatment of Mycobacterium avium complex bacteremia in AIDS; rifabutin, ethambutol, and clarithromycin versus rifampin, ethambutol, clofazimine, and ciprofloxacin. *N Engl J Med* 1996; **335:** 377–83.

### Interactions

As for Rifampicin, p.251. Rifabutin is reported to be a less potent inducer of microsomal enzymes than rifampicin, but similar interactions should nevertheless be anticipated.

Plasma concentrations of rifabutin are increased by clarithromycin (and possibly other macrolides) or fluconazole, resulting in increased rifabutin toxicity, in particular uveitis and neutropenia (see also above).

**Antiretroviral drugs.** Rifabutin interacts with *HIV-protease inhibitors*, resulting in reductions in plasma concentrations of the HIV-protease inhibitor and increases in rifabutin plasma concentrations, with a possible risk of uveitis. Most clinical experience appears to have been gained with rifabutin in combination with indinavir. The Centers for Disease Control in the USA suggest[1,2] that in patients with HIV infection who need treatment for tuberculosis, rifabutin could be used in those receiving amprenavir, atazanavir, efavirenz, fosamprenavir, indinavir, lopinavir-ritonavir, nelfinavir, nevirapine, or ritonavir; however, dose modifications are required for rifabutin in some combinations and should be substantial (150 mg every other day or three times per week) when it is given with atazanavir, lopinavir-ritonavir, or ritonavir in particular[2] (see Tuberculosis and HIV infection under Uses, below). Rifabutin should not be given with delavirdine or saquinavir alone; however, saquinavir may be given with rifabutin if ritonavir is also given.[2] Concomitant increases in doses of indinavir and nelfinavir are also required.[2]

Although rifabutin is reported to reduce the plasma concentrations of *zidovudine*, studies have shown that the effect is not marked (see p.659), and the manufacturer suggests that the reduction may not be clinically relevant.

1. Centers for Disease Control. Prevention and treatment of tuberculosis among patients infected with human immunodeficiency virus: principles of therapy and revised recommendations. *MMWR* 1998; **47** (RR-20): 1–58. Also available at: http://www.cdc.gov/mmwr/PDF/rr/rr4720.pdf (accessed 28/05/04)
2. Centers for Disease Control. Updated guidelines for the use of rifamycins for the treatment of tuberculosis among HIV-infected patients taking protease inhibitors or nonnucleoside reverse transcriptase inhibitors. *MMWR* 2004; **53:** 37. Available at: http://www.cdc.gov/nchstp/tb/tb_hiv_drugs/toc.htm (accessed 28/05/04)

**Azole antifungals.** As mentioned under Adverse Effects, above, many reports of rifabutin-associated uveitis have occurred in patients also receiving *fluconazole*. The area under the concentration-time curve for rifabutin and its active 25-deacetyl metabolite were increased by 82% and 216% respectively when fluconazole was given to 12 HIV-infected patients,[1] and elevated plasma-rifabutin concentrations were reported in a patient who developed uveitis while also receiving *itraconazole*.[2] The mechanism of the interaction remains uncertain but could involve microsomal cytochrome P450 isoenzyme CYP3A4 (see Metabolism under Pharmacokinetics, below).

1. Trapnell CB, *et al.* Increased plasma rifabutin levels with concomitant fluconazole therapy in HIV-infected patients. *Ann Intern Med* 1996; **124:** 573–6.
2. Lefort A, *et al.* Uveitis associated with rifabutin prophylaxis and itraconazole therapy. *Ann Intern Med* 1996; **125:** 939–40.

**Macrolides.** As discussed under Effects on the Eyes, above, most patients developing uveitis during rifabutin treatment are also receiving *clarithromycin*. In a study of the treatment of *Mycobacterium avium* complex infection in AIDS patients,[1] uveitis or pseudojaundice or both were noted in those receiving rifabutin, ethambutol, and clarithromycin, but not in those receiving rifabutin, ethambutol, ciprofloxacin, and clofazimine. A retrospective study following an outbreak of uveitis in a similar patient population[2] also found clarithromycin to be a risk factor, with a trend towards greater risk at higher rifabutin doses, although patient numbers were small. In 26 patients taking rifabutin with either clarithromycin or *azithromycin*,[3] the incidence and severity of adverse effects in general was similar, although the 2 patients who developed uveitis were both receiving clarithromycin.

Pharmacokinetic studies have demonstrated increased rifabutin concentrations when clarithromycin is also used. A study in healthy subjects[4] was terminated prematurely because of the high incidence of adverse effects, including neutropenia, fevers, and myalgia, particularly in subjects receiving rifabutin with azithromycin or clarithromycin. Mean serum concentrations of rifabutin and its 25-*O*-deacetyl metabolite in subjects also receiving clarithromycin were more than 4 times and 37 times those in subjects receiving rifabutin alone. Plasma concentrations were unaffected by azithromycin. Similar effects on rifabutin concentrations were found in HIV-infected subjects receiving clarithromycin[5] and reductions in clarithromycin concentrations were also noted.

1. Shafran SD, *et al.* Uveitis and pseudojaundice during a regimen of clarithromycin, rifabutin, and ethambutol. *N Engl J Med* 1994; **330:** 438–9.
2. Kelleher P, *et al.* Uveitis associated with rifabutin and macrolide therapy for Mycobacterium avium intracellulare infection in AIDS patients. *Genitourin Med* 1996; **72:** 419–21.
3. Griffith DE, *et al.* Adverse events associated with high-dose rifabutin in macrolide-containing regimens for the treatment of Mycobacterium avium complex lung disease. *Clin Infect Dis* 1995; **21:** 594–8.
4. Apseloff G, *et al.* Comparison of azithromycin and clarithromycin in their interactions with rifabutin in healthy volunteers. *J Clin Pharmacol* 1998; **38:** 830–5.
5. Hafner R, *et al.* Tolerance and pharmacokinetic interactions of rifabutin and clarithromycin in human immunodeficiency virus-infected volunteers. *Antimicrob Agents Chemother* 1998; **42:** 631–9.

### Antimicrobial Action

Rifabutin possesses a spectrum of antibacterial activity similar to that of rifampicin (p.252). However, most investigations have concentrated on its action against mycobacteria. Cross-resistance is common with rifampicin.

**Antimycobacterial action.** Rifabutin possesses activity against most species of mycobacteria. It may be more active *in vivo* than *in vitro* studies suggest, as a result of its favourable pharmacokinetic profile and prolonged postantibiotic effect.[1]

Rifabutin has been reported to be active in *animal* assays against *Mycobacterium leprae*,[2] including a rifampicin-resistant strain.[3] Synergistic activity against *M. leprae* has been reported[4] *in vitro* for rifabutin with clinafloxacin and rifabutin with sparfloxacin.

1. Kunin CM. Antimicrobial activity of rifabutin. *Clin Infect Dis* 1996; **22** (suppl 1): S3–S14.
2. Hastings RC, Jacobson RR. Activity of ansamycin against Mycobacterium leprae in mice. *Lancet* 1983; **ii:** 1079–80. Correction. *ibid.*; 1210.
3. Hastings RC, *et al.* Ansamycin activity against rifampicin-resistant Mycobacterium leprae. *Lancet* 1984; **i:** 1130.
4. Dhople AM, Ibanez MA. In-vitro activity of three new fluoroquinolones and synergy with ansamycins against Mycobacterium leprae. *J Antimicrob Chemother* 1993; **32:** 445–51.

**Resistance.** Rifampicin-resistant strains of *Mycobacterium tuberculosis* have been identified in 2 patients receiving rifabutin alone as prophylaxis against *M. avium* complex.[1,2] It is therefore important to exclude *M. tuberculosis* infection before beginning rifabutin prophylaxis.

Rifampicin-resistant *M. kansasii* has also been reported in a patient receiving rifabutin.[3]

Acquired resistance has been reported in HIV-infected persons receiving highly intermittent regimens (once- or twice-weekly) of rifabutin for the treatment of active tuberculosis,[4] and the CDC has advised that such patients receive daily treatment during the intensive phase of therapy and daily or thrice-weekly treatment during the continuation phase.

1. Weltman AC, *et al.* Rifampicin-resistant Mycobacterium tuberculosis. *Lancet* 1995; **345:** 1513.
2. Bishai WR, *et al.* Brief report: rifampin-resistant tuberculosis in a patient receiving rifabutin prophylaxis. *N Engl J Med* 1996; **334:** 1573–6.
3. Meynard JL, *et al.* Rifampin-resistant Mycobacterium kansasii infection in a patient with AIDS who was receiving rifabutin. *Clin Infect Dis* 1997; **24:** 1262–3.
4. Centers for Disease Control. Notice to readers: acquired rifamycin resistance in persons with advanced HIV disease being treated for active tuberculosis with intermittent rifamycin-based regimens. *MMWR* 2002; **51:** 214–15.

### Pharmacokinetics

Rifabutin is poorly absorbed from the gastrointestinal tract, but is widely distributed. Approximately 70% is bound to plasma proteins. Both hepatic and renal clearance occurs. A mean terminal half-life of 45 hours has been reported.

**HIV-infected patients.** The pharmacokinetics of rifabutin were studied in HIV-infected patients with normal renal and hepatic function.[1] A two-compartment open pharmacokinetic model was proposed. Rifabutin was rapidly but incompletely absorbed from the gastrointestinal tract and bioavailability was poor, being 20% on day 1 of the study and 12% on day 28. Mean peak plasma concentrations occurred 2 to 3 hours following oral doses and were about 350, 500, and 900 nanograms/mL following doses of 300, 600, and 900 mg respectively. The peak and trough concentrations following 600 mg twice daily were about 900 and 200 nanograms/mL respectively. Rifabutin was about 70% bound to plasma proteins. The area under the curve showed a decrease on repeated dosage which might be explained by the induction of drug-metabolising liver enzymes. A large volume of distribution of 8 to 9 litres/kg, indicative of extensive tissue distribution, and a mean terminal half-life of 32 to 38 hours were reported.

This study[1] also showed that the peak plasma concentration of the major metabolite, 25-deacetylrifabutin, was 10% of the parent compound. Only 4% of unchanged rifabutin was excreted in the urine following oral use and between 6 to 14% following intravenous use. Total urinary excretion of rifabutin and metabolite 72 hours after intravenous use was 44%; total faecal excretion was between 30 and 49%.

Peak and trough concentrations at steady state were reported as 900 and 200 nanograms/mL respectively in a patient with tuberculosis given rifabutin 450 mg daily.[2] While these figures were the same as those previously reported with 600 mg twice daily,[1] the earlier study showed that there was considerable interpatient variability.

CSF concentrations in 5 patients with AIDS on rifabutin 450 mg daily ranged from 36 to 70% of serum concentrations.[3]

1. Skinner MH, *et al.* Pharmacokinetics of rifabutin. *Antimicrob Agents Chemother* 1989; **33:** 1237–41.
2. Gillespie SH, *et al.* The serum rifabutin concentrations in a patient successfully treated for multi-resistant mycobacterium tuberculosis infection. *J Antimicrob Chemother* 1990; **25:** 490–1. Correction. *ibid.* 1991; **27:** 877.
3. Siegal FP, *et al.* Dose-limiting toxicity of rifabutin in AIDS-related complex: syndrome of arthralgia/arthritis. *AIDS* 1990; **4:** 433–41.

**Metabolism.** Five metabolites of rifabutin were identified in an *in-vitro* study[1] using human hepatic and enterocyte microsomes. Cytochrome P450 isoenzyme CYP3A4 was involved in the formation of all metabolites except 25-*O*-deacetylrifabutin. Deacetylation of rifabutin was apparently mediated by microsomal cholinesterase,[1] although another study[2] showed that further metabolism of 25-*O*-deacetylrifabutin is dependent on CYP3A4. The results[1] also suggested that metabolism by intestinal CYP3A4 contributes significantly to presystemic metabolism of rifabutin (and consequently its low bioavailability) and to drug interactions with azole antifungals and with macrolides (see above).

1. Iatsimirskaia E, *et al.* Metabolism of rifabutin in human enterocyte and liver microsomes: kinetic parameters, identification of enzyme systems, and drug interactions with macrolides and antifungal agents. *Clin Pharmacol Ther* 1997; **61:** 554–62.
2. Trapnell CB, *et al.* Metabolism of rifabutin and its 25-desacetyl metabolite, LM565, by human liver microsomes and recombinant human cytochrome P-450 3A4: relevance to clinical interaction with fluconazole. *Antimicrob Agents Chemother* 1997; **41:** 924–6.

## Uses and Administration

Rifabutin is a rifamycin antibiotic used for the prophylaxis of *Mycobacterium avium* complex (MAC) infection in immunocompromised patients. It is also used for the treatment of opportunistic mycobacterial infections (including those due to MAC) (p.137) and tuberculosis, including latent tuberculosis infection (p.150). When used for treatment rifabutin, like rifampicin, should be used with other antibacterials to prevent the emergence of resistant organisms.

Rifabutin is given by mouth as a single daily dose. The dose for the prophylaxis of *M. avium* complex infection is 300 mg daily. For the treatment of opportunistic mycobacterial infections the dose is 450 to 600 mg daily and for pulmonary tuberculosis the dose is 150 to 450 mg daily, in each case as part of a multidrug regimen. Doses should be reduced to 300 mg daily in patients also receiving macrolides or azole antifungals (see under Adverse Effects, Effects on the Eyes, above). Dosage alterations may also be necessary in patients receiving HIV-protease inhibitors (see under Tuberculosis, below).

◊ Reviews.

1. Brogden RN, Fitton A. Rifabutin: a review of its antimicrobial activity, pharmacokinetic properties and therapeutic efficacy. *Drugs* 1994; **47:** 983–1009.

**Cryptosporidiosis.** Rifabutin may have a potential prophylactic effect against cryptosporidiosis (p.596).

**Mycobacterium avium complex infections.** Alterations in rifabutin dosage may be necessary in patients receiving antiretrovirals for the management of HIV infection; further details are given under Tuberculosis, below.

**Toxoplasmosis.** A beneficial response to rifabutin used with pyrimethamine was reported in a patient with AIDS-related *Toxoplasma gondii* encephalitis.[1] The patient was allergic to sulfonamides and clindamycin, the drugs most commonly used (see p.598).

1. Schürmann D, *et al.* Rifabutin appears to be a promising agent for combination treatment of AIDS-related toxoplasma encephalitis. *J Infect* 1998; **36:** 352–3.

**Tuberculosis and HIV infection.** The CDC in the USA recommends that rifabutin should be used in place of rifampicin in short-course therapy for tuberculosis in patients receiving antiretroviral drugs for HIV infection.[1] However, dose modifications are often necessary;[1,2] additionally, some combinations, notably rifabutin with delavirdine or saquinavir alone, should not be employed, although rifabutin may be given with saquinavir if ritonavir is also given.

In patients receiving atazanavir, lopinavir-ritonavir, or ritonavir, the dose of rifabutin should be substantially reduced from 300 mg daily or twice weekly to 150 mg every other day or three times per week. In those receiving amprenavir, fosamprenavir, indinavir, or nelfinavir the daily dose of rifabutin should be decreased from 300 mg to 150 mg, and the dose for intermittent therapy should be 300 mg three times weekly. The doses of indinavir and nelfinavir will need to be increased. In patients receiving efavirenz, the dose of rifabutin should be increased from 300 mg daily or twice weekly to 450 mg daily or 600 mg three times per week. In patients receiving nevirapine, the dose of rifabutin should be 300 mg daily or 300 mg three times per week. In patients with a CD4 count greater than 100 cells/microlitre, twice weekly administration of rifabutin may be considered with amprenavir, efavirenz, fosamprenavir, indinavir, nelfinavir, or nevirapine.

1. Centers for Disease Control. Prevention and treatment of tuberculosis among patients infected with human immunodeficiency virus: principles of therapy and revised recommendations. *MMWR* 1998; **47** (RR-20): 1–58. Also available at: http://www.cdc.gov/mmwr/PDF/rr/rr4720.pdf (accessed 28/05/04)
2. Centers for Disease Control. Updated guidelines for the use of rifamycins for the treatment of tuberculosis among HIV-infected patients taking protease inhibitors or nonnucleoside reverse transcriptase inhibitors. *MMWR* 2004; **53:** 37. Available at: http://www.cdc.gov/nchstp/tb/tb_hiv_drugs/toc.htm (accessed 28/05/04)

## Preparations

***USP 27:*** Rifabutin Capsules.

**Proprietary Preparations** (details are given in Part 3)

***Austral.:*** Mycobutin; ***Austria:*** Mycobutin; ***Belg.:*** Mycobutin; ***Canad.:*** Mycobutin; ***Fin.:*** Ansatipin; ***Fr.:*** Ansatipine; ***Ger.:*** Alfacid; Mycobutin; ***Gr.:*** Mycobutin; ***Hong Kong:*** Mycobutin; ***Israel:*** Mycobutin; ***Ital.:*** Mycobutin; ***Neth.:*** Mycobutin; ***NZ:*** Mycobutin; ***Port.:*** Mycobutin; ***S.Afr.:*** Mycobutin; ***Spain:*** Ansatipin; ***Swed.:*** Ansatipin; ***Switz.:*** Mycobutin; ***UK:*** Mycobutin; ***USA:*** Mycobutin.

# Rifampicin *(BAN, rINN)*

Ba-41166/E; L-5103; NSC-113926; Rifaldazine; Rifampicina; Rifampicinum; Rifampin *(USAN)*; Rifamycin AMP. 3-(4-Methylpiperazin-1-yliminomethyl)rifamycin SV; (12*Z*,14*E*,24*E*)-(2*S*,16*S*,17*S*,18*R*,19*R*,20*R*,21*S*,22*R*,23*S*)-1,2-Dihydro-5,6,9,17,19-pentahydroxy-23-methoxy-2,4,12,16,18,20,22-heptamethyl-8-(4-methylpiperazin-1-yliminomethyl)-1,11-dioxo-2,7-(epoxypentadeca[1,11,13]trienimino)naphtho[2,1-*b*]furan-21-yl acetate.

$C_{43}H_{58}N_4O_{12}$ = 822.9.

*CAS — 13292-46-1.*

*ATC — J04AB02.*

**Pharmacopoeias.** In *Chin.*, *Eur.* (see p.vi), *Int.*, *Jpn*, *Pol.*, *US*, and *Viet.*

**Ph. Eur. 5.0** (Rifampicin). A reddish-brown or brownish-red, crystalline powder. Slightly soluble in water, in alcohol, and in acetone; soluble in methyl alcohol. A 1% suspension has a pH of 4.5 to 6.5. Store at a temperature not exceeding 25° in an atmosphere of nitrogen in airtight containers. Protect from light.

**USP 27** (Rifampin). A red-brown crystalline powder. Very slightly soluble in water; freely soluble in chloroform; soluble in ethyl acetate and in methyl alcohol. A 1% suspension in water has a pH of 4.5 to 6.5. Store at a temperature not exceeding 40° in airtight containers. Protect from light.

**Stability.** The method used when preparing an oral liquid from commercial rifampicin capsules influenced the dispersion of the powder and consequently the measured concentration of rifampicin in the final product.[1]

1. Nahata MC, *et al.* Effect of preparation method and storage on rifampin concentration in suspensions. *Ann Pharmacother* 1994; **28:** 182–5.

## Adverse Effects

Rifampicin is usually well tolerated. Adverse effects are more common during intermittent therapy or after restarting interrupted treatment.

Some patients may experience a cutaneous syndrome which presents 2 to 3 hours after a daily or intermittent dose as facial flushing, itching, rash, or rarely eye irritation. A 12-hour flu-like syndrome of fever, chills, headache, dizziness, bone pain, shortness of breath, and malaise has been associated with intermittent use. It usually occurs after 3 to 6 months of intermittent treatment and has a higher incidence with doses of 25 mg/kg or more given once weekly than with currently recommended regimens. Anaphylaxis or shock has occurred rarely.

Gastrointestinal adverse effects include nausea, vomiting, anorexia, diarrhoea, and epigastric distress. Administration on an empty stomach is recommended for maximal absorption, but this has to be balanced against administration after a meal to minimise gastrointestinal intolerance. Pseudomembranous colitis has been reported. Rifampicin produces transient abnormalities in liver function. Hepatitis occurs rarely. Fatalities due to hepatotoxicity have been reported occasionally (see Effects on the Liver, below).

Rifampicin can cause thrombocytopenia and purpura, usually when given as an intermittent regimen, and if this occurs further use of rifampicin is contra-indicated. Other haematological adverse effects include eosinophilia, leucopenia, and haemolytic anaemia.

Alterations in kidney function and renal failure have occurred, particularly during intermittent therapy. Menstrual disturbances have been reported.

Nervous system adverse effects include headache, drowsiness, ataxia, dizziness, and numbness.

Oedema, myopathy, and muscular weakness have been reported.

Thrombophlebitis has occurred following prolonged intravenous infusion. Extravasation during intravenous infusion may cause local irritation and inflammation.

Rifampicin causes a harmless orange-red discoloration of the urine, faeces, sweat, saliva, sputum, tears, and other body fluids.

**Effects on the blood.** Thrombocytopenia may occur in patients taking rifampicin, most commonly as intermittent therapy, and probably has an immunological basis. The platelet count may fall within 3 hours of a dose and return to normal within 36 hours, if additional doses are not given.[1] There may also be a risk of thrombocytopenia when re-introducing rifampicin to patients who have interrupted their treatment.[2] Thrombocytopenia has also been reported in a patient taking rifampicin for the first time for meningococcal prophylaxis.[3] Fatalities have occurred when rifampicin was not withdrawn once thrombocytopenic purpura had developed or when treatment with rifampicin was resumed in patients who had experienced purpura.[1] However, there is a report of the successful re-introduction of rifampicin in a patient who developed thrombocytopenia without rifampicin-dependent antibodies.[4]

Bleeding from the oral cavity not associated with thrombocytopenia has been reported in a patient taking rifampicin.[5] Leucopenia,[6,7] haemolysis or haemolytic anaemia,[8] and red cell aplasia[9] have occurred. Disseminated intravascular coagulation has been reported in a patient receiving intermittent rifampicin therapy.[10] The incidence of deep-vein thrombosis increased in one group of hospitalised tuberculosis patients when rifampicin was introduced as standard therapy,[11] but data from others have not supported a causal relationship.[12]

1. Girling DJ. Adverse effects of antituberculosis drugs. *Drugs* 1982; **23:** 56–74.
2. Burnette PK, *et al.* Rifampin-associated thrombocytopenia secondary to poor compliance. *Drug Intell Clin Pharm* 1989; **23:** 382–4.
3. Hall AP, *et al.* New hazard of meningococcal chemoprophylaxis. *J Antimicrob Chemother* 1993; **31:** 451.
4. Bhasin DK, *et al.* Can rifampicin be restarted in patients with rifampicin-induced thrombocytopenia? *Tubercle* 1991; **72:** 306–7.
5. Sule RR. An unusual reaction to rifampicin in a once monthly dose. *Lepr Rev* 1996; **67:** 227–33.
6. Van Assendelft AHW. Leucopenia in rifampicin chemotherapy. *J Antimicrob Chemother* 1985; **16:** 407–8.
7. Vijayakumaran P, *et al.* Leucocytopenia after rifampicin and ofloxacin therapy in leprosy. *Lepr Rev* 1997; **68:** 10–15.
8. Lakshminarayan S, *et al.* Massive haemolysis caused by rifampicin. *BMJ* 1973; **2:** 282–3.
9. Mariette X, *et al.* Rifampicin-induced pure red cell aplasia. *Am J Med* 1989; **87:** 459–60.
10. Souza CS, *et al.* Disseminated intravascular coagulopathy as an adverse reaction to intermittent rifampin schedule in the treatment of leprosy. *Int J Lepr* 1997; **65:** 366–71.
11. White NW. Venous thrombosis and rifampicin. *Lancet* 1989; **ii:** 434–5.
12. Cowie RL, *et al.* Deep-vein thrombosis and pulmonary tuberculosis. *Lancet* 1989; **ii:** 1397.

**Effects on the gastrointestinal tract.** In addition to symptoms of gastrointestinal intolerance, there have been reports of gastrointestinal bleeding and erosive gastritis,[1] ulcerative colitis,[2] and eosinophilic colitis[3] in patients receiving rifampicin.

1. Zargar SA, *et al.* Rifampicin-induced upper gastrointestinal bleeding. *Postgrad Med J* 1990; **66:** 310–11.
2. Tajima A, *et al.* Rifampicin-associated ulcerative colitis. *Ann Intern Med* 1992; **116:** 778–9.
3. Lange P, *et al.* Eosinophilic colitis due to rifampicin. *Lancet* 1994; **344:** 1296–7.

**Effects on the immune system.** Symptoms including malaise, arthralgia, arthritis, and oedema of the extremities, occurring in 4 patients taking rifampicin and 3 taking rifabutin, were considered to be due to drug-induced lupus syndrome.[1] Cutaneous lupus erythematosus was reported in a patient receiving rifampicin with clarithromycin and ethambutol.[2] All patients had positive anti-nuclear antibody titres.[1,2]

1. Berning SE, Iseman MD. Rifamycin-induced lupus syndrome. *Lancet* 1997; **349:** 1521–2.
2. Patel GK, Anstey AV. Rifampicin-induced lupus erythematosus. *Clin Exp Dermatol* 2001; **26:** 260–2.

**Effects on the liver.** Transient abnormalities in liver function are common during the early stages of antituberculous therapy with rifampicin and other drugs, but sometimes there is more serious hepatotoxicity that may require a change of treatment especially in patients with pre-existing liver disease.

The use of rifampicin daily with ethionamide or protionamide for the treatment of multibacillary leprosy has long been associated with a high incidence of hepatotoxicity (see under Adverse Effects of Ethionamide, p.212), and ethionamide and protionamide are no longer recommended for the treatment of leprosy because of these effects. However, hepatic reactions have also been reported with rifampicin, isoniazid, and pyrazinamide, the drugs most commonly used to treat tuberculosis, and have occasionally proved fatal. A report[1] of 4 cases of fulminant hepatic failure in patients given triple therapy with this potentially hepatotoxic combination regimen (1 patient also received ethambutol) highlighted the importance of strict liver function monitoring and this was reinforced by others.

The Joint Tuberculosis Committee of the British Thoracic Society is nevertheless anxious that fears over the safety of treatment regimens do not compromise adequate therapy of the disease itself. They make recommendations[2] for initial measurement of liver function in all patients and regular monitoring in patients with pre-existing liver disease. Tests should be repeated if symptoms of liver dysfunction occur, and details are given concerning the response to deteriorating liver function and include guidelines for prompt re-introduction of appropriate antituberculosis therapy once normal liver function is restored.

In the USA, the CDC and the American Thoracic Society now recommend that the combination of rifampicin with pyrazinamide should not generally be offered to persons with latent tuberculosis.[3]

Hepatitis and liver dysfunction have also been reported in patients taking rifampicin, in the absence of other hepatotoxic drugs, for the treatment of pruritus associated with primary biliary cirrhosis.[4]

1. Mitchell I, *et al.* Anti-tuberculous therapy and acute liver failure. *Lancet* 1995; **345:** 555–6.
2. Ormerod LP, *et al.* Hepatotoxicity of antituberculosis drugs. *Thorax* 1996; **51:** 111–13.
3. Centers for Disease Control. Update: adverse event data and revised American Thoracic Society/CDC recommendations against the use of rifampin and pyrazinamide for treatment of latent tuberculosis infection—United States, 2003. *MMWR* 2003; **52:** 735–9. Also available at: http://www.cdc.gov/mmwr/preview/mmwrhtml/mm5231a4.htm (accessed 24/05/04)
4. Prince MI, *et al.* Hepatitis and liver dysfunction with rifampicin therapy for pruritus in primary biliary cirrhosis. *Gut* 2002; **50:** 436–9.

**Effects on the lungs.** Pulmonary fibrosis[1] in one elderly man and pneumonitis[2] in another were attributed to rifampicin.

1. Umeki S. Rifampicin and pulmonary fibrosis. *Arch Intern Med* 1988; **148:** 1663, 7.
2. Kunichika N, *et al.* Pneumonitis induced by rifampicin. *Thorax* 2002; **57:** 1000–1001.

**Effects on the pancreas.** Report of chronic pancreatic insufficiency in a patient following use of rifampicin, isoniazid, ethambutol, and pyrazinamide.[1]

1. Liu BA, *et al.* Pancreatic insufficiency due to antituberculosis therapy. *Ann Pharmacother* 1997; **31:** 724–6.

**Effects on the skin.** Skin reactions to rifampicin are usually mild, irrespective of it being given daily or intermittently.[1] However, there have been a few isolated reports of severe reactions.[2-5] Contact dermatitis has been observed.[6]

1. Girling DJ. Adverse reactions to rifampicin in antituberculosis regimens. *J Antimicrob Chemother* 1977; **3:** 115–32.
2. Okano M, *et al.* Toxic epidermal necrolysis due to rifampicin. *J Am Acad Dermatol* 1987; **17:** 303–4.
3. Goldin HM, *et al.* Rifampin and exfoliative dermatitis. *Ann Intern Med* 1987; **107:** 789.
4. Mimouni A, *et al.* Fixed drug eruption following rifampin treatment. *DICP Ann Pharmacother* 1990; **24:** 947–8.
5. John SS. Fixed drug eruption due to rifampin. *Lepr Rev* 1998; **69:** 397–9.
6. Anker N, Da Gunha Bang F. Long-term intravenous rifampicin treatment: advantages and disadvantages. *Eur J Respir Dis* 1981; **62:** 84–6.

**Hypersensitivity.** References.

1. Girling DJ. Adverse reactions to rifampicin in antituberculosis regimens. *J Antimicrob Chemother* 1977; **3:** 115–32.
2. Wurtz RM, *et al.* Anaphylactoid drug reactions to ciprofloxacin and rifampicin in HIV-infected patients. *Lancet* 1989; **i:** 955–6.
3. Harland RW, *et al.* Anaphylaxis from rifampin. *Am J Med* 1992; **92:** 581–2.
4. Cnudde F, Leynadier F. The diagnosis of allergy to rifampicin confirmed by skin test. *Am J Med* 1994; **97:** 403–4.
5. Sharma VK, *et al.* Rifampicin-induced urticaria in leprosy. *Lepr Rev* 1997; **68:** 331–2.
6. Martínez E, *et al.* Shock and cerebral infarct after rifampin re-exposure in a patient infected with human immunodeficiency virus. *Clin Infect Dis* 1998; **27:** 1329–30.

**Overdosage.** Cases of skin pigmentation induced by rifampicin overdose have been reviewed.[1] Reddish-orange discoloration of the skin appeared within a few hours of drug administration; urine, mucous membranes, and sclera were also discoloured. Periorbital or facial oedema, pruritus, and gastrointestinal intolerance occurred in most patients. Treatment was supportive and clinical symptoms resolved in most patients over 3 to 4 days, although fatalities occurred with doses over 14 g.

1. Holdiness MR. A review of the redman syndrome and rifampicin overdosage. *Med Toxicol Adverse Drug Exp* 1989; **4:** 444–51.

## Precautions

Liver function should be checked before treatment with rifampicin and special care should be taken in alcoholic patients or those with pre-existing liver disease who require regular monitoring during therapy. The UK manufacturers state that its use is contra-indicated in patients with jaundice. A self-limiting hyperbilirubinaemia may occur in the first 2 or 3 weeks of treatment. Alkaline phosphatase values may be raised moderately due to rifampicin's enzyme-inducing capacity. When other liver function tests are within normal limits, hyperbilirubinaemia in the first few weeks or moderately elevated transaminase levels are not indications to withdraw rifampicin. However, dose adjustment is necessary when there is other evidence of hepatic impairment and treatment should be suspended when there is evidence of more serious liver toxicity.

Blood counts should be monitored during prolonged treatment and in patients with hepatic disorders. Should thrombocytopenia or purpura occur then rifampicin should be withdrawn permanently. The UK manufacturers also recommend such withdrawal in patients who develop haemolytic anaemia or renal failure.

Use of rifampicin following interruption of treatment has been associated with increased risk of serious adverse effects.

Patients should be advised that rifampicin may colour faeces, saliva, sputum, sweat, tears, urine, and other body-fluids orange-red. Soft contact lenses may become permanently stained.

Rifampicin should not be given by the intramuscular or subcutaneous route. When given by intravenous infusion care should be taken to avoid extravasation.

**Adrenocortical insufficiency.** Acute adrenal crisis has been precipitated by rifampicin in patients with adrenal insufficiency[1] and induction of microsomal enzymes may be enough to compromise even patients with mildly impaired cortisol production. Critical hypotension has also developed in non-Addisonian patients within a week to 10 days of starting rifampicin therapy. However, it has not been necessary to suspend the use of rifampicin if patients are treated with corticosteroids.[2] The effectiveness of corticosteroid therapy can be reduced by rifampicin.

1. Elansary EH, Earis JE. Rifampicin and adrenal crisis. *BMJ* 1983; **286:** 1861–2.
2. Boss G. Rifampicin and adrenal crisis. *BMJ* 1983; **287:** 62.

**Breast feeding.** No adverse effects have been observed in breast-fed infants whose mothers were receiving rifampicin, and the American Academy of Pediatrics considers[1] that it is therefore usually compatible with breast feeding.

1. American Academy of Pediatrics. The transfer of drugs and other chemicals into human milk. *Pediatrics* 2001; **108:** 776–89. Correction. *ibid.*; 1029. Also available at: http://aappolicy.aappublications.org/cgi/content/full/pediatrics%3b108/3/776 (accessed 28/05/04)

**Porphyria.** Rifampicin has been associated with acute attacks of porphyria and is considered unsafe in porphyric patients.

**Pregnancy.** The International Union Against Tuberculosis[1] and the WHO Expert Committee on Leprosy[2] recommend **treatment of pregnant** patients with the same rifampicin-containing multidrug regimens as would be used in non-pregnant patients. Of the standard drugs recommended for leprosy or tuberculosis, only streptomycin has proven teratogenicity.[3] While use of rifampicin in pregnant patients is generally considered to be safe, the drug does cross into the fetus[4] and malformations and bleeding tendencies have been reported.[3] A literature review[3] revealed 386 normal term infants and 29 elective terminations out of 446 pregnancies in patients who took rifampicin with other antimycobacterial drugs. A variety of malformations were reported; there were 14 abnormal infants or fetuses, 2 premature births, 9 still-births and 7 spontaneous abortions. It was considered that rifampicin did not increase the overall risk of congenital malformations.

Rifampicin treatment can increase the metabolism of vitamin K, resulting in clotting disorders associated with vitamin K deficiency. Bleeding disorders in 2 mothers shortly after delivery, and scalp haemorrhage, anaemia, and shock in one of the infants have been reported.[5] The authors recommended blood coagulation monitoring and prophylactic administration of vitamin K to mothers and neonates when the mother has received rifampicin during pregnancy.

1. Committee on Treatment of the International Union against Tuberculosis and Lung Disease. Antituberculosis regimens of chemotherapy. *Bull Int Union Tuberc Lung Dis* 1988; **63:** 60–4.
2. WHO. WHO expert committee on leprosy: sixth report. *WHO Tech Rep Ser 768* 1988.
3. Snider DE, *et al.* Treatment of tuberculosis during pregnancy. *Am Rev Respir Dis* 1980; **122:** 65–79.
4. Holdiness MR. Transplacental pharmacokinetics of the antituberculosis drugs. *Clin Pharmacokinet* 1987; **13:** 125–9.
5. Chouraqui JP, *et al.* Hémorragie par avitaminose K chez la femme enceinte et le nouveau-né: rôle éventuel de la rifampicine: a propos de 2 observations. *Therapie* 1982; **37:** 447–50.

## Interactions

Rifampicin accelerates the metabolism of some drugs by inducing microsomal liver enzymes and possibly by interfering with hepatic uptake but the clinical significance of some of these interactions remains to be determined. Although most drugs involved may require an increase in dosage to maintain effectiveness, women taking oral contraceptives should change to another form of contraception (see p.1534).

The absorption of rifampicin may be reduced by antacids, drugs that reduce gastric motility (anticholinergics and opioids), ketoconazole, or preparations containing bentonite (for example some aminosalicylic acid preparations). However, such interactions can be overcome by giving rifampicin a few hours before any of these drugs. Some other interactions affecting the activity of rifampicin are discussed below.

◊ Reviews.

1. Finch CK, *et al.* Rifampin and rifabutin drug interactions: an update. *Arch Intern Med* 2002; **162:** 985–92.
2. Yew WW. Clinically significant interactions with drugs used in the treatment of tuberculosis. *Drug Safety* 2002; **25:** 111–33.
3. Niemi M, *et al.* Pharmacokinetic interactions with rifampicin: clinical relevance. *Clin Pharmacokinet* 2003; **42:** 819–50.

**Antiretroviral drugs.** Rifamycins can induce the metabolism of zidovudine, the non-nucleoside reverse transcriptase inhibitors delavirdine, efavirenz, and nevirapine, and HIV-protease inhibitors, resulting in potentially subtherapeutic plasma concentrations. In addition HIV-protease inhibitors inhibit the metabolism of rifamycins resulting in elevated plasma-rifamycin concentrations and an increased incidence of adverse effects.[1,2] In general, rifampicin should not be used concurrently with HIV-protease inhibitors alone, with the exception of ritonavir which may be used with rifampicin without dosage adjustment. Rifampicin may be given in usual doses with saquinavir or with lopinavir-ritonavir, *but only in each case if additional ritonavir is given* and dosage adjustment is made for the HIV-protease inhibitors. Rifampicin may be given in usual doses with nevirapine or with efavirenz, although the dose of efavirenz should be increased to 800 mg daily. Rifampicin should not be given with delavirdine.

See also p.249 for comment on the interaction of antiretrovirals with rifabutin.

1. Anonymous. Clinical update: impact of HIV protease inhibitors on the treatment of HIV-infected tuberculosis patients with rifampin. *MMWR* 1996; **45:** 921–5.
2. Centers for Disease Control. Updated guidelines for the use of rifamycins for the treatment of tuberculosis among HIV-infected patients taking protease inhibitors or nonnucleoside reverse transcriptase inhibitors. *MMWR* 2004; **53:** 37. Available at: http://www.cdc.gov/nchstp/tb/tb_hiv_drugs/toc.htm (accessed 28/05/04)

**Clofazimine.** Use of clofazimine in leprosy patients receiving rifampicin with or without dapsone may decrease the rate of absorption of rifampicin and increase the time to peak plasma concentration.[1] In patients receiving clofazimine, rifampicin, and dapsone, the area under the curve for rifampicin was reduced.[1] However, a multiple dose study showed that the pharmacokinetics of rifampicin were similar after 7 days of treatment with rifampicin and dapsone or rifampicin, dapsone, and clofazimine.[2]

1. Mehta J, *et al.* Effect of clofazimine and dapsone on rifampicin (Lositril) pharmacokinetics in multibacillary and paucibacillary leprosy cases. *Lepr Rev* 1986; **57** (suppl 3): 67–76.
2. Venkatesan K, *et al.* The effect of clofazimine on the pharmacokinetics of rifampicin and dapsone in leprosy. *J Antimicrob Chemother* 1986; **18:** 715–18.

**Co-trimoxazole.** In 15 patients receiving therapy including rifampicin for tuberculosis, a course of co-trimoxazole resulted in increases in maximum plasma concentrations and in the area under the concentration-time curve for rifampicin.[1] No adverse effects were observed and the clinical implications of this observation remain unclear. In another study, significant reductions in the area under the plasma concentration-time curves for trimethoprim and sulfamethoxazole were observed after administration of therapy including rifampicin to 10 HIV-infected patients on co-trimoxazole prophylaxis.[2] Again, the clinical significance of this interaction is unclear.

1. Bhatia RS, *et al.* Drug interaction between rifampicin and cotrimoxazole in patients with tuberculosis. *Hum Exp Toxicol* 1991; **10:** 419–21.
2. Ribera E, *et al.* Rifampin reduces concentrations of trimethoprim and sulfamethoxazole in serum in human immunodeficiency virus-infected patients. *Antimicrob Agents Chemother* 2001; **45:** 3238–41.

**Isoniazid.** There is little significant pharmacokinetic interaction between rifampicin and isoniazid.[1] Although lower blood concentrations of rifampicin have been reported with isoniazid, the effect is not considered clinically significant.[2] Since both drugs are hepatotoxic, there could be an increased incidence of hepatic damage, although the benefits of using this combination are considered to outweigh any potential risks.

1. Acocella G, *et al.* Kinetics of rifampicin and isoniazid administered alone and in combination to normal subjects and patients with liver disease. *Gut* 1972; **13:** 47–53.
2. Mouton RP, *et al.* Blood levels of rifampicin, desacetylrifampicin and isoniazid during combined therapy. *J Antimicrob Chemother* 1979; **5:** 447–54.

**Ketoconazole.** Concomitant administration of rifampicin, ketoconazole, and isoniazid has produced low serum concentrations of each drug resulting in failure of antifungal treatment.[1] Rifampicin serum concentrations are reduced when rifampicin is given with ketoconazole;[2] separation of the doses by 30 minutes[3] to 12 hours[2] may result in similar rifampicin concentrations to those attained when rifampicin is given alone, although serum concentrations of ketoconazole remain depressed regardless of the time of administration.

1. Abadie-Kemmerly S, *et al.* Failure of ketoconazole treatment of Blastomyces dermatitidis due to interaction of isoniazid and rifampin. *Ann Intern Med* 1988; **109:** 844–5. Correction. *ibid.* 1989; **111:** 96.
2. Engelhard D, *et al.* Interaction of ketoconazole with rifampin and isoniazid. *N Engl J Med* 1984; **311:** 1681–3.
3. Doble N, *et al.* Pharmacokinetic study of the interaction between rifampicin and ketoconazole. *J Antimicrob Chemother* 1988; **21:** 633–5.

**Probenecid.** Although one study[1] showed that probenecid could increase serum-rifampicin concentrations, another[2] subsequently found that the effect was uncommon and inconsistent and concluded that probenecid had no place as an adjunct to routine rifampicin therapy.

1. Kenwright S, Levi AJ. Impairment of hepatic uptake of rifamycin antibiotics by probenecid and its therapeutic implications. *Lancet* 1973; **ii:** 1401–5.
2. Fallon RJ, *et al.* Probenecid and rifampicin serum levels. *Lancet* 1975; **ii:** 792–4.

## Antimicrobial Action

Rifampicin is bactericidal against a wide range of micro-organisms and interferes with their synthesis of nucleic acids by inhibiting DNA-dependent RNA polymerase. It has the ability to kill intracellular organisms. It is active against mycobacteria, including *Mycobacterium tuberculosis* and *M. leprae* and, having high sterilising activity against these organisms, it possesses the ability to eliminate semi-dormant or persisting organisms. Rifampicin is active against Gram-positive bacteria, especially staphylococci, but less active against Gram-negative organisms. The most sensitive Gram-negative bacteria include *Neisseria meningitidis, N. gonorrhoeae, Haemophilus influenzae*, and *Legionella* spp. Rifampicin also has activity against *Chlamydia trachomatis* and some anaerobic bacteria. At high concentrations it is active against some viruses. Rifampicin has no effect on fungi but has been reported to enhance the antifungal activity of amphotericin B. Use with other antimicrobials may enhance or antagonise the bactericidal activity of rifampicin.

Strains of *Mycobacterium tuberculosis, M. leprae*, and other usually susceptible bacteria have demonstrated resistance, both initially and during treatment. Thus in tuberculosis and leprosy regimens, rifampicin is used with other drugs to delay or prevent the development of rifampicin resistance. There does not appear to be cross-resistance apart from that between rifampicin and other rifamycins. However, there have been isolated reports of the emergence of multidrug-resistant strains of *M. leprae* (see below).

**Multidrug resistance.** Strains of *Mycobacterium leprae* with multiple resistance to rifampicin, ofloxacin, and dapsone have been isolated from patients who have previously received dapsone monotherapy followed by treatment with rifampicin in combination with ofloxacin.[1,2]

1. Cambau E, *et al.* Multidrug-resistance to dapsone, rifampicin, and ofloxacin in Mycobacterium leprae. *Lancet* 1997; **349:** 103–4.
2. Ji B, *et al.* High relapse rate among lepromatous leprosy patients treated with rifampicin plus ofloxacin daily for 4 weeks. *Antimicrob Agents Chemother* 1997; **41:** 1953–6.

## Pharmacokinetics

Rifampicin is readily absorbed from the gastrointestinal tract and peak plasma concentrations of about 7 to 9 micrograms/mL have been reported 2 to 4 hours after a dose of 600 mg, although there may be considerable interindividual variation. Food may reduce and delay absorption. Rifampicin is about 80% bound to plasma proteins. It is widely distributed in body tissues and fluids and diffusion into the CSF is increased when the meninges are inflamed. Rifampicin is distributed into breast milk and crosses the placenta (see Breast Feeding and Pregnancy, under Precautions, above). Half-lives for rifampicin have been reported to range initially from 2 to 5 hours, the longest elimination times occurring after the largest doses. However, as rifampicin induces its own metabolism, elimination time may decrease by up to 40% during the first 2 weeks, resulting in half-lives of about 1 to 3 hours. The half-life is prolonged in patients with severe hepatic impairment.

Rifampicin is rapidly metabolised in the liver mainly to active 25-*O*-deacetylrifampicin; rifampicin and deacetylrifampicin are excreted in the bile. Deacetylation diminishes intestinal reabsorption and increases faecal excretion, although significant enterohepatic circulation still takes place. About 60% of a dose eventually appears in the faeces. The amount excreted in the urine increases with increasing doses and up to 30% of a dose of 900 mg may be excreted in the urine, about half of it within 24 hours. The metabolite formylrifampicin is also excreted in the urine. In patients with renal impairment the half-life of rifampicin is not prolonged at doses of 600 mg or less.

**Distribution.** Rifampicin is widely distributed in most body tissues and fluids following oral or intravenous use.[1] Rifampicin is also able to penetrate into polymorphonuclear leucocytes to kill intracellular pathogens.[2] Rifampicin does not appear to diffuse well through the uninflamed meninges[3] but therapeutic concentrations have been attained in the CSF after daily doses of 600 and 900 mg when the meninges are inflamed;[4] concentrations in the CSF are about 10 to 20% of simultaneous serum concentrations, and approximately represent the fraction unbound to plasma proteins. Corticosteroids do not appear to influence the penetration of rifampicin into the CSF of patients with tuberculous meningitis.[5]

1. Holdiness MR. Clinical pharmacokinetics of the antituberculosis drugs. *Clin Pharmacokinet* 1984; **9:** 511–44.
2. Prokesch RC, Hand WL. Antibiotic entry into human polymorphonuclear leukocytes. *Antimicrob Agents Chemother* 1982; **21:** 373–80.
3. Sippel JE, *et al.* Rifampin concentrations in cerebrospinal fluid of patients with tuberculous meningitis. *Am Rev Respir Dis* 1974; **109:** 579–80.
4. D'Oliveira JJG. Cerebrospinal fluid concentrations of rifampin in meningeal tuberculosis. *Am Rev Respir Dis* 1972; **106:** 432–7.
5. Woo J, *et al.* Cerebrospinal fluid and serum levels of pyrazinamide and rifampicin in patients with tuberculous meningitis. *Curr Ther Res* 1987; **42:** 235–42.

**Intravenous administration.** Mean peak plasma concentrations of 10 micrograms/mL have been reported after rifampicin 600 mg by intravenous infusion over 3 hours. Peak plasma concentrations declined with repeated doses but to a less marked extent than occurs with oral use.[1] Mean peak plasma concentrations of 27 micrograms/mL have been reported in children following doses of 11.5 mg/kg infused over 30 minutes. Mean concentrations of 1.9 micrograms/mL were reported 8 hours after the dose.[2]

1. Acocella G, *et al.* Serum and urine concentrations of rifampicin administered by intravenous infusion in man. *Arzneimittelforschung* 1977; **27:** 1221–6.
2. Koup JR, *et al.* Pharmacokinetics of rifampin in children I. Multiple dose intravenous infusion. *Ther Drug Monit* 1986; **8:** 11–16.

**Oral administration.** Gastrointestinal absorption of rifampicin is considered good. However, analysis of serum-rifampicin concentrations in children indicated that only 50 ± 22% of a freshly prepared suspension was absorbed following oral use.[1] Also, varying oral bioavailability from capsule formulations has been reported and could result in ineffective therapy[2] or higher than needed serum concentrations.[3]

The oral bioavailability of rifampicin and isoniazid, but not of pyrazinamide, was decreased by food in one study.[4] Another report[5] also showed reduced peak serum concentrations when rifampicin was given with a high-fat meal, and it was suggested that rifampicin should preferably be given on an empty stomach.

Subtherapeutic plasma-rifampicin concentrations have been reported in some patients with HIV infection, possibly related to impaired absorption,[6-8] although others[9,10] have found that HIV infection did not affect the pharmacokinetics of rifampicin.

1. Koup JR, *et al.* Pharmacokinetics of rifampin in children II. Oral bioavailability. *Ther Drug Monit* 1986; **8:** 17–22.
2. Holdiness MR. Clinical pharmacokinetics of the antituberculosis drugs. *Clin Pharmacokinet* 1984; **9:** 511–44.
3. Ganiswarna SG, *et al.* Bioavailability of rifampicin caplets (600 mg and 450 mg) in healthy Indonesian subjects. *Int J Clin Pharmacol Ther Toxicol* 1986; **24:** 60–4.
4. Zent C, Smith P. Study of the effect of concomitant food on the bioavailability of rifampicin, isoniazid and pyrazinamide. *Tubercle Lung Dis* 1995; **76:** 109–13.
5. Peloquin CA, *et al.* Pharmacokinetics of rifampin under fasting conditions, with food, and with antacids. *Chest* 1999; **115:** 12–18.
6. Patel KB, *et al.* Drug malabsorption and resistant tuberculosis in HIV-infected patients. *N Engl J Med* 1995; **332:** 336–7.
7. Peloquin CA, *et al.* Low antituberculosis drug concentrations in patients with AIDS. *Ann Pharmacother* 1996; **30:** 919–25.
8. Sahai J, *et al.* Reduced plasma concentrations of antituberculosis drugs in patients with HIV infection. *Ann Intern Med* 1997; **127:** 289–93.
9. Choudri SH, *et al.* Pharmacokinetics of antimycobacterial drugs in patients with tuberculosis, AIDS, and diarrhea. *Clin Infect Dis* 1997; **25:** 104–11.
10. Taylor B, Smith PJ. Does AIDS impair the absorption of antituberculosis agents? *Int J Tuberc Lung Dis* 1998; **2:** 670–5.

## Uses and Administration

Rifampicin belongs to the rifamycin group of antimycobacterials (p.117) and is used in the treatment of various infections due to mycobacteria and other susceptible organisms (see Antimicrobial Action, above). It is usually given with other antibacterials to prevent the emergence of resistant organisms.

Rifampicin is used, notably with isoniazid and pyrazinamide, as a component of multidrug regimens for the treatment of tuberculosis, and with dapsone and clofazimine in the treatment of leprosy. It is a component of various regimens for the treatment of opportunistic mycobacterial infections.

Other uses include brucellosis, *Chlamydia* and *Chlamydophila* infections, the treatment of staphylococcal endocarditis, penicillin-resistant pneumococcal meningitis, prophylaxis of epiglottitis due to *Haemophilus influenzae*, Legionnaires' disease, the prophylaxis of meningococcal and *H. influenzae* meningitis, mycetoma, the eradication of pharyngeal streptococcal carriage in pharyngitis, Q fever, and in various staphylococcal infections for treatment or prophylactically to reduce staphylococcal carriage. For discussions of all these infections and their treatment, see under Choice of Antibacterial, p.120.

The usual adult dose of rifampicin is 600 mg daily by mouth, preferably on an empty stomach, or by intravenous infusion as the base or the sodium salt; higher doses are sometimes used (see below).

Rifampicin is given in the initial and continuation phases of short-course **tuberculosis** regimens (p.150) with other antimycobacterials. Rifampicin is administered orally on an empty stomach in adult doses of 10 mg/kg (maximum 600 mg) daily or two or three times weekly. Children may be given a dose of 10 to 20 mg/kg (maximum 600 mg) daily or two or three times weekly. Alternatively, doses may be expressed as follows: with daily administration, adults weighing less than 50 kg receive 450 mg and those over 50 kg receive 600 mg; with intermittent administration, adults receive 600 to 900 mg three times weekly. The maximum recommended dose is considered to be 900 mg because a greater incidence of adverse effects is associated with doses above 900 mg.

Rifampicin is also used in the chemoprophylaxis of tuberculosis.

In **leprosy** regimens (p.133), rifampicin is usually given with dapsone for paucibacillary leprosy, and with dapsone and clofazimine for multibacillary leprosy. WHO recommends that rifampicin is given once monthly in a usual adult dose of 600 mg by mouth. Single-dose treatment with rifampicin, ofloxacin, and minocycline may be an alternative in patients with single-lesion paucibacillary leprosy.

For **prophylaxis** against meningococcal meningitis and the treatment of meningococcal carriers, rifampicin is usually given in a dose of 600 mg twice daily by mouth for 2 days. Recommended doses for children in the UK are 10 mg/kg for children between

1 and 12 years of age and 5 mg/kg for children under 12 months each twice daily for 2 days; in the USA children aged 1 month or more are given 10 mg/kg and infants less then 1 month old are given 5 mg/kg, both twice daily for 2 days. For prophylaxis against meningitis due to *Haemophilus influenzae*, a dose of 600 mg daily by mouth for 4 days is given to adults. Recommended doses for children in the UK are 10 mg/kg once daily by mouth for 4 days for children aged 1 to 3 months, and 20 mg/kg once daily by mouth for 4 days for those aged over 3 months, with a maximum daily dose of 600 mg.

In the treatment of **brucellosis, Legionnaires' disease,** and serious **staphylococcal infections** a dose of 600 to 1200 mg daily in divided doses has been recommended in combination with other drugs.

Doses of rifampicin should be reduced in patients with hepatic impairment (see below).

**Administration in hepatic impairment.** Reduced doses of rifampicin are recommended for patients with hepatic impairment and a maximum of 8 mg/kg daily has been suggested. See also Precautions, above.

**Ehrlichiosis.** Beneficial responses to rifampicin have been reported[1] in 2 pregnant women with granulocytic ehrlichiosis (p.125), in whom the usual treatment with a tetracycline was contra-indicated.

1. Buitrago MI, *et al.* Human granulocytic ehrlichiosis during pregnancy treated successfully with rifampin. *Clin Infect Dis* 1998; **27:** 213–15.

**Meningitis prophylaxis.** HAEMOPHILUS INFLUENZAE MENINGITIS PROPHYLAXIS. Meningeal infection with *Haemophilus influenzae* type b (Hib) in children is associated with substantial morbidity, but the incidence has decreased since the introduction of immunisation with *H. influenzae* type b vaccine. Although a world-wide problem, the disease and its prophylaxis has been studied mainly in the USA, where it has been shown that children under 4 years of age form the highest risk group for primary infection while children under 2 years of age form the highest risk group for secondary infection.[1] The goal of prophylaxis in close contacts is to eliminate carriage of the organism to prevent spread to young children. Risk of infection to young children with recent household contact to the primary case of infection with *Haemophilus influenzae* type b is increased 600- to 800-fold,[1,2] but only increased 20-fold[3] from day-care or school contact. The risk may be higher when more than 1 index patient is identified.

Rifampicin in doses of 20 mg/kg once daily for 4 days (maximum dose 600 mg) has been shown to eradicate Hib nasopharyngeal carriage in at least 95% of contacts of the primary case.[4] There is some evidence from a study involving 68 families of patients with Hib infection that rifampicin 20 mg/kg daily for 2 days may be as effective as a 4-day course in eradicating Hib pharyngeal colonisation.[5] Rifampicin prophylaxis appears to be successful in preventing infection in household contacts, but benefit in school settings where there has been a single index case has not been established.[3]

Various recommendations have been made for rifampicin prophylaxis. Administration of rifampicin to all persons, regardless of vaccine status, with close, recent (within 2 weeks) contact to the primary case and who are likely to be exposed to susceptible children has been endorsed by the American Academy of Pediatrics;[6] similar recommendations have been made in the UK.[2] Rifampicin should also be given to the primary case since treatment of the infection does not eradicate nasopharyngeal carriage.[2,6] Rifampicin prophylaxis following exposure through day-care or school contact may be given and has been endorsed by the American Centers for Disease Control.[7]

In the UK, prophylaxis is recommended for all room contacts when 2 or more cases of *H. influenzae* disease have occurred in a playgroup or nursery within 120 days.[2]

Rifampicin prophylaxis is not recommended for pregnant women,[2,6] and in the UK prophylaxis is not recommended in breast-feeding mothers.[2]

Treatment of *H. influenzae* meningitis is discussed on p.134.

1. Casto DT, Edwards DL. Preventing Haemophilus influenzae type b disease. *Clin Pharm* 1985; **4:** 637–48.
2. Cartwright KAV, *et al.* Chemoprophylaxis for Haemophilus influenzae type b: rifampicin should be given to close contacts. *BMJ* 1991; **302:** 546–7.
3. ASHP Commission on Therapeutics. ASHP therapeutic guidelines on nonsurgical antimicrobial prophylaxis. *Clin Pharm* 1990; **9:** 423–45.
4. Band JD, *et al.* Prevention of Hemophilus influenzae type b disease. *JAMA* 1984; **251:** 2381–6.
5. Green M, *et al.* Duration of rifampin chemoprophylaxis for contacts of patients infected with Haemophilus influenzae type B. *Antimicrob Agents Chemother* 1992; **36:** 545–7.
6. American Academy of Pediatrics. Revision of recommendation for use of rifampin prophylaxis of contacts of patients with Haemophilus influenzae infection. *Pediatrics* 1984; **74:** 301–2.
7. Broome CV, *et al.* Use of chemoprophylaxis to prevent the spread of Hemophilus influenzae b in day-care facilities. *N Engl J Med* 1987; **36:** 1226–8.

MENINGOCOCCAL MENINGITIS PROPHYLAXIS. *Neisseria meningitidis* is an important cause of bacterial meningitis; all age groups are at risk during epidemics but children are usually at highest risk during endemic outbreaks. Vaccines are available for meningococci groups A and C but not for group B, therefore antimicrobial prophylaxis remains important in preventing the spread of the disease. The aim of prophylaxis is to eliminate nasopharyngeal carriage of the organism. Sulfadiazine and minocycline are no longer used because of resistance and adverse effects. The current antibacterial of choice is rifampicin; rates of 70 to 90% have been reported for eradication of nasal carriage.[1] Alternative drugs are ceftriaxone and ciprofloxacin. Once a meningococcal infection occurs, the risk of infection in household contacts increases 500- to 1200-fold.[2] Antibacterial prophylaxis should be given as soon as possible to household contacts and persons exposed to the patient's oral secretions (ideally within 24 hours of diagnosis of the index case). It is also recommended for child care or nursery school contacts in the USA,[1] but is not usually advised for this group in the UK following a single case.[2] The index patient should also receive rifampicin or other prophylaxis since treatment with penicillin does not necessarily eradicate nasopharyngeal carriage.

Treatment of meningococcal meningitis is discussed on p.134.

1. Committee on Infectious Diseases of the American Academy of Pediatrics, Infectious Diseases and Immunization Committee of the Canadian Pediatric Society. Meningococcal disease prevention and control strategies for practice-based physicians. *Pediatrics* 1996; **97:** 404–11.
2. PHLS Meningococcal Infections Working Group and Public Health Medicine Environmental Group. Control of meningococcal disease: guidance for consultants in communicable disease control. *Commun Dis Rep* 1995; **5** (review 13): R189–R195.

**Naegleria infections.** For mention of the use of rifampicin in primary amoebic meningoencephalitis, see p.595.

## Preparations

***BP 2003:*** Rifampicin Capsules; Rifampicin Oral Suspension;
***USP 27:*** Rifampin and Isoniazid Capsules; Rifampin Capsules; Rifampin for Injection; Rifampin Oral Suspension; Rifampin, Isoniazid, and Pyrazinamide Tablets; Rifampin, Isoniazid, Pyrazinamide, and Ethambutol Hydrochloride Tablets.

**Proprietary Preparations** (details are given in Part 3)
***Arg.:*** Moxina; Pharmaceutix; Rifadecina; Rifadin; ***Austral.:*** Rifadin; Rimycin; ***Austria:*** Eremfat; Rifoldin; Rimactan; ***Belg.:*** Rifadine; Rimactan†; ***Braz.:*** Monicil; Rifaldin; Rifamp; ***Canad.:*** Rifadin; Rofact; ***Denm.:*** Rimactan; ***Fin.:*** Rimapen; ***Fr.:*** Rifadine; Rimactan; ***Ger.:*** Eremfat; Rifa; Rimactan†; ***Gr.:*** Rifadin; ***Hong Kong:*** Ricin; Rifadin; Rifasynt; Rimactane; ***India:*** R-Cin; Rifacilin; Rifacom E-Z; Rifamycin; Rimactane; Siticox; ***Irl.:*** Rifadin; Rimactane; ***Israel:*** Rimactan; ***Ital.:*** Rifadin; Rifapiam; ***Malaysia:*** Ramfin; Rifasynt; Rimactane; ***Mex.:*** Eurifam†; Fampin†; Finamicina; Pestarin; Ricilin†; Rifadin; Rifamcilin†; Rimactan; Simar†; Turifam†; ***Neth.:*** Rifadin; Rimactan; ***Norw.:*** Rifadin†; Rimactan; ***NZ:*** Rifadin; ***Port.:*** Rifadin; Rifex; ***S.Afr.:*** Rifadin; Rimactane; ***Singapore:*** Rimactane; ***Spain:*** Rifagen; Rifaldin; Rifocina†; Rimactan; ***Swed.:*** Rifadin; Rimactan; ***Switz.:*** Rimactan; ***Thai.:*** Cinifa†; Manorifcin; Myrin; Myrin-P; Ramfin; Rampicin; Ricin; Rifadin; Rifagen; Rifam; Rifam-P; Rifamcin; Rifano†; Rifasynt; Rimactane; RP-Pose†; Tibirim†; ***UK:*** Rifadin; Rimactane; ***USA:*** Rifadin; Rimactane.

**Multi-ingredient:** ***Arg.:*** Bacifim; Rifaprim; Rifinah; Risoniac; Ritroprim; ***Austria:*** Rifater; Rifoldin INH; Rimactan + INH; ***Canad.:*** Rifater; ***Fr.:*** Rifater; Rifinah; ***Ger.:*** Iso-Eremfat; Rifater; Rifinah; ***Gr.:*** Oboliz; Rifinah; Rimactazid; ***Hong Kong:*** Ricinis†; Rifater; Rifinah; ***India:*** Akt-3; Akt-4; Arzide; Cx-3; Cx-4; Cx-5; Gocox Compound; Gocox-3; Ipcacin Kid; Isorifam; R-Cinex; R-Cinex Z; Rifa; Rifa E; Rimactazid + Z; Rimpazid; Siticox-INH; Tibirim INH; Tricox; Wokex-2; Wokex-3; Wokex-4; ***Irl.:*** Rifater; Rifinah; Rimactazid; ***Ital.:*** Rifanicozid†; Rifater; Rifinah; ***Malaysia:*** Rimactazid; ***Mex.:*** Finater; Rifaprim; Rifater; Rifinah; ***Neth.:*** Rifinah; ***NZ:*** Rifinah; ***Port.:*** Rifater; Rifinah; Tuberen†; ***S.Afr.:*** Myrin Plus; Myrin†; Pyrifin†; Rifafour; Rifater†; Rifinah; Rimactazid; Rimcure; ***Singapore:*** Rifater†; Rifinah†; Rimactazid; ***Spain:*** Rifater; Rifazida; Rifinah; Rimactazid; Tisobrif; ***Switz.:*** Rifater; Rifinah; Rimactazide + Z†; Rimactazide†; ***Thai.:*** Ricinis†; Rifamiso†; Rifampyzid; Rifater; Rifinah; Rimactazid; Rimcure 3-FDC; ***UK:*** Rifater; Rifinah; Rimactazid; ***USA:*** Rifamate; Rifater.

---

## Rifamycin Sodium *(BANM, rINNM)*

M-14 (rifamycin); Rifamicina sódica; Rifamycin SV Sodium; Rifamycinum Natricum. Sodium (12*Z*,14*E*,24*E*)-(2*S*,16*S*,17*S*,18*R*,19*R*,20*R*,21*S*,22*R*,23*S*)-21-acetoxy-1,2-dihydro-6,9,17,19-tetrahydroxy-23-methoxy-2,4,12,16,18,20,22-heptamethyl-1,11-dioxo-2,7-(epoxypentadeca-1,11,13-trienimino)-naphtho[2,1-*b*]furan-5-olate.

$C_{37}H_{46}NNaO_{12}$ = 719.8.
*CAS — 6998-60-3 (rifamycin); 14897-39-3 (rifamycin sodium); 15105-92-7 (rifamycin sodium).*
*ATC — J04AB03; S02AA12.*

**Pharmacopoeias.** In *Eur.* (see p.vi) and *Pol.*

**Ph. Eur. 5.0** (Rifamycin Sodium). The monosodium salt of rifamycin SV, a substance obtained by chemical transformation of rifamycin B which is produced during growth of certain strains of *Amycolatopsis mediterranei*. Rifamycin SV may also be obtained directly from certain mutants of *A. mediterranei*. The potency is not less than 900 units/mg calculated with reference to the anhydrous substance. A red, fine or slightly granular powder. Soluble in water; freely soluble in dehydrated alcohol. A 5% solution in water has a pH of 6.5 to 8.0. Store in airtight containers at a temperature of 2° to 8°. Protect from light.

### Adverse Effects and Precautions

Some gastrointestinal adverse effects have occurred following injections of rifamycin. High doses may produce alterations in liver function. Hypersensitivity reactions including rashes, pruritus, and anaphylaxis have occurred rarely, but prolonged use increases the risk of sensitisation. A reddish coloration of the urine has been reported. It should be used with care in patients with hepatic dysfunction.

### Antimicrobial Action

Rifamycin has similar antimicrobial actions to those of rifampicin (p.252).

### Pharmacokinetics

Rifamycin is not effectively absorbed from the gastrointestinal tract. Plasma concentrations of 2 micrograms/mL have been achieved 2 hours after a dose of 250 mg by intramuscular injection; concentrations of about 11 micrograms/mL have been achieved 2 hours after an intravenous dose of 500 mg. Rifamycin is reported to be about 80% bound to plasma proteins. The plasma half-life is reported to be about 1 hour.

Rifamycin is excreted mainly in the bile and only small amounts appear in the urine.

### Uses and Administration

Rifamycin is a rifamycin antibacterial that has been used in the treatment of infections caused by susceptible organisms such as staphylococci. It has been given as the sodium salt by intramuscular injection and by slow intravenous infusion and is also given by local instillation and topical application.

### Preparations

**Proprietary Preparations** (details are given in Part 3)
***Arg.:*** Plusderm ATB; Rifocina; ***Austria:*** Rifocin; ***Belg.:*** Rifocine; ***Braz.:*** Rifan; Rifocina; ***Fr.:*** Otofa; Rifocine†; ***Ital.:*** Rifocin; ***Mex.:*** Rifocyna; ***Port.:*** Otofa†; Rifocina; ***Switz.:*** Otofa.

**Multi-ingredient:** ***Braz.:*** Rifocort.

---

## Rifapentine *(BAN, USAN, rINN)*

DL-473; DL-473-IT; L-11473; MDL-473; Rifapentina. 3-[*N*-(4-Cyclopentyl-1-piperazinyl)formimidoyl]rifamycin.

$C_{47}H_{64}N_4O_{12}$ = 877.0.
*CAS — 61379-65-5.*
*ATC — J04AB05.*

### Adverse Effects

As for Rifampicin, p.250. A higher incidence of hyperuricaemia has been reported with rifapentine than with rifampicin.

### Precautions

As for Rifampicin, p.251.

Rifapentine is teratogenic in *animals*.

### Interactions

As for Rifampicin, p.251.

### Antimicrobial Action

As for Rifampicin, p.252. Cross-resistance is common between rifapentine and rifampicin in *Mycobacterium tuberculosis*.

**Antimycobacterial action.** References.

1. Mor N, *et al.* Comparison of activities of rifapentine and rifampin against Mycobacterium tuberculosis residing in human macrophages. *Antimicrob Agents Chemother* 1995; **39:** 2073–7.
2. Vernon A, *et al.* Acquired rifamycin monoresistance in patients with HIV-related tuberculosis treated with once-weekly rifapentine and isoniazid. *Lancet* 1999; **353:** 1843–7.

### Pharmacokinetics

Rifapentine is absorbed following oral doses. Absorption is enhanced when rifapentine is taken with food. Peak plasma concentrations are achieved 5 to 6 hours after a single dose of 600 mg and steady-state concentrations are achieved by day 10 during daily use. A half-life of about 13 hours has been reported. Rifapentine does not appear to induce its own metabolism. Rifapentine and its active metabolite 25-deacetylrifapentine are 98% and 93% bound to plasma proteins, respectively.

Rifapentine and 25-deacetylrifapentine are excreted mainly in the faeces with a small amount appearing in the urine.

◊ References.

1. Keung ACF, *et al.* Pharmacokinetics of rifapentine in patients with varying degrees of hepatic dysfunction. *J Clin Pharmacol* 1998; **38:** 517–24.
2. Keung AC-F, *et al.* Pharmacokinetics of rifapentine in subjects seropositive for the human immunodeficiency virus: a phase I study. *Antimicrob Agents Chemother* 1999; **43:** 1230–3.
3. Conte JE, *et al.* Single-dose intrapulmonary pharmacokinetics of rifapentine in normal subjects. *Antimicrob Agents Chemother* 2000; **44:** 985–90.

### Uses and Administration

Rifapentine is a rifamycin antibacterial (see Rifampicin, p.250) that is used, with other antimycobacterials, for the treatment of tuberculosis. It is under investigation for the treatment and prophylaxis of *Mycobacterium avium* complex infections in patients with AIDS.

Rifapentine is given by mouth in a dose of 600 mg twice weekly during the initial phase of short-course tuberculosis regimens, then once weekly during the continuation phase.

◊ Reviews.

1. Jarvis B, Lamb HM. Rifapentine. *Drugs* 1998; **56:** 607–16.
2. Temple ME, Nahata MC. Rifapentine: its role in the treatment of tuberculosis. *Ann Pharmacother* 1999; **33:** 1203–10.

### Preparations

**Proprietary Preparations** (details are given in Part 3)
***Braz.:*** Priftin†; ***USA:*** Priftin.

---

## Rifaximin *(USAN, rINN)*

L-105; Rifaxidin; Rifaximina; Rifaximine. (2S,16Z,18E,20S,21S,22R,23R,24R,25S,26S,27S,28E)-5,6,21,23,25-Pentahydroxy-27-methoxy-2,4,11,16,20,22,24,26-octamethyl-2,7-(epoxypentadeca[1,11,13]trienimino)benzofuro[4,5-e]pyrido[1,2-*a*]benzimidazole-1,15(2*H*)-dione 25-acetate.

$C_{43}H_{51}N_3O_{11}$ = 785.9.

*CAS — 80621-81-4.*

*ATC — A07AA11; D06AX11.*

NOTE. The code L-105 has also been applied to the cephalosporin cefuzonam.

### Profile

Rifaximin is a rifamycin antibacterial with antimicrobial actions similar to those of rifampicin (p.252), but which is poorly absorbed from the gastrointestinal tract. It has been given by mouth in the treatment of gastrointestinal infections, including travellers' diarrhoea, for surgical infection prophylaxis, and to reduce hyperammonaemia in hepatic encephalopathy (p.1243). Doses in adults have ranged from 10 to 15 mg/kg daily, or from 800 to 1200 mg daily, both in divided doses.

Rifaximin has also been used topically as a 5% ointment.

◊ References.

1. Gillis JC, Brogden RN. Rifaximin: a review of its antibacterial activity, pharmacokinetic properties and therapeutic potential in conditions mediated by gastrointestinal bacteria. *Drugs* 1995; **49:** 467–84.
2. DuPont HL, *et al.* Rifaximin: a nonabsorbed antimicrobial in the therapy of travelers' diarrhea. *Digestion* 1998; **59:** 708–14.
3. DuPont HL, *et al.* Rifaximin versus ciprofloxacin for the treatment of traveler's diarrhea: a randomized, double-blind clinical trial. *Clin Infect Dis* 2001; **33:** 1807–15.

### Preparations

**Proprietary Preparations** (details are given in Part 3)
***Ital.:*** Dermodis†; Normix; Redactiv†; Rifacol; ***Mex.:*** Flonorm; Redactiv.

## Rokitamycin *(rINN)*

M-19-Q; 3″-Propionyl-leucomycin $A_5$; Rikamycin; Rokitamicina; TMS-19Q. [(4R,5S,6S,7R,9R,10R,11E,13E,16R)-7-(Formylmethyl)-4,10-dihydroxy-5-methoxy-9,16-dimethyl-2-oxooxacyclohexadeca-11,13-dien-6-yl]-3,6-dideoxy-4-*O*-(2,6-dideoxy-3-*C*-methyl-α-L-*ribo*-hexopyranosyl)-3-(dimethylamino)-β-D-glucopyranoside 4″-butyrate 3″-propionate.

$C_{42}H_{69}NO_{15}$ = 828.0.

*CAS — 74014-51-0.*

*ATC — J01FA12.*

**Pharmacopoeias.** In *Jpn.*

### Profile

Rokitamycin is a macrolide antibacterial with actions and uses similar to those of erythromycin (p.208). It has been given by mouth in doses of 400 mg twice daily.

### Preparations

**Proprietary Preparations** (details are given in Part 3)
***Ital.:*** Paidocin; Rokital.

## Rolitetracycline *(BAN, USAN, rINN)*

PMT; Pyrrolidinomethyltetracycline; Rolitetraciclina; SQ-15659. $N^2$-(Pyrrolidin-1-ylmethyl)tetracycline.

$C_{27}H_{33}N_3O_8$ = 527.6.

*CAS — 751-97-3.*

*ATC — J01AA09.*

### Profile

Rolitetracycline is a tetracycline derivative with general properties similar to those of tetracycline (p.266). It is included in some topical eye preparations. It has also been given by injection, when it has been associated with shivering and, more rarely, rigor, due to a Jarisch-Herxheimer reaction. Injection has also been followed by a peculiar taste sensation, often similar to ether.

### Preparations

**Proprietary Preparations** (details are given in Part 3)
***Canad.:*** Reverin†.
**Multi-ingredient:** ***Arg.:*** Eubetal Biotic; ***Ital.:*** Colbiocin; Eubetal Antibiotico; Iducol†; Vitecaf.

## Rosoxacin *(BAN, USAN, rINN)*

Acrosoxacin; Rosoxacino; Win-35213. 1-Ethyl-1,4-dihydro-4-oxo-7-(4-pyridyl)quinoline-3-carboxylic acid.

$C_{17}H_{14}N_2O_3$ = 294.3.

*CAS — 40034-42-2.*

*ATC — J01MB01.*

### Adverse Effects and Precautions

As for Nalidixic Acid, p.234.

Dizziness, drowsiness, and visual disturbances may occur relatively frequently and patients should be advised not to drive or operate machinery if affected.

### Uses and Administration

Rosoxacin is a 4-quinolone antibacterial with actions similar to those of nalidixic acid (p.234). It is active against *Neisseria gonorrhoeae* and has been given by mouth in the treatment of gonorrhoea (p.130) as a single dose of 300 mg, preferably on an empty stomach.

### Preparations

**Proprietary Preparations** (details are given in Part 3)
***Braz.:*** Eradacil; ***Fr.:*** Eracine†; ***Mex.:*** Eradacil; ***Port.:*** Eradacil.

## Roxithromycin *(USAN, rINN)*

Roxithromycinum; Roxitromicina; RU-965; RU-28965. Erythromycin 9-{*O*-[(2-methoxyethoxy)methyl]oxime}.

$C_{41}H_{76}N_2O_{15}$ = 837.0.

*CAS — 80214-83-1.*

*ATC — J01FA06.*

**Pharmacopoeias.** In *Chin., Eur.* (see p.vi), and *Jpn.*

**Ph. Eur. 5.0** (Roxithromycin). A white crystalline powder. It exhibits polymorphism. Very slightly soluble in water; freely soluble in alcohol, in acetone, and in dichloromethane; slightly soluble in dilute hydrochloric acid. Store in airtight containers.

### Adverse Effects and Precautions

As for Erythromycin, p.208. Gastrointestinal disturbances are the most frequent adverse effect, but are less frequent than with erythromycin. Increases in liver enzyme values and hepatitis have been reported. Rashes and other hypersensitivity reactions, headache, dizziness, weakness, and changes in blood cell counts have also occurred.

**Effects on the lungs.** Acute eosinophilic pneumonia was attributed to the use of roxithromycin to treat tonsillitis in a 21-year-old woman.[1] The condition resolved after treatment with methylprednisolone.

1. Pérez-Castrillón JL, *et al.* Roxithromycin-induced eosinophilic pneumonia. *Ann Pharmacother* 2002; **36:** 1808–9.

**Effects on the pancreas.** Acute pancreatitis, with duodenal inflammation, pain, pancreatic enlargement and raised serum-amylase developed within 24 hours of substitution of roxithromycin for erythromycin ethyl succinate in a patient being treated for respiratory-tract infection.[1] Symptoms resolved rapidly once roxithromycin was withdrawn.

1. Souweine B, *et al.* Acute pancreatitis associated with roxithromycin therapy. *DICP Ann Pharmacother* 1991; **25:** 1137.

**Eosinophilia.** For a report of an eosinophilic syndrome in a patient following treatment with azithromycin or roxithromycin, see Azithromycin, p.159. See also under Effects on the Lungs, above.

### Interactions

For a discussion of drug interactions of macrolide antibacterials, see Erythromycin, p.209.

### Antimicrobial Action

As for Erythromycin, p.209. It is reported to be as active or slightly less active than erythromycin.

### Pharmacokinetics

Following oral use roxithromycin is absorbed, with a bioavailability of about 50%. Peak plasma concentrations of about 6 to 8 micrograms/mL occur around 2 hours after a single dose of 150 mg. The mean peak plasma concentration at steady state after a dose of 150 mg twice daily is 9.3 micrograms/mL. Absorption is reduced when taken after a meal. It is widely distributed in tissues and body fluids. It is reported to be about 96% bound to plasma protein (mainly $\alpha_1$-acid glycoprotein) at trough concentrations, but binding is saturable, and only about 86% is bound at usual peak concentrations. Small amounts of roxithromycin are metabolised in the liver, and the majority of a dose is excreted in the faeces as unchanged drug and metabolites; about 7 to 10% is excreted in urine, and up to 15% via the lungs. The elimination half-life is reported to range between about 8 and 13 hours, but may be more prolonged in patients with hepatic or renal impairment and in children.

◊ References.

1. Puri SK, Lassman HB. Roxithromycin: a pharmacokinetic review of a macrolide. *J Antimicrob Chemother* 1987; **20** (suppl B): 89–100.

### Uses and Administration

Roxithromycin is a macrolide antibacterial with actions and uses similar to those of erythromycin (p.210). It is given by mouth to adults in a dose of 150 mg twice daily or sometimes 300 mg once daily, before meals, in the treatment of susceptible infections. In children of up to 40 kg body-weight a dose of 5 to 8 mg/kg daily may be used.

◊ References.

1. Williams JD, Sefton AM. Comparison of macrolide antibiotics. *J Antimicrob Chemother* 1993; **31** (suppl C): 11–26.
2. Markham A, Faulds D. Roxithromycin: an update of its antimicrobial activity, pharmacokinetic properties and therapeutic use. *Drugs* 1994; **48:** 297–326.
3. Young LS, Lode H, eds. Roxithromycin: first of a new generation of macrolides: update and perspectives. *Infection* 1995; **23** (suppl 1): S1–S52.
4. Lovering AM, *et al.*, eds. Roxithromycin—additional therapeutic potential. *J Antimicrob Chemother* 1998; **41** (suppl B): 1–97.

**Ischaemic heart disease.** Macrolide antibacterials, including roxithromycin,[1,2] have been investigated in the prevention of ischaemic heart disease, based on a suggested link between atherosclerosis and *Chlamydophila pneumoniae* (*Chlamydia pneumoniae*) infection (see Ischaemic Heart Disease, under Azithromycin, p.160).

1. Gurfinkel E, *et al.* Treatment with the antibiotic roxithromycin in patients with acute non-Q-wave coronary syndromes: the final report of the ROXIS Study. *Eur Heart J* 1999; **20:** 121–7.
2. Wiesli P, *et al.* Roxithromycin treatment prevents progression of peripheral arterial occlusive disease in Chlamydia pneumoniae seropositive men: a randomized, double-blind, placebo-controlled trial. *Circulation* 2002; **105:** 2646–52.

### Preparations

**Proprietary Preparations** (details are given in Part 3)
***Arg.:*** Anuar; Delos; Klomicina; Rulid; Sinurit; ***Austral.:*** Biaxsig; Rulide; ***Austria:*** Roxithrostad; Rulide; ***Belg.:*** Claramid; Rulid; ***Braz.:*** Floxid; Rotram; Roxid; Roxina; Roxitran; Roxitricina; Roxitrom; Roxitromin; Rulid; ***Chile:*** Ramivan; ***Denm.:*** Forilin; Forimycin; Surlid; ***Fin.:*** Roxibion; Surlid; ***Fr.:*** Claramid; Rulid; ***Ger.:*** Infectoroxit; Roxi; Roxi-Puren; Roxidura; Roxigrun; Roxiklinge; Roxithro-Lich; Rulid; ***Gr.:*** Acevor; Aristomycin; Azuril; Bazuctril; Bicofen; Delitroxin; Erybros; Neo-Suxigal; Redotrin; Roxicilline; Roximin-Galenica; Roxyspes; Rulid; Seide; Thriostaxil; Tirabicin; Toscamycin-R; Uramilon; Vaselpin; ***Hong Kong:*** Roxicin; Rulid; ***India:*** Roxeptin; Roxid; Roxyrol; Unorox; ***Israel:*** Roxo; Rulid; ***Ital.:*** Assoral; Overal; Rossitrol; Rulid; ***Malaysia:*** Roxcin; Roxinox; Rulid; Uonin; ***Mex.:*** Crolix; Kensodic; Roxitrol†; Rulid; Surlid†; ***Neth.:*** Rulide; ***NZ:*** Romicin; Rulide†; ***Port.:*** Rulide; ***S.Afr.:*** Rulide; ***Singapore:*** Rulid; ***Spain:*** Macrosil; Rotesan†; Rotramin; Rulide; ***Swed.:*** Surlid; ***Switz.:*** Rulid; ***Thai.:*** Ammirox; Eroxade; Poliroxin; Rothricin; Roxcin; Roxicin; Roxilan; Roximin; Roxithroxyl; Roxitin; Roxlecon; Roxomycin; Roxthomed; Roxthrin; Roxto; Roxtrocin; Roxy; Rucin; Rulid; Uonin; Utolid.

## Rufloxacin Hydrochloride *(BANM, rINNM)*

MF-934 (rufloxacin). 9-Fluoro-2,3-dihydro-10-[4-methylpiperazin-1-yl]-7-oxo-7*H*-pyrido[1,2,3-*de*]-1,4-benzothiazine-6-carboxylic acid hydrochloride.

$C_{17}H_{18}FN_3O_3S,HCl$ = 399.9.

*CAS — 101363-10-4 (rufloxacin); 106017-08-7 (rufloxacin hydrochloride).*

*ATC — J01MA10.*

### Profile

Rufloxacin is a fluoroquinolone antibacterial with properties similar to those of ciprofloxacin (p.188). It is given by mouth as the hydrochloride in the treatment of susceptible infections in a usual initial dose of 400 mg followed by 200 mg daily. A plasma half-life of 30 hours or more has been reported.

### Preparations

**Proprietary Preparations** (details are given in Part 3)
***Braz.:*** Ruflox†; ***Ital.:*** Monos; Qari; Tebraxin; ***Mex.:*** Uroflox.

## Sarafloxacin Hydrochloride *(BANM, USAN, rINNM)*

A-57135 (sarafloxacin); A-56620 (sarafloxacin or sarafloxacin hydrochloride); Abbott-56620 (sarafloxacin or sarafloxacin hydrochloride); Hidrocloruro de sarafloxacino.

$C_{20}H_{17}F_2N_3O_3,HCl$ = 421.8.

*CAS — 98105-99-8 (sarafloxacin); 91296-87-6 (sarafloxacin hydrochloride).*

### Profile

Sarafloxacin is a fluoroquinolone antibacterial used as the hydrochloride in veterinary medicine.

## Sisomicin Sulfate *(USAN, rINNM)*

Antibiotic 6640 (sisomicin); Rickamicin Sulphate; Sch-13475 (sisomicin); Sisomicin Sulphate *(BANM)*; Sissomicin Sulphate; Sulfato de sisomicina. 4-*O*-[(2*R*,3*R*)-*cis*-3-Amino-6-aminomethyl-3,4-dihydro-2*H*-pyran-2-yl]-2-deoxy-6-*O*-(3-deoxy-4-*C*-methyl-3-methylamino-β-L-arabinopyranosyl)streptamine sulphate; 2-Deoxy-6-*O*-(3-deoxy-4-*C*-methyl-3-methylamino-β-L-arabinopyranosyl)-4-*O*-(2,6-diamino-2,3,4,6-tetradeoxy-D-*glycero*-hex-4-enopyranosyl)streptamine sulphate.

$(C_{19}H_{37}N_5O_7)_2,5H_2SO_4$ = 1385.4.

*CAS — 32385-11-8 (sisomicin); 53179-09-2 (sisomicin sulfate).*

*ATC — J01GB08.*

**Pharmacopoeias.** In *Chin., Jpn,* and *US.*

**USP 27** (Sisomicin Sulfate). It loses not more than 15% of its weight on drying. 1 mg of sisomicin sulfate has a potency equivalent to not less than 580 micrograms of sisomicin calculated on the dried basis. A 4% solution in water of sisomicin has a pH of 3.5 to 5.5. Store in airtight containers.

### Profile

Sisomicin, an antibiotic produced by *Micromonospora inyoensis* and closely related to gentamicin $C_{1A}$, is an aminoglycoside with general properties similar to those of gentamicin (p.217). It is given as the sulfate but doses are expressed in terms of the base. 1.5 g of sisomicin sulfate is approximately equivalent to 1 g of sisomicin. The usual dose for adults is 3 mg/kg daily given intramuscularly in 2 or 3 divided doses. It may be given by intravenous infusion if necessary.

### Preparations

**USP 27:** Sisomicin Sulfate Injection.

**Proprietary Preparations** (details are given in Part 3)
***India:*** Sisoptin; ***Ital.:*** Mensiso; ***Spain:*** Sisomina†.

## Sparfloxacin *(BAN, USAN, rINN)*

AT-4140; CI-978; Esparfloxacino. 5-Amino-1-cyclopropyl-7-(*cis*-3,5-dimethylpiperazin-1-yl)-6,8-difluoro-1,4-dihydro-4-oxoquinoline-3-carboxylic acid.

$C_{19}H_{22}F_2N_4O_3$ = 392.4.
*CAS — 110871-86-8.*
*ATC — J01MA09.*

### Adverse Effects and Precautions

As for Ciprofloxacin, p.188.

Concern over phototoxicity associated with sparfloxacin has led to restriction of its use in some countries; patients should be advised to avoid exposure to sunlight during, and for a few days after, sparfloxacin therapy, and to discontinue the drug immediately if phototoxicity occurs.

Sparfloxacin may prolong the QT interval and various cardiac arrhythmias have been reported.

**Photosensitivity.** In a survey[1] of the reporting rate for phototoxicity associated with sparfloxacin in France, the manufacturer or the French Pharmacovigilance System received 371 reports of severe phototoxic reactions during the first 9 months following marketing of the drug; this approximated to between 4 and 25 times the rate reported for other fluoroquinolones.

1. Pierfitte C, *et al.* The link between sunshine and phototoxicity of sparfloxacin. *Br J Clin Pharmacol* 2000; **49:** 609–12.

### Interactions

As for Ciprofloxacin, p.190.

As sparfloxacin may prolong the QT interval it should not be used with other drugs known to have this effect (such as the antihistamines astemizole and terfenadine, cisapride, erythromycin, pentamidine, phenothiazines, or tricyclic antidepressants).

Sparfloxacin does not appear to interact with theophylline or caffeine, nor with warfarin or cimetidine. Probenecid does not alter the pharmacokinetics of sparfloxacin.

### Antimicrobial Action

As for Ciprofloxacin, p.190.

Sparfloxacin is reported to be more active *in vitro* than ciprofloxacin against mycobacteria and against Gram-positive bacteria, including *Streptococcus pneumoniae* and other streptococci and staphylococci.

◊ References.

1. Richard MP, *et al.* Sensitivity to sparfloxacin and other antibiotics, of Streptococcus pneumoniae, Haemophilus influenzae and Moraxella catarrhalis strains isolated from adult patients with community-acquired lower respiratory tract infections: a European multicentre study. *J Antimicrob Chemother* 1998; **41:** 207–14.

### Pharmacokinetics

Sparfloxacin is well absorbed from the gastrointestinal tract with a reported bioavailability of about 90%. Peak plasma concentrations are achieved 3 to 6 hours after a dose. Sparfloxacin is widely distributed into body tissues and fluids, including respiratory tissues, but is only about 45% bound to plasma proteins. It is metabolised in the liver by glucuronidation and has an elimination half-life of about 20 hours. It is excreted in equal amounts in the faeces and urine as unchanged drug and as the glucuronide metabolite.

◊ References.

1. Shimada J, *et al.* Clinical pharmacokinetics of sparfloxacin. *Clin Pharmacokinet* 1993; **25:** 358–69.
2. Trautmann M, *et al.* Pharmacokinetics of sparfloxacin and serum bactericidal activity against pneumococci. *Antimicrob Agents Chemother* 1996; **40:** 776–9.
3. Dorr MB, *et al.* Pharmacokinetics of sparfloxacin in patients with renal impairment. *Clin Ther* 1999; **21:** 1202–15.

### Uses and Administration

Sparfloxacin is a fluoroquinolone antibacterial with actions similar to those of ciprofloxacin (p.191). It is used for the treatment of community-acquired pneumonia and acute bacterial exacerbations of chronic bronchitis including those caused by pneumococci. The usual dose by mouth is 400 mg initially followed by 200 mg daily.

For details of reduced doses to be used in renal impairment, see below.

◊ General references.

1. Finch RG, *et al.*, eds. Sparfloxacin: focus on clinical performance. *J Antimicrob Chemother* 1996; **37** (suppl A): 1–167.
2. Goa KL, *et al.* Sparfloxacin: a review of its antibacterial activity, pharmacokinetic properties, clinical efficacy and tolerability in lower respiratory tract infections. *Drugs* 1997; **53:** 700–25.
3. Martin SJ, *et al.* Levofloxacin and sparfloxacin: new quinolone antibiotics. *Ann Pharmacother* 1998; **32:** 320–36.
4. Schentag JJ. Sparfloxacin: a review. *Clin Ther* 2000; **22:** 372–87.

**Administration in renal impairment.** Doses of sparfloxacin should be reduced in patients with renal impairment; following the usual initial dose of 400 mg, 200 mg may be given on alternate days.

### Preparations

**Proprietary Preparations** (details are given in Part 3)
***Austria:*** Zagam; ***Fr.:*** Zagam†; ***Ger.:*** Zagam†; ***Hong Kong:*** Zagam†; ***India:*** Spardac; Sparx; ***Jpn:*** Spara; ***NZ:*** Zagam†; ***S.Afr.:*** Zagam†; ***Switz.:*** Zagam†; ***Thai.:*** Zagam†; ***USA:*** Zagam.

## Spectinomycin *(BAN, rINN)*

Actinospectacin; Espectinomicina. Perhydro-4a,7,9-trihydroxy-2-methyl-6,8-bis(methylamino)pyrano[2,3-*b*][1,4]benzodioxin-4-one.

$C_{14}H_{24}N_2O_7$ = 332.3.
*CAS — 1695-77-8.*
*ATC — J01XX04.*

**Description.** Spectinomycin is an antimicrobial substance produced by the growth of *Streptomyces spectabilis* or by any other means.

### Spectinomycin Hydrochloride *(BANM, USAN, rINNM)*

Hidrocloruro de espectinomicina; M-141; Spectinomycini Hydrochloridum; U-18409AE. Spectinomycin dihydrochloride pentahydrate.

$C_{14}H_{24}N_2O_7,2HCl,5H_2O$ = 495.3.
*CAS — 21736-83-4 (anhydrous spectinomycin hydrochloride); 22189-32-8 (spectinomycin hydrochloride pentahydrate).*
*ATC — J01XX04.*

**Pharmacopoeias.** In *Chin., Eur.* (see p.vi), *Int., Jpn,* and *US.*

**Ph. Eur. 5.0** (Spectinomycin Hydrochloride). A white or almost white, slightly hygroscopic, powder. Freely soluble in water; very slightly soluble in alcohol. A 10% solution in water has a pH of 3.8 to 5.6. Store at a temperature not exceeding 30° in airtight containers.

**USP 27** (Spectinomycin Hydrochloride). A white to pale buff crystalline powder. 1 mg of monograph substance has a potency equivalent to not less than 603 micrograms of spectinomycin. Freely soluble in water; practically insoluble in alcohol, in chloroform, and in ether. A 1% solution in water has a pH of 3.8 to 5.6. Store in airtight containers.

### Adverse Effects and Precautions

Nausea, headache, dizziness, fever and chills, insomnia, and urticaria have occasionally occurred with single doses of spectinomycin. Anaphylaxis has occurred rarely. Mild to moderate pain has been reported following intramuscular injections. Alterations in kidney and liver function and a decrease in haemoglobin and haematocrit have occasionally been observed with repeated doses. Although a reduction in urine output has been seen after single and multiple doses, spectinomycin has not been observed to produce functional changes indicative of nephrotoxicity.

Spectinomycin is ineffective in the treatment of syphilis and patients being treated for gonorrhoea should be observed for evidence of syphilis.

### Interactions

**Lithium.** For the effect of spectinomycin on lithium, see Antimicrobials, under Interactions of Lithium, p.303.

### Antimicrobial Action

Spectinomycin is an aminocyclitol antibacterial that acts by binding to the 30S subunit of the bacterial ribosome and inhibiting protein synthesis. Its activity is generally modest, particularly against Gram-positive organisms. Anaerobic organisms are mostly resistant. Various Gram-negative organisms are sensitive, including many enterobacteria and also *Haemophilus ducreyi*, and it is particularly effective against *Neisseria gonorrhoeae*. Although generally bacteriostatic, spectinomycin is bactericidal against susceptible gonococci at concentrations not much above the MIC.

Resistance may develop by chromosomal mutation or may be plasmid-mediated in some organisms; resistant gonococci have been reported clinically, notably in the Far East, but in most parts of the world resistant neisserial strains have been uncommon to date.

### Pharmacokinetics

Spectinomycin is poorly absorbed by mouth but is rapidly absorbed following the intramuscular injection of the hydrochloride. A 2-g dose produces peak plasma concentrations of about 100 micrograms/mL at 1 hour while a 4-g dose produces peak concentrations of about 160 micrograms/mL at 2 hours. Therapeutic plasma concentrations are maintained for up to 8 hours. Distribution into saliva is poor (which limits its value in pharyngeal gonorrhoea). It is poorly bound to plasma proteins. Spectinomycin is excreted in an active form in the urine and up to 100% of a dose has been recovered within 48 hours. A half-life of about 1 to 3 hours has been reported; it is prolonged in patients with renal impairment. Spectinomycin is partially removed by dialysis.

### Uses and Administration

Spectinomycin is used as an alternative to cephalosporins or fluoroquinolones in the treatment of gonorrhoea (p.130) although poor distribution into saliva limits its usefulness in pharyngeal infections. It has also been used in the treatment of chancroid (p.123).

Spectinomycin is given as the hydrochloride but doses are expressed in terms of the base. 1.5 g of spectinomycin hydrochloride is approximately equivalent to 1 g of spectinomycin. In the treatment of gonorrhoea it is given by deep intramuscular injection as a single dose equivalent to 2 g of spectinomycin, although a dose of 4 g may sometimes be required, divided between two injection sites. Multiple-dose courses have been used for the treatment of disseminated infections.

Spectinomycin is not effective against syphilis or chlamydial infections and additional therapy for these infections may be given concomitantly.

Doses equivalent to spectinomycin 40 mg/kg have been given to children.

### Preparations

**USP 27:** Spectinomycin for Injectable Suspension.

**Proprietary Preparations** (details are given in Part 3)
***Arg.:*** Togamycin; ***Austral.:*** Trobicin; ***Austria:*** Trobicin; ***Belg.:*** Trobicin; ***Braz.:*** Trobicin; ***Canad.:*** Trobicin†; ***Fr.:*** Trobicine; ***Ger.:*** Stanilo; ***Hong Kong:*** Kirin; Trobicin; ***India:*** Trobicin; ***Irl.:*** Trobicin†; ***Israel:*** Togamycin; ***Ital.:*** Trobicin; ***Malaysia:*** Kirin; ***Mex.:*** Trobicin†; ***Port.:*** Trobicin; ***S.Afr.:*** Trobicin; ***Singapore:*** Trobicin; ***Spain:*** Kempi; ***Swed.:*** Trobicin†; ***Switz.:*** Trobicin; ***Thai.:*** Trobicin; Vabicin; ***USA:*** Trobicin†.

## Spiramycin *(BAN, USAN, rINN)*

Espiramicina; IL-5902; NSC-55926; NSC-64393 (spiramycin hydrochloride); RP-5337; Spiramycinum. A mixture comprised principally of (4*R*,5*S*,6*S*,7*R*,9*R*,10*R*,16*R*)-(11*E*,13*E*)-6-[(*O*-2,6-dideoxy-3-*C*-methyl-α-L-*ribo*-hexopyranosyl)-(1→4)-(3,6-dideoxy-3-dimethylamino-β-D-glucopyranosyl)oxy]-7-formylmethyl-4-hydroxy-5-methoxy-9,16-dimethyl-10-[(2,3,4,6-tetradeoxy-4-dimethylamino-D-*erythro*-hexopyranosyl)oxy]oxacyclohexadeca-11,13-dien-2-one (Spiramycin I).

$C_{43}H_{74}N_2O_{14}$ = 843.1.
*CAS — 8025-81-8.*
*ATC — J01FA02.*

**Pharmacopoeias.** In *Eur.* (see p.vi). *Jpn* includes Acetylspiramycin.

**Ph. Eur. 5.0** (Spiramycin). A macrolide antibiotic produced by the growth of certain strains of *Streptomyces ambofaciens* or obtained by any other means. The potency is not less than 4100 units/mg, calculated with reference to the dried substance.

A white or slightly yellowish, slightly hygroscopic powder. Slightly soluble in water; freely soluble in alcohol, in acetone, and in methyl alcohol. A 0.5% solution in methyl alcohol and water has a pH of 8.5 to 10.5. Store in airtight containers.

### Adverse Effects and Precautions

As for Erythromycin, p.208. The most frequent adverse effects are gastrointestinal disturbances; skin hypersensitivity reactions have also occurred. Transient paraesthesia has been reported during parenteral use.

### Interactions

For a discussion of drug interactions of macrolide antibacterials, see Erythromycin, p.209.

◊ Spiramycin is reported to have little or no effect on hepatic cytochrome P450 isoenzymes and may therefore produce fewer interactions than erythromycin with other drugs metabolised by this enzyme system (see under Interactions of Erythromycin, Mechanism, p.209). The lack of interactions between spiramycin and theophylline (p.801) and ciclosporin (p.1354) would appear to support this. Nevertheless, a report of torsade de pointes in a patient with a congenital long QT syndrome during treatment with spiramycin and *mequitazine*[1] suggests that caution is still needed.

Reduced plasma concentrations of *levodopa* have been reported during concurrent administration of spiramycin (see p.1208).

1. Verdun F, *et al*. Torsades de pointes sous traitement par spiramycine et méquitazine: à propos d'un cas. *Arch Mal Coeur Vaiss* 1997; **90:** 103–6.

### Antimicrobial Action

As for Erythromycin, p.209, although it is somewhat less active *in vitro* against many species. It is active against *Toxoplasma gondii*.

### Pharmacokinetics

Spiramycin is incompletely absorbed from the gastrointestinal tract and is widely distributed in the tissues. An oral dose of 6 million units produces peak blood concentrations of 3.3 micrograms/mL after 1.5 to 3 hours; the half-life is reported to be about 5 to 8 hours. High tissue concentrations are achieved and persist long after the plasma concentration has fallen to low levels, but it does not diffuse into the CSF to an appreciable extent.

Spiramycin is metabolised in the liver to active metabolites; substantial amounts are excreted in the bile and about 10% in the urine. It is distributed into breast milk.

### Uses and Administration

Spiramycin is a macrolide antibacterial that has been used similarly to erythromycin (p.210) in the treatment of susceptible bacterial infections. It has also been used in the protozoal infections cryptosporidiosis (p.596) and toxoplasmosis (p.598).

Spiramycin is given by mouth as the base or rectally or intravenously as the adipate. The usual adult dose is 6 to 9 million units by mouth daily, in 2 or 3 divided doses. Doses of up to 15 million units have been given daily in divided doses for severe infections. A dose of 1.5 million units of spiramycin may be given by slow intravenous infusion every 8 hours; in severe infection the dose may be doubled. Children may be given 150 000 to 300 000 units/kg daily in divided doses by mouth.

Acetylspiramycin is also used.

◊ Reviews.

1. Rubinstein E, Keller N. Spiramycin renaissance. *J Antimicrob Chemother* 1998; **42:** 572–6.

### Preparations

**Proprietary Preparations** (details are given in Part 3)
***Arg.:*** Rovamycine; ***Austria:*** Rovamycin; ***Belg.:*** Rovamycine; ***Braz.:*** Rovamicina; ***Canad.:*** Rovamycine; ***Denm.:*** Rovamycin†; Spiravet†; ***Fr.:*** Rovamycine; ***Ger.:*** Rovamycine; Selectomycin; ***Gr.:*** Rovamycine; ***Hong Kong:*** Rovamycine; ***India:*** Rovamycin; ***Israel:*** Rovamycine; ***Ital.:*** Rovamicina; Spiromix; ***Malaysia:*** Rovamycine; ***Mex.:*** Provamicina; ***Neth.:*** Rovamycine; ***Norw.:*** Rovamycin; ***Port.:*** Rovamycine; ***Singapore:*** Rovamycine; ***Spain:*** Dicorvin; Rovamycine; ***Switz.:*** Rovamycine; ***Thai.:*** Rovamycin; Spiracin.

**Multi-ingredient:** ***Arg.:*** Estilomicin; ***Braz.:*** Periodontil; ***Fr.:*** Birodogyl; Rodogyl; ***Mex.:*** Rodogyl; ***Spain:*** Rhodogil.

## Streptomycin *(BAN, rINN)*

Estreptomicina. *O*-2-Deoxy-2-methylamino-α-L-glucopyranosyl-(1→2)-*O*-5-deoxy-3-*C*-formyl-α-L-lyxofuranosyl-(1→4)-$N^3$,$N^3$-diamidino-D-streptamine.

$C_{21}H_{39}N_7O_{12}$ = 581.6.
*CAS — 57-92-1.*
*ATC — A07AA04; J01GA01.*

**Description.** An antimicrobial organic base produced by the growth of certain strains of *Streptomyces griseus*, or by any other means.

### Streptomycin Hydrochloride *(BANM, rINNM)*

Hidrocloruro de estreptomicina.
$C_{21}H_{39}N_7O_{12}$,3HCl = 691.0.
*CAS — 6160-32-3.*
*ATC — A07AA04; J01GA01.*

### Streptomycin Sulfate *(rINNM)*

Streptomycin Sesquisulphate; Streptomycin Sulphate *(BANM)*; Streptomycini Sulfas; Sulfato de estreptomicina.

$(C_{21}H_{39}N_7O_{12})_2$,$3H_2SO_4$ = 1457.4.
*CAS — 3810-74-0.*
*ATC — A07AA04; J01GA01.*

**Pharmacopoeias.** In *Chin., Eur.* (see p.vi), *Int., Jpn, Pol., US,* and *Viet.*

**Ph. Eur. 5.0** (Streptomycin Sulphate). A white or almost white, hygroscopic powder. The potency is not less than 720 units/mg, calculated with reference to the dried substance. Very soluble in water; practically insoluble in dehydrated alcohol. A 25% solution in water has a pH of 4.5 to 7.0. Store in airtight containers.

**USP 27** (Streptomycin Sulfate). A white or practically white, hygroscopic powder; odourless or with not more than a faint odour. It has a potency equivalent to not less than 650 micrograms and not more than 850 micrograms of streptomycin per mg. Freely soluble in water; very slightly soluble in alcohol; practically insoluble in chloroform. A solution in water containing the equivalent of streptomycin 20% has a pH of 4.5 to 7.0. Store in airtight containers.

**Incompatibility.** Streptomycin sulfate is incompatible with acids and alkalis.

### Adverse Effects, Treatment, and Precautions

As for Gentamicin Sulfate, p.217. Like gentamicin the ototoxic effects of streptomycin are manifested mainly on vestibular rather than auditory function. Ototoxicity has been observed in infants whose mothers had been given streptomycin during pregnancy. However, streptomycin is reported to be somewhat less nephrotoxic than the other aminoglycosides.

Paraesthesia in and around the mouth is not uncommon after intramuscular injection of streptomycin, and other neurological symptoms, including peripheral neuropathies, optic neuritis, and scotoma have occasionally occurred. Intrathecal administration has resulted in symptoms of meningeal inflammation including radiculitis, arachnoiditis, nerve root pain, and paraplegia, and some authorities recommend that it be avoided. The risk of neurotoxic reactions is greater in patients with renal impairment or pre-renal azotaemia.

Hypersensitivity skin reactions are reported in about 5% of patients, and eosinophilia may occur. There have been reports of Stevens-Johnson syndrome, severe exfoliative dermatitis, and anaphylaxis. Sensitisation is common among those who handle streptomycin occupationally. Topical and inhalational use of streptomycin should be avoided. If necessary, hypersensitivity can usually be overcome by desensitisation. Aplastic anaemia and agranulocytosis have been reported rarely.

Although sources differ, it is usually suggested that peak plasma concentrations should be between 15 and 40 micrograms/mL, and trough concentrations below 3 to 5 micrograms/mL; in the UK the *British National Formulary* recommends that trough concentrations in excess of 1 microgram/mL should be avoided in those over 50 years of age or those with renal impairment. A total cumulative dose in excess of 100 g may be associated with a higher incidence of adverse effects and should only be exceeded in exceptional circumstances.

**Breast feeding.** No adverse effects have been observed in breast-fed infants whose mothers were receiving streptomycin, and the American Academy of Pediatrics considers[1] that it is therefore usually compatible with breast feeding.

1. American Academy of Pediatrics. The transfer of drugs and other chemicals into human milk. *Pediatrics* 2001; **108:** 776–89. Correction. *ibid.*; 1029. Also available at: http://aappolicy.aappublications.org/cgi/content/full/pediatrics%3b108/3/776 (accessed 28/05/04)

**Handling.** Streptomycin may cause severe dermatitis in sensitised persons, and pharmacists, nurses, and others who handle the drug frequently should wear masks and rubber gloves.

### Interactions

As for Gentamicin Sulfate, p.218.

### Antimicrobial Action

Streptomycin has a mode of action and antimicrobial spectrum similar to that of gentamicin (p.218), although most strains of *Pseudomonas aeruginosa* are resistant. It is effective against *Yersinia pestis, Francisella tularensis*, and *Brucella* spp. Streptomycin has particular activity against *Mycobacterium tuberculosis*.

Resistance to streptomycin has often been reported and may develop in strains which are initially sensitive within a few days or weeks of beginning therapy. The widespread emergence of resistance has largely halted its use in infections due to the common Gram-negative aerobes. Primary resistance in *M. tuberculosis* is relatively uncommon in the UK and USA but may be seen in a third or more of cases in the Far East.

Both low-level and high-level resistance have been reported; the latter is thought to be due to mutation of the ribosomal binding site of the antibiotic and cannot be overcome by the synergistic use of another drug such as a beta lactam, whereas strains with moderate resistance due to decreased uptake or permeability of streptomycin may respond to combined use.

Organisms resistant to framycetin, kanamycin, neomycin, and paromomycin usually show cross-resistance to streptomycin, although streptomycin-resistant strains sometimes respond to one of these drugs.

◊ References.

1. Cooksey RC, *et al*. Characterization of streptomycin resistance mechanisms among Mycobacterium tuberculosis isolates from patients in New York City. *Antimicrob Agents Chemother* 1996; **40:** 1186–8.
2. Ho YII, *et al*. In-vitro activities of aminoglycoside-aminocyclitols against mycobacteria. *J Antimicrob Chemother* 1997; **40:** 27–32.

### Pharmacokinetics

As for Gentamicin Sulfate, p.218. After intramuscular injection of streptomycin, maximum concentration in the blood is reached in 0.5 to 2 hours but the time taken and the concentration attained, which may be as high as about 50 micrograms/mL after a dose of 1 g, vary considerably. The half-life of streptomycin is about 2.5 hours. About one-third of streptomycin in the circulation is bound to plasma proteins. It is rapidly excreted by glomerular filtration and the concentration of streptomycin in the urine is often very high, with about 30 to 90% of a dose usually being excreted within 24 hours. It is distributed into breast milk.

### Uses and Administration

Streptomycin is an aminoglycoside antibacterial mainly used as a first-line drug, with other antimycobacterials, in the treatment of tuberculosis. It is given during the initial phase of treatment unless the risk of drug resistance is small. Streptomycin has been used, with a penicillin, as an alternative to gentamicin in the treatment of bacterial endocarditis. Streptomycin is effective in the treatment of plague, tularaemia, and, with a tetracycline, in brucellosis. It has also been used, with other drugs, in various other infections including mycetoma and Whipple's disease. For details of these infections and their treatment, see under Choice of Antibacterial, p.120.

Streptomycin is mostly used as the sulfate but doses are expressed in terms of the base. 1.25 g of streptomycin sulfate is approximately equivalent to 1 g of streptomycin. Administration is by intramuscular injection.

In the treatment of tuberculosis, streptomycin is given during the initial phase of short-course regimens in usual adult doses of 15 mg/kg daily, up to a maximum of 1 g daily. The maximum daily dose should be reduced to 500 to 750 mg in adults aged over 40 years, and in those weighing less than 50 kg. Dosage should also be reduced in those with renal impairment, in whom plasma-drug concentration should be monitored. Streptomycin may also be given as part of an intermittent regimen 2 or 3 times weekly. It has been given by the intrathecal route, together with intramuscular administration, for tuberculous meningitis, but this is no longer recommended.

Children with tuberculosis may be given streptomycin 15 to 20 mg/kg daily (to a maximum of 1 g daily).

In the treatment of non-tuberculous infections, streptomycin has been given in usual adult doses of 1 to 2 g daily in divided doses, depending on the susceptibility and severity of infection; children may be given up to 40 mg/kg daily (maximum 1 g daily), usually in divided doses.

In all patients dosage should preferably be adjusted according to plasma-streptomycin concentrations, and particularly where factors such as age, renal impairment, or prolonged therapy may predispose to toxicity. The course of treatment (other than in tuberculosis) should usually be limited to 7 to 14 days, and peak plasma concentrations should be between 15 and 40 micrograms/mL and trough concentrations below 3 to 5 micrograms/mL or below 1 microgram/mL in renal impairment or in those over 50 years of age. For discussion of the methods used to calculate aminoglycoside dosage requirements, see under Gentamicin Sulfate, p.219.

Streptomycin has also been used as the hydrochloride, the pantothenate, and as a complex with calcium chloride.

**Administration and dosage.** A report of the successful use of streptomycin 7 to 15 mg/kg as an intravenous infusion over 30 to 60 minutes in 4 patients with tuberculosis. Despite the view that streptomycin should be given intramuscularly because of the greater risk of toxicity with the intravenous route, this study was considered to indicate that intravenous use was feasible in selected patients unable to tolerate the intramuscular route.[1]

1. Driver AG, Worden JP. Intravenous streptomycin. *DICP Ann Pharmacother* 1990; **24:** 826–8.

**Ménière's disease.** Streptomycin and gentamicin have been used for medical ablation in advanced Ménière's disease (p.422). Systemic treatment has generally been limited by the development of chronic ataxia and oscillopsia (oscillating vision). However, streptomycin sulfate 1 g twice daily by intramuscular injection on 5 days each week for 2 weeks, repeated as necessary to a total dose of up to 60 g,[1,2] or 1 g twice daily for 5 days, followed if necessary by a further 3 days' treatment in the second week,[3] has produced improvements in vestibular symptoms without hearing loss in patients with Ménière's disease. Local (intratympanic) injections have also been tried,[4] but gentamicin is considered to be less toxic and is now generally preferred.

1. Shea JJ, *et al.* Long-term results of low dose intramuscular streptomycin for Ménière's disease. *Am J Otol* 1994; **15:** 540–4.
2. Balyan FR, *et al.* Titration streptomycin therapy in Meniere's disease: long-term results. *Otolaryngol Head Neck Surg* 1998; **118:** 261–6.
3. Graham MD. Bilateral Meniere's disease: treatment with intramuscular titration streptomycin sulfate. *Otolaryngol Clin North Am* 1997; **30:** 1097–1100.
4. Beck C, Schmidt CL. 10 Years of experience with intratympanally applied streptomycin (gentamycin) in the therapy of Morbus Menière. *Arch Otorhinolaryngol* 1978; **221:** 149–52.

## Preparations

***BP 2003:*** Streptomycin Injection;
***USP 27:*** Streptomycin for Injection; Streptomycin Injection.

**Proprietary Preparations** (details are given in Part 3)

***Ger.:*** Strepto-Fatol; Strepto-Hefa; ***Gr.:*** Pan-Streptomycin; ***India:*** Ambistryn-S; ***Ital.:*** Streptocol†; ***Mex.:*** Sulfestrep; ***S.Afr.:*** Novostrep; Solustrep; ***Thai.:*** Strepto.

**Multi-ingredient:** ***Arg.:*** Estreptocarbocaftiazol; ***Braz.:*** Climacilin†; Enteromicina†; Ortocilin†; ***India:*** Strepto-Erbazide; ***Port.:*** Bienterico; Trisinerge†; ***Thai.:*** Diolin†.

## Succinylsulfathiazole *(BAN, rINN)*

Succinilsolfatiazolo; Succinilsulfatiazol; Succinylsulfathiazolum; Succinylsulphathiazole. 4′-(1,3-Thiazol-2-ylsulphamoyl)succinanilic acid monohydrate.

$C_{13}H_{13}N_3O_5S_2,H_2O = 373.4.$
*CAS — 116-43-8 (anhydrous succinylsulfathiazole).*
*ATC — A07AB04.*

**Pharmacopoeias.** In *Eur.* (see p.vi).

**Ph. Eur. 5.0** (Succinylsulfathiazole). A white or yellowish-white crystalline powder. Very slightly soluble in water; slightly soluble in acetone and in alcohol; dissolves in solutions of alkali hydroxides and carbonates. Protect from light.

### Profile

Succinylsulfathiazole is a sulfonamide with properties similar to those of sulfamethoxazole (p.261). It is poorly absorbed and has been given for its antibacterial activity in the gastrointestinal tract.

## Sulbactam *(BAN, rINN)*

CP-45899. Penicillanic acid 1,1-dioxide; (2*S*,5*R*)-3,3-Dimethyl-7-oxo-4-thia-1-azabicyclo[3.2.0]heptane-2-carboxylic acid 4,4-dioxide.

$C_8H_{11}NO_5S = 233.2.$
*CAS — 68373-14-8.*
*ATC — J01CG01.*

## Sulbactam Sodium *(BANM, USAN, rINNM)*

CP-45899-2; Sulbactam sódico.

$C_8H_{10}NNaO_5S = 255.2.$
*CAS — 69388-84-7.*
*ATC — J01CG01.*

**Pharmacopoeias.** In *Chin., Jpn,* and *US.*

**USP 27** (Sulbactam Sodium). A white to off-white crystalline powder. It contains not less than 886 micrograms and not more than 941 microgram of sulbactam per mg, calculated on the anhydrous basis. Freely soluble in water and in dilute acid; sparingly soluble in acetone, in chloroform, and in ethyl acetate. Store in airtight containers.

### Profile

Sulbactam is a penicillanic acid sulfone with beta-lactamase inhibitory properties. It is active against Neisseriaceae and *Acinetobacter baumanii*, but generally has only weak antibacterial activity against other organisms. It is an irreversible inhibitor of many plasmid-mediated and some chromosomal beta-lactamases and has a similar spectrum of beta-lactamase inhibition to clavulanic acid (p.193), although it is regarded as less potent. Sulbactam can therefore enhance the activity of penicillins and cephalosporins against many resistant strains of bacteria.

It is given with ampicillin (p.157) in the treatment of various infections where beta-lactamase production is suspected. Sulbactam is poorly absorbed from the gastrointestinal tract and is given by injection as the sodium salt. The pharmacokinetics of parenteral sulbactam and ampicillin are similar. For oral use the mutual prodrug sultamicillin (p.264) is available in some countries. Sulbactam has also been given with cefoperazone.

◊ References.

1. Campoli-Richards DM, Brogden RN. Sulbactam/ampicillin: a review of its antibacterial activity, pharmacokinetic properties, and therapeutic use. *Drugs* 1987; **33:** 577–609.
2. Payne DJ, *et al.* Comparative activities of clavulanic acid, sulbactam, and tazobactam against clinically important β-lactamases. *Antimicrob Agents Chemother* 1994; **38:** 767–72.
3. Nicolas-Chanoine MH. Inhibitor-resistant β-lactamases. *J Antimicrob Chemother* 1997; **40:** 1–3.
4. Lee NLS, *et al.* β-Lactam antibiotic and β-lactamase inhibitor combinations. *JAMA* 2001; **285:** 386–8.
5. Lode H. Role of sultamicillin and ampicillin/sulbactam in the treatment of upper and lower bacterial respiratory tract infections. *Int J Antimicrob Agents* 2001; **18:** 199–209.
6. Kanra G. Experience with ampicillin/sulbactam in severe infections. *J Int Med Res* 2002; **30** (suppl 1): 20A–30A.

**Breast feeding.** Although sulbactam is distributed into breast milk in small amounts,[1] no adverse effects have been observed in breast-fed infants and the American Academy of Pediatrics considers that it is usually compatible with breast feeding.[2]

1. Foulds G, *et al.* Sulbactam kinetics and excretion into breast milk in postpartum women. *Clin Pharmacol Ther* 1985; **38:** 692–6.
2. American Academy of Pediatrics. The transfer of drugs and other chemicals into human milk. *Pediatrics* 2001; **108:** 776–89. Correction. *ibid.*; 1029. Also available at: http://aappolicy.aappublications.org/cgi/content/full/pediatrics%3b108/3/776 (accessed 28/05/04)

## Preparations

***USP 27:*** Ampicillin and Sulbactam for Injection.

**Proprietary Preparations** (details are given in Part 3)

***Austria:*** Combactam; ***Fr.:*** Betamaze†; ***Ger.:*** Combactam.

**Multi-ingredient:** ***Arg.:*** Aminoxidin Sulbactam; Ampi-Bis Plus; Ampigen SB; Darzitil SB; Prixin; Sulperazon; Trifamox IBL; Unsayna; ***Austria:*** Unasyn; ***Braz.:*** Trifamox; ***Chile:*** Sulbamox; Sulperazon; Unasyn; ***Fr.:*** Unacim; ***Ger.:*** Unacid; ***Gr.:*** Begalin-P; ***Hong Kong:*** Sulperazon; Unasyn; ***India:*** Sulbacin; ***Israel:*** Unasyn; ***Ital.:*** Bethacil; Loricin; Unasyn; ***Jpn:*** Sulperazon; Unasyn-S; ***Malaysia:*** Sulperazon; Unasyn; ***Mex.:*** Trifamox IBL; Unasyna; ***Singapore:*** Unasyn; ***Spain:*** Bacimex†; Unasyn; ***Thai.:*** Sulperazon; Unasyn; ***USA:*** Unasyn.

## Sulbenicillin Sodium *(rINNM)*

Sulbenicilina sódica; α-Sulfobenzylpenicillin Sodium; Sulfocillin Sodium. The disodium salt of (6*R*)-6-(2-phenyl-2-sulphoacetamido)penicillanic acid.

$C_{16}H_{16}N_2Na_2O_7S_2 = 458.4.$
*CAS — 34779-28-7 (sulbenicillin); 41744-40-5 (sulbenicillin).*
*ATC — J01CA16.*

**Pharmacopoeias.** In *Chin.* and *Jpn.*

### Profile

Sulbenicillin sodium has actions and uses similar to those of carbenicillin sodium (p.166). It is given by intramuscular or intravenous injection or infusion.

## Preparations

**Proprietary Preparations** (details are given in Part 3)

***Ital.:*** Kedacillina†; ***Jpn:*** Lilacillin; ***Mex.:*** Kedacillin.

## Sulfabenzamide *(BAN, USAN, rINN)*

Sulfabenzamida. *N*-Sulphanilylbenzamide.

$C_{13}H_{12}N_2O_3S = 276.3.$
*CAS — 127-71-9.*

**Pharmacopoeias.** In *US.*

**USP 27** (Sulfabenzamide). A fine, white, practically odourless powder. Insoluble in water and in ether; soluble in alcohol, in acetone, and in sodium hydroxide 4% solution. Protect from light.

### Profile

Sulfabenzamide is a sulfonamide with properties similar to those of sulfamethoxazole (p.261). It is reported to exert an optimal bacteriostatic action at pH 4.6. It is used with sulfacetamide and sulfathiazole in pessaries or a vaginal cream for the treatment of bacterial vaginosis, although its value has been questioned. The vaginal cream has also been used for the prevention of bacterial infection following cervical and vaginal surgery.

## Preparations

***USP 27:*** Triple Sulfa Vaginal Cream; Triple Sulfa Vaginal Tablets.

**Proprietary Preparations** (details are given in Part 3)

**Multi-ingredient:** ***Austral.:*** Sultrin†; ***Belg.:*** Sultrin; ***Braz.:*** Vagi-Sulfa; ***Canad.:*** Sultrin†; ***Irl.:*** Sultrin; ***Port.:*** Sultrin; ***S.Afr.:*** Sultrin; ***UK:*** Sultrin; ***USA:*** Dayto Sulf†; Gyne-Sulf†; Sultrin; Triple Sulfa†; Trysul†; VVS†.

## Sulfacarbamide *(BAN, rINN)*

Sulfacarbamida; Sulfanilcarbamide; Sulfaurea; Sulphacarbamide; Sulphanilylurea; Sulphaurea; Urosulphanum. Sulphanilylurea monohydrate.

$C_7H_9N_3O_3S,H_2O = 233.2.$
*CAS — 547-44-4 (anhydrous sulfacarbamide); 6101-35-5 (sulfacarbamide monohydrate).*

**Pharmacopoeias.** In *Pol.*

### Profile

Sulfacarbamide is a sulfonamide with properties similar to those of sulfamethoxazole (p.261). It has been used in the treatment of urinary-tract infections, sometimes with other drugs.

## Sulfacetamide *(BAN, rINN)*

Acetosulfaminum; Sulfacetamida; Sulphacetamide. *N*-Sulphanilylacetamide.

$C_8H_{10}N_2O_3S = 214.2.$
*CAS — 144-80-9.*
*ATC — S01AB04.*

**Pharmacopoeias.** In *Int.* and *US.*

**USP 27** (Sulfacetamide). A white, odourless, crystalline powder. Slightly soluble in water and in ether; soluble in alcohol; very slightly soluble in chloroform; freely soluble in dilute mineral acids and in solutions of potassium and sodium hydroxides; practically insoluble in benzene. Solutions in water are acid to litmus and sensitive to light; they are unstable when acidic or strongly alkaline. Protect from light.

## Sulfacetamide Sodium *(BANM, rINNM)*

Soluble Sulphacetamide; Sulfacetamida sódica; Sulfacetamidum Natricum; Sulfacylum; Sulphacetamide Sodium; Sulphacetamidum Sodium.

$C_8H_9N_2NaO_3S,H_2O = 254.2.$
*CAS — 127-56-0 (anhydrous sulfacetamide sodium); 6209-17-2 (sulfacetamide sodium monohydrate).*
*ATC — S01AB04.*

NOTE. SULF is a code approved by the BP 2003 for use on single unit doses of eye drops containing sulfacetamide sodium where the individual container may be too small to bear all the appropriate labelling information.

**Pharmacopoeias.** In *Chin., Eur.* (see p.vi), *Int., Pol., US,* and *Viet.*

**Ph. Eur. 5.0** (Sulfacetamide Sodium). A white or yellowish-white, crystalline powder. Freely soluble in water; slightly soluble in dehydrated alcohol. A 5% solution in water has a pH of 8.0 to 9.5. Protect from light.

**USP 27** (Sulfacetamide Sodium). A white odourless crystalline powder. Soluble 1 in 2.5 of water; sparingly soluble in alcohol; practically insoluble in chloroform and in ether. A 5% solution in water has a pH of 8.0 to 9.5. Store in airtight containers. Protect from light.

**Stability.** When solutions of sulfacetamide sodium are heated, hydrolysis occurs forming sulfanilamide which may be deposited as crystals, especially from concentrated solutions and under cold storage conditions.

## Adverse Effects, Treatment, and Precautions

As for Sulfamethoxazole, p.261.

Local application of sulfacetamide sodium to the eye may cause burning or stinging but this is rarely severe enough to necessitate discontinuation of treatment.

## Antimicrobial Action

As for Sulfamethoxazole, p.262.

### Pharmacokinetics

When sulfacetamide sodium is applied to the eye it penetrates into ocular tissues and fluids; sulfacetamide may be absorbed into the blood when the conjunctiva is inflamed.

### Uses and Administration

Sulfacetamide is a sulfonamide antibacterial that is used with sulfabenzamide and sulfathiazole in preparations for vaginal use, and is applied, as the sodium salt, in infections or injuries of the eyes, although it is rarely of much value. Eye drops containing sulfacetamide sodium 10% to 30% and eye ointments containing up to 10% have been used. The sodium salt is also applied topically in the treatment of skin infections.

### Preparations

**USP 27:** Neomycin Sulfate, Sulfacetamide Sodium, and Prednisolone Acetate Ophthalmic Ointment; Sulfacetamide Sodium and Prednisolone Acetate Ophthalmic Ointment; Sulfacetamide Sodium and Prednisolone Acetate Ophthalmic Suspension; Sulfacetamide Sodium Ophthalmic Ointment; Sulfacetamide Sodium Ophthalmic Solution; Sulfacetamide Sodium Topical Suspension; Triple Sulfa Vaginal Cream; Triple Sulfa Vaginal Tablets.

**Proprietary Preparations** (details are given in Part 3)

***Arg.:*** Dermaseb; ***Austral.:*** Acetopt; Bleph-10; Optamide†; ***Austria:*** Beocid Puroptal†; Cetazin; ***Belg.:*** Anginamide; Antebor; Isopto Cetamide†; Sulfa 10; Sulfacollyre; Ultra†; ***Braz.:*** Sulfanil†; ***Canad.:*** Bleph-10†; Cetamide; Diosulf; Ophtho-Sulf†; Sodium Sulamyd; Sulfex†; ***Fr.:*** Antebor; Vitaseptine†; ***Ger.:*** Albucid; ***Hong Kong:*** Bleph-10; Spersacet; Sulfex; Vista-Cetamide; ***India:*** Albucid; Locula; ***Israel:*** Klaron; Optisol; Sulfacid; Sulphamide†; ***Ital.:*** Optamid; Prontamid†; ***Mex.:*** Blef-10; Ceta Sulfa†; Examida; Sul 10; ***NZ:*** Acetopt; Bleph-10; ***S.Afr.:*** Bleph-10†; Covosulf; Spersamide; ***Spain:*** Sulfacet†; Sulfacetam; ***Switz.:*** Spersacet; ***Thai.:*** Bleph-10; Cetasil†; Opsar; Optal; ***USA:*** Ak-Sulf; Bleph-10; Cetamide; Isopto Cetamide; Klaron; Ocusulf-10; Sebizon†; Sodium Sulamyd; Sulf-10; Sulfac; Vanocin.

**Multi-ingredient:** ***Arg.:*** Blefamide; C-G; ***Austral.:*** Blephamide†; Sultrin†; ***Austria:*** Blephamide†; ***Belg.:*** Cetapred†; Isopto Cetapred†; Sultrin; ***Braz.:*** Isopto Cetapred; Oto-Biotic; Paraqueimol; Pyelodion†; Sulnil; Uromix†; Vagi-Sulfa; ***Canad.:*** Blephamide; Dioptimyd; Metimyd†; Sulfacet-R; Sultrin†; Vasocidin; Vasosulf†; ***Chile:*** Blefamide; ***Fr.:*** Antebor B$_6$†; ***Ger.:*** Blefcon†; Blephamide; ***Gr.:*** Sulfachloramphenicol; Sulfanicole; ***Hong Kong:*** Blephamide; Spersacet C†; ***India:*** Cortola-m; Nazalin; Nebasulf; Zinco Sulpha; ***Irl.:*** Sultrin; ***Israel:*** Blephamide; Prednisylet†; ***Ital.:*** Antisettico Astringente Sedativo; Aureomix; Brumeton Colloidale S; Cosmiciclina; Visublefarite; ***Malaysia:*** Blephamide; ***Mex.:*** Blefamide SF; Blefamide SOP; Colirio Sulvi; Deltamid; Locion Axel; Metimyd; Premid; Sulfa Cloran; Sulfa Hidro; ***NZ:*** Blephamide; ***Port.:*** Blifamol†; Meocil; Sultrin; ***S.Afr.:*** Blephamide†; Covancaine; Covosan; Spersacet C; Sultrin; ***Singapore:*** Blephamide; ***Spain:*** Betamida; Celestone S; Icolamida†; Liquipom Dexamida†; Oto Neomicin Calm†; Visublefarite†; ***Swed.:*** Blefcon†; Metimyd†; ***Switz.:*** Blephamide; Spersacet C; ***Thai.:*** Spersacet C†; ***UK:*** Sultrin; ***USA:*** Ak-Cide†; Avar; Blephamide; Cetapred†; Clenia; Dayto Sulf†; FML-S; Gyne-Sulf†; Isopto Cetapred†; Metimyd; Nicosyn; Novacet; Plexion; Rosac; Rosanil; Rosula; Sulfacet-R; Sulfamide; Sultrin; Triple Sulfa†; Trysul†; Vasocidin; Vasocine†; Vasosulf; VVS†; Zetacet.

---

## Sulfachlorpyridazine *(BAN, rINN)*

Sulfaclorpiridazina; Sulphachlorpyridazine. $N^1$-(6-Chloropyridazin-3-yl)sulphanilamide.

$C_{10}H_9ClN_4O_2S = 284.7.$

*CAS — 80-32-0.*

**Pharmacopoeias.** In *US* for veterinary use only.

**USP 27** (Sulfachlorpyridazine). Protect from light.

### Profile

Sulfachlorpyridazine is a sulfonamide antibacterial used in veterinary medicine.

### Preparations

**Proprietary Preparations** (details are given in Part 3)

**Multi-ingredient:** ***Braz.:*** Mictasol com Sulfa.

---

## Sulfachrysoidine *(rINN)*

Carboxysulfamidochrysoidine; Sulfacrisoidina. 3,5-Diamino-2-(*p*-sulfamoylphenylazo) benzoic acid.

$C_{13}H_{13}N_5O_4S = 335.3.$

*CAS — 485-41-6.*

### Profile

Sulfachrysoidine is a sulfonamide antibacterial used topically for infections of the oral mucosa.

### Preparations

**Proprietary Preparations** (details are given in Part 3)

***Braz.:*** Colubiazol†.

---

## Sulfaclozine *(rINN)*

Sulfaclozina. $N^1$-(6-Chloropyrazinyl)sulfanilamide.

$C_{10}H_9ClN_4O_2S = 284.7.$

*CAS — 102-65-8; 27890-59-1.*

### Profile

Sulfaclozine is a sulfonamide antibacterial that has been used in veterinary medicine.

---

## Sulfadiazine *(BAN, rINN)*

Solfadiazina; Solfapirimidina; Sulfadiazina; Sulfadiazinum; Sulphadiazine. $N^1$-(Pyrimidin-2-yl)sulphanilamide.

$C_{10}H_{10}N_4O_2S = 250.3.$

*CAS — 68-35-9.*

*ATC — J01EC02.*

NOTE. Compounded preparations of sulfadiazine may be represented by the following names:

- Co-tetroxazine (*BAN*)—sulfadiazine 5 parts and tetroxoprim 2 parts (see p.199)
- Co-trimazine (*BAN*)—sulfadiazine 5 parts and trimethoprim 1 part (see p.199).

**Pharmacopoeias.** In *Chin., Eur.* (see p.vi), *US,* and *Viet.*

**Ph. Eur. 5.0** (Sulfadiazine). White, yellowish-white, or pinkish-white, crystalline powder or crystals. Practically insoluble in water; very slightly soluble in alcohol; slightly soluble in acetone. It dissolves in solutions of alkali hydroxides and in dilute mineral acids. Protect from light.

**USP 27** (Sulfadiazine). White or slightly yellow, odourless or nearly odourless, powder, slowly darkening on exposure to light. Soluble 1 in 13 000 of water; sparingly soluble in alcohol and in acetone; freely soluble in dilute mineral acids and in solutions of potassium and sodium hydroxides, and ammonia. Protect from light.

## Sulfadiazine Sodium *(BANM, rINN)*

Sodium Sulfadiazine; Soluble Sulphadiazine; Sulfadiazina sódica; Sulfadiazinum Natricum; Sulphadiazine Sodium.

$C_{10}H_9N_4NaO_2S = 272.3.$

*CAS — 547-32-0.*

*ATC — J01EC02.*

**Pharmacopoeias.** In *Chin.* and *US.*

**USP 27** (Sulfadiazine Sodium). A white powder. Soluble 1 in 2 of water; slightly soluble in alcohol. On prolonged exposure to humid air it absorbs carbon dioxide with the liberation of sulfadiazine and becomes incompletely soluble in water. Store in airtight containers at a temperature of 25°, excursions permitted between 15° and 30°. Protect from light.

**Incompatibility.** Solutions of sulfadiazine sodium are alkaline, and incompatibility may reasonably be expected with acidic drugs or with preparations unstable at high pH. In the UK, the manufacturers state that sulfadiazine sodium injection is incompatible with fructose, iron salts, and salts of heavy metals.

### Adverse Effects, Treatment, and Precautions

As for Sulfamethoxazole, p.261.

Because of the low solubilities of sulfadiazine and its acetyl derivative in urine, crystalluria is more likely after use of sulfadiazine than after sulfamethoxazole.

Sulfadiazine sodium solution is strongly alkaline and it should therefore be given intravenously in a strength not exceeding 5%, over at least 10 minutes. For the same reason, intramuscular injections are painful and sulfadiazine sodium should not be given by intrathecal or subcutaneous injection.

**Carnitine deficiency.** A case of hyperammonaemia and carnitine deficiency in an immunocompromised patient receiving sulfadiazine and pyrimethamine for the treatment of toxoplasmosis.[1]

1. Sekas G, Harbhajan SP. Hyperammonemia and carnitine deficiency in a patient receiving sulfadiazine and pyrimethamine. *Am J Med* 1993; **95:** 112–13.

**Effects on the eyes.** Numerous white stone-like concretions of sulfadiazine occurred in the conjunctiva of a woman who had used sulfadiazine eye drops for about 1 year.[1]

1. Boettner EA, *et al.* Conjunctival concretions of sulfadiazine. *Arch Ophthalmol* 1974; **92:** 446–8.

**Effects on the kidneys.** Reports of crystalluria and renal failure associated with the use of sulfadiazine in patients with AIDS,[1-4] including the suggestion that such patients may be particularly prone to sulfadiazine-induced renal toxicity.[3]

1. Goadsby PJ, *et al.* Acquired immunodeficiency syndrome (AIDS) and sulfadiazine-associated acute renal failure. *Ann Intern Med* 1987; **107:** 783–4.
2. Ventura MG, *et al.* Sulfadiazine revisited. *J Infect Dis* 1989; **160:** 556–7.
3. Simon DI, *et al.* Sulfadiazine crystalluria revisited: the treatment of Toxoplasma encephalitis in patients with acquired immunodeficiency syndrome. *Arch Intern Med* 1990; **150:** 2379–84.
4. Díaz F, *et al.* Sulfadiazine-induced multiple urolithiasis and acute renal failure in a patient with AIDS and Toxoplasma encephalitis. *Ann Pharmacother* 1996; **30:** 41–2.

**Effects on the salivary glands.** Enlargement of the salivary glands (sialadenitis) has been reported[1] in a patient who received a preparation containing sulfadiazine; complete recovery followed within 3 days of stopping therapy. Rechallenge confirmed that sulfadiazine was the causative agent.

1. Añíbarro B, Fontela JL. Sulfadiazine-induced sialadenitis. *Ann Pharmacother* 1997; **31:** 59–60.

### Interactions

As for Sulfamethoxazole, p.262.

### Antimicrobial Action

As for Sulfamethoxazole, p.262.

### Pharmacokinetics

Sulfadiazine is readily absorbed from the gastrointestinal tract, peak blood concentrations being reached 3 to 6 hours after a single dose; 20 to 55% has been reported to be bound to plasma proteins. It penetrates into the CSF within 4 hours of an oral dose to produce therapeutic concentrations which may be more than half those in the blood. Up to 40% of sulfadiazine in the blood is present as the acetyl derivative. The half-life of sulfadiazine is about 10 hours; it is prolonged in renal impairment.

About 50% of a single dose of sulfadiazine given by mouth is excreted in the urine in 24 hours; 15 to 40% is excreted as the acetyl derivative.

◊ The urinary excretion of sulfadiazine and the acetyl derivative is dependent on pH. About 30% is excreted unchanged in both fast and slow acetylators when the urine is acidic whereas about 75% is excreted unchanged by slow acetylators when the urine is alkaline. The half-life of sulfadiazine ranges from 7 to 12 hours and that of its metabolite from 8 to 12 hours.[1]

1. Vree TB, *et al.* Determination of the acetylator phenotype and pharmacokinetics of some sulphonamides in man. *Clin Pharmacokinet* 1980; **5:** 274–94.

### Uses and Administration

Sulfadiazine is a short-acting sulfonamide that has been used similarly to sulfamethoxazole (p.262) in the treatment of infections due to susceptible organisms. It has been used in the treatment of nocardiosis and lymphogranuloma venereum, and has been given for the prophylaxis of rheumatic fever in penicillin-allergic patients. For details of these infections and their treatment, see Choice of Antibacterial, p.120. Sulfadiazine is also given with pyrimethamine for the treatment and prevention of relapse of toxoplasmosis (p.598) and has been tried in disseminated *Acanthamoeba* infection (p.595).

In the treatment of susceptible infections, sulfadiazine may be given by mouth in usual initial doses of 2 to 4 g, followed by up to 6 g daily in divided doses. A dose in children is 75 mg/kg initially, then 150 mg/kg daily in divided doses to a maximum of 6 g daily. Sulfadiazine is used in infants less than 2 months of age for congenital toxoplasmosis.

Immunocompromised patients who have toxoplasmosis should be given a dose of 4 to 6 g daily in 4 divided doses for at least 6 weeks, followed by a suppressive dose of 2 to 4 g daily, which should continue indefinitely. Pyrimethamine should always be given concurrently.

For the prophylaxis of rheumatic fever, patients weighing less than about 30 kg are given 500 mg once daily, while those over 30 kg may receive 1 g once daily.

Sulfadiazine is also given intravenously as the sodium salt. 1.09 g of sulfadiazine sodium is approximately equivalent to 1 g of sulfadiazine. The usual dose is the equivalent of sulfadiazine 2 to 3 g initially, followed by 1 g four times daily for 2 days; subsequent treatment is given by mouth. Children and infants over 2 months of age may be given the equivalent of 50 mg/kg initially, followed by 25 mg/kg four times daily.

Intravenous doses of sulfadiazine sodium are given by infusion or by slow intravenous injection of a solution containing up to 5% sulfadiazine. It may be diluted with sodium chloride 0.9%. Sulfadiazine sodium has been given by deep intramuscular injection, but great care must be taken to prevent damage to subcutaneous tissues; the intravenous route is preferred.

Sulfadiazine has been used with trimethoprim as co-trimazine (p.199). Sulfadiazine has also been used with other sulfonamides, particularly sulfamerazine and sulfadimidine, to reduce the problems of low solubility in urine.

### Preparations

***BP 2003:*** Sulfadiazine Injection;
***USP 27:*** Sulfadiazine Sodium Injection; Sulfadiazine Tablets; Trisulfapyrimidines Oral Suspension; Trisulfapyrimidines Tablets.

**Proprietary Preparations** (details are given in Part 3)
***Arg.:*** Silvederma; Sulfatral; ***Braz.:*** Neo Sulfazina; Sulfadiazinac; ***Fr.:*** Adiazine; ***Gr.:*** Adiazine; ***Port.:*** Labdiazina.

**Multi-ingredient:** ***Arg.:*** Afonisan; Anginotrat; Pastillas Lorbi; Sulfatral-Cerio; ***Austria:*** Ophcillin N; Rhinon; Triglobe; ***Braz.:*** Anfomicin†; Enterodina†; Enterovit†; Enterozol†; Gargosedans†; Testinfex†; Triglobe; ***Canad.:*** Coptin; Trisulfaminic†; ***Fin.:*** Ditrim; Trimetin Duplo; ***Fr.:*** Trimadiaz Antrima†; ***Ger.:*** Sterinor; Triglobe†; Urospasmon; Urospasmon sine; ***India:*** Aubril; Zad-G; ***Ital.:*** Kombinax†; Oxosint†; Sterinor†; ***Malaysia:*** Badin; Beaglobe; Triglobe; Trisulprim; ***Mex.:*** Estrefen; ***Port.:*** Broncodiazina; ***Singapore:*** Balin; Triglobe†; ***Spain:*** Bronco Aseptilex†; Broncomicin Bals†; Triglobe†; ***Swed.:*** Trimin sulfa; ***Thai.:*** Balin†; Sulfatril.

## Sulfadiazine Silver *(BANM, rINNM)*

Silver Sulfadiazine *(USAN)*; Silver Sulphadiazine; Sulfadiazina argéntica; Sulfadiazinum Argentum; Sulphadiazine Silver.

$C_{10}H_9AgN_4O_2S$ = 357.1.
*CAS — 22199-08-2.*
*ATC — D06BA01.*

**Pharmacopoeias.** In *Chin., Int., Jpn,* and *US.*

**USP 27** (Silver Sulfadiazine). A white to creamy-white, odourless or almost odourless crystalline powder. It becomes yellow on exposure to light. Practically insoluble in alcohol, in chloroform, and in ether; slightly soluble in acetone; freely soluble in 30% ammonia solution. It decomposes in moderately strong mineral acids. Protect from light.

### Adverse Effects, Treatment, and Precautions

Sulfadiazine silver may be absorbed following topical application and produce systemic effects similar to those of other sulfonamides (see Sulfamethoxazole, p.261).

Local pain or irritation are uncommon; the separation of the eschar may be delayed and fungal invasion of the wound may occur.

Transient leucopenia does not usually require withdrawal of sulfadiazine silver, but blood counts should be monitored to ensure they return to normal within a few days. Systemic absorption of silver, resulting in argyria, can occur when sulfadiazine silver is applied to large area wounds or over prolonged periods.

**Argyria.** A report of argyria, with discoloration of the skin and sensorimotor neuropathy, caused by excessive application of sulfadiazine silver 1% cream to extensive leg ulcers.[1]

1. Payne CMER, *et al.* Argyria from excessive use of topical silver sulphadiazine. *Lancet* 1992; **340:** 126.

### Interactions

As for Sulfamethoxazole, p.262.

Sulfadiazine silver is not antagonised by *p*-aminobenzoic acid or related compounds. The silver content of sulfadiazine silver may inactivate enzymatic debriding agents.

### Antimicrobial Action

Sulfadiazine silver has broad antimicrobial activity against Gram-positive and Gram-negative bacteria including *Pseudomonas aeruginosa,* and some yeasts and fungi. Sulfadiazine silver has a bactericidal action; in contrast to sulfadiazine, the silver salt acts primarily on the cell membrane and cell wall and its action is not antagonised by *p*-aminobenzoic acid. Resistance to sulfadiazine silver has been reported and may develop during therapy.

### Pharmacokinetics

Sulfadiazine silver slowly releases sulfadiazine when in contact with wound exudates. Up to about 10% of the sulfadiazine may be absorbed; concentrations in blood of 10 to 20 micrograms/mL have been reported, although higher concentrations may be achieved when extensive areas of the body are treated. Some silver may also be absorbed.

### Uses and Administration

Sulfadiazine silver is a sulfonamide that is used, in conjunction with debridement, as a 1% cream for the prevention and treatment of infection in severe burns (p.1134).

Sulfadiazine silver has also been used in other skin conditions, such as leg ulcers (p.1139), where infection may prevent healing and for the prophylaxis of infection in skin grafting. It has also been applied to the eyes in the treatment of superficial *Aspergillus* infections.

Catheters impregnated with sulfadiazine silver have been used to reduce catheter colonisation and related bloodstream infection (p.1165).

### Preparations

***USP 27:*** Silver Sulfadiazine Cream.

**Proprietary Preparations** (details are given in Part 3)
***Austria:*** Flammazine; ***Belg.:*** Flammazine; ***Braz.:*** Dermazine†; Pratazine†; Sulfaderm; ***Canad.:*** Dermazin; Flamazine; SSD; ***Denm.:*** Flamazine; ***Fin.:*** Flamazine; ***Fr.:*** Flammazine; Sicazine; ***Ger.:*** Brandiazin; Flammazine; ***Gr.:*** Flamazine; ***Hong Kong:*** Aldo-Silverderma; Dermazin; Flamazine; Silverol†; ***India:*** SSZ; ***Irl.:*** Flamazine; ***Israel:*** Silverol; ***Ital.:*** Bacternil; Sofargen; ***Mex.:*** Argental; Silvadene; ***Neth.:*** Flammazine; ***Norw.:*** Flamazine; ***Port.:*** Flamazine; Sicazine†; ***S.Afr.:*** Argent-Eze†; Bactrazine†; Flamazine; Silbecor; ***Singapore:*** Flamazine; ***Spain:*** Flammazine; Silvederma; ***Switz.:*** Flammazine; Silvertone; ***Thai.:*** Dermazin; Flamazine; Silverol; ***UAE:*** Silvadiazin; ***UK:*** Flamazine; ***USA:*** Silvadene; SSD; Thermazene.

**Multi-ingredient:** ***Arg.:*** Platsul-A; Sulfadiazina de Plata; Sulfaplat; ***Austral.:*** Silvazine; ***Belg.:*** Flammacerium; ***Braz.:*** Dermacerium†; ***Canad.:*** Flamazine C; ***Chile:*** Hebermin; Platsul A; ***Fr.:*** Flammacerium; ***India:*** Silverex; ***Israel:*** Flammacerium†; ***Ital.:*** Altergen; Connettivina Plus; ***Neth.:*** Flammacerium; ***NZ:*** Silvazine; ***Singapore:*** Silvazine; ***Spain:*** Unitul Complex; ***Switz.:*** Ialugen Plus; ***UK:*** Flammacerium.

## Sulfadicramide *(rINN)*

Sulfadicramida. *N'*-(3,3-Dimethylacroyl)sulphanilamide.

$C_{11}H_{14}N_2O_3S$ = 254.3.
*CAS — 115-68-4.*
*ATC — S01AB03.*

### Profile

Sulfadicramide is a sulfonamide with properties similar to those of sulfamethoxazole (p.261). It is applied as a 15% ointment for superficial infections of the eye.

### Preparations

**Proprietary Preparations** (details are given in Part 3)
***Denm.:*** Irgamid; ***Fin.:*** Irgamid; ***Neth.:*** Irgamid†; ***Switz.:*** Irgamid.

## Sulfadimethoxine *(BAN, rINN)*

Sulfadimetossina; Sulfadimetossipirimidina; Sulfadimetoxina; Sulphadimethoxine. $N^1$-(2,6-Dimethoxypyrimidin-4-yl)sulphanilamide.

$C_{12}H_{14}N_4O_4S$ = 310.3.
*CAS — 122-11-2.*
*ATC — J01ED01.*

**Pharmacopoeias.** In *Fr.* and *It.* In *US* for veterinary use only.

**USP 27** (Sulfadimethoxine). Practically white, crystalline powder. Practically insoluble in water; slightly soluble in alcohol, in chloroform, in ether, and in hexane; soluble in 2N sodium hydroxide; sparingly soluble in 2N hydrochloric acid. Store in airtight containers. Protect from light.

### Profile

Sulfadimethoxine is a long-acting sulfonamide with properties similar to those of sulfamethoxazole (p.261). It is used in veterinary medicine, sometimes with baquiloprim or ormetoprim. It was formerly used in humans for the treatment of urinary-tract infections.

## Sulfadimidine *(BAN, rINN)*

Solfametazina; Sulfadimerazine; Sulfadimezinum; Sulfadimidina; Sulfadimidinum; Sulfamethazine; Sulphadimethylpyrimidine; Sulphadimidine; Sulphamethazine. $N^1$-(4,6-Dimethylpyrimidin-2-yl)sulphanilamide.

$C_{12}H_{14}N_4O_2S$ = 278.3.
*CAS — 57-68-1.*
*ATC — J01EB03.*

NOTE. Sulfadimethylpyrimidine has been used as a synonym for sulfisomidine (p.264). Care should be taken to avoid confusion between the two compounds, which are isomeric.

**Pharmacopoeias.** In *Eur.* (see p.vi), *Int., US,* and *Viet.*

**Ph. Eur. 5.0** (Sulfadimidine). White or almost white powder or crystals. Very slightly soluble in water; slightly soluble in alcohol; soluble in acetone. It dissolves in solutions of alkali hydroxides and in dilute mineral acids. Protect from light.

**USP 27** (Sulfamethazine). White to yellowish-white, practically odourless, powder. It may darken on exposure to light. Very slightly soluble in water and in ether; slightly soluble in alcohol; soluble in acetone. Protect from light.

## Sulfadimidine Sodium *(BANM, rINNM)*

Soluble Sulphadimidine; Sulfadimidina sódica; Sulfamethazine Sodium; Sulphadimidine Sodium.

$C_{12}H_{13}N_4NaO_2S$ = 300.3.
*CAS — 1981-58-4.*
*ATC — J01EB03.*

**Pharmacopoeias.** In *Int.*

### Profile

Sulfadimidine is a short-acting sulfonamide with properties similar to those of sulfamethoxazole (p.261).

It is well absorbed from the gastrointestinal tract and is about 80 to 90% bound to plasma proteins. Reported half-lives have ranged from 1.5 to 4 hours in fast and 5.5 to 8.8 hours in slow acetylators. Because of the relatively high solubility of the drug and its acetyl metabolite, crystalluria may be less likely than with sulfamethoxazole.

In the treatment of susceptible infections, sulfadimidine has been given by mouth in an initial dose of 2 g, followed by 0.5 to 1.0 g every 6 to 8 hours. It has also been given parenterally as the sodium salt.

Sulfadimidine has also been used with other sulfonamides, particularly sulfamerazine and sulfadiazine. It is also used in veterinary medicine, sometimes with baquiloprim or trimethoprim.

Because its pharmacokinetics differ in fast and slow acetylators, sulfadimidine has been used to determine acetylator status.

### Preparations

***USP 27:*** Trisulfapyrimidines Oral Suspension; Trisulfapyrimidines Tablets.

**Proprietary Preparations** (details are given in Part 3)
**Multi-ingredient:** ***Canad.:*** Trisulfaminic†; ***Thai.:*** Sulfatril.

## Sulfadoxine *(BAN, USAN, rINN)*

Ro-4-4393; Sulfadoxina; Sulfadoxinum; Sulformethoxine; Sulforthomidine; Sulphormethoxine; Sulphorthodimethoxine. $N^1$-(5,6-Dimethoxypyrimidin-4-yl)sulphanilamide.

$C_{12}H_{14}N_4O_4S$ = 310.3.
*CAS — 2447-57-6.*

**Pharmacopoeias.** In *Chin., Eur.* (see p.vi), *Int., US,* and *Viet.*

**Ph. Eur. 5.0** (Sulfadoxine). White or yellowish-white crystalline powder or crystals. Very slightly soluble in water; slightly soluble in alcohol and in methyl alcohol. It dissolves in solutions of alkali hydroxides and in dilute mineral acids. Protect from light.

**USP 27** (Sulfadoxine). Protect from light.

### Adverse Effects, Treatment, and Precautions

As for Sulfamethoxazole, p.261. For reference to the adverse effects of a combination of sulfadoxine and pyrimethamine, see Pyrimethamine, p.458.

If adverse effects occur, sulfadoxine has the disadvantage that several days are required for elimination from the body.

### Interactions

As for Sulfamethoxazole, p.262.

### Antimicrobial Action

As for Sulfamethoxazole, p.262. Synergy exists between sulfadoxine and pyrimethamine, which act against folate metabolism at different points of the metabolic cycle.

Resistance to the combination of sulfadoxine and pyrimethamine in plasmodia, first noted in Thailand in the late 1970s, has become widespread in many malarious areas of the world. For further details of resistance to antimalarial drugs, see p.444.

### Pharmacokinetics

Sulfadoxine is readily absorbed from the gastrointestinal tract. High concentrations in the blood are reached in about 4 hours; the half-life in the blood is about 4 to 9 days. About 90 to 95% is reported to be bound to plasma proteins.

Sulfadoxine is widely distributed to body tissues and fluids; it passes into the fetal circulation and has been detected in low concentrations in breast milk. Sulfadoxine is excreted very slowly in urine, primarily unchanged.

### Uses and Administration

Sulfadoxine is a long-acting sulfonamide that has been used in the treatment of various infections but is now rarely used alone.

It is given as a fixed-dose combination of 20 parts sulfadoxine with 1 part pyrimethamine (Fansidar) in the treatment of falciparum malaria resistant to other therapies (p.444), usually following a course of quinine. Although the combination has been used in the prophylaxis of malaria, the risk of toxicity is now generally considered to outweigh its value.

In the treatment of malaria, the usual dose by mouth is 1.5 g of sulfadoxine with 75 mg of pyrimethamine as a single dose; this should not be repeated for at least 7 days. Oral doses for children are: 5 to 10 kg body-weight, 250 mg sulfadoxine with 12.5 mg pyrimethamine; 11 to 20 kg, 500 mg sulfadoxine with 25 mg pyrimethamine; 21 to 30 kg, 750 mg sulfadoxine with 37.5 mg pyrimethamine; 31 to 45 kg, 1 g sulfadoxine with 50 mg pyrimethamine.

The combination of sulfadoxine with pyrimethamine has also been given intramuscularly.

Sulfadoxine with pyrimethamine has also been tried in the treatment of actinomycetomas (see Mycetoma p.136), and for prophylaxis of *Pneumocystis carinii* pneumonia in immunocompromised patients (see p.389 for the more usual prophylactic regimens).

A mixture of 5 parts of sulfadoxine with 1 part trimethoprim is used in veterinary medicine.

### Preparations

***USP 27:*** Sulfadoxine and Pyrimethamine Tablets.

**Proprietary Preparations** (details are given in Part 3)
***Ital.:*** Fanasil†.

**Multi-ingredient:** ***Austral.:*** Fansidar; ***Belg.:*** Fansidar†; Malastop; ***Braz.:*** Fansidar; ***Canad.:*** Fansidar; ***Denm.:*** Fansidar; ***Fr.:*** Fansidar; ***India:*** Laridox; Pyralfin; Rimodar; ***Irl.:*** Fansidar; ***Israel:*** Fansidar; ***Malaysia:*** Madomine; ***S.Afr.:*** Fansidar; ***Singapore:*** Madomine; ***Swed.:*** Fansidar†; ***Switz.:*** Fansidar; Fansimef; ***Thai.:*** Vivaxine; ***UK:*** Fansidar; ***USA:*** Fansidar.

## Sulfafurazole *(BAN, pINN)*

Sulfafurazol; Sulfafurazolum; Sulfisoxazole; Sulphafuraz; Sulphafurazole. $N^1$-(3,4-Dimethylisoxazol-5-yl)sulphanilamide.
$C_{11}H_{13}N_3O_3S$ = 267.3.
*CAS — 127-69-5.*
*ATC — J01EB05; S01AB02.*

**Pharmacopoeias.** In *Chin., Eur.* (see p.vi), *Jpn, Pol.,* and *US.*
**Ph. Eur. 5.0** (Sulfafurazole). White or yellowish-white, crystalline powder or crystals. Practically insoluble in water; sparingly soluble in alcohol; slightly soluble in dichloromethane. It dissolves in solutions of alkali hydroxides and in dilute mineral acids. Protect from light.
**USP 27** (Sulfisoxazole). A white to slightly yellowish, odourless crystalline powder. Soluble 1 in 7700 of water and 1 in 10 of boiling alcohol; soluble in 3N hydrochloric acid. Store in airtight containers. Protect from light.

### Acetyl Sulfafurazole

Acetilsulfafurazol; Acetyl Sulphafurazole; Sulfisoxazole Acetyl. $N^1$-Acetyl Sulphafurazole; N-(3,4-Dimethylisoxazol-5-yl)-N-sulphanilylacetamide.
$C_{13}H_{15}N_3O_4S$ = 309.3.
*CAS — 80-74-0.*
*ATC — J01EB05; S01AB02.*

NOTE. Acetyl sulfafurazole is to be distinguished from the $N^4$-acetyl derivative formed from sulfafurazole by conjugation in the body.
Compounded preparations of acetyl sulfafurazole may be represented by the following name:
- Co-erynsulfisox *(PEN)*—acetyl sulfafurazole and erythromycin ethyl succinate.

**Pharmacopoeias.** In *US.*
**USP 27** (Sulfisoxazole Acetyl). A white or slightly yellow crystalline powder. Practically insoluble in water; soluble 1 in 176 of alcohol, 1 in 35 of chloroform, 1 in 1064 of ether, and 1 in 203 of methyl alcohol. Store in airtight containers. Protect from light.

### Sulfafurazole Diolamine *(pINNM)*

NU-445; Sulfafurazol diolamina; Sulfisoxazole Diolamine *(USAN)*; Sulphafurazole Diethanolamine; Sulphafurazole Diolamine. The 2,2′-iminobisethanol salt of sulphafurazole.
$C_{11}H_{13}N_3O_3S,C_4H_{11}NO_2$ = 372.4.
*CAS — 4299-60-9.*
*ATC — J01EB05; S01AB02.*

### Adverse Effects, Treatment, and Precautions

As for Sulfamethoxazole, p.261.

Sulfafurazole and its acetyl derivative are relatively soluble in urine and the risk of crystalluria is generally slight, but nevertheless adequate fluid intake is recommended.

**Breast feeding.** A study[1] in 6 women who received sulfafurazole concluded that the amount of drug secreted into breast milk poses no risk to the healthy infant beyond the immediate newborn period, but potential risk in breast-fed infants with jaundice or G6PD deficiency, or who are ill, stressed, or premature, was more difficult to evaluate. Based on this evidence, the American Academy of Pediatrics[2] has stated that sulfafurazole is usually compatible with breast feeding, but caution is required in the infants mentioned above.

1. Kauffman RE, *et al.* Sulfisoxazole secretion into human milk. *J Pediatr* 1980; **97:** 839–41.
2. American Academy of Pediatrics. The transfer of drugs and other chemicals into human milk. *Pediatrics* 2001; **108:** 776–89. Correction. *ibid.*; 1029. Also available at: http://aappolicy.aappublications.org/cgi/content/full/pediatrics%3b108/3/776 (accessed 28/05/04)

### Interactions

As for Sulfamethoxazole, p.262.

Sulfafurazole has been reported to increase the anaesthetic effect of thiopental.

Eye preparations of sulfafurazole diolamine should not be applied with preparations of silver salts.

### Antimicrobial Action

As for Sulfamethoxazole, p.262.

### Pharmacokinetics

Sulfafurazole is readily absorbed from the gastrointestinal tract with peak plasma concentrations occurring 1 to 4 hours after a dose by mouth. Acetyl sulfafurazole (the $N^1$-acetyl derivative) is broken down to sulfafurazole in the gastrointestinal tract before absorption, resulting in delayed and somewhat lower peak concentrations. Following absorption about 85 to 90% is bound to plasma proteins. Sulfafurazole readily diffuses into extracellular fluid, but very little diffuses into cells. Concentrations in the CSF are about one-third of those in the blood. It crosses the placenta into the fetal circulation and is distributed into breast milk. About 30% of sulfafurazole in the blood and in the urine is in the form of the $N^4$-acetyl derivative.

Sulfafurazole is excreted rapidly in the urine, up to 97% of a single dose being eliminated in 48 hours. The half-life is reported to range from about 5 to 8 hours. Both sulfafurazole and its $N^4$-acetyl derivative are more soluble than many other sulfonamides in urine.

### Uses and Administration

Sulfafurazole is a short-acting sulfonamide that is used similarly to sulfamethoxazole (p.262), notably in the treatment of urinary-tract infections, pneumonia due to *Chlamydophila pneumoniae* (*Chlamydia pneumoniae*), nocardiosis, and trachoma. It is also used, usually with erythromycin, in the treatment of otitis media. For details of these infections and their treatment see Choice of Antibacterial, p.120.

Sulfafurazole is usually given by mouth. In the treatment of susceptible infections, it has been given in an initial dose of 2 to 4 g, followed by 4 to 8 g daily in divided doses every 4 to 6 hours. For children and infants over 2 months of age, the dose has been 75 mg/kg initially, followed by 150 mg/kg daily in divided doses to a maximum of 6 g daily. Dosage modification may be necessary in patients with renal impairment. Acetyl sulfafurazole is tasteless and is used in liquid oral preparations of the drug; doses are expressed in terms of sulfafurazole. 1.16 g of acetyl sulfafurazole is approximately equivalent to 1 g of sulfafurazole.

Sulfafurazole diolamine has been used, as an ophthalmic ointment or solution containing the equivalent of 4% of sulfafurazole, in the topical treatment of susceptible eye infections. Sulfafurazole diolamine 1.39 g is approximately equivalent to 1 g of sulfafurazole.

Sulfafurazole diolamine has also been given parenterally.

### Preparations

***USP 27:*** Erythromycin Estolate and Sulfisoxazole Acetyl Oral Suspension; Erythromycin Ethylsuccinate and Sulfisoxazole Acetyl for Oral Suspension; Sulfisoxazole Acetyl Oral Suspension; Sulfisoxazole Tablets.

**Proprietary Preparations** (details are given in Part 3)
***Canad.:*** Novo-Soxazole†; ***Mex.:*** Sulfizax†; ***USA:*** Gantrisin.

**Multi-ingredient:** ***Arg.:*** Pediazole; ***Canad.:*** Pediazole; ***Chile:*** Bioquin; Pediazole; ***Fr.:*** Pediazole; ***Gr.:*** Pediazole; ***Hong Kong:*** Pediazole; ***Israel:*** Pediazole; ***Mex.:*** Pediazole†; ***S.Afr.:*** Pediazole†; ***USA:*** Eryzole; Pediazole.

## Sulfaguanidine *(BAN, rINN)*

Solfaguanidina; Sulfaguanidina; Sulfaguanidinum; Sulfamidinum; Sulginum; Sulphaguanidine. 1-Sulphanilylguanidine; N′-Amidinosulphanilamide.
$C_7H_{10}N_4O_2S$ = 214.2.
*CAS — 57-67-0 (anhydrous sulfaguanidine); 6190-55-2 (sulfaguanidine monohydrate).*
*ATC — A07AB03.*

**Pharmacopoeias.** In *Eur.* (see p.vi).
*Viet.* includes the monohydrate.
**Ph. Eur. 5.0** (Sulfaguanidine). A white or almost white, fine crystalline powder. Very slightly soluble in water and in alcohol; slightly soluble in acetone; practically insoluble in dichloromethane. It dissolves in dilute solutions of mineral acids. Protect from light.

### Profile

Sulfaguanidine is a sulfonamide with properties similar to those of sulfamethoxazole (p.261). It is absorbed to a limited extent from the gastrointestinal tract and may therefore be more likely to cause systemic effects than less well absorbed drugs such as phthalylsulfathiazole and succinylsulfathiazole. It is used, usually with other drugs, in the treatment of gastrointestinal infections, and has also been applied locally to the skin and throat.

### Preparations

**Proprietary Preparations** (details are given in Part 3)
***Fr.:*** Enteropathyl.

**Multi-ingredient:** ***Braz.:*** Enteroftal†; Sanadiar†; Testinfex†; ***Fr.:*** Litoxol†; ***Thai.:*** Biodan.

## Sulfamazone Sodium

Sulfamazone sodium *(rINNM)*; Sulfenazone; Sulphenazone. Sodium α-{p-[(6-methoxy-3-pyridazinyl)sulfamoyl]anilino}-2,3-dimethyl-5-oxo-1-phenyl-3-pyrazoline-4-methanesulphonate.
$C_{23}H_{24}N_6O_7S_2Na$ = 583.6.
*CAS — 65761-24-2 (sulfamazone); 13061-27-3 (sulfamazone sodium).*

### Profile

Sulfamazone is an antibacterial with antipyretic activity that is given as the sodium salt, by mouth or rectally, in infections of the upper respiratory tract.

### Preparations

**Proprietary Preparations** (details are given in Part 3)
***Ital.:*** Marespin.

## Sulfamerazine *(BAN, rINN)*

RP-2632; Solfamerazina; Sulfamerazina; Sulfamerazinum; Sulfamethyldiazine; Sulfamethylpyrimidine; Sulphamerazine. $N^1$-(4-Methylpyrimidin-2-yl)sulphanilamide.
$C_{11}H_{12}N_4O_2S$ = 264.3.
*CAS — 127-79-7.*
*ATC — J01ED07.*

**Pharmacopoeias.** In *Eur.* (see p.vi).
**Ph. Eur. 5.0** (Sulfamerazine). White, yellowish-white, or pinkish-white, crystalline powder or crystals. Very slightly soluble in water and in dichloromethane; slightly soluble in alcohol; sparingly soluble in acetone. It dissolves in solutions of alkali hydroxides and in dilute mineral acids. Protect from light.

### Sulfamerazine Sodium *(BANM, rINNM)*

Soluble Sulphamerazine; Sulfamerazina sódica; Sulfamerazinum Natricum; Sulphamerazine Sodium.
$C_{11}H_{11}N_4NaO_2S$ = 286.3.
*CAS — 127-58-2.*
*ATC — J01ED07.*

### Profile

Sulfamerazine is a short-acting sulfonamide with properties similar to those of sulfamethoxazole (p.261). It has usually been given with other sulfonamides, or with trimethoprim.

### Preparations

***USP 27:*** Trisulfapyrimidines Oral Suspension; Trisulfapyrimidines Tablets.

**Proprietary Preparations** (details are given in Part 3)

**Multi-ingredient:** ***Canad.:*** Trisulfaminic†; ***Ger.:*** Berlocombin; ***Thai.:*** Sulfatril.

## Sulfamethizole *(BAN, rINN)*

Sulfamethizolum; Sulfametizol; Sulphamethizole. $N^1$-(5-Methyl-1,3,4-thiadiazol-2-yl)sulphanilamide.
$C_9H_{10}N_4O_2S_2$ = 270.3.
*CAS — 144-82-1.*
*ATC — B05CA04; D06BA04; J01EB02; S01AB01.*

**Pharmacopoeias.** In *Eur.* (see p.vi), *Jpn,* and *US.*
**Ph. Eur. 5.0** (Sulfamethizole). White or yellowish-white crystalline powder or crystals. Very slightly soluble in water; sparingly soluble in alcohol; soluble in acetone. It dissolves in dilute solutions of alkali hydroxides and in dilute mineral acids. Protect from light.

**USP 27** (Sulfamethizole). Practically odourless, white crystals or powder. Soluble 1 in 2000 of water, 1 in 38 of alcohol, 1 in 13 of acetone, and 1 in 1900 of chloroform and of ether; freely soluble in solutions of ammonium, potassium, and sodium hydroxides; soluble in dilute mineral acids; practically insoluble in benzene. Protect from light.

### Adverse Effects, Treatment, and Precautions

As for Sulfamethoxazole, p.261.

Sulfamethizole and its acetyl derivative are relatively soluble in urine, and the risk of crystalluria is quite low, but an adequate fluid intake should generally be maintained.

### Interactions

As for Sulfamethoxazole, p.262.

### Antimicrobial Action

As for Sulfamethoxazole, p.262.

### Pharmacokinetics

Sulfamethizole is readily absorbed from the gastrointestinal tract; about 90% has been reported to be bound to plasma proteins. Its half-life has been reported to range from about 1.5 to 3 hours. It is only slightly acetylated in the body and is rapidly excreted, about 60% of a dose being eliminated in the urine in 5 hours and around 90% within 10 hours. Sulfamethizole and its acetyl derivative are readily soluble in urine over a wide pH range. Only low concentrations are achieved in blood and tissues because of its rapid excretion.

### Uses and Administration

Sulfamethizole is a short-acting sulfonamide that is given by mouth in the treatment of infections of the urinary tract, sometimes with other antibacterials; it is unsuitable for the treatment of systemic infection since only relatively low concentrations of drug are achieved in the blood and tissues.

It is given in adult doses of 1.5 to 4 g daily in 3 or 4 divided doses. A usual dose for children is 30 to 45 mg/kg daily in 4 divided doses.

Sulfamethizole monoethanolamine has also been used.

### Preparations

***USP 27:*** Sulfamethizole Oral Suspension; Sulfamethizole Tablets.

**Proprietary Preparations** (details are given in Part 3)
***Denm.:*** Lucosil; ***Fr.:*** Rufol; ***Norw.:*** Lucosil; ***Thai.:*** Luco-Oph; ***USA:*** Thiosulfil Forte†.

**Multi-ingredient:** ***Braz.:*** Uromix†; ***S.Afr.:*** Nicene†; ***Spain:*** Micturol Sedante; ***USA:*** Urobiotic-250.

---

## Sulfamethoxazole *(BAN, USAN, rINN)*

Ro-4-2130; Sulfamethoxazolum; Sulfametoxazol; Sulfisomezole; Sulphamethoxazole. $N^1$-(5-Methylisoxazol-3-yl)sulphanilamide.

$C_{10}H_{11}N_3O_3S$ = 253.3.

*CAS — 723-46-6.*

*ATC — J01EC01.*

NOTE. Compounded preparations of sulfamethoxazole may be represented by the following names:

- Co-trimoxazole *(BAN)*—sulfamethoxazole 5 parts and trimethoprim 1 part (see p.199)
- Co-trimoxazole *(PEN)*—sulfamethoxazole and trimethoprim.

**Pharmacopoeias.** In *Chin., Eur.* (see p.vi), *Int., Jpn, Pol., US,* and *Viet.*

**Ph. Eur. 5.0** (Sulfamethoxazole). A white or almost white, crystalline powder. Practically insoluble in water; sparingly soluble in alcohol; freely soluble in acetone. It dissolves in dilute solutions of sodium hydroxide and in dilute acids. Protect from light.

**USP 27** (Sulfamethoxazole). A white to off-white, practically odourless, crystalline powder. Soluble 1 in 3400 of water, 1 in 50 of alcohol, and 1 in 1000 of chloroform and of ether; slowly and usually incompletely soluble 1 in 2 of carbon disulfide; freely soluble in acetone and in dilute solutions of sodium hydroxide. Store at a temperature of 25°, excursions permitted between 15° and 30°. Protect from light.

### Adverse Effects and Treatment

Nausea, vomiting, anorexia, and diarrhoea are relatively common following the use of sulfamethoxazole and other sulfonamides.

Hypersensitivity reactions to sulfonamides have proved a problem. Fever is relatively common, and reactions involving the skin may include rashes, pruritus, photosensitivity reactions, exfoliative dermatitis, and erythema nodosum. Severe, potentially fatal, skin reactions including toxic epidermal necrolysis and the Stevens-Johnson syndrome have occurred in patients treated with sulfonamides. Dermatitis may also occur from contact of sulfonamides with the skin. Systemic lupus erythematosus, particularly exacerbation of pre-existing disease, has also been reported.

Nephrotoxic reactions including interstitial nephritis and tubular necrosis, which may result in renal failure, have been attributed to hypersensitivity to sulfamethoxazole. Lumbar pain, haematuria, oliguria, and anuria may also occur due to crystallisation in the urine of sulfamethoxazole or its less soluble acetylated metabolite. The risk of crystalluria can be reduced by giving fluids to maintain a high urine output. If necessary, alkalinisation of the urine with sodium bicarbonate may increase solubility and aid the elimination of sulfonamides.

Blood disorders have occasionally occurred during treatment with the sulfonamides including sulfamethoxazole, and include agranulocytosis, aplastic anaemia, thrombocytopenia, leucopenia, hypoprothrombinaemia, and eosinophilia. Many of these effects on the blood may result from hypersensitivity reactions. Sulfonamides may rarely cause cyanosis due to methaemoglobinaemia. Acute haemolytic anaemia is a rare complication which may be associated with G6PD deficiency.

Other adverse effects which may be manifestations of a generalised hypersensitivity reaction to sulfonamides include a syndrome resembling serum sickness, hepatic necrosis, hepatomegaly and jaundice, myocarditis, pulmonary eosinophilia and fibrosing alveolitis, and vasculitis including polyarteritis nodosa. Anaphylaxis has been reported only very rarely.

Other adverse reactions that have been reported after sulfamethoxazole or other sulfonamides include hypoglycaemia, hypothyroidism, neurological reactions including aseptic meningitis, ataxia, benign intracranial hypertension, convulsions, dizziness, drowsiness, fatigue, headache, insomnia, mental depression, peripheral or optic neuropathies, psychoses, tinnitus, vertigo, and pancreatitis.

Sulfonamides may displace serum-bound bilirubin, resulting in kernicterus in premature neonates.

As with other antimicrobials, sulfamethoxazole may cause alterations of the bacterial flora in the gastrointestinal tract. There is, therefore, the possibility, although it appears to be small, that pseudomembranous colitis may occur.

Slow acetylators of sulfamethoxazole may be at greater risk of adverse reactions than fast acetylators.

For further information on the adverse effects of sulfamethoxazole when used with trimethoprim, see Co-trimoxazole, p.199.

### Precautions

In patients receiving sulfamethoxazole, adequate fluid intake is necessary to reduce the risk of crystalluria; the daily urine output should be 1200 mL or more. The use of compounds which render the urine acidic may increase the risk of crystalluria; the risk may be reduced with alkaline urine.

Treatment with sulfonamides should be discontinued immediately a rash appears because of the danger of severe allergic reactions such as the Stevens-Johnson syndrome.

Sulfamethoxazole should be given with care to patients with renal or hepatic impairment and is contra-indicated in patients with severe renal or hepatic failure or with blood disorders. Dosage reduction may be necessary in renal impairment. Complete blood counts and urinalyses with microscopic examination should be carried out particularly during prolonged therapy. Sulfamethoxazole should not be given to patients with a history of hypersensitivity to sulfonamides as cross-sensitivity may occur between drugs of this group. Care is generally advisable in patients with a history of allergy or asthma. Caution is also needed in the elderly, who may be more likely to have other risk factors for reactions. Some consider sulfamethoxazole to be contra-indicated in lupus erythematosus as it may exacerbate the condition. Patients with glucose 6-phosphate dehydrogenase deficiency may be at risk of haemolytic reactions.

Sulfamethoxazole and other sulfonamides are not usually given to infants within 1 to 2 months of birth because of the risk of producing kernicterus; for the same reason, they are generally contra-indicated in women prior to delivery (see below).

Patients with AIDS may be particularly prone to adverse reactions, especially when sulfamethoxazole is given with trimethoprim as co-trimoxazole.

Sulfonamides have been reported to interfere with some diagnostic tests, including those for urea, creatinine, and urinary glucose and urobilinogen.

**Breast feeding.** Sulfonamides are excreted into breast milk in low concentrations and, although they are generally contra-indicated in the USA in breast-feeding women because of the risk of kernicterus, they are usually thought to pose a negligible risk to healthy neonates. However, sulfonamides should be used with caution in breast-feeding mothers of ill, stressed, or premature infants and of infants with jaundice, hyperbilirubinaemia or G6PD deficiency.

The American Academy of Pediatrics considers sulfamethoxazole, when given with trimethoprim, to be compatible with breast feeding.[1]


1. American Academy of Pediatrics. The transfer of drugs and other chemicals into human milk. *Pediatrics* 2001; **108:** 776–89. Correction. *ibid.*; 1029. Also available at: http://aappolicy.aappublications.org/cgi/content/full/pediatrics%3b108/3/776 (accessed 28/05/04)


**Immunocompromised patients.** Sulfamethoxazole is mainly conjugated in the liver to the $N^4$-acetyl derivative, but is also oxidised, to a limited extent, to the hydroxylamine metabolite.[1-5] Although this metabolite was originally implicated[6] in the development of adverse reactions to sulfonamides, recent work[7] has cast some doubt on this hypothesis. The metabolite appears to be produced through cytochrome P450 oxidative metabolism, and it has been suggested that slow acetylators of sulfamethoxazole exhibit increased oxidation compared with other metabolic routes.[1] AIDS patients also exhibit increased oxidation, since they may be depleted of substrates such as acetylcoenzyme A or glutathione necessary for acetylation or detoxification, and this may explain their susceptibility to sulfamethoxazole toxicity.[2,3]

There have been attempts to inhibit the formation of the hydroxylamine metabolite by competitive inhibition of cytochrome P450 enzymes, notably with fluconazole and ketoconazole.[4,5] Encouraging results have been obtained with fluconazole in healthy volunteers, but the potential for clinical benefit in AIDS patients requires further study.[5]

However, one successful method of overcoming adverse effects in AIDS patients has been **desensitisation**. Desensitisation by use of initial doses of 4 mg of sulfamethoxazole or 5 mg of sulfadiazine every 6 hours, doubled at 24-hour intervals until the desired dose was reached, was uneventful in 9 of 13 patients with AIDS requiring sulfonamide treatment for opportunistic infections.[8] The remaining 4 had cutaneous reactions with fever, but in 2 of these the reactions were successfully managed with an antihistamine. Although there is a risk of anaphylaxis, patients with AIDS can be successfully treated with sulfonamides if desensitisation is employed.

See also Immunocompromised Patients under Precautions of Co-trimoxazole, p.200.


1. Cribb AE, Spielberg SP. Sulfamethoxazole is metabolized to the hydroxylamine in humans. *Clin Pharmacol Ther* 1992; **51:** 522–6.
2. Lee BL, *et al.* The hydroxylamine of sulfamethoxazole and adverse reactions in patients with acquired immunodeficiency syndrome. *Clin Pharmacol Ther* 1994; **56:** 184–9.
3. van der Ven AJA, *et al.* Urinary recovery and kinetics of sulphamethoxazole and its metabolites in HIV-seropositive patients and healthy volunteers after a single oral dose of sulphamethoxazole. *Br J Clin Pharmacol* 1995; **39:** 621–5.
4. Mitra AK, *et al.* Inhibition of sulfamethoxazole hydroxylamine formation by fluconazole in human liver microsomes and healthy volunteers. *Clin Pharmacol Ther* 1996; **59:** 332–40.
5. Gill HJ, *et al.* The effect of fluconazole and ketoconazole on the metabolism of sulphamethoxazole. *Br J Clin Pharmacol* 1996; **42:** 347–53.
6. van der Ven AJAM, *et al.* Adverse reactions to co-trimoxazole in HIV infection. *Lancet* 1991; **338:** 431–3.
7. ter Hofstede HJM, *et al.* Drug reactions to cotrimoxazole in HIV infection: possibly not due to the hydroxylamine metabolites of sulphamethoxazole. *Br J Clin Pharmacol* 1999; **47:** 571–3.
8. Torgovnick J, Arsura E. Desensitization to sulfonamides in patients with HIV infection. *Am J Med* 1990; **88:** 548–9.


**Porphyria.** Sulfonamides have been associated with acute attacks of porphyria and are considered unsafe in porphyric patients.

**Pregnancy.** Some sulfonamides have been shown to cause fetal abnormalities including cleft palate in *animals*, but fears of teratogenic effects in humans do not appear to be substantiated. Sulfonamides are probably safe in the first trimester of pregnancy, although throughout pregnancy they should be used only in the absence of a suitable alternative drug.[1] Sulfonamides may displace serum-bound bilirubin and they should be avoided close to delivery because of the risk of kernicterus in the neonate. The risk of drug-induced bilirubin displacement has been reviewed.[2] The initial evidence suggesting a kernicterus-promoting effect of drugs in neonates was reported for sulfafurazole, and this drug now serves as a standard displacing agent against which other drugs are evaluated. Although all sulfonamides are highly protein bound, each has a different capacity to displace bilirubin. Sulfadiazine and sulfanilamide have been found to be the least displacing of the sulfonamides and the effects of sulfadiazine on bilirubin may not be clinically significant; an increased incidence of hyperbilirubinaemia and kernicterus has not been demonstrated following its use for prophylaxis of rheumatic fever during pregnancy. Sulfasalazine should theoretically cause significant bilirubin displacement, but studies suggest that the drug may be given to patients with Crohn's disease who are pregnant or breast feeding. Metabolites of sulfonamides have also been evaluated for kernicterus-promoting effects; glucuronide metabolites are expected to compete for binding sites less effectively than the parent compound, whereas acetylated metabolites of some sulfonamides appear to be more potent bilirubin displacers.


1. Wise R. Prescribing in pregnancy: antibiotics. *BMJ* 1987; **294:** 42–4.
2. Walker PC. Neonatal bilirubin toxicity: a review of kernicterus and the implications of drug-induced bilirubin displacement. *Clin Pharmacokinet* 1987; **13:** 26–50.


## Interactions

The action of sulfonamides may be antagonised by *p*-aminobenzoic acid and compounds derived from it, particularly potassium aminobenzoate and the procaine group of local anaesthetics.

Sulfamethoxazole and other sulfonamides may potentiate the effects of some drugs, such as oral anticoagulants (p.1024), methotrexate (p.570), and phenytoin (p.372); this may be due to displacement of the drug from plasma protein binding sites or to inhibition of metabolism. However, the clinical significance of these interactions appears to depend on the particular sulfonamide involved. The possibility of interactions with other highly protein-bound drugs, such as NSAIDs, should be considered.

High doses of sulfonamides have been reported to have a hypoglycaemic effect; the antidiabetic effect of the sulfonylurea compounds may be enhanced by sulfonamides (p.347). Some sulfonamides have been associated with a decrease in plasma-ciclosporin concentrations when used together (p.1354). Isolated reports have described possible failures of hormonal contraceptives resulting in pregnancy in patients given sulfonamides (p.1534).

The use of compounds which render the urine acidic may increase the risk of crystalluria.

## Antimicrobial Action

Sulfamethoxazole and other sulfonamides have a similar structure to *p*-aminobenzoic acid and interfere with the synthesis of nucleic acids in sensitive micro-organisms by blocking the conversion of *p*-aminobenzoic acid to the coenzyme dihydrofolic acid, a reduced form of folic acid; in man, dihydrofolic acid is obtained from dietary folic acid so sulfonamides do not affect human cells. Their action is primarily bacteriostatic, although they may be bactericidal where concentrations of thymine are low in the surrounding medium. The sulfonamides have a broad spectrum of action, but the development of widespread resistance (see below) has greatly reduced their usefulness, and susceptibility often varies widely even among nominally sensitive pathogens.

Gram-positive cocci, particularly the Group A streptococci and some strains of *Streptococcus pneumoniae*, are usually sensitive and staphylococci also demonstrate sensitivity but to a lesser extent. Enterococci and many of the clostridia are more or less resistant, although strains of *Clostridium perfringens* are moderately susceptible. Among other Gram-positive organisms that have been reported to be sensitive are *Bacillus anthracis* and many strains of Nocardia, especially *N. asteroides*.

The Gram-negative cocci *Neisseria meningitidis* and *N. gonorrhoeae* were formerly extremely susceptible to sulfonamides, but many strains are now resistant. Susceptibility is often seen in *Haemophilus influenzae* although resistance in *H. ducreyi* is increasingly common. Susceptibility varies widely among the Enterobacteriaceae: strains of *Escherichia coli, Klebsiella, Proteus, Salmonella,* and *Serratia* are sometimes sensitive, but few strains of *Shigella* are now susceptible. *Vibrio cholerae* may be sensitive.

Other organisms that have been reported to be sensitive include *Actinomyces* spp., *Brucella, Calymmatobacterium granulomatis, Legionella,* and *Yersinia pestis*. Chlamydiaceae are sensitive, but not mycoplasmas, rickettsias, or spirochaetes, nor in general the mycobacteria. *Pseudomonas aeruginosa* is resistant, although sulfonamides may be effective against *Burkholderia pseudomallei* (*Pseudomonas pseudomallei*).

Sulfonamides have some activity against the protozoa *Plasmodium falciparum* and *Toxoplasma gondii*. They are also active against *Pneumocystis carinii*, but are ineffective against most fungi.

Sulfamethoxazole and other sulfonamides demonstrate synergy with the dihydrofolate reductase inhibitors pyrimethamine and trimethoprim which inhibit a later stage in folic acid synthesis. For reports of the antimicrobial activity of sulfamethoxazole with trimethoprim, see Co-trimoxazole, p.200.

The *in-vitro* antimicrobial activity of sulfamethoxazole is very dependent on both the culture medium and size of inoculum used.

*Resistance.* Acquired resistance to sulfonamides is common and widespread among formerly susceptible organisms, particularly *Neisseria* spp., *Shigella* and some other enterobacteria, staphylococci, and streptococci.

There appear to be several mechanisms of resistance including alteration of dihydropteroate synthetase, the enzyme inhibited by sulfonamides, to a less sensitive form, or an alteration in folate biosynthesis to an alternative pathway; increased production of *p*-aminobenzoic acid; or decreased uptake or enhanced metabolism of sulfonamides.

Resistance may result from chromosomal alteration, or may be plasmid-mediated and transferable, as in many resistant strains of enterobacteria. High-level resistance is usually permanent and irreversible. There is complete cross-resistance between the different sulfonamides.

## Pharmacokinetics

Sulfamethoxazole is readily absorbed from the gastrointestinal tract and peak plasma concentrations are reached after about 2 hours. Following a single 2-g dose by mouth, blood concentrations of up to 100 micrograms/mL are achieved. About 70% is bound to plasma proteins. The plasma half-life is about 6 to 12 hours; it is prolonged in patients with severe renal impairment.

Sulfamethoxazole, like most sulfonamides, diffuses freely throughout the body tissues and may be detected in the urine, saliva, sweat, and bile, in the cerebrospinal, peritoneal, ocular, and synovial fluids, and in pleural and other effusions. It crosses the placenta into the fetal circulation and low concentrations have been detected in breast milk.

Sulfamethoxazole undergoes conjugation mainly in the liver, chiefly to the inactive $N^4$-acetyl derivative; this metabolite represents about 15% of the total amount of sulfamethoxazole in the blood. Metabolism is increased in patients with renal impairment and decreased in those with hepatic impairment. Elimination in the urine is dependent on pH. About 80 to 100% of a dose is excreted in the urine, of which about 60% is in the form of the acetyl derivative, with the remainder as unchanged drug and glucuronide.

Sulfamethoxazole is also oxidised to the hydroxylamine, a metabolite that has been implicated in adverse reactions to sulfonamides (see also Immunocompromised Patients, under Precautions, above), although some doubt has been cast upon this hypothesis.

## Uses and Administration

The use of sulfamethoxazole and other sulfonamides has been limited by the increasing incidence of resistant organisms. Their main use has been in the treatment of acute, uncomplicated urinary-tract infections, particularly those caused by *Escherichia coli*. They have also been used in nocardiosis, and in some other bacterial infections such as otitis media, *Chlamydia* and *Chlamydophila* infections, and prophylaxis of meningococcal meningitis, but have largely been replaced by other drugs: even where pathogens retain some sensitivity to sulfonamides, a combination such as co-trimoxazole (sulfamethoxazole with trimethoprim) has often been preferred. The usual treatment of these infections is discussed under Choice of Antibacterial, p.120. Sulfonamides are also used, often with pyrimethamine or trimethoprim, in the treatment of protozoal infections, particularly malaria (p.444) and toxoplasmosis (p.598). They are also used similarly in *Pneumocystis carinii* pneumonia (p.389).

Sulfamethoxazole is an intermediate-acting sulfonamide that has been given by mouth in a usual dose of 2 g initially, followed by 1 g twice daily. In severe infections 1 g three times daily has been given.

Children have been given a dose of 50 to 60 mg/kg initially, followed by 25 to 30 mg/kg twice daily, up to a maximum daily dose of 75 mg/kg.

Reduction of dosage may be required in patients with renal impairment.

For the uses and dosage of sulfamethoxazole with trimethoprim, see Co-trimoxazole, p.200.

Sulfamethoxazole lysine has also been used.

**Administration.** The US manufacturers of sulfamethoxazole recommended that blood concentrations be measured in patients receiving sulfonamides for serious infections. The following concentrations of free sulfonamide in the blood were considered to be therapeutically effective: for most infections, 50 to 150 micrograms/mL, and for serious infections, 120 to 150 micrograms/mL. Concentrations of 200 micrograms/mL should not be exceeded since the incidence of adverse reactions might be increased.

## Preparations

***BP 2003:*** Co-trimoxazole Intravenous Infusion; Co-trimoxazole Oral Suspension; Co-trimoxazole Tablets; Dispersible Co-trimoxazole Tablets; Paediatric Co-trimoxazole Oral Suspension; Paediatric Co-trimoxazole Tablets;
***USP 27:*** Sulfamethoxazole and Trimethoprim Injection; Sulfamethoxazole and Trimethoprim Oral Suspension; Sulfamethoxazole and Trimethoprim Tablets; Sulfamethoxazole Oral Suspension; Sulfamethoxazole Tablets.

**Proprietary Preparations** (details are given in Part 3)
***USA:*** Gantanol†.

**Multi-ingredient:** ***Arg.:*** Adrenol; Bacti-Uril; Bacticel; Bactrim; Bactrim Balsamico; Cotrizol-G; Danferane; Diocla; Dosulfin Bronquial; Dosulfin Fuerte; Enterobacticel; Netocur; Netocur Balsamico; Neumobacticel; Novidrine; Sulfagrand; Tritenk; Urisept NF; Uro-Bactrim; ***Austral.:*** Bactrim; Cosig; Resprim; Septrin; Trimoxazole; ***Austria:*** Bactrim; Cotribene; Cotristad; Eusaprim; Oecotrim; Supracombin; Trimetho comp; ***Belg.:*** Bactrim; Eusaprim; Steroprim; ***Braz.:*** Assepium; Assepium Balsamico; Bac Septin Balsamico†; Bac Septin†; Bac-Sulfitrin; Bacfar; Bacfar Balsamico†; Bacgen Balsamico†; Bacgen†; Bacprotin; Bacris; Bacteracin; Bacteracin Balsamico†; Bactox Balsamico†; Bactox†; Bactren†; Bactrex†; Bactricin Balsamico†; Bactricin†; Bactrim; Bactrisan; Bactrisan Balsamico†; Bactrizol; Bactropin; Bactropin Balsamico†; Baklinger†; Balsandin†; Balsiprin†; Baxapril†; Becaltrin†; Belfactrin†; Benectrin; Benectrin Balsamico; Binoctrin; Diazol; Dientrin; Dispeptrin†; Diteutrin†; Duoctrin; Duoctrin Balsamico†; Duoctrin Enterico†; Ectrin; Ectrin Balsamico; Entercal†; Entero Heractrin†; Enterone†; Espectrin; Gamactrin; Heractrin†; Ibtrim†; Imuneprim; Infecteracin†; Infectrin; Infectrin Balsamico†; Katrim Balsamico†; Katrim†; Leotrim†; Linurin; Lupectrim; Lupectrim Balsamico†; Metoprin; Metoprin Balsamico†; Mictrex†; Neotrin; Neotrin Balsamico†; Pulkrin; Qiftrin; Quimio-Ped; Quimio-Ped Balsamico†; Roytrin; Sedactrim Balsamico†; Sedactrim†; Selectrim†; Septiolan; Septiolan Balsamico†; Septoprin†; Silpin†; Sulf+Trim†; Sulfa+Trim†; Sulfatrex†; Suss Balsamico†; Suss†; Teutrin; Teutrin Balsamico†; Trimetoprim Balsamico†; Trimexazol; Trimexazol Balsamico†; Trizol Balsamico†; Urizal†; Uro Bac Septin†; Uro Bactrim†; Uro Batrox†; Uro Duoctrim†; Uro Heractrim†; Uro Septoprin†; Uro-Bacteracin†; Uro-Baxapril; Uro-Leotrim†; Uro-Septiolan†; Uro-Teutrim†; Urobactrex†; Urobioctrin†; Uroctrin; Urofar†; Uroneotrim†; Uropol; Uroxazol†; Utrim†; ***Canad.:*** Apo-Sulfatrim; Bactrim†; Novo-Trimel; Nu-Cotrimox; Roubac†; Septra; ***Chile:*** Bacterol; Bactrimel; Entero Micinovo; Introcin; Septrin; Trelibec; Uro-Micinovo; ***Denm.:*** Bactrim†; Sulfotrim; ***Fin.:*** Cotrim; ***Fr.:*** Bactrim; Cotrimazol†; Eusaprim; ***Ger.:*** Bactoreduct; Bactrim†; Berlocid; Co-trim-Tablinen†; Cotrim; Cotrim-Diolan; Cotrimhexal; Cotrimox-Wolff; Cotrimstada; Drylin; Eusaprim; Jenamoxazol†; Kepinol; Linaris†; Microtrim; Sigaprim; Supracombin; TMS; ***Gr.:*** Bactrimel; Bioprim; Septrin; ***Hong Kong:*** Apo-Sulfatrim†; Bacin†; BS†; Chemitrim; Chemoprim; Dhatrin; Letus; Septrin; ***India:*** Bactrim; Ciplin; Colizole; Oriprim; Sepmax; Septran; Trisulfose; ***Irl.:*** Bactrim†; Cotrimel†; Duobact; Septrin; Tricomox†; ***Israel:*** Diseptyl; Resprim; Septrin; Sulfatrim; ***Ital.:*** Abacin; Bacterial†; Bactrim; Chemitrim; Eusaprim; Gantrim; Isotrim†; Medixin†; Strepto-Plus†; ***Malaysia:*** Bacin; Baserin; Chemix; Cotrim; Resprim; Trimexazole; Virin; ***Mex.:*** Andoprim; Anitrim; Bacpiryl; Bactelan; Bactide; Bactilen; Bactiver; Bactrim; Bactrim Compositum; Bactropin; Bateral; Batrizol; Bioprim; Dertrin; Dibaprim;

Ectaprim; Enterobacticel†; Esteprim; Fectri; Isobac†; Kaltrim; Lidaprim†; Maxtrim; Metoxiprim; Microbactim; Octex; Octiban; Pisatrina; Polibatrin; Protaxol; Septrin; Servitrim; Sulfawal; Sulfoid Trimetho; Sulfort†; Sulprim; Sultiprim; Supristol†; Syraprim; Thriazol; Tribakin; Trim-Vit†; Trimesul†; Trimesuxol†; Trimetoger; Trimetox; Trimexazol; Trimexole; Trimexole Compositum; Trimzol†; Trinelax†; Trisufin; Urovec; Zaprin†; **Neth.:** Bactrimel; Eusaprim; Trimoxol; **Norw.:** Bactrim; Trimetoprim-Sulfa; **NZ:** Apo-Sulfatrim; Bactrim†; Trimel†; Trisul; **Port.:** Bactrim; Cotrim; Metomide; Septrin; **S.Afr.:** Acuco†; Arcanaprim†; Bactrim; Bencole; Cocydal†; Cozole; Doctrim†; Durobac; Dynazole†; Fabubac; Lagatrim; Mezenol; Purbac; Septran; Spectrim; Tri-Co†; Trimethox; Trimoks†; Trimzol†; Ultrasept†; Xerazole; Xeroprim; **Singapore:** Apo-Sulfatrim; Bacin; Bactrim†; BS; Chemix; Chemoprim; Dhatrin; Septrin; Suprim; Trimezole; **Spain:** Abactrim†; Bactifor†; Bactopumon; Balsoprim; Bridotrim†; Bronco Aseptilex Fuerte; Bronco Bactifor†; Bronco Sergo†; Broncomega; Broncoremа†; Broncovir; Brongenit†; Bronquicisteina; Bronquidiazina CR; Bronquimar; Bronquimucil; Bronquium†; Cotrazol; Eduprim; Eduprim Mucolitico; Gobens Trim; Lotusix†; Momentol; Mucorama TS†; Neumopectolina; Pulmo Menal; Pulmosterin Duo; Salvatrim†; Septrin; Soltrim; Toose†; Tosdetan†; Traquivan†; Tresium†; **Swed.:** Bactrim; Eusaprim; **Switz.:** Agoprim; Bactrim; Cotrim; Escoprim; Eusaprim†; Groprim; Helveprim†; Imexim†; Lagatrim; Mediprim; Nopil; Sigaprim; Supracombin; **Thai.:** Actin; Bacin; Bacta; Bactrim; Baczole; Chemoprim; Co-Tasian; Co-Trimed; Conprim; Cotamox; Ko-Cap; Ko-Kure; Lastrim; Letus; M-Trim; Med-Sultrim; Mega-Prim; Metrim; Metxaprim; Mycosamthong; Po-Trim; Pulvicin; Septrin; Servitrim†; Sulbacta; Sulfometh; Tampo; Toprim; Trimexazole; Trimox†; Trimoxzol†; Triprim; Trixzol; Zoleprim; **UAE:** Trimol; **UK:** Chemotrim†; Fectrim; Laratrim†; Septrin; **USA:** Bactrim; Cotrim; Septra; SMZ-TMP; Sulfatrim.

## Sulfamethoxypyridazine *(BAN, rINN)*

Solfametossipiridazina; Sulfamethoxypyridazinum; Sulfametoxipiridazina; Sulphamethoxypyridazine. $N^1$-(6-Methoxypyridazin-3-yl)sulphanilamide.

$C_{11}H_{12}N_4O_3S$ = 280.3.
*CAS — 80-35-3.*
*ATC — J01ED05.*

**Pharmacopoeias.** In *Int.* and *Viet.* In *Eur.* (see p.vi) for veterinary use only.

**Ph. Eur. 5.0** (Sulfamethoxypyridazine for Veterinary Use). A white or slightly yellowish crystalline powder which colours slowly on exposure to light. Practically insoluble in water; slightly soluble in alcohol; sparingly soluble in acetone; very slightly soluble in dichloromethane; dissolves in dilute mineral acids and solutions of alkali hydroxides. Protect from light.

### Profile

Sulfamethoxypyridazine is a long-acting sulfonamide with properties similar to those of sulfamethoxazole (p.261) and is used for the treatment of susceptible infections. It is rapidly absorbed from the gastrointestinal tract and excreted slowly in urine, partly as the $N^4$-acetyl metabolite; it remains detectable for up to 7 days after a dose. It has also been used with trimethoprim similarly to co-trimoxazole.

Acetyl sulfamethoxypyridazine, which is hydrolysed in the gastrointestinal tract forming sulfamethoxypyridazine, and sulfamethoxypyridazine sodium have also been used.

**Skin disorders.** Reference to the use of sulfamethoxypyridazine in the treatment of pemphigoid.[1] Sulfamethoxypyridazine has also been used in the treatment of dermatitis herpetiformis.[2]

1. Thornhill M, *et al.* An open clinical trial of sulphamethoxypyridazine in the treatment of mucous membrane pemphigoid. *Br J Dermatol* 2000; **143:** 117–26.
2. Fry L. Dermatitis herpetiformis. *Baillieres Clin Gastroenterol* 1995; **9:** 371–93.

### Preparations

**Proprietary Preparations** (details are given in Part 3)
**Mex.:** Dibasul†; Exasul†.
**Multi-ingredient: Braz.:** Nipactrin†; Testinfex†; Urofen; Uropac; **Ital.:** Velaten†.

## Sulfamethylthiazole

Methylsulfathiazole; Sulfametiltiazol. 4-Amino-*N*-(4-methyl-2-thiazolyl)benzenesulfonamide.

$C_{10}H_{11}N_3O_2S_2$ = 269.3.
*CAS — 515-59-3.*

### Profile

Sulfamethylthiazole is a sulfonamide with properties similar to those of sulfamethoxazole (p.261). It is applied topically with tetracycline in the treatment of eye infections.

### Preparations

**Proprietary Preparations** (details are given in Part 3)
**Multi-ingredient: Ital.:** Pensulvit.

## Sulfametopyrazine *(BAN)*

Sulfalene *(USAN, pINN)*; AS-18908; NSC-110433; Solfametopirazina; Solfametossipirazina; Sulfaleno; Sulfamethoxypyrazine; Sulfapirazinmetossina; Sulfapyrazin Methoxyne; Sulphalene. $N^1$-(3-Methoxypyrazin-2-yl)sulphanilamide.

$C_{11}H_{12}N_4O_3S$ = 280.3.
*CAS — 152-47-6.*
*ATC — J01ED02.*

**Pharmacopoeias.** In *It.*

### Adverse Effects, Treatment, and Precautions

As for Sulfamethoxazole, p.261.

If adverse effects occur, sulfametopyrazine has the disadvantage that several days are required for its elimination from the body.

### Interactions

As for Sulfamethoxazole, p.262.

### Antimicrobial Action

As for Sulfamethoxazole, p.262.

### Pharmacokinetics

Sulfametopyrazine is readily absorbed from the gastrointestinal tract; 60 to 80% is bound to plasma proteins. Only about 5% of a dose is metabolised to the acetyl derivative. It is slowly excreted in the urine. The biological half-life has been reported to be about 60 to 65 hours.

### Uses and Administration

Sulfametopyrazine is a long-acting sulfonamide that has been used in the treatment of respiratory- and urinary-tract infections due to sensitive organisms. It has been given by mouth in a single dose of 2 g once each week.

Sulfametopyrazine is given with pyrimethamine (p.459) in the treatment of malaria.

It has also been given in the ratio 4 parts of sulfametopyrazine to 5 parts of trimethoprim as a combination with uses similar to those of co-trimoxazole (p.200).

### Preparations

**Proprietary Preparations** (details are given in Part 3)
**Belg.:** Kelfizina†; Longum†; **Ger.:** Longum; **Irl.:** Kelfizine W†; **Ital.:** Kelfizina†; **UK:** Kelfizine W†.
**Multi-ingredient: Braz.:** Periodine Anti-Malarico†; **Ital.:** Kelfiprim†; Metakelfin; **Mex.:** Kelfiprim†; **Thai.:** Kelfiprim†.

## Sulfametrole *(BAN, rINN)*

Sulfametrol. $N^1$-(4-Methoxy-1,2,5-thiadiazol-3-yl)sulphanilamide.

$C_9H_{10}N_4O_3S_2$ = 286.3.
*CAS — 32909-92-5.*

### Profile

Sulfametrole is a sulfonamide with properties similar to those of sulfamethoxazole (p.261). It is given in the ratio of 5 parts of sulfametrole to 1 part of trimethoprim as a combination with uses similar to those of co-trimoxazole (p.200). Usual doses are 960 mg (800 mg of sulfametrole and 160 mg of trimethoprim) twice daily by mouth. It has also been given by intravenous infusion.

### Preparations

**Proprietary Preparations** (details are given in Part 3)
**Multi-ingredient: Austria:** Lidaprim; **Gr.:** Lidaprim; **Hong Kong:** Lidaprim; **Ital.:** Lidaprim; **Switz.:** Maderan†; **Thai.:** Lidaprim.

## Sulfamonomethoxine *(BAN, USAN, rINN)*

DJ-1550; DS-36; ICI-32525; Ro-4-3476; Sulfamonometoxina. $N^1$-(6-Methoxypyrimidin-4-yl)sulphanilamide monohydrate.

$C_{11}H_{12}N_4O_3S,H_2O$ = 298.3.
*CAS — 1220-83-3 (anhydrous sulfamonomethoxine).*

**Pharmacopoeias.** In *Jpn.*

### Profile

Sulfamonomethoxine is a sulfonamide antibacterial with properties similar to those of sulfamethoxazole (p.261). It is used in veterinary medicine.

## Sulfamoxole *(BAN, USAN, rINN)*

Sulfamoxol; Sulphadimethyloxazole; Sulphamoxole. $N^1$-(4,5-Dimethyloxazol-2-yl)sulphanilamide.

$C_{11}H_{13}N_3O_3S$ = 267.3.
*CAS — 729-99-7.*
*ATC — J01EC03.*

NOTE. Compounded preparations of sulfamoxole may be represented by the following name:

- Co-trifamole (*BAN*)—sulfamoxole 5 parts and trimethoprim 1 part (see p.199).

**Pharmacopoeias.** In *Fr.*

### Profile

Sulfamoxole is a sulfonamide antibacterial with properties similar to those of sulfamethoxazole (p.261). It has been used with trimethoprim as co-trifamole (p.199).

## Sulfanilamide *(rINN)*

Solfammide; Streptocidum; Sulfaminum; Sulfanilamida; Sulfanilamidum; Sulphanilamide. 4-Aminobenzenesulphonamide; *p*-Sulphamidoaniline.

$C_6H_8N_2O_2S$ = 172.2.
*CAS — 63-74-1.*
*ATC — J01EB06.*

**Pharmacopoeias.** In *Eur.* (see p.vi).

**Ph. Eur. 5.0** (Sulfanilamide). White or yellowish-white crystals or fine powder. Slightly soluble in water; sparingly soluble in alcohol; freely soluble in acetone; practically insoluble in dichloromethane; dissolves in solutions of alkali hydroxides and in dilute mineral acids. Protect from light.

### Profile

Sulfanilamide is a short-acting sulfonamide with properties similar to those of sulfamethoxazole (p.261). Its antibacterial activity is less than that of sulfamethoxazole. It has been used topically, including vaginally, for the treatment of susceptible infections, often with other drugs. The sodium, sodium mesilate, and camsilate salts have also been used.

### Preparations

**Proprietary Preparations** (details are given in Part 3)
**Belg.:** Astreptine†; **Canad.:** AVC; **Spain:** Azol; **USA:** AVC†.
**Multi-ingredient: Arg.:** Clinal; Iodotiazol; **Belg.:** Mucorhinyl†; Polyseptol; Pyal†; Rhinamide†; Sulfaryl†; **Braz.:** Gargotan†; Malvosulfam†; Otovix†; Yatropan†; **Port.:** Otocalma; **S.Afr.:** Achromide; AMS†; Daromide; Ung Vernleigh; **Spain:** Buco Regis; Cilinafosal; Cilinafosal DHD Estrep; Cilinafosal Hidrocort; Cilinavagin Neomicina†; Kanafosal; Kanafosal Predni; Nasopomada; Odontocromil c Sulfamida; Oto Difusor†; Otonasal†; Pental Forte; Pentalmicina†; Polvos Wilfe; Pomada Heridas; Pomada Wilfe; Quimpe Amida†; Vitavox Pastillas; **USA:** Alasulf; Deltavac; DIT I-2.

## Sulfapyridine *(BAN, rINN)*

Sulfapiridina; Sulphapyridine. $N^1$-(2-Pyridyl)sulphanilamide.

$C_{11}H_{11}N_3O_2S$ = 249.3.
*CAS — 144-83-2.*
*ATC — J01EB04.*

**Pharmacopoeias.** In *Fr.* and *US.*

**USP 27** (Sulfapyridine). White or faintly yellowish-white, odourless or practically odourless, crystals, granules, or powder. It slowly darkens on exposure to light. Soluble 1 in 3500 of water, 1 in 440 of alcohol, 1 in 65 of acetone; freely soluble in dilute mineral acids and in solutions of potassium and sodium hydroxides. Protect from light.

### Profile

Sulfapyridine is a short- or intermediate-acting sulfonamide, with properties similar to those of sulfamethoxazole (p.261). It is slowly and incompletely absorbed from the gastrointestinal tract and excreted in urine; sulfapyridine and its acetyl metabolite are poorly soluble in urine and the risk of crystalluria is relatively high. Adverse effects are common, and gastrointestinal disturbances may preclude continued therapy. Because of its toxicity, sulfapyridine is now little used except occasionally for dermatitis herpetiformis and related skin disorders where alternative treatment cannot be used; doses of up to 1 g four times daily by mouth have been given initially, reduced to the minimum effective maintenance dose once improvement occurs.

**Breast feeding.** The American Academy of Pediatrics[1] states that, although sulfapyridine is usually compatible with breast feeding, caution is required in breast-fed infants with jaundice or G6PD deficiency, or who are ill, stressed, or premature, whose mothers have received the drug.

1. American Academy of Pediatrics. The transfer of drugs and other chemicals into human milk. *Pediatrics* 2001; **108:** 776–89. Correction. *ibid.*; 1029. Also available at: http://aappolicy.aappublications.org/cgi/content/full/pediatrics%3b108/3/776 (accessed 28/05/04)

**Pemphigoid.** Benefit has been seen with sulfapyridine in ocular cicatricial pemphigoid.[1]

1. Elder MJ, *et al.* Sulphapyridine—a new agent for the treatment of ocular cicatricial pemphigoid. *Br J Ophthalmol* 1996; **80:** 549–52.

### Preparations

***USP 27:*** Sulfapyridine Tablets.
**Proprietary Preparations** (details are given in Part 3)
**Canad.:** Dagenan†.

## Sulfaquinoxaline *(BAN, rINN)*

Sulfabenzpyrazine; Sulfaquinoxalina; Sulphaquinoxalina; Sulphaquinoxaline. $N^1$-(Quinoxalin-2-yl)sulphanilamide.

$C_{14}H_{12}N_4O_2S$ = 300.3.
*CAS — 59-40-5 (sulfaquinoxaline); 967-80-6 (sulfaquinoxaline sodium).*

**Pharmacopoeias.** In *Fr.* Also in *BP(Vet)* and in *US* for veterinary use only. *Fr.* also includes Sulfaquinoxaline Sodium, $C_{14}H_{11}N_4NaO_2S$ = 322.3.

**BP(Vet) 2003** (Sulfaquinoxaline). A yellow, odourless or almost odourless, powder. Practically insoluble in water and in ether; very slightly soluble in alcohol. It dissolves in aqueous solutions of alkalis. Protect from light.

**USP 27** (Sulfaquinoxaline). Protect from light.

### Profile

Sulfaquinoxaline is a sulfonamide antibacterial used in veterinary medicine, sometimes with trimethoprim.

## Sulfasuccinamide (rINN)

Sulfasuccinamida. 4′-Sulphamoylsuccinanilic acid.

$C_{10}H_{12}N_2O_5S$ = 272.3.

*CAS — 3563-14-2.*

### Profile

Sulfasuccinamide is a sulfonamide antibacterial with properties similar to those of sulfamethoxazole (p.261). It is applied topically in the treatment of local infections of the ear, nose, and throat. It has also been given as the sodium salt.

### Preparations

**Proprietary Preparations** (details are given in Part 3)

**Multi-ingredient:** ***Fr.:*** Otoralgyl sulfamide†; RhinATP†; ***Switz.:*** Otoralgyl†.

## Sulfathiazole (BAN, rINN)

M&B-760; Norsulfazole; RP-2090; Solfatiazolo; Sulfanilamidothiazolum; Sulfathiazolum; Sulfatiazol; Sulfonazolum; Sulphathiazole. $N^1$-(1,3-Thiazol-2-yl)sulphanilamide.

$C_9H_9N_3O_2S_2$ = 255.3.

*CAS — 72-14-0.*

*ATC — D06BA02; J01EB07.*

**Pharmacopoeias.** In *Eur.* (see p.vi), *US*, and *Viet.*

**Ph. Eur. 5.0** (Sulfathiazole). A white or slightly yellowish, crystalline powder. Practically insoluble in water; slightly soluble in alcohol; practically insoluble in dichloromethane. It dissolves in dilute solutions of alkali hydroxides and in dilute mineral acids. Protect from light.

**USP 27** (Sulfathiazole). A white or faintly yellowish-white, practically odourless, fine powder. Very slightly soluble in water; slightly soluble in alcohol; soluble in acetone, in dilute mineral acids, in solutions of alkali hydroxides, and in 6N ammonium hydroxide. Protect from light.

## Sulfathiazole Sodium (BANM, rINNM)

Soluble Sulphathiazole; Sulfathiazolum Natricum; Sulfatiazol sódico; Sulphathiazole Sodium.

$C_9H_8N_3NaO_2S_2,5H_2O$ = 367.4.

*CAS — 144-74-1 (anhydrous sulfathiazole sodium); 6791-71-5 (sulfathiazole sodium pentahydrate).*

*ATC — D06BA02; J01EB07.*

**Pharmacopoeias.** In *BP(Vet)* ($1\frac{1}{2}H_2O$ or $5H_2O$).

**BP(Vet) 2003** (Sulfathiazole Sodium). A white or yellowish-white, odourless or almost odourless, crystalline powder or granules. Freely soluble in water; soluble in alcohol. A solution in water containing the equivalent of 1% of the anhydrous substance has a pH of 9.0 to 10.0. Protect from light.

### Profile

Sulfathiazole is a short-acting sulfonamide with properties similar to those of sulfamethoxazole (p.261). It is now rarely used systemically due to its toxicity.

Sulfathiazole is used with other sulfonamides, usually sulfabenzamide and sulfacetamide, in preparations for the topical treatment of vaginal infections and is also used with other drugs in the treatment of skin infections.

Sulfathiazole sodium has been applied topically with other drugs in the treatment of eye infections.

### Preparations

***USP 27:*** Triple Sulfa Vaginal Cream; Triple Sulfa Vaginal Tablets.

**Proprietary Preparations** (details are given in Part 3)

***Arg.:*** Blefarosan; Welt-Sulfazol; ***Mex.:*** Sulfagine†; ***Port.:*** Stopex.

**Multi-ingredient:** ***Arg.:*** Leroid; Otocuril; Otorinazol; ***Austral.:*** Sultrin†; ***Austria:*** Linobion-Sulfonamid†; ***Belg.:*** Pyal†; Sultrin; ***Braz.:*** Mentozil†; Otobel; Vagi-Sulfa; ***Canad.:*** Sultrin†; ***Chile:*** Gotas Otologicas; Indocalm; Polvos Antibioticos; Tru; ***Irl.:*** Sultrin; ***Ital.:*** Streptosil con Neomicina-Fher; ***Port.:*** Sultrin; ***S.Afr.:*** Sultrin; ***Spain:*** Cremsol; Polvos Wilfe; Pomada Wilfe; Sabanotropico; Salitanol Estreptomicina; ***UK:*** Sultrin; ***USA:*** Dayto Sulf†; Gyne-Sulf†; Sultrin; Triple Sulfa†; Trysul†; VVS†.

## Sulfatroxazole (BAN, rINN)

Sulfatroxazol. $N^1$-(4,5-Dimethyl-1,2-oxazol-3-yl)sulfanilamide.

$C_{11}H_{13}N_3O_3S$ = 267.3.

*CAS — 23256-23-7.*

### Profile

Sulfatroxazole is a sulfonamide antibacterial used with trimethoprim in veterinary medicine.

## Sulfisomidine (BAN, rINN)

Sulfa-isodimérazine; Sulfaisodimidine; Sulfasomidine; Sulfisomidina; Sulfisomidinum; Sulphasomidine. $N^1$-(2,6-Dimethylpyrimidin-4-yl)sulphanilamide.

$C_{12}H_{14}N_4O_2S$ = 278.3.

*CAS — 515-64-0.*

*ATC — J01EB01.*

NOTE. Sulfadimethylpyrimidine has been used as a synonym for sulfisomidine, and sulphadimethylpyrimidine is sometimes used as a synonym for sulfadimidine (p.259). Care should be taken to avoid confusion between the two compounds, which are isomeric.

**Pharmacopoeias.** In *Eur.* (see p.vi).

**Ph. Eur. 5.0** (Sulfisomidine). White or yellowish-white powder or crystals. Very slightly soluble in water; slightly soluble in alcohol and in acetone; dissolves in dilute solutions of alkali hydroxides and in dilute mineral acids. Protect from light.

### Profile

Sulfisomidine is a short-acting sulfonamide with properties similar to those of sulfamethoxazole (p.261). It has been used topically for skin or vaginal infections and has also been given by mouth. The sodium salt has also been used.

### Preparations

**Proprietary Preparations** (details are given in Part 3)

***Thai.:*** Aristamed.

## Sultamicillin (BAN, USAN, rINN)

CP-49952; Sultamicilina. Penicillanoyloxymethyl (6R)-6-(D-2-phenylglycylamino)penicillanate S′,S′-dioxide.

$C_{25}H_{30}N_4O_9S_2$ = 594.7.

*CAS — 76497-13-7.*

*ATC — J01CR04.*

## Sultamicillin Tosilate (BANM, rINNM)

Sultamicillin Tosylate. Sultamicillin toluene-4-sulphonate.

$C_{25}H_{30}N_4O_9S_2,C_7H_8O_3S$ = 766.9.

*CAS — 83105-70-8.*

**Pharmacopoeias.** In *Chin.* and *Jpn.*

### Profile

Sultamicillin is a prodrug of ampicillin (p.157) and of the beta-lactamase inhibitor sulbactam (p.257); it consists of the two compounds linked as a double ester. During absorption from the gastrointestinal tract it is hydrolysed, releasing equimolar quantities of ampicillin and sulbactam.

Sultamicillin is given by mouth as tablets containing sultamicillin tosilate or as oral suspension containing sultamicillin. It is used in the treatment of infections where beta-lactamase-producing organisms might occur, including uncomplicated gonorrhoea, otitis media, and respiratory-tract and urinary-tract infections. The usual dose is 375 to 750 mg of sultamicillin (equivalent to 147 to 294 mg of sulbactam and 220 to 440 mg of ampicillin) twice daily. A single dose of sultamicillin 2.25 g together with probenecid 1 g may be used for uncomplicated gonorrhoea.

When parenteral therapy is necessary a combined preparation of ampicillin with sulbactam is given.

◊ References.

1. Friedel HA, *et al.* Sultamicillin: a review of its antibacterial activity, pharmacokinetic properties and therapeutic use. *Drugs* 1989; **37:** 491–522.
2. Lode H. Role of sultamicillin and ampicillin/sulbactam in the treatment of upper and lower bacterial respiratory tract infections. *Int J Antimicrob Agents* 2001; **18:** 199–209.

### Preparations

**Proprietary Preparations** (details are given in Part 3)

***Arg.:*** Ampigen SB; Unsayna; ***Austria:*** Dynapen†; Unasyn; ***Chile:*** Unasyna; ***Fr.:*** Unacim†; ***Ger.:*** Unacid PD; ***Gr.:*** Begalin; ***Hong Kong:*** Unasyn; ***India:*** Sulbacin; ***Ital.:*** Bethacil†; Unasyn; ***Malaysia:*** Unasyn; ***Mex.:*** Unasyna; ***Singapore:*** Unasyn; ***Spain:*** Bacimex†; Unasyn; ***Thai.:*** Unasyn.

## Taurolidine (BAN, rINN)

Taurolidina. 4,4′-Methylenebis(perhydro-1,2,4-thiadiazine 1,1-dioxide).

$C_7H_{16}N_4O_4S_2$ = 284.4.

*CAS — 19388-87-5.*

*ATC — B05CA05.*

### Profile

Taurolidine is a broad-spectrum antimicrobial. It is hydrolysed in aqueous solution to its monomeric form taurultam and other metabolites, with the release of what was originally thought to be formaldehyde but is now considered to be activated methylene glycol or methylol groups, from which it is believed to derive its activity. Its antibacterial activity *in vitro* is modest but is reported to be enhanced in the presence of serum or urine; it is active against a variety of pathogens including *Staphylococcus aureus*, *Escherichia coli*, and *Pseudomonas aeruginosa*. Taurolidine is also reported to inactivate bacterial endotoxin.

Taurolidine is used in peritonitis; a solution containing 0.5% is used for irrigation and another containing 2% is available for instillation. It has been given experimentally as an intravenous infusion in the treatment of severe sepsis or endotoxic shock and in pancreatitis.

### Preparations

**Proprietary Preparations** (details are given in Part 3)

***Austria:*** Taurolin; ***Ger.:*** Taurolin; ***Switz.:*** Taurolin.

## Tazobactam Sodium (BANM, USAN, rINNM)

CL-307579; CL-298741 (tazobactam); Tazobactam sódico; YTR-830; YTR-830H (tazobactam). Sodium (2S,3S,5R)-3-methyl-7-oxo-3-(1H-1,2,3-triazol-1-ylmethyl)-4-thia-1-azabicyclo[3.2.0]-heptane-2-carboxylate 4,4-dioxide.

$C_{10}H_{11}N_4NaO_5S$ = 322.3.

*CAS — 89786-04-9 (tazobactam); 89785-84-2 (tazobactam sodium).*

*ATC — J01CG02.*

### Profile

Tazobactam is a penicillanic acid sulfone derivative with beta-lactamase inhibitory properties similar to those of sulbactam (p.257) although it is regarded as more potent. It has the potential to enhance the activity of beta-lactam antibacterials against beta-lactamase-producing bacteria.

Tazobactam sodium is given intravenously with piperacillin sodium (p.243) for the treatment of bacterial infections. The pharmacokinetics of tazobactam and piperacillin are similar.

◊ References.

1. Bush K, *et al.* Kinetic interactions of tazobactam with β-lactamases from all major structural classes. *Antimicrob Agents Chemother* 1993; **37:** 851–8.
2. Payne DJ, *et al.* Comparative activities of clavulanic acid, sulbactam, and tazobactam against clinically important β-lactamases. *Antimicrob Agents Chemother* 1994; **38:** 767–72.
3. Lee NLS, *et al.* β-Lactam antibiotic and β-lactamase inhibitor combinations. *JAMA* 2001; **285:** 386–8.

### Preparations

**Proprietary Preparations** (details are given in Part 3)

***Mex.:*** Tazocin.

**Multi-ingredient:** ***Arg.:*** Pipetexina; Tazonam; ***Austral.:*** Tazocin; ***Austria:*** Tazonam; ***Belg.:*** Tazocin; ***Braz.:*** Tazocin; ***Canad.:*** Tazocin; ***Chile:*** Tazonam; ***Denm.:*** Tazocin; ***Fin.:*** Tazocin; ***Fr.:*** Tazocilline; ***Ger.:*** Tazobac; ***Gr.:*** Tazocin; ***Hong Kong:*** Tazocin; ***India:*** Zosyn; ***Irl.:*** Tazocin; ***Israel:*** Tazocin; ***Ital.:*** Tazobac†; Tazocin; ***Malaysia:*** Tazocin; ***Neth.:*** Tazocin; ***Norw.:*** Tazocin; ***NZ:*** Tazocin; ***Port.:*** Tazobac; ***S.Afr.:*** Tazocin; ***Singapore:*** Tazocin; ***Spain:*** Tazocel; ***Swed.:*** Tazocin; ***Switz.:*** Tazobac; ***Thai.:*** Tazocin; ***UK:*** Tazocin; ***USA:*** Zosyn.

# Teicoplanin (BAN, USAN, rINN)

A-8327; DL-507-IT; L-12507; MDL-507; Teichomycin $A_2$; Teicoplanina.

*CAS — 61036-62-2 (teichomycin); 61036-64-4 (teichomycin $A_2$).*

*ATC — J01XA02.*

**Description.** A glycopeptide antibiotic obtained from cultures of *Actinoplanes teichomyceticus* or the same substance obtained by any other means.

**Pharmacopoeias.** In *Jpn.*

## Adverse Effects and Precautions

Fever, skin rash and pruritus, and occasional bronchospasm and anaphylaxis have been reported in patients receiving teicoplanin, but, in comparison with vancomycin (p.275), it appears to be better tolerated when given by rapid intravenous injection and, although erythema and flushing of the upper body have occurred, the 'red-man syndrome' has been reported less often. In addition, unlike vancomycin, teicoplanin does not appear to cause tissue necrosis and can be given by intramuscular injection. Other hypersensitivity reactions have included rigors, angioedema, and, rarely, severe skin reactions including exfoliative dermatitis, erythema multiforme, Stevens-Johnson syndrome, and toxic epidermal necrolysis.

Other reported reactions include gastrointestinal disturbances, dizziness, headache, thrombocytopenia (especially at high doses), leucopenia, neutropenia, eosinophilia, disturbances in liver enzyme values, and pain, erythema, and thrombophlebitis or abscess at the injection site. Rare cases of agranulocytosis have occurred. Renal impairment and ototoxicity have been reported but both appear to be less frequent than with vancomycin.

Renal and auditory function should be monitored during prolonged therapy in patients with pre-existing renal impairment, and in those receiving other ototoxic or nephrotoxic drugs, although opinions conflict as to whether increased risk of nephrotoxicity has been demonstrated from combined therapy with drugs such as the aminoglycosides. In general, periodic blood counts and liver- and renal-function tests are advised during treatment.

No relationship has yet been established between plasma concentration and toxicity, and plasma-concentration monitoring is not generally considered necessary. Dosage adjustment is required in renal impairment.

**Hypersensitivity.** Although there have been occasional reports of cross-sensitivity to teicoplanin in patients hypersensitive to vancomycin,[1-3] the majority of reports suggest that cross-sensitivity is very rare and teicoplanin can usually be used in patients intolerant of vancomycin.[4-6]


1. McElrath MJ, *et al.* Allergic cross-reactivity of teicoplanin and vancomycin. *Lancet* 1986; **i:** 47.
2. Grek V, *et al.* Allergic cross-reaction of teicoplanin and vancomycin. *J Antimicrob Chemother* 1991; **28:** 476–7.
3. Marshall C, *et al.* Glycopeptide-induced vasculitis—cross-reactivity between vancomycin and teicoplanin. *J Infect* 1998; **37:** 82–3.
4. Schlemmer B, *et al.* Teicoplanin for patients allergic to vancomycin. *N Engl J Med* 1988; **318:** 1127–8.
5. Smith SR, *et al.* Teicoplanin administration in patients experiencing reactions to vancomycin. *J Antimicrob Chemother* 1989; **23:** 810–12.
6. Wood G, Whitby M. Teicoplanin in patients who are allergic to vancomycin. *Med J Aust* 1989; **150:** 668.


**Red-man syndrome.** Although teicoplanin is believed[1,2] to be less likely than vancomycin to induce the red-man syndrome, symptoms consistent with the syndrome have nevertheless been reported following intravenous use.[3]


1. Sahai J, *et al.* Comparison of vancomycin- and teicoplanin-induced histamine release and "red man syndrome". *Antimicrob Agents Chemother* 1990; **34:** 765–9.
2. Rybak MJ, *et al.* Absence of "red man syndrome" in patients being treated with vancomycin or high-dose teicoplanin. *Antimicrob Agents Chemother* 1992; **36:** 1204–7.
3. Dubettier S, *et al.* Red man syndrome with teicoplanin. *Rev Infect Dis* 1991; **13:** 770.


## Antimicrobial Action

As for Vancomycin Hydrochloride, p.276, although in general teicoplanin is more active against susceptible strains. In particular, it may be more active *in vitro* against enterococci and some anaerobic organisms, including strains of *Clostridium*. However, some coagulase-negative staphylococci are less sensitive to teicoplanin than to vancomycin.

Acquired resistance to teicoplanin has developed in staphylococci during treatment with teicoplanin. Cross-resistance with vancomycin has occurred in staphylococci and enterococci.

## Pharmacokinetics

Teicoplanin is poorly absorbed from the gastrointestinal tract. Following a 400-mg intravenous dose, peak plasma concentrations 1 hour later are reported to be in the range 20 to 50 micrograms/mL. It is well absorbed following intramuscular injection with a bioavailability of about 90%; after administration of 3 mg/kg intramuscularly, peak plasma concentrations of 5 to 7 micrograms/mL have been reported after 2 to 4 hours.

The pharmacokinetics of teicoplanin are triphasic, with a biphasic distribution and a prolonged elimination. Penetration into the CSF is poor. It is taken up into white blood cells, and about 90 to 95% of teicoplanin in plasma is protein bound. It is excreted almost entirely by glomerular filtration in the urine, as unchanged drug. The terminal half-life is prolonged, but reported half-lives have ranged from about 30 to 190 hours or longer, depending on the sampling time; an effective clinical half-life of about 60 hours has been suggested for use in calculating dosage regimens. Half-life is increased progressively with increasing degrees of renal impairment. Teicoplanin is not removed by haemodialysis.

Teicoplanin is a mixture of several components, the pharmacokinetics of which have been shown to vary slightly, depending on their lipophilicity.

◊ Reviews.


1. Wilson APR. Clinical pharmacokinetics of teicoplanin. *Clin Pharmacokinet* 2000; **39:** 167–83.


## Uses and Administration

Teicoplanin is a glycopeptide antibiotic that may be used as an alternative to vancomycin (p.276) in the treatment of serious Gram-positive infections where other drugs cannot be used, including the treatment and prophylaxis of infective endocarditis, peritonitis associated with continuous ambulatory peritoneal dialysis, and suspected infection in neutropenic or otherwise immunocompromised patients. Teicoplanin, given orally, has been suggested as a possible alternative to vancomycin or metronidazole in antibiotic-associated colitis. For details of these infections and their treatment, see under Choice of Antibacterial, p.120.

Teicoplanin is given intravenously, as a bolus dose or by infusion over 30 minutes, or by intramuscular injection. The usual mean dose is 6 mg/kg intravenously or intramuscularly initially, followed by 3 mg/kg intravenously or intramuscularly on each subsequent day of treatment (in practice this equates to a usual dose of 400 mg initially followed by 200 mg daily, except in patients weighing more than 85 kg in whom it is adapted accordingly). In more severe infections, 6 mg/kg may be given every 12 hours for the first 3 doses, followed by 6 mg/kg daily.

For the prophylaxis of endocarditis in high-risk patients undergoing dental or other procedures who are unable to receive penicillin, teicoplanin may be given in a single dose of 400 mg by intravenous injection together with gentamicin, before the procedure. A similar dose of teicoplanin is given for prophylaxis in orthopaedic surgery at induction of anaesthesia.

In children, a loading dose of 10 mg/kg every 12 hours for 3 doses is followed by 6 to 10 mg/kg daily, depending on the severity of infection. In neonates, a loading dose of 16 mg/kg on the first day is followed by maintenance doses of 8 mg/kg daily, given by intravenous infusion.

Dosage should be adjusted in patients with impaired renal function (see Administration in Renal Impairment, below).

◊ Reviews.


1. Brogden RN, Peters DH. Teicoplanin: a reappraisal of its antimicrobial activity, pharmacokinetic properties and therapeutic efficacy. *Drugs* 1994; **47:** 823–54.
2. Murphy S, Pinney RJ. Teicoplanin or vancomycin in the treatment of Gram-positive infections? *J Clin Pharm Ther* 1995; **20:** 5–11.
3. de Lalla F, Tramarin A. A risk-benefit assessment of teicoplanin in the treatment of infections. *Drug Safety* 1995; **13:** 317–28.
4. Periti P, *et al.* Antimicrobial prophylaxis in orthopaedic surgery: the role of teicoplanin. *J Antimicrob Chemother* 1998; **41:** 329–40.
5. Schaison G, *et al.* Teicoplanin in the treatment of serious infection. *J Chemother* 2000; **12** (suppl 5): 26–33.


**Administration in renal impairment.** Doses of teicoplanin should be adjusted in patients with renal impairment, though reduction is not required until the fourth day of treatment. Teicoplanin should be given in usual doses for the first 3 days of therapy, thereafter the dose is adjusted according to creatinine clearance (CC):

- CC 40 to 60 mL/minute: half initial dose given daily or initial dose given every 2 days
- CC less than 40 mL/minute: one-third initial dose given daily or initial dose given every 3 days

## Preparations

**Proprietary Preparations** (details are given in Part 3)
***Arg.:*** Targocid; Teicox; Teiklonal; ***Austral.:*** Targocid; ***Austria:*** Targocid; ***Belg.:*** Targocid; ***Braz.:*** Targocid; ***Denm.:*** Targocid; ***Fin.:*** Targocid; ***Fr.:*** Targocid; ***Ger.:*** Targocid; ***Gr.:*** Targocid; ***Hong Kong:*** Targocid; ***India:*** Targocid; ***Irl.:*** Targocid; ***Israel:*** Targocid; ***Ital.:*** Targosid; Teicomid†; ***Jpn:*** Targocid; ***Malaysia:*** Targocid; ***Mex.:*** Targocid; ***Neth.:*** Targocid; ***Norw.:*** Targocid; ***NZ:*** Targocid; ***Port.:*** Targosid; ***S.Afr.:*** Targocid; ***Singapore:*** Targocid; ***Spain:*** Targocid; ***Swed.:*** Targocid; ***Switz.:*** Targocid; ***Thai.:*** Targocid; ***UK:*** Targocid.

# Telithromycin *(BAN, rINN)*

HMR-3647; RU-66647; Telitromicina. (3a*S*,4*R*,7*R*,9*R*,10*R*,11*R*,13*R*,15*R*,15a*R*)-4-Ethyloctahydro-11-methoxy-3a,7,9,11,13,15-hexamethyl-1-{4-[4-(3-pyridyl)imidazol-1-yl]butyl}-10-{[3,4,6-trideoxy-3-(dimethylamino)-β-D-*xylo*-hexopyranosyl]oxy}-2*H*-oxacyclotetradecino[4,3-*d*][1,3]oxazole-2,6,8,14(1*H*,7*H*,9*H*)-tetrone.

$C_{43}H_{65}N_5O_{10}$ = 812.0.
*CAS — 173838-31-8.*
*ATC — J01FA15.*

## Adverse Effects

Diarrhoea and other gastrointestinal disturbances such as nausea, vomiting, abdominal pain, and flatulence are among the most common adverse reactions following telithromycin. Elevation of liver enzymes and cholestatic jaundice have occurred. Effects on the CNS may include dizziness, headache, and, occasionally, insomnia or drowsiness. Taste disturbances may occur. Other effects less commonly reported include paraesthesia, blurred vision, eosinophilia, skin rashes, and cardiovascular effects such as arrhythmias, hypotension, and bradycardia. There have been isolated cases of erythema multiforme and pseudomembranous colitis.

## Precautions

Telithromycin should not be given to patients with known hypersensitivity to it or to the macrolide antibacterials. Patients with a congenital or family history of QT interval prolongation should not receive telithromycin; it should be used with care in patients with coronary heart disease, cardiac arrhythmias, and in patients with hypokalaemia or hypomagnesaemia, due to its potential to prolong the QT interval.

Telithromycin is not recommended in patients with myasthenia gravis, unless other therapeutic alternatives are unavailable, because it may exacerbate symptoms of the disease; a fatality has been reported in one such patient.

Reproductive toxicity has been observed in *animals*.

Reduced doses of telithromycin may be necessary in patients with renal impairment.

**Breast feeding.** Telithromycin has been shown to be excreted in the milk of lactating *animals* at concentrations 5 times greater than those in maternal plasma and the UK manufacturer states that it should not be used by breast-feeding women.

## Interactions

Telithromycin is an inhibitor of the cytochrome P450 isoenzymes CYP3A4 and CYP2D6. Although there have been few clinical reports, drug interactions with telithromycin may be expected to be similar to those seen with erythromycin (see p.209). In particular, caution is required when telithromycin is given with drugs that may prolong the QT interval; the UK manufacturers state that the use of telithromycin with cisapride, pimozide, astemizole, or terfenadine is contra-indicated. They also state that telithromycin should not be given with drugs that induce the cytochrome P450 isoenzyme CYP3A4, such as rifampicin.

## Antimicrobial Action

Telithromycin is a ketolide antibacterial with a bactericidal action and is highly active against Gram-positive bacteria such as streptococci, including erythromycin-resistant strains of *Streptococcus pneumoniae* and *S. pyogenes*. Some strains of *Staphylococcus aureus* are also sensitive.

Telithromycin also shows good activity against the Gram-negative organisms *Haemophilus influenzae* and *Moraxella catarrhalis* (*Branhamella catarrhalis*). Activity against *Mycoplasma pneumoniae* and *Chlamydophila pneumoniae* (*Chlamydia pneumoniae*) is comparable with macrolides, and it shows greater activity than erythromycin and roxithromycin against *Legionella* spp. *Mycobacterium* spp. are reported to be moderately susceptible.

Enterobacteriaceae, *Pseudomonas* spp., and *Acinetobacter* spp. are not susceptible.

◊ References.


1. Hammerschlag MR, *et al.* Activity of telithromycin, a new ketolide antibacterial, against atypical and intracellular respiratory tract pathogens. *J Antimicrob Chemother* 2001; **48** (suppl T1): 25–31.
2. Felmingham D, *et al.* Activity of the ketolide antibacterial telithromycin against typical community-acquired respiratory pathogens. *J Antimicrob Chemother* 2001; **48** (suppl T1): 33–42.


## Pharmacokinetics

Telithromycin is rapidly absorbed following an oral dose, with a bioavailability of about 60%. Peak plasma concentrations of about 2 micrograms/mL are reached around 1 to 3 hours after a dose of 800 mg. Food does not appear to affect the absorption of telithromycin.

Telithromycin is widely distributed in body fluids and tissues, including those of the respiratory tract, and plasma protein binding is reported to be 60 to 70%. Concentrations in target tissues are reported to be higher than plasma concentrations, suggesting the drug may remain active when the plasma concentration has fallen below the MIC.

About two-thirds of a dose is metabolised in the liver to inactive metabolites and the remaining third is eliminated unchanged in the urine and faeces. Metabolism is mediated both by cytochrome P450 isoenzymes (mainly CYP3A4) and non-cytochrome P450 enzymes. The pharmacokinetics of telithromycin are reported to be triphasic with a biphasic elimination phase; the elimination half-life is reported to be 2 to 3 hours and the terminal half-life approximately 10 hours.

## Uses and Administration

Telithromycin is a ketolide antibacterial used for the treatment of susceptible respiratory-tract infections. It is given by mouth in a usual dose of 800 mg once daily.

Doses may need to be reduced in patients with renal impairment (see below).

◊ Reviews.


1. Barman Balfour JA, Figgitt DP. Telithromycin. *Drugs* 2001; **61:** 815–29.
2. Yassin HM, Dever LL. Telithromycin: a new ketolide antimicrobial for treatment of respiratory tract infections. *Expert Opin Invest Drugs* 2001; **10:** 353–67.
3. Zhanel GC, *et al.* The ketolides: a critical review. *Drugs* 2002; **62:** 1771–1804.
4. Zhanel GC, Hoban DJ. Ketolides in the treatment of respiratory infections. *Expert Opin Pharmacother* 2002; **3:** 277–97.
5. Ackermann G, Rodloff AC. Drugs of the 21st century: telithromycin (HMR 3647)—the first ketolide. *J Antimicrob Chemother* 2003; **51:** 497–511.


**Administration in renal impairment.** Doses of telithromycin should be halved in patients with renal impairment who have a creatinine clearance of less than 30 mL/minute.

## Preparations

**Proprietary Preparations** (details are given in Part 3)
***Arg.:*** Ketek; ***Belg.:*** Ketek; ***Braz.:*** Ketek; ***Chile:*** Ketek; ***Fr.:*** Ketek; ***Ger.:*** Ketek; ***Irl.:*** Ketek; ***Ital.:*** Ketek; ***Norw.:*** Ketek; ***Spain:*** Ketek; Leviax; ***Swed.:*** Ketek; ***UK:*** Ketek; ***USA:*** Ketek.

# Temafloxacin *(BAN, rINN)*

A-62254; Abbott-62254; Temafloxacino. (*RS*)-1-(2,4-Difluorophenyl)-6-fluoro-1,4-dihydro-7-(3-methylpiperazin-1-yl)-4-oxoquinoline-3-carboxylic acid.
$C_{21}H_{18}F_3N_3O_3$ = 417.4.
*CAS — 108319-06-8.*
*ATC — J01MA05.*

# Temafloxacin Hydrochloride *(BANM, USAN, rINNM)*

$C_{21}H_{18}F_3\text{-}N_3O_3,HCl$ = 453.8.
*CAS — 105784-61-0.*

## Profile

Temafloxacin is a fluoroquinolone antibacterial with properties similar to those of ciprofloxacin (p.188). It was formerly given by mouth as the base or as the hydrochloride in the treatment of susceptible infections but was withdrawn worldwide in 1992 following reports of serious adverse events, mainly in the USA. These adverse effects included symptoms of severe hypoglycaemia, hepatic dysfunction, haemolytic anaemia, renal dysfunction sometimes requiring dialysis, anaphylaxis, and death.

# Temocillin *(BAN, USAN, rINN)*

(6*S*)-6-[2-carboxy-2-(3-thienyl)acetamido]-6-methoxypenicillanic acid.
$C_{16}H_{18}N_2O_7S_2$ = 414.5.
*CAS — 66148-78-5.*
*ATC — J01CA17.*

# Temocillin Sodium *(BANM, rINNM)*

BRL-17421; Temocilina sódica; Temocillin Disodium. The disodium salt of (6*S*)-6-[2-carboxy-2-(3-thienyl)acetamido]-6-methoxypenicillanic acid.
$C_{16}H_{16}N_2Na_2O_7S_2$ = 458.4.
*CAS — 61545-06-0.*
*ATC — J01CA17.*

## Profile

Temocillin is a semisynthetic penicillin that is highly resistant to a wide range of beta-lactamases and is used for the treatment of infections caused by beta-lactamase-producing strains of Gram-negative aerobic bacteria, including those resistant to third-generation cephalosporins.

It is given as the sodium salt and doses are expressed in terms of the base. 1.11 g of temocillin sodium is approximately equivalent to 1 g of temocillin. It is given by intravenous or intramuscular injection or by intravenous infusion in usual doses of 1 g every 12 hours. Intravenous doses may be doubled in severe infections.

In patients with renal impairment the interval between doses may need to be increased.

## Preparations

**Proprietary Preparations** (details are given in Part 3)
***Belg.:*** Negaban; ***Ital.:*** ISF 09338.

# Terizidone *(rINN)*

B-2360; Terizidona. 4,4′-[*p*-Phenylenebis(methyleneamino)]bis(isoxazolidin-3-one).
$C_{14}H_{14}N_4O_4$ = 302.3.
*CAS — 25683-71-0.*
*ATC — J04AK03.*

## Profile

Terizidone has been used in the treatment of infections of the urinary tract and of pulmonary and extrapulmonary tuberculosis.

## Preparations

**Proprietary Preparations** (details are given in Part 3)
***Austria:*** Terivalidin; ***Braz.:*** Fatol†.

# Tetracycline *(BAN, rINN)*

Tetraciclina; Tetracyclinum. A variably hydrated form of (4*S*,4a*S*,5a*S*,6*S*,12a*S*)-4-Dimethylamino-1,4,4a,5,5a,6,11,12a-octahydro-3,6,10,12,12a-pentahydroxy-6-methyl-1,11-dioxonaphthacene-2-carboxamide.
$C_{22}H_{24}N_2O_8$ = 444.4.
*CAS — 60-54-8 (anhydrous tetracycline); 6416-04-2 (tetracycline trihydrate).*
*ATC — A01AB13; D06AA04; J01AA07; S01AA09; S02AA08; S03AA02.*

**Pharmacopoeias.** In *Eur.* (see p.vi) and *US.*

**Ph. Eur. 5.0** (Tetracycline). A yellow crystalline powder. Very slightly soluble in water; soluble in alcohol and in methyl alcohol; sparingly soluble in acetone. It dissolves in dilute acid and alkaline solutions. A 1% suspension in water has a pH of 3.5 to 6.0. Protect from light.

**USP 27** (Tetracycline). A yellow, odourless, crystalline powder. It darkens in strong sunlight. Soluble 1 in 2500 of water and 1 in 50 of alcohol; practically insoluble in chloroform and in ether; soluble in methyl alcohol; freely soluble in dilute acids and in alkali hydroxide solutions. It loses not more than 13% of its weight on drying. A 1% suspension in water has a pH of 3.0 to 7.0. The potency of tetracycline is reduced in solutions having a pH below 2 and it is rapidly destroyed in solutions of alkali hydroxides. Store in airtight containers. Protect from light.

# Tetracycline Hydrochloride *(BANM, rINNM)*

Hidrocloruro de tetraciclina; Tetracyclini Hydrochloridum.
$C_{22}H_{24}N_2O_8,HCl$ = 480.9.
*CAS — 64-75-5.*
*ATC — A01AB13; D06AA04; J01AA07; S01AA09; S02AA08; S03AA02.*

**Pharmacopoeias.** In *Chin., Eur.* (see p.vi), *Int., Jpn, Pol., US,* and *Viet.*

*US* also includes Epitetracycline Hydrochloride.

**Ph. Eur. 5.0** (Tetracycline Hydrochloride). A yellow crystalline powder. Soluble in water; slightly soluble in alcohol; practically insoluble in acetone. It dissolves in solutions of alkali hydroxides and carbonates. Solutions in water become turbid on standing, owing to the precipitation of tetracycline. A 1% solution in water has a pH of 1.8 to 2.8. Protect from light.

**USP 27** (Tetracycline Hydrochloride). A yellow, odourless, hygroscopic, crystalline, powder. Tetracycline hydrochloride darkens in moist air when exposed to strong sunlight. Soluble 1 in 10 of water and 1 in 100 of alcohol; practically insoluble in chloroform and in ether; soluble in solutions of alkali hydroxides and carbonates, although it is rapidly destroyed by alkali hydroxide solutions. A 1% solution in water has a pH of 1.8 to 2.8. The potency of tetracycline hydrochloride is reduced in solutions having a pH below 2. Store in airtight containers. Protect from light.

# Tetracycline Phosphate Complex *(BAN)*

Tetraciclina, complejo con fosfato.
*CAS — 1336-20-5.*
*ATC — A01AB13; D06AA04; J01AA07; S01AA09; S02AA08; S03AA02.*

**Description.** A complex of sodium metaphosphate and tetracycline.

**Incompatibility.** Tetracycline injections have an acid pH and incompatibility may reasonably be expected with alkaline preparations, or with drugs unstable at low pH. Tetracyclines can chelate metal cations to produce insoluble complexes, and incompatibility has been reported with solutions containing metallic salts. Reports of incompatibility are not always consistent, and other factors, such as the strength and composition of the vehicles used, may play a role.

**Stability.** Tetracycline undergoes reversible epimerisation in solution to the less active 4-epitetracycline;[1,2] the degree of epimerisation is dependent on pH, and is greatest at a pH of about 3, with conversion of some 55% to the epimer at equilibrium.[1] The rate at which epimerisation occurs is affected by a variety of factors including temperature and the presence of phosphate or citrate ions.[1] Intravenous solutions of tetracycline hydrochloride with a pH between 3 and 5 have been reported to be stable for 6 hours, but to lose approximately 8 to 12% of their potency in 24 hours at room temperature.[3] Although epimerisation has been observed to be the dominant degradation reaction at pH 2.5 to 5, outside this pH range other reactions become important, with the pH-dependent formation of anhydrotetracycline at very low pH, and oxidation to isotetracycline at alkaline pH.[4]

In contrast to the case in solution, suspensions of tetracycline hydrochloride with a pH between 4 and 7 are stable for at least 3 months.[2] This is because epimerisation, which continues until an equilibrium is achieved between tetracycline and its epimer, depends only on the portion in solution, and the solubility of tetracycline at this pH range is low.

The stability of solid dosage forms and powder at various temperatures and humidities has also been studied; tetracycline hydrochloride was fairly stable when stored at 37° and 66% humidity for 2 months, with about a 10% loss of potency, but the phosphate was rather less stable, with potency losses of 25 to 40% and the formation of potentially toxic degradation products.[5] Comparison with other tetracyclines indicated that tetracycline was less stable than demeclocycline and more stable than rolitetracycline.[5] However, although this study, and an accelerated stability study carried out by WHO[6] indicate that there is a risk of deterioration of solid dose tetracycline, in practice a study of its stability during shipment to the tropics found that deterioration was not a problem.[7]


1. Remmers EG, *et al.* Some observations on the kinetics of the C4 epimerization of tetracycline. *J Pharm Sci* 1963; **52:** 752–6.
2. Grobben-Verpoorten A, *et al.* Determination of the stability of tetracycline suspensions by high performance liquid chromatography. *Pharm Weekbl (Sci)* 1985; **7:** 104–8.
3. Parker EA. Solution additive chemical incompatibility study. *Am J Hosp Pharm* 1967; **24:** 434–9.
4. Vej-Hansen B, Bundgaard H. Kinetic study of factors affecting the stability of tetracycline in aqueous solution. *Arch Pharm Chemi (Sci)* 1978; **6:** 201–14.
5. Walton VC, *et al.* Anhydrotetracycline and 4-epianhydrotetracycline in market tetracyclines and aged tetracycline products. *J Pharm Sci* 1970; **59:** 1160–4.
6. WHO. WHO expert committee on specifications for pharmaceutical preparations: thirty-first report. *WHO Tech Rep Ser 790* 1990.
7. Hogerzeil HV, *et al.* Stability of essential drugs during shipment to the tropics. *BMJ* 1992; **304:** 210–14.


## Adverse Effects

The adverse effects of tetracycline are common to all tetracyclines. Gastrointestinal effects including nausea, vomiting, and diarrhoea are common especially with high doses and most are attributed to irritation of the mucosa. Other effects that have been reported include dry mouth, glossitis and discoloration of the tongue, stomatitis, and dysphagia. Oesophageal ulceration has also been reported, particularly after ingestion of capsules or tablets with insufficient water at bedtime.

Oral candidiasis, vulvovaginitis, and pruritus ani occur, mainly due to overgrowth with *Candida albicans*, and there may be overgrowth of resistant coliform organisms, such as *Pseudomonas* spp. and *Proteus* spp., causing diarrhoea. More seriously, enterocolitis due to superinfection with resistant staphylococci and pseudomembranous colitis due to *Clostridium difficile* have occasionally been reported. It has been suggested that disturbances in the intestinal flora are more common with tetracycline than with better absorbed analogues such as doxycycline.

Renal dysfunction has been reported with tetracyclines, and particularly exacerbation of dysfunction in those with pre-existing renal impairment. Usual therapeutic doses given to patients with renal disease increase the severity of uraemia with increased excretion of nitrogen and losses of sodium, accompanied by acidosis and hyperphosphataemia. These effects are related to the dose and the severity of renal impairment and are probably due to the anti-anabolic effects of the tetracycline. Acute renal failure and nephritis have occurred rarely.

Increases in liver enzyme values have been reported with tetracyclines. In some cases severe and sometimes fatal hepatotoxicity, associated with fatty changes in the liver and pancreatitis, has occurred in pregnant women given tetracycline intravenously for pyelonephritis, and in patients with renal impairment or those given high doses.

Tetracyclines are deposited in deciduous and permanent teeth during their formation, causing discoloration and enamel hypoplasia. They are also deposited in calcifying areas in bone and the nails and interfere with bone growth when given in therapeutic doses to young infants or pregnant women. An increase in intracranial pressure with headache, visual disturbances, and papilloedema has been reported in patients given tetracyclines; the use of tetracyclines in infants has been associated with a bulging fontanelle. If raised intracranial pressure occurs tetracycline treatment should be stopped.

Hypersensitivity to the tetracyclines is much less common than to the beta lactams, but hypersensitivity reactions, including rashes, fixed drug eruptions, exfoliative dermatitis, toxic epidermal necrolysis, drug fever, pericarditis, angioedema, urticaria, and asthma have been reported; anaphylaxis has occurred very rarely. Photosensitivity, which has been reported with most tetracyclines but particularly with demeclocycline and other long-acting analogues, appears to be phototoxic rather than photoallergic in nature. Paraesthesia may be an early sign of impending phototoxicity. Nail discoloration and onycholysis may occur. Abnormal pigmentation of the skin and eye has occurred rarely: permanent discoloration of the cornea has been reported in infants born to mothers given tetracycline in high doses during pregnancy. Myopia in patients taking tetracyclines may be due to transient hydration of the lens. Local pain and irritation can occur when tetracyclines are given parenterally and thrombophlebitis may follow intravenous injections. A Jarisch-Herxheimer reaction occurs commonly in patients with relapsing fever treated with tetracycline.

Although rare, agranulocytosis, aplastic anaemia, haemolytic anaemia, eosinophilia, neutropenia, and thrombocytopenia have been reported. Tetracyclines may produce hypoprothrombinaemia. They have also been associated with reductions in serum-vitamin B concentrations, including a case of folate deficiency and concomitant megaloblastic anaemia.

The use of out-of-date or deteriorated tetracyclines has been associated with the development of a reversible Fanconi-type syndrome characterised by polyuria and polydipsia with nausea, glycosuria, aminoaciduria, hypophosphataemia, hypokalaemia, and hyperuricaemia with acidosis and proteinuria; these effects have been attributed to the presence of degradation products, in particular anhydroepitetracycline.

Other adverse effects that have occasionally been reported with tetracyclines include increased muscle weakness in patients with myasthenia gravis and provocation of lupus erythematosus.

## Precautions

The tetracyclines are contra-indicated in patients hypersensitive to any of this group of antibacterials, since cross-sensitivity may occur. They should be avoided in patients with systemic lupus erythematosus. In general the tetracyclines, with the exception of doxycycline and perhaps minocycline, are considered to be contra-indicated in renal impairment, particularly if severe: if they must be given, doses should be reduced.

Tetracyclines should not be used during pregnancy because of the risk of hepatotoxicity in the mother as well as the effects on the developing fetus. They should also be avoided during breast feeding and in children up to the age of 8, or some authorities say 12, years. Use in pregnancy, potentially during breast feeding, or in childhood, may result in impaired bone growth and permanent discoloration of the child's teeth.

Care should be taken if tetracyclines are given to patients with hepatic impairment and high doses should be avoided. Patients who may be exposed to direct sunlight should be warned of the risk of photosensitivity. Care is advisable in patients with myasthenia gravis, who may be at risk of neuromuscular blockade. Serum monitoring of tetracyclines may be helpful in patients with risk factors receiving parenteral therapy: it has been suggested that serum concentrations of tetracycline should not exceed 15 micrograms/mL. When given by mouth, tetracyclines (notably doxycycline, see p.206) should be taken with plenty of fluid while sitting or standing, and well before going to bed, to avoid the risk of oesophageal ulceration.

Tetracycline may interfere with some diagnostic tests including determination of urinary catecholamines or glucose.

**Breast feeding.** The American Academy of Pediatrics[1] states that, following use of tetracycline by breast-feeding mothers, there is negligible absorption by the infant and that tetracycline is therefore usually compatible with breast feeding. However, the manufacturers state that adverse effects including permanent tooth discoloration and enamel hypoplasia may occur in breast-fed infants and that breast feeding is contra-indicated during treatment with tetracyclines.

1. American Academy of Pediatrics. The transfer of drugs and other chemicals into human milk. *Pediatrics* 2001; **108:** 776–89. Correction. *ibid.*; 1029. Also available at: http://aappolicy.aappublications.org/cgi/content/full/pediatrics%3b108/3/776 (accessed 28/05/04)

**Porphyria.** Tetracyclines are considered to be probably safe in patients with porphyria, although there is conflicting experimental evidence of porphyrinogenicity. Doxycycline has been associated with acute attacks of porphyria and is considered unsafe in porphyric patients, and results from *animals* or *in-vitro* systems suggest that oxytetracycline might be porphyrinogenic.

## Interactions

The absorption of the tetracyclines is reduced by divalent and trivalent cations such as aluminium, bismuth, calcium, iron, magnesium, and zinc, and therefore use of tetracyclines with antacids, iron preparations, some foods such as milk and dairy products, or other preparations containing such cations, whether as active ingredients or excipients, may result in subtherapeutic serum concentrations of the antibacterial. Sodium **bicarbonate**, colestipol, colestyramine, and kaolin-pectin are also reported to reduce tetracycline absorption, but potential reductions due to cimetidine or sucralfate are probably of little clinical significance.

The nephrotoxic effects of tetracyclines may be exacerbated by diuretics, methoxyflurane, or other potentially nephrotoxic drugs. Potentially hepatotoxic drugs should be used with caution in patients receiving tetracyclines. An increased incidence of benign intracranial hypertension has been reported when retinoids and tetracyclines are given together. Tetracyclines have been reported to produce increased concentrations of lithium, digoxin, and theophylline (although these interactions are not strongly established); the effects of oral anticoagulants have also been increased in a few patients. There have been occasional reports of tetracyclines increasing the toxic effects of ergot alkaloids and methotrexate. Tetracyclines may decrease plasma-atovaquone concentrations. Ocular inflammation has occurred following the use of ocular preparations preserved with thiomersal in some patients receiving tetracyclines. Tetracyclines may decrease the effectiveness of oral contraceptives.

Because of possible antagonism of the action of the penicillins by predominantly bacteriostatic tetracyclines it has been recommended that the two types of drug should not be used together, especially when a rapid bactericidal action is necessary.

## Antimicrobial Action

The tetracyclines are mainly bacteriostatic, with a broad spectrum of antimicrobial activity including Chlamydiaceae, Mycoplasma spp., Rickettsia spp., spirochaetes, many aerobic and anaerobic Gram-positive and Gram-negative pathogenic bacteria, and some protozoa.

*Mechanism of action.* Tetracyclines are taken up into sensitive bacterial cells by an active transport process. Once within the cell they bind reversibly to the 30S subunit of the ribosome, preventing the binding of aminoacyl transfer RNA and inhibiting protein synthesis and hence cell growth. Although tetracyclines also inhibit protein synthesis in mammalian cells they are not actively taken up, permitting selective activity against the infecting organism.

*Spectrum of activity.* The following pathogenic organisms are usually sensitive to tetracyclines:

Gram-positive cocci including some strains of *Staphylococcus aureus* and coagulase-negative staphylococci, and streptococci including *Str. pneumoniae, Str. pyogenes* (group A), and some viridans streptococci. Enterococci are essentially resistant.

Other sensitive Gram-positive bacteria including strains of *Actinomyces israelii, Bacillus anthracis, Erysipelothrix rhusiopathiae, Listeria monocytogenes*, and among the anaerobes some *Clostridium* spp. *Nocardia* spp. are generally much less susceptible although some are sensitive to minocycline. *Propionibacterium acnes* is susceptible although the action of the tetracyclines in acne is complex and benefit may be seen even at subinhibitory concentrations.

Gram-negative cocci including *Neisseria meningitidis* (meningococci) and *N. gonorrhoeae* (gonococci), although some strains are resistant, and *Moraxella catarrhalis (Branhamella catarrhalis). Acinetobacter* spp. may be resistant to tetracycline, but most strains are susceptible to doxycycline and minocycline.

Other sensitive Gram-negative aerobes including *Bordetella pertussis, Brucella* spp., *Calymmatobacterium granulomatis, Campylobacter* spp., *Eikenella corrodens, Francisella tularensis, Haemophilus influenzae* and some strains of *Haemophilus ducreyi, Legionella* spp., *Pasteurella multocida, Streptobacillus moniliformis*, and various members of the Vibrionaceae including *Aeromonas hydrophila, Plesiomonas shigelloides, Vibrio cholerae* and *Vibrio parahaemolyticus.* Although many of the Enterobacteriaceae, including *Salmonella, Shigella*, and *Yersinia* spp., are susceptible, resistant strains are common; *Proteus* and *Providencia* spp. are not susceptible. *Pseudomonas aeruginosa* is not susceptible either, although some other species formerly classified as *Pseudomonas* respond, including *Burkholderia mallei, B. pseudomallei*, and *Stenotrophomonas maltophilia* (*Xanthomonas maltophilia*).

Among the Gram-negative anaerobes *Bacteroides fragilis* may sometimes be susceptible, although wild strains are often resistant, and *Fusobacterium* may also be sensitive.

Other organisms usually sensitive to tetracyclines include *Helicobacter pylori*, Chlamydiaceae, *Rickettsia* and *Coxiella* spp., many spirochaetes including *Borrelia burgdorferi, Leptospira* spp., and *Treponema pallidum*, atypical mycobacteria such as *Mycobacterium marinum*, and mycoplasmas including *Mycoplasma pneumoniae* and *Ureaplasma urealyticum.* In addition the tetracyclines are active against some protozoa including *Plasmodium falciparum* and *Entamoeba histolytica.*

Fungi, yeasts, and viruses are generally resistant.

*Resistance.* Resistance to the tetracyclines is usually plasmid-mediated and transferable. It is often inducible, and appears to be associated with the ability to prevent accumulation of the antibiotic within the bacterial cell, both by decreasing active transport of the drug into the cell and by increasing tetracycline efflux.

Unsurprisingly, given the widespread use of the tetracyclines (including as components of animal feeds, although this is now banned in some countries), resistant strains of the majority of sensitive species have now been reported. Resistance has increased particularly among Enterobacteriaceae such as *Escherichia coli, Enterobacter, Salmonella*, and *Shigella* spp., especially in hospital isolates, and multiple resistance is common. Staphylococci are commonly resistant, although doxycycline or minocycline are occasionally effective against tetracycline-resistant strains. Resistance is now also common among group A streptococci, and even more so among group B streptococci; there is also resistance among pneumococci, which often show multiple drug resistance. Emergence of high-level tetracycline-resistant strains of *Neisseria gonorrhoeae* is common in some areas. Frequent resistance is also seen in clostridia, and in *Bacteroides fragilis* (among more than 60% of isolates in some countries), while increasing resistance amongst *Haemophilus ducreyi* has limited the value of tetracyclines in chancroid.

## Pharmacokinetics

Most tetracyclines are incompletely absorbed from the gastrointestinal tract, about 60 to 80% of a dose of the drug usually being available. The degree of absorption is diminished by the presence of divalent and trivalent metal ions, with which tetracyclines form stable insoluble complexes, and to a variable degree by milk or food. However, the more lipophilic analogues doxycycline and minocycline are almost completely absorbed (more than 90%), and they are little affected by food. Formulation with phosphate may enhance the absorption of tetracycline.

Administration of tetracycline 500 mg by mouth every 6 hours generally produces steady-state plasma concentrations of 4 to 5 micrograms/mL, whereas with doxycycline a dose of 200 mg is sufficient to produce peak concentrations of about 3 micrograms/mL. Peak plasma concentrations occur about 1 to 3 hours after oral use. Higher concentrations can be achieved after intravenous use; concentrations may be higher in women than in men.

In the circulation, tetracyclines are bound to plasma proteins to varying degrees, but reported values differ considerably ranging from about 20 to 40% for oxytetracycline, 20 to 65% for tetracycline, about 45% for chlortetracycline, 35 to 90% for demeclocycline, 75% for minocycline, and about 80 to 95% for methacycline and for doxycycline.

The tetracyclines are widely distributed throughout the body tissues and fluids. Concentrations in CSF are relatively low, but may be raised if the meninges are inflamed. Small amounts appear in saliva, and in the fluids of the eye and lung; higher concentrations are achieved with more lipid-soluble analogues such as minocycline and doxycycline. Tetracyclines appear in breast milk, where concentrations may be 60% or more of those in the plasma. They diffuse across the placenta and appear in the fetal circulation in concentrations of about 25 to 75% of those in the maternal blood. Tetracyclines are retained at sites of new bone formation and recent calcification and in developing teeth.

The tetracyclines have been classified in terms of their duration of action in the body, although the divisions appear to overlap somewhat. Of the 'short-acting' derivatives, chlortetracycline has a reported half-life of about 6 hours, oxytetracycline 9 hours, and tetracycline 8 hours, although reported values for the latter two range from about 6 to 12 hours. The 'intermediate-acting' tetracyclines, demeclocycline and methacycline, have reported half-lives of about 12 and 14 hours respectively, although various sources cite values of 7 to 17 hours, and the 'long-acting' minocycline and doxycycline have half-lives of about 16 and 18 hours, with reported values anywhere between 11 to 26 and 12 to 24 hours respectively.

The tetracyclines are excreted in the urine and in the faeces. Renal clearance is by glomerular filtration. Up to 60% of an intravenous dose of tetracycline, and up to 55% of a dose by mouth, is eliminated unchanged in the urine; tetracycline concentrations in the urine of up to 300 micrograms/mL may be reached 2 hours after a usual dose is taken and be maintained for up to 12 hours. Usually about 40 to 70% of a dose is excreted in the urine, but for chlortetracycline, doxycycline, and minocycline, rather less is eliminated by this route since chlortetracycline and minocycline undergo metabolism, and doxycycline is excreted mainly in the faeces. Urinary excretion is increased if urine is alkalinised.

The tetracyclines are excreted in the bile, where concentrations 5 to 25 times those in plasma can occur. Since there is some enterohepatic reabsorption complete elimination is slow. Considerable quantities occur in the faeces after administration by mouth and lesser amounts after administration by injection.

## Uses and Administration

The tetracyclines are bacteriostatic antibiotics with a wide spectrum of activity and have been used in the treatment of a large number of infections caused by susceptible organisms. With the emergence of bacterial resistance and the development of other antibacterials their use has become more restricted, but they remain drugs of choice in rickettsial infections, including ehrlichiosis, Q fever, spotted fevers, and typhus; trench fever; chlamydial infections, including psittacosis, lymphogranuloma venereum, trachoma, non-gonococcal urethritis, and conjunctivitis, and also pharyngitis, sinusitis, or pneumonia due to *Chlamydophila pneumoniae* (*Chlamydia pneumoniae*); and mycoplasmal infections, especially pneumonia caused by *Mycoplasma pneumoniae*. They are widely used as part of regimens for pelvic inflammatory disease. A tetracycline is often used in the treatment of cholera, in conjunction with fluid and electrolyte replacement, and is usually the treatment of choice in relapsing fever and in the early stages of Lyme disease. They are also used in the oral treatment of acne (below) and rosacea. Tetracyclines may be of benefit in the treatment of melioidosis. They may be used for mouth infections, especially in destructive forms of periodontal disease. Tetracyclines are used, often with streptomycin or rifampicin, in the treatment of brucellosis, and may be given with streptomycin in plague, and as an alternative to streptomycin in the treatment of tularaemia. Tetracyclines are used as an alternative to other drugs in the treatment of actinomycosis, infected animal bites, anthrax, bronchitis, gastro-enteritis (due to *Campylobacter* or *Yersinia enterocolitica*), granuloma inguinale, leptospirosis, and syphilis. Opinions differ as to their value in listeriosis. There are now relatively few areas where tetracycline-resistant gonococci are uncommon, which limits the value of tetracyclines in gonorrhoea, but they are often given with antigonorrhoeal therapy to treat concomitant chlamydial infections, and they retain some value in the prophylaxis and treatment of neonatal gonococcal conjunctivitis by topical application. For details of these infections and their treatment, see under Choice of Antibacterial, p.120.

Tetracyclines have antiprotozoal actions and tetracycline or doxycycline may be given with quinine in the management of falciparum malaria resistant to chloroquine (below). Tetracyclines are the usual treatment for balantidiasis (p.596) and they have been used with an amoebicide in the treatment of severe amoebic dysentery and in *Dientamoeba fragilis* infections (p.595).

Tetracycline has been used in the management of malabsorption syndromes such as tropical sprue.

Tetracycline has been instilled as a sclerosant solution for pleurodesis and in the management of malignant effusions (p.512).

*Administration and dosage.* In the treatment of systemic infections the tetracyclines are usually given by mouth. They should be taken with plenty of fluid while sitting or standing, and well before going to bed, to avoid the risk of oesophageal ulceration. In severe acute infections they may be given by slow intravenous infusion or, rarely, by intramuscular injection; parenteral therapy should be substituted by oral administration as soon as practicable.

Doses of tetracycline base and tetracycline hydrochloride are expressed in terms of tetracycline hydrochloride. Tetracycline (anhydrous) 0.92 g is approximately equivalent to 1 g of tetracycline hydrochloride. The usual adult dosage of tetracycline hydrochloride is 250 or 500 mg every 6 hours by mouth, preferably 1 hour before or 2 hours after meals. Higher doses, up to 4 g daily have occasionally been given in severe infection, but increase the risk of adverse effects. Modified-release formulations are available in some countries.

In severe infections, tetracycline hydrochloride has been given by slow intravenous infusion every 12 hours as a solution containing not more than 0.5% in a usual total dose of 0.5 to 1 g daily, although up to 2 g daily has been given. If the intramuscular route is to be used, tetracycline hydrochloride has been given in a dosage of 250 mg once daily, or 300 mg daily in divided doses. As intramuscular injections are painful, procaine hydrochloride is usually included in the solution.

In children, the effects on teeth should be considered and tetracyclines only used when absolutely essential. Tetracycline hydrochloride has been given to older children (over 8 years) in doses of 25 to 50 mg/kg daily by mouth in divided doses.

Care is required if tetracyclines are given to the elderly. They should be avoided if possible in renal impairment (with the exception of doxycycline and minocycline) and doses reduced if they must be used. For dosage recommendations in patients with hepatic impairment, see below.

*Other routes.* Although topical application carries the risk of sensitisation and may contribute to the development of resistance, tetracycline hydrochloride has been used as a 3% ointment; a 0.2% solution has been used in acne but systemic treatment appears to produce better results. A 1% eye ointment or eye drops have been used in the treatment of ocular infections due to sensitive organisms. For the treatment of pleural effusions, 500 mg of tetracycline hydrochloride has been dissolved in 30 to 50 mL of sodium chloride 0.9% and instilled into the pleural space. For periodontal disease, fibres that release tetracycline have been inserted into the periodontal pocket.

◊ Reviews.

1. Chopra I, *et al.* Tetracyclines, molecular and clinical aspects. *J Antimicrob Chemother* 1992; **29:** 245–77.

**Administration in hepatic impairment.** The manufacturers state that the dosage of tetracycline should not exceed 1 g daily in patients with known liver disease.

**Malaria.** Tetracyclines have been used with quinine to treat malaria (p.444).[1] They are active against both blood and tissue forms of the parasite, and high cure rates have been obtained with such combinations. The action of tetracyclines is relatively slow and they should never be used alone to treat malaria.

A usual oral regimen is a 3-day course of quinine given concurrently with 7 to 10 days of the tetracycline. The dose of tetracycline hydrochloride has varied; doses of 1 to 2 g daily have been given for 7 days or 1 g daily for 7 to 10 days. The total daily dose should be divided, and that usually recommended is 250 mg four times daily, although 500 mg twice daily may be more practical in the field. If the patient is too ill for oral medication quinine should be given parenterally until oral therapy can be begun; tetracycline should not be used parenterally. Although tetracycline therapy is normally contra-indicated in pregnant women and children, it may have to be given if the risk of withholding the drug is judged to outweigh the risk to developing teeth and bones.

The dose of doxycycline given by mouth following treatment with quinine is 200 mg daily for at least 7 days.

Tetracyclines are not considered suitable for extended prophylactic use, although doxycycline 100 mg daily has been used for short-term prophylaxis in areas of high risk where other drugs are likely to be ineffective.

1. WHO. *WHO model prescribing information: drugs used in parasitic diseases.* 2nd ed. Geneva: WHO, 1995.

**Mouth ulceration.** Tetracyclines may be used as mouthwashes in recurrent aphthous stomatitis (p.1245) and reportedly reduce ulcer pain and duration,[1] but their potential for adverse effects if swallowed must be borne in mind, and their acidity can damage tooth enamel if poorly formulated. Topical application of a tetracycline has been tried for oral ulceration associated with Behçet's syndrome (p.1076).

1. Henricsson V, Axéll T. Treatment of recurrent aphthous ulcers with Aureomycin mouth rinse or Zendium dentifrice. *Acta Odontol Scand* 1985; **43:** 47–52.

**Peptic ulcer disease.** Tetracycline has been used as part of triple therapy to eradicate *Helicobacter pylori* in patients with peptic ulcer disease (p.1246). The usual dose of tetracycline in these regimens has been 500 mg four times daily for 2 weeks.

**Rheumatic disorders.** Tetracyclines, usually minocycline, are among the wide range of drugs tried in rheumatoid arthritis (p.9). Studies[1,2] indicate that minocycline can produce modest beneficial effects in patients with advanced rheumatoid arthritis, but the clinical significance of these improvements has been questioned.[3] Greater symptomatic improvements have been obtained with minocycline when it is used in patients with early rheumatoid arthritis;[4,5] continued treatment with minocycline may also reduce the need for disease-modifying antirheumatic drugs.[6] Its mechanism of action, whether antibacterial or anti-inflammatory, remains to be determined.[7] There has been speculation over the role of infection as a cause of rheumatoid arthritis.[3,8]

The role of antibacterials is also uncertain in reactive arthritis (p.122), although long-term treatment with a tetracycline in addition to an NSAID has been reported to shorten the duration of reactive arthritis resulting from *Chlamydia trachomatis* infection.[9]

1. Kloppenburg M, *et al.* Minocycline in active rheumatoid arthritis. *Arthritis Rheum* 1994; **37:** 629–36.

2. Tilley BC, *et al.* Minocycline in rheumatoid arthritis: a 48-week, double-blind, placebo-controlled trial. *Ann Intern Med* 1995; **122:** 81–9.
3. McKendry RJR. Is rheumatoid arthritis caused by an infection? *Lancet* 1995; **345:** 1319–20.
4. O'Dell JR, *et al.* Treatment of early rheumatoid arthritis with minocycline or placebo: results of a randomized double-blind, placebo-controlled trial. *Arthritis Rheum* 1997; **40:** 842–8.
5. O'Dell JR, *et al.* Treatment of early seropositive rheumatoid arthritis: a two-year, double-blind comparison of minocycline and hydroxychloroquine. *Arthritis Rheum* 2001; **44:** 2235–41.
6. O'Dell JR, *et al.* Treatment of early seropositive rheumatoid arthritis with minocycline: four-year follow-up of a double-blind, placebo-controlled trial. *Arthritis Rheum* 1999; **42:** 1691–5.
7. Paulus HE. Minocycline treatment of rheumatoid arthritis. *Ann Intern Med* 1995; **122:** 147–8.
8. O'Dell JR. Is there a role for antibiotics in the treatment of patients with rheumatoid arthritis? *Drugs* 1999; **57:** 279–82.
9. Lauhio A. Reactive arthritis: consider combination treatment. *BMJ* 1994; **308:** 1302–3.

**Skin disorders.** ACNE. Tetracyclines may be used topically or orally in the treatment of acne (p.1133). In acne, antibacterials appear to act by suppressing the growth of *Propionibacterium acnes*, but also by suppressing inflammation. Topical tetracycline is used for mild inflammatory acne and as an adjunct to systemic treatment in more severe forms. Tetracyclines, given orally, are the drugs of choice for moderate acne and may be considered, in high doses, for severe acne. Licensed doses in the UK are: doxycycline 50 mg daily; minocycline 100 mg daily; oxytetracycline 250 to 500 mg daily; and tetracycline 1 g daily. Higher doses for doxycycline of 100 mg daily and for oxytetracycline of 1 g daily are advocated in the *British National Formulary*. Treatment should be changed to another antibacterial if there has been no improvement in the first 3 months. Maximum improvement is said to occur after 3 to 6 months, but treatment may need to continue for 2 or more years.

Minocycline has been reported to have superior antibacterial activity against *P. acnes* and a reduced incidence of resistance,[1] and has also been more effective than erythromycin against oxytetracycline-resistant acne.[2] However, it can cause skin pigmentation and may be associated rarely with immunologically mediated reactions[3] and some dermatologists do not favour its use. Although the usual dose of minocycline is 100 mg daily in one or two divided doses some patients may need up to 200 mg daily.[4]

1. Eady EA, *et al.* Superior antibacterial action and reduced incidence of bacterial resistance in minocycline compared to tetracycline-treated acne patients. *Br J Dermatol* 1990; **122:** 233–44.
2. Knaggs HE, *et al.* The role of oral minocycline and erythromycin in tetracycline therapy-resistant acne—a retrospective study and a review. *J Dermatol Treat* 1993; **4:** 53–6.
3. Ferner RE, Moss C. Minocycline for acne. *BMJ* 1996; **312:** 138.
4. Goulden V, *et al.* Safety of long-term high-dose minocycline in the treatment of acne. *Br J Dermatol* 1996; **134:** 693–5.

PEMPHIGUS AND PEMPHIGOID. Corticosteroids are generally given to control the blistering in pemphigus and pemphigoid (p.1137), although there have been reports[1-3] suggesting that a tetracycline (often minocycline) may be of value in controlling the lesions associated with various types of pemphigus and pemphigoid.

1. Sawai T, *et al.* Pemphigus vegetans with oesophageal involvement: successful treatment with minocycline and nicotinamide. *Br J Dermatol* 1995; **132:** 668–70.
2. Poskitt L, Wojnarowska F. Minimizing cicatricial pemphigoid orodynia with minocycline. *Br J Dermatol* 1995; **132:** 784–9.
3. Kolbach DN, *et al.* Bullous pemphigoid successfully controlled by tetracycline and nicotinamide. *Br J Dermatol* 1995; **133:** 88–90.

ROSACEA. Tetracycline is commonly used in the treatment of rosacea (p.1138). Long-term treatment is usually necessary. Tetracycline and doxycycline have also been shown to improve ocular manifestations of rosacea.[1]

1. Frucht-Pery J, *et al.* Efficacy of doxycycline and tetracycline in ocular rosacea. *Am J Ophthalmol* 1993; **116:** 88–92.

## Preparations

***BP 2003:*** Tetracycline Capsules; Tetracycline Tablets;
***USP 27:*** Tetracycline Hydrochloride and Nystatin Capsules; Tetracycline Hydrochloride Capsules; Tetracycline Hydrochloride for Injection; Tetracycline Hydrochloride for Topical Solution; Tetracycline Hydrochloride Ointment; Tetracycline Hydrochloride Ophthalmic Ointment; Tetracycline Hydrochloride Ophthalmic Suspension; Tetracycline Hydrochloride Oral Suspension; Tetracycline Hydrochloride Tablets; Tetracycline Oral Suspension.

**Proprietary Preparations** (details are given in Part 3)
***Arg.:*** Ciclotetryl; Tancilina; ***Austral.:*** Achromycin; Achromycin V; Latycin; Mysteclin†; Tetrex; ***Austria:*** Achromycin; Actisite; Hostacyclin†; Latycin; ***Braz.:*** Ambra-Sinto T; Aureciclina; Combitrex†; Infex†; Miociclin†; Statinclyne; Teraciton; Tetracina; Tetraclin; Tetramax; Tetramicin; Tetraxil; Tetrex; Tetrib†; ***Canad.:*** Achromycin V†; Achromycin†; Apo-Tetra; Novo-Tetra; Nu-Tetra; Tetracyn†; ***Denm.:*** Achromycin†; Actisite†; Dumocyclin†; ***Fin.:*** Apocyclin; Oricyclin; ***Fr.:*** Florocycline†; ***Ger.:*** Achromycin; Actisite†; Hostacyclin†; Imex; Sagittacin N†; Supramycin; Tefilin; Tetralution; ***Gr.:*** Hostacyclin; ***Hong Kong:*** Achromycin V†; Apo-Tetra†; Medocycline; ***India:*** Achromycin; Hostacycline; Resteclin; Subamycin; ***Irl.:*** Achromycin†; Topicycline; ***Israel:*** Recycline; Tevacycline; ***Ital.:*** Acromicina†; Actisite; Ambramicina; Calociclina†; Spaciclina†; Tetrabioptal†; Tetrafosammina†; ***Malaysia:*** Beatacycline; Dhatracin; Latycyn; Tracyne; ***Mex.:*** Acromicina; Ambotetra; Berciclina; Biotricina; Cortigrin; Dibaterr; Droclina†; Forciclinе†; Imacol†; Inacol†; Istix; Laur; Macrocilin†; Miciclin†; Ofticlin; Oxi-T; Parenciclina†; Pavitron†; Quimocyclar; Rayetetra†; Senociclin†; Solclin; Te-Br; Tecyn†; Terrakal; Terranumonyl†; Tetra; Tetranovax†; Tetrapres†; Tetraprocyn†; Tetrazil†; Tetrerba†; Tetrex; Tetrim; Triclin; Tromicol†; ***NZ:*** Panmycin†; ***Port.:*** Ciclobiotico; Neociclina; ***S.Afr.:*** Achromycin†; Arcanacycline†; Hostacycline†; Tetrex†; ***Singapore:*** Beatacycline; Latycin†; ***Spain:*** Actisite; Bristaciclina†; Kinciclina†; Quimpe Antibiotico; Tetra Hubber; ***Swed.:*** Achromycin†; Actisite†; ***Switz.:*** Achromycine†; Actisite; Triphacycline†; ***Thai.:*** Achromycin; Boramycin; Hydromycin; Lenocin; Pantocycline; Servitet†; Tetra Central; Tetralim; Tetrana; Tetrano; ***UK:*** Achromycin†; Economycin†; Topicycline; ***USA:*** Achromycin V; Actisite; Panmycin†; Sumycin; Tetracap†; Topicycline†.

**Multi-ingredient:** ***Arg.:*** Dresan Biotic; Eubetal Biotic; Febrimicina; Papasine; Solustres; ***Austral.:*** Helidac†; Mysteclin-V†; ***Austria:*** Eftapan Tetra; Fluorex Plus; Mysteclin; ***Braz.:*** Acobiotic†; Anfoterin; Gino-Teracin; Monocetin†; Parenzyme Tetraciclina; Talsutin; Tericin AT; Tricangine; Trinotrex; Vagiklin; Velutrix†; ***Chile:*** Talseclin; ***Fin.:*** Helipak T; ***Fr.:*** Amphocycline; Colicort†; ***Ger.:*** Mysteclin; Polcortolon TC; ***Hong Kong:*** Talsutin; ***Irl.:*** Deteclo†; ***Ital.:*** Alfaflor; Betafloroto; Colbiocin; Dermobios†; Eubetal Antibiotico; Flumetol Antibiotico; Iducol†; Mictasone; Pensulvit; Vitecaf; ***Malaysia:*** Talsutin; ***Mex.:*** Berciclina Enzimatica; Quimotrip; Solfranicol; Trecloran; Urovec; ***Port.:*** Ciclobiotico; Neociclina Vitaminada†; ***S.Afr.:*** Riostatin; Tetrex-F†; Tritet†; Vagmycin; ***Spain:*** Bristaciclina Dental; Gine Heyden; Mucorex Ciclin†; Nasopomada; Sanicel; Tantum Ciclina†; Terranilo†; Tetra Tripsin†; ***UK:*** Deteclo; ***USA:*** Helidac.

## Tetroxoprim *(BAN, USAN, rINN)*

Tetroxoprima. 5-[3,5-Dimethoxy-4-(2-methoxyethoxy)benzyl]pyrimidine-2,4-diyldiamine.
$C_{16}H_{22}N_4O_4$ = 334.4.
*CAS — 53808-87-0.*

NOTE. Compounded preparations of tetroxoprim may be represented by the following name:

- Co-tetroxazine (*BAN*)—tetroxoprim 2 parts and sulfadiazine 5 parts (see p.199).

### Profile

Tetroxoprim is a dihydrofolate reductase inhibitor similar to, but less active than, trimethoprim (p.272). It is used, with sulfadiazine, as co-tetroxazine (p.199).

Tetroxoprim embonate has been used similarly.

### Preparations

**Proprietary Preparations** (details are given in Part 3)
**Multi-ingredient:** ***Ger.:*** Sterinor; ***Ital.:*** Oxosint†; Sterinor†.

## Thenoic Acid

Tenoic Acid; Tenoico, ácido; 2-Thiophenic Acid. Thiophene-2-carboxylic acid.
$C_5H_4O_2S$ = 128.1.
*CAS — 527-72-0.*

### Profile

Thenoic acid has been given orally, rectally, or intranasally as the sodium salt, and by mouth as the lithium salt, in the treatment of respiratory-tract infections. The monoethanolamine salt has been used as a mucolytic.

### Preparations

**Proprietary Preparations** (details are given in Part 3)
***Fr.:*** Rhinotrophyl; Soufrane.
**Multi-ingredient:** ***Fr.:*** Glossithiase; Trophires; Trophires Compose; ***Spain:*** Trophires.

## Thiamphenicol *(BAN, USAN, rINN)*

CB-8053; Dextrosulphenidol; Thiamfenicol; Thiamphenicolum; Thiophenicol; Tiamfenicolo; Tianfenicol; Win-5063-2; Win-5063 (racephenicol). (αR,βR)-2,2-Dichloro-N-(β-hydroxy-α-hydroxymethyl-4-methylsulphonylphenethyl)acetamide.
$C_{12}H_{15}Cl_2NO_5S$ = 356.2.
*CAS — 15318-45-3 (thiamphenicol); 847-25-6 (racephenicol).*
*ATC — J01BA02.*

NOTE. Racephenicol, the racemic form of thiamphenicol, is *USAN*.

**Pharmacopoeias.** In *Chin.* and *Eur.* (see p.vi).

**Ph. Eur. 5.0** (Thiamphenicol). A fine, white or yellowish-white, crystalline powder or crystals. Slightly soluble in water and in ethyl acetate; sparingly soluble in dehydrated alcohol and in acetone; freely soluble in acetonitrile and in dimethylformamide; very soluble in dimethylacetamide; soluble in methyl alcohol. Protect from light and moisture.

## Thiamphenicol Glycinate Hydrochloride

Thiamphenicol Aminoacetate Hydrochloride; Tiamfenicolo Glicinato Cloridrato; Tianfenicol, hidrocloruro del glicinato de.
$C_{14}H_{18}Cl_2N_2O_6S,HCl$ = 449.7.
*CAS — 2393-92-2 (thiamphenicol glycinate); 2611-61-2 (thiamphenicol glycinate hydrochloride).*
*ATC — J01BA02.*

**Pharmacopoeias.** In *It.*

### Adverse Effects and Precautions

As for Chloramphenicol, p.185.

Thiamphenicol is probably more liable to cause dose-dependent reversible depression of the bone marrow than chloramphenicol but it is not usually associated with aplastic anaemia. Thiamphenicol also appears to be less likely to cause the 'grey syndrome' in neonates.

Doses of thiamphenicol should be reduced in patients with renal impairment. It is probably not necessary to reduce doses in patients with hepatic impairment.

### Interactions

As for Chloramphenicol, p.186.

Although thiamphenicol is not metabolised in the liver and might not be expected to be affected by drugs which induce hepatic enzymes, it is reported to inhibit hepatic microsomal enzymes and may affect the metabolism of other drugs.

### Antimicrobial Action

Thiamphenicol has a broad spectrum of activity resembling that of chloramphenicol (p.186). Although in general it is less active than chloramphenicol it is reported to be equally effective, and more actively bactericidal, against *Haemophilus* and *Neisseria* spp.

Cross-resistance occurs between thiamphenicol and chloramphenicol. However, some strains resistant to chloramphenicol may be susceptible to thiamphenicol.

### Pharmacokinetics

Thiamphenicol is absorbed from the gastrointestinal tract following oral administration and peak serum concentrations of 3 to 6 micrograms/mL have been achieved about 2 hours after a 500-mg dose.

Thiamphenicol diffuses into the CSF, across the placenta, into breast milk, and penetrates well into the lungs. About 10% is bound to plasma proteins. The half-life of thiamphenicol is around 2 to 3 hours but unlike chloramphenicol the half-life is increased in patients with renal impairment. It is excreted in the urine, about 70% of a dose being excreted in 24 hours as unchanged drug. It undergoes little or no conjugation with glucuronic acid in the liver. A small amount is excreted in the bile and the faeces.

### Uses and Administration

Thiamphenicol has been used similarly to chloramphenicol (p.186) in the treatment of susceptible infections, including sexually transmitted diseases. The usual adult dose is 1.5 g daily by mouth in divided doses; up to 3 g daily has been given initially in severe infections. A daily dose of 30 to 100 mg/kg may be used in children. Equivalent doses, expressed in terms of thiamphenicol base, may be administered by intramuscular or intravenous injection as the more water soluble glycinate hydrochloride. 1.26 g of thiamphenicol glycinate hydrochloride is approximately equivalent to 1 g of thiamphenicol. Doses should be reduced in patients with renal impairment (see below).

For the treatment of gonorrhoea, oral doses of thiamphenicol have ranged from 2.5 g daily for 1 or 2 days through to 2.5 g on the first day followed by 2 g daily on each of 4 subsequent days. The single daily dose may be most appropriate for male patients with uncomplicated gonorrhoea.

Thiamphenicol glycinate hydrochloride may also be given by inhalation, or by endobronchial or intracavitary instillation.

Thiamphenicol has also been used as thiamphenicol glycine acetylcysteinate, thiamphenicol sodium glycinate isophthalolate, and thiamphenicol palmitate.

**Administration in renal impairment.** Doses of thiamphenicol should be reduced in patients with renal impairment according to creatinine clearance (CC):

- CC 30 to 60 mL/minute: 500 mg twice daily
- CC 10 to 30 mL/minute: 500 mg once daily

### Preparations

**Proprietary Preparations** (details are given in Part 3)
***Belg.:*** Fluimucil Antibiotic; Urfamycine; ***Braz.:*** Flogotisol†; Glitisol; ***Fr.:*** Fluimucil Antibiotic†; Thiophenicol; ***Hong Kong:*** Urfamycin; ***Ital.:*** Flogotisol†; Fluimucil Antibiotico; Glitisol; ***Mex.:*** Tiofeniclin; ***Spain:*** Fluimucil Antibiotico; Urfamycin; ***Switz.:*** Urfamycine; ***Thai.:*** Ervin†; Thiamcin; Treomycin; Urfamycin.

**Multi-ingredient:** ***Braz.:*** Acobiotic†; Fluimucil Biotic†; ***Spain:*** Flumil Antibiotico; ***Thai.:*** Fluimucil Antibiotic.

## Thioacetazone *(BAN, rINN)*

Amithiozone; TBI/698; Tebezonum; Thiacetazone; Tioacetazona. 4-Acetamidobenzaldehyde thiosemicarbazone.
$C_{10}H_{12}N_4OS$ = 236.3.
*CAS — 104-06-3.*

**Pharmacopoeias.** In *Int.*

### Adverse Effects

Gastrointestinal disturbances, hypersensitivity reactions including skin rashes, conjunctivitis, and vertigo are the adverse effects most frequently reported with thioacetazone although the incidence appears to vary between countries. Toxic epidermal necrolysis, exfoliative dermatitis, which has sometimes been fatal, and the Stevens-Johnson syndrome have been reported; the incidence of severe skin reactions is especially high in patients with HIV infection (see below). Thioacetazone may cause bone-marrow depression with leucopenia, agranulocytosis, and thrombocytopenia. Acute haemolytic anaemia may occur and a large percentage of patients will have some minor degree of anaemia. Hepatotoxicity with jaundice may also develop and acute hepatic failure has been reported. Cerebral oedema has been reported. Dose-related ototoxicity may occur rarely.

◊ In a 10-year series of 1212 patients with tuberculosis who were treated with a regimen of streptomycin, isoniazid, and thioacetazone, 171 (14%) had adverse reactions associated with thioacetazone. The most common adverse effects were giddiness (10%), occurring mainly in association with streptomycin, and skin rashes (3%) including exfoliation and the Stevens-Johnson syndrome.[1]

1. Pearson CA. Thiacetazone toxicity in the treatment of tuberculosis patients in Nigeria. *J Trop Med Hyg* 1978; **81:** 238–42.

**Effects on the nervous system.** Acute peripheral neuropathy which occurred in a 50-year-old man on 2 separate occasions within 15 minutes of administration of thioacetazone may have been due to an allergic reaction.[1]

1. Gupta PK, *et al.* Acute severe peripheral neuropathy due to thiacetazone. *Indian J Tuberc* 1984; **31:** 126–7.

**Effects on the skin.** A high incidence of severe and sometimes fatal cutaneous hypersensitivity reactions to thioacetazone has been reported in patients with HIV infection being treated for tuberculosis.[1,2] WHO advised that thioacetazone should be avoided in such patients.[3] Unfortunately, thioacetazone has been one of the mainstays of tuberculosis treatment in the developing world because of its relatively low cost.[4] Some have supported a change to rifampicin-based regimens in, for example, parts of Africa with a high incidence of HIV infection.[5] Others have found a lower frequency of fatalities from adverse cutaneous reactions to thioacetazone than reported previously and have suggested that improved management might allow retention of thioacetazone in tuberculosis programmes.[6] This was rejected by other workers who considered that better and more cost-effective regimens were available than those containing thioacetazone.[7] A pragmatic approach may be to adopt a strategy depending upon the prevailing incidence of HIV infection in the population.[8] Thus, where the incidence of HIV infection is high, ethambutol should be substituted for thioacetazone; where the incidence is moderate, routine HIV testing could be used to identify patients at risk; and where the incidence is low, education of patients on the risks of skin reaction would be adequate.

1. Nunn P, *et al.* Cutaneous hypersensitivity reactions due to thiacetazone in HIV-1 seropositive patients treated for tuberculosis. *Lancet* 1991; **337:** 627–30.
2. Chintu C, *et al.* Cutaneous hypersensitivity reactions due to thiacetazone in the treatment of tuberculosis in Zambian children infected with HIV-I. *Arch Dis Child* 1993; **68:** 665–8.
3. Raviglione MC, *et al.* HIV-associated tuberculosis in developing countries: clinical features, diagnosis, and treatment, *Bull WHO* 1992; **70:** 515–26.
4. Nunn P, *et al.* Thiacetazone—avoid like poison or use with care? *Trans R Soc Trop Med Hyg* 1993; **87:** 578–82.
5. Okwera A, *et al.* Randomised trial of thiacetazone and rifampicin-containing regimens for pulmonary tuberculosis in HIV-infected Ugandans. *Lancet* 1994; **344:** 1323–8.
6. Ipuge YAI, *et al.* Adverse cutaneous reactions to thiacetazone for tuberculosis treatment in Tanzania. *Lancet* 1995; **346:** 657–60.
7. Elliott AM, *et al.* Treatment of tuberculosis in developing countries. *Lancet* 1995; **346:** 1098–9.
8. van Gorkom J, Kibuga DK. Cost-effectiveness and total costs of three alternative strategies for the prevention and management of severe skin reactions attributable to thiacetazone in the treatment of human immunodeficiency virus positive patients with tuberculosis in Kenya. *Tubercle Lung Dis* 1996; **77:** 30–6.

**Hypertrichosis.** Hypertrichosis occurred in 2 children receiving thioacetazone.[1]

1. Nair LV, Sugathan P. Thiacetazone induced hypertrichosis. *Indian J Dermatol Venereol* 1982; **48:** 161–3.

### Precautions

The efficacy and toxicity of a regimen of treatment which includes thioacetazone should be determined in a community before it is used widely since there appear to be geographical differences.

Thioacetazone should not be given to patients with hepatic impairment. It has also been suggested that, because thioacetazone has a low therapeutic index and is excreted mainly in the urine, it should not be given to patients with renal impairment. Treatment should be discontinued if rash or other signs of hypersensitivity occur. It should probably be avoided in HIV-positive patients because they are at increased risk of severe adverse effects (see Effects on the Skin, above).

### Interactions

Thioacetazone may enhance the ototoxicity of streptomycin.

### Antimicrobial Action

Thioacetazone is bacteriostatic. It is effective against most strains of *Mycobacterium tuberculosis*, although sensitivity varies in different parts of the world.

Thioacetazone is also bacteriostatic against *Mycobacterium leprae.* Resistance to thioacetazone develops when used alone. Cross-resistance can develop between thioacetazone and ethionamide or protionamide.

### Pharmacokinetics

Thioacetazone is absorbed from the gastrointestinal tract and peak plasma concentrations of 1 to 2 micrograms/mL have been obtained about 4 to 5 hours after a 150-mg dose. About 20% of a dose is excreted unchanged in the urine. A half-life of about 12 hours has been reported.

### Uses and Administration

Thioacetazone has been used with other antimycobacterials in the initial and continuation treatment phases of tuberculosis (p.150). Thioacetazone-containing regimens are less effective than the short-course regimens recommended by WHO but are used in long-term regimens with isoniazid in some developing countries to reduce drug costs. However, thioacetazone is not generally recommended for use in HIV-positive patients because of the risk of severe adverse reactions (but see Effects on the Skin, above).

Thioacetazone has been used in the treatment of leprosy (p.133), but WHO now considers that such use is no longer justified.

In the treatment of tuberculosis, thioacetazone has been given orally in doses of 150 mg daily or 2.5 mg/kg daily. Thioacetazone may be used with isoniazid, usually in the continuation phase of some longer treatment regimens, to prevent emergence of isoniazid resistance. Thioacetazone has also been used in the initial phase in association with streptomycin and isoniazid. Daily administration is recommended as the drug is less effective when given intermittently.

### Preparations

**Proprietary Preparations** (details are given in Part 3)
**Multi-ingredient:** ***India:*** Isokin-T Forte.

---

## Thiostrepton

Tiostreptón.

$C_{72}H_{85}N_{19}O_{18}S_5$ = 1664.9.
*CAS — 1393-48-2.*

**Pharmacopoeias.** In *US* for veterinary use only.

**USP 27** (Thiostrepton). An antibacterial substance produced by the growth of strains of *Streptomyces azureus*. It has a potency of not less than 900 units/mg, calculated on the dried basis. A white to off-white crystalline solid. Practically insoluble in water, in the lower alcohols, in nonpolar organic solvents, and in dilute aqueous acids or alkalis; soluble in glacial acetic acid, in chloroform, in dimethylformamide, in dimethyl sulfoxide, in dioxan, and in pyridine. Store in airtight containers.

### Profile

Thiostrepton is an antibacterial produced by strains of *Streptomyces azureus*. It is included in topical antibacterial preparations for veterinary use.

---

## Tiamulin Fumarate *(BANM, USAN, rINNM)*

Fumarato de tiamulina; 81723-hfu; SQ-14055 (tiamulin); SQ-22947 (tiamulin fumarate); Tiamulini Hydrogenofumaras. 11-Hydroxy-6,7,10,12-tetramethyl-1-oxo-10-vinylperhydro-3a,7-pentanoinden-8-yl (2-diethylaminoethylthio)acetate hydrogen fumarate.

$C_{28}H_{47}NO_4S,C_4H_4O_4$ = 609.8.
*CAS — 55297-95-5 (tiamulin); 555297-96-6 (tiamulin fumarate).*

**Pharmacopoeias.** In *Eur.* (see p.vi) and *US* for veterinary use only. *Eur.* also includes tiamulin for veterinary use only.

**Ph. Eur. 5.0** (Tiamulin Hydrogen Fumarate for Veterinary Use). A white or light yellow, crystalline powder. Soluble in water and in methyl alcohol; freely soluble in dehydrated alcohol. A 1% solution in water has a pH of 3.1 to 4.1. Protect from light.

**USP 27** (Tiamulin Fumarate). A 1.0% solution in water has a pH of 3.1 to 4.1. Store in airtight containers. Protect from light.

### Profile

Tiamulin fumarate is an antibacterial used in veterinary medicine.

---

## Ticarcillin Monosodium *(BANM, rINNM)*

Monosodium (6*R*)-6-[2-carboxy-2-(3-thienyl)acetamido]penicillanate monohydrate.

$C_{15}H_{15}N_2NaO_6S_2,H_2O$ = 424.4.
*CAS — 34787-01-4 (ticarcillin); 3973-04-4 (ticarcillin); 74682-62-5 (ticarcillin monosodium).*

**Pharmacopoeias.** In *US.*

**USP 27** (Ticarcillin Monosodium). Store in airtight containers.

## Ticarcillin Sodium *(BANM, rINNM)*

BRL-2288; Ticarcilina sódica; Ticarcillin Disodium *(USAN)*; Ticarcillinum Natricum. Disodium (6*R*)-6-[2-carboxy-2-(3-thienyl)acetamido]penicillanate.

$C_{15}H_{14}N_2Na_2O_6S_2$ = 428.4.
*CAS — 4697-14-7; 29457-07-6.*
*ATC — J01CA13.*

**Pharmacopoeias.** In *Eur.* (see p.vi), *Jpn*, and *US.*

**Ph. Eur. 5.0** (Ticarcillin Sodium). A white or slightly yellow, hygroscopic powder. Freely soluble in water; soluble in methyl alcohol. A 5% solution in water has a pH of 5.5 to 7.5. Store in airtight containers at a temperature of 2° to 8°.

**USP 27** (Ticarcillin Disodium). A white to pale yellow powder or solid. 1 mg of monograph substance has a potency equivalent to not less than 800 micrograms of ticarcillin, calculated on the anhydrous basis. Freely soluble in water. A 1% solution in water has a pH of 6.0 to 8.0. Store in airtight containers.

**Incompatibility.** Ticarcillin sodium has been reported to be incompatible with aminoglycosides.

References.

1. Swenson E, *et al.* Compatibility of ticarcillin disodium clavulanate potassium with commonly used intravenous solutions. *Curr Ther Res* 1990; **48:** 385–94.

**Stability.** References.

1. Zhang Y, Trissel LA. Stability of piperacillin and ticarcillin in AutoDose Infusion System bags. *Ann Pharmacother* 2001; **35:** 1360–3.

### Adverse Effects and Precautions

As for Carbenicillin Sodium, p.166.

Cholestatic jaundice and hepatitis have been reported when ticarcillin was used with clavulanic acid; the clavulanic acid component has been implicated.

Ticarcillin should be given with caution to patients with renal impairment.

**Breast feeding.** Although ticarcillin is distributed into breast milk in small amounts,[1] no adverse effects have been observed in breast-fed infants and the American Academy of Pediatrics considers that it is usually compatible with breast feeding.[2]

1. von Kobyletzki D, *et al.* Ticarcillin serum and tissue concentrations in gynecology and obstetrics. *Infection* 1983; **11:** 144–9.
2. American Academy of Pediatrics. The transfer of drugs and other chemicals into human milk. *Pediatrics* 2001; **108:** 776–89. Correction. *ibid.*; 1029. Also available at: http://aappolicy.aappublications.org/cgi/content/full/pediatrics%3b108/3/776 (accessed 28/05/04)

**Effects on the bladder.** The Australian Adverse Drug Reactions Advisory Committee had received 15 reports of haemorrhagic cystitis associated with ticarcillin or ticarcillin-clavulanic acid between 1980 and June 2002, mainly in paediatric cystic fibrosis patients.[1] Almost all patients recovered quickly after the withdrawal of ticarcillin.

1. Adverse Drug Reactions Advisory Committee (ADRAC). Haemorrhagic cystitis with ticarcillin in cystic fibrosis patients. *Aust Adverse Drug React Bull* 2002; **21:** 6–7. Also available at: http://www.tga.health.gov.au/docs/html/aadrbltn/aadr0206.htm (accessed 28/05/04)

**Effects on the liver.** Cholestatic jaundice and hepatitis have been associated with combined preparations of a penicillin and clavulanic acid (see Amoxicillin, p.155) and 2 cases had been reported to the UK Committee on Safety of Medicines in association with ticarcillin and clavulanic acid.[1] It appeared that the clavulanic acid was probably responsible.

1. Committee on Safety of Medicines/Medicines Control Agency. Cholestatic jaundice with co-amoxiclav. *Current Problems* 1993; **19:** 2.

**Sodium content.** Each g of ticarcillin sodium contains about 4.7 mmol of sodium.

### Interactions

As for Benzylpenicillin, p.164.

### Antimicrobial Action

Ticarcillin is bactericidal and has a mode of action and range of activity similar to that of carbenicillin (p.166), but is reported to be 2 to 4 times more active against *Pseudomonas aeruginosa*.

Combinations of ticarcillin and aminoglycosides have been shown to be synergistic *in vitro* against *Ps. aeruginosa* and Enterobacteriaceae.

The activity of ticarcillin against organisms usually resistant because of the production of certain beta-lactamases is enhanced by clavulanic acid, a beta-lactamase inhibitor. Such organisms have included staphylococci, many Enterobacteriaceae, *Haemophilus influenzae*, and *Bacteroides* spp.; the activity of ticarcillin against *Ps. aeruginosa* is not enhanced by clavulanic acid. Resistance to ticarcillin with clavulanic acid has been reported.

There is cross-resistance between carbenicillin and ticarcillin.

◊ References.

1. Pulverer G, *et al.* In-vitro activity of ticarcillin with and without clavulanic acid against clinical isolates of Gram-positive and Gram-negative bacteria. *J Antimicrob Chemother* 1986; **17** (suppl C): 1–5.
2. Masterton RG, *et al.* Timentin resistance. *Lancet* 1987; **ii:** 975–6.
3. Fass RJ, Prior RB. Comparative in vitro activities of piperacillin-tazobactam and ticarcillin-clavulanate. *Antimicrob Agents Chemother* 1989; **33:** 1268–74.
4. Kempers J, MacLaren DM. Piperacillin/tazobactam and ticarcillin/clavulanic acid against resistant Enterobacteriaceae. *J Antimicrob Chemother* 1990; **26:** 598–9.
5. Klepser ME, *et al.* Comparison of the bactericidal activities of piperacillin-tazobactam, ticarcillin-clavulanate, and ampicillin-sulbactam against clinical isolates of Bacteroides fragilis, Enterococcus faecalis, Escherichia coli, and Pseudomonas aeruginosa. *Antimicrob Agents Chemother* 1997; **41:** 435–9.

### Pharmacokinetics

Ticarcillin is not absorbed from the gastrointestinal tract. After intramuscular injection of 1 g peak plasma concentrations in the range of 22 to 35 micrograms/mL are achieved after 0.5 to 1 hour. About 50% of ticarcillin in the circulation is bound to plasma proteins. A plasma half-life of 70 minutes has been reported. A shorter half-life in patients with cystic fibrosis (about 50 minutes in one study) has been attributed to increased renal and non-renal elimination. The half-life is prolonged in neonates and also in patients with renal impairment, especially if hepatic function is also impaired. A half-life of about 15 hours has been reported in severe renal impairment.

Distribution of ticarcillin in the body is similar to that of carbenicillin. Relatively high concentrations have been reported in bile, but ticarcillin is excreted principally by glomerular filtration and tubular secretion. Concentrations of 2 to 4 mg/mL are achieved in the urine after the intramuscular injection of 1 or 2 g. Ticarcillin is metabolised to a limited extent. Up to 90% of a dose is excreted unchanged in the urine, mostly within 6 hours after administration. Plasma concentrations are enhanced by probenecid.

Ticarcillin is removed by haemodialysis and, to some extent, by peritoneal dialysis.

Ticarcillin crosses the placenta and small amounts are distributed into breast milk.

*Ticarcillin with clavulanic acid.* The pharmacokinetics of ticarcillin and clavulanic acid are broadly similar and neither appears to affect the other to any great extent.

◊ References.


1. Staniforth DH, *et al.* Pharmacokinetics of parenteral ticarcillin formulated with clavulanic acid: Timentin. *Int J Clin Pharmacol Ther Toxicol* 1986; **24:** 123–9.
2. Brogard JM, *et al.* Biliary elimination of ticarcillin plus clavulanic acid (Claventin®): experimental and clinical study. *Int J Clin Pharmacol Ther Toxicol* 1989; **27:** 135–44.
3. de Groot R, *et al.* Pharmacokinetics of ticarcillin in patients with cystic fibrosis: a controlled prospective study. *Clin Pharmacol Ther* 1990; **47:** 73–8.
4. Wang J-P, *et al.* Disposition of drugs in cystic fibrosis IV: mechanisms for enhanced renal clearance of ticarcillin. *Clin Pharmacol Ther* 1993; **54:** 293–302.
5. Burstein AH, *et al.* Ticarcillin-clavulanic acid pharmacokinetics in preterm neonates with presumed sepsis. *Antimicrob Agents Chemother* 1994; **38:** 2024–8.


### Uses and Administration

Ticarcillin is a carboxypenicillin used in the treatment of severe Gram-negative infections, especially those due to *Pseudomonas aeruginosa*. Pseudomonal infections where ticarcillin is used include those in cystic fibrosis (respiratory-tract infections), immunocompromised patients (neutropenia), peritonitis, and septicaemia. Other infections that may be due to *Ps. aeruginosa* include bone and joint infections, meningitis, otitis media (chronic), skin infections (burns, ecthyma gangrenosum, ulceration), and urinary-tract infections. For details of these infections and their treatment, see under Choice of Antibacterial, p.120.

*Administration and dosage.* Ticarcillin is given by injection as the sodium salt. Doses are expressed in terms of the equivalent amount of ticarcillin. 1.1 g of ticarcillin sodium is approximately equivalent to 1 g of ticarcillin. Doses may need to be reduced in renal impairment (see below).

Ticarcillin is given to adults and children in a dose of 200 to 300 mg/kg daily by intravenous infusion in divided doses every 4 or 6 hours.

In adults the use of probenecid 500 mg four times daily by mouth may produce higher and more prolonged plasma concentrations of ticarcillin, but caution is advised in patients with renal impairment.

In the treatment of complicated urinary-tract infections, adults and children may be given a dose of ticarcillin 150 to 200 mg/kg daily by intravenous infusion in divided doses every 4 or 6 hours. In uncomplicated urinary-tract infections, the usual adult dose is ticarcillin 1 g every 6 hours intramuscularly or by slow intravenous injection. Children with uncomplicated urinary-tract infections may be given 50 to 100 mg/kg daily in divided doses every 6 or 8 hours. Not more than 2 g of ticarcillin should be injected intramuscularly into one site.

In patients with cystic fibrosis, ticarcillin has been given by nebuliser in the management of respiratory-tract infections.

Ticarcillin is often used with an aminoglycoside but the injections must be given separately because of possible incompatibility.

*Ticarcillin with clavulanic acid.* Ticarcillin may be used with clavulanic acid (p.193), a beta-lactamase inhibitor, to widen its antibacterial spectrum to organisms usually resistant because of the production of beta-lactamases. This combination is given by intravenous infusion in a ratio of 15 or 30 parts of ticarcillin (as the sodium salt) to 1 part of clavulanic acid (as the potassium salt). Doses are according to the content of ticarcillin, and usual adult doses range from 9 to 18 g daily in 3 to 6 divided doses.

**Administration in renal impairment.** Doses of ticarcillin may need to be reduced in patients with renal impairment. Following an initial intravenous loading dose of 3 g, the intravenous maintenance dosage should be adjusted according to the patient's creatinine clearance (CC):

- CC 30 to 60 mL/minute: 2 g every 4 hours
- CC 10 to 30 mL/minute: 2 g every 8 hours
- CC less than 10 mL/minute: 2 g every 12 hours (or 1 g intramuscularly every 6 hours)
- CC less than 10 mL/minute in presence of *hepatic impairment*: 2 g intravenously every 24 hours or 1 g intramuscularly every 12 hours
- peritoneal dialysis patients: 3 g every 12 hours
- haemodialysis patients: 2 g every 12 hours plus an additional dose of 3 g after each dialysis session

### Preparations

***USP 27:*** Ticarcillin and Clavulanic Acid for Injection; Ticarcillin and Clavulanic Acid Injection; Ticarcillin for Injection.

**Proprietary Preparations** (details are given in Part 3)
***Belg.:*** Triacilline†; ***Canad.:*** Ticar†; ***Fr.:*** Ticarpen; ***Neth.:*** Ticarpen; ***Spain:*** Ticarpen; ***USA:*** Ticar.

**Multi-ingredient:** ***Austral.:*** Timentin; ***Belg.:*** Timentin; ***Braz.:*** Timentin; ***Canad.:*** Timentin; ***Fr.:*** Claventin; ***Ger.:*** Betabactyl†; ***Gr.:*** Timentin; ***Hong Kong:*** Timentin; ***India:*** Timentin; ***Irl.:*** Timentin; ***Israel:*** Timentin; ***Ital.:*** Clavucar; Timentin; ***Mex.:*** Timentin; ***Neth.:*** Timentin; ***NZ:*** Timentin; ***Switz.:*** Timenten; ***UK:*** Timentin; ***USA:*** Timentin.

## Tilmicosin *(BAN, USAN, rINN)*

EL-870; LY-177370; Tilmicosina. 4^A^-O-De(2,6-dideoxy-3-C-methyl-α-L-*ribo*-hexopyranosyl)-20-deoxo-20-(*cis*-3,5-dimethyl-piperidino)tylosin.

$C_{46}H_{80}N_2O_{13}$ = 869.1.
*CAS — 108050-54-0.*

**Pharmacopoeias.** In *US* for veterinary use only.
**USP 27** (Tilmicosin). White to off-white amorphous solid. Slightly soluble in water and in *n*-hexane. Store at a temperature not exceeding 40°. Protect from light.

## Tilmicosin Phosphate *(BANM, USAN, rINNM)*

$C_{46}H_{80}N_2O_{13},H_3O_4P$ = 967.1.
*CAS — 137330-13-3.*

### Profile

Tilmicosin is a macrolide antibacterial used as the phosphate in veterinary medicine.

**Adverse effects.** A report[1] of accidental self-injection of tilmicosin by a farm worker, resulting in asthenia and temporary pulmonary, gastrointestinal, and neuromuscular toxicity.


1. Crown LA, Smith RB. Accidental veterinary antibiotic injection into a farm worker. *Tenn Med* 1999; **92:** 339–40.


**Handling.** Contact with tilmicosin should be avoided. It is irritating to the eyes and may cause allergic reactions.

## Tobramycin *(BAN, USAN, rINN)*

47663; Nebramycin Factor 6; Tobramicina; Tobramycinum. 6-O-(3-Amino-3-deoxy-α-D-glucopyranosyl)-2-deoxy-4-O-(2,6-diamino-2,3,6-trideoxy-α-D-*ribo*-hexopyranosyl)streptamine.

$C_{18}H_{37}N_5O_9$ = 467.5.
*CAS — 32986-56-4.*
*ATC — J01GB01; S01AA12.*

**Pharmacopoeias.** In *Chin.*, *Eur.* (see p.vi), *Jpn*, *Pol.*, and *US.*
**Ph. Eur. 5.0** (Tobramycin). A substance produced by *Streptomyces tenebrarius* or obtained by any other means. A white or almost white powder. Freely soluble in water; very slightly soluble in alcohol. A 10% solution in water has a pH of 9.0 to 11.0.
**USP 27** (Tobramycin). A white to off-white, hygroscopic powder. Freely soluble in water; very slightly soluble in alcohol; practically insoluble in chloroform and in ether. Contains not more than 8.0% w/w of water. A 10% solution in water has a pH of 9.0 to 11.0. Store in airtight containers.

## Tobramycin Sulfate *(rINNM)*

Sulfato de tobramicina; Tobramycin Sulphate *(BANM)*.

$(C_{18}H_{37}N_5O_9)_2,5H_2SO_4$ = 1425.4.
*CAS — 49842-07-1 ($C_{18}H_{37}N_5O_9,xH_2SO_4$); 79645-27-5 (($C_{18}H_{37}N_5O_9)_2,5H_2SO_4$).*
*ATC — J01GB01; S01AA12.*

**Pharmacopoeias.** In *Pol.* and *US.*
**USP 27** (Tobramycin Sulfate). It has a potency of not less than 634 micrograms and not more than 739 micrograms of tobramycin per mg. A 4% solution in water has a pH of 6.0 to 8.0. Store in airtight containers.

**Incompatibility.** For discussion of the incompatibility of aminoglycosides, including tobramycin, with beta lactams, see under Gentamicin Sulfate, p.217. Tobramycin is also reported to be incompatible with various other drugs and, as injections have an acid pH, incompatibility with alkaline preparations or with drugs unstable at acid pH may reasonably be expected.

### Adverse Effects, Treatment, and Precautions

As for Gentamicin Sulfate, p.217. Some studies suggest that tobramycin is slightly less nephrotoxic than gentamicin, but others have not found any significant difference in their effects on the kidneys.

Peak plasma-tobramycin concentrations greater than 12 micrograms/mL (the *British National Formulary* suggests 10 micrograms/mL) and trough concentrations greater than 2 micrograms/mL should be avoided.

When tobramycin is given by inhalation with other inhaled drugs, they should be given first before the dose of tobramycin. Following the initial inhaled dose of tobramycin, patients should be monitored for bronchospasm and if it occurs, the test should be repeated using a bronchodilator. Peak flow should be measured before nebulisation and again after it. Caution should be exercised in the presence of severe haemoptysis. Renal function should be monitored before treatment and every six months during use.

### Interactions

As for Gentamicin Sulfate, p.218.

### Antimicrobial Action

As for Gentamicin Sulfate, p.218. Tobramycin is reported to be somewhat more active *in vitro* than gentamicin against *Pseudomonas aeruginosa* and less active against *Serratia*, staphylococci, and enterococci; however these differences do not necessarily translate into differences in clinical effectiveness.

Cross-resistance between tobramycin and gentamicin is generally seen, but about 10% of strains resistant to gentamicin are susceptible to tobramycin.

◊ References to activity against *Pseudomonas aeruginosa*.


1. Barclay ML, *et al.* Adaptive resistance to tobramycin in Pseudomonas aeruginosa lung infection in cystic fibrosis. *J Antimicrob Chemother* 1996; **37:** 1155–64.
2. den Hollander JG, *et al.* Synergism between tobramycin and ceftazidime against a resistant Pseudomonas aeruginosa strain, tested in an in vitro pharmacokinetic model. *Antimicrob Agents Chemother* 1997; **41:** 95–100.
3. Wu YL, *et al.* Ability of azlocillin and tobramycin in combination to delay or prevent resistance development in Pseudomonas aeruginosa. *J Antimicrob Chemother* 1999; **44:** 389–92.
4. Shawar RM, *et al.* Activities of tobramycin and six other antibiotics against Pseudomonas aeruginosa isolates from patients with cystic fibrosis. *Antimicrob Agents Chemother* 1999; **43:** 2877–80.


### Pharmacokinetics

As for Gentamicin Sulfate, p.218.

Following intramuscular use of tobramycin, peak plasma concentrations are achieved within 30 to 90 minutes and concentrations of about 4 micrograms/mL have been reported following doses of 1 mg/kg. Usual doses by slow intravenous injection may result in plasma concentrations which briefly exceed 12 micrograms/mL. A plasma half-life of 2 to 3 hours has been reported.

**Inhalation.** References.


1. Touw DJ, *et al.* Pharmacokinetics of aerosolized tobramycin in adult patients with cystic fibrosis. *Antimicrob Agents Chemother* 1997; **41:** 184–7.
2. Beringer PM, *et al.* Pharmacokinetics of tobramycin in adults with cystic fibrosis: implications for once-daily administration. *Antimicrob Agents Chemother* 2000; **44:** 809–13.

### Uses and Administration

Tobramycin is an aminoglycoside antibiotic with actions and uses similar to those of gentamicin (p.219). It is used, usually as the sulfate, particularly in the treatment of pseudomonal infections.

As with gentamicin, tobramycin may be used with penicillins or cephalosporins; the injections should be administered separately.

Doses of tobramycin sulfate are expressed in terms of tobramycin base; 1.5 g of tobramycin sulfate is approximately equivalent to 1 g of tobramycin. Doses are similar to those of gentamicin, with the usual adult dose ranging from 3 to 5 mg/kg daily in 3 or 4 divided doses. In patients with cystic fibrosis, doses of 8 to 10 mg/kg daily in divided doses may be necessary to achieve therapeutic plasma concentrations.

The usual dose for children is 6 to 7.5 mg/kg daily in 3 or 4 divided doses. Premature and full-term neonates may be given 2 mg/kg every 12 hours.

For mild to moderate urinary-tract infections in adults, a dose of 2 to 3 mg/kg once daily may be effective.

See under Gentamicin Sulfate (p.219) for reference to once-daily dosage of aminoglycosides.

Tobramycin sulfate is given by intramuscular injection, or by intravenous infusion over 20 to 60 minutes in 50 to 100 mL of sodium chloride 0.9% or glucose 5% injection; proportionately less fluid should be given to children. It has also been given slowly by direct intravenous injection.

Treatment should generally be limited to 7 to 10 days, and peak plasma concentrations greater than 12 micrograms/mL (the *British National Formulary* suggests 10 micrograms/mL) or trough concentrations greater than 2 micrograms/mL should be avoided. In all patients, dosage should be adjusted according to plasma-tobramycin concentrations and particularly where factors such as age, renal impairment, or prolonged therapy may predispose to toxicity (see Uses and Administration of Gentamicin Sulfate, p.219).

Tobramycin may be used as a 0.3% eye ointment or eye drops in the treatment of eye infections. It is also given by inhalation in patients with cystic fibrosis to control *Pseudomonas aeruginosa* infections in a dose of 300 mg every 12 hours for 28 days using a suitable nebuliser. Treatment is then stopped for 28 days before being resumed for another treatment period. This cycle may be repeated indefinitely.

◊ Reviews.

1. Cheer SM, *et al.* Inhaled tobramycin (TOBI®): a review of its use in the management of pseudomonas aeruginosa infections in patients with cystic fibrosis. *Drugs* 2003; **63:** 2501–20.

### Preparations

***BP 2003:*** Tobramycin Injection;
***USP 27:*** Tobramycin and Dexamethasone Ophthalmic Ointment; Tobramycin and Dexamethasone Ophthalmic Suspension; Tobramycin and Fluorometholone Acetate Ophthalmic Suspension; Tobramycin for Injection; Tobramycin Inhalation Solution; Tobramycin Injection; Tobramycin Ophthalmic Ointment; Tobramycin Ophthalmic Solution.

**Proprietary Preparations** (details are given in Part 3)
***Arg.:*** Bioptic; Gotabiotic; Gotabiotic D; Klonamicin; Oftalbrax; Radina; Tobi; Tobragan; Tobrex; Toflamixina; Xao T; ***Austral.:*** Nebcin; Tobi; Tobrex; ***Austria:*** Brulamycin; Cromycin; Tobi; Tobrasix; Tobrex; ***Belg.:*** Obracin; Tobrex; ***Braz.:*** Tobra-M; Tobragan; Tobramina; Tobranom; Tobrex; Toflamixina; ***Canad.:*** Nebcin; Tobi; Tobrex; Tomycine; ***Chile:*** Tobragan; Tobrex; Tobrin; Xolof; ***Denm.:*** Nebcina; Tobi; Tobrex; ***Fin.:*** Nebcina; Tobi; Tobrex; Tomycin; ***Fr.:*** Nebcine; Tobi; Tobrex; ***Ger.:*** Brulamycin; Gernebcin; Tobi; Tobra-cell; Tobramaxin; ***Gr.:*** Colther; Eyebrex; Eyetobrin; Ikobel; Nebcin; Thilo-micine; Tobi; Tobrex; ***Hong Kong:*** Nebcin; Tobrex; ***India:*** Tobacin; Tobraneg; ***Irl.:*** Nebcin; Tobi; Tobralex; ***Israel:*** Nebcin; Tobi; Tobrex; ***Ital.:*** Nebicina; Tobi; Tobral; Tobrex†; ***Malaysia:*** Tobrex; ***Mex.:*** Obry; Tobra; Tobrex; Trazil; ***Neth.:*** Obracin; ***Norw.:*** Nebcina; Tobi; Tobrex; ***NZ:*** Nebcin; Tobi; Tobrex; ***Port.:*** Distobram; Tobra Gobens; Tobracil†; Tobrex; Tobridavi; ***S.Afr.:*** Mytobrin†; Nebcin; Tobrex; ***Singapore:*** Tobrex; ***Spain:*** Tobi; Tobra Gobens; Tobrabact; Tobradistin; Tobrex; ***Swed.:*** Nebcina; Tobi; Tobrex; ***Switz.:*** Obracin; Tobrex; ***Thai.:*** Tobrex; ***UK:*** Nebcin; Tobi; ***USA:*** AkTob; Nebcin; Tobi; Tobrasol; Tobrex.

**Multi-ingredient:** ***Arg.:*** Antibioptal; Bioptic DX; Gotabiotic F; Larsen; Polioftal; Radina Dex; Tobradex; Toflamixina Plus; Xao-Dex; ***Austria:*** Tobradex; ***Belg.:*** Ocubrax; Tobradex; ***Braz.:*** Orlamix†; Tobracort; Tobradex; ***Canad.:*** Tobradex; ***Chile:*** Poentobral Plus; Tobradex; Tobrin-D; Todexona; Xolof D; ***Fr.:*** Tobradex; ***Hong Kong:*** Tobradex; ***India:*** Tobazon; ***Ital.:*** Tobradex; ***Malaysia:*** Tobradex; ***Mex.:*** Obrydex; Obrypre; Tobradex; Trazidex; Trazinac†; ***NZ:*** Tobradex; Tobrasone†; ***S.Afr.:*** Tobradex; ***Singapore:*** Tobradex; ***Spain:*** Ocubrax; Tobradex; ***Switz.:*** Tobradex; Tobrafen; ***Thai.:*** Tobradex; ***UK:*** Tobradex; ***USA:*** Tobradex.

---

### Tosufloxacin *(USAN, rINN)*

Abbott-61827. (±)-7-(3-Amino-1-pyrrolidinyl)-1-(2,4-difluorophenyl)-6-fluoro-1,4-dihydro-4-oxo-1,8-naphthyridine-3-carboxylic acid.

$C_{19}H_{15}F_3N_4O_3$ = 404.3.
*CAS — 100490-36-6 (anhydrous tosufloxacin); 108138-46-1 (anhydrous tosufloxacin); 107097-79-0 (tosufloxacin monohydrate).*

### Tosufloxacin Tosilate *(rINNM)*

Tosilato de tosufloxacino; Tosufloxacin Tosylate. Tosufloxacin toluene-4-sulphonate monohydrate.

$C_{19}H_{15}F_3N_4O_3,C_7H_8O_3S,H_2O$ = 594.6.
*CAS — 115964-29-9; 144742-63-2.*

#### Profile

Tosufloxacin is a fluoroquinolone antibacterial with properties similar to those of ciprofloxacin (p.188). It is given by mouth as the tosilate in the treatment of susceptible infections in usual doses of 300 to 450 mg daily in two or three divided doses. It is also under investigation for ophthalmic use.

#### Preparations

**Proprietary Preparations** (details are given in Part 3)
***Jpn:*** Ozex.

---

## Trimethoprim *(BAN, USAN, rINN)*

BW-56-72; NSC-106568; Trimethoprimum; Trimethoxyprim; Trimetoprima. 5-(3,4,5-Trimethoxybenzyl)pyrimidine-2,4-diamine.

$C_{14}H_{18}N_4O_3$ = 290.3.
*CAS — 738-70-5.*
*ATC — J01EA01.*

NOTE. Compounded preparations of trimethoprim may be represented by the following names:

- Co-trifamole (*BAN*)—trimethoprim 1 part and sulfamoxole 5 parts (see p.199)
- Co-trimazine (*BAN*)—trimethoprim 1 part and sulfadiazine 5 parts (see p.199)
- Co-trimoxazole (*BAN*)—trimethoprim 1 part and sulfamethoxazole 5 parts (see p.199)
- Co-trimoxazole (*PEN*)—trimethoprim and sulfamethoxazole.

**Pharmacopoeias.** In *Chin., Eur.* (see p.vi), *Int., Pol., US,* and *Viet.*

**Ph. Eur. 5.0** (Trimethoprim). A white or yellowish-white powder. Very slightly soluble in water; slightly soluble in alcohol.

**USP 27** (Trimethoprim). White to cream-coloured, odourless crystals or crystalline powder. Very slightly soluble in water; slightly soluble in alcohol and in acetone; soluble in benzyl alcohol; practically insoluble in carbon tetrachloride and in ether; sparingly soluble in chloroform and in methyl alcohol. Store in airtight containers at a temperature of 25°, excursions permitted between 15° and 30°. Protect from light.

### Trimethoprim Sulfate *(USAN, rINNM)*

BW-72U; Trimethoprim Sulphate *(BANM)*.

$(C_{14}H_{18}N_4O_3)_2.H_2SO_4$ = 678.7.
*CAS — 56585-33-2.*

**Pharmacopoeias.** In *Viet.* and *US.*

**USP 27** (Trimethoprim Sulfate). A white to off-white crystalline powder. Soluble in water, in alcohol, in dilute mineral acids, and in fixed alkalis. pH of a 0.05% solution in water is between 7.5 and 8.5. Store at a temperature of 25°, excursions permitted between 15° and 30°.

**Incompatibility.** The UK manufacturers state that trimethoprim injections (containing the lactate) should not be mixed with solutions of sulfonamides because of incompatibility. Although a former such preparation stated that it should not be diluted in chloride-containing infusion solutions, because of the risk of precipitating trimethoprim hydrochloride, others are stated to be compatible with sodium chloride 0.9% and some other chloride-containing solutions including Ringer's solution. Injections are considered compatible with glucose 5% and with sodium lactate.

### Adverse Effects and Treatment

Trimethoprim is reasonably well tolerated in general, and the most frequent adverse effects at usual doses are pruritus and skin rash (in about 3 to 7% of patients) and mild gastrointestinal disturbances including nausea, vomiting, and glossitis.

Rarely, more severe effects have been reported. Sulfonamide-like skin reactions including exfoliative dermatitis, erythema multiforme, Stevens-Johnson syndrome, and toxic epidermal necrolysis have occurred. Disturbances of liver enzyme values and cholestatic jaundice have been associated with trimethoprim. Rises in serum creatinine and blood-urea nitrogen have been reported although it is unclear whether this represents genuine renal dysfunction or inhibition of tubular secretion of creatinine. Photosensitivity has been reported. Fever is not uncommon but occasionally hypersensitivity reactions may be severe and anaphylaxis and angioedema have been reported. Cases of aseptic meningitis have also occurred.

Trimethoprim may cause a depression of haematopoiesis due to interference of the drug in the metabolism of folic acid, particularly when given over a prolonged period or in high doses. This may manifest as megaloblastic anaemia, or as thrombocytopenia and leucopenia; methaemoglobinaemia has also been seen. Calcium folinate 5 to 15 mg daily by mouth may be given to counter this effect. Trimethoprim is teratogenic in *animals*.

For further information on the adverse effects of trimethoprim when used with sulfamethoxazole, see Co-trimoxazole, p.199.

**Effects on the eyes.** There have been isolated reports of bilateral anterior uveitis associated with trimethoprim. In 2 such patients,[1,2] the reaction recurred upon rechallenge with trimethoprim. A third patient developed uveitis following co-trimoxazole, and subsequently uveitis with retinal haemorrhage following trimethoprim alone.[3]

1. Gilroy N, *et al.* Trimethoprim-induced aseptic meningitis and uveitis. *Lancet* 1997; **350:** 112.
2. Arola O, *et al.* Arthritis, uveitis, and Stevens-Johnson syndrome induced by trimethoprim. *Lancet* 1998; **351:** 1102.
3. Kristinsson JK, *et al.* Bilateral anterior uveitis and retinal haemorrhages after administration of trimethoprim. *Acta Ophthalmol Scand* 1997; **75:** 314–15.

**Hyperkalaemia.** Trimethoprim has been reported to induce hyperkalaemia,[1] particularly in HIV-infected patients being treated for *Pneumocystis carinii* pneumonia or in the elderly. The hyperkalaemia may be due to amiloride-like potassium-sparing properties of trimethoprim, and may be potentiated by ACE inhibitors.

1. Perazella MA. Trimethoprim-induced hyperkalaemia: clinical data, mechanism, prevention and management. *Drug Safety* 2000; **22:** 227–36.

### Precautions

Trimethoprim should not be given to patients with a history of hypersensitivity to the drug, and it should be discontinued if a skin rash appears. Care is necessary in giving trimethoprim to patients with renal impairment to avoid accumulation and toxicity: it should not be given in severe renal impairment unless blood concentrations can be monitored. It should be used with caution in patients with severe hepatic damage as changes may occur in the absorption and metabolism of trimethoprim.

It is suggested that regular haematological examination should be made during prolonged courses of treatment although the *British National Formulary* considers evidence of their practical value to be unsatisfactory; patients or their carers should be told how to recognise signs of blood toxicity and should be advised to seek immediate medical attention if symptoms such as fever, sore throat, rash, mouth ulcers, purpura, bruising or bleeding develop. Trimethoprim should not usually be given to patients with serious haematological disorders and particularly not in megaloblastic anaemia secondary to folate depletion. Caution should be taken in patients with actual, or possible, folate deficiency and use of folinic acid should be considered. Trimethoprim should be avoided during pregnancy. Elderly patients may be more susceptible to adverse effects and a lower dosage may be advisable.

Trimethoprim may interfere with some diagnostic tests, including serum-methotrexate assay where dihydrofolate reductase is used and the Jaffé reaction for creatinine.

For further information on precautions for trimethoprim given with sulfamethoxazole, see Co-trimoxazole, p.200.

**Breast feeding.** Trimethoprim appears in breast milk and the US manufacturers have stated that care is required when it is used in breast-feeding mothers.

The American Academy of Pediatrics considers trimethoprim, when given with sulfamethoxazole, to be compatible with breast feeding.[1]

1. American Academy of Pediatrics. The transfer of drugs and other chemicals into human milk. *Pediatrics* 2001; **108:** 776–89. Correction. *ibid.*; 1029. Also available at: http://aappolicy.aappublications.org/cgi/content/full/pediatrics%3b108/3/776 (accessed 28/05/04)

**Fragile X syndrome.** A warning that trimethoprim and other folate antagonists should be avoided in children with the fragile X chromosome which is associated with mental retardation and is folate sensitive.[1]

1. Hecht F, Glover TW. Antibiotics containing trimethoprim and the fragile X chromosome. *N Engl J Med* 1983; **308:** 285–6.

**Porphyria.** Trimethoprim has been associated with acute attacks of porphyria and is considered unsafe in porphyric patients.

## Interactions

Trimethoprim may increase serum concentrations and potentiate the effect of a number of drugs, including phenytoin, digoxin, and procainamide. The effect may be due to competitive inhibition of renal excretion, decreased metabolism, or both. It has been suggested that trimethoprim may potentiate the effects of warfarin. Trimethoprim has been reported to reduce the renal excretion and increase blood concentrations of zidovudine, zalcitabine, and lamivudine. Trimethoprim and dapsone increase each other's serum concentrations, whereas rifampicin may decrease trimethoprim concentrations.

An increased risk of nephrotoxicity has been reported with the use of trimethoprim or co-trimoxazole and ciclosporin. Intravenous use of trimethoprim and sulfonamides may reduce ciclosporin concentrations in blood. In patients given trimethoprim who were also receiving diuretics, hyponatraemia has been reported (an increased risk of thrombocytopenia has been seen in elderly patients given co-trimoxazole with diuretics, although it is unclear which component is responsible).

Use of trimethoprim with other depressants of bone marrow function may increase the likelihood of myelosuppression, and there may be a particular risk of megaloblastic anaemia if it is given with other folate inhibitors, such as pyrimethamine or methotrexate.

Severe hyperkalaemia has been noted in patients given trimethoprim (or co-trimoxazole) together with an ACE inhibitor.

## Antimicrobial Action

Trimethoprim is a dihydrofolate reductase inhibitor. It inhibits the conversion of bacterial dihydrofolic acid to tetrahydrofolic acid which is necessary for the synthesis of certain amino acids, purines, thymidine, and ultimately DNA. It acts in the same metabolic pathway as the sulfonamides. It exerts its selective action because of a far greater affinity for the bacterial than the mammalian enzyme. Trimethoprim may be bacteriostatic or bactericidal depending on growth conditions; pus, for example, may inhibit the action of trimethoprim because of the presence of thymine and thymidine.

*Spectrum of activity.* Trimethoprim is active against a wide range of Gram-negative and Gram-positive aerobes, as well as some protozoa. The following species are usually susceptible (but see also Resistance, below).

Many Gram-positive cocci are sensitive, including *Staphylococcus aureus*, streptococci including *Streptococcus pyogenes*, *Str. pneumoniae*, and the viridans streptococci, and to a variable extent enterococci, although their sensitivity is reduced in the presence of folate.

Other sensitive Gram-positive organisms include strains of *Listeria*, *Corynebacterium diphtheriae*, and the Gram-positive bacilli.

Among the Gram-negative organisms, most of the Enterobacteriaceae are susceptible, or moderately so, including *Citrobacter*, *Enterobacter*, *Escherichia coli*, *Hafnia*, *Klebsiella*, *Proteus mirabilis*, *Providencia*, *Salmonella*, some *Serratia*, *Shigella*, and *Yersinia*. *Legionella* and *Vibrio* are also sensitive, and so are *Haemophilus influenzae* and *H. ducreyi*.

Anaerobic species are usually resistant, and so, to varying degrees are *Brucella*, *Neisseria*, and *Nocardia*. *Mycobacterium tuberculosis* is resistant although *M. marinum* may not be. *Pseudomonas aeruginosa* is resistant, and so are the Chlamydiaceae, Mycoplasma spp., and Rickettsia spp., as well as the spirochaetes.

Trimethoprim has some activity against *Pneumocystis carinii* and against some protozoa such as *Naegleria*, *Plasmodium*, and *Toxoplasma*.

*Activity with other antimicrobials.* Because their modes of action are complementary, affecting different stages in folate metabolism, a potent synergistic effect exists between trimethoprim and sulfonamides against many organisms *in vitro*.

Fixed-dose combinations of trimethoprim with various sulfonamides are available, of which co-trimoxazole (trimethoprim with sulfamethoxazole in a 1:5 mixture) is the most widely used. For further details on the antimicrobial action of co-trimoxazole, see p.200.

Synergy has also been reported with rifampicin, and with the polymyxins.

*Resistance.* Resistance to trimethoprim may be due to several mechanisms. Clinical resistance is often due to plasmid-mediated dihydrofolate reductases that are resistant to trimethoprim: such genes may become incorporated into the chromosome via transposons. Resistance may also be due to overproduction of dihydrofolate reductase, changes in cell permeability, or bacterial mutants which are intrinsically resistant to trimethoprim because they depend on exogenous thymine and thymidine for growth. Despite fears of a rapid increase in resistance if trimethoprim was used alone there is little evidence that this has been any worse than in areas where it has been used in combination with sulfonamides. Nonetheless, trimethoprim resistance has been reported in many species, and very high frequencies of resistance have been seen in some developing countries, particularly among the Enterobacteriaceae.

◊ References.

1. Huovinen P, *et al.* Trimethoprim and sulfonamide resistance. *Antimicrob Agents Chemother* 1995; **39:** 279–89.

## Pharmacokinetics

Trimethoprim is rapidly and almost completely absorbed from the gastrointestinal tract and peak concentrations in the circulation occur about 1 to 4 hours after an oral dose; peak plasma concentrations of about 1 microgram/mL have been reported after a single dose of 100 mg. About 45% is bound to plasma proteins. Trimethoprim is widely distributed to various tissues and fluids including kidneys, liver, lung and bronchial secretions, saliva, aqueous humour, prostatic tissue and fluid, and vaginal secretions; concentrations in many of these tissues are reported to be higher than serum concentrations but concentrations in the CSF are about one-quarter to one-half of those in serum. Trimethoprim readily crosses the placenta and it appears in breast milk. The half-life is about 8 to 10 hours in adults and somewhat less in children, but is prolonged in severe renal impairment and in neonates, whose renal function is immature.

Trimethoprim is excreted primarily by the kidneys through glomerular filtration and tubular secretion. About 10 to 20% of trimethoprim is metabolised in the liver and small amounts are excreted in the faeces via the bile, but most, about 40 to 60% of a dose, is excreted in urine, predominantly as unchanged drug, within 24 hours. Trimethoprim is removed from the blood by haemodialysis to some extent.

## Uses and Administration

Trimethoprim is a diaminopyrimidine antibacterial that is used for the treatment of infections due to sensitive organisms, including gastro-enteritis and respiratory-tract infections, and in particular for the treatment and prophylaxis of urinary-tract infections. For details of these infections and their treatment, see Choice of Antibacterial, p.120.

Trimethoprim is also used with sulfonamides. The most common combination is co-trimoxazole (trimethoprim with sulfamethoxazole) (p.199). Other combinations are co-trimazine (with sulfadiazine) and co-trifamole (with sulfamoxole); trimethoprim has also been used with sulfamerazine, sulfametopyrazine, sulfametrole, and sulfamethoxypyridazine, and, in veterinary practice, with sulfadoxine, sulfaquinoxaline, sulfatroxazole, sulfadimethoxine, sulfadimidine, or sulfafurazole.

The combination of trimethoprim with sulfamethoxazole (co-trimoxazole) or with dapsone is used in the management of *Pneumocystis carinii* pneumonia (p.389).

The usual adult dose of trimethoprim in acute infection is 100 or 200 mg twice daily by mouth; doses of 200 or 300 mg daily as a single dose are also used. For the dosage of trimethoprim when given with sulfamethoxazole, see under Co-trimoxazole, p.200. Up to 20 mg/kg daily may be given in combination with dapsone for the treatment of *Pneumocystis carinii* pneumonia.

Children may be given 6 to 8 mg/kg daily of trimethoprim in 2 divided doses: regimens for children are, 6 to 12 years, 100 mg twice daily; 6 months to 5 years, 50 mg twice daily; 6 weeks to 5 months, 25 mg twice daily.

For long-term prophylaxis the usual dose is 100 mg at night for adults; children aged 6 to 12 years may be given 50 mg at night and those aged 6 months to 5 years, 25 mg at night. Alternatively, children may be given a dose of 1 to 2 mg/kg at night.

Trimethoprim is also given intravenously by injection or infusion as the lactate although doses are in terms of the base. The usual dose is 200 mg every 12 hours in adults; children may be given 8 mg/kg daily in 2 or 3 divided doses. Initial doses may be higher or given more frequently in severely ill patients.

Care should be taken in patients with moderate to severe renal impairment and doses generally should be reduced (see below).

Trimethoprim with polymyxin B has been used topically in the treatment and prophylaxis of eye infections. Trimethoprim sulfate and trimethoprim hydrochloride are also used.

**Administration.** SINGLE-DOSE THERAPY. Although there are obvious advantages to a single-dose regimen, one study[1] found that there was about a 1 in 4 risk of recurrence of urinary-tract infection within 10 days in 50 children given, according to age, a single dose of 75 to 450 mg of trimethoprim. The problems with a single-dose regimen were confirmed by others[2] in a study involving 344 evaluated cases of cystitis in 306 women. Only 122 of 173 cases treated with trimethoprim 320 mg as a single dose were evaluated as cured after 5 weeks, compared with 149 of 171 given 160 mg twice daily for 1 week (71 versus 87%). Again, these results suggest that about 1 patient in 4 would have to be re-treated.

1. Nolan T, *et al.* Single dose trimethoprim for urinary tract infection. *Arch Dis Child* 1989; **64:** 581–6.
2. Österberg E, *et al.* Efficacy of single-dose versus seven-day trimethoprim treatment of cystitis in women: a randomized double-blind study. *J Infect Dis* 1990; **161:** 942–7.

**Administration in renal impairment.** Doses of trimethoprim should generally be reduced in patients with moderate to severe renal impairment according to creatinine clearance (CC):

- CC 15 to 27 mL/minute: normal dose for 3 days reduced to one-half thereafter
- CC below 15 mL/minute: half the normal dose from the start of treatment

Plasma concentrations should be monitored in patients with severe renal impairment.

## Preparations

***BP 2003:*** Co-trimoxazole Intravenous Infusion; Co-trimoxazole Oral Suspension; Co-trimoxazole Tablets; Dispersible Co-trimoxazole Tablets; Paediatric Co-trimoxazole Oral Suspension; Paediatric Co-trimoxazole Tablets; Trimethoprim Oral Suspension; Trimethoprim Tablets;
***USP 27:*** Polymyxin B Sulfate and Trimethoprim Ophthalmic Solution; Sulfamethoxazole and Trimethoprim Injection; Sulfamethoxazole and Trimethoprim Oral Suspension; Sulfamethoxazole and Trimethoprim Tablets; Trimethoprim Tablets.

**Proprietary Preparations** (details are given in Part 3)
***Austral.:*** Alprim; Triprim; ***Austria:*** Monoprim†; Motrim; Solotrim; Triprim; Wellcoprim; ***Belg.:*** Wellcoprim†; ***Canad.:*** Proloprim; ***Denm.:*** Monotrim; Trimopan; ***Fin.:*** Trimetin; Trimex; Trimopan; ***Fr.:*** Wellcoprim; ***Ger.:*** InfectoTrimet; TMP; Trimono†; ***Irl.:*** Ipral; Monotrim; ***Ital.:*** Abaprim†; ***Malaysia:*** Alprim; ***Neth.:*** Wellcoprim; ***NZ:*** TMP; Triprim; ***S.Afr.:*** Triprim; ***Singapore:*** Alprim; ***Spain:*** Tediprima; ***Swed.:*** Idotrim; ***Switz.:*** Monotrim; ***Thai.:*** Utisept; ***UAE:*** Trimol-A; ***UK:*** Monotrim; Tiempe†; Trimogal†; Trimopan; ***USA:*** Primsol; Proloprim; Trimpex.

**Multi-ingredient:** ***Arg.:*** Adrenol; Bacti-Uril; Bacticel; Bactrim; Bactrim Balsamico; Cotrizol-G; Danferane; Diocla; Dosulfin Bronquial; Dosulfin Fuerte; Enterobacticel; Neoftalm; Neoftalm Dexa; Netocur; Netocur Balsamico; Neumobacticel; Novidrine; Rifaprim; Ritroprim; Sulfagrand; Tritenk; Urisept NF; Uro-Bactrim; ***Austral.:*** Bactrim; Cosig; Resprim; Septrin; Trimoxazole; ***Austria:*** Bactrim; Cotribene; Cotristad; Eusaprim; Lidaprim; Oecotrim; Polytrim; Supracombin; Triglobe; Trimetho comp; ***Belg.:*** Bactrim; Eusaprim; Ophtalmotrim; Polytrim; Steroprim; ***Braz.:*** Assepium; Assepium Balsamico; Bac Septin Balsamico†; Bac Septin†; Bac-Sulfitrin; Bacfar; Bacfar Balsamico†; Bacgen Balsamico†; Bacgen†; Bacprotin; Bacris; Bacteracin; Bacteracin Balsamico†; Bactox Balsamico†; Bactox†; Bactren†; Bactrex†; Bactricin Balsamico†; Bactricin†; Bactrim; Bactrisan; Bactrisan Balsamico†; Bactrizol; Bactropin; Bactropin Balsamico†; Baklinger†; Balsandin†; Balsiprin†; Baxapril†; Becaltrin†; Belfactrin†; Benectrin; Benectrin Balsamico; Binoctrin; Diazol; Dientrin; Dispeptrin†; Diteutrin†; Duoctrin; Duoctrin Balsamico†; Duoctrin Enterico†; Ectrin; Ectrin Balsamico; Entercal†; Entero Heractrin†; Enterone†; Espectrin; Gamactrin; Heractrin†; Ibtrim†; Imuneprim; Infecteracin†; Infectrin; Infectrin Balsamico†; Katrim Balsamico†; Katrim†; Leotrim†; Linurin; Lupectrim; Lupectrim Balsamico†; Metoprin; Metoprin Balsamico†; Mictrex†; Neotrin; Neotrin Balsamico†; Pertrim†; Pulkrin; Qiftrin; Quimio-Ped; Quimio-Ped Balsamico†; Roytrin; Sedactrim Balsamico†; Sedactrim†; Selectrim†; Septiolan; Septiolan Balsamico†; Septoprin†; Silpin†; Sulf+Trim†; Sulfa+Trim†; Sulfatrex†; Suss Balsamico†; Suss†; Teutrin; Teutrin Balsamico†; Triglobe; Trimetoprim Balsamico†; Trimexazol; Trimexazol Balsamico†; Trizol Balsamico†; Urizal†; Uro Bac Septin†; Uro Bactrim†; Uro Batrox†; Uro Duoctrim†; Uro Heractrim†; Uro Septoprin†; Uro-Bacteracin†; Uro-Baxapril; Uro-Leotrim†; Uro-Septiolan†; Uro-Teutrim†; Urobactrex†; Urobioctrin†; Uroctrin; Urofar†; Uroneotrim†; Uropol; Uroxazol†; Utrim†; ***Canad.:*** Apo-Sulfatrim; Bactrim†; Coptin; Novo-Trimel; Nu-Cotrimox; PMS-Polytrimethoprim; Polytrim; Roubac†; Septra; ***Chile:*** Bacterol; Bactrimel; Entero Micinovo; Introcin; Septrin; Trelibec; Uro-Micinovo; ***Denm.:*** Bactrim†; Sulfotrim; ***Fin.:*** Cotrim; Ditrim; Trimetin Duplo; ***Fr.:*** Bactrim; Cotrimazol†; Eusaprim; Trimadiaz Antrima†; ***Ger.:*** Bactoreduct; Bactrim†; Berlocid; Berlocombin; Cotrim-Tablinen†; Cotrim; Cotrim-Diolan; Cotrimhexal; Cotrimox-Wolff; Cotrimstada; Drylin; Eusaprim; Jenamoxazol†; Kepinol; Linaris†; Microtrim; Sigaprim; Supracombin; TMS; Triglobe†; ***Gr.:*** Bactrimel; Bioprim; Lidaprim; Septrin; ***Hong Kong:*** Apo-Sulfatrim†; Bacin†; BS†; Chemitrim; Chemoprim; Dhatrin; Letus; Lidaprim; Oftalmotrim†; Septrin; ***India:*** Aubril; Bactrim; Ciplin; Colizole; Oriprim; Sepmax; Septran; Trisulfose; ***Irl.:*** Bactrim†; Cotrimel†; Duobact; Septrin; Tricomox†; ***Israel:*** Diseptyl; Resprim; Septrin; Sulfatrim; ***Ital.:*** Abacin; Bacterial†; Bactrim; Chemitrim; Eusaprim; Gantrim; Isotrim†; Kelfiprim†; Kombinax†; Lidaprim; Medixin†; Strepto-Plus†; Velaten†; ***Malaysia:*** Bacin; Balin; Baserin; Beaglobe; Chemix; Cotrim; Oftalmotrim; Resprim; Triglobe; Trimexazole; Trisulprim; Virin; ***Mex.:*** Andoprim; Anitrim; Bacpiryl; Bactelan; Bactide; Bactilen; Bactiver; Bactrim; Bactrim Compositum; Bactropin; Bateral; Batrizol; Bioprim; Dertrin; Dibaprim; Ectaprim; Enterobacticel†; Esteprim; Fectri; Isobac†; Kaltrim; Kelfiprim†; Lidaprim†; Maxtrim; Metoxiprim; Microbactim; Octex; Octiban; Pisatrina; Polibatrin; Protaxol; Rifaprim; Septrin; Servitrim; Sulfawal; Sulfoid Trimetho; Sulfort†; Sulprim; Sultiprim; Supristol†; Syraprim; Thriazol; Tribakin; Trim-Vit†; Trimesul†; Trimesuxol†; Trimetoger; Trimetox; Trimexazol; Trimexole; Trimexole Compositum; Trimzol†; Trinelax†; Trisufin; Zaprin†; ***Neth.:*** Bactrimel; Eusaprim; Polytrim; Trimoxol; ***Norw.:*** Bactrim; Trimetoprim-Sulfa; ***NZ:*** Apo-Sulfatrim; Bactrim†; Trimel†; Trisul; ***Port.:*** Bactrim; Cotrim; Metomide; Oftalmotrim; Septrin; ***S.Afr.:*** Acuco†; Arcanaprim†; Bactrim; Bencole; Cocydal†; Cozole; Doctrim†; Durobac; Dynazole†; Fabubac; Lagatrim; Mezenol; Polytrim; Purbac; Septran; Spectrim; Tri-Co†; Trimethox; Trimoks†; Trimzol†; Ultrasept†; Xerazole; Xeroprim; ***Singapore:*** Apo-Sulfatrim; Bacin; Bactrim†; Balin; BS; Chemix; Chemoprim; Dhatrin; Oftalmotrim†; Septrin; Suprim; Triglobe†; Trimezole; ***Spain:*** Abactrim†; Bactifor†; Bactopumon; Balsoprim; Bridotrim†; Bronco Aseptilex Fuerte; Bronco Bactifor†; Bronco Sergo†; Broncomega; Broncorema†; Broncovir; Brongenit†; Bronquicisteina; Bronquidiazina CR; Bronquimar; Bronquimucil; Bronquium†; Cotrazol; Eduprim; Eduprim Mucolitico; Gobens Trim; Lotusix†; Momentol; Mucorama TS†; Neumopectolina; Oftalmotrim; Oftalmotrim Dexa; Otix; Pulmo Menal; Pulmosterin Duo; Salvatrim†; Septrin; Soltrim; Toose†; Tosdetan†; Traquivan†; Tresium†; Triglobe†; ***Swed.:*** Bactrim; Eusaprim; Trimin sulfa; ***Switz.:*** Agoprim; Bactrim; Cotrim; Escoprim; Eusaprim†; Groprim; Helveprim†; Imexim†; Lagatrim; Maderan†; Mediprim; Nopil; Sigaprim; Supracombin; ***Thai.:*** Actin; Bacin; Bacta; Bactrim; Baczole; Balin†; Chemoprim; Co-Tasian; Co-Trimed; Conprim; Cotamox; Kelfiprim†; Ko-Cap; Ko-Kure; Lastrim; Letus; Lidaprim; M-Trim; Med-Sultrim; Mega-Prim; Metrim; Metxaprim; Mycosamthong; Po-Trim; Pulvicin; Septrin; Servitrim†; Sulbacta; Sulfometh; Tampo; Toprim; Trimexazole; Trimox†; Trimoxzol†; Triprim; Trixzol; Zoleprim; ***UAE:*** Trimol; ***UK:*** Chemotrim†; Fectrim; Laratrim†; Polytrim; Septrin; ***USA:*** Bactrim; Cotrim; Polytrim; Septra; SMZ-TMP; Sulfatrim.

## Troleandomycin *(BAN, USAN, rINN)*

NSC-108166; Triacetyloleandomycin; Troleandomicina. The triacetyl ester of oleandomycin.

$C_{41}H_{67}NO_{15}$ = 814.0.

*CAS — 2751-09-9.*

*ATC — J01FA08.*

**Pharmacopoeias.** In *Fr.* and *US.*

**USP 27** (Troleandomycin). A white, odourless, crystalline powder. It contains the equivalent of not less than 750 micrograms of oleandomycin per mg. Slightly soluble in water and in ether; freely soluble in alcohol; soluble in chloroform. A 10% solution in alcohol and water (1:1) has a pH of 7.0 to 8.5. Store in airtight containers.

### Adverse Effects and Precautions

As for Erythromycin, p.208. Hepatotoxicity with transient disturbances of liver function and jaundice has occurred after use of troleandomycin for 2 weeks or more, or in repeated courses, and liver function should be monitored in patients receiving such treatment. It should be used with care in patients with hepatic impairment and avoided in those who have previously developed liver toxicity on receiving it.

### Interactions

For a discussion of drug interactions of macrolide antibacterials, see Erythromycin, p.209.

◊ For the effect of troleandomycin on serum concentrations of *carbamazepine*, see p.355 and for its effect on *triazolam*, see under Diazepam, p.693. The use of troleandomycin with *cisapride* can increase plasma concentrations of cisapride, which may result in serious ventricular arrhythmias. Troleandomycin has a more potent effect on hepatic cytochrome P450 than erythromycin (see Interactions, Mechanism, p.209), and interactions reported between drugs such as *astemizole*, the *ergot alkaloids*, *terfenadine*, or *theophylline* and other macrolides are at least as likely if they are taken with troleandomycin. The administration of troleandomycin to women on *oral contraceptives* should be avoided (see p.1534).

For the effects of troleandomycin on *methylprednisolone*, see Administration in Asthma under Uses, below.

### Antimicrobial Action

Troleandomycin is hydrolysed *in vivo* to oleandomycin (p.240) which has a range of activity similar to but, in general, less effective than that of erythromycin (p.209). It has a similar pattern of resistance to erythromycin.

### Pharmacokinetics

Troleandomycin is more rapidly and completely absorbed from the gastrointestinal tract than is oleandomycin, to which it is hydrolysed *in vivo*. Peak plasma-oleandomycin concentrations of about 2 micrograms/mL are attained 2 hours after a single dose of 500 mg, and detectable amounts are present in plasma for 12 hours. It is excreted in the faeces via the bile; about 20% of the dose can be recovered in active form from the urine.

### Uses and Administration

Troleandomycin is a prodrug of the macrolide antibacterial oleandomycin that has actions similar to those of erythromycin (p.210). It has been given by mouth in the treatment of susceptible infections although more effective antibacterials are generally preferred. Doses of troleandomycin are expressed in terms of the equivalent amount of oleandomycin; 1.18 g of troleandomycin is approximately equivalent to 1 g of oleandomycin. The usual adult dose is the equivalent of 1 to 2 g daily of oleandomycin in four divided doses by mouth. Children have been given the equivalent of about 25 to 45 mg/kg daily.

**Administration in asthma.** Troleandomycin inhibits the elimination of methylprednisolone[1] and has been given to children with corticosteroid-dependent asthma (p.777), to permit a reduction in the oral dosage of methylprednisolone.[2-4] It is unclear whether troleandomycin has actions in asthma beyond its effect on methylprednisolone metabolism; there is some evidence that it may reduce airway hyperresponsiveness,[3] and there is a report of a patient who was successfully maintained on troleandomycin alone after her corticosteroid therapy was tapered to zero.[5] However, a systematic review[6] concluded that there is insufficient evidence to support its use in corticosteroid-dependent asthma.

1. Szefler SJ, *et al.* Dose- and time-related effect of troleandomycin on methylprednisolone elimination. *Clin Pharmacol Ther* 1982; **32:** 166–71.
2. Eitches RW, *et al.* Methylprednisolone and troleandomycin in treatment of steroid-dependent asthmatic children. *Am J Dis Child* 1985; **139:** 264–8.
3. Ball BD, *et al.* Effect of low-dose troleandomycin on glucocorticoid pharmacokinetics and airway hyperresponsiveness in severely asthmatic children. *Ann Allergy* 1990; **65:** 37–45.
4. Kamada AK, *et al.* Efficacy and safety of low-dose troleandomycin therapy in children with severe, steroid-requiring asthma. *J Allergy Clin Immunol* 1993; **91:** 873–82.
5. Rosenberg SM, *et al.* Use of TAO without methylprednisolone in the treatment of severe asthma. *Chest* 1991; **100:** 849–50.
6. Evans DJ, *et al.* Troleandomycin as an oral corticosteroid sparing agent in stable asthma. Available in The Cochrane Library; Issue 2. Chichester: John Wiley; 2004.

### Preparations

**USP 27:** Troleandomycin Capsules.

**Proprietary Preparations** (details are given in Part 3)
***Ital.:*** Triocetin; ***USA:*** TAO.

## Trospectomycin Sulfate *(USAN, rINNM)*

Sulfato de trospectomicina; Trospectomycin Sulphate *(BANM)*; U-63366 (trospectomycin); U-63366F. (2*R*,4a*R*,5a*R*,6*S*,7*S*,8*R*,9*S*,9a*R*,10a*S*)-2-Butyl-4a,7,9-trihydroxy-6,8-bis(methylamino)perhydropyrano[2,3-*b*][1,4]benzodioxin-4-one sulphate pentahydrate.

$C_{17}H_{30}N_2O_7,H_2SO_4,5H_2O$ = 562.6.

*CAS — 88669-04-9 (trospectomycin); 88851-61-0 (trospectomycin sulfate).*

### Profile

Trospectomycin is a water-soluble derivative of spectinomycin (p.255) but is more active against Gram-positive organisms, *Haemophilus influenzae*, and *Chlamydia trachomatis* as well as *Neisseria*. It has been investigated in various infections and given as the sulfate intravenously or intramuscularly. Reported adverse effects include perioral paraesthesia, pain at the injection site, nausea, and dizziness.

## Trovafloxacin Mesilate *(rINNM)*

CP-99219-27; CP-99219 (trovafloxacin); Mesilato de trovafloxacino; Trovafloxacin Mesylate *(USAN)*. 7-[(1*R*,5*S*,6*S*)-6-Amino-3-azabicyclo[3.1.0]hex-3-yl]-1-(2,4-difluorophenyl)-6-fluoro-1,4-dihydro-4-oxo-1,8-naphthyridine-3-carboxylic acid monomethanesulphonate.

$C_{20}H_{15}F_3N_4O_3,CH_4O_3S$ = 512.5.

*CAS — 147059-72-1 (trovafloxacin); 147059-75-4 (trovafloxacin mesilate).*

*ATC — J01MA13.*

### Adverse Effects and Precautions

As for Ciprofloxacin, p.188.

Dizziness is the most common adverse effect reported with trovafloxacin.

Trovafloxacin preparations have been withdrawn in many countries following reports of unpredictable severe hepatic adverse effects, including some fatalities. Symptomatic pancreatitis has also been reported. In countries (such as the USA) where trovafloxacin is still available, it is recommended that liver function tests and pancreatic tests should be performed when symptoms develop and, if necessary, that the drug be discontinued.

### Antimicrobial Action

As for Ciprofloxacin, p.190. It is more active against pneumococci.

### Pharmacokinetics

Trovafloxacin is readily absorbed from the gastrointestinal tract following an oral dose, peak plasma concentrations being achieved after about 1 to 2 hours. Following intravenous use, alatrofloxacin is rapidly converted to trovafloxacin. Bioavailability following oral trovafloxacin has been reported to be 88%. Trovafloxacin is widely distributed into body tissues and is about 76% bound to plasma proteins. It appears in breast milk.

The serum half-life of trovafloxacin ranges from about 9 to 12 hours. Trovafloxacin is metabolised by conjugation, 13% of a dose appearing in the urine as the glucuronide and 9% in the faeces as the *N*-acetyl metabolite; other metabolites appear in both the urine and faeces in minor amounts, but approximately 50% of an oral dose is excreted unchanged, mainly in the faeces but also in the urine.

### Uses and Administration

Trovafloxacin is a fluoroquinolone antibacterial with actions and uses similar to those of ciprofloxacin (p.191). It is given as the mesilate by mouth for the treatment of susceptible infections. The prodrug alatrofloxacin (p.154) is used as the mesilate for intravenous infusion.

Trovafloxacin and alatrofloxacin preparations have been withdrawn in many countries following reports of unpredictable severe hepatic adverse effects, including some fatalities; the use in some other countries such as the USA is restricted to specified serious conditions and usually for a treatment period of up to a maximum of 2 weeks. Doses of both trovafloxacin mesilate and alatrofloxacin mesilate are expressed in terms of trovafloxacin base. Usual daily doses are the equivalent of 200 mg of trovafloxacin by mouth or 200 to 300 mg intravenously.

◊ General references.

1. Haria M, Lamb HM. Trovafloxacin. *Drugs* 1997; **54:** 435–45.
2. Amyes SGN, *et al.* (eds.) Trovafloxacin: a novel extended spectrum quinolone. *J Antimicrob Chemother* 1997; **39** (suppl B): 1–97.
3. Alghasham AA, Nahata MC. Trovafloxacin: a new fluoroquinolone. *Ann Pharmacother* 1999; **33:** 48–60.

### Preparations

**Proprietary Preparations** (details are given in Part 3)
***Austral.:*** Trovan†; ***Braz.:*** Trovan†; ***Canad.:*** Trovan; ***Hong Kong:*** Trovan†; ***Mex.:*** Trovan†; ***USA:*** Trovan.

## Tylosin *(BAN, rINN)*

Tilosina; Tylosinum.

$C_{46}H_{77}NO_{17}$ = 916.1.

*CAS — 1401-69-0.*

**Pharmacopoeias.** In *Eur.* (see p.vi) and *US*, both for veterinary use.

**Ph. Eur. 5.0** (Tylosin for Veterinary Use; Tylosin BP 2003). A mixture of macrolide antibiotics produced by a strain of *Streptomyces fradiae* or by any other means. The main component of the mixture is tylosin A, but tylosin B (desmycosin), tylosin C (macrocin), and tylosin D (relomycin) may also be present. An almost white or slightly yellow powder. Slightly soluble in water; freely soluble in dehydrated alcohol and in dichloromethane. It dissolves in dilute solutions of mineral acids. A 2.5% suspension in water has a pH of 8.5 to 10.5. Protect from light.

**USP 27** (Tylosin). A macrolide antibiotic substance or mixture of such substances produced by the growth of *Streptomyces fradiae* or by any other means. A white to buff-coloured powder. Slightly soluble in water; soluble in alcohol, in amyl acetate, in chloroform, and in dilute mineral acids; freely soluble in methyl alcohol. It loses not more than 5% of its weight on drying. Protect from light, moisture, and temperatures exceeding 40°.

### Tylosin Tartrate *(BANM, rINNM)*

Tartrato de tilosina.

$(C_{46}H_{77}NO_{17})_2,C_4H_6O_6$ = 1982.3.

*CAS — 1405-54-5.*

**Pharmacopoeias.** In *Eur.* (see p.vi) for veterinary use.

**Ph. Eur. 5.0** (Tylosin Tartrate for Veterinary Use; Tylosin Tartrate BP 2003). An almost white or slightly yellow hygroscopic powder. Freely soluble in water and in dichloromethane; slightly soluble in dehydrated alcohol. It dissolves in dilute solutions of mineral acids. A 2.5% solution in water has a pH of 5.0 to 7.2. Store in airtight containers. Protect from light.

#### Profile

Tylosin is a macrolide antibacterial with actions similar to those of erythromycin (p.208). Tylosin and its phosphate and tartrate salts are used in veterinary medicine in the prophylaxis and treatment of various infections caused by susceptible organisms.

Tylosin and tylosin phosphate have been added to animal feeding stuffs as growth promotors for pigs.

### Tyrothricin *(BAN, rINN)*

Tirotricina; Tyrothricinum.

*CAS — 1404-88-2.*

*ATC — D06AX08; R02AB02; S01AA05.*

**Pharmacopoeias.** In *Eur.* (see p.vi) and *US.*

**Ph. Eur. 5.0** (Tyrothricin). A mixture of antimicrobial linear and cyclic polypeptides, isolated from the fermentation broth of *Bacillus brevis.* It consists mainly of gramicidins and tyrocidins; other related compounds may be present in smaller amounts. The potency is 180 to 280 units/mg, calculated with reference to the dried substance. A white or almost white powder. Practically insoluble in water; soluble in alcohol and in methyl alcohol. Store in airtight containers. Protect from light.

**USP 27** (Tyrothricin). An antibacterial substance produced by the growth of *Bacillus brevis.* It is a mixture consisting chiefly of gramicidin and tyrocidine, the latter being usually present as the hydrochloride. Store in airtight containers.

#### Adverse Effects and Precautions

Tyrothricin is too toxic to be used systemically; effects that have been reported include liver and kidney damage as well as Stevens-Johnson syndrome. It damages the sensory epithelium of the nose and instances of prolonged loss of smell have occurred after its use as a nasal spray or instillation. Tyrothricin should not be instilled into the nasal cavities or into closed body cavities.

#### Uses and Administration

Tyrothricin is unsuitable for systemic use. It is active *in vitro* against many Gram-positive bacteria and has been used either alone or with other antibacterials in the local treatment of infections mainly of the skin and mouth.

#### Preparations

**Proprietary Preparations** (details are given in Part 3)

***Fr.:*** Codetricine; ***Ger.:*** Tyrosur; ***Gr.:*** Triciderm; ***Hong Kong:*** Tyrosur; ***Israel:*** Rafathricin†; ***Ital.:*** Faringotricina; Hydrotricine; Rinotricina; ***Port.:*** Hydrotricine.

**Multi-ingredient:** ***Arg.:*** Aseptobron Caramelos; Biotaer; Biotaer Gamma; Biotaer Nebulizable; Biotaer Ultrason Nebulizable; Bucotricin; Caramelos Antibioticos; Caramelos Antibioticos Bucoangin; Fanaletas; Filotricin A; Fonergine; Gineseptina; Oralsone C; Solumerin; Suavisan; Sulfanoral T; Tavinex; Vagicural; Vagisan; Vagisan Compuesto; Vulnofilin Compuesto; ***Austria:*** Dorithricin; Gingivan; Lemocin; Limexx; Neocones; Sanoral; Tongill; Tonsicur†; Tyrothricin comp; Tyrothricin compositum; ***Belg.:*** Lemocin; Pantricine; Tricidine; Tyro-Drops; ***Braz.:*** Amidalin; Amigdagen; Amigdalol; Amigdamicin; Anapyon†; Anfomicin†; Angi-a-Mid†; Angino Tricin; Anginozetes†; Auritricin; Colpacid†; Colpagex N; Colpolase; Dermosed†; Eucament†; Filogargan†; Gargosedans†; Gargotan†; Gynax-N; Gyrol†; Higienex†; Lacto Vagin; Lacto-Gin†; Laringex; Larintil†; Malvatricin; Mentozil†; Naso Instil†; Neomicina Composta†; Otovix†; Oturga; Passilin†; Rinocron†; Sedauric†; Trivagel N; Vagitrin-N; Varigerm†; Vulgix†; ***Canad.:*** Antibiotic Cold Sore Ointment; Emercreme No 4†; Soropon; ***Fr.:*** Broncorinol rhinites; Bronpax†; Codetricine vitamine C; Collunovar; Ergix; Pharyngine a la Vitamine C†; Solutricine Tetracaine; Solutricine Vitamine C; Tyrcine†; Tyrothricine Lafran†; Veybirol-Tyrothyricine; ***Ger.:*** Anginomycin; Dori†; Dorithricin Limone; Dorithricin Original; Inspirol Halsschmerztabletten; Lemocin; Myacyne†; Nordathricin N; Pellit dermal Wund- und Heilsalbe†; Trachisan; Tyrosur; ***Hong Kong:*** Deq; Trachisan; Tyrocaine; Tyrothricin Co; ***India:*** Tytin; ***Irl.:*** Tyrozets; ***Israel:*** Acnex; Kalgaron; Lemocin; Rafathricin with Benzocaine; ***Ital.:*** Bio-Arscolloid; Deltavagin; Furotricina; Golamixin; Kinogen; Rinocidina; ***Malaysia:*** Deq; Trachisan; Upha Lozenges; ***Port.:*** Afonina†; Mebocaina; Medifon; Mentocaina R; Oralbiotico; Tyrozets†; ***Singapore:*** Beathricin; Deq; Dorithricin; Trachisan; ***Spain:*** Anginovag; Bucometasana; Cicatral; Cohortan; Cohortan Antibiotico†; Diformiltricina; Gradin Del D Andreu; Hemodren Compuesto; Miozets; Neocones; Otosedol Biotico; Oxidermiol Antihist†; Pastillas Koki Ment Tiro; Piorlis; Roberfarin; Sedofarin; Viberol Tirotricina; ***Switz.:*** Lemocin; Mebucaine; Mebucasol f; Otothricinol; Rhinothricinol; Sangerol; Solmucaine; Solutricine†; Trachisan†; Tyrocombine; Tyroqualine; Tyrothricin; Tyrothricine + Gramicidine; ***Thai.:*** Deq; Iwazin; Sigatricin; Trocacin; Troneo; ***UAE:*** B-Cool; ***UK:*** Tyrozets.

### Valnemulin *(rINN)*

Valnemulina; Valnémuline. ({2-[(*R*)-2-Amino-3-methylbutyramido]-1,1-dimethylethyl}thio)acetic acid 8-ester with (3a*S*,4*R*,5*S*,6*S*,8*R*,9*R*,9a*R*,10*R*)-octahydro-5,8-dihydroxy-4,6,9,10-tetramethyl-6-vinyl-3a,9-propano-3a*H*-cyclopentacycloocten-1(4*H*)-one.

$C_{31}H_{52}N_2O_5S$ = 564.8.

*CAS — 101312-92-9.*

#### Profile

Valnemulin is an antibacterial used as the hydrochloride in veterinary medicine.

## Vancomycin *(BAN, rINN)*

($S_a$)-(3*S*,6*R*,7*R*,22*R*,23*S*,26*S*,36*R*,38a*R*)-44-{[2-*O*-(3-Amino-2,3,6-trideoxy-3-*C*-methyl-α-L-*lyxo*-hexopyranosyl)-β-D-glucopyranosyl]oxy}-3-(carbamoylmethyl)-10,19-dichloro-2,3,4,5,6,7,23,24,25,26,36,37,38,38a-tetradecahydro-7,22,28,30,32-pentahydroxy-6-[(2*R*)-4-methyl-2-(methylamino)valeramido]-2,5,24,38,39-pentaoxo-22*H*-8,11:18,21-dietheno-23,36-(iminomethano)-13,16:31,35-dimetheno-1*H*,16*H*-[1,6,9]oxadiazacyclohexadecino[4,5-*m*][10,2,16]-benzoxadiazacyclotetracosine-26-carboxylic acid.

$C_{66}H_{75}Cl_2N_9O_{24}$ = 1449.3.

*CAS — 1404-90-6.*

*ATC — A07AA09; J01XA01.*

**Description.** A glycopeptide antimicrobial substance or mixture of glycopeptides produced by the growth of certain strains of *Amycolatopsis orientalis* (*Nocardia orientalis, Streptomyces orientalis*), or by any other means.

**Pharmacopoeias.** In *US.*

**USP 27** (Vancomycin). Store in airtight containers.

### Vancomycin Hydrochloride *(BANM, rINNM)*

Hidrocloruro de vancomicina; Vancomycini Hydrochloridum.

$C_{66}H_{75}Cl_2N_9O_{24}$,HCl = 1485.7.

*CAS — 1404-93-9.*

*ATC — A07AA09; J01XA01.*

**Pharmacopoeias.** In *Eur.* (see p.vi), *Jpn, Pol.* and *US.*

**Ph. Eur. 5.0** (Vancomycin Hydrochloride). A mixture of related glycopeptides, consisting principally of vancomycin B, a substance produced by certain strains of *Amycolatopsis orientalis* or obtained by any other means. A white or almost white, hygroscopic powder. Freely soluble in water; slightly soluble in alcohol. A 5% solution in water has a pH of 2.5 to 4.5. Store in airtight containers. Protect from light.

**USP 27** (Vancomycin Hydrochloride). A substance or mixture of substances produced by the growth of *Streptomyces orientalis.* A tan to brown, odourless, free-flowing powder. Freely soluble in water; insoluble in chloroform and in ether. A 5% solution in water has a pH of 2.5 to 4.5. Store in airtight containers.

**Incompatibility.** Solutions of vancomycin hydrochloride have an acid pH and incompatibility may reasonably be expected with alkaline preparations, or with drugs unstable at low pH. Reports of incompatibility are not always consistent, and other factors such as the strength of solution, and composition of the vehicles used, may play a part.

**Stability.** Although the manufacturers recommend storage at 2° to 8°, solutions of vancomycin hydrochloride in various diluents (sodium chloride 0.9%, glucose 5%, and peritoneal dialysis solution) have been found to be stable for at least 14 days at room temperature.[1-3]

The stability of vancomycin in ophthalmic solution has also been studied.[4]


1. Das Gupta V, *et al.* Stability of vancomycin hydrochloride in 5% dextrose and 0.9% sodium chloride injections. *Am J Hosp Pharm* 1986; **43:** 1729–31.
2. Walker SE, Birkhans B. Stability of intravenous vancomycin. *Can J Hosp Pharm* 1988; **41:** 233–8.
3. Mauhinuey WM, *et al.* Stability of vancomycin hydrochloride in peritoneal dialysis solution. *Am J Hosp Pharm* 1992; **49:** 137–9.
4. Fuhrman LC, Stroman RT. Stability of vancomycin in an extemporaneously compounded ophthalmic solution. *Am J Health-Syst Pharm* 1998; **55:** 1386–8.


### Adverse Effects

The intravenous use of vancomycin may be associated with the so-called 'red-neck' or 'red-man' syndrome, characterised by erythema, flushing, or rash over the face and upper torso, and sometimes by hypotension and shock-like symptoms. The effect appears to be due in part to the release of histamine and is usually related to rapid infusion.

Hypersensitivity reactions may occur in about 5% of patients and include rashes, fever, chills, and rarely, anaphylactoid reactions, exfoliative dermatitis, Stevens-Johnson syndrome, toxic epidermal necrolysis, and vasculitis. Many reactions have become less frequent with the availability of more highly purified preparations. Reversible neutropenia, eosinophilia, and rarely thrombocytopenia and agranulocytosis have been reported; neutropenia is stated to be more common in patients who have received a total dose of 25 g or more. Nephrotoxicity, including rare cases of interstitial nephritis, may occur, particularly at high doses or in patients with predisposing factors, but has declined in frequency with greater awareness of the problem and appropriate monitoring of plasma concentrations and renal function.

Ototoxicity is also associated with vancomycin, and is more likely in patients with high plasma concentrations, or with renal impairment or pre-existing hearing loss.. It may progress after drug withdrawal, and may be irreversible. Hearing loss may be preceded by tinnitus, which must be regarded as a sign to discontinue treatment.

Vancomycin is irritant; intravenous use may be associated with thrombophlebitis, although this can be minimised by the slow infusion of dilute solutions, and by using different infusion sites. Extravasation may cause tissue necrosis.

Because of its poor absorption, relatively few adverse effects have been reported after the oral use of vancomycin, although mild gastrointestinal disturbances have occurred.

**Effects on the ears.** Reviews[1,2] of ototoxicity associated with vancomycin therapy have indicated that the actual number of cases is quite small, and close examination suggests that in most cases where hearing loss occurred patients had also received an aminoglycoside. The degree, and the reversibility, of ototoxicity associated with vancomycin alone is uncertain.


1. Bailie GR, Neal D. Vancomycin ototoxicity and nephrotoxicity: a review. *Med Toxicol* 1988; **3:** 376–86.
2. Brummett RE, Fox KE. Vancomycin- and erythromycin-induced hearing loss in humans. *Antimicrob Agents Chemother* 1989; **33:** 791–6.


**Effects on the gastrointestinal tract.** A 25-year-old woman developed *Clostridium difficile* colitis following a course of vancomycin and metronidazole, both by mouth, for pelvic inflammatory disease.[1] The condition resolved after treatment with vancomycin given alone.


1. Bingley PJ, Harding GM. Clostridium difficile colitis following treatment with metronidazole and vancomycin. *Postgrad Med J* 1987; **63:** 993–4.


**Effects on the heart.** A report[1] of cardiac arrest associated with inadvertent and rapid intravenous administration of vancomycin 150 mg to a neonate.


1. Boussemart T, *et al.* Cardiac arrest associated with vancomycin in a neonate. *Arch Dis Child* 1995; **73:** F123.


**Effects on the kidneys.** In a study,[1] nephrotoxicity was seen in 14 of 101 patients assigned to vancomycin 1 g before and after vascular surgery for infection prophylaxis compared with 2 of 99 assigned to saline placebo, suggesting that even short regimens of vancomycin can affect renal function. In another study involving 224 patients, nephrotoxicity was seen in 8 of 168 given vancomycin alone, 14 of 63 given vancomycin with an aminoglycoside, and 11 of 103 given an aminoglycoside without vancomycin.[2] This latter study found that concomitant aminoglycoside therapy, trough serum concentrations of vancomycin greater than 10 micrograms/mL, and prolonged vancomycin therapy (for more than 21 days) were associated with an increased risk of nephrotoxicity. In both studies nephrotoxicity was defined in terms of increased serum creatinine.


1. Gudmundsson GH, Jensen LJ. Vancomycin and nephrotoxicity. *Lancet* 1989; **i:** 625.
2. Rybak MJ, *et al.* Nephrotoxicity of vancomycin, alone and with an aminoglycoside. *J Antimicrob Chemother* 1990; **25:** 679–87.


**Effects on the nervous system.** Reports of encephalopathy[1] (associated with high CSF concentrations after oral administration) and peripheral neuropathy[2] associated with vancomycin.


1. Thompson CM, *et al.* Absorption of oral vancomycin—possible associated toxicity. *Int J Pediatr Nephrol* 1983; **4:** 1–4.
2. Leibowitz G, *et al.* Mononeuritis multiplex associated with prolonged vancomycin treatment. *BMJ* 1990; **300:** 1344.


**Effects on the skin.** Rashes, erythema, or pruritus are the most common skin reactions associated with vancomycin but there have also been reports of linear IgA dermatosis,[1-4] Stevens-Johnson-like reaction,[5] bullous eruption,[6] and exfoliative dermatitis.[6] In an analysis, risk factors for adverse cutaneous reactions were suggested to be age under 40 years and duration of therapy greater than 7 days.[6]


1. Piketty C, *et al.* Linear IgA dermatosis related to vancomycin. *Br J Dermatol* 1994; **130:** 130–1.
2. Nousari HC, *et al.* Vancomycin-associated linear IgA bullous dermatosis. *Ann Intern Med* 1998; **129:** 507–8.
3. Bernstein EF, Schuster M. Linear IgA bullous dermatosis associated with vancomycin. *Ann Intern Med* 1998; **129:** 508–9.
4. Danielsen AG, Thomsen K. Vancomycin-induced linear IgA bullous disease. *Br J Dermatol* 1999; **141:** 756–7.
5. Laurencin CT, *et al.* Stevens-Johnson-like reaction with vancomycin treatment. *Ann Pharmacother* 1992; **26:** 1520–1.
6. Korman TM, *et al.* Risk factors for adverse cutaneous reactions associated with intravenous vancomycin. *J Antimicrob Chemother* 1997; **39:** 371–81.


**Red-man syndrome.** References[1-3] to the 'red-man syndrome', and evidence that pretreatment with an antihistamine can provide significant protection against it.[4,5] Similar reactions appear to be much less of a problem with teicoplanin and substitution of teicoplanin for vancomycin may be a viable alternative in patients at risk.[2,3,6] Skin tests are reported[7] to be of little value in predicting the severity of 'red-man syndrome'.

1. Wallace MR, *et al.* Red man syndrome: incidence, etiology, and prophylaxis. *J Infect Dis* 1991; **164:** 1180–5.
2. Polk RE. Anaphylactoid reactions to glycopeptide antibiotics. *J Antimicrob Chemother* 1991; **27** (suppl B): 17–29.
3. Rybak MJ, *et al.* Absence of "red man syndrome" in patients being treated with vancomycin or high-dose teicoplanin. *Antimicrob Agents Chemother* 1992; **36:** 1204–7.
4. Renz CL, *et al.* Oral antihistamines reduce the side effects from rapid vancomycin infusion. *Anesth Analg* 1998; **87:** 681–5.
5. Renz CL, *et al.* Antihistamine prophylaxis permits rapid vancomycin infusion. *Crit Care Med* 1999; **27:** 1732–7.
6. Smith SR. Vancomycin and histamine release. *Lancet* 1990; **335:** 1341.
7. Polk RE, *et al.* Vancomycin skin tests and prediction of "red man syndrome" in healthy volunteers. *Antimicrob Agents Chemother* 1993; **37:** 2139–43.

AFTER ORAL ADMINISTRATION. Reports of rash[1] and 'red-man syndrome'[2,3] following oral vancomycin.

1. McCullough JM, *et al.* Oral vancomycin-induced rash: case report and review of the literature. *DICP Ann Pharmacother* 1991; **25:** 1326–8.
2. Killian AD, *et al.* Red man syndrome after oral vancomycin. *Ann Intern Med* 1991; **115:** 410–11.
3. Bergeron L, Boucher FD. Possible red-man syndrome associated with systemic absorption of oral vancomycin in a child with normal renal function. *Ann Pharmacother* 1994; **28:** 581–4.

## Precautions

Vancomycin should not be given to patients who have experienced a hypersensitivity reaction to it. It should not be given intramuscularly, and care should be taken when it is given intravenously to avoid extravasation, because of the risk of tissue necrosis. The adverse effects of infusion may be minimised by dilution of each 500 mg of vancomycin in at least 100 mL of fluid, and by infusion of doses over not less than 60 minutes.

Because the risk of ototoxicity and nephrotoxicity is thought to be increased at high plasma concentrations it may be desirable to adjust dosage requirements according to plasma-vancomycin concentrations. It has been suggested that dosage should be adjusted to avoid peak plasma concentrations above 30 to 40 micrograms/mL and trough concentrations exceeding 10 micrograms/mL, although uncertainty about the optimum methods and sampling times for monitoring, as well as some uncertainty about the degree of risk, means that there is less general agreement than for the aminoglycosides. It is generally agreed, however, that vancomycin should be avoided in patients with a history of impaired hearing and that particular care is necessary in patients with renal impairment, in neonates (especially if premature), and in the elderly, all of whom may be at increased risk of toxicity. Renal function and blood counts should be monitored regularly in all patients, and monitoring of auditory function is advisable, especially in high-risk patients. Vancomycin should be discontinued in patients who develop tinnitus.

Since vancomycin is poorly absorbed, toxicity is much less of a problem following oral use than with the intravenous route, but care is required in patients with inflammatory gastrointestinal disorders, including antibiotic-associated colitis, in whom absorption may be enhanced.

## Interactions

Other ototoxic or nephrotoxic drugs, such as aminoglycosides, polymyxins, cisplatin, and loop diuretics, markedly increase the risk of toxicity and should be given with vancomycin only with great caution.

Some of the adverse effects of vancomycin may be enhanced by the use of general anaesthetics; it has been suggested that, where patients require both, vancomycin infusions should be completed before the induction of anaesthesia.

Vancomycin may increase neuromuscular blockade produced by drugs such as suxamethonium or vecuronium.

## Antimicrobial Action

Vancomycin is a glycopeptide antibiotic with a primarily bactericidal action against a variety of Gram-positive bacteria.

*Mechanism of action.* Vancomycin exerts its action by inhibiting the formation of the peptidoglycan polymers of the bacterial cell wall. Unlike penicillins, which act primarily to prevent the cross-linking of peptidoglycans which gives the cell wall its strength, vancomycin prevents the transfer and addition of the muramylpentapeptide building blocks that make up the peptidoglycan molecule itself. Vancomycin may also exert some effects by damaging the cytoplasmic membrane of the protoplast, and by inhibiting bacterial RNA synthesis.

*Spectrum of activity.* Staphylococci, notably *Staph. aureus* and *Staph. epidermidis* (including meticillin-resistant strains), *Streptococcus pneumoniae, Str. pyogenes*, and some strains of Group B streptococci are reported to be susceptible to vancomycin. The viridans streptococci, and enterococci such as *Enterococcus faecalis*, are often 'tolerant', i.e. inhibition, but no bactericidal effect, can be achieved at usual plasma concentrations (but see Activity with other Antimicrobials and Resistance, below).

*Clostridium difficile* is usually highly susceptible as are most other clostridia. *Actinomyces* spp., *Bacillus anthracis, Corynebacterium* spp., some lactobacilli, and *Listeria* are usually susceptible. Virtually all Gram-negative organisms, as well as mycobacteria and fungi, are intrinsically resistant.

*Activity with other antimicrobials.* Vancomycin exhibits synergy with the aminoglycosides against enterococci; such combinations are usually bactericidal, even against vancomycin-tolerant strains. The synergistic effect is reported to be greater with gentamicin than with streptomycin. Combinations with an aminoglycoside are also reported to demonstrate synergy against *Staph. aureus*; however, variable results, including antimicrobial antagonism, or lack of synergy, have been reported against strains of *Staph. aureus* when vancomycin was combined with rifampicin. Synergy has been reported with the third-generation cephalosporins against *Staph. aureus* and enterococci.

*Resistance* to vancomycin in normally susceptible organisms has until recently remained relatively uncommon, although high-level intrinsic resistance has been seen in some species of *Lactobacillus, Leuconostoc*, and *Erysipelothrix*. However, there are an increasing number of reports of high-level acquired resistance amongst enterococci, apparently plasmid-mediated and transferable to other Gram-positive organisms, notably *Staph. aureus*, which are causing considerable concern. Organisms exhibiting high-level vancomycin resistance demonstrate cross-resistance to teicoplanin. Low-level resistance has also been reported in enterococci, but these organisms remain sensitive to teicoplanin, and this form of resistance does not appear to be transferable. Low-level vancomycin resistance has also been seen rarely among some staphylococcal strains: in contrast to the enterococci, these are often cross-resistant to teicoplanin. The mechanism of acquired resistance is uncertain, although it appears to be associated with the development of novel cell-membrane proteins.

◊ Reference[1] to increasing resistance to vancomycin amongst enterococci and *Staphylococcus aureus*,[2-8] and guidelines to prevent its spread.[9,10]

1. Murray BE. Vancomycin-resistant enterococci. *Am J Med* 1997; **102:** 284–93.
2. Hiramatsu K, *et al.* Methicillin-resistant Staphylococcus aureus clinical strain with reduced vancomycin susceptibility. *J Antimicrob Chemother* 1997; **40:** 135–6.
3. Johnson AP. Intermediate vancomycin resistance in Staphylococcus aureus: a major threat or a minor inconvenience? *J Antimicrob Chemother* 1998; **42:** 289–91.
4. Ploy MC, *et al.* First clinical isolate of vancomycin-intermediate Staphylococcus aureus in a French hospital. *Lancet* 1998; **351:** 1212.
5. Smith TL, *et al.* Emergence of vancomycin resistance in Staphylococcus aureus. *N Engl J Med* 1999; **340:** 493–501.
6. Sieradzki K, *et al.* The development of vancomycin resistance in a patient with methicillin-resistant Staphylococcus aureus infection. *N Engl J Med* 1999; **340:** 517–23.
7. Hiramatsu K. Vancomycin-resistant Staphylococcus aureus: a new model of antibiotic resistance. *Lancet Infect Dis* 2001; **1:** 147–55.
8. Chang S, *et al.* Infection with vancomycin-resistant Staphylococcus aureus containing the VanA resistance gene. *N Engl J Med* 2003; **348:** 1342–7.
9. Hospital Infection Control Practices Advisory Committee (HICPAC). Recommendations for preventing the spread of vancomycin resistance. *Infect Control Hosp Epidemiol* 1995; **16:** 105–13.
10. Edmond MB, *et al.* Vancomycin-resistant Staphylococcus aureus: perspectives on measures needed for control. *Ann Intern Med* 1996; **124:** 329–34.

## Pharmacokinetics

Vancomycin is only poorly absorbed from the gastrointestinal tract, although absorption may be somewhat greater when the gastrointestinal tract is inflamed. Infusion of a 1-g dose intravenously over 60 minutes has reportedly been associated with plasma concentrations of up to about 60 micrograms/mL immediately after completion of the infusion, and about 25 micrograms/mL 2 hours later, falling to under 10 micrograms/mL after 11 hours. However, there may be considerable interindividual variation in the pharmacokinetics of vancomycin: a range of half-lives between 3 and 13 hours has been reported, with an average of about 6 hours, in patients with normal renal function. Half-life may be prolonged in patients with renal impairment, to 7 days or more in anephric patients. About 55% is bound to plasma proteins, although large variations have been reported.

Vancomycin diffuses into extracellular fluid, including pleural, pericardial, ascitic, and synovial fluid. Small amounts are found in bile. However, there is little diffusion into the CSF and even when the meninges are inflamed effective concentrations may not be achieved. Vancomycin crosses the peritoneal cavity; about 60% of an intraperitoneal dose is reported to be absorbed in 6 hours. It is reported to cross the placenta. It is also distributed into breast milk.

Little or no metabolism of vancomycin is thought to take place. It is excreted unchanged by the kidneys, mostly by glomerular filtration. Some 80 to 90% of the dose is excreted in urine within 24 hours. There appears to be a small amount of non-renal clearance, although the mechanism for this has not been determined.

The pharmacokinetics of vancomycin may be altered by conditions which affect renal clearance: clearance of vancomycin has been reported to be enhanced in burn patients, whereas in those with renal impairment, or reduced renal function (such as neonates or the elderly), clearance is reduced and plasma-concentrations and half-lives increased. Dosage adjustment is often necessary in patients with reduced or impaired renal function; ideally, this should be based on plasma-concentration monitoring. Although clearance is also altered in hepatic impairment, it has been suggested that dosage adjustment is not necessary in the absence of other factors.

Plasma concentrations of vancomycin are reported to be little affected by conventional haemodialysis, although the use of high-flux membranes may significantly reduce vancomycin concentrations. Peritoneal dialysis, although it may decrease concentrations, is also thought not to do so by significant amounts, but haemoperfusion or haemofiltration effectively removes vancomycin from the blood.

## Uses and Administration

Vancomycin is a glycopeptide antibiotic that is used in the treatment of serious staphylococcal or other Gram-positive infections when other drugs such as the penicillins cannot be used because of resistance or patient intolerance. It is used particularly in the treatment of meticillin-resistant staphylococcal infections (p.147), in conditions such as brain abscess, staphylococcal meningitis, peritonitis associated with continuous ambulatory peritoneal dialysis, and septicaemia. It is used alone, or with another drug such as an aminoglycoside, in the treatment and prophylaxis of endocarditis, for the prophylaxis of surgical infection, and in intensive care and the management of immunocompromised patients. It is also used (by mouth) in the treatment of antibiotic-associated colitis (see under Gastro-enteritis, p.128). For details of all these infections and their treatment, see under Choice of Antibacterial, p.120.

Vancomycin may be used with other antibacterials to extend the spectrum of efficacy or increase effectiveness, notably with gentamicin or other aminoglycosides, or with rifampicin (but see Antimicrobial Action, above).

*Administration and dosage.* Vancomycin is given as the hydrochloride but doses are expressed in terms of the base. 1.03 g of vancomycin hydrochloride is approximately equivalent to 1 g of vancomycin. It is given intravenously, preferably by intermittent infusion, although continuous infusion has been used. For intermittent infusion, a concentrated solution containing the equivalent of 500 mg of vancomycin in 10 mL of water is prepared and then added to glucose 5% or sodium chloride 0.9% to produce a diluted solution containing not more than 5 mg/mL; this diluted solution is then infused over at least 60 minutes for a 500-mg dose or 100 minutes for a 1-g dose. Final concentrations of up to 10 mg/mL may be used for patients requiring fluid restriction, although there is an increased risk of adverse events. For continuous intravenous infusion when intermittent infusion is not feasible, the equivalent of 1 to 2 g is added to a sufficiently large volume of glucose or sodium chloride to permit the daily dose to be given over a period of 24 hours.

The usual adult dose is the equivalent of 500 mg of vancomycin every 6 hours or 1 g every 12 hours. Response is generally seen within 48 to 72 hours in sensitive infections. In patients with staphylococcal endocarditis, treatment for at least 3 weeks has been recommended.

For the prophylaxis of endocarditis in high-risk patients undergoing dental or other procedures who are unable to receive penicillin, vancomycin may be given before the procedure in a single dose of 1 g by intravenous infusion over at least 100 minutes followed by intravenous gentamicin.

*Doses in infants and children.* Children and infants over 1 month of age may be given 10 mg/kg every 6 hours. Neonates and infants up to 1 month old may be given an initial dose of 15 mg/kg; this is followed by 10 mg/kg every 12 hours in the first week of life or by 10 mg/kg every 8 hours in those aged 1 week to 1 month.

For the prophylaxis of endocarditis in children up to 10 years, a single dose of 20 mg/kg may be used.

*Dose adjustment and monitoring.* It has been recommended that dosage should be adjusted if necessary according to plasma-vancomycin concentrations, and this is particularly important where factors such as age or renal impairment (see also below) may predispose to toxicity, or where there is a risk of subtherapeutic concentrations. There has been some dispute about the relationship between plasma concentrations and toxicity, and this, complicated by differences in the sampling time after the end of infusion and by differences in the regimens administered and assay method used, has meant that suggested peak and trough concentrations have varied considerably. However, in order to avoid toxic concentrations immediately after the end of infusion the consensus appears to be that concentrations of not more than 30 to 40 micrograms/mL should be aimed for 1 to 2 hours after completion of infusion. It is usually recommended that trough concentrations (measured just before the next dose) should be below 10 micrograms/mL.

*Other routes.* Vancomycin hydrochloride is given by mouth in the treatment of staphylococcal enterocolitis and antibiotic-associated colitis, including pseudomembranous colitis associated with the overgrowth of *Clostridium difficile*. It is given in a dose of 0.5 to 2 g daily in 3 or 4 divided doses for 7 to 10 days; the lowest dose of 500 mg daily is often considered adequate. The manufacturers' suggested dose for children is 40 mg/kg daily in 3 or 4 divided doses; the *British National Formulary* considers that half this dose is adequate.

In meningitis or other CNS infections, vancomycin has sometimes been given by the intrathecal or intraventricular route in order to ensure adequate CSF concentrations of antibiotic. Vancomycin has also been applied topically to the eye or given by subconjunctival or intravitreal injection; it has also been given by inhalation.

◊ Reviews.

1. Wilhelm MP, Estes L. Vancomycin. *Mayo Clin Proc* 1999; **74:** 928–35.

**Administration in renal impairment.** Various methods, including predictive nomograms based on creatinine clearance and pharmacokinetic methods such as those using Bayesian statistics, have been suggested for calculating vancomycin dosage requirements in patients with reduced renal function. One suggested approach has been a loading dose of 15 mg/kg followed by a daily dose in mg equivalent to about 15 times the glomerular filtration rate in mL/minute; or in anuric patients a dose of 1 g every 7 to 10 days. However, individualised dosage based on plasma concentrations is generally to be preferred.

## Preparations

***BP 2003:*** Vancomycin Injection;
***USP 27:*** Sterile Vancomycin Hydrochloride; Vancomycin Hydrochloride Capsules; Vancomycin Hydrochloride for Injection; Vancomycin Hydrochloride for Oral Solution; Vancomycin Injection.

**Proprietary Preparations** (details are given in Part 3)
***Arg.:*** Icoplax; Rivervan; Vancocin; Vancomax; Vancotenk; Varedet; ***Austral.:*** Vancocin; Vancoled†; ***Belg.:*** Vancocin; ***Braz.:*** Biovancomin; Vanclomin; Vancoabbott; Vancocid; Vancocina; Vancoplus; Vancoson; ***Canad.:*** Vancocin; ***Chile:*** Kovan; Vancocina; ***Denm.:*** Vancocin; ***Fin.:*** Orivan; Vancocin; ***Fr.:*** Vancocine; ***Ger.:*** Vanco; Vanco-saar; ***Gr.:*** Voncon; ***Hong Kong:*** Lyphocin; Vanco-Teva†; Vancocin; ***India:*** Vancocin; ***Irl.:*** Vancocin; ***Israel:*** Vanco-Teva; Vancocin; Vancoled; ***Ital.:*** Copovan; Vanco; Vancocina; Zengac; ***Malaysia:*** Vancocin; ***Mex.:*** Balcoran†; Ifavac; Vanaurus; Vancam; Vancocin; Vancox; Vanmicina†; ***Neth.:*** Vancocin; ***Norw.:*** Vancocin; ***NZ:*** Vancocin; ***Port.:*** Glipep; Vancocina; ***S.Afr.:*** Vancocin; ***Spain:*** Diatracin; ***Swed.:*** Vancocin; Vancoscand; ***Switz.:*** Vancocin; Vancoled†; ***Thai.:*** Edicin; Vancocin; ***UAE:*** Vancolan; ***UK:*** Vancocin; ***USA:*** Lyphocin; Vancocin; Vancoled.

## Virginiamycin *(BAN, USAN, rINN)*

Antibiotic 899; SKF-7988; Virgimycin; Virginiamicina.

*CAS — 11006-76-1; 21411-53-0 (virginiamycin $M_1$); 23152-29-6 (virginiamycin $S_1$).*

*ATC — D06AX10.*

### Profile

Virginiamycin is a streptogramin antibacterial mixture consisting principally of 2 antimicrobial substances, virginiamycin $M_1$, and virginiamycin $S_1$, produced by the growth of *Streptomyces virginiae*. It has been used for the treatment of infections due to sensitive organisms, particularly Gram-positive cocci. It has been given by mouth and applied locally. It may cause gastrointestinal disturbances including diarrhoea and vomiting. A few instances of hypersensitivity have been observed.

Virginiamycin has been used in animal feeding stuffs as a growth promotor.

### Preparations

**Proprietary Preparations** (details are given in Part 3)

**Multi-ingredient:** ***Belg.:*** Spitalen.

## Xibornol *(BAN, rINN)*

CP3H; 1HP; 1BX. 6-(Isoborn-2-yl)-3,4-xylenol; 6-[(1R,2S,4S)-Born-2-yl]-3,4-xylenol.

$C_{18}H_{26}O$ = 258.4.

*CAS — 38237-68-2; 13741-18-9.*

*ATC — J01XX02.*

### Profile

Xibornol is an antimicrobial that is reported to have a bacteriostatic action on Gram-positive organisms such as staphylococci and streptococci, as well as activity against *Haemophilus influenzae*. It has been given by mouth in doses of 1 to 1.5 g daily; it has also been given as an oral spray and rectally.

### Preparations

**Proprietary Preparations** (details are given in Part 3)
***Fr.:*** Nanbacine†; ***Ital.:*** Bornilene.

**Multi-ingredient:** ***Spain:*** Xibornol Prodes†.

# Antidepressants

Bipolar disorder, p.278
Depression, p.279
Mania, p.280

This chapter describes drugs used principally in the treatment of affective disorders. Affective disorders are disorders of mood that may manifest as *depression* or *mania* or, in some cases, as *mixed affective states* in which depressive and manic episodes may coexist or alternate.

- The core features of *depressive disorders* are low mood, anhedonia (the loss of interest in former pleasures or activities), pessimism, and lethargy. They were formerly classified either as *endogenous*, in which the symptoms were independent of external factors and considered to be a consequence of factors within the patient, or *reactive*, in which depressive symptoms were a result of external stressors (i.e. exogenous). It is now recognised that depressive disorders are composed of both endogenous and reactive factors. Similarly, the classification of *neurotic depression* is no longer considered useful because it encompasses several different syndromes.

  Depressive episodes are classified according to severity as mild, moderate, severe, or severe with psychosis. *Recurrent brief depression* is defined as depressive episodes of a few days' duration that recur regularly. Depression is often accompanied by characteristic *somatic* symptoms, including anorexia, weight loss, insomnia, early morning waking, and psychomotor retardation. Symptoms associated with *atypical depression* include overeating and oversleeping.
- The main symptoms of *mania* are overactivity, mood changes ranging from elation to irritability, expansive ideas, and inflated self-importance. Manic episodes are classified according to severity in a similar manner to depressive disorders: namely, mild, moderate, severe, or severe with psychosis. *Hypomania* is differentiated from mania in terms of a reduction in intensity of symptoms and social incapacity.
- Alternating episodes of mania and depression are termed *bipolar disorder*. Since it is very rare for repeated episodes of mania to occur without alternating episodes of depression, it is accepted practice to include mania without depression within the bipolar category. The term *unipolar disorder* (*unipolar depression*) is reserved for depressive disorders without mania.
- States of persistent but mild disturbances of mood exist in which the symptoms are not severe enough to meet the criteria for classification as a major depressive or hypomanic disorder, but may nevertheless cause considerable suffering to the patient. *Dysthymia* is the term used to describe a chronic depressive state whereas *cyclothymia* has some similarity to bipolar disorder, the instability characterised by long periods of milder elation and milder depression.
- The term *seasonal affective disorder* has been applied to depressive disorders repeatedly occurring seasonally, but not related to seasonal stressful life events; the depressive symptoms usually occur during the autumn and winter months. There have also been reports of patients developing seasonal bipolar disorder with hypomania or mania occurring in the summer months.
- Anxiety is often associated with depressive disorders at all levels of severity and it may be difficult to distinguish between the two conditions, especially in the milder forms. *Mixed anxiety and depressive disorder* defines a state in which anxiety and depressive symptoms coexist but neither component is severe enough to merit classification as an anxiety disorder or a depressive disorder.

**Classification of antidepressants.** Antidepressants are classified into different groups either structurally or depending on which central neurotransmitters they act upon. The older tricyclic (e.g. amitriptyline) and related cyclic antidepressants and the monoamine oxidase inhibitors (MAOIs) (e.g. phenelzine) have now been joined by the selective serotonin reuptake inhibitors (SSRIs) (e.g. fluoxetine), the reversible inhibitors of monoamine oxidase type A (RIMAs) (e.g. moclobemide), and more recently by the serotonin and noradrenaline reuptake inhibitors (SNRIs) (e.g. venlafaxine). Other antidepressants that do not fit exactly into these groups include bupropion, the herbal preparation hypericum (St John's wort), mirtazapine, nefazodone, reboxetine, and trazodone.

Lithium salts provide a source of lithium ions that compete with sodium ions at various sites in the body and thus have an action and side-effects distinct and separate from those of other antidepressants.

## Bipolar disorder

Bipolar disorder (manic depression) is a mixed affective disorder in which the patient experiences alternating episodes of hypomania or mania and depression. Although isolated episodes of mania may occur, they are more usually part of bipolar disorder; for the purposes of classification, mania without depression is therefore included in the bipolar category. Bipolar disorder is usually treated with mood-stabilising drugs, the most important of which is lithium although some antiepileptic drugs are also used. ECT is also effective and is used for example in patients for whom lithium treatment is unsuitable or in patients refractory to lithium or other drugs.

Drug therapy of the **manic phase** is directed at controlling the acute attack, maintaining that response, and preventing further attacks. Lithium is effective in acute mania but it may take a few days before an antimanic effect is seen. Treatment in acutely manic patients with coexisting psychotic features, agitation, or disruptive behaviour is therefore usually begun with an antipsychotic to produce a rapid tranquillising effect; traditionally, drugs such as the phenothiazine chlorpromazine and the butyrophenone haloperidol have been used, although the atypical antipsychotics such as olanzapine are now becoming more widely used. Clozapine may be useful in refractory mania although its use is restricted by adverse effects. Both olanzapine and clozapine are also considered to have antimanic actions. The antipsychotic may be used with lithium, and then gradually withdrawn once lithium becomes effective, but the risks from interactions between antipsychotics and lithium (see under Interactions of Lithium, p.303) should be borne in mind. Alternatively, lithium therapy may be postponed until the acute attack has been stabilised with the antipsychotic. Benzodiazepines are also used in manic patients with coexisting agitation or insomnia until lithium has achieved its full effect; they should not be used for long periods owing to the risk of dependence. Valproate is also effective in acute mania (see below).

Once the acute phase has been brought under control drug treatment should continue until it is safe to expect that the patient will not suffer a relapse; this might entail **maintaining treatment** for several months. High doses of lithium are usually required to control the acute phase, but as the margin between the therapeutic and the toxic concentration of lithium is narrow, the dose should be reduced to maintenance levels as soon as practicable. Regular monitoring of serum concentrations of lithium is essential during the initial and maintenance phases of therapy to minimise the risks of lithium toxicity (see under Pharmacokinetics of Lithium, p.304).

The treatment of the subsequent **depressive phase** of bipolar disorder depends on the severity of the depression and whether psychotic symptoms are still present. In some milder cases optimal therapy with lithium may suffice, as lithium itself possesses antidepressant activity; however in more severe cases or in those receiving only an antipsychotic, additional antidepressant therapy may be required. Treatment with antidepressants is essentially similar to that of unipolar depression (see below), but extra care is needed because antidepressants may precipitate hypomania or mania. Antidepressants have also been implicated in the induction of rapid cycling, in which there are four or more affective episodes in a year. Some recommend that, if an antidepressant is needed, it should be given in the lowest effective dose and for the shortest time possible; it should not be given long term without the cover of a mood-stabilising drug. Bupropion is the antidepressant of choice of many clinicians in the USA; SSRIs are also an alternative. Tricyclic antidepressants should only be used with caution and data for the newer antidepressants such as nefazodone and venlafaxine are limited. MAOIs may be less likely to induce mania than other antidepressants, but troublesome side-effects and safety issues have limited their use to second-line. ECT is a valuable alternative and should be considered for bipolar depression.

Patients with recurrent episodes of bipolar disorder may require **prophylactic therapy** with lithium. Sometimes prophylaxis may be instituted following treatment of a first episode where there is an expectation of repeated attacks. Lithium prophylaxis usually entails extending the maintenance treatment and continuing to monitor serum concentrations as before; it may need to be continued for a prolonged period. Some have also given antipsychotics, either alone or with lithium, for prophylaxis.

When lithium therapy is to be discontinued, withdrawal should be gradual over a period of weeks to allay any concerns about relapse.

**Alternative mood-stabilisers** to lithium are antiepileptics such as carbamazepine and valproate. Valproate is effective in the treatment of acute mania and in the maintenance and prophylactic phases. In some countries the use of valproate as first-line therapy is increasing although others still prefer to use lithium initially, despite its side-effects, as there is more reliable evidence for its use. However, it is generally agreed that valproate should be used in those who fail to respond to lithium or in whom it causes serious adverse effects; in addition valproate may be the first choice in rapid cycling bipolar disorder, for which it is particularly effective, and in mixed or dysphoric states. The efficacy of carbamazepine is not as well established although it too may have a role in those patients with non-classical features. Some commentators suggest that its use is falling out of favour with specialists treating bipolar disorder. If patients fail to respond after several weeks of therapy with a mood stabiliser then a different one should be substituted, with gradual tapering of the first drug. If there is only a partial response after several weeks then a second mood stabiliser may be added. For example carbamazepine or valproate may be added to existing lithium therapy or alternatively lithium can be added to treatment with carbamazepine or valproate. Some of the newer antiepileptics such as gabapentin, lamotrigine, and topiramate are also being investigated.

References.

1. Silverstone T, Romans S. Long term treatment of bipolar disorder. *Drugs* 1996; **51:** 367–82.
2. The Expert Consensus Panel for Bipolar Disorder. Treatment of bipolar disorder. *J Clin Psychiatry* 1996; **57:** (suppl 12A): 1–89.
3. Daly I. Mania. *Lancet* 1997; **349:** 1157–60.
4. Bauer MS, *et al.* Clinical practice guidelines for bipolar disorder from the Department of Veterans Affairs. *J Clin Psychiatry* 1999; **60:** 9–21.
5. Sachs GS, *et al.* The expert consensus guideline series: medication treatment of bipolar disorder 2000. *Postgrad Med* 2000; **Apr** (spec no): 1–104. Also available at: http://www.psychguides.com/Bipolar_2000.pdf (accessed 04/06/04)
6. Berk M, *et al.* Emerging options in the treatment of bipolar disorders. *Drugs* 2001; **61:** 1407–14.
7. Ferrier IN. Developments in mood stabilisers. *Br Med Bull* 2001; **57:** 179–92.
8. Müller-Oerlinghausen B, *et al.* Bipolar disorder. *Lancet* 2002; **359:** 241–7.
9. American Psychiatric Association. Practice guideline for the treatment of patients with bipolar disorder (revision). *Am J Psychiatry* 2002; **159** (suppl): 1–50. Also available at: http://www.psych.org/psych_pract/treatg/pg/bipolar_revisebook_index.cfm (accessed 04/06/04)
10. Grunze H, *et al.* World Federation of Societies of Biological Psychiatry (WFSBP) guidelines for biological treatment of bipolar disorders, part I: treatment of bipolar depression. *World J Biol Psychiatry* 2002; **3:** 115–24.
11. Grunze H, *et al.* World Federation of Societies of Biological Psychiatry (WFSBP) guidelines for biological treatment of bipolar disorders, part II: treatment of mania. *World J Biol Psychiatry* 2003; **4:** 5–13.
12. National Institute for Clinical Excellence. Olanzapine and valproate semisodium in the treatment of acute mania associated with bipolar I disorder (issued September 2003). Available at: http://www.nice.org.uk/pdf/66_bipolardisorder_fullguidance.pdf (accessed 04/06/04)

## Depression

Clinical depression (unipolar depression) is a disturbance of mood that is distinguishable from the usual mood fluctuations of everyday life. A depressed mood is usually the major symptom, which may be accompanied by other mental or somatic symptoms representing several depressive syndromes.

The aetiology of depression is unknown but it may represent an interaction between psychological and biochemical mechanisms rather than any single factor. The symptoms appear to be mediated through alterations in levels of some central neurotransmitters, although it is not certain that this represents a cause of the disorder. However, it is at this level that the antidepressant drugs currently in clinical use exert their action.

Approaches to the treatment of depression depend on the severity of the condition and the risks to the patient, as summarised in consensus statements and guidelines in the UK[1,2] and the USA.[3,4] Some guidelines in the UK[5] and the USA[6] have recently been revised. Although the most common form of treatment is with an antidepressant, other forms of therapy may also be of value in some situations. Psychosocial or psychotherapeutic management may be effective alone in mild depressive disorders or may be used with antidepressants[1,3] or following ECT. ECT is used in severe depression or when the patient has not responded to drug therapy; it has been given in repeated courses without evidence of brain damage.[7-9] ECT is of particular value when a rapid improvement in symptoms is essential (e.g. patients at high risk of suicide), and for patients with depressive psychosis or psychomotor retardation.[3,7] Light therapy appears to be effective in patients with seasonal affective disorder.[10] Exposure to bright artificial light may take place at any time of the day,[3] and the therapy should continue until the natural seasonal remission of the disorder; antidepressant drugs may also be used.[3]

There has been much debate about the **choice of antidepressant** therapy. Tricyclic antidepressants have long been preferred over MAOIs because of the problem of drug interactions and the need for strict dietary precautions with the latter group. Tricyclics with sedative properties may be more suitable for agitated and anxious patients, whereas those with less sedative properties may be preferred for withdrawn and apathetic patients. Unfortunately, the traditional tricyclics such as amitriptyline have antimuscarinic and cardiotoxic adverse effects that can limit their use. Their cardiotoxicity also means that they are associated with a high risk of fatality in patients taking overdoses (see toxicity in overdosage, below). Continuing development[11,12] produced lofepramine and drugs related to the tricyclic group such as mianserin that are less cardiotoxic than the earlier tricyclics.[2] The subsequent introduction of SSRIs such as fluoxetine provided a group of drugs with still fewer antimuscarinic and cardiotoxic side-effects. However, the SSRIs themselves have characteristic side-effects; gastrointestinal symptoms such as nausea and vomiting may be a problem, and sleep disturbances and anxiety may be exacerbated at the start of treatment. Moreover, those in current clinical use interact to varying degrees with cytochrome P450 isoenzymes, which carries a potential for interaction with a wide range of compounds.[11]

More recently serotonin and noradrenaline reuptake inhibitors (SNRIs) such as venlafaxine have been developed, as well as reversible inhibitors of monoamine oxidase type A (RIMAs) such as moclobemide. RIMAs offer a safer alternative to the MAOIs and fewer dietary restrictions are necessary.[13] Nefazodone, mirtazapine, and reboxetine, which have slightly different biochemical profiles from the major groups, are also more recent introductions. Bupropion, another unrelated antidepressant, is also available in some countries. Like the SSRIs, most of these newer drugs seem to be associated with fewer severe adverse effects; their efficacy is also comparable to that of the tricyclics and SSRIs.[14-16]

Other drugs used in the treatment of depression include flupentixol, the antidepressant dose of which is lower than that used for the treatment of psychoses. Ademetionine, the active derivative of methionine, has been tried in depressive disorders, and extracts of the plant hypericum (St John's Wort) are widely used in some countries for depression. Lithium may be used for the prophylaxis of recurrent unipolar depression as an alternative to standard antidepressants, although it is more commonly used in the management of bipolar disorder (see above); its role in unipolar depression is more usually to augment the effect of standard antidepressants in drug-resistant patients.

The improvement in treatment options offered by the newer antidepressants has meant that choice of therapy is increasingly tailored to individual patient requirements.[4-6]

There are arguments supporting both the first-choice use of SSRIs, because of fewer unpleasant side-effects,[17] and the tricyclics, because of wide experience with their use and familiarity with their pharmacological actions.[1,2,18] Meta-analyses[19-23] comparing the efficacy of SSRIs and tricyclics in general find no difference in efficacy although there is the suggestion of a greater efficacy for some tricyclics when given to inpatients. However, drop-out rates due to adverse effects have generally been higher in patients receiving tricyclics than in those taking SSRIs.

The sedative properties of some of the antidepressants may adversely affect the performance of potentially hazardous tasks such as driving and the operation of machinery. One of the less sedative antidepressants should be used where appropriate, although care is needed with all psychotropic drugs, especially at the start of treatment.

An area of particular concern with regard to initial choice of an antidepressant is the most appropriate drug for patients considered to be a high suicide risk.[24] Varying relative risks of **toxicity in overdosage** for different groups of antidepressant have been assessed:[25-28] older tricyclics and the tetracyclic maprotiline[29] appear to be more toxic in overdosage than the tetracyclic mianserin[30] and the SSRIs;[27] MAOIs have an intermediate risk.[31] Within the tricyclic group, desipramine[25,26] has been reported to be associated more frequently with fatal overdosage whereas lofepramine[28,32] may be one of the safer tricyclics. Although such analyses cannot determine to what extent the data reflect prescribing patterns and patient selection as opposed to drug toxicity[25,26,32] it is widely accepted that the older tricyclics are more toxic in overdosage, and that the SSRIs[33,34] and the newer tricyclic and related cyclic antidepressants are safer.[34] In practice, it is often difficult to identify patients at high risk for suicide, and it has therefore been suggested that a routine strategy should be to initiate antidepressant therapy in all patients with drugs that have low toxicity in overdose.[24,34] However, whichever antidepressant is chosen, all patients should be closely monitored during early therapy until improvement in depression has been observed and limited quantities of antidepressants should be prescribed at any one time. It is important to remember that suicide is an inherent risk in depression; it is generally accepted that with all antidepressant therapies the risk of suicide may increase in the early stages of recovery.

When **starting antidepressant therapy** a low initial dose will minimise adverse effects; this is then increased until an adequate response is observed.[1,6] When this is done with the newer antidepressants, including the SSRIs, the dose can generally be increased after a few days; for the tricyclics the increase should be more gradual.[35] Gradual introduction of treatment is of particular importance in the elderly who may be more susceptible to adverse effects. Although some adverse effects of antidepressant drugs appear soon after treatment is initiated, there is a delay of about 2 weeks before any therapeutic benefit is observed, and at least 6 weeks before maximum improvement in depressive symptoms occurs.[11] Claims of a fast onset of action have been made for several antidepressants, but in a review[36] of data relating to onset of action with currently available antidepressants, none have been shown conclusively to work faster than any other. This delay in benefit may relate to a combination of pharmacokinetic and neurochemical factors. Patients should not be considered resistant to the chosen drug until they have been maintained at an adequate dose for at least 4 weeks,[5] (the *British National Formulary* has recommended 6 weeks in the elderly). Patients with a partial response should continue for a further 2 weeks before being considered resistant.[5] Treatment failure is often due to subtherapeutic doses being used,[2] particularly with the older tricyclics whose adverse effects limit maximum tolerable doses in many patients.[37] Where lack of compliance leads to subtherapeutic doses therapeutic drug monitoring may be of value.[3]

In those who show little or no response to an adequate trial of the first-choice antidepressant two options exist: either switching to another antidepressant or adding another drug (augmentation). If switching antidepressants, a drug with a different biochemical profile may be substituted;[3] alternatively, some patients may respond preferentially to another drug within the same group.[38,39] MAOIs can be tried in patients who are refractory to or intolerant of treatment with other antidepressants.[6]

When **changing a patient from one type of antidepressant to another** an appropriate drug-free interval may be needed. An MAOI (including a RIMA) should not be started until at least one week after stopping a tricyclic antidepressant, an SSRI, or any related antidepressant; in the case of the SSRIs paroxetine and sertraline the drug-free interval is extended to 2 weeks, and for fluoxetine, to 5 weeks because of their longer half-lives. For the tricyclics clomipramine and imipramine a drug-free interval of 3 weeks should be allowed. Conversely, 2 weeks should elapse between discontinuing MAOI therapy and starting patients on a tricyclic antidepressant (3 weeks in the case of clomipramine or imipramine), an SSRI, or any related antidepressant. Although some manufacturers recommend a similar treatment-free period between stopping a reversible inhibitor of monoamine oxidase type A (RIMA) and starting an SSRI there does not seem to be any evidence to support such a requirement.

Drugs that have been used in **augmentation strategies** for resistant depression include lithium,[5] thyroid hormones (liothyronine),[5,40] and central stimulants[3,40] such as methylphenidate. Pindolol has also been studied as an augmentation agent with several SSRIs and other serotonergic antidepressants.[40] Another method is to combine different classes of antidepressants. Although this has been used successfully in the treatment of drug-resistant depression,[3,40] it may result in enhanced adverse reactions or interactions and is therefore considered unsuitable or controversial by some authorities; it should only ever be used under expert supervision. For further details of the interactions between different antidepressants, see under Interactions of Phenelzine, p.315.

If the response to treatment is good, the patient should continue with the same treatment for at least 4 to 6 months,[1-3,5] and perhaps 12 months in the elderly; symptoms are likely to recur if treatment is discontinued too soon.[41-43] It is often recommended that doses should be reduced for **maintenance treatment** but this view has been challenged and the recommendation made that the dose closest to that which achieved clinical response should be used unless adverse effects are intolerable.[1-3,5,6] Continuation of antidepressant therapy beyond this phase[44] is a matter of clinical judgement. **Prophylactic maintenance therapy** should be considered for recurrent depressive disorders,[1-3,41,43,45] and may be necessary for several years in some cases. Again, full therapeutic doses are recommended for prophylaxis rather than reduced doses.[6,42,45]

When stopping treatment, the sudden **discontinuation of antidepressant therapy** after regular administration for 8 weeks or more may precipitate withdrawal symptoms.[46-48] Common symptoms seen following antidepressant withdrawal include headache, anorexia, nausea, insomnia, and anxiety; the SSRIs have also been associated with episodes of dizziness and paraesthesia which are rarely seen with the tricyclics.[49] Withdrawal reactions may be more severe with the MAOIs especially tranylcypromine.[49] To minimise symptoms, most authorities recommend reducing the dose over a period of about 4 weeks, although considerably longer periods may be required when withdrawing maintenance therapy.[48]

Depressive disorders may arise in **childhood and adolescence**, the prevalence increasing with age.[50] Treatment generally commences with psychosocial and psychotherapeutic methods, followed by antidepressant therapy if no improvement is seen after 4 to 6 weeks.[50,51] The SSRI fluoxetine[50-53] and lofepramine[50] are considered the optimum first choices in children and adolescents because they are less toxic in overdose. However, in the UK, fluoxetine is not licensed for the treatment of depression in those under 18 years, although this may not be the case in other countries. The other SSRIs should not be used in children because of a lack of demonstrated efficacy and/or an increased risk of a harmful outcome (see Effects on Mental State under Fluoxetine, p.293 for further details). The older tricyclics are reserved for refractory cases in adolescents and may be augmented with lithium;[51] ECT may be used in severe depression.[50] Some authorities recommend avoiding desipramine because of reports of death due to cardiotoxicity in children.[52]

Depression in the **elderly** may be particularly severe and the suicide risk higher compared with younger adults.[54,55] SSRIs are often the first choice of treatment in the elderly because of their favourable adverse effect profile and low toxicity in overdose.[56] They may be especially appropriate in patients with an existing cardiovascular disease or in those taking other medications that may lower the blood pressure. Tricyclics such as amitriptyline and imipramine are probably best avoided in the elderly as their cardiotoxic, antimuscarinic, and sedative effects may be particularly troublesome. However, the tricyclics desipramine and nortriptyline are considered by some[6] to be an alternative first-choice as they are less cardiotoxic and have fewer antimuscarinic and sedative actions compared with amitriptyline or imipramine. Other antidepressants may also be useful in specific situations. As in younger patients, MAOIs may be tried in those who have failed to respond to other therapies, and bupropion has the advantage of a relative lack of cardiotoxicity and drug interactions. Lower initial doses of antidepressant drugs are often recommended in the elderly to minimise adverse effects but individual differences in metabolism and excretion may mean that some patients are undertreated.[55] The elderly tend to respond more slowly to antidepressants than younger patients and additional psychosocial or psychotherapeutic management may be warranted. ECT is safe and effective in the elderly, although temporary memory impairment after treatment in some patients may limit its use to those at high risk for suicide or who are refractory to or intolerant of antidepressant drugs. Depression late in life may require long-term antidepressant treatment beyond the recovery phase, even after first episodes of depression and should be a continuation of the treatment that was successful in the initial acute phase.[57]

Treatment of women with depressive disorders during and after **pregnancy** raises concerns about the risk of teratogenicity, fetal growth retardation, or perinatal problems; the ratio of risk to benefit must therefore be considered very carefully before antidepressants are given.[58,59] Maternal mood disorders in the immediate postpartum period are related to hormonal changes, particularly falling progesterone levels; the symptoms are mild and resolve spontaneously after several days, therefore no treatment is required.[60] Of greater concern are major depressive episodes that occur beyond this initial phase, which are clinically identical to depressive disorders in general and call for the same principles of management. These depressive episodes have been found to be related to the presence of immediate postpartum mood disorders, although no hormonal basis to this association has been identified.[61] Nevertheless, there is interest in the use of oestrogen as a treatment.

As with use of any medication in **breast feeding** mothers, the risks to the infant from drugs distributed into breast milk must be considered. The American Academy of Pediatrics[62] considers that all antidepressants are drugs whose effect on nursing infants could be of concern.

Symptoms of **anxiety and depression** often coexist, and although it may be difficult to distinguish which is the predominant disorder, especially in milder forms, patients usually require an antidepressant. Anxiolytics and antipsychotics can be useful adjuncts in agitated depression, but a sedative antidepressant might be preferable. Combination preparations of antidepressants with antipsychotics or anxiolytics should not be used because the dosage of the individual components should be adjusted separately. Also, anxiolytics should only be prescribed on a short-term basis whereas antidepressants are given for several months.

Although no randomised double-blind studies assessing the efficacy of antidepressants in **chronic fatigue syndrome** have been published it has been suggested that antidepressant therapy should be tried in patients with coexisting depression.[63] Cognitive therapy may also be useful. Controlled trials of antidepressants in non-depressed patients with chronic fatigue syndrome are particularly needed.[63]

1. Paykel ES, Priest RG. Recognition and management of depression in general practice: consensus statement. *BMJ* 1992; **305:** 1198–1202.
2. Montgomery SA, *et al.* Guidelines for treating depressive illness with antidepressants: a statement from the British Association for Psychopharmacology. *J Psychopharmacol* 1993; **7:** 19–23.
3. American Psychiatric Association. Practice guidelines for major depressive disorder in adults. *Am J Psychiatry* 1993; **150** (suppl): 1–26.
4. Snow V, *et al.* Clinical guidelines, part 1. Pharmacologic treatment of acute major depression and dysthymia. *Ann Intern Med* 2000; **132:** 738–42.
5. Anderson IM, *et al.* Evidence-based guidelines for treating depressive disorders with antidepressants: a revision of the 1993 British Association for Psychopharmacology guidelines. *J Psychopharmacol* 2000; **14:** 3–20.
6. American Psychiatric Association. Practice guideline for the treatment of patients with major depressive disorder (revision). *Am J Psychiatry* 2000; **157** (suppl): 1–45. Also available at: http://www.psych.org/psych_pract/treatg/pg/Depression2e.book.cfm (accessed 04/06/04)
7. Scott AIF. Contemporary practice of electroconvulsive therapy. *Br J Hosp Med* 1994; **51:** 334–8.
8. The UK ECT Review Group. Efficacy and safety of electroconvulsive therapy in depressive disorders: a systematic review and meta-analysis. *Lancet* 2003; **361:** 799–808.
9. National Institute for Clinical Excellence. Guidance on the use of electroconvulsive therapy (issued April 2003). Available at: http://www.nice.org.uk/pdf/59ectfullguidance.pdf (accessed 04/06/04)
10. Partonen T, Lönnqvist J. Seasonal affective disorder. *Lancet* 1998; **352:** 1369–74.
11. Richelson E. Pharmacology of antidepressants—characteristics of the ideal drug. *Mayo Clin Proc* 1994; **69:** 1069–81.
12. Möller H-J, Volz H-P. Drug treatment of depression in the 1990s: an overview of achievements and future possibilities. *Drugs* 1996; **52:** 625–38.
13. Lecrubier Y. Risk-benefit assessment of newer versus older monoamine oxidase (MAO) inhibitors. *Drug Safety* 1994; **10:** 292–300.
14. Kent JM. SNaRIs, NaSSAa, and NaRIs: new agents for the treatment of depression. *Lancet* 2000; **355:** 911–8. Correction. *ibid.*; 2000.
15. Anderson IM. Meta-analytical studies on new antidepressants. *Br Med Bull* 2001: **57:** 161–78.
16. Mulrow CD, *et al.* Efficacy of newer medications for treating depression in primary care patients. *Am J Med* 2000; **108:** 54–64.
17. Harrison G. New or old antidepressants: new is better. *BMJ* 1994; **309:** 1280–1.
18. Owens D. New or old antidepressants: benefits of new drugs are exaggerated. *BMJ* 1994; **309:** 1281–2.
19. Trindade E, Menon D. *Selective serotonin reuptake inhibitors (SSRIs) for major depression. Part 1: evaluation of the clinical literature.* Ottawa: Canadian Coordinating Office for Health Technology Assessment, 1997.
20. Anderson IM. SSRIs versus tricyclic antidepressants in depressed inpatients: a meta-analysis of efficacy and tolerability. *Depress Anxiety* 1998; **7** (suppl 1): 11–17.
21. Geddes JR, *et al.* Selective serotonin reuptake inhibitors (SSRIs) versus other antidepressants for depression. Available in The Cochrane Library; Issue 2. Chichester: John Wiley; 2004.
22. MacGillivray S, *et al.* Efficacy and tolerability of selective serotonin reuptake inhibitors compared with tricyclic antidepressants in depression treated in primary care: systematic review and meta-analysis. *BMJ* 2003; **326:** 1014–17.
23. Guaiana G, *et al.* Amitriptyline versus other types of pharmacotherapy for depression. Available in The Cochrane Library; Issue 2. Chichester: John Wiley; 2004.
24. Henry JA. Epidemiology and relative toxicity of antidepressant drugs in overdose. *Drug Safety* 1997; **16:** 374–90.
25. Beaumont G. The toxicity of antidepressants. *Br J Psychiatry* 1989; **154:** 454–8.
26. Kapur S, *et al.* Antidepressant medications and the relative risk of suicide attempt and suicide. *JAMA* 1992; **268:** 3441–5.
27. de Jonghe F, Swinkels JA. The safety of antidepressants. *Drugs* 1992; **43** (suppl 2): 40–7.
28. Mason J, *et al.* Fatal toxicity associated with antidepressant use in primary care. *Br J Gen Pract* 2000; **50:** 366–70.
29. Knudsen KAI, Heath A. Effects of self poisoning with maprotiline. *BMJ* 1984; **288:** 601–3.
30. Inman WHW. Blood disorders and suicide in patients taking mianserin or amitriptyline. *Lancet* 1988; **ii:** 90–2.
31. Cassidy S, Henry J. Fatal toxicity of antidepressant drugs in overdose. *BMJ* 1987; **295:** 1021–4.
32. Malmvik J, *et al.* Antidepressants in suicide: differences in fatality and drug utilisation. *Eur J Clin Pharmacol* 1994; **46:** 291–4.
33. Henry JA, *et al.* Relative mortality from overdose of antidepressants. *BMJ* 1995; **310:** 221–4. Correction. *ibid.*; 911.
34. Freemantle N, *et al.* Prescribing selective serotonin reuptake inhibitors as strategy for prevention of suicide. *BMJ* 1994; **309:** 249–53.
35. Spigset O, Mårtensson B. Drug treatment of depression. *BMJ* 1999; **318:** 1188–91.
36. Soares JC, Gershon S. Prospects for the development of new treatments with a rapid onset of action in affective disorders. *Drugs* 1996; **52:** 477–82.
37. Kendrick T. Prescribing antidepressants in general practice. *BMJ* 1996; **313:** 829–30.
38. Brown WA, Harrison W. Are patients who are intolerant to one serotonin selective reuptake inhibitor intolerant to another? *J Clin Psychiatry* 1995; **56:** 30–4.
39. Joffe RT, *et al.* Response to an open trial of a second SSRI in major depression. *J Clin Psychiatry* 1996; **57:** 114–15.
40. Schweitzer I, Tuckwell V. Risk of adverse events with the use of augmentation therapy for the treatment of resistant depression. *Drug Safety* 1998; **19:** 45–64.
41. Angst J. A regular review of the long term follow up of depression. *BMJ* 1997; **315:** 1143–6.
42. Paykel ES. Continuation and maintenance therapy in depression. *Br Med Bull* 2001: **57:** 145–59.
43. Geddes JR, *et al.* Relapse prevention with antidepressant drug treatment in depressive disorders: a systematic review. *Lancet* 2003; **361:** 653–61.
44. Edwards JG. Long term pharmacotherapy of depression. *BMJ* 1998; **316:** 1180–1.
45. Montgomery SA. Prophylactic treatment of depression. *Br J Hosp Med* 1994; **52:** 5–7.
46. Dilsaver SC. Withdrawal phenomena associated with antidepressant and antipsychotic agents. *Drug Safety* 1994; **10:** 103–114.
47. Haddad P, *et al.* Antidepressant discontinuation reactions. *BMJ* 1998; **316:** 1105–6.
48. Anonymous. Withdrawing patients from antidepressants. *Drug Ther Bull* 1999; **37:** 49–52.
49. Haddad PM. Antidepressant discontinuation syndromes: clinical relevance, prevention and management. *Drug Safety* 2001; **24:** 183–97.
50. Mirza KAH, Michael A. Major depression in children and adolescents. *Br J Hosp Med* 1996; **55:** 57–61.
51. Harrington R. Depressive disorder in adolescence. *Arch Dis Child* 1995; **72:** 193–5.
52. Carrey NJ, *et al.* Pharmacological treatment of psychiatric disorders in children and adolescents: focus on guidelines for the primary care practitioner. *Drugs* 1996; **51:** 750–9.
53. Renaud J, *et al.* A risk-benefit assessment of pharmacotherapies for clinical depression in children and adolescents. *Drug Safety* 1999; **20:** 59–75.
54. Wattis J. What an old age psychiatrist does. *BMJ* 1996; **313:** 101–4.
55. Waern M, *et al.* High rate of antidepressant treatment in elderly people who commit suicide. *BMJ* 1996; **313:** 1118.
56. The American Society of Health-System Pharmacists (ASHP). ASHP therapeutic position statement on the recognition and treatment of depression in older adults. *Am J Health-Syst Pharm* 1998; **55:** 2514–18.
57. Lebowitz BD, *et al.* Diagnosis and treatment of depression in late life: consensus statement update. *JAMA* 1997; **278:** 1186–90.
58. Robert E. Treating depression in pregnancy. *N Engl J Med* 1996; **335:** 1056–8.
59. Schou M. Treating recurrent affective disorders during and after pregnancy: what can be taken safely? *Drug Safety* 1998; **18:** 143–52.
60. Harris B, *et al.* Maternity blues and major endocrine changes: Cardiff puerperal mood and hormone study II. *BMJ* 1994; **308:** 949–53.
61. Cooper PJ, Murray L. Postnatal depression. *BMJ* 1998; **316:** 1884–6.
62. American Academy of Pediatrics Committee on Drugs. The transfer of drugs and other chemicals into human milk. *Pediatrics* 2001; **108:** 776–89. Correction. *ibid.*; 1029. Also available at: http://aappolicy.aappublications.org/cgi/content/full/pediatrics%3b108/3/776 (accessed 04/06/04)
63. The Royal Colleges of Physicians, Psychiatrists and General Practitioners. *Chronic Fatigue Syndrome.* London, 1997.

### Mania

Although isolated episodes of mania may occur, mania is usually followed by depression when it is considered to be part of bipolar disorder. It is accepted practice to include mania without depression within the bipolar category. The treatment and prophylaxis of acute mania are therefore described under Bipolar Disorder, above.

---

## Amineptine Hydrochloride *(rINNM)*

Hidrocloruro de amineptina; S-1694. 7-[(10,11-Dihydro-5*H*-dibenzo[*a,d*]cyclohepten-5-yl)amino]heptanoic acid hydrochloride.

$C_{22}H_{27}NO_2,HCl$ = 373.9.

*CAS — 57574-09-1 (amineptine); 30272-08-3 (amineptine hydrochloride).*

*ATC — N06AA19.*

### Profile

Amineptine hydrochloride is a tricyclic antidepressant (see Amitriptyline, below). It has been given by mouth in the treatment of depression.

Hepatic adverse effects seem to be more common than with most other tricyclic antidepressants (see Effects on the Liver, p.282). Also amineptine has been subject to abuse and withdrawal has been both prolonged and difficult; for these reasons, it is no longer marketed in many countries.

**Adverse effects.** In 5 patients very severe acne-type lesions were associated with the chronic self-increased use of high doses of amineptine (200 to 1000 mg daily).[1] The presence of an unusual lactam form of metabolites was detected in all patients and in 2 these metabolites were still present, along with the lesions, 3 months after therapy had been withdrawn.

1. Vexiau P, *et al.* Severe acne-like lesions caused by amineptine overdose. *Lancet* 1988; **i:** 585.

**Porphyria.** Amineptine is considered to be unsafe in patients with porphyria because it has been shown to be porphyrinogenic in *in-vitro* systems.

### Preparations

**Proprietary Preparations** (details are given in Part 3)
***Braz.:*** Survector; ***Ital.:*** Maneon†; ***Port.:*** Directim; Survector.

---

## Amitriptyline *(BAN, rINN)*

Amitriptilina. 3-(10,11-Dihydro-5*H*-dibenzo[*a,d*]cyclohepten-5-ylidene)propyldimethylamine; 10,11-Dihydro-*N,N*-dimethyl-5*H*-dibenzo[*a,d*]cycloheptene-$\Delta^{5,\gamma}$-propylamine.

$C_{20}H_{23}N$ = 277.4.

*CAS — 50-48-6.*

*ATC — N06AA09.*

## Amitriptyline Embonate *(BANM, rINNM)*

Embonato de amitriptilina.

$(C_{20}H_{23}N)_2,C_{23}H_{16}O_6$ = 943.2.

*CAS — 17086-03-2.*

**Pharmacopoeias.** In *Br.*

**BP 2003** (Amitriptyline Embonate). A pale yellow to brownish-yellow, odourless or almost odourless powder. Practically insoluble in water; slightly soluble in alcohol; freely soluble in chloroform. Protect from light.

## Amitriptyline Hydrochloride *(BANM, rINNM)*

Amitriptylini Hydrochloridum; Hidrocloruro de amitriptilina.

$C_{20}H_{23}N,HCl$ = 313.9.

*CAS — 549-18-8.*

**Pharmacopoeias.** In *Chin., Eur.* (see p.vi), *Int., Jpn, Pol.,* and *US.*

**Ph. Eur. 5.0** (Amitriptyline Hydrochloride). A white or almost white powder or colourless crystals. Freely soluble in water, in alcohol, and in dichloromethane. Protect from light.

**USP 27** (Amitriptyline Hydrochloride). A white or practically white, odourless or practically odourless, crystalline powder or small crystals. Freely soluble in water, in alcohol, in chloroform, and in methyl alcohol; insoluble in ether. pH of a 1% solution in water is between 5.0 and 6.0.

**Stability.** Decomposition occurred when solutions of amitriptyline hydrochloride in water or phosphate buffers were autoclaved at 115° to 116° for 30 minutes in the presence of excess oxygen.[1] The decomposition of amitriptyline as the hydrochloride in buffered aqueous solution was accelerated by metal ions particularly from amber glass ampoules.[2] Disodium edetate 0.1% significantly reduced the decomposition rate of these amitriptyline solutions but propyl gallate and hydroquinone were less effective. Sodium metabisulfite produced an initial lowering of amitriptyline concentration and subsequently an acceleration of decomposition.

Solutions of amitriptyline hydrochloride in water are stable for at least 8 weeks at room temperature if protected from light either by storage in a cupboard or in amber containers.[3] Decomposition to ketone and, to a lesser extent, other unidentified products was found to occur on exposure to light.


1. Enever RP, *et al.* Decomposition of amitriptyline hydrochloride in aqueous solution: identification of decomposition products. *J Pharm Sci* 1975; **64:** 1497–9.
2. Enever RP, *et al.* Factors influencing decomposition rate of amitriptyline hydrochloride in aqueous solution. *J Pharm Sci* 1977; **66:** 1087–9.
3. Buckles J, Walters V. The stability of amitriptyline hydrochloride in aqueous solution. *J Clin Pharm* 1976; **1:** 107–12.


## Adverse Effects

Many adverse effects of amitriptyline and similar tricyclic antidepressants are caused by their antimuscarinic actions. Antimuscarinic effects are relatively common and occur before an antidepressant effect is obtained. They include dry mouth, constipation occasionally leading to paralytic ileus, urinary retention, blurred vision and disturbances in accommodation, increased intra-ocular pressure, and hyperthermia. Tolerance is often achieved if treatment is continued and adverse effects may be less troublesome if treatment is begun with small doses and then increased gradually, although this may delay the clinical response.

Drowsiness may also be common. Conversely, a few tricyclic antidepressants possess little or no sedative potential and nervousness and insomnia may occur.

Other neurological adverse effects include headache, peripheral neuropathy, tremor, ataxia, epileptiform seizures, tinnitus, and occasional extrapyramidal symptoms including speech difficulties (dysarthria). Confusion or delirium may occur, particularly in the elderly and mania or hypomania, and behavioural disturbances (particularly in children) have been reported. Gastrointestinal complaints include sour or metallic taste, stomatitis, and gastric irritation with nausea and vomiting.

Various effects on the cardiovascular system have been reported and are discussed in more detail under Effects on the Cardiovascular System, below. Orthostatic hypotension and tachycardia may occur in patients without a history of cardiovascular disease, and may be particularly troublesome in the elderly.

Hypersensitivity reactions, such as urticaria and angioedema, and photosensitisation have been reported and, rarely, cholestatic jaundice and blood disorders, including eosinophilia, bone-marrow depression, thrombocytopenia, leucopenia, and agranulocytosis.

Endocrine effects include testicular enlargement, gynaecomastia and breast enlargement, and galactorrhoea. Sexual dysfunction may also occur. Changes in blood sugar concentrations may also occur, and, very occasionally, hyponatraemia associated with inappropriate secretion of antidiuretic hormone.

Other side-effects that have been reported are increased appetite with weight gain (or occasionally anorexia with weight loss). Sweating may be a problem.

Symptoms of **overdosage** may include excitement and restlessness with marked antimuscarinic effects, including dryness of the mouth, dilated pupils, tachycardia, urinary retention, and intestinal stasis. Severe symptoms include unconsciousness, convulsions and myoclonus, hyperreflexia, hypothermia, hypotension, metabolic acidosis, and respiratory and cardiac depression, with life-threatening cardiac arrhythmias that may recur some days after apparent recovery. Delirium, with confusion, agitation and hallucinations, is common during recovery.

**Antimuscarinic and antihistaminic properties.** Studies *in vitro* showed antidepressant affinities for human muscarinic acetylcholine receptors and therefore the likelihood of antimuscarinic effects to be, in descending order:[1]

- amitriptyline
- protriptyline
- clomipramine
- trimipramine
- doxepin
- imipramine
- nortriptyline
- desipramine
- amoxapine
- maprotiline
- trazodone

The effect of affinities for other receptor sites was less certain, although those antidepressants with high affinity for histamine $H_1$ receptors might be expected to be more sedating. Affinities for *murine* histamine $H_1$ receptors in descending order were:

- doxepin
- trimipramine
- amitriptyline
- maprotiline
- amoxapine
- nortriptyline
- imipramine
- clomipramine
- protriptyline
- trazodone
- desipramine


1. Richelson E. Antimuscarinic and other receptor-blocking properties of antidepressants. *Mayo Clin Proc* 1983; **58:** 40–6.


**Effects on the blood.** Following a case report of agranulocytosis linked with imipramine, review of the literature suggested that agranulocytosis associated with tricyclic antidepressant use was a rare idiosyncratic condition, resulting from a direct toxic effect rather than an allergic mechanism, and particularly affected the elderly from 4 to 8 weeks after beginning treatment.[1]

Between 1963 and 1993 the UK Committee on Safety of Medicines (CSM) received 912 reports of drug-induced agranulocytosis of which 38 were due to tricyclic antidepressants (12 fatal) and 1499 cases of neutropenia of which 46 were due to tricyclics (none fatal).[2] In a report[3] on a patient who developed aplastic anaemia associated with use of remoxipride and dosulepin it was noted that up to May 1993 the CSM had received 11 reports of aplastic anaemia secondary to use of dosulepin.

Neutropenia reported[4] in a patient after separate exposure to imipramine and nortriptyline, indicated that there might be cross-intolerance between the tricyclic antidepressants and if neutropenia developed with one member of the group the use of others on future occasions should be avoided.


1. Albertini RS, Penders TM. Agranulocytosis associated with tricyclics. *J Clin Psychiatry* 1978; **39:** 483–5.
2. Committee on Safety of Medicines/Medicines Control Agency. Drug-induced neutropenia and agranulocytosis. *Current Problems* 1993; **19:** 10–11.
3. Philpott NJ, *et al.* Aplastic anaemia and remoxipride. *Lancet* 1993; **342:** 1244–5.
4. Draper BM, Manoharan A. Neutropenia with cross-intolerance between two tricyclic antidepressant agents. *Med J Aust* 1987; **146:** 452–3.


**Effects on the cardiovascular system.** The cardiotoxic potential of tricyclic antidepressants after overdosage is widely acknowledged; symptoms include arrhythmias, conduction defects, and hypotension. This factor was, in part, responsible for the development of antidepressants with different chemical structures and pharmacological properties that are less cardiotoxic. It also led to some concern over whether tricyclic antidepressants had adverse effects on the heart or cardiovascular system when used in usual therapeutic doses.

Since the introduction of the tricyclic antidepressants, several reports, often anecdotal, have been published of adverse cardiovascular effects and have included malignant hypertension with amitriptyline,[1] and cardiomyopathy in a patient who had received amitriptyline and imipramine.[2] QT prolongation, which is considered a risk factor for torsade de pointes, has also been associated with the use of some tricyclics.[3] Sudden cardiac death in patients with pre-existing cardiac disease has been linked with amitriptyline[4-6] or imipramine,[5] although the Boston Collaborative Drug Surveillance Program failed to substantiate these findings.[7] There have also been reports of sudden death in children given desipramine[8-10] or imipramine;[10] in at least some of these cases plasma concentrations were not elevated and the children had no cardiac abnormality. Again, however, evaluation of much of the evidence for the association suggests it is weak;[11] nonetheless, the American Heart Association recommends baseline ECG monitoring in children who are to be treated with tricyclic antidepressants, and a repeat ECG when steady-state dosage is achieved.[12]

Re-evaluations and reviews of this topic[13,14] concluded that the only significant or serious cardiovascular side-effects, seen in *patients with no previous history* of cardiovascular disease given therapeutic doses of tricyclic antidepressants, are orthostatic hypotension and tachycardia, and that these effects may be particularly troublesome in elderly patients. However, a more recent study[15] also considers that prolongation of the QT interval may occur with therapeutic doses of tricyclics in non-risk patients.

In *patients with overt heart disease* it was considered[13] that increased risk was likely in those with intraventricular conduction abnormalities; in patients with a history of myocardial infarction or angina, but free of conduction defects, the use of tricyclics appeared to be primarily limited by the degree to and frequency with which they developed orthostatic hypotension. In a re-evaluation of the risks and benefits of tricyclics in patients with ischaemic heart disease no consensus was reached.[16] In practice the authors used SSRIs or bupropion as first-choice therapy in patients with ischaemic heart disease who were mildly or moderately depressed; tricyclics were reserved for patients not responding and were also used as first-choice therapy for patients with more severe depression despite cardiac risks. More recently an increased risk of myocardial infarction has been found in patients receiving tricyclic antidepressants (but not SSRIs) and concomitant treatment for heart disease.[17] Results of a later case-control study[18] examining the risk of ischaemic heart disease for different types of antidepressants and individual antidepressants support these findings. After adjustment for confounders and use of other antidepressants the risk of ischaemic heart disease was significantly raised in patients who had ever taken tricyclics but not in those who had received other antidepressants. When the risk was calculated for the tricyclics amitriptyline, dosulepin, and lofepramine, and confounders had been adjusted for, an increased risk of ischaemic heart disease remained only for dosulepin with evidence of a dose-response relationship.


1. Dunn FG. Malignant hypertension associated with use of amitriptyline hydrochloride. *South Med J* 1982; **75:** 1124–5.
2. Howland JS, *et al.* Cardiomyopathy associated with tricyclic antidepressants. *South Med J* 1983; **76:** 1455–6.
3. Baker B, *et al.* Electrocardiographic effects of fluoxetine and doxepin in patients with major depressive disorder. *J Clin Psychopharmacol* 1997; **17:** 15–21.
4. Coull DC, *et al.* Amitriptyline and cardiac disease. *Lancet* 1970; **ii:** 590–1.
5. Moir DC, *et al.* Cardiotoxicity of amitriptyline. *Lancet* 1972; **ii:** 561–4.
6. Moir DC, *et al.* Medicines evaluation and monitoring group: a follow-up study of cardiac patients receiving amitriptyline. *Eur J Clin Pharmacol* 1973; **6:** 98–101.
7. Boston Collaborative Drug Surveillance Program. Adverse reactions to the tricyclic-antidepressant drugs: report from Boston Collaborative Drug Surveillance Program. *Lancet* 1972; **i:** 529–31.
8. Anonymous. Sudden death in children treated with a tricyclic antidepressant. *Med Lett Drugs Ther* 1990; **32:** 53.
9. Riddle MA, *et al.* Another sudden death in a child treated with desipramine. *J Am Acad Child Adolesc Psychiatry* 1993; **32:** 792–7.
10. Varley CK, McClellan J. Case study: two additional sudden deaths with tricyclic antidepressants. *J Am Acad Child Adolesc Psychiatry* 1997; **36:** 390–4.
11. Biederman J, *et al.* Estimation of the association between desipramine and the risk for sudden death in 5- to 14-year-old children. *J Clin Psychiatry* 1995; **56:** 87–93.
12. Gutgesell H, *et al.* Cardiovascular monitoring of children and adolescents receiving psychotropic drugs: a statement for healthcare professionals from the Committee on Congenital Cardiac Defects, Council on Cardiovascular Disease in the Young, American Heart Association. *Circulation* 1999; **99:** 979–82.
13. Glassman AH. Cardiovascular effects of tricyclic antidepressants. *Annu Rev Med* 1984; **35:** 503–11.
14. Mortensen SA. Cyclic antidepressants and cardiotoxicity. *Practitioner* 1984; **228:** 1180–3.
15. Reilly JG, *et al.* QTc-interval abnormalities and psychotropic drug therapy in psychiatric patients. *Lancet* 2000; **355:** 1048–52.
16. Glassman AH, *et al.* The safety of tricyclic antidepressants in cardiac patients: risk-benefit reconsidered. *JAMA* 1993; **269:** 2673–5.
17. Cohen HW, *et al.* Excess risk of myocardial infarction in patients treated with antidepressant medications: association with use of tricyclic agents. *Am J Med* 2000; **108:** 2–8.
18. Hippisley-Cox J, *et al.* Antidepressants as risk factor for ischaemic heart disease: case-control study in primary care. *BMJ* 2001; **323:** 666–9.


EFFECTS ON THE PERIPHERAL CIRCULATION. Painful vasospastic episodes, characterised by cold and blue hands and feet, occurred in a woman each time she received imipramine 150 mg daily but with amitriptyline only when the dose was increased to 200 mg daily.[1] This suggested that the ability of tricyclic antidepressants to induce vasospasm was not limited to imipramine and that the effect might be partly dose-dependent. Additionally, acrocyanosis of the hands and feet has been reported in a child receiving imipramine for nocturnal enuresis.[2]


1. Appelbaum PS, Kapoor W. Imipramine-induced vasospasm: a case report. *Am J Psychiatry* 1983; **140:** 913–15.
2. Anderson RP, Morris BAP. Acrocyanosis due to imipramine. *Arch Dis Child* 1988; **63:** 204–5.


**Effects on the endocrine system.** The *syndrome of inappropriate antidiuretic hormone secretion with hyponatraemia* has been reported in patients receiving tricyclics and other antidepressants. The UK Committee on Safety of Medicines, commenting on reports it had received of hyponatraemia associated with antidepressants (fluoxetine, paroxetine, lofepramine, clomipramine, and imipramine), considered that it was likely to occur with any antidepressant and usually involved elderly patients.[1] Case reports of hyponatraemia in 24 patients treated with tricyclics and 20 patients treated with other antidepressants have been summarised.[2]

In a review covering the effects of drugs on *prolactin secretion*[3] it was stated that antidepressants could affect prolactin secretion by disturbing the balance of catecholaminergic inhibition and serotonergic stimulation of prolactin release, although any change is less than with antipsychotic therapy. Clomipramine and nortriptyline had been reported to stimulate prolactin release whereas amitriptyline, desipramine, and imipramine had been reported to be without effect. Such stimulation may account for symptoms of galactorrhoea or amenorrhoea reported with some tricyclics.

1. Committee on Safety of Medicines/Medicines Control Agency. Antidepressant-induced hyponatraemia. *Current Problems* 1994; **20:** 5–6.
2. Spigset O, Hedenmalm K. Hyponatraemia and the syndrome of inappropriate antidiuretic hormone secretion (SIADH) induced by psychotropic drugs. *Drug Safety* 1995; **12:** 209–25.
3. Hell K, Wernze H. Drug-induced changes in prolactin secretion: clinical implications. *Med Toxicol* 1988; **3:** 463–98.

**Effects on the gastrointestinal tract.** Rare cases of ileus and pseudo-obstruction have apparently resulted from the antimuscarinic effects of tricyclic antidepressants.[1-4] An early report[1] from the UK Committee on Safety of Medicines noted no evidence that any tricyclic was especially liable to cause ileus.

1. Committee on Safety of Medicines. *Current Problems 3* 1978.
2. McMahon AJ. Amitriptyline overdose complicated by intestinal pseudo-obstruction and caecal perforation. *Postgrad Med J* 1989; **65:** 948–9.
3. Sood A, Kumar R. Imipramine induced acute colonic pseudo-obstruction (Ogilvie's syndrome): a report of two cases. *Indian J Gastroenterol* 1996; **15:** 70–1.
4. Ross JP, *et al.* Imipramine overdose complicated by toxic megacolon. *Am Surg* 1998; **64:** 242–4.

**Effects on the kidneys and urine.** Haematuria has been observed in a patient receiving amitriptyline and carbamazepine;[1] carbamazepine had previously been taken alone for an extensive period without producing this symptom.

Amitriptyline may have produced a blue-green colour in urine,[2] although it was considered to be a rare phenomenon.

1. Gillman MA, Sandyk R. Hematuria following tricyclic therapy. *Am J Psychiatry* 1984; **141:** 463–4.
2. Beeley L. *BMJ* 1986; **293:** 750.

**Effects on the liver.** In a report of 91 cases of hepatitis due to antidepressant therapy, 63 occurred in patients receiving the tricyclic antidepressant amineptine, sometimes with other psychotropic drugs; in approximately 50% of these amineptine cases, benzodiazepines had also been taken and it was postulated that the benzodiazepines may have increased the oxidation of amineptine to a toxic metabolite.[1] Most patients presented with abdominal pain and mixed liver damage with predominant cholestasis. One died after myocardial infarction, but all the others recovered. The mean amineptine dosage was 200 mg daily. In comparison, only a few cases were attributed to other tricyclic antidepressants—amitriptyline (4), clomipramine (3), and dibenzepin (1). Cross hepatotoxicity has also been reported in one patient between amineptine and clomipramine.[2]

Hepatotoxicity has also been noted with lofepramine. The UK Committee on Safety of Medicines had by the end of 1987 received 57 reports of abnormal liver function tests associated with lofepramine.[3] They included hepatic failure (1), jaundice (9), and hepatitis (5). All reactions occurred within the first 8 weeks of treatment and all were reversible on discontinuation of the drug.

1. Lefebure B, *et al.* Hépatites aux antidépresseurs. *Therapie* 1984; **39:** 509–16.
2. Larrey D, *et al.* Cross hepatotoxicity between tricyclic antidepressants. *Gut* 1986; **27:** 726–7.
3. Committee on Safety of Medicines. Lofepramine (Gamanil) and abnormal blood tests of liver function. *Current Problems 23* 1988.

**Effects on the mouth.** The inhibition of salivation caused by tricyclic antidepressants (in this case clomipramine) has been implicated in dental caries formation.[1]

1. deVries MW, Peeters F. Dental caries with longterm use of antidepressants. *Lancet* 1995; **346:** 1640.

**Effects on the nervous system.** Effects on the nervous system attributed to tricyclic antidepressants include drowsiness (especially with those with antihistaminic activity), peripheral neuropathy, tremor, ataxia, confusion, and delirium. Of particular concern is a reduction in the seizure threshold (see Epileptogenic Effect, below). Extrapyramidal effects and neuroleptic malignant syndrome (see below) may also occasionally occur.

**Effects on sexual function.** Loss of libido and impotence are common in depression, often making the role of drugs in producing sexual dysfunction difficult to assess.[1]

Sedation due to tricyclic antidepressants may lead to loss of libido and many of the tricyclics have been reported to cause impotence.[1,2] Amitriptyline, clomipramine, desipramine, doxepin, nortriptyline, and trimipramine have been stated to delay or inhibit ejaculation, and amoxapine, imipramine, and protriptyline, also to cause painful ejaculation. However, some tricyclics have been used for their effect on ejaculation in the management of premature ejaculation (see Clomipramine, p.290).

In women, anorgasmia or delayed orgasm has been reported with amitriptyline, amoxapine, clomipramine, and imipramine,[1-3] although spontaneous orgasm associated with yawning has been reported with clomipramine.[4]

1. Beeley L. Drug-induced sexual dysfunction and infertility. *Adverse Drug React Acute Poisoning Rev* 1984; **3:** 23–42.
2. Anonymous. Drugs that cause sexual dysfunction. *Med Lett Drugs Ther* 1987; **29:** 65–70.
3. Shen WW, Sata LS. Inhibited female orgasm resulting from psychotropic drugs: a clinical review. *J Reprod Med* 1983; **28:** 497–9.
4. McLean JD, *et al.* Unusual side effects of clomipramine associated with yawning. *Can J Psychiatry* 1983; **28:** 569–70.

**Effects on the skin.** Hypersensitivity reactions to tricyclic antidepressants are said to be uncommon.[1] Urticaria and angioedema have occurred, the urticaria occasionally clearing without drug withdrawal. Pruritus is also uncommon, but may be associated with transient erythema. Photosensitivity reactions are far less common than with phenothiazines; protriptyline has been the tricyclic most frequently implicated.[2,3] Rarely exfoliative dermatitis has developed, and purpura, pigmentation, and lichen planus have been noted in isolated reports. Toxic epidermal necrolysis has been reported in a patient 2 weeks after commencing therapy with amoxapine.[4] Hypersensitivity reactions to tricyclic antidepressants usually occur between 14 and 60 days after the start of treatment.[5]

Amitriptyline and fluoxetine have been implicated in the development of atypical cutaneous lymphoid hyperplasia in 8 patients, 7 of whom either had an underlying immunosuppressant systemic disease or were also receiving immunomodulatory drugs.[6] The lesions improved or resolved on stopping the antidepressant, although in some patients other factors may have contributed to lesional resolution.

1. Almeyda J. Drug reactions XIII: cutaneous reactions to imipramine and chlordiazepoxide. *Br J Dermatol* 1971; **84:** 298–9.
2. Smith AG. Drug-induced photosensitivity. *Adverse Drug React Bull* 1989; **136** (June): 508–11.
3. Harth Y, Rapoport M. Photosensitivity associated with antipsychotics, antidepressants and anxiolytics. *Drug Safety* 1996; **14:** 252–9.
4. Camisa C, Grines C. Amoxapine: a cause of toxic epidermal necrolysis? *Arch Dermatol* 1983; **119:** 709–10.
5. Quitkin F. Cross-tolerance of tricyclic antidepressant drugs. *JAMA* 1979; **241:** 1625.
6. Crowson AN, Magro CM. Antidepressant therapy: a possible cause of atypical cutaneous lymphoid hyperplasia. *Arch Dermatol* 1995; **131:** 925–9.

**Epileptogenic effect.** Seizures have been reported after therapeutic doses of tricyclic antidepressants as well as after overdosage, although the mechanism by which the seizures are induced is unclear.[1] Seizures usually appear within a few days of starting the drug or changing to a higher dose but in patients with no previous history of epilepsy or no predisposing medical condition the frequency seems[1] to be very low with an incidence of about 1 in 1000. An incidence of 0.4 per 1000 was reported[2] based on 16 cases out of an estimated group of 42 000 patients receiving tricyclics and who had no predisposing factors, but in another review[3] a reasonable estimate of the incidence was considered to be 3 to 6 per 1000. However, it is widely agreed that tricyclics should be used very cautiously in patients with epilepsy or those with a low convulsive threshold.

In a retrospective analysis of 1313 cases[4] of overdosage involving cyclic antidepressants, seizures occurred more commonly with the tricyclics amoxapine (24.5%) and desipramine (17.9%), and the tetracyclic maprotiline (12.2%). In another analysis of 302 consecutive cases of tricyclic overdosage a higher rate of seizures was seen with dosulepin in overdosage (13%) than other tricyclics.[5]

1. Zaccara G, *et al.* Clinical features, pathogenesis and management of drug-induced seizures. *Drug Safety* 1990; **5:** 109–51.
2. Jick SS, *et al.* Antidepressants and convulsions. *J Clin Psychopharmacol* 1992; **12:** 241–5.
3. Rosenstein DL, *et al.* Seizures associated with antidepressants: a review. *J Clin Psychiatry* 1993; **54:** 289–99.
4. Wedin GP, *et al.* Relative toxicity of cyclic antidepressants. *Ann Emerg Med* 1986; **15:** 797–804.
5. Buckley NA, *et al.* Greater toxicity in overdose of dothiepin than of other tricyclic antidepressants. *Lancet* 1994: **343:** 159–62.

**Extrapyramidal effects.** Extrapyramidal effects such as orofacial and choreoathetoid movements, and dyskinesias have been attributed to treatment with tricyclic antidepressants. Some patients with panic disorder may be sensitive to imipramine, developing symptoms of insomnia, jitteriness, and irritability.[1] These symptoms have also been seen in patients with panic disorder treated with low doses of desipramine although the symptoms usually subsided when the dose of the tricyclic was gradually increased. It has been suggested[2] that these symptoms may be related to akathisia and are more likely to occur with those tricyclics that have a more potent effect on inhibition of noradrenaline reuptake.

Dysarthria has been reported[3] and was said to be not uncommon in those taking higher doses of tricyclic antidepressants, but unusual at lower doses.[4]

Reviews of adverse effects of drugs on the nervous system have also listed acute torsion dystonias and tremors[5] as being caused or exacerbated by tricyclic antidepressants.

1. Yeragani VK, *et al.* Tricyclic induced jitteriness—a form of akathisia? *BMJ* 1986; **292:** 1529.
2. Cole JO, Bodkin JA. Antidepressant drug side effects. *J Clin Psychiatry* 1990; **51** (suppl): 21–6.
3. Quader SE. Dysarthria: an unusual side effect of tricyclic antidepressants. *BMJ* 1977; **2:** 97.
4. Saunders M. Dysarthria with tricyclic antidepressants. *BMJ* 1977; **2:** 317.
5. Lane RJM, Routledge PA. Drug-induced neurological disorders. *Drugs* 1983; **26:** 124–47.

**Hypersensitivity.** See under Effects on the Skin, above.

**Hyponatraemia.** See Effects on the Endocrine System, above.

**Neuroleptic malignant syndrome.** Of 16 cases of neuroleptic malignant syndrome reported to the UK Committee on Safety of Medicines by July 1986, 3 cases occurred in patients receiving a tricyclic antidepressant; amitriptyline with perphenazine had been taken by one patient and dosulepin or clomipramine alone by 2 other patients. The clomipramine case was fatal.[1] Other reports have been associated with amoxapine,[2] and clomipramine with triazolam.[3]

1. Committee on Safety of Medicines. Neuroleptic malignant syndrome—an underdiagnosed condition? *Current Problems 18* 1986.
2. Madakasira S. Amoxapine-induced neuroleptic malignant syndrome. *DICP Ann Pharmacother* 1989; **23:** 50–1.
3. Domingo P, *et al.* Benign type of malignant syndrome. *Lancet* 1989; **i:** 50.

**Overdosage.** In a 1993 report[1] tricyclic antidepressants were associated with a higher risk of fatality after suicide attempts by drug overdose compared with the non-tricyclics available at the time. Some reports[2] have considered desipramine to be associated more frequently than other tricyclic antidepressants with fatal overdosage, although others[3] assign this status to dosulepin.

More recent reviews continue to cite tricyclic antidepressants as one of the most commonly ingested substances in fatal cases of self-poisoning.[3,4]

1. Anonymous. Antidepressant drugs and the risk of suicide. *WHO Drug Inf* 1993; **7:** 18–20.
2. Amitai Y, Frischer H. The toxicity and dose of desipramine hydrochloride. *JAMA* 1994; **272:** 1719–20.
3. Kerr GW, *et al.* Tricyclic antidepressant overdose: a review. *Emerg Med J* 2001; **18:** 236–41.
4. Glauser J. Tricyclic antidepressant poisoning. *Cleve Clin J Med* 2000; **67:** 704–19.

## Treatment of Adverse Effects

The basis of the management of tricyclic antidepressant poisoning is intensive supportive care and symptomatic therapy.

Since tricyclic antidepressants slow gastrointestinal transit time, absorption may be delayed in overdosage. Activated charcoal may be given by mouth or nasogastric tube if more than 4 mg/kg of a tricyclic antidepressant has been ingested within 1 hour; a second dose may be considered after 2 hours in patients with central features of toxicity. Gastric lavage has also been used, alone or in combination with charcoal. Multiple doses of charcoal may be appropriate in patients who have ingested modified-release preparations. The patient should be monitored for cardiac arrhythmias. UK authorities consider that although cardiac arrhythmias are of concern they are best treated by correction of hypoxia and acidosis and that the use of antiarrhythmic drugs is best avoided.

Convulsions can be managed by giving diazepam or lorazepam intravenously. Phenytoin should be avoided because it may increase the risk of arrhythmias. Diazepam by mouth is usually adequate to sedate delirious patients, although large doses may be needed.

Physostigmine salicylate may be beneficial in some forms of cardiotoxicity, and in convulsions and coma, but its routine use cannot be recommended because of the serious adverse effects it may cause (see Antimuscarinic Poisoning in Uses of Physostigmine, p.1494). Peritoneal dialysis, haemodialysis, and measures to increase urine production are not of value in tricyclic antidepressant poisoning, and charcoal haemoperfusion is of doubtful benefit.

## Precautions

The antimuscarinic effects of tricyclic antidepressants warrant care in patients with urinary retention, prostatic hyperplasia, or chronic constipation; caution has also been advised in untreated angle-closure glaucoma and in phaeochromocytoma.

The epileptogenic potential of tricyclic antidepressants requires care in patients with a history of epilepsy, and their potential cardiotoxicity needs caution in cardiovascular disease and avoidance in heart block, cardiac arrhythmias, or in the immediate recovery period after myocardial infarction. Caution has also been recommended in patients with hyperthyroidism as tricyclics may precipitate cardiac arrhythmias.

Blood-sugar concentrations may be altered in diabetic patients.

Because tricyclic antidepressants are metabolised and inactivated in the liver they should be used with caution in patients with hepatic impairment; they should be avoided in severe liver disease.

Patients should be closely monitored during early antidepressant therapy until improvement in depression is observed because suicide is an inherent risk in depressed patients. For further details, see under Depression, p.279.

If tricyclic antidepressants are used for the depressive component of bipolar disorder, mania may be precipitated; similarly, psychotic symptoms may be aggravated if tricyclics are used for a depressive component of schizophrenia.

Drowsiness often occurs, particularly at the start of therapy, and patients, if affected, should not drive or operate machinery.

Tricyclic antidepressants may inhibit salivation and regular dental check-ups are recommended for patients on long-term therapy, particularly when taking those with marked antimuscarinic actions.

Elderly patients can be particularly sensitive to the side-effects of tricyclic antidepressants and a reduced dose, especially initially, should be used.

Tricyclic antidepressants are not recommended for depression in children. If they are used for nocturnal enuresis in children they should be limited to short courses with a full physical examination before subsequent courses.

Tricyclic antidepressants should be withdrawn gradually to reduce the risk of withdrawal symptoms (see below).

It has been recommended that, where possible, tricyclic antidepressants should be stopped some days before elective surgery, and that they should be used with caution in patients requiring ECT, but see also under Anaesthesia, below.

**Anaesthesia.** Patients receiving tricyclic antidepressants are at an increased risk of developing hypotension or cardiac arrhythmias during anaesthesia. Tricyclics may also dangerously potentiate the cardiovascular effects of vasopressor drugs such as sympathomimetics that may be required during anaesthesia. Although some manufacturers recommend stopping tricyclics several days before elective surgery where possible, the *British National Formulary* advises that this is unnecessary as long as the anaesthetist is informed.

Commenting on the anaesthetic considerations relevant to ECT,[1] it was considered that therapy with tricyclic antidepressants should not be a contra-indication to anaesthesia for ECT. A major consideration, though, was said to be the interaction of tricyclics with barbiturates resulting in increased sleep time and duration of anaesthesia. This meant that lower doses of barbiturate anaesthetics should be used.

1. Gaines GY, Rees DI. Electroconvulsive therapy and anesthetic considerations. *Anesth Analg* 1986; **65:** 1345–56.

**Breast feeding.** In general, only small amounts of tricyclic antidepressants are distributed into breast milk. Nevertheless, the American Academy of Pediatrics[1] considers that all antidepressants, including tricyclics, are drugs whose effect on nursing infants is unknown but may be of concern. In addition, most manufacturers advise that tricyclics should be avoided by the mother during breast feeding.

Case reports indicate that amitriptyline and its metabolite (nortriptyline),[2,3] clomipramine,[4] desipramine and its metabolite (2-hydroxydesipramine),[5] dosulepin and its primary metabolites (nordothiepin, dothiepin-*S*-oxide, and nordothiepin-*S*-oxide),[6] doxepin and its metabolite (*N*-desmethyldoxepin),[7-9] imipramine and its metabolite (desipramine),[10] and maprotiline[11] are all present in breast milk in concentrations similar to those in maternal blood; amoxapine and its metabolite (8-hydroxyamoxapine)[12] have also been detected in breast milk but in concentrations lower than in maternal blood. In all but two of the above cases the infants were breast fed without experiencing side-effects and tricyclics were undetectable in the infant's blood or present only in minute amounts. In one of the affected infants,[8] adverse effects included sedation and shallow respiration. The infant's mother had received doxepin and, although doxepin was almost undetectable in the infant's serum, the desmethyl metabolite appeared to have accumulated. In the other infant, drowsiness, poor suckling, and difficulty in swallowing were noted.[9] In this case the levels of both doxepin and its desmethyl metabolite were below the lower level of quantification; however, it was considered that the infant may have been at a greater risk for adverse effects because he had also developed hyperbilirubinaemia. There were no data for the effects of amoxapine on breast-fed infants because the case reported[12] involved samples of milk taken from a woman experiencing galactorrhoea as an adverse effect of tricyclic administration. No adverse effects were seen during a 27-month follow-up of 14 breast-fed infants whose mothers had received imipramine 100 to 225 mg daily for 4 to 24 weeks.[13]

1. American Academy of Pediatrics Committee on Drugs. The transfer of drugs and other chemicals into human milk. *Pediatrics* 2001; **108:** 776–89. Correction. *ibid.*; 1029. Also available at: http://aappolicy.aappublications.org/cgi/content/full/pediatrics%3b108/3/776 (accessed 04/06/04)
2. Bader TF, Newman K. Amitriptyline in human breast milk and the nursing infant's serum. *Am J Psychiatry* 1980; **137:** 855–6.
3. Brixen-Rasmussen L, *et al.* Amitriptyline and nortriptyline excretion in human breast milk. *Psychopharmacology (Berl)* 1982; **76:** 94–5.
4. Schimmell MS, *et al.* Toxic neonatal effects following maternal clomipramine therapy. *Clin Toxicol* 1991; **29:** 479–84.
5. Stancer HC, Reed KL. Desipramine and 2-hydroxydesipramine in human breast milk and the nursing infant's serum. *Am J Psychiatry* 1986; **143:** 1597–1600.
6. Ilett KF, *et al.* The excretion of dothiepin and its primary metabolites in breast milk. *Br J Clin Pharmacol* 1992; **33:** 635–9.
7. Kemp J, *et al.* Excretion of doxepin and N-desmethyldoxepin in human milk. *Br J Clin Pharmacol* 1985; **20:** 497–9.
8. Matheson I, *et al.* Respiratory depression caused by N-desmethyldoxepin in breast milk. *Lancet* 1985; **ii:** 1124.
9. Frey OR, *et al.* Adverse effects in a newborn infant breast-fed by a mother treated with doxepin. *Ann Pharmacother* 1999; **33:** 690–3.
10. Sovner R, Orsulak PJ. Excretion of imipramine and desipramine in human breast milk. *Am J Psychiatry* 1979; **136:** 451–2.
11. Lloyd AH. Practical considerations in the use of maprotiline (Ludiomil) in general practice. *J Int Med Res* 1977; **5** (suppl 4): 122–38.
12. Gelenberg AJ. Amoxapine, a new antidepressant, appears in human milk. *J Nerv Ment Dis* 1979; **167:** 635–6.
13. Misri S, Sivertz K. Tricyclic drugs in pregnancy and lactation: a preliminary report. *Int J Psychiatry Med* 1991; **21:** 157–71.

**Cardiovascular disease.** For comments on the potential cardiotoxicity of tricyclic antidepressants and precautions to be observed in patients with pre-existing cardiovascular disorders, see under Effects on the Cardiovascular System in Adverse Effects, above.

**Contact lenses.** Based on reports involving amitriptyline[1] and maprotiline[2] it has been considered that the antimuscarinic action of tricyclic antidepressants may decrease tear flow enough to cause corneal drying and staining of contact lenses.[3]

1. Litovitz GL. Amitriptyline and contact lenses. *J Clin Psychiatry* 1984; **45:** 188.
2. Troiano G. Amitriptyline and contact lenses. *J Clin Psychiatry* 1985; **46:** 199.
3. Anonymous. Drugs interfering with contact lenses. *Aust J Hosp Pharm* 1987; **17:** 55–6.

**Diabetes mellitus.** The fact that tricyclic antidepressants may cause alterations in blood-glucose concentrations has led to the recommendation that these drugs be used with caution in diabetic patients. Additionally, amitriptyline has been reported[1] to cause hypoglycaemic unawareness; a patient did not experience her usual adrenergic symptoms that preceded or accompanied a hypoglycaemic episode.

1. Sherman KE, Bornemann M. Amitriptyline and asymptomatic hypoglycemia. *Ann Intern Med* 1988; **109:** 683–4.

**Driving.** While affective disorders probably adversely affect driving skill,[1,2] treatment with antidepressant drugs may also be hazardous,[1] although patients may be safer drivers with medication than without.[2] Impairment of performance is largely related to sedative and antimuscarinic effects both of which are more pronounced at the start of treatment; sedative tricyclics, such as amitriptyline and doxepin, are likely to cause greater psychomotor impairment than less sedative tricyclics such as imipramine and nortriptyline.[1] However, an epidemiological study[3] was unable to confirm any increased risk of road-traffic accidents in those drivers receiving tricyclic antidepressants or SSRIs. In healthy subjects fluoxetine (an SSRI) and dosulepin appeared to have a similar but apparently small potential for impairing psychomotor and driving performance.[4]

In the UK, the Driver and Vehicle Licensing Authority (DVLA) considers that drugs with antimuscarinic adverse effects, such as tricyclic antidepressants, should be avoided in drivers, and that care is needed when taking antidepressants with antihistamine effects, because of the risk of drowsiness.[5] Patients with severe depressive illnesses complicated by significant memory or concentration problems, agitation, behavioural disturbances or suicidal thoughts should cease driving pending the outcome of medical enquiry.

1. Ashton H. Drugs and driving. *Adverse Drug React Bull* 1983; **98:** 360–3.
2. Cremona A. Mad drivers: psychiatric illness and driving performance. *Br J Hosp Med* 1986; **35:** 193–5.
3. Barbone F, *et al.* Association of road-traffic accidents with benzodiazepine use. *Lancet* 1998; **352:** 1331–6.
4. Ramaekers JG, *et al.* A comparative study of acute and subchronic effects of dothiepin, fluoxetine and placebo on psychomotor and actual driving performance. *Br J Clin Pharmacol* 1995; **39:** 397–404.
5. Driver and Vehicle Licensing Agency. For medical practitioners: at a glance guide to the current medical standards of fitness to drive. Available at: http://www.dvla.gov.uk/at_a_glance/ch4_psychiatric.htm (accessed 04/06/04)

**Electroconvulsive therapy.** For comments concerning the precautions to be observed in patients receiving ECT, see under Anaesthesia, above.

**Epilepsy.** For comments on the epileptogenic effect of tricyclic antidepressants and the need for caution in patients with a history of epilepsy or other risk factors for development of seizures, see under Epileptogenic Effect in Adverse Effects, above.

**Food.** There has been a report of 3 patients in whom a high-fibre diet reduced or abolished the effectiveness of their tricyclic antidepressant therapy;[1] the tricyclics involved were doxepin in two patients and desipramine in one.

1. Stewart DE. High-fiber diet and serum tricyclic antidepressant levels. *J Clin Psychopharmacol* 1992; **12:** 438–40.

**Gastro-oesophageal reflux disease.** The antimuscarinic action of tricyclic antidepressants may cause relaxation of the lower oesophageal sphincter and could aggravate nocturnal symptoms of gastro-oesophageal reflux if given in the late evening.[1]

1. Atkinson M. Use and misuse of drugs in the treatment of gastro-oesophageal reflux. *Prescribers' J* 1982; **22:** 129–36.

**Glaucoma.** It has been considered by the manufacturers that tricyclic antidepressants, because of their antimuscarinic actions, should be used with caution in patients with angle-closure glaucoma or raised intra-ocular pressure. There have been few reports of glaucoma associated with tricyclics, although acute angle-closure glaucoma was reported in 4 patients with narrow angles while taking imipramine in usual doses,[1] and in another patient taking clomipramine.[2] In the latter case, the presenting sign was amaurosis fugax, caused by the combination of an abnormally large drop in blood pressure on standing with raised intra-ocular pressure.

1. Ritch R, *et al.* Oral imipramine and acute angle closure glaucoma. *Arch Ophthalmol* 1994; **112:** 67–8.
2. Schlingemann RO, *et al.* Amaurosis fugax on standing and angle-closure glaucoma with clomipramine. *Lancet* 1996; **347:** 465.

**Phaeochromocytoma.** Use of imipramine[1,2] or desipramine[3] has caused adverse effects such as seizures and cardiovascular abnormalities (tachycardia and hypertension or hypotension) in patients with previously undiagnosed phaeochromocytoma. It has been suggested[3] that imipramine and its metabolite, desipramine, may be particularly effective in unmasking phaeochromocytoma and that this may be a reflection of their relative potency in inhibiting the noradrenaline reuptake mechanism.

1. Kaufmann JS. Pheochromocytoma and tricyclic antidepressants. *JAMA* 1974; **229:** 1282.
2. Mok J, Swann I. Diagnosis of phaeochromocytoma after ingestion of imipramine. *Arch Dis Child* 1978; **53:** 676–7.
3. Achong MR, Keane PM. Pheochromocytoma unmasked by desipramine therapy. *Ann Intern Med* 1981; **94:** 358–9.

**Porphyria.** Amitriptyline has been associated with acute attacks of porphyria and is considered unsafe in porphyric patients.

**Pregnancy.** Management of depression during pregnancy may be difficult, and one report[1] on experience in 8 pregnant women being treated with a tricyclic antidepressant suggested that the antidepressant dose might need to be increased during the second half of pregnancy to achieve a response. There are obvious concerns about such treatment (see also Depression, p.279). However, although there have been isolated reports[2] attributing *congenital malformations* to the use of tricyclic antidepressants during pregnancy, large-scale studies and case-control data[3,4] have failed to substantiate any such association.

The effects of tricyclics on fetal neurodevelopment were studied[5] in 80 pregnant women by later assessing global IQ of the children; no differences were seen in those exposed to tricyclics *in utero* in the first trimester compared with those exposed to fluoxetine or no adverse developmental influences. A subsequent study indicated that exposure to tricyclic antidepressants or fluoxetine throughout gestation did not appear to adversely affect cognition.[6]

*Fetal tachyarrhythmia* detected at 37 weeks of gestation was attributed to maternal use of dosulepin during pregnancy. When this was stopped, no abnormalities in fetal heart rate were found and an uneventful labour led to a healthy infant being delivered. However, the authors expressed concern that fetal tachycardias might result in *in-utero* cardiac failure and considered that tricyclic antidepressants should be used during pregnancy only if there were compelling reasons.[7]

*Withdrawal syndromes* manifesting as hypothermia and jitteriness,[8] convulsions,[9,10] or myoclonus[11] have been reported in neonates whose mothers took clomipramine during pregnancy. Management has been with phenobarbital or clomipramine. The manufacturers advise that if it is justifiable to do so, clomipramine should be withdrawn at least 7 weeks before the calculated date of delivery.

1. Wisner KL, *et al.* Tricyclic dose requirements across pregnancy. *Am J Psychiatry* 1993; **150:** 1541–2.
2. Barson AJ. Malformed infant. *BMJ* 1972; **2:** 45.
3. Greenberg G, *et al.* Maternal drug histories and congenital abnormalities. *BMJ* 1977; **2:** 853–6.
4. Winship KA, *et al.* Maternal drug histories and central nervous system anomalies. *Arch Dis Child* 1984; **59:** 1052–60.
5. Nulman I, *et al.* Neurodevelopment of children exposed in utero to antidepressant drugs. *N Engl J Med* 1997; **336:** 258–62.
6. Nulman I, *et al.* Child development following exposure to tricyclic antidepressants or fluoxetine throughout fetal life: a prospective, controlled study. *Am J Psychiatry* 2002; **159:** 1889–95.
7. Prentice A, Brown R. Fetal tachyarrhythmia and maternal antidepressant treatment. *BMJ* 1989; **298:** 190.
8. Musa AB, Smith CS. Neonatal effects of maternal clomipramine therapy. *Arch Dis Child* 1979; **54:** 405.
9. Cowe L, *et al.* Neonatal convulsions caused by withdrawal from maternal clomipramine. *BMJ* 1982; **284:** 1837–8.
10. Bromiker R, Kaplan M. Apparent intrauterine fetal withdrawal from clomipramine hydrochloride. *JAMA* 1994; **272:** 1722–3.
11. Bloem BR, *et al.* Clomipramine withdrawal in newborns. *Arch Dis Child Fetal Neonatal Ed* 1999; **81:** F77–F79.

**Surgery.** For comments regarding the precautions to be observed in patients undergoing surgery, see under Anaesthesia, above.

**Withdrawal.** Suddenly stopping antidepressant therapy after regular use for 8 weeks or more may precipitate withdrawal symptoms. The symptoms associated with withdrawal of tricyclic antidepressants appear to form four distinct syndromes:[1]

- gastrointestinal disturbances and generalised somatic symptoms such as malaise, chills, headache, and increased perspiration, which may also be accompanied by anxiety and agitation
- sleep disturbances characterised by insomnia followed by excessive and vivid dreams
- parkinsonism or akathisia
- hypomania or mania

Tricyclic withdrawal has also resulted in cardiac arrhythmias in some patients. Withdrawal symptoms seem to be more common and more severe in children.[2]

Many of the symptoms associated with stopping tricyclics may be produced by cholinergic rebound[1] and can be minimised by a gradual reduction in antidepressant dosage. The *British National Formulary* has recommended reduction over a period of at least 4 weeks, or as much as 6 months in patients who have been receiving long-term maintenance therapy. If withdrawal symptoms do occur, they can be managed by reinstitution of the tricyclic in a dose sufficient to eliminate them, followed by gradual discontinuation thereafter.[1,2] On the occasions that it may be necessary to stop a tricyclic abruptly, the withdrawal symptoms can be treated with a centrally active antimuscarinic such as atropine or benzatropine,[1] or alternatively, an antimuscarinic that does not cross the blood-brain barrier, such as propantheline, if the only withdrawal symptoms are gastrointestinal in nature.[1] Awareness of the possibility of withdrawal syndromes helps to avoid misinterpreting new symptoms after withdrawal as evidence of relapse.

Tricyclic antidepressants have been included in some classifications as drugs of dependence because of their potential to produce withdrawal syndromes, but a review[3] of several substance abuse studies challenged this on finding no evidence of abuse or dependence of the barbiturate type developing with the tricyclics.

For reports of withdrawal symptoms in neonates born to mothers who took tricyclic antidepressants during pregnancy, and their management, see under Pregnancy, above.

1. Dilsaver SC. Withdrawal phenomena associated with antidepressant and antipsychotic agents. *Drug Safety* 1994; **10:** 103–14.
2. Anonymous. Problems when withdrawing antidepressives. *Drug Ther Bull* 1986; **24:** 29–30.
3. Lichtigfeld FJ, Gillman MA. The possible abuse of and dependence on major tranquillisers and tricyclic antidepressants. *S Afr Med J* 1994; **84:** 5–6.

## Interactions

Interactions involving tricyclic antidepressants often result from additive toxicity or from altered metabolism of one drug by the other. Drugs that inhibit the cytochrome P450 isoenzyme CYP2D6 may produce substantial decreases in tricyclic metabolism and marked increases in plasma concentrations.

Adverse effects may be enhanced by antimuscarinic drugs or CNS depressants, including alcohol. Barbiturates and other enzyme inducers such as rifampicin and some antiepileptics can increase the metabolism of tricyclic antidepressants and may lower plasma concentrations and reduce antidepressant response. Cimetidine, methylphenidate, antipsychotics, and calcium-channel blockers may reduce the metabolism of the tricyclics leading to the possibility of increased plasma concentrations and accompanying toxicity.

Patients taking thyroid preparations may show an accelerated response to tricyclic antidepressants and occasionally liothyronine has been used to produce this effect in patients with refractory depression. However, the use of tricyclics with thyroid hormone therapy may precipitate cardiac arrhythmias.

The antihypertensive effects of betanidine, debrisoquine, guanethidine, and clonidine may be reduced by tricyclic antidepressants. The pressor effects of sympathomimetics, especially those of the direct-acting drugs adrenaline and noradrenaline, can be enhanced by tricyclic antidepressants; however, there is no clinical evidence of dangerous interactions between adrenaline-containing local anaesthetics and tricyclic antidepressants. Great care should, however, be taken to avoid inadvertent intravenous injection of the local anaesthetic preparation.

Drugs that prolong the QT interval including antiarrhythmics such as quinidine, the antihistamines astemizole and terfenadine, some antipsychotics (notably pimozide, sertindole, and thioridazine), cisapride, halofantrine, and sotalol, may increase the likelihood of ventricular arrhythmias when taken with tricyclic antidepressants. The problem may be exacerbated where the interacting drug (such as quinidine or some antipsychotics) also reduces tricyclic metabolism.

Although different antidepressants have been used together under expert supervision in refractory cases of depression, severe adverse reactions including the serotonin syndrome (see p.313) may occur. For this reason an appropriate drug-free interval should elapse between stopping some types of antidepressant and starting another. Tricyclic antidepressants should not generally be given to patients receiving MAOIs or for at least 2 weeks (3 weeks if starting clomipramine or imipramine) after their withdrawal. No treatment-free period is necessary after stopping a reversible inhibitor of monoamine oxidase type A (RIMA) and starting a tricyclic. At least 1 to 2 weeks (3 weeks in the case of clomipramine or imipramine) should elapse between withdrawing a tricyclic antidepressant and starting any drug liable to provoke a serious reaction (e.g. phenelzine).

Further details concerning some of the above interactions, and others, are given below.

**Alcohol.** For reference to the effect of alcohol on amitriptyline, see under CNS depressants, below.

**Analgesics.** Doubling of plasma-doxepin concentrations with associated lethargy has been reported in a patient following the addition of *dextropropoxyphene* to the tricyclic.[1] This was consistent with previous studies indicating that dextropropoxyphene can impair the hepatic metabolism of other drugs.

For general reference to the effect of tricyclic antidepressants, notably amitriptyline and clomipramine, on opioid analgesics, see under Morphine, p.61.

1. Abernethy DR, *et al.* Impairment of hepatic drug oxidation by propoxyphene. *Ann Intern Med* 1982; **97:** 223–4.

**Antiarrhythmics.** Antiarrhythmics that prolong the QT interval may increase the likelihood of ventricular arrhythmias when given with tricyclic antidepressants.

There has been a report[1] of a patient receiving desipramine who had raised serum-desipramine concentrations and signs of toxicity after starting treatment with digoxin and *propafenone* for paroxysmal atrial fibrillation. It was considered that propafenone probably reduced the metabolism and clearance of desipramine.

1. Katz MR. Raised serum levels of desipramine with the antiarrhythmic propafenone. *J Clin Psychiatry* 1991; **52:** 432–3.

**Anticoagulants.** For the effect of tricyclic antidepressants on anticoagulants, see under Warfarin, p.1025.

**Antidepressants.** Combination therapy with differing classes of antidepressants has been used successfully in the treatment of drug-resistant depression. It should be emphasised, however, that such combinations may result in interactions or enhanced adverse reactions, and should be used only under expert supervision. This practice is considered unsuitable or controversial by some authorities. For further details of the interactions between different antidepressants when coadministered, see Phenelzine, p.315. For details of the serotonin syndrome that can arise when two serotonergic drugs with different mechanisms of action are administered, see under Adverse Effects of Phenelzine, p.313.

**Antidiabetics.** For the effect of tricyclic antidepressants on *sulfonylureas* and *insulin,* see Interactions, p.347 and p.338, respectively.

**Antiepileptics.** Antidepressants may antagonise the activity of antiepileptics by lowering the convulsive threshold.

A review[1] of drug interactions with *phenytoin* noted that although there had been a number of reports of interactions between antiepileptics and tricyclic or related antidepressants, most involved enzyme-inducing antiepileptics other than phenytoin or phenytoin with other drugs. In the only report where phenytoin could be identified as the sole antiepileptic used, 2 patients required high doses of desipramine to achieve an antidepressant effect and to maintain plasma-desipramine concentrations in the range usually associated with therapeutic efficacy.

*Carbamazepine* has been reported to induce the metabolism of a number of tricyclic antidepressants (amitriptyline, desipramine, doxepin, imipramine, and nortriptyline) and to reduce their plasma concentrations. The clinical importance of the interaction is unclear. Use of nortriptyline with carbamazepine in a patient led to a decrease in serum-nortriptyline concentration requiring an increase in nortriptyline dose.[2] In another patient a prolonged QT interval was noted following use of desipramine with carbamazepine;[3] the authors hypothesised that the accelerated metabolism of desipramine had resulted in high levels of a cardiotoxic metabolite.

*Valproate* has been reported to increase plasma concentrations of amitriptyline,[4] clomipramine,[5] and nortriptyline.[4,6]

For the effect of the cyclic antidepressants desipramine and viloxazine on carbamazepine, see p.356. For the effects of tricyclic antidepressants on phenytoin, see p.373.

1. Nation RL, *et al.* Pharmacokinetic drug interactions with phenytoin (part II). *Clin Pharmacokinet* 1990; **18:** 131–50.
2. Brøsen K, Kragh-Sørensen P. Concomitant intake of nortriptyline and carbamazepine. *Ther Drug Monit* 1993; **15:** 258–60.
3. Baldessarini RJ, *et al.* Anticonvulsant cotreatment may increase toxic metabolites of antidepressants and other psychotropic drugs. *J Clin Psychopharmacol* 1988; **8:** 381–2.
4. Wong SL, *et al.* Effects of divalproex sodium on amitriptyline and nortriptyline pharmacokinetics. *Clin Pharmacol Ther* 1996; **60:** 48–53.
5. Fehr C, *et al.* Increase in serum clomipramine concentrations caused by valproate. *J Clin Psychopharmacol* 2000; **20:** 493–4.
6. Fu C, *et al.* Valproate/nortriptyline interaction. *J Clin Psychopharmacol* 1994; **14:** 205–6.

**Antifungals.** Increased serum concentrations of nortriptyline[1] or amitriptyline[2,3] have occurred in patients also taking *fluconazole.* In some patients the use of amitriptyline with fluconazole has led to syncope[3] or torsade de pointes.[4] Raised serum concentrations of nortriptyline and associated symptoms of intoxication have been reported in 2 patients during treatment with *terbinafine;*[5,6] the interaction was confirmed on rechallenge. A study in healthy subjects indicated that terbinafine similarly inhibited the metabolism of desipramine.[7]

1. Gannon RH. Fluconazole-nortriptyline drug interaction. *Ann Pharmacother* 1992; **26:** 1456.
2. Newberry DL, *et al.* A fluconazole/amitriptyline drug interaction in three male adults. *Clin Infect Dis* 1997; **24:** 270–1.
3. Robinson RF, *et al.* Syncope associated with concurrent amitriptyline and fluconazole therapy. *Ann Pharmacother* 2000; **34:** 1406–1409.
4. Dorsey ST, Biblo LA. Prolonged QT interval and torsades de pointes caused by the combination of fluconazole and amitriptyline. *Am J Emerg Med* 2000; **18:** 227–9.
5. van der Kuy P-HM, *et al.* Nortriptyline intoxication induced by terbinafine. *BMJ* 1998; **316:** 441.
6. ven der Kuy P-HM, *et al.* Pharmacokinetic interaction between nortriptyline and terbinafine. *Ann Pharmacother* 2002; **36:** 1712–14.
7. Madani S, *et al.* Effect of terbinafine on the pharmacokinetics and pharmacodynamics of desipramine in healthy volunteers identified as cytochrome P450 2D6 (CYP2D6) extensive metabolizers. *J Clin Pharmacol* 2002; **42:** 1211–18.

**Antihypertensives.** In general, the hypotensive effect of antihypertensives is enhanced by tricyclic antidepressants, but there may be antagonism of the effect of *adrenergic neurone blockers* and of *clonidine.*

**Antimigraine drugs.** For the effect of some tricyclics on *dihydroergotamine,* see p.468.

**Antineoplastics.** For the effect of tricyclic antidepressants on *altretamine,* see p.526.

**Antiprotozoals.** *Furazolidone,* an antiprotozoal with monoamine oxidase inhibiting activity, resulted in a toxic psychosis when given with amitriptyline to a patient.[1]

1. Aderhold RM, Muniz CE. Acute psychosis with amitriptyline and furazolidone. *JAMA* 1970; **213:** 2080.

**Antipsychotics.** For a discussion of interactions between antipsychotics and tricyclic antidepressants, see *Chlorpromazine* (p.679). For details of a possible interaction between clomipramine and *clozapine,* see p.688.

**Antivirals.** HIV-protease inhibitors may increase the plasma concentrations of tricyclic antidepressants whose metabolism is mediated through common cytochrome P450 isoenzymes. *Ritonavir* has produced moderate increases in the plasma concentrations of desipramine and the manufacturer of ritonavir has warned that a similar increase may occur for other tricyclics. Monitoring of drug concentrations and/or adverse effects is recommended when tricyclics are used with ritonavir.

**Anxiolytics.** For a suggestion that *benzodiazepines* may increase the oxidation of amineptine to a toxic metabolite, see under Effects on the Liver in Adverse Effects, above. For a possible interaction of desipramine and other antidepressants with *zolpidem* see p.729.

**Barbiturates.** Barbiturates can increase the metabolism of tricyclic antidepressants and thereby produce lower plasma concentrations.

For details of the interaction of tricyclic antidepressants with barbiturate anaesthetics, see under Anaesthesia in Precautions, above.

**Beta blockers.** *Labetalol* increased the bioavailability of imipramine in healthy subjects and inhibited its metabolism.[1]

The risk of ventricular arrhythmias may be increased when tricyclic antidepressants are taken with *sotalol.*

1. Hermann DJ, *et al.* Comparison of verapamil, diltiazem, and labetalol on the bioavailability and metabolism of imipramine. *J Clin Pharmacol* 1992; **32:** 176–83.

**Calcium-channel blockers.** *Diltiazem* and *verapamil* each increased the bioavailability of imipramine in healthy subjects; second-degree heart block developed in 2 subjects.[1] Diltiazem also increased the bioavailability of nortriptyline in one patient,[2] probably by reducing the first-pass metabolism of nortriptyline. Increased serum concentrations of trimipramine have been reported when taken with diltiazem,[3] although there was no evidence of toxicity.

1. Hermann DJ, *et al.* Comparison of verapamil, diltiazem, and labetalol on the bioavailability and metabolism of imipramine. *J Clin Pharmacol* 1992; **32:** 176–83.
2. Krähenbühl S, *et al.* Pharmacokinetic interaction between diltiazem and nortriptyline. *Eur J Clin Pharmacol* 1996; **49:** 417–19.
3. Cotter PA, *et al.* Asymptomatic tricyclic toxicity associated with diltiazem. *Ir J Psychol Med* 1996; **13:** 168–9.

**CNS depressants.** Drugs with depressant actions on the CNS may be expected to enhance the drowsiness and related effects produced by the sedating type of tricyclic antidepressants. Such an interaction may occur between *alcohol* and tricyclic antidepressants and one study has shown that alcohol decreases the hepatic first-pass extraction of amitriptyline resulting in increased free plasma-amitriptyline concentrations, especially during the period of drug absorption.[1]

The problems that may be encountered with *barbiturate anaesthetics* are discussed under Anaesthesia in Precautions, above.

1. Dorian P, *et al.* Amitriptyline and ethanol: pharmacokinetic and pharmacodynamic interaction. *Eur J Clin Pharmacol* 1983; **25:** 325–31.

**Disulfiram.** Acute organic brain syndrome has been reported in 2 patients receiving disulfiram following the addition of amitriptyline to their treatment.[1] It was suspected that the syndrome was potentiated by the combined action of the two drugs and the synergistic elevation in dopamine concentration.

For a report of the enhancement of the disulfiram-alcohol reaction by amitriptyline, see p.1682.

1. Maany I, *et al.* Possible toxic interaction between disulfiram and amitriptyline. *Arch Gen Psychiatry* 1982; **39:** 743–4.

**Dopaminergics.** Serious adverse effects have been reported[1] when *selegiline*, an irreversible selective inhibitor of monoamine oxidase type B, and tricyclic antidepressants have been used concomitantly. In some instances effects resembled the potentially fatal serotonin syndromes reported when tricyclics are given with non-selective MAOIs (see under Phenelzine, p.313).

Some manufacturers of selegiline advise that tricyclic antidepressants should not generally be given at the same time, or for at least 2 weeks after it has been discontinued. Similarly, at least one week should elapse between withdrawing a tricyclic antidepressant and starting selegiline.

For reference to the effect of tricyclic antidepressants on *levodopa*, see p.1208.

1. Anonymous. Selegiline and antidepressants: risk of serious interactions. *WHO Drug Inf* 1995; **9:** 160–1.

**General anaesthetics.** For the effect of amitriptyline on *enflurane*, see p.1298. For the effects of concomitant use of tricyclic antidepressants and *barbiturates* see under Anaesthesia in Precautions, above.

**Histamine $H_2$-antagonists.** *Cimetidine* is a known inhibitor of hepatic metabolism of drugs and symptoms of tricyclic toxicity have been reported in patients receiving cimetidine with desipramine,[1] doxepin,[2] and imipramine;[1] there has been a report of psychosis developing in a patient given imipramine and cimetidine.[3] Elevated tricyclic concentrations during combined therapy or reductions in tricyclic concentrations after withdrawal of cimetidine have been reported for imipramine[4] and nortriptyline.[5] Studies in healthy subjects have also indicated increased bioavailability and/or impaired hepatic metabolism of amitriptyline,[6] doxepin,[7,8] and imipramine[9] during cimetidine therapy. Adjustment of tricyclic antidepressant dosage may therefore be required if cimetidine therapy is begun or stopped.

*Ranitidine* has been reported not to alter the pharmacokinetics of amitriptyline,[10] doxepin,[8] or imipramine.[9]

1. Miller DD, Macklin M. Cimetidine-imipramine interaction: a case report. *Am J Psychiatry* 1983; **140:** 351–2.
2. Brown BA, *et al.* Cimetidine-doxepin interaction. *J Clin Psychopharmacol* 1985; **5:** 245–7.
3. Miller ME, *et al.* Psychosis in association with combined cimetidine and imipramine treatment. *Psychosomatics* 1987; **28:** 217–19.
4. Shapiro PA. Cimetidine-imipramine interaction: case report and comments. *Am J Psychiatry* 1984; **141:** 152.
5. Miller DD, *et al.* Cimetidine's effect on steady-state serum nortriptyline concentrations. *Drug Intell Clin Pharm* 1983; **17:** 904–5.
6. Curry SH, *et al.* Cimetidine interaction with amitriptyline. *Eur J Clin Pharmacol* 1985; **29:** 429–33.
7. Abernethy DR, Todd EL. Doxepin-cimetidine interaction: increased doxepin bioavailability during cimetidine treatment. *J Clin Psychopharmacol* 1986; **6:** 8–12.
8. Sutherland DL, *et al.* The influence of cimetidine versus ranitidine on doxepin pharmacokinetics. *Eur J Clin Pharmacol* 1987; **32:** 159–64.
9. Wells BG, *et al.* The effect of ranitidine and cimetidine on imipramine disposition. *Eur J Clin Pharmacol* 1986; **31:** 285–90.
10. Curry SH, *et al.* Lack of interaction of ranitidine with amitriptyline. *Eur J Clin Pharmacol* 1987; **32:** 317–20.

**Muscle relaxants.** There has been an isolated report[1] of a patient taking *baclofen* for spasticity who experienced leg weakness and was unable to stand after starting treatment with nortriptyline. Symptoms improved on stopping nortriptyline but recurred when imipramine was given.

1. Silverglat MJ. Baclofen and tricyclic antidepressants: possible interaction. *JAMA* 1981; **246:** 1659.

**Sex hormones.** There have been anecdotal reports of interactions between tricyclic antidepressants and *oestrogens*[1-3] resulting in a lack of antidepressant response and/or tricyclic toxicity; the significance of these interactions is not, however, established.

1. Prange AJ, *et al.* Estrogen may well affect response to antidepressant. *JAMA* 1972; **219:** 143–4.
2. Khurana RC. Estrogen-imipramine interaction. *JAMA* 1972; **222:** 702–3.
3. Somani SM, Khurana RC. Mechanism of estrogen-imipramine interaction. *JAMA* 1973; **223:** 560.

**Smoking.** Tobacco smoke has been reported to reduce the plasma levels of tricyclic antidepressants.[1-3] The clinical significance is not, however, fully established as the plasma concentration of unbound drug may not be affected.[3] The mechanism is probably by stimulation of hepatic drug metabolism by components present in cigarette smoke.

1. Perel JM, *et al.* Pharmacodynamics of imipramine in depressed patients. *Psychopharmacol Bull* 1975; **11:** 16–18.
2. John VA, *et al.* Effects of age, cigarette smoking and the oral contraceptive on the pharmacokinetics of clomipramine and its desmethyl metabolite during chronic dosing. *J Int Med Res* 1980; **8** (suppl 3): 88–95.
3. Perry PJ, *et al.* Effects of smoking on nortriptyline plasma concentrations in depressed patients. *Ther Drug Monit* 1986; **8:** 279–84.

**Sympathomimetics.** The pressor effects of sympathomimetics can be enhanced by tricyclic antidepressants.

For precautions to be observed in patients on tricyclic therapy who may require sympathomimetics during anaesthesia, see under Anaesthesia in Precautions, above.

**Thyroid hormones.** An increase in receptor sensitivity to catecholamines produced by thyroid hormones has been proposed as the reason for an increase in response to tricyclic antidepressants given with *liothyronine*.[1,2]

1. Banki CM. Cerebrospinal fluid amine metabolites after combined amitriptyline-triiodothyronine treatment of depressed women. *Eur J Clin Pharmacol* 1977; **11:** 311–15.
2. Goodwin FK, *et al.* Potentiation of antidepressant effects by L-triiodothyronine in tricyclic nonresponders. *Am J Psychiatry* 1982; **139:** 34–8.

## Pharmacokinetics

Amitriptyline is readily absorbed from the gastrointestinal tract, peak plasma concentrations occurring within a few hours of oral doses.

Amitriptyline undergoes extensive first-pass metabolism and is demethylated in the liver by the cytochrome P450 isoenzymes CYP3A4, CYP2C9, and CYP2D6 to its primary active metabolite, nortriptyline. Other paths of metabolism of amitriptyline include hydroxylation (possibly to active metabolites) by CYP2D6 and *N*-oxidation; nortriptyline follows similar paths. Amitriptyline is excreted in the urine, mainly in the form of its metabolites, either free or in conjugated form.

Amitriptyline and nortriptyline are widely distributed throughout the body and are extensively bound to plasma and tissue protein. Amitriptyline has been estimated to have an elimination half-life ranging from about 9 to 25 hours, which may be considerably extended in overdosage. Plasma concentrations of amitriptyline and nortriptyline vary very widely between individuals and no simple correlation with therapeutic response has been established.

Amitriptyline and nortriptyline cross the placenta and are distributed into breast milk (see Breast Feeding under Precautions, above).

◊ References.

1. Schulz P, *et al.* Discrepancies between pharmacokinetic studies of amitriptyline. *Clin Pharmacokinet* 1985; **10:** 257–68.
2. Brøsen K, Gram LF. Clinical significance of the sparteine/debrisoquine oxidation polymorphism. *Eur J Clin Pharmacol* 1989; **36:** 537–47.
3. Caccia S, Garattini S. Formation of active metabolites of psychotropic drugs: an updated review of their significance. *Clin Pharmacokinet* 1990; **18:** 434–59.
4. Wood AJJ, Zhou HH. Ethnic differences in drug disposition and responsiveness. *Clin Pharmacokinet* 1991; **20:** 350–73.
5. Llerena A, *et al.* Debrisoquin and mephenytoin hydroxylation phenotypes and CYP2D6 genotype in patients treated with neuroleptic and antidepressant agents. *Clin Pharmacol Ther* 1993; **54:** 606–11.

## Uses and Administration

Tricyclic antidepressants such as amitriptyline were developed from phenothiazine compounds related to chlorpromazine and, as the name suggests, possess a 3-ring molecular structure. They inhibit the neuronal reuptake of noradrenaline in the CNS; some, in addition, inhibit the reuptake of serotonin (5-HT). Prevention of the reuptake of these monoamine neurotransmitters, which potentiates their action in the brain, appears to be associated with antidepressant activity. Tricyclic antidepressants also possess affinity for muscarinic and histamine $H_1$ receptors to varying degrees, see under Adverse Effects, above. Amitriptyline is one of the more sedating tricyclics. Antidepressants with one, two, or four rings have also been developed, and these share only some of the properties of the tricyclics.

While the sedative action and other adverse effects of amitriptyline and other tricyclics are soon apparent, it may be 2 to 4 weeks before any antidepressant effect is seen. After a response has been obtained, maintenance therapy should be continued at the optimum dose for at least 4 to 6 months (12 months in the elderly) to avoid relapse on discontinuation of therapy. It is important to use doses that are sufficiently high for effective treatment, but not so high as to cause toxic effects.

Amitriptyline, a dibenzocycloheptadiene, is usually given by mouth as the hydrochloride; the hydrochloride may also be given by intramuscular injection. For both these routes doses are expressed in terms of the hydrochloride. Amitriptyline may also be given by mouth as the embonate; doses of amitriptyline embonate are expressed in terms of the base. Amitriptyline embonate 112.7 mg is approximately equivalent to 75.0 mg of amitriptyline hydrochloride and 66.3 mg of amitriptyline base. Amitriptyline oxide (amitriptylinoxide) is also given by mouth.

In the treatment of **depression**, amitriptyline hydrochloride is given by mouth initially in a daily dose of 75 mg in divided doses (or as a single dose at night). Thereafter, the dose may be gradually increased, if necessary, to 150 mg daily, the additional doses being given in the late afternoon or evening. Therapy may also be begun with a single dose of 50 to 100 mg at bedtime, increased by 25 or 50 mg as necessary to a total of 150 mg daily. Doses of up to 200 mg daily and, occasionally, up to 300 mg daily have been used in severely depressed patients in hospital.

Adolescent and elderly patients often have reduced tolerance to tricyclic antidepressants and initial doses of amitriptyline hydrochloride 25 to 75 mg daily are licensed in these groups, given either as divided doses or as a single dose, preferably at bedtime. The *British National Formulary* suggests a minimum initial dose of 30 mg daily.

In the initial stages of treatment, if dosage by mouth is impracticable or inadvisable, amitriptyline hydrochloride may be given by intramuscular injection, but the oral route should be substituted as soon as possible. The dose is 20 to 30 mg four times daily. The intravenous route has also been used.

Amitriptyline is also used for the treatment of **nocturnal enuresis** in children in whom organic pathology has been excluded. However, drug therapy for nocturnal enuresis should be reserved for when other methods have failed and should preferably only be given to cover periods away from home; tricyclic antidepressants are not recommended in children under 6 years of age (the *British National Formulary* recommends that they should not be given until 7 years of age). Doses of amitriptyline hydrochloride that may be used are 10 to 20 mg at bedtime for children aged 6 to 10 years, and 25 to 50 mg at bedtime for children over 11 years of age. Treatment for enuresis, including the period of gradual withdrawal, should not continue for longer than 3 months. A full physical examination is recommended before a further course.

Tricyclic antidepressants, including amitriptyline, may be helpful in some disorders characterised by anxiety, and in the management of neuropathic pain.

Amitriptyline should be withdrawn gradually to reduce the risk of withdrawal symptoms.

**Anxiety disorders.** See under Clomipramine, p.290.

**Bulimia nervosa.** A combination of counselling, support, psychotherapy, and antidepressants is the usual treatment for bulimia nervosa. Antidepressants can help to reduce the frequency of overeating and some other symptoms of bulimia but relapse tends to occur when stopped. Many antidepressants have been tried, but the tricyclic desipramine and the SSRI fluoxetine have been the most commonly used and are considered to be well tolerated.

References.

1. Bacaltchuk J, *et al.* Antidepressants versus psychological treatments and their combination for bulimia nervosa. Available in The Cochrane Library; Issue 2. Chichester: John Wiley; 2004.
2. Bacaltchuk J, Hay P. Antidepressants versus placebo for people with bulimia nervosa. Available in The Cochrane Library; Issue 2. Chichester: John Wiley; 2004.

**Ciguatera poisoning.** Amitriptyline has relieved some of the neurological symptoms associated with ciguatera poisoning (see Mannitol, p.951).

**Cocaine dependence.** See under Desipramine, p.290.

**Depression.** As discussed on p.279, there is very little difference in efficacy between the different groups of antidepressant drugs, and choice is often made on the basis of adverse effect profile. Tricyclic antidepressants are often still chosen because of wide experience with their use and familiarity with their pharmacological actions. The more sedating tricyclics such as amitriptyline, clomipramine, dosulepin, doxepin, and trimipramine may be of value in depression with associated agitation or anxiety. The less sedating tricyclics such as amoxapine, desipramine, imipramine, lofepramine, nortriptyline, and protriptyline may be of value for withdrawn or apathetic depressed patients.

Combination therapy with differing classes of antidepressants, including the tricyclics, has been used in the treatment of refractory or drug-resistant depression. However, such therapy may result in enhanced adverse reactions or interactions and requires expert supervision; it is considered unsuitable or controversial by some. For further details, see Antidepressants under Interactions of Phenelzine, p.315.

**Headache.** Tricyclic antidepressants can be effective in the management of some types of headache and, although they are especially useful when the headache is accompanied by depression, their beneficial effects appear to be independent of their antidepressant action. They are used for the prophylaxis of migraine (p.464) when drugs such as propranolol or pizotifen have proved ineffective. Amitriptyline is the tricyclic usually used but others have been tried. It has also been investigated in children. A suggested adult dosage for amitriptyline in the prophylaxis of migraine is 10 mg at night increased to a maintenance dose of 50 to 75 mg at night; the need for continuing prophylaxis should be reviewed at intervals of about 6 months. Tricyclics are also used prophylactically in the control of chronic tension-type headache (p.465) although benefit is rarely complete. Improvement is generally seen with low doses, but full antidepressant doses are necessary in the presence of underlying depression.

References.

1. Mathew NT. Prophylaxis of migraine and mixed headache: a randomized controlled study. *Headache* 1981; **21:** 105–9.
2. Pfaffenrath V, *et al.* Combination headache: practical experience with a combination of a β-blocker and an antidepressive. *Cephalalgia* 1986; **6** (suppl 5): 25–32.
3. Wörz R, Scherhag R. Treatment of chronic tension headache with doxepin or amitriptyline—results of a double-blind study. *Headache Q* 1990; **1:** 216–23.
4. Ziegler DK, *et al.* Propranolol and amitriptyline in prophylaxis of migraine: pharmacokinetic and therapeutic effects. *Arch Neurol* 1993; **50:** 825–30.
5. Pfaffenrath V, *et al.* Efficacy and tolerability of amitriptylinoxide in the treatment of chronic tension-type headache: a multi-centre controlled study. *Cephalalgia* 1994; **14:** 149–55.
6. Hershey AD, *et al.* Effectiveness of amitriptyline in the prophylactic management of childhood headaches. *Headache* 2000; **40:** 539–49.
7. Holroyd KA, *et al.* Management of chronic tension-type headache with tricyclic antidepressant medication, stress management therapy, and their combination: a randomized controlled trial. *JAMA* 2001; **285:** 2208–15.

**Hiccup.** Amitriptyline is one of many drugs for which there are anecdotal reports[1] of success in the treatment of intractable hiccup. A protocol for the management of intractable hiccups may be found under Chlorpromazine, p.682.

1. Stalnikowicz R, *et al.* Amitriptyline for intractable hiccups. *N Engl J Med* 1986; **315:** 64–5.

**Hyperactivity.** When drug therapy is required for attention deficit hyperactivity disorder (p.1583), initial treatment is usually with a central stimulant. Tricyclic antidepressants such as imipramine or desipramine are reserved for patients who fail to respond to or who are intolerant of stimulants. They may also be of use for selected patients with certain co-existing disorders.

**Interstitial cystitis.** Tricyclic antidepressants such as amitriptyline or imipramine have been found to be of benefit in the treatment of interstitial cystitis (see Dimethyl Sulfoxide, p.1473) given at night in conjunction with methenamine hippurate during the day.[1]

1. Cardozo L. Postmenopausal cystitis. *BMJ* 1996; **313:** 129.

**Irritable bowel syndrome.** A tricyclic antidepressant may be tried in irritable bowel syndrome (p.1244), particularly where diarrhoea and abdominal pain are presenting symptoms.

**Micturition disorders.** Tricyclic antidepressants are among the drugs used as an alternative or adjunct to nonpharmacological methods for the treatment of **nocturnal enuresis** in children (p.475) in whom organic pathology has been excluded. However, because of their potentially fatal toxicity in overdosage, there has been concern over the safety of using tricyclics in households with children. Most experience in nocturnal enuresis has been with imipramine, but other tricyclics such as amitriptyline, nortriptyline, and clomipramine have also been used. Their mechanism of action in nocturnal enuresis is unclear. It may be the result of their antimuscarinic and antispasmodic actions as well as their effect on sleep patterns and possible stimulation of antidiuretic hormone secretion. Imipramine appears to be most effective in older children, but many patients develop tolerance and increasingly higher doses are required.

Tricyclic antidepressants are also sometimes used in the management of **urinary incontinence** (p.476).

References.

1. Glazener CMA, Evans JHC. Tricyclic and related drugs for nocturnal enuresis in children. Available in The Cochrane Library; Issue 2. Chichester: John Wiley; 2004.

**Narcoleptic syndrome.** Tricyclic antidepressants are the primary treatment for cataplexy and sleep paralysis associated with narcolepsy (p.1583). Imipramine appears to be one of the most widely used for these symptoms. The onset of action is quicker than when used for depression and doses required appear to be lower (typically 10 to 75 mg daily). Doses should be titrated to provide maximal protection for the time of day when symptoms usually occur. Clomipramine and protriptyline are also commonly used.

**Pain.** Tricyclic antidepressants, usually amitriptyline, are useful in alleviating some types of pain when given in subantidepressant doses. An initial dose of 10 to 25 mg at night increased gradually if necessary to about 75 mg daily has been suggested by the *British National Formulary* for the management of neuropathic pain. See also Choice of Analgesic on p.2. Chronic neuropathic pain as seen in cancer (p.5), central post-stroke pain (p.5), diabetic neuropathy (p.6), phantom limb pain (p.7), and postherpetic neuralgia (p.7) responds to therapy with tricyclics. Tricyclics are also often of benefit in the treatment of idiopathic orofacial pain (p.7), and may be of value for patients with complex regional pain syndrome (p.5). Pain and sleep quality may be improved by tricyclics in patients with fibromyalgia (see Soft-tissue Rheumatism, p.11), a condition that responds poorly to analgesics and anti-inflammatory drugs. Patients with migraine or chronic tension-type headache may also benefit from tricyclics (see Headache, above). There is little evidence for an analgesic effect of tricyclics in acute or arthritic pain.

References.

1. Onghena P, Van Houdenhove, B. Antidepressant-induced analgesia in chronic non-malignant pain: a meta-analysis of 39 placebo-controlled studies. *Pain* 1992; **49:** 205–19.
2. McQuay HJ, *et al.* A systematic review of antidepressants in neuropathic pain. *Pain* 1996; **68:** 217–27.
3. Godfrey RG. A guide to the understanding and use of tricyclic antidepressants in the overall management of fibromyalgia and other chronic pain syndromes. *Arch Intern Med* 1996; **156:** 1047–52.
4. McQuay HJ, Moore RA. Antidepressants and chronic pain. *BMJ* 1997; **314:** 763–4.
5. Joss JD. Tricyclic antidepressant use in diabetic neuropathy. *Ann Pharmacother* 1999; **33:** 996–1000.
6. Arnold LM, *et al.* Antidepressant treatment of fibromyalgia: a meta-analysis and review. *Psychosomatics* 2000; **41:** 104–13.
7. Lynch ME. Antidepressants as analgesics: a review of randomized controlled trials. *J Psychiatry Neurosci* 2001; **26:** 30–6.

**Pathological crying or laughing.** Pathological crying or laughing can result from lesions in certain areas of the brain. Attempts at treatment have mostly been with antidepressants and favourable results have been reported in double-blind studies with amitriptyline[1] and nortriptyline.[2]

1. Schiffer RB, *et al.* Treatment of pathologic laughing and weeping with amitriptyline. *N Engl J Med* 1985; **312:** 1480–2.
2. Robinson RG, *et al.* Pathological laughing and crying following stroke: validation of a measurement scale and a double-blind treatment study. *Am J Psychiatry* 1993; **150:** 286–93.

**Premenstrual syndrome.** See under Clomipramine, p.290.

**Schizophrenia.** Antidepressants such as the tricyclics are considered worth trying as an adjunct in the treatment of patients with schizophrenia (p.665) who develop depression during the recovery phase after an acute episode of psychosis. There is, however, no clear evidence that they are effective during acute psychotic episodes or for depression during periods of remission in patients with chronic schizophrenia.[1]

1. Anonymous. The drug treatment of patients with schizophrenia. *Drug Ther Bull* 1995; **33:** 81–6.

**Sexual dysfunction.** Impotence or ejaculatory problems have been reported as adverse effects of tricyclic antidepressants (see Effects on Sexual Function in Adverse Effects, above). Such properties have been studied as a potential form of treatment for men with premature ejaculation (see Clomipramine, p.290).

**Skin disorders.** See under Doxepin, p.291.

**Smoking cessation.** Tricyclic antidepressants are among the drugs that have been tried with varying degrees of success as alternatives to nicotine replacement therapy (NRT) to alleviate the withdrawal syndrome associated with smoking cessation (p.1721). Nortriptyline is recommended by some as a second-line treatment in those patients who cannot tolerate or relapse after NRT.

References.

1. Hughes JR, *et al.* Antidepressants for smoking cessation. Available in The Cochrane Library; Issue 2. Chichester: John Wiley; 2004.

## Preparations

***BP 2003:*** Amitriptyline Tablets;
***USP 27:*** Amitriptyline Hydrochloride Injection; Amitriptyline Hydrochloride Tablets; Chlordiazepoxide and Amitriptyline Hydrochloride Tablets; Perphenazine and Amitriptyline Hydrochloride Tablets.

**Proprietary Preparations** (details are given in Part 3)
***Arg.:*** Tryptanol; Uxen; ***Austral.:*** Amitrol†; Endep; Tryptanol; Tryptine†; ***Austria:*** Saroten; Tryptizol; ***Belg.:*** Redomex; Tryptizol; ***Braz.:*** Amytril; Protanol; Tripsol; Tryptanol; Tryptil†; ***Canad.:*** Elavil; Levate†; Novo-Triptyn†; ***Denm.:*** Saroten; Tryptizol; ***Fin.:*** Klotriptyl; Saroten; Triptyl; ***Fr.:*** Elavil; Laroxyl; ***Ger.:*** Amineurin; Amioxid; Equilibrin; Novoprotect; Saroten; Syneudon; ***Gr.:*** Maxivalet; Saroten; ***Hong Kong:*** Domical†; Tryptanol; ***India:*** Sarotena; Tryptomer; ***Irl.:*** Lentizol; Tryptizol†; ***Israel:*** Elatrol; Elatrolet; Tryptal; ***Ital.:*** Adepril; Amilit-IFI†; Laroxyl; Triptizol; ***Malaysia:*** Endep; Tripta; Tryptanol; ***Mex.:*** Anapsique; Tryptanol; ***Neth.:*** Sarotex; Tryptizol; ***Norw.:*** Sarotex; Tryptizol; ***NZ:*** Amitrip; Tryptanol†; ***Port.:*** ADT; Tryptizol; ***S.Afr.:*** Saroten†; Trepiline; Tryptanol; ***Singapore:*** Tripta; ***Spain:*** Deprelio; Tryptizol; ***Swed.:*** Saroten; Tryptizol; ***Switz.:*** Saroten; Tryptizol; ***Thai.:*** Polytanol; Tripsyline; Tripta; Triptyline; Tryptanol; ***UK:*** Elavil; Lentizol†; ***USA:*** Elavil†.

**Multi-ingredient:** ***Arg.:*** Mutabon D; ***Austria:*** Limbitrol; Pantrop; ***Belg.:*** Limbitrol†; ***Braz.:*** Limbitrol; ***Canad.:*** Elavil Plus†; Etrafon†; PMS-Levazine†; Triavil; ***Chile:*** Antalin; Morelin; Mutabon D; ***Fin.:*** Limbitrol; Pertriptyl; ***Ger.:*** Limbatril†; ***Gr.:*** Minitran; ***Irl.:*** Triptafen†; ***Ital.:*** Diapatol; Limbitryl; Mutabon; Sedans; ***Mex.:*** Adepsique; ***Port.:*** Mutabon; ***S.Afr.:*** Etrafon; Limbitrol; ***Spain:*** Mutabase; Nobritol; ***Switz.:*** Limbitrol; ***Thai.:*** Anxipress-D; Neuragon; ***UK:*** Triptafen; ***USA:*** Etrafon; Limbitrol; Triavil.

---

# Amoxapine *(BAN, USAN, rINN)*

Amoxapina; CL-67772. 2-Chloro-11-(piperazin-1-yl)dibenz[*b,f*]-[1,4]oxazepine.

$C_{17}H_{16}ClN_3O$ = 313.8.

*CAS — 14028-44-5.*

*ATC — N06AA17.*

**Pharmacopoeias.** In *Jpn* and *US.*

**USP 27** (Amoxapine). A white to yellowish crystalline powder. Practically insoluble in water; slightly soluble in acetone; freely soluble in chloroform; sparingly soluble in methyl alcohol and in toluene; soluble in tetrahydrofuran. Store in airtight containers.

## Adverse Effects, Treatment, and Precautions

As for tricyclic antidepressants in general (see Amitriptyline, p.281).

Rare cases of tardive dyskinesias and the neuroleptic malignant syndrome have been reported with amoxapine.

**Antidopaminergic effects.** Amoxapine is a derivative of the antipsychotic loxapine (p.705) and possesses some antipsychotic activity. It also has dopamine-receptor blocking properties as do its hydroxylated metabolites. Adverse effects that are symptoms of such blockade have been reported and reviewed[1,2] and include akinesia, akathisia, withdrawal dyskinesia, reversible tardive dyskinesia, persistent dyskinesia, elevated serum concentration of prolactin, and galactorrhoea. Chorea[3] and oculogyric crisis[4] have also been reported.

1. Tao GK, *et al.* Amoxapine-induced tardive dyskinesia. *Drug Intell Clin Pharm* 1985; **19:** 548–9.
2. Devarajan S. Safety of amoxapine. *Lancet* 1989; **ii:** 1455.
3. Patterson JF. Amoxapine-induced chorea. *South Med J* 1983; **76:** 1077.
4. Hunt-Fugate AK, *et al.* Adverse reactions due to dopamine blockade by amoxapine. *Pharmacotherapy* 1984; **4:** 35–9.

**Antimuscarinic effects.** Amoxapine therapy has been reported to produce adverse effects associated with antimuscarinic activity (such as constipation, blurred vision, and dry mouth), but such reports did not reflect *in-vitro* findings that amoxapine had considerably less affinity for muscarinic binding sites than amitriptyline;[1] this was supported by results in healthy subjects. The adverse effects described as antimuscarinic could possibly be explained by amoxapine affecting noradrenergic mechanisms.

1. Bourne M, *et al.* A comparison of the effects of single doses of amoxapine and amitriptyline on autonomic functions in healthy volunteers. *Eur J Clin Pharmacol* 1993; **44:** 57–62.

**Breast feeding.** For comments on the use of tricyclic antidepressants in breast feeding patients, see under Precautions for Amitriptyline, p.283.

**Effects on the endocrine system.** Reversible nonketotic hyperglycaemia developed in a 49-year-old woman with no history of diabetes mellitus within 5 days of therapy with amoxapine 50 mg three times daily by mouth.[1] She had previously experienced nonketotic hyperglycaemic coma after loxapine 150 mg daily. 7-Hydroxyamoxapine, a metabolite common to both amoxapine and loxapine, was implicated.

See also Antidopaminergic Effects, above, for mention of galactorrhoea and hyperprolactinaemia.

1. Tollefson G, Lesar T. Nonketotic hyperglycemia associated with loxapine and amoxapine: case report. *J Clin Psychiatry* 1983; **44:** 347–8.

**Overdosage.** In overdosage, amoxapine is reported to cause acute renal failure with rhabdomyolysis,[1,2] coma, and seizures.[3-5] Although there has been some debate as to whether the incidence of seizures and death is higher with overdosage of amoxapine than with other tricyclic antidepressants, some[6] consider that evidence does seem to favour increased neurological consequences.

It has been reported that amoxapine is not cardiotoxic in overdosage[3] but later evidence would suggest that there is cardiotoxic potential.[6,7]

1. Pumariega AJ, *et al.* Acute renal failure secondary to amoxapine overdose. *JAMA* 1982; **248:** 3141–2.
2. Jennings AE, *et al.* Amoxapine-associated acute renal failure. *Arch Intern Med* 1983; **143:** 1525–7.
3. Kulig K, *et al.* Amoxapine overdose: coma and seizures without cardiotoxic effects. *JAMA* 1982; **248:** 1092–4.
4. Litovitz TL, Troutman WG. Amoxapine overdose: seizures and fatalities. *JAMA* 1983; **250:** 1069–71.
5. Jefferson JW. Convulsions associated with amoxapine. *JAMA* 1984; **251:** 603–4.
6. Leonard BE. Safety of amoxapine. *Lancet* 1989; **ii:** 808.
7. Sørensen MR. Acute myocardial failure following amoxapine intoxication. *J Clin Psychopharmacol* 1988; **8:** 75.

## Interactions

For interactions associated with tricyclic antidepressants, see Amitriptyline, p.284.

### Pharmacokinetics

Amoxapine is readily absorbed from the gastrointestinal tract. It bears a close chemical relationship to loxapine (p.705) and is similarly metabolised by hydroxylation. It is excreted in the urine, mainly as its metabolites in conjugated form as glucuronides.

Amoxapine has been reported to have a plasma half-life of 8 hours and its major metabolite, 8-hydroxyamoxapine, has been reported to have a biological half-life of 30 hours; another metabolite, 7-hydroxyamoxapine, has a half-life of 6.5 hours. Both metabolites are pharmacologically active. Amoxapine is extensively bound to plasma proteins.

Amoxapine and its metabolite 8-hydroxyamoxapine are distributed into breast milk.

### Uses and Administration

Amoxapine, the *N*-desmethyl derivative of loxapine (p.705), is a dibenzoxazepine tricyclic antidepressant with actions and uses similar to those of amitriptyline (p.285). Amoxapine is one of the less sedating tricyclics and its antimuscarinic effects are mild; it also inhibits the reuptake of dopamine.

In the treatment of depression (p.279) amoxapine is given in oral doses of 50 mg two or three times daily initially, gradually increased up to 100 mg three times daily as necessary. In the USA, higher doses of up to 600 mg daily may also be given, if required, in severely depressed patients in hospital. A suggested dose for the elderly is 25 mg two or three times daily initially, increased after 5 to 7 days to up to 150 mg daily as necessary; in the USA further increases to a maximum of 300 mg daily are permitted, if required.

Once-daily dosage regimens, usually given at night, are suitable for amoxapine up to 300 mg daily; divided-dosage regimens are recommended for doses above 300 mg daily.

It has been claimed that, in the treatment of depression, amoxapine has a more rapid onset of action than amitriptyline or imipramine with a clinical effect possibly appearing 4 to 7 days after the initiation of therapy, although this has been disputed.

Amoxapine should be withdrawn gradually to reduce the risk of withdrawal symptoms.

◊ References.

1. Jue SG, *et al.* Amoxapine: a review of its pharmacology and efficacy in depressed states. *Drugs* 1982; **24:** 1–23.

### Preparations

***USP 27:*** Amoxapine Tablets.

**Proprietary Preparations** (details are given in Part 3)
***Canad.:*** Asendin†; ***Denm.:*** Demolox; ***Fr.:*** Defanyl; ***India:*** Demolox; ***Irl.:*** Asendis†; ***NZ:*** Asendin†; ***Spain:*** Demolox†; ***UK:*** Asendis; ***USA:*** Asendin.

## Befloxatone *(rINN)*

Befloxatona. (*R*)-5-(Methoxymethyl)-3-{*p*-[(*R*)-4,4,4-trifluoro-3-hydroxybutoxy]phenyl}-2-oxazolidinone.

$C_{15}H_{18}F_3NO_5$ = 349.3.
*CAS — 134564-82-2.*

### Profile

Befloxatone, an oxazolidinone derivative, is a reversible inhibitor of monoamine oxidase type A (RIMA) (see Moclobemide, p.308) that has been investigated for the treatment of depression.

◊ References.

1. Patat A, *et al.* Pharmacodynamics and pharmacokinetics of two dose regimens of befloxatone, a new reversible and selective monoamine oxidase inhibitor, at steady state in healthy volunteers. *J Clin Pharmacol* 1996; **36:** 216–29.
2. Rosenzweig P, *et al.* Clinical pharmacology of befloxatone: a brief review. *J Affect Disord* 1998; **51:** 305–12.

## Benactyzine Hydrochloride *(BANM, rINNM)*

Hidrocloruro de benacticina. 2-Diethylaminoethyl benzilate hydrochloride.

$C_{20}H_{25}NO_3$,HCl = 363.9.
*CAS — 302-40-9 (benactyzine); 57-37-4 (benactyzine hydrochloride).*

### Profile

Benactyzine has antidepressant and antimuscarinic activity. It has been used as the hydrochloride in the management of depression and associated anxiety. It is also used as a pharmacological tool. Methylbenactyzium bromide (p.485), the methobromide of benactyzine, has been used for its antimuscarinic activity in the treatment of gastrointestinal spasm and nocturnal enuresis.

### Preparations

**Proprietary Preparations** (details are given in Part 3)
**Multi-ingredient:** ***Arg.:*** Dimaval.

## Brofaromine *(rINN)*

Brofaromina; CGP-11305A (brofaromine hydrochloride). 4-(7-Bromo-5-methoxy-2-benzofuranyl)piperidine.

$C_{14}H_{16}BrNO_2$ = 310.2.
*CAS — 63638-91-5.*

### Profile

Brofaromine is a reversible inhibitor of monoamine oxidase type A (RIMA) (see Moclobemide, p.308). It has been studied in the treatment of depression and in anxiety disorders including social phobia.

◊ References.

1. Steiger A, *et al.* Results of an open clinical trial of brofaromine (CGP 11305 A), a competitive, selective, and short-acting inhibitor of MAO-A in major endogenous depression. *Pharmacopsychiatry* 1987; **20:** 262–9.
2. van Vliet IM, *et al.* MAO inhibitors in panic disorder: clinical effects of treatment with brofaromine: a double blind placebo controlled study. *Psychopharmacology (Berl)* 1993; **112:** 483–9.
3. Zeeh J, *et al.* Influence of age, frailty and liver function on the pharmacokinetics of brofaromine. *Eur J Clin Pharmacol* 1996; **49:** 387–91.
4. Volz H-P, *et al.* Brofaromine—a review of its pharmacological properties and therapeutic use. *J Neural Transm* 1996; **103:** 217–45.
5. Lott M, *et al.* Brofaromine for social phobia: a multicenter, placebo-controlled, double-blind study. *J Clin Psychopharmacol* 1997; **17:** 255–60.
6. Lotufo-Neto F, *et al.* Meta-analysis of the reversible inhibitors of monoamine oxidase type A moclobemide and brofaromine for the treatment of depression. *Neuropsychopharmacology* 1999; **20:** 226–47.

## Bupropion Hydrochloride

*(BANM, USAN, rINNM)*

Amfebutamone Hydrochloride; BW-323; Hidrocloruro de bupropión. (±)-2-(*tert*-Butylamino)-3′-chloropropiophenone hydrochloride.

$C_{13}H_{18}ClNO$,HCl = 276.2.
*CAS — 34911-55-2 (bupropion); 31677-93-7 (bupropion hydrochloride).*
*ATC — N07BA02.*

**Pharmacopoeias.** In *US.*

**USP 27** (Bupropion Hydrochloride). A white powder. Soluble in water, in alcohol, and in 0.1N hydrochloric acid. Protect from light.

### Adverse Effects and Treatment

Agitation, anxiety, and insomnia often occur during the initial stages of bupropion therapy. Other relatively common side-effects reported with bupropion include fever, dry mouth, headache or migraine, dizziness, urinary frequency, nausea and vomiting, constipation, tremor, sweating, and skin rashes. Hypersensitivity reactions, ranging from pruritus and urticaria to, less commonly, angioedema, dyspnoea, and anaphylactoid reactions, have occurred, as have symptoms suggestive of serum sickness. There have been rare reports of Stevens-Johnson syndrome and erythema multiforme. Tachycardia, chest pain, and hypertension (sometimes severe), or occasionally vasodilatation, postural hypotension, palpitations, and syncope have been reported. Psychotic episodes, confusion, nightmares, impaired memory, dysgeusia, anorexia with weight loss, paraesthesia, tinnitus and visual disturbances have also been reported.

Seizures, which appear to be partially dose-related, may occur with bupropion and have been particularly notable in patients with anorexia nervosa or bulimia nervosa; the risk is also increased in patients with a history of seizure disorders or other predisposing factor. The manufacturers state that the overall incidence of seizure in patients receiving bupropion at recommended doses is about 0.1 to 0.4%.

Symptoms of overdosage include hallucinations, nausea and vomiting, tachycardia, loss of consciousness, and death (following massive overdose); seizures have occurred in about one-third of all bupropion overdose cases. Gastric lavage or activated charcoal may decrease absorption if used soon after ingestion. Treatment is supportive. Benzodiazepines may be tried for seizures. Diuresis, dialysis, and haemoperfusion are unlikely to be of benefit.

**Incidence of adverse effects.** Up to 24 July 2002 (the first 25 months of marketing), the UK Committee on Safety of Medicines (CSM) had received 7630 reports of suspected adverse reactions associated with the use of bupropion.[1] Of these reports, 60 were associated with a fatal outcome although in the majority of the cases underlying conditions may provide an alternative explanation. Cardiovascular and cerebrovascular disorders such as myocardial infarction and stroke were reported as the cause of death in 70% of cases. The CSM also commented that adverse reactions were mainly recognised ones and listed in the manufacturer's product information.

1. Committee on Safety of Medicines/Medicines Control Agency. Zyban (bupropion hydrochloride) - safety update. Available at: http://medicines.mhra.gov.uk/ourwork/monitorsafequalmed/safetymessages/zyban26702.pdf (accessed 04/06/04)

**Effect on the cerebrovascular system.** A 67-year-old male experienced paraesthesia, dizziness, tinnitus, confusion, and gait impairment after taking bupropion for smoking cessation.[1] Although a transient ischaemic attack was suspected symptoms resolved on stopping bupropion and recurred on rechallenge.

1. Humma LM, Swims MP. Bupropion mimics a transient ischemic attack. *Ann Pharmacother* 1999; **33:** 305–7.

**Effects on the skin.** Erythema multiforme developed in a 31-year-old woman several weeks after starting modified-release bupropion for depression.[1] Symptoms resolved on drug withdrawal. In another report, 3 patients with controlled psoriasis experienced an exacerbation of their psoriatic symptoms after starting bupropion for smoking cessation.[2] All 3 patients required hospitalisation to control their symptoms.

1. Lineberry TW, *et al.* Bupropion-induced erythema multiforme. *Mayo Clin Proc* 2001; **76:** 664–6.
2. Cox NH, *et al.* Generalized pustular and erythrodermic psoriasis associated with bupropion treatment. *Br J Dermatol* 2002; **146:** 1061–3.

**Extrapyramidal effects.** A 44-year-old man experienced acute head and neck dystonia while taking buspirone and modified-release bupropion.[1] No recurrence was noted on rechallenge with buspirone although symptoms did develop on rechallenge with bupropion when the dose was increased from 150 mg once daily to 150 mg twice daily.

1. Detweiler MB, Harpold GJ. Bupropion-induced acute dystonia. *Ann Pharmacother* 2002; **36:** 251–4.

**Hypersensitivity.** Eosinophilia has been reported[1] in a patient 12 days after bupropion was added to her existing treatment regimen of glibenclamide and tolmetin. The eosinophil count returned to normal after all medication was stopped. Bupropion appeared to be the causative drug. Serum sickness associated with bupropion exposure has also been reported.[2,3]

See also Effects on the Skin, above.

1. Malesker MA, *et al.* Eosinophilia associated with bupropion. *Ann Pharmacother* 1995; **29:** 867–8.
2. Yolles JC, *et al.* Serum sickness induced by bupropion. *Ann Pharmacother* 1999; **33:** 931–3.
3. McCollom RA, *et al.* Bupropion-induced serum sickness-like reaction. *Ann Pharmacother* 2000; **34:** 471–3.

**Overdosage.** Unlike the tricyclic antidepressants, bupropion appears to lack any significant cardiovascular or antimuscarinic adverse effects when taken in overdose. In an early review[1] of 58 overdose cases involving immediate-release bupropion alone, the most common symptoms were sinus tachycardia, lethargy, tremor, and seizures; other effects included confusion, lightheadedness, hallucinations, paraesthesias, and vomiting. Most patients experienced minor effects or none at all. Although no deaths were reported in the review, there have been fatalities following overdose; in some cases other drugs may have been involved.[2,3] More recent case reports with modified-release preparations have highlighted that seizures are a particular feature of bupropion overdose.[4,5]

1. Spiller HA, *et al.* Bupropion overdose: a 3-year multi-center retrospective analysis. *Am J Emerg Med* 1994; **12:** 43–5.
2. Friel PN, *et al.* Three fatal drug overdoses involving bupropion. *J Anal Toxicol* 1993; **17:** 436–8.
3. Harris CR, *et al.* Fatal bupropion overdose. *J Toxicol Clin Toxicol* 1997; **35:** 321–4.
4. Bhattacharjee C, *et al.* Bupropion overdose: a potential problem with the new 'miracle' anti-smoking drug. *Int J Clin Pract* 2001; **55:** 221–2.
5. Paoloni R, Szekely I. Sustained-release bupropion overdose: a new entity for Australian emergency departments. *Emerg Med (Fremantle)* 2002; **14:** 109–12.

### Precautions

Bupropion may induce seizures and consequently its use is contra-indicated in patients with epilepsy. It is also contra-indicated in patients with a history of anorexia nervosa or bulimia nervosa, as a higher incidence of seizures has been noted in such patients treated with bupropion, and in those undergoing abrupt withdrawal from alcohol or benzodiazepines. It should be used with extreme caution, if at all, in patients with a history of seizure disorders or other predisposing factors such as severe hepatic cirrhosis or a CNS tumour. The use of bupropion in patients with other risk factors for seizures (for example, alcohol abuse, a history of head trauma, diabetes, and drugs known to lower the seizure threshold) should only be undertaken when there are compelling clinical reasons.

Bupropion should be used with caution in patients with bipolar disorder or psychoses because of the risk of precipitating mania; use for smoking cessation in such patients may be contra-indicated. It should also be used cautiously in patients with a recent history of myocardial infarction or unstable heart disease, and in hepatic or renal impairment.

When bupropion is used for depression, patients should be closely monitored during early therapy until improvement is observed because suicide is an inherent risk in depressed patients. For further details, see under Depression, p.279.

As with other CNS-active drugs, the ability to perform tasks requiring motor or cognitive skills or judgement may be impaired by bupropion, and patients, if affected, should not drive or operate machinery.

**Breast feeding.** There has been a report of accumulation of bupropion in human breast milk in concentrations higher than those in maternal plasma.[1] However, neither bupropion nor its metabolites were detected in the plasma of the infant who was breast-fed twice daily by the affected mother, and no adverse effects were noted in the infant.

Although acknowledging this study, the American Academy of Pediatrics considers[2] that the effect of bupropion on nursing infants is unknown but may be of concern.

1. Briggs GC, *et al.* Excretion of bupropion in breast milk. *Ann Pharmacother* 1993; **27:** 431–3.
2. American Academy of Pediatrics. The transfer of drugs and other chemicals into human milk. *Pediatrics* 2001; **108:** 776–89. Correction. *ibid.*; 1029. Also available at: http://aappolicy.aappublications.org/cgi/content/full/pediatrics%3b108/3/776 (accessed 04/06/04)

## Interactions

Bupropion should not be given with or within 14 days of stopping an MAOI.

The use of alcohol with bupropion should be minimised or avoided completely because it may alter the seizure threshold. Similarly, other drugs that lower the seizure threshold, such as other antidepressants, antimalarials, antipsychotics, sedating antihistamines, quinolones, tramadol, theophylline, or systemic corticosteroids, should be used with extreme caution together with bupropion.

Use of nicotine transdermal patches with bupropion has been associated with hypertension, and patients using this combination should therefore have their blood pressure monitored.

Caution has been advised in patients receiving either amantadine or levodopa with bupropion because of reports of a higher incidence of adverse effects in patients receiving these combinations.

*Animal* studies have indicated that bupropion may induce drug-metabolising enzymes and pharmacokinetic interactions with other drugs are therefore a possibility. Bupropion is itself metabolised by hepatic enzyme systems and drugs known to affect such systems may interact with bupropion. For example carbamazepine, phenobarbital, or phenytoin may induce the metabolism of bupropion while other drugs such as cimetidine or valproate may inhibit its metabolism. *In-vitro* studies have shown that bupropion is metabolised by the cytochrome P450 isoenzyme CYP2B6. Consequently interactions may occur between bupropion and drugs that affect this isoenzyme, for example orphenadrine, cyclophosphamide, and ifosfamide.

*In-vitro* studies have also shown that bupropion is an inhibitor of another isoenzyme, CYP2D6; caution should be exercised when it is given with drugs metabolised by this enzyme and they should be started at the lower end of their dose range. Such drugs include some antidepressants, antipsychotics, beta blockers, and type Ic antiarrhythmics.

**Antiepileptics.** Plasma-bupropion concentrations became undetectable in 2 patients who were also receiving carbamazepine; plasma concentrations of hydroxybupropion, an active metabolite of bupropion, were high.[1]

1. Popli AP, *et al.* Bupropion and anticonvulsant drug interactions. *Ann Clin Psychiatry* 1995; **7:** 99–101.

**Antivirals.** There is some evidence from study *in vitro* that the antivirals *efavirenz, nelfinavir,* and *ritonavir* can inhibit the cytochrome P450 isoenzyme CYP2B6,[1] and the manufacturers of ritonavir (although not those of bupropion) mention the possibility of an interaction with bupropion in the product literature. However, evidence of clinically significant interaction is lacking: a small case series of 10 patients who took bupropion with low-dose ritonavir, or efavirenz or nelfinavir, did not note any episodes of seizures.[2]

1. Hesse LM, *et al.* Ritonavir, efavirenz, and nelfinavir inhibit CYP2B6 activity in vitro: potential drug interactions with bupropion. *Drug Metab Dispos* 2001; **29:** 100–102.
2. Park-Wyllie LY, Antoniou T. Concurrent use of bupropion with CYP2B6 inhibitors, nelfinavir, ritonavir and efavirenz: a case series. *AIDS* 2003; **17:** 638–40.

**Histamine $H_2$-antagonists.** A randomised controlled study in 24 volunteers found that *cimetidine* had no effect on the pharmacokinetics of modified-release bupropion or its active metabolite, hydroxybupropion.[1]

1. Kustra R, *et al.* Lack of effect of cimetidine on the pharmacokinetics of sustained-release bupropion. *J Clin Pharmacol* 1999; **39:** 1184–8.

## Pharmacokinetics

Bupropion is well absorbed from the gastrointestinal tract but may undergo extensive first-pass metabolism. Several metabolites of bupropion are pharmacologically active and have longer half-lives, and achieve higher plasma concentrations, than the parent compound. Hydroxybupropion is the major metabolite, produced by the metabolism of bupropion by the cytochrome P450 isoenzyme CYP2B6; it is comparable in potency to bupropion. Threohydrobupropion and erythrohydrobupropion are produced by hydroxylation and/or reduction and are about one-tenth to one-half the potency of the parent compound. Bupropion is 80% or more bound to plasma proteins. The terminal plasma half-life of immediate-release bupropion is about 14 hours; the terminal plasma half-life of modified-release bupropion is about 20 hours. The metabolites of bupropion are excreted primarily in the urine; less than 1% of the parent drug is excreted unchanged. Bupropion and its metabolites cross the placenta and are distributed into breast milk.

◊ References.

1. Sweet RA, *et al.* Pharmacokinetics of single- and multiple-dose bupropion in elderly patients with depression. *J Clin Pharmacol* 1995; **35:** 876–84.

**Smoking.** No clinically significant differences were observed between the pharmacokinetics of bupropion or its metabolites in cigarette smokers and non-smokers.[1]

1. Hsyu P-H, *et al.* Pharmacokinetics of bupropion and its metabolites in cigarette smokers versus nonsmokers. *J Clin Pharmacol* 1997; **37:** 737–43.

## Uses and Administration

Bupropion is a chlorpropiophenone antidepressant chemically unrelated to other classes of antidepressants but similar in structure to the central stimulant diethylpropion (p.1587). It is a weak blocker of neuronal reuptake of serotonin and noradrenaline compared with tricyclic antidepressants; it also inhibits the neuronal reuptake of dopamine. The antidepressant effect may not be evident until after 4 weeks of therapy. Bupropion is also used as an aid to smoking cessation.

Bupropion is given by mouth as the hydrochloride. To minimise agitation, anxiety, and insomnia often experienced at the start of therapy, and to reduce the risk of seizures, doses should be increased gradually; the total daily dose should be given in equally divided doses and the maximum recommended single and total daily doses should not be exceeded. Insomnia at the start of therapy may be minimised by avoiding bedtime doses. Patients with hepatic or renal impairment should be given reduced doses and monitored for toxic effects, see below.

In the treatment of **depression** bupropion hydrochloride is given in initial doses of 100 mg twice daily increased, if necessary, after at least 3 days to 100 mg three times daily. In severe cases, if no improvement has been observed after several weeks of therapy, the dose may be increased further to a maximum of 150 mg three times daily. Bupropion hydrochloride is also available as a modified-release preparation given in an initial dose of 150 mg once daily in the morning increased, if necessary, after at least 3 days to 150 mg twice daily; in severe cases, the dose of the modified-release preparation may be increased further after several weeks to 200 mg twice daily.

Bupropion hydrochloride is given as a modified-release preparation as an aid to **smoking cessation** in an initial dose of 150 mg once daily for 6 days, increasing to 150 mg twice daily on day 7. In the USA, the dose may be increased after 3 days. In the UK, the maximum recommended dose in the elderly, or in patients with predisposing risk factors for seizure (see Precautions, above), is 150 mg daily. Treatment should be started about 1 to 2 weeks before the patient attempts to stop smoking, to allow steady-state blood levels of bupropion to be reached, and normally continues for 7 to 12 weeks; if there is no significant progress towards smoking abstinence by the seventh week, then therapy should be stopped. Use with nicotine transdermal patches may be warranted in some patients, although there is a risk of hypertension with such therapy (see Interactions, above).

**Administration in hepatic impairment.** When used as an aid to smoking cessation in patients with mild to moderate hepatic impairment, bupropion should be given at a reduced frequency; the UK manufacturers suggest a dose of 150 mg once daily. The use of bupropion in patients with severe hepatic cirrhosis is contra-indicated in the UK although doses of 150 mg every other day are permitted in the USA.

In the treatment of depression, a reduction in the frequency and/or the dose of bupropion should be considered in patients with mild to moderate impairment. In patients with severe hepatic cirrhosis the dose varies according to the preparation given; for modified-release bupropion the suggested maximum dose is 100 mg once daily or 150 mg every other day while the maximum dose of immediate-release bupropion is 75 mg once daily.

**Administration in renal impairment.** When used as an aid to smoking cessation in patients with renal impairment, bupropion should be given at a reduced frequency; the UK manufacturers suggest a dose of 150 mg once daily.

In the treatment of depression, a reduction in the frequency and/or the dose of bupropion should be considered.

**Depression.** References to the use of bupropion in patients with depression (p.279) are given below.

1. Anonymous. Bupropion for depression. *Med Lett Drugs Ther* 1989; **31:** 97–8.
2. Weisler RH, *et al.* Comparison of bupropion and trazodone for the treatment of major depression. *J Clin Psychopharmacol* 1994; **14:** 170–9.
3. Kavoussi RJ, *et al.* Double-blind comparison of bupropion sustained release and sertraline in depressed outpatients. *J Clin Psychiatry* 1997; **58:** 532–7.
4. Nieuwstraten CE, Dolovich LR. Bupropion versus selective serotonin-reuptake inhibitors for treatment of depression. *Ann Pharmacother* 2001; **35:** 1608–13.

**Hyperactivity.** When drug therapy is indicated for attention deficit hyperactivity disorder (p.1583) initial treatment is usually with a central stimulant. Antidepressants may be used for patients who fail to respond to, or who are intolerant of, central stimulants. Data from open and controlled studies involving small numbers of patients suggest that bupropion is effective in adults and children.[1,2]

1. Cantwell DP. ADHD through the life span: the role of bupropion in treatment. *J Clin Psychiatry* 1998; **59** (suppl 4): 92–4.
2. Wilens TE, *et al.* A controlled clinical trial of bupropion for attention deficit hyperactivity disorder in adults. *Am J Psychiatry* 2001; **158:** 282–8.

**Smoking cessation.** References to the use of bupropion in smoking cessation (p.1721) are given below.

1. Anonymous. Bupropion (Zyban) for smoking cessation. *Med Lett Drugs Ther* 1997; **39:** 77–8.
2. Benowitz NL. Treating tobacco addiction—nicotine or no nicotine? *N Engl J Med* 1997; **337:** 1230–1.
3. Hurt RD, *et al.* A comparison of sustained-release bupropion and placebo for smoking cessation. *N Engl J Med* 1997; **337:** 1195–1202.
4. Jorenby DE, *et al.* A controlled trial of sustained-release bupropion, a nicotine patch, or both for smoking cessation. *N Engl J Med* 1999; **340:** 685–91.
5. Holm KJ, Spencer CM. Bupropion: a review of its use in the management of smoking cessation. *Drugs* 2000; **59:** 1007–1024.
6. Tashkin DP, *et al.* Smoking cessation in patients with chronic obstructive pulmonary disease: a double-blind, placebo-controlled, randomised trial. *Lancet* 2001; **357:** 1571–5.
7. Gonzales DH, *et al.* Bupropion SR as an aid to smoking cessation in smokers treated previously with bupropion: a randomized placebo-controlled study. *Clin Pharmacol Ther* 2001; **69:** 438–44.
8. Hays JT, *et al.* Sustained-release bupropion for pharmacologic relapse prevention after smoking cessation: a randomized, controlled trial. *Ann Intern Med* 2001; **135:** 423–33.
9. National Institute for Clinical Excellence. Guidance on the use of nicotine replacement therapy (NRT) and bupropion for smoking cessation (issued March 2002). Available at: http://www.nice.org.uk/pdf/NiceNRT39GUIDANCE.pdf (accessed 04/06/04)

10. Ahluwalia JS, *et al.* Sustained-release bupropion for smoking cessation in African Americans: a randomized controlled trial. *JAMA* 2002; **288:** 468–74.
11. Fagerström K, *et al.* Smoking cessation treatment with sustained-release bupropion: optimising approaches to management. A seminar-in-print. *Drugs* 2002; **62** (suppl 2): 1–70.
12. Hughes JR, *et al.* Antidepressants for smoking cessation. Available in The Cochrane Library; Issue 2. Chichester: John Wiley; 2004.

## Preparations

**USP 27:** Bupropion Hydrochloride Extended-Release Tablets; Bupropion Hydrochloride Tablets.

**Proprietary Preparations** (details are given in Part 3)
***Arg.:*** Odranal; Wellbutrin; ***Austral.:*** Zyban; ***Austria:*** Quomem; Zyban; ***Belg.:*** Zyban; ***Braz.:*** Wellbutrin; Zyban; ***Canad.:*** Wellbutrin; Zyban; ***Chile:*** Buxon; Dosier; Mondrian; Wellbutrin; ***Denm.:*** Zyban; ***Fr.:*** Zyban; ***Ger.:*** Zyban; ***Gr.:*** Zyban; ***Hong Kong:*** Zyban; ***India:*** Zyban; ***Irl.:*** Zyban; ***Israel:*** Zyban; ***Ital.:*** Quomem; Zyban; ***Mex.:*** Wellbutrin; ***Norw.:*** Zyban; ***NZ:*** Zyban; ***Port.:*** Zyban; ***Singapore:*** Zyban; ***Spain:*** Quomem; Zyntabac; ***Swed.:*** Zyban; ***Switz.:*** Zyban; ***Thai.:*** Quomem; ***UK:*** Zyban; ***USA:*** Wellbutrin; Zyban.

---

## Butriptyline Hydrochloride *(BANM, USAN, rINNM)*

AY-62014; Hidrocloruro de butriptilina. (±)-3-(10,11-Dihydro-5*H*-dibenzo[*a,d*]cyclohepten-5-yl)-2-methylpropyldimethylamine hydrochloride.

$C_{21}H_{27}N,HCl = 329.9.$

*CAS — 35941-65-2 (butriptyline); 5585-73-9 (butriptyline hydrochloride).*

*ATC — N06AA15.*

### Profile

Butriptyline hydrochloride is a tricyclic antidepressant with actions and uses similar to those of amitriptyline (p.280). It is one of the less sedating tricyclics. It has been given by mouth as the hydrochloride in the treatment of depression.

### Preparations

**Proprietary Preparations** (details are given in Part 3)
***Austria:*** Evasidol†; ***Ital.:*** Evadene†.

---

# Citalopram *(BAN, rINN)*

Lu-10-171. 1-(3-Dimethylaminopropyl)-1-(4-fluorophenyl)-1,3-dihydroisobenzofuran-5-carbonitrile.

$C_{20}H_{21}FN_2O = 324.4.$

*CAS — 59729-33-8.*

*ATC — N06AB04.*

## Citalopram Hydrobromide *(BANM, USAN, rINNM)*

Hidrobromuro de citalopram; Lu-10-171B; Nitalapram Hydrobromide.

$C_{20}H_{21}FN_2O,HBr = 405.3.$

*CAS — 59729-32-7.*

## Citalopram Hydrochloride *(BANM, rINNM)*

Hidrocloruro de citalopram.

$C_{20}H_{21}FN_2O,HCl = 360.9.$

## Adverse Effects, Treatment, and Precautions

As for SSRIs in general (see Fluoxetine, p.292) although increased appetite and weight gain have also been reported with citalopram.

**Breast feeding.** For comments on the use of SSRIs in breast feeding patients, see under Precautions for Fluoxetine, p.294.

**Children.** In the UK the Committee on Safety of Medicines recommends that citalopram should not be used to treat depressive illness in children under 18 years of age. For details, see under Effects on Mental State in Fluoxetine, p.293.

## Interactions

For interactions associated with SSRIs, see Fluoxetine, p.295.

## Pharmacokinetics

Citalopram is readily absorbed from the gastrointestinal tract and maximum plasma concentrations are reached 2 to 4 hours after oral doses. Citalopram is widely distributed throughout the body; protein binding is low. Citalopram is metabolised by demethylation, deamination, and oxidation to active and inactive metabolites. The demethylation of citalopram to one of its active metabolites, demethylcitalopram, involves the cytochrome P450 isoenzymes CYP3A4 and CYP2C19; the metabolism of citalopram is also partly dependent on CYP2D6. The elimination half-life of citalopram is reported to be about 33 hours. It is excreted mainly via the liver (85%) with the remainder via the kidneys. About 12% of the daily dose is excreted in the urine as unchanged drug. Citalopram is distributed into breast milk in very low concentrations.

## Uses and Administration

Citalopram, a phthalane derivative, is an SSRI with actions and uses similar to those of fluoxetine (p.296). Citalopram is given by mouth as the hydrobromide or hydrochloride, usually as a single daily dose. Doses are expressed in terms of citalopram; citalopram hydrobromide 25.0 mg and citalopram hydrochloride 22.3 mg are both approximately equivalent to 20.0 mg of citalopram.

In the treatment of **depression**, the initial dose is the equivalent of 20 mg daily by mouth. After at least one week, the dose may be increased to 40 mg daily; a dose of 60 mg daily may be necessary in some patients. Citalopram hydrochloride has also been given by intravenous infusion in similar doses when the oral route is impracticable.

In the treatment of **panic disorder** with or without agoraphobia, the initial dose of citalopram is 10 mg daily by mouth increasing to 20 mg daily after one week. The dose may be increased thereafter as required up to a maximum of 60 mg daily.

Doses at the lower end of the therapeutic range, up to a maximum of 40 mg, should be used in elderly patients. For dosage in hepatic and renal impairment see below.

Citalopram should be withdrawn gradually to reduce the risk of withdrawal symptoms.

The *S*-enantiomer of citalopram, escitalopram (p.292) is given for the treatment of depression.

◊ Reviews.

1. Milne RJ, Goa KL. Citalopram: a review of its pharmacodynamic and pharmacokinetic properties, and therapeutic potential in depressive illness. *Drugs* 1991; **41:** 450–77.

**Administration in hepatic or renal impairment.** Dosage of citalopram should be restricted to the lower end of the dose range in patients with hepatic impairment; a usual dose for depression in this group would be 20 mg daily. There is no need for dose adjustment in mild to moderate renal impairment although information is lacking on appropriate dosage in severe renal impairment.

**Anxiety disorders.** Citalopram has been given in anxiety disorders (p.663) including panic attacks (p.663), obsessive-compulsive disorder (p.663), post-traumatic stress disorder (p.664), and social phobia (see under Phobic Disorders, p.663).

References.

1. Koponen H, *et al.* Citalopram in the treatment of obsessive-compulsive disorder: an open pilot study. *Acta Psychiatr Scand* 1997; **96:** 343–6.
2. Bouwer C, Skin DJ. Use of the selective serotonin reuptake inhibitor citalopram in the treatment of generalized social phobia. *J Affect Disord* 1998; **49:** 79–82.
3. Lepola UM, *et al.* A controlled, prospective, 1-year trial of citalopram in the treatment of panic disorder. *J Clin Psychiatry* 1998; **59:** 528–34.
4. Seedat S, *et al.* Open trial of citalopram in adults with post-traumatic stress disorder. *Int J Neuropsychopharmacol* 2000; **3:** 135–40.
5. Montgomery SA, *et al.* Citalopram 20 mg, 40 mg and 60 mg are all effective and well tolerated compared with placebo in obsessive-compulsive disorder. *Int Clin Psychopharmacol* 2001; **16:** 75–86.

**Depression.** As discussed on p.279, there is very little difference in efficacy between the different groups of antidepressant drugs. SSRIs such as citalopram are widely used as an alternative to the older tricyclics as they have fewer side-effects and are safer in overdosage.

References.

1. Montgomery SA, *et al.* The optimal dosing regimen for citalopram—a meta-analysis of nine placebo-controlled studies. *Int Clin Psychopharmacol* 1994; **9** (suppl 1): 35–40.
2. Keller MB. Citalopram therapy for depression: a review of 10 years of European experience and data from US trials. *J Clin Psychiatry* 2000; **61:** 896–908.
3. Parker NG, Brown CS. Citalopram in the treatment of depression. *Ann Pharmacother* 2000; **34:** 761–71.

**Pathological crying or laughing.** Inappropriate or uncontrolled crying or laughing can occur in patients with lesions in certain areas of the brain. Attempts at treatment have mostly been with antidepressant drugs, including SSRIs. Favourable results have been reported in a double-blind placebo-controlled study[1] with citalopram.

1. Andersen G, *et al.* Citalopram for post-stroke pathological crying. *Lancet* 1993; **342:** 837–9.

**Schizophrenia.** The treatment of schizophrenia consists mainly of a combination of social therapy and antipsychotic drugs (see p.665). In a preliminary placebo-controlled study[1] in 15 patients with chronic schizophrenia who exhibited signs of impulsive aggression, adding citalopram to existing antipsychotic therapy significantly reduced the frequency, but not the average severity, of aggressive incidents. In a subsequent study involving 90 patients, citalopram appeared to improve subjective well-being but had no clear effect on psychopathological symptoms.[2]

1. Vartiainen H, *et al.* Citalopram, a selective serotonin reuptake inhibitor, in the treatment of aggression in schizophrenia. *Acta Psychiatr Scand* 1995; **91:** 348–51.
2. Salokangas RKR, *et al.* Citalopram as an adjuvant in chronic schizophrenia: a double-blind placebo-controlled study. *Acta Psychiatr Scand* 1996; **94:** 175–80.

## Preparations

**Proprietary Preparations** (details are given in Part 3)
***Arg.:*** Humorap; Zentius; ***Austral.:*** Celapram; Cipramil; Talam; Talohexal; ***Austria:*** Apertia; Cipram; Sepram; Seropram; ***Belg.:*** Cipramil; ***Braz.:*** Cipramil; Denyl; ***Canad.:*** Celexa; ***Chile:*** Actipram; Cimal; Cipramil; Finap; Prisma; Semax; Setronil; Temperax; Zebrak; Zentius; ***Denm.:*** Akarin; Cipramil; ***Fin.:*** Cipramil; ***Fr.:*** Seropram; ***Ger.:*** Cipramil; Citadura; Sepram; ***Gr.:*** Seropram; ***Hong Kong:*** Cipram; ***India:*** Citopam; ***Irl.:*** Cipramil; ***Israel:*** Cipramil; Recital; ***Ital.:*** Elopram; Seropram; ***Malaysia:*** Cipram; ***Mex.:*** Seropram; ***Neth.:*** Cipramil; ***Norw.:*** Cipramil; ***NZ:*** Cipramil; ***S.Afr.:*** Cipramil; ***Singapore:*** Cipram; ***Spain:*** Genprol; Prisdal; Seropram; ***Swed.:*** Cipramil; ***Switz.:*** Seropram; ***Thai.:*** Cipram; ***UK:*** Cipramil; ***USA:*** Celexa.

---

# Clomipramine Hydrochloride

*(BANM, USAN, rINNM)*

Chlorimipramine Hydrochloride; Clomipramini Hydrochloridum; G-34586; Hidrocloruro de clomipramina; Monochlorimipramine Hydrochloride. 3-(3-Chloro-10,11-dihydro-5*H*-dibenz-[*b,f*]azepin-5-yl)propyldimethylamine hydrochloride.

$C_{19}H_{23}ClN_2,HCl = 351.3.$

*CAS — 303-49-1 (clomipramine); 17321-77-6 (clomipramine hydrochloride).*

*ATC — N06AA04.*

**Pharmacopoeias.** In *Chin., Eur.* (see p.vi), *Jpn,* and *US.*

**Ph. Eur. 5.0** (Clomipramine Hydrochloride). A white or slightly yellow, slightly hygroscopic, crystalline powder. Freely soluble in water and in dichloromethane; soluble in alcohol. A 10% solution in water has a pH of 3.5 to 5.0. Protect from light.

**USP 27** (Clomipramine Hydrochloride). A white to faintly yellow crystalline powder. Very soluble in water. pH of a 10% solution in water is between 3.5 and 5.0.

## Adverse Effects, Treatment, and Precautions

As for tricyclic antidepressants in general (see Amitriptyline, p.281).

**Breast feeding.** For comments on the use of tricyclic antidepressants in breast feeding patients, see under Precautions for Amitriptyline, p.283.

**Porphyria.** Clomipramine is considered to be unsafe in patients with porphyria because it has been shown to be porphyrinogenic in *in-vitro* systems, although there is conflicting evidence of porphyrinogenicity.

## Interactions

For interactions associated with tricyclic antidepressants, see Amitriptyline, p.284.

**MAOIs.** In relation to interactions with other antidepressants, it should be noted that the combination of clomipramine and tranylcypromine is particularly hazardous, and that the serotonin syndrome (p.313) has occurred in patients receiving clomipramine and moclobemide (see under Interactions of Antidepressants in Phenelzine, p.315).

## Pharmacokinetics

Clomipramine is readily absorbed from the gastrointestinal tract, and extensively demethylated during first-pass metabolism in the liver to its primary active metabolite, desmethylclomipramine.

Clomipramine and desmethylclomipramine are widely distributed throughout the body and are extensively bound to plasma and tissue protein. Clomipramine has been estimated to have a plasma elimination half-life of about 21 hours, which may be considerably extended in overdosage; that of desmethylclomipramine is longer (about 36 hours).

Paths of metabolism of both clomipramine and desmethylclomipramine include hydroxylation and *N*-oxidation. About two-thirds of a single dose of clomipramine is excreted in the urine, mainly in the form of its metabolites, either free or in conjugated form; the remainder of the dose is excreted in the faeces. Clomipramine crosses the placenta and is distributed into breast milk.

◊ References.

1. Gex-Fabry M, *et al.* Clomipramine metabolism: model-based analysis of variability factors from drug monitoring data. *Clin Pharmacokinet* 1990; **19:** 241–55.

2. Balant-Gorgia AE, *et al.* Clinical pharmacokinetics of clomipramine. *Clin Pharmacokinet* 1991; **20:** 447–62.
3. Nielsen KK, *et al.* Single-dose kinetics of clomipramine: relationship to the sparteine and S-mephenytoin oxidation polymorphisms. *Clin Pharmacol Ther* 1994; **55:** 518–27.
4. Herrera D, *et al.* Pharmacokinetics of a sustained-release dosage form of clomipramine. *J Clin Pharmacol* 2000; **40:** 1488–93.


## Uses and Administration

Clomipramine is a dibenzazepine tricyclic antidepressant with actions and uses similar to those of amitriptyline (p.285). It has antimuscarinic properties and is also a potent serotonin reuptake inhibitor. Clomipramine is one of the more sedating tricyclics. It is used as the hydrochloride.

In the treatment of **depression**, clomipramine hydrochloride is given by mouth in doses of 10 mg daily initially, increasing gradually to 30 to 150 mg daily if required; up to 250 mg daily may be given in severe cases. A suggested initial dose for the elderly is 10 mg daily increasing gradually to 30 to 75 mg daily if required. Clomipramine may be given in divided doses throughout the day, but since it has a prolonged half-life, once-daily dosage regimens are also suitable, usually given at night.

In the treatment of **obsessive-compulsive disorders** and **phobias**, clomipramine hydrochloride may be given by mouth in an initial dose of 25 mg daily (or 10 mg daily for elderly patients) increased gradually over two weeks to 100 to 150 mg daily. In some countries, maximum doses of 250 mg daily have been used. Similar doses have also been used in the management of **panic attacks**. In some countries clomipramine hydrochloride is also used for the treatment of obsessive-compulsive disorders in children and adolescents aged 10 years and over. Initial doses are 25 mg daily, increased gradually during the first 2 weeks to a maximum daily dose of 3 mg/kg or 100 mg, whichever is smaller. Further increases are permitted, over several weeks to a maximum of 3 mg/kg or 200 mg, whichever is smaller.

In the adjunctive treatment of **cataplexy associated with narcolepsy**, clomipramine hydrochloride is given by mouth in an initial dose of 10 mg daily and gradually increased until a satisfactory response occurs, usually within the range of 10 to 75 mg daily.

In some countries clomipramine may be given by the intramuscular or intravenous routes if administration by mouth is impracticable or inadvisable. The initial dose of clomipramine hydrochloride by intramuscular injection is 25 to 50 mg daily, increasing to a maximum of 100 to 150 mg daily; oral administration should be substituted as soon as possible. Clomipramine hydrochloride may also be given by intravenous infusion in doses of 50 to 75 mg daily diluted in 250 to 500 mL of sodium chloride 0.9% or glucose 5% and infused over 1.5 to 3 hours. When a satisfactory response to intravenous infusion has been obtained oral therapy should be substituted, initially giving double the maximum intravenous dose by mouth and subsequently adjusting if necessary. Patients must be carefully supervised during intravenous infusion of clomipramine hydrochloride and the blood pressure carefully monitored owing to the risk of hypotension.

Clomipramine should be withdrawn gradually to reduce the risk of withdrawal symptoms.

**Anxiety disorders.** Tricyclic antidepressants that inhibit serotonin reuptake, such as clomipramine and imipramine, have been given in the management of anxiety disorders (p.663) including obsessive-compulsive disorder (p.663), panic attacks (p.663), post-traumatic stress disorder (p.664) and trichotillomania.

References.


1. Swedo SE, *et al.* A double-blind comparison of clomipramine and desipramine in the treatment of trichotillomania (hair pulling). *N Engl J Med* 1989; **321:** 497–501.
2. McTavish D, Benfield P. Clomipramine: an overview of its pharmacological properties and a review of its therapeutic use in obsessive compulsive disorder and panic disorder. *Drugs* 1990; **39:** 136–53.
3. Kelly MW, Myers CW. Clomipramine: a tricyclic antidepressant effective in obsessive compulsive disorder. *DICP Ann Pharmacother* 1990; **24:** 739–44.
4. Papp LA, *et al.* Clomipramine treatment of panic disorder: pros and cons. *J Clin Psychiatry* 1997; **58:** 423–5.


**Autism.** Clomipramine reduced adventitious movements when tried in 5 boys with autistic disorder.[1] However, in a small study in 7 children no improvement in symptoms was noted and adverse effects were common and serious.[2]


1. Brasic JR, *et al.* Clomipramine ameliorates adventitious movements and compulsions in prepubertal boys with autistic disorder and severe mental retardation. *Neurology* 1994; **44:** 1309–12.
2. Sanchez LE, *et al.* A pilot study of clomipramine in young autistic children. *J Am Acad Child Adolesc Psychiatry* 1996; **35:** 537–44.


**Premenstrual syndrome.** Clomipramine reduced premenstrual irritability and depressed mood when given during the luteal phase in a controlled study.[1] Doses of clomipramine ranged from 25 to 75 mg daily. It was postulated that the efficacy of clomipramine in relieving premenstrual symptoms is related to its serotonin reuptake inhibitor activity. For the overall management of premenstrual syndrome, see p.1551.


1. Sundblad C, *et al.* Clomipramine administered during the luteal phase reduces the symptoms of premenstrual syndrome: a placebo-controlled trial. *Neuropsychopharmacology* 1993; **9:** 133–45.


**Sexual dysfunction.** Clomipramine has been used for its inhibitory effect on ejaculation in the management of premature ejaculation.[1-4] Any benefits may relate to its effect as a serotonin reuptake inhibitor; other antidepressants with serotonin reuptake inhibiting actions, such as fluoxetine and sertraline, have also been tried in this condition.[4]


1. Hawton K. Erectile dysfunction and premature ejaculation. *Br J Hosp Med* 1988; **40:** 428–36.
2. Althof SE, *et al.* A double-blind crossover trial of clomipramine for rapid ejaculation in 15 couples. *J Clin Psychiatry* 1995; **56:** 402–7.
3. Haensel SM, *et al.* Clomipramine and sexual function in men with premature ejaculation and controls. *J Urol (Baltimore)* 1996; **156:** 1310–15.
4. Kim SC, Seo KK. Efficacy and safety of fluoxetine, sertraline and clomipramine in patients with premature ejaculation: a double-blind, placebo controlled study. *J Urol (Baltimore)* 1998; **159:** 425–7.


**Stuttering.** Clomipramine was of modest success in a controlled study[1] of 17 patients with developmental stuttering (p.702). It was suggested that its efficacy may be related to its serotonin reuptake inhibitor activity.


1. Gordon CT, *et al.* A double-blind comparison of clomipramine and desipramine in the treatment of developmental stuttering. *J Clin Psychiatry* 1995; **56:** 238–42.


## Preparations

***BP 2003:*** Clomipramine Capsules;
***USP 27:*** Clomipramine Hydrochloride Capsules.

**Proprietary Preparations** (details are given in Part 3)
***Arg.:*** Anafranil; ***Austral.:*** Anafranil; Clopram; Placil; ***Austria:*** Anafranil; ***Belg.:*** Anafranil; ***Braz.:*** Anafranil; ***Canad.:*** Anafranil; Novo-Clopamine; ***Chile:*** Anafranil; Atenual; Ausentron; ***Denm.:*** Anafranil; ***Fin.:*** Anafranil; ***Fr.:*** Anafranil; ***Ger.:*** Anafranil; Hydiphen; ***Gr.:*** Anafranil; ***Hong Kong:*** Anafranil; Zoiral; ***India:*** Anafranil; ***Irl.:*** Anafranil; ***Israel:*** Anafranil; Maronil; ***Ital.:*** Anafranil; ***Malaysia:*** Anafranil; Clopress; ***Mex.:*** Anafranil; ***Neth.:*** Anafranil; ***Norw.:*** Anafranil; ***NZ:*** Anafranil; Clopress; ***Port.:*** Anafranil; ***S.Afr.:*** Anafranil; Equinorm; ***Singapore:*** Anafranil; ***Spain:*** Anafranil; ***Swed.:*** Anafranil; ***Switz.:*** Anafranil; ***Thai.:*** Anafranil; Clofranil; ***UK:*** Anafranil; ***USA:*** Anafranil.

---

# Desipramine Hydrochloride *(BANM, USAN, rINNM)*

Desipramini Hydrochloridum; Desmethylimipramine Hydrochloride; DMI; EX-4355; G-35020; Hidrocloruro de desipramina; JB-8181; NSC-114901; RMI-9384A. 3-(10,11-Dihydro-5*H*-dibenz[*b,f*]azepin-5-yl)propyl(methyl)amine hydrochloride.

$C_{18}H_{22}N_2,HCl = 302.8.$

*CAS — 50-47-5 (desipramine); 58-28-6 (desipramine hydrochloride).*

*ATC — N06AA01.*

**Pharmacopoeias.** In *Eur.* (see p.vi), *Pol.*, and *US.*

**Ph. Eur. 5.0** (Desipramine Hydrochloride). A white or almost white crystalline powder. Soluble in water and in alcohol. Protect from light.

**USP 27** (Desipramine Hydrochloride). A white to off-white crystalline powder. Soluble 1 in 12 of water, 1 in 14 of alcohol, and 1 in 3.5 of chloroform; insoluble in ether; freely soluble in methyl alcohol. Store in airtight containers.

## Adverse Effects, Treatment, and Precautions

As for tricyclic antidepressants in general (see Amitriptyline, p.281).

**Breast feeding.** For comments on the use of tricyclic antidepressants in breast feeding patients, see under Precautions for Amitriptyline, p.283.

## Interactions

For interactions associated with tricyclic antidepressants, see Amitriptyline, p.284.

## Pharmacokinetics

Desipramine is the principal active metabolite of imipramine (p.300).

## Uses and Administration

Desipramine, the principal active metabolite of imipramine (p.300), is a dibenzazepine tricyclic antidepressant with actions and uses similar to those of amitriptyline (p.285). It is one of the less sedating tricyclics and its antimuscarinic effects are mild. Desipramine is used as the hydrochloride.

In the treatment of depression, desipramine hydrochloride is given by mouth in daily doses of 100 to 200 mg; higher doses of up to 300 mg daily may be required in severely depressed patients in hospital. Lower doses should be used in adolescents and the elderly and are usually 25 to 100 mg daily; higher doses of up to 150 mg daily may be required for severe depression. Initial doses should be at a lower level and gradually increased according to tolerance and clinical response. Therapy may initially be given as a single daily dose or in divided doses; maintenance therapy may be given as a single daily dose usually at night.

Desipramine should be withdrawn gradually to reduce the risk of withdrawal symptoms.

**Cocaine dependence.** Since dopamine depletion may be the cause of the depression often associated with cocaine craving and with relapse, drugs such as desipramine that interact with dopaminergic systems have been tried in managing cocaine withdrawal symptoms (p.1375). However, a systematic review[1] was unable to find evidence to support the use of antidepressants in the treatment of cocaine dependence although the efficacy of desipramine was suggested in some individual studies.


1. Lima MS, *et al.* Antidepressants for cocaine dependence. Available in The Cochrane Library; Issue 2. Chichester: John Wiley; 2004.


**Hyperactivity.** When drug therapy is required for attention deficit hyperactivity disorder (see p.1583) tricyclic antidepressants such as imipramine or desipramine[1-4] are usually reserved for patients who fail to respond to, or who are intolerant of, stimulants. They may also be of use for selected patients with co-existing disorders such as Tourette's syndrome, anxiety, and enuresis.


1. Rapport MD, *et al.* Methylphenidate and desipramine in hospitalized children: I. separate and combined effects on cognitive function. *J Am Acad Child Adolesc Psychiatry* 1993; **32:** 333–42.
2. Pataki CS, *et al.* Side effects of methylphenidate and desipramine alone and in combination in children. *J Am Acad Child Adolesc Psychiatry* 1993; **32:** 1065–72.
3. Singer HS, *et al.* The treatment of attention-deficit hyperactivity disorder in Tourette's syndrome: a double-blind placebo-controlled study with clonidine and desipramine. *Pediatrics* 1995; **95:** 74–81.
4. Spencer T, *et al.* A double-blind comparison of desipramine and placebo in children and adolescents with chronic tic disorder and comorbid attention-deficit/hyperactivity disorder. *Arch Gen Psychiatry* 2002; **59:** 649–56.


**Pain.** Antidepressants, usually amitriptyline or another tricyclic, are useful in alleviating some types of pain (see Choice of Analgesic, p.2) when given in subantidepressant doses.

References to the use of desipramine.


1. Kishore-Kumar R, *et al.* Desipramine relieves postherpetic neuralgia. *Clin Pharmacol Ther* 1990; **47:** 305–12.
2. Max MB, *et al.* Effects of desipramine, amitriptyline, and fluoxetine on pain in diabetic neuropathy. *N Engl J Med* 1992; **326:** 1250–6.
3. Coquoz D, *et al.* Central analgesic effects of desipramine, fluvoxamine, and moclobemide after single oral dosing: a study in healthy volunteers. *Clin Pharmacol Ther* 1993; **54:** 339–44.
4. Gordon NC, *et al.* Temporal factors in the enhancement of morphine analgesia by desipramine. *Pain* 1993; **53:** 273–6.


## Preparations

***BP 2003:*** Desipramine Tablets;
***USP 27:*** Desipramine Hydrochloride Tablets.

**Proprietary Preparations** (details are given in Part 3)
***Arg.:*** Nebril; ***Austral.:*** Pertofran†; ***Austria:*** Pertofran; ***Belg.:*** Pertofran; ***Canad.:*** Norpramin; ***Chile:*** Distonal; ***Fr.:*** Pertofran; ***Ger.:*** Pertofran; Petylyl; ***Israel:*** Deprexan; ***Ital.:*** Nortimil; ***Mex.:*** Norpramin; ***Neth.:*** Pertofran; ***NZ:*** Pertofran; ***USA:*** Norpramin.

**Multi-ingredient:** ***Arg.:*** Plafonyl.

---

# Dibenzepin Hydrochloride *(BANM, USAN, rINNM)*

HF-1927; Hidrocloruro de dibenzepina. 10-(2-Dimethylaminoethyl)-5,10-dihydro-5-methyl-dibenzo[*b,e*][1,4]diazepin-11-one hydrochloride.

$C_{18}H_{21}N_3O,HCl = 331.8.$

*CAS — 4498-32-2 (dibenzepin); 315-80-0 (dibenzepin hydrochloride).*

*ATC — N06AA08.*

## Profile

Dibenzepin hydrochloride is a tricyclic antidepressant (see Amitriptyline, p.280).

In the treatment of depression dibenzepin hydrochloride is given by mouth in doses of 240 to 480 mg daily; higher doses of up to 720 mg daily may be required in some patients with severe depression.

Dibenzepin hydrochloride has also been given in doses of up to 360 mg daily by intravenous infusion.

Dibenzepin should be withdrawn gradually to reduce the risk of withdrawal symptoms.

◊ References.


1. Wirtheim E, Bloch Y. Dibenzepin overdose causing pulmonary edema. *Ann Pharmacother* 1996; **30:** 789–90.


## Preparations

**Proprietary Preparations** (details are given in Part 3)
***Austria:*** Noveril; ***Ger.:*** Noveril; ***Israel:*** Noveril; Victoril; ***Switz.:*** Noveril.

## Dosulepin Hydrochloride (BANM, rINNM)

Dosulepini Hydrochloridum; Dothiepin Hydrochloride (USAN); Hidrocloruro de dosulepina. 3-(Dibenzo[b,e]thiepin-11-ylidene)propyldimethylamine hydrochloride.

$C_{19}H_{21}NS,HCl = 331.9.$

*CAS — 113-53-1 (dosulepin); 897-15-4 (dosulepin hydrochloride).*

*ATC — N06AA16.*

**Pharmacopoeias.** In *Eur.* (see p.vi).

**Ph. Eur. 5.0** (Dosulepin Hydrochloride). A white or faintly yellow crystalline powder. It consists chiefly of the *E*-isomer. Freely soluble in water, in alcohol, and in dichloromethane. A 10% solution in water has a pH of 4.2 to 5.2. Protect from light.

### Adverse Effects, Treatment, and Precautions

As for tricyclic antidepressants in general (see Amitriptyline, p.281).

**Breast feeding.** For comments on the use of tricyclic antidepressants in breast feeding patients, see under Precautions for Amitriptyline, p.283.

**Effects on the cardiovascular system.** For reference to an increased risk of ischaemic heart disease in patients treated with dosulepin, see under Amitriptyline, p.281.

**Overdosage.** Following an overdose of 1 g of dosulepin, the ECG of a 41-year-old man showed cardiac abnormalities mimicking an acute myocardial infarction.[1] However, as cardiac enzymes did not confirm an ischaemic event, the abnormalities were thought to be due to either the quinidine-like effect of dosulepin or changes in potassium membrane permeability.

1. Steeds RP, Muthusamy R. Abnormal ventricular conduction following dothiepin overdose simulating acute myocardial infarction. *Heart* 2000; **83:** 289.

**Porphyria.** Dosulepin hydrochloride is considered to be unsafe in patients with porphyria because it has been shown to be porphyrinogenic in *animals*.

### Interactions

For interactions associated with tricyclic antidepressants, see Amitriptyline, p.284.

### Pharmacokinetics

Dosulepin hydrochloride is readily absorbed from the gastrointestinal tract, and extensively demethylated by first-pass metabolism in the liver to its primary active metabolite, desmethyldothiepin (also termed northiaden). Paths of metabolism also include *S*-oxidation.

Dosulepin is excreted in the urine, mainly in the form of its metabolites; small amounts are also excreted in the faeces. Elimination half-lives of about 14 to 24 and 23 to 46 hours have been reported for dosulepin and its metabolites, respectively.

Dosulepin is distributed into breast milk (see Breast Feeding under Precautions in Amitriptyline, p.283).

◊ References.

1. Maguire KP, *et al.* Clinical pharmacokinetics of dothiepin: single-dose kinetics in patients and prediction of steady-state concentrations. *Clin Pharmacokinet* 1983; **8:** 179–85.
2. Yu DK, *et al.* Pharmacokinetics of dothiepin in humans: a single dose dose-proportionality study. *J Pharm Sci* 1986; **75:** 582–5.
3. Ilett KF, *et al.* The excretion of dothiepin and its primary metabolites in breast milk. *Br J Clin Pharmacol* 1992; **33:** 635–9.

### Uses and Administration

Dosulepin hydrochloride is a tricyclic antidepressant with actions and uses similar to those of amitriptyline (p.285). It is one of the more sedating tricyclics.

In the treatment of depression, dosulepin hydrochloride is given by mouth in doses of 25 mg three times daily initially, gradually increased to 50 mg three times daily if necessary; alternatively a single dose at night may be given. Higher doses of up to 225 mg daily have been given to severely depressed patients in hospital. The recommended initial dose for the elderly is 50 to 75 mg daily.

Dosulepin should be withdrawn gradually to reduce the risk of withdrawal symptoms.

### Preparations

***BP 2003:*** Dosulepin Capsules; Dosulepin Tablets.

**Proprietary Preparations** (details are given in Part 3)
***Austral.:*** Dothep; Prothiaden; ***Austria:*** Xerenal; ***Belg.:*** Prothiaden; ***Denm.:*** Prothiaden; ***Fr.:*** Prothiaden; ***Ger.:*** Idom; ***Hong Kong:*** Prothiaden; ***India:*** Prothiaden; ***Irl.:*** Dothep; Prothiaden; ***Ital.:*** Protiaden; ***Malaysia:*** Dothep; Prothiaden; ***Neth.:*** Prothiaden; ***NZ:*** Dopress; Prothiaden; ***Port.:*** Protiadene; ***S.Afr.:*** Prothiaden; Thaden; ***Singapore:*** Espin; Prothiaden; ***Spain:*** Prothiaden; ***Switz.:*** Protiaden; ***Thai.:*** Dopin; Prothiaden; ***UK:*** Dothapax; Prepadine; Prothiaden; Thaden†.
**Multi-ingredient:** ***Austria:*** Harmomed.

## Doxepin Hydrochloride

(BANM, USAN, rINNM)

Doxepini Hydrochloridum; Hidrocloruro de doxepina; NSC-108160; P-3693A. (*E*)-3-(Dibenz[b,e]oxepin-11-ylidene)propyldimethylamine hydrochloride.

$C_{19}H_{21}NO,HCl = 315.8.$

*CAS — 1668-19-5 (doxepin); 1229-29-4 (doxepin hydrochloride); 4698-39-9 (doxepin hydrochloride, E-isomer); 25127-31-5 (doxepin hydrochloride, Z-isomer).*

*ATC — N06AA12.*

**Pharmacopoeias.** In *Chin., Eur.* (see p.vi), *Pol.,* and *US.*

**Ph. Eur. 5.0** (Doxepin Hydrochloride). A white or almost white crystalline powder. Freely soluble in water, in alcohol, and in dichloromethane. Protect from light.

**USP 27** (Doxepin Hydrochloride). It consists of a mixture of *Z*- and *E*-isomers.

### Adverse Effects, Treatment, and Precautions

As for tricyclic antidepressants in general (see Amitriptyline, p.281). Drowsiness and other systemic effects can also occur following topical application.

**Breast feeding.** For comments on the use of tricyclic antidepressants in breast feeding patients, see under Precautions for Amitriptyline, p.283.

**Overdosage.** An infant became difficult to arouse following the application of doxepin cream 5% to approximately 50% of her body-surface; an entire 30-g tube of the cream was used in only 2 applications.[1] The cream is not recommended for use in children.

1. Zell-Kanter M, *et al.* Doxepin toxicity in a child following topical application. *Ann Pharmacother* 2000; **34:** 328–9.

### Interactions

For interactions associated with tricyclic antidepressants, see Amitriptyline, p.284.

### Pharmacokinetics

Doxepin is readily absorbed from the gastrointestinal tract after oral doses, and is extensively demethylated by first-pass metabolism in the liver, to its primary active metabolite, desmethyldoxepin. Doxepin is also absorbed through the skin following topical application.

Paths of metabolism of both doxepin and desmethyldoxepin include hydroxylation and *N*-oxidation. Doxepin is excreted in the urine, mainly in the form of its metabolites, either free or in conjugated form.

Doxepin and desmethyldoxepin are widely distributed throughout the body and are extensively bound to plasma and tissue protein. Doxepin has been estimated to have a plasma elimination half-life ranging from 8 to 24 hours, which may be considerably extended in overdosage; that of desmethyldoxepin is longer.

Doxepin crosses the blood-brain barrier and the placenta. It is distributed into breast milk (see Breast Feeding under Precautions in Amitriptyline, p.283).

◊ References.

1. Faulkner RD, *et al.* Multiple-dose doxepin kinetics in depressed patients. *Clin Pharmacol Ther* 1983; **34:** 509–15.
2. Joyce PR, Sharman JR. Doxepin plasma concentrations in clinical practice: could there be a pharmacokinetic explanation for low concentrations? *Clin Pharmacokinet* 1985; **10:** 365–70.

### Uses and Administration

Doxepin is a dibenzoxepine tricyclic antidepressant with actions and uses similar to those of amitriptyline (p.285). It has moderate antimuscarinic and marked sedative properties and has serotonin reuptake inhibitor activity.

In the treatment of depression doxepin is given by mouth as the hydrochloride although doses are expressed in terms of the base; doxepin hydrochloride 84.8 mg is approximately equivalent to 75 mg of doxepin. The initial dose is 75 mg daily, gradually adjusted according to individual response. Doses of up to 300 mg daily may be required in severely depressed patients; mildly affected patients may respond to as little as 25 to 50 mg daily. Daily doses up to 100 mg may be given in divided doses or as a single dose at bedtime. If the total daily dose exceeds 100 mg, it should be given in divided doses, although the largest portion, up to a maximum of 100 mg, may be given at bedtime. In the USA, the maximum single dose is 150 mg. A suggested starting dose in the elderly is 10 to 50 mg daily.

Doxepin hydrochloride has also been given by intramuscular or intravenous injection.

Doxepin should be withdrawn gradually to reduce the risk of withdrawal symptoms.

Doxepin has histamine $H_1$- and $H_2$-antagonist activity and is used topically in a cream containing 5% of the hydrochloride for the short-term (up to 8 days) relief of moderately severe pruritus associated with various types of dermatitis (see below).

**Headache.** Tricyclic antidepressants can be effective in the management of some types of headache—see p.286.

References to the use of doxepin.

1. Wörz R, Scherhag R. Treatment of chronic tension headache with doxepin or amitriptyline—results of a double-blind study. *Headache Q* 1990; **1:** 216–23.

**Skin disorders.** Tricyclic antidepressants have a wide range of pharmacological activity and some members of the group have notable antihistaminic actions. Doxepin in particular has very potent antihistaminic activity. It has been shown to be an effective oral alternative to conventional antihistamines in the treatment of chronic urticaria,[1-3] and to be an effective oral treatment for idiopathic cold urticaria.[4,5] In the case of cold urticaria doxepin may act by inhibiting release of a platelet-activating factor-like lipid.[5]

For an overview of the possible treatments for the various urticarias, including mention of the use of doxepin, see p.1138.

Like standard antihistamines (p.422) doxepin has also been used topically for the relief of pruritus (see also p.1137) associated with various types of allergic and inflammatory skin disorders[6,7] although some authorities remain to be convinced of its efficacy.[8,9] Topical application of doxepin can also produce contact dermatitis and drowsiness and other systemic effects.

1. Greene SL, *et al.* Double-blind crossover study comparing doxepin with diphenhydramine for the treatment of chronic urticaria. *J Am Acad Dermatol* 1985; **12:** 669–75.
2. Harto A, *et al.* Doxepin in the treatment of chronic urticaria. *Dermatologica* 1985; **170:** 90–3.
3. Goldsobel AB, *et al.* Efficacy of doxepin in the treatment of chronic idiopathic urticaria. *J Allergy Clin Immunol* 1986; **78:** 867–73.
4. Neittaanmäki H, *et al.* Comparison of cinnarizine, cyproheptadine, doxepin, and hydroxyzine in treatment of idiopathic cold urticaria: usefulness of doxepin. *J Am Acad Dermatol* 1984; **11:** 483–9.
5. Grandel KE, *et al.* Association of platelet-activating factor with primary acquired cold urticaria. *N Engl J Med* 1985; **313:** 405–9.
6. Drake LA, *et al.* Relief of pruritus in patients with atopic dermatitis after treatment with topical doxepin cream. *J Am Acad Dermatol* 1994; **31:** 613–16.
7. Smith PF, Corelli RL. Doxepin in the management of pruritus associated with allergic cutaneous reactions. *Ann Pharmacother* 1997; **31:** 633–5.
8. Anonymous. Doxepin cream for pruritus. *Med Lett Drugs Ther* 1994; **36:** 99–100.
9. Anonymous. Doxepin cream for eczema? *Drug Ther Bull* 2000; **38:** 31–2.

### Preparations

***BP 2003:*** Doxepin Capsules;
***USP 27:*** Doxepin Hydrochloride Capsules; Doxepin Hydrochloride Oral Solution.

**Proprietary Preparations** (details are given in Part 3)
***Arg.:*** Doxederm; ***Austral.:*** Deptran; Sinequan; ***Austria:*** Sinequan; ***Belg.:*** Quitaxon†; Sinequan; ***Canad.:*** Sinequan; Triadapin†; Zonalon; ***Denm.:*** Quitaxon†; Sinequan; ***Fin.:*** Doxal; ***Fr.:*** Quitaxon; ***Ger.:*** Aponal; Desidoxepin†; Doneurin; Doxepia; Mareen; Sinquan; ***Gr.:*** Sinequan; ***Hong Kong:*** Sinequan; ***India:*** Spectra; ***Irl.:*** Sinequan; Xepin; ***Israel:*** Gilex; Zonalon; ***Mex.:*** Sinequan; ***Neth.:*** Sinequan; ***Norw.:*** Sinequan; ***NZ:*** Anten; ***Spain:*** Sinequan; ***Switz.:*** Sinquane; ***Thai.:*** Sinequan; ***UK:*** Sinequan; Xepin; ***USA:*** Sinequan; Zonalon.

## Duloxetine Hydrochloride (BANM, USAN, rINNM)

Hidrocloruro de duloxetina; LY-248686 (duloxetine). (+)-(*S*)-*N*-Methyl-γ-(1-naphthyloxy)-2-thiophenepropylamine hydrochloride.

$C_{18}H_{19}NOS,HCl = 333.9.$

*CAS — 116539-59-4 (duloxetine); 136434-34-9 (duloxetine hydrochloride).*

### Profile

Duloxetine hydrochloride is a serotonin and noradrenaline reuptake inhibitor (SNRI) under investigation for the treatment of depression. It is also being studied in the management of urinary incontinence.

◊ References.

1. Sharma A, *et al.* Pharmacokinetics and safety of duloxetine, a dual-serotonin and norepinephrine reuptake inhibitor. *J Clin Pharmacol* 2000; **40:** 161–7.
2. Goldstein DJ, *et al.* Duloxetine in the treatment of major depressive disorder: a double-blind clinical trial. *J Clin Psychiatry* 2002; **63:** 225–31.

3. Detke MJ, *et al.* Duloxetine, 60 mg once daily, for major depressive disorder: a randomized double-blind placebo-controlled trial. *J Clin Psychiatry* 2002; **63:** 308–15.
4. Norton PA, *et al.* Duloxetine versus placebo in the treatment of stress urinary incontinence. *Am J Obstet Gynecol* 2002; **187:** 40–8.


## Escitalopram Oxalate *(BANM, USAN, rINNM)*

S-Citalopram Oxalate; Lu-26-054/0. (+)-(S)-1-[3-(dimethylamino)propyl]-1-(p-fluorophenyl)-5-phthalancarbonitrile oxalate.

$C_{20}H_{21}FN_2O,C_2H_2O_4$ = 414.4.

*CAS — 128196-01-0 (escitalopram); 219861-08-2 (escitalopram oxalate).*

*ATC — N06AB10.*

### Profile

Escitalopram, the *S*-enantiomer of citalopram (p.289), is an SSRI with actions and uses similar to those of fluoxetine (p.292). It is given by mouth as the oxalate although doses are expressed in terms of the base; escitalopram oxalate 12.8 mg is approximately equivalent to 10 mg of escitalopram base.

In the treatment of **depression**, the usual dose is 10 mg once daily increased to a maximum of 20 mg once daily if necessary.

Escitalopram is also used in the treatment of **panic disorder** with or without agoraphobia. Initial doses are 5 mg once daily increased after one week to 10 mg once daily; further increases up to a maximum of 20 mg daily may be necessary in some patients.

Doses of escitalopram used in the treatment of **generalised anxiety disorder** and **social phobia** are similar to those used in depression.

Initial treatment with half the usual recommended dose and a lower maximum dose should be considered in elderly patients. Patients with hepatic impairment or those who are poor metabolisers with respect to the cytochrome P450 isoenzyme CYP2C19 should also receive an initial dose of 5 mg daily; the dose may be increased to 10 mg daily after two weeks depending on patient response.

Escitalopram should be withdrawn gradually to reduce the risk of withdrawal symptoms.

**Use.** References.


1. Burke WJ, *et al.* Fixed-dose trial of the single isomer SSRI escitalopram in depressed outpatients. *J Clin Psychiatry* 2002; **63:** 331–6.
2. Wade A, *et al.* Escitalopram 10mg/day is effective and well tolerated in a placebo-controlled study in depression in primary care. *Int Clin Psychopharmacol* 2002; **17:** 95–102.


CHILDREN. In the UK the Committee on Safety of Medicines recommends that escitalopram should not be used to treat depressive illness in children under 18 years of age. For details, see under Effects on Mental State in Fluoxetine, p.293.

### Preparations

**Proprietary Preparations** (details are given in Part 3)

***Austral.:*** Lexapro; ***Chile:*** Lexapro; ***Irl.:*** Lexapro; ***Norw.:*** Cipralex; ***UK:*** Cipralex; ***USA:*** Lexapro.

## Etoperidone Hydrochloride *(USAN, rINNM)*

Clopradone Hydrochloride; Hidrocloruro de etoperidona; McN-A-2673-11; ST-1191 (etoperidone). 2-{3-[4-(3-Chlorophenyl)piperazin-1-yl]propyl}-4,5-diethyl-2,4-dihydro-3H-1,2,4-triazol-3-one hydrochloride.

$C_{19}H_{28}ClN_5O,HCl$ = 414.4.

*CAS — 52942-31-1 (etoperidone); 57775-22-1 (etoperidone hydrochloride).*

*ATC — N06AB09.*

### Profile

Etoperidone hydrochloride is a triazolopyridine antidepressant related structurally to trazodone (p.319). It has been used in the treatment of depression.

### Preparations

**Proprietary Preparations** (details are given in Part 3)

***Spain:*** Depraser†.

# Fluoxetine Hydrochloride

*(BANM, USAN, rINNM)*

Fluoxetini Hydrochloridum; Hidrocloruro de fluoxetina; LY-110140. (±)-N-Methyl-3-phenyl-3-(α,α,α-trifluoro-p-tolyloxy)-propylamine hydrochloride.

$C_{17}H_{18}F_3NO,HCl$ = 345.8.

*CAS — 54910-89-3 (fluoxetine); 59333-67-4 (fluoxetine hydrochloride).*

*ATC — N06AB03.*

**Pharmacopoeias.** In *Eur.* (see p.vi), *Pol.*, and *US.*

**Ph. Eur. 5.0** (Fluoxetine Hydrochloride). A white or almost white crystalline powder. Sparingly soluble in water and in dichloromethane; freely soluble in methyl alcohol. A 1% solution in water has a pH of 4.5 to 6.5.

**USP 27** (Fluoxetine Hydrochloride). A white to off-white crystalline powder. Sparingly soluble in water and in dichloromethane; freely soluble in alcohol and in methyl alcohol; practically insoluble in ether. Store in airtight containers.

**Stability.** References.


1. Peterson JA, *et al.* Stability of fluoxetine hydrochloride in fluoxetine solution diluted with common pharmaceutical diluents. *Am J Hosp Pharm* 1994; **51:** 1342–5.


## Adverse Effects

SSRIs such as fluoxetine are less sedative than tricyclic antidepressants and have fewer antimuscarinic or cardiotoxic effects. Adverse effects reported with SSRIs include dry mouth and gastrointestinal disturbances such as nausea, vomiting, dyspepsia, constipation, and diarrhoea. Anorexia and weight loss may also occur. Neurological side-effects have included either anxiety, restlessness, nervousness, and insomnia, or drowsiness and fatigue; headache, tremor, dizziness, convulsions, hallucinations, confusion, agitation, extrapyramidal effects, depersonalisation, panic attacks, sexual dysfunction, and symptoms suggestive of a serotonin syndrome (p.313) have also occurred. The concern that some SSRIs may be associated with increased suicidal ideation is discussed under Effects on Mental State, below.

Excessive sweating, pruritus, skin rashes, photosensitivity, and urticaria have also been reported. Angioedema and anaphylactoid reactions have occurred. In some patients who have developed rashes while taking fluoxetine, systemic hypersensitivity reactions involving the lungs, kidneys, or liver, and possibly related to vasculitis, have developed; it has therefore been advised that fluoxetine therapy should be stopped in any patient who develops a skin rash.

Hyponatraemia, possibly due to inappropriate secretion of antidiuretic hormone, has been associated with the use of antidepressants, particularly in the elderly. Hyperprolactinaemia and galactorrhoea have occurred, as have changes in blood sugar, in patients receiving SSRIs.

Arthralgia and myalgia have been reported and there have also been cases of abnormal vision, orthostatic hypotension, and urinary retention. Abnormal liver function tests have been reported rarely. SSRIs have occasionally been associated with bleeding disorders and other effects on the blood.

In overdosage nausea, vomiting, and excitation of the CNS are considered to be prominent features; death has been reported.

**Incidence of adverse effects.** In June 1992 the UK Committee on Safety of Medicines (CSM) had received 1236 reports of adverse effects with fluvoxamine (from about 280 000 prescriptions) compared with 2422 for fluoxetine (from about 480 000 prescriptions).[1] The overall adverse reactions profiles were similar but dermatological reactions were more likely with fluoxetine and gastrointestinal reactions with fluvoxamine. Reports of attempted suicide increased after adverse publicity about SSRIs in 1990, and the number of reports per million prescriptions were similar for the 2 drugs (25 for fluoxetine and 20 for fluvoxamine); such figures were not considered disconcerting given that features of depression, including attempted suicide, can worsen after the introduction of any antidepressant. A more recent review[2] by the CSM of the 5 SSRIs available in the UK (citalopram, fluoxetine, fluvoxamine, paroxetine, and sertraline) found that the SSRIs were broadly similar with respect to their safety profile. A list of adverse reactions common to all SSRIs was provided.

A review[3] of 1861 adverse reactions to citalopram, fluoxetine, fluvoxamine, paroxetine, or sertraline reported to the Swedish Adverse Drug Reactions Advisory Committee found that the most commonly reported reactions were neurological (22.4% of all reports), psychiatric (19.5%), and gastrointestinal (18.0%). Compared with other SSRIs, gastrointestinal symptoms were more common with fluvoxamine, psychiatric symptoms with sertraline, and dermatological symptoms with fluoxetine.


1. Committee on Safety of Medicines. Safety of fluoxetine (Prozac): comparison with fluvoxamine (Faverin). *Current Problems 34* 1992.
2. Committee on Safety of Medicines/Medicines Control Agency. Selective serotonin reuptake inhibitors (SSRIs). *Current Problems* 2000; **26:** 11–12. Also available at: http://www.mca.gov.uk/ourwork/monitorsafequalmed/currentproblems/cpsept2000.pdf (accessed 10/06/04)
3. Spigset O. Adverse reactions of selective serotonin reuptake inhibitors: reports from a spontaneous reporting system. *Drug Safety* 1999; **20:** 277–87.


**Effects on the blood.** Abnormalities in platelet aggregation were associated with fluoxetine given to a severely underweight patient.[1] Platelet activity returned to normal when fluoxetine was discontinued. Fluoxetine was also suspected of being the cause of bruising in a patient whose blood clotting parameters were within normal limits.[2] Purpura and bruising have been reported to be the commonest adverse blood effects associated with fluoxetine, paroxetine, or sertraline although cases of thrombocytopenia have been recorded for all three antidepressants.[3] The suggested mechanism was inhibition of uptake of serotonin into platelets, thereby disrupting platelet aggregation; caution was recommended when treating patients with a history of bleeding disorders with SSRIs. However, a subsequent cohort study based on prescription event monitoring provided only weak evidence of a link between the use of SSRIs and the development of bleeding disorders.[4] A similar study[5] found no evidence of a major increased risk of intracranial haemorrhage with the use of SSRIs, although smaller increases in risk could not be ruled out.

For mention of a possibly increased risk of gastrointestinal bleeding, see Effects on the Gastrointestinal Tract, below.


1. Alderman CP, *et al.* Abnormal platelet aggregation associated with fluoxetine therapy. *Ann Pharmacother* 1992; **26:** 1517–19.
2. Pai VB, Kelly MW. Bruising associated with the use of fluoxetine. *Ann Pharmacother* 1996; **30:** 786–8.
3. Anonymous. Bruising and bleeding with SSRIs. *Aust Adverse Drug React Bull* 1998; **17:** 10. Also available at: http://www.tga.gov.au/docs/html/aadrbltn/aadr9808.htm (accessed 10/06/04)
4. Layton D, *et al.* Is there an association between selective serotonin reuptake inhibitors and risk of abnormal bleeding? Results from a cohort study based on prescription event monitoring in England. *Eur J Clin Pharmacol* 2001; **57:** 167–76.
5. de Abajo FJ, *et al.* Intracranial haemorrhage and use of selective serotonin reuptake inhibitors. *Br J Clin Pharmacol* 2000; **50:** 43–7.


**Effects on the cardiovascular system.** SSRIs are not associated with the same degree of cardiotoxicity as the tricyclic antidepressants (see p.281), although orthostatic hypotension has been reported in some patients. A decrease in heart rate with ECG changes has been noted with fluvoxamine. However, a study[1] on long-term fluvoxamine treatment in 311 patients followed for 1 year revealed no significant effect on ECG findings compared with patients given placebo.

Concern over the use of sertraline in patients with coronary heart disease was raised following a report[2] of a 53-year-old man with a history of coronary heart disease who experienced attacks of sudden precordial chest pain after starting treatment with sertraline. The pain responded to glyceryl trinitrate. The manufacturers[3] pointed out that there had been no ECG changes confirming an ischaemic origin of the disorder in this patient and that in studies sertraline had had no demonstrable clinical effects on intraventricular conduction or ECG intervals. Furthermore, no significant changes in cardiovascular indices had been recorded in patients who had taken overdoses of up to 6 g of sertraline. It was suggested that this might have been an effect on the gastrointestinal tract possibly at the oesophageal level.


1. Hochberg HM, *et al.* Electrocardiographic findings during extended clinical trials of fluvoxamine in depression: one years experience. *Pharmacopsychiatry* 1995; **28:** 253–6.
2. Iruela LM. Sudden chest pain with sertraline. *Lancet* 1994; **343:** 1106.
3. Berti CA, Doogan DP. Sudden chest pain with sertraline. *Lancet* 1994; **343:** 1510–11.


**Effects on the endocrine system.** The *syndrome of inappropriate antidiuretic hormone secretion (SIADH)* with *hyponatraemia* has been reported in patients receiving antidepressants. The UK Committee on Safety of Medicines, commenting on reports it had received of hyponatraemia associated with antidepressants (fluoxetine, paroxetine, lofepramine, clomipramine, and imipramine), considered that it was likely to occur with any antidepressant, and usually involved elderly patients.[1] However, the results of a later study[2] have suggested that cases are more likely to occur with serotonergic antidepressants such as the SSRIs, clomipramine, and venlafaxine. Case reports of hyponatraemia in 16 patients treated with SSRIs have been summarised.[3] A further review[4] of reports on 15 patients with hyponatraemia with SIADH induced by fluoxetine (12 cases), fluvoxamine (2 cases), and paroxetine (1 case) showed that the risk was greatest during the early treatment phase. This is borne out by single-case reports[5-11] of hyponatraemia with SIADH in elderly patients receiving either citalopram, paroxetine, or sertraline. A retrospective study[12] of hyponatraemia associated with either fluoxetine or paroxetine use also showed the early onset of the condition and identified low body-weight as being another risk factor for developing hyponatraemia. Not unexpectedly, replacing one SSRI with another has resulted in a recurrence of hyponatraemia; however, in one report,[13] the symptoms of hyponatraemia did not recur until about 16 months after switching SSRIs.

SSRI-associated *hyperprolactinaemia* has been reported.[14] Lactation and raised prolactin levels occurred in a teenager 3 days after fluoxetine was added to her existing therapy which included pimozide. Stopping fluoxetine had no effect on lactation, which only ceased after withdrawing pimozide. In another report,[15] hyperprolactinaemia and galactorrhoea in an elderly woman receiving fluoxetine resolved on discontinuing the drug.

Although SSRIs may be favoured for the management of depression in patients with diabetes, there is some evidence that sertraline and fluoxetine can induce *hypoglycaemia*.[16,17]


1. Committee on Safety of Medicines/Medicines Control Agency. Antidepressant-induced hyponatraemia. *Current Problems* 1994; **20:** 5–6.
2. Movig KLL, *et al.* Serotonergic antidepressants associated with an increased risk for hyponatraemia in the elderly. *Eur J Clin Pharmacol* 2002; **58:** 143–8.

3. Spigset O, Hedenmalm K. Hyponatraemia and the syndrome of inappropriate antidiuretic hormone secretion (SIADH) induced by psychotropic drugs. *Drug Safety* 1995; **12:** 209–25.
4. Canadian Medical Association. Hyponatraemia and selective serotonin reuptake inhibitors. *Can Med Assoc J* 1996; **154:** 63.
5. Bluff DD. SIADH in a patient receiving sertraline. *Ann Intern Med* 1995; **123:** 811.
6. Adverse Drug Reactions Advisory Committee. Selective serotonin reuptake inhibitors and SIADH. *Med J Aust* 1996; **164:** 562.
7. Kessler J, Samuels SC. Sertraline and hyponatremia. *N Engl J Med* 1996; **335:** 524.
8. Robinson D, *et al.* SIADH—compulsive drinking or SSRI influence? *Ann Pharmacother* 1996; **30:** 885.
9. Monmany J, *et al.* Syndrome of inappropriate secretion of antidiuretic hormone induced by paroxetine. *Arch Intern Med* 1999; **159:** 2089–90.
10. Odeh M, *et al.* Severe life-threatening hyponatremia during paroxetine therapy. *J Clin Pharmacol* 1999; **39:** 1290–1.
11. Barclay TS, Lee AJ. Citalopram-associated SIADH. *Ann Pharmacother* 2002; **36:** 1558–63.
12. Wilkinson TJ, *et al.* Incidence and risk factors for hyponatraemia following treatment with fluoxetine or paroxetine in elderly people. *Br J Clin Pharmacol* 1999; **47:** 211–17.
13. Arinzon ZH, *et al.* Delayed recurrent SIADH associated with SSRIs. *Ann Pharmacother* 2002; **36:** 1175–7.
14. Arya DK, *et al.* Lactation associated with fluoxetine treatment. *Aust N Z J Psychiatry* 1995; **29:** 697.
15. Peterson MC. Reversible galactorrhea and prolactin elevation related to fluoxetine use. *Mayo Clin Proc* 2001; **76:** 215–16.
16. Deeg MA, Lipkin EW. Hypoglycemia associated with the use of fluoxetine. *West J Med* 1996; **164:** 262–3.
17. Pollak PT, *et al.* Sertraline-induced hypoglycemia. *Ann Pharmacother* 2001; **35:** 1371–4.

**Effects on the eyes.** Symptoms of glaucoma that developed in a patient receiving fluoxetine subsided within 2 days of drug withdrawal.[1] Similar symptoms have been reported with citalopram,[2] fluvoxamine,[3] paroxetine,[2,4] and sertraline.[2] In some cases, the SSRI may have aggravated pre-existing glaucoma.[2,3] Intra-ocular pressure after doses of fluoxetine was recorded in 20 patients in a placebo-controlled crossover double-blind study.[5] Significant increases were found in all patients 2 hours after receiving fluoxetine by mouth; some patients still had raised intra-ocular pressure after 8 hours.

There has been a report[6] of anisocoria (uneven pupillary dilatation) in a patient taking paroxetine and in another taking sertraline. It was noted that the UK Committee on Safety of Medicines had received 21 reports of mydriasis associated with paroxetine but it appeared that noticeably asymmetrical mydriasis as seen in these 2 patients had not previously been reported.

1. Ahmad S. Fluoxetine and glaucoma. *DICP Ann Pharmacother* 1991; **25:** 436.
2. Anonymous. SSRIs and increased intraocular pressure. *Aust Adverse Drug React Bull* 2001; **20:** 3. Also available at: http://www.tga.gov.au/docs/html/aadrbltn/aadr0102.htm (accessed 10/06/04)
3. Jiménez-Jiménez FJ, *et al.* Aggravation of glaucoma with fluvoxamine. *Ann Pharmacother* 2001; **35:** 1565–6.
4. Eke T, Carr S. Acute glaucoma, chronic glaucoma, and serotoninergic drugs. *Br J Ophthalmol* 1998; **82:** 976–7.
5. Costagliola C, *et al.* Fluoxetine oral administration increases intraocular pressure. *Br J Ophthalmol* 1996; **80:** 678.
6. Barrett J. Anisocoria associated with selective serotonin reuptake inhibitors. *BMJ* 1994; **309:** 1620.

**Effects on the gastrointestinal tract.** A case-control study[1] has suggested that treatment with SSRIs produces a moderately increased risk of upper gastrointestinal bleeding (adjusted relative risk 3.0). The risk was greatly increased if SSRIs were given with NSAIDs (relative risk 15.6). Treatment with SSRIs did not appear to increase the risk of ulcer perforation. The absolute risk of bleeding was estimated at one case per 8000 prescriptions, a risk similar to that of low-dose ibuprofen. Others, however, have questioned whether such an association exists.[2] A later retrospective cohort study[3] in elderly patients found that there was an increasing risk of upper gastrointestinal bleeding as the extent of inhibition of serotonin reuptake by the antidepressant used increased. The effect was considered to be clinically important for patients with a high risk of such bleeding, namely the very elderly and those with a history of previous upper gastrointestinal bleeding.

1. de Abajo FJ, *et al.* Association between selective serotonin reuptake inhibitors and upper gastrointestinal bleeding: population based case-control study. *BMJ* 1999; **319:** 1106–9.
2. Dunn NR, *et al.* Association between SSRIs and upper gastrointestinal bleeding. *BMJ* 2000; **320:** 1405–6.
3. van Walraven C, *et al.* Inhibition of serotonin reuptake by antidepressants and upper gastrointestinal bleeding in elderly patients: retrospective cohort study. *BMJ* 2001; **323:** 655–8.

**Effects on the hair.** A report[1] on 2 patients who experienced hair loss associated with the use of fluoxetine noted 4 other published cases and stated that, up to the end of 1991, the US manufacturers had received 498 reports of fluoxetine-associated alopecia.

1. Ogilvie AD. Hair loss during fluoxetine treatment. *Lancet* 1993; **342:** 1423.

**Effects on the liver.** Acute hepatitis occurred in 2 patients after several months of fluoxetine treatment;[1] it was noted that 5 other cases of acute hepatitis with fluoxetine had been reported. Abnormal liver function tests were seen in a patient after a suicide attempt with sertraline and cefalexin.[2] The patient was then started on venlafaxine but, again abnormal liver function tests were noted. When these abnormal values had decreased, sertraline was restarted at therapeutic doses, with a subsequent increase in liver function tests. Values returned to normal once all medications were stopped. Hepatotoxicity has also been rarely associated with paroxetine.[3]

1. Cai Q, *et al.* Acute hepatitis due to fluoxetine therapy. *Mayo Clin Proc* 1999; **74:** 692–4.
2. Kim KY, *et al.* Acute liver damage possibly related to sertraline and venlafaxine ingestion. *Ann Pharmacother* 1999; **33:** 381–2.
3. Azaz-Livshits T, *et al.* Paroxetine associated hepatotoxicity: a report of 3 cases and a review of the literature. *Pharmacopsychiatry* 2002; **35:** 112–15.

**Effects on mental state.** There has been concern that fluoxetine increases *suicidal ideation* and there have been suggestions that there may be a link with akathisia[1] or dosage.[2] Meta-analyses[3,4] (criticism of statistical power notwithstanding[5]) have not confirmed an increased risk and this appears to be supported by the results of prescription event monitoring,[6] and is the view of various regulatory authorities. Nevertheless some reviewers consider that under certain conditions all antidepressants and antipsychotics can induce suicidal ideation in some individuals and comment that there does appear to be enough anecdotal evidence to indicate that fluoxetine may induce suicidal ideation on rare occasions.[7,8] It has been suggested that as suicidal ideation has been associated with induction of akathisia, agitation, or panic by fluoxetine, propranolol might be added to therapy to control these effects.[7,8] There has also been concern that fluvoxamine, like fluoxetine, may increase suicidal ideation and a suggestion that it might be dose-related.[9]

In 2003 the UK Committee on Safety of Medicines (CSM) recommended that paroxetine should not be used to treat depressive illness in **children under 18**. Data from trials received by CSM in May 2003 failed to demonstrate that paroxetine was effective in depressive illness in this age group and indicated that the risk of harmful outcome, including self-harm and potentially suicidal behaviour, was 1.5 to 3.2 times greater in those who received paroxetine when compared with placebo.[10] Following a further review,[11] the CSM extended their recommendation to include the SSRIs citalopram, escitalopram, and sertraline; subsequent analysis had also associated these antidepressants with an unfavourable risk to benefit ratio in the treatment of depression in children under 18. The CSM also included fluvoxamine in their recommendation as its risk to benefit ratio was unassessable. Fluoxetine was not included and the CSM acknowledged that clinical trials have shown a favourable risk to benefit ratio for fluoxetine in the treatment of depression in young patients; however the drug is not licensed for depression in children and adolescents in the UK, and the *British National Formulary* does not recommend such use.

Other regulatory authorities such as the FDA have not issued advice contra-indicating the use of these antidepressants in those under 18, although they have stressed that all patients, including adolescents and children, should be closely monitored for worsening depression or suicidal behaviour, especially at the beginning of treatment.[12] They also comment that, apart from fluoxetine, the SSRIs are not licensed in the USA for the treatment of depression in young patients.

For a discussion of the choice of antidepressant with respect to safety in overdosage, see under Depression, p.279.

For further effects on mental function, see also under Withdrawal and under Mania in Precautions, below.

There have also been suggested links between the use of fluoxetine and *irritability, hostility, and aggression.*[13] However, one review[8] noted that an unpublished analysis had indicated that patients taking fluoxetine for a variety of disorders were not more likely to be aggressive than those taking placebo. Prescription event monitoring has also found no evidence to suggest that fluoxetine increases the frequency of aggression.[6]

Initiation of antidepressant therapy with paroxetine or sertraline has been associated with either worsening or a new onset of *flashback syndrome* in 2 patients with a history of lysergide abuse.[14]

1. Rothschild AJ, Locke CA. Reexposure to fluoxetine after serious suicide attempts by three patients: the role of akathisia. *J Clin Psychiatry* 1991; **52:** 491–3.
2. Fichtner CG, *et al.* Does fluoxetine have a therapeutic window? *Lancet* 1991; **338:** 520–1.
3. Beasley CM, *et al.* Fluoxetine and suicide: a meta-analysis of controlled trials of treatment for depression. *BMJ* 1991; **303:** 685–92. Correction. *ibid.*; 968.
4. Goldstein DJ, *et al.* Analyses of suicidality in double-blind, placebo-controlled trials of pharmacotherapy for weight reduction. *J Clin Psychiatry* 1993; **54:** 309–16.
5. Li Wan Po A. Fluoxetine and suicide: meta-analysis and Monte-Carlo simulations. *Pharmacoepidemiol Drug Safety* 1993; **2:** 79–84.
6. Nakielny J. Fluoxetine and suicide. *Lancet* 1994; **343:** 1359.
7. Healy D. The fluoxetine and suicide controversy: a review of the evidence. *CNS Drugs* 1994; **1:** 223–31.
8. Power AC, Cowen PJ. Fluoxetine and suicidal behaviour; some clinical and theoretical aspects of a controversy. *Br J Psychiatry* 1992; **161:** 735–41.
9. Pitchot W, *et al.* Therapeutic window for 5-HT reuptake inhibitors. *Lancet* 1992; **339:** 689.
10. Safety of Seroxat (paroxetine) in children and adolescents under 18 years - contraindication in the treatment of depressive illness - Epinet message from Professor G Duff, Chairman of Committee on Safety of Medicines (CSM) (issued 10/06/03). Available at: http://medicines.mhra.gov.uk/ourwork/monitorsafequalmed/safetymessages/seroxat18.pdf (accessed 10/06/04)
11. Selective Serotonin Reuptake Inhibitors - use in children and adolescents with major depressive disorder - Epinet message from Professor G Duff, Chairman of Committee on Safety of Medicines (CSM) (issued 10/12/03). Available at: http://www.mca.gov.uk/ourwork/monitorsafequalmed/safetymessages/cemssri_101203.pdf (accessed 10/06/04)
12. The FDA Public Health Advisory. Worsening depression and suicidality in patients being treated with antidepressant medications (issued 22/03/04). Available at: http://www.fda.gov/cder/drug/antidepressants/AntidepressanstPHA.htm (accessed 10/06/04)
13. Anonymous. Fluoxetine, suicide and aggression. *Drug Ther Bull* 1992; **30:** 5–6.
14. Markel H, *et al.* LSD flashback syndrome exacerbated by selective serotonin reuptake inhibitor antidepressants in adolescents. *J Pediatr* 1994; **125:** 817–19.

**Effects on sexual function.** It has been considered that sexual dysfunction occurs in up to 1.9% of patients taking fluoxetine, with impotence or ejaculatory problems occurring in less than 1% of patients.[1] These figures were based on information supplied by the US manufacturer for the data sheet but have been disputed.[2,3] Earlier studies and anecdotal reports quoted rates of 7.8 to 75% for sexual dysfunction with fluoxetine but it appears that only small numbers of men were studied.[4] A more recent review[5] also estimated the incidence of SSRI-induced sexual dysfunction at between 10 and 75%. The reported frequency of sexual dysfunction is usually higher in men taking SSRIs than in women; complaints include a decrease in or loss of libido, delayed ejaculation, erectile difficulty, or anorgasmia.[6] However, loss of libido, delayed orgasm, or anorgasmia have also been reported in women.[6,7]

Suggested[6,8] strategies for managing SSRI-induced sexual dysfunction include reducing the dosage of the SSRI or altering the timing of doses, or changing to another antidepressant. Evidence of efficacy for drug treatments is mainly anecdotal. Cyproheptadine seems to have been tried most often, but the SSRI may become less effective (see Antihistamines, under Interactions, below) and patients should be monitored for worsening symptoms of depression.

The effects of the SSRIs on sexual function have been studied as a potential form of treatment for men with premature ejaculation (see Sexual Dysfunction in Uses, below).

1. Hollander JB. Fluoxetine and sexual dysfunction. *JAMA* 1994; **272:** 242.
2. Balon R. Fluoxetine and sexual dysfunction. *JAMA* 1995; **273:** 1489.
3. Hopkins HS, Gelenberg AJ. Fluoxetine and sexual dysfunction. *JAMA* 1995; **273:** 1489–90.
4. Hollander JB. Fluoxetine and sexual dysfunction. *JAMA* 1995; **273:** 1490.
5. Gregorian RS, *et al.* Antidepressant-induced sexual dysfunction. *Ann Pharmacother* 2002; **36:** 1577–89.
6. Frye CB, Berger JE. Treatment of sexual dysfunction induced by selective serotonin-reuptake inhibitors. *Am J Health-Syst Pharm* 1998; **55:** 1167–9.
7. Feiger A, *et al.* Nefazodone versus sertraline in outpatients with major depression: focus on efficacy, tolerability, and effects on sexual function and satisfaction. *J Clin Psychiatry* 1996; **57** (suppl 2): 53–62.
8. Woodrum ST, Brown CS. Management of SSRI-induced sexual dysfunction. *Ann Pharmacother* 1998; **32:** 1209–15.

**Effects on the skin.** *Toxic epidermal necrolysis* developed in a 16-year-old girl 8 days after beginning fluvoxamine therapy.[1] Other drugs, which included metoclopramide, clorazepate, and clomipramine were discounted as possible causes.

Amitriptyline and fluoxetine have been implicated in the development of *atypical cutaneous lymphoid hyperplasia* in 8 patients, 7 of whom either had an underlying immunosuppressant systemic disease or were receiving concomitant therapy with immunomodulatory drugs.[2] The lesions improved or resolved on stopping the antidepressant, although in some patients other factors may have contributed to the improvement.

*Bullous pemphigoid* induced by fluoxetine has been reported in a 75-year-old woman.[3] Spontaneous resolution followed within 3 weeks of discontinuing the drug.

1. Wolkenstein P, *et al.* Toxic epidermal necrolysis after fluvoxamine. *Lancet* 1993; **342:** 304–5.
2. Crowson AN, Magro CM. Antidepressant therapy: a possible cause of atypical cutaneous lymphoid hyperplasia. *Arch Dermatol* 1995; **131:** 925–9.
3. Rault S, *et al.* Bullous pemphigoid induced by fluoxetine. *Br J Dermatol* 1999; **141:** 755–6.

**Epileptogenic effect.** Generalised seizures have been reported in 2 patients with no previous history of seizures following initiation of fluoxetine therapy.[1,2] Although convulsions have been noted in patients receiving fluvoxamine (see p.298), a small clinical study involving 35 depressed epileptic patients[3] found no change in the number of seizures or in their nature when fluvoxamine was given in doses of up to 200 mg daily.

1. Weber JJ. Seizure activity associated with fluoxetine therapy. *Clin Pharm* 1989; **8:** 296–8.
2. Ware MR, Stewart RB. Seizures associated with fluoxetine therapy. *DICP Ann Pharmacother* 1989; **23:** 428.
3. Harmant J, *et al.* Fluvoxamine: an antidepressant with low (or no) epileptogenic effect. *Lancet* 1990; **336:** 386.

**Extrapyramidal effects.** Extrapyramidal effects, such as tics[1] and akathisia,[2,3] have been reported with fluoxetine. By 1993, the UK Committee on Safety of Medicines had received 39 reports of extrapyramidal reactions with paroxetine including 15 of dystonia of the face and mouth.[4] It was noted that, although extrapyramidal effects may occur with other SSRIs, orofacial dystonias appeared to be more common with paroxetine. However, evidence from monitoring prescriptions within the UK has shown that the overall incidence of extrapyramidal effects is the same for paroxetine as for other SSRIs.[5] Orofacial dystonias (teeth clenching) or dyskinesias (teeth grinding), with resultant severe damage to teeth and gums in the majority of cases, have been reported[6] in 6 patients receiving fluoxetine, fluvoxamine, paroxetine, or sertraline. The authors concluded that these adverse effects were not specific for any particular SSRI. Analysis of spontaneous adverse reaction reports received by the national pharmacovigilance centre in The Netherlands found that there had been 41 reports of extrapyramidal effects associated with the SSRIs over a period of nearly 15 years;[7] parkinsonism and dystonia were the most frequently reported effects. Over the same time period, 14 reports had been received in total for other antidepressants. The authors commented that the difference in reporting may be biased particularly by the selective reporting of adverse reactions to the SSRIs.

Dyskinesia associated with withdrawal of citalopram and risperidone has been reported in a patient.[8]


1. Eisenhauer G, Jermain DM. Fluoxetine and tics in an adolescent. *Ann Pharmacother* 1993; **27:** 725–6.
2. Lipinski JF, *et al.* Fluoxetine-induced akathisia: clinical and theoretical implications. *J Clin Psychiatry* 1989; **50:** 339–42.
3. Rothschild AJ, Locke CA. Reexposure to fluoxetine after serious suicide attempts by three patients: the role of akathisia. *J Clin Psychiatry* 1991; **52:** 491–3.
4. Committee on Safety of Medicines/Medicines Control Agency. Dystonia and withdrawal symptoms with paroxetine (Seroxat). *Current Problems* 1993; **19:** 1.
5. Choo V. Paroxetine and extrapyramidal reactions. *Lancet* 1993; **341:** 624.
6. Fitzgerald K, Healy D. Dystonias and dyskinesias of the jaw associated with the use of SSRIs. *Hum Psychopharmacol Clin Exp* 1995; **10:** 215–19.
7. Schillevoort I, *et al.* Extrapyramidal syndromes associated with selective serotonin reuptake inhibitors: a case-control study using spontaneous reports. *Int Clin Psychopharmacol* 2002; **17:** 75–9.
8. Miller LJ. Withdrawal-emergent dyskinesia in a patient taking risperidone/citalopram. *Ann Pharmacother* 2000; **34:** 269.


**Hypersensitivity.** Hypersensitivity reactions to SSRIs are well documented. Interestingly, despite structural dissimilarities, there have been a few reports of cross-sensitivity between SSRIs. A young man who had previously developed a maculopapular rash while taking paroxetine suffered a similar reaction after starting sertraline;[1] both episodes resolved after the SSRI was withdrawn.


1. Warnock CA, Azadian AG. Cross-sensitivity between paroxetine and sertraline. *Ann Pharmacother* 2002; **36:** 631–3.


**Hyponatraemia.** See Effects on the Endocrine System, above.

**Overdosage.** SSRIs are generally regarded as being less toxic in overdosage than tricyclic antidepressants or MAOIs. A review[1] of SSRI overdosage, covering the period 1985 to 1997, noted that there had been remarkably few fatal overdoses when taken alone. Moderate overdoses (up to about 30 times the usual daily dose) were generally associated with minor symptoms at most; only at very high doses (more than 75 times the usual daily dose) did more serious effects such as seizures, ECG abnormalities, and decreased consciousness tend to occur. Toxicity was greatly increased, however, when overdoses of SSRIs were taken with alcohol or other drugs. There was no evidence of a difference in the various SSRIs with respect to safety in overdosage.

A report involving 87 cases in which fluoxetine was taken in overdosage without other drugs found that the main symptoms were tachycardia, drowsiness, tremor, and nausea and vomiting.[2] These were considered relatively minor, and were of short duration, and supportive care was considered to be the only intervention necessary. Of 41 cases of self-poisoning with fluvoxamine, only one patient died and even here fluvoxamine was not implicated.[3] Prolonged cerebral depression occurred in a patient following fluvoxamine overdose,[3] but this may have been due to an interaction with temazepam which the patient also took in overdose. One hour after taking 2 g of sertraline in a suicide attempt a 42-year-old woman was flushed, angry, emotionally labile, and easily distracted but not psychotic.[4] Apart from watery bowel movements recovery was mainly uneventful following treatment with gastric lavage, oral activated charcoal with sorbitol, and intravenous hydration. Abnormal liver function tests have also been noted after a suicide attempt with sertraline (see Effects on the Liver, above).

Fatal overdose has been reported with citalopram in 6 patients,[5] although the suggested cause of death as cardiac dysfunction rather than seizures was disputed.[6]

For a discussion of choice of antidepressant with respect to toxicity in overdosage, see under Depression, p.279.


1. Barbey JT, Roose SP. SSRI safety in overdose. *J Clin Psychiatry* 1998; **59** (suppl 15): 42–8.
2. Borys DJ, *et al.* Acute fluoxetine overdose: a report of 234 cases. *Am J Emerg Med* 1992; **10:** 115–20.
3. Banerjee AK. Recovery from prolonged cerebral depression after fluvoxamine overdose. *BMJ* 1988; **296:** 1774.
4. Brown DF, Kerr HD. Sertraline overdose. *Ann Pharmacother* 1994; **28:** 1307.
5. Öström M, *et al.* Fatal overdose with citalopram. *Lancet* 1996; **348:** 339–40.
6. Brion F, *et al.* Fatal overdose with citalopram? *Lancet* 1996; **348:** 1380.


## Treatment of Adverse Effects

Treatment of overdosage with an SSRI involves appropriate symptomatic and supportive therapy. Activated charcoal may be given by mouth if the amount ingested was large (see below) and treatment is within an hour of ingestion. Gastric lavage is generally unnecessary as overdose is rarely life-threatening (see Overdosage, above). Dialysis, haemoperfusion, exchange transfusion, and measures to increase urine production are considered unlikely to be of benefit.

**Activated charcoal.** The UK Poisons Information Service considers the benefit of gastric decontamination in the management of overdosage with SSRIs to be uncertain. However, it is suggested that oral activated charcoal may be considered if this is given within 1 hour of ingestion and the quantity of SSRI exceeds the following amount:

- citalopram: 5 mg/kg (adult); 5 mg/kg (child)
- escitalopram: 2.5 mg/kg (adult); 2.5 mg/kg (child)
- fluoxetine: 500 mg (adult); 5 mg/kg (child)
- fluvoxamine: 1 g (adult); 100 mg (child)
- paroxetine: 600 mg (adult); 5 mg/kg (child)
- sertraline: 1 g (adult); 10 mg/kg (child)

## Precautions

Because of their epileptogenic effect SSRIs should be used with caution in patients with epilepsy or a history of such disorders (and should be avoided if the epilepsy is poorly controlled). Treatment should be stopped if seizures develop or when there is an increase in seizure frequency. Care is advised in patients receiving ECT. SSRIs should also be used with caution in patients with cardiac disease or a history of bleeding disorders. Although SSRIs are preferred to tricyclics for the treatment of depression in patients with diabetes, they may alter glycaemic control and therefore caution is also warranted in diabetic subjects. Fluoxetine should be discontinued in patients who develop a rash since systemic effects, possibly related to vasculitis, have occurred in such patients. Fluoxetine undergoes hepatic metabolism and should be used with caution and in reduced doses in patients with impaired hepatic function.

Patients should be closely monitored during early therapy until improvement in depression is observed because suicide is an inherent risk in depressed patients. For further details, see under Depression, p.279. For a discussion of the concern that SSRIs, particularly fluoxetine, may increase suicidal ideation, and concerns about their use for depression in children and adolescents, see Effects on Mental State in Adverse Effects, above.

If SSRIs are given for the depressive component of bipolar disorder, mania may be precipitated.

SSRIs may impair performance of skilled tasks and, if affected, patients should not drive or operate machinery.

Some manufacturers recommend reduced or less frequent dosage of SSRIs for elderly patients.

Significant amounts of fluoxetine are distributed into breast milk and the manufacturers have reported that adverse effects have been observed in a breast-fed infant; consequently fluoxetine is not recommended for nursing mothers. Similarly, the manufacturers of some other SSRIs (citalopram, fluvoxamine, paroxetine, and sertraline) have recommended that they should be avoided during breast feeding.

SSRIs should generally be withdrawn gradually to reduce the risk of withdrawal symptoms although this may be unnecessary for fluoxetine because of its long half-life.

**Abuse.** There have been occasional reports of individuals abusing fluoxetine.[1,2]


1. Pagliaro LA, Pagliaro AM. Fluoxetine abuse by an intravenous drug user. *Am J Psychiatry* 1993; **150:** 1898.
2. Tinsley JA, *et al.* Fluoxetine abuse. *Mayo Clin Proc* 1994; **69:** 166–8.


**Blood disorders.** For a reference recommending cautious use of fluoxetine in patients with thrombocytopenia or platelet dysfunction, see Effects on the Blood in Adverse Effects, above.

**Breast feeding.** The American Academy of Pediatrics[1] considers that all antidepressants, including SSRIs (fluoxetine, fluvoxamine, paroxetine, and sertraline) are drugs whose effect on nursing infants is unknown but may be of concern.

- *Citalopram* and its metabolites have been detected in breast milk; however, plasma concentrations in exposed infants were either very low or undetectable and no adverse effects were reported.[2]
- Symptoms of colic were reported[3] in a 6-week-old infant whose mother was taking *fluoxetine* 20 mg daily. The concentrations of fluoxetine and its active metabolite norfluoxetine were 69 nanograms/mL and 90 nanograms/mL respectively in breast milk, and 340 nanograms/mL and 208 nanograms/mL respectively in the infant's plasma. The infant's symptoms resolved when he was formula fed. Post-natal weight gain has been reduced in infants exposed to fluoxetine during breast feeding, although in all cases the reduction was less than 2 standard deviations below the norm.[4] In another report,[5] several seizure-like episodes occurred in a breast-fed infant whose mother was taking fluoxetine in addition to carbamazepine and buspirone; however, plasma drug concentrations in the infant were significant only for fluoxetine and norfluoxetine. In a study[6] of 10 women taking fluoxetine while breast feeding 11 infants, breast milk concentrations of fluoxetine ranged from 17.4 to 293 nanograms/mL and of norfluoxetine from 23.4 to 379.1 nanograms/mL. No adverse effects were noted in the infants. Similar levels have occurred in other breast-fed infants without any apparent drug-induced adverse effects.[7-9] Fluoxetine and norfluoxetine were detected in the milk of 14 nursing women.[10] Blood samples were taken from 9 of the infants in the study, and of these, fluoxetine was detected in the plasma of 5 and norfluoxetine in 7. Although it was felt that many infants would tolerate the mean combined dose of fluoxetine and norfluoxetine transmitted to infants via breast milk in this study, there was considerable interpatient variability in estimated infant dose and caution should be exercised; neonates in particular exhibited higher concentrations of norfluoxetine than older infants. Moreover, since both fluoxetine and norfluoxetine have long half-lives, neonates already exposed *in utero* may have an additional risk of adverse effects during breast feeding.
- The excretion of *fluvoxamine* into breast milk was studied[11] in a woman who had been receiving fluvoxamine maleate 100 mg twice daily for 2 weeks. The concentration of fluvoxamine base 4.75 hours after a dose was 310 nanograms/mL in maternal plasma and 90 nanograms/mL in breast milk. It was estimated that an infant would ingest only 0.5% of the daily maternal intake. It was considered that these data supported the notion that the use of fluvoxamine by nursing mothers posed little risk to the infant. A subsequent study[12] found no detectable drug levels in the plasma of breast-fed infants exposed to fluvoxamine; the authors suggested that fluvoxamine was a reasonable choice for nursing mothers requiring treatment for depression.
- Although *paroxetine* was detected in measurable concentrations in the breast milk of a group of 10 nursing mothers receiving paroxetine no adverse effects were reported in any of their breast-fed infants.[13] Paroxetine could not be detected in the plasma of 7 of the 8 infants from whom samples were obtained and in the other infant, concentrations were not quantifiable. Another study involving 7 women suggested that the dose of paroxetine to suckling infants would be 0.7 to 2.9% of the weight-adjusted maternal dose.[14] A more recent study[12] also found no detectable drug levels in the plasma of breast-fed infants exposed to paroxetine; the authors suggested that paroxetine was a reasonable choice for nursing mothers requiring treatment for depression.
- Plasma concentrations of *sertraline* were undetectable in a breast-fed infant despite the presence of concentrations in the mother's breast milk ranging from 8.8 to 43 nanograms/mL over a 24-hour period.[15] However, the authors pointed out that metabolite levels were not measured and that sertraline may have been present in the infant at a concentration below the level of sensitivity of the assay. Other studies[12,16-18] have detected desmethylsertraline in breast milk, which was also detected in the plasma of some of the infants in a number of the studies[12,16,18] but not all.[17] The authors of at least one study[12] suggested that sertraline was a reasonable choice for nursing mothers requiring treatment for depression.


1. American Academy of Pediatrics. The transfer of drugs and other chemicals into human milk. *Pediatrics* 2001; **108:** 776–89. Correction. *ibid.*; 1029. Also available at: http://aappolicy.aappublications.org/cgi/content/full/pediatrics%3b108/3/776 (accessed 10/06/04)
2. Heikkinen T, *et al.* Citalopram in pregnancy and lactation. *Clin Pharmacol Ther* 2002; **72:** 184–91.
3. Lester BM, *et al.* Possible association between fluoxetine hydrochloride and colic in an infant. *J Am Acad Child Adolesc Psychiatry* 1993; **32:** 1253–5.
4. Chambers CD, *et al.* Weight gain in infants breastfed by mothers who take fluoxetine. *Pediatrics* 1999; **104:** 1120–1.
5. Brent NB, Wisner KL. Fluoxetine and carbamazepine concentrations in a nursing mother/infant pair. *Clin Pediatr (Phila)* 1998; **37:** 41–4.
6. Taddio A, *et al.* Excretion of fluoxetine and its metabolite, norfluoxetine, in human breast milk. *J Clin Pharmacol* 1996; **36:** 42–7.
7. Isenberg KE. Excretion of fluoxetine in human breast milk. *J Clin Psychiatry* 1990; **51:** 169.
8. Burch KJ, Wells BG. Fluoxetine/norfluoxetine concentrations in human milk. *Pediatrics* 1992; **89:** 676–7.
9. Yoshida K, *et al.* Fluoxetine in breast-milk and developmental outcome of breast-fed infants. *Br J Psychiatry* 1998; **172:** 175–9.
10. Kristensen JH, *et al.* Distribution and excretion of fluoxetine and norfluoxetine in human milk. *Br J Clin Pharmacol* 1999; **48:** 521–7.
11. Wright S, *et al.* Excretion of fluvoxamine in breast milk. *Br J Clin Pharmacol* 1991; **31:** 209.
12. Hendrick V, *et al.* Use of sertraline, paroxetine and fluvoxamine by nursing women. *Br J Psychiatry* 2001; **179:** 163–6.
13. Begg EJ, *et al.* Paroxetine in human milk. *Br J Clin Pharmacol* 1999; **48:** 142–7.
14. Öhman R, *et al.* Excretion of paroxetine into breast milk. *J Clin Psychiatry* 1999; **60:** 519–23.
15. Altshuler LL, *et al.* Breastfeeding and sertraline: a 24-hour analysis. *J Clin Psychiatry* 1995; **56:** 243–5.
16. Stowe ZN, *et al.* Sertraline and desmethylsertraline in human breast milk and nursing infants. *Am J Psychiatry* 1997; **154:** 1255–60.

17. Kristensen JH, *et al.* Distribution and excretion of sertraline and N-desmethylsertraline in human milk. *Br J Clin Pharmacol* 1998; **45:** 453–7.
18. Epperson N, *et al.* Maternal sertraline treatment and serotonin transport in breast-feeding mother-infant pairs. *Am J Psychiatry* 2001; **158:** 1631–7.

**Children.** For precautions on the use of SSRIs for the treatment of depression in patients under 18 years old, see under Effects on Mental State, above.

**Diabetes mellitus.** A report of the loss of hypoglycaemic awareness in a patient with type 1 diabetes mellitus following the start of treatment with fluoxetine.[1] Awareness returned following reduction and discontinuation of fluoxetine dosage. Changes in blood sugar concentrations may occur in patients with diabetes treated for depression with SSRIs (see also Effects on the Endocrine System, above); however, these may represent an improvement in glycaemic control.[2]

1. Sawka AM, *et al.* Loss of hypoglycemia awareness in an adolescent with type 1 diabetes mellitus during treatment with fluoxetine hydrochloride. *J Pediatr* 2000; **136:** 394–6.
2. Lustman PJ, *et al.* Fluoxetine for depression in diabetes: a randomized double-blind placebo-controlled trial. *Diabetes Care* 2000; **23:** 618–23.

**Driving.** While affective disorders probably adversely affect driving skill,[1,2] treatment with antidepressants can also be hazardous,[1] although patients may be safer drivers with medication than without.[2] Impairment of performance is largely related to sedative and antimuscarinic effects. These are more pronounced with older antidepressants such as the tricyclic antidepressants than with the SSRIs, but a comparative study[3] of fluoxetine (an SSRI) and dosulepin (a tricyclic) in healthy subjects demonstrated a similar but apparently small potential for impairing psychomotor and driving performance. A later epidemiological study[4] was unable to confirm any increased risk of road-traffic accidents in those drivers receiving tricyclic antidepressants or SSRIs.

In the UK, the Driver and Vehicle Licensing Authority considers that SSRIs, MAOIs, and noradrenaline reuptake inhibitors have fewer adverse effects on drivers than antidepressants with antimuscarinic or antihistaminic adverse effects, such as tricyclic antidepressants. However some patients have idiosyncratic responses and should be advised accordingly.[5] Patients with severe depressive illnesses complicated by significant memory or concentration problems, agitation, behavioural disturbances or suicidal thoughts should cease driving pending the outcome of medical enquiry.

1. Ashton H. Drugs and driving. *Adverse Drug React Bull* 1983; **98:** 360–3.
2. Cremona A. Mad drivers: psychiatric illness and driving performance. *Br J Hosp Med* 1986; **35:** 193–5.
3. Ramaekers JG, *et al.* A comparative study of acute and subchronic effects of dothiepin, fluoxetine and placebo on psychomotor and actual driving performance. *Br J Clin Pharmacol* 1995; **39:** 397–404.
4. Barbone F, *et al.* Association of road-traffic accidents with benzodiazepine use. *Lancet* 1998; **352:** 1331–6.
5. Driver and Vehicle Licensing Agency. For medical practitioners: at a glance guide to the current medical standards of fitness to drive. Available at: http://www.dvla.gov.uk/at_a_glance/ch4_psychiatric.htm (accessed 10/06/04)

**Gastrointestinal disorders.** For the opinion that the SSRIs may produce a clinically important increase in the risk of upper gastrointestinal bleeding in patients with a high risk of such bleeding, see under Effects on the Gastrointestinal Tract, above.

**Glaucoma.** For reference to SSRIs precipitating or exacerbating symptoms of glaucoma, see Effects on the Eyes, above.

**Mania.** Hypomania or mania have been reported with some of the SSRIs.

Fluvoxamine was associated with manic behaviour in 8 patients who were being treated for major depression;[1] 3 also had concurrent obsessive-compulsive disorder. Daily doses of fluvoxamine ranged from 75 to 300 mg and duration of therapy to development of manic behaviour from 2 to 6 weeks. The authors were unable to determine whether fluvoxamine had induced mania or unmasked latent bipolar disorder in these patients. However, they recommended that fluvoxamine-treated patients should be monitored for manic behaviour.

1. Dorevitch A, *et al.* Fluvoxamine-associated manic behavior: a case series. *Ann Pharmacother* 1993; **27:** 1455–7.

**Pregnancy.** In an early prospective study[1] comparing 128 pregnant women exposed to a mean daily dose of about 26 mg of fluoxetine during their first trimester with control groups receiving tricyclic antidepressants or non-teratogens, the incidence of neonatal malformations was similar in all groups and did not exceed that in the general population. However, there was a tendency to a higher incidence of miscarriages in the groups receiving fluoxetine or tricyclics. A more recent prospective study[2] comparing 228 pregnant women taking fluoxetine with a control group taking non-teratogens also failed to find a significant increased incidence in major fetal abnormalities in the fluoxetine group; it also did not reveal an increased risk of miscarriage. There was an increase in the incidence of minor fetal abnormalities in infants exposed to fluoxetine during the first trimester. Also, infants exposed to fluoxetine during the third trimester experienced more perinatal complications such as prematurity, low full-term birth-weight and length, and poor neonatal adaptation compared with infants exposed only during the first and second trimesters. However, the design of this study was criticised[3] because of several methodological problems such as unmatched controls and a higher maternal age in the fluoxetine group, which may partly explain the excess of poor perinatal outcomes.

The manufacturer evaluated the outcome of 796 pregnancies in which the mother received fluoxetine during the first trimester and considered that it was unlikely that fluoxetine increased the risk of miscarriage or fetal malformation.[4] A prospective controlled study[5] on pregnancy outcome in women exposed to fluvoxamine, paroxetine, or sertraline also found that, when used in recommended doses, there appeared to be no increase in the risk of major congenital malformations, miscarriages, or still-births when compared with women exposed to non-teratogens.

The effects of fluoxetine on fetal neurodevelopment were studied[6] in 55 pregnant women by later assessing global IQ of the children; no differences were seen in those exposed to fluoxetine *in utero* during the first trimester compared with those exposed to tricyclic antidepressants or adverse developmental influences. A subsequent study indicated that exposure to fluoxetine or tricyclic antidepressants throughout gestation did not appear to affect cognition adversely.[7]

CNS toxicity and an increased heart rate were reported in a neonate whose mother had received 20 mg of fluoxetine daily throughout most of her pregnancy.[8] The neonate's symptoms resolved 96 hours after delivery. In another neonate whose mother took up to 30 mg daily of fluoxetine throughout the third trimester cardiac arrhythmias were noted.[9] A number of reports[2,10,11] have described symptoms such as jitteriness, irritability, and altered muscle tone in neonates who had been exposed to SSRIs *in utero*. However, it is unclear whether this represents a withdrawal syndrome or perhaps a serotonin syndrome.[12] In a matched-control study[13] the rate of complications after delivery in 55 infants exposed to paroxetine during the third trimester was higher than in a control group who had been exposed to paroxetine or non-teratogenic agents during the first or second timesters. Complications that occurred in the infants exposed in the third trimester included respiratory distress (9), hypoglycaemia (2), bradycardia (1), jaundice (1), and suckling problems (1).

1. Pastuszak A, *et al.* Pregnancy outcome following first-trimester exposure to fluoxetine (Prozac). *JAMA* 1993; **269:** 2246–8.
2. Chambers CD, *et al.* Birth outcomes in pregnant women taking fluoxetine. *N Engl J Med* 1996; **335:** 1010–15.
3. Robert E. Treating depression in pregnancy. *N Engl J Med* 1996; **335:** 1056–8.
4. Goldstein DJ, *et al.* Effects of first-trimester fluoxetine exposure on the newborn. *Obstet Gynecol* 1997; **89:** 713–18.
5. Kulin NA, *et al.* Pregnancy outcome following maternal use of the new selective serotonin reuptake inhibitors: a prospective controlled multicenter study. *JAMA* 1998; **279:** 609–10.
6. Nulman I, *et al.* Neurodevelopment of children exposed in utero to antidepressant drugs. *N Engl J Med* 1997; **336:** 258–62.
7. Nulman I, *et al.* Child development following exposure to tricyclic antidepressants or fluoxetine throughout fetal life: a prospective, controlled study. *Am J Psychiatry* 2002; **159:** 1889–95.
8. Spencer MJ. Fluoxetine hydrochloride (Prozac) toxicity in a neonate. *Pediatrics* 1993; **92:** 721–2.
9. Abebe-Campino G, *et al.*. Cardiac arrhythmia in a newborn infant associated with fluoxetine use during pregnancy. *Ann Pharmacother* 2002; **36:** 533–4.
10. Nijhuis IJM, *et al.* Withdrawal reactions of a premature neonate after maternal use of paroxetine. *Arch Dis Child Fetal Neonatal Ed* 2001; **84:** F77–F78.
11. Stiskal JA, *et al.* Neonatal paroxetine withdrawal syndrome. *Arch Dis Child Fetal Neonatal Ed* 2001; **84:** F134–F135.
12. Isbister GK, *et al.* Neonatal paroxetine withdrawal syndrome or actually serotonin syndrome? *Arch Dis Child Fetal Neonatal Ed* 2001; **85:** F147–F148.
13. Costei AM, *et al.* Perinatal outcome following third trimester exposure to paroxetine. *Arch Pediatr Adolesc Med* 2002; **156:** 1129–32.

**Withdrawal.** Withdrawal symptoms have been reported for SSRIs,[1-6] although the number of cases is greatest for paroxetine. Up to July 1994 the UK Committee on Safety of Medicines (CSM) had received 430 reports of symptoms occurring on withdrawal of paroxetine, including dizziness, sweating, nausea, insomnia, tremor, and confusion. The reactions, which had been reported more often with paroxetine than with other SSRIs, tended to start 1 to 4 days after stopping paroxetine and resolved in some patients on re-instating treatment. An update[6] by the CSM in September 2000 confirmed that in most cases the symptoms occurred within 3 days of stopping treatment with the most common symptoms being dizziness, headache, nausea, and paraesthesia. A retrospective analysis[5] has also found that withdrawal symptoms occur more frequently in patients treated with the shorter half-life SSRIs, such as paroxetine, than in those receiving an SSRI with a longer half-life metabolite, such as fluoxetine. There has also been a report[2] of 2 patients without a history of major psychiatric disorder who developed severe behavioural symptoms when paroxetine was withdrawn. Discontinuation was abrupt in one patient and gradual, over a 12-day period, in the other. Symptoms were predominantly hypomanic over the first few days, followed by a period of escalated ego-dystonic aggression, behavioural dyscontrol, and suicidal intention.

The *British National Formulary* recommends that any antidepressant, including an SSRI, that has been administered regularly for 8 weeks or more should be discontinued gradually over a period of about 4 weeks, or as much as 6 months in patients who have been receiving long-term maintenance therapy.

The withdrawal syndrome of the SSRIs is not considered to be a consequence of dependence.[6] See also Extrapyramidal Effects under Adverse Effects, above. For debate about whether a withdrawal syndrome exists in neonates whose mothers have received SSRIs see Pregnancy, above.

1. Price JS, *et al.* A comparison of the post-marketing safety of four selective serotonin re-uptake inhibitors including the investigation of symptoms occurring on withdrawal. *Br J Clin Pharmacol* 1996; **42:** 757–63.
2. Bloch M, *et al.* Severe psychiatric symptoms associated with paroxetine withdrawal. *Lancet* 1995; **346:** 57.
3. Szabadi E. Fluvoxamine withdrawal syndrome. *Br J Psychiatry* 1992; **160:** 283–4.
4. Adverse Drug Reactions Advisory Committee (ADRAC). SSRI's and withdrawal syndrome. *Aust Adverse Drug React Bull* 1996; **15:** 3. Also available at: http://www.tga.gov.au/docs/html/aadrbltn/aadr9602.htm (accessed 10/06/04)
5. Coupland NJ, *et al.* Serotonin reuptake inhibitor withdrawal. *J Clin Psychopharmacol* 1996; **16:** 356–62.
6. Committee on Safety of Medicines/Medicines Control Agency. Selective serotonin reuptake inhibitors (SSRIs). *Current Problems* 2000; **26:** 11–12. Also available at: http://www.mca.gov.uk/ourwork/monitorsafequalmed/currentproblems/cpsept2000.pdf (accessed 10/06/04)

## Interactions

SSRIs interact with a range of other drugs mainly as a result of their inhibitory activity on hepatic cytochrome P450 isoenzymes. Individual SSRIs do not all exhibit the same degree of inhibition nor do they react with the same isoenzymes. The range of drugs inhibited by specific SSRIs varies according to which isoenzyme is affected.

As SSRIs have occasionally been associated with bleeding disorders and other effects on the blood, caution is advised when they are given with drugs known to affect platelet function.

Although different antidepressants have been used together under expert supervision in refractory cases of depression, severe adverse reactions including the *serotonin syndrome* (see p.313) may occur. Sequential prescribing of different types of antidepressant may also produce adverse reactions, and an appropriate drug-free interval should elapse between stopping one type of antidepressant and starting another. SSRIs should not generally be given to patients receiving MAOIs or for at least 2 weeks after their use. Although some manufacturers recommend a similar treatment-free period between stopping a reversible inhibitor of monoamine oxidase type A (RIMA) and starting an SSRI there does not seem to be any evidence to support such a requirement. At least one week should elapse between withdrawing an SSRI and starting any drug liable to provoke a serious reaction (e.g. phenelzine); in the case of the SSRIs paroxetine and sertraline the drug-free interval is extended to 2 weeks, and for fluoxetine 5 weeks, because of their longer half-lives. Adverse effects such as the serotonin syndrome may also occur when the SSRIs are given with other drugs known to act on the same neurotransmitter, a consequence of synergistic interaction.

Further details concerning some of these interactions, and others, are given below.

◊ References.

1. Mitchell PB. Drug interactions of clinical significance with selective serotonin reuptake inhibitors. *Drug Safety* 1997; **17:** 390–406.
2. Sproule BA, *et al.* Selective serotonin reuptake inhibitors and CNS drug interactions: a critical review of the evidence. *Clin Pharmacokinet* 1997; **33:** 454–71.

**Antibacterials.** Rapid development of delirium was reported[1] in a patient when *clarithromycin* was added to his existing regimen of fluoxetine and nitrazepam. It was suggested that his delirium was a result of increased plasma-fluoxetine concentrations produced by the inhibition of cytochrome P450 enzymes by clarithromycin. A report[2] of a serotonin syndrome in a patient given *erythromycin* in addition to sertraline was attributed to inhibition of CYP3A4 by the antibacterial, resulting in accumulation of the SSRI.

1. Pollak PT, *et al.* Delirium probably induced by clarithromycin in a patient receiving fluoxetine. *Ann Pharmacother* 1995; **29:** 486–8.
2. Lee DO, Lee CD. Serotonin syndrome in a child associated with erythromycin and sertraline. *Pharmacotherapy* 1999; **19:** 894–6.

**Anticoagulants.** SSRIs may increase the anticoagulant activity of *warfarin* (see p.1025).

**Antidepressants.** Combination therapy with differing classes of antidepressants has been used successfully in the treatment of drug-resistant depression. It should be emphasised, however, that such combinations may result in enhanced adverse reactions or interactions, and should be used only under expert supervision. This practice is considered unsuitable or controversial by some authorities. For further details of the interactions between different antidepressants when given together, see Phenelzine, p.315. For details of the serotonin syndrome that can arise when two serotonergic drugs with different mechanisms of action are given, see under Adverse Effects of Phenelzine, p.313.

**Antiepileptics.** Antidepressants may antagonise the activity of antiepileptics by lowering the convulsive threshold.

There has been a report of the serotonin syndrome (see p.313) developing in a patient 14 days after fluoxetine had been added to *carbamazepine* therapy.[1]

*Phenobarbital* has been reported to reduce serum concentrations of paroxetine.[2] Steady-state serum concentrations of paroxetine were found to be lower in patients taking *phenytoin* than in those taking carbamazepine or valproate.[3]

Low serum concentrations of citalopram have been reported in 2 patients also taking carbamazepine.[4] Serum concentrations increased when carbamazepine was changed to oxcarbazepine.

Some SSRIs have been reported to increase plasma concentrations of carbamazepine (see p.356) and phenytoin (see p.373).

1. Dursun SM, *et al.* Toxic serotonin syndrome after fluoxetine plus carbamazepine. *Lancet* 1993; **342:** 442–3.
2. Greb WH, *et al.* The effect of liver enzyme inhibition by cimetidine and enzyme induction by phenobarbitone on the pharmacokinetics of paroxetine. *Acta Psychiatr Scand* 1989; **80** (suppl 350): 95–8.
3. Andersen BB, *et al.* No influence of the antidepressant paroxetine on carbamazepine, valproate and phenytoin. *Epilepsy Res* 1991; **10:** 201–4.
4. Leinonen E, *et al.* Substituting carbamazepine with oxcarbazepine increases citalopram levels. A report on two cases. *Pharmacopsychiatry* 1996; **29:** 156–8.

**Antihistamines.** *Cyproheptadine* given to male and female patients as treatment for sexual dysfunction induced by fluoxetine or paroxetine has produced re-emergence of previously controlled depressive symptoms[1,2] or bulimia nervosa[3] in some patients.

Citalopram, fluoxetine, and fluvoxamine may increase plasma concentrations of *astemizole* or *terfenadine* by inhibition of their hepatic cytochrome P450 metabolism, increasing the risk of ventricular arrhythmias; use together should be avoided.

1. Feder R. Reversal of antidepressant activity of fluoxetine by cyproheptadine in three patients. *J Clin Psychiatry* 1991; **52:** 163–4.
2. Christensen RC. Adverse interaction of paroxetine and cyproheptadine. *J Clin Psychiatry* 1995; **56:** 433–4.
3. Goldbloom DS, Kennedy SH. Adverse interaction of fluoxetine and cyproheptadine in two patients with bulimia nervosa. *J Clin Psychiatry* 1991; **52:** 261–2.

**Antimalarials.** For mention of the effect of the SSRI fluvoxamine on the metabolism of *proguanil*, see p.457.

**Antimigraine drugs.** There may be an increased risk of CNS toxicity with SSRIs and serotonin ($5HT_1$) agonists such as *sumatriptan* (see p.472). Fluvoxamine may inhibit the metabolism of *zolmitriptan* (see p.473). For the effect of some SSRIs on *dihydroergotamine*, see p.468.

**Antimuscarinics.** For the effect of SSRIs on *benzatropine*, see p.479.

**Antipsychotics.** For reports of adverse effects in patients treated with SSRIs and antipsychotics, see under Chlorpromazine, p.679. Interactions between SSRIs and atypical antipsychotics are also mentioned under clozapine, p.688, sertindole, p.722, and zotepine, p.730.

**Antivirals.** Plasma concentrations of fluoxetine and other SSRIs are possibly increased by *HIV-protease inhibitors*.

For the effect of fluoxetine on *delavirdine*, see p.630.

**Anxiolytics.** Fluoxetine and fluvoxamine increase plasma concentrations of some *benzodiazepines* (see under Diazepam, p.693). There is a report of hyponatraemia and serotonin syndrome developing in a patient who received high doses of citalopram and *buspirone*.[1]

1. Spigset O, Adielsson G. Combined serotonin syndrome and hyponatraemia caused by a citalopram-buspirone interaction. *Int Clin Psychopharmacol* 1997; **12:** 61–3.

**Beta blockers.** For the effect of fluoxetine and fluvoxamine on beta blockers, see p.871.

**Ciclosporin.** For the effect of fluoxetine and fluvoxamine on ciclosporin, see p.1354.

**Cough suppressants.** For the effect of fluoxetine and paroxetine on *dextromethorphan*, see p.1118.

**Dopaminergics.** *Selegiline* is an irreversible selective inhibitor of monoamine oxidase type B. Serious adverse effects have been reported when selegiline and SSRIs have been used concomitantly (see p.1214). In some instances, these reactions resemble the potentially fatal serotonin syndromes reported when SSRIs are given with non-selective MAOIs (see p.313).

SSRIs should not generally be given to patients receiving selegiline, or for at least 2 weeks after it has been discontinued. Similarly, at least one week should elapse between withdrawing an SSRI and starting selegiline; this interval should be increased to 2 weeks for paroxetine and sertraline, and to 5 weeks for fluoxetine because of their longer half-lives.

**Gastrointestinal drugs.** Acute dystonia has been noted in a patient given fluvoxamine and *metoclopramide*.[1] Similar reports have been published for other SSRIs (fluoxetine[2] or sertraline[3]) and metoclopramide. Involuntary twitching, tremor, and stiffness of the jaw and tongue occurred on both occasions following the use of intravenous metoclopramide in a patient also taking sertraline.[4] The authors considered the adverse effects to be features of the serotonin syndrome.

1. Palop V, *et al.* Acute dystonia associated with fluvoxamine-metoclopramide. *Ann Pharmacother* 1999; **33:** 382.
2. Coulter DM, Pillans PI. Fluoxetine and extrapyramidal side effects. *Am J Psychiatry* 1995; **152:** 122–5.
3. Christensen RC, Byerly MJ. Mandibular dystonia associated with the combination of sertraline and metoclopramide. *J Clin Psychiatry* 1996; **57:** 596.
4. Fisher AA, Davis MW. Serotonin syndrome caused by selective serotonin reuptake-inhibitors–metoclopramide interaction. *Ann Pharmacother* 2002; **36:** 67–71.

**General anaesthetics.** For a report of a generalised tonic-clonic seizure in a patient receiving paroxetine and *methohexital sodium*, see p.1303.

**Hypnotics.** For reference to visual hallucinations in patients receiving an SSRI concomitantly with *zolpidem*, see p.729.

**Levothyroxine.** For mention of a decreased effect of levothyroxine in patients given sertraline concomitantly, see p.1601.

**Local anaesthetics.** For the effect of fluvoxamine on *ropivacaine*, see p.1384.

**Muscle relaxants.** For a report of QT prolongation in a patient taking fluoxetine and *cyclobenzaprine*, see p.1393.

**NSAIDs.** For reference to an increased risk of upper gastrointestinal bleeding in patients taking SSRIs and NSAIDs together, see under Effects on the Gastrointestinal Tract, above.

**Opioid analgesics.** A possible case of serotonin syndrome (p.313) has been reported with *tramadol* and sertraline,[1] and another when sertraline was given with high doses of *oxycodone*.[2] There have also been occasional reports of the syndrome in patients given tramadol with fluoxetine[3] or paroxetine.[4,5] For reference to SSRIs enhancing the effects and toxicity of *methadone*, see p.58.

1. Mason BJ, Blackburn KH. Possible serotonin syndrome associated with tramadol and sertraline coadministration. *Ann Pharmacother* 1997; **31:** 175–7.
2. Rosebraugh CJ, *et al.* Visual hallucination and tremor induced by sertraline and oxycodone in a bone marrow transplant patient. *J Clin Pharmacol* 2001; **41:** 224–7.
3. Kesavan S, Sobala GM. Serotonin syndrome with fluoxetine plus tramadol. *J R Soc Med* 1999; **92:** 474–5.
4. Egberts ACG, *et al.* Serotonin syndrome attributed to tramadol addition to paroxetine therapy. *Int Clin Psychopharmacol* 1997; **12:** 181–2.
5. Lantz MS, *et al.* Serotonin syndrome following the administration of tramadol with paroxetine. *Int J Geriatr Psychiatry* 1998; **13:** 343–5.

**Parasympathomimetics.** For the effect of fluvoxamine on *tacrine*, see p.1497.

**Sibutramine.** There is a risk of CNS toxicity due to synergistic serotonergic actions when an SSRI is given with sibutramine.

**Smoking.** Serum concentrations of fluvoxamine were lower in smokers than non-smokers in a single-dose study.[1] It was proposed that the polycyclic hydrocarbons present in cigarette smoke stimulated hepatic metabolism of fluvoxamine by cytochrome P450 enzymes.

1. Spigset O, *et al.* Effect of cigarette smoking on fluvoxamine pharmacokinetics in humans. *Clin Pharmacol Ther* 1995; **58:** 399–403.

**Theophylline.** For the effect of fluvoxamine on theophylline, see p.802.

## Pharmacokinetics

Fluoxetine is readily absorbed from the gastrointestinal tract with peak plasma concentrations appearing about 6 to 8 hours after oral doses. Systemic bioavailability does not appear to be affected by food. Fluoxetine is extensively metabolised, by demethylation, in the liver to its primary active metabolite norfluoxetine. Excretion is mainly via the urine. Protein binding is reported to be about 95%.

Fluoxetine used clinically is a racemic mixture consisting of *R* and *S* enantiomers in equal amounts. Both enantiomers are active according to *animal* studies, but *S*-fluoxetine is eliminated more slowly. Metabolism is believed to be mediated by cytochrome P450 isoenzyme CYP2D6 (but see below), and leads to *R* and *S* enantiomers of norfluoxetine, with the *S* enantiomer being considered as active as the parent drug; the *R* enantiomer is considered to be much less active. This metabolism is subject to genetic polymorphism. While the small proportion of the population known as slow metabolisers do show a different spectrum of parent drug and metabolite, the overall activity does not appear to be altered.

Fluoxetine is widely distributed throughout the body. Fluoxetine has a relatively long elimination half-life of about 1 to 3 days after acute use and 4 to 6 days after long-term use; that of its metabolite, norfluoxetine, is even longer, being about 4 to 16 days. These long half-lives have clinical implications. Steady-state plasma concentrations will only be attained after several weeks. Additionally, fluoxetine and its metabolites may persist for a considerable time after treatment, and this has led to precautions concerning the subsequent use of other serotonergic drugs (see Interactions, above).

Fluoxetine and norfluoxetine are distributed into breast milk (see Breast Feeding under Precautions, above).

◊ References.

1. van Harten J. Clinical pharmacokinetics of selective serotonin reuptake inhibitors. *Clin Pharmacokinet* 1993; **24:** 203–20.
2. Altamura AC, *et al.* Clinical pharmacokinetics of fluoxetine. *Clin Pharmacokinet* 1994; **26:** 201–14.
3. Baumann P. Pharmacokinetic-pharmacodynamic relationship of the selective serotonin reuptake inhibitors. *Clin Pharmacokinet* 1996; **31:** 444–69.
4. Greenblatt DJ, *et al.* Inhibition of human cytochrome P450-3A isoforms by fluoxetine and norfluoxetine: in vitro and in vivo studies. *J Clin Pharmacol* 1996; **36:** 792–8.
5. Hamelin BA, *et al.* The disposition of fluoxetine but not sertraline is altered in poor metabolizers of debrisoquin. *Clin Pharmacol Ther* 1996; **60:** 512–21.
6. Preskorn SH. Clinically relevant pharmacology of selective serotonin reuptake inhibitors: an overview with emphasis on pharmacokinetics and effects on oxidative drug metabolism. *Clin Pharmacokinet* 1997; **32** (suppl 1): 1–21.

**Metabolism.** Although fluoxetine is stated by the manufacturers to be metabolised by the cytochrome P450 isoenzyme CYP2D6, which is supported by studies[1] indicating that its disposition is altered in poor metabolisers of debrisoquine (a substrate for this enzyme), others have suggested that CYP2C19, and perhaps CYP2C9, play an important role.[2]

1. Hamelin BA, *et al.* The disposition of fluoxetine but not sertraline is altered in poor metabolizers of debrisoquin. *Clin Pharmacol Ther* 1996; **60:** 512–21.
2. Liu Z-Q, *et al.* Effect of the CYP2C19 oxidation polymorphism on fluoxetine metabolism in Chinese healthy subjects. *Br J Clin Pharmacol* 2001; **52:** 96–9.

## Uses and Administration

Prevention of the reuptake of monoamine transmitters such as serotonin, which potentiates their action in the brain, appears to be associated with antidepressant activity. SSRIs such as fluoxetine preferentially inhibit the reuptake of serotonin compared with noradrenaline, and have limited direct action at other neurotransmitter sites, including muscarinic receptors. They therefore cause fewer antimuscarinic or sedative side-effects than the tricyclic antidepressants and are less cardiotoxic. Citalopram is the most selective of the SSRIs currently available, whereas paroxetine is the most potent.

SSRIs provide an alternative to the tricyclics for the treatment of depression. As with the tricyclics, it may be several weeks before an antidepressant effect is seen. Once depression has then resolved, maintenance therapy should be continued for at least 4 to 6 months (12 months in the elderly) to avoid relapse on discontinuation of therapy.

Some SSRIs are also used as part of the management of generalised anxiety disorder, obsessive-compulsive disorder, panic disorders with or without agoraphobia, social phobia, and post-traumatic stress disorder, and as part of the management of bulimia nervosa. Fluoxetine is also used in the treatment of premenstrual dysphoric disorder.

Fluoxetine, a phenylpropylamine derivative, is given by mouth as the hydrochloride; doses are expressed in terms of fluoxetine. Fluoxetine hydrochloride 22.4 mg is approximately equivalent to 20 mg of fluoxetine base.

In the treatment of **depression** the usual initial dose of fluoxetine is 20 mg daily; the US manufacturers recommend giving this dose in the morning. If no clinical response is seen after several weeks, the daily dose may be gradually increased, up to a maximum of 80 mg daily (60 mg in the elderly). Doses above 20 mg daily may be administered in 2 divided doses, for example in the morning and at noon, or as a once daily dose. A once-weekly, modified-release preparation equivalent to 90 mg of fluoxetine is available in the USA for use in patients whose depressive symptoms have stabilised, and who require long-term treatment; it is recommended that weekly dosing is started 7 days after the last daily dose of fluoxetine.

The USA also allows fluoxetine to be given at an initial dose of 10 to 20 mg daily for the treatment of depression in children aged 8 years and over. Initial doses of 10 mg should be increased to 20 mg daily after 1 week except in low-weight children when such increases should not be made for several weeks and only if the clinical response is insufficient. For concerns about the use of SSRIs in children see Effects on Mental State, above.

Fluoxetine is used in doses of 60 mg daily in the management of **bulimia nervosa**.

In the management of **obsessive-compulsive disorder** the initial dose of fluoxetine is 20 mg daily increased after several weeks if there is no response to up to 60 mg daily. Up to 80 mg daily has been used in the USA, sometimes divided into 2 doses. Fluoxetine is also licensed there for use in children aged 7 years and over for obsessive-compulsive disorder. The starting dose is 10 mg daily; in low-weight children this is increased after several weeks to 20 to 30 mg daily, if required. Adolescents and higher-weight children may be increased to 20 mg daily after 2 weeks; further increases to 60 mg daily may be made after several weeks, as necessary.

Fluoxetine may be used in the treatment of **panic disorder** in initial doses of 10 mg daily. After a week the dose should be increased to 20 mg daily; further increases to 60 mg daily may be considered after several weeks if no improvement is seen.

A dose of 20 mg daily is used in the USA in the treatment of **premenstrual dysphoric disorder**. Intermittent dosing is also permitted: for each new cycle, fluoxetine should be started 14 days before the onset of menstruation and continued until the first full day of menstruation. Treatment may be continued for 6 months; benefit should then be reassessed before continuing further.

A lower or less frequent dosage is recommended in elderly patients. For dosage in hepatic or renal impairment see below.

It should be noted that because fluoxetine and norfluoxetine have prolonged half-lives several weeks of therapy are required before steady-state concentrations are attained; similarly after dosage adjustments a time lag will occur before steady-state concentrations are again achieved. Although SSRIs should generally be withdrawn gradually to reduce the risk of withdrawal symptoms the long half-life may reduce the need for dose tapering with fluoxetine.

◊ References.


1. Gram LF. Fluoxetine. *N Engl J Med* 1994; **331:** 1354–61.
2. Finley PR. Selective serotonin reuptake inhibitors: pharmacologic profiles and potential therapeutic distinctions. *Ann Pharmacother* 1994; **28:** 1359–69.
3. Hyttel J. Pharmacological characterization of selective serotonin reuptake inhibitors (SSRIs). *Int Clin Psychopharmacol* 1994; **9** (suppl 1): 19–26.
4. Edwards JG, Anderson I. Systematic review and guide to selection of selective serotonin reuptake inhibitors. *Drugs* 1999; **57:** 507–33.


**Administration in hepatic or renal impairment.** Fluoxetine is subject to hepatic metabolism, and, therefore, lower doses, such as alternate-day dosing, have been recommended in patients with significant hepatic impairment.

It is also excreted by the kidneys and some manufacturers recommend a similar dose reduction in patients with mild to moderate renal impairment and that fluoxetine should be avoided in those with severe impairment. However, another manufacturer has stated that plasma concentrations of fluoxetine or its metabolite norfluoxetine in patients with severe renal impairment requiring dialysis did not differ from those in controls with normal renal function when given fluoxetine 20 mg daily for 2 months.

**Anorexia nervosa.** Counselling and psychotherapy form the major part of treatment of anorexia nervosa and there is little or no role for specific drug therapy. Antidepressants may be indicated when there is co-existing depression but malnourished anorexic patients may be more susceptible to adverse effects and less responsive than other patients with depression. Fluoxetine has been tried with some success, although the efficacy and safety of SSRIs has been questioned.

References.


1. Bergh C, *et al.* Selective serotonin reuptake inhibitors in anorexia. *Lancet* 1996; **348:** 1459–60.
2. Mayer LES, Walsh BT. The use of selective serotonin reuptake inhibitors in eating disorders. *J Clin Psychiatry* 1998; **59:** (suppl 15): 28–34.
3. Kaye WH, *et al.* Double-blind placebo-controlled administration of fluoxetine in restricting- and restricting-purging-type anorexia nervosa. *Biol Psychiatry* 2001; **49:** 644–52.


**Anxiety disorders.** SSRIs have been given in a variety of anxiety disorders but their role in these disorders is most well established in the treatment of *obsessive-compulsive disorder* (p.663). Efficacy in obsessive-compulsive disorder appears to have been best demonstrated for fluvoxamine and fluoxetine but other SSRIs are also effective and patients unresponsive to one SSRI may respond to another. SSRIs are also of use in the treatment of *generalised anxiety disorder* (p.663), *panic attacks* (p.663), and *post-traumatic stress disorder* (p.664). SSRIs are considered to be the first choice for the treatment of *social phobia* (see under Phobic Disorders, p.663). Fluoxetine is one of the SSRIs that has been tried in the treatment of *trichotillomania*.

References.


1. Montgomery SA, *et al.* A double-blind, placebo-controlled study of fluoxetine in patients with DSM-III-R obsessive-compulsive disorder. *Eur Neuropsychopharmacol* 1993; **3:** 143–52.
2. Wood A, *et al.* Pharmacotherapy of obsessive compulsive disorder—experience with fluoxetine. *Int Clin Psychopharmacol* 1993; **8:** 301–6.
3. Van Ameringen M, *et al.* Fluoxetine efficacy in social phobia. *J Clin Psychiatry* 1993; **54:** 27–32.
4. Tollefson GD, *et al.* A multicenter investigation of fixed-dose fluoxetine in the treatment of obsessive-compulsive disorder. *Arch Gen Psychiatry* 1994; **51:** 559–67.
5. Yanchick JK, *et al.* Efficacy of fluoxetine in trichotillomania. *Ann Pharmacother* 1994; **28:** 1245–6.
6. Boyer W. Serotonin uptake inhibitors are superior to imipramine and alprazolam in alleviating panic attacks: a meta-analysis. *Int Clin Psychopharmacol* 1995; **10:** 45–9.
7. Michelson D, *et al.* Continuing treatment of panic disorder after acute response: randomised, placebo-controlled trial with fluoxetine. *Br J Psychiatry* 1999; **174:** 213–18.
8. Connor KM, *et al.* Fluoxetine in post-traumatic stress disorder: randomised, double-blind study. *Br J Psychiatry* 1999; **175:** 17–22.
9. Meltzer-Brody S, *et al.* Symptom-specific effects of fluoxetine in post-traumatic stress disorder. *Int Clin Psychopharmacol* 2000; **15:** 227–31.
10. Geller DA, *et al.* Fluoxetine treatment for obsessive-compulsive disorder in children and adolescents: a placebo-controlled clinical trial. *J Am Acad Child Adolesc Psychiatry* 2001; **40:** 773–9.


**Bipolar disorder.** Treatment of the depressive phase of bipolar disorder (p.278) with antidepressants needs caution since these drugs may precipitate mania or hypomania. SSRIs such as fluoxetine have nonetheless been used in bipolar disorder with some success. In some countries, fluoxetine is also available as a fixed-dose combination with the atypical antipsychotic olanzapine for use in the depressive phase of bipolar disorder.

References.


1. Amsterdam JD, *et al.* Efficacy and safety of fluoxetine in treating bipolar II major depressive episode. *J Clin Psychopharmacol* 1998; **18:** 435–40.
2. Megna JL, Devitt PJ. Treatment of bipolar depression with twice-weekly fluoxetine: management of antidepressant-induced mania. *Ann Pharmacother* 2001; **35:** 45–7.


**Bulimia nervosa.** A combination of counselling, support, psychotherapy, and antidepressants is the usual treatment for bulimia nervosa. Fluoxetine and the tricyclic desipramine have been suggested as the antidepressants of choice because they have been used extensively and are considered to be well tolerated. Other SSRIs that have been tried include sertraline, fluvoxamine, and paroxetine. Antidepressants in general do not appear to alter the patient's disturbed self-image, although disturbed attitudes might improve during short-term therapy with fluoxetine.

References.


1. Goldbloom DS, Olmsted MP. Pharmacotherapy of bulimia nervosa with fluoxetine: assessment of clinically significant attitudinal change. *Am J Psychiatry* 1993; **150:** 770–4.
2. Mayer LES, Walsh BT. The use of selective serotonin reuptake inhibitors in eating disorders. *J Clin Psychiatry* 1998; **59** (suppl 15): 28–34.
3. Bacaltchuk J, *et al.* Antidepressants versus psychological treatments and their combination for bulimia nervosa. Available in The Cochrane Library; Issue 2. Chichester: John Wiley; 2004.
4. Bacaltchuk J, Hay P. Antidepressants versus placebo for people with bulimia nervosa. Available in The Cochrane Library; Issue 2. Chichester: John Wiley; 2004.


**Depression.** As discussed on p.279, there is very little difference in efficacy between the different groups of antidepressant drugs, and choice is often made on the basis of adverse effect profile. SSRIs such as fluoxetine are widely used as an alternative to the older tricyclics as they have fewer unpleasant side-effects and are safer in overdosage.

Combination therapy with differing classes of antidepressants, including the SSRIs, has been used in the treatment of drug-resistant depression. However, such therapy may result in enhanced adverse reactions or interactions and is considered unsuitable or controversial by some workers. For further details see Antidepressants, under Interactions of Phenelzine, p.315.

References to the use of SSRIs in general and to the use of fluoxetine are given below.


1. Roose SP, *et al.* Comparative efficacy of selective serotonin reuptake inhibitors and tricyclics in the treatment of melancholia. *Am J Psychiatry* 1994; **151:** 1735–9.
2. Lam RW, *et al.* Multicenter, placebo-controlled study of fluoxetine in seasonal affective disorder. *Am J Psychiatry* 1995; **152:** 1765–70.
3. Anderson IM, Tomenson BM. Treatment discontinuation with selective serotonin reuptake inhibitors compared with tricyclic antidepressants: a meta-analysis. *BMJ* 1995; **310:** 1433–8.
4. Brown WA, Harrison W. Are patients who are intolerant to one serotonin selective reuptake inhibitor intolerant to another? *J Clin Psychiatry* 1995; **56:** 30–4.
5. Fava M, *et al.* Relapse in patients on long-term fluoxetine treatment: response to increased fluoxetine dose. *J Clin Psychiatry* 1995; **56:** 52–5.
6. Joffe RT, *et al.* Response to an open trial of a second SSRI in major depression. *J Clin Psychiatry* 1996; **57:** 114–15.
7. Nobler MS, *et al.* Fluoxetine treatment of dysthymia in the elderly. *J Clin Psychiatry* 1996; **57:** 254–6.
8. Mourilhe P, Stokes PE. Risks and benefits of selective serotonin reuptake inhibitors in the treatment of depression. *Drug Safety* 1998; **18:** 57–82.
9. Trindade E, Merion D. *Selective serotonin reuptake inhibitors (SSRIs) for major depression. Part 1. Evaluation of the clinical literature.* Ottawa: Canadian Coordinating Office for Health Technology Assessment, 1997.
10. Anderson IM. SSRIs versus tricyclic antidepressants in depressed inpatients: a meta-analysis of efficacy and tolerability. *Depress Anxiety* 1998; **7** (suppl 1): 11–17.
11. Cheer SM, Goa KL. Fluoxetine: a review of its therapeutic potential in the treatment of depression associated with physical illness. *Drugs* 2001; **61:** 81–110.
12. Sampson SM. Treating depression with selective serotonin reuptake inhibitors: a practical approach. *Mayo Clin Proc* 2001; **76:** 739–44.
13. Wagstaff AJ, Goa KL. Once-weekly fluoxetine. *Drugs* 2001; **61:** 2221–8.
14. Bull SA, *et al.* Discontinuing or switching selective serotonin-reuptake inhibitors. *Ann Pharmacother* 2002 **36:** 578–84.
15. Geddes JR, *et al.* Selective serotonin reuptake inhibitors (SSRIs) versus other antidepressants for depression. Available in The Cochrane Library; Issue 2. Chichester: John Wiley; 2004.


**Disturbed behaviour.** SSRIs appear to have been of some benefit in controlling symptoms such as impulsiveness and aggression[1-3] when tried in various disorders for the management of disturbed behaviour (see p.665). There have been several case reports of fluoxetine being used with some success in the control of fantasies associated with various paraphilias.[4]


1. Cornelius JR, *et al.* Fluoxetine trial in borderline personality disorder. *Psychopharmacol Bull* 1990; **26:** 151–4.
2. Vartiainen H, *et al.* Citalopram, a selective serotonin reuptake inhibitor, in the treatment of aggression in schizophrenia. *Acta Psychiatr Scand* 1995; **91:** 348–51.
3. Coccaro EF, Kavoussi RJ. Fluoxetine and impulsive aggressive behavior in personality-disordered subjects. *Arch Gen Psychiatry* 1997; **54:** 1081–8.
4. Richer M, Crismon ML. Pharmacotherapy of sexual offenders. *Ann Pharmacother* 1993; **27:** 316–19.


**Headache.** The results of several studies have suggested that SSRIs may be of benefit in the treatment of chronic tension-type headache (p.465); however, results in the prophylaxis of migraine (p.464) have been conflicting.

References.


1. Sosin D. Clinical efficacy of fluoxetine vs sertraline in a headache clinic population. *Headache* 1993; **33:** 284.
2. Solomon GD, Pearson E. Sertraline in the management of headache. *Clin Pharmacol Ther* 1994; **55:** 130.
3. Jung AC, *et al.* The efficacy of selective serotonin reuptake inhibitors for the management of chronic pain. *J Gen Intern Med* 1997; **12:** 384–9.
4. d'Amato CC, *et al.* Fluoxetine for migraine prophylaxis: a double-blind trial. *Headache* 1999; **39:** 716–19.


**Hyperactivity.** When drug therapy is indicated for attention deficit hyperactivity disorder (ADHD—p.1583) initial treatment is usually with a central stimulant. SSRIs such as fluoxetine have produced beneficial effects as an adjunct to central stimulants in small numbers of patients with comorbid disorders such as depression or obsessive-compulsive disorder;[1-3] although there is insufficient evidence to assess their efficacy in ADHD alone.


1. Gammon GD, Brown TE. Fluoxetine and methylphenidate in combination for treatment of attention deficit disorder and comorbid depressive disorder. *J Child Adolesc Psychopharmacol* 1993; **3:** 1–10.
2. Bussing R, Levin GM. Methamphetamine and fluoxetine treatment of a child with attention-deficit hyperactivity disorder and obsessive-compulsive disorder. *J Child Adolesc Psychopharmacol* 1993; **3:** 53–8.
3. Finding RL. Open-label treatment of comorbid depression and attentional disorders with co-administration of serotonin reuptake inhibitors and psychostimulants in children, adolescents and adults: a case series. *J Child Adolesc Psychopharmacol* 1996; **6:** 165–75.


**Hypochondriasis.** SSRIs may be of benefit in patients with hypochondriasis.[1] Fluoxetine in an initial dose of 20 mg daily gradually increased up to 80 mg daily produced some beneficial results in 10 of 14 patients with hypochondriasis (p.664) who completed 12 weeks of treatment.[2] Fluvoxamine[3] and paroxetine[4] have also been tried.


1. Fallon BA, *et al.* The pharmacotherapy of hypochondriasis. *Psychopharmacol Bull* 1996; **32:** 607–11.
2. Fallon BA, *et al.* Fluoxetine for hypochondriacal patients without major depression. *J Clin Psychopharmacol* 1993; **13:** 438–41.
3. Fallon BA, *et al.* An open trial of fluvoxamine for hypochondriasis. *Psychosomatics* 2003; **44:** 298–303.
4. Oosterbaan DB, *et al.* An open study of paroxetine in hypochondriasis. *Prog Neuropsychopharmacol Biol Psychiatry* 2001; **25:** 1023–33.


**Hypotension.** SSRIs have been suggested for patients with neurally mediated hypotension refractory to standard treatment (see p.828).

See also Orthostatic Hypotension, below.

**Obesity.** Fluoxetine has been tried with some success as part of the management of obesity (p.1583). Fluoxetine's mechanism of action in obesity is unknown. Serotonin is believed to be involved in the regulation of satiety[1] but fluoxetine has also been shown to increase resting energy expenditure and raise basal body temperature.[2] A common dose for fluoxetine in the management of obesity has been 60 mg daily; it appears that fluoxetine has a dose-related effect on weight loss.[3] Reviews[1,4,5] agree that fluoxetine can aid weight reduction in the short term but after 16 to 20 weeks some patients have started to regain weight and its long-term efficacy remains to be established. Troublesome adverse effects can occur.[1] Some patients treated with fluoxetine for depression have experienced an increase of appetite and some have gained weight. There has been a report[6] of a patient who lost weight during treatment with fluoxetine for depression despite an increased appetite and food intake.


1. Anonymous. Fluoxetine (Prozac) and other drugs for treatment of obesity. *Med Lett Drugs Ther* 1994; **36:** 107–8.
2. Bross R, Hoffer LJ. Fluoxetine increases resting energy expenditure and basal body temperature in humans. *Am J Clin Nutr* 1995; **61:** 1020–5.
3. Levine LR, *et al.* Use of fluoxetine, a selective serotonin-uptake inhibitor, in the treatment of obesity: a dose-response study. *Int J Obes* 1989; **13:** 635–45.
4. Bray GA. Use and abuse of appetite-suppressant drugs in the treatment of obesity. *Ann Intern Med* 1993; **119:** 707–13.
5. Mayer LE, Walsh BT. The use of selective serotonin reuptake inhibitors in eating disorders. *J Clin Psychiatry* 1998; **59** (suppl 15): 28–34.
6. Fichtner CG, Braun BG. Hyperphagia and weight loss during fluoxetine treatment. *Ann Pharmacother* 1994; **28:** 1350–2.


**Orthostatic hypotension.** Although orthostatic hypotension has been reported in some patients taking SSRIs, there has been a report[1] that fluoxetine 20 mg daily for 6 to 8 weeks produced beneficial effects in 4 of 5 patients with chronic symptomatic orthostatic hypotension (p.1100) refractory to other treatment. Modest benefits have also been seen in patients with orthostatic hypotension associated with parkinsonism.[2]


1. Grubb BP, *et al.* Fluoxetine hydrochloride for the treatment of severe refractory orthostatic hypotension. *Am J Med* 1994; **97:** 366–8.
2. Montastruc JL, *et al.* Fluoxetine in orthostatic hypotension of Parkinson's disease: a clinical and experimental pilot study. *Fundam Clin Pharmacol* 1998; **12:** 398–402.


**Pain.** SSRIs have been tried in the treatment of painful disorders including fibromyalgia and diabetic neuropathy.

See also Headache, above.

References.


1. Goldenberg D, *et al.* A randomized, double-blind crossover trial of fluoxetine and amitriptyline in the treatment of fibromyalgia. *Arthritis Rheum* 1996; **39:** 1852–9.
2. Jung AC, *et al.* The efficacy of selective serotonin reuptake inhibitors for the management of chronic pain. *J Gen Intern Med* 1997; **12:** 384–9.
3. Smith AJ. The analgesic effects of selective serotonin reuptake inhibitors. *J Psychopharmacol* 1998; **12:** 407–13.
4. Arnold LM, *et al.* A randomized, placebo-controlled, double-blind, flexible-dose study of fluoxetine in the treatment of women with fibromyalgia. *Am J Med* 2002; **112:** 191–7.


**Parkinsonism.** It has been suggested that fluoxetine might be of use in the management of selected patients with Parkinson's disease (p.1196) who have levodopa-induced dyskinesias unresponsive to other measures.[1] However, although fluoxetine has been reported to have produced beneficial results in such patients[2] there has also been a report of increased disability in patients with Parkinson's disease given fluoxetine.[3] Extrapyramidal effects have also been reported in other patients taking fluoxetine (see under Adverse Effects, above). Fluoxetine has been tried in parkinsonism-related orthostatic hypotension (above).


1. Giron LT, Koller WC. Methods of managing levodopa-induced dyskinesias. *Drug Safety* 1996; **14:** 365–74.
2. Durif F, *et al.* Levodopa-induced dyskinesias are improved by fluoxetine. *Neurology* 1995; **45:** 1855–8.
3. Steur ENHJ. Increase of Parkinson disability after fluoxetine medication. *Neurology* 1993; **43:** 211–3.


**Pathological crying or laughing.** Inappropriate or uncontrolled crying or laughing can occur in patients with lesions in certain areas of the brain. Attempts at treatment have mostly been with antidepressant drugs, including SSRIs. Beneficial effects have been claimed for fluoxetine in a number of uncontrolled studies and reports.[1-4]


1. Seliger GM, *et al.* Fluoxetine improves emotional incontinence. *Brain Inj* 1992; **6:** 267–70.
2. Sloan RL, *et al.* Fluoxetine as a treatment for emotional lability after brain injury. *Brain Inj* 1992; **6:** 315–19.
3. Hanger HC. Emotionalism after stroke. *Lancet* 1993; **342:** 1235–6.
4. Tsai WC, *et al.* Treatment of emotionalism with fluoxetine during rehabilitation. *Scand J Rehabil Med* 1998; **30:** 145–9.


**Peripheral vascular disease.** Anecdotal reports[1,2] and a small pilot study[3] of fluoxetine (in a daily dose of 20 to 60 mg) suggest it may produce favourable therapeutic responses in patients with Raynaud's syndrome (p.833).


1. Bolte MA, Avery D. Case of fluoxetine-induced remission of Raynaud's phenomenon—a case report. *Angiology* 1993; **44:** 161–3.
2. Jaffe IA. Serotonin reuptake inhibitors in Raynaud's phenomenon. *Lancet* 1995; **345:** 1378.
3. Coleiro B, *et al.* Treatment of Raynaud's phenomenon with the selective serotonin reuptake inhibitor fluoxetine. *Rheumatology (Oxford)* 2001; **40:** 1038–43.


**Premenstrual syndrome.** Fluoxetine is used to control both the psychological and somatic symptoms of women with premenstrual syndrome (p.1551). Other SSRIs also appear to be useful, although evidence is so far more limited.

References.


1. Romano S, *et al.* The role of fluoxetine in the treatment of premenstrual dysphoric disorder. *Clin Ther* 1999; **21:** 615–33.
2. Eriksson E. Serotonin reuptake inhibitors for the treatment of premenstrual dysphoria. *Int Clin Psychopharmacol* 1999; **14** (suppl 2): S27–S33.
3. Dimmock PW, *et al.* Efficacy of selective serotonin-reuptake inhibitors in premenstrual syndrome: a systematic review. *Lancet* 2000; **356:** 1131–6.
4. Carr RR, Ensom MHH. Fluoxetine in the treatment of premenstrual dysphoric disorder. *Ann Pharmacother* 2002; **36:** 713–17.
5. Pearlstein T. Selective serotonin reuptake inhibitors for premenstrual dysphoric disorder: the emerging gold standard. *Drugs* 2002; **62:** 1869–85.


**Sexual dysfunction.** Impotence or ejaculatory problems have been reported as adverse effects of SSRIs (see Effects on Sexual Function in Adverse Effects, above). Such properties of the SSRIs have been studied as a potential form of treatment for men with premature ejaculation.[1,2] The relative effects of the SSRIs on delaying ejaculation have also been studied.[3] Paroxetine was found to cause the strongest delay, followed by fluoxetine and then sertraline; fluvoxamine caused a slight increase in the delay although the effect was not significantly different from that seen with placebo. (Citalopram was unavailable at the time of the study.)


1. Waldinger MD, *et al.* Paroxetine treatment of premature ejaculation: a double-blind, randomized, placebo-controlled study. *Am J Psychiatry* 1994; **151:** 1377–9.
2. Mendels J, *et al.* Sertraline treatment for premature ejaculation. *J Clin Psychopharmacol* 1995; **15:** 341–6.
3. Waldinger MD, *et al.* Effect of SSRI antidepressants on ejaculation: a double-blind, randomized, placebo-controlled study with fluoxetine, fluvoxamine, paroxetine and sertraline. *J Clin Psychopharmacol* 1998; **18:** 274–81.


## Preparations

***BP 2003:*** Fluoxetine Capsules; Fluoxetine Oral Solution;
***USP 27:*** Fluoxetine Capsules; Fluoxetine Oral Solution; Fluoxetine Tablets.

**Proprietary Preparations** (details are given in Part 3)
***Arg.:*** Alental; Animex-On; Captaton; Eburnate; Equilibrane; Fluopiram; Foxetin; Lapsus; Mitilase; Nervosal; Neupax; Prozac; Saurat; ***Austral.:*** Auscap; Erocap; Fluohexal; Lovan; Prozac; Zactin; ***Austria:*** Felicium; Fluctine; Fluoxibene; Fluoxistad; Fluoxityrol; Flux; Fluxil; FluxoMed; Mutan; Positivum; ***Belg.:*** Fontex; Prozac; ***Braz.:*** Daforin; Deprax; Depress; Eufor; Fluxene; Nortec; Prozac; Prozen; Psiquial; Verotina; ***Canad.:*** Prozac; ***Chile:*** Actan; Anisimol; Clinium; Dominium; Pragmaten; Prozac; Sostac; Tremafarm; ***Denm.:*** Afeksin; Flutin; Fluxantin; Folizol; Fondur; Fonigen; Fontex; Fonzac; Nycoflox†; ***Fin.:*** Fluxantin; Fontex; Seromex; Seronil; ***Fr.:*** Prozac; ***Ger.:*** Fluctin; Fluneurin; Fluox; Fluox-Puren; Fluoxa; Fluoxemerck; Fluoxgamma; Fluxet; Fysionorm; Motivone†; ***Gr.:*** Dagrilan; Dinalexin; Exostrept; Flonital; Fluxadir; Fokeston; Ladose; Orthon; Sartuzin; Stephadilat-S; ***Hong Kong:*** Deprexin; Fluxil; Magrilan; Nopres; Provatine; Prozac; ***India:*** Fludac; Flufran; Platin; ***Irl.:*** Affex; Biozac; Gerozac; Norzac; Prozac; Prozamel; Prozatan; Prozit; ***Israel:*** Affectine; Flutine; Prizma; Prozac; ***Ital.:*** Deprexen; Diesan; Flotina; Fluoxeren; Fluoxin; Grinflux; Prozac; Serezac; Zafluox; ***Malaysia:*** Prozac; ***Mex.:*** Auroken; Axtin; Flocet; Florexal; Fluoxac; Prozac; Siquial; ***Neth.:*** Prozac; ***Norw.:*** Fontex; Nycoflox†; ***NZ:*** Fluox; Lovan†; Plinzene; Prozac; ***Port.:*** Digassim; Nodepe; Prozac; Psipax; Salipax; Selectus; Tuneluz; ***S.Afr.:*** Lorien; Nuzak; Prohexal; Prozac; Prozyn†; Sanzur; ***Singapore:*** Deprexin; Fluxetil; Fluxetin; Magrilan; Prodep†; Prozac; Zactin; ***Spain:*** Adofen; Astrin; Lecimar; Nodepe; Prozac; Reneuron; ***Swed.:*** Fluxantin; Fontex; Seroscand; ***Switz.:*** Fluctine; Fluocim; fluoxbasan; Fluoxifar; Flusol; ***Thai.:*** Actisac; Anzac; Atd; Deproxin; Flumed; Fluoxine; Flusac; Flutine; Fluxetil; Fluxetin; Fluzac; Hapilux; Loxetine; Magrilan; Oxetine; Oxsac; Prodep; Prozac; Unprozy; ***UAE:*** Flutin; ***UK:*** Felicium†; Prozac; Prozit; ***USA:*** Prozac; Sarafem.

**Multi-ingredient:** ***USA:*** Symbyax.

---

# Fluvoxamine Maleate *(BANM, USAN, rINNM)*

DU-23000; Maleato de fluvoxamina. (*E*)-5-Methoxy-4′-trifluoromethylvalerophenone *O*-2-aminoethyloxime maleate.

$C_{15}H_{21}F_3N_2O_2,C_4H_4O_4 = 434.4.$

*CAS — 54739-18-3 (fluvoxamine); 61718-82-9 (fluvoxamine maleate).*

*ATC — N06AB08.*

**Pharmacopoeias.** In *Br.*

**BP 2003** (Fluvoxamine Maleate). A white to almost white crystalline powder. Sparingly soluble in water; freely soluble in alcohol and in methyl alcohol.

## Adverse Effects, Treatment, and Precautions

As for SSRIs in general (see Fluoxetine, p.292).

Bradycardia with ECG changes has been noted with fluvoxamine (but see also Effects on the Cardiovascular System in Adverse Effects of Fluoxetine, p.292).

It is recommended that fluvoxamine should be withdrawn in patients who have an increase in serum concentrations of liver enzymes.

Fluvoxamine should be given in low initial dosage to patients with hepatic impairment. US and UK manufacturers vary in that they recommend similar reductions in the elderly and those with renal impairment, respectively.

**Incidence of adverse effects.** The UK Committee on Safety of Medicines has reported[1] that between 25 September 1986 and 23 March 1988 it had received 961 reports of adverse reactions associated with the use of fluvoxamine and that these included 5 deaths. The most frequently reported reactions were nausea (183) and vomiting (101). Other reactions included dizziness, somnolence, agitation, headache, tremor, and, during the first few days, worsening of anxiety. There were 13 reports of convulsions. Reports of appetite stimulation and antimuscarinic reactions were unusual. The effects sometimes resolved with time or dose reduction.

The safety profile of fluvoxamine has been reviewed.[2] For a comparison of the adverse reaction profiles of other SSRIs including fluoxetine with that of fluvoxamine, see under Adverse Effects of Fluoxetine, p.292.


1. Committee on Safety of Medicines. Fluvoxamine (Faverin): adverse reaction profile. *Current Problems 22* 1988.
2. Wagner W, *et al.* Fluvoxamine: a review of its safety profile in world-wide studies. *Int Clin Psychopharmacol* 1994; **9:** 223–7.


**Breast feeding.** For comments on the use of SSRIs in breast feeding patients, see under Precautions for Fluoxetine, p.294.

**Children.** In the UK the Committee on Safety of Medicines recommends that fluvoxamine should not be used to treat depressive illness in children under 18 years of age. For details, see under Effects on Mental State in Fluoxetine, p.293.

## Interactions

For interactions associated with SSRIs, see Fluoxetine, p.295.

Fluvoxamine can greatly increase plasma concentrations of theophylline (see p.802), and they should not be given together, or, if this is unavoidable, the dose of theophylline should be halved and plasma-theophylline concentrations monitored more closely.

◊ References.


1. Wagner W, Vause EW. Fluvoxamine: a review of global drug-drug interaction data. *Clin Pharmacokinet* 1995; **29** (suppl 1): 26–32.


## Pharmacokinetics

Fluvoxamine is readily absorbed from the gastrointestinal tract with peak plasma concentrations occurring 3 to 8 hours after a dose. Systemic bioavailability does not appear to be affected by food. It is extensively metabolised in the liver by oxidative demethylation and deamination, to inactive metabolites. Excretion is mainly in the urine. Fluvoxamine is widely distributed throughout the body and protein binding is reported to be about 80%; it has a plasma-elimination half-life of about 15 hours. Fluvoxamine is distributed into breast milk (see Breast Feeding under Precautions in Fluoxetine, p.294).

◊ References.


1. De Bree H, *et al.* Fluvoxamine maleate: disposition in man. *Eur J Drug Metab Pharmacokinet* 1983; **8:** 175–9.
2. Overmars H, *et al.* Fluvoxamine maleate: metabolism in man. *Eur J Drug Metab Pharmacokinet* 1983; **8:** 269–80.
3. van Harten J, *et al.* Pharmacokinetics of fluvoxamine maleate in patients with liver cirrhosis after single-dose oral administration. *Clin Pharmacokinet* 1993; **24:** 177–82.
4. Perucca E, *et al.* Clinical pharmacokinetics of fluvoxamine. *Clin Pharmacokinet* 1994; **27:** 175–90.
5. van Harten J. Overview of the pharmacokinetics of fluvoxamine. *Clin Pharmacokinet* 1995; **29** (suppl 1): 1–9.
6. Xu Z-H, *et al.* In vivo inhibition of CYP2C19 but not CYP2D6 by fluvoxamine. *Br J Clin Pharmacol* 1996; **42:** 518–21.
7. Spigset O, *et al.* Non-linear fluvoxamine disposition. *Br J Clin Pharmacol* 1998; **45:** 257–63.


## Uses and Administration

Fluvoxamine, an aralkylketone derivative, is an SSRI with actions and uses similar to those of fluoxetine (p.296). It is used as the maleate and doses are expressed in terms of this salt.

In the treatment of **depression** fluvoxamine maleate is given by mouth in an initial dose of 50 or 100 mg daily; in some patients the dose may need to be gradually increased up to a maximum of 300 mg daily. It is recommended that daily dosages exceeding 150 mg should be given in divided doses.

Fluvoxamine maleate is also used in the management of **obsessive-compulsive disorder**. In the UK, doses are similar to those used in the treatment of depression. The recommended starting dose in the USA is 50 mg once daily; this dose may be increased by increments of 50 mg every 4 to 7 days to a maximum of 300 mg daily. Doses above 100 mg daily should be given in two divided doses. In both countries the drug may also be used in children of 8 years and over with obsessive-compulsive disorder. The recommended starting dose is 25 mg once daily, which may be increased in increments of 25 mg every 3 to 7 days to a maximum daily dose of 200 mg (in the USA adolescents over 11 years may be given a maximum dose of 300 mg daily). Daily doses of more than 50 mg should be given as two divided doses. It is recommended that if no improvement is observed within 10 weeks, treatment with fluvoxamine should be re-assessed.

The US manufacturer recommends that dosage modification be considered in elderly patients, in whom clearance may be decreased. For dosage in renal and hepatic impairment, see below.

Fluvoxamine should be withdrawn gradually to reduce the risk of withdrawal symptoms.

◊ Reviews.


1. Mendlewicz J. Efficacy of fluvoxamine in severe depression. *Drugs* 1992; **43** (suppl 2): 32–9.
2. Wilde ME, *et al.* Fluvoxamine: an updated review of its pharmacology, and therapeutic use in depressive illness. *Drugs* 1993; **46:** 895–924.
3. Palmer KJ, Benfield P. Fluvoxamine: an overview of its pharmacological properties and review of its therapeutic potential in non-depressive disorders. *CNS Drugs* 1994; **1:** 57–87.


**Administration in hepatic or renal impairment.** The UK manufacturer recommends that patients with hepatic or renal impairment should begin therapy with a low dose of fluvoxamine maleate and be carefully monitored; the US manufacturer only recommends that dosage modification be considered in hepatic impairment, since it considers evidence of accumulation in renal impairment to be lacking.

**Anxiety disorders.** Fluvoxamine has been given in a variety of anxiety disorders including obsessive-compulsive disorder (p.663), panic attacks (p.663), and social phobia (see under Phobic Disorders, p.663).

References.


1. Jenike MA, *et al.* A controlled trial of fluvoxamine in obsessive-compulsive disorder: implications for a serotonergic theory. *Am J Psychiatry* 1990; **147:** 1209–15.
2. Mallya GK, *et al.* Short- and long-term treatment of obsessive-compulsive disorder with fluvoxamine. *Ann Clin Psychiatry* 1992; **4:** 77–80.
3. Black DW, *et al.* A comparison of fluvoxamine, cognitive therapy, and placebo in the treatment of panic disorder. *Arch Gen Psychiatry* 1993; **50:** 44–50.
4. Hoehn-Saric R, *et al.* Effect of fluvoxamine on panic disorder. *J Clin Psychopharmacol* 1993; **13:** 321–6.
5. van Vliet IM, *et al.* Psychopharmacological treatment of social phobia: a double blind placebo controlled study with fluvoxamine. *Psychopharmacology (Berl)* 1994; **115:** 128–34.
6. Freeman CPL, *et al.* Fluvoxamine versus clomipramine in the treatment of obsessive compulsive disorder: a multicenter, randomized, double-blind, parallel group comparison. *J Clin Psychiatry* 1994; **55:** 301–5.
7. Greist JH, *et al.* Efficacy of fluvoxamine in obsessive-compulsive disorder: results of a multicentre, double blind, placebo-controlled trial. *Eur J Clin Res* 1995; **7:** 195–204.
8. Stein MB, *et al.* Fluvoxamine treatment of social phobia (social anxiety disorder): a double-blind placebo-controlled study. *Am J Psychiatry* 1999; **156:** 756–60.
9. Figgitt DP, McClellan KJ. Fluvoxamine: an updated review of its use in the management of adults with anxiety disorders. *Drugs* 2000; **60:** 925–54.
10. The Research Unit on Pediatric Psychopharmacology Anxiety Study Group. Fluvoxamine for the treatment of anxiety disorders in children and adolescents. *N Engl J Med* 2001; **344:** 1279–85.


**Hypochondriasis.** For reference to the use of SSRIs, including fluvoxamine, in hypochondriasis, see under Fluoxetine, p.297.

## Preparations

**BP 2003:** Fluvoxamine Tablets.

**Proprietary Preparations** (details are given in Part 3)
***Arg.:*** Luvox; ***Austral.:*** Faverin; Luvox; Movox; ***Austria:*** Felixsan; Floxyfral; ***Belg.:*** Dumirox; Floxyfral; ***Braz.:*** Luvox; ***Canad.:*** Luvox; ***Chile:*** Luvox; ***Denm.:*** Fevarin; ***Fin.:*** Fevarin; Fluvosol; ***Fr.:*** Floxyfral; ***Ger.:*** Desifluvoxamin; Fevarin; Fluvohexal; Fluvoxadura; ***Gr.:*** Dumyrox; ***Hong Kong:*** Faverin; ***India:*** Fluvoxin; ***Irl.:*** Faverin; ***Israel:*** Favoxil; ***Ital.:*** Dumirox; Fevarin; Maveral; ***Malaysia:*** Luvox; ***Mex.:*** Luvox; ***Neth.:*** Fevarin; ***Norw.:*** Fevarin; ***Port.:*** Dumyrox; ***S.Afr.:*** Luvox; ***Singapore:*** Faverin; ***Spain:*** Dumirox; ***Swed.:*** Fevarin; ***Switz.:*** Flox-ex; Floxyfral; ***Thai.:*** Faverin; ***UK:*** Faverin; ***USA:*** Luvox.

## Hypericum

Hipérico; Hyperici Herba; Johanniskraut; Millepertuis; St. John's Wort.

*CAS — 548-04-9 (hypericin).*

**Pharmacopoeias.** In *Eur.* (see p.vi) and *Pol.* Also in *USNF.*
*Eur.* also includes a form for homoeopathic preparations.
*Swiss* also includes monographs for hypericum (fresh flowering tops) and hypericum oil.

**Ph. Eur. 5.0** (St. John's Wort). The whole or cut, dried flowering tops of *Hypericum perforatum* gathered during flowering. It contains not less than 0.08% of total hypericins, expressed as hypericin ($C_{30}H_{16}O_8$ = 504.4) calculated with reference to the dried drug. Protect from light.

**Ph. Eur. 5.0** (Hypericum for Homoeopathic Preparations; Hypericum Perforatum ad Praeparationes Homoeopathicas). The whole, fresh plant of *Hypericum perforatum*, at the beginning of the flowering period. Protect from light.

**USNF 22** (St. John's Wort). The dried flowering tops or aerial parts of *Hypericum perforatum* (Hypericaceae), gathered shortly before or during flowering. It contains not less than 0.04% of the combined total of hypericin ($C_{30}H_{16}O_8$ = 504.4) and pseudohypericin ($C_{30}H_{16}O_9$ = 520.4) and not less than 0.6% of hyperforin ($C_{35}H_{52}O_4$ = 536.8). Store in airtight containers. Protect from light.

### Adverse Effects and Precautions

Adverse effects reported with hypericum have included gastrointestinal symptoms, allergic reactions, and fatigue. Photosensitivity has also been reported; hypericin and pseudohypericin are the constituents of hypericum thought to be responsible for this reaction.

**Effects on the nervous system.** Subacute polyneuropathy following sun exposure developed in a woman who had taken hypericum for mild depression; she improved following drug withdrawal.[1]


1. Bove GM. Acute neuropathy after exposure to sun in a patient treated with St John's Wort. *Lancet* 1998; **352:** 1121–2.


**Effects on the skin.** In addition to photosensitivity reactions associated with hypericum use,[1] there has been a report of severe erythroderma in a patient who supplemented his regular antidepressant medication (dosulepin) with hypericum.[2] The reaction was seen on both light-exposed and non-exposed areas, and was thought to be due to the hypericum although there remained a possibility that it was due to an interaction between the 2 drugs.


1. Lane-Brown MM. Photosensitivity associated with herbal preparations of St John's wort (Hypericum perforatum). *Med J Aust* 2000; **172:** 302.
2. Holme SA, Roberts DL. Erythroderma associated with St John's wort. *Br J Dermatol* 2000; **143:** 1127–8.


### Interactions

Hypericum has been shown to induce several drug metabolising enzymes including some cytochrome P450 isoenzymes (in particular CYP3A4) and the transport protein P-glycoprotein. Clinically important interactions resulting in decreased plasma concentrations of the interacting drug have been reported with ciclosporin, digoxin, HIV-protease inhibitors such as indinavir, oral contraceptives, tacrolimus, theophylline, and warfarin. There is also a theoretical possibility of an interaction between hypericum and antiepileptics such as carbamazepine (p.356), phenobarbital (p.368), and phenytoin (p.373), and non-nucleoside reverse transcriptase inhibitors. In addition, stopping hypericum may result in increased, and possibly toxic, concentrations of the interacting drug.

In many countries, including the UK, preparations of hypericum are not required to be licensed, and the amount of active ingredient may vary widely between preparations. Changing preparations may therefore alter the degree of enzyme induction.

Use of hypericum with drugs known to act on serotonergic neurotransmitters may result in synergistic interactions and an increased risk of adverse effects may also occur. Examples include the SSRIs and nefazodone (see p.315) and the selective serotonin ($5-HT_1$) agonists (see p.472) used to treat migraine.

◊ References.


1. Roby CA, *et al.* St John's Wort: effect on CYP3A4 activity. *Clin Pharmacol Ther* 2000; **67:** 451–7.
2. Committee on Safety of Medicines/Medicines Control Agency. Reminder: St John's Wort (Hypericum perforatum) interactions. *Current Problems* 2000; **26:** 6–7. http://www.mca.gov.uk/ourwork/monitorsafequalmed/currentproblems/cpmay2000.pdf (accessed 10/06/04)
3. Dürr D, *et al.* St John's Wort induces intestinal p-glycoprotein/MDR1 and intestinal and hepatic CYP3A4. *Clin Pharmacol Ther* 2000; **68:** 598–604.
4. Wang Z, *et al.* The effects of St John's wort (*Hypericum perforatum*) on human cytochrome P450 activity. *Clin Pharmacol Ther* 2001: **70:** 317–26.
5. Hennessy M, *et al.* St John's Wort increases expression of P-glycoprotein: implications for drug interactions. *Br J Clin Pharmacol* 2002 **53:** 75–82.
6. Henderson L, *et al.* St John's wort (*Hypericum perforatum*): drug interactions and clinical outcomes. *Br J Clin Pharmacol* 2002; **54:** 349–56.


**Anticoagulants.** For mention of a possible interaction between hypericum and *warfarin*, see p.1027.

**Antineoplastics.** For mention of a possible interaction between hypericum and *aminolevulinic acid* or *irinotecan*, see p.527 and p.564, respectively.

**Antivirals.** For details of a possible interaction between hypericum and *HIV-protease inhibitors* such as indinavir, see p.639.

**Cardiac glycosides.** For details of a possible interaction between hypericum and *digoxin*, see p.897.

**Immunosuppressants.** For details of possible interactions between hypericum and *ciclosporin* or *tacrolimus*, see p.1354 and p.1364, respectively.

**Oral contraceptives.** For reports of a possible interaction between hypericum and oral contraceptives, see p.1534.

**Xanthines.** For details of a possible interaction between hypericum and *theophylline*, see p.802.

### Uses and Administration

Herbal preparations containing hypericum are used, frequently for self-medication, in the treatment of depression. Such preparations are also promoted for the treatment of other nervous disorders such as insomnia and anxiety, particularly if associated with the menopause. Hypericum oil has also been used as an astringent. Hypericin, a major constituent of hypericum, has been investigated as an antiviral in the treatment of HIV infection and AIDS (but see below).

The amount of active constituents can vary between different preparations and doses depend on the preparation being used.

Hypericum has been used in homoeopathic preparations.

◊ References.


1. McIntyre M. A review of the benefits, adverse events, drug interactions, and safety of St. John's Wort (Hypericum perforatum): the implications with regard to the regulation of herbal medicines. *J Altern Complement Med* 2000; **6:** 115–24.


**Antiviral action.** A study involving 30 HIV-infected patients suggested that hypericin, given intravenously or by mouth, produced significant phototoxicity and had no effect on virological markers or CD4 cell count.[1]


1. Gulick RM, *et al.* Phase I studies of hypericin, the active compound in St John's Wort, as an antiretroviral agent in HIV-infected adults. *Ann Intern Med* 1999; **130:** 510–14.


**Depression.** Hypericum extracts are widely used in some countries for the treatment of depression (p.279).

Two systematic reviews[1,2] of randomised trials found hypericum extracts to be more effective than placebo in mild to moderately severe depressive disorders. There was insufficient evidence available to establish relative efficacy and tolerability compared with standard antidepressants,[1] although experience from those populations in whom hypericum extracts are widely used suggests that the herb may offer an advantage in terms of relative safety and tolerability.[3] Two multicentre randomised controlled trials found hypericum extract to be ineffective in patients with major depression.[4,5] Further studies are required before the herb can be recommended in major depression.[2,3,5]

The mechanism of action of hypericum extracts in the treatment of depression remains unclear. Extracts contain at least 10 active principles. Hypericin, one of the major constituents of hypericum, was first thought responsible for the antidepressant effect since it had an inhibitory action on monoamine oxidase *in vitro*. However it was later shown that this action was, at best, weak and it is now generally believed that monoamine oxidase inhibition is not responsible for the antidepressant effect of hypericum. More recent studies have suggested that hyperforin may be one of the major constituents responsible for the antidepressant effect.[6] Although the evidence is mainly from *in vitro* studies, hyperforin inhibits the reuptake of several major neurotransmitters including serotonin, dopamine, and noradrenaline.[7]


1. Linde K, Mulrow CD. St John's wort for depression. Available in The Cochrane Library; Issue 2. Chichester: John Wiley; 2004.
2. Stevinson C, Ernst E. Hypericum for depression: an update of the clinical evidence. *Eur Neuropsychopharmacol* 1999; **9:** 501–5.
3. de Smet PAGM, Nolen WA. St John's wort as an antidepressant. *BMJ* 1996; **313:** 241–2.
4. Shelton RC, *et al.* Effectiveness of St John's Wort in major depression: a randomized controlled trial. *JAMA* 2001; **285:** 1978–86.
5. Hypericum Depression Trial Study Group. Effect of *Hypericum perforatum* (St John's wort) in major depressive disorder. *JAMA* 2002; **287:** 1807–14.
6. Laakmann G, *et al.* St. John's Wort in mild to moderate depression: the relevance of hyperforin for the clinical efficacy. *Pharmacopsychiatry* 1998: **31** (suppl.): 54–9.
7. Chatterjee SS, *et al.* Hyperforin as a possible antidepressant component of hypericum extracts. *Life Sci* 1998; **63:** 499–510.


## Preparations

**Proprietary Preparations** (details are given in Part 3)
***Arg.:*** Amenicil; Felis; Herbaccion Motivante; Hipax; Remotiv; ***Austral.:*** Bioglan Stress-Relax†; Hyperiforte†; Remotiv; ***Austria:*** Esbericum; Felis; Hyperiforce; Jarsin; Johanicum; Kira; Perikan; Psychotonin; Remotiv; ***Braz.:*** Adprex; Emotival; Equilibra; Fiotan; Hiperex; Hipericin; Hiperico; Hiperil; Hipersac; Hyperico; Iperisan; Jarsin; Motiven; Prazen; Triativ; ***Canad.:*** Kira; Movana; ***Chile:*** Anxium; Ciplazin; Edual; Remotiv; ***Fr.:*** Bains Romains; Dermum; ***Ger.:*** aar brain N; Aristo; Aristoforat; Cesradyston; Cesran†; dysto-lux; Esbericum; Felis; Futuran†; Helarium; Herbaneurin; Hewepsychon uno; Hyperforat; Hypericaps; Hyperimerck; Hyperpur; Jarsin; Jukunda Rotöl†; Kira; Kytta-Modal; Laif; Libertin; Lomahypericum; mct Psycho Dragees N†; Nervei; Neuroplant; Neurotisan†; Neurovegetalin; Psychotonin; Psychotonin M; Remotiv†; Rephahyval†; Rotöl†; Sedovegan; Spilan†; Syxal; Texx; Tonizin; Turineurin; Viviplus; ***Ital.:*** Nervaxon; Quiens; Remotive; ***Mex.:*** Hiperikan; Nutegen H; Remotiv; ***S.Afr.:*** Remotiv; ***Singapore:*** Lomahypericum†; ***Spain:*** Animic; Arkocapsulas Hiperico; Hiperico; Hyneurin; Kajel†; Quetzal; Tolecen†; Vitalium; ***Switz.:*** Felis†; Hypericettes; Hyperiforce; HyperiMed; Hyperiplant; Hyperval; Jarsin; Lucilium; Mandal 425†; Movina†; ReBalance; Remotiv; Solevita; Valverde Hyperval†; ***UK:*** Kira.

**Multi-ingredient:** ***Austral.:*** Anti-Flamme†; Bioglan 3B Beer Belly Buster†; Feminine Herbal Complex†; Infant Tonic†; Irontona†; Joint & Muscle Relief Cream†; Nappy Rash Relief Cream†; Skin Healing Cream†; Vitatona†; ***Austria:*** Eryval; Magentee EF-EM-ES; Nerventee EF-EM-ES; Species nervinae; Vulpuran; Wechseltee EF-EM-ES; ***Braz.:*** Eugynol†; ***Fr.:*** Cicaderma†; ***Ger.:*** Allya; anabol-loges; Anisan; Arthrodynat P; Befelka-Oel; Cefaktivon†; Cheiranthol; Discmigon†; Dolo-cyl; Gastritol; Gastrol S; Gutnacht; Hewepsychon duo†; Hocura-Spondylose novo†; Hyperesa; Hyperforat-forte; JuCholan S†; JuDorm; JuNeuron S†; JuViton; Kneipp Herz- und Kreislauf-Tee†; Kneipp Krauter Taschenkur Nerven und Schlaf N†; Marianon; Neurapas; Oxacant N; Phytogran; Presselin Arterien K 5 P; Presselin Nerven K I N; Psychotonin-sed†; Remifemin plus; Rhoival; Salus Nerven-Schlaf-Tee Nr.22†; Salusan†; Sedariston; Sedariston Konzentrat; Sinedyston†; Valena N†; Venacton; ***Ital.:*** Elisir Depurativo Ambrosiano†; Hiperogyn; Mithen; Neumoral†; ***Port.:*** Cicaderma; ***Spain:*** Natusor Gastrolen; Natusor Somnisedan; ***Switz.:*** Alpina Gel a la consoude†; Drosana Hyperflorin†; Gel a la consoude; Huile de millepertuis A. Vogel (huile de St. Jean); Hyperiforce comp; Keppur; Malvedrin; Phytoberidin†; Pommade Po-Ho N A Vogel†; Saltrates; Saltrates Rodell; Tai Ginseng N†; Yakona

N†; **UK:** Amileve; Savlon Natural First Aid for Burns; Savlon Natural First Aid for Cuts & Sores; Savlon Natural First Aid for Insect Bites & Stings; St Johnswort Compound.

## Imipramine *(BAN, rINN)*

Imipramina. 3-(10,11-Dihydro-5*H*-dibenz[*b,f*]azepin-5-yl)propyldimethylamine.

$C_{19}H_{24}N_2$ = 280.4.
*CAS — 50-49-7.*
*ATC — N06AA02.*

### Imipramine Embonate *(BANM, rINNM)*

Embonato de imipramina; Imipramine Pamoate.

$(C_{19}H_{24}N_2)_2,C_{23}H_{16}O_6$ = 949.2.
*CAS — 10075-24-8.*

### Imipramine Hydrochloride *(BANM, rINNM)*

Hidrocloruro de imipramina; Impiram. Hydrochlor.; Imipramini Chloridum; Imipramini Hydrochloridum; Imizine.

$C_{19}H_{24}N_2,HCl$ = 316.9.
*CAS — 113-52-0.*

**Pharmacopoeias.** In *Chin., Eur.* (see p.vi), *Int., Jpn, Pol.,* and *US.*

**Ph. Eur. 5.0** (Imipramine Hydrochloride). A white or slightly yellow crystalline powder. Freely soluble in water and in alcohol. A 10% solution in water has a pH of 3.6 to 5.0. Protect from light.

**USP 27** (Imipramine Hydrochloride). A white to off-white, odourless or practically odourless, crystalline powder. Freely soluble in water and in alcohol; soluble in acetone; insoluble in ether and in benzene. Store in airtight containers.

## Adverse Effects, Treatment, and Precautions

As for tricyclic antidepressants in general (see Amitriptyline, p.281).

**Breast feeding.** For comments on the use of tricyclic antidepressants in breast feeding patients, see under Precautions for Amitriptyline, p.283.

**Porphyria.** Imipramine has been associated with acute attacks of porphyria and is considered unsafe in porphyric patients.

## Interactions

For interactions associated with tricyclic antidepressants, see Amitriptyline, p.284.

## Pharmacokinetics

Imipramine is readily absorbed from the gastrointestinal tract, and extensively demethylated by first-pass metabolism in the liver, to its primary active metabolite, desipramine.

Paths of metabolism of both imipramine and desipramine include hydroxylation and *N*-oxidation. Imipramine is excreted in the urine, mainly in the form of its metabolites, either free or in conjugated form; small amounts are excreted in the faeces via the bile.

Imipramine and desipramine are widely distributed throughout the body and are extensively bound to plasma and tissue protein. Imipramine has been estimated to have an elimination half-life ranging from 9 to 28 hours, which may be considerably extended in overdosage. Plasma concentrations of imipramine and desipramine vary very widely between individuals but some correlation with therapeutic response has been established.

Imipramine and desipramine cross the blood-brain barrier and placenta and are distributed into breast milk (see Breast Feeding under Precautions in Amitriptyline, p.283).

◊ References.

1. Sallee FR, Pollock BG. Clinical pharmacokinetics of imipramine and desipramine. *Clin Pharmacokinet* 1990; **18:** 346–64.

## Uses and Administration

Imipramine is a dibenzazepine tricyclic antidepressant with actions and uses similar to those of amitriptyline (p.285). Imipramine is one of the less sedating tricyclics and has moderate antimuscarinic activity. Imipramine is usually given by mouth as the hydrochloride or embonate, with doses expressed in terms of the hydrochloride. Imipramine embonate 149.8 mg and imipramine base 88.5 mg are both approximately equivalent to 100 mg of imipramine hydrochloride.

In the treatment of **depression**, the usual daily dose of imipramine hydrochloride is up to 75 mg in divided doses initially, gradually increased to 150 to 200 mg daily as necessary; higher doses of up to 300 mg daily may be required in severely depressed patients in hospital. A suggested initial dose for the elderly in the UK is 10 mg at night, gradually increasing to 30 to 50 mg daily. In the USA, daily doses of 25 to 50 mg are recommended for initial therapy in the elderly and adolescents, increasing to a maximum of 100 mg daily as required. Since imipramine has a prolonged half-life, once-daily dosage regimens may also be suitable, usually given at night.

In the initial stages of treatment, if dosage by mouth is impracticable or inadvisable, up to 100 mg of imipramine hydrochloride may be given daily in divided doses by intramuscular injection, but oral doses should be substituted as soon as possible.

Imipramine is also used for the treatment of **nocturnal enuresis** in children in whom organic pathology has been excluded. However, drug therapy for nocturnal enuresis should be reserved for those in whom other methods have failed and should preferably only be given to cover periods away from home; tricyclic antidepressants are not recommended in children under 6 years of age (the *British National Formulary* recommends that they should not be given until 7 years of age). Suggested doses of imipramine hydrochloride are 25 mg for children aged 6 to 7 years (20 to 25 kg), 25 to 50 mg for children aged 8 to 11 years (25 to 35 kg), and 50 to 75 mg for children aged over 11 years (35 to 54 kg). The dose should be taken just before bedtime and treatment, including the gradual period of withdrawal, should not continue for longer than 3 months. A full physical examination is recommended before a further course.

Imipramine oxide hydrochloride (imipraminoxide hydrochloride) is also used as an antidepressant and for nocturnal enuresis.

Imipramine should be withdrawn gradually to reduce the risk of withdrawal symptoms.

**Anxiety disorders.** See under Clomipramine, p.290.

Some references to the use of imipramine in anxiety disorders are given below.

1. Cross-National Collaborative Panic Study, Second Phase Investigators. Drug treatment of panic disorder: comparative efficacy of alprazolam, imipramine, and placebo. *Br J Psychiatry* 1992; **160:** 191–202.
2. Lepola UM, *et al.* Three-year follow-up of patients with panic disorder after short-term treatment with alprazolam and imipramine. *Int Clin Psychopharmacol* 1993; **8:** 115–18.
3. Rickels K, *et al.* Antidepressants for the treatment of generalised anxiety disorder: a placebo-controlled comparison of imipramine, trazodone, and diazepam. *Arch Gen Psychiatry* 1993; **50:** 884–95.
4. Clark DM, *et al.* A comparison of cognitive therapy, applied relaxation and imipramine in the treatment of panic disorder. *Br J Psychiatry* 1994; **164:** 759–69.
5. Barlow DH, *et al.* Cognitive-behavioral therapy, imipramine, or their combination for panic disorder: a randomized controlled trial. *JAMA* 2000; **283:** 2529–36. Correction. *ibid.*; **284:** 2597.

**Hyperactivity.** See under Desipramine, p.290.

**Pain.** Antidepressants, usually amitriptyline or another tricyclic, are useful in alleviating some types of pain (see Choice of Analgesic, p.2) when given in subantidepressant doses.

Some references to the use of imipramine are given below.

1. Walsh TD. Controlled study of imipramine and morphine in chronic pain due to advanced cancer. *Proc Am Soc Clin Oncol* 1986; **5:** 237.
2. Sindrup SH, *et al.* Concentration-response relationship in imipramine treatment of diabetic neuropathy symptoms. *Clin Pharmacol Ther* 1990; **47:** 509–15.
3. Hummel T, *et al.* A comparison of the antinociceptive effects of imipramine, tramadol and anpirtoline. *Br J Clin Pharmacol* 1994; **37:** 325–33.
4. Cannon RO, *et al.* Imipramine in patients with chest pain despite normal coronary angiograms. *N Engl J Med* 1994; **330:** 1411–17.
5. Godfrey RG. A guide to the understanding and use of tricyclic antidepressants in the overall management of fibromyalgia and other chronic pain syndromes. *Arch Intern Med* 1996; **156:** 1047–52.
6. Minotti V, *et al.* Double-blind evaluation of short-term analgesic efficacy of orally administered diclofenac, diclofenac plus codeine, and diclofenac plus imipramine in chronic cancer pain. *Pain* 1998; **74:** 133–7.

## Preparations

***BP 2003:*** Imipramine Tablets;
***USP 27:*** Imipramine Hydrochloride Injection; Imipramine Hydrochloride Tablets.

**Proprietary Preparations** (details are given in Part 3)
***Arg.:*** Elepsin; Tofranil; ***Austral.:*** Melipramine; Tofranil; ***Austria:*** Tofranil; ***Belg.:*** Tofranil; ***Braz.:*** Depramina; Imipra; Praminan; Tofranil; ***Canad.:*** Impril†; Novo-Pramine†; Tofranil; ***Fr.:*** Tofranil; ***Ger.:*** Pryleugan; Tofranil; ***Hong Kong:*** Tofranil; ***India:*** Antidep; Depsonil; ***Irl.:*** Tofranil; ***Israel:*** Primonil; Tofranil; ***Ital.:*** Tofranil; ***Mex.:*** Talpramin; Tofranil; ***Neth.:*** Tofranil; ***NZ:*** Tofranil; ***Port.:*** Tofranil; ***S.Afr.:*** Ethipramine; Tofranil; ***Spain:*** Tofranil; ***Swed.:*** Tofranil; ***Switz.:*** Tofranil; ***Thai.:*** Antidep†; Celamine; Sermonil; Tofranil†; Topramine; ***UK:*** Tofranil; ***USA:*** Tofranil; Tofranil-PM.

**Multi-ingredient:** ***India:*** Depsonil-DZ.

## Iproniazid Phosphate *(BANM, rINNM)*

Fosfato de iproniazida. 2'-Isopropylisonicotinohydrazide phosphate.

$C_9H_{13}N_3O,H_3PO_4$ = 277.2.
*CAS — 54-92-2 (iproniazid); 305-33-9 (iproniazid phosphate).*
*ATC — N06AF05.*

### Adverse Effects, Treatment, and Precautions

As for MAOIs in general (see Phenelzine, p.312).

**Effects on the liver.** Of 91 cases of hepatitis due to antidepressant therapy, cytolytic reactions occurred in 11 treated with iproniazid.[1] Five patients died, 3 of them after involuntary rechallenge. High levels of antimitochondrial antibody were found in 5 patients.

1. Lefebure B, *et al.* Hépatites aux antidépresseurs. *Therapie* 1984; **39:** 509–16.

**Porphyria.** Iproniazid has been associated with acute attacks of porphyria and is considered unsafe in porphyric patients.

### Interactions

For interactions associated with MAOIs, see Phenelzine, p.314.

### Uses and Administration

Iproniazid, a hydrazine derivative, is an irreversible inhibitor of both monoamine oxidase types A and B with actions and uses similar to those of phenelzine (p.316).

Iproniazid is used in the treatment of depression, but as discussed on p.279 the risks associated with irreversible non-selective MAOIs usually mean that other antidepressants are preferred. It is given by mouth as the phosphate although doses are expressed in terms of the base; iproniazid phosphate 77.3 mg is approximately equivalent to 50 mg of iproniazid base. The usual initial dose is the equivalent of 50 to 150 mg daily. Once a response has been obtained the dosage may be gradually reduced for maintenance therapy; some patients may respond to 25 to 50 mg daily or every other day.

Iproniazid should be withdrawn gradually to reduce the risk of withdrawal symptoms.

Iproniazid is the isopropyl derivative of isoniazid (see p.222) and was developed for use in tuberculosis, but owing to its toxicity is no longer used for this purpose.

### Preparations

**Proprietary Preparations** (details are given in Part 3)
***Fr.:*** Marsilid.

## Isocarboxazid *(BAN, rINN)*

Isocarboxazida; Ro-5083I. 2'-Benzyl-5-methylisoxazole-3-carbohydrazide.

$C_{12}H_{13}N_3O_2$ = 231.3.
*CAS — 59-63-2.*
*ATC — N06AF01.*

**Pharmacopoeias.** In *Chin.*

### Adverse Effects, Treatment, and Precautions

As for MAOIs in general (see Phenelzine, p.312).

### Interactions

For interactions associated with MAOIs, see Phenelzine, p.314.

### Pharmacokinetics

Isocarboxazid is readily absorbed from the gastrointestinal tract reaching peak plasma concentrations 3 to 5 hours after ingestion. It is metabolised by the liver, and is excreted in the urine mainly in the form of metabolites.

### Uses and Administration

Isocarboxazid, a hydrazine derivative, is an irreversible inhibitor of both monoamine oxidase types A and B with actions and uses similar to those of phenelzine (p.316).

Isocarboxazid is used in the treatment of depression but as discussed on p.279 the risks associated with irreversible non-selective MAOIs usually mean that other antidepressants are preferred. It is given by mouth in an initial dose of 30 mg daily in single or divided doses. If no improvement occurs after 4 weeks, doses of up to 60 mg daily can be tried for up to 4 to 6 weeks. Once a response has been obtained the dosage may be gradually reduced to a maintenance dose of 10 to 20 mg daily, although doses of up to 40 mg daily may be needed in some patients. Half the normal maintenance dose may be adequate in the elderly.

Isocarboxazid should be withdrawn gradually to reduce the risk of withdrawal symptoms.

### Preparations

**Proprietary Preparations** (details are given in Part 3)
***Chile:*** Marplan; ***Denm.:*** Marplan; ***USA:*** Marplan.

## Lithium Carbonate *(USAN)*

CP-15467-61; Dilithium Carbonate; Lithii Carbonas; Lithium Carb.; Litio, carbonato de; NSC-16895. Carbonic acid, dilithium salt.

$Li_2CO_3$ = 73.89.
*CAS — 554-13-2.*
*ATC — N05AN01.*

NOTE. Commercially available lithium materials have atomic weights ranging from 6.939 to 6.996. The molecular weight of lithium carbonate of 73.89 given above has been calculated using the lowest atomic weight; using the highest figure would give a molecular weight of 74.00. This difference does not affect the figure of 27 mmol of lithium being provided by 1 g of lithium carbonate and is unlikely to contribute noticeably to any variations in serum concentration. Nor should it affect the outcome of assays of serum-lithium concentrations given the limits of error of the assay methods.

**Pharmacopoeias.** In *Chin.*, *Eur.* (see p.vi), *Int.*, *Jpn*, *Pol.*, and *US.*

**Ph. Eur. 5.0** (Lithium Carbonate). A white powder. Slightly soluble in water; practically insoluble in alcohol.

**USP 27** (Lithium Carbonate). A white odourless granular powder. Sparingly soluble in water, very slightly soluble in alcohol; dissolves, with effervescence, in dilute mineral acids.

### Lithium Citrate

Lithii Citras; Litio, citrato de.

$C_6H_5Li_3O_7,4H_2O$ = 282.0.
*CAS — 919-16-4 (anhydrous lithium citrate); 6080-58-6 (lithium citrate tetrahydrate).*

NOTE. Commercially available lithium materials have atomic weights ranging from 6.939 to 6.996. The molecular weight of lithium citrate of 282.0 given above has been calculated using the lowest atomic weight; using the highest figure would give a molecular weight of 282.1. This difference does not affect the figure of 10.6 mmol of lithium being provided by 1 g of lithium citrate and is unlikely to contribute noticeably to any variations in serum concentration. Nor should it affect the outcome of assays of serum-lithium concentrations given the limits of error of the assay methods.

**Pharmacopoeias.** In *Eur.* (see p.vi) and *US.*
*US* also includes lithium hydroxide.

**Ph. Eur. 5.0** (Lithium Citrate). A white or almost white fine crystalline powder. Freely soluble in water; slightly soluble in alcohol.

**USP 27** (Lithium Citrate). A white odourless deliquescent powder or granules. Freely soluble in water; slightly soluble in alcohol. pH of a 5% solution in water is between 7.0 and 10.0. Store in airtight containers.

## Adverse Effects

Many of the side-effects of lithium are dose-related and the margin between the therapeutic and toxic dose is narrow.

Initial adverse effects of lithium therapy include nausea, diarrhoea, vertigo, muscle weakness, and a dazed feeling; these effects often abate with continued therapy. Fine hand tremors, polyuria, and polydipsia may, however, persist. Other adverse effects that may occur at therapeutic serum-lithium concentrations include weight gain and oedema (which should not be treated with diuretics). Hypercalcaemia, hypermagnesaemia, and hyperparathyroidism have been reported. Skin disorders such as acne, psoriasis, and rashes may be exacerbated by lithium therapy. Leucocytosis is a relatively common adverse effect. Long-term adverse effects include hypothyroidism and/or goitre, rarely hyperthyroidism, and mild cognitive and memory impairment. Histological and functional changes in the kidney have been noted following long-term use of therapeutic concentrations of lithium (but see under Effects on the Kidneys, below).

Toxic effects may be expected at serum-lithium concentrations of about 1.5 mmol/litre, although they can appear at lower concentrations. They call for immediate withdrawal of treatment and should always be considered very seriously.

Signs of lithium toxicity include increasing diarrhoea, vomiting, anorexia, muscle weakness, lethargy, giddiness with ataxia, lack of coordination, tinnitus, blurred vision, coarse tremor of the extremities and lower jaw, muscle hyperirritability, choreoathetoid movements, dysarthria, and drowsiness. Symptoms of severe overdosage at serum-lithium concentrations above 2 mmol/litre include hyperreflexia and hyperextension of limbs, syncope, toxic psychosis, seizures, polyuria, renal failure, electrolyte imbalance, dehydration, circulatory failure, coma, and occasionally death.

The hazards of lithium in pregnant patients are discussed under Pregnancy in Precautions, below.

**Effects on the blood.** A patient developed thrombocytopenia after restarting lithium therapy following a gap of some weeks.[1] Withdrawing the lithium led to an improvement in platelet count, but the count fell when lithium therapy was tried again. Leucocytosis is a recognised effect of lithium which this patient also experienced. Although concerns about leukaemia induction have not been verified, the author noted earlier reports of aplastic and megaloblastic anaemia and a case of fatal haemolytic anaemia reported to the UK Committee on Safety of Medicines.


1. Collings S. Thrombocytopenia associated with lithium carbonate. *BMJ* 1992; **305:** 159.


**Effects on the cardiovascular system.** Reports of adverse effects on the heart associated with lithium have included bradycardia due to sinus node dysfunction,[1] which has persisted after stopping lithium,[2] premature ventricular contractions,[3] atrioventricular block,[4] and T-wave depression.[5] For the adverse cardiac effects associated with lithium intoxication, see under Overdosage, below.

For mention of myocarditis associated with lithium therapy, see under Effects on the Musculoskeletal System, below.


1. Montalescot G, *et al.* Serious sinus node dysfunction caused by therapeutic doses of lithium. *Int J Cardiol* 1984; **5:** 94–6.
2. Palileo EV, *et al.* Persistent sinus node dysfunction secondary to lithium therapy. *Am Heart J* 1983; **106:** 1443–4.
3. Tangedahl TN, Gau GT. Myocardial irritability associated with lithium carbonate therapy. *N Engl J Med* 1972; **287:** 867–9.
4. Martin CA, Piascik MT. First degree A-V block in patients on lithium carbonate. *Can J Psychiatry* 1985; **30:** 114–16.
5. Demers RG, Heninger GR. Electrocardiographic T-wave changes during lithium carbonate treatment. *JAMA* 1971; **218:**381–6.


**Effects on the endocrine system.** Although the published prevalence figures have varied widely there is a small, but definite, risk that patients taking lithium in therapeutic doses will develop clinical *goitre*, *hypothyroidism*, or, rarely, both; the risk appears to be greatest during the first 2 years of lithium therapy.[1] However, some authors[2] suggest that the incidence of clinical hypothyroidism is no more frequent in patients taking lithium than in the general population. Early goitre and lithium-induced hypothyroidism are both reversible if lithium is discontinued; if continued treatment with lithium is desirable the patient should be treated with levothyroxine.

There have been rare reports of *hyperthyroidism* in lithium-treated patients and the association may only be one of coincidence, although it is important to realise that hyperthyroidism can precipitate mania and can also be mistaken for an attack of mania.

*Increases in serum concentrations of calcium and parathyroid hormone* have been described in patients receiving lithium therapy. Although generally considered to be slight, some patients have experienced *parathyroid hyperplasia*.[3,4]

Cases of *diabetes mellitus* developing in patients treated with lithium have been reported but may not be attributable to lithium.[5]


1. Vincent A, *et al.* Lithium-associated hypothyroidism: a practical review. *Lithium* 1994; **5:** 73–4.
2. Bocchetta A, *et al.* Six-year follow-up of thyroid function during lithium treatment. *Acta Psychiatr Scand* 1996; **94:** 45–8.
3. Nordenström J, *et al.* Hyperparathyroidism associated with treatment of manic-depressive disorders by lithium. *Eur J Surg* 1992; **158:** 207–11.
4. Taylor JW, Bell AJ. Lithium-induced parathyroid dysfunction: a case report and review of the literature. *Ann Pharmacother* 1993; **27:** 1040–3.
5. Pandit MK, *et al.* Drug-induced disorders of glucose tolerance. *Ann Intern Med* 1993; **118:** 529–39.


**Effects on the eyes.** Decrease in accommodation has been reported in up to 10% of patients taking lithium but mainly younger patients are affected.[1] Blurred vision can also occur, most commonly early in therapy, but this may improve with time. Lithium can affect extra-ocular muscles and produce diplopia. A reduction in dosage or discontinuation of therapy may be required. It reduces lachrymal secretions and is excreted in tears in increased concentrations. In rare cases this may result in ocular irritation but this usually causes few problems when artificial tears are used. Photophobia, which occurs rarely with lithium therapy, may also be associated with the excretion of lithium in tears. Lithium can reduce dark adaptation due to a direct neural effect but whether this can progress further to cause irreversible macular or retinal degeneration is not proven. There are some rare but poorly documented reports of deposits in the cornea or conjunctiva. It was considered unlikely that lithium increased the risk of developing senile cataracts.

Lithium can cause nystagmus, many forms of which are reversible on reducing the dose or withdrawal of the drug. However, downbeat nystagmus is a serious adverse effect and is often irreversible. Irreversible oscillopsia can occur rarely secondary to nystagmus. Oculogyric crisis has been associated with lithium therapy and may be exacerbated by haloperidol.

Some ocular effects may be secondary to the effects of lithium on other systems. Exophthalmos and other thyroid-related eye disorders may occur rarely as a secondary effect of lithium on the thyroid. Lithium can also cause pseudotumour cerebri with papilloedema (benign intracranial hypertension). Most cases have occurred a few years after starting therapy but there has been a report of this condition after only 7 months of treatment. Ptosis has been reported, mainly associated with unmasking of myasthenia gravis.


1. Fraunfelder FT, *et al.* The effects of lithium on the human visual system. *J Toxicol Cutan Ocul Toxicol* 1992; **11:** 97–169.


**Effects on the kidneys.** Polyuria with associated polydipsia, due to drug-induced nephrogenic diabetes insipidus, is the most common result of the effects of lithium on the kidney; an early review[1] stated that the incidence ranged from 4 to 50%. In some patients, irreversible kidney damage, associated with renal histological changes that included tubular atrophy, focal interstitial nephropathy and focal fibrosis, and impairment of glomerular filtration rate, was reported. However, although patients on long-term maintenance lithium therapy did appear to be susceptible to the development of progressive impairment of urinary concentrating ability it was most noticeable in patients with a history of acute lithium toxicity. The risk of renal damage and impaired glomerular filtration rate was thought to be extremely small in patients on stable maintenance lithium therapy without prior episodes of acute lithium intoxication.[1]

A similar review considered that, although it was necessarily an oversimplified view, many, and perhaps all, of the renal side-effects of lithium were induced by excessive dosage.[2] Others have also defended lithium with respect to its renal toxicity and stated that long-term therapy, if properly controlled, does not necessarily lead to chronic or irreversible renal damage.[3-5]


1. Walker RG, Kincaid-Smith P. Kidneys and the fluid regulatory system. In: Johnson FN, ed. *Depression & mania: modern lithium therapy.* Oxford: IRL Press, 1987: 206–13.
2. George CRP. Renal aspects of lithium toxicity. *Med J Aust* 1989; **150:** 291–2.
3. Schou M. Serum lithium monitoring of prophylactic treatment: critical review and updated recommendations. *Clin Pharmacokinet* 1988; **15:** 283–6.
4. Schou M. Lithium treatment of manic-depressive illness: past, present, and perspectives. *JAMA* 1988; **259:** 1834–6.
5. Gitlin M. Lithium and the kidney: an updated review. *Drug Safety* 1999; **20:** 231–43.


**Effects on the musculoskeletal system.** The effects of lithium on skeletal muscle are represented mainly by varying degrees of weakness and tremor (for further details see under Effects on the Nervous and Neuromuscular Systems, below). Aggravation of myasthenia gravis has been reported. Acute or subacute painful proximal myopathy causing myalgia, cramps, myokymia, or weakness has also been described. An association with myocarditis has been proposed[1] but it is unclear whether this is causal.


1. Coulter DM, *et al.* Antipsychotic drugs and heart muscle disorder in international pharmacovigilance: data mining study. *BMJ* 2001; **322:** 1207–9.


**Effects on the nervous and neuromuscular systems.** Neurotoxicity has long been recognised as a potential adverse effect of lithium. Minor effects of lithium on the nervous system can be minimised by reduction of lithium dose during maintenance therapy but severe effects warrant immediate and complete withdrawal of the drug.[1] Minor effects have been considered to include impaired concentration, comprehension, and short-term memory, restlessness and anxiety, depression, fine rapid tremors, and easy fatigue. Serious or severe effects might include declining cognition and mental status, gait disturbances, movement disorders such as choreoathetosis, myoclonus, and parkinsonism, seizures, cerebellar signs, pseudotumour cerebri (although this was rare), neuroleptic malignant syndrome, myopathy, axonal neuropathy, a myasthenic syndrome, and exacerbation of underlying neuromuscular disease.

There are 2 types of lithium-induced tremor.[2] The first is a coarse tremor occurring with impending and actual lithium toxicity and appears to have both cerebellar and parkinsonian components. It is often associated with incoordination, facial spasms, twitching of muscles and limbs, hyperactive reflexes, and more general systemic signs of toxicity. With this type of tremor it was mandatory to stop or decrease the dose of lithium. The second type, which is more common, is a fine tremor, usually occurring within normal therapeutic concentrations, either transiently within a few days of starting treatment or later as a long-standing side-effect. With this type of fine tremor there was evidence to show that a slight decrease in dose may be beneficial.

In addition to the effects mentioned above, impairment of taste perception (mainly involving butter and celery)[3] and speech disturbances with few other signs of toxicity[4-7] have been reported.

For further details of the effects of lithium on the nervous system, see under Effects on the Eyes above, Effects on the Musculoskeletal System, above, and under Epileptogenic Effect, below.


1. Sansone ME, Ziegler DK. Brain and nervous system. In: Johnson FN, ed. *Depression & mania: modern lithium therapy.* Oxford: IRL Press, 1987: 240–5.
2. Johns S, Harris B. Tremor. *BMJ* 1984; **288:** 1309.
3. Himmelhoch JM, Hanin I. Side effects of lithium carbonate. *BMJ* 1974; **4:** 233.
4. Solomon K, Vickers R. Dysarthria resulting from lithium carbonate: a case report. *JAMA* 1975; **231:** 280.
5. Worrall EP, Gillham RA. Lithium-induced constructional dyspraxia. *BMJ* 1983; **286:** 189.
6. McGovern GP. Lithium induced constructional dyspraxia. *BMJ* 1983; **286:** 646.
7. Netski AL, Piasecki M. Lithium-induced exacerbation of stutter. *Ann Pharmacother* 2001; **35:** 961.


**Effects on respiration.** Lithium is not generally recognised as a respiratory depressant but an episode of reversible respiratory failure about 3 weeks after the start of lithium therapy has been described in a patient with stable chronic airways obstruction.[1] Recovery of consciousness and resolution of hypercapnia occurred within 24 to 36 hours of lithium discontinuation.

1. Weiner M, *et al.* Effect of lithium on the responses to added respiratory resistances. *N Engl J Med* 1983; **308:** 319–22.

**Effects on sexual function and fertility.** Lithium does not seem to interfere with sexual function in most patients, but there have been isolated reports of impotence and loss of libido attributed to lithium therapy.[1]

Studies *in vitro* have demonstrated that in concentrations comparable with those reported to be achieved in semen lithium can inhibit sperm motility,[2] but concentrations found in cervicovaginal mucus were considered unlikely to affect motility.[3]

1. Beeley L. Drug-induced sexual dysfunction and infertility. *Adverse Drug React Acute Poisoning Rev* 1984; **3:** 23–42.
2. Raoof NT, *et al.* Lithium inhibits human sperm motility in vitro. *Br J Clin Pharmacol* 1989; **28:** 715–17.
3. Salas IG, *et al.* Lithium carbonate concentration in cervico-vaginal mucus and serum after repeated oral dose administration. *Br J Clin Pharmacol* 1989; **28:** 751P.

**Effects on the skin and hair.** Patients taking lithium may develop skin disorders, though these are not necessarily serious or severe.[1,2] Although the onset varies from 2 or 3 weeks to 7 or more years, many reactions start to appear once optimal serum-lithium concentrations have been attained. Effects reported include psoriasis which may be severe and require lithium withdrawal. Seborrhoeic dermatitis and follicular keratosis are also encountered and can improve spontaneously or after stopping lithium. Acneform eruptions are found in areas not usually affected by acne vulgaris; in general the face is less affected or not affected at all.

Hair loss, not always severe, is more frequent than cutaneous effects. About 6% of patients may be affected and all kinds of alopecias have been found. The onset occurs several weeks or months after the start of lithium therapy. The hair usually regrows despite continuing therapy but in some cases regrowth only occurs after withdrawal of lithium. In a review[3] of the effects on the ocular system, loss of eyebrows and eyelashes was noted as a rare event. Hair loss due to lithium-induced hypothyroidism can be corrected by thyroid replacement therapy.

For references to the association of lithium with lupus, see under Lupus, below.

1. Lambert D, Dalac S. Skin, hair and nails. In: Johnson FN, ed. *Depression & mania: modern lithium therapy.* Oxford: IRL Press, 1987: 232–4.
2. Gupta AK, *et al.* Lithium therapy associated with hidradenitis suppurativa: case report and a review of the dermatologic side effects of lithium. *J Am Acad Dermatol* 1995; **32:** 382–6.
3. Fraunfelder FT, *et al.* The effects of lithium on the human visual system. *J Toxicol Cutan Ocul Toxicol* 1992; **11:** 97–169.

**Epileptogenic effect.** Seizures during lithium therapy usually indicate toxicity or impending toxicity. There have, however, been a few isolated reports describing seizures in patients with serum-lithium concentrations within the normally accepted therapeutic range.[1,2]

1. Demers R, *et al.* Convulsion during lithium therapy. *Lancet* 1970; **ii:** 315–16.
2. Massey EW, Folger WN. Seizures activated by therapeutic levels of lithium carbonate. *South Med J* 1984; **77:** 1173–5.

**Lupus.** Studies have found that antinuclear antibodies were more common in patients taking lithium carbonate than in controls.[1,2] The absence of anti-DNA antibodies indicated that they did not have true systemic lupus erythematosus but it was considered that patients ingesting lithium might be at risk. Dermatological manifestations of lupus together with antinuclear antibodies have been reported in a patient taking lithium.[3]

1. Johnstone EC, Whaley K. Antinuclear antibodies in psychiatric illness: their relationship to diagnosis and drug treatment. *BMJ* 1975; **2:** 724–5.
2. Presley AP, *et al.* Antinuclear antibodies in patients on lithium carbonate. *BMJ* 1976; **2:** 280–1.
3. Shukla VR, Borison RL. Lithium and lupuslike syndrome. *JAMA* 1982; **248:** 921–2.

**Overdosage.** Nausea, vomiting, and diarrhoea are common early features of lithium toxicity, and are followed by coarse tremor, increased muscle tone, cogwheel rigidity, fasciculation, and myoclonus.[1] Coma and convulsions may occur in serious cases and cardiac effects (first-degree heart block and QRS and QT prolongation) have been described rarely. A patient may appear to be aware with open eyes but have an expressionless face and be unable to move or speak (coma vigil). Acute renal failure and nephrogenic diabetes insipidus may develop.

One reviewer considered that the great majority of lithium intoxications reported had occurred in patients with renal impairment or in patients who had been given too high a dose.[2] The patient usually experiences a prodromal period of days to a few weeks with minor 'nervous' symptoms which are signs of a manifest slight intoxication. At an unpredictable point renal function starts to deteriorate and within hours or at the most within a few days, the patient will become severely intoxicated. By this point lithium should have been discontinued and efficient detoxification measures (see Treatment of Adverse Effects, below) instituted if the patient is to make a complete recovery.

Serum concentrations should be measured to ensure that values for lithium do not rise to levels associated with toxicity. Some patients may have concentrations considered to be toxic without showing any symptoms; unfortunately other patients may develop signs of toxicity at therapeutic serum concentrations.[3]

In acute overdosage[2] vomiting often occurs within an hour of ingestion due to the high concentration of lithium in the stomach, but significant amounts of lithium can still reach the systemic circulation. The typical clinical symptoms often appear after a latency period and gastrointestinal symptoms can re-appear at a later time. The symptoms of overdosage are reported to be mainly related to the alimentary and nervous systems and include abdominal pain, anorexia, nausea, and vomiting, occasionally mild diarrhoea, giddiness, tremor, ataxia, slurring speech, myoclonus, twitching, asthenia, and depression; renal symptoms have also been noted by some investigators. Again efficient detoxification procedures (see Treatment of Adverse Effects, below) should be instituted as rapidly as possible.

In a series of 28 patients with lithium self-poisoning or therapeutic intoxication many of the features and symptoms mentioned above were noted.[4] Other workers[5] have also reported cases which illustrate the differences between acute and chronic toxicity encountered clinically.

Other symptoms that have been noted in case reports of lithium intoxication in individual patients include photophobia,[6] acute polyarthritis involving several large joints,[7] severe hypertension,[8] deep venous thrombophlebitis,[9] reduction of central temperature,[10] and severe leucopenia.[11]

1. Proudfoot AT. Acute poisoning with antidepressants and lithium. *Prescribers' J* 1986; **26:** 97–106.
2. Amdisen A. Clinical features and management of lithium poisoning. *Med Toxicol* 1988; **3:** 18–32.
3. Stern R. Lithium in the treatment of mood disorders. *N Engl J Med* 1995; **332:** 127–8.
4. Dyson EH, *et al.* Self-poisoning and therapeutic intoxication with lithium. *Hum Toxicol* 1987; **6:** 325–9.
5. Ananth J, *et al.* Acute and chronic lithium toxicity: case reports and a review. *Lithium* 1992; **3:** 139–45.
6. Caplan RP, Fry AH. Photophobia in lithium intoxication. *BMJ* 1982; **285:** 1314–15.
7. Black DW, Waziri R. Arthritis associated with lithium toxicity: case report. *J Clin Psychiatry* 1984; **45:** 135–6.
8. Michaeli J, *et al.* Severe hypertension and lithium intoxication. *JAMA* 1984; **251:** 1680.
9. Lyles MR. Deep venous thrombophlebitis associated with lithium toxicity. *J Natl Med Assoc* 1984; **76:** 633–4.
10. Follézou J-Y, Bleibel J-M. Reduction of temperature and lithium poisoning. *N Engl J Med* 1985; **313:** 1609.
11. Green ST, Dunn FG. Severe leucopenia in fatal lithium poisoning. *BMJ* 1985; **290:** 517.

## Treatment of Adverse Effects

In recent acute overdosage with lithium, consideration should be given to emptying the stomach if ingestion has occurred within 1 hour of presentation. However gastric lavage may be of limited value following overdosage with modified-release preparations, which do not disintegrate in the stomach and may be too large to pass through a lavage tube. Activated charcoal is of no value. Whole bowel irrigation has been suggested although there do not appear to be clinical studies to confirm efficacy.

Further measures may involve procedures to enhance the renal clearance of lithium or its active removal. Adequate hydration should be ensured and any electrolyte imbalance corrected, but forced diuresis or diuretics are contra-indicated. Appropriate supportive care may include measures to control hypotension and convulsions. Maintenance of fluid and electrolyte balance is particularly important because of the risk of hypernatraemia. The ECG should be monitored in symptomatic patients.

In severe poisoning, haemodialysis is the treatment of choice (particularly if there is renal impairment). Although effective in reducing serum-lithium concentrations, substantial rebound increases can be expected when dialysis is stopped, and prolonged or repeated treatments may be required. Peritoneal dialysis is less effective and only appropriate if haemodialysis facilities are not available. Haemofiltration has been tried to good effect.

Serum lithium concentrations should be monitored regularly throughout treatment. Once the serum and dialysis fluid are free of lithium, it has been recommended that serum-lithium concentrations should be monitored for at least another week so that allowance can be made for delayed diffusion from body tissues.

As a result of the narrow margin between therapeutic and toxic serum concentrations, lithium poisoning may also develop during the course of therapy. In some instances temporary withdrawal of lithium therapy and giving generous amounts of sodium and fluid may be all that is required while adverse effects abate. In any serious or severe case of intoxication active measures such as dialysis and supportive measures outlined above may need to be instituted.

◊ References.

1. Smith SW, *et al.* Whole-bowel irrigation as a treatment for acute lithium overdose. *Ann Emerg Med* 1991; **20:** 536–9.
2. Okusa MD, *et al.* Clinical manifestations and management of acute lithium intoxication. *Am J Med* 1994; **97:** 383–9.
3. Swartz CM, Jones P. Hyperlithemia correction and persistent delirium. *J Clin Pharmacol* 1994; **34:** 865–70.
4. Tyrer SP. Lithium intoxication: appropriate treatment. *CNS Drugs* 1996; **6:** 426–39.

## Precautions

The margin between the therapeutic and the toxic concentration of lithium is narrow so therapy usually requires specialist advice, and serum concentrations should be monitored regularly under controlled conditions. Patients receiving lithium therapy should be taught to recognise the symptoms of early toxicity (see Adverse Effects, above) and, should these occur, to stop therapy and request medical aid at once. They should be warned not to compensate for an omitted dose by subsequently taking a double dose. Additionally, patients should not be switched between different formulations or preparations of lithium without therapeutic monitoring, as bioavailability may be different.

Lithium should be avoided in patients with cardiac disease or renal impairment; cardiac and renal function should be monitored regularly during treatment. It should also be avoided in Addison's disease or other conditions with a sodium imbalance and in severely debilitated or dehydrated patients.

Patients receiving lithium should be examined periodically for abnormal thyroid function, since goitre and hypothyroidism may develop. Lithium should be avoided in untreated hypothyroidism. Lithium should be used with caution in patients with myasthenia gravis because exacerbation of this disorder has been reported (see Effects on the Musculoskeletal System in Adverse Effects, above).

Lithium should be used with special care in the elderly since this group may be particularly susceptible to toxicity owing to reduced renal function.

Impaired driving performance or machine operating skills may occur in patients receiving lithium (see Driving, below).

It may be necessary to temporarily reduce or stop lithium therapy in patients suffering from vomiting, diarrhoea, excessive sweating, or any other condition that causes excessive sodium loss and hence increased serum-lithium concentrations. Conversely, increased sodium levels are likely to reduce serum-lithium concentrations. Patients taking lithium should therefore maintain an adequate fluid intake and should avoid increasing or decreasing sodium intake through dietary changes or ingestion of sodium-containing medicaments. Significant changes in caffeine intake may affect serum-lithium concentrations (see Xanthines under Interactions, below).

Lithium therapy should, where possible, be withdrawn slowly over a period of weeks to allay any concerns about relapse (see below).

The risks of using lithium in pregnant patients are described under Pregnancy, below. If lithium is used during pregnancy then dose adjustments will be required to compensate for the altered renal handling.

Lithium should be temporarily discontinued 24 hours before major surgery to safeguard the patient from accumulation (see under Anaesthesia, below).

**Anaesthesia.** The *British National Formulary* states that lithium should be stopped 24 hours before major surgery, but the normal dose can be continued for minor surgery if fluids and electrolytes are carefully monitored.

There is no clinical evidence of interaction between lithium and anaesthetics, although lithium may prolong the action of neuromuscular blockers.[1] Lithium may accumulate because of reduced renal clearance associated with anaesthesia; treatment should be resumed as soon as possible after surgery, when kidney function and fluid-electrolyte balance have become normal. Patients are often not allowed fluids or foods by mouth the night before surgery but patients with lithium-induced polyuria should be given fluids parenterally during the night before the operation, if they vomit copiously, or if they are unconscious for several hours.

1. Schou M, Hippus H. Guidelines for patients receiving lithium treatment who require major surgery. *Br J Anaesth* 1987; **59:** 809–10.

**Breast feeding.** Lithium is distributed into breast milk. Early reports suggested that serum concentrations in breast-fed infants were approximately one-third to one-half of those measured in mothers.[1] However, advice regarding the decision to breast feed remains equivocal. The American Academy of Pediatrics[2] considers that lithium should be given with caution to breast-feeding women but does not contra-indicate such use, and this is supported by some authors.[3,4] Conversely, most manufacturers in the UK and other authors[5,6] suggest that mothers receiving lithium should bottle feed their infants. It has been recommended[5] that if a mother did want to breast feed this should be done at times to avoid peak blood concentrations of lithium and the infant carefully monitored. Medication should be withheld or breast feeding stopped if the infant developed an infection or dehydration as they would be more susceptible to the adverse effects of lithium.

1. Schou M, Amdisen A. Lithium and pregnancy—III, lithium ingestion by children breast-fed by women on lithium treatment. *BMJ* 1973; **2:** 138.
2. American Academy of Pediatrics. The transfer of drugs and other chemicals into human milk. *Pediatrics* 2001; **108:** 776–89. Correction. *ibid.*; 1029. Also available at: http://aappolicy.aappublications.org/cgi/content/full/pediatrics%3b108/3/776 (accessed 11/06/04)
3. Schou M. Lithium treatment during pregnancy, delivery, and lactation: an update. *J Clin Psychiatry* 1990; **51:** 410–13.
4. Sykes PA, *et al.* Lithium carbonate and breast-feeding. *BMJ* 1976; **2:** 1299.
5. Ananth J. Lithium during pregnancy and lactation. *Lithium* 1993; **4:** 231–7.
6. Llewellyn A, *et al.* The use of lithium and management of women with bipolar disorder during pregnancy and lactation. *J Clin Psychiatry* 1998; **59** (suppl 6): 57–64.

**Cystic fibrosis.** Reduced renal excretion of lithium was demonstrated in 8 patients with cystic fibrosis compared with healthy subjects.[1] The authors recommended caution when prescribing standard doses of lithium to patients with cystic fibrosis until more definitive data were available.

1. Brager NPD, *et al.* Reduced renal fractional excretion of lithium in cystic fibrosis. *Br J Clin Pharmacol* 1996; **41:** 157–9.

**Driving.** In the UK, the Driver and Vehicle Licensing Authority considers that patients with severe depressive illnesses complicated by significant memory or concentration problems, agitation, behavioural disturbances or suicidal thoughts should cease driving pending the outcome of medical enquiry.[1] Mania or hypomania is particularly dangerous and may require a longer period off driving if the illness cycles rapidly.

Treatment with antidepressant drugs, including lithium, may also be hazardous,[2] although patients may be safer drivers with medication than without.[3] Lithium has been reported[2] to adversely affect the choice reaction time (a test to assess the time taken to respond correctly to some signals but not others) to a level considered dangerous for driving.

1. Driver and Vehicle Licensing Agency. For medical practitioners: at a glance guide to the current medical standards of fitness to drive. Available at: http://www.dvla.gov.uk/at_a_glance/ch4_psychiatric.htm (accessed 11/06/04)
2. Ashton H. Drugs and driving. *Adverse Drug React Bull* 1983; **98:** 360–3.
3. Cremona A. Mad drivers: psychiatric illness and driving performance. *Br J Hosp Med* 1986; **35:** 193–5.

**Pregnancy.** Case reports of mothers taking lithium during pregnancy pointed to an increased risk of congenital abnormalities with the heart being mainly affected.[1] Support for this increased risk came from a study[2] of the records of 59 children born to women who had taken lithium during pregnancy. However, a later study[3] prospectively followed 138 pregnant women being treated with lithium and did not identify any difference in pregnancy outcome between them and a control group. The authors considered that lithium was not a major teratogen and felt that women with major affective disorders could continue lithium treatment during pregnancy provided that adequate fetal screening tests were carried out. A subsequent review[4] considered that the teratogenic risk was lower than previously thought, but that it would still be wise for women who wished to become pregnant to discontinue lithium if at all possible, at least during the period of embryogenesis.

There is limited evidence that lithium treatment during pregnancy may increase the risk of fetal macrosomia, premature delivery, and perinatal mortality.[1,5]

The renal clearance of lithium by the mother is not constant during pregnancy; in the second half of the pregnancy clearance rises gradually by 30 to 50% but falls abruptly and significantly after delivery to pre-pregnancy values.[1,6] The increased doses of lithium that may be given during pregnancy to compensate for this increased clearance may result in lithium toxicity.[6] It is generally considered[1,7] advisable to stop lithium during the last few days of pregnancy to reduce the risk of maternal lithium toxicity due to accumulation of lithium but it should be started again a few days later after delivery at reduced dosage because of the increased postpartum risk of manic and depressive relapse.[1] Polyhydramnios (an excess of amniotic fluid) in the last trimester of pregnancy has been reported and has been attributed to fetal lithium toxicity (polyuria and diabetes insipidus).[8,9]

Reducing the dosage during the last few days of pregnancy also helps to reduce lithium concentrations in the neonate and avoid associated adverse effects.[1,7] Adverse effects that have been reported in neonates exposed *in utero* to lithium include cyanosis, lethargy, flaccidity, hypotonia, poor gag and sucking reflexes, feeding problems, bradycardia, tachycardia, goitre, hypothyroidism, nephrogenic diabetes, and jaundice;[7] withdrawal symptoms have also been observed.

1. Schou M. Lithium treatment during pregnancy, delivery, and lactation: an update. *J Clin Psychiatry* 1990; **51:** 410–13.
2. Källén B, Tandberg A. Lithium and pregnancy: a cohort study on manic-depressive women. *Acta Psychiatr Scand* 1983; **68:** 134–9.
3. Jacobson SJ, *et al.* Prospective multicentre study of pregnancy outcome after lithium exposure during first trimester. *Lancet* 1992; **339:** 530–3.
4. Cohen LS, *et al.* A reevaluation of risk of in utero exposure to lithium. *JAMA* 1994; **271:** 146–50.
5. Troyer WA, *et al.* Association of maternal lithium exposure and premature delivery. *J Perinatol* 1993; **XIII:** 123–7.
6. Lemoine J-M. Pregnancy, delivery and lactation. In: Johnson FN, ed. *Depression & mania: modern lithium therapy.* Oxford: IRL Press, 1987: 139–46.
7. Ananth J. Lithium during pregnancy and lactation. *Lithium* 1993; **4:** 231–7.
8. Krause S, *et al.* Polyhydramnios with maternal lithium treatment. *Obstet Gynecol* 1990; **75:** 504–6.
9. Ang MS, *et al.* Maternal lithium therapy and polyhydramnios. *Obstet Gynecol* 1990; **76:** 517–19.

**Surgery.** For comments regarding the precautions to be observed in patients undergoing surgery, see under Anaesthesia, above.

**Withdrawal.** A withdrawal syndrome consisting of symptoms such as anxiety, tremor, fatigue, nausea, sweating, headache, sleep disturbances, diarrhoea, or blurred vision, usually develops within days of sudden cessation of treatment with lithium.[1] These may simply be a recurrence of symptoms of mood change. Uncontrolled studies of withdrawal symptoms have raised the possibility of a lithium-withdrawal state but controlled studies have been convincingly negative. It is, however, wise to reduce lithium dosage gradually rather than stop high-dosage treatment abruptly.

A frequent worry associated with stopping lithium therapy is that of relapse. Most evidence has supported the view that any relapses occurring in the first weeks after lithium withdrawal are simply part of a pattern of recurrence of bipolar disorder in general and are not indicative of a higher rate of recurrence. Some,[2] however, have found the proportion of patients relapsing on sudden withdrawal of lithium therapy to be 50%, a figure they consider to be too high to be accounted for by the natural history of the disease process. They and others[3] advise that this risk should be considered when prescribing lithium for bipolar disorder. In patients who previously had been stable on lithium for at least 18 months, the risk of early recurrence of bipolar disorder was higher when therapy was withdrawn rapidly in less than 2 weeks than when it was withdrawn gradually over 2 to 4 weeks.[4]

1. Goodnick PJ. Terminating treatment. In: Johnson FN, ed. *Depression & mania: modern lithium therapy.* Oxford: IRL Press, 1987: 115–17.
2. Mander AJ, Loudon JB. Rapid recurrence of mania following abrupt discontinuation of lithium. *Lancet* 1988; **ii:** 15–17.
3. Goodwin GM. Recurrence of mania after lithium withdrawal. *Br J Psychiatry* 1994; **164:** 149–52.
4. Faedda GL, *et al.* Outcome after rapid vs gradual discontinuation of lithium treatment in bipolar disorders. *Arch Gen Psychiatry* 1993; **50:** 448–55.

## Interactions

Some diuretics may reduce lithium excretion and result in toxicity (see below for further details). Thiazide diuretics may also show a paradoxical antidiuretic effect. Consequently diuretics should be avoided or used with great caution in those receiving lithium. Further interactions reported with lithium are discussed below.

◊ Reviews of drug interactions with lithium.

1. Amdisen A. Lithium and drug interactions. *Drugs* 1982; **24:** 133–9.
2. Beeley L. Drug interactions with lithium. *Prescribers' J* 1986; **26:** 160–2.
3. Harvey NS, Merriman S. Review of clinically important drug interactions with lithium. *Drug Safety* 1994; **10:** 455–63.
4. Finley PR, *et al.* Clinical relevance of drug interactions with lithium. *Clin Pharmacokinet* 1995; **29:** 172–91.

**ACE inhibitors.** Giving lithium with ACE inhibitors has been reported[1-5] to increase serum-lithium concentrations. ACE inhibitors such as *captopril*,[2] *enalapril*,[1,3,5] and *lisinopril*[4,5] have been implicated, although in a study[6] of enalapril and lithium in healthy subjects, the lithium levels remained unchanged. The mechanism is unclear but it has been suggested[7] that suppression of the renin-angiotensin-aldosterone system by ACE inhibitors may be responsible. Lithium excretion by the kidney is dependent on both glomerular filtration and sodium concentration in the proximal tubule, both of which are reduced by ACE inhibitors. It has also been suggested[5] that inhibition of angiotensin II production may lead to reduced fluid intake through lack of activation of the thirst stimulus and this would enhance the tendency to volume depletion caused by natriuresis. Patients considered[7] to be at risk from this reaction would include those whose renal function is largely dependent on the effect of angiotensin II, those with congestive heart failure, and those with volume depletion.

1. Douste-Blazy P, *et al.* Angiotensin converting enzyme inhibitors and lithium treatment. *Lancet* 1986; **i:** 1448.
2. Pulik M, Lida H. Interaction lithium-inhibiteurs de l'enzyme de conversion. *Presse Med* 1988; **17:** 755.
3. Navis GJ, *et al.* Volume homeostasis, angiotensin converting enzyme inhibition, and lithium therapy. *Am J Med* 1989; **86:** 621.
4. Baldwin CM, Safferman AZ. A case of lisinopril-induced lithium toxicity. *DICP Ann Pharmacother* 1990; **24:** 946–7.
5. Correa FJ, Eiser AR. Angiotensin-converting enzyme inhibitors and lithium toxicity. *Am J Med* 1992; **93:** 108–9.
6. DasGupta K, *et al.* The effect of enalapril on serum lithium levels in healthy men. *J Clin Psychiatry* 1992; **53:** 398–400.
7. Mignat C, Unger T. Ace inhibitors: drug interactions of clinical significance. *Drug Safety* 1995; **12:** 334–47.

**Analgesics.** See NSAIDs and opioid analgesics, below.

**Angiotensin II receptor antagonists.** There have been case reports of lithium intoxication occurring in patients following the addition of *candesartan*,[1] *losartan*,[2] or *valsartan*[3] to their therapy. The mechanism may be similar to that for ACE inhibitors (above).

1. Zwanzger P, *et al.*. Lithium intoxication after administration of $AT_1$ blockers. *J Clin Psychiatry* 2001; **62:** 208–9.
2. Blanche P, *et al.* Lithium intoxication in an elderly patient after combined treatment with losartan. *Eur J Clin Pharmacol* 1997; **52:** 501.
3. Leung M, Remick RA. Potential drug interaction between lithium and valsartan. *J Clin Psychopharmacol* 2000; **20:** 392–3.

**Antidepressants.** Lithium has been used to augment the effect of other antidepressants in refractory depression. However, there have been reports of adverse reactions with some of these combinations. For further details, see Antidepressants under Interactions of Phenelzine, p.315.

**Antiepileptics.** Severe CNS toxicity despite 'normal' serum-lithium concentrations has been described in a patient also taking *phenytoin* together with *phenobarbital*.[1] Symptoms indicative of lithium toxicity have also been reported in a patient taking it with *phenytoin* alone;[2] again concentrations were not abnormal.

For reports of neurotoxicity in patients receiving *carbamazepine* and lithium, see p.356. Carbamazepine-induced renal failure has also resulted in toxic serum-lithium concentrations.[3]

1. Speirs J, Hirsch SR. Severe lithium toxicity with "normal" serum concentrations. *BMJ* 1978; **1:** 815–16.
2. MacCallum WAG. Interaction of lithium and phenytoin. *BMJ* 1980; **280:** 610–11.
3. Mayan H, *et al.* Lithium intoxication due to carbamazepine-induced renal failure. *Ann Pharmacother* 2001; **35:** 560–2.

**Antimicrobials.** Lithium toxicity has been reported on isolated occasions in patients receiving *metronidazole*,[1] *spectinomycin*,[2] and *tetracycline*.[3]

However, it has been noted that lithium and tetracycline have been used together without serious problems in many patients and that additionally tetracycline has been used to treat the acneform skin eruptions induced by lithium.[4] These same authors investigating healthy subjects found that lithium concentrations were decreased, rather than increased, following the addition of tetracycline but considered this was probably of no clinical significance.

1. Teicher MH, *et al.* Possible nephrotoxic interaction of lithium and metronidazole. *JAMA* 1987; **257:** 3365–6.
2. Anonymous. Possible adverse drug-drug interaction report: lithium intoxication in a spectinomycin-treated patient. *Int Drug Ther Newslett* 1978; **13:** 15.
3. McGennis AJ. Lithium carbonate and tetracycline interaction. *BMJ* 1978; **1:** 1183.
4. Fankhauser MP, *et al.* Evaluation of lithium-tetracycline interaction. *Clin Pharm* 1988; **7:** 314–17.

**Antimigraine drugs.** For comment on the suggestion that there may be a risk of increased CNS toxicity when *sumatriptan* and lithium are given together, see p.472.

**Antineoplastics.** Transient decreases in serum-lithium concentration occurred in a patient given *cisplatin*.[1] The relative contributions of cisplatin itself, or the fluid loading procedure involving intravenous fluids and mannitol, or their combined effects were unclear. The interaction, however, had no apparent clinical significance in this patient although a risk of undertreatment with lithium may occur in other patients.

1. Pietruszka LJ, *et al.* Evaluation of cisplatin-lithium interaction. *Drug Intell Clin Pharm* 1985; **19:** 31–2.

**Antipsychotics and anxiolytics.** In the control of acute mania lithium is often too slow in onset to be used alone and therefore additional therapy with an antipsychotic may be necessary. It should be noted, however, that such combinations should be used with care as interactions and adverse reactions have occurred.

The renal excretion of lithium is increased by *chlorpromazine* treatment,[1] which means that subsequent withdrawal of chlorpromazine can result in an abrupt rise in serum-lithium concentrations.[2] The serum concentration of chlorpromazine can also be reduced by lithium,[3] and chlorpromazine toxicity may be precipitated by the abrupt withdrawal of lithium in patients previously stabilised on the two drugs together. Ventricular fibrillation has been described following withdrawal of lithium in a patient concurrently taking chlorpromazine;[4] it was suggested that the chlorpromazine dose should be reduced if lithium is to be stopped.

There have been isolated reports of neurotoxicity or brain damage, characterised by delirium, seizures, encephalopathy, or an increased incidence of extrapyramidal symptoms in patients receiving lithium with *flupentixol decanoate*,[5] *fluphenazine decanoate*,[6] or high-dose *haloperidol*,[7-9] although two earlier retrospective studies of patients taking lithium with antipsychotics had failed to detect such adverse reactions.[10,11] Neurological reactions have continued to be reported in patients receiving lithium with *thioridazine*,[12,13] *sulpiride*,[14] *clozapine*,[15] and *risperidone*.[16] Although a causal relationship between these events and use of lithium with antipsychotics has not been fully established, patients should be monitored for signs of neurotoxicity if receiving such combinations.

It has been noted that the neurotoxicity induced by lithium and antipsychotics was a rare entity.[17] Whether the combination produced any greater risk than either drug alone, and whether the neurotoxicity was a distinct diagnostic entity or simply represented atypical cases of lithium toxicity or the neuroleptic malignant syndrome, was debatable. The interaction between lithium and haloperidol might represent a form of neuroleptic malignant syndrome and that between lithium and the phenothiazines, especially thioridazine, a form of lithium toxicity. It was concluded that the risk from combination therapy was very small but that the clinician should, nevertheless, be aware of it.

Although lithium has been reported to interact with *diazepam* resulting in hypothermic episodes,[18] some authors[17] considered that this was more likely to be an idiosyncratic response rather than a true drug interaction; in general it was considered quite safe to use lithium and benzodiazepines in combination.

1. Sletten I, *et al.* The effect of chlorpromazine on lithium excretion in psychiatric subjects. *Curr Ther Res* 1966; **8:** 441–6.
2. Pakes GE. Lithium toxicity with phenothiazine withdrawal. *Lancet* 1979; **ii:** 701.
3. Rivera-Calimlim L, *et al.* Effect of lithium on plasma chlorpromazine levels. *Clin Pharmacol Ther* 1978; **23:** 451–5.
4. Stevenson RN, *et al.* Ventricular fibrillation due to lithium withdrawal—an interaction with chlorpromazine? *Postgrad Med J* 1989; **65:** 936–8.
5. West A. Adverse effects of lithium treatment. *BMJ* 1977; **2:** 642.
6. Singh SV. Lithium carbonate/fluphenazine decanoate producing irreversible brain damage. *Lancet* 1982; **ii:** 278.
7. Cohen WJ, Cohen NH. Lithium carbonate, haloperidol, and irreversible brain damage. *JAMA* 1974; **230:** 1283–7.
8. Loudon JB, Waring H. Toxic reactions to lithium and haloperidol. *Lancet* 1976; **ii:** 1088.
9. Thomas C, *et al.* Lithium/haloperidol combinations and brain damage. *Lancet* 1982; **i:** 626.
10. Baastrup PC, *et al.* Adverse reactions in treatment with lithium carbonate and haloperidol. *JAMA* 1976; **236:** 2645–6.
11. Prakash R. Lithium-haloperidol combination and brain damage. *Lancet* 1982; **i:** 1468–9.
12. Standish-Barry HMAS, Shelly MA. Toxic neurological reaction to lithium/thioridazine. *Lancet* 1983; **i:** 771.
13. Cantor CH. Encephalopathy with lithium and thioridazine in combination. *Med J Aust* 1986; **144:** 164–5.
14. Dinan TG, O'Keane V. Acute extrapyramidal reactions following lithium and sulpiride co-administration: two case reports. *Hum Psychopharmacol Clin Exp* 1991; **6:** 67–9.
15. Blake LM, *et al.* Reversible neurologic symptoms with clozapine and lithium. *J Clin Psychopharmacol* 1992; **12:** 297–9.
16. Swanson CL, *et al.* Effects of concomitant risperidone and lithium treatment. *Am J Psychiatry* 1995; **152:** 1096.
17. Ross DR, Coffey CE. Neuroleptics and anti-anxiety agents. In: Johnson FN, ed. *Depression & mania: modern lithium therapy.* Oxford: IRL Press, 1987: 167–71.
18. Naylor GJ, McHarg A. Profound hypothermia on combined lithium carbonate and diazepam treatment. *BMJ* 1977; **2:** 22.

**Benzodiazepines.** See Antipsychotics and Anxiolytics, above.

**Calcium-channel blockers.** Neurotoxicity has been reported in a patient receiving lithium following the addition of *verapamil*.[1] Serum-lithium concentrations were still inside the accepted therapeutic range and it was considered that the similar actions of lithium and verapamil on neurosecretory processes may have been responsible. Verapamil has also been reported to decrease serum-lithium concentrations.[2] Neurotoxicity has also been reported in a patient receiving lithium and *diltiazem*[3] as well as other drugs. Psychosis, possibly induced by the use of diltiazem and lithium together, has been reported in another patient.[4]

1. Price WA, Giannini AJ. Neurotoxicity caused by lithium-verapamil synergism. *J Clin Pharmacol* 1986; **26:** 717–19.
2. Weinrauch LA, *et al.* Decreased serum lithium during verapamil therapy. *Am Heart J* 1984; **108:** 1378–80.
3. Valdiserri EV. A possible interaction between lithium and diltiazem: case report. *J Clin Psychiatry* 1985; **46:** 540–1.
4. Binder EF, *et al.* Diltiazem-induced psychosis and a possible diltiazem-lithium interaction. *Arch Intern Med* 1991; **151:** 373–4.

**Central stimulants.** There is a report of a woman who had been stabilised on lithium treatment for 15 months developing lithium toxicity within a few days of being given *mazindol*.[1]

There is a risk of CNS toxicity due to synergistic serotonergic actions when lithium is given with *sibutramine*.

1. Hendy MS, *et al.* Mazindol-induced lithium toxicity. *BMJ* 1980; **280:** 684–5.

**Diuretics.** *Thiazide diuretics* produce sodium depletion by inhibiting distal tubular sodium reabsorption. The consequent increase in proximal tubular reabsorption frequently results in an increase in serum-lithium concentrations.[1] Patients who are stabilised on lithium therapy and begin taking thiazide diuretics are at significant risk of developing lithium toxicity. Toxic lithium concentrations may be seen within 3 to 5 days of diuretic initiation. *Loop diuretics* (*furosemide, bumetanide,* and *etacrynic acid*) seem less likely to cause lithium retention, although caution is warranted, especially with patients in whom dietary sodium is restricted.[1] *Amiloride*, and probably other potassium-sparing diuretics, have no effect on lithium excretion, but *acetazolamide* increases lithium excretion. However, the diuretic action of acetazolamide is short-lived and the interaction may therefore be transient.[1]

It has therefore been suggested that if diuretic therapy is necessary in patients stabilised on lithium, the lithium dose should be reduced by 25 to 50%,[1,2] lithium concentrations measured twice weekly until re-stabilisation occurs, and that perhaps loop diuretics such as bumetanide or furosemide would be preferable.

The topic of lithium-diuretic interaction and precautions to be observed has also been discussed.[3]

1. Beeley L. Drug interactions with lithium. *Prescribers' J* 1986; **26:** 160–3.
2. Ramsay LE. Interactions that matter: diuretics and antihypertensive drugs. *Prescribers' J* 1984; **24:** 60–5.
3. Grau E. Diuretics. In: Johnson FN, ed. *Depression & mania: modern lithium therapy.* Oxford: IRL Press, 1987: 180–3.

**Gastrointestinal drugs.** Giving *sodium bicarbonate* with lithium has led to reduced blood-lithium concentrations, attributed to increased renal excretion of the lithium cation in response to the extra load of bicarbonate anion to be excreted.[1] *Antacids* containing combinations of *aluminium and magnesium hydroxides* and *simeticone* had no effect on the dissolution and solubility of lithium carbonate *in vitro*[2] nor on its bioavailability *in vivo*.[3]

There has been a case report describing a possible interaction between lithium and *ispaghula* where low serum concentrations of lithium may have been due to ispaghula inhibiting intestinal absorption of lithium.[4]

There is an increased risk of extrapyramidal effects and the possibility of neurotoxicity when drugs such as *metoclopramide* are given to patients receiving lithium.

Concomitant use of *cisapride* and lithium may increase the risk of ventricular arrhythmias.

1. McSwiggan C. A significant drug interaction. *Aust J Pharm* 1978; **59:** 6.
2. Schiessler DM, *et al.* Effect of antacids on lithium carbonate dissolution and solubility in vitro. *Am J Hosp Pharm* 1983; **40:** 825–8.
3. Goode DL, *et al.* Effect of antacid on the bioavailability of lithium carbonate. *Clin Pharm* 1984; **3:** 284–7.
4. Perlman BB. Interaction between lithium salts and ispaghula husk. *Lancet* 1990; **335:** 416.

**Methyldopa.** Lithium toxicity induced by methyldopa has been described on a number of occasions.[1-3] Symptoms of toxicity may occur even though serum-lithium concentrations remain within the therapeutic range.

1. Byrd GJ. Methyldopa and lithium carbonate: suspected interaction. *JAMA* 1975; **233:** 320.
2. O'Regan JB. Adverse interaction of lithium carbonate and methyldopa. *Can Med Assoc J* 1976; **115:** 385–6.
3. Osanloo E, Deglin JH. Interaction of lithium and methyldopa. *Ann Intern Med* 1980; **92:** 433–4.

**Muscle relaxants.** For reports of hypothermic episodes occurring with lithium and *diazepam* see under Antipsychotics and Anxiolytics, above.

Severe aggravation of hyperkinetic symptoms occurred in 2 patients with Huntington's chorea when *baclofen* was added to their treatment with lithium and haloperidol.[1]

1. Andén N-E, *et al.* Baclofen and lithium in Huntington's chorea. *Lancet* 1973; **ii:** 93.

**Neuromuscular blockers.** For reports of prolongation of neuromuscular blockade by lithium see under Atracurium, p.1401. For further comments relating to surgery and anaesthesia, see under Anaesthesia in Precautions, above.

**NSAIDs.** Decreased clearance and increased serum concentrations of lithium, resulting in toxicity on some occasions, have been reported after use of lithium with *celecoxib*,[1] *diclofenac*,[2] *ibuprofen*,[3,4] *indometacin*,[5,6] *ketorolac*,[7,8] *mefenamic acid*,[9,10] *naproxen*,[11] *piroxicam*,[12,13] *rofecoxib*,[14,15] and *tiaprofenic acid*;[16] secondary sources have also implicated *azapropazone, ketoprofen*,[17] and *phenylbutazone*.[17] However, serum-lithium concentration is not increased by *sulindac*.[11,18,19] Although serum-lithium concentrations were increased in one patient receiving *aspirin*[20] this has not been substantiated in others and an interaction is considered unlikely;[6,21] it has also been pointed out that control of sodium balance is necessary in such studies[21] and in the report purporting to demonstrate an interaction the diet had not been controlled.

It has been stated that for mild occasional aches, pains, and fever paracetamol was the preferred analgesic in patients receiving lithium, although occasional doses of aspirin were acceptable.[17] Sulindac appeared to be the safest NSAID for long-term use. Diclofenac, ibuprofen, indometacin, ketoprofen, naproxen, phenylbutazone, and piroxicam should be avoided where possible but if it was necessary to use one of these drugs the maintenance dose of lithium should be reduced. It was also considered that perhaps other NSAIDs, for which no information was available at that time, should be regarded as having the potential to cause a rise in serum-lithium concentrations.

1. Slørdal L, *et al.* A life-threatening interaction between lithium and celecoxib. *Br J Clin Pharmacol* 2003; **55:** 413–14.
2. Reimann IW, Frölich JC. Effects of diclofenac on lithium kinetics. *Clin Pharmacol Ther* 1981; **30:** 348–52.
3. Kristoff CA, *et al.* Effect of ibuprofen on lithium plasma and red blood cell concentrations. *Clin Pharm* 1986; **5:** 51–5.
4. Ragheb M. Ibuprofen can increase serum lithium level in lithium-treated patients. *J Clin Psychiatry* 1987; **48:** 161–3.
5. Frölich JC, *et al.* Indomethacin increases plasma lithium. *BMJ* 1979; **1:** 1115–16.
6. Reimann IW, *et al.* Indomethacin but not aspirin increases plasma lithium ion levels. *Arch Gen Psychiatry* 1983; **40:** 283–6.
7. Langlois R, Paquette D. Increased serum lithium levels due to ketorolac therapy. *Can Med Assoc J* 1994; **150:** 1455–6.
8. Iyer V. Ketorolac (Toradol®) induced lithium toxicity. *Headache* 1994; **34:** 442–4.
9. Shelley RK. Lithium toxicity and mefenamic acid: a possible interaction and the role of prostaglandin inhibition. *Br J Psychiatry* 1987; **151:** 847–8.
10. MacDonald J, Neale TJ. Toxic interaction of lithium carbonate and mefenamic acid. *BMJ* 1988; **297:** 1339.
11. Ragheb M, Powell AL. Lithium interaction with sulindac and naproxen. *J Clin Psychopharmacol* 1986; **6:** 150–4.
12. Kerry RJ, *et al.* Possible toxic interaction between lithium and piroxicam. *Lancet* 1983; **i:** 418–19.
13. Walbridge DG, Bazire SR. An interaction between lithium carbonate and piroxicam presenting as lithium toxicity. *Br J Psychiatry* 1985; **147:** 206–7.
14. Sajbel TA, *et al.* Pharmacokinetic effects of rofecoxib therapy on lithium. *Pharmacotherapy* 2001; **21:** 380.
15. Lundmark J, *et al.* A possible interaction between lithium and rofecoxib. *J Clin Pharmacol* 2002; **53:** 403–4.
16. Alderman CP, Lindsay KSW. Increased serum lithium concentration secondary to treatment with tiaprofenic acid and fosinopril. *Ann Pharmacother* 1996; **30:** 1411–3.
17. Furnell MM. Non-steroidal anti-inflammatory drugs. In: Johnson FN, ed. *Depression & mania: modern lithium therapy.* Oxford: IRL Press, 1987: 183–6.
18. Furnell MM, Davies J. The effect of sulindac on lithium therapy. *Drug Intell Clin Pharm* 1985; **19:** 374–6.
19. Ragheb MA, Powell AL. Failure of sulindac to increase serum lithium levels. *J Clin Psychiatry* 1986; **47:** 33–4.
20. Bendz H, Feinberg M. Aspirin increases serum lithium ion levels. *Arch Gen Psychiatry* 1984; **41:** 310–11.
21. Reimann I. Aspirin increases serum lithium ion levels. *Arch Gen Psychiatry* 1984; **41:** 311.

**Opioid analgesics.** There is a risk of CNS toxicity due to synergistic serotonergic actions when lithium is given with *tramadol*.

**Parasympathomimetics.** For the effect of lithium on parasympathomimetics, see Interactions, p.1492.

**Xanthines.** It has been reported[1] that *theophylline* enhances the renal clearance of lithium, thus tending to reduce serum-lithium concentrations. Lithium blood concentrations increased by 24% when *caffeine* was eliminated from the diet of 11 patients taking lithium.[2] No toxicity was observed but these patients had been maintained on low baseline lithium concentrations; toxicity might occur in patients maintained at higher concentrations.

1. Cook BL, *et al.* Theophylline-lithium interaction. *J Clin Psychiatry* 1985; **46:** 278–9.
2. Mester R, *et al.* Caffeine withdrawal increases lithium blood levels. *Biol Psychiatry* 1995; **37:** 348–50.

## Pharmacokinetics

Lithium is readily and completely absorbed from the gastrointestinal tract when taken as one of its salts. Absorption can be affected by the formulation of the preparation taken. Peak serum concentrations are obtained between 0.5 and 3 hours after ingestion from conventional tablets or capsules; following modified-release formulations peak concentrations are delayed and may occur between 2 and 12 hours after a dose. Lithium is distributed throughout the body and distribution is complete within about 6 to 10 hours; higher concentrations occur in the bones, the thyroid gland, and portions of the brain, than in the serum.

Lithium is excreted mainly in the urine; only a small amount can be detected in the faeces, saliva, and sweat. It is not bound to plasma proteins. It crosses the placenta and is distributed into breast milk. The elimination half-life in patients with normal renal function is about 20 to 24 hours, but increases with decreasing renal function; half-lives of up to 36 hours have been reported for elderly patients and 40 to 50 hours for patients with renal impairment. Steady-state concentrations may not, therefore, be attained until 4 to 7 days after starting treatment.

There is wide intersubject variation in the serum concentrations obtained following a given dose, and also in those required for therapeutic effect. Concentrations also vary considerably according to factors such as the dosage regimen (whether given in single or divided daily doses), renal function, the dietary regimen of the patient, the patient's state of health, the time at which the blood sample is taken, and other medication, such as sodium salts or diuretics, as well as by formulation and bioavailability. Moreover, there is only a narrow margin between the therapeutic and the toxic serum concentration of lithium. Therefore, not only is individual titration of lithium dosage essential to ensure constant appropriate concentrations for the patient, but the conditions under which the blood samples are taken for monitoring must be carefully controlled. In practice, a blood sample drawn 12 hours after the last dose of lithium following a consistent dosing schedule for 4 to 7 days is used for measurement of serum-lithium concentrations. Under these conditions the distribution of the last dose of lithium is complete, and steady-state concentrations will have been attained. The usual maintenance therapeutic serum concentrations of lithium are 0.4 to 1 mmol/litre; toxic effects may be expected at concentrations exceeding 1.5 mmol/litre. For further details regarding monitoring of serum concentrations of lithium, see under Uses and Administration, below. Estimation of lithium concentrations in other body fluids such as saliva has been investigated as a less invasive method of monitoring. However, results have been equivocal and these methods have not replaced serum monitoring in general practice.

◊ References.


1. Ward ME, *et al.* Clinical pharmacokinetics of lithium. *J Clin Pharmacol* 1994; **34:** 280–5.
2. Reiss RA, *et al.* Lithium pharmacokinetics in the obese. *Clin Pharmacol Ther* 1994; **55:** 392–8.
3. Thomsen K, Schou M. Avoidance of lithium intoxication: advice based on knowledge about the renal lithium clearance under various circumstances. *Pharmacopsychiatry* 1999; **32:** 83–6.
4. Sproule BA, *et al.* Differential pharmacokinetics of lithium in elderly patients. *Drugs Aging* 2000; **16:** 165–77.


**Administration.** References concerning the pharmacokinetic methods of predicting lithium dosage requirements.


1. Marken PA, *et al.* Preliminary comparison of predictive and empiric lithium dosing: impact on patient outcome. *Ann Pharmacother* 1994; **28:** 1148–52.
2. Taright N, *et al.* Nonparametric estimation of population characteristics of the kinetics of lithium from observational and experimental data: individualization of chronic dosing regimen using a new Bayesian approach. *Ther Drug Monit* 1994 **16:** 258–69.
3. Sproule BA, *et al.* Fuzzy logic pharmacokinetic modeling: application to lithium concentration prediction. *Clin Pharmacol Ther* 1997; **62:** 29–40.
4. Wright R, Crimson ML. Comparison of three a priori methods and one empirical method in predicting lithium dosage requirements. *Am J Health-Syst Pharm* 2000; **57:** 1698–1702.


**Cystic fibrosis.** For a reference to reduced renal excretion of lithium in patients with cystic fibrosis, see Precautions, above.

**Distribution into breast milk.** For references to the distribution of lithium into breast milk, see Precautions, above.

**Pregnancy.** For references to changes in renal clearance of lithium during pregnancy, see Precautions, above.

## Uses and Administration

Lithium, given as one of its salts, provides a source of lithium ions, which compete with sodium ions at various sites in the body. It thus has an action and side-effects distinct and separate from those of other antidepressants. Its mode of action is not understood, but it is effective in the treatment and prophylaxis of **mania**, and prophylaxis of **bipolar disorder** and **recurrent unipolar depression**. Since the margin between therapeutic and toxic serum concentrations is narrow the decision to give lithium is usually based on specialist advice; lithium should not be prescribed unless facilities for monitoring serum concentrations are available.

Treatment with lithium needs to be monitored by measurement of serum concentrations, which must be adjusted for each patient to those that give a clinical response without evidence of toxicity. There is evidence that patients are most likely to respond to concentrations of 0.8 mmol/litre or above, but individual patients may respond to concentrations as low as 0.4 mmol/litre, and it is impossible to identify these patients beforehand. Because toxic effects are associated with concentrations above 1.5 mmol/litre, and may occur with concentrations as low as 1 mmol/litre in susceptible patients such as the elderly, it is therefore recommended that doses are adjusted to provide a serum-lithium concentration of 0.4 to 1 mmol/litre (at the lower end of this range for maintenance therapy and elderly patients). Patients must be taught to recognise the symptoms of early lithium intoxication in order to omit further doses of lithium and seek medical care should it be impending.

The dose of lithium given depends on the preparation chosen since different preparations of lithium salts vary widely in bioavailability. Recommended doses for some UK preparations are as follows:

- *Camcolit* tablets (Norgine, UK) containing lithium carbonate; for treatment, initially 1 to 1.5 g daily; for prophylaxis, initially 300 to 400 mg daily
- *Li-Liquid* oral solution (Rosemont, UK) containing lithium citrate; for treatment and prophylaxis, initially 1.018 to 3.054 g daily in two divided doses (elderly or patients less than 50 kg, 0.509 g twice daily)
- *Liskonum* tablets (GlaxoSmithKline, UK) containing lithium carbonate; for treatment, initially 450 to 675 mg twice daily (elderly, 225 mg twice daily); for prophylaxis, initially 450 mg twice daily (elderly, 225 mg twice daily)
- *Priadel* tablets (Sanofi Synthelabo, UK) containing lithium carbonate; for treatment and prophylaxis, initially 0.4 to 1.2 g daily as a single dose or in two divided doses (elderly or patients less than 50 kg, 0.4 g daily)
- *Priadel* syrup (Sanofi Synthelabo, UK) containing lithium citrate; for treatment and prophylaxis, initially 1.04 to 3.12 g daily in two divided doses (elderly or patients less than 50 kg, 0.52 g twice daily)

Lithium is not recommended for use in children.

The initial dose given is adjusted after 4 to 7 days according to the results of serum-lithium estimations obtained under controlled conditions (samples being taken 12 hours after the preceding dose). Serum-lithium concentrations are then checked once a week until the dosage has remained constant for 4 weeks. The frequency of estimations can then be reduced to about once every 3 months. Should the patient's circumstances change such that the lithium pharmacokinetics or requirements might be affected, close control of serum concentrations should be reinstated until the concentrations stabilise once more. Such circumstances could involve a change of lithium preparation, an intercurrent illness (including a urinary-tract infection), a manic or depressive phase, a change in dietary regimen or body temperature, pregnancy, or concomitant administration of medication (in particular, sodium-containing preparations and diuretics). For further details see under Precautions and Interactions, above. Long-term use of lithium has been associated with thyroid disorders and mild cognitive and memory impairment. Therefore, long-term treatment should only be undertaken if it is definitely indicated. Patients need to be carefully reassessed after a period of 3 to 5 years and lithium continued only if the benefit persists.

Lithium is also used for the management of **aggressive or self-mutilating behaviour**. The doses are similar to those used in the prophylaxis of recurrent affective disorders described above.

Lithium therapy should, where possible, be withdrawn slowly over a period of weeks to allay any concerns about relapse. For further details, see Withdrawal under Precautions, above.

Other lithium salts have been used in the treatment of psychiatric disorders and these include the acetate, gluconate, glutamate, and sulfate.

Lithium carbonate is used in homoeopathic medicines.

**Anxiety disorders.** Lithium has been tried as augmentation therapy in the treatment of obsessive-compulsive disorder (p.663).

**Bipolar disorder.** Lithium's main role in the management of bipolar disorder is for prophylaxis (see p.278). It is sometimes used in the control of the acute manic stage, but, because of its slow onset of action, usually in conjunction with an antipsychotic.

References.


1. Aronson JK, Reynolds DJM. Lithium. *BMJ* 1992; **305:** 1273–6.
2. Birch NJ, *et al.* Lithium prophylaxis: proposed guidelines for good clinical practice. *Lithium* 1993; **4:** 225–30.
3. Peet M, Pratt JP. Lithium: current status in psychiatric disorders. *Drugs* 1993; **46:** 7–17.
4. Price LH, Heninger GR. Lithium in the treatment of mood disorders. *N Engl J Med* 1994; **331:** 591–8.
5. Jensen HV, *et al.* Lithium prophylaxis of manic-depressive disorder: daily lithium dosing schedule versus every second day. *Acta Psychiatr Scand* 1995; **92:** 69–74.
6. Moncrieff J. Lithium revisited: a re-examination of the placebo-controlled trials of lithium prophylaxis in manic-depressive disorder. *Br J Psychiatry* 1995; **167:** 569–74.
7. Jensen HV, *et al.* Twelve-hour brain lithium concentration in lithium maintenance treatment of manic-depressive disorder: daily versus alternate-day dosing schedule. *Psychopharmacology (Berl)* 1996; **124:** 275–8.
8. Maj M, *et al.* Late non-responders to lithium prophylaxis in bipolar patients: prevalence and predictors. *J Affect Disord* 1996; **39:** 39–42.
9. Anonymous. Using lithium safely. *Drug Ther Bull* 1999; **37:** 22–4.
10. Sproule B. Lithium in bipolar disorder: can drug concentrations predict therapeutic effect? *Clin Pharmacokinet* 2002; **41:** 639–60.
11. Burgess S, *et al.* Lithium for maintenance treatment of mood disorders. Available in The Cochrane Library; Issue 2. Chichester: John Wiley; 2004.


**Depression.** Lithium may be used in the treatment and prophylaxis of recurrent unipolar depression, usually when standard antidepressants have failed (p.279). Lithium is also used to augment the efficacy of other antidepressants in refractory cases.

References.


1. Heit S, Nemeroff CB. Lithium augmentation of antidepressants in treatment-refractory depression. *J Clin Psychiatry* 1998; **59** (suppl 6): 28–33.
2. Bauer M, Dopfmer S. Lithium augmentation in treatment-resistant depression: meta-analysis of placebo-controlled studies. *J Clin Psychopharmacol* 1999; **19:** 427–34. Correction. *ibid.* 2000; **20:** 287.
3. Sackeim HA, *et al.* Continuation pharmacotherapy in the prevention of relapse following electroconvulsive therapy; a randomized controlled trial. *JAMA* 2001; **285:** 1299–1307.


**Headache.** Lithium is one of a number of drugs tried in cluster headache (p.464) to prevent headache attacks during cluster periods when ergotamine is ineffective or has had to be withdrawn. In a double-blind study[1] lithium and verapamil were found to be of similar efficacy for cluster headache prophylaxis although verapamil appeared to produce fewer adverse effects. However, in a more recent placebo-controlled trial[2] lithium was found to be no more effective than the placebo and the trial was stopped early.


1. Bussone G, *et al.* Double blind comparison of lithium and verapamil in cluster headache prophylaxis. *Headache* 1990; **30:** 411–17.
2. Steiner TJ, *et al.* Double-blind placebo-controlled trial of lithium in episodic cluster headache. *Cephalalgia* 1997; **17:** 673–5.


**Hyperthyroidism.** Lithium has been tried in hyperthyroidism (p.1594), though its practical value is a matter of debate and, rarely, it may even cause hyperthyroidism (see Effects on the Endocrine System in Adverse Effects, above). Pretreatment with lithium has also been reported to prolong the exposure of the thyroid to radioactive iodine in patients with Graves' thyrotoxicosis.[1]


1. Bogazzi F, *et al.* Treatment with lithium prevents serum thyroid hormone increase after thionamide withdrawal and radioiodine therapy in patients with Graves' disease. *J Clin Endocrinol Metab* 2002; **87:** 4490–5.


**Schizophrenia.** The addition of lithium to antipsychotic treatment may be worthwhile in patients with schizophrenia (p.665) or schizoaffective disorders who fail to respond to an antipsychotic alone, but the danger of an interaction between the drugs should be borne in mind (see under Interactions, above). Although affective symptoms need not be present for patients with schizophrenia to respond to adjunctive lithium, their presence does appear to predict a greater likelihood of response.[1]


1. Christison GW, *et al.* When symptoms persist: choosing among alternative somatic treatments for schizophrenia. *Schizophr Bull* 1991; **17:** 217–45.


### Preparations

***BP 2003:*** Lithium Carbonate Tablets; Lithium Citrate Oral Solution; Slow Lithium Carbonate Tablets;
***USP 27:*** Lithium Carbonate Capsules; Lithium Carbonate Extended-release Tablets; Lithium Carbonate Tablets; Lithium Citrate Syrup.

**Proprietary Preparations** (details are given in Part 3)
***Arg.:*** Ceglution; Karlit; Lithiun; ***Austral.:*** Lithicarb; Quilonum; ***Austria:*** Neurolepsin; Quilonorm; ***Belg.:*** Camcolit; Maniprex; Priadel; ***Braz.:*** Acolitium†; Carbolim; Carbolitium; Litiocar; Neurolithium; ***Canad.:*** Carbolith; Duralith; Lithane; Lithizine†; ***Chile:*** Carbolit; Carboron; ***Denm.:*** Litarex; ***Fin.:*** Lito; ***Fr.:*** Neurolithium; Teralithe; ***Ger.:*** Hypnorex; leukominerase; Li 450; Quilonum; ***Gr.:*** Lithiofor; Milithin; ***Hong Kong:*** Camcolit; Lithicarb; Lithiofor; ***India:*** Licab; ***Irl.:*** Camcolit; Priadel; ***Israel:*** Licarbium; ***Ital.:*** Carbolithium; ***Malaysia:*** Priadel; ***Mex.:*** Carbolit; Litheum; ***Neth.:*** Priadel; ***Norw.:*** Litarex†; Lithionit; ***NZ:*** Lithicarb; Priadel; ***Port.:*** Priadel; ***S.Afr.:*** Camcolit; Lentolith; Quilonum; ***Singapore:*** Camcolit; Lithosun†; Priadel; ***Spain:*** Plenur; ***Swed.:*** Lithionit; ***Switz.:*** Litarex; Lithiofor; Neurolithium; Priadel; Quilonorm; ***Thai.:*** Licab†; Licarb; Limed; Lit-300; Phanate; ***UK:*** Camcolit; Li-Liquid; Liskonum; Litarex†; Lithonate; Priadel; ***USA:*** Eskalith; Lithobid.

**Multi-ingredient:** ***Austral.:*** Caprilate†; ***Austria:*** Togal†; ***Ger.:*** NeyDop N (Revitorgan-Dilutionen N Nr 97); Togal; ***Spain:*** Citinoides.

---

## Lofepramine Hydrochloride *(BANM, USAN, rINNM)*

Hidrocloruro de lofepramina; Leo-640; Lopramine Hydrochloride; WHR-2908A. 5-{3-[N-(Chlorophenacyl)-N-methylamino]propyl}-10,11-5*H*-dihydrodibenz[*b,f*]azepine hydrochloride.

$C_{26}H_{27}ClN_2O,HCl$ = 455.4.
*CAS — 23047-25-8 (lofepramine); 26786-32-3 (lofepramine hydrochloride).*
*ATC — N06AA07.*

**Pharmacopoeias.** In *Br.*

**BP 2003** (Lofepramine Hydrochloride). A fine, yellowish-white to green-yellow powder with a faint characteristic odour. It exhibits polymorphism. Very slightly soluble in alcohol and in methyl alcohol; slightly soluble in acetone. Store in airtight containers. Protect from light.

### Adverse Effects, Treatment, and Precautions

As for tricyclic antidepressants in general (see Amitriptyline, p.281). Lofepramine should be avoided in patients with severe hepatic or severe renal impairment.

**Effects on the liver.** See under Amitriptyline, p.282.

**Overdosage.** Lofepramine may be less toxic in overdosage than earlier tricyclics.[1] An analysis of data from the Office of National Statistics in England and Wales has also shown that the risk of death following an overdose with lofepramine was not significantly different from that associated with the SSRIs which, as a group, are considered to be safer in overdose than the tricyclics.[2]


1. Reid F, Henry JA. Lofepramine overdosage. *Pharmacopsychiatry* 1990; **23:** 23–27.
2. Mason J, *et al.* Fatal toxicity associated with antidepressant use in primary care. *Br J Gen Pract* 2000; **50:** 366–70.

### Interactions

For interactions associated with tricyclic antidepressants, see Amitriptyline, p.284.

### Pharmacokinetics

Lofepramine is readily absorbed from the gastrointestinal tract, and extensively demethylated by first-pass metabolism in the liver to its active, primary metabolite, desipramine (p.290). Since lofepramine slows gastrointestinal transit time absorption can, however, be delayed, particularly in overdosage. Paths of metabolism also include *N*-oxidation and hydroxylation. Lofepramine is mainly excreted in the urine, chiefly in the form of its metabolites. It is highly bound to plasma proteins. Lofepramine is distributed into breast milk.

### Uses and Administration

Lofepramine is a dibenzazepine tricyclic antidepressant with actions and uses similar to those of amitriptyline (p.285). One of its metabolites is desipramine (p.290). Lofepramine is one of the less sedating tricyclics.

In the treatment of depression lofepramine is given by mouth as the hydrochloride although doses are expressed in terms of the base. Lofepramine hydrochloride 76.1 mg is approximately equivalent to 70 mg of lofepramine base. The usual dose is the equivalent of 70 mg two or three times daily.

Lofepramine should be withdrawn gradually to reduce the risk of withdrawal symptoms.

◊ References.

1. Lancaster SG, Gonzalez JP. Lofepramine: a review of its pharmacodynamic and pharmacokinetic properties, and therapeutic efficacy in depressive illness. *Drugs* 1989; **37:** 123–40.

**Administration in the elderly.** The UK manufacturer has suggested that some elderly patients may respond to lower than usual doses of lofepramine, but in a study[1] involving 46 elderly patients with various grades of depression lofepramine 70 mg once daily was no more effective than placebo at the end of 28 days of treatment.

1. Tan RSH, *et al.* The effect of low dose lofepramine in depressed elderly patients in general medical wards. *Br J Clin Pharmacol* 1994; **37:** 321–4.

### Preparations

**BP 2003:** Lofepramine Tablets.

**Proprietary Preparations** (details are given in Part 3)
***Austria:*** Tymelyt; ***Belg.:*** Tymelyt†; ***Denm.:*** Tymelyt; ***Ger.:*** Gamonil; ***Irl.:*** Gamanil; ***Ital.:*** Timelit†; ***Port.:*** Deprimil; ***S.Afr.:*** Emdalen; ***Spain:*** Deftan; ***Swed.:*** Tymelyt; ***Switz.:*** Gamonil; ***UK:*** Feprapax; Gamanil; Lomont†.

## Maprotiline *(BAN, USAN, rINN)*

3-(9,10-Dihydro-9,10-ethanoanthracen-9-yl)propyl(methyl)amine; *N*-Methyl-9,10-ethanoanthracene-9(10*H*)-propylamine.

$C_{20}H_{23}N$ = 277.4.
*CAS — 10262-69-8.*
*ATC — N06AA21.*

## Maprotiline Hydrochloride *(BANM, rINNM)*

Ba-34276; Hidrocloruro de maprotilina; Maprotilini Hydrochloridum.

$C_{20}H_{23}N,HCl$ = 313.9.
*CAS — 10347-81-6.*

**Pharmacopoeias.** In *Chin., Eur.* (see p.vi), *Jpn,* and *US.*

**Ph. Eur. 5.0** (Maprotiline Hydrochloride). A white or almost white crystalline powder. It shows polymorphism. Slightly soluble in water; soluble in alcohol; very slightly soluble in acetone; sparingly soluble in dichloromethane; freely soluble in methyl alcohol.

**USP 27** (Maprotiline Hydrochloride). A fine white to off-white, practically odourless, crystalline powder. Slightly soluble in water; freely soluble in chloroform and in methyl alcohol; practically insoluble in isooctane. Store in airtight containers.

### Adverse Effects, Treatment, and Precautions

Adverse effects with maprotiline, a tetracyclic antidepressant, are broadly similar to those with tricyclic antidepressants (see Amitriptyline, p.281) but antimuscarinic effects are less frequent.

Skin rashes seem more common with maprotiline than with tricyclic antidepressants. Seizures have occurred in patients with no prior history of such disorders as well as in those with a history of epilepsy and the risk is increased if high doses of maprotiline are employed. It should not be used in patients with epilepsy or a lowered seizure threshold.

**Incidence of adverse effects.** By March 1985 the UK Committee on Safety of Medicines[1] had received reports of the following adverse reactions associated with maprotiline from a cumulative total of 2.5 million prescriptions: convulsions (124), hepatic reactions (4), and haematological reactions (8). There had also been 454 reports of skin rashes.

1. Committee on Safety of Medicines. Dangers of newer antidepressants. *Current Problems 15* 1985.

**Effects on the skin.** In addition to many recorded instances of skin rashes with maprotiline (see above) cutaneous vasculitis, which resolved on discontinuation of therapy, has also been observed.[1]

1. Oakley AMM, Hodge L. Cutaneous vasculitis from maprotiline. *Aust N Z J Med* 1985; **15:** 256–7.

**Epileptogenic effect.** In a retrospective review of 186 psychiatric patients with no history of seizures, 5 of 32 patients receiving maprotiline developed generalised tonic-clonic seizures, compared with 1 of 45 receiving a tricyclic antidepressant.[1] There were no seizures in the remaining patients who received other medications, or no drug treatment. Two of the 5 patients experiencing seizures with maprotiline were receiving doses of 75 to 150 mg daily, 2 were receiving daily doses of 200 to 300 mg, and one patient experienced partial complex seizures with a daily dose of 150 mg and generalised tonic-clonic seizures after increasing the daily dose to 300 mg.

1. Jabbari B, *et al.* Incidence of seizures with tricyclic and tetracyclic antidepressants. *Arch Neurol* 1985; **42:** 480–1.

**Overdosage.** Apart from seizures being more common with maprotiline, features of overdosage are similar to those experienced with tricyclic antidepressant poisonings (see under Adverse Effects of Amitriptyline, p.281).

For a discussion of choice of antidepressant with respect to toxicity in overdosage, see under Depression, p.279.

References.

1. Crome P, Newman B. Poisoning with maprotiline and mianserin. *BMJ* 1977; **2:** 260.
2. Curtis RA, *et al.* Fatal maprotiline intoxication. *Drug Intell Clin Pharm* 1984; **18:** 716–20.
3. Knudsen K, Heath A. Effects of self poisoning with maprotiline. *BMJ* 1984; **288:** 601–3.
4. Crome P, Ali C. Clinical features and management of self-poisoning with newer antidepressants. *Med Toxicol* 1986; **1:** 411–20.

**Porphyria.** Maprotiline hydrochloride is considered to be unsafe in patients with porphyria because it has been shown to be porphyrinogenic in *animals.*

### Interactions

Interactions associated with maprotiline are similar to those associated with tricyclic antidepressants (see Amitriptyline, p.284).

### Pharmacokinetics

Maprotiline is slowly but completely absorbed from the gastrointestinal tract. It is widely distributed throughout the body and is extensively bound to plasma protein.

Maprotiline is extensively demethylated in the liver to its principal active metabolite, desmethylmaprotiline; paths of metabolism of both maprotiline and desmethylmaprotiline include *N*-oxidation, aliphatic and aromatic hydroxylation, and the formation of aromatic methoxy derivatives. In addition to desmethylmaprotiline, maprotiline-*N*-oxide is also reported to be pharmacologically active. The average elimination half-life of maprotiline is reported to be about 43 hours and that of its active metabolite even longer (range 60 to 90 hours). Maprotiline is excreted in the urine, mainly in the form of its metabolites, either in free or in conjugated form; appreciable amounts are also excreted in the faeces.

Maprotiline is distributed into breast milk (see Breast Feeding under Precautions of Amitriptyline, p.283).

◊ References.

1. Maguire KP, *et al.* An evaluation of maprotiline: intravenous kinetics and comparison of two oral doses. *Eur J Clin Pharmacol* 1980; **18:** 249–54.
2. Alkalay D, *et al.* Bioavailability and kinetics of maprotiline. *Clin Pharmacol Ther* 1980; **27:** 697–703.
3. Firkusny L, Gleiter H. Maprotiline metabolism appears to cosegregate with the genetically-determined CYP2D6 polymorphic hydroxylation of debrisoquine. *Br J Clin Pharmacol* 1994; **37:** 383–8.

### Uses and Administration

Maprotiline is a tetracyclic antidepressant with actions and uses similar to those of tricyclic antidepressants (see Amitriptyline, p.285). It is one of the more sedating antidepressants but antimuscarinic effects are less marked. Like the tricyclics, maprotiline is an inhibitor of the reuptake of noradrenaline; it also has weak affinity for central adrenergic ($\alpha_1$) receptors.

Maprotiline is usually given by mouth as the hydrochloride but it has also been given by injection as the mesilate and in oral drops as the resinate.

In the treatment of depression (p.279) maprotiline hydrochloride is given by mouth in doses of 25 to 75 mg daily in three divided doses, gradually increased to 150 mg daily if necessary; up to 225 mg daily may be required in severely depressed patients in hospital. The dosage should be adjusted after 1 or 2 weeks according to response. Because of the prolonged half-life of maprotiline the total daily dose may also be given as a single dose, usually at night. A suggested initial dose for elderly patients is 10 mg three times daily or 30 mg at night gradually increased according to response over a period of 1 to 2 weeks to 25 mg three times daily or 75 mg at night.

Maprotiline should be withdrawn gradually to reduce the risk of withdrawal symptoms.

### Preparations

**USP 27:** Maprotiline Hydrochloride Tablets.

**Proprietary Preparations** (details are given in Part 3)
***Austria:*** Ludiomil; ***Belg.:*** Ludiomil; ***Braz.:*** Ludiomil; ***Canad.:*** Ludiomil; ***Denm.:*** Ludiomil; Maludil; ***Fr.:*** Ludiomil; ***Ger.:*** Aneural†; Deprilept; Ludiomil; Mapro-GRY†; Maprolu; Mirpan†; Psymion†; ***Gr.:*** Ludiomil; ***Hong Kong:*** Ludiomil; ***Israel:*** Ludiomil†; Melodil; ***Ital.:*** Ludiomil; ***Malaysia:*** Ludiomil; ***Mex.:*** Ludiomil; ***Neth.:*** Ludiomil; ***NZ:*** Ludiomil; ***Port.:*** Ludiomil; ***S.Afr.:*** Ludiomil; ***Singapore:*** Ludiomil; ***Spain:*** Ludiomil; ***Swed.:*** Ludiomil; ***Switz.:*** Ludiomil; ***Thai.:*** Ludiomil; ***UK:*** Ludiomil; ***USA:*** Ludiomil†.

## Melitracen Hydrochloride *(USAN, rINNM)*

Hidrocloruro de melitraceno; N7001; U-24973A. 3-(9,10-Dihydro-10,10-dimethyl-9-anthrylidene)propyldimethylamine hydrochloride.

$C_{21}H_{25}N,HCl$ = 327.9.
*CAS — 5118-29-6 (melitracen); 10563-70-9 (melitracen hydrochloride).*
*ATC — N06AA14.*

### Profile

Melitracen is a tricyclic antidepressant (see Amitriptyline, p.280).

In the treatment of depression melitracen is given by mouth as the hydrochloride although doses are expressed in terms of the base. Melitracen hydrochloride 28.1 mg is approximately equivalent to 25 mg of melitracen base. The recommended initial dose is the equivalent of 25 mg two or three times daily gradually increased to a total of 225 mg daily if necessary. Elderly patients should generally be given reduced doses of 25 mg daily initially.

Melitracen should be withdrawn gradually to reduce the risk of withdrawal symptoms.

### Preparations

**Proprietary Preparations** (details are given in Part 3)
***Austria:*** Dixeran; ***Belg.:*** Dixeran.

**Multi-ingredient:** ***Austria:*** Deanxit; ***Belg.:*** Deanxit; ***Hong Kong:*** Deanxit; ***Ital.:*** Deanxit; ***Singapore:*** Deanxit; ***Spain:*** Deanxit; ***Switz.:*** Deanxit; ***Thai.:*** Deanxit.

## Mianserin Hydrochloride *(BANM, USAN, rINNM)*

Hidrocloruro de mianserina; Mianserini Hydrochloridum; Org-GB-94. 1,2,3,4,10,14b-Hexahydro-2-methyldibenzo[*c,f*]pyrazino[1,2-*a*]azepine hydrochloride.

$C_{18}H_{20}N_2,HCl$ = 300.8.
*CAS — 24219-97-4 (mianserin); 21535-47-7 (mianserin hydrochloride).*
*ATC — N06AX03.*

**Pharmacopoeias.** In *Eur.* (see p.vi) and *Pol.*

**Ph. Eur. 5.0** (Mianserin Hydrochloride). A white or almost white crystalline powder or crystals. Sparingly soluble in water; slightly soluble in alcohol; soluble in dichloromethane. A 1% solution in water has a pH of 4.0 to 5.5. Protect from light.

### Adverse Effects

Antimuscarinic and cardiac side-effects are fewer and milder with mianserin, a tetracyclic antidepressant, than with tricyclic antidepressants but effects are otherwise broadly similar (see Amitriptyline, p.281); mianserin may be associated with a lower risk of cardiotoxicity in overdosage.

The most common adverse effect associated with mianserin is drowsiness. Mianserin also causes bone-marrow depression usually presenting as leucopenia, granulocytopenia, or agranulocytosis; aplastic anaemia has been reported. These adverse haematological reactions generally occur during the first few weeks of therapy and especially in the elderly.

Other side-effects reported include disturbances of liver function and jaundice, breast disorders (gynaecomastia, nipple tenderness, and non-puerperal lactation), and polyarthropathy.

**Effects on the blood.** Between 1976 and the end of 1988 the UK Committee on Safety of Medicines (CSM) had received 239 reports of adverse haematological reactions associated with mianserin.[1] The reports included 68 of agranulocytosis and 84 of granulocytopenia or leucopenia where mianserin was considered to be the probable or possible cause; there had been 17 fatalities. Allowing for the pattern of prescribing there was a greater number of reports of white blood cell disorders in patients over 65 years of age but there was no sex difference. The data also indicated that the adverse reactions were most likely to develop during the first 3 months of therapy. By the end of 1992 the number of reports of mianserin-induced agranulocytosis or neutropenia received by the CSM[2] had risen to 79 and 105, respectively.

A case of fatal aplastic anaemia associated with mianserin has also been reported.[3]

Proposed mechanisms of mianserin haematotoxicity have included a direct toxicity[4] and an immunologically-mediated mechanism.[5] There is evidence from *in vitro* studies of a significant correlation between the desmethyl metabolite and cytotoxicity. Mianserin is given as a racemic preparation and the formation of metabolites was greater with the *R*(−)-enantiomer than with the *S*(+)-enantiomer.[6]

1. Committee on Safety of Medicines. Mianserin and white blood cell disorders in the elderly. *Current Problems 25* 1989.
2. Committee on Safety of Medicines/Medicines Control Agency. Drug-induced neutropenia and agranulocytosis. *Current Problems* 1993; **19:** 10–11.
3. Durrant S, Read D. Fatal aplastic anaemia associated with mianserin. *BMJ* 1982; **285:** 437.
4. O'Donnell JL, *et al.* Possible mechanism for mianserin induced neutropenia associated with saturable elimination kinetics. *BMJ* 1985; **291:** 1375–6.

5. Stricker BHC, *et al.* Thrombocytopenia and leucopenia with mianserin-dependent antibodies. *Br J Clin Pharmacol* 1985; **19:** 102–4.
6. Riley RJ, *et al.* A stereochemical investigation of the cytotoxicity of mianserin metabolites in vitro. *Br J Clin Pharmacol* 1989; **27:** 823–30.


**Effects on the cardiovascular system.** Although mianserin is considered to be less cardiotoxic than the tricyclic antidepressants adverse effects have been noted in individual patients. Two elderly patients developed signs of disturbed cardiac function (cardiac failure, atrial and ventricular fibrillation, bradycardia, and frequent ventricular ectopic beats) which resolved after the drug was discontinued.[1] One of the patients also developed hypokalaemia which was possibly caused by mianserin. It was suggested that persons most likely to experience problems were the elderly with a past history of cardiovascular disorders. Further reports of mianserin-induced cardiac effects include recurrent ventricular fibrillation in a 61-year-old man after an overdose of mianserin[2] and bradycardia in a 50-year-old woman following a therapeutic dose.[3]


1. Whiteford H, *et al.* Disturbed cardiac function possibly associated with mianserin therapy. *Med J Aust* 1984; **140:** 166–7.
2. Haefeli WE, *et al.* Recurrent ventricular fibrillation in mianserin intoxication. *BMJ* 1991; **302:** 415–16.
3. Carcone B, *et al.* Symptomatic bradycardia caused by mianserin at therapeutic doses. *Hum Exp Toxicol* 1991; **10:** 383–4.


**Effects on the liver.** By March 1985 the UK Committee on Safety of Medicines had received 57 reports of hepatic reactions associated with mianserin from a total of 5 million prescriptions. Reactions had included jaundice and other abnormalities of liver function, but no fatalities had been reported.[1]

Case reports have also been published concerning jaundice;[2-5] liver function returned to normal after stopping mianserin or lowering the dose.


1. Committee on Safety of Medicines. Dangers of newer antidepressants. *Current Problems 15* 1985.
2. Adverse Drug Reactions Advisory Committee. Mianserin: a possible cause of neutropenia and agranulocytosis. *Med J Aust* 1980; **2:** 673–4.
3. Goldstraw PW, *et al.* Mianserin and jaundice. *N Z Med J* 1983; **96:** 985.
4. Zarski J-P, *et al.* Toxicité hépatique des nouveaux anti-dépresseurs: a propos d'une observation. *Gastroenterol Clin Biol* 1983; **7:** 220–1.
5. Otani K, *et al.* Hepatic injury caused by mianserin. *BMJ* 1989; **299:** 519.


**Effects on the musculoskeletal system.** A patient developed an acute polyarthritis affecting the hands and feet 6 days after commencing therapy with mianserin;[1] the authors of the report also mentioned that the UK Committee on Safety of Medicines had received 19 reports of arthritis and arthralgia associated with mianserin.


1. Hughes A, Coote J. Arthropathy associated with treatment with mianserin. *BMJ* 1986; **292:** 1050.


**Effects on the skin.** Reports of adverse dermatological reactions in individual patients related to mianserin therapy have included toxic epidermal necrolysis[1] and erythema multiforme.[2,3]


1. Randell P. Tolvon and toxic epidermal necrolysis. *Med J Aust* 1979; **2:** 653.
2. Quraishy E. Erythema multiforme during treatment with mianserin—a case report. *Br J Dermatol* 1981; **104:** 481.
3. Cox NH. Erythema multiforme due to mianserin—a case against generic prescribing. *Br J Clin Pract* 1985; **39:** 293–4.


**Effects on the tongue.** Glossitis associated with mianserin therapy was reported in 2 patients.[1] Additionally, glossitis accompanied by severe facial oedema has been noted in another patient.[2] In all cases symptoms resolved after withdrawal of mianserin.


1. de la Fuente JR, Berlanga C. Glossitis associated with mianserin. *Lancet* 1984; **i:** 233.
2. Leibovitch G, *et al.* Severe facial oedema and glossitis associated with mianserin. *Lancet* 1989; **ii:** 871–2.


**Epileptogenic effect.** By March 1985 the UK Committee on Safety of Medicines had received 64 reports of convulsions associated with mianserin from a total of 5 million prescriptions.[1] In a previous review[2] concerning 40 of these cases it was considered that a causal connection could be established only in a minority. It was suggested that mianserin is no more epileptogenic than tricyclic antidepressants, an opinion that was also shared by other reviewers.[3]


1. Committee on Safety of Medicines. Dangers of newer antidepressants. *Current Problems 15* 1985.
2. Edwards JG, Glen-Bott M. Mianserin and convulsive seizures. *Br J Clin Pharmacol* 1983; **15:** 299S–311S.
3. Richens A, *et al.* Antidepressant drugs, convulsions and epilepsy. *Br J Clin Pharmacol* 1983; **15:** 295S–298S.


**Overdosage.** Experience with 100 consecutive cases of intoxication with mianserin[1] revealed that when it was the only drug ingested symptoms were mild and neither deep coma nor convulsions occurred. More serious symptoms were seen in patients who had taken multiple drug overdoses and there were 2 fatalities. The results suggested that following an acute overdose mianserin is less toxic than the tricyclic antidepressants. This conclusion was also supported by a large follow-up study[2] comparing the outcome of suicide attempts among patients who had taken mianserin in overdose with those who had taken amitriptyline.


1. Chand S, *et al.* One hundred cases of acute intoxication with mianserin hydrochloride. *Pharmakopsychiatrie* 1981; **14:** 15–17.
2. Inman WHW. Blood disorders and suicide in patients taking mianserin or amitriptyline. *Lancet* 1988; **ii:** 90–2.


## Precautions

As for tricyclic antidepressants in general (see Amitriptyline, p.282). Although mianserin is less cardiotoxic than the tricyclic antidepressants, it still should be used with caution in patients with cardiovascular disorders, such as heart block, or after recent myocardial infarction. Similarly, patients with angle-closure glaucoma or prostatic hyperplasia should be monitored even though antimuscarinic effects are rare. Mianserin should be used with caution in patients with diabetes mellitus, epilepsy, and hepatic or renal impairment; it should be avoided in severe hepatic disease.

Patients should be carefully monitored during early antidepressant therapy until improvement in depression is observed because suicide is an inherent risk in depressed patients. For further details, see under Depression, p.279.

A full blood count is recommended every 4 weeks during the first 3 months of treatment with mianserin, because of the risk of bone-marrow depression. Similarly, if a patient receiving mianserin develops fever, sore throat, stomatitis, or other signs of infection, treatment should be stopped and a full blood count obtained. The elderly are considered to be at special risk of blood disorders from mianserin. For further details see Effects on the Blood under Adverse Effects, above.

The UK manufacturers recommend that mianserin should not be given during breast feeding, but the *British National Formulary* considers the amount distributed into breast milk too small to be harmful.

**Porphyria.** Mianserin hydrochloride is considered to be unsafe in patients with porphyria because it has been shown to be porphyrinogenic in *animals*.

## Interactions

It is recommended that mianserin should not be given to patients receiving MAOIs or for at least 14 days afterwards. At least one week should elapse between withdrawing mianserin and starting any drug liable to provoke a serious reaction (e.g. phenelzine). Unlike the tricyclics (p.284), mianserin does not diminish the effects of the antihypertensives guanethidine, hydralazine, propranolol, clonidine, or betanidine. However, it is still recommended that blood pressure be monitored when mianserin is prescribed with antihypertensive therapy. Plasma-phenytoin concentrations should be monitored carefully in patients also treated with mianserin; phenytoin has also been reported to reduce concentrations of mianserin (see below). There may be potentiation of effects when mianserin is given with CNS depressants such as alcohol, anxiolytics, or antipsychotics.

**Antiepileptics.** Reduced plasma concentrations and half-lives of mianserin and desmethylmianserin were observed in 6 patients also receiving antiepileptic therapy consisting of *phenytoin* with either *carbamazepine* or *phenobarbital*.[1] Carbamazepine alone may also reduce the plasma concentration of mianserin.[2,3]

Mianserin may antagonise the action of antiepileptics by lowering the convulsive threshold.


1. Nawishy S, *et al.* Kinetic interaction of mianserin in epileptic patients on anticonvulsant drugs. *Br J Clin Pharmacol* 1982; **13:** 612P–13P.
2. Leinonen E, *et al.* Effects of carbamazepine on serum antidepressant concentrations in psychiatric patients. *J Clin Psychopharmacol* 1991; **11:** 313–18.
3. Eap CB, *et al.* Effects of carbamazepine coadministration on plasma concentrations of the enantiomers of mianserin and of its metabolites. *Ther Drug Monit* 1999; **21:** 166–70.


## Pharmacokinetics

Mianserin is readily absorbed from the gastrointestinal tract, but its bioavailability is reduced by extensive first-pass metabolism in the liver.

Paths of metabolism of mianserin include aromatic hydroxylation, *N*-oxidation, and *N*-demethylation. Desmethylmianserin and 8-hydroxymianserin are pharmacologically active.

Mianserin is excreted in the urine, almost entirely as its metabolites, either free or in conjugated form; some is also found in the faeces.

Mianserin is widely distributed throughout the body and is extensively bound to plasma proteins. It has been found to have a biphasic plasma half-life with the duration of the terminal phase ranging from about 6 to 40 hours. Mianserin crosses the blood-brain barrier and the placenta. It is distributed into breast milk.

◊ References.


1. Hrdina PD, *et al.* Mianserin kinetics in depressed patients. *Clin Pharmacol Ther* 1983; **33:** 757–62.
2. Pinder RM, Van Delft AML. The potential therapeutic role of enantiomers and metabolites of mianserin. *Br J Clin Pharmacol* 1983; **15:** 269S–276S.
3. Timmer CJ, *et al.* Absolute bioavailability of mianserin tablets and solution in healthy humans. *Eur J Drug Metab Pharmacokinet* 1985; **10:** 315–23.
4. Begg EJ, *et al.* Variability in the elimination of mianserin in elderly patients. *Br J Clin Pharmacol* 1989; **27:** 445–51.
5. Buist A, *et al.* Mianserin in breast milk. *Br J Clin Pharmacol* 1993; **36:** 133–4.
6. Dahl M-L, *et al.* Stereoselective disposition of mianserin is related to debrisoquin hydroxylation polymorphism. *Clin Pharmacol Ther* 1994; **56:** 176–83.


## Uses and Administration

Mianserin is a tetracyclic antidepressant. It does not appear to have significant antimuscarinic properties, but has a marked sedative action. Unlike the tricyclic antidepressants (see Amitriptyline, p.285), mianserin does not prevent the peripheral reuptake of noradrenaline; it blocks presynaptic adrenergic ($\alpha_2$) receptors and increases the turnover of brain noradrenaline. Mianserin is also an antagonist of serotonin receptors in some parts of the brain.

In the treatment of depression (p.279) mianserin hydrochloride is given by mouth in initial doses of 30 to 40 mg daily increased gradually thereafter as necessary. The effective daily dosage is usually between 30 and 90 mg. The daily dosage may be divided throughout the day or given as a single dose at night. Divided daily dosages of up to 200 mg have been given. The recommended initial daily dose in the elderly is not more than 30 mg, which may be slowly increased if necessary.

Mianserin should be withdrawn gradually to reduce the risk of withdrawal symptoms.

## Preparations

**BP 2003:** Mianserin Tablets.

**Proprietary Preparations** (details are given in Part 3)
***Arg.:*** Lerivon; ***Austral.:*** Lerivon†; Lumin; Tolvon; ***Austria:*** Miabene; Tolvon; ***Belg.:*** Lerivon; ***Braz.:*** Tolvon; ***Chile:*** Athimil; Prevalina; ***Denm.:*** Tolmin; Tolvon; ***Fin.:*** Miaxan; Tolvon; ***Fr.:*** Athymil; ***Ger.:*** Hopacem; Mianeurin; Prisma; Tolvin; ***Hong Kong:*** Tolvon; ***India:*** Depnon; ***Irl.:*** Tolvon; ***Israel:*** Bolvidon†; Bonserin; ***Ital.:*** Lantanon; ***Mex.:*** Tolvon; ***Neth.:*** Tolvon; ***Norw.:*** Tolvon; ***NZ:*** Tolvon; ***Port.:*** Tolvon; ***S.Afr.:*** Lantanon; ***Singapore:*** Tolvon†; ***Spain:*** Lantanon; ***Swed.:*** Tolvon; ***Switz.:*** Tolvon; ***Thai.:*** Mealin; Servin; Tolimed; Tolvon.

# Milnacipran Hydrochloride *(BANM, rINNM)*

F-2207 (milnacipran); Hidrocloruro de milnaciprán; Midalcipran Hydrochloride. (±)-*cis*-2-(Aminomethyl)-*N*,*N*-diethyl-1-phenylcyclopropanecarboxamide hydrochloride.

$C_{15}H_{22}N_2O,HCl$ = 282.8.

*CAS — 92623-85-3 (milnacipran); 101152-94-7 (milnacipran hydrochloride); 175131-61-0 (milnacipran hydrochloride).*

*ATC — N06AX17.*

## Profile

Milnacipran hydrochloride is a serotonin and noradrenaline reuptake inhibitor (SNRI) used for the treatment of depression (p.279). It is given by mouth in doses of 100 mg daily.

◊ References.


1. Ansseau M, *et al.* Controlled comparison of milnacipran and fluoxetine in major depression. *Psychopharmacology (Berl)* 1994; **114:** 131–7.
2. Leinonen E, *et al.* Long-term efficacy and safety of milnacipran compared to clomipramine in patients with major depression. *Acta Psychiatr Scand* 1997; **96:** 497–504.
3. Tignol J, *et al.* Double-blind study of the efficacy and safety of milnacipran and imipramine in elderly patients with major depressive episode. *Acta Psychiatr Scand* 1998; **97:** 157–65.
4. Spencer CM, Wilde MI. Milnacipran: a review of its use in depression. *Drugs* 1998; **56:** 405–27.
5. Rouillon F, *et al.* Milnacipran efficacy in the prevention of recurrent depression: a 12-month placebo-controlled study. *Int Clin Psychopharmacol* 2000; **15:** 133–40.
6. Clerc G. Antidepressant efficacy and tolerability of milnacipran, a dual serotonin and noradrenaline reuptake inhibitor: a comparison with fluvoxamine. *Int Clin Psychopharmacol* 2001; **16:** 145–51.
7. Fukuchi T, Kanemoto K. Differential effects of milnacipran and fluvoxamine, especially in patients with severe depression and agitated depression: a case-control study. *Int Clin Psychopharmacol* 2002; **17:** 53–8.


## Preparations

**Proprietary Preparations** (details are given in Part 3)
***Arg.:*** Dalcipran; Ixel; ***Austria:*** Dalcipran; Ixel; ***Fin.:*** Ixel; ***Fr.:*** Ixel; ***Israel:*** Ixel; ***Port.:*** Ixel.

# Mirtazapine *(BAN, USAN, rINN)*

Mirtazapina; Org-3770. (*RS*)-1,2,3,4,10,14b-Hexahydro-2-methylpyrazino-[2,1-*a*]pyrido[2,3-*c*][2]benzazepine.

$C_{17}H_{19}N_3$ = 265.4.

*CAS — 61337-67-5.*

*ATC — N06AX11.*

## Adverse Effects

Side-effects commonly reported with mirtazapine are an increase in appetite and weight; drowsiness or sedation generally occur during the first few weeks of treatment. Dizziness, headache, oedema, and increases in liver enzyme levels have been reported less commonly; jaundice may occur. Other rarely reported side-effects include postural hypotension, exanthema, nightmares, agitation, mania, hallucinations, paraesthesia, convulsions, tremor, myoclonus, restless legs syndrome, arthralgia, myalgia, and reversible agranulocytosis, leucopenia, and granulocytopenia.

Hyponatraemia, possibly due to inappropriate secretion of antidiuretic hormone, has been associated with the use of antidepressants, particularly in the elderly.

**Extrapyramidal effects.** Akathisia that developed in 2 patients given mirtazapine 30 mg at night[1] resolved in one after being treated with clonazepam and in the other patient after reducing the dose of mirtazapine to 15 mg at night.

1. Girishchandra BG, *et al.* Mirtazapine-induced akathisia. *Med J Aust* 2002; **176:** 242.

**Serotonin syndrome.** The serotonin syndrome (p.313) is most commonly due to the additive adverse effects of two or more drugs that enhance serotonin activity at central receptors; rarely, a single serotonergic drug has caused the syndrome. One such case[1] occurred in an elderly patient given mirtazapine 15 mg daily; he was also taking salbutamol, ipratropium, and nimodipine, although none of these are known to have serotonergic effects.

1. Hernández JL, *et al.* Severe serotonin syndrome induced by mirtazapine monotherapy. *Ann Pharmacother* 2002; **36:** 641–3.

## Precautions

Mirtazapine should be used with caution in patients with epilepsy, hepatic or renal impairment, and cardiac disorders such as conduction disturbances, angina pectoris, and recent myocardial infarction, and also in patients with hypotension, diabetes mellitus, psychoses, and in those with a history of bipolar disorder. Treatment should be stopped if jaundice develops. Although mirtazapine has only weak antimuscarinic activity, caution should nevertheless be exercised in patients with micturition disturbances, angle-closure glaucoma, and raised intra-ocular pressure.

Patients should be advised to report any of the following symptoms during treatment: fever, sore throat, stomatitis, or other signs of infection; treatment should be stopped and a blood count performed.

Drowsiness is often experienced at the start of therapy and patients, if affected, should not drive or operate machinery.

Patients should be closely monitored during early therapy until improvement in depression is observed because suicide is an inherent risk in depressed patients. For further details, see under Depression, p.279.

Mirtazapine should be withdrawn gradually to reduce the risk of withdrawal symptoms.

## Interactions

Mirtazapine should not be used with or within 2 weeks of stopping an MAOI; at least one week should elapse between stopping mirtazapine and starting any drug liable to provoke a serious reaction (e.g. phenelzine). Use of mirtazapine with alcohol or benzodiazepines may potentiate sedative effects.

## Pharmacokinetics

Mirtazapine is well absorbed from the gastrointestinal tract with peak plasma levels occurring after about 2 hours. Plasma protein binding is about 85%. Mirtazapine is extensively metabolised in the liver and the major biotransformation pathways are demethylation and oxidation followed by glucuronide conjugation; cytochrome P450 isoenzymes involved are CYP2D6, CYP1A2, and CYP3A4. The *N*-desmethyl metabolite is pharmacologically active. Elimination is via urine (75%) and faeces (15%). The mean plasma elimination half-life is 20 to 40 hours. Data from *animal* studies indicate that mirtazapine crosses the placenta and is distributed into breast milk.

◊ References.

1. Timmer CJ, *et al.* Clinical pharmacokinetics of mirtazapine. *Clin Pharmacokinet* 2000; **38:** 461–74.

## Uses and Administration

Mirtazapine, a piperazinoazepine, is an analogue of mianserin (p.306); it is a noradrenergic and specific serotonergic antidepressant. It enhances the release of noradrenaline and, indirectly, serotonin through blockade of central presynaptic adrenergic ($\alpha_2$) receptors. The effects of released serotonin are mediated via 5-$HT_1$ receptors as mirtazapine blocks both 5-$HT_2$ and 5-$HT_3$ receptors. Mirtazapine is given as a racemic mixture: the S(+)-enantiomer blocks $\alpha_2$ and 5-$HT_2$ receptors whereas the R(−)-enantiomer blocks 5-$HT_3$ receptors. Mirtazapine is also a potent antagonist at histamine ($H_1$) receptors which gives it sedative properties; it has very little antimuscarinic activity.

In the treatment of depression (p.279), mirtazapine is given by mouth in an initial daily dose of 15 mg, which may be increased gradually according to clinical response. Changes in dose should be made at intervals of at least 1 to 2 weeks because of the long half-life. The usual effective daily dose lies within the range of 15 to 45 mg. Daily doses may be given as a single dose, preferably at bedtime, or in 2 equally divided doses. Mirtazapine should be withdrawn gradually to reduce the risk of withdrawal symptoms.

◊ References.

1. Sitsen JMA, Moors J. Mirtazapine, a novel antidepressant, in the treatment of anxiety symptoms: results from a placebo-controlled trial. *Drug Invest* 1994; **8:** 339–44.
2. Kasper S, *et al.* A risk-benefit assessment of mirtazapine in the treatment of depression. *Drug Safety* 1997; **17:** 251–64.
3. Puzantian T. Mirtazapine, an antidepressant. *Am J Health-Syst Pharm* 1998; **55:** 44–9.
4. Holm KJ, Markham A. Mirtazapine: a review of its use in major depression. *Drugs* 1999; **57:** 607–31.

## Preparations

**Proprietary Preparations** (details are given in Part 3)
***Arg.:*** Comenter; Remeron; ***Austral.:*** Avanza; Mirtazon; Remeron; ***Austria:*** Remeron; ***Belg.:*** Remergon; ***Braz.:*** Remeron; ***Canad.:*** Remeron; ***Chile:*** Ciblex; Divaril; Promyrtil; Zuleptan; ***Denm.:*** Remeron; ***Fin.:*** Remeron; ***Fr.:*** Norset; ***Ger.:*** Remergil; ***Gr.:*** Remeron; ***Hong Kong:*** Remeron; ***India:*** Mirtaz; ***Irl.:*** Zispin; ***Israel:*** Remeron; ***Ital.:*** Remeron; ***Malaysia:*** Remeron; ***Mex.:*** Remeron; ***Neth.:*** Remeron; ***Norw.:*** Remeron; ***Port.:*** Remeron; ***S.Afr.:*** Remeron; ***Singapore:*** Remeron; ***Spain:*** Rexer; ***Swed.:*** Remeron; ***Switz.:*** Remeron; ***Thai.:*** Remeron; ***UK:*** Zispin; ***USA:*** Remeron.

# Moclobemide *(BAN, USAN, rINN)*

Moclobemida; Ro-11-1163; Ro-11-1163/000. 4-Chloro-N-(2-morpholinoethyl)benzamide.
$C_{13}H_{17}ClN_2O_2$ = 268.7.
*CAS — 71320-77-9.*
*ATC — N06AG02.*

**Pharmacopoeias.** In *Swiss.*

## Adverse Effects

Adverse effects reported to occur with moclobemide include sleep disturbances, dizziness, agitation, feelings of anxiety, restlessness, irritability, and headache. Gastrointestinal disturbances include dry mouth, diarrhoea, constipation, and nausea and vomiting. Paraesthesia, visual disturbances, and oedema have also been reported, and skin reactions include rash, pruritus, urticaria, and flushing. Confusional states have been observed that disappear rapidly on stopping the drug. Raised liver enzymes have been reported.

Hyponatraemia, possibly due to inappropriate secretion of antidiuretic hormone, has been associated with the use of antidepressants, particularly in the elderly.

**Effects on the cardiovascular system.** Hypertension has been reported[1,2] rarely in patients taking moclobemide, some of whom were also taking other drugs although moclobemide was suspected to be the cause. Blood pressure usually returned to normal after stopping moclobemide.

1. Coulter DM, Pillans PI. Hypertension with moclobemide. *Lancet* 1995; **346:** 1032.
2. Boyd IW. Hypertension with moclobemide. *Lancet* 1995; **346:** 1498.

**Effects on the endocrine system.** A prescription-event monitoring study found that galactorrhoea is significantly associated with the use of moclobemide.[1]

1. Dunn NR, *et al.* Galactorrhoea with moclobemide. *Lancet* 1998; **351:** 802.

**Overdosage.** Symptoms that have been reported with overdosage of moclobemide include agitation, aggression, behavioural disturbances, and gastrointestinal irritation.

References.

1. Hetzel W. Safety of moclobemide taken in overdose for attempted suicide. *Psychopharmacology (Berl)* 1992; **106:** S127–S129.
2. Hackett LP, *et al.* Disposition and clinical effects of moclobemide and three of its metabolites following overdose. *Drug Invest* 1993; **5:** 281–4.
3. Myrenfors PG, *et al.* Moclobemide overdose. *J Intern Med* 1993; **233:** 113–15.

## Precautions

Moclobemide is contra-indicated in patients with acute confusional states and in those with phaeochromocytoma. It should be avoided in excited or agitated patients, unless used with a sedative. Manic episodes may be provoked in patients with bipolar disorder. Care is also required in patients with thyrotoxicosis as moclobemide may theoretically precipitate a hypertensive reaction. Reduced doses should be used in patients with severe hepatic impairment.

Patients should be closely monitored during early antidepressant therapy until improvement in depression is observed because suicide is an inherent risk in depressed patients. For further details, see under Depression, p.279.

Although impairment of mental alertness is generally not expected with moclobemide, caution should be exercised with respect to driving or operating machinery until individual reactions have been assessed.

Antidepressants, particularly MAOIs, should be withdrawn gradually to reduce the risk of withdrawal symptoms.

**Breast feeding.** In a study[1] of the distribution of moclobemide into the breast milk of 6 lactating mothers given a single 300-mg dose of moclobemide, a mean of 0.057% of the dose appeared in breast milk as moclobemide and 0.031% as its major metabolite Ro-12-8095 within 24 hours of administration. It was considered that this small amount of moclobemide was unlikely to be hazardous to suckling infants. The manufacturers advise caution and consideration of the benefits of moclobemide therapy to the mother against possible risks to the infant.

1. Pons G, *et al.* Moclobemide excretion in human breast milk. *Br J Clin Pharmacol* 1990; **29:** 27–31.

## Interactions

The dietary restrictions that need to be followed with selective reversible inhibitors of monoamine oxidase type A such as moclobemide are less stringent than those for non-selective inhibitors of monoamine oxidase types A and B (see under Interactions of Phenelzine, p.314). However, the manufacturers of moclobemide recommend that since some patients may be especially sensitive to tyramine, consumption of large amounts of tyramine-rich food should be avoided.

Medicines containing *sympathomimetics, dextromethorphan,* or *anorectics* should not be taken with moclobemide. Moclobemide should not be given with *other antidepressants* although, owing to its short duration of action, a treatment-free period is generally considered unnecessary following its cessation. For further details, see Antidepressants under Interactions of Phenelzine, p.315. Therapy with moclobemide should not be started until at least a week following cessation of a tricyclic or related antidepressant or an SSRI or related antidepressant (2 weeks in the case of paroxetine and sertraline; at least 5 weeks in the case of fluoxetine) or for at least a week after stopping treatment with non-selective MAOIs. CNS excitation or depression may occur if moclobemide is taken with *opioid analgesics,* and there is also a risk of CNS toxicity if taken with *serotonin (5-$HT_1$) agonists.* The metabolism of moclobemide is inhibited by *cimetidine,* leading to increased plasma concentrations and a need for reduced dosage (see below).

**Antimigraine drugs.** For the effects of moclobemide on *serotonin (5-$HT_1$) agonists,* see under Sumatriptan, p.472.

**Cimetidine.** Cimetidine 1 g daily for 2 weeks increased the mean maximum plasma concentration of moclobemide in 8 healthy subjects from 575 nanograms/mL to 787 nanograms/mL; several other parameters associated with moclobemide absorption and disposition were also affected.[1] It was suggested that a reduction in the dosage of moclobemide might be required. The manufacturers of moclobemide recommend reducing its dose by half in patients also receiving cimetidine.

1. Schoerlin M-P, *et al.* Cimetidine alters the disposition kinetics of the monoamine oxidase-A inhibitor moclobemide. *Clin Pharmacol Ther* 1991; **49:** 32–8.

**Dopaminergics.** Adverse effects including nausea, vomiting, and dizziness were noted in healthy subjects given moclobemide and *levodopa with benserazide;*[1] however, no significant hypertensive reactions were seen.

Caution is also required when *selegiline* and moclobemide are given together.[1] Dietary restrictions with this combination (see under Phenelzine, p.314) are recommended by one manufacturer of selegiline, whereas another advises that this combination should be avoided (as does the manufacturer of moclobemide).

See also under Selegiline, p.1214.

1. Dingemanse J. An update of recent moclobemide interaction data. *Int Clin Psychopharmacol* 1993; **7:** 167–80.

**Omeprazole.** Omeprazole, which is an inhibitor of cytochrome P450 isoenzyme CYP2C19, increased plasma concentrations and elimination half-life of moclobemide in extensive metabolisers of the drug towards values seen in poor metabolisers.[1] It had little effect on pharmacokinetic parameters in poor metabolisers. The clinical effects were uncertain but extra care might be warranted if the 2 drugs are given together.

1. Yu K-S, *et al.* Effect of omeprazole on the pharmacokinetics of moclobemide according to the genetic polymorphism of CYP2C19. *Clin Pharmacol Ther* 2001; **69:** 266–73.

**Opioid analgesics.** Symptoms suggestive of a mild serotonin syndrome (p.313) developed in a 73-year-old woman taking moclobemide, nortriptyline, and lithium after she was given *pethidine* intravenously.[1]

1. Gillman PK. Possible serotonin syndrome with moclobemide and pethidine. *Med J Aust* 1995; **162:** 554.

**Sympathomimetics.** Symptoms resembling phaeochromocytoma occurred in an elderly woman who was receiving the reversible MAOI toloxatone;[1] the woman had also been taking a preparation containing *phenylephrine* without ill-effect but the symptoms occurred after addition of *terbutaline* therapy. It was noted that such an interaction is more typical of older, irreversible, less selective MAOIs.

1. Lefebvre H, *et al.* Life-threatening pseudo-phaeochromocytoma after toloxatone, terbutaline, and phenylephrine. *Lancet* 1993; **341:** 555–6.

## Pharmacokinetics

Moclobemide is readily absorbed from the gastrointestinal tract, peak plasma concentrations occurring within about 1 hour of ingestion. Absorption is virtually complete but first-pass metabolism reduces bioavailability of the drug. Moclobemide is widely distributed throughout the body and undergoes extensive metabolism in the liver, in part by the cytochrome P450 isoenzymes CYP2C19 and CYP2D6. Metabolites of moclobemide and a small amount of unchanged drug are excreted in the urine. Moclobemide has a plasma elimination half-life of 2 to 4 hours. Moclobemide is distributed into breast milk.

◊ References.

1. Mayersohn M, Guentert TW. Clinical pharmacokinetics of the monoamide oxidase-A inhibitor moclobemide. *Clin Pharmacokinet* 1995; **29:** 292–332.
2. Gram LF, *et al.* Moclobemide: a substrate of CYP2C19 and an inhibitor of CYP2C19, CYP2D6, and CYP1A2: a panel study. *Clin Pharmacol Ther* 1995; **57:** 670–7.

## Uses and Administration

Moclobemide, a benzamide derivative, is a reversible inhibitor of monoamine oxidase type A (RIMA) (see under Phenelzine, p.316) used for the treatment of depression and of social phobia.

In the treatment of **depression** the usual initial daily dose of moclobemide is 300 mg by mouth in divided doses. This may be increased to up to 600 mg daily according to response. In some patients, a maintenance dose of 150 mg daily may be sufficient.

In the treatment of **social phobia**, the initial daily dose of moclobemide is 300 mg increased after 3 days to 600 mg given in 2 divided doses. Treatment should be continued for 8 to 12 weeks to assess efficacy; patients should be periodically re-evaluated thereafter to determine the need for further treatment.

Moclobemide should be taken after food.

Reduced doses should be given in hepatic impairment (see below) and in patients also taking cimetidine (see above).

Antidepressants, particularly MAOIs, should be withdrawn gradually to reduce the risk of withdrawal symptoms.

◊ Reviews.

1. Fulton B, Benfield P. Moclobemide: an update of its pharmacological properties and therapeutic use. *Drugs* 1996; **52:** 450–74.

**Administration in hepatic impairment.** Doses of moclobemide in patients with severe hepatic impairment may need to be reduced to half or one-third.

**Anxiety disorders.** The use of MAOIs in general in the management of anxiety disorders is discussed under Phenelzine on p.316. For a discussion of the overall treatment of anxiety disorders, see p.663.

References.

1. Noyes R, *et al.* Moclobemide in social phobia: a controlled dose-response trial. *J Clin Psychopharmacol* 1997; **17:** 247–54.
2. Neal LA, *et al.* An open trial of moclobemide in the treatment of post-traumatic stress disorder. *Int Clin Psychopharmacol* 1997; **12:** 231–7.
3. Schneier FR, *et al.* Placebo-controlled trial of moclobemide in social phobia. *Br J Psychiatry* 1998; **172:** 70–7.
4. Tiller JW, *et al.* Moclobemide and fluoxetine for panic disorder. *Eur Arch Psychiatry Clin Neurosci* 1999; **249** (suppl 1): S7–S10.
5. Stein DJ, *et al.* Moclobemide is effective and well tolerated in the long-term pharmacotherapy of social anxiety disorder with or without comorbid anxiety disorder. *Int Clin Psychopharmacol* 2002; **17:** 161–70.

**Depression.** As discussed on p.279 there is very little difference in efficacy between the different groups of antidepressant drugs, and choice is often made on the basis of adverse effects. The traditional MAOIs such as phenelzine are rarely used as first-choice antidepressants because of the dangers of dietary and drug interactions. Reversible inhibitors of monoamine oxidase type A (RIMAs) such as moclobemide offer a safer alternative to the irreversible non-selective MAOIs and fewer dietary restrictions are necessary.

References.

1. Fitton A, *et al.* Moclobemide: a review of its pharmacological properties and therapeutic use in depressive illness. *Drugs* 1992; **43:** 561–96.
2. Angst J, Stabl M. Efficacy of moclobemide in different patient groups: a meta-analysis of studies. *Psychopharmacology (Berl)* 1992; **106** (suppl): S109–S113.
3. Freeman H. Moclobemide. *Lancet* 1993; **342:** 1528–32.
4. Lonnqvist J, *et al.* Moclobemide and fluoxetine in atypical depression: a double-blind trial. *J Affect Disord* 1994; **32:** 169–77.
5. Anonymous. Moclobemide for depression. *Drug Ther Bull* 1994; **32:** 6–8.
6. Norman TR, Burrows GD. A risk-benefit assessment of moclobemide in the treatment of depressive disorders. *Drug Safety* 1995; **12:** 46–54.
7. Roth M, *et al.* Moclobemide in elderly patients with cognitive decline and depression: an international double-blind, placebo-controlled trial. *Br J Psychiatry* 1996; **168:** 149–57.
8. Lotufo-Neto F, *et al.* Meta-analysis of the reversible inhibitors of monoamine oxidase type A moclobemide and brofaromine for the treatment of depression. *Neuropsychopharmacology* 1999; **20:** 226–47.

**Smoking cessation.** In a preliminary double-blind, placebo-controlled parallel-group study in 88 smokers, moclobemide facilitated smoking cessation (p.1721) in highly dependent smokers.[1]

1. Berlin I, *et al.* A reversible monoamine oxidase A inhibitor (moclobemide) facilitates smoking cessation and abstinence in heavy, dependent smokers. *Clin Pharmacol Ther* 1995; **58:** 444–52.

## Preparations

**Proprietary Preparations** (details are given in Part 3)

***Arg.:*** Aurorix; ***Austral.:*** Arima; Aurorix; Clobemix; Maosig; Mohexal; ***Austria:*** Aurorix; ***Belg.:*** Aurorix; ***Braz.:*** Aurorix; ***Canad.:*** Manerix; ***Chile:*** Aurorix; Inpront; ***Denm.:*** Aurorix; ***Fin.:*** Aurorix; ***Fr.:*** Moclamine; ***Ger.:*** Aurorix; Moclix; Moclodura; ***Gr.:*** Aurorix; ***Hong Kong:*** Aurorix; ***India:*** Rimarex; ***Irl.:*** Manerix; ***Israel:*** Mobemide; ***Ital.:*** Aurorix†; ***Mex.:*** Aurorex; Feraken; ***Neth.:*** Aurorix; ***Norw.:*** Aurorix; ***NZ:*** Aurorix; ***Port.:*** Aurorix; ***S.Afr.:*** Aurorix; Depnil; ***Singapore:*** Aurorix; ***Spain:*** Manerix; ***Swed.:*** Aurorix; ***Switz.:*** Aurorix; Moclo A; ***Thai.:*** Aurorix; ***UK:*** Manerix.

---

## Nefazodone Hydrochloride *(BANM, USAN, rINNM)*

BMY-13754; Hidrocloruro de nefazodona; MJ-13754-1. 2-{3-[4-(3-Chlorophenyl)piperazin-1-yl]propyl}-5-ethyl-2,4-dihydro-4-(2-phenoxyethyl)-1,2,4-triazol-3-one monohydrochloride.

$C_{25}H_{32}ClN_5O_2,HCl = 506.5.$

*CAS — 83366-66-9 (nefazodone); 82752-99-6 (nefazodone hydrochloride).*

### Adverse Effects and Treatment

The most common adverse effects seen with nefazodone are weakness, dry mouth, nausea, constipation, somnolence, dizziness, and lightheadedness. Other effects which have occurred less frequently include chills, fever, orthostatic hypotension, incoordination, vasodilatation, arthralgia, paraesthesia, confusion, memory impairment, abnormal dreams, ataxia, and amblyopia and other visual disturbances. Syncope has occurred rarely and there have been reports of sinus bradycardia. Hepatotoxicity has occurred (see below).

Hyponatraemia, possibly due to inappropriate secretion of antidiuretic hormone, has been associated with the use of antidepressants, particularly in the elderly.

In overdosage, the symptoms that have been reported most frequently include hypotension, nausea, vomiting, and drowsiness. The value of gastric decontamination in the treatment of overdosage is uncertain. Activated charcoal should be considered if more than 1.5 g (in an adult) or 20 mg/kg (in a child) has been taken and treatment is within 1 hour of ingestion. The manufacturers recommend gastric lavage, although this technique is seldom practicable and should not be attempted unless the airway is protected. Supportive therapy should be given as necessary.

◊ Reviews.

1. Robinson DS, *et al.* The safety profile of nefazodone. *J Clin Psychiatry* 1996; **57** (suppl 2): 31–8.

**Effects on the liver.** Subfulminant hepatic failure developed in 3 women given nefazodone for depression.[1] Two patients required liver transplantation although this was unsuccessful in one case and the patient died. Hepatitis, positive on rechallenge, has also been reported with nefazodone.[2]

The US manufacturers of nefazodone state that rare events of raised liver enzymes, hepatitis, hepatic failure and necrosis have been reported since marketing but no causal relationship has been established. In the USA, a reported rate of about 1 case of hepatic failure resulting in death or transplantation per 250 000 to 300 000 patient years of nefazodone treatment has been estimated by the manufacturer; this rate is about 3 to 4 times greater than the background rate of hepatic failure.[3] Onset times for such cases ranged from 2 weeks to 6 months. The Canadian manufacturers have indicated[4] that as of June 2001 there had been 109 reports of serious hepatic adverse events associated with nefazodone from postmarketing surveillance worldwide. These included 23 cases of hepatic failure, of which 16 led to transplantation and/or death. Most cases occurred within 4 months of beginning treatment although a few were after continuous use for up to 2 years. Following a review[5] of the data available to December 2002, it was decided to withdraw nefazodone from the Canadian market in November 2003. Subsequently, one manufacturer (Bristol-Myers Squibb) has withdrawn nefazodone worldwide.

1. Aranda-Michel J, *et al.* Nefazodone-induced liver failure: report of three cases. *Ann Intern Med* 1999; **130:** 285–8.
2. Schrader GD, Roberts-Thompson IC. Adverse effect of nefazodone: hepatitis. *Med J Aust* 1999; **170:** 452.
3. Jody DM [Bristol-Myers Squibb]. Important drug warning including black box information. Available at: http://www.fda.gov/medwatch/SAFETY/2002/serzone_deardoc.PDF (accessed 11/06/04)
4. Bristol-Myers Squibb Canada Inc/Linson Pharama Inc. Important safety information on nefazodone HCl: severe and serious hepatic events (issued June 2001). Available at: http://www.hc-sc.gc.ca./hpfb-dgpsa/tpd-dpt/nefazodone_e.pdf (accessed 11/06/04)
5. Bristol-Myers Squibb Canada. Important safety information regarding the discontinuation of sales of nefazodone in Canada (issued October 2003). Available at: http://www.hc-sc.gc.ca/hpfb-dgpsa/tpd-dpt/bms_nefazodone_2_hpc_e.pdf (accessed 11/06/04)

**Overdosage.** A 27-year-old woman developed no serious toxicity after taking 3 g of nefazodone in a suicide attempt.[1] Somnolence was the most severe effect noted. In another case, a 31-year-old woman attempted suicide with 16.8 g of nefazodone and an unknown quantity of verapamil.[2] The patient was lethargic, and developed significant bradycardia and hypotension; she recovered after supportive therapy. The authors reported that among the 7 cases of overdose occurring during clinical trials, there were no fatalities or permanent sequelae.

1. Gaffney PW, *et al.* Nefazodone overdose. *Ann Pharmacother* 1998; **32:** 1249–50.
2. Catalano G, *et al.* Nefazodone overdose: a case report *Clin Neuropharmacol* 1999; **22:** 63–5.

### Precautions

Treatment with nefazodone should not generally be started in patients with active hepatic disease or elevated baseline serum transaminases. Patients who develop signs or symptoms of hepatic impairment such as jaundice, anorexia, abdominal pain, elevated transaminase levels, or malaise during treatment should be evaluated with regard to possible hepatic damage and withdrawn from nefazodone if necessary. Nefazodone is contra-indicated in patients previously withdrawn from the drug because of hepatotoxicity.

Nefazodone should be used with caution in patients with epilepsy, a history of hypomania or mania, or severe renal impairment. It should also be used with caution in cardiovascular or cerebrovascular disease that could be exacerbated by hypotension (for example recent history of myocardial infarction, unstable heart disease, angina, or ischaemic stroke), and in any condition such as dehydration or hypovolaemia that may predispose patients to hypotension.

Since nefazodone is structurally related to trazodone which is known to have caused priapism (see p.319), the US manufacturer recommends that any patient developing inappropriate or prolonged penile erections should discontinue nefazodone immediately.

Patients should be closely monitored during early antidepressant therapy until improvement in depression is observed because suicide is an inherent risk in depressed patients. For further details, see under Depression, p.279.

Nefazodone may impair performance of skilled tasks and, if affected, patients should not drive or operate machinery.

Antidepressants should be withdrawn gradually to reduce the risk of withdrawal symptoms.

**Breast feeding.** A study[1] in 2 nursing mothers receiving nefazodone for postpartum depression indicated that nefazodone, but not its major active metabolites, was distributed into breast milk in variable amounts; the quantity present did not seem to be dose related. The calculated exposure of the two women's offspring was 2.2% and 0.4% of the maternal dose respectively. Another report suggested that even such low exposures might result in clinically significant effects:[2] drowsiness, inability to maintain normal body temperature, and poor feeding were reported in the breast-fed infant of a woman receiving nefazodone. After breast feeding was stopped the symptoms resolved, suggesting an association between the two despite a calculated exposure in the infant of only 0.45% of the maternal dose.

1. Dodd S, *et al.* Nefazodone in the breast milk of nursing mothers: a report of two patients. *J Clin Psychopharmacol* 2000; **20:** 717–18.
2. Yapp P, *et al.* Drowsiness and poor feeding in a breast-fed infant: association with nefazodone and its metabolites. *Ann Pharmacother* 2000; **34:** 1269–72.

### Interactions

Nefazodone should not be given to patients receiving MAOIs or for at least 14 days after their discontinuation; it has also been recommended that any drug liable to provoke a serious reaction (e.g. phenelzine) should not be given within one week of stopping nefazodone therapy. For further details on the coadministration of antidepressants, see Antidepressants under Interactions of Phenelzine, p.315.

Orthostatic hypotension can be a problem with nefazodone, and therefore a dose reduction may be required for any antihypertensive therapy.

Nefazodone is an inhibitor of the cytochrome P450 isoenzyme CYP3A4 responsible for the metabolism of some benzodiazepines, and consequently it may produce clinically important increases in their plasma concentrations. Use with astemizole, cisapride, pimozide, and terfenadine (which are metabolised by the same isoenzyme) is best avoided because the potential also exists for increased plasma concentrations of these drugs, with the risk of inducing ventricular arrhythmias. Other substrates for this isoenzyme may also interact with nefazodone: atorvastatin, lovastatin, and simvastatin should be used with caution with nefazodone since there have been rare reports of rhabdomyolysis with such combinations. Increased serum levels of ciclosporin or tacrolimus, both substrates for CYP3A4, have been reported in patients also receiving nefazodone. Monitoring of serum ciclosporin or tacrolimus levels is recommended when either of these two drugs is given with nefazodone.

Plasma concentrations of digoxin are increased by nefazodone and it is recommended that, because of digoxin's narrow therapeutic index, plasma concentrations of digoxin should be monitored if use with nefazodone is necessary.

Caution should be exercised when haloperidol is given with nefazodone as the clearance of haloperidol may be reduced. Plasma concentrations of carbamazepine are also increased when used with nefazodone. More importantly, carbamazepine may reduce nefazodone plasma concentrations to subtherapeutic levels and therefore use together is not recommended. Giving buspirone with nefazodone significantly increases the serum concentrations of buspirone; the manufacturers of nefazodone recommend that the initial dose of buspirone is reduced if these drugs are given together.

The potential for interaction between nefazodone and general anaesthetics exists and the manufacturer recommends that nefazodone should be stopped before elective surgery for as long as clinically feasible.

### Pharmacokinetics

Nefazodone is readily absorbed from the gastrointestinal tract and peak plasma concentrations have been obtained 1 to 3 hours after oral doses. Absorption is delayed and reduced by food but this is not considered to be clinically significant. Nefazodone undergoes extensive first-pass metabolism and is more than 99% bound to plasma proteins; it is widely distributed. It is extensively metabolised by N-dealkylation and hydroxylation in the liver to several metabolites, two of which, hydroxynefazodone and *m*-chlorophenylpiperazine, are known to be pharmacologically active. Excretion is predominately as metabolites via the urine (approximately 55%) and the faeces (20 to 30%). The plasma elimination half-life is 2 to 4 hours. Pharmacokinetic parameters are reported to be non-linear with increasing doses. Nefazodone is distributed in small amounts into breast milk (see Precautions, above).

◊ Reviews.

1. Greene DS, Barbhaiya RH. Clinical pharmacokinetics of nefazodone. *Clin Pharmacokinet* 1997; **33:** 260–75.

### Uses and Administration

Nefazodone is a phenylpiperazine antidepressant structurally related to trazodone (see p.319). It blocks the reuptake of serotonin at presynaptic neurones and is an antagonist at postsynaptic 5-$HT_2$ receptors. Unlike trazodone, nefazodone inhibits the reuptake of noradrenaline. It blocks $\alpha_1$-adrenoceptors but has no apparent effect on dopamine receptors. Nefazodone does not appear to have very significant antimuscarinic properties compared with tricyclic antidepressants.

Nefazodone hydrochloride is given by mouth for the treatment of depression in a usual initial dose of 100 mg twice daily. The daily dose may be increased if necessary, in increments of 100 to 200 mg at intervals of no less than a week, to a maximum of 300 mg twice daily. Elderly patients, especially females, or debilitated patients, may have higher plasma concentrations, and initial doses should be restricted to 50 mg twice daily. For dosage recommendations in patients with hepatic impairment, see below.

Antidepressants should be withdrawn gradually to reduce the risk of withdrawal symptoms.

**Administration in hepatic impairment.** The manufacturers recommend that nefazodone treatment should not be started in patients with active liver disease or elevated liver enzyme values; they note that although there is no evidence that pre-existing liver disease increases the risk of developing hepatic failure, baseline abnormalities may complicate the monitoring of liver function.

**Anxiety disorders.** Nefazodone has been tried in a variety of anxiety disorders including panic attacks (p.663) with or without associated depression, social phobia (see under Phobic Disorders, p.663), and post-traumatic stress disorder (p.664).

References.

1. DeMartinis NA, *et al.* An open-label trial of nefazodone in high comorbidity panic disorder. *J Clin Psychiatry* 1996; **57:** 245–8.
2. Hidalgo R, *et al.* Nefazodone in post-traumatic stress disorder: results from six open-label trials. *Int Clin Psychopharmacol* 1999; **14:** 61–8.
3. Van Ameringen M, *et al.* Nefazodone in social phobia. *J Clin Psychiatry* 1999; **60:** 96–100.
4. Papp LA, *et al.* Efficacy of open-label nefazodone treatment in patients with panic disorder. *J Clin Psychopharmacol* 2000; **20:** 544–6.
5. Gillin JC, *et al.* An open-label, 12-week clinical and sleep EEG study of nefazodone in chronic combat-related posttraumatic stress disorder. *J Clin Psychiatry* 2001; **62:** 789–96.

**Depression.** As discussed on p.279, there is very little difference in efficacy between the different groups of antidepressant drugs, and choice is often made on the basis of adverse effect profile. Nefazodone has a different biochemical profile from both the tricyclics and the SSRIs.

References.

1. Rickels K, *et al.* Nefazodone and imipramine in major depression: a placebo-controlled trial. *Br J Psychiatry* 1994; **164:** 802–5.
2. Fontaine R, *et al.* A double-blind comparison of nefazodone, imipramine, and placebo in major depression. *J Clin Psychiatry* 1994; **55:** 234–41.
3. Ansseau M, *et al.* Controlled comparison of nefazodone and amitriptyline in major depressive inpatients. *Psychopharmacology (Berl)* 1994; **115:** 254–60.
4. Ellingrod VL, Perry PJ. Nefazodone: a new antidepressant. *Am J Health-Syst Pharm* 1995; **52:** 2799–2812.
5. Baldwin DS, *et al.* A multicenter double-blind comparison of nefazodone and paroxetine in the treatment of outpatients with moderate-to-severe depression. *J Clin Psychiatry* 1996; **57** (suppl 2): 46–52.
6. Feiger A, *et al.* Nefazodone versus sertraline, in outpatients with major depression: focus on efficacy, tolerability, and effects on sexual function and satisfaction. *J Clin Psychiatry* 1996; **57** (suppl 2): 53–62.
7. Cyr M, Brown CS. Nefazodone: its place among antidepressants. *Ann Pharmacother* 1996; **30:** 1006–12.
8. Davis R, *et al.* Nefazodone: a review of its pharmacology and clinical efficacy in the management of major depression. *Drugs* 1997; **53:** 608–36.
9. Feighner J, *et al.* A double-blind, placebo-controlled trial of nefazodone in the treatment of patients hospitalized for major depression. *J Clin Psychiatry* 1998; **59:** 246–53.
10. Baldwin DS, *et al.* A randomized, double-blind controlled comparison of nefazodone and paroxetine in the treatment of depression: safety, tolerability and efficacy in continuation phase treatment. *J Psychopharmacol* 2001; **15:** 161–5.
11. Schatzberg AF, *et al.* Clinical use of nefazodone in major depression: a 6-year perspective. *J Clin Psychiatry* 2002; **63:** 18–31.

### Preparations

**Proprietary Preparations** (details are given in Part 3)
***Arg.:*** Deprefax; ***Austral.:*** Serzone†; ***Austria:*** Dutonin†; ***Braz.:*** Serzone†; ***Canad.:*** Serzone†; ***Denm.:*** Nefadar†; ***Fin.:*** Nefadar†; ***Ger.:*** Nefadar†; ***Gr.:*** Nefirel†; ***Hong Kong:*** Serzone†; ***Irl.:*** Dutonin†; ***Israel:*** Serzonil†; ***Ital.:*** Reseril†; ***Mex.:*** Serzone†; ***Neth.:*** Dutonin†; ***Norw.:*** Nefadar†; ***NZ:*** Serzone†; ***S.Afr.:*** Serzone†; ***Singapore:*** Serzone†; ***Spain:*** Dutonin†; Menfazona†; Rulivan†; ***Swed.:*** Nefadar†; ***Switz.:*** Nefadar†; ***Thai.:*** Serzone†; ***UK:*** Dutonin†; ***USA:*** Serzone†.

---

## Nialamide *(BAN, rINN)*

Nialamida. *N'*-(2-Benzylcarbamoylethyl)isonicotinohydrazide.

$C_{16}H_{18}N_4O_2$ = 298.3.

*CAS — 51-12-7.*

*ATC — N06AF02.*

### Profile

Nialamide, a hydrazine derivative, is an irreversible inhibitor of monoamine oxidase types A and B (see Phenelzine, p.312). It has been used in the treatment of depression and is sometimes used as a pharmacological tool.

---

# Nortriptyline Hydrochloride

*(BANM, USAN, rINNM)*

38489; Hidrocloruro de nortriptilina; Nortriptylini Hydrochloridum. 3-(10,11-Dihydro-5*H*-dibenzo[*a*,*d*]cyclohepten-5-ylidene)-propyl(methyl)amine hydrochloride.

$C_{19}H_{21}N,HCl$ = 299.8.

*CAS — 72-69-5 (nortriptyline); 894-71-3 (nortriptyline hydrochloride).*

*ATC — N06AA10.*

**Pharmacopoeias.** In *Eur.* (see p.vi), *Jpn*, and *US*.

**Ph. Eur. 5.0** (Nortriptyline Hydrochloride). A white or almost white powder. Sparingly soluble in water; soluble in alcohol and in dichloromethane. Protect from light.

**USP 27** (Nortriptyline Hydrochloride). A white to off-white powder having a slight characteristic odour. Soluble 1 in 90 of water, 1 in 30 of alcohol, 1 in 20 of chloroform, and 1 in 10 of methyl alcohol; practically insoluble in ether, in benzene, and in most other organic solvents. pH of a 1% solution in water is about 5. Store in airtight containers. Protect from light.

### Adverse Effects, Treatment, and Precautions

As for tricyclic antidepressants in general (see Amitriptyline, p.281).

**Breast feeding.** For comments on the use of tricyclic antidepressants in breast feeding patients, see under Precautions for Amitriptyline, p.283.

**Effects on ventilation.** Severe hyperventilation developed in a 61-year-old man with end-stage renal disease after receiving nortriptyline 125 mg daily;[1] mechanical ventilation was necessary to correct severe respiratory alkalosis.

1. Sunderrajan S, *et al.* Nortriptyline-induced severe hyperventilation. *Arch Intern Med* 1985; **145:** 746–7.

**Porphyria.** Nortriptyline is considered to be unsafe in patients with porphyria although there is conflicting experimental evidence of porphyrinogenicity.

### Interactions

For interactions associated with tricyclic antidepressants, see Amitriptyline, p.284.

### Pharmacokinetics

Nortriptyline is the principal active metabolite of amitriptyline (p.285). Nortriptyline has been reported to have a longer plasma half-life than amitriptyline. Nortriptyline is subject to extensive first-pass metabolism in the liver to 10-hydroxynortriptyline, which is active.

**Metabolism.** Individuals with a poor debrisoquine hydroxylation phenotype may be at greater risk of confusional states when taking nortriptyline.[1] This was thought to be because the polymorphic hydroxylation of debrisoquine and nortriptyline are mediated by similar enzymatic mechanisms, with poor oxidisers having higher plasma nortriptyline concentrations.[2,3] A nonlinear (dose-dependent) relationship between dose and plasma-nortriptyline concentrations has been observed during therapeutic drug monitoring[4] in subjects who were considered to be extensive metabolisers of debrisoquine; nonlinearity did not appear to occur in poor metabolisers. There was no significant correlation between hydroxylation phenotype and amitriptyline concentrations, suggesting that demethylation and hydroxylation of tricyclic antidepressants are mediated by different cytochrome P450 isoenzymes.[5]

The pharmacokinetics and pharmacological actions of 10-hydroxynortriptyline, the major active metabolite of nortriptyline, have been reviewed.[3]

1. Park BK, Kitteringham NR. Adverse reactions and drug metabolism. *Adverse Drug React Bull* 1987; **122:** 456–9.
2. Nordin C, *et al.* Plasma concentrations of nortriptyline and its 10-hydroxy metabolite in depressed patients—relationship to the debrisoquine hydroxylation metabolic ratio. *Br J Clin Pharmacol* 1985; **19:** 832–5.
3. Nordin C, Bertilsson L. Active hydroxymetabolites of antidepressants: emphasis on E-10-hydroxy-nortriptyline. *Clin Pharmacokinet* 1995; **28:** 26–40.
4. Jerling M, Alván G. Nonlinear kinetics of nortriptyline in relation to nortriptyline clearance as observed during therapeutic drug monitoring. *Eur J Clin Pharmacol* 1994; **46:** 67–70.
5. Bertilsson L, *et al.* Metabolism of various drugs in subjects with different debrisoquine and sparteine oxidation phenotypes. *Br J Clin Pharmacol* 1982; **14:** 602P.

**Plasma concentrations.** Nortriptyline appears to have an optimum antidepressant effect at plasma concentrations between 50 and 150 nanograms/mL. Outside this range, there is a poor clinical response. Plasma concentration measurements are unequivocally useful in problem patients who do not respond to usual oral doses or in high-risk patients for whom, because of age or medical illness, it is especially important to use the lowest possible effective dose of the drug.[1]

It has been suggested[2] that within this window of total nortriptyline concentrations there is a probability of an antidepressant response of 68% or more with free concentrations of 7 to 10 nanograms/mL.

For reference to dose-dependent kinetics of nortriptyline observed in individuals with an extensive debrisoquine hydroxylation phenotype, see under Metabolism, above.

1. Task Force on the Use of Laboratory Tests in Psychiatry. Tricyclic antidepressants—blood level measurements and clinical outcome: an APA task force report. *Am J Psychiatry* 1985; **142:** 155–62.
2. Perry PJ, *et al.* The relationship of free nortriptyline levels to antidepressant response. *Drug Intell Clin Pharm* 1984; **18:** 510.

### Uses and Administration

Nortriptyline is a dibenzocycloheptadiene tricyclic antidepressant with actions and uses similar to those of amitriptyline (p.285). It is the principal active metabolite of amitriptyline. Nortriptyline is one of the less sedating tricyclics and its antimuscarinic effects are mild.

Nortriptyline is given by mouth as the hydrochloride although doses are expressed in terms of the base; nortriptyline hydrochloride 113.8 mg is approximately equivalent to 100 mg of nortriptyline base. In the treatment of **depression** a low starting dose is given gradually increasing to the equivalent of 75 to 100 mg daily in divided doses. Up to a maximum of 150 mg daily may be required in patients with severe depression. The manufacturers recommend that plasma concentrations of nortriptyline should be monitored when doses above 100 mg daily are given. Adolescents and the elderly may be given 30 to 50 mg daily in divided doses.

Since nortriptyline has a prolonged half-life, once-daily dosage regimens are also suitable, usually given at night.

Nortriptyline is also used for the treatment of **nocturnal enuresis** in children in whom organic pathology has been excluded. However, drug therapy for nocturnal enuresis should be reserved for those in whom other methods have failed and should preferably only be given to cover periods away from home; tricyclic antidepressants are not recommended in children under 6 years of age (the *British National Formulary* recommends that they should not be given until 7 years of age). Suggested doses are 10 mg for children aged 6 to 7 years, 10 to 20 mg for children aged 8 to 11 years, and 25 to 35 mg for children aged over 11 years. The dose should be given 30 minutes before bedtime and treatment should not continue for longer than 3 months, which should include a period of gradual withdrawal. A full physical examination is recommended before a further course.

An initial dose of 10 to 25 mg at night has been suggested by the *British National Formulary* for the management of **neuropathic pain.**

Nortriptyline should be withdrawn gradually to reduce the risk of withdrawal symptoms.

**Smoking cessation.** For reference to the use of nortriptyline in management of smoking cessation, see p.286.

### Preparations

***BP 2003:*** Nortriptyline Capsules; Nortriptyline Tablets;
***USP 27:*** Nortriptyline Hydrochloride Capsules; Nortriptyline Hydrochloride Oral Solution.

**Proprietary Preparations** (details are given in Part 3)
***Arg.:*** Ateben; ***Austral.:*** Allegron; ***Austria:*** Nortrilen; ***Belg.:*** Nortrilen; ***Braz.:*** Pamelor; ***Canad.:*** Aventyl; Norventyl; ***Denm.:*** Noritren; ***Fin.:*** Noritren; ***Ger.:*** Nortrilen; ***Gr.:*** Nortrilen; ***Hong Kong:*** Nortrilen; ***India:*** Sensival; ***Irl.:*** Aventyl†; ***Israel:*** Nortylin; ***Ital.:*** Noritren; Vividyl†; ***Neth.:*** Nortrilen; ***Norw.:*** Noritren; ***NZ:*** Allegron†; Norpress; ***Port.:*** Norterol; Nortrix; ***S.Afr.:*** Aventyl†; ***Spain:*** Martimil†; Norfenazin; Paxtibi; ***Swed.:*** Sensaval; ***Switz.:*** Nortrilen; ***Thai.:*** Norline; Nortrilen; Nortyline; Ortrip; ***UK:*** Allegron; ***USA:*** Aventyl; Pamelor.

**Multi-ingredient:** ***Arg.:*** Karile; ***Chile:*** Motitrel; ***Hong Kong:*** Motival†; ***Irl.:*** Motival; ***Ital.:*** Dominans; ***S.Afr.:*** Motival; ***Spain:*** Tropargal; ***Thai.:*** Motival†; ***UK:*** Motipress†; Motival.

## Opipramol Hydrochloride *(BANM, USAN, rINNM)*

G-33040; Hidrocloruro de opipramol. 2-[4-(3-5*H*-Dibenz-[*b,f*]azepin-5-ylpropyl)piperazin-1-yl]ethanol dihydrochloride.
$C_{23}H_{29}N_3O,2HCl = 436.4.$
*CAS — 315-72-0 (opipramol); 909-39-7 (opipramol dihydrochloride).*
*ATC — N06AA05.*

**Pharmacopoeias.** In *Pol.*

### Profile

Opipramol hydrochloride is a tricyclic antidepressant (see Amitriptyline, p.280) given by mouth in doses of 50 to 300 mg daily in the treatment of depression.

It should be withdrawn gradually to reduce the risk of withdrawal symptoms.

### Preparations

**Proprietary Preparations** (details are given in Part 3)
***Austria:*** Insidon; ***Belg.:*** Insidon†; ***Ger.:*** Insidon; ***Irl.:*** Insidon†; ***Israel:*** Oprimol; ***Ital.:*** Insidon†; ***Neth.:*** Insidon†; ***Switz.:*** Insidon.

## Oxitriptan *(rINN)*

5-HTP; L-5-Hydroxytryptophan; Ro-0783/B. L-2-Amino-3-(5-hydroxy-1*H*-indol-3-yl)propionic acid.
$C_{11}H_{12}N_2O_3 = 220.2.$
*CAS — 4350-09-8 (oxitriptan); 56-69-9 (DL-5-hydroxytryptophan).*
*ATC — N06AX01.*

### Profile

Oxitriptan is the L form of 5-hydroxytryptophan, a precursor of serotonin. Like tryptophan (p.320) it is used in the treatment of depression; it is given in doses of up to 600 mg daily by mouth.

Oxitriptan is also used in doses of up to 1 g daily in myoclonic disorders, especially posthypoxic myoclonus (p.353). It has also been used in various neurological conditions including migraine, pain syndromes, and sleep disorders, and as an adjunct in epilepsy and parkinsonism.

DL-Oxitriptan has also been used as an antidepressant.

### Preparations

**Proprietary Preparations** (details are given in Part 3)
***Fr.:*** Levotonine; ***Ger.:*** Levothym; ***Ital.:*** Tript-OH; ***Port.:*** Cincofarm; ***Spain:*** Cincofarm; Telesol†; ***Switz.:*** Tript-OH.

## Paroxetine *(BAN, USAN, rINN)*

BRL-29060; FG-7051. (−)-*trans*-5-(4-*p*-Fluorophenyl-3-piperidylmethoxy)-1,3-benzodioxole.
$C_{19}H_{20}FNO_3 = 329.4.$
*CAS — 61869-08-7.*
*ATC — N06AB05.*

## Paroxetine Hydrochloride *(BANM, rINNM)*

BRL-29060A; Hidrocloruro de paroxetina; Paroxetine Hydrochloride Hemihydrate; Paroxetini Hydrochloridum Hemihydricum.
$C_{19}H_{20}FNO_3,HCl,\frac{1}{2}H_2O = 374.8.$
*CAS — 78246-49-8 (paroxetine hydrochloride); 110429-35-1 (paroxetine hydrochloride hemihydrate).*

**Pharmacopoeias.** In *Eur.* (see p.vi) and *US*, which permits the anhydrous and hemihydrate forms.

**Ph. Eur. 5.0** (Paroxetine Hydrochloride Hemihydrate). A white or almost white, crystalline powder. It exhibits pseudopolymorphism. Slightly soluble in water; sparingly soluble in alcohol and in dichloromethane; freely soluble in methyl alcohol. Protect from light.

**USP 27** (Paroxetine Hydrochloride). It is anhydrous or contains one-half molecule of water of hydration. A white to off-white solid. Slightly soluble in water; soluble in alcohol and in methyl alcohol. Store the anhydrous form in airtight containers. Both forms should be stored at a temperature of 15° to 30°.

## Paroxetine Mesilate *(BANM, rINNM)*

Paroxetine Mesylate *(USAN)*.
$C_{19}H_{20}FNO_3,CH_4O_3S = 425.5.$
*CAS — 217797-14-3.*
*ATC — N06AB05.*

### Adverse Effects, Treatment, and Precautions

As for SSRIs in general (see Fluoxetine, p.292).

Extrapyramidal reactions (including orofacial dystonias) and withdrawal symptoms associated with paroxetine have been reported to the UK Committee on Safety of Medicines more commonly than with other SSRIs. For further details, see Extrapyramidal Effects under Adverse Effects of Fluoxetine, p.293 and Withdrawal under Precautions, p.295.

There is a potential for worsening of panic symptoms during the initial treatment of panic disorder with paroxetine.

**Breast feeding.** For comments on the use of SSRIs in breast feeding patients, see under Precautions for Fluoxetine, p.294.

**Children.** In the UK the Committee on Safety of Medicines recommends that paroxetine should not be used to treat depressive illness in children under 18 years of age. For details, see under Effects on Mental State in Fluoxetine, p.293.

### Interactions

For interactions associated with SSRIs, see Fluoxetine, p.295.

### Pharmacokinetics

Paroxetine is readily absorbed from the gastrointestinal tract with peak plasma concentrations occurring within about 5 hours of ingestion. It undergoes extensive first-pass metabolism in the liver. The main metabolic pathway is oxidation followed by methylation and formation of glucuronide and sulfate conjugates. The cytochrome P450 isoenzyme CYP2D6 is partly responsible for the metabolism of paroxetine. Paroxetine is widely distributed throughout body tissues and is about 95% bound to plasma proteins. The elimination half-life of paroxetine is reported to be about 21 hours. Excretion is via the urine (approximately 64%) and the faeces (approximately 36%), mainly as metabolites in both cases. Paroxetine is distributed into breast milk (see Breast Feeding under Precautions in Fluoxetine, p.294).

◊ References.


1. Dalhoff K, *et al.* Pharmacokinetics of paroxetine in patients with cirrhosis. *Eur J Clin Pharmacol* 1991; **41:** 351–4.


### Uses and Administration

Paroxetine, a phenylpiperidine derivative, is an SSRI with actions and uses similar to those of fluoxetine (p.296). It is given by mouth usually as paroxetine hydrochloride, as a single dose in the morning; it is also given as the mesilate. Doses are expressed in terms of paroxetine base; paroxetine hydrochloride 22.8 mg or paroxetine mesilate 25.8 mg are approximately equivalent to 20 mg of paroxetine. The doses given below refer to preparations containing paroxetine hydrochloride; similar doses are also used when paroxetine is given as the mesilate.

In the treatment of **depression**, the usual dose of paroxetine is 20 mg daily, increased gradually, if necessary, in weekly increments of 10 mg to a maximum of 50 mg daily.

In the treatment of **obsessive-compulsive disorder**, the initial dose is 20 mg daily increased weekly in 10-mg increments to a usual maintenance dose of 40 mg daily; some patients may require up to 60 mg daily.

In the treatment of **panic disorder** with or without agoraphobia, the initial dose is 10 mg daily increased weekly in 10-mg increments according to clinical response; the usual recommended maintenance dose is 40 mg daily, although some patients may benefit from 50 or 60 mg daily.

The initial dose for the treatment of **social phobia** is 20 mg daily increased after at least 2 weeks, if necessary, by increments of 10 mg at weekly intervals to a maximum of 50 or 60 mg daily.

In the treatment of **generalised anxiety disorder**, the initial dose is 20 mg daily; in the USA further increases in weekly increments of 10 mg to a maximum of 50 mg have been given.

The recommended starting dose for the treatment of **post-traumatic stress disorder** is 20 mg daily. If necessary this may be increased in increments of 10 mg up to a maximum of 50 mg daily.

A suggested maximum daily dose in elderly or debilitated patients is 40 mg; the US manufacturers also recommend a starting dose of 10 mg daily in such patients. Reduced doses should be given to patients with hepatic or renal impairment, see below.

A modified-release preparation (as the hydrochloride) is also available in the USA for the treatment of depression, panic disorder, and social phobia; the maximum doses with this preparation may be slightly greater than those recommended with the normal-release preparation. The modified-release preparation may also be used in the treatment of **premenstrual dysphoric disorder**. The initial dose is 12.5 mg once daily, usually in the morning, which may be increased to 25 mg once daily, if necessary, after an interval of at least one week. Treatment may be given throughout the menstrual cycle or limited to the luteal phase.

Paroxetine should be withdrawn gradually to reduce the risk of withdrawal symptoms. For further details, see Withdrawal under Precautions of Fluoxetine, p.295.

◊ Reviews.


1. Caley CF, Weber SS. Paroxetine: a selective serotonin reuptake inhibiting antidepressant. *Ann Pharmacother* 1993; **27:** 1212–22.
2. Gunasekara NS, *et al.* Paroxetine: an update of its pharmacology and therapeutic use in depression and a review of its use in other disorders. *Drugs* 1998; **55:** 85–120.
3. Wagstaff AJ, *et al.* Paroxetine: an update of its use in psychiatric disorders in adults. *Drugs* 2002; **62:** 655–703. Correction. *ibid.*; 1461.


**Administration in hepatic or renal impairment.** A recommended dose of paroxetine for patients with severe renal or severe hepatic impairment is 10 mg daily in the USA, and 20 mg daily in the UK; incremental dosage if required should be restricted to the lower end of the range.

**Anxiety disorders.** Paroxetine is used in a variety of anxiety disorders including generalised anxiety disorder (p.663), obsessive-compulsive disorder (p.663), panic attacks (p.663), post-traumatic stress disorder (p.664), and social phobia (see under Phobic Disorders, p.663). It has also been tried for adult night terrors (see under Parasomnias, p.667).

References.


1. Oehrberg S, *et al.* Paroxetine in the treatment of panic disorder: a randomised, double-blind, placebo-controlled study. *Br J Psychiatry* 1995; **167:** 374–9.
2. Zohar J, *et al.* Paroxetine versus clomipramine in the treatment of obsessive-compulsive disorder. *Br J Psychiatry* 1996; **169:** 468–74.
3. Lecrubier Y, *et al.* Long-term evaluation of paroxetine, clomipramine and placebo in panic disorder. *Acta Psychiatr Scand* 1997; **95:** 153–60.
4. Wilson SJ, *et al.* Adult night terrors and paroxetine. *Lancet* 1997; **350:** 185.
5. Stein MB, *et al.* Paroxetine treatment of generalized social phobia (social anxiety disorder). *JAMA* 1998; **280:** 708–13.

6. Baldwin D, *et al.* Paroxetine in social phobia/social anxiety disorder: randomised, double-blind, placebo-controlled study. *Br J Psychiatry* 1999; **175:** 120–6.
7. Baldwin DS. Clinical experience with paroxetine in social anxiety disorder. *Int Clin Psychopharmacol* 2000; **15** (suppl): S19–24.
8. Marshall RD, *et al.* Efficacy and safety of paroxetine treatment for chronic PTSD: a fixed-dose, placebo-controlled study. *Am J Psychiatry* 2001; **158:** 1982–8.
9. Tucker P, *et al.* Paroxetine in the treatment of chronic posttraumatic stress disorder: results of a placebo-controlled, flexible-dosage trial. *J Clin Psychiatry* 2001; **62:** 860–8.
10. Liebowitz MR, *et al.* A randomized, double-blind, fixed-dose comparison of paroxetine and placebo in the treatment of generalized social anxiety disorder. *J Clin Psychiatry* 2002; **63:** 66–74.


**Depression.** As discussed on p.279, there is very little difference in efficacy between the different groups of antidepressant drugs, and choice is often made on the basis of adverse effect profile. SSRIs such as paroxetine are widely used as an alternative to the older tricyclics as they have fewer unpleasant side-effects and are safer in overdosage.

References.


1. Leyman S, *et al.* Paroxetine: post-marketing experience on 4024 depressed patients in Belgium. *Eur J Clin Res* 1995; **7:** 287–96.
2. Rodríguez-Ramos P, *et al.* Effects of paroxetine in depressed adolescents. *Eur J Clin Res* 1996; **8:** 49–61.
3. Franchini L, *et al.* Dose-response efficacy of paroxetine in preventing depressive recurrences: a randomized, double-blind study. *J Clin Psychiatry* 1998; **59:** 229–32.
4. Williams JW, *et al.* Treatment of dysthymia and minor depression in primary care: a randomized controlled trial in older adults. *JAMA* 2000; **284:** 1519–26.
5. Keller MB, *et al.* Efficacy of paroxetine in the treatment of adolescent major depression: a randomized, controlled trial. *J Am Acad Child Adolesc Psychiatry* 2001; **40:** 762–72.
6. Golden RN, *et al.* Efficacy and tolerability of controlled-release and immediate-release paroxetine in the treatment of depression. *J Clin Psychiatry* 2002; **63:** 577–84.


**Hypochondriasis.** For mention of the use of SSRIs, including paroxetine, in hypochondriasis, see under Fluoxetine, p.297.

**Premenstrual syndrome.** Paroxetine in doses ranging from 10 to 30 mg daily throughout the menstrual cycle has produced beneficial effects in controlling both the psychological and somatic symptoms of premenstrual syndrome;[1] it was more effective than the tetracyclic antidepressant maprotiline.

For a discussion of the overall management of premenstrual syndrome, see p.1551.


1. Eriksson E, *et al.* The serotonin reuptake inhibitor paroxetin is superior to the noradrenaline reuptake inhibitor maprotiline in the treatment of premenstrual syndrome. *Neuropsychopharmacology* 1995; **12:** 167–76.


**Sexual dysfunction.** Impotence or ejaculatory problems have been reported as adverse effects of SSRIs; for the potential use of these effects in the management of premature ejaculation see Fluoxetine, p.298.

## Preparations

*USP 27:* Paroxetine Tablets.

**Proprietary Preparations** (details are given in Part 3)
***Arg.:*** Aropax; Pamoxet; Psicoasten; ***Austral.:*** Aropax; Oxetine; Paxtine; Roxatine†; ***Austria:*** Seroxat; ***Belg.:*** Aropax; Seroxat; ***Braz.:*** Aropax; Cebrilin; Pondera; ***Canad.:*** Paxil; ***Chile:*** Aroxat; Bectam; Posivyl; Seretran; Traviata; ***Denm.:*** Oxetine; Seroxat; ***Fin.:*** Seroxat; ***Fr.:*** Deroxat; Divarius; ***Ger.:*** Euplix; Paroxat; Paroxedura; Seroxat; Tagonis; ***Gr.:*** Seroxat; ***Hong Kong:*** Seroxat; ***India:*** Xet; ***Irl.:*** Meloxat; Parox; Seroxat; ***Israel:*** Paxxet; Seroxat; ***Ital.:*** Sereupin; Seroxat; ***Malaysia:*** Seroxat; ***Mex.:*** Aropax; Paxil; ***Neth.:*** Seroxat; ***Norw.:*** Seroxat; ***NZ:*** Aropax; ***Port.:*** Paxetil; Seroxat; ***S.Afr.:*** Aropax; ***Singapore:*** Seroxat; ***Spain:*** Casbol; Frosinor; Motivan; Seroxat; ***Swed.:*** Seroxat; ***Switz.:*** Deroxat; ***Thai.:*** Seroxat; ***UK:*** Seroxat; ***USA:*** Paxil; Pexeva.

# Phenelzine Sulfate *(pINNM)*

Phenelzine Sulphate *(BANM)*; Sulfato de fenelzina. Phenethylhydrazine hydrogen sulphate.

$C_8H_{12}N_2,H_2SO_4 = 234.3.$

*CAS — 51-71-8 (phenelzine); 156-51-4 (phenelzine sulfate).*

*ATC — N06AF03.*

**Pharmacopoeias.** In *Br.* and *US.*

**BP 2003** (Phenelzine Sulphate). A white powder or pearly platelets with a pungent odour. Freely soluble in water; practically insoluble in alcohol, in chloroform, and in ether. Protect from light.

**USP 27** (Phenelzine Sulfate). A white to yellowish-white powder having a characteristic odour. Freely soluble in water; practically insoluble in alcohol, in chloroform, and in ether. pH of a 1% solution in water is between 1.4 and 1.9. Store in airtight containers. Protect from heat and light.

## Adverse Effects

Adverse effects commonly associated with phenelzine and other MAOIs include orthostatic hypotension and attacks of dizziness. Other common side-effects include headache, dry mouth, constipation and other gastrointestinal disturbances (including nausea and vomiting), and oedema. Drowsiness, weakness, and fatigue are reported frequently although CNS stimulation may occur and symptoms include agitation, nervousness, euphoria, restlessness, insomnia, and convulsions. Psychotic episodes, with manic reactions, or toxic delirium, may be induced in susceptible persons. Sweating and muscle tremors, twitching, or hyperreflexia may occur, which in overdosage may present as extreme hyperpyrexia and neuromuscular irritability. Other reported reactions include blurred vision, urinary retention or difficulty in micturition, skin rashes, leucopenia, sexual disturbances, and weight gain with inappropriate appetite. Jaundice has been reported with hydrazine MAOIs and, on rare occasions, fatal progressive hepatocellular necrosis. Peripheral neuropathies associated with the hydrazine derivatives may be caused by pyridoxine deficiency. Hyponatraemia, possibly due to inappropriate secretion of antidiuretic hormone, has been associated with the use of antidepressants, particularly in the elderly.

Symptoms of overdosage may be mild initially and progress over the ensuing 24 to 48 hours. Following mild overdosage and symptomatic and supportive therapy, recovery may occur in 3 to 4 days, but following massive overdosage symptoms may persist for up to 2 weeks. Symptoms of CNS depression including drowsiness have been observed with overdosage, but CNS stimulation is more common and is manifested by irritability, hyperactivity, agitation, hallucinations, or convulsions. Respiratory depression and coma may ultimately occur. Cardiovascular effects include hypertension, sometimes with severe headache, although hypotension is more frequently observed; cardiac arrhythmias and peripheral collapse can also develop. Profuse sweating, hyperpyrexia, and neuromuscular excitation with hyperreflexia are also prominent features of overdosage.

MAOIs have been the most commonly implicated drugs in the serotonin syndrome (see below). A severe hypertensive crisis, sometimes fatal, may occur if an MAOI is taken with some other drugs or certain foods (see Interactions, below). These reactions are characterised by severe headache and a rapid and sometimes prolonged rise in blood pressure followed by intracranial haemorrhage or acute cardiac failure.

For the adverse effects of reversible inhibitors of monoamine oxidase type A (RIMAs), see Moclobemide, p.308.

◊ A suspicion that the reported side-effects of MAOIs were both exaggerated and overemphasised prompted a comparative study in patients receiving phenelzine or imipramine.[1] The report noted that the dosages of phenelzine used were at the upper end of the usual therapeutic range (mean 77 mg daily) while those of imipramine were in the middle of the usual therapeutic range (mean 139 mg daily). A very similar profile of side-effects in the two groups was observed. With the exception of significantly increased incidence of drowsiness in the phenelzine-treated group, the 2 groups did not differ in the frequency of autonomic, CNS, cardiovascular, or psychological side-effects. However, a significantly greater number of phenelzine-treated patients had to discontinue their treatment because of the severity of the side-effects. Nonetheless it was considered that phenelzine was reasonably well-tolerated when compared with imipramine.

Others have also studied the side-effect profile of phenelzine and made comparisons with tranylcypromine and imipramine.[2,3] A retrospective review involving 198 patients led them to believe that although phenelzine was more likely than the other two drugs to induce side-effects, drug discontinuation because of side-effects was less likely to occur. This was probably because phenelzine showed clear-cut clinical efficacy resulting in prescribers being reluctant to discontinue therapy.


1. Evans DL, *et al.* Early and late side effects of phenelzine. *J Clin Psychopharmacol* 1982; **2:** 208–10.
2. Rabkin J, *et al.* Adverse reactions to monoamine oxidase inhibitors. Part I: a comparative study. *J Clin Psychopharmacol* 1984; **4:** 270–8.
3. Rabkin JG, *et al.* Adverse reactions to monoamine oxidase inhibitors. Part II: treatment correlates and clinical management. *J Clin Psychopharmacol* 1985; **5:** 2–9.


**Effects on the cardiovascular system.** MAOIs are generally considered to be relatively free of adverse cardiovascular effects. The hypertensive reaction that may follow interactions of MAOIs with foods or other drugs is well known (see Interactions, below) but orthostatic hypotension may occur when these drugs are used on their own.

In one study[1] involving 14 patients it was found that phenelzine produced both a significant decrease in systolic blood pressure while lying, and significant orthostatic hypotension; in 2 patients these effects on blood pressure meant treatment had to be altered. Differences between the effects of phenelzine and those reported for the tricyclic antidepressants were noted. Tricyclics were not known to affect lying systolic blood pressure and although both tricyclics and phenelzine could cause orthostatic hypotension, that occurring with the tricyclics typically reaches a maximum within the first week of treatment whereas with phenelzine the maximum effect was noted after 4 weeks. Additionally, the study provided some indication that the blood pressure effects of phenelzine may attenuate with time, a phenomenon that is not known to occur with the tricyclics.


1. Kronig MH, *et al.* Blood pressure effects of phenelzine. *J Clin Psychopharmacol* 1983; **3:** 307–10.


**Effects on the endocrine system.** MAOIs may induce *hyperprolactinaemia*[1] and this has led to galactorrhoea in women.[2] Occasionally, MAOIs may cause *dilutional hyponatraemia* due to a reduction in the renal excretion of free water mediated by both enhanced vasopressin release and increased antidiuretic action on the renal tubule.[3] The UK Committee on Safety of Medicines, commenting on reports[4] it had received of hyponatraemia with antidepressants (fluoxetine, paroxetine, lofepramine, clomipramine, and imipramine), considered that it was likely to occur with any antidepressant and usually involved elderly patients.


1. Slater SL, *et al.* Elevation of plasma-prolactin by monoamine-oxidase inhibitors. *Lancet* 1977; **ii:** 275–6.
2. Segal M, Heys RF. Inappropriate lactation. *BMJ* 1969; **4:** 236.
3. Baylis PH. Drug-induced endocrine disorders. *Adverse Drug React Bull* 1986; No 116: 432–5.
4. Committee on Safety of Medicines/Medicines Control Agency. Antidepressant-induced hyponatraemia. *Current Problems* 1994; **20:** 5–6.


**Effects on the liver.** Published case reports of hepatotoxic reactions to MAOIs have included jaundice in 4 patients[1] and hepatic failure progressing to encephalopathy in 2 patients;[2] this latter reaction was attributed to a hypersensitivity reaction.

Of 91 cases of hepatitis associated with antidepressants reported to French pharmacovigilance centres during the years 1977 to 1983 an MAOI (iproniazid) was implicated in 11. These 11 cases were associated with cytolytic reactions and 5 patients died.[3]

Two cases of fulminant hepatic failure have been reported[4] following use of phenelzine for 4 months; all other causes of acute liver damage were ruled out. Both patients recovered after emergency liver transplantation.


1. Holdsworth CD, *et al.* Hepatitis caused by the newer amine-oxidase-inhibiting drugs. *Lancet* 1961; **ii:** 621–3.
2. Wilkinson SP, *et al.* Frequency and type of renal and electrolyte disorders in fulminant hepatic failure. *BMJ* 1974; **1:** 186–9.
3. Lefebure B, *et al.* Hépatites aux antidépresseurs. *Therapie* 1984; **39:** 509–16.
4. Gómez-Gil E, *et al.* Phenelzine-induced fulminant hepatic failure. *Ann Intern Med* 1996; **124:** 692–3.


**Effects on the nervous system.** MAOIs produce a variety of effects on the nervous system. Drowsiness is frequently reported but symptoms of CNS stimulation, including agitation, nervousness, and euphoria may also occur; psychotic episodes may be induced in susceptible individuals. Further adverse neurological reactions are described under Epileptogenic Effect and Extrapyramidal Effects, below.

Peripheral neuropathies, sometimes associated with a documented pyridoxine deficiency, have been reported in patients receiving phenelzine.[1,2] In most of the patients the neuropathies developed 6 weeks to 4 months after starting phenelzine,[2] although in one case symptoms did not occur for 11 years.[1] The symptoms also generally disappeared when pyridoxine was given together with continued phenelzine therapy.[2] The possibility that the dietary restrictions imposed on persons taking phenelzine might have contributed to a low pyridoxine intake was considered unlikely. The most probable mechanism for the induced pyridoxine deficiency was combination of the hydrazine moiety with the pyridoxal form of the vitamin to form an inactive compound.

Many drugs can inhibit transmission at the myoneural junction under experimental conditions and it has been said that phenelzine may cause postoperative respiratory depression, possibly through a combined action with neuromuscular blockers.[3] For further details, see Anaesthesia under Precautions, below.


1. Heller CA, Friedman PA. Pyridoxine deficiency and peripheral neuropathy associated with long-term phenelzine therapy. *Am J Med* 1983; **75:** 887–8.
2. Stewart JW, *et al.* Phenelzine-induced pyridoxine deficiency. *J Clin Psychopharmacol* 1984; **4:** 225–6.
3. Lane RJM, Routledge PA. Drug-induced neurological disorders. *Drugs* 1983; **26:** 124–47.


**Effects on sexual function.** MAOIs such as phenelzine and tranylcypromine have been implicated in producing both impotence and failure of ejaculation.[1,2] Priapism has been reported with phenelzine.[3] There have also been several reports of anorgasmia in women attributed to MAOIs, an effect which appears to be dose-related.[4] It should be remembered that loss of libido and impotence are common symptoms of depression, often making the role of drugs in producing sexual dysfunction difficult to assess.


1. Simpson GM, *et al.* Effects of anti-depressants on genito-urinary function. *Dis Nerv Syst* 1965; **26:** 787–9.
2. Wyatt RJ, *et al.* Treatment of intractable narcolepsy with a monoamine oxidase inhibitor. *N Engl J Med* 1971; **285:** 987–91.
3. Yeragani VK, Gershon S. Priapism related to phenelzine therapy. *N Engl J Med* 1987; **317:** 117–18.
4. Shen WW, Sata LS. Inhibited female orgasm resulting from psychotropic drugs: a clinical review. *J Reprod Med* 1983; **28:** 497–9.

**Epileptogenic effect.** Convulsions represent one of the less common adverse effects of MAOIs; they may be a feature of overdosage.

A typical grand-mal seizure with tonic-clonic convulsions has been reported in a patient with no history of epilepsy or predisposing factors shortly after the start of phenelzine therapy.[1] The point was made that phenelzine-induced seizures had rarely been observed.

1. Bhugra DK, Kaye N. Phenelzine induced grand mal seizure. *Br J Clin Pract* 1986; **40:** 173–4.

**Extrapyramidal effects.** A parkinsonian syndrome developed in a patient about 5 weeks after the start of therapy with phenelzine. Symptoms gradually resolved over 10 days following the withdrawal of phenelzine. The mechanisms by which phenelzine could have induced these effects were discussed.[1]

1. Gillman MA, Sandyk R. Parkinsonism induced by a monoamine oxidase inhibitor. *Postgrad Med J* 1986; **62:** 235–6.

**Hyponatraemia.** See Effects on the Endocrine System, above.

**Lupus.** A reversible lupus-like reaction has been reported in a patient who had been taking phenelzine sulfate for 8 months.[1]

1. Swartz C. Lupus-like reaction to phenelzine. *JAMA* 1978; **239:** 2693.

**Overdosage.** MAOIs in overdose rarely produce severe hypertension; the blood pressure may be high or low, or may alternate between the two. More commonly the patient gradually develops widespread muscle spasms, trismus, and opisthotonus with widely dilated pupils and a hot and sweating skin. About 16 to 24 hours after ingestion potentially fatal hyperthermia may develop; temperatures of 42.1 to 43.8° have been recorded immediately before death. Disseminated intravascular coagulation, rhabdomyolysis, and acute tubular necrosis can also occur.[1]

1. Henry JA. Specific problems of drug intoxication. *Br J Anaesth* 1986; **58:** 223–33.

**Serotonin syndrome.** The serotonin syndrome is a drug-induced excess in serotonergic activity at central receptors, usually due to an additive effect of 2 or more serotonergic drugs; the pathogenesis and management have been reviewed.[1-8] It is characterised by the development of *at least three* of the following clinical features after a recent change in a treatment regimen involving serotonergic drugs:

- agitation
- ataxia
- diaphoresis
- diarrhoea
- fever
- hyperreflexia
- myoclonus
- shivering
- changes in mental status

The onset of the syndrome may occur within minutes of altering the regimen, or several weeks later.[3] The occurrence and severity of the syndrome do not appear to be dose-related,[3] but to depend on the extent and duration of the rise in intrasynaptic serotonin.[6] The syndrome should be distinguished from the hypertensive crises produced by the interaction between MAOIs and tyramine (see Interactions of MAOIs with Foods, below), and from the neuroleptic malignant syndrome (see p.677).[4]

The serotonin syndrome is relatively uncommon and symptoms are usually mild. However, severe complications, including disseminated intravascular coagulation, severe hyperthermia, respiratory failure, and seizures have been reported; there have also been fatalities.

**MAOIs** have been the most commonly implicated drugs in this syndrome, including cases with other antidepressants such as the tricyclics, SSRIs, serotonin and noradrenaline reuptake inhibitors (SNRIs), trazodone, lithium, and tryptophan. (The use of combination therapy with serotonergic antidepressant drugs is discussed under Interactions of MAOIs with other Drugs, below.) MAOIs combined with the opioids dextromethorphan and pethidine have also produced the serotonin syndrome. The interaction can occur with both irreversible and reversible MAOIs, and with those selective for monoamine oxidase type A such as moclobemide as well as with non-selective MAOIs.[9] The selective inhibitor of monoamine oxidase type B, selegiline, may also pose problems at high doses as its selectivity starts to diminish.

As usage of the **SSRIs** has increased, so too has the number of reports of adverse reactions when these drugs have been combined with other serotonergic drugs, including the herbal preparation hypericum.

**Other drugs** that may potentially cause serotonin syndrome in certain circumstances include buspirone, carbamazepine, dihydroergotamine, methylenedioxyamfetamine, selective serotonin ($5\text{-}HT_1$) agonists such as sumatriptan, and tramadol.[2,6] Rarely, a single serotonergic drug has produced the serotonin syndrome.[3]

Serotonergic potentiation may also occur if one serotonergic drug is used after another without allowing a sufficient **drug-free interval** after stopping the first. This is a particular problem when the first drug is an irreversible MAOI or a drug with a long half-life such as the SSRI fluoxetine.

Most cases of serotonin syndrome resolve within 24 hours following withdrawal of the offending drugs and administration of supportive **therapy**,[1-5] including appropriate management of fever and hyperthermia (p.8). Benzodiazepines may be of value to control myoclonus and seizures. The non-specific serotonin antagonists cyproheptadine and methysergide have been used with some success.[3,4,7] Other drugs that have been tried include propranolol, chlorpromazine, and dantrolene.[3,4,7]

1. Sternbach H. The serotonin syndrome. *Am J Psychiatry* 1991; **148:** 705–13.
2. Nierenberg DW, Semprebon M. The central nervous system serotonin syndrome. *Clin Pharmacol Ther* 1993; **53:** 84–8.
3. Sporer KA. The serotonin syndrome: implicated drugs, pathophysiology and management. *Drug Safety* 1995; **13:** 94–104.
4. Corkeron MA. Serotonin syndrome—a potentially fatal complication of antidepressant therapy. *Med J Aust* 1995; **163:** 481–2.
5. Brown TM, *et al.* Pathophysiology and management of the serotonin syndrome. *Ann Pharmacother* 1996; **30:** 527–33.
6. Gillman PK. Serotonin syndrome: history and risk. *Fundam Clin Pharmacol* 1998; **12:** 482–91.
7. Gillman PK. The serotonin syndrome and its treatment. *J Psychopharmacol* 1999; **13:** 100–109.
8. Mason PJ, *et al.* Serotonin syndrome. Presentation of 2 cases and review of the literature. *Medicine (Baltimore)* 2000; **79:** 201–9.
9. Livingston MG. Interactions with selective MAOIs. *Lancet* 1995; **345:** 533–4.

## Treatment of Adverse Effects

In cases of overdosage with MAOIs in patients who present within 1 hour activated charcoal may be given by mouth, or the stomach may be emptied by lavage. Management then largely involves intensive symptomatic and supportive therapy with particular attention being given to CNS effects, raised body temperature (which may develop into malignant hyperthermia), and cardiovascular effects. Delayed effects may develop some time after the overdose even in patients who are initially asymptomatic, and therefore prolonged monitoring is warranted. Other drugs taken with an overdose of MAOIs may complicate the features and result in the need for an even longer period of monitoring. Special care should be observed with any drug therapy used in the management of MAOI overdosage in view of the many known interactions which occur with this class of drugs.

Muscle spasm, agitation, and convulsions should be treated with diazepam. Severe neuromuscular irritability may call for the use of a competitive neuromuscular blocker such as pancuronium and intubation with assisted ventilation. Hyperthermia may be a particular problem; if simple antipyretics such as paracetamol and external cooling measures fail a competitive neuromuscular blocker has often been advocated; dantrolene has also been suggested.

Hypotension, which is a fairly common feature, should be managed by intravenous fluid therapy and volume expansion; vasopressors should be avoided. Conversely, a hypertensive crisis may occasionally occur following an overdose with MAOIs and can be managed with phentolamine given by slow intravenous injection. A short-acting beta blocker such as esmolol has also been advocated for persistent tachycardia and hypertension.

## Precautions

Phenelzine and other MAOIs should not be given to patients with liver disease or, because of their effects on blood pressure, to patients with cerebrovascular disease or phaeochromocytoma. (Blood pressure should be monitored in all patients.) MAOIs should be avoided or only used with great caution in patients with blood disorders or cardiovascular disease, and in elderly or agitated patients who may be particularly susceptible to their adverse effects. They should be given with caution to epileptic patients. Caution has also been advised in diabetic patients because of conflicting evidence whether glucose metabolism is altered or requirements for hypoglycaemics changed. MAOIs should be used with caution in patients with hyperthyroidism because of increased sensitivity to pressor amines.

Patients should be closely monitored during early antidepressant therapy until improvement in depression is observed because suicide is an inherent risk in depressed patients. For further details, see under Depression, p.279.

Mania may be precipitated if MAOIs are used for the depressive component of bipolar disorder, and they are not usually indicated; similarly psychotic symptoms may be aggravated if they are used for a depressive component of schizophrenia.

MAOIs have a prolonged action so patients should not take any of the foods or drugs known to cause reactions (see Interactions, below) for at least 14 days after stopping treatment. A similar drug-free period has been advised before any patient undergoes surgery since it may involve the use of drugs that can interact with MAOIs, although not all agree that this is necessary; caution has been advised in patients requiring MAOIs with ECT; for further details see under Anaesthesia, below. Patients should carry cards giving details of their MAOI therapy; they and their relatives should be fully conversant with the implications of food and drug interactions and the precautions to be taken.

Patients liable to take charge of vehicles or other machinery should be warned that MAOIs may modify behaviour and state of alertness. Patients affected by drowsiness should not drive or operate machinery.

MAOIs should be withdrawn gradually to reduce the risk of withdrawal symptoms (see below).

For the precautions to be observed with reversible inhibitors of monoamine oxidase A (RIMAs), see Moclobemide, p.308.

**Anaesthesia.** The considerations given to patients receiving tricyclic antidepressants before receiving anaesthesia for ECT or surgery (see Amitriptyline, p.283) are also generally applicable to patients being treated with MAOIs; the manufacturer of phenelzine also warns that cardiovascular depression following ECT has been reported. The interactions of other drugs with MAOIs may be more numerous or more severe than those with tricyclics and the interaction with pethidine should not be forgotten.

A review[1] of the potential problems of anaesthesia in patients receiving MAOIs considered that stopping MAOIs about 2 weeks before anaesthesia was unreasonable, as there was a wide range of safe and suitable anaesthetics available, although the dangers of sympathetic overactivity must always be remembered. This view, that it is safe to continue MAOIs throughout the period of anaesthesia and surgery, has also been advocated by others[2,3] although some disagree.[4]

Regardless of any decision, the anaesthetist should be informed of all drugs that the patient is or has been taking; this is particularly important when emergency surgery is required in a patient receiving MAOI therapy.

- It has been stated[1] that the interaction between MAOIs and *opioid analgesics* has two distinct forms: an excitatory form [serotonin syndrome—see above]; and a depressive form consisting of respiratory depression, hypotension, and coma as a result of the inhibition of hepatic microsomal enzymes by the MAOI leading to accumulation of free opioid analgesic. *Pethidine* is the only commonly used opioid analgesic in anaesthesia to have elicited the excitatory response, which has frequently been severe and often fatal. For this reason, pethidine should never be given to patients receiving MAOIs. *Morphine* does not block neuronal serotonin uptake but its narcotic effects may be potentiated in the presence of MAOIs and a single case report of the depressive type of reaction has been described. Thus, morphine is the opioid analgesic of choice but must be given in reduced dosage and the dosage carefully titrated against clinical response. *Phenoperidine* is probably best avoided as its metabolites are norpethidine and, to a lesser extent, pethidine. *Papaveretum* would appear to have no advantage over morphine. Although interactions of MAOIs with *pentazocine* have occurred in *animals*, it is not clear if this occurs in man. *Methadone* has been used in a patient without mishap and there is also anecdotal evidence to support the safety of *fentanyl*. A case report[5] described the successful use of *alfentanil* (together with propofol and atracurium) mentioning that this was the first report of such use in patients receiving MAOIs. A further case report[6] described a patient who underwent successful anaesthesia with *sufentanil* (together with thiopental, lidocaine, and vecuronium) while continuing to take an MAOI (tranylcypromine) as well as a tricyclic antidepressant (imipramine) and lorazepam.
- With regard to induction agents,[1] the use of *ketamine* in patients receiving MAOIs should be avoided on theoretical grounds, although no interactions have been reported. Potentiation of *barbiturates* may be expected.
- With neuromuscular blockers, phenelzine has been shown to decrease plasma cholinesterase concentrations and there have been case reports of a prolonged effect with *suxamethonium*; additionally this prolongation of the effect of suxamethonium may lead to apnoea and modification of the convulsion during ECT. There appeared to be a theoretical hazard with *pancuronium* since it releases stored adrenaline (although its use has been advocated in the treatment of symptoms of overdosage with MAOIs, see above), but *alcuronium*, *atracurium*, or *vecuronium* would all appear to be suitable alternatives.
- *Enflurane*, *halothane*, *isoflurane*, and *nitrous oxide* are all safe in the presence of MAOIs, although there is a theoretical possibility of an increased risk of hepatic damage with halothane.

- *Indirect-acting sympathomimetics* pose the risk of a serious and possibly lethal hypertensive interaction but *direct-acting sympathomimetics*, such as *adrenaline*, *isoprenaline*, and *noradrenaline*, are reliable vasopressors in the presence of MAOIs although great care should be taken with their use because of enhanced receptor sensitivity.

1. Stack CG, *et al.* Monoamine oxidase inhibitors and anaesthesia: a review. *Br J Anaesth* 1988; **60:** 222–7.
2. Hirshman CA, Lindeman K. MAO inhibitors: must they be discontinued before anesthesia? *JAMA* 1988; **260:** 3507–8.
3. Hirshman CA, Lindeman KS. Anesthesia and monoamine oxidase inhibitors. *JAMA* 1989; **261:** 3407–8.
4. Gevirtz C. Anesthesia and monoamine oxidase inhibitors. *JAMA* 1989; **261:** 3407.
5. Powell H. Use of alfentanil in a patient receiving monoamine oxidase inhibitor therapy. *Br J Anaesth* 1990; **64:** 528.
6. O'Hara JF, *et al.* Sufentanil-isoflurane-nitrous oxide anesthesia for a patient treated with monoamine oxidase inhibitor and tricyclic antidepressant. *J Clin Anesth* 1995; **7:** 148–50.

**Driving.** While affective disorders probably adversely affect driving skill,[1,2] treatment with antidepressant drugs may also be hazardous,[1] although patients may be safer drivers with medication than without.[2] Impairment of performance is largely related to sedative properties and some MAOIs can adversely affect psychomotor performance.[1,2]

In the UK, the Driver and Vehicle Licensing Authority (DVLA) considers that SSRIs, MAOIs, and noradrenaline reuptake inhibitors have fewer adverse effects on drivers than antidepressants with antimuscarinic or antihistaminic adverse effects, such as tricyclic antidepressants. However some patients have idiosyncratic responses and should be advised accordingly.[3] Patients with severe depressive illnesses complicated by significant memory or concentration problems, agitation, behavioural disturbances or suicidal thoughts should cease driving pending the outcome of medical enquiry.

1. Ashton H. Drugs and driving. *Adverse Drug React Bull* 1983; **98:** 360–3.
2. Cremona A. Mad drivers: psychiatric illness and driving performance. *Br J Hosp Med* 1986; **35:** 193–5.
3. Driver and Vehicle Licensing Agency. For medical practitioners: at a glance guide to the current medical standards of fitness to drive. Available at: http://www.dvla.gov.uk/at_a_glance/ch4_psychiatric.htm (accessed 11/06/04)

**Electroconvulsive therapy.** For comments concerning the precautions to be observed in patients receiving ECT, see under Anaesthesia, above.

**Porphyria.** Phenelzine is considered to be unsafe in patients with porphyria because it has been shown to be porphyrinogenic in *animals*.

**Surgery.** For comments regarding the precautions to be observed in patients undergoing surgery, see under Anaesthesia, above.

**Withdrawal.** Suddenly stopping antidepressant therapy after regular use for 8 weeks or more can precipitate withdrawal symptoms which may be very severe.

Symptoms associated with withdrawal of MAOIs[1,2] include gastrointestinal disturbances and generalised somatic symptoms such as nausea and vomiting, anorexia, chills, headache, and giddiness; sleep disturbances characterised by insomnia, severe nightmares, and somnolence; and a range of CNS symptoms including panic, anxiety, restlessness, agitation, cognitive impairment, mood swings, depression and suicidal ideation, hypomania, delusions, and hallucinations. Some of the above may be ameliorated by reinstitution of the MAOI in low doses, but the best management is considered to be prevention by gradually discontinuing the drug.[2] The *British National Formulary* recommends reducing the dose over a period of 4 weeks, or as much as 6 months in patients who have been receiving long-term maintenance therapy.

The pathophysiology of the MAOI withdrawal syndrome is not fully known, although it has been hypothesised that some of the symptoms represent adrenergic hyperactivity[1] produced by the release of excessive amounts of dopamine and noradrenaline.[2]

With the exception of tranylcypromine, the withdrawal syndrome of MAOIs is not a consequence of drug dependence.[1] Tranylcypromine has been reported to produce dependence and tolerance in patients receiving high doses irrespective of whether or not they had a previous history of substance abuse. Tranylcypromine is similar in structure to amfetamine, which may be responsible for its addictive properties.[1]

1. Anonymous. Problems when withdrawing antidepressives. *Drug Ther Bull* 1986; **24:** 29–30.
2. Dilsaver SC. Withdrawal phenomena associated with antidepressant and antipsychotic agents. *Drug Safety* 1994; **10:** 103–14.

## Interactions of MAOIs with Foods

A major disadvantage of MAOIs such as phenelzine is that by inhibiting monoamine oxidase they cause an accumulation of amine neurotransmitters. This means that the pressor effects of *tyramine*, which occurs in a number of common foods and is also metabolised by monoamine oxidase, can be dangerously enhanced. Reactions to foods rich in pressor amines such as tyramine can therefore occur in patients being treated with MAOIs, producing hypertensive crises. Cheese, especially aged or matured cheeses, meat or yeast extracts, pickled herrings, smoked foods, and broad bean pods have caused such reactions. Patients should be warned not to eat any of these foods while being treated with an MAOI and for at least 14 days after its discontinuation. Some foods will only cause a reaction if large amounts are eaten, and foods may vary in tyramine content depending upon methods of manufacture and storage. Any protein-containing food such as meat, fish, or game subject to hydrolysis, fermentation, pickling, smoking, or spoilage could contain tyramine derived from tyrosine as a result of these processes or of deterioration. Patients taking MAOIs should therefore be advised to eat protein-containing foods only if fresh.

Alcoholic beverages, including wines, beers, and drinks that are de-alcoholised or are low in alcohol, contain variable amounts of tyramine and are best avoided.

The above dietary restrictions that need to be observed with MAOIs may be less stringent for reversible inhibitors of monoamine oxidase type A (RIMAs) such as moclobemide (see p.308), although the manufacturers recommend that since some patients may be especially sensitive to tyramine, consumption of large amounts of tyramine-rich food should be avoided.

◊ MAOIs can, when taken with certain foodstuffs, cause a potentially fatal hypertensive reaction. This effect is accepted and well documented and has led to the publication of many lists of prohibited foods and drinks. Some workers have expressed the opinion that the dangers of the interaction may have been slightly overemphasised or exaggerated and that the published lists may have been overinclusive;[1-3] this may have led to reduced compliance in a number of patients.

A review and discussion[1] of the MAOI interaction with tyramine made the following observations and recommendations:

- the hyperadrenergic state resulting from this interaction consisted of three syndromes although significant overlap between them existed: paroxysmal headache of great severity; cardiovascular symptoms with paroxysmal hypertension; and intracerebral haemorrhage and death
- the most common offending drug reported had been tranylcypromine at doses of 20 to 50 mg daily although a few reports had involved phenelzine
- only 4 foodstuffs clearly warranted total prohibition: aged cheese, pickled herring or fish, concentrated yeast extracts, and broad bean pods
- the ingestion of cheese was said to have been associated with 80% of all case reports and with virtually all fatalities. It was agreed that aged cheese should not be permitted, although cottage and cream cheese required no restriction. There was less agreement concerning dairy products such as yogurt and sour cream and it was suggested that limited amounts were permissible
- pickled herring or smoked fish were to be avoided because of several well-documented cases of hypertensive crisis as well as detection of high levels of tyramine. Any meat may become dangerous unless consumed while fresh as tyramine is formed from bacterial protein degradation
- concentrated yeast extracts have a significant tyramine content and yeast vitamin supplements may also constitute a hazard; baker's yeast was considered to be safe
- broad bean pods contain dopamine although the beans were stated to have little pressor activity and carried no prohibition
- other foods which had been reported to have caused a hypertensive reaction but for which these authors considered that there was insufficient evidence to warrant dietary restriction were chocolate and caffeine-containing beverages, soy sauce, fresh fish, wild game, and fruits although caution was necessary with avocados and bananas.

Other reviews of foods[2,4] give broadly similar recommendations.

The consumption of alcoholic beverages, and in particular Chianti wine, has frequently been advised against. However, sources have differed on whether particular types of drink (white wine, red wine, spirits, or beer) are safe or not. One study[5] demonstrated no significant differences in mean free tyramine concentration between white wine, red wine, Chianti, and beer although within each category of wine there could be up to a fiftyfold variation even if from the same grape stock. Mention has also been made[6,7] that alcohol-free or low-alcohol beers are likely to contain similar amounts of tyramine to alcoholic beers. The consumption of alcoholic drinks with MAOIs still appears to be controversial with some advocating total abstinence while others permit a modest intake.

1. Brown C, *et al.* The monoamine oxidase inhibitor-tyramine interaction. *J Clin Pharmacol* 1989; **29:** 529–32.
2. Lippman SB, Nash K. Monoamine oxidase inhibitor update: potential adverse food and drug interactions. *Drug Safety* 1990; **5:** 195–204.
3. Folks DG. Monoamine oxidase inhibitors: reappraisal of dietary considerations. *J Clin Psychopharmacol* 1983; **3:** 249–52.
4. Anonymous. Foods interacting with MAO inhibitors. *Med Lett Drugs Ther* 1989; **31:** 11–12.
5. Hannah P, *et al.* Tyramine in wine and beer. *Lancet* 1988; **i:** 879.
6. Sandler M. Monoamine oxidase inhibitors and low alcohol or alcohol free drinks. *BMJ* 1990; **300:** 1527.
7. Beswick DT, Rogers ML. Monoamine oxidase inhibitors and low alcohol or alcohol free drinks. *BMJ* 1990; **301:** 179–80.

## Interactions of MAOIs with other Drugs

MAOIs inhibit the metabolism of some *amine drugs* (notably indirect-acting sympathomimetics), which can lead to dangerous enhancement of their pressor effects. MAOIs also inhibit other drug-metabolising enzymes and are therefore responsible for a large number of *other drug interactions*. Moreover, they have an additive effect with serotonergic drugs which may result in the *serotonin syndrome* (see under Adverse Effects, above). As in the case of foods, the danger of an interaction persists for at least 14 days after treatment with an MAOI has been discontinued.

Severe hypertensive reactions due to enhancement of pressor activity have followed the use of sympathomimetics such as *amfetamines, dopamine, ephedrine, levodopa, phenylephrine, phenylpropanolamine*, and *pseudoephedrine*. Reactions may also follow the use of anorectics and stimulants with sympathomimetic activity such as *fenfluramine, methylphenidate, pemoline*, and *phentermine*. There have been case reports of fatalities in patients who took cough preparations containing *dextromethorphan*. There is no clinical evidence of dangerous interactions between *local anaesthetic preparations containing adrenaline* and MAOIs but great care should be taken to avoid inadvertent intravenous administration of the local anaesthetic. Significant rises in blood pressure have been reported following the use of *buspirone* with MAOIs.

Inhibition of drug-metabolising enzymes by MAOIs may enhance the effects of *barbiturates* and possibly other *hypnotics, hypoglycaemics*, and possibly *antimuscarinics*. *Alcohol* metabolism may be altered and its effects enhanced; see also under Interactions of MAOIs with Foods, above. *Antihypertensives* including *guanethidine, reserpine*, and *methyldopa* should be given with caution; hypotensive and hypertensive reactions have been suggested; the hypotensive effects of *beta blockers* and *thiazide diuretics* may be enhanced.

Giving *pethidine* and possibly other *opioid analgesics* to patients taking an MAOI has also been associated with very severe and sometimes fatal reactions. When it is considered essential to use an opioid analgesic a test dose of morphine should be given. It has been suggested that the test dose should be one-tenth to one-fifth of the normal dose and if this produces no untoward reaction, the dose of morphine can be gradually and carefully increased over a period of 2 to 3 hours. The use of opioid analgesics and other drugs used during general anaesthesia in patients continuing to take MAOIs is discussed in Anaesthesia under Precautions, above.

*Clozapine* may enhance the CNS effects of MAOIs.

Although different antidepressants have been used together under expert supervision in refractory cases of depression, severe adverse reactions may occur. MAOIs should not generally be given to patients receiving *tricyclic antidepressants, SSRIs, serotonin and noradrenaline reuptake inhibitors (SNRIs)*, or *nefazodone* or *trazodone*. An appropriate drug-free interval should elapse between stopping one type of antidepressant and starting another. An MAOI should not be started until at least 1 or 2 weeks after stopping a tricyclic antidepressant. For the tricyclic antidepressants clomipramine and imipramine a drug-free interval of 3 weeks should be allowed. For an SSRI, an SNRI, nefazodone, trazodone, or any related antidepressant the drug-free interval should be at least one week; in the case of the SSRIs paroxetine and sertraline, the interval is extended to 2 weeks, and for fluoxetine, 5 weeks because of their longer half-lives. Conversely, 2 weeks should elapse between discontinuing MAOI therapy and starting patients on a tricyclic antidepressant (3 weeks in the case of clomipramine or imipramine), an SSRI, an SNRI, or any related antidepressant. For further warnings on the combined use of antidepressants, see below. Interactions can also occur between MAOIs themselves.

For details of the less severe interactions associated with reversible inhibitors of monoamine oxidase A (RIMAs), see Interactions of Moclobemide, p.308.

◊ References.


1. Lippman SB, Nash K. Monoamine oxidase inhibitor update: potential adverse food and drug interactions. *Drug Safety* 1990; **5:** 195–204.
2. Blackwell B. Monoamine oxidase inhibitor interactions with other drugs. *J Clin Psychopharmacol* 1991; **11:** 55–9.
3. Livingston MC, Livingston HM. Monoamine oxidase inhibitors: an update on drug interactions. *Drug Safety* 1996; **14:** 219–27.


**Antidepressants.** Combination therapy with differing classes of antidepressants may result in interactions or enhanced adverse reactions such as the serotonin syndrome (see under Adverse Effects, above), and is therefore considered unsuitable or controversial by some authorities. Despite these drawbacks certain combinations of drugs have been found to be beneficial in the treatment of drug-resistant depression, although others are considered unsuitable; absence of information documenting unsuitability or hazard does not necessarily imply that the two drugs may be used safely together but may merely reflect an untried combination. Because combination therapy poses increased risks it should be used only under expert supervision.

MAOIs have been used fairly frequently under expert supervision with tricyclics in refractory depression and it has been stated[1] that the risk of serious problems in combining *tricyclic antidepressant and MAOI* antidepressant therapy is almost exclusively limited to sequential prescribing, in particular the addition of a tricyclic to established treatment with an MAOI. The recommended procedure was said to be to allow a drug-free interval of at least one week and then to start both drugs together at a low dosage. The dosage of both drugs is then gradually increased to around half that normally prescribed for the drugs when given on their own. The dietary restrictions for MAOIs alone apply equally to the combined antidepressant regimen.

Amitriptyline and trimipramine were considered to be the tricyclics least likely to produce side-effects with MAOIs, while phenelzine and isocarboxazid were the safest MAOIs. In contrast, clomipramine, a tricyclic with serotonin reuptake inhibiting activity, and imipramine are unsuitable for such use.[2,3] The combination of clomipramine with tranylcypromine is particularly dangerous. Symptoms suggestive of the serotonin syndrome occurred in an elderly patient due to an interaction between clomipramine and moclobemide, a reversible inhibitor of monoamine oxidase type A (RIMA).[4] Two fatalities due to serotonin syndrome have been reported following overdosage with clomipramine and moclobemide.[5] The syndrome has also developed when a patient was switched from clomipramine to moclobemide with no suitable drug-free interval.[6] A 39-year-old woman developed the serotonin syndrome while taking imipramine with moclobemide, although it was suggested that an excessive dose of the tricyclic may have been ingested accidentally.[7]

The UK Committee on Safety of Medicines (CSM) has warned[8] that enhanced serotonergic effects may result from using *SSRIs with MAOIs* or other antidepressants. Although such an enhancement may be beneficial in some instances it can produce a life-threatening serotonin syndrome. Such reactions were later reported in patients taking sertraline with MAOIs.[9-11] Three fatalities due to serotonin syndrome have been reported following overdosage with citalopram and moclobemide.[5] A case of serotonin syndrome has been reported after switching from fluoxetine to moclobemide with no suitable drug-free interval.[6] Some authors[12] have reported good efficacy and tolerability with combinations of moclobemide and SSRIs. However, others[13] reported a high rate of adverse events although, as significant improvement in depressive symptoms was observed in some patients, it was suggested that the combination of moclobemide with SSRIs deserved consideration as an option for the treatment of refractory depression.

Combination therapy with a *tricyclic antidepressant and an SSRI* has sometimes been used to treat resistant depression. Fluvoxamine[14] and fluoxetine[15] have been reported to increase plasma concentrations of the tricyclic, although to varying degrees. Fluoxetine has been reported to produce three- to fourfold increases in plasma concentrations of desipramine and imipramine. Fluvoxamine has a minimal effect on desipramine plasma levels but produces a three- to fourfold increase in concentrations of imipramine.[16] Plasma-desipramine concentrations are elevated threefold by paroxetine but increases of only 30% are produced by sertraline.[16] However, an inadequate interval of one day between stopping desipramine and starting paroxetine resulted in a case of serotonin syndrome.[6] Serotonin syndrome has also been reported[17] in a patient who received paroxetine and imipramine together and in another given sertraline and amitriptyline.[18] A threefold increase in concentrations of trimipramine resulting in sedation and orthostatic hypotension has been reported[19] in 2 patients also given paroxetine. Additionally, norfluoxetine, the active metabolite of fluoxetine, has a long half-life and is responsible for the continuing interaction with tricyclics for several days or weeks after fluoxetine has been withdrawn. Citalopram was reported to have no effect on plasma-tricyclic concentrations in a patient although antidepressant effects were augmented.[20]

*Lithium* and *tryptophan* have been used to augment the effect of other antidepressants in refractory depression. Phenelzine has been used successfully in combination with lithium and tryptophan[21] in patients with treatment-resistant chronic depression although such a regimen has probably been used less since the reports of the eosinophilia-myalgia syndrome associated with tryptophan (see p.321). There have, however, been several case reports of reactions similar to the serotonin syndrome in patients receiving MAOIs together with tryptophan.[22,23] Although lithium is often added to tricyclic antidepressant therapy in patients with refractory depression, epileptic seizures have been reported in a patient receiving amitriptyline when lithium was added.[24] Serotonin syndrome has been reported[25] in a patient given clomipramine and lithium. Severe neurotoxicity has been reported[26,27] in some patients receiving lithium and tricyclic or tetracyclic antidepressants together; adverse effects included tremor, memory impairment, disorganised thinking, and auditory hallucinations. One manufacturer of lithium preparations also reports symptoms of nephrogenic diabetes in patients receiving these combinations. By 1989 the CSM had received 19 reports of adverse reactions in patients treated with fluvoxamine and lithium; 5 reports concerned convulsions and 1 hyperthermia.[8] Tremor has been reported when lithium was given with paroxetine,[28] and in general the risk of CNS toxicity is increased when lithium is given with fluoxetine, fluvoxamine, paroxetine, or sertraline. There has been a report[29] of a fatality when fluoxetine was replaced by tranylcypromine and tryptophan with no drug-free period; the patient was also receiving other drugs concurrently.

Use of the serotonin and noradrenaline reuptake inhibitor (SNRI) *venlafaxine with tricyclic antidepressants* has been associated with increased antimuscarinic adverse effects.[30,31] Seizures have also been reported with venlafaxine and trimipramine[32] and serotonin syndrome developed in a patient given amitriptyline, venlafaxine, and pethidine.[33] Similar antimuscarinic adverse effects have occurred in patients given *venlafaxine and the SSRI* fluoxetine;[31] serotonin syndrome has been reported in a patient who received venlafaxine and paroxetine.[6] The use of *venlafaxine with MAOIs* is contra-indicated by the manufacturers of venlafaxine because of the risk of life-threatening adverse reactions. Serious adverse reactions have been reported when venlafaxine was combined with isocarboxazid,[34] moclobemide,[6] phenelzine,[35] or tranylcypromine.[36]

*Trazodone* is chemically unrelated to other antidepressants but does have serotonergic actions. Serotonin syndrome has been reported when trazodone was combined with the SSRI paroxetine.[37]

Serotonin syndrome has been reported[38] in a patient who took *nefazodone* and *fluoxetine* together. There has been a similar report[39] in a patient who received *paroxetine* 2 days after finishing gradual withdrawal from over 6 months of treatment with nefazodone.

Symptoms resembling serotonin syndrome have occurred in a patient taking the noradrenergic and specific serotonergic antidepressant, *mirtazapine* with *fluvoxamine*;[40] another report[41] suggests that the plasma concentrations of mirtazapine may be increased as much as fourfold by fluvoxamine.

Raised *nortriptyline* levels were noted in a patient also taking *bupropion*; the effect recurred on rechallenge.[42]

In a report[43] of an interaction between *hypericum* and *paroxetine*, a 50-year-old woman was found incoherent, groggy, and slow-moving after self-administering a single dose of paroxetine while taking hypericum; recovery was uneventful. Concomitant administration of hypericum and the SSRIs may potentiate their serotonergic effects and increase the incidence of adverse reactions. The CSM has advised that patients should stop taking hypericum if treatment with an SSRI is necessary.[44] Symptoms of serotonin syndrome have also been reported when *hypericum* and *nefazodone* were taken.[45]


1. Katona CLE, Barnes TRE. Pharmacological strategies in depression. *Br J Hosp Med* 1985; **34:** 168–71.
2. Beaumont G. Drug interactions with clomipramine (Anafranil). *J Int Med Res* 1973; **1:** 480–4.
3. Graham PM, *et al.* Combination monoamine oxidase inhibitor/tricyclic antidepressant interaction. *Lancet* 1982; **ii:** 440.
4. Spigset O, *et al.* Serotonin syndrome caused by a moclobemide-clomipramine interaction. *BMJ* 1993; **306:** 248.
5. Neuvonen PJ, *et al.* Five fatal cases of serotonin syndrome after moclobemide-citalopram or moclobemide-clomipramine overdoses. *Lancet* 1993; **342:** 1419.
6. Chan BSH, *et al.* Serotonin syndrome resulting from drug interactions. *Med J Aust* 1998; **169:** 523–5.
7. Brodribb TR, *et al.* Efficacy and adverse effects of moclobemide. *Lancet* 1994; **343:** 475.
8. Committee on Safety of Medicines. Fluvoxamine and fluoxetine-interaction with monoamine oxidase inhibitors, lithium and tryptophan. *Current Problems 26* 1989. Correction. *ibid. 27* 1989 [hypothermia should have read hyperthermia].
9. Brannan SK, *et al.* Sertraline and isocarboxazid cause a serotonin syndrome. *J Clin Psychopharmacol* 1994; **14:** 144–5.
10. Graber MA, *et al.* Sertraline-phenelzine drug interaction: a serotonin syndrome reaction. *Ann Pharmacother* 1994; **28:** 732–5.
11. Corkeron MA. Serotonin syndrome — a potentially fatal complication of antidepressant therapy. *Med J Aust* 1995; **163:** 481–2.
12. Bakish D, *et al.* Moclobemide and specific serotonin re-uptake inhibitor combination treatment of resistant anxiety and depressive disorders. *Hum Psychopharmacol Clin Exp* 1995; **10:** 105–9.
13. Hawley CJ, *et al.* Combining SSRIs and moclobemide. *Pharm J* 1996; **257:** 506.
14. Bertschy G, *et al.* Fluvoxamine-tricyclic antidepressant interaction: an accidental finding. *Eur J Clin Pharmacol* 1991; **40:** 119–20.
15. Westermeyer J. Fluoxetine-induced tricyclic toxicity: extent and duration. *J Clin Pharmacol* 1991; **31:** 388–92.
16. Ereshefsky L, *et al.* Antidepressant drug interactions and the cytochrome P450 system: the role of cytochrome P450 2D6. *Clin Pharmacokinet* 1995; **29** (suppl 1): 10–19.
17. Weiner AL, *et al.* Serotonin syndrome: case report and review of the literature. *Conn Med* 1997; **61:** 717–21.
18. Alderman CP, Lee PC. Serotonin syndrome associated with combined sertraline-amitriptyline treatment. *Ann Pharmacother* 1996; **30:** 1499–1500.
19. Leinonen E, *et al.* Paroxetine increases serum trimipramine concentration: a report of two cases. *Hum Psychopharmacol Clin Exp* 1995; **10:** 345–7.
20. Baettig D, *et al.* Tricyclic antidepressant plasma levels after augmentation with citalopram: a case study. *Eur J Clin Pharmacol* 1993; **44:** 403–5.
21. Barker WA, *et al.* The Newcastle chronic depression study: results of a treatment regime. *Int Clin Psychopharmacol* 1987; **2;** 261–72.
22. Pare CMB. Potentiation of monoamine oxidase inhibitors by tryptophan. *Lancet* 1963; **ii:** 527–8.
23. Price WA, *et al.* Serotonin syndrome: a case report. *J Clin Pharmacol* 1986; **26:** 77–8.
24. Solomon JG. Seizures during lithium-amitriptyline therapy. *Postgrad Med* 1979; **66:** 145–8.
25. Kojima H, *et al.* Serotonin syndrome during clomipramine and lithium treatment. *Am J Psychiatry* 1993; **150:** 1897.
26. Austin LS, *et al.* Toxicity resulting from lithium augmentation of antidepressant treatment in elderly patients. *J Clin Psychiatry* 1990; **51:** 344–5.
27. Lafferman J, *et al.* Lithium augmentation for treatment-resistant depression in the elderly. *J Geriatr Psychiatry Neurol* 1988; **1:** 49–52.
28. Zaninelli R, *et al.* Changes in quantitatively assessed tremor during treatment of major depression with lithium augmented by paroxetine or amitriptyline. *J Clin Psychopharmacol* 2001; **21:** 190–8.
29. Kline SS, *et al.* Serotonin syndrome versus neuroleptic malignant syndrome as a cause of death. *Clin Pharm* 1989; **8:** 510–14.
30. Benazzi F. Anticholinergic toxic syndrome with venlafaxine-desipramine combination. *Pharmacopsychiatry* 1998; **31:** 36–7.
31. Benazzi F. Venlafaxine drug-drug interactions in clinical practice. *J Psychiatry Neurosci* 1998; **23:** 181–2.
32. Schlienger RG, *et al.* Seizures associated with therapeutic doses of venlafaxine and trimipramine. *Ann Pharmacother* 2000; **34:** 1402–5.
33. Dougherty JA, *et al.* Serotonin syndrome induced by amitriptyline, meperidine, and venlafaxine. *Ann Pharmacother* 2002; **36:** 1647–8.
34. Klysner R, *et al.* Toxic interaction of venlafaxine and isocarboxazid. *Lancet* 1995; **346:** 1298–9.
35. Heister MA, *et al.* Serotonin syndrome induced by administration of venlafaxine and phenelzine. *Ann Pharmacother* 1996; **30:** 84.
36. Hodgman MJ. Serotonin syndrome due to venlafaxine and maintenance tranylcypromine therapy. *Hum Exp Toxicol* 1997; **16:** 14–17.
37. Reeves RR, *et al.* Serotonin syndrome produced by paroxetine and low-dose trazodone. *Psychosomatics* 1995; **36:** 159.
38. Smith DL, Wenegrat BG. A case report of serotonin syndrome associated with combined nefazodone and fluoxetine. *J Clin Psychiatry* 2000; **61:** 146.
39. John L, *et al.* Serotonin syndrome associated with nefazodone and paroxetine. *Ann Emerg Med* 1997; **29:** 287–9.
40. Demers J, Malone M. Serotonin syndrome induced by fluvoxamine and mirtazapine. *Ann Pharmacother* 2001; **35:** 1217–20.
41. Anttila SAK, *et al.* Fluvoxamine augmentation increases serum mirtazapine concentrations three- to fourfold. *Ann Pharmacother* 2001; **35:** 1221–3.
42. Weintraub D. Nortriptyline toxicity secondary to interaction with bupropion sustained-release. *Depress Anxiety* 2001; **13:** 50–2.
43. Gordon JB. SSRIs and St. John's Wort: possible toxicity? *Am Fam Physician* 1998; **57:** 950, 953.
44. Committee on Safety of Medicines/Medicines Control Agency. Reminder: St John's wort (Hypericum perforatum) interactions. *Current Problems* 2000; **26:** 6–7. Also available at: http://www.mca.gov.uk/ourwork/monitorsafequalmed/currentproblems/cpmay2000.pdf (accessed 05/07/04)
45. Lantz MS, *et al.* St. John's Wort and antidepressant drug interactions in the elderly. *J Geriatr Psychiatry Neurol* 1999; **12:** 7–10.


**Antiepileptics.** Antidepressants may antagonise the activity of antiepileptics by lowering the convulsive threshold. Treatment with *carbamazepine* should be avoided with or within 2 weeks of MAOIs.

**Antimigraine drugs.** For the effect of MAOIs on *serotonin (5-HT₁) agonists*, see under Sumatriptan, p.472.

**Antineoplastics.** For the effect of MAOIs on *altretamine*, see p.526.

**Dopaminergics.** For the effect of MAOIs with *amantadine*, see p.1198, with *levodopa*, see p.1208, and with *selegiline*, see p.1214.

**General anaesthetics.** The problems that may occur when patients receiving MAOIs are also given general anaesthetics are discussed under Anaesthesia in Precautions, above.

**Ginseng.** There have been 2 reports[1,2] of adverse effects, including headaches, insomnia, tremulousness, and irritability when ginseng was taken with phenelzine.


1. Shader RI, Greenblatt DJ. Phenelzine and the dream machine—ramblings and reflections. *J Clin Psychopharmacol* 1985; **5:** 65.
2. Jones BD, Runikis AM. Interaction of ginseng with phenelzine. *J Clin Psychopharmacol* 1987; **7:** 201–2.


**Insulin.** For the effect of MAOIs on Insulin, see p.338.

**Neuromuscular blockers.** For the effects of MAOIs on *suxamethonium*, see p.1408. Problems that may be encountered with MAOIs and neuromuscular blockers used during anaesthesia are discussed under Precautions, above.

**Opioid analgesics.** The problems that may occur with MAOIs and opioid analgesics used during anaesthesia are discussed under Precautions, above.

**Respiratory stimulants.** For the effect of MAOIs on *doxapram*, see p.1587.

## Pharmacokinetics

Phenelzine is readily absorbed from the gastrointestinal tract reaching peak plasma concentrations 2 to 4 hours after ingestion. It is metabolised in the liver and is excreted in the urine almost entirely in the form of metabolites.

## Uses and Administration

Monoamine oxidase inhibitors (MAOIs) inhibit the action of monoamine oxidase, the enzyme responsible for the metabolism of several biogenic amines. Monoamine oxidase exists in two forms: type A and type B. Monoamine oxidase type A preferentially deaminates adrenaline, noradrenaline, and serotonin whereas monoamine oxidase type B preferentially metabolises benzylamine and phenylethylamine; dopamine and tyramine are de-aminated by both forms of the enzyme.

- The traditional MAOIs such as phenelzine, iproniazid, isocarboxazid, nialamide, and tranylcypromine are inhibitors of both types; apart from tranylcypromine, which produces a less prolonged inhibition of the enzyme than phenelzine, all are hydrazine derivatives and bind irreversibly
- Selective inhibitors include selegiline (p.1214), an irreversible inhibitor of monoamine oxidase type B used in the treatment of Parkinson's disease. Clorgiline, an irreversible selective type A inhibitor, was investigated for use as an antidepressant
- Reversible inhibitors of monoamine oxidase type A (RIMAs) include brofaromine, moclobemide, and toloxatone

Antidepressant activity appears to reside predominantly with inhibition of monoamine oxidase type A although the mode of action of these drugs in depression is not fully understood. Advantages claimed for selective inhibitors are fewer or less severe adverse effects than those experienced with non-selective inhibitors. As tyramine is de-aminated by both monoamine oxidase types A and B, inhibiting only one of the enzymes allows for continued, albeit reduced, de-amination. Thus the dietary precautions that need to be observed with non-selective inhibitors of both monoamine oxidase types A and B are less stringent with the selective inhibitors.

Phenelzine and other antidepressant MAOIs are used in the treatment of atypical depression, particularly where phobic features or associated anxiety are present, or in patients who have not responded to other antidepressants. However, the risks associated with irreversible non-selective MAOIs usually mean that other antidepressants are preferred. Up to a month may elapse before an antidepressant response is obtained with MAOIs. After a response has been obtained maintenance therapy may need to be continued for at least 4 to 6 months to avoid relapse on discontinuation of therapy. MAOI therapy is not generally indicated for children. Care should be taken in elderly patients because of an increased susceptibility to adverse effects. Moreover, therapy with the non-selective inhibitors is particularly unsuitable for patients considered unable to adhere to the strict dietary requirements necessary for safe usage.

Phenelzine is given by mouth as the sulfate although doses are expressed in terms of the base. Phenelzine sulfate 25.8 mg is approximately equivalent to 15 mg of phenelzine. The usual initial dose is equivalent to phenelzine 15 mg three times daily; if no response has been obtained after 2 weeks the dosage may be increased to 15 mg four times daily; severely depressed patients in hospital may be given up to 30 mg three times daily. Once a response has been obtained the dosage may be gradually reduced for maintenance therapy; some patients may continue to respond to 15 mg on alternate days.

Phenelzine should be withdrawn gradually to reduce the risk of withdrawal symptoms.

**Anxiety disorders.** MAOIs have been used in the treatment of *anxiety disorders*. MAOIs appear to be effective in blocking *panic attacks* (p.663). They also appear to be effective in *social phobia* (see under Phobic Disorders, p.663) and can improve anticipatory anxiety and functional disability. The major treatment for *post-traumatic stress disorder* (p.664) is psychotherapy but MAOIs can help to reduce traumatic recollections and nightmares and to repress flashbacks.

References.

1. Buigues J, Vallejo J. Therapeutic response to phenelzine in patients with panic disorder and agoraphobia with panic attacks. *J Clin Psychiatry* 1987; **48:** 55–9.
2. Frank JB, *et al.* A randomized clinical trial of phenelzine and imipramine for posttraumatic stress disorder. *Am J Psychiatry* 1988; **145:** 1289–91.
3. Heimberg RG, *et al.* Cognitive behavioural group therapy vs phenelzine therapy for social phobia: 12 week outcome. *Arch Gen Psychiatry* 1998; **55:** 1133–41.

**Depression.** As discussed on p.279 there is very little difference in efficacy between the different groups of antidepressant drugs, and choice is often made on the basis of adverse effects. MAOIs are rarely used as first-choice antidepressants because of the dangers of dietary and drug interactions. Even in depressed patients with atypical, hypochondriacal, hysterical, or phobic features, for which MAOIs are particularly effective, it is often recommended that another antidepressant type should be tried first. Reversible inhibitors of monoamine oxidase type A (RIMAs) offer an alternative to the MAOIs and less strict dietary restrictions are necessary. They may be an effective first choice in a wide range of depressive disorders, although their relative efficacy in atypical depression remains to be established.

Combination therapy with differing classes of antidepressants, including the MAOIs, has been used in the treatment of drug-resistant depression. However, such therapy may result in enhanced adverse reactions or interactions and is considered unsuitable or controversial by some workers. For further details, see Antidepressants under Interactions, above.

**Hyperactivity.** When drug therapy is required for attention deficit hyperactivity disorder (p.1583), initial treatment is usually with a central stimulant. MAOIs have been used successfully but problems with dietary restriction and potential drug interactions have limited their use.

**Migraine.** A number of drugs have been used for the prophylaxis of migraine (p.464), although propranolol or pizotifen are generally preferred. Antidepressants such as the tricyclics can be useful alternatives when these drugs are ineffective or unsuitable. MAOIs are best reserved for severe cases refractory to other forms of prophylactic treatment.

## Preparations

**BP 2003:** Phenelzine Tablets;
**USP 27:** Phenelzine Sulfate Tablets.

**Proprietary Preparations** (details are given in Part 3)
**Austral.:** Nardil; **Belg.:** Nardelzine; **Canad.:** Nardil; **Irl.:** Nardil; **Israel:** Nardil†; **NZ:** Nardil†; **UK:** Nardil; **USA:** Nardil.

---

## Pirlindole *(rINN)*

Pirlindol. 2,3,3a,4,5,6-Hexahydro-8-methyl-1*H*-pyrazino[3,2,1-*jk*]carbazole.

$C_{15}H_{18}N_2$ = 226.3.
*CAS — 60762-57-4.*

### Profile

Pirlindole has been given by mouth in the treatment of depression.

### Preparations

**Proprietary Preparations** (details are given in Part 3)
**Port.:** Implementor; **Spain:** Lifril†.

---

## Protriptyline Hydrochloride *(BANM, USAN, rINNM)*

Hidrocloruro de protriptilina; MK-240. 3-(5*H*-Dibenzo[*a,d*]cyclohept-5-enyl)propyl(methyl)amine hydrochloride.

$C_{19}H_{21}N,HCl$ = 299.8.
*CAS — 438-60-8 (protriptyline); 1225-55-4 (protriptyline hydrochloride).*
*ATC — N06AA11.*

**Pharmacopoeias.** In *Br.* and *US.*

**BP 2003** (Protriptyline Hydrochloride). A white to yellowish-white, odourless or almost odourless, powder. Freely soluble in water; in alcohol, and in chloroform; practically insoluble in ether. A 1% solution in water has a pH of 5.0 to 6.5.

**USP 27** (Protriptyline Hydrochloride). A white to yellowish powder. Is odourless or has not more than a slight odour. Soluble 1 in 2 of water, 1 in 3.5 of alcohol, and 1 in 2.5 of chloroform; practically insoluble in ether. pH of a 1% solution in water is between 5.0 and 6.5.

### Adverse Effects, Treatment, and Precautions

As for tricyclic antidepressants in general (see Amitriptyline, p.281).

Since protriptyline may have some stimulant properties anxiety and agitation can occur more frequently; cardiovascular effects such as tachycardia and hypotension may also be more frequent than with other tricyclics. Photosensitivity rashes have been noted more commonly with protriptyline than with other tricyclic antidepressants and patients taking it should avoid direct sunlight.

### Interactions

For interactions associated with tricyclic antidepressants, see Amitriptyline, p.284.

### Pharmacokinetics

Protriptyline is well but slowly absorbed after oral doses, peak plasma concentrations being achieved after several hours.

Paths of metabolism of protriptyline include *N*-oxidation and hydroxylation. Protriptyline is excreted in the urine, mainly in the form of its metabolites, either free or in conjugated form.

Protriptyline is widely distributed throughout the body and extensively bound to plasma and tissue protein. Protriptyline has been estimated to have a very prolonged elimination half-life ranging from 55 to 198 hours, which may be further prolonged in overdosage.

### Uses and Administration

Protriptyline is a dibenzocycloheptatriene tricyclic antidepressant with actions and uses similar to those of amitriptyline (p.285). It has considerably less sedative properties than other tricyclics and may have a stimulant effect, thus making it particularly suitable for apathetic and withdrawn patients; its antimuscarinic properties are moderate.

In the treatment of depression, protriptyline hydrochloride is given by mouth in doses of 5 to 10 mg three or four times daily. It has been suggested that, because of its potential stimulant activity, any dosage increases should be added to the morning dose first and if insomnia occurs the last dose should be given no later than mid-afternoon. Higher doses of up to 60 mg daily may be required in severely depressed patients. A suitable initial dose for adolescents and the elderly is 5 mg three times daily; close monitoring of the cardiovascular system has been recommended if the dose exceeds a total of 20 mg daily in elderly subjects.

Protriptyline should be withdrawn gradually to reduce the risk of withdrawal symptoms.

### Preparations

**BP 2003:** Protriptyline Tablets;
**USP 27:** Protriptyline Hydrochloride Tablets.

**Proprietary Preparations** (details are given in Part 3)
**Canad.:** Triptil†; **Denm.:** Concordin†; **Irl.:** Concordin†; **Swed.:** Concordin†; **UK:** Concordin†; **USA:** Vivactil.

---

## Quinupramine *(rINN)*

LM-208; Quinupramina. 10,11-Dihydro-5-(quinuclidin-3-yl)-5*H*-dibenz[*b,f*]azepine.

$C_{21}H_{24}N_2$ = 304.4.
*CAS — 31721-17-2.*
*ATC — N06AA23.*

### Profile

Quinupramine is a tricyclic antidepressant (see Amitriptyline, p.280) that has been used in the treatment of depression.

### Preparations

**Proprietary Preparations** (details are given in Part 3)
**Austria:** Kevopril†; **Fr.:** Kinupril†.

---

## Reboxetine Mesilate *(BANM, rINNM)*

FCE-20124 (reboxetine or reboxetine mesilate); Mesilato de reboxetina; PNU-155950E; Reboxetine Mesylate *(USAN)*. (±)-(2*RS*)-2-[(α*RS*)-α-(2-Ethoxyphenoxy)benzyl]morpholine methanesulphonate.

$C_{19}H_{23}NO_3,CH_4O_3S$ = 409.5.
*CAS — 71620-89-8; 98769-81-4 (both reboxetine); 98769-82-5; 98769-84-7 (both reboxetine mesilate).*
*ATC — N06AX18.*

### Adverse Effects

Adverse effects most commonly seen with reboxetine include insomnia, dry mouth, constipation, and increased sweating. Disturbance of visual accommodation, loss of appetite, vertigo, tachycardia, palpitations, vasodilatation, postural hypotension, urinary hesitancy or retention (mainly in men), and erectile dysfunction including ejaculatory delay are also reported as being common adverse reactions. There have been reports of allergic dermatitis, convulsions, and nausea and vomiting. Reduced plasma-potassium concentrations have been observed in elderly patients following prolonged use.

Hyponatraemia, possibly as a result of inappropriate secretion of antidiuretic hormone, has been associated with the use of antidepressants, particularly in the elderly.

**Effects on the endocrine system.** A report[1] of *hyponatraemia*, thought to be associated with reboxetine therapy and to be due to the syndrome of inappropriate antidiuretic hormone secretion, in an elderly patient.

1. Ranieri P, *et al.* Reboxetine and hyponatremia. *N Engl J Med* 2000; **342:** 215–16.

## Treatment of Adverse Effects

Symptomatic and supportive therapy should be given as required; activated charcoal may be given to adults who have ingested more than 40 mg of reboxetine, and to children, who present within 1 hour of ingestion. Heart rhythm should be monitored if changes in blood pressure occur.

**Genito-urinary disorders.** Tamsulosin has been used successfully in the treatment of urinary hesitancy and painful ejaculation associated with reboxetine (see p.1009).

## Precautions

Reboxetine should be used with caution in patients with renal or hepatic impairment. It should also be used under close supervision in patients with bipolar disorder, urinary retention, benign prostatic hyperplasia, glaucoma, or a history of epilepsy or cardiac disorders.

Patients should be closely monitored during early therapy until improvement in depression is observed because suicide is an inherent risk in depressed patients. For further details, see under Depression, p.279.

Ability to perform tasks requiring motor or cognitive skills or judgement may be impaired by reboxetine and patients, if affected, should not drive or operate machinery.

## Interactions

Reboxetine should not be taken with, or within 2 weeks of stopping, an MAOI; at least one week should elapse after stopping reboxetine therapy before starting any drug liable to provoke a serious reaction (e.g. phenelzine). Caution should be exercised when reboxetine is given with other drugs that lower blood pressure because postural hypotension has occurred with reboxetine. The possibility of hypokalaemia if reboxetine is given with potassium-depleting diuretics should also be considered.

Reboxetine is primarily metabolised by the cytochrome P450 isoenzyme CYP3A4 and potent inhibitors of this isoenzyme may limit the elimination of reboxetine. Consequently, reboxetine should not be given with drugs known to inhibit CYP3A4 such as azole antifungals (e.g. ketoconazole), macrolide antibiotics (e.g. erythromycin) or fluvoxamine. Reboxetine in high concentrations has also been shown *in vitro* to inhibit CYP3A4 and CYP2D6; however *in vivo* studies have suggested that interactions with drugs metabolised by these isoenzymes are unlikely.

**Antifungals.** Plasma levels of reboxetine were significantly increased when given with *ketoconazole*.[1] The interaction was said to have involved the inhibition of the cytochrome P450 isoenzyme CYP3A4 by ketoconazole.

1. Herman BD, *et al.* Ketoconazole inhibits the clearance of the enantiomers of the antidepressant reboxetine in humans. *Clin Pharmacol Ther* 1999; **66:** 374–9.

## Pharmacokinetics

Reboxetine is well absorbed from the gastrointestinal tract with peak plasma levels occurring after about 2 hours. Plasma protein binding is about 97% (92% in elderly subjects). Reboxetine is metabolised *in vivo* by the cytochrome P450 isoenzyme CYP3A4; the main metabolic pathways identified are dealkylation, hydroxylation, and oxidation followed by glucuronide or sulfate conjugation. Elimination is mainly via urine (78%) with 10% excreted as unchanged drug. The plasma elimination half-life is 13 hours. Data from *animal* studies indicate that reboxetine crosses the placenta and is distributed into breast milk.

◊ References.

1. Dostert P, *et al.* Review of the pharmacokinetics and metabolism of reboxetine, a selective noradrenaline reuptake inhibitor. *Eur Neuropsychopharmacol* 1997; **7** (suppl 1): S23–S35.
2. Fleishaker JC. Clinical pharmacokinetics of reboxetine, a selective norepinephrine reuptake inhibitor for the treatment of patients with depression. *Clin Pharmacokinet* 2000; **39:** 413–27.
3. Coulomb F, *et al.* Pharmacokinetics of single-dose reboxetine in volunteers with renal insufficiency. *J Clin Pharmacol* 2000; **40:** 482–7.
4. Poggesi I, *et al.* Pharmacokinetics of reboxetine in elderly patients with depressive disorders. *Int J Clin Pharmacol Ther* 2000; **38:** 254–9.

## Uses and Administration

Reboxetine is a selective and potent inhibitor of the reuptake of noradrenaline; it also has a weak effect on serotonin reuptake. Reboxetine has no significant affinity for muscarinic receptors. It is given by mouth as the mesilate for the treatment of depression with doses expressed as reboxetine base. Reboxetine mesilate 5.2 mg is approximately equivalent to 4 mg of reboxetine. The dose of reboxetine is 4 mg twice daily, which may be increased after 3 to 4 weeks, if necessary, to 10 mg daily; the maximum daily dose should not exceed 12 mg. Reduced doses should be given in hepatic or renal impairment, see below.

Antidepressants should be withdrawn gradually to reduce the risk of withdrawal symptoms.

**Administration in hepatic or renal impairment.** Lower initial doses equivalent to 2 mg of reboxetine twice daily are recommended in hepatic or renal impairment; doses may be increased thereafter according to tolerance.

**Depression.** As discussed on p.279, there is very little difference in efficacy between the different groups of antidepressant drugs, and choice is often made on the basis of adverse effect profile. Reboxetine, a selective inhibitor of noradrenaline reuptake, has a slightly different biochemical profile from both the tricyclics and the SSRIs; however, like the SSRIs, reboxetine appears to have fewer unpleasant side-effects and to be safer in overdosage in comparison with the older tricyclics.

References.

1. Anonymous. Reboxetine—another new antidepressant. *Drug Ther Bull* 1998; **36:** 86–8.
2. Montgomery SA. The place of reboxetine in antidepressant therapy. *J Clin Psychiatry* 1998; **59** (suppl 14): 26–9.
3. Versiani M, *et al.* Reboxetine, a unique selective NRI, prevents relapse and recurrence in long-term treatment of major depressive disorder. *J Clin Psychiatry* 1999; **60:** 400–406.
4. Holm KJ, Spencer CM. Reboxetine: a review of its use in depression. *CNS Drugs* 1999; **12:** 65–83.
5. Scates AC, Doraiswamy PM. Reboxetine: a selective norepinephrine reuptake inhibitor for the treatment of depression. *Ann Pharmacother* 2000; **34:** 1302–12.
6. Versiani M, *et al.* Double-blind, placebo-controlled study with reboxetine in inpatients with severe major depressive disorder. *J Clin Psychopharmacol* 2000; **20:** 28–34.
7. Ferguson JM, *et al.* Effects of reboxetine on Hamilton Depression Rating Scale factors from randomized, placebo-controlled trials in major depression. *Int Clin Psychopharmacol* 2002; **17:** 45–51.
8. Andreoli V, *et al.* Reboxetine, a new noradrenaline selective antidepressant, is at least as effective as fluoxetine in the treatment of depression. *J Clin Psychopharmacol* 2002; **22:** 393–9.
9. Montgomery S, *et al.* The antidepressant efficacy of reboxetine in patients with severe depression. *J Clin Psychopharmacol* 2003; **23:** 45–50.

## Preparations

**Proprietary Preparations** (details are given in Part 3)
***Arg.:*** Prolift; ***Austral.:*** Edronax; ***Austria:*** Edronax; ***Belg.:*** Edronax; ***Braz.:*** Prolift; ***Chile:*** Prolift; ***Denm.:*** Edronax; ***Fin.:*** Edronax; ***Ger.:*** Edronax; Solvex; ***Irl.:*** Edronax; ***Israel:*** Edronax; ***Ital.:*** Davedax; Edronax; ***Mex.:*** Edronax; ***Norw.:*** Edronax; ***NZ:*** Edronax; ***Port.:*** Edronax; ***S.Afr.:*** Edronax; ***Spain:*** Irenor; Norebox; ***Swed.:*** Edronax; ***Switz.:*** Edronax; ***UK:*** Edronax.

# Sertraline Hydrochloride

*(BANM, USAN, rINNM)*

CP-51974-01; CP-51974-1; Hidrocloruro de sertralina. (1S,4S)-4-(3,4-Dichlorophenyl)-1,2,3,4-tetrahydro-1-naphthyl(methyl)-amine hydrochloride.

$C_{17}H_{17}Cl_2N,HCl = 342.7.$

*CAS — 79617-96-2 (sertraline); 79559-97-0 (sertraline hydrochloride).*

*ATC — N06AB06.*

## Adverse Effects, Treatment, and Precautions

As for SSRIs in general (see Fluoxetine, p.292). Menstrual irregularities and, rarely, erythema multiforme and pancreatitis have also been reported.

Sertraline should be used with caution in patients with hepatic or renal impairment; reduced doses should be considered in patients with hepatic impairment.

**Breast feeding.** For comments on the use of SSRIs in breast feeding patients, see under Precautions for Fluoxetine, p.294.

**Children.** In the UK the Committee on Safety of Medicines recommends that sertraline should not be used to treat depressive illness in children under 18 years of age. For details, see under Effects on Mental State in Fluoxetine, p.293.

## Interactions

For interactions associated with SSRIs, see Fluoxetine, p.295.

## Pharmacokinetics

Sertraline is slowly absorbed from the gastrointestinal tract with peak plasma concentrations occurring about 4.5 to 8.5 hours after ingestion. It undergoes extensive first-pass metabolism in the liver. The main pathway is demethylation to *N*-desmethylsertraline which is inactive; further metabolism and glucuronide conjugation occurs. Sertraline is widely distributed throughout body tissues and is about 98% bound to plasma proteins. The plasma elimination half-life of sertraline is reported to be about 26 hours. Sertraline is excreted in approximately equal amounts in the urine and faeces, mainly as metabolites. Sertraline is distributed into breast milk (see Breast Feeding under Precautions in Fluoxetine, p.294).

◊ References.

1. Démolis J-L, *et al.* Influence of liver cirrhosis on sertraline pharmacokinetics. *Br J Clin Pharmacol* 1996; **42:** 394–7.
2. Preskorn SH, ed. Sertraline: a pharmacokinetic profile. *Clin Pharmacokinet* 1997; **32** (suppl 1): 1–55.
3. DeVane CL, *et al.* Clinical pharmacokinetics of sertraline. *Clin Pharmacokinet* 2002; **41:** 1247–66.

## Uses and Administration

Sertraline, a naphthaleneamine derivative, is an SSRI with actions and uses similar to those of fluoxetine (p.296). It is given by mouth as sertraline hydrochloride as a single dose in the morning or evening. Doses are expressed in terms of sertraline base; sertraline hydrochloride 56 mg is approximately equivalent to 50 mg of sertraline.

In the treatment of **depression**, the usual initial dose of sertraline is 50 mg daily increased, if necessary, in increments of 50 mg at intervals of at least a week to a maximum of 200 mg daily.

In the treatment of **obsessive-compulsive disorder** the usual initial dose of sertraline is 50 mg daily. In the treatment of **panic disorder** with or without agoraphobia, **social phobia**, and **post-traumatic stress disorder**, the usual initial dose is 25 mg daily increased after one week to 50 mg daily. Thereafter, doses in all these disorders may be increased, if necessary, in increments of 50 mg at intervals of at least a week to a maximum of 200 mg daily.

Sertraline is also given for the treatment of obsessive-compulsive disorder in *children and adolescents* aged 6 years and over. In children aged 6 to 12 years the usual initial dose is 25 mg once daily; adolescents may be started on 50 mg once daily. Increases in doses, if necessary, are similar to those in adults; however, the lower body-weights of children should be considered in order to avoid excessive doses.

In the treatment of **premenstrual dysphoric disorder**, sertraline is given in an initial dose of 50 mg daily either throughout the menstrual cycle or during the luteal phase only, as appropriate. Doses may be increased by 50 mg each menstrual cycle up to a maximum of 150 mg for continuous dosing or 100 mg daily when dosing during the luteal phase only. Those patients who require 100 mg daily during luteal phase-only dosing should initially be given 50 mg daily for the first 3 days of each luteal phase dosing period.

Once the optimal therapeutic response is obtained dosage should be reduced to the lowest effective level for maintenance.

Reduced doses are recommended in patients with hepatic impairment, see below.

Sertraline should be withdrawn gradually to reduce the risk of withdrawal symptoms.

**Administration in hepatic impairment.** Sertraline should be used with caution in patients with hepatic impairment; lower or less frequent doses are recommended. No specific guidance is given on dosage reduction by the manufacturers, although US product information notes that exposure to sertraline in patients with chronic mild hepatic impairment given 50 mg daily was about 3 times that in subjects with normal hepatic function.

**Anxiety disorders.** Sertraline has been given in a variety of anxiety disorders (p.663) including obsessive-compulsive disorder (p.663), panic attacks (p.663), social phobia (see under Phobic Disorders, p.663), and post-traumatic stress disorder (p.664).

References.


1. Greist J, *et al.* Double-blind parallel comparison of three dosages of sertraline and placebo in outpatients with obsessive-compulsive disorder. *Arch Gen Psychiatry* 1995; **52:** 289–95.
2. Katzelnick DJ, *et al.* Sertraline for social phobia: a double-blind, placebo-controlled crossover study. *Am J Psychiatry* 1995; **152:** 1368–71.
3. Brady KT, *et al.* Sertraline treatment of comorbid posttraumatic stress disorder and alcohol dependence. *J Clin Psychiatry* 1995; **56:** 502–5.
4. March JS, *et al.* Sertraline in children and adolescents with obsessive-compulsive disorder: a multicenter randomized controlled trial. *JAMA* 1998; **280:** 1752–6.
5. Londborg PD, *et al.* Sertraline in the treatment of panic disorder. A multi-site, double-blind, placebo-controlled, fixed-dose investigation. *Br J Psychiatry* 1998; **173:** 54–60.
6. Brady K, *et al.* Efficacy and safety of sertraline treatment of posttraumatic stress disorder: a randomized controlled trial. *JAMA* 2000; **283:** 1837–44.
7. Walker JR, *et al.* Prevention of relapse in generalized social phobia: results of a 24-week study in responders to 20 weeks of sertraline treatment. *J Clin Psychopharmacol* 2000; **20:** 636–44.
8. Rynn MA, *et al.* Placebo-controlled trial of sertraline in the treatment of children with generalized anxiety disorder. *Am J Psychiatry* 2001; **158:** 2008–14.
9. Rapaport MH, *et al.* Sertraline treatment of panic disorder: results of a long-term study. *Acta Psychiatr Scand* 2001; **104:** 289–98.
10. Rapaport MH, *et al.* Posttraumatic stress disorder and quality of life: results across 64 weeks of sertraline treatment. *J Clin Psychiatry* 2002; **63:** 59–65.
11. Koran LM, *et al.* Efficacy of sertraline in the long-term treatment of obsessive-compulsive disorder. *Am J Psychiatry* 2002; **159:** 88–95.


**Depression.** As discussed on p.279, there is very little difference in efficacy between the different groups of antidepressant drugs, and choice is often made on the basis of adverse effect profile. SSRIs such as sertraline are widely used as an alternative to the older tricyclics as they have fewer unpleasant side-effects and are safer in overdosage.

References.


1. Haider A, *et al.* Clinical effect of converting antidepressant therapy from fluoxetine to sertraline. *Am J Health-Syst Pharm* 1995; **52:** 1317–19.
2. Bennie EH, *et al.* A double-blind multicenter trial comparing sertraline and fluoxetine in outpatients with major depression. *J Clin Psychiatry* 1995; **56:** 229–37.
3. Stowe ZN, *et al.* Sertraline in the treatment of women with postpartum major depression. *Depression* 1995; **3:** 49–55.
4. Keller MB, *et al.* Maintenance phase efficacy of sertraline for chronic depression: a randomized controlled trial. *JAMA* 1998; **280:** 1665–72.
5. Baca E, *et al.* Sertraline is more effective than imipramine in the treatment of non-melancholic depression: results from a multicentre, randomized study. *Prog Neuropsychopharmacol Biol Psychiatry* 2003; **27:** 493–500.
6. Wagner KD, *et al.* Efficacy of sertraline in the treatment of children and adolescents with major depressive disorder: two randomized controlled trials. *JAMA* 2003; **290:** 1033–41.
7. Lepine JP, et al. A randomized, placebo-controlled trial of sertraline for prophylactic treatment of highly recurrent major depressive disorder. *Am J Psychiatry* 2004; **161:** 836–42.
8. Moscovitch A, *et al.* A placebo-controlled study of sertraline in the treatment of outpatients with seasonal affective disorder. *Psychopharmacology (Berl)* 2004; **171:** 390–7.


**Headache.** For reference to the use of SSRIs, including sertraline, in the management of various types of headache, see under Fluoxetine, p.297.

**Premenstrual syndrome.** Sertraline throughout the menstrual cycle has produced beneficial effects in controlling both the psychological and somatic symptoms of women with premenstrual syndrome.[1-3] Giving sertraline solely during the luteal phase was also of benefit.[4,5]

For a discussion of the overall management of premenstrual syndrome, see p.1551.


1. Freeman EW, *et al.* Sertraline versus desipramine in the treatment of premenstrual syndrome: an open-label trial. *J Clin Psychiatry* 1996; **57:** 7–11.
2. Yonkers KA, *et al.* Sertraline in the treatment of premenstrual dysphoric disorder. *Psychopharmacol Bull* 1996; **32:** 41–6.
3. Yonkers KA, *et al.* Symptomatic improvement of premenstrual dysphoric disorder with sertraline treatment: a randomized controlled trial. *JAMA* 1997; **278:** 983–8.
4. Young SA, *et al.* Treatment of premenstrual dysphoric disorder with sertraline during the luteal phase: a randomized, double-blind, placebo-controlled crossover trial. *J Clin Psychiatry* 1998; **59:** 76–80.
5. Jermain DM, *et al.* Luteal phase sertraline treatment for premenstrual dysphoric disorder: results of a double-blind, placebo-controlled, crossover study. *Arch Fam Med* 1999; **8:** 328–32.


**Sexual dysfunction.** Impotence or ejaculatory problems have been reported as adverse effects of SSRIs; for the use of these effects as a potential form of management for premature ejaculation see Fluoxetine, p.298.

## Preparations

**Proprietary Preparations** (details are given in Part 3)

***Arg.:*** Anilar; Atenix; Bicromil; Insertec; Irradial; Zoloft; ***Austral.:*** Zoloft; ***Austria:*** Gladem; Tresleen; ***Belg.:*** Serlain; ***Braz.:*** Novativ; Sercerin; Tolrest; Zoloft; ***Canad.:*** Zoloft; ***Chile:*** Altruline; Deprax; Eleval; Emergen; Implicane; Lowfin; Sedoran; Serivo; ***Denm.:*** Zoloft; ***Fin.:*** Zoloft; ***Fr.:*** Zoloft; ***Ger.:*** Gladem; Zoloft; ***Gr.:*** Zoloft; ***Hong Kong:*** Zoloft; ***India:*** Serta; ***Irl.:*** Lustral; ***Israel:*** Lustral; ***Ital.:*** Serad†; Tatig; Zoloft; ***Malaysia:*** Zoloft; ***Mex.:*** Altruline; ***Neth.:*** Zoloft; ***Norw.:*** Zoloft; ***NZ:*** Zoloft; ***Port.:*** Zoloft; ***S.Afr.:*** Zoloft; ***Singapore:*** Zoloft; ***Spain:*** Aremis; Besitran; Sealdin; ***Swed.:*** Zoloft; ***Switz.:*** Gladem; Zoloft; ***Thai.:*** Zoloft; ***UK:*** Lustral; ***USA:*** Zoloft.

---

## Tianeptine Sodium *(rINNM)*

Tianeptina sódica; Tianeptinum Natricum. The sodium salt of 7-[(3-chloro-6,11-dihydro-6-methyldibenzo[*c,f*][1,2]thiazepin-11-yl)amino]heptanoic acid *S,S*-dioxide.

$C_{21}H_{24}ClN_2NaO_4S$ = 458.9.

*CAS — 66981-73-5 (tianeptine).*

*ATC — N06AX14.*

**Pharmacopoeias.** In *Eur.* (see p.vi).

**Ph. Eur. 5.0** (Tianeptine Sodium). A white or yellowish, very hygroscopic, powder. Freely soluble in water, in dichloromethane, and in methyl alcohol. Store in airtight containers.

### Profile

Tianeptine sodium is an antidepressant reported to act by increasing (rather than inhibiting) the presynaptic reuptake of serotonin. It is given by mouth in doses of 12.5 mg three times daily in the treatment of depression (p.279). Doses should be reduced to a total of 25 mg daily in elderly patients and those with renal impairment, but it has been stated that no dose modification is necessary in patients with chronic alcoholism or cirrhosis.

Isolated cases of hepatitis have been reported during treatment with tianeptine.

◊ References.


1. Royer RJ, *et al.* Tianeptine and its main metabolite: pharmacokinetics in chronic alcoholism and cirrhosis. *Clin Pharmacokinet* 1989; **16:** 186–91.
2. Carlhant D, *et al.* Pharmacokinetics and bioavailability of tianeptine in the elderly. *Drug Invest* 1990; **2:** 167–72.
3. Demotes-Mainard F, *et al.* Pharmacokinetics of the antidepressant tianeptine at steady state in the elderly. *J Clin Pharmacol* 1991; **31:** 174–8.
4. Wilde MI, Benfield P. Tianeptine: a review of its pharmacodynamic and pharmacokinetic properties, and therapeutic efficacy in depression and coexisting anxiety and depression. *Drugs* 1995; **49:** 411–39.
5. Ginestet D. Efficacy of tianeptine in major depressive disorders with or without melancholia. *Eur Neuropsychopharmacol* 1997; **7** (suppl 3): S341–S345.
6. Wagstaff AJ, *et al.* Tianeptine: a review of its use in depressive disorders. *CNS Drugs* 2001; **15:** 231–59.


**Asthma.** Tianeptine has been reported to improve symptoms in patients with asthma.[1] It was thought that reduction of raised levels of free serotonin found in such patients contributed to the beneficial effect of tianeptine.


1. Lechin F, *et al.* The serotonin uptake-enhancing drug tianeptine suppresses asthmatic symptoms in children: a double-blind, crossover, placebo-controlled study. *J Clin Pharmacol* 1998; **38:** 918–25.


### Preparations

**Proprietary Preparations** (details are given in Part 3)

***Arg.:*** Stablon; ***Austria:*** Stablon; ***Braz.:*** Stablon; ***Fr.:*** Stablon; ***India:*** Stablon; ***Malaysia:*** Stablon; ***Mex.:*** Stablon†; ***Port.:*** Stablon; ***Singapore:*** Stablon; ***Thai.:*** Stablon.

---

## Toloxatone *(rINN)*

Toloxatona. 5-(Hydroxymethyl)-3-*m*-tolyl-2-oxazolidinone.

$C_{11}H_{13}NO_3$ = 207.2.

*CAS — 29218-27-7.*

*ATC — N06AG03.*

### Profile

Toloxatone is a reversible inhibitor of monoamine oxidase type A (RIMA) (see Moclobemide, p.308). It is used as an antidepressant in doses of 200 mg three times daily by mouth.

◊ References.


1. Benedetti MS, *et al.* Pharmacokinetics of toloxatone in man following intravenous and oral administrations. *Arzneimittelforschung* 1982; **32:** 276–80.
2. Lemoine P, Mirabaud C. A double-blind comparison of moclobemide and toloxatone in out-patients presenting a major depressive disorder. *Psychopharmacology (Berl)* 1992; **106** (suppl): S118–S119.


### Preparations

**Proprietary Preparations** (details are given in Part 3)

***Fr.:*** Humoryl†; ***Ital.:*** Umoril†.

---

## Tranylcypromine Sulfate *(rINNM)*

SKF-385; Sulfato de tranilcipromina; Transamine Sulphate; Tranylcypromine Sulphate *(BANM)*. (±)-*trans*-2-Phenylcyclopropylamine sulphate.

$(C_9H_{11}N)_2,H_2SO_4$ = 364.5.

*CAS — 155-09-9 (tranylcypromine); 13492-01-8 (tranylcypromine sulfate).*

*ATC — N06AF04.*

**Pharmacopoeias.** In *Br.*

**BP 2003** (Tranylcypromine Sulphate). A white or almost white crystalline powder; odourless or with a faint odour of cinnamaldehyde. Soluble in water; very slightly soluble in alcohol and in ether; insoluble in chloroform.

### Adverse Effects, Treatment, and Precautions

As for MAOIs in general (see Phenelzine, p.312).

Tranylcypromine has a stimulant action and insomnia is a common side-effect if it is taken in the evening.

Hypertensive reactions are more likely to occur with tranylcypromine than with other MAOIs, but severe liver damage occurs less frequently.

**Dependence.** Dependence on tranylcypromine with tolerance has been reported in patients receiving high doses with or without a history of previous substance abuse. For further details, see Withdrawal under Precautions in Phenelzine, p.314.

**Effects on the cardiovascular system.** Although orthostatic hypotension is more common, hypertension can occur with MAOIs. A hypertensive crisis has been described in 2 patients after only one dose of tranylcypromine.[1,2] In the first case it was thought possible that an autointeraction may have occurred between tranylcypromine and amfetamine to which it is partly metabolised. In the second case the provocation of hypertension led to the finding of a previously undiagnosed phaeochromocytoma and it was suggested this may have been a possibility in previous reports of hypertension induced by MAOIs.


1. Gunn J, *et al.* Hypertensive crisis and broad complex bradycardia after a single dose of monoamine oxidase inhibitor. *BMJ* 1989; **298:** 964.
2. Cook RF, Katritsis D. Hypertensive crisis precipitated by a monoamine oxidase inhibitor in a patient with phaeochromocytoma. *BMJ* 1990; **300:** 614.


**Porphyria.** Tranylcypromine is considered to be unsafe in patients with porphyria because it has been shown to be porphyrinogenic in *animals*.

### Interactions

For interactions associated with MAOIs, see Phenelzine, p.314.

The use of clomipramine with tranylcypromine is particularly hazardous.

### Pharmacokinetics

Tranylcypromine is readily absorbed from the gastrointestinal tract, peak plasma concentrations occurring about 1 to 3 hours after ingestion. It is excreted in the urine mainly in the form of metabolites. Tranylcypromine has a reported plasma elimination half-life of about 2.5 hours.

◊ In 9 depressed patients, tranylcypromine absorption was rapid after oral dosing.[1] Absorption was biphasic in 7. Elimination was also rapid, with an elimination half-life of 1.54 to 3.15 hours. From 2 to 7 hours after dosing, standing systolic and diastolic blood pressures were lowered, and standing pulse was raised. The onset of the effect on standing systolic blood pressure correlated with the time of peak plasma tranylcypromine concentration. Maximum orthostatic drop of blood pressure and rise in pulse rate occurred 2 hours after dosing. Mean plasma-tranylcypromine concentrations correlated with mean orthostatic drop of systolic blood pressure and rise of pulse rate. Patients experiencing clinically significant hypotensive reactions to tranylcypromine may benefit from changes in their dose regimen aimed at minimising peak concentrations.


1. Mallinger AG, *et al.* Pharmacokinetics of tranylcypromine in patients who are depressed: relationship to cardiovascular effects. *Clin Pharmacol Ther* 1986; **40:** 444–50.


### Uses and Administration

Tranylcypromine, a cyclopropylamine derivative, is an MAOI with actions and uses similar to those of phenelzine (p.316). It produces a less prolonged inhibition of the enzymes than phenelzine.

Tranylcypromine is used in the treatment of depression, but as discussed on p.279 the risks associated with traditional non-selective MAOIs such as tranylcypromine usually mean that other antidepressants are preferred. It is given by mouth as the sulfate although doses are expressed in terms of tranylcypromine base. Tranylcypromine sulfate 13.7 mg is approximately equivalent to 10 mg of tranylcypromine.

The usual initial dose is equivalent to tranylcypromine 10 mg in the morning and 10 mg in the afternoon; if the response is inadequate after a week, 10 mg may be given additionally at midday; a dosage of 30 mg daily should only be exceeded with caution, although in the USA a maximum dose of 60 mg daily is allowed. Once a satisfactory response has been obtained the dosage may be gradually reduced for maintenance; some patients may continue to respond to 10 mg daily.

Tranylcypromine should be withdrawn gradually to reduce the risk of withdrawal symptoms.

### Preparations

**BP 2003:** Tranylcypromine Tablets.

**Proprietary Preparations** (details are given in Part 3)
**Arg.:** Parnate; **Austral.:** Parnate; **Braz.:** Parnate; **Canad.:** Parnate; **Ger.:** Jatrosom N; Parnate†; **Irl.:** Parnate; **NZ:** Parnate; **S.Afr.:** Parnate; **Spain:** Parnate; **UK:** Parnate†; **USA:** Parnate.

**Multi-ingredient: Arg.:** Cuait D; Stelapar; **Braz.:** Stelapar; **Irl.:** Parstelin†; **Ital.:** Parmodalin.

## Trazodone Hydrochloride

*(BANM, USAN, rINNM)*

AF-1161; Hidrocloruro de trazodona. 2-[3-(4-*m*-Chlorophenylpiperazin-1-yl)propyl]-1,2,4-triazolo[4,3-*a*]pyridin-3(2*H*)-one hydrochloride.

$C_{19}H_{22}ClN_5O,HCl$ = 408.3.

*CAS — 19794-93-5 (trazodone); 25332-39-2 (trazodone hydrochloride).*

*ATC — N06AX05.*

**Pharmacopoeias.** In *Br.* and *US.*

**BP 2003** (Trazodone Hydrochloride). A white or almost white crystalline powder. Soluble in water; sparingly soluble in alcohol; practically insoluble in ether. A 1% solution in water has a pH of 3.9 to 4.5. Store in airtight containers. Protect from light.

**USP 27** (Trazodone Hydrochloride). A white to off-white crystalline powder. Sparingly soluble in water and in chloroform. Store in airtight containers. Protect from light.

### Adverse Effects and Treatment

Trazodone has sedative properties and drowsiness may initially occur but usually disappears on continuing treatment. Other side-effects occasionally reported include dizziness, headache, nausea and vomiting, weakness, weight loss, tremor, dry mouth, bradycardia or tachycardia, orthostatic hypotension, oedema, constipation, diarrhoea, blurred vision, restlessness, confusional states, insomnia, and skin rash. Although some of these effects are typical of antimuscarinic activity it is reported that trazodone has little antimuscarinic activity compared with tricyclic antidepressants. *Animal* studies have also indicated that trazodone is less cardiotoxic than the tricyclics. Priapism has been reported on a number of occasions.

Agranulocytosis, thrombocytopenia, and anaemia have been reported rarely. Adverse effects on hepatic function, including jaundice and hepatocellular damage, which may sometimes be severe, have also been reported rarely.

Hyponatraemia possibly due to inappropriate secretion of antidiuretic hormone has been associated with the use of antidepressants, particularly in the elderly.

Symptoms of overdosage include drowsiness, dizziness, vomiting, priapism, respiratory arrest, seizures, and ECG changes. Treatment of overdosage may involve gastric lavage followed by the administration of activated charcoal and symptomatic and supportive therapy.

**Effects on the cardiovascular system.** Although trazodone is considered to cause fewer adverse cardiovascular reactions than the tricyclic antidepressants, they have, nevertheless, been reported in individual patients. In therapeutic doses it has been associated with heart block in a patient with pre-existing cardiovascular disease,[1] as well as in a patient with no ECG abnormalities.[2] Similarly, ventricular arrhythmias have been associated with therapeutic doses of trazodone both in patients with a history of cardiac problems,[3,4] and with no history of cardiac abnormalities.[5] Atrial fibrillation has been reported in a patient with ischaemic heart disease.[6]

1. Rausch JL, *et al.* Complete heart block following a single dose of trazodone. *Am J Psychiatry* 1984; **141:** 1472–3.
2. Lippmann S, *et al.* Trazodone cardiotoxicity. *Am J Psychiatry* 1983; **140:** 1383.
3. Janowsky D, *et al.* Ventricular arrhythmias possibly aggravated by trazodone. *Am J Psychiatry* 1983; **140:** 796–7.
4. Vlay SC, Friedling S. Trazodone exacerbation of VT. *Am Heart J* 1983; **106:** 604.
5. Johnson BA. Trazodone toxicity. *Br J Hosp Med* 1985; **33:** 298.
6. White WB, Wong SHY. Rapid atrial fibrillation associated with trazodone hydrochloride. *Arch Gen Psychiatry* 1985; **42:** 424.

**Effects on the eyes.** A patient receiving clomipramine and trazodone by mouth noted excessive blinking whenever the dose of trazodone exceeded or equalled that of clomipramine.[1] When trazodone, but not clomipramine, was withdrawn, blinking became normal within 3 weeks.

1. Cooper MA, Dening TR. Excessive blinking associated with combined antidepressants. *BMJ* 1986; **293:** 1243.

**Effects on the liver.** A mixed hepatocellular-cholestatic liver enzyme pattern has been reported in a patient after about 3 weeks of treatment with trazodone in doses of up to 500 mg daily.[1] The enzyme abnormalities returned to normal 4 weeks after trazodone was stopped but it was suggested that liver enzyme values should be monitored during the first 4 weeks of therapy. A similar case apparently presenting as obstructive jaundice and hepatocellular inflammation, in which the patient had only been receiving 50 mg daily for 2 weeks, has also been described.[2] It was believed that the patient suffered an idiosyncratic drug reaction to trazodone. Further reports of trazodone-induced liver injury include an elderly patient who developed chronic active hepatitis after receiving trazodone 150 mg daily for approximately 8 months.[3] A case of fatal hepatic necrosis reported in another elderly patient was considered to be due to treatment with trazodone and antipsychotics.[4] The authors of the report[4] noted that up to August 1991 the UK Committee on Safety of Medicines had received 14 reports of adverse effects on the liver associated with trazodone including one episode of fatal hepatic necrosis. In one of 2 more recent reports of trazodone-induced hepatotoxicity,[5] a female patient with rheumatoid arthritis developed jaundice 18 months after trazodone was added to her existing medications. All drugs were stopped and the patient improved; however, an inadvertent rechallenge with trazodone (without any other medication) led to a recurrence of her symptoms which again resolved following trazodone withdrawal. The second case[6] involved a HIV-positive male who was started on methadone, clonidine, and trazodone as part of a detoxification program; 4 days later acute hepatitis and cholestasis was noted and trazodone and clonidine were withdrawn with subsequent resolution of symptoms. The authors considered that trazodone was probably the causative agent.

1. Chu AG, *et al.* Trazodone and liver toxicity. *Ann Intern Med* 1983; **99:** 128–9.
2. Sheikh KH, Nies AS. Trazodone and intrahepatic cholestasis. *Ann Intern Med* 1983; **99:** 572.
3. Beck PL, *et al.* Chronic active hepatitis associated with trazodone therapy. *Ann Intern Med* 1993; **118:** 791–2.
4. Hull M, *et al.* Fatal hepatic necrosis associated with trazodone and neuroleptic drugs. *BMJ* 1994; **309:** 378.
5. Fernandes NF, *et al.* Trazodone-induced hepatotoxicity: a case report with comments on drug-induced hepatotoxicity. *Am J Gastroenterol* 2000; **95:** 532–5.
6. Rettman KS, McClintock C. Hepatotoxicity after short-term trazodone therapy. *Ann Pharmacother* 2001; **35:** 1559–61.

**Effects on mental state.** There have been reports of mania,[1,2] and paranoid psychosis with hallucinations[3] associated with the use of trazodone in depressed patients; delirium[4] in patients with bulimia nervosa; and possible psychosis or hypomania[5] in a patient receiving trazodone-tryptophan treatment for aggression.

1. Warren M, Bick PA. Two case reports of trazodone-induced mania. *Am J Psychiatry* 1984; **141:** 1103–4.
2. Arana GW, Kaplan GB. Trazodone-induced mania following desipramine-induced mania in major depressive disorders. *Am J Psychiatry* 1985; **142:** 386.
3. Kraft TB. Psychosis following trazodone administration. *Am J Psychiatry* 1983; **140:** 1383–4.
4. Damlouji NF, Ferguson JM. Trazodone-induced delirium in bulimic patients. *Am J Psychiatry* 1984; **141:** 434–5.
5. Patterson BD, Srisopark MM. Severe anorexia and possible psychosis or hypomania after trazodone-tryptophan treatment of aggression. *Lancet* 1989; **i:** 1017.

**Effects on sexual function.** Trazodone is notable for the number of reports of priapism associated with its use.[1,2] In most cases, priapism occurred during treatment with standard doses after 1 to 3 weeks of therapy. Several patients required surgery and recovery was not always complete.[1] A review[3] of priapism induced by psychotropic drugs proposed that the effect was related to blockade of alpha-adrenoceptors in the absence of sufficient antimuscarinic activity, criteria which the pharmacological profile of trazodone fulfills.

Inhibition of ejaculation has also been reported in a man[4] and an increase in libido in women[5] and men.[6] There has also been a report of trazodone-associated priapism of the clitoris.[7]

1. Committee on Safety of Medicines. Priapism and trazodone (Molipaxin). *Current Problems 13* 1984.
2. Anonymous. Priapism with trazodone (Desyrel). *Med Lett Drugs Ther* 1984; **26:** 35.
3. Patel AG, *et al.* Priapism associated with psychotropic drugs. *Br J Hosp Med* 1996; **55:** 315–19.
4. Jones SD. Ejaculatory inhibition with trazodone. *J Clin Psychopharmacol* 1984; **4:** 279–81.
5. Gartrell N. Increased libido in women receiving trazodone. *Am J Psychiatry* 1986; **143:** 781–2.
6. Sullivan G. Increased libido in three men treated with trazodone. *J Clin Psychiatry* 1988; **49:** 202–3.
7. Pescatori ES, *et al.* Priapism of the clitoris: a case report following trazodone use. *J Urol (Baltimore)* 1993; **149:** 1557–9.

**Effects on the skin.** Individual reports of adverse dermatological reactions to trazodone have included leucocytoclastic vasculitis,[1] erythema multiforme,[2] and exacerbation of psoriasis.[3]

1. Mann SC, *et al.* Leukocytoclastic vasculitis secondary to trazodone treatment. *J Am Acad Dermatol* 1984; **10:** 699–70.
2. Ford HE, Jenike MA. Erythema multiforme associated with trazodone therapy: case report. *J Clin Psychiatry* 1985; **46:** 294–5.
3. Barth JH, Baker H. Generalized pustular psoriasis precipitated by trazodone in the treatment of depression. *Br J Dermatol* 1986; **115:** 629–30.

**Epileptogenic effect.** Tonic-clonic seizures related to trazodone therapy have been reported in 2 patients[1,2] with no previous history of seizure disorders.

1. Bowdan ND. Seizure possibly caused by trazodone hydrochloride. *Am J Psychiatry* 1983; **140:** 642.
2. Lefkowitz D, *et al.* Seizures and trazodone therapy. *Arch Gen Psychiatry* 1985; **42:** 523.

**Overdosage.** Reviews have indicated that the incidence of serious toxicity from trazodone overdose alone was low compared with tricyclic antidepressant overdose.[1-4]

In a review covering 149 overdose cases,[1] only 10 deaths had been reported and in only 1 case was trazodone the sole agent reported to be ingested; in this case autopsy revealed an acute myocardial infarction after the patient was stable. The remaining 9 patients also had histories of ingestion of unknown quantities of alcohol, benzodiazepines, or other sedative-hypnotics that may have contributed to their demise. In the surviving 139 patients, 2 cases of respiratory arrest, 2 cases of right bundle branch block, and one case each of priapism, seizure, atrioventricular block, and T-wave inversion were reported. The remaining patients had minor CNS-depressant effects.

In a second review[2] of 88 cases of overdose, no fatalities occurred in the 39 cases where trazodone alone was ingested. However 9 deaths occurred in the remaining 49 cases where trazodone was ingested with other drugs or alcohol.

For a discussion of choice of antidepressant with respect to toxicity in overdosage, see under Depression, p.279.

1. Hassan E, Miller DD. Toxicity and elimination of trazodone after overdose. *Clin Pharm* 1985; **4:** 97–100.
2. Gamble DE, Peterson LG. Trazodone overdose: four years of experience from voluntary reports. *J Clin Psychiatry* 1986; **47:** 544–6.
3. Crome P, Ali C. Clinical features and management of self-poisoning with newer antidepressants. *Med Toxicol* 1986; **1:** 411–20.
4. Gallant DM. Antidepressant overdose: symptoms and treatment. *Psychopathology* 1987; **20** (suppl 1): 75–81.

### Precautions

Trazodone should be used with caution in patients with cardiovascular disorders, such as ischaemic heart disease, and its use is not recommended in the immediate recovery phase after myocardial infarction. Similarly, it should be used with caution in patients with epilepsy and severe hepatic or renal impairment. Trazodone should be stopped immediately if patients develop signs of hepatic dysfunction or blood dyscrasias. Patients developing inappropriate or prolonged penile erections should also stop trazodone immediately.

Patients should be closely monitored during early antidepressant therapy until improvement in depression is observed because suicide is an inherent risk in depressed patients. For further details, see under Depression, p.279.

Drowsiness is often experienced at the start of trazodone antidepressant therapy and patients, if affected, should not drive or operate machinery.

As with other antidepressants, trazodone therapy should be withdrawn gradually.

**Breast feeding.** The American Academy of Pediatrics[1] considers that, although the effect of trazodone on breast-feeding infants is unknown, its use by mothers during breast feeding may be of concern since antidepressant drugs do appear in breast milk and thus could conceivably alter CNS function in the infant both in the short and long term.

In a study of 6 lactating women each given a single 50-mg dose of trazodone, it was concluded that exposure of infants to trazodone via breast milk is very small.[2] However, trazodone has been reported to form an active metabolite and it was not known to what extent this metabolite distributed into breast milk.

1. American Academy of Pediatrics. The transfer of drugs and other chemicals into human milk. *Pediatrics* 2001; **108:** 776–89. Correction. *ibid.*; 1029. Also available at: http://aappolicy.aappublications.org/cgi/content/full/pediatrics%3b108/3/776 (accessed 14/06/04)
2. Verbeeck RK, *et al.* Excretion of trazodone in breast milk. *Br J Clin Pharmacol* 1986; **22:** 367–70.

**Porphyria.** Trazodone hydrochloride is considered to be unsafe in patients with porphyria because it has been shown to be porphyrinogenic in *animals*.

### Interactions

Trazodone should not be given to patients receiving MAOIs or for at least 14 days afterwards. It has also been recommended that any drug liable to provoke a serious reaction (e.g. phenelzine) should not be given within one week of stopping trazodone therapy. For further details, see Antidepressants under Interactions of Phenelzine, p.315.

It is considered unlikely that trazodone will alter the effects of antihypertensives such as guanethidine; some interaction may, however, occur with clonidine. The dose of other antihypertensives may need to be reduced if used with trazodone.

The sedative effects of trazodone may be enhanced by alcohol or other CNS depressants. The potential for interaction between trazodone and general anaesthetics or muscle relaxants exists and some manufacturers recommend that trazodone should be stopped before elective surgery for as long as clinically feasible.

Trazodone may increase plasma concentrations of digoxin or phenytoin and some manufacturers recommend monitoring concentrations if used with trazodone.

Trazodone is metabolised by the cytochrome P450 isoenzyme CYP3A4 and inhibitors of this isoenzyme may limit the elimination of trazodone. Consequently, trazodone may need to be given in reduced doses with drugs known to be potent inhibitors of CYP3A4 such as the azole antifungals itraconazole and ketoconazole, and the protease inhibitors indinavir and ritonavir. CYP3A4 inducers such as carbamazepine may reduce the plasma concentrations of trazodone.

**Anticoagulants.** For the effect of trazodone on *warfarin*, see p.1025.

**Antiepileptics.** Antidepressants may antagonise the activity of antiepileptics by lowering the convulsive threshold.

Trazodone may increase plasma concentrations of *carbamazepine* (see p.356) and *phenytoin* (see p.373). Some manufacturers recommend monitoring concentrations of phenytoin if used with trazodone.

## Pharmacokinetics

Trazodone is readily absorbed from the gastrointestinal tract although absorption is affected by food. When trazodone is taken shortly after a meal there may be an increase in the amount absorbed, a decrease in the maximum concentration, and a lengthening in the time to maximum concentration compared with the fasting state; peak plasma concentrations occur about one hour after a dose when taken on an empty stomach and after about 2 hours when taken with food. Protein binding is reported to be about 89 to 95%.

Trazodone is extensively metabolised in the liver and paths of metabolism include *N*-oxidation and hydroxylation. It is metabolised to its active metabolite *m*-chlorophenylpiperazine via the cytochrome P450 isoenzyme CYP3A4. Trazodone is excreted mainly in the urine almost entirely in the form of its metabolites, either in free or in conjugated form: some is excreted in the faeces via biliary elimination. The elimination of trazodone from the plasma is biphasic, with a terminal elimination half-life of 5 to 9 hours.

Small amounts of trazodone are distributed into breast milk.

◊ References.

1. Bayer AJ, *et al.* Pharmacokinetic and pharmacodynamic characteristics of trazodone in the elderly. *Br J Clin Pharmacol* 1983; **16:** 371–6.
2. Nilsen OG, Dale O. Single dose pharmacokinetics of trazodone in healthy subjects. *Pharmacol Toxicol* 1992; **71:** 150–3.
3. Nilsen OG, *et al.* Pharmacokinetics of trazodone during multiple dosing to psychiatric patients. *Pharmacol Toxicol* 1993; **72:** 286–9.

## Uses and Administration

Trazodone is a triazolopyridine antidepressant chemically unrelated to other classes of antidepressants. It blocks the reuptake of serotonin at presynaptic neurones and also has an action at $5\text{-HT}_1$ receptors. Unlike the tricyclic antidepressants, trazodone does not inhibit the peripheral reuptake of noradrenaline, although it may indirectly facilitate neuronal release. Trazodone blocks central $\alpha_1$-adrenoceptors and appears to have no effect on the central reuptake of dopamine. It does not appear to have very significant antimuscarinic properties, but has a marked sedative action.

For the treatment of **depression** trazodone hydrochloride is given by mouth in doses of 150 mg daily initially; total daily dosage may be increased by 50 mg every 3 or 4 days up to 300 to 400 mg daily if necessary. The daily dosage may be divided throughout the day after food or be given as a single dose at night. Divided daily dosages of up to 600 mg may be given in severe depression in hospitalised patients. A suggested initial dose in elderly and other susceptible patients is 100 mg daily, and total daily doses above 300 mg are unlikely to be needed in these patients.

In the treatment of **anxiety** (p.663), trazodone hydrochloride is given in an initial dose of 75 mg daily by mouth increasing to 300 mg daily if necessary.

As with other antidepressants, trazodone should be withdrawn gradually.

**Depression.** As discussed on p.279, there is very little difference in efficacy between the different groups of antidepressant drugs, and choice is often made on the basis of adverse effect profile. Trazodone has a different biochemical profile from both the tricyclics and the SSRIs.

References.

1. Weisler RH, *et al.* Comparison of bupropion and trazodone for the treatment of major depression. *J Clin Psychopharmacol* 1994; **14:** 170–9.

**Disturbed behaviour.** Trazodone has produced beneficial results[1-3] when tried in various disorders for the control of symptoms such as agitation, aggression, and disruptive behaviour (see p.665). Although adverse effects such as sedation and orthostatic hypotension can occur with trazodone and may be particularly problematical in the elderly, some[4] consider that, in the management of dementia, trazodone might be worth trying in nonpsychotic patients with disturbed behaviour, especially those with mild symptoms or those intolerant of or unresponsive to antipsychotics.

1. Pasion RC, Kirby SG. Trazodone for screaming. *Lancet* 1993; **341:** 970.
2. Lebert F, *et al.* Behavioral effects of trazodone in Alzheimer's disease. *J Clin Psychiatry* 1994; **55:** 536–8.
3. Sultzer DL, *et al.* A double-blind comparison of trazodone and haloperidol for treatment of agitation in patients with dementia. *Am J Geriatr Psychiatry* 1997; **5:** 60–9.
4. American Psychiatric Association. Practice guideline for the treatment of patients with Alzheimer's disease and other dementias of late life. *Am J Psychiatry* 1997; **154** (suppl): 1–39. Also available at: http://www.psych.org/psych_pract/treatg/pg/pg_dementia_32701.cfm (accessed 14/06/04)

**Sexual dysfunction.** Priapism can occur as an adverse effect of trazodone (see Effects on Sexual Function in Adverse Effects, above) and this has led to trials of oral trazodone for the treatment of erectile dysfunction (p.1745). Positive responses have been reported, either in conjunction with yohimbine[1] or alone.[2] However, there appear to have been few controlled studies and a recent systematic review[3] considered some of these to be either small, brief, or methodologically weak. Meta-analysis[3] of data from 6 studies did not find trazodone to be superior to placebo but subgroup analysis possibly suggested a better outcome in patients with psychogenic erectile dysfunction and in those given doses of 150 to 200 mg daily.

1. Montorsi F, *et al.* Effect of yohimbine-trazodone on psychogenic impotence: a randomized, double-blind, placebo-controlled study. *Urology* 1994; **44:** 732–6.
2. Lance R, *et al.* Oral trazodone as empirical therapy for erectile dysfunction: a retrospective review. *Urology* 1995; **46:** 117–20.
3. Fink HA, *et al.* Trazodone for erectile dysfunction: a systematic review and meta-analysis. *BJU Int* 2003; **92:** 441–6.

**Substance dependence.** The antidepressant and anxiolytic properties of trazodone have been reported to have been useful when tried in patients experiencing withdrawal syndromes from cocaine (p.1375)[1] or benzodiazepines (p.690).[2]

1. Small GW, Purcell JJ. Trazodone and cocaine abuse. *Arch Gen Psychiatry* 1985; **42:** 524.
2. Ansseau M, De Roeck J. Trazodone in benzodiazepine dependence. *J Clin Psychiatry* 1993; **54:** 189–91.

## Preparations

***USP 27:*** Trazodone Hydrochloride Tablets.

**Proprietary Preparations** (details are given in Part 3)

***Arg.:*** Taxagon; ***Austria:*** Trittico; ***Belg.:*** Trazolan; ***Braz.:*** Donaren; ***Canad.:*** Desyrel; Trazorel; ***Chile:*** Trittico; ***Fin.:*** Azona; ***Ger.:*** Thombran; ***Gr.:*** Trittico; ***Hong Kong:*** Trittico; ***Irl.:*** Molipaxin; ***Israel:*** Depyrel; Trazodil; ***Ital.:*** Trittico; ***Mex.:*** Sideril†; ***Neth.:*** Trazolan; ***Port.:*** Trazone; Triticum; ***S.Afr.:*** Molipaxin; ***Spain:*** Deprax; ***Switz.:*** Trittico; ***Thai.:*** Desirel; ***UK:*** Molipaxin; ***USA:*** Desyrel.

# Trimipramine *(BAN, USAN, rINN)*

IL-6001; 7162-RP; Trimeprimine; Trimipramina. Dimethyl{3-(10,11-dihydro-5*H*-dibenz[*b*,*f*]azepin-5-yl-2-methyl)propyl}-amine.

$C_{20}H_{26}N_2$ = 294.4.

*CAS — 739-71-9.*

*ATC — N06AA06.*

## Trimipramine Maleate *(BANM, USAN, rINNM)*

Maleato de trimipramina; Trimipramine Hydrogen Maleate; Trimipramini Maleas.

$C_{20}H_{26}N_2,C_4H_4O_4$ = 410.5.

*CAS — 521-78-8.*

**Pharmacopoeias.** In *Eur.* (see p.vi).

**Ph. Eur. 5.0** (Trimipramine Maleate). A white or almost white crystalline powder. Slightly soluble in water and in alcohol. Protect from light.

## Adverse Effects, Treatment, and Precautions

As for tricyclic antidepressants in general (see Amitriptyline, p.281).

**Porphyria.** Trimipramine is considered to be unsafe in patients with porphyria although there is conflicting experimental evidence of porphyrinogenicity.

## Interactions

For interactions associated with tricyclic antidepressants, see Amitriptyline, p.284.

## Pharmacokinetics

Trimipramine is readily absorbed after oral doses, peak plasma concentrations being obtained in 2 hours. It is metabolised in the liver to its major metabolite desmethyltrimipramine, which is active. Trimipramine is excreted in the urine mainly in the form of its metabolites. It is extensively bound to plasma proteins. The plasma elimination half-life is reported to be about 23 hours.

◊ References.

1. Maurer H. Metabolism of trimipramine in man. *Arzneimittelforschung* 1989; **39:** 101–3.
2. Musa MN. Nonlinear kinetics of trimipramine in depressed patients. *J Clin Pharmacol* 1989; **29:** 746–7.

## Uses and Administration

Trimipramine is a dibenzazepine tricyclic antidepressant with actions and uses similar to those of amitriptyline (p.285). It has marked antimuscarinic and sedative properties.

Trimipramine is given by mouth as the maleate although doses are expressed in terms of trimipramine base. Trimipramine maleate 34.9 mg is approximately equivalent to 25 mg of trimipramine. In the treatment of depression, the usual initial dose is the equivalent of trimipramine 50 to 75 mg daily, gradually increased as necessary to 150 to 300 mg daily. The recommended initial dose for the elderly in the UK is 30 to 75 mg daily, gradually increased as necessary. In the USA, the elderly and adolescents may be given 50 mg daily initially followed by gradual increments as necessary up to a maximum of 100 mg daily. Trimipramine may be given in divided doses during the day, but since it has a prolonged half-life, once-daily dosage regimens are also suitable and usually given at night.

Trimipramine has also been given orally as the hydrochloride and intramuscularly as the mesilate.

Trimipramine should be withdrawn gradually to reduce the risk of withdrawal symptoms.

## Preparations

***BP 2003:*** Trimipramine Tablets.

**Proprietary Preparations** (details are given in Part 3)

***Austral.:*** Surmontil; ***Austria:*** Stangyl†; ***Belg.:*** Surmontil†; ***Canad.:*** Apo-Trimip; Novo-Tripramine; Rhotrimine; Surmontil; ***Denm.:*** Surmontil; ***Fin.:*** Surmontil; ***Fr.:*** Surmontil; ***Ger.:*** Herphonal; Stangyl; Trimidura; Trimineurin; Trimipramin; ***Hong Kong:*** Apo-Trimip†; Surmontil; ***India:*** Surmontil; ***Irl.:*** Surmontil; ***Israel:*** Surmontil; ***Ital.:*** Surmontil; ***Neth.:*** Surmontil; ***Norw.:*** Surmontil; ***NZ:*** Surmontil; Tripress; ***Port.:*** Surmontil; ***S.Afr.:*** Surmontil; Tydamine; ***Spain:*** Surmontil; ***Swed.:*** Surmontil; ***Switz.:*** Surmontil; ***UK:*** Surmontil; ***USA:*** Surmontil.

# Tryptophan *(USAN, rINN)*

Triptófano; L-Tryptophan; Tryptophanum; W. L-2-Amino-3-(indol-3-yl)propionic acid.

$C_{11}H_{12}N_2O_2$ = 204.2.

*CAS — 73-22-3.*

*ATC — N06AX02.*

**Pharmacopoeias.** In *Chin., Eur.* (see p.vi), *Jpn,* and *US.*

**Ph. Eur. 5.0** (Tryptophan). A white or almost white crystalline or amorphous powder. Sparingly soluble in water; slightly soluble in alcohol; dissolves in dilute mineral acids and in dilute solutions of alkali hydroxides. Protect from light.

**USP 27** (Tryptophan). White to slightly yellowish-white crystals or crystalline powder. Soluble in hot alcohol and in dilute hydrochloric acid. pH of a 1% solution in water is between 5.5 and 7.0.

## Adverse Effects

Tryptophan-containing products have been associated with the eosinophilia-myalgia syndrome; for further details, see below.

Other side-effects that have been reported include nausea, headache, lightheadedness, and drowsiness.

An increased incidence of bladder tumours has been reported in *mice* given L-tryptophan orally as well as in cholesterol pellets embedded in the bladder lumen. However, there was no increase in tumour incidence when only high-dose, oral tryptophan was given.

**Eosinophilia-myalgia syndrome.** In late 1989 the first notification linking the eosinophilia-myalgia syndrome with the use of tryptophan-containing products was made in the USA.[1] There followed a number of similar published case reports from the USA, Europe, and Japan. Reviews of tryptophan-associated eosinophilia-myalgia syndrome have noted that by early 1990 over 1500 cases were known in the USA.[2,3]

In early 1990 the Centers for Disease Control in the USA summarised the features and known reports concerning the syndrome.[4] As the name implies the characteristic features are an intense eosinophilia together with disabling fatigue and muscle pain, although multisystem organ involvement and inflammatory disorders affecting the joints, skin, connective tissue, lungs, heart, and liver have also been recorded. Symptoms have generally developed over several weeks and the syndrome has occurred in patients who had been receiving tryptophan for many years previously with no untoward effect. In most patients slow and gradual improvement in the degree of eosinophilia and other clinical manifestations has followed the withdrawal of tryptophan, but in some patients the disease has progressed despite withdrawal and there have been fatalities.[5-7] The inflammatory condition has necessitated the use of corticosteroids in some patients.

The eosinophilia-myalgia syndrome has been reported in patients taking both tryptophan-containing prescription products for depression and non-prescription dietary supplements for a number of disorders including insomnia, the premenstrual syndrome, and stress; it does not appear to have occurred in patients receiving amino-acid preparations containing tryptophan as part of total parenteral nutrition regimens. The recognition of this syndrome led to the withdrawal of tryptophan-containing products or severe restrictions being imposed upon their use in many countries during 1990.

Various theories were proposed as to the reason for the association of tryptophan with this syndrome. Confusion existed because the reports implicated a very wide range of products from different manufacturers. More recent evidence, however, appears to have confirmed that contaminated tryptophan has originated from a single manufacturer in Japan.[8-10] Bulk tryptophan is imported from Japan for manufacture into finished pharmaceutical dosage forms and it was noted in one of these reports[9] that a single product was often found to contain two or more lots of powdered tryptophan that were blended together during the production of tablets or capsules. Many trace contaminants have been found in batches of tryptophan associated with the syndrome.[11] One contaminant has been identified as 1,1′-ethylidenebis(tryptophan).[12] Its inclusion in bulk tryptophan powder appeared to coincide with alterations in the manufacturing conditions that involved a change in the strain of *Bacillus amyloliquefaciens* used in the fermentation process and a reduction in the amount of charcoal used for purification.[9] Other investigations indicated the presence of bacitracin-like peptides in batches of the contaminated tryptophan.[13] However, further work[14] has provided only weak support for an association between the syndrome and any one particular contaminant and the causative agent remains to be confirmed. Nonetheless, since the syndrome only appeared to be associated with tryptophan from one manufacturer, tryptophan preparations were reintroduced in the UK in 1994 for restricted use under carefully monitored conditions.[15]


1. Anonymous. Eosinophilia-myalgia syndrome—New Mexico. *MMWR* 1989; **38:** 765–7.
2. Troy JL. Eosinophilia-myalgia syndrome. *Mayo Clin Proc* 1991; **66:** 535–8.
3. Milburn DS, Myers CW. Tryptophan toxicity: a pharmacoepidemiologic review of eosinophilia-myalgia syndrome. *DICP Ann Pharmacother* 1991; **25:** 1259–62.
4. Kilbourne EM, *et al.* Interim guidance on the eosinophilia-myalgia syndrome. *Ann Intern Med* 1990; **112:** 85–6.
5. Anonymous. Eosinophilia-myalgia syndrome associated with ingestion of L-tryptophan—United States, through August 24, 1990. *JAMA* 1990; **264:** 1655.
6. Kaufman LD, *et al.* Clinical follow-up and immunogenetic studies of 32 patients with eosinophilia-myalgia syndrome. *Lancet* 1991; **337:** 1071–4.
7. Hertzman PA, *et al.* The eosinophilia-myalgia syndrome: status of 205 patients and results of treatment 2 years after onset. *Ann Intern Med* 1995; **122:** 851–5.
8. Slutsker L, *et al.* Eosinophilia-myalgia syndrome associated with exposure to tryptophan from a single manufacturer. *JAMA* 1990; **264:** 213–17.
9. Belongia EA, *et al.* An investigation of the cause of the eosinophilia-myalgia syndrome associated with tryptophan use. *N Engl J Med* 1990; **323:** 357–65.
10. Varga J, *et al.* The cause and pathogenesis of the eosinophilia-myalgia syndrome. *Ann Intern Med* 1992; **116:** 140–7.
11. Hill RH, *et al.* Contaminants in L-tryptophan associated with eosinophilia myalgia syndrome. *Arch Environ Contam Toxicol* 1993; **25:** 134–42.
12. Mayeno AN, *et al.* Characterization of "peak E", a novel amino acid associated with eosinophilia-myalgia syndrome. *Science* 1990; **250:** 1707–8.
13. Barnhart ER, *et al.* Bacitracin-associated peptides and contaminated L-tryptophan. *Lancet* 1990; **336:** 742.
14. Philen RM, *et al.* Tryptophan contaminants associated with eosinophilia-myalgia syndrome. *Am J Epidemiol* 1993; **138:** 154–9.
15. Committee on Safety of Medicines/Medicines Control Agency. L-Tryptophan (Optimax): limited availability for resistant depression. *Current Problems* 1994; **20:** 2.


### Precautions

As tryptophan has been associated with eosinophilia-myalgia syndrome, patients taking it should be closely monitored, with particular care being paid to eosinophil counts, haematological changes, and muscle symptomatology.

Patients taking tryptophan may experience drowsiness and, if affected, they should not drive or operate machinery. For further details of the effects of antidepressant therapy on driving see under Amitriptyline, p.283.

Abnormal metabolism of tryptophan may occur in patients with pyridoxine deficiency and tryptophan is thus sometimes given with pyridoxine supplements.

### Interactions

Although tryptophan has been given to patients receiving MAOIs in the belief that clinical efficacy may be improved, it should be noted that the adverse effects of either drug may also be potentiated. For further details, see Antidepressants under Interactions of Phenelzine, p.315.

Use of tryptophan with drugs that inhibit the reuptake of serotonin may exacerbate the adverse effects of the latter and precipitate the serotonin syndrome (p.313).

There have been occasional reports of sexual disinhibition in patients taking tryptophan with phenothiazines or benzodiazepines.

For a report of tryptophan reducing blood concentrations of levodopa, see Nutritional Agents under Interactions for Levodopa, p.1208.

### Pharmacokinetics

Tryptophan is readily absorbed from the gastrointestinal tract. Tryptophan is extensively bound to plasma albumin. It is metabolised in the liver by tryptophan pyrrolase and tryptophan hydroxylase. Metabolites include hydroxytryptophan, which is then converted to serotonin, and kynurenine derivatives. Some tryptophan is converted to nicotinic acid and nicotinamide. Pyridoxine and ascorbic acid are cofactors in the decarboxylation and hydroxylation, respectively of tryptophan; pyridoxine apparently prevents the accumulation of the kynurenine metabolites.

◊ References.


1. Green AR, *et al.* The pharmacokinetics of L-tryptophan following its intravenous and oral administration. *Br J Clin Pharmacol* 1985; **20:** 317–21.


### Uses and Administration

Tryptophan is an amino acid which is an essential constituent of the diet. Tryptophan and DL-tryptophan have been used as dietary supplements.

Tryptophan is a precursor of serotonin. Because CNS depletion of serotonin is considered to be involved in depression, tryptophan has been used in its treatment. Although it has been given alone, evidence of effectiveness is scant and tryptophan has generally been used as adjunctive therapy in depression. Pyridoxine and ascorbic acid are involved in the metabolism of tryptophan to serotonin (see Pharmacokinetics, above) and have sometimes been given concomitantly.

In many countries preparations containing tryptophan have either been withdrawn from the market or their availability severely restricted or limited because of its association with the eosinophilia-myalgia syndrome. In the UK, tryptophan is restricted to use only as an adjunct to other antidepressant medication for patients with severe and disabling depressive illness of more than 2 years' continuous duration who have failed to respond to an adequate trial of standard antidepressant drug treatment. Therapy should be started by hospital specialists; thereafter tryptophan may be prescribed in the community.

In the treatment of depression the usual dose of tryptophan is 1 g given three times daily, but some patients may require up to 6 g daily in divided doses. Lower doses may be required in the elderly especially those with renal or hepatic impairment.

**Depression.** Evidence of benefit for tryptophan when given alone for depression (p.279) is lacking, though there is some suggestion of a weak antidepressant effect.[1] It has therefore mainly been used with other antidepressants in the belief that it would potentiate their effects. Although beneficial effects have been reported in some patients given tryptophan with tricyclic antidepressants or MAOIs, alone or with lithium, evidence of efficacy is mainly limited to case reports and small controlled studies.[2,3]

Since the publication of reports linking the use of tryptophan with the eosinophilia-myalgia syndrome (see under Adverse Effects, above) preparations containing tryptophan for depression have either been withdrawn from the market or their use severely restricted as in the UK[4] and many other countries. For details of UK restrictions see Uses and Administration, above.


1. Shaw K, *et al.* Tryptophan and 5-hydroxytryptophan for depression. Available in The Cochrane Library; Issue 2. Chichester: John Wiley; 2004.
2. Barker WA, *et al.* The Newcastle chronic depression study: results of a treatment regime. *Int Clin Psychopharmacol* 1987; **2:** 261–72.
3. Smith S. Tryptophan in the treatment of resistant depression—a review. *Pharm J* 1998; **261:** 819–21.
4. Committee on Safety of Medicines/Medicines Control Agency. L-Tryptophan (Optimax): limited availability for resistant depression. *Current Problems* 1994; **20:** 2.


**Dietary supplementation.** The use of tryptophan as a dietary supplement has been reviewed.[1] However, because of its association with the eosinophilia-myalgia syndrome (see under Adverse Effects, above), the addition of tryptophan to food intended for human consumption is prohibited in some countries.


1. Li Wan Po A, Maguire T. Tryptophan: useful dietary supplement or a health hazard? *Pharm J* 1990; **244:** 484–5.


**Insomnia.** Tryptophan, sometimes in the form of dietary supplements, has enjoyed some popularity for the treatment of insomnia (p.667). However, in comparison with other hypnotics such as the benzodiazepines, the effects of tryptophan have been difficult to substantiate, and enthusiasm for tryptophan has waned considerably amongst sleep researchers.[1] It should also be noted that since the publication of reports linking the use of tryptophan with the eosinophilia-myalgia syndrome (see under Adverse Effects, above) preparations indicated for insomnia have been withdrawn from the market in many countries.


1. Lahmeyer HW. Tryptophan for insomnia. *JAMA* 1989; **262:** 2748.


### Preparations

**Proprietary Preparations** (details are given in Part 3)

***Austria:*** Kalma; ***Canad.:*** Tryptan; ***Ger.:*** Ardeydorm; Ardeytropin; Kalma; ***UK:*** Optimax.

**Multi-ingredient:** ***Fr.:*** Vita-Dermacide; ***Irl.:*** Optimax†; ***Spain:*** Calcioretard†; ***USA:*** PDP Liquid Protein.

## Venlafaxine Hydrochloride

*(BANM, USAN, rINNM)*

Hidrocloruro de venlafaxina; Wy-45030. (*RS*)-1-(2-Dimethylamino-1-*p*-methoxyphenylethyl)cyclohexanol hydrochloride.

$C_{17}H_{27}NO_2,HCl = 313.9.$

*CAS — 93413-69-5 (venlafaxine); 99300-78-4 (venlafaxine hydrochloride).*

*ATC — N06AX16.*

### Adverse Effects and Treatment

Adverse effects that have been reported most frequently with venlafaxine include nausea, headache, insomnia, somnolence, dry mouth, dizziness, constipation, sexual dysfunction, asthenia, sweating, and nervousness. Other common adverse effects have included anorexia, diarrhoea, dyspepsia, abdominal pain, anxiety, urinary frequency, visual disturbances, vasodilatation, vomiting, tremor, paraesthesia, chills or fever, palpitations, weight gain or loss, increased serum cholesterol, agitation, abnormal dreams, confusion, arthralgia, myalgia, tinnitus, pruritus, dyspnoea, and skin rashes. Dose-related increases in blood pressure have also been observed in some patients. Less commonly reported side-effects have included reversible increases in liver enzymes, orthostatic hypotension, syncope, arrhythmias, tachycardia, ecchymosis, hallucinations, urinary retention, angioedema, and photosensitivity reactions. Convulsions, galactorrhoea, haemorrhage including gastrointestinal bleeding, anaphylaxis, hepatitis, erythema multiforme, Stevens-Johnson syndrome, ataxia, dysarthria, extrapyramidal disorders, and activation of mania or hypomania have been reported rarely. Very rare adverse effects include blood dyscrasias such as agranulocytosis, aplastic anaemia, neutropenia, and pancytopenia, prolongation of the QT interval, pancreatitis, and pulmonary eosinophilia. Suicidal ideation has been reported, particularly in children (see under Effects on Mental State, below).

Hyponatraemia possibly due to inappropriate secretion of antidiuretic hormone has been associated with the use of antidepressants, particularly in the elderly.

In overdosage, the symptoms that have been reported include lethargy, somnolence, ECG changes, cardiac arrhythmias, and seizures. Treatment of overdosage includes consideration of the use of activated charcoal or gastric lavage followed by symptomatic and supportive therapy. Dialysis, haemoperfusion, exchange perfusion, and measures to increase urine production are considered unlikely to be of benefit.

**Effects on the eyes.** Acute angle-closure glaucoma developed in a 45-year-old woman 3 days after starting venlafaxine;[1] she recovered following iridotomy.


1. Ng B, *et al.* Venlafaxine and bilateral acute angle closure glaucoma. *Med J Aust* 2002; **176:** 241.


**Effects on the liver.** Acute hepatitis developed in a 44-year-old woman approximately 6 months after starting venlafaxine;[1] she recovered once venlafaxine was withdrawn. In another report,[2] acute hepatitis developed in a 78-year-old man about a month after venlafaxine was added to therapy. Again, symptoms resolved when the drug was discontinued.

For a report of hepatotoxicity in patients taking venlafaxine subsequent to an attempted overdose with sertraline, see p.293.

1. Horsmans Y, *et al.* Venlaxafine-associated [sic] hepatitis. *Ann Intern Med* 1999; **130:** 944.
2. Cardona X, *et al.* Venlafaxine-associated hepatitis. *Ann Intern Med* 2000; **132:** 417.

**Effects on mental state.** Data from trials received by the UK Committee on Safety of Medicine (CSM) failed to demonstrate that venlafaxine was effective in the treatment of depressive illness in those under 18 years and indicated that the risk of harmful outcome including self-harm and suicidal ideation was increased in those receiving venlafaxine when compared with placebo.[1] The CSM recommended that venlafaxine should not be used to treat depressive illness in children under 18 years. Similar warnings have also been issued in Canada.[2]

1. Safety of venlafaxine in children and adolescents under 18 years in the treatment of depressive illness - Epinet message issued September 2003 from Professor G Duff, Chairman of Committee on Safety of Medicines (CSM). Available at: http://medicines.mhra.gov.uk/ourwork/monitorsafequalmed/safetymessages/efexor0903.pdf (accessed 14/06/04)
2. Wyeth Canada. Important safety information regarding the use of Effexor (venlafaxine HCl) tablets and Effexor XR (venlafaxine HCl) capsules in children and adolescents (issued September 2003). Available at: http://www.hc-sc.gc.ca/hpfb-dgpsa/tpd-dpt/effexor_prof_e.pdf (accessed 14/06/04)

**Neuroleptic malignant syndrome.** For mention of neuroleptic malignant syndrome developing when venlafaxine was added to treatment with antipsychotics, see under Interactions in Chlorpromazine, p.679.

**Overdosage.** Rare serious events including seizures and ECG changes[1-3] have occurred following venlafaxine overdoses; in some cases, death has ensued.[4]

Venlafaxine may not be as safe in overdose as some other serotonergic antidepressants. A review[5] of UK data recording the number of deaths due to acute poisoning by a single drug, with or without alcohol, found the number of fatalities per million prescriptions (the fatal toxicity index) was higher for venlafaxine than for other serotonergic antidepressants, and was similar to that for some of the less toxic tricyclic antidepressants.

1. White CM, *et al.* Seizure resulting from a venlafaxine overdose. *Ann Pharmacother* 1997; **31:** 178–80.
2. Coorey AN, Wenck DJ. Venlafaxine overdose. *Med J Aust* 1998; **168:** 523.
3. Blythe D, Hackett LP. Cardiovascular and neurological toxicity of venlafaxine. *Hum Exp Toxicol* 1999; **18:** 309–13.
4. Banham NDG. Fatal venlafaxine overdose. *Med J Aust* 1998; **169:** 445, 448.
5. Buckley NA, McManus PR. Fatal toxicity of serotoninergic and other antidepressant drugs: analysis of United Kingdom mortality data. *BMJ* 2002; **325:** 1332–3.

## Precautions

Venlafaxine should be used with caution in patients with moderate to severe hepatic or renal impairment and dosage adjustment may be necessary. Caution is also advised in those with a recent history of myocardial infarction or unstable heart disease, or whose condition might be exacerbated by an increase in heart rate. Due to the risk of dose-related hypertension, blood pressure monitoring may be advisable. Measurement of serum-cholesterol levels should also be considered with long-term treatment. Venlafaxine should also be used with caution in patients with a history of epilepsy and should be discontinued in any patient developing a seizure. It should also be used cautiously in patients with a history of bleeding disorders or of hypomania or mania. Patients with raised intra-ocular pressure or at risk of angle-closure glaucoma should be monitored closely. Patients who develop a rash, urticaria, or related allergic reaction with venlafaxine should be advised to contact their doctor.

Patients should be closely monitored during early antidepressant therapy until improvement in depression is observed because suicide is an inherent risk in depressed patients. For further details, see under Depression, p.279.

As with other antidepressants, venlafaxine may impair performance of skilled tasks and, if affected, patients should not drive or operate machinery. Patients, especially the elderly, should be warned of the risk of dizziness or unsteadiness due to orthostatic hypotension.

Symptoms reported on abrupt discontinuation or dose reduction of venlafaxine therapy include fatigue, somnolence, headache, nausea, vomiting, anorexia, dizziness, dry mouth, diarrhoea, insomnia, agitation, anxiety, nervousness, confusion, hypomania, paraesthesia, sweating, and vertigo. It is therefore recommended that venlafaxine should be withdrawn gradually over at least one week after more than one week's therapy and the patient monitored to minimise the risk of withdrawal reactions.

**Abuse.** Report of a patient who took crushed modified-release tablets of venlafaxine in doses of up to 3600 mg daily to obtain an amphetamine-like "high".[1] He continued to ingest increasing amounts of venlafaxine until a 4050-mg dose produced chest pain. On evaluation he had a raised pulse and blood pressure but these returned to normal within a few days.

1. Sattar SP, *et al.* A case of venlafaxine abuse. *N Engl J Med* 2003; **348:** 764–5.

**Breast feeding.** The manufacturers recommend that venlafaxine should not be used in women who are breast feeding.

In a study[1] both venlafaxine and its metabolite *O*-desmethylvenlafaxine were detected in breast milk in significant quantities and there were measurable concentrations of desmethylvenlafaxine in the infants' plasma. In another study[2] by the same group the milk-to-plasma ratio in 7 breast-fed infants was calculated to be 2.5 for venlafaxine and 2.74 for *O*-desmethylvenlafaxine. Detectable plasma levels of venlafaxine were found only in 1 infant while 4 infants had detectable *O*-desmethylvenlafaxine levels; no adverse effects were reported in the infants. Nonetheless, the authors recommended caution when giving venlafaxine to breast-feeding women particularly for those feeding premature or very young neonates.

1. Ilett KF, *et al.* Distribution and excretion of venlafaxine and O-desmethylvenlafaxine in human milk. *Br J Clin Pharmacol* 1998; **45:** 459–62.
2. Ilett KF, *et al.* Distribution of venlafaxine and its O-desmethyl metabolite in human milk and their effects in breastfed infants. *Br J Clin Pharmacol* 2002; **53:** 17–22.

**Children.** The use of venlafaxine for the treatment of depression in patients under 18 years of age is contra-indicated in some countries (see under Effects on Mental State, above).

**Pregnancy.** The manufacturers recommend that venlafaxine should not be used during pregnancy unless clearly necessary. In addition, if used shortly before birth, withdrawal effects may be seen in the neonate after delivery.

In a study of 150 women who took venlafaxine in the first trimester of pregnancy there were 125 live births, 18 spontaneous abortions, 7 therapeutic abortions and 2 reports of major malformations (hypospadias and neural tube defect with club foot).[1] Although the rate of spontaneous abortions was non-significantly higher in the venlafaxine group than in historical controls, the rate of major malformations was not greater than the baseline rate of 1 to 3%.

1. Einarson A, *et al.* Pregnancy outcome following gestational exposure to venlafaxine: a multicenter prospective controlled study. *Am J Psychiatry* 2001; **158:** 1728–30.

**Renal impairment.** The mean terminal disposition half-life of venlafaxine was prolonged from a mean of 3.8 hours in 18 healthy subjects to 5.8 hours in 12 patients with mild to moderate renal impairment (creatinine clearance 10 to 70 mL/minute) and 10.6 hours in patients requiring haemodialysis;[1] corresponding values for *O*-desmethylvenlafaxine, the active major metabolite of venlafaxine, were 11.8, 16.8, and 28.5 hours, respectively. Because of the large intersubject variability, the change in disposition for venlafaxine and its active metabolite was evident only in patients with a creatinine clearance of less than 30 mL/minute; drug clearance in these patients was reduced by about 55% and half-life more than doubled. It was calculated that for these patients half the usually daily dose could be given once daily.

Similar recommendations are made by the manufacturer, see under Uses and Administration, below.

1. Troy SM, *et al.* The effect of renal disease on the disposition of venlafaxine. *Clin Pharmacol Ther* 1994; **56:** 14–21.

**Withdrawal.** Case reports[1,2] of withdrawal reactions to venlafaxine.

1. Anonymous. Venlafaxine withdrawal reactions. *Med J Aust* 1998; **169:** 91–2.
2. Johnson H, *et al.* Withdrawal reaction associated with venlafaxine. *BMJ* 1998; **317:** 787.

## Interactions

Venlafaxine should not be used with MAOIs and at least 14 days should elapse between stopping an MAOI and starting treatment with venlafaxine. At least 7 days should elapse between stopping venlafaxine and starting any drug liable to provoke a serious reaction (e.g. phenelzine). For further details, see Antidepressants under Interactions of Phenelzine, p.315.

Although cimetidine inhibits the hepatic metabolism of venlafaxine, it has no effect on the active metabolite of venlafaxine, *O*-desmethylvenlafaxine, which is present in the plasma in much greater concentrations. The manufacturer, therefore, recommends that when cimetidine and venlafaxine are used together, clinical monitoring may only be necessary in elderly patients and in those with hepatic impairment or pre-existing hypertension.

◊ Conversion of venlafaxine to its equally active metabolite *O*-desmethylvenlafaxine is mediated by the cytochrome P450 isoenzyme CYP2D6. Although the potential exists for drugs that inhibit or act as a substrate for this enzyme to affect plasma concentrations of venlafaxine and its active metabolite, the manufacturers consider that, as the total amount of active compounds is unaffected, no dosage adjustment is usually necessary for venlafaxine. Venlafaxine itself is considered to be a relatively weak inhibitor of CYP2D6.

**Antipsychotics.** For mention of neuroleptic malignant syndrome developing in patients who received venlafaxine with antipsychotics see under Interactions in Chlorpromazine, p.679.

**Selegiline.** Although it is generally recommended that venlafaxine should not be started for at least 14 days after discontinuation of an MAOI, there is a report[1] of serotonin syndrome developing when a patient began venlafaxine treatment 15 days after stopping selegiline, which is an MAO type B inhibitor.

1. Gitlin MJ. Venlafaxine, monoamine oxidase inhibitors, and the serotonin syndrome. *J Clin Psychopharmacol* 1997; **17:** 66–7.

## Pharmacokinetics

Venlafaxine is readily absorbed from the gastrointestinal tract. After oral doses it undergoes extensive first-pass metabolism in the liver mainly to the active metabolite *O*-desmethylvenlafaxine; formation of *O*-desmethylvenlafaxine is mediated by the cytochrome P450 isoenzyme CYP2D6. The isoenzyme CYP3A4 is also involved in the metabolism of venlafaxine. Other metabolites include *N*-desmethylvenlafaxine and *N,O*-didesmethylvenlafaxine. Peak plasma concentrations of venlafaxine and *O*-desmethylvenlafaxine appear about 2 and 4 hours after a dose, respectively. Protein binding of venlafaxine and *O*-desmethylvenlafaxine is low. The mean elimination half-life of venlafaxine and *O*-desmethylvenlafaxine is about 5 and 11 hours, respectively. Venlafaxine is excreted predominately in the urine, mainly in the form of its metabolites, either free or in conjugated form; about 2% is excreted in the faeces.

◊ References.

1. Troy SM, *et al.* The pharmacokinetics of venlafaxine when given in a twice-daily regimen. *J Clin Pharmacol* 1995; **35:** 404–9.
2. Troy SM, *et al.* Pharmacokinetics and effect of food on the bioavailability of orally administered venlafaxine. *J Clin Pharmacol* 1997; **37:** 954–61.
3. Ball SE, *et al.* Venlafaxine: in vitro inhibition of CYP2D6 dependent imipramine and desipramine metabolism; comparative studies with selected SSRIs, and effects on human hepatic CYP3A4, CYP2C9 and CYP1A2. *Br J Clin Pharmacol* 1997; **43:** 619–26.

## Uses and Administration

Venlafaxine, a phenylethylamine derivative, is a serotonin and noradrenaline reuptake inhibitor (SNRI); it also weakly inhibits dopamine reuptake. It is reported to have little affinity for muscarinic, histaminergic, or $\alpha_1$-adrenergic receptors *in vitro*.

Venlafaxine is used in the treatment of **depression**. It is given by mouth as the hydrochloride; doses are expressed in terms of venlafaxine base. Venlafaxine hydrochloride 28.3 mg is approximately equivalent to 25 mg of venlafaxine. The initial daily dose is equivalent to venlafaxine 75 mg in two or three divided doses with food. In the USA, it is suggested that some patients may be best started on 37.5 mg daily for the first 4 to 7 days before increasing the dose to 75 mg daily. The dose may be increased, if necessary, after several weeks to 150 mg daily. Further increases, to a maximum daily dose of 225 mg, may be made at intervals of not less than 4 days. Severely depressed or hospitalised patients may require an initial daily dose of 150 mg increased, if necessary, by up to 75 mg every 2 to 3 days to a maximum daily dose of 375 mg; the dosage should then be gradually reduced. Modified-release preparations are available for once daily dosing.

Venlafaxine is also used, as a modified-release preparation, in the treatment of **generalised anxiety disorder**. The recommended initial dose is 75 mg once daily by mouth. In the USA it is suggested that some patients may be best begun with 37.5 mg daily for 4 to 7 days initially; dosage may subsequently be adjusted, at intervals of at least 4 days, up to a maximum of 225 mg daily. Venlafaxine should be withdrawn gradually if there is no response after 8 weeks.

In the USA, modified-release venlafaxine is also licensed for the treatment of **social phobia** in doses similar to those used for generalised anxiety disorder.

Reduced doses may need to be given in hepatic or renal impairment, see below.

Venlafaxine should be withdrawn gradually to reduce the risk of withdrawal symptoms (see Precautions, above).

**Administration in hepatic or renal impairment.** Patients with mild renal or hepatic impairment do not require a change in dose of venlafaxine. For those with moderate renal or hepatic impairment, the dose should be reduced by half and given once daily. There are insufficient data to make any recommendations for patients with severe renal or hepatic impairment.

**Anxiety disorders.** Venlafaxine is used in the treatment of generalised anxiety disorder; it may also be of use in a variety of other types of anxiety disorders (p.663) including the treatment of obsessive-compulsive disorder (p.663), panic attacks (p.663), social phobia (see under Phobic Disorders, p.663), and post-traumatic stress disorder (p.664).

References.


1. Ananth J, *et al.* Venlafaxine for treatment of obsessive-compulsive disorder. *Am J Psychiatry* 1995; **152:** 1832.
2. Geracioti TD. Venlafaxine treatment of panic disorder: a case series. *J Clin Psychiatry* 1995; **56:** 408–10.
3. Rauch SL, *et al.* Open treatment of obsessive-compulsive disorder with venlafaxine: a series of ten cases. *J Clin Psychopharmacol* 1996; **16:** 81–4.
4. Pollack MH, *et al.* Venlafaxine for panic disorder: results from a double-blind, placebo-controlled study. *Psychopharmacol Bull* 1996; **32:** 667–70.
5. Altamura AC, *et al.* Venlafaxine in social phobia: a study in selective serotonin reuptake inhibitor non-responders. *Int Clin Psychopharmacol* 1999; **14:** 239–45.
6. Sheehan DV. Attaining remission in generalized anxiety disorder: venlafaxine extended release comparative data. *J Clin Psychiatry* 2001; **62** (suppl 19): 26–31.
7. Katz IR, *et al.* Venlafaxine ER as a treatment for generalized anxiety disorder in older adults: pooled analysis of five randomised placebo-controlled clinical trials. *J Am Geriatr Soc* 2002; **50:** 18–25.
8. Denys D, *et al.* A double-blind switch study of paroxetine and venlafaxine in obsessive-compulsive disorder. *J Clin Psychiatry* 2004; **65:** 37–43.


**Depression.** As discussed on p.279, there is very little difference in efficacy between the different groups of antidepressant drugs, and choice is often made on the basis of adverse effect profile. SSRIs are widely used as an alternative to the older tricyclics as they have fewer unpleasant side-effects and are safer in overdosage. Similar properties also favour the use of serotonin and noradrenaline reuptake inhibitors such as venlafaxine.

References.


1. Ellingrod VL, Perry PJ. Venlafaxine: a heterocyclic antidepressant. *Am J Hosp Pharm* 1994; **51:** 3033–46.
2. Holliday SM, Benfield P. Venlafaxine: a review of its pharmacology and therapeutic potential in depression. *Drugs* 1995; **49:** 280–94.
3. Morton WA, *et al.* Venlafaxine: a structurally unique and novel antidepressant. *Ann Pharmacother* 1995; **29:** 387–95.
4. Derivan A, *et al.* Venlafaxine: measuring the onset of antidepressant action. *Psychopharmacol Bull* 1995; **31:** 439–47.
5. Anonymous. Three new antidepressants. *Drug Ther Bull.* 1996; **34:** 65–8.
6. Baldwin DS. Venlafaxine. *Prescribers' J* 1999; **39:** 242–7.
7. Wellington K, Perry CM. Venlafaxine extended-release: a review of its use in the management of major depression. *CNS Drugs* 2001; **15:** 643–69.
8. Cohen LS, *et al.* Venlafaxine in the treatment of postpartum depression. *J Clin Psychiatry* 2001; **62:** 592–6.
9. Montgomery SA, *et al.* Venlafaxine versus placebo in the prevention treatment of recurrent major depression. *J Clin Psychiatry* 2004; **65:** 328–36.


**Hyperactivity.** When drug therapy is indicated for attention deficit hyperactivity disorder (p.1583) initial treatment is usually with a central stimulant. Antidepressants may be used for patients who fail to respond to, or who are intolerant of, central stimulants and venlafaxine has been reported[1,2] to be effective in a small number of adult patients.


1. Hedges D, *et al.* An open trial of venlafaxine in adult patients with attention deficit hyperactivity disorder. *Psychopharmacol Bull* 1995; **31:** 779–83.
2. Adler LA, *et al.* Open-label trial of venlafaxine in adults with attention deficit disorder. *Psychopharmacol Bull* 1995; **31:** 785–8.


**Migraine.** Retrospective analysis[1] in patients with tension-type headache (p.465) or migraine (p.464) indicated that venlafaxine, as a modified-release preparation, had potential for headache prophylaxis.


1. Adelman LC, *et al.* Venlafaxine extended release (XR) for the prophylaxis of migraine and tension-type headache: a retrospective study in a clinical setting. *Headache* 2000; **40:** 572–80.


**Pain.** There are reports of benefit from the use of venlafaxine in patients with painful diabetic neuropathy,[1,2] or neuropathic pain of unknown cause.[3]


1. Davis JL, Smith RL. Painful peripheral diabetic neuropathy treated with venlafaxine HCl extended release capsules. *Diabetes Care* 1999; **22:** 1909–10.
2. Kiayias JA, *et al.* Venlafaxine HCl in the treatment of painful peripheral diabetic neuropathy. *Diabetes Care* 2000; **23:** 699.
3. Sumpton JE, Moulin DE. Treatment of neuropathic pain with venlafaxine. *Ann Pharmacother* 2001; **35:** 557–9.


## Preparations

**Proprietary Preparations** (details are given in Part 3)

***Arg.:*** Efexor; Elafax; ***Austral.:*** Efexor; ***Austria:*** Efectin; Efexor†; Trewilor†; ***Belg.:*** Efexor; ***Braz.:*** Efexor; ***Canad.:*** Effexor; ***Chile:*** Depurol; Efexor; Norpilen; Sentidol; Venlax; ***Denm.:*** Efexor; ***Fin.:*** Efexor; ***Fr.:*** Effexor; ***Ger.:*** Trevilor; ***Gr.:*** Efexor; ***Hong Kong:*** Efexor; ***India:*** Flavix; Venlor; ***Irl.:*** Efexor; ***Israel:*** Efexor; ***Ital.:*** Efexor; ***Malaysia:*** Efexor; ***Mex.:*** Efexor; ***Neth.:*** Efexor; ***Norw.:*** Efexor; ***NZ:*** Efexor; ***Port.:*** Efexor; ***S.Afr.:*** Efexor; ***Singapore:*** Efexor; ***Spain:*** Dobupal; Vandral; ***Swed.:*** Efexor; ***Switz.:*** Efexor; ***Thai.:*** Efexor; ***UK:*** Efexor; ***USA:*** Effexor.

# Viloxazine Hydrochloride *(BANM, USAN, rINNM)*

Hidrocloruro de viloxazina; ICI-58834. 2-(2-Ethoxyphenoxymethyl)morpholine hydrochloride.

$C_{13}H_{19}NO_3,HCl = 273.8.$

*CAS — 46817-91-8 (viloxazine); 35604-67-2 (viloxazine hydrochloride).*

*ATC — N06AX09.*

## Profile

Viloxazine is a bicyclic antidepressant. Like the tricyclic antidepressants (see Amitriptyline, p.280), viloxazine is an inhibitor of the reuptake of noradrenaline; it may also enhance the release of serotonin from neuronal stores. However, it does not have marked antimuscarinic, cardiotoxic, or sedative properties.

Viloxazine is given for the treatment of depression (p.279) by mouth as the hydrochloride although doses are expressed in terms of viloxazine base; viloxazine hydrochloride 57.7 mg is approximately equivalent to 50 mg of viloxazine. The usual dose is equivalent to viloxazine 300 mg daily increased, if necessary, to 600 mg daily as tolerated. The initial dose for the elderly or patients with hepatic or renal impairment is 100 mg daily cautiously increased if necessary. Viloxazine hydrochloride may also be given by intravenous infusion.

Viloxazine should be withdrawn gradually to reduce the risk of withdrawal symptoms.

**Porphyria.** Viloxazine hydrochloride is considered to be unsafe in patients with porphyria because it has been shown to be porphyrinogenic in *animals.*

## Preparations

**Proprietary Preparations** (details are given in Part 3)

***Belg.:*** Vivalan; ***Fr.:*** Vivalan; ***Ger.:*** Vivalan; ***Ital.:*** Vicilan†; ***Port.:*** Vivalan; ***Spain:*** Vivarint†; ***UK:*** Vivalan†.

# Antidiabetics

This chapter describes diabetes mellitus and its management with antidiabetics. The oral drugs included in this chapter are classified in Table 1, below; insulin, which is given parenterally, is discussed on p.333 and classified in Table 2, p.336.

## Diabetes mellitus

Diabetes mellitus is a group of disorders of carbohydrate metabolism in which the action of insulin is diminished or absent through altered secretion, decreased insulin activity, or a combination of both factors. It is characterised by hyperglycaemia. As the disease progresses tissue or vascular damage ensues leading to severe complications such as retinopathy, nephropathy, neuropathy, cardiovascular disease, and foot ulceration.

Diabetes mellitus may be categorised into several types but the two major types are type 1 (insulin-dependent diabetes mellitus; IDDM) and type 2 (non-insulin-dependent diabetes mellitus; NIDDM). The term juvenile-onset diabetes has sometimes been used for type 1 and maturity-onset diabetes for type 2. Malnutrition-related diabetes is no longer considered a separate entity (see Effects of Cassava, under Starch, p.1449).

**Type 1 diabetes mellitus** is present in patients who have little or no endogenous insulin secretory capacity and who therefore require exogenous insulin therapy for survival. This form of the disease has an auto-immune basis in most cases, and usually develops before adulthood. The associated hypoinsulinaemia and hyperglucagonaemia put such patients at risk of ketosis and ketoacidosis.

In **type 2 diabetes mellitus** the disease typically develops in later life. Insulin secretion may appear normal or even excessive (and type 2 patients are thus less prone to ketosis) but it is insufficient to compensate for insulin resistance (p.339). Obesity is present in the majority of type 2 patients; non-obese patients tend to have low insulin secretory capacity (although not as low as in type 1 diabetes) rather than appreciable insulin resistance.

**Diagnosis of diabetes mellitus.** Diagnosis is based upon blood-glucose concentrations exceeding set values under specified conditions.[1-4] Diabetes mellitus is likely if the glucose concentration in a random sample of venous plasma is 11.1 mmol/litre or more. If there are accompanying symptoms of increased thirst and urine volume, recurrent infections and weight loss, the presence of marked hyperglycaemia is considered diagnostic of diabetes. In the absence of symptoms or if the elevation of blood-glucose concentration is less marked (more often the case with type 2 than with type 1 diabetes), the diagnosis needs to be confirmed either by repeated sampling or by an **oral glucose tolerance test** (OGTT). This test consists of an overnight fast followed by measurement of the fasting blood-glucose concentration, then the administration of a 75-g oral glucose load (in children 1.75 g/kg up to a maximum of 75 g), and further measurement of the blood-glucose concentration two hours later. Diagnostic values for measurements in venous whole blood are greater than or equal to 6.1 mmol/litre for the fasting state and 10.0 mmol/litre after the glucose load. The corresponding values for capillary whole blood are 6.1 and 11.1 mmol/litre, and for venous plasma 7.0 and 11.1 mmol/litre.[2] There has been some confusion at an international level as to whether the glucose load should be 75 g of the anhydrous form or the monohydrate. Sources at WHO have therefore suggested that the form should be standardised as 75 g of anhydrous glucose (anhydrous dextrose), which would be equivalent to 82.5 g of the monohydrate (Glucose BP; dextrose monohydrate). The threshold for the diagnosis of diabetes has recently been lowered from a fasting plasma glucose concentration of 7.8 mmol/litre,[5] to reflect an increased risk of microvascular disease in patients with concentrations of 7.0 mmol/litre or more. However, there has been some concern about the lack of agreement between these newer criteria and the previous ones, which may result in alterations in prevalence of diabetes.[6,7]

Other diagnostic methods, such as measurement of glycosylated haemoglobin, have been investigated.[8] There is also some interest in using antibodies to insulin, to islet cells, or to the enzyme glutamic acid decarboxylase, as predictive tests for those patients likely to develop diabetes mellitus.[9]

Once the presence of diabetes has been confirmed the distinction between type 1 and type 2 is made on clinical grounds.

**Table 1.** Classification of oral antidiabetics.

| | |
|---|---|
| *Aldose Reductase Inhibitors* | *Sulfonylureas* |
| Epalrestat | Acetohexamide |
| Sorbinil | Carbutamide |
| | Chlorpropamide |
| *Alpha Glucosidase Inhibitors* | Glibenclamide |
| Acarbose | Glibornuride |
| Miglitol | Gliclazide |
| Voglibose | Glimepiride |
| | Glipizide |
| *Biguanides* | Gliquidone |
| Buformin | Glisentide |
| Metformin | Glisolamide |
| Phenformin | Glisoxepide |
| | Glyclopyramide |
| *Meglitinides* | Glycyclamide |
| Nateglinide | Tolazamide |
| Repaglinide | Tolbutamide |
| | |
| *Miscellaneous* | *Thiazolidinediones* |
| Glybuzole | Pioglitazone |
| Glymidine | Rosiglitazone |
| Guar Gum | Troglitazone |
| Midaglizole | |

**Management of diabetes mellitus.**

- DIETARY MODIFICATION. Dietary control is important in both type 1 and type 2 diabetes.[10] The goals of dietary modification are to maintain glucose concentrations in the normal range or as close to normal as possible, and a lipid and lipoprotein profile and blood pressure that reduce the risk of macrovascular disease (see Diabetic Complications, below). Correction of obesity is desirable in all patients, and weight loss in patients with type 2 diabetes can decrease insulin resistance, improve glycaemic and lipid measures, and reduce blood pressure. Anorectic drugs are not effective in promoting weight loss in these patients,[11] although orlistat, a gastric and pancreatic lipase inhibitor, can be used as an adjunctive treatment to reduce weight and improve blood glucose control in overweight patients with type 2 diabetes.[12-14] A high fibre intake may also lower blood-glucose concentrations and additional fibre is sometimes taken in the form of guar gum (see p.333). The influence of diet on diabetes is such that all diabetic patients need to be aware of the composition of foods and to be able to make adjustments to their diet, especially to counteract treatment-induced hypoglycaemia. Controversy continues, however, as to the optimum composition of the diet in diabetics, and in particular the relative contribution of calories from fat and from carbohydrate.
- EXERCISE. All diabetic patients should be encouraged to exercise, according to their age and physical capability.[5] Exercise improves carbohydrate metabolism, insulin sensitivity,[15,16] and cardiovascular function.[17] It is also a useful component of any weight reduction programme although diet is more effective in promoting weight loss and metabolic control.[11]
- ORAL ANTIDIABETICS. If patients with type 2 diabetes have not achieved suitable control after about 3 months of dietary modification and increased physical activity, then oral antidiabetics (oral hypoglycaemics) may be tried. The two major classes are the *sulfonylureas* and the *biguanides.* Sulfonylureas act mainly by increasing endogenous insulin secretion, while biguanides act chiefly by decreasing hepatic gluconeogenesis and increasing peripheral utilisation of glucose. Both types function only in the presence of some endogenous insulin production. More recently developed classes of oral antidiabetics include the *alpha-glucosidase inhibitors,* the *meglitinides,* and the *thiazolidinediones* (see Table 1, p.324). Alpha-glucosidase inhibitors act by delaying the absorption of glucose from the gastrointestinal tract; meglitinides increase endogenous insulin secretion; and thiazolidinediones appear to increase insulin sensitivity.

  Oral treatment of type 2 diabetes in non-obese patients is usually begun with a sulfonylurea. Chlorpropamide and glibenclamide have long half-lives and hence an increased tendency to cause hypoglycaemia, although a large study[18] reported that hypoglycaemic episodes were less frequent with chlorpropamide than glibenclamide. These 2 drugs are best avoided in the elderly; a sulfonylurea with a short half-life, such as gliclazide, gliquidone, or tolbutamide, should be used instead.

  There is evidence that the use of low-dose sulfonylurea therapy in patients with diagnosed type 2 diabetes but near-normoglycaemia due to early remission (the so-called honeymoon period) can delay the onset of hyperglycaemia.[19]

  Sulfonylureas can cause weight gain and obese patients are preferably treated with the biguanide metformin rather than with a sulfonylurea. Results from the UK Prospective Diabetes Study (UKPDS) have suggested that the use of metformin to provide intensive blood-glucose control in overweight diabetic patients substantially reduced the risk of diabetes-related end-points such as myocardial infarction, stroke, amputation, renal failure, blindness, and death.[20] Metformin is as effective as the sulfonylureas in terms of blood-glucose control and is less likely to cause hypoglycaemia,[20] but has a rare tendency to cause lactic acidosis in patients with renal impairment, in whom it should not be used.

  Drug treatment may also involve an alpha-glucosidase inhibitor such as acarbose or miglitol. These have a small but significant effect in lowering blood glucose and do not cause hypoglycaemia when used alone, but they can cause intolerable gastrointestinal effects. Meglitinides such as repaglinide and nateglinide are a new chemical class of antidiabetics which act similarly to sulfonylureas; repaglinide has a rapid onset and short duration of action and is administered with meals. The thiazolidinediones, such as pioglitazone or rosiglitazone, appear to increase insulin sensitivity and have been the subject of much interest for type 2 diabetes and insulin resistance.

  Should treatment with one of the oral antidiabetics fail then a different type or in some instances combinations of different types may produce improvement. Alarming evidence[20] of an increased risk of death in UKPDS patients given intensive therapy with metformin plus a sulfonylurea was not borne out by further analysis, and this combination is widely used. In patients in whom such combinations fail or are contra-indicated, pioglitazone or rosiglitazone may be combined with metformin or a sulfonylurea as an alternative to progressing to insulin. Biguanides may also be added to meglitinide therapy. Alpha-glucosidase inhibitors may improve diabetes control when used as an adjunct to sulfonylureas or biguanides. Guar gum may also be used as an adjunct to any of the oral hypoglycaemics to enhance the improvement in blood-glucose control.

  Patients with type 2 diabetes who cannot be controlled adequately by oral therapy and diet need insulin either in addition to or in place of oral therapy. Type 2 diabetes is a progressive disease, and about 30% of those on sulfonylureas will be transferred to insulin treatment within 4 years, a change which now tends to be made earlier owing to increasingly strict criteria for glycaemic control (tight control of blood glucose has now been shown to decrease the risk of complications, see Diabetic Complications, below). However, as insulin therapy is associated with more hypoglycaemic episodes and a greater tendency to weight gain it remains reasonable to begin with oral therapy in type 2 diabetes before proceeding to insulin.[21] There is evidence that therapy with insulin and a sulfonylurea is more effective than therapy with insulin alone in type 2 patients,[22] and in general, as the disease progresses, the majority of patients need multiple therapies to achieve glycaemic control.[23] Biguanides and alpha-glucosidase inhibitors may also be combined with insulin.

  Insulin is also substituted for oral treatment to provide cover during periods of severe stress, as in severe infection, trauma, or major surgery. Type 2 patients who become pregnant should also be switched from oral therapy to insulin (see Pregnancy, below).
- INSULIN THERAPY. While insulin may not be a necessary part of the treatment of type 2 diabetes, it is essential in the treatment of patients with type 1, since they have little or no endogenous insulin secretory capacity.

  The aim of insulin therapy is to achieve the best possible control of blood-glucose concentrations without the risk of the hypoglycaemia that can occur if too fine a degree of control is attempted. Tight control of blood-glucose concentrations can reduce the long-term complications of diabetes such as retinopathy, nephropathy, and neuropathy (see Diabetic Complications, below) but in some patients (such as the elderly, or those who lack motivation) it may be better merely to alleviate symptoms rather than attempt tight control. Exercise and dietary discipline are necessary to maintain normal sensitivity to insulin.

Insulin may be of beef or pork origin, or it may be human insulin produced by gene technology or by modification of porcine insulin. Human and porcine insulin are less immunogenic than bovine insulin and where possible most newly diagnosed type 1 patients are now given human insulin. Modified insulin analogues such as insulin lispro, insulin aspart, insulin detemir, and insulin glargine are now available.

Insulin is available in preparations offering a short, intermediate, or long action. It may be given intramuscularly but the subcutaneous route is usually preferred. Soluble insulin can also be given intravenously. Details of insulin administration are given on p.340. Insulin dosage schedules make use of the varying durations of action, for example by incorporating a short-acting and intermediate-acting insulin into a daily schedule. Most patients with type 1 diabetes require two or three injections of insulin daily, or with intensive regimens even more. A once-daily regimen can be used if the patient is simply to be kept asymptomatic; this may also be successful in patients with type 2 diabetes not satisfactorily controlled by oral antidiabetics.

- IMMUNOSUPPRESSION. Many patients with type 1 diabetes experience a temporary improvement in pancreatic beta-cell function soon after initial treatment with insulin. This produces a period of remission known as the honeymoon period during which a small dose of insulin is sufficient to maintain good control. Attempts to prolong the honeymoon period have included tight control immediately following diagnosis and also, given the probable auto-immune nature of the condition, use of an immunosuppressant.[24-30]
- PANCREATIC TRANSPLANTATION. Transplantation of the whole pancreas in patients with type 1 diabetes poorly controlled by insulin therapy has led to insulin-independence, and has usually been carried out with kidney transplantation (see also Pancreatic Transplantation, p.1347).[31] Transplantation of pancreatic islet cells has been investigated as an alternative. In early reports, few patients remained independent of insulin within a year of islet-cell transplantation.[31] However, more experienced centres are now reporting greater success, and studies are underway to determine the most effective protocol.[32] Results in *animals* have suggested that a reasonable degree of glycaemic control may be achievable long term without immunosuppression, using a vascularised 'artificial pancreas' containing allogeneic or even xenogeneic islet cells.[33]
- OTHER DRUG TREATMENTS. Various other drugs have been tried for diabetes mellitus, particularly when conventional therapy has proved unsuccessful. Addition of the amylin analogue *pramlintide* to insulin therapy has improved glycaemic control in patients with type 1 and type 2 diabetes.[34,35] Other approaches under investigation include inhibition of fatty acid oxidation or the use of $\beta_3$-adrenoceptor agonists (selective agonists of β-receptors thought to be associated with lipolysis and thermogenesis) to stimulate energy expenditure.[36]

  *Mecasermin* (insulin-like growth factor I; IGF-1) has been shown to improve metabolic control in patients with type 1 diabetes and insulin resistance (and in some type 2 patients).[37,38] *Glucagon-like peptide 1* (GLP-1; insulinotropin) improves glycaemic control in type 2 patients.[39,40] *Exenatide* (synthetic exendin-4) has actions similar to GLP-1, and is also under investigation in type 2 diabetes. Improvements in insulin sensitivity have also been seen in insulin-resistant type 2 patients treated with a haemodialysate of calf blood,[41] while in other studies improved insulin sensitivity was seen following treatment with the *vanadium* salt, vanadyl sulfate.[42,43] Adjunctive *chromium* supplementation may reduce serum-glucose in type 2 diabetes, but high doses may be required and long-term safety and efficacy have not been established.[44]
- PROPHYLAXIS. Because overt diabetes is the culmination of a prolonged process, methods to delay or prevent its development are being investigated, either by modifying risk factors in populations or groups, or by targeting individuals thought to be at high risk. Strategies under consideration for the prevention of type 1 diabetes include avoidance of cows' milk proteins (thought to be a possible environmental trigger) during infancy;[45] giving free radical scavengers such as nicotinamide;[46] prophylactic insulin[47-49] (or possibly oral antidiabetics) to allow 'beta cell rest'; encouraging the development of antigen tolerance, for example by taking oral antigens such as insulin, glutamic acid decarboxylase, or heat shock protein[48,50,51] (a similar approach using subcutaneous antigen has apparently extended the honeymoon period in *animal* studies[52]); or by immunosuppression (see above) or immunomodulation with agents such as BCG vaccine,[53] although some have found the latter ineffective.[54] Preventive strategies for insulin resistance and type 2 diabetes have tended to focus on weight loss, dietary modification, and exercise. However, prophylactic drug therapy may be possible. In a study[55] of patients with impaired glucose tolerance and at high risk of developing type 2 diabetes, acarbose delayed progression to diabetes by 25% over about 3 years and increased the probability of reversion to normal glucose tolerance. Orlistat, given in a 4-year study,[56] reduced the risk of developing diabetes by about 37% in obese patients; in those with impaired glucose tolerance the risk was reduced by at least 45%. Orlistat also improved weight loss irrespective of glucose tolerance. There is also some data from studies of cardiovascular risk reduction to suggest that ramipril[57] and pravastatin[58] may reduce the onset of diabetes. However, a study[59] of patients at high risk of developing diabetes found that although prophylactic metformin reduced the incidence of diabetes, lifestyle intervention was more effective. Guidelines[60] for the prevention of type 2 diabetes recommend that individuals with pre-diabetes (impaired fasting glucose or impaired glucose tolerance) should be counselled on weight loss and exercise, and that drug therapy should not be routinely used until more information becomes available. Screening for diabetes has been encouraged, particularly for those patients with risk factors.[61]

**Monitoring of therapy.** Monitoring of therapy is an integral part of the management of the diabetic patient.[62] Detection of urinary glucose has generally been superseded by the monitoring of blood glucose (see Glucose Tests, p.1694). For adequate diabetic control, the aim is to reduce fasting blood-glucose concentrations to within the range 3.3 to 5.6 mmol/litre of venous whole blood, and postprandial concentrations to below 10 mmol/litre.[5] Many patients monitor their blood-glucose concentrations regularly at home and this is essential for intensified insulin regimens when tight control is required. Although the value of self-monitoring of blood-glucose concentrations in type 2 patients is less clear, the results of a large cohort study[63] suggest that such monitoring can improve glycaemic control in these patients. Detection of urinary ketones is useful in diabetics prone to ketosis; this is usually performed in clinics. Diabetic clinics also measure the degree of haemoglobin glycosylation (HbA$_1$ or HbA$_{1c}$) as an indicator of longer term blood-glucose control and hence the risk of complications (see Diabetic Complications, below). UK guidelines[64] recommend that a target of 6.5 to 7.5% should be set for HbA$_{1c}$ in individuals with type 2 diabetes, the lower value being preferred for those at risk of macrovascular complications. More recently the advanced glycation end-product (AGE) of haemoglobin has also been found to be a useful indicator of long-term blood glucose control.[65] Measurement of glycated serum proteins, particularly albumin, is also used to give an indication of glucose control, but for a shorter period than haemoglobin. Other techniques that have been developed for monitoring blood-glucose concentrations include continuous monitoring by a subcutaneous system, and a minimally invasive device that uses reverse iontophoresis through the skin.

**Pregnancy.** Adverse pregnancy outcomes, including spontaneous abortion and congenital malformation, are more common in diabetic than in nondiabetic women. Improved management of the pregnant diabetic patient, particularly early in pregnancy, lessens the incidence of such events,[66,67] but an increased risk still exists.[68] Diabetic women are advised to plan their pregnancies so that glycaemic control can be improved before conception.[69] Some may need to avoid pregnancy (most commonly because of renal disease),[70] but management has improved sufficiently for this to be rare.[67]

Insulin is the preferred treatment in pregnancy,[71] even in women with type 2 diabetes; patients taking oral antidiabetics should therefore be switched to insulin. Insulin regimens are similar to those in nonpregnant patients, the dose being adjusted according to regular blood-glucose measurements. Insulin requirements may decrease during the first trimester but they increase during the latter two, reaching about twice prepregnancy requirements at term; they then fall once labour has begun and fall again after delivery.[71]

Pregnant diabetic patients are at risk of nocturnal hypoglycaemia owing to continued fetal glucose consumption while the mother is in a relatively fasting state. They are also prone to diabetic ketoacidosis which must be treated with great urgency because of the high risk of fetal loss.

Gestational diabetes mellitus is defined as glucose intolerance with onset or first recognition during pregnancy.[72-74] Many women with gestational diabetes may be managed by diet alone or, if necessary, also with insulin. However, giving prophylactic insulin to women who could be managed by diet alone has been suggested, in view of the metabolic effects of insulin.[75] Dietary management of gestational diabetes can improve maternal and fetal outcomes, and insulin therapy reduces fetal macrosomia and perinatal morbidity.[73,74] There has been much debate about the benefits of screening for gestational diabetes, and both universal[72] and selective screening based on risk factors[74] have been promoted.

**Surgery.** Insulin-dependent diabetics who require surgery may be managed with a continuous intravenous insulin infusion.[76] Insulin is given as normal the night before operation, and switched to either a variable-rate infusion via a syringe pump, with a 5 or 10% glucose drip (with potassium chloride, provided the patient is not hyperkalaemic), or to a combined insulin-glucose infusion, on the day of operation. (Many anaesthetists prefer insulin and a sodium chloride infusion if blood glucose is already high.[77]) Subsequent conversion back to subcutaneous insulin should be undertaken before breakfast, giving the first subcutaneous dose 30 minutes before stopping continuous infusion. Non-insulin-dependent patients should have any oral treatment omitted on the day of operation, and may be given insulin by a similar regimen if control is poor or deteriorates as can happen with major surgery.


1. Meltzer S, *et al.* 1998 clinical practice guidelines for the management of diabetes in Canada. *Can Med Assoc J* 1998; **159** (suppl 8): S1–S29.
2. WHO. *Definition, diagnosis and classification of diabetes mellitus and its complications.* Geneva: WHO, 1999.
3. Colman PG, *et al.* New classification and criteria for diagnosis of diabetes mellitus. *Med J Aust* 1999; **170:** 375–8.
4. American Diabetes Association. Diagnosis and classification of diabetes mellitus. *Diabetes Care* 2004; **27** (suppl 1): S5–S10. Also available at: http://care.diabetesjournals.org/cgi/reprint/27/suppl_1/s5.pdf (accessed 07/07/04)
5. WHO. Diabetes mellitus: report of a WHO study group. *WHO Tech Rep Ser 727* 1985.
6. DECODE Study Group. Will new diagnostic criteria for diabetes mellitus change phenotype of patients with diabetes? Reanalysis of European epidemiological data. *BMJ* 1998; **317:** 371–5.
7. Wahl PW, *et al.* Diabetes in older adults: comparison of 1997 American Diabetes Association classification of diabetes mellitus with 1985 WHO classification. *Lancet* 1998; **352:** 1012–15.
8. McCance DR, *et al.* Comparison of tests for glycated haemoglobin and fasting and two hour plasma glucose concentrations as diagnostic methods for diabetes. *BMJ* 1994; **308:** 1323–8.
9. Palmer JP. What is the best way to predict IDDM? *Lancet* 1994; **343:** 1377–8.
10. American Diabetes Association. Nutrition principles and recommendations in diabetes. *Diabetes Care* 2004; **27** (suppl 1): S36–S46. Also available at: http://care.diabetesjournals.org/cgi/reprint/27/suppl_1/s36.pdf (accessed 07/07/04)
11. Brown SA, *et al.* Promoting weight loss in type II diabetes. *Diabetes Care* 1996; **19:** 613–24.
12. Hollander PA, *et al.* Role of orlistat in the treatment of obese patients with type 2 diabetes: a 1-year randomized double-blind study. *Diabetes Care* 1998; **21:** 1288–94.
13. Kelley DE, *et al.* Clinical efficacy of orlistat therapy in overweight and obese patients with insulin-treated type 2 diabetes: a 1-year randomized controlled trial. *Diabetes Care* 2002; **25:** 1033–41.
14. Miles JM, *et al.* Effect of orlistat in overweight and obese patients with type 2 diabetes treated with metformin. *Diabetes Care* 2002; **25:** 1123–8.
15. Boulé NG, *et al.* Effects of exercise on glycemic control and body mass in type 2 diabetes mellitus: a meta-analysis of controlled clinical trials. *JAMA* 2001; **286:** 1218–27.
16. American Diabetes Association. Physical activity/exercise and diabetes. *Diabetes Care* 2004; **27** (suppl 1): S58–S62. Also available at: http://care.diabetesjournals.org/cgi/reprint/27/suppl_1/s58.pdf (accessed 07/07/04)
17. Stewart KJ. Exercise training and the cardiovascular consequences of type 2 diabetes and hypertension: plausible mechanisms for improving cardiovascular health. *JAMA* 2002; **288:** 1622–31.
18. United Kingdom Prospective Diabetes Study Group. United Kingdom prospective diabetes study (UKPDS) 13: relative efficacy of randomly allocated diet, sulphonylurea, insulin, or metformin in patients with newly diagnosed non-insulin dependent diabetes followed for three years. *BMJ* 1995; **310:** 83–8.
19. Banerji MA, *et al.* Prolongation of near-normoglycemic remission in black NIDDM subjects with chronic low-dose sulfonylurea treatment. *Diabetes* 1995; **44:** 466–70.
20. UK Prospective Diabetes Study Group. Effect of intensive blood-glucose control with metformin on complications in overweight patients with type 2 diabetes (UKPDS 34). *Lancet* 1998; **352:** 854–65. Correction. *ibid.*; 1558.

21. United Kingdom Prospective Diabetes Study Group. United Kingdom Prospective Diabetes Study 24: a 6-year, randomized, controlled trial comparing sulfonylurea, insulin, and metformin therapy in patients with newly diagnosed type 2 diabetes that could not be controlled with diet therapy. *Ann Intern Med* 1998; **128:** 165–75.
22. Johnson JL, *et al.* Efficacy of insulin and sulfonylurea combination therapy in type II diabetes: a meta-analysis of the randomized placebo-controlled trials. *Arch Intern Med* 1996; **156:** 259–64.
23. Turner RC, *et al.* Glycemic control with diet, sulfonylurea, metformin, or insulin in patients with type 2 diabetes mellitus: progressive requirement for multiple therapies (UKPDS 49). *JAMA* 1999; **281:** 2005–12.
24. Pozzilli P, Maclaren NK. Immunotherapy at clinical diagnosis of insulin-dependent diabetes: an approach still worth considering. *Trends Endocrinol Metab* 1993; **4:** 101–5.
25. Bougneres PF, *et al.* Factors associated with early remission of type I diabetes in children treated with cyclosporine. *N Engl J Med* 1988; **318:** 663–70.
26. The Canadian-European Randomized Control Trial Group. Cyclosporin-induced remission of IDDM after early intervention: association of 1 yr of cyclosporin treatment with enhanced insulin secretion. *Diabetes* 1988; **37:** 1574–82.
27. Harrison LC, *et al.* Increase in remission rate in newly diagnosed type I diabetic subjects treated with azathioprine. *Diabetes* 1985; **34:** 1306–8.
28. Yilmaz MT, *et al.* Immunoprotection in spontaneous remission of type 1 diabetes: long-term follow-up results. *Diabetes Res Clin Pract* 1993; **19:** 151–62.
29. Herold KC, *et al.* Anti-CD3 monoclonal antibody in new-onset type 1 diabetes mellitus. *N Engl J Med* 2002; **346:** 1692–8.
30. Carel JC, *et al.* Cyclosporine delays but does not prevent clinical onset in glucose intolerant pre-type 1 diabetic children. *J Autoimmun* 1996; **9:** 739–45.
31. Robertson RP, *et al.* Pancreas and islet transplantation for patients with diabetes. *Diabetes Care* 2000; **23:** 112–16.
32. Robertson RP. Islet transplantation as a treatment for diabetes—a work in progress. *N Engl J Med* 2004; **350:** 694–705.
33. Maki T, *et al.* Novel delivery of pancreatic islet cells to treat insulin-dependent diabetes mellitus. *Clin Pharmacokinet* 1995; **28:** 471–82.
34. Thompson RG, *et al.* Effects of pramlintide, an analog of human amylin, on plasma glucose profiles in patients with IDDM: results of a multicenter trial. *Diabetes* 1997; **46:** 632–6.
35. Thompson RG, *et al.* Pramlintide, a synthetic analog of human amylin, improves the metabolic profile of patients with type 2 diabetes using insulin. *Diabetes Care* 1998; **21:** 987–93.
36. Petrie JR, Donnelly R. New pharmacological approaches to insulin and lipid metabolism. *Drugs* 1994; **47:** 701–10.
37. Moses AC, *et al.* Insulin-like growth factor I (rhIGF-I) as a therapeutic agent for hyperinsulinemic insulin-resistant diabetes mellitus. *Diabetes Res Clin Pract* 1995; **28** (suppl): S185–S194.
38. Acerini CL, *et al.* Randomised placebo-controlled trial of human recombinant insulin-like growth factor I plus intensive insulin therapy in adolescents with insulin-dependent diabetes mellitus. *Lancet* 1997; **350:** 1199–1204.
39. Todd JF, *et al.* Glucagon-like peptide-1 (GLP-1): a trial of treatment in non-insulin-dependent diabetes mellitus. *Eur J Clin Invest* 1997; **27:** 533–6.
40. Zander M, *et al.* Effect of 6-week course of glucagon-like peptide 1 on glycaemic control, insulin sensitivity, and β-cell function in type 2 diabetes: a parallel-group study. *Lancet* 2002; **359:** 824–30.
41. Jacob S, *et al.* Improvement of glucose metabolism in patients with type II diabetes after treatment with a hemodialysate. *Arzneimittelforschung* 1996; **46:** 269–72.
42. Cohen N, *et al.* Oral vanadyl sulfate improves hepatic and peripheral insulin sensitivity in patients with non-insulin-dependent diabetes mellitus. *J Clin Invest* 1995; **95:** 2501–9.
43. Cusi K, *et al.* Vanadyl sulfate improves hepatic and muscle insulin sensitivity in type 2 diabetes. *J Clin Endocrinol Metab* 2001; **86:** 1410–7.
44. Ryan GJ, *et al.* Chromium as adjunctive treatment for type 2 diabetes. *Ann Pharmacother* 2003; **37:** 876–85.
45. Åkerblom HK. Diabetes and cows' milk. *Lancet* 1996; **348:** 1656–7.
46. Pozzilli P, *et al.* Meta-analysis of nicotinamide treatment in patients with recent-onset IDDM. *Diabetes Care* 1996; **19:** 1357–63.
47. Keller RJ, *et al.* Insulin prophylaxis in individuals at high risk of type 1 diabetes. *Lancet* 1993; **341:** 927–8.
48. Alberti KGMM. Preventing insulin dependent diabetes mellitus. *BMJ* 1993; **307:** 1435–6.
49. Diabetes Prevention Trial—Type 1 Diabetes Study Group. Effects of insulin in relatives of patients with type 1 diabetes mellitus. *N Engl J Med* 2002; **346:** 1685–91.
50. Williams G. IDDM: long honeymoon, sweet ending. *Lancet* 1994; **343:** 684–5.
51. Jones DB, Armstrong NW. Peptide therapy for diabetes. *Lancet* 1994; **343:** 1168–9.
52. Elias D, Cohen IR. Peptide therapy for diabetes in NOD mice. *Lancet* 1994; **343:** 704–6.
53. Shehadeh N, *et al.* Effect of adjuvant therapy on development of diabetes in mouse and man. *Lancet* 1994; **343:** 706–7.
54. Pozzilli P, *et al.* BCG vaccine in insulin-dependent diabetes mellitus. *Lancet* 1997; **349:** 1520–1.
55. Chiasson J-L, *et al.* Acarbose for prevention of type 2 diabetes mellitus: the STOP-NIDDM randomised trial. *Lancet* 2002; **359:** 2072–7.
56. Torgerson JS, *et al.* Xenical in the prevention of diabetes in obese subjects (XENDOS) study: a randomized study of orlistat as an adjunct to lifestyle changes for the prevention of type 2 diabetes in obese patients. *Diabetes Care* 2004; **27:** 155–61.
57. Yusuf S, *et al.* Ramipril and the development of diabetes. *JAMA* 2001; **286:** 1882–5.
58. Freeman DJ, *et al.* Pravastatin and the development of diabetes mellitus: evidence for a protective treatment effect in the West of Scotland Coronary Prevention Study. *Circulation* 2001; **103:** 357–62.
59. Diabetes Prevention Program Research Group. Reduction in the incidence of type 2 diabetes with lifestyle intervention or metformin. *N Engl J Med* 2002; **346:** 393–403.
60. American Diabetes Association, National Institute of Diabetes and Digestive and Kidney Diseases. Prevention or delay of type 2 diabetes. *Diabetes Care* 2004; **27** (suppl 1): S47–S54. Also available at: http://care.diabetesjournals.org/cgi/reprint/27/suppl_1/s47.pdf (accessed 07/07/04)
61. American Diabetes Association. Screening for type 2 diabetes. *Diabetes Care* 2004; **27** (suppl 1): S11–S14. Also available at: http://care.diabetesjournals.org/cgi/reprint/27/suppl_1/s11.pdf (accessed 07/07/04)
62. American Diabetes Association. Tests of glycemia in diabetes. *Diabetes Care* 2004; **27** (suppl 1): S91–S93. Also available at: http://care.diabetesjournals.org/cgi/reprint/27/suppl_1/s91.pdf (accessed 07/07/04)
63. Karter AJ, *et al.* Self-monitoring of blood glucose levels and glycemic control: the Northern California Kaiser Permanente Diabetes registry. *Am J Med* 2001; **111:** 1–9.
64. National Institute for Clinical Excellence. Management of type 2 diabetes: management of blood glucose (issued September 2002). Available at: http://www.nice.org.uk/pdf/NICE_INHERITEG_guidelines.pdf (accessed 07/07/04)
65. Wolffenbuttel BHR, *et al.* Long-term assessment of glucose control by haemoglobin-AGE measurement. *Lancet* 1996; **347:** 513–15.
66. Steel JM, *et al.* Can prepregnancy care of diabetic women reduce the risk of abnormal babies? *BMJ* 1990; **301:** 1070–4.
67. Steel JM, Johnstone FD. Guidelines for the management of insulin-dependent diabetes mellitus in pregnancy. *Drugs* 1996; **52:** 60–70.
68. Casson IF, *et al.* Outcomes of pregnancy in insulin dependent diabetic women: results of a five year population cohort study. *BMJ* 1997; **315:** 275–8.
69. American Diabetes Association. Preconception care of women with diabetes. *Diabetes Care* 2004; **27** (suppl 1): S76–S78. Also available at: http://care.diabetesjournals.org/cgi/reprint/27/suppl_1/s76.pdf (accessed 07/07/04)
70. Pearson JF. Pregnancy and complicated diabetes. *Br J Hosp Med* 1993; **49:** 739–42.
71. Crombach G, *et al.* Insulin use in pregnancy: clinical pharmacokinetic considerations. *Clin Pharmacokinet* 1993; **24:** 89–100.
72. Hoffman L, *et al.* Gestational diabetes mellitus—management guidelines [of] the Australasian Diabetes in Pregnancy Society. *Med J Aust* 1998; **169:** 93–7.
73. Kjos SL, Buchanan TA. Gestational diabetes mellitus. *N Engl J Med* 1999; **341:** 1749–56.
74. American Diabetes Association. Gestational diabetes mellitus. *Diabetes Care* 2004; **27** (suppl 1): S88–S90. Also available at: http://care.diabetesjournals.org/cgi/reprint/27/suppl_1/s88.pdf (accessed 07/07/04)
75. Thompson DJ, *et al.* Prophylactic insulin in the management of gestational diabetes. *Obstet Gynecol* 1990; **75:** 960–4.
76. Jacober SJ, Sowers JR. An update on perioperative management of diabetes. *Arch Intern Med* 1999; **159:** 2405–11.
77. Eldridge AJ, Sear JW. Peri-operative management of diabetic patients: any changes for the better since 1985? *Anaesthesia* 1996; **51:** 45–51.

## Diabetic complications

Much of the increased mortality and morbidity seen in diabetic patients is the result of various complications which develop with increasing duration of disease, particularly when glycaemic control is poor. Such complications may originate from increased glycation of proteins and other biological macromolecules in the hyperglycaemic environment, or from increased accumulation of sorbitol and other polyols via the aldose reductase pathway, but other factors play an important role in determining susceptibility. At the *macrovascular* level, diabetics are prone to hypertension and ischaemic heart disease, and heart disease is a major cause of death; control of blood pressure is now seen as being as important as glycaemic control in patients with type 2 diabetes. *Microvascular* tissue damage is an important factor in the development of diabetic nephropathy and retinopathy; it may also contribute to the other major complication, diabetic neuropathy. Collagen abnormalities are also seen. Diabetics with poor glycaemic control also have an increased liability to severe bacterial or fungal infection. Sometimes several factors may interact; thus neuropathy, infection, and impaired blood flow due to macro- or microvascular disease may all play a role in the development of diabetic foot disease, a complication which can ultimately lead to amputation.

**Prevention of diabetic complications.** Much attention has been focused on whether strict or tight glycaemic control can modify the development or progression of diabetic complications. In general, the longer-term studies have provided more encouraging results than initial results indicated, and meta-analysis of such studies[1] has suggested that intensive regimens may prevent microvascular complications.

The Diabetes Control and Complications Trial (DCCT)[2] confirmed this view in type 1 diabetes. It compared in selected patients the effects of conventional insulin therapy with those of continuous subcutaneous insulin infusion or multiple-injection regimens, on the development and progression of complications. The intensive treatment was aimed at keeping preprandial blood-glucose concentrations between 3.9 and 6.7 mmol/litre, postprandial concentrations at less than 10 mmol/litre, a weekly 3 a.m. measurement at greater than 3.6 mmol/litre, and the monthly glycosylated haemoglobin measurement at less than 6.05%. Intensive insulin therapy reduced the development and progression of retinopathy; it also reduced the occurrence of microalbuminuria, albuminuria, and clinical neuropathy. The major disadvantage of intensive insulin therapy was a threefold greater risk of hypoglycaemia; weight gain was also significantly greater.

While it is accepted that some patients will benefit from intensive insulin regimens, this approach requires caution in patients at risk of hypoglycaemia. Also such intensive treatment may not always be necessary, for example in patients known to maintain good control by conventional dosage schedules, or where improvement can be obtained by setting achievable targets and improving patient education.[3] However, intensive therapy can help sustain endogenous insulin secretion in type 1 diabetes, which is associated with improved metabolic control;[4] this would support initiation of intensive insulin therapy at an early stage.

The reports of the UK Prospective Diabetes Study (UKPDS) have provided similar evidence in patients with type 2 diabetes. This study has examined the benefits of intensive therapy, using a variety of drugs with diet and exercise. Intensive therapy, which aimed at producing fasting plasma-glucose concentrations of below 6 mmol/litre, substantially decreased the risk of microvascular complications (particularly retinopathy). There was no difference in benefit between intensive therapy with sulfonylureas and with insulin.[5] Metformin also produced benefit in the overweight patients who received it.[6] The UKPDS did not provide unequivocal evidence of a reduction in macrovascular disease with improved glycaemic control, although there was some suggestion of a reduction in risk of myocardial infarction (in line with a small earlier Japanese study[7]). However, it did show that vigorous control of blood pressure, using captopril or atenolol as the first-line drugs, reduced the risk of both macrovascular and microvascular complications,[8,9] suggesting that this should have a high priority in the treatment of type 2 diabetes.

**Diabetic eye disease**. Diabetic patients are prone to potentially blinding eye disease, usually in the form of cataract or diabetic retinopathy. Cataract generally requires surgical extraction, particular care being taken to avoid infection. Diabetic retinopathy may take a 'background', nonproliferative form, or become a more serious proliferative retinopathy associated with neovascularisation, vitreous haemorrhage and retinal detachment.

Although strict glycaemic control has been shown to reduce the risk of developing retinopathy,[2,5] once proliferative retinopathy has developed, glycaemic control is not adequate to prevent worsening.[10] Moreover, transient early worsening may occur in patients transferred to more intensive regimens.[11]

Aldose reductase inhibitors such as epalrestat and sorbinil have been investigated for the prevention of retinopathy, but despite some benefits results have generally been unimpressive.[12] The benefits of antiplatelet drugs are also unclear; aspirin, dipyridamole, and ticlopidine appear to reduce the development of microaneurysms in diabetic patients,[13,14] but aspirin has not been shown to prevent the development of retinopathy.[15]

Once severe nonproliferative or proliferative retinopathy has developed, photocoagulation using an argon laser or a xenon arc is effective in limiting progression, while vitrectomy may be helpful for vitreous haemorrhage and retinal detachment.[16] Interferon alfa-2a has been reported to slow the progression of proliferative diabetic retinopathy in 3 patients,[17] although all 3 experienced haemorrhage within 6 weeks of stopping the drug. Epoetin has also proved of benefit in a few patients,[18] and it has been suggested that pentoxifylline should be investigated.[19] Results from a large European study (EUCLID) demonstrated a reduction in the progression of retinopathy in patients with type 1 diabetes treated with an ACE inhibitor, lisinopril.[20] Improvement in retinal hard exudates has been seen in patients given the low-molecular-weight heparinoid danaparoid sodium.[21]

**Diabetic nephropathy**. Nephropathic changes associated with microvascular disease develop in up to 30% of patients with type 1 diabetes and up to 40% of those with type 2 disease; diabetic nephropathy, of which the first clinical sign is albuminuria, is one of the major causes of end-stage renal disease (p.1222).

Results from the DCCT indicate that strict glycaemic control reduces the incidence of microalbuminuria in type 1 diabetes,[2] and a smaller reduction was seen in the UKPDS in patients with type 2 diabetes.[5] However, while good control may prevent development of the initial lesion, it is not clear whether it can prevent progression in patients who are already microalbuminuric. Some studies, including the DCCT, have suggested that this is the case;[2,7] others have failed to confirm it.[22]

Another approach is dietary protein restriction (see Renal Failure, p.1418), which appears from a number of small studies to have a beneficial effect on disease progression.[23,24]

The most important approach to slowing the progression of diabetic nephropathy is aggressive antihypertensive control.[8,25-28] Although meta-analysis[29] has suggested that ACE inhibitors have an antiproteinuric effect over and above their antihypertensive properties, results from the UKPDS showed no difference between the effects of an ACE inhibitor and a beta blocker in reducing microalbuminuria in type 2 diabetics with hypertension.[9] Nonetheless, UK guidelines consider ACE inhibitors the drug class of first choice in this group, although most patients will require combination therapy.[28] Beneficial effects have also been reported when ACE inhibitors are given to patients with microalbuminuria but without hypertension,[30-33] and it has been recommended that such patients receive ACE inhibitors, initially in small doses, to slow the progression of renal disease.[25] Some consider that small decreases in blood pressure associated with such therapy may be responsible for the benefit.[9] ACE inhibition also had a modest renal protective effect in normotensive diabetics with normal urinary albumin excretion,[34] and such use requires further study.

The effect of angiotensin II receptor antagonists on diabetic nephropathy has also been investigated. In patients with type 2 diabetes, microalbuminuria, and hypertension, irbesartan reduced the rate of progression to nephropathy, independently of any effect on blood pressure.[35] In further studies of patients with type 2 diabetes and hypertension, who had already developed nephropathy, the use of irbesartan[36] and losartan[37] slowed the progression of renal disease.

The aldose reductase inhibitors have been investigated for their effects on nephropathy, but results have been, at best, ambiguous; a study in microalbuminuric patients given tolrestat (now withdrawn worldwide) did show a decrease in urinary albumin excretion but this was concomitant with a decrease in the (initially raised) glomerular filtration rate.[38] Pimagedine, which inhibits the formation of glycosylated end products, is also under investigation.

**Diabetic neuropathy.** A variety of peripheral neuropathies are common complications of diabetes mellitus. The intensity and extent of neurological abnormalities are proportional to the degree and duration of hyperglycaemia. Neuropathic symptoms include symmetrical sensory loss, particularly in the feet and lower limbs; the various features of autonomic neuropathy including gastroparesis, orthostatic hypotension, erectile dysfunction, and gustatory sweating; pain and cranial nerve palsy associated with mononeuropathies; and acute, painful, sensory neuropathy.

Results from the DCCT indicated that strict glycaemic control could substantially reduce the occurrence of clinical neuropathy in patients with type 1 diabetes,[2,39] a result which was not duplicated in the UKPDS in patients with type 2 diabetes.[5]

Although some studies have suggested that aldose reductase inhibitors such as epalrestat[40] can reduce the severity of diabetic neuropathy, larger scale analysis has apparently failed to demonstrate any benefit. Interesting preliminary results have suggested that ACE inhibitors may also have benefits in diabetic neuropathy.[41,42] An analysis[43] of 4 studies using the antoxidant thioctic acid found variable results, but an overall benefit, in symptomatic diabetic polyneuropathy. Results from another study[44] have suggested some improvement in cardiac autonomic neuropathy.

Other management of diabetic neuropathy is essentially symptomatic. The pain, which can be severe, may be managed with tricyclic antidepressants; mexiletine, antiepileptics including carbamazepine, and topical capsaicin may also be tried, as discussed on p.6.

Diabetic gastroparesis may respond to prokinetic drugs such as metoclopramide, cisapride, domperidone, or erythromycin,[45] but their effects can be variable and long-term use may be limited by adverse effects. Endoscopic or surgical interventions may be needed when symptoms cannot be controlled. Diarrhoea may respond to tetracycline (see below), while orthostatic hypotension should be managed conventionally (see p.1100) although care may be required in the use of elastic stockings in patients with impaired blood flow to the feet. For the management of erectile dysfunction, see p.1745.

**Diarrhoea.** Diabetic patients may develop intermittent bouts of watery diarrhoea, increasing in frequency as the condition worsens; autonomic neuropathy and abnormalities of digestion and bowel flora may play a role.[46] Beneficial results have been reported from the use of clonidine,[47,48] and of octreotide,[49,50] but a conventional antidiarrhoeal drug (usually codeine or diphenoxylate) or a broad spectrum antibacterial (especially tetracycline) may also be effective. The mechanism of action of tetracycline in diabetic diarrhoea is uncertain, but it has been suggested that one or two doses of tetracycline should be the first line of treatment.[51]

**Foot disease.** Various types of diabetic tissue damage, including circulatory impairment, neuropathy, collagen changes, and increased susceptibility to infection, may contribute to the foot lesions to which diabetics are prone. Ulceration and tissue necrosis at pressure-points may be followed by infection, gangrene, and sepsis. Management involves drainage and debridement of dead and infected tissue, and the use of antibiotics if necessary:[52] broad spectrum cover should be given intravenously if there is systemic infection, and adapted once the results of bacteriological culture are available.[53] Local antiseptic therapy may be helpful, especially for infections with *Pseudomonas* or *Proteus* spp. Neuropathic skin ulcers of the lower extremities have responded to a platelet-derived growth factor, becaplermin.[54] Granulocyte colony-stimulating factors have been used as adjunctive therapy with antibacterials in severe foot infections. Strict control of blood glucose is important and insulin should be given as required. Effective pain relief and bed rest may be required, and surgical reconstruction to improve blood supply may be helpful in some cases. Ultimately, some patients require amputation of all or part of the foot. Preventive care, with regular visits to a chiropodist, is therefore particularly important.

**Heart disease.** Most damage to the cardiac tissue in diabetic patients is due to accelerated ischaemic heart disease. Hypertension and hyperlipidaemias, both of which are prevalent in diabetes mellitus, contribute to this process. Symptoms of angina pectoris may be less marked or absent in diabetic patients. Management of ischaemic heart disease is, however, similar in diabetic and non-diabetic patients (see Angina Pectoris, p.813), except that if a beta blocker is given it should be a selective one. Diabetic patients are more likely than non-diabetics to die after myocardial infarction, but it has been shown that treatment with an insulin-glucose infusion after myocardial infarction, followed by subcutaneous insulin for at least 3 months, improves long-term survival in patients with both type 1 and type 2 diabetes.[55] Despite concerns about the use of aspirin in diabetics there is evidence for its value for the secondary prevention of cardiovascular disease and for primary prevention in patients at high risk.[56-58] There is some suggestion that higher than usual doses (300 mg rather than 75 to 100 mg daily) may be required in diabetics.[56]

Diabetics may also develop a form of restrictive cardiomyopathy in the absence of ischaemic heart disease. Again, the condition is managed similarly to cardiomyopathy in non-diabetic patients (see p.818).

Cardiac autonomic neuropathy has been reported to be improved by thioctic acid (see Diabetic Neuropathy, above).

**Hyperlipidaemias.** Insulin plays an important role in lipid metabolism and deficient insulin action means that diabetics are prone to hypertriglyceridaemia and have a blood-lipid profile associated with an increased risk of atherosclerosis, and hence of macrovascular complications. To reduce the risk of such complications good glycaemic control, dietary advice and where necessary the use of lipid regulating drugs are necessary (see also Cardiovascular Risk Reduction, p.819 and Hyperlipidaemias, p.823). The American Diabetes Association recommends that LDL cholesterol concentrations should be below 2.6 mmol/litre, HDL cholesterol concentrations more than 1.15 mmol/litre, and triglyceride concentrations less than 1.7 mmol/litre.[59] Similarly, UK guidelines require only annual monitoring in patients with cholesterol 5 mmol/litre or less (LDL cholesterol 3 mmol/litre or lower) and triglycerides less than 2.3 mmol/litre.[60] When necessary statins, such as simvastatin,[61] should be used to lower LDL cholesterol. Nicotinic acid has been used to raise HDL cholesterol concentrations,[62] but high doses can have an adverse effect on glycaemic control.[59] Fibrates may therefore be used as an alternative, and can also be used to lower triglyceride concentrations.[59]

**Hypertension.** Hypertension is twice as common in the diabetic as in the non-diabetic population, and is associated with both macrovascular complications and microvascular disease (especially diabetic nephropathy). Management of hypertension in diabetics follows the same principles as in the general population, but it should be treated aggressively with a view to retarding development of complications,[8,28,60,63,64] and the threshold for drug treatment and the treatment goal are lower than in non-diabetic patients (see Hypertension, p.825). All of the main groups of antihypertensive drugs may be used although an ACE inhibitor,[65] such as ramipril,[66] or a beta blocker may be effective in reducing complications.[8,9] Low-dose diuretic therapy has also been shown to be beneficial.[67] The calcium-channel blocker felodipine was effective in the subset of diabetics in one study[68] but other studies have suggested that calcium-channel blockers are less effective than ACE inhibitors, or may even increase cardiovascular adverse events (see under Nifedipine, p.968). In the UK, guidelines recommend that long-acting calcium-channel blockers may be used as second-line treatment or as part of combination therapy, but that short-acting calcium-channel blockers should not be prescribed to patients with type 2 diabetes.[60]


1. Wang PH, *et al.* Meta-analysis of effects of intensive blood-glucose control on late complications of type I diabetes. *Lancet* 1993; **341:** 1306–9.
2. The Diabetes Control and Complications Trial Research Group. The effect of intensive treatment of diabetes on the development and progression of long-term complications in insulin-dependent diabetes mellitus. *N Engl J Med* 1993; **329:** 977–86.
3. Short R. Implementing the lessons of DCCT. *Diabet Med* 1994; **11:** 220–8.
4. The Diabetes Control and Complications Trial Research Group. Effect of intensive therapy on residual β-cell function in patients with type 1 diabetes in the Diabetes Control and Complications Trial: a randomized, controlled trial. *Ann Intern Med* 1998; **128:** 517–23.
5. UK Prospective Diabetes Study Group. Intensive blood-glucose control with sulphonylureas or insulin compared with conventional treatment and risk of complications in patients with type 2 diabetes (UKPDS 33). *Lancet* 1998; **352:** 837–53. Correction. *ibid.* 1999; **354:** 602.
6. UK Prospective Diabetes Study (UKPDS) Group. Effect of intensive blood-glucose control with metformin on complications in overweight patients with type 2 diabetes (UKPDS 34). *Lancet* 1998; **352:** 854–65. Correction. *ibid.*; 1558.
7. Ohkubo Y, *et al.* Intensive insulin therapy prevents the progression of diabetic microvascular complications in Japanese patients with non-insulin-dependent diabetes mellitus: a randomized prospective 6-year study. *Diabetes Res Clin Pract* 1995; **28:** 103–17.
8. UK Prospective Diabetes Study Group. Tight blood pressure control and risk of macrovascular and microvascular complications in type 2 diabetes: UKPDS 38. *BMJ* 1998; **317:** 703–13.
9. UK Prospective Diabetes Study Group. Efficacy of atenolol and captopril in reducing risk of macrovascular and microvascular complications in type 2 diabetes: UKPDS 39. *BMJ* 1998; **317:** 713–20.
10. Esmatjes E, *et al.* Long-term evolution of diabetic retinopathy and renal function after pancreas transplantation. *Transplant Proc* 1992; **24:** 12–13.
11. Henricsson M, *et al.* The effect of glycaemic control and the introduction of insulin therapy on retinopathy in non-insulin-dependent diabetes mellitus. *Diabet Med* 1997; **14:** 123–31.
12. Sorbinil Retinopathy Trial Research Group. A randomized trial of sorbinil, an aldose reductase inhibitor, in diabetic retinopathy. *Arch Ophthalmol* 1990; **108:** 1234–44.
13. The DAMAD Study Group. Effect of aspirin alone and aspirin plus dipyridamole in early diabetic retinopathy: a multicenter randomized controlled clinical trial. *Diabetes* 1989; **38:** 491–8.
14. The TIMAD Study Group. Ticlopidine treatment reduces the progression of nonproliferative diabetic retinopathy. *Arch Ophthalmol* 1990; **108:** 1577–83.
15. Early Treatment Diabetic Retinopathy Study Research Group. Effects of aspirin treatment on diabetic retinopathy: ETDRS report number 8. *Ophthalmology* 1991; **98** (suppl): 757–65.
16. Ferris FL, *et al.* Treatment of diabetic retinopathy. *N Engl J Med* 1999; **341:** 667–78.
17. Skowsky WR, *et al.* A pilot study of chronic recombinant interferon-alfa 2a for diabetic proliferative retinopathy: metabolic effects and ophthalmologic effects. *J Diabetes Complications* 1996; **10:** 94–9.
18. Friedman EA, *et al.* Erythropoietin in diabetic macular edema and renal insufficiency. *Am J Kidney Dis* 1995; **26:** 202–8.
19. Sebag J, *et al.* Effects of pentoxifylline on choroidal blood flow in nonproliferative diabetic retinopathy. *Angiology* 1994; **45:** 429–33.
20. Chaturvedi N, *et al.* Effect of lisinopril on progression of retinopathy in normotensive people with type 1 diabetes. *Lancet* 1998; **351:** 28–31.
21. van der Pijl JW, *et al.* Effect of danaparoid sodium on hard exudates in diabetic retinopathy. *Lancet* 1997; **350:** 1743–5.
22. Microalbuminuria Collaborative Study Group, United Kingdom. Intensive therapy and progression to clinical albuminuria in patients with insulin dependent diabetes mellitus and microalbuminuria. *BMJ* 1995; **311:** 973–7.
23. Pedrini MT, *et al.* The effect of dietary protein restriction on the progression of diabetic and nondiabetic renal diseases: a meta-analysis. *Ann Intern Med* 1996; **124:** 627–32.
24. Waugh NR, Robertson AM. Protein restriction for diabetic renal disease. Available in The Cochrane Library; Issue 2. Chichester: John Wiley; 2004.
25. Mogensen CE, *et al.* Prevention of diabetic renal disease with special reference to microalbuminuria. *Lancet* 1995; **346:** 1080–4.
26. Savage MW, *et al.* Therapeutic options in diabetic renal disease and hypertension. *Br J Hosp Med* 1995; **54:** 429–34.
27. Bakris GL, *et al.* Preserving renal function in adults with hypertension and diabetes: a consensus approach. *Am J Kidney Dis* 2000; **36:** 646–61.
28. National Institute for Clinical Excellence. Management of type 2 diabetes: renal disease—prevention and early management (issued February 2002). Available at: http://www.nice.org.uk/pdf/diabetesrenalguideline.pdf (accessed 07/07/04)
29. Kasiske BL, *et al.* Effect of antihypertensive therapy on the kidney in patients with diabetes: a meta-regression analysis. *Ann Intern Med* 1993; **118:** 129–38.
30. Mathiesen ER, *et al.* Randomised controlled trial of long term efficacy of captopril on preservation of kidney function in normotensive patients with insulin dependent diabetes and microalbuminuria. *BMJ* 1999; **319:** 24–5.

31. The EUCLID Study Group. Randomised placebo-controlled trial of lisinopril in normotensive patients with insulin-dependent diabetes and normoalbuminuria or microalbuminuria. *Lancet* 1997; **349:** 1787–92.
32. Lovell HG. Angiotensin converting enzyme inhibitors in normotensive diabetic patients with microalbuminuria. Available in The Cochrane Library; Issue 2. Chichester: John Wiley; 2004.
33. The ACE inhibitors in diabetic nephropathy trialist group. Should all patients with type 1 diabetes mellitus and microalbuminuria receive angiotensin-converting enzyme inhibitors? A meta-analysis of individual patient data. *Ann Intern Med* 2001; **134:** 370–9.
34. Ravid M, *et al.* Use of enalapril to attenuate decline in renal function in normotensive, normoalbuminuric patients with type 2 diabetes mellitus: a randomized controlled trial. *Ann Intern Med* 1998; **128:** 982–8.
35. Parving H-H, *et al.* The effect of irbesartan on the development of diabetic nephropathy in patients with type 2 diabetes. *N Engl J Med* 2001; **345:** 870–8.
36. Lewis EJ, *et al.* Renoprotective effect of the angiotensin-receptor antagonist irbesartan in patients with nephropathy due to type 2 diabetes. *N Engl J Med* 2001; **345:** 851–60.
37. Brenner BM, *et al.* Effects of losartan on renal and cardiovascular outcomes in patients with type 2 diabetes and nephropathy. *N Engl J Med* 2001; **345:** 861–9.
38. Passariello N, *et al.* Effect of aldose reductase inhibitor (tolrestat) on urinary albumin excretion rate and glomerular filtration rate in IDDM subjects with nephropathy. *Diabetes Care* 1993; **16:** 789–95.
39. The Diabetes Control and Complications Trial Research Group. The effect of intensive diabetes therapy on measures of autonomic nervous system function in the Diabetes Control and Complications Trial (DCCT). *Diabetologia* 1998; **41:** 416–23.
40. Uchida K, *et al.* Effect of 24 weeks of treatment with epalrestat, an aldose reductase inhibitor, on peripheral neuropathy in patients with non-insulin-dependent diabetes mellitus. *Clin Ther* 1995; **17:** 460–6.
41. Reja A, *et al.* Is ACE inhibition with lisinopril helpful in diabetic neuropathy? *Diabet Med* 1995; **12:** 307–9.
42. Malik RA, *et al.* Effect of angiotensin-converting-enzyme (ACE) inhibitor trandolapril on human diabetic neuropathy: randomised double-blind controlled trial. *Lancet* 1998; **352:** 1978–81.
43. Ziegler D, *et al.* Treatment of symptomatic diabetic polyneuropathy with the antioxidant α-lipoic acid: a meta-analysis. *Diabet Med* 2004; **21:** 114–21.
44. Ziegler D, *et al.* Effects of treatment with the antioxidant α-lipoic acid on cardiac autonomic neuropathy in NIDDM patients: a 4-month randomized controlled multicenter trial (DEKAN study). *Diabetes Care* 1997; **20:** 369–73.
45. Smith DS, Ferris CD. Current concepts in diabetic gastroparesis. *Drugs* 2003; **63:** 1339–58.
46. Ogbonnaya KI, Arem R. Diabetic diarrhea: pathophysiology, diagnosis, and management. *Arch Intern Med* 1990; **150:** 262–7.
47. Fedorak RN, *et al.* Treatment of diabetic diarrhea with clonidine. *Ann Intern Med* 1985; **102:** 197–9.
48. Sacerdote A. Topical clonidine for diabetic diarrhea. *Ann Intern Med* 1986; **105:** 139.
49. Michaels PE, Cameron RB. Octreotide is cost-effective therapy in diabetic diarrhea. *Arch Intern Med* 1991; **151:** 2469.
50. Mourad FH, *et al.* Effective treatment of diabetic diarrhoea with somatostatin analogue, octreotide. *Gut* 1992; **33:** 1578–80.
51. Clark CM, Lee DA. Prevention and treatment of the complications of diabetes mellitus. *N Engl J Med* 1995; **332:** 1210–17.
52. National Institute for Clinical Excellence. Type 2 diabetes: prevention and management of foot problems (January 2004). Available at: http://www.nice.org.uk/pdf/CG010NICEguideline.pdf (accessed 07/07/04)
53. West NJ. Systemic antimicrobial treatment of foot infections in diabetic patients. *Am J Health-Syst Pharm* 1995; **52:** 1199–1207.
54. Wieman TJ, *et al.* Efficacy and safety of a topical gel formulation of recombinant human platelet-derived growth factor-BB (becaplermin) in patients with chronic neuropathic diabetic ulcers: a phase III randomized placebo-controlled double-blind study. *Diabetes Care* 1998; **21:** 822–7.
55. Malmberg K, *et al.* Prospective randomised study of intensive insulin treatment on long term survival after acute myocardial infarction in patients with diabetes mellitus. *BMJ* 1997; **314:** 1512–15.
56. Yudkin JS. Which diabetic patients should be taking aspirin? *BMJ* 1995; **311:** 641–2.
57. Grundy SM, *et al.* Diabetes and cardiovascular disease: a statement for healthcare professionals from the American Heart Association. *Circulation* 1999; **100:** 1134–46.
58. American Diabetes Association. Aspirin therapy in diabetes. *Diabetes Care* 2004; **27** (suppl 1): S72–S73. Also available at: http://care.diabetesjournals.org/cgi/reprint/27/suppl_1/s72.pdf (accessed 07/07/04)
59. American Diabetes Association. Dyslipidemia management in adults with diabetes. *Diabetes Care* 2004; **27** (suppl 1): S68–S71. Also available at: http://care.diabetesjournals.org/cgi/reprint/27/suppl_1/s68.pdf (accessed 07/07/04)
60. National Institute for Clinical Excellence. Management of type 2 diabetes: management of blood pressure and blood lipids (issued October 2002). Available at: http://www.nice.org.uk/pdf/NICE_INHERITEd_Hv8.pdf (accessed 07/07/04)
61. Haffner SM, *et al.* Reduced coronary events in simvastatin-treated patients with coronary heart disease and diabetes or impaired fasting glucose levels: subgroup analyses in the Scandinavian Simvastatin Survival Study. *Arch Intern Med* 1999; **159:** 2661–7.
62. Elam MB, *et al.* Effect of niacin on lipid and lipoprotein levels and glycemic control in patients with diabetes and peripheral arterial disease. The ADMIT study: a randomized trial. *JAMA* 2000; **284:** 1263–70.
63. Kaplan NM. Management of hypertension in patients with type 2 diabetes mellitus: guidelines based on current evidence. *Ann Intern Med* 2001; **135:** 1079–83.
64. American Diabetes Association. Hypertension management in adults with diabetes. *Diabetes Care* 2004; **27** (suppl 1): S65–S67. Also available at: http://care.diabetesjournals.org/cgi/reprint/27/suppl_1/s65.pdf (accessed 07/07/04)
65. Pahor M, *et al.* Therapeutic benefits of ACE inhibitors and other antihypertensive drugs in patients with type 2 diabetes. *Diabetes Care* 2000; **23:** 888–92.
66. Heart Outcomes Prevention Evaluation (HOPE) study investigators. Effects of ramipril on cardiovascular and microvascular outcomes in people with diabetes mellitus: results of the HOPE study and MICRO-HOPE substudy. *Lancet* 2000; **355:** 253–9. Correction. *ibid.*; **356:** 860.
67. Curb JD, *et al.* Effect of diuretic-based antihypertensive treatment on cardiovascular disease risk in older diabetic patients with isolated systolic hypertension. *JAMA* 1996; **276:** 1886–92. Correction. *ibid.* 1997; **277:** 1356.
68. Hansson L, *et al.* Effects of intensive blood-pressure lowering and low-dose aspirin in patients with hypertension: principal results of the Hypertension Optimal Treatment (HOT) randomised trial. *Lancet* 1998; **351:** 1755–62.

### Diabetic emergencies

**Hypoglycaemia.** The most frequent complication of insulin therapy is hypoglycaemia and patients taking insulin need to be educated about its cause, symptoms, and treatment. Most patients can recognise the early warning signs of hypoglycaemia and by taking sugar immediately can prevent more serious symptoms developing. Comatose patients need to be given intravenous glucose or, if this is not practicable, subcutaneous, intramuscular, or intravenous glucagon (although glucose is still required if there is no response within 10 minutes). Hypoglycaemia can also develop in patients taking oral antidiabetics, notably the sulfonylureas.

Some patients report loss of the warning signs of hypoglycaemia after transferring from animal to human insulin and these patients, if appropriate, may need to be transferred back to animal insulin. However, the most significant factor in loss of hypoglycaemic warning signs may be exposure to hypoglycaemia itself; a study found that total avoidance of hypoglycaemic episodes for 3 weeks while maintaining glycaemic control restored awareness.[1] Loss of hypoglycaemic awareness, which appears to be due to an adaptive conservation of glucose uptake in the brain,[2] is liable to be a particular problem in patients receiving intensive therapy. There is limited data to suggest that caffeine can improve awareness of hypoglycaemia.[3,4]

For further details on the treatment of insulin-induced hypoglycaemia, see p.335.

**Diabetic ketoacidosis** is caused by an absolute or relative lack of insulin and commonly occurs after noncompliance or failure to adjust insulin dosage in the presence of factors such as infection that increase insulin requirements (see Precautions for Insulin, p.338). Failure of an insulin pump can be a cause.[5] Also pregnant diabetic women are more prone to development of diabetic ketoacidosis.

Diabetic ketoacidosis is characterised by hyperglycaemia, hyperketonaemia, and acidaemia, with subsequent dehydration and electrolyte abnormalities. Onset may be rapid, or insidious over many days. Initial presenting symptoms such as thirst, polyuria, fatigue, and weight loss are those of any newly presenting type 1 diabetic; they then progress to nausea, vomiting, abdominal pain, and impaired consciousness or coma, and, if untreated, death.[5,6]

Diabetic ketoacidosis is a medical emergency and should be treated immediately with fluid replacement and insulin.[5-8] Fluid requirements depend on the needs of the individual; overvigorous fluid replacement without severe dehydration carries the risk of precipitating cerebral oedema.[6-8]

Soluble insulin should also be administered immediately. Large doses were formerly thought necessary, but lower dose regimens accompanied by adequate hydration have since been shown to be preferable.[5] Insulin resistance in diabetic ketoacidosis is generally exacerbated by hyperosmolarity and other confounding factors, and insulin therapy is therefore most effective when preceded or accompanied by adequate fluid and electrolyte replacement.[5] In the UK, the *British National Formulary* considers that insulin should preferably be given by intravenous infusion, with the intramuscular route used if facilities for intravenous infusion are not available. However, in the USA some consider that an intravenous bolus followed by subcutaneous injection may be appropriate in certain patients.[5] Intramuscular or subcutaneous injection are not appropriate in patients with hypovolaemic shock, due to poor tissue perfusion.[5] Where the response to insulin is inadequate the intravenous route is generally required[5] and the rate of infusion may be doubled on an hourly basis until an appropriate response is seen. A case report has suggested that mecasermin may be useful if there is insulin resistance.[9]

When the blood-glucose concentration has fallen to about 12.5 mmol/litre the dose of insulin may be reduced by about half and glucose given intravenously,[5] usually in a strength of 5% with saline although in rare cases a glucose strength of 10% may be necessary.[5] The use of glucose enables insulin to be continued in order to clear ketone bodies without inducing hypoglycaemia. Once glucose concentrations have been controlled and acidosis has completely cleared, subcutaneous injections of insulin can begin;[6] but intravenous insulin should not be stopped until subcutaneous dosage has begun.

Total body stores of potassium are depleted in patients with diabetic ketoacidosis. Insulin deficiency appears to be the main initiating factor for hyperkalaemia in diabetic ketoacidosis.[10] Although patients may present with raised, normal, or decreased serum-potassium concentrations, the concentrations will start to fall with the correction of acidosis. Potassium is added to the infusion fluid after initial fluid expansion and once insulin therapy is commenced.[5] In hyperkalaemic patients, potassium is given once serum concentrations have fallen to within normal limits.[5,6] In the rare patient presenting with hypokalaemia potassium replacement should be begun before insulin therapy and the latter withheld until potassium concentrations have risen to normal values.[5]

Intravenous bicarbonate is now generally reserved for patients with severe acidaemia; a common practice[5,6] is to give isotonic bicarbonate to those with a pH of less than 7.0 with the aim of raising the pH to 7.1.

Phosphate concentrations are affected in a similar manner to potassium concentrations in the ketoacidotic state, but there is less agreement on the need for routine doses of phosphate. Phosphate concentrations should be monitored and phosphate given if clinically significant hypophosphataemia occurs.[5,6]

The precipitating cause of diabetic ketoacidosis should also be identified and managed appropriately.

**Hyperosmolar hyperglycaemic state** or hyperosmolar hyperglycaemic nonketotic coma (HONK) occurs mainly in elderly patients with type 2 diabetes and though much less common than diabetic ketoacidosis it carries a higher mortality. Patients may present in coma with severe hyperglycaemia but with minimal ketosis; dehydration and renal impairment are common.[5] Treatment is similar to that of diabetic ketoacidosis (see above), although potassium requirements are lower and large amounts of fluid and less insulin may be required; some suggest the use of hypotonic fluid if necessary.[11] There is an increased likelihood of thrombotic events, so prophylactic anticoagulation should be considered.

1. Cranston I, *et al.* Restoration of hypoglycaemia awareness in patients with long-duration insulin-dependent diabetes. *Lancet* 1994; **344:** 283–7.
2. Boyle PJ, *et al.* Brain glucose uptake and unawareness of hypoglycemia in patients with insulin-dependent diabetes mellitus. *N Engl J Med* 1995; **333:** 1726–31.
3. Debrah K, *et al.* Effect of caffeine on recognition of and physiological responses to hypoglycaemia in insulin-dependent diabetes. *Lancet* 1996; **347:** 19–24.
4. Watson JM, *et al.* Influence of caffeine on the frequency and perception of hypoglycemia in free-living patients with type 1 diabetes. *Diabetes Care* 2000; **23:** 455–9.
5. Kitabchi AE, *et al.* Management of hyperglycemic crises in patients with diabetes. *Diabetes Care* 2001; **24:** 131–53.
6. Lebovitz HE. Diabetic ketoacidosis. *Lancet* 1995; **345:** 767–72.
7. Adrogué HJ, *et al.* Salutary effects of modest fluid replacement in the treatment of adults with diabetic ketoacidosis: use in patients without extreme volume deficit. *JAMA* 1989; **262:** 2108–13.
8. Johnston C. Fluid replacement in diabetic ketoacidosis. *BMJ* 1992; **305:** 522.
9. Usala A-L, *et al.* Brief report: treatment of insulin-resistant diabetic ketoacidosis with insulin-like growth factor I in an adolescent with insulin-dependent diabetes. *N Engl J Med* 1992; **327:** 853–7.
10. Anonymous. Hyperkalaemia in diabetic ketoacidosis. *Lancet* 1986; **ii:** 845–6.
11. Wright AD. Diabetic emergencies in adults. *Prescribers' J* 1989; **29:** 147–54.

## Acarbose *(BAN, USAN, rINN)*

Acarbosa; Bay-g-5421. *O*-{4-Amino-4,6-dideoxy-*N*-[(1*S*,4*R*,5*S*,6*S*)-4,5,6-trihydroxy-3-hydroxymethylcyclohex-2-enyl]-α-D-glucopyranosyl}-(1→4)-*O*-α-D-glucopyranosyl-(1→4)-D-glucopyranose.

$C_{25}H_{43}NO_{18}$ = 645.6.
*CAS — 56180-94-0.*
*ATC — A10BF01.*

### Adverse Effects

Acarbose often causes gastrointestinal disturbances, particularly flatulence due to bacterial action on nonabsorbed carbohydrate in the colon. Abdominal distension, diarrhoea, and pain may occur. Ileus has been reported very rarely. A decreased dosage of acarbose and improved dietary habits may reduce these adverse effects. Hepatotoxicity may occur and may necessitate a reduction in dosage or withdrawal of the drug. Skin reactions have occurred rarely. Very rarely oedema has been reported.

◊ The manufacturers reported that the incidence of adverse effects with acarbose was lower in a postmarketing surveillance study than in previous clinical trials;[1] this was held to represent better tailoring of individual doses to patient tolerability.

1. Spengler M, Cagatay M. The use of acarbose in the primary-care setting: evaluation of efficacy and tolerability of acarbose by postmarketing surveillance study. *Clin Invest Med* 1995; **18:** 325–31.

**Effects on the liver.** Hepatocellular liver damage, with jaundice and elevated serum aminotransferases, have been reported in patients receiving acarbose.[1-3] Symptoms resolved on discontinuation of the drug.

1. Andrade RJ, *et al.* Hepatic injury caused by acarbose. *Ann Intern Med* 1996; **124:** 931.
2. Carrascosa M, *et al.* Acarbose-induced acute severe hepatotoxicity. *Lancet* 1997; **349:** 698–9.
3. Fujimoto Y, *et al.* Acarbose-induced hepatic injury. *Lancet* 1998; **351:** 340.

**Effects on the skin.** Generalised erythema multiforme and eosinophilia occurred in a male diabetic patient 13 days after starting acarbose.[1] The hypersensitivity reaction was confirmed by rechallenge.

1. Kono T, *et al.* Acarbose-induced generalised erythema multiforme. *Lancet* 1999; **354:** 396–7.

## Precautions

Acarbose is contra-indicated in inflammatory bowel disease, particularly where there is associated ulceration, and in gastrointestinal obstruction or patients predisposed to it. It should be avoided in patients with chronic intestinal diseases that significantly affect digestion or absorption, and in conditions which may deteriorate as a result of increased gas formation, such as hernia.

Acarbose is also contra-indicated in patients with hepatic impairment and liver enzyme values should be monitored, particularly at high doses.

If hypoglycaemia should develop in a patient receiving acarbose it needs to be treated with glucose, since the action of acarbose inhibits the hydrolysis of disaccharides.

**Breast feeding.** In the absence of evidence, the manufacturers recommend that acarbose should be avoided during breast feeding.

## Interactions

Acarbose may enhance the effects of other antidiabetics, including insulin, and a reduction in their dosage may be needed. Use with gastrointestinal adsorbents and digestive enzyme preparations can diminish the effects of acarbose and should be avoided. Neomycin and colestyramine may enhance the effects of acarbose and a reduction in its dosage may be required. Acarbose may inhibit the absorption of digoxin (see Antidiabetics, under Interactions of Digoxin, p.897).

## Pharmacokinetics

After ingestion of acarbose, the majority of active unchanged drug remains in the lumen of the gastrointestinal tract to exert its pharmacological activity and is metabolised by intestinal enzymes and by the microbial flora. Ultimately about 35% of a dose is absorbed in the form of metabolites. Acarbose is excreted in the urine and faeces.

## Uses and Administration

Acarbose is an inhibitor of alpha glucosidases, especially sucrase. This retards the digestion and absorption of carbohydrates in the small intestine and hence reduces the increase in blood-glucose concentrations after a carbohydrate load. It is given by mouth in the treatment of type 2 diabetes mellitus (p.324) either alone or combined with a sulfonylurea, biguanide, or insulin. Acarbose treatment may be started with a low dose of 25 or 50 mg daily to minimise gastrointestinal disturbance. It is then gradually increased to a usual dose of 25 or 50 mg three times daily, immediately before food. Doses up to 100 to 200 mg three times daily may be given if necessary. Some benefit has also been demonstrated when acarbose is used to supplement insulin therapy in type 1 diabetes mellitus.

Acarbose has also been studied for the treatment of reactive hypoglycaemia, the dumping syndrome, and certain types of hyperlipoproteinaemia.

◊ References.

1. Chiasson J-L, *et al.* The efficacy of acarbose in the treatment of patients with non-insulin-dependent diabetes mellitus: a multicenter controlled clinical trial. *Ann Intern Med* 1994; **121:** 928–35.
2. Coniff RF, *et al.* Multicenter, placebo-controlled trial comparing acarbose (BAY g 5421) with placebo, tolbutamide, and tolbutamide-plus-acarbose in non-insulin-dependent diabetes mellitus. *Am J Med* 1995; **98:** 443–51.
3. Spengler M, Cagatay M. The use of acarbose in the primary-care setting: evaluation of efficacy and tolerability of acarbose by postmarketing surveillance study. *Clin Invest Med* 1995; **18:** 325–31.
4. Salvatore T, Giugliano D. Pharmacokinetic-pharmacodynamic relationships of acarbose. *Clin Pharmacokinet* 1996; **30:** 94–106.
5. Anonymous. Acarbose for diabetes mellitus. *Med Lett Drugs Ther* 1996; **38:** 9–10.
6. Hoffman J, Spengler M. Efficacy of 24-week monotherapy with acarbose, metformin, or placebo in dietary-treated NIDDM patients: the Essen-II study. *Am J Med* 1997; **103:** 483–90.
7. Hollander P, *et al.* Acarbose in the treatment of type I diabetes. *Diabetes Care* 1997; **20:** 248–53.
8. Buse J, *et al.* The PROTECT study: final results of a large multicenter postmarketing study in patients with type 2 diabetes. *Clin Ther* 1998; **20:** 257–69.
9. Holman RR, *et al.* A randomized double-blind trial of acarbose in type 2 diabetes shows improved glycemic control over 3 years (UK Prospective Diabetes Study 44). *Diabetes Care* 1999; **22:** 960–4.
10. Riccardi G, *et al.* Efficacy and safety of acarbose in the treatment of type 1 diabetes mellitus: a placebo-controlled, double-blind, multicentre study. *Diabet Med* 1999; **16:** 228–32.
11. Chiasson J-L, *et al.* Acarbose for prevention of type 2 diabetes mellitus: the STOP-NIDDM randomised trial. *Lancet* 2002; **359:** 2072–7.

## Preparations

**Proprietary Preparations** (details are given in Part 3)
***Arg.:*** Glucobay; ***Austral.:*** Glucobay; ***Austria:*** Glucobay; ***Belg.:*** Glucobay; ***Braz.:*** Glucobay; ***Canad.:*** Prandase; ***Chile:*** Glucobay; ***Denm.:*** Glucobay; ***Fin.:*** Glucobay†; ***Fr.:*** Glucor; ***Ger.:*** Glucobay; ***Gr.:*** Glucobay; ***Hong Kong:*** Glucobay; ***India:*** Asucrose; Glucobay; ***Irl.:*** Glucobay; ***Israel:*** Prandase; ***Ital.:*** Glicobase; Glucobay; ***Malaysia:*** Glucobay; ***Mex.:*** Glucobay; ***Neth.:*** Glucobay; ***Norw.:*** Glucobay; ***NZ:*** Glucobay; ***Port.:*** Glucobay; ***S.Afr.:*** Glucobay; ***Singapore:*** Glucobay; ***Spain:*** Glucobay; Glumida; ***Swed.:*** Glucobay; ***Switz.:*** Glucobay; ***Thai.:*** Glucobay; ***UK:*** Glucobay; ***USA:*** Precose.

---

# Acetohexamide *(BAN, USAN, rINN)*

Acetohexamida; Compound 33006. 1-(4-Acetylbenzenesulphonyl)-3-cyclohexylurea.

$C_{15}H_{20}N_2O_4S = 324.4.$
*CAS — 968-81-0.*
*ATC — A10BB31.*

**Pharmacopoeias.** In *Jpn* and *US.*

**USP 27** (Acetohexamide). A white, practically odourless, crystalline powder. Practically insoluble in water and in ether; soluble 1 in 230 of alcohol and 1 in 210 of chloroform; soluble in pyridine and in dilute solutions of alkali hydroxides.

## Profile

Acetohexamide is a sulfonylurea antidiabetic (p.346). Its duration of action is 12 hours or more. It is given by mouth in the treatment of type 2 diabetes mellitus (p.324) in a usual initial dose of 250 mg daily before breakfast. The daily dose may then be increased by 250 to 500 mg at intervals of 5 to 7 days, to a maintenance dose of up to 1.5 g daily; increasing the dose above 1.5 g does not usually lead to further benefit. Doses in excess of 1 g daily may be taken in 2 divided doses, before the morning and evening meals.

## Preparations

***USP 27:*** Acetohexamide Tablets.

**Proprietary Preparations** (details are given in Part 3)
***Canad.:*** Dimelor†; ***Hong Kong:*** Dimelor†; ***S.Afr.:*** Dimelor†; ***USA:*** Dymelor.

---

# Biguanide Antidiabetics

Antidiabéticos biguanídicos.

## Adverse Effects

Gastrointestinal adverse effects including anorexia, nausea, and diarrhoea may occur with biguanides; patients may experience a metallic taste and there may be weight loss. Absorption of various substances including vitamin $B_{12}$ may be impaired.

Hypoglycaemia is rare with a biguanide given alone, although it may occur if other contributing factors or drugs are present.

Lactic acidosis, sometimes fatal, has occurred with biguanides, primarily with phenformin. When it has occurred with metformin most cases have been in patients whose condition contra-indicated the use of the drug, particularly those with renal impairment.

Phenformin has been implicated in the controversial reports of excessive cardiovascular mortality associated with oral hypoglycaemic therapy (see under Sulfonylureas, Effects on the Cardiovascular System, p.346).

◊ Reviews.

1. Paterson KR, *et al.* Undesired effects of biguanide therapy. *Adverse Drug React Acute Poisoning Rev* 1984; **3:** 173–82.
2. Howlett HCS, Bailey CJ. A risk-benefit assessment of metformin in type 2 diabetes mellitus. *Drug Safety* 1999; **20:** 489–503.

**Effects on the blood.** Megaloblastic anaemia has occurred with biguanide therapy (see Malabsorption, under Effects on the Gastrointestinal Tract, below). A few cases of metformin-induced haemolysis resulting in hyperbilirubinaemia and jaundice have also been described.[1,2]

1. Lin K-D, *et al.* Metformin-induced hemolysis with jaundice. *N Engl J Med* 1998; **339:** 1860–1.
2. Meir A, *et al.* Metformin-induced hemolytic anemia in a patient with glucose-6-phosphate dehydrogenase deficiency. *Diabetes Care* 2003; **26:** 956–7.

**Effects on the gastrointestinal tract.** DIARRHOEA. In a retrospective survey,[1] 30 of 265 diabetic patients reported diarrhoea or alternating diarrhoea and constipation, comprising: 11 of 54 taking metformin; 9 of 45 taking metformin with a sulfonylurea; 3 of 53 taking a sulfonylurea only; 5 of 78 on insulin therapy; 2 of 35 on diet alone. Among 150 nondiabetic controls 12 reported diarrhoea. Chronic diarrhoea described as watery, often explosive, and frequently causing faecal incontinence, has been reported as an adverse effect of late onset in patients receiving metformin. Some patients had been on stable metformin therapy for several years before the onset of diarrhoea. Symptoms ceased upon withdrawal of metformin, and recurred in cases of rechallenge.[2,3]

1. Dandona P, *et al.* Diarrhea and metformin in a diabetic clinic. *Diabetes Care* 1983; **6:** 472–4.
2. Raju B, *et al.* Metformin and late gastrointestinal complications. *Am J Med* 2000; **109:** 260–1.
3. Foss MT, Clement KD. Metformin as a cause of late-onset chronic diarrhea. *Pharmacotherapy* 2001; **21:** 1422–4.

MALABSORPTION. Megaloblastic anaemia due to vitamin $B_{12}$ malabsorption in a 58-year-old woman was associated with long-term treatment with metformin.[1]

In a survey of diabetic patients receiving biguanide therapy,[2] malabsorption of vitamin $B_{12}$ was observed in 14 of 46 diabetics taking metformin or phenformin; metformin was more commonly to blame. Withdrawal of the drug resulted in normal absorption in only 7 of the 14. In a series of 10 patients[3] with vitamin $B_{12}$ deficiency associated with metformin, vitamin $B_{12}$ concentrations and blood count abnormalities were reported to have been corrected within 3 months of starting treatment with intramuscular or oral cyanocobalamin; 2 patients were transferred to treatment with other antidiabetic agents.

1. Callaghan TS, *et al.* Megaloblastic anaemia due to vitamin $B_{12}$ malabsorption associated with long-term metformin treatment. *BMJ* 1980; **280:** 1214–15.
2. Adams JF, *et al.* Malabsorption of vitamin $B_{12}$ and intrinsic factor secretion during biguanide therapy. *Diabetologia* 1983; **24:** 16–18.
3. Andrès E, *et al.* Metformin-associated vitamin $B_{12}$ deficiency. *Arch Intern Med* 2002; **162:** 2251–2.

**Effects on the liver.** Severe cholestatic hepatitis attributed to metformin has been reported.[1]

1. Babich MM, *et al.* Metformin-induced acute hepatitis. *Am J Med* 1998; **104:** 490–2.

**Hypersensitivity.** Vasculitis and pneumonitis in a 59-year-old woman was associated with administration of metformin.[1] Symptoms improved on withdrawal of metformin, but reappeared on its reintroduction.

1. Klapholz L, *et al.* Leucocytoclastic vasculitis and pneumonitis induced by metformin. *BMJ* 1986; **293:** 483.

**Hypoglycaemia.** The UK manufacturers of metformin state that hypoglycaemia does not occur with metformin alone, even in overdosage, although it may occur if given with alcohol or other hypoglycaemics. Interim results from the UK Prospective Diabetes Study,[1] however, indicate that metformin therapy was associated with fewer hypoglycaemic episodes than sulfonylurea or insulin treatment, but more than with diet alone. One or more hypoglycaemic episodes were reported in 6% of the patients receiving the biguanide in this study, although only 1 patient had a severe episode.

1. United Kingdom Prospective Diabetes Study Group. United Kingdom prospective diabetes study (UKPDS) 13: relative efficacy of randomly allocated diet, sulphonylurea, insulin, or metformin in patients with newly diagnosed non-insulin dependent diabetes followed for 3 years. *BMJ* 1995; **310:** 83–8.

**Lactic acidosis.** There is a small but definite risk of lactic acidosis associated with use of biguanide antidiabetics. Most early reports involved phenformin, which was consequently removed from the market in many countries although cases of phenformin-associated lactic acidosis still occur.[1-3] There has therefore been concern about the risks of lactic acidosis with metformin, which is still in wide use. However, lactic acidosis with metformin appears to be much less common: a review suggested that the incidence was of the order of 3 cases per 100 000 patient years, which was 20 times less frequent than with phenformin.[4] This concurs with the findings of the FDA following the introduction of metformin to the US market: in the year following the marketing of metformin in the USA, the FDA had received reports of metformin-associated lactic acidosis in 66 patients,[5] the diagnosis being confirmed in 47. This represented a rate of about 5 cases per 100 000. Most patients who do develop lactic acidosis with metformin have one or more precipitating risk factors such as renal impairment, congestive heart failure, or other conditions predisposing to hypoxaemia or acute renal failure, including septicaemia, acute hepatic decompensation, alcohol abuse, acute myocardial infarction, and shock.[4] A systematic review,[6] which considered results comprising over 35 000 patient years of treatment with metformin, concluded that provided metformin was prescribed taking into account the proper contra-indications, there was no evidence of an increased risk of lactic acidosis. Nonetheless, there have been a few reports of lactic acidosis developing in metformin-treated patients without apparent risk factors.[4]

1. Rosand J, *et al.* Fatal phenformin-associated lactic acidosis. *Ann Intern Med* 1997; **127:** 170.
2. Enia G, *et al.* Lactic acidosis induced by phenformin is still a public health problem in Italy. *BMJ* 1997; **315:** 1466–7.
3. Kwong SC, Brubacher J. Phenformin and lactic acidosis: a case report and review. *J Emerg Med* 1998; **16:** 881–6.
4. Chan NN, *et al.* Metformin-associated lactic acidosis: a rare or very rare clinical entity? *Diabet Med* 1999; **16:** 273–81.
5. Misbin RI, *et al.* Lactic acidosis in patients with diabetes treated with metformin. *N Engl J Med* 1998; **338:** 265–6.
6. Salpeter S, *et al.* Risk of fatal and nonfatal lactic acidosis with metformin use in type 2 diabetes mellitus. Available in The Cochrane Library; Issue 2. Chichester: John Wiley; 2004.

**Pancreatitis.** References to acute pancreatitis associated with phenformin.[1,2]

1. Wilde H. Pancreatitis and phenformin. *Ann Intern Med* 1972; **77:** 324.
2. Chase HS, Mogan GR. Phenformin-associated pancreatitis. *Ann Intern Med* 1977; **87:** 314–15.

### Treatment of Adverse Effects

Acute poisoning with biguanides may lead to the development of lactic acidosis (p.1217) and calls for intensive supportive therapy. Glucose or glucagon may be required for hypoglycaemia, the general management of which is outlined in Insulin, p.335.

### Precautions

Biguanides are inappropriate for patients with diabetic coma and ketoacidosis, or for those with severe infection, trauma, or other severe conditions where the biguanide is unlikely to control the hyperglycaemia; insulin should be administered in such situations. Biguanides should not be given to patients with even mild renal impairment, as it may predispose patients to lactic acidosis, and renal function should be monitored throughout therapy. Dehydration may contribute to renal impairment. Conditions associated with hypoxia, such as acute heart failure, recent myocardial infarction, or shock, may increase the risk of lactic acidosis. Other conditions that may also predispose to lactic acidosis in a patient taking a biguanide include excessive alcohol intake and hepatic impairment. Biguanides should be temporarily stopped 48 hours before examinations using contrast media because of the risk of contrast media-induced renal impairment; biguanides should be withheld for at least 48 hours after the examination, and until normal renal function is confirmed.

Insulin is preferred for the treatment of diabetes in pregnancy.

Owing to the possibility of decreased vitamin $B_{12}$ absorption, annual monitoring of vitamin $B_{12}$ concentrations is advisable during long-term treatment.

**Driving.** In the UK, patients with diabetes mellitus treated with insulin or oral hypoglycaemics are required to notify their condition to the Driver and Vehicle Licensing Agency, who then assess their fitness to drive. Patients treated with oral hypoglycaemics are generally allowed to retain standard driving licences; those treated with insulin receive restricted licences which must be renewed (with appropriate checks) every 1 to 3 years. Patients should be warned of the dangers of hypoglycaemic attacks while driving, and should be counselled in appropriate management of the situation (stopping driving as soon as it is safe to do so, taking carbohydrate immediately, and quitting the driving seat and removing the ignition key from the car) should such an event occur. Patients who have lost hypoglycaemic awareness, or have frequent hypoglycaemic episodes, should not drive. In addition, eyesight must be adequate (field of vision of at least 120°) for a licence to be valid. Patients treated with diet or oral hypoglycaemics are normally allowed to hold vocational driving licences for heavy goods vehicles or passenger carrying vehicles; those treated with insulin may not drive such vehicles, and are restricted in driving some other vehicles such as small lorries and minibuses.

References.

1. British Diabetic Association (Diabetes UK). Information sheet: driving and diabetes: August 2003. Available at: http://www.diabetes.org.uk/infocentre/inform/downloads/drive.doc (accessed 07/07/04)
2. Driver and Vehicle Licensing Agency. For medical practitioners: at a glance guide to the current medical standards of fitness to drive (February 2004). Available at: http://www.dvla.gov.uk/at_a_glance/AAG2004feb.pdf (accessed 07/07/04)

### Interactions

Use of a biguanide with other drugs that lower blood-glucose concentrations increases the risk of hypoglycaemia, while drugs that increase blood glucose may reduce the effect of biguanide therapy.

In general fewer drug interactions have been reported with biguanides than with sulfonylureas. Alcohol may increase the risk of lactic acidosis as well as of hypoglycaemia. Care should be taken if biguanides are given with drugs that may impair renal function.

**Anticoagulants.** For the effect of metformin on *phenprocoumon*, see Antidiabetics, p.1025.

**Antivirals.** Fatal lactic acidosis has been reported[1] in a patient who received metformin with *didanosine*, *stavudine*, and *tenofovir*.

1. Worth L, *et al.* A cautionary tale: fatal lactic acidosis complicating nucleoside analogue and metformin therapy. *Clin Infect Dis* 2003; **37:** 315–16.

**Cimetidine.** Cimetidine increased plasma-metformin concentrations in 7 healthy subjects.[1] The renal clearance of metformin was reduced; competition for proximal tubular secretion was considered responsible. A reduction in metformin dosage may be required in patients taking metformin and cimetidine, in order to reduce the risk of lactic acidosis.

1. Somogyi A, *et al.* Reduction of metformin renal tubular secretion by cimetidine in man. *Br J Clin Pharmacol* 1987; **23:** 545–51.

**Ketotifen.** Platelet counts in 10 diabetic patients receiving biguanides fell (markedly in 3 patients) when they were also given ketotifen.[1] Counts returned to normal a few days after the end of ketotifen therapy. However, the investigators did not consider the effect clinically significant.

1. Doleček R. Ketotifen in the treatment of diabetics with various allergic conditions. *Pharmatherapeutica* 1981; **2:** 568–74.

**Sulfonylureas.** For reference to an apparent increase in mortality with an intensive regimen of metformin plus a sulfonylurea, see p.347.

### Uses and Administration

The biguanide antidiabetics are a class of antidiabetic drugs given by mouth in the treatment of type 2 diabetes mellitus (p.324). They are used to supplement treatment by diet modification when such modification has not proved effective on its own. In addition, because biguanides are not associated with weight gain they are preferred in obese patients. Although sulfonylureas (p.346) may be preferred in non-obese patients, a biguanide is often added or given instead to patients who are not responding to a sulfonylurea.

The mode of action of biguanides is not clear. They do not stimulate insulin release but require that some insulin be present in order to exert their antidiabetic effect. Possible mechanisms of action include delay in the absorption of glucose from the gastrointestinal tract, an increase in insulin sensitivity and glucose uptake into cells, and inhibition of hepatic gluconeogenesis. Biguanides do not usually lower blood-glucose concentrations in non-diabetic subjects.

**Hyperlipidaemias.** The effect of biguanides on lipid metabolism is unclear, although some studies have demonstrated a beneficial effect on serum-lipid profiles in both obese and lean patients with type 2 diabetes, hypertension and/or hyperlipidaemia.[1] Reductions in concentrations of total cholesterol, low-density and very low-density-lipoprotein cholesterol have been reported, as well as modest increases in high-density-lipoprotein cholesterol. Some studies have also reported a reduction in serum-triglyceride levels. Such effects may be beneficial in the long-term treatment of type 2 diabetes mellitus with concomitant lipid disorders.

1. Dunn CJ, Peters DH. Metformin: a review of its pharmacological properties and therapeutic use in non-insulin-dependent diabetes mellitus. *Drugs* 1995; **49:** 721–49.

**Polycystic ovary syndrome.** For discussion of the potential of metformin in polycystic ovary syndrome, see p.343.

### Preparations

**Proprietary Preparations** (details are given in Part 3)
**Multi-ingredient: *Mex.*:** Glinorboral.

## Buformin (USAN, pINN)

Buformina; DBV; W-37. 1-Butylbiguanide.
$C_6H_{15}N_5$ = 157.2.
*CAS — 692-13-7 (buformin); 1190-53-0 (buformin hydrochloride).*
*ATC — A10BA03.*

### Profile

Buformin is a biguanide antidiabetic (p.329). It is given by mouth in the treatment of type 2 diabetes mellitus (p.324) in doses of up to 300 mg daily. Buformin is also used as the hydrochloride.

### Preparations

**Proprietary Preparations** (details are given in Part 3)
***Spain:*** Silubin; ***Switz.:*** Silubin.

## Carbutamide (BAN, rINN)

BZ-55; Ca-1022; Carbutamida; Glybutamide; U-6987. 1-Butyl-3-sulphanilylurea.
$C_{11}H_{17}N_3O_3S$ = 271.3.
*CAS — 339-43-5.*
*ATC — A10BB06.*

### Profile

Carbutamide is a sulfonylurea antidiabetic (p.346). It is given by mouth in the treatment of type 2 diabetes mellitus (p.324) in single daily doses of 0.5 to 1 g, but is more toxic than chlorpropamide.

### Preparations

**Proprietary Preparations** (details are given in Part 3)
***Fr.:*** Glucidoral.

# Chlorpropamide (BAN, rINN)

Chlorpropamidum; Clorpropamida. 1-(4-Chlorobenzenesulphonyl)-3-propylurea.
$C_{10}H_{13}ClN_2O_3S$ = 276.7.
*CAS — 94-20-2.*
*ATC — A10BB02.*

**Pharmacopoeias.** In *Chin.*, *Eur.* (see p.vi), *Jpn*, *Pol.*, and *US.*
**Ph. Eur. 5.0** (Chlorpropamide). A white, crystalline powder. It exhibits polymorphism. Practically insoluble in water; soluble in alcohol; freely soluble in acetone and in dichloromethane; dissolves in dilute solutions of alkali hydroxides. Protect from light.
**USP 27** (Chlorpropamide). A white crystalline powder having a slight odour. Practically insoluble in water; soluble in alcohol; sparingly soluble in chloroform.

### Adverse Effects and Treatment

As for sulfonylureas in general, p.346.

Chlorpropamide may be more likely than other sulfonylureas to induce a syndrome of inappropriate secretion of antidiuretic hormone characterised by water retention, hyponatraemia, and CNS effects. Patients receiving chlorpropamide may develop facial flushing after drinking alcohol.

### Precautions

As for sulfonylureas in general, p.346.

Chlorpropamide should be avoided in the elderly and in renal or hepatic impairment because its long half-life increases the risk of hypoglycaemia. The antidiuretic effect of chlorpropamide may cause problems in patients with conditions associated with fluid retention.

**Porphyria.** Chlorpropamide has been associated with acute attacks of porphyria and is considered unsafe in porphyric patients.

**Thyroid disorders.** Some manufacturers recommend that chlorpropamide should not be used in patients with impaired thyroid function, but see under Sulfonylureas, p.346.

### Interactions

As for sulfonylureas in general, p.347.

Chlorpropamide may produce profound facial flushing associated with alcohol ingestion.

### Pharmacokinetics

Chlorpropamide is readily absorbed from the gastrointestinal tract and is extensively bound to plasma proteins. The half-life is about 35 hours. About 80% of a dose is metabolised in the liver; metabolites and unchanged drug are excreted in the urine. Chlorpropamide crosses the placenta and has been detected in breast milk.

### Uses and Administration

Chlorpropamide is a sulfonylurea antidiabetic (p.346). It has a duration of action of at least 24 hours, and is given by mouth in the treatment of type 2 **diabetes mellitus** (p.324) in an initial daily dose of 250 mg as a single dose with breakfast. It is usual to adjust this dose after 5 to 7 days to achieve an optimum maintenance dose which is usually in the range 100 to 500 mg daily; increasing the dose above 500 mg is unlikely to produce further benefit. Although a reduced dose range has been proposed for the elderly, use of chlorpropamide is inadvisable in this group.

Chlorpropamide, though not the other sulfonylureas, is also sometimes used in cranial **diabetes insipidus** (p.1314). It has been reported to act by sensitising the renal tubules to antidiuretic hormone. The dose has to be carefully adjusted to minimise the risk of hypoglycaemia. An initial dose of 100 mg daily, adjusted if necessary to a maximum of 350 mg daily has been recommended, although doses of up to 500 mg daily have been used.

**Diabetes mellitus.** Patients with type 2 diabetes whose blood glucose is adequately controlled at first by sulfonylureas often eventually experience treatment failure and loss of diabetic control. Results from the UK Prospective Diabetes Study[1] have suggested that the 6-year failure rate was higher in patients treated with glibenclamide (48%) than in those given chlorpropamide (40%). This difference was equivalent to delaying the requirement for additional therapy for a year in chlorpropamide-treated patients.

1. Matthews DR, *et al.* UKPDS 26: sulphonylurea failure in non-insulin-dependent diabetic patients over six years. *Diabet Med* 1998; **15:** 297–303.

### Preparations

***BP 2003:*** Chlorpropamide Tablets;
***USP 27:*** Chlorpropamide Tablets.

**Proprietary Preparations** (details are given in Part 3)

***Arg.:*** Diabinese; Idle; Trane; ***Austral.:*** Diabinese†; ***Belg.:*** Diabinese; ***Braz.:*** Diabecontrol; Diabinese; Glicoben; Glicorp; ***Canad.:*** Diabinese†; Novo-Propamide†; ***Chile:*** Diabinese; ***Gr.:*** Diabinese; ***Hong Kong:*** Diabinese; ***India:*** Copamide; ***Irl.:*** Diabinese†; ***Israel:*** Diabinese; Diabitex; ***Ital.:*** Diabemide; Diabexan†; ***Malaysia:*** Anti-D; Diabinese; Propamide; ***Mex.:*** Deavynfar†; Diabiclor; Diabinese; Insogen; ***Norw.:*** Diabinese†; ***S.Afr.:*** Diabinese†; Diabitex†; Hypomide; ***Singapore:*** Anti-D; Chlomide; Diabinese; Propamide; ***Spain:*** Diabinese; ***Swed.:*** Diabines†; ***Switz.:*** Diabinese†; ***Thai.:*** Diabeedol; Diabinese; Dibecon; Glycemin; Propamide; ***UK:*** Glymese†; ***USA:*** Diabinese.

**Multi-ingredient:** ***India:*** Chlorformin; ***Ital.:*** Bidiabe; Pleiamide; ***Mex.:*** Insogen Plus; Mellitron; Obinese; ***Switz.:*** Diabiformine.

---

## Epalrestat *(rINN)*

ONO-2235. 5-[(*Z,E*)-β-Methylcinnamylidene]-4-oxo-2-thioxo-3-thiazolidineacetic acid.

$C_{15}H_{13}NO_3S_2$ = 319.4.

*CAS — 82159-09-9.*

### Profile

Epalrestat inhibits the enzyme aldose reductase which catalyses the conversion of glucose to sorbitol. It has been suggested that accumulation of sorbitol in certain cells, occurring only in conditions of hyperglycaemia and resulting in a hyperosmotic effect, may be involved in the pathogenesis of some diabetic complications. Aldose reductase inhibitors have no influence on blood-glucose concentrations. Epalrestat is given by mouth for the treatment of diabetic complications including neuropathy (p.326), in a usual dose of 50 mg three times daily before meals.

◊ References.

1. Goto Y, *et al.* A placebo-controlled double-blind study of epalrestat (ONO-2235) in patients with diabetic neuropathy. *Diabet Med* 1993; **10** (suppl 2): 39S–43S.
2. Uchida K, *et al.* Effect of 24 weeks of treatment with epalrestat, an aldose reductase inhibitor, on peripheral neuropathy in patients with non-insulin-dependent diabetes mellitus. *Clin Ther* 1995; **17:** 460–6.
3. Hotta N, *et al.* Clinical investigation of epalrestat, an aldose reductase inhibitor, on diabetic neuropathy in Japan: multicenter study. *J Diabetes Complications* 1996; **10:** 168–72.
4. Ikeda T, *et al.* Long-term effect of epalrestat on cardiac autonomic neuropathy in subjects with non-insulin dependent diabetes mellitus. *Diabetes Res Clin Pract* 1999; **43:** 193–8.
5. Iso K, *et al.* Long-term effect of epalrestat, an aldose reductase inhibitor, on the development of incipient diabetic nephropathy in type 2 diabetic patients. *J Diabetes Complications* 2001; **15:** 241–4.

### Preparations

**Proprietary Preparations** (details are given in Part 3)

***Jpn:*** Kinedak.

---

## Glibenclamide *(BAN, rINN)*

Glibenclamida; Glibenclamidum; Glybenclamide; Glybenzcyclamide; Glyburide *(USAN)*; HB-419; U-26452. 1-{4-[2-(5-Chloro-2-methoxybenzamido)ethyl]benzenesulphonyl}-3-cyclohexylurea.

$C_{23}H_{28}ClN_3O_5S$ = 494.0.

*CAS — 10238-21-8.*

*ATC — A10BB01.*

NOTE. The name glibornuride has frequently but erroneously been applied to glibenclamide.

**Pharmacopoeias.** In *Chin., Eur.* (see p.vi), *Int., Jpn, Pol.,* and *US.*

**Ph. Eur. 5.0** (Glibenclamide). A white or almost white, crystalline powder. Practically insoluble in water; slightly soluble in alcohol and in methyl alcohol; sparingly soluble in dichloromethane.

**USP 27** (Glyburide). Store in airtight containers.

### Adverse Effects, Treatment, and Precautions

As for sulfonylureas in general, p.346.

◊ For a suggestion that the failure rate in type 2 diabetics treated with glibenclamide may be higher than that for those treated with chlorpropamide, see Diabetes Mellitus under Uses and Administration of Chlorpropamide, p.331.

**Effects on the blood.** References.

1. Nataas OB, Nesthus I. Immune haemolytic anaemia induced by glibenclamide in selective IgA deficiency. *BMJ* 1987; **295:** 366–7.
2. Israeli A, *et al.* Glibenclamide causing thrombocytopenia and bleeding tendency: case reports and a review of the literature. *Klin Wochenschr* 1988; **66:** 223–4.
3. Meloni G, Meloni T. Glyburide-induced acute haemolysis in a G6PD-deficient patient with NIDDM. *Br J Haematol* 1996; **92:** 159–60.
4. Noto H, *et al.* Glyburide-induced hemolysis in myelodysplastic syndrome. *Diabetes Care* 2000; **23:** 129.

**Hypoglycaemia.** Severe hypoglycaemia may occur in any patient treated with any sulfonylurea (see p.346); this potentially life-threatening complication requires prolonged and energetic treatment.[1] Glibenclamide has a relatively prolonged duration of action and appears to cause severe hypoglycaemia more often than shorter-acting sulfonylureas such as tolbutamide.

In a review[2] of 57 instances of hypoglycaemia associated with glibenclamide the median age of patients affected was 70 years; only one was less than 60 years old. Median daily dosage was 10 mg. Coma or disturbed consciousness was observed in 46 patients. Ten of these remained comatose despite alleviation of their hypoglycaemia and died up to 20 days after presentation. In discussing their review, the authors reported that, including the present series of 57 cases, there had been published reports on 101 severe hypoglycaemias with glibenclamide, 14 with a fatal outcome.

There has been a report[3] of hypoglycaemic coma associated with the inhalation of glibenclamide by a worker at a pharmaceutical plant.

1. Ferner RE, Neil HAW. Sulphonylureas and hypoglycaemia. *BMJ* 1988; **296:** 949–50.
2. Asplund K, *et al.* Glibenclamide-associated hypoglycaemia: a report on 57 cases. *Diabetologia* 1983; **24:** 412–17.
3. Albert F, *et al.* Hypoglycaemia by inhalation. *Lancet* 1993; **342:** 47–8.

**Porphyria.** Glibenclamide has been associated with acute attacks of porphyria and is considered unsafe in porphyric patients.

### Interactions

As for sulfonylureas in general, p.347.

### Pharmacokinetics

Glibenclamide is readily absorbed from the gastrointestinal tract, peak plasma concentrations usually occurring within 2 to 4 hours, and is extensively bound to plasma proteins. Absorption may be slower in hyperglycaemic patients and may differ according to the particle size of the preparation used. It is metabolised, almost completely, in the liver, the principal metabolite being only very weakly active. Approximately 50% of a dose is excreted in the urine and 50% via the bile into the faeces.

◊ References.

1. Coppack SW, *et al.* Pharmacokinetic and pharmacodynamic studies of glibenclamide in non-insulin dependent diabetes mellitus. *Br J Clin Pharmacol* 1990; **29:** 673–84.
2. Jaber LA, *et al.* The pharmacokinetics and pharmacodynamics of 12 weeks of glyburide therapy in obese diabetics. *Eur J Clin Pharmacol* 1993; **45:** 459–63.
3. Hoffman A, *et al.* The effect of hyperglycaemia on the absorption of glibenclamide in patients with non-insulin-dependent diabetes mellitus. *Eur J Clin Pharmacol* 1994; **47:** 53–5.
4. Rydberg T, *et al.* Concentration-effect relations of glibenclamide and its active metabolites in man: modelling of pharmacokinetics and pharmacodynamics. *Br J Clin Pharmacol* 1997; **43:** 373–81.

### Uses and Administration

Glibenclamide is a sulfonylurea antidiabetic (p.346). It is given by mouth in the treatment of type 2 diabetes mellitus (p.324) and has a duration of action of up to 24 hours.

The usual initial dose of conventional formulations in type 2 diabetes mellitus is 2.5 to 5 mg daily with breakfast, adjusted every 7 days by increments of 2.5 or 5 mg daily up to 15 mg daily. Although increasing the dose above 15 mg is unlikely to produce further benefit, doses of up to 20 mg daily have been given. Doses greater than 10 mg daily may be given in 2 divided doses. Because of the relatively long duration of action of glibenclamide, it is best avoided in the elderly.

In some countries micronised preparations of glibenclamide are available, in which the drug is formulated with a smaller particle size, and which have enhanced bioavailability. The usual initial dose of one such preparation (Glynase, USA) is 1.5 to 3 mg daily, adjusted every 7 days by increments of 1.5 mg, up to a usual maximum of 12 mg daily. Doses greater than 6 mg daily may be given in 2 divided doses.

**Action.** Proceedings of a symposium on the mechanism of action of glibenclamide.[1]

1. Gavin JR, ed. Glyburide: new insights into its effects on the beta cell and beyond. *Am J Med* 1990; **89** (suppl 2A): 1–53S.

EFFECTS ON THE HEART. A reduced incidence of ventricular fibrillation has been reported in diabetics treated with glibenclamide who develop myocardial infarction, compared with those receiving other treatments or with nondiabetic patients with myocardial infarction.[1] However, some evidence has also suggested that sulfonylureas may impair the adaptive responses of the heart to ischaemia—see p.346.

1. Lomuscio A, *et al.* Effects of glibenclamide on ventricular fibrillation in non-insulin-dependent diabetes with acute myocardial infarction. *Coron Artery Dis* 1994; **5:** 767–71.

### Preparations

***BP 2003:*** Glibenclamide Tablets;
***USP 27:*** Glyburide Tablets.

**Proprietary Preparations** (details are given in Part 3)

***Arg.:*** Daonil; Diabemin; Euglucon; Gardoton; Glibediab; Glidanil; Glitral; Gon; Pira; ***Austral.:*** Daonil; Glimel; Semi-Daonil; ***Austria:*** Daonil; Dia-Eptal; Euglucon; Gewaglucon; Gilemal; Glucobene; Glucostad; Neoglu-conin†; Normoglucon; Semi-Euglucon; ***Belg.:*** Bevoren; Daonil; Euglucon; ***Braz.:*** Aglucil; Benclamin; Clamiben; Daonil; Di-Solvente†; Diaben; Diabexil; Euglucon; Gliben; Glibenclamon; Glibexil; Glionil; Lisaglucon; Uni Gliben; ***Canad.:*** DiaBeta; Euglucon; Gen-Glybe; ***Chile:*** Daonil; Euglusid; ***Denm.:*** Daonil; Euglucon†; Hexaglucon; Regulin; ***Fin.:*** Daonil; Euglamin; Euglucon; Origlucon; Semi-Euglucon; ***Fr.:*** Daonil; Euglucan; Hemi-Daonil; Miglucan; ***Ger.:*** Azuglucon; Bastiverit; Dia-BASF†; duraglucon N; Euglucon N; Glib; Glib-ratiopharm; Gliben; Gliben-Azu; Gliben-Puren N; Glibenbeta; Glibendoc; Glibenhexal; Glimidstada; Gluco-Tablinen†; Gluconorm†; Glucoremed; Glukoreduct; Glukovital; glycolande N; Humedia; Maninil; Praeciglucon; Semi-Euglucon N; Semi-Gliben-Puren N†; ***Gr.:*** Daonil; Deroctyl; ***Hong Kong:*** Calabren; Clamide; Daonil; Euglucon; GBN†; Gliben; Gliboral; Glimel; Melix†; Semi-Daonil; Semi-Euglucon; Xeltic; ***India:*** Daonil; Euglucon; Semi-Daonil; Semi-Euglucon; ***Irl.:*** Daonil; Melbetese†; Semi-Daonil; ***Israel:*** Daonil; Glibetic; Gluben; ***Ital.:*** Daonil; Euglucon; Gliben; Gliboral; ***Malaysia:*** Claben; Daonil; Debtan; Dibelet; Gliben; Glibesyn; Glimide; ***Mex.:*** Abuglib; Biostin; Daonil; Dibetid†; Diglexol; Euglucon; Glemicid; Glibenil; Glibenval; Glicoxem†; Glifarcal; Glikeyer; Glucal; Glucoven; Nadib; Norboral; Reglusan; Saluglibent†; ***Neth.:*** Daonil; Euglucon†; Hemi-Daonil; Semi-Euglucon†; ***Norw.:*** Daonil; Euglucon†; ***NZ:*** Daonil†; Gliben; Semi-Daonil†; ***Port.:*** Daonil; Euglucon; Semi-Daonil; Semi-Euglucon; ***S.Afr.:*** Daonil; Diacare; Euglucon; Glycomin; ***Singapore:*** Clamide; Daonil; Dibelet; Euglucon†; GBN; Glibemid; Glibesyn†; Glimide; ***Spain:*** Daonil; Euglucon; Glucolon; Norglicem; ***Swed.:*** Daonil; Euglucon; ***Switz.:*** Daonil; Euglucon; gli-basan; Glibesifar; Melix; Semi-Daonil; Semi-Euglucon; ***Thai.:*** Benclamin; BNIL; Cytagon; Daonil; Daono; Debtan; Diabenol; Dibelet; Diclanil; Euglucon; Glencamide; Gliben; Glibesyn†; Glibetic; Glibic; Gluconil; Gluzo; Locose; Manoglucon; Med-Glionil; Semi-Euglucon; Sugril; ***UAE:*** Glynase; Mini-Glynase; ***UK:*** Calabren†; Daonil; Diabetamide; Euglucon; Malix†; Semi-Daonil; ***USA:*** DiaBeta; Glynase; Micronase.

**Multi-ingredient:** ***Chile:*** Bi-Euglucon M; Glucovance; ***Gr.:*** Normell; ***Ital.:*** Bi-Euglucon; Bi-Euglucon M; Gliben F; Glibomet; Gliconorm; Glicorest; Gliformin; Glucomide; Suguan; Suguan M; ***Mex.:*** Bi-Euglucon M; Dabex G†; Glinorboral; Sil-Norboral; ***Port.:*** Glucovance; ***USA:*** Diofen; Glucovance.

---

## Glibornuride *(BAN, USAN, rINN)*

Glibornurida; Ro-6-4563. 1-[(2*S*,3*R*)-2-Hydroxyborn-3-yl]-3-tosylurea; 1-[(2*S*,3*R*)-2-Hydroxyborn-3-yl]-3-*p*-tolylsulphonylurea.

$C_{18}H_{26}N_2O_4S$ = 366.5.

*CAS — 26944-48-9.*

*ATC — A10BB04.*

NOTE. The name glibornuride has frequently but erroneously been applied to glibenclamide.

### Profile

Glibornuride is a sulfonylurea antidiabetic (p.346). It is given by mouth in the treatment of type 2 diabetes mellitus (p.324) in doses of 12.5 to 75 mg daily. Daily doses of 50 mg or more are given in 2 divided doses.

## Preparations

**Proprietary Preparations** (details are given in Part 3)
***Austria:*** Gluborid†; Glutril; ***Fr.:*** Glutril; ***Ger.:*** Gluborid; Glutril; ***Switz.:*** Gluborid; Glutril.

## Gliclazide *(BAN, rINN)*

Gliclazida; Gliclazidum; Glyclazide; SE-1702. 1-(3-Azabicyclo[3.3.0]oct-3-yl)-3-tosylurea; 1-(3-Azabicyclo[3.3.0]oct-3-yl)-3-*p*-tolylsulphonylurea.

$C_{15}H_{21}N_3O_3S$ = 323.4.
*CAS — 21187-98-4.*
*ATC — A10BB09.*

**Pharmacopoeias.** In *Chin.* and *Eur.* (see p.vi).

**Ph. Eur. 5.0** (Gliclazide). A white or almost white powder. Practically insoluble in water; slightly soluble in alcohol; sparingly soluble in acetone; freely soluble in dichloromethane.

### Adverse Effects, Treatment, and Precautions

As for sulfonylureas in general, p.346.

The *British National Formulary* suggests that gliclazide may be suitable for use in patients with renal impairment, but careful monitoring of blood-glucose concentration is essential. The UK manufacturers recommend that it should not be used in patients with severe renal impairment.

### Interactions

As for sulfonylureas in general, p.347.

### Pharmacokinetics

Gliclazide is readily absorbed from the gastrointestinal tract. It is extensively bound to plasma proteins. The half-life is about 10 to 12 hours. Gliclazide is extensively metabolised in the liver to metabolites that have no significant hypoglycaemic activity. Metabolites and a small amount of unchanged drug are excreted in the urine.

◊ References.


1. Kobayashi K, *et al.* Pharmacokinetics of gliclazide in healthy and diabetic subjects. *J Pharm Sci* 1984; **73:** 1684–7.


### Uses and Administration

Gliclazide is a sulfonylurea antidiabetic (p.346). It is given by mouth in the treatment of type 2 diabetes mellitus (p.324) and has a duration of action of 12 to 24 hours. Because its effects are less prolonged than those of chlorpropamide or glibenclamide it may be more suitable for elderly patients, who are prone to hypoglycaemia with longer-acting sulfonylureas. The usual initial dose is 40 to 80 mg daily, gradually increased, if necessary, up to 320 mg daily. Doses of more than 160 mg daily are given in 2 divided doses. A modified-release tablet is also available: the usual initial dose is 30 mg once daily, increased if necessary up to a maximum of 120 mg daily.

◊ References.


1. Palmer KJ, Brogden RN. Gliclazide: an update of its pharmacological properties and therapeutic efficacy in non-insulin-dependent diabetes mellitus. *Drugs* 1993; **46:** 92–125.
2. Mailhot J. Efficacy and safety of gliclazide in the treatment of non-insulin-dependent diabetes mellitus: a Canadian multicenter study. *Clin Ther* 1993; **15:** 1060–8.
3. Ziegler O, Drouin P. Hemobiological properties of gliclazide. *J Diabetes Complications* 1994; **8:** 235–9.
4. Jennings PE. Vascular benefits of gliclazide beyond glycemic control. *Metabolism* 2000; **49** (suppl 2): 17–20.
5. Crepaldi G, Fioretto P. Gliclazide modified release: its place in the therapeutic armamentarium. *Metabolism* 2000; **49** (suppl 2): 21–5.
6. McGavin JK, *et al.* Gliclazide modified release. *Drugs* 2002; **62:** 1357–64.


### Preparations

***BP 2003:*** Gliclazide Tablets.

**Proprietary Preparations** (details are given in Part 3)
***Arg.:*** Aglucide; Diamicron; Unava; ***Austral.:*** Diamicron; Glyade; Nidem; ***Austria:*** Diamicron; ***Belg.:*** Diamicron; ***Braz.:*** Diamicron; ***Canad.:*** Diamicron; ***Chile:*** Dianormax; ***Denm.:*** Diamicron; ***Fr.:*** Diamicron; Glycemirex†; ***Ger.:*** Diamicron; ***Gr.:*** Diamicron; ***Hong Kong:*** Diamicron; Diamitex; Glimicron; Glupozide; ***India:*** Diamicron; Gliza; Lycazid; ***Irl.:*** Diabrezide; Diaclide; Diamicron; ***Ital.:*** Diabrezide; Diamicron; ***Malaysia:*** Diacron; Diamicron; Dianid; Glimicron; Glucozide; Glyade; Melicron; Sun-Glizide; ***Mex.:*** Diamicron; ***Neth.:*** Diamicron; ***NZ:*** Diamicron; ***Port.:*** Diamicron; ***S.Afr.:*** Diaglucide; Diamicron; Glucomed; Glycron; Ziclin; ***Singapore:*** Diamicron; Glimicron; Glucozide; Medoclazide†; Melicron; Sun-Glizide†; ***Spain:*** Diamicron; ***Switz.:*** Diamicron; ***Thai.:*** Cadicon; Diabeside; Diaclaron; Dialoc†; Diamaze; Diamexon; Diamicron; Dianid; Glicron; Glucocron; Glucozide†; Glycon; Medoclazide; Serviclazide; ***UAE:*** Glyzide; ***UK:*** Diaglyk; Diamicron.

## Glimepiride *(BAN, USAN, rINN)*

Glimepirida; Hoe-490. 1-({*p*-[2-(3-Ethyl-4-methyl-2-oxo-3-pyrroline-1-carboxamido)ethyl]phenyl}sulfonyl)-3-(*trans*-4-methylcyclohexyl)urea.

$C_{24}H_{34}N_4O_5S$ = 490.6.
*CAS — 93479-97-1.*
*ATC — A10BB12.*

### Adverse Effects, Treatment, and Precautions

As for sulfonylureas in general, p.346. In some countries hepatic and haematological monitoring is recommended in patients receiving glimepiride; in the UK the *British National Formulary* considers the practical value of such monitoring unproven.

### Interactions

As for sulfonylureas in general, p.347.

### Pharmacokinetics

Glimepiride is completely absorbed from the gastrointestinal tract. Peak plasma concentrations occur in 2 to 3 hours, and it is highly protein bound. The drug is extensively metabolised to two main metabolites, a hydroxy derivative and a carboxy derivative. The half-life after multiple doses is about 9 hours. Approximately 60% of a dose is eliminated in the urine and 40% in the faeces.

### Uses and Administration

Glimepiride is a sulfonylurea antidiabetic (p.346). It is given by mouth for the treatment of type 2 diabetes mellitus (p.324). Doses of 1 to 2 mg daily by mouth initially may be increased if necessary to 4 mg daily for maintenance. The maximum recommended dose is 6 mg in the UK and 8 mg in the USA.

◊ References.


1. Langtry HD, Balfour JA. Glimepiride: a review of its use in the management of type 2 diabetes mellitus. *Drugs* 1998; **55:** 563–84.
2. Campbell RK. Glimepiride: role of a new sulfonylurea in the treatment of type 2 diabetes mellitus. *Ann Pharmacother* 1998; **32:** 1044–52.
3. McCall AL. Clinical review of glimepiride. *Expert Opin Pharmacother* 2001; **2:** 699–713.
4. Massi-Benedetti M. Glimepiride in type 2 diabetes mellitus: a review of the worldwide therapeutic experience. *Clin Ther* 2003; **25:** 799–816.
5. Weitgasser R, *et al.* Effects of glimepiride on HbA(1c) and body weight in type 2 diabetes: results of a 1.5-year follow-up study. *Diabetes Res Clin Pract* 2003; **61:** 13–19.
6. Feinbock C, *et al.* Prospective multicentre trial comparing the efficacy of, and compliance with, glimepiride or acarbose treatment in patients with type 2 diabetes not controlled with diet alone. *Diabetes Nutr Metab* 2003; **16:** 214–21.


### Preparations

**Proprietary Preparations** (details are given in Part 3)
***Arg.:*** Amaryl; Endial; Glemaz; Gluceride; Glucopirida; Islopir; ***Austral.:*** Amaryl; Dimirel; ***Austria:*** Amaryl; ***Belg.:*** Amarylle; ***Braz.:*** Amaryl; Glimepil; Glimesec; ***Chile:*** Amaryl; ***Denm.:*** Amaryl; ***Fin.:*** Amaryl; ***Fr.:*** Amarel; ***Ger.:*** Amaryl; ***Gr.:*** Solosa; ***Hong Kong:*** Amaryl; ***India:*** Amaryl; Euglim; ***Irl.:*** Amaryl; ***Ital.:*** Amaryl; Solosa; ***Malaysia:*** Amaryl; ***Mex.:*** Amaryl; ***Neth.:*** Amaryl; ***Norw.:*** Amaryl; ***Port.:*** Amaryl; Glimial; ***S.Afr.:*** Amaryl; ***Singapore:*** Amaryl; ***Spain:*** Amaryl; Roname; ***Swed.:*** Amaryl; ***Switz.:*** Amaryl; ***Thai.:*** Amaryl; ***UK:*** Amaryl; ***USA:*** Amaryl.

## Glipizide *(BAN, USAN, pINN)*

CP-28720; Glipizida; Glipizidum; Glydiazinamide; K-4024. 1-Cyclohexyl-3-{4-[2-(5-methylpyrazine-2-carboxamido)ethyl]benzenesulphonyl}urea.

$C_{21}H_{27}N_5O_4S$ = 445.5.
*CAS — 29094-61-9.*
*ATC — A10BB07.*

**Pharmacopoeias.** In *Chin., Eur.* (see p.vi), and *US.*

**Ph. Eur. 5.0** (Glipizide). A white or almost white crystalline powder. Practically insoluble in water and in alcohol; sparingly soluble in acetone; soluble in dichloromethane. It dissolves in dilute solutions of alkali hydroxides.

**USP 27** (Glipizide). Store in airtight containers. Protect from light.

### Adverse Effects, Treatment, and Precautions

As for sulfonylureas in general, p.346.

**Porphyria.** Glipizide has been associated with acute attacks of porphyria and is considered unsafe in porphyric patients.

### Interactions

As for sulfonylureas in general, p.347.

**Antacids.** *Magnesium hydroxide* and *sodium bicarbonate* have been reported to increase the rate of absorption, although not the total amount absorbed, of a dose of glipizide in healthy subjects.[1,2] No such effect was seen with *aluminium hydroxide.*[2]


1. Kivisto KT, Neuvonen PJ. Enhancement of absorption and effect of glipizide by magnesium hydroxide. *Clin Pharmacol Ther* 1991; **49:** 39–43.
2. Kivisto KT, Neuvonen PJ. Differential effects of sodium bicarbonate and aluminium hydroxide on the absorption and activity of glipizide. *Eur J Clin Pharmacol* 1991; **40:** 383–6.


### Pharmacokinetics

Glipizide is readily absorbed from the gastrointestinal tract with peak plasma concentrations occurring 1 to 3 hours after a single dose. It is extensively bound to plasma proteins and has a half-life of approximately 2 to 4 hours. It is metabolised mainly in the liver and excreted chiefly in the urine, largely as inactive metabolites.

### Uses and Administration

Glipizide is a sulfonylurea antidiabetic (p.346). It is given by mouth in the treatment of type 2 diabetes mellitus (p.324) and has a duration of action of up to 24 hours. The usual initial dose is 2.5 to 5 mg daily given as a single dose about 30 minutes before breakfast. Dosage may be adjusted at intervals of several days by amounts of 2.5 to 5 mg daily, to a maximum of 20 mg daily. Doses up to 40 mg daily have been used, but see below. Doses larger than 15 mg daily are given in two divided doses before meals. Modified-release formulations of glipizide are available in some countries; one such preparation (Glucotrol XL, USA) is given in doses of 5 to 10 mg daily as a single dose with breakfast.

**Administration.** Although glipizide may be given in doses up to a maximum of 40 mg daily, evidence for the benefits of high doses is scanty. A small study in patients with type 2 diabetes mellitus found that not only did increases in glipizide doses to more than 10 mg daily produce little or no benefit, but that the higher doses were associated with reduced rises in plasma-insulin concentrations and a lesser reduction in plasma-glucose concentrations.[1] There is, however, some evidence that glycaemic control and insulin sensitivity can be improved by the use of a modified-release rather than a conventional formulation of glipizide.[2,3]


1. Stenman S, *et al.* What is the benefit of increasing the sulfonylurea dose? *Ann Intern Med* 1993; **118:** 169–72.
2. Berelowitz M, *et al.* Comparative efficacy of once-daily controlled-release formulation of glipizide and immediate-release glipizide in patients with NIDDM. *Diabetes Care* 1994; **17:** 1460–4.
3. Leaf E, King JO. Patient outcomes after formulary conversion from immediate-release to extended-release glipizide tablets. *Am J Health-Syst Pharm* 1999; **56:** 454–6.


### Preparations

***BP 2003:*** Glipizide Tablets;
***USP 27:*** Glipizide Tablets.

**Proprietary Preparations** (details are given in Part 3)
***Arg.:*** Minodiab; ***Austral.:*** Melizide; Minidiab; ***Austria:*** Glibenese; Minidiab; ***Belg.:*** Glibenese; Minidiab; ***Braz.:*** Glipgen; Minidiab; ***Chile:*** Minidiab; Xiprine; ***Denm.:*** Glibenese; Mindiab; ***Fin.:*** Apamid; Glibenese; Melizid; Mindiab; ***Fr.:*** Glibenese; Minidiab; Ozidia; ***Ger.:*** Glibenese†; ***Gr.:*** Glibenese; Minodiab; ***Hong Kong:*** Diasef; Glidiab†; Glucotrol; Minidiab; ***India:*** Glide; Glipicontin; Glucolip; Glynase; Glyzip; ***Irl.:*** Glibenese; ***Israel:*** Glucorite; ***Ital.:*** Minidiab; ***Malaysia:*** Glix; Melizide; ***Mex.:*** Glupitel; Luditec; Minodiab; ***Neth.:*** Glibenese; Minidiab; ***Norw.:*** Apamid; Mindiab; ***NZ:*** Glipid; Minidiab; ***Port.:*** Minidiab; ***S.Afr.:*** Minidiab; ***Singapore:*** Beapizide; Diasef; Melizide; Minidiab; ***Spain:*** Glibenese; Minodiab; ***Swed.:*** Apamid; Glipiscand; Mindiab; ***Switz.:*** Glibenese; ***Thai.:*** Apamid; Depizide; Diasef; Dipazide; Gipzide; Glizide; Glucodiab; Glygen; Melizide; Minibit; Minidiab; ***UK:*** Glibenese; Minodiab; ***USA:*** Glucotrol.

**Multi-ingredient:** ***USA:*** Metaglip.

## Gliquidone *(BAN, rINN)*

ARDF-26; Gliquidona. 1-Cyclohexyl-3-{4-[2-(3,4-dihydro-7-methoxy-4,4-dimethyl-1,3-dioxo-2(1*H*)-isoquinolyl)ethyl]benzenesulphonyl}urea.

$C_{27}H_{33}N_3O_6S$ = 527.6.
*CAS — 33342-05-1.*
*ATC — A10BB08.*

**Pharmacopoeias.** In *Br.*

**BP 2003** (Gliquidone). A white or almost white powder. Practically insoluble in water; slightly soluble in alcohol and in methyl alcohol; soluble in acetone; freely soluble in dimethylformamide.

### Adverse Effects, Treatment, and Precautions

As for sulfonylureas in general, p.346.

Since renal excretion plays little part in the elimination of gliquidone, it has been suggested by the *British National Formulary* that it may be suitable in patients with renal impairment, but careful monitoring of blood-glucose concentration is essential. The UK manufacturers recommend that it should not be used in patients with severe renal impairment.

### Interactions

As for sulfonylureas in general, p.347.

### Pharmacokinetics

Gliquidone is readily absorbed from the gastrointestinal tract. It is extensively bound to plasma proteins and has a half-life of approximately 1.5 hours. It is extensively metabolised in the liver, the metabolites having no significant hypoglycaemic effect, and is eliminated chiefly in the faeces via the bile; only about 5% of a dose is excreted in the urine.

### Uses and Administration

Gliquidone is a sulfonylurea antidiabetic (p.346). It is given by mouth in the treatment of type 2 diabetes mellitus (p.324) in a usual initial dosage of 15 mg daily given as a single dose up to

30 minutes before breakfast. Dosage may be adjusted by increments of 15 mg to a usual dose of 45 to 60 mg daily in 2 or 3 unequally divided doses, the largest dose being taken in the morning with breakfast. Single doses above 60 mg and daily doses above 180 mg are not recommended.

### Preparations

**BP 2003:** Gliquidone Tablets.

**Proprietary Preparations** (details are given in Part 3)
***Austria:*** Glurenorm; ***Belg.:*** Glurenorm; ***Ger.:*** Glurenorm; ***Ital.:*** Glurenor; ***Port.:*** Glurenor; ***Spain:*** Glurenor; ***Thai.:*** Glurenor; ***UK:*** Glurenorm.

---

## Glisentide *(rINN)*

Glipentide; Glisentida. 1-Cyclopentyl-3-[*p*-(2-o-anisamidoethyl)benzenesulphonyl]urea.

$C_{22}H_{27}N_3O_5S$ = 445.5.
*CAS — 32797-92-5.*

### Profile

Glisentide is a sulfonylurea antidiabetic (p.346). It is given by mouth in the treatment of type 2 diabetes mellitus (p.324) in doses of 2.5 to 20 mg daily.

### Preparations

**Proprietary Preparations** (details are given in Part 3)
***Spain:*** Staticum.

---

## Glisolamide *(rINN)*

Glisolamida. 1-Cyclohexyl-3-{*p*-[2-(5-methylisoxazole-3-carboxamido)ethyl]benzenesulphonyl}urea.

$C_{20}H_{26}N_4O_5S$ = 434.5.
*CAS — 24477-37-0.*

### Profile

Glisolamide is a sulfonylurea antidiabetic (p.346). It is given by mouth in the treatment of type 2 diabetes mellitus (p.324) in doses of 5 to 20 mg daily.

### Preparations

**Proprietary Preparations** (details are given in Part 3)
***Ital.:*** Diabenor.

---

## Glisoxepide *(BAN, rINN)*

Bay-b-4231; FBB-4231; Glisoxepid; Glisoxepida; RP-22410. 1-(Perhydroazepin-1-yl)-3-{4-[2-(5-methylisoxazole-3-carboxamido)ethyl]benzenesulphonyl}urea.

$C_{20}H_{27}N_5O_5S$ = 449.5.
*CAS — 25046-79-1.*
*ATC — A10BB11.*

### Profile

Glisoxepide is a sulfonylurea antidiabetic (p.346). It is given by mouth in the treatment of type 2 diabetes mellitus (p.324) in a usual initial dose of 2 to 4 mg daily at breakfast, increased if necessary up to 16 mg daily in divided doses.

### Preparations

**Proprietary Preparations** (details are given in Part 3)
***Austria:*** Pro-Diaban; ***Ger.:*** Pro-Diaban†.

---

## Glybuzole *(rINN)*

AN-1324; Désaglybuzole; Glibuzol; RP-7891. *N*-(5-*tert*-Butyl-1,3,4-thiadiazol-2-yl)benzenesulphonamide.

$C_{12}H_{15}N_3O_2S_2$ = 297.4.
*CAS — 1492-02-0.*

### Profile

Glybuzole is an oral antidiabetic with a structure distinct from that of the sulfonylureas, biguanides, or sulfonamidopyrimidines.

---

## Glyclopyramide *(rINN)*

Gliclopiramida. 1-(4-Chlorobenzenesulphonyl)-3-(pyrrolidin-1-yl)urea.

$C_{11}H_{14}ClN_3O_3S$ = 303.8.
*CAS — 631-27-6.*

### Profile

Glyclopyramide is a sulfonylurea antidiabetic (p.346). It has been given by mouth in the treatment of type 2 diabetes mellitus.

---

## Glycyclamide *(rINN)*

Gliciclamida; Gliciclamide; K-38; K-386; Tolcyclamide. 1-Cyclohexyl-3-tosylurea; 1-Cyclohexyl-3-*p*-tolylsulphonylurea.

$C_{14}H_{20}N_2O_3S$ = 296.4.
*CAS — 664-95-9.*

### Profile

Glycyclamide is a sulfonylurea antidiabetic (p.346). It is given by mouth in the treatment of type 2 diabetes mellitus.

The symbol † denotes a preparation no longer actively marketed

### Preparations

**Proprietary Preparations** (details are given in Part 3)
***Ital.:*** Diaborale.

---

## Glymidine Sodium *(BAN, USAN, rINN)*

Glimidina sódica; Glycodiazine; Glymidine; SH-717. *N*-[5-(2-Methoxyethoxy)pyrimidin-2-yl]benzenesulphonamide sodium.

$C_{13}H_{14}N_3NaO_4S$ = 331.3.
*CAS — 3459-20-9 (glymidine sodium); 339-44-6 (glymidine).*
*ATC — A10BC01.*

### Profile

Glymidine sodium is a sulfonamidopyrimidine antidiabetic; its actions and uses are similar to those of the sulfonylureas (p.346) and it has been given by mouth in the treatment of type 2 diabetes mellitus.

---

# Guar Gum

E412; Goma guar; Guar Flour; Guar Galactomannan; Jaguar Gum.
*CAS — 9000-30-0.*
*ATC — A10BX01.*

**Pharmacopoeias.** In *Eur.* (see p.vi). Also in *USNF.*

**Ph. Eur. 5.0** (Guar). Guar is obtained by grinding the endosperms of the seeds of *Cyamopsis tetragonolobus*. It consists mainly of guar galactomannan. Guar is a white or almost white powder, yielding a mucilage of variable viscosity when dissolved in water. Practically insoluble in alcohol.

**Ph. Eur. 5.0** (Guar Galactomannan). A yellowish-white powder. It is soluble in cold and hot water; practically insoluble in organic solvents. Its main components are polysaccharides composed of D-galactose and D-mannose at molecular ratios of 1:1.4 to 1:2. The molecules consist of a linear main chain of β-(1→4)-glycosidically linked mannopyranoses and single α-(1→6)-glycosidically linked galactopyranoses.

**USNF 22** (Guar Gum). A gum obtained from the ground endosperms of *Cyamopsis tetragonolobus* (Leguminosae). It consists chiefly of a high-molecular-weight hydrocolloidal polysaccharide, a galactomannan, composed of galactan and mannan units combined through glycosidic linkages. It is a white to yellowish-white, practically odourless, powder. Dispersible in hot or cold water forming a colloidal solution.

## Adverse Effects and Precautions

Guar gum can cause gastrointestinal disturbance with flatulence, diarrhoea, or nausea, particularly at the start of treatment.

Because guar gum swells on contact with liquid it should always be washed down carefully with water and should not be taken immediately before going to bed. It should not be used in patients with dysphagia, oesophageal disease, or intestinal obstruction.

## Interactions

Guar gum may retard the absorption of other drugs; where this is likely to pose a problem the other drug should be taken at least an hour before guar gum.

## Uses and Administration

Guar gum is used in diabetes mellitus (p.324) as an adjunct to treatment with diet, insulin, or oral antidiabetics since it results in some reduction in both postprandial and fasting blood-glucose concentrations. It is given with or immediately before meals in doses of 5 g usually three times daily. Adverse gastrointestinal effects may be reduced by using a lower initial dose. Each dose of guar gum granules should be taken stirred in about 200 mL of a cold drink. Alternatively it can be sprinkled over or mixed with food which must be taken with about 200 mL of fluid. Guar gum has also been incorporated into various foods.

Guar gum is also used to slow gastric emptying in some patients with the dumping syndrome (p.1242). It is also used as an adjunct in the treatment of hyperlipidaemias.

Guar gum is also used as a thickening and suspending agent, and as a tablet binder.

◊ Guar gum is an example of a soluble fibre.[1] On contact with water it forms a highly viscous gel, the viscosity of which varies with such factors as its plant source or the form in which it is administered.[2]

Fibres such as guar gum reduce postprandial and fasting blood-glucose concentrations as well as plasma-insulin concentrations in healthy subjects and diabetic patients.[1,3,4] Such reductions in blood-glucose concentrations and in glycosylated haemoglobin have been demonstrated in both type 1 and type 2 **diabetes**, but they have generally been small.[3] Possible mechanisms for these effects of guar gum include a delay in gastric emptying,[1,3-5] decreased small-bowel motility,[1,4] decreased glucose absorption resulting from increased viscosity of the contents of the gastrointestinal tract,[1,3] or inhibition of gastrointestinal hormones.[3]

Guar gum also lowers serum total cholesterol and low-density-lipoprotein (LDL) cholesterol concentrations; high-density-lipoprotein (HDL) cholesterol and triglyceride concentrations appear to be unaffected.[4] The most likely mechanism is binding of bile acids, reducing their enterohepatic circulation in a similar way to bile-acid sequestrants.[3,4] When used alone in patients with **hypercholesterolaemia** guar gum has generally produced a modest reduction in plasma-cholesterol and LDL-cholesterol concentrations although some studies have been unable to demonstrate an effect. A few studies have suggested that the cholesterol-lowering effect is attenuated after 8 to 12 weeks of treatment but a long-term study observed a 17% decrease in total serum cholesterol that was maintained for 24 months.[6] Some studies have shown further reductions in cholesterol and LDL-cholesterol concentrations on addition of guar gum to therapy with other lipid regulating drugs.[4] The usual treatment of hyperlipidaemias is discussed on p.823.

There have been suggestions that guar gum reduces appetite by promoting a feeling of fullness, but a meta-analysis has indicated that it is not effective for reducing body-weight.[7] Products containing guar gum have, however, been promoted as **slimming aids**. Their use cannot be advocated because of the risk of tablets swelling before reaching the stomach and causing oesophageal obstruction.


1. Hockaday TDR. Fibre in the management of diabetes 1: natural fibre useful as part of total dietary prescription. *BMJ* 1990; **300:** 1334–6.
2. Ellis PR, *et al.* Guar gum: the importance of reporting data on its physico-chemical properties. *Diabet Med* 1986; **3:** 490–1.
3. Anonymous. Guar gum: of help to diabetics? *Drug Ther Bull* 1987; **25:** 65–7.
4. Todd PA, *et al.* Guar gum: a review of its pharmacological properties, and use as a dietary adjunct in hypercholesterolaemia. *Drugs* 1990; **39:** 917–28.
5. Tattersall R, Mansell P. Fibre in the management of diabetes 2: benefits of fibre itself are uncertain. *BMJ* 1990; **300:** 1336–7.
6. Salenius J-P, *et al.* Long term effects of guar gum on lipid metabolism after carotid endarterectomy. *BMJ* 1995; **310:** 95–6.
7. Pittler MH, Ernst E. Guar gum for body weight reduction: meta-analysis of randomized trials. *Am J Med* 2001; **110:** 724–30.


### Preparations

**Proprietary Preparations** (details are given in Part 3)
***Arg.:*** Regudig; ***Austral.:*** Benefiber; ***Braz.:*** Benefiber; Biofiber; ***Fin.:*** Guarem; ***Ger.:*** Glucotard†; Guar Verlan; Lejguar†; ***Hong Kong:*** Guarem; ***Irl.:*** Guarem; ***Israel:*** Guarem†; ***Spain:*** Biotropic†; Fibraguar; Plantaguar; ***Switz.:*** Leiguar; Lubo†; ***UK:*** Guarem†; Resource Benefiber; ***USA:*** Benefiber.

**Multi-ingredient: *Belg.:*** Mucipulgite†; ***Fr.:*** Moxydar; Mucipulgite; Mulkine; ***Ital.:*** Cruscasohn; Resource Gelificata; ***Switz.:*** Demosvelte N†; Mucipulgite; ***UK:*** Lipolest†.

---

# Insulin

Insulina; Insulinum.

*CAS — 9004-10-8 (insulin; neutral insulin); 11070-73-8 (bovine insulin); 12584-58-6 (porcine insulin); 11061-68-0 (human insulin); 8063-29-4 (biphasic insulin); 9004-21-1 (globin zinc insulin); 68859-20-1 (insulin argine); 8049-62-5 (insulin zinc suspensions); 53027-39-7 (isophane insulin); 9004-17-5 (protamine zinc insulin); 116094-23-6 (insulin aspart); 9004-12-0 (dalanated insulin); 51798-72-2 (bovine insulin defalan); 11091-62-6 (porcine insulin defalan); 160337-95-1 (insulin glargine); 133107-64-9 (insulin lispro).*
*ATC — A10AB01 (human); A10AB02 (beef); A10AB03 (pork); A10AB04 (lispro); A10AB05 (aspart); A10AC01 (human); A10AC02 (beef); A10AC03 (pork); A10AC04 (lispro); A10AD01 (human); A10AD02 (beef); A10AD03 (pork); A10AD04 (lispro); A10AE01 (human); A10AE02 (beef); A10AE03 (pork); A10AE04 (glargine).*

**Pharmacopoeias.** Most pharmacopoeias have monographs for insulin and a variety of insulin preparations.

**Ph. Eur. 5.0** (Insulin, Bovine). The natural antidiabetic principle obtained from beef pancreas and purified. A white or almost white powder. Practically insoluble in water and in dehydrated alcohol. It dissolves in dilute mineral acids and, with decomposition, in dilute solutions of alkali hydroxides. Store in airtight containers. Protect from light. It should be stored at −20° until released by the manufacturer. When thawed, insulin may be stored at 2° to 8° and used for manufacturing purposes within a short period of time. To avoid absorption of humidity from the air during weighing, the insulin must be at room temperature.

**Ph. Eur. 5.0** (Insulin, Porcine). The natural antidiabetic principle obtained from pork pancreas and purified. A white or almost white powder. Practically insoluble in water and in dehydrated alcohol. It dissolves in dilute mineral acids and, with decomposition, in dilute solutions of alkali hydroxides. Store in airtight containers. Protect from light. It should be stored at −20° until released by the manufacturer. When thawed, insulin may be stored at 2° to 8° and used for manufacturing purposes within a short period of time. To avoid absorption of humidity from the air during weighing, the insulin must be at room temperature.

**Ph. Eur. 5.0** (Insulin, Human). A protein having the structure of the antidiabetic hormone produced by the human pancreas. It is produced either by enzymatic modification and suitable purification of insulin obtained from the pancreas of the pig or by a method based on recombinant DNA (rDNA) technology. A white or almost white powder. Practically insoluble in water and in alcohol. It dissolves in dilute mineral acids and, with decomposition, in dilute solutions of alkali hydroxides. Store in airtight containers. Protect from light. It should be stored at −18° or below until released by the manufacturer. When thawed, insulin is stored at 2° to 8° and used for manufacturing preparations within a short period of time. To avoid absorption of humidity from the air during weighing, the insulin must be at room temperature.

**Ph. Eur. 5.0** (Insulin Aspart; Insulinum Aspartum). It is a 2-chain peptide containing 51 amino acids. The A-chain is composed of 21 amino acids and the B-chain is composed of 30 amino acids. It is identical in primary structure to human insulin, except that it has aspartic acid instead of proline at position 28 of the B-chain. As in human insulin, insulin aspart contains 2 interchain disulfide bonds and 1 intrachain disulfide bond. It is produced by a method based on recombinant DNA (rDNA) technology. A white or almost white powder. Practically insoluble in aqueous solutions with a pH around 5.1. In aqueous solutions below pH 3.5 or above pH 6.5, the solubility is greater than or equal to 25 mg/mL. Store in airtight containers. Protect from light. It should be stored at −18° until released by the manufacturer. When thawed, insulin aspart may be stored at 2° to 8° and used for manufacturing purposes within a short period of time. To avoid absorption of humidity from the air during weighing, insulin aspart must be at room temperature before opening the container.

**Ph. Eur. 5.0** (Insulin Lispro; Insulinum Lisprum). It is a 2-chain peptide containing 51 amino acids. The A-chain is composed of 21 amino acids and the B-chain is composed of 30 amino acids. It is identical in primary structure to human insulin, only differing in amino acid sequence at positions 28 and 29 of the B-chain. Human insulin is Pro(B28), Lys(B29), whereas insulin lispro is Lys(B28), Pro(B29). As in human insulin, insulin lispro contains 2 interchain disulfide bonds and 1 intrachain disulfide bond. It is produced by a method based on recombinant DNA (rDNA) technology. A white or almost white powder. Practically insoluble in water and in alcohol. It dissolves in dilute mineral acids and with decomposition in dilute solutions of alkali hydroxides. Store in airtight containers. Protect from light. It should be stored at or below −18°. When thawed, insulin lispro is used for manufacturing purposes within a short period of time. To avoid absorption of humidity from the air during weighing, insulin aspart must be at room temperature before opening the container.

**USP 27** (Insulin). A protein that affects the metabolism of glucose obtained from the pancreas of healthy bovine or porcine animals, or both, used for food by humans. White or practically white crystals. Soluble in solutions of dilute acids and alkalis. Store in airtight containers. Protect from light. It should be stored at −10° to −25°.

**USP 27** (Insulin Human). A protein corresponding to the active principle elaborated in the human pancreas that affects the metabolism of carbohydrate (particularly glucose), fat, and protein. It is derived by enzymatic modification of insulin from pork pancreas in order to change its amino acid sequence appropriately, or produced by microbial synthesis via a recombinant DNA process. Store in airtight containers. Protect from light. It should be stored at −10° to −25°.

**USP 27** (Insulin Lispro). Insulin Lispro is identical in structure to Insulin Human, except that it has lysine and proline at positions 28 and 29, respectively, of chain B, whereas this sequence is reversed in Insulin Human. It is produced by microbial synthesis via a recombinant DNA process. White or practically white crystals. Soluble in solutions of dilute acids and alkalis. Store in airtight containers. Protect from light. It should be stored at −10° to −25°.

## Definitions and Terminology

Insulin is a hormone produced by the beta cells of the islets of Langerhans of the pancreas and consists of 2 chains of amino acids, the A and B chains, connected by 2 disulfide bridges. Insulin produced by different species conforms to the same basic structure but has different sequences of amino acids in the chains. **Porcine insulin** ($C_{256}H_{381}N_{65}O_{76}S_6$ = 5777.5) differs from **human insulin** ($C_{257}H_{383}N_{65}O_{77}S_6$ = 5807.6) in only one amino acid in the B chain, whereas **bovine insulin** ($C_{254}H_{377}N_{65}O_{75}S_6$ = 5733.5) differs from human insulin not only in this same amino acid in the B chain but also in 2 amino acids in the A chain.

The precursor of insulin in the pancreas is proinsulin which is a single polypeptide chain incorporating both the A and B chains of insulin connected by a peptide termed the C-peptide (or connecting-peptide). Although the insulins of various species may be similar in composition the proinsulins are not, in that the sequence and number of amino acids in the C-peptide may vary considerably.

Early commercial insulins were obtained by extraction from bovine or porcine or mixed bovine and porcine pancreases and were purified by recrystallisation only. Insulins obtained by such methods were often termed **'conventional insulins'** to distinguish them from insulins which have undergone further purification processes. An extract which has been recrystallised only once can be separated into 3 components or fractions termed the 'a', 'b', and 'c' components. The 'a' component consists of high molecular weight substances and is only usually found in very impure preparations since repeated recrystallisation will remove most of it. The 'b' component consists largely of proinsulin and insulin dimers, and the 'c' component consists of insulin, insulin esters, arginine insulin, and desamidoinsulin. Other pancreatic peptides such as glucagon, pancreatic polypeptide, somatostatin, and vasoactive intestinal peptide are also usually found in products which have not undergone further purification. Gel filtration will substantially reduce the content of proinsulin but will not significantly reduce the content of insulin derivatives or pancreatic peptides; products purified by gel filtration are often termed **'single-peak insulins'**. Addition of ion-exchange chromatography to the purification methods will further reduce the proinsulin content and also reduce the contamination by insulin derivatives and pancreatic peptides. In the UK **'highly purified insulins'** and **'monocomponent insulins'** are terms sometimes applied to insulins which have undergone both gel filtration and ion-exchange chromatography. In the USA the FDA has designated the term **'purified insulins'** for preparations similarly prepared and containing less than 10 ppm of proinsulin.

Much of the insulin now produced has an amino-acid sequence identical to that of human insulin. **Human insulin (emp)** is produced by the enzymatic modification of insulin obtained from the porcine pancreas; it is also sometimes called **semisynthetic human insulin.** The term **human insulin (crb)** is used for insulin produced by the chemical combination of A and B chains which have been obtained from bacteria genetically modified by recombinant DNA technology. **Human insulin (prb)** is produced from proinsulin obtained from bacteria genetically modified by recombinant DNA technology. **Human insulin (pyr)** is insulin produced from a precursor obtained from a yeast genetically modified by recombinant DNA technology. Human insulin obtained by recombinant DNA technology is sometimes termed **biosynthetic human insulin.**

Insulin or human insulin is supplied in a variety of forms in solution or suspension for injection (see Table 2, p.336). Crystalline insulin may be prepared for therapeutic use merely by making a solution, either of acidic or neutral pH. **Soluble insulin** or **'neutral insulin'** is a short-acting preparation that can be given intravenously if necessary to cover emergencies. Soluble formulations are sometimes referred to as **'regular insulin'** or **'unmodified insulin'**; these names reflect the fact that the preparation has not been formulated in order to prolong the duration of action of the insulin.

In order to prolong the duration of action of insulin, preparations may be formulated as suspensions in 2 general ways. The first involves complexing insulin with a protein from which it is slowly released; examples are **protamine zinc insulin**, which contains an excess of protamine, and **isophane insulin** (NPH insulin), which contains equimolecular amounts of insulin and protamine. The second method of prolonging the action of insulin is to modify the particle size and the various **insulin zinc suspensions** are in this category.

**Biphasic insulins** are mixtures providing for both immediate and prolonged action.

Chemical modification of the insulin molecule has resulted in insulins such as **dalanated insulin** (prepared by the removal of the C-terminal alanine from the B chain of insulin), **insulin defalan** (prepared by the removal of the terminal phenylalanine), and **sulfated insulin**, but these insulins have not been widely used.

More recently, recombinant DNA technology has enabled production of *insulin analogues* with altered pharmacokinetic profiles. **Insulin lispro** is one such analogue, in which the B28 and B29 amino acid residues of human insulin are replaced with lysine and proline. It is available as a rapidly acting alternative to soluble insulin and as an intermediate-acting complex with protamine. **Insulin aspart** is another rapidly acting analogue. **Insulin glargine** (HOE-901) is a long-acting form used for once-daily administration, and **insulin detemir** is used once or twice daily. Further information on these can be found under the heading Insulin Analogues and Proinsulin, in Uses, below.

### Stability and Storage

Insulin in powder form should be stored in airtight containers and protected from light. Storage at a low temperature is also recommended. The Ph. Eur. 5.0 advises storage at a temperature of −20° while the USP 27 requires storage at −10° to −25°. It is stressed that this temperature is for the powder and not for the preparations; preparations should not be subjected to storage conditions that lead to freezing.

Both the Ph. Eur. 5.0 and the USP 27 recommend that insulin preparations be stored in a refrigerator at 2° to 8° and not be allowed to freeze. The Ph. Eur. 5.0 directs that insulin preparations should be protected from light, and the USP 27 that they should be protected from sunlight. It is recognised that patients may not follow such stringent storage guidelines and most manufacturers of commercial insulin preparations consider that storage by the patient at a temperature of up to 25° would be acceptable for up to one month. Patients should still be advised not to expose their vials or cartridges to excessive heat or sunlight.

It is advisable to shake suspensions gently before a dose is withdrawn.

**Adsorption.** The adsorption of insulin onto glass and plastics used in giving sets has been decreased by the addition of albumin or polygeline to insulin solutions but it has been stated[1,2] that in practice this was unnecessary since insulin adsorption was not a major problem. However, in studies of insulin infusions used in neonatal hyperglycaemia, various methods have been investigated and found to reduce the amount of insulin lost by adsorption to the administration set. These included flushing[3] or priming[4] the system with the insulin infusion, or using a concentrated insulin solution to prime the tubing.[5] A study[6] that compared different methods found wide variation in insulin delivery depending on solution concentration, flow rate, addition of albumin, catheter type, and priming or flushing of the system.


1. Alberti KGMM. Diabetic emergencies. *Br Med Bull* 1989; **45:** 242–63.
2. Sanson TH, Levine SN. Management of diabetic ketoacidosis. *Drugs* 1989; **38:** 289–300.
3. Simeon PS, *et al.* Continuous insulin infusions in neonates: pharmacologic availability of insulin in intravenous solutions. *J Pediatr* 1994; **124:** 818–20.
4. Avent M, Whitfield J. Insulin infusions in extremely low birth weight infants. *Pediatrics* 2000; **105:** 915.
5. Fuloria M, *et al.* Effect of flow rate and insulin priming on the recovery of insulin from microbore infusion tubing. *Pediatrics* 1998; **102:** 1401–6.
6. Hewson MP, *et al.* Insulin infusions in the neonatal unit: delivery variation due to adsorption. *J Paediatr Child Health* 2000; **36:** 216–20.


**Aggregation.** For discussion of the problems of insulin aggregation, see Intensive Administration Regimens under Uses, below.

## Units

One unit of *bovine insulin* is contained in 0.03891 mg of the first International Standard (1986). One unit of *porcine insulin* is contained in 0.03846 mg of the first International Standard (1986). One unit of *human insulin* is contained in 0.03846 mg of the first International Standard (1986).

## Adverse Effects

The most frequent complication of insulin therapy is hypoglycaemia, the speed of onset and duration of which may vary according to the type of preparation used and the route of administration. It is usually associated with an excessive dosage of insulin, the omission of a meal by the patient, or increased physical activity. Patients, especially the elderly or those with tightly controlled diabetes or diabetes of long standing, may not experience the typical early warning symptoms of a hypoglycaemic attack. There have been reports of hypoglycaemia, sometimes with decreased warning symptoms, in patients changing from animal (especially bovine) to human insulin (see under Hypoglycaemia, below). Symptoms of hypoglycaemia resulting from increased sympathetic activity include hunger, pallor, sweating, palpitations, anxiety, and tremulousness. Other symptoms include headache, visual disturbances such as blurred or double vision, slurred speech, paraesthesia of the mouth and fingers, alterations in behaviour, and impaired mental or intellectual ability. If untreated, hypoglycaemia may lead to convulsions and coma which should not be confused with hyperglycaemic coma.

Insulin, given subcutaneously, may cause either lipoatrophy or lipohypertrophy. Lipoatrophy appears to occur less frequently with purified insulins than with conventional insulins; if it has occurred, it may be reversed by the injection of a purer animal insulin or human insulin into and around the atrophied site. Lipohypertrophy is usually associated with repeated injections at the same site and may usually be overcome by rotating the site of injection, although absorption of insulin may vary from different anatomical areas. Prolonged insulin therapy may result in weight gain.

Insulin occasionally causes local or systemic hypersensitivity reactions. Local reactions, characterised by erythema and pruritus at the injection site, usually disappear with continued use. Generalised hypersensitivity may produce urticaria, angioedema, and very rarely anaphylactic reactions; if continued therapy with insulin is essential hyposensitisation may be needed. Again, hypersensitivity reactions occur less frequently with purified than with conventional insulins and porcine insulin is less immunogenic than bovine insulin. Although hypersensitivity reactions have been reported in patients transferred from animal to human insulins, there are only isolated reports of such reactions in patients treated exclusively with human insulin.

Many patients treated with insulin, either animal or human insulin, develop antibodies but the clinical significance of this is not entirely clear.

◊ Of patients who received intensive insulin therapy for type 1 diabetes as part of the Diabetes Control and Complications Trial, those who experienced the greatest weight gain also had increased blood concentrations of triglycerides and low-density-lipoprotein cholesterol, and lowered high-density-lipoprotein cholesterol.[1] These lipid changes, together with higher blood pressure, increased waist-to-hip ratio, and greater insulin requirements, were held to be similar to the symptoms of insulin resistance and to indicate a possible increased risk of macrovascular disease. Results from the UK Prospective Diabetes Study indicated that type 2 diabetic patients treated with insulin had greater weight gain than those managed with other therapies,[2] but demonstrated no evidence of harmful cardiovascular effects.

For discussion of some of the specific problems associated with continuous infusion of insulin, see Intensive Administration Regimens under Uses, below.


1. Purnell JQ, *et al.* Effect of excessive weight gain with intensive therapy of type 1 diabetes on lipid levels and blood pressure: results from the DCCT. *JAMA* 1998; **280:** 140–6. Correction. *ibid.*; 1484.
2. UK Prospective Diabetics Study (UKPDS) Group. Intensive blood-glucose control with sulphonylureas or insulin compared with conventional treatment and risk of complications in patients with type 2 diabetes (UKPDS 33). *Lancet* 1998; **352:** 837–53. Correction. *ibid.* 1999; **354:** 602.


**Effects on the liver.** For a report of hepatomegaly occurring after insulin overdosage, see under Abuse, in Precautions, below.

**Effects on the skin.** Delayed pressure urticaria, in the form of large wheals occurring 4 to 6 hours after prolonged pressure, and lasting for up to 24 hours, was seen in a patient with type 1 diabetes within 6 months of changing from animal to human insulin.[1] The condition improved following a switch back to insulin of animal origin, and became aggravated again following a second attempt to switch to human insulin. Intermittent urticaria simultaneously affecting previous injection sites was reported in a child receiving human insulin, who had never received animal insulin.[2]


1. Payne CMER, *et al.* True delayed pressure urticaria induced by human Monotard insulin. *Br J Dermatol* 1996; **134:** 184.
2. Sackey AH. Recurrent generalised urticaria at insulin injection sites. *BMJ* 2000; **321:** 1449.


**Hypersensitivity.** Hypersensitivity reactions to insulin preparations may be caused not only by the insulin itself, but also by other components of the formulation such as zinc[1-3] or protamine.[4-9] Hypersensitivity reactions and lipoatrophy (which is also thought to have an immune basis) have become rare since the introduction of highly purified and human insulins.[10]

See also Adverse Effects, above and under Precautions, below.


1. Feinglos MN, Jegasothy BV. "Insulin" allergy due to zinc. *Lancet* 1979; **i:** 122–4.
2. Bruni B, *et al.* Case of generalized allergy due to zinc and protamine in insulin preparation. *Diabetes Care* 1986; **9:** 552.
3. Gin H, Aubertin J. Generalized allergy due to zinc and protamine in insulin preparation treated with insulin pump. *Diabetes Care* 1987; **10:** 789–90.
4. Sánchez MB, *et al.* Protamine as a cause of generalised allergic reactions to NPH insulin. *Lancet* 1982; **i:** 1243.
5. Hulshof MM, *et al.* Granulomatous hypersensitivity to protamine as a complication of insulin therapy. *Br J Dermatol* 1992; **127:** 286–8.
6. Kim R. Anaphylaxis to protamine masquerading as an insulin allergy. *Del Med J* 1993; **65:** 17–23.
7. Dykewicz MS, *et al.* Immunologic analysis of anaphylaxis to protamine component in neutral protamine Hagedorn human insulin. *J Allergy Clin Immunol* 1994; **93:** 117–25.
8. Blanco C, *et al.* Anaphylaxis to subcutaneous neutral protamine Hagedorn insulin with simultaneous sensitization to protamine and insulin. *Allergy* 1996; **51:** 421–4.
9. Bollinger ME, *et al.* Protamine allergy as a complication of insulin hypersensitivity: a case report. *J Allergy Clin Immunol* 1999; **104:** 462–5.
10. Schernthaner G. Immunogenicity and allergenic potential of animal and human insulins. *Diabetes Care* 1993; **16** (suppl 3): 155–65.


HYPOSENSITISATION. Following failure of standard hyposensitisation measures in a patient with cutaneous hypersensitivity to insulin, hyposensitisation was attempted by giving insulin by mouth.[1] Aspirin 1.3 g three times daily by mouth was also given to antagonise vascular mediators of the reaction. After one week subsequent hyposensitisation using insulin by injection was successful. When the patient stopped taking aspirin after 6 months the original hypersensitivity reactions recurred; aspirin was then given permanently in a dose of 1.3 g twice daily.


1. Holdaway IM, Wilson JD. Cutaneous insulin allergy responsive to oral desensitisation and aspirin. *BMJ* 1984; **289:** 1565–6.


**Hypoglycaemia.** Hypoglycaemia is the major adverse effect of insulin treatment with severe hypoglycaemic episodes occurring in up to a third of all insulin-treated patients at some point in their lives. Moves towards more intensive insulin therapy, in order to reduce the development of diabetic complications, increase the risk of hypoglycaemic episodes.[1,2] This may be connected with the fact that patients maintaining strict glycaemic control are prone to 'hypoglycaemia unawareness' in which the normal adrenergic counter-response to hypoglycaemia (characterised by symptoms such as pallor, sweating, and tremor) is reduced or lost,[3] so that hypoglycaemia can develop without warning. Such a loss of awareness of impending hypoglycaemia also seems to develop in diabetics as disease duration increases.[4] One of the primary factors in reducing awareness of hypoglycaemia is that repeated hypoglycaemic episodes seem to trigger an adaptive conservation of glucose concentrations in the brain, resulting in higher central than peripheral blood glucose values;[5] avoidance of hypoglycaemia helps restore awareness.

When recombinant human insulin became generally available in the late 1980s a number of patients complained of a loss of awareness of impending hypoglycaemia following transfer to human insulin,[6,7] and there were reports of severe or even fatal hypoglycaemia occurring in patients who had been well stabilised on animal insulins.[6-8]

This was, and remains, a somewhat controversial area. Despite some small studies suggesting a problem, others failed to find evidence of a difference between animal and human insulins, and a systematic review[9] concluded that the available evidence did not support the suggestion that human insulin increased the frequency or severity of hypoglycaemia, or affected the symptoms of hypoglycaemia, compared with animal insulins. However, most commentators appear to consider that patients should continue to have access to animal insulins if desired, and that those well maintained on animal insulin should not be transferred to human insulin without appropriate clinical grounds,[4,8,10-12] and then only with careful monitoring.

There has also been concern about possible long-term sequelae of hypoglycaemic episodes on the CNS. However, a report on patients participating in the Diabetes Control and Complications Trial (DCCT) suggested that the increased risk of hypoglycaemia seen with intensive therapy was not associated with neuropsychological impairment.[13]

For the treatment of insulin-induced hypoglycaemia, see below.


1. The Diabetes Control and Complications Trial Research Group. The effect of intensive treatment of diabetes on the development and progression of long-term complications in insulin-dependent diabetes mellitus. *N Engl J Med* 1993; **329:** 977–86.
2. Egger M, *et al.* Risk of adverse effects of intensified treatment in insulin-dependent diabetes mellitus: a meta-analysis. *Diabet Med* 1997; **14:** 919–28.
3. Widom B, Simonson DC. Glycemic control and neuropsychologic function during hypoglycemia in patients with insulin-dependent diabetes mellitus. *Ann Intern Med* 1990; **112:** 904–12.
4. Everett J, Kerr D. Changing from porcine to human insulin. *Drugs* 1994; **47:** 286–96.
5. Cranston I, *et al.* Restoration of hypoglycaemia awareness in patients with long-duration insulin-dependent diabetes. *Lancet* 1994; **344:** 283–7.
6. Teuscher A, Berger WG. Hypoglycaemia unawareness in diabetics transferred from beef/porcine insulin to human insulin. *Lancet* 1987; **ii:** 382–5.
7. Pickup J. Human insulin: problems with hypoglycaemia in a few patients. *BMJ* 1989; **299:** 991–3.
8. Gale EAM. Hypoglycaemia and human insulin. *Lancet* 1989; **ii:** 1264–6.
9. Airey CM, *et al.* Hypoglycaemia induced by exogenous insulin - 'human' and animal insulin compared. *Diabet Med* 2000; **17:** 416–32.
10. Gerich JE. Unawareness of hypoglycaemia and human insulin. *BMJ* 1992; **305:** 324–5.
11. Williams G, Patrick AW. Human insulin and hypoglycaemia: burning issue or hot air? *BMJ* 1992; **305:** 355–7.
12. Teuscher A, Kiln MR. Patient-empowerment and free insulin market. *Lancet* 1994; **344:** 1299–1300.
13. The Diabetes Control and Complications Trial Research Group. Effects of intensive diabetes therapy on neuropsychological function in adults in the Diabetes Control and Complications Trial. *Ann Intern Med* 1996; **124:** 379–88.


**Oedema.** Severe, acute oedema is a rare adverse effect of insulin treatment, occurring most often at the initiation of therapy.[1-4] It should be distinguished from chronic and subacute forms of oedema which may be complications of the diabetic disease process.[2,3] Possible mechanisms of acute oedema are sodium retention resulting from a direct action of insulin on the renal tubule or an effect of insulin on vascular permeability.[1,3] The oedema is usually self-limiting,[2,4] but does respond to a decrease in insulin dosage, or diuretic therapy.[1,3]


1. Bleach NR, *et al.* Insulin oedema. *BMJ* 1979; **2:** 177–8.
2. Lawrence JR, Dunnigan MG. Diabetic (insulin) oedema. *BMJ* 1979; **2:** 445.
3. Evans DJ, *et al.* Insulin oedema. *Postgrad Med J* 1986; **62:** 665–8.
4. Hirshberg B, *et al.* Natural course of insulin edema. *J Endocrinol Invest* 2000; **23:** 187–8.


## Treatment of Insulin-induced Hypoglycaemia

In the conscious and cooperative patient hypoglycaemia is treated by giving a readily absorbable form of carbohydrate by mouth, such as sugar lumps or a glucose-based drink; all diabetics should always carry a suitable sugar source by way of precaution.

If the patient is drowsy or unconscious, then glucose must be given parenterally. Doses of 50 mL of a 20% solution of glucose or 25 to 50 mL of glucose 50% can be given intravenously; the higher concentration is more viscous and irritant to the veins. Lower concentrations are equally effective, and carry less risk of irritant effects, but larger volumes are required, e.g. up to 500 mL of glucose 5%, or 250 mL of 10%, titrated to patient response. Smaller quantities (e.g. 5 to 10 mL/kg of a 10% solution) are required in children. Bolus doses may need to be repeated, or a maintenance infusion started, to prevent persistent hypoglycaemia. If the patient has not regained consciousness within a few minutes after a bolus dose of glucose, the possibility of cerebral oedema should be considered.

In situations where the intravenous administration of glucose is impractical or not feasible, glucagon 0.5 to 1 mg by subcutaneous, intramuscular, or intravenous injection may arouse the patient sufficiently to allow oral glucose to be given. If the patient fails to respond to glucagon within about 10 to 15 minutes, then glucose has to be given intravenously despite any impracticalities.

Following a return to consciousness, carbohydrates by mouth may need to be given until the action of insulin has ceased which, for preparations with a relatively long duration of action such as isophane insulin, some insulin zinc suspensions, and protamine zinc insulin, may be several hours.

**Carbohydrate.** A comparative study[1] of 7 different preparations of oral carbohydrate for the treatment of hypoglycaemia in the conscious patient found no significant difference in effectiveness between glucose or sucrose in solution or tablet form; a hydrolysed polysaccharide solution containing glucose, maltose, and various more complex saccharides (Glucidex 19) was also roughly comparable. However, a glucose gel and orange juice were each less effective than the other formulations in treating hypoglycaemia.


1. Slama G, *et al.* The search for an optimized treatment of hypoglycemia: carbohydrates in tablets, solution, or gel for the correction of insulin reactions. *Arch Intern Med* 1990: **150:** 589–93.


**Glucagon.** A discussion of the relative merits of parenteral glucose and glucagon in unconscious hypoglycaemic patients[1] suggested that glucagon should be encouraged as first-line treatment, although in practice (see above) parenteral glucose is usually preferred. The effect of glucagon relies upon the patient having adequate liver glycogen stores, which may not always be the case.


1. Gibbins RL. Treating hypoglycaemia in general practice. *BMJ* 1993; **306:** 600–601.


**Overdose.** The requirements for glucose are greater and more prolonged when hypoglycaemia is caused by insulin overdosage rather than therapeutic doses.[1] Correction of insulin-induced hypokalaemia may also be required. Surgical excision of tissue at

**Table 2.** Ph. Eur., BP, and USP insulin preparations.

| Type | Ph. Eur./BP/USP Title | Synonyms | Description | pH | Common classification | Approximate action profile after subcutaneous administration | | |
|---|---|---|---|---|---|---|---|---|
| | | | | | | Onset | Time to peak | Duration |
| Soluble insulins (also known as regular or unmodified insulin) | Soluble Insulin Injection (Ph. Eur. 5.0) | Neutral Insulin<br>Neutral Insulin Injection<br>Soluble Insulin<br>Insulin Injection | Solution of bovine, porcine, or human insulin | 6.9 to 7.8 | | | | |
| | Insulin Injection (USP 27) | | Solution of bovine or porcine, or a mixture of bovine and porcine, insulin | 7.0 to 7.8 | Short-acting | 30 minutes to 1 hour | 2 to 5 hours | 6 to 8 hours |
| | Insulin Human Injection (USP 27) | | Solution of human insulin | 7.0 to 7.8 | | | | |
| Insulin analogues, rapid | Insulin Lispro Injection (USP 27) | | Modified human insulin with lysine and proline at positions 28 and 29 respectively of chain B | 7.0 to 7.8 | Short-acting | 5 to 20 minutes | 1 to 3 hours | 2 to 5 hours |
| Biphasic insulins | Biphasic Insulin Injection (Ph. Eur. 5.0) | Biphasic Insulin | Suspension of crystals containing bovine insulin in a solution of porcine insulin | 6.6 to 7.2 | | | | |
| | Biphasic Isophane Insulin Injection (Ph. Eur. 5.0) | Biphasic Isophane Insulin | Buffered suspension of porcine insulin or human insulin complexed with protamine sulfate or other suitable protamine, in a solution of porcine insulin or human insulin respectively. | 6.9 to 7.8 | | | | |
| Insulin suspensions | Isophane Insulin Injection (Ph. Eur. 5.0) | Isophane Insulin<br>Isophane Insulin (NPH)<br>Isophane Protamine Insulin Injection | Suspension of bovine, porcine, or human insulin complexed with protamine sulfate or another suitable protamine. Contains 300 to 600 micrograms of protamine sulfate per 100 units of insulin | 6.9 to 7.8 | | | | |
| | Isophane Insulin Suspension (USP 27) | | Buffered aqueous suspension of zinc-insulin (bovine or porcine) crystals and protamine sulfate, combined in a manner such that the solid phase of the suspension consists of crystals composed of insulin, protamine, and zinc | 7.0 to 7.8 | Intermediate-acting | Within 2 hours | 4 to 12 hours | Up to 24 hours |
| | Isophane Insulin Human Suspension (USP 27) | | Buffered aqueous suspension of zinc-insulin human crystals and protamine sulfate, combined in such a manner that the solid phase of the suspension consists of crystals composed of insulin human, protamine, and zinc | 7.0 to 7.5 | | | | |
| | Insulin Zinc Injectable Suspension (Amorphous) (Ph. Eur. 5.0) | Amorph. I.Z.S.<br>Insulin Semilente<br>Insulin Zinc Suspension (Amorphous) | Suspension of bovine, porcine, or human insulin complexed with a suitable zinc salt; the insulin is in a form practically insoluble in water | 6.9 to 7.8 | | | | |
| | Prompt Insulin Zinc Suspension (USP 27) | | Buffered aqueous suspension of bovine or porcine, or a mixture of bovine and porcine, insulin modified by the addition of a suitable zinc salt in a manner such that the solid phase is amorphous | 7.0 to 7.8 | | | | |

**Table 2.** Ph. Eur., BP, and USP insulin preparations.

| Type | Ph. Eur./BP/USP Title | Synonyms | Description | pH | Common classification | Approximate action profile after subcutaneous administration | | |
|---|---|---|---|---|---|---|---|---|
| | | | | | | Onset | Time to peak | Duration |
| Insulin suspensions *cont* | Insulin Zinc Injectable Suspension (Ph. Eur. 5.0) | Insulin Lente<br>I.Z.S.<br>I.Z.S. (Mixed)<br>Insulin Zinc Suspension (Mixed)<br>Insulin Zinc Suspension | Suspension of bovine or porcine, or a mixture of bovine and porcine, or human insulin with a suitable zinc salt; the insulin is in a form practically insoluble in water. It may be produced by mixing Insulin Zinc Injectable Suspension (Amorphous) (Ph. Eur. 5.0) and Insulin Zinc Injectable Suspension (Crystalline) (Ph. Eur. 5.0) in a ratio of 3 to 7 | 6.9 to 7.8 | | | | |
| | Insulin Zinc Suspension (USP 27) | Insulin Zinc | Buffered aqueous suspension of bovine or porcine, or a mixture of bovine and porcine, insulin modified by the addition of a suitable zinc salt in a manner such that the solid phase of the suspension consists of a mixture of approximately 3 parts of amorphous insulin to 7 parts of crystalline insulin | 7.0 to 7.8 | Intermediate or long-acting | 2 to 3 hours | 6 to 15 hours | Up to 30 hours |
| | Insulin Human Zinc Suspension (USP 27) | | Buffered aqueous suspension of human insulin modified by the addition of a suitable zinc salt in a manner such that the solid phase of the suspension consists of a mixture of approximately 3 parts of amorphous insulin to 7 parts of crystalline insulin | 7.0 to 7.8 | | | | |
| | Insulin Zinc Injectable Suspension (Crystalline) (Ph. Eur. 5.0) | Cryst. I.Z.S.<br>Insulin Ultralente<br>Insulin Zinc Suspension (Crystalline) | Suspension of bovine, porcine, or human insulin complexed with a suitable zinc salt; the insulin is in a form practically insoluble in water | 6.9 to 7.8 | | | | |
| | Protamine Zinc Insulin Injection (BP 2003) | Protamine Zinc Insulin | Buffered suspension of bovine, porcine, or human insulin complexed with protamine sulfate or another suitable protamine and zinc chloride or another suitable zinc salt | 6.9 to 7.8 | | | | |
| | Extended Insulin Zinc Suspension (USP 27) | | Buffered aqueous suspension of bovine or porcine, or a mixture of bovine and porcine, insulin modified by the addition of a suitable zinc salt in a manner such that the solid phase is predominantly crystalline | 7.0 to 7.8 | Long-acting | 4 hours | 10 to 20 hours | Up to 36 hours |
| | Extended Insulin Human Zinc Suspension (USP 27) | | Buffered aqueous suspension of human insulin modified by the addition of a suitable zinc salt in a manner such that the solid phase of the suspension is predominantly crystalline | 7.0 to 7.8 | | | | |

the site of injection has been used for massive overdose of a long-acting insulin.[2,3]


1. Roberge RJ, *et al.* Intentional massive insulin overdosage: recognition and management. *Ann Emerg Med* 1993; **22:** 228–34.
2. Campbell IW, Ratcliffe JG. Suicidal insulin overdose managed by excision of insulin injection site. *BMJ* 1982; **285:** 408–9.
3. Levine DF, Bulstrode C. Managing suicidal insulin overdose. *BMJ* 1982; **285:** 974–5.


## Precautions

Dosage requirements of insulin may be altered by many factors. Increased doses are usually necessary during infection, emotional stress, accidental or surgical trauma, puberty, and the latter two trimesters of pregnancy. Decreased doses are usually necessary in patients with impaired renal or hepatic function or during the first trimester of pregnancy. On initiation and stabilisation of therapy in newly diagnosed diabetic patients, a temporary decrease in requirements may also occur (the so-called honeymoon period).

Because of the possibility of differing responses to insulins from different species, care is recommended to avoid the inadvertent change from insulin of one species to another. Reduction in insulin dosage may be required on transfer from animal (especially bovine) to human insulin. Hypoglycaemic problems associated with a change to human insulin are discussed under Adverse Effects, above. Care is also necessary during excessive exercise; hypoglycaemia caused by metabolic effects and increased insulin absorption is the usual response, but hyperglycaemia may sometimes occur.

The use of insulin requires monitoring of therapy, such as testing blood or urine for glucose concentrations and the urine for ketones, by the patient.

Drugs which have an effect on blood-glucose concentrations may alter glycaemic control with consequent need for a change in insulin dose (see under Interactions, below).

CAUTION. *Biphasic insulin, insulin zinc suspensions, isophane insulin, protamine zinc insulin, and insulin glargine should never be given intravenously and they are not suitable for the emergency treatment of diabetic ketoacidosis.*

**Abuse.** Transient recurrent hepatomegaly associated with hypoglycaemia was associated with the surreptitious injection of additional insulin doses in an insulin-dependent diabetic. Increased storage of glycogen in the liver resulting from insulin excess was considered responsible for the hepatomegaly.[1]

Decreased plasma C-peptide concentrations or the presence of anti-insulin antibodies may be used to confirm insulin abuse as a cause of hypoglycaemia in patients who have never been treated with insulin medically.[2] Insulin has been abused by bodybuilders and other sportspersons;[3,4] severe brain damage after prolonged neuroglycopenia has resulted.[3] There are rare reports of the misuse of insulin to induce mind-altering effects of hypoglycaemia.[5]


1. Asherov J, *et al.* Hepatomegaly due to self-induced hyperinsulinism. *Arch Dis Child* 1979; **54:** 148–9.
2. Grunberger G, *et al.* Factitious hypoglycemia due to surreptitious administration of insulin: diagnosis, treatment, and long-term follow-up. *Ann Intern Med* 1988; **108:** 252–7.
3. Elkin SL, *et al.* Bodybuilders find it easy to obtain insulin to help them in training. *BMJ* 1997; **314:** 1280.
4. Honour JW. Misuse of natural hormones in sport. *Lancet* 1997; **349:** 1786.
5. Cassidy EM, *et al.* Insulin as a substance of misuse in a patient with insulin dependent diabetes mellitus. *BMJ* 1999; **319:** 1417–8.


**Accelerated absorption.** Factors such as a hot bath, sauna, or use of a sunbed have been reported to accelerate the absorption of subcutaneous injection, presumably by an increase in skin blood flow.[1-4] There may, therefore, be a risk of hypoglycaemia.[4]


1. Koivisto VA. Sauna-induced acceleration in insulin absorption from subcutaneous injection site. *BMJ* 1980; **280:** 1411–13.
2. Cüppers HJ, *et al.* Sauna-induced acceleration in insulin absorption? *BMJ* 1980; **281:** 307.
3. Koivisto VA. Sauna-induced acceleration in insulin absorption. *BMJ* 1980; **281:** 621–2.
4. Husband DJ, Gill GV. "Sunbed seizures": a hypoglycaemic hazard for insulin-dependent diabetics. *Lancet* 1984; **ii:** 1477.


**Adrenocortical insufficiency.** Recurrent severe hypoglycaemia, which occurred in 2 patients with type 1 diabetes, persisted despite a reduction in insulin doses and proved to be due to Addison's disease.[1] Insulin requirements rose again in both patients following replacement therapy with fludrocortisone and hydrocortisone.


1. Armstrong L, Bell PM. Addison's disease presenting as reduced insulin requirement in insulin dependent diabetes. *BMJ* 1996; **312:** 1601–2.


**Driving.** In the UK, patients with diabetes mellitus treated with insulin or oral hypoglycaemics are required to notify their condition to the Driver and Vehicle Licensing Agency, who then assess their fitness to drive. Patients treated with oral hypoglycaemics are generally allowed to retain standard driving licences; those treated with insulin receive restricted licences which must be renewed (with appropriate checks) every 1 to 3 years. Patients should be warned of the dangers of hypoglycaemic attacks while driving, and should be counselled in appropriate management of the situation (stopping driving as soon as it is safe to do so, taking carbohydrate immediately, and quitting the driving seat and removing the ignition key from the car) should such an event occur. Patients who have lost hypoglycaemic awareness, or have frequent hypoglycaemic episodes, should not drive. In addition, eyesight must be adequate (field of vision of at least 120°) for a licence to be valid. Patients treated with diet or oral hypoglycaemics are normally allowed to hold vocational driving licences for heavy goods vehicles or passenger carrying vehicles; those treated with insulin may not drive such vehicles, and are restricted in driving some other vehicles such as small lorries and minibuses.[1,2]

Regulations in other countries differ widely.[3]


1. British Diabetic Association (Diabetes UK). Information sheet: driving and diabetes: August 2003. Available at: http://www.diabetes.org.uk/infocentre/inform/downloads/drive.doc (accessed 08/07/04)
2. Driver and Vehicle Licensing Agency. For medical practitioners: at a glance guide to the current medical standards of fitness to drive (February 2004). Available at: http://www.dvla.gov.uk/at_a_glance/AAG2004feb.pdf (accessed 08/07/04)
3. DiaMond Project Group on Social Issues. Global regulations on diabetics treated with insulin and their operation of commercial motor vehicles. *BMJ* 1993; **307:** 250–3.


**Exercise.** Discussions[1,2] of the metabolic effects of exercise and the precautions to be taken by the exercising type 1 diabetic.


1. Greenhalgh PM. Competitive sport and the insulin-dependent diabetic patient. *Postgrad Med J* 1990; **66:** 803–6.
2. American Diabetes Association. Physical activity/exercise and diabetes. *Diabetes Care* 2004; **27** (suppl 1): S58–S62. Also available at: http://care.diabetesjournals.org/cgi/reprint/27/suppl_1/s58.pdf (accessed 08/07/04)


**Hypersensitivity to protamine.** Retrospective surveys have indicated that patients receiving isophane insulin, which contains protamine, have an increased risk of severe anaphylactoid reactions when protamine is used to reverse systemic heparinisation after cardiac catheterisation or cardiac surgery. The degree of increase in risk is unclear, however, as it has been reported as both large[1] and small.[2,3] A review of the literature suggested that surgical patients may be at greater risk because of a higher rate of prior sensitisation to protamine and the larger doses used.[3] A mechanism involving IgE and IgG antibodies to protamine has been proposed.[4]

See also Hypersensitivity under Adverse Effects, above.


1. Stewart WJ, *et al.* Increased risk of severe protamine reactions in NPH insulin-dependent diabetics undergoing cardiac catheterization. *Circulation* 1984; **70:** 788–92.
2. Levy JH, *et al.* Evaluation of patients at risk for protamine reactions. *J Thorac Cardiovasc Surg* 1989; **98:** 200–204.
3. Vincent GM, *et al.* Protamine allergy reactions during cardiac catheterization and cardiac surgery: risk in patients taking protamine-insulin preparations. *Cathet Cardiovasc Diagn* 1991; **23:** 164–8.
4. Weiss ME, *et al.* Association of protamine IgE and IgG antibodies with life-threatening reactions to intravenous protamine. *N Engl J Med* 1989; **320:** 886–92.


**Infections.** Decreased requirements of insulin, added to the dialysate, occurred in 6 diabetic patients undergoing continuous ambulatory peritoneal dialysis for chronic renal failure during episodes of severe bacterial peritonitis.[1] This was contrary to the increased insulin requirements exhibited by most diabetic patients during severe infections and probably resulted from increased absorption of insulin due to mesothelial damage.


1. Henderson IS, *et al.* Decreased intraperitoneal insulin requirements during peritonitis on continuous ambulatory peritoneal dialysis. *BMJ* 1985; **290:** 1474.


**Menstruation.** Changes in glycaemic control associated with the menstrual cycle have been recorded in women with type 1 diabetes mellitus. In a retrospective review of 124 women,[1] 61% reported perimenstrual changes in glucose concentrations and 36% made adjustments to their insulin dose, usually a small increase in the premenstrual insulin dose followed by a small decrease at the onset of menstruation. Based on mean glycosylated haemoglobin measurements, there was no evidence of improved glycaemic control in women adjusting their insulin dose compared with those leaving it unchanged despite changes in capillary glucose measurements. Changes in appetite and food consumption associated with the menstrual cycle may affect variations in glucose concentrations and insulin requirements.


1. Lunt H, Brown LJ. Self-reported changes in capillary glucose and insulin requirements during the menstrual cycle. *Diabet Med* 1996; **13:** 525–30.


**Morning hyperglycaemia.** Morning hyperglycaemia may be the result of mere waning of subcutaneously injected insulin. It may also be rebound hyperglycaemia (posthypoglycaemic hyperglycaemia or the Somogyi phenomenon) occurring after an episode of nocturnal hypoglycaemia. Morning hyperglycaemia has also been observed without antecedent hypoglycaemia even during constant intravenous infusion of insulin, when the waning of previously injected insulin would not be a factor and this is commonly referred to as the dawn phenomenon. Clinically, it is important to distinguish between the dawn phenomenon, simple waning of previously injected insulin, and rebound hyperglycaemia as a cause of early-morning hyperglycaemia because their treatment differs. Management of the dawn phenomenon and insulin waning generally consists of adjusting the evening dose of insulin to provide additional coverage between 4 a.m. and 7 a.m. Management of rebound hyperglycaemia consists of reducing insulin doses or providing additional late-evening carbohydrate, or both, to avoid nocturnal hypoglycaemia. Mistaking rebound hyperglycaemia for the dawn phenomenon or mere waning of injected insulin could result in more serious nocturnal hypoglycaemia, if evening doses of insulin were increased.[1]


1. Cryer PE, Gerich JE. Glucose counterregulation, hypoglycemia, and intensive insulin therapy in diabetes mellitus. *N Engl J Med* 1985; **313:** 232–41.


**Pregnancy.** For discussion of the precautions necessary in the management of diabetes mellitus during pregnancy, see p.324.

There has been a report of 2 cases of fetal malformation in the offspring of well-controlled diabetic women who received *insulin lispro*.[1] However, the incidence of fetal malformation is increased in infants of women with diabetes. Although the use of insulin lispro is not recommended during pregnancy the manufacturers were aware of 19 live births among women treated with insulin lispro, 1 of which exhibited a congenital abnormality.[2]


1. Diamond T, Kormas N. Possible adverse fetal effect of insulin lispro. *N Engl J Med* 1997; **337:** 1009.
2. Anderson JH, *et al.* Possible adverse fetal effect of insulin lispro. *N Engl J Med* 1997; **337:** 1010.


**Renal impairment.** See under Infections, above.

**Smoking.** Smoking has been reported to decrease the absorption of insulin and dosage adjustment may be necessary, although glycaemic control does not seem to be significantly affected.[1]


1. Zevin S, Benowitz NL. Drug interactions with tobacco smoking: an update. *Clin Pharmacokinet* 1999; **36:** 425–38.


**Surgery.** For a discussion of the management of diabetes mellitus during surgery, see p.324.

**Transmission of prion disease.** Studies of cattle with proven bovine spongiform encephalopathy (BSE) have not detected infectivity in the pancreas, from which bovine insulin is derived.[1]


1. Wickham EA. Potential transmission of BSE via medicinal products. *BMJ* 1996; **312:** 988–9.


**Travelling.** Advice for the diabetic patient when travelling, including adjustment of insulin dosage when crossing time zones.[1-3] Since insulin solution or suspension must not be frozen, it should not be carried in the luggage hold of an aircraft.


1. Barry M, Bia F. Advice for the traveling diabetic. *JAMA* 1989; **261:** 1799.
2. Sane T, *et al.* Adjustment of insulin doses of diabetic patients during long distance flights. *BMJ* 1990; **301:** 421–2.
3. Dewey CM, Riley WJ. Have diabetes, will travel. *Postgrad Med* 1999; **105:** 111–13, 117–18, 124–6.


## Interactions

Many drugs have an effect on blood-glucose concentrations and may alter insulin requirements. Drugs with hypoglycaemic activity or which may decrease insulin requirements include ACE inhibitors, alcohol, anabolic steroids, aspirin, beta blockers (which may also mask the warning signs of hypoglycaemia), disopyramide, fenfluramine, guanethidine, some MAOIs, mebendazole, octreotide, some tetracyclines, and the tricyclic antidepressant amitriptyline.

On the other hand, increased requirements of insulin may possibly be seen with chlordiazepoxide, chlorpromazine, some calcium-channel blockers such as diltiazem or nifedipine, corticosteroids, diazoxide, lithium, thiazide diuretics, and thyroid hormones.

Both increased and decreased requirements may occur with cyclophosphamide, isoniazid, and oral contraceptives.

**ACE inhibitors.** Although ACE inhibitors are favoured for use in diabetic patients with hypertension or evidence of incipient nephropathy or both, they may increase insulin sensitivity and thus decrease insulin requirements when given concomitantly.[1,2] A study[3] of hospital admissions found that ACE inhibitors increased the risk of severe hypoglycaemia in patients receiving insulin. However, an analysis of pharmacovigilance data[4] and a case-control study[5] have both found no such increase in risk.


1. Ferriere M, *et al.* Captopril and insulin sensitivity. *Ann Intern Med* 1985; **102:** 134–5.
2. McMurray J, Fraser DM. Captopril, enalapril, and blood glucose. *Lancet* 1986; **i:** 1035.
3. Morris AD, *et al.* ACE inhibitor use is associated with hospitalization for severe hypoglycemia in patients with diabetes. *Diabetes Care* 1997; **20:** 1363–7.
4. Moore N, *et al.* Reports of hypoglycaemia associated with the use of ACE inhibitors and other drugs: a case/non-case study in the French pharmacovigilance system database. *Br J Clin Pharmacol* 1997; **44:** 513–8.
5. Thamer M, *et al.* Association between antihypertensive drug use and hypoglycemia: a case-control study of diabetic users of insulin or sulfonylureas. *Clin Ther* 1999; **21:** 1387–1400.


**Alcohol.** Severe hypoglycaemic episodes have been reported in type 1 diabetics following heavy drinking episodes.[1,2] Alcohol inhibits gluconeogenesis, and its effects are therefore likely to be greatest if taken without food; however, it seems to be generally agreed that diabetics need not abstain from a moderate alcohol intake with meals.


1. Arky RA, *et al.* Irreversible hypoglycemia. *JAMA* 1968; **206:** 575–8.
2. Potter J, *et al.* Insulin induced hypoglycaemia in an accident and emergency department: the tip of an iceberg. *BMJ* 1982; **285:** 1180–2.

**Aspirin.** Aspirin produces a modest decrease in blood-glucose concentrations but a significant interaction at conventional analgesic doses appears to be unlikely. One study in children with type 1 diabetes found an average 15% decrease in blood glucose values following treatment with aspirin 1.2 to 2.4 g daily for 3 days, but there were no significant changes in insulin requirements.[1] However, high doses of aspirin can reduce or even replace the insulin dose required.[2] Other salicylates might be expected to have similar properties.


1. Kaye R, *et al.* Antipyretics in patients with juvenile diabetes mellitus. *Am J Dis Child* 1966; **112:** 52–5.
2. Reid J, Lightbody TD. The insulin equivalence of salicylate. *BMJ* 1959; **1:** 897.


**Beta blockers.** There are a few reports of severe hypoglycaemia in patients, including insulin-treated diabetics, who were given *propranolol* or *pindolol*;[1-3] there is also a report of an interaction with *timolol* given as eye drops.[4] Some evidence exists of an interaction with *metoprolol*,[5] but little evidence for some of the more selective beta blockers. Because of the effects of beta blockers on the sympathetic nervous system the usual premonitory signs of hypoglycaemia may not occur, allowing a severe episode to develop before the patient is aware and able to counter it.


1. Kotler MN, *et al.* Hypoglycaemia precipitated by propranolol. *Lancet* 1966; **ii:** 1389–90.
2. McMurtry RJ. Propranolol, hypoglycemia, and hypertensive crisis. *Ann Intern Med* 1974; **80:** 669–70.
3. Samii K, *et al.* Severe hypoglycaemia due to beta-blocking drugs in haemodialysis patients. *Lancet* 1976; **i:** 545–6.
4. Angelo-Nielsen K. Timolol topically and diabetes mellitus. *JAMA* 1980; **244:** 2263.
5. Newman RJ. Comparison of propranolol, metoprolol, and acebutolol on insulin-induced hypoglycaemia. *BMJ* 1976; **2:** 447–9.


**Calcium-channel blockers.** Diabetes worsened in an insulin-treated diabetic when given *diltiazem*.[1] The resultant intractable hyperglycaemia improved when the drug was withdrawn, and recurred, although at a more manageable level, when diltiazem was restarted at a lower dose. There are also reports of a diabetogenic effect of *nifedipine*.[2,3] However, reports of significant disturbances of metabolic control appear to be uncommon.


1. Pershadsingh HA, *et al.* Association of diltiazem therapy with increased insulin resistance in a patient with type I diabetes mellitus. *JAMA* 1987; **257:** 930–1.
2. Bhatnagar SK, *et al.* Diabetogenic effects of nifedipine. *BMJ* 1984; **289:** 19.
3. Heyman SN, *et al.* Diabetogenic effect of nifedipine. *DICP Ann Pharmacother* 1989; **23:** 236–7.


**Interferons.** Markedly increased insulin requirements developed in a previously well controlled diabetic following treatment with *interferon alfa 2a*.[1] Insulin requirements rapidly fell once interferon therapy was discontinued.


1. Campbell S, *et al.* Rapidly reversible increase in insulin requirement with interferon. *BMJ* 1996; **313:** 92.


**Oral contraceptives.** Both increases and decreases (mainly the former) in insulin requirements have been reported in insulin-dependent diabetics given various oral contraceptives.[1] However, it appears that in most cases the effects of a hormonal contraceptive on diabetic control are modest or insignificant: limited data suggest that progestogen-only and combined oral contraceptives in general have little effect.[2,3]


1. Zeller WJ, *et al.* Verträglichkeit von hormonalen Ovulationskemmern bei Diabetikerinnen. *Arzneimittelforschung* 1974; **24:** 351–7.
2. Rådberg T, *et al.* Oral contraception in diabetic women: diabetes control, serum and high density lipoprotein lipids during low-dose progestogen, combined oestrogen/progestogen and non-hormonal contraception. *Acta Endocrinol (Copenh)* 1981; **98:** 246–51.
3. Lunt H, Brown LJ. Self-reported changes in capillary glucose and insulin requirements during the menstrual cycle. *Diabet Med* 1996; **13:** 525–30.


## Pharmacokinetics

Insulin has no hypoglycaemic effect when administered by mouth since it is inactivated in the gastrointestinal tract.

It is fairly rapidly absorbed from subcutaneous tissue following injection and although the half-life of unmodified insulin in blood is very short (being only a matter of minutes), the duration of action of most preparations is considerably longer due to their formulation (for further details see Uses and Administration, below). The rate of absorption from different anatomical sites depends on local blood flow, with absorption from the abdomen being faster than that from the arm, and that from the arm faster than from buttock or thigh. Absorption may also be increased by exercise. The absorption of insulin after intramuscular injection is more rapid than that following subcutaneous doses. Human insulin may be absorbed slightly faster from subcutaneous tissue than porcine or bovine insulin.

Insulin is rapidly metabolised, mainly in the liver but also in the kidneys and muscle tissue. In the kidneys it is reabsorbed in the proximal tubule and either returned to venous blood or metabolised, with only a small amount excreted unchanged in the urine.

◊ For discussion of factors which may affect the absorption of insulin, see under Precautions, Accelerated Absorption, above, and Uses, Administration Routes, below.

## Resistance to Insulin

The term insulin resistance has traditionally been used to describe a state in which diabetic patients exhibit considerably increased insulin requirements. It is now used in a much wider sense, and is for instance also applied to patients in whom a subnormal biological response to insulin can be demonstrated, although many of these patients do not apparently present difficulties in their clinical management. Insulin resistance is found particularly in obese patients; resistance to endogenous insulin is thought to be linked to the development of type 2 diabetes in such patients. Insulin resistance is frequently associated with lipid disorders, hypertension, and ischaemic heart disease. In women, it may also be linked to polycystic ovary syndrome.

Insulin resistance of the type manifested by greatly increased insulin requirements may be due to a variety of factors, including antibody formation and inadequate absorption of insulin from subcutaneous sites. A few patients with severe insulin resistance have responded to insulin lispro (see Insulin Analogues and Proinsulin under Uses, below).

Mecasermin (insulin-like growth factor) has been observed to reverse hyperglycaemia and ketoacidosis in patients with insulin resistance (see p.1339).

◊ References.


1. Moller DE, Flier JS. Insulin resistance—mechanisms, syndromes, and implications. *N Engl J Med* 1991; **325:** 938–48.
2. Eckel RH. Insulin resistance: an adaptation for weight maintenance. *Lancet* 1992; **340:** 1452–3.
3. Clausen JO, *et al.* Insulin resistance: interactions between obesity and a common variant of insulin receptor substrate-1. *Lancet* 1995; **346:** 397–402.
4. Davidson MB. Clinical implications of insulin resistance syndromes. *Am J Med* 1995; **99:** 420–6.
5. Krentz AJ. Insulin resistance. *BMJ* 1996; **313:** 1385–9. Correction. *ibid.* 1997; **314:** 134.


## Uses and Administration

Insulin is a hormone that plays a key role in regulating carbohydrate, protein, and fat metabolism. The main stimulus for its secretion is glucose, although many other factors including amino acids, catecholamines, glucagon, and somatostatin, are involved in its regulation. The secretion of insulin is not constant and peaks occur in response to the intake of food.

The major effects of insulin on carbohydrate homoeostasis follow its binding to specific cell-surface receptors on insulin-sensitive tissues, notably the liver, muscles, and adipose tissue. It inhibits hepatic glucose production and enhances peripheral glucose disposal thereby reducing blood-glucose concentration. It also inhibits lipolysis thereby preventing the formation of ketone bodies.

Therapy with insulin is essential for the long-term survival of all patients with type 1 diabetes mellitus. It may also be necessary in some patients with type 2 disease. The management of diabetes mellitus and the role of insulin in type 1 and type 2 disease is discussed on p.324. Insulin is generally the treatment chosen for all types of diabetes mellitus during pregnancy.

**Choice of insulin.** The different types of insulin and their formulations are described under Definitions, above. In some countries including the UK the commercially available preparations have been standardised to a single **strength** containing 100 units/mL; a strength of 40 units/mL is still available in some other countries, and in others concentrated injections (500 units/mL) are available to enable high doses to be given subcutaneously in a small volume. All formulations can be given by subcutaneous injection, most by intramuscular injection, but only soluble insulins can be given by the intravenous **route**. The long-term management of diabetic patients usually involves the subcutaneous route. Syringes and needles for subcutaneous injection are preferably disposable. Pen-injector devices which hold the insulin in cartridge form and meter the required dose are becoming increasingly popular. Soluble insulin is often given by the intraperitoneal route to patients on continuous ambulatory peritoneal dialysis.

The various formulations of insulin are classified, according to their **duration of action** after subcutaneous injection, as short-, intermediate-, or long-acting. The exact duration of action for any particular preparation, however, is variable and may depend upon factors such as interindividual variation, the patient's antibody status, whether the insulin is of human or animal origin, the dose, and the site of injection. *Short-acting* insulins are the soluble insulins, which have an onset after about 30 minutes to 1 hour, a peak activity at about 2 to 5 hours, and a duration of about 6 to 8 hours. Some analogues, such as insulins lispro and aspart, are also short-acting, with a faster onset and shorter duration of action than soluble insulin and are sometimes known as rapid-acting insulins. *Intermediate-acting* insulins include biphasic insulins, isophane insulins, and amorphous insulin zinc suspensions. In general these have an onset within about 2 hours, peak activity after about 4 to 12 hours, and a duration of up to 24 hours. Commercially available mixtures of soluble insulins and isophane insulins have activities which would normally place them within the intermediate-acting category. Mixed insulin zinc suspensions may be classified as either *intermediate- or long-acting* as the duration of action may be up to 30 hours; the onset of action is generally 2 to 3 hours and the time to peak activity 6 to 15 hours. *Long-acting* insulins include crystalline insulin zinc suspensions and protamine zinc insulins. These generally have an onset after about 4 hours, a peak activity at about 10 to 20 hours, and a duration of up to 36 hours. The insulin analogues insulin glargine and insulin detemir are also long-acting. After intramuscular injection, the onset of action of all insulins is generally more rapid and the duration of action shorter.

The type of formulation, its dose, and the frequency of administration are chosen to suit the needs of the individual patient. Whatever the formulation, human insulin is generally used for all newly diagnosed diabetics.

**Control.** The **dosage** of insulin must be determined for each patient and although a precise dose range cannot be given a total dose in excess of about 80 units daily would be unusual and may indicate the presence of a form of insulin resistance. The dose should be adjusted as necessary according to the results of regular monitoring of blood concentrations (or occasionally urine concentrations) of glucose by the patient.

The WHO has recommended that the glucose concentration of venous whole blood under fasting conditions should be kept within the range of 3.3 to 5.6 mmol/litre (60 to 100 mg per 100 mL) and after meals should not be allowed to exceed 10 mmol/litre (180 mg per 100 mL); blood-glucose concentrations should not be allowed to fall below 3 mmol/litre (55 mg per 100 mL). In practice it seems to be generally acceptable for patients to aim for blood-glucose concentrations between 4 and 10 mmol/litre, with the understanding that occasional variations outside this range may occur. It should be remembered that the glucose concentrations in venous plasma, venous whole blood, and capillary whole blood may be slightly different. Control may also be determined by monitoring of glycosylated haemoglobin concentrations; ideally the aim is an $HbA_{1c}$ level of less than 7% or an $HbA_1$ of less than 8.8%, compared with normal ranges of 4 to 6% and 5 to 7.5% respectively. Insulin requirements may be altered by various factors (see Precautions, above). The aim of any regimen should be to achieve the best possible control of blood glucose by attempting to mimic as closely as possible the pattern of optimum endogenous insulin secretion. Many **regimens** involve the use of a short-acting soluble insulin with an intermediate-acting insulin, such as isophane insulin or mixed insulin zinc suspension, often given twice daily.

It may sometimes be necessary, though, to give 3 or 4 injections daily to achieve good control and this typically involves giving a soluble insulin before meals and an intermediate- or long-acting insulin in the evening. A once-daily injection of an intermediate- or long-acting insulin is now generally considered to be acceptable only for those patients with type 2 diabetes mellitus who still retain some endogenous insulin secretion but nevertheless require insulin therapy, or for those patients with type 1 disease unable to cope satisfactorily with more intensive regimens. If a more intensive regimen is desired, **continuous subcutaneous infusion** may be employed using soluble insulin in an infusion pump. This delivers a constant basal infusion of insulin supplying about half of the total daily requirements, the remainder being provided by patient-activated bolus doses before each meal. The technique has a limited place in the management of diabetes; patients using it need to be well-motivated, reliable, and able to monitor their own blood glucose, and must have access to expert advice at all times. Formulations in which the insulin is in suspension are not suitable for continuous subcutaneous infusion and some brands of soluble insulin are unsuitable for this purpose because of the risk of precipitation in the pump catheter.

**Ketoacidosis.** Insulin is also an essential part of the emergency management of diabetic ketoacidosis. Only short-acting soluble insulins should be used. Treatment includes adequate fluid replacement, usually by infusing sodium chloride 0.9% initially, and the use of potassium salts to prevent or correct hypokalaemia. Insulin should be given by continuous intravenous infusion if possible, although other routes have also been used—for details of regimens see Diabetic Emergencies, under Diabetes Mellitus, below. Since insulin normally corrects hyperglycaemia before ketosis it is usually necessary to continue giving insulin once normoglycaemia has been achieved but to change the rehydration fluid to glucose-saline so that the additional glucose prevents the development of hypoglycaemia.

◊ General reviews of insulin and its use.[1-3] It has been suggested that the plethora of insulin preparations available might sensibly be reduced,[2] although others dispute this.[4]


1. MacPherson JN, Feely J. Insulin. *BMJ* 1990; **300:** 731–6.
2. Anonymous. Insulin preparations—time to rationalise. *Drug Ther Bull* 1996; **34:** 11–14.
3. American Diabetes Association. Insulin administration. *Diabetes Care* 2004; **27** (suppl 1): S106–S109. Also available at: http://care.diabetesjournals.org/cgi/reprint/27/suppl_1/s106.pdf (accessed 08/07/04)
4. von Kriegstein E, *et al.* Need for many types of insulin. *Lancet* 1996; **347:** 1045.


**Administration.** ADMINISTRATION ROUTES. The long-term management of diabetic patients usually involves injection by the **subcutaneous** route. The advice to diabetics has been to inject their insulin using a full-depth perpendicular injection.[1] In many non-obese patients, however, such a technique can result in inadvertent intramuscular injection.[1,2] Since insulin is absorbed more rapidly after intramuscular than subcutaneous injection, this may lead to greater day-to-day variability in blood-glucose control. In particular, overnight control may be inadequate if intermediate-acting preparations such as isophane insulin are used.[1] Some therefore consider that extended-action insulins should be injected at an angle into a raised skin fold. Although injection of soluble insulin into muscle may produce a more physiological action profile, until more data are available a technique that ensures subcutaneous injection may be prudent with soluble insulins as well.[1]

The anatomic *site* of subcutaneous insulin injection is usually rotated in an attempt to decrease local adverse effects (see Adverse Effects, above). However, the rate of absorption varies between sites and such a practice may also contribute to day-to-day variability in blood-glucose concentrations.[3] For example, large variations in blood-glucose concentrations have been reported on subcutaneous injection into the thigh.[4] Some have suggested rotation of injection sites within an anatomic region, or possibly use of the same anatomic region for injections given at a specific time of day.[3]

*Jet injectors* deliver insulin at high pressure across the skin into the subcutaneous tissue without use of a needle.[5,6] The greater dispersion obtained gives more rapid absorption of short- and intermediate-acting insulins and consequently reduces the total duration of action.[5] Mild pain, bruising, and bleeding may be a problem.[5-7] Despite having been available for some years, there is little information about their benefits and risks and they are not widely used.[6] However, results in a small study in women with gestational diabetes have suggested that jet injection may be associated with less variation in postprandial blood-glucose concentration and a lower incidence of insulin antibodies.[8]

Insulin preparations may also be given by **intramuscular** injection. Absorption is more rapid than from a subcutaneous injection. However, exercise may produce considerable variations in insulin absorption after intramuscular injection.[1] Soluble insulins may be given **intravenously**; this route is used in diabetic ketoacidosis, and also in surgery and labour.[9] Intermittent pulsed intravenous insulin therapy added to a conventional subcutaneous regimen has been reported to improve symptoms of orthostatic hypotension[10] and hypertension.[11]

The subcutaneous and intravenous routes, and, rarely, the intramuscular route have all been used for the continuous administration of insulin (see Intensive Administration Regimens, below).

Formulations of insulin for **intranasal** use are under investigation.[7,12,13] They have been tried in both type 1 and type 2 diabetes, but bioavailability is low and variable. Absorption enhancers have been used to facilitate uptake of insulin from the nasal mucosa and local adverse effects are dependent, in part, on their irritancy. Similarly, **buccal** formulations are under investigation.[7]

Devices for delivering insulin to the lungs via oral **inhalation** are being developed.[7] Studies[14-17] in patients with type 1 or type 2 diabetes have shown promising results, but long-term safety and efficacy remain to be established.

Endogenous insulin is delivered into the portal venous system, and then passes immediately to the liver where a large fraction of the insulin is extracted. The above routes of administration all deliver insulin into the peripheral circulation, with the risk of peripheral hyperinsulinaemia which has been considered a risk factor for atherosclerotic complications.[18] Giving insulin via the **intraperitoneal** or **oral** routes may overcome this problem to some extent. Peritoneal insulin is used routinely in diabetics undergoing chronic ambulatory peritoneal dialysis, but has also been used for continuous administration (see Intensive Administration Regimens, below). Various formulations of insulin for oral delivery are also under investigation.[7,13,19] **Rectal**[13] or transdermal[7] insulin has also been tried.


1. Thow J, Home P. Insulin injection technique: depth of injection is important. *BMJ* 1990; **301:** 3–4.
2. Frid A, Linden B. Where do lean diabetics inject their insulin? A study using computed tomography. *BMJ* 1986; **292:** 1638.
3. Bantle JP, *et al.* Rotation of the anatomic regions used for insulin injections and day-to-day variability of plasma glucose in type 1 diabetic subject. *JAMA* 1990; **263:** 1802–6.
4. Henriksen JE, *et al.* Impact of injection sites for soluble insulin on glycaemic control in type 1 (insulin-dependent) diabetic patients treated with a multiple insulin injection regimen. *Diabetologia* 1993; **36:** 752–8.
5. MacPherson JN, Feely J. Insulin. *BMJ* 1990; **300:** 731–6.
6. Bremseth DL, Pass F. Delivery of insulin by jet injection: recent observations. *Diabetes Technol Ther* 2001; **3:** 225–32.
7. Cefalu WT. Concept, strategies, and feasibility of noninvasive insulin delivery. *Diabetes Care* 2004; **27:** 239–46.
8. Jovanovic-Peterson L, *et al.* Jet-injected insulin is associated with decreased antibody production and postprandial glucose variability when compared with needle-injected insulin in gestational diabetic women. *Diabetes Care* 1993; **16:** 1479–84.
9. Home PD, *et al.* Insulin treatment: a decade of change. *Br Med Bull* 1989; **45:** 92–110.
10. Aoki TT, *et al.* Chronic intermittent intravenous insulin therapy corrects orthostatic hypotension of diabetes. *Am J Med* 1995; **99:** 683–4.
11. Aoki TT, *et al.* Effect of chronic intermittent intravenous insulin therapy on antihypertensive medication requirements in IDDM subjects with hypertension and nephropathy. *Diabetes Care* 1995; **18:** 1260–5.
12. Illum L, Davis SS. Intranasal insulin: clinical pharmacokinetics. *Clin Pharmacokinet* 1992; **23:** 30–41.
13. Hoffman A, Ziv E. Pharmacokinetic considerations of new insulin formulations and routes of administration. *Clin Pharmacokinet* 1997; **33:** 285–301.
14. Skyler JS, *et al.* Efficacy of inhaled human insulin in type 1 diabetes mellitus: a randomised proof-of-concept study. *Lancet* 2001; **357:** 331–5.
15. Cefalu WT, *et al.* Inhaled human insulin treatment in patients with type 2 diabetes mellitus. *Ann Intern Med* 2001; **134:** 203–7.
16. Gerber RA, *et al.* Treatment satisfaction with inhaled insulin in patients with type 1 diabetes: a randomized controlled trial. *Diabetes Care* 2001; **24:** 1556–9.
17. Cappelleri JC, *et al.* Treatment satisfaction in type 2 diabetes: a comparison between an inhaled insulin regimen and a subcutaneous insulin regimen. *Clin Ther* 2002; **24:** 552–64.
18. Zinman B. The physiologic replacement of insulin: an elusive goal. *N Engl J Med* 1989; **321:** 363–70.
19. Kipnes M, *et al.* Control of postprandial plasma glucose by an oral insulin product (HIM2) in patients with type 2 diabetes. *Diabetes Care* 2003; **26:** 421–6.


INSULIN ANALOGUES AND PROINSULIN. Recombinant-DNA technology has enabled the production of insulin analogues with altered pharmacokinetic profiles.[1,2] Most of the insulin in pharmaceutical preparations is in the form of hexamers, which require time to dissociate before absorption from a subcutaneous site. Substitution of amino-acid residues at the monomer-monomer interface has produced monomeric insulin analogues that retain the biological activity of insulin. Good results have been reported with an analogue, **insulin lispro**, in which the B28 and B29 residues are replaced with lysine and proline. This analogue is commercially available and has been widely reviewed.[3-7] In comparative studies of insulin lispro versus soluble insulin given before meals to patients also receiving a long-acting insulin, insulin lispro was reported to result in good glycaemic control, and could be given immediately before meals (5 to 15 minutes) rather than 20 to 40 minutes before as with soluble insulin. There is a suggestion that it may result in fewer severe hypoglycaemic episodes in such regimens.[8] However, an analysis of 10 clinical trials did not find any difference between insulin lispro and neutral insulin (Humulin R) with respect to overall adverse effects or development of long-term diabetic complications.[9] A few cases of response to insulin lispro in patients with severe insulin resistance have been reported.[10,11] Insulin lispro has been complexed with protamine to produce an intermediate-acting form, which is available as a biphasic preparation. **Insulin aspart** is another short-acting insulin analogue, with aspartic acid substituted for proline at position B28.[12-15] It is also used immediately before meals and controls postprandial blood glucose concentrations at least as well as regular human insulin, and may cause fewer hypoglycaemic episodes. Insulin glulisine is another insulin analogue, with asparagine at position B3 replaced by lysine, and lysine at B29 replaced by glutamic acid. It also has a rapid onset and short duration of action.

Recombinant-DNA technology has also been used to produce a long-acting basal insulin analogue, **insulin glargine**, suitable for once-daily use.[16-19] It is available as a solution at pH 4; on subcutaneous injection and neutralisation by tissue buffering processes, microprecipitates are formed that slowly release insulin glargine over 24 hours with no pronounced peak in concentration or in metabolic activity. Controlled studies have reported insulin glargine to be more effective than human isophane insulin in producing glycaemic control as part of a basal-bolus regimen, and to be associated with fewer hypoglycaemic episodes. **Insulin detemir** (NN-304) is another long-acting insulin analogue that may have some benefit over isophane insulin.[20,21]

Proinsulin (the natural precursor of insulin) appears to be more active than insulin in suppressing the hepatic production rather than the peripheral uptake of glucose.[22,23] It has therefore been studied particularly in patients with type 2 diabetes mellitus. However, development by some manufacturers has been suspended because of a higher rate of adverse cardiac effects in patients treated with proinsulin than in controls.[22]


1. Barnett AH, Owens DR. Insulin analogues. *Lancet* 1997; **349:** 47–51. Correction. *ibid.*; 656.
2. Owens DR, *et al.* Insulins today and beyond. *Lancet* 2001; **358:** 739–46. Correction. *ibid*; 1374.
3. Anonymous. Lispro, a rapid-onset insulin. *Med Lett Drugs Ther* 1996; **38:** 97–8.
4. Campbell RK, *et al.* Insulin lispro: its role in the treatment of diabetes mellitus. *Ann Pharmacother* 1996; **30:** 1263–71.
5. Holleman F, Hoekstra JBL. Insulin lispro. *N Engl J Med* 1997; **337:** 176–83. Correction. *ibid.* 2003; **349:** 1487.
6. Anonymous. Humalog—a new insulin analogue. *Drug Ther Bull* 1997; **35:** 57–8.
7. Wilde MI, McTavish D. Insulin Lispro: a review of its pharmacological properties and therapeutic use in the management of diabetes mellitus. *Drugs* 1997; **54:** 597–614.
8. Brunelle RL, *et al.* Meta-analysis of the effect of insulin lispro on severe hypoglycemia in patients with type 1 diabetes. *Diabetes Care* 1998; **21:** 1726–31.
9. Glazer NB, *et al.* Safety of insulin lispro: pooled data from clinical trials. *Am J Health-Syst Pharm* 1999; **56:** 542–7.
10. Henrichs HR, *et al.* Severe insulin resistance treated with insulin lispro. *Lancet* 1996; **348:** 1248.
11. Lahtela JT, *et al.* Severe antibody-mediated human insulin resistance: successful treatment with the insulin analog lispro. *Diabetes Care* 1997; **20:** 71–3.
12. Setter SM, *et al.* Insulin aspart: a new rapid-acting insulin analog. *Ann Pharmacother* 2000; **34:** 1423–31.
13. Lindholm A, Jacobsen LV. Clinical pharmacokinetics and pharmacodynamics of insulin aspart. *Clin Pharmacokinet* 2001; **40:** 641–59.
14. Anonymous. Insulin aspart, a new rapid-acting insulin. *Med Lett Drugs Ther* 2001; **43:** 89–90.
15. Chapman TM, *et al.* Insulin aspart: a review of its use in the management of type 1 and 2 diabetes mellitus. *Drugs* 2002; **62:** 1945–81. Correction. *ibid.* 2003; **63:** 512.
16. Anonymous. Insulin glargine (Lantus), a new long-acting insulin. *Med Lett Drugs Ther* 2001; **43:** 65–6.
17. McKeage K, Goa KL. Insulin glargine: a review of its therapeutic use as a long-acting agent for the management of type 1 and 2 diabetes mellitus. *Drugs* 2001; **61:** 1599–1624.
18. Levien TL, *et al.* Insulin glargine: a new basal insulin. *Ann Pharmacother* 2002; **36:** 1019–27.
19. Dunn CJ, *et al.* Insulin glargine: an updated review of its use in the management of diabetes mellitus. *Drugs* 2003; **63:** 1743–78.
20. Vague P, *et al.* Insulin detemir is associated with more predictable glycemic control and reduced risk of hypoglycemia than NPH insulin in patients with type 1 diabetes on a basal-bolus regimen with premeal insulin aspart. *Diabetes Care* 2003; **26:** 590–6.
21. Home P, *et al.* Insulin detemir offers improved glycemic control compared with NPH insulin in people with type 1 diabetes: a randomized clinical trial. *Diabetes Care* 2004; **27:** 1081–7.
22. Zinman B. The physiologic replacement of insulin: an elusive goal. *N Engl J Med* 1989; **321:** 363–70.
23. Goran EA. Human proinsulin—a new therapeutic agent? *Pharm J* 1986; **236:** 667.


INTENSIVE ADMINISTRATION REGIMENS. Intensive regimens for insulin administration aim to mimic more closely the physiological insulin pattern in which a basal insulin concentration is supplemented by a preprandial boost of insulin. Such intensive regimens are used to provide tight control in an attempt to avoid long-term complications (see p.326).

Intensified insulin regimens have the advantage of improving the patient's lifestyle and allowing flexibility in timing of meals. However, careful dietary control must still be maintained and regular monitoring of blood-glucose concentrations is an important component of such regimens. Therefore patients must be well-motivated, reliable, and able to monitor their own blood glucose, and must have access to expert 24-hour help. Although there are reports of success with intensive regimens in brittle (labile) diabetics,[1] these patients are generally unlikely to benefit from such regimens.

In **multiple-injection regimens**, the basal insulin is provided by an injection of intermediate- or long-acting insulin given usually at night, and soluble insulin is administered before each main meal. Systems for **continuous administration** may be designed on an open-loop or closed-loop delivery system. *Open-loop systems* comprise an infusion pump with the infusion rate programmed or controlled manually according to manual blood-glucose monitoring. *Closed-loop systems* (the 'artificial pancreas') consist of an insulin pump, a glucose sensor, and a computer for analysis of blood-glucose data. Systems for continuous administration have most commonly used the subcutaneous route, but intraperitoneal, intravenous, or intramuscular infusion have also been used.

The most extensively used **open-loop** system is *continuous subcutaneous insulin infusion* (CSII) using an external pump. A battery-powered pump infuses soluble insulin via a subcutaneous catheter which is resited every 2 to 3 days. A background infusion is given at a predetermined rate, and preprandial bolus doses given using an override switch or manual drive.[2] CSII provides better glycaemic control than conventional injection therapy, but may be only slightly more effective than optimised multiple daily injection therapy.[3] Complications include erythema, abscess, or cellulitis at the injection site and, rarely, contact dermatitis to components of the giving set, pump malfunction, or precipitation of insulin and catheter obstruction.[2] Pump therapy increases the risk of ketoacidosis and intensive regimens are associated with decreased hypoglycaemic awareness and more severe hypoglycaemic episodes compared with conventional therapy,[4] although there is some suggestion that CSII might reduce the risk of severe hypoglycaemia compared with multiple daily injection therapy.[2] If the pump fails or there is an acute increase in insulin requirements, the onset of ketoacidosis may be more rapid and more likely to be associated with dangerous hyperkalaemia than with conventional regimens because there is no depot of insulin.[2,5]

Further development of open-loop delivery systems has been in the design of *implantable insulin pumps*. The first pumps delivered insulin at a constant basal rate, but variable-rate models are now available. Studies[6,7] have shown that intravenous or intraperitoneal delivery of insulin from an implantable pump can produce excellent glycaemic control, and fewer episodes of severe hypoglycaemia than are associated with intensive subcutaneous multiple-injection regimens. The main problems associated with such therapy are pump slow-down or catheter obstruction due to aggregation of insulin within the device; these can normally be corrected by procedures to flush the pump and catheter,[7,8] although alternative insulin formulations (e.g. with poloxamer) have been investigated. Other problems may include fibrinous obstruction of the catheter or local intolerance of the pump.[8]

**Closed-loop** continuous infusion systems are generally confined to research and experimental work because glucose sensors suitable for implantation are still being developed.[8] However, results in *animals* have suggested that an alternative to such systems may be a vascularised artificial pancreas containing islet cells.[9]


1. Wood DF, *et al.* Management of "brittle" diabetes with a preprogrammable implanted pump delivering intraperitoneal insulin. *BMJ* 1990; **301:** 1143–4.
2. Lenhard MJ, Reeves GD. Continuous subcutaneous insulin infusion: a comprehensive review of insulin pump therapy. *Arch Intern Med* 2001; **161:** 2293–2300.
3. Pickup J, *et al.* Glycaemic control with continuous subcutaneous insulin infusion compared with intensive insulin injections in patients with type 1 diabetes: meta-analysis of randomised controlled trials. *BMJ* 2002; **324:** 705–8.
4. Egger M, *et al.* Risk of adverse effects of intensified treatment in insulin-dependent diabetes mellitus: a meta-analysis. *Diabet Med* 1997; **14:** 919–28.
5. Knight G. Risks with continuous subcutaneous insulin infusion can be serious. *BMJ* 2001; **323:** 693–4.
6. Broussolle C, *et al.* French multicentre experience of implantable insulin pumps. *Lancet* 1994; **343:** 514–15.
7. Dunn FL, *et al.* Long-term therapy of IDDM with an implantable insulin pump. *Diabetes Care* 1997; **20:** 59–63.
8. Selam JL. Implantable insulin pumps. *Lancet* 1999; **354:** 178–9.
9. Maki T, *et al.* Novel delivery of pancreatic islet cells to treat insulin-dependent diabetes mellitus. *Clin Pharmacokinet* 1995; **28:** 471–82.


MIXING OF INSULINS. Mixtures of insulin with differing durations of action may be used in order to produce a more normal pattern of blood glucose variation than can be achieved with a single insulin. However, physicochemical changes in the mixture may occur, either immediately on mixing or over time, and the physiological response to the mixture may therefore be different than if the components were given separately. An early review[1] suggested that insulins from different manufacturers should not be mixed, since formulation differences might render them incompatible. It is important that a consistent routine is followed in preparing and using such mixtures, and manufacturers advise that the shorter-acting insulin should be drawn into the syringe first, to avoid contamination of the vial with the longer-acting component. Pre-prepared mixtures are available from many manufacturers and may be preferable provided that the proportions are suited to the patient's needs.

The American Diabetes Association has issued guidelines[2] for mixing of insulins, including:

- patients well controlled on a particular mixed regimen should maintain their standard procedure for preparing doses
- no other medication or diluent should be mixed with insulin unless approved by the prescriber
- insulin glargine should not be mixed with other forms of insulin because of the low pH of its diluent
- currently available isophane and short-acting insulin formulations when mixed may be used immediately or stored for future use
- rapid-acting insulins (insulin aspart, insulin lispro) can be mixed with isophane, lente, and ultralente insulins. Ultralente insulins do not affect the onset of action of the rapid-acting component; a slight decrease in absorption rate but not bioavailability is seen if rapid-acting insulins are mixed with isophane insulin but postprandial blood-glucose response is similar to that seen with mixtures of rapid-acting and ultralente insulin
- mixtures of rapid-acting insulin with an intermediate- or long-acting insulin should be injected within 15 minutes before a meal
- mixing of short-acting (soluble) and lente or ultralente insulin is not recommended, as zinc ions present in the lente insulin may bind with the short-acting insulin and delay its effects. The degree and rate of binding vary with the insulins used, and may not reach equilibrium for 24 hours; if such mixtures are used the patient should standardise the interval between mixing and injection
- phosphate-buffered insulins (e.g. isophane insulin) should not be mixed with zinc-containing (lente or ultralente) insulins, as zinc phosphate may be precipitated, and the longer acting insulin may be partially and unpredictably converted to a short-acting form

Insulin formulations may change and the manufacturers should be consulted if their recommendations differ from those in the guidelines.


1. Fisher BM. Choosing an insulin. *Prescribers' J* 1988; **28:** 138–43. Correction. *ibid.*; 169.
2. American Diabetes Association. Insulin administration. *Diabetes Care* 2004; **27** (suppl 1): S106–S109. Also available at: http://care.diabetesjournals.org/cgi/reprint/27/suppl_1/s106.pdf (accessed 08/07/04)


**Diabetes mellitus.** Insulin is the mainstay of the treatment of **type 1 diabetes mellitus**. For a discussion of the treatment of diabetes mellitus, including the contexts in which insulin is used, see p.324. The possible role of tight glycaemic control with insulin to prevent the development of microvascular and macrovascular complications in patients with type 1 diabetes is discussed on p.326, while further discussion of specific regimens and approaches to insulin therapy is given under Administration, above.

DIABETIC EMERGENCIES. As discussed on p.328, **diabetic ketoacidosis** and hyperosmolar hyperglycaemic state are medical emergencies and should be treated immediately with fluid replacement and insulin. Potassium, and possibly phosphate, replacement may also be required, but bicarbonate should not be given unless acidaemia is very severe. In the *UK* the *British National Formulary* recommends that insulin be given by intravenous infusion for diabetic ketoacidosis, as a solution of soluble insulin 1 unit/mL via an infusion pump. An infusion rate of 6 units/hour in adults and 0.1 units/kg per hour in children is recommended initially, with the rate doubled or quadrupled if the blood glucose concentration fails to decrease by about 5 mmol/litre per hour. When blood glucose concentrations have fallen to 10 mmol/litre the infusion rate can be reduced to 3 units/hour in adults or about 0.02 units/kg per hour in children, and continued, with glucose 5% to prevent hypoglycaemia, until ketone bodies have been cleared and the patient is ready to take food by mouth. The insulin infusion should not be stopped before subcutaneous insulin has been started. Potassium chloride is included in the infusion as appropriate to prevent insulin-induced hypokalaemia. If facilities for intravenous infusion are not available the insulin is given by intramuscular injection: in adults an initial loading dose of 20 units intramuscularly is followed by 6 units intramuscularly every hour until the blood glucose concentration falls to 10 mmol/litre, when the dose is given every 2 hours. Late hypoglycaemia due to insulin accumulation should be watched for and managed appropriately.

In the *USA* the intramuscular or the subcutaneous route have been used as alternatives to intravenous insulin, together with other appropriate management. One successful set of protocols for insulin dosage in diabetic ketoacidosis is as follows:[1] an initial intravenous bolus of 0.15 units/kg is followed by infusion of 0.1 units/kg per hour; if blood glucose does not fall by about 2.5 to 3.5 mmol/litre in the first hour the infusion rate is doubled every hour until this rate of decline is achieved. (A similar insulin regimen has proved effective in patients with hyperosmolar hyperglycaemic state.[1]) When given by the intramuscular or subcutaneous routes an initial bolus of 0.4 units/kg is divided and given half by the intravenous route and half either intramuscularly or subcutaneously as appropriate. This is followed by 0.1 units/kg every hour intramuscularly or subcutaneously; if response is inadequate it is replaced by an intravenous bolus of 10 units until blood glucose falls by 2.5 to 3.5 mmol/litre. In children intravenous infusion of 0.1 units/kg per hour is recommended, or if intravenous infusion is impractical an initial intramuscular bolus of 0.1 units/kg followed by 0.1 units/kg per hour either intramuscularly or subcutaneously. Treatment is continued at this rate until a serum-glucose concentration of about 12.5 mmol/litre is reached (or about 15 mmol/litre for hyperosmolar hyperglycaemic state), when the rate is decreased to 0.05 to 0.1 units/kg per hour until acidosis is controlled and subcutaneous insulin replacement treatment can be started.


1. American Diabetes Association. Hyperglycemic crises in diabetes. *Diabetes Care* 2004; **27** (suppl 1): S94–S102. Also available at: http://care.diabetesjournals.org/cgi/reprint/27/suppl_1/s94.pdf (accessed 26/05/04)


TYPE 2 DIABETES MELLITUS. Traditionally the use of insulin in patients with type 2 diabetes has tended to be reserved for those who cannot be controlled by diet and oral antidiabetics alone.[1,2] Given the possible association between circulating insulin and atherosclerotic cardiovascular symptoms[3] there has been some concern about the use of exogenous insulin in insulin-resistant patients who are already hyperinsulinaemic. Furthermore, patients switched to insulin tend to gain weight[2] which is undesirable in a frequently obese patient group.

Insulin is nonetheless being used more frequently in type 2 patients. This is largely because of a trend toward more intensive regimens designed to produce tighter glycaemic control, on the hypothesis that, as in patients with type 1 disease, this will reduce the development and progression of diabetic complications. Results from the UK Prospective Diabetes Study,[4-6] show that insulin is an effective option in type 2 diabetes, and confirm both the value of intensive therapy in retarding microvascular complications,[6] and that oral therapy should be used before insulin in patients with primary diet failure.[7]

In order to minimise the dose of insulin required, and any risks it may entail, it has been suggested that insulin therapy in type 2 diabetes should be combined with other measures including oral hypoglycaemic drugs.[8] There has long been debate about the value of combined therapy, but a meta-analysis indicated that glycaemic control was better, and insulin requirements lower, in type 2 diabetics who received insulin with a sulfonylurea.[9]

For further discussion of the management of type 2 diabetes mellitus see p.324.


1. Tattersall RB, Scott AR. When to use insulin in the maturity onset diabetic. *Postgrad Med J* 1987; **63:** 859–64.
2. Taylor R. Insulin for the non-insulin dependent? *BMJ* 1988; **296:** 1015–16.
3. Stern MP. Do non-insulin-dependent diabetes mellitus and cardiovascular disease share common antecedents? *Ann Intern Med* 1996; **124** (suppl): 110–16.
4. United Kingdom Prospective Diabetes Study Group. United Kingdom prospective diabetes study (UKPDS) 13: relative efficacy of randomly allocated diet, sulphonylurea, insulin, or metformin in patients with newly diagnosed non-insulin-dependent diabetes followed for three years. *BMJ* 1995; **310:** 83–8.
5. Turner R, *et al.* United Kingdom Prospective Diabetes Study 17: a 9-year update of a randomized, controlled trial on the effect of improved metabolic control on complications in non-insulin-dependent diabetes mellitus. *Ann Intern Med* 1996; **124** (suppl): 136–45.
6. UK Prospective Diabetes Study Group. Intensive blood-glucose control with sulphonylureas or insulin compared with conventional treatment and risk of complications in patients with type 2 diabetes (UKPDS 33). *Lancet* 1998; **352:** 837–53. Correction. *ibid.* 1999; **354:** 602.
7. United Kingdom Prospective Diabetes Study Group. United Kingdom Prospective Diabetes Study 24: a 6-year, randomized, controlled trial comparing sulfonylurea, insulin, and metformin therapy in patients with newly diagnosed type 2 diabetes that could not be controlled with diet therapy. *Ann Intern Med* 1998; **128:** 165–75.
8. Henry RR. Glucose control and insulin resistance in non-insulin-dependent diabetes mellitus. *Ann Intern Med* 1996; **124** (suppl): 97–103.
9. Johnson JL, *et al.* Efficacy of insulin and sulfonylurea combination therapy in type II diabetes: a meta-analysis of the randomized placebo-controlled trials. *Arch Intern Med* 1996; **156:** 259–64.


**Diagnosis and testing.** PITUITARY FUNCTION. Insulin-induced hypoglycaemia has been used to provide a stressful stimulus in order to assess hypothalamic-pituitary function. The insulin stress or insulin-tolerance test has been used as a standard test for assessment of growth hormone or corticotropin deficiency. However, it is unpleasant, expensive, and not without risk, and is contra-indicated in patients with angina, heart failure, cerebrovascular disease, or epilepsy; some recommend its use only when results of alternative tests are equivocal,[1-3] and it should only be performed in specialist units under strict surveillance.[4]


1. Clayton RN. Diagnosis of adrenal insufficiency. *BMJ* 1989; **298:** 271–2.
2. Stewart PM, *et al.* A rational approach for assessing the hypothalamic-pituitary-adrenal axis. *Lancet* 1988; **1:** 1208–10.
3. Lindholm J. The insulin hypoglycaemia test for the assessment of the hypothalamic–pituitary–adrenal function. *Clin Endocrinol (Oxf)* 2001; **54:** 283–6.
4. Hindmarsh PC, Swift PGF. An assessment of growth hormone provocation tests. *Arch Dis Child* 1995; **72:** 362–8.


**Hyperkalaemia.** Insulin promotes the intracellular uptake of potassium. It is therefore used in the management of moderate to severe hyperkalaemia, when it is given with glucose (see p.1219).

**Liver disorders.** There have been reports[1,2] of benefit from the use of insulin and glucagon in the treatment of liver disorders, based on their reported hepatotrophic effect. However, randomised studies have found no benefit from insulin and glucagon infusions in fulminant hepatic failure[3] and acute alcoholic hepatitis.[4]


1. Baker AL, *et al.* A randomized clinical trial of insulin and glucagon infusion for treatment of alcoholic hepatitis: progress report in 50 patients. *Gastroenterology* 1981; **80:** 1410–14.
2. Jaspan JB, *et al.* Insulin and glucagon infusion in the treatment of liver failure. *Arch Intern Med* 1984; **144:** 2075–8.

3. Harrison PM, *et al.* Failure of insulin and glucagon infusion to stimulate liver regeneration in fulminant hepatic failure. *J Hepatol* 1990; **10:** 332–6.
4. Bird G, *et al.* Insulin and glucagon infusion in acute alcoholic hepatitis: a prospective randomized controlled trial. *Hepatology* 1991; **14:** 1097–1101.


**Myocardial infarction.** Discussions on the effects of insulin with glucose and potassium in the ischaemic heart, including its effect in reducing blood free fatty acids, have emphasised its potential benefits in left ventricular failure and cardiogenic shock.[1,2] Glucose-insulin-potassium solutions have been investigated in only small numbers of patients with acute myocardial infarction although a meta-analysis[3] of randomised controlled studies performed before the widespread use of thrombolytics found a reduction in mortality in recipients of these solutions; following a small pilot study with similar findings,[4] a larger study is now underway. Insulin-glucose infusion followed by multiple daily subcutaneous insulin injections has been reported to reduce mortality in diabetics who suffered a myocardial infarction.[5,6]

For the conventional management of myocardial infarction, see p.828.


1. Opie LH. Glucose and the metabolism of ischaemic myocardium. *Lancet* 1995; **345:** 1520–1.
2. Taegtmeyer H, *et al.* Metabolic support for the postischaemic heart. *Lancet* 1995; **345:** 1552–5.
3. Fath-Ordoubadi F, Beatt KJ. Glucose-insulin-potassium therapy for treatment of acute myocardial infarction: an overview of randomized placebo-controlled trials. *Circulation* 1997; **96:** 1152–6.
4. Díaz R, *et al.* Metabolic modulation of acute myocardial infarction: the ECLA Glucose-Insulin-Potassium Pilot Trial. *Circulation* 1998; **98:** 2227–34.
5. Malmberg K, *et al.* Randomized trial of insulin-glucose infusion followed by subcutaneous insulin treatment in diabetic patients with acute myocardial infarction (DIGAMI Study): effects on mortality at 1 year. *J Am Coll Cardiol* 1995; **26:** 57–65.
6. Malmberg K, *et al.* Prospective randomised study of intensive insulin treatment on long term survival after acute myocardial infarction in patients with diabetes mellitus. *BMJ* 1997; **314:** 1512–15.


**Neonatal hyperglycaemia.** Hyperglycaemia is common in very immature neonates because of delayed or reduced insulin production. It can be treated by glucose restriction until glucose tolerance improves. However, this may not provide enough glucose to meet basal metabolic needs, and the use of an insulin infusion can allow sufficient glucose to be given. It has been suggested that insulin is best given intravenously in a separate, easily titratable solution because of the frequent fluctuations of requirement in these infants.[1]


1. Ditzenberger GR, *et al.* Continuous insulin intravenous infusion therapy for VLBW infants. *J Perinat Neonatal Nurs* 1999; **13:** 70–82.


**Overdosage with calcium-channel blockers.** Continuous infusion of insulin 0.5 units/kg per hour, with glucose as required to maintain euglycaemia, has been reported to be of value in the management of overdosage with calcium-channel blockers when conventional therapy has failed.[1]


1. Boyer EW, Shannon M. Treatment of calcium-channel-blocker intoxication with insulin infusion. *N Engl J Med* 2001; **344:** 1721–2.


## Preparations

***BP 2003:*** Protamine Zinc Insulin Injection;
***Ph. Eur.:*** Biphasic Insulin Injection; Biphasic Isophane Insulin Injection; Insulin Zinc Injectable Suspension; Insulin Zinc Injectable Suspension (Amorphous); Insulin Zinc Injectable Suspension (Crystalline); Isophane Insulin Injection; Soluble Insulin Injection;
***USP 27:*** Extended Insulin Human Zinc Suspension; Extended Insulin Zinc Suspension; Insulin Human Injection; Insulin Human Zinc Suspension; Insulin Injection; Insulin Lispro Injection; Insulin Zinc Suspension; Isophane Insulin Human Suspension; Isophane Insulin Suspension; Prompt Insulin Zinc Suspension.

**Proprietary Preparations** (details are given in Part 3)
***Arg.:*** Actrapid HM; Actrapid MC; Biohulin Humana; Humalog; Humulin 70/30; Humulin L; Humulin N; Humulin R; Humulin U; Insulatard HM; Insulatard MC; Insuman N; Insuman R; Mixtard 10, 20, 30, 40, and 50 HM; Monotard HM; Monotard MC; ***Austral.:*** Actrapid; Humalog; Humalog Mix 25; Humulin 20/80, 30/70 and 50/50; Humulin L; Humulin NPH; Humulin R; Humulin UL; Hypurin Isophane; Hypurin Neutral; Insulin 2†; Isotard MC†; Lantus; Lente MC†; Mixtard 20/80, 30/70, 50/50; Monotard; NovoMix 30; NovoRapid; Protaphane; Ultralente MC†; Ultratard; ***Austria:*** Actrapid HM; Depot-Insulin; Humalog; Humalog Mix 25 and 50; Huminsulin Basal; Huminsulin Long; Huminsulin Normal; Huminsulin Profil I, II, III, and IV; Huminsulin Ultralong; Insulatard HM; Insuman Basal; Insuman Comb 15, 25, and 50; Insuman Infusat; Insuman komb Typ 15, Typ 25, and Typ 50†; Insuman Rapid; Komb-Insulin; Lente MC†; Mixtard HM 10/90, 20/80, 30/70, 40/60, and 50/50; Monotard HM; Ultratard HM; Velosulin HM†; ***Belg.:*** Actrapid HM; Humaject 20/80, 30/70, 40/60, 50/50; Humaject NPH; Humaject Regular; Humalog; Humuline 20/80, 30/70, 40/60, 50/50; Humuline Long; Humuline NPH; Humuline Regular; Humuline Ultralong; Insulatard HM; Lente MC†; Mixtard HM 30/70, 10/90, 20/80, 40/60, 50/50; Monotard HM; Ultratard HM; Velosuline Humanum; ***Braz.:*** Actrapid MC; Biohulin 70/30, 80/20, and 90/10; Biohulin L; Biohulin NPH; Biohulin R; Biohulin Ultralenta; Humalog; Humalog Mix 25; Humulin 70/30; Humulin Lenta; Humulin NPH; Humulin Regular; Insuman Comb 85N/15R and 75N/25R; Insuman N; Insuman R; Iolin NPH†; Iolin Regular†; Monolin NPH†; Monolin Regular†; Monotard MC; Neosulin Lenta†; Neosulin NPH†; Neosulin Regular†; Novolin 90/10, 80/20, 70/30, and 60/40; Novolin L; Novolin N; Novolin R; Novolin U; Protaphane MC; ***Canad.:*** Humalog; Humalog Mix 25; Humulin 20/80, 30/70; Humulin L; Humulin N; Humulin R; Humulin U; Iletin II Pork Lente; Iletin II Pork NPH; Iletin II Pork Regular; Iletin Lente†; Iletin NPH†; Iletin Regular†; Novolin 10/90, 20/80, 30/70, 40/60, 50/50; Novolin Lente; Novolin NPH; Novolin Toronto; Novolin Ultralente; ***Chile:*** Actrapid; Actrapid HM; Humalog; Humulin 70/30; Humulin L; Humulin N; Humulin R; Insulatard; Insulatard HM; Insuman N; Insuman R; Lenta; Mixtard HM; Monotard HM; ***Denm.:*** Actrapid; Humalog; Humalog Mix 25 and 50; Humulin Mix 30/70; Humulin NPH; Humulin Regular; Humutard Ultra†; Insulatard; Insuman Basal; Insuman Comb 25; Insuman Rapid; Mixtard 10/90, 20/80, 30/70, 40/60, and 50/50; Monotard; NovoRapid; Velosulin†; ***Fin.:*** Actrapid; Humalog; Humalog Mix 25 and 50; Humulin Mix 30/70†; Humulin NPH; Humulin Regular; Humutard; Humutard Ultra†; Insulin Lente MC†; Insulin Lyhyt; Insulin Pitka; Insuman Basal; Insuman Comb 25; Insuman Infusat; Insuman Rapid; Mixtard 10/90, 20/80, 30/70, 40/60, and 50/50; Monotard; NovoRapid; Protaphan; Ultratard; Velosulin; ***Fr.:*** Actrapid HM; Endopancrine 100†; Endopancrine 40†; Endopancrine Protamine†; Endopancrine Zinc Protamine†; Humalog; Humalog Mix 25 and 50; Insulatard; Insuline Semi Tardum†; Insuline Tardum MX†; Insuline Ultra Tardum†; Insuman Basal; Insuman Comb 15, 25, and 50; Insuman Infusat; Insuman Intermediaire 100%†; Insuman Intermediaire 25/75†; Insuman Rapid; Lantus; Lillypen Profil 10, 20, 30, and 40†; Lillypen Protamine Isophane†; Lillypen Rapide; Mixtard 10, 20, 30, 40, and 50 HM; Monotard; NovoMix 30; NovoRapid; Orgasuline 30/70†; Orgasuline NPH†; Orgasuline Rapide†; Ultratard HM; Umuline Profil 20and 30; Umuline Protamine Isophane (NPH); Umuline Rapide; Umuline Zinc; Umuline Zinc Compose; ***Ger.:*** Actraphane HM 10/90, 20/80, 30/70, 40/60, 50/50; Actrapid; B-Insulin†; Basal-H-Insulin†; Berlinsulin H 20/80, 30/70; Berlinsulin H Basal; Berlinsulin H Normal; Depot-H-Insulin†; Depot-H15-Insulin†; Depot-Insulin; Depot-Insulin S; H-Insulin†; H-Tronin; Humalog; Humalog Mix 25 and 50; Huminsulin Basal; Huminsulin Long†; Huminsulin Normal; Huminsulin Profil II and III; Huminsulin Ultralong†; Insulatard Human; Insulatard MC†; Insulin S; Insulin SNC; Insuman Basal; Insuman Comb 15, 25, and 50; Insuman Infusat; Insuman Rapid; Komb-H-Insulin†; Komb-Insulin; Komb-Insulin S; L-Insulin SNC†; L-Insulin†; Lantus; Lente†; Mixtard†; Monotard HM; NovoMix 30; NovoRapid; Protaphan; Semilente; Ultratard HM; Velasulin Human†; Velasulin MC†; Velasulin†; ***Gr.:*** Actraphane HM; Actrapid HM; Humalog; Humulin (NPH); Humulin L (Lente); Humulin M1, M2, M3, M4, M5; Humulin Regular; Humulin UL (Utralente); Monotard HM; PenMix 10, 20, 30, 40, or 50; Protaphane HM; ***Hong Kong:*** Actrapid HM; Actrapid MC; Humalog; Humulin 70/30; Humulin L; Humulin N; Humulin R; Insulatard MC; Mixtard 10, 20, 30, 40, and 50 HM; Monotard HM; Monotard MC; NovoRapid; Protaphane HM; Protaphane MC†; Ultratard HM; ***India:*** Actrapid; Human Actrapid; Human Insultard; Human Mixtard 30 and 50; Human Monotard; Lentard; Rapidica; Rapimix; Zinulin; ***Irl.:*** Actrapid; Humalog; Humalog Mix 25 and 50; Humulin I; Humulin Lente; Humulin M2, M3, M4; Humulin S; Humulin Zn; Insulatard; Insuman Basal; Insuman Comb 15, 25, and 50; Insuman Rapid; Lantus; Mixtard 10, 20, 30, 40, and 50; Monotard; NovoMix 30; NovoRapid; Ultratard; ***Israel:*** Humalog; Humalog Mix 25; Humulin 70/30, 80/20; Humulin N; Humulin R; Humulin U; NovoRapid; ***Ital.:*** Actraphane HM 10/90, 20/80, 30/70, 40/60, 50/50; Actrapid HM; Bio-Insulin 30/70 and 50/50; Bio-Insulin I; Bio-Insulin L; Bio-Insulin R; Bio-Insulin U; Humalog; Humalog Mix 25; Humulin 10/90, 20/80, 30/70, 40/60, and 50/50; Humulin I; Humulin L; Humulin R; Humulin U; Monotard HM; NovoRapid; Protaphane HM; Ultratard HM; ***Jpn:*** Humacart 3/7; InnoLet 30R; InnoLet N; InnoLet R; Monotard; NovoLet 10R,20R, 30R, 40R, 50R; NovoLet N; NovoLet R; Novolin 30R; Novolin N; Novolin R; Novolin U; NovoRapid; Penfill N; Penfill R; Penfill 10R, 20R, 30R, 40R, 50R; Velosulin; ***Malaysia:*** Actrapid; Humalog; Humulin 30/70; Humulin L; Humulin N; Humulin R; Insulatard; Mixtard 30 HM; Monotard HM; Ultratard HM; ***Mex.:*** Anilusin†; Humalog; Humalog Mix 25; Humanilusin; Humulin 70/30, 80/20; Humulin L; Humulin N; Humulin R; Insulex; Novolin 30/70; Novolin L; Novolin N; Novolin R; ***Neth.:*** Actrapid; Humaject 10/90, 20/80, 30/70, 40/60, 50/50†; Humaject NPH†; Humaject Regular†; Humalog; Humalog Mix 25; Humuline; Humuline NPH; Humuline 20/80, 30/70; Insulatard; Insuman Basal; Insuman Comb 15, 25, and 50; Insuman Rapid; Isuhuman Basal†; Isuhuman Comb 15, Comb 25, Comb 50†; Isuhuman Infusat; Isuhuman Rapid†; Mixtard 10/90, 20/80, 30/70, 40/60, 50/50; Monotard; NovoRapid; Ultratard; Velosulin; ***Norw.:*** Actrapid; Humalog; Humalog Mix 25; Humulin Mix 30/70†; Humulin NPH; Humulin Regular†; Insulatard; Insulin Basal†; Insulin Infusat†; Insulin Komb 25/75†; Insulin Rapid†; Insuman Basal; Insuman Comb 25; Insuman Infusat; Insuman Rapid; Lantus; Mixtard 10/90, 20/80, 30/70, 40/60, 50/50; Monotard; NovoRapid; Ultratard; Velosulin; ***NZ:*** Actrapid; Humalog; Humalog Mix 25; Humulin 70/30 and 80/20; Humulin L; Humulin N; Humulin R; Humulin U; Mixtard 30/70 or 50/50; Monotard; NovoRapid; PenMix 10, 20, 30, 40, or 50; Protaphane; Ultratard; ***Port.:*** Actrapid; Humalog†; Humulin Lenta; Humulin M1, M2, M3, M4, M5; Humulin NPH; Humulin Regular; Humulin Ultralenta; Insulatard; Isuhuman Basal; Isuhuman Comb 25; Isuhuman Rapid; Mixtard 10, 20, 30, 40, and 50 HM; Monotard; Ultratard; ***S.Afr.:*** Actraphane HM; Actrapid HM; Humalog; Humalog Mix 25; Humulin 30/70; Humulin L; Humulin N; Humulin R; Humulin U†; Mixtard 20/80; Monotard HM; NovoRapid; Protaphane HM; Ultratard HM; ***Singapore:*** Actrapid HM; Humalog; Humalog Mix 25; Humulin 30/70; Humulin L; Humulin N; Humulin R; Insulatard HM; Mixtard 20, 30, 50 HM; Monotard HM; NovoRapid; Ultratard HM; ***Spain:*** Actrapid; Humalog; Humalog Mix 25 and 50; Humalog NPL; Humaplus NPH; Humaplus Regular; Humaplus 20/80, 30/70; Humulina 20:80, 30:70, 50:50; Humulina Lenta; Humulina NPH; Humulina Regular; Humulina Ultralenta; Insulatard NPH; Lente MC†; Mixtard 10, 20, 30, 40, and 50; Mixtard 30/70; Monotard; NovoMix 30; NovoRapid; Ultratard; ***Swed.:*** Actrapid; Humalog; Humalog Mix 25 and 50; Humulin Mix 30/70; Humulin NPH; Humulin Regular; Humutard†; Insulatard; Insuman Basal; Insuman Comb 25; Insuman Infusat; Insuman Rapid; Isuhuman Basal†; Isuhuman Comb 25/75, 50/50†; Isuhuman Infusat†; Isuhuman Rapid†; Mixtard 10/90, 20/80, 30/70, 40/60, 50/50; Monotard; NovoRapid; Ultratard; Velosulin†; ***Switz.:*** Actrapid HM; Actrapid MC; Humalog; Huminsulin Basal (NPH); Huminsulin Long; Huminsulin Normal; Huminsulin Profil I, II, III, and IV; Huminsulin Ultralong; Hypurin 30/70 Mix; Hypurin Isophane; Hypurin Neutral; Insulatard HM; Insulatard MC; Insuman Basal; Insuman Comb 15, 25, and 50; Insuman Infusat; Insuman Rapid; Lente MC; Mixtard 30 MC; Mixtard HM 10, 20, 30, 40, 50; Monotard HM; NovoRapid; Rapitard MC†; Semilente MC; Ultralente MC†; Ultratard HM; Velosulin HM; Velosulin MC†; ***Thai.:*** Actrapid HM; Humalog; Humalog Mix 25; Humulin 70/30; Humulin N; Humulin R; Insulatard; Mixtard 20, 30, 50 HM; Monotard HM; Ultratard HM†; ***UAE:*** Jusline 70/30†; Jusline N†; Jusline R†; ***UK:*** Actrapid; Humaject I†; Humaject M1, M2, M3, M4, M5†; Humaject S; Humalog; Humalog Mix 25 and 50; Humulin I; Humulin Lente†; Humulin M3; Humulin S; Humulin Zn†; Hypurin 30/70; Hypurin Isophane; Hypurin Lente; Hypurin Neutral; Hypurin Protamine Zinc; Insulatard; Insuman Basal; Insuman Comb 15, 25, and 50; Insuman Rapid; Lantus; Lentard MC†; Mixtard 10, 20, 30, 40, and 50; Monotard; NovoMix 30; NovoRapid; Pork Actrapid; Pork Insulatard; Pork Mixtard 30; Ultratard; Velosulin; ***USA:*** Humalog; Humalog Mix 75/25 and 50/50; Humulin 70/30, 50/50; Humulin L; Humulin N; Humulin R; Humulin U Ultralente; Lantus; Lente; Lente Iletin I†; Lente Iletin II; Lente L†; Novolin 70/30; Novolin L†; Novolin N; Novolin R; NovoLog; NovoLog Mix 70/30; NPH Iletin I†; NPH Iletin II; Regular Iletin I†; Regular Iletin II; Ultralente; Velosulin Human BR.

# Metformin Hydrochloride

*(BANM, USAN, rINNM)*

Hidrocloruro de metformina; LA-6023 (metformin or metformin hydrochloride); Metformini Hydrochloridum. 1,1-Dimethylbiguanide hydrochloride.

$C_4H_{11}N_5,HCl = 165.6$.

*CAS — 657-24-9 (metformin); 1115-70-4 (metformin hydrochloride).*

*ATC — A10BA02.*

**Pharmacopoeias.** In *Chin.* and *Eur.* (see p.vi).

**Ph. Eur. 5.0** (Metformin Hydrochloride). White crystals. Freely soluble in water; slightly soluble in alcohol; practically insoluble in acetone and in dichloromethane.

## Adverse Effects, Treatment, and Precautions

As for biguanides in general, p.329.

**Breast feeding.** Based on *animal* studies the UK and US manufacturers warn that metformin may be distributed into breast milk, and that the possible effects on the infant should be considered if women wish to breast feed while receiving the drug. However, a study in 7 breast-feeding women receiving metformin at a median dose of 1.5 g daily found the concentrations in milk to be about a third of those in maternal plasma, resulting in a mean calculated dose to the infants of 40 micrograms/kg daily. Blood samples were taken from 4 of the infants: metformin concentrations were undetectable in 2, and were very low (10 to 15% of maternal values) in the others. Given these results the authors considered that women receiving metformin need not be discouraged from breast feeding.[1]


1. Hale TW, *et al.* Transfer of metformin into human milk. *Diabetologia* 2002; **45:** 1509–14.


## Interactions

As for biguanides in general, p.330.

## Pharmacokinetics

Metformin hydrochloride is slowly and incompletely absorbed from the gastrointestinal tract; the absolute bioavailability of a single 500-mg dose is reported to be about 50 to 60%, although this is reduced somewhat if taken with food. Once absorbed plasma protein binding is negligible, and it is excreted unchanged in the urine. The plasma elimination half-life is reported to range from about 2 to 6 hours after oral doses. Metformin is distributed into breast milk in small amounts.

◊ References.


1. Scheen AJ. Clinical pharmacokinetics of metformin. *Clin Pharmacokinet* 1996; **30:** 359–71.
2. Sambol NC, *et al.* Pharmacokinetics and pharmacodynamics of metformin in healthy subjects and patients with noninsulin-dependent diabetes mellitus. *J Clin Pharmacol* 1996; **36:** 1012–21.


## Uses and Administration

Metformin hydrochloride is a biguanide antidiabetic (p.329). It is given by mouth in the treatment of type 2 diabetes mellitus (p.324), and is the drug of first choice in obese patients. Initial dosage is 500 mg two or three times daily or 850 mg once or twice daily with or after meals, gradually increased if necessary to 2 to 3 g daily; doses above 2 g daily are associated with an increased incidence of gastrointestinal adverse effects. Gastrointestinal effects are also common on beginning therapy, and the *British National Formulary* recommends starting therapy more gradually with 500 mg at breakfast for at least 1 week, then increasing to 500 mg twice daily for at least 1 week, with further increases as required, up to the maximum of 2 to 3 g daily.

Metformin is also used as the chlorophenoxyacetate and as the embonate.

◊ General references.


1. Dunn CJ, Peters DH. Metformin: a review of its pharmacological properties and therapeutic use in non-insulin-dependent diabetes mellitus. *Drugs* 1995; **49:** 721–49.
2. Anonymous. Metformin for non-insulin-dependent diabetes mellitus. *Med Lett Drugs Ther* 1995; **37:** 41–2.
3. Bailey CJ, Turner RC. Metformin. *N Engl J Med* 1996; **334:** 574–9.
4. Melchior WR, Jaber LA. Metformin: an antihyperglycemic agent for treatment of type II diabetes. *Ann Pharmacother* 1996; **30:** 158–64.
5. Davidson MB, Peters AL. An overview of metformin in the treatment of type 2 diabetes mellitus. *Am J Med* 1997; **102:** 99–110.
6. Klepser TB, Kelly MW. Metformin hydrochloride: an antihyperglycemic agent. *Am J Health-Syst Pharm* 1997; **54:** 893–903. Correction. *ibid.*; 1335.
7. Kirpichnikov D, *et al.* Metformin: an update. *Ann Intern Med* 2002; **137:** 25–33.


**Action.** A review of the action of metformin[1] considered that although a number of possible mechanisms have been suggested (see p.330), the major action of metformin lay in increasing glucose transport across the cell membrane in skeletal muscle. There is also some evidence *in vitro* that it can inhibit the formation of advanced glycosylation end-products.[2]


1. Klip A, Leiter LA. Cellular mechanism of action of metformin. *Diabetes Care* 1990; **13:** 696–704.
2. Tanaka Y, *et al.* Inhibitory effect of metformin on formation of advanced glycation end products. *Curr Ther Res* 1997; **58:** 693–7.


**Diabetes mellitus.** Results of the United Kingdom Prospective Diabetes Study (UKPDS) demonstrated that intensive blood glucose control with metformin reduces the risk of diabetic complications and death in overweight patients with type 2 diabetes.[1] The study also generated some concern regarding intensive therapy with metformin plus a sulfonylurea (see Uses and Administration of Biguanide Antidiabetics, p.347) but this was not borne out on further analysis and such combinations are widely used. Metformin is also used with the thiazolidinediones,[2,3] or with insulin[4] in patients requiring combined or more intensive therapy.


1. UK Prospective Diabetes Study Group. Effect of intensive blood-glucose control with metformin on complications in overweight patients with type 2 diabetes (UKPDS 34). *Lancet* 1998; **352:** 854–65.
2. Fonseca V, *et al.* Effect of metformin and rosiglitazone combination therapy in patients with type 2 diabetes mellitus: a randomized controlled trial. *JAMA* 2000; **283:** 1695–1702. Correction. *ibid.*; **284:** 1384.
3. Einhorn D, *et al.* Pioglitazone hydrochloride in combination with metformin in the treatment of type 2 diabetes mellitus: a randomized, placebo-controlled study. *Clin Ther* 2000; **22:** 1395–1409.
4. Avilés-Santa L, *et al.* Effects of metformin in patients with poorly controlled, insulin-treated type 2 diabetes mellitus: a randomized, double-blind, placebo-controlled trial. *Ann Intern Med* 1999; **131:** 182–88.


**Polycystic ovary syndrome.** It has been suggested that hyperinsulinism may play a pathogenetic role in stimulating the abnormal androgen production from the ovary seen in women with polycystic ovary syndrome (PCOS, p.1317). Most early studies of metformin in PCOS were small, observational, and of short duration, with mixed results. Although there were reports of reduced insulin levels, increased insulin sensitivity, and improved androgen concentrations, other studies failed to confirm these effects.[1] Later randomised studies were also small, but some were of longer duration. These reported reductions in body-weight of obese patients,[2] reductions in insulin levels[2-4] and increased sensitivity,[5] improved androgen and other hormonal measures,[2,3,5] improved menstrual patterns,[2,4,5] and reduced hirsutism,[2] but again, not consistently. Combination of metformin with clomifene appeared to improve ovulatory response, compared with clomifene alone, in studies of women with PCOS,[6,7] though there is also a report of no apparent benefit.[8] Metformin has also been reported to increase the rate of spontaneous ovulation,[6,9] and may improve the outcome of *in-vitro* fertilisation procedures.[10]

Some consider that current evidence supports a trial of metformin in patients with anovulation, androgen excess, and vascular risk factors, but because of the lack of data on long-term safety such use should be supervised by an endocrinologist or a physician with suitable expertise.[1]


1. Norman RJ, *et al.* Metformin and intervention in polycystic ovary syndrome. *Med J Aust* 2001; **174:** 580–3.
2. Pasquali R, *et al.* Effect of long-term treatment with metformin added to hypocaloric diet on body composition, fat distribution, and androgen and insulin levels in abdominally obese women with and without the polycystic ovary syndrome. *J Clin Endocrinol Metab* 2000; **85:** 2767–74.
3. Nestler JE, Jakubowicz DJ. Decreases in ovarian cytochrome P450c17α activity and serum free testosterone after reduction of insulin secretion in polycystic ovary syndrome. *N Engl J Med* 1996; **335:** 617–23.
4. Morin-Papunen LC, *et al.* Endocrine and metabolic effects of metformin versus ethinyl estradiol-cyproterone acetate in obese women with polycystic ovary syndrome: a randomized study. *J Clin Endocrinol Metab* 2000; **85:** 3161–8.
5. Moghetti P, *et al.* Metformin effects on clinical features, endocrine and metabolic profiles, and insulin sensitivity in polycystic ovary syndrome: a randomized, double-blind, placebo-controlled 6-month trial, followed by open, long-term clinical evaluation. *J Clin Endocrinol Metab* 2000; **85:** 139–46.
6. Nestler JE, *et al.* Effects of metformin on spontaneous and clomiphene-induced ovulation in the polycystic ovary syndrome. *N Engl J Med* 1998; **338:** 1876–80.
7. Kocak M, *et al.* Metformin therapy improves ovulatory rates, cervical scores, and pregnancy rates in clomiphene citrate-resistant women with polycystic ovary syndrome. *Fertil Steril* 2002; **77:** 101–6.
8. Sturrock NDC, *et al.* Metformin does not enhance ovulation induction in clomiphene resistant polycystic ovary syndrome in clinical practice. *Br J Clin Pharmacol* 2002; **53:** 469–73.
9. Fleming R, *et al.* Ovarian function and metabolic factors in women with oligomenorrhea treated with metformin in a randomized double blind placebo-controlled trial. *J Clin Endocrinol Metab* 2002; **87:** 569–74.
10. Stadtmauer LA, *et al.* Metformin treatment of patients with polycystic ovary syndrome undergoing in vitro fertilization improves outcomes and is associated with modulation of the insulin-like growth factors. *Fertil Steril* 2001; **75:** 505–9.


## Preparations

***BP 2003:*** Metformin Tablets.

**Proprietary Preparations** (details are given in Part 3)
***Arg.:*** DBI AP; Glucaminol; Glucophage; Islotin; Metfori; ***Austral.:*** Diabex; Diaformin; Glucohexal; Glucomet; Glucophage; Novomet; ***Austria:*** Diabetex; Glucomin; Glucophage; Meglucon; Orabet; ***Belg.:*** Glucophage; Metformax; ***Braz.:*** Dimefor; Glifage; Glucoformin; Teutoformin; ***Canad.:*** Glucophage; Glycon; ***Chile:*** Fintaxim; Glafornil; Glifortex; Glucophage; Hipoglucin; Menarini-Metforal; ***Denm.:*** Glucophage; Orabet; ***Fin.:*** Diformin; Glucophage; Metforem; Oramet; ***Fr.:*** Diabamyl; Eddia†; Glucinan†; Glucophage; Glymax†; Metfirex†; Stagid; ***Ger.:*** Biocos; Diabesin; Diabetase; espa-formin; Glucobon; Glucophage; Mediabet; Meglucon; Mescorit; Met; Metfogamma; Metfor; Metform; Siofor; Thiabet; ***Gr.:*** Glucophage; ***Hong Kong:*** Diabetmin; Diaformin; Glucophage; Glumet; Melbin; ***India:*** Formin; Glyciphage; Walaphage; ***Irl.:*** Glucophage; ***Israel:*** Apophage; Glucomin; Glucophage; Glufor; ***Ital.:*** Glucophage; Metbay; Metforal; Metiguanide; ***Jpn:*** Melbin; ***Malaysia:*** Diabemet; Diabetmin; Glucophage; Glumet; ***Mex.:*** Anglucid; Dabex; Dimefor; Glucophage; ***Neth.:*** Glucophage; ***Norw.:*** Glucophage; Orabet†; ***NZ:*** Glucomet; Glucophage; Metomin; ***Port.:*** Glucophage; Risidon; Stagid; ***S.Afr.:*** Glucophage; ***Singapore:*** Diabetmin; Diamin; Glucophage; Glycoran; Metforal; ***Spain:*** Dianben; Glucophage†; ***Swed.:*** Glucophage; ***Switz.:*** Glucophage; Metfin; ***Thai.:*** Ammiformin; Deson; Diamet; Formin; Glucoles-500; Glucomet; Glucophage; Gluformin; Glustress; Gluzolyte; Macromin; Maformin; ME-F; Meformed; Metfor-500; Metfron; Miformin; Pocophage; Poli-Formin; Prophage; Serformin; Siamformet; ***UAE:*** Dialon; ***UK:*** Glucamet†; Glucophage; Orabet†; ***USA:*** Glucophage; Riomet.

**Multi-ingredient:** ***Chile:*** Bi-Euglucon M; Glucovance; ***Gr.:*** Normell; ***Ital.:*** Bi-Euglucon M; Glibomet; Gliconorm; Glicorest; Glucomide; Glucosulfa†; Pleiamide; Suguan M; ***Mex.:*** Bi-Euglucon M; Dabex G†; Insogen Plus; Mellitron; Obinese; Sil-Norboral; ***Port.:*** Glucovance; ***Switz.:*** Diabiformine; ***UK:*** Avandamet; ***USA:*** Avandamet; Diofen; Glucovance; Metaglip.

## Midaglizole *(rINN)*

DG-5128; Midaglizol. (±)-2-[α-(2-Imidazolin-2-ylmethyl)benzyl]pyridine.

$C_{16}H_{17}N_3 = 251.3.$

*CAS — 66529-17-7.*

### Profile

Midaglizole has been investigated as an antidiabetic. A proposed mode of action is stimulation of insulin secretion by antagonism of alpha$_2$-adrenoceptors. Midaglizole has also been investigated as a bronchodilator in asthma.

◊ References.


1. Kawazu S, *et al.* Initial phase II clinical studies on midaglizole (DG-5128). *Diabetes* 1987; **36:** 221–6.
2. Yoshie Y, *et al.* The inhibitory effect of a selective α$_2$-adrenergic receptor antagonist on moderate- to severe-type asthma. *J Allergy Clin Immunol* 1989; **84:** 747–52.
3. Nomura H, *et al.* Pharmacokinetics of midaglizole, a new hypoglycaemic agent in healthy subjects. *Biopharm Drug Dispos* 1990; **11:** 701–13.
4. Sakai H, *et al.* Protective effect of an alpha 2-adrenoceptor antagonist, midaglizole, against allergen-provoked late asthmatic responses. *J Asthma* 1995; **32:** 221–6.
5. Sakai H, *et al.* Effect of an alpha 2-adrenoceptor antagonist, midaglizole, on bronchial responsiveness to histamine in patients with mild asthma. *J Asthma* 1995; **32:** 259–64.


## Miglitol *(BAN, USAN, pINN)*

Bay-m-1099. (2R,3R,4R,5S)-1-(2-Hydroxyethyl)-2-(hydroxymethyl)piperidine-3,4,5-triol.

$C_8H_{17}NO_5 = 207.2.$

*CAS — 72432-03-2.*

*ATC — A10BF02.*

### Adverse Effects and Precautions

As for alpha-glucosidase inhibitors in general (see Acarbose, p.328). Skin rash may occur. Miglitol should be used with caution in patients with renal impairment.

### Interactions

As for alpha-glucosidase inhibitors in general (see Acarbose, p.329). Miglitol may reduce the bioavailability of propranolol and ranitidine.

### Pharmacokinetics

Miglitol is completely absorbed at a dose of 25 mg, but only 50 to 70% is absorbed at a dose of 100 mg. It is not metabolised, and is excreted unchanged in the urine with a plasma elimination half-life of about 2 hours.

### Uses and Administration

Miglitol is an alpha-glucosidase inhibitor similar in action to acarbose (p.329). It is given by mouth in the management of type 2 diabetes mellitus (p.324), alone or with a sulfonylurea. Usual initial doses are 25 mg three times daily with meals, increased if necessary to a maximum of 100 mg three times daily.

◊ References.


1. Campbell LK, *et al.* Miglitol: assessment of its role in the treatment of patients with diabetes mellitus. *Ann Pharmacother* 2000; **34:** 1291–1301.
2. Scott LJ, Spencer CM. Miglitol: a review of its therapeutic potential in type 2 diabetes mellitus. *Drugs* 2000; **59:** 521–49.
3. Standl E, *et al.* Improved glycaemic control with miglitol in inadequately-controlled type 2 diabetics. *Diabetes Res Clin Pract* 2001; **51:** 205–13.
4. Chiasson JL, *et al.* The synergistic effect of miglitol plus metformin combination therapy in the treatment of type 2 diabetes. *Diabetes Care* 2001; **24:** 989–94.
5. Van Gaal L, *et al.* Miglitol combined with metformin improves glycaemic control in type 2 diabetes. *Diabetes Obes Metab* 2001; **3:** 326–31.
6. Drent ML, *et al.* Dose-dependent efficacy of miglitol, an alpha-glucosidase inhibitor, in type 2 diabetic patients on diet alone: results of a 24-week double-blind placebo-controlled study. *Diabetes Nutr Metab* 2002; **15:** 152–9.


### Preparations

**Proprietary Preparations** (details are given in Part 3)
***Austria:*** Diastabol; ***Braz.:*** Diastabol†; ***Fin.:*** Diastabol†; ***Fr.:*** Diastabol; ***Ger.:*** Diastabol; ***Mex.:*** Diastabol; ***Port.:*** Diastabol†; ***Spain:*** Diastabol; Plumarol; ***Swed.:*** Diastabol; ***Switz.:*** Diastabol; ***USA:*** Glyset.

## Nateglinide *(USAN, rINN)*

A-4166; AY-4166; DJN-608; Nateglinida; SDZ-DJN-608; Senaglinide; YM-026. (−)-N-[(*trans*-4-Isopropylcyclohexyl)carbonyl]-D-phenylalanine.

$C_{19}H_{27}NO_3 = 317.4.$

*CAS — 105816-04-4.*

*ATC — A10BX03.*

### Adverse Effects and Precautions

As for Repaglinide, p.344.

### Interactions

As with other oral antidiabetics, the efficacy of nateglinide may be affected by drugs independently increasing or decreasing blood glucose concentrations (see Sulfonylureas, p.347).

**Antibacterials.** In a study[1] of healthy subjects, *rifampicin* reduced the plasma concentrations and half-life of nateglinide, probably by induction of its metabolism by the cytochrome P450 isoenzyme CYP2C9. The glucose-lowering effect of nateglinide was not affected, but there was a marked interindividual variation in the pharmacokinetic changes, and the authors suggested that some diabetic patients could be affected.


1. Niemi M, *et al.* Effect of rifampicin on the pharmacokinetics and pharmacodynamics of nateglinide in healthy subjects. *Br J Clin Pharmacol* 2003; **56:** 427–32.


**Antifungals.** In a study[1] of healthy subjects, *fluconazole* raised the plasma concentrations and prolonged the half-life of nateglinide, probably by inhibition of its metabolism by the cytochrome P450 isoenzyme CYP2C9. The glucose-lowering effect of nateglinide was not affected, but a low dose of nateglinide had been used and the authors suggested that in diabetic patients fluconazole may enhance and prolong the effects of nateglinide.


1. Niemi M, *et al.* Effect of fluconazole on the pharmacokinetics and pharmacodynamics of nateglinide. *Clin Pharmacol Ther* 2003; **74:** 25–31.


### Pharmacokinetics

Nateglinide is rapidly absorbed after oral doses, with peak plasma concentrations occurring within one hour and an absolute bioavailability of 73%. Nateglinide is 98% bound to plasma proteins. It is predominantly metabolised by cytochrome P450 isoenzyme CYP2C9, and to a lesser extent by CYP3A4. The parent drug and metabolites are mainly excreted in the urine but about 10% is eliminated in the faeces. The elimination half-life is about 1.5 hours.

◊ References.


1. Choudhury S, *et al.* Single-dose pharmacokinetics of nateglinide in subjects with hepatic cirrhosis. *J Clin Pharmacol* 2000; **40:** 634–40.
2. Devineni D, *et al.* Pharmacokinetics of nateglinide in renally impaired diabetic patients. *J Clin Pharmacol* 2003; **43:** 163–70.
3. McLeod JF. Clinical pharmacokinetics of nateglinide: a rapidly-absorbed, short-acting insulinotropic agent. *Clin Pharmacokinet* 2004; **43:** 97–120.


### Uses and Administration

Nateglinide, like repaglinide (p.345), is a meglitinide antidiabetic used in the treatment of type 2 diabetes mellitus (p.324). It is given by mouth within the 30 minutes before meals in doses of 60 or 120 mg three times daily. This may be increased to 180 mg three times daily if necessary. Nateglinide is also given in similar doses with metformin or a thiazolidinedione in type 2 diabetes not adequately controlled by these drugs alone.

◊ References.


1. Dunn CJ, Faulds D. Nateglinide. *Drugs* 2000; **60:** 607–15.
2. Hanefeld M, *et al.* Rapid and short-acting mealtime insulin secretion with nateglinide controls both prandial and mean glycemia. *Diabetes Care* 2000; **23:** 202–7.
3. Horton ES, *et al.* Nateglinide alone and in combination with metformin improves glycemic control by reducing mealtime glucose levels in type 2 diabetes. *Diabetes Care* 2000; **23:** 1660–5.
4. Levien TL, *et al.* Nateglinide therapy for type 2 diabetes mellitus. *Ann Pharmacother* 2001; **35:** 1426–34.
5. Fonseca V. *et al.* Addition of nateglinide to rosiglitazone monotherapy suppresses mealtime hyperglycemia and improves overall glycemic control. *Diabetes Care* 2003; **26:** 1685–90.


### Preparations

**Proprietary Preparations** (details are given in Part 3)
***Arg.:*** Nateglin; Starlix; ***Braz.:*** Starlix; ***Chile:*** Starlix; ***Denm.:*** Starlix; ***Fin.:*** Starlix; ***Ger.:*** Starlix; ***Gr.:*** Starlix; ***Hong Kong:*** Starlix; ***India:*** Glinate; ***Irl.:***

Starlix; **Malaysia:** Starlix; **Norw.:** Starlix; **NZ:** Starlix; **S.Afr.:** Starlix; **Singapore:** Starlix; **Spain:** Starlix; **Swed.:** Starlix; **Switz.:** Starlix; **UK:** Starlix; **USA:** Starlix.

## Phenformin Hydrochloride *(BANM, pINNM)*

Fenformina Cloridrato; Hidrocloruro de fenformina. 1-Phenethylbiguanide hydrochloride.

$C_{10}H_{15}N_5,HCl = 241.7.$

*CAS — 114-86-3 (phenformin); 834-28-6 (phenformin hydrochloride).*

*ATC — A10BA01.*

**Pharmacopoeias.** In *Chin.*

### Profile

Phenformin hydrochloride is a biguanide antidiabetic (p.329). Although it is generally considered to be associated with an unacceptably high incidence of lactic acidosis, often fatal, it is still available in some countries for the treatment of type 2 diabetes mellitus.

Phenformin was implicated in the controversial reports of excess cardiovascular mortality associated with oral hypoglycaemic therapy (see under Sulfonylureas, Effects on the Cardiovascular System, p.346).

### Preparations

**Proprietary Preparations** (details are given in Part 3)
**Braz.:** Debei†; **India:** DBI; **Mex.:** Azucaps; Debeone; **Port.:** Debeina.
**Multi-ingredient:** **India:** Chlorformin; **Ital.:** Bi-Euglucon; Bidiabe; Gliben F; Gliformin; Suguan.

## Pimagedine *(rINN)*

GER-11 (pimagedine hydrochloride); Pimagedina. Aminoguanidine.

$CH_6N_4 = 74.09.$

*CAS — 79-17-4.*

NOTE. Pimagedine Hydrochloride is *USAN.*

### Profile

Pimagedine reportedly inhibits the formation of glycosylated proteins (advanced glycosylation end-products) and has other actions including inhibition of aldose reductase. It is under investigation for the prevention of diabetic complications (p.326).

◊ References.


1. Corbett JA, *et al.* Aminoguanidine, a novel inhibitor of nitric oxide formation, prevents diabetic vascular dysfunction. *Diabetes* 1992; **41:** 552–6.
2. Wolffenbuttel BHR, Huijberts MSP. Aminoguanidine, a potential drug for the treatment of diabetic complications. *Neth J Med* 1993; **42:** 205–8.


# Pioglitazone Hydrochloride

*(BANM, USAN, rINNM)*

AD-4833 (pioglitazone); Hidrocloruro de pioglitazona; U-72107A; U-72107E (pioglitazone). (±)-5-{*p*-[2-(5-Ethyl-2-pyridyl)ethoxy]benzyl}-2,4-thiazolidinedione hydrochloride.

$C_{19}H_{20}N_2O_3S,HCl = 392.9.$

*CAS — 111025-46-8 (pioglitazone); 112529-15-4 (pioglitazone hydrochloride).*

*ATC — A10BG03.*

### Adverse Effects and Precautions

As for Rosiglitazone Maleate, p.345. The effects of pioglitazone on serum lipid concentrations appear to differ from those of rosiglitazone, see below. Other adverse effects reported include upper respiratory-tract infections, haematuria, myalgia, and visual disturbances. Liver function should be monitored periodically as there have been isolated reports of liver dysfunction, and the drug should be used with caution in patients with hepatic impairment (see below). For a suggestion that use with insulin may contribute to heart failure see Administration, below. See also Effects on the Heart, under Rosiglitazone, p.345.

**Effects on lipids.** Thiazolidinediones are reported to affect serum concentrations of lipids. Compared with placebo,[1,2] pioglitazone has been found to reduce triglycerides, increase high-density lipoprotein (HDL)-cholesterol, and have little or no effect on low-density lipoprotein (LDL)- and total cholesterol. In a study[3] of patients being transferred from troglitazone to either pioglitazone or rosiglitazone, there were decreases in concentrations of triglycerides, LDL- and total cholesterol, and an increase in HDL-cholesterol in those patients on pioglitazone, whereas the opposite occurred for rosiglitazone. Whether these effects of pioglitazone reduce cardiovascular risk in patients with type 2 diabetes is yet to be established.


1. Kipnes MS, *et al.* Pioglitazone hydrochloride in combination with sulfonylurea therapy improves glycemic control in patients with type 2 diabetes mellitus: a randomized, placebo-controlled study. *Am J Med* 2001; **111:** 10–17.
2. Rosenblatt S, *et al.* The impact of pioglitazone on glycemic control and atherogenic dyslipidemia in patients with type 2 diabetes mellitus. *Coron Artery Dis* 2001; **12:** 413–23.
3. Gegick CG, Altheimer MD. Comparison of effects of thiazolidinediones on cardiovascular risk factors: observations from a clinical practice. *Endocr Pract* 2001; **7:** 162–9.


**Effects on the liver.** There have been isolated reports of hepatocellular injury in patients receiving pioglitazone.[1-3]

The UK and US manufacturers recommend that liver enzymes should be checked before starting therapy with pioglitazone; patients with aminotransferase (ALT) concentrations more than 2.5 times the upper limit of normal should not be given pioglitazone. ALT concentrations should then be monitored every 2 months during the first 12 months of treatment and periodically thereafter. If ALT concentrations rise to more than 3 times the upper limit of normal and remain so after retesting then treatment with pioglitazone should be discontinued; treatment should also be discontinued if jaundice develops.


1. Maeda K. Hepatocellular injury in a patient receiving pioglitazone. *Ann Intern Med* 2001; **135:** 306.
2. May LD, *et al.* Mixed hepatocellular-cholestatic liver injury after pioglitazone therapy. *Ann Intern Med* 2002; **136:** 449–52.
3. Pinto AG, *et al.* Severe but reversible cholestatic liver injury after pioglitazone therapy. *Ann Intern Med* 2002; **137:** 857.


### Interactions

**Antibacterials.** For a report of hypoglycaemia when *gatifloxacin* was given to a patient already receiving glibenclamide and pioglitazone, see p.216.

### Pharmacokinetics

Pioglitazone is rapidly absorbed after oral doses. Peak plasma concentrations are obtained within 2 hours and bioavailability exceeds 80%. Pioglitazone is more than 99% bound to plasma proteins. It is extensively metabolised by cytochrome P450 isoenzymes CYP3A4 and CYP2C9 to both active and inactive metabolites. It is excreted in urine and faeces and has a plasma half-life of up to 7 hours. The active metabolites have a half-life of up to 24 hours.

### Uses and Administration

Pioglitazone is a thiazolidinedione oral antidiabetic similar to rosiglitazone (p.345). It is used in the management of type 2 diabetes mellitus (p.324). It is given as pioglitazone hydrochloride but doses are expressed in terms of the base; pioglitazone hydrochloride 1.1 mg is approximately equivalent to 1 mg of pioglitazone. It is given orally as monotherapy, particularly in patients who are overweight and for whom metformin is contra-indicated or not tolerated. Pioglitazone may also be added to metformin, a sulfonylurea, or insulin, when single-agent therapy is inadequate (but see Administration, below). The usual dose is 15 or 30 mg once daily. This may be increased to a maximum of 45 mg once daily if necessary, when used as monotherapy or with metformin or a sulfonylurea. Pioglitazone may be taken with or without food.

◊ References.


1. Gillies PS, Dunn CJ. Pioglitazone. *Drugs* 2000; **60:** 333–43.
2. Anonymous. Pioglitazone and rosiglitazone for diabetes. *Drug Ther Bull* 2001; **39:** 65–8.
3. Parulkar AA, *et al.* Nonhypoglycemic effects of thiazolidinediones. *Ann Intern Med* 2001; **134:** 61–71.
4. O'Moore-Sullivan TM, Prins JB. Thiazolidinediones and type 2 diabetes: new drugs for an old disease. *Med J Aust* 2002; **176:** 381–6. Correction. *ibid.*; **177:** 396.
5. Diamant M, Heine RJ. Thiazolidinediones in type 2 diabetes mellitus: current clinical evidence. *Drugs* 2003; **63:** 1373–1405.


**Administration.** Although pioglitazone is licensed for use in combination with other antidiabetic drugs, the specifics of licensing and use may vary from country to country. In the UK, use of pioglitazone with insulin is considered to be contra-indicated, because of an increased risk of heart failure. Furthermore, although it is licensed for use in combination therapy with metformin or a sulfonylurea in patients who do not respond to monotherapy with one of these drugs, the National Institute for Clinical Excellence recommends such use of pioglitazone or rosiglitazone only in patients who cannot be given combination therapy with metformin plus a sulfonylurea.[1] However, in the USA, pioglitazone is licensed for combination therapy with insulin (with appropriate monitoring), metformin, or a sulfonylurea in any patient in whom single agent therapy is inadequate.


1. National Institute for Clinical Excellence. Guidance on the use of glitazones for the treatment of type 2 diabetes (issued August 2003). Available at: http://www.nice.org.uk/pdf/TA63_Glitazones_Review_Guidance.pdf (accessed 08/07/04)


### Preparations

**Proprietary Preparations** (details are given in Part 3)
**Arg.:** Actos; Cereluc; Pioglit; **Austral.:** Actos; **Braz.:** Actos; **Canad.:** Actos; **Chile:** Actos; Diabestat; **Denm.:** Actos; **Fin.:** Actos; **Fr.:** Actos; **Ger.:** Actos; **Gr.:** Actos; **Hong Kong:** Actos; **India:** G-Tase; Glizone; Opam; **Ital.:** Actos; **Jpn:** Actos; **Mex.:** Zactos; **Norw.:** Actos; **NZ:** Actos; **Port.:** Actos; **S.Afr.:** Actos; **Spain:** Actos; **Swed.:** Actos; **Switz.:** Actos; **Thai.:** Actos; **UK:** Actos; **USA:** Actos.

## Pramlintide *(BAN, USAN, rINN)*

AC-137; AC-0137 (pramlintide or pramlintide acetate); Pramlintida; Tripro-amylin.

*CAS — 151126-32-8 (pramlintide); 196078-30-5 (pramlintide acetate).*

### Profile

Pramlintide is an analogue of amylin, a pancreatic peptide thought to play a role in the regulation of glucose homoeostasis. Pramlintide is under investigation in the management of diabetes mellitus (p.324).

◊ References.


1. Thompson RG, *et al.* Pramlintide: a human amylin analogue reduced postprandial plasma glucose, insulin, and C-peptide concentrations in patients with type 2 diabetes. *Diabet Med* 1997; **14:** 547–55.
2. Thompson RG, *et al.* Effects of pramlintide, an analog of human amylin, on plasma glucose profiles in patients with IDDM: results of a multicenter trial. *Diabetes* 1997; **46:** 632–6.
3. Thompson RG, *et al.* Pramlintide, a synthetic analog of human amylin, improves the metabolic profile of patients with type 2 diabetes using insulin. *Diabetes Care* 1998; **21:** 987–93.
4. Whitehouse F, *et al.* A randomized study and open-label extension evaluating the long-term efficacy of pramlintide as an adjunct to insulin therapy in type 1 diabetes. *Diabetes Care* 2002; **25:** 724–30.
5. Ratner RE, *et al.* Adjunctive therapy with the amylin analogue pramlintide leads to a combined improvement in glycemic and weight control in insulin-treated subjects with type 2 diabetes. *Diabetes Technol Ther* 2002; **4:** 51–61.
6. Hollander PA, *et al.* Pramlintide as an adjunct to insulin therapy improves long-term glycemic and weight control in patients with type 2 diabetes: a 1-year randomized controlled trial. *Diabetes Care* 2003; **26:** 784–90.


# Repaglinide *(BAN, USAN, rINN)*

AG-EE-6232W; AG-EE-623-ZW; Repaglinida. (+)-2-Ethoxy-α-{[(*S*)-α-isobutyl-*o*-piperidinobenzyl]carbamoyl}-*p*-toluic acid; (*S*)-2-Ethoxy-4-{[1-(*o*-piperidinophenyl)-3-methylbutyl]carbamoylmethyl}benzoic acid.

$C_{27}H_{36}N_2O_4 = 452.6.$

*CAS — 135062-02-1.*

*ATC — A10BX02.*

**Pharmacopoeias.** In *US.*

**USP 27** (Repaglinide). A white to off-white solid. Soluble in methyl alcohol. Store in airtight containers.

### Adverse Effects and Precautions

Repaglinide may cause gastrointestinal adverse effects including abdominal pain, diarrhoea, constipation, nausea, and vomiting. Hypoglycaemia (usually mild), back and joint pain, hypersensitivity reactions including pruritus, rashes and urticaria, and elevated liver enzyme values may occur.

Precautions are similar to those which apply with the shorter-acting sulfonylurea hypoglycaemics (p.346). Repaglinide should not be given to patients with severe hepatic impairment.

**Hypoglycaemia.** Mild hypoglycaemia has been reported in patients receiving repaglinide,[1] although in a study comparing flexible repaglinide dosing with fixed glibenclamide dosing, all hypoglycaemic events recorded were in the glibenclamide group.[2] Other studies have found rates of hypoglycaemia in patients receiving repaglinide to be less than, or similar to, sulfonylureas.[3] The risk of hypoglycaemia may be reduced as patients can omit a dose of repaglinide if a meal is missed.


1. Moses RG, *et al.* Flexible meal-related dosing with repaglinide facilitates glycemic control in therapy-naive type 2 diabetes. *Diabetes Care* 2001; **24:** 11–15.
2. Damsbo P, *et al.* A double-blind randomized comparison of meal-related glycemic control by repaglinide and glyburide in well-controlled type 2 diabetic patients. *Diabetes Care* 1999; **22:** 789–94.
3. Culy CR, Jarvis B. Repaglinide: a review of its therapeutic use in type 2 diabetes mellitus. *Drugs* 2001; **61:** 1625–60.


### Interactions

As with other oral antidiabetics, the efficacy of repaglinide may be affected by drugs independently increasing or decreasing blood glucose concentrations (see Sulfonylureas, p.347).

Cytochrome P450 isoenzyme CYP3A4 inducers such as rifampicin and carbamazepine may decrease the effect of repaglinide. *In vitro* studies suggest that drugs that inhibit CYP3A4 may reduce the metabolism of repaglinide. Although study of healthy subjects has found no interaction with ketoconazole, clarithromycin may increase plasma concentrations of repaglinide. Use of repaglinide with the CYP2C8 inhibitor gemfibrozil has resulted in marked reduction in repaglinide clearance, and severe hypoglycaemia; the combination is contra-indicated.

For a report of hypoglycaemia when gatifloxacin was given to a patient already receiving repaglinide, see p.216.

◊ References.


1. Hatorp V, Thomsen MS. Drug interaction studies with repaglinide: repaglinide on digoxin or theophylline pharmacokinetics and cimetidine on repaglinide pharmacokinetics. *J Clin Pharmacol* 2000; **40:** 184–92.
2. Niemi M, *et al.* Rifampin decreases the plasma concentrations and effects of repaglinide. *Clin Pharmacol Ther* 2000; **68:** 495–500.
3. Niemi M, *et al.* The cytochrome P4503A4 inhibitor clarithromycin increases the plasma concentrations and effects of repaglinide. *Clin Pharmacol Ther* 2001; **70:** 58–65.
4. Niemi M, *et al.* Effects of gemfibrozil, itraconazole, and their combination on the pharmacokinetics and pharmacodynamics of repaglinide: potentially hazardous interaction between gemfibrozil and repaglinide. *Diabetologia* 2003; **46:** 347–51.


### Pharmacokinetics

Repaglinide is rapidly absorbed from the gastrointestinal tract, with peak plasma concentrations occurring within 1 hour. The mean bioavailability is about 60%. Repaglinide is highly bound to plasma proteins, and has a plasma elimination half-life of about 1 hour. It undergoes almost complete hepatic metabolism involving the cytochrome P450 isoenzyme CYP3A4. The metabolites, which are inactive, are excreted in the bile. Higher plasma concentrations and prolonged half-life of repaglinide may occur in patients with severe renal impairment or chronic liver disease.

◊ References.


1. Marbury TC, *et al.* Pharmacokinetics of repaglinide in subjects with renal impairment. *Clin Pharmacol Ther* 2000; **67:** 7–15.
2. Hatorp V, *et al.* Single-dose pharmacokinetics of repaglinide in subjects with chronic liver disease. *J Clin Pharmacol* 2000; **40:** 142–52.
3. Hatorp V. Clinical pharmacokinetics and pharmacodynamics of repaglinide. *Clin Pharmacokinet* 2002; **41:** 471–83.


### Uses and Administration

Repaglinide is a meglitinide antidiabetic used for the treatment of type 2 diabetes mellitus (p.324). It has a chemical structure different from that of the sulfonylureas, but appears to have a similar mode of action.

Repaglinide is given by mouth up to 30 minutes before meals, in usual initial doses of 0.5 mg; initial doses of 1 or 2 mg are usually given to patients who have had previous hypoglycaemic treatment. The dose may be adjusted, at intervals of 1 to 2 weeks, up to a maximum of 4 mg before meals; a total of 16 mg daily should not be exceeded. Repaglinide is also given with metformin or a thiazolidinedione in type 2 diabetes not adequately controlled by metformin alone.

◊ References.


1. Anonymous. Repaglinide for type 2 diabetes mellitus. *Med Lett Drugs Ther* 1998; **40:** 55–6.
2. Moses R, *et al.* Effect of repaglinide addition to metformin monotherapy on glycemic control in patients with type 2 diabetes. *Diabetes Care* 1999; **22:** 119–24.
3. Wolffenbuttel BH, Landgraf R. A 1-year multicenter randomized double-blind comparison of repaglinide and glyburide for the treatment of type 2 diabetes. *Diabetes Care* 1999; **22:** 463–7.
4. Moses RG, *et al.* Flexible meal-related dosing with repaglinide facilitates glycemic control in therapy-naive type 2 diabetes. *Diabetes Care* 2001; **24:** 11–15.
5. Dornhorst A. Insulinotropic meglitinide analogues. *Lancet* 2001; **358:** 1709–16.
6. Culy CR, Jarvis B. Repaglinide: a review of its therapeutic use in type 2 diabetes mellitus. *Drugs* 2001; **61:** 1625–60.
7. Moses R. Repaglinide in combination therapy. *Diabetes Nutr Metab* 2002; **15** (suppl): 33–8.
8. Derosa G, *et al.* Comparison between repaglinide and glimepiride in patients with type 2 diabetes mellitus: a one-year, randomized, double-blind assessment of metabolic parameters and cardiovascular risk factors. *Clin Ther* 2003; **25:** 472–84.
9. Raskin P, *et al.* Combination therapy for type 2 diabetes: repaglinide plus rosiglitazone. *Diabet Med* 2004; **21:** 329–35.


### Preparations

***USP 27:*** Repaglinide Tablets.

**Proprietary Preparations** (details are given in Part 3)
***Arg.:*** NovoNorm; Sestrine; ***Austral.:*** NovoNorm; ***Austria:*** NovoNorm; ***Belg.:*** NovoNorm; ***Braz.:*** Gluconorm; NovoNorm; Prandin; ***Canad.:*** Gluconorm; ***Chile:*** Novonorm; ***Denm.:*** NovoNorm; ***Fin.:*** NovoNorm; ***Fr.:*** NovoNorm; ***Ger.:*** NovoNorm; ***Gr.:*** NovoNorm; ***Hong Kong:*** NovoNorm; ***India:*** Rapilin; ***Irl.:*** NovoNorm; ***Israel:*** NovoNorm; ***Ital.:*** NovoNorm; ***Malaysia:*** NovoNorm; ***Neth.:*** NovoNorm; ***Norw.:*** NovoNorm; ***NZ:*** NovoNorm; ***S.Afr.:*** NovoNorm; ***Singapore:*** NovoNorm; ***Spain:*** NovoNorm; Prandin; ***Swed.:*** NovoNorm; ***Switz.:*** NovoNorm; ***Thai.:*** NovoNorm; ***UK:*** NovoNorm; ***USA:*** Prandin.

## Rosiglitazone Maleate *(BANM, USAN, rINNM)*

BRL-49653-C; Maleato de rosiglitazona. (±)-5-{*p*-[2-(Methyl-2-pyridylamino)ethoxy]benzyl}-2,4-thiazolidinedione maleate (1:1).

$C_{18}H_{19}N_3O_3S,C_4H_4O_4$ = 473.5.

*CAS — 122320-73-4 (rosiglitazone); 155141-29-0 (rosiglitazone maleate).*

*ATC — A10BG02.*

### Adverse Effects and Precautions

Rosiglitazone may cause hypoglycaemia, headache, weight gain, and anaemia. It may also cause dizziness, gastrointestinal disturbances, muscle cramps, dyspnoea, paraesthesia, alopecia, pruritus, and hypercholesterolaemia. Very rarely angioedema and urticaria have been reported.

Rosiglitazone can cause oedema, which may worsen or precipitate heart failure. It should therefore be used with caution in patients with oedema, and should not be used in those with a history of heart failure (see also below). Liver function should be monitored periodically as there have been isolated reports of liver dysfunction, and the drug should be used with caution in patients with hepatic impairment (see below).

In women who are anovulatory because of insulin resistance, rosiglitazone therapy may result in a resumption of ovulation.

**Effects on the heart.** Both pioglitazone and rosiglitazone can cause peripheral and pulmonary oedema, which can worsen or precipitate heart failure; a number of cases have been described.[1,2] A large retrospective cohort study[3] also found that the use of thiazolidinediones increased the risk of heart failure. The incidence of peripheral oedema with monotherapy has been reported[4] to range from 3 to 5%, and this increases slightly when a thiazolidinedione is used with another oral antidiabetic. The incidence is about 15% when a thiazolidinedione is used with insulin. The incidence of heart failure is lower, but has been reported to be 2 to 3% when a thiazolidinedione is used with insulin. The American Heart Association and American Diabetes Association have recommended[4] that patients with risk factors for heart disease or a depressed ejection fraction but without symptoms, and patients with NYHA class I or II heart failure, should start with a low dose of a thiazolidinedione that is only increased gradually as necessary and with careful monitoring. Patients with more severe heart failure (class III and IV) should not receive these drugs.

For restrictions on combination therapy see Administration, below.


1. Page RL, *et al.* Possible heart failure exacerbation associated with rosiglitazone: case report and literature review. *Pharmacotherapy* 2003; **23:** 945–54.
2. Cheng AYY, Fantus IG. Thiazolidinedione-induced congestive heart failure. *Ann Pharmacother* 2004; **38:** 817–20.
3. Delea TE, *et al.* Use of thiazolidinediones and risk of heart failure in people with type 2 diabetes: a retrospective cohort study. *Diabetes Care* 2003; **26:** 2983–9.
4. Nesto RW, *et al.* Thiazolidinedione use, fluid retention, and congestive heart failure: a consensus statement from the American Heart Association and American Diabetes Association. *Circulation* 2003; **108:** 2941–8. Also published in *Diabetes Care* 2004; **27:** 256–63.


**Effects on the liver.** Several cases of hepatotoxicity have been described[1-5] in patients receiving rosiglitazone. Most of these occurred within a few weeks or months of starting rosiglitazone therapy. However, the causality of some of these cases has been debated[6,7] because of coexisting disease and concomitant medication.

The UK and US manufacturers recommend that liver enzymes should be checked before starting therapy with rosiglitazone; patients with aminotransferase (ALT) concentrations more than 2.5 times the upper limit of normal should not be given rosiglitazone. ALT concentrations should then be monitored every 2 months during the first 12 months of treatment and periodically thereafter. If ALT concentrations rise to more than 3 times the upper limit of normal and remain so after retesting then treatment with rosiglitazone should be discontinued; treatment should also be discontinued if jaundice develops.


1. Forman LM, *et al.* Hepatic failure in a patient taking rosiglitazone. *Ann Intern Med* 2000; **132:** 118–21.
2. Al-Salman J, *et al.* Hepatocellular injury in a patient receiving rosiglitazone: a case report. *Ann Intern Med* 2000; **132:** 121–4.
3. Ravinuthala RS, Nori U. Rosiglitazone toxicity. *Ann Intern Med* 2000; **133:** 658.
4. Hachey DM, *et al.* Isolated elevation of alkaline phosphatase level associated with rosiglitazone. *Ann Intern Med* 2000; **133:** 752.
5. Gouda HE, *et al.* Liver failure in a patient treated with long-term rosiglitazone therapy. *Am J Med* 2001; **111:** 584–5.
6. Freid J, *et al.* Rosiglitazone and hepatic failure. *Ann Intern Med* 2000; **132:** 164.
7. Isley WL, Oki JC. Rosiglitazone and liver failure. *Ann Intern Med* 2000; **133:** 393.


### Pharmacokinetics

Rosiglitazone is well absorbed from the gastrointestinal tract following oral dosing. Peak plasma concentrations are achieved within 1 hour and the bioavailability is 99%. It is 99.8% bound to plasma proteins. Rosiglitazone is extensively metabolised, almost exclusively by the cytochrome P450 isoenzyme CYP2C8. It is excreted in the urine and faeces, and has a half-life of 3 to 4 hours.

◊ References.


1. Baldwin SJ, *et al.* Characterization of the cytochrome P450 enzymes involved in the in vitro metabolism of rosiglitazone. *Br J Clin Pharmacol* 1999; **48:** 424–32.


### Uses and Administration

Rosiglitazone is a thiazolidinedione oral antidiabetic that improves insulin sensitivity and is used for the treatment of type 2 diabetes mellitus (p.324). It is given as rosiglitazone maleate but doses are expressed in terms of the base; rosiglitazone maleate 1.32 mg is approximately equivalent to 1 mg of rosiglitazone. It is given orally as monotherapy, particularly in patients who are overweight and for whom metformin is contra-indicated or not tolerated. Rosiglitazone may also be added to metformin, a sulfonylurea, or insulin, when single-agent therapy is inadequate (but see Administration, below). The usual initial dose is 4 mg daily, given in a single dose or two divided doses. The dose may be increased to a maximum of 8 mg daily if necessary after 8 to 12 weeks in patients receiving monotherapy or combination therapy with metformin. Rosiglitazone may be taken with or without food.

◊ References.


1. Nolan JJ, *et al.* Rosiglitazone taken once daily provides effective glycaemic control in patients with type 2 diabetes mellitus. *Diabet Med* 2000; **17:** 287–94.
2. Fonseca V, *et al.* Effect of metformin and rosiglitazone combination therapy in patients with type 2 diabetes mellitus: a randomized controlled trial. *JAMA* 2000; **283:** 1695–1702. Correction. *ibid.*; **284:** 1384.
3. Lebovitz HE, *et al.* Rosiglitazone monotherapy is effective in patients with type 2 diabetes. *J Clin Endocrinol Metab* 2001; **86:** 280–8.
4. Anonymous. Pioglitazone and rosiglitazone for diabetes. *Drug Ther Bull* 2001; **39:** 65–8.
5. Parulkar AA, *et al.* Nonhypoglycemic effects of thiazolidinediones. *Ann Intern Med* 2001; **134:** 61–71.
6. Raskin P, *et al.* A randomized trial of rosiglitazone therapy in patients with inadequately controlled insulin-treated type 2 diabetes. *Diabetes Care* 2001; **24:** 1226–32.
7. O'Moore-Sullivan TM, Prins JB. Thiazolidinediones and type 2 diabetes: new drugs for an old disease. *Med J Aust* 2002; **176:** 381–6. Correction. *ibid.*; **177:** 396.
8. Wagstaff AJ, Goa KL. Rosiglitazone: a review of its use in the management of type 2 diabetes mellitus. *Drugs* 2002; **62:** 1805–37.
9. Diamant M, Heine RJ. Thiazolidinediones in type 2 diabetes mellitus: current clinical evidence. *Drugs* 2003; **63:** 1373–1405.


**Administration.** Although rosiglitazone is licensed for use in combination with other antidiabetic drugs the specifics of licensing and use may vary from country to country. In the UK the use of rosiglitazone with insulin is considered to be contra-indicated, because of an increased risk of heart failure and other cardiac events (see Effects on the Heart, above). Furthermore, although it is licensed for use in combination therapy with metformin or a sulfonylurea in patients who do not respond to monotherapy with one of these drugs, the National Institute for Clinical Excellence recommends such use only in patients who cannot be given combination therapy with metformin plus a sulfonylurea.[1] However, in the USA, rosiglitazone is licensed for combination therapy with insulin (with appropriate monitoring), metformin, or a sulfonylurea in patients in whom single agent therapy is inadequate.


1. National Institute for Clinical Excellence. Guidance on the use of glitazones for the treatment of type 2 diabetes (issued August 2003). Available at: http://www.nice.org.uk/pdf/TA63_Glitazones_Review_Guidance.pdf (accessed 08/07/04)


### Preparations

**Proprietary Preparations** (details are given in Part 3)
***Arg.:*** Avandia; Glimide; ***Austral.:*** Avandia; ***Belg.:*** Avandia; ***Braz.:*** Avandia; Tiltab†; ***Canad.:*** Avandia; ***Chile:*** Avandia; ***Denm.:*** Avandia; ***Fin.:*** Avandia; ***Fr.:*** Avandia; ***Ger.:*** Avandia; ***Gr.:*** Avandia; ***Hong Kong:*** Avandia; ***India:*** Rezult; ***Irl.:*** Avandia; ***Israel:*** Avandia; ***Ital.:*** Avandia; ***Malaysia:*** Avandia; ***Mex.:*** Avandia; ***Neth.:*** Avandia; ***Norw.:*** Avandia; ***NZ:*** Avandia; ***Port.:*** Avandia; ***S.Afr.:*** Avandia; ***Singapore:*** Avandia; ***Spain:*** Avandia; ***Swed.:*** Avandia; ***Switz.:*** Avandia; ***Thai.:*** Avandia; ***UK:*** Avandia; ***USA:*** Avandia.

**Multi-ingredient:** ***UK:*** Avandamet; ***USA:*** Avandamet.

## Sorbinil *(BAN, USAN, rINN)*

CP-45634; Sorbinilo. (*S*)-6-Fluorospiro(chroman-4,4′-imidazolidine)-2′,5′-dione.

$C_{11}H_9FN_2O_3$ = 236.2.

*CAS — 68367-52-2.*

### Profile

Sorbinil is an aldose reductase inhibitor similar in action to epalrestat (p.331). It was tried mainly in the treatment of diabetic retinopathy and neuropathy, with conflicting results.

Severe skin reactions have been reported.

◊ References.

1. Sorbinil Retinopathy Trial Research Group. A randomized trial of sorbinil, an aldose reductase inhibitor, in diabetic retinopathy. *Arch Ophthalmol* 1990; **108:** 1234–44.
2. Sorbinil Retinopathy Trial Research Group. The sorbinil retinopathy trial; neuropathy results. *Neurology* 1993; **43:** 1141–9.

## Sulfonylurea Antidiabetics

Antidiabéticos sulfonilureas.

### Adverse Effects

Gastrointestinal disturbances such as nausea, vomiting, heartburn, anorexia, diarrhoea, and a metallic taste may occur with sulfonylureas and are usually mild and dose-dependent; increased appetite and weight gain may occur. Skin rashes and pruritus may occur and photosensitivity has been reported. Rashes are usually hypersensitivity reactions and may progress to more serious disorders (see below). Facial flushing may develop in patients receiving sulfonylureas, particularly chlorpropamide, when alcohol is consumed (see under Interactions, below).

Mild hypoglycaemia may occur; severe hypoglycaemia is usually an indication of overdosage and is relatively uncommon. Hypoglycaemia is more likely with long-acting sulfonylureas such as chlorpropamide and glibenclamide, which have been associated with severe, prolonged, and sometimes fatal hypoglycaemia.

Other severe effects may be manifestations of a hypersensitivity reaction. They include altered liver enzyme values, hepatitis and cholestatic jaundice, leucopenia, thrombocytopenia, aplastic anaemia, agranulocytosis, haemolytic anaemia, erythema multiforme or the Stevens-Johnson syndrome, exfoliative dermatitis, and erythema nodosum.

The sulfonylureas, particularly chlorpropamide, occasionally induce a syndrome of inappropriate secretion of antidiuretic hormone (SIADH) characterised by water retention, hyponatraemia, and CNS effects. However, some sulfonylureas, such as glibenclamide, glipizide, and tolazamide are also stated to have mild diuretic actions.

Work on tolbutamide has suggested that the sulfonylureas might be associated with an increase in cardiovascular mortality; this has been the subject of considerable debate (see Effects on the Cardiovascular System, below).

◊ Reviews.

1. Paice BJ, *et al.* Undesired effects of the sulphonylurea drugs. *Adverse Drug React Acute Poisoning Rev* 1985; **4:** 23–36.
2. Harrower ADB. Comparative tolerability of sulphonylureas in diabetes mellitus. *Drug Safety* 2000; **22:** 313–20.

**Effects on the cardiovascular system.** A multicentre study carried out under the University Group Diabetes Program (UGDP) reported an increased incidence in mortality from cardiovascular complications in diabetic patients given tolbutamide as compared with those treated with diet alone or insulin;[1] a similar increase was also noted in patients given phenformin.[2] The reports from the UGDP aroused prolonged controversy which was not entirely settled by detailed reassessment of relevant studies.[3] Eventually in 1984 the FDA made it a requirement that sulfonylurea oral antidiabetics be labelled with a specific warning about the possibility of increased cardiovascular mortality associated with the use of these drugs.[4] Subsequently the cardiovascular effects of the sulfonylureas were reviewed.[5] More recently it has been hypothesised that the action of the sulfonylureas in preventing the opening of ATP-sensitive potassium channels in the myocardium may abolish adaptive changes (ischaemic preconditioning) that protect the heart against ischaemic insult.[6] However, results from the UK Prospective Diabetes Study did not demonstrate any adverse cardiovascular effects associated with sulfonylurea therapy.[7]

1. University Group Diabetes Program. Effects of hypoglycemic agents on vascular complications in patients with adult-onset diabetes III: clinical implications of UGDP results. *JAMA* 1971; **218:** 1400–10.
2. University Group Diabetes Program. Effects of hypoglycemic agents on vascular complications in patients with adult-onset diabetes IV: a preliminary report on phenformin results. *JAMA* 1971; **217:** 777–84.
3. Report of the Committee for the Assessment of Biometric Aspects of Controlled Trials of Hypoglycemic Agents. *JAMA* 1975; **231:** 583–600.
4. FDA. Class labeling for oral hypoglycemics. *FDA Drug Bull* 1984; **14:** 16–17.
5. Huupponen R. Adverse cardiovascular effects of sulphonylurea drugs: clinical significance. *Med Toxicol* 1987; **2:** 190–209.
6. Yellon DM, *et al.* Angina reassessed: pain or protector? *Lancet* 1996; **347:** 1159–62.
7. UK Prospective Diabetes Study (UKPDS) Group. Intensive blood-glucose control with sulphonylureas or insulin compared with conventional treatment and risk of complications in patients with type 2 diabetes (UKPDS 33). *Lancet* 1998; **352:** 837–53. Correction. *ibid.* 1999; **354:** 602.

**Effects on the eyes.** When a diabetic patient who had experienced bilateral visual loss for several months and who had been taking chlorpropamide for one year stopped treatment, visual acuity improved and colour vision rapidly returned.[1] A 5-day challenge with chlorpropamide resulted in a mild decrease in acuity followed by return to baseline values when treatment was again stopped. Drug-induced optic neuropathy was considered to have occurred. There is also a report of a patient with type 2 diabetes mellitus who developed myopia two days after starting treatment with glibenclamide 10 mg daily.[2] Visual difficulties resolved a few days after stopping glibenclamide.

1. Wymore J, Carter JE. Chlorpropamide-induced optic neuropathy. *Arch Intern Med* 1982; **142:** 381.
2. Teller J, *et al.* Accommodation insufficiency induced by glybenclamide. *Ann Ophthalmol* 1989; **21:** 275–6.

**Effects on the kidneys.** The nephrotic syndrome has been reported in a patient treated with chlorpropamide.[1] Serological testing and renal biopsy demonstrated that the glomerular lesions were of an immune-complex nature. Both the nephrotic syndrome and the glomerulonephritis resolved after treatment was stopped. The patient also developed a skin eruption, hepatitis, and eosinophilia.

1. Appel GB, *et al.* Nephrotic syndrome and immune complex glomerulonephritis associated with chlorpropamide therapy. *Am J Med* 1983; **74:** 337–42.

**Effects on the liver.** Chlorpropamide was implicated[1] in 8 of 53 cases of drug-induced acute liver disease admitted to a hospital in Jamaica over the years 1973 to 1988. Hepatocanalicular cholestasis occurred in 5 cases and diffuse necrosis in 3. One patient with massive hepatic necrosis died. Intrahepatic cholestasis,[2-4] an acute hepatitis-like syndrome,[5] and a combination of both[6] have been described in patients receiving glibenclamide.

1. Lee MG, *et al.* Drug-induced acute liver disease. *Postgrad Med J* 1989; **65:** 367–70.
2. Wongpaitoon V, *et al.* Intrahepatic cholestasis and cutaneous bullae associated with glibenclamide therapy. *Postgrad Med J* 1981; **57:** 244–6.
3. Krivoy N, *et al.* Fatal toxic intrahepatic cholestasis secondary to glibenclamide. *Diabetes Care* 1996; **19:** 385–6.
4. Tholakanahalli VN, *et al.* Glibenclamide-induced cholestasis. *West J Med* 1998; **168:** 274–7.
5. Goodman RC, *et al.* Glyburide-induced hepatitis. *Ann Intern Med* 1987; **106:** 837–9.
6. Petrogiannopoulos C, Zacharof A. Glibenclamide and liver disease. *Diabetes Care* 1997; **20:** 1215.

**Effects on the thyroid.** See under Precautions, below.

**Hypoglycaemia.** Severe hypoglycaemia may occur in any patient treated with any sulfonylurea; this potentially life-threatening complication requires prolonged and energetic treatment.[1] Sulfonylureas with a prolonged duration of action such as chlorpropamide and glibenclamide appear to cause severe hypoglycaemia more often than shorter-acting drugs such as tolbutamide. Experience with newer drugs is limited.

A review of 1418 cases of drug-induced hypoglycaemia reported since 1940 showed that sulfonylureas (especially chlorpropamide and glibenclamide), either alone or with a second antidiabetic or potentiating agent, accounted for 63% of all cases.[2] A study of sulfonylurea use in nearly 14,000 patients aged 65 years or older confirmed that chlorpropamide and glibenclamide were associated with hypoglycaemia. However, glipizide caused significantly fewer cases than glibenclamide.[3]

An analysis,[4] of 185 children reported to 10 regional poison centres in the USA after ingesting sulfonylureas found that hypoglycaemia developed only in 56. A lack of hypoglycaemia during the first 8 hours after ingestion was predictive of a benign outcome, and it was recommended that suspected cases be observed for 8 hours with frequent blood glucose monitoring. Children who developed signs of hypoglycaemia, or in whom blood glucose fell below 3.3 mmol/litre could be given intravenous glucose if necessary.

See also under Abuse, below.

1. Ferner RE, Neil HAW. Sulphonylureas and hypoglycaemia. *BMJ* 1988; **296:** 949–50.
2. Seltzer HS. Drug-induced hypoglycemia. *Endocrinol Metab Clin North Am* 1989; **18:** 163–83.
3. Shorr RI, *et al.* Individual sulfonylureas and serious hypoglycemia in older people. *J Am Geriatr Soc* 1996; **44:** 751–5.
4. Spiller HA, *et al.* Prospective multicenter study of sulfonylurea ingestion in children. *J Pediatr* 1997; **131:** 141–6.

### Treatment of Adverse Effects

In acute poisoning with sulfonylureas, if the patient is conscious and presents within 1 hour of ingestion, the stomach should be emptied and/or activated charcoal given. Hypoglycaemia should be treated with urgency; the general management of hypoglycaemia is described under insulin (see p.335). The patient should be observed over several days in case hypoglycaemia recurs. Octreotide has been used in the treatment of severe refractory cases of sulfonylurea-induced hypoglycaemia.

◊ References.

1. Spiller HA. Management of antidiabetic medication in overdose. *Drug Safety* 1998; **19:** 411–24.
2. McLaughlin SA, *et al.* Octreotide: an antidote for sulfonylurea-induced hypoglycemia. *Ann Emerg Med* 2000; **36:** 133–8.
3. Carr R, Zed PJ. Octreotide for sulfonylurea-induced hypoglycemia following overdose. *Ann Pharmacother* 2002; **36:** 1727–32.

### Precautions

Sulfonylureas should not be used in type 1 diabetes mellitus. Use in type 2 diabetes mellitus is contra-indicated in patients with ketoacidosis and in those with severe infection, trauma, or other severe conditions where the sulfonylurea is unlikely to control the hyperglycaemia; insulin should be used in such situations. Insulin is also preferred for therapy during pregnancy.

Sulfonylureas with a long half-life such as chlorpropamide or glibenclamide are associated with an increased risk of hypoglycaemia. They should therefore be avoided in patients with impairment of renal or hepatic function, and a similar precaution would tend to apply in other groups with an increased susceptibility to this effect, such as the elderly, debilitated or malnourished patients, and those with adrenal or pituitary insufficiency. Irregular mealtimes, missed meals, changes in diet, or prolonged exercise may also provoke hypoglycaemia. Where a sulfonylurea needs to be used in patients at increased risk of hypoglycaemia, a short-acting drug such as tolbutamide, gliquidone, or gliclazide may be preferred; these three sulfonylureas, being principally inactivated in the liver, are perhaps particularly suitable in renal impairment, although careful monitoring of blood-glucose concentration is essential.

**Abuse.** Severe hypoglycaemia, at first thought to be due to insulinoma but later found to be due to nesidioblastosis [proliferation of the islet cells], was reported in a woman covertly taking chlorpropamide.[1]

1. Rayman G, *et al.* Hyperinsulinaemic hypoglycaemia due to chlorpropamide-induced nesidioblastosis. *J Clin Pathol* 1984; **37:** 651–4.

**Administration.** It has been suggested that continuously high plasma concentrations of sulfonylureas may lead to the development of tolerance, and that therefore the maximum recommended doses should be reduced.[1]

1. Melander A, *et al.* Is there a concentration-effect relationship for sulphonylureas? *Clin Pharmacokinet* 1998; **34:** 181–8.

**Breast feeding.** Some sulfonylureas are distributed into breast milk and the class of drugs should be avoided during breast feeding.

**Driving.** In the UK, patients with diabetes mellitus treated with insulin or oral hypoglycaemics are required to notify their condition to the Driver and Vehicle Licensing Agency, who then assess their fitness to drive. Patients treated with oral hypoglycaemics are generally allowed to retain standard driving licences; those treated with insulin receive restricted licences which must be renewed (with appropriate checks) every 1 to 3 years. Patients should be warned of the dangers of hypoglycaemic attacks while driving, and should be counselled in appropriate management of the situation (stopping driving as soon as it is safe to do so, taking carbohydrate immediately, and quitting the driving seat and removing the ignition key from the car) should such an event occur. Patients who have lost hypoglycaemic awareness, or have frequent hypoglycaemic episodes, should not drive. In addition, eyesight must be adequate (field of vision of at least 120°) for a licence to be valid. Patients treated with diet or oral hypoglycaemics are normally allowed to hold vocational driving licences for heavy goods vehicles or passenger carrying vehicles; those treated with insulin may not drive such vehicles, and are restricted in driving some other vehicles such as small lorries and minibuses.

References.

1. British Diabetic Association (Diabetes UK). Information sheet: driving and diabetes: August 2003. Available at: http://www.diabetes.org.uk/infocentre/inform/downloads/drive.doc (accessed 08/07/04)
2. Driver and Vehicle Licensing Agency. For medical practitioners: at a glance guide to the current medical standards of fitness to drive (February 2004). Available at: http://www.dvla.gov.uk/at_a_glance/AAG2004feb.pdf (accessed 08/07/04)

**Porphyria.** Sulfonylureas have been associated with acute attacks of porphyria and are considered unsafe in porphyric patients.

**Thyroid disorders.** There are conflicting reports concerning the effects of sulfonylureas on thyroid function, with some studies suggesting an increased incidence of thyroid dysfunction in patients treated with tolbutamide or chlorpropamide,[1] while other suggest no antithyroid action.[2,3] Some manufacturers consequently recommend that chlorpropamide should be avoided in patients with impaired thyroid function. Changes in thyroid function may conversely affect glycaemic control—for mention of the possible effects of thyroid hormones on sulfonylurea requirements see under Interactions, below.

1. Hunton RB, *et al.* Hypothyroidism in diabetics treated with sulphonylurea. *Lancet* 1965; **ii:** 449–51.
2. Burke G, *et al.* Effect of long-term sulfonylurea therapy on thyroid function in man. *Metabolism* 1967; **16:** 651–7.
3. Feely J, *et al.* Antithyroid effect of chlorpropamide? *Hum Toxicol* 1983; **2:** 149–53.

## Interactions

Numerous interactions have been reported with the sulfonylureas, largely representing either pharmacokinetic interactions (due to the displacement of the antidiabetic from plasma proteins or alteration in its metabolism or excretion) or pharmacological interactions with drugs having an independent effect on blood glucose. In the former class most reports concern older sulfonylureas such as chlorpropamide and tolbutamide, although the possibility of such reactions with newer drugs should be borne in mind.

A diminished hypoglycaemic effect, possibly requiring an increased dose of sulfonylurea, has been seen or might be expected on theoretical grounds with adrenaline, aminoglutethimide, chlorpromazine, corticosteroids, diazoxide, oral contraceptives, rifamycins, thiazide diuretics, and thyroid hormones.

An increased hypoglycaemic effect has occurred or might be expected with ACE inhibitors, alcohol, allopurinol, some analgesics (notably azapropazone, phenylbutazone, and the salicylates), azole antifungals (fluconazole, ketoconazole, and miconazole), chloramphenicol, cimetidine, clofibrate and related compounds, coumarin anticoagulants, fluoroquinolones, heparin, MAOIs, octreotide (although this may also produce hyperglycaemia), ranitidine, sulfinpyrazone, sulfonamides (including co-trimoxazole), tetracyclines, and tricyclic antidepressants.

Beta blockers have been reported both to increase hypoglycaemia and to mask the typical sympathetic warning signs. There are sporadic and conflicting reports of a possible interaction with calcium-channel blockers, but overall any effect seems to be of little clinical significance.

In addition to producing hypoglycaemia alcohol can interact with chlorpropamide to produce an unpleasant flushing reaction. Such an effect is rare with other sulfonylureas and alcohol.

◊ General references.

1. O'Byrne S, Feely J. Effects of drugs on glucose tolerance in non-insulin-dependent diabetics (part I). *Drugs* 1990; **40:** 6–18.
2. O'Byrne S, Feely J. Effects of drugs on glucose tolerance in non-insulin-dependent diabetics (part II). *Drugs* 1990; **40:** 203–19.
3. Girardin E, *et al.* Hypoglycémies induites par les sulfamides hypoglycémiants. *Ann Med Interne (Paris)* 1992; **143:** 11–17.

**ACE inhibitors.** There are sporadic reports of marked hypoglycaemia developing in patients taking a sulfonylurea who are given an ACE inhibitor (mainly *captopril* or *enalapril*),[1-3] and 2 case-control studies have indicated that the combination is associated with an increased risk of developing severe hypoglycaemia.[4,5] However, other studies have failed to find much evidence of a problem.[6-9]

1. McMurray J, Fraser DM. Captopril, enalapril, and blood glucose. *Lancet* 1986; **i:** 1035.
2. Rett K, *et al.* Hypoglycemia in hypertensive diabetic patients treated with sulfonylureas, biguanides, and captopril. *N Engl J Med* 1988; **319:** 1609.
3. Arauz-Pacheco C, *et al.* Hypoglycemia induced by angiotensin-converting enzyme inhibitors in patients with non-insulin-dependent diabetes receiving sulfonylurea therapy. *Am J Med* 1990; **89:** 811–13.
4. Herings RMC, *et al.* Hypoglycaemia associated with use of inhibitors of angiotensin converting enzyme. *Lancet* 1995; **345:** 1195–8.
5. Morris AD, *et al.* ACE inhibitor use is associated with hospitalization for severe hypoglycemia in patients with diabetes. *Diabetes Care* 1997; **20:** 1363–7.
6. Ferriere M, *et al.* Captopril and insulin sensitivity. *Ann Intern Med* 1985; **102:** 134–5.
7. Passa P, *et al.* Enalapril, captopril, and blood glucose. *Lancet* 1986; **i:** 1447.
8. Winocour P, *et al.* Captopril and blood glucose. *Lancet* 1986; **ii:** 461.
9. Shorr RI, *et al.* Antihypertensives and the risk of serious hypoglycemia in older persons using insulin or sulfonylureas. *JAMA* 1997; **278:** 40–3.

**Alcohol.** Sulfonylurea-induced alcohol intolerance is seen mainly but not exclusively with chlorpropamide; this is similar to the disulfiram-alcohol interaction, although it is not clear whether the mechanism is the same. Since the main symptom of the reaction (facial flushing) appears to occur more commonly in diabetic than non-diabetic subjects, it has been proposed that this symptom could be used as a diagnostic test for a certain subset of patients with type 2 diabetes mellitus.[1,2] However, some have not considered the test to be sufficiently specific[3-6] and despite a great deal having been published on the chlorpropamide-alcohol flushing test (CPAF), its value remains poorly defined. Alcohol, as well as provoking a flushing reaction with chlorpropamide, has been reported both to increase and to decrease the half-life of tolbutamide depending on whether the alcohol administration was acute or chronic.[7] Alcohol may also have a variable effect of its own on blood-glucose concentrations; there is a general tendency to increased hypoglycaemia when alcohol and sulfonylureas are taken concurrently.[6]

1. Leslie RDG, Pyke DA. Chlorpropamide-alcohol flushing: a dominantly inherited trait associated with diabetes. *BMJ* 1978; **2:** 1519–21.
2. Pyke DA, Leslie RDG. Chlorpropamide-alcohol flushing: a definition of its relation to non-insulin-dependent diabetes. *BMJ* 1978; **2:** 1521–2.
3. de Silva NE, *et al.* Low incidence of chlorpropamide-alcohol flushing in diet-treated, non-insulin-dependent diabetes. *Lancet* 1981; **i:** 128–31.
4. Fui SNT, *et al.* Epidemiological study of prevalence of chlorpropamide alcohol flushing in insulin dependent diabetes, non-insulin dependent diabetics, and non-diabetics. *BMJ* 1983; **287:** 1509–12.
5. Fui SNT, *et al.* Test for chlorpropamide-alcohol flush becomes positive after prolonged chlorpropamide treatment in insulin-dependent and non-insulin-dependent diabetics. *N Engl J Med* 1983; **309:** 93–6.
6. Lao B, *et al.* Alcohol tolerance in patients with non-insulin-dependent (type 2) diabetes treated with sulphonylurea derivatives. *Arzneimittelforschung* 1994; **44:** 727–34.
7. Sellers EM, Holloway MR. Drug kinetics and alcohol ingestion. *Clin Pharmacokinet* 1978; **3:** 440–52.

**Analgesics.** *Phenylbutazone*[1,2] and related drugs such as *azapropazone*[3] have been associated with acute hypoglycaemic episodes when given to patients receiving sulfonylureas (in most reports, tolbutamide). Other analgesics may enhance the hypoglycaemic effect of sulfonylureas, including *indobufen*,[4] *fenclofenac*,[5] and the *salicylates*.[6,7] Although a study in healthy subjects found no interaction,[7] there has been a report of hypoglycaemia with *ibuprofen* in a diabetic patient who had been stabilised on glibenclamide.[8]

1. Tannenbaum H, *et al.* Phenylbutazone-tolbutamide drug interaction. *N Engl J Med* 1974; **290:** 344.
2. Dent LA, Jue SG. Tolbutamide-phenylbutazone interaction. *Drug Intell Clin Pharm* 1976; **10:** 711.
3. Andreasen PB, *et al.* Hypoglycaemia induced by azapropazone-tolbutamide interaction. *Br J Clin Pharmacol* 1981; **12:** 581–3.
4. Elvander-Ståhl E, *et al.* Indobufen interacts with the sulphonylurea, glipizide, but not with the β-adrenergic receptor antagonists, propranolol and atenolol. *Br J Clin Pharmacol* 1984; **18:** 773–8.
5. Allen PA, Taylor RT. Fenclofenac and thyroid function tests. *BMJ* 1980; **281:** 1642.
6. Richardson T, *et al.* Enhancement by sodium salicylate of the blood glucose lowering effect of chlorpropamide—drug interaction or summation of similar effects? *Br J Clin Pharmacol* 1986; **22:** 43–8.
7. Kubacka RT, *et al.* Effects of aspirin and ibuprofen on the pharmacokinetics and pharmacodynamics of glyburide in healthy subjects. *Ann Pharmacother* 1996; **30:** 20–6.
8. Sone H, *et al.* Ibuprofen-related hypoglycemia in a patient receiving sulfonylurea. *Ann Intern Med* 2001; **134:** 344.

**Antibacterials.** *Chloramphenicol* markedly inhibits the metabolism of tolbutamide and increases its half-life,[1] which can result in hypoglycaemia. Sulfonamides,[2] including *co-trimoxazole*,[3-5] may also enhance the hypoglycaemic effects of the sulfonylureas. There have been rare reports of elevated glibenclamide concentrations and hypoglycaemia when *ciprofloxacin* was given to patients who were on stable glibenclamide therapy.[6] For reports of hypoglycaemia when *gatifloxacin* was given to patients already receiving a sulfonylurea (glimepiride in one case, and glibenclamide plus pioglitazone in another), see p.216. There have also been a few cases of severe hypoglycaemia when *clarithromycin* was added to glibenclamide or glipizide; renal impairment may have played a role in these cases.[7] *Rifampicin* (and probably other rifamycins) can enhance the metabolism and decrease the effect of tolbutamide, chlorpropamide,[8,9] and glibenclamide[10] and dosage of the hypoglycaemic drug may need to be increased. The effects on glipizide[10] and glimepiride[11] appear to be less pronounced.

1. Christensen LK, Skovsted L. Inhibition of drug metabolism by chloramphenicol. *Lancet* 1969; **ii:** 1397–9.
2. Soeldner JS, Steinke J. Hypoglycemia in tolbutamide-treated diabetes: report of two cases with measurement of serum insulin. *JAMA* 1965; **193:** 148–9.
3. Wing LMH, Miners JO. Cotrimoxazole as an inhibitor of oxidative drug metabolism: effects of trimethoprim and sulphamethoxazole separately and combined on tolbutamide disposition. *Br J Clin Pharmacol* 1985; **20:** 482–5.
4. Johnson JF, Dobmeier ME. Symptomatic hypoglycemia secondary to a glipizide-trimethoprim/sulfamethoxazole drug interaction. *DICP Ann Pharmacother* 1990; **24:** 250–1.
5. Abad S, *et al.* Possible interaction between gliclazide, fluconazole and sulfamethoxazole resulting in severe hypoglycaemia. *Br J Clin Pharmacol* 2001; **52:** 456–7.
6. Roberge RJ, *et al.* Glyburide-ciprofloxacin interaction with resistant hypoglycemia. *Ann Emerg Med* 2000; **36:** 160–3.
7. Bussing R, Gende A. Severe hypoglycemia from clarithromycin-sulfonylurea drug interaction. *Diabetes Care* 2002; **25:** 1659–61.
8. Syvälahti EKG, *et al.* Rifampicin and drug metabolism. *Lancet* 1974; **ii:** 232–3.
9. Self TH, Morris T. Interaction of rifampin and chlorpropamide. *Chest* 1980; **77:** 800–1.
10. Niemi M, *et al.* Effects of rifampin on the pharmacokinetics and pharmacodynamics of glyburide and glipizide. *Clin Pharmacol Ther* 2001; **69:** 400–406.
11. Niemi M, *et al.* Effect of rifampicin on the pharmacokinetics and pharmacodynamics of glimepiride. *Br J Clin Pharmacol* 2000; **50:** 591–5.

**Anticoagulants.** *Dicoumarol* increases serum concentrations and therefore the hypoglycaemic effects of tolbutamide, and possibly chlorpropamide. In addition, sulfonylureas may affect anticoagulant function (p.1025).

**Antiepileptics.** For references to *phenytoin* toxicity when tolbutamide or tolazamide was given, see under Phenytoin p.373.

**Antifungals.** Increased plasma concentrations of tolbutamide have been reported when *fluconazole* was given,[1] but there was no evidence of hypoglycaemia, and no hypoglycaemic symptoms were seen in 29 women receiving gliclazide or glibenclamide who were given fluconazole or *clotrimazole* for vulvovaginitis.[2] A study in healthy volunteers found that fluconazole increased plasma concentrations of glimepiride, but again there was no significant effect on glucose concentrations.[3] However, there are reports of hypoglycaemia in a patient who took fluconazole with glipizide,[4] and another who took fluconazole and co-trimoxazole with gliclazide.[5] Similar interactions have been reported for *ketoconazole* (with tolbutamide, in healthy subjects)[6] and *miconazole* (with tolbutamide, in a diabetic),[7] suggesting that such combinations should be regarded with caution.

1. Lazar JD, Wilner DK. Drug interactions with fluconazole. *Rev Infect Dis* 1990; **12** (suppl 3): S327–S333.
2. Rowe BR, *et al.* Safety of fluconazole in women taking oral hypoglycaemic agents. *Lancet* 1992; **339:** 255–6.
3. Niemi M, *et al.* Effects of fluconazole and fluvoxamine on the pharmacokinetics and pharmacodynamics of glimepiride. *Clin Pharmacol Ther* 2001; **69:** 194–200.
4. Fournier JP, *et al.* Coma hypoglycémique chez une patiente traitée par glipizide et fluconazole: une possible interaction? *Therapie* 1992; **47:** 446–7.
5. Abad S, *et al.* Possible interaction between gliclazide, fluconazole and sulfamethoxazole resulting in severe hypoglycaemia. *Br J Clin Pharmacol* 2001; **52:** 456–7.
6. Krishnaiah YSR, *et al.* Interaction between tolbutamide and ketoconazole in healthy subjects. *Br J Clin Pharmacol* 1994; **37:** 205–7.
7. Meurice JC, *et al.* Interaction miconazole et sulfamides hypoglycémiants. *Presse Med* 1983; **12:** 1670.

**Metformin.** Results apparently suggesting increased mortality in patients who received intensive drug therapy with metformin and a sulfonylurea were reported by the UK Prospective Diabetes Study.[1] This was considered to be artefactual, since it was not confirmed by epidemiological analysis, and such combinations are widely used in practice, but some concern remains and further study is needed.

1. UK Prospective Diabetes Study Group. Effect of intensive blood-glucose control with metformin on complications in overweight patients with type 2 diabetes (UKPDS 34). *Lancet* 1998; **352:** 854–65. Correction. *ibid.*; 1558.

**Thyroid hormones.** It has been suggested that initiation of thyroid replacement therapy may increase the requirement for insulin or oral antidiabetic drugs in diabetic patients, which would not seem unreasonable given the stimulant effects of thyroid hormones on metabolic function. For a discussion of the mooted effects of sulfonylureas on thyroid function, see Precautions, above.

## Pharmacokinetics

◊ Reviews.

1. Marchetti P, Navalesi R. Pharmacokinetic-pharmacodynamic relationships of oral hypoglycaemic agents: an update. *Clin Pharmacokinet* 1989; **16:** 100–28.
2. Marchetti P, *et al.* Pharmacokinetic optimisation of oral hypoglycaemic therapy. *Clin Pharmacokinet* 1991; **21:** 308–17.
3. Harrower AD. Pharmacokinetics of oral antihyperglycaemic agents in patients with renal insufficiency. *Clin Pharmacokinet* 1996; **31:** 111–19.

## Uses and Administration

The sulfonylurea antidiabetics are a class of antidiabetic drugs given by mouth in the treatment of type 2 diabetes mellitus (p.324). They are used to supplement treatment by diet modification when such modification has not proved effective on its own, although metformin is preferred in patients who are obese.

Sulfonylureas appear to have several modes of action, apparently mediated by inhibition of ATP-sensitive potassium channels. Initially, secretion of insulin by functioning islet beta cells is increased. However, insulin secretion subsequently falls again but the hypoglycaemic effect persists and may be due to inhibition of hepatic glucose production and increased sensitivity to any available insulin; this may explain the observed clinical improvement in glycaemic control. The duration of action of sulfonylureas is variable; drugs such as tolbutamide are relatively short-acting (approximately 6 to 12 hours) while chlorpropamide has a prolonged action (over 24 hours).

Sulfonylurea therapy may be combined with metformin or other oral hypoglycaemics in patients who fail to respond to a single type of drug; such combination therapy is usually tried (in the absence of contra-indications) before considering the addition of, or transfer to, insulin therapy.

## Tolazamide (BAN, USAN, rINN)

NSC-70762; Tolazamida; U-17835. 1-(Perhydroazepin-1-yl)-3-tosylurea; 1-(Perhydroazepin-1-yl)-3-p-tolylsulphonylurea.
$C_{14}H_{21}N_3O_3S$ = 311.4.
*CAS — 1156-19-0.*
*ATC — A10BB05.*

**Pharmacopoeias.** In *Br., Jpn*, and *US*.

**BP 2003** (Tolazamide). A white or almost white, odourless or almost odourless, crystalline powder. Very slightly soluble in water; slightly soluble in alcohol; soluble in acetone; freely soluble in chloroform.

**USP 27** (Tolazamide). A white or off-white crystalline powder, odourless or having a slight odour. Very slightly soluble in water; slightly soluble in alcohol; soluble in acetone; freely soluble in chloroform.

### Adverse Effects, Treatment, and Precautions

As for sulfonylureas in general, p.346.

**Porphyria.** Tolazamide has been associated with acute attacks of porphyria and is considered unsafe in porphyric patients.

### Interactions

As for sulfonylureas in general, p.347.

### Pharmacokinetics

Tolazamide is slowly absorbed from the gastrointestinal tract, peak plasma concentrations occurring 4 to 8 hours after a dose by mouth, and is extensively bound to plasma proteins. It has a half-life of about 7 hours. It is metabolised in the liver to metabolites with some hypoglycaemic activity. About 85% of an oral dose is excreted in the urine, chiefly as metabolites.

### Uses and Administration

Tolazamide is a sulfonylurea antidiabetic (p.346). It is given by mouth in the treatment of type 2 diabetes mellitus (p.324) and has a duration of action of at least 10 hours and sometimes up to 20 hours. The usual initial dose is 100 to 250 mg daily given as a single dose with breakfast. Dosage may be increased if necessary at weekly intervals by 100 to 250 mg, usually to a maximum of 1 g daily; no further benefit is likely to be gained with higher doses. Doses of more than 500 mg daily may be given in divided doses.

### Preparations

***BP 2003:*** Tolazamide Tablets;
***USP 27:*** Tolazamide Tablets.

**Proprietary Preparations** (details are given in Part 3)
***Irl.:*** Tolanase†; ***Swed.:*** Tolinase†; ***UK:*** Tolanase†; ***USA:*** Tolinase.

## Tolbutamide (BAN, rINN)

Butamidum; Tolbutamida; Tolbutamidum; Tolglybutamide. 1-Butyl-3-tosylurea; 1-Butyl-3-p-tolylsulphonylurea.
$C_{12}H_{18}N_2O_3S$ = 270.3.
*CAS — 64-77-7 (tolbutamide); 473-41-6 (tolbutamide sodium).*
*ATC — A10BB03; V04CA01.*

**Pharmacopoeias.** In *Chin., Eur.* (see p.vi), *Int., Jpn, Pol.*, and *US*.

**Ph. Eur. 5.0** (Tolbutamide). A white crystalline powder. Practically insoluble in water; soluble in alcohol and in acetone. It dissolves in dilute solutions of alkali hydroxides.

**USP 27** (Tolbutamide). A white or practically white, practically odourless, crystalline powder. Practically insoluble in water; soluble in alcohol and in chloroform.

### Adverse Effects, Treatment, and Precautions

As for sulfonylureas in general, p.346. Tolbutamide was implicated in the controversial reports of excess cardiovascular mortality associated with oral hypoglycaemic therapy (see under Sulfonylureas, Effects on the Cardiovascular System, p.346).

Thrombophlebitis with thrombosis has occurred following the intravenous injection of tolbutamide sodium, but this is usually painless and the vein gradually recovers. Rapid injection may cause a transient mild pain or sensation of heat in the vein.

The *British National Formulary* has suggested that tolbutamide may be suitable for use in patients with renal impairment, but careful monitoring of blood-glucose concentration is essential. The UK manufacturers recommend that it should not be used in patients with severe renal impairment.

**Breast feeding.** Tolbutamide is distributed into breast milk in relatively low quantities.[1] The American Academy of Pediatrics[2] states that, although usually compatible with breast feeding, use of tolbutamide by breast-feeding mothers may possibly result in jaundice in the infant.

1. Moiel RH, Ryan JR. Tolbutamide orinase in human breast milk. *Clin Pediatr (Phila)* 1967; **6:** 480.
2. American Academy of Pediatrics. The transfer of drugs and other chemicals into human milk. *Pediatrics* 2001; **108:** 776–89. Correction. *ibid.*; 1029. Also available at: http://aappolicy.aappublications.org/cgi/content/full/pediatrics%3b108/3/776 (accessed 08/07/04)

**Porphyria.** Tolbutamide has been associated with acute attacks of porphyria and is considered unsafe in porphyric patients.

### Interactions

As for sulfonylureas in general, p.347.

### Pharmacokinetics

Tolbutamide is readily absorbed from the gastrointestinal tract and is extensively bound to plasma proteins; the half-life is generally within the range of 4 to 7 hours but may be considerably longer. Tolbutamide is metabolised in the liver by hydroxylation mediated by the cytochrome P450 isoenzyme CYP2C9. It is excreted in the urine chiefly as metabolites with little hypoglycaemic activity. Tolbutamide has been detected in breast milk.

### Uses and Administration

Tolbutamide is a sulfonylurea antidiabetic (p.346). It is given by mouth in the treatment of type 2 diabetes mellitus (p.324) and has a duration of action of about 10 hours.

The usual initial dose by mouth in type 2 diabetes mellitus may range from 1 to 2 g daily, given either as a single dose with breakfast or, more usually, in divided doses. Maintenance doses usually range from 0.25 to 2 g daily. Although it is unlikely that the response will be improved by increasing the dose further, daily doses of 3 g have been given.

Tolbutamide sodium ($C_{12}H_{17}N_2NaO_3S$ = 292.3) has sometimes been used in the diagnosis of insulinoma as well as other pancreatic disorders including diabetes mellitus. The equivalent of 1 g of tolbutamide is given by intravenous injection as a 5% solution usually over 2 to 3 minutes. Tolbutamide sodium 1.08 g is approximately equivalent to 1 g of tolbutamide.

**Diagnosis and testing.** References.

1. McMahon MM, *et al.* Diagnostic interpretation of the intravenous tolbutamide test for insulinoma. *Mayo Clin Proc* 1989; **64:** 1481–8.
2. Marks V. Diagnosis and differential diagnosis of hypoglycemia. *Mayo Clin Proc* 1989; **64:** 1558–61.

### Preparations

***BP 2003:*** Tolbutamide Tablets;
***USP 27:*** Tolbutamide for Injection; Tolbutamide Tablets.

**Proprietary Preparations** (details are given in Part 3)
***Austral.:*** Rastinon; ***Austria:*** Rastinon†; ***Canad.:*** Novo-Butamide†; Orinase†; ***Denm.:*** Arcosal; ***Ger.:*** Artosin†; Orabet; Rastinon†; ***Hong Kong:*** Diatol; Rastinon†; ***Israel:*** Orsinon; ***Ital.:*** Rastinon†; ***Mex.:*** Bioglusil; Dabetil; Diatelan†; Diaval; Flusan; Ifumelus; Ipoglusan†; Rastinon; ***Neth.:*** Artosin†; Rastinon†; ***NZ:*** Diatol; ***S.Afr.:*** Rastinon†; ***Spain:*** Rastinon†; ***UK:*** Glyconon†; ***USA:*** Orinase; Orinase Diagnostic.

**Multi-ingredient:** ***Ital.:*** Glucosulfa†.

## Troglitazone (BAN, USAN, rINN)

CI-991; CS-045; GR-92132X; Troglitazona. (±)-all-rac-5-{p-[(6-Hydroxy-2,5,7,8-tetramethyl-2-chromanyl)methoxy]benzyl}-2,4-thiazolidinedione.
$C_{24}H_{27}NO_5S$ = 441.5.
*CAS — 97322-87-7.*
*ATC — A10BG01.*

### Adverse Effects and Precautions

Troglitazone has been associated with severe hepatic reactions, sometimes fatal, which has led to its withdrawal in most countries. Regular monitoring of liver function during therapy, and withdrawal of the drug in any patient who develops jaundice or signs of liver dysfunction, is required. It should not be given to patients with pre-existing moderate or severe elevations of liver enzyme values, or active liver disease. Increased plasma volume has been reported in healthy subjects given troglitazone: it should be used with caution in patients with heart failure. Other adverse effects reported in patients receiving troglitazone include dizziness, headache, fatigue, musculoskeletal pain, and nausea and vomiting. There is no evidence of hypoglycaemia associated with the use of troglitazone alone.

**Effects on the liver.** The UK Committee on Safety of Medicines[1] was aware of over 130 cases of hepatic reactions to troglitazone worldwide as of December 1997, although only 1 had been in the UK. There had been 6 deaths. The average time to the onset of the reaction was 3 months, but the frequency of these reactions, and the existence of risk factors predisposing to them, were unclear. The manufacturers had voluntarily withdrawn the drug in the UK.

The US manufacturer and the FDA recommended[2] a schedule for routine monitoring of liver function in November 1997 and revised this again in December 1997. It was estimated that 2% of patients treated with troglitazone would have elevated liver enzyme values necessitating discontinuation of the drug. The FDA[3] had received 560 reports of troglitazone-associated hepatotoxicity by June 1998. There were 24 cases of hepatic failure which were likely to have been caused by the drug; 21 patients died and 3 patients received transplants. More intensive liver function monitoring recommendations were made by the US manufacturer again in July 1998 and in June 1999. Subsequently the manufacturer withdrew the drug in Australia, Japan, and the USA in March 2000.

1. Committee on Safety of Medicines/Medicines Control Agency. Troglitazone (Romozin) withdrawn. *Current Problems* 1997; **23:** 13. Also available at: http://www.mca.gov.uk/ourwork/monitorsafequalmed/currentproblems/first.htm (accessed 13/07/04)
2. Anonymous. Troglitazone and liver injury. *WHO Drug Inf* 1998; **12:** 13.
3. Misbin RI. Troglitazone-associated hepatic failure. *Ann Intern Med* 1999; **130:** 330.

### Interactions

Troglitazone may enhance the hypoglycaemic effects of sulfonylureas; dosage adjustment may be necessary. There is a possibility that troglitazone may enhance the metabolism of drugs metabolised by cytochrome P450 isoenzyme CYP3A4, including some oral contraceptives and terfenadine.

**Ciclosporin.** For the effect of troglitazone on blood concentrations of ciclosporin see Hypoglycaemic Drugs, p.1356.

**Colestyramine.** Colestyramine markedly impaired the absorption of troglitazone.[1]

1. Young MA, *et al.* Concomitant administration of cholestyramine influences the absorption of troglitazone. *Br J Clin Pharmacol* 1998; **45:** 37–40.

### Pharmacokinetics

Troglitazone is rapidly absorbed after oral doses, with peak plasma concentrations 1 to 3 hours after a dose. Bioavailability is about 53%; absorption is markedly increased in the presence of food. In the body, troglitazone is more than 99% bound to plasma albumin. It is extensively metabolised in the liver and excreted largely in faeces as metabolites; small amounts of metabolites are excreted in urine. Plasma elimination half-life ranges from 10 to 39 hours.

◊ Reviews.

1. Loi C-M, *et al.* Clinical pharmacokinetics of troglitazone. *Clin Pharmacokinet* 1999; **37:** 91–104.

### Uses and Administration

Troglitazone is a thiazolidinedione oral antidiabetic (see Rosiglitazone Maleate, p.345). It has been given by mouth for the treatment of type 2 diabetes mellitus (p.324) although as mentioned above it has been withdrawn in most countries owing to hepatotoxicity.

◊ Reviews.

1. Anonymous. Troglitazone for non-insulin-dependent diabetes mellitus. *Med Lett Drugs Ther* 1997; **39:** 49–51.
2. Spencer CM, Markham A. Troglitazone. *Drugs* 1997; **54:** 89–101.
3. Chen C. Troglitazone: an antidiabetic agent. *Am J Health-Syst Pharm* 1998; **55:** 905–25.
4. Plosker GL, Faulds D. Troglitazone: a review of its use in the management of type 2 diabetes mellitus. *Drugs* 1999; **57:** 409–38.
5. Parulkar AA, *et al.* Nonhypoglycemic effects of thiazolidinediones. *Ann Intern Med* 2001; **134:** 61–71.

### Preparations

**Proprietary Preparations** (details are given in Part 3)
***Austral.:*** Rezulin†; ***Jpn:*** Noscal†; ***Mex.:*** Rezulin†; ***USA:*** Rezulin†.

## Voglibose (USAN, rINN)

A-71100; AO-128; Voglibosa. 3,4-Dideoxy-4-{[2-hydroxy-1-(hydroxymethyl)ethyl]amino}-2-C-(hydroxymethyl)-D-epi-inositol.
$C_{10}H_{21}NO_7$ = 267.3.
*CAS — 83480-29-9.*
*ATC — A10BF03.*

### Profile

Voglibose is an inhibitor of alpha-glucosidase with general properties similar to those of acarbose (p.328). It is used in the treatment of diabetes mellitus (p.324) in doses of 200 to 300 micrograms by mouth three times daily before meals.

**Hepatic encephalopathy.** Voglibose has been investigated[1] in the management of hepatic encephalopathy (p.1243).

1. Uribe M, *et al.* Beneficial effect of carbohydrate maldigestion induced by a disaccharidase inhibitor (AO-128) in the treatment of chronic portal systemic encephalopathy: a double-blind, randomized controlled trial. *Scand J Gastroenterol* 1998; **33:** 1099–1106.

### Preparations

**Proprietary Preparations** (details are given in Part 3)
***Braz.:*** Voglisan†; ***Jpn:*** Basen; ***Thai.:*** Basen.

# Antiepileptics

Epilepsy, p.349
Epilepsy and breast feeding, p.351
Epilepsy and cognition, p.351
Epilepsy and driving, p.351
Epilepsy and pregnancy, p.351
Status epilepticus, p.352
Other convulsive disorders, p.352
Alcohol withdrawal syndrome, p.352
Eclampsia and pre-eclampsia, p.352
Febrile convulsions, p.353
Myoclonus, p.353
Neonatal seizures, p.353
Porphyria, p.353

This chapter describes drugs whose chief use is in the management of epilepsy, status epilepticus, and other convulsive disorders.

## Epilepsy

Epilepsy is a common neurological disorder. An individual's lifetime risk of developing epilepsy is between 3 and 5%; neonates, children, and the elderly are at the highest risk of developing the disorder.

**Definitions and classification**. An epileptic seizure has been defined as a paroxysmal discharge of cerebral neurones accompanied by clinical phenomena apparent to the patient or to an observer. The phenomena may be of a motor, sensory, or autonomic nature and there may also be impairment or complete loss of consciousness. Motor disturbances may include convulsions—which are involuntary, violent, and spasmodic—or prolonged contraction of skeletal muscles. The word 'fit' is often used colloquially to describe an epileptic seizure. Epilepsy is defined as a condition characterised by a recurrence of such seizures. A patient should not be described as having epilepsy until a second non-febrile seizure occurs.

The following is a broad account of the classification of seizures, epilepsies, and epileptic syndromes based on the views of the Commission on Classification and Terminology of the International League Against Epilepsy in 1981[1] and 1989.[2]

- **Partial seizures** (focal seizures or localisation-related seizures) are epileptic seizures in which the neuronal discharges remain localised in one area of the brain. The phenomena associated with such a seizure depend on the site of origin of the discharge. If there is no loss of consciousness, the seizure is known as a *simple partial seizure* and includes Jacksonian epilepsy, which may be associated with motor or sensory disturbances. If there is impaired consciousness the seizure is referred to as a *complex partial seizure*. Partial seizures were formerly referred to as psychomotor epilepsy or temporal lobe epilepsy, but the terms are not synonymous and should be avoided. Partial seizures may become *secondarily generalised seizures* if the neuronal discharge spreads to involve the entire brain.
- **Generalised seizures** are characterised by neuronal discharges involving both cerebral hemispheres simultaneously from the outset. Subclassifications are based on the presence or absence of different types of convulsions. *Absences* (petit mal) are generalised seizures occurring in children characterised by a sudden loss of consciousness lasting for a few seconds. There is usually accompanying motor activity which may vary in degree from eyelid blinking to more extensive clonic body movements. *Atypical absence seizures* are those with a slower onset and longer duration. *Myoclonic seizures* are epileptic seizures in which the motor manifestation is myoclonus (see below). *Clonic seizures* are characterised by loss of consciousness, autonomic symptoms, and rhythmic clonic contractions of all muscles. *Tonic seizures* are also associated with loss of consciousness and autonomic symptoms accompanied by tonic contractions of the limbs. *Tonic-clonic seizures* (grand mal) are characterised by disordered contraction of muscles. During the tonic phase, all the muscles go into spasm followed up to a minute later by rhythmic clonic contractions. Finally, the patient enters a deep stupor followed by a period of confusion as consciousness is regained. *Atonic seizures* are characterised by loss of postural tone; the head sags or the patient falls down.

  Within the categories of partial and generalised epilepsies, seizures have also been classified as idiopathic, symptomatic (in which the seizures are associated with diagnosable underlying disorders), or cryptogenic (in which the epilepsies are known or suspected to be symptomatic but the cause is not clear). Partial syndromes include Rolandic and occipital epilepsies (both idiopathic), while generalised idiopathic syndromes include childhood absence epilepsies, juvenile myoclonic epilepsy, and the cryptogenic or symptomatic generalised syndromes include infantile spasms (as for example in West's syndrome), Lennox-Gastaut syndrome, and epilepsy with myoclonic absences.
- A third **unclassified** category covers undetermined epilepsies and epileptic syndromes.
- **Special syndromes** include conditions such as febrile convulsions (see below) in which seizures are related to specific situations.

It has been suggested that classification based on seizure type is the most useful in choice of antiepileptic drug whereas the syndrome classification has more benefits in deciding an overall therapeutic strategy and assessing long-term prognosis.

**Status epilepticus** is generally recognised as a seizure lasting more than 30 minutes or several distinct episodes without restoration of consciousness in between (see below).

Other convulsive disorders include alcohol withdrawal syndrome, eclampsia and pre-eclampsia, myoclonus, neonatal seizures, and porphyria, and are discussed below.

**Starting antiepileptic therapy**. A single seizure does not constitute epilepsy and therefore does not necessarily warrant immediate treatment with antiepileptics. The decision to start antiepileptic therapy should be based on whether the risks of further seizures outweigh the risks of treatment.

- Starting antiepileptic therapy *too early* means that the patient may be unnecessarily exposed to the adverse effects of the drugs used, and may have social implications if erroneously diagnosed, such as the loss of a patient's driving licence
- However, the implications of *delaying* treatment must also be considered. Although there has long been concern that seizures may damage the brain and intellectual capabilities, or even cause death, there are insufficient data to support these claims. Status epilepticus, rather than individual or frequent seizures, may be the factor associated with brain injury or death, but the risks of a newly diagnosed epileptic patient developing status epilepticus are unknown. The most compelling reasons for treatment are risk of personal injury or causing injury to others during a seizure, and the psychosocial consequences of untreated epilepsy such as low self-esteem, anxiety, and domestic and employment difficulties

There has been a long-held belief that seizures beget seizures. This is not necessarily borne out by epidemiological studies,[3] and there is evidence in children[4] and adults[5] that the risk of recurrence after a first unprovoked seizure may be 50% or less. Furthermore, a decelerating disease process with successively longer intervals between seizures has been shown[6] in untreated children with newly diagnosed tonic-clonic seizures followed up for 2 years. Results from another study[7] suggested that seizure control or the prospects for and success of eventual withdrawal of therapy is little influenced by the number of pretreatment seizures up to 10 seizures; above this number there was a reduced chance of completely controlling seizures. Similarly, although patients treated immediately after a first tonic-clonic seizure had a lower 2-year risk of recurrence than patients who were only started on treatment after a recurrence, immediate treatment did not affect the probability of achieving longer-term seizure control.[5]

However, epilepsy is a heterogeneous disorder and there is some experimental evidence[8] that certain seizure types can have a detrimental effect on prognosis. Differences in reported risks in seizure recurrence may be attributable to differences in methodology as well as different important risk factors in the populations studied; also, few studies have followed up patients for more than 2 to 4 years.

Whether antiepileptic therapy should be started early to improve prognosis or delayed or avoided altogether therefore remains contentious.[9,10] Some neurologists do not treat a first seizure but prefer to wait for evidence of recurrence unless clinical features such as more than one seizure type or a neurological deficit predispose to poor seizure control. However, a first non-convulsive seizure may go undetected. Furthermore, as single partial seizures appear to occur less frequently than single generalised tonic-clonic seizures, many neurologists assume that the first detected attack of a non-convulsive seizure is in fact one of multiple seizures and institute treatment.

**Choice of antiepileptic**. Once a decision to treat has been made, the choice of antiepileptic is determined primarily by its effectiveness against the type of seizures experienced and its potential adverse effects.[11-25]

- Monotherapy is preferable to a multiple-drug regimen and treatment is therefore initiated with a single drug, increasing the dose gradually until seizures are brought under control or adverse effects become unacceptable
- If treatment with the first drug fails, it is preferable to try alternative single first-line antiepileptics before giving combinations of drugs
- The change-over from one antiepileptic to another should be made cautiously, withdrawing the first drug only when the new regimen has been largely established
- If combinations are necessary in intractable cases, regimens should avoid the inclusion, where possible, of sedating drugs such as the barbiturates or benzodiazepines
- Drugs with different modes of action should be selected for combined therapy, to reduce the risk that adverse effects will be additive
- Many antiepileptics interact with each other through complex mechanisms and dosage adjustments may be necessary to maintain plasma concentrations within the therapeutic range; plasma monitoring is often advisable with combination therapy

Patients who fail to respond to adequate medical treatment may be considered for resective surgery; vagus nerve stimulation by means of an implanted device has also proved effective in those with severe intractable epilepsy who experience an aura before the onset of a seizure.[19,20]

Simple and complex **partial seizures** with or without **secondary generalisation** may be treated with *carbamazepine*, *phenytoin* or *valproate*; the response rate is somewhat lower than for tonic-clonic seizures associated with primary generalised epilepsy (see below). There is some evidence in favour of carbamazepine rather than valproate in the treatment of partial seizures.[26] However, there is no evidence of any significant difference between phenytoin and carbamazepine[27] or valproate[28] in partial seizures. *Lamotrigine* has been shown to be of equal efficacy to carbamazepine as monotherapy for partial seizures with or without secondary generalisation. In some countries *oxcarbazepine* is becoming more widely accepted as an effective and safe alternative to carbamazepine.[29] *Phenobarbital* or *primidone* are used less often; sedation can be a problem. In the UK *topiramate* is available for monotherapy; it is also used as an adjunct to other treatments. *Acetazolamide, clobazam,* or *clonazepam*, or one of the newer antiepileptics such as *gabapentin, levetiracetam, tiagabine, vigabatrin,* or *zonisamide*, may be tried as adjunctive therapy in refractory cases. Calcium-channel blockers such as *flunarizine* have been studied with equivocal results in patients with refractory epilepsy, particularly those with partial seizures.

The drugs used most often to treat **generalised** tonic-clonic seizures are *carbamazepine, lamotrigine, phenytoin,* or *valproate*. For tonic-clonic seizures as part of the syndrome of primary generalised epilepsy, valproate is the drug of choice, although systematic reviews were unable to establish evidence for this.[26,28] *Phenobarbital* and *primidone* may also be used, but sedation might be a problem, and *topiramate* is also available. In refractory cases, *vigabatrin* may be tried, or a combination of valproate and lamotrigine has been proposed.[19]

The drugs of choice for **absence seizures** are *ethosuximide* or *valproate*, both of which appear to be equally effective.[30] Since absence seizures occur primarily in children the precautions concerning valproate hepatotoxicity apply, and some prefer ethosuximide despite its potentially serious adverse effects (see p.360). However, where absence seizures are associated with tonic-clonic seizures valproate is the drug of choice since it is effective in both conditions; valproate is also preferred for atypical absence seizures. Lamotrigine may also be tried for absence seizures.[31,32]

*Valproate* is normally the drug of choice for **myoclonic seizures**, including those associated with juvenile myoclonic epilepsy.[33,34] *Clonazepam* is also used alone or in combination with valproate[35] but its sedative side-effects and the development of tolerance limit its use.[36] *Ethosux-*

*imide* and *mesuximide* have also been used. Some forms of myoclonus may respond to *lamotrigine* but others may be exacerbated.[34]

In **catamenial epilepsy** (epilepsy associated with menstruation) seizures can be predicted and intermittent therapy with *clobazam* may be useful.

The **Lennox-Gastaut syndrome** begins in early childhood and is particularly difficult to treat because multiple seizure types co-exist; seizures rarely remit entirely. *Valproate* is most frequently used[37] because of its broad spectrum of activity and *lamotrigine* is also effective. *Phenytoin, phenobarbital,* and *carbamazepine* may be useful for tonic or tonic-clonic seizures, but they may exacerbate absence or myoclonic seizures. *Benzodiazepines* have also been used although development of tolerance is a problem. *Felbamate, topiramate,* and *vigabatrin* have also been shown to be effective.

Conventional antiepileptics are generally ineffective in **infantile spasms** (as for example in **West's syndrome**).[38-40] *Corticotropin* and *corticosteroids* have been commonly used but they are associated with frequent and severe adverse effects, and there is controversy over whether they have a better effect on long-term outcome than antiepileptics. *Vigabatrin* is effective either as adjunctive treatment or monotherapy. Many consider that it should replace corticotropin or corticosteroids as the treatment of choice,[31,41-45] despite the risk of visual field defects,[46] although others disagree.[47,48] However, vigabatrin may offer the best first option in the treatment of infantile spasms due to tuberous sclerosis.[49] Other drugs that have been used include *nitrazepam* and *valproate*.[31] *Felbamate* and *lamotrigine* have also been shown to be effective for infantile spasms,[40,50] as has *topiramate*.[51]

**Choice of antiepileptics in children**. The use of antiepileptics in general in children has been reviewed.[50,52-56] Again, appropriate treatment depends on seizure type, but there is a lack of evidence to support many therapeutic choices,[53,57] in part because of the difficulties in undertaking trials in this population. In addition, children may be particularly susceptible to some adverse effects, including effects on behaviour, cognition, and development; behavioural problems have been associated particularly with phenobarbital.[58] Where control is not achieved with one antiepileptic others should be tried,[53,59] although the chances of remission are reduced somewhat.[59] Dietary modification (the ketogenic diet) may also be tried.[60,61]

**Withdrawal of antiepileptic therapy**. Concern over the potential adverse effects of antiepileptic therapy clearly makes withdrawal attractive in patients who achieve prolonged seizure-free periods; however, the practical and social consequences of seizure recurrence may be considerable (for example, loss of driving licence and restricted employment prospects).

Long-term follow-up in *children* whose therapy was withdrawn after seizures had been controlled for several years found that about 25 to 30% had seizure recurrence, in most cases within 2 years of withdrawal.[62,63] Another group reported a higher relapse rate when therapy was withdrawn after 1 year (46%) compared with 3 years (29%);[64] analysis by seizure type suggested that this was due particularly to a difference in outcome in children with complex partial seizures.[65] Another prospective study found that the remission rate may be as high as 80% among the general population of epileptic children (containing fewer refractory cases than those seen in epilepsy centres).[66]

There has been some uncertainty as to whether these results can be extrapolated to *adults*.[67] A meta-analysis[68] that included 25 studies and 5354 patients (children and adults) found the overall rate of relapse in seizure-free patients following discontinuation of antiepileptic therapy was 25% at 1 year and 29% at 2 years. There was a higher risk for relapse in adolescent- and adult-onset epilepsy compared with childhood-onset epilepsy.

Although these findings indicate that it is often possible to withdraw therapy successfully, it is more difficult to offer an individual *prognosis*. Some consider that most adult patients whose livelihood or lifestyle depends on being seizure-free would be ill advised to contemplate drug withdrawal.[69] Factors that may increase the risk of relapse include epilepsy of long duration before remission is achieved,[62,70] refractory epilepsy[70] or combined seizure types,[62] cerebral pathology[71] or mental or neurological deficit[72] and there is a greater likelihood of relapse in adolescent- and adult-onset epilepsy. Seizure type also seems to be important in most studies, with partial seizures associated with a higher risk of relapse,[70] particularly if secondarily generalised;[70] the risk may also be increased in patients with a history of tonic-clonic seizures but the findings of studies are conflicting.[69] Withdrawal of treatment in juvenile myoclonic epilepsy is generally considered inappropriate as up to 90% of patients who are in remission will relapse if treatment is withdrawn.[73,74] Abnormal EEG before withdrawal is also reported in many studies, including the previously quoted meta-analysis,[68] to be prognostic of a poor outcome but this is not universally accepted.[71] One group[64] found that in children who demonstrated abnormal EEG activity the overall risk of relapse on discontinuation of therapy was only slightly higher than in patients with no such activity, although certain patterns were associated with higher relapse rates than others.

Treatment with more than one antiepileptic is a risk factor for poor prognosis on withdrawal.[69,75] One study has suggested that the type of drug withdrawn is significant, with a poorer prognosis for patients on valproate.[70] Interestingly, however, another study in patients receiving combination antiepileptic therapy, as opposed to monotherapy, indicated that a significant increase in seizures was more likely when the carbamazepine component was withdrawn.[76] It should be remembered that withdrawal of hepatic enzyme-inducing antiepileptics can result in changes in serum concentrations of other concomitantly administered antiepileptics.[77]

Limited data suggest that the longer the duration of remission before withdrawal, the lower the risk of relapse.[75] In practice, seizure control for at least 2 to 3 years before withdrawal is attempted appears to be considered mandatory,[71,78] although some suggest that this may not be necessary with all seizure types.[65]

Several strategies for predicting the likely outcome after withdrawal of antiepileptic therapy in individuals have been published.[74,79,80] Recognising that epilepsy is a heterogeneous disorder, scoring systems to allow for various risk factors have been devised.[74,79]

When a decision to withdraw is made, it is agreed that the *withdrawal regimen* should be gradual to reduce the risk of provoking withdrawal seizures. Drugs should be withdrawn one at a time but there is no agreement on the optimum rate of withdrawal for individual drugs. It has been suggested that withdrawal of carbamazepine, barbiturates, benzodiazepines, or zonisamide should be carried out slowly whereas it may be possible to discontinue phenytoin or valproate quickly (over a few days in hospital) if necessary. Exacerbation of seizures may be brought under control by re-establishing the drug being withdrawn. Although it has been suggested that withdrawal over a long period may reduce the relapse rate, one study in children indicated no significant difference in seizure recurrence rate when various antiepileptics including barbiturates were withdrawn over 6 weeks or 9 months.[81]


1. Commission on Classification and Terminology of the International League against Epilepsy. Proposal for revised clinical and electroencephalographic classification of epileptic seizures. *Epilepsia* 1981; **22:** 489–501.
2. Commission on Classification and Terminology of the International League against Epilepsy. Proposal for revised classification of epilepsies and epileptic syndromes. *Epilepsia* 1989; **30:** 389–99.
3. Sadzot B. Epilepsy: a progressive disease? *BMJ* 1997; **314:** 391–2.
4. Shinnar S, *et al.* The risk of seizure recurrence after a first unprovoked afebrile seizure in childhood: an extended follow-up. *Pediatrics* 1996; **98:** 216–25.
5. First Seizure Trial Group. Treatment of first tonic-clonic seizure does not improve the prognosis of epilepsy. *Neurology* 1997; **49:** 991–8.
6. van Donselaar CA, *et al.* Clinical course of untreated tonic-clonic seizures in childhood: prospective, hospital based study. *BMJ* 1997; **314:** 401–4.
7. Camfield C, *et al.* Does the number of seizures before treatment influence ease of control or remission of childhood epilepsy?: not if the number is 10 or less. *Neurology* 1996; **46:** 41–4.
8. O'Donoghue M, Sander JWAS. Does early anti-epileptic drug treatment alter the prognosis for remission of the epilepsies? *J R Soc Med* 1996; **89:** 245–8.
9. Reynolds EH. Do anticonvulsants alter the natural course of epilepsy?: treatment should be started as early as possible. *BMJ* 1995; **310:** 176–7.
10. Chadwick D. Do anticonvulsants alter the natural course of epilepsy?: case for early treatment is not established. *BMJ* 1995; **310:** 177–8.
11. Sabers A, Gram L. Drug treatment of epilepsy in the 1990s: achievements and new developments. *Drugs* 1996; **52:** 483–93.
12. Brodie MJ, Dichter MA. Antiepileptic drugs. *N Engl J Med* 1996; **334:** 168–75.
13. Britton JW, So EL. Selection of antiepileptic drugs: a practical approach. *Mayo Clin Proc* 1996; **71:** 778–86.
14. Wallace SJ, *et al.* Epilepsy—a guide to medical treatment 1: antiepileptic drugs. *Hosp Med* 1998; **59:** 379–87.
15. Dichter MA, Brodie MJ. New antiepileptic drugs. *N Engl J Med* 1996; **334:** 1583–90.
16. Stephen LJ, Brodie MJ. New drug treatments for epilepsy. *Prescribers' J* 1998; **38:** 98–106.
17. Devinsky O. Patients with refractory seizures. *N Engl J Med* 1999; **340:** 1565–70.
18. Feely M. Drug treatment of epilepsy. *BMJ* 1999; **318:** 106–9.
19. Smith D, Chadwick D. The management of epilepsy. *J Neurol Neurosurg Psychiatry* 2001; **70** (suppl 2): ii15–ii21.
20. Brodie MJ, French JA. Management of epilepsy in adolescents and adults. *Lancet* 2000; **356:** 323–9.
21. Brodie MJ. Management strategies for refractory localization-related seizures. *Epilepsia* 2001; **42** (suppl 3): 27–30.
22. Anonymous. Drugs for epilepsy. *Treatment Guidelines* 2003; **1:** 57–64.
23. National Institute for Clinical Excellence. Newer drugs for epilepsy in adults (issued March 2004). Available at: http://www.nice.org.uk/pdf/TA076fullguidance.pdf (accessed 12/05/04)
24. French JA, *et al.* Efficacy and tolerability of the new antiepileptic drugs, I: Treatment of new-onset epilepsy: report of the TTA and QSS Subcommittees of the American Academy of Neurology and the American Epilepsy Society. *Epilepsia* 2004; **45:** 401–9. Also available at: http://www.neurology.org/cgi/reprint/62/8/1252.pdf (accessed 09/06/04)
25. French JA, *et al.* Efficacy and tolerability of the new antiepileptic drugs, II: Treatment of refractory epilepsy: report of the TTA and QSS Subcommittees of the American Academy of Neurology and the American Epilepsy Society. *Epilepsia* 2004; **45:** 410–23. Also available at: http://www.neurology.org/cgi/reprint/62/8/1261.pdf (accessed 09/06/04)
26. Marson AG, *et al.* Carbamazepine versus valproate monotherapy for epilepsy. Available in The Cochrane Library; Issue 1. Chichester: John Wiley; 2004.
27. Tudur Smith C, *et al.* Carbamazepine versus phenytoin monotherapy for epilepsy. Available in The Cochrane Library; Issue 1. Chichester: John Wiley; 2004.
28. Tudur Smith C, *et al.* Phenytoin versus valproate monotherapy for partial onset seizures and generalized onset tonic-clonic seizures. Available in The Cochrane Library; Issue 1. Chichester: John Wiley; 2004.
29. Perucca E. The new generation of antiepileptic drugs: advantages and disadvantages. *Br J Clin Pharmacol* 1996; **42:** 531–43.
30. Mikati MA, Browne TR. Comparative efficacy of antiepileptic drugs. *Clin Neuropharmacol* 1988; **11:** 130–40.
31. Anonymous. Managing childhood epilepsy. *Drug Ther Bull* 2001; **39:** 12–16.
32. Panayiotopoulos CP. Typical absence seizures and their treatment. *Arch Dis Child* 1999; **81:** 351–5.
33. Timmings PL, Richens A. Juvenile myoclonic epilepsy. *BMJ* 1992; **305:** 4–5.
34. Wallace SJ. Myoclonus and epilepsy in childhood: a review of treatment with valproate, ethosuximide, lamotrigine and zonisamide. *Epilepsy Res* 1998; **29:** 147–54.
35. Anonymous. Diagnosing juvenile myoclonic epilepsy. *Lancet* 1992; **340:** 759–60.
36. Ashton H. Guidelines for the rational use of benzodiazepines: when and what to use. *Drugs* 1994; **48:** 25–40.
37. Schmidt D, Bourgeois B. A risk-benefit assessment of therapies for Lennox-Gastaut syndrome. *Drug Safety* 2000; **22:** 467–77.
38. Appleton RE. Infantile spasms. *Arch Dis Child* 1993; **69:** 614–18.
39. Haines ST, Casto DT. Treatment of infantile spasms. *Ann Pharmacother* 1994; **28:** 779–91.
40. Nabbout R. A risk-benefit assessment of treatments for infantile spasms. *Drug Safety* 2001; **24:** 813–28.
41. Vigevano F, Cilio MR. Vigabatrin versus ACTH as first-line treatment for infantile spasms: a randomized, prospective study. *Epilepsia* 1997; **38:** 1270–4.
42. Granstrom ML, *et al.* Treatment of infantile spasms: results of a population-based study with vigabatrin as the first drug for spasms. *Epilepsia* 1999; **40:** 950–7.
43. Cossette P, *et al.* ACTH versus vigabatrin therapy in infantile spasms: a retrospective study. *Neurology* 1999; **52:** 1691–4.
44. Appleton RE. Guideline may help in prescribing vigabatrin. *BMJ* 1998; **317:** 1322. Full version: http://www.bmj.com/cgi/content/full/317/7168/1322 (accessed 13/05/04)
45. Appleton RE, *et al.* Randomised, placebo-controlled study of vigabatrin as first-line treatment of infantile spasms. *Epilepsia* 1999; **40:** 1627–33.
46. Vigabatrin Paediatric Advisory Group. Guideline for prescribing in children has been revised. *BMJ* 2000; **320:** 1404–5.
47. Lux AL, *et al.* Revised guideline for prescribing vigabatrin in children: guideline's claim about infantile spasms is not based on appropriate evidence. *BMJ* 2001; **322:** 236–7.
48. Riikonen RS. Steroids or vigabatrin in the treatment of infantile spasms? *Pediatr Neurol* 2000; **23:** 403–8.
49. Hancock E, Osborne JP. Vigabatrin in the treatment of infantile spasms in tuberous sclerosis: literature review. *J Child Neurol* 1999; **14:** 71–4.
50. Morton LD, Pellock JM. Diagnosis and treatment of epilepsy in children and adolescents. *Drugs* 1996; **51:** 399–414.
51. Glauser TA, *et al.* Long-term response to topiramate in patients with West syndrome. *Epilepsia* 2000; **41** (suppl 1): 591–4.
52. Zupanc ML. Update on epilepsy in pediatric patients. *Mayo Clin Proc* 1996; **71:** 899–916.
53. Neville BGR. Epilepsy in childhood. *BMJ* 1997; **315:** 924–30.
54. Pellock JM. Managing pediatric epilepsy syndromes with new antiepileptic drugs. *Pediatrics* 1999; **104:** 1106–16.
55. National Institute for Clinical Excellence. Newer drugs for epilepsy in children (issued April 2004). Available at: http://www.nice.org.uk/pdf/ta079fullguidance.pdf (accessed 12/05/04)
56. Hirtz D, *et al.* Practice parameter: Treatment of the child with a first unprovoked seizure: report of the Quality Standards Subcommittee of the American Academy of Neurology and the Practice Committee of the Child Neurology Society. *Neurology* 2003; **60:** 166–75. Also available at: http://www.neurology.org/cgi/reprint/60/2/166.pdf (accessed 09/06/04)
57. Appleton RE. The new antiepileptic drugs. *Arch Dis Child* 1996; **75:** 256–62. Correction. *ibid.* 1997; **76:** 81.
58. de Silva M, *et al.* Randomised comparative monotherapy trial of phenobarbitone, phenytoin, carbamazepine, or sodium valproate for newly diagnosed childhood epilepsy. *Lancet* 1996; **347:** 709–13.
59. Camfield PR, *et al.* If a first antiepileptic drug fails to control a child's epilepsy, what are the chances of success with the next drug? *J Pediatr* 1997; **131:** 821–4.
60. Hemingway C, *et al.* The ketogenic diet: a 3- to 6-year follow-up of 150 children enrolled prospectively. *Pediatrics* 2001; **108:** 898–905.
61. Kassoff EH, *et al.* Efficacy of the ketogenic diet for infantile spasms. *Pediatrics* 2002; **109:** 780–3.
62. Thurston JH, *et al.* Prognosis in childhood epilepsy. *N Engl J Med* 1982; **306:** 831–6.
63. Shinnar S, *et al.* Discontinuing antiepileptic medication in children with epilepsy after two years without seizures. *N Engl J Med* 1985; **313:** 976–80.
64. Andersson T, *et al.* A comparison between one and three years of treatment in uncomplicated childhood epilepsy: a prospective study: II: the EEG as predictor of outcome after withdrawal of treatment. *Epilepsia* 1997; **38:** 225–32.

65. Braathen G, *et al.* Comparison between one and three years of treatment in uncomplicated childhood epilepsy: a prospective study: I: outcome in different seizure types. *Epilepsia* 1996; **37:** 822–32.
66. Bouma PAD, *et al.* Discontinuation of antiepileptic therapy: a prospective study in children. *J Neurol Neurosurg Psychiatry* 1987; **50:** 1579–83.
67. Pedley TA. Discontinuing antiepileptic drugs. *N Engl J Med* 1988; **318:** 982–4.
68. Berg AT, Shinnar S. Relapse following discontinuation of antiepileptic drugs: a meta-analysis. *Neurology* 1994; **44:** 601–8.
69. Anonymous. Antiepileptic drug withdrawal—hawks or doves? *Lancet* 1991; **337:** 1193–4.
70. Callaghan N, *et al.* Withdrawal of anticonvulsant drugs in patients free of seizures for two years: a prospective study. *N Engl J Med* 1988; **318:** 942–6.
71. Chadwick D. Drug withdrawal and epilepsy: when and how? *Drugs* 1988; **35:** 579–83.
72. Emerson R, *et al.* Stopping medication in children with epilepsy: predicators of outcome. *N Engl J Med* 1981; **304:** 1125–9.
73. Anonymous. Diagnosing juvenile myoclonic epilepsy. *Lancet* 1992; **340:** 759–60.
74. Medical Research Council Antiepileptic Drug Withdrawal Study Group. Prognostic index for recurrence of seizures after remission of epilepsy. *BMJ* 1993; **306:** 1374–8.
75. Medical Research Council Antiepileptic Drug Withdrawal Study Group. Randomised study of antiepileptic drug withdrawal in patients in remission. *Lancet* 1991; **337:** 1175–80.
76. Duncan JS, *et al.* Discontinuation of phenytoin, carbamazepine, and valproate in patients with active epilepsy. *Epilepsia* 1990; **31:** 324–33.
77. Duncan JS, *et al.* Effects of discontinuation of phenytoin, carbamazepine, and valproate on concomitant antiepileptic medication. *Epilepsia* 1991; **32:** 101–15.
78. Anonymous. Withdrawing antiepileptic drugs. *Drug Ther Bull* 1989; **27:** 29–30.
79. Camfield C, *et al.* Outcome of childhood epilepsy: a population-based study with a simple predictive scoring system for those treated with medication. *J Pediatr* 1993; **122:** 861–8.
80. Shinnar S, *et al.* Discontinuing antiepileptic drugs in children with epilepsy: a prospective study. *Ann Neurol* 1994; **35:** 534–45.
81. Tennison MB, *et al.* Discontinuing antiepileptic drugs in children with epilepsy: a comparison of a six-week and a nine-month taper period. *N Engl J Med* 1994; **330:** 1407–10.

**Epilepsy and breast feeding.** Antiepileptics are generally distributed into breast milk (although this information is not always known for the newer ones), but for most of the older established drugs, the concentrations are lower than in maternal plasma, and breast feeding is considered to be safe for these antiepileptics when given in usual doses.[1-7] The American Academy of Pediatrics[8] also considers that most of the older antiepileptics, specifically carbamazepine, ethosuximide, phenytoin, and valproate, are usually compatible with breast feeding; however, they also recommend that phenobarbital and primidone should be used with caution as significant adverse effects have occurred in nursing infants. Problems of neonatal sedation may occur with the *benzodiazepines* and *barbiturates* (including *primidone*).[1] *Ethosuximide* is distributed in significant amounts into breast milk; hyperexcitability and poor suckling have been reported in the infant. There is little data for the new antiepileptics regarding breast feeding (the manufacturers and the UK Drugs in Lactation Advisory Service[9] generally recommend that breast feeding should be avoided). There is a possibility that *lamotrigine* may accumulate in breast-fed infants as the metabolic pathway for lamotrigine may not be fully developed in newborns;[5] the American Academy of Pediatrics[8] considers that the use of lamotrigine during breast feeding may be of concern.

1. Brodie MJ. Management of epilepsy during pregnancy and lactation. *Lancet* 1990; **336:** 426–7.
2. Delgado-Escueta AV, Janz D. Consensus guidelines: preconception counseling, management, and care of the pregnant woman with epilepsy. *Neurology* 1992; **42** (suppl 5): 149–160.
3. Anonymous. Epilepsy and pregnancy. *Drug Ther Bull* 1994; **32:** 49–51.
4. Hägg S, Spigset O. Anticonvulsant use during lactation. *Drug Safety* 2000; **22:** 425–40.
5. Crawford P. Epilepsy and pregnancy. *Seizure* 2001; **10:** 212–19.
6. Scottish Obstetric Guidelines and Audit Project. The management of pregnancy in women with epilepsy: a clinical practice guideline for professionals involved in maternity care. Available at http://www.show.scot.nhs.uk/sign/guidelines/sogap/sogap1.html (accessed 13/05/04)
7. Bar-Oz B, *et al.* Anticoagulants and breast feeding: a critical review. *Paediatr Drugs* 2000; **2:** 113–26.
8. American Academy of Pediatrics. The transfer of drugs and other chemicals into human milk. *Pediatrics* 2001; **108:** 776–89. Correction. *ibid.*; 1029. Also available at: http://aappolicy.aappublications.org/cgi/content/full/pediatrics%3b108/3/776 (accessed 13/05/04)
9. UK Drugs in Lactation Advisory Service. Drugs in lactation guidance: anticonvulsants. Available at: http://www.ukmicentral.nhs.uk/drugpreg/anticonvulsants.asp (accessed 12/05/04)

**Epilepsy and cognition.** The relationship between cognitive impairment, antiepileptic drugs, and epilepsy is complex and poorly understood; psychosocial and environmental factors may also contribute.[1-3] Children are particularly vulnerable to cognitive impairment, which can develop insidiously and therefore be overlooked. Many studies, including comparative studies, have assessed the effects of antiepileptics on cognitive function, but the results have often been variable. A major difficulty has been to distinguish subtle effects of drug therapy on mental function, if they exist, from those of sedation or the effect of the disease itself or its underlying pathology.[1,4]

Although subtle effects on cognition have been most commonly reported with barbiturate antiepileptics such as phenobarbital, they may also occur with other antiepileptics, and in adults as well as children. Benzodiazepines, phenobarbital, and primidone are most frequently linked to sedative effects and behavioural problems whereas phenytoin, carbamazepine, and valproate are less problematic. Studies of effects on cognition have been conducted in healthy adults in an effort to separate any confounding factors of epilepsy and seizures, and standard antiepileptics have been shown to impair cognition in people with and without epilepsy. Results from studies in both groups have demonstrated that at therapeutic serum concentrations phenobarbital, phenytoin, carbamazepine, oxcarbazepine, and valproate have similar adverse effects on cognitive function,[1,5] although there is also evidence that phenobarbital has the greatest potential for adverse cognitive and behavioural effects.[1] Most of the newer antiepileptics appear to be better tolerated, although zonisamide and topiramate produce some cognitive impairment. There is also limited evidence that gabapentin, lamotrigine, and vigabatrin may enhance cognitive function. However, further data are required for the newer antiepileptics before a definitive assessment can be made.[1-3,6]

There is wide interindividual variation in the cognitive effects of antiepileptics; in some patients the effects may become apparent at low serum levels, whereas others tolerate high serum levels without apparent untoward effect.[6] Variable results from studies mean that it is difficult to make comparisons. It is, however, generally agreed that phenobarbital is less desirable for use in children than other antiepileptics.

Most studies on the adverse effects of antiepileptics on cognitive function have had methodological flaws and have involved small numbers of patients; recommendations for future research have been made.[7] Future studies should assess antiepileptic use in different epileptic patient populations.[6]

In view of the potential effect of antiepileptics on cognition, the recommendations of the Committee on Drugs of the American Academy of Pediatrics[8] include:

- the relative influence of each antiepileptic on cognitive and behavioural function should be considered along with all other potential adverse effects;
- the child's behaviour and academic progress should be monitored through routine questioning of parents and teachers as well as by the physician's own observations of cognitive function, mood, and behaviour;
- should behavioural or cognitive changes occur in relation to starting antiepileptic therapy, the need for medication and/or possible alteration of medication must be reassessed.

1. Kwan P, Brodie MJ. Neuropsychological effects of epilepsy and antiepileptic drugs. *Lancet* 2001; **357:** 216–22.
2. Meador KJ. Current discoveries on the cognitive effects of antiepileptic drugs. *Pharmacotherapy* 2000; **20:** 185S–190S.
3. Brunbech L, Sabers A. Effect of antiepileptic drugs on cognitive function in individuals with epilepsy: a comparative review of newer versus older agents. *Drugs* 2002; **62:** 593–604.
4. Prevey ML, *et al.* Complex partial and secondarily generalized seizure patients: cognitive functioning prior to treatment with antiepileptic medication. *Epilepsy Res* 1998; **30:** 1–9.
5. Kälviäinen R, *et al.* Cognitive adverse effects of antiepileptic drugs: incidence, mechanisms and therapeutic implications. *CNS Drugs* 1996; **5:** 358–68.
6. Devinsky O. Cognitive and behavioral effects of antiepileptic drugs. *Epilepsia* 1995; **36** (suppl 2): S46–S65.
7. Aldenkamp AP, Vermeulen J. Phenytoin and carbamazepine: differential effects on cognitive function. *Seizure* 1995; **4:** 95–104.
8. Committee on Drugs of the American Academy of Pediatrics. Behavioral and cognitive effects of anticonvulsant therapy. *Pediatrics* 1995; **96:** 538–40. Also available at: http://aappolicy.aappublications.org/cgi/reprint/pediatrics;96/3/538.pdf (accessed 07/06/04)

**Epilepsy and driving.** Driving by patients with epilepsy is generally regulated[1,2] and restricted to those whose seizures are adequately controlled. Also, antiepileptic drugs may produce CNS-related adverse effects, including dizziness and drowsiness, that could impair a patient's ability to drive a vehicle or operate machinery, particularly during the initial stages of therapy.

In the UK,[3] patients suffering from epilepsy may drive a motor vehicle (but not a heavy goods or public service vehicle) provided that they have had a seizure-free period of 1 year, or, if subject to attacks only while asleep, have established a 3-year period without awake attacks. It is recommended that patients should not drive during withdrawal of antiepileptic drugs, or for 6 months afterwards.

1. Berg AT, Engel J. Restricted driving for people with epilepsy. *Neurology* 1999; **52:** 1306–7.
2. Ooi WW, Gutrecht JA. International regulations for automobile driving and epilepsy. *J Travel Med* 2000; **7:** 1–4.
3. Driver and Vehicle Licensing Agency. At a glance: a guide for medical practitioners. Available at: http://www.dvla.gov.uk/at_a_glance/ch1_neurological.htm (accessed 13/05/04)

**Epilepsy and pregnancy.** The management of epilepsy during pregnancy may present problems for both the mother and the fetus.[1-8]

The incidence of spontaneous abortion, preterm delivery, still-births, and low birth-weights increases in women with epilepsy although the reasons are unknown. A single generalised seizure does not usually pose clinical problems for the fetus, but both mother and fetus are at risk of serious trauma from maternal falls and intra-uterine deaths have been reported. Status epilepticus is associated with significant mortality in mother and fetus. The frequency of seizures may increase during pregnancy in some women; this may be related to hormonal or other factors such as lack of sleep, but one of the main reasons is likely to be decreased plasma-antiepileptic concentrations due to changes in drug clearance and binding as pregnancy progresses.

Although the vast majority of pregnant women receiving antiepileptic therapy will deliver normal infants, unequivocal teratogenic risks have been identified for all the major antiepileptics.[9,10] The risk appears to increase when 2 or more drugs are given together especially if valproate is part of the combination.

A variety of syndromes, including craniofacial and digital abnormalities and, less commonly, cleft lip and palate, have been described with *carbamazepine, oxcarbazepine, phenobarbital, phenytoin, primidone, trimethadione,* and *valproate*; congenital heart disease, microcephaly, and developmental delay may also occur with some antiepileptics. Specific syndromes have previously been ascribed to individual antiepileptics such as the 'fetal hydantoin syndrome' with phenytoin, but now it is recognised that there is some degree of overlap between the effects seen with different drugs, and the broader term 'fetal antiepileptic drug syndrome' is therefore considered to be more appropriate by some.[11] In some cases, the milder dysmorphic features become less apparent as the child grows older. It is difficult to establish whether one antiepileptic is more teratogenic than another although data from the UK pregnancy register has shown that valproate is significantly more teratogenic than carbamazepine. Consequently some authors have recommended that valproate should be avoided in pregnancy[7] (but see below). Neural tube defects are associated with valproate and carbamazepine and the risk of spina bifida has been calculated[12-14] to be about 1%, which is about 20 times the rate in the general population. Analysis of data[15] from 5 prospective studies showed that there was a dose-response relationship between maternal use of valproate and the development of major congenital abnormalities; in particular, daily doses above 1 g or high peak concentrations were associated with a significantly increased risk. Such a relationship is not, in general, seen with the other antiepileptics. Additional problems that may occur with some antiepileptic therapies include neonatal sedation and drug dependence with phenobarbital (see p.368) and benzodiazepines if given close to term. Neonatal bleeding is associated with the enzyme-inducing antiepileptics carbamazepine, phenobarbital, and phenytoin, and has also been reported with valproate and other antiepileptics. Little is known of the effects of the newer antiepileptics on the fetus, although the manufacturers have reported congenital anomalies in the offspring of some mothers using *vigabatrin* during pregnancy and teratogenicity with *topiramate, vigabatrin* and *zonisamide* in *animals*. From the limited data available there is little to suggest that *lamotrigine* is a major teratogen although there is a theoretical risk because like valproate, it is a folate antagonist. There also appears to be little evidence of teratogenic potential for *felbamate* or *gabapentin* in *animal* studies to date.

Untreated epilepsy itself has been associated with an increase in fetal abnormalities such as cleft palate and spina bifida,[7,11] although to a lesser degree than with antiepileptics. This does not appear to be associated with maternal seizures during pregnancy and, since some of these effects were also described before the use of antiepileptics became widespread, there may be a relationship with a genetic component of epilepsy.[11]

Patients with epilepsy who present for pre-conception advice should be seen by a specialist. Withdrawal of antiepileptic therapy may be an option if the patient has been seizure-free for at least 2 years (for further details of drug withdrawal, see above); resumption of therapy may be considered after the end of the first trimester. If antiepileptics are to be continued throughout pregnancy, monotherapy is preferred using the lowest possible effective dose, although doses may have to be increased in response to changes in drug disposition during pregnancy, with the necessary readjustments being made after delivery. Since there is a risk of fetal malformations with all the established antiepileptics, and a lack of data for the newer ones, it is generally considered that as long as there is good seizure control there is little to be gained from changing a pregnant patient's antiepileptic. However high daily doses of valproate (more than 1 g daily) should be avoided if possible, and peak plasma concentrations may be reduced by dividing the daily dose over 3 or 4 administrations or by giving a modified-release preparation. For those patients who first present when already pregnant there is probably little to be gained in altering potentially teratogenic antiepileptics as the time for intervention has almost certainly passed.[7,8] If a patient becomes pregnant while taking carbamazepine, phenytoin, or valproate she should be counselled regarding the risk of neural tube and other defects and should be offered antenatal screening. Adequate supplementation of folic acid is advised before pregnancy and during the first trimester to counteract the risk of neural tube defects; it has been suggested that women receiving antiepileptics should be given folic acid in similar doses to those used in women who have previously given birth to an infant with neural tube defects (for further details, see Neural Tube Defects under Folic Acid, p.1430). Although folic acid can reduce serum-phenytoin concentrations this does not appear to be a problem in practice (see p.375).

To counteract the risk of neonatal bleeding associated with carbamazepine, oxcarbazepine, phenobarbital, phenytoin, and topiramate, prophylactic vitamin $K_1$ is recommended for the mother from 36 weeks' gestation, and then for the neonate after delivery (for further details, see under Vitamin K deficiency bleeding, p.1468), although the justification of prophylactic maternal administration has been challenged[16] in the face of available evidence. Patients with epilepsy have also a higher risk of preterm delivery and antenatal corticosteroid therapy may, therefore, be warranted. High doses of corticosteroid may be required in those women receiving enzyme-inducing antiepileptics.[7]

Status epilepticus occurring during pregnancy should be treated in the same way as for the general population (see below). First seizures occurring during the second half of pregnancy may be part of eclampsia (see below) and should be differentiated from epilepsy.


1. Brodie MJ. Management of epilepsy during pregnancy and lactation. *Lancet* 1990; **336:** 426–7.
2. Delgado-Escueta AV, Janz D. Consensus guidelines: preconception counseling, management, and care of the pregnant woman with epilepsy. *Neurology* 1992; **42** (suppl 5): 149–160.
3. Anonymous. Epilepsy and pregnancy. *Drug Ther Bull* 1994; **32:** 49–51.
4. Cleland PG. Management of pre-existing disorders in pregnancy: epilepsy. *Prescribers' J* 1996; **36:** 102–109.
5. Quality Standards Subcommittee of the American Academy of Neurology. Practice parameter: management issues for women with epilepsy (summary statement). *Neurology* 1998; **51:** 944–8. Also available at: http://aan.com/professionals/practice/pdfs/pdf_1995_thru_1998/1998.51.944.pdf (accessed 07/06/04)
6. Nulman I, *et al.* Treatment of epilepsy in pregnancy. *Drugs* 1999; **57:** 535–44.
7. Crawford P. Epilepsy and pregnancy. *Seizure* 2001; **10:** 212–19.
8. Scottish Obstetric Guidelines and Audit Project. The management of pregnancy in women with epilepsy: a clinical practice guideline for professionals involved in maternity care. Available at: http://www.show.scot.nhs.uk/sign/guidelines/sogap/sogap1.html (accessed 13/05/04)
9. Morrell MJ. Antiepileptic drug use in women. In: Levy RH, *et al.*, eds. *Antiepileptic drugs.* 5th ed. Philadelphia: Lippincott Williams & Wilkins, 2002; 132–48.
10. McAuley JW, Anderson GD. Treatment of epilepsy in women of reproductive age: pharmacokinetic considerations. *Clin Pharmacokinet* 2002; **41:** 559–79.
11. Gaily E, *et al.* Minor anomalies in offspring of epileptic mothers. *J Pediatr* 1988; **112:** 520–9.
12. Lindhout D, Schmidt D. In-utero exposure to valproate and neural tube defects. *Lancet* 1986; **i:** 1392–3.
13. Oakeshott P, Hunt GM. Valproate and spina bifida. *BMJ* 1989; **298:** 1300–1.
14. Rosa FW. Spina bifida in infants of women treated with carbamazepine during pregnancy. *N Engl J Med* 1991; **324:** 674–7.
15. Samrén EB, *et al.* Maternal use of antiepileptic drugs and the risk of major congenital malformations: a joint European prospective study of human teratogenesis associated with maternal epilepsy. *Epilepsia* 1997; **38:** 981–90.
16. Hey E. Effect of maternal anticonvulsant treatment on neonatal blood coagulation. *Arch Dis Child Fetal Neonatal Ed* 1999; **81:** F208–F210.


### Status epilepticus

Status epilepticus has been arbitrarily defined as a prolonged seizure, or a period of repeated seizures without restoration of normal consciousness in between, lasting for more than 30 minutes;[1] in practice, prolonged or repeated seizure activity lasting more than 5 to 10 minutes may be regarded as status epilepticus and should be treated appropriately.[2-5] Any type of seizure can lead to status epilepticus but generalised tonic-clonic status epilepticus is the most common and most dangerous type.[2,3] The longer seizures continue, the more difficult they are to control and the higher the morbidity and mortality; permanent neuronal damage can occur after 30 minutes of seizure activity.

Initial treatment consists of positioning the patient to avoid injury, supporting respiration, including the provision of oxygen, correcting any hypoglycaemia, and maintaining blood pressure. The aim is then to terminate the seizures as quickly as possible. Antiepileptic treatment differs slightly between centres and countries,[1-12] but in the early stages of an attack, control is generally attempted with a *benzodiazepine*. *Diazepam* by intravenous injection or as a rectal solution has traditionally been used. (Rectal diazepam has also been used in the home setting to treat acute repetitive seizures,[13] which may evolve into status epilepticus.) However, *lorazepam* is increasingly preferred to diazepam as the initial benzodiazepine[4,5,11,12] because it combines rapid onset with prolonged duration of antiepileptic action. Other benzodiazepines used include *clonazepam* and *midazolam*. Patients who respond to treatment should be started on maintenance antiepileptic treatment; failure to do this may lead to the recurrence of seizures.

If, after 30 minutes, the above measures fail to control the seizures or the seizures recur, then phenytoin sodium, fosphenytoin, or phenobarbital should be tried; repeat doses may be required. *Phenytoin sodium* may be given intravenously with monitoring of blood pressure and ECG. Phenytoin may also be more appropriate than a benzodiazepine for the management of status epilepticus or recurrent seizures in patients with head injuries or other acute neurological lesions; phenytoin carries a lower risk of respiratory failure or loss of consciousness, and results in a longer-lasting control of seizures.[14] *Fosphenytoin sodium* is a prodrug of phenytoin sodium and has the advantage that it may be administered at a faster rate of intravenous infusion although monitoring is still required. Alternatively, intravenous *phenobarbital sodium* may be given if the patient has not recently received oral phenobarbital or primidone; careful observation of respiration is mandatory as a large dose of diazepam may have been given previously.[1] Some have suggested that using phenobarbital for the initial treatment of convulsive status epilepticus might be at least as effective, safe, and practical as using diazepam with phenytoin,[15] but others consider that phenytoin is again to be preferred as causing less CNS and respiratory depression.[4] More recent reviews suggest that phenobarbital should be reserved for seizures that do not respond to repeat doses of phenytoin or fosphenytoin.[5,11,12] Other alternatives have included *paraldehyde* rectally or by deep intramuscular injection, and intravenous *clomethiazole edisilate* was formerly available. Intravenous *valproate* may also be tried. Another option is to give *lidocaine* intravenously.

Status epilepticus may be considered refractory if the seizures fail to respond to the above measures after 60 to 90 minutes. At this point, anaesthesia should be instituted with a short-acting barbiturate such as *thiopental*, and the patient ventilated;[1,6] *pentobarbital* is used similarly.[2,3,8] Other anaesthetics have been tried in the treatment of intractable convulsive status epilepticus including *etomidate, isoflurane, midazolam,* and *propofol*.[3,5,6,8,11,12]

If cerebral neoplasm or arteritis is suspected high-dose *dexamethasone* therapy is started, provided meningitis or cerebral abscess is absent.[1] Alcoholics are given intravenous *thiamine*.[1,6] Pyridoxine may be tried in children under 3 years of age with established convulsive status epilepticus, in case the seizures are pyridoxine dependent or responsive.[4]

The treatment of partial status epilepticus is similar to that of generalised tonic-clonic status epilepticus.[3] However, epilepsia partialis continua (continuous clonic movements of a limited part of the body) may be refractory to standard antiepileptics; it may respond to treatment with high doses of *corticosteroids*.[1]

Intravenous benzodiazepines are usually used for the initial treatment of absence status epilepticus[3] followed by oral administration of valproate or *ethosuximide*. Valproate is considered to be the drug of choice to prevent recurrence of absence status epilepticus.[16]


1. Brodie MJ. Status epilepticus in adults. *Lancet* 1990; **336:** 551–2.
2. Working Group on Status Epilepticus. Treatment of convulsive status epilepticus: recommendations of the Epilepsy Foundation of America's Working Group on Status Epilepticus. *JAMA* 1993; **270:** 854–9.
3. Bauer J, Elger CE. Management of status epilepticus in adults. *CNS Drugs* 1994; **i:** 26–44.
4. The Status Epilepticus Working Party. The treatment of convulsive status epilepticus in children. *Arch Dis Child* 2000; **83:** 415–19.
5. Manno EM. New management strategies in the treatment of status epilepticus. *Mayo Clin Proc* 2003; **78:** 508–18.
6. Anonymous. Stopping status epilepticus. *Drug Ther Bull* 1996; **34:** 73–5.
7. Rylance GW. Treatment of epilepsy and febrile convulsions in children. *Lancet* 1990; **336:** 488–91.
8. Cascino GD. Generalized convulsive status epilepticus. *Mayo Clin Proc* 1996; **71:** 787–92.
9. Tasker RC. Emergency treatment of acute seizures and status epilepticus. *Arch Dis Child* 1998; **79:** 78–83.
10. Lowenstein DH, Alldredge BK. Status epilepticus. *N Engl J Med* 1998; **338:** 970–6.
11. Smith BJ. Treatment of status epilepticus. *Neurol Clin North Am* 2001; **19:** 347–69.
12. Chapman MG, *et al.* Status epilepticus. *Anaesthesia* 2001; **56:** 648–59.
13. Akinbi MS, Welty TE. Benzodiazepines in the home treatment of acute seizures. *Ann Pharmacother* 1999; **33:** 99–102.
14. Eldridge PR, Punt JAG. Risks associated with giving benzodiazepines to patients with acute neurological injuries. *BMJ* 1990; **300:** 1189–90.
15. Shaner DM, *et al.* Treatment of status epilepticus: a prospective comparison of diazepam and phenytoin versus phenobarbital and optional phenytoin. *Neurology* 1988; **38:** 202–7.
16. Berkovic SF, *et al.* Valproate prevents the recurrence of absence status. *Neurology* 1989; **39:** 1294–7.


### Other convulsive disorders

Disorders that feature convulsions or epileptic seizures but are not considered to be forms of epilepsy are described below.

**Alcohol withdrawal syndrome.** For a discussion of the management of seizures associated with alcohol withdrawal syndrome, see p.1166.

**Eclampsia and pre-eclampsia.** Pre-eclampsia is a hypertensive disorder occurring in pregnancy that entails increased blood pressure together with proteinuria, and sometimes abnormal coagulation, liver dysfunction, and oedema; rarely the disorder may progress to eclampsia, which is a convulsive phase. It is difficult to identify those patients who will experience eclamptic seizures. The treatment of pre-eclampsia and eclampsia is primarily aimed at reducing hypertension (see Hypertension in Pregnancy, under Hypertension, p.825) and treating or preventing resultant seizures. However, the treatment of the hypertension alone may not be sufficient to prevent the progression of pre-eclampsia to eclampsia.[1]

Eclampsia in the UK was traditionally **treated** with *diazepam, clomethiazole,* or *phenytoin. 'Lytic cocktails'* consisting of chlorpromazine, pethidine, and/or promethazine have also been used in some countries in the management of pre-eclampsia and imminent eclampsia but they result in heavy sedation and the use of phenothiazines is generally not recommended late in pregnancy. Nowadays most in the UK consider *magnesium sulfate* to be the preferred drug for the treatment of eclampsia;[2-6] it has been the preferred treatment of eclampsia in the USA for many years. Studies[7-9] have shown magnesium sulfate to be more effective and to cause fewer adverse effects than other antiepileptics. A meta-analysis[10] of 9 randomised trials involving 2390 patients with pre-eclampsia and 1743 patients with eclampsia concluded that magnesium sulfate was more effective than phenytoin or no therapy in prevention of seizures in pre-eclamptic patients. In eclamptic patients, magnesium sulfate was superior to phenytoin, diazepam, or a lytic cocktail in terms of seizure recurrence.

Until recently there has been insufficient evidence to establish the benefits and hazards of antiepileptics in the **prevention** of eclampsia in pre-eclamptic patients although it was considered that magnesium sulfate was the best choice if an antiepileptic was needed.[11] The significant benefits of magnesium sulfate in the prevention of eclampsia have now been confirmed in a large, international trial.[12] However, some commentators have suggested,[13] in the light of evidence of possible neonatal toxicity, that magnesium sulfate should be restricted to use in more severe pre-eclampsia or eclampsia.


1. Ramsay MM, *et al.* Are anticonvulsants necessary to prevent eclampsia. *Lancet* 1994; **343:** 540–1.
2. Anthony J, *et al.* Role of magnesium sulfate in seizure prevention in patients with eclampsia and pre-eclampsia. *Drug Safety* 1996; **15:** 188–99.
3. Robson SC. Magnesium sulphate: the time of reckoning. *Br J Obstet Gynaecol* 1996; **103:** 99–102.
4. Duley L. Magnesium sulphate regimens for women with eclampsia: messages from the Collaborative Eclampsia Trial. *Br J Obstet Gynaecol* 1996; **103:** 103–5.
5. Gülmezoglu AM, Duley L. Use of anticonvulsants in eclampsia and pre-eclampsia: survey of obstetricians in the United Kingdom and Republic of Ireland. *BMJ* 1998; **316:** 975–6.
6. Walker JJ. Pre-eclampsia. *Lancet* 2000; **356:** 1260–5.
7. Dommisse J. Phenytoin sodium and magnesium sulphate in the management of eclampsia. *Br J Obstet Gynaecol* 1990; **97:** 104–9.
8. The Eclampsia Trial Collaborative Group. Which anticonvulsant for women with eclampsia?: evidence from the Collaborative Eclampsia Trial. *Lancet* 1995; **345:** 1455–63. Correction. *ibid.*; **346:** 258.

9. Lucas MJ, *et al.* A comparison of magnesium sulfate with phenytoin for the prevention of eclampsia. *N Engl J Med* 1995; **333:** 201–5.
10. Chien PFW, *et al.* Magnesium sulphate in the treatment of eclampsia and pre-eclampsia: an overview of the evidence from randomised trials. *Br J Obstet Gynaecol* 1996; **103:** 1085–91.
11. Duley L, *et al.* Magnesium sulphate and other anticonvulsants for women with pre-eclampsia. Available in The Cochrane Library; Issue 2. Chichester: John Wiley; 2004.
12. The Magpie Trial Collaborative Group. Do women with pre-eclampsia, and their babies, benefit from magnesium sulphate? The Magpie Trial: a randomised placebo-controlled trial. *Lancet* 2002; **359:** 1877–90.
13. Bennett P, Edwards D. Use of magnesium sulphate in obstetrics. *Lancet* 1997; **350:** 1491.

**Febrile convulsions.** Febrile convulsions have been defined[1] as epileptic seizures occurring between the ages of 6 months to 5 years and associated with a fever arising from an infectious illness outside the CNS. They usually occur during the rising phase of fever early in the course of the infection and are not considered to be a form of epilepsy.[2]

Febrile convulsions are considered to be benign if limited to a single tonic or tonic-clonic seizure lasting less than 15 minutes without any focal characteristics.[2] About one-third of children who have a benign febrile convulsion will experience a recurrence.[1-3] Risk factors for recurrence include a young onset age, a history of epilepsy or febrile seizures in a first-degree relative, subsequent episodes of fever, and a first complex febrile seizure.[3] The risk of developing epilepsy is low, but nevertheless it is 2 to 3 times greater than the risk in the population as a whole.[2] Unless they are recurrent, benign febrile convulsions need only simple treatment to lower body temperature[1,2] such as that described under Fever and Hyperthermia, p.8.

Prolonged febrile convulsions lasting longer than 15 minutes and associated with some focal characteristics are not considered to be benign and further increase the risk of developing epilepsy.[2] When they are prolonged or recurrent they are treated with *diazepam* intravenously, or as a rectal solution, to prevent possible brain damage resulting from continued seizure activity, although any such effect appears to be rare.[4]

The prophylactic administration of *antiepileptics* to children thought to be at risk of recurrence of febrile convulsions remains controversial. Many consider that even if recurrences can be prevented there is no evidence that the risk of developing epilepsy is reduced.[1-3] A working group of the Royal College of Physicians and the British Paediatric Association considered that pooled analyses of studies of the prophylactic use of *phenobarbital* or *sodium valproate* showed that long-term prophylaxis was rarely indicated.[1] Although some workers have demonstrated that intermittent prophylaxis with phenobarbital or diazepam[5] given at the onset of and during fever could prevent recurrence of febrile convulsions, the working group did not recommend their routine use in this way.[1] Other workers have found that administration of paracetamol as an antipyretic and the use of diazepam for intermittent prophylaxis failed to prevent recurrences of febrile convulsions.[6] A later meta-analysis[7] concluded that neither continuous nor intermittent prophylaxis could be recommended as the benefits did not outweigh the potential adverse effects, a view endorsed by the American Academy of Pediatrics.[8]

1. Joint Working Group of the Research Unit of the Royal College of Physicians and the British Paediatric Association. Guidelines for the management of convulsions with fever. *BMJ* 1991; **303:** 634–6.
2. Smith MC. Febrile seizures: recognition and management. *Drugs* 1994; **47:** 933–44.
3. Knudsen FU. Febrile seizures: treatment and prognosis. *Epilepsia* 2000; **41:** 2–9.
4. Verity CM. Do seizures damage the brain? The epidemiological evidence. *Arch Dis Child* 1998; **78:** 78–84.
5. Rosman NP, *et al.* A controlled trial of diazepam administered during febrile illnesses to prevent recurrence of febrile seizures. *N Engl J Med* 1993; **329:** 79–84.
6. Uhari M, *et al.* Effect of acetaminophen and of low intermittent doses of diazepam on prevention of recurrences of febrile seizures. *J Pediatr* 1995; **126:** 991–5.
7. Rantala H, *et al.* A meta-analytic review of the preventative treatment of recurrences of febrile seizures. *J Pediatr* 1997; **131:** 922–5.
8. American Academy of Pediatrics. Practice parameter: long-term treatment of the child with simple febrile seizures. *Pediatrics* 1999; **103:** 1307–9. Also available at: http://aappolicy.aappublications.org/cgi/reprint/pediatrics;103/6/1307.pdf (accessed 07/06/04)

**Myoclonus.** Myoclonus consists of brief, involuntary, jerky movements of sudden onset which may be focal, segmental, or generalised, and are caused by muscular contractions (positive myoclonus) or inhibitions/pauses (negative myoclonus). The term 'myoclonus' is non-specific and classification is important in order to decide on treatment:[1,2] physiological (in normal subjects); essential (no known cause); epileptic (seizures dominate); or symptomatic (encephalopathy dominates and there are many causes including storage diseases, neurodegenerative syndromes, toxic and drug-induced syndromes, and hypoxia). Myoclonus may also be subdivided into cortical, reticular, or spinal forms. Cortical myoclonus is considered to be a subset of epilepsy and responds best to antiepileptics, usually *valproate* and/or *clonazepam*; *piracetam* is also used, usually as adjunctive therapy. In epileptic myoclonus, epileptic seizures (myoclonic seizures in which the motor manifestation is myoclonus) dominate. Their treatment is discussed under Epilepsy, above. Reticular myoclonus is usually caused by anoxia or acute encephalopathy and may be treated with clonazepam; *serotonin* or serotonergic agonists have also been tried. Posthypoxic myoclonus occurring after hypoxic coma may respond to *oxitriptan* or serotonin combined with *carbidopa*; antiepileptics may help. Essential myoclonus may benefit from clonazepam.

1. Caviness JN. Myoclonus. *Mayo Clin Proc.* 1996; **71:** 679–88.
2. Blindauer K. Myoclonus and its disorders. *Neurol Clin North Am* 2001; **19:** 723–34.

**Neonatal seizures.** Neonatal seizures differ from epilepsy and the definitions in the international classification of epilepsy and epileptic syndromes (see above) do not apply. They are frequently subtle and difficult to recognise. Causes include asphyxia, glucose or electrolyte imbalance, infection, CNS or cerebrovascular lesions, inborn errors of metabolism, and drug withdrawal or intoxication.

Neonatal seizures represent a neurological emergency in the newborn and rapid diagnosis and treatment is essential. Infusion of glucose or electrolytes may be of benefit. Current practice involves administration of antiepileptic drugs to control seizures, although there is no consensus on their use. *Phenobarbital* and *phenytoin* are the most widely used. Some consider phenobarbital to be the mainstay of treatment for all types of seizures in neonates, although response rates are variable. If seizures persist, phenytoin may be added to therapy. Other drugs that have been tried include *carbamazepine, benzodiazepines*, and *primidone*. Pyridoxine-dependent seizures can be abolished by regular administration of large doses of the vitamin (see p.1457).

References.

1. Zupanc ML. Update on epilepsy in pediatric patients. *Mayo Clin Proc* 1996; **71:** 899–916.
2. Morton LD, Pellock JM. Diagnosis and treatment of epilepsy in children and adolescents. *Drugs* 1996; **51:** 399–414.
3. Singh B, *et al.* Treatment of neonatal seizures with carbamazepine. *J Child Neurol* 1996; **11:** 378–82.
4. Evans D, Levene M. Neonatal seizures. *Arch Dis Child Fetal Neonatal Ed* 1998; **78:** F70–F75.
5. Painter MJ, *et al.* Phenobarbital compared with phenytoin for the treatment of neonatal seizures. *N Engl J Med* 1999; **341:** 485–9.
6. Hill A. Neonatal seizures. *Pediatr Rev* 2000; **21:** 117–21.
7. Painter MJ, Alvin J. Neonatal seizures. *Curr Treat Options Neurol* 2001; **3:** 237–48.

**Porphyria.** Convulsions may occur at the peak of an attack of acute porphyria (p.1040) but usually disappear as the attack resolves and therapy should be aimed at the underlying disease. However, some patients continue to experience convulsions while in remission and their management poses a major therapeutic problem as all the first-line antiepileptics have been associated with acute attacks.[1] Barbiturates (*phenobarbital, primidone*), hydantoins (*phenytoin, ethotoin*), and *carbamazepine* are considered unsafe, as are *sultiame* and *progabide*. There is limited evidence that the *benzodiazepines, sodium valproate*, and probably *valpromide* are porphyrinogenic but status epilepticus has been treated successfully with intravenous *diazepam*. Seizure prophylaxis may be undertaken as a calculated risk using valproate or *clonazepam* if considered essential. *Magnesium sulfate* is safe. *Clomethiazole* is also probably safe. *Gabapentin* and *vigabatrin* have each been tried in a few patients without ill-effect, although there has been a report of a bullous skin eruption in a patient with porphyria cutanea tarda given vigabatrin.[2] Other antiepileptics such as the succinimides (*ethosuximide, mesuximide, phensuximide*) and oxazolidinediones (*trimethadione*) are considered to be unsafe.

1. Gorchein A. Drug treatment in acute porphyria. *Br J Clin Pharmacol* 1997; **44:** 427–34.
2. Hommel L, *et al.* Acute bullous skin eruption after treatment with vigabatrine. *Dermatology* 1995; **191:** 181.

## 4-Amino-3-hydroxybutyric Acid

Buxamin; Gabob.

$C_4H_9NO_3$ = 119.1.

*CAS — 352-21-6.*

### Profile

Aminohydroxybutyric acid has been claimed to be of value in a variety of neurological disorders including use as an adjunct in the treatment of epilepsy. It should be distinguished from its isomer 3-amino-4-hydroxybutyric acid (Gobab) which is reported to possess anti-inflammatory and antifungal activity.

### Preparations

**Proprietary Preparations** (details are given in Part 3)
***Arg.:*** Gabimex; ***Braz.:*** Gamibetal; ***Ital.:*** Gamibetal; ***Mex.:*** Gamibetal; ***Port.:*** Gabomade; Gamibetal; ***Spain:*** Bogil†.

**Multi-ingredient:** ***Arg.:*** Gabimex Plus; ***Braz.:*** Gamibetal Complex; ***Ital.:*** Gamibetal Complex; Gamibetal Plus; Parvisedil; ***Port.:*** Gabisedil; Gamibetal Compositum; ***Spain:*** Cefabol; Disfil†; Dorken; Gamalate B6; Pertranquil†; Redutona.

## Barbexaclone (*rINN*)

Barbexaclona. Compound of (−)-*N*,α-Dimethylcyclohexaneethylamine with 5-ethyl-5-phenylbarbituric acid.

$C_{12}H_{12}N_2O_3,C_{10}H_{21}N$ = 387.5.

*CAS — 4388-82-3.*

*ATC — N03AA04.*

### Profile

Barbexaclone is a compound of levopropylhexedrine (see under Propylhexedrine, p.1593) with phenobarbital (p.367). It is used in the treatment of various types of epilepsy (p.349). Usual adult doses are 200 to 400 mg daily given by mouth in divided doses.

### Preparations

**Proprietary Preparations** (details are given in Part 3)
***Austria:*** Maliasin; ***Braz.:*** Maliasin; ***Ger.:*** Maliasin†; ***Ital.:*** Maliasin; ***Switz.:*** Maliasin.

## Beclamide (*BAN, rINN*)

Beclamida; Benzchlorpropamide; Chlorethylphenamide. *N*-Benzyl-3-chloropropionamide.

$C_{10}H_{12}ClNO$ = 197.7.

*CAS — 501-68-8.*

*ATC — N03AX30.*

### Profile

Beclamide has been used as an antiepileptic for the control of tonic-clonic and simple partial seizures. It has also been used for the management of behaviour disorders.

## Benzobarbital (*rINN*)

Benzobarbitone; Benzonal; Benzonalum. 1-Benzoyl-5-ethyl-5-phenylbarbituric acid.

$C_{19}H_{16}N_2O_4$ = 336.3.

*CAS — 744-80-9.*

**Pharmacopoeias.** In *Int.*

### Profile

Benzobarbital is a barbiturate used in the treatment of epilepsy.

# Carbamazepine (*BAN, USAN, rINN*)

Carbamazepina; Carbamazepinum; G-32883. 5*H*-Dibenz[*b,f*]azepine-5-carboxamide.

$C_{15}H_{12}N_2O$ = 236.3.

*CAS — 298-46-4.*

*ATC — N03AF01.*

**Pharmacopoeias.** In *Chin., Eur.* (see p.vi), *Int., Jpn, Pol.*, and *US.*

**Ph. Eur. 5.0** (Carbamazepine). A white or almost white crystalline powder. It exhibits polymorphism. Very slightly soluble in water; sparingly soluble in alcohol and in acetone; freely soluble in dichloromethane. Store in airtight containers.

**USP 27** (Carbamazepine). A white or off-white powder. Practically insoluble in water; soluble in alcohol and in acetone. Store in airtight containers.

**Incompatibility.** Carbamazepine suspension should be mixed with an equal volume of diluent before nasogastric administration as undiluted suspension is adsorbed onto PVC nasogastric tubes.[1]

The FDA have received a report of a patient who passed an orange rubbery mass in his faeces the day after taking a carbamazepine suspension (Tegretol) followed immediately by chlorpromazine solution (Thorazine). Subsequent testing showed that mixing the same carbamazepine suspension with a thioridazine hydrochloride solution (Mellaril) also resulted in the precipitation of a rubbery orange mass.

1. Clark-Schmidt AL, *et al.* Loss of carbamazepine suspension through nasogastric feeding tubes. *Am J Hosp Pharm* 1990; **47:** 2034–7.

**Stability.** FDA studies indicate that carbamazepine tablets could lose up to one-third of their effectiveness if stored in humid conditions.[1] This appears to be due to formation of a dihydrate form which leads to hardening of the tablet and poor dissolution and absorption.[2,3] As the dihydrate has also been detected after storage under ambient conditions some suggest that storage with silica gel sachets may be necessary to avoid physical deterioration of carbamazepine tablets.[2]

1. Anonymous. Moisture hardens carbamazepine tablets, FDA finds. *Am J Hosp Pharm* 1990; **47:** 958.

2. Lowes MMJ. More information on hardening of carbamazepine tablets. *Am J Hosp Pharm* 1991; **48:** 2130–1.
3. Wang JT, *et al.* Effects of humidity and temperature on in vitro dissolution of carbamazepine tablets. *J Pharm Sci* 1993; **82:** 1002–5.

## Adverse Effects

Fairly common side-effects of carbamazepine, particularly in the initial stages of therapy, include dizziness, drowsiness, and ataxia. These effects may be minimised by starting therapy with a low dose. Drowsiness and disturbances of cerebellar and oculo-motor function (with ataxia, nystagmus, and diplopia) are also symptoms of excessive plasma concentrations of carbamazepine, and may disappear with continued treatment at reduced dosage.

Gastrointestinal symptoms are reported to be less common, and include dry mouth, abdominal pain, nausea and vomiting, anorexia, and diarrhoea or constipation.

Generalised erythematous rashes may be severe and may necessitate withdrawal of treatment. Photosensitivity reactions, urticaria, alopecia, exfoliative dermatitis, toxic epidermal necrolysis, erythema multiforme and Stevens-Johnson syndrome, and systemic lupus erythematosus (but see below) have also been reported.

Occasional reports of blood disorders include agranulocytosis, aplastic anaemia, eosinophilia, persistent leucopenia, leucocytosis, thrombocytopenia, and purpura. Lymphadenopathy, splenomegaly, pneumonitis, abnormalities of liver and kidney function, hepatitis, and cholestatic jaundice have occurred. Some or all of these symptoms as well as fever and rashes may represent a generalised hypersensitivity reaction to carbamazepine.

Hyponatraemia, and sometimes oedema, have occurred. Other adverse effects reported include paraesthesia, headache, arrhythmias and heart block, heart failure, impotence, male infertility, gynaecomastia, galactorrhoea, and dystonias and dyskinesias with asterixis. Rectal administration has resulted in local irritation.

Overdosage may be manifested by many of the adverse effects listed above, especially those on the CNS, and may result in stupor, coma, convulsions, respiratory depression, and death.

In rare cases, carbamazepine has been reported to exacerbate seizures in patients suffering from mixed-type epilepsy—see Precautions, below.

Congenital malformations have been reported in infants born to women who received carbamazepine during pregnancy.

**Effects on the blood.** Occasional reports of fatal haematological reactions associated with carbamazepine led the manufacturers to recommend extensive blood monitoring during therapy. However, because of the rarity of such reactions these recommendations were questioned and the manufacturers subsequently modified their guidelines (see Precautions, below).

Case reports and studies of carbamazepine's haematological effects have been reviewed.[1] The incidence of haematological reactions to carbamazepine has been estimated to range between 1:10 800 and 1:38 000 per year while one group reported the rate of bone marrow suppression to be between 1:10 000 and 1:50 000 cases. The incidence of aplastic anaemia has been calculated to be 1:200 000 per year. Another investigator indicated that 2.2 deaths per million exposures were associated with aplastic anaemia and agranulocytosis. However, of 27 reports of aplastic anaemia (16 fatal) associated with carbamazepine many were found to have had co-incidental disease or were receiving multiple-drug therapy. Benign or clinically insignificant leucopenia has occurred, usually during the first 3 months of treatment, in about 12% of children and 7% of adults but in most patients this resolved despite continuation of therapy. Mild transient thrombocytopenia has occurred in about 2% of patients; transient eosinophilia has also occurred.

The reviewers[1] suggested that all patients should have blood and platelet counts before treatment. Patients with low white cell and neutrophil counts were at risk of developing leucopenia and should be monitored every 2 weeks for the first 1 to 3 months. If counts fell further the dose should be reduced or treatment discontinued. It should be noted that the *British National Formulary* doubts the practical value of routine monitoring: in particular, aplastic anaemia, agranulocytosis, and thrombocytopenia have a rapid onset and are best monitored by instructing the patient to report warning symptoms (see Precautions, below).

For a discussion of the effects of antiepileptics, including carbamazepine, on serum folate, see Folic Acid Deficiency, under Phenytoin, p.370.

1. Sobotka JL, *et al.* A review of carbamazepine's hematologic reactions and monitoring recommendations. *DICP Ann Pharmacother* 1990; **24:** 1214–19.

**Effects on bone.** For the effects of antiepileptics including carbamazepine on bone and on calcium and vitamin D metabolism, see under Phenytoin, p.371.

**Effects on the endocrine system.** There have been a number of reports of *hyponatraemia* or *water intoxication* in patients receiving carbamazepine.[1-6] One review[7] states that although hyponatraemia occurs in 10 to 15% of patients taking carbamazepine, it is seldom symptomatic or severe enough to cause fluid retention. However, care should be taken to distinguish the confusion, dizziness, nausea and headache of water intoxication from the central and gastrointestinal effects of the drug.[2] The mechanism is uncertain; although some studies suggest an increase in secretion of antidiuretic hormone in subjects given carbamazepine,[3,4,6] others indicate the reverse,[5,8] and the fact that the hyponatraemic effects of carbamazepine can be partly reversed by demeclocycline[5] is cited as evidence for an effect on the kidney, either directly upon the distal tubule or by increasing sensitivity to the effects of antidiuretic hormone.

Carbamazepine may reduce serum concentrations of *thyroid* hormones through enzyme induction—see under Interactions of Levothyroxine, p.1601.

For mention of the effects of antiepileptics on *sexual function* in male epileptic patients, see under Phenytoin, p.371.

1. Henry DA, *et al.* Hyponatraemia during carbamazepine treatment. *BMJ* 1977; **1:** 83–4.
2. Stephens WP, *et al.* Water intoxication due to carbamazepine. *BMJ* 1977; **1:** 754–5.
3. Ashton MG, *et al.* Water intoxication associated with carbamazepine treatment. *BMJ* 1977; **1:** 1134–5.
4. Smith NJ, *et al.* Raised plasma arginine vasopressin concentration in carbamazepine-induced water intoxication. *BMJ* 1977; **2:** 804.
5. Ballardie FW, Mucklow JC. Partial reversal of carbamazepine-induced water intolerance by demeclocycline. *Br J Clin Pharmacol* 1984; **17:** 763–5.
6. Sørensen PS, Hammer M. Effects of long-term carbamazepine treatment on water metabolism and plasma vasopressin concentration. *Eur J Clin Pharmacol* 1984; **26:** 719–22.
7. Mucklow J. Selected side-effects 2: carbamazepine and hyponatraemia. *Prescribers' J* 1991; **31:** 61–4.
8. Stephens WP, *et al.* Plasma arginine vasopressin concentrations and antidiuretic action of carbamazepine. *BMJ* 1978; **1:** 1445–7.

**Effects on the eyes.** On rare occasions lenticular opacities have been associated with carbamazepine.[1] Retinotoxicity associated with long-term carbamazepine use has been reported[2] in 2 patients. Following discontinuation of the drug visual function and retinal morphological changes improved.

1. Anonymous. Adverse ocular effects of systemic drugs. *Med Lett Drugs Ther* 1976; **18:** 63–4.
2. Nielsen NV, Syversen K. Possible retinotoxic effect of carbamazepine. *Acta Ophthalmol (Copenh)* 1986; **64:** 287–90.

**Effects on the heart.** A review[1] of reports of cardiac effects associated with carbamazepine revealed that patients could be divided into 2 distinct groups based on their symptoms. One group consisted mainly of young patients with non life-threatening sinus tachycardia following carbamazepine overdosage while the other group was composed of older female patients with potentially life-threatening bradycardia or atrioventricular block associated with therapeutic or modestly raised blood concentrations of carbamazepine. However, there has been a report of fatal syncope, probably due to ventricular asystole, in a 20-year-old patient.[2] Carbamazepine should be avoided in patients who develop conduction abnormalities, or who have conditions such as myotonic dystrophy in which conduction abnormalities are likely.[1]

Elevation of ventricular and atrial stimulation thresholds was reported in a 59-year-old man with a permanent dual-chamber pacemaker, 5 days after starting carbamazepine for mania.[3]

For a report of carbamazepine producing fatal eosinophilic myocarditis, see under Hypersensitivity, below.

1. Kasarkis EJ, *et al.* Carbamazepine-induced cardiac dysfunction: characterization of two distinct clinical syndromes. *Arch Intern Med* 1992; **152:** 186–91.
2. Stone S, Lange LS. Syncope and sudden unexpected death attributed to carbamazepine in a 20-year-old epileptic. *J Neurol Neurosurg Psychiatry* 1986; **49:** 1460–1.
3. Ambrosi P, *et al.* Carbamazepine and pacing threshold. *Lancet* 1993; **342:** 365.

**Effects on the immune system.** A report of hypogammaglobulinaemia associated with carbamazepine.[1] The authors stated that this was a recognised but rare adverse effect of carbamazepine and noted that the UK Committee on Safety of Medicines had 9 reports on file of hypogammaglobulinaemia or gammaglobulin abnormalities related to the use of carbamazepine; there were also a few other reports in the literature.

1. Hayman G, Bansal A. Antibody deficiency associated with carbamazepine. *BMJ* 2002; **325:** 1213.

**Effects on the liver.** A report in 1990 commented that of 499 reports of unwanted effects of carbamazepine on the liver about half comprised only abnormal results from liver function tests;[1] however, deaths have occurred from liver failure[1,2] or hepatic necrosis.[3]

Hepatotoxicity may form part of the antiepileptic hypersensitivity syndrome reported with carbamazepine (see below).

1. Hadžić N, *et al.* Acute liver failure induced by carbamazepine. *Arch Dis Child* 1990; **65:** 315–17.
2. Zucker P, *et al.* Fatal carbamazepine hepatitis. *J Pediatr* 1977; **91:** 667–8.
3. Smith DW, *et al.* Fatal hepatic necrosis associated with multiple anticonvulsant therapy. *Aust N Z J Med* 1988; **18:** 575–81.

**Effects on mental function.** Carbamazepine therapy has been associated in a few patients with the development of acute psychotic and paranoid symptoms[1-3] and with phobias[2] and mood disturbances, including mania[4] and melancholia.[5] One case of acute paranoid psychosis was associated with the addition of carbamazepine to long-term sodium valproate therapy in a patient subsequently diagnosed as having a schizotypal personality.[3] The problems of antiepileptic therapy adversely affecting cognition are discussed on p.351.

1. Berger H. An unusual manifestation of Tegretol® (carbamazepine) toxicity. *Ann Intern Med* 1971; **74:** 449–50.
2. Mathew G. Psychiatric symptoms associated with carbamazepine. *BMJ* 1988; **296:** 1071.
3. McKee RJW, *et al.* Acute psychosis with carbamazepine and sodium valproate. *Lancet* 1989; **i:** 167.
4. Reiss AL, O'Donnell DJ. Carbamazepine-induced mania in two children: case report. *J Clin Psychiatry* 1984; **45:** 272–4.
5. Gardner DL, Cowdry RW. Development of melancholia during carbamazepine treatment in borderline personality disorder. *J Clin Psychopharmacol* 1986; **6:** 236–9.

**Effects on the nervous system.** ASEPTIC MENINGITIS. Aseptic meningitis has developed in a patient with Sjögren's syndrome given carbamazepine. It abated when the drug was withdrawn and symptoms recurred on rechallenge.[1] Aseptic meningitis has also been associated with carbamazepine in patients without Sjögren's syndrome.[2-4]

1. Hilton E, Stroh EM. Aseptic meningitis associated with administration of carbamazepine. *J Infect Dis* 1989; **159:** 363–4.
2. Simon LT, *et al.* Carbamazepine-induced aseptic meningitis. *Ann Intern Med* 1990; **112:** 627–8.
3. Hemet C, *et al.* Aseptic meningitis secondary to carbamazepine treatment of manic-depressive illness. *Am J Psychiatry* 1994; **151:** 1393.
4. Dang CT, Riley DK. Aseptic meningitis secondary to carbamazepine therapy. *Clin Infect Dis* 1996; **22:** 729–30.

EXTRAPYRAMIDAL EFFECTS. References to extrapyramidal effects associated with carbamazepine.

1. Schwartzman MJ, Leppik IE. Carbamazepine-induced dyskinesia and ophthalmoplegia. *Cleve Clin J Med* 1990; **57:** 367–72.
2. Soman P, *et al.* Dystonia—a rare manifestation of carbamazepine toxicity. *Postgrad Med J* 1994; **70:** 54–5.
3. Lee JW. Persistent dystonia associated with carbamazepine therapy: a case report. *N Z Med J* 1994; **107:** 360–1.
4. Stryjer R, *et al.* Segmental dystonia as the sole manifestation of carbamazepine toxicity. *Gen Hosp Psychiatry* 2002; **24:** 114–15.

**Effects on the skin.** Rashes occurring with carbamazepine may form part of an antiepileptic hypersensitivity syndrome (see below). In one report,[1] erythema multiforme followed substitution of a generic for a proprietary brand of carbamazepine. Skin lesions resolved when the patient stopped taking the generic formulation and did not recur when the proprietary brand was restarted. In another report, a 6-year-old boy developed Stevens-Johnson syndrome 5 weeks after carbamazepine was added to valproic acid, which he had been taking as sole antiepileptic therapy for several weeks.[2] Carbamazepine was discontinued and the patient eventually made a full recovery; valproic acid was continued because it was not thought to be the causative agent (but see under Valproate, p.381).

1. Busch RL. Generic carbamazepine and erythema multiforme: generic-drug nonequivalency. *N Engl J Med* 1989; **321:** 692–3.
2. Keating A, Blahunka P. Carbamazepine-induced Stevens-Johnson syndrome in a child. *Ann Pharmacother* 1995; **29:** 538–9.

**Hypersensitivity.** An antiepileptic hypersensitivity syndrome, comprising fever, rash, and lymphadenopathy and less commonly hepatosplenomegaly and eosinophilia, has been associated with some antiepileptic drugs including carbamazepine.[1-3] Although a literature search[1] was only able to find 20 published cases to 1986, 22 cases had been reported to the Australian Adverse Drug Reactions Advisory Committee between 1975 and 1990. Some have estimated the incidence at 1 in 1000 to 1 in 10 000 new exposures to aromatic anticonvulsants,[2,3] but the true incidence is uncertain due to variations in presentation and reporting. Most reactions occurred within 30 days of the start of carbamazepine administration,[1] although symptoms may occur anywhere between 1 and 8 weeks after exposure.[2] In previously sensitised individuals the reactions may occur within 1 day of rechallenge. The potential for cross-reactivity between carbamazepine, phenobarbital, and phenytoin is approximately 75%, and patients who develop the syndrome, and their close relatives, should be warned of the risk associated with use of these antiepileptics.[2]

Carbamazepine antibodies were detected in an 8-year-old child who developed symptoms of serum sickness including fever, skin rash, oedema, and lymphadenopathy during treatment with carbamazepine.[4] Hypersensitivity to carbamazepine with multisystem effects clinically resembling a mononucleosis syndrome was reported in a 15-year-old boy 2 weeks after starting monotherapy with carbamazepine.[5] All symptoms resolved after discontinuation of carbamazepine and treatment with prednisone.

A hypersensitivity reaction producing fatal eosinophilic myocarditis has been reported in a 13-year-old patient; initial symptoms mimicked scarlet fever.[6]

Generalised erythroderma with renal, hepatic, and bone-marrow failure (characterised by hypercellularity and dyserythropoiesis) has been reported[7] in an 81-year-old man 50 days after starting carbamazepine therapy. Symptoms recurred following an inadvertent rechallenge. The presence of underlying lymphoproliferative disease may have potentiated the severe drug-induced reaction.

If the antiepileptic hypersensitivity syndrome develops, immediate withdrawal of carbamazepine is recommended. In most cases this is all that is required and does not seem to precipitate an increase in seizures, compared with gradual withdrawal.[8]

Successful desensitisation to carbamazepine was reported[9] in a 12-year-old boy who was sensitive to carbamazepine, sodium valproate, and phenytoin. Starting with a low dose of carbamazepine 0.1 mg daily the dose was doubled, generally every 2 days, up to 100 mg daily. The dose was then gradually increased over 4 weeks to a maintenance dose of 200 mg twice daily. The same technique was used to desensitise 7 patients, all of whom developed dramatic skin rashes when first exposed to carbamazepine.[10] Carbamazepine therapy in full doses was achieved without problem in about 6 weeks. Some[11] consider that desensitisation is not to be recommended in patients with full-blown antiepileptic hypersensitivity syndrome.

1. Anonymous. Anticonvulsants and lymphadenopathy. *WHO Drug Inf* 1991; **5:** 11.
2. Knowles SR, *et al.* Anticonvulsant hypersensitivity syndrome: incidence, prevention and management. *Drug Safety* 1999; **21:** 489–501.
3. Bessmertny O, *et al.* Antiepileptic hypersensitivity syndrome in children. *Ann Pharmacother* 2001; **35:** 533–8.
4. Hosoda N, *et al.* Anticarbamazepine antibody induced by carbamazepine in a patient with severe serum sickness. *Arch Dis Child* 1991; **66:** 722–3.
5. Merino N, *et al.* Multisystem hypersensitivity reaction to carbamazepine. *Ann Pharmacother* 1994; **28:** 402–3.
6. Salzman MB, *et al.* Carbamazepine and fatal eosinophilic myocarditis. *N Engl J Med* 1997; **336:** 878–9.
7. Lombardi SM, *et al.* Severe multisystemic hypersensitivity reaction to carbamazepine including dyserythropoietic anemia. *Ann Pharmacother* 1999; **33:** 571–5.
8. Pirmohamed M, *et al.* Hypersensitivity to carbamazepine and lamotrigine: clinical considerations. *Br J Clin Pharmacol* 2000; **49:** 519P–520P.
9. Smith H, Newton R. Adverse reactions to carbamazepine managed by desensitisation. *Lancet* 1985; **i:** 753.
10. Eames P. Adverse reactions to carbamazepine managed by desensitisation. *Lancet* 1989; **i:** 509–10.
11. Knowles SR, *et al.* Anticonvulsant hypersensitivity syndrome: incidence, prevention and management. *Drug Safety* 1999; **21:** 489–501.

**Sudden unexplained death in epilepsy.** Sudden unexplained death in epilepsy (SUDEP) is a common cause of seizure-related mortality in patients with chronic epilepsy. Risk factors may include early onset of epilepsy, frequent generalised tonic-clonic seizures, intractability, and polytherapy. *Carbamazepine* use has also been implicated but the evidence is insufficient to recommend one antiepileptic regimen over another.[1] Although the FDA in the USA had required data about the specific risk of SUDEP to be included in the prescribing information for the newer antiepileptic drugs *gabapentin, lamotrigine, tiagabine, topiramate,* and *zonisamide*, some commentators[2] consider that none of these antiepileptics have shown an associated change in the risk of SUDEP. It was mooted that the incidence of SUDEP was related to the disease rather than a specific drug effect.

1. Pedley TA, Hauser WA. Sudden death in epilepsy: a wake-up call for management. *Lancet* 2002; **359:** 1790–1.
2. Lathers CM, Schraeder PL. Clinical pharmacology: drugs as a benefit and/or risk in sudden unexpected death in epilepsy? *J Clin Pharmacol* 2002; **42:** 123–36.

**Systemic lupus erythematosus.** A review[1] of 80 cases of systemic lupus erythematosus-like syndromes associated with carbamazepine that had been reported to the manufacturer suggested that the frequency of reports (less than 0.001%) was below that for idiopathic lupus. The symptoms due to carbamazepine usually resolved on discontinuation of treatment.

1. Jain KK. Systemic lupus erythematosus (SLE)-like syndromes associated with carbamazepine therapy. *Drug Safety* 1991; **6:** 350–60.

## Treatment of Adverse Effects

In the treatment of carbamazepine overdosage repeated doses of activated charcoal may be given by mouth to adults and children who have ingested more than 20 mg/kg; the aim is not only to prevent absorption but also to aid elimination. Gastric lavage may be considered if undertaken within 1 hour of ingestion. Supportive and symptomatic therapy alone may then suffice, with particular attention to correcting hypoxia and hypotension; haemoperfusion has been suggested for severe poisoning (see Overdosage, below).

**Hypersensitivity reactions.** For reference to successful desensitisation in patients sensitive to carbamazepine, see Hypersensitivity under Adverse Effects, above.

**Overdosage.** Carbamazepine poisoning and its management has been reviewed.[1] Management is primarily supportive, with prompt attention to airway management and seizure control. Activated charcoal should be given; although multiple dose activated charcoal has been recommended for carbamazepine overdosage, care must be taken to protect the airway since carbamazepine inhibits intestinal motility and there is a significant risk of aspiration. In patients with seizures unresponsive to benzodiazepines phenobarbital should be used; phenytoin is not a drug of choice in this situation. Hypotension is rare, and should be managed with fluid and vasopressor support; the combination of hypotension and refractory seizures should be treated aggressively as it has led to permanent neurological disability and death.

Haemodialysis or haemoperfusion may be warranted in patients with unstable cardiac status or status epilepticus complicated by bowel hypomotility and unresponsive to more conventional therapy. However, a report[2] of the use of plasmapheresis in the treatment of an acute overdose of carbamazepine concluded that plasmapheresis removed a very small percentage of the total body load of carbamazepine and could not be recommended.

For a further review of the features and management of poisoning with some antiepileptics, including carbamazepine, see under Phenytoin, p.371.

1. Spiller HA. Management of carbamazepine overdose. *Pediatr Emerg Care* 2001; **17:** 452–6.
2. Kale PB, *et al.* Evaluation of plasmapheresis in the treatment of an acute overdose of carbamazepine. *Ann Pharmacother* 1993; **27:** 866–70.

## Precautions

Carbamazepine should be avoided in patients with atrioventricular conduction abnormalities. It should not be given to patients with a history of bone marrow depression. Carbamazepine should be given with caution to patients with a history of blood disorders or haematological reactions to other drugs, or of cardiac, hepatic, or renal disease. Patients or their carers should be told how to recognise signs of blood, liver, and skin toxicity and they should be advised to seek immediate medical attention if symptoms such as fever, sore throat, rash, mouth ulcers, bruising, or bleeding develop. Carbamazepine should be withdrawn, if necessary under cover of a suitable alternative antiepileptic, if leucopenia which is severe, progressive, or associated with clinical symptoms develops. The manufacturers recommend blood counts and hepatic and renal-function tests before starting carbamazepine therapy and periodically during treatment, but the *British National Formulary* considers the evidence of practical value unsatisfactory. Clinical monitoring is of primary importance throughout treatment.

Care is required in identifying patients with mixed seizure disorders that include generalised absence or atypical absence seizures, who may be at risk of an increase in generalised seizures if given carbamazepine. Carbamazepine may also exacerbate absence and myoclonic seizures.

Care is required when withdrawing carbamazepine therapy—see also under Uses and Administration, below.

Since carbamazepine has mild antimuscarinic properties caution should be observed in patients with glaucoma or raised intra-ocular pressure; scattered punctate lens opacities occur rarely with carbamazepine and it has been suggested that patients should be examined periodically for eye changes.

**Abuse.** Overdosage requiring hospital admission has been reported following abuse of carbamazepine.[1]

1. Crawford PJ, Fisher BM. Recreational overdosage of carbamazepine in Paisley drug abusers. *Scott Med J* 1997; **42:** 44–5.

**Breast feeding.** No adverse effects have been seen in breast-fed infants whose mothers were receiving carbamazepine, and the American Academy of Pediatrics considers[1] that it is therefore usually compatible with breast feeding.

For further comment on antiepileptic therapy and breast feeding, see p.351.

1. American Academy of Pediatrics. The transfer of drugs and other chemicals into human milk. *Pediatrics* 2001; **108:** 776–89. Correction. *ibid.*; 1029. Also available at: http://aappolicy.aappublications.org/cgi/content/full/pediatrics%3b108/3/776 (accessed 13/05/04)

**Driving.** For comment on antiepileptic drugs and driving, see p.351.

**Multiple sclerosis.** Exacerbation of symptoms of multiple sclerosis has been reported[1] in 5 patients following initiation of carbamazepine therapy for paroxysmal neurological symptoms and pain. There was a close temporal association between starting carbamazepine and worsening of symptoms, followed by resolution when it was discontinued.

1. Ramsaransing G, *et al.* Worsening of symptoms of multiple sclerosis associated with carbamazepine. *BMJ* 2000; **320:** 1113.

**Porphyria.** Carbamazepine has been associated with acute attacks of porphyria and is considered unsafe in porphyric patients.

**Pregnancy.** For comments on the management of epilepsy during pregnancy, see p.351.

There is an increased risk of neural tube defects in infants exposed *in utero* to antiepileptics including carbamazepine and a variety of syndromes such as craniofacial and digital abnormalities and, less commonly, cleft lip and palate have been described. Exposure to carbamazepine has been calculated to carry a 1% risk of spina bifida.[1] A 'carbamazepine syndrome' characterised by facial dysmorphic features and mild mental retardation has been described.[2] There is also a risk of neonatal bleeding.

1. Rosa FW. Spina bifida in infants of women treated with carbamazepine during pregnancy. *N Engl J Med* 1991; **324:** 674–7.
2. Ornoy A, Cohen E. Outcome of children born to epileptic mothers treated with carbamazepine during pregnancy. *Arch Dis Child* 1996; **75:** 517–20.

## Interactions

There are complex interactions between antiepileptics and toxicity may be enhanced without a corresponding increase in antiepileptic activity. Such interactions are very variable and unpredictable and plasma monitoring is often advisable with combination therapy.

The metabolism of carbamazepine is reported to be less susceptible to inhibition by other drugs than that of phenytoin but a few drugs are reported to inhibit its metabolism by the cytochrome P450 isoenzyme CYP3A4, resulting in raised plasma concentrations and associated toxicity. Conversely, drugs that induce CYP3A4 may increase the metabolism of carbamazepine, leading to reduced plasma concentrations and potentially a decrease in therapeutic effect. The manufacturers advise that, in such situations, the dose of carbamazepine should be adjusted accordingly and/or the plasma concentrations monitored.

Carbamazepine is itself a hepatic enzyme inducer, and induces its own metabolism as well as that of a number of other drugs including some antibacterials (notably, doxycycline), anticoagulants, and sex hormones (notably, oral contraceptives). Carbamazepine and phenytoin may also mutually enhance one another's metabolism. The metabolism of carbamazepine is similarly enhanced by enzyme inducers such as phenobarbital.

◊ General references.

1. Spina E, *et al.* Clinically significant pharmacokinetic drug interactions with carbamazepine: an update. *Clin Pharmacokinet* 1996; **31:** 198–214.

**Alcohol.** Alcohol may exacerbate the CNS side-effects of carbamazepine.

**Analgesics.** *Dextropropoxyphene* has been reported to cause substantial elevation of serum-carbamazepine concentrations[1] and carbamazepine toxicity,[1,2] probably due to inhibition of carbamazepine metabolism.[1]

The concurrent use of enzyme-inducing antiepileptics such as carbamazepine affects the administration of antidote in the treatment of *paracetamol* poisoning, see p.78.

For the effect of carbamazepine on *tramadol*, see p.95.

1. Dam M, Christiansen J. Interaction of propoxyphene with carbamazepine. *Lancet* 1977; **ii:** 509.
2. Yu YL, *et al.* Interaction between carbamazepine and dextropropoxyphene. *Postgrad Med J* 1986; **62:** 231–3.

**Anthelmintics.** For the effect of carbamazepine on *mebendazole* and *praziquantel*, see p.108 and p.112, respectively.

**Antibacterials.** The antimycobacterial *isoniazid*[1,2] and macrolides such as *troleandomycin*[3,4] and *erythromycin*[4-7] have been reported to cause substantial elevations of serum concentrations of carbamazepine and symptoms of carbamazepine toxicity.[1-4,6,7] *Clarithromycin* has also been reported to increase serum concentrations of carbamazepine.[8]

Carbamazepine may enhance the metabolism of *doxycycline*.[9]

Use of carbamazepine with isoniazid may increase the risk of isoniazid-induced hepatotoxicity.

1. Valsalan VC, Cooper GL. Carbamazepine intoxication caused by interaction with isoniazid. *BMJ* 1982; **285:** 261–2.
2. Wright JM, *et al.* Isoniazid-induced carbamazepine toxicity and vice versa. *N Engl J Med* 1982; **307:** 1325–7.
3. Dravet C, *et al.* Interaction between carbamazepine and triacetyloleandomycin. *Lancet* 1977; **i:** 810–11.
4. Mesdjian E, *et al.* Carbamazepine intoxication due to triacetyloleandomycin administration in epileptic patients. *Epilepsia* 1980; **21:** 489–96.
5. Wong YY, *et al.* Effect of erythromycin on carbamazepine kinetics. *Clin Pharmacol Ther* 1983; **33:** 460–4.
6. Hedrick R, *et al.* Carbamazepine-erythromycin interaction leading to carbamazepine toxicity in four epileptic children. *Ther Drug Monit* 1983; **5:** 405–7.
7. Mitsch RA. Carbamazepine toxicity precipitated by intravenous erythromycin. *Drug Intell Clin Pharm* 1989; **23:** 878–9.
8. Albani F, *et al.* Clarithromycin-carbamazepine interaction: a case report. *Epilepsia* 1993; **34:** 161–2.
9. Neuvonen PJ, *et al.* Effect of antiepileptic drugs on the elimination of various tetracycline derivatives. *Eur J Clin Pharmacol* 1975; **9:** 147–54.

**Anticoagulants.** For the effect of carbamazepine on *warfarin*, see p.1025.

**Antidepressants.** As with all antiepileptics, antidepressants may antagonise the antiepileptic activity of carbamazepine by lowering the convulsive threshold.

Antidepressants such as *desipramine*,[10] *fluoxetine*,[1] *fluvoxamine*,[2] *nefazodone*[3] (and perhaps *trazodone*[4]), and *viloxazine*[5] increase plasma concentrations of carbamazepine and may induce carbamazepine toxicity. A toxic serotonin syndrome (see p.313) has been reported in a patient who received fluoxetine with carbamazepine.[6] Severe neurotoxicity reported during therapy with *lithium* and carbamazepine[7,8] may be due to a synergistic effect as reports indicate that either drug was tolerated when not administered with the other and measured plasma concentrations did not indicate overdosage.[8] However, toxic serum concentrations of lithium have also been reported, due to carbamazepine-induced acute renal failure (see p.303).

Because of the structural similarity to tricyclic antidepressants the manufacturers have suggested that carbamazepine should not be given to patients taking an *MAOI* or within 14 days of stopping such treatment.

*Hypericum* has been shown to induce several drug metabolising enzymes (see p.299) and consequently it might reduce the blood concentrations of carbamazepine leading to an increased risk of seizure.[9]

For the effect of carbamazepine on antidepressants, see Bupropion (p.288), Mianserin (p.307), Fluoxetine (p.296), and Amitriptyline (p.284).

1. Pearson HJ. Interaction of fluoxetine with carbamazepine. *J Clin Psychiatry* 1990; **51:** 126.
2. Fritze J, *et al.* Interaction between carbamazepine and fluvoxamine. *Acta Psychiatr Scand* 1991; **84:** 583–4.
3. Ashton AK, Wolin RE. Nefazodone-induced carbamazepine toxicity. *Am J Psychiatry* 1996; **153:** 733.
4. Sánchez Romero A, *et al.* Interaction between trazodone and carbamazepine. *Ann Pharmacother* 1999; **33:** 1370.
5. Scarpello JHB, Cottrell N. Overuse of monitoring of blood concentrations of antiepileptic drugs. *BMJ* 1987; **294:** 1355.
6. Dursun SM, *et al.* Toxic serotonin syndrome after fluoxetine plus carbamazepine. *Lancet* 1993; **342:** 442–3.
7. Andrus PF. Lithium and carbamazepine. *J Clin Psychiatry* 1984; **45:** 525.
8. Chaudhry RP, Waters BGH. Lithium and carbamazepine interaction: possible neurotoxicity. *J Clin Psychiatry* 1983; **44:** 30–1.
9. Committee on Safety of Medicines/Medicines Control Agency. Reminder: St John's wort (Hypericum perforatum) interactions. *Current Problems* 2000; **26:** 6–7. Also available at: http://www.mca.gov.uk/ourwork/monitorsafequalmed/currentproblems/cpmay2000.pdf (accessed 13/05/04)
10. Lesser I. Carbamazepine and desipramine: a toxic reaction. *J Clin Psychiatry* 1984; **45:** 360.

**Antiepileptics.** Interactions of varying degrees of clinical significance have been reported between carbamazepine and other antiepileptics.

Serum concentrations of carbamazepine are reported to be reduced by *phenobarbital*, but without loss of seizure control;[1,2] this reduction is probably due to induction of carbamazepine metabolism.

The interaction with *phenytoin* is somewhat more complex and the consequences vary. There is evidence of a lowering of serum-carbamazepine concentrations, presumably due to induction of metabolism by phenytoin;[1-3] in return carbamazepine has been reported both to lower and increase serum phenytoin—see p.373. Again, these reports do not indicate a loss of seizure control or toxicity resulting from the interaction, although the possibility presumably exists. Gradually withdrawing phenytoin from 2 patients who had been receiving carbamazepine and phenytoin resulted in a dramatic increase in plasma-carbamazepine concentrations;[4] one patient exhibited neurotoxic symptoms. The authors recommended that plasma-carbamazepine monitoring should be carried out whenever phenytoin is discontinued in patients receiving these two drugs together.

*Valproic acid* produces an increase in serum concentrations of the active epoxide metabolite of carbamazepine. This is usually attributed to inhibition of its hydrolysis by epoxide hydrolase, although an additional proposed mechanism[5] is inhibition of the glucuronidation of carbamazepine-10,11-trans-diol, the compound to which the epoxide is converted under normal circumstances. Adverse effects may be a problem if unusually high epoxide concentrations arise but, in general, this interaction is of limited clinical significance. However, *valpromide*, the amide derivative, is a much more powerful inhibitor of epoxide hydrolase than valproic acid,[6-8] and therefore produces greater increases in epoxide plasma concentrations with clinical signs of toxicity.[7] Switching from sodium valproate to valpromide has resulted in toxicity in patients also receiving carbamazepine.[7] Neither valproic acid nor valpromide have any significant effect on plasma concentrations of the parent drug, carbamazepine. *Valnoctamide*, an isomer of valpromide, appears to be at least as potent as valpromide in inhibiting the elimination of the epoxide metabolite of carbamazepine.[9] Valnoctamide has been used as an anxiolytic, although it does appear to possess some antiepileptic activity. For a report of acute psychosis associated with the combination of carbamazepine and sodium valproate, see Effects on Mental Function under Adverse Effects, above. For the effects of carbamazepine on valproate, see p.381.

Of the other antiepileptics *stiripentol*[10] has been reported to inhibit carbamazepine metabolism, while *felbamate* causes a significant fall in plasma-carbamazepine concentrations which may require an increase in the dose of carbamazepine.[11] However, another study[12] has shown a significant increase in plasma-concentrations of the active epoxide metabolite, which may counteract the effect of the decrease in plasma concentrations of the parent compound. Neurotoxicity has been observed following use of carbamazepine with *lamotrigine*.[13] The suggestion that this was due to raised concentrations of carbamazepine epoxide was not confirmed in a controlled study in which the 2 drugs were used together safely and effectively.[14] *Progabide* has been reported to increase plasma concentrations of the epoxide metabolite, probably due to inhibition of microsomal epoxide hydrolase.[15] For the effects of carbamazepine on *clonazepam*, see p.359, on *ethosuximide*, see p.360, on *lamotrigine*, see p.364, on *oxcarbazepine*, see p.367, on *primidone*, see p.377, on *tiagabine*, see p.378, and on *topiramate*, see p.379.

For interactions with benzodiazepines, see below.

1. Cereghino JJ, *et al.* The efficacy of carbamazepine combinations in epilepsy. *Clin Pharmacol Ther* 1975; **18:** 733–41.
2. Rane A, *et al.* Kinetics of carbamazepine and its 10,11-epoxide metabolite in children. *Clin Pharmacol Ther* 1976; **19:** 276–83.
3. Christiansen J, Dam M. Influence of phenobarbital and diphenylhydantoin on plasma carbamazepine levels in patients with epilepsy. *Acta Neurol Scand* 1973; **49:** 543–6.
4. Chapron DJ, *et al.* Unmasking the significant enzyme-inducing effects of phenytoin on serum carbamazepine concentrations during phenytoin withdrawal. *Ann Pharmacother* 1993; **27:** 708–11.
5. Bernus I, *et al.* The mechanism of the carbamazepine-valproate interaction in humans. *Br J Clin Pharmacol* 1997; **44:** 21–7.
6. Levy RH, *et al.* Inhibition of carbamazepine epoxide elimination by valpromide and valproic acid. *Epilepsia* 1986; **27:** 592.
7. Meijer JWA, *et al.* Possible hazard of valpromide-carbamazepine combination therapy in epilepsy. *Lancet* 1984; **i:** 802.
8. Pisani F, *et al.* Effect of valpromide on the pharmacokinetics of carbamazepine-10,11-epoxide. *Br J Clin Pharmacol* 1988; **25:** 611–13.
9. Pisani F, *et al.* Impairment of carbamazepine-10,11-epoxide elimination by valnoctamide, a valpromide isomer, in healthy subjects. *Br J Clin Pharmacol* 1992; **34:** 85–7.
10. Levy RH, *et al.* Stiripentol level-dose relationship and interaction with carbamazepine in epileptic patients. *Epilepsia* 1985; **26:** 544–5.
11. Albani F, *et al.* Effect of felbamate on plasma levels of carbamazepine and its metabolites. *Epilepsia* 1991; **32:** 130–2.
12. Wagner ML, *et al.* Effect of felbamate on carbamazepine and its major metabolites. *Clin Pharmacol Ther* 1993; **53:** 536–43.
13. Warner T, *et al.* Lamotrigine-induced carbamazepine toxicity: an interaction with carbamazepine-10,11-epoxide. *Epilepsy Res* 1992; **11:** 147–50.
14. Stolarek I, *et al.* Vigabatrin and lamotrigine in refractory epilepsy. *J Neurol Neurosurg Psychiatry* 1994; **57:** 921–4.
15. Kroetz DL, *et al.* In vivo and in vitro correlation of microsomal epoxide hydrolase inhibition by progabide. *Clin Pharmacol Ther* 1993; **54:** 485–97.

**Antifungals.** Malaise, myoclonus, and trembling are reported[1] to have developed in a patient receiving carbamazepine following the addition of *miconazole* to therapy. *Ketoconazole* was associated with a significant increase in plasma-carbamazepine concentrations in 8 epileptic patients stabilised on carbamazepine;[2] plasma concentrations of the epoxide metabolite were unchanged.

For the effect of carbamazepine on *itraconazole*, see p.402.

1. Loupi E, *et al.* Interactions médicamenteuses et miconazole. *Therapie* 1982; **37:** 437–41.
2. Spina E, *et al.* Elevation of plasma carbamazepine concentrations by ketoconazole in patients with epilepsy. *Ther Drug Monit* 1997; **19:** 535–8.

**Antihistamines.** *Terfenadine* and carbamazepine are both highly protein bound and therefore may compete for protein binding sites. An 18-year-old woman receiving carbamazepine as an antiepileptic experienced symptoms of neurotoxicity shortly after starting treatment with terfenadine for rhinitis.[1] The concentration of free carbamazepine in the plasma was higher than normal and returned to normal on discontinuation of terfenadine.

1. Hirschfeld S, Jarosinski P. Drug interaction of terfenadine and carbamazepine. *Ann Intern Med* 1993; **118:** 907–8.

**Antimalarials.** *Chloroquine* and *mefloquine* may antagonise the antiepileptic activity of carbamazepine by lowering the convulsive threshold.

**Antiprotozoals.** A patient receiving carbamazepine for bipolar disorder developed dizziness, diplopia, and nausea 4 days after the addition of *metronidazole* for diverticulitis.[1]

1. Patterson BD. Possible interaction between metronidazole and carbamazepine. *Ann Pharmacother* 1994; **28:** 1303–4.

**Antipsychotics.** As with all antiepileptics, antipsychotics may antagonise the antiepileptic activity of carbamazepine by lowering the convulsive threshold. Increased plasma concentrations of carbamazepine epoxide have been reported to occur during therapy with carbamazepine and *loxapine*, possibly due to induction of carbamazepine metabolism or inhibition of metabolism of the epoxide.[1] Raised serum concentrations of carbamazepine have also been reported in patients receiving *haloperidol*.[2] For the effect of carbamazepine on antipsychotics, see under Chlorpromazine, p.679.

1. Collins DM, *et al.* Potential interaction between carbamazepine and loxapine: case report and retrospective review. *Ann Pharmacother* 1993; **27:** 1180–3.
2. Iwahashi K, *et al.* The drug-drug interaction effects of haloperidol on plasma carbamazepine levels. *Clin Neuropharmacol* 1995; **18:** 233–6.

**Antivirals.** *Ritonavir* inhibits several microsomal liver enzymes and therefore may potentially increase plasma concentrations of carbamazepine. The manufacturer of ritonavir advises that such combinations may require monitoring or should be avoided. Carbamazepine toxicity has been reported[1] in a patient following a severe interaction with ritonavir.

For the effect of carbamazepine on HIV-protease inhibitors, see p.639.

1. Mateu-de Antonio J, Grau S. Ritonavir-induced carbamazepine toxicity. *Ann Pharmacother* 2001; **35:** 125–6.

**Anxiolytics.** For a discussion of the potential interaction between carbamazepine and the anxiolytic *valnoctamide*, an isomer of the antiepileptic valpromide, see under Antiepileptics, above.

See also under Benzodiazepines, below.

**Benzodiazepines.** The metabolism of benzodiazepines may be enhanced due to induction of hepatic drug-metabolising enzymes in patients who have received long-term therapy with carbamazepine; benzodiazepine plasma concentrations are reduced, half-life is shorter, and clearance is increased.[1,2] Some benzodiazepines may also affect carbamazepine. One group of workers reported that after addition of *clobazam* to carbamazepine therapy a dose reduction for the latter was required due to increased blood concentrations.[3] In a later study[4] it appeared that clobazam could produce a moderate increase in the metabolism of carbamazepine. The plasma ratio of metabolites of carbamazepine, including carbamazepine-10,11-epoxide, to parent compound was increased in patients taking clobazam and carbamazepine.

1. Dhillon S, Richens A. Pharmacokinetics of diazepam in epileptic patients and normal volunteers following intravenous administration. *Br J Clin Pharmacol* 1981; **12:** 841–4.
2. Lai AA, *et al.* Time-course of interaction between carbamazepine and clonazepam in normal man. *Clin Pharmacol Ther* 1978; **24:** 316–23.
3. Franceschi M, *et al.* Clobazam in drug-resistant and alcoholic withdrawal seizures. *Clin Trials J* 1983; **20:** 119–25.
4. Muñoz JJ, *et al.* The effect of clobazam on steady state plasma concentrations of carbamazepine and its metabolites. *Br J Clin Pharmacol* 1990; **29:** 763–5.

**Calcium-channel blockers.** Six patients with steady-state carbamazepine concentrations experienced symptoms of neurotoxicity consistent with carbamazepine intoxication within 36 to 96 hours of the first dose of *verapamil*.[1] In 5 patients, in whom plasma concentrations were measured, there was a mean increase of 46% in total carbamazepine and 33% in free carbamazepine; no effect on the plasma protein binding of carbamazepine was observed. The results suggested that verapamil inhibits the metabolism of carbamazepine to an extent likely to have important clinical repercussions. There has also been a report[2] of a patient in whom *diltiazem*, but not *nifedipine*, precipitated carbamazepine neurotoxicity.

For the effect of carbamazepine on dihydropyridine calcium-channel blockers, see under Nifedipine, p.969.

1. Macphee GJA, *et al.* Verapamil potentiates carbamazepine neurotoxicity: a clinically important inhibitory interaction. *Lancet* 1986; **i:** 700–703.
2. Brodie MJ, Macphee GJA. Carbamazepine neurotoxicity precipitated by diltiazem. *BMJ* 1986; **292:** 1170–1.

**Ciclosporin.** For the effect of carbamazepine on ciclosporin, see p.1355.

**Corticosteroids.** For the effect of carbamazepine on corticosteroids, see p.1072.

**Danazol.** Co-administration of *danazol* with carbamazepine has been reported to increase the half-life and decrease clearance of carbamazepine,[1] resulting in increases in plasma-carbamazepine concentrations of up to 100%[1,2] and resultant toxicity in a number of patients.[2]

1. Krämer G, *et al.* Carbamazepine-danazol drug interaction: its mechanism examined by a stable isotope technique. *Ther Drug Monit* 1986; **8:** 387–92.
2. Zielinski JJ, *et al.* Clinically significant danazol-carbamazepine interaction. *Ther Drug Monit* 1987; **9:** 24–7.

**Dermatological drugs.** In a patient stabilised on carbamazepine therapy addition of *isotretinoin* appeared to reduce plasma concentrations of carbamazepine and its active epoxide metabolite.[1] However, no adverse events were noted during a 6-week period of treatment with isotretinoin. Nonetheless, the manufacturers of carbamazepine recommend that the levels of carbamazepine are monitored during concomitant therapy.

1. Marsden JR. Effect of isotretinoin on carbamazepine pharmacokinetics. *Br J Dermatol* 1988; **119:** 403–4.

**Diuretics.** There has been a report of symptomatic hyponatraemia associated with use of carbamazepine and a diuretic (*hydrochlorothiazide* or *furosemide*—see under Interactions in Furosemide, p.920). Carbamazepine serum concentrations are increased by *acetazolamide*.[1]

1. McBride MC. Serum carbamazepine levels are increased by acetazolamide. *Ann Neurol* 1984; **16:** 393.

**Gastrointestinal drugs.** *Cimetidine* is reported to produce a transient increase in plasma-carbamazepine concentrations, followed by a return to pre-cimetidine values within about a week;[1] some increase in side-effects was seen. *Ranitidine* does not appear to affect plasma-carbamazepine concentrations.[2] Neurotoxicity has been observed in a patient receiving carbamazepine and *metoclopramide*.[3]

1. Dalton MJ, *et al.* Cimetidine and carbamazepine: a complex drug interaction. *Epilepsia* 1986; **27:** 553–8.

2. Dalton MJ, *et al.* Ranitidine does not alter single-dose carbamazepine pharmacokinetics in healthy adults. *Drug Intell Clin Pharm* 1985; **19:** 941–4.
3. Sandyk R. Carbamazepine and metoclopramide interaction: possible neurotoxicity. *BMJ* 1984; **288:** 830.

**Grapefruit juice.** The bioavailability and plasma concentrations of carbamazepine have been reported[1] to be increased by grapefruit juice.

1. Garg SK, *et al.* Effect of grapefruit juice on carbamazepine bioavailability in patients with epilepsy. *Clin Pharmacol Ther* 1998; **64:** 286–8.

**Levothyroxine.** For the effect of carbamazepine on levothyroxine, see p.1601.

**Neuromuscular blockers.** For the effect of carbamazepine on *suxamethonium*, see p.1408 and on *competitive neuromuscular blockers*, see under Atracurium, p.1400.

**Sex hormones.** For the effect of carbamazepine on *oral contraceptives*, see p.1534 and for the possible effect on *tibolone*, see p.1573.

**Theophylline.** A decrease in serum-carbamazepine concentrations of about 50% was reported[1] in an epileptic patient given theophylline. The patient experienced seizures and the proposed mechanism was that theophylline had increased the metabolism of carbamazepine.

For the effect of carbamazepine on theophylline, see p.802.

1. Mitchell EA, *et al.* Interaction between carbamazepine and theophylline. *N Z Med J* 1986; **99:** 69–70.

**Vitamins.** The plasma concentration of carbamazepine was increased in 2 patients given *nicotinamide*.[1] For the effect of antiepileptics, including carbamazepine, on *vitamin D* concentrations, see Effects on Bone under the Adverse Effects of Phenytoin, p.371.

1. Bourgeois BFD, *et al.* Interactions between primidone, carbamazepine, and nicotinamide. *Neurology* 1982; **32:** 1122–6.

## Pharmacokinetics

Carbamazepine is slowly and irregularly absorbed from the gastrointestinal tract. It is extensively metabolised in the liver, notably by the cytochrome P450 isoenzymes CYP3A4 and CYP2C8. One of its primary metabolites, carbamazepine-10,11-epoxide is also active. Carbamazepine is excreted in the urine almost entirely in the form of its metabolites; some is also excreted in faeces. Elimination of carbamazepine is reported to be more rapid in children and accumulation of the active metabolite may often be higher than in adults.

Carbamazepine is widely distributed throughout the body and is about 75% bound to plasma proteins. It induces its own metabolism so that the plasma half-life may be considerably reduced after repeated administration. The mean plasma half-life of carbamazepine on repeated administration is about 5 to 26 hours; it appears to be considerably shorter in children than in adults. Moreover, the metabolism of carbamazepine is readily induced by drugs which induce hepatic microsomal enzymes (see under Interactions, above).

Monitoring of plasma concentrations may be performed as an aid in assessing control and the therapeutic range of total plasma-carbamazepine is usually quoted as being about 4 to 12 micrograms/mL (17 to 50 micromoles/litre), although this is subject to considerable variation. It has been suggested by some, but not all investigators, that measurement of free carbamazepine concentrations in plasma may prove more reliable, and measurement of concentrations in saliva or tears, which contain only free carbamazepine, has also been performed.

Carbamazepine crosses the placental barrier and is distributed into breast milk.

The pharmacokinetics of carbamazepine are affected by the concomitant administration of other antiepileptics (see under Interactions, above).

◊ References.

1. Schmidt D, Haenel F. Therapeutic plasma levels of phenytoin, phenobarbital, and carbamazepine: individual variation in relation to seizure frequency and type. *Neurology* 1984; **34:** 1252–5.
2. Bertilsson L, Tomson T. Clinical pharmacokinetics and pharmacological effects of carbamazepine and carbamazepine-10,11-epoxide: an update. *Clin Pharmacokinet* 1986; **11:** 177–98.
3. Gilman JT. Carbamazepine dosing for pediatric seizure disorders: the highs and lows. *DICP Ann Pharmacother* 1991; **25:** 1109–12.
4. Kodama Y, *et al.* In vivo binding characteristics of carbamazepine and carbamazepine-10,11-epoxide to serum proteins in paediatric patients with epilepsy. *Eur J Clin Pharmacol* 1993; **44:** 291–3.
5. Bernus I, *et al.* Early stage autoinduction of carbamazepine metabolism in humans. *Eur J Clin Pharmacol* 1994; **47:** 355–60.
6. Caraco Y, *et al.* Carbamazepine pharmacokinetics in obese and lean subjects. *Ann Pharmacother* 1995; **29:** 843–7.
7. Mahmood I, Chamberlin N. A limited sampling method for the estimation of AUC and $C_{max}$ of carbamazepine and carbamazepine epoxide following a single and multiple dose of a sustained-release product. *Br J Clin Pharmacol* 1998; **45:** 241–6.
8. Cohen H, *et al.* Feasibility and pharmacokinetics of carbamazepine oral loading doses. *Am J Health-Syst Pharm* 1998; **55:** 1134–40.

## Uses and Administration

Carbamazepine is a dibenzazepine derivative with antiepileptic and psychotropic properties. It is used to control secondarily generalised tonic-clonic seizures and partial seizures, and in some primary generalised seizures. Carbamazepine is also used in the treatment of trigeminal neuralgia and has been tried with variable success in glossopharyngeal neuralgia and other severe pain syndromes associated with neurological disorders such as tabes dorsalis and multiple sclerosis. Another use of carbamazepine is in the prophylaxis of bipolar disorder unresponsive to lithium.

In the treatment of **epilepsy**, the dose of carbamazepine should be adjusted to the needs of the individual patient to achieve adequate control of seizures; this usually requires total plasma-carbamazepine concentrations of about 4 to 12 micrograms/mL (17 to 50 micromoles/litre). A low initial dose of carbamazepine is recommended to minimise side-effects. The suggested initial oral dose is 100 to 200 mg once or twice daily gradually increased by increments of 100 to 200 mg every 2 weeks to a usual maintenance dose of 0.8 to 1.2 g daily in divided doses; up to 2 g daily may occasionally be necessary. The usual oral dosage in children is 10 to 20 mg/kg daily in divided doses. Alternatively the dose may be expressed in terms of the age of the child and suggested daily doses are: up to 1 year of age, 100 to 200 mg; 1 to 5 years, 200 to 400 mg; 5 to 10 years, 400 to 600 mg; 10 to 15 years, 0.6 to 1 g.

Oral carbamazepine is usually given in divided doses 2 to 4 times daily. A twice-daily regimen may be associated with improved compliance but may produce widely fluctuating plasma-carbamazepine concentrations leading to intermittent side-effects. However, twice-daily administration may be suitable for patients receiving carbamazepine as monotherapy, and without peak-related side-effects. Also modified-release formulations can minimise fluctuations in plasma concentration and may allow effective twice-daily administration. Different preparations vary in bioavailability and it may be prudent to avoid changing the formulation.

The time and manner of taking carbamazepine should be standardised for the patient since variations might affect absorption with consequent fluctuations in the plasma concentrations.

Carbamazepine may be given by the rectal route in doses up to a maximum of 250 mg every 6 hours to patients for whom oral treatment is temporarily not possible. The dosage should be increased by about 25% when changing from an oral formulation to suppositories, and it is recommended that the rectal route should not be used for longer than 7 days.

As with other antiepileptics, withdrawal of carbamazepine therapy or transition to or from another type of antiepileptic therapy should be made gradually to avoid precipitating an increase in the frequency of seizures. For a discussion on whether or not to withdraw antiepileptic therapy in seizure-free patients, see p.349.

In the treatment of **trigeminal neuralgia** the initial dose of carbamazepine is 100 mg once or twice daily by mouth (although higher initial doses may be required in some patients) increased gradually as necessary. The usual maintenance dose is 400 to 800 mg daily in 2 to 4 divided doses but up to 1.6 g daily may be required. When pain relief has been obtained attempts should be made to reduce and ultimately discontinue the therapy, until another attack occurs.

For the prophylaxis of **bipolar disorder**, carbamazepine is given in an initial oral dose of 400 mg daily in divided doses, increased gradually as necessary up to a maximum of 1.6 g daily; the usual maintenance dose range is 400 to 600 mg daily.

**Administration.** A modified-release formulation of carbamazepine can reduce fluctuations in carbamazepine concentrations,[1] and tolerability and seizure control in patients with epilepsy may be improved.[2,3] Such formulations should be considered in patients receiving high doses who suffer intermittent adverse effects, and might also permit a reduction to twice- or even, in some patients, once-daily administration.[2,4] However, bioavailability appears to be slightly less than conventional preparations and dosage adjustments may be required when changing between formulations.[1]

1. McKee PJW, *et al.* Monotherapy with conventional and controlled-release carbamazepine: a double-blind, double-dummy comparison in epileptic patients. *Br J Clin Pharmacol* 1991; **32:** 99–104.
2. Anonymous. Carbamazepine update. *Lancet* 1989; **ii:** 595–7.
3. Ryan SW, *et al.* Slow release carbamazepine in treatment of poorly controlled seizures. *Arch Dis Child* 1990; **65:** 930–5.
4. McKee PJW, *et al.* Double dummy comparison between once and twice daily dosing with modified-release carbamazepine in epileptic patients. *Br J Clin Pharmacol* 1993; **36:** 257–61.

**Bipolar disorder.** Carbamazepine has been given as an alternative to lithium in patients with bipolar disorder (p.278). Studies of its efficacy have been conflicting; although clearly effective in some patients, at least one early study suggested that short-term benefit was not sustained in the longer term.[1] More recent results[2] have suggested that lithium is more effective in patients with classical bipolar disorder, but that carbamazepine may conceivably have a role in patients with nonclassical features. Carbamazepine has also been used in combination with lithium, particularly in patients unresponsive to either drug alone; although there are suggestions that the combination may be more effective than monotherapy, particularly in patients with a history of rapid cycling,[3] it is associated with a potential risk of serious neurotoxicity—see Antidepressants, under Interactions, above—and some commentators suggest that carbamazepine is falling out of favour with specialists prescribing for bipolar disorder.[4]

1. Frankenburg FR, *et al.* Long-term response to carbamazepine: a retrospective study. *J Clin Psychopharmacol* 1988; **8:** 130–2.
2. Kleindienst N, Greil W. Differential efficacy of lithium and carbamazepine in the prophylaxis of bipolar disorder: results of the MAP study. *Neuropsychobiology* 2000; **42** (suppl 1): 2–10.
3. Denicoff KD, *et al.* Comparative prophylactic efficacy of lithium, carbamazepine, and the combination in bipolar disorder. *J Clin Psychiatry* 1997; **58:** 470–8.
4. Ferrier IN. Developments in mood stabilisers. *Br Med Bull* 2001; **57:** 179–92.

**Depression.** Carbamazepine has been tried[1,2] for the augmentation of antidepressant therapy in the treatment of resistant depression (p.279). However, such combined therapy may lead to interactions—see also Antidepressants under Interactions, above.

1. De la Fuente JM, Mendlewicz J. Carbamazepine addition in tricyclic antidepressant-resistant unipolar depression. *Biol Psychiatry* 1992; **32:** 369–74.
2. Otani K, *et al.* Carbamazepine augmentation therapy in three patients with trazodone-resistant depression. *Int Clin Psychopharmacol* 1996; **11:** 55–7.

**Diabetes insipidus.** Cranial diabetes insipidus is usually treated by replacement therapy with antidiuretic hormone (ADH) in the form of desmopressin (see p.1314). Carbamazepine is one of a variety of other drugs that have been tried to promote ADH secretion, although some consider that it is usually ineffective and has unwanted effects.[1,2] Doses of 200 to 400 mg daily by mouth have been given. See also Effects on the Endocrine System under Adverse Effects, above.

1. Seckl J, Dunger D. Postoperative diabetes insipidus. *BMJ* 1989; **298:** 2–3.
2. Singer I, *et al.* The management of diabetes insipidus in adults. *Arch Intern Med* 1997; **157:** 1293–1301.

**Epilepsy.** Carbamazepine is one of the drugs of choice for partial seizures with or without secondary generalisation (see p.349). It has been used for some primary generalised seizures, although valproate is the drug of choice, but may exacerbate absence and myoclonic seizures.

**Hemifacial spasm.** Carbamazepine has been reported to have been of help in the treatment of hemifacial spasm (p.1390).

**Hiccup.** A protocol for the management of intractable hiccups can be found under Chlorpromazine, p.682. Carbamazepine may be of value for the treatment of neurogenic hiccups such as those that occur in multiple sclerosis.[1] Carbamazepine has also been reported to have been of benefit in 3 patients with diaphragmatic flutter,[2] a rare disorder associated with involuntary contractions of the diaphragm.

1. McFarling DA, Susac JO. Hoquet diabolique: intractable hiccups as a manifestation of multiple sclerosis. *Neurology* 1979; **29:** 797–801.
2. Vantrappen G, *et al.* High-frequency diaphragmatic flutter: symptoms and treatment by carbamazepine. *Lancet* 1992; **339:** 265–7.

**Hyperactivity.** When drugs are indicated for attention deficit hyperactivity disorder (p.1583) initial treatment is usually with a central stimulant but meta-analysis of a small number of trials has provided preliminary evidence that carbamazepine may be an effective alternative.[1]

1. Silva RR, *et al.* Carbamazepine use in children and adolescents with features of attention-deficit hyperactivity disorder: a meta-analysis. *J Am Acad Child Adolesc Psychiatry* 1996; **35:** 352–8.

**Lesch-Nyhan syndrome.** The severe self-mutilation that occurs in patients with Lesch-Nyhan syndrome (p.682) has been reported to improve in those given antiepileptics such as carbamazepine.[1]

1. Roach ES, *et al.* Carbamazepine trial for Lesch-Nyhan self-mutilation. *J Child Neurol* 1996; **11:** 476–8.

**Movement disorders.** Carbamazepine is one of many drugs that have been tried in the symptomatic treatment of *chorea* (p.664); there have been anecdotal reports of benefit in both non-hereditary[1] and hereditary choreas.[2] Carbamazepine is also among the drugs that have been tried in the treatment of *dystonias* that have not responded to levodopa or antimuscarinics (p.1209). Although some patients may benefit from carbamazepine, it is not generally recommended because of a relatively low success rate and the possibility of adverse effects.[3]

Carbamazepine has also been used in resistant cases of *tardive dyskinesia* (see under Extrapyramidal Disorders, p.677).

1. Roig M, *et al.* Carbamazepine: an alternative drug for the treatment of nonhereditary chorea. *Pediatrics* 1988; **82:** 492–5.
2. Roulet E, Deonna T. Successful treatment of hereditary dominant chorea with carbamazepine. *Pediatrics* 1989; **83:** 1077.
3. Anonymous. Dystonia: underdiagnosed and undertreated? *Drug Ther Bull* 1988; **26:** 33–6.

**Neonatal seizures.** Carbamazepine has been tried in the management of neonatal seizures (p.353).

**Neuropathic pain.** As well as being used to ease the pain of trigeminal neuralgia (see below) carbamazepine may be of use in other neuropathic pain including that associated with diabetic neuropathy (p.6). Chronic burning pain in the feet of a former prisoner of war, a result of neuropathic beriberi, was virtually abolished by treatment with carbamazepine 200 mg three times daily.[1]

Carbamazepine has been tried in an attempt to prevent the painful sensory neuropathy associated with oxaliplatin treatment (p.577); results of preliminary studies have been conflicting.[2,3]

1. Skelton WP. Neuropathic beriberi and carbamazepine. *Ann Intern Med* 1988; **109:** 598–9.
2. Eckel F, *et al.* Prophylaxe der Oxaliplatin-induzierten Neuropathie mit Carbamazepin: eine Pilotstudie. *Dtsch Med Wochenschr* 2002; **127:** 78–82.
3. Wilson RH, *et al.* Acute oxaliplatin-induced peripheral nerve hyperexcitability. *J Clin Oncol* 2002; **20:** 1767–74.

**Psychiatric disorders.** Carbamazepine has psychotropic properties and has been tried in the management of several psychiatric disorders, particularly in patients with *bipolar disorder* (see above). Carbamazepine has also been used with mixed results in various disorders for the control of symptoms such as agitation, aggression, and rage[1-4] (see Disturbed Behaviour, p.665). It may produce modest benefit when used as an adjunct to antipsychotics in the management of refractory schizophrenia (p.665) but any improvement appears to be related to its mood stabilising effect.[5] However, carbamazepine also has the potential to reduce serum concentrations of antipsychotics, resulting in clinical deterioration (see under Interactions for Chlorpromazine, p.679). Carbamazepine has also been tried[6] in *post-traumatic stress disorder* (p.664).

1. Mattes JA. Comparative effectiveness of carbamazepine and propranolol for rage outbursts. *J Neuropsychiatr Clin Neurosci* 1990; **2:** 159–64.
2. Gleason RP, Schneider LS. Carbamazepine treatment of agitation in Alzheimer's outpatients refractory to neuroleptics. *J Clin Psychiatry* 1990; **51:** 115–18.
3. Tariot PN, *et al.* Carbamazepine treatment of agitation in nursing home patients with dementia: a preliminary study. *J Am Geriatr Soc* 1994; **42:** 1160–6.
4. Cueva JE, *et al.* Carbamazepine in aggressive children with conduct disorder: a double-blind and placebo-controlled study. *J Am Acad Child Adolesc Psychiatry* 1996; **35:** 480–90.
5. Okuma T. Use of antiepileptic drugs in schizophrenia: a review of efficacy and tolerability. *CNS Drugs* 1994; **1:** 269–84.
6. Wolf ME, *et al.* Posttraumatic stress disorder in Vietnam veterans: clinical and EEG findings; possible therapeutic effects of carbamazepine. *Biol Psychiatry* 1988; **23:** 642–4.

**Restless legs syndrome.** The aetiology of restless legs syndrome (see Parasomnias, p.667) is obscure and treatment has been largely empirical. In a double-blind study involving 174 patients carbamazepine appeared to be more effective than placebo.[1]

1. Telstad W, *et al.* Treatment of the restless legs syndrome with carbamazepine: a double blind study. *BMJ* 1984; **288:** 444–6.

**Tinnitus.** Treatment of tinnitus (p.1381) is difficult, and many drugs have been tried. Although carbamazepine has been reported to be effective in some patients, it is rarely used because of its adverse effects.

**Trigeminal neuralgia.** Carbamazepine is the drug of choice in the treatment of the acute stages of trigeminal neuralgia (p.8). Satisfactory pain relief may be achieved in 70% or more of patients, although increasingly larger doses may be required and side-effects can be troublesome.

**Withdrawal syndromes.** Carbamazepine has been tried in the prophylaxis and treatment of various withdrawal syndromes. Reduction in *cocaine use* associated with carbamazepine treatment was demonstrated in one short-term controlled study,[1] although a systematic review[2] of data from later studies concluded that there was no evidence to support the use of carbamazepine in the treatment of cocaine dependence (p.1375). It has been reported[3,4] to be of benefit in some patients during *benzodiazepine withdrawal* but such adjunct therapy is not usually indicated (see p.690). Carbamazepine has been shown[5,6] to be effective in the treatment of symptoms of the *alcohol withdrawal syndrome* (p.1166) but as there are limited data on its efficacy in preventing associated delirium tremens and seizures it is usually recommended that it should only be used as an adjunct to benzodiazepine therapy. Carbamazepine has also been studied[7] as an aid in the treatment of alcohol dependence.

1. Halikas JA, *et al.* Cocaine reduction in unmotivated crack users using carbamazepine versus placebo in a short-term, double-blind crossover design. *Clin Pharmacol Ther* 1991; **50:** 81–95.
2. Lima AR, *et al.* Carbamazepine for cocaine dependence. Available in The Cochrane Library; Issue 2. Chichester: John Wiley; 2004.
3. Schweizer E, *et al.* Carbamazepine treatment in patients discontinuing long-term benzodiazepine therapy: effects on withdrawal severity and outcome. *Arch Gen Psychiatry* 1991; **48:** 448–52.
4. Klein E, *et al.* Alprazolam withdrawal in patients with panic disorder and generalized anxiety disorder: vulnerability and effect of carbamazepine. *Am J Psychiatry* 1994; **151:** 1760–6.
5. Malcolm R, *et al.* Double-blind controlled trial comparing carbamazepine to oxazepam treatment of alcohol withdrawal. *Am J Psychiatry* 1989; **146:** 617–21.
6. Stuppaeck CH, *et al.* Carbamazepine versus oxazepam in the treatment of alcohol withdrawal: a double-blind study. *Alcohol Alcohol* 1992; **27:** 153–8.
7. Mueller TI, *et al.* A double-blind, placebo-controlled pilot study of carbamazepine for the treatment of alcohol dependence. *Alcohol Clin Exp Res* 1997; **21:** 86–92.

## Preparations

***BP 2003:*** Carbamazepine Tablets;
***USP 27:*** Carbamazepine Extended-Release Tablets; Carbamazepine Oral Suspension; Carbamazepine Tablets.

**Proprietary Preparations** (details are given in Part 3)
***Arg.:*** Actinerval; Carbagramon; Carbamat; CMP; Conformal; Tegretol; ***Austral.:*** Carbium†; Tegretol; Teril; ***Austria:*** Deleptin; Neurotop; Sirtal; Tegretol; ***Belg.:*** Tegretol; ***Braz.:*** Carmazin; Convulsan; Karbac†; Tegretard; Tegretol; Tegrex; Tegrezin; Uni Carbamaz; ***Canad.:*** Novo-Carbamaz; Tegretol; ***Chile:*** Carbactol Retard; Eposal; Tegretal; ***Denm.:*** Nordotol; Tardotol†; Tegretol; Trimonil; ***Fin.:*** Neurotol; Tegretol; Trimonil†; ***Fr.:*** Tegretol; ***Ger.:*** Carba; Carbabeta; Carbadura; Carbaflux; Carbagamma; Carbium; espa-lepsin; Finlepsin; Fokalepsin; Sirtal; Tegretal; Timonil; ***Gr.:*** Tegretol; ***Hong Kong:*** Tegretol; Teril; Timonil†; ***India:*** Mazetol; Tegrital; ***Irl.:*** Gericarb; Tegretol; Temporol; ***Israel:*** Carbi; Tegretol; Teril; Timonil; ***Ital.:*** Tegretol; ***Malaysia:*** Taver; Tegretol; ***Mex.:*** Adepril†; Bioneuryl; Bioreunil; Carbalan; Carbaval; Carbazep; Carbazina; Carpin; Clostedal; Kezepin†; Neugeron; Neurolep†; Tegretol; Trantil†; Volutol; Zepiken†; ***Neth.:*** Tegretol; ***Norw.:*** Tegretol; Trimonil; ***NZ:*** Tegretol; Teril; ***Port.:*** Tegretol; ***S.Afr.:*** Degranol; Tegretol; ***Singapore:*** Neurotop; Tegretol; ***Spain:*** Tegretol; ***Swed.:*** Hermolepsin; Tegretol; Trimonil; ***Switz.:*** Tegretol; Timonil; ***Thai.:*** Antafit; Carbazene; Carmapine; Carpine; Carzepine; Mapezine; Panitol; Taver; Tegretol; ***UAE:*** Fitzecalm; ***UK:*** Arbil; Carbagen; Epimaz; Tegretol; Teril; Timonil; ***USA:*** Atretol†; Carbatrol; Epitol; Tegretol; Teril.

# Clobazam *(BAN, USAN, rINN)*

Clobazamum; H-4723; HR-376; LM-2717. 7-Chloro-1,5-dihydro-1-methyl-5-phenyl-1,5-benzodiazepine-2,4(3*H*)-dione.
$C_{16}H_{13}ClN_2O_2 = 300.7$.
*CAS — 22316-47-8.*
*ATC — N05BA09.*

**Pharmacopoeias.** In *Eur.* (see p.vi).

**Ph. Eur. 5.0** (Clobazam). A white or almost white crystalline powder. Slightly soluble in water; sparingly soluble in alcohol; freely soluble in dichloromethane.

## Dependence and Withdrawal

As for Diazepam, p.690.

## Adverse Effects, Treatment, and Precautions

As for Diazepam, p.690.

**Effects on menstruation.** Occasionally the use of clobazam before menstruation for catamenial epilepsy appeared to delay the period.[1]

1. Feely M. Prescribing anticonvulsant drugs 3: clonazepam and clobazam. *Prescribers' J* 1989; **29:** 111–15.

**Effects on the skin.** Report[1] of toxic epidermal necrolysis that developed in light-exposed areas in a patient being treated with clobazam.

1. Redondo P, *et al.* Photo-induced toxic epidermal necrolysis caused by clobazam. *Br J Dermatol* 1996; **135:** 999–1002.

**Porphyria.** Clobazam is considered to be unsafe in patients with porphyria although there is conflicting evidence of porphyrinogenicity.

## Interactions

As for Diazepam, p.692.

## Pharmacokinetics

Clobazam is well absorbed from the gastrointestinal tract and peak plasma concentrations have been reached 1 to 4 hours after oral administration. It is about 85% bound to plasma proteins. Clobazam is highly lipophilic and rapidly crosses the blood-brain barrier. It is metabolised in the liver by demethylation and hydroxylation but unlike the 1,4-benzodiazepines such as diazepam, clobazam, a 1,5-benzodiazepine, is hydroxylated at the 4-position rather than the 3-position (see also Metabolism under Diazepam, p.695). Clobazam is excreted unchanged and as metabolites mainly in the urine. Mean half-lives of 18 hours and 42 hours have been reported for clobazam and its main active metabolite *N*-desmethylclobazam, respectively.

◊ References.

1. Greenblatt DJ, *et al.* Clinical pharmacokinetics of the newer benzodiazepines. *Clin Pharmacokinet* 1983; **8:** 233–52.
2. Ochs HR, *et al.* Single and multiple dose kinetics of clobazam, and clinical effects during multiple dosage. *Eur J Clin Pharmacol* 1984; **26:** 499–503.

## Uses and Administration

Clobazam is a long-acting 1,5-benzodiazepine with uses similar to those of diazepam (a 1,4-benzodiazepine; see p.695). It may be used as an adjunct in the treatment of epilepsy in association with other antiepileptics, although its use may be limited by the development of tolerance or sedation (but see below). It is also used in the short-term treatment of acute anxiety.

As an adjunct in **epilepsy** usual adult doses in the UK are 20 to 30 mg daily by mouth, increased if necessary to a maximum of 60 mg daily; in some countries smaller initial doses of 5 to 15 mg, and higher maxima (up to 80 mg daily) are suggested. Children over 3 years of age may be given no more than half the adult dose.

As with other antiepileptics, withdrawal of clobazam therapy or transition to or from another type of antiepileptic therapy should be made gradually to avoid precipitating an increase in the frequency of seizures. For a discussion on whether or not to withdraw antiepileptic therapy in seizure-free patients, see p.349 and under Clonazepam, above.

For the short-term management of acute **anxiety** usual doses of 10 to 30 mg daily may be taken by mouth; up to 80 mg daily has been used in hospitalised patients with severe anxiety states. Low initial doses and cautious incrementation to a usual dose of 10 to 20 mg are recommended in elderly or debilitated patients.

**Epilepsy.** Benzodiazepines are sometimes employed in the management of epilepsy (p.349), but their long-term use is limited by problems of sedation, dependence, and tolerance to the antiepileptic effects.

Clobazam, along with clonazepam, is one of the benzodiazepines most commonly used as an oral antiepileptic. Sedation appears to be less of a problem with clobazam than with clonazepam, and this advantage may make it more appropriate as adjunctive therapy for adults.[1] Clobazam is active against partial and generalised seizures in epilepsy of widely differing aetiology in patients of all ages but is usually only indicated for adjunctive therapy. Intermittent therapy with clobazam has been used successfully in women with catamenial epilepsy (seizures associated with menstruation). Short-term therapy may also be useful for patients whose epileptic attacks occur in clusters or as cover for special events. Clobazam has also been tried with some success in children, including those with refractory epilepsy.[2-4]

1. Feely M. Prescribing anticonvulsant drugs 3: clonazepam and clobazam. *Prescribers' J* 1989; **29:** 111–15.
2. Munn R, Farrell K. Open study of clobazam in refractory epilepsy. *Pediatr Neurol* 1993; **9:** 465–9.
3. Sheth RD, *et al.* Clobazam for intractable pediatric epilepsy. *J Child Neurol* 1995; **10:** 205–8.
4. Canadian Study Group for Childhood Epilepsy. Clobazam has equivalent efficacy to carbamazepine and phenytoin as monotherapy for childhood epilepsy. *Epilepsia* 1998; **39:** 952–9.

**Phantom limb pain.** There has been a mention[1] of the complete relief of phantom limb pain refractory to other therapy in an elderly patient given clobazam 10 mg three times daily.

1. Rice-Oxley CP. The limited list: clobazam for phantom limb pain. *BMJ* 1986; **293:** 1309.

## Preparations

***BP 2003:*** Clobazam Capsules.

**Proprietary Preparations** (details are given in Part 3)
***Arg.:*** Karidium; ***Austral.:*** Frisium; ***Austria:*** Frisium; ***Belg.:*** Frisium; ***Braz.:*** Frisium; Urbanil; ***Canad.:*** Frisium; ***Chile:*** Frisin; Grifoclobam; ***Denm.:*** Frisium; ***Fin.:*** Frisium; ***Fr.:*** Urbanyl; ***Ger.:*** Frisium; ***Gr.:*** Frisium; ***Hong Kong:*** Frisium; ***India:*** Frisium; ***Irl.:*** Frisium; ***Israel:*** Frisium†; ***Ital.:*** Frisium; ***Malaysia:*** Frisium; ***Mex.:*** Frisium; Urbadan†; ***Neth.:*** Frisium; ***NZ:*** Frisium; ***Port.:*** Castilium; Urbanil; ***S.Afr.:*** Urbanol; ***Singapore:*** Frisium†; ***Spain:*** Noiafren; ***Switz.:*** Urbanyl; ***Thai.:*** Frisium; ***UK:*** Frisium.

## Clonazepam (BAN, USAN, rINN)

Clonazepamum; Ro-5-4023. 5-(2-Chlorophenyl)-1,3-dihydro-7-nitro-1,4-benzodiazepin-2-one.

$C_{15}H_{10}ClN_3O_3$ = 315.7.

*CAS — 1622-61-3.*

*ATC — N03AE01.*

**Pharmacopoeias.** In *Chin., Eur.* (see p.vi), *Jpn, Pol.,* and *US.*

**Ph. Eur. 5.0** (Clonazepam). A slightly yellowish, crystalline powder. Practically insoluble in water; slightly soluble in alcohol and in methyl alcohol. Protect from light.

**USP 27** (Clonazepam). A light yellow powder having a faint odour. Insoluble in water; slightly soluble in alcohol and in ether; sparingly soluble in acetone and in chloroform. Store in airtight containers. Protect from light.

### Dependence and Withdrawal

As for Diazepam, p.690.

**Withdrawal.** A study[1] of the withdrawal of clonazepam therapy in 40 epileptic children found that 19 had withdrawal symptoms of increased seizure frequency, either alone or with other symptoms but that this effect was transient. Withdrawal seizures and status may become an obstacle to the removal of useless or even deleterious therapy with clonazepam because the transient nature of these effects is not always recognised. Clonazepam should not be prescribed for more than 3 to 6 months and should be discontinued if clear and lasting therapeutic benefit cannot be demonstrated.

See also under Uses and Administration, below.

1. Specht U, *et al.* Discontinuation of clonazepam after long-term treatment. *Epilepsia* 1989; **30:** 458–63.

### Adverse Effects, Treatment, and Precautions

As for Diazepam, p.690.

The principal adverse effect of clonazepam is drowsiness, which occurs in about 50% of all patients on starting therapy. Salivary or bronchial hypersecretion may cause respiratory problems in children.

Care is required when withdrawing clonazepam therapy—see above.

**Breast feeding.** Benzodiazepines, such as clonazepam, given to the mother may cause neonatal sedation and breast feeding should be avoided. For comments on antiepileptic therapy and breast feeding, see p.351.

**Driving.** For a comment on antiepileptic drugs and driving, see p.351.

**Effects on the endocrine system.** Precocious development of secondary sexual characteristics occurred in a 15-month-old girl 2 months after starting treatment with clonazepam 500 micrograms twice daily for convulsions.[1] Symptoms regressed upon withdrawal of clonazepam.

1. Choonara IA, *et al.* Clonazepam and sexual precocity. *N Engl J Med* 1985; **312:** 185.

**Effects on mental function.** For a review of the effects of antiepileptic therapy, including clonazepam, on *cognition*, see p.351.

**Effects on the mouth.** A 52-year-old woman developed burning mouth syndrome after starting clonazepam;[1] some improvement was noted when the dose was reduced but symptoms were still intolerable and, therefore, clonazepam was withdrawn. Subsequently, symptoms resolved within 3 weeks.

1. Culhane NS, Hodle AD. Burning mouth syndrome after taking clonazepam. *Ann Pharmacother* 2001; **35:** 874–6.

**Effects on sexual function.** Sexual dysfunction was reported[1] in 18 of 42 male patients receiving clonazepam for the treatment of post-traumatic stress disorder; symptoms resolved when therapy was changed to diazepam in 17 patients and lorazepam in the remaining patient.

1. Fossey MD, Hamner MB. Clonazepam-related sexual dysfunction in male veterans with PTSD. *Anxiety* 1994-95; **1:** 233–6.

**Extrapyramidal disorders.** For reference to extrapyramidal disorders associated with the administration of benzodiazepines including clonazepam, see under Effects on the Nervous System in Diazepam, p.691. However, clonazepam is also used in the treatment of some extrapyramidal disorders as discussed under Uses and Administration, below.

**Porphyria.** Clonazepam is considered to be unsafe in patients with porphyria although there is conflicting evidence of porphyrinogenicity.

For comments on the use of benzodiazepines in porphyria, see p.353.

**Pregnancy.** For comments on the management of epilepsy during pregnancy, see p.351.

### Interactions

Hepatic enzyme inducers, such as carbamazepine, phenobarbital, or phenytoin, may accelerate the metabolism of clonazepam. Alcohol may affect the patient's response to clonazepam. Clonazepam may be expected to have the sedative interactions associated with benzodiazepines in general (see under Interactions of Diazepam, p.692).

**Antiarrhythmics.** For reference to an interaction between clonazepam and amiodarone, see under Diazepam, p.693.

**Antiepileptics.** Serum-clonazepam concentrations fell markedly in 4 of 8 children who had *lamotrigine* added to their therapy.[1] For reference to possible interactions between clonazepam and other antiepileptics, see under Diazepam, p.693 and Benzodiazepines under Interactions of Phenytoin, p.374.

1. Eriksson A-S, *et al.* Pharmacokinetic interactions between lamotrigine and other antiepileptic drugs in children with intractable epilepsy. *Epilepsia* 1996; **37:** 769–73.

### Pharmacokinetics

Clonazepam is well absorbed following oral administration and peak plasma concentrations have been reported to occur within 4 hours. It is extensively metabolised in the liver, its principal metabolite being 7-aminoclonazepam, which probably has little antiepileptic activity; minor metabolites are the 7-acetamido- and 3-hydroxy- derivatives. It is excreted mainly in the urine almost entirely as its metabolites in free or conjugated form. It is about 86% bound to plasma protein and estimations of its plasma half-life range from about 20 to 40 hours, and occasionally more.

A therapeutic range of plasma concentrations has not been established.

Clonazepam crosses the placental barrier and is distributed into breast milk.

**Bioavailability.** It has been suggested, on the basis of anecdotal evidence,[1] that there may be differences in bioavailability, and hence in clinical effect, between formulations of clonazepam.

1. Rapaport MH. Clinical differences between the generic and non-generic forms of clonazepam. *J Clin Psychopharmacol* 1997; **17:** 424.

### Uses and Administration

Clonazepam is a benzodiazepine derivative similar to diazepam (p.695), with marked antiepileptic properties.

It may be used in the treatment of all types of epilepsy and seizures (p.349) but its usefulness is sometimes limited by the development of tolerance and by sedation, and other antiepileptics are often preferred. It may also be used in myoclonus (p.353) and associated abnormal movements. Clonazepam is also employed for the treatment of panic disorders.

For **epilepsy** and **myoclonus** treatment is started with small doses that are progressively increased to an optimum dose according to the response of the patient. In the UK the initial adult dose is 1 mg (500 micrograms in the elderly) by mouth at night for 4 nights gradually increased over 2 to 4 weeks to a usual maintenance dose of 4 to 8 mg daily; it is recommended that the total dose should not exceed 20 mg daily. Total daily doses are taken in 3 or 4 divided doses; however, once the maintenance dose has been reached, the daily amount may be given as a single dose at night. In the UK initial daily doses in children are 250 micrograms for children up to 5 years of age and 500 micrograms for children 5 to 12 years of age; usual daily maintenance doses, given in 3 or 4 divided doses, are: infants up to 1 year, 0.5 to 1 mg; children 1 to 5 years, 1 to 3 mg; children 5 to 12 years, 3 to 6 mg. In the USA it is recommended that the total dose in children should not exceed 200 micrograms/kg daily. There is little value in routinely monitoring plasma-clonazepam concentrations.

Clonazepam is also used as an alternative to other benzodiazepines in the emergency management of **status epilepticus** (p.352). The usual dose is 1 mg given by intravenous injection over about 30 seconds or by intravenous infusion, repeated if necessary; the dose in infants and children is 500 micrograms.

As with other antiepileptics, withdrawal of clonazepam therapy or transition to or from another type of antiepileptic therapy should be made gradually to avoid precipitating an increase in the frequency of seizures. For a discussion on whether or not to withdraw antiepileptic therapy in seizure-free patients, see p.349 and above.

In the treatment of **panic disorders**, clonazepam is given in an initial dose of 250 micrograms twice daily by mouth. This may be increased after 3 days to a total of 1 mg daily; a few patients may benefit from further increases, up to a maximum of 4 mg daily. In order to minimise drowsiness, clonazepam may be taken as a single dose at bedtime. Withdrawal should again be gradual.

**Administration.** Serum concentrations of clonazepam after administration via the buccal, intranasal, or intravenous routes were measured in a crossover study[1] in 7 healthy males. The results showed that intranasal clonazepam may offer an alternative to buccal administration in patients with serial seizures but the initial concentrations were too low to recommend its use as an alternative to intravenous clonazepam in the management of status epilepticus. The nasal formulation used in this study contained dimethyl-β-cyclodextrin as a solubiliser and absorption enhancer.

1. Schols-Hendriks MWG, *et al.* Absorption of clonazepam after intranasal and buccal administration. *Br J Clin Pharmacol* 1995; **39:** 449–51.

**Anxiety disorders.** Clonazepam is used for the treatment of panic attacks with or without agoraphobia (p.663), and a beneficial response has been reported in such patients,[1] suggesting a similar action to alprazolam.

1. Davidson JRT, Moroz G. Pivotal studies of clonazepam in panic disorder. *Psychopharmacol Bull* 1998; **34:** 169–74.

**Depression.** Short-term use of clonazepam in low doses has been tried[1,2] with beneficial results for the augmentation of conventional antidepressant therapy in the treatment of depression (p.279). One study[1] found that augmentation was significantly more effective with a daily dose of 3 mg of clonazepam than with lower doses.

1. Morishita S, Aoki S. Clonazepam in the treatment of prolonged depression. *J Affect Disord* 1999; **53:** 275–8.
2. Londborg PD, *et al.* Short-term cotherapy with clonazepam and fluoxetine: anxiety, sleep disturbance and core symptoms of depression. *J Affect Disord* 2000; **61:** 73–9.

**Extrapyramidal disorders.** Clonazepam may be of benefit in some extrapyramidal disorders. It has been tried in the management of patients with *tic disorders* such as *Tourette's syndrome* (p.664) but evidence of efficacy from controlled studies is limited.[1] Some use clonazepam in preference to haloperidol[2] since it does not carry the risk of tardive dyskinesia associated with such antipsychotics. There is also limited evidence of benefit with clonazepam in antipsychotic-induced *akathisia*[3,4] and *tardive dyskinesia*[5,6] (see under Extrapyramidal Disorders, p.677), and of improvement in *dysarthria* in a study in patients with parkinsonism.[7]

1. Goetz CG. Clonidine and clonazepam in Tourette syndrome. *Adv Neurol* 1992; **58:** 245–51.
2. Truong DD, *et al.* Clonazepam, haloperidol, and clonidine in tic disorders. *South Med J* 1988; **81:** 1103–5.
3. Kutcher S, *et al.* Successful clonazepam treatment of neuroleptic-induced akathisia in older adolescents and young adults: a double-blind, placebo-controlled study. *J Clin Psychopharmacol* 1989; **9:** 403–6.
4. Pujalte D, *et al.* A double-blind comparison of clonazepam and placebo in the treatment of neuroleptic-induced akathisia. *Clin Neuropharmacol* 1994; **17:** 236–42.
5. Thaker GK, *et al.* Clonazepam treatment of tardive dyskinesia: a practical GABAmimetic strategy. *Am J Psychiatry* 1990; **147:** 445–51.
6. Shapleske J, *et al.* Successful treatment of tardive dystonia with clozapine and clonazepam. *Br J Psychiatry* 1996; **168:** 516–18.
7. Biary N, *et al.* A double-blind trial of clonazepam in the treatment of parkinsonian dysarthria. *Neurology* 1988; **38:** 255–8.

**Hiccup.** A protocol for the management of intractable hiccups can be found under Chlorpromazine, p.682. Clonazepam might also be of value, especially in neurogenic hiccups.

**Parasomnias.** Treatment of parasomnias (p.667) including sleep behaviour disorder, restless legs syndrome, and periodic limb movements in sleep is largely empirical, but benzodiazepines such as clonazepam are often used.[1] Small studies have provided some evidence for benefit with clonazepam therapy.[2-4]

1. Schenck CH, Mahowald MW. Long-term, nightly benzodiazepine treatment of injurious parasomnias and other disorders of disrupted nocturnal sleep in 170 adults. *Am J Med* 1996; **100:** 333–7.
2. Montagna P, *et al.* Clonazepam and vibration in restless legs syndrome. *Acta Neurol Scand* 1984; **69:** 428–30.
3. Peled R, Lavie P. Double-blind evaluation of clonazepam on periodic leg movements in sleep. *J Neurol Neurosurg Psychiatry* 1987; **50:** 1679–81.
4. Saletu M, *et al.* Restless legs syndrome (RLS) and periodic limb movement disorder (PLMD): acute placebo-controlled sleep laboratory studies with clonazepam. *Eur Neuropsychopharmacol* 2001; **11:** 153–61.

**Phantom limb pain.** The management of phantom limb pain (p.7) can be difficult, and tricyclic antidepressants and antiepileptics are used for the neuropathic components of the pain. Rapid and marked pain relief was achieved in 2 patients with lancinating phantom limb pain following treatment with clonazepam with or without amitriptyline.[1]

1. Bartusch SL, *et al.* Clonazepam for the treatment of lancinating phantom limb pain. *Clin J Pain* 1996; **12:** 59–62.

**Stiff-man syndrome.** Clonazepam has been used as an alternative to diazepam in the management of stiff-man syndrome (see under Muscle Spasm, p.696) and is reported[1] to be effective for familial startle disease, a rare congenital form of stiff-man syndrome.

1. Ryan SG, *et al.* Startle disease, or hyperekplexia: response to clonazepam and assignment of the gene (STHE) to chromosome 5q by linkage analysis. *Ann Neurol* 1992; **31:** 663–8.

**Trigeminal neuralgia.** Although carbamazepine is the drug of choice in the treatment of trigeminal neuralgia (p.8), clonazepam may be used in carbamazepine-intolerant patients.

## Preparations

***BP 2003:*** Clonazepam Injection;
***USP 27:*** Clonazepam Tablets.

**Proprietary Preparations** (details are given in Part 3)
***Arg.:*** Clonagin; Clonax; Diocam; Neuryl; Rivotril; Solfidin; ***Austral.:*** Paxam; Rivotril; ***Austria:*** Rivotril; ***Belg.:*** Rivotril; ***Braz.:*** Rivotril; ***Canad.:*** Clonapam; Rivotril; ***Chile:*** Acepran; Clonapam; Clozanil; Crismol; Neuryl; Ravotril; Valpax; ***Denm.:*** Rivotril; ***Fin.:*** Rivatril; ***Fr.:*** Rivotril; ***Ger.:*** Antelepsin; Rivotril; ***Gr.:*** Rivotril; ***Hong Kong:*** Rivotril; ***India:*** Epitril; ***Irl.:*** Rivotril; ***Israel:*** Clonex; Rivotril; ***Ital.:*** Rivotril; ***Mex.:*** Kenoket; Kriadex; Rivotril; ***Neth.:*** Rivotril; ***Norw.:*** Rivotril; ***NZ:*** Rivotril; ***Port.:*** Rivotril; ***S.Afr.:*** Rivotril; ***Singapore:*** Rivotril†; ***Spain:*** Rivotril; ***Swed.:*** Iktorivil; ***Switz.:*** Rivotril; ***Thai.:*** Rivotril; ***UK:*** Rivotril; ***USA:*** Klonopin.

## Ethadione

Etadiona. 3-Ethyl-5,5-dimethyl-2,4-oxazolidinedione.
$C_7H_{11}NO_3$ = 157.2.
*CAS — 520-77-4.*
*ATC — N03AC03.*

### Profile

Ethadione is an oxazolidinedione antiepileptic with actions and uses similar to those of trimethadione (p.379); like trimethadione it appears to owe its action to metabolism to dimethadione. It has been used to treat epilepsy (p.349) in patients with absence seizures resistant to other therapy. Usual initial doses are 500 mg daily by mouth, increased gradually to up to 2 g daily if necessary.

### Preparations

**Proprietary Preparations** (details are given in Part 3)
***Austria:*** Petidion; ***Switz.:*** Petidion†.

# Ethosuximide *(BAN, USAN, rINN)*

CI-366; CN-10395; Etosuximida; NSC-64013; PM-671. 2-Ethyl-2-methylsuccinimide.
$C_7H_{11}NO_2$ = 141.2.
*CAS — 77-67-8.*
*ATC — N03AD01.*

**Pharmacopoeias.** In *Chin., Eur.* (see p.vi), *Int., Jpn,* and *US.*

**Ph. Eur. 5.0** (Ethosuximide). A white or almost white powder or waxy solid. It exhibits polymorphism. Freely soluble in water; very soluble in alcohol and in dichloromethane. Protect from light.

**USP 27** (Ethosuximide). A white to off-white crystalline powder or waxy solid, having a characteristic odour. Freely soluble in water and in chloroform; very soluble in alcohol and in ether; very slightly soluble in petroleum spirit. Store in airtight containers.

## Adverse Effects and Treatment

Gastrointestinal adverse effects including nausea, vomiting, anorexia, gastric upset, and abdominal pain occur fairly frequently with ethosuximide. Other effects that may occur include headache, fatigue, lethargy, drowsiness, dizziness, ataxia, hiccup, and mild euphoria.

More rarely dyskinesias, personality changes, depression, psychosis, sleep disturbances including night terrors, skin rashes, erythema multiforme or Stevens-Johnson syndrome, systemic lupus erythematosus, photophobia, gum hypertrophy, tongue swelling, myopia, increased libido, and vaginal bleeding have been reported. There are a few reports of blood disorders including eosinophilia, leucopenia, agranulocytosis, thrombocytopenia, pancytopenia, and aplastic anaemia; fatalities have occurred.

Abnormal renal and liver function values have been recorded.

**Overdosage.** For a review of the features and management of poisoning with some antiepileptics, including ethosuximide, see under Phenytoin, p.371.

## Precautions

Ethosuximide should be used with caution in patients with impaired hepatic or renal function. The manufacturers recommend regular hepatic and renal-function tests (and some suggest blood counts) during treatment with ethosuximide, although the *British National Formulary* questions the practical value of such monitoring. Patients or their carers should be told how to recognise signs of blood toxicity and they should be advised to seek immediate medical attention if symptoms such as fever, sore throat, mouth ulcers, bruising, or bleeding develop.

Care is required when withdrawing ethosuximide therapy—see also under Uses and Administration, below.

**Breast feeding.** Ethosuximide is distributed in significant amounts into breast milk; hyperexcitability and poor suckling have been reported in the infant. Although the manufacturers recommend that breast feeding should be avoided, the American Academy of Pediatrics[1] considers that ethosuximide is usually compatible with breast feeding.

For further comment on antiepileptic therapy and breast feeding, see p.351.

1. American Academy of Pediatrics. The transfer of drugs and other chemicals into human milk. *Pediatrics* 2001; **108:** 776–89. Correction. *ibid.*; 1029. Also available at: http://aappolicy.aappublications.org/cgi/content/full/pediatrics%3b108/3/776 (accessed 13/05/04)

**Driving.** For a comment on antiepileptic drugs and driving, see p.351.

**Porphyria.** Ethosuximide has been associated with acute attacks of porphyria and is considered unsafe in porphyric patients.

**Pregnancy.** For comments on the management of epilepsy during pregnancy, see p.351.

## Interactions

There are complex interactions between antiepileptics and toxicity may be enhanced without a corresponding increase in antiepileptic activity. Such interactions are very variable and unpredictable and plasma monitoring is often advisable with combination therapy.

**Antibacterials.** *Isoniazid* raises the plasma concentration and increases the risk of toxicity of ethosuximide. Psychotic behaviour has been reported[1] in a patient stabilised on ethosuximide and sodium valproate, after the introduction of isoniazid. Serum-ethosuximide concentrations rose substantially until both ethosuximide and isoniazid were discontinued.

1. van Wieringen A, Vrijlandt CM. Ethosuximide intoxication caused by interaction with isoniazid. *Neurology* 1983; **33:** 1227–8.

**Antidepressants.** As with all antiepileptics, antidepressants may antagonise the antiepileptic activity of ethosuximide by lowering the convulsive threshold.

**Antiepileptics.** Since ethosuximide has a limited spectrum of antiepileptic action, patients with mixed seizure syndromes may require addition of other antiepileptics. *Carbamazepine, phenobarbital,* and *phenytoin* have all been shown[1] to increase the clearance of ethosuximide and thus reduce plasma concentrations. This interaction is likely to be clinically relevant and higher ethosuximide dosages may be necessary to achieve therapeutic drug levels. The effect of *valproic acid* on ethosuximide concentrations is unclear. One study[2] showed a marked increase in serum ethosuximide concentrations once valproate was added to combination therapies; increases in ethosuximide concentrations have also been noted in healthy subjects when taken with valproic acid.[3] Conversely, other studies have reported reductions[4] or no significant changes in serum ethosuximide concentrations[5,6] with valproic acid.

1. Giaccone M, *et al.* Effect of enzyme inducing anticonvulsants on ethosuximide pharmacokinetics in epileptic patients. *Br J Clin Pharmacol* 1996; **41:** 575–9.
2. Mattson RH, Cramer JA. Valproic acid and ethosuximide interaction. *Ann Neurol* 1980; **7:** 583–4.
3. Pisani F, *et al.* Valproic acid-ethosuximide interaction: a pharmacokinetic study. *Epilepsia* 1984; **25:** 229–33.
4. Battino D, *et al.* Ethosuximide plasma concentrations: influence of age and associated concomitant therapy. *Clin Pharmacokinet* 1982; **7:** 176–80.
5. Fowler GW. Effect of dipropylacetate on serum levels of anticonvulsants in children. *Proc West Pharmacol Soc* 1978; **21:** 37–40.
6. Bauer LA, *et al.* Ethosuximide kinetics: possible interaction with valproic acid. *Clin Pharmacol Ther* 1982; **31:** 741–5.

**Antipsychotics.** As with all antiepileptics, antipsychotics may antagonise the antiepileptic activity of ethosuximide by lowering the convulsive threshold.

## Pharmacokinetics

Ethosuximide is readily absorbed from the gastrointestinal tract and extensively hydroxylated in the liver to its principal metabolite which is reported to be inactive. Ethosuximide is excreted in the urine mainly in the form of its metabolite, either free or conjugated, but about 12 to 20% is also excreted unchanged.

Ethosuximide is widely distributed throughout the body, but is not significantly bound to plasma proteins. A half-life of about 40 to 60 hours has been reported for adults with a shorter half-life of about 30 hours in children.

Monitoring of plasma concentrations has been suggested as an aid in assessing control and the therapeutic range of ethosuximide is usually quoted as being 40 to 100 micrograms/mL (about 300 to 700 micromoles/litre); measurement of concentrations in saliva and tears has also been performed.

Ethosuximide crosses the placental barrier, and is distributed into breast milk.

The pharmacokinetics of ethosuximide are affected by the concomitant administration of other antiepileptics (see under Interactions, above).

## Uses and Administration

Ethosuximide is a succinimide antiepileptic used in the treatment of absence seizures. It may also be used for myoclonic seizures. Ethosuximide is ineffective against tonic-clonic seizures and may unmask them if given alone in mixed seizure types.

A plasma-ethosuximide concentration of 40 to 100 micrograms/mL (about 300 to 700 micromoles/litre) appears to be generally necessary. The initial dose for adults and children aged 6 years and over is 500 mg daily by mouth. The dosage is then adjusted by increments, usually of 250 mg every 4 to 7 days, according to the response of the patient. Control of seizures is usually produced with a daily dose of 1 to 1.5 g, although some patients may require doses of up to 2 g; strict supervision is necessary when the dose exceeds 1.5 g. In the UK, children up to 6 years of age may be given an initial dose of 250 mg daily, increased gradually in small increments every few days to a usual dose of 20 mg/kg; one manufacturer in the UK recommends that the dose should not exceed 1 g. Similar dosages are recommended in the USA for children aged between 3 to 6 years.

As with other antiepileptics, withdrawal of ethosuximide therapy or transition to or from another type of antiepileptic therapy should be made gradually to avoid precipitating an increase in the frequency of seizures. For a discussion on whether or not to withdraw antiepileptic therapy in seizure-free patients, see p.349.

**Epilepsy.** Ethosuximide is a drug of choice in the treatment of absence seizures; it may also be used for myoclonic, atonic, and tonic seizures but is ineffective in other forms of epilepsy (p.349). Ethosuximide may be given with other antiepileptics in the treatment of mixed-seizure syndromes that include absences. It has been suggested that ethosuximide may provoke tonic-clonic seizures, but there is not a great deal of evidence for this. One early report indicated that 22 of 85 patients receiving a regimen of ethosuximide, mesuximide, and trimethadione for absence seizures developed tonic-clonic seizures[1] and another of similar vintage reported exacerbation of mixed-seizure types in 7 patients receiving ethosuximide.[2] However, it is recognised that patients with absence seizures have a high incidence of generalised tonic-clonic seizures[3] and it would presumably be difficult to distinguish such attacks from any putative effect of ethosuximide. Furthermore, ethosuximide is not effective against tonic-clonic seizures, and in patients with mixed-seizure types it might be expected to unmask the non-absence components of the disease.

Ethosuximide has also been tried in the management of absence status epilepticus (p.352).

1. Friedel B, Lempp R. Grand-mal-Provokation bei der Behandlung kindlicher petit-mal mit Oxazolidinen oder Succinimiden und ihre therapeutischen Konsequenzen. *Z Kinderheilk* 1962; **87:** 42–51.
2. de Haas AML, Kuilman M. Ethosuximide (α-ethyl-α-methylsuccinimide) and grand mal. *Epilepsia* 1964; **5:** 90–6.
3. Glauser TA. Succinimides: Adverse Effects. In: Levy RG, *et al.*, eds. *Antiepileptic drugs* 5th ed. Philadelphia: Lippincott Williams & Wilkins, 2002; 658–64.

## Preparations

***BP 2003:*** Ethosuximide Capsules; Ethosuximide Oral Solution;
***USP 27:*** Ethosuximide Capsules; Ethosuximide Oral Solution.

**Proprietary Preparations** (details are given in Part 3)
***Arg.:*** Zarontin; ***Austral.:*** Zarontin; ***Austria:*** Petinimid; Simatin†; Suxinutin; ***Belg.:*** Zarontin; ***Canad.:*** Zarontin; ***Denm.:*** Zarondan; ***Fin.:*** Suxinutin; ***Fr.:*** Zarontin; ***Ger.:*** Petnidan; Suxilep; Suxinutin; ***Gr.:*** Zarontin; ***Irl.:*** Zarontin; ***Israel:*** Zarontin; ***Ital.:*** Zarontin; ***Mex.:*** Zarontin†; ***Neth.:*** Zarontin; ***Norw.:*** Zarondan†; ***NZ:*** Zarontin; ***S.Afr.:*** Zarontin; ***Spain:*** Zarontin; ***Swed.:*** Suxinutin; ***Switz.:*** Petinimid; Suxinutin; ***UK:*** Emeside; Zarontin; ***USA:*** Zarontin.

**Multi-ingredient:** ***Austria:*** Acrisuxin†; ***Switz.:*** Acrisuxin†.

## Ethotoin (BAN, rINN)

Etotoína. 3-Ethyl-5-phenylhydantoin.

$C_{11}H_{12}N_2O_2$ = 204.2.

*CAS — 86-35-1.*

*ATC — N03AB01.*

**Pharmacopoeias.** In *US.*

**USP 27** (Ethotoin). A white crystalline powder. Insoluble in water; freely soluble in dehydrated alcohol and in chloroform; soluble in ether. Store in airtight containers.

### Profile

Ethotoin is a hydantoin antiepileptic with actions similar to those of phenytoin (p.370), but it is reported to be both less toxic and less effective; it is not one of the main drugs used to treat epilepsy (p.349).

Ethotoin has been given by mouth in an initial dosage of up to 1 g daily, increased gradually at intervals of several days to 2 to 3 g daily, given in 4 to 6 divided doses after meals.

**Administration.** A study[1] of the pharmacokinetics of ethotoin given at more convenient intervals of every 8 hours.

1. Browne TR, Szabo GK. A pharmacokinetic rationale for three times daily administration of ethotoin (Peganone). *J Clin Pharmacol* 1989; **29:** 270–1.

**Porphyria.** Ethotoin has been associated with acute attacks of porphyria and is considered unsafe in porphyric patients.

### Preparations

***USP 27:*** Ethotoin Tablets.

**Proprietary Preparations** (details are given in Part 3)

***USA:*** Peganone.

## Felbamate (USAN, rINN)

AD-03055; Felbamato; W-554. 2-Phenyl-1,3-propanediol dicarbamate.

$C_{11}H_{14}N_2O_4$ = 238.2.

*CAS — 25451-15-4.*

*ATC — N03AX10.*

### Adverse Effects

The most frequently reported adverse effects with felbamate are anorexia, weight loss, nausea and vomiting, rash, insomnia, headache, dizziness, somnolence, and diplopia. Aplastic anaemia or acute liver failure, sometimes fatal, have occurred rarely, and there have been reports of Stevens-Johnson syndrome.

**Effects on the kidneys.** A 15-year-old boy receiving up to 3 g of felbamate daily developed urethral obstruction due to formation of urethral stones composed of felbamate.[1] Records revealed that unidentified urinary crystals had been found in the patient's urine 2 years before presentation with acute urolithiasis.

For a report of crystalluria associated with felbamate overdosage, see below.

1. Sparagana SP, *et al.* Felbamate urolithiasis. *Epilepsia* 2001; **42:** 682–5.

**Effects on the skin.** Toxic epidermal necrolysis has been reported[1] in a patient 16 days after she started monotherapy with felbamate for partial complex seizures.

1. Travaglini MT, *et al.* Toxic epidermal necrolysis after initiation of felbamate therapy. *Pharmacotherapy* 1995; **15:** 260–4.

**Overdosage.** A 20-year-old woman presented with slurred speech and nausea 4 hours after ingesting 18 g of felbamate and 12 to 25 g of sodium valproate.[1] Over the next 4 to 5 hours she became combative, uncooperative, and progressively obtunded and eventually required endotracheal intubation and assisted ventilation. Peak plasma concentrations of 200 micrograms/mL for felbamate and 470 micrograms/mL for sodium valproate occurred 12 and 14 hours respectively after ingestion. Large quantities of macroscopic crystals, identified as containing felbamate, were noted in the urine 18 hours after ingestion and the patient developed renal failure. The crystalluria and renal failure responded to parenteral hydration.

1. Rengstorff DS, *et al.* Felbamate overdose complicated by massive crystalluria and acute renal failure. *Clin Toxicol* 2000; **38:** 667–9.

### Precautions

Felbamate is contra-indicated in patients with a history of blood disorders or hepatic impairment. It should be used only in the treatment of severe epilepsy refractory to other antiepileptics because of the risk of fatal aplastic anaemia or acute liver failure. Patients or their carers should be advised of the symptoms of aplastic anaemia and be told to report immediately should any such symptoms develop. Complete blood counts should be carried out before the patient starts treatment and regularly during treatment (but see Epilepsy, under Uses and Administration, below). Aplastic anaemia may occur after felbamate has been discontinued so patients should continue to be monitored for some time. Liver function tests are also recommended before commencing and regularly (at 1- to 2-week intervals) during treatment. Felbamate should be discontinued if there is any evidence of bone marrow depression or liver abnormalities.

Felbamate should be used with caution in patients with renal impairment (see Uses and Administration, below). Felbamate may cause photosensitivity reactions and patients should be advised to take protective measures against exposure to UV radiation.

Care is required when withdrawing felbamate therapy—see also under Uses and Administration, below.

**Breast feeding.** For comment on antiepileptic therapy and breast feeding, see p.351.

**Driving.** For a comment on antiepileptic drugs and driving, see p.351.

**The elderly.** Felbamate may need to be given with care in elderly patients (see Administration in the Elderly, below).

**Pregnancy.** For comments on the management of epilepsy during pregnancy, see p.351.

### Interactions

There are complex interactions between antiepileptics and toxicity may be enhanced without a corresponding increase in antiepileptic activity. Such interactions are very variable and unpredictable and plasma monitoring is often advisable with combination therapy. The metabolism of felbamate is enhanced by enzyme inducers such as phenytoin, phenobarbital, or carbamazepine. In contrast, the half-life of felbamate may be prolonged by gabapentin. Felbamate inhibits or enhances the metabolism of several other antiepileptics and care is required when it is added to therapy.

**Anticoagulants.** For the effect of felbamate on *warfarin*, see p.1025.

**Antiepileptics.** For some references to the effect of felbamate on other antiepileptics, see under *Carbamazepine*, p.356, *Phenobarbital*, p.368, *Phenytoin*, p.373, and *Valproate* p.381.

**Sex hormones.** For the effect of felbamate on *oral contraceptives* see under Gestodene, p.1556.

### Pharmacokinetics

Felbamate is well absorbed from the gastrointestinal tract and peak plasma concentrations have been reported 1 to 6 hours after oral administration. Protein binding is reported to be about 22 to 25%. It is partly metabolised in the liver by hydroxylation and conjugation to inactive metabolites. Felbamate is excreted mainly in the urine as metabolites and unchanged drug (40 to 50%); less than 5% appears in the faeces. The elimination half-life is reported to be between 14 and 23 hours. Felbamate is distributed into breast milk.

The pharmacokinetics of felbamate are reported to be linear at the doses used clinically. Therapeutic plasma concentrations have been reported to be between 30 and 80 micrograms/mL.

The pharmacokinetics of felbamate are affected by the concomitant administration of other antiepileptics (see under Interactions, above).

◊ See under Uses and Administration (below) for mention of pharmacokinetic studies of felbamate in the elderly and in patients with renal impairment.

### Uses and Administration

Felbamate is a carbamate structurally related to meprobamate (p.706). It is used in the treatment of epilepsy; however, because of its toxicity, it should only be used in severe cases unresponsive to other drugs.

Felbamate is given to adults as monotherapy or adjunctive therapy for refractory partial seizures with or without secondary generalisation. It is used in children as adjunctive therapy in controlling the seizures associated with the Lennox-Gastaut syndrome.

The initial adult dose of felbamate when given as *monotherapy* is 1.2 g daily by mouth in 3 or 4 divided doses. The daily dose should be increased gradually under close supervision; increments of 600 mg every 2 weeks are given according to response, up to 2.4 g daily. Thereafter doses may be further increased to a maximum of 3.6 g daily if necessary.

Similar initial doses are given as *adjunctive* therapy, but the doses of concomitant antiepileptics should be decreased as necessary. Incremental increases of adjunctive felbamate are 1200 mg at weekly intervals. The initial dose in children 2 to 14 years of age is 15 mg/kg daily in 3 or 4 divided doses increased gradually in increments of 15 mg/kg per day at weekly intervals up to a maximum of 45 mg/kg daily.

As with other antiepileptics, withdrawal of felbamate therapy or transition to or from another type of antiepileptic therapy should be made gradually to avoid precipitating an increase in the frequency of seizures. For a discussion on whether or not to withdraw antiepileptic therapy in seizure-free patients, see p.349.

**Administration in the elderly.** The elderly may require lower initial doses of felbamate and slower dose titration. Following single doses of felbamate, plasma concentrations and half-lives were greater and mean clearance lower in elderly than in young subjects, whereas pharmacokinetic parameters following multiple dosing schedules were similar.[1]

1. Richens A, *et al.* Single and multiple dose pharmacokinetics of felbamate in the elderly. *Br J Clin Pharmacol* 1997; **44:** 129–34.

**Administration in renal impairment.** A single-dose pharmacokinetic study[1] indicated that in patients with renal impairment the initial dose of felbamate may need to be lower and increases made more cautiously than in patients with normal renal function.

1. Glue P, *et al.* Single-dose pharmacokinetics of felbamate in patients with renal dysfunction. *Br J Clin Pharmacol* 1997; **44:** 91–3.

**Epilepsy.** Although felbamate was well tolerated in clinical trials, rare but serious adverse effects were noted during early post-marketing use.[1,2] Aplastic anaemia and serious hepatotoxic reactions, sometimes with fatal outcomes, developed in some patients. Patients taking felbamate should have frequent blood counts and monitoring of liver enzymes. However there is no evidence that such monitoring will prevent adverse outcomes; in addition, the risk of aplastic anaemia is thought to decrease after the first year of therapy, and the need for ongoing blood counts is still less clear.[3] Even if detected early, aplastic anaemia and hepatic impairment may not be reversible.[1] Usage in the USA is restricted to patients with refractory partial seizures with or without secondary generalisation or for adjunctive therapy for children with Lennox-Gastaut syndrome. Guidelines on appropriate use have been issued.[3]

The overall management of epilepsy is discussed on p.349.

1. Dichter MA, Brodie MJ. New antiepileptic drugs. *N Engl J Med* 1996; **334:** 1583–90.
2. Appleton RE. The new antiepileptic drugs. *Arch Dis Child* 1996; **75:** 256–62.
3. French J, *et al.* The use of felbamate in the treatment of patients with intractable epilepsy. Report of the Quality Standards Subcommittee of the American Academy of Neurology and the American Epilepsy Society. *Epilepsia* 1999; **40:** 803–8.

### Preparations

**Proprietary Preparations** (details are given in Part 3)

***Arg.:*** Felbamyl; ***Austria:*** Taloxa; ***Belg.:*** Taloxa; ***Fr.:*** Taloxa; ***Ger.:*** Taloxa; ***Ital.:*** Taloxa; ***Neth.:*** Taloxa; ***Norw.:*** Taloxa; ***Port.:*** Taloxa; ***Spain:*** Taloxa†; ***Swed.:*** Taloxa; ***Switz.:*** Taloxa; ***USA:*** Felbatol.

## Fosphenytoin Sodium (BANM, USAN, rINNM)

ACC-9653; ACC-9653-010; CI-982 (fosphenytoin or fosphenytoin sodium); Fosfenitoína sódica; PD-135711-15B. 5,5-Diphenyl-3-[(phosphonooxy)methyl]-2,4-imidazolidinedione, disodium salt; 3-(Hydroxymethyl)-5,5-diphenylhydantoin, disodium phosphate (ester); 2,5-Dioxo-4,4-diphenylimidazolidin-1-ylmethyl phosphate disodium.

$C_{16}H_{13}N_2Na_2O_6P$ = 406.2.

*CAS — 93390-81-9 (fosphenytoin); 92134-98-0 (fosphenytoin sodium).*

*ATC — N03AB05.*

**Pharmacopoeias.** In *US.*

**USP 27** (Fosphenytoin Sodium). A white to pale yellow solid. Freely soluble in water. pH of a 7.5% solution in water is between 8.5 and 9.5. Store in airtight containers.

**Stability.** References.

1. Fischer JH, *et al.* Stability of fosphenytoin sodium with intravenous solutions in glass bottles, polyvinyl chloride bags, and polypropylene syringes. *Ann Pharmacother* 1997; **31:** 553–9.

### Adverse Effects and Precautions

As for Phenytoin, p.370.

Severe cardiovascular reactions, sometimes fatal, have been reported following intravenous administration of fosphenytoin. Therefore, continuous monitoring of ECG, blood pressure, and respiratory function is recommended during the infusion, and the patient should be kept under observation for at least 30 minutes after the end of the infusion. Hypotension may occur with recommended doses and rates of infusion; a reduction in the infusion rate or discontinuation of therapy may be necessary.

Burning, itching, and paraesthesia, particularly in the groin area, have also been reported following intravenous administration of fosphenytoin; reducing the rate of, or temporarily stopping, the infusion may relieve the discomfort.

Caution should be exercised when giving fosphenytoin to patients in whom phosphate restriction is necessary. The rate of metabolism of fosphenytoin to phenytoin may be increased after intravenous administration to patients with hepatic or renal disease, or in those with hypoalbuminaemia, and consequently there is an increased risk of adverse effects in such patients.

**Effects on the cardiovascular system.** The UK Committee on the Safety of Medicines[1] stated in May 2000 that worldwide there had been reports of 21 cases of asystole, ventricular fibrillation, or cardiac arrest associated with intravenous administration of fosphenytoin. Of these, 5 cases had received doses or infusion rates greater than recommended. There had also been 34 reports of hypotension, 15 of bradycardia, and 10 of varying degrees of heart block. Most reactions had occurred within 30 minutes of the infusion.

ECG changes consistent with hypocalcaemia have occurred in a patient who received 1500 mg-equivalents of phenytoin over 85 minutes as an intravenous infusion of fosphenytoin.[2] The patient had initially been normocalcaemic and it was suggested that the effect may have been due to acute inorganic phosphate toxicity.

1. Committee on Safety of Medicines/Medicines Control Agency. Fosphenytoin sodium (Pro-Epanutin): serious arrhythmias and hypotension. *Current Problems* 2000; **26:** 1. Also available at: http://www.mca.gov.uk/ourwork/monitorsafequalmed/currentproblems/cpmay2000.pdf (accessed 13/05/04)
2. Keegan MT, *et al.* Hypocalcemia-like electrocardiographic changes after administration of intravenous fosphenytoin. *Mayo Clin Proc* 2002; **77:** 584–6.

**Porphyria.** Phenytoin is considered unsafe in porphyric patients; it would be prudent to assume that this consideration also applied to its prodrug, fosphenytoin.

## Interactions

As for Phenytoin, p.372.

## Pharmacokinetics

Plasma concentrations of fosphenytoin are maximal at the end of intravenous infusion and about 30 minutes after intramuscular injection. Protein binding of fosphenytoin is high (95 to 99%) and is saturable; fosphenytoin displaces phenytoin from protein binding sites. Fosphenytoin is hydrolysed to phenytoin; one mmol of fosphenytoin yields one mmol of phenytoin. Other metabolites produced during the conversion include phosphate and formaldehyde. Metabolites of phenytoin are excreted in the urine. For the pharmacokinetics of phenytoin, see p.375.

## Uses and Administration

Fosphenytoin is a prodrug of phenytoin (p.370) used similarly as part of the emergency treatment of status epilepticus (p.352). It is also used for the prevention and treatment of post-traumatic seizures (p.376) associated with neurosurgery or head trauma and as a short-term parenteral substitute for oral phenytoin in the management of epilepsy (p.349).

Fosphenytoin is administered in the form of the sodium salt and doses of fosphenytoin sodium are expressed as phenytoin sodium equivalents (PSE); therefore no adjustment in dosage is necessary when substituting fosphenytoin for phenytoin or vice versa. Fosphenytoin may be given by intramuscular injection or intravenous infusion; only the intravenous route is recommended in children.

The maximum rate of intravenous infusion in PSE is 150 mg/minute (or in children aged 5 years and over, 3 mg/kg per minute) and should not be exceeded. Continuous monitoring of ECG, blood pressure, and respiratory function is recommended during intravenous infusion. Patients should also be observed for at least 30 minutes after the end of infusion.

In the treatment of tonic-clonic status epilepticus in the UK, the loading dose in PSE is 15 mg/kg by intravenous infusion at a rate of 100 to 150 mg/minute (or in children aged 5 years and over, 2 to 3 mg/kg per minute). The intramuscular route is not appropriate for the management of status epilepticus because peak phenytoin concentrations will not be reached quickly enough. The loading dose in PSE for seizures other than in status epilepticus is 10 to 15 mg/kg, given by intramuscular injection or by intravenous infusion at a rate of 50 to 100 mg/minute (or in children aged 5 years and over, 1 to 2 mg/kg per minute). Initial maintenance doses in PSE for status epilepticus and other seizures are 4 to 5 mg/kg daily given by intramuscular injection or by intravenous infusion at a rate of 50 to 100 mg/minute (or in children aged 5 years and over, 1 to 2 mg/kg per minute). Subsequent doses are dependent on patient response and trough plasma-phenytoin concentrations.

Fosphenytoin given intramuscularly or by intravenous infusion at a rate of 50 to 100 mg/minute may be substituted for oral phenytoin at the same equivalent total daily dose for up to 5 days.

In the USA, loading doses in PSE of up to 20 mg/kg are permitted, and maintenance doses are 4 to 6 mg/kg daily.

A lower loading dose and/or infusion rate, and lower or less frequent maintenance dosing may be necessary for elderly patients; the UK manufacturer suggests a reduction in dose or rate of 10 to 25%. Similar reductions are suggested for patients with renal or hepatic impairment (see also below) or in those with hypoalbuminaemia, except in the treatment of status epilepticus.

◊ References.

1. Wilder BJ, *et al.* Safety and tolerance of multiple doses of intramuscular fosphenytoin substituted for oral phenytoin in epilepsy or neurosurgery. *Arch Neurol* 1996; **53:** 764–8.
2. Meek PD, *et al.* Guidelines for nonemergency use of parenteral phenytoin products: proceedings of an expert panel consensus process. *Arch Intern Med* 1999; **159:** 2639–44.
3. Heafield MTE. Managing status epilepticus: new drug offers real advantages. *BMJ* 2000: **320:** 953–4.
4. DeToledo JC, Ramsay RE. Fosphenytoin and phenytoin in patients with status epilepticus: improved tolerability versus increased costs. *Drug Safety* 2000; **22:** 459–66.

**Administration in hepatic or renal impairment.** The rate and extent of conversion of fosphenytoin to phenytoin in patients with hepatic cirrhosis or renal impairment requiring dialysis was not found to be significantly different from those for healthy controls.[1] However, there was a trend towards an increase in fosphenytoin clearance and a decrease in the time to peak phenytoin concentrations in those with hepatic or renal impairment. Consequently, the authors recommended that fosphenytoin may need to be given at lower doses or infused more slowly (see above for the manufacturer's recommendations).

1. Aweeka FT, *et al.* Pharmacokinetics of fosphenytoin in patients with hepatic or renal disease. *Epilepsia* 1999; **40:** 777–82.

## Preparations

***USP 27:*** Fosphenytoin Sodium Injection.

**Proprietary Preparations** (details are given in Part 3)
***Austral.:*** Pro-Epanutin†; ***Austria:*** Pro-Epanutin; ***Canad.:*** Cerebyx; ***Denm.:*** Pro-Epanutin; ***Fin.:*** Pro-Epanutin; ***Fr.:*** Prodilantin; ***Gr.:*** Pro-Epanutin; ***Irl.:*** Pro-Epanutin; ***Neth.:*** Pro-Epanutin; ***Norw.:*** Pro-Epanutin; ***Port.:*** Pro-Epanutin†; ***Spain:*** Cereneu; ***Swed.:*** Pro-Epanutin; ***UK:*** Pro-Epanutin; ***USA:*** Cerebyx.

# Gabapentin *(BAN, USAN, rINN)*

CI-945; Gabapentina; GOE-3450. 1-(Aminomethyl)cyclohexaneacetic acid.

$C_9H_{17}NO_2$ = 171.2.
*CAS — 60142-96-3.*
*ATC — N03AX12.*

## Adverse Effects and Precautions

The most commonly reported adverse effects associated with gabapentin are somnolence, dizziness, ataxia, and fatigue. Nystagmus, tremor, diplopia, amblyopia, pharyngitis, dysarthria, weight gain, dyspepsia, amnesia, weakness, paraesthesia, arthralgia, purpura, leucopenia, anxiety, and urinary-tract infection may occur less frequently. Rarely, pancreatitis, altered liver function tests, erythema multiforme, Stevens-Johnson syndrome, rhinitis, nervousness, myalgia, headache, oedema, nausea and vomiting, and blood glucose fluctuations in diabetics have been reported. Rare CNS effects include confusion, depression, hallucinations, and psychoses.

Gabapentin should be used with caution in patients with a history of psychotic illness. It should also be used with caution in renal impairment; the manufacturer recommends dosage reduction in patients with reduced renal function or those undergoing haemodialysis. False positive readings have been reported with some urinary protein tests in patients taking gabapentin.

Care is required when withdrawing gabapentin therapy—see also under Uses and Administration, below.

**Breast feeding.** For comment on antiepileptic therapy and breast feeding, see p.351.

**Carcinogenicity.** It had been reported[1] that studies on gabapentin had been temporarily stopped in 1990 when pancreatic tumours were seen in *rodent* studies. However, the tumours were benign, occurred only with large doses, and were not thought to relate to humans.

1. Ramsay RE. Clinical efficacy and safety of gabapentin. *Neurology* 1994; **44** (suppl 5): S23–S30.

**Driving.** For a comment on antiepileptic drugs and driving, see p.351.

**Effects on bone.** For the effects of antiepileptics on bone and on calcium and vitamin D metabolism, see under Phenytoin, p.371.

**Effects on the liver.** A report[1] of a patient who developed cholestatic jaundice 2 weeks after starting therapy with gabapentin 300 mg three times daily for diabetic neuropathy. Clinical symptoms and liver function tests improved on withdrawal of gabapentin.

1. Richardson CE, *et al.* Gabapentin induced cholestasis. *BMJ* 2002; **325:** 635.

**Effects on mental function.** For a review of the effects of antiepileptic therapy including gabapentin on *cognition*, see p.351.

**Overdosage.** A 16-year-old girl complained of dizziness 6 hours after ingesting 48.9 g of gabapentin and was lethargic but arousable 2 hours later.[1] Her gabapentin plasma concentration was 62 micrograms/mL 8.5 hours after ingestion. By 18 hours she was alert and had no further complaints of lethargy or dizziness. In another report[2] a patient with renal failure inadvertently received inappropriately high doses of gabapentin for 3 weeks and had a serum gabapentin concentration of 85 micrograms/mL without serious adverse effects.

1. Fischer JH, *et al.* Lack of serious toxicity following gabapentin overdose. *Neurology* 1994; **44:** 982–3.
2. Verma A, *et al.* A case of sustained massive gabapentin overdose without serious side effects. *Ther Drug Monit* 1999; **21:** 615–17.

**Pregnancy.** For comments on the management of epilepsy during pregnancy, see p.351.

## Interactions

The absorption of gabapentin from the gastrointestinal tract is reduced by antacids containing aluminium with magnesium; it is recommended that gabapentin is taken at least 2 hours after the administration of such an antacid. Cimetidine has been reported to reduce the renal clearance of gabapentin but the manufacturers do not consider this to be of clinical importance. For references to possible interactions with other antiepileptics, see under Phenytoin, p.373 and under Felbamate, p.361.

## Pharmacokinetics

Gabapentin is absorbed from the gastrointestinal tract by means of a saturable mechanism. Following multiple dosing peak plasma concentrations are usually achieved within 2 hours of administration and steady state achieved within 1 to 2 days. Gabapentin is not appreciably metabolised and most of a dose is excreted unchanged in the urine with the remainder appearing in the faeces. Gabapentin is widely distributed throughout the body but binding to plasma proteins is minimal. The elimination half-life has been reported to be about 5 to 7 hours. Gabapentin is distributed into breast milk.

◊ References.

1. Blum RA, *et al.* Pharmacokinetics of gabapentin in subjects with various degrees of renal function. *Clin Pharmacol Ther* 1994; **56:** 154–9.
2. Elwes RDC, Binnie CD. Clinical pharmacokinetics of newer antiepileptic drugs: lamotrigine, vigabatrin, gabapentin and oxcarbazepine. *Clin Pharmacokinet* 1996; **30:** 403–15.

**In children.** A study[1] of the pharmacokinetics of gabapentin following single doses in children aged 1 month to 12 years found that peak plasma concentrations occurred 2 to 3 hours after the dose in all age groups but that the mean value was higher in those older than 5 years than in younger children, and the exposure was calculated to be about 30% less in the younger age group. As a result it was suggested that the initial dose of gabapentin in studies of safety and efficacy should be 40 mg/kg daily in children aged from 1 month up to 5 years, and 30 mg/kg daily in children aged 5 to 12 years. (For licensed doses, see Uses and Administration, below.)

1. Haig GM, *et al.* Single-dose gabapentin pharmacokinetics and safety in healthy infants and children. *J Clin Pharmacol* 2001; **41:** 507–14.

## Uses and Administration

Gabapentin is an antiepileptic effective in the treatment of partial seizures with or without secondary generalisation and is used as adjunctive therapy in patients unresponsive to or intolerant of standard antiepileptic drugs. It is not generally considered effective for absence seizures. Although gabapentin is an analogue of gamma-aminobutyric acid (GABA), it is neither a GABA agonist nor antagonist and its mechanism of action is unknown. Gabapentin is also used in the treatment of neuropathic pain.

The initial adult dose of gabapentin for the treatment of **epilepsy** is 300 mg by mouth on the first day of treatment, 300 mg twice daily on the second day, and 300 mg three times daily on the third day; thereafter the dose may be increased in increments of 300 mg daily until effective antiepileptic control is achieved, which is usually within the range of 0.9 to 1.2 g daily. Higher doses up to a maximum of 2.4 g daily may be required in some patients; in the USA, doses of up to 3.6 g daily administered for a short period have been reported to be well tolerated. The total daily dose should be taken in three equally divided doses and the maximum dosage interval should not exceed 12 hours. The initial dose for children 6 to 12 years of age for the treatment of epilepsy is 10 mg/kg on the first day of treatment, 20 mg/kg on the second day, and 25 to 35 mg/kg on the third day. Recommended maintenance doses are 900 mg daily for children weighing 26 to 36 kg and 1200 mg daily for those weighing 37 to 50 kg. In the USA, gabapentin is licensed for adjunctive use in children from 3 years of age. An initial dose of 10 to 15 mg/kg daily is recommended, increased over about 3 days to doses of about 40 mg/kg daily in those aged 3 to 4 years, or 25 to 35 mg/kg daily in those 5 years of age or older. The total daily dose should be taken in three divided doses.

In the treatment of **neuropathic pain** in adults, doses should be titrated to a usual maximum of 1.8 g daily in three divided doses, in a similar manner to that recommended for the treatment of epilepsy in adults given above, although the doses do not need to be equally divided.

As with other antiepileptics, withdrawal of gabapentin therapy or transition to or from another type of antiepileptic therapy should be made gradually to avoid precipitating an increase in the frequency of seizures. The manufacturers recommend reducing the dose gradually over at least 7 days. For a discussion on whether or not to withdraw antiepileptic therapy in seizure-free patients, see p.349.

Dosage of gabapentin should be reduced in patients with renal impairment—see below.

**Administration in renal impairment.** Reduced doses of gabapentin are recommended for patients with renal impairment or those undergoing haemodialysis. Suitable maintenance doses based on creatinine clearance (CC) and given as 3 divided doses are:

- CC 50 to 79 mL/minute: 600 to 1200 mg daily
- CC 30 to 49 mL/minute: 300 to 600 mg daily
- CC 15 to 29 mL/minute: 300 mg on alternate days to 300 mg daily
- CC less than 15 mL/minute: 300 mg on alternate days

For those undergoing haemodialysis who have never received gabapentin, the recommended loading dose is 300 to 400 mg followed by 200 to 300 mg after each 4 hours of haemodialysis.

**Bipolar disorder.** Although early open studies[1] found that gabapentin may be of benefit in patients with bipolar disorder (p.278), randomised controlled trials have so far failed to confirm this effect.[2,3]

1. Maidment ID. Gabapentin treatment for bipolar disorders. *Ann Pharmacother* 2001; **35:** 1264–9.
2. Pande AC, *et al.* Gabapentin in bipolar disorder: a placebo-controlled trial of adjunctive therapy. *Bipolar Disord* 2000; **2:** 249–55.
3. Frye MA, *et al.* A placebo-controlled study of lamotrigine and gabapentin monotherapy in refractory mood disorders. *J Clin Psychopharmacol* 2000; **20:** 607–14.

**Ciguatera poisoning.** Gabapentin has relieved some of the neurological symptoms associated with ciguatera poisoning (see Mannitol, p.951).

**Depression.** Gabapentin has been tried[1] for the augmentation of antidepressant therapy in the treatment of resistant depression (p.279).

1. Yasmin S, *et al.* Adjunctive gabapentin in treatment-resistant depression: a retrospective chart review. *J Affect Disord* 2001; **63:** 243–7.

**Epilepsy.** Gabapentin is used in epilepsy (p.349) as adjunctive therapy for partial seizures with or without secondary generalisation in patients refractory to standard antiepileptics. In double-blind placebo-controlled studies[1-4] in such patients seizure frequency was reduced when gabapentin was added to treatment. Long-term efficacy has been encouraging,[5-7] and its lack of potential for interactions with other antiepileptics is considered to make it particularly suitable for adjunctive treatment. Dosage is adjusted against clinical response rather than by monitoring blood concentrations. Experience of its use as monotherapy in partial epilepsy[8-10] is limited and its efficacy as adjunctive treatment in generalised seizures also remains to be determined.

Although experience with gabapentin in children is also limited it has been found to be effective as adjunctive therapy in children with refractory partial seizures.[11]

1. UK Gabapentin Study Group. Gabapentin in partial epilepsy. *Lancet* 1990; **335:** 1114–17.
2. Sivenius J, *et al.* Double-blind study of gabapentin in the treatment of partial seizures. *Epilepsia* 1991; **32:** 539–42.
3. US Gabapentin Study Group. Gabapentin as add-on therapy in refractory partial epilepsy: a double-blind, placebo-controlled, parallel-group study. *Neurology* 1993; **43:** 2292–8.
4. Anhut H, *et al.* International Gabapentin Study Group. Gabapentin (Neurontin) as add-on therapy in patients with partial seizures: a double-blind, placebo-controlled study. *Epilepsia* 1994; **35:** 795–801.
5. US Gabapentin Study Group. The long-term safety and efficacy of gabapentin (Neurontin®) as add-on therapy in drug-resistant partial epilepsy. *Epilepsy Res* 1994; **18:** 67–73.
6. Sivenius J, *et al.* Long-term study with gabapentin in patients with drug-resistant epileptic seizures. *Arch Neurol* 1994; **51:** 1047–50.
7. Anhut H, *et al.* Long-term safety and efficacy of gabapentin (Neurontin) as add-on therapy in patients with refractory partial seizures. *J Epilepsy* 1995; **8:** 44–50.
8. Ojemann LM, *et al.* Long-term treatment with gabapentin for partial epilepsy. *Epilepsy Res* 1992; **13:** 159–65.
9. Beydoun A, *et al.* Gabapentin monotherapy II: a 26-week, double-blind, dose-controlled multicenter study of conversion from polytherapy in outpatients with refractory complex partial or secondarily generalized seizures. *Neurology* 1997; **49:** 746–52.
10. Chadwick DW, *et al.* A double-blind trial of gabapentin monotherapy for newly diagnosed partial seizures. *Neurology* 1998; **51:** 1282–8.
11. Appleton R, *et al.* Gabapentin as add-on therapy in children with refractory partial seizures: a 12-week, multicentre, double-blind, placebo-controlled study. *Epilepsia* 1999; **40:** 1147–54.

**Headache.** Benefit has been reported[1] from the use of gabapentin in the prophylaxis of *migraine* (p.464). Gabapentin may also be effective[2] in the management of *cluster headache* (p.464).

1. Mathew NT, *et al.* Efficacy of gabapentin in migraine prophylaxis. *Headache* 2001; **41:** 119–128.
2. Leandri M, *et al.* Drug-resistant cluster headache responding to gabapentin: a pilot study. *Cephalalgia* 2001; **21:** 744–6.

**Lesch-Nyhan syndrome.** The severe self-mutilation that occurs in patients with Lesch-Nyhan syndrome (p.682) has been reported to improve in those given antiepileptics such as gabapentin.[1]

1. McManaman J, Tam DA. Gabapentin for self-injurious behavior in Lesch-Nyhan syndrome. *Pediatr Neurol* 1999; **20:** 381–2.

**Motor neurone disease.** Interest has been shown in gabapentin as a potential therapy for amyotrophic lateral sclerosis (see Motor Neurone Disease, p.1739) because it may inhibit glutamate formation. Results from an early study[1] demonstrated a trend towards a beneficial effect; however, a randomised trial[2] failed to confirm any benefit from gabapentin on disease progression or symptoms.

1. Miller RG, *et al.* Placebo-controlled trial of gabapentin in patients with amyotrophic lateral sclerosis. *Neurology* 1996; **47:** 1383–8.
2. Miller RG, *et al.* Phase III randomized trial of gabapentin in patients with amyotrophic lateral sclerosis. *Neurology* 2001; **56:** 843–8.

**Multiple sclerosis.** Gabapentin has been found to control pain, spasm, and spasticity in patients with multiple sclerosis (p.646).

References.

1. Mueller ME, *et al.* Gabapentin for relief of upper motor neuron symptoms in multiple sclerosis. *Arch Phys Med Rehabil* 1997; **78:** 521–4.
2. Samkoff LM, *et al.* Amelioration of refractory dysesthetic limb pain in multiple sclerosis by gabapentin. *Neurology* 1997; **49:** 304–5.
3. Solaro C, *et al.* An open-label trial of gabapentin treatment of paroxysmal symptoms in multiple sclerosis patients. *Neurology* 1998; **51:** 609–11.
4. Dunevsky A, Perel AB. Gabapentin for relief of spasticity associated with multiple sclerosis. *Am J Phys Med Rehabil* 1998; **77:** 451–4.
5. Cutter NC, *et al.* Gabapentin effect on spasticity in multiple sclerosis: a placebo-controlled, randomized trial. *Arch Phys Med Rehabil* 2000; **81:** 164–9.
6. Solaro C, *et al.* Gabapentin is effective in treating nocturnal painful spasms in multiple sclerosis. *Multiple Sclerosis* 2000; **6:** 192–3.

**Neuropathic pain.** Antiepileptics are among the drugs used to manage neuropathic pain, which is often insensitive to opioid analgesics (see Choice of Analgesic, p.2). Although carbamazepine appears to be the antiepileptic most frequently used, gabapentin is also given in the treatment of neuropathic pain,[1,2] including central pain[3] (see p.5), complex regional pain syndrome (see p.5), postherpetic neuralgia[4-6] (see p.7), trigeminal neuralgia (see p.8), and painful diabetic neuropathy[7,8] (see also p.6).

1. Rose MA, Kam PC. Gabapentin: pharmacology and its use in pain management. *Anaesthesia* 2002; **57:** 451–62.
2. Backonja M, Glanzman RL. Gabapentin dosing for neuropathic pain: evidence from randomized, placebo-controlled clinical trials. *Clin Ther* 2003; **25:** 81–104.
3. Schachter SC, Sauter MK. Treatment of central pain with gabapentin: case reports. *J Epilepsy* 1996; **9:** 223–5.
4. Rowbotham M, *et al.* Gabapentin for the treatment of postherpetic neuralgia: a randomized controlled trial. *JAMA* 1998; **280:** 1837–42.
5. Rice ASC, Maton S. Gabapentin in postherpetic neuralgia: a randomised, double blind, placebo controlled study. *Pain* 2001; **94:** 215–24.
6. Singh D, Kennedy DH. The use of gabapentin for the treatment of postherpetic neuralgia. *Clin Ther* 2003; **25:** 852–89.
7. Backonja M, *et al.* Gabapentin for the symptomatic treatment of painful neuropathy in patients with diabetes mellitus: a randomized controlled trial. *JAMA* 1998; **280:** 1831–6.
8. Morello CM, *et al.* Randomized double-blind study comparing the efficacy of gabapentin with amitriptyline on diabetic peripheral neuropathy pain. *Arch Intern Med* 1999; **159:** 1931–7.

**Parkinsonism.** While some overall ratings of Parkinson's disease (p.1196) appeared to be improved by gabapentin in a double-blind study involving 19 patients with advanced parkinsonism, improvements in individual signs and symptoms were not significant.[1] It was also reported that 5 of 6 other patients with progressive supranuclear palsy had experienced worsening of their disease when given gabapentin.

1. Olson WL, *et al.* Gabapentin for parkinsonism: a double-blind, placebo-controlled, crossover trial. *Am J Med* 1997; **102:** 60–6.

**Restless legs syndrome.** The aetiology of restless legs syndrome (see Parasomnias, p.667) is obscure and treatment has been largely empirical. Two small randomised double-blind crossover studies[1,2] found 6 weeks' treatment with gabapentin to produce improvement in symptoms; in patients undergoing haemodialysis the effects were seen with a dose of 300 mg after each of the 3 dialysis sessions per week,[1] although in patients with idiopathic disease the mean effective dose was 1.855 g daily.[2]

1. Thorp ML, *et al.* A crossover study of gabapentin in treatment of restless legs syndrome among hemodialysis patients. *Am J Kidney Dis* 2001; **38:** 104–8.
2. Garcia-Borreguero D, *et al.* Treatment of restless legs syndrome with gabapentin: a double-blind, cross-over study. *Neurology* 2002; **59:** 1573–9.

**Stiff-man syndrome.** Gabapentin may improve the symptoms of stiff-man syndrome (p.696) in patients unable to tolerate benzodiazepine therapy.

## Preparations

**Proprietary Preparations** (details are given in Part 3)

***Arg.:*** Neurontin; ***Austral.:*** Gantin; Neurontin; Pendine; ***Austria:*** Neurontin; ***Belg.:*** Neurontin; ***Braz.:*** Neurontin; Progresse; ***Canad.:*** Neurontin; ***Chile:*** Dineurin; Normatol; ***Fin.:*** Neurontin; ***Fr.:*** Neurontin; ***Ger.:*** Neurontin; ***Gr.:*** Neurontin; ***Hong Kong:*** Neurontin; ***India:*** Neurontin; ***Irl.:*** Neurontin; Neurostil; ***Israel:*** Neurontin; ***Ital.:*** Aclonium†; Neurontin; ***Malaysia:*** Neurontin; ***Mex.:*** Neurontin; ***Neth.:*** Neurontin; ***Norw.:*** Neurontin; ***NZ:*** Neurontin; ***Port.:*** Neurontin; ***S.Afr.:*** Neurontin; ***Singapore:*** Neurontin; ***Spain:*** Equipax†; Neurontin; ***Swed.:*** Neurontin; ***Switz.:*** Neurontin; ***Thai.:*** Neurontin; ***UK:*** Neurontin; ***USA:*** Neurontin.

# Lamotrigine *(BAN, USAN, rINN)*

BW-430C; Lamotrigina. 6-(2,3-Dichlorophenyl)-1,2,4-triazine-3,5-diyldiamine.

$C_9H_7Cl_2N_5$ = 256.1.

*CAS — 84057-84-1.*

*ATC — N03AX09.*

## Adverse Effects and Treatment

Skin rashes may occur during therapy with lamotrigine; severe skin reactions including Stevens-Johnson syndrome and toxic epidermal necrolysis have been reported, especially in children, and usually occur within 8 weeks of starting lamotrigine. Symptoms such as fever, malaise, flu-like symptoms, drowsiness, lymphadenopathy, facial oedema and, rarely, hepatic dysfunction, leucopenia, and thrombocytopenia have also been reported in conjunction with rashes as part of a hypersensitivity syndrome.

Other adverse effects include angioedema and photosensitivity; diplopia, blurred vision, and conjunctivitis; and dizziness, drowsiness, insomnia, headache, ataxia, nystagmus, tremor, tiredness, nausea and vomiting, irritability and aggression, hallucinations, agitation, and confusion.

◊ The manufacturers report that there have been rare instances of death following a rapidly progressive illness with status epilepticus, multi-organ dysfunction, and disseminated intravascular coagulation in patients receiving therapy with multiple antiepileptics including lamotrigine, although the role of lamotrigine remains to be established. It has been suggested[1] that multi-organ failure and disseminated intravascular coagulation, with associated rhabdomyolysis, are complications of severe convulsive seizures rather than of lamotrigine therapy. However, there has been a report[2] of a patient with no history of generalised seizures who developed a syndrome of disseminated intravascular coagulation, rhabdomyolysis, renal failure, maculopapular rash, and ataxia 14 days after lamotrigine was added to her antiepileptic regimen. Two cases of disseminated intravascular coagulation were found in a cohort of 11316 patients involved in prescription-event monitoring of lamotrigine therapy in general practice.[3]

1. Yuen AWC, Bihari DJ. Multiorgan failure and disseminated intravascular coagulation in severe convulsive seizures. *Lancet* 1992; **340:** 618.
2. Schaub JEM, *et al.* Multisystem adverse reaction to lamotrigine. *Lancet* 1994; **344:** 481.
3. Mackay FJ, *et al.* Safety of long-term lamotrigine in epilepsy. *Epilepsia* 1997; **38:** 881–6.

**Effects on the blood.** Septic shock secondary to leucopenia occurred in a patient when lamotrigine was added to therapy with sodium valproate.[1] There has also been a report of agranulocytosis in a child given high initial doses of monotherapy with lamotrigine.[2] The fall in the blood count was noted several days after lamotrigine had been discontinued due to skin rash. The UK Committee on Safety of Medicines (CSM) subsequently reported[3] that 7 cases of aplastic anaemia, 12 of bone-marrow depression, and 20 of pancytopenia associated with lamotrigine had been received worldwide. Given the extensive usage of lamotrigine the CSM considered the risk of aplastic anaemia to be small and routine blood monitoring was not recommended.

However, prescribers were warned to be alert for symptoms and signs suggestive of bone-marrow depression.

1. Nicholson RJ, *et al.* Leucopenia associated with lamotrigine. *BMJ* 1995; **310:** 504.
2. de Camargo OAK, Bode H. Agranulocytosis associated with lamotrigine. *BMJ* 1999; **318:** 1179.
3. Committee on Safety of Medicines/Medicines Control Agency. Lamotrigine (Lamictal): rare blood dyscrasias. *Current Problems* 2000; **26:** 4. Also available at: http://www.mca.gov.uk/ourwork/monitorsafequalmed/currentproblems/cpmay2000.pdf (accessed 13/05/04)

**Effects on bone.** For the effects of antiepileptics including lamotrigine on bone and on calcium and vitamin D metabolism, see under Phenytoin, p.371.

**Effects on the liver.** Fatal fulminant hepatic failure has been reported[1] in a patient following addition of lamotrigine to an antiepileptic regimen comprising sodium valproate and carbamazepine.

1. Makin AJ, *et al.* Fulminant hepatic failure induced by lamotrigine. *BMJ* 1995; **311:** 292.

**Effects on mental function.** For a review of the effects of antiepileptic therapy including lamotrigine on *cognition*, see p.351.

**Effects on the skin.** Rashes account for withdrawal from therapy in about 2% of those given lamotrigine,[1,2] and serious skin reactions including Stevens-Johnson syndrome and toxic epidermal necrolysis occur in about 1 in 1000 adult patients.[3,4] The main risk factors appear to be concomitant use with valproate, and exceeding the recommended initial dose of lamotrigine or the recommended rate of dose escalation. The risk appears to be greater in children[1,4,5] and has been estimated to be between 1 in 300 and 1 in 50. These skin reactions usually occur within 8 weeks of starting therapy with lamotrigine, but onset as early as the first day and as late as 2 years has been noted.[6] Following continuing reports of serious skin reactions in children, UK recommended dosage regimens for children have been revised to further reduce the risk of such reactions.[7]

1. Mackay FJ, *et al.* Safety of long-term lamotrigine in epilepsy. *Epilepsia* 1997; **38:** 881–6.
2. Messenheimer J, *et al.* Safety review of adult clinical trial experience with lamotrigine. *Drug Safety* 1998; **18:** 281–96.
3. Committee on Safety of Medicines/Medicines Control Agency. Lamotrigine (Lamictal) and serious skin reactions. *Current Problems* 1996; **22:** 12. Also available at: http://www.mca.gov.uk/ourwork/monitorsafequalmed/currentproblems/volume22.htm (accessed 04/06/04)
4. Committee on Safety of Medicines/Medicines Control Agency. Lamotrigine (Lamictal): increased risk of serious skin reactions in children. *Current Problems* 1997; **23:** 8. Also available at: http://www.mca.gov.uk/ourwork/monitorsafequalmed/currentproblems/volume24.htm (accessed 04/06/04)
5. Mitchell P. Paediatric lamotrigine use hit by rash reports. *Lancet* 1997; **349:** 1080.
6. Adverse Drug Reactions Advisory Committee (ADRAC). Lamotrigine and severe skin reactions. *Aust Adverse Drug React Bull* 1997; **16:** 3. Also available at: http://www.tga.health.gov.au/docs/html/aadrbltn/aadr9702.htm (accessed 07/06/04)
7. Committee on Safety of Medicines/Medicines Control Agency. Lamotrigine (Lamictal): revised doses for children. *Current Problems* 2000; **26:** 3. Also available at: http://www.mca.gov.uk/ourwork/monitorsafequalmed/currentproblems/cpmay2000.pdf (accessed 13/05/04)

**Overdosage.** No serious toxicity was observed in a patient who deliberately took an overdose of 1.35 g of lamotrigine and was subsequently treated with gastric lavage and activated charcoal.[1] Symptoms at presentation one hour after ingestion had included nystagmus and muscle hypertonicity. ECG monitoring had revealed widening of the QRS interval. Low-grade fever, erythema, and periorbital oedema suggestive of a hypersensitivity syndrome developed in another patient who inadvertently received lamotrigine 2.7 g daily for 4 days.[2] The patient recovered following corticosteroid treatment and discontinuation of lamotrigine. Generalised tonic-clonic seizures, tremor, muscle weakness, ataxia, and hypertonia were reported[3] in a 2-year-old child following ingestion of 800 mg of lamotrigine. Symptoms resolved within 24 hours following treatment with gastric lavage and activated charcoal, midazolam, and fluids. Plasma-lamotrigine concentrations were in the high adult therapeutic range (3.8 micrograms/mL) with a slow elimination rate.

For a further review of the features and management of poisoning with some antiepileptics, including lamotrigine, see under Phenytoin, p.371.

1. Buckley NA, *et al.* Self-poisoning with lamotrigine. *Lancet* 1993; **342:** 1552–3.
2. Mylonakis E, *et al.* Lamotrigine overdose presenting as anticonvulsant hypersensitivity syndrome. *Ann Pharmacother* 1999; **33:** 557–9.
3. Briassoulis G, *et al.* Lamotrigine childhood overdose. *Pediatr Neurol* 1998; **19:** 239–42.

## Precautions

Lamotrigine should be given with caution to patients with hepatic or renal impairment. Patients receiving lamotrigine should be closely monitored, especially for changes in hepatic, renal, and clotting functions. Children's body-weight should also be monitored and the dose reviewed if necessary. All patients should be warned to see their doctor immediately if rashes or flu-like symptoms associated with hypersensitivity develop. To minimise the risk of developing serious skin reactions, dosage recommendations should not be exceeded. Particular care is needed in patients also receiving valproate—see under Interactions, below.

Withdrawal of lamotrigine should be considered if rash, fever, flu-like symptoms, drowsiness, or worsening of seizure control occurs. Care is required when withdrawing lamotrigine therapy—see also under Uses and Administration, below. Abrupt withdrawal should be avoided unless serious skin reactions have occurred.

**Breast feeding.** The American Academy of Pediatrics[1] considers that the use of lamotrigine by mothers during breast feeding may be of concern, since there is the potential for therapeutic serum concentrations to occur in the infant. A case report[2] gave an estimated milk-to-plasma ratio for lamotrigine of 0.6, but although the authors considered such a value might be associated with pharmacological effects, no adverse effects were noted in the breast-fed infant in this case.

For further comment on antiepileptic therapy and breast feeding, see p.351.

1. American Academy of Pediatrics. The transfer of drugs and other chemicals into human milk. *Pediatrics* 2001; **108:** 776–89. Correction. *ibid.*; 1029. Also available at: http://aappolicy.aappublications.org/cgi/content/full/pediatrics%3b108/3/776 (accessed 13/05/04)
2. Tomson T, *et al.* Lamotrigine in pregnancy and lactation: a case report. *Epilepsia* 1997; **38:** 1039–41.

**Driving.** For a comment on antiepileptic drugs and driving, see p.351.

**Hepatic impairment.** The pharmacokinetics of lamotrigine were not significantly altered in patients with moderate cirrhosis;[1] however, those with severe cirrhosis showed significantly lower oral clearance and longer elimination half-lives than those in healthy subjects.

The manufacturers' recommended doses in patients with hepatic impairment are given in Uses and Administration, below.

1. Marcellin P, *et al.* Influence of cirrhosis on lamotrigine pharmacokinetics. *Br J Clin Pharmacol* 2001; **51:** 410–14.

**Intellectual impairment.** Aggressive behaviour has been reported in intellectually impaired patients given lamotrigine.[1] Of 19 such patients given lamotrigine, aggressive behaviour developed in 9; the drug was discontinued in 5, and stopped but reintroduced in a further 2, together with psychiatric management. One patient responded to a reduction in lamotrigine dosage.

1. Beran RG, Gibson RJ. Aggressive behaviour in intellectually challenged patients with epilepsy treated with lamotrigine. *Epilepsia* 1998; **39:** 280–2.

**Pregnancy.** For comments on the management of epilepsy during pregnancy, see p.351. There is a theoretical risk of teratogenicity with lamotrigine because, like valproate, it is a folate antagonist. In 2002 the manufacturer of lamotrigine, GlaxoSmithKline, reported[1] that it had follow-up information on 395 outcomes of pregnancies exposed to lamotrigine between September 1992 and September 2001. Major birth defects were found in 13 infants but no distinctive pattern of abnormalities suggestive of a common cause could be identified. Of the 168 who had been exposed to lamotrigine monotherapy during the first trimester, birth defects were reported in 3 (1.8%). The frequency of major birth defects in pregnancies exposed to polytherapy containing lamotrigine with valproate was 10% compared with 4.3% in lamotrigine polytherapy without valproate. Although it was considered that the sample sizes were too small to rule out a small increase in the frequency of major birth defects it was noted that the frequency of malformations after lamotrigine monotherapy did not differ from that reported in the literature for women with epilepsy receiving antiepileptic monotherapy.

1. Tennis P, *et al.* Preliminary results on pregnancy outcomes in women using lamotrigine. *Epilepsia* 2002; **43:** 1161–7.

**Renal impairment.** Results from a pharmacokinetic study[1] indicated that impaired renal function was likely to have little effect on plasma concentrations of lamotrigine. The drug is mainly cleared by metabolism and although the glucuronide metabolite accumulates it is inactive. Nevertheless, there is limited clinical experience with lamotrigine in such patients and caution was recommended.

1. Wootton R, *et al.* Comparison of the pharmacokinetics of lamotrigine in patients with chronic renal failure and healthy volunteers. *Br J Clin Pharmacol* 1997; **43:** 23–7.

## Interactions

There are complex interactions between antiepileptics and toxicity may be enhanced without a corresponding increase in antiepileptic activity. Such interactions are very variable and unpredictable and plasma monitoring is often advisable with combination therapy. The metabolism of lamotrigine is enhanced by the enzyme inducers carbamazepine, phenytoin, phenobarbital, and primidone, and inhibited by valproate (see below).

**Analgesics.** *Paracetamol* affects the metabolic disposition of lamotrigine but the clinical significance of this interaction remains to be determined.[1] Paracetamol reduced the area under the plasma concentration-time curve for lamotrigine, reduced lamotrigine's half-life, and increased the percentage of lamotrigine recovered in the urine.

1. Depot M, *et al.* Kinetic effects of multiple oral doses of acetaminophen on a single oral dose of lamotrigine. *Clin Pharmacol Ther* 1990; **48:** 346–55.

**Antibacterials.** Use with *rifampicin* significantly increased the clearance of lamotrigine.[1] The total urinary excretion of lamotrigine and the amount excreted as glucuronide were significantly higher compared with placebo.

1. Ebert U, *et al.* Effects of rifampicin and cimetidine on pharmacokinetics and pharmacodynamics of lamotrigine in healthy subjects. *Eur J Clin Pharmacol* 2000; **56:** 299–304.

**Antidepressants.** An epileptic patient maintained on lamotrigine 200 mg daily complained[1] of increasing confusion and cognitive impairment after starting *sertraline* 25 mg daily for post-traumatic disorder; after 6 weeks her lamotrigine blood concentrations had risen from 2.5 to 5.1 micrograms/mL during this period. The adverse effects cleared and blood concentrations of lamotrigine fell to 3.1 micrograms/mL within 3 weeks of changing the daily dosage to lamotrigine 100 mg and sertraline 50 mg. A poorly controlled epileptic patient who initially had been receiving lamotrigine 450 mg and sertraline 75 mg together daily for 6 weeks without adverse effects had marked sedation, fatigue, and decreased cognition 6 weeks after the daily dosage of lamotrigine was increased to 600 mg. Her lamotrigine blood concentration was 19.3 micrograms/mL. The patient was subsequently stabilised on lamotrigine 800 mg and sertraline 50 mg daily and had less sedation and fatigue and clearer cognition; blood concentrations of lamotrigine fell to 9.8 micrograms/mL.

1. Kaufman KR, Gerner R. Lamotrigine toxicity secondary to sertraline. *Seizure* 1998; **7:** 163–5.

**Antiepileptics.** *Valproate* can inhibit the metabolism of lamotrigine resulting in increased concentrations of lamotrigine. This effect can be beneficial in the control of certain seizures, although careful monitoring is required as toxicity may occur. Disabling tremor occurred in 3 patients receiving such a combination which resolved when the dose of lamotrigine or valproate was reduced.[1]

Other reported symptoms of toxicity, that resolved on reduction of the lamotrigine dose, were sedation, ataxia, and fatigue.[2] Reversible encephalopathy has been reported[3] when sodium valproate was substituted for phenytoin in a patient also receiving lamotrigine, although her clinical condition had been satisfactory on this new regimen for several months. Symptoms improved when the doses of both valproate and lamotrigine were reduced. Pharmacokinetic studies[4,5] in healthy adults have attempted to elucidate the mechanism of the interaction between lamotrigine and valproate. The clearance of lamotrigine was found to be reduced, and the area under the curve and elimination half-life increased when valproate was administered concomitantly. Renal elimination was not affected and the investigators[4] suggested that there was hepatic competition for glucuronidation between valproate and lamotrigine. However, there was no substantial alteration in the linear kinetics of lamotrigine in the presence of therapeutic plasma concentrations of valproate.[5] Similar observations were made when lamotrigine was added to existing antiepileptic regimens in children,[6] although the clinical relevance of the influence of age on the pharmacokinetics remains to be determined. Both young age and concomitant administration of valproate are risk factors for lamotrigine-induced dermatological toxicity—see Effects on the Skin, above.

For details of dosage reductions required for lamotrigine used with valproate, see Uses and Administration, below.

Other antiepileptics also affect plasma concentrations of lamotrigine. In contrast to valproate, *carbamazepine, phenytoin*, or *phenobarbital* all markedly induced the elimination of lamotrigine.[7] Others have confirmed a reduction in plasma-lamotrigine concentrations when given with phenytoin and other enzyme-inducing antiepileptics,[8] but analysis of results from another study[9] suggested that the increase in lamotrigine clearance by phenytoin and carbamazepine was of minimal clinical significance. Plasma-lamotrigine concentrations were also significantly reduced when given with *mesuximide* in 16 young patients (aged 9 to 19 years) with a variety of seizure types and syndromes.[10]

For the effect of lamotrigine on carbamazepine or clonazepam concentrations, see p.356 and p.359, respectively. For a report of severe toxicity occurring with concomitant use of lamotrigine and *oxcarbazepine*, see p.367.

1. Reutens DC, *et al.* Disabling tremor after lamotrigine with sodium valproate. *Lancet* 1993; **342:** 185–6.
2. Pisani F, *et al.* Interaction of lamotrigine with sodium valproate. *Lancet* 1993; **341:** 1224.
3. Hennessy MJ, Wiles CM. Lamotrigine encephalopathy. *Lancet* 1996; **347:** 974–5.
4. Yuen AWC, *et al.* Sodium valproate acutely inhibits lamotrigine metabolism. *Br J Clin Pharmacol* 1992; **33:** 511–13.
5. Anderson GD, *et al.* Bidirectional interaction of valproate and lamotrigine in healthy subjects. *Clin Pharmacol Ther* 1996; **60:** 145–56.
6. Vauzelle-Kervroëdan F, *et al.* Influence of concurrent antiepileptic medication on the pharmacokinetics of lamotrigine as add-on therapy in epileptic children. *Br J Clin Pharmacol* 1996; **41:** 325–30.
7. May TW, *et al.* Serum concentrations of lamotrigine in epileptic patients: the influence of dose and comedication. *Ther Drug Monit* 1996; **18:** 523–31.
8. Battino D, *et al.* Lamotrigine plasma concentrations in children and adults: influence of age and associated therapy. *Ther Drug Monit* 1997; **19:** 620–7.

9. Grasela TH, *et al.* Population pharmacokinetics of lamotrigine adjunctive therapy in adults with epilepsy. *J Clin Pharmacol* 1999; **39:** 373–84.
10. Besag FM, *et al.* Methsuximide lowers lamotrigine blood levels: a pharmacokinetic antiepileptic drug interaction. *Epilepsia* 2000; **41:** 624–7.

## Pharmacokinetics

Lamotrigine is well absorbed from the gastrointestinal tract and peak plasma concentrations occur approximately 2.5 hours after oral administration. It is widely distributed in the body and is reported to be about 55% bound to plasma protein. It is extensively metabolised in the liver and excreted almost entirely in urine, principally as a glucuronide conjugate. It slightly induces its own metabolism and the half-life at steady state is reported to be about 24 hours. Lamotrigine is distributed into breast milk.

The pharmacokinetics of lamotrigine are affected by other antiepileptics (see Interactions, above).

◊ General references.

1. Rambeck B, Wolf P. Lamotrigine clinical pharmacokinetics. *Clin Pharmacokinet* 1993; **25:** 433–43.
2. Elwes RDC, Binnie CD. Clinical pharmacokinetics of newer antiepileptic drugs: lamotrigine, vigabatrin, gabapentin and oxcarbazepine. *Clin Pharmacokinet* 1996; **30:** 403–15.

**Renal impairment.** See under Precautions, above.

**Therapeutic drug monitoring.** A literature review[1] concluded that a clear relationship between lamotrigine concentrations and toxicity or antiepileptic efficacy has not been demonstrated. Routine therapeutic drug monitoring was therefore not recommended and clinical end-points rather than plasma concentrations remained the best guide for dosage adjustment of lamotrigine.

1. Chong E, Dupuis LL. Therapeutic drug monitoring of lamotrigine. *Ann Pharmacother* 2002; **36:** 917–20.

## Uses and Administration

Lamotrigine, a phenyltriazine compound, is an antiepileptic used as monotherapy and as an adjunct to treatment with other antiepileptics for partial seizures and primary and secondarily generalised tonic-clonic seizures. It is also used for seizures associated with the Lennox-Gastaut syndrome. Another use of lamotrigine is in the prophylaxis of bipolar disorder.

The doses given below for the use of lamotrigine in **epilepsy** are those licensed in the UK; similar doses are given in the USA although the use of lamotrigine is more limited than in the UK.

- The initial **adult** dose for use as *monotherapy* is 25 mg once daily by mouth for 2 weeks followed by 50 mg once daily for 2 weeks; thereafter the dose is increased by a maximum of 50 to 100 mg every 1 to 2 weeks to usual maintenance doses of 100 to 200 mg daily, given as a single dose or in 2 divided doses. Some patients have required up to 500 mg daily.
- The initial adult dose of lamotrigine for use as an *adjunct* to therapy with enzyme-inducing antiepileptics (but *not with valproate*) is 50 mg once daily for 2 weeks followed by 50 mg twice daily for 2 weeks; thereafter the dose is increased by a maximum of 100 mg every 1 to 2 weeks to usual maintenance doses of 200 to 400 mg daily given in 2 divided doses. Some patients have required up to 700 mg daily.
- In adults *taking valproate* the initial dose of lamotrigine is 25 mg every other day for 2 weeks followed by 25 mg once daily for 2 weeks; thereafter the dose is increased by a maximum of 25 to 50 mg every 1 to 2 weeks to usual maintenance doses of 100 to 200 mg daily given as a single dose or in 2 divided doses.

The doses above are also permitted in **children** over 12 years of age; the use of lamotrigine as *monotherapy* is not recommended for children under 12 years of age.

- For children aged 2 to 12 years the initial dose of lamotrigine as an *adjunct* to therapy with enzyme-inducing antiepileptics (but *not with valproate*) is 600 micrograms/kg daily in 2 divided doses for 2 weeks followed by 1.2 mg/kg daily in 2 divided doses for 2 weeks; thereafter the dose is increased by a maximum of 1.2 mg/kg every 1 to 2 weeks to usual maintenance doses of 5 to 15 mg/kg daily given in 2 divided doses.
- In children *taking valproate*, the initial dose of lamotrigine is 150 micrograms/kg once daily for 2 weeks followed by 300 micrograms/kg once daily for 2 weeks; thereafter the dose is increased by a maximum of 300 micrograms/kg every 1 to 2 weeks to usual maintenance doses of 1 to 5 mg/kg, which may be given once daily or in 2 divided doses.
- If the calculated dose for children lies between 1 and 2 mg then 2 mg may be given on alternate days for the first 2 weeks of therapy. Lamotrigine should not be administered if the calculated dose is less than 1 mg.

If the potential for interaction with adjunctive antiepileptics is unknown, treatment with lamotrigine should be started with lower doses such as those used with valproate.

In the management of **bipolar disorder**, the target dose of lamotrigine is 200 mg daily as *monotherapy*; for patients *taking valproate* the target dose is 100 mg daily and in those taking enzyme-inducing drugs (but *not with valproate*) the target dose is 400 mg daily. Lamotrigine should be started at a reduced dose and increased gradually to the target dose in a regimen similar to that used in the treatment of epilepsy (see above).

Doses should be reduced in patients with hepatic impairment regardless of indication (see below).

As with other antiepileptics, withdrawal of lamotrigine therapy or transition to or from another type of antiepileptic therapy should be made gradually to avoid precipitating an increase in the frequency of seizures. For a discussion on whether or not to withdraw antiepileptic therapy in seizure-free patients, see p.349. The manufacturers recommend that regardless of indication the withdrawal of lamotrigine should be tapered over at least 2 weeks.

**Administration in hepatic impairment.** The manufacturers of lamotrigine recommend that doses should be reduced by about 50% in patients with moderate hepatic impairment, and by about 75% in severe hepatic impairment.

**Anxiety disorders.** Small studies have suggested that lamotrigine may relieve some of the symptoms of post-traumatic stress disorder (p.664).

References.

1. Hertzberg MA, *et al.* A preliminary study of lamotrigine for the treatment of posttraumatic stress disorder. *Biol Psychiatry* 1999; **45:** 1226–9.
2. Hageman I, *et al.* Post-traumatic stress disorder: a review of psychobiology and pharmacotherapy. *Acta Psychiatr Scand* 2001; **104:** 411–22.

**Bipolar disorder.** In a multicentre placebo-controlled study involving 195 patients, lamotrigine 50 or 200 mg daily by mouth produced dose-related improvement in patients with bipolar disorder (p.278) experiencing a major depressive episode.[1] A review[2] of this controlled study as well as earlier case reports and small open trials concluded that lamotrigine is a promising option for the treatment of refractory bipolar disorder. Further data from randomised controlled trials[3-6] and a more recent review[7] continue to suggest benefit.

1. Calabrese JR, *et al.* A double-blind placebo-controlled study of lamotrigine monotherapy in outpatients with bipolar I depression. *J Clin Psychiatry* 1999; **60:** 79–88.
2. Engle PM, Heck AM. Lamotrigine for the treatment of bipolar disorder. *Ann Pharmacother* 2000; **34:** 258–62.
3. Bowden CL, *et al.* Lamotrigine in the treatment of bipolar depression. *Eur Neuropsychopharmacol* 1999; **9** (suppl 4): S113–S117.
4. Calabrese JR, *et al.* A double-blind, placebo-controlled, prophylaxis study of lamotrigine in rapid-cycling bipolar disorder. *J Clin Psychiatry* 2000; **61:** 841–50.
5. Ichim L, *et al.* Lamotrigine compared with lithium in mania: a double-blind randomized controlled trial. *Ann Clin Psychiatry* 2000; **12:** 5–10.
6. Obrocea GV, *et al.* Clinical predictors of response to lamotrigine and gabapentin monotherapy in refractory affective disorders. *Biol Psychiatry* 2002; **51:** 253–60.
7. Hurley SC. Lamotrigine update and its use in mood disorders. *Ann Pharmacother* 2002; **36:** 860–73.

**Epilepsy.** Lamotrigine is used in the treatment of epilepsy (p.349) refractory to standard antiepileptic therapy. It has been used for both partial and secondarily generalised tonic-clonic seizures. A systematic review[1] of randomised, placebo-controlled trials concluded that lamotrigine is effective in reducing the seizure frequency when added to current antiepileptic regimens in patients with refractory partial seizures. About 30% of patients may experience a 50% reduction in seizure frequency and a relatively small percentage will become seizure-free.[2] Lamotrigine has shown comparable efficacy to carbamazepine as monotherapy for partial seizures with or without secondary generalisation and primary generalised tonic-clonic seizures in newly diagnosed patients.[3] It also appears to be an effective adjunctive treatment in children with the Lennox-Gastaut syndrome.[4,5] Lamotrigine has also been used for myoclonic seizures.

There are anecdotal reports suggesting efficacy in patients with other types of seizures including atypical absence seizures, atonic seizures, primary generalised tonic-clonic seizures, and status epilepticus; preliminary studies of lamotrigine given with valproate for absence seizures[6] and infantile spasms[7] showed promising results. Lamotrigine as adjunctive therapy has been found to be effective and well tolerated in paediatric patients with refractory epilepsy including those with developmental impairment;[8] it was particularly effective in absence and atypical seizures in this open-label study. However, despite all these encouraging views concerning the role of lamotrigine, the authors of a follow-up study[9] were less optimistic. They followed up 124 patients who had participated in an open-label trial of lamotrigine as adjunctive therapy for refractory epilepsy 6 to 8 years earlier and concluded that lamotrigine had only marginal benefit on the long-term prognosis of severe refractory epilepsy.

1. Ramaratnam S, *et al.* Lamotrigine add-on for drug-resistant partial epilepsy. Available in The Cochrane Library, Issue 2. Chichester: John Wiley; 2004.
2. Brodie MJ. Drugs in focus: 10. Lamotrigine. *Prescribers' J* 1993; **33:** 212–16.
3. Brodie MJ, *et al.* UK Lamotrigine/Carbamazepine Monotherapy Trial Group. Double-blind comparison of lamotrigine and carbamazepine in newly diagnosed epilepsy. *Lancet* 1995; **345:** 476–9.
4. Donaldson JA, *et al.* Lamotrigine adjunctive therapy in childhood epileptic encephalopathy (the Lennox Gastaut Syndrome). *Epilepsia* 1997; **38:** 68–73.
5. Motte J, *et al.* Lamotrigine for generalized seizures associated with the Lennox-Gastaut syndrome. *N Engl J Med* 1997; **337:** 1807–12. Correction. *ibid.* 1998; **339:** 851–2.
6. Ferrie CD, *et al.* Lamotrigine as an add-on drug in typical absence seizures. *Acta Neurol Scand* 1995; **91:** 200–202.
7. Veggiotti P, *et al.* Lamotrigine in infantile spasms. *Lancet* 1994; **344:** 1375–6.
8. Besag FMC, *et al.* Lamotrigine for the treatment of epilepsy in childhood. *J Pediatr* 1995; **127:** 991–7.
9. Walker MC, *et al.* Long term use of lamotrigine and vigabatrin in severe refractory epilepsy: audit of outcome. *BMJ* 1996; **313:** 1184–5.

**Motor neurone disease.** Lamotrigine has been tried as a potential therapy for amyotrophic lateral sclerosis (see Motor Neurone Disease, p.1739) but with disappointing results.[1]

1. Ryberg H, *et al.* A double-blind randomized clinical trial in amyotrophic lateral sclerosis using lamotrigine: effects on CSF glutamate, aspartate, branched-chain amino acid levels and clinical parameters. *Acta Neurol Scand* 2003; **108:** 1–8.

**Movement disorders.** Symptomatic improvement and a trend towards decreased chorea was reported[1] with lamotrigine in a double-blind, placebo-controlled study of 64 patients with Huntington's chorea (p.664) with motor signs of less than 5 years' duration. There was, however, no clear evidence that lamotrigine retarded the progression of early Huntington disease over a period of 30 months.

1. Kremer B, *et al.* Influence of lamotrigine on progress of early Huntington disease: a randomized clinical trial. *Neurology* 1999; **53:** 1000–11.

**Neuropathic pain.** There is growing evidence that lamotrigine is of use in the management of neuropathic pain.[1] It was effective when used in conjunction with carbamazepine or phenytoin in the treatment of refractory trigeminal neuralgia[2] (p.8), and has also shown promise in the treatment of pain associated with HIV-related distal sensory neuropathy[3] (p.623). Some benefit has been found[4] in the treatment of diabetic neuropathy (see p.6). Case reports[5] and a placebo-controlled trial[6] have also indicated that lamotrigine may be effective in central post-stroke pain (p.5).

1. McCleane GJ. Lamotrigine in the management of neuropathic pain: a review of the literature. *Clin J Pain* 2000; **16:** 321–6.
2. Zakrewska JM, *et al.* Lamotrigine (Lamictal) in refractory trigeminal neuralgia: results from a double-blind placebo controlled crossover study. *Pain* 1997; **73:** 223–30.
3. Simpson DM, *et al.* Lamotrigine for HIV-associated painful sensory neuropathies: a placebo-controlled trial. *Neurology* 2003; **60:** 1508–14.
4. Eisenberg E, *et al.* Lamotrigine reduces painful diabetic neuropathy: a randomized, controlled study. *Neurology* 2001; **57:** 505–9.
5. Canavero S, Bonicalzi V. Lamotrigine control of central pain. *Pain* 1996; **68:** 179–81.
6. Vestergaard K, *et al.* Lamotrigine for central post-stroke pain: a randomized controlled trial. *Neurology* 2001; **56:** 184–90.

## Preparations

**Proprietary Preparations** (details are given in Part 3)

***Arg.:*** Lamictal; ***Austral.:*** Lamictal; ***Austria:*** Lamictal; ***Belg.:*** Lamictal; ***Braz.:*** Lamictal; Neurium; ***Canad.:*** Lamictal; ***Chile:*** Lafigin; Lamictal; Tradox; ***Denm.:*** Lamictal; ***Fin.:*** Lamictal; ***Fr.:*** Lamictal; ***Ger.:*** Lamictal; ***Gr.:*** Lamictal; ***Hong Kong:*** Lamictal; ***India:*** Lametec; ***Irl.:*** Lamictal; ***Israel:*** Lamictal; ***Ital.:*** Lamictal; ***Malaysia:*** Lamictal; ***Mex.:*** Lamictal; ***Neth.:*** Lamictal; ***Norw.:*** Lamictal; ***NZ:*** Lamictal; ***Port.:*** Lamictal; ***S.Afr.:*** Lamictin; ***Singapore:*** Lamictal; ***Spain:*** Crisomet; Labileno; Lamictal; ***Swed.:*** Lamictal; ***Switz.:*** Lamictal; ***Thai.:*** Lamictal; ***UK:*** Lamictal; ***USA:*** Lamictal.

## Levetiracetam *(BAN, USAN, rINN)*

S-Etiracetam; UCB-22059; UCB-L059. (S)-2-(2-Oxopyrrolidin-1-yl)butanamide.

$C_8H_{14}N_2O_2$ = 170.2.
*CAS — 102767-28-2.*
*ATC — N03AX14.*

### Adverse Effects and Precautions

The most commonly reported adverse effects associated with levetiracetam are somnolence, weakness, and dizziness. Anorexia, diarrhoea, dyspepsia, nausea, ataxia, headache, amnesia, depression, emotional lability, insomnia, aggression, nervousness, tremor, vertigo, diplopia, and rash may occur less frequently. A raised incidence of mild infections, such as the common cold and upper respiratory-tract infections, has been reported.

Other adverse effects reported include abnormal behaviour, aggression, anger, anxiety, confusion, hallucinations, irritability, psychotic disorders, neutropenia, pancytopenia, and thrombocytopenia.

Levetiracetam should be used with caution and in reduced doses in patients with renal impairment, those undergoing haemodialysis, and in patients with severe hepatic impairment.

Care is required when withdrawing levetiracetam therapy—see also under Uses and Administration, below.

**Breast feeding.** For comment on antiepileptic therapy and breast feeding, see p.351.

**Driving.** For a comment on antiepileptic drugs and driving, see p.351.

**Pregnancy.** For comments on the management of epilepsy during pregnancy, see p.351.

### Pharmacokinetics

Levetiracetam is readily absorbed from the gastrointestinal tract and peak plasma concentrations are usually achieved within 1.3 hours of oral doses and steady state achieved after 2 days. Plasma protein binding is minimal. Levetiracetam is not extensively metabolised; approximately 25% of the dose is metabolised by hydroxylation to inactive metabolites. About 95% of a dose is excreted as unchanged drug and metabolites in the urine. The plasma elimination half-life has been reported to be about 7 hours.

◊ References.

1. Radtke RA. Pharmacokinetics of levetiracetam. *Epilepsia* 2001; **42** (suppl 4): 24–7.

### Uses and Administration

Levetiracetam is an analogue of piracetam (p.1732) used as adjunctive therapy in the treatment of partial seizures with or without secondary generalisation.

The daily dose of levetiracetam is given by mouth in two divided doses. The initial adult dose is 1 g on the first day of treatment; thereafter, the daily dose may be increased in increments of 1 g every 2 to 4 weeks until effective antiepileptic control is achieved, up to a maximum dose of 3 g daily. Reduced doses are recommended in renal and severe hepatic impairment (see below).

As with other antiepileptics, withdrawal of levetiracetam therapy or transition to or from another type of antiepileptic therapy should be made gradually to avoid precipitating an increase in the frequency of seizures. The manufacturers recommend reducing the daily dose by 1 g every 2 to 4 weeks. For a discussion on whether or not to withdraw antiepileptic therapy in seizure-free patients, see p.349.

**Administration in hepatic impairment.** No dose adjustment is needed in patients with mild to moderate hepatic impairment. In patients with severe liver impairment, creatinine clearance may underestimate concomitant renal impairment, and the usual adult maintenance dose (see above) should be reduced by 50% in those with creatinine clearance of less than 70 mL/minute.

**Administration in renal impairment.** Reduced doses of levetiracetam are recommended for patients with renal impairment. Suitable daily doses based on creatinine clearance (CC) and given in 2 divided doses are:

- CC 50 to 79 mL/minute: 1 to 2 g
- CC 30 to 49 mL/minute: 0.5 to 1.5 g
- CC less than 30 mL/minute: 0.5 to 1 g

Patients receiving dialysis may be given a loading dose of 750 mg when starting levetiracetam followed by doses of 500 to 1000 mg once daily; a supplemental dose of 250 to 500 mg is recommended after dialysis.

See also above for dosage recommendations in those patients with severe hepatic impairment and concomitant renal impairment.

**Epilepsy.** Levetiracetam is one of the newer drugs used in the treatment of epilepsy (p.349). Efficacy has been shown as adjunctive therapy in the treatment of drug-resistant partial seizures.[1-3]

1. Dooley M, Plosker GL. Levetiracetam: a review of its adjunctive use in the management of partial onset seizures. *Drugs* 2000; **60:** 871–93.
2. Chaisewikul R, *et al.* Levetiracetam add-on for drug-resistant localization related (partial) epilepsy. Available in The Cochrane Library; Issue 2. Chichester: John Wiley; 2004.
3. Welty TE, *et al.* Levetiracetam: a different approach to the pharmacotherapy of epilepsy. *Ann Pharmacother* 2002; **36:** 296–304.

### Preparations

**Proprietary Preparations** (details are given in Part 3)
***Arg.:*** Keppra; ***Austral.:*** Keppra; ***Belg.:*** Keppra; ***Denm.:*** Keppra; ***Fin.:*** Keppra; ***Fr.:*** Keppra; ***Ger.:*** Keppra; ***Gr.:*** Kepra; ***Hong Kong:*** Keppra; ***Irl.:*** Keppra; ***Ital.:*** Keppra; ***Norw.:*** Keppra; ***Port.:*** Keppra; ***Singapore:*** Keppra; ***Spain:*** Keppra; ***Swed.:*** Keppra; ***Switz.:*** Keppra; ***Thai.:*** Keppra; ***UK:*** Keppra; ***USA:*** Keppra.

## Losigamone *(rINN)*

AO-33; Losigamona. (5R*)-5-[(αS*)-o-Chloro-α-hydroxybenzyl]-4-methoxy-2(5H)-furanone.

$C_{12}H_{11}ClO_4$ = 254.7.
*CAS — 112856-44-7.*

### Profile

Losigamone is an antiepileptic that has been investigated as adjunctive therapy in the treatment of partial seizures.

◊ References

1. Bauer J, *et al.* Losigamone add-on therapy in partial epilepsy: a placebo-controlled study. *Acta Neurol Scand* 2001; **103:** 226–30.

## Mephenytoin *(BAN, USAN, rINN)*

Mefenitoína; Mephenetoin; Methantoin; Methoin; NSC-34652; Phenantoin. 5-Ethyl-3-methyl-5-phenylhydantoin.

$C_{12}H_{14}N_2O_2$ = 218.3.
*CAS — 50-12-4.*
*ATC — N03AB04.*

**Pharmacopoeias.** In *US.*

**USP 27** (Mephenytoin). Store in airtight containers.

### Profile

Mephenytoin is a hydantoin antiepileptic with actions similar to those of phenytoin (p.370), but it is more toxic. Because of its potential toxicity it is not one of the main drugs used in the treatment of epilepsy (p.349) and is given only to patients unresponsive to other treatment. Some of the side-effects of mephenytoin may be due to the metabolite, 5-ethyl-5-phenylhydantoin (also termed nirvanol). Like phenytoin the rate of metabolism of mephenytoin is subject to genetic polymorphism.

Mephenytoin is given in an initial daily dose by mouth of 50 to 100 mg for one week; thereafter the daily dose is increased by 50 to 100 mg at weekly intervals until the optimum dose is reached, which is usually between 200 and 600 mg daily for an adult and 100 and 400 mg daily for a child; daily maintenance doses are usually taken in 3 divided doses.

**Porphyria.** Mephenytoin has been associated with acute attacks of porphyria and is considered unsafe in porphyric patients.

### Preparations

***USP 27:*** Mephenytoin Tablets.

**Proprietary Preparations** (details are given in Part 3)
***Austria:*** Epilan; ***USA:*** Mesantoin†.

## Mesuximide *(BAN, rINN)*

Mesuximida; Methsuximide; PM-396. N,2-Dimethyl-2-phenylsuccinimide.

$C_{12}H_{13}NO_2$ = 203.2.
*CAS — 77-41-8.*
*ATC — N03AD03.*

**Pharmacopoeias.** In *US.*

**USP 27** (Methsuximide). A white to greyish-white crystalline powder. Is odourless or has a slight odour. Soluble 1 in 350 of water, 1 in 3 of alcohol, 1 in less than 1 of chloroform, and 1 in 2 of ether. Store in airtight containers.

### Profile

Mesuximide is a succinimide antiepileptic with actions similar to those of ethosuximide (p.360); although it also has some activity in complex partial seizures it is reported to be less well tolerated than ethosuximide, and is usually only given to patients unresponsive to other antiepileptic treatment. It is thought to owe its activity to its major metabolite *N*-desmethylmesuximide.

The usual initial dosage is a single dose of 300 mg daily by mouth for the first week, and this is increased by 300 mg at weekly intervals to an optimum dosage, according to the patient's response. The suggested maximum daily dose is 1.2 g in divided doses.

**Epilepsy.** Mesuximide is used for absence seizures that are refractory to less toxic antiepileptics such as ethosuximide or valproate, which are the usual drugs to try (see p.349). Mesuximide has also been tried in complex partial seizures and myoclonic seizures.

References.

1. Tennison MB, *et al.* Methsuximide for intractable childhood seizures. *Pediatrics* 1991; **87:** 186–9.
2. Sigler M, *et al.* Effective and safe but forgotten: methsuximide in intractable epilepsies in childhood. *Seizure* 2001; **10:** 120–4.

**Interactions.** For the effect of mesuximide on lamotrigine, see p.364.

**Porphyria.** Mesuximide has been associated with acute attacks of porphyria and is considered unsafe in porphyric patients.

### Preparations

***USP 27:*** Methsuximide Capsules.

**Proprietary Preparations** (details are given in Part 3)
***Austria:*** Petinutin; ***Canad.:*** Celontin; ***Ger.:*** Petinutin; ***Israel:*** Celontin; ***Neth.:*** Celontin; ***Switz.:*** Petinutin; ***USA:*** Celontin.

## Methylphenobarbital *(BAN, rINN)*

Enphenemalum; Mephobarbital; Methylphenobarbitalum; Methylphenobarbitone; Metilfenobarbital; Phemitone. 5-Ethyl-1-methyl-5-phenylbarbituric acid.

$C_{13}H_{14}N_2O_3$ = 246.3.
*CAS — 115-38-8.*
*ATC — N03AA01.*

**Pharmacopoeias.** In *Eur.* (see p.vi) and *US.*

**Ph. Eur. 5.0** (Methylphenobarbital). A white, crystalline powder or colourless crystals. Practically insoluble in water; very slightly soluble in dehydrated alcohol. It forms water-soluble compounds with alkali hydroxides and carbonates, and with ammonia.

**USP 27** (Mephobarbital). A white, odourless, crystalline powder. Slightly soluble in water, in alcohol, and in ether; soluble in chloroform and in solutions of fixed alkali hydroxides and carbonates. Its saturated solution in water is acid to litmus.

### Dependence and Withdrawal, Adverse Effects, Treatment, and Precautions

As for Phenobarbital, p.368.

### Interactions

As for Phenobarbital, p.368.

### Pharmacokinetics

Methylphenobarbital is incompletely absorbed from the gastrointestinal tract. It is demethylated to phenobarbital (p.369) in the liver.

### Uses and Administration

Methylphenobarbital is used similarly to phenobarbital (p.369) in the treatment of epilepsy (p.349). It is given in doses of up to 600 mg daily by mouth. It has also been used as a sedative.

### Preparations

***BP 2003:*** Methylphenobarbital Tablets;
***USP 27:*** Mephobarbital Tablets.

**Proprietary Preparations** (details are given in Part 3)
***Austral.:*** Prominal†; ***Spain:*** Prominal†; ***UK:*** Prominal†; ***USA:*** Mebaral.

**Multi-ingredient:** ***Arg.:*** Cumatil L; ***Belg.:*** Mathoine†; ***Ital.:*** Dintoinale; Metinal-Idantoina; Metinal-Idantoina L; ***Port.:*** Comital L†; ***Spain:*** Comital L.

## Oxcarbazepine *(BAN, USAN, rINN)*

GP-47680; KIN-493; Oxcarbazepina. 10,11-Dihydro-10-oxo-5H-dibenz[b,f]azepine-5-carboxamide.

$C_{15}H_{12}N_2O_2$ = 252.3.
*CAS — 28721-07-5.*
*ATC — N03AF02.*

### Adverse Effects, Treatment, and Precautions

As for Carbamazepine, p.354.

Hypersensitivity reactions such as skin rashes occur less frequently with oxcarbazepine than with carbamazepine. However, cross-sensitivity does occur and about 25 to 30% of patients hypersensitive to carbamazepine may experience such reactions with oxcarbazepine. Reductions in plasma-sodium levels have also been observed with oxcarbazepine (see Hyponatraemia, below). Patients with cardiac insufficiency and secondary heart failure should be weighed regularly to detect fluid retention.

Dosage reductions are recommended in renal impairment.

**Breast feeding.** For comment on antiepileptic therapy and breast feeding, see p.351.

**Driving.** For a comment on antiepileptic drugs and driving, see p.351.

**Effects on the blood.** Although it would appear that oxcarbazepine is less likely than carbamazepine to cause leucopenia, individual cases have been reported. In one such case leucopenia and hyponatraemia developed in a 57-year-old woman while taking oxcarbazepine;[1] she recovered after treatment with filgrastim. It was noted that the patient had experienced a similar reaction when taking carbamazepine.

1. Ryan M, *et al.* Hyponatremia and leukopenia associated with oxcarbazepine following carbamazepine therapy. *Am J Health-Syst Pharm* 2001; **58:** 1637–9.

**Effects on mental function.** For a review of the effects of antiepileptic therapy including oxcarbazepine on *cognition,* see p.351.

**Hyponatraemia.** Hyponatraemia appears to be more pronounced at clinical doses of oxcarbazepine than with carbamazepine. Hyponatraemia was reported[1] in 12 of 15 patients in whom oxcarbazepine was substituted for carbamazepine therapy. The fall in plasma-sodium concentrations appeared to be related to the dose of oxcarbazepine. In another report[2] hyponatraemia occurred in 23% of 350 patients whose serum-sodium concentrations were monitored. The manufacturers state that in 14 controlled studies sodium levels of less than 125 mmol/litre occurred in 2.5% of 1524 patients treated with oxcarbazepine compared to no such patients in the control groups. Most patients remain asymptomatic but some may experience drowsiness, increase in seizure frequency, and impaired consciousness.[3]

It has been suggested that serum-sodium concentrations should be measured before the start of therapy but routine repeated determinations may be indicated only in elderly patients or if a high dosage is used.[4] The manufacturers themselves recommend that monitoring be considered in those with pre-existing conditions associated with low sodium levels and in those taking other medications known to interfere with sodium levels, for example NSAIDs and diuretics. Severe hyponatraemia has been reported[5] in a 12-year-old child during treatment with oxcarbazepine. On reviewing the case notes of 48 other children who had received oxcarbazepine in the same centre, 9 were found to have had hyponatraemia, and the authors suggested that sodium levels should be monitored in paediatric patients.


1. Pendlebury SC, *et al.* Hyponatraemia during oxcarbazepine therapy. *Hum Toxicol* 1989; **8:** 337–44.
2. Friis ML, *et al.* Therapeutic experiences with 947 epileptic outpatients in oxcarbazepine treatment. *Acta Neurol Scand* 1993; **87:** 224–7.
3. Steinhoff BJ, *et al.* Hyponatraemic coma under oxcarbazepine therapy. *Epilepsy Res* 1992; **11;** 67–70.
4. Kälviäinen R, *et al.* Place of newer antiepileptic drugs in the treatment of epilepsy. *Drugs* 1993; **46:** 1009–24.
5. Borusiak P, *et al.* Hyponatremia induced by oxcarbazepine in children. *Epilepsy Res* 1998; **30:** 241–6.


**Pregnancy.** For comments on the management of epilepsy during pregnancy, see p.351.

## Interactions

There are complex interactions between antiepileptics and toxicity may be enhanced without a corresponding increase in antiepileptic activity. Such interactions are very variable and unpredictable and plasma monitoring is often advisable with combination therapy. Plasma concentrations of the active monohydroxy metabolite of oxcarbazepine may be reduced by strong inducers of cytochrome P450 isoenzymes, such as carbamazepine, phenytoin, or phenobarbital. Oxcarbazepine appears to induce hepatic enzymes to a lesser extent than carbamazepine. However, oxcarbazepine and its active metabolite do inhibit the cytochrome P450 isoenzyme CYP2C19, and in high doses may raise plasma concentrations of phenobarbital or phenytoin. Oxcarbazepine and its metabolite also have the capacity to induce CYP3A4 and CYP3A5 with the possibility of reducing plasma concentrations of drugs such as carbamazepine (but see below), dihydropyridine calcium-channel blockers and oral contraceptives.

**Antiepileptics.** In a study[1] of epileptic patients receiving monotherapy the area under the concentration-time curve (AUC) for *carbamazepine, phenytoin,* or *valproate* was unchanged when oxcarbazepine was added to treatment; only carbamazepine affected the pharmacokinetics of oxcarbazepine, producing a reduction in the AUC for the active metabolite hydroxycarbazepine. It was considered that there was unlikely to be any clinically relevant pharmacokinetic interaction if oxcarbazepine was used with any of these antiepileptics, including carbamazepine. However, increases in plasma-phenytoin concentration have been reported after use with oxcarbazepine (see p.373).

There is a case-report of severe toxicity occurring with concomitant use of oxcarbazepine and *lamotrigine.*[2]


1. McKee PJW, *et al.* A double-blind, placebo-controlled interaction study between oxcarbazepine and carbamazepine, sodium valproate and phenytoin in epileptic patients. *Br J Clin Pharmacol* 1994; **37:** 27–32.
2. Alving J. Case of severe acute intoxication with oxcarbazepine combined with lamotrigine. *Epilepsia* 1994; **35** (suppl 7): 72.


**Sex hormones.** The manufacturers state that oxcarbazepine may reduce the effectiveness of *oral contraceptives.*

## Pharmacokinetics

Oxcarbazepine is well absorbed from the gastrointestinal tract. It is rapidly and extensively metabolised in the liver to the principal metabolite 10,11-dihydro-10-hydroxy-carbamazepine, which also possesses antiepileptic activity. The plasma half-life has been reported to be about 2 hours for oxcarbazepine, and about 9 hours for the monohydroxy metabolite; consequently the latter provides most of the antiepileptic activity. The monohydroxy metabolite is widely distributed in the body and is about 40% bound to plasma protein. Oxcarbazepine is excreted in the urine mainly as metabolites; less than 1% is excreted as unchanged drug.

Oxcarbazepine and its monohydroxy metabolite cross the placental barrier and are distributed into breast milk.

The pharmacokinetics of oxcarbazepine and its monohydroxy metabolite are affected by the concomitant administration of other antiepileptics (see under Interactions, above).

◊ References.


1. Dickinson RG, *et al.* First dose and steady-state pharmacokinetics of oxcarbazepine and its 10-hydroxy metabolite. *Eur J Clin Pharmacol* 1989; **37:** 69–74.
2. Patsalos PN, *et al.* Protein binding of oxcarbazepine and its primary active metabolite, 10-hydroxycarbazepine, in patients with trigeminal neuralgia. *Eur J Clin Pharmacol* 1990; **39:** 413–15.
3. Kumps A, Wurth C. Oxcarbazepine disposition: preliminary observations in patients. *Biopharm Drug Dispos* 1990; **11:** 365–70.
4. van Heiningen PNM, *et al.* The influence of age on the pharmacokinetics of the antiepileptic agent oxcarbazepine. *Clin Pharmacol Ther* 1991; **50:** 410–19.
5. Elwes RDC, Binnie CD. Clinical pharmacokinetics of newer antiepileptic drugs: lamotrigine, vigabatrin, gabapentin and oxcarbazepine. *Clin Pharmacokinet* 1996; **30:** 403–15.


## Uses and Administration

Oxcarbazepine is a derivative of carbamazepine (p.357) with similar actions. It is used as monotherapy or adjunctive therapy in the treatment of partial seizures with or without secondarily generalised tonic-clonic seizures. The initial dose for monotherapy and adjunctive therapy in adults is 600 mg daily by mouth, given in 2 divided doses. The dose may be increased thereafter, if necessary, in maximum increments of 600 mg daily at approximately weekly intervals until the desired clinical response has been achieved. Maintenance doses are usually in the range of 600 to 1200 mg daily or up to 2400 mg daily if given as adjunctive therapy or in refractory patients switched from other antiepileptics. The recommended initial dose for children aged 6 years and over (as monotherapy or adjunctive therapy) is 8 to 10 mg/kg by mouth daily, given in 2 divided doses. This may be increased as necessary in maximum increments of 10 mg/kg daily at approximately weekly intervals to a maximum dose of 46 mg/kg daily; usual maintenance doses in adjunctive therapy are around 30 mg/kg daily. In the USA, similar dosage recommendations are given for monotherapy or adjunctive therapy in children aged 4 years and over.

Reduced initial doses are recommended in patients with renal impairment (see below).

As with other antiepileptics, withdrawal of oxcarbazepine therapy or transition to or from another type of antiepileptic therapy should be made gradually to avoid precipitating an increase in the frequency of seizures. For a discussion on whether or not to withdraw antiepileptic therapy in seizure-free patients, see p.349.

**Administration in renal impairment.** Initial doses for patients with a creatinine clearance of less than 30 mL/minute should be 300 mg daily in adults (half the usual starting dose, above), increased at weekly intervals or longer.

**Epilepsy.** Oxcarbazepine is used in the treatment of epilepsy (p.349) and may be a useful alternative in patients unable to tolerate carbamazepine.

In a double-blind trial[1] involving newly diagnosed adult patients, oxcarbazepine was of similar efficacy and tolerability to valproate for partial or generalised tonic-clonic seizures. Oxcarbazepine was of similar efficacy to phenytoin, but was better tolerated in adults and children with newly diagnosed partial or generalised tonic-clonic seizures.[2,3] Further randomised controlled trials (and a small systematic review[4]) have also confirmed the efficacy and tolerability of oxcarbazepine as adjunctive therapy[4,5] or monotherapy[6,7] in refractory partial seizures in children and adults.


1. Christe W, *et al.* A double-blind controlled clinical trial: oxcarbazepine versus sodium valproate in adults with newly diagnosed epilepsy. *Epilepsy Res* 1997; **26:** 451–60.
2. Bill PA, *et al.* A double-blind controlled clinical trial of oxcarbazepine versus phenytoin in adults with previously untreated epilepsy. *Epilepsy Res* 1997; **27:** 195–204.
3. Guerreiro MM, *et al.* A double-blind controlled clinical trial of oxcarbazepine versus phenytoin in children and adolescents with epilepsy. *Epilepsy Res* 1997; **27:** 205–13.
4. Castillo S, *et al.* Oxcarbazepine add-on for drug-resistant partial epilepsy. Available in The Cochrane Library; Issue 2. Chichester: John Wiley; 2004.
5. Glauser TA, *et al.* Adjunctive therapy with oxcarbazepine in children with partial seizures. *Neurology* 2000; **54:** 2237–44.
6. Beydoun A, *et al.* Oxcarbazepine monotherapy for partial-onset seizures: a multicenter, double-blind, clinical trial. *Neurology* 2000; **54:** 2245–51.
7. Sachdeo R, *et al.* Oxcarbazepine (Trileptal) as monotherapy in patients with partial seizures. *Neurology* 2001; **57:** 864–71.


## Preparations

**Proprietary Preparations** (details are given in Part 3)
***Arg.:*** Atoxecar; Aurene; Oxcazen; Trileptal; ***Austral.:*** Trileptal; ***Austria:*** Trileptal; ***Belg.:*** Trileptal; ***Braz.:*** Auram; Trileptal; ***Chile:*** Alox; Oxicodal; Trileptal; ***Denm.:*** Apydan; Trileptal; ***Fin.:*** Apydan; Trileptal; ***Fr.:*** Trileptal; ***Ger.:*** Timox; Trileptal; ***Gr.:*** Trileptal; ***Hong Kong:*** Trileptal; ***India:*** Oxrate; ***Irl.:*** Trileptal; ***Israel:*** Trileptin; ***Ital.:*** Tolep; Trileptal†; ***Malaysia:*** Trileptal; ***Mex.:*** Trileptal; ***Neth.:*** Trileptal; ***Norw.:*** Trileptal; ***NZ:*** Trileptal; ***S.Afr.:*** Trileptal; ***Spain:*** Trileptal; ***Swed.:*** Trileptal; ***Switz.:*** Trileptal; ***UK:*** Trileptal; ***USA:*** Trileptal.

## Phenacemide *(BAN, rINN)*

Carbamidum Phenylaceticum; Fenacemida. (Phenylacetyl)urea.

$C_9H_{10}N_2O_2$ = 178.2.
*CAS — 63-98-9.*
*ATC — N03AX07.*

### Profile

Phenacemide is an acetylurea antiepileptic that is the straight-chain analogue of a hydantoin. It has been used in the treatment of epilepsy (p.349), especially in complex partial seizures; because of its potential toxicity it was given only to patients unresponsive to other antiepileptics.

Severe adverse effects reported with phenacemide have included psychoses and personality changes, blood disorders including aplastic anaemia, and liver and kidney damage; extreme caution has been advised in giving phenacemide to patients with a history of such disorders.

**Administration in renal impairment.** Serum-creatinine concentrations should not be used as a measure of renal function in patients receiving phenacemide as it can increase creatinine concentrations in the absence of renal impairment.[1]


1. Cahen R, *et al.* Creatinine metabolism impairment by an anticonvulsant drug, phenacemide. *Ann Pharmacother* 1994; **28:** 49–51.


## Pheneturide *(BAN, rINN)*

Ethylphenacemide; Feneturida; S-46. (2-Phenylbutyryl)urea.

$C_{11}H_{14}N_2O_2$ = 206.2.
*CAS — 90-49-3.*
*ATC — N03AX13.*

### Profile

Pheneturide is an acetylurea antiepileptic used in the treatment of epilepsy (p.349). It is given by mouth in usual daily doses of 300 to 600 mg in 2 or 3 divided doses, up to a maximum of 1.2 g daily.

### Preparations

**Proprietary Preparations** (details are given in Part 3)
***Belg.:*** Laburide.

## Phenobarbital *(BAN, rINN)*

Fenobarbital; Phenemalum; Phenobarbitalum; Phenobarbitone; Phenylethylbarbituric Acid; Phenylethylmalonylurea. 5-Ethyl-5-phenylbarbituric acid.

$C_{12}H_{12}N_2O_3$ = 232.2.
*CAS — 50-06-6.*
*ATC — N03AA02.*

**Pharmacopoeias.** In *Chin., Eur.* (see p.vi), *Int., Jpn, Pol., US,* and *Viet.*

**Ph. Eur. 5.0** (Phenobarbital). A white, crystalline powder or colourless crystals. Very slightly soluble in water; freely soluble in alcohol. It forms water-soluble compounds with alkali hydroxides and carbonates, and with ammonia.

**USP 27** (Phenobarbital). White, odourless, glistening, small crystals or a white crystalline powder. It may exhibit polymorphism. Soluble 1 in 1000 of water and 1 in 10 of alcohol; sparingly soluble in chloroform; soluble in ether and in solutions of fixed alkali hydroxides and carbonates. A saturated solution in water has a pH of about 5.

## Phenobarbital Sodium *(BANM, rINN)*

Fenobarbital sódico; Phenemalnatrium; Phenobarbitalum Natricum; Phenobarbitone Sodium; Sodium Phenylethylbarbiturate; Soluble Phenobarbitone. Sodium 5-ethyl-5-phenylbarbiturate.

$C_{12}H_{11}N_2NaO_3$ = 254.2.
*CAS — 57-30-7.*
*ATC — N03AA02.*

**Pharmacopoeias.** In *Chin., Eur.* (see p.vi), *Int., Pol.,* and *US.*

**Ph. Eur. 5.0** (Phenobarbital Sodium). A white, hygroscopic, crystalline powder. Freely soluble in carbon dioxide-free water (a small amount may be insoluble); soluble in alcohol; practically insoluble in dichloromethane. A 10% solution in water has a pH not greater than 10.2. Store in airtight containers.

**USP 27** (Phenobarbital Sodium). Flaky crystals, or white crystalline granules, or a white powder. It is odourless and hygroscopic. Very soluble in water; soluble in alcohol; practically insoluble in chloroform and in ether. pH of a 10% solution in water is between 9.2 and 10.2. Solutions decompose on standing. Store in airtight containers.

**Incompatibility.** Phenobarbital sodium is incompatible with many other drugs and phenobarbital may be precipitated from mixtures containing phenobarbital sodium. This precipitation is dependent upon the concentration and the pH, and also on the presence of other solvents.

## Dependence and Withdrawal

As for the barbiturates (see Amobarbital, p.670).

## Adverse Effects

The most frequent adverse effect associated with phenobarbital is sedation, but this often becomes less marked with continued administration. Like some of the other antiepileptics, phenobarbital may produce subtle mood changes and impairment of cognition and memory that may not be apparent without testing. Depression may occur.

Prolonged administration may occasionally result in folate deficiency; rarely, megaloblastic anaemia has been reported. There is some evidence that phenobarbital interferes with vitamin D metabolism.

At high doses nystagmus and ataxia may occur and the typical barbiturate-induced respiratory depression may become severe. Overdosage can prove fatal; toxic effects include coma, severe respiratory and cardiovascular depression, with hypotension and shock leading to renal failure. Hypothermia may occur, with associated pyrexia during recovery. Skin blisters (bullae) reportedly occur in about 6% of patients with barbiturate overdose.

Sodium salts of barbiturates have a very high pH in solution, and necrosis has followed subcutaneous injection or extravasation. Intravenous injections can be hazardous and cause hypotension, shock, laryngospasm, and apnoea.

Hypersensitivity reactions occur in a small proportion of patients; skin reactions are reported in 1 to 3% of patients receiving phenobarbital, and are most commonly maculopapular, morbilliform, or scarlatiniform rashes. More severe reactions such as exfoliative dermatitis, Stevens-Johnson syndrome, and toxic epidermal necrolysis are extremely rare. Hepatitis and disturbances of liver function have been reported.

Paradoxical excitement, restlessness, and confusion may sometimes occur in the elderly, and irritability and hyperactivity may occur in children.

Neonatal drug dependence and symptoms resembling vitamin K deficiency have been reported in infants born to mothers who received phenobarbital during pregnancy. Congenital malformations have been reported in children of women who received phenobarbital during pregnancy but the causal role of the drug is a matter of some debate.

**Effects on the blood.** For the effects of antiepileptics including phenobarbital on serum folate, see under Phenytoin, p.370.

**Effects on bone.** For the effects of antiepileptics including phenobarbital on bone and on calcium and vitamin D metabolism, see under Phenytoin, p.371.

**Effects on connective tissue.** The use of phenobarbital and primidone has been associated with the development of Dupuytren's contracture, frozen shoulder, Ledderhose's syndrome, Peyronie's disease, fibromas, and general joint pain.[1]

1. Mattson RH, *et al.* Barbiturate-related connective tissue disorders. *Arch Intern Med* 1989; **149:** 911–14.

**Effects on the endocrine system.** For mention of the effects of antiepileptics on *sexual function* in male epileptic patients, see under Phenytoin, p.371.

Barbiturates may reduce serum concentrations of *thyroid* hormones through enzyme induction—see under Interactions of Levothyroxine, p.1601.

**Effects on the liver.** For mention of the effects of phenobarbital on the liver, see under Phenytoin, p.371.

**Effects on mental function.** For a review of the effects of antiepileptics, including phenobarbital, on *cognition*, see p.351.

DEPRESSION. Follow-up of 28 patients aged 6 to 16 who had received phenobarbital or carbamazepine for epilepsy indicated that the rate of major depression was significantly higher in those receiving phenobarbital.[1] It was recommended that treatment with phenobarbital should be avoided particularly in patients with a personal or family history of an affective disorder; patients who do receive it should be monitored for symptoms of depression.

1. Brent DA, *et al.* Phenobarbital treatment and major depressive disorder in children with epilepsy: a naturalistic follow-up. *Pediatrics* 1990; **85:** 1086–91.

**Hypersensitivity.** An antiepileptic hypersensitivity syndrome, comprising fever, rash, and lymphadenopathy and less commonly lymphocytosis, and liver and other organ involvement, has been associated with some antiepileptics including phenobarbital.[1,2] Some have estimated the incidence at 1 in 1000 to 1 in 10 000 new exposures to aromatic anticonvulsants,[1,2] but the true incidence is unknown due to variations in presentation and reporting. The syndrome occurs most frequently on first exposure to the drug, with initial symptoms starting anywhere between 1 and 8 weeks after exposure. In previously sensitised individuals the reaction may occur within 1 day of rechallenge. The potential for cross-reactivity between carbamazepine, phenobarbital, and phenytoin is about 75%, and patients who develop the syndrome, and their close relatives, should be warned of the risk associated with use of these antiepileptics.[1]

1. Knowles SR, *et al.* Anticonvulsant hypersensitivity syndrome: incidence, prevention and management. *Drug Safety* 1999; **21:** 489–501.
2. Bessmertny O, *et al.* Antiepileptic hypersensitivity syndrome in children. *Ann Pharmacother* 2001; **35:** 533–8.

## Treatment of Adverse Effects

After an overdose of a barbiturate, gastric lavage may be considered if undertaken within about 1 hour. Repeated doses of activated charcoal should be given by mouth with the aim of preventing absorption and also aiding elimination; care should be taken to protect the airway. The prime objectives of management are then intensive symptomatic and supportive therapy with particular attention being paid to the maintenance of cardiovascular, respiratory, and renal functions and to the maintenance of electrolyte balance.

Charcoal haemoperfusion may be considered for patients with severe refractory poisoning; other methods aimed at the active removal of barbiturates with a long elimination half-life (such as phenobarbital) include forced diuresis, haemodialysis, and peritoneal dialysis, but the hazards of such procedures are generally considered to outweigh any purported benefits.

## Precautions

Phenobarbital and other barbiturates should be used with care in children and in elderly or debilitated patients, in those in acute pain, and in those with depressive disorders. Phenobarbital should be used with caution in patients with impaired hepatic, renal, or respiratory function; its use is contra-indicated in those with severe respiratory depression.

Care is required when withdrawing phenobarbital therapy—see also Uses and Administration, below.

Phenobarbital and other barbiturates cause drowsiness and patients receiving them, if affected, should not take charge of vehicles or machinery where loss of attention could cause accidents.

**Breast feeding.** The American Academy of Pediatrics[1] considers that phenobarbital should be given with caution to breast-feeding mothers, since there have been significant adverse effects including sedation and methaemoglobinaemia in nursing infants. The *British National Formulary* recommends that phenobarbital should be avoided where possible during breast feeding. Both authorities make similar recommendations for primidone.

For further comment on antiepileptic therapy and breast feeding, see p.351.

1. American Academy of Pediatrics. The transfer of drugs and other chemicals into human milk. *Pediatrics* 2001; **108:** 776–89. Correction. *ibid.*; 1029. Also available at: http://aappolicy.aappublications.org/cgi/content/full/pediatrics%3b108/3/776 (accessed 13/05/04)

**Driving.** For a comment on antiepileptic drugs and driving, see p.351.

**Neonates.** Care should be taken when giving phenobarbital orally as the elixir to neonates because regular dosing could result in alcohol toxicity [the BP 2003 formulation contains 38% v/v alcohol].[1] Aqueous preparations are more readily made using the sodium salt than the acid.[2]

1. Colquhoun-Flannery W, Wheeler R. Treating neonatal jaundice with phenobarbitone: the inadvertent administration of significant doses of ethyl alcohol. *Arch Dis Child* 1992; **67:** 152.
2. Leach F. Treating neonatal jaundice with phenobarbitone: the inadvertent administration of significant doses of ethyl alcohol. *Arch Dis Child* 1992; **67:** 152.

**Porphyria.** Phenobarbital has been associated with acute attacks of porphyria and is considered unsafe in porphyric patients.

**Pregnancy.** For comments on the management of epilepsy during pregnancy, see p.351.

Congenital craniofacial and digital abnormalities and, less commonly, cleft lip and palate have been described with antiepileptics including phenobarbital. *In utero* exposure to phenobarbital might result in neonatal sedation and drug dependence and also in neonatal bleeding due to vitamin K deficiency.

## Interactions

There are complex interactions between antiepileptics, and toxicity may be enhanced without a corresponding increase in antiepileptic activity. Such interactions are very variable and unpredictable and plasma monitoring is often advisable with combination therapy. Valproate and phenytoin have been reported to cause rises in phenobarbital (and primidone) concentrations in plasma.

The effects of phenobarbital and other barbiturates are enhanced by other CNS depressants including alcohol.

Phenobarbital and other barbiturates may reduce the activity of many drugs by increasing the rate of metabolism through induction of drug-metabolising enzymes in liver microsomes.

**Analgesics.** Administration of *dextropropoxyphene* 65 mg three times daily to 4 epileptic patients stabilised on phenobarbital therapy resulted in increases in serum-phenobarbital concentration ranging from 8 to 29% but the increase was not considered of major importance in the light of the normally accepted therapeutic range for phenobarbital.[1]

For the effect of phenobarbital on *fenoprofen, methadone,* and *pethidine*, see p.39, p.58, and p.81, respectively. Use of enzyme-inducing antiepileptics such as phenobarbital also affects the administration of antidote in the treatment of *paracetamol* poisoning, see p.78.

1. Hansen BS, *et al.* Influence of dextropropoxyphene on steady state serum levels and protein binding of three anti-epileptic drugs in man. *Acta Neurol Scand* 1980; **61:** 357–67.

**Antiarrhythmics.** For the effect of phenobarbital on *disopyramide, lidocaine* and *quinidine*, see p.905, p.1378, and p.992, respectively.

**Antibacterials.** Serum concentrations of phenytoin and phenobarbital in a previously stabilised patient were increased when he took *chloramphenicol*.[1] Subsequent monitoring revealed a similar effect when chloramphenicol was taken with phenobarbital alone. In turn, phenobarbital may affect serum concentrations of chloramphenicol (see p.186).

Barbiturates such as phenobarbital and primidone may enhance the metabolism of *doxycycline*.[2]

1. Koup JR, *et al.* Interaction of chloramphenicol with phenytoin and phenobarbital. *Clin Pharmacol Ther* 1978; **24:** 571–5.
2. Neuvonen PJ, *et al.* Effect of antiepileptic drugs on the elimination of various tetracycline derivatives. *Eur J Clin Pharmacol* 1975; **9:** 147–54.

**Anticoagulants.** For the effect of barbiturates such as phenobarbital and primidone on *warfarin* and other coumarins, see p.1025.

**Antidepressants.** As with all antiepileptics, antidepressants may antagonise the antiepileptic activity of phenobarbital by lowering the convulsive threshold.

*Hypericum* has been shown to induce several drug metabolising enzymes (see p.299) and consequently it might reduce the blood concentrations of phenobarbital leading to an increased risk of seizure.[1]

For the effect of phenobarbital on antidepressants, see under *bupropion* (p.288), *fluoxetine* (p.296), *lithium* (p.303), and *mianserin* (p.307).

Inhibition of drug-metabolising enzymes by *MAOIs* may enhance the effects of barbiturates.

1. Committee on Safety of Medicines/Medicines Control Agency. Reminder: St John's wort (Hypericum perforatum) interactions. *Current Problems* 2000; **26:** 6–7. Also available at: http://www.mca.gov.uk/ourwork/monitorsafequalmed/currentproblems/cpmay2000.pdf (accessed 13/05/04)

**Antiepileptics.** Interactions may occur if phenobarbital is given with other antiepileptics, of which probably the most significant is the interaction with *valproate*. Valproate results in an increase in plasma-phenobarbital concentration that has been reported to range from 17 to 48%,[1] and it may be necessary to reduce the dose of phenobarbital in some patients.[1,2] The mechanism for the increase appears to be inhibition of the metabolism of phenobarbital, resulting in reduced clearance;[2,3] valproate appears to inhibit both the direct *N*-glucosidation of phenobarbital and the *O*-glucuronidation of *p*-hydroxyphenobarbital.[4] However, it is worthy of note that phenobarbital reciprocally increases the clearance of valproate, thus potentially requiring the valproate dose to be adjusted too.[5]

A similarly complex interaction exists between phenobarbital and *phenytoin*. Phenytoin may cause a rise in plasma concentrations of phenobarbital in some patients[6] since the two drugs compete for metabolism by the same enzyme system, but other evidence suggests that where this occurs it is rarely of significant magnitude.[7] Similarly, although phenobarbital induces the metabolism of phenytoin it is also, as stated, a competitive inhibitor and in practice the two effects appear to balance out, with rarely any need for dose adjustment.[7-9] However, dosage adjustment of phenobarbital may be crucial for some patients.[10] Measurement of serum concentrations of phenytoin and phenobarbital in one patient[10] showed that, in her case, large increases in serum-phenobarbital concentrations resulted from concomitant administration of phenytoin; the increases were concentration-dependent.

The GABA-agonist, *progabide* has also been reported to cause a significant increase in phenobarbital concentrations when the two were given together to healthy subjects,[11] and the possibility exists that dosage adjustment might be necessary if progabide were added to phenobarbital therapy.

Neurotoxicity, attributed to an increase in plasma concentrations of phenobarbital, has been observed[12] in one patient receiving phenobarbital and sodium valproate when *felbamate* was added to treatment. The dosage of phenobarbital had already been reduced before treatment with felbamate was started. Data from a pharmacokinetic study[13] indicated that the interaction may result from the inhibition of phenobarbital hydroxylation by felbamate.

*Vigabatrin* has been reported to lower plasma concentrations of phenobarbital in some patients,[14] although dosage changes were not necessary in these patients.

High dose of *oxcarbazepine* may increase the plasma concentrations of phenobarbital but this was thought unlikely to be clinically significant;[15] conversely phenobarbital may reduce the plasma concentrations of the active metabolite of oxcarbazepine (p.367).

For the effect of phenobarbital on the metabolism of other antiepileptics, see under *Carbamazepine*, p.356, *Clonazepam*, p.359, *Ethosuximide*, p.360, *Lamotrigine*, p.364, *Tiagabine*, p.378, and *Zonisamide*, p.385.

1. Richens A, Ahmad S. Controlled trial of sodium valproate in severe epilepsy. *BMJ* 1975; **4:** 255–6.
2. Patel IH, *et al.* Phenobarbital-valproic acid interaction. *Clin Pharmacol Ther* 1980; **27:** 515–21.
3. Kapetanović IM, *et al.* Mechanism of valproate-phenobarbital interaction in epileptic patients. *Clin Pharmacol Ther* 1981; **29:** 480–6.
4. Bernus I, *et al.* Inhibition of phenobarbitone N-glucosidation by valproate. *Br J Clin Pharmacol* 1994; **38:** 411–16.
5. Perucca E, *et al.* Disposition of sodium valproate in epileptic patients. *Br J Clin Pharmacol* 1978; **5:** 495–9.
6. Morselli PL, *et al.* Interaction between phenobarbital and diphenylhydantoin in animals and in epileptic patients. *Ann N Y Acad Sci* 1971; **179:** 88–107.
7. Eadie MJ, *et al.* Factors influencing plasma phenobarbitone levels in epileptic patients. *Br J Clin Pharmacol* 1977; **4:** 541–7.
8. Cucinell SA, *et al.* Drug interactions in man: lowering effect of phenobarbital on plasma levels of bishydroxycoumarin (Dicumarol) and diphenylhydantoin (Dilantin). *Clin Pharmacol Ther* 1965; **6:** 420–9.
9. Booker HE, *et al.* Concurrent administration of phenobarbital and diphenylhydantoin: lack of an interference effect. *Neurology* 1971; **21:** 383–5.
10. Kuranari M, *et al.* Effect of phenytoin on phenobarbital pharmacokinetics in a patient with epilepsy. *Ann Pharmacother* 1995; **29:** 83–4.
11. Bianchetti G, *et al.* Pharmacokinetic interactions of progabide with other antiepileptic drugs. *Epilepsia* 1987; **28:** 68–73.
12. Gidal BE, Zupanc ML. Potential pharmacokinetic interaction between felbamate and phenobarbital. *Ann Pharmacother* 1994; **28:** 455–8.
13. Reidenberg P, *et al.* Effects of felbamate on the pharmacokinetics of phenobarbital. *Clin Pharmacol Ther* 1995; **58:** 279–87.
14. Browne TR, *et al.* A multicentre study of vigabatrin for drug-resistant epilepsy. *Br J Clin Pharmacol* 1989; **27** (suppl): 95S–100S.
15. Hossain M, *et al.* Drug-drug interaction profile of oxcarbazepine in children and adults. *Neurology* 1999; **52** (suppl 2): A525.

**Antifungals.** For the effect of phenobarbital on *griseofulvin*, see p.401, and on *itraconazole*, see p.402.

**Antineoplastics.** For the effect of phenobarbital on *teniposide*, see p.587.

**Antiprotozoals.** For the effect of phenobarbital on *metronidazole*, see p.608.

**Antipsychotics.** As with all antiepileptics, antipsychotics may antagonise the antiepileptic activity of phenobarbital by lowering the convulsive threshold.

For the effect of phenobarbital on antipsychotics, see under Chlorpromazine, p.679.

**Antivirals.** For the possible effect of phenobarbital on *HIV-protease inhibitors*, see p.639.

**Beta blockers.** For the effect of barbiturates on beta blockers, see under Anxiolytics and Antipsychotics, p.871.

**Calcium-channel blockers.** For the effect of phenobarbital on *dihydropyridine calcium-channel blockers*, see under Nifedipine, p.969, and on *verapamil*, see p.1020.

**Cardiac glycosides.** Phenobarbital may greatly accelerate the metabolism of *digitoxin* (p.894).

**Ciclosporin.** For the effect of phenobarbital on ciclosporin, see p.1355.

**Corticosteroids.** For the effect of phenobarbital on corticosteroids, see p.1072.

**Diuretics.** Serum-phenobarbital concentrations were raised in 8 of 10 epileptic patients taking phenobarbital and additional antiepileptics when given *furosemide* 40 mg three times daily for 4 weeks.[1] This might have been the cause of drowsiness in 5 of 14 patients, 3 of whom had to discontinue furosemide.

1. Ahmad S, *et al.* Controlled trial of frusemide as an antiepileptic drug in focal epilepsy. *Br J Clin Pharmacol* 1976; **3:** 621–5.

**Levothyroxine.** For the effects of barbiturates on levothyroxine, see p.1601.

**Montelukast.** For the effect of phenobarbital on montelukast, see p.789.

**Sex hormones.** For the effect of phenobarbital on sex hormones in oral contraceptives, see p.1534.

**Theophylline.** For the effect of phenobarbital on theophylline, see p.802.

**Vaccines.** *Influenza vaccination* can cause prolonged rises in serum-phenobarbital concentrations in some patients.[1]

1. Jann MW, Fidone GS. Effect of influenza vaccine on serum anticonvulsant concentrations. *Clin Pharm* 1986; **5:** 817–20.

**Vitamins.** *Pyridoxine* reduced serum-phenobarbital concentrations in 5 patients.[1] Plasma concentrations of phenobarbital and primidone are possibly reduced by *folic acid* and *folinic acid*. For the effect of antiepileptics, including phenobarbital, on *vitamin D* concentrations, see Effects on Bone under Adverse Effects of Phenytoin, p.371.

1. Hansson O, Sillanpaa M. Pyridoxine and serum concentration of phenytoin and phenobarbitone. *Lancet* 1976; **i:** 256.

## Pharmacokinetics

Like other barbiturates phenobarbital is readily absorbed from the gastrointestinal tract, although it is relatively lipid-insoluble; peak concentrations are reached in about 2 hours after oral administration and within 4 hours of intramuscular administration.

Phenobarbital is about 45 to 60% bound to plasma proteins and is only partly metabolised in the liver. About 25% of a dose is excreted in the urine unchanged at normal urinary pH. The plasma half-life is about 75 to 120 hours in adults but is greatly prolonged in neonates, and shorter (about 21 to 75 hours) in children. There is considerable interindividual variation in phenobarbital kinetics.

Monitoring of plasma concentrations has been performed as an aid in assessing control and the therapeutic range of plasma-phenobarbital is usually quoted as 15 to 40 micrograms/mL (65 to 170 micromoles/litre).

Phenobarbital crosses the placental barrier and is distributed into breast milk.

The pharmacokinetics of phenobarbital are affected if given with other antiepileptics (see under Interactions, above).

## Uses and Administration

Phenobarbital is a barbiturate that may be used as an antiepileptic to control partial and generalised tonic-clonic seizures.

The dose should be adjusted to the needs of the individual patient to achieve adequate control of seizures; this usually requires plasma concentrations of 15 to 40 micrograms/mL (65 to 170 micromoles/litre). The usual dose by mouth is 60 to 180 mg daily, taken at night, and a suggested dose for children is up to 8 mg/kg daily.

Phenobarbital sodium may be given parenterally as part of the emergency management of acute seizures. Doses of 200 mg have been given by intramuscular or subcutaneous injection to adults, repeated after 6 hours if necessary. Children may be given 15 mg/kg intramuscularly as a loading dose, which may be followed by 5 mg/kg daily by mouth in divided doses if appropriate. Doubts have been expressed about the efficacy of the intramuscular route owing to the delay in achieving adequate blood concentrations, and the subcutaneous route may cause tissue necrosis.

For the control of status epilepticus in adults, doses of 10 mg/kg may be given intravenously. Injections for intravenous administration should be diluted 1 in 10 and given at a rate not exceeding 100 mg/minute.

As with other antiepileptics, withdrawal of phenobarbital therapy or transition to or from another type of antiepileptic therapy should be made gradually to avoid precipitating an increase in the frequency of seizures. For a discussion on whether or not to withdraw antiepileptic therapy in seizure-free patients, see p.349.

Phenobarbital has also been used as a hypnotic and sedative but drugs such as the benzodiazepines are preferred.

Phenobarbital stimulates the enzymes in hepatic microsomes responsible for the metabolism of some drugs and normal body constituents including bilirubin, and for this reason it has been used to reduce hyperbilirubinaemia in neonatal jaundice.

Phenobarbital magnesium and phenobarbital diethylamine have also been used.

Tetrabamate is a complex of phenobarbital, difebarbamate, and febarbamate but its use has been associated with the development of hepatitis.

**Alcohol withdrawal syndrome.** Phenobarbital is used in some centres for the management of alcohol withdrawal syndrome (p.1166), but has a lower safety profile than benzodiazepines (the treatment of choice) and creates the potential for multiple drug interactions. Additionally, a lack of well-defined studies make its role difficult to assess.[1]

1. Rodgers JE, Crouch MA. Phenobarbital for alcohol withdrawal syndrome. *Am J Health-Syst Pharm* 1999; **56:** 175–8.

**Cerebral malaria.** Phenobarbital has been used to prevent convulsions in patients with cerebral malaria (p.444) but a systematic review[1] concluded that, although it was an effective anticonvulsant, it should not be given routinely to patients with cerebral malaria as it might increase mortality. The optimal dose, particularly in children, has yet to be confirmed. In an early study[2] a single intramuscular injection of phenobarbital sodium 3.5 mg/kg, or 200 mg in patients over 60 kg was effective. A dose of 10 to 15 mg/kg was later suggested.[3] Although a single intramuscular dose of phenobarbital 20 mg/kg markedly reduced seizure frequency in young children with cerebral malaria, it was also associated with a doubling of mortality.[4] The frequency of respiratory arrest was higher in the phenobarbital group than in controls given placebo, and mortality was greatly increased in those given phenobarbital who required 3 or more doses of diazepam.

1. Meremikwu M, Marson AG. Routine anticonvulsants for treating cerebral malaria. Available in The Cochrane Library: Issue 2. Chichester: John Wiley: 2004.
2. White NJ, *et al.* Single dose phenobarbitone prevents convulsions in cerebral malaria. *Lancet* 1988; **ii:** 64–6.
3. Gilles HM. *Management of severe and complicated malaria.* Geneva: WHO, 1991.
4. Crawley J, *et al.* Effect of phenobarbitone on seizure frequency and mortality in childhood cerebral malaria: a randomized, controlled intervention study. *Lancet* 2000; **355:** 701–6.

**Epilepsy.** Phenobarbital is used in the treatment of epilepsy (p.349) for partial seizures with or without secondary generalisation and for primary generalised tonic-clonic seizures. It may also be tried for atypical absence, atonic, and tonic seizures but is not effective in absence seizures. However, the usefulness of phenobarbital is limited by problems of sedation in adults and paradoxical excitement in children. There is also concern about its effects on behaviour and cognition in children. Phenobarbital is therefore usually reserved for use in cases unresponsive to other antiepileptics, although some have suggested that its low cost and broad efficacy make it a suitable first-line drug in developing countries.

References.

1. Pal DK, *et al.* Randomised controlled trial to assess acceptability of phenobarbital for childhood epilepsy in rural India. *Lancet* 1998; **351:** 19–23.

**Febrile convulsions.** Phenobarbital has been used prophylactically in children thought to be at risk of recurrence of febrile convulsions (p.353), but routine use of antiepileptics is no longer recommended.

References.

1. Newton RW. Randomised controlled trials of phenobarbitone and valproate in febrile convulsions. *Arch Dis Child* 1988; **63:** 1189–91.
2. Farwell JR, *et al.* Phenobarbital for febrile seizures: effects on intelligence and on seizure recurrence. *N Engl J Med* 1990; **322:** 364–9. Correction. *ibid.* 1992; **326:** 144.

**Neonatal abstinence syndrome.** For reference to the use of phenobarbital for the treatment of neonates with opioid abstinence syndrome, see p.72.

**Neonatal intraventricular haemorrhage.** Phenobarbital is one of several drugs that has been tried to prevent the development of neonatal intraventricular haemorrhage (p.740). Initial studies[1-3] of antenatal administration to the mother were promising, but a larger randomised study[4] in 610 women failed to show any effect of antenatal phenobarbital on incidence or severity of intraventricular haemorrhage. A systematic review[5] of these and other studies concluded that administration of phenobarbital before preterm birth cannot be recommended for routine clinical practice; strategies for future trials were suggested to improve methodology. Studies of administration to neonates have also shown inconsistent results. A systematic review[6] of studies of phenobarbital for prophylaxis of intraventricular haemorrhage in preterm neonates concluded that postnatal administration cannot be recommended either, and is associated with an increased need for mechanical ventilation.

1. Kaempf JW, *et al.* Antenatal phenobarbital for the prevention of periventricular and intraventricular hemorrhage: a double-blind, randomized, placebo-controlled, multihospital trial. *J Pediatr* 1990; **117:** 933–8.
2. Barnes ER, Thompson DF. Antenatal phenobarbital to prevent or minimize intraventricular hemorrhage in the low-birthweight neonate. *Ann Pharmacother* 1993; **27:** 49–52.

3. Thorp JA, *et al.* Antepartum vitamin K and phenobarbital for preventing intraventricular hemorrhage in the premature newborn: a randomized, double-blind, placebo-controlled trial. *Obstet Gynecol* 1994; **83:** 70–6.
4. Shankaran S, *et al.* The effect of antenatal phenobarbital therapy on neonatal intracranial hemorrhage in preterm infants. *N Engl J Med* 1997; **337:** 466–71.
5. Crowther CA, Henderson-Smart DJ. Phenobarbital prior to preterm birth for preventing neonatal periventricular haemorrhage. Available in The Cochrane Library; Issue 2. Chichester: John Wiley; 2004.
6. Whitelaw A. Postnatal phenobarbitone for the prevention of intraventricular hemorrhage in preterm infants. Available in The Cochrane Library; Issue 2. Chichester: John Wiley; 2004.


**Neonatal seizures.** Some consider phenobarbital to be the mainstay of treatment for all types of neonatal seizures (p.353). In a study[1] in 120 neonates with clinical seizure activity of varying aetiology, 48 were controlled by an initial intravenous loading dose of phenobarbital 15 to 20 mg/kg over 10 to 15 minutes, and a further 37 were controlled by sequential bolus doses of phenobarbital 5 to 10 mg/kg every 20 to 30 minutes up to a serum concentration of 40 micrograms/mL. Of the remaining 35 neonates only 7 responded when the serum-phenobarbital concentration was increased to 100 micrograms/mL, 13 required addition of a second antiepileptic (phenytoin or lorazepam) and 4 were controlled by addition of a third drug. Phenobarbital alone can effectively control seizures in the majority of neonates with recurrent seizure activity.

Phenobarbital administered prophylactically as a single dose of about 40 mg/kg intravenously over one hour has also been shown to be effective in reducing the incidence of seizures in 15 infants with severe perinatal asphyxia compared with a control group who only received phenobarbital if there was clinical evidence of seizures.[2] Subsequent follow-up over 3 years suggested that prophylactic phenobarbital might also improve later neurological outcome.[2]


1. Gilman JT, *et al.* Rapid sequential phenobarbital treatment of neonatal seizures. *Pediatrics* 1989; **83:** 674–8.
2. Hall RT, *et al.* High-dose phenobarbital therapy in term newborn infants with severe perinatal asphyxia: a randomized, prospective study with three-year follow-up. *J Pediatr* 1998; **132:** 345–8.


**Status epilepticus.** Phenobarbital given intravenously is an alternative to intravenous phenytoin in the management of status epilepticus (p.352). It should not be used in patients who have recently received oral phenobarbital or primidone.

Although one study[1] suggested that phenobarbital might be at least as effective, safe, and practical as diazepam with phenytoin for the initial treatment of convulsive status epilepticus, it tends to be reserved for patients who do not respond to benzodiazepines or phenytoin.


1. Shaner DM, *et al.* Treatment of status epilepticus: a prospective comparison of diazepam and phenytoin versus phenobarbital and optional phenytoin. *Neurology* 1988; **38:** 202–7.


## Preparations

***BP 2003:*** Phenobarbital Elixir; Phenobarbital Injection; Phenobarbital Sodium Tablets; Phenobarbital Tablets;
***USP 27:*** Phenobarbital Elixir; Phenobarbital Sodium for Injection; Phenobarbital Sodium Injection; Phenobarbital Tablets; Theophylline, Ephedrine Hydrochloride, and Phenobarbital Tablets.

**Proprietary Preparations** (details are given in Part 3)
***Arg.:*** Alepsal; Gardenal; Luminal; Luminaletas; ***Belg.:*** Gardenal; ***Braz.:*** Barbitron; Edhanol; Fenocris; Gardenal; Unifenobarb; ***Denm.:*** Fenemal; ***Fr.:*** Aparoxal; Gardenal; Kaneuron; ***Ger.:*** Lepinal†; Lepinaletten†; Luminal; Luminaletten; Phenaemal†; Phenaemaletten†; ***Gr.:*** Gardenal; Kaneuron; Lumidrops; ***Hong Kong:*** Gardenal†; ***India:*** Gardenal; Luminal; Luminalettes; ***Israel:*** Luminal; ***Ital.:*** Comizial; Gardenale; Luminale; Luminalette; Neurobiol; ***Mex.:*** Alepsal; Fenocriz†; Sevenal†; Sevenaleta†; ***Norw.:*** Fenemal; ***NZ:*** Gardenal; ***Port.:*** Bialminal; Luminal; Luminaletas; ***S.Afr.:*** Gardenal; Lethyl; Sedabarb†; ***Spain:*** Gardenal; Gratusminal; Luminal; Luminaletas; Sevrium†; ***Swed.:*** Fenemal; ***Switz.:*** Aphenylbarbit; Luminal; ***Thai.:*** Gardenal; Menobarb; Phenobarb; Phenotal; ***UK:*** Gardenal; ***USA:*** Luminal; Solfoton†.

**Multi-ingredient:** ***Arg.:*** Cumatil L; Lotoquis; Trixol; ***Belg.:*** Epipropane; Spasmosedine†; Vethoine; ***Braz.:*** Bromosedan†; Espasmalgon; Filinasma†; Gamibetal Complex; Gratusminal†; Piptalake P†; Vagostesyl; ***Canad.:*** Bellergal; Dilantin with Phenobarbital†; Donnatal†; Phenaphen with Codeine†; Tedral†; ***Chile:*** Abalgin; Baldmin; Bellergal Retardado; Belupan; Bufacyl; Dispasmol; Ergobelan; Immediat; Sinpasmon; Valpin; ***Fr.:*** Alepsal; Atrium†; Dinacode; Enuretine†; Natisedine†; Nuidor†; Ortenal†; Prenoxan au phenobarbital†; Sedatonyl†; Sedibaine†; Spasmidenal†; ***Hung.:*** Triospan; ***India:*** Alergin; Asmapax; Asthmino; Cadiphylate; Dilantin with Phenobarbital; Epilan; Garoin; ***Israel:*** Pacetal; Philinal; Philinet; ***Ital.:*** Bellergil†; Gamibetal Complex; Metinal-Idantoina L; ***Jpn:*** Trancolon P; ***Mex.:*** Alepsal Compuesto; Paliatil; ***Port.:*** Anti-Asmatico; Comital L†; Cosmaxil; Fluidin Antiasmatico†; Fluidin Nocturno†; Hidantina Composta; Prelus; ***S.Afr.:*** Adco-Phenobarbitone Vitalet; Analgen-SA; Bellatard†; Bellergal†; Depain Plus†; Donnatal; Garoin†; Menoflush + ¼†; Millerspas; Pedriachol†; Propain Forte; ***Spain:*** Comital L; Disfil†; Distovagal†; Epilantin; Redutona; Solufilina Sedante†; Winasma†; ***Switz.:*** Atrium†; Bellergal†; ***Thai.:*** Bellergal; Benera; Donnatal; Neuramizone; ***USA:*** Antispasmodic Elixir; Antrocol†; Arco-Lase Plus†; Barbidonna; Bel-Phen-Ergot S; Bellacane; Bellamine; Bellatal; Bellergal-S; Donnatal†; Folergot-DF; Gustase Plus†; Hyosophen; Lufyllin-EPG; Mudrane GG†; Mudrane†; Phenerbel-S; Quadrinal; Susano; Tedrigen; Theodrine.

# Phensuximide *(BAN, rINN)*

Fensuximida. *N*-Methyl-2-phenylsuccinimide.
$C_{11}H_{11}NO_2$ = 189.2.
*CAS — 86-34-0.*
*ATC — N03AD02.*

**Pharmacopoeias.** In *US.*

**USP 27** (Phensuximide). A white to off-white crystalline powder. Is odourless or has not more than a slight odour. Slightly soluble in water; soluble in alcohol; very soluble in chloroform. Store in airtight containers.

## Profile

Phensuximide is a succinimide antiepileptic with actions similar to those of ethosuximide (p.360), but it is reported to be less effective.

**Porphyria.** Phensuximide has been associated with acute attacks of porphyria and is considered unsafe in porphyric patients.

## Preparations

***USP 27:*** Phensuximide Capsules.

# Phenytoin *(BAN, USAN, rINN)*

Diphenylhydantoin; Fenitoína; Phenantoinum; Phenytoinum. 5,5-Diphenylhydantoin; 5,5-Diphenylimidazolidine-2,4-dione.
$C_{15}H_{12}N_2O_2$ = 252.3.
*CAS — 57-41-0.*
*ATC — N03AB02.*

**Pharmacopoeias.** In *Eur.* (see p.vi), *Int., Jpn, Pol., US,* and *Viet.*

**Ph. Eur. 5.0** (Phenytoin). A white or almost white, crystalline powder. Practically insoluble in water; sparingly soluble in alcohol; very slightly soluble in dichloromethane. It dissolves in dilute solutions of alkali hydroxides.

**USP 27** (Phenytoin). A white, odourless powder. Practically insoluble in water; soluble in hot alcohol; slightly soluble in cold alcohol, in chloroform, and in ether. Store in airtight containers.

## Phenytoin Sodium *(BANM, rINNM)*

Diphenin; Fenitoína sódica; Phenytoinum Natricum; Soluble Phenytoin.
$C_{15}H_{11}N_2NaO_2$ = 274.2.
*CAS — 630-93-3.*
*ATC — N03AB02.*

**Pharmacopoeias.** In *Chin., Eur.* (see p.vi), *Int., Jpn, Pol.,* and *US.*

**Ph. Eur. 5.0** (Phenytoin Sodium). A white, slightly hygroscopic, crystalline powder. Soluble in water and in alcohol; practically insoluble in dichloromethane. Store in airtight containers.

**USP 27** (Phenytoin Sodium). A white, odourless powder. Is somewhat hygroscopic and on exposure to air gradually absorbs carbon dioxide. Freely soluble in water, the solution usually being somewhat turbid due to partial hydrolysis and absorption of carbon dioxide; soluble in alcohol; practically insoluble in chloroform and in ether. Store in airtight containers.

**Incompatibility.** Phenytoin sodium only remains in solution when the pH is considerably alkaline (about 10 to 12) and there have been reports of loss of clarity or precipitation of phenytoin crystals when solutions of phenytoin sodium for injection have been mixed with a variety of drugs[1-6] or added to intravenous infusion fluids,[7-10] while binding has been reported following addition to enteral nutrition solutions.[11] A phenytoin precipitate has been reported to occlude implanted central venous access devices following the inadvertent admixture of phenytoin sodium with glucose 5% or glucose in sodium chloride (pH 4);[12,13] it may be successfully cleared by the local instillation of sodium bicarbonate 8.4% to increase the pH of the medium.


1. Misgen R. Compatibilities and incompatibilities of some intravenous solution admixtures. *Am J Hosp Pharm* 1965; **22:** 92–4.
2. Patel JA, Phillips GL. A guide to physical compatibility of intravenous drug admixtures. *Am J Hosp Pharm* 1966; **23:** 409–11.
3. Klamerus KJ, *et al.* Stability of nitroglycerin in intravenous admixtures. *Am J Hosp Pharm* 1984; **41:** 303–5.
4. Hasegawa GR, Eder JF. Visual compatibility of dobutamine hydrochloride with other injectable drugs. *Am J Hosp Pharm* 1984; **41:** 949–51.
5. Gayed AA, *et al.* Visual compatibility of diltiazem injection with various diluents and medications during simulated Y-site injection. *Am J Health-Syst Pharm* 1995; **52:** 516–20.
6. Trissel LA, *et al.* Compatibility of propofol injectable emulsion with selected drugs during simulated Y-site administration. *Am J Health-Syst Pharm* 1997; **54:** 1287–92.
7. Bauman JL, *et al.* Phenytoin crystallization in intravenous fluids. *Drug Intell Clin Pharm* 1977; **11:** 646–9.
8. Bauman JL, Siepler JK. Intravenous phenytoin (concluded). *N Engl J Med* 1977; **296:** 111.
9. Cloyd JC, *et al.* Concentration-time profile of phenytoin after admixture with small volumes of intravenous fluids. *Am J Hosp Pharm* 1978; **35:** 45–8.
10. Giacona N, *et al.* Crystallization of three phenytoin preparations in intravenous solutions. *Am J Hosp Pharm* 1982; **39:** 630–4.
11. Miller SW, Strom JG. Stability of phenytoin in three enteral nutrient formulas. *Am J Hosp Pharm* 1988; **45:** 2529–32.
12. Akinwande KI, Keehn DM. Dissolution of phenytoin precipitate with sodium bicarbonate in an occluded central various access device. *Ann Pharmacother* 1995; **29:** 707–9.
13. Tse CST, Abdullah R. Dissolving phenytoin precipitate in central venous access device. *Ann Intern Med* 1998; **128:** 1049.


## Adverse Effects

Side-effects are fairly frequent in patients receiving phenytoin, but some remit with dose reduction or continued use. Often reported are lack of appetite, headache, dizziness, tremor, transient nervousness, insomnia, and gastrointestinal disturbances such as nausea, vomiting, and constipation. Tenderness and hyperplasia of the gums often occurs, particularly in younger patients. Acne, hirsutism, and coarsening of the facial features may be associated with phenytoin therapy, and may be particularly undesirable in adolescents and women.

Phenytoin toxicity may be manifested as a syndrome of cerebellar, vestibular, and ocular effects, notably nystagmus, diplopia, slurred speech, and ataxia. Mental confusion, sometimes severe, may occur, and dyskinesias and exacerbations of seizure frequency have been noted. Hyperglycaemia has been associated with toxic concentrations.

Overdosage may result in hypotension, coma, and respiratory depression. Hypotension and CNS depression may also follow intravenous administration, if too rapid, as may cardiac arrhythmias and impaired cardiac conduction. Solutions for injection are very alkaline and may result in irritation at the injection site or phlebitis.

Prolonged therapy may produce subtle effects on mental function and cognition, especially in children. In addition there is some evidence that phenytoin interferes with vitamin D and folate metabolism. Rickets and osteomalacia have occurred in a few patients not exposed to adequate sunlight, although the causal role of phenytoin is debatable. A proportion of patients develop peripheral neuropathies, usually mild, and occasional cases of megaloblastic anaemia have been seen.

Mild hypersensitivity reactions are common, with skin rashes, often morbilliform, sometimes accompanied by fever. Bullous, exfoliative, or purpuric rashes may be symptoms of rare but severe reactions such as lupus erythematosus, erythema multiforme, Stevens-Johnson syndrome, or toxic epidermal necrolysis. Eosinophilia, lymphadenopathy, hepatitis, polyarteritis nodosa, and blood disorders such as aplastic anaemia, leucopenia, thrombocytopenia, and agranulocytosis, have occurred rarely; some of these conditions may also represent hypersensitivity reactions.

Hypoprothrombinaemia of the newborn following administration of phenytoin during pregnancy has been reported. Congenital malformations have been seen in the offspring of mothers receiving phenytoin during pregnancy (see under Precautions, below).

**Effects on the blood.** AGRANULOCYTOSIS. Fatal agranulocytosis has been reported[1] in a patient 17 years after starting therapy with phenytoin and primidone. In the report it was stated that since 1963 the UK Committee on Safety of Medicines had received reports of 3 previous cases of fatal agranulocytosis associated with phenytoin and none associated with primidone. The most likely cause was considered to be a direct toxic effect of phenytoin although other possible mechanisms included the ability of both drugs to produce folate deficiency. For a discussion of the effect of antiepileptics on serum folate, see below.


1. Laurenson IF, *et al.* Delayed fatal agranulocytosis in an epileptic taking primidone and phenytoin. *Lancet* 1994, **344:** 332–3.


FOLIC ACID DEFICIENCY. Antiepileptic therapy has long been associated with folate deficiency: early studies suggested that more than half of all patients on long-term therapy with drugs such as phenytoin, phenobarbital, and primidone had subnormal serum-folate concentrations.[1,2] Megaloblastic haematopoiesis is often present,[3] but clinical megaloblastic anaemia appears to be rare.

The relative importance of individual antiepileptics in causing folate deficiency and macrocytosis has been difficult to establish, because of the tendency to use combination regimens; with greater emphasis on single drug therapy there is evidence that monotherapy may produce less significant changes.[4,5] Despite suggestions that carbamazepine has relatively little effect on folic acid concentrations, its effects have been found to be comparable with those of phenytoin;[5] in this study only valproate had little or no effect on red cell folate concentrations.

The mechanism by which phenytoin and similar antiepileptics reduce serum folate is uncertain; there is good evidence for a reduction in absorption of glutamate both *in vitro*[6] and *in vivo*,[7] but the drugs associated with subnormal serum folate are all enzyme inducers and it has been suggested that enzyme induction and enhanced folate metabolism may also play a role.[2,5,8] Adverse blood changes also result from hypersensitivity (see below).


1. Horwitz SJ, *et al.* Relation of abnormal folate metabolism to neuropathy developing during anticonvulsant drug therapy. *Lancet* 1968; **i:** 563–5.
2. Maxwell JD, *et al.* Folate deficiency after anticonvulsant drugs: an effect of hepatic enzyme induction? *BMJ* 1972; **1:** 297–9.
3. Wickramasinghe SN, *et al.* Megaloblastic erythropoiesis and macrocytosis in patients on anticonvulsants. *BMJ* 1975; **4:** 136–7.

4. Dellaportas DI, *et al.* Chronic toxicity in epileptic patients receiving single-drug treatment. *BMJ* 1982; **285:** 409–10.
5. Goggin T, *et al.* A comparative study of the relative effects of anticonvulsant drugs and dietary folate on the red cell folate status of patients with epilepsy. *Q J Med* 1987; **NS65** (247): 911–9.
6. Hoffbrand AV, Necheles TF. Mechanism of folate deficiency in patients receiving phenytoin. *Lancet* 1968; **ii:** 528–30.
7. Rosenberg IH, *et al.* Impairment of intestinal deconjugation of dietary folate. *Lancet* 1968; **ii:** 530–2.
8. Kishi T, *et al.* Mechanism for reduction of serum folate by antiepileptic drugs during prolonged therapy. *J Neurol Sci* 1997; **145:** 109–12.

**Effects on bone.** The effects of phenytoin and other antiepileptics on the skeletal system are a matter of some debate. There are numerous reports indicating effects on bone and on calcium and vitamin D metabolism. Therapy with *carbamazepine, phenobarbital,* or *phenytoin* has been associated with reduction in serum-calcium concentration to hypocalcaemic values, significant reduction in 25-hydroxycholecalciferol concentrations, and elevated alkaline phosphatase.[1] In this study, involving 226 outpatients with epilepsy, the association was not seen with *valproate*. The effects were significantly greater in the group of patients receiving polytherapy, and there was limited evidence that these biochemical changes were exacerbated by reduced exposure to sunlight. In contrast, measurements of bone mineral density in one study of 26 children,[2] and in another of 19 children,[3] receiving antiepileptic monotherapy revealed a reduction in density in those taking *valproate* but no reduction with *carbamazepine*. Another study[4] in 54 male patients followed for 12 to 29 months revealed that treatment with antiepileptics was associated with bone loss at the hip in the absence of vitamin D deficiency. There was no evidence that any particular drug produced more bone loss than another.

Nonetheless, reports of associated clinical osteomalacia are rare.[5] A study in 20 epileptic outpatients who had received antiepileptic therapy for a mean of 14½ years failed to show any clinical evidence of osteomalacia although there was some evidence of altered calcium metabolism.[6] Similarly osteomalacia was seen in only 1 of 19 elderly inpatients in another study,[7] a rate similar to that previously seen in elderly patients with acute illness not receiving antiepileptic therapy.

A recent review[8] stated that there have been no significant reports of altered bone metabolism associated with the newer antiepileptics (*gabapentin, lamotrigine, topiramate,* and *vigabatrin*). However, short stature, low bone mineral density, and reduced bone formation have been reported with long-term lamotrigine treatment, particularly in combination with valproate;[9] further study is needed.

1. Gough H, *et al.* A comparative study of the relative influence of different anticonvulsant drugs, UV exposure and diet on vitamin D and calcium metabolism in out-patients with epilepsy. *Q J Med* 1986; **NS59** (230): 569–77.
2. Sheth RD, *et al.* Effect of carbamazepine and valproate on bone mineral density. *J Pediatr* 1995; **127:** 256–62.
3. Kafalı G, *et al.* Effect of antiepileptic drugs on bone mineral density in children between ages 6 and 12 years. *Clin Pediatr (Phila)* 1999; **38:** 93–8.
4. Andress DL, *et al.* Antiepileptic drug-induced bone loss in young male patients who have seizures. *Arch Neurol* 2002; **59:** 781–6.
5. Beghi E, *et al.* Adverse effects of anticonvulsant drugs: a critical review. *Adverse Drug React Acute Poisoning Rev* 1986; **2:** 63–86.
6. Fogelman I, *et al.* Do anticonvulsant drugs commonly induce osteomalacia? *Scott Med J* 1982; **27:** 136–42.
7. Harrington MG, Hodkinson HM. Anticonvulsant drugs and bone disease in the elderly. *J R Soc Med* 1987; **80:** 425–7.
8. Pack AM, Morrell MJ. Adverse effects of antiepileptic drugs on bone structure: epidemiology, mechanisms and therapeutic indications. *CNS Drugs* 2001; **15:** 633–42.
9. Guo C-Y, *et al.* Long-term valproate and lamotrigine treatment may be a marker for reduced growth and bone mass in children with epilepsy. *Epilepsia* 2001; **42:** 1141–7.

**Effects on the endocrine system and metabolism.** Antiepileptics diminish *sexual potency* and *fertility* in young male epileptics.[1] Phenytoin is excreted in human semen in small quantities and might affect sperm morphology and motility. Reduced plasma concentrations of free testosterone have been detected in male epileptic patients receiving one or more of the following: carbamazepine, phenytoin, primidone, and sodium valproate.[2] *Gynaecomastia* has been reported[3] in 5 men receiving long-term antiepileptic treatment; one also complained of impotence but libido was stated to be normal in all 5. Phenytoin was a component of therapy in all patients and was the sole drug used in one.

Phenytoin may cause reversible *hyperglycaemia* at toxic doses but it does not appear to produce long-term effects on glucose tolerance when used in therapeutic doses.[4] Paradoxically, phenytoin has also been reported to improve insulin resistance in some patients.

Phenytoin may reduce serum concentrations of *thyroid* hormones through enzyme induction—see under Interactions of Levothyroxine, p.1601.

1. Anonymous. [A brief summary]. *BMJ* 1979; **2:** 1118.
2. Dana-Haeri J, *et al.* Reduction of free testosterone by antiepileptic drugs. *BMJ* 1982; **284:** 85–6.
3. Monson JP, Scott DF. Gynaecomastia induced by phenytoin in men with epilepsy. *BMJ* 1987; **294:** 612.
4. Hurel SJ, Taylor R. Drugs and glucose tolerance. *Adverse Drug React Bull* 1995; **174:** 659–62.

**Effects on the liver.** There have been occasional reports of liver damage, probably due to hypersensitivity (see below), associated with phenobarbital and phenytoin; the authors of an early study suggested that such drugs need not be withdrawn if there were merely transient elevations in transaminase values,[1] but care is needed to distinguish such effects from the early symptoms of the antiepileptic hypersensitivity syndrome (see below).

1. Aiges HW, *et al.* The effects of phenobarbital and diphenylhydantoin on liver function and morphology. *J Pediatr* 1980; **97:** 22–6.

**Effects on the lungs.** Pulmonary eosinophilia and acute respiratory failure requiring mechanical ventilation have been reported[1] in a patient receiving phenytoin; other pulmonary symptoms associated with phenytoin were reviewed.

1. Mahatma M, *et al.* Phenytoin-induced acute respiratory failure with pulmonary eosinophilia. *Am J Med* 1989; **87:** 93–4.

**Effects on mental function.** For a review of the effects of antiepileptic therapy including phenytoin on cognition, see p.351.

**Effects on the skin.** Skin reactions produced by phenytoin are discussed under Hypersensitivity, below. Rare, but severe reactions such as Stevens-Johnson syndrome and toxic epidermal necrolysis have also occurred.

For reference to cutaneous manifestations of zinc deficiency, possibly due to chelation with phenytoin, see under Valproate, p.381.

**Gingival hyperplasia.** Gingival hyperplasia, characterised by inflammation and a marked fibrotic response, may affect up to 50% of patients receiving phenytoin. It usually becomes apparent within the first few months of therapy and is observed more frequently in children; there is no increase in alveolar bone loss. The mechanism underlying its development is unknown, although the main metabolite of phenytoin, 5-(4-hydroxyphenyl)-5-phenylhydantoin, has been implicated.[1-3]

1. Ball DE, *et al.* Plasma and saliva concentrations of phenytoin and 5-(4-hydroxyphenyl)-5-phenylhydantoin (HPPH) in relation to gingival overgrowth in epileptic patients. *Br J Clin Pharmacol* 1995; **39:** 539P–588P.
2. Ieiri I, *et al.* Effect of 5-(p-hydroxyphenyl)-5-phenylhydantoin (p-HPPH) enantiomers, major metabolites of phenytoin, on the occurrence of chronic-gingival hyperplasia: in vivo and in vitro study. *Eur J Clin Pharmacol* 1995; **49:** 51–6.
3. Zhou LX, *et al.* Metabolism of phenytoin by the gingiva of normal humans: the possible role of reactive metabolites of phenytoin in the initiation of gingival hyperplasia. *Clin Pharmacol Ther* 1996; **60:** 191–8.

**Hypersensitivity.** An antiepileptic hypersensitivity syndrome, comprising fever, rash, and lymphadenopathy and less commonly lymphocytosis, and liver and other organ involvement, has been associated with some antiepileptic drugs including phenytoin.[1-3] Clinical manifestations may include interstitial nephritis, anaemia, interstitial pulmonary infiltrates, thrombocytopenia, eosinophilia, myopathy, and diffuse intravascular coagulation.[1,2] Some have estimated the incidence at 1 in 1000 to 1 in 10 000 new exposures to aromatic anticonvulsants,[2,3] but the true incidence is unknown due to variations in presentation and reporting. The syndrome occurs most frequently on first exposure to the drug, with initial symptoms starting anywhere between 1 and 8 weeks after exposure. The mean interval to onset is 17 to 21 days with phenytoin. In previously sensitised individuals the reaction may occur within 1 day of rechallenge. The potential for cross-reactivity between carbamazepine, phenobarbital, and phenytoin is approximately 75%, and patients who develop the syndrome, and their close relatives, should be warned of the risk associated with use of these antiepileptics.[2] An early review[1] of the syndrome in patients taking phenytoin commented that it occurred mainly in black male patients and should not be confused with more common mild general hypersensitivity reactions. More recent evidence does not suggest that ethnic origin predicts differences in risk.[2]

Most cases resolve spontaneously following withdrawal of the drug and symptomatic management. The use of corticosteroids in the management of severe cases remains controversial in the absence of controlled studies of their effectiveness.[1,2]

Phenytoin-induced pseudolymphoma mimicking cutaneous T-cell lymphoma has also been reported.[2,4] In most cases, symptoms resolve within 7 to 14 days of drug discontinuation, and the condition is not considered premalignant.[2] However, in one report[4] the cutaneous eruption and lymphadenopathy persisted after withdrawal of phenytoin for one year when the patient eventually became asymptomatic.

In a prospective study[5] of 306 patients given phenytoin there was an overall incidence of 8.5% of morbilliform rash, but there was a marked seasonal incidence with most reactions occurring during the summer months. The results did not appear to be due to photosensitivity and might represent seasonal alterations in the immune system.

1. Flowers FP, *et al.* Phenytoin hypersensitivity syndrome. *J Emerg Med* 1987; **5:** 103–8.
2. Knowles SR, *et al.* Anticonvulsant hypersensitivity syndrome: incidence, prevention and management. *Drug Safety* 1999; **21:** 489–501.
3. Bessmertny O, *et al.* Antiepileptic hypersensitivity syndrome in children. *Ann Pharmacother* 2001; **35:** 533–8.
4. Harris DWS, *et al.* Phenytoin-induced pseudolymphoma: a report of a case and review of the literature. *Br J Dermatol* 1992; **127:** 403–6.
5. Leppik IE, *et al.* Seasonal incidence of phenytoin allergy unrelated to plasma levels. *Arch Neurol* 1985; **42:** 120–2.

**Peripheral neuropathies.** Electrophysiological abnormalities following prolonged phenytoin treatment are common, but clinically significant peripheral neuropathy is rare.[1] The neuropathy usually involves sensory nerves and lesions are generally mild and asymptomatic.[2] Much of the reported clinical neuropathy has been associated with multiple drug therapy of epilepsy and with exposure to toxic concentrations of phenytoin.[1] Although an association with folate deficiency has been suggested, a study in 52 patients receiving long-term antiepileptic therapy failed to find any convincing evidence of a relationship between serum-folate concentration and peripheral neuropathy.[3]

1. Bruni J. Phenytoin and other hydantoins: adverse effects. In: Levy RH, *et al.*, eds. *Antiepileptic drugs*. 5th ed. Philadelphia: Lippincott Williams & Wilkins, 2002; 605–10.
2. Argov Z, Mastaglia FL. Drug-induced peripheral neuropathies. *BMJ* 1979; **1:** 663–6.
3. Horwitz SJ, *et al.* Relation of abnormal folate metabolism to neuropathy developing during anticonvulsant drug therapy. *Lancet* 1968; **i:** 563–5.

## Treatment of Adverse Effects

Treatment of poisoning with phenytoin tends to be supportive. Repeated doses of activated charcoal should be given by mouth with the aim not only of preventing absorption but also of aiding elimination. If vomiting is severe, charcoal may be given by nasogastric tube. Gastric lavage may be considered if a very large amount has been taken within 1 hour.

◊ Multiple oral doses of activated charcoal may reduce the absorption of phenytoin[1,2] but the degree of clinical benefit is unclear.[3] The value of charcoal haemoperfusion in the management of phenytoin overdosage is debatable. A review of haemoperfusion included data from 2 patients who ingested phenytoin[4] but, although it was suggested that haemoperfusion should contribute significantly to drug removal, results are difficult to evaluate in these patients who had also ingested phenobarbital. An evaluation in a patient who had also taken primidone[5] suggested that, although initial clearance of phenytoin was promising, the system rapidly became saturated and there was little overall benefit. Neither haemodialysis[6] nor peritoneal dialysis[7] is considered worthwhile. A review[3] of the features and management of poisoning with the antiepileptics carbamazepine, ethosuximide, lamotrigine, phenytoin, valproate, and vigabatrin concluded that meticulous supportive care is required; gastric lavage and activated charcoal should be administered within 1 to 2 hours of overdose. Haemodialysis and haemoperfusion are kinetically unfavourable and of doubtful clinical efficacy.

1. Weidle PJ, *et al.* Multiple-dose activated charcoal as adjunct therapy after chronic phenytoin intoxication. *Clin Pharm* 1991; **10:** 711–14.
2. Dolgin JG, *et al.* Pharmacokinetic simulation of the effect of multiple-dose activated charcoal in phenytoin poisoning—report of two pediatric cases. *DICP Ann Pharmacother* 1991; **25:** 646–9.
3. Jones AL, Proudfoot AT. Features and management of poisoning with modern drugs used to treat epilepsy. *Q J Med* 1998; **91:** 325–32.
4. Pond S, *et al.* Pharmacokinetics of haemoperfusion for drug overdose. *Clin Pharmacokinet* 1979; **4:** 329–54.
5. Baehler RW, *et al.* Charcoal hemoperfusion in the therapy for methsuximide and phenytoin overdose. *Arch Intern Med* 1980; **140:** 1466–8.
6. Rubinger D, *et al.* Inefficiency of haemodialysis in acute phenytoin intoxication. *Br J Clin Pharmacol* 1979; **7:** 405–7.
7. Czajka PA, *et al.* A pharmacokinetic evaluation of peritoneal dialysis for phenytoin intoxication. *J Clin Pharmacol* 1980; **20:** 565–9.

## Precautions

Phenytoin is metabolised in the liver and should be given with care to patients with impaired liver function. Caution is also advocated in diabetic patients because of the potential effects of phenytoin on blood sugar.

Protein binding may be reduced in certain disease states such as uraemia, and in certain patient populations such as neonates, pregnant women, and the elderly. Although phenytoin is extensively protein bound this may be of little clinical significance in itself, provided that hepatic function is not impaired, because the concentration of free (pharmacologically active) drug in the plasma often remains more or less unchanged, due to distribution, metabolism, and excretion. Thus, an alteration in protein binding would not necessarily require a change in dosage of phenytoin to be made although, when plasma concentrations are being monitored, relatively lower total plasma-phenytoin concentrations will be found to be effective since there is less bound (pharmacologically inactive) phenytoin available for measurement.

Intravenous phenytoin must be given slowly and extravasation and intra-arterial administration must be avoided. Phenytoin should not be given intravenously to patients with sinus bradycardia, heart block, or Stokes-Adams syndrome, and should be used with caution in patients with hypotension, heart failure, or myocardial infarction; monitoring of blood pressure and the ECG is recommended during intravenous use.

Patients or their carers should be told how to recognise signs of blood or skin toxicity and they should be advised to seek immediate medical attention if symptoms such as fever, sore throat, rash, mouth ulcers, bruising, or bleeding develop. Phenytoin should be withdrawn, if necessary under cover of a suitable alternative antiepileptic, if leucopenia which is severe, progressive, or associated with clinical symptoms develops. It should also be discontinued if a skin rash develops; in the case of mild rashes phenytoin may be reintroduced cautiously, but should be discontinued immediately and permanently if the rash recurs.

Care is required when withdrawing phenytoin therapy—see also under Uses and Administration, below.

Phenytoin may interfere with some tests of thyroid function as it can reduce free and circulating concentrations of levothyroxine, mainly by enhanced conversion to tri-iodothyronine, and it may also produce lower than normal values for dexamethasone and metyrapone suppression tests.

**Breast feeding.** The American Academy of Pediatrics[1] considers that phenytoin is usually compatible with breast feeding, although there had been an early case report of methaemoglobinaemia in a breast-fed infant.

For further comment on antiepileptic therapy and breast feeding, see p.351.

1. American Academy of Pediatrics. The transfer of drugs and other chemicals into human milk. *Pediatrics* 2001; **108:** 776–89. Correction. *ibid.*; 1029. Also available at: http://aappolicy.aappublications.org/cgi/content/full/pediatrics%3b108/3/776 (accessed 14/05/04)

**Driving.** For comment on antiepileptic drugs and driving, see p.351.

**Infections.** A 52-year-old woman previously well-controlled on phenytoin 400 mg daily suffered phenytoin toxicity after a viral infection;[1] her plasma-phenytoin concentration had increased from 16 to 51 micrograms/mL. Six weeks later she had recovered and was re-stabilised on phenytoin 400 mg daily.

1. Levine M, Jones MW. Toxic reaction to phenytoin following a viral infection. *Can Med Assoc J* 1983; **128:** 1270–1.

AIDS. Renal abnormalities or hypoalbuminaemia associated with AIDS may increase the risk of elevated free phenytoin concentrations and subsequent toxicity. Altered protein binding resulted in marked phenytoin toxicity, with lethargy and seizure-like activity, in an HIV-positive patient with profound hypoalbuminaemia and moderate renal insufficiency.[1] Therapeutic drug monitoring in 21 patients with AIDS indicated that although total serum concentrations of phenytoin were lower than in a reference population, the fraction of unbound drug was higher.[2] These changes might be attributed to hypoalbuminaemia and it was suggested that free rather than total phenytoin concentrations should be measured in HIV-infected patients with hypoalbuminaemia.

Phenytoin itself was associated with reversible hypogammaglobulinaemia in an HIV-positive patient who previously had borderline hypergammaglobulinaemia.[3]

1. Toler SM, *et al.* Severe phenytoin intoxication as a result of altered protein binding in AIDS. *DICP Ann Pharmacother* 1990; **24:** 698–700.
2. Burger DM, *et al.* Therapeutic drug monitoring of phenytoin in patients with the acquired immunodeficiency syndrome. *Ther Drug Monit* 1994; **16:** 616–20.
3. Britigan BE. Diphenylhydantoin-induced hypogammaglobulinemia in a patient infected with human immunodeficiency virus. *Am J Med* 1991; **90:** 524–7.

**Porphyria.** Phenytoin has been associated with acute attacks of porphyria and is considered unsafe in porphyric patients.

**Pregnancy.** For comments on the management of epilepsy during pregnancy, see p.351.

There is an increased risk of neural tube defects in infants exposed *in utero* to antiepileptics including phenytoin and a variety of syndromes such as craniofacial and digital abnormalities and, less commonly, cleft lip and palate have been described. Specific syndromes such as the 'fetal hydantoin syndrome' with phenytoin have been linked to individual antiepileptics. However, there is overlap between the effects seen with different antiepileptics and some consider the broader term 'fetal antiepileptic drug syndrome' to be more appropriate. There is also a risk of neonatal bleeding with phenytoin.

## Interactions

There are complex interactions between antiepileptics, and toxicity may be enhanced without a corresponding increase in antiepileptic activity. Such interactions are very variable and unpredictable and plasma monitoring is often advisable with combination therapy.

Since phenytoin is extensively bound to plasma proteins it can be displaced by drugs competing for protein-binding sites, thus liberating more free (pharmacologically active) phenytoin into the plasma. However, elevation of free phenytoin is reported to be of little clinical significance provided hepatic function is not impaired (see Precautions, above). A potentially more serious type of interaction may occur because phenytoin metabolism is saturable: toxic concentrations of phenytoin can develop in patients given drugs that inhibit phenytoin metabolism even to quite a minor degree. Phenytoin itself is also a potent enzyme inducer, and induces the metabolism of a number of drugs, including some antibacterials, anticoagulants, corticosteroids, quinidine, and sex hormones (notably, oral contraceptives).

The hypotensive properties of dopamine and the cardiac depressant properties of drugs such as lidocaine may be dangerously enhanced by intravenous administration of phenytoin.

◊ General references.

1. Nation RL, *et al.* Pharmacokinetic drug interactions with phenytoin. *Clin Pharmacokinet* 1990; **18:** 37–60 and 131–150.

**Anaesthetics.** A 10-year-old girl with epilepsy who had been treated with phenytoin 100 mg three times daily for 5 years and who had lateral nystagmus developed symptoms of phenytoin intoxication following anaesthesia with *halothane*.[1] The plasma concentration of phenytoin 72 hours after anaesthesia was 41 microgram/mL. It was suggested that temporary liver dysfunction was responsible for impaired metabolism of phenytoin.

1. Karlin JM, Kutt H. Acute diphenylhydantoin intoxication following halothane anesthesia. *J Pediatr* 1970; **76:** 941–4.

**Analgesics.** Various analgesics may interact with phenytoin. *Aspirin* is reported to displace phenytoin from plasma binding[1,2] but there is no evidence of any effect on metabolism and effects are unlikely to be clinically significant.[3,4] *Paracetamol* is reported to have no significant effect on serum-phenytoin concentrations.[4] (However, the use of enzyme-inducing antiepileptics such as phenytoin affects the administration of antidote in the treatment of paracetamol poisoning, see p.78.) Alterations of the pharmacokinetics of phenytoin have been reported with *bromfenac*, but it was thought unlikely that a change in phenytoin dose would be necessary.[5]

Other analgesic and anti-inflammatory drugs may have clinically significant effects. *Phenylbutazone* has been reported to cause an initial decrease in serum phenytoin, followed by an increase;[4] in addition to effects on protein binding it inhibits phenytoin metabolism[6] and severe phenytoin toxicity may result.[7] *Azapropazone* appears to be a competitive inhibitor of phenytoin metabolism and has also been implicated in interactions resulting in toxicity.[8,9] Substantial increases in serum phenytoin have been demonstrated in healthy subjects given the analgesic and muscle relaxant *fenyramidol*,[10] indicating a potential for toxicity. There is a single report of toxicity in a patient receiving *ibuprofen* with phenytoin[11] but in a study in 9 healthy subjects, ibuprofen had no effect on the pharmacokinetics of phenytoin.[12]

The opioid analgesic *dextropropoxyphene* has also been reported to affect phenytoin metabolism, with the resultant development of toxic blood-phenytoin concentrations;[13] however, the patient in this case was taking relatively high doses of dextropropoxyphene (650 mg daily). For the effect of phenytoin on *methadone* and *pethidine*, see p.58 and p.81, respectively.

1. Fraser DG, *et al.* Displacement of phenytoin from plasma binding sites by salicylate. *Clin Pharmacol Ther* 1980; **27:** 165–9.
2. Paxton JW. Effects of aspirin on salivary and serum phenytoin kinetics in healthy subjects. *Clin Pharmacol Ther* 1980; **27:** 170–8.
3. Leonard RF, *et al.* Phenytoin-salicylate interaction. *Clin Pharmacol Ther* 1981; **29:** 56–60.
4. Neuvonen PJ, *et al.* Antipyretic analgesics in patients on antiepileptic drug therapy. *Eur J Clin Pharmacol* 1979; **15:** 263–8.
5. Gumbhir-Shah K, *et al.* Evaluation of pharmacokinetic interaction between bromfenac and phenytoin in healthy males. *J Clin Pharmacol* 1997; **37:** 160–8.
6. Andreasen PB, *et al.* Diphenylhydantoin half-life in man and its inhibition by phenylbutazone: the role of genetic factors. *Acta Med Scand* 1973; **193:** 561–4.
7. Kristensen MB. Drug interactions and clinical pharmacokinetics. *Clin Pharmacokinet* 1976; **1:** 351–72.
8. Roberts CJC, *et al.* Anticonvulsant intoxication precipitated by azapropazone. *Postgrad Med J* 1981; **57:** 191–2.
9. Geaney DP, *et al.* Interaction of azapropazone with phenytoin. *BMJ* 1982; **284:** 1373.
10. Solomon HM, Schrogie JJ. The effect of phenyramidol on the metabolism of diphenylhydantoin. *Clin Pharmacol Ther* 1967; **8:** 554–6.
11. Sandyk R. Phenytoin toxicity induced by interaction with ibuprofen. *S Afr Med J* 1982; **62:** 592.
12. Townsend RJ, *et al.* The effects of ibuprofen on phenytoin pharmacokinetics. *Drug Intell Clin Pharm* 1985; **19:** 447–8.
13. Kutt H. Interactions between anticonvulsants and other commonly prescribed drugs. *Epilepsia* 1984; **25** (suppl 2): S118–S131.

**Anthelmintics.** For report of an interaction between phenytoin and *levamisole* with fluorouracil, see under Antineoplastics, below. For the effect of phenytoin on *mebendazole* and *praziquantel*, see p.108 and p.112, respectively.

**Antiarrhythmics.** There have been reports of phenytoin toxicity associated with substantial rises in serum-phenytoin concentrations following addition of *amiodarone* to the therapeutic regimen.[1,2] For the effect of phenytoin on amiodarone, see p.861. For the effect of phenytoin on other antiarrhythmics, see p.905 (disopyramide), p.958 (mexiletine), p.992 (quinidine), and p.1378 (lidocaine).

1. Gore JM, *et al.* Interaction of amiodarone and diphenylhydantoin. *Am J Cardiol* 1984; **54:** 1145.
2. McGovern B, *et al.* Possible interaction between amiodarone and phenytoin. *Ann Intern Med* 1984; **101:** 650.

**Antibacterials.** Interactions, some clinically significant, may occur between phenytoin and various antibacterials. Giving *chloramphenicol* with phenytoin has resulted in moderate[1] to marked[2] elevation of serum-phenytoin concentrations due to inhibition of phenytoin metabolism;[2] toxicity has resulted.[3,4] In turn, phenytoin may affect serum concentrations of chloramphenicol (see p.186).

Phenytoin may enhance the metabolism of *doxycycline*.[5]

There is limited evidence that *erythromycin* decreases phenytoin clearance[6] but this was subject to considerable interindividual variation and is of unknown clinical significance. Results from another study[7] suggested that *clarithromycin* might also raise phenytoin levels.

The interaction with *isoniazid* is well documented and potentially significant in slow acetylators of isoniazid who may develop raised phenytoin concentrations and signs of toxicity;[8,9] in at least one case, death has resulted.[10] Plasma-isoniazid concentrations may become sufficiently raised in slow acetylators of isoniazid to produce marked inhibition of the hepatic microsomal enzymes responsible for the metabolism of phenytoin.

There have been conflicting reports of the effect of *ciprofloxacin* on serum concentrations of phenytoin. While some report no effect[11] others have reported reduced[12-16] or increased[17,18] concentrations of phenytoin in patients given ciprofloxacin. A fall in serum-phenytoin concentrations, and resultant loss of seizure control has been reported in a patient in whom *nitrofurantoin* was added to therapy.[19] The mechanism of this interaction is unknown although a combination of impaired absorption and increased metabolism of the phenytoin was suggested. Something similar was reported in a patient given *oxacillin* in whom plasma-phenytoin concentrations dropped markedly and status epilepticus developed.[20] This effect was thought to be due to impaired phenytoin absorption.

*Rifampicin* can also reduce plasma-phenytoin concentrations and markedly increase its clearance;[21,22] this is in marked contrast to the effects of isoniazid, and when given together it overrides the effects of isoniazid on phenytoin, even in slow acetylators.[22]

Various sulfonamides are reported to interact with phenytoin, reducing clearance and prolonging half-life: *sulfaphenazole* is reportedly the strongest inhibitor of phenytoin metabolism but *sulfamethizole* also inhibits phenytoin metabolism and the latter has been implicated in producing phenytoin toxicity.[23] *Co-trimoxazole* reportedly inhibits phenytoin metabolism to a modest degree; a case of phenytoin toxicity in a child given co-trimoxazole has been reported[24] but the role of the co-trimoxazole is uncertain since the patient was also receiving sultiame.

See also under Antiprotozoals, below.

1. Koup JR, *et al.* Interaction of chloramphenicol with phenytoin and phenobarbital. *Clin Pharmacol Ther* 1978; **24:** 571–5.
2. Christensen LK, Skovsted L. Inhibition of drug metabolism by chloramphenicol. *Lancet* 1969; **ii:** 1397–9.
3. Ballek RE, *et al.* Inhibition of diphenylhydantoin metabolism by chloramphenicol. *Lancet* 1973; **i:** 150.
4. Rose JQ, *et al.* Intoxication caused by interaction of chloramphenicol and phenytoin. *JAMA* 1977; **237:** 2630–1.
5. Neuvonen PJ, *et al.* Effect of antiepileptic drugs on the elimination of various tetracycline derivatives. *Eur J Clin Pharmacol* 1975; **9:** 147–54.
6. Bachmann K, *et al.* Single dose phenytoin clearance during erythromycin treatment. *Res Commun Chem Pathol Pharmacol* 1984; **46:** 207–17.
7. Burger DM, *et al.* Therapeutic drug monitoring of phenytoin in patients with the acquired immunodeficiency syndrome. *Ther Drug Monit* 1994; **16:** 616–20.
8. Brennan RW, *et al.* Diphenylhydantoin intoxication attendant to slow inactivation of isoniazid. *Neurology* 1970; **20:** 687–93.
9. Kutt H, *et al.* Diphenylhydantoin intoxication: a complication of isoniazid therapy. *Am Rev Respir Dis* 1970; **101:** 377–84.
10. Johnson J, Freeman HL. Death due to isoniazid (INH) and phenytoin. *Br J Psychiatry* 1976; **129:** 511.
11. Slavich IL, *et al.* Grand mal epileptic seizures during ciprofloxacin therapy. *JAMA* 1989; **261:** 558–9.
12. Dillard ML, *et al.* Ciprofloxacin-phenytoin interaction. *Ann Pharmacother* 1992; **26:** 263.
13. Pollak PT, Slayter KL. Hazards of doubling phenytoin dose in the face of an unrecognized interaction with ciprofloxacin. *Ann Pharmacother* 1997; **31:** 61–4.
14. Brouwers PJ, *et al.* Ciprofloxacin-phenytoin interaction. *Ann Pharmacother* 1997; **31:** 498.
15. McLeod R, Trinkle R. Unexpectedly low phenytoin concentration in a patient receiving ciprofloxacin. *Ann Pharmacother* 1998; **32:** 1110–11.
16. Otero M-J, *et al.* Interaction between phenytoin and ciprofloxacin. *Ann Pharmacother* 1999; **33:** 251–2.
17. Schroeder D, *et al.* Effect of ciprofloxacin on serum phenytoin concentrations in epileptic patients. *Pharmacotherapy* 1991; **11:** 276.
18. Hull RL. Possible phenytoin-ciprofloxacin interaction. *Ann Pharmacother* 1993; **27:** 1283.
19. Heipertz R, Pilz H. Interaction of nitrofurantoin with diphenylhydantoin. *J Neurol* 1978; **218:** 297–301.
20. Fincham RW, *et al.* Use of phenytoin serum levels in a case of status epilepticus. *Neurology* 1976; **26:** 879–81.
21. Wagner JC, Slama TG. Rifampin-phenytoin drug interaction. *Drug Intell Clin Pharm* 1984; **18:** 497.
22. Kay L, *et al.* Influence of rifampicin and isoniazid on the kinetics of phenytoin. *Br J Clin Pharmacol* 1985; **20:** 323–6.

23. Siersbaek-Nielsen K, *et al.* Sulfamethizole-induced inhibition of diphenylhydantoin and tolbutamide metabolism in man. *Clin Pharmacol Ther* 1973; **14:** 148.
24. Gillman MA, Sandyk R. Phenytoin toxicity and co-trimoxazole. *Ann Intern Med* 1985; **102:** 559.

**Anticoagulants.** Serum-phenytoin concentrations have been reported to be markedly elevated by *dicoumarol*[1,2] and elevated to a lesser extent by *phenprocoumon*;[2] however, although *warfarin* has been implicated in a report of phenytoin toxicity,[3] other evidence suggests that it has no effect on serum-phenytoin concentrations in most patients.[2]

For the effect of phenytoin on anticoagulants such as dicoumarol and warfarin, see p.1025.

1. Hansen JM, *et al.* Dicoumarol-induced diphenylhydantoin intoxication. *Lancet* 1966; **ii:** 265–6.
2. Skovsted L, *et al.* The effect of different oral anticoagulants on diphenylhydantoin and tolbutamide metabolism. *Acta Med Scand* 1976; **199:** 513–5.
3. Rothermich NO. Diphenylhydantoin intoxication. *Lancet* 1966; **ii:** 640.

**Antidepressants.** As with all antiepileptics, antidepressants may antagonise the antiepileptic activity of phenytoin by lowering the convulsive threshold.

Plasma-phenytoin concentrations rose in 2 epileptic patients also receiving *imipramine* 75 mg daily for about 3 months for depression.[1] In one patient the concentration gradually increased over several weeks to more than twice the pretreatment figure and he showed mild signs of phenytoin intoxication which remitted after imipramine was stopped. Increased serum-phenytoin concentration and phenytoin toxicity possibly precipitated by addition of *trazodone* has been described;[2] the manufacturers of trazodone recommend monitoring serum-phenytoin concentrations in patients receiving these two drugs. Elevated plasma-phenytoin concentrations, in some cases accompanied by signs and symptoms of phenytoin toxicity, have also been reported with *fluoxetine*,[3] *fluvoxamine*,[4] *sertraline*,[5] or *viloxazine*.[6] The manufacturer of *mianserin* recommends that plasma concentrations of phenytoin should be monitored carefully during concomitant therapy.

*Hypericum* has been shown to induce several drug metabolising enzymes (see p.299) and consequently it might reduce the blood concentrations of phenytoin leading to an increased risk of seizure.[7] One UK manufacturer of phenytoin (Parke, Davis) therefore recommends that phenytoin and hypericum should not be used together and warns that the effects of hypericum may persist for at least 2 weeks after it was last used.

For the effects of phenytoin on antidepressants, see under Amitriptyline (p.284), Fluoxetine (p.296), and Lithium (p.303).

1. Perucca E, Richens A. Interaction between phenytoin and imipramine. *Br J Clin Pharmacol* 1977; **4:** 485–6.
2. Dorn JM. A case of phenytoin toxicity possibly precipitated by trazodone. *J Clin Psychiatry* 1986; **47:** 89–90.
3. Nightingale SL. Fluoxetine labeling revised to identify phenytoin interaction and to recommend against use in nursing mothers. *JAMA* 1994; **271:** 1067.
4. Feldman D, *et al.* Cas clinique d'interaction médicamenteuse entre phénytoïne et fluvoxamine. *J Pharm Clin* 1995; **14:** 296–7.
5. Haselberger MB, *et al.* Elevated serum phenytoin concentrations associated with coadministration of sertraline. *J Clin Psychopharmacol* 1997; **17:** 107–9.
6. Pisani F, *et al.* Elevation of plasma phenytoin by viloxazine in epileptic patients: a clinically significant interaction. *J Neurol Neurosurg Psychiatry* 1992; **55:** 126–7.
7. Committee on Safety of Medicines/Medicines Control Agency. Reminder: St John's wort (Hypericum perforatum) interactions. *Current Problems* 2000; **26:** 6–7. Also available at: http://www.mca.gov.uk/ourwork/monitorsafequalmed/currentproblems/cpmay2000.pdf (accessed 14/05/04)

**Antidiabetics.** Transient rises in the amount of non-protein-bound phenytoin were observed in 17 patients when *tolbutamide* was given in addition to phenytoin, but none developed signs of intoxication.[1] Toxic symptoms were reported in another patient given phenytoin with tolbutamide, although she had tolerated this combination on a previous occasion.[2]

Symptoms of phenytoin toxicity are known to have occurred[1] in one patient receiving *tolazamide* and phenytoin.

1. Wesseling H, Mols-Thürkow I. Interaction of diphenylhydantoin (DPH) and tolbutamide in man. *Eur J Clin Pharmacol* 1975; **8:** 75–8.
2. Beech E, *et al.* Phenytoin toxicity produced by tolbutamide. *BMJ* 1988; **297:** 1613–14.

**Antiepileptics.** Interactions may occur when phenytoin is used with other antiepileptics, but these are often variable in their effect and difficult to predict.

For a discussion of the effect of *benzodiazepines* on plasma concentrations of phenytoin, see under Benzodiazepines, below.

*Carbamazepine* has been generally reported to lower serum-phenytoin concentrations,[1,2] although reports exist of elevated serum-phenytoin concentrations when the two were given concurrently.[3] It should be noted that phenytoin also reduces serum-carbamazepine values—see p.356. These studies have not indicated any loss of seizure control due to this interaction.

For the effects of phenytoin on *ethosuximide*, see p.360.

*Felbamate* has caused increases in serum-phenytoin concentrations, and in some cases toxicity requiring a reduction in phenytoin dose.[4,5]

Increased plasma concentrations of phenytoin with symptoms of toxicity have been reported in a patient receiving phenytoin, carbamazepine, and clobazam after *gabapentin* was added to treatment.[6]

Phenytoin reduces plasma concentrations of *lamotrigine* as described on p.364.

Phenytoin plasma concentrations may be increased by high doses of *oxcarbazepine*;[7] the US manufacturer of oxcarbazepine suggests that doses of phenytoin may need to be reduced when high doses of oxcarbazepine are given.

*Phenobarbital* both induces the metabolism of phenytoin and competes with it for metabolism by the same enzyme system; in practice there is rarely sufficient alteration for a change in phenytoin dosage to be necessary.[8-10] For the effect of phenytoin on phenobarbital, see p.368. Phenytoin has also been reported to enhance the metabolism of *primidone* to phenobarbital, see p.377.

*Progabide* may increase blood-phenytoin concentrations[11] and *stiripentol* appears to produce a dose-dependent reduction in phenytoin clearance.[12]

*Sultiame* causes substantial increases in plasma-phenytoin concentrations, in some cases resulting in phenytoin toxicity;[13] the dose of phenytoin may therefore require adjustment if these drugs are given together.

Modest increases in plasma-phenytoin concentrations have been observed in some patients when *topiramate* was added to therapy, but it was considered that dosage adjustments were unlikely to be necessary.[14] For the effect of phenytoin on topiramate, see p.379.

The interaction between phenytoin and *valproate* is complex. Valproate displaces phenytoin from serum binding sites and may inhibit its metabolism;[15] the former effect increases the concentration of free drug but reduces total serum phenytoin.[16,17] Most studies seem to suggest that the dose of phenytoin need only rarely be adjusted, but the possibility of loss of seizure control, or phenytoin toxicity, does exist.[15] Interestingly there is some evidence that the interactions may be affected by circadian variations in valproate concentrations.[18] Total plasma-phenytoin concentrations rose significantly in 9 of 11 patients, 2 of whom developed toxic symptoms, when the formulation of sodium valproate that they were taking with phenytoin was changed from a standard tablet to a slow-release form.[19] The authors hypothesised that reduced diurnal fluctuations in plasma-valproate concentrations due to the use of slow-release tablets reduced the displacement interaction between phenytoin and valproate, thereby increasing total plasma-phenytoin concentrations. Phenytoin may also cause a fall in serum concentrations of valproate—see p.381.

Gradual or delayed reductions in plasma-phenytoin concentrations have been seen in several studies in patients given *vigabatrin*;[20] a review[20] states that concentrations have been reduced by 20 to 30%. The manufacturer of vigabatrin considers that this is unlikely to be of clinical significance although in a study the reduction was considered to compromise seizure control.[21]

1. Hansen JM, *et al.* Carbamazepine-induced acceleration of diphenylhydantoin and warfarin metabolism in man. *Clin Pharmacol Ther* 1971; **12:** 539–43.
2. Windorfer A, Sauer W. Drug interactions during anticonvulsant therapy in childhood: diphenylhydantoin, primidone, phenobarbitone, clonazepam, nitrazepam, carbamazepin, and dipropylacetate. *Neuropadiatrie* 1977; **8:** 29–41.
3. Zielinski JJ, *et al.* Carbamazepine-phenytoin interaction: elevation of plasma phenytoin concentrations due to carbamazepine comedication. *Ther Drug Monit* 1985; **7:** 51–3.
4. Sheridan PH, *et al.* Open pilot study of felbamate (ADD03055) in partial seizures. *Epilepsia* 1986; **27:** 649.
5. Wilensky AJ, *et al.* Pharmacokinetics of W-554 (ADD 03055) in epileptic patients. *Epilepsia* 1985; **26:** 602–6.
6. Tyndel F. Interaction of gabapentin with other antiepileptics. *Lancet* 1994; **343:** 1363–4.
7. Hossain M, *et al.* Drug-drug interaction profile of oxcarbazepine in children and adults. *Neurology* 1999; **52** (suppl 2): A525.
8. Morselli PL, *et al.* Interaction between phenobarbital and diphenylhydantoin in animals and in epileptic patients. *Ann N Y Acad Sci* 1971; **179:** 88–107.
9. Cucinell SA, *et al.* Drug interactions in man: 1. lowering effect of phenobarbital on plasma levels of bishydroxycoumarin (Dicumarol) and diphenylhydantoin (Dilantin). *Clin Pharmacol Ther* 1965; **6:** 420–9.
10. Booker HE, *et al.* Concurrent administration of phenobarbital and diphenylhydantoin: lack of an interference effect. *Neurology* 1971; **21:** 383–5.
11. Bianchetti G, *et al.* Pharmacokinetic interactions of progabide with other antiepileptic drugs. *Epilepsia* 1987; **28:** 68–73.
12. Levy RH, *et al.* Stiripentol kinetics in epileptic patients: nonlinearity and interactions. *Epilepsia* 1984; **25:** 657.
13. Hansen JM, *et al.* Sulthiame (Ospolot) as inhibitor of diphenylhydantoin metabolism. *Epilepsia* 1968; **9:** 17–22.
14. Bourgeois BFD. Drug interaction profile of topiramate. *Epilepsia* 1996; **37** (suppl 2): S14–S17.
15. Levy RH, Koch KM. Drug interactions with valproic acid. *Drugs* 1982; **24:** 543–56.
16. Monks A, Richens A. Effect of single doses of sodium valproate on serum phenytoin levels and protein binding in epileptic patients. *Clin Pharmacol Ther* 1980; **27:** 89–95.
17. Perucca E, *et al.* Interaction between phenytoin and valproic acid: plasma protein binding and metabolic effects. *Clin Pharmacol Ther* 1980; **28:** 779–89.
18. Riva R, *et al.* Time-dependent interaction between phenytoin and valproic acid. *Neurology* 1985; **35:** 510–15.
19. Suzuki Y, *et al.* Interaction between valproate formulation and phenytoin concentrations. *Eur J Clin Pharmacol* 1995; **48:** 61–3.
20. Grant SM, Heel RC. Vigabatrin: a review of its pharmacodynamic and pharmacokinetic properties, and therapeutic potential in epilepsy and disorders of motor control. *Drugs* 1991; **41:** 889–926.
21. Browne TR, *et al.* Vigabatrin for refractory complex partial seizures: multicenter single-blind study with long-term follow-up. *Neurology* 1987; **37:** 184–9.

**Antifungals.** There have been several reports of interactions, sometimes resulting in phenytoin toxicity, between imidazole antifungals and phenytoin. The drug most frequently implicated is *miconazole*.[1-3] The related triazole antifungal *fluconazole* is also reported to interact with phenytoin,[4-6] possibly due to dose-related inhibition of cytochrome P450 by fluconazole.[4]

Phenytoin can decrease plasma concentrations of azole antifungals such as *ketoconazole* and *itraconazole*.

1. Bourgoin B, *et al.* Interaction pharmacocinétique possible phénytoïne-miconazole. *Therapie* 1981; **36:** 347–9.
2. Loupi E, *et al.* Interactions médicamenteuses et miconazole. *Therapie* 1982; **37:** 437–41.
3. Rolan PE, *et al.* Phenytoin intoxication during treatment with parenteral miconazole. *BMJ* 1983; **287:** 1760.
4. Mitchell AS, Holland JT. Fluconazole and phenytoin: a predictable interaction. *BMJ* 1989; **298:** 1315.
5. Howitt KM, Oziemski MA. Phenytoin toxicity induced by fluconazole. *Med J Aust* 1989; **151:** 603–4.
6. Cadle RM, *et al.* Fluconazole-induced symptomatic phenytoin toxicity. *Ann Pharmacother* 1994; **28:** 191–5.

**Antigout drugs.** The manufacturer of *sulfinpyrazone* states that it displaces phenytoin from its protein-binding sites, and also inhibits microsomal liver enzymes. The net result is an increase in plasma-phenytoin concentrations and a prolonged half-life, which is potentially hazardous.

A case has been described[1] in which reduced doses of phenytoin were necessary to avoid toxicity when *allopurinol* was added to the therapy of a child with the Lesch-Nyhan syndrome. Although the authors thought caution was advisable in using these two drugs together, they did emphasise that overgeneralisation may be dangerous since the child also received other antiepileptics and the contribution his disease may have played was unknown.

1. Yokochi K, *et al.* Phenytoin-allopurinol interaction: Michaelis-Menten kinetic parameters of phenytoin with and without allopurinol in a child with Lesch-Nyhan syndrome. *Ther Drug Monit* 1982; **4:** 353–7.

**Antihistamines.** A young woman developed drowsiness, ataxia, diplopia, tinnitus, and episodes of occipital headaches associated with vomiting after taking phenytoin sodium and *chlorphenamine*.[1] Chlorphenamine might have delayed the hepatic metabolism of phenytoin thereby increasing the plasma concentrations.

1. Pugh RNH, *et al.* Interaction of phenytoin with chlorpheniramine. *Br J Clin Pharmacol* 1975; **2:** 173–5.

**Antihypertensives.** In 2 patients with hypoglycaemia associated with hyperinsulinism, therapeutic serum-phenytoin concentrations could not be achieved while they were also receiving *diazoxide*.[1] It was suggested that an increased rate of metabolism, and possibly a decreased binding, of phenytoin induced by diazoxide might have been responsible.

1. Roe TF, *et al.* Drug interaction: diazoxide and diphenylhydantoin. *J Pediatr* 1975; **87:** 480–4.

**Antimalarials.** Antimalarials may antagonise the antiepileptic activity of phenytoin by lowering the convulsive threshold.

**Antineoplastics.** There have been reports of decreased plasma-phenytoin concentrations associated with cancer chemotherapy,[1-4] resulting in some cases in loss of seizure control.[2-4] The effect appears to be due to impaired absorption of phenytoin arising from antineoplastic damage to the gastrointestinal mucosa. In a patient a mean of 32% of an oral dose of phenytoin was absorbed after therapy with *cisplatin*, *vinblastine*, and *bleomycin*; this compared with a reported oral bioavailability of 80% or more.[3]

The US manufacturer of levamisole reports that increased plasma-phenytoin concentrations have been observed in patients taking phenytoin with *levamisole* given as an adjuvant to *fluorouracil* therapy. Treatment with fluorouracil (taken once weekly in combination with calcium leucovorin) has also resulted in phenytoin toxicity in a patient on long-term antiepileptic therapy.[5] Similar interactions have occurred with *doxifluridine*[6] and *capecitabine*, both prodrugs of fluorouracil. For the effect of phenytoin on *busulfan* see under Effects on the Nervous System under Adverse Effects of Busulfan, p.532. For the effect of phenytoin on *streptozocin* and on *teniposide* see p.584 and p.587, respectively.

1. Fincham RW, Schottelius DD. Decreased phenytoin levels in antineoplastic therapy. *Ther Drug Monit* 1979; **1:** 277–83.
2. Bollini P, *et al.* Decreased phenytoin level during antineoplastic therapy: a case report. *Epilepsia* 1983; **24:** 75–8.
3. Sylvester RK, *et al.* Impaired phenytoin bioavailability secondary to cisplatinum, vinblastine, and bleomycin. *Ther Drug Monit* 1984; **6:** 302–5.
4. Grossman SA, *et al.* Decreased phenytoin levels in patients receiving chemotherapy. *Am J Med* 1989; **87:** 505–10.
5. Gilbar PJ, Brodribb TR. Phenytoin and fluorouracil interaction. *Ann Pharmacother* 2001; **35:** 1367–70.
6. Konishi H, *et al.* Probable metabolic interaction of doxifluridine with phenytoin. *Ann Pharmacother* 2002; **36:** 831–4.

**Antiprotozoals.** Conflicting results have been reported with *metronidazole*: while one study has suggested only minimal effects on phenytoin concentrations and metabolism,[1] another has indicated inhibition of the metabolism of phenytoin.[2] For the effect of phenytoin on metronidazole, see p.608.

1. Jensen JC, Gugler R. Interaction between metronidazole and drugs eliminated by oxidative metabolism. *Clin Pharmacol Ther* 1985; **37:** 407–10.
2. Blyden GT, *et al.* Metronidazole impairs clearance of phenytoin but not of alprazolam or lorazepam. *Clin Pharmacol Ther* 1986; **39:** 181.

**Antipsychotics.** As with all antiepileptics, antipsychotics may antagonise the antiepileptic activity of phenytoin by lowering the convulsive threshold. Two cases of phenytoin toxicity and elevated plasma-phenytoin concentrations associated with the phenothiazine *thioridazine* have been reported;[1] but another study indicated that *thioridazine*, *chlorpromazine*, or *mesoridazine* reduced serum-phenytoin concentrations.[2]

The non-phenothiazine antipsychotic *loxapine* has also been implicated as producing a fall in serum-phenytoin concentration.[3]

For the effect of phenytoin on antipsychotics in general, see under Chlorpromazine, p.679. For the effect of phenytoin on *clozapine*, see p.688.

1. Vincent FM. Phenothiazine-induced phenytoin intoxication. *Ann Intern Med* 1980; **93:** 56–7.
2. Haidukewych D, Rodin EA. Effect of phenothiazines on serum antiepileptic drug concentrations in psychiatric patients with seizure disorder. *Ther Drug Monit* 1985; **7:** 401–4.
3. Ryan GM, Matthews PA. Phenytoin metabolism stimulated by loxapine. *Drug Intell Clin Pharm* 1977; **11:** 428–9.

**Antivirals.** *Zidovudine* may possibly reduce or increase plasma concentrations of phenytoin. There has been a report[1] of markedly decreased serum-phenytoin concentrations resulting in a recurrence of seizure activity in an epileptic patient following initiation of *nelfinavir* as part of antiretroviral therapy.

For the possible effect of phenytoin on HIV-protease inhibitors, see p.639.

1. Honda M, *et al.* A generalized seizure following initiation of nelfinavir in a patient with human immunodeficiency virus type 1 infection, suspected due to interaction between nelfinavir and phenytoin. *Intern Med* 1999; **38:** 302–3.

**Anxiolytics.** See under Benzodiazepines, below.

**Benzodiazepines.** The metabolism of benzodiazepines may be enhanced as a result of induction of hepatic drug-metabolising enzymes following long-term therapy with phenytoin. In comparison with healthy subjects, half-lives have been shorter and clearance increased.[1,2]

There are sporadic reports of interactions between phenytoin and benzodiazepines, but the evidence is conflicting. One group of workers[3] found some evidence of elevated plasma concentrations of phenytoin in patients given *diazepam* or *chlordiazepoxide* but, in contrast, another study suggested that these drugs produced a significant fall in serum-phenytoin concentrations.[4] There have been reports suggesting that phenytoin intoxication could result from the impaired metabolism associated with the combination[3,5] but in practice this seems to be very rare. There are similar conflicting reports for *clonazepam*.[6-8]

1. Dhillon S, Richens A. Pharmacokinetics of diazepam in epileptic patients and normal volunteers following intravenous administration. *Br J Clin Pharmacol* 1981; **12:** 841–4.
2. Scott AK, *et al.* Oxazepam pharmacokinetics in patients with epilepsy treated long-term with phenytoin alone or in combination with phenobarbitone. *Br J Clin Pharmacol* 1983; **16:** 441–4.
3. Vajda FJE, *et al.* Interaction between phenytoin and the benzodiazepines. *BMJ* 1971; **1:** 346.
4. Houghton GW, Richens A. The effect of benzodiazepines and pheneturide on phenytoin metabolism in man. *Br J Clin Pharmacol* 1974; **1:** 344P–345P.
5. Kutt H, McDowell F. Management of epilepsy with diphenylhydantoin sodium: dosage regulation for problem patients. *JAMA* 1968; **203:** 969–72.
6. Eeg-Oloffson O. Experiences with Rivotril® in treatment of epilepsy—particularly minor motor epilepsy—in mentally retarded children. *Acta Neurol Scand* 1973; **49** (suppl 53): 29–31.
7. Johannessen SI, *et al.* Lack of effect of clonazepam on serum levels of diphenylhydantoin, phenobarbital and carbamazepine. *Acta Neurol Scand* 1977; **55:** 506–12.
8. Saavedra IN, *et al.* Phenytoin/clonazepam interaction. *Ther Drug Monit* 1985; **7:** 481–4.

**Calcium-channel blockers.** Raised serum-phenytoin concentration with phenytoin toxicity developed in a patient who had been taking *nifedipine* in addition to phenytoin for 3 weeks;[1] symptoms resolved completely after nifedipine withdrawal. The mechanism of interaction appeared to be complex. Similar effects have been reported with *diltiazem*[2] and *isradipine*.[3]

For the effect of phenytoin on dihydropyridine calcium-channel blockers, see under Nifedipine, p.969, and on verapamil, see p.1020.

1. Ahmad S. Nifedipine-phenytoin interaction. *J Am Coll Cardiol* 1984; **3:** 1582.
2. Bahls FH, *et al.* Interactions between calcium channel blockers and the anticonvulsants carbamazepine and phenytoin. *Neurology* 1991; **41:** 740–2.
3. Cachat F, Tufro A. Phenytoin/isradipine interaction causing severe neurologic toxicity. *Ann Pharmacother* 2002; **36:** 1399–1402.

**Cardiac glycosides.** For the effect of phenytoin on cardiac glycosides, see under Digoxin, p.897.

**Corticosteroids.** Serum concentrations of phenytoin have been elevated[1] or reduced[2,3] by *dexamethasone* and adjustment of phenytoin dosage may be required.[2,3] For the effect of phenytoin on corticosteroids, see p.1072.

1. Lawson LA, *et al.* Phenytoin-dexamethasone interaction: a previously unreported observation. *Surg Neurol* 1981; **16:** 23–4.
2. Wong DD, *et al.* Phenytoin-dexamethasone: a possible drug-drug interaction. *JAMA* 1985; **254:** 2062–3.
3. Recuenco I, *et al.* Effect of dexamethasone on the decrease of serum phenytoin concentrations. *Ann Pharmacother* 1995; **29:** 935.

**Dermatological drugs.** For the effect of phenytoin on *methoxsalen*, see p.1153.

**Disulfiram.** A well-documented interaction exists between phenytoin and *disulfiram*, which may result in clinical phenytoin toxicity.[1,2] The effect appears to be due to non-competitive inhibition of the metabolism of phenytoin by disulfiram,[2] which results in a substantial increase in phenytoin half-life and a decrease in its clearance.[3]

1. Dry J, Pradalier A. Intoxication par la phénytoïne au cours d'une association thérapeutique avec le disulfirame. *Therapie* 1973; **28:** 799–802.
2. Taylor JW, *et al.* Mathematical analysis of a phenytoin-disulfiram interaction. *Am J Hosp Pharm* 1981; **38:** 93–5.
3. Svendsen TL, *et al.* The influence of disulfiram on the half-life and metabolic clearance rate of diphenylhydantoin and tolbutamide in man. *Eur J Clin Pharmacol* 1976; **9:** 439–41.

**Diuretics.** Severe osteomalacia in 2 previously active young women taking *acetazolamide* in association with phenytoin or primidone and phenobarbital has been reported.[1]

For the effect of antiepileptics such as phenytoin on *furosemide*, see p.920.

1. Mallette LE. Anticonvulsants, acetazolamide and osteomalacia. *N Engl J Med* 1975; **293:** 668.

**Dopaminergics.** For the effect of phenytoin on *levodopa*, see p.1208.

**Enteral and parenteral nutrition.** Therapeutic plasma concentrations of phenytoin may be difficult to achieve in patients receiving enteral or total parenteral nutrition.[1,2] Incompatibility studies indicate that phenytoin probably binds to components of the feed (see under Incompatibility, above), which might explain this interaction when both are given together nasogastrically, but the same effect has also been reported when they were given separately by the intravenous route.[2] A review[3] of case reports and studies concluded that the exact role of enteral feeding in this interaction still remained unclear because of a lack of prospective, randomised, controlled trials performed in patients, rather than in healthy subjects. However, because of the amount of literature describing such a phenomenon, it was considered unlikely to occur just by chance. Monitoring of serum-phenytoin concentrations to guide therapy was recommended, and measures such as staggering phenytoin and enteral feed administration might be considered to minimise the occurrence of this reaction.

1. Summers VM, Grant R. Nasogastric feeding and phenytoin interaction. *Pharm J* 1989; **243:** 181.
2. Messahel FM, *et al.* Does total parenteral nutrition lower serum phenytoin levels? *Curr Ther Res* 1990; **47:** 1017–20.
3. Au Yeung SC, Ensom MH. Phenytoin and enteral feedings: does evidence support an interaction? *Ann Pharmacother* 2000 **34:** 896–905.

**Gastrointestinal drugs.** Evidence for an interaction between phenytoin and *antacids* is conflicting. Some studies have shown a decrease in the bioavailability of phenytoin given with various antacid mixtures[1,2] but others have failed to find any evidence of reduced absorption.[3] Furthermore even those studies which recorded decreased absorption varied in their results with regard to particular drugs, suggesting for example that calcium carbonate both does[1] and does not[2] reduce phenytoin bioavailability. The clinical significance of this data is uncertain but it has been suggested that if antacids and phenytoin are both required administration should be spaced several hours apart.[4,5] *Sucralfate* is also reported to reduce phenytoin absorption.[6]

A well documented interaction exists between phenytoin and *cimetidine*, which produces a dose-dependent reduction in phenytoin clearance[7] and a significant elevation of serum-phenytoin concentration.[8] There are reports of phenytoin toxicity when cimetidine was given to epileptic patients[9,10] including a report of severe granulocytopenia.[11] Although some studies have found that neither *ranitidine*[12] nor *famotidine*[13] appear to affect the pharmacokinetics of phenytoin significantly, there have been isolated reports of raised plasma concentrations of phenytoin associated with use of ranitidine[14-16] or famotidine.[17]

*Omeprazole* 40 mg daily can decrease the plasma clearance of phenytoin[18] and increase the area under the serum-phenytoin concentration-time curve,[19] but one study[20] suggests that the dosage of 20 mg daily usually used for peptic ulcer disease is unlikely to produce a clinically significant effect on the steady-state plasma concentrations of phenytoin in patients with epilepsy.

1. Garnett WR, *et al.* Bioavailability of phenytoin administered with antacids. *Ther Drug Monit* 1979; **1:** 435–6.
2. Kulshrestha VK, *et al.* Interaction between phenytoin and antacids. *Br J Clin Pharmacol* 1978; **6:** 177–9.
3. O'Brien LS, *et al.* Failure of antacids to alter the pharmacokinetics of phenytoin. *Br J Clin Pharmacol* 1978; **6:** 176–7.
4. Cacek AT. Review of alterations in oral phenytoin bioavailability associated with formulation, antacids, and food. *Ther Drug Monit* 1986; **8:** 166–71.
5. D'Arcy PF, McElnay JC. Drug-antacid interactions: assessment of clinical importance. *Drug Intell Clin Pharm* 1987; **21:** 607–17.
6. Smart HL, *et al.* The effects of sucralfate upon phenytoin absorption in man. *Br J Clin Pharmacol* 1985; **20:** 238–40.
7. Bartle WR, *et al.* Dose-dependent effect of cimetidine on phenytoin kinetics. *Clin Pharmacol Ther* 1983; **33:** 649–55.
8. Iteogu MO, *et al.* Effect of cimetidine on single-dose phenytoin kinetics. *Clin Pharm* 1983; **2:** 302–4.
9. Phillips P, Hansky J. Phenytoin toxicity secondary to cimetidine administration. *Med J Aust* 1984; **141:** 602.
10. Hetzel DJ, *et al.* Cimetidine interaction with phenytoin. *BMJ* 1981; **282:** 1512.
11. Sazie E, Jaffe JP. Severe granulocytopenia with cimetidine and phenytoin. *Ann Intern Med* 1980; **93:** 151–2.
12. Watts RW, *et al.* Lack of interaction between ranitidine and phenytoin. *Br J Clin Pharmacol* 1983; **15:** 499–500.
13. Sambol NC, *et al.* A comparison of the influence of famotidine and cimetidine on phenytoin elimination and hepatic blood flow. *Br J Clin Pharmacol* 1989; **27:** 83–7.
14. Bramhall D, Levine M. Possible interaction of ranitidine with phenytoin. *Drug Intell Clin Pharm* 1988; **22:** 979–80.
15. Tse CST, *et al.* Phenytoin concentration elevation subsequent to ranitidine administration. *Ann Pharmacother* 1993; **27:** 1448–51.
16. Tse CST, Iagmin P. Phenytoin and ranitidine interaction. *Ann Intern Med* 1994; **120:** 892–3.
17. Shinn AF. Unrecognized drug interactions with famotidine and nizatidine. *Arch Intern Med* 1991; **151:** 814.
18. Gugler R, Jensen JC. Omeprazole inhibits oxidative drug metabolism: studies with diazepam and phenytoin in vivo and 7-ethoxycoumarin in vitro. *Gastroenterology* 1985; **89:** 1235–41.
19. Prichard PJ, *et al.* Oral phenytoin pharmacokinetics during omeprazole therapy. *Br J Clin Pharmacol* 1987; **24:** 543–5.
20. Andersson T, *et al.* A study of the interaction between omeprazole and phenytoin in epileptic patients. *Ther Drug Monit* 1990; **12:** 329–33.

**Immunosuppressants.** Increased plasma-phenytoin concentrations were reported[1] in one patient when *tacrolimus* was added to existing therapy. Phenytoin was discontinued until levels were within the therapeutic range and then restarted at a lower dose, tacrolimus therapy continuing throughout; phenytoin levels remained stable thereafter.

For the effect of phenytoin on *ciclosporin*, see p.1355.

1. Thompson PA, Mosley CA. Tacrolimus-phenytoin interaction. *Ann Pharmacother* 1996; **30:** 544.

**Levothyroxine.** For the effects of phenytoin on levothyroxine, see p.1601.

**Muscle relaxants.** An increase in serum concentrations of phenytoin has been reported[1] in a patient when *tizanidine* was added to therapy.

1. Ueno K, *et al.* Phenytoin-tizanidine interaction. *DICP Ann Pharmacother* 1991; **25:** 1273.

**Neuromuscular blockers.** For the effect of phenytoin on *suxamethonium*, see p.1408 and on *competitive neuromuscular blockers*, see under Atracurium, p.1400.

**Sex hormones.** For the effect of phenytoin on *oral contraceptives*, see p.1534. Similar effects may also be noted in patients receiving *HRT*, see p.1539.

**Stimulants and anorectics.** Although there has been a report of elevated phenytoin and primidone serum concentrations in a 5-year-old following addition of *methylphenidate* to therapy[1] there was no similar elevation in 2 other children receiving phenobarbital and phenytoin in the same report, nor in 11 patients of varying ages given methylphenidate with antiepileptic therapy as part of a controlled study.[2] The likelihood of an interaction seems small in the majority of patients.

1. Garrettson LK, *et al.* Methylphenidate interaction with both anticonvulsants and ethyl biscoumacetate. *JAMA* 1969; **207:** 2053–6.
2. Kupferberg HJ, *et al.* Effect of methylphenidate on plasma anticonvulsant levels. *Clin Pharmacol Ther* 1972; **13:** 201–4.

**Theophylline.** Although most reports of an interaction between phenytoin and *theophylline* concern effects on theophylline concentrations, one study in 14 healthy subjects suggested that concurrent administration of the two could produce lowered serum-phenytoin concentrations, with a subsequent rise in concentration on discontinuing theophylline.[1] The mechanism was suggested to be enzyme induction by the xanthine resulting in increased phenytoin metabolism.

For the effect of phenytoin on theophylline, see p.802.

1. Taylor JW, *et al.* The interaction of phenytoin and theophylline. *Drug Intell Clin Pharm* 1980; **14:** 638.

**Ticlopidine.** Acute phenytoin toxicity has been reported in a well-stabilised 44-year-old patient following introduction of ticlopidine to prevent restenosis after placement of a coronary stent.[1] The patient also received metoprolol, aspirin, and for a short period lovastatin, but inhibition of the cytochrome P450 isoenzyme CYP2C19 by ticlopidine was considered the most likely cause of the patient's elevated serum phenytoin. A later report[2] by the same authors found that ticlopidine inhibited the clearance of phenytoin in 6 patients receiving phenytoin monotherapy; the involvement of CYP2C19 was also supported. The authors recommended that dosage adjustment of phenytoin should be considered if ticlopidine is also given.

A similar interaction occurred in a 72-year-old patient,[3] and the authors postulated that, since steady-state plasma concentrations of ticlopidine are almost twofold higher in elderly patients than those in younger patients, the higher ticlopidine concentrations may have played a role in this drug interaction.

1. Donahue SR, *et al.* Ticlopidine inhibition of phenytoin metabolism mediated by potent inhibition of CYP2C19. *Clin Pharmacol Ther* 1997; **62:** 572–7.
2. Donahue S,*et al.* Ticlopidine inhibits phenytoin clearance. *Clin Pharmacol Ther* 1999; **66:** 563–8.
3. Klaassen SL. Ticlopidine-induced phenytoin toxicity. *Ann Pharmacother* 1998; **32:** 1295–8.

**Vaccines.** Contradictory results have been reported for the effects of *influenza vaccine* on serum-phenytoin concentrations. A significant elevation in total phenytoin concentration has been reported[1] following vaccination, and was suggested to be due to interferon induction and concomitant inhibition of cytochrome P450. In contrast, other reports have suggested that any increase in serum-phenytoin concentration was temporary and not significant overall[2] or even that there was a slight fall in serum-phenytoin concentration.[3] One study reported a significant increase in total phenytoin concentration two days after vaccination, followed by a return to previous values but this was accompanied by evidence of a gradual and prolonged fall in free phenytoin concentrations.[4] The possibility of either phenytoin toxicity or loss of seizure control may exist in some epileptic patients given influenza vaccine during phenytoin therapy.[5]

1. Jann MW, Fidone GS. Effect of influenza vaccine on serum anticonvulsant concentrations. *Clin Pharm* 1986; **5:** 817–20.
2. Levine M, *et al.* Increased serum phenytoin concentration following influenza vaccination. *Clin Pharm* 1984; **3:** 505–9.
3. Sawchuk RJ, *et al.* Effect of influenza vaccination on plasma phenytoin concentrations. *Ther Drug Monit* 1979; **1:** 285–8.
4. Smith CD, *et al.* Effect of influenza vaccine on serum concentrations of total and free phenytoin. *Clin Pharm* 1988; **7:** 828–32.
5. Grabenstein JD. Drug interactions involving immunologic agents, part 1. vaccine-vaccine, vaccine-immunoglobulin, and vaccine-drug interactions. *DICP Ann Pharmacother* 1990; **24:** 67–81.

**Vitamins.** *Pyridoxine* given in large doses produced a reduction in serum-phenytoin concentrations in 7 patients,[1] perhaps reflecting increased activity by pyridoxal phosphate-dependent enzymes involved in phenytoin metabolism.

Correction of antiepileptic-associated folate deficiency with *folic acid* has been reported to result in a decrease in serum-phenytoin concentrations and an increase in seizure frequency.[2,3] The effect has been reported to be most marked in subjects with high initial serum-phenytoin concentrations[4] and is associated with an increased phenytoin metabolism.[5] However, in the majority of patients the effect is unlikely to assume clinical significance,[2,4] and there is some evidence that very low doses of folic acid may be used to maintain normal serum-folate values without an increase in seizure frequency.[3] Information regarding the dual and interdependent interaction between phenytoin and folic acid has been reviewed.[6] Although limited numbers of patients and healthy subjects were involved, evaluation of the data suggested that initiation of phenytoin and folic acid concomitantly prevents decreased folate levels and steady-state concentrations of phenytoin are reached sooner. Plasma concentrations of phenytoin are also possibly reduced by *folinic acid.*

For the effect of antiepileptics, including phenytoin, on *vitamin D* concentrations, see Effects on Bone under Adverse Effects, above.

1. Hansson O, Sillanpaa M. Pyridoxine and serum concentration of phenytoin and phenobarbitone. *Lancet* 1976; **i:** 256.
2. Baylis EM, *et al.* Influence of folic acid on blood-phenytoin levels. *Lancet* 1971; **i:** 62–4.
3. Inoue F. Clinical implications of anticonvulsant-induced folate deficiency. *Clin Pharm* 1982; **1:** 372–3.
4. Furlanut M, *et al.* Effects of folic acid on phenytoin kinetics in healthy subjects. *Clin Pharmacol Ther* 1978; **24:** 294–7.
5. Berg MJ, *et al.* Phenytoin and folic acid interaction: a preliminary report. *Ther Drug Monit* 1983; **5:** 389–94.
6. Lewis DP, *et al.* Phenytoin-folic acid interaction. *Ann Pharmacother* 1995; **29:** 726–35.

## Pharmacokinetics

Phenytoin is slowly but almost completely absorbed from the gastrointestinal tract. It is largely insoluble at the acid pH of the stomach, most being absorbed from the upper intestine; the rate of absorption is variable and is reported to be affected by the presence of food. Absorption after intramuscular injection is slower than that from the gastrointestinal tract.

Phenytoin is extensively metabolised in the liver to inactive metabolites, chiefly 5-(4-hydroxyphenyl)-5-phenylhydantoin. The rate of metabolism appears to be subject to genetic polymorphism and may also be influenced by racial characteristics; it is reported to be increased during pregnancy and menstruation and to decrease with age. Phenytoin hydroxylation is saturable and is therefore readily inhibited by drugs that compete for its metabolic pathways; this is also the reason why small increments in dose may produce large rises in plasma concentration. Phenytoin undergoes enterohepatic recycling and is excreted in the urine, mainly as its hydroxylated metabolite, in either free or conjugated form.

Phenytoin is widely distributed throughout the body. It is about 90% bound to plasma protein, although this may be reduced in certain disease states and in certain patient populations (see under Precautions, above). It has a very variable, dose-dependent half-life, but the mean plasma half-life appears to be about 22 hours at steady state; because phenytoin inhibits its own metabolism it may sometimes be several weeks before a steady-state plasma-phenytoin concentration is attained.

Monitoring of plasma concentrations may be performed as an aid in assessing control, and the therapeutic range of total plasma-phenytoin concentrations is usually quoted as 10 to 20 micrograms/mL (40 to 80 micromoles/litre); some patients, however, achieve control at concentrations outside this range. It has been suggested that, because of differences in protein binding, measurement of free phenytoin concentrations in plasma may prove more reliable; measurement of concentrations in saliva, which contains only free phenytoin, has also been performed.

Phenytoin crosses the placental barrier and small amounts are distributed into breast milk.

The pharmacokinetics of phenytoin are affected by other antiepileptics (see Interactions, above).

## Uses and Administration

Phenytoin is a hydantoin antiepileptic used to control partial and generalised tonic-clonic seizures. It is also used as part of the emergency treatment of status epilepticus and has been used for the prophylactic control of seizures associated with neurosurgery or severe traumatic injury to the head. Phenytoin has also been used in the treatment of trigeminal neuralgia. It is a class Ib antiarrhythmic and has been used to treat cardiac arrhythmias.

Doses may be expressed in terms of phenytoin or phenytoin sodium; although phenytoin 92 mg is approximately equivalent to 100 mg of phenytoin sodium these molecular equivalents are not necessarily biologically equivalent. In the UK an oral suspension of phenytoin 90 mg in 15 mL may be considered approximately equivalent in therapeutic effect to capsules or tablets containing phenytoin sodium 100 mg. In the USA a suspension containing phenytoin 125 mg in 5 mL is available.

For **epilepsy** the dose of phenytoin should be adjusted to the needs of the individual patient to achieve adequate control of seizures, preferably with monitoring of plasma concentrations; in many patients control requires total plasma-phenytoin concentrations of 10 to 20 micrograms/mL (40 to 80 micromoles/litre), but some are controlled at concentrations outside this range. A suggested initial dose by mouth of phenytoin or phenytoin sodium given as a single dose or in divided doses is 3 to 4 mg/kg daily or 150 to 300 mg daily progressively increased with care to 600 mg daily if necessary; the suggested minimum interval between increments has ranged from about 7 to 10 days. Particular care is needed at higher doses, where saturation of metabolism may mean that a small increment produces a large rise in plasma concentrations. A usual maintenance dose is 200 to 500 mg daily.

A suggested initial dose for children is 5 mg/kg daily in 2 or 3 divided doses up to a maximum of 300 mg daily; a suggested maintenance dose is 4 to 8 mg/kg daily in divided doses. Young children may require a higher dose per kg body-weight than adults due to more rapid metabolism.

The practice of starting phenytoin therapy with initial small doses means that more than a week may be required before therapeutic plasma concentrations are attained; it has been reported that it may even be several weeks before a steady-state concentration is established. An initial loading dose may therefore be given, with the usual maintenance dosage being instituted 24 hours after the loading dose. Once the patient is stabilised the long half-life of phenytoin may permit the total daily dose to be given in two daily divisions or as a single dose, usually at night.

Although clinical evidence is lacking, different brands of phenytoin, as well as different formulations from the same manufacturer, may vary in their bioavailability and patients may need to be restabilised in the event of a change.

In order to lessen gastric irritation, phenytoin should be taken with or after food. The time and manner of taking phenytoin should be standardised for the patient since variations might affect absorption with consequent fluctuations in the plasma concentrations.

As with other antiepileptics, withdrawal of phenytoin therapy or transition to or from another type of antiepileptic therapy should be made gradually to avoid precipitating an increase in the frequency of seizures. For a discussion on whether or not to withdraw antiepileptic therapy in seizure-free patients, see p.349.

In the treatment of tonic-clonic **status epilepticus** a benzodiazepine such as diazepam is usually given initially intravenously or rectally followed by the administration of phenytoin sodium intravenously. A suggested dose of phenytoin sodium has been 10 to 15 mg/kg given by slow intravenous injection or by intermittent infusion at a uniform rate of not more than 50 mg/minute. Thereafter maintenance doses of 100 mg by mouth or intravenously are given every 6 to 8 hours; the rate and dose should be reduced according to body-weight. The intravenous dose for neonates is 15 to 20 mg/kg at a rate not exceeding 1 to 3 mg/kg per minute. A suggested dose in children is 15 mg/kg given at a rate of 1 mg/kg per minute, not to exceed 50 mg/minute. Deaths have been caused by the over-rapid intravenous injection of phenytoin sodium and continuous monitoring of the ECG and blood pressure is recommended whenever phenytoin sodium is given intravenously.

Phenytoin sodium is absorbed slowly and erratically from the intramuscular site and therefore intramuscular injections are not appropriate for the emergency arrest of status epilepticus. They may, however, be used in certain situations to maintain or establish therapeutic plasma concentrations of phenytoin in patients who are unconscious or otherwise unable to take phenytoin by mouth. Owing to the slower absorption of phenytoin from intramuscular sites, patients stabilised on the oral route require an increase in the intramuscular dose of about 50%; it is recommended that, if possible, intramuscular injections of phenytoin sodium should not be continued for longer than one week. On transfer back to the oral route the patient should receive 50% of the original oral dose for the same period of time as intramuscular injections were given, to allow for continued absorption of the residual phenytoin in the intramuscular sites. In a patient who has not previously received phenytoin sodium, a suggested intramuscular dose is 100 to 200 mg.

**Administration.** IN CHILDREN AND NEONATES. A comparison of methods[1] for the prediction of required phenytoin dosage in paediatric patients indicated that all methods produced a sizeable number of predictions with an error of more than 10% and that close monitoring of serum concentrations and clinical status was recommended regardless of the method chosen to adjust dosage. Similar conclusions have been made regarding the need to monitor plasma concentrations of phenytoin in the newborn and young infants.[2]

1. Yuen GJ, *et al.* Phenytoin dosage predictions in paediatric patients. *Clin Pharmacokinet* 1989; **16:** 254–60.
2. Loughnan PM, *et al.* Pharmacokinetic observations of phenytoin disposition in the newborn and young infant. *Arch Dis Child* 1977; **52:** 302–9.

IN THE ELDERLY. Pharmacokinetic studies in elderly patients have shown reduced binding to plasma protein which was not itself an indication for dosage change,[1] but a study showing a decreased metabolism[2] did indicate that elderly patients may need lower doses of phenytoin than younger adults to maintain similar serum concentrations.

1. Patterson M, *et al.* Plasma protein binding of phenytoin in the aged: in vivo studies. *Br J Clin Pharmacol* 1982; **13:** 423–5.
2. Bauer LA, Blouin RA. Age and phenytoin kinetics in adult epileptics. *Clin Pharmacol Ther* 1982; **31:** 301–4.

**Cardiac arrhythmias.** Phenytoin has been given intravenously in the treatment of ventricular arrhythmias (p.816), especially those caused by overdosage with cardiac glycosides. Although this use now appears to be obsolete, in the UK the licensed dose of phenytoin sodium is 3.5 to 5 mg/kg administered by slow intravenous injection at a uniform rate of not more than 50 mg/minute, repeated once if necessary.

**Eclampsia and pre-eclampsia.** Phenytoin has been used for eclampsia but now treatment with magnesium sulfate is preferred, see p.352.

**Epidermolysis bullosa.** There have been reports[1,2] of a favourable but variable clinical response to phenytoin in patients with recessive dystrophic epidermolysis bullosa (p.1135), a condition for which there is no truly effective treatment. However, a double-blind placebo-controlled study[3] concluded that phenytoin is not an effective treatment and offered no overall benefit when compared with placebo.

1. Bauer EA, *et al.* Phenytoin therapy of recessive dystrophic epidermolysis bullosa. *N Engl J Med* 1980; **303:** 776–81.
2. Cooper TW, Bauer EA. Therapeutic efficacy of phenytoin in recessive dystrophic epidermolysis. *Arch Dermatol* 1984; **120:** 490–5.
3. Caldwell-Brown D, *et al.* Lack of efficacy of phenytoin in recessive dystrophic epidermolysis bullosa. *N Engl J Med* 1992; **327:** 163–7.

**Epilepsy.** Phenytoin is one of the drugs of choice in the treatment of partial seizures with or without secondary generalisation and in primarily generalised tonic-clonic seizures (see p.349). It is also effective in other forms of epilepsy with the exception of absence and myoclonic seizures.

The non-linear pharmacokinetics of phenytoin make it difficult to use, particularly at higher doses, because small increases in doses may produce large rises in plasma concentrations. Phenytoin may be unsuitable for adolescents or for women because of potential coarsening of the facial features, acne, or hirsutism. Gingival hyperplasia and tenderness can also be a problem.

**Hiccup.** Phenytoin may be of value for the treatment of intractable hiccups,[1] especially those of neurogenic origin. A protocol for the management of intractable hiccups may be found under Chlorpromazine, p.682.

1. Petroski D, Patel AN. Diphenylhydantoin for intractable hiccups. *Lancet* 1974; **i:** 739.

**Intracerebral haemorrhage.** For reference to the use of antiepileptic prophylaxis, usually with phenytoin, in patients following intracerebral haemorrhage, see under Stroke, p.836.

**Myotonia.** A review[1] of myotonia congenita, a hereditary muscular disorder characterised by symptoms of muscle stiffness especially after rest and when initiating movement. Where treatment is necessary it is usually with phenytoin or procainamide, the former being preferred as being better tolerated.

1. Gutmann L, *et al.* Myotonia congenita. *Semin Neurol* 1991; **11:** 244–8.

**Neonatal seizures.** Phenytoin is one of the antiepileptics that may be used in the management of neonatal seizures (p.353).

**Neuropathic pain.** Phenytoin is used alone or added to treatment in trigeminal neuralgia (p.8) in patients unresponsive to or intolerant of carbamazepine. It has also been used in the treatment of painful diabetic neuropathy (p.6).

**Post-traumatic seizures.** About 12% of patients with severe traumatic brain injury develop seizures and the rate may be more than 50% for those with penetrating missile injuries.[1] The use of antiepileptics to treat such seizures is standard but there has been some debate about prophylactic use. Evidence suggests that prophylaxis with phenytoin (and perhaps carbamazepine) is effective in preventing early seizures (arbitrarily defined as those occurring up to 7 days after trauma) but prophylaxis with these or other antiepileptics such as phenobarbital or valproate, has not been shown to be effective for preventing late seizures, disability, or death.[1-4] Guidelines and recommendations for such use have been issued.[1,5] Children with severe, acute neurotrauma were found to have markedly altered protein binding and phenytoin metabolism, and therefore may require increased doses.[6]

1. Chang BS, Lowenstein DH. Practice parameter: antiepileptic drug prophylaxis in severe traumatic brain injury. Report of the Quality Standards Subcommittee of the American Academy of Neurology. *Neurology* 2003; **60:** 10–16. Also available at: http://www.neurology.org/cgi/reprint/60/1/10.pdf (accessed 08/06/04)
2. Schierhout G, Roberts I. Anti-epileptic drugs for preventing seizures following acute traumatic brain injury. Available in the Cochrane Library; Issue 2. Chichester: John Wiley; 2004.
3. Chadwick D. Seizures and epilepsy after traumatic brain injury. *Lancet* 2000; **355:** 334–5.
4. Temkin NR. Antiepileptogenesis and seizure prevention trials with antiepileptic drugs: meta-analysis of controlled trials. *Epilepsia* 2001; **42:** 515–24.
5. Meek PD, *et al.* Guidelines for nonemergency use of parenteral phenytoin products. *Arch Intern Med* 1999; **159:** 2639–44.
6. Stowe CD, *et al.* Altered phenytoin pharmacokinetics in children with severe, acute traumatic brain injury. *J Clin Pharmacol* 2000; **40:** 1452–61.

**Status epilepticus.** A benzodiazepine is the usual choice to abort an attack of status epilepticus (p.352). If this fails to control the seizures or the seizures recur, then intravenous phenytoin may be given. Phenytoin may also be more appropriate than a benzodiazepine for the management of status epilepticus in patients with head injuries or other acute neurological lesions.[1]

Once seizures have been brought under control, maintenance antiepileptic therapy may be started.

1. Eldridge PR, Punt JAG. Risks associated with giving benzodiazepines to patients with acute neurological injuries. *BMJ* 1990; **300:** 1189–90.

**Syndrome of inappropriate ADH secretion.** Phenytoin has been used occasionally to inhibit pituitary antidiuretic hormone (ADH) secretion in patients with the syndrome of inappropriate ADH secretion (SIADH), the management of which is discussed on p.1318.

**Tinnitus.** Phenytoin is one of many drugs that have been tried in tinnitus (p.1381), but although it has been reported to be effective in some patients it is rarely used because of problems with adverse effects.

**Withdrawal syndromes.** Phenytoin has little place in the management of seizures associated with the *alcohol withdrawal syndrome* (p.1166). Prophylaxis with phenytoin has been shown[1,2] to be ineffective for prevention of recurrent alcohol-related seizures and therefore drugs such as the benzodiazepines or clomethiazole, which are effective both for the treatment and prophylaxis of such seizures, are preferred.

Results from a double-blind study[3] indicated that phenytoin was associated with a reduction in *cocaine abuse* compared with placebo. The abuse of cocaine is discussed on p.1374 and treatment of cocaine withdrawal on p.1375.

1. Chance JF. Emergency department treatment of alcohol withdrawal seizures with phenytoin. *Ann Emerg Med* 1991; **20:** 520–2.
2. Rathlev NK, *et al.* The lack of efficacy of phenytoin in the prevention of recurrent alcohol-related seizures. *Ann Emerg Med* 1994; **23:** 513–8.
3. Crosby RD, *et al.* Phenytoin in the treatment of cocaine abuse: a double-blind study. *Clin Pharmacol Ther* 1996; **59:** 458–68.

**Wounds and ulcers.** Phenytoin has been used to promote wound healing (p.1139). Topical application of phenytoin has produced encouraging results in the healing of various types of ulcers[1-5] and large abscess cavities.[6] It has been suggested that phenytoin may reduce bacterial colonisation by changing the pH or by a direct antibacterial effect.[2] The enhanced wound healing may also be due to increased fibroblast proliferation and increased collagen content.[2] Limited absorption from the wound site may occur[7,8] and patients may need to be monitored for signs of toxicity.

1. Muthukumarasamy MG, *et al.* Topical phenytoin in diabetic foot ulcers. *Diabetes Care* 1991; **14:** 909–11.
2. Pendse AK, *et al.* Topical phenytoin in wound healing. *Int J Dermatol* 1993; **32:** 214–17.
3. Anstead GM, *et al.* Phenytoin in wound healing. *Ann Pharmacother* 1996; **30:** 768–75.
4. Adjei O, *et al.* Phenytoin in the treatment of Buruli ulcer. *Trans R Soc Trop Med Hyg* 1998; **92:** 108–9.
5. Rhodes RS, *et al.* Topical phenytoin treatment of stage II decubitus ulcers in the elderly. *Ann Pharmacother* 2001; **35:** 675–81.
6. Lodha SC, *et al.* Role of phenytoin in healing of large abscess cavities. *Br J Surg* 1991; **78:** 105–8.
7. Gore R, *et al.* Topical phenytoin. *Pharm J* 1991; **247:** 620.
8. Lewis WG, Rhodes RS. Systemic absorption of topical phenytoin sodium. *Ann Pharmacother* 1994; **28:** 961.

## Preparations

***BP 2003:*** Phenytoin Capsules; Phenytoin Injection; Phenytoin Oral Suspension; Phenytoin Tablets;
***USP 27:*** Extended Phenytoin Sodium Capsules; Phenytoin Oral Suspension; Phenytoin Sodium Injection; Phenytoin Tablets; Prompt Phenytoin Sodium Capsules.

**Proprietary Preparations** (details are given in Part 3)
***Arg.:*** Epamin; Etoina; Fenigramon; Fenitenk; Lotoquis Simple; Opliphon; ***Austral.:*** Dilantin; ***Austria:*** Epanutin; Epilan-D; Phenhydan; ***Belg.:*** Di-Hydan†; Diphantoine; Epanutin; ***Braz.:*** Dantalin; Epelin; Fenidantal†; Fenital; Feniton; Hidantal; ***Canad.:*** Dilantin; ***Chile:*** Epamin; ***Fin.:*** Hydantin; ***Fr.:*** Di-Hydan†; Dilantin; Pyoredol†; ***Ger.:*** Epanutin; Phenhydan; Zentropil†; ***Gr.:*** Epanutin; ***Hong Kong:*** Dilantin; Ditoin; ***India:*** Dilantin; Epsolin; Eptoin; ***Irl.:*** Epanutin; ***Israel:*** Dilantin; Epanutin; ***Ital.:*** Aurantin; Dintoina; ***Malaysia:*** Dilantin; Ditoin; ***Mex.:*** Biodan; Epamin; Fenidantoin S; Fenitron; Hidantil†; Hidantoina; Nuctane; ***Neth.:*** Epanutin; ***Norw.:*** Epinat; ***NZ:*** Dilantin; ***Port.:*** Hidantina; ***S.Afr.:*** Epanutin; ***Singapore:*** Dilantin; ***Spain:*** Epanutin; Neosidantoina; Sinergina; ***Swed.:*** Epanutin; Fenantoin; Lehydan; ***Switz.:*** Epanutin; Epilantine; Phenhydan; ***Thai.:*** Dilantin; Ditoin; Ditomed; Pepsytoin; ***UK:*** Epanutin; ***USA:*** Dilantin; Phenytek.

**Multi-ingredient:** ***Arg.:*** Cumatil L; Lotoquis; ***Belg.:*** Mathoine†; Vethoine; ***Braz.:*** Dialudon; Gamibetal Complex; Taludon; ***Canad.:*** Dilantin with Phenobarbital†; ***India:*** Dilantin with Phenobarbital; Epilan; Garoin; ***Ital.:*** Dintoinale; Gamibetal Complex; Metinal-Idantoina; Metinal-Idantoina L; ***Mex.:*** Alepsal Compuesto; ***Port.:*** Comital L†; Hidantina Composta; ***S.Afr.:*** Garoin†; ***Spain:*** Comital L; Disfil†; Epilantin; Redutona.

# Pregabalin *(USAN, rINN)*

CI-1008; Pregabalina. (S)-3-(Aminomethyl)-5-methylhexanoic acid.

$C_8H_{17}NO_2$ = 159.2.
*CAS — 148553-50-8.*

## Adverse Effects

The most common adverse effects reported during therapy with pregabalin are dizziness and somnolence. Other common adverse effects include blurred vision, diplopia, increased appetite and weight gain, dry mouth, constipation, vomiting, flatulence, euphoria, confusion, reduced libido, erectile dysfunction, irritability, vertigo, ataxia, tremor, dysarthria, paraesthesia, fatigue, and oedema. Disturbances of attention, memory, coordination, and gait also occur frequently.

## Precautions

Dizziness, somnolence, and blurred vision may impair a patient's ability to perform skilled tasks such as driving.

The manufacturer states that care is required when withdrawing pregabalin therapy, regardless of the indication—see also under Uses and Administration, below.

## Pharmacokinetics

Pregabalin is rapidly absorbed after oral administration and peak plasma concentrations are achieved after 1 hour. Oral bioavailability is about 90%. The rate but not the extent of absorption is reduced by administration with food but this is not clinically significant. Steady state is achieved after 1 to 2 days. Pregabalin is not bound to plasma proteins and undergoes negligible metabolism. About 98% of a dose is excreted in the urine as unchanged drug. The mean elimination half-life is 6.3 hours. Pregabalin is removed by haemodialysis.

## Uses and Administration

Pregabalin is an antiepileptic used as an adjunct in the treatment of partial seizures with or without secondary generalisation (p.349). It is also used in the treatment of neuropathic pain (see Choice of Analgesic, p.2).

Pregabalin is given by mouth in two or three divided doses daily. The manufacturer states that if pregabalin therapy has to be stopped, this should be done gradually over a minimum of 1 week, regardless of indication.

The initial adult dose in the treatment of **epilepsy** is 150 mg daily increased after 1 week according to response to 300 mg daily and then to 600 mg daily after another week.

For **neuropathic pain** the initial adult dose is 150 mg daily increased after 3 to 7 days according to response to 300 mg and then to 600 mg daily after another 7 days.

Dosage of pregabalin should be reduced in patients with renal impairment—see below.

◊ References.

1. Beydoun AA, *et al.* Pregabalin add-on trial: a double-blind, multicenter study in patients with partial epilepsy: results from the interim analysis (N = 129). *Epilepsia* 1999; **40** (suppl 7): 108.
2. French JA, *et al.* Pregabalin adjunctive therapy in patients with partial seizures. *Epilepsia* 1999: **40** (suppl 7): 106.
3. Arroyo S, *et al.* Pregabalin add-on treatment: a randomized, double-blind, placebo-controlled, dose-response study in adults with partial seizures. *Epilepsia* 2004; **45:** 20–7.
4. Sabatowski R, *et al.* Pregabalin reduces pain and improves sleep and mood disturbances in patients with post-herpetic neuralgia: results of a randomised, placebo-controlled clinical trial. *Pain* 2004; **109:** 26–35.

**Administration in renal impairment.** The dose of pregabalin for patients with renal impairment should be reduced according to creatinine clearance (CC):

- CC 30 to less than 60 mL/minute: starting daily dose: 75 mg; maximum daily dose: 300 mg; daily dose given in 2 or 3 divided doses
- CC 15 to less than 30 mL/minute: starting daily dose: 25 to 50 mg; maximum daily dose: 150 mg; daily dose given in 2 divided doses or once daily
- CC less than 15 mL/minute: starting daily dose: 25 mg; maximum daily dose: 75 mg; daily dose given as one dose
- haemodialysis patients should receive in addition to the daily dose a supplementary dose of 25 to 100 mg immediately after each 4-hour haemodialysis session.

## Preparations

**Proprietary Preparations** (details are given in Part 3)
***UK:*** Lyrica.

# Primidone *(BAN, rINN)*

Hexamidinum; Primaclone; Primidona; Primidonum. 5-Ethyl-5-phenylperhydropyrimidine-4,6-dione.

$C_{12}H_{14}N_2O_2$ = 218.3.
*CAS — 125-33-7.*
*ATC — N03AA03.*

**Pharmacopoeias.** In *Chin., Eur.* (see p.vi), *Jpn, Pol.,* and *US.*
**Ph. Eur. 5.0** (Primidone). A white or almost white, crystalline powder. Very slightly soluble in water; slightly soluble in alcohol. It dissolves in alkaline solutions.
**USP 27** (Primidone). A white, odourless, crystalline powder. Soluble 1 in 2000 of water and 1 in 200 of alcohol; very slightly soluble in most organic solvents.

## Adverse Effects, Treatment, and Precautions

As for Phenobarbital, p.368. Adverse effects may be more frequent than with phenobarbital. Most patients rapidly develop tolerance to the adverse effects of primidone, including ataxia, dizziness, drowsiness, headache, nausea and vomiting, nystagmus, skin rashes, and visual disturbances.

Care is required when withdrawing primidone therapy—see also under Uses and Administration, below.

**Effects on the blood.** For a report of delayed agranulocytosis in a patient treated with phenytoin and primidone, see p.370.

**Effects on the endocrine system.** For mention of the effects of antiepileptics on *sexual function* in male epileptic patients, see under Phenytoin, p.371.

**Overdosage.** Crystalluria has been reported[1] following acute overdosage of primidone and 7 other reported cases were also reviewed. Based on these few reports, crystalluria appears to be associated with serum-primidone concentrations in excess of 80 micrograms/mL. There is evidence from 2 reports of renal damage associated with crystal formation *in vivo.* Vigorous hydration is recommended in patients at risk, in order to lessen the potential for renal toxicity and improve elimination.

1. Lehmann DF. Primidone crystalluria following overdose: a report of a case and an analysis of the literature. *Med Toxicol* 1987; **2:** 383–7.

**Porphyria.** Primidone has been associated with acute attacks of porphyria and is considered unsafe in porphyric patients.

**Tremor.** It was noted that patients receiving primidone for essential tremor have a high incidence of acute adverse reactions following small initial doses.[1] This could be due to the absence of induced hepatic enzymes in these patients previously not exposed to antiepileptics.

1. Findley LJ, *et al.* Primidone in essential tremor of the hands and head: a double blind controlled clinical study. *J Neurol Neurosurg Psychiatry* 1985; **48:** 911–15.

## Interactions

Primidone is metabolised in the body in part to phenobarbital, and interactions recorded for phenobarbital (p.368) might potentially occur in patients receiving primidone. In addition, enzyme-inducing drugs enhance this metabolism and have the potential to produce elevated phenobarbital concentrations.

**Antiepileptics.** Both *phenytoin*[1] and *carbamazepine*[2] have been reported to enhance the metabolism of primidone to phenobarbital and when primidone was combined with phenytoin there have been instances of phenobarbital toxicity.[3] *Vigabatrin* has been reported[4] to lower plasma concentrations of primidone in some patients, although it is unlikely that dosage changes would be necessary. *Valproate* may increase plasma concentrations of primidone and phenobarbital, but patient response seems to be inconsistent.

1. Reynolds EH, *et al.* Interaction of phenytoin and primidone. *BMJ* 1975; **2:** 594–5.
2. Baciewicz AM. Carbamazepine drug interactions. *Ther Drug Monit* 1986; **8:** 305–17.
3. Galdames D, *et al.* Interacción fenitoína-primidona: intoxicación por fenobarbital, en un adulto tratado con ambas drogas. *Rev Med Chil* 1980; **108:** 716–20.
4. Browne TR, *et al.* A multicentre study of vigabatrin for drug-resistant epilepsy. *Br J Clin Pharmacol* 1989; **27** (suppl 1): 95S–100S.

## Pharmacokinetics

Primidone is readily absorbed from the gastrointestinal tract and is reported to have a plasma half-life ranging from 10 to 15 hours, which is shorter than those of its principal metabolites phenylethylmalonamide and phenobarbital, both of which are active. Therapeutic plasma concentrations of primidone have been suggested to be between 5 and 12 micrograms/mL. It is excreted in urine as unchanged drug (40%) and metabolites.

Primidone is widely distributed but is only partially bound to plasma protein; it has been suggested that it exhibits variable binding of up to about 20%. It crosses the placenta and is distributed into breast milk.

## Uses and Administration

Primidone is an antiepileptic that is partially metabolised to phenobarbital (p.369), but is also considered to have some antiepileptic activity in its own right. It may be given to control partial (especially complex partial) and generalised tonic-clonic seizures. Primidone is also used in the management of essential tremor.

In the treatment of **epilepsy** the dose of primidone should be adjusted according to the response of the patient; a limited correlation with plasma concentrations has suggested that concentrations of 5 to 12 micrograms/mL (23 to 55 micromoles/litre) are usually necessary, but the *British National Formulary* recommends monitoring of phenobarbital concentrations instead.

Suggested initial doses are 125 mg daily by mouth at bedtime increased, if necessary, by 125 mg every 3 days to a total of 500 mg daily given in 2 divided doses. If necessary, the daily dose may be increased further every 3 days by 250 mg in adults up to a maximum of 1.5 g daily given in divided doses; in children under 9 years of age the dose may be increased by increments of 125 mg. Usual maintenance doses in adults and children over 9 years of age are 0.75 to 1.5 g daily. Suggested maintenance doses for children are: up to 2 years, 250 to 500 mg daily; 2 to 5 years, 500 to 750 mg daily; 6 to 9 years, 0.75 to 1 g daily. Maintenance doses are usually given as 2 divided doses.

As with other antiepileptics, withdrawal of primidone or transition to or from another type of antiepileptic therapy should be made gradually to avoid precipitating an increase in the frequency of seizures. For a discussion on whether or not to withdraw antiepileptic therapy in seizure-free patients, see p.349.

For **essential tremor** primidone is given in usual initial doses of 50 mg daily by mouth, increased gradually over 2 to 3 weeks if necessary, to a maximum of 750 mg daily.

**Epilepsy.** Primidone, like its metabolite phenobarbital, is used in the treatment of epilepsy (p.349) for partial seizures with or without secondary generalisation and for primary generalised tonic-clonic seizures. However, because of problems of sedation, it is usually reserved for use in cases unresponsive to other antiepileptics.

**Neonatal apnoea.** Results from a preliminary study suggested that adjunctive treatment with primidone[1] might be of value in neonatal apnoea (p.806) resistant to first-line therapy with xanthines alone, but subsequent confirmatory studies seem to be lacking.

1. Miller CA, *et al.* The use of primidone in neonates with theophylline-resistant apnea. *Am J Dis Child* 1993; **147:** 183–6.

**Neonatal seizures.** Primidone has been tried in the management of neonatal seizures (p.353).

**Tremor.** A beta blocker is often the first drug used in patients with essential tremor who require regular treatment (p.872) but primidone[1] may also be tried. A high incidence of acute adverse reactions has been reported following initial doses (see Tremor, under Adverse Effects, above). There has been concern that long-term use may produce tolerance to primidone's effects, although a small study has found a reduced response in only a few patients.[2] A later study[3] found a dose of 250 mg daily to be as or more effective than 750 mg daily without there being evidence of loss of efficacy during a 12-month follow-up.

1. Koller WC, Royse VL. Efficacy of primidone in essential tremor. *Neurology* 1986; **36:** 121–4.
2. Sasso E, *et al.* Primidone in the long-term treatment of essential tremor: a prospective study with computerized quantitative analysis. *Clin Neuropharmacol* 1990; **13:** 67–76.
3. Serrano-Dueñas M. Use of primidone in low doses (250 mg/day) versus high doses (750 mg/day) in the management of essential tremor: double-blind comparative study with one-year follow-up. *Parkinsonism Relat Disord* 2003; **10:** 29–33.

## Preparations

***BP 2003:*** Primidone Oral Suspension; Primidone Tablets;
***USP 27:*** Primidone Oral Suspension; Primidone Tablets.

**Proprietary Preparations** (details are given in Part 3)
***Arg.:*** Mysoline; ***Austral.:*** Mysoline; ***Austria:*** Cyral; Mysoline; ***Belg.:*** Mysoline; ***Braz.:*** Epidona; Mysoline; ***Canad.:*** Mysoline; ***Chile:*** Mysoline; ***Denm.:*** Mysoline; ***Fin.:*** Mysoline; ***Fr.:*** Mysoline; ***Ger.:*** Liskantin; Mylepsinum; Resimatil; ***Gr.:*** Mysoline; ***Hong Kong:*** Mysoline†; ***India:*** Mysoline; ***Irl.:*** Mysoline; ***Israel:*** Prysoline; ***Ital.:*** Mysoline; ***Mex.:*** Mysoline; ***Neth.:*** Mysoline†; ***Norw.:*** Mysoline; ***NZ:*** Mysoline†; ***Port.:*** Mysoline; ***S.Afr.:*** Mysoline; ***Singapore:*** Mysoline†; ***Spain:*** Mysoline; ***Swed.:*** Mysoline; ***Switz.:*** Mysoline; ***UK:*** Mysoline; ***USA:*** Mysoline.

## Progabide *(BAN, USAN, rINN)*

Halogabide; Progabida; SL-76-002. 4-(4′-Chloro-5-fluoro-2-hydroxybenzhydrylideneamino)butyramide.
$C_{17}H_{16}ClFN_2O_2$ = 334.8.
*CAS — 62666-20-0.*
*ATC — N03AG05.*

### Profile

Progabide is an analogue of gamma-aminobutyric acid (GABA) and is believed to owe its antiepileptic properties to its action as an agonist at central GABA receptors. It has been used in the treatment of partial and generalised tonic-clonic seizures resistant to other therapy and for myoclonic seizures and in the Lennox-Gastaut and West's syndromes.

Liver disorders, indicated by elevation of liver enzyme values, have been reported to occur in about 9% of patients receiving progabide, usually in the first few months of treatment, and have progressed to jaundice, hepatitis, encephalopathy and death in some patients.

**Interactions.** For the effects of progabide on other antiepileptics, see *Carbamazepine*, p.356; *Phenobarbital*, p.368; and *Phenytoin*, p.373.

**Porphyria.** Progabide is considered to be unsafe in patients with porphyria because it has been shown to be porphyrinogenic in *in-vitro* systems.

### Preparations

**Proprietary Preparations** (details are given in Part 3)
***Fr.:*** Gabrene†.

## Remacemide Hydrochloride *(USAN, pINNM)*

FPL-12924AA (remacemide or remacemide hydrochloride); Hidrocloruro de remacemida; PR-934-423 (remacemide); PR-934423 (remacemide); PR-934-423A (remacemide or remacemide hydrochloride). (±)-2-Amino-N-(1-methyl-1,2-diphenylethyl)acetamide.
$C_{17}H_{20}N_2O$ = 268.4.
*CAS — 128298-28-2 (remacemide); 111686-79-4 (remacemide hydrochloride).*

### Profile

Remacemide is an NMDA antagonist that has been investigated as adjunctive treatment for refractory epilepsy. It has also been investigated for the treatment of Parkinson's disease and as a neuroprotective drug in ischaemic stroke and for intra-operative cerebral ischaemia.

◊ References.

1. Dyker AG, Lees KR. Remacemide hydrochloride: a double-blind, placebo-controlled, safety and tolerability study in patients with acute ischaemic stroke. *Stroke* 1999; **30:** 1796–1801.
2. Parkinson Study Group. A multicenter randomized controlled trial of remacemide hydrochloride as monotherapy for PD. *Neurology* 2000; **54:** 1583–8.
3. Schachter SC, Tarsy D. Remacemide: current status and clinical applications. *Expert Opin Invest Drugs* 2000; **9:** 871–83.
4. Richens A, *et al.* A placebo-controlled, double-blind cross-over trial of adjunctive one month remacemide hydrochloride treatment in patients with refractory epilepsy. *Seizure* 2000; **9:** 537–43.
5. Chadwick D, *et al.* Remacemide hydrochloride: a placebo-controlled, one month, double-blind assessment of its safety, tolerability and pharmacokinetics as adjunctive therapy in patients with epilepsy. *Seizure* 2000; **9:** 544–50.
6. Shoulson I, *et al.* A randomized, controlled trial of remacemide for motor fluctuations in Parkinson's disease. *Neurology* 2001; **56:** 455–62.
7. Jones MW, *et al.* Remacemide hydrochloride as an add-on therapy in epilepsy: a randomized, placebo-controlled trial of three dose levels (300, 600 and 800 mg/day) in a b.i.d. regimen. *Seizure* 2002; **11:** 104–13.
8. Chadwick DW, *et al.* Remacemide hydrochloride as an add-on therapy in epilepsy: a randomized, placebo-controlled trial of three dose levels (300, 600 and 1200 mg/day) in a q.i.d. regimen. *Seizure* 2002; **11:** 114–23.
9. Leach JP, *et al.* Remacemide for drug-resistant localization related epilepsy. Available in The Cochrane Library; Issue 2. Chichester: John Wiley; 2004.

## Rufinamide *(BAN, USAN, rINN)*

CGP-33101; RUF-331; Rufinamida. 1-(2,6-Difluorobenzyl)-1*H*-1,2,3-triazole-4-carboxamide.
$C_{10}H_8F_2N_4O$ = 238.2.
*CAS — 106308-44-5.*

### Profile

Rufinamide is an antiepileptic under investigation as adjunctive therapy in the treatment of partial and primary generalised tonic-clonic seizures.

◊ References.

1. Jain KK. An assessment of rufinamide as an anti-epileptic in comparison with other drugs in clinical development. *Expert Opin Invest Drugs* 2000; **9:** 829–40.
2. Pålhagen S, *et al.* Rufinamide: a double-blind, placebo-controlled proof of principle trial in patients with epilepsy. *Epilepsy Res* 2001; **43:** 115–24.

## Stiripentol *(USAN, rINN)*

BCX-2600; Estiripentol. 4,4-Dimethyl-1-[(3,4-methylenedioxy)phenyl]-1-penten-3-ol.
$C_{14}H_{18}O_3$ = 234.3.
*CAS — 49763-96-4.*

### Profile

Stiripentol has been investigated for the treatment of various types of epilepsy, in particular severe myoclonic epilepsy in infancy. It is thought to be less potent than some conventional antiepileptics, but may reduce their adverse effects when used adjunctively. Adverse effects of stiripentol itself may include insomnia, gastrointestinal disturbances, and occasional psychotic reactions. It is a potent inhibitor of hepatic cytochrome P450 isoenzymes.

**Epilepsy.** A 24-week study[1] in 10 children demonstrated that stiripentol might be effective as adjunctive therapy for the treatment of atypical absence seizures (p.349). Further studies suggested benefit from adjunctive use in children with partial epilepsy[2] and severe myoclonic epilepsy.[2,3]

For interactions of stiripentol with other antiepileptics, see under Carbamazepine, p.356 and Phenytoin, p.373.

1. Farwell JR, *et al.* Stiripentol in atypical absence seizures in children: an open trial. *Epilepsia* 1993; **34:** 305–11.
2. Perez J, *et al.* Stiripentol: efficacy and tolerability in children with epilepsy. *Epilepsia* 1999; **40:** 1618–26.
3. Chiron C, *et al.* Stiripentol in severe myoclonic epilepsy in infancy: a randomised placebo-controlled syndrome-dedicated trial. *Lancet* 2000; **356:** 1638–42.

## Sultiame *(BAN, rINN)*

Riker-594; Sulthiame *(USAN)*; Sultiamo. 4-(Tetrahydro-2*H*-1,2-thiazin-2-yl)benzenesulphonamide *S,S*-dioxide.
$C_{10}H_{14}N_2O_4S_2$ = 290.4.
*CAS — 61-56-3.*
*ATC — N03AX03.*

**Pharmacopoeias.** In *Jpn.*

### Profile

Sultiame is a carbonic anhydrase inhibitor that has been used as an antiepileptic in most forms of epilepsy (p.349) except absence seizures. It has usually been given with other antiepileptics and it is believed that much of its activity is due to the inhibition of metabolism of the other drugs.

Sultiame has been given by mouth in initial doses of 100 mg twice daily or 50 mg three times daily gradually increased according to response to 200 mg three times daily. A dose of 5 to 10 mg/kg daily, adjusted according to response, has been recommended in Rolandic epilepsy.

**Interactions.** For the effect of sultiame on *phenytoin*, see p.373.

**Porphyria.** Sultiame has been associated with acute attacks of porphyria and is considered unsafe in porphyric patients.

## Preparations

**Proprietary Preparations** (details are given in Part 3)
***Austral.:*** Ospolot; ***Austria:*** Ospolot; ***Ger.:*** Ospolot; ***Israel:*** Ospolot.

# Tiagabine Hydrochloride

*(BANM, USAN, rINNM)*

Abbott-70569.1; ABT-569; Hidrocloruro de tiagabina; NNC-05-0328; NO-05-0328. (−)-(R)-1-[4,4-Bis(3-methyl-2-thienyl)-3-butenyl]nipecotic acid hydrochloride.

$C_{20}H_{25}NO_2S_2,HCl = 412.0.$

*CAS — 115103-54-3 (tiagabine); 145821-59-6 (tiagabine hydrochloride).*

*ATC — N03AG06.*

**Pharmacopoeias.** In *US.*

**USP 27** (Tiagabine Hydrochloride). A white to off-white powder. Sparingly soluble in water; very slightly soluble in chloroform; practically insoluble in *n*-heptane. Store in airtight containers at a temperature not exceeding 30°. Protect from light.

## Adverse Effects

The most common adverse effects include dizziness, nervousness, tiredness, somnolence, and tremor. Other reported adverse effects include irritability, confusion, depression, psychosis, difficulties in concentration, diarrhoea, abdominal pain, nausea, ataxia, emotional lability, and nystagmus. Bruising, rashes, speech difficulties, and an flu-like syndrome of chills, fever, myalgia, and headache have also been reported. Visual field defects have been reported rarely and decreased white blood cell counts have been noted at routine screenings.

**Incidence of adverse effects.** A systematic review[1] of 5 double-blind trials involving approximately 1000 patients of whom 675 were receiving tiagabine as adjunctive therapy for refractory partial seizures has been reported. Discontinuation due to adverse effects was infrequent and occurred in 15% of patients receiving tiagabine compared with 5% receiving placebo. Adverse effects were usually associated with dose titration, and were generally mild to moderate in severity, and transient. Another review[2] by the same author on data from all clinical trials (52 trials involving nearly 3100 patients) reported discontinuations for adverse effects in 21% of patients receiving tiagabine, with most occurring during the first 6 months of therapy. Sub-analysis showed that figures for placebo-controlled, adjunctive studies were similar to those of the earlier review.

1. Leppik IE. Tiagabine: the safety landscape. *Epilepsia* 1995; **36** (suppl 6): S10–S13.
2. Leppik IE, *et al.* Safety of tiagabine: summary of 53 trials. *Epilepsy Res* 1999; **33:** 235–46.

**Effects on the eyes.** Unlike vigabatrin (see p.383), there have been very few reports of visual field defects in patients taking tiagabine, another GABAergic antiepileptic. In a case report[1] a 39-year-old patient was noted to have visual field defects while receiving long-term tiagabine therapy for bipolar disorder. The defects reversed after tiagabine was withdrawn.

1. Kaufman KR, *et al.* Visual fields and tiagabine: a quandary. *Seizure* 2001; **10:** 525–9.

**Effects on mental function.** For a review of the effects of antiepileptic therapy on *cognition*, see p.351.

**Effects on the nervous system.** Acute dystonic reactions occurred in 3 patients when tiagabine was added to their existing carbamazepine treatment;[1] the reactions were associated with an increase in the dose of tiagabine to 20 mg or more. In all cases the dystonias disappeared despite continuing tiagabine therapy at the same dose, although in one patient carbamazepine was withdrawn.

There have been case reports of nonconvulsive status epilepticus, particularly of a complex partial nature, occurring with tiagabine.[2] However, the authors of one such report noted that, in placebo-controlled trials, the incidence of such an event was no higher in the tiagabine group than in the placebo group.

1. Wolańczyk T, Grabowska-Grzyb A. Transient dystonias in three patients treated with tiagabine. *Epilepsia* 2001; **42:** 944–6.
2. Fitzek S, *et al.* Drug-induced nonconvulsive status epilepticus with low dose of tiagabine. *Epileptic Disord* 2001; **3:** 147–50.

**Overdosage.** A 30-year-old man who took 320 mg of tiagabine in overdose together with 400 mg of phenytoin showed no serious signs of toxicity other than significantly depressed levels of consciousness from which he quickly recovered.[1] Plasma levels of tiagabine measured 4 hours after ingestion were 30 times higher than those seen with therapeutic doses; phenytoin levels just exceeded the therapeutic range.

1. Leach JP, *et al.* Deliberate overdose with the novel anticonvulsant tiagabine. *Seizure* 1995; **4:** 155–7.

## Precautions

Hepatic metabolism of tiagabine is reduced in patients with hepatic impairment, and dosage should therefore be reduced and/or the intervals between doses increased. It should not be used in patients with severely impaired hepatic function.

Care is required when withdrawing tiagabine therapy—see Uses and Administration, below.

**Breast feeding.** For comment on antiepileptic therapy and breast feeding, see p.351.

**Driving.** For comment on antiepileptic drugs and driving, see p.351.

**Pregnancy.** For comments on the management of epilepsy during pregnancy, see p.351.

## Interactions

There are complex interactions between antiepileptics and toxicity may be enhanced without a corresponding increase in antiepileptic activity. Such interactions are very variable and unpredictable and plasma monitoring is often advisable with combination therapy. The hepatic metabolism of tiagabine is accelerated by antiepileptics that induce enzymes of the cytochrome P450 system such as carbamazepine, phenobarbital, phenytoin, or primidone. Plasma concentrations of tiagabine may be reduced by up to threefold by concomitant use.

## Pharmacokinetics

Tiagabine is readily absorbed after oral doses. Food reduces the rate but not the extent of absorption. The absorption and elimination pharmacokinetics of tiagabine are linear within the therapeutic dosage range.

Tiagabine is widely distributed throughout the body and plasma protein binding is 96%.

Tiagabine is extensively metabolised in the liver and excreted as metabolites in the faeces or, to a lesser extent, in the urine; less than 2% of a dose is eliminated as unchanged drug. The plasma-elimination half-life is 7 to 9 hours, although this may be reduced to 2 to 3 hours by liver enzyme-inducing drugs (see also Interactions, above).

◊ References.

1. Gustavson LE, Mengel HB. Pharmacokinetics of tiagabine, a γ-aminobutyric acid-uptake inhibitor, in healthy subjects after single and multiples doses. *Epilepsia* 1995; **36:** 605–11.
2. So EL, *et al.* Pharmacokinetics of tiagabine as add-on therapy in patients taking enzyme-inducing antiepilepsy drugs. *Epilepsy Res* 1995; **22:** 221–6.
3. Snel S, *et al.* The pharmacokinetics of tiagabine in healthy elderly volunteers and elderly patients with epilepsy. *J Clin Pharmacol* 1997; **37:** 1015–20.
4. Cato A, *et al.* Effect of renal impairment on the pharmacokinetics and tolerability of tiagabine. *Epilepsia* 1998; **39:** 43–7.
5. Samara EE, *et al.* Population analysis of the pharmacokinetics of tiagabine in patients with epilepsy. *Epilepsia* 1998; **39:** 868–73.

## Uses and Administration

Tiagabine is a nipecotic acid derivative used in the treatment of epilepsy (p.349) as adjunctive therapy for refractory partial seizures with or without secondary generalisation. It inhibits the uptake of GABA into neuronal and glial cells, and therefore increases the availability of GABA at receptor sites.

UK licensing information states that tiagabine hydrochloride is given as the monohydrate, but doses are described in terms of tiagabine; dose forms providing the equivalent of 5, 10, and 15 mg of tiagabine are available. In the USA, however, the licensed product is stated to contain anhydrous tiagabine hydrochloride, and doses are described in terms of this substance; dose forms providing 2, 4, 12, 16, and 20 mg are available. As a result, the doses in the UK and US literature may not be directly comparable.

In the UK, the initial dose as adjunctive therapy in adults and children over 12 years of age is the equivalent of tiagabine 5 mg twice daily by mouth for 1 week, increased weekly as necessary by increments of 5 to 10 mg. The usual maintenance dose is 30 to 45 mg daily, in three divided doses, in patients receiving enzyme-inducing antiepileptics; in patients *not* taking enzyme-inducing drugs an initial maintenance dosage of 15 to 30 mg daily is suggested. Lower initial doses of the hydrochloride are recommended in the USA. Doses should be taken with food to avoid rapid rises in plasma concentrations, thereby reducing the incidence of adverse effects. Reduced doses should be given in hepatic impairment—see below.

As with other antiepileptics, withdrawal of tiagabine therapy or transition to or from another type of antiepileptic therapy should be made gradually to avoid precipitating an increase in the frequency of seizures. The UK manufacturer recommends gradual withdrawal over a period of 2 to 3 weeks. For a discussion on whether or not to withdraw antiepileptic therapy in seizure-free patients, see p.349.

**Administration in hepatic impairment.** The initial daily maintenance dosage of tiagabine in patients with mild to moderate hepatic impairment should be reduced to 5 to 10 mg given as a single dose or in 2 divided doses. Tiagabine should not be given to patients with severe hepatic impairment.

**Epilepsy.** Tiagabine is one of a number of drugs that may be used as adjunctive therapy in patients with partial seizures (with or without secondary generalisation) refractory to standard treatment (p.349). It appears to be reasonably well tolerated.

References.

1. Leach JP, Brodie MJ. Tiagabine. *Lancet* 1998; **351:** 203–7.
2. Adkins JC, Noble S. Tiagabine: a review of its pharmacodynamic and pharmacokinetic properties and therapeutic potential in the management of epilepsy. *Drugs* 1998; **55:** 437–60.
3. Luer MS, Rhoney DH. Tiagabine: a novel antiepileptic drug. *Ann Pharmacother* 1998; **32:** 1173–80.
4. Loiseau P. Review of controlled trials of gabitril (tiagabine): a clinician's viewpoint. *Epilepsia* 1999; **40** (suppl 9): S14–19.
5. Anonymous. Tiagabine: add-on treatment for partial seizures. *Drug Ther Bull* 2000; **38:** 47–8.
6. Dodrill CB, *et al.* Tiagabine versus phenytoin and carbamazepine as add-on therapies: effects on abilities, adjustment, and mood. *Epilepsy Res* 2000; **42:** 123–32.
7. Crawford P, *et al.* Tiagabine: efficacy and safety in adjunctive treatment of partial seizures. *Epilepsia* 2001; **42:** 531–8.
8. Biraben A, *et al.* Comparison of twice- and three times daily tiagabine for the adjunctive treatment of partial seizures in refractory patients with epilepsy: an open label, randomised, parallel-group study. *Epileptic Disord* 2001; **3:** 91–100.

**Stiff-man syndrome.** There have been anecdotal reports[1] of improvement of stiff-man syndrome (p.696) with tiagabine in patients unable to tolerate benzodiazepine therapy.

1. Murinson BB, Rizzo M. Improvement of stiff-person syndrome with tiagabine. *Neurology* 2001; **57:** 366.

## Preparations

**Proprietary Preparations** (details are given in Part 3)
***Austral.:*** Gabitril; ***Austria:*** Gabitril; ***Belg.:*** Gabitril; ***Braz.:*** Gabitril†; ***Denm.:*** Gabitril; ***Fin.:*** Gabitril; ***Fr.:*** Gabitril; ***Ger.:*** Gabitril; ***Gr.:*** Gabitril; ***Irl.:*** Gabitril; ***Ital.:*** Gabitril; ***Mex.:*** Gabatril; ***Port.:*** Gabitril; ***Spain:*** Gabitril; ***Switz.:*** Gabitril; ***UK:*** Gabitril; ***USA:*** Gabitril.

# Topiramate *(BAN, USAN, rINN)*

McN-4853; RWJ-17021; Topiramato. 2,3:4,5-Di-*O*-isopropylidene-β-D-fructopyranose sulphamate.

$C_{12}H_{21}NO_8S = 339.4.$

*CAS — 97240-79-4.*

*ATC — N03AX11.*

## Adverse Effects

Adverse effects associated with topiramate therapy include ataxia, impaired concentration, confusion, dizziness, fatigue, paraesthesia or hypoaesthesia, drowsiness, and difficulties with memory or cognition. Agitation, anxiety, nervousness, emotional lability (with mood disorders), and depression may also occur. Other reported adverse effects include abdominal pain, anorexia, asthenia, diplopia, leucopenia, nausea, nystagmus, insomnia, psychomotor retardation, impaired speech, altered taste, visual disturbances, and weight loss. The risk of developing renal calculi is increased, especially in predisposed patients. Reduced sweating with hyperthermia has occurred particularly in children. Rare cases of acute myopia with secondary angle-closure glaucoma have been reported.

**Effects on bone.** For the effects of antiepileptics on bone and on calcium and vitamin D metabolism, see under Phenytoin, p.371.

**Effects on electrolytes.** Metabolic acidosis has been associated with topiramate treatment. Data from clinical trials estimate that the incidence of persistently decreased serum bicarbonate levels ranges from 23 to 67% with topiramate compared with 1 to 10% with placebo;[1] children, in particular, may be at a greater risk than adults.[1,2] Generally, the decreases in serum bicarbonate are mild to moderate and occur soon after starting topiramate. Clinical signs such as hyperventilation may develop.

Some authorities including the US manufacturer recommend that baseline and periodic serum bicarbonate levels should be monitored during topiramate treatment. If metabolic acidosis develops or persists, it may be necessary to reduce the dose or discontinue topiramate although, in some cases, correcting the acidosis with alkali therapy may be more appropriate.

1. Janssen-Ortho Canada. Important drug safety information: Topamax (topiramate) use is associated with metabolic acidosis. Available at: http://www.hc-sc.gc.ca/hpfb-dgpsa/tpd-dpt/topamax_3_hpc_e.pdf (accessed 14/05/04)
2. Philippi H, *et al.* Topiramate and metabolic acidosis in infants and toddlers. *Epilepsia* 2002; **43:** 744–7.

**Effects on the eyes.** There have been rare reports of acute myopia with secondary angle-closure glaucoma in adults and children receiving topiramate:[1-3] as of April 2002 the Committee on Safety of Medicines in the UK was aware of 23 cases worldwide.[4] Symptoms include decreased visual acuity and ocular pain which generally appear within one month of starting treatment; hyperaemia and raised intra-ocular pressure may be present with or without mydriasis. Choroidal effusions resulting in anterior displacement of lens and iris have been reported. Appropriate measures to reduce intra-ocular pressure should be taken, and topiramate stopped as rapidly as is clinically feasible.[4]

1. Gubbay SS. *Epilepsia* 1998; **39:** 451.
2. Sen HA, *et al.* Topiramate-induced acute myopia and retinal striae. *Arch Ophthalmol* 2001; **119:** 775–7.
3. Rhee DJ, *et al.* Bilateral angle-closure glaucoma and ciliary body swelling from topiramate. *Arch Ophthalmol* 2001; **119:** 1721–3.
4. Committee on Safety of Medicines/Medicines Control Agency. Topiramate (Topamax): acute myopia and raised intraocular pressure. *Current Problems* 2002; **28:** 4. Also available at: http://www.mca.gov.uk/ourwork/monitorsafequalmed/currentproblems/cpapril2002.pdf (accessed 14/05/04)

**Effects on the liver.** Fulminant liver failure has been reported[1] following an increase in adjunctive topiramate dose in a patient maintained on carbamazepine.

1. Bjøro K, *et al.* Topiramate and fulminant liver failure. *Lancet* 1998; **352:** 1119.

**Effects on mental function.** For a review of the effects of antiepileptic therapy including topiramate on *cognition*, see p.351.

**Effects on the nervous system.** Decreased sweating and hyperthermia have been reported in patients given topiramate; some cases were reported after exposure to high ambient temperatures. The manufacturer noted that children appeared to be at an increased risk of developing these adverse reactions and should be monitored closely for such effects especially during warm or hot weather. Caution was also advised when topiramate was given with other drugs known to cause similar effects, for example, carbonic anhydrase inhibitors and antimuscarinics.

Hemiparesis that resolved on withdrawal of topiramate has been reported[1] in 2 patients, although both already had compromised neurological function.

1. Stephen LJ, *et al.* Transient hemiparesis with topiramate. *BMJ* 1999; **318:** 845.

## Precautions

Topiramate should be used with caution in patients with renal or hepatic impairment. Adequate hydration is recommended to reduce the risk of developing renal calculi, especially in predisposed patients.

Care is required when withdrawing topiramate therapy—see also under Uses and Administration, below.

**Breast feeding.** For comment on antiepileptic therapy and breast feeding, see p.351.

**Driving.** For a comment on antiepileptic drugs and driving, see p.351.

**Pregnancy.** For comments on the management of epilepsy during pregnancy, see p.351.

## Interactions

There are complex interactions between antiepileptics and toxicity may be enhanced without a corresponding increase in antiepileptic activity. Such interactions are very variable and unpredictable and plasma monitoring is often advisable with combination therapy.

**Antiepileptics.** In pharmacokinetic studies[1] *phenytoin* and *carbamazepine* both decreased the plasma concentration of topiramate.

For the effect of topiramate on phenytoin, see p.373.

1. Bourgeois BFD. Drug interaction profile of topiramate. *Epilepsia* 1996; **37:** (suppl 2): S14–S17.

**Cardiac glycosides.** For the effect of topiramate on *digoxin*, see p.897.

**Sex hormones.** For the effects of antiepileptics including topiramate on *oral contraceptives*, see p.1534.

## Pharmacokinetics

Topiramate is readily absorbed after oral doses, with peak plasma concentrations achieved after about 2 hours. Bioavailability is not affected by the presence of food. Protein binding is about 9 to 17%. The volume of distribution in women is approximately half that in men. Topiramate crosses the placental barrier and is distributed into breast milk.

In healthy subjects topiramate is not extensively metabolised; however, up to 50% of a dose may undergo metabolism in the liver in patients receiving enzyme-inducing drugs concomitantly. It is eliminated chiefly in urine, as unchanged drug and metabolites; mean plasma elimination half-life is about 21 hours. Steady-state concentrations are achieved after about 4 to 8 days in patients with normal renal function. Clearance is decreased in patients with impaired renal or hepatic function, and steady-state plasma concentrations may not be achieved for 10 to 15 days in the former. Children exhibit a higher clearance and shorter elimination half-life than adults.

The pharmacokinetics of topiramate may be affected by the concurrent administration of other antiepileptics (see under Interactions, above).

◊ References.

1. Perucca E, Bialer M. The clinical pharmacokinetics of the newer antiepileptic drugs: focus on topiramate, zonisamide, and tiagabine. *Clin Pharmacokinet* 1996; **31:** 29–46.
2. Glauser TA, *et al.* Topiramate pharmacokinetics in infants. *Epilepsia* 1999; **40:** 788–91.

## Uses and Administration

Topiramate, a sulfamate-substituted monosaccharide, is an antiepileptic used as adjunctive therapy in adults and children over 2 years for refractory partial seizures with or without secondary generalisation, seizures associated with the Lennox-Gastaut syndrome, and primary generalised tonic-clonic seizures. In the UK, topiramate may also be used as monotherapy in adults and children aged 6 years and over with newly diagnosed epilepsy who have generalised tonic-clonic seizures or partial seizures.

For *both adjunctive and monotherapy*, the initial dose of topiramate in **adults** is 25 mg once daily by mouth for one week increased thereafter by increments of 25 to 50 mg at intervals of one to two weeks until the effective dose is reached. Daily doses of more than 25 mg should be taken in 2 divided doses. The usual daily dose for *adjunctive therapy* is 200 to 400 mg although some patients may require up to 800 mg daily. When used as *monotherapy*, usual doses range from 100 mg daily to a maximum of 400 mg daily.

The initial dose as *adjunctive therapy* for **children** aged 2 to 16 years is 25 mg nightly for the first week, increased at intervals of one to two weeks by increments of 1 to 3 mg/kg daily, according to response. The recommended dose thereafter is about 5 to 9 mg/kg daily given in 2 divided doses, though up to 30 mg/kg may be given. For *monotherapy*, children aged 6 years and over may be started on 0.5 to 1 mg/kg at night for the first week, increased at intervals of one to two weeks by increments of 0.5 to 1 mg/kg daily. The usual dose is 3 to 6 mg/kg daily in 2 divided doses, although higher doses have been tolerated.

Smaller increments or longer intervals between increments may be necessary if patients cannot tolerate the above regimen; US product information suggests that doses should be halved in patients with moderate to severe renal impairment (see also below).

As with other antiepileptics, withdrawal of topiramate therapy or transition to or from another type of antiepileptic therapy should be made gradually to avoid precipitating an increase in the frequency of seizures. For a discussion on whether or not to withdraw antiepileptic therapy in seizure-free patients, see p.349. The UK manufacturers have suggested decreasing the dose by 100 mg daily at weekly intervals.

**Administration in renal impairment.** Patients with moderate to severe renal impairment take longer to reach steady-state plasma concentrations of topiramate than patients with normal renal function (see under Pharmacokinetics, above) and the dosage regimen may need adjusting; US product information recommends that usual adult doses (see above) be halved in such patients.

In patients undergoing haemodialysis a supplemental dose equal to about one-half of the daily dose should be given in divided doses (at the start and finish of the procedure).

**Bipolar disorder.** Mood-stabilising antiepileptics such as carbamazepine and valproate are alternatives to lithium in the management of bipolar disorder (p.278). Some of the newer antiepileptics such as topiramate are also being investigated.[1-3]

1. Teter CJ, *et al.* Treatment of affective disorder and obesity with topiramate. *Ann Pharmacother* 2000; **34:** 1262–5.
2. Erfurth A, Kuhn G. Topiramate monotherapy in the maintenance treatment of bipolar I disorder: effects on mood, weight and serum lipids. *Neuropsychobiology* 2000; **42** (suppl 1): 50–1.
3. McElroy SL, *et al.* Open-label adjunctive topiramate in the treatment of bipolar disorders. *Biol Psychiatry* 2000; **47:** 1025–33.

**Epilepsy.** Topiramate is used[1-3] in epilepsy (p.349) as adjunctive therapy for refractory partial seizures; monotherapy with topiramate may also be safe and effective. Gradual initiation of topiramate therapy improves tolerability without delaying therapeutic response.[4]

Topiramate is also used in patients with the Lennox-Gastaut syndrome[5] and with primary generalised tonic-clonic seizures.[6] It has also been investigated in children with infantile spasms (as for example in West's syndrome)[7] and severe myoclonic epilepsy.[8] A retrospective review[9] of the use of topiramate in such drug-resistant childhood epilepsies concluded that it was efficacious and well tolerated.

1. Langtry HD, *et al.* Topiramate: a review of its pharmacodynamic and pharmacokinetic properties and clinical efficacy in the management of epilepsy. *Drugs* 1997; **54:** 752–73.
2. Sachdeo RC, *et al.* Topiramate: clinical profile in epilepsy. *Clin Pharmacokinet* 1998; **34:** 335–46.
3. Garnett WR. Clinical pharmacology of topiramate: a review. *Epilepsia* 2000; **41** (suppl 1): S61–S65.
4. Biton V, *et al.* Topiramate titration and tolerability. *Ann Pharmacother* 2001; **35:** 173–9.
5. Sachdeo RC, *et al.* A double-blind, randomized trial of topiramate in Lennox-Gastaut syndrome. *Neurology* 1999; **52:** 1882–7.
6. Biton V. A randomized, placebo-controlled study of topiramate in primary generalized tonic-clonic seizures. *Neurology* 1999; **52:** 1330–7.
7. Glauser TA, *et al.* Long-term response to topiramate in patients with West syndrome. *Epilepsia* 2000; **41** (suppl 1): S91–S94.
8. Nieto-Barrera M, *et al.* Topiramate in the treatment of severe myoclonic epilepsy in infancy. *Seizure* 2000; **9:** 590–4.
9. Yeung S, *et al.* Topiramate for drug-resistant epilepsies. *Eur J Paediatr Neurol* 2000; **4:** 31–3.

**Migraine.** Results from placebo-controlled studies[1,2] have shown a significant reduction in migraine frequency in those patients receiving prophylactic topiramate.

1. Storey JR, *et al.* Topiramate in migraine prevention: a double-blind, placebo-controlled study. *Headache* 2001; **41:** 968–75.
2. Brandes JL, *et al.* Topiramate for migraine prevention: a randomized controlled trial. *JAMA* 2004; **291:** 965–73.

**Motor neurone disease.** Topiramate has been tried as a potential therapy for amyotrophic lateral sclerosis (see Motor Neurone Disease, p.1739) but with disappointing results.[1]

1. Cudkowicz ME, *et al.* A randomized, placebo-controlled trial of topiramate in amyotrophic lateral sclerosis. *Neurology* 2003; **61:** 456–64.

**Neuropathic pain.** Although carbamazepine is the drug of choice in the treatment of trigeminal neuralgia (p.8), topiramate has also been tried successfully.[1] It has also been tried in the treatment of diabetic neuropathy (p.6).

1. Zvartau-Hind M, *et al.* Topiramate relieves refractory trigeminal neuralgia in MS patients. *Neurology* 2000; **55:** 1587–8.

**Psychiatric disorders.** Topiramate would appear to have psychotropic properties and has been tried in the management of several psychiatric disorders, including *bipolar disorder* (see above). It has also been tried in binge-eating.[1]

1. Shapira NA, *et al.* Treatment of binge-eating disorder with topiramate: a clinical case series. *J Clin Psychiatry* 2000; **61:** 368–72.

**Tremor.** Topiramate has been tried in the treatment of tremor.[1]

1. Galvez-Jimenez N, Hargreave M. Topiramate and essential tremor. *Ann Neurol* 2000; **47:** 837–8.

## Preparations

**Proprietary Preparations** (details are given in Part 3)
***Arg.:*** Topamac; ***Austral.:*** Topamax; ***Austria:*** Topamax; ***Belg.:*** Topamax; ***Braz.:*** Topamax; ***Canad.:*** Topamax; ***Chile:*** Topamax; Toprel; ***Denm.:*** Topimax; ***Fin.:*** Topimax; ***Fr.:*** Epitomax; ***Ger.:*** Topamax; ***Gr.:*** Topamac; ***Hong Kong:*** Topamax; ***India:*** Topamac; ***Irl.:*** Topamax; ***Israel:*** Topamax; ***Ital.:*** Topamax; ***Malaysia:*** Topamax; ***Mex.:*** Topamax; ***Neth.:*** Topamax; ***Norw.:*** Topimax; ***NZ:*** Topamax; ***Port.:*** Topamax; ***S.Afr.:*** Topamax; ***Singapore:*** Topamax; ***Spain:*** Topamax; ***Swed.:*** Topimax; ***Switz.:*** Topamax; ***Thai.:*** Topamax; ***UK:*** Topamax; ***USA:*** Topamax.

---

## Trimethadione *(BAN, rINN)*

Trimetadiona; Trimethadionum; Trimethinum; Troxidone. 3,5,5-Trimethyl-1,3-oxazolidine-2,4-dione.

$C_6H_9NO_3$ = 143.1.
*CAS — 127-48-0.*
*ATC — N03AC02.*

**Pharmacopoeias.** In *Eur.* (see p.vi), *Int.*, and *Jpn.*

**Ph. Eur. 5.0** (Trimethadione). Colourless or almost colourless crystals. Soluble in water; very soluble in alcohol. Protect from light.

### Profile

Trimethadione is an oxazolidinedione antiepileptic that has been given in the treatment of absence seizures refractory to other antiepileptics. However, because of its potential toxicity, other antiepileptics are preferred (see under Epilepsy, p.349).

**Porphyria.** Trimethadione has been associated with acute attacks of porphyria and is considered unsafe in porphyric patients.

**Pregnancy.** Characteristic congenital malformations, termed the fetal trimethadione syndrome, have been associated with the use of trimethadione in pregnancy.

For comments on the management of epilepsy during pregnancy, see p.351.

## Valproate

Valproato.

Valproate is a generic term applied to valproic acid, its salts and esters.

### Valproic Acid *(BAN, USAN, rINN)*

Abbott-44089; Ácido valproico; Acidum Valproicum. 2-Propylvaleric acid; 2-Propylpentanoic acid.

$C_8H_{16}O_2$ = 144.2.
*CAS — 99-66-1.*
*ATC — N03AG01.*

**Pharmacopoeias.** In *Eur.* (see p.vi) and *US.*

**Ph. Eur. 5.0** (Valproic Acid). A colourless or very slightly yellow, slightly viscous, clear liquid. Very slightly soluble in water; miscible with alcohol and with dichloromethane. It dissolves in dilute solutions of alkali hydroxides. Store in airtight containers.

**USP 27** (Valproic Acid). A colourless to pale yellow, slightly viscous, clear liquid having a characteristic odour. Slightly soluble in water; freely soluble in alcohol, in acetone, in chloroform, in ether, in methyl alcohol, in benzene, in *n*-heptane, and in 1N sodium hydroxide; slightly soluble in 0.1N hydrochloric acid. Store in airtight glass, stainless steel, or polyethylene containers.

### Sodium Valproate *(BANM, rINNM)*

Abbott-44090; Natrii Valproas; Valproate Sodium *(USAN)*; Valproato sódico. Sodium 2-propylvalerate; Sodium 2-propylpentanoate.

$C_8H_{15}NaO_2$ = 166.2.
*CAS — 1069-66-5.*
*ATC — N03AG01.*

**Pharmacopoeias.** In *Chin., Eur.* (see p.vi), *Int.*, and *Jpn.*

**Ph. Eur. 5.0** (Sodium Valproate). A white or almost white, hygroscopic, crystalline powder. Very soluble in water; slightly to freely soluble in alcohol. Store in airtight containers.

### Valproate Pivoxil *(rINN)*

Valproato de pivoxilo. Hydroxymethyl 2-propylvalerate pivalate.

$C_{14}H_{26}O_4$ = 258.4.
*CAS — 77372-61-3.*
*ATC — N03AG01.*

### Valproate Semisodium *(rINN)*

Abbott-50711; Divalproex Sodium *(USAN)*; Semisodium Valproate *(BAN)*; Valproato semisódico. 2-Propylvaleric acid—Sodium 2-propylvalerate (1:1); Sodium hydrogen bis(2-propylvalerate) oligomer.

$C_{16}H_{31}NaO_4$ = 310.4.
*CAS — 76584-70-8.*
*ATC — N03AG01.*

### Valpromide *(rINN)*

Dipropylacetamide; Valpromida. 2-Propylvaleramide.

$C_8H_{17}NO$ = 143.2.
*CAS — 2430-27-5.*
*ATC — N03AG02.*

### Adverse Effects

The most frequently reported adverse effects associated with valproate therapy are gastrointestinal disturbances, particularly at the start of therapy; enteric-coated formulations, taking doses with meals, and starting with low doses may minimise symptoms. There may be increased appetite, and weight gain is common.

Less common adverse effects include oedema, headache, reversible prolongation of bleeding time, and thrombocytopenia. Leucopenia and bone marrow depression have been reported. Neurological adverse effects including ataxia, tremor, sedation, lethargy, confusion, and more rarely encephalopathy and coma, have occasionally been reported, although these are often associated with too high a starting dose, increasing doses too rapidly, or use with other antiepileptics. Very rare cases of extrapyramidal symptoms or reversible dementia associated with cerebral atrophy have been reported. Increased alertness may occur, which is generally considered beneficial, but occasionally aggression, hyperactivity, and behavioural disturbances have been reported. Hearing loss has been noted. There may occasionally be rashes, and, rarely, hirsutism, acne, toxic epidermal necrolysis and Stevens-Johnson syndrome or erythema multiforme. Transient hair loss, sometimes with regrowth of curly hair, has occurred. Irregular periods, amenorrhoea, and gynaecomastia have been reported rarely.

Liver dysfunction including hepatic failure has occasionally been reported, usually in the first few months of treatment, and necessitates valproate withdrawal; there have been fatalities. Elevation of liver enzyme values is common but normally transient and dose-related. Hyperammonaemia has occurred, even in the absence of overt hepatic failure, and is sometimes associated with neurological symptoms; hyperglycinaemia has also been reported. Pancreatitis has also been reported rarely; plasma amylase should be measured if there is acute abdominal pain. In a few patients there have been reports of reversible defects in renal tubular function (Fanconi's syndrome).

Congenital malformations have been reported in infants born to women who had received antiepileptics including valproate during pregnancy.

Inflammatory reactions and pain have been reported at the injection site following intravenous administration.

**Incidence of adverse effects.** Side-effects were present in 71 of 88 children receiving sodium valproate monotherapy[1] and, although average doses in these patients were significantly higher than in the 17 with no side-effects, no difference in the plasma concentrations was observed between the 2 groups.

- Behavioural alterations seen in 56 included irritability, longer and deeper sleep, superficial sleep, hyperactivity, being more alert, lassitude, drowsiness, being more sociable, calmness, being happier, absent mindedness, being sadder, aggressiveness, being more skillful, and docility; it was emphasised that stimulatory reactions were as frequent as depressant effects
- Digestive disorders occurred in 43 children with anorexia, abdominal pain, and nausea and vomiting being the most frequent; diarrhoea, constipation, an increase in appetite, and a gain in weight also occurred. With the exception of a temporary increase in plasma transaminase concentrations in 2 patients, hepatic or pancreatic dysfunction was not seen
- Neurological changes in the form of tremor, paraesthesia, or ataxia, occurring in only 4 patients, were less frequent than either behavioural or digestive reactions
- Miscellaneous reactions including polydipsia, polyuria, diaphoresis, enuresis, hair loss, change in hair colour or texture, and rash were seen in 23 children
- Of the 71 children experiencing reactions therapy continued unchanged in 56, was changed in 3 either by altering the pharmaceutical formulation (syrup, tablets, granules), by changing the frequency of dosing, or by reducing the dose in 6, and in the remaining 9 children valproate therapy was discontinued.

1. Herranz JL, *et al.* Side effects of sodium valproate in monotherapy controlled by plasma levels: a study in 88 pediatric patients. *Epilepsia* 1982; **23:** 203–14.

**Carnitine deficiency.** Carnitine deficiency (p.1424) may occasionally arise during long-term use of valproate; although it is unclear whether carnitine supplementation is of value in children receiving valproate, some neurologists consider it justified in selected cases.[1]

1. De Vivo DC, *et al.* L-Carnitine supplementation in childhood epilepsy: current perspectives. *Epilepsia* 1998; **39:** 1216–25.

**Effects on the blood.** A number of reports have implicated valproate as a cause of occasional neutropenia,[1,2] leucopenia,[3] and thrombocytopenia.[2] A 1-year prospective study involving 45 patients found that absolute neutropenia developed in 12 and thrombocytopenia in 15, but that the disorders were transient and self-limiting.[2] However, neutropenia has occasionally been sufficiently severe to warrant withdrawal of valproate.[4] Red cell aplasia has also been associated with valproate therapy.[5,6] A study[7] involving 30 children indicated that valproate might produce symptoms similar to those of von Willebrand's disease; 19 of the 30 had a history of minor haemorrhage during therapy, and 7 had abnormal bleeding times. Factor VIII therapy might need to be given in patients receiving valproate who undergo surgery or in whom bleeding was severe.

For a discussion of the effects of antiepileptics, including valproate, on serum folate, see under Phenytoin, p.370.

1. Jaeken J, *et al.* Neutropenia during sodium valproate treatment. *Arch Dis Child* 1979; **54:** 986–7.
2. Barr RD, *et al.* Valproic acid and immune thrombocytopenia. *Arch Dis Child* 1982; **57:** 681–4.
3. Coulter DL, *et al.* Valproic acid therapy in childhood epilepsy. *JAMA* 1980; **244:** 785–8.
4. Symon DNK, Russell G. Sodium valproate and neutropenia. *Arch Dis Child* 1983; **58:** 235.
5. MacDougall LG. Pure red cell aplasia associated with sodium valproate therapy. *JAMA* 1982; **247:** 53–4.
6. Watts RG, *et al.* Valproic acid-induced cytopenias: evidence for a dose-related suppression of hematopoiesis. *J Pediatr* 1990; **117:** 495–9.
7. Kreuz W, *et al.* Induction of von Willebrand disease type I by valproic acid. *Lancet* 1990; **335:** 1350–1.

**Effects on bone.** For the effects of antiepileptics including valproate on bone and on calcium and vitamin D metabolism, see under Phenytoin, p.371.

**Effects on the endocrine system.** *Menstrual disturbances* occurred more frequently with valproate than other antiepileptics in a study of 238 women with epilepsy.[1] The disturbances were attributed to valproate-associated reproductive endocrine disorders, namely polycystic ovaries and elevated serum-testosterone concentrations.

For mention of the effects of antiepileptics on *sexual function* in male epileptic patients, see under Phenytoin, p.371.

1. Isojärvi JIT, *et al.* Polycystic ovaries and hyperandrogenism in women taking valproate for epilepsy. *N Engl J Med* 1993; **329:** 1383–8.

**Effects on the liver.** An early review[1] of the hepatotoxicity of valproate included an analysis of 42 cases with fatal hepatitis, 3 cases with a Reye's-like syndrome, and 22 instances of hyperammonaemia:

- In 19 clinical trials the incidence of *abnormal serum aminotransferase* activity ranged from 0 to 44% with an overall incidence of 11% in the 1197 patients monitored; in the non-fatal cases activity was usually between one and three times the upper limit of normal and was not usually, except in the most severe cases, accompanied by rises in serum bilirubin or alkaline phosphatase
- In the 42 cases of *hepatitis* with a fatal outcome the age at presentation ranged from 2.5 months to 34 years with 69% aged 10 years or less. Below the age of 15 years the proportion of males was 62.5% but above this age it was 30%; the disproportionate vulnerability of young individuals, particularly boys, did not appear to be a reflection of prescribing habits in that age group. In more than two-thirds of these patients with a fatal outcome, prodromal symptoms comprised anorexia and vomiting, loss of epilepsy control, impaired consciousness, and ataxia; in about one-third there were signs of liver damage with fever, jaundice, ascites, peripheral oedema, and easy bruising. In all of the patients hepatic coma developed. In 36 patients on whom data were available the onset of hepatic illness in one-third occurred between 1 and 2 months and in only 2 patients did the onset occur after more than 5 months. Of these 42 patients with fatal hepatotoxicity 36 had received other drugs, mostly antiepileptics, concurrently
- The 3 children with a *Reye's-like syndrome* all died within 3 weeks of the first occurrence of symptoms as a result of cerebral oedema (2) or aspiration pneumonia (1)
- In the 22 patients with symptomatic *hyperammonaemia*, characterised usually by impaired consciousness and ataxia, but without overt liver disease, withdrawal of valproate resulted in all becoming asymptomatic and biochemical abnormalities returned to normal. Hyperammonaemia has also been reported in asymptomatic patients

Various hypotheses for the cause of valproate hepatotoxicity have been discussed in detail.[2]

Analysis of deaths in the USA attributed to valproate liver toxicity identified a decline in the incidence of fatalities as use in young children and use concurrently with other antiepileptics declined.[3]

1. Powell-Jackson PR, *et al.* Hepatotoxicity to sodium valproate: a review. *Gut* 1984; **25:** 673–81.
2. Eadie MJ, *et al.* Valproate-associated hepatotoxicity and its biochemical mechanisms. *Med Toxicol* 1988; **3:** 85–106.
3. Dreifuss FE, *et al.* Valproic acid hepatic fatalities: II US experience since 1984. *Neurology* 1989; **39:** 201–7.

**Effects on mental function.** For a review of the effects of antiepileptic therapy including valproate on cognition, see p.351.

**Effects on the nervous system.** An *extrapyramidal* syndrome of tremor and rigidity, unresponsive to benzatropine or trihexyphenidyl, developed in a 52-year-old man with schizophrenia given a therapeutic trial of sodium valproate 1 to 2 g daily.[1] Administration of sodium valproate to a man with dystonic movements of the neck and spine produced a severe subjective and objective deterioration in his symptoms which returned to their previous severity on withdrawal of the drug.[2]

A *stuporous state* associated with EEG abnormalities has been described[3,4] during valproate therapy for complex partial or mixed seizure types and it was suggested that in certain forms of epilepsy valproate may exhibit a paradoxical epileptogenic effect. Other findings[5] have argued against an epileptic origin for valproate-induced stupor.

1. Lautin A, *et al.* Extrapyramidal syndrome with sodium valproate. *BMJ* 1979; **2:** 1035–6.
2. Dick DJ, Saunders M. Extrapyramidal syndrome with sodium valproate. *BMJ* 1980; **280:** 189.
3. Marescaux C, *et al.* Stuporous episodes during treatment with sodium valproate: report of seven cases. *Epilepsia* 1982; **23:** 297–305.
4. Stecker MM, Kita M. Paradoxical response to valproic acid in a patient with a hypothalamic hamartoma. *Ann Pharmacother* 1998; **32:** 1168–72.
5. Aguglia U, *et al.* Negative myoclonus during valproate-related stupor: neurophysiological evidence of a cortical non-epileptic origin. *Electroencephalogr Clin Neurophysiol* 1995; **94:** 103–8.

**Effects on the pancreas.** An early report of 4 cases of pancreatitis associated with valproic acid therapy also reviewed 10 previously published cases.[1] None of the 14 patients, 2 of whom died, suffered other symptoms of a toxic reaction to valproic acid. Pancreatitis was not dose-related and had developed as early as one week and as late as 4.5 years following the introduction of therapy. Symptoms recurred on rechallenge in 6 of 7 patients. However, routine monitoring of serum-amylase concentrations in asymptomatic patients did not seem necessary. In February 1994 the UK Committee on Safety of Medicines commented[2] in a review of drug-induced pancreatitis that they had received 29 reports of pancreatitis, including 2 fatalities, associated with sodium valproate.

1. Wyllie E, *et al.* Pancreatitis associated with valproic acid therapy. *Am J Dis Child* 1984; **138:** 912–14.
2. Committee on Safety of Medicines/Medicines Control Agency. Drug-induced pancreatitis. *Current Problems* 1994; **20:** 2–3.

**Effects on the skin and hair.** Five of 250 patients developed curly hair during treatment with sodium valproate 1 g daily;[1] in 3 patients this effect followed temporary alopecia. Another report of hair curling in a patient who received sodium valproate in doses up to 3 g daily for 30 months commented that her hair started to revert to the former straight style 9 months after discontinuing the drug.[2]

Valproate-induced nicotinic-acid deficiency with an associated pellagra-like syndrome has been reported in a young boy;[3] the condition responded dramatically to the administration of nicotinamide.

Reduced serum-zinc concentrations and cutaneous manifestations of zinc deficiency were found in 2 patients receiving antiepileptic drugs.[4] It was postulated that deficiency occurred as a result of chelation by sodium valproate, and possibly phenytoin, in association with malabsorption and that, in one case, malabsorption was initiated by valproate.

Cutaneous vasculitis has been reported[5] in 2 patients taking sodium valproate. The reaction recurred on rechallenge.

Valproate might share the same order of risk as other antiepileptics for the development of Stevens-Johnson syndrome and toxic epidermal necrolysis,[6] although it had previously been regarded as safer in this respect.

1. Jeavons PM, *et al.* Valproate and curly hair. *Lancet* 1977; **i:** 359.
2. Gupta AK. 'Perming' effects associated with chronic valproate therapy. *Br J Clin Pract* 1988; **42:** 75–7.
3. Gillman MA, Sandyk R. Nicotinic acid deficiency induced by sodium valproate. *S Afr Med J* 1984; **65:** 986.
4. Lewis-Jones MS, *et al.* Cutaneous manifestations of zinc deficiency during treatment with anticonvulsants. *BMJ* 1985; **290:** 603–4.
5. Kamper AM, *et al.* Cutaneous vasculitis induced by sodium valproate. *Lancet* 1991; **337:** 497–8.
6. Anonymous. Drugs as risk factors in severe cutaneous diseases. *WHO Drug Inf* 1996; **10:** 33–5.

**Enuresis.** Nocturnal enuresis associated with sodium valproate therapy has been reported[1] in 2 children. Remission of the enuresis was achieved either by reducing or redistributing the doses. Several studies have recorded enuresis as a side-effect of valproate in children,[2] the frequency being between 1 and 7%. The most likely explanations are that either it is secondary to a central effect on the thirst centre resulting in polydipsia or it is a consequence of the increased depth of sleep associated with valproate.

1. Panayiotopoulos CP. Nocturnal enuresis associated with sodium valproate. *Lancet* 1985; **i:** 980–1.
2. Choonara IA. Sodium valproate and enuresis. *Lancet* 1985; **i:** 1276.

## Treatment of Adverse Effects

The value of gastric decontamination following overdose is uncertain since valproic acid and its salts are rapidly absorbed. Activated charcoal may be tried if the patient presents within 1 hour of a potentially life-threatening overdose; alternatively gastric lavage may be considered in similar circumstances. Supportive therapy alone may then suffice although haemodialysis should be considered in very severe poisoning.

◊ Although a variety of active treatments including forced diuresis, naloxone, and haemodialysis or haemoperfusion have been advocated for valproate overdose, supportive measures provided sufficient treatment for a patient who had taken 25 g of sodium valproate.[1] For a further review of the features and management of poisoning with some antiepileptics, including valproate, see under Phenytoin, p.371.

1. Lakhani M, McMurdo MET. Survival after severe self poisoning with sodium valproate. *Postgrad Med J* 1986; **62:** 409–10.

## Precautions

Valproate is contra-indicated in patients with pre-existing liver disease or a family history of severe hepatic dysfunction. Children under 3 years of age and those with congenital metabolic or degenerative disorders, organic brain disease, or severe seizure disorders associated with mental retardation may be at particular risk of hepatotoxicity and the drug should be used with particular caution in these groups. Combination with other antiepileptics, which may also increase the risks of liver damage, should be avoided if possible. Liver function tests should be carried out, particularly in those most at risk, before and during the first 6 months of therapy. Raised liver enzymes are not uncommon during treatment and are usually transient or respond to reduction in dosage, but patients should be reassessed clinically and liver function, including prothrombin time, monitored until they return to normal. An abnormally prolonged prothrombin time, particularly in association with other relevant abnormalities, requires discontinuation of treatment. Any concomitant use of salicylates should also be stopped. Treatment should also be discontinued if pancreatitis is diagnosed.

Patients or their carers should be told how to recognise signs of blood and liver toxicity or pancreatitis, and they should be advised to seek immediate medical attention if symptoms develop.

Patients should be monitored for potential bleeding complications before major elective surgery; some manufacturers suggest regular monitoring before and during therapy.

Valproate should be used with caution if systemic lupus erythematosus is suspected.

Patients should be warned of the risk of weight gain and appropriate strategies adopted to minimise the effect.

Care is required when withdrawing valproate therapy—see also under Uses and Administration, below.

It should be noted that the protein binding of valproate is saturable and thus shows concentration dependency with significant increases in free drug occurring at high total plasma concentrations.

Because valproate is partly excreted in the form of ketone bodies, it may cause false positives in urine tests for diabetes mellitus.

Dosage adjustments may be necessary in severe renal impairment in accordance with free serum valproate levels.

**Breast feeding.** Thrombocytopenic purpura and anaemia occurred in a breast-fed infant whose mother was being treated with valproic acid.[1] The baby recovered when breast feeding was stopped. Low serum-valproate levels were detected[2] in 6 breast-fed infants whose mothers had been taking valproate semisodium post partum; no adverse effects were observed in the infants. Similar results have previously been obtained for patients taking sodium valproate[3] or valproic acid.[4] The American Academy of Pediatrics considers[5] that valproate is, therefore, usually compatible with breast feeding.

For further comment on antiepileptic therapy and breast feeding, see p.351.

1. Stahl MMS, *et al.* Thrombocytopenic purpura and anemia in a breast-fed infant whose mother was treated with valproic acid. *J Pediatr* 1997; **130:** 1001–3.
2. Piontek CM, *et al.* Serum valproate levels in 6 breastfeeding mother-infant pairs. *J Clin Psychiatry* 2000; **61:** 170–2.
3. Alexander FW. Sodium valproate and pregnancy. *Arch Dis Child* 1979; **54:** 240.
4. von Unruh GE, *et al.* Valproic acid in breast milk: how much is really there? *Ther Drug Monit* 1984; **6:** 272–6.
5. American Academy of Pediatrics. The transfer of drugs and other chemicals into human milk. *Pediatrics* 2001; **108:** 776–89. Correction. *ibid.*; 1029. Also available at: http://aappolicy.aappublications.org/cgi/content/full/pediatrics%3b108/3/776 (accessed 14/05/04)

**Driving.** For a comment on antiepileptic drugs and driving, see p.351.

**HIV infection and AIDS.** The use of valproic acid in HIV-positive patients has been reviewed.[1] Limited data from several small *in-vitro* studies have demonstrated that valproic acid may induce viral replication of HIV; some clinicians have therefore suggested increased monitoring of viral load in HIV-positive patients treated with valproic acid.

1. Jennings HR, Romanelli F. The use of valproic acid in HIV-positive patients. *Ann Pharmacother* 1999; **33:** 1113–16.

**Porphyria.** Valproate is considered to be unsafe in patients with porphyria because it has been shown to be porphyrinogenic in *animals* or *in-vitro* systems. There is conflicting evidence of the porphyrinogenicity of valpromide, although it has also been shown to be porphyrinogenic in *in-vitro* systems.

For comments on the use of valproate in porphyria, see p.353.

**Pregnancy.** For comments on the management of epilepsy during pregnancy see p.351.

There is an increased risk of neural tube defects in infants exposed *in utero* to antiepileptics including valproate and a variety of syndromes such as craniofacial and digital abnormalities and, less commonly, cleft lip and palate have been described. In an unselected series[1] of 17 infants whose epileptic mothers had received valproate during pregnancy, 9 had minor abnormalities and of these 5 also had major abnormalities, including congenital heart defect in 4. Neonatal bleeding, attributed to fibrinogen depletion and sometimes fatal, has been reported following exposure *in utero* to valproate.[2,3] Hypoglycaemia was recorded[4] in 13 of 22 neonates whose mothers had taken valproate during pregnancy. Valproate-withdrawal symptoms, including irritability, jitteriness, hypertonia, seizures, and feeding problems were also noted.

1. Thisted E, Ebbesen F. Malformations, withdrawal manifestations, and hypoglycaemia after exposure to valproate in utero. *Arch Dis Child* 1993; **69:** 288–91.
2. Majer RV, Green PJ. Neonatal afibrinogenaemia due to sodium valproate. *Lancet* 1987; **ii:** 740–1.
3. Bavoux F, *et al.* Neonatal fibrinogen depletion caused by sodium valproate. *Ann Pharmacother* 1994; **28:** 1307.
4. Ebbesen F, *et al.* Neonatal hypoglycaemia and withdrawal symptoms after exposure in utero to valproate. *Arch Dis Child Fetal Neonatal Ed* 2000; **83:** F124–F129.

## Interactions

There are complex interactions between antiepileptics and toxicity may be enhanced without a corresponding increase in antiepileptic activity. Such interactions are very variable and unpredictable and plasma monitoring is often advisable with combination therapy. Caution is recommended when giving valproate with other drugs liable to interfere with blood coagulation, such as aspirin or warfarin. Use with other hepatotoxic drugs should be avoided. Use of highly protein bound drugs with valproate may increase free valproate plasma concentrations.

◊ General references.

1. Levy RH, Koch KM. Drug interactions with valproic acid. *Drugs* 1982; **24:** 543–56.

**Analgesics.** The valproic acid free fraction was reported to be increased, as was the half-life, when *aspirin* was given in a study in 6 epileptic children;[1] this suggests that salicylates may inhibit the metabolism of valproate in addition to displacing it from protein binding sites. Furthermore, salicylates have been associated with an increased risk of Reye's syndrome (p.16) in children, and combination with another hepatotoxic drug such as valproate is clearly undesirable. In addition, both aspirin and valproate affect blood coagulation and platelet function.

*Naproxen* has also been reported to produce a slight displacement of protein-bound valproic acid but the effect is probably not sufficiently marked for it to have a clinical effect.[2]

1. Orr JM, *et al.* Interaction between valproic acid and aspirin in epileptic children: serum protein binding and metabolic effects. *Clin Pharmacol Ther* 1982; **31:** 642–9.
2. Grimaldi R, *et al.* In vivo plasma protein binding interaction between valproic acid and naproxen. *Eur J Drug Metab Pharmacokinet* 1984; **9:** 359–63.

**Antibacterials.** Raised valproate blood concentrations and symptoms consistent with valproate toxicity have been reported in a patient also given *erythromycin*.[1]

There is a theoretical possibility that carnitine deficiency may be increased in patients receiving *pivampicillin* and valproate. Hyperammonaemic encephalopathy developed in a 72-year-old woman who had been taking valproate for 10 months when she was given *pivmecillinam* for a urinary-tract infection. It was suggested that valproate's propensity to produce hyperammonaemia had been exacerbated by a secondary hyperammonaemia induced by both drugs reducing carnitine concentrations.[2]

Decreases in plasma concentrations of valproic acid to subtherapeutic levels have been noted in 2 patients during therapy with *meropenem* and amikacin.[3] Meropenem was regarded as the likely cause of the interaction with valproic acid. Marked reductions in valproate concentrations have also been reported in 3 children given *panipenem* (with betamipron).[4]

Increased serum-valproate concentrations resulting in signs of valproate toxicity occurred in a child after beginning therapy with *isoniazid*;[5] the child was a slow acetylator of isoniazid and valproate dosage had to be reduced by about 60% to maintain satisfactory concentrations. When isoniazid was subsequently stopped, valproate dosage had to be increased to its previous value in order to maintain a therapeutic effect.

1. Redington K, *et al.* Erythromycin and valproate interaction. *Ann Intern Med* 1992; **116:** 877–8.
2. Lokrantz C-M, *et al.* Hyperammonemic encephalopathy induced by a combination of valproate and pivmecillinam. *Acta Neurol Scand* 2004; **109:** 297–301.
3. De Turck BJG, *et al.* Lowering of plasma valproic acid concentrations during concomitant therapy with meropenem and amikacin. *J Antimicrob Chemother* 1998; **42:** 563–4.
4. Nagai K, *et al.* Decrease in serum levels of valproic acid during treatment with a new carbapenem, panipenem/betamipron. *J Antimicrob Chemother* 1997; **39:** 295–6.
5. Jonville AP, *et al.* Interaction between isoniazid and valproate: a case of valproate overdosage. *Eur J Clin Pharmacol* 1991; **40:** 197–8.

**Antidepressants.** As with all antiepileptics, antidepressants may antagonise the antiepileptic activity of valproate by lowering the convulsive threshold. For the effect of valproate on *amitriptyline*, see p.284.

**Antiepileptics.** The barbiturate antiepileptic *phenobarbital* is reported to decrease serum-valproate concentrations when given concomitantly,[1] apparently by induction of valproate metabolism.[2] This effect is overshadowed, however, by the marked increase in serum-phenobarbital concentrations caused by valproate inhibition of phenobarbital metabolism—see p.368.

*Carbamazepine* and *phenytoin* are also enzyme-inducing drugs and, as might be expected, are reported to increase the metabolism and decrease the serum concentration of valproate.[3-5] The effect may be clinically significant.[6] The reciprocal effects of valproate on both drugs are complex, with conflicting effects on metabolism and protein binding, and the clinical outcome is difficult to predict. For more details see under Carbamazepine, p.356 and Phenytoin, p.373.

Raised serum concentrations of valproic acid have been reported in patients given *felbamate.*[7]

Valproate inhibits the metabolism of *lamotrigine* which may result in serious toxic reactions—see p.364. There is limited evidence that valproic acid may inhibit the metabolism of *ethosuximide* in some patients—see p.360. Valproate reduces the half-life of *zonisamide*—see p.385.

For interactions with benzodiazepines, see under Diazepam, p.693.

1. Perucca E. Pharmacokinetic interactions with antiepileptic drugs. *Clin Pharmacokinet* 1982; **7:** 57–84.
2. Levy RH, Koch KM. Drug interactions with valproic acid. *Drugs* 1982; **24:** 543–56.
3. Panesar SK, *et al.* The effect of carbamazepine on valproic acid disposition in adult volunteers. *Br J Clin Pharmacol* 1989; **27:** 323–8.
4. Reunanen MI, *et al.* Low serum valproic acid concentrations in epileptic patients on combination therapy. *Curr Ther Res* 1980; **28:** 456–62.
5. Cramer JA, *et al.* Variable free and total valproic acid concentrations in sole- and multi-drug therapy. *Ther Drug Monit* 1986; **8:** 411–15.
6. Jann MW, *et al.* Increased valproate serum concentrations upon carbamazepine cessation. *Epilepsia* 1988; **29:** 578–81.
7. Wagner ML, *et al.* The effect of felbamate on valproic acid disposition. *Clin Pharmacol Ther* 1994; **56:** 494–502.

**Antimalarials.** Low serum concentrations of valproate have been reported[1] in patients taking *mefloquine.* Also, mefloquine and *chloroquine* may antagonise the antiepileptic activity of valproate by lowering the convulsive threshold.

1. Anonymous. Mefloquine for malaria. *Med Lett Drugs Ther* 1990; **32:** 13–14.

**Antineoplastics.** A marked reduction in serum-valproate concentration occurred in a 6-year-old child following a high-dose 24-hour infusion of *methotrexate.*[1]

1. Schrøder H, Østergaard JR. Interference of high-dose methotrexate in the metabolism of valproate? *Pediatr Hematol Oncol* 1994; **11:** 445–9.

**Antipsychotics.** As with all antiepileptics, antipsychotics may antagonise the antiepileptic activity of valproate by lowering the convulsive threshold. For the effect of valproate on *clozapine,* see p.688.

**Antivirals.** For the effect of valproate on *zidovudine,* see p.659.

**Benzodiazepines.** For interactions between valproate and benzodiazepines, see under Diazepam, p.693.

**Calcium-channel blockers.** For the effect of sodium valproate on *nimodipine,* see under Nifedipine, p.969.

**Colestyramine.** Colestyramine may decrease the absorption of valproate.

**Gastrointestinal drugs.** Administration with an *antacid* (aluminium and magnesium hydroxides) has been shown to increase significantly the bioavailability of a valproic acid preparation in healthy subjects;[1] other antacids in this study (calcium carbonate and an aluminium magnesium trisilicate mixture) had a lesser, insignificant effect.

*Cimetidine* significantly increased the half-life and decreased the clearance of sodium valproate in another study;[2] *ranitidine* had no effect on valproate pharmacokinetics.[2]

These interactions have not been reported to be of clinical significance, although the possibility must exist, particularly in patients on high-dose therapy.

1. May CA, *et al.* Effects of three antacids on the bioavailability of valproic acid. *Clin Pharm* 1982; **1:** 244–7.
2. Webster LK, *et al.* Effect of cimetidine and ranitidine on carbamazepine and sodium valproate pharmacokinetics. *Eur J Clin Pharmacol* 1984; **27:** 341–3.

## Pharmacokinetics

Valproic acid and its salts are rapidly and completely absorbed from the gastrointestinal tract; the rate, but not the extent, of absorption is delayed by administration with or after food.

Valproic acid is extensively metabolised in the liver, a large part by glucuronidation and the rest by a variety of complex pathways. It does not appear to enhance its own metabolism, but metabolism may be enhanced by other drugs which induce hepatic microsomal enzymes. It is excreted in the urine almost entirely in the form of its metabolites; small amounts are excreted in faeces and expired air.

Valproic acid is extensively bound to plasma protein. The extent of protein binding is concentration dependent and is stated to be about 90 to 95% at total concentrations of 50 micrograms/mL, falling to about 80 to 85% at 100 micrograms/mL. Reported half-lives for valproic acid have ranged from about 5 to 20 hours; the shorter half-lives have generally been recorded in epileptic patients receiving multiple drug therapy.

The 'target' range of total plasma-valproic acid is usually quoted as being 40 to 100 micrograms/mL (280 to 700 micromoles/litre) but routine monitoring of plasma concentrations is not generally considered to be of use as an aid to assessing control.

Valproic acid crosses the placental barrier and small amounts are distributed into breast milk.

Valpromide is an amide derivative of valproic acid and its absorption is slower and its bioavailability somewhat less than that of valproic acid. Valpromide is rapidly and almost completely metabolised in the liver to valproic acid.

The pharmacokinetics of valproate are affected other antiepileptics (see under Interactions, above).

◊ References.

1. Zaccara G, *et al.* Clinical pharmacokinetics of valproic acid—1988. *Clin Pharmacokinet* 1988; **15:** 367–89.
2. Bialer M. Clinical pharmacology of valpromide. *Clin Pharmacokinet* 1991; **20:** 114–22.
3. Cloyd JC, *et al.* Valproic acid pharmacokinetics in children IV: effects of age and antiepileptic drugs on protein binding and intrinsic clearance. *Clin Pharmacol Ther* 1993; **53:** 22–9.
4. Yukawa E, *et al.* Population-based investigation of valproic acid relative clearance using nonlinear mixed effects modeling: influence of drug-drug interaction and patient characteristics. *J Clin Pharmacol* 1997; **37:** 1160–7.

## Uses and Administration

Valproate is an antiepileptic used particularly in the treatment of primary generalised seizures, and notably absence and myoclonic seizures, and also for partial seizures. Its actions are complex and its mode of action in epilepsy is not fully understood. Valproate is also used to treat the acute manic phase of bipolar disorder and for the prophylaxis of migraine.

It can be given in a variety of forms including the sodium salts (valproate semisodium and sodium valproate), the amide derivative (valpromide), or as valproic acid. Magnesium valproate has also been tried as has calcium valproate. Valproate should preferably be taken with or after food.

In the treatment of **epilepsy** the dose should be adjusted to the needs of the individual patient to achieve adequate control of seizures. Plasma concentrations of valproate (see Pharmacokinetics, above) are not considered to be a useful index of efficacy and thus their routine monitoring is generally not helpful. A suggested initial oral dose of *sodium valproate* for *adults* is 600 mg daily in 2 divided doses. This may be increased by 200 mg every 3 days to a usual range of 1 to 2 g daily (20 to 30 mg/kg daily); up to a maximum of 2.5 g daily may be necessary if adequate control has not been achieved.

A suggested initial oral dose of sodium valproate for *children* weighing more than 20 kg is 400 mg daily (irrespective of weight) in 2 divided doses, gradually increased until control is achieved, with a usual range of 20 to 30 mg/kg daily; further increases to a maximum of 35 mg/kg daily may be necessary if adequate control has not been achieved. Children weighing less than 20 kg may be given 20 mg/kg daily in 2 divided doses, which may be increased to 40 mg/kg daily in severe cases, but only if it is possible to monitor the patient's plasma-valproate concentrations; it has been recommended that if the dose exceeds 40 mg/kg daily, the patient's clinical chemistry and haematological parameters should also be monitored.

When oral administration is not possible, sodium valproate may be given *intravenously* to initiate therapy or to continue therapy previously given orally. A suggested dose to *initiate* therapy in *adults* is up to 10 mg/kg by intravenous injection over 3 to 5 minutes followed by intravenous infusion, as necessary, up to a maximum of 2.5 g daily. The usual intravenous dose for *children* is in the range of 20 to 30 mg/kg daily. If doses in excess of this are required, plasma-valproate concentrations must be monitored, and if the dose exceeds 40 mg/kg daily, clinical chemistry and haematological parameters should also be monitored. To *continue* therapy intravenously doses are the same as the patient's previous oral dose. In the USA, intravenous sodium valproate is given in doses equivalent to those used for valproic acid by mouth (see below).

A suggested initial oral dose of *valproic acid* in *adults and children* is 15 mg/kg daily increased at one-week intervals by 5 to 10 mg/kg. The maximum recommended dose of valproic acid in the UK is 30 mg/kg daily whereas in the USA it is 60 mg/kg daily. Valproic acid may be given in 2 to 4 divided doses.

*Valproate semisodium* is given by mouth in doses equivalent to those used for valproic acid by mouth (see above).

The amide derivative of valproic acid, *valpromide,* is also used in some countries. Usual doses have ranged from 600 mg to 1.8 g by mouth daily, in divided doses.

As with other antiepileptics, withdrawal of valproate or transition to or from another type of antiepileptic therapy should be made gradually to avoid precipitating an increase in the frequency of seizures. For a discussion on whether or not to withdraw antiepileptic therapy in seizure-free patients, see p.349.

In the treatment of acute manic episodes of **bipolar disorder,** valproate semisodium is given by mouth in an initial dose equivalent to valproic acid 750 mg daily in divided doses. Thereafter, the dose is increased as rapidly as possible to achieve the optimal response, up to a maximum of 60 mg/kg daily. Patients receiving doses higher than 45 mg/kg daily should be carefully monitored.

In the prophylaxis of **migraine** valproate semisodium is given by mouth in a dose equivalent to valproic acid 250 mg twice daily; up to 1 g daily may be necessary in some patients.

**Bipolar disorder.** Valproate, usually as valproate semisodium, is increasingly being used as an alternative to lithium in patients with bipolar disorder (p.278).[1-10] Some consider it to be particularly effective in those who have rapid cycling disease with 4 or more affective episodes a year and in those with mixed or dysphoric states. However, a recent systematic review[11] considered that any shift in prescribing practice in favour of valproate was not based on reliable evidence of efficacy.

1. Pope HG, *et al.* Valproate in the treatment of acute mania: a placebo-controlled study. *Arch Gen Psychiatry* 1991; **48:** 62–8.
2. Keck PE, *et al.* Valproate oral loading in the treatment of acute mania. *J Clin Psychiatry* 1993; **54:** 305–8.
3. Joffe RT. Valproate in bipolar disorder: the Canadian perspective. *Can J Psychiatry* 1993; **38** (suppl 2): S46–S50.
4. Schaff MR, *et al.* Divalproex sodium in the treatment of refractory affective disorders. *J Clin Psychiatry* 1993; **54:** 380–4.
5. Nurnberg HG, *et al.* Response to anticonvulsant substitution among refractory bipolar manic patients. *J Clin Psychopharmacol* 1994; **14:** 207–9.
6. Anonymous. Valproate for bipolar disorder. *Med Lett Drugs Ther* 1994; **36:** 74–5.
7. Bowden CL, *et al.* Efficacy of divalproex vs lithium and placebo in the treatment of mania. *JAMA* 1994; **271:** 918–24. Correction. *ibid.*; 1830.
8. Stoll AL, *et al.* Neurologic factors predict a favorable valproate response in bipolar and schizoaffective disorders. *J Clin Psychopharmacol* 1994; **14:** 311–13.
9. Swann AC, *et al.* Depression during mania: treatment response to lithium or divalproex. *Arch Gen Psychiatry* 1997; **54:** 37–42.
10. Müller-Oerlinghausen B, *et al.* Valproate as adjunct to neuroleptic medication for the treatment of acute episodes of mania: a prospective, randomized, double-blind, placebo-controlled, multicenter study. *J Clin Psychopharmacol* 2000; **20:** 195–203.
11. Macritchie KAN, *et al.* Valproic acid, valproate and divalproex in the maintenance treatment of bipolar disorder. Available in The Cochrane Library; Issue 2. Chichester: John Wiley; 2004.

**Cushing's syndrome.** Sodium valproate has been used in the management of Cushing's syndrome (p.1313).

**Depression.** Valproate has been added as a mood stabiliser for augmentation of antidepressant therapy in the treatment of resistant depression (p.279).

**Epilepsy.** Valproate is one of the drugs of choice in primary generalised tonic-clonic seizures, absence seizures, and myoclonic seizures (see p.349), although evidence for some of these is lacking. It is also the drug of choice in epileptic syndromes such as the Lennox-Gastaut syndrome because of its wide therapeutic spectrum, and it may be useful in infantile spasms. It is often used in partial seizures and controlled trials have suggested similar efficacy to the first-line drugs carbamazepine and phenytoin.

References.

1. Mattson RH, *et al.* A comparison of valproate with carbamazepine for the treatment of complex partial seizures and secondarily generalized tonic-clonic seizures in adults. *N Engl J Med* 1992; **327:** 765–71.
2. Richens A, *et al.* A multicentre trial of sodium valproate and carbamazepine in adult onset epilepsy. *J Neurol Neurosurg Psychiatry* 1994; **57:** 682–7.
3. Verity CM, *et al.* A multicentre comparative trial of sodium valproate and carbamazepine in paediatric epilepsy. *Dev Med Child Neurol* 1995; **37:** 97–108.
4. Beydoun A, *et al.* and the Depakote Monotherapy for Partial Seizures Study Group. Safety and efficacy of divalproex sodium monotherapy in partial epilepsy: a double-blind, concentration-response design clinical trial. *Neurology* 1997; **48:** 182–8.
5. Brodie MJ, Mumford JP. Double-blind substitution of vigabatrin and valproate in carbamazepine-resistant partial epilepsy. *Epilepsy Res* 1999; **34:** 199–205.

**Extrapyramidal disorders.** Valproate is one of several drugs with GABAergic action that has been tried with encouraging results in the management of tardive dyskinesia (see under Extrapyramidal Disorders on p.677).

**Febrile convulsions.** Sodium valproate has been used prophylactically in children thought to be at risk of recurrence of febrile convulsions (p.353), but routine use of antiepileptics is no longer recommended.

References.


1. Newton RW. Randomised controlled trials of phenobarbitone and valproate in febrile convulsions. *Arch Dis Child* 1988; **63:** 1189–91.


**Headache.** Valproate, as valproate semisodium, may be used for the prophylaxis of *migraine* (p.464) in patients refractory to drugs such as propranolol or pizotifen; success has been demonstrated in several studies.[1-6] It has also been tried for prevention of *cluster headache* (p.464). Valproate has also been shown to be effective and well-tolerated for the prophylaxis of migraine in children aged between 7 and 16 years.[7] Preliminary data from open-label studies suggest that intravenous valproate is effective and well-tolerated in the treatment of acute migraine attacks.[8,9] However, a double-blind study found it to be less effective than prochlorperazine.[10]

Valproate has also been tried in the prophylaxis of persistent chronic daily headache including *tension-type headache* (p.465) unresponsive to other drugs.[11]


1. Sørensen KV. Valproate: a new drug in migraine prophylaxis. *Acta Neurol Scand* 1988; **78:** 346–8.
2. Hering R, Kuritzky A. Sodium valproate in the prophylactic treatment of migraine: a double-blind study versus placebo. *Cephalalgia* 1992; **12:** 81–4.
3. Coria F, *et al.* Low-dose sodium valproate in the prophylaxis of migraine. *Clin Neuropharmacol* 1994; **17:** 569–73.
4. Mathew NT, *et al.* Migraine prophylaxis with divalproex. *Arch Neurol* 1995; **52:** 281–6.
5. Kaniecki RG. A comparison of divalproex with propranolol and placebo for the prophylaxis of migraine without aura. *Arch Neurol* 1997; **54:** 1141–5.
6. Erdemoglu AK, Ozbakir S. Valproic acid in prophylaxis of refractory migraine. *Acta Neurol Scand* 2000; **102:** 354–8.
7. Caruso JM, *et al.* The efficacy of divalproex sodium in the prophylactic treatment of children with migraine. *Headache* 2000; **40:** 672–6.
8. Mathew NT, *et al.* Intravenous valproate sodium (Depacon) aborts migraine rapidly: a preliminary report. *Headache* 2000; **40:** 720–3.
9. Stillman MJ, *et al.* Treatment of primary headache disorders with intravenous valproate: initial outpatient experience. *Headache* 2004; **44:** 65–9.
10. Tanen DA, *et al.* Intravenous sodium valproate versus prochlorperazine for the emergency department treatment of acute migraine headaches: a prospective, randomized, double-blind trial. *Ann Emerg Med* 2003; **41:** 847–53.
11. Mathew NT, Ali S. Valproate in the treatment of persistent chronic daily headache: an open label study. *Headache* 1991; **31:** 71–4.


**Hiccup.** Valproic acid may be of value in the treatment of intractable hiccups,[1] especially those of neurogenic origin. A protocol for the management of intractable hiccups may be found under Chlorpromazine, p.682.


1. Jacobson PL, *et al.* Treatment of intractable hiccups with valproic acid. *Neurology* 1981; **31:** 1458–60.


**Migraine.** See under Headache, above.

**Muscle spasm.** The mainstay of management of *spasticity* is physiotherapy and an antispastic drug (see p.1386). Valproate has been tried for its GABAergic activity and case reports[1] of 4 patients with spastic conditions of various aetiologies indicated that the addition of valproate to the existing regimen of antispastic drugs might produce improvements in spasticity and pain; further studies are warranted.

Valproate has also been tried[2] in the management of *stiff-man syndrome* (see under Muscle Spasm, p.696) unresponsive to diazepam.


1. Zachariah SB, *et al.* Positive response to oral divalproex sodium (Depakote) in patients with spasticity and pain. *Am J Med Sci* 1994; **308:** 38–40.
2. Spehlmann R, *et al.* Improvement of stiff-man syndrome with sodium valproate. *Neurology* 1981; **31:** 1162–3.


**Myoclonus.** Valproate is used alone or in combination with clonazepam for cortical myoclonus (see p.353).

**Psychiatric disorders.** Valproate has psychotropic properties and has been used in the management of depression and bipolar disorder (see above). Valproate has also been tried in various disorders for the control of symptoms such as agitation, aggression, and rage[1,2] (see Disturbed Behaviour, p.665). It has also been reported[3,4] to be efficacious as adjunctive therapy to antipsychotics. It has also been tried in anxiety disorders such as panic attacks[5-7] (p.663), and post-traumatic stress disorder[8,9] (p.664).


1. Geracioti TD. Valproic acid treatment of episodic explosiveness related to brain injury. *J Clin Psychiatry* 1994; **55:** 416–17.
2. Narayan M, *et al.* Treatment of dementia with behavioral disturbances using divalproex or a combination of divalproex and a neuroleptic. *J Clin Psychiatry* 1997; **58:** 351–4.
3. Wassef AA, *et al.* Randomized, placebo-controlled pilot study of divalproex sodium in the treatment of acute exacerbations of chronic schizophrenia. *J Clin Psychopharmacol* 2000; **20:** 357–61.
4. Grove VE, *et al.* Improvement of Huntington's disease with olanzapine and valproate. *N Engl J Med* 2000; **343:** 973–4.
5. Primeau F, *et al.* Valproic acid and panic disorder. *Can J Psychiatry* 1990; **35:** 248–50.
6. Keck PE, *et al.* Valproate treatment of panic disorder and lactate-induced panic attacks. *Biol Psychiatry* 1993; **33:** 542–6.
7. Woodman CL, Noyes R. Panic disorder: treatment with valproate. *J Clin Psychiatry* 1994; **55:** 134–6.
8. Fesler FA. Valproate in combat-related posttraumatic stress disorder. *J Clin Psychiatry* 1991; **52:** 361–4.
9. Petty F, *et al.* Valproate therapy for chronic, combat-induced posttraumatic stress disorder. *J Clin Psychopharmacol* 2002; **22:** 100–101.


**Status epilepticus.** Valproate has been used in *absence* status epilepticus once the initial attack has been brought under control with intravenous benzodiazepines[1] and has been considered to be the drug of choice to prevent its recurrence.[2] It is not usually given in the management of *convulsive* status epilepticus (p.352) but it has been tried as an alternative to phenytoin derivatives or phenobarbital. In a small study it was effective in controlling status epilepticus associated with generalised tonic-clonic and myoclonic seizures.[3] Intravenous valproate decreased clinical seizures in 2 children with refractory generalised convulsive and 1 with nonconvulsive status epilepticus, although one of the former continued to exhibit electrical activity consistent with seizures.[4]


1. Bauer J, Elger CE. Management of status epilepticus in adults. *CNS Drugs* 1994; **1:** 26–44.
2. Berkovic SF, *et al.* Valproate prevents the recurrence of absence status. *Neurology* 1989; **39:** 1294–7.
3. Giroud M, *et al.* Use of injectable valproic acid in status epilepticus: a pilot study. *Drug Invest* 1993; **5:** 154–9.
4. Hovinga CA, *et al.* Use of intravenous valproate in three pediatric patients with nonconvulsive or convulsive status epilepticus. *Ann Pharmacother* 1999; **33:** 579–84.


**Trigeminal neuralgia.** Although carbamazepine is the drug of choice in the treatment of trigeminal neuralgia (p.8), sodium valproate is an alternative antiepileptic that may be used in carbamazepine-intolerant patients.

## Preparations

***BP 2003:*** Sodium Valproate Enteric-coated Tablets; Sodium Valproate Oral Solution; Sodium Valproate Tablets;
***USP 27:*** Divalproex Sodium Delayed-Release Tablets; Valproic Acid Capsules; Valproic Acid Syrup.

**Proprietary Preparations** (details are given in Part 3)
***Arg.:*** Depakene; Exibral; Logical; Tekaval; Valcote; Valnar; ***Austral.:*** Epilim; Valpro; ***Austria:*** Convulex; Depakine; Depakine Chrono; Leptilanil; ***Belg.:*** Convulex; Depakine; ***Braz.:*** Depakene; Depakote; Epilenil; Valpakine; Valprene; ***Canad.:*** Depakene; Deproic†; Epiject; Epival; ***Chile:*** Atemperator; Depakene; Leptilan; Neuractin; Valcote; ***Denm.:*** Deleptsine; Deprakine; Leptilan†; Orfiril; ***Fin.:*** Absenor; Deprakine; Deprakine Depot; Orfiril; ***Fr.:*** Depakine; Depakine Chrono; Depakote; Depamide; ***Ger.:*** Convulex; Convulsofin; Ergenyl; Ergenyl Chrono; Espa-Valept; Leptilan; Mylproin†; Orfiril; Valpro; Valpro Beta; Valprodura; Valproflux; Valprolept; ValproNa; ***Gr.:*** Depakine; Depakine Chrono; ***Hong Kong:*** Epilim; Orfiril†; Valpro; ***India:*** Epilex; Valparin; ***Irl.:*** Epilim; Epilim Chrono; ***Israel:*** Depalept; Depalept Chrono; Orfiril; Valporal; ***Ital.:*** Depakin; Depakin Chrono; Depamag; Depamide; ***Jpn:*** Depakene; ***Malaysia:*** Epilim; Orfiril; ***Mex.:*** Atemperator; Criam; Cryoval†; Depakene; Epival; Leptilan; Pimiken; Proteval†; Provetal†; Valcaps†; Valken†; Valprosid; ***Neth.:*** Convulex; Depakine; Depakine Chrono; ***Norw.:*** Deprakine; Orfiril; ***NZ:*** Epilim; ***Port.:*** Depakine; Depakine Chrono; Diplexil; Diplexil-R; ***S.Afr.:*** Convulex; Epilim; ***Singapore:*** Convulex; Encorate†; Epilim; Orfiril; ***Spain:*** Depakine; Depakine Crono; Depamide; ***Swed.:*** Absenor; Ergenyl; Orfiril; ***Switz.:*** Convulex; Depakine; Depakine Chrono; Orfiril; ***Thai.:*** Depakine; Valparin; ***UAE:*** Valopin; ***UK:*** Convulex; Depakote; Epilim; Epilim Chrono; Orlept; ***USA:*** Depacon; Depakene; Depakote.

---

# Vigabatrin *(BAN, USAN, rINN)*

4-Amino-5-hexenoic Acid; MDL-71754; RMI-71754; Vigabatrina; γ-Vinyl Aminobutyric Acid; γ-Vinyl-GABA. 4-Aminohex-5-enoic acid.

$C_6H_{11}NO_2$ = 129.2.

*CAS — 60643-86-9.*

*ATC — N03AG04.*

**Pharmacopoeias.** In *Br.*

**BP 2003** (Vigabatrin). A white to almost white powder. Very soluble in water.

## Adverse Effects, Treatment, and Precautions

About half of all patients experience adverse effects with vigabatrin. The most common are drowsiness and fatigue, although in children excitation and agitation occur more frequently. Other CNS-related adverse effects include dizziness, nervousness, irritability, headache, nystagmus, ataxia, paraesthesia, tremor, and impaired concentration. Less commonly, confusion and memory disturbances have been reported. Other reported adverse effects include weight gain, gastrointestinal disturbances, oedema, alopecia, angioedema, urticaria, and skin rash. Haemoglobin and liver enzyme values may be decreased. Rarely marked sedation, stupor and confusion, together with other symptoms suggestive of encephalopathy, have occurred.

About one-third of all patients receiving vigabatrin have developed irreversible visual field defects, ranging from mild to severe and usually occurring after months or years of therapy. Blurred vision, diplopia, or nystagmus are somewhat less common. Retinal disorders such as peripheral retinal atrophy, or very rarely optic neuritis or atrophy have also been reported (see also below). Visual field function should be assessed before beginning treatment and during routine follow-up (ideally at 6-month intervals), and patients should be warned to report any new visual symptoms that develop during therapy. Vigabatrin should not be used in patients with pre-existing visual field defects.

Psychiatric reactions such as agitation, aggression, depression, and paranoid reactions have occurred in patients with or without a psychiatric history; psychosis or mania have been reported rarely. Patients receiving vigabatrin should be observed carefully for any signs of adverse effects on neurological function. Caution is warranted in patients with a history of psychosis, depression, or behavioural problems.

Vigabatrin may exacerbate myoclonic or absence seizures.

Vigabatrin should be given with caution to the elderly and patients with renal impairment.

Care is required when withdrawing vigabatrin therapy—see also under Uses and Administration, below.

**Breast feeding.** The manufacturers state that breast feeding is not recommended in women receiving vigabatrin. For comment on antiepileptic therapy and breast feeding, see p.351.

**Driving.** For a comment on antiepileptic drugs and driving, see p.351.

Particular care should be taken in view of the possible effects of vigabatrin on visual acuity.

**Effects on bone.** For the effects of antiepileptics on bone and on calcium and vitamin D metabolism, see under Phenytoin, p.371.

**Effects on the eyes.** A report of 3 patients who developed bilateral severely constricted visual fields 2 to 3 years after vigabatrin was added to their antiepileptic regimens[1] prompted publication of similar anecdotal reports.[2-5] Peripheral retinal atrophy rather than optic nerve damage appeared to be the cause. Symptoms showed no improvement on discontinuation of the drug, although there was no further deterioration. At that time (1997) the manufacturers replied[6] stating that it was a rare occurrence (less than 0.1%) and was being monitored in further clinical trials. The UK Committee on Safety of Medicines (CSM) subsequently stated[7] (in March 1998) that it had received 41 reports of visual field defects since December 1989, which persisted in most cases despite discontinuation of treatment. The evidence suggested that the onset of symptoms varied from 1 month to several years after starting vigabatrin. In most cases, visual field defects have persisted despite discontinuation of vigabatrin.[8,9] Interim results of a Prescription Event Monitoring Study[10] in the UK stated that vigabatrin was considered to be probably or possibly associated with objective evidence of a visual field defect in 0.2% of patients. However, subsequent evidence appears to have confirmed that the incidence of visual field defects is much higher;[11-14] revised product literature issued by the manufacturers in late 1999 indicated that visual field defects occurred in about one-third of all patients receiving vigabatrin. Males were also noted to be at an increased risk of developing defects.[15]

Cases of visual field defects with vigabatrin continue to be published including those seen in children.[16,17]

The CSM now considers[14] that vigabatrin should only be prescribed by a specialist, and only where all other combination therapies have failed. Ophthalmological consultation and visual field assessment should be undertaken before starting vigabatrin and visual field screening repeated at 6-monthly intervals during treatment. Conventional perimetry is unsuitable in patients under 9 years of age, in whom alternative methods should be employed. Opinion amongst some paediatricians[18] was that the risk of developing visual field defects had to be weighed against the potential benefit of seizure control. In very young patients, in whom monitoring of vision was impossible, the benefits of vigabatrin in the treatment of infantile spasms were felt by some to outweigh this risk.[19]

Vigabatrin should not be used in patients with pre-existing visual field defects.[14,18]


1. Eke T, *et al.* Severe persistent visual field constriction associated with vigabatrin. *BMJ* 1997; **314:** 180–1.
2. Wilson EA, Brodie MJ. Severe persistent visual field constriction associated with vigabatrin. *BMJ* 1997; **314:** 1693.
3. Wong ICK, *et al.* Severe persistent visual field constriction associated with vigabatrin. *BMJ* 1997; **314:** 1693–4.
4. Blackwell N, *et al.* Severe persistent visual field constriction associated with vigabatrin. *BMJ* 1997; **314:** 1694.
5. Harding GFA. Severe persistent visual field constriction associated with vigabatrin. *BMJ* 1997; **314:** 1694.
6. Backstrom JT, *et al.* Severe persistent visual field constriction associated with vigabatrin. *BMJ* 1997; **314:** 1694–5.
7. Committee of Safety of Medicines/Medicines Control Agency. Vigabatrin (Sabril) and visual field defects. *Current Problems* 1998; **24:** 1. Also available at: http://www.mca.gov.uk/ourwork/monitorsafequalmed/currentproblems/volume24a.htm (accessed 14/05/04)
8. Hardus P, *et al.* Long term changes in the visual fields of patients with temporal lobe epilepsy using vigabatrin. *Br J Ophthalmol* 2000; **84:** 788–90.

9. Johnson MA, *et al.* Visual function loss from vigabatrin: effect of stopping the drug. *Neurology* 2000; **55:** 40–5.
10. Wilton LV, *et al.* Interim report on the incidence of visual field defects in patients on long term vigabatrin therapy. *Pharmacoepidemiol Drug Safety* 1999; **8** (suppl): S9–S14.
11. Wilton LV, *et al.* Visual field defect associated with vigabatrin: observational cohort study. *BMJ* 1999; **319:** 1165–6.
12. Kälviäinen R, *et al.* Vigabatrin, a gabaergic antiepileptic drug, causes concentric visual defects. *Neurology* 1999; **53:** 922–6.
13. Lawden MC, *et al.* Visual field defects associated with vigabatrin therapy. *J Neurol Neurosurg Psychiatry* 1999; **67:** 716–22.
14. Committee on Safety of Medicines/Medicines Control Agency. Vigabatrin (Sabril): visual field defects. *Current Problems* 1999; **25:** 13. Also available at: http://www.mca.gov.uk/ourwork/monitorsafequalmed/currentproblems/volume25nov.htm (accessed 14/05/04)
15. Kälviäinen R, Nousiainen I. Visual field defects with vigabatrin: epidemiology and therapeutic implications. *CNS Drugs* 2001; **15:** 217–30.
16. Russell-Eggitt IM, *et al.* Vigabatrin-associated visual field defects in children. *Eye* 2000; **14:** 334–9.
17. Koul R, *et al.* Vigabatrin associated retinal dysfunction in children with epilepsy. *Arch Dis Child* 2001; **85:** 469–73.
18. Appleton RE. Guideline may help in prescribing vigabatrin. *BMJ* 1998; **317:** 1322.
19. Harding GFA. Severe persistent visual field constriction associated with vigabatrin. *BMJ* 1998; **316:** 232–3.

**Effects on the liver.** Vigabatrin has demonstrated *in-vivo* and *in-vitro* inhibition of plasma-alanine transaminase activity, which may mask signs of early underlying hepatic disease if only transaminase levels are evaluated.[1]

1. Richens A, *et al.* Evidence for both in vivo and in vitro interaction between vigabatrin and alanine transaminase. *Br J Clin Pharmacol* 1997; **43:** 163–8.

**Effects on mental function.** Behavioural disturbances ranging from irritability and confusion to psychotic reactions have been reported in patients receiving vigabatrin.[1-7] An analysis[8] of adverse effect reports from double-blind controlled studies found that the incidence of psychotic reactions was about 2.5% in vigabatrin treated patients; however, the most common psychiatric reaction was depression, which occurred in 8 to 12% of patients. Symptoms of psychiatric disturbance were often relatively mild. Psychiatric reactions are generally reversible when doses are reduced or gradually discontinued. In 2 patients[9,10] psychosis developed following sudden withdrawal of vigabatrin; mental state improved when the drug was reinstated. It is not clear whether patients with a history of previous psychiatric disturbances are at greater risk when given vigabatrin.[8,11] Also, using low doses of vigabatrin to start therapy did not reduce the incidence of disturbances.[11]

The problems of antiepileptic therapy adversely affecting cognition are discussed on p.351.

1. Sander JWAS, Hart YM. Vigabatrin and behaviour disturbances. *Lancet* 1990; **335:** 57.
2. Dam M. Vigabatrin and behaviour disturbances. *Lancet* 1990; **335:** 605.
3. Betts T, Thomas L. Vigabatrin and behaviour disturbances. *Lancet* 1990; **335:** 605–6.
4. Johnston SJ. Vigabatrin and behaviour disturbances. *Lancet* 1990; **335:** 606.
5. Robinson MK, *et al.* Vigabatrin and behaviour disturbances. *Lancet* 1990; **336:** 504.
6. Martínez AC, *et al.* Vigabatrin-associated reversible acute psychosis in a child. *Ann Pharmacother* 1995; **29:** 1115–17.
7. Naumann M, *et al.* Bipolar affective psychosis after vigabatrin. *Lancet* 1994; **343:** 606–7.
8. Levinson DF, Devinsky O. Psychiatric adverse events during vigabatrin therapy. *Neurology* 1999; **53:** 1503–11.
9. Ring HA, Reynolds EH. Vigabatrin and behaviour disturbance. *Lancet* 1990; **335:** 970.
10. Brodie MJ, McKee PJW. Vigabatrin and psychosis. *Lancet* 1990; **335:** 1279.
11. Wong ICK. Retrospective study of vigabatrin and psychiatric behavioural disturbances. *Epilepsy Res* 1995; **21:** 227–30.

**Effects on the nervous system.** Two patients developed disturbances of motor behaviour associated with the addition of vigabatrin to therapy for intractable seizures.[1]

Acute encephalopathy was reported[2] in two patients after starting vigabatrin in addition to carbamazepine; symptoms of stupor, dysphoria, and irritability were present in both and their EEG background activity was slowed. Clinical symptoms could not be related to intoxication with carbamazepine or its epoxide but it was not known whether an interaction between carbamazepine and vigabatrin had caused the acute encephalopathy. In a further report[3] vigabatrin was associated with the development of encephalopathy in 3 patients already receiving a variety of antiepileptic drugs other than carbamazepine; withdrawal of vigabatrin led to full recovery. The authors suggested that acute encephalopathy after vigabatrin may be related to a pre-existing cerebral abnormality. Other predisposing factors suggested by the manufacturers include higher than recommended initial doses, faster dose increases at greater increments than those recommended, and renal failure.

1. Jongsma MJ, *et al.* Reversible motor disturbances induced by vigabatrin. *Lancet* 1991; **338:** 893.
2. Sälke-Kellermann A, Baier H. Acute encephalopathy with vigabatrin. *Lancet* 1993; **342:** 185.
3. Sharief MK, *et al.* Acute encephalopathy with vigabatrin. *Lancet* 1993; **342:** 619.

**Interference with diagnostic tests.** Vigabatrin can cause changes in the urinary excretion of amino acids which could be potentially misleading in patients undergoing investigation for metabolic disorders.[1,2]

1. Bonham JR, *et al.* Pyroglutamicaciduria from vigabatrin. *Lancet* 1989; **i:** 1452–3.
2. Shih VE, Tenanbaum A. Aminoaciduria due to vinyl-gaba administration. *N Engl J Med* 1990; **323:** 1353.

**Overdosage.** For a review of the features and management of poisoning with some antiepileptics, including vigabatrin, see under Phenytoin, p.371.

**Porphyria.** For comment on the use of vigabatrin in porphyria, see p.353.

**Pregnancy.** For comments on the management of epilepsy in pregnancy, see p.351.

Little is known of the effects of newer antiepileptics such as vigabatrin on the fetus, although congenital anomalies have been reported in the offspring of some mothers using vigabatrin during pregnancy.

## Interactions

There are complex interactions between antiepileptics and toxicity may be enhanced without a corresponding increase in antiepileptic activity. Such interactions are very variable and unpredictable and plasma monitoring is often advisable with combination therapy.

**Antiepileptics.** For the effect of vigabatrin on plasma concentrations of other antiepileptics, see *Phenobarbital*, p.368; *Phenytoin*, p.373; and *Primidone*, p.377.

## Pharmacokinetics

Vigabatrin is well absorbed following oral doses of the racemate; the inactive *R*(−)-enantiomer is reported to be present at much higher plasma concentrations than the active *S*(+)-enantiomer, perhaps indicating a difference in bioavailability. About 60 to 80% of an oral dose is excreted in urine as unchanged drug. The elimination half-life is reported to be 5 to 8 hours. Vigabatrin is not significantly bound to plasma proteins.

There does not appear to be any correlation between plasma concentrations of vigabatrin and its efficacy or toxicity.

Vigabatrin is distributed into breast milk.

◊ References.

1. Rey E, *et al.* Vigabatrin: clinical pharmacokinetics. *Clin Pharmacokinet* 1992; **23:** 267–78.
2. Hoke JF, *et al.* Pharmacokinetics of vigabatrin following single and multiple oral doses in normal volunteers. *J Clin Pharmacol* 1993; **33:** 458–62.
3. Elwes RDC, Binnie CD. Clinical pharmacokinetics of newer antiepileptic drugs: lamotrigine, vigabatrin, gabapentin and oxcarbazepine. *Clin Pharmacokinet* 1996; **30:** 403–15.
4. Vauzelle-Kervroëdan F, *et al.* Pharmacokinetics of the individual enantiomers of vigabatrin in neonates with uncontrolled seizures. *Br J Clin Pharmacol* 1996; **42:** 779–81.
5. Jacqz-Aigrain E, *et al.* Pharmacokinetics of the S(+) and R(−) enantiomers of vigabatrin during chronic dosing in a patient with renal failure. *Br J Clin Pharmacol* 1997; **44:** 183–5.
6. Tran A, *et al.* Vigabatrin: placental transfer in vivo and excretion into breast milk of the enantiomers. *Br J Clin Pharmacol* 1998; **45:** 409–11.

## Uses and Administration

Vigabatrin is an analogue of gamma-aminobutyric acid (GABA) that acts as an irreversible inhibitor of GABA-transaminase, the enzyme responsible for the catabolism of GABA. It is used as an adjunctive antiepileptic in patients with resistant partial epilepsy with or without secondary generalisation, unresponsive to other therapy. It is also used as monotherapy for infantile spasms (as for example in West's syndrome).

The recommended initial dose of vigabatrin as *adjunctive therapy* in adults is 1 g daily by mouth, increased if necessary in increments of 500 mg at weekly intervals to a maximum of 3 g daily. A recommended initial dose in children is 40 mg/kg daily. Maintenance recommendations according to body-weight range are: 10 to 15 kg, 0.5 to 1 g daily; 15 to 30 kg, 1 to 1.5 g daily; 30 to 50 kg, 1.5 to 3 g daily; and 50 kg or more, 2 to 3 g daily. For infantile spasms the initial dose of vigabatrin as *monotherapy* is 50 mg/kg daily, adjusted according to response over 7 days. Up to 150 mg/kg daily has been used in some infants.

Doses may be divided and given twice daily or taken as a single daily dose. Dosage reductions may be required in the elderly and in patients with renal impairment.

As with other antiepileptics, withdrawal of vigabatrin therapy or transition to or from another type of antiepileptic therapy should be made gradually to avoid precipitating an increase in the frequency of seizures. For a discussion on whether or not to withdraw antiepileptic therapy in seizure-free patients, see p.349. It has been recommended that the dose of vigabatrin should be gradually reduced over 2 to 4 weeks.

**Epilepsy.** Vigabatrin is used in the treatment of epilepsy (p.349) as adjunctive therapy for refractory seizures. Reviews[1-3] of vigabatrin have considered it to be most effective in the treatment of complex partial seizures with or without secondary generalisation; it may, however, exacerbate myoclonic or absence seizures. Efficacy as adjunctive therapy in refractory partial seizures was demonstrated by 2 multicentre studies[4,5] involving 228 patients (including 46 children) and a study[6] involving 52 patients being assessed for epilepsy surgery. However, in a follow-up study[7] of 120 patients who had participated in an open-label trial of vigabatrin as adjunctive therapy for refractory epilepsy 6 to 8 years earlier, it was considered that vigabatrin had had only marginal benefit on the long-term prognosis of severe refractory epilepsy, despite favourable results from the original trial.

Vigabatrin is also of value in infantile spasms (as for example in West's syndrome). In an assessment of vigabatrin as monotherapy in 192 infants with infantile spasms who were followed up for an average of 7.6 months,[8] there was complete cessation of spasms in 131 patients, a decrease in cluster frequency in 37, and no improvement in 24 (including deterioration in one infant). A crossover study comparing vigabatrin with corticotropin in 42 infants found that both drugs produced some benefit.[9] A review of the literature suggested that vigabatrin was particularly effective in infantile spasms associated with tuberous sclerosis;[10] the authors considered that its efficacy might be less in other forms of infantile spasm.[10]

1. French JA. Vigabatrin. *Epilepsia* 1999; **40** (suppl 5): S11–S16.
2. Gidal BE, *et al.* Vigabatrin: a novel therapy for seizure disorders. *Ann Pharmacother* 1999; **33:** 1277–86.
3. Lewis H, Wallace SJ. Vigabatrin. *Dev Med Child Neurol* 2001 **43:** 833–5.
4. Dalla Bernadina B, *et al.* Efficacy and tolerability of vigabatrin in children with refractory partial seizures: a single-blind dose-increasing study. *Epilepsia* 1995; **36:** 687–91.
5. French JA, *et al.* A double-blind, placebo-controlled study of vigabatrin three g/day in patients with uncontrolled complex partial seizures. *Neurology* 1996; **46:** 54–61.
6. Malmgren K, *et al.* Cost analysis of epilepsy surgery and of vigabatrin treatment in patients with refractory partial epilepsy. *Epilepsy Res* 1996; **25:** 199–207.
7. Walker MC, *et al.* Long term use of lamotrigine and vigabatrin in severe refractory epilepsy: audit of outcome. *BMJ* 1996; **313:** 1184–5.
8. Aicardi J, *et al.* Sabril IS Investigator and Peer Review Groups. Vigabatrin as initial therapy for infantile spasms: a European retrospective survey. *Epilepsia* 1996; **37:** 638–42.
9. Vigevano F, Cilio MR. Vigabatrin versus ACTH as first-line treatment for infantile spasms: a randomized, prospective study. *Epilepsia* 1997; **38:** 1270–4.
10. Hancock E, Osborne JP. Vigabatrin in the treatment of infantile spasms in tuberous sclerosis. *J Child Neurol* 1999; **14:** 71–4.

**Metabolic disorders.** Vigabatrin, an irreversible inhibitor of GABA-transaminase, has been tried in GABA metabolic disorders not accompanied by epilepsy,[1-4] with ambivalent results. Data from 23 case reports of patients with succinic semialdehyde dehydrogenase deficiency indicated that vigabatrin was clinically beneficial in only about one-third of patients.[4]

1. Jaeken J, *et al.* Vigabatrin in GABA metabolism disorders. *Lancet* 1989; **i:** 1074.
2. Gibson KM, *et al.* Vigabatrin therapy in patient with succinic semialdehyde dehydrogenase deficiency. *Lancet* 1989; **ii:** 1105–6.
3. Stephenson JBP. Vigabatrin for startle-disease with altered cerebrospinal-fluid free gamma-aminobutyric acid. *Lancet* 1992; **340:** 430–1.
4. Gibson KM, *et al.* The clinical phenotype of succinic semialdehyde dehydrogenase deficiency (4-hydroxybutyric aciduria): case reports of 23 new patients. *Pediatrics* 1997; **99:** 567–74.

**Stiff-man syndrome.** There have been anecdotal reports[1-3] of improvement of stiff-man syndrome (see under Muscle Spasm, p.696) with vigabatrin in patients unable to tolerate benzodiazepine therapy.

1. Vermeij FH, *et al.* Improvement of stiff-man syndrome with vigabatrin. *Lancet* 1996; **348:** 612.
2. Prevett MC, *et al.* Improvement of stiff-man syndrome with vigabatrin. *Neurology* 1997; **48:** 1133–4.
3. Sharoqi IA. Improvement of stiff-man syndrome with vigabatrin. *Neurology* 1998; **50:** 833–4.

## Preparations

***BP 2003:*** Vigabatrin Oral Powder; Vigabatrin Tablets.

**Proprietary Preparations** (details are given in Part 3)
***Arg.:*** Sabril; ***Austral.:*** Sabril; ***Austria:*** Sabril; ***Belg.:*** Sabril; ***Braz.:*** Sabril; ***Canad.:*** Sabril; ***Chile:*** Sabril; ***Denm.:*** Sabrilex; ***Fin.:*** Sabrilex; ***Fr.:*** Sabril; ***Ger.:*** Sabril; ***Hong Kong:*** Sabril; ***Irl.:*** Sabril; ***Israel:*** Sabrilan; ***Ital.:*** Sabril; ***Mex.:*** Sabril; ***Neth.:*** Sabril; ***Norw.:*** Sabrilex; ***NZ:*** Sabril; ***Port.:*** Sabril; ***S.Afr.:*** Sabril; ***Singapore:*** Sabril; ***Spain:*** Sabrilex; ***Swed.:*** Sabrilex; ***Switz.:*** Sabril; ***UK:*** Sabril.

---

## Zonisamide *(BAN, USAN, rINN)*

AD-810; CI-912; PD-110843; Zonisamida. 1-(1,2-Benzoxazol-3-yl)methanesulphonamide.

$C_8H_8N_2O_3S$ = 212.2.
*CAS — 68291-97-4.*
*ATC — N03AX15.*

### Adverse Effects

The most common adverse effects with zonisamide have included anorexia, nausea, somnolence, dizziness, headache, and agitation or irritability. Severe skin reactions including Stevens-Johnson syndrome and toxic epidermal necrolysis have occurred rarely, and consideration should be given to withdrawing zonisamide in patients who develop unexplained rash. There have been isolated reports of aplastic anaemia or agranulocytosis. Other adverse effects have included renal calculi (see below), depression, psychosis, psychomotor slowing, reduced concentration, speech or language difficulties, ataxia, paraesthesia, nystagmus, diplopia, gastrointestinal disorders, and fatigue. Reduced sweating with hyperthermia has occurred in children.

**Effects on mental function.** For a review of the effects of antiepileptic therapy including zonisamide on *cognition*, see p.351.

**Effects on the nervous system.** Decreased sweating and hyperthermia have been reported in patients given zonisamide. By the end of December 2001 the manufacturers in the USA were aware of 40 such cases; of these, 38 had occurred in the first 11 years of marketing in Japan and 2 in the first year of marketing in the USA. Many cases were reported after exposure to high ambient temperatures and some progressed to heat stroke, but none had led to death.

The manufacturer noted that children appeared to be at an increased risk of developing these adverse reactions and should be monitored closely for such effects especially during warm or hot weather. Caution was also advised when zonisamide was given with other drugs known to cause similar effects, for example, carbonic anhydrase inhibitors and antimuscarinics.[1]

1. O'Brien C [Elan Pharmaceuticals]. Important drug warning. Available at: http://www.fda.gov/medwatch/SAFETY/2002/Zonegran_deardoc.pdf (accessed 14/05/04)

**Renal calculi.** Patients treated with zonisamide in the USA and Europe may have had a higher incidence of renal calculi than those treated in Japan. In one US study, 4 of 113 patients (3.5%) receiving long-term treatment with zonisamide developed renal calculi,[1] but a familial relationship was found for 2. In pooled data from earlier studies, renal calculi had been reported in 13 of 700 patients (1.9%) treated in the USA and Europe compared with 2 of 1008 patients (0.2%) in Japan.[2] Another review, involving information from more than 750 patients, considered the risk of renal calculi in zonisamide-treated patients to be 5 to 9 times greater than that in the general population.[3]

1. Patsalos PN, Sander JWAS. Newer antiepileptic drugs: towards an improved risk-benefit ratio. *Drug Safety* 1994; **11:** 37–67.
2. Peters DH, Sorkin EM. Zonisamide: a review of its pharmacodynamic and pharmacokinetic properties, and therapeutic potential in epilepsy. *Drugs* 1993; **45:** 760–87.
3. Bennett WM. Risk of kidney stones in patients treated with zonisamide. *Neurology* 2002; **58** (suppl 3): A298–A299.

## Precautions

Zonisamide is a sulfonamide derivative and is therefore contraindicated in patients with a history of hypersensitivity to sulfonamides. It should be used with care in patients with hepatic or renal impairment. Adequate hydration is recommended to increase urine output and try to reduce the risk of developing renal calculi, especially in predisposed patients.

Care is required when withdrawing zonisamide therapy—see also under Uses and Administration below.

Zonisamide has been found to be teratogenic in *animal* studies.

**Breast feeding.** Zonisamide is distributed into breast milk;[1] in view of the potential for serious adverse effects in infants from zonisamide, the manufacturers recommend that it should only be used in nursing mothers if the benefits outweigh the risks. For comment on antiepileptic therapy and breast feeding, see p.351.

1. Kawada K, *et al.* Pharmacokinetics of zonisamide in perinatal period. *Brain Dev* 2002; **24:** 95–7.

**Driving.** For a comment on antiepileptic drugs and driving, see p.351.

**Pregnancy.** Zonisamide crosses the placenta.[1] For comments on the management of epilepsy during pregnancy, see p.351.

1. Kawada K, *et al.* Pharmacokinetics of zonisamide in perinatal period. *Brain Dev* 2002; **24:** 95–7.

## Interactions

There are complex interactions between antiepileptics and toxicity may be enhanced without a corresponding increase in antiepileptic activity. Such interactions are very variable and unpredictable and plasma monitoring is often advisable with combination therapy. Use with drugs that induce or inhibit the cytochrome P450 isoenzyme CYP3A4 may alter plasma concentrations of zonisamide. Carbamazepine, phenytoin, or phenobarbital reduce the half-life of zonisamide; reductions have also been noted with valproate but to a lesser degree.

## Pharmacokinetics

Zonisamide is absorbed from the gastrointestinal tract and peak plasma concentrations are achieved within 2 to 6 hours of oral administration. The presence of food does not affect the bioavailability of zonisamide but the time to reach peak plasma concentrations is delayed. Steady-state concentrations are achieved within 14 days. Plasma protein binding is low but zonisamide is extensively bound to erythrocytes. The plasma elimination half-life is about 63 hours.

Zonisamide undergoes acetylation to *N*-acetylzonisamide and reduction mediated by the cytochrome P450 isoenzyme CYP3A4 to 2-sulfamoylacetylphenol (SMAP). Excretion is mainly in the urine, 35% appearing as unchanged drug, 15% as *N*-acetylzonisamide, and 50% as the glucuronide of SMAP.

Zonisamide crosses the placenta and is distributed into breast milk, see above.

The pharmacokinetics of zonisamide are affected by the concomitant administration of other antiepileptics (see under Interactions, above).

◊ References.

1. Kochak GM, *et al.* Steady-state pharmacokinetics of zonisamide, an antiepileptic agent for treatment of refractory complex partial seizures. *J Clin Pharmacol* 1998; **38:** 166–71.
2. Mimaki T. Clinical pharmacology and therapeutic drug monitoring of zonisamide. *Ther Drug Monit* 1998; **20:** 593–7.

## Uses and Administration

Zonisamide, a benzisoxazole derivative, is used as an adjunctive antiepileptic in the treatment of partial seizures. The usual initial dose in adults and adolescents over 16 years of age is 100 mg given once daily by mouth, increased after at least 2 weeks to 200 mg daily given as a single dose or in two divided doses. Thereafter, if necessary, the dose may be further increased by increments of 100 mg at intervals of at least 2 weeks up to 400 mg daily. Doses up to 600 mg daily have been used, but there is no current evidence of an increase in response above 400 mg daily; many of the adverse effects of zonisamide are reported to be more frequent at doses of 300 mg daily and above.

As with other antiepileptics, withdrawal of zonisamide therapy or transition to or from another type of antiepileptic therapy should be made gradually to avoid precipitating an increase in the frequency of seizures. For a discussion on whether or not to withdraw antiepileptic therapy in seizure-free patients, see p.349.

**Epilepsy.** Zonisamide is used in the treatment of refractory epilepsy (p.349). Many studies have been conducted in Japan where clinical experience demonstrated its efficacy mainly in the treatment of partial seizures with or without secondary generalisation.[1,2] Data from studies[3-5] conducted outside Japan have confirmed the efficacy of zonisamide as an adjunct in the treatment of partial epilepsies. Efficacy in primary generalised and mixed-seizure epilepsies appears to be more variable, although it may be of value in refractory myoclonic seizures.[6] Zonisamide might also be of use in the treatment of epileptic syndromes such as Lennox-Gastaut syndrome and infantile spasms (as for example in West's syndrome), although only a small number of patients with the latter condition have been studied.[7]

1. Peters DH, Sorkin EM. Zonisamide: a review of its pharmacodynamic and pharmacokinetic properties, and therapeutic potential in epilepsy. *Drugs* 1993; **45:** 760–87.
2. Patsalos PN, Sander JWAS. Newer antiepileptic drugs: towards an improved risk-benefit ratio. *Drug Safety* 1994; **11:** 37–67.
3. Leppik IE, *et al.* Efficacy and safety of zonisamide: results of a multicenter study. *Epilepsy Res* 1993; **14:** 165–73.
4. Schmidt D, *et al.* Zonisamide for add-on treatment of refractory partial epilepsy: a European double-blind trial. *Epilepsy Res* 1993; **15:** 67–73.
5. Chadwick DW, Marson AG. Zonisamide add-on for drug-resistant partial epilepsy. Available in The Cochrane Library; Issue 2. Chichester: John Wiley; 2004.
6. Kyllerman M, Ben-Menachen E. Zonisamide for progressive myoclonus epilepsy: long-term observations in seven patients. *Epilepsy Res* 1998; **29:** 109–14.
7. Yanai S, *et al.* Treatment of infantile spasms with zonisamide. *Brain Dev* 1999; **21:** 157–61.

## Preparations

**Proprietary Preparations** (details are given in Part 3)
***Jpn:*** Excegran; ***USA:*** Zonegran.

# Antifungals

Aspergillosis, p.386
Blastomycosis, p.386
Candidiasis, p.386
Chromoblastomycosis, p.387
Coccidioidomycosis, p.387
Cryptococcosis, p.387
Dermatophytoses, p.388
Endocarditis, p.388
Eye infections, p.388
Histoplasmosis, p.388
Infections in immunocompromised patients, p.388
Meningitis, p.388
Mucormycosis, p.388
Mycetoma, p.388
Nail infections, p.389
Paracoccidioidomycosis, p.389
Peritonitis, p.389
Pityriasis versicolor, p.389
Pneumocystis carinii pneumonia, p.389
Protothecosis, p.390
Respiratory-tract infections, p.390
Skin infections, p.390
Sporotrichosis, p.391
Tinea, p.391

This chapter describes those drugs that are used mainly in the treatment and prophylaxis of fungal infections (mycoses). They include the azole derivatives, including imidazoles (such as ketoconazole) and triazoles (such as fluconazole and itraconazole), the allylamines (naftifine and terbinafine), several polyene antibiotics (including amphotericin B and nystatin), other antifungal antibiotics (for example griseofulvin), and a number of other compounds among them amorolfine, ciclopirox olamine, flucytosine, haloprogin, tolnaftate, and undecenoic acid and its salts.

## Choice of Antifungal

Fungi may be classified as either yeasts or moulds according to their appearance and means of growth. Yeast-like fungi involved in infections include *Blastomyces dermatitidis*, *Candida* spp., *Coccidioides immitis*, *Histoplasma capsulatum*, *Sporothrix schenckii*, and the infective agents of chromoblastomycosis. Examples of pathogenic moulds include *Aspergillus* spp., the dermatophytes, and the Mucorales fungi.

Some fungi are true pathogens and can cause disease in any individual. Other fungi such as *Candida* species and *Pneumocystis carinii* (once thought to be a protozoan but now considered to be a fungus) are of low pathogenicity and require an alteration in the normal defence mechanisms for disease to occur; such disease is called opportunistic.

Fungal infections may be classified as **superficial**, affecting only the skin, hair, nails, or mucous membranes, or **systemic**, affecting the body as a whole; systemic infections tend to occur more frequently in immunocompromised individuals such as those with AIDS. Fungal infections may also be described as **local** when they are restricted to one body area, as **invasive** when there is spread into the tissues, or as **disseminated** when the infection has spread from the primary site to other organs throughout the body.

Ideally antifungal treatment should be chosen after the infecting organism has been identified, but it is often necessary to start treatment before the pathogen can be cultured and identified, especially in immunocompromised patients in whom infections are often rapidly progressive.

The choice of treatment for the important fungal diseases is described below.

### Aspergillosis

Aspergillosis is an infection caused by fungi of the genus *Aspergillus*, usually *A. fumigatus* although *A. flavus* and *A. niger* are also important. Aspergillosis is usually acquired by inhalation and most commonly causes non-invasive disease of the respiratory tract. Other sites of infection include the eye following trauma or cataract surgery. Invasive disease of tissues adjacent to the site of infection, for example spread from the paranasal sinus to the orbit, and dissemination to distant organs may occur, predominantly in immunocompromised patients. In severely immunocompromised patients aspergillosis usually presents as severe acute pneumonia. Other organs affected may include the heart (particularly damaged or prosthetic valves), kidneys, bone, brain, liver, and skin.

In general the response of **invasive** aspergillosis to treatment is poor and early initiation of treatment is essential. Surgical excision may be necessary. High intravenous doses of amphotericin B remain the antifungal treatment of choice.[1-4] However, the overall response rate to conventional amphotericin B is reported[2] to be only 30 to 35%, although this may be improved by the use of liposomal amphotericin B.[5-7] Combination therapy with amphotericin B and flucytosine has also been suggested[8] and may be useful in cerebral, meningeal, or endocardial infections.[2] Itraconazole by mouth[3,9] has been used as the main alternative to amphotericin B. Voriconazole is emerging as a promising alternative in the treatment of invasive aspergillosis in immunocompromised patients;[4,10] at least one study has found it to be superior to amphotericin B.[11] Caspofungin may be used in patients who are refractory to, or intolerant of, other antifungals.[4]

Approaches to reducing the incidence of aspergillosis in immunocompromised patients have included chemoprophylaxis with either low-dose intravenous, intranasal, or nebulised amphotericin B, or oral itraconazole,[12,13] or a combination of these.[14]

**Non-invasive** forms of aspergillosis include allergic bronchopulmonary aspergillosis, a hypersensitivity reaction to *Aspergillus* usually occurring in asthmatic patients, and aspergilloma, a fungal mass or ball developing within the pulmonary cavity or paranasal sinus. **Allergic bronchopulmonary aspergillosis** is usually treated with corticosteroids although oral itraconazole may be a useful adjunct.[3,15] A systematic review[16] has concluded that itraconazole modifies the immunological activation associated with allergic bronchopulmonary aspergillosis in asthmatic patients and improves clinical outcome in the first 4 months of treatment. The treatment of **aspergilloma** depends on the severity of symptoms, and includes conservative management, antifungal therapy, or surgical resection. Oral itraconazole or intravenous amphotericin B are the most effective drugs. Direct intracavitary instillation of antifungals may also be useful[3] and has been advocated for patients at particularly high risk of complications.[17] Inhaled amphotericin B aerosol was reported to be poorly tolerated and of little value in preventing invasive pulmonary aspergillosis in granulocytopenic patients.[18]

**Chronic locally invasive infections** have been reported to respond to prolonged treatment with itraconazole; in a small study in 3 patients,[19] treatment for 5 to 12 months with itraconazole produced clinical improvements but not mycological cure.

Aspergillosis of the **eye**, like other fungal eye infections, is difficult to treat; antifungals are generally not well absorbed following topical application and infections extending into the vitreous or anterior chamber require subconjunctival, intra-ocular, and/or systemic treatment. Systemic treatment is necessary for ocular manifestations of disseminated disease. When systemic therapy is required intravenous amphotericin B is usually given; an oral azole compound may be given for less severe infections. For superficial eye infections a number of drugs including natamycin, amphotericin B, azole compounds, and sulfadiazine silver have been applied topically alone or as an adjunct to systemic therapy. Surgical excision of infected tissue may be necessary in severe infections.

1. Anonymous. Essential drugs: systemic mycoses. *WHO Drug Inf* 1991; **5:** 129–36.
2. Denning DW. Treatment of invasive aspergillosis. *J Infect* 1994; **28** (suppl 1): 25–33.
3. Stevens DA, *et al.* Practice guidelines for diseases caused by Aspergillus. *Clin Infect Dis* 2000; **30:** 696–709.
4. Anonymous. Systemic antifungal drugs. In: *Handbook of antimicrobial therapy.* 16th ed. New York: The Medical Letter, 2002: 111–119.
5. Ringdén O, *et al.* Efficacy of amphotericin B encapsulated in liposomes (AmBisome) in the treatment of invasive fungal infections in immunocompromised patients. *J Antimicrob Chemother* 1991; **28** (suppl B): 73–82.
6. Chopra R, *et al.* Liposomal amphotericin B (AmBisome) in the treatment of fungal infections in neutropenic patients. *J Antimicrob Chemother* 1991; **28** (suppl B): 93–104.
7. Mills W, *et al.* Liposomal amphotericin B in the treatment of fungal infections in neutropenic patients: a single-centre experience of 133 episodes in 116 patients. *Br J Haematol* 1994; **86:** 754–60.
8. Saral R. Candida and aspergillus infections in immunocompromised patients: an overview. *Rev Infect Dis* 1991; **13:** 487–92.
9. Denning DW, *et al.* NIAID mycoses study group multicenter trial of oral itraconazole therapy for invasive aspergillosis. *Am J Med* 1994; **97:** 135–44. Correction. *ibid.*; 497.
10. Denning DW, *et al.* Efficacy and safety of voriconazole in the treatment of acute invasive aspergillosis. *Clin Infect Dis* 2002; **34:** 563–71.
11. Herbrecht R, *et al.* Voriconazole versus amphotericin B for primary therapy of invasive aspergillosis. *N Engl J Med* 2002; **347:** 408–15.
12. Beyer J, *et al.* Strategies in prevention of invasive pulmonary aspergillosis in immunosuppressed or neutropenic patients. *Antimicrob Agents Chemother* 1994; **38:** 911–17.
13. Cafferkey MT. Chemoprophylaxis of invasive pulmonary aspergillosis. *J Antimicrob Chemother* 1994; **33:** 917–24.
14. Todeschini G, *et al.* Oral itraconazole plus nasal amphotericin B for prophylaxis of invasive aspergillosis in patients with hematological malignancies. *Eur J Clin Microbiol Infect Dis* 1993; **12:** 614–18.
15. Vlahakis NE, Aksamit TR. Diagnosis and treatment of allergic bronchopulmonary aspergillosis. *Mayo Clin Proc* 2001; **76:** 930–8.
16. Wark PAB, *et al.* Azoles for allergic bronchopulmonary aspergillosis associated with asthma. Available in The Cochrane Library; Issue 2. Chichester: John Wiley; 2004.
17. Kauffman CA. Quandary about treatment of aspergillomas persists. *Lancet* 1996; **347:** 1640.
18. Erjavec Z, *et al.* Tolerance and efficacy of amphotericin B inhalations for prevention of invasive pulmonary aspergillosis in haematological patients. *Eur J Clin Microbiol Infect Dis* 1997; **16:** 364–8.
19. Caras WE, Pluss JL. Chronic necrotizing pulmonary aspergillosis: pathologic outcome after itraconazole therapy. *Mayo Clin Proc* 1996; **71:** 25–30.

### Blastomycosis

Blastomycosis (not to be confused with South American blastomycosis, see Paracoccidioidomycosis, below) is an infection caused by the fungus *Blastomyces dermatitidis.* Infection may be through the lungs and is usually followed by dissemination; the skin, skeleton, and genito-urinary system often become infected. Blastomycosis has been reported only rarely in patients with AIDS, but when it occurs it may be widely disseminated with CNS involvement and a high mortality.[1]

Intravenous amphotericin B, once the mainstay of treatment, is reserved for severe cases, CNS disease, cases unresponsive to other treatment, and infections in immunocompromised patients.[2] Mild to moderate disease is treated with an oral azole,[2] usually itraconazole, although fluconazole, or ketoconazole may also be effective. Patients with AIDS may require prolonged suppressive treatment, preferably with an oral azole, after a clinical response has been achieved.[1]

1. Pappas PG, *et al.* Blastomycosis in patients with the acquired immunodeficiency syndrome. *Ann Intern Med* 1992; **116:** 847–53.
2. Chapman SW, *et al.* Practice guidelines for the management of patients with blastomycosis. *Clin Infect Dis* 2000; **30:** 679–83.

### Candidiasis

*Candida* spp. are commensal fungi commonly found in the gastrointestinal tract, mouth, and vagina; they become pathogenic only when natural defence mechanisms fail. *C. albicans* is the species most commonly associated with infection although infections with other species, notably *C. glabrata (Torulopsis glabrata), C. krusei, C. lusitaniae, C. parapsilosis,* and *C. tropicalis*, also occur. Predisposing factors for pathogenic *Candida* infection include antibacterial therapy, skin trauma, debility, diabetes mellitus, pregnancy, and immunodeficiency; candidiasis often occurs in patients with HIV infection.

Candidiasis (or candidosis), the general term for pathogenic infection with *Candida* spp., can be superficial, deep local invasive, or disseminated.

**Superficial** candidiasis includes infection of the oropharynx, vagina, and skin. Oropharyngeal and vulvovaginal infections are commonly known as thrush. Superficial infections can usually be treated topically with an antifungal although the rare chronic mucocutaneous candidiasis syndrome normally requires systemic treatment. Antifungals used topically include amphotericin B, ciclopirox olamine, natamycin, nystatin, terbinafine, and several azole derivatives such as clotrimazole, econazole, and miconazole. The choice of drug is determined by the availability of a suitable formulation for the site of infection as well as by toxicity and duration of treatment.

Antiseptics including chlorhexidine and povidone-iodine have anticandidal activity and have been used in **oropharyngeal** infections, although they can be toxic if swallowed.[1] Methylrosanilinium chloride has also been used,[2,3] but as well as being cosmetically less acceptable its use has become restricted due to fears over possible carcinogenicity.

Infection involving the **nails** and surrounding tissue is difficult to treat. Chronic paronychia (infection affecting the tissue around the nails) is often resistant to treatment but may respond to prolonged application of topical imidazoles.[1] Onychomycosis (infection affecting the nail itself) generally requires systemic treatment with oral itraconazole.[4]

**Oesophageal** infections are not normally accessible to topical therapy and should be treated with oral azoles.

**Vulvovaginal** candidiasis responds well to short courses of treatment (typically 3 to 14 days) with a topical antifungal as a cream or pessary. Single-dose preparations are also available for local treatment.[5] In general, uncomplicated vulvovaginal infections in immunocompetent patients will respond to a course of treatment of 7 days or less, while patients with complicated infections usually require treatment for 10 to 14 days.[4,6] In pregnancy, a topical imidazole appears to be more effective than nystatin.[7] Treatment for 7 days may be necessary. Single-dose or short-course oral therapy with fluconazole or itraconazole is also effective, but oral treatment of such superficial infections may be reserved for patients who do not respond to, or are intolerant of, topical therapy. Vulvovaginal infections with non-*albicans* species may not respond to azoles but may respond to topical boric acid or topical flucytosine.[4]

Topical therapy of superficial candidiasis may not be adequate in immunocompromised patients and oral azole therapy should also be considered in these patients.[8] Patients who neither respond to nor tolerate oral therapy, or those at risk of developing disseminated disease, may require intravenous amphotericin B.[2,3,8]

Relapse after treatment of superficial candidiasis is common, especially in patients with predisposing factors for infection. Recurrence may result from inadequate initial treatment. (In recurrent vulvovaginal candidiasis re-infection from other body sites or by sexual transmission from an untreated partner is not thought to be implicated.[9,10]) Patients with frequent recurrences usually require systemic treatment. Although long-term or intermittent administration of oral antifungals, usually fluconazole, has been recommended to reduce recurrences in immunocompromised patients,[8,11] and 6-month maintenance therapy has been used in immunocompetent patients with recurrent infections,[5,6,10] there is concern over the increasing incidence of drug resistance.[12-16] This may be a consequence of the selection of resistant strains of *C. albicans* or of intrinsically less sensitive species such as *C. krusei*.[14,17-20] Secondary prophylaxis in immunocompromised patients is now largely restricted to those with frequent or severe recurrences, including oesophageal infections.[21] Primary prophylaxis against candidiasis is not recommended for patients with advanced HIV infection.[21]

Preparations, such as yogurt, containing *Lactobacillus* spp. have been used in the treatment and prevention of vaginal candidiasis in an attempt to displace *Candida* from the vagina but evidence to support their use is limited. Other novel treatments have included the adjuvant use of granulocyte-macrophage colony-stimulating factors.[22,23]

**Deep local invasive** and **disseminated** candidiasis require systemic antifungal treatment. Intravenous amphotericin B, with or without flucytosine, has been regarded as the initial treatment of choice in most infections, although there has been some concern regarding the use of flucytosine in AIDS patients because of its bone-marrow toxicity. Treatment with an azole such as fluconazole or itraconazole may be an effective alternative. Fluconazole has been shown to be as effective as intravenous amphotericin B.[24,25] Caspofungin may also be as effective as intravenous amphotericin B for invasive candidiasis and, more specifically, for candidaemia.[26] Fluconazole may be used as a first-line option for clinically stable patients with uncomplicated candidaemia, provided that they have not recently been treated with an azole.[27] There has been debate over how to treat patients in an unstable clinical condition or those with non-*albicans* candidal infections,[28] although amphotericin B is often preferred.[4] Fluconazole is preferred for infections with *C. lusitaniae* since many strains are resistant to amphotericin B.[4] As with superficial infections, the emergence of resistant *Candida* is causing concern, especially in intensive care settings and in severely immunocompromised patients.[29] Prophylactic antifungal treatment is not recommended routinely[27,30] although some would consider it in critically ill patients or those receiving bone-marrow transplants at high risk of infection.[4,27] Empirical treatment before confirmation of disseminated candidiasis has been recommended for patients with heavy colonisation and a deteriorating condition.[27,30]


1. WHO. *WHO model prescribing information: drugs used in skin diseases*. Geneva: WHO, 1997.
2. WHO. *Global programme on AIDS: guidelines for the clinical management of HIV infection in children*. Geneva: WHO, 1993.
3. Garber GE. Treatment of oral candida mucositis infections. *Drugs* 1994; **47:** 734–40.
4. Pappas PG, *et al.* Infectious Diseases Society of America. Guidelines for treatment of candidiasis. *Clin Infect Dis* 2004; **38:** 161–89.
5. Anonymous. Drugs for sexually transmitted infections. In: *Handbook of antimicrobial therapy*. 16th ed. New York: The Medical Letter, 2002: 99–110.
6. Centers for Disease Control. Sexually transmitted diseases treatment guidelines 2002. *MMWR* 2002; **51** (RR-6): 1–80.
7. Young GL, Jewell D. Topical treatment for vaginal candidiasis (thrush) in pregnancy. Available in The Cochrane Library; Issue 2. Chichester: John Wiley; 2004.
8. British Society for Antimicrobial Chemotherapy Working Party. Antifungal chemotherapy in patients with acquired immunodeficiency syndrome. *Lancet* 1992; **340:** 648–51.
9. Working Group of the British Society for Medical Mycology. Management of genital candidiasis. *BMJ* 1995; **310:** 1241–4.
10. Clinical Effectiveness Group, Association of Genitourinary Medicine and the Medical Society for the Study of Venereal Diseases. National guideline for the management of vulvovaginal candidiasis. Available at: http://www.bashh.org/guidelines/2002/candida%2006%2001.PDF (accessed 12/05/04)
11. Working Party of the British Society for Antimicrobial Chemotherapy. Chemoprophylaxis for candidosis and aspergillosis in neutropenia and transplantation: a review and recommendations. *J Antimicrob Chemother* 1993; **32:** 5–21.
12. Powderly WG. Resistant candidiasis. *AIDS Res Hum Retroviruses* 1994; **10:** 925–9.
13. Sangeorzan JA, *et al.* Epidemiology of oral candidiasis in HIV-infected patients: colonization, infection, treatment, and emergence of fluconazole resistance. *Am J Med* 1994; **97:** 339–46.
14. Johnson EM, Warnock DW. Azole drug resistance in yeasts. *J Antimicrob Chemother* 1995; **36:** 751–5.
15. Baily G. Weekly fluconazole for preventing mucosal candidiasis in HIV infection. *Ann Intern Med* 1997; **127:** 1131.
16. Goldman M, *et al.* Does long-term itraconazole prophylaxis result in in vitro azole resistance in mucosal Candida albicans isolates from persons with advanced human immunodeficiency virus infection? *Antimicrob Agents Chemother* 2000; **44:** 1585–7.
17. Millon L, *et al.* Émergence de Candida glabrata et Candida krusei chez des patients séropositifs pour le VIH atteints de candidose oropharyngée, traités de façon prolongée par le fluconazole. *J Mycol Med* 1994; **4:** 90–2.
18. Law D, *et al.* High prevalence of antifungal resistance in Candida spp from patients with AIDS. *J Antimicrob Chemother* 1994; **34:** 659–68.
19. Denning DW. Can we prevent azole resistance in fungi? *Lancet* 1995; **346:** 454–5.
20. Lewis RE, Klepser ME. The changing face of nosocomial candidemia: epidemiology, resistance, and drug therapy. *Am J Health-Syst Pharm* 1999; **56:** 525–33.
21. Centers for Disease Control and Prevention. Guidelines for preventing opportunistic infections among HIV-infected persons—2002: recommendations of the US Public Health Service and the Infectious Diseases Society of America. *MMWR* 2002; **51** (RR-8): 1–52. Also available at: http://www.cdc.gov/mmwr/PDF/rr/rr5108.pdf (accessed 12/05/04)
22. Shahar E, *et al.* White cell enhancement in the treatment of severe candidosis. *Lancet* 1995; **346:** 974–5.
23. Capetti A, *et al.* Employment of recombinant human granulocyte-macrophage colony stimulating factor in oesophageal candidiasis in AIDS patients. *AIDS* 1995; **9:** 1378–9.
24. Rex JH, *et al.* A randomized trial comparing fluconazole with amphotericin B for the treatment of candidemia in patients without neutropenia. *N Engl J Med* 1994; **331:** 1325–30.
25. Anaissie EJ, *et al.* Management of invasive candidal infections: results of a prospective, randomized, multicenter study of fluconazole versus amphotericin B and review of the literature. *Clin Infect Dis* 1996; **23:** 964–72.
26. Mora-Duarte J, *et al.* Comparison of caspofungin and amphotericin B for invasive candidiasis. *N Engl J Med* 2002; **347:** 2020–9.
27. Edwards JE, *et al.* International conference for the development of a consensus on the management and prevention of severe candidal infections. *Clin Infect Dis* 1997; **25:** 43–59.
28. Graybill JR. Editorial response: can we agree on the treatment of candidiasis? *Clin Infect Dis* 1997; **25:** 60–2.
29. Nguyen MH, *et al.* The changing face of candidemia: emergence of non-Candida albicans species and antifungal resistance. *Am J Med* 1996; **100:** 617–23.
30. British Society for Antimicrobial Chemotherapy Working Party. Management of deep Candida infection in surgical and intensive care unit patients. *Intensive Care Med* 1994; **20:** 522–8.


## Chromoblastomycosis

Chromoblastomycosis (chromomycosis) is an infection caused by a number of opportunistic fungi, including *Fonsecaea compacta (Phialophora compacta), F. pedrosoi (P. pedrosoi), Phialophora verrucosa, Cladosporium carrionii,* and *Rhinocladiella aquaspersa*, following invasion of skin trauma sites. It occurs worldwide but is more common in tropical and subtropical climates. The disease is characterised by chronic cutaneous and subcutaneous lesions. In its early stages, when lesions are small, surgical excision or cryotherapy are the treatments of choice, although it has been suggested that there is some risk of spreading the lesion during surgery. Drug treatment with itraconazole, alone or with flucytosine, may be used.[1] Saperconazole[2] and terbinafine[3] have also been used with some success. However, recurrence and drug resistance has been a problem with monotherapy. Local heat treatment aids healing and may be useful.


1. WHO. *WHO model prescribing information: drugs used in skin diseases*. Geneva: WHO, 1997.
2. Franco L, *et al.* Saperconazole in the treatment of systemic and subcutaneous mycoses. *Int J Dermatol* 1992; **31:** 725–9.
3. Esterre P, *et al.* Treatment of chromomycosis with terbinafine: preliminary results of an open pilot study. *Br J Dermatol* 1996; **134** (suppl 46): 33–6.


## Coccidioidomycosis

Coccidioidomycosis is an infection caused by inhalation of the spores of *Coccidioides immitis*, a fungus found in the soil in arid and semi-desert areas mainly of North, Central, and South America. Patients may experience acute or chronic lung infections, meningitis, and disseminated disease although many infections are subclinical. Common names for the infection include valley fever, desert fever, and desert rheumatism. In endemic areas, coccidioidomycosis is a common opportunistic infection in immunocompromised patients.

Acute pulmonary coccidioidomycosis is usually self-limiting and resolves spontaneously without specific chemotherapy; in 60% of cases the infection is asymptomatic or mild. In some patients the infection progresses to chronic pulmonary coccidioidomycosis with granulomatous lesions, fibrosis, and cavitation. A small proportion of patients develop acute progressive pneumonia (which is commonly fatal if untreated) or disseminated disease (usually involving the skin, bone, meninges, and joints). Severe pulmonary and disseminated infections are more likely in pregnant women, certain ethnic groups, diabetics, and immunocompromised patients.

Antifungal therapy is with either intravenous amphotericin B or an oral azole.[1,2] Treatment is usually reserved for severe or complicated infections or for patients with concurrent risk factors, especially immunosuppression.[2] Ketoconazole, itraconazole, and fluconazole have all been reported to be at least moderately effective in non-meningeal infections. Amphotericin B is generally used for rapidly progressive disease.[2] Fluconazole is effective in meningeal infections and is the most frequently recommended antifungal for this indication,[2] although itraconazole has also produced beneficial responses; intrathecal amphotericin B may also be used, especially in aggressive infections.[2,3] The incidence of relapses following treatment is high, and lifelong therapy is recommended following coccidioidal meningitis.[4] In patients with HIV infection, lifelong suppressive therapy with fluconazole or itraconazole is recommended following treatment of either meningeal or non-meningeal coccidioidomycosis.[5]


1. Stevens DA. Coccidioidomycosis. *N Engl J Med* 1995; **332:** 1077–82.
2. Galgiani JN, *et al.* Infectious Diseases Society of America. Practice guidelines for the treatment of coccidioidomycosis. *Clin Infect Dis* 2000; **30:** 658–61.
3. Anonymous. Systemic antifungal drugs. In: *Handbook of antimicrobial therapy*. 16th ed. New York: The Medical Letter, 2002: 111–119.
4. Dewsnup DH, *et al.* Is it ever safe to stop azole therapy for Coccidioides immitis meningitis? *Ann Intern Med* 1996; **124:** 305–10.
5. Centers for Disease Control and Prevention. Guidelines for preventing opportunistic infections among HIV-infected persons—2002: recommendations of the US Public Health Service and the Infectious Diseases Society of America. *MMWR* 2002; **51** (RR-8): 1–52. Also available at: http://www.cdc.gov/mmwr/PDF/rr/rr5108.pdf (accessed 12/05/04)


## Cryptococcosis

Cryptococcosis is an infection caused by inhalation of the fungus *Cryptococcus neoformans*. It is rare in immunocompetent individuals, but is an important life-threatening disease in immunocompromised patients, especially those with AIDS, in whom it occurs principally as cryptococcal meningitis.

Mild infections in immunocompetent patients may resolve without treatment, but oral fluconazole is usually effective if treatment is necessary.[1] Itraconazole is a suitable alternative in patients unable to take fluconazole. In either case, treatment should continue for several months. For more severe disease, amphotericin B may be given alone, or, especially if there is CNS involvement, with flucytosine. Patients may be transferred to oral fluconazole after induction therapy with amphotericin B and flucytosine or may continue on amphotericin B and flucytosine for 6 to 10 weeks.[1] Intrathecal or intraventricular amphotericin B may be used in refractory cases.

Any infection in immunocompromised patients should be treated as for CNS infections in immunocompetent patients, although AIDS-related cryptococcal pneumonia may be treated with oral fluconazole or itraconazole, continued indefinitely. Fluconazole plus flucytosine is another alternative, but the toxicity of this regimen limits its usefulness.[1] Immunocompromised patients require long-term suppressive treatment, preferably with oral fluconazole, after a primary course of antifungal therapy, and in patients with HIV infection this should generally be life-long.[1,2] However, it may be possible to discontinue secondary prophylaxis in patients with HIV infection in whom there is a sustained response to highly active antiretroviral therapy, and who remain asymptomatic with respect to cryptococcosis. US guidelines[2] recommend re-starting secondary prophylaxis if the CD4+ T lymphocyte count falls below 100 to 200 cells/microlitre. Oral itraconazole or intermittent intravenous amphotericin B are alternatives but are generally reserved for patients who cannot take fluconazole.

Primary prophylaxis in patients with HIV infection is not generally recommended since it has not been shown to be more beneficial than treating cryptococcal infections when they occur and may increase the risk of resistance.[2]

1. Saag MS, *et al.* Infectious Diseases Society of America. Practice guidelines for the management of cryptococcal disease. *Clin Infect Dis* 2000; **30:** 710–18.
2. Centers for Disease Control and Prevention. Guidelines for preventing opportunistic infections among HIV-infected persons—2002: recommendations of the US Public Health Service and the Infectious Diseases Society of America. *MMWR* 2002; **51** (RR-8): 1–52. Also available at: http://www.cdc.gov/mmwr/PDF/rr/rr5108.pdf (accessed 12/05/04)

## Dermatophytoses

See under Skin Infections, below.

## Endocarditis

Infective endocarditis caused by fungi such as *Aspergillus* or *Candida* is much less common than that caused by bacteria (p.125). Fungal endocarditis is usually treated with intravenous amphotericin B; surgical removal of an infected valve is often required.[1,2] Long-term survival was reported[3] in a patient with endocarditis due to *C. parapsilosis* who was not suitable for surgery. Treatment was initially with amphotericin B, replaced by fluconazole after 27 days because of renal dysfunction. The patient had remained free of disease having received fluconazole for 26 months.

1. Ellis M. Fungal endocarditis. *J Infect* 1997; **35:** 99–103.
2. Ellis ME, *et al.* Fungal endocarditis: evidence in the world literature, 1965-1995. *Clin Infect Dis* 2001; **32:** 50–62.
3. Czwerwiec FS, *et al.* Long-term survival after fluconazole therapy of candidal prosthetic valve endocarditis. *Am J Med* 1993; **94:** 545–6.

## Eye infections

Fungal infections of the eye are less common than infections with bacteria or viruses, but are usually severe and may lead to loss of vision. Diagnosis may be delayed due to a gradual onset of symptoms and empirical treatment with antibacterials. Patients with impaired host resistance such as diabetics or immunocompromised patients are particularly at risk. The most common fungi causing eye infections are *Aspergillus, Candida,* and *Fusarium*; others include *Blastomyces*, *Cryptococcus*, and *Sporothrix*. Infections of the orbit usually occur by spread from an infection of the paranasal sinus, commonly mucormycosis or aspergillosis.

Fungal infections of the eye are difficult to treat. Antifungals are generally not well absorbed following topical application and infections extending to the vitreous or anterior chamber require subconjunctival, intra-ocular, and/or systemic treatment. Systemic treatment is necessary for ocular manifestations of disseminated disease. When systemic therapy is required intravenous amphotericin B is usually given; an oral azole compound may be given for less severe infections. Superficial infections may respond to topical treatment. Amphotericin B or natamycin are most commonly used. An azole compound such as miconazole is sometimes used, or flucytosine in combination with another antifungal. Chlorhexidine has also produced promising results. Topical treatment may also be used as an adjunct to systemic therapy. Surgical excision of infected tissue may be necessary in severe infections.

## Histoplasmosis

Histoplasmosis is a systemic infection caused by *Histoplasma capsulatum,* a fungus found in the soil in endemic areas, particularly at sites with heavy accumulations of bird or bat excrement. Infection is by inhalation of spores. Two types of histoplasmosis occur: classic histoplasmosis due to infection with *H. capsulatum* var. *capsulatum* and African histoplasmosis due to infection with *H. capsulatum* var. *duboisii.*

The major endemic area for *H. capsulatum* var. *capsulatum* is central USA. In endemic regions most of the population is infected and mild infections are generally asymptomatic. However, acute pulmonary infection can occur. Massive infection can be fatal. Chronic pulmonary histoplasmosis can result in lung fibrosis and cavitation. Histoplasmosis may also present as an acute or chronic disseminated infection involving widespread infiltration of the reticuloendothelial system, which is primarily seen in immunodeficient or immunocompromised patients.

*Histoplasma capsulatum* var. *duboisii* is found in central Africa and causes a chronic disseminated form of histoplasmosis with focal lesions predominantly in skin and bone.

Antifungal therapy for classic or African histoplasmosis is necessary in patients with severe pulmonary infections, chronic fibrotic or cavitary disease, or disseminated infection. Infections which are not life-threatening may be treated with an oral azole in both immunocompetent and immunocompromised patients.[1] Itraconazole is the preferred drug.[1] Ketoconazole is moderately effective but more toxic. Fluconazole is less effective than either itraconazole or ketoconazole but may be the preferred azole in CNS infections where its better penetration may be an advantage.[1] Patients with life-threatening infections or those not responding to oral treatment are given amphotericin B intravenously. Patients with HIV infection should continue maintenance therapy with itraconazole daily or amphotericin B weekly;[1,2] the use of fluconazole for maintenance should be discouraged.[1] Primary prophylaxis with itraconazole is not recommended routinely but may be considered for patients with advanced AIDS at especially high risk of infection due to occupational exposure or residence in a hyperendemic area.[2]

1. Wheat J, *et al.* Infectious Diseases Society of America. Practice guidelines for the management of patients with histoplasmosis. *Clin Infect Dis* 2000; **30:** 688–95.
2. Centers for Disease Control and Prevention. Guidelines for preventing opportunistic infections among HIV-infected persons—2002: recommendations of the US Public Health Service and the Infectious Diseases Society of America. *MMWR* 2002; **51** (RR-8): 1–52. Also available at: http://www.cdc.gov/mmwr/PDF/rr/rr5108.pdf (accessed 12/05/04)

## Infections in immunocompromised patients

Patients with a defective immune system are at special risk of infections, including those caused by fungi. Primary immune deficiency is rare, whereas secondary deficiency is more common; immunosuppressive therapy, cancer and its treatment, HIV infection, and splenectomy may all cause neutropenia and impaired humoral and cellular immunity in varying degrees. Fungi most commonly associated with infection in these patients include *Cryptococcus neoformans* and species of *Aspergillus* and *Candida*. *Pneumocystis carinii*, now considered to have characteristics of fungi, is an important cause of pneumonia in patients with AIDS. In areas in which they are endemic, coccidioidomycosis, histoplasmosis, and *Penicillium marneffei* infections are also more common in immunocompromised patients and a growing number of uncommon organisms including *Fusarium*, *Scedosporium*, and *Trichosporon* species has been reported to cause invasive infections.

A fungal cause of infection should be considered in immunocompromised patients with fever of unknown origin who have not responded to broad spectrum antibacterials. Fungal infection in patients with immune deficiency usually occurs as a widely disseminated disease and treatment should be commenced as early as possible. If the infection has not been identified, empirical treatment with intravenous amphotericin B has been attempted but the effects of this on overall mortality remain uncertain.

Long-term suppression of fungal infection has been recommended for immunocompromised patients although this might allow development of resistance and the overgrowth of species not susceptible to the antifungals used. This is of particular concern with fluconazole (see Resistance, p.398), one of the drugs that has been most widely used for this purpose. Antifungals are also used in selective digestive tract decontamination (see Intensive Care, p.132).

Treatment and prophylaxis of specific fungal infections in immunocompromised patients is discussed under the appropriate headings—see Aspergillosis, Candidiasis, Coccidioidomycosis, Cryptococcosis, and Histoplasmosis (above), and *Pneumocystis carinii* Pneumonia (below).

References.

1. British Society for Antimicrobial Chemotherapy Working Party. Antifungal chemotherapy in patients with acquired immunodeficiency syndrome. *Lancet* 1992; **340:** 648–51.
2. Working Party of the British Society for Antimicrobial Chemotherapy. Chemoprophylaxis for candidosis and aspergillosis in neutropenia and transplantation: a review and recommendations. *J Antimicrob Chemother* 1993; **32:** 5–21.
3. American Thoracic Society. Fungal infection in HIV-infected persons. *Am J Respir Crit Care Med* 1995; **152:** 816–22.
4. Warnock DW. Fungal complications of transplantation: diagnosis, treatment and prevention. *J Antimicrob Chemother* 1995; **36** (suppl B): 73–90.
5. Meunier F. Targeting fungi: a challenge. *Am J Med* 1995; **99** (suppl 6A): 60S–67S.
6. Hood S, Denning DW. Treatment of fungal infections in AIDS. *J Antimicrob Chemother* 1996; **37** (suppl B): 71–85.
7. Working Party of the British Society for Antimicrobial Chemotherapy. Therapy of deep fungal infection in haematological malignancy. *J Antimicrob Chemother* 1997; **40:** 779–88.
8. Warnock DW. Fungal infections in neutropenia: current problems and chemotherapeutic control. *J Antimicrob Chemother* 1998; **41** (suppl D): 95–105.
9. Centers for Disease Control and Prevention. Guidelines for preventing opportunistic infections among hematopoietic stem cell transplant recipients: recommendations of CDC, the Infectious Disease Society of America, and the American Society of Blood and Marrow Transplantation. *MMWR* 2000; **49** (RR-10): 1–128. Also available at: http://www.cdc.gov/mmwr/PDF/rr/rr4910.pdf (accessed 21/06/04)
10. Centers for Disease Control and Prevention. Guidelines for preventing opportunistic infections among HIV-infected persons—2002: recommendations of the US Public Health Service and the Infectious Diseases Society of America. *MMWR* 2002; **51** (RR-8): 1–52. Also available at: http://www.cdc.gov/mmwr/PDF/rr/rr5108.pdf (accessed 12/05/04)
11. Johansen HK, Gøtzsche PC. Amphotericin B versus fluconazole for controlling fungal infections in neutropenic cancer patients. Available in The Cochrane Library; Issue 2. Chichester: John Wiley; 2004.
12. Gøtzsche PC, Johansen HK. Routine versus selective antifungal administration for control of fungal infections in patients with cancer. Available in The Cochrane Library; Issue 2. Chichester: John Wiley; 2004.

## Meningitis

Fungal diseases associated with meningitis include aspergillosis, candidiasis, coccidioidomycosis, cryptococcosis, and histoplasmosis (see above), although many disseminated fungal infections can involve the CNS, especially in immunocompromised patients. The treatment of each infection is discussed under the appropriate heading, but in general the initial drug of choice in fungal meningitis is intravenous amphotericin B, sometimes with flucytosine.

## Mucormycosis

Mucormycosis, a rare but serious infection caused by Mucorales fungi, is a type of zygomycosis, a term which is sometimes used synonymously. Mucormycosis usually occurs in poorly controlled diabetic patients or in immunocompromised patients. Patients receiving desferrioxamine may also be at increased risk of infection (see p.1034). Infections of the mucosa of the respiratory tract or gastrointestinal tract, or of abraded skin, usually with *Rhizopus* or *Rhizomucor* spp., can result in local invasion of deeper tissues including bone and the CNS with extensive tissue destruction. Disseminated disease may also occur.

Intravenous amphotericin B can be effective in mucormycosis and is usually combined with aggressive surgical debridement of infected tissue. Invasive disease is difficult to treat and is usually fatal.

References.

1. Boelaert JR. Mucormycosis (zygomycosis): is there news for the clinician? *J Infect* 1994; **28** (suppl 1): 1–6.
2. Lee FY, *et al.* Pulmonary mucormycosis: the last 30 years. *Arch Intern Med* 1999; **159:** 1301–9.

## Mycetoma

Mycetoma is seen especially in the tropics and subtropics and involves subcutaneous tissue, bone, and skin. The term Madura foot is used for mycetoma affecting the foot. Organisms enter the tissues via local skin trauma. Mycetomas caused by fungi such as *Madurella mycetomatis, M. grisea,* or *Pseudallescheria boydii* are called eumycetomas. Those caused by the filamentous bacteria, actinomycetes, are called actinomycetomas and are discussed on p.136. Eumycetomas are often unresponsive to treatment. Some infections have responded to prolonged use of ketoconazole[1,2] and itraconazole has also been tried.[2] Surgical excision may be necessary.

1. Mahgoub ES, Gumaa SA. Ketoconazole in the treatment of eumycetoma due to Madurella mycetomii. *Trans R Soc Trop Med Hyg* 1984; **78:** 376–9.
2. Restrepo A. Treatment of tropical mycoses. *J Am Acad Dermatol* 1994; **31:** S91–S102.

#### Nail infections

See under Skin Infections, below.

#### Paracoccidioidomycosis

Paracoccidioidomycosis (South American blastomycosis) is caused by an infection with the fungus *Paracoccidioides brasiliensis.* The disease occurs mainly in inhabitants or former inhabitants of regions of Central and South America and may remain dormant for long periods. Infection is thought to be by inhalation. While most primary infections are subclinical, some may be progressive and severe, particularly in immunocompromised patients. The lungs may be affected, the disease usually presenting as a chronic infection. Disseminated disease affects the skin, mucous membranes, gastrointestinal tract, reticuloendothelial system, and adrenals, and may be either acute or chronic.

Treatment is usually with itraconazole, ketoconazole, or, for patients with severe infection, intravenous amphotericin B.[1] Sulfonamides are now rarely used. Other azole derivatives may prove effective. There has been a case report describing successful treatment with terbinafine when access to azoles was not possible.[2] Treatment may need to be continued for months or years to prevent relapse.

1. Anonymous. Systemic antifungal drugs. In: *Handbook of antimicrobial therapy.* 16th ed. New York: The Medical Letter, 2002: 111–119.
2. Ollague JM, *et al.* Paracoccidioidomycosis (South American blastomycosis) successfully treated with terbinafine: first case report. *Br J Dermatol* 2000; **143:** 188–91.

#### Peritonitis

Fungal peritonitis occasionally occurs in patients undergoing continuous ambulatory peritoneal dialysis or abdominal surgery, or in trauma. It is usually caused by yeasts such as *Candida*. Amphotericin B may be the treatment of choice;[1,2] intravenous administration has been preferred to intraperitoneal administration since the latter route is painful.[3] Fluconazole or other azole antifungals or flucytosine may also be effective.[1,4] However, fungal peritonitis is a difficult infection to treat and it has a high morbidity and mortality.[3]

1. Keane WF, *et al.* Peritoneal dialysis-related peritonitis treatment recommendations: 1996 update. *Perit Dial Int* 1996; **16:** 557–73.
2. Johnson CC, *et al.* Peritonitis: update on pathophysiology, clinical manifestations, and management. *Clin Infect Dis* 1997; **24:** 1035–47.
3. Working Party of the British Society for Antimicrobial Chemotherapy. Diagnosis and management of peritonitis in continuous ambulatory peritoneal dialysis. *Lancet* 1987; **i:** 845–9.
4. Aguado JM, *et al.* Successful treatment of candida peritonitis with fluconazole. *J Antimicrob Chemother* 1994; **34:** 847.

#### Pityriasis versicolor

See under Skin Infections, below.

#### Pneumocystis carinii pneumonia

*Pneumocystis carinii* is an opportunistic unicellular pathogen which has been classified both with the protozoa and with the fungi, although more recent evidence suggests that it is probably a fungus. Although *Pneumocystis carinii* has recently been renamed *Pneumocystis jiroveci*, this term has not been widely adopted in the medical literature and in *Martindale* the name *P. carinii* is still used. It appears to be acquired by the airborne route. In persons with normally functioning immune systems, clinical infection resolves spontaneously, but in immunosuppressed patients it can produce interstitial pneumonia with progressive damage to the alveolar walls and accumulation of exudate in the air spaces. If untreated, the disease is almost always fatal. With the advent of AIDS (p.621), *Pneumocystis carinii* pneumonia (PCP) has become an increasing problem.

Co-trimoxazole, dapsone, and pentamidine are currently the most effective drugs for both treatment and prophylaxis. However, there is evidence of the emergence of strains of *P. carinii* potentially resistant to both sulfonamides and dapsone,[1,2] emphasising the need for continuing development of alternative regimens.

**Treatment** of acute disease is primarily with either co-trimoxazole or pentamidine. Co-trimoxazole is the preferred drug,[3-5] given intravenously in severe infections and orally in mild infections. Intravenous pentamidine is generally reserved for patients who do not respond to, or cannot tolerate, co-trimoxazole. Combination therapy with co-trimoxazole and pentamidine is not more effective and is potentially more toxic than either drug alone.[6] Although it has been suggested that folinic acid could be administered with co-trimoxazole to reduce the risk of haematotoxicity,[4] increased therapeutic failure has been reported in patients receiving this combination.[7]

Some centres have given trimethoprim with dapsone for second-line therapy[4] although the combination is only effective in patients with mild or moderately severe infections.[5] Dapsone should probably not be used alone for treatment of PCP,[4] but may be useful for prophylaxis (see below). Other alternatives include primaquine plus clindamycin,[8-10] and trimetrexate plus folinic acid.[11,12] A comparison of oral co-trimoxazole with trimethoprim plus dapsone or primaquine plus clindamycin found them equally effective in initial treatment of mild to moderate infection.[10] Atovaquone may be used to treat mild to moderate infections.[5,13,14] Nebulised pentamidine is occasionally suggested for mild infections but is now generally reserved for prophylaxis (see below). A meta-analysis[15] involving 27 studies and 497 patients concluded that primaquine plus clindamycin appeared to be the most effective alternative treatment for patients with *Pneumocystis carinii* pneumonia unresponsive to conventional first-line treatment.

Prompt additional treatment with a corticosteroid is now of established value for patients with moderate or severe disease (see p.1085) and is started at the same time as the antipneumocystis treatment is begun.[5] Adjuvant treatment with corticosteroids reduces morbidity and mortality[5] and concerns over corticosteroid-induced immunosuppression have generally not been borne out in practice.

**Prophylaxis** is used in high-risk patients, especially among those with compromised immunity due to HIV infection. Primary prophylaxis is attempted in all HIV-infected adults with a CD4+ T lymphocyte count below 200 cells/microlitre or those with a history of oropharyngeal candidiasis regardless of CD4+ T lymphocyte count.[16] In infants and young children, in whom PCP commonly occurs at higher CD4+ T lymphocyte counts of greater than 200 cells/microlitre, guidelines in the USA propose prophylaxis at age-specific CD4+ T lymphocyte count thresholds.[16] US guidelines recommend that infants of HIV-positive mothers should receive prophylaxis beginning at 4 to 6 weeks of age and continuing until they are shown to be seronegative, or for at least 1 year initially.[16] In Europe, clinicians have tended to have a less aggressive approach to prophylaxis, with only one-third of clinics offering prophylaxis routinely to all children exposed to HIV while the remaining two-thirds only offer prophylaxis once HIV infection is confirmed or opportunistic infection occurs.[17]

Secondary prophylaxis is given to all patients with a history of PCP. Recommendations for prophylaxis in patients without HIV infection are not widely publicised, but it has been suggested that prophylaxis should be considered for patients who are immunosuppressed due to an underlying disorder or to immunosuppressant drug therapy.[18,19]

Co-trimoxazole by mouth is currently preferred for primary and secondary prophylaxis.[5,16] Pentamidine administered by an appropriate jet nebuliser, dapsone (alone or with pyrimethamine), or atovaquone, are the usual alternatives in patients unable to tolerate co-trimoxazole.[5,16] A meta-analysis found that co-trimoxazole was more effective than dapsone or pentamidine[20] but because it is not well tolerated, long-term studies suggest that, on an intention-to-treat basis, dapsone[21] or inhaled pentamidine[21,22] may be as good, at least in patients with CD4+ T lymphocyte counts of more than 100 cells/microlitre. Atovaquone appears to be as effective as dapsone or inhaled pentamidine.[16] For secondary prophylaxis, dapsone was found to be less effective than nebulised pentamidine in a study in patients with AIDS,[23] but the efficacy of regimens for secondary prophylaxis has not yet been fully evaluated. Regimens containing co-trimoxazole also protect against toxoplasmosis, an increasingly common opportunistic infection in AIDS patients;[16,24,25] alternatives in patients who cannot tolerate co-trimoxazole include dapsone plus pyrimethamine or atovaquone with or without pyrimethamine.[16]

Co-trimoxazole and dapsone are usually administered daily for prophylaxis of PCP,[16] but intermittent administration has been tried in an attempt to improve tolerance without compromising efficacy. Doses of co-trimoxazole have usually been 960 mg given on three days of each week, although 960 mg twice daily on three days each week has also been used; a low dose of 480 mg daily on every day each week is said to be better tolerated than a dose of 960 mg daily on every day each week and equally effective (see under Co-trimoxazole, p.201). Intermittent use of dapsone has involved administration with pyrimethamine on two days each week,[26] although such intermittent use may be less effective than other regimens.[27,28] Response to inhaled pentamidine can be influenced by the choice of nebuliser;[29] commonly used nebulisers include the Fisoneb and Respirgard II. Patients receiving inhaled pentamidine may be prone to extrapulmonary *Pneumocystis* infection.[30,31] Other prophylactic regimens include intermittent parenteral administration of pentamidine, pyrimethamine with sulfadoxine, clindamycin with primaquine, and trimetrexate but are not recommended unless the more usual drugs cannot be used.[5,16]

A meta-analysis[32] indicated that it may be possible to discontinue primary and secondary prophylaxis in patients with HIV infection who obtain a sustained response to combination antiretroviral therapy with at least partial recovery of immune function and US guidelines[16] recommend this approach. Restarting primary and secondary prophylaxis is recommended in patients whose CD4+ T lymphocyte count falls to below 200 cells/microlitre, and in those in whom PCP recurs at a count of greater than 200 cells/microlitre.[16] However, a study of solid organ transplant recipients[33] suggested that lung transplant recipients were at continued risk of developing PCP and that prophylaxis may need to be continued indefinitely in this group.

1. Mei Q, *et al.* Failure of co-trimoxazole in Pneumocystis carinii infection and mutations in dihydropteroate synthase gene. *Lancet* 1998; **351:** 1631–2.
2. Helweg-Larsen J, *et al.* Effects of mutations in Pneumocystis carinii dihydropteroate synthase gene on outcome of AIDS-associated P carinii pneumonia. *Lancet* 1999; **354:** 1347–51.
3. Medical Letter on Drugs and Therapeutics. Drugs for parasitic infections (issued April 2002). Available at: http://www.medicalletter.com/freedocs/parasitic.pdf (accessed 12/05/04)
4. Peters BS, *et al.* Adverse effects of drugs used in the management of opportunistic infections associated with HIV infection. *Drug Safety* 1994; **10:** 439–54.
5. Miller RF, *et al.* Pneumocystis carinii infection: current treatment and prevention. *J Antimicrob Chemother* 1996; **37** (suppl B): 33–53.
6. Glatt AE, Chirgwin K. Pneumocystis carinii pneumonia in human immunodeficiency virus-infected patients. *Arch Intern Med* 1990; **150:** 271–9.
7. Safrin S, *et al.* Adjunctive folinic acid with trimethoprim-sulfamethoxazole for Pneumocystis carinii pneumonia in AIDS patients is associated with an increased risk of therapeutic failure and death. *J Infect Dis* 1994; **170:** 912–17.
8. Toma E, *et al.* Clindamycin/primaquine versus trimethoprim-sulfamethoxazole as primary therapy for Pneumocystis carinii pneumonia in AIDS: a randomized, double-blind pilot trial. *Clin Infect Dis* 1993; **17:** 178–84.
9. Black JR, *et al.* Clindamycin and primaquine therapy for mild-to-moderate episodes of Pneumocystis carinii pneumonia in patients with AIDS: AIDS Clinical Trials Group 044. *Clin Infect Dis* 1994; **18:** 905–13.
10. Safrin S, *et al.* Comparison of three regimens for treatment of mild to moderate Pneumocystis carinii pneumonia in patients with AIDS: a double-blind, randomized trial of oral trimethoprim-sulfamethoxazole, dapsone-trimethoprim, and clindamycin-primaquine. *Ann Intern Med* 1996; **124:** 792–802.
11. Amsden GW, *et al.* Trimetrexate for Pneumocystis carinii pneumonia in patients with AIDS. *Ann Pharmacother* 1992; **26:** 218–26.
12. Sattler FR, *et al.* Trimetrexate with leucovorin versus trimethoprim-sulfamethoxazole for moderate to severe episodes of Pneumocystis carinii pneumonia in patients with AIDS: a prospective, controlled multicenter investigation of the AIDS Clinical Trials Group Protocol 029/031. *J Infect Dis* 1994; **170:** 165–72.
13. Hughes W, *et al.* Comparison of atovaquone (566C80) with trimethoprim-sulfamethoxazole to treat Pneumocystis carinii pneumonia in patients with AIDS. *N Engl J Med* 1993; **328:** 1521–7.
14. Dohn MN, *et al.* Oral atovaquone compared with intravenous pentamidine for Pneumocystis carinii pneumonia in patients with AIDS. *Ann Intern Med* 1994; **121:** 174–80.
15. Smego RA, *et al.* A meta-analysis of salvage therapy for Pneumocystis carinii pneumonia. *Arch Intern Med* 2001; **161:** 1529–33.
16. Centers for Disease Control and Prevention. Guidelines for preventing opportunistic infections among HIV-infected persons—2002: recommendations of the US Public Health Service and the Infectious Diseases Society of America. *MMWR* 2002; **51** (RR-8): 1–52. Also available at: http://www.cdc.gov/mmwr/PDF/rr/rr5108.pdf (accessed 12/05/04)
17. Bernardi S, *et al.* Variable use of therapeutic interventions for children with human immunodeficiency virus type 1 infection in Europe. *Eur J Pediatr* 2000; **159:** 170–5.
18. Sepkowitz KA, *et al.* Pneumocystis carinii pneumonia without acquired immunodeficiency syndrome: more patients, same risk. *Arch Intern Med* 1995; **155:** 1125–8.
19. Yale SH, Limper AH. Pneumocystis carinii pneumonia in patients without acquired immunodeficiency syndrome: associated illnesses and prior corticosteroid therapy. *Mayo Clin Proc* 1996; **71:** 5–13.
20. Ioannidis JP, *et al.* A meta-analysis of the relative efficacy and toxicity of Pneumocystis carinii prophylactic regimens. *Arch Intern Med* 1996; **156:** 177–88.
21. Bozzette SA, *et al.* A randomised trial of three antipneumocystis agents in patients with advanced human immunodeficiency virus infection. *N Engl J Med* 1995; **332:** 693–9.
22. Rizzardi GP, *et al.* Risks and benefits of aerosolized pentamidine and cotrimoxazole in primary prophylaxis of Pneumocystis carinii pneumonia in HIV-1-infected patients: a two-year Italian multicentric randomized controlled trial. *J Infect* 1996; **32:** 123–31.
23. Salmon-Ceron D, *et al.* Lower survival in AIDS patients receiving dapsone compared with aerosolized pentamidine for secondary prophylaxis of Pneumocystis carinii pneumonia. *J Infect Dis* 1995; **172:** 656–64.
24. Girard P-M, *et al.* Dapsone–pyrimethamine compared with aerosolized pentamidine as primary prophylaxis against Pneumocystis carinii pneumonia and toxoplasmosis in HIV infection. *N Engl J Med* 1993; **328:** 1514–20.
25. Torres RA, *et al.* Randomized trial of dapsone and aerosolized pentamidine for the prophylaxis of Pneumocystis carinii pneumonia and toxoplasmosis encephalitis. *Am J Med* 1993; **95:** 573–83.

26. Podzamczer D, *et al.* Intermittent trimethoprim-sulfamethoxazole compared with dapsone-pyrimethamine for the simultaneous primary prophylaxis of pneumocystis pneumonia and toxoplasmosis in patients infected with HIV. *Ann Intern Med* 1995; **122:** 755–61.
27. Souza JP, *et al.* High rates of Pneumocystis carinii pneumonia in allogeneic blood and marrow transplant recipients receiving dapsone prophylaxis. *Clin Infect Dis* 1999; **29:** 1467–71.
28. McIntosh K, *et al.* Toxicity and efficacy of daily vs weekly dapsone for prevention of Pneumocystis carinii pneumonia in children infected with human immunodeficiency virus. *Pediatr Infect Dis J* 1999; **18:** 432–9.
29. Miller R, Steel S. Nebulized pentamidine as prophylaxis for Pneumocystis carinii pneumonia. *J Antimicrob Chemother* 1991; **27:** 153–7.
30. Witt K, *et al.* Dissemination of Pneumocystis carinii in patients with AIDS. *Scand J Infect Dis* 1991; **23:** 691–5.
31. Sha BE, *et al.* Pneumocystis carinii choroiditis in patients with AIDS: clinical features, response to therapy, and outcome. *J Acquir Immune Defic Syndr Hum Retrovirol* 1992; **5:** 1051–8.
32. Trikalinos TA, Ioannidis JPA. Discontinuation of Pneumocystis carinii prophylaxis in patients infected with human immunodeficiency virus: a meta-analysis and decision analysis. *Clin Infect Dis* 2001; **33:** 1901–9.
33. Gordon SM, *et al.*. Should prophylaxis for Pneumocystis carinii pneumonia in solid organ transplant recipients ever be discontinued? *Clin Infect Dis* 1999; **28:** 240–6.

## Protothecosis

Protothecosis is an infection with algae of the *Prototheca* spp., usually *P. wickerhamii.* Infection may follow minor trauma or surgery leading to a chronic skin lesion and occasionally dissemination. There are case reports of amphotericin B with tetracycline[1] or of itraconazole[2,3] being used successfully in protothecosis. Fluconazole has been used successfully[4] to treat a case unresponsive to itraconazole therapy.

1. Venezio FR, *et al.* Progressive cutaneous protothecosis. *Am J Clin Pathol* 1982; **77:** 485–93.
2. Tang WYM, *et al.* Cutaneous protothecosis: report of a case in Hong Kong. *Br J Dermatol* 1995; **133:** 479–82.
3. Okuyama Y, *et al.* A human case of protothecosis successfully treated with itraconazole. *Jpn J Med Mycol* 2001; **42:** 143–7.
4. Kim S-T, *et al.* Successful treatment with fluconazole of protothecosis developing at the site of an intralesional corticosteroid injection. *Br J Dermatol* 1996; **135:** 803–6.

## Respiratory-tract infections

A number of pathogenic fungi enter the body by inhalation and colonise the respiratory tract. Fungal infections of the respiratory tract include aspergillosis, blastomycosis, coccidioidomycosis, cryptococcosis, histoplasmosis, and paracoccidioidomycosis (see above). *Pneumocystis carinii,* now considered to have characteristics of fungi, is an important cause of pneumonia in HIV-infected patients (see above). Other fungi reported to produce respiratory-tract infections mainly in immunocompromised patients include *Candida* spp., *Fusarium* spp., *Penicillium marneffei, Pseudoallescheria boydii,* and Zygomycetes such as *Rhizopus arrhizus.* Acute pulmonary fungal infections in immunocompetent individuals are mostly self-limiting conditions that resolve without treatment. Severe, persistent, or progressive infections, or infections in immunocompromised patients, require treatment. Intravenous amphotericin B is usually the drug of choice but mild to moderate infection can be treated with an oral azole such as fluconazole, itraconazole, or ketoconazole. Pulmonary granulomas may require surgical removal. Chronic suppressive treatment is recommended for patients with immunosuppression due to HIV infection.

## Skin infections

The most common fungal skin infections are the dermatophytoses, pityriasis versicolor, and candidiasis. The first two are described here; candidiasis is described on p.386. Other fungal skin infections are discussed under the appropriate headings: blastomycosis, chromoblastomycosis, mycetoma, mucormycosis, protothecosis (above), and sporotrichosis (below). Fungal infections that may involve the skin by dissemination include aspergillosis, coccidioidomycosis, cryptococcosis, histoplasmosis, and paracoccidioidomycosis (above). Less common fungi causing skin infections include *Penicillium marneffei.* Sometimes a fungal infection may affect mucous membranes, nails, or subcutaneous tissue, and there can be spread to deeper tissue and dissemination especially in immunosuppressed patients. The term superficial fungal infections includes those involving the skin, nails, and mucous membranes. Antifungal treatment may be topical or systemic.[1,2]

**Dermatophytoses** (ringworm, tinea) are infections by dermatophytes, a group of fungi which includes soil-dwelling organisms and human and animal pathogens from 3 genera — *Epidermophyton, Microsporum,* and *Trichophyton.* Dermatophytoses are encouraged by hot and humid conditions and poor hygiene and occur throughout tropical and temperate regions of the world.

Dermatophytoses are classified according to the body site affected. They include

- tinea barbae (beard)
- tinea capitis (scalp)
- tinea corporis (body)
- tinea cruris (groin)
- tinea manuum (hand)
- tinea pedis (athlete's foot)
- tinea unguium (nail)

A chronic infection most commonly seen in the tropics is known as favus (tinea favosa) and a variant of tinea corporis is known as tinea imbricata (tokelau) is caused by *T. concentricum* and is endemic in parts of the Far East and Central and South America. A severe form of dermatophytosis caused by animal pathogens with deep, suppurant, inflammatory lesions is known as kerion.

Deep infections may occur rarely in immunocompromised patients and may spread to involve lymph nodes, liver, and brain, and may be fatal.

Mild localised superficial dermatophytoses of hairless skin sites will often respond to *topical* therapy.[3-5] Non-specific agents with a long history of topical use include benzoic acid, methylrosanilinium chloride, selenium sulfide, and salicylic acid. Many of these agents are effective, and while some older preparations such as Compound Benzoic Acid Ointment may be less cosmetically acceptable than modern products, they still have a role in the treatment of minor infections, particularly in the tropics.[6] However, the use of methylrosanilinium chloride is restricted due to fears over possible carcinogenicity (see p.1186). There are a number of specific topical antifungals that are active against dermatophytes. The azoles used topically include clotrimazole, econazole, ketoconazole, and miconazole. Ciclopirox olamine[7] and the allylamine antifungals naftifine and terbinafine[5] appear to have similar activity to the azoles. Chlorphenesin, tolnaftate, and undecenoic acid salts are all effective in uncomplicated dermatophytoses, but there are few comparative studies of their relative efficacy. Amorolfine has also been shown to be effective in skin infections, although its major application is in nail infections (see below).

Infections of some body sites respond poorly to topical therapy, as do extensive infections or those in heavily keratinised areas.[4,8] *Systemic* therapy may be appropriate in these cases as well as in disseminated disease. Griseofulvin, ketoconazole, and itraconazole have been the drugs most widely used, although terbinafine has been reported to be more effective than itraconazole in some forms of tinea[9,10] and also requires only short-duration therapy.[11,12] However, efficacy of terbinafine is reported to depend on the infecting organism.[13] Griseofulvin has proved to have few major toxic effects during long-term therapy and is useful for tinea capitis, extensive or disseminated infections, and nail infections in selected patients. However, since it has a narrow spectrum of activity largely confined to the dermatophytes, accurate diagnosis is essential, particularly before embarking on a prolonged treatment course when no immediate response is anticipated. Ketoconazole has a broader spectrum of activity, but severe adverse effects can occur on prolonged administration and its place is likely to be taken by itraconazole which appears to produce a rapid response and thus requires shorter treatment periods.[4] Other azoles such as fluconazole may also be effective.[14] Selenium sulfide and povidone-iodine shampoos may be useful adjuncts to oral therapy for tinea capitis to improve efficacy and limit the spread of infection.[15,16] A suitable topical antifungal is used in individuals suspected of carrying infection.[17]

Infections of the **nails (onychomycoses)** are notoriously difficult to treat.[5,18] Infections of the fingernails take up to 6 months to respond to oral griseofulvin and those of the toenails, a year or longer, but about 60% of nail infections fail to respond or relapse after the initial treatment course. The oral antifungals, terbinafine, itraconazole, and fluconazole, produce persistent antifungal concentrations in the nail more rapidly than griseofulvin.[18,19] Terbinafine and itraconazole have been most widely studied. Both are reported to produce clinical and mycological cures in a high proportion of patients more quickly than griseofulvin, generally after 12 weeks' treatment or less. Long-term follow-up has demonstrated that the response to terbinafine is maintained.[20-22] Terbinafine has been reported to be more effective than itraconazole,[23-26] although neither is effective in all patients. Although topical treatments have generally been ineffective in nail infections, ciclopirox nail lacquer has been shown to be effective.[27] Amorolfine applied as a lacquer has also produced encouraging results.[28] Another approach has been the dissolution of the nail plate with 40% urea paste, usually in combination with bifonazole.[29] Guidelines for the treatment of onychomycosis have been published in the UK.[30]

**Pityriasis versicolor** (tinea versicolor) is a superficial infection caused by the commensal yeast *Malassezia furfur (Pityrosporum orbiculare).* It is more common in tropical than in temperate latitudes and sun exposure may trigger the infection. Pityriasis versicolor will often respond to topical treatment with an azole antifungal or with selenium sulfide. Terbinafine administered topically (but not orally) is an alternative. Immunocompromised patients, including those receiving corticosteroids, may develop extensive infections. In addition, these fungi have caused septicaemia in patients receiving parenteral nutrition.[31] Severe infections require oral treatment with an azole.[32] Griseofulvin is not effective.

Other infections in which *Malassezia* yeasts are implicated include seborrhoeic dermatitis (p.1138) and pityrosporum folliculitis, both of which may present in a more severe form in patients with AIDS. Topical or systemic azole antifungals are effective in these conditions and are the main drugs used. However, relapses are common.[33]

1. Gupta AK, *et al.* Antifungal agents: an overview, part II. *J Am Acad Dermatol* 1994; **30:** 911–33.
2. Piérard GE, *et al.* Treatment and prophylaxis of tinea infections. *Drugs* 1996; **52:** 209–24.
3. Smith EB. Topical antifungal drugs in the treatment of tinea pedis, tinea cruris, and tinea corporis. *J Am Acad Dermatol* 1993; **28:** S24–S28.
4. Degreef HJ, DeDoncker PRG. Current therapy of dermatophytosis. *J Am Acad Dermatol* 1994; **31:** S25–S30.
5. Crawford F, *et al.* Topical treatments for fungal infections of the skin and nails of the foot. Available in The Cochrane Library; Issue 2. Chichester: John Wiley; 2004.
6. Gooskens V, *et al.* Treatment of superficial mycoses in the tropics: Whitfield's ointment versus clotrimazole. *Int J Dermatol* 1994; **33:** 738–42.
7. Bogaert H, *et al.* Multicentre double-blind clinical trials of ciclopirox olamine cream 1% in the treatment of tinea corporis and tinea cruris. *J Int Med Res* 1986; **14:** 210–16.
8. Higgins EM, *et al.* Guidelines for the management of tinea capitis. *Br J Dermatol* 2000; **143:** 53–8.
9. Budimulja U, *et al.* A double-blind, randomized, stratified controlled study of the treatment of tinea imbricata with oral terbinafine or itraconazole. *Br J Dermatol* 1994; **130** (suppl 43): 29–31.
10. De Keyser P, *et al.* Two-week oral treatment of tinea pedis, comparing terbinafine (250 mg/day) with itraconazole (100 mg/day): a double-blind, multicentre study. *Br J Dermatol* 1994; **130** (suppl 43): 22–25.
11. Farag A, *et al.* One-week therapy with oral terbinafine in cases of tinea cruris/corporis. *Br J Dermatol* 1994; **131:** 684–6.
12. Hay RJ, *et al.* A comparison of 2 weeks of terbinafine 250 mg/day with 4 weeks of itraconazole 100 mg/day in plantar-type tinea pedis. *Br J Dermatol* 1995; **132:** 604–8.
13. Baudraz-Rosselet F, *et al.* Efficacy of terbinafine treatment of tinea capitis in children varies according to the dermatophyte species. *Br J Dermatol* 1996; **135:** 1011–12.
14. Faergemann J, *et al.* A multicentre (double-blind) comparative study to assess the safety and efficacy of fluconazole and griseofulvin in the treatment of tinea corporis and tinea cruris. *Br J Dermatol* 1997; **136:** 575–7.
15. Allen HB, *et al.* Selenium sulfide: adjunctive therapy for tinea capitis. *Pediatrics* 1982; **69:** 81–3.
16. Givens TG, *et al.* Comparison of 1% and 2.5% selenium sulfide in the treatment of tinea capitis. *Arch Pediatr Adolesc Med* 1995; **149:** 808–11.
17. Anonymous. Management of scalp ringworm. *Drug Ther Bull* 1996; **34:** 5–6.
18. Denning DW, *et al.* Fungal nail disease: a guide to good practice (report of a working group of the British Society for Medical Mycology). *BMJ* 1995; **311:** 1277–81.
19. Gupta AK, Scher RK. Oral antifungal agents for onychomycosis. *Lancet* 1998; **351:** 541–2.
20. De Cuyper C. Long-term evaluation of terbinafine 250 and 500 mg daily in a 16-week oral treatment for toenail onychomycosis. *Br J Dermatol* 1996; **135:** 156–7.
21. Bräutigam M, *et al.* Successful treatment of toenail mycosis with terbinafine and itraconazole gives long term benefits. *BMJ* 1998; **317:** 1084.
22. De Cuyper C, Hindryckx PHFB. Long-term outcomes in the treatment of toenail onychomycosis. *Br J Dermatol* 1999; **141** (suppl 56): 15–20.
23. De Backer M, *et al.* A 12-week treatment for dermatophyte toe onychomycosis: terbinafine 250 mg/day vs itraconazole 200 mg/day—a double-blind comparative trial. *Br J Dermatol* 1996; **134** (suppl 46): 16–17.
24. Bräutigam M, *et al.* Randomised double blind comparison of terbinafine and itraconazole for treatment of toenail tinea infection. *BMJ* 1995; **311:** 919–22. Correction. *ibid.*; 1350.
25. Evans EGV, Sigurgeirsson B. Double blind, randomised study of continuous terbinafine compared with intermittent itraconazole in treatment of toenail onychomycosis. *BMJ* 1999; **318:** 1031–5.
26. Heikkilä H, Stubb S. Long-term results in patients with onychomycosis treated with terbinafine or itraconazole. *Br J Dermatol* 2002; **146:** 250–3.
27. Gupta AK, *et al.* Ciclopirox nail lacquer topical solution 8% in the treatment of toenail onychomycosis. *J Am Acad Dermatol* 2000; **43:** S70–S80.
28. Reinel D. Topical treatment of onychomycosis with amorolfine 5% nail lacquer: comparative efficacy and tolerability of once and twice weekly use. *Dermatology* 1992; **184** (suppl 1): 21–4.
29. Roberts DT, *et al.* Topical treatment of onychomycosis using bifonazole 1% urea/40% paste. *Ann N Y Acad Sci* 1988; **544:** 586–7.
30. Roberts DT, *et al.* Guidelines for treatment of onychomycosis. *Br J Dermatol* 2003; **148:** 402–10.
31. Dankner WM, *et al.* Malassezia fungemia in neonates and adults: complication of hyperalimentation. *Rev Infect Dis* 1987; **9:** 743–53.

32. Goodless DR, *et al.* Ketoconazole in the treatment of pityriasis versicolor: international review of clinical trials. *DICP Ann Pharmacother* 1991; **25:** 395–8.
33. McGrath J, Murphy GM. The control of seborrhoeic dermatitis and dandruff by antipityrosporal drugs. *Drugs* 1991: **41:** 178–84.


### Sporotrichosis

Sporotrichosis is a disease caused by *Sporothrix schenckii*, a fungus found in soil and vegetation. The disease occurs in the Americas and Africa, and may be divided into cutaneous or extracutaneous infection. The cutaneous form is the more common. It probably follows entry of the organism through skin abrasions and usually presents as a single skin lesion, although infection may spread along lymphatic channels causing a series of skin lesions. Extracutaneous sporotrichosis usually presents as osteoarticular infection. Pulmonary infections are occasionally seen and, rarely, CNS and ocular infections.

Potassium iodide by mouth has traditionally been used for cutaneous infections although the mode of action is unclear since potassium iodide does not demonstrate antifungal activity *in vitro*. Itraconazole by mouth is also effective[1-3] and is regarded by some[4] as the treatment of choice. Oral treatment with terbinafine[5,6] or fluconazole[7] has been tried and may be effective.

Extracutaneous sporotrichosis is treated with amphotericin B given intravenously or with itraconazole by mouth;[4] fluconazole is an alternative although it is mainly reserved for patients who cannot tolerate amphotericin B or itraconazole.[4]

Lifelong maintenance therapy with itraconazole may be beneficial in patients with AIDS following treatment of a primary infection.[4]


1. Anonymous. Systemic antifungal drugs. In: *Handbook of antimicrobial therapy*. 16th ed. New York: The Medical Letter, 2002: 111–119.
2. Sharkey-Mathis PK, *et al.* Treatment of sporotrichosis with itraconazole. *Am J Med* 1993; **95:** 279–85.
3. Restrepo A, *et al.* Itraconazole therapy in lymphangitic and cutaneous sporotrichosis. *Arch Dermatol* 1986; **122:** 413–17.
4. Kauffman CA, *et al.* Infectious Diseases Society of America. Practice guidelines for the management of patients with sporotrichosis. *Clin Infect Dis* 2000; **30:** 684–7.
5. Hull PR, Vismer HP. Treatment of cutaneous sporotrichosis with terbinafine. *J Dermatol Treat* 1992; **3** (suppl 1): 35–8.
6. Kudoh K, *et al.* Successful treatment of cutaneous sporotrichosis with terbinafine. *J Dermatol Treat* 1996; **7:** 33–5.
7. Castro LGM, *et al.* Successful treatment of sporotrichosis with oral fluconazole: a report of three cases. *Br J Dermatol* 1993; **128:** 352–6.


### Tinea

See under Skin Infections, above.

## Amorolfine *(BAN, USAN, rINN)*

Ro-14-4767/000. (±)-*cis*-2,6-Dimethyl-4-[2-methyl-3-(*p-tert*-pentylphenyl)propyl]morpholine.

$C_{21}H_{35}NO = 317.5$.

*CAS — 78613-35-1.*

*ATC — D01AE16.*

### Amorolfine Hydrochloride *(BANM, rINNM)*

Hidrocloruro de amorolfina; Ro-14-4767/002.

$C_{21}H_{35}NO,HCl = 354.0$.

*CAS — 78613-38-4.*

*ATC — D01AE16.*

### Adverse Effects

Skin irritation, presenting as erythema, pruritus, or a burning sensation, and, rarely, more severe skin reactions have been reported following topical application of amorolfine.

### Antimicrobial Action

Amorolfine is a morpholine derivative with antifungal activity. It appears to act by interfering with the synthesis of sterols essential for the functioning of fungal cell membranes.

Amorolfine is active *in vitro* against a wide variety of pathogenic and opportunistic fungi including dermatophytes, *Blastomyces dermatitidis*, *Candida* spp., *Histoplasma capsulatum*, and *Sporothrix schenckii*. It also has variable activity against *Aspergillus* spp. However, despite its *in vitro* activity, amorolfine is inactive when given systemically and this limits its use to topical application for superficial infections.

### Uses and Administration

Amorolfine is a morpholine derivative applied topically as the hydrochloride in the treatment of fungal nail and skin infections (p.390). After topical application, systemic absorption of amorolfine is negligible.

For the treatment of nail infections caused by dermatophytes, yeasts, and moulds a lacquer containing the equivalent of 5% amorolfine is painted onto the affected nail once or sometimes twice weekly until the nail has regenerated. Treatment generally needs to be continued for 6 to 12 months.

For skin infections, including dermatophyte infections, a cream containing the equivalent of 0.25% amorolfine is applied once daily for at least 2 to 3 weeks (up to 6 weeks for foot infections) and continued for 3 to 5 days after clinical cure is achieved.

◊ Reviews.


1. Haria M, Bryson HM. Amorolfine: a review of its pharmacological properties and therapeutic potential in the treatment of onychomycosis and other superficial fungal infections. *Drugs* 1995; **49:** 103–20.


### Preparations

**Proprietary Preparations** (details are given in Part 3)
***Arg.:*** Locetar; ***Austral.:*** Loceryl; ***Austria:*** Loceryl; ***Belg.:*** Loceryl; ***Braz.:*** Loceryl; ***Chile:*** Loceryl; ***Denm.:*** Loceryl; ***Fin.:*** Loceryl; ***Fr.:*** Loceryl; ***Ger.:*** Loceryl; ***Gr.:*** Loceryl; ***Hong Kong:*** Loceryl; ***Irl.:*** Loceryl; ***Ital.:*** Locetar; ***Jpn:*** Pekiron; ***Malaysia:*** Loceryl; ***Mex.:*** Loceryl; ***Norw.:*** Loceryl; ***NZ:*** Loceryl; ***Port.:*** Locetar; ***S.Afr.:*** Loceryl; ***Singapore:*** Loceryl; ***Spain:*** Locetar; Odenil Unas; ***Swed.:*** Loceryl; ***Switz.:*** Loceryl; ***UK:*** Loceryl.

## Amphotericin B *(BANM, rINN)*

Amfotericina B; Amphotericin; Anfotericina B.

$C_{47}H_{73}NO_{17} = 924.1$.

*CAS — 1397-89-3.*

*ATC — A01AB04; A07AA07; G01AA03; J02AA01.*

**Pharmacopoeias.** In *Chin., Eur.* (see p.vi), *Int., Jpn, Pol.,* and *US.*

**Ph. Eur. 5.0** (Amphotericin B; Amphotericin BP 2003). A mixture of antifungal polyenes produced by the growth of certain strains of *Streptomyces nodosus* or by any other means. It consists largely of amphotericin B. It occurs as a yellow or orange powder. The potency is not less than 750 units per mg with reference to the dried substance. It contains not more than 10% of tetraenes, or not more than 5% if intended for use in parenteral dosage forms. Practically insoluble in water and in alcohol; soluble in dimethyl sulfoxide and in propylene glycol; slightly soluble in dimethylformamide; very slightly soluble in methyl alcohol. Amphotericin B is inactivated at low pH values. Store at 2° to 8° in airtight containers. Protect from light.

**USP 27** (Amphotericin B). A yellow to orange, odourless or practically odourless, powder. It contains not less than 750 micrograms of $C_{47}H_{73}NO_{17}$ per mg, and, for material intended for oral or topical use, not more than 15% of amphotericin A, both calculated on the dried substance. Insoluble in water, in dehydrated alcohol, in ether, in benzene, and in toluene; soluble in dimethylformamide, in dimethyl sulfoxide, and in propylene glycol; slightly soluble in methyl alcohol. Store at a temperature not exceeding 8° in airtight containers. Protect from light.

◊ References.


1. Kintzel PE, Smith GH. Practical guidelines for preparing and administering amphotericin B. *Am J Hosp Pharm* 1992; **49:** 1156–64.


**Formulation.** Conventional formulations of amphotericin B injection are typically a complex of amphotericin B and deoxycholate with suitable buffers which form a colloidal dispersion when reconstituted. Other formulations of amphotericin B for injection include liposomal amphotericin B, a colloidal dispersion of an amphotericin B and sodium cholesteryl sulfate complex, and a phospholipid complex.

**Incompatibility.** Because of the wide range of incompatibilities reported with conventional amphotericin B preparations, it is generally advisable not to mix them with any other drug. Most incompatibilities are caused by precipitation of amphotericin B due to a change in pH or by the disruption of the colloidal suspension. Precipitation can occur if amphotericin B is added to sodium chloride 0.9% or to electrolyte solutions.

Although heparin is generally reported to be compatible with conventional amphotericin B injection, care should be taken if heparin flush solutions, which are diluted with sodium chloride solution, are used to maintain the patency of intravenous lines in patients receiving amphotericin B. Flushing the intravenous line with 5% glucose solution has been suggested.

Mixtures of conventional amphotericin B in commercial lipid emulsions have been reported to be unstable,[1-3] although others have reported satisfactory stability.[4-6] In one study,[6] vigorous agitation of the mixtures enhanced their stability when compared with gentle mixing.


1. Ericsson O, *et al.* Amphotericin B is incompatible with lipid emulsions. *Ann Pharmacother* 1996; **30:** 298.
2. Ranchère JY, *et al.* Amphotericin B intralipid formulation: stability and particle size. *J Antimicrob Chemother* 1996; **37:** 1165–9.
3. Heide PE. Precipitation of amphotericin B from iv fat emulsion. *Am J Health-Syst Pharm* 1997; **54:** 1449.
4. Lopez RM, *et al.* Stability of amphotericin B in an extemporaneously prepared iv fat emulsion. *Am J Health-Syst Pharm* 1996; **53:** 2724–7.
5. Owens D, *et al.* Stability of amphotericin B 0.05 and 0.5 mg/mL in 20% fat emulsion. *Am J Health-Syst Pharm* 1997; **54:** 683–6.
6. Shadkhan Y, *et al.* The use of commercially available lipid emulsions for the preparation of amphotericin B-lipid admixtures. *J Antimicrob Chemother* 1997; **39:** 655–8. Correction. *ibid.* 1998; **42:** 413.


**Preparation of solutions for injection.** Conventional amphotericin B formulations for injection are prepared by reconstitution of amphotericin B with sterile water for injection without preservatives, then dilution with glucose injection 5% with a pH above 4.2 to the desired final concentration. Mixture with sodium chloride injection 0.9% would precipitate the amphotericin B.

**Stability of oral suspensions.** An oral suspension of amphotericin B 100 mg/mL, prepared from powder and a cherry-flavoured vehicle and maintained at pH 5.3, was found to be stable at 22 to 25° for 93 days.[1]


1. Dentinger PJ, *et al.* Stability of amphotericin B in an extemporaneously compounded oral suspension. *Am J Health-Syst Pharm* 2001; **58:** 1021–4.


### Adverse Effects

Amphotericin B for intravenous use was originally only available in a conventional colloidal form; liposomal and other formulations have been developed to reduce toxicity. The following adverse effects apply to the **conventional** form. Common adverse effects which occur during or following intravenous infusion of amphotericin B include headache, nausea, vomiting, chills, fever, malaise, muscle and joint pains, anorexia, diarrhoea, and gastrointestinal cramp. Hypertension, hypotension, cardiac arrhythmias including ventricular fibrillation and cardiac arrest, skin rashes, flushing, anaphylactoid reactions including bronchospasm and dyspnoea, blurred vision, tinnitus, hearing loss, vertigo, gastrointestinal bleeding, liver disorders, peripheral neuropathy, and convulsions have been reported occasionally.

Nephrotoxicity occurs in almost all patients receiving amphotericin B intravenously. Both tubular and glomerular damage occur; there may be improvement on cessation of therapy, but there is a risk of permanent renal impairment, particularly in patients receiving large cumulative doses (over 5 g). Renal tubular acidosis without systemic acidosis may develop. Use of amphotericin B is associated with increased urinary excretion of potassium and magnesium resulting in hypokalaemia and hypomagnesaemia respectively. Uric acid excretion is increased and nephrocalcinosis can occur. Limited data indicate that renal toxicity may be associated with sodium depletion; for strategies to improve sodium load see Nephrotoxicity, under Treatment of Adverse Effects, below.

A reversible, normocytic, normochromic anaemia develops in most patients receiving amphotericin B, possibly due to a direct suppressive effect on erythropoietin production. There are rare reports of thrombocytopenia, leucopenia, agranulocytosis, eosinophilia, and coagulation defects.

Leukoencephalopathy has been reported rarely in patients also receiving total body irradiation.

Solutions of amphotericin B irritate the venous endothelium and may cause pain and thrombophlebitis at the injection site. Extravasation may cause tissue damage.

After intrathecal injection amphotericin B may also cause irritation of the meninges, neuropathy with pain, impaired vision, and retention of urine.

Topical application may produce local irritation, pruritus, and skin rash.

In general, adverse effects of **nonconventional** amphotericin B have been similar to those of conventional amphotericin B, but are less frequent and less severe. Brief reversible episodes of renal impairment have been observed but nonconventional formulations have been considered to be safe enough to use in patients with renal impairment who could not be given conventional amphotericin B. Anaphylaxis has been reported rarely.

**Effects on the cardiovascular system.** Ventricular arrhythmias in 2 patients, resulting in fatal sudden cardiac arrest in 1, were associated with both conventional and liposomal formulations of amphotericin B at conventional doses and infusion rates,[1] but cardiac toxicity is more commonly associated with high doses or rapid infusion rates (see Infusion Rate, under Administration, below). Cardiac arrests in 5 infants and children, fatal in 4 cases, were associated[2] with overdoses of conventional amphotericin B of between 3.8 and 40.8 mg/kg. An increased risk of arrhythmia and cardiac arrest has been reported in patients with evidence of antimony-induced myocardial damage who were switched to amphotericin B treatment for visceral leishmaniasis.[3] A rest period of at least 10 days was advised before beginning amphotericin B in such patients.

Severe hypertension was associated with infusion of phospholipid-amphotericin B complex in 1 patient.[4]

1. Aguado JM, *et al.* Ventricular arrhythmias with conventional and liposomal amphotericin. *Lancet* 1993; **342:** 1239.
2. Cleary JD, *et al.* Amphotericin B overdose in pediatric patients with associated cardiac arrest. *Ann Pharmacother* 1993; **27:** 715–19.
3. Thakur CP. Sodium antimony gluconate, amphotericin, and myocardial damage. *Lancet* 1998; **351:** 1928–9.
4. Rowles DM, Fraser SL. Amphotericin B lipid complex (ABLC)-associated hypertension: case report and review. *Clin Infect Dis* 1999; **29:** 1564–5.

**Effects on the eyes.** Rapid loss of vision resulting in permanent bilateral blindness occurred in a patient with lupus erythematosus and cryptococcal meningitis after a 1-mg test dose of amphotericin B.[1] Amphotericin B was considered to be the cause as visual disturbances associated with cryptococcal meningitis are usually progressive in nature and acute blindness with normal funduscopic appearance had not previously been reported.

1. Li PKT, Lai KN. Amphotericin B induced ocular toxicity in cryptococcal meningitis. *Br J Ophthalmol* 1989; **73:** 397–8.

**Effects on the liver.** Amphotericin B has only rarely been associated with adverse effects on the liver. Fatal liver failure was reported in a patient after administration of a total dose of 4.82 g given intermittently over 1 year.[1] The patient had been given a potentially incompatible intravenous admixture of amphotericin B and diphenhydramine.

There have been a few reports of abnormal liver-function tests during amphotericin B therapy;[2,3] in such cases amphotericin B should be discontinued.

1. Carnecchia BM, Kurtzke JF. Fatal toxic reaction to amphotericin B in cryptococcal meningo-encephalitis. *Ann Intern Med* 1960; **53:** 1027–36.
2. Miller MA. Reversible hepatotoxicity related to amphotericin B. *Can Med Assoc J* 1984; **131:** 1245–7.
3. Abajo FJ, Carcas AJ. Amphotericin B hepatotoxicity. *BMJ* 1986; **293:** 1243.

**Effects on the lungs.** Reports implicating use of leucocytes[1] or other blood products[2] in the development of pulmonary reactions in patients receiving amphotericin B have been refuted,[3,4] and a report has indicated that amphotericin B can produce pulmonary toxicity in the absence of blood products.[5] An increased incidence of pulmonary symptoms was noted in patients receiving amphotericin B in lipid emulsion,[6] including acute respiratory distress after initiation of the infusion.

1. Wright DG, *et al.* Lethal pulmonary reactions associated with the combined use of amphotericin B and leukocyte transfusions. *N Engl J Med* 1981; **304:** 1185–9.
2. Haber RH, *et al.* Acute pulmonary decompensation due to amphotericin B in the absence of granulocyte transfusions. *N Engl J Med* 1986; **315:** 836.
3. Forman SJ, *et al.* Pulmonary reactions associated with amphotericin B and leukocyte transfusions. *N Engl J Med* 1981; **305:** 584–5.
4. Bow EJ, *et al.* Pulmonary complications in patients receiving granulocyte transfusions and amphotericin B. *Can Med Assoc J* 1984; **130:** 593–7.
5. Roncoroni AJ, *et al.* Bronchiolis obliterans possibly associated with amphotericin B. *J Infect Dis* 1990; **161:** 589.
6. Schöffski P, *et al.* Safety and toxicity of amphotericin B in glucose 5% or intralipid 20% in neutropenic patients with pneumonia or fever of unknown origin: randomised study. *BMJ* 1998; **317:** 379–84.

**Effects on potassium homoeostasis.** In addition to the hypokalaemia known to be associated with amphotericin B and due to increased urinary excretion of potassium, hyperkalaemia has been reported in a patient with severe renal impairment who received a rapid infusion of amphotericin B (see Infusion Rate, under Administration, below).

**Hypersensitivity.** Anaphylactoid reactions have occurred with conventional amphotericin B, but have also been associated with liposomal amphotericin B,[1,2] including a report in 2 patients who subsequently tolerated conventional formulations.[1]

1. Laing RBS, *et al.* Anaphylactic reactions to liposomal amphotericin. *Lancet* 1994; **344:** 682.
2. Torre I, *et al.* Anaphylactic reaction to liposomal amphotericin B in children. *Ann Pharmacother* 1996; **30:** 1036–7.

**Red man syndrome.** Red man syndrome (see Vancomycin, p.275) occurred in a patient on 2 occasions following a 1-mg test dose of amphotericin B.[1]

1. Ellis ME, Tharpe W. Red man syndrome associated with amphotericin B. *BMJ* 1990; **300:** 1468.

## Treatment of Adverse Effects

To reduce febrile reactions antipyretics and antihistamines may be given before the intravenous infusion of conventional amphotericin B. Hydrocortisone given intravenously before or during amphotericin B infusion may also reduce febrile reactions. However, corticosteroids should not be given indiscriminately to patients receiving amphotericin B (see Interactions, below) and dosage should be kept to a minimum. In the UK the advice is to give antipyretics or hydrocortisone prophylactically, but only to patients who have previously experienced acute adverse reactions and in whom continued treatment with intravenous amphotericin B is essential. Pethidine has been given intravenously to treat amphotericin B-induced shaking chills. Antiemetics may also be required. Amphotericin B is not removed by haemodialysis. Hypokalaemia and hypomagnesaemia should be corrected, and adequate hydration and sodium supplements may reduce the severity of renal impairment. Liposomal, phospholipid-complexed, or nonconventional colloidal amphotericin B can be substituted for conventional amphotericin B if the latter cannot be tolerated.

Heparin has been added to conventional amphotericin B infusions to reduce the incidence of thrombophlebitis.

**Anaemia.** Amphotericin B appears to produce a normochromic, normocytic anaemia by suppression of erythropoietin production.[1,2] Discontinuation of amphotericin B reverses the suppression but if the anaemia is severe, or treatment with amphotericin B cannot be stopped, blood transfusions may be required. Recombinant erythropoietin may prove an alternative to blood transfusions in patients who need to continue treatment with amphotericin B.

1. MacGregor RR, *et al.* Erythropoietin concentrations in amphotericin B-induced anemia. *Antimicrob Agents Chemother* 1978; **14:** 270–3.
2. Lin AC, *et al.* Amphotericin B blunts erythropoietin response to anemia. *J Infect Dis* 1990; **161:** 348–51.

**Electrolyte disturbances.** It has been suggested[1] that amiloride could ameliorate the hypokalaemia and hypomagnesaemia associated with amphotericin B. However, since amiloride may produce sodium depletion and its own associated renal toxicity this strategy is potentially hazardous. Another report[2] has suggested that spironolactone may be a safe and effective method of preventing hypokalaemia.

1. Wazny LD, Brophy DF. Amiloride for the prevention of amphotericin B-induced hypokalemia and hypomagnesemia. *Ann Pharmacother* 2000; **34:** 94–7.
2. Ural AU. Comment: spironolactone prevents amphotericin B-induced hypokalemia in neutropenic patients. *Ann Pharmacother* 2000; **34:** 1488.

**Nephrotoxicity.** A review of strategies for limiting the toxicity of amphotericin B concluded that sodium balance should be monitored and sodium replacement implemented if necessary and that, where possible, salt restriction and drugs which potentiate sodium loss or nephrotoxicity should be avoided.[1] Correction of sodium depletion may reverse amphotericin B-induced nephrotoxicity.[2] However, assessment of sodium status and correction of deficiency should precede amphotericin B administration.[3,4] Some have recommended supplementation with 150 mmol sodium for suitable patients.[4] However, routine prophylactic use of sodium is not advised.[5] A randomised study in a small number of patients has suggested that prophylactic sodium supplementation could be beneficial, but that it enhances potassium loss.[6] Diuretics in general should be avoided[7] although there have been suggestions that potassium-sparing diuretics such as amiloride or spironolactone may be useful in preventing hypokalaemia (see Electrolyte Disturbances, above). Use of mannitol as a protective agent is controversial and is not recommended.[3,4,8] Administration of amphotericin B on alternate days is widely practised although it has never been proven to reduce nephrotoxicity.[3,4]

More recently, liposomal, nonconventional colloidal, and phospholipid-complex formulations have been reported to overcome most problems of chronic nephrotoxicity, even in patients with renal impairment following previous treatment with conventional amphotericin B (see Alternative Formulations, under Administration, below).

1. Khoo SH, *et al.* Administering amphotericin B—a practical approach. *J Antimicrob Chemother* 1994; **33:** 203–13.
2. Heidemann HT, *et al.* Amphotericin B nephrotoxicity in humans decreased by salt repletion. *Am J Med* 1983; **75:** 476–81.
3. Warda J, Barriere SL. Amphotericin B nephrotoxicity. *Drug Intell Clin Pharm* 1985; **19:** 25–6.
4. Sabra R, Branch RA. Amphotericin B nephrotoxicity. *Drug Safety* 1990; **5:** 94–108.
5. Gardner ML, *et al.* Sodium loading treatment for amphotericin B-induced nephrotoxicity. *DICP Ann Pharmacother* 1990; **24:** 940–6.
6. Llanos A, *et al.* Effect of salt supplementation on amphotericin B nephrotoxicity. *Kidney Int* 1991; **40:** 302–8.
7. Fisher MA, *et al.* Risk factors for amphotericin B-associated nephrotoxicity. *Am J Med* 1989; **87:** 547–52.
8. Bullock WE, *et al.* Can mannitol reduce amphotericin B nephrotoxicity? Double-blind study and description of a new vascular lesion in kidneys. *Antimicrob Agents Chemother* 1976; **10:** 555–63.

**Prophylaxis.** The value of prophylaxis against generalised reactions to amphotericin B infusion was questioned after a retrospective study in 397 patients.[1] The most commonly used drugs were diphenhydramine, corticosteroids, paracetamol, and heparin. It was concluded that patients who had experienced an adverse reaction following amphotericin B should receive appropriate premedication before subsequent amphotericin B infusions, but that routine premedication was not justified.

1. Goodwin SD, *et al.* Pretreatment regimens for adverse events related to infusion of amphotericin B. *Clin Infect Dis* 1995; **20:** 755–61.

## Precautions

Although anaphylaxis is rare following intravenous amphotericin B, it is advisable to give a test dose and then to observe the patient carefully for about 30 minutes before starting treatment. Patients experiencing acute toxic reactions in whom treatment is essential may be given prophylactic treatment, as mentioned under Treatment of Adverse Effects, above, to ameliorate the reactions. To reduce the risk of vein irritation and infusion-related adverse effects, the rate of intravenous infusion of conventional amphotericin B should be slow (see Infusion Rate, under Administration, below). Patients receiving any parenteral form of amphotericin B should be monitored for changes in renal function, liver function, serum electrolytes, and haematological status. If the BUN or creatinine concentrations increase to clinically significant levels amphotericin B therapy should be interrupted or the dose reduced until renal function improves. Alternatively, a nonconventional amphotericin B preparation may be substituted. Treatment should be discontinued if liver function tests are abnormal. Acute pulmonary reactions have been noted in patients receiving amphotericin B during or shortly after leucocyte transfusions. Although the association is contested (see Effects on the Lungs, above), manufacturers of some amphotericin B products consider it advisable to separate administration and to monitor pulmonary function in these patients.

Care should be taken not to confuse the dosage regimens for individual preparations, and in particular those of conventional and nonconventional formulations.

**Pregnancy.** There are case reports of amphotericin B having been used successfully to treat fungal infections in pregnant women without any adverse effects on the infant.[1,2] A review[3] of the use of antifungal drugs in pregnancy concluded that parenteral amphotericin B was the drug of first choice in the treatment of serious fungal infections in pregnancy. The safety of the newer amphotericin formulations in pregnancy is not yet clear.

1. Ismail MA, Lerner SA. Disseminated blastomycosis in a pregnant woman. *Am Rev Respir Dis* 1982; **126:** 350–3.
2. Peterson CM, *et al.* Coccidiodal meningitis and pregnancy: a case report. *Obstet Gynecol* 1989; **73:** 835–6.
3. Sobel JD. Use of antifungal drugs in pregnancy: a focus on safety. *Drug Safety* 2000; **23:** 77–85.

## Interactions

Most interactions involving amphotericin B have been observed during treatment with conventional formulations. Since nonconventional formulations appear to be less toxic, it may be anticipated that they will produce fewer serious interactions.

Use of nephrotoxic antibacterials, ciclosporin or other nephrotoxic immunosuppressants, or parenteral pentamidine may lead to an increased risk of nephrotoxicity. If possible, amphotericin B should not be given to patients receiving antineoplastics. Diuretics should generally be avoided in patients taking amphotericin B. If a diuretic has to be given then volume and electrolyte depletion should be monitored carefully. The potassium-depleting effect of amphotericin B may enhance the effects of neuromuscular blocking drugs and may increase the toxicity of digitalis glycosides; corticosteroids may enhance the depletion of potassium and their immunosuppressive effects may be detrimental in patients with severe fungal infections.

Amphotericin B may increase the toxicity of flucytosine, but the combination is used in severe infections for its synergistic activity. For information on synergistic and antagonistic effects with other antimicrobials, see under Antimicrobial Action, below. Renal excretion of zalcitabine may be reduced by amphotericin B.

For an increased risk of cardiac arrhythmias and arrest when amphotericin B was given to patients with myocardial damage induced by an antimony compound, see Effects on the Cardiovascular System, under Adverse Effects, above.

## Antimicrobial Action

Amphotericin B is a polyene antifungal antibiotic which appears to act mainly by interfering with the permeability of the cell membrane of sensitive fungi by binding to sterols, chiefly ergosterol. It is reported to be fungistatic at concentrations achieved clinically. It is active against *Absidia* spp., *Aspergillus* spp., *Basidiobolus* spp., *Blastomyces dermatitidis, Candida* spp., *Coccidioides immitis, Conidiobolus* spp., *Cryptococcus neoformans, Histoplasma capsulatum, Mucor* spp., *Paracoccidioides brasiliensis, Rhizopus* spp., *Rhodotorula* spp., and *Sporothrix schenckii*. Other organisms that have been reported to be sensitive to amphotericin B include the algal *Prototheca* spp. and the protozoa *Leishmania* and *Naegleria* spp. It is inactive against bacteria (including rickettsia) and viruses.

Some resistant strains of *Candida* have been isolated from immunocompromised patients receiving prolonged treatment with amphotericin B.

**Microbiological interactions.** Until recently, assessment of antifungal activity has depended largely upon empirical observations based on clinical experience. The development of a standard *in-vitro* method of susceptibility testing should improve the comparability of test results obtained from different laboratories, but the correlation of *in-vitro* results with clinical outcome has still to be determined, especially in relation to drug combinations.[1]

*Azoles.* Although there have been occasional reports of synergy between amphotericin B and the azole antifungals,[2] greater emphasis has been placed on possible antagonism. Studies *in vitro* have supported theoretical concerns that the action of amphotericin B (which depends on binding to ergosterol in the fungal cell membrane) would be antagonised by azoles (which inhibit ergosterol synthesis).[3,4] *Animal* studies appear to have confirmed antagonism between amphotericin B and the imidazole ketoconazole, but not between amphotericin B and the triazoles fluconazole or itraconazole.[1] Available clinical evidence seems to indicate that azoles given concurrently, or as continuation therapy after induction therapy with amphotericin B, are effective in severe infections, although reduced plasma concentrations of itraconazole have been reported in some patients while receiving amphotericin B.[5] However, strains of *Candida albicans* resistant to both amphotericin B and fluconazole have emerged in patients who have received repeated or prolonged courses of fluconazole.[6,7]

*Flucytosine.* Despite the results of an *in-vitro* study which found antagonism between amphotericin B and flucytosine,[3] this combination is used clinically in severe systemic fungal infections and is generally considered to be synergistic.

*Rifamycins.* Studies *in vitro* have shown rifampicin[8] or rifabutin[9] to increase the antifungal activity of amphotericin B against various *Aspergillus* spp.[8,9] and *Fusarium*.[9]

*Tetracyclines.* Minocycline may enhance amphotericin B's activity against *Aspergillus* spp. *in vitro*.[10]

*Zidovudine.* Amphotericin B may inhibit the metabolism of zidovudine (see p.660).

1. Sugar AM. Use of amphotericin B with azole antifungal drugs: what are we doing? *Antimicrob Agents Chemother* 1995; **39:** 1907–12.
2. Smith D, *et al.* Effect of ketoconazole and amphotericin B on encapsulated and non-encapsulated strains of Cryptococcus neoformans. *Antimicrob Agents Chemother* 1983; **24:** 851–5.
3. Martin E, *et al.* Antagonistic effects of fluconazole and 5-fluorocytosine on candidacidal action of amphotericin B in human serum. *Antimicrob Agents Chemother* 1994; **38:** 1331–8.
4. Sud IJ, Feingold DS. Effect of ketoconazole on the fungicidal action of amphotericin B in Candida albicans. *Antimicrob Agents Chemother* 1983; **23:** 185–7.
5. Pennick GJ, *et al.* Concomitant therapy with amphotericin B and itraconazole: does this combination affect the serum concentration of itraconazole? *Intersci Conf Antimicrob Agents Chemother* 1994; **34:** 39 (A34).
6. Kelly SL, *et al.* Resistance to fluconazole and amphotericin in Candida albicans from AIDS patients. *Lancet* 1996; **348:** 1523–4.
7. Nolte FS, *et al.* Isolation and characterization of fluconazole- and amphotericin B-resistant Candida albicans from blood of two patients with leukemia. *Antimicrob Agents Chemother* 1997; **44:** 196–9.
8. Hughes CE, *et al.* In vitro activities of amphotericin B in combination with four antifungal agents and rifampin against Aspergillus spp. *Antimicrob Agents Chemother* 1984; **25:** 560–2.
9. Clancy CJ, *et al.* Inhibition of RNA synthesis as a therapeutic strategy against Aspergillus and Fusarium: demonstration of in vitro synergy between rifabutin and amphotericin B. *Antimicrob Agents Chemother* 1998; **42:** 509–13.
10. Hughes CE, *et al.* Enhancement of the in vitro activity of amphotericin B against Aspergillus spp. by tetracycline analogs. *Antimicrob Agents Chemother* 1984; **26:** 837–40.

## Pharmacokinetics

There is little or no absorption of amphotericin B from the gastrointestinal tract. When administered intravenously in the conventional colloidal form and in the usual increasing dosage regimens, peak plasma concentrations of 0.5 to 4 micrograms/mL have been reported; the average plasma concentration with maintenance doses of 400 to 600 micrograms/kg daily tends to be 500 nanograms/mL. Amphotericin B is reported to be highly bound to plasma proteins and is widely distributed, but passes into the CSF only in small quantities. The plasma half-life has been reported to be about 24 hours; with long-term administration the terminal half-life increases to 15 days.

Unchanged amphotericin B is excreted in small amounts slowly in the urine. Traces have been reported to be present in the serum and urine several weeks after completion of treatment. Amphotericin B is not removed by haemodialysis.

The pharmacokinetics of the nonconventional formulations differ considerably from the conventional formulation and from each other:

- at clinical doses of 1 to 7.5 mg/kg, *liposomal amphotericin B* produces peak plasma concentrations of around 8 to 80 micrograms/mL, around 20 times those with conventional formulations
- after doses of 0.5 to 8 mg/kg, an *amphotericin B-sodium cholesteryl sulfate complex* is reported to produce peak plasma concentrations of about 0.7 to 6.2 micrograms/mL
- at a dose of 5 mg/kg daily, *amphotericin B phospholipid complex* produces maximum plasma concentrations of about 1.7 micrograms/mL

Studies in *animals* have shown that concentrations in the kidney are several times lower following nonconventional formulations than with conventional ones.

**Children and neonates.** Serum-amphotericin B concentrations ranged from 0.78 to 10.02 micrograms/mL in 12 children (many with leukaemia) aged 4 months to 14 years following the intravenous infusion of conventional amphotericin B 0.25 to 1.5 mg/kg daily. Serum concentrations did not correlate with dose. The elimination half-life was 18.1 ± 6.65 hours. There was an inverse relationship between age and total clearance, suggesting that children older than 9 years may require lower doses.[1]

The pharmacokinetics of amphotericin B have also been studied in a group of 13 neonates with systemic fungal infections.[2] Conventional amphotericin B was infused over 4 to 6 hours every 24 hours. Ten of the infants started treatment with 100 micrograms/kg increased over 4 to 6 days to 500 micrograms/kg. Three infants were started on a dose of 800 to 1000 micrograms/kg reduced to 500 micrograms/kg daily. All infants were maintained on 500 micrograms/kg daily; total doses ranged from 17.3 to 28.6 mg/kg. Serum-amphotericin B concentrations were measured after the first dose in 3 infants in the first group and 2 in the second; no serum-amphotericin B could be detected in the 3 infants who had received 100 micrograms/kg. After 5 days' treatment peak serum-amphotericin B concentrations ranged from 0.5 to 4.0 micrograms/mL and this was considered to be the range that could be achieved with the daily maintenance dose of 500 micrograms/kg. The elimination half-life was 14.8 hours. Drug elimination between doses was not detected in 4 of the infants; one was in oliguric renal failure and the other 3 had developed increases in serum-creatinine concentrations. CSF-amphotericin B concentrations in 5 of the neonates ranged from 40 to 90% of simultaneous serum concentrations. It was considered that an initial dose of 500 micrograms/kg was well tolerated and could produce therapeutic serum concentrations more quickly than a regimen which consisted of 100 micrograms/kg on day one increased over 4 to 6 days to 500 micrograms/kg daily.

1. Benson JM, Nahata MC. Pharmacokinetics of amphotericin B in children. *Antimicrob Agents Chemother* 1989; **33:** 1989–93.
2. Baley JE, *et al.* Pharmacokinetics, outcome of treatment, and toxic effects of amphotericin B and 5-fluorocytosine in neonates. *J Pediatr* 1990; **116:** 791–7.

**Distribution.** Amphotericin B concentrations in various organs and tissues were determined in 13 cancer patients who had received conventional amphotericin B before death.[1] Concentrations were determined by high-pressure liquid chromatography (HPLC) and bioassay. Mean recovery by HPLC reported as a percentage of total dose given was liver 27.5%, spleen 5.2%, lungs 3.2%, kidney 1.5%, heart 0.4%, brain 0.3%, and pancreas 0.2%; each organ had a specific accumulation pattern. The mean total recovery was 38.8%. Reported median bile concentration was 7.3 micrograms/mL. The drug concentrations obtained by bioassay were much lower than those measured by HPLC. As the HPLC-determined concentrations of amphotericin B were higher than the MICs for the pathogens in patients with candidiasis or aspergillosis, the poor clinical outcome in these patients suggested that amphotericin B in the tissue lacked antifungal activity.

In another study,[2] amphotericin B was not detected in the CSF of 4 AIDS patients with cryptococcal meningitis on intravenous maintenance conventional doses of 350 to 1890 micrograms/kg given 1 to 7 times weekly. The clinical success of amphotericin B for this indication could not be explained by measurable CSF drug concentrations.

Concentrations of amphotericin B have been measured in fetal-cord serum in an infant and were 37.5% of maternal serum concentration.[3]

1. Collette N, *et al.* Tissue concentrations and bioactivity of amphotericin B in cancer patients treated with amphotericin B-deoxycholate. *Antimicrob Agents Chemother* 1989; **33:** 362–8.
2. Dugoni BM, *et al.* Amphotericin B concentrations in cerebrospinal fluid of patients with AIDS and cryptococcal meningitis. *Clin Pharm* 1989; **8:** 220–1.
3. Ismail MA, Lerner SA. Disseminated blastomycosis in a pregnant woman. *Am Rev Respir Dis* 1982; **126:** 350–3.

**Half-life.** The terminal half-life for amphotericin B was 15 days in 2 patients on completion of conventional amphotericin B infusion therapy for disseminated histoplasmosis.[1] In another study,[2] the half-life was 21.5 hours (based on the exponential phase of disappearance from the blood) in a 65-year-old patient on a maintenance conventional dose of 500 micrograms/kg infused over 1 hour every other day. Serum concentrations appeared to plateau at about 600 nanograms/mL 36 to 48 hours after each dose. This suggested that alternate-day administration might be effective.

1. Atkinson AJ, Bennett JE. Amphotericin B pharmacokinetics in humans. *Antimicrob Agents Chemother* 1978; **13:** 271–6.
2. Hoeprich PD. Elimination half-life of amphotericin B. *J Infect* 1990; **20:** 173–5.

**Non-conventional formulations.** References.

1. Janknegt R, *et al.* Liposomal and lipid formulations of amphotericin B: clinical pharmacokinetics. *Clin Pharmacokinet* 1992; **23:** 279–91.
2. Adedoyin A, *et al.* Pharmacokinetic profile of ABELCET (amphotericin B lipid complex injection): combined experience from phase I and phase II studies. *Antimicrob Agents Chemother* 1997; **41:** 2201–8.
3. Adedoyin A, *et al.* A pharmacokinetic study of amphotericin B lipid complex injection (Abelcet) in patients with definite or probable systemic fungal infections. *Antimicrob Agents Chemother* 2000; **44:** 2900–2.
4. Bekersky I, *et al.* Pharmacokinetics, excretion, and mass balance of liposomal amphotericin B (AmBisome) and amphotericin B deoxycholate in humans. *Antimicrob Agents Chemother* 2002; **46:** 828–33.

## Uses and Administration

Amphotericin B is a polyene antifungal antibiotic. It is reported to be fungistatic at concentrations achieved clinically. Amphotericin B is given by intravenous infusion in the treatment of severe *systemic* fungal infections including aspergillosis, blastomycosis, candidiasis, coccidioidomycosis, cryptococcosis, histoplasmosis, mucormycosis, paracoccidioidomycosis, and sporotrichosis, and is the usual treatment of choice in fungal endocarditis, meningitis, peritonitis, or severe respiratory-tract infections. Many of these infections are most likely to occur in immunocompromised patients. Amphotericin may be given in combination with flucytosine (p.399) in severe infections.

Amphotericin B is also used for the *local* treatment of superficial candidiasis. It is taken by mouth for intestinal candidiasis, sometimes as part of regimens for selective decontamination of the digestive tract in patients at special risk of infection, such as those in intensive care (see p.132).

The role of amphotericin B in the treatment of the above systemic and local infections is discussed under Choice of Antifungal, p.386.

Amphotericin B also has antiprotozoal activity. It is used for primary amoebic meningoencephalitis caused by *Naegleria* spp. and for the treatment of visceral and mucocutaneous leishmaniasis.

**Administration and dosage.** Amphotericin B is given by *intravenous* infusion conventionally as a colloidal complex with sodium deoxycholate. There is also a liposomal form and other complexes of amphotericin B available for use by infusion when conventional amphotericin B is contra-indicated because of toxicity, especially nephrotoxicity. Before starting therapy with any form of intravenous amphotericin B a test dose is usually advised and the patient observed carefully for about 30 minutes.

Details of intravenous administration and dosage vary according to the formulation being used. Therapy has sometimes continued for several months depending on the infection. Doses are expressed in terms of amphotericin B.

- *Conventional amphotericin B* (e.g. Fungizone, UK). After an initial test dose (1 mg infused over 20 to 30 minutes) treatment usually starts with a daily dose of 250 micrograms/kg, increased gradually to a maximum of 1 mg/kg daily; in seriously ill patients up to 1.5 mg/kg daily or on alternate days may be necessary. If treatment is stopped for longer than 7 days, it should be resumed at a dose of 250 micrograms/kg daily and increased gradually. The daily dose is infused over 2 to 4 hours at a concentration of 100 micrograms/mL in glucose 5%. Slower infusion, over up to 6 hours, may be necessary to reduce the incidence of acute toxic effects.
- *Liposomal amphotericin B* (e.g. AmBisome, UK). After an initial test dose (1 mg infused over 10 minutes), the usual dose is 1 mg/kg daily, increased gradually to 3 mg/kg if necessary. The daily dose is infused over 30 to 60 minutes at a concentration of 200 to 2000 micrograms/mL in glucose 5%.
- *Amphotericin B-sodium cholesteryl sulfate complex* (e.g. Amphocil, UK). After an initial test dose (2 mg infused over 10 minutes) the usual dose is 1 mg/kg daily, increased gradually to 3 to 4 mg/kg daily if necessary; doses of up to 6 mg/kg daily have been given. The daily dose is infused at a rate of 1 to 2 mg/kg per hour at a concentration of 625 micrograms/mL in glucose 5%.
- *Amphotericin B-phospholipid complex* (e.g. Abelcet, UK). After an initial test dose (1 mg infused over 15 minutes) the usual dose is 5 mg/kg daily. The daily dose is infused at a rate of 2.5 mg/kg per hour as a diluted suspension containing 1 mg/mL in glucose 5%.

Conventional amphotericin B may be given by *intrathecal* injection to patients with severe meningitis especially when intravenous therapy has been ineffective. Starting with 25 micrograms, the dose is gradually increased to the maximum that can be tolerated without excessive discomfort. The usual dosage is 0.25 to 1 mg given two to four times each week.

Amphotericin B is also used *orally* as 10-mg lozenges or as a suspension containing 100 mg/mL for oral or perioral candidiasis. The suspension is given in a dose of 1 mL four times daily; it should be retained in the mouth for as long as possible before swallowing. The lozenges are intended to be dissolved in the mouth and are given four times daily, increased to 8 lozenges daily if necessary. Doses of 100 to 200 mg are given four times daily by mouth as tablets or suspension to suppress intestinal *Candida*.

Amphotericin B has been given for candiduria by *continuous bladder irrigation* daily at a suggested concentration of 50 mg in 1000 mL of sterile water. Intermittent irrigation has also been tried.

Amphotericin B has also been administered into the lung by nebulised solution, into the eye topically or by subconjunctival or intravitreal injection, to the skin by topical application, into body cavities by instillation, and into joint spaces by intra-articular injection.

**Administration.** ALTERNATIVE FORMULATIONS. A number of lipid formulations of amphotericin B have been developed in an attempt to minimise renal toxicity and acute toxic reactions. Three lipid-based formulations of amphotericin B available commercially in some countries are: liposomes (e.g. AmBisome);[1] a lipid complex with L-α-dimyristoylphosphatidylcholine and L-α-dimyristoylphosphatidylglycerol (e.g. Abelcet); and a colloidal dispersion with sodium cholesteryl sulfate (e.g. Amphocil). The aim of reducing renal toxicity has largely been achieved, and in some cases patients unable to tolerate conventional amphotericin B have subsequently been successfully treated with one of the lipid-based formulations. Experience with these formulations suggests that they also produce fewer acute toxic reactions. Clinical studies with these formulations are generally encouraging,[2-4] but they differ in their pharmacokinetics and dosage and there are few formal comparisons of their efficacy.[5]

Conventional amphotericin B dispersed in lipid emulsions (such as Intralipid) has been tried as a less expensive alternative to these commercial formulations.[6] However, such dispersions require vigorous mixing to incorporate the amphotericin B into the lipid phase and several have been shown to be unstable (see Incompatibility, above). While some clinical successes have been achieved, reduced renal toxicity or improved tolerability have not been convincingly demonstrated. There is currently insufficient evidence to recommend their use.[7]

Other novel formulations under investigation include an aggregated form produced by heating conventional amphotericin B injection,[8] a lipid nanosphere-encapsulated form (NS-718),[9,10] and a conjugate with the polysaccharide arabinogalactan.[11]


1. Barnes RA, *et al.*, eds. AmBisome: an international workshop. *J Antimicrob Chemother* 2002; **49** (suppl S1): 1–86.
2. Coukell AJ, Brogden RN. Liposomal amphotericin B: therapeutic use in the management of fungal infections and visceral leishmaniasis. *Drugs* 1998; **55:** 585–612.
3. Brogden RN, *et al.* Amphotericin-B colloidal dispersion: a review of its use against systemic fungal infections and visceral leishmaniasis. *Drugs* 1998; **56:** 365–83.
4. Johansen HK, Gøtzsche PC. Amphotericin B lipid soluble formulations versus amphotericin B in cancer patients with neutropenia. Available in The Cochrane Library; Issue 2. Chichester: John Wiley; 2004.
5. Robinson RF, Nahata MC. A comparative review of conventional and lipid formulations of amphotericin B. *J Clin Pharm Ther* 1999; **24:** 249–57.
6. Cleary JD. Amphotericin B formulated in a lipid emulsion. *Ann Pharmacother* 1996; **30:** 409–12.
7. Sievers TM, *et al.* Safety and efficacy of Intralipid emulsions of amphotericin B. *J Antimicrob Chemother* 1996; **38:** 333–47.
8. Petit C, *et al.* Activity of a heat-induced reformulation of amphotericin B deoxycholate (Fungizone) against Leishmania donovani. *Antimicrob Agents Chemother* 1999; **43:** 390–2.
9. Hossain MA, *et al.* Efficacy of NS-718, a novel lipid nanosphere-encapsulated amphotericin B, against Cryptococcus neoformans. *Antimicrob Agents Chemother* 1998; **42:** 1722–5.
10. Hossain MA, *et al.* Attenuation of nephrotoxicity by a novel lipid nanosphere (NS-718) incorporating amphotericin B. *J Antimicrob Chemother* 2000; **46:** 263–8.
11. Falk R, *et al.* A novel injectable water-soluble amphotericin B-arabinogalactan conjugate. *Antimicrob Agents Chemother* 1999; **43:** 1975–81.


INFUSION RATE. Conventional amphotericin B is usually given by intravenous infusion over 2 to 6 hours. A long infusion time is inconvenient for outpatients and often impractical in patients receiving other intravenous medications. This may be overcome by using one of the nonconventional formulations that can be infused over 30 to 120 minutes. Shorter infusion times have been tried with conventional amphotericin B with varying results. In small numbers of patients without pre-existing renal impairment, rapid infusion over 1 hour was generally no more toxic than infusion over 4 hours in two studies,[1,2] whereas another[3] found infusion over 45 minutes to be more toxic than a 4-hour infusion during the first 5 to 7 days of treatment. Cardiac toxicity reported in patients receiving rapid infusions includes atrial fibrillation in a patient with pre-existing cardiac disease,[2] ventricular fibrillation associated with hyperkalaemia in a patient with severe renal impairment,[4] and bradycardia[5] and dilated cardiomyopathy[6] in patients without apparent risk factors. Ventricular dysrhythmias were not observed in 27 patients with adequate renal function.[7] In general, there is not sufficient evidence to justify reducing infusion times for conventional amphotericin B to below 2 hours.

Conversely, continuous administration of amphotericin B over 24 hours has resulted in fewer adverse effects and a significant reduction in nephrotoxicity compared with infusion over 4 hours.[8]


1. Oldfield EC, *et al.* Randomized, double-blind trial of 1- versus 4-hour amphotericin B infusion durations. *Antimicrob Agents Chemother* 1990; **34:** 1402–6.
2. Cruz JM, *et al.* Rapid intravenous infusion of amphotericin B: a pilot study. *Am J Med* 1992; **93:** 123–30.
3. Ellis ME, *et al.* Double-blind randomized study of the effect of infusion rates on toxicity of amphotericin B. *Antimicrob Agents Chemother* 1992; **36:** 172–9.
4. Craven PC, Gremillion DH. Risk factors of ventricular fibrillation during rapid amphotericin B infusion. *Antimicrob Agents Chemother* 1985; **27:** 868–71.
5. Soler JA, *et al.* Bradycardia after rapid intravenous infusion of amphotericin B. *Lancet* 1993; **341:** 372–3.
6. Arswa EL, *et al.* Amphotericin B-induced dilated cardiomyopathy. *Am J Med* 1994; **97:** 560–2.
7. Bowler WA, *et al.* Risk of ventricular dysrhythmias during 1-hour infusions of amphotericin B in patients with preserved renal function. *Antimicrob Agents Chemother* 1992; **36:** 2542–3.
8. Eriksson U, *et al.* Comparison of effects of amphotericin B deoxycholate infused over 4 or 24 hours: randomised controlled trial. *BMJ* 2001; **322:** 579–82.


**Administration in neonates.** Although the most appropriate dose of lipid formulations of amphotericin B for low-birth-weight preterm infants has yet to be firmly established reports suggest that it may be safe and effective at doses similar to those used in adults, relative to body weight.[1-3]


1. Scarcella A, *et al.* Liposomal amphotericin B treatment for neonatal fungal infections. *Pediatr Infect Dis J* 1998; **17:** 146–8.
2. Weitkamp J-H, *et al.* Candida infection in very low birth-weight infants: outcome and nephrotoxicity of treatment with liposomal amphotericin B (AmBisome). *Infection* 1998; **26:** 11–15.
3. Walsh TJ, *et al.* Amphotericin B lipid complex in pediatric patients with invasive fungal infections. *Pediatr Infect Dis J* 1999; **18:** 702–8.


**Leishmaniasis.** The treatment of visceral and mucocutaneous leishmaniasis including the use of amphotericin B is described on p.597.

VISCERAL LEISHMANIASIS. Evidence of declining responsiveness to pentavalent antimonials has led to the evaluation of intravenous amphotericin B as an alternative for first-line therapy. WHO has included liposomal amphotericin B 3 mg/kg daily on each of 5 consecutive days and a sixth dose 6 days later among the regimens suggested for first-line therapy of Mediterranean visceral leishmaniasis in immunocompetent patients.[1] Similar doses are recommended by the manufacturers, who recommend 3 mg/kg for 5 days with further doses on days 14 and 21. Amphotericin B is also being evaluated in other parts of the world. In India, conventional amphotericin B in modest doses (500 micrograms/kg on alternate days) produced good responses both in patients unresponsive to antimonials[2,3] and as first-line therapy.[4] Experience with a higher dose of 1 mg/kg daily for 20 days achieved a 99% cure rate in 938 patients.[5] Liposomal amphotericin B 2 mg/kg daily on 3, 5 or 7 days over a 10-day period all produced clinical cures and minimal toxicity,[6] as did 5 mg/kg as a single infusion or as once-daily infusions of 1 mg/kg for 5 days.[7] Amphotericin B lipid complex 1, 2, or 3 mg/kg daily for 5 days,[8] or 5 mg/kg given once or twice (5 days apart),[9] has been used successfully although relapses occurred in some patients taking the lower doses in these latter studies. In Brazil, colloidal amphotericin B with sodium cholesteryl sulfate in a dose of 2 mg/kg daily for 5 days produced cures in 10 patients although 1 subsequently relapsed.[10] A study by WHO[11] suggested that more intensive courses of treatment may be needed in Brazil compared with India and Kenya. Responses to liposomal amphotericin B were reported to be slower in immunocompromised patients, and relapses occurred in 8 of 11 patients despite treatment with liposomal amphotericin B 1.38 to 1.85 mg/kg daily for 21 days.[12] Increasing the dose to 4 mg/kg daily given on 10 days over a 38-day period did not improve the long-term outcome, although initial responses were good[13] and this regimen is now that recommended by the manufacturers. Conventional amphotericin B mixed with a commercial fat emulsion preparation has been tried as a less expensive alternative to the newer formulations and was found to be effective and well tolerated when given in a dose of 2 mg/kg on alternate days for 5 doses.[14] However, there are doubts about such formulation (see Administration, above).

MUCOCUTANEOUS LEISHMANIASIS. Amphotericin B is used in mucocutaneous leishmaniasis unresponsive to antimonials. Successful treatment with liposomal amphotericin B has been reported.[15]


1. Gradoni L, *et al.* Treatment of Mediterranean visceral leishmaniasis. *Bull WHO* 1995; **73:** 191–7.
2. Giri OP. Amphotericin B therapy in kala-azar. *J Indian Med Assoc* 1993; **91:** 91–3.
3. Mishra M, *et al.* Amphotericin versus pentamidine in antimony-unresponsive kala-azar. *Lancet* 1992; **340:** 1256–7.
4. Mishra M, *et al.* Amphotericin versus sodium stibogluconate in first-line treatment of Indian kala-azar. *Lancet* 1994; **344:** 1599–1600.
5. Thakur CP, *et al.* Amphotericin B deoxycholate treatment of visceral leishmaniasis with newer modes of administration and precautions: a study of 938 cases. *Trans R Soc Trop Med Hyg* 1999; **93:** 319–23.
6. Thakur CP, *et al.* Comparison of three treatment regimens with liposomal amphotericin B (AmBisome) for visceral leishmaniasis in India: a randomized dose-finding study. *Trans R Soc Trop Med Hyg* 1996; **90:** 319–22.
7. Sundar S, *et al.* Treatment of Indian visceral leishmaniasis with single or daily infusions of low dose liposomal amphotericin B: randomised trial. *BMJ* 2001; **323:** 419–22.
8. Sundar S, *et al.* Short-course, low-dose amphotericin B lipid complex therapy for visceral leishmaniasis unresponsive to antimony. *Ann Intern Med* 1997; **127:** 133–7.
9. Sundar S, *et al.* Treatment of antimony-unresponsive Indian visceral leishmaniasis with ultra-short courses of amphotericin-B-lipid complex. *Ann Trop Med Parasitol* 1998; **92:** 755–64.
10. Dietze R, *et al.* Treatment of kala-azar in Brazil with Amphocil (amphotericin B cholesterol dispersion) for 5 days. *Trans R Soc Trop Med Hyg* 1995; **89:** 309–11.
11. Berman JD, *et al.* Efficacy and safety of liposomal amphotericin B (AmBisome) for visceral leishmaniasis in endemic developing countries. *Bull WHO* 1998; **76:** 25–32.
12. Davidson RN, *et al.* Liposomal amphotericin B (AmBisome) in Mediterranean visceral leishmaniasis: a multi-centre trial. *Q J Med* 1994; **87:** 75–81.
13. Russo R, *et al.* Visceral leishmaniasis in HIV infected patients: treatment with high dose liposomal amphotericin B (AmBisome). *J Infect* 1996; **32:** 133–7.
14. Sundar S, *et al.* Short-course, cost-effective treatment with amphotericin B-fat emulsion cures visceral leishmaniasis. *Trans R Soc Trop Med Hyg* 2000; **94:** 200–4.
15. Sampaio RNR, Marsden PD. Mucosal leishmaniasis unresponsive to glucantime therapy successfully treated with AmBisome. *Trans R Soc Trop Med Hyg* 1997; **91:** 77.


**Primary amoebic meningoencephalitis.** Although amphotericin B is active *in vitro* against *Naegleria fowleri* and has been recommended for the treatment of primary amoebic meningoencephalitis (p.595) caused by this amoeba, there have been few reports of survival after its use. One patient who survived was treated with intravenous and intrathecal amphotericin B.[1] Another survivor received both amphotericin B and miconazole by the intravenous and intrathecal routes, and rifampicin and sulfafurazole by mouth.[2] In a third, aggressive therapy with intravenous and intrathecal amphotericin B together with high-dose oral rifampicin was successful.[3] A fourth patient received a combination of intravenous, subarachnoid, and intrathecal administration of amphotericin B.[4]


1. Anderson K, Jamieson A. Primary amoebic meningoencephalitis. *Lancet* 1972; **i:** 902–3.
2. Seidel JS, *et al.* Successful treatment of primary amebic meningoencephalitis. *N Engl J Med* 1982; **306:** 346–8.
3. Brown RL. Successful treatment of primary amebic meningoencephalitis. *Arch Intern Med* 1991; **151:** 1201–2.
4. Loschiavo F, *et al.* Acute primary meningoencephalitis from entamoeba Naegleria fowleri: report of a clinical case with a favourable outcome. *Acta Neurol (Napoli)* 1993; **15:** 333–40.

### Preparations

**BP 2003:** Amphotericin Lozenges; Amphotericin Oral Suspension;
**USP 27:** Amphotericin B Cream; Amphotericin B for Injection; Amphotericin B Lotion; Amphotericin B Ointment.

**Proprietary Preparations** (details are given in Part 3)
***Arg.:*** Abelcet; AmBisome; Amfostat; Amphotec; ***Austral.:*** Abelcet; AmBisome; Amphocil; Fungilin; Fungizone; ***Austria:*** Abelcet; AmBisome; Ampho-Moronal; Amphocil; ***Belg.:*** Abelcet; AmBisome†; Fungizone; ***Braz.:*** Abelcet; AmBisome†; Amphocil; Anforicin B; Fungi B; Fungizon; ***Canad.:*** Abelcet; AmBisome; Fungizone; ***Chile:*** Fungizon; ***Denm.:*** Abelcet; AmBisome; Amphocil†; Fungilin; ***Fin.:*** Abelcet; AmBisome; Fungizone; ***Fr.:*** Abelcet; AmBisome; Fungizone; ***Ger.:*** AmBisome; Ampho-Moronal; ***Gr.:*** Abelcet; Ambisome; Amphocil; Fungizone; ***Hong Kong:*** Abelcet†; AmBisome; Amphocil; Fungilin†; Fungizone; ***India:*** Fungizone; ***Irl.:*** Abelcet; AmBisome; Amphocil; Fungizone; ***Israel:*** AmBisome; Amphocil; Fungilin; Fungizone; ***Ital.:*** Abelcet; AmBisome; Amphocil†; Fungilin; Fungizone; ***Malaysia:*** Amphocil; Fungizone; ***Mex.:*** Amfostat; Amphocil; Candipres†; ***Neth.:*** AmBisome; Amphocil†; Fungizone; ***Norw.:*** Abelcet; AmBisome; Fungizone; ***NZ:*** AmBisome; Fungilin; Fungizone; ***Port.:*** Abelcet; Amphocil†; ***S.Afr.:*** Fungizone; ***Singapore:*** Abelcet; Amphocil; Fungizone; ***Spain:*** Abelcet; AmBisome; Amphocil; Funganiline; Fungizona; ***Swed.:*** Abelcet; AmBisome; Amphocil†; Fungizone; ***Switz.:*** Abelcet; AmBisome; Ampho-Moronal; Fungizone; ***Thai.:*** AmBisome; Fungizone; ***UK:*** Abelcet; AmBisome; Amphocil; Fungilin; Fungizone; ***USA:*** Abelcet; AmBisome; Amphotec; Fungizone.

**Multi-ingredient:** ***Austria:*** Mysteclin; ***Braz.:*** Anfoterin; Gino-Teracin; Talsutin; Tericin AT; Vagiklin; ***Chile:*** Talseclin; ***Fr.:*** Amphocycline; ***Ger.:*** Ampho-Moronal V L†; Ampho-Moronal V†; Mysteclin; ***Hong Kong:*** Talsutin; ***Ital.:*** Anfocort; ***Malaysia:*** Talsutin; ***S.Afr.:*** Vagmycin; ***Spain:*** Gine Heyden; Sanicel; Trigon Topico.

## Anidulafungin *(USAN, rINN)*

LY-303366; V-Echinocandin. (4*R*,5*R*)-4,5-Dihydroxy-$N^2$-{[4″-(pentyloxy)-*p*-terphenyl-4-yl]carbonyl}-L-ornithyl-L-threonyl-*trans*-4-hydroxy-L-prolyl-(*S*)-4-hydroxy-4-(*p*-hydroxyphenyl)-L-threonyl-L-threonyl-(3*S*,4*S*)-3-hydroxy-4-methyl-L-proline cyclic (6→1)-peptide; 1-((4*R*,5*R*)-4,5-Dihydroxy-$N^2$-{[4″-(pentyloxy)(1,1′:4′,1″-terphenyl)-4-yl]carbonyl}-L-ornithine)-echinocandin B.

$C_{58}H_{73}N_7O_{17}$ = 1140.2.
*CAS — 166663-25-8.*

### Profile

Anidulafungin is an antifungal under investigation for the treatment of candidiasis and aspergillosis.

## Bifonazole *(BAN, USAN, rINN)*

Bay-h-4502; Bifonazol; Bifonazolum. 1-(α-Biphenyl-4-ylbenzyl)imidazole.

$C_{22}H_{18}N_2$ = 310.4.
*CAS — 60628-96-8.*
*ATC — D01AC10.*

**Pharmacopoeias.** In *Chin., Eur.* (see p.vi), and *Jpn.*

**Ph. Eur. 5.0** (Bifonazole). A white or almost white crystalline powder. It exhibits polymorphism. Practically insoluble in water; sparingly soluble in dehydrated alcohol.

### Profile

Bifonazole is an imidazole antifungal with a broad spectrum of activity; sensitive fungi include dermatophytes, *Malassezia furfur*, and *Candida* spp. It also has antibacterial activity *in vitro* against some Gram-positive cocci.

Bifonazole is mainly used by topical application in the treatment of fungal skin and nail infections (p.390). It is applied once daily as a 1% cream, powder, solution, or gel. Treatment is usually continued for 2 to 4 weeks. More prolonged treatment is necessary for nail infections and bifonazole may be applied initially with a 40% urea paste to soften the nail.

Local reactions including burning and itching have been reported.

For a discussion of the caution needed when using azole antifungals during pregnancy, see under Pregnancy in Precautions of Fluconazole, p.398.

◊ Reviews.

1. Lackner TE, Clissold SP. Bifonazole: a review of its antimicrobial activity and therapeutic use in superficial mycoses. *Drugs* 1989; **38:** 204–25.

### Preparations

**Proprietary Preparations** (details are given in Part 3)
***Arg.:*** Bifonal; Bimicot; Micosol; Mycospor; ***Austral.:*** Canesten Once Daily; Mycospor; ***Austria:*** Fungiderm; ***Belg.:*** Mycospor; ***Braz.:*** Mycospor; ***Chile:*** Biocitronil; Micotopic; Multifung; Mycosporan; ***Denm.:*** Mycospor†; ***Fr.:*** Amycor; ***Ger.:*** Bifomyk; Bifon; Canesten Extra; Mycospor; ***Gr.:*** Bifized; Bifon; Fungiderm; Myco-flusemidon; Mycospor; Rye; ***Hong Kong:*** Mycospor; ***Israel:*** Agispor; ***Ital.:*** Azolmen; Bifazol; ***Mex.:*** Mycospor; ***Neth.:*** Mycospor; ***Norw.:*** Mycospor†; ***Port.:*** Mycospor; Topical†; ***S.Afr.:*** Mycospor; ***Spain:*** Bifokey; Levelina; Moldina; Monostop†; Mycospor; ***Swed.:*** Mycosporan; ***Thai.:*** Mycospor†; ***UK:*** Canesten AF Once Daily.

**Multi-ingredient:** ***Arg.:*** Prurisedan Antimicotico; ***Austria:*** Fungiderm comp; ***Chile:*** Mycosporan Onycoset; ***Denm.:*** Mycospor Carbamid†; ***Fr.:*** Amycor Onychoset; ***Ger.:*** Mycospor Nagelset; ***Israel:*** Agispor Onychoset; Comagis; Keratospor; ***Mex.:*** Mycospor Onicoset; ***Norw.:*** Mycospor Carbamid†; ***Port.:*** Mycospor; ***Spain:*** Mycospor Onicoset; ***Swed.:*** Mycosporan Karbamid†.

## Bromochlorosalicylanilide

Bromoclorosalicilanilida. 5-Bromo-4′-chlorosalicylanilide; 5-Bromo-*N*-(4-chlorophenyl)-2-hydroxybenzamide.

$C_{13}H_9BrClNO_2$ = 326.6.
*ATC — D01AE01.*

### Profile

Bromochlorosalicylanilide is a bromsalan antifungal that has been applied topically. Photosensitivity may occur. See also Bromsalans, p.1171.

### Preparations

**Proprietary Preparations** (details are given in Part 3)
***Austria:*** Multifungin.

**Multi-ingredient:** ***Austria:*** Multifungin; ***India:*** Multifungin; Multifungin H.

## Buclosamide *(BAN, rINN)*

Buclosamida. *N*-Butyl-4-chlorosalicylamide; *N*-Butyl-4-chloro-2-hydroxybenzamide.

$C_{11}H_{14}ClNO_2$ = 227.7.
*CAS — 575-74-6.*

### Profile

Buclosamide is an antifungal that has been applied topically in association with salicylic acid in the treatment of fungal skin infections. Photosensitivity has occurred.

### Preparations

**Proprietary Preparations** (details are given in Part 3)
**Multi-ingredient:** ***Braz.:*** Jadit†.

## Butenafine Hydrochloride *(BANM, USAN, rINNM)*

Hidrocloruro de butenafina; KP-363. *N*-(*p*-*tert*-Butylbenzyl)-*N*-methyl-1-naphthalenemethylamine hydrochloride; 4-*tert*-Butylbenzyl(methyl)(1-naphthalenemethyl)amine hydrochloride.

$C_{23}H_{27}N,HCl$ = 353.9.
*CAS — 101828-21-1 (butenafine); 101827-46-7 (butenafine hydrochloride).*
*ATC — D01AE23.*

### Profile

Butenafine is a benzylamine antifungal with actions similar to those of the allylamine antifungal terbinafine (p.408). The hydrochloride is used topically as a 1% cream for the treatment of superficial dermatophyte infections (p.390).

◊ Reviews.

1. McNeely W, Spencer CM. Butenafine. *Drugs* 1998; **55:** 405–12.

### Preparations

**Proprietary Preparations** (details are given in Part 3)
***Arg.:*** Buticrem; ***Braz.:*** Mentax†; ***Canad.:*** Scholl Athlete's Foot; ***Israel:*** Mentax; ***Jpn:*** Mentax; ***USA:*** Lotrimin Ultra; Mentax.

## Butoconazole Nitrate *(BANM, USAN, rINNM)*

Nitrato de butoconazol; RS-35887; RS-35887-00-10-3. 1-[4-(4-Chlorophenyl)-2-(2,6-dichlorophenylthio)butyl]imidazole mononitrate.

$C_{19}H_{17}Cl_3N_2S,HNO_3$ = 474.8.
*CAS — 64872-76-0 (butoconazole); 64872-77-1 (butoconazole nitrate).*
*ATC — G01AF15.*

**Pharmacopoeias.** In *US.*

**USP 27** (Butoconazole Nitrate). A white to off-white crystalline powder. Practically insoluble in water; slightly soluble in acetone, in acetonitrile, in dichloromethane, and in tetrahydrofuran; very slightly soluble in ethyl acetate; sparingly soluble in methyl alcohol. Protect from light.

### Adverse Effects and Precautions

Local reactions including burning and irritation may occur when butoconazole is applied vaginally.

Intravaginal preparations of butoconazole may damage latex contraceptives and additional contraceptive measures are therefore necessary during local administration.

For a discussion of the caution needed when using azole antifungals during pregnancy, see under Pregnancy in Precautions of Fluconazole, p.398.

**Effects on the blood.** Severe reversible thrombocytopenia was associated with treatment with intravaginal butoconazole.[1] The patient had previously experienced a drop in white cell count following treatment with intravaginal clotrimazole, suggestive of an idiosyncratic reaction to imidazoles.

1. Maloley PA, *et al.* Severe reversible thrombocytopenia resulting from butoconazole cream. *DICP Ann Pharmacother* 1990; **24:** 143–4.

### Antimicrobial Action

Butoconazole is an imidazole antifungal with antimicrobial activity similar to that of ketoconazole (p.404) including activity against *Candida* spp.

### Pharmacokinetics

Approximately 5% of a dose of butoconazole is absorbed following vaginal administration. The plasma half-life is 21 to 24 hours.

### Uses and Administration

Butoconazole nitrate is an imidazole antifungal used locally in the treatment of vulvovaginal candidiasis (p.386). It is administered intravaginally as a 100-mg pessary or as 5 g of a 2% cream for 3 consecutive nights; a single application of the cream has also been used.

### Preparations

**USP 27:** Butoconazole Nitrate Vaginal Cream.

**Proprietary Preparations** (details are given in Part 3)
***Belg.:*** Gynomyk; ***Fr.:*** Gynomyk; ***Mex.:*** Femstal†; ***Neth.:*** Gynomyk; ***USA:*** Femstat†; Gynazole; Mycelex-3.

## Candicidin *(BAN, USAN, rINN)*

Candicidina; NSC-94219.
*CAS — 1403-17-4.*
*ATC — G01AA04.*

### Profile

Candicidin is a mixture of antifungal heptaenes produced by *Streptomyces griseus*. It has been used in the treatment of vaginal candidiasis.

## Caspofungin Acetate *(BANM, USAN, rINNM)*

Acetato de caspofungina; L-743873; MK-0991. (4*R*,5*S*)-5-[(2-Aminoethyl)amino]-$N^2$-(10,12-dimethyltetradecanoyl)-4-hydroxy-L-ornithyl-L-threonyl-*trans*-4-hydroxy-L-prolyl-(*S*)-4-hydroxy-4-(*p*-hydroxyphenyl)-L-threonyl-*threo*-3-hydroxy-L-ornithyl-*trans*-3-hydroxy-L-proline cyclic (6→1)-peptide diacetate.

$C_{52}H_{88}N_{10}O_{15},2C_2H_4O_2$ = 1213.4.
*CAS — 179463-17-3.*
*ATC — J02AX04.*

### Adverse Effects and Precautions

Adverse experiences reported with caspofungin have included nausea and vomiting, flushing, fever, and venous complications around the infusion site. Possible histamine-mediated symptoms have been rash, facial swelling, pruritus, or sensation of warmth. Anaphylaxis has occurred.

Caspofungin may need to be given in reduced doses to patients with hepatic impairment.

### Interactions

Caspofungin concentrations may be reduced if it is administered with other drugs that can increase its clearance. Such effects have been noted with carbamazepine, dexamethasone, efavirenz, nelfinavir, nevirapine, phenytoin, and rifampicin, and an increase in the dose of caspofungin to 70 mg daily should be considered in patients who are also taking these drugs and who are not clinically responding.

When caspofungin has been given with ciclosporin, an increase in the area under the concentration-time curve for caspofungin, as well as increases in hepatic enzymes, were observed and use of the two drugs together is not recommended.

Caspofungin has resulted in decreased blood concentrations of tacrolimus and therapeutic drug monitoring and appropriate dosage adjustments to tacrolimus are recommended.

### Pharmacokinetics

Plasma concentrations of caspofungin decline in a polyphasic manner following intravenous infusion. The initial short α-phase occurs immediately post-infusion and is followed by a β-phase with a half-life of 9 to 11 hours; an additional longer γ-phase also occurs with a half-life of 40 to 50 hours. Plasma clearance is dependent on distribution rather than on biotransformation or excretion. There is slow metabolism of caspofungin by hydrolysis and *N*-acetylation and excretion in faeces and urine.

### Uses and Administration

Caspofungin is an antifungal used in the treatment of invasive aspergillosis (p.386) in patients who are refractory to, or intolerant of, other therapy. It is also used in the treatment of invasive candidiasis in non-neutropenic patients. It acts by inhibiting the synthesis of β-(1,3)-D-glucan, an essential component of the cell wall of susceptible filamentous fungi.

Caspofungin is used as the acetate but doses are expressed in terms of the base; 77.7 mg of caspofungin acetate is equivalent to 70 mg of caspofungin. It is given by slow intravenous infusion over about 1 hour. A loading dose of 70 mg is given on the first day and is followed by 50 mg daily or 70 mg daily in patients weighing more than 80 kg. Doses may need to be reduced in patients with hepatic impairment (see below).

◊ Reviews.

1. Letscher-Bru V, Herbrecht R. Caspofungin: the first representative of a new antifungal class. *J Antimicrob Chemother* 2003; **51:** 513–21.
2. Deresinski SC, Stevens DA. Caspofungin. *Clin Infect Dis* 2003; **36:** 1445–57.
3. Keating GM, Figgitt DP. Caspofungin: a review of its use in oesophageal candidiasis, invasive candidiasis and invasive aspergillosis. *Drugs* 2003; **63:** 2235–63.

**Administration in hepatic impairment.** Patients with mild hepatic impairment do not require dosage adjustment. In patients with moderate hepatic impairment, a daily dose of caspofungin 35 mg should be used after the initial dose of 70 mg; appropriate doses for patients with severe hepatic impairment have not been established.

#### Preparations

**Proprietary Preparations** (details are given in Part 3)
***Arg.:*** Cancidas; ***Austral.:*** Cancidas; ***Chile:*** Cancidas; ***Hong Kong:*** Cancidas; ***NZ:*** Cancidas; ***Singapore:*** Cancidas; ***UK:*** Cancidas; ***USA:*** Cancidas.

## Chlormidazole Hydrochloride *(BANM, rINNM)*

Clomidazole Hydrochloride; Hidrocloruro de clormidazol. 1-(4-Chlorobenzyl)-2-methylbenzimidazole hydrochloride.
$C_{15}H_{13}ClN_2,HCl$ = 293.2.
*CAS — 3689-76-7 (chlormidazole); 54118-67-1 (chlormidazole hydrochloride).*

#### Profile

Chlormidazole hydrochloride is an imidazole antifungal used topically in the treatment of fungal infections of the skin.

For a discussion of the caution needed when using azole antifungals during pregnancy, see under Pregnancy in Precautions of Fluconazole, p.398.

#### Preparations

**Proprietary Preparations** (details are given in Part 3)

**Multi-ingredient:** ***Austria:*** Myco-Synalar; ***Spain:*** Myco-Synalar†; ***Switz.:*** Myco-Synalar.

## Chlorphenesin *(BAN, pINN)*

Clorfenesina. 3-(4-Chlorophenoxy)propane-1,2-diol.
$C_9H_{11}ClO_3$ = 202.6.
*CAS — 104-29-0.*
*ATC — D01AE07.*

#### Profile

Chlorphenesin has antifungal and antibacterial properties. It is applied locally in mild uncomplicated dermatophyte and other cutaneous infections and in vaginal infections.

Chlorphenesin carbamate (p.1392) is used as a skeletal muscle relaxant.

#### Preparations

**Proprietary Preparations** (details are given in Part 3)
***Austral.:*** Nappy Rash Powder†; ***Austria:*** Adermykon†; ***Canad.:*** Mycil; ***Ger.:*** Soorphenesin.

**Multi-ingredient:** ***Austral.:*** ZSC; ***Austria:*** Aleot; ***Braz.:*** Adermykon-C†; Oto Betnovate; ***Canad.:*** Anivy†.

## Ciclopirox *(BAN, USAN, rINN)*

Ciclopiroxum; Hoe-296b. 6-Cyclohexyl-1-hydroxy-4-methyl-2-pyridone.
$C_{12}H_{17}NO_2$ = 207.3.
*CAS — 29342-05-0.*
*ATC — D01AE14; G01AX12.*

**Pharmacopoeias.** In *Eur.* (see p.vi) and *US.*

**Ph. Eur. 5.0** (Ciclopirox). A white or yellowish-white, crystalline powder. Slightly soluble in water; freely soluble in alcohol and in dichloromethane. Protect from light.

**USP 27** (Ciclopirox). A white to slightly yellowish white, crystalline powder. Slightly soluble in water; freely soluble in dehydrated alcohol and in dichloromethane; soluble in ether. Store at a temperature of 15° to 30°. Protect from light.

## Ciclopirox Olamine *(BANM, USAN, rINNM)*

Ciclopirox olamina; Ciclopiroxolamine; Hoe-296. The 2-aminoethanol salt of 6-Cyclohexyl-1-hydroxy-4-methyl-2-pyridone.
$C_{12}H_{17}NO_2,C_2H_7NO$ = 268.4.
*CAS — 41621-49-2.*
*ATC — D01AE14; G01AX12.*

**Pharmacopoeias.** In *Chin., Eur.* (see p.vi), and *US.*

**Ph. Eur. 5.0** (Ciclopirox Olamine). A white or pale yellow crystalline powder. It exhibits polymorphism. Slightly soluble in water; very soluble in alcohol and in dichloromethane; slightly soluble in ethyl acetate; practically insoluble in cyclohexane. A 1% solution in water has a pH of 8.0 to 9.0. Protect from light.

**USP 27** (Ciclopirox Olamine). A white to slightly yellowish-white, crystalline powder. Slightly soluble in water; very soluble in alcohol and in dichloromethane; practically insoluble in cyclohexane. pH of a 1% solution in water is between 8.0 and 9.0. Store in airtight containers at a temperature of 5° to 25°. Protect from light.

#### Adverse Effects

Irritation and pruritus have been reported after topical application of ciclopirox.

#### Antimicrobial Action

Ciclopirox has a wide spectrum of antifungal activity. It inhibits most *Candida, Epidermophyton, Microsporum,* and *Trichophyton* spp. and is also active against *Malassezia furfur.* It has some antibacterial activity.

#### Uses and Administration

Ciclopirox is an antifungal which is applied topically in the treatment of fungal skin and nail infections, including cutaneous candidiasis (p.386), dermatophytosis, pityriasis versicolor (p.390), and seborrhoeic dermatitis (p.1138). It has also been used in the treatment of vaginal candidiasis.

It is applied twice daily for skin infections, as a cream, gel, lotion, solution, or powder; both the base and the olamine salt have been used, with products containing the equivalent of 0.77% ciclopirox base.

A lacquer containing 8% ciclopirox base is applied once daily for nail infections.

◊ References.

1. Jue SG, *et al.* Ciclopirox olamine 1% cream: a preliminary review of its antimicrobial activity and therapeutic use. *Drugs* 1985; **29:** 330–41.
2. Gupta AK, *et al.* Ciclopirox nail lacquer topical solution 8% in the treatment of toenail onychomycosis. *J Am Acad Dermatol* 2000; **43** (suppl 4): S70–S80.
3. Dupuy P, *et al.* Randomized, placebo-controlled, double-blind study on clinical efficacy of ciclopiroxolamine 1% cream in facial seborrhoeic dermatitis. *Br J Dermatol* 2001; **144:** 1033–7.

#### Preparations

***USP 27:*** Ciclopirox Olamine Cream; Ciclopirox Olamine Topical Suspension.

**Proprietary Preparations** (details are given in Part 3)
***Arg.:*** Dermaflor; Loprox; Micopirox; ***Austria:*** Batrafen; ***Braz.:*** Fungirox; Gino Loprox; Loprox; Micoliv; Stiprox; ***Canad.:*** Loprox; ***Chile:*** Batrafen; Fungopirox; Mikium; Stiprox; ***Denm.:*** Mycofen; ***Fr.:*** Mycosquam; Mycoster; Stiprox; ***Ger.:*** Batrafen; Inimur Myko; Nagel Batrafen; Sebiprox; ***Gr.:*** Candimyc; Neo-botacreme; Neo-mycodermol; ***Hong Kong:*** Batrafen; ***India:*** Olamin; ***Irl.:*** Batrafen; Stieprox; ***Israel:*** Batrafen; Cicloderm; ***Ital.:*** Batrafen; Biroxol; Brumixol; Dafnegin; Miclast; Micomicen; Micoxolamina; Stiprox; ***Mex.:*** Loprox; Stiprox; ***Neth.:*** Loprox; ***NZ:*** Batrafen; ***Port.:*** Mycoster; ***Singapore:*** Stieprox; ***Spain:*** Aquomin†; Batrafen; Ciclochem; Fungowas; Rimafungol; Sebiprox; ***Switz.:*** Batrafen; Dafnegil Neo; ***Thai.:*** Cicloderm; Loprox; Stieprox; ***UK:*** Oilatum Shampoo; ***USA:*** Loprox; Penlac.

**Multi-ingredient:** ***Fr.:*** Stiproxal; ***India:*** Flucort-C; ***Israel:*** Cicloderm-C.

## Climbazole *(BAN, rINN)*

Bay-e-6975; MEB-6401. 1-(p-Chlorophenoxy)-1-imidazol-1-yl-3,3-dimethyl-2-butanone.
$C_{15}H_{17}ClN_2O_2$ = 292.8.
*CAS — 38083-17-9.*

#### Profile

Climbazole is an azole antifungal included in preparations for the topical treatment of seborrhoeic dermatitis.

For a discussion of the caution needed when using azole antifungals during pregnancy, see under Pregnancy in Precautions of Fluconazole, p.398.

#### Preparations

**Proprietary Preparations** (details are given in Part 3)
***Mon.:*** Hegor Climbazole.

**Multi-ingredient:** ***Arg.:*** Mencogrin; Micocert; ***Fr.:*** Item Alphazole; Node DS; Node P; Sebosquam†; ***Port.:*** Alphazole; Efluvium Anti-caspa.

## Clodantoin *(BAN, rINN)*

Chlordantoin *(USAN)*; Clodantoína. 5-(1-Ethylpentyl)-3-(trichloromethylthio)hydantoin; 5-(1-Ethylpentyl)-3-(trichloromethylthio)imidazolidine-2,4-dione.
$C_{11}H_{17}Cl_3N_2O_2S$ = 347.7.
*CAS — 5588-20-5.*
*ATC — G01AX01.*

#### Profile

Clodantoin is an antifungal that has been included in preparations used locally for vulvovaginal infections.

## Clotrimazole *(BAN, USAN, rINN)*

Bay-5097; Clotrimazol; Clotrimazolum; FB-5097. 1-(α-2-Chlorotrityl)imidazole.
$C_{22}H_{17}ClN_2$ = 344.8.
*CAS — 23593-75-1.*
*ATC — A01AB18; D01AC01; G01AF02.*

NOTE. Compounded preparations of clotrimazole may be represented by the following names:

- Co-climasone *(PEN)*—clotrimazole and betamethasone dipropionate.

**Pharmacopoeias.** In *Chin., Eur.* (see p.vi), *Jpn, Pol.,* and *US.*

**Ph. Eur. 5.0** (Clotrimazole). A white or pale yellow crystalline powder. Practically insoluble in water; soluble in alcohol and in dichloromethane. Protect from light.

**USP 27** (Clotrimazole). A white to pale yellow, crystalline powder. Practically insoluble in water; freely soluble in alcohol, in acetone, in chloroform, and in methyl alcohol. Store in airtight containers.

### Adverse Effects and Precautions

Gastrointestinal disturbance, elevation of liver enzymes, dysuria, and mental depression have been reported after administration of clotrimazole by mouth. Local reactions including irritation and a burning sensation may occur in patients treated topically; contact allergic dermatitis has been reported.

Intravaginal preparations of clotrimazole may damage latex contraceptives and additional contraceptive measures are therefore necessary during local administration. For a discussion of the caution needed when using azole antifungals during pregnancy, see under Pregnancy in Precautions of Fluconazole, p.398.

### Antimicrobial Action

Clotrimazole is an imidazole antifungal with antimicrobial activity similar to that of ketoconazole (p.404).

### Pharmacokinetics

When applied topically clotrimazole penetrates the epidermis but there is little if any systemic absorption. Absorption of 3 to 10% of a dose has been reported following vaginal administration. Clotrimazole is metabolised in the liver to inactive compounds and excreted in the faeces and urine.

### Uses and Administration

Clotrimazole is an imidazole antifungal used topically in superficial candidiasis (p.386), and in the skin infections pityriasis versicolor and dermatophytosis (p.390). Topical preparations containing an imidazole such as clotrimazole, ketoconazole, or miconazole, usually together with hydrocortisone, are used in the management of seborrhoeic dermatitis (see p.1138). Clotrimazole may also be used occasionally for symptomatic relief of the protozoal infection trichomoniasis when other drugs are contra-indicated (see p.599).

Clotrimazole is applied topically two or three times daily for 2 to 4 weeks as a 1% cream, lotion, or solution in the treatment of fungal skin infections; a 1% powder may be used in conjunction with the cream or solution and has been applied to prevent re-infection. The 1% solution is also used topically for fungal otitis externa. Clotrimazole is given as pessaries in dosage regimens of 100 mg for 6 days, 200 mg for 3 days, or a single dose of 500 mg in the treatment of vulvovaginal candidiasis; similar doses are given as a 1, 2, or 10% vaginal cream. It may be necessary to treat balanitis in male partners concurrently.

Lozenges of clotrimazole 10 mg are dissolved in the mouth for treatment or prophylaxis of oral candidiasis and may be used five times daily for 14 days. Clotrimazole has also been given by mouth but has now been largely superseded by other azole drugs.

**Sickle-cell disease.** Oral clotrimazole has been investigated[1] in the treatment of sickle-cell disease (p.734).

1. Brugnara C, *et al.* Therapy with oral clotrimazole induces inhibition of the Gardos channel and reduction of erythrocyte dehydration in patients with sickle cell disease. *J Clin Invest* 1996; **97:** 1227–34.

### Preparations

***BP 2003:*** Clotrimazole Cream; Clotrimazole Pessaries;
***USP 27:*** Clotrimazole and Betamethasone Dipropionate Cream; Clotrimazole Cream; Clotrimazole Lotion; Clotrimazole Lozenges; Clotrimazole Topical Solution; Clotrimazole Vaginal Tablets.

**Proprietary Preparations** (details are given in Part 3)
***Arg.:*** Empecid; Ikolan; Klomazole; Livomonil; Medifungol; Micomazol; Micomazol Deo; Micotrim; Panmicol; ***Austral.:*** Canesten; Chemists Own Clozole; Clofeme; Clonea; Clotreme; Clozole†; Gyne-Lotrimin; Hiderm†; Tinaderm Extra; ***Austria:*** Candibene; Canesten; Myko Cordes; Pedikurol; ***Belg.:*** Canestene; Gyno-Canestene; ***Braz.:*** Canesten; Clogen†; Clomazen; Clonasten†; Clotren; Clotrimix; Clotrizan; Dermobene; Gino Clotrimix; Gino-Canesten; Kinasten; Miclonazol; Micosten; Micotrat; Micotrizol†; Neo Clotrimazyl; Tricosten†; ***Canad.:*** Canesten; Clotrimaderm; Myclo-Derm†; Myclo-Gyne†; Neo-Zol; ***Chile:*** Arnela; Axasol; Canesten; Cestop; Clotrimin; Cotrisan; Creminem; Funzal; Gynocanesten; Konifungil; Laboterol; Novacetol; Telugren; ***Denm.:*** Canazol†; Canesten; ***Fin.:*** Canesten; Klotricid†; ***Ger.:*** Antifungol; Antimyk†; Apocanda†; Aru C; Azutrimazol; Benzoderm Myco; Candazol; Canesten; Canifug; Cloderm; Clotri OPT†; Clotrifug†; Clotrigalen; cutistad; Dignotrimazol†; durafungol; Fungiderm; Fungizid; Gilt; Gyno-Canesten; Holfungin; Jenamazol; Kade-Fungin; Lokalicid†; Mycofug; Mycohaug C†; Myko Cordes; Mykofungin; Mykohaug; Ovis Neu; Pedisafe†; Radikal†; SD-Hermal; Uromykol; ***Gr.:*** Canesten; Factodin; ***Hong Kong:*** Canesten; Clocreme; Clotri-Denk; Clozole; Cotren; Fungizid; Gyne-Lotremin; Lotremin; Mycoril; Tricloderm; Warimazol; ***India:*** Imidil; Mycocid; Mycoderm-C; Surfaz; ***Irl.:*** Canesten; ***Israel:*** Agisten; Baby Agisten; Clotrimaderm; Myco-Hermal; Oralten Troche; ***Ital.:*** Antimicotico; Canesten; Gyno-Canesten; ***Malaysia:*** Candazole; Canesten; Cotren; Gyne-Lotremin; Loriderm; Lotremin; Trimazol; ***Mex.:*** Baycuten; Candimon; Canesten†; Cinabel†; Dermasten; Lonestin; Lotrimin; ***Neth.:*** Canesten; ***Norw.:*** Canesten; Fungisten†; ***NZ:*** Canesten; Clocreme; Clotrihexal; Clotrimaderm; Fungizid†; ***Port.:*** Candid; Canesten; Diomicete; Gino-Canesten; Gino-Lotremine; Lotremine; Pan-Fungex; ***S.Afr.:*** A-Por; Canalba; Candaspor; Candizole; Canesten; Canex; Clomaderm†; Closcript; Covospor; Dynaspor†; Gynezol†; Gyno-Trimaze; Medaspor; Micomisan; Mycoban; Mycohexal; Normospor; Trimaze; Xeraspor; ***Singapore:*** Candazole; Canesten; Clozole†; Cotren; Cristan; Gyne-Lotremin; Lotremin; Myco-Hermal; Mycoril; Sastid Anti-Fungal; Vanesten; ***Spain:*** Canesten; Fungidermo; Gine Canesten; Ictan†; ***Swed.:*** Canesten; ***Switz.:*** Acnecolor; Canestene; Clocim†; Corisol; cutis-

tad†; Eurosan; Fungotox; Gromazol; Gyno-Canestene; Imazol; Undex; **Thai.:** Caginal; Canadine; Canazol; Candid; Candinox; Canesten; Chingazol; Clotri; Clotricin; Comat; Cotren; CST; Defungo; Fungicon; Fungiderm; Gynebo; Klamacin; Mycozole; Nestic; Taraten; Vamazole; Vanesten; **UK:** Abtrim; Athletes Foot Cream†; Candiden; Canesten; Canesten Combi; Fungederm; Masnoderm†; Medisport Athlete's Foot†; Mycil Gold†; Privacom; **USA:** Fungoid†; Gyne-Lotrimin; Lotrimin; Lotrimin AF; Mycelex; Mycelex-7; Mycelex-G†.

**Multi-ingredient: Arg.:** Becortin; Cortispec; Dermovit; Empecid Cort; Lotricomb; Micomazol B; Quadriderm CD; Quiacort G Plus; Vagarne; Vagisan Compuesto; Vitacortil; **Austral.:** Hydrozole; **Austria:** Myko Cordes; **Belg.:** Lotriderm; **Braz.:** Baycuten; Floregin Composto†; **Canad.:** Lotriderm; **Chile:** B-Laboterol; Baycuten; Cestop B; Clotrimin-B; Creminem-B; Cutanil; Donomix; Locrim; Lotriderm; Novadrel; Novamela; Telugren Plus; Tribesona; **Denm.:** Clotrason; **Ger.:** Baycuten; Canesten HC; Fungidexan; Imazol; Imazol comp; Lotricomb; Myko Cordes Plus; **Hong Kong:** Canesten HC; Clotrinolon; Lozopin; Synco-CFN; Triderm; **India:** Cloben-G; Clomycin; Sofradex-F; Surfaz; Surfaz-SN; **Irl.:** Canesten HC; Lotriderm; **Israel:** Hydroagisten; Polycutan; Tevacutan; Triderm; **Ital.:** Desamix Effe; Meclon; **Malaysia:** Baycuten N; Candacort; Dermal C; Triderm-C; **Mex.:** Baycuten N; Gelmicin; Miclobet; Quadriderm NF; Triderm; **NZ:** Lotricomb; **Port.:** Baycuten; Flotiran; Quadriderme; **S.Afr.:** Lotriderm; **Singapore:** Canesten HC; Clotrasone; Combiderm; Gentrisone; Neoderm; Triderm; **Spain:** Beta Micoter; Clotrasone; **Switz.:** Imacort; Imazol; Triderm; **Thai.:** Canasone; Canazol-BE; Clotrasone; Derzid-C; Fungiderm-B; Gynesten-B; Gynestin; Twina; **UK:** Canesten HC; Lotriderm†; **USA:** Lotrisone.

## Cloxiquine *(rINN)*

Cloxyquin *(USAN)*. 5-Chloroquinolin-8-ol.

$C_9H_6ClNO$ = 179.6.

*CAS — 130-16-5.*

### Profile

Cloxiquine has been included in preparations used topically for the treatment of fungal and bacterial skin infections.

### Preparations

**Proprietary Preparations** (details are given in Part 3)

**Multi-ingredient: Austria:** Decoderm trivalent; **Spain:** Decoderm Trivalente†; **Thai.:** Supracortin 3.

## Copper Naphthenate

Naftenato de cobre.

*CAS — 1338-02-9.*

### Profile

Copper naphthenate is a topical antifungal that has been used in veterinary medicine.

## Croconazole Hydrochloride *(rINNM)*

Cloconazole Hydrochloride; Hidrocloruro de croconazol; 710674-S (croconazole). 1-(1-{*o*-[(*m*-Chlorobenzyl)oxy]phenyl}vinyl)imidazole hydrochloride.

$C_{18}H_{15}ClN_2O,HCl$ = 347.2.

*CAS — 77175-51-0 (croconazole).*

**Pharmacopoeias.** In *Jpn.*

### Profile

Croconazole hydrochloride is an imidazole antifungal used topically in the treatment of superficial cutaneous candidiasis, dermatophytosis, and pityriasis versicolor.

For a discussion of the caution needed when using azole antifungals during pregnancy, see under Pregnancy in Precautions of Fluconazole, p.398.

### Preparations

**Proprietary Preparations** (details are given in Part 3)

**Austria:** Pilzcin; **Ger.:** Pilzcin; **Jpn:** Pilzcin.

## Eberconazole *(rINN)*

Eberconazol; WAS-2160. (±)-1-(2,4-Dichloro-10,11-dihydro-5*H*-dibenzo[*a*,*d*]cyclohepten-5-yl)imidazole.

$C_{18}H_{14}Cl_2N_2$ = 329.2.

*CAS — 128326-82-9.*

### Profile

Eberconazole is an imidazole antifungal under investigation for the topical treatment of superficial fungal skin infections.

# Econazole *(BAN, USAN, rINN)*

Econazolum; SQ 13050. 1-[2,4-Dichloro-β-(4-chlorobenzyloxy)phenethyl]imidazole.

$C_{18}H_{15}Cl_3N_2O$ = 381.7.

*CAS — 27220-47-9.*

*ATC — D01AC03; G01AF05.*

**Pharmacopoeias.** In *Eur.* (see p.vi).

**Ph. Eur. 5.0** (Econazole). A white or almost white powder. M.p. 88° to 92°. Practically insoluble in water; very soluble in alcohol and in dichloromethane. Protect from light.

## Econazole Nitrate *(BANM, USAN, rINNM)*

C-C2470; Econazoli Nitras; Nitrato de econazol; R-14827; SQ-13050. (±)-1-[2,4-Dichloro-β-(4-chlorobenzyloxy)phenethyl]imidazole nitrate.

$C_{18}H_{15}Cl_3N_2O,HNO_3$ = 444.7.

*CAS — 24169-02-6 (econazole nitrate); 68797-31-9 ((±)-econazole nitrate).*

*ATC — D01AC03; G01AF05.*

**Pharmacopoeias.** In *Chin., Eur.* (see p.vi), and *US.*

**Ph. Eur. 5.0** (Econazole Nitrate). A white or almost white crystalline powder. Very slightly soluble in water; slightly soluble in alcohol; sparingly soluble in dichloromethane; soluble in methyl alcohol. Protect from light.

**USP 27** (Econazole Nitrate). A white or practically white, crystalline powder, with not more than a slight odour. Very slightly soluble in water and in ether; slightly soluble in alcohol; sparingly soluble in chloroform; soluble in methyl alcohol. Protect from light.

### Adverse Effects and Precautions

Local reactions including burning and irritation may occur when econazole nitrate is applied topically. Contact dermatitis has been reported rarely.

Intravaginal preparations of econazole may damage latex contraceptives and additional contraceptive measures are therefore necessary during local administration.

For a discussion of the caution needed when using azole antifungals during pregnancy, see under Pregnancy in Precautions of Fluconazole, p.398.

**Porphyria.** Econazole nitrate has been associated with acute attacks of porphyria and is considered unsafe in porphyric patients.

### Antimicrobial Action

Econazole is an imidazole antifungal with antimicrobial activity similar to that of ketoconazole (p.404).

### Pharmacokinetics

Absorption is not significant when econazole nitrate is applied to the skin or vagina.

### Uses and Administration

Econazole is an imidazole antifungal used topically in the treatment of superficial candidiasis (see p.386) and in dermatophytosis and pityriasis versicolor (see Skin Infections, p.390).

Econazole nitrate is applied topically up to 3 times daily as a 1% cream, lotion, powder, or solution in the treatment of fungal skin infections. Treatment is continued for 2 to 4 weeks. It is also used in the treatment of vaginal candidiasis as pessaries of 150 mg once daily at bedtime for 3 consecutive nights; a single dose of 150 mg in a long-acting formulation has also been used. Intravaginal administration of 5 g of a 1% cream once daily at night has been given for 2 weeks. A 1% cream may be used concurrently for the treatment of vulval infections or for the treatment of balanitis in a male partner.

In the treatment of fungal infections of the nails, a 1% cream or lotion is applied once daily and covered with an occlusive dressing.

Econazole nitrate has also been used as eye or ear drops.

Econazole sulfosalicylate has also been used.

### Preparations

**BP 2003:** Econazole Cream; Econazole Pessaries.

**Proprietary Preparations** (details are given in Part 3)

**Arg.:** Micocide; Micofitex; Micolis; Novo Paramicon; Sinamida Econazol; **Austral.:** Dermazole; Ecostatin†; Pevaryl; **Austria:** Gyno-Pevaryl; Pevalip†; Pevaryl; **Belg.:** Gyno-Pevaryl; Pevaryl; **Braz.:** Dermazol; Limpele†; Micostyl; **Canad.:** Ecostatin; **Chile:** Micolis; **Denm.:** Pevaryl; **Fin.:** Pevaryl; **Fr.:** Dermazol; Fongeryl; Gyno-Pevaryl; Mycoapaisyl; Pevaryl; **Ger.:** Epi-Pevaryl; Epi-Pevaryl Pv; Gyno-Pevaryl; **Gr.:** Bismultin; Mycobacter; Pevaryl; **Hong Kong:** Dermazole; Gyno-Pevaryl; Heads Shampoo; Pevaryl; **India:** Ecanol; **Irl.:** Ecostatin; Gyno-Pevaryl; Pevaryl; **Israel:** Gyno-Pevaryl; Pevaryl; **Ital.:** Amicel†; Chemionazolo; Eccelium; Eco Mi; Ecodergin; Ecorex; Ecosteril; Ganazolo; Ifenec; Micogin†; Micos; Pargin†; Pevaryl; Polinazolo; **Malaysia:** Ecoderm; Gyno-Pevaryl; Pevaryl; Zoliderm; **Mex.:** Micostyl; Pevaryl; **Neth.:** Pevaryl; **Norw.:** Pevaryl; **NZ:** Dermazole; Ecostatin†; Ecreme; Gyno-Pevaryl; Pevaryl; **Port.:** Gyno-Pevaryl; Pevaryl; **S.Afr.:** Gyno-Pevaryl; Pevaryl; **Singapore:** Dermazole; Ecoderm†; Gyno-Pevaryl; Pevaryl; **Spain:** Ecotam; Etramon†; Gyno-Pevaryl; Micoespec; Pevaryl; **Swed.:** Pevaryl; **Switz.:** Gyno-Pevaryl; Pevaryl; Sebolith; **Thai.:** Econ; **UK:** Ecostatin; Gyno-Pevaryl; Pevaryl; **USA:** Spectazole.

**Multi-ingredient: Arg.:** Filoderma Plus; Griseocrem; Griseoplus; Novo Bacticort Complex; **Austria:** Pevaryl; Pevisone; **Belg.:** Pevisone; **Denm.:** Pevisone; **Fin.:** Pevisone; **Fr.:** Pevisone; **Ger.:** Epi-Pevaryl Heilpaste; Epipevisone; **Gr.:** Pevison; **Hong Kong:** Pevisone; **India:** Cobederm-H; Ecodax; **Israel:** Pevisone; **Ital.:** Pevisone; **Malaysia:** Ecocort; Econazine; Pevisone; **Norw.:** Pevisone; **Port.:** Pevisone; **S.Afr.:** Pevisone; **Singapore:** Ecocort; Econazine; Pevisone; **Swed.:** Pevisone; **Switz.:** Pevaryl; Pevisone; **Thai.:** Ecoderm; Pevisone; **UK:** Econacort; Pevaryl TC†.

## Enilconazole *(BAN, USAN, rINN)*

Enilconazol; Enilconazolum; R-23979. (±)-1-(β-Allyloxy-2,4-dichlorophenethyl)imidazole.

$C_{14}H_{14}Cl_2N_2O$ = 297.2.

*CAS — 35554-44-0.*

**Pharmacopoeias.** In *Eur.* (see p.vi) for veterinary use only.

**Ph. Eur. 5.0** (Enilconazole for Veterinary Use). A clear, yellowish, oily liquid or solid mass. Very slightly soluble in water; freely soluble in alcohol, in methyl alcohol, and in toluene. Store in airtight containers. Protect from light.

### Profile

Enilconazole is an imidazole antifungal used topically in veterinary medicine for the treatment of fungal skin infections in cattle, horses, and dogs. It is also used by inhalation for the treatment of aspergillosis in ostriches.

## Fenticlor *(BAN, USAN, rINN)*

D-25; Fenticloro; HL-1050; NSC-4112; Ph-549; S-7. 2,2′-Thiobis(4-chlorophenol).

$C_{12}H_8Cl_2O_2S$ = 287.2.

*CAS — 97-24-5.*

### Profile

Fenticlor is an antifungal that has been applied topically in the treatment of dermatophyte infections.

Photosensitivity reactions have been reported.

### Preparations

**Proprietary Preparations** (details are given in Part 3)

**Multi-ingredient: Spain:** Dermisdin.

# Fenticonazole Nitrate *(BANM, USAN, rINNM)*

Fenticonazoli Nitras; Nitrato de fenticonazol; Rec-15/1476. (±)-1-[2,4-Dichloro-β-{[*p*-(phenylthio)benzyl]oxy}phenethyl]imidazole mononitrate.

$C_{24}H_{20}Cl_2N_2OS,HNO_3$ = 518.4.

*CAS — 72479-26-6 (fenticonazole); 73151-29-8 (fenticonazole nitrate).*

*ATC — D01AC12; G01AF12.*

**Pharmacopoeias.** In *Eur.* (see p.vi).

**Ph. Eur. 5.0** (Fenticonazole Nitrate). A white or almost white, crystalline powder. Practically insoluble in water; sparingly soluble in dehydrated alcohol; freely soluble in dimethylformamide and in methyl alcohol. Protect from light.

### Adverse Effects and Precautions

Burning and itching have been reported following the application of fenticonazole nitrate.

Intravaginal preparations of fenticonazole may damage latex contraceptives and additional contraceptive measures are therefore necessary during local administration.

For a discussion of the caution needed when using azole antifungals during pregnancy, see under Pregnancy in Precautions of Fluconazole, p.398.

### Antimicrobial Action

Fenticonazole is an imidazole antifungal active against a range of organisms including dermatophyte pathogens, *Malassezia furfur,* and *Candida albicans.*

### Uses and Administration

Fenticonazole nitrate is an imidazole antifungal used locally in the treatment of vulvovaginal candidiasis (p.386). A 200-mg pessary is inserted into the vagina at bedtime for 3 nights or a 600-mg pessary is inserted once only at bedtime. Fenticonazole nitrate is also applied topically as a 2% cream or solution for the treatment of fungal skin infections.

### Preparations

**Proprietary Preparations** (details are given in Part 3)

**Arg.:** Lomexin; **Austria:** Fenizolan†; Lomexin; **Braz.:** Fentizol; Lomexin; **Fr.:** Lomexin; Terlomexin; **Ger.:** Fenizolan; Lomexin; **Gr.:** Lomexin; **Ital.:** Falvin; Fentiderm; Fentigyn; Lomexin; **S.Afr.:** Lomexin; **Singapore:** Lomexin; **Spain:** Laurimic; Lomexin; Micofulvin; **Switz.:** Mycodermil; **UK:** Lomexin.

## Fluconazole (BAN, USAN, rINN)

Fluconazol; UK-49858. 2-(2,4-Difluorophenyl)-1,3-bis(1H-1,2,4-triazol-1-yl)propan-2-ol.

$C_{13}H_{12}F_2N_6O$ = 306.3.

CAS — 86386-73-4.

ATC — D01AC15; J02AC01.

**Pharmacopoeias.** In *Chin.*

**Incompatibility and stability.** References.


1. Lor E, *et al.* Visual compatibility of fluconazole with commonly used injectable drugs during simulated Y-site administration. *Am J Hosp Pharm* 1991; **48:** 744–6.
2. Couch P, *et al.* Stability of fluconazole and amino acids in parenteral nutrient solutions. *Am J Hosp Pharm* 1992; **49:** 1459–62.
3. Hunt-Fugate AK, *et al.* Stability of fluconazole in injectable solutions. *Am J Hosp Pharm* 1993; **50:** 1186–7.
4. Ishisaka DY. Visual compatibility of fluconazole with drugs given by continuous infusion. *Am J Hosp Pharm* 1994; **51:** 2290 and 2292.


### Adverse Effects

Adverse effects reported with fluconazole most commonly affect the gastrointestinal tract and include abdominal pain, diarrhoea, flatulence, nausea and vomiting, and taste disturbance. Other adverse effects include headache, dizziness, leucopenia, thrombocytopenia, hyperlipidaemias, and raised liver enzyme values. Serious hepatotoxicity has been reported in patients with severe underlying disease such as AIDS or malignancy. Anaphylaxis and angioedema have been reported rarely.

Skin reactions are rare but exfoliative cutaneous reactions such as toxic epidermal necrolysis and Stevens-Johnson syndrome have occurred, more commonly in patients with AIDS.

**Alopecia.** Alopecia has occasionally been reported in patients receiving fluconazole, especially during prolonged treatment.[1,2]


1. Weinroth SE, Tuazon CU. Alopecia associated with fluconazole treatment. *Ann Intern Med* 1993; **119:** 637.
2. Pappas PG, *et al.* Alopecia associated with fluconazole therapy. *Ann Intern Med* 1995; **123:** 354–7.


**Effect on electrolyte balance.** Hypokalaemia was associated with fluconazole administration in 3 patients with acute myeloid leukaemia.[1]


1. Kidd D, *et al.* Hypokalaemia in patients with acute myeloid leukaemia after treatment with fluconazole. *Lancet* 1989; **i:** 1017.


**Effects on the heart.** Prolonged QT interval and torsade de pointes have been reported in 2 patients receiving fluconazole.[1,2]


1. Wassmann S, *et al.* Long QT syndrome and torsade de pointes in a patient receiving fluconazole. *Ann Intern Med* 1999; **131:** 797.
2. Tholakanahalli VN, *et al.* Fluconazole-induced torsade de pointes. *Ann Pharmacother* 2001; **35:** 432–4.


**Effects on the liver.** Although severe hepatic reactions to fluconazole are rare they have been reported, especially in patients with severe underlying diseases or hepatic dysfunction.[1,2] Elevation of liver enzymes is commonly encountered and there have been reports of jaundice associated with fluconazole treatment.[3,4] Hepatic necrosis has been found rarely post mortem in patients with severe underlying disease who had received fluconazole. In one such patient, hepatotoxicity was concluded to be dose-dependent.[5]


1. Wells C, Lever AML. Dose-dependent fluconazole hepatotoxicity proven on biopsy and rechallenge. *J Infect* 1992; **24:** 111–12.
2. Jacobson MA, *et al.* Fatal acute hepatic necrosis due to fluconazole. *Am J Med* 1994; **96:** 188–90.
3. Holmes J, Clements D. Jaundice in HIV positive haemophiliac. *Lancet* 1989; **i:** 1027.
4. Franklin IM, *et al.* Fluconazole-induced jaundice. *Lancet* 1990; **336:** 565.
5. Bronstein J-A, *et al.* Fatal acute hepatic necrosis due to dose-dependent fluconazole hepatotoxicity. *Clin Infect Dis* 1997; **25:** 1266–7.


**Hypersensitivity.** Desensitisation has been successfully carried out in a patient with AIDS who exhibited hypersensitivity to both fluconazole and itraconazole.[1] Gradually increasing oral doses of fluconazole (starting at 5 mg daily) were administered over 7 days; thereafter dosage was maintained at 400 mg daily. No adverse reactions were noted during the desensitisation period or in the 3 months up to the publication of the report.


1. Takahashi T, *et al.* Desensitization to fluconazole in an AIDS patient. *Ann Pharmacother* 2001; **35:** 642–3.


### Precautions

Fluconazole should be used with caution in patients with impaired renal or hepatic function. Abnormalities in haematological, hepatic, and renal function tests have been observed in patients with serious underlying diseases such as AIDS or malignancy.

Teratogenicity has occurred in *animals* given high doses of fluconazole and its use is not recommended in pregnancy (see under Pregnancy, below).

**Breast feeding.** Fluconazole is distributed into breast milk, achieving concentrations similar to those found in maternal plasma,[1] and its use in women who are breast feeding is not recommended by the manufacturer.

In one report,[2] no untoward effects, other than a slight increase in lactase dehydrogenase level, were observed in an infant who was exposed to fluconazole in breast milk for 6 weeks.

The American Academy of Pediatrics considers that the use of fluconazole is usually compatible with breast feeding.[3]


1. Force RW. Fluconazole concentrations in breast milk. *Pediatr Infect Dis J* 1995; **14:** 235–6.
2. Bodley V, Powers D. Long-term treatment of a breastfeeding mother with fluconazole-resolved nipple pain caused by yeast: a case study. *J Hum Lact* 1997; **13:** 307–11.
3. American Academy of Pediatrics. The transfer of drugs and other chemicals into human milk. *Pediatrics* 2001; **108:** 776–89. Correction. *ibid.*; 1029. Also available at: http://aappolicy.aappublications.org/cgi/content/full/pediatrics%3b108/3/776 (accessed 12/05/04)


**Pregnancy.** High (toxic) doses of *fluconazole, itraconazole,* and *ketoconazole* have been reported to be teratogenic in *rodents.* Although there is little information about the use of these drugs in human pregnancy, there is a report of a woman who had received fluconazole 400 mg daily throughout pregnancy and who gave birth to an infant with severe craniofacial and limb abnormalities.[1] The abnormalities resembled those associated with the Antley-Bixler syndrome, a genetic disorder, but a teratogenic effect could not be excluded. Although prescription-event-monitoring studies of fluconazole did not reveal adverse effects on the fetus,[2-4] congenital abnormalities have occurred in infants whose mothers had received high doses of fluconazole for 3 months or more. Data collected by the manufacturer,[5] relating to 198 women exposed to itraconazole during the first trimester of pregnancy, indicated that the malformation rate for both exposed women and matched controls was within the expected baseline risk for the general population. Nevertheless, the manufacturers recommend that fluconazole, itraconazole, and ketoconazole should be avoided during pregnancy.

*Other azole antifungals* including butoconazole, clotrimazole, econazole, miconazole, sulconazole, terconazole, and tioconazole are reported to be embryotoxic but not teratogenic in *rodents* given high doses. Many of these drugs are used topically or intravaginally and the systemic absorption from these routes of administration varies. While these drugs may not necessarily be contra-indicated in pregnancy, consideration should be given to these potential risks when choosing antifungal therapy for such patients.


1. Lee BE, *et al.* Congenital malformations in an infant born to a woman treated with fluconazole. *Pediatr Infect Dis J* 1992; **11:** 1062–4.
2. Rubin PC, *et al.* Fluconazole and pregnancy: results of a prescription event-monitoring study. *Int J Gynecol Obstet* 1992; **37** (suppl): 25–7.
3. Inman W, *et al.* Safety of fluconazole in the treatment of vaginal candidiasis: a prescription-event monitoring study, with special reference to the outcome of pregnancy. *Eur J Clin Pharmacol* 1994; **46:** 115–18.
4. Sørensen HT, *et al.* Risk of malformations and other outcomes in children exposed to fluconazole in utero. *Br J Clin Pharmacol* 1999; **48:** 234–8.
5. Bar-Oz B, *et al.* Pregnancy outcome after in utero exposure to itraconazole: a prospective cohort study. *Am J Obstet Gynecol* 2000; **183:** 617–20.


**Renal impairment.** For dose adjustments in renal impairment, see Administration in Renal Impairment, under Uses and Administration, below.

### Interactions

In general, fewer interactions are considered to occur with fluconazole than with either itraconazole or ketoconazole.

Use of rifampicin with fluconazole results in reduced plasma concentrations of fluconazole. Use of hydrochlorothiazide and fluconazole has resulted in clinically insignificant increases in plasma-fluconazole concentrations.

Fluconazole may interfere with the metabolism of some drugs if given concomitantly, mainly through inhibition of the cytochrome P450 isoenzymes CYP3A4 and CYP2C9. This may account for the reported increases in plasma concentrations of ciclosporin, midazolam, nortriptyline, phenytoin, rifabutin, sulfonylurea hypoglycaemics and nateglinide, tacrolimus, triazolam, warfarin, and zidovudine; fluconazole may inhibit the formation of a toxic metabolite of sulfamethoxazole.

Increases in terfenadine concentrations following high doses of fluconazole have been associated with ECG abnormalities. A similar effect may be anticipated with astemizole. Use of fluconazole with cisapride could result in increased cisapride concentrations and associated toxicity. The use of fluconazole with astemizole, cisapride, or terfenadine should therefore be avoided because of the risk of cardiac arrhythmias. Syncope attributed to increased amitriptyline concentrations has occurred when amitriptyline was given with fluconazole.

Fluconazole may also reduce the clearance of theophylline. The concentration of contraceptive steroids has been reported to be both increased and decreased in patients receiving fluconazole and the efficacy of oral contraceptives may be affected.

◊ Reviews of drug interactions with azole antifungals.


1. Baciewicz AM, Baciewicz FA. Ketoconazole and fluconazole drug interactions. *Arch Intern Med* 1993; **153:** 1970–6.
2. Lomaestro BM, Piatek MA. Update on drug interactions with azole antifungal agents. *Ann Pharmacother* 1998; **32:** 915–28.
3. Venkatakrishnan K, *et al.* Effects of the antifungal agents on oxidative drug metabolism: clinical relevance. *Clin Pharmacokinet* 2000; **38:** 111–80.


### Antimicrobial Action

Fluconazole is a triazole antifungal drug which in sensitive fungi inhibits cytochrome P450-dependent enzymes, resulting in impairment of ergosterol synthesis in fungal cell membranes. It is active against *Blastomyces dermatitidis, Candida* spp., *Coccidioides immitis, Cryptococcus neoformans, Epidermophyton* spp., *Histoplasma capsulatum, Microsporum* spp., and *Trichophyton* spp.

Resistance has developed in some *Candida* spp. following long-term prophylaxis with fluconazole, and cross-resistance with other azoles has been reported.

**Microbiological interactions.** A synergistic antifungal effect was seen *in vitro* with terbinafine and fluconazole against strains of *Candida albicans.*[1] For effects on the antifungal activity of fluconazole when given with amphotericin B, see p.393.


1. Barchiesi F, *et al.* In vitro activities of terbinafine in combination with fluconazole and itraconazole against isolates of Candida albicans with reduced susceptibility to azoles. *Antimicrob Agents Chemother* 1997; **41:** 1812–14.


**Resistance.** The emergence of strains of *Candida* spp. resistant to fluconazole has become increasingly important, particularly in immunocompromised patients receiving long-term prophylaxis with fluconazole.[1] In addition to resistance in *C. albicans,*[2-4] infections with *C. dubliniensis,*[4] *C. glabrata,* and *C. krusei,* all of which may be less sensitive to fluconazole than *C. albicans,* have been noted in these patients,[5,6] and secondary resistance of *C. glabrata* has been reported during fluconazole therapy.[7,8] Resistance to fluconazole has been reported to occur more frequently than resistance to either ketoconazole or itraconazole and may be related to the widespread use of this drug.[3,6] Cross-resistance with other azoles[9,10] and with amphotericin B[11,12] has been reported.

Fluconazole resistance has also been reported in *Cryptococcus neoformans*[13] and *Histoplasma capsulatum.*[14] Histoplasmosis developed during treatment with fluconazole in a patient with HIV infection.[15] Fluconazole-resistant *C. neoformans* has been isolated from an immunocompetent patient who had not been exposed to azole antifungals previously.[16]


1. Rex JH, *et al.* Resistance of Candida species to fluconazole. *Antimicrob Agents Chemother* 1995; **39:** 1–8.
2. Sandven P, *et al.* Susceptibilities of Norwegian Candida albicans strains to fluconazole: emergence of resistance. *Antimicrob Agents Chemother* 1993; **37:** 2443–8.
3. Johnson EM, *et al.* Emergence of azole drug resistance in Candida species from HIV-infected patients receiving prolonged fluconazole therapy for oral candidosis. *J Antimicrob Chemother* 1995; **35:** 103–14.
4. Ruhnke M, *et al.* Development of simultaneous resistance to fluconazole in Candida albicans and Candida dubliniensis in a patient with AIDS. *J Antimicrob Chemother* 2000; **46:** 291–5.
5. Price MF, *et al.* Fluconazole susceptibilities of Candida species and distribution of species recovered from blood cultures over a 5-year period. *Antimicrob Agents Chemother* 1994; **38:** 1422–4.
6. Odds FC. Resistance of yeasts to azole-derivative antifungals. *J Antimicrob Chemother* 1993; **31:** 463–71.
7. Hitchcock CA, *et al.* Fluconazole resistance in Candida glabrata. *Antimicrob Agents Chemother* 1993; **37:** 1962–5.
8. Miyazaki H, *et al.* Fluconazole resistance associated with drug efflux and increased transcription of a drug transporter gene, PDH1, in Candida glabrata. *Antimicrob Agents Chemother* 1998; **42:** 1695–1701.
9. Martinez-Suarez JV, Rodriguez-Tudela JL. Patterns of in vitro activity of itraconazole and imidazole antifungal agents against Candida albicans with decreased susceptibility to fluconazole from Spain. *Antimicrob Agents Chemother* 1995; **39:** 1512–16.
10. Goldman M, *et al.* Does long-term itraconazole prophylaxis result in in vitro azole resistance in mucosal Candida albicans isolates from persons with advanced human immunodeficiency virus infection? *Antimicrob Agents Chemother* 2000; **44:** 1585–7.
11. Kelly SL, *et al.* Resistance to fluconazole and amphotericin in Candida albicans from AIDS patients. *Lancet* 1996; **348:** 1523–4.
12. Nolte FS, *et al.* Isolation and characterization of fluconazole- and amphotericin B-resistant Candida albicans from blood of two patients with leukemia. *Antimicrob Agents Chemother* 1997; **41:** 196–9.
13. Venkateswarlu K, *et al.* Fluconazole tolerance in clinical isolates of Cryptococcus neoformans. *Antimicrob Agents Chemother* 1997; **41:** 748–51.
14. Wheat J, *et al.* Hypothesis on the mechanism of resistance to fluconazole in Histoplasma capsulatum. *Antimicrob Agents Chemother* 1997; **41:** 410–14.

15. Pottage JC, Sha BE. Development of histoplasmosis via human immunodeficiency virus infected patient receiving fluconazole. *J Infect Dis* 1991; **164:** 622–3.
16. Omi-Wasserlauf R, *et al.* Fluconazole-resistant Cryptococcus neoformans isolated from an immunocompetent patient without prior exposure to fluconazole. *Clin Infect Dis* 1999; **29:** 1592–3.

## Pharmacokinetics

Fluconazole is well absorbed following oral administration, bioavailability from the oral route being 90% or more of that from the intravenous route. Mean peak plasma concentrations of 6.72 micrograms/mL have been reported in healthy subjects following a 400-mg oral dose. Peak concentrations are reached within 1 to 2 hours of oral administration. Plasma concentrations are proportional to the dose over a range of 50 to 400 mg. Multiple dosing leads to increases in peak plasma concentrations; steady-state concentrations are reached in 5 to 10 days but may be attained on day 2 if a loading dose is given.

Fluconazole is widely distributed and the apparent volume of distribution is close to that of total body water. Concentrations in breast milk, joint fluid, saliva, sputum, vaginal fluids, and peritoneal fluid are similar to those achieved in plasma. Concentrations in the CSF range from 50 to 90% of plasma concentrations, even in the absence of meningeal inflammation. Protein binding is only about 12%.

About 80% of a dose is excreted unchanged in the urine and about 11% as metabolites. The elimination half-life of fluconazole is about 30 hours and is increased in patients with renal impairment. Fluconazole is removed by dialysis.

◊ Reviews.

1. Debruyne D, Ryckelynek J-P. Clinical pharmacokinetics of fluconazole. *Clin Pharmacokinet* 1993; **24:** 10–27.
2. Debruyne D. Clinical pharmacokinetics of fluconazole in superficial and systemic mycoses. *Clin Pharmacokinet* 1997; **33:** 52–77.

**Burns.** The mean half-life of fluconazole was decreased to 24.4 hours in 9 patients with burns.[1] Fluconazole clearance was 27.5 mL/minute which was 30% higher than that reported in healthy subjects.

1. Boucher BA, *et al.* Fluconazole pharmacokinetics in burn patients. *Antimicrob Agents Chemother* 1998; **42:** 930–3.

**Children and neonates.** References.

1. Saxén H, *et al.* Pharmacokinetics of fluconazole in very low birth weight infants during the first two weeks of life. *Clin Pharmacol Ther* 1993; **54:** 269–77.
2. Nahata MC, Brady MT. Pharmacokinetics of fluconazole after oral administration in children with human immunodeficiency virus infection. *Eur J Clin Pharmacol* 1995; **48:** 291–3.

**Distribution.** Salivary concentrations of fluconazole following oral administration should be adequate for the treatment of oropharyngeal and oesophageal candidiasis[1,2] even in patients with AIDS who may have decreased salivation.[3] Treatment failures are more likely to be due to inadequate dosage or resistant organisms than to decreased salivary secretion.[3]

Pharmacologically active concentrations of fluconazole have been detected in scalp hair[4] and nails[5] following oral treatment with conventional daily administration and with once-weekly administration.

1. Force RW, Nahata MC. Salivary concentrations of ketoconazole and fluconazole: implications for drug efficacy in oropharyngeal and esophageal candidiasis. *Ann Pharmacother* 1995; **29:** 10–15.
2. Koks CHW, *et al.* Pharmacokinetics of fluconazole in saliva and plasma after administration of an oral suspension and capsules. *Antimicrob Agents Chemother* 1996; **40:** 1935–7.
3. Garcia-Hermoso D, *et al.* Fluconazole concentrations in saliva from AIDS patients with oropharyngeal candidosis refractory to treatment with fluconazole. *Antimicrob Agents Chemother* 1995; **39:** 656–60.
4. Yeates R, *et al.* Accumulation of fluconazole in scalp hair. *J Clin Pharmacol* 1998; **38:** 138–43.
5. Faergemann J. Pharmacokinetics of fluconazole in skin and nails. *J Am Acad Dermatol* 1999; **40** (suppl): S14–S20.

**HIV-infected patients.** Plasma clearance of fluconazole may be lower in patients with HIV infection than in immunocompetent patients, and the half-life may be prolonged.[1,2]

1. Tett S, *et al.* Pharmacokinetics and bioavailability of fluconazole in two groups of males with human immunodeficiency virus (HIV) infection compared with those in a group of males without HIV infection. *Antimicrob Agents Chemother* 1995; **39:** 1835–41.
2. McLachlan AJ, Tett SE. Pharmacokinetics of fluconazole in people with HIV infection: a population analysis. *Br J Clin Pharmacol* 1996; **41:** 291–8.

## Uses and Administration

Fluconazole is a triazole antifungal used for superficial mucosal (oropharyngeal, oesophageal, or vaginal) candidiasis and for fungal skin infections. It is also given for systemic infections including systemic candidiasis, coccidioidomycosis, and cryptococcosis, and has been tried in blastomycosis, chromoblastomycosis, histoplasmosis, and sporotrichosis. The place of fluconazole in the treatment of fungal infections is discussed in the various sections under Choice of Antifungal, p.386.

Fluconazole is given by mouth or intravenous infusion in similar doses. For intravenous infusion it is given as a solution containing 2 mg/mL at a rate of 5 to 10 mL/minute (300 to 600 mL/hour). In the USA, a maximum infusion rate of 100 mL/hour is recommended.

For superficial mucosal candidiasis (other than genital candidiasis), the usual dose of fluconazole in the UK is 50 mg daily by mouth, although 100 mg daily may be given if necessary. Treatment usually continues for 7 to 14 days in oropharyngeal candidiasis (except in severely immunocompromised patients), for 14 days in atrophic oral candidiasis associated with dentures, and for 14 to 30 days in other mucosal candidal infections including oesophagitis. Higher doses are recommended in the USA where an initial dose of fluconazole 200 mg is followed by 100 mg daily and where the minimum treatment period is 14 days for oropharyngeal infection, or a minimum of 21 days and at least 14 days after resolution of symptoms for oesophageal infections; doses of up to 400 mg daily may be used for oesophageal candidiasis if necessary.

Fluconazole 150 mg by mouth as a single dose may be used for vaginal candidiasis or candidal balanitis.

Dermatophytosis, pityriasis versicolor, and *Candida* infections of the skin may be treated with fluconazole 50 mg daily by mouth for up to 6 weeks.

Systemic candidiasis, cryptococcal meningitis, and other cryptococcal infections may be treated with fluconazole by mouth or by intravenous infusion; the initial dose is 400 mg followed by 200 to 400 mg daily. Duration of therapy is based on clinical and mycological response, but is usually at least 6 to 8 weeks in cryptococcal meningitis; in the USA, treatment for 10 to 12 weeks after the CSF cultures become negative is recommended. Fluconazole may also be used in daily doses of 100 to 200 mg orally or intravenously to prevent relapse following a primary course of antifungal treatment for acute cryptococcal meningitis in patients with AIDS.

In immunocompromised patients at risk of fungal infections, fluconazole may be given prophylactically in a dose of 50 to 400 mg daily by mouth or by intravenous infusion, although long-term prophylaxis has been associated with the emergence of resistant organisms (see under Intermittent Doses, below).

Doses for children over 4 weeks of age are 3 mg/kg daily for superficial infections (a loading dose of 6 mg/kg may be used on the first day if necessary), and 6 to 12 mg/kg daily for systemic infections. For prophylaxis in immunocompromised children, a dose of 3 to 12 mg/kg daily may be given. For infants under 2 weeks of age, all these doses should be given once every 72 hours; for those aged between 2 and 4 weeks, the doses should be given every 48 hours. A maximum dose of 400 mg daily should not be exceeded in children, or 12 mg/kg at appropriate intervals in infants.

Dosage may need to be reduced in patients with renal impairment (see below).

◊ Reviews.

1. Grant SM, Clissold SP. Fluconazole: a review of its pharmacodynamic and pharmacokinetic properties, and therapeutic potential in superficial and systemic mycoses. *Drugs* 1990; **39:** 877–916. Correction. *ibid.* **40:** 862.
2. Kowalsky SF, Dixon DM. Fluconazole: a new antifungal agent. *Clin Pharm* 1991; **10:** 179–94.
3. Goa KL, Barradell LB. Fluconazole: an update of its pharmacodynamic and pharmacokinetic properties and therapeutic use in major superficial and systemic mycoses in immunocompromised patients. *Drugs* 1995; **50:** 658–90.

**Administration.** HIGH DOSES. Doses of fluconazole of up to 1000 mg daily have been tried in the treatment of cryptococcal meningitis. In a study of 11 patients who received fluconazole 800 to 1000 mg daily intravenously for 3 weeks then orally until the CSF culture became negative, 6 patients had responded at 10 weeks and another 2 improved clinically.[1] Daily doses of up to 800 mg have been used in blastomycosis[2] and coccidioidomycosis,[3] and doses of 10 mg/kg daily have been tried in disseminated candidiasis.[4]

1. Menichetti F, *et al.* High-dose fluconazole therapy for cryptococcal meningitis in patients with AIDS. *Clin Infect Dis* 1996; **22:** 838–40.
2. Pappas PG, *et al.* Treatment of blastomycosis with higher doses of fluconazole. *Clin Infect Dis* 1997; **25:** 200–5.
3. Galgiani JN, *et al.* Infectious Diseases Society of America. Practice guidelines for the treatment of coccidioidomycosis. *Clin Infect Dis* 2000; **30:** 658–61.
4. Graninger W, *et al.* Treatment of Candida albicans fungaemia with fluconazole. *J Infect* 1993; **26:** 133–46.

INTERMITTENT DOSES. Concern has been expressed about the increasingly widespread use of fluconazole[1] and, in particular, about the impact of continuous fluconazole therapy in immunocompromised patients on the development of resistance (see under Antimicrobial Action, above). Nevertheless, fluconazole remains popular for primary and secondary prophylaxis. Some investigators have suggested the use of intermittent doses[2,3] although this could further increase the risk of infections with resistant organisms.

Once-weekly treatment with fluconazole has been tried in onychomycosis[4] and tinea capitis.[5]

1. Mangino JE, *et al.* When to use fluconazole. *Lancet* 1995; **345:** 6–7.
2. Singh N, *et al.* Low-dose fluconazole as primary prophylaxis for cryptococcal infection in AIDS patients with CD4 cell counts of ≤ 100/mm³: demonstration of efficacy in a prospective, multicenter trial. *Clin Infect Dis* 1996; **23:** 1282–6.
3. Schuman P, *et al.* Weekly fluconazole for the prevention of mucosal candidiasis in women with HIV infection: a randomized, double-blind, placebo-controlled trial. *Ann Intern Med* 1997; **126:** 689–96.
4. Scher RK, *et al.* Once-weekly fluconazole (150 mg, 300 mg, or 450 mg) in the treatment of distal subungual onychomycosis of the toenail. *J Am Acad Dermatol* 1998; **38:** S77–S86.
5. Gupta AK, *et al.* Once weekly fluconazole is effective in children in the treatment of tinea capitis: a prospective, multicentre study. *Br J Dermatol* 2000; **142:** 965–8.

**Administration in renal impairment.** Patients with renal impairment may require dosage reduction. Normal loading or initial doses of fluconazole should be given on the first day of treatment and subsequent doses should be adjusted according to creatinine clearance. If the creatinine clearance is more than 50 mL/minute, the standard dose can be given. If the creatinine clearance is less than 50 mL/minute and the patient is not receiving dialysis, half the standard dose can be given. Patients on regular haemodialysis should receive a standard dose of fluconazole after every dialysis session. No dosage adjustment is needed in patients with renal impairment given single-dose therapy.

**Leishmaniasis.** Fluconazole has been tried in the treatment of cutaneous leishmaniasis (p.597) caused by *Leishmania major.* In a randomised, double-blind, placebo-controlled study,[1] 80 patients received a six-week course of oral fluconazole 200 mg daily, of whom 63 had complete healing of lesions after 3 months, compared with 22 of 65 patients who received placebo.

1. Alrajhi AA, *et al.* Fluconazole for the treatment of cutaneous leishmaniasis caused by Leishmania major. *N Engl J Med* 2002; **346:** 891–5.

## Preparations

**Proprietary Preparations** (details are given in Part 3)

***Arg.:*** Femixol; Fluzol; Fungocina; Honguil Plus; Klonazol; Micolis Novo; Mutum; Naxo C; Nifurtox; Periplum; Ponaris; Triflucan; ***Austral.:*** Diflucan; ***Austria:*** Diflucan; Fungata; ***Belg.:*** Diflucan; ***Braz.:*** Candizol; Flucanol; Flucazol; Flucoltrix†; Fluconal; Fluconax; Fluconeo; Flucozen; Flunazol; Fluotec†; Flusan†; Flutec; Glyfucan; Helmicin; Lertus†; Monipax; Pantec†; Pronazol; Riconazol; Teczol†; Triazol; Unizol; Zelix; Zolanix; Zolmic; Zolstatin; Zoltec; Zoltren; ***Canad.:*** Diflucan; ***Chile:*** Diflucan; Felsol; Flucoxan; Fluctin; Ibarin; Micofin; Plusgin; Tavor; ***Denm.:*** Diflucan; ***Fin.:*** Diflucan; ***Fr.:*** Beagyne; Triflucan; ***Ger.:*** Diflucan; Fungata; ***Gr.:*** Figalol; Fluseníl; Fungustatin; Fungusteril; Hadlinol; Rifagen; Stabilanol; Tierlite; Zidonil; ***Hong Kong:*** Diflucan; Flucozal; ***India:*** Forcan; Logican; Syscan; ***Irl.:*** Diflucan; ***Israel:*** Diflucan; Flucanol; Trican; Triflucan; ***Ital.:*** Biozolene; Diflucan; Elazor; ***Jpn:*** Diflucan; ***Malaysia:*** Diflucan; ***Mex.:*** Afungil; Bioxel; Candizol; Diflucan; Flukazol; Flukenol†; Fluzor; Neofomiral; Oxifungol; Waynazol†; Zoldicam; Zonal†; ***Neth.:*** Diflucan; ***Norw.:*** Diflucan; ***NZ:*** Diflucan; ***Port.:*** Azoflune; Diflucan; Fludocel; Reforce; Supremase; ***S.Afr.:*** Diflucan; ***Singapore:*** Diflucan; ***Spain:*** Diflucan; Lavisa; Loitin; Solacap; ***Swed.:*** Diflucan; ***Switz.:*** Diflucan; ***Thai.:*** Biozole; Diflucan; Flucozole; Fludizol; Flunco; Funa; Stalene; ***UK:*** Canesten Oral; Diflucan; ***USA:*** Diflucan.

# Flucytosine *(BAN, USAN, rINN)*

5-FC; Flucitosina; Flucytosinum; Ro-2-9915. 5-Fluorocytosine; 4-Amino-5-fluoropyrimidin-2(1*H*)-one.

$C_4H_4FN_3O$ = 129.1.

*CAS — 2022-85-7.*

*ATC — D01AE21; J02AX01.*

**Pharmacopoeias.** In *Chin., Eur.* (see p.vi), *Int., Jpn, Pol.,* and *US.*

**Ph. Eur. 5.0** (Flucytosine). A white or almost white crystalline powder. Sparingly soluble in water; slightly soluble in dehydrated alcohol. Protect from light.

**USP 27** (Flucytosine). A white to off-white crystalline powder, odourless or with a slight odour. Sparingly soluble in water; slightly soluble in alcohol; practically insoluble in chloroform and in ether. Store in airtight containers. Protect from light.

**Stability.** A solution of flucytosine for intravenous infusion should be stored between 18° and 25°. Precipitation may occur at lower temperatures and decomposition, with the formation of fluorouracil, at higher temperatures.

## Adverse Effects

Side-effects of flucytosine include nausea, vomiting, diarrhoea, and skin rashes. Less frequently reported adverse effects include confusion, hallucinations, convulsions, headache, sedation, and vertigo, and also allergic reactions, toxic epidermal necrolysis, and cardiotoxicity. Alterations in liver function tests are generally dose-related and reversible; hepatotoxicity may also occur. Hypokalaemia may occur. There have been a few reports of peripheral neuropathy.

Bone-marrow depression, especially leucopenia and thrombocytopenia, is associated with blood concentrations of flucytosine greater than 100 micrograms/mL, with concurrent amphotericin B administration, and with renal impairment. Fatal agranulocytosis and aplastic anaemia have been reported.

**Effects on the blood.** Bone marrow toxicity associated with flucytosine has been attributed to its conversion to fluorouracil, possibly by intestinal flora.[1]

1. Pirmohamed M, *et al.* The role of active metabolites in drug toxicity. *Drug Safety* 1994; **11:** 114–44.

## Precautions

Flucytosine should be administered with great care to patients with renal impairment, or with blood disorders or bone marrow depression. Renal and hepatic function and blood counts should be monitored during therapy (at least weekly in patients with renal impairment or blood disorders). In patients with renal impairment, doses should be reduced and trough blood concentrations of flucytosine should be checked regularly from blood samples taken just before an injection of flucytosine. Care should be taken in patients receiving radiation therapy or other drugs which depress bone marrow.

Flucytosine is teratogenic in *rats*.

**AIDS.** High incidences of bone marrow toxicity have been reported in patients with AIDS during flucytosine therapy.[1] However, in a study in 381 patients, no additional haematotoxicity was reported in patients receiving amphotericin B plus flucytosine compared with those receiving amphotericin B alone.[2] The toxicity could be minimised by monitoring serum concentrations[3] and the British Society for Antimicrobial Chemotherapy has suggested that these should be maintained within 25 to 50 micrograms/mL in patients with AIDS.[4]

1. Chuck SL, Sande MA. Infections with Cryptococcus neoformans in the acquired immunodeficiency syndrome. *N Engl J Med* 1989; **321:** 794–9.
2. van der Horst CM, *et al.* Treatment of cryptococcal meningitis associated with the acquired immunodeficiency syndrome. *N Engl J Med* 1997; **337:** 15–21.
3. Viviani MA. Flucytosine—what is its future? *J Antimicrob Chemother* 1995; **35:** 241–4.
4. British Society for Antimicrobial Chemotherapy Working Party. Antifungal chemotherapy in patients with acquired immunodeficiency syndrome. *Lancet* 1992; **340:** 648–51.

**Renal impairment.** For dosage recommendations, see Administration in Renal Impairment under Uses and Administration, below.

## Interactions

Flucytosine is commonly used with amphotericin B. Amphotericin B can cause a deterioration in renal function, which can result in raised flucytosine blood concentrations and increased toxicity. However, the two drugs are generally regarded as having synergistic antifungal activity. Cytarabine has been claimed to reduce blood concentrations of flucytosine and to antagonise its antifungal activity, although the evidence is limited.

## Antimicrobial Action

Flucytosine is a fluorinated pyrimidine antifungal. In susceptible fungi it is converted by cytosine deaminase to fluorouracil which is then incorporated in place of uracil into fungal RNA and disrupts protein synthesis. The activity of thymidilate synthetase is also inhibited and this effect interferes with fungal DNA synthesis.

Flucytosine is active against *Candida* spp., *Cryptococcus neoformans*, *Cladosporium* spp., and *Fonsecaea* spp. Some *Aspergillus* spp. have also been reported to be sensitive. There is synergy between flucytosine and amphotericin B against *Candida* spp. and *Cryptococcus neoformans*.

There is a high incidence of primary resistance to flucytosine among isolates of *Candida* spp. and *Cryptococcus neoformans*. Resistance also develops during treatment with flucytosine and has been reported rarely from combination therapy with flucytosine and amphotericin B.

**Microbiological interactions.** Although flucytosine is generally regarded as having synergistic activity with *amphotericin B*, antagonism of the *in vitro* antifungal activity of amphotericin B against *Candida* spp. by flucytosine has been reported.[1]

Enhanced antifungal activity against *Cryptococcus neoformans* has been reported using flucytosine with *fluconazole* in *animal* studies.[2,3]

1. Martin E, *et al.* Antagonistic effects of fluconazole and 5-fluorocytosine on candidacidal action of amphotericin B in human serum. *Antimicrob Agents Chemother* 1994; **38:** 1331–8.
2. Larsen RA, *et al.* Effect of fluconazole on fungicidal activity of flucytosine in murine cryptococcal meningitis. *Antimicrob Agents Chemother* 1996; **40:** 2178–82.
3. Nguyen MH, *et al.* Combination therapy with fluconazole and flucytosine in the murine model of cryptococcal meningitis. *Antimicrob Agents Chemother* 1997; **41:** 1120–3.

## Pharmacokinetics

Flucytosine is absorbed rapidly and almost completely from the gastrointestinal tract. Bioavailability is reported to be 78 to 89%. After oral doses of 37.5 mg/kg every 6 hours, peak plasma concentrations of 70 to 80 micrograms/mL have been achieved within 2 hours; similar concentrations have been achieved but more rapidly, after an intravenous dose. The plasma-flucytosine concentration for optimum response is 25 to 50 micrograms/mL. Flucytosine is widely distributed through the body tissues and fluids; concentrations in the CSF have been reported to be 65 to 90% of those in serum. About 2 to 4% of flucytosine is protein bound.

About 90% of a dose is excreted unchanged by glomerular filtration; a small amount of flucytosine may be metabolised to fluorouracil. The small amount of an oral dose of flucytosine not absorbed from the gastrointestinal tract is eliminated unchanged in the faeces. The elimination half-life is 2.5 to 6 hours in patients with normal renal function but increases with decreasing renal function. Flucytosine is removed by haemodialysis or peritoneal dialysis.

◊ References.

1. Daneshmend TK, Warnock DW. Clinical pharmacokinetics of systemic antifungal agents. *Clin Pharmacokinet* 1983; **8:** 17–42.
2. Baley JE, *et al.* Pharmacokinetics, outcome of treatment, and toxic effects of amphotericin B and 5-fluorocytosine in neonates. *J Pediatr* 1990; **116:** 791–7.

## Uses and Administration

Flucytosine is a fluorinated pyrimidine antifungal used in the treatment of systemic fungal infections, the treatments for which are discussed under Choice of Antifungal, p.386. It is mainly used with amphotericin B or fluconazole in the treatment of severe systemic candidiasis and cryptococcal meningitis. It has also been tried in other infections due to susceptible fungi including chromoblastomycosis.

Flucytosine is given by *intravenous infusion* as a 1% solution over 20 to 40 minutes. The usual dose is 200 mg/kg daily in 4 divided doses; a dose of 100 to 150 mg/kg daily may be sufficient in some patients. Dosage should be adjusted to produce trough plasma concentrations of 25 to 50 micrograms/mL. This is particularly important in patients with AIDS who are at increased risk of bone marrow toxicity. Parenteral treatment is rarely given for more than 7 days, except for cryptococcal meningitis when it is continued for at least 4 months. For intravenous doses to be used in patients with renal impairment, see below.

Flucytosine is given by *mouth* in usual doses of 50 to 150 mg/kg daily in 4 divided doses. Again, blood concentrations should be monitored and dosage adjusted in patients with renal impairment to avoid accumulation of the drug.

Flucytosine has been used *topically*, but such use may increase problems of resistance.

◊ Reviews.

1. Viviani MA. Flucytosine—what is its future? *J Antimicrob Chemother* 1995; **35:** 241–4.
2. Summers KK, *et al.* Therapeutic drug monitoring of systemic antifungal therapy. *J Antimicrob Chemother* 1997; **40:** 753–64.
3. Vermes A, *et al.* Flucytosine: a review of its pharmacology, clinical indications, pharmacokinetics, toxicity and drug interactions. *J Antimicrob Chemother* 2000; **46:** 171–9.

**Administration in renal impairment.** Flucytosine is mainly excreted by the kidneys and the dose must be adjusted in patients with renal impairment.

Intravenous doses of 50 mg/kg every 12 hours should be used in patients with a creatinine clearance of 20 to 40 mL/minute and similar doses every 24 hours in patients with a creatinine clearance of 10 to 20 mL/minute. Patients with a creatinine clearance of less than 10 mL/minute may be given a single dose of 50 mg/kg; further doses should then be based on plasma concentrations which should not exceed 80 micrograms/mL.

Initial oral doses should be at the lower end of the recommended range (see above) and dosage should be adjusted subsequently to avoid accumulation.

## Preparations

***BP 2003:*** Flucytosine Tablets;
***USP 27:*** Flucytosine Capsules.

**Proprietary Preparations** (details are given in Part 3)
***Austral.:*** Ancotil; ***Austria:*** Ancotil; ***Braz.:*** Ancotil†; ***Denm.:*** Ancotil; ***Fr.:*** Ancotil; ***Ger.:*** Ancotil; ***Hong Kong:*** Ancotil; ***Irl.:*** Alcobon†; Ancotil; ***Ital.:*** Ancotil; ***Malaysia:*** Ancotil; ***Neth.:*** Ancotil; ***Norw.:*** Ancotil†; ***NZ:*** Alcobon; ***Singapore:*** Ancotil†; ***Swed.:*** Ancotil; ***Switz.:*** Ancotil; ***UK:*** Ancotil; ***USA:*** Ancobon.

---

## Flutrimazole *(BAN, rINN)*

Flutrimazol; Flutrimazolum; UR-4056. 1-[*o*-Fluoro-α-(*p*-fluorophenyl)-α-phenylbenzyl]imidazole; (*RS*)-1-(2,4′-Difluorotrityl)imidazole.

$C_{22}H_{16}F_2N_2$ = 346.4.
*CAS — 119006-77-8.*
*ATC — D01AC16.*

**Pharmacopoeias.** In *Eur.* (see p.vi).

**Ph. Eur. 5.0** (Flutrimazole). A white or almost white powder. Practically insoluble in water; soluble in methyl alcohol; freely soluble in tetrahydrofuran. Protect from light.

### Profile

Flutrimazole is an imidazole antifungal used topically in the treatment of superficial fungal infections.

For a discussion of the caution needed when using azole antifungals during pregnancy, see under Pregnancy in Precautions of Fluconazole, p.398.

### Preparations

**Proprietary Preparations** (details are given in Part 3)
***Arg.:*** Flusporan; ***Chile:*** Micetal; ***Spain:*** Cutimian†; Flusporan; Funcenal; Micetal.

---

## Genaconazole

Genaconazol; Sch-39304; SM-8668. [*R*-(*R**,*R**)]-α-(2,4-Difluorophenyl)-α[1-(methylsulphonyl)ethyl]-1*H*-1,2,4-triazole-1-ethanol.

$C_{13}H_{15}F_2N_3O_3S$ = 331.3.
*CAS — 121650-83-7.*

### Profile

Genaconazole is a triazole antifungal that has been investigated for systemic use.

---

## Griseofulvin *(BAN, rINN)*

Curling Factor; Griseofulvina; Griseofulvinum. (2*S*,4′*R*)-7-Chloro-2′,4,6-trimethoxy-4′-methylspiro[benzofuran-2(3*H*),3′-cyclohexene]-3,6′-dione.

$C_{17}H_{17}ClO_6$ = 352.8.
*CAS — 126-07-8.*
*ATC — D01AA08; D01BA01.*

**Pharmacopoeias.** In *Chin.*, *Eur.* (see p.vi), *Int.*, *Jpn*, *Pol.*, *US*, and *Viet.*

**Ph. Eur. 5.0** (Griseofulvin). An antifungal substance produced by the growth of certain strains of *Penicillium griseofulvum*, or by any other means. It is a white or yellowish-white powder. The particles of the powder are generally up to 5 micrometres in maximum dimension, though larger particles, which may occasionally exceed 30 micrometres, may be present. It contains 97 to 102% of $C_{17}H_{17}ClO_6$, calculated on the dried substance. Practically insoluble in water; slightly soluble in dehydrated alcohol and in methyl alcohol; freely soluble in dimethylformamide and in tetrachloroethane.

**USP 27** (Griseofulvin). A white to creamy-white, odourless powder, in which particles of the order of 4 micrometres in diameter predominate. It has a potency of not less than 900 micrograms of $C_{17}H_{17}ClO_6$ per mg. Very slightly soluble in water; sparingly soluble in alcohol; soluble in acetone, in chloroform, and in dimethylformamide. Store in airtight containers.

### Adverse Effects

Adverse effects are usually mild and transient and consist of headache, skin rashes and urticaria, dry mouth, an altered sensation of taste, and gastrointestinal disturbances. Angioedema, erythema multiforme, toxic epidermal necrolysis, proteinuria, leucopenia and other blood dyscrasias, oral candidiasis, peripheral neuropathy, photosensitisation, and severe headache have been reported occasionally. Depression, confusion, dizziness, impaired coordination, insomnia, and fatigue have also been reported. Griseofulvin may precipitate or aggravate systemic lupus erythematosus.

There have been a few reports of hepatotoxicity attributed to griseofulvin.

**Effects on the skin.** A report of fatal toxic epidermal necrolysis in a 19-year-old woman.[1] The reaction was attributed to griseofulvin that she had taken for 6 days; she had also received metronidazole for 1 day. Erythema multiforme occurred in 3 patients taking griseofulvin for 3 to 10 days.[2]

1. Mion G, *et al.* Fatal toxic epidermal necrolysis after griseofulvin. *Lancet* 1989; **ii:** 1331.
2. Rustin MHA, *et al.* Erythema multiforme due to griseofulvin. *Br J Dermatol* 1989; **120:** 455–8.

### Precautions

Griseofulvin is contra-indicated in patients with severe liver disease or systemic lupus erythematosus.

Griseofulvin is embryotoxic and teratogenic in *rats.* There have been isolated cases of conjoined twins following griseofulvin treatment during the first trimester of pregnancy. Griseofulvin is therefore contra-indicated in pregnancy and women should not become pregnant during, or within 1 month of stopping, griseofulvin treatment. Since griseofulvin may reduce the effectiveness of oral contraceptives, additional contraceptive precautions should be taken during this time. Data from *in-vitro* and *in-vivo* studies using mammalian cells which demonstrated aneuploidy have led to the warning that men receiving griseofulvin should not father children within 6 months of treatment.

Griseofulvin may impair the ability to drive or operate machinery, and has been reported to enhance the effects of alcohol.

**Porphyria.** Griseofulvin has been associated with acute attacks of porphyria and is considered unsafe in porphyric patients.

### Interactions

Phenobarbital has been reported to decrease the gastrointestinal absorption of griseofulvin. Plasma concentrations of griseofulvin have also been reported to be reduced by drugs that induce metabolising enzymes such as phenylbutazone and hypnotics.

Griseofulvin may increase the rate of metabolism and diminish the effects of some drugs such as coumarin anticoagulants and oral contraceptives.

Griseofulvin may enhance the effects of alcohol.

**Alcohol.** In addition to reports of griseofulvin enhancing the effects of alcohol, a severe disulfiram-like reaction to alcohol has been reported in a patient taking griseofulvin.[1]

1. Fett DL, Vukov LF. An unusual case of severe griseofulvin-alcohol interaction. *Ann Emerg Med* 1994; **24:** 95–7.

**Bromocriptine.** For a report that griseofulvin can block the response to bromocriptine, see p.1202.

**Salicylates.** Griseofulvin has been reported to reduce plasma concentrations of salicylate in a patient taking aspirin, see p.17.

### Antimicrobial Action

Griseofulvin is a fungistatic antibiotic which inhibits fungal cell division by disruption of the mitotic spindle structure. It may also interfere with DNA production. It is active against the common dermatophytes, including some species of *Epidermophyton, Microsporum,* or *Trichophyton.*

### Pharmacokinetics

Absorption of griseofulvin from the gastrointestinal tract is variable and incomplete, but is enhanced by reducing the particle size and by administration with a fatty meal. Peak plasma concentrations are reached within 4 hours and are maintained for 10 to 20 hours. Griseofulvin is about 84% bound to plasma proteins. It is deposited in keratin precursor cells and is concentrated in the stratum corneum of the skin and in the nails and hair, thus preventing fungal invasion of newly formed cells. Concentrations of 12 to 25 micrograms/g are maintained in skin during long-term administration, while concurrent plasma concentrations remain at about 1 to 2 micrograms/mL. Griseofulvin has an elimination half-life of 9 to 24 hours, and is metabolised by the liver mainly to 6-demethylgriseofulvin and its glucuronide conjugate which are excreted in the urine. A large amount of a dose of griseofulvin of reduced particle size appears unchanged in the faeces; less than 1% is excreted unchanged in the urine; some is excreted in the sweat.

### Uses and Administration

Griseofulvin is an antifungal used by mouth in the treatment of dermatophyte infections. It is generally given for such infections that involve the scalp, hair, nails, and skin and which do not respond to topical treatment (see p.390); infections of the soles of the feet, the palms of the hands, and the nails respond slowly.

The usual dose of griseofulvin is 0.5 to 1 g daily in single or divided doses; children may be given 10 mg/kg daily. These doses are for preparations of griseofulvin of reduced particle size, sometimes known as microcrystalline or microsize griseofulvin, but the doses have been reduced by about one-third when preparations, available in some countries, containing ultramicrocrystalline or ultramicrosize griseofulvin are used. Griseofulvin should be given with or after meals.

The duration of treatment depends on the thickness of the keratin layer: 2 to 8 weeks for infections of the hair and skin, up to 6 months for infections of the fingernails, and 12 months or more for infections of the toenails.

**Administration.** Although griseofulvin is usually given systemically, beneficial responses have been reported with some topical formulations[1,2] in fungal skin infections.

1. Macasaet EN, Pert P. Topical (1%) solution of griseofulvin in the treatment of tinea corporis. *Br J Dermatol* 1991; **124:** 110–11.
2. Aly R, *et al.* Topical griseofulvin in the treatment of dermatophytoses. *Clin Exp Dermatol* 1994; **19:** 43–6.

**Non-infective skin disorders.** Lichen planus is usually treated with corticosteroids, ciclosporin, or retinoids (see p.1136) but griseofulvin has been suggested as an alternative to topical corticosteroids in erosive disease.[1] However, some researchers have found it to be of no value.[2]

Dramatic responses of pigmented purpuric dermatoses to griseofulvin 500 to 750 mg daily have been reported in 5 patients.[3]

1. Lamey P-J, Lewis MAO. Oral medicine in practice: white patches. *Br Dent J* 1990; **168:** 147–52.
2. Bagan JV, *et al.* Treatment of lichen planus with griseofulvin. *Oral Surg Oral Med Oral Pathol* 1985; **60:** 608–10.
3. Tamaki K, *et al.* Successful treatment of pigmented purpuric dermatosis with griseofulvin. *Br J Dermatol* 1995; **132:** 159–60.

### Preparations

***BP 2003:*** Griseofulvin Tablets;
***USP 27:*** Griseofulvin Capsules; Griseofulvin Oral Suspension; Griseofulvin Tablets; Ultramicrosize Griseofulvin Tablets.

**Proprietary Preparations** (details are given in Part 3)
***Arg.:*** Grisovin; ***Austral.:*** Fulcin†; Griseostatin; Grisovin; ***Austria:*** Griseomed; Grisovin; ***Braz.:*** Fulcin; Sporostatin; ***Canad.:*** Fulvicin; Grisovin FP†; ***Chile:*** Fulvistatin P/G; ***Denm.:*** Fulcin†; ***Fin.:*** Fulcin†; ***Fr.:*** Fulcine†; Griséfuline; ***Ger.:*** Fulcin S; Gricin; Griseo; Likuden M; ***Hong Kong:*** Fulcin†; Griseostatin†; Grisovin†; ***India:*** Grisactin; Walavin; ***Irl.:*** Fulcin; ***Israel:*** Grifulin; ***Ital.:*** Fulcin; Grisovina FP; ***Malaysia:*** Grisuvin; Grivin; Krisovin; Medofulvin; Myconil; ***Mex.:*** Fulcin; Fulsivin; Fulvina; Griseoful†; Grisovin; ***Norw.:*** Fulcin†; Lamoryl†; ***NZ:*** Grisovin†; ***Port.:*** Fulcin; Grisomicon; Grisovin; ***S.Afr.:*** Fulcin†; Microcidal; ***Singapore:*** Erlivin†; Fulcin†; Grivin; Krisovin; Medofulvin†; ***Spain:*** Fulcin; Greosin; ***Swed.:*** Fulcin†; ***Switz.:*** Fulcin†; Grisol; ***Thai.:*** Aofen; Fulcin†; Grifulvin; Grisflavin; Grisovin†; Grivin; Neofulvin; Trivanex; ***UK:*** Fulcin†; Grisovin; ***USA:*** Fulvicin†; Grifulvin V†; Gris-PEG; Grisactin†.

**Multi-ingredient:** ***Arg.:*** Griseoplus.

## Haloprogin (USAN, rINN)

Haloprogina; M-1028; NSC-100071. 3-Iodoprop-2-ynyl 2,4,5-trichlorophenyl ether.

$C_9H_4Cl_3IO$ = 361.4.
*CAS — 777-11-7.*
*ATC — D01AE11.*

### Adverse Effects

Local reactions may occur and include irritation, pruritus, and vesiculation.

### Antimicrobial Action

Haloprogin is reported to inhibit *Epidermophyton, Microsporum, Trichophyton,* and *Candida* spp. and *Malassezia furfur.*

### Uses and Administration

Haloprogin is an antifungal used in the treatment of dermatophytosis and pityriasis versicolor. It is applied topically as a 1% cream or solution twice daily for 2 to 4 weeks.

### Preparations

**Proprietary Preparations** (details are given in Part 3)
***USA:*** Halotex†.

## Isoconazole (BAN, USAN, rINN)

Isoconazol; Isoconazolum. 1-[2,4-Dichloro-β-(2,6-dichlorobenzyloxy)phenethyl]imidazole.

$C_{18}H_{14}Cl_4N_2O$ = 416.1.
*CAS — 27523-40-6.*
*ATC — D01AC05; G01AF07.*

**Pharmacopoeias.** In *Eur.* (see p.vi).

**Ph. Eur. 5.0** (Isoconazole). A white or almost white powder. Practically insoluble in water; freely soluble in alcohol; very soluble in methyl alcohol. Protect from light.

## Isoconazole Nitrate (BANM, rINNM)

Isoconazoli Nitras; Nitrato de isoconazol; R-15454.

$C_{18}H_{14}Cl_4N_2O,HNO_3$ = 479.1.
*CAS — 24168-96-5 (isoconazole mononitrate); 40036-10-0 (isoconazole nitrate).*
*ATC — D01AC05; G01AF07.*

**Pharmacopoeias.** In *Eur.* (see p.vi).

**Ph. Eur. 5.0** (Isoconazole Nitrate). A white or almost white powder. Very slightly soluble in water; slightly soluble in alcohol; soluble in methyl alcohol. Protect from light.

### Adverse Effects and Precautions

Local reactions including burning or itching may occur following the application of isoconazole.

Intravaginal preparations of azole antifungals may damage latex contraceptives and additional contraceptive measures are therefore necessary during local administration of isoconazole.

For a discussion of the caution needed when using azole antifungals during pregnancy, see under Pregnancy in Precautions of Fluconazole, p.398.

### Antimicrobial Action

Isoconazole is an imidazole antifungal active against a wide spectrum of fungi including *Candida* spp., dermatophytes, and *Malassezia furfur.* It is also active against some Gram-positive bacteria.

### Uses and Administration

Isoconazole nitrate is an imidazole antifungal used locally in the treatment of vaginal mycoses, particularly due to *Candida* spp. (p.386) and in fungal skin infections (p.390). For vaginal infections it is usually given as pessaries in a single dose of 600 mg or 300 mg daily for 3 days, or as a 1% vaginal cream daily for 7 days. For skin infections a 2% cream or other topical formulation has been used.

### Preparations

***BP 2003:*** Isoconazole Pessaries.

**Proprietary Preparations** (details are given in Part 3)
***Arg.:*** Mupaten; ***Austria:*** Gyno-Travogen; Travogen; ***Belg.:*** Gyno-Travogen†; Travogen; ***Braz.:*** Gino Monipax; Ginotrax; Gyno Icaden; Gyno-Mycel; Gynoplus†; Icaden; Mycel; Neo Isocaden; ***Chile:*** Ufarin; ***Fr.:*** Fazol; Fazol G; ***Ger.:*** Travogen; ***Gr.:*** Travogen; ***Hong Kong:*** Gyno-Travogen; Travogen; ***Israel:*** Gyno-Travogen; Isogen; ***Ital.:*** Isogyn; Travogen; ***Malaysia:*** Travogen; ***Mex.:*** Icaden; ***NZ:*** Gyno-Travogen†; ***Port.:*** Gino-Travogen; ***Singapore:*** Gyno-Travogen; Travogen; ***Switz.:*** Gyno-Travogen; Travogen; ***Thai.:*** Nacozil; Travogen.

**Multi-ingredient:** ***Arg.:*** Scheriderm; ***Austria:*** Travocort; ***Belg.:*** Travocort; ***Ger.:*** Bi-Vaspit; Travocort; ***Gr.:*** Travocort; ***Hong Kong:*** Travocort; ***Irl.:*** Travocort; ***Israel:*** Isocort; ***Ital.:*** Travocort; ***Malaysia:*** Isoradin; Travocort; ***Mex.:*** Scheriderm; ***Port.:*** Travocort; ***S.Afr.:*** Travocort; ***Singapore:*** Travocort; ***Switz.:*** Travocort; ***Thai.:*** Travocort.

## Itraconazole (BAN, USAN, rINN)

Itraconazol; Itraconazolum; Oriconazole; R-51211. (±)-2-sec-Butyl-4-[4-(4-{4-[(2R*,4S*)-2-(2,4-dichlorophenyl)-2-(1H-1,2,4-triazol-1-ylmethyl)-1,3-dioxolan-4-ylmethoxy]phenyl}-piperazin-1-yl)phenyl]-2,4-dihydro-1,2,4-triazol-3-one.

$C_{35}H_{38}Cl_2N_8O_4$ = 705.6.
*CAS — 84625-61-6.*
*ATC — J02AC02.*

**Pharmacopoeias.** In *Eur.* (see p.vi).

**Ph. Eur. 5.0** (Itraconazole). A white or almost white powder. Practically insoluble in water; very slightly soluble in alcohol; freely soluble in dichloromethane; sparingly soluble in tetrahydrofuran. Protect from light.

### Adverse Effects

The most common adverse effects associated with itraconazole include dyspepsia, abdominal pain, nausea, constipation, diarrhoea (with the oral liquid), headache, and dizziness. Others include allergic reactions such as pruritus, rash, urticaria, and angioedema. Isolated cases of the Stevens-Johnson syndrome have been associated with itraconazole.

An increase in liver enzyme values has occurred in some patients and cases of hepatitis and cholestatic jaundice have been observed, especially in those treated for more than one month. There have been rare cases of liver failure and death.

Heart failure and pulmonary oedema have been reported rarely and serious cardiovascular events including arrhythmias and sudden death have been attributed to drug interactions in patients receiving itraconazole (see Interactions, below).

Alopecia, oedema, and hypokalaemia have also been associated with prolonged treatment. Menstrual disorders and peripheral neuropathy have been reported in a few patients.

**Incidence of adverse effects.** Itraconazole 50 to 400 mg daily for a median of 5 months was considered to be well tolerated in 189 patients with systemic fungal infections.[1] Of 86 patients with underlying disease, including 49 with AIDS, 16 with diabetes, and 23 with malignancy, nausea and vomiting occurred in 19 patients, hypertriglyceridaemia in 16, hypokalaemia in 11, and elevated liver enzyme values in 13. The role of itraconazole in hypertriglyceridaemia could not be assessed because all the samples were not drawn in the fasting state and hypertriglyceridaemia is a complication of HIV infection. Gynaecomastia occurred in 2 patients, 1 receiving concurrent spironolactone. Rash occurred in 4 patients.

Of 49 patients receiving itraconazole 100 to 400 mg daily for up to 39 months, 23 did not experience adverse effects during treatment,[2] while 6 had nausea and vomiting, 5 developed oedema, and 2 developed hypertension; 3 of the patients who developed oedema and 1 who became hypertensive were diabetic. Three patients discontinued itraconazole, 1 due to vomiting, 1 to leucopenia, and 1 to nephrotic syndrome. The patient with nephrotic syndrome had pre-existing oedema and hypertension; the syndrome cleared when itraconazole was discontinued.

1. Tucker RM, *et al.* Adverse events associated with itraconazole in 189 patients on chronic therapy. *J Antimicrob Chemother* 1990; **26:** 561–6.
2. Graybill JR, *et al.* Itraconazole treatment of coccidioidomycosis. *Am J Med* 1990; **89:** 282–90.

**Effects on the heart.** Between September 1992, when itraconazole was approved in the USA, and April 2001, the FDA had received 58 reports of potential cases of heart failure associated with itraconazole.[1] There had been 28 patients admitted to hospital, and 13 had died. However, a causal relationship was difficult to prove. Overall, 43 patients had risk factors or diseases which might confound an association between the use of itraconazole and development of heart failure. Unpublished studies in *dogs* and humans had suggested a negative inotropic effect with intravenous itraconazole.

In August 2001, the UK Committee on Safety of Medicines (CSM) published a similar alert.[2] By this time, approximately 67 million patients worldwide had received itraconazole and there had been 75 spontaneously reported cases of suspected heart failure and an additional 63 reports of oedema suggestive of heart failure associated with oral formulations; there had been only 1 report of suspected heart failure in the UK. The CSM considered that the risk of heart failure with itraconazole was low, especially in young healthy patients receiving short courses of treatment (e.g. for vulvovaginal candidiasis). However, the risks appeared to be higher for older patients, patients with pre-existing heart disease or risk factors for heart failure, and for those receiving high doses and longer treatment courses (e.g. for onychomycosis).

The CSM[2] therefore advised caution when prescribing itraconazole to patients at risk of heart failure, whereas the FDA[1] contra-indicated it for the treatment of onychomycosis in patients with evidence of ventricular dysfunction.

1. Ahmad SR, *et al.* Congestive heart failure associated with itraconazole. *Lancet* 2001; **357:** 1766–7.
2. Committee on Safety of Medicines. Cardiodepressant effect of itraconazole (Sporanox). *Current Problems* 2001; **27:** 11–12. Also available at: http://www.mca.gov.uk/ourwork/monitorsafequalmed/currentproblems/cpaug2001.pdf (accessed 02/07/04)

## Precautions

Itraconazole has caused abnormalities in fetal development in *rodents* and is therefore contra-indicated in pregnancy. For further information, see Pregnancy, under Precautions of Fluconazole, p.398.

Itraconazole should be avoided in patients with hepatic impairment. Liver function should be monitored if treatment lasts more than one month or if there are symptoms suggestive of hepatitis. Treatment should be stopped if abnormal liver function is detected. Plasma-itraconazole concentrations should be monitored in patients with active liver disease and the dosage adjusted if necessary.

Dose adjustments may also be required in some patients with renal impairment, for example those receiving continuous ambulatory peritoneal dialysis. Intravenous administration is not recommended in patients with a creatinine clearance of less than 30 mL/minute. Itraconazole should be discontinued if neuropathy develops.

Itraconazole should not be used for the treatment of less severe fungal infections such as onychomycosis in patients with evidence of, or a history of, ventricular dysfunction such as heart failure.

Hypochlorhydria, which may be present in patients with AIDS, can reduce absorption of itraconazole. In this case absorption may be improved by administering itraconazole with an acidic drink, such as a cola beverage.

**Breast feeding.** Breast feeding while receiving itraconazole is not recommended by the manufacturer although only small amounts of itraconazole are distributed into breast milk.

## Interactions

Enzyme-inducing drugs such as carbamazepine, isoniazid, nevirapine, phenobarbital, phenytoin, rifabutin, or rifampicin may decrease plasma concentrations of itraconazole. Conversely, enzyme inhibitors such as clarithromycin, erythromycin, indinavir, or ritonavir may increase plasma concentrations of itraconazole. Use of drugs that reduce stomach acidity, such as antimuscarinics, antacids, proton pump inhibitors, and histamine $H_2$-receptor antagonists, may reduce the absorption of itraconazole.

Itraconazole may interfere with drugs metabolised by hepatic microsomal enzymes, especially the cytochrome P450 isoenzyme CYP3A4, hence the warnings that plasma concentrations of astemizole, ciclosporin, cisapride, dihydropyridine calcium-channel blockers such as felodipine, dofetilide, midazolam, mizolastine, pimozide, quinidine, sildenafil, sirolimus, statins such as atorvastatin, lovastatin or simvastatin, tacrolimus, terfenadine, triazolam, verapamil, and warfarin may be increased. Concentrations of HIV-protease inhibitors such as indinavir, ritonavir, and saquinavir may also be increased; itraconazole plasma concentrations may be increased in turn by indinavir or ritonavir (but not by saquinavir). Other drugs that may be affected include alfentanil, alprazolam, buspirone, busulfan, carbamazepine, diazepam, digoxin, docetaxel, methylprednisolone, oral hypoglycaemics, rifabutin, trimetrexate, and the vinca alkaloids. The efficacy of oral contraceptives might be reduced.

There is a risk of cardiac arrhythmias if itraconazole is used with astemizole, cisapride, dofetilide, pimozide, quinidine, or terfenadine and such combinations should be avoided.

◊ For reviews of drug interactions with azole antifungals, see Fluconazole, p.398.

**Metal ions.** Didanosine in a formulation containing aluminium and magnesium ion buffering agents could reduce the absorption of itraconazole due to the resultant increase in gastric pH.[1]

1. Moreno F, *et al.* Itraconazole-didanosine excipient interaction. *JAMA* 1993; **269:** 1508.

## Antimicrobial Action

Itraconazole is a triazole antifungal drug which in sensitive fungi inhibits cytochrome P450-dependent enzymes resulting in impairment of ergosterol synthesis in fungal cell membranes. It has a slightly wider spectrum of activity than ketoconazole. It is active against *Aspergillus* spp., *Blastomyces dermatitidis*, *Candida* spp., *Coccidioides immitis*, *Cryptococcus neoformans*, *Epidermophyton* spp., *Histoplasma capsulatum*, *Malassezia furfur*, *Microsporum* spp., *Paracoccidioides brasiliensis*, *Sporothrix schenckii*, and *Trichophyton* spp. Itraconazole also has some antiprotozoal activity against *Leishmania* spp.

Acquired resistance to itraconazole is rare but ketoconazole-resistant strains of *Candida albicans* have been found to be cross resistant to itraconazole.

**Microbiological interactions.** Synergistic antifungal effects were seen *in vitro* with terbinafine and itraconazole against strains of *Candida albicans*[1] and *Scedosporium prolificans*.[2] For effects on the antifungal activity of azoles when given with amphotericin B, see p.393.

1. Barchiesi F, *et al.* In vitro activities of terbinafine in combination with fluconazole and itraconazole against isolates of Candida albicans with reduced susceptibility to azoles. *Antimicrob Agents Chemother* 1997; **41:** 1812–14.
2. Meletiadis J, *et al.* In vitro interaction of terbinafine with itraconazole against clinical isolates of Scedosporium prolificans. *Antimicrob Agents Chemother* 2000; **44:** 470–2.

**Resistance.** For a discussion of increasing resistance of *Candida* spp. to azoles see Fluconazole, Antimicrobial Action, p.398. Decreased susceptibility to itraconazole and cross-resistance to fluconazole has been reported in *C. albicans* isolated from patients with AIDS receiving long-term prophylaxis with itraconazole.[1] *Aspergillus fumigatus* resistant to itraconazole has also been identified.[2,3]

1. Goldman M, *et al.* Does long-term itraconazole prophylaxis result in in vitro azole resistance in mucosal Candida albicans isolates from persons with advanced human immunodeficiency virus infection? *Antimicrob Agents Chemother* 2000; **44:** 1585–7.
2. Denning DW, *et al.* Itraconazole resistance in Aspergillus fumigatus. *Antimicrob Agents Chemother* 1997; **41:** 1364–8.
3. Dannaoui E, *et al.* Acquired itraconazole resistance in Aspergillus fumigatus. *J Antimicrob Chemother* 2001; **47:** 333–340.

## Pharmacokinetics

Itraconazole is absorbed from the gastrointestinal tract when administered by mouth either as capsules containing itraconazole coated onto sugar spheres or as an oral liquid formulated with hydroxypropyl-β-cyclodextrin. Absorption from the capsule formulation is enhanced by an acidic gastric environment and is greatest when doses are taken with food; absorption from the oral liquid is not dependent on an acid environment, and absorption is greatest in the fasting state. Peak plasma concentrations are achieved between 1.5 and 5 hours after a dose of either formulation, and steady state is reached within 15 days during daily dosing. Peak plasma concentrations at steady state of about 2 micrograms/mL have been reported following daily doses of 200 mg.

Bioavailability increases with doses of 100 to 400 mg in such a manner as to suggest that itraconazole undergoes saturable metabolism. Itraconazole is highly protein bound; only 0.2% circulates as free drug. Itraconazole is widely distributed but only small amounts diffuse into the CSF. Concentrations attained in the skin, sebum, pus, and many organs and tissues are several times higher than simultaneous plasma concentrations. Therapeutic concentrations of itraconazole remain in the skin and mucous membranes for 1 to 4 weeks after the drug is discontinued. Small amounts are distributed into breast milk.

Itraconazole is metabolised in the liver mainly by cytochrome P450 isoenzyme CYP3A4. The major metabolite, hydroxyitraconazole, has antifungal activity comparable with that of itraconazole. Itraconazole is also excreted as inactive metabolites in the bile or urine; 3 to 18% is excreted in the faeces as unchanged drug. Small amounts are eliminated in the stratum corneum and hair. Itraconazole is not removed by dialysis.

The elimination half-life following a single 100-mg dose has been reported as 20 hours; the half-life increases to 30 to 40 hours with continued administration.

◊ References.

1. Baelaert J, *et al.* Itraconazole pharmacokinetics in patients with renal dysfunction. *Antimicrob Agents Chemother* 1988; **32:** 1595–7.
2. Cauwenbergh G, *et al.* Pharmacokinetic profile of orally administered itraconazole in human skin. *J Am Acad Dermatol* 1988; **18:** 263–8.
3. Zimmermann T, *et al.* Influence of concomitant food intake on the oral absorption of two triazole antifungal agents, itraconazole and fluconazole. *Eur J Clin Pharmacol* 1994; **46:** 147–50.
4. Coronel B, *et al.* Itraconazole concentrations during continuous haemodiafiltration. *J Antimicrob Chemother* 1994; **34:** 448–9.
5. Patterson TF, *et al.* Systemic availability of itraconazole in lung transplantation. *Antimicrob Agents Chemother* 1996; **40:** 2217–20.
6. Zhou H, *et al.* A pharmacokinetic study of intravenous itraconazole followed by oral administration of itraconazole capsules in patients with advanced human immunodeficiency virus infection. *J Clin Pharmacol* 1998; **38:** 593–602.
7. Poirier J-M, Cheymol G. Optimisation of itraconazole therapy using target drug concentrations. *Clin Pharmacokinet* 1998; **35:** 461–73.
8. Sermet-Gaudelus I, *et al.* Sputum itraconazole concentrations in cystic fibrosis patients. *Antimicrob Agents Chemother* 2001; **45:** 1937–8.

**Bioavailability.** The bioavailability of extemporaneously prepared oral liquid formulations of itraconazole has generally been poor.[1-3] However, a formulation with hydroxypropyl-β-cyclodextrin, which is available commercially, has been shown to have good bioavailability in both healthy subjects[4] and patients.[5-8]


1. Kintzel PE, *et al.* Low itraconazole serum concentrations following administration of itraconazole suspension to critically ill allogeneic bone marrow transplant recipients. *Ann Pharmacother* 1995; **29:** 140–3.
2. Villarreal JD, Erush SC. Bioavailability of itraconazole from oral liquids in question. *Am J Health-Syst Pharm* 1995; **52:** 1707–8.
3. Christensen KJ, *et al.* Relative bioavailability of itraconazole from an extemporaneously prepared suspension and from the marketed capsules. *Am J Health-Syst Pharm* 1998; **55:** 261–5.
4. Barone JA, *et al.* Enhanced bioavailability of itraconazole in hydroxypropyl-β-cyclodextrin solution versus capsules in healthy volunteers. *Antimicrob Agents Chemother* 1998; **42:** 1862–5.
5. Prentice AG, *et al.* Multiple dose pharmacokinetics of an oral solution of itraconazole in autologous bone marrow transplant recipients. *J Antimicrob Chemother* 1994; **34:** 247–52.
6. Prentice AG, *et al.* Multiple dose pharmacokinetics of an oral solution of itraconazole in patients receiving chemotherapy for acute myeloid leukaemia. *J Antimicrob Chemother* 1995; **36:** 657–63.
7. Reynes J, *et al.* Pharmacokinetics of itraconazole (oral solution) in two groups of human immunodeficiency virus-infected adults with oral candidiasis. *Antimicrob Agents Chemother* 1997; **41:** 2554–8.
8. de Repentigny L, *et al.* Repeated-dose pharmacokinetics of an oral solution of itraconazole in infants and children. *Antimicrob Agents Chemother* 1998; **42:** 404–8.


## Uses and Administration

Itraconazole is a triazole antifungal given by mouth for the treatment of oropharyngeal and vulvovaginal candidiasis, for pityriasis versicolor, for dermatophytoses unresponsive to topical treatment, for onychomycosis, and for systemic infections including aspergillosis, blastomycosis, candidiasis, chromoblastomycosis, coccidioidomycosis, cryptococcosis, histoplasmosis, paracoccidioidomycosis, and sporotrichosis. It is also given for the prophylaxis of fungal infections in immunocompromised patients. The place of itraconazole in the treatment of fungal infections is discussed in the various sections under Choice of Antifungal, p.386.

When given by mouth, doses of itraconazole oral liquid and capsules are not equivalent and may not be used interchangeably.

In the UK, itraconazole **oral liquid** is licensed for use in oral and oesophageal candidiasis in a dose of 200 mg daily for 1 week; it may be taken as a single daily dose, or, preferably, in 2 divided doses, the liquid being retained in the mouth for 20 seconds before swallowing. If there is no response after a week, treatment may be continued for a further week. In the USA, a similar regimen is licensed for oropharyngeal candidiasis, but in oesophageal candidiasis an alternative regimen of 100 mg daily for at least 3 weeks is preferred, although the dose may be increased to 200 mg daily if necessary.

For patients with fluconazole-resistant infections the dose in the UK is 100 to 200 mg twice daily for 2 weeks; if there is no response, 100 mg twice daily may be given for a further 2 weeks. In the USA the recommended dose is 100 mg twice daily.

Itraconazole oral liquid is also licensed in the UK for prophylaxis of susceptible fungal infections in immunocompromised patients, in doses of 5 mg/kg daily, in 2 divided doses.

The following doses all apply to itraconazole **capsules**. The dose in oropharyngeal candidiasis is 100 mg (or 200 mg in patients with AIDS or neutropenia) daily by mouth for 15 days. Vulvovaginal candidiasis may be treated with itraconazole 200 mg by mouth twice daily for one day. Pityriasis versicolor may be treated with itraconazole 200 mg daily for 7 days. For dermatophytoses the dose is 100 mg daily for 15 days or 200 mg daily for 7 days in tinea corporis or tinea cruris; doses are 100 mg daily for 30 days or 200 mg twice daily for 7 days in tinea pedis or tinea manuum. For nail infections the dose is 200 mg daily for 3 months or pulse therapy with 200 mg twice daily for 7 days repeated once (for fingernails) or twice (for toenails) after drug-free intervals of 21 days.

For systemic infections, itraconazole is given by mouth in usual doses of 100 to 200 mg once daily, increased to 200 mg twice daily for invasive or disseminated infections, including cryptococcal meningitis. In life-threatening infections a loading dose of 200 mg three times daily for 3 days has been given. A dose of 200 mg daily is used for primary or secondary prophylaxis in neutropenic patients or those with AIDS. Absorption may be impaired in these patients and monitoring of plasma concentrations is advised with an increase in dose to 200 mg twice daily if necessary. This higher dose is recommended routinely by some authorities in the USA.

Itraconazole may also be given by **intravenous infusion** in a dose of 200 mg given twice daily over 1 hour for two days, then 200 mg daily thereafter.

◊ Reviews.


1. Haria M, *et al.* Itraconazole: a reappraisal of its pharmacological properties and therapeutic use in the management of superficial fungal infections. *Drugs* 1996; **51:** 585–620.
2. Stevens DA (ed). Managing fungal infections in the 21st century: focus on itraconazole. *Drugs* 2001; **61** (suppl 1): 1–56.
3. Slain D, *et al.* Intravenous itraconazole. *Ann Pharmacother* 2001; **35:** 720–9.


**Administration.** HIGH DOSES. Doses of itraconazole 600 mg daily in two divided doses for 3 to 16 months were used in 8 patients with systemic mycoses resistant to conventional therapy.[1] Two patients with AIDS and cryptococcal meningitis failed to respond and two who responded initially later relapsed or developed progressive disease when the dose was reduced. The main adverse effects were hypokalaemia, hypertension, and oedema possibly associated with adrenal suppression.

In a patient with cerebral aspergillosis, itraconazole 800 mg daily for 5 months then 400 mg daily for a further 4½ months produced complete resolution of cerebral lesions.[2]


1. Sharkey PK, *et al.* High-dose itraconazole in the treatment of severe mycoses. *Antimicrob Agents Chemother* 1991; **35:** 707–13.
2. Sánchez C, *et al.* Treatment of cerebral aspergillosis with itraconazole: do high doses improve the prognosis? *Clin Infect Dis* 1995; **21:** 1485–7.


**Administration in children and neonates.** Itraconazole has been used in children in the treatment of tinea capitis.[1] Doses were 50 mg daily by mouth for those below 20 kg and 100 mg daily for those weighing 20 kg or more.

Itraconazole was administered to two premature infants with disseminated candidiasis in a dose of 10 mg/kg daily in two divided doses for 3 or 4 weeks without adverse effects.[2] Treatment was successful in both infants.


1. Möhrenschlager M, *et al.* Optimizing the therapeutic approach in tinea capitis of childhood with itraconazole. *Br J Dermatol* 2000; **143:** 1011–15.
2. Bhandari V, Narang A. Oral itraconazole therapy for disseminated candidiasis in low birth weight infants. *J Pediatr* 1992; **120:** 330.


**Amoebic infections.** Itraconazole has been suggested for *Acanthamoeba* keratitis (p.595), when it is given orally in combination with topical miconazole.

**Leishmaniasis.** When systemic therapy is required for the treatment of cutaneous leishmaniasis (p.597), pentavalent antimonials are most commonly used. The successful use of itraconazole has been reported in a few patients[1-3] but infections with *Leishmania aethiopica* may not respond.[4]


1. Albanese G, *et al.* Cutaneous leishmaniasis: treatment with itraconazole. *Arch Dermatol* 1989; **125:** 1540–2.
2. Pialoux G, *et al.* Cutaneous leishmaniasis in an AIDS patient: cure with itraconazole. *J Infect Dis* 1990; **162:** 1221–2.
3. Dogra J, Saxena VN. Itraconazole and leishmaniasis: a randomised double-blind trial in cutaneous disease. *Int J Parasitol* 1996; **26:** 1413–15.
4. Akuffo H, *et al.* The use of itraconazole in the treatment of leishmaniasis caused by Leishmania aethiopica. *Trans R Soc Trop Med Hyg* 1990; **84:** 532–4.


**Trypanosomiasis.** Itraconazole, in combination with allopurinol, may produce beneficial responses in American trypanosomiasis (p.600).

## Preparations

**Proprietary Preparations** (details are given in Part 3)

***Arg.:*** ITC; Micotenk; Nitridazol; Salimidin; Sporanox; ***Austral.:*** Sporanox; ***Austria:*** Sporanox; ***Belg.:*** Sporanox; ***Braz.:*** Itracotan; Itranax; Itraspor; Itrazol; Neo Itrax; Sporanox; Spozol; Traconal; Tracozon; Tranazol; ***Canad.:*** Sporanox; ***Chile:*** Itodal; Sporanox; Teramic; ***Denm.:*** Sporanox; ***Fin.:*** Sporanox; ***Fr.:*** Sporanox; ***Ger.:*** Sempera; Siros; ***Gr.:*** Sporanox; ***Hong Kong:*** Sporanox; ***India:*** Candistat; ***Irl.:*** Sporanox; ***Israel:*** Sporanox; ***Ital.:*** Sporanox; Triasporin; ***Malaysia:*** Sporanox; ***Mex.:*** Carexan; Fulzoltec; Fuzoltec; Isox; Itranax; Sinozol; Sporanox; Zolken†; ***Neth.:*** Trisporal; ***Norw.:*** Sporanox; ***NZ:*** Sporanox; ***Port.:*** Sporanox; ***S.Afr.:*** Sporanox; ***Singapore:*** Canditral; Sporanox; ***Spain:*** Canadiol; Hongoseril; Sporanox; ***Swed.:*** Sporanox; ***Switz.:*** Sporanox; ***Thai.:*** Itra; Itracon; Norspor; Spazol; Sporal; Sporlab; Spornar; ***UK:*** Sporanox; ***USA:*** Sporanox.

**Multi-ingredient:** ***Mex.:*** Sporasec.

## Ketoconazole *(BAN, USAN, rINN)*

Ketoconazol; Ketoconazolum; R-41400. (±)-*cis*-1-Acetyl-4-{4-[2-(2,4-dichlorophenyl)-2-imidazol-1-ylmethyl-1,3-dioxolan-4-ylmethoxy]phenyl}piperazine.

$C_{26}H_{28}Cl_2N_4O_4$ = 531.4.

*CAS — 65277-42-1.*

*ATC — D01AC08; G01AF11; J02AB02.*

**Pharmacopoeias.** In *Chin., Eur.* (see p.vi), *Int., Pol.,* and *US.*

**Ph. Eur. 5.0** (Ketoconazole). A white or almost white powder. Practically insoluble in water; sparingly soluble in alcohol; freely soluble in dichloromethane; soluble in methyl alcohol. Protect from light.

## Adverse Effects

Gastrointestinal disturbances are the most frequently reported adverse effect following the oral use of ketoconazole. Nausea and vomiting have been reported in about 3% of patients, and abdominal pain in about 1%. These adverse effects are dose-related and may be minimised by giving ketoconazole with food. Asymptomatic, transient elevations in serum concentrations of liver enzymes may occur in about 10% of patients. Hepatitis has been reported and the risk appears to increase if treatment with ketoconazole is continued for longer than 2 weeks; it is usually reversible on discontinuation of ketoconazole but fatalities have occurred. Ketoconazole interferes with steroid biosynthesis and reported adverse endocrine effects include gynaecomastia, oligospermia, menstrual irregularities, and adrenal cortex suppression, especially at high doses.

Other adverse effects include allergic reactions such as urticaria and angioedema, and rare cases of anaphylaxis have been reported. Pruritus, rash, alopecia, headache, dizziness, impotence, and somnolence may also occur. Thrombocytopenia, paraesthesia, raised intracranial pressure, and photophobia have been reported rarely.

After topical administration of ketoconazole, irritation, dermatitis, or a burning sensation has occurred.

**Effects on the blood.** A case of fatal aplastic anaemia was reported[1] in a 23-year-old woman who had taken ketoconazole for 4 days for the treatment of vaginal discharge.


1. Duman D, *et al.* Fatal aplastic anemia during treatment with ketoconazole. *Am J Med* 2001; **111:** 737.


**Effects on endocrine function.** References.


1. DeFelice R, *et al.* Gynecomastia with ketoconazole. *Antimicrob Agents Chemother* 1981; **19:** 1073–4.
2. Pont A, *et al.* High-dose ketoconazole therapy and adrenal and testicular function in humans. *Arch Intern Med* 1984; **144:** 2150–3.
3. White MC, Kendall-Taylor P. Adrenal hypofunction in patients taking ketoconazole. *Lancet* 1985; **i:** 44–5.
4. Dandona P, *et al.* Non-suppression of cortisol secretion by long term treatment with ketoconazole in patients with acute leukaemia. *J Clin Pathol* 1985; **38:** 677–8.
5. Pillans PI, *et al.* Hyponatraemia and confusion in a patient taking ketoconazole. *Lancet* 1985; **i:** 821–2.
6. McCance DR, *et al.* Acute hypoadrenalism and hepatotoxicity after treatment with ketoconazole. *Lancet* 1987; **i:** 573.
7. Best TR, *et al.* Persistent adrenal insufficiency secondary to low-dose ketoconazole therapy. *Am J Med* 1987; **82:** 676–80.
8. Khosla S, *et al.* Adrenal crisis in the setting of high-dose ketoconazole therapy. *Arch Intern Med* 1989; **149:** 802–4.


**Effects on the liver.** Transient minor elevations of liver enzymes without clinical signs or symptoms of hepatic disease occur in about 10% of patients given ketoconazole and may occur at any stage of treatment. Although this reaction is not usually clinically important it may signal the onset of more serious hepatic injury and indicates the need for close monitoring of liver function. Symptomatic hepatic reactions are much rarer occurring in less than 0.1% of patients but are potentially fatal. There is usually a hepatocellular pattern of damage and sometimes cholestasis. Patients at increased risk of hepatic injury include those with a history of liver disease, those aged over 50, especially women, and those requiring prolonged treatment. It is important to monitor liver function during treatment as well as to limit the length of treatment. If liver enzyme values continue to rise or jaundice or hepatitis occur, ketoconazole should be withdrawn immediately since fatalities have occurred in patients who continued treatment after signs of hepatic injury developed.

References.


1. Janssen PA, Symoens JE. Hepatic reactions during ketoconazole treatment. *Am J Med* 1983; **74:** 80–5.
2. Lewis JH, *et al.* Hepatic injury associated with ketoconazole therapy. *Gastroenterology* 1984; **86:** 503–13.
3. Lake-Bakaar G, *et al.* Hepatic reactions associated with ketoconazole in the United Kingdom. *BMJ* 1987; **294:** 419–21.
4. García Rodríguez LA, *et al.* A cohort study on the risk of acute liver injury among users of ketoconazole and other antifungal drugs. *Br J Clin Pharmacol* 1999; **48:** 847–52.

## Precautions

Since ketoconazole has been reported to cause hepatotoxicity it should not be given to patients with pre-existing liver disease. Patients receiving ketoconazole should be monitored for symptoms of hepatitis; also, liver function tests should be performed before starting treatment with ketoconazole lasting for more than 14 days and then at least monthly throughout treatment.

Ketoconazole has been shown to be teratogenic in *animal* studies and its use is generally not recommended during pregnancy. For a discussion of the caution needed when using azole antifungals during pregnancy, see under Pregnancy in Precautions of Fluconazole, p.398.

Hypochlorhydria, which may be present in patients with AIDS, can reduce absorption of ketoconazole. In this case absorption may be improved by administering ketoconazole with an acidic drink, such as a cola beverage.

**Breast feeding.** Ketoconazole is excreted in breast milk and the manufacturers state that its use should be avoided during breast feeding. However, no adverse effects have been observed in a breast-fed infant whose mother was receiving ketoconazole;[1] it was calculated that the infant was exposed to about 0.4% of the dose of ketoconazole that would be used therapeutically in this age group. The American Academy of Pediatrics considers[2] that use of ketoconazole is therefore usually compatible with breast feeding.

1. Moretti ME, *et al.* Disposition of maternal ketoconazole in breast milk. *Am J Obstet Gynecol* 1995; **173:** 1625–6.
2. American Academy of Pediatrics. The transfer of drugs and other chemicals into human milk. *Pediatrics* 2001; **108:** 776–89. Correction. *ibid.*; 1029. Also available at: http://aappolicy.aappublications.org/cgi/content/full/pediatrics%3b108/3/776 (accessed 12/05/04)

**Porphyria.** Ketoconazole is considered to be unsafe in patients with porphyria because it has been shown to be porphyrinogenic in *in-vitro* systems.

## Interactions

Use of drugs that reduce stomach acidity, such as antimuscarinics, antacids, histamine $H_2$-antagonists, and proton pump inhibitors, may reduce the absorption of ketoconazole. Absorption of ketoconazole may also be reduced by sucralfate. Use of ketoconazole with enzyme-inducing drugs such as rifampicin, isoniazid, or phenytoin may reduce plasma-ketoconazole concentrations. Concentrations of isoniazid and rifampicin may also be reduced by ketoconazole.

Ketoconazole inhibits certain hepatic oxidase enzymes, especially the cytochrome P450 isoenzyme CYP3A4, and may account for increases in plasma concentrations of some hepatically metabolised drugs such as alfentanil, the antihistamines astemizole, mizolastine, and terfenadine, the benzodiazepines midazolam and triazolam, ciclosporin, cisapride, dihydropyridine calcium-channel blockers, HIV-protease inhibitors such as indinavir or ritonavir (which may increase plasma concentrations of ketoconazole in turn), immunosuppressants such as sirolimus and tacrolimus, methylprednisolone, non-nucleoside reverse transcriptase inhibitors including delavirdine and nevirapine, oral anticoagulants, pimozide, quinidine, sertindole, sildenafil, statins such as lovastatin or simvastatin, tolbutamide, and verapamil. Other drugs that may be affected include buspirone, busulfan, carbamazepine, digoxin, docetaxel, dofetilide, reboxetine, rifabutin, trimetrexate, and the vinca alkaloids.

There is a risk of cardiac arrhythmias if ketoconazole is used with astemizole, cisapride, pimozide, quinidine or terfenadine and such combinations should be avoided.

A disulfiram-like reaction may occur in patients taking ketoconazole after drinking alcohol. The efficacy of oral contraceptives may be reduced.

◊ For reviews of drug interactions with azole antifungals, see Fluconazole, p.398.

## Antimicrobial Action

Ketoconazole is an imidazole antifungal which interferes with ergosterol synthesis and therefore alters the permeability of the cell membrane of sensitive fungi. It is reported to be fungistatic at concentrations achieved clinically. Ketoconazole has a wide spectrum of antimicrobial activity including activity against *Blastomyces dermatitidis, Candida* spp., *Coccidioides immitis, Epidermophyton floccosum, Histoplasma capsulatum, Malassezia* spp., *Microsporum canis, Paracoccidioides brasiliensis, Trichophyton mentagrophytes,* and *T. rubrum*. Some strains of *Aspergillus* spp., *Cryptococcus neoformans,* and *Sporothrix schenckii* are sensitive.

Ketoconazole has activity against some Gram-positive bacteria and some antiprotozoal activity against *Leishmania* spp.

There are rare reports of *Candida albicans* acquiring resistance to ketoconazole.

**Microbiological interactions.** For the effect of imidazoles and amphotericin B on each other's antimicrobial activity, see Amphotericin B, p.393.

**Resistance.** For a discussion of increasing resistance of *Candida* spp. to azoles see Fluconazole, Antimicrobial Action, p.398.

## Pharmacokinetics

The absorption of ketoconazole from the gastrointestinal tract is variable and increases with decreasing stomach pH. Mean peak plasma concentrations of about 3.5 micrograms/mL have been obtained 2 hours after administration of 200 mg by mouth. Systemic absorption following topical or vaginal application in healthy subjects is minimal. Ketoconazole is more than 90% bound to plasma proteins, mainly albumin. It is widely distributed and appears in breast milk. Penetration into the CSF is poor. The elimination of ketoconazole is reported to be biphasic, with an initial half-life of 2 hours and a terminal half-life of about 8 hours.

Ketoconazole is metabolised in the liver to inactive metabolites. It is excreted as metabolites and unchanged drug chiefly in the faeces; some is excreted in the urine.

◊ References.

1. Daneshmend TK, Warnock DW. Clinical pharmacokinetics of ketoconazole. *Clin Pharmacokinet* 1988; **14:** 13–34.
2. Lelawongs P, *et al.* Effect of food and gastric acidity on absorption of orally administered ketoconazole. *Clin Pharm* 1988; **7:** 228–35.
3. Lake-Bakaar G, *et al.* Gastropathy and ketoconazole malabsorption in the acquired immunodeficiency syndrome (AIDS). *Ann Intern Med* 1988; **109:** 471–3.
4. Daneshmend TK. Diseases and drugs but not food decrease ketoconazole 'bioavailability'. *Br J Clin Pharmacol* 1990; **29:** 783–4.

## Uses and Administration

Ketoconazole is an imidazole antifungal administered topically or by mouth. It is given by mouth in chronic mucocutaneous candidiasis, in fungal infections of the gastrointestinal tract, in dermatophyte infections of the skin and fingernails not responding to topical treatment, and in systemic infections including blastomycosis, candidiasis, coccidioidomycosis, histoplasmosis, and paracoccidioidomycosis. It has been given for the prophylaxis of fungal infections in immunocompromised patients, although fluconazole or itraconazole are usually preferred. It has been recommended that, because of its erratic absorption and slow therapeutic response, ketoconazole should not be used for the treatment of life-threatening fungal infections, including fungal meningitis, or for severe infections in immunocompromised patients. Also, because of the risk of hepatotoxicity with ketoconazole, its use in non-systemic fungal infections tends to be restricted to serious infections resistant to other treatment.

The place of ketoconazole in the treatment of fungal infections is discussed in the various sections under Choice of Antifungal, p.386.

The usual oral dose for treatment and prophylaxis of fungal infections is 200 mg once daily taken with food. This may be increased to 400 mg daily if an adequate response is not obtained; in some infections even higher doses have been used. Children may be given approximately 3 mg/kg daily, or 50 mg for those aged 1 to 4 years and 100 mg for children aged 5 to 12 years. Treatment should usually be continued for 14 days and for at least one week after symptoms have cleared and cultures have become negative. Some infections may require several months' treatment and administering ketoconazole for such prolonged periods may increase the risk of liver toxicity.

A dose of 400 mg once daily for 5 days is used for the treatment of chronic vaginal candidiasis.

Ketoconazole is applied topically as a 2% cream in the treatment of candidal or dermatophyte infections of the skin, or in the treatment of pityriasis versicolor. It is applied once or twice daily and continued for at least a few days after the disappearance of symptoms. A shampoo containing 1 or 2% ketoconazole is used twice weekly for 2 to 4 weeks (or occasionally longer) in the treatment of dandruff or seborrhoeic dermatitis. The 2% shampoo is used once daily for up to 5 days in pityriasis versicolor. For prophylaxis of seborrhoeic dermatitis the 2% shampoo is used once every 1 to 2 weeks; for prophylaxis of pityriasis versicolor it may be used once daily for a maximum of 3 days before exposure to sunshine.

**Acanthamoeba infections.** Although there is currently no established treatment for granulomatous amoebic encephalitis, ketoconazole may have some activity against the *Acanthamoeba* spp. responsible for this infection and has been applied topically to skin lesions. Ketoconazole has also been suggested for *Acanthamoeba* keratitis (p.595), when it has been given orally with topical miconazole.

**Acute respiratory distress syndrome.** In two small double-blind, controlled trials,[1,2] the development of acute respiratory distress syndrome (ARDS—p.1075) and mortality rates were lower in high-risk patients who received ketoconazole than in those who received placebo. An accompanying editorial[3] commented that adequate blood concentrations appeared to be essential. The mode of action could be associated with inhibition of leukotriene and thromboxane synthesis.[2,3] Nevertheless, in a study in 234 patients,[4] ketoconazole failed to reduce mortality or improve clinical outcomes when given early in the course of ARDS. Some centres have developed guidelines for ketoconazole prophylaxis in patients at risk of ARDS.[5]

1. Slotman GJ, *et al.* Ketoconazole prevents acute respiratory failure in critically ill surgical patients. *J Trauma* 1988; **28:** 648–54.
2. Yu M, Tomasa G. A double-blind, prospective, randomized trial of ketoconazole, a thromboxane synthetase inhibitor, in the prophylaxis of the adult respiratory distress syndrome. *Crit Care Med* 1993; **21:** 1635–42.
3. Slotman GJ. Ketoconazole: maybe it isn't the magic potion, but ... *Crit Care Med* 1993; **21:** 1642–4.
4. The ARDS Network Authors for the ARDS Network. Ketoconazole for early treatment of acute lung injury and acute respiratory distress syndrome: a randomized controlled trial. *JAMA* 2000; **283:** 1995–2002.
5. Sinuff T, *et al.* Development, implementation, and evaluation of a ketoconazole practice guideline for ARDS prophylaxis. *J Crit Care* 1999; **14:** 1–6.

**Blastomycosis.** Although ketoconazole has been replaced by itraconazole as the azole of choice in the treatment of blastomycosis (p.386), it has been used as an alternative in doses of 400 to 800 mg daily.[1]

1. Chapman SW, *et al.* Practice guidelines for the management of patients with blastomycosis. *Clin Infect Dis* 2000; **30:** 679–83.

**Endocrine disorders and malignant neoplasms.** Ketoconazole has been reported to impair steroid hormone synthesis[1] and to blunt the response of cortisone to adrenocorticotrophic hormone (ACTH)[2] and has been tried in the management of a number of endocrine disorders.

In **Cushing's syndrome** (p.1313), ketoconazole in doses of up to 1200 mg daily has been used successfully as an alternative or adjuvant to definitive therapies such as surgery or radiotherapy.[3-6]

Treatment of **hirsutism** is usually with an anti-androgen (see p.1545), but ketoconazole has been tried in small numbers of women at a dose of 300 mg daily[7] or 400 mg daily,[8,9] with variable results.

Ketoconazole has been reported to produce a beneficial response in some forms of **precocious puberty** (p.1318) that do not generally respond to gonadorelin analogues.[10,11]

The anti-androgenic effects of ketoconazole have also been found useful in the management of **prostatic cancer** (p.521) in selected patients,[12-16] although there have been some concerns about its tolerability,[15] and it is not generally used as a first-line treatment.

1. Pont A, *et al.* Ketoconazole blocks adrenal steroid synthesis. *Ann Intern Med* 1982; **97:** 370–2.
2. White MC, Kendall-Taylor P. Adrenal hypofunction in patients taking ketoconazole. *Lancet* 1985; **i:** 44–5.
3. Winquist EW, *et al.* Ketoconazole in the management of paraneoplastic Cushing's syndrome secondary to ectopic adrenocorticotropin production. *J Clin Oncol* 1995; **13:** 157–64.
4. Estrada J, *et al.* The long-term outcome of pituitary irradiation after unsuccessful transsphenoidal surgery in Cushing's disease. *N Engl J Med* 1997; **336:** 172–7.
5. Berwaerts JJ, *et al.* Corticotropin-dependent Cushing's syndrome in older people: presentation of five cases and therapeutical use of ketoconazole. *J Am Geriatr Soc* 1998; **46:** 880–4.
6. Chou SC, Lin JD. Long-term effects of ketoconazole in the treatment of residual or recurrent Cushing's disease. *Endocr J* 2000; **47:** 401–6.
7. Venturoli S, *et al.* A prospective randomized trial comparing low dose flutamide, finasteride, ketoconazole, and cyproterone acetate-estrogen regimens in the treatment of hirsutism. *J Clin Endocrinol Metab* 1999; **84:** 1304–10.
8. Sonino N, *et al.* Low-dose ketoconazole treatment in hirsute women. *J Endocrinol Invest* 1990; **13:** 35–40.

9. Venturoli S, *et al.* Ketoconazole therapy for women with acne and/or hirsutism. *J Clin Endocrinol Metab* 1990; **71:** 335–9.
10. Bertelloni S, *et al.* Long-term outcome of male-limited gonadotropin-independent precocious puberty. *Horm Res* 1997; **48:** 235–9.
11. Syed FA, Chalew SA. Ketoconazole treatment of gonadotropin independent precocious puberty in girls with McCune-Albright syndrome: a preliminary report. *J Pediatr Endocrinol Metab* 1999; **12:** 81–3.
12. Lowe FC, Bamberger MH. Indications for use of ketoconazole in management of metastatic prostate cancer. *Urology* 1990; **36:** 541–5.
13. Mahler C, *et al.* Ketoconazole and liarozole in the treatment of advanced prostatic cancer. *Cancer* 1993; **71:** 1068–73.
14. Small EJ, *et al.* Ketoconazole retains activity in advanced prostate cancer patients with progression despite flutamide withdrawal. *J Urol (Baltimore)* 1997; **157:** 1204–7.
15. Bok RA, Small EJ. The treatment of advanced prostate cancer with ketoconazole: safety issues. *Drug Safety* 1999; **20:** 451–8.
16. Pettaway CA, *et al.* Neoadjuvant chemotherapy and hormonal therapy followed by radical prostatectomy: feasibility and preliminary results. *J Clin Oncol* 2000; **18:** 1050–7.

**Hypercalcaemia.** Ketoconazole has been used[1,2] in the treatment of hypercalcaemia (p.1218). It acts by reducing 1,25-dihydroxycholecalciferol concentrations by inhibiting cytochrome P450-dependent 1α-hydroxylation of vitamin D.

1. Yavuz H. Familiar drugs for the treatment of hypercalcemia. *J Pediatr* 1998; **133:** 311.
2. Young C, *et al.* Hypercalcaemia in sarcoidosis. *Lancet* 1999; **353:** 374.

**Leishmaniasis.** As discussed on p.597, ketoconazole has been tried as an alternative to conventional first- and second-line therapy for visceral leishmaniasis,[1,2] although reports of treatment have not all been favourable.[3,4]

It has also been tried in cutaneous leishmaniasis. A cure rate of 70% was reported in over 100 patients with *Leishmania major* infections treated with ketoconazole 200 to 400 mg daily by mouth for 4 to 6 weeks. Ketoconazole was not considered to be effective in infections due to *L. tropica*, *L. aethiopica*,[5] or *L. guyanensis*.[6] Ketoconazole 600 mg daily for 28 days has produced similar results to sodium stibogluconate intramuscularly for 20 days in patients with cutaneous leishmaniasis due to *L. panamensis*.[7] In another study,[8] ketoconazole was less effective than sodium stibogluconate when cutaneous leishmaniasis was due to *L. braziliensis*, but more effective when *L. mexicana* was the cause.

1. Wali JP, *et al.* Ketoconazole in treatment of visceral leishmaniasis. *Lancet* 1990; **330:** 810–11.
2. Wali JP, *et al.* Ketoconazole in the treatment of antimony- and pentamidine-resistant Kala-azar. *J Infect Dis* 1992; **166:** 215–16.
3. Sundar S, *et al.* Ketoconazole in visceral leishmaniasis. *Lancet* 1990; **336:** 1582–3.
4. Rashid JR, *et al.* The efficacy and safety of ketoconazole in visceral leishmaniasis. *East Afr Med J* 1994; **71:** 392–5.
5. Weinrauch L, *et al.* Ketoconazole in cutaneous leishmaniasis. *Br J Dermatol* 1987; **117:** 666–7.
6. Dedet J-P, *et al.* Failure to cure Leishmania braziliensis guyanensis cutaneous leishmaniasis with oral ketoconazole. *Trans R Soc Trop Med Hyg* 1986; **80:** 176.
7. Saenz RE, *et al.* Efficacy of ketoconazole against Leishmania braziliensis panamensis cutaneous leishmaniasis. *Am J Med* 1990; **89:** 147–55.
8. Navin TR, *et al.* Placebo-controlled clinical trial of sodium stibogluconate (Pentostam) versus ketoconazole for treating cutaneous leishmaniasis in Guatemala. *J Infect Dis* 1992; **165:** 528–34.

## Preparations

***USP 27:*** Ketoconazole Oral Suspension; Ketoconazole Tablets.

**Proprietary Preparations** (details are given in Part 3)

***Arg.:*** C-86; Cetonil; Faction; Fangan; Fitonal; Fungicil; Grenfung; Keduo; Ketogel; Ketonazol; Ketozol; Krol; Micoral; Orifungal; Perative; Quadion; Socosep; Tersoderm Plus; Tikl; Triatop; ***Austral.:*** Daktagold; Hexal Konazol Shampoo; Nizoral; Sebizole; ***Austria:*** Fungoral; Nizoral; Triatop; ***Belg.:*** Nizoral; ***Braz.:*** Aciderm; Arcolan; Candiderm; Candoral; Cetohexal; Cetomed; Cetonax; Cetoneo; Cetonil; Cetozan; Cetozol; Fungoral; Ketocon†; Ketomicol; Ketonan; Ketonazol; Konazil†; Lozan; Miconan; Micoral; Nizoral; Nizoretic; Noriderm; Norizal†; Noronal; Zanoc; ***Canad.:*** Nizoral; ***Chile:*** Arcolane; Biogel; Eprofil; Fungarest; Fungium; Ketonil; Soridermal; TKC; ***Denm.:*** Nizoral; ***Fin.:*** Nizoral; ***Fr.:*** Ketoderm; Nizoral; ***Ger.:*** Nizoral; Terzolin; ***Gr.:*** Abba; Adenosan; Aquarius; Botaderm; Cezolin; Ebersept; Fungoral; Ilgem; Mycofebrin; Neo-egmol; Scalpin; Sostatin; Vafluson; ***Hong Kong:*** Diazon; Fungazol; Nizoral; Pristine; Pristinex; Sebizole; Synizoral; ***India:*** Danruf; Funazole; Fungicide; ***Irl.:*** Nizoral; ***Israel:*** Nizoral; ***Ital.:*** Nizoral; Triatop; ***Malaysia:*** Dezor; Fungazol; Funginox; Kezoral; Nizoral; Pristine; Pristinex; Yucomy; Ziconal; ***Mex.:*** Akorazol; Biozoral; Conazol; Cremosan; Ehlifung†; Ergomicon; Eurolat†; Fungamizol†; Fungazol†; Fungoral; Honzil†; Keprobiozol; Kestomicol; Ketofar; Ketomizol†; Ketone†; Konaderm; Konaturil; Lizovag; Lornazol; Luperzol†; Mi-Ke-Sons; Micogal†; Micoser; Miketos†; Mycodib; Nastil; Nazolfarm†; Nikorazol†; Nizoral; Onofin-K; Prenalon; Termizol; Tiniazol; Tocomizol†; Toconal; Vagmicor†; ***Neth.:*** Nizoral; ***Norw.:*** Fungoral; ***NZ:*** Daktagold; Nizoral; Sebizole; ***Port.:*** Cesol†; Frisol; Frisolac; Nizale; Nizoral; Rapamic; Tedol; ***S.Afr.:*** Adco-Dermed; Ketazol; Nizcreme; Nizoral; Nizorelle; Nizovules; Nizshampoo; ***Singapore:*** Antanazol; Beatoconazole; Dezoral; Diazon; Ketozole; Mycoral†; Nizoral; Pristine; Pristinex; Profungal; Sebizole; Spozal†; Yucomy; Zorinax†; ***Spain:*** Fungarest; Fungo Hubber; Ketoisdin; Micoticum; Panfungol; ***Swed.:*** Fundan; Fungoral; Ketoson; ***Switz.:*** Ketozol; Nizoral; Terzolin; ***Thai.:*** AC-FA†; Chintaral; Diazon; Fungazol; Fungicide†; Fungiderm-K; Funginox; Kara; Katsin; Kazinal; Kenalyn; Kenazol; Kenazole; Kenoral; Ketazol; Ketazon; Ketocine; Ketolan; Ketomed; Ketonazole; Ketoral; Ketosil; Ketozal; Kezon; Konazol; Lama; Larry; Manoketo; Masarol; Mizoron; Mycella; Ninazol; Nizoral; Nora; Pasalen; Sporoxyl; Triatop; ***UK:*** Daktarin Gold; Dandrazol; Dandrid; Nizoral; ***USA:*** Nizoral.

**Multi-ingredient: *Arg.:*** Aeromicrosona C; Ciprocort; Duo Minoxi; Gynerium; Ketohair; Micozol Compuesto; Microsona C; Prurisedan Biotic; Start NP; Tridermal; Triefect; ***Braz.:*** Betazol Cort; Candicort; Capel; Cetobeta; Cetocort; Novacort; ***Chile:*** Kpl; ***Mex.:*** Femisan.

## Lanoconazole *(rINN)*

Lanoconazol; Latoconazole; NND-318; TJN-318. (±)-α-[(E)-4-(o-Chlorophenyl)-1,3-dithiolan-2-ylidene]imidazole-1-acetonitrile.

$C_{14}H_{10}ClN_3S_2$ = 319.8.

*CAS — 101530-10-3.*

### Profile

Lanoconazole is an imidazole antifungal used topically in the treatment of fungal skin infections as a 1% cream, ointment, or solution, applied once daily. For a discussion of the caution needed when using azole antifungals during pregnancy, see under Pregnancy in Precautions of Fluconazole, p.398.

### Preparations

**Proprietary Preparations** (details are given in Part 3)

***Jpn:*** Astat.

## Mepartricin *(BAN, USAN, rINN)*

Mepartricina; Methylpartricin; SN-654; SPA-S-160.

*CAS — 11121-32-7.*

*ATC — A01AB16; D01AA06; G01AA09; G04CX03.*

### Profile

Mepartricin is a mixture of the methyl esters of 2 related polyene antibiotics that may be obtained from a strain of *Streptomyces aureofaciens*. It has antifungal and antiprotozoal activity and has been used in vaginal candidiasis and trichomoniasis as pessaries or as a vaginal cream. A cream is also available for the treatment of superficial candidiasis. Mepartricin sodium laurilsulfate is also used.

**Benign prostatic hyperplasia.** Mepartricin has been given by mouth in the treatment of benign prostatic hyperplasia (see under Finasteride p.1555 for the more usual treatment).

References.

1. Tosto A, *et al.* A double-blind study of the effects of mepartricin in the treatment of obstruction due to benign prostatic hyperplasia. *Curr Ther Res* 1995; **56:** 1270–75.
2. Denis L, *et al.* Double-blind, placebo-controlled trial to assess the efficacy and tolerability of mepartricin in the treatment of BPH. *Prostate* 1998; **37:** 246–52.

### Preparations

**Proprietary Preparations** (details are given in Part 3)

***Austria:*** Iperplasin; Prostec; ***Belg.:*** Tricandil; ***Braz.:*** Montricin; Orofungin†; ***Chile:*** Normoprost; ***Ital.:*** Ipertrofan; Montricin†; Tricandil; ***Port.:*** Tricandil.

**Multi-ingredient: *Braz.:*** Tricangine.

## Micafungin Sodium *(USAN, rINNM)*

FK-463. 5-((1*S*,2*S*)-2-{(2*R*,6*S*,9*S*,11*R*,12*R*,14a*S*,15*S*,16*S*,20*S*,23*S*,25a*S*)-20-[(1*R*)-3-Amino-1-hydroxy-3-oxopropyl]-2,11,12,15-tetrahydroxy-6-[(1*R*)-1-hydroxyethyl]-16-methyl-5,8,14,19,22,25-hexaoxo-9-[(4-{5-[4-(pentyloxy)phenyl]isoxazol-3-yl}benzoyl)amino]tetracosahydro-1*H*-dipyrrolo[2,1-*c*:2′,1′-*l*][1,4,7,10,13,16]hexaazacyclohenicosin-23-yl}-1,2-dihydroxyethyl)-2-hydroxyphenyl sodium sulfate.

$C_{56}H_{70}N_9NaO_{23}S$ = 1292.3.

*CAS — 235114-32-6 (micafungin); 208538-73-2 (micafungin sodium).*

### Profile

Micafungin is an antifungal used for the treatment of candidiasis and aspergillosis. It is given as the sodium salt by intravenous infusion in doses of 50 mg once daily for candidiasis or 50 to 150 mg once daily for aspergillosis. Doses may be increased to 300 mg daily in severe or refractory disease.

## Miconazole *(BAN, rINN)*

Miconazol; Miconazolum; R-18134. 1-[2,4-Dichloro-β-(2,4-dichlorobenzyloxy)phenethyl]imidazole.

$C_{18}H_{14}Cl_4N_2O$ = 416.1.

*CAS — 22916-47-8.*

*ATC — A01AB09; A07AC01; D01AC02; G01AF04; J02AB01; S02AA13.*

**Pharmacopoeias.** In *Eur.* (see p.vi), *Jpn*, and *US*.

**Ph. Eur. 5.0** (Miconazole). A white or almost white powder. It exhibits polymorphism. M.p. 83° to 87°. Very slightly soluble in water; soluble in alcohol; freely soluble in methyl alcohol. Protect from light.

**USP 27** (Miconazole). A white to pale cream powder. It may exhibit polymorphism. M.p. 78° to 88°. Insoluble in water; soluble 1 in 9.5 of alcohol, 1 in 2 of chloroform, 1 in 15 of ether, 1 in 4 of isopropyl alcohol, 1 in 5.3 of methyl alcohol, and 1 in 9 of propylene glycol; freely soluble in acetone and in dimethylformamide. Store at a temperature of 25°, excursions permitted between 15° and 30°. Protect from light.

## Miconazole Nitrate *(BANM, USAN, rINNM)*

Miconazoli Nitras; Nitrato de miconazol; R-14889.

$C_{18}H_{14}Cl_4N_2O,HNO_3$ = 479.1.

*CAS — 22832-87-7.*

*ATC — A01AB09; A07AC01; D01AC02; G01AF04; J02AB01; S02AA13.*

**Pharmacopoeias.** In *Chin., Eur.* (see p.vi), *Int., Jpn, Pol.*, and *US*.

**Ph. Eur. 5.0** (Miconazole Nitrate). A white or almost white powder. Very slightly soluble in water; slightly soluble in alcohol; sparingly soluble in methyl alcohol. Protect from light.

**USP 27** (Miconazole Nitrate). A white or practically white, crystalline powder, with not more than a slight odour. Soluble 1 in 6250 of water, 1 in 312 of alcohol, 1 in 75 of methyl alcohol, 1 in 525 of chloroform, 1 in 1408 of isopropyl alcohol, 1 in 119 of propylene glycol; freely soluble in dimethyl sulfoxide; soluble in dimethylformamide; insoluble in ether. Protect from light.

### Adverse Effects

After oral use of miconazole, nausea and vomiting have been reported, and also diarrhoea (usually on long-term treatment). There have been allergic reactions, rarely, and isolated reports of hepatitis.

Local irritation and sensitivity reactions may occur when miconazole nitrate is used topically; contact dermatitis has been reported.

After the intravenous infusion of miconazole, phlebitis, nausea, vomiting, diarrhoea, anorexia, pruritus, rash, febrile reactions, flushes, drowsiness, and hyponatraemia have been reported. Other effects include hyperlipidaemia, aggregation of erythrocytes, anaemia, and thrombocytosis. Transient tachycardia and other cardiac arrhythmias have followed the rapid intravenous injection of miconazole (but see also Effects on the Heart, below). Rare adverse effects include acute psychosis, arthralgia, and anaphylaxis. Many of these adverse effects have been associated with the injection vehicle which contains polyethoxylated castor oil (see Polyoxyl Castor Oils, p.1414).

**Effects on the heart.** Bradycardia, progressing to fatal ventricular fibrillation and cardiac arrest, occurred in a heart transplant patient during intravenous infusion of miconazole for an invasive fungal infection.[1]

1. Coley KC, Crain JL. Miconazole-induced fatal dysrhythmia. *Pharmacotherapy* 1997; **17:** 379–82.

**Overdosage.** A report[1] of a generalised tonic-clonic convulsion that occurred in an infant 10 to 15 minutes after the inadvertent infusion of miconazole 500 mg instead of 50 mg.

1. Coulthard K, *et al.* Convulsions after miconazole overdose. *Med J Aust* 1987; **146:** 57–8.

### Precautions

Miconazole should be avoided in patients with hepatic impairment.

Intravaginal preparations of miconazole may damage latex contraceptives and additional contraceptive measures are therefore necessary during local administration.

Miconazole has been fetotoxic at high doses in *animals* and its use is generally not recommended during pregnancy. For a discussion of the caution needed when using azole antifungals during pregnancy, see under Pregnancy in Precautions of Fluconazole, p.398.

**Porphyria.** Miconazole is considered to be unsafe in patients with porphyria because it has been shown to be porphyrinogenic in *in-vitro* systems.

### Interactions

Miconazole can inhibit the metabolism of drugs metabolised by the cytochrome P450 isoenzymes CYP3A4 and CYP2C9, and may thus have effects similar to those of fluconazole (p.398). Miconazole may enhance the activity of oral anticoagulants, sulfonylurea hypoglycaemics, or phenytoin. Adverse effects have been reported when miconazole was given with carbamazepine.

There is a risk of cardiac arrhythmias if miconazole is used with astemizole, cisapride, or terfenadine and such combinations should be avoided.

**Anticoagulants.** The anticoagulant activity of coumarin anticoagulants can be potentiated by miconazole administered orally[1] or intravaginally.[2]

1. Ortín M, *et al.* Miconazole oral gel enhances acenocoumarol anticoagulant activity: a report of three cases. *Ann Pharmacother* 1999; **33:** 175–7.
2. Lansdorp D, *et al.* Potentiation of acenocoumarol during vaginal administration of miconazole. *Br J Clin Pharmacol* 1999; **47:** 225–26.

## Antimicrobial Action

Miconazole is an imidazole antifungal with similar antimicrobial activity to that of ketoconazole (p.404). It also has some activity against *Aspergillus* spp., *Cryptococcus neoformans, Pseudallescheria boydii,* and some Gram-positive bacteria including staphylococci and streptococci.

**Microbiological interactions.** A study *in vitro* indicating antimicrobial synergism of miconazole and benzoyl peroxide against *Staphylococcus* spp. and *Propionibacterium acnes*.[1]

For the effect on antifungal activity of giving azoles and amphotericin B together, see p.393.

1. Vanden Bossche H, *et al.* Synergism of the antimicrobial agents miconazole and benzoyl peroxide. *Br J Dermatol* 1982; **107:** 343–8.

## Pharmacokinetics

Miconazole is incompletely absorbed from the gastrointestinal tract. Peak plasma concentrations of 1 microgram/mL are achieved about 4 hours after a dose of 1 g daily. Over 90% is reported to be bound to plasma proteins.

Miconazole is metabolised in the liver to inactive metabolites. From 10 to 20% of an oral dose is excreted in the urine, mainly as metabolites, within 6 days. About 50% of an oral dose may be excreted unchanged in the faeces. The elimination pharmacokinetics of miconazole have been described as triphasic, with a biological half-life of about 24 hours.

Very little miconazole is removed by haemodialysis.

There is little absorption through skin or mucous membranes when miconazole nitrate is applied topically.

◊ Reviews.

1. Daneshmend TK, Warnock DW. Clinical pharmacokinetics of systemic antifungal drugs. *Clin Pharmacokinet* 1983; **8:** 17–42.

## Uses and Administration

Miconazole is an imidazole antifungal used as miconazole base or nitrate in the treatment of superficial candidiasis (p.386), and of the skin infections dermatophytosis and pityriasis versicolor (p.390). It has also been given intravenously by infusion in the treatment of disseminated fungal infections, but other azoles are now more commonly used.

Miconazole may be given by mouth as an oral gel containing 20 mg/g (24 mg/mL) for the treatment of oropharyngeal and intestinal candidiasis. The usual adult dose is 5 to 10 mL four times daily (approximately equivalent to a total of 15 mg/kg daily). Children under the age of 2 years may be given the oral gel in a dose of 2.5 mL twice daily; those aged between 2 and 6 years, 5 mL twice daily; and those aged over 6 years, 5 mL four times daily. For the treatment of oral lesions the oral gel is applied directly. A sustained release lacquer is available for dentures.

Miconazole nitrate is usually applied twice daily as a 2% cream, lotion, or powder in the treatment of fungal infections of the skin including candidiasis, dermatophytosis, and pityriasis versicolor. In the treatment of vaginal candidiasis, 5 g of a 2% intravaginal cream is inserted into the vagina once daily for 10 to 14 days or twice daily for 7 days. Miconazole nitrate pessaries may be inserted in dosage regimens of 100 mg once daily for 7 or 14 days, 100 mg twice daily for 7 days, 200 or 400 mg daily for 3 days, or in a single dose of 1200 mg.

**Acanthamoeba keratitis.** Miconazole has been applied topically in *Acanthamoeba* keratitis (p.595) in combination with systemic treatment with either ketoconazole or itraconazole.

**Skin disorders.** Topical preparations containing an imidazole such as clotrimazole, ketoconazole, or miconazole usually together with hydrocortisone are used in the management of *seborrhoeic dermatitis* (p.1138). A cream containing miconazole nitrate 2% and benzoyl peroxide 5% has been used topically in the treatment of *acne* (p.1133).

## Preparations

***BP 2003:*** Miconazole Cream; Miconazole Oromucosal Gel;
***USP 27:*** Miconazole Injection; Miconazole Nitrate Cream; Miconazole Nitrate Topical Powder; Miconazole Nitrate Vaginal Suppositories.

**Proprietary Preparations** (details are given in Part 3)
***Arg.:*** Daktarin; Deralbine; Miconol; Micotral; Micotrim P; Micotrim S; Nedis; Salicrem Miconazol; ***Austral.:*** Chemists Own Zapazole†; Daktarin; Eulactol Antifungal; Gyno-Daktarin†; Monistat; Resolve; Resolve Thrush; ***Austria:*** Daktarin; Gyno-Daktarin; ***Belg.:*** Albistat†; Daktar; Daktarin; Gyno-Daktarin; ***Braz.:*** Amicose†; Ciconazol; Daktarin; Daktazol; Ginedak; Ginotarin; Gyno-Daktarin; Micofim; Micogyn; Micoless†; Miconax†; Micotarin†; Micozen; Mycosin; Vodol; ***Canad.:*** Micatin; Micozole; Monazole; Monistat; ***Chile:*** Daktarin; Fungos; ZeaSorb AF; ***Denm.:*** Brenazol; Brentan; Dumicoat†; ***Fin.:*** Daktarin; Dumicoat†; Gyno-Daktarin; Medizol; ***Fr.:*** Britane†; Daktarin; Gyno-Daktarin; ***Ger.:*** Amykon; Castellani mit Miconazol; Daktar; Derma-Mykotral; Dumicoat†; Epi-Monistat†; Fungur M; Gyno-Daktar; Gyno-Monistat†; Gyno-Mykotral; InfectoSoor; Micotar; Mykoderm Mund-Gel; Mykotin; Vobamyk; ***Gr.:*** Daktarin; Medacter; Mezolitan; Untano; ***Hong Kong:*** Daktarin; Dermon; Funga; Fungo; Gyno-Daktarin; ***India:*** Daktarin; Gyno-Daktarin; Micogel; Zole; ***Irl.:*** Daktarin; Gyno-Daktarin; ***Israel:*** Daktarin; Gyno-Daktarin; Pitrion; ***Ital.:*** Andergin†; Daktarin; Fungiderm†; Micoderm†; Micomax†; Miconal; Micotef; Miderm; Nizacol; Pivanozolo; Prilagin†; ***Malaysia:*** Antifungal; Becarin; Daktarin; Decozol; Fungo; Setarin; Uniderm; Zarin; ***Mex.:*** Aloid; Daktarin; Dermifun; Fungicrem; Fungiquim; Gyno-Daktarin†; K-Mizol†; Lotrimin AF; Micoffen; Micosid†; Mindosan V; Neomicol; Nimicon†; Piat; ***Neth.:*** Daktarin; Dermacure; Gyno-Daktarin; ***Norw.:*** Daktar; Dumicoat†; ***NZ:*** Daktarin; Fungo; Gyno-Daktarin†; Hairscience Antidandruff; Micozole†; Micreme; ***Port.:*** Daktarin; Gyno-Daktarin; Micane; ***S.Afr.:*** Covarex; Daktarin; Gyno-Daktarin; Gynospor; ***Singapore:*** Antifungal; Candiplas†; Daktarin; Decozol; Fungo; Hairscience; Liconar; Zarin; ***Spain:*** Daktarin; Fungisdin; Medefungin†; Pasedon; Tremix; ***Swed.:*** Daktar; Dumicoat†; ***Switz.:*** Daktarin; Dumicoat; Monistat; ***Thai.:*** Candiplas†; Daktarin; Funcort; Fungi-M; Fungisil; Liconar; Micazin; Minaza†; Misone; Mysocort; Neomite†; Nikarin; Noxraxin; Ranozol; Skindure; Tara; ***UAE:*** Gyno-Mikozal; Mikozal; ***UK:*** Daktarin; Dumicoat†; Femeron†; Gyno-Daktarin; ***USA:*** Absorbine Antifungal Foot Powder; Breezee Mist Antifungal; Femizol-M; Fungoid; Lotrimin AF; M-Zole; Maximum Strength Desenex Antifungal; Micatin; Monistat; Ony-Clear†; Podactin; Ting; ZeaSorb AF.

**Multi-ingredient: *Arg.:*** Adenil; Ciprocort; Daktozin; Denvercrem; Dermizol Trio; Dermosona; Factor Dermico; Gentasol; Ginal Cent; Ginkan; Gynormal; Hifamonil Crema; Ladylen; Macril; Miklogen; Protiderm; Triplex; Vagicural Plus; ***Austral.:*** Daktozin; Resolve; Resolve Plus; ***Austria:*** Acne Plus; Acnidazil†; Daktacort†; ***Belg.:*** Acnidazil†; Daktacort; Daktozin; ***Braz.:*** Amplium-G; Daktozin†; Facyl M; Gino Pletil; Ginosutin M; Trinizol M; ***Chile:*** Doxifen; Famidal; Famidal Ad; Ginecopast; Ginedazol Dual; Mizonase; ***Denm.:*** Acnidazil†; Brentacort; ***Fin.:*** Daktacort; ***Fr.:*** Daktacort†; ***Ger.:*** Acne Plus; Acnidazil†; Decoderm tri; InfectoSoor; Vobaderm; ***Gr.:*** Daktodor; Micogen; Verdal; ***Hong Kong:*** Daktacort; Hydro-Funga; ***India:*** Betamil-M; Betnovate-GM; Betnovate-M; Candizole-T; Daktacort; Flucort-MZ; Flucreme NM; Lobate-GM; Lobate-M; Stecort-NM; Tenovate M; Valbet; Zole-F; ***Irl.:*** Daktacort; ***Israel:*** Daktacort; ***Ital.:*** Acnidazil; ***Malaysia:*** Becacort; Daktacort; Decocort; Setarin H; Zaricort; ***Mex.:*** Daktacort; ***Neth.:*** Acnecure; Acnidazil; Daktacort; ***Norw.:*** Daktacort; ***NZ:*** Daktacort; Daktozin; Fungocort; Micreme H; ***Port.:*** Daktacort; ***S.Afr.:*** Acneclear; Acnidazil; Daktacort; Trialone; ***Singapore:*** Betnovate-GM†; Betnovate-M†; Conazole; Daktacort; Decocort; Neo-Penotran; Tri-Micon; Zaricort; ***Spain:*** Bexicortil; Blastoestimulina; Brentan; Dermisdin; Nutracel; ***Swed.:*** Cortimyk; Daktacort; ***Switz.:*** Acne Creme Plus; Daktacort; Decoderm bivalent; ***Thai.:*** Daktacort; Fungisil-T; Kelaplus; Ladocort; Tara-Plus; Timi; Trimicon; ***UK:*** Acnidazil†; Daktacort; Daktacort HC; ***USA:*** Fungoid HC.

---

# Naftifine Hydrochloride *(BANM, USAN, rINNM)*

AW-105-843; Hidrocloruro de naftifina; Naftifungin Hydrochloride; SN-105-843 (naftifine). (*E*)-*N*-Cinnamyl-*N*-methyl(1-naphthylmethyl)amine hydrochloride.

$C_{21}H_{21}N,HCl = 323.9.$

*CAS — 65472-88-0 (naftifine); 65473-14-5 (naftifine hydrochloride).*

*ATC — D01AE22.*

**Pharmacopoeias.** In *US.*

**USP 27** (Naftifine Hydrochloride). Store in airtight containers.

## Profile

Naftifine hydrochloride is an allylamine derivative (see Terbinafine Hydrochloride, p.408) which is reported to be fungicidal against dermatophytes, but only fungistatic against *Candida* spp.

Naftifine hydrochloride 1% is applied topically once or twice daily for fungal skin infections, particularly dermatophytosis (p.390).

Local reactions such as burning or stinging may occur.

## Preparations

***USP 27:*** Naftifine Hydrochloride Cream; Naftifine Hydrochloride Gel.

**Proprietary Preparations** (details are given in Part 3)
***Austria:*** Benecut; Exoderil; ***Canad.:*** Naftin; ***Ger.:*** Exoderil; ***Hong Kong:*** Exoderil; ***Israel:*** Exoderil; ***Ital.:*** Suadian; ***Malaysia:*** Exoderil; ***Singapore:*** Exoderil; ***Spain:*** Micosona; ***USA:*** Naftin.

---

# Natamycin *(BAN, USAN, pINN)*

Antibiotic A-5283; CL-12625; E235; Natamicina; Pimaricin.

$C_{33}H_{47}NO_{13} = 665.7.$

*CAS — 7681-93-8.*

*ATC — A01AB10; A07AA03; D01AA02; G01AA02; S01AA10.*

**Pharmacopoeias.** In *Jpn, Pol.,* and *US.*

**USP 27** (Natamycin). An off-white to cream-coloured powder. It may contain up to 3 moles of water. Practically insoluble in water; soluble in glacial acetic acid and in dimethylformamide; slightly soluble in methyl alcohol. A 1% suspension in water has a pH of 5.0 to 7.5. Store in airtight containers. Protect from light.

## Adverse Effects and Precautions

Gastrointestinal disturbances have occurred after the administration of natamycin by mouth. Local application of natamycin has sometimes produced irritation.

**Porphyria.** Natamycin has been associated with acute attacks of porphyria and is considered unsafe in porphyric patients.

## Antimicrobial Action

Natamycin is a polyene antifungal active against *Candida* and *Fusarium* spp. In addition it is active against the protozoan *Trichomonas vaginalis.*

## Pharmacokinetics

Natamycin is poorly absorbed from the gastrointestinal tract. It is not absorbed through the skin or mucous membranes when applied topically. Following ocular administration, natamycin is present in therapeutic concentrations in corneal stroma but not in intra-ocular fluid; systemic absorption does not usually occur.

## Uses and Administration

Natamycin is a polyene antifungal antibiotic produced by the growth of *Streptomyces natalensis*. It is used for the local treatment of candidiasis (p.386) and fungal keratitis (see Eye Infections, p.388). It has also been used in vaginal trichomoniasis (p.599).

A 5% ophthalmic suspension or a 1% ointment of natamycin is used in the treatment of blepharitis, conjunctivitis, or keratitis due to susceptible fungi, including *Fusarium solani*.

Natamycin is given by mouth for the treatment of intestinal candidiasis in a dose of up to 400 mg daily in divided doses, and as 10-mg lozenges for oral candidiasis.

Natamycin is used topically as a 2% cream for fungal skin infections and for candidal and trichomonal infections of the vagina. Natamycin pessaries have been used.

## Preparations

***USP 27:*** Natamycin Ophthalmic Suspension.

**Proprietary Preparations** (details are given in Part 3)
***Arg.:*** Natacyn; ***Belg.:*** Pimafucin†; ***Fin.:*** Pimafucin; ***Ger.:*** Deronga Heilpaste; Pima Biciron N; Pimafucin; ***Ital.:*** Natafucin; ***Mex.:*** Miconacina; ***S.Afr.:*** Natacyn; ***Singapore:*** Natacyn; ***Thai.:*** Natacyn; ***USA:*** Natacyn.

**Multi-ingredient: *Belg.:*** Pimafucort†; ***Fin.:*** Pimafucort; ***Ger.:*** Pimafucort†; ***NZ:*** Pimafucort; ***Port.:*** Pimafucort.

---

# Neticonazole Hydrochloride *(rINNM)*

Hidrocloruro de neticonazol; SS-717. (*E*)-1-{2-(Methylthio)-1-[*o*-(pentyloxy)phenyl]vinyl}imidazole hydrochloride.

$C_{17}H_{22}N_2OS,HCl = 338.9.$

*CAS — 130726-68-0 (neticonazole); 130773-02-3 (neticonazole hydrochloride).*

## Profile

Neticonazole hydrochloride is an imidazole antifungal that has been used topically in the treatment of superficial fungal infections.

## Preparations

**Proprietary Preparations** (details are given in Part 3)
***Jpn:*** Atolant.

---

# Nifuroxime *(rINN)*

Nifuroxima. 5-Nitro-2-furaldehyde oxime.

$C_5H_4N_2O_4 = 156.1.$

*CAS — 6236-05-1.*

## Profile

Nifuroxime is a nitrofuran antimicrobial that has been used with furazolidone to treat vaginal candidiasis and trichomoniasis.

## Preparations

**Proprietary Preparations** (details are given in Part 3)
**Multi-ingredient: *Ital.:*** Ginecofuran†.

---

# Nystatin *(BAN, USAN, rINN)*

Fungicidin; Nistatina; Nystatinum.

*CAS — 1400-61-9.*

*ATC — A07AA02; D01AA01; G01AA01.*

**Pharmacopoeias.** In *Eur.* (see p.vi), *Int., Jpn, Pol., US,* and *Viet.*

**Ph. Eur. 5.0** (Nystatin). An antifungal substance obtained by fermentation using certain strains of *Streptomyces noursei*. It contains mainly tetraenes, the principal component being nystatin $A_1$. The potency is not less than 4400 units/mg and not less than 5000 units/mg if intended for oral use, calculated with reference to the dried substance. It is a yellow or slightly brownish hygroscopic powder. Practically insoluble in water and in alcohol; freely soluble in dimethylformamide and in dimethyl sulfoxide; slightly soluble in methyl alcohol. Store in airtight containers. Protect from light.

**USP 27** (Nystatin). A substance, or a mixture of two or more substances, produced by the growth of *Streptomyces noursei* (Streptomycetaceae). It has a potency of not less than 4400 units/mg, or, where intended for use in extemporaneous preparation of oral suspensions, not less than 5000 units/mg. A yellow to light tan, hygroscopic powder, with an odour suggestive of cereals; it is affected by long exposure to light, heat, and air. Practically insoluble in water and in alcohol; insoluble in chloroform and in ether; freely soluble in dimethylformamide and in dimethyl sulfoxide; slightly to sparingly soluble in methyl alcohol, in n-butyl alcohol, and in n-propyl alcohol. A 3% suspension in water has a pH of 6.0 to 8.0. Store in airtight containers. Protect from light.

## Adverse Effects

Nausea, vomiting, and diarrhoea have occasionally been reported after oral use of nystatin. Oral irritation or sensitisation may occur. Rashes, including urticaria, have occurred and Stevens-Johnson syndrome has been reported rarely. Irritation may occur rarely after the topical use of nystatin.

**Effects on the skin.** Generalised pustular eruptions were reported in 3 patients following oral nystatin.[1] Subsequent sensitivity testing revealed delayed (type IV) hypersensitivity to nystatin.

1. Küchler A, *et al.* Acute generalized exanthematous pustulosis following oral nystatin therapy: a report of three cases. *Br J Dermatol* 1997; **137:** 808–11.

## Precautions

Intravaginal preparations of nystatin may damage latex contraceptives and additional contraceptive precautions are necessary during treatment.

## Antimicrobial Action

Nystatin is a polyene antifungal antibiotic which interferes with the permeability of the cell membrane of sensitive fungi by binding to sterols, chiefly ergosterol. Its main action is against *Candida* spp.

## Pharmacokinetics

Nystatin is poorly absorbed from the gastrointestinal tract. It is not absorbed through the skin or mucous membranes when applied topically.

**Administration.** In a study in 5 healthy subjects high salivary nystatin concentrations were maintained throughout a 2-hour period during which a controlled-release delivery system was retained in the mouth; concentrations exceeded those achieved with a nystatin pastille.[1] However, a further study[2] found that fungicidal nystatin concentrations were maintained in saliva 5 hours after nystatin pastilles had been used, whereas concentrations were undetectable 2 hours after using an oral suspension.

1. Encarnacion M, Chin I. Salivary nystatin concentrations after administration of an osmotic controlled release tablet and a pastille. *Eur J Clin Pharmacol* 1994; **46:** 533–5.
2. Millns B, Martin MV. Nystatin pastilles and suspension in the treatment of oral candidosis. *Br Dent J* 1996; **181:** 209–11.

## Uses and Administration

Nystatin is a polyene antifungal antibiotic used for the prophylaxis and treatment of candidiasis of the skin and mucous membranes (see p.386). It has been used with antibacterials in various regimens to suppress the overgrowth of gastrointestinal flora and as part of selective decontamination regimens (see Intensive Care, p.132).

For the treatment of intestinal or oesophageal candidiasis, nystatin is given in doses of 500 000 or 1 000 000 units by mouth 3 or 4 times daily. In infants and children a dosage of 100 000 units or more may be given 4 times daily.

For the treatment of lesions of the mouth, pastilles or a suspension may be given in a dosage of 100 000 units 4 times daily. Higher doses of, for example, 500 000 units 4 times daily, may be needed in immunocompromised patients (but see also Candidiasis, below). The formulation should be kept in contact with the affected area for as long as possible, and patients should avoid taking food or drink for one hour after a dose. In the USA, doses of 400 000 to 600 000 units 4 times daily of the suspension, or 200 000 to 400 000 units 4 or 5 times daily as lozenges, are used.

For prophylaxis of intestinal candidiasis in patients receiving broad-spectrum antibacterials, a total dose of 1 000 000 units daily may be given. A prophylactic dose for infants born to mothers with vaginal candidiasis is 100 000 units daily.

For the treatment of vaginal infections, nystatin is given in a dosage of 100 000 to 200 000 units daily for 14 days or longer as pessaries or vaginal cream. For cutaneous lesions, ointment, gel, cream, or dusting powder containing 100 000 units/g may be applied 2 to 4 times daily.

A liposomal formulation of nystatin for *parenteral* administration is under investigation.

**Candidiasis.** A systematic review[1] of 12 studies (10 of prophylaxis, 2 of treatment) considered that nystatin could not be recommended for prophylaxis or treatment of *Candida* infections in patients with immunosuppression. In practice, fluconazole is usually preferred in such patients (see p.386).

1. Gøtzsche PC, Johansen HK. Nystatin prophylaxis and treatment in severely immunodepressed patients. Available in The Cochrane Library; Issue 2. Chichester: John Wiley; 2004.

### Preparations

**BP 2003:** Nystatin Ointment; Nystatin Oral Suspension; Nystatin Pastilles; Nystatin Pessaries; Nystatin Tablets;
**USP 27:** Nystatin and Triamcinolone Acetonide Cream; Nystatin and Triamcinolone Acetonide Ointment; Nystatin Cream; Nystatin for Oral Suspension; Nystatin Lotion; Nystatin Lozenges; Nystatin Ointment; Nystatin Oral Suspension; Nystatin Tablets; Nystatin Topical Powder; Nystatin Vaginal Suppositories; Nystatin Vaginal Tablets; Nystatin, Neomycin Sulfate, Gramicidin, and Triamcinolone Acetonide Cream; Nystatin, Neomycin Sulfate, Gramicidin, and Triamcinolone Acetonide Ointment; Oxytetracycline and Nystatin Capsules; Oxytetracycline and Nystatin for Oral Suspension; Tetracycline Hydrochloride and Nystatin Capsules.

**Proprietary Preparations** (details are given in Part 3)
**Arg.:** Candermil; Dipni; Micostatin; Nistagrand; Nistat; **Austral.:** Mycostatin; N-Statin; Nilstat; **Austria:** Candio; Mycostatin; **Belg.:** Nilstat; Sterostatine; **Braz.:** Albistin; Candistatin; Kandistat; Micostatin; Neo Mistatin; Neostatin; Nidazolin; Nistagyn; Nistanil; Nistaval; Nistax; Tricocet; **Canad.:** Candistatin; Mycostatin; Nadostine; Nilstat; Nyaderm; **Chile:** Micostatin; Nistoral; **Denm.:** Mycostatin; **Fin.:** Mycostatin; **Fr.:** Mycostatine; **Ger.:** Adiclair; Biofanal; Candio; Cordes Nystatin Soft†; Fungireduct; Lederlind; Moronal; Mykoderm Heilsalbe; MykoPosterine N; Mykundex; Mykundex mono; Nystaderm; **Gr.:** Nystamont; **Hong Kong:** Lystin; Mycostatin; Nadostine†; **India:** Mycostatin; **Irl.:** Mycostatin; **Ital.:** Mycostatin; **Malaysia:** Mycostatin; Uphastatin; **Mex.:** Bistatin V; Micostatin†; Nistan†; Nistaquim; Nystasan†; **Norw.:** Mycostatin; **NZ:** Mycostatin; Nilstat; **Port.:** Mycostatin; **S.Afr.:** Candacide; Canstat†; Mycostatin; Nystacid; **Singapore:** Mycostatin; **Spain:** Mycostatin; **Swed.:** Mycostatin; **Switz.:** Candio†; Mycostatine; Rivostatin†; **Thai.:** Lystin; Mycostatin; **UAE:** Mikostat; **UK:** Nyspes†; Nystamont; Nystan; Nystatin-Dome†; **USA:** Mycostatin; Nilstat; Nystex†; Nystop; Pedi-Dri.

**Multi-ingredient: Arg.:** Bacticort Complex; Bexon; Biotaer Nebulizable; Dermadex NN; Farm-X Duo; Fasigyn Nistatina; Flagystatin; Kenacomb; Linfol; Min O; Naxo TV; O-Biol; O-Biol P; Polygynax; Terra-Cortril Nistatina; **Austral.:** Kenacomb; Mysteclin-V†; Otocomb Otic; **Austria:** Mycostatin V; Mycostatin-Zinkoxid; Topsym polyvalent; **Belg.:** Eoline; Flogocid†; Mycolog; Polygynax; **Braz.:** Benzevit; Bio-Vagin; Colpagex N; Colpanist†; Colpatrin; Colpist; Colpistar; Colpistatin; Colpolase; Dermodex; Dermokin; Donnagel; Flagyl Nistatina; Fungimax; Ginec; Ginestatin; Ginometrim†; Gynax-N; Halcicomb†; Londerm-N; Minegyl C/Nistatina; Naxogin Composto; Neolon-D; Nistazol; Omcilon A M; Onciplus; Poliginax; Tricolpex; Trisdazol†; Trivagel N; Vagi Biotic†; Vagimax; Vagitrin-N; **Canad.:** Flagystatin; Kenacomb; Triacomb; Viaderm-KC; **Chile:** Multilind; Naxogin Compositum; Naxogin Dos; Nistaglos; **Denm.:** Kenalog Comp med Mycostatin; **Fin.:** Flagyl Comp; **Fr.:** Auricularum; Myco-Ultralan†; Mycolog; Polygynax; Polygynax Virgo; Tergynan†; **Ger.:** Aureomycin N; Candio-Hermal Plus; Halog Tri; Jellin polyvalent; Lokalison-antimikrobiell Creme N; Moronal V; Multilind; mykoproct sine; Mykundex Heilsalbe; Nystaderm comp; Nystalocal; Penanyst; Polygynax; Topsym polyvalent; Volonimat Plus N; **Hong Kong:** Kenacomb; Macmiror Complex†; Polygynax; Triacomb; **India:** Kenacomb; **Irl.:** Flagyl Compak†; Kenacomb; Nystaform; Nystaform-HC; Terra-Cortril Nystatin†; Timodine; Tinaderm-M; **Israel:** Auricularum; Dermacombin; Kenacomb; **Ital.:** Assocort; Fasigin N; Macmiror Complex; **Malaysia:** Kenacomb; **Mex.:** Decadron con Nistatina; Dermalog-C; Flagystatin V; Kenacomb; Macmiror Complex V; Metrofur; Promibasol-Plus; Vagitrol-V; **Neth.:** Mycolog; **NZ:** Kenacomb; Kenoid†; **Port.:** Dafnegil; Dermovate-NN; Kenacomb; Polygynax†; **S.Afr.:** Duoderm; Hiconcil-NS†; Kenacomb; Riostatin; Tetrex-F†; **Singapore:** Flagystatin; Kenacomb; Polygynax; **Spain:** Interderm; Intradermo Cort Ant Fung; Milrosina Nistatina; Positon; **Swed.:** Kenacombin Novum; **Switz.:** Dafnegil†; Dermovate-NN; Flogocid NN†; Korticoid polyvalent†; Multilind; Mycolog; Nystacortone; Nystalocal; Topsym polyvalent; **Thai.:** Dermacombin; Gynecon; Gynoco; Gynova; Gyracon; Kenacomb; Nystin; Quinradon-N; Vagicin; **UAE:** Mikostat Baby Ointment; Panderm; **UK:** Dermovate-NN; Flagyl Compak†; Gregoderm; Nystadermal†; Nystaform; Nystaform-HC; Terra-Cortril Nystatin†; Timodine; Tinaderm-M; Tri-Adcortyl; Trimovate; **USA:** Myco-Biotic II; Myco-Triacet II; Mycogen II; Mycolog-II; Myconel; Mytrex†; NGT; Tri-Statin II.

## Omoconazole Nitrate *(USAN, rINNM)*

10-80-07; Nitrato de omoconazol. (Z)-1-{2,4-Dichloro-β-[2-(p-chlorophenoxy)ethoxy]-α-methylstyryl}imidazole nitrate.

$C_{20}H_{17}Cl_3N_2O_2,HNO_3 = 486.7.$

*CAS — 74512-12-2 (omoconazole); 83621-06-1 (omoconazole nitrate).*

*ATC — D01AC13; G01AF16.*

### Profile

Omoconazole nitrate is an imidazole antifungal used locally for fungal skin infections (p.390) and for vaginal candidiasis (p.386). It is applied topically as a 1% cream, powder, or solution in the treatment of cutaneous candidiasis, dermatophytosis, and pityriasis versicolor. For vaginal candidiasis, omoconazole nitrate is given as pessaries in doses of 150 mg daily for 6 days, 300 mg daily for 3 days, or 900 mg as a single dose.

Intravaginal preparations of azoles may damage latex contraceptives.

For a discussion of the caution needed when using azole antifungals during pregnancy, see under Pregnancy in Precautions of Fluconazole, p.398.

### Preparations

**Proprietary Preparations** (details are given in Part 3)
**Austria:** Afongan; **Belg.:** Fongarex†; **Fr.:** Fongamil; Fongarex; **Ger.:** Fungisan†; **Gr.:** Fongamil; **Ital.:** Afongan†; **Mex.:** Afongan†; **Port.:** Afongan; **Spain:** Fongamil†; **Switz.:** Azameno†.

## Oxiconazole Nitrate *(BANM, USAN, rINNM)*

Nitrato de oxiconazol; Ro-13-8996; Ro-13-8996/001; Ro-13-8996/000 (oxiconazole); SGD-301-76; ST-813. 2′,4′-Dichloro-2-imidazol-1-ylacetophenone (Z)-O-(2,4-dichlorobenzyl)oxime mononitrate.

$C_{18}H_{13}Cl_4N_3O,HNO_3 = 492.1.$

*CAS — 64211-45-6 (oxiconazole); 64211-46-7 (oxiconazole nitrate).*

*ATC — D01AC11; G01AF17.*

### Profile

Oxiconazole nitrate is an imidazole antifungal applied topically as a cream, solution, or powder equivalent to oxiconazole 1% in the treatment of fungal infections of the skin (p.390). It is also given as a pessary in a single dose equivalent to 600 mg of oxiconazole in the treatment of vaginal candidiasis (p.386).

Local reactions including burning and itching have been reported. Intravaginal preparations of azoles may damage latex contraceptives.

For a discussion of the caution needed when using azole antifungals during pregnancy, see under Pregnancy in Precautions of Fluconazole, p.398.

◊ Reviews.

1. Jegasothy BV, Pakes GE. Oxiconazole nitrate: pharmacology, efficacy, and safety of a new imidazole antifungal agent. *Clin Ther* 1991; **13:** 126–41.

### Preparations

**Proprietary Preparations** (details are given in Part 3)
**Arg.:** Oxistat; **Austria:** Gyno Oceral†; Gyno-Liderman; Liderman; Oceral; **Braz.:** Oceral; Oxitrat; **Canad.:** Oxizole; **Fr.:** Fonx; **Ger.:** Myfungar; Oceral GB; **Mex.:** Gyno-Myfungar; Myfungar; Oxistat; **Spain:** Salongo; **Switz.:** Gyno-Myfungar†; Myfungar†; Oceral; **USA:** Oxistat.

## Parconazole Hydrochloride *(USAN, rINNM)*

Hidrocloruro de parconazol; R-39500. *cis*-1-{[2-(2,4-Dichlorophenyl)-4-[(2-propynyloxy)methyl]-1,3-dioxolan-2-yl]methyl}-1*H*-imidazole hydrochloride.

$C_{17}H_{16}Cl_2N_2O_3.\ HCl = 403.7.$

*CAS — 68685-54-1 (parconazole); 62973-77-7 (parconazole hydrochloride).*

### Profile

Parconazole is an antifungal that has been used as the hydrochloride in the treatment of gastrointestinal candidiasis in veterinary medicine.

## Pentamycin

Pentamicina.

$C_{35}H_{58}O_{12} = 670.8.$

*CAS — 6834-98-6.*

*ATC — G01AA11.*

### Profile

Pentamycin is a polyene antifungal antibiotic obtained from *Streptomyces pentaticus*. It is used in the treatment of vaginal candidiasis and for the protozoal infection trichomoniasis. A 3-mg vaginal pessary is inserted once or twice daily for 5 to 10 days.

### Preparations

**Proprietary Preparations** (details are given in Part 3)
**Switz.:** Pentacine†.

## Posaconazole *(BAN, USAN, rINN)*

Sch-56592. 4-{p-[4-(p-{[(3R,5R)-5-(2,4-Difluorophenyl)tetrahydro-5-(1H-1,2,4-triazol-1-ylmethyl)-3-furyl]methoxy}phenyl)-1-piperazinyl]phenyl}-1-[(1S,2S)-1-ethyl-2-hydroxypropyl]-$\Delta^2$-1,2,4-triazolin-5-one.

$C_{37}H_{42}F_2N_8O_4 = 700.8.$

*CAS — 171228-49-2.*

### Profile

Posaconazole is a triazole antifungal under investigation for the treatment of opportunistic fungal infections in immunocompromised patients.

## Propionic Acid

E280; E282 (calcium propionate); E283 (potassium propionate); Propanoico, ácido. Propanoic acid.

$C_2H_5.CO_2H = 74.08.$

*CAS — 79-09-4.*

*ATC — S01AX10.*

**Pharmacopoeias.** In *Fr.* Also in *USNF.*

**USNF 22** (Propionic Acid). An oily liquid having a slight pungent, rancid odour. Miscible with water, with alcohol, and with various other organic solvents. Store in airtight containers.

## Sodium Propionate

E281; Natrii Propionas; Propionato de sodio. Sodium propanoate.

$C_3H_5NaO_2$ = 96.06.
*CAS — 137-40-6 (anhydrous sodium propionate); 6700-17-0 (sodium propionate hydrate).*
*ATC — S01AX10.*

**Pharmacopoeias.** In *Eur.* (see p.vi). Also in *USNF.*

**Ph. Eur. 5.0** (Sodium Propionate). Slightly hygroscopic colourless crystals or white powder. Freely soluble in water; sparingly soluble in alcohol; practically insoluble in dichloromethane. A 2% solution in water has a pH of 7.8 to 9.2. Store in airtight containers.

**USNF 22** (Sodium Propionate). Colourless transparent crystals or a granular crystalline powder; odourless or with a faint acetic-butyric odour. Deliquescent in moist air. Soluble 1 in 1 of water, 1 in 0.65 of boiling water, and 1 in 24 of alcohol; practically insoluble in chloroform and in ether. Store in airtight containers.

### Profile

Propionic acid and its salts are antifungals. Sodium propionate has been used topically, usually in combination with other antimicrobial agents for the treatment of dermatophyte infections. Eye drops containing sodium propionate have also been used. Propionic acid and its calcium, sodium, and potassium salts are used in the baking industry as inhibitors of moulds.

### Preparations

**Proprietary Preparations** (details are given in Part 3)
***Ital.:*** Propionat.

**Multi-ingredient: *Arg.:*** Cicatrol; Farm-X; Fungicida; Hipoglos Cicatrizante; Piecidex; Plusderm; ***Austral.:*** Mycoderm; ***Austria:*** Dermowund; ***Braz.:*** Andriodermol; Colpagex N; Gynax-N; Micotox†; Otosulf†; Vagitrin-N; ***Canad.:*** Amino-Cerv; ***Chile:*** Fittig; ***Fr.:*** Angispray†; Dermacide; Otoralgyl a la phenylephrine; Rhinyl†; ***Hong Kong:*** Mycoderm; ***Israel:*** Otomycin; ***Malaysia:*** Mycoderm; ***S.Afr.:*** Neopan; ***USA:*** Amino-Cerv; Prophyllin.

## Pyrrolnitrin *(USAN, rINN)*

52230; NSC-107654; Pirrolnitrina. 3-Chloro-4-(3-chloro-2-nitrophenyl)pyrrole.

$C_{10}H_6Cl_2N_2O_2$ = 257.1.
*CAS — 1018-71-9.*
*ATC — D01AA07.*

**Pharmacopoeias.** In *Jpn.*

### Profile

Pyrrolnitrin is an antifungal antibiotic isolated from *Pseudomonas pyrrocinia* and applied topically in the treatment of superficial fungal infections.

### Preparations

**Proprietary Preparations** (details are given in Part 3)
***Ital.:*** Micutrin.

**Multi-ingredient: *Ital.:*** Micutrin Beta; ***Port.:*** Pirrolfungin.

## Saperconazole *(BAN, USAN, rINN)*

R-66905; Saperconazol. 2-sec-Butyl-4-[4-(4-{4-[(2*RS*,4*SR*)-2-(2,4-difluorophenyl)-2-(1*H*-1,2,4-triazol-1-ylmethyl)-1,3-dioxolan-4-ylmethoxy]phenyl}piperazin-1-yl)phenyl]-2,4-dihydro-1,2,4-triazol-3-one.

$C_{35}H_{38}F_2N_8O_4$ = 672.7.
*CAS — 110588-57-3.*

### Profile

Saperconazole is a triazole derivative that has been investigated for the treatment of systemic fungal infections.

◊ References.

1. Odds FC. Antifungal activity of saperconazole (R66905) in vitro. *J Antimicrob Chemother* 1989; **24:** 533–7.
2. Franco L, *et al.* Saperconazole in the treatment of systemic and subcutaneous mycoses. *Int J Dermatol* 1992; **31:** 725–9.
3. Khoo SH, Denning DW. Cure of chronic invasive sinus aspergillosis with oral saperconazole. *J Med Vet Mycol* 1995; **33:** 63–6.

## Sertaconazole Nitrate *(BANM, rINNM)*

Nitrato de sertaconazol; Sertaconazoli Nitras. (±)-1-{2,4-Dichloro-β-[(7-chlorobenzo[*b*]thien-3-yl)methoxy]phenethyl}imidazole nitrate.

$C_{20}H_{15}Cl_3N_2OS,HNO_3$ = 500.8.
*CAS — 99592-32-2 (sertaconazole); 99592-39-9 (sertaconazole nitrate).*
*ATC — D01AC14.*

**Pharmacopoeias.** In *Eur.* (see p.vi).

**Ph. Eur. 5.0** (Sertaconazole Nitrate). A white or almost white powder. Practically insoluble in water; sparingly soluble in alcohol and in dichloromethane; soluble in methyl alcohol. Protect from light.

### Profile

Sertaconazole nitrate is an imidazole antifungal used topically as a 2% cream, gel, solution, or powder in the treatment of superficial candidiasis, dermatophytosis, seborrhoeic dermatitis, and pityriasis versicolor. In the treatment of vaginal candidiasis it is used as a 2% vaginal cream daily for 7 or 8 days or as a single dose of a 300-mg or 500-mg pessary.

For a discussion of the caution needed when using azole antifungals during pregnancy, see under Pregnancy in Precautions of Fluconazole, p.398.

### Preparations

**Proprietary Preparations** (details are given in Part 3)
***Arg.:*** Zalain; ***Braz.:*** Gyno Zalain; Zalain; ***Chile:*** Tromderm; Zalain; ***Ger.:*** Mykosert; Zalain; ***Ital.:*** Sertacream; Sertadie; Sertagyn; Zalain; ***Malaysia:*** Zalain; ***Mon.:*** Monazol; ***Port.:*** Dermofix; Sertopic; ***Singapore:*** Zalain†; ***Spain:*** Dermofix; Dermoseptic; Gine Zalain†; Ginedermofix; Zalain; ***USA:*** Ertaczo.

## Sulconazole Nitrate *(BANM, USAN, rINNM)*

Nitrato de sulconazol; RS-44872; RS-44872-00-10-3. 1-[2,4-Dichloro-β-(4-chlorobenzyl)thiophenethyl]imidazole nitrate.

$C_{18}H_{15}Cl_3N_2S,HNO_3$ = 460.8.
*CAS — 61318-90-9 (sulconazole); 61318-91-0 (sulconazole nitrate).*
*ATC — D01AC09.*

**Pharmacopoeias.** In *Fr.* and *US.*

**USP 27** (Sulconazole Nitrate). A white to off-white crystalline powder. Soluble 1 in 3333 of water, 1 in 100 of alcohol, 1 in 130 of acetone, 1 in 333 of chloroform, 1 in 286 of dichloromethane, 1 in 2000 of dioxan, 1 in 71 of methyl alcohol, 1 in 10 of pyridine, and 1 in 2000 of toluene. Protect from light.

### Adverse Effects and Precautions

Local reactions including blistering, burning, itching, and erythema have been reported following sulconazole use.

For a discussion of the caution needed when using azole antifungals during pregnancy, see under Pregnancy in Precautions of Fluconazole, p.398.

### Antimicrobial Action

Sulconazole is an imidazole antifungal with activity against dermatophytes, *Candida* spp., and *Malassezia furfur.*

### Uses and Administration

Sulconazole nitrate is an imidazole antifungal applied topically once or twice daily as a 1% cream or solution in the treatment of fungal skin infections including dermatophyte infections and pityriasis versicolor (p.390), and candidiasis (p.386).

◊ Reviews.

1. Benfield P, Clissold SP. Sulconazole: a review of its antimicrobial activity and therapeutic use in superficial dermatomycoses. *Drugs* 1988; **35:** 143–53.

### Preparations

**Proprietary Preparations** (details are given in Part 3)
***Arg.:*** Minot; ***Belg.:*** Myk-1; ***Fr.:*** Myk†; ***Irl.:*** Exelderm; ***Ital.:*** Exelderm†; ***Mex.:*** Exelderm†; ***Neth.:*** Myk-1; ***UK:*** Exelderm; ***USA:*** Exelderm.

# Terbinafine *(BAN, USAN, rINN)*

SF-86-327; SF-86327. (*E*)-6,6-Dimethylhept-2-en-4-ynl(methyl)-(1-naphthylmethyl)amine.

$C_{21}H_{25}N$ = 291.4.
*CAS — 91161-71-6.*
*ATC — D01AE15; D01BA02.*

## Terbinafine Hydrochloride *(BANM, rINNM)*

Hidrocloruro de terbinafina.

$C_{21}H_{26}ClN$ = 327.9.
*CAS — 78628-80-5.*
*ATC — D01AE15; D01BA02.*

### Adverse Effects

The most frequent adverse effects after oral use of terbinafine hydrochloride are gastrointestinal disturbances such as nausea, diarrhoea, and mild abdominal pain. Loss or disturbance of taste may occur and occasionally may be severe enough to lead to anorexia and weight loss. Other frequent adverse effects include headache and skin reactions, including rash or urticaria, sometimes with arthralgia or myalgia. Severe skin reactions including photosensitivity, Stevens-Johnson syndrome, and toxic epidermal necrolysis have occurred rarely. Liver dysfunction with isolated reports of cholestasis, hepatitis, and jaundice, has occurred and there have also been rare cases of liver failure, sometimes leading to death or necessitating liver transplantation, in patients both with and without pre-existing liver disease. Other rare adverse effects include paraesthesia, hypoaesthesia, dizziness, malaise, fatigue, and alopecia. Haematological disorders including neutropenia, thrombocytopenia, and agranulocytosis, and psychiatric disturbances such as depression and anxiety, have been reported very rarely.

There may be local reactions after topical use of terbinafine.

**Incidence of adverse effects.** Postmarketing surveillance of about 10 000 patients[1] suggested the following incidences of adverse effects to oral terbinafine: gastrointestinal symptoms, 4.7%; dermatological effects, 3.3%; CNS symptoms (commonly headache), 1.8%; taste disturbances, 0.6%; and transient disturbances in liver function, 0.1%. Serious adverse effects possibly or probably related to terbinafine included angioedema, bronchospasm, erythema multiforme, extended stroke, and unilateral leg oedema. Combined data from 25 884 patients from this and 3 further studies[2] generally confirmed these results. Overall, adverse effects were reported in 10.5% of patients and caused treatment to be discontinued in 5.3%. Serious adverse effects probably or possibly related to terbinafine occurred in 12 patients (0.046%).

1. O'Sullivan DP, *et al.* Postmarketing surveillance of oral terbinafine in the UK: report of a large cohort study. *Br J Clin Pharmacol* 1996; **42:** 559–65.
2. O'Sullivan DP. Terbinafine: tolerability in general medical practice. *Br J Dermatol* 1999; **141** (suppl 56): 21–5.

**Effects on the eyes.** The US manufacturer has noted that changes in the lens and retina of the eye have sometimes been associated with oral terbinafine, although the significance of these changes was not known.

**Effects on the salivary glands.** Bilateral parotid swelling was associated with terbinafine in a 38-year-old man.[1] Information from the manufacturer and the UK Committee on Safety of Medicines indicated that this effect had occurred in other patients but was very rare.

1. Torrens JK, McWhinney PH. Parotid swelling and terbinafine. *BMJ* 1998; **316:** 440–1.

**Effects on the skin.** Serious skin reactions are occasionally reported in patients receiving terbinafine and have included erythema multiforme,[1,2] erythroderma,[1] severe urticaria,[1] pityriasis rosea,[1] worsening of pre-existing psoriasis,[1] acute generalised exanthematous pustulosis,[3] and lupus erythematosus.[4-6] Several of these patients had a history of auto-immune disease[2,6] and it has been suggested that this could be a risk factor for developing severe reactions.[2]

1. Gupta AK, *et al.* Cutaneous adverse effects associated with terbinafine therapy: 10 case reports and a review of the literature. *Br J Dermatol* 1998; **138:** 529–32.
2. Goeteyn V, *et al.* Is systemic autoimmune disease a risk factor for terbinafine-induced erythema multiforme? *Br J Dermatol* 2000; **142:** 578–9.
3. Condon CA, *et al.* Terbinafine-induced acute generalized exanthematous pustulosis. *Br J Dermatol* 1998; **138:** 709–10.
4. Murphy M, Barnes L. Terbinafine-induced lupus erythematosus. *Br J Dermatol* 1998; **138:** 708–9.
5. Brooke R, *et al.* Terbinafine-induced subacute cutaneous lupus erythematosus. *Br J Dermatol* 1998; **139:** 1132–3.
6. Holmes S, Kemmett D. Exacerbation of systemic lupus erythematosus induced by terbinafine. *Br J Dermatol* 1998; **139:** 1133.

**Effects on taste.** Disturbance and loss of taste have been reported in about 0.6% of patients receiving terbinafine. While this usually resolves gradually once the drug is withdrawn, persistent impairment of taste has been reported.[1,2]

1. Bong JL, *et al.* Persistent impairment of taste resulting from terbinafine. *Br J Dermatol* 1998; **139:** 747–8.
2. Duxbury AJ, *et al.* Persistent impairment of taste associated with terbinafine. *Br Dent J* 2000; **188:** 295–6.

### Precautions

Terbinafine should not be used in patients with existing liver disease and liver function tests should be performed in all patients before starting oral therapy. Terbinafine should be discontinued if clinical or biochemical evidence of hepatotoxicity develops; it should also be discontinued if any progressive skin rash occurs.

It should be used with caution in patients with psoriasis (see below).

Terbinafine should be given in reduced doses to patients with renal impairment (see Administration in Renal Impairment, under Uses and Administration, below).

**Breast feeding.** Terbinafine is excreted in breast milk and it should be avoided during breast feeding.

**Psoriasis.** It has been suggested that terbinafine may provoke or exacerbate psoriasis[1] (see also under Effects on the Skin, above), and that it should be avoided in patients with this disorder.

1. Wilson NJE, Evans S. Severe pustular psoriasis provoked by oral terbinafine. *Br J Dermatol* 1998; **139:** 168.

### Interactions

Plasma concentrations of terbinafine may be increased by drugs that inhibit its metabolism by cytochrome P450, such as cimetidine, and decreased by drugs that induce cytochrome P450, such as rifampicin. Menstrual disturbances including breakthrough bleeding have been reported in patients taking oral contraceptives and terbinafine.

Terbinafine has been shown *in vitro* to inhibit metabolism mediated by the cytochrome P450 isoenzyme CYP2D6. Hence it may affect the plasma concentrations of drugs predominantly metabolised by this enzyme such as tricyclic antidepressants, beta-blockers, SSRIs, and type B MAOIs.

For the effects of terbinafine on some other drugs, see under ciclosporin (p.1355), nortriptyline (p.284), and warfarin (p.1025).

## Antimicrobial Action

Terbinafine is an allylamine derivative reported to have a broad spectrum of antifungal activity. It is considered to act through inhibition of fungal sterol synthesis. Terbinafine is fungicidal against dermatophytes and some yeasts.

◊ References.

1. Petranyi G, *et al.* Antifungal activity of the allylamine derivative terbinafine in vitro. *Antimicrob Agents Chemother* 1987; **31:** 1365–8.
2. Schuster I, Ryder NS. Allylamines—mode and selectivity of action compared to azole antifungals and biological fate in mammalian organisms. *J Dermatol Treat* 1990; **1** (suppl 2): 7–9.
3. Clayton YM. Relevance of broad-spectrum and fungicidal activity of antifungals in the treatment of dermatomycoses. *Br J Dermatol* 1994; **130** (suppl 43): 7–8.
4. Leeming JP, *et al.* Susceptibility of Malassezia furfur subgroups to terbinafine. *Br J Dermatol* 1997; **137:** 764–7.
5. Ryder NS, *et al.* In vitro activities of terbinafine against cutaneous isolates of Candida albicans and other pathogenic yeasts. *Antimicrob Agents Chemother* 1998; **42:** 1057–61.
6. McGinnis MR, *et al.* In vitro comparison of terbinafine and itraconazole against Penicillium marneffei. *Antimicrob Agents Chemother* 2000; **44:** 1407–8.
7. Moore CB, *et al.* In vitro activities of terbinafine against Aspergillus species in comparison with those of itraconazole and amphotericin B. *Antimicrob Agents Chemother* 2001; **45:** 1882–5.

**Microbiological interactions.** Additive and synergistic activity was reported with terbinafine in combination with fluconazole or itraconazole against strains of *Candida albicans* that had reduced susceptibility to azoles *in vitro*.[1] Terbinafine was also reported to enhance the activity of azoles against *Scedosporium prolificans*[2] and against the protozoan *Leishmania braziliensis*.[3]

1. Barchiesi F, *et al.* In vitro activities of terbinafine in combination with fluconazole and itraconazole against isolates of Candida albicans with reduced susceptibility to azoles. *Antimicrob Agents Chemother* 1997; **41:** 1812–14.
2. Meletiadis J, *et al.* In vitro interaction of terbinafine with itraconazole against clinical isolates of Scedosporium prolificans. *Antimicrob Agents Chemother* 2000; **44:** 470–2.
3. Rangel H, *et al.* Naturally azole-resistant Leishmania braziliensis promastigotes are rendered susceptible in the presence of terbinafine: comparative study with azole-susceptible Leishmania mexicana promastigotes. *Antimicrob Agents Chemother* 1996; **40:** 2785–91. Correction. *ibid.* 1997; **41:** 496.

## Pharmacokinetics

Terbinafine hydrochloride is well absorbed from the gastrointestinal tract. The bioavailability is about 40% because of first-pass hepatic metabolism. Mean peak plasma concentrations of about 1 microgram/mL are reported within 2 hours of a single oral dose of 250 mg. Steady state concentrations are about 25% higher than those seen after a single dose and are reached in 10 to 14 days. Terbinafine is extensively bound to plasma proteins. Terbinafine is distributed into the stratum corneum of the skin, the nail plate, and hair where it reaches concentrations considerably higher than those found in plasma. It appears in breast milk. Less than 5% of a topical dose of terbinafine hydrochloride is absorbed.

Terbinafine is metabolised in the liver to inactive metabolites which are excreted mainly in the urine. A plasma elimination half-life varying from 17 to 36 hours has been reported and a terminal elimination half-life of up to 400 hours in patients receiving prolonged therapy, probably representing elimination from skin and adipose tissue. Fungicidal concentrations in nails are maintained for several weeks after therapy is discontinued. The elimination rate may be altered in patients with liver or kidney disease.

◊ References.

1. Kovarik JM, *et al.* Multiple-dose pharmacokinetics and distribution in tissue of terbinafine and metabolites. *Antimicrob Agents Chemother* 1995; **39:** 2738–41.

## Uses and Administration

Terbinafine is an allylamine antifungal given by mouth as the hydrochloride in the treatment of dermatophyte infections of the skin and nails (p.390). Oral doses are stated in terms of the base. Terbinafine hydrochloride 1.13 g is approximately equivalent to 1 g of terbinafine. It is also applied to the skin in dermatophytoses, in pityriasis versicolor (p.390), and in cutaneous candidiasis (p.386).

A dose of 250 mg is given once daily by mouth for 2 to 4 weeks for tinea cruris; treatment may be continued for up to 6 weeks for tinea pedis infections; a 4-week course is used in tinea corporis infections. A cream or solution containing 1% terbinafine hydrochloride is applied once or twice daily for 1 to 2 weeks to treat tinea corporis and tinea cruris; a 1-week course is recommended for tinea pedis. A 2-week course of treatment is used in cutaneous candidiasis and pityriasis versicolor.

Dermatophyte infections of the nails are treated with the equivalent of terbinafine 250 mg by mouth once daily for 6 to 12 weeks although longer treatment may be necessary in toe-nail infections.

Dosage should be reduced in patients with renal impairment (see below).

◊ Reviews.

1. Balfour JA, Faulds D. Terbinafine: a review of its pharmacodynamic and pharmacokinetic properties, and therapeutic potential in superficial mycoses. *Drugs* 1992; **43:** 259–84.
2. Abdel-Rahman SM, Nahata MC. Oral terbinafine: a new antifungal agent. *Ann Pharmacother* 1997; **31:** 445–56.
3. McClellan KJ, *et al.* Terbinafine: an update of its use in superficial mycoses. *Drugs* 1999; **58:** 179–202.

**Administration in children.** Although terbinafine is not currently licensed in the UK for use in children, the *British National Formulary* suggests the following doses for the treatment of tinea capitis in children over 1 year of age (usually as a 2-week course):

- in those weighing 10 to 20 kg: the equivalent of terbinafine 62.5 mg once daily by mouth
- in those weighing 20 to 40 kg: 125 mg once daily
- in those weighing over 40 kg: 250 mg once daily

Similar regimens have been reported in the literature.[1,2]

1. Jones TC. Overview of the use of terbinafine (Lamisil) in children. *Br J Dermatol* 1995; **132:** 683–9.
2. Fuller LC, *et al.* A randomized comparison of 4 weeks of terbinafine vs 8 weeks of griseofulvin for the treatment of tinea capitis. *Br J Dermatol* 2001; **144:** 321–7.

**Administration in renal impairment.** The UK manufacturer recommends that in patients with renal impairment (creatinine clearance less than 50 mL/minute or serum creatinine greater than 300 micromol/litre) usual oral doses should be halved to the equivalent of 125 mg of terbinafine daily.

**Leishmaniasis.** An inadvertent beneficial response has been reported[1] in an HIV-positive patient with cutaneous leishmaniasis (p.597) who was receiving terbinafine 250 mg daily for tinea corporis and onychomycosis. Beneficial results were also reported in a pilot study[2] in which patients with cutaneous leishmaniasis received either terbinafine 125 mg twice daily (those aged 5 to 15 years), or terbinafine 250 mg twice daily (those over 15 years), for 4 weeks.

1. González-Rupérez J, *et al.* Remission of localized cutaneous leishmaniasis in a HIV-positive patient using systemic terbinafine. *Dermatology* 1997; **194:** 85–6.
2. Bahamdan KA, *et al.* Terbinafine in the treatment of cutaneous leishmaniasis: a pilot study. *Int J Dermatol* 1997; **36:** 59–60.

**Non-dermatophyte fungal infections.** Beneficial responses to oral terbinafine have been reported in candidal nail infections,[1,2] aspergillosis,[3] chromoblastomycosis,[4] paracoccidioidomycosis,[5] and sporotrichosis.[6,7]

1. Nolting S, *et al.* Terbinafine in onychomycosis with involvement by non-dermatophytic fungi. *Br J Dermatol* 1994; **130** (suppl 43): 16–21.
2. Segal R, *et al.* Treatment of Candida nail infection with terbinafine. *J Am Acad Dermatol* 1996; **35:** 958–61.
3. Schiraldi GF, *et al.* Refractory pulmonary aspergillosis: compassionate trial with terbinafine. *Br J Dermatol* 1996; **134** (suppl 46): 25–9.
4. Esterre P, *et al.* Treatment of chromomycosis with terbinafine: preliminary results of an open pilot study. *Br J Dermatol* 1996; **134** (suppl 46): 33–6.
5. Okague JM, *et al.* Paracoccidioidomycosis (South American blastomycosis) successfully treated with terbinafine: first case report. *Br J Dermatol* 2000; **143:** 188–91.
6. Hull PR, Vismer HP. Treatment of cutaneous sporotrichosis with terbinafine. *J Dermatol Treat* 1992; **3** (suppl 1): 35–8.
7. Kudoh K, *et al.* Successful treatment of cutaneous sporotrichosis with terbinafine. *J Dermatol Treat* 1996; **7:** 33–5.

**Seborrhoeic dermatitis.** Terbinafine has been tried in the treatment of seborrhoeic dermatitis (p.1138). In one study, 60 patients were randomised to receive oral terbinafine 250 mg daily or a placebo cream applied twice daily for 4 weeks.[1] Clinical improvement, maintained 8 weeks after completing treatment, in the terbinafine group led the investigators to conclude that oral terbinafine is an effective treatment for seborrhoeic dermatitis, and to suggest that this might be due to its activity against *Malassezia ovalis* (*Pityrosporum ovale*) as well as to some anti-inflammatory action. However, the methodology of this study has been questioned[2] and further investigation is needed.

1. Scaparro E, *et al.* Evaluation of the efficacy and tolerability of oral terbinafine (Daskil®) in patients with seborrhoeic dermatitis: a multicentre, randomized, investigator-blinded, placebo-controlled trial. *Br J Dermatol* 2001; **144:** 854–7.
2. Faergemann J. Treatment of seborrhoeic dermatitis with oral terbinafine? *Lancet* 2001; **358:** 170.

## Preparations

**Proprietary Preparations** (details are given in Part 3)
***Arg.:*** Lamisil; Maditez; Terekol; ***Austral.:*** Lamisil; ***Austria:*** Daskil; Lamisil; ***Belg.:*** Lamisil; ***Braz.:*** Alamil†; Finex; Lamisil; Micosil; ***Canad.:*** Lamisil; ***Chile:*** Dermoxyl; Finex; Lamisil; Micoset; Micostop; Terfex; ***Denm.:*** Lamisil; ***Fin.:*** Lamisil; ***Fr.:*** Lamisil; ***Ger.:*** Lamisil; ***Gr.:*** Lamisil; Romiver; ***Hong Kong:*** Lamisil; ***India:*** Lamisil; ***Irl.:*** Lamisil; ***Israel:*** Lamisil; ***Ital.:*** Daskil; Lamisil; ***Malaysia:*** Lamisil; ***Mex.:*** Lamisil; ***Neth.:*** Lamisil; ***Norw.:*** Lamisil; ***NZ:*** Lamisil; ***Port.:*** Daskyl; Lamisil; ***S.Afr.:*** Lamisil; ***Singapore:*** Lamisil; ***Spain:*** Lamisil; ***Swed.:*** Lamisil; ***Switz.:*** Lamisil; ***Thai.:*** Lamisil; ***UK:*** Lamisil; ***USA:*** DesenexMax; Lamisil.

---

# Terconazole *(BAN, USAN, rINN)*

R-42470; Terconazol; Terconazolum; Triaconazole. 1-{4-[[2-(2,4-Dichlorophenyl)-*r*-2-(1*H*-1,2,4-triazol-1-ylmethyl)-1,3-dioxolan-*c*-4-yl]methoxy]phenyl}-4-isopropylpiperazine.

$C_{26}H_{31}Cl_2N_5O_3$ = 532.5.
*CAS — 67915-31-5.*
*ATC — G01AG02.*

**Pharmacopoeias.** In *Eur.* (see p.vi).

**Ph. Eur. 5.0** (Terconazole). A white or almost white powder. It exhibits polymorphism. Practically insoluble in water; sparingly soluble in alcohol; soluble in acetone; freely soluble in dichloromethane. Protect from light.

## Adverse Effects

Local reactions including burning and itching have been reported with vaginal use of terconazole. Other adverse effects have included dysmenorrhoea and abdominal pain. A flu-like syndrome with headache, fever, chills, and hypotension has been reported in some patients and may be more prevalent with vaginal pessaries providing doses larger than 80 mg.

**Flu-like syndrome.** References.

1. Moebius UM. Influenza-like syndrome after terconazole. *Lancet* 1988; **ii:** 966–7.

## Precautions

Intravaginal preparations of terconazole may damage latex contraceptives and additional contraceptive measures are therefore necessary during local administration.

For a discussion of the caution needed when using azole antifungals during pregnancy, see under Pregnancy in Precautions of Fluconazole, p.398.

## Antimicrobial Action

Terconazole is a triazole derivative that binds to fungal cytochrome P450, thus disrupting ergosterol synthesis. Terconazole is active *in vitro* against *Candida* spp. and other fungi. It has some antibacterial activity *in vitro* but not against usual vaginal flora such as lactobacilli.

## Pharmacokinetics

Following intravaginal administration, 5 to 16% of terconazole is absorbed. Systemically absorbed drug is metabolised by the liver and excreted in urine and faeces.

## Uses and Administration

Terconazole is a triazole antifungal used in the local treatment of vulvovaginal candidiasis (p.386). Intravaginal dosage regimens are terconazole 40 mg (as 0.8% vaginal cream) or 80 mg (as a pessary) at bedtime for 3 nights or 20 mg (as 0.4% cream) at bedtime for 7 nights.

## Preparations

**Proprietary Preparations** (details are given in Part 3)
***Belg.:*** Gyno-Terazol†; ***Braz.:*** Ginconazol; Gyno-Fungistat†; Gyno-Fungix; ***Canad.:*** Terazol; ***Denm.:*** Terazol†; ***Mex.:*** Fungistat; ***Neth.:*** Gyno-Terazol; ***S.Afr.:*** Terazol†; ***Swed.:*** Terazol†; ***Switz.:*** Gyno-Terazol; ***USA:*** Terazol.

---

# Tioconazole *(BAN, USAN, rINN)*

Tioconazol; Tioconazolum; UK-20349. 1-[2,4-Dichloro-β-(2-chloro-3-thenyloxy)phenethyl]imidazole.

$C_{16}H_{13}Cl_3N_2OS$ = 387.7.
*CAS — 65899-73-2.*
*ATC — D01AC07; G01AF08.*

**Pharmacopoeias.** In *Eur.* (see p.vi) and *US.*

**Ph. Eur. 5.0** (Tioconazole). A white or almost white crystalline powder. Very slightly soluble in water; freely soluble in alcohol; very soluble in dichloromethane. Protect from light.

**USP 27** (Tioconazole). Store in airtight containers.

## Adverse Effects and Precautions

Local reactions to tioconazole including burning, itching, and erythema have been reported.

Intravaginal preparations of tioconazole may damage latex contraceptives and additional contraceptive measures are therefore necessary during local administration.

For a discussion of the caution needed when using azole antifungals during pregnancy, see under Pregnancy in Precautions of Fluconazole, p.398.

**Hypersensitivity.** Tioconazole, an imidazole antifungal widely used in Finland, appeared to be an important cause of contact allergy in that country, since an incidence of more than 1% was reported in patients undergoing routine patch testing.[1] There may be cross-reactivity with other commonly used imidazole derivatives.

1. Heikkilä H, *et al.* A study of 72 patients with contact allergy to tioconazole. *Br J Dermatol* 1996; **134:** 678–80.

## Antimicrobial Action

Tioconazole is an imidazole antifungal with a broad spectrum of activity including action against dermatophytes, *Malassezia furfur*, and *Candida albicans*. Tioconazole is active *in vitro* against some Gram-positive bacteria.

## Uses and Administration

Tioconazole is an imidazole antifungal used in the treatment of superficial candidiasis (p.386), and dermatophytoses and pityriasis versicolor (p.390).

For vaginal candidiasis it is used as pessaries or vaginal cream or ointment usually as a single 300-mg dose.

It has been applied topically as a 1% cream, lotion, or powder in the treatment of superficial fungal infections. Tioconazole has also been used for nail infections as a 28% w/w topical solution, although systemic treatment is generally preferred.

## Preparations

**BP 2003:** Tioconazole Cream; Tioconazole Nail Solution.

**Proprietary Preparations** (details are given in Part 3)
***Arg.:*** Honguil; Tiomicol; Trosyd; ***Austria:*** Trosyd; ***Braz.:*** Dezol†; Gino Conazol; Gino Tralen; Neo Tionazol; Tinazol†; Tioconax; Tionazen; Tralen; ***Canad.:*** Gynecure; Trosyd; ***Chile:*** Telset; ***Fin.:*** Gyno-Trosyd; Trosyd; ***Fr.:*** Gyno-Trosyd; Trosyd; ***Ger.:*** Fungibacid†; Mykontral; ***Gr.:*** Cotinazin; ***Hong Kong:*** Gyno-Trosyd; Trosyd; ***Irl.:*** Trosyl; ***Ital.:*** Trosyd; ***Malaysia:*** Gyno-Trosyd; Trosyd; ***NZ:*** Gyno-Trosyd; Trosyd†; ***Port.:*** Gino-Trosyd; Trosyd; ***S.Afr.:*** Gyno-Trosyd†; Trosyd; ***Singapore:*** Gyno-Trosyd; Trosyd; ***Spain:*** Trosderm; Trosid; ***Switz.:*** Gyno-Trosyd; Trosyd; ***Thai.:*** Trosyd; ***UK:*** Trosyl; ***USA:*** Vagistat.

**Multi-ingredient:** ***Braz.:*** Cartrax; Duozol; Gynomax; Seczol; Takil; Travogyn; ***Fin.:*** Trosycort; ***Mex.:*** Fasigyn VT.

# Tolciclate *(USAN, rINN)*

K-9147; KC-9147; Tolciclato. *O*-(1,2,3,4-Tetrahydro-1,4-methano-6-naphthyl) *m,N*-dimethylthiocarbanilate.

$C_{20}H_{21}NOS = 323.5.$
*CAS — 50838-36-3.*
*ATC — D01AE19.*

## Profile

Tolciclate is an antifungal with activity against *Epidermophyton, Microsporum*, and *Trichophyton* spp. It is used topically as a 1% cream, lotion, or ointment, or as a 0.5% powder in the treatment of various dermatophyte infections and in pityriasis versicolor.

## Preparations

**Proprietary Preparations** (details are given in Part 3)
***Braz.:*** Tolmicol; ***Ger.:*** Fungifos; ***Gr.:*** Tolmicil; ***Hong Kong:*** Tolmicen†; ***Ital.:*** Tolmicen; ***Mex.:*** Kilmicen†; ***NZ:*** Tolmicen; ***Port.:*** Tolmicen.

# Tolnaftate *(BAN, USAN, rINN)*

Sch-10144; Tolnaftato; Tolnaftatum. *O*-2-Naphthyl *m,N*-dimethylthiocarbanilate.

$C_{19}H_{17}NOS = 307.4.$
*CAS — 2398-96-1.*
*ATC — D01AE18.*

**Pharmacopoeias.** In *Eur.* (see p.vi), *Jpn*, and *US*.

**Ph. Eur. 5.0** (Tolnaftate). A white or yellowish-white powder. Practically insoluble in water; very slightly soluble in alcohol; freely soluble in acetone and in dichloromethane. Protect from light.

**USP 27** (Tolnaftate). A white to creamy-white, fine powder, with a slight odour. Practically insoluble in water; slightly soluble in alcohol; freely soluble in acetone and in chloroform; sparingly soluble in ether. Store in airtight containers.

## Adverse Effects

Skin reactions occur rarely with tolnaftate and include irritation and contact dermatitis.

## Antimicrobial Action

Tolnaftate inhibits the growth of the dermatophytes *Epidermophyton, Microsporum, Trichophyton* spp., and *Malassezia furfur*, but is not active against *Candida* spp. or bacteria.

## Uses and Administration

Tolnaftate is an antifungal used topically as a 1% gel, solution, powder, ointment, or cream in the treatment or prophylaxis of superficial dermatophyte infections and of pityriasis versicolor (see p.390). Tolnaftate is applied twice daily for 2 to 6 weeks. Repeat treatment may be required.

## Preparations

**USP 27:** Tolnaftate Cream; Tolnaftate Gel; Tolnaftate Topical Aerosol; Tolnaftate Topical Powder; Tolnaftate Topical Solution.

**Proprietary Preparations** (details are given in Part 3)
***Arg.:*** Athletes Foot; Tinaderm; ***Austral.:*** Antifungal Foot Deodorant†; Curatin†; Ringworm Ointment; Tinaderm; Tineafax; ***Austria:*** Sorgoran†; ***Braz.:*** Trinaderm†; ***Canad.:*** Absorbine Antifungal†; Absorbine Jr Antifungal; Avon Footworks†; Footworks; Pitrex; Scholl Athlete's Foot Preparations; Tinactin; ZeaSorb AF; ***Chile:*** Tinaderm; ***Fr.:*** Sporiline; ***Ger.:*** Sorgoa†; Tinatox; Tonoftal; ***Hong Kong:*** Aftate; ***India:*** Tinaderm; Tolnaderm; ***Irl.:*** Mycil; Tinaderm; ***Israel:*** Athletes Foot; Pitrex; Tinasol†; ***Ital.:*** Tinaderm; ***Malaysia:*** Dermoplex Antifungal; Myco-Aid; Tinaderm; ***Mex.:*** Excelsior; Tinaderm; Tolnaderm†; ***NZ:*** Tinaderm; ***Port.:*** Tinaderme; ***S.Afr.:*** Tinaderm; ***Singapore:*** Tinaderm; ***Spain:*** Devorfungi†; Micoisdin; Tinaderm†; ***Thai.:*** Ezon-T; Tono; ***UK:*** Mycil; Scholl Athlete's Foot; Tinaderm; ***USA:*** Aftate; Blis-To-Sol; Breezee Mist Antifungal; Dr Scholl's Athlete's Foot; Genaspor; Podactin; Quinsana Plus; Tinactin.

**Multi-ingredient:** ***Arg.:*** Bacticort Complex; Cevaderm; Quadriderm; ***Austral.:*** Mycil Healthy Feet; ***Braz.:*** Cremederme; Poliderms; Quadriderm; Quadrikin; Quadrilon; Quadriplus; Tetraderm; ***Hong Kong:*** Alber T; Mycil; Quadriderm; Triditol-G; ***India:*** Quiss; ***Irl.:*** Mycil; Tinaderm-M; ***Israel:*** Phytoderm Compositum; ***Malaysia:*** Elan-Forte; ***S.Afr.:*** Duoderm; Quadriderm; ***Singapore:*** Quadriderm; ***Spain:*** Cuatroderm; ***Switz.:*** Quadriderm; ***Thai.:*** Alber T; Ezon-T; Quadriderm†; ***UK:*** Mycil; Tinaderm-M; ***USA:*** Absorbine Athletes Foot Care; Dermasept Antifungal.

# Triacetin *(rINN)*

E1518; Glycerol Triacetate; Glycerolum Triacetas; Glyceryl Triacetate; Triacetina; Triacetinum. 1,2,3-Propanetriol triacetate.

$C_9H_{14}O_6 = 218.2.$
*CAS — 102-76-1.*

**Pharmacopoeias.** In *Eur.* (see p.vi) and *US*.

**Ph. Eur. 5.0** (Triacetin). A clear, colourless, slightly viscous, oily liquid. Soluble in water; miscible with dehydrated alcohol and with toluene. Store in well-filled containers.

**USP 27** (Triacetin). A colourless, somewhat oily liquid with a slight, fatty odour. Soluble in water; slightly soluble in carbon disulfide; miscible with alcohol, with chloroform, and with ether. Store in airtight containers.

## Profile

Triacetin is reported to possess fungistatic properties based on the liberation of acetic acid. It has been applied topically in the treatment of superficial dermatophyte infections. It has also been used as a plasticiser in oral preparations.

Triacetin may destroy rayon fabric. It should not come into contact with metals.

## Preparations

**Proprietary Preparations** (details are given in Part 3)

**Multi-ingredient:** ***Braz.:*** Acident†; Micosan†; ***Hong Kong:*** Alber T; ***Thai.:*** Alber T; Ezon-T.

# Trimetrexate Glucuronate *(BANM, USAN, rINNM)*

CI-898 (trimetrexate); Glucuronato de trimetrexato; JB-11 (trimetrexate); NSC-352122; NSC-249008 (trimetrexate). 5-Methyl-6-(3,4,5-trimethoxyanilinomethyl)quinazolin-2,4-diyldiamine mono-D-glucuronate.

$C_{19}H_{23}N_5O_3,C_6H_{10}O_7 = 563.6.$
*CAS — 52128-35-5 (trimetrexate); 82952-64-5 (trimetrexate glucuronate).*
*ATC — P01AX07.*

**Incompatibility.** Trimetrexate is reported to be incompatible with foscarnet. Trimetrexate should not be mixed with folinic acid or chloride ions, since precipitation occurs instantly.

## Adverse Effects, Treatment, and Precautions

As for Methotrexate, p.568. Trimetrexate must be given with folinic acid, which should be continued for 72 hours after the last dose of trimetrexate.

## Interactions

Studies in *animals* suggest that cimetidine and imidazole antifungals such as clotrimazole and ketoconazole may inhibit trimetrexate metabolism, and there is a risk of possible interactions with all drugs that affect hepatic cytochrome P450 systems.

## Pharmacokinetics

The pharmacokinetics of trimetrexate have not been well characterised. Following intravenous administration of trimetrexate glucuronate the pharmacokinetics have been described as both biphasic and triphasic, with a terminal elimination half-life of about 16 to 18 hours. Following administration with folinic acid a biphasic disposition with a terminal half-life of 11 hours has also been reported. It is extensively protein bound; reports suggest that it is 95 to 98% bound at low serum concentrations, but that binding is saturable, with free fraction increasing at plasma concentrations above 1 microgram/mL. Trimetrexate is excreted mainly in the urine, as unchanged drug and metabolites, some of which may be active. The major metabolic pathway appears to be oxidative O-demethylation followed by conjugation to the sulfate or glucuronide.

## Uses and Administration

Trimetrexate is a dihydrofolate reductase inhibitor with general properties similar to those of methotrexate (p.571). It is used in the management of *Pneumocystis carinii* pneumonia in immunocompromised patients, notably patients with AIDS, where other therapy has proved ineffective (see also p.389). It has also been tried as an antineoplastic in the management of various solid tumours.

Trimetrexate is given as the glucuronate but doses are stated in terms of trimetrexate. Trimetrexate glucuronate 1.53 mg is approximately equivalent to 1 mg of trimetrexate. It is given by intravenous infusion, over 60 to 90 minutes. A suggested schedule in *Pneumocystis carinii* pneumonia is 45 mg/m² daily for 21 days, in association with folinic acid rescue for 24 days. The dosage of trimetrexate and folinic acid should be adjusted according to the results of blood tests, which should be performed at least twice a week during therapy. Renal and hepatic function and haemoglobin values should also be monitored. It is recommended that treatment with zidovudine and other myelosuppressive drugs should be interrupted to allow full doses of trimetrexate to be given.

Doses of 8 mg/m² daily for 5 days at 3-week intervals, or 150 to 220 mg/m² every 28 days, have been given in the management of neoplastic disease, usually with folinic acid rescue.

◊ Trimetrexate is a non-classical antifolate which is a potent inhibitor of dihydrofolate reductase but differs from methotrexate in two important aspects.[1] It is taken up avidly by most mammalian tumour cells by a process independent of the folate carrier system, and within the cell it does not undergo polyglutamylation. In consequence, cell lines resistant to methotrexate may retain sensitivity to trimetrexate, particularly where resistance is due to polyglutamylation defects, uptake defects, or low level gene amplification. Only methotrexate resistant cells with altered dihydrofolate reductase have been shown to be insensitive to trimetrexate while those with high level amplification of the dihydrofolate reductase gene are partially cross resistant. A few cell lines have shown trimetrexate resistance of unknown cause.

1. Bertino JR. Folate antagonists: toward improving the therapeutic index and development of new analogs. *J Clin Pharmacol* 1990; **30:** 291–5.

◊ Further reviews.

1. Marshall JL, DeLap RJ. Clinical pharmacokinetics and pharmacology of trimetrexate. *Clin Pharmacokinet* 1994; **26:** 190–200.
2. Fulton B, *et al.* Trimetrexate: a review of its pharmacodynamic and pharmacokinetic properties and therapeutic potential in the treatment of Pneumocystis carinii pneumonia. *Drugs* 1995; **49:** 563–76.

## Preparations

**Proprietary Preparations** (details are given in Part 3)
***Canad.:*** Neutrexin†; ***Denm.:*** Neutrexin†; ***Fr.:*** Neutrexin†; ***Hong Kong:*** Neutrexin; ***Irl.:*** Neutrexin; ***Ital.:*** Neutrexin†; ***Spain:*** Neutrexin; ***Swed.:*** Neutrexin†; ***Thai.:*** Neutrexin; ***UK:*** Neutrexin†; ***USA:*** Neutrexin.

# Undecenoic Acid

Acidum Undecylenicum; 10-Hendecenoic Acid; Undecilénico, ácido; Undecylenic Acid. Undec-10-enoic acid.

$C_{11}H_{20}O_2 = 184.3.$
*CAS — 112-38-9.*
*ATC — D01AE04.*

**Pharmacopoeias.** In *Chin., Eur.* (see p.vi), and *US*.

**Ph. Eur. 5.0** (Undecylenic Acid; Undecenoic Acid BP 2003). A colourless or pale yellow liquid or a white or very pale yellow crystalline mass. Practically insoluble in water; freely soluble in alcohol and in fatty and essential oils. Store in nonmetallic containers. Protect from light.

**USP 27** (Undecylenic Acid). A clear, colourless to pale yellow liquid with a characteristic odour. Practically insoluble in water; miscible with alcohol, with chloroform, with ether, with benzene, and with fixed and volatile oils. Store in airtight containers. Protect from light.

# Calcium Undecenoate

Calcium Undecylenate *(USAN)*; Undecilenato de calcio. Calcium di(undec-10-enoate).

$(C_{11}H_{19}O_2)_2Ca = 406.6.$
*ATC — D01AE04.*

**Pharmacopoeias.** In *US*.

**USP 27** (Calcium Undecylenate). A fine white powder with a characteristic odour and no grit. Practically insoluble in water, in cold alcohol, in acetone, in chloroform, and in ether; slightly soluble in hot alcohol.

## Zinc Undecenoate

Undecilenato de zinc; Undecilinato de Zinco; Zinc Undecylenate; Zinci Undecylenas. Zinc di(undec-10-enoate).

$(C_{11}H_{19}O_2)_2Zn = 431.9$.

*CAS — 557-08-4.*

*ATC — D01AE04.*

**Pharmacopoeias.** In *Chin., Eur.* (see p.vi), and *US.*

**Ph. Eur. 5.0** (Zinc Undecylenate; Zinc Undecenoate BP 2003). A fine white or almost white powder. Practically insoluble in water and in alcohol. Protect from light.

**USP 27** (Zinc Undecylenate). A fine, white powder. Practically insoluble in water and in alcohol.

### Adverse Effects

Irritation may rarely occur after the topical application of undecenoic acid or its salts.

### Antimicrobial Action

Undecenoic acid and its derivatives are active against some pathogenic fungi, including the dermatophytes *Epidermophyton, Trichophyton,* and *Microsporum* spp.

### Uses and Administration

Undecenoic acid and its zinc salt are applied topically in the prophylaxis and treatment of superficial dermatophytoses, particularly tinea pedis (p.390). Typical concentrations are undecenoic acid 2 to 5% and zinc undecenoate 20%. They are used in creams, ointments, solutions, or powders, often in conjunction with each other. Calcium undecenoate is used as a 10 or 15% powder.

Several other salts and derivatives of undecenoic acid including methyl and propyl undecenoate, sodium sulfosuccinated undecenoic acid monoethanolamide, and undecenoic acid monoethanolamide are used similarly.

◊ A systematic review[1] of topical treatments for fungal skin or nail infections considered undecenoates to be effective, although comparative studies with other classes of topical antifungal were lacking.

1. Crawford F, *et al.* Topical treatments for fungal infections of the skin and nails of the foot. Available in The Cochrane Library; Issue 2. Chichester: John Wiley; 2004.

### Preparations

*USP 27:* Compound Undecylenic Acid Ointment.

**Proprietary Preparations** (details are given in Part 3)
***Arg.:*** Sinamida Pies; Umasam; ***Austria:*** Mayfung; Pelsana Med; ***Braz.:*** Anti-Micot†; ***Canad.:*** Caldesene†; Cruex†; Desenex; ***Fr.:*** Mycodecyl; ***Hong Kong:*** Mycota†; ***Irl.:*** Caldesene; Desenex; ***Israel:*** Undecyl; ***Mex.:*** Cruex†; ***S.Afr.:*** Mycota; Pedil†; ***Switz.:*** Fungex; Lubex; Turexan Creme; Turexan Douche; ***UK:*** Mycota; ***USA:*** Blis-To-Sol; Caldesene; Cruex; Decylenes; Desenex; Fungoid AF†; Protectol; Undelenic.

**Multi-ingredient:** ***Arg.:*** Bacteroskin; Champuacid; Cicatrol; Clevosan; Farm-X; Fungicida; Fungocop; Hipoglos Cicatrizante; Novofarma Champu; Piecidex; Plusderm; ***Austral.:*** Acnederm†; Egomycol†; Mycoderm; Pedoz; Sebitar; Seborrol†; ***Austria:*** Crino Cordes; Dequafungan; Mycopol; Pelsana Med; Salvyl; ***Belg.:*** Pelsano†; ***Braz.:*** Acidern†; Andriodermol; Micosan†; Micotox†; Micoz; ***Canad.:*** Athletes Foot Antifungal†; ***Chile:*** Fittig; Hansaplast Footcare; Lady Fittig; ***Fr.:*** Micaveen†; Paps; ***Ger.:*** Gehwol Fungizid; Gehwol Nagelpilz; Skinman Soft; ***Hong Kong:*** Acnederm; Fungifax; Mycoderm; Sebitar; Seborrol†; ***Irl.:*** Ceanel; Genisol†; ***Israel:*** Fungimon; Pedisol; Pitrisan; ***Ital.:*** Balta Intimo; Foot Zeta; Genisol; Micofoot; Neo Zeta-Foot†; Propast; ***Malaysia:*** Acnederm; ***NZ:*** Acnederm; Egomycol; Grans Remedy; Sebitar; Seborrol; ***Port.:*** Edoltar; Micaveen†; ***S.Afr.:*** AF; Ceanel†; Mycota; ***Singapore:*** Acnederm; Sebitar; ***Spain:*** Acnosan†; ***Switz.:*** Fungex; Pelsano; Pruri-med; Sebo Shampooing; Turexan Emulsion; ***UK:*** Ceanel; Healthy Feet; Monphytol; Mycota; ***USA:*** Dermasept Antifungal; Gordochom; Pedi-Pro; Phicon-F.

## Voriconazole *(BAN, USAN, rINN)*

UK-109496; Voriconazol. (2*R*,3*S*)-2-(2,4-Difluorophenyl)-3-(5-fluoropyrimidin-4-yl)-1-(1,2,4-triazol-1-yl)butan-2-ol.

$C_{16}H_{14}N_5F_3O = 349.3$.

*CAS — 137234-62-9.*

*ATC — J02AC03.*

### Adverse Effects

The most commonly reported adverse effects with voriconazole are visual disturbances, fever, rashes, nausea, vomiting, diarrhoea, abdominal pain, headache, and peripheral oedema. There have been some serious hepatic reactions including fatalities. Skin reactions have included rare cases of erythema multiforme, Stevens-Johnson syndrome, toxic epidermal necrolysis, and photosensitivity reactions.

### Precautions

Voriconazole should be used with caution in patients with hepatic impairment and doses may need to be adjusted (see under Uses and Administration, below). Patients should avoid sunlight during treatment as photosensitivity reactions have been reported. Visual disturbances may occur and patients affected should not drive or operate hazardous machinery.

### Interactions

Voriconazole is metabolised by cytochrome P450 isoenzymes CYP2C19, CYP2C9, and CYP3A4. Use of drugs that are either inhibitors or inducers of these isoenzymes may increase or decrease plasma concentrations of voriconazole. Rifampicin has been shown to decrease voriconazole plasma concentrations and a similar effect may be expected with carbamazepine or phenobarbital; use of voriconazole with these drugs is therefore not recommended.

Concentrations of other drugs that are metabolised by CYP2C19, CYP2C9, or CYP3A4 may be increased by voriconazole. Increased plasma concentrations of astemizole, cisapride, pimozide, quinidine, and terfenadine could be expected and concomitant use is contra-indicated because of the risk of cardiac arrhythmias including torsade de pointes. Use with ergot alkaloids such as ergotamine and dihydroergotamine is also contra-indicated because of the possible risk of ergotism. Increased plasma concentrations of sirolimus and tacrolimus have been noted; use with sirolimus is contra-indicated, although tacrolimus may be used providing its dose is reduced and concentrations monitored. Similarly, reduced dose with monitoring is recommended for ciclosporin. Concentrations of oral anticoagulants may be affected and increased prothrombin time has occurred with warfarin; monitoring should therefore be carried out. Close monitoring of blood glucose is necessary if voriconazole is used with oral hypoglycaemics such as the sulfonylureas. Dose reductions may be needed for some statins and some benzodiazepines (such as midazolam and triazolam) if their plasma concentrations are increased.

Interactions may occur where both voriconazole and the other drug are affected. Examples are phenytoin and rifabutin (where concentrations of voriconazole are reduced but those of phenytoin or rifabutin are increased). If it is essential to give either drug with voriconazole, then an increase in the dose of voriconazole is recommended. With omeprazole, the plasma concentration of both drugs may be increased and a reduced dose of omeprazole is recommended.

### Pharmacokinetics

Voriconazole exhibits non-linear pharmacokinetics due to saturable metabolism. It is rapidly and almost completely absorbed from the gastrointestinal tract. Peak plasma concentrations occur about 1 to 2 hours after an oral dose. Plasma protein binding of voriconazole is estimated to be about 58%. Voriconazole diffuses into CSF.

Voriconazole is metabolised by hepatic cytochrome P450 isoenzyme CYP2C19; the major metabolite is the inactive *N*-oxide. Metabolism via isoenzymes CYP2C9 and CYP3A4 has also been demonstrated *in vitro*. About 80% of voriconazole is excreted in the urine.

### Uses and Administration

Voriconazole is a triazole antifungal used mainly in immunocompromised patients for the treatment of invasive aspergillosis (p.386), fluconazole-resistant serious invasive *Candida* infections (p.386), and serious fungal infections due to *Scedosporium* and *Fusarium* spp.

Voriconazole may be given orally or intravenously. Loading doses of voriconazole are given every 12 hours for the first 24 hours. By mouth, these are 400 mg in adults weighing more than 40 kg and 200 mg in those weighing under 40 kg; a dose of 6 mg/kg every 12 hours may be given to children aged 2 to 12 years. Subsequent oral doses are 200 mg twice daily for adults over 40 kg, 100 mg twice daily for adults under 40 kg, and 4 mg/kg twice daily for children aged 2 to 12 years. Oral doses should be taken at least 1 hour before, or 1 hour after, a meal.

Intravenous doses of voriconazole for both adults and children are: loading doses of 6 mg/kg every 12 hours for the first 24 hours followed by maintenance doses of 4 mg/kg twice daily. Intravenous infusions should be administered at a maximum rate of 3 mg/kg per hour over 1 to 2 hours.

Doses of voriconazole should be reduced in patients with hepatic impairment (see below).

◊ Reviews.

1. Muijsers RBR, *et al.* Voriconazole: in the treatment of invasive aspergillosis. *Drugs* 2002; **62:** 2655–64.
2. Johnson LB, Kauffman CA. Voriconazole: a new triazole antifungal agent. *Clin Infect Dis* 2003; **36:** 630–7.
3. Pearson MM, *et al.* Voriconazole: a new triazole antifungal agent. *Ann Pharmacother* 2003; **37:** 420–32.

**Administration in hepatic impairment.** Patients with mild to moderate hepatic cirrhosis should receive the standard loading doses of voriconazole (see above) but maintenance doses should be halved. Doses for patients with severe disease have not been established.

### Preparations

**Proprietary Preparations** (details are given in Part 3)
***Austral.:*** Vfend; ***Fr.:*** Vfend; ***Irl.:*** Vfend; ***Port.:*** Vfend; ***Spain:*** Vfend; ***UK:*** Vfend; ***USA:*** Vfend.

# Antigout Drugs

This chapter deals with the treatment of gout and hyperuricaemia and the drugs used mainly for these disorders.

## Gout and hyperuricaemia

Uric acid is the final product of the metabolism of endogenous and exogenous purine in man. An excess of uric acid, measured in the plasma as sodium urate, constitutes **hyperuricaemia**. This excess may be caused by an overproduction or underexcretion of urate. It is influenced by genetic and environmental factors and may be classified as primary (mainly idiopathic) or secondary. An increase in urate production may be caused by an excessive dietary intake of purines, certain cancers or their treatment, or, more rarely, enzyme defects of purine metabolism. Reduced urate excretion may be caused by renal disease, hypertension, or the intake of certain drugs such as thiazide diuretics. Other factors contributing to hyperuricaemia include hyperlipidaemia, obesity, alcohol consumption, and lead exposure.

A patient is usually considered to be hyperuricaemic when plasma-urate concentrations exceed 0.42 mmol/litre (7 mg per 100 mL) in men and 0.36 mmol/litre (6 mg per 100 mL) in women. At these high concentrations there is a risk of crystals of monosodium urate monohydrate being formed and deposited in synovial fluid and various tissues. However, some subjects may have supersaturated plasma-urate concentrations without any crystal deposits, while others may suffer from deposits in the absence of apparent hyperuricaemia.

The presence of urate crystals in the synovial fluid leads to an inflammatory response in the affected joint, commonly at the base of the big toe (podagra). The ensuing exquisite pain, tenderness, erythema, and swelling constitute the clinical manifestations of **acute inflammatory gouty arthritis**. Repeated acute attacks may be associated with a visible or palpable build up of crystal deposits (**tophi**) at various sites including in and around the affected joint. Tophi release urate crystals into the synovial fluid following various stimuli and so cause further acute attacks, leading to **chronic tophaceous gout**. Intra-articular and periarticular tophi may cause gradual joint erosion, which, without treatment, results in disabling **chronic gouty arthritis**. Rarely, the kidney can be affected by urate deposits producing a gouty nephropathy or by uric acid calculi or stones (uric acid nephrolithiasis or urolithiasis).

**Treatment** aims to alleviate the acute attack, prevent future attacks, and lower plasma-urate concentration.

Plasma-urate concentrations may be reduced by control of obesity and modification of diet and alcohol intake. Drug treatment can relieve the pain of acute attacks but more prolonged therapy for hyperuricaemia is generally only considered if there are recurrent attacks of gout or there is renal involvement (see under Chronic Gout, below).

**Acute gout**. An attack of acute inflammatory gouty arthritis is best treated as soon as possible with an NSAID. Aspirin or other salicylates are not suitable since they may increase plasma-urate concentrations. Treatment is started with high doses of an NSAID, the doses being reduced as the patient responds. Usually treatment can be withdrawn within a week. Colchicine has a role in treating patients in whom NSAIDs are contra-indicated. Patients who do not respond to NSAIDs or colchicine, or for whom these drugs are contra-indicated, may be treated with a systemic corticosteroid. Intra-articular corticosteroids are effective in acute monoarticular gout. Drugs used for chronic gout (allopurinol or the uricosurics) should not be started during an acute attack since they can exacerbate and prolong it (see below).

**Chronic gout**. If the patient suffers frequent acute attacks or develops tophaceous gout, or has renal complications as a result of urate overproduction, then long-term treatment of hyperuricaemia may be needed. Such **urate-lowering therapy** should not be started during an acute attack, or for 2 to 3 weeks thereafter, as fluctuations in urate concentration may prolong the existing attack or initiate a new one. Treatment involves inhibiting the production of uric acid or enhancing its urinary excretion. Hyperuricaemia due to overproduction of urate is treated with allopurinol which inhibits the enzyme xanthine oxidase, involved in purine metabolism. Hyperuricaemia associated with underexcretion of uric acid can be treated with either allopurinol or a uricosuric such as benzbromarone, probenecid or sulfinpyrazone. Allopurinol is most commonly given as first-line therapy, but may be combined with or replaced by uricosurics if treatment fails. Allopurinol should also be used for patients with renal urate deposits or with uric acid renal calculi as it reduces urolithiasis.

With either treatment there is mobilisation of urate crystals from established tophi, as the plasma-urate concentration falls, which can trigger further acute attacks of gout. Patients are thus also given **prophylaxis** with an NSAID or colchicine from the start of urate-lowering treatment until at least a month after the plasma-urate has been reduced to an acceptable concentration; 3 or 4 months of prophylactic cover appears to be common.

Once the hyperuricaemia is corrected, the patient continues to receive therapy with allopurinol or uricosurics indefinitely. If an acute attack occurs during such maintenance therapy, this therapy should be continued to avoid fluctuations in urate concentration, and the acute attack treated in its own right.

Surgery may have to be considered for patients severely affected by chronic tophaceous gout.

General references to gout and its management are given below.


1. Emmerson BT. The management of gout. *N Engl J Med* 1996; **334:** 445–51.
2. Wood J. Gout and its management. *Pharm J* 1999; **262:** 808–11.
3. Davis JC. A practical approach to gout: current management of an 'old' disease. *Postgrad Med* 1999; **106:** 115–16, 119–23.
4. Agudelo CA, Wise CM. Gout: diagnosis, pathogenesis, and clinical manifestations. *Curr Opin Rheumatol* 2001; **13:** 234–9.
5. Schlesinger N, Schumacher HR. Gout: can management be improved? *Curr Opin Rheumatol* 2001; **13:** 240–4.
6. Terkeltaub RA. Gout. *N Engl J Med* 2003; **349:** 1647–55.
7. Snaith ML, Adebajo AO. Gout and hyperuricaemia. In: Snaith ML, ed. *ABC of rheumatology*. 3rd ed. London: BMJ Publishing Group, 2004: 39–44.


## Allopurinol *(BAN, USAN, rINN)*

Allopurinolum; Alopurinol; BW-56-158; HPP; NSC-1390.
1*H*-Pyrazolo[3,4-*d*]pyrimidin-4-ol; 1,5-Dihydro-4*H*-pyrazolo[3,4-*d*]pyrimidin-4-one.

$C_5H_4N_4O$ = 136.1.

*CAS — 315-30-0 (allopurinol); 17795-21-0 (allopurinol sodium).*

*ATC — M04AA01.*

**Description.** Allopurinol is a tautomeric mixture of 1*H*-pyrazolo[3,4-*d*]pyrimidin-4-ol and 1,5-dihydro-4*H*-pyrazolo[3,4-*d*]pyrimidin-4-one.

**Pharmacopoeias.** In *Chin.*, *Eur.* (see p.vi), *Int.*, *Jpn*, *Pol.*, and *US.*

**Ph. Eur. 5.0** (Allopurinol). A white or almost white powder. Very slightly soluble in water and in alcohol; dissolves in dilute solutions of alkali hydroxides.

**USP 27** (Allopurinol). A fluffy white to off-white powder having only a slight odour. Very slightly soluble in water and in alcohol; practically insoluble in chloroform and in ether; soluble in solutions of potassium and sodium hydroxides.

**Incompatibility.** Allopurinol sodium as a 3 mg/mL solution in 0.9% sodium chloride was visually incompatible with amikacin sulfate, amphotericin B, carmustine, cefotaxime sodium, chlormethine hydrochloride, chlorpromazine hydrochloride, cimetidine hydrochloride, clindamycin phosphate, cytarabine, dacarbazine, daunorubicin hydrochloride, diphenhydramine hydrochloride, doxorubicin hydrochloride, doxycycline hyclate, droperidol, floxuridine, gentamicin sulfate, haloperidol lactate, hydroxyzine hydrochloride, idarubicin hydrochloride, imipenem with cilastatin sodium, methylprednisolone sodium succinate, metoclopramide hydrochloride, minocycline hydrochloride, nalbuphine hydrochloride, netilmicin sulfate, ondansetron hydrochloride, pethidine hydrochloride, prochlorperazine edisilate, promethazine hydrochloride, sodium bicarbonate, streptozocin, tobramycin sulfate, and vinorelbine tartrate.[1]


1. Trissel LA, Martinez JF. Compatibility of allopurinol sodium with selected drugs during simulated Y-site administration. *Am J Hosp Pharm* 1994; **51:** 1792–9.


### Adverse Effects

The most common side-effect of allopurinol is skin rash. Rashes are generally maculopapular or pruritic, sometimes purpuric, but more serious hypersensitivity reactions may occur and include exfoliative rashes, the Stevens-Johnson syndrome, and toxic epidermal necrolysis. It is therefore recommended that allopurinol be withdrawn immediately if a rash occurs (see Precautions, below). Further symptoms of hypersensitivity include fever and chills, lymphadenopathy, leucopenia or leucocytosis, eosinophilia, arthralgia, and vasculitis leading to renal and hepatic damage and, very rarely, seizures. These hypersensitivity reactions may be severe, even fatal, and patients with hepatic or renal impairment are at special risk.

Hepatotoxicity and signs of altered liver function may also be found in patients not exhibiting hypersensitivity. Haematological effects include thrombocytopenia, aplastic anaemia, agranulocytosis, and haemolytic anaemia.

Many other side-effects have been noted rarely and include paraesthesia, peripheral neuropathy, alopecia, gynaecomastia, hypertension, taste disturbances, nausea, vomiting, abdominal pain, diarrhoea, headache, malaise, drowsiness, vertigo, and visual disturbances.

Patients with gout may experience an increase in acute attacks on beginning treatment with allopurinol, although attacks usually subside after several months.

**Incidence of adverse effects.** A Boston Collaborative Drug Surveillance Program of 29 524 hospitalised patients revealed that, with the exception of skin reactions, of 1835 patients treated with allopurinol 33 (1.8%) experienced adverse effects. These effects were dose-related and the most frequent were haematological (11 patients, 0.6%), diarrhoea (5 patients, 0.3%), and drug fever (5 patients, 0.3%). Hepatotoxicity was reported in 3 patients (0.2%). Two patients developed possible hypersensitivity reactions to allopurinol.[1]

A further analysis involving 1748 outpatients indicated no instances of acute blood disorders, skin diseases, or hypersensitivity that warranted hospital treatment. Liver disease, although found, was considered to be unassociated with allopurinol. There were only 2 patients in whom renal disease could possibly have been caused by allopurinol.[2]


1. McInnes GT, *et al.* Acute adverse reactions attributed to allopurinol in hospitalised patients. *Ann Rheum Dis* 1981; **40:** 245–9.
2. Jick H, Perera DR. Reactions to allopurinol. *JAMA* 1984; **252:** 1411.


**Effects on the blood.** In addition to the haematological abnormalities of leucopenia, thrombocytopenia, haemolytic anaemia, and clotting abnormalities noted in the Boston Collaborative Drug Surveillance Program,[1] aplastic anaemia has also been reported, sometimes in patients with renal impairment.[2] One case of pure red cell aplasia has been reported.[3]


1. McInnes GT, *et al.* Acute adverse reactions attributed to allopurinol in hospitalised patients. *Ann Rheum Dis* 1981; **40:** 245–9.
2. Anonymous. Allopurinol and aplastic anaemia. *WHO Drug Inf* 1989; **3:** 26.
3. Lin Y-W *et al.* Acute pure red cell aplasia associated with allopurinol therapy. *Am J Hematol* 1999; **61:** 209–11.


**Effects on the eyes.** Some case reports have suggested an association between allopurinol use and the development of cataracts,[1] but a detailed ophthalmological survey involving 51 patients who had taken allopurinol failed to confirm this.[2] However, a large retrospective case-control study in elderly patients concluded that long-term, or high-dose, allopurinol therapy did increase the risk of cataract extraction.[3]


1. Fraunfelder FT, *et al.* Cataracts associated with allopurinol therapy. *Am J Ophthalmol* 1982; **94:** 137–40.
2. Clair WK, *et al.* Allopurinol use and the risk of cataract formation. *Br J Ophthalmol* 1989; **73:** 173–6.
3. Garbe E, *et al.* Exposure to allopurinol and the risk of cataract extraction in elderly patients. *Arch Ophthalmol* 1998; **116:** 1652–6.


**Effects on the skin.** Skin reactions are the most common side-effects of allopurinol.

One report calculated that of 215 adverse effects noted over a 16-year period 188 (87.4%) were related to the skin or mucous membranes.[1] An analysis by the Boston Collaborative Drug Surveillance Program of data on 15 438 patients hospitalised between 1975 and 1982 detected 6 allergic skin reactions attributed to allopurinol among 784 recipients of the drug.[2] Desensitisation protocols[3] and alternative drugs[4] have been used following cutaneous reactions to allopurinol.

Serious skin reactions to allopurinol may occur as part of a generalised hypersensitivity reaction. A review of the literature between 1970 and the end of 1990 revealed 101 cases of allopurinol hypersensitivity syndrome, 94 of which involved the skin.[5] Skin reactions included erythema multiforme, Stevens-Johnson syndrome, toxic epidermal necrolysis, or a diffuse maculopapular or exfoliative dermatitis; 27 of the 101 patients died. The relative risk of toxic epidermal necrolysis or Stevens-Johnson syndrome occurring with allopurinol was high (calculated to be 5.5) in a case-control study including 13 patients with these cutaneous reactions who had received allopurinol.[6] This risk was not constant over time, being higher during the first 2 months of treatment. During these 2 months the estimated excess risk was 1.5 cases per million users per week.


1. Vinciullo C. Allopurinol hypersensitivity. *Med J Aust* 1984; **141:** 449–50.
2. Bigby M, *et al.* Drug-induced cutaneous reactions. *JAMA* 1986; **256:** 3358–63.

3. Fam AG, *et al.* Efficacy and safety of desensitization to allopurinol following cutaneous reactions. *Arthritis Rheum* 2001; **44:** 231–8.
4. Fam AG. Difficult gout and new approaches for control of hyperuricemia in the allopurinol-allergic patient. *Curr Rheumatol Rep* 2001; **3:** 29–35.
5. Arellano F, Sacristán JA. Allopurinol hypersensitivity syndrome: a review. *Ann Pharmacother* 1993; **27:** 337–43.
6. Roujeau J-C, *et al.* Medication use and the risk of Stevens-Johnson syndrome or toxic epidermal necrolysis. *N Engl J Med* 1995; **333:** 1600–1607.

## Precautions

Allopurinol should not be used for the treatment of an acute attack of gout; additionally, allopurinol therapy should not be initiated for any purpose during an acute attack. However, allopurinol is continued when acute attacks occur in patients already receiving the drug, and the acute attack is treated separately.

Treatment should be stopped immediately if any skin reactions or other signs of hypersensitivity develop. A cautious reintroduction at a low dose may be attempted when mild skin reactions have cleared (see Effects on the Skin, above); allopurinol should not be reintroduced in those patients who have experienced other forms of hypersensitivity reaction. Dosage should be reduced in renal impairment (see below) and in hepatic impairment. Care is advised in patients being treated for hypertension or cardiac insufficiency, who may have concomitant renal impairment.

To reduce the risk of renal xanthine deposition an adequate fluid intake (2 to 3 litres daily) is required. In addition, a neutral or slightly alkaline urine may be desirable.

**Breast feeding.** Allopurinol and its metabolite, oxipurinol, are distributed into breast milk, and the manufacturers recommend that allopurinol should be given with caution to breast feeding women. Although oxipurinol was detected in the plasma of a breast-fed infant, no adverse effects were noted in the infant during 6 weeks of maternal treatment with allopurinol.[1] The American Academy of Pediatrics noted that there had been no documented problems with allopurinol and considered its use to be usually compatible with breast feeding.[2]

1. Kamilli I, Gresser U. Allopurinol and oxypurinol in human breast milk. *Clin Investig* 1993; **71:** 161–4.
2. American Academy of Pediatrics. The transfer of drugs and other chemicals into human milk. *Pediatrics* 2001; **108:** 776–89. Correction. *ibid.*; 1029. Also available at: http://aappolicy.aappublications.org/cgi/content/full/pediatrics%3b108/3/776 (accessed 26/05/04)

## Interactions

Drugs that can increase uric acid concentrations may decrease the efficacy of allopurinol. Aspirin and the salicylates possess this activity and should generally be avoided in hyperuricaemia and gout. An increase in hypersensitivity reactions, and possibly also other adverse effects, has been reported in patients receiving allopurinol with ACE inhibitors or thiazide diuretics, particularly in patients with impaired renal function.

The metabolism of azathioprine and mercaptopurine is inhibited by allopurinol and their doses should be markedly reduced when either of them is given with allopurinol to avoid potentially life-threatening toxicity. There have also been reports of allopurinol enhancing the activity of, and possibly increasing the toxicity of, a number of other drugs including some antibacterials, some anticoagulants, some antineoplastics, ciclosporin, some sulfonylurea antidiabetics, theophylline, and vidarabine.

**ACE inhibitors.** An apparent interaction between allopurinol and *captopril* has been reported in patients with chronic renal failure. In one patient fatal Stevens-Johnson syndrome developed and it was suggested that the reaction was secondary to the introduction of allopurinol potentiated by the presence of captopril.[1] In the second patient hypersensitivity, characterised by fever, arthralgia, and myalgia, occurred and in this case the cause was believed to be captopril, or one of its metabolites, potentiated by the addition of allopurinol.[2] The authors of both reports considered that the combination of allopurinol and captopril should be prescribed with care, especially in patients with chronic renal failure.

1. Pennell DJ, *et al.* Fatal Stevens-Johnson syndrome in a patient on captopril and allopurinol. *Lancet* 1984; **i:** 463.
2. Samanta A, Burden AC. Fever, myalgia, and arthralgia in a patient on captopril and allopurinol. *Lancet* 1984; **i:** 679.

**Antacids.** Allopurinol failed to reduce blood-uric-acid concentrations when administered at the same time as *aluminium hydroxide* in 3 patients on chronic haemodialysis. However, if allopurinol was given 3 hours before aluminium hydroxide the expected decrease in uric acid concentration did occur.[1]

1. Weissman I, Krivoy N. Interaction of aluminium hydroxide and allopurinol in patients on chronic hemodialysis. *Ann Intern Med* 1987; **107:** 787.

**Antibacterials.** Although an increased incidence of skin rashes has been noted when allopurinol has been used with *ampicillin* or *amoxicillin*, data currently available are insufficient to confirm whether this is due to allopurinol or not. For further details, see Ampicillin, p.157.

**Anticoagulants.** For the effect of allopurinol on *dicoumarol, phenprocoumon,* or *warfarin*, see Warfarin, p.1025.

**Antiepileptics.** For a report of allopurinol possibly inhibiting the metabolism of *phenytoin*, see under Antigout Drugs, p.373.

**Antigout drugs.** Uricosuric drugs are likely to increase the renal elimination of oxipurinol (the major active metabolite of allopurinol). For example, use of allopurinol with *benzbromarone* was found to lower plasma concentrations of oxipurinol by some 40%, although plasma concentrations of allopurinol itself were not affected.[1] The interaction was not clinically significant, since the combination was more effective than allopurinol alone in lowering serum concentrations of uric acid. The manufacturer recommends reassessing the dosage of allopurinol on an individual basis when a uricosuric drug is added.

*Probenecid* has been reported to decrease the clearance of orally administered allopurinol riboside.[2]

1. Müller FO, *et al.* The effect of benzbromarone on allopurinol/oxypurinol kinetics in patients with gout. *Eur J Clin Pharmacol* 1993; **44:** 69–72.
2. Were JBO, Shapiro TA. Effects of probenecid on the pharmacokinetics of allopurinol riboside. *Antimicrob Agents Chemother* 1993; **37:** 1193–6.

**Antineoplastics.** Allopurinol inhibits the metabolism of *mercaptopurine* and marked dosage reduction of this drug to one-quarter to one-third of the usual dose is required if it is used with allopurinol. There are also reports of interactions between allopurinol and other antineoplastics. Mild chronic allopurinol-induced hepatotoxicity has been reported in one male patient to have been exacerbated by *tamoxifen*.[1] Hypersensitivity vasculitis resulting in the death of one patient receiving allopurinol and *pentostatin* has been described. Although it could not be ascertained whether this effect was due to one of the drugs alone or to an interaction it was believed that this combination should not be used.[2]

For a report of an increased incidence of bone-marrow toxicity in patients given allopurinol with *cyclophosphamide*, see p.541.

1. Shah KA, *et al.* Allopurinol hepatotoxicity potentiated by tamoxifen. *N Y State J Med* 1982; **82;** 1745–6.
2. Steinmetz JC, *et al.* Hypersensitivity vasculitis associated with 2-deoxycoformycin and allopurinol therapy. *Am J Med* 1989; **86:** 499.

**Antivirals.** For the effect of allopurinol on *didanosine*, see p.631.

**Immunosuppressants.** Allopurinol inhibits the metabolism of *azathioprine* and marked dosage reduction of this drug is required if it is given with allopurinol (see p.1349). The effects of allopurinol on *ciclosporin* concentrations (a marked increase) are reported on p.1354.

**Xanthines.** For the effect of allopurinol on the pharmacokinetics of *caffeine* and *theophylline*, see p.782 and p.802 respectively.

## Pharmacokinetics

Up to 90% of a dose of allopurinol is absorbed from the gastrointestinal tract after oral administration; its plasma half-life is about 1 to 2 hours. Allopurinol's major metabolite is oxipurinol (alloxanthine) which is also an inhibitor of xanthine oxidase with a plasma half-life of about 15 or more hours in patients with normal renal function, although this is greatly prolonged by renal impairment. Both allopurinol and oxipurinol are conjugated to form their respective ribonucleosides. Allopurinol and oxipurinol are not bound to plasma proteins.

Excretion is mainly through the kidney, but it is slow since oxipurinol undergoes tubular reabsorption. About 70% of a daily dose may be excreted in the urine as oxipurinol and up to 10% as allopurinol; prolonged administration may alter these proportions, as allopurinol inhibits its own metabolism. The remainder of the dose is excreted in the faeces. Allopurinol and oxipurinol have also been detected in breast milk.

◊ References.

1. Murrell GAC, Rapeport WG. Clinical pharmacokinetics of allopurinol. *Clin Pharmacokinet* 1986; **11:** 343–53.
2. McGaurn SP, *et al.* The pharmacokinetics of injectable allopurinol in newborns with the hypoplastic left heart syndrome. *Pediatrics* 1994; **94:** 820–3.
3. Turnheim K, *et al.* Pharmacokinetics and pharmacodynamics of allopurinol in elderly and young subjects. *Br J Clin Pharmacol* 1999; **48:** 501–9.

## Uses and Administration

Allopurinol is used to treat hyperuricaemia (p.412) associated with chronic gout, acute uric acid nephropathy, recurrent uric acid stone formation, enzyme disorders, or cancer and its treatment (see Tumour Lysis Syndrome, p.495). It is not used for asymptomatic hyperuricaemia. Allopurinol is also used in the management of renal calculi caused by the deposition of calcium oxalate (in the presence of hyperuricosuria) and of 2,8-dihydroxyadenine (see Renal Calculi, below). It may have the potential to reduce oxidative stress by blocking the production of free radicals and is an ingredient of kidney preservation solutions. In addition allopurinol has antiprotozoal activity and has been used in leishmaniasis and American trypanosomiasis.

Allopurinol is used in **gout and hyperuricaemia** to inhibit the enzyme xanthine oxidase, thus preventing the oxidation of hypoxanthine to xanthine and xanthine to uric acid. The urinary purine load, normally almost entirely uric acid, is thereby divided between hypoxanthine, xanthine, and uric acid, each with its independent solubility. This results in the reduction of urate and uric acid concentrations in plasma and urine, ideally to such an extent that deposits of monosodium urate monohydrate or uric acid are dissolved or prevented from forming. At low concentrations allopurinol acts as a competitive inhibitor of xanthine oxidase and at higher concentrations as a non-competitive inhibitor. However, most of its activity is due to the metabolite oxipurinol which is a non-competitive inhibitor of xanthine oxidase.

Allopurinol is used in chronic gout to correct hyperuricaemia, reduce the likelihood of acute attacks, and prevent the sequelae of chronic gout. Initially, it may increase plasma-concentrations of urate and uric acid by dissolving deposits. This can trigger or exacerbate acute attacks, hence allopurinol should not be started until an acute attack has completely subsided, and treatment should be started with a low dose increased gradually; an NSAID or colchicine should also be given during the first few months.

A suggested starting dose of allopurinol is 100 mg daily by mouth, gradually increased by 100 mg for example at weekly intervals until the concentration of urate in plasma is reduced to 0.36 mmol/litre (6 mg per 100 mL) or less. A daily dose range of 100 to 300 mg may be adequate for those with mild gout and up to 600 mg for those with moderately severe tophaceous gout. The maximum recommended daily dose is 800 mg in the USA and 900 mg in the UK. Up to 300 mg may be taken as a single daily dose; larger amounts should be taken in divided doses to reduce the risk of gastric irritation. Taking allopurinol after food will also minimise gastric irritation. Patients should maintain an adequate fluid intake to prevent renal xanthine deposition.

Doses of allopurinol should be reduced in patients with renal impairment (see below)

When used for the prevention of uric acid nephropathy associated with cancer therapy 600 to 800 mg may be given daily generally for 2 or 3 days before starting the cancer treatment. A high fluid intake is essential. In hyperuricaemia secondary to cancer or cancer chemotherapy, maintenance doses of allopurinol are similar to those used in gout and are given according to the response.

The main use of allopurinol in children is for hyperuricaemia associated with cancer or cancer chemotherapy or with enzyme disorders. The dosage used may vary: in the UK a dose of 10 to 20 mg/kg daily up to a maximum of 400 mg daily is recommended for children under 15 years of age, while in the USA the dose is 150 mg daily for children under 6 years of age and 300 mg daily for those aged 6 to 10 years, adjusted if necessary after 48 hours.

Allopurinol sodium has been given by intravenous infusion in sodium chloride 0.9% or glucose 5% to patients (usually cancer patients) unable to take allopurinol by mouth. The recommended dose in adults is the equivalent of allopurinol 200 to 400 mg/m$^2$ daily up to a maximum of 600 mg daily. Allopurinol sodium 116.2 mg is equivalent to 100 mg of allopurinol.

**Administration in renal impairment.** Excretion of allopurinol and its active metabolite oxipurinol is primarily via the kidneys and therefore the dosage should be reduced in renal impairment according to creatinine clearance (CC).

In the USA the manufacturer suggests the following:

- CC 10 to 20 mL/minute: 200 mg daily
- CC less than 10 mL/minute: no more than 100 mg daily
- CC less than 3 mL/minute: consider a longer dosage interval

In the UK the manufacturer recommends a maximum initial daily dosage of 100 mg for those with impaired renal function, increased only if the response is inadequate. Doses less than 100 mg daily or 100 mg at intervals longer than 1 day are recommended for those with severe renal insufficiency. Because of the imprecision of low creatinine clearance values, they suggest that, if facilities are available for monitoring, the allopurinol dose should be adjusted to maintain plasma-oxipurinol concentrations below 100 micromoles/litre (15.2 micrograms/mL). A suggested alternative dose for patients requiring dialysis two or three times a week is 300 to 400 mg allopurinol immediately after dialysis only.

**Diagnosis and testing.** Deficiency of the enzyme ornithine carbamoyltransferase can result in severe CNS dysfunction or even in death, and identification of women at risk of being carriers of this genetic enzyme deficiency has been described.[1] The enzyme deficiency causes carbamoyl phosphate to accumulate, which stimulates the synthesis of orotidine. The test relies on the administration of a single dose of allopurinol, which will, in carriers, greatly increase the urinary excretion of orotidine.

1. Hauser ER, *et al.* Allopurinol-induced orotidinuria. *N Engl J Med* 1990; **322:** 1641–5. Correction. *ibid.* 1997; **336:** 1335.

**Duchenne muscular dystrophy.** Allopurinol has been used in an attempt to increase the ATP levels in muscle which are depleted in Duchenne muscular dystrophy (p.1083). Although some have reported favourable results,[1-3] double-blind studies[4-6] failed to show any benefit from treatment. Despite these findings, some interest in the use of allopurinol for this disorder has continued.[7]

1. Thomson WHS, Smith I. X-linked recessive (Duchenne) muscular dystrophy (DMD) and purine metabolism: effects of oral allopurinol and adenylate. *Metabolism* 1978; **27:** 151–63.
2. Thomson WHS, Smith I. Allopurinol in Duchenne's muscular dystrophy. *N Engl J Med* 1978; **299:** 101.
3. Castro-Gago M, *et al.* Allopurinol in Duchenne muscular dystrophy. *Lancet* 1980; **i;** 1358–9.
4. Stern LM, *et al.* The progression of Duchenne muscular dystrophy: clinical trial of allopurinol therapy. *Neurology* 1981; **31:** 422–6.
5. Hunter JR, *et al.* Effects of allopurinol in Duchenne's muscular dystrophy. *Arch Neurol* 1983; **40:** 294–9.
6. Bertorini TE, *et al.* Chronic allopurinol and adenine therapy in Duchenne muscular dystrophy: effects on muscle function, nucleotide degradation, and muscle ATP and ADP content. *Neurology* 1985; **35:** 61–5.
7. Castro-Gago M, *et al.* Long-term effects of xanthine-oxidase inhibitor (allopurinol) in Duchenne muscular dystrophy. *Int Pediatr* 1994; **9:** 15–20.

**Epilepsy.** Reduction in the frequency of seizures has been described in some patients with severe or intractable epilepsy (p.349) when allopurinol was added to their existing antiepileptic therapy.[1-3] Although the mode of action was not known it was noted that the patients were not hyperuricaemic and that allopurinol did not affect plasma concentrations of existing antiepileptics.[1]

1. DeMarco P, Zagnoni P. Allopurinol and severe epilepsy. *Neurology* 1986; **36:** 1538–9.
2. Tada H, *et al.* Clinical effects of allopurinol on intractable epilepsy. *Epilepsia* 1991; **32:** 279–83.
3. Zagnoni PG, *et al.* Allopurinol as an add-on therapy in refractory epilepsy—a double-blind placebo-controlled randomised study. *Epilepsia* 1994; **35:** 107–12.

**Organ and tissue transplantation.** Allopurinol 25 mg on alternate days has been added to the immunosuppressive treatment for renal transplantation,[1] and is reported to reduce the frequency of acute rejection. One possible explanation for this effect is allopurinol's ability to suppress the production of free radicals (see Oxidative Stress, below). Organ and tissue transplantation, and the more usual drugs used in immunosuppressive regimens are discussed on p.1344. It should be noted that allopurinol interacts with azathioprine (see Immunosuppressants, under Interactions, above) and ciclosporin (p.1354).

1. Chocair P, *et al.* Low-dose allopurinol plus azathioprine/cyclosporin/prednisolone, a novel immunosuppressive regimen. *Lancet* 1993; **342:** 83–4.

**Oxidative stress.** Allopurinol, through its inhibition of xanthine oxidase, can block the development of superoxide free radicals during reperfusion after an ischaemic episode. Consequently, the ability of allopurinol to reduce oxidative stress has been investigated in a number of clinical situations.

In a small study[1] of patients with idiopathic dilated cardiomyopathy, short-term intracoronary administration of allopurinol improved myocardial efficiency by decreasing the oxygen demand of left ventricular contraction. In patients undergoing coronary artery bypass graft surgery, perioperative allopurinol administration reduced the number of ischaemic events and reduced the amount of dopamine required.[2,3] A large study[4] in neonates undergoing cardiac surgery found that allopurinol caused a reduction in seizures and cardiac events in those with hypoplastic left heart syndrome. No benefit was found in neonates with less severe forms of congenital heart disease, considered to be at lower risk of adverse surgical outcome or reperfusion injury. Allopurinol also failed to reduce the incidence of periventricular leucomalacia (thought to represent ischaemic infarction of the developing brain) in preterm infants compared with placebo in a large study.[5] Similarly, allopurinol did not reduce the incidence of infarct extension in patients with acute myocardial infarction.[6]

The possibility that allopurinol limits the production of free radicals has also led to allopurinol sodium being included as an ingredient of the University of Wisconsin solution [UW Solution; Belzer Solution], which is used for the preservation of organs for transplantation.[7]

A pilot study using allopurinol showed a beneficial effect on free radical formation, cerebral blood volume, and electrical brain activity in severely asphyxiated newborns.[8]

1. Cappola TP, *et al.* Allopurinol improves myocardial efficiency in patients with idiopathic dilated cardiomyopathy. *Circulation* 2001; **104:** 2407–11.
2. Sisto T, *et al.* Pretreatment with antioxidants and allopurinol diminishes cardiac onset events in coronary artery bypass grafting. *Ann Thorac Surg* 1995; **59:** 1519–23.
3. Coghlan JG, *et al.* Allopurinol pretreatment improves postoperative recovery and reduces lipid peroxidation in patients undergoing coronary artery bypass grafting. *J Thorac Cardiovasc Surg* 1994; **107:** 248–56.
4. Clancy RR, *et al.* Allopurinol neurocardiac protection trial in infants undergoing heart surgery using deep hypothermic circulatory arrest. *Pediatrics* 2001; **108:** 61–70.
5. Russell GAB, Cooke RWI. Randomised controlled trial of allopurinol prophylaxis in very preterm infants. *Arch Dis Child Fetal Neonatal Ed* 1995; **73:** F27–F31.
6. Parmley LF, *et al.* Allopurinol therapy of ischemic heart disease with infarct extension. *Can J Cardiol* 1992; **8:** 280–6.
7. Southard JH, Belzer FO. Organ preservation. *Annu Rev Med* 1995; **46:** 235–47.
8. Van Bel F, *et al.* Effect of allopurinol on postasphyxial free radical formation, cerebral haemodynamics, and electrical brain activity. *Pediatrics* 1998; **101:** 185–93.

**Protozoal infections.** Beneficial results have been reported in patients with *visceral leishmaniasis* (p.597) when allopurinol was added to their therapy;[1,2] these studies involved patients who had either little or no response to antimonial drugs, or included untreated patients from areas where unresponsive cases were frequent. Positive results in leishmaniasis have also been described in patients with AIDS.[3,4] Variable responses in American *cutaneous leishmaniasis* have been reported.[5-7]

Some beneficial results have been noted in indeterminate and chronic Chagas' disease (*American trypanosomiasis,* p.600).[8-10]

The selective antiparasitic action of allopurinol is believed to be due to its incorporation into the protozoal, but not the mammalian, purine salvage pathway. This leads to the formation of 4-aminopyrazolopyrimidine ribonucleotide triphosphate, a highly toxic analogue of adenosine triphosphate, that is incorporated into ribonucleic acid. This action of allopurinol is shared by allopurinol riboside, one of the minor metabolites in man, but not by oxipurinol, the major human metabolite. Thus, some studies have been conducted with allopurinol riboside, rather than allopurinol, in an attempt to enhance activity by avoiding host-mediated inactivation.[11]

1. Chunge CN, *et al.* Visceral leishmaniasis unresponsive to antimonial drugs: successful treatment using a combination of sodium stibogluconate plus allopurinol. *Trans R Soc Trop Med Hyg* 1985; **79:** 715–18.
2. di Martino L, *et al.* Low dosage combination of meglumine antimoniate plus allopurinol as first choice treatment of infantile visceral leishmaniasis in Italy. *Trans R Soc Trop Med Hyg* 1990; **84:** 534–5.
3. Dellamonica P, *et al.* Allopurinol for treatment of visceral leishmaniasis in patients with AIDS. *J Infect Dis* 1989; **160:** 904–5.
4. Smith D, *et al.* Visceral leishmaniasis (kala azar) in a patient with AIDS. *AIDS* 1989; **3:** 41–3.
5. Martinez S, Marr JJ. Allopurinol in the treatment of American cutaneous leishmaniasis. *N Engl J Med* 1992; **326:** 741–4.
6. Velez I, *et al.* Inefficacy of allopurinol as monotherapy for Colombian cutaneous leishmaniasis: a randomized, controlled trial. *Ann Intern Med* 1997; **126:** 232–6.
7. Martinez S, *et al.* Treatment of cutaneous leishmaniasis with allopurinol and stibogluconate. *Clin Infect Dis* 1997; **24:** 165–9.
8. Gallerano RH, *et al.* Therapeutic efficacy of allopurinol in patients with chronic Chagas' disease. *Am J Trop Med Hyg* 1990; **43:** 159–66.
9. Sánchez G, *et al.* Treatment with allopurinol and itraconazole changes lytic activity in patients with chronic, low grade Trypanosoma cruzi infection. *Trans R Soc Trop Med Hyg* 1995; **89:** 438–9.
10. Apt W, *et al.* Treatment of chronic Chagas' disease with itraconazole and allopurinol. *Am J Trop Med Hyg* 1998; **59:** 133–8.
11. Shapiro TA, *et al.* Pharmacokinetics and metabolism of allopurinol riboside. *Clin Pharmacol Ther* 1991; **49:** 506–14.

**Renal calculi.** Patients with recurrent calcium oxalate stones are usually treated with thiazide diuretics (p.936). Allopurinol has been suggested[1] as an alternative where there is also hyperuricosuria. The recommended dose of allopurinol is 200 to 300 mg daily adjusted on the basis of subsequent 24-hour urinary urate excretion. Allopurinol is also advocated for the management of 2,8-dihydroxyadenine (2,8-DHA) renal stones associated with deficient activity of the enzyme adenine phosphoribosyltransferase.

1. Ettinger B, *et al.* Randomized trial of allopurinol in the prevention of calcium oxalate calculi. *N Engl J Med* 1986; **315:** 1386–9.

**Sarcoidosis.** Although corticosteroids remain the mainstay of drug therapy for sarcoidosis (p.1087), and other drugs are very much second line, there are reports[1,2] of benefit in cutaneous disease from the use of allopurinol.

1. Brechtel B, *et al.* Allopurinol: a therapeutic alternative for disseminated cutaneous sarcoidosis. *Br J Dermatol* 1996; **135:** 307–9.
2. Antony F, Layton AM. A case of cutaneous acral sarcoidosis with response to allopurinol. *Br J Dermatol* 2000; **142:** 1052–3.

## Preparations

***BP 2003:*** Allopurinol Tablets;
***USP 27:*** Allopurinol Oral Suspension; Allopurinol Tablets.

**Proprietary Preparations** (details are given in Part 3)
***Arg.:*** Alloboxal; Gotir; Puritenk; ***Austral.:*** Allohexal; Allorin; Capurate; Progout; Zyloprim; ***Austria:*** Allostad; Allotyrol; Apurin; Gewapurol; Gichtex; Purinol; Urosin; Zyloric; ***Belg.:*** Zyloric; ***Braz.:*** Lopurax; Uricemil; Zyloric; ***Canad.:*** Novo-Purol†; Zyloprim; ***Chile:*** Talol; Urogotan A; Zyloric; ***Denm.:*** Abopur; Apurin; Hexanurat; ***Fin.:*** Allonol; Apurin; Arturic; Zyloric; ***Fr.:*** Zyloric; ***Ger.:*** Allo; Allo-300-Tablinen†; Allo-Efeka; Allo-Puren; Allobeta; Allohexal†; Allpargin†; Bleminol; Cellidrin; dura AL; Epidropal; Foligan; Jenapurinol; Milurit; Pureduct; Remid; Uribenz; Uripurinol; Urosin†; Urtias†; Zyloric; ***Gr.:*** Soluric; Zylapour; Zyloric; ***Hong Kong:*** Allnol; Allorin†; Caplenal†; Mephanol; Milurit; Progout; Zyloric; ***India:*** Zyloric; ***Irl.:*** Caplenal†; Purinol; Tipuric; Zyloric; ***Israel:*** Allori; Zylol; Zyloric; ***Ital.:*** Allurit; Uricemil; Zyloric; ***Malaysia:*** Harpagin; Uritab; Zyloric; ***Mex.:*** Acyprin; Atisuril; Aurigen; Etindrax; Labypurol†; Oloprim†; Unizuric; Zyloprim; ***Neth.:*** Zyloric; ***Norw.:*** Allopur; Arturic; Zyloric; ***NZ:*** Allorin; Progout; Z 300†; Zyloprim†; ***Port.:*** Alosfar; Uriprim; Zurim; Zyloric; ***S.Afr.:*** Be-Uric†; Lonol; Puricos; Ranpuric†; Redurate; Urozyl-SR†; Zyloprim; ***Singapore:*** Allorin†; Erloric; Progout; Valeric; Zyloric; ***Spain:*** Allural†; Zyloric; ***Swed.:*** Zyloric; ***Switz.:*** allo-basan; Allopur; Cellidrine; Foligan†; Lysuron†; Mephanol; Sigapurol; Uriconorme; Zyloric; ***Thai.:*** Alinol; Allopin; Allorin†; Apnol; Apurol; Loporic; Medoric; Mephanol†; Puricin; Puride; Sigapurol†; Uricad; Valeric; Xanol; Zyloric; ***UK:*** Aloral†; Caplenal; Cosuric; Progout†; Rimapurinol; Xanthomax; Zyloric; ***USA:*** Aloprim; Zyloprim.

**Multi-ingredient:** ***Arg.:*** Artrex; Colpuril; ***Austria:*** Allobenz; Duovitan; Gichtex plus; ***Belg.:*** Comburic; ***Fr.:*** Desatura†; ***Ger.:*** Acifugan†; Allo.comp.; Allomaron; Harpagin; ***Ital.:*** Uricodue; ***Port.:*** Acifugan; ***S.Afr.:*** Allomaron; ***Spain:*** Acifugan; Facilit; ***Switz.:*** Acifugan†; ***Thai.:*** Allomaron.

---

## Benzbromarone *(BAN, USAN, rINN)*

Benzbromarona; Benzbromaronum; L-2214; MJ-10061. 3,5-Dibromo-4-hydroxyphenyl 2-ethylbenzofuran-3-yl ketone.

$C_{17}H_{12}Br_2O_3$ = 424.1.
*CAS — 3562-84-3.*
*ATC — M04AB03.*

**Pharmacopoeias.** In *Eur.* (see p.vi) and *Jpn.*

**Ph. Eur. 5.0** (Benzbromarone). A white or almost white crystalline powder. Practically insoluble in water; sparingly soluble in alcohol; freely soluble in acetone and in dichloromethane. Protect from light.

### Adverse Effects

Benzbromarone may cause gastrointestinal side-effects, especially diarrhoea. It may precipitate an acute attack of gout and cause uric acid renal calculi and renal colic. Hepatotoxicity has occurred and monitoring of liver function has been recommended.

**Effects on the liver.** Benzbromarone-induced liver damage has been reported.[1-3]

1. Van Der Klauw MM, *et al.* Hepatic injury caused by benzbromarone. *J Hepatol* 1994; **20:** 376–9.
2. Anonymous. Benzbromarone and hepatitis. *WHO Drug Inf* 2000; **14:** 29.
3. Arai M, *et al.* Fulminant hepatic failure associated with benzbromarone treatment: a case report. *J Gastroenterol Hepatol* 2002; **17:** 625–6.

### Precautions

Benzbromarone should be avoided in patients with moderate or severe renal impairment, in those with uric acid renal calculi, and in those with urinary uric acid excretion rates of greater than 700 mg per 24 hours. Like other uricosurics, treatment with benzbromarone should not be started during an acute attack of gout. Similarly, an adequate fluid intake should be maintained to reduce the risk of uric acid renal calculi; additionally, alkalinisation of the urine may be considered.

**Porphyria.** Benzbromarone is considered to be unsafe in patients with porphyria because it has been shown to be porphyrinogenic in *in-vitro* systems.

### Interactions

Aspirin and other salicylates antagonise the effect of benzbromarone. Benzbromarone may increase the anticoagulant activity of coumarin oral anticoagulants.

**Antigout drugs.** For mention of the effects of benzbromarone on the clearance of oxipurinol, the major active metabolite of *allopurinol*, and the view that this was not clinically significant, see under Interactions of Allopurinol, p.413.

### Pharmacokinetics

Benzbromarone is only partially absorbed from the gastrointestinal tract, reaching peak plasma concentrations about 2 to 4 hours after a dose by mouth. Benzbromarone is extensively bound to plasma proteins. It is metabolised in the liver, and is excreted mainly in the faeces; a small amount appears in the urine.

◊ References.

1. Maurer H, Wollenberg P. Urinary metabolites of benzbromarone in man. *Arzneimittelforschung* 1990; **40:** 460–2.
2. Walter-Sack I, *et al.* Variation of benzbromarone elimination in man—a population study. *Eur J Clin Pharmacol* 1990; **39:** 173–6.

### Uses and Administration

Benzbromarone is a uricosuric drug that reduces plasma concentrations of uric acid by blocking renal tubular reabsorption. It has been suggested that benzbromarone may also increase the intestinal elimination of uric acid. It has been used to treat hyperuricaemia including that associated with chronic gout (p.412) although it has been withdrawn in many countries due to reports of hepatotoxicity.

Benzbromarone is not used to treat acute attacks of gout and may exacerbate and prolong them if given during an attack; treatment should not start therefore until an acute attack has subsided.

The usual dose has been 50 to 300 mg daily by mouth. An NSAID or colchicine should be given initially to reduce the risk of precipitating acute gout. An adequate fluid intake should be maintained. Lower doses of benzbromarone (20 mg) have also been used in the form of a combination product with allopurinol.

### Preparations

**Proprietary Preparations** (details are given in Part 3)
***Arg.:*** Max Uric; ***Austria:*** Uricovac; ***Belg.:*** Desuric; ***Braz.:*** Narcaricina; ***Fr.:*** Desuric†; ***Ger.:*** Narcaricin; ***Hong Kong:*** Narcaricin†; ***Malaysia:*** Harpagin; ***Mex.:*** Desuric; ***Neth.:*** Desuric; ***S.Afr.:*** Minuric; ***Singapore:*** Narcaricin; ***Spain:*** Urinorm; ***Switz.:*** Desuric; Obaron; ***Thai.:*** Narcaricin.

**Multi-ingredient:** ***Austria:*** Allobenz; Duovitan; Gichtex plus; ***Belg.:*** Comburic; ***Fr.:*** Desatura†; ***Ger.:*** Acifugan†; Allo.comp.; Allomaron; Harpagin; ***Port.:*** Acifugan; ***S.Afr.:*** Allomaron; ***Spain:*** Acifugan; Facilit; ***Switz.:*** Acifugan†; ***Thai.:*** Allomaron.

## Benziodarone (BAN, rINN)

Benciodarona; L-2329. 2-Ethylbenzofuran-3-yl 4-hydroxy-3,5-diiodophenyl ketone.

$C_{17}H_{12}I_2O_3$ = 518.1.
*CAS — 68-90-6.*
*ATC — C01DX04.*

### Profile

Benziodarone is a uricosuric drug structurally related to benzbromarone (see above) that is used to reduce hyperuricaemia in chronic gout. It was formerly used as a vasodilator.

Benziodarone has been associated with jaundice and thyroid disorders.

### Preparations

**Proprietary Preparations** (details are given in Part 3)
***Spain:*** Dilafurane.
**Multi-ingredient:** ***Ital.:*** Uricodue.

## Colchicine

Colchicina; Colchicinum. (*S*)-*N*-(5,6,7,9-Tetrahydro-1,2,3,10-tetramethoxy-9-oxobenzo[α]heptalen-7-yl)acetamide.

$C_{22}H_{25}NO_6$ = 399.4.
*CAS — 64-86-8.*
*ATC — M04AC01.*

**Description.** Colchicine is an alkaloid obtained from various *Colchicum* spp.

**Pharmacopoeias.** In *Chin., Eur.* (see p.vi), *Int., Jpn,* and *US. Chin.* also has a monograph for colchicine amide.

**Ph. Eur. 5.0** (Colchicine). A yellowish-white amorphous or crystalline powder. Very soluble in water, rapidly recrystallising from concentrated solutions as the sesquihydrate; freely soluble in alcohol and in chloroform. Protect from light.

**USP 27** (Colchicine). Pale yellow to pale greenish-yellow amorphous scales, or powder or crystalline powder. Is odourless or nearly so, and darkens on exposure to light. Soluble 1 in 25 of water and 1 in 220 of ether; freely soluble in alcohol and in chloroform. Store in airtight containers. Protect from light.

### Adverse Effects and Treatment

The most frequent adverse effects of oral colchicine are those involving the gastrointestinal tract and may be associated with its antimitotic action. Diarrhoea, nausea, vomiting, and abdominal pain are often the first signs of toxicity and are usually an indication that colchicine therapy should be stopped or the dose reduced. Larger doses may cause profuse diarrhoea, gastrointestinal haemorrhage, skin rashes, and renal and hepatic damage.

Rarely, bone marrow depression with agranulocytosis, thrombocytopenia, and aplastic anaemia have occurred on prolonged treatment as have peripheral neuropathy, myopathy, rashes, and alopecia.

Adverse effects after intravenous administration include cardiac arrhythmias and local reactions such as thrombophlebitis and neuritis. Extravasation may cause tissue necrosis.

Symptoms of acute **overdosage** with oral colchicine often do not appear for 2 to 12 hours. The first signs of toxicity are nausea, vomiting and diarrhoea; a burning sensation of the throat, stomach, and skin may also occur. The diarrhoea may be severe and haemorrhagic and, coupled with vascular damage, and paralytic ileus can lead to dehydration, hypotension, and shock. Multiple organ failure may occur, manifest as CNS toxicity (confusion, delirium, sometimes coma), bone marrow depression, hepatocellular damage, muscle damage, neuropathy, respiratory distress, myocardial depression, and renal damage. A toxic epidermal necrolysis-like reaction has also been reported. Death may be due to respiratory depression, cardiovascular collapse, or sepsis following pancytopenia. In surviving patients, alopecia, rebound leucocytosis, and stomatitis may occur about 10 days after the acute overdose. The lethal dose varies: 7 mg of colchicine has caused death, yet recovery has occurred after much larger doses.

When treating colchicine overdosage or acute poisoning patients should be carefully monitored for some time to take account of the delayed onset of symptoms. In acute poisoning the stomach may be emptied by lavage; multiple dose activated charcoal should be given. Treatment is primarily symptomatic and supportive with attention being given to the control of respiration, maintenance of blood pressure and the circulation, and correction of fluid and electrolyte imbalance.

**Effects on the neuromuscular system.** Colchicine-induced myoneuropathy may be a common but unrecognised condition in patients with *reduced* renal function who receive usual doses of colchicine.[1] Although both skeletal muscles and peripheral nerves are affected, myopathy is most prominent and associated axonal neuropathy is mild. The condition usually presents with proximal muscle weakness and is always accompanied by elevations in serum creatine kinase concentrations. Withdrawal of colchicine leads to spontaneous remission of these symptoms within a few weeks but resolution of the polyneuropathy is slow. Examination of proximal muscles shows marked abnormal spontaneous activity and, because of the features of the condition, it is often initially misdiagnosed as probable polymyositis or uraemic myopathy.

There has been a report of a patient with *normal* renal function but chronic alcohol-induced liver disease who developed an unusual form of myoneuropathy after receiving only a short course of colchicine. This patient was also taking tolbutamide, the microsomal enzyme-inhibiting activity of which may have exacerbated the toxicity of colchicine.[2] Rhabdomyolysis has also been reported.[3,4]


1. Kuncl RW, *et al.* Colchicine myopathy and neuropathy. *N Engl J Med* 1987; **316:** 1562–8.
2. Besana C, *et al.* Colchicine myoneuropathy. *Lancet* 1987; **ii:** 1271–2.
3. Chattopadhyay I, *et al.* Colchicine induced rhabdomyolysis. *Postgrad Med J* 2001; **77:** 191–2.
4. Boomershine KH. Colchicine induced rhabdomyolysis. *Ann Pharmacother* 2002; **36:** 824–6.


**Overdosage.** References.


1. McIntyre IM, *et al.* Death following colchicine poisoning. *J Forensic Sci* 1994; **39:** 280–6.
2. Hood RL. Colchicine poisoning. *J Emerg Med* 1994; **12:** 171–7.
3. Baud FJ, *et al.* Brief report: treatment of severe colchicine overdose with colchicine-specific Fab fragments. *N Engl J Med* 1995; **332:** 642–5.
4. Critchley JAJH, *et al.* Granulocyte-colony stimulating factor in the treatment of colchicine poisoning. *Hum Exp Toxicol* 1997; **16:** 229–32.
5. Milne ST, Meek PD. Fatal colchicine overdose: report of a case and review of the literature. *Am J Emerg Med* 1998; **16:** 603–8.
6. Kubler PA. Fatal colchicine toxicity. *Med J Aust* 2000; **172:** 498–9.
7. Harris R, *et al.* Colchicine-induced bone marrow suppression: treatment with granulocyte colony-stimulating factor. *J Emerg Med* 2000; **18:** 435–40.
8. Mullins ME, *et al.* Fatal cardiovascular collapse following acute colchicine ingestion. *J Toxicol Clin Toxicol* 2000; **38:** 51–4.


### Precautions

Colchicine should be given with great care to elderly or debilitated patients who may be particularly susceptible to cumulative toxicity. It should also be used with caution in patients with cardiac, hepatic, renal, or gastrointestinal disease (for dosage in renal impairment see below). Colchicine should generally be avoided in pregnancy since it is known to be teratogenic in *animals* and there have also been some suggestions of a risk of fetal chromosome damage (trisomy 21) in humans.

Colchicine should not be given by subcutaneous or intramuscular injection as it causes severe local irritation.

**Breast feeding.** Colchicine is distributed into breast milk,[1-3] and recommendations have been made to wait for 8 hours[2] or 12 hours[3] after a dose before breast feeding to minimise exposure of the infant. However, since no adverse effects on the infant have been noted in these reports, the American Academy of Pediatrics considered its use to be usually compatible with breast feeding.[4]


1. Milunsky JM, Milunsky A. Breast-feeding during colchicine therapy for familial Mediterranean fever. *J Pediatr* 1991; **119:** 164.
2. Guillonneau M, *et al.* Colchicine is excreted at high concentrations in human breast milk. *Eur J Obstet Gynecol Reprod Biol* 1995; **61:** 177–8.
3. Ben-Chetrit E, *et al.* Colchicine in breast milk of patients with familial Mediterranean fever. *Arthritis Rheum* 1996; **39:** 1213–17.
4. American Academy of Pediatrics. The transfer of drugs and other chemicals into human milk. *Pediatrics* 2001; **108:** 776–89. Correction. *ibid.*; 1029. Also available at: http://aappolicy.aappublications.org/cgi/content/full/pediatrics%3b108/3/776 (accessed 26/05/04)


**Pregnancy.** Colchicine is considered to be contra-indicated in pregnancy because of *animal* teratogenicity. However, colchicine has been used during pregnancy in women with familial Mediterranean fever (see under Uses, below).[1] There was no increase in abnormality rate of the newborns and no problems were detected in 130 offspring.


1. Rabinovitch O, *et al.* Colchicine treatment in conception and pregnancy: two hundred thirty-one pregnancies in patients with familial Mediterranean fever. *Am J Reprod Immunol* 1992; **28:** 245–6.


### Interactions

**Ciclosporin.** There is a need for caution if colchicine is used with ciclosporin. Myopathies or rhabdomyolysis[1] may be a problem, especially in transplant patients[2] or those with renal impairment.[3] In addition, increased blood-ciclosporin concentrations and nephrotoxicity developed in a renal transplant patient after the introduction of colchicine therapy.[4]


1. Arellano F, Krupp P. Muscular disorders associated with cyclosporin. *Lancet* 1991; **337:** 915.
2. Simkin PA, Gardner GC. Colchicine use in cyclosporine treated transplant recipients: how little is too much? *J Rheumatol* 2000; **27:** 1334–7.
3. Rumpf KW, Henning HV. Is myopathy in renal transplant patients induced by cyclosporin or colchicine? *Lancet* 1990; **335:** 800–1.
4. Menta R, *et al.* Reversible acute cyclosporin nephrotoxicity induced by colchicine administration. *Nephrol Dial Transplant* 1987; **2:** 380–1.


**Macrolides.** Life-threatening colchicine toxicity has been described after use for 2 weeks with *erythromycin* in a patient with hepatic and renal impairment.[1] In a patient with end-stage renal disease, but no hepatic impairment, fatal colchicine toxicity developed after 4 days of *clarithromycin* therapy.[2]


1. Caraco Y, *et al.* Acute colchicine intoxication—possible role of erythromycin administration. *J Rheumatol* 1992; **19:** 494–6.
2. Dogukan A, *et al.* Acute fatal colchicine intoxication in a patient on continuous ambulatory peritoneal dialysis (CAPD): possible role of clarithromycin administration. *Clin Nephrol* 2001; **55:** 181–2.


**Tolbutamide.** For a suggestion that tolbutamide may have exacerbated the toxicity of colchicine in a patient with liver disease, see under Effects on the Neuromuscular System, above.

### Pharmacokinetics

Peak plasma concentrations of colchicine are reached within 2 hours of oral administration. Colchicine is partially deacetylated in the liver and the unchanged drug and its metabolites are excreted in the bile and undergo intestinal reabsorption. Colchicine is found in high concentrations in leucocytes, kidneys, the liver, and spleen. Most of the drug is excreted in the faeces but 10 to 20% is excreted in the urine and this proportion rises in patients with liver disorders. Colchicine is distributed into breast milk.

◊ References.


1. Rochdi M, *et al.* Toxicokinetics of colchicine in humans: analysis of tissue, plasma and urine data in ten cases. *Hum Exp Toxicol* 1992; **11:** 510–16.
2. Chappey ON, *et al.* Colchicine disposition in human leukocytes after single and multiple oral administration. *Clin Pharmacol Ther* 1993; **54:** 360–7.
3. Rochdi M, *et al.* Pharmacokinetics and absolute bioavailability of colchicine after iv and oral administration in healthy human volunteers and elderly subjects. *Eur J Clin Pharmacol* 1994; **46:** 351–4.
4. Ferron GM, *et al.* Oral absorption characteristics and pharmacokinetics of colchicine in healthy volunteers after single and multiple doses. *J Clin Pharmacol* 1996; **36:** 874–83.


### Uses and Administration

Colchicine is used for the relief of acute gout (p.412) and for the prophylaxis of acute attacks, particularly during the first few months of treatment with allopurinol or uricosurics. Colchicine produces a dramatic response in acute gout, probably by reducing the inflammatory reaction to urate crystals; this effect might be due to several actions including decreased leucocyte mobility. It is not an analgesic and has no effect on blood concentrations of uric acid, or on the excretion of uric acid. Colchicine also has an antimitotic action.

Colchicine has also been used in several other conditions including amyloidosis, Behçet's syndrome, familial Mediterranean fever, idiopathic thrombocytopenic purpura, pericarditis, primary biliary cirrhosis, and pyoderma gangrenosum.

If colchicine is used for acute attacks of **gout**, then treatment should be started as soon as possible and an effect may be expected within 12 hours. The recommended oral dose in the UK is 1 mg initially, then 500 micrograms every 2 to 3 hours until pain relief is obtained or gastrointestinal adverse effects occur (but see also Administration, below). Although licensed doses allow up to a maximum of 10 mg, the *British National Formulary* considers that the total dose should not exceed 6 mg. At least 3 days should elapse before another course is given. In the USA the dose by mouth is 0.5 to 1.2 mg initially, then 500 or 600 micrograms every 1 to 2 hours, or 1 or 1.2 mg every 2 hours, until pain is relieved or gastrointestinal adverse effects occur; the maximum total dose is 6 mg.

Colchicine has sometimes been given intravenously in a dose of 1 or 2 mg over 2 to 5 minutes with additional doses of 0.5 or 1 mg every 6 to 24 hours as required to a total dose of not more than 4 mg in one course; once this amount of colchicine has been given further doses should not then be given by any route for at least 7 days. For the view that intravenous administration should be avoided see below.

When used for the short-term prophylaxis of gout doses by mouth are 500 or 600 micrograms one to three times daily.

Consideration should be given to using reduced dosages in patients with renal impairment, see below.

◊ References.

1. Lange U, *et al.* Current aspects of colchicine therapy: classical indications and new therapeutic uses. *Eur J Med Res* 2001; **6:** 150–60.

**Administration.** Although colchicine 1 mg initially by mouth, followed by 500 micrograms every 2 to 3 hours, is recommended in the UK for the treatment of acute gout, many rheumatologists consider this excessive; a low-dose regimen of 500 micrograms no more than 3 times daily has been advocated in preference.[1] It has also been suggested that intravenous colchicine, although undoubtedly effective, should not be used because of the risk of severe or fatal adverse effects.[2]

1. Morris I, *et al.* Colchicine in acute gout. *BMJ* 2003; **327:** 1275–6.
2. Morris I, *et al.* Colchicine in acute gout. *BMJ* 2004; **328:** 289.

**Administration in renal impairment.** The manufacturers in the UK recommend that the dose of colchicine given *orally* should be reduced by up to 50% in patients with mild to moderate renal impairment, and should not be used in those with severe impairment. In the USA, it has been recommended that the *intravenous* dose of colchicine be reduced by 50% in patients with a creatinine clearance of between 10 and 50 mL/minute, and that the cumulative maximum dose should not exceed 2 mg; use is contra-indicated in those patients with a creatinine clearance less than 10 mL/minute.

**Amyloidosis.** Colchicine is well known to have a useful role in amyloidosis (p.567) secondary to familial Mediterranean fever, where results have unexpectedly suggested the possibility of reversing nephropathic changes due to renal amyloid deposition (see below). However, combination therapy with melphalan and prednisone was found to be more effective than colchicine alone in primary amyloidosis,[1] and a later trial[2] found no benefit in adding colchicine to the standard therapy. The mechanism of the anti-amyloid effect of colchicine is not clear.

1. Skinner M, *et al.* Treatment of 100 patients with primary amyloidosis: a randomised trial of melphalan, prednisone, and colchicine versus colchicine only. *Am J Med* 1996; **100:** 290–8.
2. Kyle RA, *et al.* A trial of three regimens for primary amyloidosis: colchicine alone, melphalan and prednisone, and melphalan, prednisone, and colchicine. *N Engl J Med* 1997; **336:** 1202–7.

**Behçet's syndrome.** Behçet's syndrome (p.1076) has been treated with numerous drugs. Where possible, topical treatment of local lesions should be attempted before embarking on systemic therapy. Corticosteroids are favoured for systemic treatment in many countries, but colchicine has also been widely employed. Beneficial responses have been described for most of the symptoms including the arthritic,[1] ocular, and cutaneous manifestations,[2-5] although a systematic review has questioned colchicine's efficacy.[6] The mechanism of action in this condition is believed to be based on the effect on polymorphonuclear leucocytes and other cellular effects.[7] Colchicine has also been used with corticosteroids for acute exacerbations, followed by colchicine maintenance;[8] colchicine with aspirin has also been recommended in acute disease,[9] and colchicine with benzathine benzylpenicillin has been tried.[10]

1. Yurdakul S, *et al.* A double-blind trial of colchicine in Behçet's syndrome. *Arthritis Rheum* 2001; **44:** 2686–92.
2. Mizushima Y, *et al.* Colchicine in Behçet's disease. *Lancet* 1977; **ii:** 1037.
3. Miyachi Y, *et al.* Colchicine in the treatment of the cutaneous manifestations of Behçet's disease. *Br J Dermatol* 1981; **104:** 67–9.
4. Benezra D, Cohen E. Treatment and visual prognosis in Behçet's disease. *Br J Ophthalmol* 1986; **70:** 589–92.
5. Masuda K, *et al.* Double-masked trial of cyclosporin versus colchicine and long term open study of cyclosporin in Behçet's disease. *Lancet* 1989; **i:** 1093–6.
6. Saenz A, *et al.* Pharmacotherapy for Behcet's syndrome. Available in The Cochrane Library; Issue 2. Chichester: John Wiley; 2004.
7. Schattner A. Colchicine—expanding horizons. *Postgrad Med J* 1991; **67:** 223–6.
8. Rakover Y, *et al.* Behcet disease: long-term follow-up of three children and review of the literature. *Pediatrics* 1989; **83:** 986–92.
9. Wechsler B, Piette JC. Behçet's disease. *BMJ* 1992; **304:** 1199–1200.
10. Çalgüneri M, *et al.* Effect of prophylactic benzathine penicillin on mucocutaneous symptoms of Behçet's disease. *Dermatology* 1996; **192:** 125–8.

**Diffuse parenchymal lung disease.** Colchicine is a potential alternative to corticosteroid therapy in patients with cryptogenic fibrosing alveolitis (see Diffuse Parenchymal Lung Disease, p.1079). However the degree of benefit, if any, is unclear.

References.

1. Douglas WW, *et al.* Colchicine versus prednisolone as treatment of usual interstitial pneumonia. *Mayo Clin Proc* 1997; **72:** 201–9.
2. Douglas WW, *et al.* Colchicine versus prednisone in the treatment of idiopathic pulmonary fibrosis: a randomized prospective study. *Am J Respir Crit Care Med* 1998; **158:** 220–5.
3. Douglas WW, *et al.* Idiopathic pulmonary fibrosis: impact of oxygen and colchicine, prednisone, or no therapy on survival. *Am J Respir Crit Care Med* 2000; **161:** 1172–8.

**Familial Mediterranean fever.** Familial Mediterranean fever (recurrent or paroxysmal polyserositis; periodic disease) is an inherited disorder that primarily affects Sephardic Jews or persons of Arab, Armenian, and Turkish ancestry.[1,2] It is characterised by attacks of acute abdominal pain, fever, and signs of peritonitis, which resolve spontaneously, usually in 24 to 48 hours. Pleuritic chest pain, arthritis, skin rash, pericarditis, and headache may occur. The most dangerous complication, however, is type AA amyloidosis (see also p.567), which can lead to nephrotic syndrome, renal failure, and death.

Familial Mediterranean fever is treated with colchicine.[1,2] Colchicine cannot stop an established attack, but, given prophylactically in doses of 1 to 3 mg daily, it reduces the frequency of attacks, prevents amyloidosis and reverses proteinuria. Anecdotal evidence has suggested that prazosin may also be of benefit,[3] but initial reports of improvement with interferon alfa have not been borne out.[2]

1. Ben-Chetrit E, Levy M. Familial Mediterranean fever. *Lancet* 1998; **351:** 659–63.
2. Drenth JPH, van der Meer JWM. Hereditary periodic fever. *N Engl J Med* 2001; **345:** 1748–57.
3. Kataoka H, *et al.* Treating familial Mediterranean fever with prazosin hydrochloride. *Ann Intern Med* 1998; **129:** 424–5.

**Idiopathic thrombocytopenic purpura.** In idiopathic thrombocytopenic purpura (p.1082), refractory to standard therapy, a few patients have had partial or complete response to colchicine[1,2] and further studies have been suggested.[2,3]

1. Strother SV, *et al.* Colchicine therapy for refractory idiopathic thrombocytopenic purpura. *Arch Intern Med* 1984; **144:** 2198–2200.
2. Bonnotte B, *et al.* Efficacy of colchicine alone or in combination with vinca alkaloids in severe corticoid-resistant thrombocytopenic purpura: six cases. *Am J Med* 1999; **107:** 645–6.
3. McMillian R. Therapy for adults with refractory chronic immune thrombocytopenic purpura. *Ann Intern Med* 1997; **126:** 307–14.

**Pericarditis.** Mild cases of recurrent pericarditis may be treated with colchicine, as an adjunct to NSAID therapy.[1-3] It may also provide effective prophylaxis, allowing the tapering of corticosteroids, which are usually reserved for the treatment of severe acute attacks.[2,3] The drug has also been used successfully in children.[4]

1. Millaire A, *et al.* Treatment of recurrent pericarditis with colchicine. *Eur Heart J* 1994; **15:** 120–4.
2. Adler Y, *et al.* Colchicine treatment for recurrent pericarditis: a decade of experience. *Circulation* 1998; **97:** 2183–5.
3. Oakley CM. Myocarditis, pericarditis and other pericardial diseases. *Heart* 2000; **84:** 449–54.
4. Yazigi A, *et al.* Colchicine for recurrent pericarditis in children. *Acta Paediatr Scand* 1998; **87:** 603–4.

**Primary biliary cirrhosis.** Primary biliary cirrhosis (p.1761) is a chronic progressive liver disease with no specific treatment, and in general drug therapy has been poor or largely ineffective. Reviewers have noted[1,2] that several trials have been conducted with colchicine, and, although biochemical parameters were improved, a beneficial effect on clinical symptoms or liver histology was not found. A comparative study of colchicine and methotrexate therapy showed that while both drugs improved biochemical test results and symptoms, the response to methotrexate was greater.[3] Some consider that combination therapy with colchicine, methotrexate, and ursodeoxycholic acid may be more promising than monotherapy.[2]

1. Heathcote EJ. Evidence-based therapy of primary biliary cirrhosis. *Eur J Gastroenterol Hepatol* 1999; **11:** 607–15.
2. Holtmeier J, Leuschner U. Medical treatment of primary biliary cirrhosis and primary sclerosing cholangitis. *Digestion* 2001; **64:** 137–50.
3. Kaplan MM, *et al.* A prospective trial of colchicine and methotrexate in the treatment of primary biliary cirrhosis. *Gastroenterology* 1999; **117:** 1173–80.

**Pyoderma gangrenosum.** Pyoderma gangrenosum (p.1138) associated with inflammatory bowel disease has been successfully treated with colchicine in 2 patients.[1,2] Colchicine was also of benefit in 3 patients with pyoderma associated with familial Mediterranean fever.[3]

1. Paolini O, *et al.* Treatment of pyoderma gangrenosum with colchicine. *Lancet* 1995; **345:** 1057–8.
2. Rampal P, *et al.* Colchicine in pyoderma gangrenosum. *Lancet* 1998; **351:** 1134–5.
3. Lugassy G, Ronnen M. Severe pyoderma associated with familial Mediterranean fever: favourable response to colchicine in three patients. *Am J Med Sci* 1992; **304:** 29–31.

## Preparations

**BP 2003:** Colchicine Tablets;
**USP 27:** Colchicine Injection; Colchicine Tablets; Probenecid and Colchicine Tablets.

**Proprietary Preparations** (details are given in Part 3)
***Austral.:*** Colgout; ***Braz.:*** Colchis; Reugot†; ***Hong Kong:*** Colgout; ***India:*** Goutnil; ***Malaysia:*** Goutnil; ***Mex.:*** Colchiquim; Ticolcin; ***Thai.:*** Colchily; Colcine; Goutichine; Tolchicine.

**Multi-ingredient:** ***Arg.:*** Artrex; Colpuril; ***Fr.:*** Colchimax; ***Mex.:*** Butayonacol; ***Spain:*** Colchimax; ***USA:*** ColBenemid.

## Colchicum

Colchico; Colchique.

### Profile

Colchicum, the dried ripe seeds or dried corm of the meadow saffron, *Colchicum autumnale*, contains colchicine (p.415) and has been used similarly for the relief of acute gout.

It is also included in several herbal and homoeopathic preparations.

### Preparations

**Proprietary Preparations** (details are given in Part 3)
***Ger.:*** Colchysat.

**Multi-ingredient:** ***Fr.:*** Antigoutteux Rezall†; ***Ger.:*** Unguentum lymphaticum.

## Isobromindione *(rINN)*

Isobromindiona. 5-Bromo-2-phenyl-indan-1,3-dione.
$C_{15}H_9BrO_2$ = 301.1.
*CAS — 1470-35-5.*
*ATC — M04AB04.*

### Profile

Isobromindione is a uricosuric drug that has been used by mouth in gout and hyperuricaemia. Bromindione was formerly used as an anticoagulant.

## Probenecid *(BAN, rINN)*

Probenecidum. 4-(Dipropylsulphamoyl)benzoic acid.
$C_{13}H_{19}NO_4S$ = 285.4.
*CAS — 57-66-9.*
*ATC — M04AB01.*

**Pharmacopoeias.** In *Chin., Eur.* (see p.vi), *Int., Jpn,* and *US.*

**Ph. Eur. 5.0** (Probenecid). A white or almost white crystalline powder or small crystals. Practically insoluble in water; sparingly soluble in dehydrated alcohol; soluble in acetone.

**USP 27** (Probenecid). A white or practically white, fine, practically odourless, crystalline powder. Practically insoluble in water and in dilute acids; soluble in alcohol, in acetone, in chloroform, and in dilute alkali.

### Adverse Effects

Probenecid may cause nausea, vomiting, anorexia, headache, sore gums, flushing, alopecia, dizziness, anaemia, and urinary frequency. Hypersensitivity reactions, with fever, dermatitis, pruritus, urticaria, and, rarely, anaphylaxis, and Stevens-Johnson syndrome have occurred. There have been reports of leucopenia, hepatic necrosis, nephrotic syndrome, and aplastic anaemia. Haemolytic anaemia has also occurred, and may be associated with G6PD deficiency.

When used in chronic gout, and particularly during the first few months of therapy, probenecid may precipitate acute attacks. Uric acid renal calculi, with or without haematuria, costovertebral pain and renal colic may occur.

In massive overdosage probenecid causes stimulation of the CNS, with convulsions and death from respiratory failure. Severe overdosage should be managed by lavage and symptomatic treatment.

### Precautions

Probenecid therapy should not be started during an acute attack of gout; however treatment is usually continued when acute attacks occur in patients already receiving the drug, and the acute attack is treated separately. Probenecid should not be given to patients with a history of uric acid renal calculi or blood disorders. It is not recommended for children under 2 years of age. Probenecid is also unsuitable for the control of hyperuricaemia secondary to cancer or cancer chemotherapy. It should be used with caution in patients with a history of peptic ulceration. Probenecid should not be used as an antibacterial adjunct in patients with known renal impairment, and it is ineffective in gout in patients with severe renal impairment.

To reduce the risk of uric acid renal calculi in patients with gout an adequate fluid intake (2 to 3 litres daily) is required, and, if necessary, especially during the first few months of treatment, sodium bicarbonate or potassium citrate may be given to render the urine alkaline.

A reducing substance has been found in the urine of some patients taking probenecid, and may give false positive results with some tests for glucose in the urine. Probenecid reduces the excretion of some iodinated contrast media and may interfere with laboratory tests by decreasing the excretion of aminohippuric acid, phenolsulfonphthalein, and sulfobromophthalein.

**Abuse.** It has been alleged that some athletes using banned anabolic steroids have also been taking probenecid in an attempt to inhibit the urinary excretion of steroid metabolites in order to avoid detection by urine screening tests.[1]

1. Anonymous. Does probenecid mask steroid use? *Pharm J* 1987; **239:** 299.

**Porphyria.** Probenecid is considered to be unsafe in patients with porphyria although there is conflicting experimental evidence of porphyrinogenicity.

## Interactions

The dose of probenecid may need to be increased if patients are also given drugs such as *diuretics* or *pyrazinamide* that increase the blood concentration of uric acid. Salicylates, including *aspirin*, and probenecid are mutually antagonistic and should not be given together.

Probenecid may also affect many other drugs. By inhibiting renal tubular secretion, it has the potential to increase the toxicity and/or to enhance the therapeutic efficacy of drugs excreted by that route. In some instances a reduction in dose is essential to counteract an increase in toxicity, as is the case with *methotrexate*. Some combinations, such as that with *ketorolac*, should be avoided. Conversely, probenecid may be given with some *antibacterials* such as the penicillins and cephalosporins to increase their effects.

Altered excretion may also increase serum concentrations of other antibacterials (aminosalicylic acid, conjugated sulfonamides, dapsone, meropenem, some quinolones, rifampicin), some *antivirals* (aciclovir, ganciclovir, zalcitabine, zidovudine, and possibly famciclovir), some *benzodiazepines* (lorazepam and possibly nitrazepam), *captopril*, some *NSAIDs* (diflunisal, indometacin, ketoprofen, meclofenamate, naproxen), *paracetamol*, and *sulfonylurea hypoglycaemic drugs*. The clinical significance of such interactions is not entirely clear although the possibility of the need for a reduction in dosage of these drugs should be borne in mind.

It has been reported that patients receiving probenecid require lower doses of *thiopental* for induction of anaesthesia; induction of anaesthesia may be quicker with *midazolam*.

Reducing the urinary concentration of some drugs could diminish their activity in certain diseases as might happen with *nitrofurantoin* or some *quinolones* in urinary-tract infections and *penicillamine* in cystinuria.

## Pharmacokinetics

Probenecid is completely absorbed from the gastrointestinal tract with peak plasma concentrations achieved 2 to 4 hours after a dose. It is extensively bound to plasma proteins (85 to 95%). The plasma half-life is dose-dependent and ranges from less than 5 to more than 8 hours. Probenecid crosses the placenta. It is metabolised by the liver, and excreted in the urine mainly as metabolites. Excretion is increased in alkaline urine.

◊ References.

1. Ho JC, *et al.* Probenecid disposition by parallel Michaelis-Menten and dose-dependent pseudo-first-order processes. *J Pharm Sci* 1986; **75:** 664–8.
2. Emanuelsson B-M, *et al.* Non-linear elimination and protein binding of probenecid. *Eur J Clin Pharmacol* 1987; **32:** 395–401.

## Uses and Administration

Probenecid is a uricosuric drug used to treat hyperuricaemia (p.412) associated with chronic gout; it has also been used to treat hyperuricaemia caused by diuretic therapy. It is also used as an adjunct to some antibacterials to reduce their renal tubular excretion and has been given with the antiviral cidofovir (p.630) to reduce nephrotoxicity.

Probenecid is used in **chronic gout and hyperuricaemia** to inhibit the renal tubular reabsorption of uric acid so increasing the urinary excretion of uric acid, lowering plasma-urate concentrations, and eventually reducing urate deposits in the tissues. Probenecid is therefore of value in hyperuricaemia caused by decreased uric acid excretion rather than increased urate production, and is not used for hyperuricaemia associated with cancer or cancer therapy.

Probenecid has no analgesic or anti-inflammatory action and is of no value in acute gout. Initially it may increase plasma concentrations of urate and uric acid by dissolving deposits. This can trigger or exacerbate acute attacks, hence probenecid should not be started until an acute attack has completely subsided, and an NSAID or colchicine may be given during the first few months.

It is usual to start treatment for gout with doses of 250 mg twice daily by mouth increased after a week to 500 mg twice daily and later, if the therapeutic effects are inadequate, by increments of 500 mg every 4 weeks, up to 2 g daily. Probenecid may not be effective in chronic renal impairment particularly when the glomerular filtration rate is less than 30 mL/minute. An adequate fluid intake is required to reduce the risk of uric acid renal calculi.

When the patient has been free from acute attacks for at least 6 months, and provided that the plasma-urate concentration is within acceptable limits, the daily dose may be gradually reduced, by 500 mg every 6 months, to the lowest effective maintenance dose which is then given indefinitely.

Probenecid may also be used as an **adjunct to antibacterial therapy** particularly when treating severe or resistant infections. It reduces the tubular excretion of penicillins and most cephalosporins and may increase their plasma concentrations up to fourfold. The usual dosage for reducing tubular excretion of penicillins and cephalosporins is 500 mg four times daily, or less in elderly patients with suspected renal impairment. When renal impairment is sufficient to retard the excretion of antibacterials, probenecid should not be given concurrently.

The dosage for children over 2 years of age and weighing less than 50 kg is 25 mg/kg (700 mg/m$^2$) initially, followed by 10 mg/kg (300 mg/m$^2$) every 6 hours.

Single doses of probenecid 1 g are given by mouth with an oral antibacterial, or at least 30 minutes before an injected antibacterial, in the single-dose treatment of gonorrhoea.

## Preparations

***BP 2003:*** Probenecid Tablets;
***USP 27:*** Ampicillin and Probenecid for Oral Suspension; Probenecid and Colchicine Tablets; Probenecid Tablets.

**Proprietary Preparations** (details are given in Part 3)
***Austral.:*** Benemid†; Pro-Cid; ***Canad.:*** Benemid†; Benuryl; ***Fin.:*** Probecid; ***Fr.:*** Benemide; ***India:*** Bencid; ***Irl.:*** Benemid†; ***Mex.:*** Benecid; ***Norw.:*** Probecid; ***NZ:*** Benemid†; ***S.Afr.:*** Benemid†; Proben; ***Swed.:*** Probecid; ***Switz.:*** Benemid†; ***Thai.:*** Bencid; Benemid; ***UK:*** Benemid†; ***USA:*** Benemid.

**Multi-ingredient:** ***USA:*** ColBenemid.

*Used as an adjunct in:* ***Braz.:*** Ampicler com Probenecide†; Degonat†; Emicilin; Gonocilin†; Gonol; Gonorrels†; Probecilin†; ***Spain:*** Blenox.

# Sulfinpyrazone *(BAN, rINN)*

G-28315; Sulfinpirazona; Sulfinpyrazonum; Sulphinpyrazone; Sulphoxyphenylpyrazolidine. 1,2-Diphenyl-4-(2-phenylsulphinylethyl)pyrazolidine-3,5-dione.

$C_{23}H_{20}N_2O_3S$ = 404.5.

*CAS — 57-96-5.*

*ATC — M04AB02.*

**Pharmacopoeias.** In *Eur.* (see p.vi), *Jpn*, and *US*.

**Ph. Eur. 5.0** (Sulfinpyrazone). A white or almost white powder. Very slightly soluble in water; sparingly soluble in alcohol; dissolves in dilute solutions of alkali hydroxides. Protect from light

**USP 27** (Sulfinpyrazone). A white to off-white powder. Practically insoluble in water and in petroleum spirit; soluble in alcohol and in acetone; sparingly soluble in dilute alkali.

## Adverse Effects

The most frequent adverse effects of sulfinpyrazone involve the gastrointestinal tract, and include nausea, vomiting, and abdominal pain. It may cause gastric bleeding or aggravate existing peptic ulcers. Skin rashes have been reported, and may be associated with a hypersensitivity reaction. Anaemia, agranulocytosis, leucopenia, and thrombocytopenia have been reported rarely as have raised liver enzyme values, jaundice, and hepatitis, impaired renal function, salt and water retention, and acute renal failure.

When used in chronic gout, particularly during the first few months of treatment, sulfinpyrazone may precipitate acute attacks and there is a risk of uric acid renal calculi developing.

Symptoms of overdosage include hypotension, acute renal failure, arrhythmias, respiratory disorders, convulsions, and coma, as well as gastrointestinal effects. Treatment of overdose may involve gastric lavage if a substantial amount has been ingested within 1 hour of presentation, followed by symptomatic and supportive therapy.

**Effects on the kidneys.** Although renal failure has been reported occasionally in patients receiving sulfinpyrazone for gout[1] many of the cases have occurred in patients given the drug after a myocardial infarction.[2,3] Acute renal failure may also occur after overdose or in patients with intravascular volume depletion.[4,5]

1. Durham DS, Ibels LS. Sulphinpyrazone-induced acute renal failure. *BMJ* 1981; **282:** 609.
2. Boelaert J, *et al.* Sulphinpyrazone-induced decrease in renal function: a review of reports with discussion of pathogenesis. *Acta Clin Belg* 1982; **37:** 368–75.
3. Lijnen P, *et al.* Decrease in renal function due to sulphinpyrazone treatment early after myocardial infarction. *Clin Nephrol* 1983; **19:** 143–6.
4. Florkowski CM, *et al.* Acute non-oliguric renal failure secondary to sulphinpyrazone overdose. *J Clin Pharm Ther* 1992; **17:** 71.
5. Walls M, *et al.* Acute renal failure due to sulfinpyrazone. *Am J Med Sci* 1998; **315:** 319–21.

## Precautions

Sulfinpyrazone should not be started during an acute attack of gout; however, treatment is usually continued when acute attacks occur in patients already receiving the drug, and the acute attack is treated separately. Sulfinpyrazone is not suitable for the control of hyperuricaemia associated with cancer or cancer chemotherapy. It should not be given to patients with uric acid renal calculi or peptic ulcer disease or a history of such disorders; use is also contra-indicated in patients with blood dyscrasias or blood coagulation disorders, and in those with severe kidney or liver damage. It should be given with care to patients whose renal function is impaired and to those with heart failure.

Sulfinpyrazone should not be given to patients hypersensitive to it or to other pyrazole derivatives such as phenylbutazone; nor should it be given to patients in whom hypersensitivity reactions (including bronchospastic reactions in asthmatics) have been provoked by aspirin or by other drugs with prostaglandin-synthetase inhibiting activity.

To reduce the risk of uric acid renal calculi an adequate fluid intake (2 to 3 litres daily) is required; alkalinising the urine with sodium bicarbonate or potassium citrate may also be considered. It is recommended that patients have periodic full blood counts to detect any haematological abnormalities.

Renal-function tests involving aminohippuric acid or phenolsulfonphthalein may be invalidated.

**Porphyria.** Sulfinpyrazone is considered to be unsafe in patients with porphyria because it has been shown to be porphyrinogenic in *in-vitro* systems.

## Interactions

Doses of sulfinpyrazone may need to be increased if it is given with other drugs such as *diuretics* or *pyrazinamide* that increase uric acid concentrations. Sulfinpyrazone and salicylates including *aspirin* are mutually antagonistic and should not be used together. There may also be an increased risk of bleeding when sulfinpyrazone is used with other drugs such as aspirin that inhibit platelet function.

Sulfinpyrazone's renal tubular secretion is inhibited by probenecid although with little clinical effect. Since sulfinpyrazone, like probenecid, inhibits the tubular secretion of weak organic acids, interactions can be expected with penicillins although the effect is not considered to be clinically useful.

Sulfinpyrazone can potentiate the action of some drugs. The most significant interaction of this type involves *warfarin, acenocoumarol*, and possibly other coumarin anticoagulants (p.1025). Patients receiving sulfinpyrazone and such an anticoagulant should have their prothrombin times monitored and the anticoagulant dosage reduced as appropriate. Similarly, sulfinpyrazone may potentiate the effects of *phenytoin* (see Antigout Drugs, p.373), and possibly some *sulfonamides* and *sulfonylureas*.

In contrast, sulfinpyrazone may increase the metabolism of *theophylline* (p.802) and diminish its activity.

## Pharmacokinetics

Sulfinpyrazone is readily absorbed from the gastrointestinal tract. It is about 98% bound to plasma proteins. It has been reported to have a plasma half-life of about 2 to 4 hours. Sulfinpyrazone is partly metabolised in the liver and some of the metabolites are active. On long-term therapy, sulfinpyrazone appears to induce its own metabolism. Unchanged drug and metabolites are mainly excreted in the urine.

◊ References.


1. Bradbrook ID, *et al.* Pharmacokinetics of single doses of sulphinpyrazone and its major metabolites in plasma and urine. *Br J Clin Pharmacol* 1982; **13:** 177–85.
2. Schlicht F, *et al.* Pharmacokinetics of sulphinpyrazone and its major metabolites after a single dose and during chronic treatment. *Eur J Clin Pharmacol* 1985; **28:** 97–103.


## Uses and Administration

Sulfinpyrazone is a uricosuric drug used to treat hyperuricaemia associated with chronic gout (p.412). It also has some antiplatelet activity.

Sulfinpyrazone is used in chronic gout to inhibit the renal tubular reabsorption of uric acid so increasing the urinary excretion of uric acid, lowering plasma-urate concentrations, and eventually reducing urate deposits in the tissues. It is therefore of value in hyperuricaemia caused by decreased uric acid excretion rather than increased urate production and is not used for hyperuricaemia associated with cancer or cancer therapy.

Sulfinpyrazone has little analgesic or anti-inflammatory action and is of no value in acute gout. Initially, it may increase plasma concentrations of urate and uric acid by dissolving deposits. This can trigger or exacerbate acute attacks, hence sulfinpyrazone should not be given until an acute attack has completely subsided, and an NSAID or colchicine may be given during the first few months.

The initial dose of sulfinpyrazone is 100 to 200 mg once or twice daily, taken with meals or milk. This may be gradually increased over 1 to 3 weeks until a daily dosage of 600 mg is reached; up to 800 mg daily may be given if necessary. After the plasma-urate concentration has been controlled, the daily maintenance dose may be reduced to as low as 200 mg. An adequate fluid intake is required to prevent formation of uric acid renal calculi.

**Antiplatelet therapy.** Sulfinpyrazone inhibits platelet function, thereby inhibiting thrombosis. It has been given after myocardial infarction, at a maintenance dose of 200 mg four times daily. For other antithrombotic indications the drug may be given at a dose of 600 to 800 mg daily in 3 or 4 divided doses. A meta-analysis of trials, conducted by the Antiplatelet Trialists' Collaboration, has shown that sulfinpyrazone reduces the risk of myocardial infarction, stroke, or vascular death in patients at high risk of occlusive vascular disease.[1] Similarly, sulfinpyrazone reduces the risk of occlusion in patients undergoing arterial reperfusion and revascularisation procedures.[2] However, aspirin is the most widely used antiplatelet therapy, as discussed on p.819.


1. Antiplatelet Trialists' Collaboration. Collaborative overview of randomised trials of antiplatelet therapy—I: prevention of death, myocardial infarction, and stroke by prolonged antiplatelet therapy in various categories of patients. *BMJ* 1994; **308:** 81–106.
2. Antiplatelet Trialists' Collaboration. Collaborative overview of randomised trials of antiplatelet therapy—II: maintenance of vascular graft or arterial patency by antiplatelet therapy. *BMJ* 1994; **308:** 159–68.


## Preparations

***BP 2003:*** Sulfinpyrazone Tablets;
***USP 27:*** Sulfinpyrazone Capsules; Sulfinpyrazone Tablets.

**Proprietary Preparations** (details are given in Part 3)
***Austral.:*** Anturan†; ***Austria:*** Anturan†; ***Canad.:*** Novo-Pyrazone†; ***Israel:*** Anturan†; ***Ital.:*** Enturen; ***NZ:*** Anturan†; SPZ†; ***Port.:*** Sulfinona; ***Switz.:*** Anturan†; ***UK:*** Anturan; ***USA:*** Anturane.

---

# Tisopurine *(rINN)*

MPP; Tisopurina. 1*H*-Pyrazolo[3,4-*d*]pyrimidine-4-thiol.

$C_5H_4N_4S = 152.2$.

*CAS — 5334-23-6.*

*ATC — M04AA02.*

## Profile

Tisopurine, an analogue of allopurinol, is an inhibitor of uric acid synthesis. It is used in the treatment of disorders associated with hyperuricaemia (p.412), including gout, in doses of 100 to 400 mg daily.

## Preparations

**Proprietary Preparations** (details are given in Part 3)
***Austria:*** Exuracid.

---

# Urate Oxidase

CB-8129; Uricasa; Uricase.
*CAS — 9002-12-4.*
*ATC — M04AX01.*

# Rasburicase *(BAN, USAN, rINN)*

Rasburicasa; SR-29142.
*CAS — 134774-45-1.*
*ATC — V03AF07.*

## Profile

Rasburicase is a recombinant form of the enzyme urate oxidase, which oxidises uric acid to allantoin. It is used in the treatment and prophylaxis of severe hyperuricaemia associated with the treatment of malignancy. It is given by intravenous infusion before and during the initiation of chemotherapy, in a dose of 150 or 200 micrograms/kg daily over 30 minutes. Duration of treatment may vary from 5 to 7 days. Adverse effects reported during treatment with rasburicase include fever, gastrointestinal disturbances, and headache. Hypersensitivity reactions, including anaphylaxis, have occurred. Haemolysis and methaemoglobinaemia have been reported rarely. Rasburicase is contra-indicated in patients with G6PD deficiency or other cellular metabolic disorders known to cause haemolytic anaemia; hydrogen peroxide, which is produced during oxidation of uric acid to allantoin, can induce haemolytic anaemia in these patients.

The native enzyme has also been used.

**Tumour lysis syndrome.** The tumour lysis syndrome (p.495) represents a biochemical disturbance following massive release of cellular breakdown products from tumour cells sensitive to therapy; hyperuricaemia is a cardinal feature. Rasburicase was effective in the prophylaxis or treatment of hyperuricaemia in children and young adults with leukaemia or lymphoma who either presented with abnormally high plasma concentrations of uric acid or had large tumour cell burdens.[1] Treatment was mostly well tolerated; one patient developed nausea and vomiting and one experienced bronchospasm and hypoxaemia 3 hours after infusion. Antibodies to rasburicase were seen in 17 of 121 assessable patients. Safety and efficacy were confirmed in further studies of children[2] and adults[2,3] considered to be at particularly high risk of tumour lysis syndrome. In children[4] with haematologic malignancies at high risk for tumour lysis, rasburicase given intravenously achieved more rapid control and lower levels of plasma uric acid than oral allopurinol. No antibodies to rasburicase were detected at day 14. In 3 children with acute lymphoblastic leukaemia, hyperuricaemia was reportedly controlled with oral allopurinol and a single dose of rasburicase, although subclinical tumour lysis was apparent.[5]


1. Pui C-H, *et al.* Recombinant urate oxidase for the prophylaxis or treatment of hyperuricemia in patients with leukaemia or lymphoma. *J Clin Oncol* 2001; **19:** 697–704.
2. Pui C-H, *et al.* Recombinant urate oxidase (rasburicase) in the prevention and treatment of malignancy-associated hyperuricemia in pediatric and adult patients: results of a compassionate-use trial. *Leukemia* 2001; **15:** 1505–9.
3. Coiffier B, *et al.* Efficacy and safety of rasburicase (recombinant urate oxidase) for the prevention and treatment of hyperuricemia during induction chemotherapy of aggressive non-Hodgkin's lymphoma: results of the GRAAL1 (Groupe d'Etude des Lymphomes de l'Adulte Trial on Rasburicase Activity in Adult Lymphoma) study. *J Clin Oncol* 2003; **21:** 4402–6.
4. Goldman SC, *et al.* A randomized comparison between rasburicase and allopurinol in children with lymphoma or leukemia at high risk for tumor lysis. *Blood* 2001; **97:** 2998–3003.
5. Lee ACW, *et al.* Treatment of impending tumor lysis with single-dose rasburicase. *Ann Pharmacother* 2003; **37:** 1614–17.


## Preparations

**Proprietary Preparations** (details are given in Part 3)
***Austral.:*** Fasturtec; ***Belg.:*** Fasturtec; ***Chile:*** Fasturtec; ***Denm.:*** Fasturtec; ***Fin.:*** Fasturtec; ***Fr.:*** Fasturtec; Uricozyme†; ***Ger.:*** Fasturtec; ***Gr.:*** Fasturtec; ***Hong Kong:*** Fasturtec; ***Ital.:*** Fasturtec; Uricozyme; ***Norw.:*** Fasturtec; ***NZ:*** Fasturtec; ***Port.:*** Fasturtec; ***Spain:*** Fasturtec; ***Swed.:*** Fasturtec; ***Switz.:*** Fasturtec; ***UK:*** Fasturtec; ***USA:*** Elitek.

# Antihistamines

Adverse Effects of Antihistamines, p.419
Precautions for Antihistamines, p.420
Interactions of Antihistamines, p.421
Uses of Antihistamines, p.421
Anaesthesia, p.421
Anaphylaxis, p.421
Angioedema, p.421
Asthma, p.421
Conjunctivitis, p.421
Coughs and colds, p.421
Food allergy, p.422
Hay fever, p.422
Insomnia, p.422
Ménière's disease, p.422
Migraine, p.422
Nausea and vomiting, p.422
Otitis media, p.422
Pruritus, p.422
Rhinitis, p.422
Urticaria and angioedema, p.423
Vertigo, p.423

The peripheral effects of histamine are chiefly mediated by 2 sets of receptors termed $H_1$ and $H_2$. Effects mediated by the $H_1$ receptors include the contraction of smooth muscle and the dilatation and increased permeability of the capillaries. The effects of histamine on vascular smooth muscle are mediated by $H_2$ as well as $H_1$ receptors. Other effects that are mediated by $H_2$ receptors include cardiac accelerating effects and, in particular, the stimulating action of histamine on the secretion of gastric acid. An $H_3$ receptor has also been identified in a number of systems including the CNS and peripheral nerves. It is thought that $H_3$ receptors are involved in the autoregulation of the release of histamine and other neurotransmitters from neurones.

The term 'antihistamines' is normally reserved for histamine $H_1$-antagonists and this is the convention used in *Martindale*. $H_2$-antagonists, typified by cimetidine (p.1255), are described in the chapter on Gastrointestinal Drugs. $H_3$-antagonists are under investigation.

The older antihistamines are associated with troublesome sedative and antimuscarinic effects, and are often termed 'sedating antihistamines'. The newer antihistamines, which are essentially devoid of these effects, are correspondingly termed 'non-sedating antihistamines' and include acrivastine, astemizole, cetirizine, loratadine, and terfenadine.

On the basis of their chemical structure most antihistamines can be classified into one of 6 groups:

- *Alkylamines:* drugs within this group typically possess significant sedative actions, although paradoxical stimulation can occur, especially in children. They are highly potent $H_1$-antagonists. Brompheniramine and chlorphenamine are typical alkylamines; acrivastine is a non-sedating alkylamine antihistamine.
- *Monoethanolamines:* monoethanolamine derivatives have pronounced sedative and antimuscarinic actions but a low incidence of gastrointestinal effects. Examples include clemastine and diphenhydramine.
- *Ethylenediamines:* these antihistamines are selective $H_1$-antagonists. They cause moderate sedation (despite having weak CNS effects), gastric disturbances, and skin sensitisation. Antazoline and mepyramine are examples.
- *Phenothiazines:* phenothiazine antihistamines have significant sedative, and pronounced antiemetic and antimuscarinic effects. Photosensitivity reactions have occurred. Promethazine is a typical phenothiazine.
- *Piperazines:* this group of antihistamines possesses moderate sedative and significant antiemetic actions. Piperazine derivatives include cetirizine, cyclizine, and hydroxyzine. Cetirizine causes less sedation than other members of this group.
- *Piperidines:* piperidines cause moderate or low sedation and are highly selective for $H_1$ receptors. Examples include azatadine, cyproheptadine, and the non-sedating antihistamines astemizole, loratadine, and terfenadine.

Although characteristic pharmacological properties have been described for members of each group it should be noted that many of the effects of antihistamines vary as much with each patient as with each drug and that, in particular, some of the newer non-sedating antihistamines may share the chemical structure of a group in which the other members have sedative effects.

◊ References.

1. Hill SJ, *et al.* International Union of Pharmacology. XIII. Classification of histamine receptors. *Pharmacol Rev* 1997; **49:** 253–78.
2. Leurs R, *et al.* Therapeutic potential of histamine $H_3$ receptor agonists and antagonists. *Trends Pharmacol Sci* 1998; **19:** 177–83.

**Hypersensitivity.** Hypersensitivity may be defined as an exaggerated or inappropriate immune response causing tissue damage. Hypersensitivity reactions are generally classified into 4 types (types I to IV) although this may be considered an over simplification and more than one type can often be postulated for a patient's hypersensitivity. In each of the 4 types, prior sensitisation of the patient to the specific antigen is required. The term *'allergy'* by definition originally covered all types of hypersensitivity reactions as well as the induction of immunity in an individual. Nowadays, the term is more commonly applied to type I hypersensitivity reactions.

**Type I**, immediate hypersensitivity reactions occur after exposure to an antigen (the allergen) in a sensitised subject; that is, one in whom the initial exposure to the antigen has caused the production of specific antibodies, mainly IgE (immunoglobulin E), which are bound to the surface of mast cells and basophils. At subsequent exposure, antigen binds to antibody resulting in degranulation of mast cells and basophils with release of mediators. These include preformed mediators such as histamine and chemotactic factors, and newly synthesised mediators such as leukotrienes, platelet-activating factor, and prostaglandins. Although type I reactions are usually described as being acute and short-lived, clinically there may often also be a late-phase and more prolonged reaction affecting the skin and bronchi. Examples of type I hypersensitivity reactions discussed below include allergic conjunctivitis, allergic rhinitis, urticaria and angioedema, and anaphylactic shock.

**Type II**, cell-surface hypersensitivity reactions are caused by the interaction of circulating antibodies, mainly IgG (immunoglobulin G) and IgM (immunoglobulin M), with antigens that are on the surface of specific cells or tissues. This interaction results in activation of complement and of phagocytic and killer cells leading to cell damage or lysis. Type II reactions are responsible for blood transfusion reactions, some drug-induced blood disorders, and many auto-immune disorders.

**Type III**, immune complex hypersensitivity reactions, are caused by the interaction of fixed or circulating antigens with circulating antibodies, mainly IgG and IgM (either soluble or particulate), resulting in formation of immune complexes. The immune complexes trigger a variety of inflammatory processes including complement activation, mediator release from mast cells and basophils, and platelet aggregation. Examples of type III reactions include serum sickness, some auto-immune and neoplastic disorders, type 2 lepra reactions (p.133), and reactions, particularly in the lung, to some particulate antigens such as micro-organisms.

**Type IV**, cell-mediated or delayed hypersensitivity reactions, are caused by interaction of an antigen with sensitised T lymphocytes; lymphokines are released by T lymphocytes and inflammation ensues. Type IV reactions usually occur at least 24 hours after contact with the antigen. A type IV reaction is responsible for tuberculin reactions used for sensitivity testing, contact dermatitis, and some reactions to chronic infectious disease for example type 1 lepra reactions (p.133).

An **anaphylactoid** (pseudoallergic) reaction produces similar symptoms to those of anaphylaxis (see below), but is caused by direct release of histamine provoked by an unclear, non-immune mechanism. There is thus no requirement for prior exposure to the triggering factor, commonly a drug.

## Adverse Effects of Antihistamines

The most common side-effect of the *sedating antihistamines* is CNS depression, with effects varying from slight drowsiness to deep sleep, and including lassitude, dizziness, and incoordination (although paradoxical stimulation may occasionally occur, especially at high doses and in children or the elderly). These sedative effects, when they occur, may diminish after a few days of treatment. A major advantage of the *non-sedating antihistamines* is that they generally cause little or no drowsiness (but see Sedation, below).

Other side-effects that are more common with the *sedating antihistamines* include headache, psychomotor impairment, and antimuscarinic effects, such as dry mouth, thickened respiratory-tract secretions, blurred vision, urinary difficulty or retention, constipation, and increased gastric reflux. Another major advantage of the *non-sedating antihistamines* is that most have little or no antimuscarinic effect.

Occasional gastrointestinal side-effects of antihistamines include nausea, vomiting, diarrhoea, or epigastric pain. Those with antiserotonin actions, such as cyproheptadine, may cause an increase in appetite with resultant weight gain, whereas anorexia has been reported with some other antihistamines.

Palpitations and arrhythmias have been reported occasionally with most antihistamines, but a major disadvantage of the *non-sedating antihistamines* astemizole and terfenadine is the rare occurrence of hazardous ventricular arrhythmias which has led to important restrictions on their use (see under Precautions, below).

Antihistamines may sometimes cause rashes and hypersensitivity reactions (including bronchospasm, angioedema, and anaphylaxis) and cross-sensitivity to related drugs may occur. Photosensitivity can be a problem, particularly with the phenothiazine antihistamines.

Blood disorders, including agranulocytosis, leucopenia, haemolytic anaemia, and thrombocytopenia, although rare, have been reported. Jaundice has also been observed, particularly with the phenothiazine antihistamines.

Other adverse effects that have been reported with the antihistamines include convulsions, sweating, myalgia, paraesthesias, extrapyramidal effects, tremor, sleep disturbances, depression, confusion, tinnitus, hypotension, and hair loss.

Despite reports suggesting a possibility of human fetal abnormalities resulting from the use of some antihistamines, especially the piperazine derivatives, a causal relationship has largely been rejected; for details see under Precautions, below.

Some antihistamines have been abused for their mental effects.

Antihistamines available as preparations for application to the skin may occasionally cause skin sensitisation; systemic side-effects have been reported after topical application to large areas of the skin.

**Overdosage** with *sedating antihistamines* is associated with antimuscarinic, extrapyramidal, and CNS effects. When CNS stimulation predominates over CNS depression, which is more likely in children or the elderly, it causes ataxia, excitement, tremors, psychoses, hallucinations, and convulsions; hyperpyrexia may also occur. Deepening coma and cardiorespiratory collapse may follow. In adults, CNS depression is more common with drowsiness, coma, and convulsions, progressing to respiratory failure and cardiovascular collapse. In the case of the *non-sedating antihistamines*, antimuscarinic effects are less marked, but hazardous ventricular arrhythmias (below) may be a special problem with astemizole and terfenadine, even in modest overdoses, and have led to restrictions on their use.

◊ Reviews.


1. Simons FER. $H_1$-receptor antagonists: comparative tolerability and safety. *Drug Safety* 1994; **10:** 350–80.
2. Horak F, Stübner UP. Comparative tolerability of second generation antihistamines. *Drug Safety* 1999; **20:** 385–401.


**Arrhythmias.** Ventricular arrhythmias have been reported rarely with astemizole and terfenadine particularly in association with increased blood concentrations. For full details and specific warnings see under Astemizole, p.424, and Terfenadine, p.441.

The suspicion that such life-threatening arrhythmias may be a class effect of the non-sedating antihistamines has so far proven unfounded. Data[1] from the WHO adverse drug reaction database showed that cardiac events had been reported with the 5 most widely prescribed non-sedating antihistamines at that time (acrivastine, astemizole, cetirizine, loratadine, and terfenadine), and an attempt to quantify the risk[2] suggested that use of these drugs was associated overall with a fourfold increase in likelihood of developing ventricular arrhythmias, although the absolute risk remained low. However, other centres[3] have argued that definitive causality has only been proven for astemizole and terfenadine. In addition, a possible mechanism for drug-induced cardiac toxicity has only been demonstrated with astemizole and terfenadine;[4] both drugs have been shown to block cardiac potassium channels *in vitro*, a phenomenon that results in prolongation of the QT interval, which is a risk factor for developing ventricular arrhythmias. Studies[5] with loratadine and cetirizine have demonstrated that neither drug blocked potassium channels *in vitro*, and similar lack of activity might be expected with desloratadine and levocetirizine, but there is some evidence that mizolastine can block potassium channels at high concentrations *in vitro*[6] (although a small study in healthy subjects noted no adverse effects on cardiac conduction at doses up to 4 times those normally given).[7] A case report[8] of arrhythmias in a patient with pre-existing QT-prolongation given fexofenadine, did not appear to be associated with blocking of potassium channels.[9]


1. Lindquist M, Edwards IR. Risks of non-sedating antihistamines. *Lancet* 1997; **349:** 1322. Correction. *ibid.;* 1482.
2. de Abajo FJ, García Rodrígues LA. Risk of ventricular arrhythmias associated with nonsedating antihistamine drugs. *Br J Clin Pharmacol* 1999; **47:** 307–13.
3. Himmel MH, *et al.* Dangers of non-sedating antihistamines. *Lancet* 1997; **350:** 69.
4. Salata JJ, *et al.* Cardiac electrophysiological actions of the histamine $H_1$-receptor antagonists astemizole and terfenadine compared with chlorpheniramine and pyrilamine. *Circ Res* 1995; **76:** 110–19.
5. Woosley RL. Cardiac actions of antihistamines. *Ann Rev Pharmacol Toxicol* 1996; **36:** 233–52.
6. Taglialatela M, *et al.* Inhibition of HERG1 $K^+$ channels by the novel second-generation antihistamine mizolastine. *Br J Clin Pharmacol* 2000; **131:** 1081–8.
7. Chaufour S, *et al.* Study of cardiac repolarization in healthy volunteers performed with mizolastine, a new $H_1$-receptor antagonist. *Br J Clin Pharmacol* 1999; **47:** 515–20.
8. Pinto YM, *et al.* QT lengthening and life-threatening arrhythmias associated with fexofenadine. *Lancet* 1999; **353:** 980.
9. Scherer CR, *et al.* The antihistamine fexofenadine does not affect $I_{Kr}$ currents in a case report of drug-induced cardiac arrhythmia. *Br J Clin Pharmacol* 2002; **137:** 892–900.


**Reye's syndrome.** For criticism of a suggested link in children between antihistamines and Reye's syndrome, see p.16.

**Sedation.** CNS depression is a common adverse effect of the sedating antihistamines and sedative effects can range from slight drowsiness to deep sleep. Daytime sedation can be a problem especially for those who have to drive or operate machinery. When sedative effects do occur they are most apparent at the start of treatment and often diminish after a few days despite continued administration. Sedation caused by alcohol or other CNS depressants is enhanced. Many studies have attempted to quantify and compare the sedative effects of the older antihistamines, but results vary widely and classifications are difficult to make. Theoretically, the onset, degree, and persistence of sedation depend on factors such as penetration of the blood-brain barrier and on the relative affinity for central and peripheral histamine $H_1$ receptors. In general, antihistamines of the monoethanolamine and phenothiazine classes cause the most sedation.

In view of these problems, non-sedating antihistamines have been developed. These compounds have poor penetration into the CNS and/or higher affinity for peripheral rather than central histamine $H_1$ receptors. Studies with acrivastine,[1] astemizole,[2] fexofenadine,[3] loratadine,[4] and terfenadine[5] have generally indicated a lower incidence of sedation and related CNS effects than that observed with older antihistamines and comparable with that of placebo; prescription-event monitoring suggested that sedation was lower with fexofenadine and loratadine than with acrivastine or cetirizine, although the risk was low with all 4 drugs.[6] In a study[7] to compare the effects of acrivastine, terfenadine, and diphenhydramine on driving performance, terfenadine had no significant effect on driving performance. Acrivastine's effects were dose-related, but with little effect at the normal therapeutic dose, whereas diphenhydramine profoundly impaired all the measures of driving performance. In another study,[8] the effects of fexofenadine on driving performance were comparable to placebo. Studies with terfenadine[5] suggest that the incidence of sedation does not increase significantly with increased dose or duration of administration. Cetirizine appears to be more sedating than loratadine or terfenadine but less sedating than older antihistamines; the effect appears to be dose dependent.[9] Limited data with azelastine[10] indicate a similar incidence of drowsiness to that with terfenadine. An incidence of sedation comparable with that caused by terfenadine has also been observed for mequitazine when given in the recommended dosage of 5 mg twice daily.[5] Sedation has, however, occurred after doses of 10 mg twice daily.[11] Other newer antihistamines claimed to produce no troublesome sedation include ebastine, epinastine, mizolastine, and setastine.

A number of studies have indicated that the non-sedating antihistamines do not seem to enhance the effects of alcohol and other CNS depressants.

*A few patients treated with non-sedating antihistamines have experienced drowsiness. Therefore it is prudent to exercise caution before driving or operating machinery; the effect of a drug on a particular patient can be ascertained after the first few doses.*


1. Bojkowski CJ, *et al.* Acrivastine in allergic rhinitis: a review of clinical experience. *J Int Med Res* 1989; **17** (suppl 2): 54B–68B.
2. Anonymous. Astemizole—another non-sedating antihistamine. *Med Lett Drugs Ther* 1989; **31:** 43–4.
3. Hindmarch I, *et al.* A double-blind, placebo-controlled investigation of the effects of fexofenadine, loratadine and promethazine on cognitive and psychomotor function. *Br J Clin Pharmacol* 1999; **48:** 200–206.
4. Clissold SP, *et al.* Loratadine: a preliminary review of its pharmacodynamic properties and therapeutic efficacy. *Drugs* 1989; **37:** 42–57.
5. McTavish D, *et al.* Terfenadine: an updated review of its pharmacological properties and therapeutic efficacy. *Drugs* 1990; **39:** 552–74.
6. Mann RD, *et al.* Sedation with "non-sedating" antihistamines: four prescription-event monitoring studies in general practice. *BMJ* 2000; **320:** 1184–6.
7. Ramaekers JG, O'Hanlon JF. Acrivastine, terfenadine and diphenhydramine effects on driving performance as a function of dose and time after dosing. *Eur J Clin Pharmacol* 1994; **47:** 261–6.
8. Weiler JM, *et al.* Effects of fexofenadine, diphenhydramine, and alcohol on driving performance: a randomized, placebo-controlled trial in the Iowa driving simulator. *Ann Intern Med* 2000; **132:** 354–63.
9. Spencer CM, *et al.* Cetirizine: a reappraisal of its pharmacological properties and therapeutic use in selected allergic disorders. *Drugs* 1993; **46:** 1055–80.
10. McTavish D, Sorkin EM. Azelastine: a review of its pharmacodynamic and pharmacokinetic properties, and therapeutic potential. *Drugs* 1989; **38:** 778–800.
11. Brandon ML. Newer non-sedating antihistamines: will they replace older agents? *Drugs* 1985; **30:** 377–81.


## Precautions for Antihistamines

Drowsiness is a major problem with the *sedating antihistamines* and those affected should not drive or operate machinery; alcohol should be avoided. In the case of *non-sedating antihistamines*, although drowsiness is rare, it can occur and may affect the performance of skilled tasks.

Because of their antimuscarinic actions the *sedating antihistamines* should be used with care in conditions such as angle-closure glaucoma, urinary retention, prostatic hyperplasia, or pyloroduodenal obstruction; antimuscarinic side-effects are not a significant problem with the *non-sedating antihistamines*.

Occasional reports of convulsions in patients taking antihistamines suggest a need for caution in patients with epilepsy.

Many antihistamines are excreted in the urine in the form of active metabolites so that dosage reduction may be necessary in renal impairment (see individual monographs for specific advice). Caution is also needed in hepatic impairment, notably with phenothiazine antihistamines (for further details, see Effects on the Liver, under Chlorpromazine, p.676) and, above all, with the *non-sedating antihistamines*, astemizole and terfenadine (hazardous ventricular arrhythmias may occur in the presence of excessive blood concentrations). Other important cautions for astemizole and terfenadine include avoidance of concomitant use of drugs liable to interfere with their hepatic metabolism or otherwise increase the risk of arrhythmias, and contra-indication in patients with cardiac disease, known or suspected prolongation of the QT interval, or hypokalaemia or other electrolyte imbalances. For full details see under Astemizole, p.424, and Terfenadine, p.441.

Antihistamines should not be given to neonates owing to their increased susceptibility to antimuscarinic effects. It has also been recommended that antihistamines, in particular phenothiazines (see Promethazine, p.439 and Alimemazine, p.423), should be avoided in young children. Elderly patients are also more susceptible to many of the adverse effects of antihistamines and, in particular, their inappropriate use for postural giddiness should be avoided (see Vertigo, below).

Topical preparations containing antihistamines should not be used on broken or eczematous skin.

A number of large studies have failed to demonstrate any strong associations between fetal abnormalities and antihistamines taken during pregnancy (see under Pregnancy, below).

**Asthma.** Antihistamines are not considered effective in the management of asthma[1] and their use has often been contra-indicated in patients with asthma because of fears that they may cause airway obstruction. However, antihistamine-induced airway obstruction has rarely been noted clinically and many patients with asthma tolerate concurrent treatment with antihistamines without obvious adverse effects. Therefore the American Academy of Allergy and Immunology has recommended that antihistamines are not contra-indicated in patients with asthma, unless an adverse reaction has previously been demonstrated, and the FDA no longer warns against the use of over-the-counter antihistamines by people with asthma.[2]


1. Meltzer EO. To use or not to use antihistamines in patients with asthma. *Ann Allergy* 1990; **64:** 183–6.
2. Food and Drug Administration. Cold, cough, allergy, bronchodilator, and antiasthmatic drug products for over-the-counter human use: final monograph for OTC antihistamine drug products: final rule. *Fed Regist* 1992; **57:** 58369–70.


**Pregnancy.** Considerable anxiety has surrounded the issue of whether there is any risk to the fetus from antiemetic therapy during pregnancy. The most widely studied preparation was Debendox which contained doxylamine, dicycloverine, and pyridoxine, and was known as Bendectin in some countries. Dicycloverine was removed from the preparation in 1976 in the USA and subsequently in other countries, and the product was withdrawn from the market in 1983 because of threatened litigation.[1] By that time Debendox had been used for over 27 years and in over 33 million pregnancies worldwide.[1]

Initial concern came from anecdotal reports of malformations in infants whose mothers had taken Debendox during pregnancy.[2,3] Evidence was found[4] of an association between prenatal exposure to the 3-component formulation of Bendectin and an increased risk of pyloric stenosis and possibly also defective heart valves in a study of 1369 malformed infants and 2968 healthy control cases. Other studies have suggested an increased incidence of oral clefts,[5] gastrointestinal atresia,[6] and genital tract disorders,[7] but generally such increases have been small. No overall pattern of malformations appears to have emerged, and many large studies have failed to confirm an association between doxylamine use and congenital malformations.[8-13]

A prospective study of 11 481 pregnancies found no increased incidence of either severe congenital abnormalities or perinatal mortality rates in women who had been prescribed prochlorperazine, meclozine, cyclizine, or Bendectin during pregnancy, although there was some evidence of an excess number of congenital abnormalities in patients taking trimethobenzamide.[14]

The Collaborative Perinatal Project[15] monitored the mothers of 50 282 children between 1958 and 1965. Of these, 5401 were exposed to antihistamines and 1309 to phenothiazines during the first 4 months of pregnancy. There was no evidence to suggest that exposure to these drugs was related to malformations, although there were slight suggestions of associations between respiratory malformations and pheniramine, inguinal hernia and meclozine, inguinal hernia or genito-urinary malformations and diphenhydramine, and cardiovascular deformities and phenothiazines. A report[16] on the same study found no effects of phenothiazines on perinatal mortality, birth-weight, or IQ scores at the age of 4 years. The Collaborative Perinatal Project also noted a relationship between cardiovascular defects and inguinal hernia and dimenhydrinate exposure.[15]

Both the UK Committee on Safety of Medicines[17] and the FDA in the USA[18] reviewed the literature in 1981 and concluded that while the scientific evidence did not demonstrate an increase in birth defects with Debendox, the risk of teratogenicity could not be completely excluded. A subsequent review[19] by the FDA in 1999 into the reasons for withdrawal stated that the evidence supported the conclusion that the combination had not been withdrawn from the market for reasons of safety or efficacy. In some countries a combination preparation of doxylamine and pyridoxine remains available for the treatment of nausea and vomiting in pregnancy. There has been a study indicating that vomiting itself is not teratogenic.[20]

A number of other studies have been carried out on meclozine prompted by reports of fetal abnormalities in 10 patients associated with a preparation of meclozine and pyridoxine;[21] these studies have not supported the original reports.[22-24]


1. Merrell Pharmaceuticals. Production of Debendox to stop. *Lancet* 1983; **i:** 1395.
2. Paterson DC. Congenital deformities associated with Bendectin. *Can Med Assoc J* 1977; **116:** 1348.
3. Donnai D, Harris R. Unusual fetal malformations after antiemetics in early pregnancy. *BMJ* 1978; **1:** 691–2.
4. Eskenazi B, Bracken MB. Bendectin (Debendox) as a risk factor for pyloric stenosis. *Am J Obstet Gynecol* 1982; **144:** 919–24.
5. Golding J, *et al.* Maternal anti-nauseants and clefts of lip and palate. *Hum Toxicol* 1983; **2:** 63–73.
6. Jick H, *et al.* First-trimester drug use and congenital disorders. *JAMA* 1981; **246:** 343–6.
7. Gibson GT, *et al.* Congenital anomalies in relation to the use of doxylamine/dicyclomine and other antenatal factors: an ongoing prospective study. *Med J Aust* 1981; **i:** 410–4.

8. Shapiro S, *et al.* Antenatal exposure to doxylamine succinate and dicyclomine hydrochloride (Bendectin) in relation to congenital malformations: perinatal mortality rate, birth weight, and intelligence quotient score. *Am J Obstet Gynecol* 1977; **128:** 480–5.
9. Harron DWG, *et al.* Debendox and congenital malformations in Northern Ireland. *BMJ* 1980; **281:** 1379–81.
10. Fleming DM, *et al.* Debendox in early pregnancy and fetal malformation. *BMJ* 1981; **283:** 99–101.
11. Mitchell AA, *et al.* Birth defects related to Bendectin use in pregnancy 1: Oral clefts and cardiac defects. *JAMA* 1981; **245:** 2311–14.
12. Mitchell AA, *et al.* Birth defects in relation to Bendectin use in pregnancy. *Am J Obstet Gynecol* 1983; **147:** 737–42.
13. Winship KA, *et al.* Maternal drug histories and central nervous system anomalies. *Arch Dis Child* 1984; **59:** 1052–9.
14. Milkovich L, van den Berg BJ. An evaluation of the teratogenicity of certain antinauseant drugs. *Am J Obstet Gynecol* 1976; **125:** 244–8.
15. Heinonen OP, *et al. Birth defects and drugs in pregnancy.* Massachusetts: Publishing Sciences Group, 1977.
16. Slone D, *et al.* Antenatal exposure to the phenothiazines in relation to congenital malformations, perinatal mortality rate, birth weight, and intelligence quotient score. *Am J Obstet Gynecol* 1977; **128:** 486–8.
17. Committee on Safety of Medicines. Data sheet change—Debendox. *Current Problems 6* 1981.
18. Food and Drugs Administration. Indications for Bendectin narrowed. *FDA Drug Bull* 1981; **11** (1).
19. Food and Drug Administration. Determination that Bendectin was not withdrawn from sale for reasons of safety or effectiveness. Available at: http://www.fda.gov/OHRMS/DOCKETS/98fr/080999e.pdf (accessed 08/04/04)
20. Klebanoff MA, Mills JL. Is vomiting during pregnancy teratogenic? *BMJ* 1986; **292:** 724–6.
21. Watson GI. Meclozine ("Ancoloxin") and foetal abnormalities: preliminary report by the epidemic observation unit of the College of General Practitioners. *BMJ* 1962; **ii:** 1446.
22. Lenz W. How can the teratogenic action of a factor be established in man? *South Med J* 1971; **64** (suppl 1): 41–7.
23. Greenberg G, *et al.* Maternal drug histories and congenital abnormalities. *BMJ* 1977; **2:** 853–6.
24. Shapiro S, *et al.* Meclizine in pregnancy in relation to congenital malformations. *BMJ* 1978; **i:** 483.


## Interactions of Antihistamines

*Sedating antihistamines* may enhance the sedative effects of CNS depressants including alcohol, barbiturates, hypnotics, opioid analgesics, anxiolytic sedatives, and antipsychotics. Sedative interactions apply to a lesser extent with the *non-sedating antihistamines*; they do not appear to potentiate the effects of alcohol, but it should be avoided in excess.

*Sedating antihistamines* have an additive antimuscarinic action with other antimuscarinic drugs, such as atropine and some antidepressants (both tricyclics and MAOIs).

Potentially hazardous ventricular arrhythmias have occurred when the *non-sedating antihistamines* astemizole and terfenadine have been given with drugs liable to interfere with their hepatic metabolism, with other potentially arrhythmogenic drugs including those that prolong the QT interval, or with those likely to cause electrolyte imbalance. For full details see under Astemizole, p.424, and Terfenadine, p.441.

It has been suggested that some *sedating antihistamines* could mask the warning signs of damage caused by ototoxic drugs such as aminoglycoside antibiotics.

Antihistamines may suppress the cutaneous histamine response to allergen extracts and should be stopped several days before skin testing.

## Uses of Antihistamines

Histamine $H_1$-antagonists (termed 'antihistamines' in *Martindale*) diminish or abolish the major actions of histamine in the body by competitive, reversible blockade of histamine $H_1$-receptor sites on tissues; they do not inactivate histamine or prevent its synthesis, nor, in most cases, its release (although some are claimed to have mast-cell stabilising properties). Histamine $H_1$ receptors are responsible for vasodilatation, increased capillary permeability, flare and itch reactions in the skin, and to some extent for contraction of smooth muscle in the bronchi and gastrointestinal tract.

Many of the *sedating antihistamines* also possess antimuscarinic, adrenaline-antagonising, serotonin-antagonising, and local anaesthetic effects. Some have calcium-channel blocking activity.

Antihistamines are used primarily for the alleviation of conditions such as urticarial **rashes** and **nasal allergy** that are characterised by type I hypersensitivity (see above), but by virtue of their associated pharmacological actions they are also used to alleviate the symptoms of a wide range of other conditions (such as pruritus and nausea and vomiting).

The antihistamines can improve or relieve the symptoms of **seasonal allergic rhinitis** ('hay fever') in many patients. They alleviate rhinorrhoea and sneezing (and ocular symptoms such as conjunctivitis) but may be less effective for nasal congestion. The relief obtained is dependent on the severity and nature of the symptoms, being greater in the milder stages. The *non-sedating antihistamines* are preferred for daytime control, but a *sedating antihistamine* may be preferred at night. Antihistamines may also be of value in **vasomotor rhinitis**, despite the fact that this is not primarily an allergic condition. *Sedating antihistamines* are widely marketed, often with a decongestant, in compound preparations for the symptomatic treatment of coughs and **colds** although there is little evidence of value.

Antihistamines are of value in preventing **urticaria** and are used to treat urticarial rashes and mild **angioedema**. They are also used as adjuncts to adrenaline in the emergency treatment of **anaphylaxis** and severe angioedema. However, the use of an antihistamine is not appropriate for the control of blood transfusion reactions caused by ABO incompatibility.

The *sedating antihistamines* are of value in the alleviation of **pruritus** both of allergic and of non-allergic origin; they have a major role in pruritus associated with atopic eczema. The *non-sedating antihistamines* do not alleviate pruritus of non-allergic origin owing to their poor penetration of the blood-brain barrier.

*Sedating antihistamines* have marked antiemetic activity and are used to control **nausea and vomiting** caused by a variety of vestibular disorders. In the case of motion sickness a sedating antihistamine, such as dimenhydrinate or promethazine, is used if severe drowsiness (or even sleep) is not considered undesirable, but generally a less sedative antihistamine, such as cyclizine, cinnarizine, or meclozine may be preferred. Sedating antihistamines are similarly used to control the vertigo and nausea associated with **Ménière's disease** and related conditions, with cinnarizine promoted as a specific treatment. Sedating antihistamines also have an important role in the alleviation of the nausea and vomiting of **migraine**, and buclizine or cyclizine are marketed in some countries in a combination preparation for this purpose; cyproheptadine, which has serotonin antagonist and calcium-channel blocking activity, may be of value in the prophylaxis of migraine. Sedating antihistamines have a very limited role in the short-term management of vomiting of pregnancy but are no longer considered appropriate for nausea alone. *Sedating antihistamines* have also been widely used for **premedication** in anaesthetic practice and still have a major role in the prevention of postoperative nausea and vomiting.

Some of the antihistamines with very pronounced sedative effects, such as diphenhydramine and promethazine, have been marketed for treatment of occasional **insomnia** but their long duration of action can cause hangover effects. Some antihistamines are also available as preparations for topical application for the alleviation of **insect bites**, but there is little evidence of any real value and such use may be associated with sensitisation.

◊ General references.


1. Simons FER, Simons KJ. Clinical pharmacology of new histamine $H_1$ receptor antagonists. *Clin Pharmacokinet* 1999; **36:** 329–52.
2. Slater JW, *et al.* Second-generation antihistamines: a comparative review. *Drugs* 1999; **57:** 31–47.


### Anaesthesia

Phenothiazine antihistamines have been used for anaesthetic premedication (p.1296) and to relieve anxiety during surgical and obstetric procedures, but benzodiazepines are now used more routinely. However, sedating antihistamines such as promethazine and cyclizine do have a role in the control of postoperative vomiting (below). Alimemazine is licensed for premedication in children, although when given alone it may cause postoperative restlessness if pain is present.

### Anaphylaxis

Anaphylaxis is commonly a type I (immediate) hypersensitivity reaction (see above) to various allergens such as drugs, foods, and insect venoms. A clinically identical reaction can, however, be provoked by some other immune mechanisms, or by non-immune mechanisms (an anaphylactoid reaction). Symptoms of anaphylaxis and anaphylactoid reactions include erythema, pruritus, urticaria, and angioedema; respiratory obstruction may result from oedema of the larynx or epiglottis. Gastrointestinal disturbances, bronchospasm, hypotension, and coma can occur in severe reactions.

Patients with severe anaphylactic or anaphylactoid reactions should be given immediate treatment with adrenaline (see Anaphylactic Shock, p.855). Addition of a parenteral antihistamine such as chlorphenamine maleate or diphenhydramine hydrochloride and a corticosteroid such as hydrocortisone after the acute episode may decrease the duration and severity of symptoms and prevent relapse. The use of antihistamines in treating the symptoms of milder forms of anaphylaxis is discussed under individual symptoms such as Pruritus (below) and Urticaria and Angioedema (below).

### Angioedema

See under Urticaria and Angioedema, below.

### Asthma

Antihistamines appear to have no place in the treatment of asthma (p.777). A meta-analysis[1] of double-blind randomised placebo-controlled trials published since 1980 did not support the use of antihistamines in the treatment of asthma, although the quality of the studies was generally considered to be poor.


1. Van Ganse E, *et al.* Effects of antihistamines in adult asthma: a meta-analysis of clinical trials. *Eur Respir J* 1997; **10:** 2216–24.


### Conjunctivitis

Allergic conjunctivitis is a type I hypersensitivity reaction (above). It is usually seasonal but perennial attacks due to allergens such as house dust mites can occur. Itching, tears, and burning are common symptoms and frequently rhinitis (below) will co-exist. Conjunctivitis can also be caused by pathogenic micro-organisms (see Eye Infections, p.127).

Avoidance of unnecessary exposure to aeroallergens is of prime importance in the management of allergic conjunctivitis. Since a large number of inflammatory mediators are involved in its pathogenesis no single drug will be completely effective. Systemic sedating and non-sedating antihistamines are effective in reducing allergic symptoms and preventing attacks; the choice of drug depends on the degree of sedation required. Ophthalmic antihistamine preparations such as antazoline, azelastine, emedastine, levocabastine, and olopatadine may also be used for acute attacks. Ophthalmic corticosteroids may reduce inflammation, but use should be restricted to severe cases only and limited to 5 to 7 days' duration because of the risk of local adverse effects such as cataract or raised intra-ocular pressure. Mast-cell stabilisers including ketotifen, lodoxamide, nedocromil, and sodium cromoglicate have been widely used for prophylaxis; some antihistamines also have mast-cell stabilising properties. Diclofenac and ketorolac eye drops are available for the treatment of allergic conjunctivitis. Combined preparations of astringents such as zinc sulfate and sympathomimetics such as naphazoline may also be used for symptomatic relief.

References.


1. Ciprandi G, *et al.* Drug treatment of allergic conjunctivitis: a review of the evidence. *Drugs* 1992; **43:** 154–76.
2. Hingorani M, Lightman S. Therapeutic options in ocular allergic disease. *Drugs* 1995; **50:** 208–21.
3. McGill JI, *et al.* Allergic eye disease mechanisms. *Br J Ophthalmol* 1998; **82:** 1203–14.
4. Bielory L. Ocular allergy guidelines: a practical treatment algorithm. *Drugs* 2002; **62:** 1611–34.


### Coughs and colds

Sedating antihistamines are frequently used in combination preparations for the treatment of coughs and colds (p.1112 and p.618 respectively). The mechanism of their antitussive action may involve reduction in cholinergic nerve transmission or may simply result from their sedative effects; reduction of nasal secretions may be of value in treating cough caused by postnasal drip. Antihistamines should not be used to treat productive coughs because reduction in bronchial secretions may cause formation of viscid mucus plugs. The sedative effects of antihistamines may prove troublesome for daytime use but may be a short-term advantage for night coughs.

### Food allergy

The term food allergy (food hypersensitivity) should be reserved for instances in which an immune mechanism for the reaction is proven, as may occur, for example, with nuts; food intolerance is used to describe a non-immune reaction. Food allergy may be the result of a type I (immediate), or possibly a type III (immune complex), hypersensitivity reaction (see above). Management revolves around the identification of the provoking food allergen and its subsequent avoidance. Individualised diets are designed and patients are educated about possible hidden sources of the allergen. Drug therapy has a very limited role in the prevention of food allergy; oral sodium cromoglicate has been used but efficacy has not been unequivocally established.

Inadvertent exposure to an allergen resulting in anaphylactic shock (p.855) requires immediate treatment with adrenaline. Milder symptoms may be controlled by antihistamines and corticosteroids. Allergen immunotherapy plays no role in the routine management of food allergy (see p.1650).

References.

1. Hunter JO. Food allergy and intolerance. *Prescribers' J* 1997; **37:** 193–8.
2. Sampson HA. Food allergy. *JAMA* 1997; **278:** 1888–94.
3. Bindslev-Jensen C. Food allergy. *BMJ* 1998; **316:** 1299–1302.
4. Høst A, *et al.* Dietary products used in infants for treatment and prevention of food allergy: joint statement of the European Society for Paediatric Allergology and Clinical Immunology (ESPACI) Committee on Hypoallergenic Formulas and the European Society for Paediatric Gastroenterology, Hepatology and Nutrition (ESPGHAN) Committee on Nutrition. *Arch Dis Child* 1999; **81:** 80–4.
5. David TJ. Adverse reactions and intolerance to foods. *Br Med Bull* 2000; **56:** 34–50.
6. Sicherer SH. Food allergy. *Lancet* 2002; **360:** 701–10.

### Hay fever

Hay fever is a seasonal form of allergic rhinitis in which symptoms of conjunctivitis are also present. Management is symptomatic and therapies used are discussed under Conjunctivitis, above and Rhinitis, below.

### Insomnia

Some of the older sedating antihistamines including diphenhydramine and promethazine, have been promoted to the public for occasional insomnia (p.667), although their long duration of action may cause hangover effects. Promethazine was formerly popular for children but the use of hypnotics in this age group is not usually justified. Moreover a possible association between phenothiazines and sudden infant death syndrome (see under the Adverse Effects of Promethazine, p.439) contributed to the recommendation that such antihistamines should not be used in young children.

### Ménière's disease

Ménière's disease is a disorder of the labyrinth (the inner ear) characterised by recurrent attacks of vertigo, progressive hearing loss, and worsening tinnitus (p.1381). It usually presents in middle age and may equally affect men and women. The predominant pathological feature is an excess of endolymph fluid producing an increase in pressure in the membranous labyrinth (endolymphatic hydrops). Attacks occur in clusters over a few weeks with periods of remission lasting weeks or months.

The aims of treatment are to alleviate symptoms and preserve hearing if possible. It is therefore important to assess how far the disease has progressed, particularly in terms of hearing loss. In addition to conventional hearing tests, cochlear dysfunction may be assessed pharmacologically. Hypertonic glycerol has been given orally to reduce the endolymphatic fluid volume by osmotic diuresis, any temporary improvement in hearing indicating reversible impairment. However, this test is associated with side-effects that some consider unacceptable. Urea has been used as an alternative to glycerol. Intravenous acetazolamide has been used diagnostically to increase endolymphatic pressure temporarily in order to produce transient hearing loss in patients in the reversible stages of the disease.

Acute attacks of vertigo in the early stages may be treated with the same drugs used for vertigo of any cause (see below).

Vasodilators have been advocated for maintenance treatment because ischaemia of the labyrinth has been postulated as a factor in the aetiology. Betahistine, a histamine analogue, is used. Restriction of dietary sodium and administration of diuretics, such as chlortalidone, furosemide, and hydrochlorothiazide, has also been used traditionally to reduce the amount of fluid in the endolymphatic spaces.

As the disease progresses, vestibular ablation with aminoglycosides may be indicated. Systemic streptomycin has been used but the risk of further hearing loss and other serious adverse effects has limited its use. Intratympanic administration of gentamicin is now preferred, and can improve vertigo in up to 90% of patients, although exacerbation of hearing loss is still a risk, albeit at a lower incidence than that with systemic streptomycin.

Surgical treatment remains an option for patients with Ménière's disease refractory to medical interventions.

References.

1. Saeed SR, *et al.* Ménière's disease. *Br J Hosp Med* 1994; **51:** 603–12.
2. Brookes GB. The pharmacological treatment of Ménière's disease. *Clin Otolaryngol* 1996; **21:** 3–11.
3. Claes J, Van de Heyning PH. Medical treatment of Ménière's disease: a review of literature. *Acta Otolaryngol* 1997; suppl 526: 37–42.
4. Saeed SR. Diagnosis and treatment of Ménière's disease. *BMJ* 1998; **316:** 368–72.
5. Thai-Van H, *et al.* Ménière's disease: pathophysiology and treatment. *Drugs* 2001; **61:** 1089–1102.

### Migraine

Antihistamines have a number of uses in the management of migraine (p.464). Those with antiemetic activity such as buclizine and cyclizine are used to alleviate the nausea and vomiting associated with migraine; they are common ingredients of compound analgesic preparations given for the initial treatment of migraine.

Those antihistamines with antiserotonin actions, including cyproheptadine and flunarizine, have been used for the prophylaxis of migraine.

### Nausea and vomiting

The management of various types of nausea and vomiting is discussed in detail on p.1245.

The older antihistamines such as cinnarizine, cyclizine, dimenhydrinate, meclozine, and promethazine are among the principal drugs used for **motion sickness**. They are all of similar efficacy but may differ in onset and duration of action and in the extent of side-effects such as drowsiness. If a sedative effect is desired dimenhydrinate and promethazine are useful, otherwise a slightly less sedating antihistamine such as cinnarizine, cyclizine, or meclozine may be preferred. The aim is prevention of motion sickness since antiemetics are more effective for prophylaxis than for treatment. Antihistamines may be slightly less effective against motion sickness than the antimuscarinic hyoscine (p.483), but are often better tolerated. Non-sedating antihistamines such as terfenadine, which penetrate poorly into the CNS, do not appear to be effective against motion sickness.

Diphenhydramine has been included in antiemetic regimens for the control of nausea and vomiting associated with **cancer chemotherapy** to reduce the extrapyramidal reactions associated with metoclopramide; it may also improve overall antiemetic control. Cyclizine is used as an antiemetic in **palliative care**.

Cyclizine is given as a supplement to opioids for premedication and has been effective prophylactically as well as in established **postoperative nausea and vomiting**. Promethazine has also been used for the prevention and treatment of postoperative nausea and vomiting, but has marked sedative effects.

Nausea in the first trimester of **pregnancy** does not require drug therapy, but on rare occasions if vomiting is severe an antihistamine such as promethazine may be required pending specialist advice. See under Precautions for Antihistamines, above, for a discussion of the risks of antiemetic therapy during pregnancy.

### Otitis media

Acute otitis media (p.138) and otitis media with effusion may resolve without treatment although antibacterials are often given. Antihistamines and decongestants, alone or in combination, have been widely given to children for symptomatic management of acute otitis media and associated respiratory symptoms, studies[1-3] have failed to show benefit, and their use is not recommended.[4] Indeed in one study,[3] adjunctive treatment with chlorphenamine was found to prolong the duration of middle ear effusion.

1. Cantekin EI, *et al.* Lack of efficacy of a decongestant-antihistamine combination for otitis media with effusion ("secretory" otitis media) in children. *N Engl J Med* 1983; **308:** 297–301.
2. Mandel EM, *et al.* Efficacy of amoxicillin with and without decongestant-antihistamine for otitis media with effusion in children: results of a double-blind, randomized trial. *N Engl J Med* 1987; **316:** 432–7.
3. Chonmaitree T, *et al.* A randomized, placebo-controlled trial of the effect of antihistamine or corticosteroid treatment in acute otitis media. *J Pediatr* 2003; **143:** 377–85.
4. The Otitis Media Guideline Panel. Managing otitis media with effusion in young children. *Pediatrics* 1994; **94:** 766–73.

### Pruritus

The sedating antihistamines are commonly used to relieve pruritus (itching) (p.1137) from a variety of causes. They are effective in relieving pruritus associated with urticaria (below) but are also used for itching associated with dermatoses such as atopic eczema (p.1135), where the degree of benefit is less certain. They are given in the latter to control nocturnal itching and for severe pruritus associated with relapse.

The exact pathophysiology of itching remains unclear.[1-3] Although histamine release is associated with itching in atopic eczema different inflammatory mediators are involved in other dermatoses. The CNS is also thought to play a part in the perception of itch. Hence, the relative roles of CNS sedation and peripheral histamine-receptor blockade in the mode of action of antihistamines in these conditions is a matter of debate. Although sedation has generally been considered the more important, the benefits of sedating antihistamines appear to be less in eczema than in urticaria. In addition, clemastine has been reported to provide no antipruritic benefit, yet it induces significant sedation. Studies with non-sedating antihistamines have been inconclusive; most found no benefit in pruritus associated with atopic eczema, although one early study has shown a slight benefit from the addition of acrivastine or terfenadine to treatment with a topical corticosteroid and an emollient.[4] Some have questioned whether any antihistamine offers much benefit in pruritus.[5]

1. Krause L, Shuster S. Mechanism of action of antipruritic drugs. *BMJ* 1983; **287:** 1199–1200.
2. Advenier C, Queille-Roussel C. Rational use of antihistamines in allergic dermatological conditions. *Drugs* 1989; **38:** 634–44.
3. Greaves MW, Wall PD. Pathophysiology of itching. *Lancet* 1996; **348:** 938–40.
4. Doherty V, *et al.* Treatment of itching in atopic eczema with antihistamines with a low sedative profile. *BMJ* 1989; **298:** 96.
5. Anonymous. Oral antihistamines for allergic disorders. *Drug Ther Bull* 2002; **40:** 59–62. Correction. *ibid.*; 2003; **41:** 24.

### Rhinitis

Rhinitis may be allergic or non-allergic in origin. Allergic rhinitis is a type I hypersensitivity reaction (see above); both early (sneezing, rhinorrhoea and nasal congestion) and late (nasal congestion) reactions may be provoked. It may be seasonal (as in hay fever) or perennial and, in some patients, will frequently co-exist with conjunctivitis (above). Non-allergic rhinitis may be divided into eosinophilic non-allergic rhinitis or non-eosinophilic non-allergic rhinitis. The term vasomotor rhinitis has been used to describe the latter although its use is best avoided since no vasomotor dysfunction has been clearly identified.

In the management of **allergic rhinitis**, avoidance of unnecessary exposure to aeroallergens is of prime importance. However, in most sufferers this is not possible and some form of drug therapy will be necessary. A large number of inflammatory mediators are involved in the pathogenesis of rhinitis and no single drug is completely effective in the alleviation of symptoms.

- Some antihistamines may nonetheless be useful in reducing secretions, nasal itching, sneezing, and ocular symptoms such as conjunctivitis, but are less effective for relief of nasal congestion. Non-sedating antihistamines such as acrivastine, cetirizine, ebastine, fexofenadine, loratadine, and mizolastine are now considered the first-choice treatment for mild and/or intermittent allergic rhinitis. They are also used for the management of breakthrough symptoms in those sufferers using prophylactic intranasal corticosteroids or sodium cromoglicate (see below). Since the maximum effect of antihistamines occurs several hours after peak serum concentrations have been obtained, they should be given in anticipation of a reaction to achieve the maximum response. Most antihistamines are unsuitable for topical use in the nose or eye since they are generally ineffective at the concentrations suitable for local therapy; also there is the potential for sensitisation. However, the antazoline salts, azelastine, and levocabastine have been used topically in the nose for control of symptoms. Such preparations are considered less effective than intra-nasal corticosteroids but probably more effective than cromoglicate.

- The actions of topical corticosteroids in allergic rhinitis include relief of inflammation, a decrease in capillary permeability and in mucus production, and vasoconstriction; they inhibit both the early and late response to allergen exposure. Corticosteroids are first-line treatment for the prophylaxis of moderate and/or persistent allergic rhinitis. In seasonal allergic rhinitis, they should be started at least 2 weeks before the pollen season and taken regularly throughout the season. Those applied intranasally include beclometasone, budesonide, flunisolide, fluticasone, mometasone, and triamcinolone. At recommended dosage, local adverse effects are mild and transient and systemic effects are not a risk; aqueous sprays may cause less local effects than pressurised aerosols. Treatment of allergic rhinitis with oral or parenteral corticosteroids has been reserved for short-term treatment in special circumstances only, although some have contested even this practice.
- Mast-cell stabilisers such as ketotifen, nedocromil, and sodium cromoglicate are thought to act primarily by preventing release of inflammatory mediators from sensitised mast cells through stabilisation of mast-cell membranes. They are an alternative to corticosteroids in the prophylactic treatment of allergic rhinitis and may be preferred for therapy in children. They may also be useful in controlling mild to moderate symptoms.
- The leukotriene receptor antagonist montelukast has produced benefits comparable to those seen with antihistamines, and is licensed in some countries for management of seasonal allergic rhinitis.
- Intranasal sympathomimetics such as phenylephrine, naphazoline, oxymetazoline, and xylometazoline may be useful for short-term treatment of allergic rhinitis to relieve severe nasal congestion which can be painful and may impede delivery of sodium cromoglicate or a corticosteroid to the mucosal surfaces. Oral sympathomimetic decongestants such as pseudoephedrine and phenylpropanolamine are less effective than topical sympathomimetics and adverse effects may be troublesome.
- Ipratropium bromide given intranasally may be useful as adjunctive therapy in patients with rhinorrhoea as it has a localised parasympathetic blocking action which reduces watery hypersecretion from nasal mucosa.

Allergen immunotherapy (see p.1650) is generally only indicated in severe allergic rhinitis when sensitivity testing demonstrates sensitivity to one allergen and when exposure to the allergen is unavoidable or symptomatic treatment has failed.

The management of **non-allergic rhinitis** is similar to that of allergic rhinitis despite different mechanisms being involved in its aetiology. Topical corticosteroids are often first-line therapy especially if nasal congestion is a dominant feature. The role of antihistamines is more limited; sedating antihistamines are useful in reducing nasal secretions because of their antimuscarinic actions; however, non-sedating antihistamines are relatively ineffective. In patients in whom rhinorrhoea is a particular problem, intranasal administration of the antimuscarinic ipratropium is of value. Although intranasal sympathomimetics have also been used they should generally be avoided because of the risk of rebound congestion. Oral sympathomimetics are largely ineffective.

Other therapies tried include topical capsaicin, to induce local desensitisation, and nasal douching with a saline and sodium bicarbonate solution.

References.


1. Horak F. Seasonal allergic rhinitis: newer treatment approaches. *Drugs* 1993; **45:** 518–27.
2. International Rhinitis Management Working Group. International consensus report on the diagnosis and management of rhinitis. *Allergy* 1994; **49** (suppl 19): 1–34.
3. Scadding GK. Chronic non-infectious, non-allergic rhinitis. *Prescribers' J* 1996; **36:** 93–101.
4. Parikh A, Scadding GK. Seasonal allergic rhinitis. *BMJ* 1997; **314:** 1392–5.
5. Naclerio R, Soloman W. Rhinitis and inhalant allergens. *JAMA* 1997; **278:** 1842–8.
6. Durham S. Summer hay fever. *BMJ* 1998; **316:** 843–5.
7. Mackay IS, Durham SR. Perennial rhinitis. *BMJ* 1998; **316:** 917–20.
8. van Cauwenberge P, *et al.* Consensus statement on the treatment of allergic rhinitis. *Allergy* 2000; **55:** 116–34.
9. Bousquet J, *et al.* The management of allergic rhinitis symptoms in the pharmacy. Available at: http://www.whiar.com/pharmguide/pharm.pdf (accessed 05/05/04)


**Urticaria and angioedema**

Most patients with urticaria or angioedema (p.1138) derive some benefit from oral antihistamines, especially in relief of pruritus. However, patients who are severely affected, particularly those with laryngeal oedema, are allergic emergencies and require immediate treatment with adrenaline (see Anaphylactic Shock, p.855). Also, large doses of antihistamines are sometimes required and urticarias with a type I immunological origin and iatrogenic urticarias respond better than physical urticarias. If attacks of urticaria are frequent, antihistamines may be given prophylactically. Sedating antihistamines such as chlorphenamine and diphenhydramine have been widely used in the treatment of urticaria but non-sedating antihistamines are now generally preferred. Hydroxyzine has been used particularly in dermographism and cholinergic urticaria. Cyproheptadine has generally been considered the drug of choice for cold urticaria, although appetite stimulation may be a problem.

Some drugs with both $H_1$-antagonist and mast-cell stabilising actions, such as ketotifen, oxatomide, and azatadine have shown efficacy in the treatment of urticaria; the role of mast-cell stabilisation is unknown.

Topical treatment is rarely effective except for cases of mild urticaria; topical antihistamines carry a risk of sensitisation.

References.


1. Monroe EW. Chronic urticaria: review of nonsedating $H_1$ antihistamines in treatment. *J Am Acad Dermatol* 1988; **19:** 842–9.
2. Theoharides TC. Histamine$_2$ ($H_2$)-receptor antagonists in the treatment of urticaria. *Drugs* 1989; **37:** 345–55.
3. Advenier C, Queille-Roussel C. Rational use of antihistamines in allergic dermatological conditions. *Drugs* 1989; **38:** 634–44.
4. Mann KV, *et al.* Nonsedating histamine $H_1$-receptor antagonists. *Clin Pharm* 1989; **8:** 331–44.
5. Greaves MW, Sabroe RA. Allergy and the skin: urticaria. *BMJ* 1998; **316:** 1147–50.


**Vertigo**

Vertigo is a symptom of vestibular disorders. It is characterised by a sensation of rotation of the surroundings or of movement of static objects. Dizziness is considered to be a wider term, although some use it as a synonym for vertigo.

A variety of disorders may affect the vestibular system and produce vertigo, including cerebrovascular disorders, epilepsy, head injury, malignant neoplasms, Ménière's disease (above), migraine, multiple sclerosis, and infections. Motion sickness can induce vertigo. Ototoxic drugs may also cause vestibular damage and precipitate vertigo.

Patients suffering from vertigo should undergo thorough investigations to identify any underlying cause. Simple measures to improve the integration of sensory input from visual, proprioceptive, and vestibular receptors may prove effective, especially in the elderly, in whom the inappropriate prescribing of drugs for postural instability needs to be avoided. Such measures include improving visual acuity, balance exercises, and the use of walking aids.

The most widely used drugs for acute vertigo are the antihistamines. They may have a direct action on the inner ear besides acting centrally. Antimuscarinic actions may contribute to their activity; antimuscarinics, especially hyoscine, have a long history of use in vertigo. Antihistamines used in the treatment of vertigo include buclizine, cyclizine, dimenhydrinate, diphenhydramine, meclozine, and promethazine. Cinnarizine and flunarizine are also used for vertigo although they are devoid of any significant antimuscarinic actions; their activity may be due to calcium-channel blockade. Phenothiazines such as prochlorperazine are also used to control any associated vomiting. Benzodiazepines including diazepam have been given in acute severe attacks. However their prolonged use in those with chronic symptoms is of questionable value.

Vasodilators may be of benefit in the treatment of vertigo of vascular aetiology. Parenteral or sublingual histamine was formerly widely used, and betahistine is still advocated especially for vertigo associated with Ménière's disease. Nicotinyl alcohol has also been used.

References.


1. Rascol O, *et al.* Antivertigo medications and drug-induced vertigo: a pharmacological review. *Drugs* 1995; **50:** 777–91.
2. Luxon LM. Vertigo: new approaches to diagnosis and management. *Br J Hosp Med* 1996; **56:** 519–20 and 537–41.
3. Luxon LM. Assessment and management of vertigo. *Prescribers' J* 1998; **38:** 87–97.
4. Baloh RW. Vertigo. *Lancet* 1998; **352:** 1841–6.


## Acrivastine *(BAN, USAN, rINN)*

Acrivastina; BW-825C. (*E*)-3-{6-[(*E*)-3-Pyrrolidin-1-yl-1-*p*-tolylprop-1-enyl]-2-pyridyl}acrylic acid.

$C_{22}H_{24}N_2O_2$ = 348.4.

*CAS — 87848-99-5.*

*ATC — R06AX18.*

### Adverse Effects and Precautions

As for the non-sedating antihistamines in general, p.419. Acrivastine should be given with care in mild renal impairment and the UK manufacturer recommends it be avoided in those with a creatinine clearance of less than 50 mL/minute. The UK manufacturer also states that acrivastine should not be used in patients hypersensitive to triprolidine.

**Sedation.** For a discussion of the sedative effects of antihistamines see p.420.

### Interactions

As for the non-sedating antihistamines in general, p.421.

### Pharmacokinetics

Acrivastine is well absorbed from the gastrointestinal tract; peak plasma concentrations are achieved in about 1.5 hours. The plasma half-life of acrivastine is about 1.5 hours and the drug does not appear to cross the blood-brain barrier to a significant extent. Acrivastine along with an active metabolite is excreted principally in the urine.

### Uses and Administration

Acrivastine is a non-sedating antihistamine structurally related to triprolidine. It does not have any significant sedative or antimuscarinic actions. It is used for the symptomatic relief of allergic conditions such as rhinitis (p.422) and various types of urticaria (p.423) when it is given by mouth in doses of 8 mg three times daily. It is also used with a decongestant such as pseudoephedrine hydrochloride.

**Administration in renal impairment.** See Precautions, above

### Preparations

**Proprietary Preparations** (details are given in Part 3)

***Austria:*** Semprex; ***Denm.:*** Benadryl; Semprex†; ***Fin.:*** Semprex; ***Hong Kong:*** Semprex; ***Ital.:*** Semprex; ***Malaysia:*** Semprex; ***Neth.:*** Semprex; ***S.Afr.:*** Semprex; ***Singapore:*** Semprex; ***Swed.:*** Semprex; ***Switz.:*** Semprex; ***Thai.:*** Semprex; ***UK:*** Benadryl Allergy Relief; Semprex†.

**Multi-ingredient:** ***Austria:*** Duact; ***Denm.:*** Duact; ***Fin.:*** Duact; ***UK:*** Benadryl Plus; ***USA:*** Semprex-D.

## Alimemazine Tartrate *(BANM, rINNM)*

Tartrato de alimemazina; Trimeprazine Tartrate. *NN*-Dimethyl-2-methyl-3-(phenothiazin-10-yl)propylamine tartrate.

$(C_{18}H_{22}N_2S)_2,C_4H_6O_6$ = 747.0.

*CAS — 84-96-8 (alimemazine); 4330-99-8 (alimemazine tartrate).*

*ATC — R06AD01.*

**Pharmacopoeias.** In *Br., Fr., Jpn,* and *US.*

**BP 2003** (Alimemazine Tartrate). A white or slightly cream, odourless or almost odourless powder. It darkens on exposure to light. Freely soluble in water and in chloroform; sparingly soluble in alcohol; very slightly soluble in ether. A 2% solution in water has a pH of 5.0 to 6.5. Protect from light.

**USP 27** (Trimeprazine Tartrate). A white to off-white, odourless, crystalline powder. Soluble 1 in 2 of water, 1 in 20 of alcohol, 1 in 5 of chloroform, and 1 in 1800 of ether; very slightly soluble in benzene. Store in airtight containers. Protect from light.

### Adverse Effects and Precautions

As for the sedating antihistamines in general, p.419.

**Children.** There have been reports of adverse effects in children given alimemazine tartrate by mouth. Fatal malignant hyperthermia[1] and severe cardiovascular depression[2] have occurred after its use for premedication, and severe respiratory and CNS depression[3] after use as a postoperative sedative. Doses in these 3 reports ranged from 2.4 to 4.4 mg/kg. A possible association between phenothiazine sedatives and sudden infant death syndrome has also been suggested, but has not been confirmed (see Promethazine Hydrochloride, p.439). Alimemazine tartrate is no longer licensed in the UK for short-term sedation in children and it is recommended that it should not be used in infants less than 2 years of age. The maximum recommended dose for premedication for children aged 2 to 7 years is 2 mg/kg by mouth. There has been a warning[4] that the use of alimemazine for deep sedation in diagnostic and therapeutic procedures in children is associated with prolonged drowsiness and that standards of monitoring, starvation, and postprocedural care should be similar to those with general anaesthesia.

1. Moyes DG. Malignant hyperpyrexia caused by trimeprazine. *Br J Anaesth* 1973; **45:** 1163–4.
2. Loan WB, Cuthbert D. Adverse cardiovascular response to oral trimeprazine in children. *BMJ* 1985; **290:** 1548–9.
3. Mann NP. Trimeprazine and respiratory depression. *Arch Dis Child* 1981; **56:** 481–2.
4. Cray SH, Hinton W. Sedation for investigations: prolonged effect of chloral and trimeprazine. *Arch Dis Child* 1994; **71:** 179.

**Pregnancy.** For a discussion of the use of antihistamines in pregnancy, including studies involving phenothiazines, see p.420.

## Interactions

As for the sedating antihistamines in general, p.421.

## Uses and Administration

Alimemazine, a phenothiazine derivative, is a sedating antihistamine with antiemetic activity and pronounced sedative effects. It also has some antimuscarinic actions. It is used mainly for the relief of urticaria (p.423) and pruritus (p.422), and, in the UK, for pre-operative medication in children. Alimemazine may also be used in compound preparations for the symptomatic treatment of coughs (p.421).

Alimemazine tartrate is administered by mouth; doses in the UK are given as the amount of alimemazine tartrate; those in the USA are expressed in terms of the equivalent amount of alimemazine. Alimemazine tartrate 25 mg is approximately equivalent to 20 mg of alimemazine. Even allowing for this, lower doses are used in the USA.

- The adult dose of alimemazine tartrate used for the relief of **urticaria** and **pruritus** in the *UK* is 10 mg two or three times daily; up to 100 mg daily has been given in refractory cases. Elderly patients are given 10 mg once or twice daily and children over 2 years of age 2.5 to 5 mg three or four times daily.
- In the *USA* the adult dose is the equivalent of alimemazine 2.5 mg four times daily, or 5 mg twice daily as a modified-release preparation. Children in the USA between 2 and 3 years of age have been given 1.25 mg at night or three times daily; for older children this dose has been increased to 2.5 mg.
- The usual recommended dose in the UK for **premedication** in children aged 2 to 7 years is up to 2 mg/kg given by mouth about one to two hours before the operation.

**Anaesthesia.** Alimemazine tartrate may be used for anaesthetic premedication (see p.421) in children when the oral route of administration is preferred to the more usual parenteral route of other phenothiazine antihistamines. Adverse effects have, however, been reported in children (see under Adverse Effects and Precautions, above), and in the UK alimemazine tartrate is not licensed for use in infants less than 2 years of age.

**Insomnia.** Antihistamines such as alimemazine tartrate have been used as alternatives to benzodiazepines for the short-term treatment of insomnia (p.422), particularly for children. However, their antimuscarinic side-effects may prove troublesome.

Regimens involving a short course of alimemazine tartrate in high dosage were tried in order to alter the sleep pattern of children with sleeping difficulties.[1,2] Adverse effects have, however, been reported in children (see under Adverse Effects and Precautions, above). The UK product is no longer indicated for short-term sedation in children and should not be used in infants less than 2 years of age.

1. Valman HB. ABC of 1 to 7 (revised): sleep problems. *BMJ* 1987; **294:** 828–30.
2. Anonymous. What can be done for night waking in children? *Lancet* 1987; **ii:** 948–9.

## Preparations

***BP 2003:*** Alimemazine Tablets; Paediatric Alimemazine Oral Solution; Strong Paediatric Alimemazine Oral Solution;
***USP 27:*** Trimeprazine Tartrate Syrup; Trimeprazine Tartrate Tablets.

**Proprietary Preparations** (details are given in Part 3)
***Austral.:*** Chemists Own Peetalix; Vallergan; ***Belg.:*** Theralene; ***Canad.:*** Panectyl; ***Denm.:*** Vallergan†; ***Fr.:*** Theralene; ***Ger.:*** Repeltin; ***Hong Kong:*** Vallergan†; ***Irl.:*** Vallergan; ***Neth.:*** Nedeltran; ***Norw.:*** Vallergan; ***NZ:*** Vallergan; ***S.Afr.:*** Vallergan; ***Spain:*** Variargil; ***Swed.:*** Theralen; ***UK:*** Vallergan.

**Multi-ingredient:** ***Belg.:*** Theralene Pectoral†; ***Fr.:*** Theralene Pectoral Nourrisson; ***Singapore:*** Walekof†.

## Antazoline Hydrochloride *(BANM, rINNM)*

Antazolini Hydrochloridum; Antazolinium Chloride; Hidrocloruro de antazolina; Imidamine Hydrochloride; Phenazolinum. *N*-Benzyl-*N*-(2-imidazolin-2-ylmethyl)aniline hydrochloride.
$C_{17}H_{19}N_3,HCl = 301.8.$
*CAS — 91-75-8 (antazoline); 2508-72-7 (antazoline hydrochloride).*
*ATC — R01AC04; R06AX05.*

**Pharmacopoeias.** In *Chin., Eur.* (see p.vi), and *Pol.*

**Ph. Eur. 5.0** (Antazoline Hydrochloride). A white or almost white crystalline powder. Sparingly soluble in water; soluble in alcohol; slightly soluble in dichloromethane.

## Antazoline Mesilate *(BANM, rINNM)*

Antazoline Mesylate; Antazoline Methanesulphonate; Imidamine Mesylate; Mesilato de antazolina.
$C_{17}H_{19}N_3,CH_3SO_3H = 361.5.$
*CAS — 3131-32-6.*
*ATC — R01AC04; R06AX05.*

**Pharmacopoeias.** In *Pol.*

## Antazoline Phosphate *(BANM, rINNM)*

Fosfato de antazolina; Imidamine Phosphate.
$C_{17}H_{19}N_3,H_3PO_4 = 363.3.$
*CAS — 154-68-7.*
*ATC — R01AC04; R06AX05.*

**Pharmacopoeias.** In *US.*

**USP 27** (Antazoline Phosphate). A white to off-white crystalline powder. Soluble in water; practically insoluble in ether and in benzene; sparingly soluble in methyl alcohol. pH of a 2% solution in water is between 4.0 and 5.0. Store in airtight containers.

## Antazoline Sulfate *(rINNM)*

Antazoline Sulphate *(BANM)*; Imidamine Sulphate; Sulfato de antazolina.
$(C_{17}H_{19}N_3)_2H_2SO_4,2H_2O = 664.8.$
*CAS — 24359-81-7 (anhydrous antazoline sulfate).*
*ATC — R01AC04; R06AX05.*

NOTE. The above molecular formula is that provided in the *It. P.* Other sources give a molecular formula of $C_{17}H_{19}N_3,H_2SO_4$.

**Pharmacopoeias.** In *It.*

### Adverse Effects and Precautions

As for the antihistamines in general, p.419.

**Hypersensitivity.** Reports of acute interstitial pneumonitis (with fever, rash, and dyspnoea)[1] and of immune thrombocytopenic purpura[2] were attributed to hypersensitivity reactions following the oral administration of antazoline.

1. Pahissa A, *et al.* Antazoline-induced allergic pneumonitis. *BMJ* 1979; **2:** 1328.
2. Nielsen JL, *et al.* Immune thrombocytopenia due to antazoline (Antistina). *Allergy* 1981; **36:** 517–19.

### Uses and Administration

Antazoline, an ethylenediamine derivative, is an antihistamine used topically for the treatment of allergic conjunctivitis (p.421). It is used as the hydrochloride, phosphate, or sulfate in eye drops, most commonly in a concentration of 0.5%; the mesilate has also been used. Antazoline salts are often used with a vasoconstrictor such as naphazoline hydrochloride or nitrate or xylometazoline hydrochloride.

Antazoline hydrochloride has been used in a strength of up to 2% in a cream or ointment for the treatment of minor skin irritations, but as with other antihistamines there is a risk of sensitisation. The hydrochloride has also been given by mouth.

### Preparations

**Proprietary Preparations** (details are given in Part 3)
***Denm.:*** Antistina-Privin; ***Singapore:*** Antistin-Privin; ***UK:*** Wasp-Eze†.

**Multi-ingredient:** ***Austral.:*** Albalon-A; Allergy Eyes†; Antistine-Privine; In A Wink Allergy†; Murine Allergy†; ***Austria:*** Histophtal†; ***Belg.:*** Zincfrin Antihistaminicum; ***Braz.:*** Albassol†; Neo Vastrictol†; ***Canad.:*** Albalon-A; Cooper AR†; Ophtrivin-A†; Vasocon-A; Zincfrin-A; ***Chile:*** Albasol A; Bacitopic Compuesto; Nasomin; Oftalirio; Red Off Plus; Rinobanedif; Spersallerg; ***Denm.:*** Sesal; ***Fin.:*** Antistin-Privin; Zincfrin-A; ***Ger.:*** Allergopos N; Antistin-Privin; Ophtalmin†; Spersallerg; ***Hong Kong:*** Spersallerg; ***Irl.:*** Otrivine-Antistin; RBC; ***Israel:*** Antistin-Privin; ***Ital.:*** Antistin-Privina; Eubetal†; ***Malaysia:*** Alergoftal; Spersallerg; ***Mex.:*** Oftalirio; ***Norw.:*** Spersallerg; ***NZ:*** Albalon-A; Otrivine-Antistin; ***Port.:*** Alergiftalmina; ***S.Afr.:*** Albalon-A; Antistin-Privin; Covosan; Gemini; Safyr Bleu Antihistamine; Spersallerg; ***Singapore:*** Alergoftal†; Spersallerg; ***Spain:*** Alergoftal; ***Swed.:*** Antasten-Privin; ***Switz.:*** Antistin-Privin; Spersallerg; ***Thai.:*** Antazallerge; Histaoph; Opsa-His; Opsil-A; Spersallerg; ***UK:*** Modantis†; Otrivine-Antistin; ***USA:*** Antazoline-V; Vasocon-A.

## Astemizole *(BAN, USAN, rINN)*

Astemizol; Astemizolum; MJD-30. 1-(4-Fluorobenzyl)-2-{[1-(4-methoxyphenethyl)-4-piperidyl]amino}benzimidazole.
$C_{28}H_{31}FN_4O = 458.6.$
*CAS — 68844-77-9.*
*ATC — R06AX11.*

NOTE. The code R-43512 has been used to describe both astemizole and its metabolite tecastemizole (norastemizole).

**Pharmacopoeias.** In *Eur.* (see p.vi) and *US.*

**Ph. Eur. 5.0** (Astemizole). A white or almost white powder. Practically insoluble in water; soluble in alcohol; freely soluble in dichloromethane and in methyl alcohol. Protect from light.

**USP 27** (Astemizole). Store in airtight containers.

### Adverse Effects and Precautions

As for the non-sedating antihistamines in general, p.419. Increased appetite and weight gain have been reported with astemizole.

Ventricular arrhythmias, including torsade de pointes, have occurred rarely with astemizole, particularly in association with raised blood concentrations (see Arrhythmias below) and as a result the drug has been withdrawn from the market in most countries. To reduce the risk of developing such arrhythmias recommendations were that licensed doses should **not** be exceeded, and that it should be **avoided** in patients with cardiac or significant hepatic disease, with hypokalaemia or other electrolyte imbalance, or with known or suspected prolonged QT interval. The concomitant use of drugs liable to interfere with the hepatic metabolism of astemizole, of other potentially arrhythmogenic drugs including those that prolong the QT interval, and of drugs likely to cause electrolyte imbalance is **contra-indicated** (see under Interactions below).

**Arrhythmias.** Although severe life-threatening cardiovascular effects including torsade de pointes and other ventricular arrhythmias were initially reported mainly after substantial overdoses of astemizole, such reactions have also occurred rarely with doses as low as 20 to 30 mg daily and even as low as 10 mg daily in those with possible predisposing factors. There has been a report[1] of astemizole-induced torsade de pointes in a 15-year-old girl who claimed to have taken 10 mg daily for 10 weeks but pharmacokinetic data were more consistent with acute ingestion of higher doses. There have also been several reports of cardiotoxicity following accidental overdosage with astemizole in children.[2-4]

Although the drug is now withdrawn in the UK, recommendations were made by the UK Committee on Safety of Medicines to reduce the risk of developing serious arrhythmias[5-7] (see Adverse Effects above for details). It was considered that astemizole should be discontinued immediately in patients who experience syncope, and appropriate clinical evaluation including ECG monitoring instituted because syncope has preceded or accompanied severe arrhythmias in some cases. Convulsions in patients taking astemizole may also be related to cardiovascular effects.[8]

Studies have suggested that astemizole induces ventricular arrhythmias by inhibiting cardiac potassium channels which results in prolongation of the QT interval, a risk factor for developing arrhythmias.[9] For further discussion, see p.420.

1. Simons FER, *et al.* Astemizole-induced torsade de pointes. *Lancet* 1988; **ii:** 624.
2. Hoppu K, *et al.* Accidental astemizole overdose in young children. *Lancet* 1991; **338:** 538–40.
3. Tobin JR, *et al.* Astemizole-induced cardiac conduction disturbances in a child. *JAMA* 1991; **266:** 2737–40.
4. Wiley JF, *et al.* Cardiotoxic effects of astemizole overdose in children. *J Pediatr* 1992; **120:** 799–802.
5. Committee on Safety of Medicines. Ventricular arrhythmias due to terfenadine and astemizole. *Current Problems 35* 1992.
6. Committee on Safety of Medicines/Medicines Control Agency. Drug-induced prolongation of the QT interval. *Current Problems* 1996; **22:** 2.
7. Committee on Safety of Medicines/Medicines Control Agency. Astemizole (Hismanal): only available on prescription. *Current Problems* 1999; **25:** 2. Also available at: http://www.mca.gov.uk/ourwork/monitorsafequalmed/currentproblems/volume25feb.htm (accessed 08/04/04)
8. Clark A, Love H. Astemizole-induced ventricular arrhythmias: an unexpected cause of convulsions. *Int J Cardiol* 1991; **33:** 165–7.
9. Rankin AC. Non-sedating antihistamines and cardiac arrhythmia. *Lancet* 1997; **350:** 1115–16.

**Overdosage.** Severe cardiac events have been associated with astemizole overdosage (see under Arrhythmias, above); management is mainly supportive. The absorption of astemizole from the gastrointestinal tract can be prevented by administration of activated charcoal[1] but because astemizole is rapidly absorbed it would need to be given as soon as possible after poisoning. Haemodialysis does not appear to increase the clearance of astemizole.

1. Laine K, *et al.* The effect of activated charcoal on the absorption and elimination of astemizole. *Hum Exp Toxicol* 1994; **13:** 502–5.

**Porphyria.** Astemizole is considered to be unsafe in patients with porphyria because it has been shown to be porphyrinogenic in *in-vitro* systems.

**Sedation.** For discussion of the sedative effects of antihistamines see p.420.

### Interactions

As for the non-sedating antihistamines in general, p.421.

Astemizole should not be given with drugs that inhibit its hepatic metabolism because of the increased risk of serious ventricular arrhythmias. These drugs include the *imidazole and triazole antifungals* such as *ketoconazole* and *itraconazole*, and the macrolide antibacterials *clarithromycin, erythromycin, troleandomycin*, and possibly other *macrolides*. Others, similarly to terfenadine (p.441), may include *serotonin reuptake inhibitors, HIV-protease inhibitors, non-nucleoside reverse transcriptase inhibitor antiretrovirals*, and *zileuton*. The metabolism of astemizole may also be inhibited by *grapefruit juice* and concomitant use should be avoided.

Use with other potentially arrhythmogenic drugs (including those that prolong the QT interval) such as *antiarrhythmics, tricyclic antidepressants*, the antimalarials *halofantrine* and *quinine, antipsychotics, cisapride*, and the beta blocker *sotalol* should be avoided, as should co-administration of *diuretics* that cause electrolyte imbalances such as hypokalaemia. The use of *terfenadine* and astemizole together is not recommended.

### Pharmacokinetics

Absorption of astemizole from the gastrointestinal tract is rapid and is reduced by food. First-pass metabolism is extensive, therefore plasma concentrations of unchanged drug are very low. The plasma concentration of astemizole plus metabolites takes about 4 to 8 weeks to reach steady state. The metabolism of astemizole is mediated through the cytochrome P450 enzyme system by the isoenzymes CYP3A4, CYP2D6, and CYP2A6. The elimination half-life of astemizole and its metabolites at steady state is about 19 days. Unchanged astemizole is highly bound to plasma proteins and does not appear to cross the blood-brain barrier to a significant extent. Desmethylastemizole, the major metabolite of astemizole, has histamine $H_1$-receptor-blocking activity; tecastemizole (norastemizole) is another active metabolite. The metabolites of astemizole are excreted slowly in the urine and faeces, and undergo enterohepatic recycling. Virtually none of an oral dose is excreted as unchanged drug.

### Uses and Administration

Astemizole, a piperidine derivative, is a non-sedating antihistamine with a very long duration of action. It does not have significant sedative or antimuscarinic actions. Astemizole has been used for the symptomatic relief of allergic conditions including rhinitis (p.422) and conjunctivitis (p.421), and skin disorders such as urticaria (p.423). Preparations of astemizole have now been withdrawn from the market in most countries because of the risk of adverse effects.

Astemizole has been given by mouth in a dose of 10 mg once daily, or 5 mg daily in children aged 6 to 12 years. These doses must not be exceeded because of the risk of cardiac arrhythmias with higher doses.

The active metabolite of astemizole, tecastemizole (norastemizole) has been investigated for the treatment of allergic rhinitis.

### Preparations

**USP 27:** Astemizole Tablets.

**Proprietary Preparations** (details are given in Part 3)
***Arg.:*** Alermizol; Astezol; Cezane; Mudantil; Vagran; ***Braz.:*** Cilergil†; Hisnot†; Histabloc†; ***Gr.:*** Tulipe-R; Tyrenol; Waruzol; ***India:*** Stemiz; ***Ital.:*** Histamen†; ***Mex.:*** Alerfur; Alerken†; Aleztem; Antagon 1; Astemina; Astesen; Aztemin†; Aztil; Biostan; Dexodin; Emdar; Emizol†; Farmidal S†; Fustermizol; Ginomizol†; Henofin†; Histalino†; Histaser; Novasten; Practizol; Ulcoid-Zol; Urtigen; ***Port.:*** Perifer H1; ***Spain:*** Alermizol; Esmacen; Histaminos†; Hubermizol; Laridal†; Narvizol; Paralergin†; Retolen†; Rifedot; Rimbol†; Romadin†; Simprox; Urdrim; ***Thai.:*** Anhisnon†; Astahis†; Astem†; Astmazol†; Dayamin†; Hismacon†; Hismizol†; Hisno†; Histema†; Irene†; Tenon†; ***USA:*** Hismanal†.

**Multi-ingredient:** ***Arg.:*** Bio Cabal; Bronco Biotaer; Cor-Tagrip; Dallamizol-D; Dexaprof D; Doma Grip NF; Factor Antigripal; Gentiabron; Ideogrip; Muco Cortos; Mucoprednibron; Novo-Nastizol; Predual; Predual Descongestivo; Qura; Vagran Descongestivo; Wilpan C; ***Austria:*** Hismadrin†.

## Azatadine Maleate *(BANM, USAN, rINNM)*

Maleato de azatadina; Sch-10649. 6,11-Dihydro-11-(1-methyl-4-piperidylidene)-5*H*-benzo[5,6]cyclohepta[1,2-*b*]pyridine dimaleate.

$C_{20}H_{22}N_2,2C_4H_4O_4$ = 522.5.

*CAS — 3964-81-6 (azatadine); 3978-86-7 (azatadine maleate).*

*ATC — R06AX09.*

**Pharmacopoeias.** In *US.*

**USP 27** (Azatadine Maleate). A white to light cream-coloured, odourless powder. Freely soluble in water, in alcohol, in chloroform, and in methyl alcohol; practically insoluble in ether and in benzene.

### Adverse Effects and Precautions

As for the sedating antihistamines in general, p.419.

**Extrapyramidal effects.** An acute dystonic reaction was reported in a patient who had taken azatadine maleate 20 to 30 mg by mouth over a 24-hour period.[1] The condition was reversed by intravenous injection of benzatropine 2 mg.

1. Joske DJL. Dystonic reaction to azatadine. *Med J Aust* 1984; **141:** 449.

### Interactions

As for the sedating antihistamines in general, p.421.

### Pharmacokinetics

Azatadine maleate is readily absorbed from the gastrointestinal tract and is partly metabolised. Peak plasma concentrations are achieved in about 4 hours. The elimination half-life has been reported to be 9 to 12 hours. Excretion of unchanged drug and metabolites is via the urine.

### Uses and Administration

Azatadine maleate is a piperidine derivative closely related to cyproheptadine. It is a sedating antihistamine with a long duration of action; it also has antimuscarinic and antiserotonin properties.

Azatadine maleate is used for the symptomatic relief of allergic conditions including rhinitis (p.422) and urticaria (p.423); it is also used for other pruritic skin disorders as well as reactions to insect bites and stings. It is given by mouth, usually in doses of 1 mg twice daily; if necessary 2 mg twice daily may be given. Children aged 6 to 12 years may be given 0.5 to 1 mg twice daily.

### Preparations

**USP 27:** Azatadine Maleate Tablets.

**Proprietary Preparations** (details are given in Part 3)
***Austral.:*** Zadine; ***Belg.:*** Optimine†; ***Canad.:*** Optimine; ***Hong Kong:*** Zadine; ***Irl.:*** Optimine†; ***Malaysia:*** Zadine; ***Mex.:*** Idulamine; ***NZ:*** Zadine; ***S.Afr.:*** Optimine†; ***Singapore:*** Zadine; ***Spain:*** Lergocil; ***UK:*** Optimine†; ***USA:*** Optimine†.

**Multi-ingredient:** ***Braz.:*** Cedrin; ***Canad.:*** Trinalin; ***Mex.:*** Trinalin; ***Spain:*** Atiramin; Idulanex; ***USA:*** Rynatan; Trinalin.

## Azelastine Hydrochloride

*(BANM, USAN, rINNM)*

A-5610 (azelastine or azelastine hydrochloride); Azelastini Hydrochloridum; E-0659 (azelastine or azelastine hydrochloride); Hidrocloruro de azelastina; W-2979M (azelastine or azelastine hydrochloride). 4-(*p*-Chlorobenzyl)-2-(hexahydro-1-methyl-1*H*-azepin-4-yl)-1(2*H*)-phthalazinone monohydrochloride.

$C_{22}H_{24}ClN_3O,HCl$ = 418.4.

*CAS — 58581-89-8 (azelastine); 79307-93-0 (azelastine hydrochloride).*

*ATC — R01AC03; R06AX19; S01GX07.*

**Pharmacopoeias.** In *Eur.* (see p.vi).

**Ph. Eur. 5.0** (Azelastine Hydrochloride). A white or almost white, crystalline powder. Sparingly soluble in water; soluble in dehydrated alcohol and in dichloromethane.

### Adverse Effects and Precautions

As for the antihistamines in general, p.419.

When given intranasally, irritation of the nasal mucosa and taste disturbances have been reported; somnolence, headache, and dry mouth have also been noted in some patients. Taste disturbance can occur after use in the eye.

**Sedation.** For discussion of the sedative effects of antihistamines see p.420.

### Pharmacokinetics

About 40% of an intranasal dose of azelastine reaches the systemic circulation. Elimination is via hepatic metabolism with excretion mainly in the faeces.

◊ Azelastine is rapidly and almost completely absorbed after administration *by mouth*, peak plasma concentrations being achieved in 4 to 5 hours. Azelastine undergoes hepatic metabolism; the major metabolite, demethylazelastine, has antihistamine activity. The elimination half-life of azelastine is about 25 hours, increasing to 35.5 hours after multiple oral doses, possibly as a result of accumulation of the demethyl metabolite. Azelastine and its metabolites are excreted predominantly in the faeces and also in urine.

### Uses and Administration

Azelastine hydrochloride is an antihistamine that, in addition to its histamine $H_1$-receptor-blocking activity, appears to inhibit the release of inflammatory mediators from mast cells. It is used topically in the symptomatic relief of allergic conditions including rhinitis (p.422) and conjunctivitis (p.421). It is also used in the treatment of non-allergic (vasomotor) rhinitis.

In the treatment of allergic **rhinitis** in adults and children aged 5 years and over, the usual dose in the UK is 140 micrograms by nasal spray into each nostril twice daily. In the USA, however, 2 sprays of a similar preparation (supplying 137 micrograms per spray) may be given into each nostril twice daily; children aged 5 years and over may be given 1 spray into each nostril twice daily. In the USA, azelastine is also used in the treatment of non-allergic rhinitis in adults and children aged 12 years and over. The dose is 2 sprays into each nostril twice daily. In the treatment of **conjunctivitis**, azelastine is licensed in the UK for the treatment of seasonal allergic conjunctivitis in adults and children aged 4 years and over and for the treatment of perennial allergic conjunctivitis in adults and children aged 12 years and over. In the USA, it is licensed for the treatment of allergic conjunctivitis in adults and children aged 3 years and over. Regardless of the age and indication, a 0.05% solution is instilled into each eye twice daily; this may be increased to four times daily in severe conditions.

Azelastine hydrochloride has also been given by mouth.

◊ References.

1. Busse WW, *et al.* Corticosteroid-sparing effect of azelastine in the management of bronchial asthma. *Am J Respir Crit Care Med* 1996; **153:** 122–7 (oral).
2. Wober W, *et al.* Efficacy and tolerability of azelastine nasal spray in the treatment of allergic rhinitis: large scale experience in community practice. *Curr Med Res Opin* 1997; **13:** 617–26 (nasal).
3. McNeely W, Wiseman LR. Intranasal azelastine: a review of its efficacy in the management of allergic rhinitis. *Drugs* 1998; **56:** 91–114.
4. Lenhard G, *et al.* Double-blind, randomised, placebo-controlled study of two concentrations of azelastine eye drops in seasonal allergic conjunctivitis or rhinoconjunctivitis. *Curr Med Res Opin* 1997; **14:** 21–8.
5. Sabbah A, Marzetto M. Azelastine eye drops in the treatment of seasonal allergic conjunctivitis or rhinoconjunctivitis in young children. *Curr Med Res Opin* 1998; **14:** 161–70.
6. Duarte C, *et al.* Treatment of severe seasonal rhinoconjunctivitis by a combination of azelastine nasal spray and eye drops: a double-blind, double-placebo study. *J Investig Allergol Clin Immunol* 2001; **11:** 34–40.
7. Canonica GW, *et al.* Topical azelastine in perennial allergic conjunctivitis. *Curr Med Res Opin* 2003; **19:** 321–9.

### Preparations

**Proprietary Preparations** (details are given in Part 3)
***Arg.:*** Allergodil; Brixia; ***Austral.:*** Azep; ***Austria:*** Allergodil; Lasticom; Oculastin; ***Belg.:*** Allergodil; Otrivine Anti-Allergic; ***Braz.:*** Azelast; Rino-Azetin; Rino-Lastin; ***Chile:*** Allergodil; Az Ofteno; Brixia; ***Denm.:*** Allergodil; ***Fin.:*** Lastin; ***Fr.:*** Allergodil; ***Ger.:*** Allergodil; Loxin; Rhinolast†; ***Hong Kong:*** Azep; ***India:*** Azep; ***Irl.:*** Rhinolast; ***Israel:*** Optilast; Rhinolast; ***Ital.:*** Allergodil; Lasticom; ***Malaysia:*** Azep; ***Mex.:*** Astelin; Az; ***Neth.:*** Allergodil; ***Norw.:*** Lastin; ***NZ:*** Rhinolast†; ***Port.:*** Allergodil; Azep; ***S.Afr.:*** Rhinolast; ***Singapore:*** Azep; ***Spain:*** Afluon; Alferos†; Corifina; ***Swed.:*** Lastin; ***Switz.:*** Allergodil; ***Thai.:*** Azep; ***UK:*** Aller-Eze; Optilast; Rhinolast; ***USA:*** Astelin; Optivar.

## Bamipine *(BAN, rINN)*

Bamipina. *N*-Benzyl-*N*-(1-methyl-4-piperidyl)aniline.

$C_{19}H_{24}N_2$ = 280.4.

*CAS — 4945-47-5.*

*ATC — D04AA15; R06AX01.*

### Profile

Bamipine is a sedating antihistamine (p.419) with pronounced sedative effects.

Bamipine and its salts are used mainly for the symptomatic relief of allergic conditions such as urticaria (p.423) and in pruritic skin disorders. Bamipine hydrochloride has been given by mouth. Bamipine, bamipine lactate, and bamipine salicylate have all been applied topically.

### Preparations

**Proprietary Preparations** (details are given in Part 3)
***Austria:*** Soventol; ***Ger.:*** Soventol; ***Mex.:*** Soventol†.

**Multi-ingredient:** ***Austria:*** Multifungin; ***India:*** Multifungin; Multifungin H; Soventol.

## Bepotastine *(rINN)*

Bepotastina; TAU-284 (bepotastine besilate). (+)-4-{[(*S*)-*p*-Chloro-α-2-pyridylbenzyl]oxy}-1-piperidinebutyric acid.

$C_{21}H_{25}ClN_2O_3$ = 388.9.

*CAS — 125602-71-3.*

### Profile

Bepotastine is an antihistamine (p.419) used in the treatment of allergic rhinitis. It is also used for the symptomatic relief of urticaria and pruritic skin disorders.

### Preparations

**Proprietary Preparations** (details are given in Part 3)
***Jpn:*** Talion.

## Bromazine Hydrochloride *(BANM, rINNM)*

Bromodiphenhydramine Hydrochloride; Hidrocloruro de bromazina. 2-(4-Bromobenzhydryloxy)-*NN*-dimethylethylamine hydrochloride.

$C_{17}H_{20}BrNO,HCl$ = 370.7.

*CAS — 118-23-0 (bromazine); 1808-12-4 (bromazine hydrochloride).*

*ATC — R06AA01.*

**Pharmacopoeias.** In *US.*

**USP 27** (Bromodiphenhydramine Hydrochloride). A white to pale buff-coloured, crystalline powder having no more than a faint odour. Soluble 1 in less than 1 of water, 1 in 2 of alcohol and of chloroform, 1 in 3500 of ether, and 1 in 31 of isopropyl alcohol; insoluble in petroleum spirit. Store in airtight containers.

### Profile

Bromazine hydrochloride, a monoethanolamine derivative, is a sedating antihistamine (p.419) with antimuscarinic and marked sedative actions. It is used in combination preparations for the symptomatic treatment of coughs and the common cold (p.421) in a dose by mouth of 12.5 to 25 mg every 4 to 6 hours. The recommended maximum dose in such preparations is 150 mg daily. Children over 6 years of age may be given 6.25 to 12.5 mg every 6 hours.

**Preparations**

***USP 27:*** Bromodiphenhydramine Hydrochloride and Codeine Phosphate Oral Solution; Bromodiphenhydramine Hydrochloride Elixir.

**Proprietary Preparations** (details are given in Part 3)

**Multi-ingredient:** ***Canad.:*** Ambenyl†; ***USA:*** Ambenyl Cough Syrup; Amgenal Cough; Bromotuss with Codeine.

---

## Brompheniramine Maleate

*(BANM, rINNM)*

Brompheniramini Maleas; Maleato de bromfeniramina; Parabromdylamine Maleate. (±)-3-(4-Bromophenyl)-*NN*-dimethyl-3-(2-pyridyl)propylamine hydrogen maleate.

$C_{16}H_{19}BrN_2,C_4H_4O_4$ = 435.3.

*CAS — 86-22-6 (brompheniramine); 980-71-2 (brompheniramine maleate).*

*ATC — R06AB01.*

**Pharmacopoeias.** In *Eur.* (see p.vi) and *US.*

**Ph. Eur. 5.0** (Brompheniramine Maleate). A white or almost white, crystalline powder. Soluble in water; freely soluble in alcohol, in dichloromethane, and in methyl alcohol. A 1% solution in water has a pH of 4.0 to 5.0. Protect from light.

**USP 27** (Brompheniramine Maleate). A white, odourless, crystalline powder. Soluble 1 in 5 of water, 1 in 15 of alcohol and of chloroform; slightly soluble in ether and in benzene. pH of a 1% solution in water is between 4.0 and 5.0. Store in airtight containers. Protect from light.

**Incompatibility.** Brompheniramine maleate has been reported to be incompatible with some amidotrizoate, adipiodone, and iotalamate salts.

### Dexbrompheniramine Maleate *(BANM, rINNM)*

Maleato de dexbromfeniramina.

*CAS — 2391-03-9.*

*ATC — R06AB06.*

**Pharmacopoeias.** In *US.*

**USP 27** (Dexbrompheniramine Maleate). A white, odourless, crystalline powder. It exists in two polymorphic forms, one melting between 106° and 107°, and the other between 112° and 113°; a mixture of the two forms may melt between 105° and 113°. Soluble 1 in 1.2 of water, 1 in 2.5 of alcohol, 1 in 2 of chloroform, and 1 in 3000 of ether. pH of a 1% solution in water is about 5. Store in airtight containers. Protect from light.

### Adverse Effects and Precautions

As for the sedating antihistamines in general, p.419.

**Breast feeding.** The American Academy of Pediatrics[1] states that, although usually compatible with breast feeding, preparations used by breast-feeding mothers which contain dexbrompheniramine maleate with pseudoephedrine have resulted in crying, irritability, and poor sleep patterns in the infant.

1. American Academy of Pediatrics. The transfer of drugs and other chemicals into human milk. *Pediatrics* 2001; **108:** 776–89. Correction. *ibid.*; 1029. Also available at: http://aappolicy.aappublications.org/cgi/content/full/pediatrics%3b108/3/776 (accessed 08/04/04)

**Effects on the blood.** A report[1] that agranulocytosis in a 34-year-old alcoholic man was possibly associated with brompheniramine therapy.

1. Hardin AS, Padilla F. Agranulocytosis during therapy with a brompheniramine-medication. *J Arkansas Med Soc* 1978; **75:** 206–8.

**Extrapyramidal disorders.** Facial dyskinesias have been reported[1,2] after administration of antihistamines including brompheniramine or dexbrompheniramine maleate.

1. Thach BT, *et al.* Oral facial dyskinesia associated with prolonged use of antihistaminic decongestants. *N Engl J Med* 1975; **293:** 486–7 (brompheniramine maleate, chlorpheniramine maleate, and phenindamine tartrate).
2. Barone DA, Raniolo J. Facial dyskinesia from overdose of an antihistamine. *N Engl J Med* 1980; **303:** 107 (dexbrompheniramine maleate).

**Withdrawal.** Withdrawal symptoms have been reported[1] following discontinuation of long-term therapy with brompheniramine maleate. A patient had been taking 48 mg almost every day for 20 years and developed tremor, nausea, depression, and apyrexial sweating within 48 hours of stopping treatment; symptoms resolved over the following weeks.

1. Kavanagh GM, *et al.* Withdrawal symptoms after discontinuation of long-acting brompheniramine maleate. *Br J Dermatol* 1994; **131:** 913–14.

### Interactions

As for the sedating antihistamines in general, p.421.

### Pharmacokinetics

After oral administration brompheniramine maleate appears to be well absorbed from the gastrointestinal tract. Peak plasma concentrations are achieved within about 5 hours. An elimination half-life of about 25 hours has been reported. Unchanged drug and metabolites are excreted primarily in the urine.

◊ References.

1. Simons FER, *et al.* The pharmacokinetics and antihistaminic effects of brompheniramine. *J Allergy Clin Immunol* 1982; **70:** 458–64.
2. Paton DM, Webster DR. Clinical pharmacokinetics of $H_1$-receptor antagonists (the antihistamines). *Clin Pharmacokinet* 1985; **10:** 477–97.

### Uses and Administration

Brompheniramine maleate, an alkylamine derivative, is a sedating antihistamine with antimuscarinic and moderate sedative actions.

Brompheniramine is a racemic mixture; dexbrompheniramine, the dextrorotatory isomer, has approximately twice the activity of brompheniramine by weight. Brompheniramine maleate and dexbrompheniramine maleate are used for the symptomatic relief of allergic conditions, mainly rhinitis (p.422) and conjunctivitis (p.421). They are common ingredients of compound preparations for the symptomatic treatment of coughs and the common cold (p.421).

*Brompheniramine maleate* is given by mouth usually in doses of 4 to 8 mg three or four times daily. Children up to 3 years of age are given 0.4 to 1 mg/kg over 24 hours in four divided doses. Children aged 3 to 6 years are given 1 to 2 mg three or four times daily and those aged 6 to 12 years 2 to 4 mg three or four times daily.

Brompheniramine maleate has also been given by subcutaneous, intramuscular, or slow intravenous injection; the dose is usually 10 mg every 8 to 12 hours as necessary and the total parenteral dose should not exceed 40 mg in 24 hours.

*Dexbrompheniramine maleate* is normally given as an ingredient of decongestant preparations containing pseudoephedrine. The dose of dexbrompheniramine maleate by mouth in these combinations is 2 mg up to four times daily. Children over 6 years can be given 1 mg up to four times a day.

*Modified-release* oral preparations of brompheniramine maleate or dexbrompheniramine maleate are available in some countries; dosage is specific to a particular formulation.

### Preparations

***BP 2003:*** Brompheniramine Tablets;
***USP 27:*** Brompheniramine Maleate Elixir; Brompheniramine Maleate Injection; Brompheniramine Maleate Tablets; Dexbrompheniramine Maleate and Pseudoephedrine Sulfate Oral Solution.

**Proprietary Preparations** (details are given in Part 3)
***Canad.:*** Dimetane†; ***Fr.:*** Dimegan; ***Ger.:*** Dimegan†; ***Irl.:*** Dimotane†; ***Malaysia:*** Bomex; ***Singapore:*** Bomex; Neo-Meton†; ***Thai.:*** Dimetane; ***UK:*** Dimotane; ***USA:*** Dimetane; Lodrane 12; Oraminic II.

**Multi-ingredient:** ***Arg.:*** Factus; ***Austral.:*** Dimetapp; Dimetapp DM; ***Austria:*** Disophrol†; ***Belg.:*** Nasapert†; Rinafort†; ***Braz.:*** Bialerge; Decongex Plus; Decongex Plus Expectorante; Dimetapp; Dimetapp Expectorante†; Disofrol†; Migral†; Winter AP; ***Canad.:*** Centracol†; Cold & Allergy Relief†; Cold & Allergy†; Cough, Cold & Allergy Relief†; Decongestant Antihistaminic Syrup†; Dimetane Expectorant C; Dimetane Expectorant DC; Dimetane Expectorant†; Dimetapp Chewables†; Dimetapp Clear†; Dimetapp Cold; Dimetapp Cough & Cold Liqui-Gels†; Dimetapp DM; Dimetapp Liqui-Gels†; Dimetapp Oral Infant Drops; Dimetapp Quick Dissolve†; Dimetapp-C; Dimetapp†; Drixoral; Drixoral Day/Night; Drixtab†; Pharmetapp†; Tantapp†; ***Chile:*** Disofrin; ***Fin.:*** Dimetane Expect DC†; Dimetane Expect†; Disofrol; Lunerin†; ***Fr.:*** Dimetane; Dimetane Expectorant Enfant; Martigene; Rupton Chronules†; Sebrane Rhume†; ***Ger.:*** Ilvico N†; ***Gr.:*** Dimetapp New; ***Hong Kong:*** Brom-PP; Brom-Ramine Compound; Bromhexine Compound; Bromphenex; DF Multi-Symptom; Dimaxin; Dime-Time†; Dimetapp; Disobrom†; Drixoral; ENT; Neosed†; Vidatapp; ***Irl.:*** Dimotane Co; Dimotane Expectorant†; Dimotapp†; Ilvico†; ***Malaysia:*** Drixoral; Rinafort; ***Mex.:*** Afrinex; Dimetapp; ***NZ:*** Dimetapp; Dimetapp DM Cold & Cough; ***Port.:*** Constipal; Ilvico N†; ***S.Afr.:*** Dimetapp; Ilvico; ***Singapore:*** Bromanate†; Dimetapp; Drixoral; Rinafort; ***Spain:*** Disofrol; Ilvico; ***Swed.:*** Disofrol; Lunerin†; ***Switz.:*** Dimetapp†; Disofrol; Rupton Chronules; ***Thai.:*** AA Cold†; Aorinyl†; Asiatapp; Bepeno; Bepeno-G; Bluco; Bromavon†; Bromesep Elixir†; Bromesep Expectorant†; Bromped†; Bromtussia; Bromtussia DC; Bromtussin†; Centapp; Coldate†; Daminate; Dimetane Expectorant DC†; Dimetane Expectorant†; Dimetapp; Medimegen†; Meditapp; Meditapp Expectorant; Minra; Nartap; Nasorest; Nasosil†; Polydine; Postap; Postap Expectorant; Rhinadine; Rhinophen-C; Rupton†; Stobcon†; ***UK:*** Dimotane Co; Dimotane Expectorant; Dimotane Plus; Dimotapp†; Robitussin Night-Time†; ***USA:*** 12 Hour Antihistamine Nasal Decongestant; 12 Hour Cold; Accuhist; Accuhist DM Pediatric; Accuhist PDX; Alacol DM; Alka-Seltzer Plus Night-Time Cold†; Alka-Seltzer Plus Sinus Allergy†; Allent; Anaplex DM; Anaplex HD; Andehist; Andehist DM; Brofed; Bromadine-DM; Bromaline Plus†; Bromaline†; Bromanate†; Bromarest DX; Bromatane DX; Bromatapp†; Bromfed; Bromfed-DM; Bromfed-PD; Bromfenex; Bromhist; Bromhist-DM; Bromophen TD†; Bromphen DX Cough; Brompheniramine Cough; Brompheniramine DC Cough†; Carbodex DM; Coldec DM; Dexaphen-SA; Dimaphen†; Dimetane DC†; Dimetane Decongestant; Dimetane DX†; Dimetapp; Dimetapp Cold & Allergy Chewable†; Dimetapp Cold & Fever; Dimetapp Cold & Flu†; Dimetapp DM; Dimetapp Nighttime Flu; Disobrom; Disophrol; Dristan Allergy; Dristan Cold Maximum Strength Multi-symptom Formula; Drixomed; Drixoral; Drixoral Cold & Allergy; Drixoral Cold & Flu; Drixoral Plus; Drocon-CS; Endafed; Histine DM†; Histinex DM†; Iofed; Iohist DM†; Liqui-Histine DM†; Lodrane; Lodrane 12D; Lortuss DM; Maximum Strength Dristan Cold; Myphetane DC†; Myphetane DX; Poly-Histine CS†; Poly-Histine DM†; Respahist; Rondamine-DM; Rondec; Sildec-DM; Siltapp†; Sinadrin Plus; Tamine SR†; Touro A & H; Touro Allergy; Trihist-CS†; Trihist-DM†; ULTRAbrom; Vicks DayQuil Allergy Relief†.

---

## Buclizine Hydrochloride *(BANM, USAN, rINNM)*

Hidrocloruro de buclizina; NSC-25141; UCB-4445. (*RS*)1-(4-*tert*-Butylbenzyl)-4-(4-chlorobenzhydryl)piperazine dihydrochloride.

$C_{28}H_{33}ClN_2,2HCl$ = 505.9.

*CAS — 82-95-1 (buclizine); 129-74-8 (buclizine hydrochloride).*

*ATC — R06AE01.*

**Pharmacopoeias.** In *Br.*

**BP 2003** (Buclizine Hydrochloride). A white or slightly yellowish, crystalline powder. Practically insoluble in water; very slightly soluble in alcohol; sparingly soluble in chloroform and in propylene glycol.

### Adverse Effects and Precautions

As for the sedating antihistamines in general, p.419.

### Interactions

As for the sedating antihistamines in general, p.421.

### Uses and Administration

Buclizine hydrochloride, a piperazine derivative, is a sedating antihistamine with antimuscarinic and moderate sedative actions. It is used mainly for its antiemetic action, particularly in the prevention of motion sickness (p.422) and in the treatment of migraine in combination with analgesics (p.464). In some countries it is given in the management of allergic conditions and in pruritic skin disorders (p.422). Buclizine has also been used in the treatment of vertigo (p.423) associated with disorders of the vestibular system, although its value in these conditions remains to be established.

To prevent motion sickness, buclizine hydrochloride is given at least 30 minutes before travelling in a dose of 25 or 50 mg by mouth, which may be repeated, if necessary, after 4 to 6 hours. The usual dose to alleviate nausea is 25 or 50 mg daily up to a maximum of 100 mg daily.

In the treatment of migraine, buclizine hydrochloride is given in usual doses of 12.5 mg at the start of an attack or when one is known to be imminent.

In pruritic skin disorders the usual dose of buclizine hydrochloride is 25 to 50 mg daily.

### Preparations

**Proprietary Preparations** (details are given in Part 3)
***Belg.:*** Longifene; ***Braz.:*** Buclina; Postafen; ***Fr.:*** Aphilan; ***Hong Kong:*** Longifene; ***Malaysia:*** Buchzine; Longifene; Longimin; ***Mex.:*** Postavit-B†; ***Port.:*** Buclina; Postafeno; ***S.Afr.:*** Longifene; ***Singapore:*** Longifene; Panzimine; ***USA:*** Bucladin-S Softab.

**Multi-ingredient:** ***Braz.:*** Apetibe; Apetil; Buclamin; Bucliamin†; Buclifen-Vit†; Bucliplex; Buclitina†; Carnabol; Carnizin†; Complevit†; Kelavitam†; Klizin; Lisinvitan†; Nutri-Ped; Nutrimaiz SM; Pepsivit; Pondusvitam; Profol; Propan; Stin†; Useton†; Vitaler; Vitalisin†; Vitamil†; ***Ger.:*** Migralave N; ***Hong Kong:*** Propan†; ***Irl.:*** Migraleve; ***Israel:*** Migraleve; ***Port.:*** Migraleve; ***S.Afr.:*** Vomifene; ***Singapore:*** Migraleve†; ***Spain:*** Migraleve; ***Switz.:*** Hexafene†; Migraleve; ***UK:*** Migraleve.

---

## Carbinoxamine Maleate *(BANM, rINNM)*

Maleato de carbinoxamina. 2-[4-Chloro-α-(2-pyridyl)benzyloxy]-*NN*-dimethylethylamine hydrogen maleate.

$C_{16}H_{19}ClN_2O,C_4H_4O_4$ = 406.9.

*CAS — 486-16-8 (carbinoxamine); 3505-38-2 (carbinoxamine maleate).*

*ATC — R06AA08.*

**Pharmacopoeias.** In *US.*

**USP 27** (Carbinoxamine Maleate). A white, odourless, crystalline powder. Soluble 1 in less than 1 of water, 1 in 1.5 of alcohol and of chloroform, and 1 in 8300 of ether. pH of a 1% solution in water is between 4.6 and 5.1. Store in airtight containers. Protect from light.

### Adverse Effects and Precautions

As for the sedating antihistamines in general, p.419.

### Interactions

As for the sedating antihistamines in general, p.421.

### Uses and Administration

Carbinoxamine maleate, a monoethanolamine derivative, is a sedating antihistamine with antimuscarinic, significant sedative, and serotonin antagonist effects. Carbinoxamine maleate is used for the relief of allergic conditions such as rhinitis (p.422), and is a common ingredient of compound preparations for symptomatic treatment of coughs and the common cold (p.421).

The usual dose of carbinoxamine maleate by mouth in adults and children aged 6 and over, used alone or in combination preparations, ranges from 4 to 16 mg daily in divided doses. Younger children may be given half the adult dose. Carbinoxamine polistirex has also been given by mouth.

**Preparations**

**USP 27:** Carbinoxamine Maleate Tablets; Pseudoephedrine Hydrochloride, Carbinoxamine Maleate, and Dextromethorphan Hydrobromide Oral Solution.

**Proprietary Preparations** (details are given in Part 3)
***Arg.:*** Omega 100; ***Fr.:*** Allergefon; ***Ger.:*** Polistin Pad†; Polistin T-Caps†; ***Thai.:*** Histin; Sinumine; ***USA:*** Carboxine; Histex CT; Histex PD; Pediatex.

**Multi-ingredient: *Arg.:*** Aseptobron C; Cobenzil Compuesto; Rondec; Rondec Compositum; Torfan H; ***Austria:*** Capramin†; Co-Tylenol†; Rhinopront; ***Belg.:*** Rhinopront; ***Braz.:*** Afebrin; Coficold-Ped†; Fluviral†; Gegrip; Gripenil†; Iodeto de Potassio Composto; Naldecon; Naldecon Pediatrico; Resprin; Xarope de Iodeto de Potassio Composto†; ***Chile:*** Rhinopront; Rinofrim; ***Fin.:*** Tinaroc-Combi†; ***Fr.:*** Humex†; ***Ger.:*** Rhinopront; Rhinotussal; ***Hong Kong:*** Coritussal; Metoplex; Rhinopront; ***India:*** Clistin; ***Israel:*** Rhinovis; ***Ital.:*** Rondec†; Torfan†; ***Malaysia:*** Became; Rhinopront; ***Mex.:*** Prindex; ***Singapore:*** Became; Coritussal†; Metussa†; Rhinopront; ***Spain:*** Rhinocap; Rinomax; Rinoretard†; Rondec†; Toscal Compuesto†; Toscal†; ***Switz.:*** Rhinopront; Rhinotussal; ***Thai.:*** Nasalgen†; Rhinar; Rhinohist; Rhinopront; Rhinotussal†; Rondec-DM; ***UAE:*** Fluzal†; ***USA:*** Andehist; Andehist DM; Carbinoxamine Compound; Carbiset; Carbodec; Carbodec DM; Carbodex DM; Carboxine-PSE; Cardec DM†; Cardec-S†; Coldec D; Cydec; Cydec DM; Decahist-DM; DMax; Histex HC; Palgic DS; Palgic-D; Pediatex-D; Pediatex-DM; Pseudo-Car DM; Rondec; Rondec-DM; Sildec-DM; Tussafed.

## Cetirizine Hydrochloride

*(BANM, USAN, rINNM)*

Cetirizini Dihydrochloridum; Hidrocloruro de cetirizina; P-071; UCB-P071. The dihydrochloride of 2-[4-(4-chlorobenzhydryl)piperazin-1-yl]ethoxyacetic acid.

$C_{21}H_{25}ClN_2O_3,2HCl = 461.8.$

*CAS — 83881-51-0 (cetirizine); 83881-52-1 (cetirizine hydrochloride).*

*ATC — R06AE07.*

**Pharmacopoeias.** In *Eur.* (see p.vi).

**Ph. Eur. 5.0** (Cetirizine Dihydrochloride; Cetirizine Hydrochloride BP 2003). A white or almost white powder. Freely soluble in water; practically insoluble in acetone and in dichloromethane. A 5% solution in water has a pH of 1.2 to 1.8. Protect from light.

### Adverse Effects and Precautions

As for the non-sedating antihistamines in general, p.419. Reduced dosage is recommended for patients with hepatic or renal impairment (see under Uses and Administration, below).

**Arrhythmias.** The ECG effects of cetirizine were studied[1] in normal subjects and administration of doses of up to six times the usual recommended dose did not prolong the QT interval. Additionally, workers from the FDA[2] in the USA and representatives of the manufacturers[3] in Belgium have not found any association so far between cetirizine and the development of ventricular arrhythmias. See also p.420.

1. Sale ME, *et al.* The electrocardiographic effects of cetirizine in normal subjects. *Clin Pharmacol Ther* 1994; **56:** 295–301.
2. Himmel MH, *et al.* Dangers of non-sedating antihistamines. *Lancet* 1997; **350:** 69.
3. Coulie P, *et al.* Non-sedating antihistamines and cardiac arrhythmias. *Lancet* 1998; **351:** 451.

**Effects on the liver.** Life-threatening hepatitis developed in a 23-year-old man who had been taking cetirizine long-term for atopic dermatitis.[1] He recovered following treatment with prednisolone.

1. Watanabe M, *et al.* Severe hepatitis in a patient taking cetirizine. *Ann Intern Med* 2001; **135:** 142–3.

**Hypersensitivity.** Hypersensitivity reactions manifest as urticaria[1,2] and fixed drug eruptions[3] have been reported with cetirizine.

1. Karamfilov T, *et al.* Cetirizine-induced urticarial reaction. *Br J Dermatol* 1999; **140:** 979–80.
2. Calista D, *et al.* Urticaria induced by cetirizine. *Br J Dermatol* 2001; **144:** 196.
3. Inamadar AC, *et al.* Multiple fixed drug eruptions due to cetirizine. *Br J Dermatol* 2002; **147:** 1025–6.

**Sedation.** For discussion of the sedative effects of antihistamines see p.420.

### Interactions

As for the non-sedating antihistamines in general, p.421. However, some interactions are less likely with cetirizine than with non-sedating antihistamines such as astemizole and terfenadine, since cetirizine appears to have low hepatic metabolism and little arrhythmogenic potential (see Arrhythmias, above).

**Anticoagulants.** For a report of an interaction between cetirizine and acenocoumarol, see under Interactions in Warfarin, p.1025.

### Pharmacokinetics

Cetirizine is rapidly absorbed from the gastrointestinal tract after oral administration, peak plasma concentrations being attained within about one hour. Food delays the time to peak plasma concentrations but does not decrease the amount of drug absorbed. It is highly bound to plasma proteins and has an elimination half-life of about 10 hours. Cetirizine has been detected in breast milk. Cetirizine is excreted primarily in the urine mainly as unchanged drug. Cetirizine does not appear to cross the blood-brain barrier to a significant extent.

◊ References.

1. Awni WM, *et al.* Effect of haemodialysis on the pharmacokinetics of cetirizine. *Eur J Clin Pharmacol* 1990; **38:** 67–9.
2. Desager JP, *et al.* A pharmacokinetic evaluation of the second-generation $H_1$-receptor antagonist cetirizine in very young children. *Clin Pharmacol Ther* 1993; **53:** 431–5.

### Uses and Administration

Cetirizine hydrochloride, a piperazine derivative and metabolite of hydroxyzine (p.434), is described as a non-sedating antihistamine which is long-acting and has some mast-cell stabilising activity. It appears to have a low potential for drowsiness in usual doses and to be virtually free of antimuscarinic activity. It is used for the symptomatic relief of allergic conditions including rhinitis (p.422) and chronic urticaria (p.423).

In adults and children aged 6 years and over, cetirizine hydrochloride is given by mouth in a dose of 10 mg once daily or 5 mg twice daily. Children aged 2 to 5 years may be given cetirizine 5 mg once daily or 2.5 mg twice daily. In the USA, children aged 6 months to 2 years may be given a dose of 2.5 mg once daily, increased to a maximum of 2.5 mg twice daily in those aged 12 months and over, for the treatment of perennial allergic rhinitis and chronic urticaria.

It is also used with a decongestant such as pseudoephedrine hydrochloride.

Dosage of cetirizine should be reduced in patients with hepatic or renal impairment, see below.

◊ References.

1. Spencer CM, *et al.* Cetirizine: a reappraisal of its pharmacological properties and therapeutic use in selected allergic disorders. *Drugs* 1993; **46:** 1055–80.
2. Barnes CL, *et al.* Cetirizine: a new, nonsedating antihistamine. *Ann Pharmacother* 1993; **27:** 464–70.
3. Breneman D, *et al.* Cetirizine and astemizole therapy for chronic idiopathic urticaria: a double-blind placebo-controlled, comparative trial. *J Am Acad Dermatol* 1995; **33:** 192–8.
4. Breneman DL. Cetirizine versus hydroxyzine and placebo in chronic idiopathic urticaria. *Ann Pharmacother* 1996; **30:** 1075–9.
5. Anonymous. Cetirizine—a new antihistamine. *Med Lett Drugs Ther* 1996; **38:** 21–3.

**Administration in hepatic or renal impairment.** In patients with hepatic impairment, the US manufacturers recommend that the dosage of cetirizine may need to be reduced to half the usual daily dose. Similarly in patients with renal impairment, both the UK and US manufacturers recommend a dosage reduction to half the usual daily dose.

### Preparations

**Proprietary Preparations** (details are given in Part 3)
***Arg.:*** Cabal; Cetriler; Salvalerg; Stopaler; Zyrtec; ***Austral.:*** Zyrtec; ***Austria:*** Alerid; Rigix; Virlix; Zirtek; Zyrtec; ***Belg.:*** Zyrtec; ***Braz.:*** Aletir; Cetrizin; Zetalerg; Zetir; Zinetrin; Zyrtec; ***Canad.:*** Allergy Relief; Reactine; Zyrtec†; ***Chile:*** Alertop; Coolips; Findaler; Histalen; Histax; Remitex; Rigotax; Sanaler; Zyrtec; ***Denm.:*** Alnok; Benaday; Zyrtec; ***Fin.:*** Zyrtec; ***Fr.:*** Virlix; Zyrtec; ***Ger.:*** Alerid; Ceti; Cetidura; Cetirlan; Zetir; Zyrtec; ***Gr.:*** Agelmin; Alenstran; Blezamont; Cetiram; Gentiran; Histafren; Telarix; Zepholin; Zirtek; Znupril; ***Hong Kong:*** Zyrtec; ***India:*** Alerid; Cetriwal; Cetrizet; Zyrtec; ***Irl.:*** Zirpine; Zirtek; Zynor; ***Israel:*** Histazine; Zyllergy; Zyrtec†; ***Ital.:*** Formistin; Virlix; Zirtec; ***Jpn:*** Zyrtec; ***Malaysia:*** Adezio; Simtec; Zyrtec; ***Mex.:*** Virlix; Zyrtec; ***Neth.:*** Zyrtec; ***Norw.:*** Reactine; Virlix; Zyrtec; ***NZ:*** Razene; Zyrtec; ***Port.:*** Virlix; Zyrtec; ***S.Afr.:*** Zyrtec; ***Singapore:*** Zyrtec; ***Spain:*** Alerlisin; Virlix; Voltric; Zyrtec; ***Swed.:*** Zyrlex; ***Switz.:*** Zyrtec; ***Thai.:*** Cetihis; Cetrimed; Cetrine; Cetrizet; Cetrizin; Cistamine; Cyzine; Fatec; Histica; Incidal-OD; Sutac; Terzine; Triz; Zensil; Zermed; Zertine; Zyrazine; Zyrcon; Zyrex; Zyrtec; Zyrzine†; Zytine†; ***UAE:*** Cetralon; ***UK:*** AllerTek; Benadryl Allergy Oral Solution; Benadryl One A Day; Cetirocol†; Hayfever & Allergy Relief; Hayfever Relief; Piriteze; Zirtek; ***USA:*** Zyrtec.

**Multi-ingredient: *Arg.:*** Cetriler D; Zyrtec-D; ***Austria:*** Cirrus; ***Belg.:*** Cirrus; ***Braz.:*** Zetir-D†; Zyrtec-D; ***Canad.:*** Reactine Plus†; ***Chile:*** Findaler-D; Remitex D; Sanaler-D; Zyrtec-D; ***Fin.:*** Cirrus; ***Hong Kong:*** Cirrus; ***Ital.:*** Naristar; Pronose; ***Malaysia:*** Cirrus; ***Mex.:*** Virlix-D; Zyrtec-D; ***NZ:*** Zyrtec Decongestant; ***Singapore:*** Cirrus; ***Spain:*** Naristar; Stopcold; ***USA:*** Zyrtec-D.

## Chlorcyclizine Hydrochloride *(BANM, rINNM)*

Chlorcyclizini Hydrochloridum; Chlorcyclizinium Chloride; Hidrocloruro de clorciclizina. 1-(4-Chlorobenzhydryl)-4-methylpiperazine hydrochloride.

$C_{18}H_{21}ClN_2,HCl = 337.3.$

*CAS — 82-93-9 (chlorcyclizine); 1620-21-9 (chlorcyclizine hydrochloride).*

*ATC — R06AE04.*

**Pharmacopoeias.** In *Eur.* (see p.vi).

**Ph. Eur. 5.0** (Chlorcyclizine Hydrochloride). A white, crystalline powder. Freely soluble in water and in dichloromethane; soluble in alcohol. A 1% solution in water has a pH of 5.0 to 6.0. Protect from light.

### Profile

Chlorcyclizine hydrochloride, a piperazine derivative, is a sedating antihistamine (p.419). It is given by mouth in doses of 50 to 100 mg once or twice daily for the symptomatic relief of hypersensitivity reactions; it is also used as an antiemetic. It has been used in topical preparations, although as with other antihistamines, there is a risk of sensitisation.

Chlorcyclizine dibunate (naftoclizine) has been used as a cough suppressant similarly to sodium dibunate (p.1130).

### Preparations

**Proprietary Preparations** (details are given in Part 3)
***Denm.:*** Trihistan; ***Norw.:*** Trihistan.

**Multi-ingredient: *Fin.:*** Anervan; ***Israel:*** Temigran; ***Neth.:*** Primatour; ***Norw.:*** Anervan; ***Spain:*** Diminex Antitusigeno; Diminex Balsamico†; ***Swed.:*** Anervan; Exolyt.

## Chloropyramine Hydrochloride *(BANM, rINNM)*

Halopyramine Hydrochloride; Hidrocloruro de cloropiramina. *N*-(4-Chlorobenzyl)-*N′N′*-dimethyl-*N*-(2-pyridyl)ethylenediamine hydrochloride.

$C_{16}H_{20}ClN_3,HCl = 326.3.$

*CAS — 59-32-5 (chloropyramine); 6170-42-9 (chloropyramine hydrochloride).*

*ATC — D04AA09; R06AC03.*

### Profile

Chloropyramine hydrochloride, an ethylenediamine derivative, is an antihistamine (p.419). It has been given by mouth and by injection.

### Preparations

**Proprietary Preparations** (details are given in Part 3)
***Hung.:*** Suprastin; ***Mex.:*** Avapena.

## Chlorphenamine Maleate *(BANM, rINNM)*

Chlorphenamini Maleas; Chlorpheniramine Maleate; Chlorprophenpyridamine Maleate; Maleato de clorfenamina. (±)-3-(4-Chlorophenyl)-*NN*-dimethyl-3-(2-pyridyl)propylamine hydrogen maleate.

$C_{16}H_{19}ClN_2,C_4H_4O_4 = 390.9.$

*CAS — 132-22-9 (chlorphenamine); 113-92-8 (chlorphenamine maleate).*

*ATC — R06AB04.*

**Pharmacopoeias.** In *Chin., Eur.* (see p.vi), *Int., Jpn, US,* and *Viet.*

**Ph. Eur. 5.0** (Chlorphenamine Maleate). A white, crystalline powder. Freely soluble in water; soluble in alcohol. Protect from light.

**USP 27** (Chlorpheniramine Maleate). A white, odourless, crystalline powder. Soluble 1 in 4 of water and 1 in 10 of alcohol and of chloroform; slightly soluble in ether and in benzene. Its solutions in water have a pH between 4 and 5. Store in airtight containers. Protect from light.

**Incompatibility.** Chlorphenamine maleate has been reported to be incompatible with calcium chloride, kanamycin sulfate, noradrenaline acid tartrate, pentobarbital sodium, and meglumine adipiodone.

### Dexchlorpheniramine Maleate *(BANM, rINNM)*

Dexchlorphenamine Maleate; Dexchlorpheniramini Maleas; Maleato de dexclorfeniramina.

*CAS — 25523-97-1 (dexchlorpheniramine); 2438-32-6 (dexchlorpheniramine maleate).*

*ATC — R06AB02.*

**Pharmacopoeias.** In *Eur.* (see p.vi), *Jpn,* and *US.*

**Ph. Eur. 5.0** (Dexchlorpheniramine Maleate). A white crystalline powder. Very soluble in water; freely soluble in alcohol, in dichloromethane, and in methyl alcohol. A 1% solution in water has a pH of 4.5 to 5.5. Protect from light.

**USP 27** (Dexchlorpheniramine Maleate). A white, odourless, crystalline powder. Soluble 1 in 1.1 of water, 1 in 2 of alcohol, 1 in 1.7 of chloroform, and 1 in 2500 of ether; slightly soluble in benzene. pH of a 1% solution in water is between 4.0 and 5.0. Store in airtight containers. Protect from light.

### Adverse Effects and Precautions

As for the sedating antihistamines in general, p.419. Exfoliative dermatitis may develop. Injections may be irritant and cause transient hypotension or stimulation of the CNS.

**Effects on the blood.** There are several old and isolated reports of blood dyscrasias after administration of chlorphenamine maleate; these include agranulocytosis,[1,2] thrombocytopenia,[3] pancytopenia,[4] and aplastic anaemia.[5] Haemolytic anaemia has occurred after administration of dexchlorpheniramine maleate.[6]

The association with antihistamine administration has been questioned in some of these cases.[7]


1. Shenfield G, Spry CJF. Unusual cause of agranulocytosis. *BMJ* 1968; **ii:** 52–3.
2. Hardin AS. Chlorpheniramine and agranulocytosis. *Ann Intern Med* 1988; **108:** 770.
3. Eisner EV, *et al.* Chlorpheniramine-dependent thrombocytopenia. *JAMA* 1975; **231:** 735–6.
4. Deringer PM, Maniatis A. Chlorpheniramine-induced bone-marrow suppression. *Lancet* 1976; **i:** 432.
5. Kanoh T, *et al.* Aplastic anaemia after prolonged treatment with chlorpheniramine. *Lancet* 1977; **i:** 546–7.
6. Duran-Suarez JR, *et al.* The I antigen as an immune complex receptor in a case of haemolytic anaemia induced by an antihistaminic agent. *Br J Haematol* 1981; **49:** 153–4.
7. Spry CJF. Chlorpheniramine-induced bone-marrow suppression. *Lancet* 1976; **i:** 545.


**Effects on the senses.** Chlorphenamine has been reported to affect the senses of smell and taste.[1]


1. Schiffman SS. Taste and smell in disease. *N Engl J Med* 1983; **308:** 1275–9.


**Extrapyramidal disorders.** Facial dyskinesias have been reported[1,2] after administration of chlorphenamine maleate by mouth.


1. Thach BT, *et al.* Oral facial dyskinesia associated with prolonged use of antihistaminic decongestants. *N Engl J Med* 1975; **293:** 486–7.
2. Davis WA. Dyskinesia associated with chronic antihistamine use. *N Engl J Med* 1976; **294:** 113.


## Interactions

As for the sedating antihistamines in general, p.421.

**Antiepileptics.** For a report of the effect of chlorphenamine on phenytoin, see p.373.

## Pharmacokinetics

Chlorphenamine maleate is absorbed relatively slowly from the gastrointestinal tract, peak plasma concentrations occurring about 2.5 to 6 hours after oral administration. Bioavailability is low, values of 25 to 50% having been reported. Chlorphenamine appears to undergo considerable first-pass metabolism. About 70% of chlorphenamine in the circulation is bound to plasma proteins. There is wide interindividual variation in the pharmacokinetics of chlorphenamine; values ranging from 2 to 43 hours have been reported for the half-life. Chlorphenamine is widely distributed in the body, and enters the CNS.

Chlorphenamine maleate is extensively metabolised. Metabolites include desmethyl- and didesmethylchlorphenamine. Unchanged drug and metabolites are excreted primarily in the urine; excretion is dependent on urinary pH and flow rate. Only trace amounts have been found in the faeces.

A duration of action of 4 to 6 hours has been reported; this is shorter than may be predicted from pharmacokinetic parameters.

More rapid and extensive absorption, faster clearance, and a shorter half-life have been reported in children.

◊ References.


1. Rumore MM. Clinical pharmacokinetics of chlorpheniramine. *Drug Intell Clin Pharm* 1984; **18:** 701–7.
2. Paton DM, Webster DR. Clinical pharmacokinetics of $H_1$-receptor antagonists (the antihistamines). *Clin Pharmacokinet* 1985; **10:** 477–97.
3. Yasuda SU, *et al.* The roles of CYP2D6 and stereoselectivity in the clinical pharmacokinetics of chlorpheniramine. *Br J Clin Pharmacol* 2002; **53:** 519–25.


## Uses and Administration

Chlorphenamine maleate, an alkylamine derivative, is a sedating antihistamine that causes a moderate degree of sedation; it also has antimuscarinic activity.

Chlorphenamine is a racemic mixture; the dextrorotatory isomer, dexchlorpheniramine, has approximately twice the activity of chlorphenamine by weight.

Chlorphenamine maleate and dexchlorpheniramine maleate are used for the symptomatic relief of allergic conditions including urticaria and angioedema (p.423), rhinitis (p.422), and conjunctivitis (p.421), and in pruritic skin disorders (p.422). They are common ingredients of compound preparations for symptomatic treatment of coughs and the common cold (p.421). Chlorphenamine may be administered intravenously as an adjunct in the emergency treatment of anaphylactic shock (p.421).

*Chlorphenamine maleate* is given by mouth in doses of 4 mg every 4 to 6 hours up to a maximum of 24 mg daily. Doses for children are: 1 to 2 years, 1 mg twice daily; 2 to 5 years, 1 mg every 4 to 6 hours (maximum 6 mg daily); 6 to 12 years, 2 mg every 4 to 6 hours (maximum 12 mg daily).

Chlorphenamine maleate may be given by intramuscular, by subcutaneous, or by slow intravenous injection over a period of 1 minute. The usual dose is 10 to 20 mg and the total dose given by these routes in 24 hours should not normally exceed 40 mg. For children, doses of 87.5 micrograms/kg subcutaneously four times daily have been suggested. The following intravenous doses may be used in children: the usual dose in children under 1 year is 250 micrograms/kg; those aged 1 to 5 years may be given a dose of 2.5 to 5 mg and those aged 6 to 12 years, 5 to 10 mg.

*Dexchlorpheniramine maleate* is given by mouth in doses of 2 mg every 4 to 6 hours up to a maximum of 12 mg daily. Children aged 2 to 5 years may be given 0.5 mg every 4 to 6 hours (maximum 3 mg daily), and those aged 6 to 12 years, 1 mg every 4 to 6 hours (maximum 6 mg daily).

*Modified-release* oral preparations of chlorphenamine maleate or dexchlorpheniramine maleate are available in some countries; dosage is specific to a particular formulation.

Dexchlorpheniramine maleate has been applied topically in some countries, although as with other antihistamines there is a risk of sensitisation. Chlorphenamine polistirex (a sulfonated diethenylbenzene-ethenylbenzene copolymer complex), chlorphenamine tannate, and dexchlorpheniramine tannate are given by mouth and are used similarly to the maleate.

**Malaria.** Chlorphenamine may be tried in patients with malaria who experience chloroquine-induced pruritus (see Effects on the Skin, p.449), but additionally it has been shown to have some promise as an adjunct in the treatment of chloroquine-resistant malaria itself. Early studies indicated that chlorphenamine was only one of a number of drugs that reversed chloroquine resistance *in vitro* in isolates of *Plasmodium falciparum*. Later clinical studies in children in Nigeria demonstrated enhanced efficacy when chlorphenamine was given with chloroquine.[1-5] The overall management of malaria is discussed on p.444.


1. Sowunmi A, *et al.* Enhanced efficacy of chloroquine-chlorpheniramine combination in acute uncomplicated falciparum malaria in children. *Trans R Soc Trop Med Hyg* 1997; **91:** 63–7.
2. Sowunmi A, Oduola AMJ. Comparative efficacy of chloroquine/chlorpheniramine combination and mefloquine for the treatment of chloroquine-resistant Plasmodium falciparum malaria in Nigerian children. *Trans R Soc Trop Med Hyg* 1997; **91:** 689–93.
3. Sowunmi A, *et al.* Comparative efficacy of chloroquine plus chlorpheniramine and pyrimethamine/sulfadoxine in acute uncomplicated falciparum malaria in Nigerian children. *Trans R Soc Trop Med Hyg* 1998; **92:** 77–81.
4. Sowunmi A, *et al.* Comparative efficacy of chloroquine plus chlorpheniramine and halofantrine in acute uncomplicated falciparum malaria in Nigerian children. *Trans R Soc Trop Med Hyg* 1998; **92:** 441–5.
5. Okonkwo CA, *et al.* Effect of chlorpheniramine on the pharmacokinetics of and response to chloroquine of Nigerian children with falciparum malaria. *Trans R Soc Trop Med Hyg* 1999; **93:** 306–11.


## Preparations

***BP 2003:*** Chlorphenamine Injection; Chlorphenamine Oral Solution; Chlorphenamine Tablets;
***USP 27:*** Chlorpheniramine Maleate and Phenylpropanolamine Hydrochloride Extended-release Capsules; Chlorpheniramine Maleate and Phenylpropanolamine Hydrochloride Extended-release Tablets; Chlorpheniramine Maleate and Pseudoephedrine Hydrochloride Extended-release Capsules; Chlorpheniramine Maleate and Pseudoephedrine Hydrochloride Oral Solution; Chlorpheniramine Maleate Extended-release Capsules; Chlorpheniramine Maleate Injection; Chlorpheniramine Maleate Syrup; Chlorpheniramine Maleate Tablets; Dexchlorpheniramine Maleate Syrup; Dexchlorpheniramine Maleate Tablets.

**Proprietary Preparations** (details are given in Part 3)
***Arg.:*** Afeme; Alergidryl; Alergitrat; Isomerine; ***Austral.:*** Polaramine; ***Austria:*** Polaramin; Polaronil†; ***Belg.:*** Bronchalene†; Polaramine; ***Braz.:*** Alergovalle; Alergyo; Alermine; Dexclor; Dexlerg; Dexmin†; Histamin; Polamin; Polaramine; ***Canad.:*** Chlor-Tripolon; Histalon†; Novo-Pheniram; Polaramine†; ***Chile:*** Asafen Nueva Formula; Clorprimeton; Prodel; Scadan; ***Denm.:*** Polaramin; ***Fr.:*** Polaramine; ***Ger.:*** Polaronil; ***Gr.:*** Istamex; Polaramine; ***Hong Kong:*** Apomin; Chlorpyrimine; Medifen; Pirimat; Piriton; Polaramine; Sprinsol; Uni-Ramine; ***Irl.:*** Anti-Hist†; Piriton; ***Israel:*** Ahiston; Anaphyl; ***Ital.:*** Polamin†; Polaramin; Trimeton; ***Malaysia:*** Chloramine; Chlorpyramine; D-Antihist; Dex-Antihist; Dexchloramine; Polamine; Polaramine; Somin; ***Mex.:*** Alerdil; Blendox; Cloro-Trimeton; Cronal; Polaramine; ***Neth.:*** Polaramine; ***Norw.:*** Phenamin; Polaramin; ***NZ:*** Histafen; Polaramine; ***Port.:*** Trenelone; ***S.Afr.:*** Allergex; Chlor-Trimeton; Chlorhist; Histamed†; Polaramine; ***Singapore:*** Allerphen; Chlorpyrimine; Piriton; Polaramine; Rhiniramine; Somin; ***Spain:*** Antihistaminico; Polaramine; ***Swed.:*** Polaramin; ***Switz.:*** Polaramine; ***Thai.:*** Allergin; Chlorleate; Chlorpheno; Chlorpyrimine; Cohistan; Histatapp; Nasamine; Piriton; ***UAE:*** Chlorohistol; ***UK:*** Allergy Relief; Allerief; Calimal; Hayleve; Piriject†; Piriton; Pollenase Antihistamine; Rimarin†; ***USA:*** Aller-Chlor; Allergy; Allergy Relief; Chlo-Amine; Chlor-Pro; Chlor-Trimeton; Efidac 24 Chlorpheniramine; PediaCare Allergy Formula; Polaramine†; Teldrin.

**Multi-ingredient:** numerous preparations are listed in Part 3.

## Chlorphenoxamine Hydrochloride *(BANM, rINNM)*

Hidrocloruro de clorfenoxamina. 2-(4-Chloro-α-methylbenzhydryloxy)-*NN*-dimethylethylamine hydrochloride.

$C_{18}H_{22}ClNO,HCl = 340.3.$

*CAS — 77-38-3 (chlorphenoxamine); 562-09-4 (chlorphenoxamine hydrochloride).*

*ATC — D04AA34; R06AA06.*

### Profile

Chlorphenoxamine, a congener of diphenhydramine (p.431), has antimuscarinic and antihistaminic properties. It has been used in nausea, vomiting, and vertigo, and was formerly used in the symptomatic treatment of parkinsonism. Chlorphenoxamine has also been used in hypersensitivity reactions.

### Preparations

**Proprietary Preparations** (details are given in Part 3)
***Austria:*** Systral†; ***Braz.:*** Clorevan†; ***Ger.:*** Systral; ***Hong Kong:*** Systral; ***Port.:*** Systral; ***Thai.:*** Systral.

**Multi-ingredient:** ***Austria:*** Calcilin compositum†; Spirbon; Systral C†; Systrason†; ***Ger.:*** Rodavan†; Systral C; ***S.Afr.:*** Analgen-SA.

## Cinnarizine *(BAN, USAN, rINN)*

Cinarizina; Cinnarizinum; 516-MD; R-516; R-1575. 1-Benzhydryl-4-cinnamylpiperazine; (*E*)-1-(Diphenylmethyl)-4-(3-phenylprop-2-enyl)piperazine.

$C_{26}H_{28}N_2 = 368.5.$

*CAS — 298-57-7.*

*ATC — N07CA02.*

**Pharmacopoeias.** In *Chin., Eur.* (see p.vi), and *Pol.*

**Ph. Eur. 5.0** (Cinnarizine). A white or almost white powder. Practically insoluble in water; slightly soluble in alcohol and in methyl alcohol; soluble in acetone; freely soluble in dichloromethane. Protect from light.

### Adverse Effects and Precautions

As for the sedating antihistamines in general, p.419.

There have been rare reports of extrapyramidal symptoms after cinnarizine, sometimes associated with depressive feelings.

High doses of cinnarizine should be used with caution in patients with hypotension because of the possibility of decreasing blood pressure further.

**Extrapyramidal disorders.** For reference to extrapyramidal disorders associated with the use of cinnarizine, see Flunarizine, p.434.

**Hypersensitivity.** A report[1] of immunologically-defined lichen planus pemphigoides in a 72-year-old woman taking cinnarizine. Lesions began to clear when treatment was stopped but challenge with cinnarizine provoked severe itching and reactivation of pigmented lesions.


1. Miyagawa S, *et al.* Lichen planus pemphigoides-like lesions induced by cinnarizine. *Br J Dermatol* 1985; **112:** 607–13.


**Porphyria.** Cinnarizine is considered to be unsafe in patients with porphyria because it has been shown to be porphyrinogenic in *animals*.

**Tinnitus.** The Spanish System of Pharmacovigilance had received reports[1] of tinnitus associated with calcium-channel blockers; some of the reports, including the one relating to cinnarizine, were in patients also receiving other ototoxic drugs. WHO was said to have additional reports of tinnitus associated with calcium-channel blockers including cinnarizine.


1. Narváez M, *et al.* Tinnitus with calcium-channel blockers. *Lancet* 1994; **343:** 1229–30.


**Weight gain.** There has been a report[1] of weight gain in 4 patients who had taken cinnarizine for 1 to 2 years; in all cases the weight gain was associated with increased appetite.


1. Navarro-Badenes J, *et al.* Weight-gain associated with cinnarizine. *Ann Pharmacother* 1992; **26:** 928–30.


### Interactions

As for the sedating antihistamines in general, p.421.

### Pharmacokinetics

Cinnarizine is absorbed from the gastrointestinal tract, peak plasma concentrations occurring 2 to 4 hours after oral administration. It undergoes metabolism and has a half-life of 3 to 6 hours. Cinnarizine is excreted in the faeces mainly as unchanged drug, and in the urine predominantly as metabolites.

### Uses and Administration

Cinnarizine is a piperazine derivative with antihistamine, sedative, and calcium-channel blocking activity. It is used for the symptomatic treatment of nausea and vertigo caused by Ménière's disease and other vestibular disorders (p.423) and for the prevention and treatment of motion sickness (p.422). It is also used in the management of various peripheral and cerebral vascular disorders.

In the UK, the usual dose for vertigo and vestibular disorders is 30 mg three times daily by mouth. For motion sickness a dose of 30 mg is taken 2 hours before the start of the journey and 15 mg every 8 hours during the journey if necessary. Children aged 5 to 12 years are given half the adult dose for both indications. In other European countries, a dose of 75 mg once or twice daily has been given for vertigo and vestibular disorders. Doses of 75 mg may also be given 1 to 3 times daily for cerebrovascular disorders and 2 or 3 times daily for peripheral vascular disorders.

◊ References.

1. Shupak A, *et al.* Cinnarizine in the prophylaxis of seasickness: laboratory vestibular evaluation and sea study. *Clin Pharmacol Ther* 1994; **55:** 670–80.

### Preparations

**Proprietary Preparations** (details are given in Part 3)

***Arg.:*** Dismaren; Fabracin; Folcodal; Iroplex; Natropas; Stugeron; ***Austria:*** Cinnabene; Pericephal; Stutgeron; ***Belg.:*** Stugeron; ***Braz.:*** Antigeron; Cinageron†; Cinaran; Cinarix; Cinarizina-Cinarin†; Cinazon; Cronogeron; Labigeron; Nerizina†; Stugerina; Stugeron; Verzum; Vessel; ***Chile:*** Cinergil; Siridone; Stugeron; ***Denm.:*** Sepan; ***Ger.:*** Cinnacet†; Stutgeron†; ***Gr.:*** Derozin; Stugeron; ***Hong Kong:*** Celenid; Corathiem†; Medozine; Stugeron; ***India:*** Cintigo; Stugeron; ***Irl.:*** Stugeron; ***Israel:*** Stunarone; ***Ital.:*** Cinazyn; Stugeron; Toliman; ***Malaysia:*** Celenid; Cereron; Cinna; Cinnaron; Stugeron; Uphageron; ***Mex.:*** Cisaken; Stugeron; ***Neth.:*** Cinnipirine†; ***Port.:*** Cinon; Stugeron; ***S.Afr.:*** Stugeron; ***Singapore:*** Celenid; Cinna; Cinnar; Cinnaron; Stugeron; Urizine; ***Spain:*** Pervasum†; Stugeron; ***Switz.:*** Cerepar; Cinnageron; Cinnamed; Stugeron; ***Thai.:*** C-Pela; Celenid; Cenai; Cerebroad; Ceremin; Cinerine; Cinnar; Cinnaza; Cinrizine; CN-25; Linazine; Manoron; Med-Circuron; Medozine; Siarizine; Silicin; Sorebral; Stugeron; Stuno; Urizine; Vernarin; ***UK:*** Cinaziere; Stugeron.

**Multi-ingredient:** ***Arg.:*** Cadencial Plus; Cinacris; Difusil; Ribex; Vasodual; ***Austria:*** Cinnarplus; ***Belg.:*** Touristil; ***Braz.:*** Coldrin; Exit; Forgrip†; Sureptil; ***Fin.:*** Rinomar; ***Fr.:*** Sureptil†; ***Ger.:*** Arlevert; ***Hong Kong:*** C-Sik; ***Neth.:*** Primatour; ***Norw.:*** Rinomar†; ***Spain:*** Clinadil; Clinadil Compositum; Diclamina; Ederal†; Ornade†; ***Swed.:*** Rinomar.

## Clemastine Fumarate *(BANM, USAN, rINNM)*

Clemastini Fumaras; Fumarato de clemastina; HS-592 (clemastine); Meclastine Fumarate; Mecloprodine Fumarate. (+)-(2*R*)-2-{2-[(*R*)-4-Chloro-α-methylbenzhydryloxy]ethyl}-1-methylpyrrolidine hydrogen fumarate.

$C_{21}H_{26}ClNO,C_4H_4O_4$ = 460.0.

*CAS — 15686-51-8 (clemastine); 14976-57-9 (clemastine fumarate).*

*ATC — D04AA14; R06AA04.*

**Pharmacopoeias.** In *Chin., Eur.* (see p.vi), *Jpn, Pol.,* and *US.*

**Ph. Eur. 5.0** (Clemastine Fumarate). A white or almost white, crystalline powder. Very slightly soluble in water; sparingly soluble in alcohol (70%); slightly soluble in alcohol (50%) and in methyl alcohol. A 10% suspension in water has a pH of 3.2 to 4.2.

**USP 27** (Clemastine Fumarate). A colourless to faintly yellow, odourless, crystalline powder. Very slightly soluble in water; very slightly soluble in chloroform; slightly soluble in methyl alcohol. pH of a 10% suspension in water is between 3.2 to 4.2. Store in airtight containers at a temperature not exceeding 25°. Protect from light.

### Adverse Effects and Precautions

As for the sedating antihistamines in general, p.419.

**Breast feeding.** The American Academy of Pediatrics[1] considers that clemastine should be given with caution to breast-feeding mothers, since it has been associated with adverse effects in the infant. Drowsiness, irritability, a high-pitched cry, neck stiffness, and refusal to feed in a 10-week-old breast-fed baby occurred 12 hours after her mother started treatment with clemastine.[2] Clemastine was detected in the mother's breast milk. The baby recovered and was feeding normally on the day after the drug was stopped.

1. American Academy of Pediatrics. The transfer of drugs and other chemicals into human milk. *Pediatrics* 2001; **108:** 776–89. Correction. *ibid.*; 1029. Also available at: http://aappolicy.aappublications.org/cgi/content/full/pediatrics%3b108/3/776 (accessed 08/04/04)
2. Kok THHG, *et al.* Drowsiness due to clemastine transmitted in breast milk. *Lancet* 1982; **i:** 914–15.

**Porphyria.** Clemastine has been associated with acute attacks of porphyria and is considered unsafe in porphyric patients.

### Interactions

As for the sedating antihistamines in general, p.421.

### Pharmacokinetics

Clemastine fumarate is rapidly and almost completely absorbed from the gastrointestinal tract; peak plasma concentrations are achieved in 2 to 4 hours. Unchanged drug and metabolites are excreted principally in the urine. An elimination half-life of about 21 hours has been reported. Clemastine is distributed into breast milk.

◊ References.

1. Schran HF, *et al.* The pharmacokinetics and bioavailability of clemastine and phenylpropanolamine in single-component and combination formulations. *J Clin Pharmacol* 1996; **36:** 911–22.

### Uses and Administration

Clemastine fumarate, a monoethanolamine derivative, is a sedating antihistamine with antimuscarinic and moderate sedative properties. It has been reported to have a duration of action of about 10 to 12 hours. It is used for the symptomatic relief of allergic conditions including urticaria and angioedema (p.423), rhinitis (p.422) and conjunctivitis (p.421), and in pruritic skin disorders (p.422).

Clemastine is given as the fumarate although doses are expressed in terms of the equivalent amount of clemastine base. Clemastine fumarate 1.34 mg is approximately equivalent to 1 mg of clemastine base. The usual dose by mouth is 1 mg twice daily. Up to 6 mg daily has been given, particularly for urticaria and angioedema. Children aged 1 to 3 years may be given 250 to 500 micrograms twice daily; those aged 3 to 6 years, 500 micrograms twice daily; and those aged 6 to 12 years 0.5 to 1 mg twice daily.

Clemastine fumarate may be given by intramuscular or slow intravenous injection in a total daily dose equivalent to 4 mg of clemastine for acute allergic reactions; for prophylaxis 2 mg is given by intravenous injection. The dose for children is 25 micrograms/kg daily in two divided doses by intramuscular injection.

Clemastine fumarate has also been used topically, although as with other antihistamines, there is a risk of sensitisation.

### Preparations

***BP 2003:*** Clemastine Oral Solution; Clemastine Tablets;
***USP 27:*** Clemastine Fumarate Tablets.

**Proprietary Preparations** (details are given in Part 3)

***Austria:*** Tavegyl; ***Braz.:*** Agasten; ***Canad.:*** Tavist†; ***Denm.:*** Tavegyl; ***Ger.:*** Tavegil; ***India:*** Clamist; ***Irl.:*** Tavegil†; ***Ital.:*** Tavegil; ***Mex.:*** Tavist; ***Neth.:*** Tavegil; ***Port.:*** Tavegyl; Tavist; ***S.Afr.:*** Tavegyl; ***Spain:*** Tavegil; ***Swed.:*** Tavegyl; ***Switz.:*** Tavegyl; ***UK:*** Aller-Eze†; Tavegil; ***USA:*** Antihist-1†; Contac 12 Hour Allergy; Dayhist-1; Tavist Allergy; Tavist†.

**Multi-ingredient:** ***Braz.:*** Emistin; ***Canad.:*** Tavist-D†; ***Ger.:*** Corto-Tavegil; ***Mex.:*** Tavist-D; ***Spain:*** Dexa Tavegil; ***UK:*** Aller-Eze Plus†; ***USA:*** Antihist-D†; Tavist-D†.

## Clemizole Hydrochloride *(BANM, rINNM)*

AL-20; Hidrocloruro de clemizol. 1-(4-Chlorobenzyl)-2-(pyrrolidin-1-ylmethyl)benzimidazole hydrochloride.

$C_{19}H_{20}ClN_3,HCl$ = 362.3.

*CAS — 442-52-4 (clemizole); 1163-36-6 (clemizole hydrochloride).*

### Profile

Clemizole hydrochloride is a sedating antihistamine (p.419). It has been used for the symptomatic relief of allergic conditions, in pruritic skin disorders, and in combination preparations for the treatment of symptoms of the common cold. Clemizole has also been applied topically as the hexachlorophene, the sodium sulfate, and the undecylate derivatives in topical and rectal preparations combined with corticosteroids and local anaesthetics, although as with other antihistamines, there is a risk of sensitisation.

See p.194 for the use of clemizole penicillin.

### Preparations

**Proprietary Preparations** (details are given in Part 3)

**Multi-ingredient:** ***Arg.:*** Apracur; ***Austria:*** Apracur†; ***Braz.:*** Ultraproct; ***Hong Kong:*** Ultraproct; ***Thai.:*** Apracur; Scheriproct.

## Clocinizine Hydrochloride *(rINNM)*

Chlorcinnazine Dihydrochloride; Hidrocloruro de clonizina. 1-(4-Chlorobenzhydryl)-4-cinnamylpiperazine dihydrochloride.

$C_{26}H_{27}ClN_2,2HCl$ = 475.9.

*CAS — 298-55-5 (clocinizine).*

### Profile

Clocinizine hydrochloride, a piperazine derivative, is an antihistamine (p.419) given by mouth in combination preparations for the symptomatic treatment of upper respiratory-tract disorders, often with a decongestant.

### Preparations

**Proprietary Preparations** (details are given in Part 3)

**Multi-ingredient:** ***Belg.:*** Denoral†; ***Fr.:*** Denoral; ***Hong Kong:*** Denoral†; ***Ital.:*** Denoral; ***Spain:*** Senioral†.

## Cyclizine *(BAN, rINN)*

Ciclizina. 1-Benzhydryl-4-methylpiperazine.

$C_{18}H_{22}N_2$ = 266.4.

*CAS — 82-92-8.*

*ATC — R06AE03.*

**Pharmacopoeias.** In *Br.*

**BP 2003** (Cyclizine). A white or creamy white, crystalline powder. Practically insoluble in water. It dissolves in most organic solvents and in dilute acids. M.p. about 107°. A saturated solution in water has a pH of 7.6 to 8.6.

## Cyclizine Hydrochloride *(BANM, rINNM)*

Cyclizini Hydrochloridum; Hidrocloruro de ciclizina.

$C_{18}H_{22}N_2,HCl$ = 302.8.

*CAS — 303-25-3.*

*ATC — R06AE03.*

**Pharmacopoeias.** In *Eur.* (see p.vi) and *US.*

**Ph. Eur. 5.0** (Cyclizine Hydrochloride). A white, crystalline powder. Slightly soluble in water and in alcohol. A 2% solution in alcohol 2 vol. and water 3 vol. has a pH of 4.5 to 5.5. Protect from light.

**USP 27** (Cyclizine Hydrochloride). A white, odourless, crystalline powder or small colourless crystals. Soluble 1 in 115 of water and of alcohol and 1 in 75 of chloroform; insoluble in ether. pH of a 2% solution in alcohol 2 vol. and water 3 vol. is between 4.5 and 5.5. Store in airtight containers. Protect from light.

## Cyclizine Lactate *(BANM, rINNM)*

Lactato de ciclizina.

$C_{18}H_{22}N_2,C_3H_6O_3$ = 356.5.

*CAS — 5897-19-8.*

*ATC — R06AE03.*

**Pharmacopoeias.** *Br.* includes an injection of cyclizine lactate.

**Incompatibility.** Cyclizine lactate is reported to be incompatible with oxytetracycline hydrochloride, chlortetracycline hydrochloride, benzylpenicillin, and solutions with a pH of 6.8 or more.

## Cyclizine Tartrate *(BANM, rINNM)*

Tartrato de ciclizina.

$C_{18}H_{22}N_2,C_4H_6O_6$ = 416.5.

*ATC — R06AE03.*

### Adverse Effects and Precautions

As for the sedating antihistamines in general, p.419. Cyclizine may aggravate severe heart failure. Hypotension may occur on injection.

**Abuse.** Cyclizine tablets have been abused either alone or with opioids for their euphoric effects.[1-7] They have been taken by mouth or used to make injections. It has been suggested that cyclizine dependence may occur when it is used with opioids in the treatment of chronic pain.[8]

1. Gott PH. Cyclizine toxicity—intentional drug abuse of a proprietary antihistamine. *N Engl J Med* 1968; **279:** 596.
2. Kahn A, Harvey GJ. Increasing misuse of cyclizine. *Pharm J* 1985; **235:** 706.
3. Atkinson MK. Misuse of cyclizine. *Pharm J* 1985; **235:** 773.
4. Halpin D. Misuse of cyclizine. *Pharm J* 1985; **235:** 773.
5. Council of the Pharmaceutical Society of Great Britain. Sales of preparations containing cyclizine. *Pharm J* 1985; **235:** 797.
6. Ruben SM, *et al.* Cyclizine abuse among a group of opiate dependents receiving methadone. *Br J Addict* 1989; **84:** 929–34.
7. Bassett KE, *et al.* Cyclizine abuse by teenagers in Utah. *Am J Emerg Med* 1996; **14:** 472–4.
8. Hughes AM, Coote J. Cyclizine dependence. *Pharm J* 1986; **236:** 130.

**Effects on the blood.** Agranulocytosis occurred in a patient after 6 weeks of treatment with cyclizine 50 mg three times daily.[1] The blood count returned to normal once cyclizine was withdrawn.

1. Collier PM. Agranulocytosis associated with oral cyclizine. *BMJ* 1986; **292:** 174.

**Effects on the heart.** In a study[1] of 11 patients with severe heart failure, cyclizine produced detrimental haemodynamic effects including increased systemic and pulmonary artery pressures and ventricular filling pressures, and negated the vasodilator effects of diamorphine. It was suggested that the use of cyclizine should be avoided in patients with acute myocardial infarction or severe heart failure.

1. Tan LB, *et al.* Detrimental haemodynamic effects of cyclizine in heart failure. *Lancet* 1988; **i:** 560–1.

**Effects on the liver.** An 8-year-old girl developed jaundice on 2 occasions after taking cyclizine hydrochloride 25 mg daily by mouth. 'Hypersensitivity hepatitis' was considered responsible.[1]

1. Kew MC, *et al.* "Hypersensitivity hepatitis" associated with administration of cyclizine. *BMJ* 1973; **2:** 307.

**Pregnancy.** For discussion of the use of antihistamines in pregnancy, including studies involving cyclizine, see p.420.

## Interactions

As for the sedating antihistamines in general, p.421. Cyclizine may counteract the haemodynamic benefits of opioids (see Effects on the Heart, above) and this should be considered before using preparations that contain a combination of cyclizine and an opioid analgesic.

**General anaesthetics.** For a possible interaction between cyclizine premedication and *barbiturate anaesthetics* see under Thiopental, p.1309.

## Pharmacokinetics

Cyclizine is absorbed from the gastrointestinal tract and has an onset of action within 2 hours. The duration of action is reported to be about 4 hours. Cyclizine is metabolised in the liver to the relatively inactive metabolite, norcyclizine. Both cyclizine and norcyclizine have plasma elimination half-lives of 20 hours. Less than 1% of the total oral dose is eliminated in the urine in 24 hours.

## Uses and Administration

Cyclizine, a piperazine derivative, is a sedating antihistamine with antimuscarinic activity, although the sedative effects are not marked.

It is used as an antiemetic in the management of nausea and vomiting (p.422) including motion sickness, postoperative nausea and vomiting, after radiotherapy, and in drug-induced nausea and vomiting. It is included as an antiemetic with some opioids, and in combination preparations for the treatment of migraine attacks (p.464). Cyclizine is also used for the symptomatic treatment of vertigo (p.423) caused by Ménière's disease and other vestibular disturbances.

In the management of nausea and vomiting, cyclizine hydrochloride is given by mouth in a usual dose of 50 mg up to three times daily, although up to 200 mg may be given in 24 hours if necessary. For the prevention of motion sickness, the first dose should be given about 30 minutes before travelling. Children aged 6 to 12 years may be given 25 mg up to three times daily.

Cyclizine is given intramuscularly or intravenously as the lactate. Doses of cyclizine lactate are similar to those of cyclizine hydrochloride given orally. For the prevention of postoperative nausea and vomiting the first dose of cyclizine lactate should be given about 20 minutes before the anticipated end of surgery.

Cyclizine salts are used as antiemetics in combination with morphine or dipipanone; the use of such fixed-combination opioid preparations is considered to be unsuitable for the prolonged treatment that may be required in palliative care. See also under Interactions, above.

## Preparations

***BP 2003:*** Cyclizine Injection; Cyclizine Tablets; Dipipanone and Cyclizine Tablets;
***USP 27:*** Cyclizine Hydrochloride Tablets.

**Proprietary Preparations** (details are given in Part 3)
***Austria:*** Echnatol; Fortravel; ***Canad.:*** Marzine†; ***Denm.:*** Marzine; ***Fin.:*** Marzine; ***Hong Kong:*** Marzine; Valoid; ***Irl.:*** Valoid†; ***Norw.:*** Marzine; ***NZ:*** Marzine; Valoid; ***S.Afr.:*** Aculoid†; Covamet; Emitex; Medazine; Nauzine; Norizine; Ryccard†; Triazine†; Valoid; ***Singapore:*** Marzine; ***Swed.:*** Marzine; ***Switz.:*** Marzine; ***UK:*** Valoid; ***USA:*** Marezine.

**Multi-ingredient:** ***Austral.:*** Migral†; ***Austria:*** Echnatol B$_6$; Migril; ***Canad.:*** Megral†; ***Fin.:*** Vertipam; ***Fr.:*** Migwell†; ***Hong Kong:*** Migril; Wellconal; ***Irl.:*** Cyclimorph; Diconal; Migril; ***NZ:*** Migril†; ***S.Afr.:*** Cyclimorph; Migril; Wellconal; ***Singapore:*** Migril†; ***Spain:*** Igril†; ***Switz.:*** Migril†; ***UK:*** Cyclimorph; Diconal; Migril.

---

# Cyproheptadine Hydrochloride

*(BANM, rINNM)*

Cyproheptadini Hydrochloridum; Hidrocloruro de ciproheptadina. 4-(5*H*-Dibenzo[*a*,*d*]cyclohepten-5-ylidene)-1-methylpiperidine hydrochloride sesquihydrate.

$C_{21}H_{21}N,HCl,1\frac{1}{2}H_2O$ = 350.9.

*CAS — 129-03-3 (cyproheptadine); 969-33-5 (anhydrous cyproheptadine hydrochloride); 41354-29-4 (cyproheptadine hydrochloride sesquihydrate).*
*ATC — R06AX02.*

**Pharmacopoeias.** In *Chin., Eur.* (see p.vi), *Jpn,* and *US.*

**Ph. Eur. 5.0** (Cyproheptadine Hydrochloride). A white or slightly yellow, crystalline powder. Slightly soluble in water; sparingly soluble in alcohol; freely soluble in methyl alcohol. Protect from light.

**USP 27** (Cyproheptadine Hydrochloride). A white to slightly yellow, odourless or practically odourless, crystalline powder. Soluble 1 in 275 of water, 1 in 35 of alcohol, 1 in 26 of chloroform, and 1 in 1.5 of methyl alcohol; practically insoluble in ether.

## Adverse Effects and Precautions

As for the sedating antihistamines in general, p.419. Increased appetite and weight gain may occur with cyproheptadine.

**Abuse.** A report[1] of dependence developing in a patient who had taken about 180 mg of cyproheptadine daily by mouth for 5 years.

1. Craven JL, Rodin GM. Cyproheptadine dependence associated with an atypical somatoform disorder. *Can J Psychiatry* 1987; **32:** 143–5.

**Effects on the nervous system.** Antimuscarinic toxicity manifest by hallucinations and agitation developed in a 9-year-old child taking cyproheptadine 4 mg twice daily for migraine prophylaxis.[1]

1. Watemberg NM, *et al.* Central anticholinergic syndrome on therapeutic doses of cyproheptadine. *Pediatrics* 1999; **103:** 158–60.

**Interference with diagnostic tests.** Cyproheptadine reduced hypoglycaemia-induced growth hormone secretion by between 5 and 97% in 8 healthy subjects.[1] It was suggested that if patients receiving cyproheptadine were given a pituitary function test that used growth hormone response to insulin-induced hypoglycaemia, then cyproheptadine therapy should be stopped before the test.

The UK manufacturer states that cyproheptadine may cause a false positive test result for tricyclic antidepressants in urine.

1. Bivens CH, *et al.* Inhibition of hypoglycaemia-induced growth hormone secretion by the serotonin antagonists cyproheptadine and methysergide. *N Engl J Med* 1973; **289:** 236–9.

## Interactions

As for the sedating antihistamines in general, p.421.

**Antidepressants.** For reports suggesting that cyproheptadine can reduce the effectiveness of *SSRIs,* see under Fluoxetine, p.296.

## Pharmacokinetics

After absorption from the gastrointestinal tract, cyproheptadine hydrochloride undergoes almost complete metabolism. Metabolites are excreted principally in the urine as conjugates, and also in the faeces.

## Uses and Administration

Cyproheptadine, a piperidine derivative, is a sedating antihistamine with antimuscarinic, serotonin-antagonist, and calcium-channel blocking actions. It is used as the hydrochloride for the symptomatic relief of allergic conditions including urticaria and angioedema (p.423), rhinitis (p.422) and conjunctivitis (p.421), and in pruritic skin disorders (p.422). Other uses include the management of migraine (p.422). Cyproheptadine hydrochloride is given as the sesquihydrate although doses are expressed in terms of the anhydrous substance. Anhydrous cyproheptadine hydrochloride 10 mg is approximately equivalent to 11 mg of cyproheptadine hydrochloride sesquihydrate.

For allergic conditions and pruritus the dose in adults is initially 4 mg three times daily by mouth, adjusted as necessary. The average dose requirement is 12 to 16 mg daily in three or four divided doses, but up to 32 mg daily may occasionally be necessary. The dose for children aged 2 to 6 years is 2 mg two or three times daily increasing to a maximum of 12 mg daily and for children aged 7 to 14 years, 4 mg two or three times daily up to a maximum of 16 mg daily. Cyproheptadine is not recommended in debilitated elderly patients.

A dose of 4 mg is used for both prophylaxis and treatment of migraine and other vascular headaches and may be repeated after 30 minutes; patients who respond usually obtain relief with 8 mg, and this dose should not be exceeded within a 4- to 6-hour period. A maintenance dose of 4 mg may be given every 4 to 6 hours.

Other cyproheptadine salts that have been given by mouth include the acetylaspartate, aspartate, cyclamate, orotate, acefyllinate (7-theophyllineacetate), and the pyridoxal phosphate salt (dihexazine).

**Abdominal migraine.** Cyproheptadine has been tried in the treatment of children with abdominal migraine (see Pizotifen, p.470).

**Angina pectoris.** Cyproheptadine was used successfully to treat 2 patients with Prinzmetal's angina (p.813) refractory to standard treatment with calcium-channel blockers and nitrates.[1] Serotonin is an important endocrine mediator of coronary vasospasm and the beneficial effects of cyproheptadine were attributed to its activity as a serotonin antagonist.

1. Schecter AD, *et al.* Refractory Prinzmetal angina treated with cyproheptadine. *Ann Intern Med* 1994; **121:** 113–14.

**Appetite disorders.** Cyproheptadine has been widely used as an appetite stimulant, including for anorexia nervosa and cachexia (see under Megestrol, p.1558), but in the long-term appears to have little value in producing weight gain and such use is no longer generally recommended. There has been concern that cyproheptadine was being promoted and used inappropriately as an appetite stimulant in some developing countries.[1]

1. Anonymous. Cyproheptadine: no longer promoted as an appetite stimulant. *WHO Drug Inf* 1994; **8:** 66.

**Carcinoid syndrome.** The management of carcinoid tumours (p.504) is largely symptomatic. Cyproheptadine hydrochloride, a serotonin antagonist, has had limited success in relieving symptoms such as diarrhoea but somatostatin analogues may now be preferred.[1] It has been used successfully with fenclonine, aprotinin, methylprednisolone, and antibacterials to prevent complications arising from release of tumour metabolites during hepatic embolisation, a procedure sometimes used to relieve the symptoms of carcinoid syndrome.[2] There have been a few reports of tumour regression, in addition to symptomatic control, after treatment of carcinoid tumours with cyproheptadine.[3,4]

1. Caplin ME, *et al.* Carcinoid tumour. *Lancet* 1998; **352:** 799–805.
2. Maton PN, *et al.* Role of hepatic arterial embolisation in the carcinoid syndrome. *BMJ* 1983; **287:** 932–5. Correction to dosage. ibid.; 1664.
3. Harris AL, Smith IE. Regression of carcinoid tumour with cyproheptadine. *BMJ* 1982; **285:** 475.
4. Leitner SP, *et al.* Partial remission of carcinoid tumor in response to cyproheptadine. *Ann Intern Med* 1989; **111:** 760–1.

**Serotonin syndrome.** Cyproheptadine has been successfully used to treat the serotonin syndrome (p.313) in patients who have developed the syndrome following overdoses involving serotonergic drugs or who have had their antidepressant therapy changed without an adequate wash-out period.[1,2]

1. Lappin RI, Auchincloss EL. Treatment of the serotonin syndrome with cyproheptadine. *N Engl J Med* 1994; **331:** 1021–2.
2. McDaniel WW. Serotonin syndrome: early management with cyproheptadine. *Ann Pharmacother* 2001; **35:** 870–3.

**Sexual dysfunction.** Cyproheptadine has been tried in the management of sexual dysfunction induced by SSRIs (see Effects on Sexual Function under Fluoxetine, p.293) but may possibly reduce the effectiveness of the SSRI.

## Preparations

***BP 2003:*** Cyproheptadine Tablets;
***USP 27:*** Cyproheptadine Hydrochloride Syrup; Cyproheptadine Hydrochloride Tablets.

**Proprietary Preparations** (details are given in Part 3)
***Austral.:*** Periactin; ***Austria:*** Periactin; ***Belg.:*** Periactin; ***Braz.:*** Periatin; Preptin; ***Canad.:*** Periactin; ***Chile:*** Viternum; ***Denm.:*** Periactin; ***Fr.:*** Periactine; ***Ger.:*** Peritol; ***Hong Kong:*** Cyprogin; Periactin†; ***India:*** Ciplactin; Peritol; Practin; ***Irl.:*** Periactin; ***Ital.:*** Periactin; ***Mex.:*** Viternum; ***Neth.:*** Periactin; ***NZ:*** Periactin; ***Port.:*** Periactin†; Supersan†; Trimetabol; Viternum; ***S.Afr.:*** Periactin; ***Spain:*** Klarivitina; Periactin; Viternum; ***Swed.:*** Periactin; ***Switz.:*** Periactin; ***Thai.:*** Cyheptine; Cyprogin; Cyprono; Cyprosian; Periactin; Polytab; ***UK:*** Periactin; ***USA:*** Periactin†.

**Multi-ingredient:** ***Arg.:*** Apetitol Forte; Ciprocort; Ciprovit Calcio; Ciprovit Energizante; Ciprovit Magnesico; Mikesan; Nipiol; Potencil; Sudevil Vita; ***Braz.:*** Apevitin BC; Ativit†; Bonapetit†; Cobactin; Cobaglobal; Cobavital; Periatin BC†; Periavita†; Trimetabol; ***Chile:*** Apetrol; Grisetin Con Carnitina; Orodina; Peracon; Revil; Rodepan; Viternum Vitaminado; ***Hong Kong:*** Lybovit†; Petina Compound; Tres Orix Forte; ***Ital.:*** Carpantin; ***Mex.:*** Ciprodexol; Ciprolisina; Pangavit Pediatrico; ***Spain:*** Actilevol Orex†; Anti Anorex Triple; Childrevit; Covitasa B12; Desarrol; Enoton; Glotone; Medenorex; Pantobamin; Pranzo; Stolina; Tonico Juventus; Tres Orix Forte; Trimetabol; Troforex Pepsico; Vita Menal.

---

# Deptropine Citrate *(BANM, rINNM)*

Citrato de deptropina; Deptropini Citras; Dibenzheptropine Citrate. (1*R*,3*r*,5*S*)-3-(10,11-Dihydro-5*H*-dibenzo[*a*,*d*]cyclohepten-5-yloxy)tropane dihydrogen citrate.

$C_{23}H_{27}NO,C_6H_8O_7$ = 525.6.

*CAS — 604-51-3 (deptropine); 2169-75-7 (deptropine citrate).*
*ATC — R06AX16.*

**Pharmacopoeias.** In *Eur.* (see p.vi).

**Ph. Eur. 5.0** (Deptropine Citrate). A white or almost white, microcrystalline powder. Very slightly soluble in water and in dehydrated alcohol; practically insoluble in dichloromethane. A saturated solution in water has a pH of 3.7 to 4.5. Protect from light.

**Profile**

Deptropine citrate is a sedating antihistamine (p.419) with a marked antimuscarinic action. It was given by mouth mainly in the treatment of respiratory-tract disorders.

## Desloratadine *(BAN, USAN, rINN)*

Descarboethoxyloratadine; Desloratadina; Sch-34117. 8-Chloro-6,11-dihydro-11-(4-piperidylidene)-5*H*-benzo[5,6]cyclohepta[1,2-*b*]pyridine.

$C_{19}H_{19}ClN_2$ = 310.8.

*CAS — 100643-71-8.*

*ATC — R06AX27.*

**Profile**

Desloratadine, the major, active metabolite of loratadine (p.436), is a non-sedating antihistamine. Desloratadine is used in the symptomatic relief of allergic conditions including rhinitis (p.422) and chronic urticaria (p.423).

Desloratadine is given by mouth in a dose of 5 mg once daily. Children aged 2 to 5 years may be given 1.25 mg once daily and those aged 6 to 11 years may be given 2.5 mg once daily.

For dosage in hepatic or renal impairment, see below.

◊ References.

1. McClellan K, Jarvis B. Desloratadine. *Drugs* 2001; **61:** 789–96.
2. Simons FER, ed. Desloratadine: clinical pharmacokinetics of a novel $H_1$ receptor antagonist. *Clin Pharmacokinet* 2002; **41** (suppl 1): 1–44.
3. Limon L, Kockler DR. Desloratadine: a nonsedating antihistamine. *Ann Pharmacother* 2003; **37:** 237–46. Correction. *ibid.*; 454.

**Administration in hepatic or renal impairment.** The US manufacturer recommends that patients with hepatic or renal impairment should be given desloratadine 5 mg on alternate days initially.

**Pregnancy.** The UK manufacturers do not recommend the use of desloratadine in pregnancy. For a discussion of the use of loratadine in pregnancy, see under Adverse Effects and Precautions, p.436.

**Preparations**

**Proprietary Preparations** (details are given in Part 3)

***Arg.:*** Aerius; Azomyr; ***Belg.:*** Aerius; ***Braz.:*** Desalex; ***Canad.:*** Aerius; ***Chile:*** Aerius; Neoclaritine; ***Denm.:*** Aerius; ***Fin.:*** Aerius; ***Fr.:*** Aerius; ***Ger.:*** Aerius; ***Gr.:*** Aerius; ***Hong Kong:*** Aerius; ***India:*** Deslor; ***Irl.:*** Neoclarityn; ***Ital.:*** Azomyr; ***Neth.:*** Aerius; ***Norw.:*** Aerius; ***NZ:*** Claramax; ***Port.:*** Aerius; Azomyr; ***S.Afr.:*** Deselex; ***Singapore:*** Aerius; ***Spain:*** Aerius; ***Swed.:*** Aerius; ***Switz.:*** Aerius; ***Thai.:*** Aerius; ***UK:*** Neoclarityn; ***USA:*** Clarinex.

# Dimenhydrinate *(BAN, rINN)*

Chloranautine; Dimenhidrinato; Dimenhydrinatum; Diphenhydramine Teoclate; Diphenhydramine Theoclate. The diphenhydramine salt of 8-chlorotheophylline .

$C_{17}H_{21}NO,C_7H_7ClN_4O_2$ = 470.0.

*CAS — 523-87-5.*

*ATC — R06AA02.*

**Pharmacopoeias.** In *Chin., Eur.* (see p.vi), *Jpn, Pol.,* and *US.*

**Ph. Eur. 5.0** (Dimenhydrinate). A white, crystalline powder or colourless crystals. M.p. 102° to 106°. Slightly soluble in water; freely soluble in alcohol. A saturated solution in water has a pH of 7.1 to 7.6.

**USP 27** (Dimenhydrinate). A white, odourless, crystalline powder. Slightly soluble in water; freely soluble in alcohol and in chloroform; sparingly soluble in ether.

**Incompatibility.** Dimenhydrinate has been reported to be incompatible in solution with a wide range of compounds; those most likely to be encountered include: aminophylline, glycopyrronium bromide, hydrocortisone sodium succinate, hydroxyzine hydrochloride, meglumine adipiodone, some phenothiazines, and some soluble barbiturates.

## Adverse Effects and Precautions

As for the sedating antihistamines in general, p.419.

**Effects on the eyes.** Dimenhydrinate 100 mg, given at 4-hourly intervals for 3 doses, was found to affect colour discrimination, night vision, reaction time, and stereopsis.[1]

1. Luria SM, *et al.* Effects of aspirin and dimenhydrinate (Dramamine) on visual processes. *Br J Clin Pharmacol* 1979; **7:** 585–93.

**Porphyria.** Dimenhydrinate has been associated with acute attacks of porphyria and is considered unsafe in porphyric patients.

**Pregnancy.** For discussion of the use of antihistamines in pregnancy, including a suggestion of a relationship between cardiovascular defects or inguinal hernia and dimenhydrinate exposure, see p.420.

## Interactions

As for the sedating antihistamines in general, p.421.

## Uses and Administration

Dimenhydrinate, a monoethanolamine derivative, is a sedating antihistamine with antimuscarinic and significant sedative effects. It is used mainly as an antiemetic in the prevention and treatment of motion sickness (p.422). It is also used for the symptomatic treatment of nausea and vertigo caused by Ménière's disease and other vestibular disturbances (p.423).

The usual dose of dimenhydrinate by mouth is 50 to 100 mg, given 3 or 4 times daily. For the prevention of motion sickness, the first dose should be given at least 30 minutes before travelling. Typical doses for children are: 2 to up to 6 years, 12.5 to 25 mg every 6 to 8 hours to a maximum of 75 mg daily (in some countries lower doses of 6.25 to 12.5 mg are given two or three times daily); 6 to 12 years, 25 to 50 mg every 6 to 8 hours to a maximum of 150 mg daily (again lower doses are used in some countries).

Dimenhydrinate may be given parenterally in usual doses of 50 mg, a concentration of 5% being used for intramuscular injection and 0.5% for slow intravenous injection (usually over 2 minutes). Children have been given dimenhydrinate by intramuscular or slow intravenous injection in a dose of 1.25 mg/kg four times daily to a maximum of 300 mg daily.

Dimenhydrinate has also been administered by the rectal route.

## Preparations

***BP 2003:*** Dimenhydrinate Tablets;
***USP 27:*** Dimenhydrinate Injection; Dimenhydrinate Syrup; Dimenhydrinate Tablets.

**Proprietary Preparations** (details are given in Part 3)

***Arg.:*** Dramamine; Marine; ***Austral.:*** Andrumin†; Dramamine; ***Austria:*** Emedyl; Nausex; Travel-Gum; Vertirosan; ***Belg.:*** Dramamine†; Vagomine; ***Braz.:*** Draituss-Ped†; Dramavit; Dramin; ***Canad.:*** Anti-Nauseant; Childrens Motion Sickness Liquid; Dinate; Gravol; Nauseatol; Nausex†; Novo-Dimenate; Travamine; Travel Aid; Travel Tabs†; Travelmate†; Traveltabs; ***Chile:*** Mareamin; ***Fr.:*** Dramamine; Nausicalm; ***Ger.:*** Dimen; Mandros Reise†; Monotrean†; Reisegold; Reisetabletten; RubieMen; Superpep; Vertigo-Vomex; Vomacur; Vomex A; ***Gr.:*** Drimen; Travelgum; Vomex A; ***Hong Kong:*** Dimate; Dimenate; Dramamine†; Gravol; Novomin; Travelgum†; ***India:*** Dramnate; Gravol; ***Irl.:*** Dramamine; ***Israel:*** Dramamine; Travamin; ***Ital.:*** Lomarin; Motozina; Travelgum; Valontan; Xamamina; ***Malaysia:*** Dramamine; Hydrinate; Novomin; Setmenate; ***Mex.:*** Dimetin-F; Dimicaps†; Dramamine; Unitril†; Vomisin; ***Neth.:*** Dramamine; ***NZ:*** Dramamine; ***Port.:*** Dramamine; Enjomin; Travel-Gum†; Viabom; Vomidrine; ***Singapore:*** Dimenate; Dramamine; Novomin†; ***Spain:*** Biodramina; Cinfamar; Contramareo; Travel Well; ***Swed.:*** Amosyt; ***Switz.:*** Antemin; Demodenal†; Dramamine; Reise Superpep-K†; Superpep†; Trawell; ***Thai.:*** Denim; Dimeno; Dramamine; Gravol; Motivan; Nausamine; Navamed†; Navamin; Vominar; ***UAE:*** Dizinil; ***UK:*** Dramamine†; ***USA:*** Calm-X; Dimetabs; Dinate; Dramamine; Dramanate; Dymenate; Hydrate; Triptone.

**Multi-ingredient:** ***Austral.:*** Travacalm; ***Austria:*** Neo-Emedyl; Synkapton; Vertirosan Vitamin $B_6$; ***Belg.:*** R Calm + B6†; ***Braz.:*** Dramavit B6; Dramin B-6; Dramin B-6 DL; Nausicalm; Nausilon B6†; ***Canad.:*** Gravergol; ***Fr.:*** Mercalm; ***Ger.:*** Arlevert; Migraeflux N; Migraeflux orange N; ***Hong Kong:*** Gravergol; Rhinocap; ***Spain:*** Acetuber; Biodramina Cafeina; Cinfamar Cafeina; Saldeva; Salvarina; Sin Mareo x 4; ***Switz.:*** Agorhino; Antemin compositum; Demodenal compositum†; Dragees contre les maux de voyage no 537; Dramamine-compositum; Medramine retard†; Medramine-$B_6$ Rectocaps†; Rhinocap; Viaggio†.

## Dimetindene Maleate *(BANM, rINNM)*

Dimethindene Maleate *(USAN)*; Dimethpyrindene Maleate; Dimethylpyrindene Maleate; Dimetindeni Maleas; Maleato de dimetindeno; NSC-107677; Su-6518. *NN*-Dimethyl-2-{3-[1-(2-pyridyl)ethyl]-1*H*-inden-2-yl}ethylamine hydrogen maleate.

$C_{20}H_{24}N_2,C_4H_4O_4$ = 408.5.

*CAS — 5636-83-9 (dimetindene); 3614-69-5 (dimetindene maleate).*

*ATC — D04AA13; R06AB03.*

**Pharmacopoeias.** In *Eur.* (see p.vi).

**Ph. Eur. 5.0** (Dimetindene Maleate). A white to almost white, crystalline powder. Slightly soluble in water; soluble in methyl alcohol. Protect from light.

**Profile**

Dimetindene maleate, an alkylamine derivative, is a sedating antihistamine (p.419); it is mildly sedative and is reported to have mast-cell stabilising properties. It is used for the symptomatic relief of allergic conditions including urticaria and angioedema (p.423) and rhinitis (p.422), and in pruritic skin disorders (p.422). It is also used in compound preparations for the symptomatic treatment of coughs and the common cold (p.421).

Dimetindene maleate is given by mouth in a dose of 1 to 2 mg three times daily; modified-release preparations are also available. It may also be given by the intravenous route. Dimetindene maleate is applied topically as a 0.1% gel or lotion although, as with other antihistamines, there is a risk of sensitisation. It is used in a strength of 0.025% in compound nasal preparations.

**Preparations**

**Proprietary Preparations** (details are given in Part 3)

***Austria:*** Fenistil; ***Belg.:*** Fenistil; ***Ger.:*** Fenistil; ***Gr.:*** Fenistil; ***India:*** Foristal; ***Israel:*** Fenistil; ***Ital.:*** Fenistil; ***Neth.:*** Fenistil; ***Norw.:*** Fenistil; ***Port.:*** Fenistil; Neostil; ***Spain:*** Fenistil; ***Switz.:*** Fenistil; ***Thai.:*** Fenistil.

**Multi-ingredient:** ***Arg.:*** Vibragel; ***Austria:*** Trimedil; Vibrocil; ***Belg.:*** Vibrocil; ***Braz.:*** Gripen; Trimedal; ***Ger.:*** Vibrocil; ***Hong Kong:*** Vibrocil; ***Israel:*** Vibrocil NF; ***Ital.:*** Vibrocil; ***Port.:*** Vibrocil; ***S.Afr.:*** Vibrocil; Vibrocil-S; ***Switz.:*** Vibrocil.

## Dimetotiazine Mesilate *(BANM, rINNM)*

Dimethothiazine Mesylate; Fonazine Mesylate *(USAN)*; IL-6302 (dimetotiazine); Mesilato de dimetotiazina; 8599-RP (dimetotiazine). 10-(2-Dimethylaminopropyl)-*NN*-dimethylphenothiazine-2-sulphonamide methanesulphonate.

$C_{19}H_{25}N_3O_2S_2,CH_3SO_3H$ = 487.7.

*CAS — 7456-24-8 (dimetotiazine); 7455-39-2 (dimetotiazine mesilate).*

*ATC — N02CX05.*

**Profile**

Dimetotiazine mesilate, a phenothiazine derivative, is a sedating antihistamine (p.419). It has been used for the symptomatic relief of hypersensitivity reactions, in pruritic skin disorders, and in the management of headaches including migraine.

**Preparations**

**Proprietary Preparations** (details are given in Part 3)

***Mex.:*** Migristene; ***Spain:*** Migristene†.

# Diphenhydramine *(BAN, rINN)*

Benzhydramine; Difenhidramina. 2-Benzhydryloxy-*NN*-dimethylethylamine.

$C_{17}H_{21}NO$ = 255.4.

*CAS — 58-73-1.*

*ATC — D04AA32; R06AA02.*

**Pharmacopoeias.** In *Jpn.*

## Diphenhydramine Citrate *(BANM, rINNM)*

Benzhydramine Citrate; Citrato de difenhidramina.

$C_{17}H_{21}NO,C_6H_8O_7$ = 447.5.

*CAS — 88637-37-0.*

*ATC — D04AA32; R06AA02.*

**Pharmacopoeias.** In *US.*

**USP 27** (Diphenhydramine Citrate). Store in airtight containers. Protect from light.

## Diphenhydramine Di(acefyllinate) *(rINNM)*

Benzhydramine Di(acefyllinate); Bietanautine; Difenhidramina, di(acefilinato) de; Diphenhydramine Di(acephyllinate). Diphenhydramine bis(theophyllin-7-ylacetate).

$C_{17}H_{21}NO,2C_9H_{10}N_4O_4$ = 731.8.

*CAS — 6888-11-5.*

*ATC — D04AA32; R06AA02.*

NOTE. The name Etanautine has been applied both to diphenhydramine monoacefyllinate and to ethylbenzhydramine, an antimuscarinic formerly used in the symptomatic treatment of parkinsonism.

## Diphenhydramine Hydrochloride *(BANM, rINNM)*

Benzhydramine Hydrochloride; Dimedrolum; Diphenhydramini Hydrochloridum; Diphenhydraminium Chloride; Hidrocloruro de difenhidramina.

$C_{17}H_{21}NO,HCl$ = 291.8.

*CAS — 147-24-0.*

*ATC — D04AA32; R06AA02.*

**Pharmacopoeias.** In *Chin., Eur.* (see p.vi), *Jpn, Pol.,* and *US. Jpn* also includes Diphenhydramine Tannate.

**Ph. Eur. 5.0** (Diphenhydramine Hydrochloride). A white or almost white, crystalline powder. Very soluble in water; freely soluble in alcohol. A 5% solution in water has a pH of 4.0 to 6.0. Protect from light.

**USP 27** (Diphenhydramine Hydrochloride). A white, odourless, crystalline powder. It slowly darkens on exposure to light. Soluble 1 in 1 of water, 1 in 2 of alcohol and of chloroform, and 1 in 50 of acetone; very slightly soluble in ether and in benzene. Its solutions are neutral to litmus. Store in airtight containers. Protect from light.

**Incompatibility.** Diphenhydramine hydrochloride has been reported to be incompatible with amphotericin B, cefmetazole sodium, cefalotin sodium, hydrocortisone sodium succinate, some soluble barbiturates, some contrast media, and solutions of alkalis or strong acids.

## Adverse Effects and Precautions

As for the sedating antihistamines in general, p.419.

**Abuse.** Reports of the abuse of diphenhydramine hydrochloride.

1. Anonymous. Is there any evidence that Benylin syrup is addictive? *BMJ* 1979; **1:** 459.

2. Smith SG, Davis WM. Nonmedical use of butorphanol and diphenhydramine. *JAMA* 1984; **252:** 1010.
3. Feldman MD, Behar M. A case of massive diphenhydramine abuse and withdrawal from use of the drug. *JAMA* 1986; **255:** 3119–20.
4. de Nesnera AP. Diphenhydramine dependence: a need for awareness. *J Clin Psychiatry* 1996; **57:** 136–7.
5. Dinndorf PA, *et al.* Risk of abuse of diphenhydramine in children and adolescents with chronic illnesses. *J Pediatr* 1998; **133:** 293–5.


**Extrapyramidal disorders.** Reports of dystonic extrapyramidal reactions to diphenhydramine.


1. Lavenstein BL, Cantor FK. Acute dystonia: an unusual reaction to diphenhydramine. *JAMA* 1976; **236:** 291.
2. Santora J, Rozek S. Diphenhydramine-induced dystonia. *Clin Pharm* 1989; **8:** 471.
3. Roila F, *et al.* Diphenhydramine and acute dystonia. *Ann Intern Med* 1989; **111:** 92–3.


**Overdosage.** In an evaluation of 136 cases, one fatal, of intoxication with diphenhydramine, the plasma concentration was correlated with frequency or extent of symptoms.[1] The most common symptom was impaired consciousness; psychosis, seizures, antimuscarinic symptoms such as mydriasis, tachycardia, and tachyarrhythmias, and respiratory failure were also observed. The positive association between dose and frequency and severity of symptoms was confirmed in a more recent study;[2] it was also found that severe symptoms were more likely to occur when 1 g or more of diphenhydramine had been taken.

There have been reports[3,4] of rhabdomyolysis as an effect of oral diphenhydramine overdosage. The liberal application of a lotion containing diphenhydramine produced acute delirium with visual and auditory hallucinations in a 9-year-old boy[5] and similar effects were seen in 3 children with varicella-zoster infection following the topical application of diphenhydramine (2 of these children also received oral diphenhydramine).[6]


1. Köppel C, Tenczer J. Clinical symptomatology of diphenhydramine overdose: an evaluation of 136 cases in 1982 to 1985. *Clin Toxicol* 1987; **25:** 53–70.
2. Radovanovic D, *et al.* Dose-dependent toxicity of diphenhydramine overdose. *Hum Exp Toxicol* 2000; **19:** 489–95.
3. Hampel G, *et al.* Myoglobinuric renal failure due to drug-induced rhabdomyolysis. *Hum Toxicol* 1983; **2:** 197–203.
4. Haas CE, *et al.* Rhabdomyolysis and acute renal failure following an ethanol and diphenhydramine overdose. *Ann Pharmacother* 2003; **37:** 538–42.
5. Filloux F. Toxic encephalopathy caused by topically applied diphenhydramine. *J Pediatr* 1986; **108:** 1018–20.
6. Chan CYJ, Wallander KA. Diphenhydramine toxicity in three children with varicella-zoster infection. *DICP Ann Pharmacother* 1991; **25:** 130–2.


**Porphyria.** Diphenhydramine has been associated with acute attacks of porphyria and is considered unsafe in porphyric patients.

**Pregnancy.** A pregnant woman who was receiving diphenhydramine hydrochloride 150 mg daily for a pruritic rash gave birth to an infant who developed diarrhoea and generalised tremulousness 5 days later.[1] The delay in appearance of withdrawal symptoms was considered to be due to reduced activity of glucuronyl conjugating enzymes in the first few days of life.

For discussion of the use of antihistamines in pregnancy, including a suggestion of a relationship between inguinal hernia or genito-urinary malformations and diphenhydramine exposure, see p.420. See also under Interactions, below, for a report of perinatal death possibly associated with temazepam and diphenhydramine.


1. Parkin DE. Probable Benadryl withdrawal manifestations in a new-born infant. *J Pediatr* 1974; **85:** 580.


## Interactions

As for the sedating antihistamines in general, p.421. Diphenhydramine inhibits the cytochrome P450 isoenzyme CYP2D6 that is partly responsible for the metabolism of some beta blockers including metoprolol and the antidepressant venlafaxine.

**Benzodiazepines.** There has been a report[1] suggesting that a reduction in *temazepam* metabolism caused by diphenhydramine may have contributed to perinatal death after ingestion of these drugs by the mother.


1. Kargas GA, *et al.* Perinatal mortality due to interaction of diphenhydramine and temazepam. *N Engl J Med* 1985; **313:** 1417–18.


## Pharmacokinetics

Diphenhydramine hydrochloride is well absorbed from the gastrointestinal tract, although high first-pass metabolism appears to affect systemic availability. Peak plasma concentrations are achieved about 1 to 4 hours after oral administration. Diphenhydramine is widely distributed throughout the body including the CNS. It crosses the placenta and has been detected in breast milk. Diphenhydramine is highly bound to plasma proteins. Metabolism is extensive. Diphenhydramine is excreted mainly in the urine as metabolites; little is excreted as unchanged drug. The elimination half-life has been reported to range from 2.4 to 9.3 hours.

◊ References.


1. Glazko AJ, *et al.* Metabolic disposition of diphenhydramine. *Clin Pharmacol Ther* 1974; **16:** 1066–76.
2. Paton DM, Webster DR. Clinical pharmacokinetics of $H_1$-receptor antagonists (the antihistamines). *Clin Pharmacokinet* 1985; **10:** 477–97 (includes studies indicating a correlation between plasma concentrations and both antihistaminic and sedative effects).
3. Simons KJ, *et al.* Diphenhydramine: pharmacokinetics and pharmacodynamics in elderly adults, young adults, and children. *J Clin Pharmacol* 1990; **30:** 665–71.
4. Scavone JM, *et al.* Pharmacokinetics and pharmacodynamics of diphenhydramine 25 mg in young and elderly volunteers. *J Clin Pharmacol* 1998; **38:** 603–9.


## Uses and Administration

Diphenhydramine, a monoethanolamine derivative, is a sedating antihistamine with antimuscarinic and pronounced sedative properties. It is used for the symptomatic relief of allergic conditions including urticaria and angioedema (p.423), rhinitis (p.422) and conjunctivitis (p.421), and in pruritic skin disorders (p.422). It is also used for its antiemetic properties in the treatment of nausea and vomiting (p.422), particularly in the prevention and treatment of motion sickness (when it should be given at least 30 minutes before travelling), and in the treatment of vertigo of various causes (p.423). Diphenhydramine is used for its antimuscarinic properties in the control of parkinsonism (p.1196) and drug-induced extrapyramidal disorders (p.677) (although the possibility that diphenhydramine itself may cause extrapyramidal symptoms should be remembered). Diphenhydramine has pronounced central sedative properties and may be used as a hypnotic in the short-term management of insomnia (p.422). It is a common ingredient of compound preparations for symptomatic treatment of coughs and the common cold (p.421). It may also be given in combination preparations containing analgesics, particularly paracetamol. Diphenhydramine may be used parenterally as an adjunct in the emergency treatment of anaphylactic shock (p.421) or when oral therapy is not feasible.

For most indications, diphenhydramine hydrochloride is given by mouth in usual doses of 25 to 50 mg three or four times daily. The dose for children is 6.25 to 25 mg three or four times daily, or a total daily dose of 5 mg/kg may be given in divided doses. The maximum dose in adults and children is 300 mg daily. A dose of 20 to 50 mg may be used as a hypnotic in adults and children over 12 years old.

When oral therapy is not feasible, diphenhydramine hydrochloride may be given by deep intramuscular injection or by intravenous injection using concentrations of 1% or 5%. Usual doses are 10 to 50 mg, although doses of 100 mg have been given. No more than 400 mg should be given in 24 hours. Children may be given 5 mg/kg daily in divided doses to a maximum of 300 mg in 24 hours. Diphenhydramine hydrochloride is applied topically, usually in preparations containing 1 to 2% although, as with other antihistamines, there is a risk of sensitisation.

Diphenhydramine citrate is given by mouth in a dose of 76 mg at night in combination preparations for its hypnotic action. Diphenhydramine di(acefyllinate) is given by mouth as an antiemetic for the prevention and treatment of motion sickness and of nausea and vomiting; the usual dose is 90 to 135 mg. Other diphenhydramine salts that have been used include the polistirex, the salicylate, and the tannate administered by mouth, the methylbromide given rectally, and the metilsulfate applied topically.

Dimenhydrinate (p.431) is diphenhydramine teoclate and mefenidramium metilsulfate is diphenhydramine methylsulfomethylate.

## Preparations

***BP 2003:*** Diphenhydramine Oral Solution;
***USP 27:*** Acetaminophen and Diphenhydramine Citrate Tablets; Acetaminophen, Diphenhydramine Hydrochloride, and Pseudoephedrine Hydrochloride Tablets; Diphenhydramine and Pseudoephedrine Capsules; Diphenhydramine Hydrochloride Capsules; Diphenhydramine Hydrochloride Elixir; Diphenhydramine Hydrochloride Injection.

**Proprietary Preparations** (details are given in Part 3)
***Arg.:*** Benadryl; Benadryl Antialergico; Drepatil; Histaler; Klonadryl; Mudantos H; ***Austral.:*** Nytol†; Unisom; ***Austria:*** Calmaben; Dermodrin; Dibondrin; Histaxin; Noctor; Prurex; Sleepia; ***Belg.:*** Azaron; Benylin Antihistaminicum; Diphamine; Nuicalm; Nustasium; R Calm; ***Braz.:*** Difenidrin; ***Canad.:*** Aller-Aide; Allerdryl; Allergy Elixir; Allergy Formula; Allergy Tablets; Allernix; Benadryl; Calmex; Children's Allergy Formula; Dormex; Dormiphen; Insomnal; Jack & Jill Bedtime; Nytol; Simply Sleep; Sleep Aid; Sleep-Eze D; Sominex; Unisom; Unisom-C†; ***Chile:*** Jaquedryl; Pasifen; Somol; ***Fin.:*** Benylan†; ***Fr.:*** Butix; Nautamine; ***Ger.:*** Benadryl N; Dolestan; Dormigoa N†; Dormutil N; Emesan; Halbmond; Hevert-Dorm; Lupovalin†; Medapur†; nervo OPT N; Nytol†; Pellit Insektenstich, Pellit Sonnenallergie†; Pheramin N†; ratioAllerg; S.8; Sedativum-Hevert; Sediat; Sedopretten; Sedovegan Novo†; Sleepia; Vivinox Stark†; ***Gr.:*** Benadryl; ***Hong Kong:*** Benadryl; Calox; Hydramine Cream; Unisom; ***India:*** Benadryl; Dimiril; ***Ital.:*** Allergan; Benadryl†; Nytol; ***Mex.:*** Bionaril; Difedram†; Difenhistat†; Nytol; Sontedril†; Tzoali; Ulcoid; Unisom; ***NZ:*** Unisom; ***Port.:*** Benaderma; Codilergi; ***S.Afr.:*** Betasleep; Nytol†; Sleepeze PM; ***Singapore:*** Benocten; Paxidorm; ***Spain:*** Benadryl; Dormplus†; Neosayomol; Nytol; Sonodor; ***Swed.:*** Benylan†; Desentol; ***Switz.:*** Bedorma; Benocten; Comprimes somniferes "S"; Comprimes somniferes formule 533†; Dobacen; Neo-Synodorm†; Sleepia; ***Thai.:*** Benadryl; ***UAE:*** Amydramine II; ***UK:*** Adult Chesty Cough; Aller-Eze†; Child Chesty Cough; Dreemon; Histergan; Mandalyn Paediatric; Nightcalm; Nytol; Paxidorm; Sleep Aid; Sleepeaze; ***USA:*** 40 Winks; Aler-Dryl; AllerMax; Banophen Allergy; Benadryl; Benadryl Childrens Allergy; Benadryl Itch; Compoz Night-time Sleep Aid; Dermamycin; Diphen AF; Diphen Cough†; Diphenhist; Dormin; Dytan; Dytuss; Genahist; Hyrexin†; Maximum Strength Sleepinal; Maximum Strength Unisom SleepGels; Miles Nervine; MouthKote P/R; Nytol; Scot-Tussin Allergy; Siladryl; Silphen; Simply Sleep; Sleep-Ettes D; Sleepeze 3†; Sleepwell 2-nite; Snooze Fast; Sominex; Tusstat; Twilite; Uni-Bent Cough†.

**Multi-ingredient:** numerous preparations are listed in Part 3.

---

## Diphenylpyraline Hydrochloride *(BANM, rINNM)*

Hidrocloruro de difenilpiralina. 4-Benzhydryloxy-1-methylpiperidine hydrochloride.

$C_{19}H_{23}NO,HCl$ = 317.9.

*CAS — 147-20-6 (diphenylpyraline); 132-18-3 (diphenylpyraline hydrochloride).*

*ATC — R06AA07.*

**Pharmacopoeias.** In *Br.*

**BP 2003** (Diphenylpyraline Hydrochloride). A white or almost white, odourless or almost odourless powder. Freely soluble in water, in alcohol, and in chloroform; practically insoluble in ether.

### Adverse Effects and Precautions

As for the sedating antihistamines in general, p.419.

### Interactions

As for the sedating antihistamines in general, p.421.

### Pharmacokinetics

◊ References.


1. Graham G, Bolt AG. Half-life of diphenylpyraline in man. *J Pharmacokinet Biopharm* 1974; **2:** 191–5 (ranged from 24 to 40 hours).


### Uses and Administration

Diphenylpyraline hydrochloride, a piperidine derivative, is a sedating antihistamine with antimuscarinic and significant sedative properties.

It has been given for the symptomatic relief of allergic conditions including rhinitis (p.422), and in pruritic skin disorders (p.422). It has also been used in compound preparations for the symptomatic treatment of coughs and the common cold (p.421).

Diphenylpyraline hydrochloride has been given by mouth in a dose of up to 6 mg daily in 3 or 4 divided doses. Diphenylpyraline and diphenylpyraline hydrochloride have been applied topically although, as with other antihistamines, there is a risk of sensitisation.

Diphenylpyraline teoclate is piprinhydrinate (p.439).

### Preparations

**Proprietary Preparations** (details are given in Part 3)
***Ger.:*** Arbid N; ***Mex.:*** Flumil.

**Multi-ingredient:** ***Austria:*** Arbid; Astronautal; Eucillin; Prurimix; Tropoderm; ***Belg.:*** Bicold; Rhinamide†; Tri-Cold†; ***Braz.:*** Ornatrol; Pelmic†; ***Canad.:*** Biohisdex DM†; Biohisdine DM†; Creo-Rectal; Emercreme No 4†; Sinugex†; Vito Bronches; ***Ger.:*** Perdiphen; Proctospre; Tempil N; Topoderm N†; ***India:*** Eskold; Eskold Expectorant; ***S.Afr.:*** Actophlem; Eskornade†; Solphyllex; Theophen Comp; ***Switz.:*** Arbid; Proctospre†; ***UK:*** Eskornade†.

---

## Doxylamine Succinate *(BANM, rINNM)*

Doxylamine Hydrogen Succinate; Doxylamini Hydrogenosuccinas; Doxylaminium Succinate; Histadoxylamine Succinate; Succinato de doxilamina. *NN*-Dimethyl-2-[α-methyl-α-(2-pyridyl)benzyloxy]ethylamine hydrogen succinate.

$C_{17}H_{22}N_2O,C_4H_6O_4$ = 388.5.

*CAS — 469-21-6 (doxylamine); 562-10-7 (doxylamine succinate).*

*ATC — R06AA09.*

**Pharmacopoeias.** In *Eur.* (see p.vi) and *US.*

**Ph. Eur. 5.0** (Doxylamine Hydrogen Succinate; Doxylamine Succinate BP 2003). A white or almost white powder. Very soluble in water; freely soluble in alcohol.

**USP 27** (Doxylamine Succinate). A white or creamy-white powder having a characteristic odour. Soluble 1 in 1 of water, 1 in 2 of alcohol and of chloroform, and 1 in 370 of ether; very slightly soluble in benzene. Protect from light.

### Adverse Effects and Precautions

As for the sedating antihistamines in general, p.419. The controversy surrounding the use in pregnancy of combination products of doxylamine is discussed on p.420.

**Overdosage.** In an evaluation of 109 cases of intoxication with doxylamine,[1] no correlation was found between the amount ingested or plasma concentration and the frequency or extent of symptoms. The most common symptom was impaired consciousness. Psychotic behaviour, seizures, and antimuscarinic symptoms such as tachycardia and mydriasis were also observed. Rhabdomyolysis occurred in one patient and was accompanied by transient impairment of renal function. The same group commented[2] that rhabdomyolysis had been noted in 7 of 442 cases of doxylamine overdosage, with an associated rise in plasma creatine kinase and myoglobinuria, and suggested that doxylamine has a direct toxic effect on striated muscle.

1. Köppel C, *et al.* Poisoning with over-the-counter doxylamine preparations: an evaluation of 109 cases. *Hum Toxicol* 1987; **6:** 355–9.
2. Köppel C, *et al.* Rhabdomyolysis in doxylamine overdose. *Lancet* 1987; **i:** 442–3.

### Interactions

As for the sedating antihistamines in general, p.421.

### Pharmacokinetics

Following oral administration of doxylamine succinate peak plasma concentrations occur after 2 to 3 hours. An elimination half-life of about 10 hours has been reported.

◊ References.

1. Friedman H, *et al.* Clearance of the antihistamine doxylamine: reduced in elderly men but not in elderly women. *Clin Pharmacokinet* 1989; **16:** 312–16.

### Uses and Administration

Doxylamine succinate, a monoethanolamine derivative, is a sedating antihistamine with antimuscarinic and pronounced sedative effects.

Doxylamine succinate is given by mouth for the symptomatic relief of hypersensitivity reactions, in pruritic skin disorders (p.422), as a hypnotic in the short-term treatment of insomnia (p.422), and as an ingredient of compound preparations for symptomatic treatment of coughs and the common cold (p.421).

In general it is no longer used in the management of nausea and vomiting of early pregnancy (see p.420 for the controversy that has surrounded the use in pregnancy of combination products of doxylamine).

Doses of up to 25 mg of doxylamine succinate have been given every 4 to 6 hours to a maximum of 150 mg daily. The usual hypnotic dose is 25 mg at night.

### Preparations

***USP 27:*** Acetaminophen, Dextromethorphan Hydrobromide, Doxylamine Succinate, and Pseudoephedrine Hydrochloride Oral Solution; Doxylamine Succinate Syrup; Doxylamine Succinate Tablets.

**Proprietary Preparations** (details are given in Part 3)
***Austral.:*** Dozile; Restavit; ***Canad.:*** Unisom-2; ***Chile:*** Calmex; Dorminoctil; Nocpaz; Trimepaz; Zarcop; ***Fr.:*** Donormyl; Lidene; Mereprine†; Noctyl; ***Ger.:*** Gittalun; Hewedormir doxyl intens; Hoggar N; Mereprine; Munleit; SchlafTabs; Sedaplus; ***India:*** Doxinate; ***Israel:*** Unisom; ***NZ:*** Dozile; ***S.Afr.:*** Equi-Sleep; Restwel; Somnil; ***Spain:*** Donormyl†; Dormidina; Duebien†; Unisom†; ***Switz.:*** Sanalepsi N; ***USA:*** Unisom SleepTabs.

**Multi-ingredient:** ***Austral.:*** Analgesic/Calmative; Codalgin Plus; Dimetapp Cold, Cough & Flu; Dolased Analgesic Calmative; Dolased Day/Night Pain Relief; Fiorinal; Mersyndol; Ordov Migradol†; Panadeine Plus†; Panalgesic; SBPA Analgesic/Calmative†; ***Austria:*** Wick Erkaltungs-Saft fur die Nacht; Wick Hustensaft; ***Belg.:*** Pholco-Mereprine; ***Braz.:*** Bisolvon Complex†; Bronco-Ped†; Broncolex; EMS Expectorante; Hytos Plus; Night Time Liquigels†; Revenil; Revenil Dospan; Revenil Expectorante†; Silencium; Silomat Plus; ***Canad.:*** Calmydone; Dalmacol; Diclectin; Mercodol with Decapryn†; Mersyndol with Codeine; Night-Time; Night-time Cold & Flu; NyQuil; Tylenol Sinus (Nighttime Relief); ***Ger.:*** Paedisup; Wick Medinait; ***Irl.:*** Syndol; ***Ital.:*** Vicks Medinait; ***NZ:*** Dimetapp Cold, Cough & Flu Day & Night; Mersyndol; Pryndette; ***Port.:*** Nausefe; ***S.Afr.:*** Abflex; Acurate; Adco-Dol; Asic; B-Dol; Betapyn; Cepacol; Forpyn; Lenapain; Nethaprin Dospan; Nethaprin Expectorant; Nomopain; Paxidal; Pynclear; Pynstop; Sedapain; Sedinol; Syndette†; Syndol; Tensopyn†; Xerotens; ***Spain:*** Cariban; Upsadex†; Vicks Medinait; ***Switz.:*** Vicks Medinait; ***UK:*** Boots Tension Headache Relief†; Painex; Propain Plus; Syndol; Vicks Medinite; ***USA:*** Alka-Seltzer Plus Night-Time Cold; All-Nite Cold Formula; Genite; Night Time Cold/Flu Relief; Nite Time Cold Formula; NyQuil Hot Therapy; NyQuil Nighttime Cold/Flu; Nytcold Medicine; Vicks NyQuil LiquiCaps; Vicks NyQuil Multi-Symptom Cold Flu Relief.

## Ebastine *(BAN, USAN, rINN)*

Ebastina; Ebastinum; LAS-W-090; W-090. 4′-*tert*-Butyl-4-[4-(diphenylmethoxy)piperidino]butyrophenone.

$C_{32}H_{39}NO_2$ = 469.7.
*CAS — 90729-43-4.*
*ATC — R06AX22.*

**Pharmacopoeias.** In *Eur.* (see p.vi).

**Ph. Eur. 5.0** (Ebastine). A white or almost white crystalline powder. M.p. about 86°. Practically insoluble in water; very soluble in dichloromethane; sparingly soluble in methyl alcohol. Protect from light.

### Profile

Ebastine, a piperidine derivative, is a non-sedating antihistamine (p.419) with a long duration of action. It does not have significant sedative or antimuscarinic actions.

Ebastine is given by mouth for the symptomatic relief of allergic conditions including rhinitis (p.422) and in pruritic skin disorders (p.422). The usual dose is 10 to 20 mg daily. It is also used with a decongestant such as pseudoephedrine hydrochloride.

◊ References.

1. Murris-Espin M, *et al.* Comparison of efficacy and safety of cetirizine and ebastine in patients with perennial allergic rhinitis. *Ann Allergy Asthma Immunol* 1998; **80:** 399–403.
2. Luria X. Comparative clinical studies with ebastine: efficacy and tolerability. *Drug Safety* 1999; **21** (suppl 1): 63–7.
3. Hurst M, Spencer CM. Ebastine: an update of its use in allergic disorders. *Drugs* 2000; **59:** 981–1006.

### Preparations

**Proprietary Preparations** (details are given in Part 3)
***Arg.:*** Ebastel; ***Belg.:*** Estivan; ***Braz.:*** Bastilong†; Ebastel; ***Chile:*** Ebastel; ***Denm.:*** Kestine; ***Fin.:*** Kestine; ***Fr.:*** Kestin; ***Hong Kong:*** Kestine; ***Israel:*** Kestine†; ***Ital.:*** Clever; ***Jpn:*** Ebastel; ***Mex.:*** Evastel; ***Neth.:*** Kestine; ***Norw.:*** Kestine; ***Port.:*** Kestine; ***S.Afr.:*** Kestine; ***Singapore:*** Kestine; ***Spain:*** Bactil; Bromselon†; Busidril; Ebastel; ***Swed.:*** Kestine.

**Multi-ingredient:** ***Arg.:*** Ebastel D; ***Braz.:*** Ebastel D; ***Spain:*** Rino Ebastel; Rinobactil; Tundrax†.

## Embramine Hydrochloride *(BANM, rINNM)*

Embraminium Chloratum; Hidrocloruro de embramina; Mebrophenhydramine Hydrochloride; Mebrophenhydraminium Chloratum. 2-(4-Bromo-α-methylbenzhydryloxy)-*NN*-dimethylethylamine hydrochloride.

$C_{18}H_{22}BrNO,HCl$ = 384.7.
*CAS — 3565-72-8 (embramine); 13977-28-1 (embramine hydrochloride).*

### Profile

Embramine hydrochloride, a monoethanolamine derivative, is a sedating antihistamine (p.419). Embramine hydrochloride and embramine teoclate have been administered by mouth for their antihistamine and antiemetic properties.

### Preparations

**Proprietary Preparations** (details are given in Part 3)
***India:*** Mebryl.

## Emedastine Fumarate *(BANM, rINNM)*

AL-3432A; Emedastine Difumarate *(USAN)*; Fumarato de emedastina; KB-2413; KG-2413; LY-188695. 1-(2-Ethoxyethyl)-2-(hexahydro-4-methyl-1*H*-1,4-diazepin-1-yl)benzimidazole fumarate (1:2).

$C_{17}H_{26}N_4O,2C_4H_4O_4$ = 534.6.
*CAS — 87233-61-2 (emedastine); 87233-62-3 (emedastine fumarate).*
*ATC — S01GX06.*

**Pharmacopoeias.** In *US.*

**USP 27** (Emedastine Difumarate). A white to faintly yellow crystalline powder. Soluble in water. pH of a 0.2% solution in water is between 3.0 and 4.5. Store in airtight containers. Protect from light.

### Adverse Effects and Precautions

As for the antihistamines in general, p.419.

Ocular corneal infiltrates, local irritation, photophobia, rhinitis, and headaches have been reported following use of emedastine eye drops. Treatment should be discontinued if corneal infiltrates develop.

### Pharmacokinetics

Emedastine is absorbed from the gastrointestinal tract, peak plasma concentrations being attained about 3 hours after administration by mouth. It is mainly metabolised in the liver to two primary metabolites 5- and 6-hydroxyemedastine which are excreted in the urine along with a small amount of unchanged drug. Small amounts of emedastine are absorbed following application to the eye. The elimination half-life is reported to be 7 hours after an oral dose and 10 hours following topical use.

### Uses and Administration

Emedastine is an antihistamine. It is instilled twice daily as the fumarate as eye drops containing the equivalent of 0.05% of emedastine for the symptomatic relief of allergic conjunctivitis (p.421). It is also given by mouth in usual doses of 2 to 4 mg of the fumarate daily in two divided doses for allergic rhinitis (p.422), urticaria (p.423), and pruritic skin disorders (p.422).

### Preparations

***USP 27:*** Emedastine Ophthalmic Solution.

**Proprietary Preparations** (details are given in Part 3)
***Austria:*** Emadine; ***Belg.:*** Emadine; ***Braz.:*** Emadine; ***Canad.:*** Emadine; ***Denm.:*** Emadine; ***Fin.:*** Emadine; ***Fr.:*** Emadine; ***Ger.:*** Emadine; ***Gr.:*** Emadine; ***Hong Kong:*** Emadine; ***Irl.:*** Emadine; ***Israel:*** Emadine; ***Ital.:*** Emadine; ***Jpn:*** Daren; ***Norw.:*** Emadine; ***Port.:*** Emadine; ***S.Afr.:*** Emadine; ***Spain:*** Emadine; ***Swed.:*** Emadine; ***Switz.:*** Emadine; ***Thai.:*** Emadine; ***UK:*** Emadine; ***USA:*** Emadine.

## Epinastine Hydrochloride *(rINNM)*

Hidrocloruro de epinastina; WAL-801-Cl. 3-Amino-9,13b-dihydro-1*H*-dibenz[*c,f*]imidazo[1,5-*a*]azepine hydrochloride.

$C_{16}H_{15}N_3,HCl$ = 285.8.
*CAS — 80012-43-7 (epinastine).*
*ATC — R06AX24; S01GX10.*

### Profile

Epinastine hydrochloride is an antihistamine (p.419) reported to have no significant sedative activity. It has been given by mouth in the management of asthma, allergic rhinitis, and pruritic skin disorders. It is also used twice daily as eye drops, usually in a concentration of 0.05%, in the symptomatic relief of allergic conjunctivitis.

### Preparations

**Proprietary Preparations** (details are given in Part 3)
***Arg.:*** Flurinol; ***Braz.:*** Talerc; ***Chile:*** Flurinol; ***Jpn:*** Alesion; ***Mex.:*** Flurinol; ***UK:*** Relestat; ***USA:*** Elestat.

## Fexofenadine Hydrochloride

*(BANM, USAN, rINNM)*

Hidrocloruro de fexofenadina; MDL-16455A; Terfenadine Carboxylate Hydrochloride. (±)-*p*-{1-Hydroxy-4-[4-(hydroxydiphenylmethyl)-piperidino]butyl}-α-methylhydratropic acid hydrochloride.

$C_{32}H_{39}NO_4,HCl$ = 538.1.
*CAS — 138452-21-8.*
*ATC — R06AX26.*

### Adverse Effects and Precautions

As for the non-sedating antihistamines in general, p.419.

**Arrhythmias.** A 67-year-old man suffered syncope after taking fexofenadine 180 mg daily for two months.[1] His ECG showed an abnormally prolonged QT interval which shortened once fexofenadine was discontinued, although the interval tended to be long even without drug therapy. Nonetheless rechallenge was positive. The manufacturers of fexofenadine have commented[2] that the patient was at risk of developing arrhythmias before taking the drug.

The ECG effects of fexofenadine have been studied[3] in normal subjects and administration of doses of up to 480 mg daily [4 times the recommended dose for seasonal allergic rhinitis] did not prolong the QT interval. See also p.420.

1. Pinto YM, *et al.* QT lengthening and life-threatening arrhythmias associated with fexofenadine. *Lancet* 1999; **353:** 980.
2. Giraud T. QT lengthening and arrhythmias associated with fexofenadine. *Lancet* 1999; **353:** 2072.
3. Pratt CM, *et al.* Cardiovascular safety of fexofenadine HCl. *Am J Cardiol* 1999; **83:** 1451–4.

**Breast feeding.** No adverse effects have been observed in breast-feeding infants whose mothers were receiving fexofenadine, and the American Academy of Pediatrics[1] considers that it is therefore usually compatible with breast feeding.

See also under Adverse Effects and Precautions, in Terfenadine, p.441.

1. American Academy of Pediatrics. The transfer of drugs and other chemicals into human milk. *Pediatrics* 2001; **108:** 776–89. Correction. *ibid.*; 1029. Also available at: http://aappolicy.aappublications.org/cgi/content/full/pediatrics%3b108/3/776 (accessed 08/04/04)

### Interactions

As for the non-sedating antihistamines in general, p.421.

Plasma concentrations of fexofenadine have been increased after the concomitant administration of erythromycin or ketoconazole, but, unlike terfenadine, the manufacturer has stated that this was not associated with adverse effects on the QT interval.

Antacids containing aluminium and magnesium hydroxide have reduced the absorption of fexofenadine.

### Pharmacokinetics

Fexofenadine is rapidly absorbed after oral administration with peak plasma concentrations being reached in 2 to 3 hours. It is about 60 to 70% bound to plasma proteins. About 5% of the total dose is metabolised, mostly by the intestinal mucosa, with only 0.5 to 1.5% of the dose undergoing hepatic biotransformation by the cytochrome P450 system. Elimination half-life of about 14 hours has been reported although this may be prolonged in patients with renal impairment. Excretion is mainly in the faeces with only 10% being present in the urine. Fexofenadine does not appear to cross the blood-brain barrier.

Fexofenadine is a metabolite of terfenadine and as such has been detected in breast milk after the administration of terfenadine.

◊ References.

1. Russell T, *et al.* Pharmacokinetics, pharmacodynamics, and tolerance of single- and multiple-dose fexofenadine hydrochloride in healthy male volunteers. *Clin Pharmacol Ther* 1998; **64:** 612–21.

## Uses and Administration

Fexofenadine, an active metabolite of terfenadine (p.441), is a non-sedating antihistamine. It does not possess significant sedative or antimuscarinic actions. Fexofenadine is used as the hydrochloride in the symptomatic relief of allergic conditions including seasonal allergic rhinitis (p.422) and chronic urticaria (p.423).

Fexofenadine hydrochloride is given by mouth in a dose of 120 mg daily either as a single dose or in two divided doses. Higher doses of 180 mg daily are recommended in the UK for chronic idiopathic urticaria and in the USA for seasonal allergic rhinitis. Children aged 6 to 11 years may be given fexofenadine in doses of 30 mg twice daily for the treatment of allergic rhinitis or urticaria.

For dosage in renal impairment, see below.

◊ References.

1. Markham A, Wagstaff AJ. Fexofenadine. *Drugs* 1998; **55:** 269–74.
2. Simpson K, Jarvis B. Fexofenadine: a review of its use in the management of seasonal allergic rhinitis and chronic idiopathic urticaria. *Drugs* 2000; **59:** 301–21.

**Administration in renal impairment.** The US manufacturer recommends that initial doses of fexofenadine hydrochloride in patients with renal impairment should be halved to 60 mg once daily.

### Preparations

**Proprietary Preparations** (details are given in Part 3)
***Arg.:*** Alerfedine; Allegra; Fexofen; ***Austral.:*** Telfast; ***Austria:*** Telfast; ***Belg.:*** Telfast; ***Braz.:*** Allegra; ***Canad.:*** Allegra; ***Chile:*** Alexia; Allegra; Fenax; ***Denm.:*** Telfast; ***Fin.:*** Telfast; ***Fr.:*** Telfast; ***Ger.:*** Telfast; ***Hong Kong:*** Telfast; ***India:*** Alernex; Allegra; ***Irl.:*** Telfast; ***Israel:*** Telfast; ***Ital.:*** Kalicet; Telfast; ***Mex.:*** Allegra; ***Neth.:*** Telfast; ***Norw.:*** Telfast; ***NZ:*** Telfast; ***Port.:*** Telfast; ***S.Afr.:*** Telfast; ***Singapore:*** Telfast; ***Spain:*** Telfast; ***Swed.:*** Telfast; ***Switz.:*** Telfast; ***Thai.:*** Telfast; ***UK:*** Telfast; ***USA:*** Allegra.

**Multi-ingredient:** ***Arg.:*** Alerfedine D; Allegra-D; ***Austral.:*** Telfast Decongestant; ***Braz.:*** Allegra-D; ***Canad.:*** Allegra-D; ***Chile:*** Alexia D; Allegra D; ***Hong Kong:*** Telfast-D; ***Mex.:*** Allegra-D; ***NZ:*** Telfast Decongestant; ***USA:*** Allegra-D.

## Flunarizine Hydrochloride *(BANM, USAN, rINNM)*

Flunarizini Dihydrochloridum; Hidrocloruro de flunarizina; R-14950. *trans*-1-Cinnamyl-4-(4,4′-difluorobenzhydryl)piperazine dihydrochloride.

$C_{26}H_{26}F_2N_2,2HCl = 477.4.$

*CAS — 52468-60-7 (flunarizine); 30484-77-6 (flunarizine hydrochloride).*

*ATC — N07CA03.*

**Pharmacopoeias.** In *Chin.* and *Eur.* (see p.vi).

**Ph. Eur. 5.0** (Flunarizine Dihydrochloride). A white or almost white hygroscopic powder. Slightly soluble in water, in alcohol, and in dichloromethane; sparingly soluble in methyl alcohol. Store in airtight containers. Protect from light.

### Adverse Effects and Precautions

As for the sedating antihistamines in general, p.419. Adverse effects also seen with flunarizine include weight gain, extrapyramidal symptoms (sometimes associated with depression), and, rarely, galactorrhoea.

**Extrapyramidal disorders.** Extrapyramidal motor signs (including parkinsonism, orofacial tardive dyskinesia, and akathisia) have been reported in 12 patients given flunarizine 10 to 40 mg daily for between 3 weeks and 15 months; 11 also had mental depression.[1] Partial or complete improvement of symptoms occurred after withdrawal of flunarizine. There have been other reports of similar effects,[2-4] but the association with flunarizine has not always been certain. Some workers have commented that flunarizine is often used in patients at increased risk of depression (migraine and geriatric patients) or extrapyramidal symptoms (geriatric patients)[2,5] or that flunarizine may unmask subclinical idiopathic Parkinson's disease.[5,6]

Extrapyramidal signs, including parkinsonism, have also been associated with the related drug, cinnarizine.[3,4] It has been suggested that such effects may be less likely to occur with cinnarizine than with flunarizine because of its shorter half-life and lower lipophilicity.[3]

1. Chouza C, *et al.* Parkinsonism, tardive dyskinesia, akathisia, and depression induced by flunarizine. *Lancet* 1986; **i:** 1303–4.
2. Meyboom RHB, *et al.* Parkinsonism, tardive dyskinesia, akathisia, and depression induced by flunarizine. *Lancet* 1986; **ii:** 292.
3. Laporte J-R, Capella D. Useless drugs are not placebos: lessons from flunarizine and cinnarizine. *Lancet* 1986; **ii:** 853–4.
4. Laporte J-R, Capella D. Useless drugs are not placebos. *Lancet* 1987; **i:** 1324.
5. Amery W. Side-effects of flunarizine. *Lancet* 1986; **i:** 1497.
6. Benvenuti F, *et al.* Side-effects of flunarizine. *Lancet* 1986; **ii:** 464.

**Porphyria.** Flunarizine hydrochloride is considered to be unsafe in patients with porphyria because it has been shown to be porphyrinogenic in *in-vitro* systems.

### Interactions

As for the sedating antihistamines in general, p.421.

Hepatic enzyme inducers such as carbamazepine, phenytoin, and valproate may interact with flunarizine by increasing its metabolism; an increase in dosage of flunarizine may be required.

### Pharmacokinetics

Flunarizine hydrochloride is well absorbed from the gastrointestinal tract, peak plasma concentrations occurring 2 to 4 hours after oral administration. Flunarizine hydrochloride is very lipophilic and is more than 90% bound to plasma proteins. It appears to undergo extensive metabolism; metabolites are excreted principally in the bile. Flunarizine hydrochloride has an elimination half-life of about 18 days.

### Uses and Administration

Flunarizine is the difluorinated derivative of cinnarizine. It has antihistamine, sedative, and calcium-channel blocking activity. Flunarizine hydrochloride is used for migraine prophylaxis, for vertigo and vestibular disorders, and for peripheral and cerebral vascular disorders. It has also been used as adjunctive antiepileptic therapy in patients refractory to standard regimens.

Flunarizine is given by mouth as the hydrochloride although doses are expressed in terms of the equivalent amount of flunarizine. Flunarizine hydrochloride 11.8 mg is approximately equivalent to 10 mg of flunarizine. The usual dose is 5 to 10 mg daily, usually given at night to minimise the effects of drowsiness.

**Epilepsy.** Flunarizine has demonstrated antiepileptic activity in *animal* models, but the mechanism of action is unclear; calcium entry blockade or an effect on sodium channels has been postulated.[1] Most clinical studies have evaluated its use as adjunctive therapy in epileptic patients with partial seizures resistant to conventional treatment (see p.349). Doses of flunarizine of 15 to 20 mg daily by mouth appeared to provide the best response when given as part of multiple-drug antiepileptic regimens.[1] However, studies using fixed doses of flunarizine have been considered unsatisfactory because of its variable clearance and long elimination half-life. A study using a parallel group design and adjusting doses to achieve a constant plasma concentration of 60 nanograms/mL found flunarizine to have modest antiepileptic efficacy as adjunctive therapy for partial seizures.[2] Even so, others[3] have concluded that the pharmacokinetic profile of flunarizine is too complex for its clinical use as an antiepileptic.

1. Todd PA, Benfield P. Flunarizine: a reappraisal of its pharmacological properties and therapeutic use in neurological disorders. *Drugs* 1989; **38:** 481–99.
2. Pledger GW, *et al.* Flunarizine for treatment of partial seizures: results of a concentration-controlled trial. *Neurology* 1994; **44:** 1830–6.
3. Hoppu K, *et al.* Flunarizine of limited value in children with intractable epilepsy. *Pediatr Neurol* 1995; **13:** 143–7.

**Migraine.** Flunarizine reduces the frequency of migraine attacks in both adult and paediatric patients and is used for the prophylaxis of migraine (p.464) in some countries. Its effects are comparable with several other prophylactic antimigraine drugs, including those generally preferred, pizotifen and propranolol,[1-4] but it is more likely to be reserved for use when first-line drugs have proved to be ineffective or unsuitable. Its mode of action in migraine is unclear; possible mechanisms are inhibition of vasospasm induced by mediators such as serotonin and prostaglandins, inhibition of cellular hypoxia, and improved blood viscosity and erythrocyte deformability. Calcium-channel blocking activity might have a role, but evidence for the efficacy of other calcium-channel blockers in migraine prophylaxis (see Nifedipine, p.971) is less convincing than for flunarizine.

Case reports have indicated benefit with flunarizine in the prophylaxis of the rare disorder of alternating hemiplegia in childhood[5,6] but a subsequent study[7] in 12 children did not produce conclusive findings. A later long-term study[8] reported that 7 of 9 children given flunarizine for up to 5 years for hemiplegia showed a reduction in the duration of attacks, and 3 had a reduction in frequency, but only 1 of these obtained a complete cessation of episodes.

The role of antihistamines in general in the management of migraine is discussed briefly on p.422.

1. Todd PA, Benfield P. Flunarizine: a reappraisal of its pharmacological properties and therapeutic use in neurological disorders. *Drugs* 1989; **38:** 481–99.
2. Andersson K-E, Vinge E. β-Adrenoceptor blockers and calcium antagonists in the prophylaxis and treatment of migraine. *Drugs* 1990; **3:** 355–73.
3. Soelberg Sørensen P, *et al.* Flunarizine versus metoprolol in migraine prophylaxis: a double-blind, randomized parallel group study of efficacy and tolerability. *Headache* 1991; **31:** 650–7.
4. Gawel MJ, *et al.* Comparison of the efficacy and safety of flunarizine to propranolol in the prophylaxis of migraine. *Can J Neurol Sci* 1992; **19:** 340–5.
5. Casaer P, Azou M. Flunarizine in alternating hemiplegia in childhood. *Lancet* 1984; **ii:** 579.
6. Curatolo P, Cusmai R. Drugs for alternating hemiplegic migraine. *Lancet* 1984; **ii:** 980.
7. Casaer P. Flunarizine in alternating hemiplegia in childhood. An international study in 12 children. *Neuropediatrics* 1987; **18:** 191–5.
8. Silver K, Andermann F. Alternating hemiplegia of childhood: a study of 10 patients and results of flunarizine treatment. *Neurology* 1993; **43:** 36–41.

**Tourette's syndrome.** A small unblinded study[1] involving 7 patients has suggested that flunarizine is more effective than placebo in the treatment of Tourette's syndrome (see Tics, p.664).

1. Micheli F, *et al.* Treatment of Tourette's syndrome with calcium antagonists. *Clin Neuropharmacol* 1990; **13:** 77–83.

**Vertigo.** Antihistamines are the mainstay of the treatment of vertigo (p.423). However, their antimuscarinic side-effects may prove troublesome, particularly in the elderly, and they produce central sedation. Flunarizine is devoid of antimuscarinic properties, although it may produce central sedation.

### Preparations

**Proprietary Preparations** (details are given in Part 3)
***Arg.:*** Bercetina; Coromert; Flufenal; Mondus; Niflucan; Sibelium; Vasculoflex; ***Austria:*** Amalium; Flunarium; Sibelium; ***Belg.:*** Sibelium; ***Braz.:*** Flunarin; Fluvert; Fluzix; Sibelium; Vertix; ***Canad.:*** Sibelium; ***Chile:*** Flerox; Fluxus; Irrigor; Sibelium; Zentralin; ***Denm.:*** Sibelium; ***Fr.:*** Sibelium; ***Ger.:*** Flunavert; Sibelium; ***Hong Kong:*** Fludan; Sibelium; ***India:*** Nomigrain; ***Irl.:*** Sibelium; ***Ital.:*** Flugeral; Flunagen; Fluxarten; Gradient; Issium; Sibelium; Vasculene; ***Malaysia:*** Fludan; Forknow; Sibelium; ***Mex.:*** Axilin; Fasolan; Nafluryl; Sibelium; ***Neth.:*** Sibelium; ***Port.:*** Sibelium; Vasilium; Zinasen; ***S.Afr.:*** Sibelium; ***Singapore:*** Forknow; Narizine; Sibelium; ***Spain:*** Flerudin; Flurpax; Sibelium; ***Switz.:*** Sibelium; ***Thai.:*** Cedelate; Finelium; Floxin; Fludan; Flulium; Flunarium; Flunaza; Flunazine; Fluricin; FNZ†; Hexilium; Liberal; Medilium; Poli-Flunarin; Seabell; Sibelium; Simoyiam; Sobelin; Zelium.

**Multi-ingredient:** ***Arg.:*** Angiolit; CCK Flunarizina; Sibelium Plus; ***Braz.:*** Vertizine D.

## Homochlorcyclizine Hydrochloride *(BANM, rINNM)*

Hidrocloruro de homoclorciclizina. 1-(4-Chlorobenzhydryl)perhydro-4-methyl-1,4-diazepine dihydrochloride.

$C_{19}H_{23}ClN_2,2HCl = 387.8.$

*CAS — 848-53-3 (homochlorcyclizine); 1982-36-1 (homochlorcyclizine hydrochloride).*

**Pharmacopoeias.** In *Jpn.*

### Profile

Homochlorcyclizine hydrochloride, a piperazine derivative, is a sedating antihistamine (p.419) with antimuscarinic and moderate sedative properties. It is used for the symptomatic relief of allergic conditions including urticaria (p.423) and rhinitis (p.422), and in pruritic skin disorders (p.422). It is given by mouth in doses of 10 to 20 mg three times daily.

### Preparations

**Proprietary Preparations** (details are given in Part 3)
***Hong Kong:*** Homoclomin; ***Jpn:*** Homoclomin; ***Thai.:*** Homoclomin.

## Hydroxyzine Embonate *(BANM, rINNM)*

Embonato de hidroxizina; Hydroxyzine Pamoate. 2-{2-[4-(4-Chlorobenzhydryl)piperazin-1-yl]ethoxy}ethanol 4,4′-methylenebis(3-hydroxy-2-naphthoate).

$C_{21}H_{27}ClN_2O_2,C_{23}H_{16}O_6 = 763.3.$

*CAS — 68-88-2 (hydroxyzine); 10246-75-0 (hydroxyzine embonate).*

*ATC — N05BB01.*

**Pharmacopoeias.** In *Jpn* and *US.*

**USP 27** (Hydroxyzine Pamoate). A light yellow, practically odourless powder. Soluble 1 in more than 1000 of water, of chloroform, and of ether, 1 in 700 of alcohol, 1 in 10 of dimethylformamide, and 1 in 3.5 of 10M sodium hydroxide solution; practically insoluble in methyl alcohol. Store in airtight containers.

## Hydroxyzine Hydrochloride *(BANM, rINNM)*

Hidrocloruro de hidroxizina; Hydroxyzini Hydrochloridum.

$C_{21}H_{27}ClN_2O_2,2HCl = 447.8.$

*CAS — 2192-20-3.*

*ATC — N05BB01.*

**Pharmacopoeias.** In *Eur.* (see p.vi), *Jpn*, and *US.*

**Ph. Eur. 5.0** (Hydroxyzine Hydrochloride). A white or almost white, crystalline, hygroscopic powder. Freely soluble in water and in alcohol; very slightly soluble in acetone. Store in airtight containers. Protect from light.

**USP 27** (Hydroxyzine Hydrochloride). A white, odourless, powder. Soluble 1 in 1 of water, 1 in 4.5 of alcohol, and 1 in 13 of chloroform; slightly soluble in acetone; practically insoluble in ether. Store in airtight containers.

**Incompatibility.** Hydroxyzine hydrochloride has been reported to be incompatible with aminophylline, benzylpenicillin salts, chloramphenicol sodium succinate, dimenhydrinate, doxorubicin hydrochloride (in a liposomal formulation), thioridazine, and some soluble barbiturates.

**Stability.** A mixture of hydroxyzine hydrochloride, chlorpromazine hydrochloride, and pethidine hydrochloride stored in glass or plastic syringes was found[1] to be stable for 366 days at 4° and 25°.

1. Conklin CA, *et al.* Stability of an analgesic-sedative combination in glass and plastic single-dose syringes. *Am J Hosp Pharm* 1985; **42:** 339–42.

### Adverse Effects and Precautions

As for the sedating antihistamines in general, p.419.

Intramuscular injection of hydroxyzine has been reported to cause marked local discomfort. Intravenous administration has been associated with haemolysis.

**Amputation.** Accidental intra-arterial injection of hydroxyzine has led to necrosis of the extremity requiring amputation of the digits of the affected limb.[1]

1. Hardesty WH. Inadvertent intra-arterial injection. *JAMA* 1970; **213:** 872.

**Arrhythmias.** ECG abnormalities, particularly alterations in T-waves, were associated with anxiolytic doses of hydroxyzine hydrochloride and were similar to those produced by thioridazine and tricyclic antidepressants.[1]

1. Hollister LE. Hydroxyzine hydrochloride: possible adverse cardiac interactions. *Psychopharmacol Comm* 1975; **1:** 61–5.

**Effects on sexual function.** A 32-year-old man experienced prolonged penile erections (priapism) after taking two separate doses of hydroxyzine for a skin rash.[1] It was suggested that the effect might be due to a hydroxyzine metabolite that was found to be structurally similar to a metabolite of trazodone, a drug known to induce penile erections.

1. Thavundayil JX. *et al.* Prolonged penile erections induced by hydroxyzine: possible mechanism of action. *Neuropsychobiology* 1994; **30:** 4–6.

**Effects on the skin.** Four children given hydroxyzine hydrochloride for restlessness developed a fixed drug eruption of the penis.[1] All recovered on drug withdrawal and subsequently had positive rechallenges.

1. Cohen HA, *et al.* Fixed drug eruption of the penis due to hydroxyzine hydrochloride. *Ann Pharmacother* 1997; **31:** 327–9.

**Liver disorders.** A study[1] has suggested that hydroxyzine should only be administered once daily for the relief of pruritus in patients with primary biliary cirrhosis. The mean serum elimination half-lives of hydroxyzine and its metabolite cetirizine in 8 patients with primary biliary cirrhosis were 36.6 and 25.0 hours respectively.

1. Simons FER, *et al.* The pharmacokinetics and pharmacodynamics of hydroxyzine in patients with primary biliary cirrhosis. *J Clin Pharmacol* 1989; **29:** 809–15.

**Porphyria.** Hydroxyzine has been associated with acute attacks of porphyria and is considered unsafe in porphyric patients.

### Interactions

As for the sedating antihistamines in general, p.421.

### Pharmacokinetics

Hydroxyzine is rapidly absorbed from the gastrointestinal tract and is metabolised. Metabolites include cetirizine (p.427), which has antihistaminic activity. An elimination half-life of about 20 hours has been reported.

◊ References.

1. Paton DM, Webster DR. Clinical pharmacokinetics of $H_1$-receptor antagonists (the antihistamines). *Clin Pharmacokinet* 1985; **10:** 477–97.

**Liver disorders.** For reference to a prolonged half-life of hydroxyzine in patients with primary biliary cirrhosis, see under Adverse Effects and Precautions, above.

### Uses and Administration

Hydroxyzine, a piperazine derivative, is a sedating antihistamine with antimuscarinic and significant sedative properties; it is also an antiemetic. Its main use is as an anxiolytic (p.663). It is also used as an adjunct to pre- and postoperative medication (see Anaesthesia, p.421) and in the management of pruritus (p.422) and urticaria (p.423) and has been used as an adjunct to opioid analgesia in the management of cancer pain (p.5).

Hydroxyzine may be given orally as the hydrochloride or the embonate; doses are expressed in terms of the equivalent amount of hydroxyzine hydrochloride. Hydroxyzine embonate 170 mg is approximately equivalent to 100 mg of hydroxyzine hydrochloride.

The usual doses by mouth in adults are: 50 to 100 mg four times daily for the short-term management of anxiety; for pruritus an initial dose of 25 mg given at night, increased if necessary to 25 mg three or four times daily; and 50 to 100 mg for pre- or postoperative sedation. For pruritus in children over 6 years the initial dose is 15 to 25 mg daily increased if necessary to 50 to 100 mg daily in divided doses; for children 6 months to 6 years old the initial dose is 5 to 15 mg daily increased if necessary to 50 mg daily in divided doses. The pre- or postoperative sedative dose in children is 600 micrograms/kg. Dosage should be reduced in patients with hepatic or renal impairment, see below.

Hydroxyzine hydrochloride may also be given by deep intramuscular injection. For prompt control of anxiety or agitation in adults 50 to 100 mg is injected intramuscularly initially, and the dose may be repeated every four to six hours as required. For other indications when oral administration is not practical, the intramuscular dose is 25 to 100 mg for adults and 1.1 mg/kg for children. Hydroxyzine should not be given by intravenous injection since haemolysis may result.

**Administration in hepatic or renal impairment.** In patients with hepatic impairment, the UK manufacturers recommend a 33% reduction in the total daily dose of hydroxyzine by mouth. In patients with moderate or severe renal impairment, a dose reduction of 50% is recommended.

### Preparations

***USP 27:*** Hydroxyzine Hydrochloride Injection; Hydroxyzine Hydrochloride Syrup; Hydroxyzine Hydrochloride Tablets; Hydroxyzine Pamoate Capsules; Hydroxyzine Pamoate Oral Suspension.

**Proprietary Preparations** (details are given in Part 3)
***Arg.:*** Ataraxone; Hidroxina; Hyderax; ***Austral.:*** Atarax†; ***Austria:*** Atarax; ***Belg.:*** Atarax; ***Braz.:*** Hixizine†; Prurizin; Zinalerg†; ***Canad.:*** Atarax; Multipax†; ***Chile:*** Dalun; Fasarax; Nexit; ***Denm.:*** Atarax; ***Fin.:*** Atarax; ***Fr.:*** Atarax; ***Ger.:*** AH 3 N; Atarax; Elroquil N; ***Gr.:*** Atarax; Iremofar; ***Hong Kong:*** Atarax; ***India:*** Atarax; ***Irl.:*** Atarax†; ***Israel:*** Otarex; ***Ital.:*** Atarax; ***Malaysia:*** Atarax; ***Mex.:*** Atarax†; ***Neth.:*** Atarax; Navicalm; ***Norw.:*** Atarax; ***NZ:*** Serecid; ***Port.:*** Atarax; ***S.Afr.:*** Aterax; ***Singapore:*** Atarax; Phymorax; ***Spain:*** Atarax; ***Swed.:*** Atarax; ***Switz.:*** Atarax; ***Thai.:*** Abacus; Antizine; Atano; Atarax; Cerax; Darax; Drazine; Hadarax; Histan; Hizin; Honsa; Hydroxin; Masarax; Med-Xyzarax; Polizine; Postarax; R-Rax; Taraxin; Trandrozine; Unamine; ***UK:*** Atarax; Ucerax; ***USA:*** Atarax; Vistaril; Vistazine†.

**Multi-ingredient:** ***Austria:*** Diligan; ***Belg.:*** Vesparax†; ***Braz.:*** Marax; ***Ger.:*** Diligan; ***India:*** Marax; ***Neth.:*** Vesparax†; ***Port.:*** Diligan; Vesparax; ***S.Afr.:*** Geratar†; Vesparax†; ***Spain:*** Calmoplex; Difilina Asmorax†; Dolodens; Somatarax†; ***Swed.:*** Histilos†; ***Switz.:*** Hexafene†; ***USA:*** Hydrophed; Marax; Theomax DF.

---

## Isothipendyl Hydrochloride *(BANM, rINNM)*

Hidrocloruro de isotipendil. *NN*-Dimethyl-1-(pyrido[3,2-*b*][1,4]-benzothiazin-10-ylmethyl)ethylamine hydrochloride.

$C_{16}H_{19}N_3S,HCl$ = 321.9.
*CAS — 482-15-5 (isothipendyl); 1225-60-1 (isothipendyl hydrochloride).*
*ATC — D04AA22; R06AD09.*

### Profile

Isothipendyl hydrochloride, an azaphenothiazine derivative, is an antihistamine (p.419) that has been applied topically for hypersensitivity and pruritic skin disorders although as with any antihistamine there is a risk of sensitisation. It has also been administered by mouth and by the rectal route.

### Preparations

**Proprietary Preparations** (details are given in Part 3)
***Arg.:*** Actapront; ***Belg.:*** Andantol†; ***Braz.:*** Andantol; ***Fr.:*** Apaisyl†; Istamyl†; Sedermyl; ***Israel:*** Thiodantol; ***Ital.:*** Calmogel; ***Mex.:*** Andantol.

---

## Levocabastine Hydrochloride

*(BANM, USAN, rINNM)*

Hidrocloruro de levocabastina; Levocabastini Hydrochloridum; R-50547. (−)-*trans*-1-[*cis*-4-Cyano-4-(*p*-fluorophenyl)cyclohexyl]-3-methyl-4-phenylisonipecotic acid hydrochloride.

$C_{26}H_{29}FN_2O_2,HCl$ = 457.0.
*CAS — 79516-68-0 (levocabastine); 79547-78-7 (levocabastine hydrochloride); 79449-98-2 (cabastine).*
*ATC — R01AC02; S01GX02.*

NOTE. Cabastine *(rINN)* is the racemate of levocabastine.

**Pharmacopoeias.** In *Eur.* (see p.vi).

**Ph. Eur. 5.0** (Levocabastine Hydrochloride). A white or almost white powder. Practically insoluble in water; slightly soluble in alcohol and in a 0.2% solution of sodium hydroxide; sparingly soluble in methyl alcohol. Protect from light.

### Adverse Effects and Precautions

As for the antihistamines in general, p.419. The most common adverse effects reported with levocabastine eye drops are transient stinging and burning of the eyes, urticaria, dyspnoea, drowsiness, and headache. Following nasal administration headache, nasal irritation, somnolence, and fatigue have been noted. The use of levocabastine nasal spray is not recommended in those with significant renal impairment.

### Pharmacokinetics

Levocabastine is absorbed following both nasal and ocular administration. Systemic availability has been estimated at 60 to 80% after nasal administration and 30 to 60% after ocular application. However absolute peak plasma concentrations are low. Plasma protein binding is about 55%. An elimination half-life of 35 to 40 hours has been reported for all routes of delivery. Elimination of levocabastine is primarily renal with 70% excreted as unchanged drug and 10% as an inactive acetylglucuronide metabolite; the remaining 20% is excreted unchanged in the faeces.

Trace amounts of levocabastine have been found in breast milk after ocular and nasal administration.

◊ References.

1. Heykants J, *et al.* The pharmacokinetic properties of topical levocabastine: a review. *Clin Pharmacokinet* 1995; **29:** 221–30.

### Uses and Administration

Levocabastine, a piperidine derivative, is a long-acting and potent antihistamine with a rapid onset of action. Levocabastine hydrochloride equivalent to 0.05% levocabastine is used topically twice daily as eye drops or as nasal spray in the treatment of allergic conjunctivitis (p.421) and rhinitis (p.422), respectively in adults and children aged 9 years and over. The frequency of the dose in both conditions may be increased to 3 or 4 times daily if necessary. In conjunctivitis it is recommended that treatment should be discontinued if there is no improvement within 3 days.

◊ References.

1. Noble S, McTavish D. Levocabastine: an update of its pharmacology, clinically efficacy and tolerability in the topical treatment of allergic rhinitis and conjunctivitis. *Drugs* 1995; **50:** 1032–49.
2. Doughty MJ. Levocabastine, a topical ocular antihistamine available as a pharmacy medicine – a literature review. *Pharm J* 2002; **268:** 367–70.

### Preparations

**Proprietary Preparations** (details are given in Part 3)
***Arg.:*** Histimet; ***Austral.:*** Livostin; ***Austria:*** Livostin; ***Belg.:*** Livostin; ***Braz.:*** Livostin; ***Canad.:*** Livostin; ***Denm.:*** Livostin; ***Fin.:*** Livostin; ***Fr.:*** Levophta; ***Ger.:*** Levophta; Livocab; ***Gr.:*** Livostin; ***Israel:*** Livostin; ***Ital.:*** Levostab; Livocab; Livostin; ***Jpn:*** Livostin; ***Mex.:*** Livostin; ***Neth.:*** Livocab; ***Norw.:*** Livostin; ***NZ:*** Livostin; ***S.Afr.:*** Livostin; ***Spain:*** Bilina; Livocab; ***Swed.:*** Livostin; ***Switz.:*** Livostin; ***Thai.:*** Livostin; ***UK:*** Livostin; ***USA:*** Livostin.

**Multi-ingredient:** ***Chile:*** Livostin.

---

## Levocetirizine *(BAN, rINN)*

Levocetirizina. (2-{4-[(*R*)-*p*-Chloro-α-phenylbenzyl]-1-piperazinyl}ethoxy)acetic acid.

$C_{21}H_{25}ClN_2O_3$ = 388.9.
*CAS — 130018-77-8.*
*ATC — R06AE09.*

## Levocetirizine Hydrochloride *(BANM, rINNM)*

$C_{21}H_{25}ClN_2O_3,2HCl$ = 461.8.
*CAS — 130018-87-0.*
*ATC — R06AE09.*

### Profile

Levocetirizine is the *R*-enantiomer of cetirizine (p.427) and is used similarly, as the hydrochloride, for the symptomatic relief of allergic conditions including rhinitis (p.422) and chronic urticaria (p.423).

In adults and children aged 6 years and over, levocetirizine hydrochloride is given by mouth in a dose of 5 mg once daily.

The dose should be reduced in patients with renal impairment, see below.

◊ Reviews.

1. Scheinfeld N. The new antihistamines—desloratadine and levocetirizine: a review. *J Drugs Dermatol* 2002; **1:** 311–16.
2. Tillement JP, *et al.* Compared pharmacological characteristics in humans of racemic cetirizine and levocetirizine, two histamine H1-receptor antagonists. *Biochem Pharmacol* 2003; **66:** 1123–6.

**Administration in renal impairment.** The dosage of levocetirizine should be reduced in patients with renal impairment according to creatinine clearance (CC):

- CC 30 to 49 mL/minute: 5 mg every other day
- CC 10 to 29 mL/minute: 5 mg every 3 days
- CC less than 10 mL/minute: contra-indicated.

### Preparations

**Proprietary Preparations** (details are given in Part 3)
***Denm.:*** Xyzal; ***Fin.:*** Xyzal; ***Fr.:*** Xyzall; ***Ger.:*** Xusal; ***Hong Kong:*** Xyzal; ***Irl.:*** Xyzal; ***Port.:*** Xyzal; ***UK:*** Xyzal.

---

## Loratadine (BAN, USAN, rINN)

Loratadina; Sch-29851. Ethyl 4-(8-chloro-5,6-dihydro-11H-benzo[5,6]cyclohepta[1,2-b]pyridin-11-ylidene)piperidine-1-carboxylate.

$C_{22}H_{23}ClN_2O_2$ = 382.9.

*CAS — 79794-75-5.*

*ATC — R06AX13.*

**Pharmacopoeias.** In *Pol.* and *US.*

**USP 27** (Loratadine). A white to off-white powder. Insoluble in water; freely soluble in acetone, in chloroform, in methyl alcohol, and in toluene.

### Adverse Effects and Precautions

As for the non-sedating antihistamines in general, p.419.

**Breast feeding.** No adverse effects have been observed in breast-feeding infants whose mothers were receiving loratadine, and the American Academy of Pediatrics[1] considers that it is therefore usually compatible with breast feeding. However, the UK manufacturers recommend that loratadine should not be used in breast-feeding mothers.

A study[2] in 6 lactating women reported that about 0.03% of a single 40-mg oral dose of loratadine was distributed into breast milk over 48 hours as loratadine and its active metabolite, desloratadine.

1. American Academy of Pediatrics. The transfer of drugs and other chemicals into human milk. *Pediatrics* 2001; **108:** 776–89. Correction. *ibid.*; 1029. Also available at: http://aappolicy.aappublications.org/cgi/content/full/pediatrics%3b108/3/776 (accessed 08/04/04)
2. Hilbert J, *et al.* Excretion of loratadine in human breast milk. *J Clin Pharmacol* 1988; **28:** 234–9.

**Effects on the liver.** Two patients[1] developed severe necroinflammatory liver injury after receiving loratadine 10 mg daily for allergic rhinitis. Although both recovered after drug withdrawal, one patient required a liver transplantation and recovery was prolonged.

The manufacturers note that abnormal hepatic function including jaundice, hepatitis, and hepatic necrosis have been reported rarely.

1. Schiano TD, *et al.* Subfulminant liver failure and severe hepatotoxicity caused by loratadine use. *Ann Intern Med* 1996; **125:** 738–40.

**Pregnancy.** The UK manufacturers do not recommend the use of loratadine in pregnancy.

Analysis of data collected by the Swedish Medical Birth Registry between 1994 and 2001 revealed 15 cases of hypospadias among a cohort of 2780 newborns exposed to loratadine during the first trimester of pregnancy.[1] The authors noted that the individual risk for having an infant with hypospadias after loratadine use is small (less than 1%) and the attributive risk of extra cases in the population is low. The US Centers for Disease Control and Prevention has also analysed data from the National Birth Defects Prevention study;[2] they found no increase in the risk of second- or third-degree hypospadias in the infants of women who used loratadine in early pregnancy. In addition, an earlier prospective multicentre study[3] in 161 women taking a median dose of loratadine 10 mg daily in the first trimester of pregnancy suggested that its use was not associated with a significant risk of major congenital malformations.

1. Källén B, Olausson PO. Monitoring of maternal drug use and infant congenital malformations: does loratadine cause hypospadias? *Int J Risk Safety Med* 2001; **14:** 115–19.
2. Centers for Disease Control and Prevention. Evaluation of an association between loratadine and hypospadias — United States, 1997-2001. *MMWR* 2004; **53:** 219–21. Also available at: http://www.cdc.gov/mmwr/PDF/wk/mm5310.pdf (accessed 11/05/04)
3. Moretti ME, *et al.* Fetal safety of loratadine use in the first trimester of pregnancy: a multicenter study. *J Allergy Clin Immunol* 2003; **111:** 479–83.

**Sedation.** For discussion of the sedative effects of antihistamines see p.420.

### Interactions

As for the non-sedating antihistamines in general, p.421.

Loratadine is metabolised by cytochrome P450 isoenzymes CYP3A4 and CYP2D6. Therefore use with other drugs that inhibit or are metabolised by these hepatic enzymes may result in changes in plasma concentrations of either drug and, possibly, adverse effects. Drugs known to inhibit one or other of these enzymes include cimetidine, erythromycin, ketoconazole, quinidine, fluconazole, and fluoxetine.

**Antibacterials.** Data held on file by the manufacturer show that *erythromycin* can inhibit the metabolism of loratadine. However, even when given in large doses loratadine does not appear to cause the cardiac conduction disorders associated with the non-sedating antihistamines astemizole (see p.424) and terfenadine (see p.441).[1] Similarly, *clarithromycin* seemed to inhibit the metabolism of loratadine and its active metabolite desloratadine.[2]

1. Affrime MB, *et al.* Three month evaluation of electrocardiographic effects of loratadine in humans. *J Allergy Clin Immunol* 1993; **91:** 259.
2. Carr RA, *et al.* Steady-state pharmacokinetics and electrocardiographic pharmacodynamics of clarithromycin and loratadine after individual or concomitant administration. *Antimicrob Agents Chemother* 1998; **42:** 1176–80.

**Antifungals.** *Ketoconazole* also appears to be able to inhibit the metabolism of loratadine and at therapeutic doses, is about 3 times more inhibitory than erythromycin.[1] However, the concentrations of ketoconazole required are reported to be much higher than those required to inhibit the metabolism of astemizole or terfenadine. Clearance of the active metabolite desloratadine is also reduced.

1. Brannan MD, *et al.* Effects of various cytochrome P450 inhibitors on the metabolism of loratadine. *Clin Pharmacol Ther* 1995; **57:** 193.

**Gastrointestinal drugs.** *Cimetidine* appears to have an inhibitory effect on the metabolism of loratadine and also attenuates the clearance of its active metabolite desloratadine although no clinically significant consequences have been observed.[1]

1. Brannan MD, *et al.* Effects of various cytochrome P450 inhibitors on the metabolism of loratadine. *Clin Pharmacol Ther* 1995; **57:** 193.

### Pharmacokinetics

Loratadine is rapidly absorbed from the gastrointestinal tract after oral administration, peak plasma concentrations being attained in about 1 hour. Bioavailability is increased and time to peak plasma concentrations is delayed when taken with food. Loratadine undergoes extensive metabolism. The major metabolite, desloratadine (p.431), has potent antihistaminic activity. Reported mean elimination half-lives for loratadine and desloratadine are 8.4 and 28 hours, respectively. Loratadine is about 98% bound to plasma proteins; desloratadine is less extensively bound. Loratadine and its metabolites have been detected in breast milk, but do not appear to cross the blood-brain barrier to a significant extent. Most of a dose is excreted equally in the urine and faeces, mainly in the form of metabolites.

**Renal impairment.** The disposition of loratadine does not appear to be significantly altered in patients with severe renal impairment and haemodialysis does not appear to be an effective means of removing loratadine or its metabolite desloratadine from the body.[1]

1. Matzke GR, *et al.* Pharmacokinetics of loratadine in patients with renal insufficiency. *J Clin Pharmacol* 1990; **30:** 364–71.

### Uses and Administration

Loratadine, a piperidine derivative related to azatadine, is a long-acting, non-sedating antihistamine with no significant antimuscarinic activity. It is used for the symptomatic relief of allergic conditions including rhinitis (p.422) and chronic urticaria (p.423).

Loratadine is given by mouth in a dose of 10 mg once daily. Children aged 2 to 5 years may be given 5 mg once daily and those aged 6 to 12 years may be given 10 mg once daily for seasonal allergic rhinitis and chronic idiopathic urticaria.

For dosage in hepatic or renal impairment, see below.

◊ References.

1. Haria M, *et al.* Loratadine: a reappraisal of its pharmacological properties and therapeutic use in allergic disorders. *Drugs* 1994; **48:** 617–37.

**Administration in hepatic or renal impairment.** The US manufacturer recommends that patients with hepatic failure or mild renal insufficiency should be given loratadine 10 mg on alternate days initially.

### Preparations

***USP 27:*** Loratadine Oral Solution; Loratadine Tablets.

**Proprietary Preparations** (details are given in Part 3)

***Arg.:*** Aerotina; Alerpriv; Bedix; Biloina; Bioaler; Clarityne; Lertamine; Lisaler; Loisan; Nastizol Antialergico; Negalerg L; Novo Vagran; Nularef; Omega 100 L; Sinaler; ***Austral.:*** Claratyne; Lorastyne; ***Austria:*** Clarityn; Loratyn; ***Belg.:*** Claritine; Sanelor; ***Braz.:*** Alergaliv; Alertal†; Atinac; Clarilerg; Claritin; Clistin; Histadin; Histalor†; Histamix; Loradine; Loralerg; Loranil; Loratamed; Loremix; Neo Loratadin; ***Canad.:*** Claritin; ***Chile:*** Allergan; Alledryl; Clarityne; Frenaler; Histaplus; Hysticlar; Larmax; Lontadex; ***Denm.:*** Clarityn; Versal; ***Fin.:*** Clarityn; ***Fr.:*** Clarityne; ***Ger.:*** Lisino; Lobeta; Lora; Lora-Lich; Lora-Puren; Loraclar; Loragalen; Loragamma; Lorano; Loratadura; Vividrin Loratadin; ***Gr.:*** Allergofact; Biliranin; Bollinol; Clarityne; Difmedol; Helporigin; Horestyl; Latoren; Lora; Loratab; Novacloxab; Ralinet; Zelmar; ***Hong Kong:*** Clarityne; Lotadine; ***India:*** Lorfast; Loridin; ***Irl.:*** Clarityn; Histaclar; ***Israel:*** Lorastine; ***Ital.:*** Alorin; Clarityn; Fristamin; ***Malaysia:*** Carin; Clarityne; Ezede; Lorastyne; ***Mex.:*** Antilergal; Clarityne; Curyken; Lertamine; Lovarin; Lowadina†; Rodakin†; Rokadin; Sensibit; ***Neth.:*** Allerfre; Claritine; ***Norw.:*** Clarityn; Versal; ***NZ:*** Claratyne; Lora-Tabs; ***Port.:*** Alertrin†; Claritine; ***S.Afr.:*** Clarityne; Demazin Anti-Allergy; Loratyne; Polaratyne; ***Singapore:*** Ardin; Clarityne; Histalor; Ridamin; ***Spain:*** Civeran; Clarityne; Fadina; Optimin; Velodan; Viatine†; ***Swed.:*** Clarityn; Versal; ***Switz.:*** Claritine; ***Thai.:*** Aller-Tab; Allerdine; Allersil; Carinose; Clarityne; Halodin; Loranox; Lorita; Lorityne; Lorsedin; Lortadine; Ridamin; Rityne; Tiradine; Tirlor; ***UAE:*** Loratin; ***UK:*** Clarityn; ***USA:*** Alavert; Claritin; Tavist ND.

**Multi-ingredient:** ***Arg.:*** Alerpriv D; Bedix-D; Celestamine-L; Ciprocort D; Ciprocort L; Clarifriol; Clarityne Cort; Clarityne D; Cortistamin L; Decidex Plus; Histamino Corteroid L; Lertamine D; Lisaler Beta; Loisan-D; Loremex; Nastizol-L; Negalerg; Novo Vagran D; Nularef Cort; Nularef-D; Sinaler B; ***Austral.:*** Clarinase; Sinease; ***Austria:*** Clarinase; ***Belg.:*** Clarinase; ***Braz.:*** Claritin-D; Loralerg-D; Loranil D; Loremix D; ***Canad.:*** Chlor-Tripolon ND; Claritin Extra; ***Chile:*** Clarinase; Frenaler-D; Lertamine; Lertamine Extra; Lontadex D; Rinomex; ***Denm.:*** Clarinase; Clarinex†; ***Fin.:*** Clarinase; ***Fr.:*** Clarinase; ***Hong Kong:*** Clariflu; Clarinase; ***India:*** Loridin-D; ***Israel:*** Clarinase; ***Malaysia:*** Clarinase; ***Mex.:*** Alvium; Celestamine NS; Claricort; Clariflu; Clarifriol; Clarinase; Clarityne D; Coricidin Expec; Lertamine D; Lovarin P; Sensibit D; ***NZ:*** Claratyne Decongestant†; Clarinase; Demazin Non-Drowsy; ***Port.:*** Claridon; ***S.Afr.:*** Clarityne D; Demazin NS; Polaratyne D; ***Singapore:*** Clarinase; ***Spain:*** Clarinase†; Logradin†; Narine; ***Thai.:*** Clarinase; ***USA:*** Alavert Allergy & Sinus D; Claritin-D.

## Mebhydrolin (BAN, rINN)

Mebhidrolina. 5-Benzyl-1,2,3,4-tetrahydro-2-methyl-γ-carboline.

$C_{19}H_{20}N_2$ = 276.4.

*CAS — 524-81-2.*

*ATC — R06AX15.*

## Mebhydrolin Napadisilate (BANM, rINNM)

Diazolinum; Mebhydrolin Napadisylate; Mebhydrolin Naphthalenedisulphonate; Napadisilato de mebhidrolina. Mebhydrolin naphthalene-1,5-disulphonate.

$(C_{19}H_{20}N_2)_2,C_{10}H_8O_6S_2$ = 841.0.

*CAS — 6153-33-9.*

*ATC — R06AX15.*

### Profile

Mebhydrolin, an ethylenediamine derivative, is a sedating antihistamine (p.419) with antimuscarinic and sedative properties. It has been given by mouth as the base or as the napadisilate salt for the symptomatic relief of allergic conditions including urticaria and rhinitis, and in pruritic skin disorders. Granulocytopenia and agranulocytosis have been reported.

### Preparations

**Proprietary Preparations** (details are given in Part 3)

***Hong Kong:*** Incidal†; ***Israel:*** Cidalin; ***Thai.:*** Dayhist; Incidal†; Posidol.

## Meclozine Hydrochloride (BAN, pINNM)

Hidrocloruro de meclozina; Meclizine Hydrochloride; Meclizinium Chloride; Meclozini Hydrochloridum; Parachloramine Hydrochloride. 1-(4-Chlorobenzhydryl)-4-(3-methylbenzyl)piperazine dihydrochloride.

$C_{25}H_{27}ClN_2,2HCl$ = 463.9.

*CAS — 569-65-3 (meclozine); 1104-22-9 (anhydrous meclozine hydrochloride); 31884-77-2 (meclozine hydrochloride monohydrate).*

*ATC — R06AE05.*

**Pharmacopoeias.** In *Chin.* and *Eur.* (see p.vi).
*US* specifies the monohydrate.

**Ph. Eur. 5.0** (Meclozine Hydrochloride). A yellow or yellowish-white, crystalline powder. Slightly soluble in water; soluble in alcohol and in dichloromethane. Store in airtight containers.

**USP 27** (Meclizine Hydrochloride). The monohydrate is white or slightly yellowish crystalline powder that has a slight odour. Practically insoluble in water and in ether; freely soluble in chloroform, in pyridine, and in acid-alcohol-water mixtures; slightly soluble in dilute acids and in alcohol. Store in airtight containers.

### Adverse Effects and Precautions

As for the sedating antihistamines in general, p.419. For reports of the use of antihistamines, including meclozine, in pregnancy, see p.420.

### Interactions

As for the sedating antihistamines in general, p.421.

### Uses and Administration

Meclozine hydrochloride, a piperazine derivative, is a sedating antihistamine with antimuscarinic and moderate sedative properties. It is mainly used for its antiemetic action, which may last for up to 24 hours. Meclozine hydrochloride is used in the prevention and treatment of nausea and vomiting associated with a variety of conditions including motion sickness (p.422) and for the symptomatic treatment of vertigo (p.423) caused by Ménière's disease and other vestibular disorders. Meclozine hydrochloride has also been used for the symptomatic relief of hypersensitivity reactions and pruritic skin disorders (p.422).

The usual dose of meclozine hydrochloride for motion sickness is 25 to 50 mg by mouth taken about one hour before travelling and repeated every 24 hours if necessary; up to 100 mg daily in divided doses has been given for the treatment of vertigo and vestibular disorders. In the prevention and treatment of motion sickness in children aged 6 to 12 years, 12.5 mg is given once daily; for children aged 2 to 6 years the dose is 6.25 mg once daily.

Both meclozine hydrochloride and meclozine base have been administered by the rectal route; doses are similar to those given by mouth.

### Preparations

***USP 27:*** Meclizine Hydrochloride Tablets.

**Proprietary Preparations** (details are given in Part 3)
***Belg.:*** Agyrax; Postafene; ***Canad.:*** Antivert†; Bonamine; ***Chile:*** Bonamina; ***Denm.:*** Postafen; ***Fin.:*** Postafen; ***Fr.:*** Agyrax; ***Ger.:*** Bonamine†; Peremesin; Peremesin N; Postadoxin N; Postafen; ***Gr.:*** Emetostop; Postafene; ***Hong Kong:*** Postafene; ***Neth.:*** Suprimal†; ***Norw.:*** Peremesin; Postafen; ***NZ:*** Sea-Legs; ***Port.:*** Navicalm; ***Spain:*** Chiclida; Dramine; Marevit†; Navicalm; ***Swed.:*** Postafen; ***Switz.:*** Duremesan; ***Thai.:*** Bonamine†; ***UK:*** Sea-Legs; ***USA:*** Antivert; Antrizine; Bonine; Dizmiss; Dramamine II; Meni-D; Vergon.

**Multi-ingredient: *Austria:*** Contravert $B_6$; Diligan; ***Belg.:*** Postadoxine†; ***Ger.:*** Diligan; ***Hong Kong:*** Navidoxine; ***India:*** Diligan; Pregnidoxin; ***Malaysia:*** Becoloxin; Navidoxine; ***Mex.:*** Bonadoxina; Bonazin; Emediba; Liatriz; Meclifar; Vo-Remi; ***Neth.:*** Emesafene; ***Port.:*** Diligan; ***S.Afr.:*** Geratar†; ***Singapore:*** Navidoxine; ***Swed.:*** Histilos†; ***Switz.:*** Duremesan; Itinerol $B_6$; ***UK:*** Traveleeze.

---

## Mepyramine Hydrochloride

*(BANM, rINNM)*

Hidrocloruro de mepiramina; Pyranisamine Hydrochloride; Pyrilamine Hydrochloride. *N-p*-Anisyl-*N'N'*-dimethyl-*N*-(2-pyridyl)-ethylenediamine hydrochloride.

$C_{17}H_{23}N_3O,HCl$ = 321.8.

*CAS — 91-84-9 (mepyramine); 6036-95-9 (mepyramine hydrochloride).*

*ATC — D04AA02; R06AC01.*

### Mepyramine Maleate *(BANM, rINNM)*

Maleato de mepiramina; Mepyramini Maleas; Pyranisamine Maleate; Pyrilamine Maleate. Mepyramine hydrogen maleate.

$C_{17}H_{23}N_3O,C_4H_4O_4$ = 401.5.

*CAS — 59-33-6.*

*ATC — D04AA02; R06AC01.*

**Pharmacopoeias.** In *Eur.* (see p.vi) and *US.*

**Ph. Eur. 5.0** (Mepyramine Maleate). A white or slightly yellowish, crystalline powder. Very soluble in water; freely soluble in alcohol. M.p. 99° to 103°. A 2% solution in water has a pH of 4.9 to 5.2. Protect from light.

**USP 27** (Pyrilamine Maleate). A white crystalline powder usually having a faint odour. Soluble 1 in 0.5 of water, 1 in 3 of alcohol, 1 in 15 of dehydrated alcohol, and 1 in 2 of chloroform; slightly soluble in ether and in benzene. Its solutions are acid to litmus. Store in airtight containers. Protect from light.

### Adverse Effects and Precautions

As for the sedating antihistamines in general, p.419.

### Interactions

As for the sedating antihistamines in general, p.421.

### Uses and Administration

Mepyramine, an ethylenediamine derivative, is a sedating antihistamine with antimuscarinic and sedative properties. Mepyramine maleate is used for the symptomatic relief of hypersensitivity reactions and in pruritic skin disorders (p.422). Mepyramine maleate is also a common ingredient of compound preparations for the symptomatic treatment of coughs and the common cold (p.421).

Mepyramine maleate has been given by mouth in a dose of 50 mg at night as a hypnotic in the short-term management of insomnia (p.422).

A cream containing 2% mepyramine maleate is used locally for insect bites or stings, and for hypersensitivity and pruritic skin conditions but, as with any antihistamine, there is a risk of sensitisation. It has also been used in eye drops.

In some countries mepyramine maleate is available for parenteral use. Mepyramine hydrochloride has also been given parenterally or by the rectal route. Mepyramine tannate and mepyramine acefyllinate have been used orally.

### Preparations

***BP 2003:*** Mepyramine Tablets;
***USP 27:*** Pyrilamine Maleate Tablets.

**Proprietary Preparations** (details are given in Part 3)
***Austral.:*** Anthisan†; Relaxa-Tabs; ***Braz.:*** Alergitanil; ***Hong Kong:*** Anthisan; ***Irl.:*** Anthisan; ***Ital.:*** Antemesyl†; ***Mex.:*** Fluidasa; ***NZ:*** Anthisan; ***S.Afr.:*** Anthisan; Mepyraderm; Mepyrimal; ***Spain:*** Fluidasa; ***UK:*** Anthisan.

**Multi-ingredient: *Arg.:*** Bajumol; Drynisan; Fadanasal; Piracalamina; Polipectol; Rynatanic; ***Austral.:*** Neo-Diophen†; ***Austria:*** Prefrin A†; ***Belg.:*** Nortussine; ***Braz.:*** Adegripan†; Alergitrat†; Alergo Glucalbet; Analgex C†; Atagripe†; Beclase†; Benistina†; Benzomel; Cefunk†; Conidrin; Engov†; Enjoy†; Expectussin†; Ginometrim Oral; Gripanil; Gripefago C†; Gripefin†; Gripol C†; Gripol Composto†; Gripsay; Killgrip; Naricin†; Naridrin; Nasogrip; Nasopan†; Plenogripe†; Posdrink; Prenefrin†; Subitan†; ***Canad.:*** Antitussive Decongestant Antihistamine Syrup†; Bronchodex DM†; Bronchosirum†; Caldomine-DH†; Centracol DM†; Extra Strength Multi-Symptom PMS Relief; Hycomine; IDM Solution†; Jack and Jill; Lemon Time; Midol Extra Strength; Midol Multi-Symptom†; Midol PMS Extra Strength; Pamprin; Pharmacol DM†; Pharminicol DM†; Prefrin A; Relievol PMS; Tantacol DM†; Theo-Bronc; Trendar PMS; Triaminic Expectorant DH†; Triaminic†; Triaminicin†; Trisulfaminic†; Tussaminic C†; Tussaminic DH†; Tylenol Menstrual; ***Chile:*** Alerzona; Kitadol Periodo Menstrual; Minfaden; Predual; Rinolergan; Tapsin Periodo Menstrual; ***Fr.:*** Nortussine; ***Hong Kong:*** Easiko; ***Israel:*** Aforinol; Alnase; Phenyphrine-Azol; ***Ital.:*** Antemesyl†; Balsamina Kroner; Triaminic; Vasofen; ***Malaysia:*** Prefrin A; ***Mex.:*** LM6; ***Port.:*** Naso-Prieulina; Profrin-A; Solpic; Ugrilon†; ***S.Afr.:*** Antiflu; Bronchiflu; Cetamine†; Codef; Codomill; Colcaps; Coughcod; Docsed; Dykatuss Co†; Expectotussin C; Flucol†; Histodor; Kiddiekof†; Meditus; Metaxol; Monotussin†; Triaminic†; ***Singapore:*** Prefrin A; ***Spain:*** Amplidermis; Pectobal Dextro; ***Switz.:*** Calpred; Demoderhin†; Demostan N; Escogripp sans codeine; Euceta Pic; Histacyl Compositum; Histacylettes; No Grip†; Stilex; ***Thai.:*** Antergan; ***UK:*** Anthisan Plus; Wasp-Eze; ***USA:*** 4-Way Fast Acting; AlleRx; Atrohist Pediatric†; C-Tanna 12D; Calamycin; Codal-DH; Codal-DM; Codimal DH; Codimal DM; Codimal PH; Covangesic†; De-Chlor MR; Derma-Pax; Duonate; Gelhist; HC Derma-Pax; Histalet Forte†; Histosal†; Iohist D†; Midol Maximum Strength Multi-Symptom Menstrual; Midol Pre-Menstrual Syndrome; Myci-Spray; ND-Gesic; P-Tanna; Pamprin; Phanadex Cough†; Poly-Histine; Poly-Histine D†; Premsyn PMS; Quadra-Hist D†; R-Tanna; R-Tannamine; R-Tannate; R-Tannic-S; Rectagene Medicated Rectal Balm; Rhinatate; Robitussin Night Relief; Rolatuss with Hydrocodone†; Ru-Tuss with Hydrocodone†; Ryna-12; Soothaderm; Statuss Green†; Tanoral; Theracaps†; Tri-P†; Tri-Tannate; Triaminic Expectorant DH†; Triaminic Oral Infant†; Tricodene Cough & Cold; Trihist-D†; Triotann; Tritan; Tussi-12 D; Tussi-12D S; Vanex Forte†; Vetuss HC†; Viravan; Viravan-DM; Z-Xtra.

---

## Mequitazine *(BAN, rINN)*

LM-209; Mequitazina. 10-(Quinuclidin-3-ylmethyl)phenothiazine.

$C_{20}H_{22}N_2S$ = 322.5.

*CAS — 29216-28-2.*

*ATC — R06AD07.*

**Pharmacopoeias.** In *Jpn.*

### Adverse Effects and Precautions

As for the sedating antihistamines in general, p.419.

**Sedation.** For discussion of the sedative effects of antihistamines, see p.420. When mequitazine is given in the recommended dosage of 5 mg twice daily the incidence of sedation appears comparable with that of terfenadine. Sedation has, however, occurred after doses of 10 mg twice daily.

### Interactions

As for the sedating antihistamines in general, p.421.

**Antibacterials.** For a report of torsade de pointes in a patient taking *spiramycin* and mequitazine, see p.256.

### Pharmacokinetics

After absorption from the gastrointestinal tract, mequitazine is metabolised. Unchanged drug and metabolites are excreted principally in the bile.

### Uses and Administration

Mequitazine, a phenothiazine derivative, is a sedating antihistamine with antimuscarinic and mild sedative properties.

Mequitazine is used for the symptomatic relief of allergic conditions including urticaria (p.423), rhinitis (p.422) and conjunctivitis (p.421), and in pruritic skin disorders (p.422). It has been given in usual doses of 5 mg twice daily by mouth.

### Preparations

**Proprietary Preparations** (details are given in Part 3)
***Arg.:*** Primalan; ***Austria:*** Metaplexan†; ***Belg.:*** Mircol†; ***Braz.:*** Primasone†; ***Chile:*** Mircol; ***Fr.:*** Butix†; Primalan; Quitadrill; ***Ger.:*** Metaplexan; ***Ital.:*** Primalan; ***Port.:*** Primalan; ***Spain:*** Mircol; ***Thai.:*** Primalan†; ***UK:*** Primalan†.

---

## Methdilazine *(BAN, rINN)*

Metodilazina. 10-(1-Methylpyrrolidin-3-ylmethyl)phenothiazine.

$C_{18}H_{20}N_2S$ = 296.4.

*CAS — 1982-37-2.*

*ATC — R06AD04.*

### Methdilazine Hydrochloride *(BANM, rINNM)*

Hidrocloruro de metodilazina.

$C_{18}H_{20}N_2S,HCl$ = 332.9.

*CAS — 1229-35-2.*

*ATC — R06AD04.*

**Pharmacopoeias.** In *US.*

**USP 27** (Methdilazine Hydrochloride). A light tan crystalline powder having a slight characteristic odour. Soluble 1 in 2 of water and of alcohol, 1 in 6 of chloroform, and 1 in 1 of 0.1N hydrochloric acid and of 0.1N sodium hydroxide solution; practically insoluble in ether. pH of a 1% solution in water is between 4.8 and 6.0. Store in airtight containers. Protect from light.

### Adverse Effects and Precautions

As for the sedating antihistamines in general, p.419.

### Interactions

As for the sedating antihistamines in general, p.421.

### Uses and Administration

Methdilazine, a phenothiazine derivative, is a sedating antihistamine with antimuscarinic and sedative activity. Methdilazine is also reported to have serotonin-antagonist properties.

Methdilazine hydrochloride is used for the symptomatic relief of hypersensitivity reactions and particularly for the control of pruritic skin disorders (p.422). A dose of 8 mg has been given by mouth 2 to 4 times daily. Children 3 years and over have been given half the adult dose. Methdilazine base has been used in similar doses.

### Preparations

***USP 27:*** Methdilazine Hydrochloride Syrup; Methdilazine Hydrochloride Tablets.

**Proprietary Preparations** (details are given in Part 3)
***Austral.:*** Dilosyn; ***Denm.:*** Tacryl; ***India:*** Dilosyn.

**Multi-ingredient: *India:*** Dilosyn Expectorant.

---

## Mizolastine *(BAN, rINN)*

Mizolastina; SL-85.0324-00. 2-{1-[1-(4-Fluorobenzyl)-1*H*-benzimidazol-2-yl]-4-piperidyl(methyl)amino}pyrimidin-4(1*H*)-one.

$C_{24}H_{25}FN_6O$ = 432.5.

*CAS — 108612-45-9.*

*ATC — R06AX25.*

### Adverse Effects and Precautions

As for the non-sedating antihistamines in general, p.419. Mizolastine has only a weak potential to prolong the QT interval (see also Arrhythmias, p.420) and has not been associated with arrhythmias. However, the manufacturers have warned against the use of mizolastine in patients with significant cardiac or hepatic disease, with hypokalaemia or other electrolyte imbalance, or with known or suspected QT prolongation. The concomitant administration of drugs liable to interfere with the hepatic metabolism of mizolastine and of other potentially arrhythmogenic drugs should also be avoided (see under Interactions, below).

### Interactions

As for the non-sedating antihistamines in general, p.421. Moderate increases in plasma concentrations of mizolastine have been reported following administration of *erythromycin* and *ketoconazole*; the concurrent use of macrolide antibacterials or systemic imidazole antifungals is contra-indicated by the manufacturer. They also advise against the concurrent use of drugs known to prolong the QT interval, such as *class I and III antiarrhythmics*, with mizolastine.

Other potent inhibitors of or substrates for the hepatic metabolism of mizolastine include *cimetidine, ciclosporin,* and *nifedipine*; caution is advised with concurrent administration.

### Pharmacokinetics

Mizolastine is rapidly absorbed from the gastrointestinal tract with peak plasma concentrations being reached after about 1.5 hours. Plasma protein binding is about 98%. The mean elimination half-life is approximately 13 hours. Mizolastine is mainly metabolised by glucuronidation although other metabolic pathways are involved, including metabolism by the cytochrome P450 isoenzyme CYP3A4, with the formation of inactive hydroxylated metabolites.

◊ References.

1. Rosenzweig P, *et al.* Pharmacodynamics and pharmacokinetics of mizolastine (SL 85.0324), a new nonsedative $H_1$ antihistamine. *Ann Allergy* 1992; **69:** 135–9.
2. Lebrun-Vignes B, *et al.* Clinical pharmacokinetics of mizolastine. *Clin Pharmacokinet* 2001; **40:** 501–7.

### Uses and Administration

Mizolastine is a non-sedating antihistamine with a long duration of action. It does not have significant antimuscarinic actions; it is reported to have mast-cell stabilising properties. Mizolastine is used for the symptomatic relief of allergic conditions including rhinitis (p.422), conjunctivitis (p.421), and skin disorders such as urticaria (p.423). The dose, by mouth, is 10 mg daily.

◊ References.

1. Leynadier F, *et al.* Efficacy and safety of mizolastine in seasonal allergic rhinitis. *Ann Allergy Asthma Immunol* 1996; **76:** 163–8.
2. Brostoff J, *et al.* Efficacy of mizolastine, a new antihistamine, compared with placebo in the treatment of chronic idiopathic urticaria. *Allergy* 1996; **51:** 320–5.
3. Stern MA, *et al.* Can an antihistamine delay appearance of hayfever symptoms when given prior to pollen season? *Allergy* 1997; **52:** 440–4.

### Preparations

**Proprietary Preparations** (details are given in Part 3)
***Arg.:*** Mistamine; ***Austria:*** Mistamin; Mizollen; ***Belg.:*** Mistamine; Mizollen; ***Braz.:*** Mizolen†; ***Chile:*** Mistamine; ***Denm.:*** Mistamine†; Mizollen; ***Fin.:*** Mizollen; ***Fr.:*** Mistaline†; Mizollen; ***Ger.:*** Mizollen; Zolim; ***Gr.:*** Mizollen; Oriens; ***India:*** Elina; ***Irl.:*** Mistamine; ***Israel:*** Mizollen; ***Ital.:*** Mizollen; Zolistam; ***Mex.:*** Mistamine; ***Neth.:*** Mistalin; Mizollen; ***Port.:*** Mistamine; Mizollen; Zolistam; ***S.Afr.:*** Mizollen; ***Spain:*** Mistamine; Mizolen; Zolistan; ***Swed.:*** Mistamine†; Mizollen; ***Switz.:*** Mistamine; Mizollen; ***UK:*** Mistamine†; Mizollen.

---

## Niaprazine *(rINN)*

1709-CERM; Niaprazina. *N*-[3-(4-*p*-Fluorophenylpiperazin-1-yl)-1-methylpropyl]nicotinamide.

$C_{20}H_{25}FN_4O$ = 356.4.
*CAS — 27367-90-4.*
*ATC — N05CM16.*

### Profile

Niaprazine, a piperazine derivative, is an antihistamine (p.419) used in children for its sedative and hypnotic properties. The usual dose by mouth is 1 mg/kg at night.

### Preparations

**Proprietary Preparations** (details are given in Part 3)
***Fr.:*** Nopron†; ***Ital.:*** Nopron.

---

## Olopatadine Hydrochloride *(BANM, USAN, pINNM)*

ALO-4943A; Hidrocloruro de olopatadina; KW-4679. 11-[(*Z*)-3-(Dimethylamino)propylidene]-6,11-dihydrodibenz[*b*,*e*]oxepin-2-acetic acid hydrochloride.

$C_{21}H_{23}NO_3,HCl$ = 373.9.
*CAS — 113806-05-6 (olopatadine); 140462-76-6 (olopatadine hydrochloride).*
*ATC — S01GX09.*

### Adverse Effects and Precautions

As for the antihistamines in general, p.419. Headache and stinging or burning of the eye have occurred after ocular administration.

### Uses and Administration

Olopatadine hydrochloride is an antihistamine with mast-cell stabilising properties. It is used twice daily as eye drops containing the equivalent of 0.1% of olopatadine base in the treatment of allergic conjunctivitis (p.421) in adults and children aged three years and over.

◊ References.

1. Anonymous. Olopatadine for allergic conjunctivitis. *Med Lett Drugs Ther* 1997; **39:** 108–9.

### Preparations

**Proprietary Preparations** (details are given in Part 3)
***Arg.:*** Patanol; ***Austral.:*** Patanol; ***Braz.:*** Patanol; ***Canad.:*** Patanol; ***Chile:*** Patanol; ***Denm.:*** Opatanol; ***Fr.:*** Opatanol; ***Mex.:*** Patanol; ***Singapore:*** Patanol; ***Thai.:*** Patanol; ***UK:*** Opatanol; ***USA:*** Patanol.

---

## Oxatomide *(BAN, USAN, rINN)*

Oxatomida; R-35443. 1-[3-(4-Benzhydrylpiperazin-1-yl)propyl]benzimidazolin-2-one.

$C_{27}H_{30}N_4O$ = 426.6.
*CAS — 60607-34-3.*
*ATC — R06AE06.*

### Profile

Oxatomide, a piperazine derivative, is a sedating antihistamine (p.419) that has also been reported to have mast-cell stabilising properties. It is used for the symptomatic relief of allergic conditions including urticaria (p.423), rhinitis (p.422), and conjunctivitis (p.421). Oxatomide is given by mouth as the anhydrous substance or as the monohydrate; doses are expressed as the anhydrous substance. Oxatomide monohydrate 1.04 mg is approximately equivalent to 1 mg of anhydrous oxatomide. The usual dose is 30 mg twice daily. The hydrate has also been applied topically but, as with other antihistamines, there is a risk of sensitisation.

**Effects on the CNS.** Acute dystonic reactions and long-lasting impaired consciousness were associated with oxatomide therapy in 6 children.[1] Impaired consciousness varied from lethargy and somnolence to a clinical picture resembling encephalitis and persisted for 2 days or more in 3 patients. Plasma-oxatomide concentrations were measured in 3 patients and found to be high, although 2 of these had been given the recommended dose.

1. Casteels-Van Daele M, *et al.* Acute dystonic reactions and long-lasting impaired consciousness associated with oxatomide in children. *Lancet* 1986; **i:** 1204–5.

### Preparations

**Proprietary Preparations** (details are given in Part 3)
***Arg.:*** Cenacert; Fensedyl; Tinset; ***Austria:*** Tinset; ***Belg.:*** Tinset; ***Chile:*** Tinset; ***Fr.:*** Tinset; ***Ger.:*** Tinset†; ***Gr.:*** Tinset; ***Hong Kong:*** Tinset; ***Ital.:*** Tinset; ***Mex.:*** Tinset; ***Neth.:*** Tinset; ***Port.:*** Tinset; ***S.Afr.:*** Tinset; ***Spain:*** Cobiona; Oxatokey; Tanzal†; ***Thai.:*** Tinset.

**Multi-ingredient:** ***Arg.:*** Causalon Bronquial; Causalon Grip; Letondal.

---

## Oxomemazine *(rINN)*

Oxomemazina; RP-6847; Trimeprazine *SS*-Dioxide. 10-(3-Dimethylamino-2-methylpropyl)phenothiazine 5,5-dioxide.

$C_{18}H_{22}N_2O_2S$ = 330.4.
*CAS — 3689-50-7.*
*ATC — R06AD08.*

## Oxomemazine Hydrochloride *(rINNM)*

Hidrocloruro de oxomemazina.

$C_{18}H_{22}N_2O_2S,HCl$ = 366.9.
*CAS — 4784-40-1.*
*ATC — R06AD08.*

**Pharmacopoeias.** In *Fr.*

### Profile

Oxomemazine, a phenothiazine derivative, is a sedating antihistamine (p.419) used for the symptomatic relief of hypersensitivity reactions and in pruritic skin disorders (p.422). It is also an ingredient of compound preparations for the symptomatic treatment of coughs and the common cold (p.421).

Oxomemazine has been given by mouth in doses of 10 to 40 mg daily. It may also be administered by the rectal route. Oxomemazine hydrochloride has been used similarly by mouth.

### Preparations

**Proprietary Preparations** (details are given in Part 3)
***Belg.:*** Doxergan†; ***Fr.:*** Rectoplexil†; Toplexil.

**Multi-ingredient:** ***Austria:*** Aplexil†; ***Belg.:*** Rectoplexil†; Toplexil; ***Braz.:*** Expec; Iodesin; Iodeto de Potassium Composto; Iodobec†; Kl-Expectorante; Tiratosse†; Toplexil; Tussol†; ***Israel:*** Oxacatin; Toplexil; ***Neth.:*** Toplexil; ***Switz.:*** Toplexil.

---

## Phenindamine Tartrate *(BANM, USAN, rINNM)*

Phenindamine Acid Tartrate; Phenindamini Tartras; Phenindaminium Tartrate; Tartrato de fenindamina. 1,2,3,4-Tetrahydro-2-methyl-9-phenyl-2-azafluorene hydrogen tartrate; 2,3,4,9-Tetrahydro-2-methyl-9-phenyl-1*H*-indeno[2,1-*c*]pyridine hydrogen tartrate.

$C_{19}H_{19}N,C_4H_6O_6$ = 411.4.
*CAS — 82-88-2 (phenindamine); 569-59-5 (phenindamine tartrate).*
*ATC — R06AX04.*

**Pharmacopoeias.** In *Br.*

**BP 2003** (Phenindamine Tartrate). A white or almost white, odourless or almost odourless, voluminous powder. Sparingly soluble in water; slightly soluble in alcohol; practically insoluble in chloroform and in ether. A 1% solution in water has a pH of 3.4 to 3.9. Protect from light.

### Adverse Effects and Precautions

As for the sedating antihistamines in general, p.419. Phenindamine tartrate may have a stimulant effect in certain individuals; to avoid the possibility of insomnia patients may be advised to take the last dose of the day several hours before retiring.

### Interactions

As for the sedating antihistamines in general, p.421.

### Uses and Administration

Phenindamine, a piperidine derivative, is a sedating antihistamine; however it may be mildly stimulating in certain individuals. It is used as the tartrate for the symptomatic relief of allergic conditions including urticaria (p.423) and rhinitis (p.422), and as an ingredient of compound preparations for coughs and the common cold (p.421).

Phenindamine tartrate is given by mouth in doses of 25 mg every 4 to 6 hours, up to a maximum of 150 mg daily. Children over 6 years of age have been given half these doses.

### Preparations

**Proprietary Preparations** (details are given in Part 3)
***Irl.:*** Thephorin†; ***USA:*** Nolahist.

**Multi-ingredient:** ***USA:*** Nolamine†; P-V-Tussin.

---

## Pheniramine *(BAN, rINN)*

Feniramina; Prophenpyridamine. *NN*-Dimethyl-3-phenyl-3-(2-pyridyl)propylamine.

$C_{16}H_{20}N_2$ = 240.3.
*CAS — 86-21-5.*
*ATC — R06AB05.*

## Pheniramine Aminosalicylate

Feniramina, aminosalicilato de; Pheniramine *p*-Aminosalicylate; Pheniramine 4-Aminosalicylate; Pheniramine Para-aminosalicylate. Pheniramine 4-amino-2-hydroxybenzoate.

$C_{16}H_{20}N_2,C_7H_7NO_3$ = 393.5.
*CAS — 3269-83-8.*
*ATC — R06AB05.*

## Pheniramine Maleate *(BANM, USAN, rINNM)*

Maleato de feniramina; Pheniramini Maleas; Pheniraminium Maleate; Prophenpyridamine Maleate. Pheniramine hydrogen maleate.

$C_{16}H_{20}N_2,C_4H_4O_4$ = 356.4.
*CAS — 132-20-7.*
*ATC — R06AB05.*

**Pharmacopoeias.** In *Eur.* (see p.vi) and *US.*

**Ph. Eur. 5.0** (Pheniramine Maleate). A white, crystalline powder. Very soluble in water; freely soluble in alcohol, in dichloromethane, and in methyl alcohol. M.p. 106° to 109°. A 1% solution in water has a pH of 4.5 to 5.5. Protect from light.

**USP 27** (Pheniramine Maleate). A white crystalline powder having a faint amine-like odour. Soluble in water and in alcohol. pH of a 1% solution in water is between 4.5 and 5.5.

### Adverse Effects and Precautions

As for the sedating antihistamines in general, p.419.

**Abuse.** References to the abuse of pheniramine by mouth.

1. Jones IH, *et al.* Pheniramine as an hallucinogen. *Med J Aust* 1973; **1:** 382–6.
2. Csillag ER, Landauer AA. Alleged hallucinogenic effect of a toxic overdose of an antihistamine preparation. *Med J Aust* 1973; **1:** 653–4.
3. Buckley NA, *et al.* Pheniramine—a much abused drug. *Med J Aust* 1994; **160:** 188–92.

**Pregnancy.** For discussion of the use of antihistamines, including pheniramine, in pregnancy, see p.420.

### Interactions

As for the sedating antihistamines in general, p.421.

### Pharmacokinetics

◊ The pharmacokinetics of pheniramine and its metabolites, *N*-desmethylpheniramine and *N*-didesmethylpheniramine, were investigated in 6 healthy subjects.[1] After oral administration of pheniramine aminosalicylate, peak-plasma pheniramine concentrations were reached in 1 to 2.5 hours. The terminal half-life ranged between 8 and 17 hours after intravenous administration (pheniramine maleate) and 16 and 19 hours after oral administration. The total recovery of pheniramine as unchanged drug and metabolites from the urine was 68 to 94% of the intravenous dose and 70 to 83% of the oral dose.

1. Witte PU, *et al.* Pharmacokinetics of pheniramine (Avil®) and metabolites in healthy subjects after oral and intravenous administration. *Int J Clin Pharmacol Ther Toxicol* 1985; **23:** 59–62.

### Uses and Administration

Pheniramine, an alkylamine derivative, is a sedating antihistamine with antimuscarinic and moderate sedative properties.

It is used as the maleate for the symptomatic relief of allergic conditions including urticaria and angioedema (p.423), rhinitis (p.422), and conjunctivitis (p.421), and in pruritic skin disorders (p.422). It has also been used for its antiemetic properties in the prevention and control of motion sickness (p.422). Pheniramine maleate is used as an ingredient of compound preparations for the symptomatic treatment of coughs and the common cold (p.421). It is also used in combination with a decongestant in eye and nasal preparations.

Pheniramine maleate is given by mouth as a syrup in usual doses of 15 to 30 mg two or three times daily. It may also be given as a tablet in doses up to about 45 mg three times daily. In some countries pheniramine maleate has been given parenterally.

The aminosalicylate, the hydrochloride, and the tannate have also been used.

### Preparations

***USP 27:*** Naphazoline Hydrochloride and Pheniramine Maleate Ophthalmic Solution.

**Proprietary Preparations** (details are given in Part 3)
***Austral.:*** Avil; Fenamine; ***Austria:*** Avil; ***Braz.:*** Histalerg Profen†; ***Ger.:*** Avil†; ***India:*** Avil; ***Irl.:*** Daneral†; ***Ital.:*** Inhiston; ***Mex.:*** Histatex; ***NZ:*** Avil; ***UAE:*** Histol.

**Multi-ingredient:** ***Arg.:*** Mira Klonal; Mirus; Refenax Colirio; ***Austral.:*** Avil Decongestant; Naphcon-A; Visine Allergy with Antihistamine; ***Austria:*** Neo Citran; Peremin†; ***Braz.:*** Claril; Gripefin†; ***Canad.:*** Ak-Vernacon; Antitussive Decongestant Antihistamine Syrup†; Bronchodex D†; Bronchodex Pediatrique†; Bronchosirum†; Caldomine-DH†; Calmylin Ace; Centracol DM†; Centracol Pediatrique†; Citron Chaud DM; Citron Chaud†; Cold Decongestant†; Diopticon A; Dristan; Hot Lemon; Hot Lemon Relief; Naphcon-A; Neo Citran; Neo Citran A; Neo Citran Calorie Reduced; Neo Citran DM; Neo Citran Extra Strength; Opcon-A; Pharmacol DM†; Pharminicol DM†; Pulmorphan; Pulmorphan Pediatrique; Robitussin AC; Robitussin with Codeine; Tantacol DM†; Triaminic Expectorant DH†; Triaminic†; Triaminicin†; Trisulfaminic†; Tussaminic C†; Tussaminic DH†; ***Chile:*** Clarimir F; Dessolets; Miral; Mirus; Naphcon-A;

**Fr.:** Fervex; Triaminic†; **Ger.:** Konjunktival Thilo; Rhinosovil; **Hong Kong:** Konjunktival; Naphcon-A; **India:** Avil Expectorant; Cosavil; Dristan Nasal Drops; Triaminic; **Irl.:** Triominic†; **Israel:** Tussosedan; **Ital.:** Medramil†; Nafcon A; Senodin-AN; Tetramil; Triaminic; Triaminicflu; **Malaysia:** Naphcon-A; **Mex.:** Solutina; **NZ:** Naphcon-A†; Visine Allergy with Antihistamine; **S.Afr.:** Allertac†; Calasthetic; Coff-Up†; Degoran; Triaminic†; **Singapore:** Naphcon-A; **Switz.:** Neo Citran Grippe/refroidissement; **Thai.:** Naphcon-A; **UK:** Triominic†; **USA:** Dristan Nasal Spray; Iohist D†; Nafazair A; Naphazoline Plus; Naphcon-A; Naphoptic-A; Ocuhist; Opcon-A; Poly-Histine; Poly-Histine D†; Quadra-Hist D†; Rolatuss with Hydrocodone†; Ru-Tuss with Hydrocodone†; S-T Forte†; Scot-Tussin Original 5-Action; Statuss Green†; Tri-P†; Triaminic Expectorant DH†; Triaminic Oral Infant†; Trihist-D†; Tussirex; Vetuss HC†.

## Phenyltoloxamine Citrate *(BANM, rINNM)*

C-5581H (phenyltoloxamine); Citrato de feniltoloxamina; Phenyltolyloxamine Citrate; PRN (phenyltoloxamine). 2-(2-Benzylphenoxy)-*NN*-dimethylethylamine dihydrogen citrate.

$C_{17}H_{21}NO,C_6H_8O_7$ = 447.5.

*CAS — 92-12-6 (phenyltoloxamine); 1176-08-5 (phenyltoloxamine citrate).*

### Profile

Phenyltoloxamine citrate, a monoethanolamine derivative, is a sedating antihistamine (p.419). It is usually given by mouth in combination preparations with a decongestant or analgesic. Phenyltoloxamine citrate has been used in nasal preparations. Phenyltoloxamine polistirex has also been administered by mouth.

### Preparations

**Proprietary Preparations** (details are given in Part 3)

**Multi-ingredient: Arg.:** Sinutab; **Austria:** Codipront; **Belg.:** Sinutab; **Braz.:** Afebrin; Setux; Setux Expectorante; Sinutab†; **Canad.:** Omni-Tuss; Sinutab Sinus & Allergy 12 Hour†; Tussionex; **Chile:** Rinofrim; Sinutab; Tossin; **Fr.:** Biocidan; Netux; Rinurel†; Rinutan†; **Ger.:** Codipront; **Hong Kong:** Codipront; Codipront cum Expectorans†; Sinutab†; **Israel:** Codivis; **Ital.:** Codipront; **Port.:** Codipront; **S.Afr.:** Adco-Sinal Co; Dequa-Flu; Pholtex; Sinutab; Sinutab with Codeine; Suncodin; **Singapore:** Codipront; **Spain:** Codipront; **Switz.:** Codipront; Codipront cum Expectorans; Ergosanol special a la cafeine†; Ergosanol special†; **Thai.:** Codipront; **UK:** Sinutab Nightime†; **USA:** Aceta-Gesic; Anabar; Chlorex-A; Comhist LA; Decongestabs†; Decongestant SR†; Decongestant†; Flextra; Hyflex; Iohist D†; Lobac; Magsal†; Major-gesic; Menoplex†; Mobigesic; Momentum; Naldecon†; Nalex-A; Nalgest†; New Decongestant Pediatric†; Norel Plus†; Percogesic; Phenylgesic; Poly-Histine; Poly-Histine D†; Quadra-Hist D†; Tetra-Mag; Tri-Phen-Chlor TR†; Trihist-D†; Uni-Decon†.

## Pimethixene *(rINN)*

BP-400; Pimetixene; Pimetixeno. 9-(1-Methyl-4-piperidylidene)thioxanthene.

$C_{19}H_{19}NS$ = 293.4.

*CAS — 314-03-4.*

*ATC — R06AX23.*

### Profile

Pimethixene is reported to be a sedating antihistamine (p.419) and an inhibitor of serotonin. It is given by mouth to children in usual doses of about 1.8 to 5.5 mg daily for coughs. It has been used as a sedative and for the treatment of respiratory disorders.

### Preparations

**Proprietary Preparations** (details are given in Part 3)

**Braz.:** Ansiotex; Muricalm; Sonin; **Fr.:** Calmixene; **Switz.:** Sedosil†.

**Multi-ingredient: Braz.:** Santussal.

## Piprinhydrinate *(BAN, rINN)*

Diphenylpyraline Teoclate; Diphenylpyraline Theoclate; Piprinhidrinato. The diphenylpyraline salt of 8-chlorotheophylline; 4-Benzhydryloxy-1-methylpiperidine salt of 8-chlorotheophylline.

$C_{19}H_{23}NO,C_7H_7ClN_4O_2$ = 496.0.

*CAS — 606-90-6.*

### Profile

Piprinhydrinate, a piperidine derivative, is an antihistamine (p.419) given by mouth as an ingredient of compound preparations for the symptomatic relief of coughs and the common cold.

### Preparations

**Proprietary Preparations** (details are given in Part 3)

**Hong Kong:** Plokon; **Thai.:** Plokon.

**Multi-ingredient: Austria:** Influvidon; **Ger.:** Kolton grippale N.

# Promethazine *(BAN, rINN)*

Prometazina. Dimethyl (1-methyl-2-phenothiazin-10-ylethyl)amine.

$C_{17}H_{20}N_2S$ = 284.4.

*CAS — 60-87-7.*

*ATC — D04AA10; R06AD02.*

## Promethazine Hydrochloride *(BANM, rINNM)*

Diprazinum; Hidrocloruro de prometazina; Proazamine Chloride; Promethazini Hydrochloridum; Promethazinium Chloride.

$C_{17}H_{20}N_2S,HCl$ = 320.9.

*CAS — 58-33-3.*

*ATC — D04AA10; R06AD02.*

**Pharmacopoeias.** In *Chin., Eur.* (see p.vi), *Int., Jpn, Pol., US,* and *Viet.*

**Ph. Eur. 5.0** (Promethazine Hydrochloride). A white or faintly yellowish, crystalline powder. Very soluble in water; freely soluble in alcohol and in dichloromethane. A 10% solution in water has a pH of 4.0 to 5.0. Protect from light.

**USP 27** (Promethazine Hydrochloride). A white to faint yellow, practically odourless, crystalline powder. Slowly oxidises and acquires a blue colour on prolonged exposure to air. Freely soluble in water, in hot dehydrated alcohol, and in chloroform; practically insoluble in acetone, in ether, and in ethyl acetate. pH of a 5% solution in water is between 4.0 to 5.0. Store in airtight containers. Protect from light.

**Adsorption.** References[1-4] to studies of the adsorption of promethazine hydrochloride onto various glass and plastic containers and infusion systems. Factors affecting the degree of adsorption included the particular material tested and the pH of the solution.

1. Kowaluk EA, *et al.* Interactions between drugs and polyvinyl chloride infusion bags. *Am J Hosp Pharm* 1981; **38:** 1308–14.
2. Kowaluk EA, *et al.* Interactions between drugs and intravenous delivery systems. *Am J Hosp Pharm* 1982; **39:** 460–7.
3. Rhodes RS, *et al.* Stability of meperidine hydrochloride, promethazine hydrochloride, and atropine sulfate in plastic syringes. *Am J Hosp Pharm* 1985; **42:** 112–5.
4. Martens HJ, *et al.* Sorption of various drugs in polyvinyl chloride, glass, and polyethylene-lined infusion containers. *Am J Hosp Pharm* 1990; **47:** 369–73.

**Incompatibility.** Solutions of promethazine hydrochloride are incompatible with alkaline substances, which precipitate the insoluble promethazine base. Compounds reported to be incompatible with promethazine hydrochloride include aminophylline, barbiturates, benzylpenicillin salts, carbenicillin sodium, chloramphenicol sodium succinate, chlorothiazide sodium, cefmetazole sodium, cefoperazone sodium, cefotetan disodium, dimenhydrinate, doxorubicin hydrochloride (in a liposomal formulation), furosemide, heparin sodium, hydrocortisone sodium succinate, meticillin sodium, morphine sulfate, nalbuphine hydrochloride, and some contrast media and parenteral nutrient solutions.

## Promethazine Teoclate *(BAN, rINN)*

Promethazine Theoclate; Teoclato de prometazina. The promethazine salt of 8-chlorotheophylline .

$C_{17}H_{20}N_2S,C_7H_7ClN_4O_2$ = 499.0.

*CAS — 17693-51-5.*

*ATC — D04AA10; R06AD02.*

**Pharmacopoeias.** In *Br.*

**BP 2003** (Promethazine Teoclate). A white or almost white, odourless or almost odourless powder. Very slightly soluble in water; sparingly soluble in alcohol; freely soluble in chloroform; practically insoluble in ether. Protect from light.

## Adverse Effects

As for the sedating antihistamines in general, p.419.

Cardiovascular side-effects are more commonly seen after injection, and bradycardia, tachycardia, transient minor increases in blood pressure, and occasional hypotension have all been reported with promethazine hydrochloride. Jaundice and blood dyscrasias have been reported, and extrapyramidal effects may occur at high doses.

Venous thrombosis has been reported at the site of intravenous injections, and arteriospasm and gangrene may follow inadvertent intra-arterial injection.

**Overdosage.** A toxic neurological syndrome which included CNS depression, acute excitomotor manifestations, ataxia and visual hallucinations, plus peripheral antimuscarinic effects developed in 2 children aged 44 months and 16 months after topical application of a 2% promethazine cream providing between 12.9 and 26 mg/kg.[1] The older child had also received hydroxyzine 10 mg by mouth 1 hour earlier.

1. Shawn DH, McGuigan MA. Poisoning from dermal absorption of promethazine. *Can Med Assoc J* 1984; **130:** 1460–1.

**Sudden infant death syndrome.** Although some early reports raised the possibility of an association between the use of phenothiazine antihistamines and the sudden infant death syndrome (SIDS) this has not been confirmed. Following an initial report that 4 of 7 infants with SIDS had been given alimemazine before death and that a series of severe apnoeic crises had been observed in the twin of a SIDS victim given promethazine,[1] the same workers studied 52 SIDS victims, 36 near-miss infants (those who had experienced severe unexplained episodes of cyanosis or pallor during sleep), and 175 control subjects to investigate the role of nasopharyngitis and phenothiazines in this syndrome.[2] They found that there was no difference in the incidence of nasopharyngitis between the 3 groups, but the proportion of infants given phenothiazines was higher in both the SIDS group (23%) and the near-miss group (22%) than in the control group (2%). In a subsequent study,[3] they found that the incidence of central and obstructive sleep apnoeas was increased in 4 healthy infants given promethazine for 3 days, although the duration of the attacks was unaltered and generally short, with a range of 3 to 10 seconds. A report on behalf of the European Commission,[4] stated that no link between sudden deaths in infants and drug administration had been confirmed by national drug monitoring centres. It was likely that the risk of apnoea was associated with all sedative drugs, especially in overdose.[4] Previously, phenothiazine-induced hyperthermia had been proposed as a contributory factor in SIDS.[5]

As recently as 1994 concern has been expressed[6] that promethazine was frequently prescribed for children under 2 years despite recommendations to the contrary. The current view in the UK and USA is that phenothiazine antihistamines such as promethazine and alimemazine should not be given to children under 2 years of age, primarily because the safety of such use has not been established.

1. Kahn A, Blum D. Possible role of phenothiazines in sudden infant death. *Lancet* 1979; **ii:** 364–5.
2. Kahn A, Blum D. Phenothiazines and sudden infant death syndrome. *Pediatrics* 1982; **70:** 75–8.
3. Kahn A, *et al.* Phenothiazine-induced sleep apneas in normal infants. *Pediatrics* 1985; **75:** 844–7.
4. Cockfield. Phenergan, Theralene, Algotropyl—drugs responsible for the death of new-born babies. *Off J EC* 1986; **29:** C130/25–6.
5. Stanton AN. Sudden infant death syndrome and phenothiazines. *Pediatrics* 1983; **71:** 986–7.
6. Pollard AJ, Rylance G. Inappropriate prescribing of promethazine in infants. *Arch Dis Child* 1994; **70:** 357.

## Precautions

As for the sedating antihistamines in general, p.420.

Intravenous injections of promethazine hydrochloride must be given slowly and extreme care must be taken to avoid extravasation or inadvertent intra-arterial injection, due to the risk of severe irritation. Intramuscular injection may be painful, and it should not be given by subcutaneous injection.

False negative and positive results have been reported with some pregnancy tests.

**Anaesthesia.** In 8 healthy subjects promethazine 25 mg intravenously decreased lower oesophageal sphincter pressure and increased the incidence of gastro-oesophageal reflux.[1] It might, therefore, increase the risk of regurgitation and aspiration of gastric contents during induction of and recovery from anaesthesia. The effect was attributed to the antimuscarinic properties of promethazine.

1. Brock-Utne JG, *et al.* The action of commonly used antiemetics on the lower oesophageal sphincter. *Br J Anaesth* 1978; **50:** 295–8.

**Children.** A possible association between phenothiazine sedatives and sudden infant death syndrome has been suggested, but has not been confirmed (see under Adverse Effects, above). The current view in the UK and USA is that promethazine should not be given to children under 2 years of age, primarily because the safety of such use has not been established.

**Porphyria.** Promethazine is considered to be unsafe in patients with porphyria because it has been shown to be porphyrinogenic in *animals* or *in-vitro* systems.

**Pregnancy.** For discussion of the use of antihistamines in pregnancy, including studies involving phenothiazines, see p.420.

**Renal impairment.** Phenothiazine-induced toxic psychosis occurred in a patient with chronic renal failure who had been given promethazine.[1]

1. McAllister CJ, *et al.* Toxic psychosis induced by phenothiazine administration in patients with chronic renal failure. *Clin Nephrol* 1978; **10:** 191–5.

## Interactions

As for the sedating antihistamines in general, p.421.

## Pharmacokinetics

Promethazine is well absorbed after oral or intramuscular administration. Peak plasma concentrations have been observed 2 to 3 hours after administration by these routes, although there is low systemic bioavailability after oral administration, due to high first-pass metabolism in the liver. Promethazine crosses the blood-brain barrier and the placenta, and is distributed into breast milk. Values ranging from 76 to 93% have been reported for plasma-protein binding. Promethazine undergoes extensive metabolism, predominantly to promethazine sulfoxide, and also to *N*-desmethylpromethazine. It is excreted slowly via the urine and bile, chiefly as metabolites. Elimination half-lives of 5 to 14 hours have been reported.

◊ References.

1. Taylor G, *et al.* Pharmacokinetics of promethazine and its sulphoxide metabolite after intravenous and oral administration to man. *Br J Clin Pharmacol* 1983; **15:** 287–93.
2. Paton DM, Webster DR. Clinical pharmacokinetics of $H_1$-receptor antagonists (the antihistamines). *Clin Pharmacokinet* 1985; **10:** 477–97.

3. Stavchansky S, *et al.* Bioequivalence and pharmacokinetic profile of promethazine hydrochloride suppositories in humans. *J Pharm Sci* 1987; **76:** 441–5.
4. Strenkoski-Nix LC, *et al.* Pharmacokinetics of promethazine hydrochloride after administration of rectal suppositories and oral syrup to healthy subjects. *Am J Health-Syst Pharm* 2000; **57:** 1499–1505.

## Uses and Administration

Promethazine, a phenothiazine derivative, is a sedating antihistamine with antimuscarinic, significant sedative, and some serotonin-antagonist properties. It is usually given as the hydrochloride or teoclate. Promethazine embonate and promethazine maleate have also been given orally. Promethazine dioxide (dioxopromethazine) has been used as the hydrochloride in eye and nasal drops. The antihistamine action has been reported to last for between 4 and 12 hours.

Promethazine hydrochloride is used for the symptomatic relief of allergic conditions including urticaria and angioedema (p.423), rhinitis (p.422) and conjunctivitis (p.421), and in pruritic skin disorders (p.422). It may be given intravenously as an adjunct in the emergency treatment of anaphylactic shock (p.421).

Promethazine hydrochloride and promethazine teoclate are used for their antiemetic action in the prevention and treatment of nausea and vomiting in conditions such as motion sickness, drug-induced vomiting, and postoperative vomiting (p.422). They are also used for the symptomatic treatment of nausea and vertigo caused by Ménière's disease and other vestibular disorders (see Vertigo, p.423). Promethazine hydrochloride is also employed pre- and postoperatively in surgery and obstetrics for its sedative effects and for the relief of apprehension (see Anaesthesia, p.421); it is often given with pethidine hydrochloride. Promethazine hydrochloride may be used for night-time sedation (p.422).

Promethazine hydrochloride is a common ingredient of compound preparations for the symptomatic treatment of coughs and the common cold (p.421).

The following doses have been given **by mouth**.

- For the treatment of *allergic conditions* promethazine hydrochloride is usually given in a dose of 25 mg at night increased to 25 mg twice daily if necessary; owing to its pronounced sedative effect it is preferably given at night but an alternative dose is 10 to 20 mg two or three times daily.
- Promethazine hydrochloride is given in doses of 20 to 50 mg at night for the short-term management of *insomnia* although its prolonged duration of action can lead to considerable drowsiness the following day.
- For the prevention of *motion sickness* promethazine hydrochloride can be given in a dose of 20 or 25 mg the night before travelling followed by a similar dose the following morning if necessary. The teoclate is used similarly. For the prevention of motion sickness the dose of promethazine teoclate is 25 mg at night or 25 mg one to two hours before travelling.
- For nausea and vomiting arising from causes such as *labyrinthitis* a dose of 25 mg at night is usually adequate; this may be increased to 50 or 75 mg at night or to 25 mg two or three times daily if necessary to a maximum of 100 mg daily.
- For *severe vomiting in pregnancy* the *British National Formulary* recommends a dose of 25 mg at night, increased if necessary to a maximum of 100 mg.

In *children* the following oral doses of promethazine hydrochloride have been recommended.

- For allergic conditions: 2 to 5 years, 5 to 15 mg daily in one or two divided doses; 5 to 10 years, 10 to 25 mg daily in one or two divided doses.
- For night sedation or premedication: 2 to 5 years, 15 to 20 mg; 5 to 10 years, 20 to 25 mg.
- For the prevention of motion sickness the following doses of promethazine hydrochloride may be given the night before the journey and repeated on the following morning if necessary: 2 to 5 years, 5 mg; 5 to 10 years, 10 mg. Promethazine teoclate may also be given to children aged 5 to 10 years for the prevention of motion sickness in a dose of 12.5 mg daily, starting either on the night before travelling for long journeys or one to two hours before short journeys.
- Children aged 5 to 10 years may also receive promethazine teoclate for nausea and vomiting from causes such as labyrinthitis in a dose of 12.5 to 37.5 mg daily.

Promethazine hydrochloride is also administered by the **rectal** route as suppositories. Doses are similar to those given by mouth.

Promethazine hydrochloride is given **parenterally** by deep intramuscular injection as a solution of 25 or 50 mg/mL. It may also be given by slow intravenous injection or injected into the tubing of a freely running infusion in a concentration of not more than 25 mg/mL, although it is usually diluted to 2.5 mg/mL. The rate of infusion should not exceed 25 mg/minute. The usual parenteral dose for all indications apart from nausea and vomiting is 25 to 50 mg; a dose of 100 mg should not be exceeded. Doses of 12.5 to 25 mg, repeated at intervals of not less than 4 hours, may be given for the treatment of nausea and vomiting, although not more than 100 mg is usually given in 24 hours.

*Children* aged 5 to 10 years may be given 6.25 to 12.5 mg of promethazine hydrochloride by deep intramuscular injection.

Promethazine has been used **topically** to provide relief in hypersensitivity disorders of the skin and for burns but, as with other antihistamines, it may produce skin sensitisation.

**Sedation.** For reference to the use of lytic cocktails of chlorpromazine, promethazine, and pethidine, and the view that alternatives should be considered in children, see under Pethidine, p.82.

## Preparations

***BP 2003:*** Promethazine Hydrochloride Tablets; Promethazine Injection; Promethazine Oral Solution; Promethazine Teoclate Tablets;
***USP 27:*** Promethazine Hydrochloride Injection; Promethazine Hydrochloride Suppositories; Promethazine Hydrochloride Syrup; Promethazine Hydrochloride Tablets.

**Proprietary Preparations** (details are given in Part 3)

***Arg.:*** Fenergan; ***Austral.:*** Avomine; Gold Cross Antihistamine Elixir; Insomn-Eze; Nyal Plus+ Allergy Relief; Phenergan; ***Austria:*** Phenergan†; ***Belg.:*** Phenergan; ***Braz.:*** Alergiderm; Alergosan; Fenergan; Pamergan; Profergan; ***Canad.:*** Histantil; Phenergan; ***Denm.:*** Phenergan; ***Fr.:*** Phenergan; ***Ger.:*** Atosil; Closin; Eusedon mono; Promethawern; Proneurin; Prothanon; Prothazin; ***Gr.:*** Phenergan; Titanox; ***Hong Kong:*** Avomine†; Phenergan†; Synvomin; ***India:*** Avomine; Phenergan; ***Irl.:*** Phenergan; ***Israel:*** Prothiazine; ***Ital.:*** Allerfen; Duplamin†; Fargan; Farganesse; Fenazil; ***Malaysia:*** Prothazine; ***Neth.:*** Phenergan†; ***Norw.:*** Phenergan; ***NZ:*** Avomine; Goodnight†; Phenergan; ***Port.:*** Fenergan; ***S.Afr.:*** Avomine; Brunazine; Daralix; Lenazine; Phenergan; Prohist; Receptozine; ***Singapore:*** Phenergan†; Xepagan†; ***Spain:*** Fenergan Topico; Frinova; Sayomol†; ***Swed.:*** Lergigan; ***Switz.:*** Phenergan†; ***Thai.:*** Phenergan; ***UAE:*** Histaloc; ***UK:*** Avomine; Phenergan; Phenhalal†; Sominex; Ziz; ***USA:*** Anergan†; Phenadoz; Phenergan.

**Multi-ingredient:** ***Austral.:*** Painstop; Panquil; Phensedyl; Tixylix Nightime; ***Belg.:*** Phenergan Expectorant†; ***Braz.:*** Fenergan Expectorante; Lisador; ***Canad.:*** Phenergan Expectorant with Codeine†; Phenergan Expectorant†; Phenergan VC Expectorant with Codeine†; Phenergan VC Expectorant†; Promatussin DM; ***Fr.:*** Algotropyl; Fluisedal; Paxeladine Noctee†; Quintopan Enfant†; Rhinathiol Promethazine; Transmer; Tussisedal; ***Ger.:*** Thesit P†; ***Hong Kong:*** Dhasedyl; Ephedyl; Fendyl; PEC; Procodine; Promethazine Compound Linctus; Rhinathiol Promethazine; Sedilix DM†; Super Cough; Tixylix Nightime†; Tripe P; ***India:*** Tixylix; ***Irl.:*** Night Nurse; Tixylix†; ***Israel:*** Promethazine Expectorants; Prothiazine Expectorant; ***Ital.:*** Bronconait; Difmetus Compositum†; Nuleron; ***Malaysia:*** Dextrodyl; Metofen Compound; Phensedyl; Promedyl; Rhinathiol Promethazine; Russedyl; SCMC Promethazine; Sedilix; Sedilix DM; Tixylix; ***NZ:*** Coldrex Night Relief†; Phensedyl Dry Family Cough; Tixylix; ***S.Afr.:*** Acustop†; Adco-Kiddipayne; Antituss†; Ban Pain; Brunacod; Colcaps; Darosed†; Dequa-Coff; Dynapayne†; Go-Pain; Goldgesic; Histodor; Infapain Forte; Kid-Eeze; Lenazine Forte; Lentogesic; Lesspain; Maxadol†; Megapyn; Mepromol; Painagon; Pedigesic†; Pedpain; Phensedyl; Propain; Pynmed; Salterpyn; Stilpane; Stopayne; Synaleve†; Tenston; Tixylix; Vacudol; Xeramax; ***Singapore:*** Delix†; Dhasedyl; Dhasedyl DM; PCL; Phensedyl; Procodin; Promedyl; Rhinathiol Promethazine†; Sedilix; Sedilix DM; Unisedyl; Walsedyl†; ***Spain:*** Actithiol Antihist; Antihemorroidal; Fenergan Expectorante; Psicosoma Solucion; Sugarceton†; ***Swed.:*** Lergigan comp; ***Switz.:*** Broncatar†; Linervidol; Lysedil; Lysedil compositum†; Nardyl; Phenergan Expectorant†; Rectoquintyl-Promethazine†; Rhinathiol Promethazine; ***Thai.:*** Conadyl†; Decos; Nordyl; Nortuss; Phencodin; Phensedyl; Teradyl; ***UAE:*** Flukit; ***UK:*** Day & Night Nurse; Medised†; Night Nurse; Pamergan P100; Phensedyl Plus†; Ronpirin Cold Remedy†; Tixylix Night-Time; ***USA:*** Mepergan†; Pentazine VC with Codeine; Phenameth DM; Phenergan VC with Codeine†; Phenergan VC†; Phenergan with Codeine†; Phenergan with Dextromethorphan†; Pherazine DM; Pherazine VC; Pherazine VC with Codeine; Pherazine with Codeine; Prometh VC Plain; Prometh with Dextromethorphan; Promethazine VC with Codeine.

---

## Propiomazine *(BAN, USAN, rINN)*

CB-1678 (propiomazine or propiomazine maleate); Wy-1359 (propiomazine or propiomazine maleate). 1-[10-(2-Dimethylaminopropyl)phenothiazin-2-yl]propan-1-one.

$C_{20}H_{24}N_2OS$ = 340.5.
*CAS — 362-29-8.*
*ATC — N05CM06.*

## Propiomazine Hydrochloride *(BANM, rINNM)*

Hidrocloruro de propiomazina.

$C_{20}H_{24}N_2OS,HCl$ = 376.9.
*CAS — 362-29-8 (propiomazine); 1240-15-9 (propiomazine hydrochloride).*
*ATC — N05CM06.*

## Propiomazine Maleate *(BANM, rINNM)*

CB-1678 (propiomazine or propiomazine maleate); Maleato de propiomazina; Propiomazine Hydrogen Maleate; Wy-1359 (propiomazine or propiomazine maleate).

$C_{20}H_{24}N_2OS,C_4H_4O_4$ = 456.6.
*CAS — 3568-23-8.*
*ATC — N05CM06.*

### Adverse Effects and Precautions

As for the sedating antihistamines in general, p.419. Local irritation may occur at the site of intravenous injection of propiomazine hydrochloride and there may be thrombophlebitis.

### Interactions

As for the sedating antihistamines in general, p.421.

### Uses and Administration

Propiomazine, a phenothiazine derivative, is a sedating antihistamine used for its sedative and antiemetic properties in insomnia (p.422) and nausea and vomiting (p.422).

Propiomazine is given by mouth as the maleate and parenterally as the hydrochloride. Doses of the maleate are expressed in terms of the equivalent amount of propiomazine base; propiomazine maleate 1.3 mg is approximately equivalent to 1 mg of propiomazine. Doses of the hydrochloride are expressed in terms of this salt.

The maleate is given by mouth as a hypnotic in doses equivalent to 25 to 50 mg at night.

Propiomazine hydrochloride has been given by intramuscular or slow intravenous injection in doses ranging from 10 to 40 mg for anaesthetic premedication and during surgical and obstetric procedures (p.421). Children weighing up to 27 kg have been given 0.55 to 1.1 mg/kg intramuscularly or intravenously. Alternatively, those aged 2 to 4 years have been given 10 mg; 4 to 6 years, 15 mg; 6 to 12 years, 25 mg.

### Preparations

**Proprietary Preparations** (details are given in Part 3)
***Swed.:*** Propavan; ***USA:*** Largon†.

---

## Quifenadine Hydrochloride *(rINNM)*

α,α-Diphenyl-3-quinuclidinemethanol hydrochloride.

$C_{20}H_{23}NO,HCl$ = 329.9.
*CAS — 10447-39-9 (quifenadine); 10447-38-8 (quifenadine hydrochloride).*

### Profile

Quifenadine is an antihistamine given orally as the hydrochloride.

---

## Rupatadine *(rINN)*

UR-12592 (rupatadine fumarate). 8-Chloro-6,11-dihydro-11-{1-[(5-methyl-3-pyridyl)methyl]-4-piperidylidene}-5*H*-benzo[5,6]cyclohepta[1,2-*b*]pyridine.

$C_{26}H_{26}ClN_3$ = 416.0.
*CAS — 158876-82-5 (rupatadine); 182349-12-8 (rupatadine fumarate).*
*ATC — R06AX28.*

### Profile

Rupatadine is an antihistamine with platelet-activating factor (PAF) antagonist activity that is used for the treatment of allergic rhinitis (p.422). It is given as the fumarate although doses are expressed in terms of the base. The usual dose by mouth is the equivalent of 10 mg once daily of rupatadine.

◊ References.

1. Izquierdo I, *et al.* Rupatadine: a new selective histamine H1 receptor and platelet-activating factor (PAF) antagonist: a review of pharmacological profile and clinical management of allergic rhinitis. *Drugs Today* 2003; **39:** 451–68.

### Preparations

**Proprietary Preparations** (details are given in Part 3)
***Spain:*** Alergoliber.

## Setastine Hydrochloride *(rINNM)*

EGIS-2062; EGYT-2062; Hidrocloruro de setastina. 1-{2-[(*p*-Chloro-α-methyl-α-phenylbenzyl)oxy]ethyl}hexahydro-1*H*-azepine hydrochloride.

$C_{22}H_{28}ClNO,HCl = 394.4.$

*CAS — 64294-95-7 (setastine).*

### Profile

Setastine hydrochloride, a derivative of clemastine, is an antihistamine (p.419) claimed to have no sedative activity. It has been given by mouth for the symptomatic relief of hypersensitivity disorders.

### Preparations

**Proprietary Preparations** (details are given in Part 3)

***Hung.:*** Loderix.

---

## Terfenadine *(BAN, USAN, rINN)*

MDL-9918; RMI-9918; Terfenadina; Terfenadinum. 1-(4-*tert*-Butylphenyl)-4-[4-(α-hydroxybenzhydryl)piperidino]butan-1-ol.

$C_{32}H_{41}NO_2 = 471.7.$

*CAS — 50679-08-8.*

*ATC — R06AX12.*

**Pharmacopoeias.** In *Eur.* (see p.vi).

**Ph. Eur. 5.0** (Terfenadine). A white, crystalline powder. It shows polymorphism. Very slightly soluble in water and in dilute hydrochloric acid; freely soluble in dichloromethane; soluble in methyl alcohol. Protect from light.

### Adverse Effects and Precautions

As for the non-sedating antihistamines in general, p.419. Erythema multiforme and galactorrhoea have also been reported.

Ventricular arrhythmias, including torsade de pointes, have occurred rarely with terfenadine, particularly in association with raised blood concentrations (see Arrhythmias, below). To *reduce the risk* of developing such arrhythmias the recommended dose should **not** be exceeded and terfenadine should be **avoided** in patients with cardiac or significant hepatic disease, with hypokalaemia or other electrolyte imbalance, or with known or suspected prolonged QT interval. The concomitant administration of drugs liable to interfere with the hepatic metabolism of terfenadine, of other potentially arrhythmogenic drugs including those that prolong the QT interval, and of drugs likely to cause electrolyte imbalance is **contra-indicated** (see under Interactions, below). If palpitations, dizziness, syncope, or convulsions occur terfenadine should be withdrawn and the patient investigated for potential arrhythmias.

**Alopecia.** Hair loss was associated with terfenadine treatment in a 24-year-old patient.[1] Regrowth occurred when treatment was stopped.


1. Jones SK, Morley WN. Terfenadine causing hair loss. *BMJ* 1985; **291:** 940.


**Arrhythmias.** Ventricular arrhythmias including torsade de pointes have occurred with terfenadine at doses greater than those recommended[1] and also at normal doses in patients whose metabolism of terfenadine is impaired by drugs or by liver disease. Generalised convulsions and a quinine-like effect on the ECG have also been reported after a presumed overdose of terfenadine.[2] Consequently a number of recommendations have been made to *reduce the risk* of developing serious arrhythmias, including those from the UK Committee on Safety of Medicines[3,4] (see Adverse Effects and Precautions, above, for details). Terfenadine should be discontinued immediately, and the patient evaluated for potential arrhythmias, in those who experience syncope, palpitations, dizziness, or convulsions after taking terfenadine.

Studies[5] have suggested that the ventricular arrhythmias are due to terfenadine itself rather than its active metabolite fexofenadine (p.433). Terfenadine has been shown to inhibit cardiac potassium channels which results in prolongation of the QT interval, a risk factor for developing arrhythmias, while the non-sedating antihistamines cetirizine, fexofenadine, and loratadine have had no demonstrable effect[5,6] (see also p.420).


1. MacConnell TJ, Stanners AJ. Torsades de pointes complicating treatment with terfenadine. *BMJ* 1991; **302:** 1469.
2. Davies AJ, *et al.* Cardiotoxic effect with convulsions in terfenadine overdose. *BMJ* 1989; **298:** 325.
3. Committee on Safety of Medicines. Ventricular arrhythmias due to terfenadine and astemizole. *Current Problems 35* 1992.
4. Committee on Safety of Medicines/Medicines Control Agency. Drug-induced prolongation of the QT interval. *Current Problems* 1996; **22:** 2.
5. Woolsey RL, *et al.* Mechanism of the cardiotoxic actions of terfenadine. *JAMA* 1993; **269:** 1532–6.
6. Rankin AC. Non-sedating antihistamines and cardiac arrhythmia. *Lancet* 1997; **350:** 1115–16.


**Breast feeding.** No adverse effects have been observed in breast-feeding infants whose mothers were receiving terfenadine, and the American Academy of Pediatrics[1] considers that it is therefore usually compatible with breast feeding.

In a study[2] of 4 healthy lactating women given 60 mg of terfenadine every 12 hours for 48 hours, terfenadine was undetected in breast milk; its active metabolite, fexofenadine, was excreted in limited amounts.


1. American Academy of Pediatrics. The transfer of drugs and other chemicals into human milk. *Pediatrics* 2001; **108:** 776–89. Correction. *ibid.*; 1029. Also available at: http://aappolicy.aappublications.org/cgi/content/full/pediatrics%3b108/3/776 (accessed 08/04/04)
2. Lucas BD, *et al.* Terfenadine pharmacokinetics in breast milk in lactating women. *Clin Pharmacol Ther* 1995; **57:** 398–402.


**Effects on the liver.** Three episodes of acute hepatitis with jaundice occurred in a patient taking terfenadine intermittently over a period of 17 months.[1] Liver function tests returned to normal after the drug was stopped. Two further cases[2] of cholestatic hepatitis associated with terfenadine have been reported. Again, liver function tests returned to normal after drug withdrawal. A study[3] by the Boston Collaborative Drug Surveillance Program of 210 683 patients who had received prescriptions for terfenadine concluded that the use of terfenadine was rarely associated with important idiopathic liver disease. The investigators found only 3 cases of acute liver disease where a causal connection to terfenadine could not be ruled out; all these patients had received a concomitant hepatotoxic drug and had made a full recovery.


1. Larrey D, *et al.* Terfenadine and hepatitis. *Ann Intern Med* 1985; **103:** 634.
2. Sahai A, Villeneuve JP. Terfenadine-induced cholestatic hepatitis. *Lancet* 1996; **348:** 552–3.
3. Myers MW, Jick H. Terfenadine and risk of acute liver disease. *Br J Clin Pharmacol* 1998; **46:** 251–3.


**Effects on the nervous system.** Non-sedating effects on the CNS have been reported after a single dose of terfenadine;[1] these have included anxiety, palpitations, and insomnia. The UK manufacturers commented that clinical studies suggest that the incidence of such effects is similar to that seen after placebo.[2]

Workers who had described a generalised tonic-clonic seizure in a patient taking terfenadine[3] later reported that the patient had subsequently had a second unprovoked seizure[4] and now considered that terfenadine may not have been the cause of his original seizure. Convulsions have been reported following overdosage with terfenadine (see under Arrhythmias, above).

The sedative effects of the older antihistamines and the lack of such effects with the non-sedating antihistamines including terfenadine are discussed under Sedation on p.420.


1. Napke E, Biron P. Nervous reactions after first dose of terfenadine in adults. *Lancet* 1989; **ii:** 615–16.
2. Masheter HC. Nervous reactions to terfenadine. *Lancet* 1989; **ii:** 1034.
3. Tidswell P, d'Assis-Fonseca A. Generalised seizure due to terfenadine. *BMJ* 1993; **307:** 241.
4. Tidswell P, d'Assis-Fonseca A. Generalised seizure due to terfenadine. *BMJ* 1993; **307:** 736.


**Hypersensitivity.** Terfenadine administration was associated with 108 reports of skin reactions, including rashes, urticaria, angioedema, photosensitivity reactions and peeling of the skin of the hands or feet.[1]


1. Stricker BHCh, *et al.* Skin reactions to terfenadine. *BMJ* 1986; **293:** 536.


**Porphyria.** Terfenadine has been associated with acute attacks of porphyria and is considered unsafe in porphyric patients.

### Interactions

As for the non-sedating antihistamines in general, p.421.

Terfenadine should not be given with drugs that inhibit its hepatic metabolism because of the increased risk of serious ventricular arrhythmias. These drugs include the *triazole* and *imidazole antifungals* such as *itraconazole* and *ketoconazole*, the *macrolide antibacterials* including *clarithromycin*, *erythromycin*, *josamycin*, and *troleandomycin*, the streptogramin antibacterial *quinupristin/dalfopristin*, the serotonin reuptake inhibitors *citalopram*, *fluoxetine*, *fluvoxamine*, *nefazodone*, and *paroxetine*, the HIV-protease inhibitors *indinavir*, *nelfinavir*, *ritonavir*, and *saquinavir*, the non-nucleoside reverse transcriptase inhibitor antiretroviral *efavirenz*, and *zileuton*. The metabolism of terfenadine may also be inhibited by grapefruit juice and concomitant use should be avoided.

Use with other potentially arrhythmogenic drugs (including those that prolong the QT interval) such as *antiarrhythmics*, *tricyclic antidepressants*, the antimalarials *halofantrine* and *quinine*, *antipsychotics*, *cisapride*, *probucol*, *pentamidine isetionate*, and the beta blocker *sotalol* should be avoided as should co-administration of *diuretics* that cause electrolyte imbalances especially hypokalaemia. The use of terfenadine and *astemizole* together is not recommended.

◊ General references.


1. Kivistö KT, *et al.* Inhibition of terfenadine metabolism: pharmacokinetic and pharmacodynamic consequences. *Clin Pharmacokinet* 1994; **27:** 1–5.


**Antibacterials.** Pharmacokinetic studies have shown that the macrolide antibiotics *erythromycin*[1] and *clarithromycin*[2] interfere with the metabolism of terfenadine leading to its accumulation. A high plasma-terfenadine concentration is associated with prolongation of the QT interval, and arrhythmias such as torsade de pointes have been reported in patients given terfenadine with erythromycin[3] or *troleandomycin*.[4]


1. Honig PK, *et al.* Changes in the pharmacokinetics and electrocardiographic pharmacodynamics of terfenadine with concomitant administration of erythromycin. *Clin Pharmacol Ther* 1992; **52:** 231–8.
2. Honig P, *et al.* Effect of erythromycin, clarithromycin and azithromycin on the pharmacokinetics of terfenadine. *Clin Pharmacol Ther* 1993; **53:** 161.
3. Biglin KE, *et al.* Drug-induced torsades de pointes: a possible interaction of terfenadine and erythromycin. *Ann Pharmacother* 1994; **28:** 282.
4. Fournier P, *et al.* Une nouvelle cause de torsades de pointes: association terfenadine et troleandomycine. *Ann Cardiol Angeiol (Paris)* 1993; **42:** 249–52.


**Antidepressants.** Cardiac abnormalities have been reported in 2 patients taking *fluoxetine* with terfenadine.[1,2] Similarly, the use of *nefazodone* with terfenadine has resulted in prolongation of the QT interval.[3]


1. Swims MP. Potential terfenadine-fluoxetine interaction. *Ann Pharmacother* 1993; **27:** 1404–5.
2. Marchiando RJ, Cook MD. Probable terfenadine-fluoxetine-associated cardiac toxicity. *Ann Pharmacother* 1995; **29:** 937–8.
3. Abernethy DR, *et al.* Loratadine and terfenadine interaction with nefazodone: both antihistamines are associated with QTc prolongation. *Clin Pharmacol Ther* 2001; **69:** 96–103.


**Antiepileptics.** For reference to an interaction between terfenadine and *carbamazepine*, see p.356.

**Antifungals.** Pharmacokinetic studies have shown that *itraconazole*[1] and *ketoconazole*[2] interfere with the metabolism of terfenadine leading to its accumulation. A high plasma-terfenadine concentration is associated with prolongation of the QT interval, and arrhythmias such as torsade de pointes have been reported in patients given terfenadine with ketoconazole[3] or itraconazole.[1,4] While there has been a pharmacokinetic study[5] that suggested that the interaction between terfenadine and *fluconazole* might not be clinically significant, as the mechanism of the interaction appeared to involve the metabolite of terfenadine and did not lead to accumulation of the cardiotoxic parent compound, this may not always be the case. Studies in a small group of patients who exhibited abnormal patterns of terfenadine metabolism found increases in terfenadine concentrations associated with ECG abnormalities when terfenadine was given with high doses of fluconazole.[6]


1. Pohjola-Sintonen S, *et al.* Itraconazole prevents terfenadine metabolism and increases risk of torsades de pointes ventricular tachycardia. *Eur J Clin Pharmacol* 1993; **45:** 191–3.
2. Honig PK, *et al.* Terfenadine-ketoconazole interaction: pharmacokinetic and electrocardiographic consequences. *JAMA* 1993; **269:** 1513–18.
3. Monahan BP, *et al.* Torsades de pointes occurring in association with terfenadine use. *JAMA* 1990; **264:** 2788–90.
4. Crane JK, *et al.* Syncope and cardiac arrhythmia due to an interaction between itraconazole and terfenadine. *Am J Med* 1993; **95:** 445–6.
5. Honig PK, *et al.* The effect of fluconazole on the steady-state pharmacokinetics and electrocardiographic pharmacodynamics of terfenadine in humans. *Clin Pharmacol Ther* 1993; **53:** 630–6.
6. Cantilena LR, *et al.* Fluconazole alters terfenadine pharmacokinetics and electrocardiographic pharmacodynamics. *Clin Pharmacol Ther* 1995; **57:** 185.


**Calcium-channel blockers.** For reference to an interaction between terfenadine and *nifedipine*, see p.969.

**Grapefruit juice.** A study[1] in healthy subjects given terfenadine and *grapefruit juice* for 7 days demonstrated raised plasma-terfenadine concentrations and prolongation of the QT interval. These effects were less pronounced when terfenadine was given 2 hours before grapefruit juice, but were nevertheless quantifiable in some subjects. In another study QT interval changes were not found in healthy subjects given single doses of terfenadine and grapefruit juice.[2] However the highly variable pharmacokinetics between individuals led the authors to conclude that prolongation of the QT interval was possible following single doses. The probable mechanism of the interaction is inhibition of the metabolism of terfenadine by the cytochrome P450 isoenzyme CYP3A4.


1. Benton RE, *et al.* Grapefruit juice alters terfenadine pharmacokinetics, resulting in prolongation of repolarization on the electrocardiogram. *Clin Pharmacol Ther* 1996; **59:** 383–8.
2. Rau SE, *et al.* Grapefruit juice-terfenadine single-dose interaction: magnitude, mechanism, and relevance. *Clin Pharmacol Ther* 1997; **61:** 401–9.


### Pharmacokinetics

Terfenadine is rapidly absorbed from the gastrointestinal tract; peak plasma concentrations are achieved within about 2 hours. It is a prodrug and undergoes extensive first-pass metabolism in the liver to its active metabolite the carboxylic acid derivative fexofenadine (p.433). The other main metabolite is an inactive piperidine-carbinol derivative. About 97% of terfenadine is bound to plasma proteins; fexofenadine is reported to be less extensively bound. Terfenadine does not appear to cross the blood-brain barrier to a significant extent; limited amounts of fexofenadine, but not the parent drug, have been detected in breast milk. An elimination half-life of 16 to 23 hours has been reported for terfenadine. The metabolites, and traces of unchanged drug, are excreted in the urine and the faeces.

◊ References.


1. Eller MG, *et al.* Pharmacokinetics of terfenadine in healthy elderly subjects. *J Clin Pharmacol* 1992; **32:** 267–71.


### Uses and Administration

Terfenadine, a piperidine derivative, is a non-sedating antihistamine. It does not have significant antimuscarinic actions. It is used for the symptomatic relief of allergic conditions including rhinitis (p.422) and conjunctivitis (p.421) and skin disorders such as urticaria (p.423).

The maximum adult dose of terfenadine is 120 mg daily by mouth given either as 60 mg twice daily or 120 mg in the morning; a starting dose of 60 mg daily in a single dose or in two divided doses is recommended for rhinitis and conjunctivitis.

Children who are over 12 years of age and weigh more than 50 kg may receive the usual adult dosage.

For dosage in renal impairment see below.

**Administration in renal impairment.** Half the usual daily dose of terfenadine has been suggested for patients with creatinine clearance less than 40 mL/minute.

### Preparations

***BP 2003:*** Terfenadine Oral Suspension; Terfenadine Tablets.

**Proprietary Preparations** (details are given in Part 3)
***Arg.:*** Terfemax; ***Austral.:*** Teldane†; ***Austria:*** Terlane†; Triludan; ***Belg.:*** Triludan†; ***Braz.:*** Fenasil†; Histadane†; Pridinol†; Teldane†; ***Canad.:*** Allergy Relief†; Contac Allergy Formula†; Seldane†; ***Denm.:*** Teldanex; Tenadin; Terfin; ***Fin.:*** Teldanex†; ***Fr.:*** Teldane†; ***Ger.:*** Balkis Spezial†; Fomos†; Hisfedin; Histaterfen†; Teldane†; Terfedura; Terfemundin; Terfium†; Vividrin mit Terfenadin†; ***Hong Kong:*** Fenason; Hisdane; Histafen; Tamagon; Teldane†; Vida Fenadine; ***India:*** Trexyl; ***Irl.:*** Triludan†; ***Israel:*** Apoterfin†; Ternalin†; ***Ital.:*** Allerzil; ***Malaysia:*** Neutramine; Tamagon; ***Mex.:*** Teldane; ***Neth.:*** Triludan; ***Norw.:*** Teldanex; ***Port.:*** Triludan; ***S.Afr.:*** Fendin†; Terfenor†; Triludan; ***Spain:*** Aldira†; Alergist†; Cyater; Rapidal; Ternadin; ***Swed.:*** Teldanex; ***Thai.:*** Centerfen†; Fenason†; Servinadine†; Tamagon†; Teranic†; Terden†; Terdine†; Terfadine†; Terfegen†; Terfen†; Trexyl†; ***UK:*** Antihistamine Forte†; Boots Hayfever Relief Antihistamine†; Histafen†; Terfenor Antihistamine†.

**Multi-ingredient:** ***Arg.:*** Cortaler Novo; Cortistamin NF; Sinlergia; Terfenadina DG; Vixidone T; ***Braz.:*** Teldafen†; ***India:*** Alpha-Zedex; Teguphen; Tusant; ***Israel:*** Ternalin-D†; ***Malaysia:*** Trexydin; ***Mex.:*** Teldane D; ***Port.:*** Trilufen†.

## Thenyldiamine Hydrochloride *(BANM, rINNM)*

Hidrocloruro de tenildiamina; Thenyldiaminium Chloride. *NN*-Dimethyl-*N'*-(2-pyridyl)-*N'*-(3-thenyl)ethylenediamine hydrochloride.

$C_{14}H_{19}N_3S,HCl = 297.8.$

*CAS — 91-79-2 (thenyldiamine); 958-93-0 (thenyldiamine hydrochloride).*

### Profile

Thenyldiamine hydrochloride, an ethylenediamine derivative, is an antihistamine (p.419). It is given by mouth as an ingredient of compound preparations for the symptomatic treatment of coughs and the common cold.

### Preparations

**Proprietary Preparations** (details are given in Part 3)
**Multi-ingredient:** ***Braz.:*** Asafen†; ***Ital.:*** NTR; ***Spain:*** Sinefricol†.

## Thiethylperazine *(BAN, USAN, rINN)*

Tietilperazina. 2-Ethylthio-10-[3-(4-methylpiperazin-1-yl)-propyl]phenothiazine.

$C_{22}H_{29}N_3S_2 = 399.6.$

*CAS — 1420-55-9.*

*ATC — R06AD03.*

## Thiethylperazine Malate *(BANM, rINNM)*

Malato de tietilperazina.

$C_{22}H_{29}N_3S_2,2C_4H_6O_5 = 667.8.$

*CAS — 52239-63-1.*

*ATC — R06AD03.*

## Thiethylperazine Maleate *(BANM, USAN, rINNM)*

GS-95; Maleato de tietilperazina; NSC-130044; Thiethylperazine Dimaleate.

$C_{22}H_{29}N_3S_2,2C_4H_4O_4 = 631.8.$

*CAS — 1179-69-7.*

*ATC — R06AD03.*

**Pharmacopoeias.** In *Swiss* and *US.*

**USP 27** (Thiethylperazine Maleate). A yellowish granular powder, odourless or has not more than a slight odour. Soluble 1 in 1700 of water and 1 in 530 of alcohol; practically insoluble in chloroform and in ether; slightly soluble in methyl alcohol. pH of a 0.1% solution in water is between 2.8 and 3.8. Store in airtight containers. Protect from light.

**Incompatibility.** Incompatibility has been reported between injections of thiethylperazine maleate and nalbuphine hydrochloride.[1]

1. Jump WG, *et al.* Compatibility of nalbuphine hydrochloride with other preoperative medications. *Am J Hosp Pharm* 1982; **39:** 841–3.

### Adverse Effects and Precautions

As for the sedating antihistamines in general, p.419.

### Interactions

As for the sedating antihistamines in general, p.421.

### Uses and Administration

Thiethylperazine, a phenothiazine derivative with a piperazine side-chain, is a sedating antihistamine used as an antiemetic for the control of nausea and vomiting (p.422) associated with surgical procedures and cancer therapy. It has also been used for the management of vertigo (p.423) and motion sickness although there is some doubt over its efficacy for these indications.

Thiethylperazine is given as the maleate or malate and doses are expressed in terms of the appropriate salt. Thiethylperazine maleate 10 mg is approximately equivalent to thiethylperazine malate 10.53 mg.

*Thiethylperazine maleate* is given in usual doses of 10 mg up to three times daily by mouth; the maleate has also been given rectally. Where oral administration is impractical similar doses of the *malate* may be given by deep intramuscular injection. Thiethylperazine is not recommended for use in children.

### Preparations

***USP 27:*** Thiethylperazine Maleate Suppositories; Thiethylperazine Maleate Tablets.

**Proprietary Preparations** (details are given in Part 3)
***Austria:*** Torecan; ***Chile:*** Torecan; ***Ger.:*** Torecan†; ***Ital.:*** Torecan; ***Mex.:*** Torecan; ***Spain:*** Torecan; ***Swed.:*** Torecan; ***Switz.:*** Torecan; ***USA:*** Torecan.

## Thonzylamine Hydrochloride *(BANM, USAN, rINNM)*

Hidrocloruro de tonzilamina. *N-p*-Anisyl-*N'N'*-dimethyl-*N*-(pyrimidin-2-yl)ethylenediamine hydrochloride.

$C_{16}H_{22}N_4O,HCl = 322.8.$

*CAS — 91-85-0 (thonzylamine); 63-56-9 (thonzylamine hydrochloride).*

*ATC — D04AA01; R01AC06; R06AC06.*

### Profile

Thonzylamine hydrochloride, an ethylenediamine derivative, is an antihistamine (p.419) given for the symptomatic relief of hypersensitivity disorders in doses of 50 to 100 mg daily by mouth; a 0.1% nasal solution and 2.5% ointment are also available. As with other antihistamines, there is a risk of skin sensitisation with the ointment. It is also used in eye drops with a vasoconstrictor such as naphazoline nitrate for allergic conjunctivitis.

### Preparations

**Proprietary Preparations** (details are given in Part 3)
***Ital.:*** Tonamil.

**Multi-ingredient:** ***Ital.:*** Ascotodin; Collirio Alfa Antistaminico; Imidazyl Antistaminico; Iristamina; Narlisim; Pupilla Antistaminico; ***Port.:*** Narizima; ***Spain:*** Normo Nar.

## Tolpropamine Hydrochloride *(BANM, rINNM)*

Hidrocloruro de tolpropamina. *NN*-Dimethyl-3-phenyl-3-*p*-tolylpropylamine hydrochloride.

$C_{18}H_{23}N,HCl = 289.8.$

*CAS — 5632-44-0 (tolpropamine); 3339-11-5 (tolpropamine hydrochloride).*

*ATC — D04AA12.*

### Profile

Tolpropamine hydrochloride, an alkylamine derivative, is an antihistamine (p.419). It has been used topically for the symptomatic relief of hypersensitivity and pruritic skin disorders although, as with other antihistamines, there is a risk of skin sensitisation.

### Preparations

**Proprietary Preparations** (details are given in Part 3)
***Austria:*** Pragman†.

## Trimethobenzamide Hydrochloride *(rINNM)*

Hidrocloruro de trimetobenzamida. *N*-[4-(2-Dimethylaminoethoxy)benzyl]-3,4,5-trimethoxybenzamide hydrochloride.

$C_{21}H_{28}N_2O_5,HCl = 424.9.$

*CAS — 138-56-7 (trimethobenzamide); 554-92-7 (trimethobenzamide hydrochloride).*

**Pharmacopoeias.** In *US.*

**USP 27** (Trimethobenzamide Hydrochloride). A white crystalline powder having a slight phenolic odour. Soluble 1 in 2 of water, 1 in 59 of alcohol, 1 in 67 of chloroform, and 1 in 720 of ether; insoluble in benzene.

### Adverse Effects and Precautions

As for the sedating antihistamines in general, p.419.

Pain at the site of intramuscular injection and local irritation after rectal administration have been noted.

**Pregnancy.** For discussion of the use of antihistamines in pregnancy, including some evidence of an excess number of congenital abnormalities in infants born to mothers exposed to trimethobenzamide, see p.420.

### Interactions

As for the sedating antihistamines in general, p.421.

### Uses and Administration

Trimethobenzamide hydrochloride, a monoethanolamine derivative, is a sedating antihistamine used as an antiemetic in the control of nausea and vomiting (p.422) including postoperative nausea and vomiting.

The usual dose is 250 or 300 mg by mouth or 200 mg by deep intramuscular injection or rectally three or four times daily. Children weighing more than about 15 kg have been given 100 to 200 mg three or four times daily by the oral or rectal route. Children weighing less than this have been given 100 mg three or four times daily by the rectal route.

### Preparations

***USP 27:*** Trimethobenzamide Hydrochloride Capsules; Trimethobenzamide Hydrochloride Injection.

**Proprietary Preparations** (details are given in Part 3)
***Mex.:*** Tigan†; ***USA:*** Arrestin†; T-Gen; Tebamide; Ticon; Tigan; Trimazide.

**Multi-ingredient:** ***USA:*** Emergent-Ez; Tigan; Triban.

## Tripelennamine Citrate *(BANM, rINNM)*

Citrato de tripelenamina; Tripelennaminium Citrate. *N*-Benzyl-*N'N'*-dimethyl-*N*-(2-pyridyl)ethylenediamine dihydrogen citrate.

$C_{16}H_{21}N_3,C_6H_8O_7 = 447.5.$

*CAS — 91-81-6 (tripelennamine); 6138-56-3 (tripelennamine citrate).*

*ATC — D04AA04; R06AC04.*

## Tripelennamine Hydrochloride *(BANM, rINNM)*

Hidrocloruro de tripelenamina; Tripelennaminium Chloride.

$C_{16}H_{21}N_3,HCl = 291.8.$

*CAS — 154-69-8.*

*ATC — D04AA04; R06AC04.*

**Pharmacopoeias.** In *US.*

**USP 27** (Tripelennamine Hydrochloride). A white crystalline powder. It slowly darkens on exposure to light. Soluble 1 in 1 of water, 1 in 6 of alcohol and of chloroform, and 1 in 350 of acetone; insoluble in ether, in ethyl acetate, and in benzene. Its solutions are practically neutral to litmus. Protect from light.

### Profile

Tripelennamine, an ethylenediamine derivative, is a sedating antihistamine (p.419) with antimuscarinic and moderate sedative properties. It has been used for the symptomatic relief of hypersensitivity reactions. It may also be used in compound preparations for the symptomatic treatment of coughs and the common cold (p.421).

Tripelennamine has been given by mouth as the citrate or the hydrochloride. Tripelennamine hydrochloride has also been applied topically to the skin, although, as with other antihistamines, there is a risk of sensitisation.

**Abuse.** References to the intravenous abuse of tripelennamine alone[1] or with pentazocine in the combination known as T's and blues.[2-4]

1. Addington J, el-Guebaly N. Intravenous tripelennamine abuse in schizophrenia. *Can J Psychiatry* 1996; **41:** 63.
2. Showalter CV. T's and blues: abuse of pentazocine and tripelennamine. *JAMA* 1980; **244:** 1224–5.
3. von Almen WF, Miller JM. "Ts and Blues" in pregnancy. *J Reprod Med* 1986; **31:** 236–9.
4. McGwier BW, *et al.* Acute myocardial infarction associated with intravenous injection of pentazocine and tripelennamine. *Chest* 1992; **101:** 1730–2.

**Overdosage.** A severe toxic reaction, including agitation, hallucinations, and myoclonic jerks occurred in an 8-year-old child who was sprayed over the trunk and extremities with tripelennamine hydrochloride 2.1375 g in the treatment of severe poison ivy poisoning.[1] It was likely that inhalation of the fine mist of the aerosol spray contributed to the reaction but in this patient the initial reaction began 3 hours after exposure suggesting that percutaneous absorption through the multiple skin lesions probably contributed significantly. The original reaction was inadvertently prolonged by subsequent treatment with diphenhydramine hydrochloride and promethazine hydrochloride.

1. Schipior PG. An unusual case of antihistamine intoxication. *J Pediatr* 1967; **71:** 589–91.

### Preparations

***USP 27:*** Tripelennamine Hydrochloride Tablets.

**Proprietary Preparations** (details are given in Part 3)
***Austria:*** Azaron; ***Canad.:*** Pyribenzamine†; Vaginex†; ***Fin.:*** Etono; ***Ger.:*** Azaron; Fenistil; ***Neth.:*** Azaron†; ***Spain:*** Azaron; ***USA:*** PBZ†; Vaginex.

**Multi-ingredient:** ***Braz.:*** Alergitrat†; Asmosterona†; Gripionex†; ***Ital.:*** Anticorizza; ***Spain:*** Oxidermiol Antihist†; ***USA:*** Di-Delamine.

# Triprolidine Hydrochloride

*(BANM, rINNM)*

Hidrocloruro de triprolidina. (*E*)-2-[3-(Pyrrolidin-1-yl)-1-*p*-tolylprop-1-enyl]pyridine hydrochloride monohydrate.

$C_{19}H_{22}N_2,HCl,H_2O = 332.9.$

*CAS — 486-12-4 (triprolidine); 550-70-9 (anhydrous triprolidine hydrochloride); 6138-79-0 (triprolidine hydrochloride monohydrate).*

*ATC — R06AX07.*

**Pharmacopoeias.** In *Br.* and *US.*

**BP 2003** (Triprolidine Hydrochloride). A white, odourless or almost odourless, crystalline powder. Freely soluble in water and in alcohol; very soluble in chloroform; practically insoluble in ether.

**USP 27** (Triprolidine Hydrochloride). A white crystalline powder, having no more than a slight, but unpleasant, odour. Soluble 1 in 2.1 of water, 1 in 1.8 of alcohol, 1 in 1 of chloroform, and 1 in 2000 of ether. Its solutions are alkaline to litmus. Store in airtight containers. Protect from light.

### Adverse Effects and Precautions

As for the sedating antihistamines in general, p.419. The UK manufacturer of acrivastine has warned that acrivastine should not be used in patients hypersensitive to triprolidine.

**Breast feeding.** No adverse effects have been observed in breast-feeding infants whose mothers were receiving triprolidine, and the American Academy of Pediatrics[1] considers that it is therefore usually compatible with breast feeding.

In a study[2] in 3 women of the excretion of triprolidine and pseudoephedrine, taken by mouth in a combined preparation, triprolidine was found to reach concentrations in breast milk similar to those found in plasma in one subject, and slightly lower than in plasma in the others. It was calculated that 0.06 to 0.2% of the ingested dose was distributed into breast milk over 24 hours. Concentrations of pseudoephedrine in breast milk exceeded those in plasma in all 3 women.

1. American Academy of Pediatrics. The transfer of drugs and other chemicals into human milk. *Pediatrics* 2001; **108:** 776–89. Correction. *ibid.*; 1029. Also available at: http://aappolicy.aappublications.org/cgi/content/full/pediatrics%3b108/3/776 (accessed 30/01/04)
2. Findlay JWA, *et al.* Pseudoephedrine and triprolidine in plasma and breast milk of nursing mothers. *Br J Clin Pharmacol* 1984; **18:** 901–6.

### Interactions

As for the sedating antihistamines in general, p.421.

### Pharmacokinetics

After absorption from the gastrointestinal tract, triprolidine is metabolised; a carboxylated derivative accounts for about half the dose excreted in the urine. Reported half-lives vary from 3 to 5 hours or more. Triprolidine is distributed into breast milk.

◊ General references.

1. Paton DM, Webster DR. Clinical pharmacokinetics of $H_1$-receptor antagonists (the antihistamines). *Clin Pharmacokinet* 1985; **10:** 477–97.
2. Miles MV, *et al.* Pharmacokinetics of oral and transdermal triprolidine. *J Clin Pharmacol* 1990; **30:** 572–5.

### Uses and Administration

Triprolidine hydrochloride, an alkylamine derivative, is a sedating antihistamine with antimuscarinic and mild sedative effects. It is used for the symptomatic relief of allergic conditions including urticaria (p.423) and rhinitis (p.422), and in pruritic skin disorders (p.422). It is often used in combination with pseudoephedrine hydrochloride for rhinitis and in other compound preparations for the symptomatic treatment of coughs and the common cold (p.421).

It is given by mouth, the usual dose for adults being 2.5 mg up to four times daily.

Triprolidine hydrochloride has also been applied topically to the skin although, as with other antihistamines, there is a risk of sensitisation.

### Preparations

***BP 2003:*** Triprolidine Tablets;
***USP 27:*** Triprolidine and Pseudoephedrine Hydrochlorides Syrup; Triprolidine and Pseudoephedrine Hydrochlorides Tablets; Triprolidine Hydrochloride Syrup; Triprolidine Hydrochloride Tablets.

**Proprietary Preparations** (details are given in Part 3)
***Austria:*** Actidil†; Pro-Actidil†; ***Israel:*** Pro-Actidil; ***Ital.:*** Actidil; ***Spain:*** Pro-Actidil; ***UAE:*** Sedofan T; ***USA:*** Zymine.

**Multi-ingredient:** ***Arg.:*** Actifedrin; ***Austral.:*** Actifed; Actifed CC Junior†; Codral Daytime/Nightime; Sudafed Daytime/Nightime Relief; Sudafed Sinus Pain & Allergy Relief; ***Belg.:*** Actifed; ***Braz.:*** Actifedrin; Trifedrin; ***Canad.:*** Actifed; Actifed DM†; Actifed Plus; CoActifed; Cotridin; Cotridin Expectorant; Covan; Triprofed†; ***Chile:*** Actifedrin; Actifedrin Antitusivo; ***Fr.:*** Actifed; Actifed Toux Seche; Tussifed†; ***Ger.:*** Actifed†; Olynth Kombi†; ***Hong Kong:*** Actifed; Actifed Compound; Actifed DM; Actihist-Co; Cough-EN; Fedac; Fedac Compound; Setprodine; Uni-Fedra Compound; Vidaldine; ***India:*** Actifed; Actifed DM; Actifed Plus; Deletus; Deletus D; ***Irl.:*** Actifed; Actifed Chesty; Actifed Compound; Benylin Childrens Cough and Cold; ***Israel:*** Actifed; Actifed Compound; Actifed DM; Actifed Expectorant; Histafed; Histafed Comp; Histafed Expectorant; Sinufed Kid Night; ***Ital.:*** Actifed; Actifed Composto; Actigrip; ***Malaysia:*** Actifed; Actifed DM; Actifed Expectorant; Actihist; Actihist Expectorant; Actihist-Co; Beatafed; Beatafed Compound; Cough-EN; Fedac; Peace; Rinafed; ***NZ:*** Actifed; Actifed CC Junior†; Codral Daytime/Nightime; Sudafed Day/Nightime Relief; Sudafed Sinus Pain & Allergy Relief; ***Port.:*** Actifed; Dinaxil; ***S.Afr.:*** Actifed; Actifed Cold & Fever; Actifed Dry Cough Regular; Actifed Dry Cough Sugar Free; Acuflu-P†; Acugest Co†; Acugest Expect†; Acugest†; Acutussive†; Adco-Flupain; Adco-Muco Expect†; Adco-Tussend; Arcana Expectorant†; Arcanafed†; Betafed; Coff-Rest; Coryx; Emprazil-A†; Endcol Cough Linctus; Endcol DM; Endcol Expectorant; Fludactil; Fludactil Co; Fludactil Expectorant; Linctifed; Medifed; Merck-Cough Linctus; Merck-Expectorant; Merck-Fed; Neofed; Phendex†; Sinuclear P; Tixylix Flu; Trifen; ***Singapore:*** 3P; Actifed; Actifed Compound; Actifed DM; Actifed Expectorant; Beactafed; Cough-EN; Fedac; Fedac Compound; Peacef; Trodrine; Unitifed; ***Spain:*** Iniston; Iniston Antitusivo; Iniston Expectorante; ***Thai.:*** Actifed; Actifed Compound; Actifed DM; Actil; Clinikold; Cofed; Consudine; Hiscifed; Med-Actigen; Milafed; Nanafed; Nasolin; Nostrilet; Policol; Policold; Pondactil; Profed; Prophedin; Sinusaid; Trifed; Triofed; Tripo; Triprodrine; Vefed; ***UAE:*** Sedofan; Sedofan DM; ***UK:*** Benylin Childrens Coughs & Colds; Multi-Action Actifed; Multi-Action Actifed Chesty Coughs Expectorant; Multi-Action Actifed Dry Coughs; Sudafed Plus; ***USA:*** Actagen; Actagen-C Cough; Actifed; Actifed Cold & Allergy; Actifed Cold & Sinus; Actifed Plus; Allercon; Allerfrim; Allerfrim with Codeine; Allerphed; Aprodine; Aprodine with Codeine; Bayer Select Night Time Cold; Cenafed Plus; Genac; Silafed; Triafed with Codeine†; Trifed-C Cough; Triofed; Triposed.

## Tritoqualine (*rINN*)

L-554; Tritocualina. 7-Amino-4,5,6-triethoxy-3-(5,6,7,8-tetrahydro-4-methoxy-6-methyl-1,3-dioxolo[4,5-g]isoquinolin-5-yl)phthalide.

$C_{26}H_{32}N_2O_8$ = 500.5.

*CAS — 14504-73-5.*

*ATC — R06AX21.*

### Profile

Tritoqualine is stated to inhibit histidine decarboxylase which catalyses the conversion of histidine to histamine. It has the uses of antihistamines (p.419) and has been given by mouth in usual doses of 200 to 600 mg daily for the symptomatic relief of hypersensitivity reactions and in pruritic skin disorders.

### Preparations

**Proprietary Preparations** (details are given in Part 3)

***Austria:*** Hypostamin; ***Fr.:*** Hypostamine; ***Ger.:*** Inhibostamin.

# Antimalarials

This chapter describes the principal drugs used in the treatment and prophylaxis of malaria, one of the most serious protozoal infections in man. An estimated 40% of the world's population may be at risk of malaria; more than 500 million develop clinical infection, which is often very severe, and 1 to 3 million die each year. WHO produces guidelines for its strategic control and the management of malaria is under constant review. In 1998, WHO initiated the 'Roll Back Malaria' project to coordinate action to control the disease, the main objective being to significantly reduce the global malaria burden and to halve the number of deaths due to malaria by 2010. Measures to control malaria include *protection* from mosquito bites, *prophylaxis* with antimalarial drugs, and prompt *treatment* of any infection that develops. They also involve *vector control*; it is now recognised that for many countries vector eradication is an unrealistic aim.

## Malaria

Malaria is caused by infection by any of 4 species of *Plasmodium* protozoa. *P. falciparum* causes falciparum (malignant tertian or subtertian) malaria, which is the most serious form and can be rapidly fatal in non-immune individuals if not treated promptly. The other 3 species cause what are often termed 'benign' malarias: *P. vivax* causes vivax (benign tertian) malaria, which is widespread but rarely fatal, although symptoms during the primary attack can be severe; *P. malariae* causes quartan malaria, which is generally mild, but can cause fatal nephrosis; and *P. ovale* causes ovale (ovale tertian) malaria, which is the least common type of malaria and produces clinical features similar to *P. vivax*.

The life cycle of *Plasmodium* is complex, comprising a sexual phase (sporogony) in the mosquito (vector) and an asexual phase (schizogony) in man (see Figure 1, below). Infection in man is usually caused by injection of *sporozoites* by the bite of an infected female anopheline mosquito. It may rarely be acquired in other ways, such as through blood transfusion, congenitally via the placenta, through needlestick injuries, or after organ transplantation. Following an infected mosquito bite, some of the sporozoites rapidly enter liver parenchymal cells, where they undergo *exoerythrocytic* or *pre-erythrocytic schizogony* forming *tissue schizonts* which mature and release thousands of *merozoites* into the blood on rupture of the cell. Some of these merozoites enter erythrocytes where they transform into *trophozoites*. These produce *blood schizonts* which, as they mature, rupture and release merozoites into the circulation, which can infect other erythrocytes. This is termed the *erythrocytic cycle* and it is this periodic release of merozoites that is responsible for the characteristic periodicity of the fever in malaria. After several erythrocytic cycles, depending on the type of malaria, some erythrocytic forms develop into sexual *gametocytes*. It is ingestion of infected blood containing gametocytes by a biting female mosquito which allows the life cycle to be completed with the sexual phase in the mosquito. In *P. vivax* and *P. ovale* infections, some of the sporozoites entering the liver cells are thought to enter a latent tissue stage in the form of *hypnozoites* which are responsible for recurrence of malaria caused by these organisms. Recurrences resulting from the persistence of latent tissue forms are often referred to as *relapses* while renewed attacks caused by persistent residual erythrocytic forms are termed *recrudescences*. True relapses do not occur with falciparum or quartan malarias. Patients may sometimes be classified as *non-immune* if they have not previously or recently been exposed to *Plasmodium* infection and as *semi-immune* or *immune* if they have a history of prolonged exposure.

**Clinical manifestations of malaria**

The clinical symptoms of malaria are varied and non-specific but commonly include fever, fatigue, malaise, headache, myalgia, and sweating. Anaemia is a common complication due to haemolysis and in falciparum malaria serious complications such as acute renal failure, pulmonary oedema, and cerebral dysfunction can occur. Since none of the clinical features of malaria are diagnostic, a definitive diagnosis depends upon the demonstration of parasites in stained blood films. However, antimalarial drug treatment should not be withheld in the absence of positive blood films if there is clinical suspicion of malaria.

**Antimalarial drugs**

Antimalarial drugs can be classified by the stage of the parasitic life cycle they affect. Thus:

*Blood schizontocides* act on the erythrocytic stages of the parasite that are directly responsible for the clinical symptoms of the disease. They can produce a clinical cure or suppression of infection by susceptible strains of all 4 species of malaria parasite but, since they have no effect on exoerythrocytic forms, do not produce a radical cure of relapsing forms of ovale or vivax malarias.

*Tissue schizontocides* act on the exoerythrocytic stages of the parasite and are used for causal prophylaxis to prevent invasion of the blood cells, or as anti-relapse drugs to produce radical cures of vivax and ovale malarias.

*Gametocytocides* destroy the sexual forms of the parasite to interrupt transmission of the infection to the mosquito vector.

*Sporontocides* have no direct effect on the gametocytes in the human host but prevent sporogony in the mosquito.

Antimalarial drugs can also be classified by the chemical group to which they belong, which in turn determines the stage of the life cycle they affect. The principal antimalarial drugs, classified according to *drug group* and *activity*, are listed in Table 1 p.445.

The naphthyridine derivative pyronaridine is under investigation for its use as an antimalarial. The quinolone antibacterials, and the 4-piperazinoquinoline derivatives, piperaquine and hydroxypiperaquine, have also been studied for their antimalarial activity. The 9-aminoacridines, such as mepacrine, are no longer used in the treatment of malaria.

The differing mechanisms of action of antimalarial drugs sometimes allow the use of combinations of antimalarials to improve efficacy. Such combinations may have a simple additive effect or, more commonly, the drugs used may potentiate each other, for instance by acting at sequential steps in the parasite's folic acid pathway (e.g. pyrimethamine with sulfadoxine or dapsone). Alternatively, a combination may be complementary, when the drugs involved act against different stages in the life cycle of the parasite (e.g. the use of chloroquine with primaquine to produce radical cure of *P. vivax* or *P. ovale* infections). The rationale behind the use of such combinations may be to enhance efficacy, particularly when drug resistance is a problem (see below), or it may be an attempt to delay the development of resistance to one or more of the drugs concerned.

**Resistance** of *Plasmodium* to antimalarial drugs, in particular the spread of strains of *P. falciparum* resistant to chloroquine, is of great concern. Chloroquine resistance in *P. falciparum* now occurs virtually everywhere that *P. falciparum* malaria is transmitted, with the exception of certain parts of Central America and limited areas of the Middle East and Central Asia.[1] Resistance in *P. falciparum* to proguanil and pyrimethamine is apparent in many endemic areas. Cross-resistance between proguanil and pyrimethamine may also occur. Resistance in *P. falciparum* to the combination pyrimethamine-sulfadoxine (Fansidar) has spread rapidly in South-East Asia, but also occurs in other parts of the world including parts of South America and Africa.[1] Mefloquine resistance is frequent in some areas of South-East Asia; it has also occurred in the Amazon region of South America and, sporadically, in Africa.[1] Resistance to quinine, halofantrine, and artemisinin derivatives has also been noted. Cross-resistance between halofantrine and mefloquine may occur, as evidenced by reduced responses to halofantrine in some patients who have experienced treatment failure with mefloquine.[1] The emergence of multiple drug resistance in *P. falciparum* makes the selection of effective prophylaxis and treatment difficult.

Resistance in *P. vivax* to chloroquine and primaquine has also been reported in several parts of the world.[1,2]

A knowledge of the extent of resistance in terms of the geographical distribution and degree of resistance is important for the selection of appropriate control measures and for the development of policies for the rational use of antimalarial drugs. Effective drugs and drug combinations need to be selected according to local patterns of drug resistance. Indiscriminate and uncontrolled use of drugs should be prevented and adequate doses should be given to delay the selection of resistant strains. Malaria control strategies also need to involve other measures such as vector control and health education.

**Treatment of malaria**

Malaria is a serious and potentially fatal disease, particularly in the case of falciparum malaria (see below) and especially in non-immune individuals. It is such a problem in many parts of the world that a global partnership named Roll Back Malaria[3] has been founded by WHO, United Nations Development Programme, UNICEF, and the World Bank with the aim of significantly reducing the world's malaria burden and halving the number of deaths due to malaria by 2010. Prompt diagnosis and effective treatment of malaria are crucial.[4-6] Treatment is with a *blood schizontocide*, selected with due regard to the prevalence of specific patterns of drug resistance in the area of infection. In the case of vivax and ovale malarias (see below) subsequent treatment with a *tissue schizontocide* is needed where it is considered appropriate to prevent relapse.

Antimalarials are generally given by mouth, although in order to obtain a rapid response in patients with severe or complicated falciparum malaria (see below) it may be nec-

**Figure 1.** Life cycle of the malaria parasite *Plasmodium*.

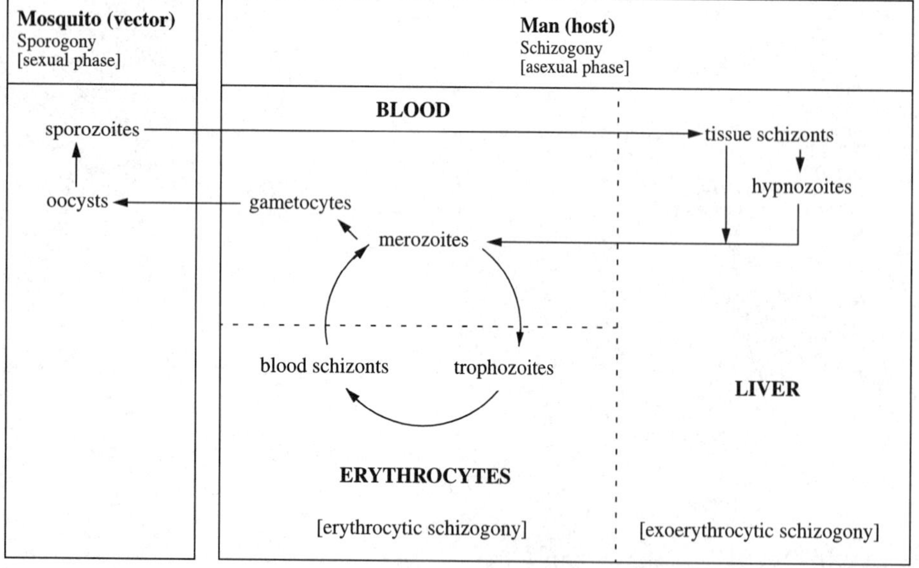

**Table 1.** Principal antimalarial drugs.

| Antimalarial groups | Principal drugs | Activity |
|---|---|---|
| 4-Methanolquinolines | Cinchona alkaloids<br>Quinine<br>Quinidine | Rapid-acting blood schizontocides. Some gametocytocidal activity. |
| | Mefloquine | Blood schizontocide. |
| 4-Aminoquinolines | Chloroquine<br>Hydroxychloroquine<br>Amodiaquine | Rapid-acting blood schizontocides. Some gametocytocidal activity. |
| 8-Aminoquinolines | Primaquine<br>Tafenoquine | Tissue schizontocide. Also gametocytocidal activity and some activity at other stages of the parasite's life-cycle. |
| Biguanides | Proguanil<br>Chlorproguanil | Tissue schizontocides and slow-acting blood schizontocides. Some sporontocidal activity. Dihydrofolate reductase inhibitors. |
| Diaminopyrimidines | Pyrimethamine | Tissue schizontocide and slow-acting blood schizontocide. Some sporontocidal activity. Dihydrofolate reductase inhibitor. Usually used with antimalarials that inhibit different stages of folate synthesis (sulfonamides or sulfones) to form synergistic combinations. |
| Dichlorobenzylidines | Lumefantrine | Blood schizontocide. |
| Hydroxynaphthoquinones | Atovaquone | Blood schizontocide. Usually given in combination with proguanil. |
| 9-Phenanthrenemethanols | Halofantrine | Blood schizontocide. |
| Sesquiterpene lactones | Artemisinin and its derivatives | Blood schizontocide. |
| Sulfonamides | Sulfadoxine<br>Sulfametopyrazine | Blood schizontocides. Dihydropteroate and folate synthesis inhibitors. Usually given in combination with pyrimethamine. |
| Tetracyclines | Doxycycline<br>Tetracycline | Blood schizontocides. Some tissue schizontocidal activity. |
| Lincosamides | Clindamycin | Blood schizontocides. Some tissue schizontocidal activity. |
| Sulfones | Dapsone | Blood schizontocide. Folate synthesis inhibitor. Usually given in combination with pyrimethamine. |

essary to give parenteral therapy initially, the patient being transferred to oral therapy when feasible.[6]

**Treatment of falciparum malaria**. In most parts of the world *P. falciparum* is now resistant to chloroquine and therefore, apart from the rare circumstance of exposure in one of the few remaining areas of chloroquine sensitivity, chloroquine is **not** suitable for treatment. Instead, in the UK, **uncomplicated falciparum malaria** is treated with one of the following:

- quinine *and* (if quinine resistance is known or suspected) followed by *either* pyrimethamine-sulfadoxine (Fansidar) *or* (if Fansidar-resistant) by doxycycline (or clindamycin in children)
- mefloquine
- atovaquone-proguanil (Malarone)
- artemether-lumefantrine (Riamet)

For malaria-endemic areas where there is chloroquine resistance, WHO recommends pyrimethamine-sulfadoxine (Fansidar) or amodiaquine as treatment of choice in uncomplicated malaria (although cross-resistance between chloroquine and amodiaquine has been reported). If either of these options is, or becomes, unsatisfactory then mefloquine, or alternatively quinine, may be used; quinine is usually given with tetracycline or doxycycline to ensure a high cure rate. Increasingly, however, *P. falciparum* is developing resistance to these conventional therapies and, in such circumstances, WHO recommends the use of combination therapies containing artemisinin derivatives (artemisinin-based combination therapies, also known as ACTs). The following combination therapies are recommended:

- artemether-lumefantrine
- artesunate plus amodiaquine
- artesunate plus pyrimethamine-sulfadoxine (Fansidar) (in areas where susceptibility to pyrimethamine-sulfadoxine remains high)
- artesunate plus mefloquine (reserved for areas of low transmission)
- in countries unable to introduce ACTs, amodiaquine plus pyrimethamine-sulfadoxine (Fansidar) may be used if susceptibility to them remains high (mainly limited to West Africa)

Additional ACTs recommended by WHO for accelerated development are piperaquine-dihydroartemisinin, chlorproguanil-dapsone-artesunate, and pyronaridine-artesunate.

In **severe or complicated falciparum malaria** including cerebral malaria, parenteral treatment is required to produce adequate blood concentrations as quickly as possible.[4,6-9] The importance of achieving therapeutic concentrations of antimalarial drugs as early as possible has been emphasised.[10] Chloroquine should be given if the infection is known to be sensitive to it. In chloroquine-resistant malaria, or where sensitivity to chloroquine is not known, quinine is usually given intravenously, starting with a loading dose; intravenous artesunate or intramuscular artemether may alternatively be used; intravenous quinidine may be used if parenteral quinine or artemisinin derivatives are not available. Patients of all ages need to be closely monitored while undergoing parenteral therapy and treatment is changed to an orally administered antimalarial as soon as the patient's condition permits. When there are only minimal health care facilities and parenteral therapy is not possible, artemisinin or artesunate suppositories may be given; the nasogastric route may also be used.[4,6] Supportive therapy in patients with severe or complicated malaria needs to be directed at reducing hyperpyrexia, controlling convulsions, maintaining fluid balance, and correcting hypoglycaemia.[4,6,7] Since iron might be involved in the pathogenesis of cerebral malaria, the iron chelator desferrioxamine has been tried in addition to standard antimalarial therapy, but any benefit is yet to be established and WHO advises against its use.[6] Anecdotal reports of the value of corticosteroids in cerebral malaria have not been substantiated by controlled studies and they have no place in the management of this condition.[6,11] Other approaches such as the use of hyperimmune serum or monoclonal antibody to tumour necrosis factor have also been unsuccessful.

**Treatment of benign malarias**. Benign malarias, which are usually caused by *P. vivax* or, less commonly, by *P. ovale* or *P. malariae*, can be debilitating but are usually less severe than falciparum malaria. Chloroquine is still the drug of choice (but chloroquine-resistant vivax infection has been reported from some areas—notably Papua New Guinea, Indonesia, Myanmar, and Vanuatu). Chloroquine alone is adequate for *P. malariae* infections, but in the case of those caused by *P. vivax* or *P. ovale* a subsequent *radical cure* with a tissue schizontocide, usually primaquine, is needed to avoid the risk of relapse (caused by the presence of latent hypnozoites) months or years after the primary infection. Radical cure is inappropriate for patients living within an endemic area since re-infection is likely and therefore WHO recommends that it should be limited to patients resident in areas where transmission is *very low* or *absent* and to those treated *during an epidemic*; other patients should simply be treated with a further course of chloroquine in the event of relapse or re-infection. *P. vivax* cases that fail to respond to chloroquine may be treated with quinine or mefloquine.

**Treatment of malaria during pregnancy**. Malaria is especially dangerous during pregnancy and the seriousness of the disease usually outweighs any potential risk from treatment. Although fetal abnormalities have been associated with the use of high doses of chloroquine, extensive clinical experience suggests it is safe; its use may be limited however, due to resistance. Quinine may be used for chloroquine-resistant malaria but care should be taken that patients do not become hypoglycaemic.[7] Artemisinin derivatives are the drugs of choice for treatment of severe malaria in the second and third trimester; data regarding their use in the first trimester is at present limited.[5] There may be difficulty if other drugs are required as opinion varies over their suitability. Intermittent treatment with pyrimethamine-sulfadoxine (Fansidar) (one dose in the second and one dose in the third trimester) may reduce the risk of severe anaemia in late pregnancy in malaria-endemic areas,[12] although there are some concerns over emerging resistance. Moreover, some consider that pyrimethamine combinations should be avoided, especially during the first trimester (see under Pregnancy in Precautions of Pyrimethamine, p.459). The tetracyclines are contra-indicated on dental grounds but the *British National Formulary* considers that a combination of clindamycin with quinine may be used. The safety of mefloquine, halofantrine, or atovaquone has not been fully assessed, although mefloquine is now suggested for prophylactic use from the fourth month of pregnancy. For patients with vivax or ovale malaria during pregnancy radical cure with primaquine should be postponed until after delivery;[7,8] weekly chloroquine can be given during the remaining weeks of pregnancy.

**Treatment of splenomegaly syndrome**. A small number of individuals infected with *Plasmodium* develop chronic hyperreactive malarial splenomegaly syndrome, an aberrant immunological response formerly known as the tropical splenomegaly syndrome. Traditionally, patients have first received a full course of antimalarial chemotherapy appropriate to the causative species followed by lengthy and probably lifelong chemoprophylaxis; however, a study in 312 patients suggested that pyrimethamine given with folinic acid for 30 days could produce a rapid reduction of splenomegaly which persisted for at least 3 months.[13]

**Prophylaxis of malaria**

Chemoprophylaxis of malaria may refer to absolute prevention of infection (*causal prophylaxis*) or to suppression of parasitaemia and its symptoms (*clinical prophylaxis*). Causal prophylaxis is provided by tissue schizontocides which destroy the exoerythrocytic forms of the parasite. Clinical prophylaxis is provided by blood schizontocides which, if continued until all exoerythrocytic forms of the parasite are destroyed, will ultimately produce a *suppressive cure*. In *P. falciparum* infections this would be achieved by about a month after the last infected bite, but relapses with *P. vivax* and *P. ovale* may still occur after standard clinical prophylactic regimens due to the presence of latent exoerythrocytic forms (hypnozoites).

The continuing increase in the prevalence of strains of *P. falciparum* resistant to chloroquine and other antimalarials, along with growing evidence of toxicity of some regimens, make recommendations for malaria prophylaxis increasingly difficult. Absolute protection cannot be guaranteed by any chemoprophylactic regimen currently in use and the importance and effectiveness of methods of avoiding bites from infected mosquitoes, such as the use of *protective clothing, bed netting, insect repellents*, and *insecticides* must be stressed.[4,5] WHO recommends the following measures to protect against mosquito bites:

- application of an effective insect repellent to exposed skin between dusk and dawn when mosquitoes commonly bite
- accommodation in buildings with screens over doors and windows
- use of mosquito nets at night, preferably impregnated with pyrethroid insecticides such as permethrin or deltamethrin
- and use of anti-mosquito sprays or insecticide dispensers, or mosquito coils in bedrooms at night

Studies have demonstrated that pyrethroid-impregnated mosquito nets can reduce mortality substantially.[14] In addition to these measures, travellers should be advised, even if chemoprophylaxis has been taken regularly, to regard **any** fever *after the first week (especially within 3 months)* and for *up to 1 year following possible exposure* as being caused by malaria and to seek medical advice **immediately**. Some authorities advise that travellers should also have antimalarial drugs ready for emergency self-treatment (*standby treatment*) when prompt medical attention is not available.

Chemoprophylaxis should be reserved for those at high risk, notably *non-immune visitors*; widespread chemoprophylaxis in *immune or semi-immune* populations is no longer recommended except for women who are *pregnant*. For the elderly, pregnant women, and children, careful consideration should be given as to whether travel to areas where falciparum malaria occurs is absolutely necessary. WHO specifically advises pregnant women not to travel to areas where transmission of *P. falciparum* occurs and also advises against taking babies and young children to malarious areas (particularly where there is transmission of *P. falciparum*).[5] Advice on chemoprophylaxis must be based on a knowledge of the occurrence and susceptibility of *Plasmodium* strains in specific geographical areas. Local variations due to altitude, seasonal variations in temperature and rainfall, the degree of urbanisation, and many other factors further complicate the issue. WHO collates information provided by national health administrations and regularly publishes this information to assist in advising international travellers on the current situation; similar information is provided at national level by local institutes specialising in tropical diseases. However, the situation is so complex that advice differs. Recommendations issued by various authorities are usually for short-term stays and expert advice should be sought if long-term cover is required.

It is generally recommended that chemoprophylaxis should start about 1 week (or longer for mefloquine) before exposure to malaria, or if this is not possible at the earliest opportunity up to 1 or 2 days before exposure; this is partly to ensure that the patient is able to tolerate the drug. Chemoprophylaxis should continue throughout exposure and for at least 4 weeks after leaving the malarious area, with the exception of atovaquone-proguanil (Malarone) which may be stopped one week after leaving.

**Prophylactic regimens**. Depending upon the risk of infection and the availability and standard of local medical care, WHO has made various recommendations concerning chemoprophylaxis and/or standby treatment for non-immune travellers:

- in areas where *P. falciparum* is *absent* or still *sensitive to chloroquine*, travellers can either take chloroquine for prophylaxis or, if the infection risk is *very low*, not take prophylaxis at all
- in areas where *P. falciparum* is *resistant to chloroquine* but with a low risk of infection, chloroquine with proguanil is recommended as it may give some protection against *P. falciparum* and may alleviate the symptoms if an attack does occur; chloroquine given alone will only protect against *P. vivax* in these areas. Mefloquine is recommended as second choice. Again if the infection risk is very low travellers may do without prophylaxis
- in areas of high risk or where there is multidrug resistance, mefloquine is recommended as first choice for prophylaxis; doxycycline or atovaquone-proguanil are recommended second choices, and chloroquine with proguanil third choice. Again if the infection risk is very low travellers may do without prophylaxis. These recommendations are subject to the local patterns of drug resistance

WHO also recommends that for the small number of travellers who would be unable to obtain prompt medical attention when malaria is suspected (within 24 hours of the onset of symptoms), it may be necessary to provide a course of treatment for self-administration (*standby treatment*). Clear instructions must be given and persons taking standby medication must seek medical advice as soon as possible. Also having completed the standby course they should resume any prophylaxis. The basis upon which the choice of prophylaxis is made (as detailed above) in turn broadly determines the appropriate choice of standby treatment. Thus:

- where *no prophylaxis* is deemed necessary, chloroquine is given for standby treatment in areas where there is chloroquine sensitivity, otherwise standby treatment is with mefloquine, or quinine, or artemether-lumefantrine, or atovaquone-proguanil
- where prophylaxis is *with chloroquine* (either alone or with proguanil), standby treatment is with mefloquine or with quinine
- where prophylaxis is *with mefloquine*, standby treatment is with quinine alone, or with quinine plus doxycycline or tetracycline
- where prophylaxis is *with doxycycline*, standby treatment is with mefloquine or with quinine plus tetracycline

In each instance, prophylaxis should be resumed 1 week after the *first* standby treatment dose, except for mefloquine prophylaxis which should be resumed 1 week after the *last* treatment dose of quinine.

In the USA, recommendations for prophylaxis are provided by the Centers for Disease Control (CDC)[15] and other sources.[8] The recommendations for chloroquine-sensitive malaria are similar to those of WHO in that chloroquine alone is advised; hydroxychloroquine is suggested as an alternative. For all areas with chloroquine-resistant malaria, the use of mefloquine alone is recommended with alternatives being either doxycycline or atovaquone-proguanil (Malarone). Atovaquone-proguanil (Malarone) is recommended for emergency standby treatment. The use of primaquine is also advocated during the last 2 weeks of prophylaxis to prevent relapses due to *P. vivax* or *P. ovale* in persons returning from prolonged exposure in areas where relapsing malaria is endemic.

UK experts[16] have also published guidelines for the prophylaxis of malaria and these are in broad agreement with those of WHO. A further option recommended for standby treatment is the combined use of quinine with pyrimethamine-sulfadoxine (Fansidar).[16]

VACCINES. Malaria vaccines are under development and several are currently undergoing clinical evaluation (see p.1622).

**Prophylaxis during pregnancy**. The choice of drugs for prophylaxis during pregnancy is limited and whenever possible women who are pregnant or likely to become so should avoid travelling to malarious areas (see also above). In pregnant women who cannot avoid travelling to endemic areas, chloroquine may be given alone for prophylaxis in the few areas where *P. falciparum* is sensitive to chloroquine, or in combination with proguanil where resistance exists.[5] Folate supplements (folic acid 5 mg daily) need to be taken with proguanil. Mefloquine is normally avoided during the first trimester but may be given from the fourth month onwards although WHO now advise[5] that it may be used *with caution* in the first trimester. Doxycycline, atovaquone-proguanil (Malarone), or primaquine are contra-indicated in pregnant women by most experts. In non-pregnant women of child-bearing potential, pregnancy needs to be avoided for 3 months after completing mefloquine prophylaxis and for one week following doxycycline prophylaxis.

Pregnant women living in endemic areas commonly receive malaria chemoprophylaxis as a matter of policy since their susceptibility to the disease, especially among primigravidas, is believed to be increased. Routine prophylaxis has been shown to reduce anaemia and produce a trend towards higher birth-weights and lower perinatal mortality.[17-19] A study of chemoprophylaxis in 1049 pregnancies[20] suggested that multigravidas obtained less benefit than primigravidas, and a follow-up study[21] found that the outcome of subsequent pregnancies was similar regardless of whether chemoprophylaxis or placebo had been given in the first pregnancy. This result suggested that it may be possible to restrict chemoprophylaxis to first pregnancies in endemic areas. A review of randomised studies[22] came to a similar conclusion. However, WHO[4] more recently suggested that antimalarial therapy should be made available in highly endemic areas to women in both their first and second pregnancies.

**Prophylaxis during breast feeding**. Breast feeding by mothers taking mefloquine is usually contra-indicated, although the amount ingested by the nursing infant may be too small to produce adverse effects. Doxycycline and atovaquone-proguanil (Malarone) are contra-indicated during breast feeding. For other antimalarials it is generally accepted that the amount distributed into breast milk and consumed by nursing infants is too small to be harmful. However, these amounts are also too small to provide adequate protection and breast-fed infants still require chemoprophylaxis.

**Prophylaxis in children**. Chloroquine and proguanil may be given in scaled down doses to children of all ages but the choice of alternative drugs may be restricted, especially in very young children, and consideration should be given to whether their travel to malarious areas is absolutely necessary (see also above).

**Prophylaxis in epilepsy**. In subjects with a history of epilepsy, the UK guidelines[16] advise that both chloroquine and mefloquine are unsuitable for prophylaxis. In areas without chloroquine resistance, proguanil alone is recommended. In areas with a high risk of chloroquine resistance, atovaquone-proguanil (Malarone) or doxycycline may be considered, but the metabolism of doxycycline may be influenced by antiepileptics.

**Prophylaxis in HIV-infected travellers**. HIV-infected travellers may take chloroquine routinely for antimalarial prophylaxis but its potential immunosuppressive effects should be recognised; proguanil, mefloquine, or doxycycline can also be used. Although patients with AIDS may be at increased risk of adverse effects to sulfonamides, a combination such as pyrimethamine-sulfadoxine (Fansidar) can be used for standby treatment if an alternative is not available.


1. Bloland PB. *Drug resistance in malaria*. Geneva: WHO, 2001.
2. Whitby M. Drug resistant Plasmodium vivax malaria. *J Antimicrob Chemother* 1997; **40:** 749–52.
3. WHO. Roll Back Malaria: a global partnership. Available at: http://rbm.who.int (accessed 16/04/04)
4. WHO. WHO expert committee on malaria: twentieth report. *WHO Tech Rep Ser 892* 2000.
5. WHO. *International travel and health*. Geneva: WHO, 2003.
6. WHO. *Management of severe malaria: a practical handbook*. Geneva: WHO, 2000.
7. Molyneux M, Fox R. Diagnosis and treatment of malaria in Britain. *BMJ* 1993; **306:** 1175–80.
8. Medical Letter on Drugs and Therapeutics. Drugs for parasitic infections (issued April 2002). Available at: http://www.medicalletter.com/freedocs/parasitic.pdf (accessed 16/04/04)
9. WHO. Severe falciparum malaria. *Trans R Soc Trop Med Hyg* 2000; **94** (suppl 1): S1/1–S1/90.
10. White NJ. Not much progress in treatment of cerebral malaria. *Lancet* 1998; **352:** 594–5.
11. Prasad K, Garner P. Steroids for treating cerebral malaria. Available in The Cochrane Library; Issue 1. Chichester: John Wiley; 2004.
12. Shulman CE, *et al.* Intermittent sulphadoxine-pyrimethamine to prevent severe anaemia secondary to malaria in pregnancy: a randomised placebo-controlled trial. *Lancet* 1999; **353:** 632–6.
13. Manenti F, *et al.* Treatment of hyperreactive malarial splenomegaly syndrome. *Lancet* 1994; **343:** 1441–2.
14. Lengeler C. Insecticide-treated bednets and curtains for preventing malaria. Available in The Cochrane Library; Issue 1. Chichester: John Wiley; 2004.
15. CDC. Malaria. In: *The Yellow Book: Health Information for International Travel; 2003-2004*. Available at: http://www.cdc.gov/travel/diseases/malaria/index.htm (accessed 16/04/04)
16. Bradley DJ, Bannister B. Guidelines for malaria prevention in travellers from the United Kingdom for 2001. *Commun Dis Public Health* 2001; **4:** 84–101. Also available at: http://www.hpa.org.uk/cdph/issues/CDPHVol4/no2/malaria_guidelinesp.pdf (accessed 16/04/04)
17. Greenwood AM, *et al.* The distribution of birth weights in Gambian women who received malaria chemoprophylaxis during their first pregnancy and in control women. *Trans R Soc Trop Med Hyg* 1994; **88:** 311–12.
18. Schultz LJ, *et al.* The efficacy of antimalarial regimens containing sulfadoxine-pyrimethamine and/or chloroquine in preventing peripheral and placental Plasmodium falciparum infection among pregnant women in Malawi. *Am J Trop Med Hyg* 1994; **51:** 515–22.
19. Nosten F, *et al.* Mefloquine prophylaxis prevents malaria during pregnancy: a double-blind, placebo-controlled study. *J Infect Dis* 1994; **169:** 595–603.
20. Greenwood BM, *et al.* The effects of malaria chemoprophylaxis given by traditional birth attendants on the course and outcome of pregnancy. *Trans R Soc Trop Med Hyg* 1989; **83:** 589–94.
21. Greenwood AM, *et al.* Can malaria chemoprophylaxis be restricted to first pregnancies? *Trans R Soc Trop Med Hyg* 1994; **88:** 681–2.
22. Garner P, Brabin B. A review of randomized controlled trials of routine antimalarial drug prophylaxis during pregnancy in endemic malarious areas. *Bull WHO* 1994; **72:** 89–99.


## Amodiaquine *(BAN, rINN)*

Amodiaquina. 4-(7-Chloro-4-quinolylamino)-2-(diethylaminomethyl)phenol.

$C_{20}H_{22}ClN_3O$ = 355.9.
*CAS — 86-42-0.*
*ATC — P01BA06.*

**Pharmacopoeias.** In *Int.* and *US.*

**USP 27** (Amodiaquine). Very pale yellow to light tan-yellow, odourless, powder. Practically insoluble in water; slightly soluble in alcohol; sparingly soluble in 1.0N hydrochloric acid. Store in airtight containers.

## Amodiaquine Hydrochloride *(BANM, rINNM)*

Amodiaquini Hydrochloridum; Hidrocloruro de amodiaquina. 4-(7-Chloro-4-quinolylamino)-2-(diethylaminomethyl)phenol dihydrochloride dihydrate.

$C_{20}H_{22}ClN_3O,2HCl,2H_2O$ = 464.8.
*CAS — 69-44-3 (anhydrous amodiaquine hydrochloride); 6398-98-7 (amodiaquine hydrochloride dihydrate).*
*ATC — P01BA06.*

**Pharmacopoeias.** In *Fr., Int.,* and *US.*

**USP 27** (Amodiaquine Hydrochloride). A yellow, odourless, crystalline powder. Soluble 1 in 25 of water and 1 in 78 of alcohol; very slightly soluble in chloroform, in ether, and in benzene. Store in airtight containers.

**Sorption.** For reference to loss of amodiaquine hydrochloride from solutions during membrane filtration, see Chloroquine, p.448.

### Adverse Effects and Precautions

As for Chloroquine, p.448, although amodiaquine was associated with hepatitis and a much higher incidence of agranulocytosis when it was used for the prophylaxis of malaria.

◊ Early isolated reports of amodiaquine causing severe neutropenia were usually when it had been used in anti-inflammatory doses for rheumatoid arthritis, but there was a cluster of cases in 1986 associated with its use in malaria prophylaxis.[1] In all, 23 cases of agranulocytosis, 7 of which were fatal, were reported in the UK, USA, and Switzerland during a 12-month period ending March 1986. Nearly all of these patients had used the drug at a dosage of 400 mg weekly and the periods of exposure ranged from 3 to 24 weeks.[1] Some of these patients also had evidence of liver damage[1] and there have been other reports of hepatotoxicity associated with the prophylactic use of amodiaquine.[2] Examination of data submitted to the UK Committee on Safety of Medicines[3] suggested that the frequency of adverse reactions to amodiaquine was about 1 in 1700 for serious reactions, 1 in 2200 for blood disorders, 1 in 15 650 for serious hepatic disorders, and 1 in 15 650 for fatal reactions. In contrast the frequency of agranulocytosis in users in France[4] has been estimated to be 1 in 25 000. Worldwide[4] the risk of severe reactions appears to be between 1 in 1000 and 1 in 5000. The manufacturers reportedly had 42 cases of serious adverse effects during amodiaquine prophylaxis, between 1985 and 1991; there were 28 cases of agranulocytosis (9 deaths) and 14 of hepatitis (3 deaths).[5] Whether there was significantly less risk when amodiaquine was given for treatment of malaria rather than prophylaxis was not certain.[6]

It has been suggested that an immunological reaction to amodiaquine quinone imine, which can be produced by autoxidation among other processes, may partially account for amodiaquine's greater tendency to induce agranulocytosis compared with chloroquine.[7,8]

The acute toxicity of amodiaquine appears to differ from that of chloroquine in that there have been no reports of cardiovascular symptoms following overdosage with amodiaquine[9] but intoxication with amodiaquine is also far less frequent than chloroquine poisoning. However, large doses of amodiaquine have been reported to produce syncope, spasticity, convulsions, and involuntary movements.[9]

1. Anonymous. Amodiaquine and agranulocytosis. *WHO Drug Inf* 1987; **1:** 5–6.
2. Larrey D, *et al.* Amodiaquine-induced hepatitis. *Ann Intern Med* 1986; **104:** 801–3.
3. Phillips-Howard PA, West LJ. Serious adverse drug reactions to pyrimethamine–sulphadoxine, pyrimethamine–dapsone and to amodiaquine in Britain. *J R Soc Med* 1990; **83:** 82–5.
4. Anonymous. Development of recommendations for the protection of short-stay travellers to malaria endemic areas: memorandum from two WHO meetings. *Bull WHO* 1988; **66:** 177–96.
5. Olliaro P, *et al.* Systematic review of amodiaquine treatment in uncomplicated malaria. *Lancet* 1996; **348:** 1196–1201.
6. White NJ. Can amodiaquine be resurrected? *Lancet* 1996; **348:** 1184–5.
7. Winstanley PA, *et al.* The toxicity of amodiaquine and its principal metabolites towards mononuclear leucocytes and granulocyte/monocyte colony forming units. *Br J Clin Pharmacol* 1990; **29:** 479–85.
8. Park BK, Kitteringham NR. Drug–protein conjugation and its immunological consequences. *Drug Metab Rev* 1990; **22:** 87–144.
9. Jaeger A, *et al.* Clinical features and management of poisoning due to antimalarial drugs. *Med Toxicol* 1987; **2:** 242–73.

### Pharmacokinetics

Amodiaquine hydrochloride is readily absorbed from the gastrointestinal tract. Amodiaquine is rapidly converted in the liver to the active metabolite desethylamodiaquine, only a negligible amount of amodiaquine being excreted unchanged in the urine. The plasma elimination half-life of desethylamodiaquine has varied from 1 to 10 days or more. Amodiaquine and desethylamodiaquine have been detected in the urine several months after administration.

◊ References.

1. Winstanley P, *et al.* The disposition of amodiaquine in man after oral administration. *Br J Clin Pharmacol* 1987; **23:** 1–7.
2. White NJ, *et al.* Pharmacokinetics of intravenous amodiaquine. *Br J Clin Pharmacol* 1987; **23:** 127–35.
3. Winstanley PA, *et al.* The disposition of amodiaquine in Zambians and Nigerians with malaria. *Br J Clin Pharmacol* 1990; **29:** 695–701.
4. Krishna S, White NJ. Pharmacokinetics of quinine, chloroquine and amodiaquine: clinical implications. *Clin Pharmacokinet* 1996; **30:** 263–99.

### Uses and Administration

Amodiaquine is a 4-aminoquinoline antimalarial with an action similar to that of chloroquine (p.451). It is as effective as chloroquine against chloroquine-sensitive strains of *Plasmodium falciparum* and is also effective against some chloroquine-resistant strains, although resistance to amodiaquine has developed and there may be partial cross-resistance between amodiaquine and chloroquine. Amodiaquine is not recommended for the prophylaxis of malaria because of resistance and the risk of major toxicity.

Amodiaquine is given by mouth as the hydrochloride, but doses are expressed in terms of amodiaquine base; amodiaquine hydrochloride 260 mg is approximately equivalent to 200 mg of amodiaquine base. For the treatment of falciparum malaria a total dose of 35 mg/kg has been given over 3 days.

◊ References.

1. Olliaro P, Mussano P. Amodiaquine for treating malaria. Available in The Cochrane Library; Issue 1. Chichester: John Wiley; 2004.
2. McIntosh HM. Chloroquine or amodiaquine combined with sulfadoxine-pyrimethamine for treating uncomplicated malaria. Available in The Cochrane Library; Issue 1. Chichester: John Wiley; 2004.

### Preparations

***USP 27:*** Amodiaquine Hydrochloride Tablets.

**Proprietary Preparations** (details are given in Part 3)
***Fr.:*** Flavoquine; ***India:*** Basoquin; Camoquin.

## Artemisinin Derivatives

Artemisinina, derivados.

### Artemether *(BAN, rINN)*

Artemeter; Artemetherum; Dihydroartemisinin Methyl Ether; Dihydroqinghaosu Methyl Ether; *o*-Methyldihydroartemisinin; SM-224. (3*R*,5a*S*,6*R*,8a*S*,9*R*,10*S*,12*R*,12a*R*)-Decahydro-10-methoxy-3,6,9-trimethyl-3,12-epoxy-12*H*-pyrano[4,3-*j*]-1,2-benzodioxepin.

$C_{16}H_{26}O_5$ = 298.4.
*CAS — 71963-77-4.*
*ATC — P01BE02.*

**Pharmacopoeias.** In *Chin.* and *Int.*

### Artemisinin *(rINN)*

Arteannuin; Artemisinina; Artemisinine; Artemisininum; Huanghuahaosu; Qinghaosu. (3*R*,5a*S*,6*R*,8a*S*,9*R*,12*S*,12a*R*)-Octahydro-3,6,9-trimethyl-3,12-epoxy-12*H*-pyrano[4,3-*j*]-1,2-benzodioxepin-10(3*H*)-one.

$C_{15}H_{22}O_5$ = 282.3.
*CAS — 63968-64-9.*
*ATC — P01BE01.*

**Pharmacopoeias.** In *Chin.*, *Int.*, and *Viet.*

### Artemotil *(rINN)*

Arteether; Artemotilo; Artemotilum; Dihydroartemisinin Ethyl Ether; Dihydroqinghaosu Ethyl Ether; SM-227. (3*R*,5a*S*,6*R*,8a*S*,9*R*,10*S*,12*R*,12a*R*)-Decahydro-10-ethoxy-3,6,9-trimethyl-3,12-epoxy-12*H*-pyrano[4,3-*j*]-1,2-benzodioxepin.

$C_{17}H_{28}O_5$ = 312.4.
*CAS — 75887-54-6.*
*ATC — P01BE04.*

**Pharmacopoeias.** In *Int.*

### Artesunate *(USAN, rINN)*

Artesunatum. (3*R*,5a*S*,6*R*,8a*S*,9*R*,10*S*,12*R*,12a*R*)-Decahydro-3,6,9-trimethyl-3,12-epoxy-12*H*-pyrano-[4,3-*j*]-1,2-benzodioxepin-10-ol hydrogen succinate.

$C_{19}H_{28}O_8$ = 384.4.
*CAS — 83507-69-1; 88495-63-0.*
*ATC — P01BE03.*

**Pharmacopoeias.** In *Int.* and *Viet.*

### Sodium Artesunate *(rINNM)*

Artesunato sódico; Dihydroartemisinin Hemisuccinate Sodium; Dihydroqinghaosu Hemisuccinate Sodium; SM-804. (3*R*,5a*S*,6*R*,8a*S*,9*R*,10*S*,12*R*,12a*R*)-Decahydro-3,6,9-trimethyl-3,12-epoxy-12*H*-pyrano-[4,3-*j*]-1,2-benzodioxepin-10-ol hydrogen succinate sodium.

$C_{19}H_{27}O_8Na$ = 406.4.

### Adverse Effects and Precautions

Artemisinin and its derivatives appear to be generally well tolerated, although there have been reports of mild gastrointestinal disturbance including nausea, vomiting, diarrhoea, and abdominal pain, dizziness, headache, tinnitus, neutropenia, elevated liver enzyme values, and ECG abnormalities including prolongation of the QT interval.

Evidence of severe neurotoxicity has been seen in *animals* given high doses.

◊ General references to adverse effects associated with artemisinin derivatives.

1. Price R, *et al.* Adverse effects in patients with acute falciparum malaria treated with artemisinin derivatives. *Am J Trop Med Hyg* 1999; **60:** 547–55.

**Effects on the heart.** Bradycardia was reported in 10 of 34 patients who received artemether orally for 4 days.[1]

1. Karbwang J, *et al.* Comparison of oral artemether and mefloquine in acute uncomplicated falciparum malaria. *Lancet* 1992; **340:** 1245–8.

**Effects on the nervous system.** Neurotoxicity has been reported in *animals* given artemotil or artemether.[1] An *in-vitro* study[2] has shown that dihydroartemisinin, the metabolite common to all artemisinin derivatives currently used, is neurotoxic. There has been a report[3] of acute cerebellar dysfunction manifesting as ataxia and slurred speech in a patient who took a 5-day course of artesunate by mouth.

1. Brewer TG, *et al.* Neurotoxicity in animals due to arteether and artemether. *Trans R Soc Trop Med Hyg* 1994; **88** (suppl 1): 33–6.
2. Wesche DL, *et al.* Neurotoxicity of artemisinin analogs in vitro. *Antimicrob Agents Chemother* 1994; **38:** 1813–19.
3. Miller LG, Panosian CB. Ataxia and slurred speech after artesunate treatment for falciparum malaria. *N Engl J Med* 1997; **336:** 1328.

**Pregnancy.** Artesunate or artemether was used to treat multidrug-resistant falciparum malaria in 83 pregnant women in Thailand; of 73 pregnancies resulting in live births none showed evidence of any congenital abnormality.[1] Sixteen of the women had received artesunate during the first trimester; of these, 12 had normal deliveries, 1 was lost to study, and 3 had spontaneous abortions.

No undue adverse effects on the neonates occurred in a study[2] involving 45 women treated for multidrug-resistant malaria during their second or third trimester of pregnancy with either artemether or artemether plus mefloquine.

A WHO report[3] assessing the safety of artemisinin derivatives in pregnancy concluded that these drugs should continue to be available for the treatment of malaria in pregnancy, irrespective of the trimester. However, WHO also stressed that further study was needed and recommended that a clinical monitoring programme be established to assess outcome of pregnancy in women treated with artemisinin derivatives and other antimalarials.

1. McGready R, *et al.* Artemisinin derivatives in the treatment of falciparum malaria in pregnancy. *Trans R Soc Trop Med Hyg* 1998; **92:** 430–3.
2. Sowunmi A, *et al.* Randomised trial of artemether versus artemether and mefloquine for the treatment of chloroquine/sufadoxine[sic]-pyrimethamine-resistant falciparum malaria during pregnancy. *J Obstet Gynaecol* 1998; **18:** 322–7.
3. WHO. Assessment of the safety of artemisinin compounds in pregnancy: report of two informal consultations convened by WHO in 2002 (Roll Back Malaria and the UNDP/World Bank/WHO Special Programme for Research and Training in Tropical Diseases). Geneva: WHO, 2003.

### Interactions

Use of artemisinin derivatives with drugs that prolong the QT interval should be avoided if possible; caution is advised when artemisinin derivatives are given with other antimalarials that have this propensity.

**Grapefruit juice.** The oral bioavailability of artemether may be increased by concomitant administration of grapefruit juice.

1. van Agtmael MA, *et al.* The effect of grapefruit juice on the time-dependent decline of artemether plasma levels in healthy subjects. *Clin Pharmacol Ther* 1999; **66:** 408–14.

### Pharmacokinetics

Peak plasma concentrations have been achieved in about 3 hours after oral administration of artemether, in about 6 hours after intramuscular injection of artemether, and in about 11 hours after rectal administration of artemisinin. Artemisinin and its derivatives are all rapidly hydrolysed to the active metabolite dihydroartemisinin. Reported elimination half-lives have been about 45 minutes after intravenous administration of artesunate, about 4 hours after rectal artemisinin, and about 4 to 11 hours after intramuscular or oral artemether. There are very few published data on the pharmacokinetics of artemotil, but its elimination half-life appears to be longer than that of artemether.

◊ Reviews.

1. White NJ, *et al.* Clinical pharmacokinetics and pharmacodynamics of artemether-lumefantrine. *Clin Pharmacokinet* 1999; **37:** 105–25.
2. Navaratnam V, *et al.* Pharmacokinetics of artemisinin-type compounds. *Clin Pharmacokinet* 2000; **39:** 255–70.

### Uses and Administration

Artemisinin is a sesquiterpene lactone isolated from *Artemisia annua*, a herb that has traditionally been used in China for the treatment of malaria. It is a potent and rapidly acting blood schizontocide active against *Plasmodium vivax* and against both chloroquine-sensitive and chloroquine-resistant strains of *P. falciparum*.

Artemisinin and its derivatives are used usually with other antimalarials for the treatment of malaria.

The following doses are those suggested by WHO. For oral administration in uncomplicated falciparum malaria, artemisinin may be given in a dose of 25 mg/kg on the first day with 12.5 mg/kg on the second and the third days. For artesunate, the dose is 4 mg/kg daily for 3 days when given with mefloquine or, if artesunate is used alone, 4 mg/kg on the first day followed by 2 mg/kg daily for 6 days.

For oral treatment of uncomplicated falciparum malaria, artemether is given, with lumefantrine 480 mg, over a period of 60 hours in a dose of 80 mg administered at diagnosis and repeated after 8, 24, 36, 48 and 60 hours (total dose of 480 mg of artemether and

2.88 g of lumefantrine). If the oral artemisinin compounds have to be used alone they should be given for a minimum of 5 days.

For parenteral administration in severe malaria, artemether or artesunate are used. The loading dose of artemether is 3.2 mg/kg intramuscularly, followed by 1.6 mg/kg daily for 6 days. The loading dose of artesunate is 2.4 mg/kg intravenously, followed at 12 and 24 hours by a dose of 1.2 mg/kg, and then 1.2 mg/kg daily for 6 days. For both drugs the patient should be transferred to oral therapy as soon as possible.

◊ Reviews.

1. McIntosh HM, Olliaro P. Artemisinin derivatives for treating uncomplicated malaria. Available in The Cochrane Library; Issue 1. Chichester: John Wiley; 2004.
2. McIntosh HM, Olliaro P. Artemisinin derivatives for treating severe malaria. Available in The Cochrane Library; Issue 1. Chichester: John Wiley; 2004.
3. Omari AAA, *et al.* Artemether-lumefantrine for treating uncomplicated falciparum malaria. Available in The Cochrane Library; Issue 1. Chichester: John Wiley; 2004.

**Administration of artemisinin derivatives.** To overcome the poor solubility of *artemisinin* in water a number of dosage forms and routes of administration have been tried. Also, several more potent derivatives with more suitable pharmaceutical properties have been developed, notably the methyl ether derivative, *artemether*, and the ethyl ether derivative, *artemotil*, which are more lipid soluble; the sodium salt of the hemisuccinate ester, *sodium artesunate*, which is soluble in water but appears to have poor stability in aqueous solutions; and *sodium artelinate*, which is both soluble and stable in water. Other derivatives that have been studied include *arteflene*. Several preparations of artemisinin derivatives are available either commercially or for studies organised by bodies such as WHO. These include oral formulations of artemether, artesunate, artemisinin itself, and *dihydroartemisinin*; intramuscular formulations of artemotil, artemether, and artesunate; intravenous formulations of *artelinic acid* and artesunate; and suppositories of artemisinin, artesunate, and dihydroartemisinin.

**Malaria.** The overall management of malaria and the place of artemisinin derivatives in current recommendations are discussed on p.444. In an attempt to delay the development of resistance to these compounds, WHO at one time recommended that their use be restricted to the treatment of malaria in areas of documented multidrug resistance and that they should not be used at all for prophylaxis. However, the development of resistance to conventional therapies has now led WHO to recommend the use in such circumstances of combination therapies containing artemisinin derivatives (artemisinin-based combination therapies, also known as ACTs). The following combination therapies are recommended:

- artemether-lumefantrine
- artesunate plus amodiaquine
- artesunate plus pyrimethamine-sulfadoxine (Fansidar) (in areas where susceptibility to pyrimethamine-sulfadoxine remains high)
- artesunate plus mefloquine (reserved for areas of low transmission)

Additional ACTs recommended by WHO for accelerated development are piperaquine-dihydroartemisinin, chlorproguanil-dapsone-artesunate, and pyronaridine-artesunate.

Artemether-lumefantrine is now also recommended in the UK as an alternative to quinine-based therapy for uncomplicated falciparum malaria.

In acute uncomplicated malaria artemisinin derivatives are usually given by mouth. Those used have been artemisinin, artemether, or artesunate. Artemotil may be given intramuscularly in acute malaria. Parenteral therapy is generally necessary in severe malaria and good results in multidrug-resistant areas have been obtained with artemether, artemotil, or artesunate intramuscularly, usually followed by oral mefloquine. Artesunate has also been given intravenously, and WHO recommends[1] intravenous artesunate or intramuscular artemether as alternatives to quinine for severe malaria. Rectal administration of artesunate or artemisinin, followed by oral mefloquine, has been successful and is recommended by WHO[1] if parenteral therapy is not possible. The nasogastric route may also be used.[1]

1. WHO. *Management of severe malaria: a practical handbook.* Geneva: WHO, 2000.

**Schistosomiasis.** Findings of a reduced intensity of *Schistosoma mansoni* infection in patients treated with sodium artesunate for malaria[1] prompted further investigation into the use of artemisinin derivatives for the control of schistosomiasis (p.100). A double-blind placebo-controlled study[2] in children negative for *S. mansoni* found a significantly lower incidence of infection in those given artemether orally. There was also a significant reduction in the prevalence of *Plasmodium falciparum* infection.

1. De Clercq D, *et al.* Efficacy of artesunate against Schistosoma mansoni infections in Richard Toll, Senegal. *Trans R Soc Trop Med Hyg* 2000; **94:** 90–1.
2. Utzinger J, *et al.* Oral artemether for prevention of Schistosoma mansoni infection: randomised controlled trial. *Lancet* 2000; **355:** 1320–5.

## Preparations

**Proprietary Preparations** (details are given in Part 3)
***Braz.:*** Paluther; Plasmotrim; ***Fr.:*** Paluther†; ***India:*** E Mal; Falcigo; Larither; ***Thai.:*** Plasmotrim.

**Multi-ingredient:** ***Austral.:*** Riamet; ***Austria:*** Riamet; ***Ger.:*** Riamet; ***Hong Kong:*** Riamet; ***Norw.:*** Riamet; ***S.Afr.:*** Coartem; ***Switz.:*** Riamet; ***Thai.:*** Coartem; ***UK:*** Riamet.

# Chloroquine *(BAN, rINN)*

Cloroquina. 4-(7-Chloro-4-quinolylamino)pentyldiethylamine; 7-Chloro-4-(4-diethylamino-1-methylbutylamino)quinoline.

$C_{18}H_{26}ClN_3$ = 319.9.
*CAS — 54-05-7.*
*ATC — P01BA01.*

**Pharmacopoeias.** In *US.*

**USP 27** (Chloroquine). A white or slightly yellow, odourless, crystalline powder. M.p. 87° to 92°. Very slightly soluble in water; soluble in chloroform, in ether, and in dilute acids. Store at a temperature of 25°, excursions permitted between 15° and 30°.

## Chloroquine Hydrochloride *(BANM, rINNM)*

Hidrocloruro de cloroquina.

$C_{18}H_{26}ClN_3,2HCl$ = 392.8.
*CAS — 3545-67-3.*
*ATC — P01BA01.*

**Pharmacopoeias.** *US* includes an injection.

## Chloroquine Phosphate *(BANM, rINNM)*

Chingaminum; Chlorochinium Phosphoricum; Chlorochinum Diphosphoricum; Chloroquini Diphosphas; Chloroquini Phosphas; Fosfato de cloroquina; Fosfato de Cloroquina; Quingamine; SN-7618.

$C_{18}H_{26}ClN_3,2H_3PO_4$ = 515.9.
*CAS — 50-63-5.*
*ATC — P01BA01.*

**Pharmacopoeias.** In *Chin., Eur.* (see p.vi), *Int., Pol., US,* and *Viet.*

**Ph. Eur. 5.0** (Chloroquine Phosphate). A white or almost white, hygroscopic, crystalline powder. It exists in two forms, one melting at about 195° and the other at about 218°. Freely soluble in water; very slightly soluble in alcohol and in methyl alcohol. A 10% solution in water has a pH of 3.8 to 4.3. Store in airtight containers. Protect from light.

**USP 27** (Chloroquine Phosphate). A white, odourless, crystalline powder, which slowly discolours on exposure to light. It exists in two polymorphic forms, one melting between 193° and 195° and the other between 210° and 215°; mixture of the two forms melts between 193° and 215°. Freely soluble in water; practically insoluble in alcohol, in chloroform, and in ether. Its solutions have a pH of about 4.5.

## Chloroquine Sulfate *(rINNM)*

Chloroquine Sulphate *(BANM)*; Chloroquini Sulfas; RP-3377; Sulfato de Cloroquina; Sulfato de cloroquina.

$C_{18}H_{26}ClN_3,H_2SO_4,H_2O$ = 436.0.
*CAS — 132-73-0 (anhydrous chloroquine sulfate).*
*ATC — P01BA01.*

**Pharmacopoeias.** In *Eur.* (see p.vi) and *Int.*

**Ph. Eur. 5.0** (Chloroquine Sulphate). A white or almost white crystalline powder. Freely soluble in water and in methyl alcohol; very slightly soluble in alcohol. An 8% solution in water has a pH of 4.0 to 5.0. Store in airtight containers. Protect from light.

**Sorption.** Various studies using low concentrations of chloroquine phosphate or chloroquine sulfate indicate that chloroquine exhibits pH-dependent binding to several materials used in medical equipment and membrane filters, including soda glass and various plastics such as cellulose acetate, cellulose propionate, methacrylate butadiene styrene, polypropylene, PVC, ethylvinyl acetate, and polyethylene.[1-3] Although this effect may not be of relevance at doses used clinically,[4] it is considered critical that laboratory workers undertaking assays and sensitivity testing should recognise that significant reductions in concentrations can occur when chloroquine is prepared or stored in equipment made from these materials.[2,3] As the effect of borosilicate glass or polystyrene appears to be minimal, it has been suggested that they may be suitable for use in such procedures.[2,3]

Similar sorption has also been reported during membrane filtration of solutions of amodiaquine hydrochloride, mefloquine hydrochloride, or quinine sulfate.[1]

1. Baird JK, Lambros C. Effect of membrane filtration of antimalarial drug solutions on in vitro activity against Plasmodium falciparum. *Bull WHO* 1984; **62:** 439–44.
2. Yahya AM, *et al.* Binding of chloroquine to glass. *Int J Pharmaceutics* 1985; **25:** 217–23.
3. Yahya AM, *et al.* Investigation of chloroquine binding to plastic materials. *Int J Pharmaceutics* 1986; **34:** 137–43.
4. Martens HJ, *et al.* Sorption of various drugs in polyvinyl chloride, glass, and polyethylene-lined infusion containers. *Am J Hosp Pharm* 1990; **47:** 369–73.

## Adverse Effects

Adverse effects experienced with dosage regimens of chloroquine used in the treatment and prophylaxis of malaria are generally less common and less severe than those associated with the higher doses used for prolonged periods in rheumatoid arthritis.

Frequent adverse effects of chloroquine include headache, various skin eruptions, pruritus, and gastrointestinal disturbances such as nausea, vomiting, and diarrhoea. More rarely, mental changes including psychotic episodes, agitation, and personality changes may occur. Convulsions have been reported. Visual disturbances such as blurred vision and difficulties in focusing have occurred but these are more common with higher doses, when they may be associated with keratopathy or retinopathy, as discussed under Effects on the Eyes, below. Keratopathy usually occurs in the form of corneal opacities and is normally reversible when chloroquine is withdrawn. Retinopathy is the most serious adverse effect of chloroquine on the eyes and it can result in severe visual impairment. Changes may be irreversible and can even progress after chloroquine is discontinued. Those taking high doses of chloroquine for prolonged periods appear to be at greatest risk of developing retinopathy. Other uncommon adverse effects from prolonged use include loss of hair, bleaching of hair pigment, bluish-black pigmentation of the mucous membranes and skin, photosensitivity, tinnitus, reduced hearing, nerve deafness, neuromyopathy, and myopathy, including cardiomyopathy.

Blood disorders have been reported rarely. They include aplastic anaemia, reversible agranulocytosis, thrombocytopenia, and neutropenia.

There have also been rare reports of changes in liver function, including hepatitis and abnormal liver function tests.

Parenteral therapy with chloroquine can be hazardous and rapid intravenous administration or the use of high doses can result in cardiovascular toxicity and other symptoms of acute overdosage.

Acute overdosage with chloroquine is extremely dangerous and death can occur within a few hours. Initial effects include headache, gastrointestinal disturbances, drowsiness, and dizziness. Hypokalaemia may occur within a few hours of ingestion of chloroquine. Visual disturbances may be dramatic with a sudden loss of vision. However, the main effect of overdosage with chloroquine is cardiovascular toxicity with hypotension and cardiac arrhythmias progressing to cardiovascular collapse, convulsions, cardiac and respiratory arrest, coma, and death.

**Effects on the blood.** Aplastic anaemia was associated with the use of chloroquine in 3 patients.[1] Two patients had received treatment over several months and one of these was later found to have acute myeloblastic leukaemia after receiving chloroquine treatment initially for discoid lupus erythematosus, and later for cerebral malaria. In the third patient aplastic anaemia developed 3 weeks after a short course of chloroquine for malaria.

1. Nagaratnam N, *et al.* Aplasia and leukaemia following chloroquine therapy. *Postgrad Med J* 1978; **54:** 108–12.

**Effects on the eyes.** The main adverse effects of chloroquine and hydroxychloroquine on the eye are keratopathy and retinopathy.

*Keratopathy,* characterised by corneal deposits, may occur within a few weeks of starting treatment. However, patients are often asymptomatic and fewer than 50% of affected patients complain of visual symptoms such as photophobia, haloes around lights, or blurred vision. Keratopathy is completely reversible on withdrawal of treatment and is not usually considered to be a contra-indication to continued treatment.[1]

*Retinopathy* is potentially more serious. The outcome following discontinuation of treatment is unpredictable and changes may be irreversible or may even progress.[2,3] Delayed-onset retinopathy has also been reported in patients many years after cessation of treatment.[4] The reported incidence of retinopathy varies according to the methodology and criteria used.[1,5,6] From studies in patients on long-term antimalarial treatment, it was reported[1] that an accumulation of 100 g of chloroquine [phosphate] (250 mg daily for 1 year) might cause retinopathy; the risk was significantly increased as the total dosage exceeded 300 g. Experience in rheumatology also indicates that the incidence of retinal toxicity is dose-related. While the total cumulative dose, the duration of treatment, and the age of the patient might all affect the incidence of retinal toxicity,[7,8] the daily dose might be the most important factor.[9] It has been suggested that the risk of retinal damage is small with daily doses of up to 4.0 mg of chloroquine phosphate per kg body-weight (= chloroquine base approximately 2.5 mg per kg daily) or up to 6.5 mg of hydroxychloroquine sulfate per kg.[9] In obese patients, excessive dosage should be avoided by calculating dosage on the basis of lean body-weight. It appears that retinopathy is rarely, if ever, associated with the weekly dosages of chloroquine recommended for the prophylaxis of malaria.[10,11]

In the UK, the Royal College of Ophthalmologists has made recommendations regarding use by rheumatologists and dermatologists. Chloroquine should only be used if hydroxychloroquine or other preferred drugs have failed as there is inadequate data to advise on a safe maximum dose; thus the following recommendations relate only to hydroxychloroquine as no guidelines have been published for chloroquine. Baseline assessment before treatment with hydroxychloroquine is commenced (maximum daily dosage 6.5 mg/kg lean body-weight) should consist of checking renal and hepatic function, questioning the patient about visual impairment not corrected by glasses, and recording near visual acuity. Thereafter, patients should be monitored annually with enquiry about visual symptomatology, rechecking of acuity, and assessment for blurred vision. Patients should be referred to an ophthalmologist if problems are detected either before or during treatment. Those taking long-term hydroxychloroquine should be subject to occasional ophthalmological review after 5 years' continuous treatment.

The UK manufacturers of chloroquine recommend ophthalmic examination at 3 to 6 monthly intervals in patients receiving continuous high doses for more than a year, or weekly treatment for more than 3 years, or for those in whom total consumption exceeds 100 g or 1.6 g/kg.

1. Bernstein HN. Ophthalmologic considerations and testing in patients receiving long-term antimalarial therapy. *Am J Med* 1983; **75** (suppl 1A): 25–34.
2. Ogawa S, *et al.* Progression of retinopathy long after cessation of chloroquine therapy. *Lancet* 1979; **i:** 1408.
3. Easterbrook M. Ocular effects and safety of antimalarial agents. *Am J Med* 1988; **85** (suppl 4A): 23–9.
4. Ehrenfeld M, *et al.* Delayed-onset chloroquine retinopathy. *Br J Ophthalmol* 1986; **70:** 281–3.
5. Finbloom DS, *et al.* Comparison of hydroxychloroquine and chloroquine use and the development of retinal toxicity. *J Rheumatol* 1985; **12:** 692–4.
6. Morsman CDG, *et al.* Screening for hydroxychloroquine retinal toxicity: is it necessary? *Eye* 1990; **4:** 572–6.
7. Elman A, *et al.* Chloroquine retinopathy in patients with rheumatoid arthritis. *Scand J Rheumatol* 1976; **5:** 161–6.
8. Marks JS, Power BJ. Is chloroquine obsolete in treatment of rheumatic disease? *Lancet* 1979; **i:** 371–3.
9. Mackenzie AH. Dose refinements in long-term therapy of rheumatoid arthritis with antimalarials. *Am J Med* 1983; **75** (suppl 1A): 40–5.
10. Breckenridge A. Risks and benefits of prophylactic antimalarial drugs. *BMJ* 1989; **299:** 1057–8.
11. Lange WR, *et al.* No evidence for chloroquine-associated retinopathy among missionaries on long-term malaria chemoprophylaxis. *Am J Trop Med Hyg* 1994; **51:** 389–92.

**Effects on glucose metabolism.** While hypoglycaemia has occurred with quinine (see p.460), it was not generally thought to be associated with chloroquine; however, there has been a report of its occurrence in a patient with reactive hypoglycaemia.[1]

1. Abu-Shakra M, Lee P. Hypoglycemia: an unusual adverse reaction to chloroquine. *Clin Exp Rheumatol* 1994; **12:** 95.

**Effects on the heart.** Studies in patients with malaria[1] and in healthy subjects[2] indicate that the acute cardiovascular toxicity that may be associated with parenteral use of chloroquine is related to transiently high plasma concentrations produced during the early part of the distribution phase; these findings appear to confirm that the rate of administration is a major determinant of this toxicity. Cardiac conduction abnormalities, including heart block, have also occurred in patients receiving long-term oral therapy with chloroquine,[3] including use in lupus erythematosus,[4,5] as well as after chloroquine overdosage or abuse.[6] Histological changes in endomyocardial biopsy specimens from 2 patients with cardiomyopathy associated with chloroquine or hydroxychloroquine therapy were found to be virtually identical to those seen in the skeletal muscle of patients with chloroquine-induced myopathy[7] (see also Effects on the Muscles, below).

1. White NJ, *et al.* Parenteral chloroquine for treating falciparum malaria. *J Infect Dis* 1987; **155:** 192–201.
2. Looareesuwan S, *et al.* Cardiovascular toxicity and distribution kinetics of intravenous chloroquine. *Br J Clin Pharmacol* 1986; **22:** 31–6.
3. Ogola ESN, *et al.* Chloroquine related complete heart block with blindness: case report. *East Afr Med J* 1992; **69:** 50–2.
4. Piette J-C, *et al.* Chloroquine cardiotoxicity. *N Engl J Med* 1987; **317:** 710–11.
5. Baguet J-P, *et al.* Chloroquine cardiomyopathy with conduction disorders. *Heart* 1999; **81:** 221–3.
6. Ihenacho HNC, Magulike E. Chloroquine abuse and heart block in Africans. *Aust N Z J Med* 1989; **19:** 17–21.
7. Ratliff NB, *et al.* Diagnosis of chloroquine cardiomyopathy by endomyocardial biopsy. *N Engl J Med* 1987; **316:** 191–3.

**Effects on the muscles.** The myopathy induced by chloroquine is characterised by progressive weakness and atrophy of proximal muscles and can develop insidiously after periods of therapy ranging from a few weeks to a few years.[1] There are often mild sensory changes, depression of tendon reflexes, and abnormal nerve conduction studies suggestive of an associated peripheral neuropathy. The myopathy is reversible on withdrawal of treatment but recovery may take several months. Cardiomyopathy may also occur (see under Effects on the Heart, above). Similar effects have been reported with hydroxychloroquine.[2] In a retrospective review of 4405 patients with rheumatic disorders, 214 had received chloroquine or hydroxychloroquine and, of these, 3 developed myopathy.[3]

1. Mastaglia FL. Adverse effects of drugs on muscle. *Drugs* 1982; **24:** 304–21.
2. Estes ML, *et al.* Chloroquine neuromyotoxicity. *Am J Med* 1987; **82:** 447–55.
3. Avina-Zubieta JA, *et al.* Incidence of myopathy in patients treated with antimalarials: a report of three cases and a review of the literature. *Br J Rheumatol* 1995; **34:** 166–70.

**Effects on the nervous system.** Apart from neuropathies (see Effects on the Muscles, above) other adverse effects of chloroquine on the nervous system have included isolated reports of extrapyramidal symptoms and other involuntary movements[1,2] (in patients being treated for malaria), nystagmus[3] (in a patient on prolonged treatment for rheumatoid arthritis), and convulsions[4,5] and nonconvulsive status epilepticus[6] (in patients on malaria prophylaxis).

1. Umez-Eronini EM, Eronini EA. Chloroquine induced involuntary movements. *BMJ* 1977; **1:** 945–6.
2. Singhi S, *et al.* Chloroquine-induced involuntary movements. *BMJ* 1977; **2:** 520.
3. Marks JS. Motor polyneuropathy and nystagmus associated with chloroquine phosphate. *Postgrad Med J* 1979; **55:** 569.
4. Fish DR, Espir MLE. Convulsions associated with prophylactic antimalarial drugs: implications for people with epilepsy. *BMJ* 1988; **297:** 526–7.
5. Fish DR, Espri MLE. Malaria prophylaxis and epilepsy. *BMJ* 1988; **297:** 1267.
6. Mülhauser P, *et al.* Chloroquine and nonconvulsive status epilepticus. *Ann Intern Med* 1995; **123:** 76–7.

**Effects on the skin.** *Pruritus* is frequently reported in patients receiving chloroquine for the treatment of malaria and it may become so severe as to compromise treatment. The onset of itching occurs a few hours after administration but usually remits spontaneously within 72 hours. Although most workers consider that antihistamines are generally ineffective,[1,2] some patients may obtain some relief.[3] The incidence of pruritus is purported to be higher in black patients, but this may only reflect the greater number of black patients surveyed. The aetiology of this reaction is unknown, but this apparent higher incidence has prompted suggestions that it may have a genetic basis[4] or be related to the affinity of chloroquine for melanin.[2] Chloroquine's main metabolite, monodesethylchloroquine, has also been implicated.[5] A survey[1] in Nigeria found that, of 1100 patients, 74% had pruritus during antimalarial therapy; 61% of these reacted to chloroquine, 30% reacted to amodiaquine, 2.5% to Fansidar (pyrimethamine-sulfadoxine), and, 6.5% reacted to all three. In another study in Nigeria,[4] the incidence of pruritus was reported to be 14% (8 of 56 patients) for chloroquine, 27% (14 of 52) for amodiaquine, and 13% (7 of 53) for halofantrine; none of 58 patients receiving quinine or 82 patients receiving mefloquine experienced pruritus.

There have been rare reports of more severe cutaneous reactions associated with chloroquine, including *toxic epidermal necrolysis*,[6,7] *erythema multiforme*,[8] and *Stevens-Johnson syndrome*,[9] although the causal role of chloroquine is not always clear as some of these patients also received other antimalarials, sometimes at an inappropriate dosage. In a more recent case of toxic epidermal necrolysis,[10] chloroquine given alone for malaria prophylaxis was the probable cause. For a discussion including the possible effect of chloroquine on the incidence of erythema multiforme in patients taking pyrimethamine with sulfadoxine, see Adverse Effects with Sulfonamides, under Pyrimethamine, p.458.

1. Ajayi AA, *et al.* Epidemiology of antimalarial-induced pruritus in Africans. *Eur J Clin Pharmacol* 1989; **37:** 539–40.
2. Osifo NG. Chloroquine-induced pruritus among patients with malaria. *Arch Dermatol* 1984; **120:** 80–2.
3. Okor RS. Responsiveness of chloroquine-induced pruritus to antihistamine therapy—clinical survey. *J Clin Pharm Ther* 1990; **15:** 147–50.
4. Sowunmi A, *et al.* Pruritus and antimalarial drugs in Africans. *Lancet* 1989; **ii:** 213.
5. Essien EE, *et al.* Chloroquine disposition in hypersensitive and non-hypersensitive subjects and its significance in chloroquine-induced pruritus. *Eur J Drug Metab Pharmacokinet* 1989; **14:** 71–7.
6. Kanwar AJ, Singh OP. Toxic epidermal necrolysis—drug induced. *Indian J Dermatol* 1976; **21:** 73–7.
7. Phillips-Howard PA, Warwick Buckler J. Idiosyncratic reaction resembling toxic epidermal necrolysis caused by chloroquine and Maloprim. *BMJ* 1988; **296:** 1605.
8. Steffen R, Somaini B. Severe cutaneous adverse reactions to sulfadoxine-pyrimethamine in Switzerland. *Lancet* 1986; **i:** 610.
9. Bamber MG, *et al.* Fatal Stevens-Johnson syndrome associated with Fansidar and chloroquine. *J Infect* 1986; **13:** 31–3.
10. Boffa MJ, Chalmers RJG. Toxic epidermal necrolysis due to chloroquine phosphate. *Br J Dermatol* 1994; **131:** 444–5.

**Overdosage.** For adverse effects associated with chloroquine overdosage, see Treatment of Adverse Effects, below.

## Treatment of Adverse Effects

*Acute overdosage with chloroquine can be rapidly lethal and intensive symptomatic supportive treatment should be started immediately.* The first steps should be to maintain adequate respiration and to correct any cardiovascular disturbances. Early administration of adrenaline with diazepam (see below) may minimise the cardiotoxicity of chloroquine and control arrhythmias. Activated charcoal may be given by mouth to adults or children who present within 1 hour of ingesting more than the equivalent of 15 mg/kg of chloroquine base; activated charcoal may be left in the stomach to limit any further absorption. Intravenous sodium bicarbonate should be given to correct metabolic acidosis. Other methods to increase the elimination of chloroquine, such as dialysis, are probably of little use.

◊ Chloroquine overdosage is the most severe and frequent cause of intoxication with antimalarial drugs and chloroquine is often used for suicide attempts. Severe toxic manifestations may occur within 1 to 3 hours and fatal outcomes usually occur within 2 to 3 hours of drug ingestion. The major clinical symptoms are of neurological, respiratory, and cardiovascular toxicity;[1] death is usually due to cardiac arrest related to the direct effect of chloroquine on the myocardium.[2] Chloroquine has a low safety margin: doses of 20 mg/kg are considered toxic and 30 mg/kg may be lethal. The mortality rate in some published studies has ranged from 10 to 30%.[1] If gastric lavage is attempted it should be preceded by correction of severe cardiovascular disturbances and institution of artificial ventilation because insertion of the stomach tube may induce sudden cardiac arrest or convulsions; induction of emesis is contra-indicated because of the risk of lung aspiration. Activated charcoal has been recommended to limit absorption of chloroquine that may be left in the gut.[3] There is no evidence to indicate that attempts to increase chloroquine elimination such as acidification of the urine, haemodialysis, peritoneal dialysis, or exchange transfusion, are effective in overdosage. Elimination in the urine is more dependent on haemodynamic status than on infusion of osmotic solutions or acidification. Any clearance achieved by haemoperfusion or haemodialysis is low in comparison with the normal total body clearance.[1]

It is not clear if correction of hypokalaemia is essential, but administration of potassium should be avoided in the initial phases of intoxication when conduction disturbances still exist. The degree of hypokalaemia may be correlated with the severity of chloroquine intoxication and might be useful diagnostically.[4] However, chloroquine-induced hypokalaemia may be due to a transport-dependent mechanism rather than to true potassium depletion and overzealous correction could result in hyperkalaemia.[4]

Since there had been no effective treatment for severe chloroquine poisoning, one group of workers tried using early mechanical ventilation, together with adrenaline and high doses of diazepam, both given intravenously, to counteract cardiotoxicity, with encouraging results.[2] Diazepam had earlier been shown to decrease the cardiotoxicity of chloroquine in *animal* studies and there had been several clinical reports of beneficial responses. It was considered that routine use of adrenaline before the onset of cardiac arrhythmia might be beneficial in the treatment of severe chloroquine poisoning.[2] The manufacturers of chloroquine have suggested giving adrenaline by intravenous infusion in a dose of 250 nanograms/kg per minute initially, with increments of 250 nanograms/kg per minute until adequate systolic blood pressure is restored, and diazepam by intravenous infusion in a dose of 2 mg/kg over 30 minutes as a loading dose, followed by 1 to 2 mg/kg per day for up to 2 to 4 days.

Overdosage with hydroxychloroquine has responded to measures similar to those used in the management of chloroquine overdosage.[5]

1. Jaeger A, *et al.* Clinical features and management of poisoning due to antimalarial drugs. *Med Toxicol* 1987; **2:** 242–73.
2. Riou B, *et al.* Treatment of severe chloroquine poisoning. *N Engl J Med* 1988; **318:** 1–6.
3. Neuvonen PJ, *et al.* Prevention of chloroquine absorption by activated charcoal. *Hum Exp Toxicol* 1992; **11:** 117–20.
4. Clemessy J-L, *et al.* Hypokalaemia related to acute chloroquine ingestion. *Lancet* 1995; **346:** 877–80.
5. Jordan P, *et al.* Hydroxychloroquine overdose: toxicokinetics and management. *J Toxicol Clin Toxicol* 1999; **37:** 861–4.

## Precautions

Excessive doses of chloroquine and hydroxychloroquine are associated with retinal or visual field changes and the precautions to be observed in order to minimise such toxicity are discussed under Effects on the Eyes in Adverse Effects, above. There may be a temporary effect on visual accommodation.

Care is necessary in administering chloroquine to patients with hepatic or renal impairment, or to those with severe gastrointestinal disorders, a history of psoriasis, or neurological disorders, especially a history of epilepsy (see below for advice not to use for malaria prophylaxis). Chloroquine should be used with caution in patients with myasthenia gravis as it may aggravate the condition. Patients with G6PD deficiency should be observed for haemolytic anaemia during chloroquine treatment. Full blood counts should be performed at regular intervals during extended treatment with chloroquine. Although there have been reports of fetal abnormalities associated with the use of chloroquine during pregnancy, the risks of malaria are considered to be greater and there appears to be no justification for withholding chloroquine for the treatment or prophylaxis of malaria.

It is important that when chloroquine is given intravenously it should be by slow infusion otherwise severe cardiotoxicity may develop.

**Breast feeding.** Chloroquine is distributed into breast milk, but not in an amount adequate to provide chemoprophylaxis against malaria for the infant (see under Pharmacokinetics, below). Furthermore, no adverse effects have been observed in breast-feeding infants whose mothers were receiving chloroquine, and the American Academy of Pediatrics considers[1] that it is therefore usually compatible with breast feeding.

1. American Academy of Pediatrics. The transfer of drugs and other chemicals into human milk. *Pediatrics* 2001; **108:** 776–89. Correction. *ibid.*: 1029. Also available at: http://aappolicy.aappublications.org/cgi/content/full/pediatrics%3b108/3/776 (accessed 16/04/04)

**Epilepsy.** Following reports[1,2] of convulsions associated with the use of chloroquine for malaria prophylaxis in 4 previously healthy patients and in 2 patients with a history of seizures, it has been suggested that prospective travellers who have a history of epilepsy should be warned of the risk. Although it was initially considered[3] that this should not restrict the use of chloroquine, UK malaria experts have recommended that it should be avoided for malaria prophylaxis in epileptic patients.[4]

1. Fish DR, Espir MLE. Convulsions associated with prophylactic antimalarial drugs: implications for people with epilepsy. *BMJ* 1988; **297:** 526–7.
2. Fish DR, Espir MLE. Malaria prophylaxis and epilepsy. *BMJ* 1988; **297:** 1267.
3. Hellgren U, Rombo L. Malaria prophylaxis and epilepsy. *BMJ* 1988; **297:** 1267.
4. Bradley DJ, Bannister B. Guidelines for malaria prevention in travellers from the United Kingdom for 2001. *Commun Dis Public Health* 2001; **4:** 84–101.

**Porphyria.** Although chloroquine is probably safe in porphyric patients, some authorities consider its use to be contentious. Pyrimethamine is also probably safe in porphyric patients. Other drugs used for prophylaxis, such as dapsone and sulfadoxine and combinations containing them, are definitely contra-indicated in porphyric patients. Quinine is of proven safety in patients with porphyria and cell-culture tests have suggested that proguanil and mefloquine may also be safe.

Chloroquine has been tried in the treatment of porphyria cutanea tarda, but this is considered by some to be hazardous (see under Uses, below).

**Pregnancy.** There has been concern about the potential teratogenic effects of chloroquine because of a few case reports including defects in hearing and vision.[1] Two of 169 infants born to women who had received chloroquine 300 mg weekly throughout pregnancy had birth defects compared with 4 of 454 control infants whose mothers had not been exposed to antimalarials; the difference was not significant. The data suggested that chloroquine in the recommended prophylactic doses is not a strong teratogen and that its proved antimalarial benefits outweigh any possible risk of low-grade teratogenicity. Also it has been reported that chloroquine prophylaxis during pregnancy did not affect the birth-weight of neonates, compared with a control group.[2]

1. Wolfe MS, Cordero JF. Safety of chloroquine in chemosuppression of malaria during pregnancy. *BMJ* 1985; **290:** 1466–7.
2. Cot M, *et al.* Effect of chloroquine chemoprophylaxis during pregnancy on birth weight: results of a randomized trial. *Am J Trop Med Hyg* 1992; **46:** 21–7.

**Psoriatic arthritis.** It is recommended that chloroquine and hydroxychloroquine should not be used in the treatment of psoriatic arthritis as exacerbations of skin lesions can occur. Some patients may go on to develop generalised erythroderma with subsequent exfoliative dermatitis.[1] However, there has been controversy over the reported incidence of this adverse effect.[2,3]

1. Slagel GA, James WD. Plaquenil-induced erythroderma. *J Am Acad Dermatol* 1985; **12:** 857–62.
2. Luzar MJ. Hydroxychloroquine in psoriatic arthropathy: exacerbations of psoriatic skin lesions. *J Rheumatol* 1982; **9:** 462–4.
3. Sayers ME, Mazanec DJ. Use of antimalarial drugs for the treatment of psoriatic arthritis. *Am J Med* 1992; **93:** 474–5.

**Renal impairment.** Although the elimination of chloroquine is prolonged in renal impairment no dosage adjustment is required in the treatment of malaria. Similarly, dosage reduction is not required for chloroquine prophylaxis except in those with severe renal impairment. Doses tend to be reduced when it is given for longer periods to patients with renal impairment.

## Interactions

There is an increased risk of inducing ventricular arrhythmias if chloroquine is used with halofantrine (see p.452) or other arrhythmogenic drugs such as amiodarone and moxifloxacin. There is an increased risk of convulsions when chloroquine is given with mefloquine. The absorption of chloroquine can be reduced by antacids or kaolin and its metabolism may be inhibited by cimetidine.

**Agalsidase.** For the effect of concomitant administration of chloroquine and *agalsidase alfa* or *beta*, see p.1651.

**Antiepileptics.** Chloroquine may antagonise the antiepileptic activity of *carbamazepine* (see p.356) and *valproate* (see p.382).

**Antimalarials.** Chloroquine should not be used with *halofantrine* since the latter prolongs the QT interval and therefore there is an increased potential to induce arrhythmias (see p.452). Use of chloroquine with *mefloquine* increases the risk of convulsions. Also concurrent use of chloroquine and *proguanil* may increase the incidence of proguanil-associated mouth ulceration.[1] The activity of chloroquine may be affected when it is given with other *antimalarials. Quinine* and chloroquine when used together may be antagonistic.[2] Mixtures of chloroquine with *quinine, mefloquine, amodiaquine, artemisinin*, or *pyrimethamine-sulfadoxine* were antagonistic *in vitro* against *Plasmodium falciparum.*[3]

1. Drysdale SF, *et al.* Proguanil, chloroquine, and mouth ulcers. *Lancet* 1990; **335:** 164.
2. Hall AP. Quinine and chloroquine antagonism in falciparum malaria. *Trans R Soc Trop Med Hyg* 1973; **67:** 425.
3. Stahel E, *et al.* Antagonism of chloroquine with other antimalarials. *Trans R Soc Trop Med Hyg* 1988; **82:** 221.

**Antimicrobials.** Acute dystonic reactions occurred during concomitant therapy with chloroquine and *metronidazole* in a woman who had previously tolerated chloroquine alone.[1] Chloroquine may also reduce the gastrointestinal absorption of *ampicillin* (see p.157).

1. Achumba JI, *et al.* Chloroquine-induced acute dystonic reactions in the presence of metronidazole. *Drug Intell Clin Pharm* 1988; **22:** 308–10.

**Ciclosporin.** Chloroquine has been reported to increase plasma concentrations of ciclosporin (see p.1355).

**Digoxin.** Hydroxychloroquine has been reported to increase plasma concentrations of digoxin (see p.897).

**Gastrointestinal drugs.** Patients often wish to take chloroquine with food, antacids, or other gastrointestinal drugs to alleviate gastrointestinal irritation. Administration with *food* may be beneficial as it appears to improve the absorption of chloroquine.[1,2] However, *antacids* or *kaolin* can reduce the absorption of chloroquine and it is therefore recommended that they should be given at least 4 hours apart.[3,4]

Cimetidine and chloroquine should be used with caution as *cimetidine* can significantly reduce the metabolism and elimination of chloroquine and increase its volume of distribution;[5] *ranitidine*, however, appears to have little effect on the pharmacokinetics of chloroquine.[6]

1. Tulpule A, Krishnaswamy K. Effect of food on bioavailability of chloroquine. *Eur J Clin Pharmacol* 1982; **23:** 271–3.
2. Lagrave M, *et al.* The influence of various types of breakfast on chloroquine levels. *Trans R Soc Trop Med Hyg* 1985; **79:** 559.
3. McElnay JC, *et al.* In vitro experiments on chloroquine and pyrimethamine absorption in the presence of antacid constituents or kaolin. *J Trop Med Hyg* 1982; **85:** 153–8.
4. McElnay JC, *et al.* The effect of magnesium trisilicate and kaolin on the in vivo absorption of chloroquine. *J Trop Med Hyg* 1982; **85:** 159–63.
5. Ette EI, *et al.* Chloroquine elimination in humans: effect of low-dose cimetidine. *J Clin Pharmacol* 1987; **27:** 813–16.
6. Ette EI, *et al.* Effect of ranitidine on chloroquine disposition. *Drug Intell Clin Pharm* 1987; **21:** 732–4.

**Levothyroxine.** For a report of a possible interaction of chloroquine with levothyroxine, see p.1601.

**Praziquantel.** For mention of possible reduced bioavailability of praziquantel when given with chloroquine, see p.112.

**Vaccines.** Although chloroquine has been reported to reduce the antibody response to *human diploid rabies vaccine* (see p.1636), the immune response to other vaccines used in routine immunisation schedules (tetanus, diphtheria, measles, poliomyelitis, typhoid, and BCG) has not been found to be altered by chloroquine prophylaxis.[1,2]

1. Greenwood BM. Chloroquine prophylaxis and antibody response to immunisation. *Lancet* 1984; **ii:** 402–3.
2. Wolfe MS. Precautions with oral live typhoid (Ty 21a) vaccine. *Lancet* 1990; **336:** 631–2.

## Pharmacokinetics

Chloroquine is rapidly and almost completely absorbed from the gastrointestinal tract when given by mouth. Absorption is also rapid following intramuscular or subcutaneous administration. It is widely distributed into body tissues and has a large apparent volume of distribution. It accumulates in high concentrations in some tissues, such as the kidneys, liver, lungs, and spleen and is strongly bound in melanin-containing cells such as those in the eyes and the skin. It also crosses the placenta. Chloroquine is eliminated very slowly from the body and it may persist in tissues for months or even years after discontinuation of therapy.

Chloroquine is extensively metabolised in the liver, mainly to monodesethylchloroquine with smaller amounts of bisdesethylchloroquine (didesethylchloroquinine) and other metabolites being formed. Monodesethylchloroquine has been reported to have some activity against *Plasmodium falciparum*. Chloroquine and its metabolites are excreted in the urine, with about half of a dose appearing as unchanged drug and about 10% as the monodesethyl metabolite. Chloroquine and its monodesethyl metabolite are both distributed into breast milk.

◊ General references.

1. Krishna S, White NJ. Pharmacokinetics of quinine, chloroquine and amodiaquine; clinical implications. *Clin Pharmacokinet* 1996; **30:** 263–99.
2. Ducharme J, Farinotti R. Clinical pharmacokinetics and metabolism of chloroquine: focus on recent advancements. *Clin Pharmacokinet* 1996; **31:** 257–74.

◊ Chloroquine is rapidly absorbed from the gastrointestinal tract but peak plasma concentrations following oral administration can vary considerably.[1] A mean peak plasma concentration of 76 nanograms/mL has been obtained in healthy adults a mean of 3.6 hours after administration of the equivalent of 300 mg of chloroquine base by mouth as tablets.[2] In children with uncomplicated malaria given the equivalent of 10 mg/kg peak plasma concentrations of 250 nanograms/mL have been reached after 2 hours;[3] a mean peak of 134 nanograms/mL has been obtained after 5 hours in healthy children given a similar dose.[4] Nasogastric administration has also produced therapeutic concentrations in children with severe falciparum malaria.[5]

Oral bioavailability is increased if chloroquine is taken with food[6,7] and some beverages[8] and may also be affected by the state of health of the patient; mean values have ranged from about 70% in patients with malaria[9] to 78 or 89% in healthy adults.[2] Although oral bioavailability appears to be unaltered in moderately undernourished adults[10] it has been reported that it may be significantly reduced in children with kwashiorkor.[4]

Preliminary studies with chloroquine suppositories indicated that, although rectal bioavailability is less than half of that of oral chloroquine, sustained therapeutic concentrations may be achieved.[11]

Absorption is also rapid following subcutaneous or intramuscular injection and mean peak plasma concentrations of chloroquine have been obtained within about 30 minutes.[5,9,12]

Chloroquine has a large apparent volume of distribution. A multicompartmental model appears to be necessary to describe the distribution kinetics of chloroquine.[2,13] Following intravenous administration there is a multi-exponential decline in plasma concentrations as chloroquine distributes out of a central compartment that has been estimated to be several orders of magnitude smaller than the total volume of distribution.[5,14] This slow distribution out of the central compartment produces transiently high cardiotoxic concentrations of chloroquine if the overall rate of parenteral delivery is not carefully controlled.

Reported mean values for protein binding have ranged from about 58 to 64%.[15,16] Chloroquine is also bound to platelets and granulocytes so that the plasma concentration is only 10 to 15% of that in whole blood.[17] If these cells are not removed by gentle centrifugation during analysis, erroneously high plasma concentrations will be reported. Furthermore, as chloroquine concentrations determined in serum are higher than those in plasma, probably due to release of chloroquine from platelets during coagulation, it is crucial to state whether analysis has been done on whole blood, serum, or properly separated plasma.

About 50% of a dose of chloroquine is metabolised in the liver, mainly to the *N*-dealkylated metabolite monodesethylchloroquine; smaller amounts of bisdesethylchloroquine, 7-chloro-4-aminoquinoline, and *N*-oxidation products are formed. Some of these metabolites may contribute to the cardiotoxicity associated with chloroquine. In one study, peak plasma concentrations of 7-chloro-4-aminoquinoline were found to be twice those of unchanged chloroquine despite the fact that only relatively small amounts are formed; this appears to be due to its fast rate of formation and long elimination half-life.[18]

A mean of 42 to 47% of a dose has been reported to be excreted in the urine as unchanged chloroquine and 7 to 12% as monodesethylchloroquine.[2] Various estimates of the terminal elimination half-life of chloroquine range from several days to up to 2 months, but its slow release from tissues ensures that small amounts may still be detected after a year.[18,19]

1. Hellgren U, *et al.* On the question of interindividual variations in chloroquine concentrations. *Eur J Clin Pharmacol* 1993; **45:** 383–5.
2. Gustafsson LL, *et al.* Disposition of chloroquine in man after single intravenous and oral doses. *Br J Clin Pharmacol* 1983; **15:** 471–9.
3. Adelusi SA, *et al.* Kinetics of the uptake and elimination of chloroquine in children with malaria. *Br J Clin Pharmacol* 1982; **14:** 483–7.
4. Walker O, *et al.* Single dose disposition of chloroquine in kwashiorkor and normal children—evidence for decreased absorption in kwashiorkor. *Br J Clin Pharmacol* 1987; **23:** 467–72.
5. White NJ, *et al.* Chloroquine treatment of severe malaria in children: pharmacokinetics, toxicity, and new dosage recommendations. *N Engl J Med* 1988; **319:** 1493–1500.
6. Tulpule A, Krishnaswamy K. Effect of food on bioavailability of chloroquine. *Eur J Clin Pharmacol* 1982; **23:** 271–3.
7. Lagrave M, *et al.* The influence of various types of breakfast on chloroquine levels. *Trans R Soc Trop Med Hyg* 1985; **79:** 559.
8. Mahmoud BM, *et al.* Significant reduction in chloroquine bioavailability following coadministration with the Sudanese beverages aradaib, karkadi and lemon. *J Antimicrob Chemother* 1994; **33:** 1005–9.
9. White NJ, *et al.* Parenteral chloroquine for treating falciparum malaria. *J Infect Dis* 1987; **155:** 192–201.
10. Tulpule A, Krishnaswamy K. Chloroquine kinetics in the undernourished. *Eur J Clin Pharmacol* 1983; **24:** 273–6.
11. WHO. Severe and complicated malaria. 2nd ed. *Trans R Soc Trop Med Hyg* 1990; **84** (suppl 2): 1–65.

12. Phillips RE, *et al.* Divided dose intramuscular regimen and single dose subcutaneous regimen for chloroquine: plasma concentrations and toxicity in patients with malaria. *BMJ* 1986; **293:** 13–16.
13. Frisk-Holmberg M, *et al.* The single dose kinetics of chloroquine and its major metabolite desethylchloroquine in healthy subjects. *Eur J Clin Pharmacol* 1984; **26:** 521–30.
14. Looareesuwan S, *et al.* Cardiovascular toxicity and distribution kinetics of intravenous chloroquine. *Br J Clin Pharmacol* 1986; **22:** 31–6.
15. Walker O, *et al.* Characterization of chloroquine plasma protein binding in man. *Br J Clin Pharmacol* 1983; **15:** 375–7.
16. Ofori-Adjei D, *et al.* Protein binding of chloroquine enantiomers and desethylchloroquine. *Br J Clin Pharmacol* 1986; **22:** 356–8.
17. Gustafsson LL, *et al.* Pitfalls in the measurement of chloroquine concentrations. *Lancet* 1983; **i:** 126.
18. Ette EI, *et al.* Pharmacokinetics of chloroquine and some of its metabolites in healthy volunteers: a single dose study. *J Clin Pharmacol* 1989; **29:** 457–62.
19. Gustafsson LL, *et al.* Chloroquine excretion following malaria prophylaxis. *Br J Clin Pharmacol* 1987; **24:** 221–4.

**Distribution into breast milk.** Studies[1,2] have suggested that it is safe for mothers to breast feed when they are receiving chloroquine for treatment of malaria. Although chloroquine and its monodesethyl metabolite are distributed into breast milk, it has been estimated that the amount that would be consumed by an infant is well below the therapeutic range and separate chemoprophylaxis for the infant is required.

There appears to be no data on the excretion of hydroxychloroquine in milk after doses appropriate for the prevention or treatment of malaria, but hydroxychloroquine has been detected in breast milk from 2 mothers receiving doses of 400 mg daily for systemic lupus erythematosus or rheumatoid arthritis.[3,4] One group of workers estimated that, calculated on a body-weight basis, a 9-month-old infant could receive about 2% of a maternal dose via breast feeding.[3]

1. Ogunbona FA, *et al.* Excretion of chloroquine and desethylchloroquine in human milk. *Br J Clin Pharmacol* 1987; **23:** 473–6.
2. Akintonwa A, *et al.* Placental and milk transfer of chloroquine in humans. *Ther Drug Monit* 1988; **10:** 147–9.
3. Nation RL, *et al.* Excretion of hydroxychloroquine in human milk. *Br J Clin Pharmacol* 1984; **17:** 368–9.
4. Østensen M, *et al.* Hydroxychloroquine in human breast milk. *Eur J Clin Pharmacol* 1985; **28:** 357.

## Uses and Administration

Chloroquine is a 4-aminoquinoline antimalarial used in the treatment and prophylaxis of malaria. It has also been used in the treatment of hepatic amoebiasis, lupus erythematosus, light-sensitive skin eruptions, and rheumatoid arthritis.

Chloroquine is used for the prophylaxis and treatment of malaria due to susceptible strains of *Plasmodium falciparum, P. ovale, P. vivax*, and *P. malariae*, but widespread resistance in *P. falciparum* has greatly limited its value. It is a rapid-acting blood schizontocide with some gametocytocidal activity against *P. ovale, P. vivax, P. malariae*, and immature gametocytes of *P. falciparum*. Since it has no activity against exo-erythrocytic forms, chloroquine does not produce a radical cure of vivax or ovale malarias. The mechanism of action of chloroquine against blood schizonts remains unclear, but it may influence haemoglobin digestion by raising intravesicular pH in malaria parasite cells. It also interferes with synthesis of nucleoproteins by the parasite.

Chloroquine may be given as the phosphate, sulfate, or hydrochloride. Doses are normally expressed in terms of chloroquine base, and as a general guide:

- chloroquine base 300 mg is approximately equivalent to chloroquine phosphate 500 mg or chloroquine sulfate 400 mg
- chloroquine base 40 mg is approximately equivalent to chloroquine hydrochloride 50 mg

Oral bioavailability is increased when chloroquine is taken with food.

For the *treatment of malaria* caused by *P. vivax, P. ovale, P. malariae*, and the few remaining strains of chloroquine-sensitive *P. falciparum*, the usual total oral dose for adults and children is the equivalent of a total of about 25 mg of chloroquine base per kg body-weight given over 3 days. This total dose is given in a variety of ways. One way is to give 10 mg/kg, followed after 6 to 8 hours by 5 mg/kg, then 5 mg/kg daily for the next 2 days; alternatively, 10 mg/kg may be given daily for the first 2 days and 5 mg/kg on the third day. Sometimes the adult doses are not expressed in terms of body-weight but as 600 mg followed after 6 to 8 hours by 300 mg, then 300 mg daily for the next 2 days. In severe and complicated malaria when the patient is unable to take oral medication and when chloroquine is to be used, then it can be given by injection. The intravenous route is preferred and a slow rate of infusion is essential, the required dose of 25 mg/kg being given in several infusions over 30 to 32 hours as described in further detail under Malaria, below. Should the patient recover sufficiently to be able to take chloroquine by mouth then the intravenous regimen should be halted and oral therapy started. It is important to bear in mind that in the majority of the world *P. falciparum* is now resistant to chloroquine, which should *not* therefore be given for treatment.

For *prophylaxis of malaria* in areas where *P. falciparum* is absent or in one of the few remaining areas where it is still sensitive to chloroquine, a dose equivalent to 300 mg of chloroquine base is given once each week, beginning about one week before exposure and continuing throughout, and for at least 4 weeks after, exposure. For children, a weekly dose of 5 mg/kg has been recommended (but see also under Malaria, below). In areas of chloroquine-resistant malaria, but with a low risk of infection, chloroquine is given with proguanil; where there is a high risk of infection alternative antimalarial regimens are recommended.

In the treatment of *hepatic amoebiasis*, chloroquine is used with an intestinal amoebicide. The usual dose is the equivalent of 600 mg of chloroquine base daily for 2 days then 300 mg daily for 2 or 3 weeks. A dose of 6 mg/kg daily up to a maximum of 300 mg daily has been suggested for children.

When chloroquine is used for long-term therapy in conditions such as *rheumatoid arthritis* or *lupus erythematosus*, the dosage in obese patients should be calculated on the basis of lean body-weight in order to avoid excessive dosage.

In *rheumatoid arthritis*, response to treatment may not be apparent for up to 6 months, but if there is no improvement by then treatment should be discontinued. The usual dose is the equivalent of chloroquine base 150 mg daily (maximum 2.5 mg/kg daily) or up to 3 mg/kg daily in children. For further details see under Effects on the Eyes, above.

In discoid and systemic *lupus erythematosus* (p.1088), chloroquine is used in a dose equivalent to 150 mg (maximum 2.5 mg/kg) of base daily; children are given a dose of up to 3 mg/kg daily.

In the management of *light-sensitive skin eruptions*, adults have been given the equivalent of 150 to 300 mg of chloroquine base daily during periods of intense light exposure; children have been given up to 3 mg/kg.

**Amoebiasis.** For a discussion of the treatment of amoebiasis with mention of chloroquine for hepatic amoebiasis, see p.595.

**Inflammatory disorders.** Chloroquine and hydroxychloroquine possess anti-inflammatory properties and they have been tried or used with some benefit in a range of inflammatory conditions which often have an immunological basis, although they rarely constitute first-line therapy in these disorders. Such conditions include rheumatoid arthritis (see under Hydroxychloroquine, p.453), ulcerative colitis,[1] infantile interstitial pneumonitis,[2,3] asthma,[4] giant cell arteritis,[5] and various skin disorders (see below). The mode of action in these conditions is unclear. Results of studies have been conflicting but it does appear that chloroquine and hydroxychloroquine might have some immunosuppressive effects.[6,7]

1. Mayer L, Sachar DB. Efficacy of chloroquine in the treatment of inflammatory bowel disease. *Gastroenterology* 1988; **94:** A293.
2. Springer C, *et al.* Chloroquine treatment in desquamative interstitial pneumonia. *Arch Dis Child* 1987; **62:** 76–7.
3. Kerem E, *et al.* Sequential pulmonary function measurements during treatment of infantile chronic interstitial pneumonitis. *J Pediatr* 1990; **116:** 61–7.
4. Charous BL. Open study of hydroxychloroquine in the treatment of severe symptomatic or corticosteroid-dependent asthma. *Ann Allergy* 1990; **65:** 53–8.
5. Le Guennec P, *et al.* Management of giant cell arteritis: value of synthetic antimalarial agents: a retrospective study of thirty six patients. *Rev Rhum* 1994; **61:** 423–8.
6. Bygbjerg IC, Flachs H. Effect of chloroquine on human lymphocyte proliferation. *Trans R Soc Trop Med Hyg* 1986; **80:** 231–5.
7. Prasad RN, *et al.* Immunopharmacology of chloroquine. *Trans R Soc Trop Med Hyg* 1987; **81:** 168–9.

**Malaria.** The overall treatment and prophylaxis of malaria and the place of chloroquine in current recommendations are discussed on p.444.

TREATMENT. In the treatment of patients with chloroquine-sensitive falciparum malaria studies have found chloroquine to be at least as effective as quinine in both uncomplicated and severe infections. However, very few areas exist where *Plasmodium falciparum* remains sensitive to chloroquine. There are also reports of resistance to chloroquine in *P. vivax*.[1]

Treatment with chloroquine is usually by mouth, adults and children being given the equivalent of 25 mg of chloroquine base per kg body-weight over 3 days. Any chloroquine lost through vomiting needs to be replaced by additional doses.[2] Encouraging results have also been obtained in a limited number of patients given the equivalent of 30 mg of chloroquine base per kg by mouth over 2 days in the form of a loading dose of 10 mg/kg followed by two doses of 5 mg/kg at intervals of 6 hours on the first day and two doses of 5 mg/kg at intervals of 12 hours on the second day.[3]

Parenteral therapy may be used if the infection is severe or oral administration is not possible. The parenteral regimen for adults and children recommended by WHO[4] consists of a loading dose equivalent to 10 mg of chloroquine base per kg given by constant rate intravenous infusion in sodium chloride 0.9% over a period of at least 8 hours and followed by a further three 8-hour infusions each of 5 mg/kg during the next 24 hours. Alternatively the entire course may be given over 30 hours, each infusion of 5 mg/kg being given over 6 hours. There should be close monitoring for hypotension and other signs of cardiovascular toxicity.

The intramuscular or subcutaneous routes have been used if intravenous administration is not possible. Intramuscular or subcutaneous doses for adults and children are 3.5 mg/kg every 6 hours[2,4] or 2.5 mg/kg every 4 hours to a total dose equivalent to 25 mg of the base per kg.[2]

Whichever parenteral route is used, patients should be transferred to oral therapy as soon as possible and administration continued until a total dose equivalent to 25 mg of the base per kg has been given.

If injections cannot be given a chloroquine suspension or syrup appears to be well absorbed when given by nasogastric tube even in comatose patients. Rectal administration in young children has also produced beneficial responses.[5,6]

PROPHYLAXIS. The widespread prevalence of strains of *P. falciparum* resistant to chloroquine has considerably diminished the value of chloroquine for malaria chemoprophylaxis and has made recommendations increasingly complex (see p.444). If chloroquine is used for prophylaxis it is usually given with proguanil. For **adults** a dose equivalent to 300 mg of chloroquine base is given by mouth once each week, beginning about one week before exposure and continuing throughout, and for at least 4 weeks after, exposure. Some countries advise the use of 100 mg daily for 6 days a week. For **children**, a weekly dose of chloroquine base 5 mg/kg has been recommended, although UK malaria experts[7] have suggested the following prophylactic doses for children based on fractions of the adult dose of 300 mg weekly:

- under 6.0 kg (0 to 12 weeks of age), one-eighth the adult dose
- 6.0 to 9.9 kg (3 to 11 months), one-quarter the adult dose
- 10.0 to 15.9 kg (1 year to 3 years 11 months), three-eighths the adult dose
- 16.0 to 24.9 kg (4 years to 7 years 11 months), half the adult dose
- 25.0 to 44.9 kg (8 years to 12 years 11 months), three-quarters the adult dose
- over 45 kg (13 years and over), the adult dose

They noted that body-weight was a better guide to dosage than age for children over 6 months.

1. Whitby M. Drug resistant Plasmodium vivax malaria. *J Antimicrob Chemother* 1997; **40:** 749–52.
2. WHO. *WHO model prescribing information: drugs used in parasitic diseases.* 2nd ed. Geneva: WHO, 1995.
3. Pussard E, *et al.* Efficacy of a loading dose of oral chloroquine in a 36-hour treatment schedule for uncomplicated Plasmodium falciparum malaria. *Antimicrob Agents Chemother* 1991; **35:** 406–9.
4. WHO. *Management of severe malaria: a practical handbook.* Geneva: WHO 2000.
5. Westman L, *et al.* Rectal administration of chloroquine for treatment of children with malaria. *Trans R Soc Trop Med Hyg* 1994; **88:** 446.
6. Antia-Obong OE, *et al.* Chloroquine phosphate suppositories in the treatment of childhood malaria in Calabar, Nigeria. *Curr Ther Res* 1995; **56:** 928–35.
7. Bradley DJ, Bannister B. Guidelines for malaria prevention in travellers from the United Kingdom for 2001. *Commun Dis Public Health* 2001; **4:** 84–101. Also available at: http://www.hpa.org.uk/cdph/issues/CDPHVol4/no2/malaria_guidelinesp.pdf (accessed 16/04/04)

**Porphyria cutanea tarda.** Chloroquine and hydroxychloroquine have been used with some benefit in the treatment of porphyria cutanea tarda (p.1040) and low doses (such as chloroquine phosphate 125 mg or hydroxychloroquine sulfate 200 mg given twice weekly) have been considered by some to be useful in patients unsuitable for phlebotomy[1-3] (but see under Porphyria in Precautions, above). However, the acute increase in urinary porphyrins and fall in hepatic porphyrin content produced by these drugs have been associated with a variable degree of hepatotoxicity[4] and others prefer to use desferrioxamine.[5]

1. Grossman ME, *et al.* Porphyria cutanea tarda. *Am J Med* 1979; **67:** 277–86.
2. Cainelli T, *et al.* Hydroxychloroquine versus phlebotomy in the treatment of porphyria cutanea tarda. *Br J Dermatol* 1983; **108:** 593–600.

3. Ashton RE, *et al.* Low-dose oral chloroquine in the treatment of porphyria cutanea tarda. *Br J Dermatol* 1984; **111:** 609–13.
4. Scholnick PL, *et al.* The molecular basis of the action of chloroquine in porphyria cutanea tarda. *J Invest Dermatol* 1973; **61:** 226–32.
5. Rocchi E. Treatment of porphyria cutanea tarda. *Br J Dermatol* 1987; **116:** 139–40.

**Rheumatoid arthritis.** For reference to the use of chloroquine in the treatment of rheumatoid arthritis, see under Hydroxychloroquine, p.453.

**Sarcoidosis.** Chloroquine and hydroxychloroquine have been tried in the management of sarcoidosis (p.1087) as alternatives or adjuncts to corticosteroid therapy.

References.

1. O'Leary TJ, *et al.* The effects of chloroquine on serum 1,25-dihydroxyvitamin D and calcium metabolism in sarcoidosis. *N Engl J Med* 1986; **315:** 727–30.
2. Adams JS, *et al.* Effective reduction in the serum 1,25-dihydroxyvitamin D and calcium concentration in sarcoidosis-associated hypercalcemia with short-course chloroquine therapy. *Ann Intern Med* 1989; **111:** 437–8.
3. DeSimone DP, *et al.* Granulomatous infiltration of the talus and abnormal vitamin D and calcium metabolism in a patient with sarcoidosis: successful treatment with hydroxychloroquine. *Am J Med* 1989; **87:** 694–6.
4. Jones E, Callen JP. Hydroxychloroquine is effective therapy for control of cutaneous sarcoidal granulomas. *J Am Acad Dermatol* 1990; **23:** 487–9.
5. Zic JA, *et al.* Treatment of cutaneous sarcoidosis with chloroquine: review of the literature. *Arch Dermatol* 1991; **127:** 1034–40.
6. Baltzan M, *et al.* Randomized trial of prolonged chloroquine therapy in advanced pulmonary sarcoidosis. *Am J Respir Crit Care Med* 1999; **160:** 192–7.

**Skin disorders.** In addition to their use in lupus erythematosus hydroxychloroquine and chloroquine have been tried in a number of other skin disorders including polymorphic light eruptions,[1] lichen planus[2,3] (p.1136), cutaneous symptoms of dermatomyositis (p.1086), erythema nodosum,[4,5] and recurrent erythema multiforme (p.1135).

1. Murphy GM, *et al.* Hydroxychloroquine in polymorphic light eruption: a controlled trial with drug and visual sensitivity monitoring. *Br J Dermatol* 1987; **116:** 379–86.
2. Mostafa WZ. Lichen planus of the nail: treatment with antimalarials. *J Am Acad Dermatol* 1989; **20:** 289–90.
3. De Argila D, *et al.* Isolated lichen planus of the lip successfully treated with chloroquine phosphate. *Dermatology* 1997; **195:** 284–5.
4. Alloway JA, Franks LK. Hydroxychloroquine in the treatment of chronic erythema nodosum. *Br J Dermatol* 1995; **132:** 661–2.
5. Jarrett P, Goodfield MJD. Hydroxychloroquine and chronic erythema nodosum. *Br J Dermatol* 1996; **134:** 373.

## Preparations

***BP 2003:*** Chloroquine Phosphate Tablets; Chloroquine Sulphate Injection; Chloroquine Sulphate Tablets;
***USP 27:*** Chloroquine Hydrochloride Injection; Chloroquine Phosphate Tablets.

**Proprietary Preparations** (details are given in Part 3)
***Arg.:*** Nivaquine; ***Austral.:*** Chlorquin; ***Austria:*** Resochin; ***Belg.:*** Nivaquine; ***Braz.:*** Diclokin; Difosquin†; Palux†; ***Canad.:*** Aralen; ***Denm.:*** Malarex; ***Fin.:*** Heliopar; ***Fr.:*** Nivaquine; ***Ger.:*** Arthrabas†; Resochin; Weimerquin; ***Hong Kong:*** Chlorquin†; Syncoquin; ***India:*** Clo-Kit; Emquin; Lariago; Melubrin; Nivaquine-P; Resochin; ***Irl.:*** Avloclor; ***Israel:*** Aralen†; Avloclor; ***Mex.:*** Aralen; Klorokin†; Paluken†; ***Neth.:*** Nivaquine; ***NZ:*** Nivaquine; ***Port.:*** Resochina; ***S.Afr.:*** Daramal; Mirquin; Nivaquine; Plasmoquine; ***Singapore:*** Avloclor†; ***Spain:*** Resochin; ***Switz.:*** Chlorochin; Nivaquine; Resochine†; ***Thai.:*** Diroquine; Genocin; P-Roquine; ***UK:*** Avloclor; Malaviron; Nivaquine; ***USA:*** Aralen.

**Multi-ingredient:** ***Arg.:*** Tri-Emcortina; ***Braz.:*** Clopirim; ***Fr.:*** Savarine; ***S.Afr.:*** Daramal-Paludrine.

## Chlorproguanil Hydrochloride *(BANM, rINNM)*

Hidrocloruro de clorproguanil; M-5943. 1-(3,4-Dichlorophenyl)-5-isopropylbiguanide hydrochloride.

$C_{11}H_{15}Cl_2N_5,HCl = 324.6.$

*CAS — 537-21-3 (chlorproguanil); 15537-76-5 (chlorproguanil hydrochloride).*

### Profile

Chlorproguanil is a biguanide antimalarial used for malaria prophylaxis similarly to proguanil (p.457). It is sometimes given with dapsone. Combination with both dapsone and artesunate is also being investigated for malaria treatment.

◊ References.

1. Keuter M, *et al.* Comparison of chloroquine, pyrimethamine and sulfadoxine, and chlorproguanil and dapsone as treatment for falciparum malaria in pregnant and non-pregnant women, Kakamega district, Kenya. *BMJ* 1990; **301:** 466–70.
2. Rooth I, *et al.* Proguanil daily or chlorproguanil twice weekly are efficacious against falciparum malaria in a holoendemic area of Tanzania. *J Trop Med Hyg* 1991; **94:** 45–9.
3. Nevill CG, *et al.* Daily chlorproguanil is an effective alternative to daily proguanil in the prevention of Plasmodium falciparum malaria in Kenya. *Trans R Soc Trop Med Hyg* 1994; **88:** 319–20.
4. Winstanley P, *et al.* Chlorproguanil/dapsone for uncomplicated Plasmodium falciparum malaria in young children: pharmacokinetics and therapeutic range. *Trans R Soc Trop Med Hyg* 1997; **91:** 322–7.
5. Amukoye E, *et al.* Chlorproguanil-dapsone: effective treatment for uncomplicated falciparum malaria. *Antimicrob Agents Chemother* 1997; **41:** 2261–4.
6. Winstanley P. Chlorproguanil-dapsone (LAPDAP) for uncomplicated falciparum malaria. *Trop Med Int Health* 2001; **6:** 952–4.
7. Mutabingwa T, *et al.* Chlorproguanil-dapsone for treatment of drug-resistant falciparum malaria in Tanzania. *Lancet* 2001; **358:** 1218–23. Correction. *ibid.:* 1556.
8. Sulo J, *et al.* Chlorproguanil-dapsone versus sulfadoxine-pyrimethamine for sequential episodes of uncomplicated falciparum malaria in Kenya and Malawi: a randomised clinical trial. *Lancet* 2002; **360:** 1136–43.

## Halofantrine Hydrochloride *(BANM, USAN, rINNM)*

Halofantrini Hydrochloridum; Hidrocloruro de halofantrina; WR-171669. (*RS*)-3-Dibutylamino-1-(1,3-dichloro-6-trifluoromethyl-9-phenanthryl)propan-1-ol hydrochloride; 1,3-Dichloro-α-[2-(dibutylamino)ethyl]-6-trifluoromethyl-9-phenanthrenemethanol hydrochloride.

$C_{26}H_{30}Cl_2F_3NO,HCl = 536.9.$

*CAS — 69756-53-2 (halofantrine); 36167-63-2 (halofantrine hydrochloride); 66051-63-6 (±-halofantrine).*

*ATC — P01BX01.*

**Pharmacopoeias.** In *Eur.* (see p.vi).

**Ph. Eur. 5.0** (Halofantrine Hydrochloride). A white or almost white powder. It exhibits polymorphism. Practically insoluble in water; sparingly soluble in alcohol; freely soluble in methyl alcohol. Protect from light.

### Adverse Effects and Precautions

Adverse effects associated with halofantrine include diarrhoea, abdominal pain, nausea, vomiting, pruritus, and skin rash. Transient elevation of serum transaminases, intravascular haemolysis, and hypersensitivity reactions have also been reported.

Halofantrine can adversely affect the heart and this is mainly seen as a prolongation of QT interval. Serious ventricular arrhythmias have been reported and fatalities have occurred. As a result it is contra-indicated in patients known to have a prolonged QT interval or those with cardiac disease or a family history of congenital QT prolongation, and also in those with unexplained syncopal attacks, thiamine deficiency, or electrolyte disturbances, or taking other arrhythmogenic drugs (see also under Effects on the Heart, below, and under Interactions, below).

Halofantrine is not recommended during pregnancy or breast feeding. It should not be taken on a full stomach since this increases its bioavailability and thus the risk of toxicity; after taking halofantrine, fatty food should be avoided for 24 hours.

**Effects on the blood.** Halofantrine has been associated with acute intravascular haemolysis.[1,2]

1. Vachon F, *et al.* Halofantrine and acute intravascular haemolysis. *Lancet* 1992; **340:** 909–10.
2. Mojon M, *et al.* Intravascular haemolysis following halofantrine intake. *Trans R Soc Trop Med Hyg* 1994; **88:** 91.

**Effects on the heart.** Prolonged PR[1,2] and QT[1-5] intervals have been reported in patients given halofantrine and there are individual reports of fatal cardiac arrest[1,5] and of torsade de pointes.[4] In 1994, the UK Committee on Safety of Medicines[6] noted that QT interval prolongation occurred at recommended doses of halofantrine in the majority of patients and that worldwide there had been 14 reports of cardiac arrhythmias associated with halofantrine; 8 patients were known to have died. To reduce the risk of arrhythmias they stressed that halofantrine should *not* be taken with meals, with other drugs that may induce arrhythmias (e.g. quinine, chloroquine, and mefloquine; tricyclic antidepressants; antipsychotics; certain antiarrhythmics; and the antihistamines terfenadine and astemizole), or with drugs causing electrolyte disturbances. They also stated that it should *not* be given to patients known to have prolongation of the QT interval or with any form of cardiac disease associated with QT interval prolongation or ventricular arrhythmia (e.g. coronary heart disease, cardiomyopathy, or congenital heart disease). Some workers[2] have suggested ECG screening of all patients before starting treatment with halofantrine. Others[7] found pretreatment ECGs to be poorly predictive of QT lengthening during treatment. Children may experience serious cardiac effects at standard doses.[8]

1. Nosten F, *et al.* Cardiac effects of antimalarial treatment with halofantrine. *Lancet* 1993; **341:** 1054–6.
2. Monlun E, *et al.* Cardiac complications of halofantrine: a prospective study of 20 patients. *Trans R Soc Trop Med Hyg* 1995; **89:** 430–3.
3. Castot A, *et al.* Prolonged QT interval with halofantrine. *Lancet* 1993; **341:** 1541.
4. Monlun E, *et al.* Prolonged QT interval with halofantrine. *Lancet* 1993; **341:** 1541–2.
5. Anonymous. Halofantrine: revised data sheet. *WHO Drug Inf* 1993; **7:** 66–7.
6. Committee on Safety of Medicines/Medicines Control Agency. Cardiac arrhythmias with halofantrine (Halfan). *Current Problems* 1994; **20:** 6.
7. Matson PA, *et al.* Cardiac effects of standard-dose halofantrine therapy. *Am J Trop Med Hyg* 1996; **54:** 229–31.
8. Sowunmi A, *et al.* Cardiac effects of halofantrine in children suffering from acute uncomplicated falciparum malaria. *Trans R Soc Trop Med Hyg* 1998; **92:** 446–8.

**Effects on the skin.** For a comparison of the incidence of pruritus associated with halofantrine and other antimalarials, see Effects on the Skin under Adverse Effects of Chloroquine, p.449.

### Interactions

Halofantrine prolongs the QT interval and should not be used with other drugs that have the potential to induce cardiac arrhythmias, in particular the antimalarials mefloquine, chloroquine, and quinine, and also tricyclic antidepressants, phenothiazine antipsychotics, some antiarrhythmics (including amiodarone, disopyramide, flecainide, procainamide, quinidine, and the beta blocker sotalol), cisapride, and the antihistamines astemizole and terfenadine. Also, halofantrine should not be given with drugs that cause electrolyte disturbances (such as diuretics).

**Grapefruit juice.** In a study in 12 healthy patients, the bioavailability of halofantrine was reported to be increased by administration with grapefruit juice and was found to accentuate halofantrine-associated QT prolongation.[1] It was suggested that grapefruit juice should be contra-indicated during use of halofantrine.

1. Charbit B, *et al.* Pharmacokinetic and pharmacodynamic interaction between grapefruit juice and halofantrine. *Clin Pharmacol Ther* 2002; **72:** 514–23.

### Pharmacokinetics

Halofantrine is slowly and erratically absorbed following administration by mouth, although it appears in the circulation within about 1 hour, peak concentrations occurring in 3 to 7 hours. Bioavailability of halofantrine is increased by administration with or after food, particularly food high in fat content, and it must therefore be taken on an empty stomach because of the risk of cardiac toxicity. The elimination half-life of halofantrine varies considerably between individuals, but is generally about 1 to 2 days. Halofantrine is metabolised in the liver, its major metabolite being desbutylhalofantrine which appears to be as active as the parent compound. Excretion of halofantrine is primarily via the faeces.

◊ References.

1. Karbwang J, Na Bangchang K. Clinical pharmacokinetics of halofantrine. *Clin Pharmacokinet* 1994; **27:** 104–19.
2. Watkins WM, *et al.* Halofantrine pharmacokinetics in Kenyan children with non-severe and severe malaria. *Br J Clin Pharmacol* 1995; **39:** 283–7.
3. Ohrt C, *et al.* Pharmacokinetics of an extended-dose halofantrine regimen in patients with malaria and in healthy volunteers. *Clin Pharmacol Ther* 1995; **57:** 525–32.

### Uses and Administration

Halofantrine is a 9-phenanthrenemethanol antimalarial that has been used in the *treatment* of uncomplicated chloroquine-resistant falciparum and of chloroquine-resistant vivax malaria. Halofantrine is a blood schizontocide but has no activity against exoerythrocytic forms. Its value is limited by its unpredictable bioavailability and by cardiotoxicity. It should *not* be used where mefloquine has been used for prophylaxis (for cardiac hazard, see Effects on the Heart, above). Halofantrine should also *not* be used for malaria prophylaxis and is no longer recommended for standby treatment.

In the treatment of malaria, halofantrine hydrochloride has been given by mouth as 3 doses of 500 mg at intervals of 6 hours, on an empty stomach. Dosage for children is based on 24 mg/kg divided into 3 doses. The following doses have been recommended: 23 to 31 kg body-weight, 3 doses of 250 mg at intervals of 6 hours; 32 to 37 kg, 3 doses of 375 mg at intervals of 6 hours; over 37 kg, adult dose. A second course should be given after a week to patients with little or no previous exposure to malaria.

### Preparations

**Proprietary Preparations** (details are given in Part 3)
***Belg.:*** Halfan; ***Fr.:*** Halfan; ***Ger.:*** Halfan; ***Neth.:*** Halfan; ***Port.:*** Halfan; ***S.Afr.:*** Halfan; ***Spain:*** Halfan; ***Switz.:*** Halfan; ***UK:*** Halfan†; ***USA:*** Halfan†.

## Hydroxychloroquine Sulfate *(rINNM)*

Hydroxychloroquine Sulphate *(BANM)*; Oxichlorochin Sulphate; Sulfato de Hidroxicloroquina; Sulfato de hidroxicloroquina; Win-1258-2. 2-{*N*-[4-(7-Chloro-4-quinolylamino)pentyl]-*N*-ethylamino}ethanol sulphate.

$C_{18}H_{26}ClN_3O,H_2SO_4 = 434.0.$

*CAS — 118-42-3 (hydroxychloroquine); 747-36-4 (hydroxychloroquine sulfate).*

*ATC — P01BA02.*

**Pharmacopoeias.** In *Br.* and *US.*

**BP 2003** (Hydroxychloroquine Sulphate). A white or almost white, odourless or almost odourless, crystalline powder. Freely soluble in water; practically insoluble in alcohol, in chloroform, and in ether. A 1% solution in water has a pH of 3.5 to 5.5. Protect from light.

**USP 27** (Hydroxychloroquine Sulfate). A white or practically white, odourless, crystalline powder. It exists in two forms, the usual form melting at about 240° and the other form at about 198°. Freely soluble in water; practically insoluble in alcohol, in chloroform, and in ether. Its solutions in water have a pH of about 4.5. Protect from light.

### Adverse Effects, Treatment, and Precautions

As for Chloroquine, p.448.

**Breast feeding.** Hydroxychloroquine has been detected in human breast milk[1,2] but no adverse effects have been observed in breast-fed infants and the American Academy of Pediatrics considers[3] that it is therefore usually compatible with breast feeding.

1. Nation RL, *et al.* Excretion of hydroxychloroquine in human milk. *Br J Clin Pharmacol* 1984; **17:** 368–9.

2. Østensen M, *et al.* Hydroxychloroquine in human breast milk. *Eur J Clin Pharmacol* 1985; **28:** 357.
3. American Academy of Pediatrics. The transfer of drugs and other chemicals into human milk. *Pediatrics* 2001; **108:** 776–89. Correction. *ibid.*: 1029. Also available at: http://aappolicy.aappublications.org/cgi/content/full/pediatrics%3b108/3/776 (accessed 19/04/04)

**Effects on the eyes.** The main adverse effects of chloroquine and hydroxychloroquine on the eye are keratopathy and retinopathy. With respect to retinopathy, precautions should be observed in patients undergoing long-term treatment, as described under Chloroquine on p.448.

**Pregnancy.** In a study[1] of 133 pregnancies in 90 women treated with hydroxychloroquine, no statistical difference in pregnancy outcome was found compared with a control group consisting of 70 pregnancies in 53 women. It was concluded that the findings supported preliminary evidence for the safety of hydroxychloroquine treatment in pregnancy, and that treatment should probably therefore be maintained during pregnancy in patients with systemic lupus erythematosus.

1. Costedoat-Chalumeau N, *et al.* Safety of hydroxychloroquine in pregnant patients with connective tissue diseases: a study of one hundred thirty-three cases compared with a control group. *Arthritis Rheum* 2003; **48:** 3207–11.

## Interactions

As for Chloroquine, p.450.

## Pharmacokinetics

The pharmacokinetics of hydroxychloroquine are similar to those of chloroquine (see p.450).

◊ References.

1. Tett SE, *et al.* Bioavailability of hydroxychloroquine tablets in healthy volunteers. *Br J Clin Pharmacol* 1989; **27:** 771–9.
2. Miller DR, *et al.* Steady-state pharmacokinetics of hydroxychloroquine in rheumatoid arthritis. *DICP Ann Pharmacother* 1991; **25:** 1302–5.
3. Ducharme J, *et al.* Enantioselective disposition of hydroxychloroquine after a single oral dose of the racemate to healthy subjects. *Br J Clin Pharmacol* 1995; **40:** 127–33.

## Uses and Administration

Hydroxychloroquine sulfate is a 4-aminoquinoline antimalarial with actions similar to those of chloroquine (p.451), but is mainly used in the treatment of systemic and discoid lupus erythematosus and rheumatoid arthritis. It is also used in the treatment of light-sensitive skin eruptions.

Hydroxychloroquine sulfate is given by mouth.

In *lupus erythematosus* and *rheumatoid arthritis*, response to treatment may not be apparent for up to 6 months but if there is no improvement by then, treatment should be discontinued. In the UK, treatment is usually started with 400 mg daily in divided doses with meals. In the USA, recommended initial doses are 400 to 600 mg daily for rheumatoid arthritis and 400 mg once or twice daily for lupus erythematosus. Doses are reduced to the minimum effective dose for maintenance; this is usually 200 to 400 mg daily but should not exceed 6.5 mg/kg daily (or 400 mg daily whichever is the smaller). To avoid excessive dosage in obese patients, special care is needed to calculate the dosage on the basis of lean body-weight. For further details, see under Effects on the Eyes in Chloroquine, p.448. In children, the minimum effective dose should be used up to a maximum of 6.5 mg/kg daily (or 400 mg daily whichever is the smaller).

Hydroxychloroquine sulfate is also used in similar doses for the treatment of *light-sensitive skin eruptions*, but treatment should only be given during periods of maximum exposure to light.

Hydroxychloroquine sulfate may be used in *malaria* both for treatment and prophylaxis, when chloroquine is not available, with the same limitations as for chloroquine. In the USA, the manufacturers recommend for *prophylaxis* of malaria a dose of 400 mg every 7 days; children may be given a weekly prophylactic dose of 6.5 mg/kg (up to a maximum of 400 mg). In *treating* an acute malarial attack, a dose of 800 mg has been used, followed after 6 to 8 hours by 400 mg and a further 400 mg on each of the 2 following days; alternatively, a single dose of 800 mg has been given. In children, an initial dose of 13 mg/kg may be given, followed by 6.5 mg/kg after 6 hours and again on the second and third days.

**Inflammatory disorders.** For the use of hydroxychloroquine and chloroquine in a range of inflammatory conditions, see under Chloroquine, p.451 and under Rheumatoid Arthritis, below.

**Lupus erythematosus.** For the use of hydroxychloroquine in lupus erythematosus, see p.1088.

**Malaria.** The role of chloroquine and potentially therefore of hydroxychloroquine in the treatment and prophylaxis of malaria is discussed on p.444.

**Porphyria cutanea tarda.** For reference to the use of hydroxychloroquine in the treatment of porphyria cutanea tarda, see under the Uses and Administration of Chloroquine, p.451.

**Rheumatoid arthritis.** Hydroxychloroquine and chloroquine are used as antirheumatic drugs in the management of *rheumatoid arthritis* (p.9) in an attempt to suppress the rate of cartilage erosion or alter the course of the disease.[1] They are considered to be less effective than the other disease-modifying antirheumatic drugs (DMARDs) but they are usually better tolerated and so may be preferred in patients with milder forms of the disease.[2] Additional benefit has been obtained using antimalarials with other DMARDs especially methotrexate and sulfasalazine,[3-5] although adverse effects may be more common. For reference to precautions to reduce the incidence of retinopathy, see under Effects on the Eyes in Adverse Effects of Chloroquine, p.448.

Generally the lowest effective dose should be used for maintenance to minimise toxicity; for hydroxychloroquine sulfate this should not exceed 6.5 mg/kg lean body-weight daily. Daily doses of 200 or 400 mg are commonly used but one study indicates that there is little advantage in using the higher dose.[6]

Experience with antimalarials to treat *juvenile idiopathic arthritis* (p.9) is limited and the results have been variable.[7,8]

Chloroquine and hydroxychloroquine have also been reported to be of use in *palindromic rheumatism.*[9-11]

1. Suarez-Almazor ME, *et al.* Antimalarials for treating rheumatoid arthritis. Available in The Cochrane Library; Issue 1. Chichester: John Wiley; 2004.
2. HERA Study Group. A randomized trial of hydroxychloroquine in early rheumatoid arthritis: the HERA study. *Am J Med* 1995; **98:** 156–68.
3. Clegg DO, *et al.* Safety and efficacy of hydroxychloroquine as maintenance therapy for rheumatoid arthritis after combination therapy with methotrexate and hydroxychloroquine. *J Rheumatol* 1997; **24:** 1896–1902.
4. O'Dell JR. Triple therapy with methotrexate, sulfasalazine, and hydroxychloroquine in patients with rheumatoid arthritis. *Rheum Dis Clin North Am* 1998; **24:** 465–77.
5. O'Dell JR, *et al.* Treatment of rheumatoid arthritis with methotrexate and hydroxychloroquine, methotrexate and sulfasalazine, or a combination of the three medications: results of a two-year, randomized, double-blind, placebo-controlled trial. *Arthritis Rheum* 2002; **46:** 1164–70.
6. Pavelka K, *et al.* Hydroxychloroquine sulphate in the treatment of rheumatoid arthritis: a double blind comparison of two dose regimens. *Ann Rheum Dis* 1989; **48:** 542–6.
7. Brewer EJ, *et al.* Penicillamine and hydroxychloroquine in the treatment of severe juvenile rheumatoid arthritis. *N Engl J Med* 1986; **314:** 1269–76.
8. Grondin C, *et al.* Slow-acting antirheumatic drugs in chronic arthritis of childhood. *Semin Arthritis Rheum* 1988; **18:** 38–47.
9. Richardson MR, Zalin AM. Treatment of palindromic rheumatism with chloroquine. *BMJ* 1987; **294:** 741.
10. Hanonen P, *et al.* Treatment of palindromic rheumatism with chloroquine. *BMJ* 1987; **294:** 1289.
11. Youssef W, *et al.* Palindromic rheumatism: a response to chloroquine. *J Rheumatol* 1991; **18:** 35–7.

**Sarcoidosis.** Chloroquine and hydroxychloroquine have been tried in the management of sarcoidosis (p.1087) as alternatives or adjuncts to corticosteroid therapy. For references to the use of hydroxychloroquine, see under Chloroquine, p.452.

**Skin disorders.** For reference to the use of hydroxychloroquine in a variety of skin disorders, see under Chloroquine, p.452.

**Venous thromboembolism.** Standard prophylaxis for surgical patients at high risk of venous thromboembolism (p.839) is usually with an anticoagulant. Hydroxychloroquine has been described by some as an antiplatelet agent[1] and although its mechanism of action is uncertain the incidence of fatal pulmonary embolism has been reduced in patients given hydroxychloroquine prophylactically after total hip replacement;[2] the usual daily divided dose was about 800 mg from the day before surgery until discharge; larger doses had been used.

1. Antiplatelet Trialists' Collaboration. Collaborative overview of randomised trials of antiplatelet therapy—III: reduction in venous thrombosis and pulmonary embolism by antiplatelet prophylaxis among surgical and medical patients. *BMJ* 1994; **308:** 235–46.
2. Loudon JR. Hydroxychloroquine and postoperative thromboembolism after total hip replacement. *Am J Med* 1988; **85:** (suppl 4A): 57–61.

## Preparations

***BP 2003:*** Hydroxychloroquine Tablets;
***USP 27:*** Hydroxychloroquine Sulfate Tablets.

**Proprietary Preparations** (details are given in Part 3)

***Arg.:*** Evoquin; Metirel; Plaquenil; Polirreumin; ***Austral.:*** Plaquenil; ***Austria:*** Plaquenil; ***Belg.:*** Plaquenil; ***Braz.:*** Plaquinol; ***Canad.:*** Plaquenil; ***Chile:*** Plaquinol; ***Denm.:*** Ercoquin; Plaquenil; ***Fin.:*** Oxiklorin; Plaquenil; ***Fr.:*** Plaquenil; ***Ger.:*** Quensyl; ***Gr.:*** Plaquenil; ***Hong Kong:*** Plaquenil; ***Irl.:*** Plaquenil; ***Israel:*** Plaquenil; ***Ital.:*** Plaquenil; ***Malaysia:*** Plaquenil; ***Mex.:*** Plaquenil; ***Neth.:*** Plaquenil; ***Norw.:*** Ercoquin†; Plaquenil; ***NZ:*** Plaquenil; ***Port.:*** Plaquinol; ***Singapore:*** Plaquenil; ***Spain:*** Dolquine; ***Swed.:*** Plaquenil; ***Switz.:*** Plaquenil; ***Thai.:*** Plaquenil; ***UK:*** Plaquenil; ***USA:*** Plaquenil.

# Lumefantrine *(BAN, rINN)*

Benflumelol; Benflumetol; Lumefantrina. 2,7-Dichloro-9-[(4-chlorophenyl)methylene]-α-[(dibutylamino)methyl]-9H-fluorene-4-methanol.

$C_{30}H_{32}Cl_3NO$ = 528.9.

*CAS — 82186-77-4.*

**Pharmacopoeias.** In *Chin.*

## Adverse Effects and Precautions

Adverse effects associated with lumefantrine in combination with artemether commonly include headache, dizziness, sleep disturbance, palpitations, gastrointestinal disturbances, anorexia, pruritus, rash, cough, arthralgia, myalgia, and fatigue. Lumefantrine-artemether should be given with caution in severe hepatic or renal impairment and ECG and blood potassium monitored.

## Pharmacokinetics

The bioavailability of lumefantrine after oral administration is variable; absorption begins after a lag-time of up to 2 hours and bioavailability is substantially increased by administration with food, particularly meals high in fat. Peak plasma concentrations occur after about 6 to 8 hours. Lumefantrine is almost completely protein bound. It is considered to be metabolised mainly in the liver and is excreted in the faeces. The elimination half-life is reported to be between 4 to 6 days in patients with malaria.

◊ References.

1. White NJ, *et al.* Clinical pharmacokinetics and pharmacodynamics of artemether-lumefantrine. *Clin Pharmacokinet* 1999; **37:** 105–25.
2. Ezzet F, *et al.* Pharmacokinetics and pharmacodynamics of lumefantrine (benflumetol) in acute falciparum malaria. *Antimicrob Agents Chemother* 2000; **44:** 697–704.

## Uses and Administration

Lumefantrine is a dichlorobenzylidine derivative given by mouth in combination with artemether (p.447) for the treatment of uncomplicated falciparum malaria. It is a blood schizontocide with a relatively slow onset of action but it has a longer duration of action than artemether.

Lumefantrine is given over a period of 60 hours in a dose of 480 mg, in combination with artemether 80 mg, administered at diagnosis and repeated after 8, 24, 36, 48, and 60 hours (total dose 2.88 g and 0.48 g respectively).

◊ References.

1. Omari AAA, *et al.* Artemether-lumefantrine for treating uncomplicated falciparum malaria. Available in The Cochrane Library; Issue 1. Chichester: John Wiley; 2004.

## Preparations

**Proprietary Preparations** (details are given in Part 3)

**Multi-ingredient:** ***Austral.:*** Riamet; ***Austria:*** Riamet; ***Ger.:*** Riamet; ***Hong Kong:*** Riamet; ***Norw.:*** Riamet; ***S.Afr.:*** Coartem; ***Switz.:*** Riamet; ***Thai.:*** Coartem; ***UK:*** Riamet.

# Mefloquine Hydrochloride

*(BANM, USAN, rINNM)*

Hidrocloruro de mefloquina; Mefloquini Hydrochloridum; Ro-21-5998 (mefloquine); Ro-21-5998/001 (mefloquine hydrochloride); WR-142490 (mefloquine). (RS)-[2,8-Bis(trifluoromethyl)-4-quinolyl]-(SR)-(2-piperidyl)methanol hydrochloride.

$C_{17}H_{16}F_6N_2O,HCl$ = 414.8.

*CAS — 53230-10-7 (mefloquine); 51773-92-3 (mefloquine hydrochloride).*

*ATC — P01BC02.*

**Pharmacopoeias.** In *Eur.* (see p.vi) and *Int.*

**Ph. Eur. 5.0** (Mefloquine Hydrochloride). A white or slightly yellow, crystalline powder. It shows polymorphism. Very slightly soluble in water; soluble in alcohol; freely soluble in methyl alcohol. Protect from light.

**Sorption.** For reference to loss of mefloquine hydrochloride from solutions during membrane filtration, see Chloroquine, p.448.

**Stability.** A report of the photolytic degradation of mefloquine hydrochloride in water.[1]

1. Tønnesen HH, Grislingaas A-L. Photochemical stability of biologically active compounds II: photochemical decomposition of mefloquine in water. *Int J Pharmaceutics* 1990; **60:** 157–62.

### Adverse Effects

Since mefloquine has a long elimination half-life, adverse effects may occur or persist up to several weeks after the last dose.

The most frequent adverse effects of mefloquine are nausea, diarrhoea, vomiting, abdominal pain, anorexia, headache, dizziness, loss of balance, somnolence, and sleep disorders, notably insomnia and abnormal dreams.

Neurological or psychiatric disturbances have also been reported with mefloquine and include sensory and motor neuropathies, tremor, ataxia, visual disturbances, tinnitus and hearing impairment, convulsions, anxiety, depression, confusion, hallucinations, panic attacks, emotional instability, aggression and agitation, and acute psychosis. There have been rare reports of suicidal ideation.

Other adverse effects include skin rashes, pruritus and urticaria, hair loss, muscle weakness, myalgia, liver function disturbances, and very rarely thrombocytopenia and leucopenia. There have been rare occurrences of erythema multiforme and Stevens-Johnson syndrome. Anaphylaxis has occurred rarely. Cardiovascular effects have included hypotension, hypertension, tachycardia or palpitations, bradycardia, and other minor ECG changes. There have been isolated cases of atrioventricular block.

◊ The frequencies of adverse effects reported[1] in 134 soldiers who received mefloquine hydrochloride 250 mg weekly for malaria chemoprophylaxis were: diarrhoea (48%), nausea (13%), vomiting (2%), headache (13%), and dizziness (7%). All of 7 healthy subjects who received a dose of mefloquine hydrochloride 15 mg/kg had symptoms that included vertigo, nausea, dizziness, and lightheadedness.[2] The manufacturers reported that dizziness occurred in 24% of patients with malaria treated with 750 mg of mefloquine, in 38% treated with 1000 mg, and in 96% treated with 1500 mg; splitting a dose into two doses given 8 hours apart can reduce the incidence of dizziness.[3] A prospective study involving 3673 patients found that anorexia, nausea, vomiting, dizziness, and sleep disorders were 1.1 to 1.4 times more frequent in patients receiving mefloquine 25 mg/kg for treatment of malaria than in those receiving 15 mg/kg, and that vomiting could be reduced by 40% if the higher dose was split and given as 15 mg/kg followed by a further 10 mg/kg after 16 to 24 hours.[4] The frequency of adverse effects is reported to be higher in subjects who become dehydrated.[5]

There has been concern that the adverse effects of mefloquine, especially neuropsychiatric reactions, might limit its use for the prophylaxis of malaria but, as discussed under Effects on the Nervous System, below, the incidence of adverse effects does not appear to be greater than with other prophylactic schedules.

1. Arthur JD, *et al.* Mefloquine prophylaxis. *Lancet* 1990; **335:** 972.
2. Patchen LC, *et al.* Neurologic reactions after a therapeutic dose of mefloquine. *N Engl J Med* 1989; **321:** 1415.
3. Stürchler D, *et al.* Neuropsychiatric side effects of mefloquine. *N Engl J Med* 1990; **322:** 1752–3.
4. ter Kuile FO, *et al.* Mefloquine treatment of acute falciparum malaria: a prospective study of non-serious adverse effects in 3673 patients. *Bull WHO* 1995; **73:** 631–42.
5. Perry IC. Malaria prophylaxis. *BMJ* 1995; **310:** 1673.

**Effects on the blood.** Agranulocytosis was reported[1] in a patient with malaria 48 hours after treatment with a 1250-mg course of mefloquine. The patient had previously taken 250 mg of mefloquine weekly for 7 weeks without side-effects.

1. Hennequin C, *et al.* Agranulocytosis during treatment with mefloquine. *Lancet* 1991; **337:** 984.

**Effects on the liver.** Acute fatty liver was reported[1] in a patient who had recently received mefloquine 250 mg weekly for 5 weeks for malaria prophylaxis. Symptoms resolved with fluid, electrolyte, and albumin replacement, following discontinuation of mefloquine. In another report,[2] acute elevation of liver transaminases, associated with severe acute hepatitis, occurred in a patient with pre-existing mild hepatic impairment following a 6-week course of mefloquine 250 mg weekly.

1. Grieco A, *et al.* Acute fatty liver after malaria prophylaxis with mefloquine. *Lancet* 1999; **353:** 295–6.
2. Gotsman I, *et al.* Mefloquine-induced acute hepatitis. *Pharmacotherapy* 2000; **20:** 1517–19.

**Effects on the nervous system.** Neuropsychiatric reactions have been associated with the use of mefloquine although various figures have been reported for their frequency. The UK Committee on Safety of Medicines has quoted[1] figures of 1 in 10 000 to 1 in 20 000 for severe reactions to *prophylactic* doses and similarly the manufacturers report that 1 in 10 000 patients receiving mefloquine prophylaxis will experience serious problems. Others consider that the incidence of serious reactions is extremely low,[2] with a frequency of about 1 in 80 000. The manufacturers have also reported that most reactions in patients taking mefloquine for prophylaxis appear to occur after the first dose and have suggested that monitoring after the first dose could identify 40% of those at risk of neuropsychiatric effects.[3] Some authorities consider that over 75% of such reactions to mefloquine are apparent by the third dose.[4] This may allow for tolerability problems with mefloquine prophylaxis to be identified before travel. There has been much discussion on the comparative tolerability of antimalarials used for chemoprophylaxis. The incidence of adverse events, including neuropsychiatric events, was comparable for mefloquine and chloroquine in 2 uncontrolled questionnaire studies, one in tourists[5] and one in US Peace Corps volunteers.[6] However, in a more recent questionnaire in travellers,[7] although the incidence of reported adverse events was similar for mefloquine and chloroquine plus proguanil, neuropsychiatric adverse events were significantly more common in mefloquine recipients. In two randomised controlled trials,[8,9] both in military personnel, there was no difference between CNS symptoms in those receiving weekly mefloquine and those receiving chloroquine (with or without proguanil). In one of these studies,[9] a subgroup receiving a loading dose of mefloquine daily for 3 days initially had a higher incidence of CNS events. A review[10] of 10 controlled trials found no significant difference in the rates of withdrawal and overall incidence of adverse effects for mefloquine and alternative prophylactic regimens, but mefloquine was more likely than other drugs to cause insomnia and fatigue. Women may be at greater risk of adverse effects than men, and WHO has commented that the occurrence of such adverse effects may mean that only highly motivated occupational subgroups or individuals at high risk of infection with chloroquine-resistant malaria will be willing to continue with mefloquine prophylaxis.[11]

Neuropsychiatric reactions are more frequent following the higher doses of mefloquine used for *treatment* than those used for prophylaxis. Some workers have estimated that overall 1 in 8000 mefloquine users suffers from such reactions, with the incidence 60 times higher after treatment than after prophylaxis.[12] Other workers who have used mefloquine in nearly 14 000 treatments calculated that the overall frequency of serious neuropsychiatric reactions was 1 per 1754 treatments; it therefore appeared that serious neuropsychiatric reactions were 10 times more probable after treatment than with prophylactic use of mefloquine.[13]

A severe neurological syndrome associated with mefloquine treatment, with agitation, delirium, stupor, hyperpyrexia, mydriasis, and generalised rigors responded rapidly to treatment with physostigmine, suggesting a central anticholinergic aetiology.[14]

A discrete post-malaria neurological syndrome (including an acute confusional state or acute psychosis, convulsions, and tremor) has been observed following recovery from falciparum malaria and there appeared to be a strong association with mefloquine although it was not the only risk factor.[15] Nevertheless the risk was considered unacceptable and the recommendation made[15] that, where there was an effective alternative drug, mefloquine should not be used after initial treatment of severe malaria.

Emergence delirium during recovery from general anaesthesia after mefloquine prophylaxis has been reported in 3 cases.[16]

1. Committee on Safety of Medicines. Mefloquine (Lariam) and neuropsychiatric reactions. *Current Problems* 1996; **22:** 6.
2. Croft AMJ, World MJ. Neuropsychiatric reactions with mefloquine chemoprophylaxis. *Lancet* 1996; **347:** 326.
3. Stürchler D, *et al.* Neuropsychiatric side effects of mefloquine. *N Engl J Med* 1990; **322:** 1752–3.
4. Bradley DJ, Bannister B. Guidelines for malaria prevention in travellers from the United Kingdom for 2001. *Commun Dis Public Health* 2001; **4:** 84–101.
5. Steffen R, *et al.* Mefloquine compared with other malaria chemoprophylactic regimens in tourists visiting East Africa. *Lancet* 1993; **341:** 1299–1303.
6. Lobel HO, *et al.* Long-term malaria prophylaxis with weekly mefloquine. *Lancet* 1993; **341:** 848–51.
7. Barrett PJ, *et al.* Comparison of adverse events associated with use of mefloquine and combination of chloroquine and proguanil as antimalarial prophylaxis: postal and telephone survey of travellers. *BMJ* 1996; **313:** 525–8. Correspondence. *ibid.*; 1552–4.
8. Croft AMJ, *et al.* Side effects of mefloquine prophylaxis for malaria: an independent randomized controlled trial. *Trans R Soc Trop Med Hyg* 1997; **91:** 199–203.
9. Boudreau E, *et al.* Tolerability of prophylactic Lariam regimens. *Trop Med Parasitol* 1993; **44:** 257–65.
10. Croft A, Garner P. Mefloquine to prevent malaria: a systematic review of trials. *BMJ* 1997; **315:** 1412–16. Correspondence. *ibid.* 1998; **316:** 1980–1.
11. Anonymous. Mefloquine effectiveness impaired by high withdrawal rates. *WHO Drug Inf* 1998; **12:** 7–8.
12. Weinke T, *et al.* Neuropsychiatric side effects after the use of mefloquine. *Am J Trop Med Hyg* 1991; **45:** 86–91.
13. Luxemburger C, *et al.* Mefloquine for multidrug-resistant malaria. *Lancet* 1991; **338:** 1268.
14. Speich R, Haller A. Central anticholinergic syndrome with the antimalarial drug mefloquine. *N Engl J Med* 1994; **331:** 57–8.
15. Mai NTH, *et al.* Post-malaria neurological syndrome. *Lancet* 1996; **348:** 917–21.
16. Gullahorn GM, *et al.* Anaesthesia emergence delirium after mefloquine prophylaxis. *Lancet* 1993; **341:** 632.

**Effects on the oesophagus.** Oesophageal ulceration in one patient and discomfort in another 4 was attributed to swallowing mefloquine tablets with insufficient fluid.[1]

1. Phillips M. Antimalarial mefloquine. *Med J Aust* 1994; **161:** 227–8.

**Effects on the skin.** Isolated cases of Stevens-Johnson syndrome,[1] severe facial lesions,[2] exfoliative dermatitis,[3] toxic epidermal necrolysis,[4] and cutaneous vasculitis[5] have been associated with use of mefloquine for malaria prophylaxis.

For a comparison of the incidence of pruritus induced by various antimalarials, see under Chloroquine, p.449.

1. Van den Enden E, *et al.* Mefloquine-induced Stevens-Johnson syndrome. *Lancet* 1991; **337:** 683.
2. Shlim DR. Severe facial rash associated with mefloquine. *JAMA* 1991; **266:** 2560.
3. Martin GJ, *et al.* Exfoliative dermatitis during malarial prophylaxis with mefloquine. *Clin Infect Dis* 1993; **16:** 341–2.
4. McBride SR, *et al.* Fatal toxic epidermal necrolysis associated with mefloquine antimalarial prophylaxis. *Lancet* 1997; **349:** 101.
5. White AC, *et al.* Cutaneous vasculitis associated with mefloquine. *Ann Intern Med* 1995; **123:** 894.

**Overdosage.** Cardiac, hepatic, and neurological symptoms have been reported in a patient who inadvertently received 5.25 g of mefloquine over 6 days.[1] All symptoms disappeared rapidly when mefloquine was discontinued.

1. Bourgeade A, *et al.* Intoxication accidentelle à la méfloquine. *Presse Med* 1990; **19:** 1903.

### Precautions

Tasks requiring fine coordination such as driving should not be undertaken during treatment with mefloquine or for at least 3 weeks afterwards; in the case of prophylactic use, care should be exercised while taking mefloquine and for at least 3 weeks after stopping it. The use of mefloquine for malaria prophylaxis is contra-indicated in patients with a history of psychiatric (including depression) or convulsive disorders. Increased plasma concentrations may occur in patients with hepatic impairment. Mefloquine should be discontinued should symptoms suggestive of psychiatric disturbance occur during prophylaxis, and an alternative antimalarial substituted. Mefloquine is teratogenic in *animals* and its use during pregnancy is best avoided; however, in areas of chloroquine-resistant *Plasmodium falciparum*, mefloquine may normally be taken for malaria prophylaxis from the fourth month of pregnancy and WHO have advised that it may be used with caution during the first trimester. It is recommended that women should also avoid becoming pregnant during, and for 3 months after, mefloquine use and that mothers should not breast feed while taking mefloquine. Mefloquine should be used with caution in patients with renal impairment and in those with cardiac conduction disorders.

**Porphyria.** For a discussion of the problems of the use of antimalarials in patients with porphyria and a comment that mefloquine may be safe for use in such patients, see under Precautions for Chloroquine, p.450.

**Pregnancy.** The manufacturers of mefloquine report that it is teratogenic in *rodents*. There is limited information on its effects in humans. One study in Thailand cited by WHO[1] found no difference between mefloquine and quinine in pregnancy outcome, but the numbers of treated patients who were in their first trimester were very small and its use should be kept to a minimum in that stage of pregnancy. Further spontaneous reports of exposure to mefloquine during the first trimester of pregnancy collected by the manufacturer revealed 24 fetal abnormalities and 17 spontaneous or missed abortions in 358 pregnancies, although a causal relationship was not established,[2] and a later study by the manufacturer involving 1627 reports of exposure during pregnancy appeared to show a similar incidence of congenital malformation to that in offspring of unexposed women.[3] In 53 army service women who inadvertently used mefloquine in pregnancy, and for whom pregnancy outcome was known, there were 17 elective abortions, 12 spontaneous abortions, one molar pregnancy, and 23 healthy live births, with no major congenital malformations.[4] The rate of spontaneous abortions was considered high.[4] A prospective cohort study involving 236 pregnant women who received an antimalarial in the first trimester did not demonstrate an increased risk of spontaneous abortion or anomaly in women who took mefloquine compared with other antimalarials, and the rate of spontaneous abortion was comparable with background rates.[5]

Confidence in the safety of mefloquine has increased, and mefloquine is now considered suitable for malaria prophylaxis in the second and third trimesters by both WHO[6] and authorities in the UK.[7] WHO have also advised[6] that mefloquine may be used *with caution* in the first trimester.

Pregnancy should be avoided during and for 3 months after prophylactic use.

1. WHO. Practical chemotherapy of malaria: report of a WHO scientific group. *WHO Tech Rep Ser 805* 1990.
2. Palmer KJ, *et al.* Mefloquine: a review of its antimalarial activity, pharmacokinetic properties and therapeutic efficacy. *Drugs* 1993; **45:** 430–75.
3. Vanhauwere B, *et al.* Post-marketing surveillance of prophylactic mefloquine (Lariam®) use in pregnancy. *Am J Trop Med Hyg* 1998; **58:** 17–21.

4. Smoak BL, *et al.* The effects of inadvertent exposure of mefloquine chemoprophylaxis on pregnancy outcomes and infants of US Army service women. *J Infect Dis* 1997; **176:** 831–3.
5. Phillips-Howard PA, *et al.* Safety of mefloquine and other antimalarial agents in the first trimester of pregnancy. *J Travel Med* 1998; **5:** 121–6.
6. WHO. *International travel and health.* Geneva: WHO, 2003.
7. Bradley DJ, Bannister B. Guidelines for malaria prevention in travellers from the United Kingdom for 2001. *Commun Dis Public Health* 2001; **4:** 84–101.

## Interactions

Halofantrine should not be given with or after mefloquine because of the increased potential to induce hazardous cardiac arrhythmias, as discussed on p.452. There is an increased risk of convulsions when mefloquine is used with chloroquine, quinidine, or quinine.

**Alcohol.** There has been a case report[1] of a patient who had neuropsychiatric disturbances after consuming a large quantity of alcohol in conjunction with mefloquine; subsequent abstinence from alcohol led to complete reversal of the reactions.

1. Wittes RC, Saginur R. Adverse reaction to mefloquine associated with ethanol ingestion. *Can Med Assoc J* 1995; **152:** 515–17.

**Antibacterials.** Studies in healthy subjects have indicated that *ampicillin*[1] or *tetracycline*,[2] could increase blood concentrations of mefloquine. Convulsions have been precipitated in 3 non-epileptic patients who were receiving mefloquine and the quinolone antibacterials *ciprofloxacin, ofloxacin,* or *sparfloxacin*.[3]

1. Karbwang J, *et al.* Effect of ampicillin on mefloquine pharmacokinetics in Thai males. *Eur J Clin Pharmacol* 1991; **40:** 631–3.
2. Karbwang J, *et al.* Effect of tetracycline on mefloquine pharmacokinetics in Thai males. *Eur J Clin Pharmacol* 1992; **43:** 567–9.
3. Mangalvedhekar SS, *et al.* Convulsions in non-epileptics due to mefloquine-fluoroquinolone co-administration. *Natl Med J India* 2000; **13:** 47.

**Antidepressants.** The manufacturers of mefloquine state that theoretically in patients taking tricyclic antidepressants use of mefloquine may contribute to prolongation of the QT interval.

**Antiepileptics.** The manufacturers state that mefloquine may reduce seizure control by lowering the plasma concentration of concomitantly administered antiepileptics, including carbamazepine, phenobarbital, and phenytoin. For the effect of mefloquine on *valproate*, see p.382. For its effect on *carbamazepine*, see p.356.

**Antihistamines.** The co-administration of mefloquine with antihistamines may theoretically contribute to the prolongation of QT intervals; however, this is not considered to be an absolute contra-indication.

**Antimalarials.** It is well established that the use of *halofantrine* with or after mefloquine is contra-indicated because of the risk of hazardous cardiac arrhythmias. Mefloquine and other related compounds such as *quinine, quinidine,* and *chloroquine* may be given concomitantly only under close medical supervision because of possible additive cardiac toxicity; there is also an increased risk of convulsions.

A study in healthy subjects indicated that use of *primaquine* could increase blood concentrations of mefloquine and might increase the incidence of adverse effects due to mefloquine,[1] but others reported no such interaction.[2]

1. MacLeod CM, *et al.* Interaction of primaquine with mefloquine in healthy males. *J Clin Pharmacol* 1990; **30:** 841.
2. Karbwang J, *et al.* Pharmacokinetics of mefloquine in the presence of primaquine. *Eur J Clin Pharmacol* 1992; **42:** 559–60.

**Antipsychotics.** The use of mefloquine with *phenothiazines* or *pimozide* may theoretically contribute to prolonged QT intervals, although this is not considered to be an absolute contra-indication.

**Cardiovascular drugs.** It has been recommended that mefloquine should be used with extreme caution in patients also taking *antiarrhythmics, beta blockers, calcium-channel blockers,* or *digitalis*, until more was known about the risks of cardiotoxicity, since theoretically these drugs might contribute to prolongation of the QT interval. An increased risk of ventricular arrhythmias has been reported when mefloquine is given with *amiodarone*.

Cardiopulmonary arrest has occurred after a single dose of mefloquine in a patient who was taking *propranolol*.[1]

1. Anonymous. Mefloquine for malaria. *Med Lett Drugs Ther* 1990; **32:** 13–14.

**Metoclopramide.** Concomitant administration of metoclopramide may increase plasma concentrations of mefloquine.[1]

1. Na Bangchang K, *et al.* The effect of metoclopramide on mefloquine pharmacokinetics. *Br J Clin Pharmacol* 1991; **32:** 640–1.

**Vaccines.** The manufacturers state that mefloquine-induced attenuation of immunisation produced by oral live *typhoid vaccines* cannot be excluded and therefore vaccination with such live vaccines should be completed at least 3 days before taking mefloquine.

## Pharmacokinetics

The pharmacokinetics of mefloquine may be altered by malaria infection in a manner similar to those of quinine, the main effects being reductions in both its volume of distribution and its overall clearance.

Mefloquine is well absorbed from the gastrointestinal tract but there is marked interindividual variation in the time required to achieve peak plasma concentrations. Mefloquine is about 98% bound to plasma proteins and high concentrations have been reported in red blood cells. It is widely distributed throughout the body. Mefloquine has a long elimination half-life; mean values of about 21 days have been reported for some patients, although like other pharmacokinetic data on mefloquine there is considerable variation in reported figures. Subtherapeutic concentrations of mefloquine may persist in the blood for several months. Mefloquine is metabolised in the liver. Little of a dose is excreted in the urine and animal studies suggest excretion of mefloquine and its metabolites is mainly in the bile and faeces.

Mefloquine is distributed into breast milk in small amounts.

◊ Reviews of pharmacokinetic studies of mefloquine reveal considerable interindividual variation for several pharmacokinetic parameters and some evidence that there might be pharmacokinetic differences between ethnic groups.[1,2] Mefloquine is well absorbed by healthy subjects and by patients with uncomplicated malaria following oral administration.[3,4] In patients with complicated malaria adequate blood concentrations have been obtained using nasogastric administration but this route cannot be relied upon for seriously ill patients[5] as absorption may be incomplete.[1] Mefloquine has a large apparent volume of distribution but this is reduced in the presence of malaria.[6,7] In children who received mefloquine with sulfadoxine and pyrimethamine as tablets crushed and mixed with a glucose syrup, maximum blood-mefloquine concentrations were higher and reached in a shorter time compared with equivalent doses in adults.[8] In pregnant women with uncomplicated malaria blood concentrations were lower than in non-pregnant women and the apparent volume of distribution was larger.[9] Once-weekly prophylactic doses of mefloquine resulted in steady-state conditions at about 10 doses with no evidence of subsequent accumulation.[10] The manufacturer has stated that mefloquine is about 98% bound to plasma proteins.

Mefloquine is metabolised in the liver[11] largely into 2,8-bis(trifluoromethyl)-4-quinoline carboxylic acid [Ro-21-5104][12] but this metabolite appears to be inactive against *Plasmodium falciparum*.[13] Only a small percentage of a dose is excreted in the urine[14] and studies in *animals* suggest excretion of mefloquine and its metabolites is primarily in the bile and faeces.[1] Mefloquine has an extremely long plasma elimination half-life; again there is considerable interindividual variation and mean values ranging from 13.9 to 27.5 days have been quoted, the smaller figure of the range referring to a formulation that did not provide as good absorption as the preparation now in use.[1]

Mefloquine is distributed into breast milk, but a single dose study in 2 women[15] indicated that the concentration of mefloquine in milk was only a small proportion of that seen in plasma.

1. Karbwang J, White NJ. Clinical pharmacokinetics of mefloquine. *Clin Pharmacokinet* 1990; **19:** 264–79.
2. Palmer KJ, *et al.* Mefloquine: a review of its antimalarial activity, pharmacokinetic properties and therapeutic efficacy. *Drugs* 1993; **45:** 430–75.
3. Karbwang J, *et al.* The pharmacokinetics of mefloquine when given alone or in combination with sulphadoxine and pyrimethamine in Thai male and female subjects. *Eur J Clin Pharmacol* 1987; **32:** 173–7.
4. Looareesuwan S, *et al.* Studies of mefloquine bioavailability and kinetics using a stable isotope technique: a comparison of Thai patients with falciparum malaria and healthy caucasian volunteers. *Br J Clin Pharmacol* 1987; **24:** 37–42.
5. Chanthavanich P, *et al.* Intragastric mefloquine is absorbed rapidly in patients with cerebral malaria. *Am J Trop Med Hyg* 1985; **34:** 1028–36.
6. Juma FD, Ogeto JO. Mefloquine disposition in normals and in patients with severe Plasmodium falciparum malaria. *Eur J Drug Metab Pharmacokinet* 1989; **14:** 15–17.
7. Karbwang J, *et al.* A comparison of the pharmacokinetics of mefloquine in healthy Thai volunteers and in Thai patients with falciparum malaria. *Eur J Clin Pharmacol* 1988; **35:** 677–80.
8. Singhasivanon V, *et al.* Pharmacokinetic study of mefloquine in Thai children aged 5-12 years suffering from uncomplicated falciparum malaria treated with MSP or MSP plus primaquine. *Eur J Drug Metab Pharmacokinet* 1994; **19:** 27–32.
9. Na Bangchang K, *et al.* Mefloquine pharmacokinetics in pregnant women with acute falciparum malaria. *Trans R Soc Trop Med Hyg* 1994; **88:** 321–3.
10. Pennie RA, *et al.* Steady state pharmacokinetics of mefloquine in long-term travellers. *Trans R Soc Trop Med Hyg* 1993; **87:** 459–62.
11. WHO. Severe and complicated malaria. 2nd ed. *Trans R Soc Trop Med Hyg* 1990; **84** (suppl 2): 1–65.
12. Panisko DM, Keystone JS. Treatment of malaria—1990. *Drugs* 1990; **39:** 160–89.
13. Håkanson A, *et al.* Comparison of the activity in vitro of mefloquine and two metabolites against Plasmodium falciparum. *Trans R Soc Trop Med Hyg* 1990; **84:** 503–4.
14. Schwartz DE, *et al.* Urinary excretion of mefloquine and some of its metabolites in African volunteers at steady state. *Chemotherapy* 1987; **33:** 305–8.
15. Edstein MD, *et al.* Excretion of mefloquine in human breast milk. *Chemotherapy* 1988; **34:** 165–9.

## Uses and Administration

Mefloquine is a 4-methanolquinoline antimalarial related to quinine. It is a blood schizontocide effective against all forms of malaria including chloroquine- or multidrug-resistant strains of *Plasmodium falciparum*, although some strains are naturally resistant to mefloquine. It is used for the treatment of uncomplicated falciparum malaria and chloroquine-resistant vivax malaria, and also for malaria prophylaxis. Mefloquine is also used following treatment with an artemisinin derivative for acute uncomplicated malaria, to reduce the risk of recrudescence.

Mefloquine is given orally as the hydrochloride but variation in the way doses are expressed could lead to confusion. In the UK and elsewhere, doses are expressed in terms of the base and a dose of 250 mg base is approximately equivalent to 274 mg of mefloquine hydrochloride. In the USA, doses are expressed in terms of the hydrochloride and a dose of 250 mg is therefore approximately equivalent to only 228 mg of mefloquine base. Doses in the USA could therefore be about 10% less than elsewhere.

Doses recommended in the UK are as follows. For the *treatment of malaria*, mefloquine base 20 to 25 mg/kg (up to a maximum of 1.5 g) as a single dose or preferably in 2 or 3 divided doses 6 to 8 hours apart. For the *prophylaxis of malaria*, a dose of mefloquine base 250 mg once weekly in adults and children over 45 kg. Children weighing 5 to 19 kg may be given one-quarter the adult dose; those weighing 20 to 30 kg, half the adult dose; and those weighing 31 to 45 kg three-quarters the adult dose. Prophylaxis should be started 1 to 3 weeks before exposure and continued for 4 weeks after leaving the malarious area.

For other dosage recommendations, see under Malaria, below.

**Malaria.** The overall treatment and prophylaxis of malaria and the place of mefloquine in current recommendations are discussed on p.444.

TREATMENT. Clinical studies have shown mefloquine to be effective in the treatment of chloroquine- or multidrug-resistant falciparum malaria. It is also effective in benign malarias, but is not normally required since they usually respond to chloroquine.

Mefloquine is widely considered to be a suitable alternative to regimens using quinine for the treatment of chloroquine-resistant or multidrug-resistant strains of *Plasmodium falciparum*.[1-4] It may also be used in combination with an artemisinin derivative in regions of greatest multidrug resistance (see p.448).

As there is no parenteral formulation of mefloquine currently available it can only be used in patients who can take oral medication and is therefore unsuitable for sole treatment in severe infections. Mefloquine has produced adequate blood concentrations following nasogastric administration, but this route cannot be relied upon in seriously ill patients.[5] If mefloquine is given to patients after parenteral administration of quinine, it is recommended that a period of 12 hours should be allowed after the last dose of quinine to avoid toxicity.

In the UK, the recommended dose for the treatment of malaria is the equivalent of 20 to 25 mg of mefloquine base per kg bodyweight, as a single dose or preferably in two or three divided doses 6 to 8 hours apart, to a maximum of 1.5 g. The manufacturers recommend a lower dose of 15 mg/kg for the partially immune. In the USA, the manufacturers recommend 1250 mg of mefloquine hydrochloride given as a single dose. WHO has recommended a dose of mefloquine base of 15 mg/kg (up to a maximum of 1000 mg).[2] However, in areas of multidrug-resistant malaria a dose of 25 mg/kg has been shown[6,7] to improve the response, and this dose is now recommended by WHO[8] for standby treatment in such areas (see below).

Mefloquine is one of the antimalarial drugs recommended by some experts to be carried as a *standby* for the emergency treatment of malaria. The adult dose recommended by WHO[8] for self-treatment is 15 mg/kg as a single dose, or 25 mg/kg (given as 15 mg/kg followed by 10 mg/kg 6 to 24 hours later) in areas of mefloquine resistance. In the USA, mefloquine is not recommended for self-treatment.[9]

PROPHYLAXIS. It had been hoped that mefloquine could be reserved for the treatment of malaria, but increasing drug resistance to chemoprophylactic regimens has led to it being widely used for malaria prophylaxis. WHO recommends[8] that mefloquine should only be used in high-risk areas where chloroquine-resistant malaria is prevalent and authorities in the UK[10] and USA[9] endorse this. For **adults** the equivalent of 250 mg of mefloquine base is given every week, starting 1 to 3 weeks before departure, and continuing throughout the period of exposure and for 4 weeks after leaving the malarious area. Starting mefloquine prophylaxis 2 to 3 weeks before exposure allows for detection of possible adverse effects before travelling (see Effects on the

Nervous System, above, for concerns about neurotoxicity). It is now considered that mefloquine prophylaxis can be given for periods of up to one year instead of the previous limit of 3 months. Mefloquine is considered to be suitable[8] for prophylaxis in women from the fourth month of pregnancy. WHO have also advised[8] that mefloquine may be used *with caution* in the first trimester. Pregnancy should be avoided during and for three months after stopping the drug.

Recommended dosages of mefloquine for prophylaxis in **children** have generally been based on 5 mg/kg as a single weekly dose in children over 15 kg and above the age of 2 years.[2] However, the doses now usually used in the UK[10] for infants and children over 5 kg and above 3 months of age are as follows:

- 6 to 15.9 kg (3 months to 3 years 11 months), one-quarter the adult dose
- 16 to 24.9 kg (4 years to 7 years 11 months), half the adult dose
- 25 to 44.9 kg (8 years to 12 years 11 months), three-quarters the adult dose

Similarly, WHO has recommended:

- 5 to 12 kg (3 to 23 months), one-quarter the adult dose
- 13 to 16 kg (2 to 3 years), one-third the adult dose
- 17 to 24 kg (4 to 7 years), half the adult dose
- 25 to 35 kg (8 to 10 years), three-quarters the adult dose
- 36 to 50 kg (11 to 13 years), the adult dose

In the event of breakthrough malaria during malaria prophylaxis there may be a delay of up to several months before the onset of symptoms in contrast to that seen with other forms of prophylaxis.[11] Mefloquine should not be used for treatment if it has been used for prophylaxis.


1. Molyneux M, Fox R. Diagnosis and treatment of malaria in Britain. *BMJ* 1993; **306:** 1175–80.
2. WHO. *WHO model prescribing information: drugs used in parasitic diseases.* 2nd ed. Geneva: WHO, 1995.
3. WHO. WHO expert committee on malaria: twentieth report. *WHO Tech Rep Ser 892* 2000.
4. Medical Letter on Drugs and Therapeutics. Drugs for parasitic infections (issued April 2002). Available at: http://www.medicalletter.com/freedocs/parasitic.pdf (accessed 19/04/04)
5. Chanthavanich P, *et al.* Intragastric mefloquine is absorbed rapidly in patients with cerebral malaria. *Am J Trop Med Hyg* 1985; **34:** 1028–36.
6. ter Kuile FO, *et al.* High-dose mefloquine in the treatment of multidrug-resistant falciparum malaria. *J Infect Dis* 1992; **166:** 1393–1400.
7. Smithuis FM, *et al.* Comparison of two mefloquine regimens for treatment of Plasmodium falciparum malaria on the northeastern Thai-Cambodian border. *Antimicrob Agents Chemother* 1993; **37:** 1977–81.
8. WHO. *International travel and health.* Geneva: WHO, 2003.
9. CDC. Malaria. In: *The Yellow Book. Health Information for International Travel, 2003-2004.* Available at: http://www.cdc.gov/travel/diseases/malaria/index.htm (accessed 19/04/04)
10. Bradley DJ, Bannister B. Guidelines for malaria prevention in travellers from the United Kingdom for 2001. *Commun Dis Public Health* 2001; **4:** 84–101. Also available at: http://www.hpa.org.uk/cdph/issues/CDPHVol4/no2/malaria_guidelinesp.pdf (accessed 16/04/04)
11. Day JH, Behrens RH. Delay in onset of malaria with mefloquine prophylaxis. *Lancet* 1995; **345:** 398.


## Preparations

**Proprietary Preparations** (details are given in Part 3)

***Arg.:*** Tropicur; ***Austral.:*** Lariam; ***Austria:*** Lariam; ***Belg.:*** Lariam; ***Braz.:*** Lariamar†; Mephaquin; ***Canad.:*** Lariam; ***Chile:*** Lariam; ***Denm.:*** Lariam; ***Fin.:*** Lariam; ***Fr.:*** Lariam; ***Ger.:*** Lariam; ***Gr.:*** Lariam; ***Hong Kong:*** Lariam; Mephaquin; ***India:*** Meflotas; ***Irl.:*** Lariam; ***Israel:*** Lariam; Mephaquin; ***Ital.:*** Lariam; ***Malaysia:*** Mephaquin; ***Neth.:*** Lariam; ***Norw.:*** Lariam; ***NZ:*** Lariam; ***Port.:*** Mephaquin; ***S.Afr.:*** Lariam; Mefliam; ***Singapore:*** Lariam; Mephaquin; ***Swed.:*** Lariam; ***Switz.:*** Lariam; Mephaquine; ***Thai.:*** Mephaquin; Mequin; ***UK:*** Lariam; ***USA:*** Lariam.

**Multi-ingredient:** ***Switz.:*** Fansimef.

## Piperaquine Phosphate

Piperaquina, fosfato de; Piperaquini Phosphas; 13228-RP. 1,3-Bis[1-(7-chloro-4-quinolyl)-4′-piperazinyl]propane.

$C_{29}H_{32}Cl_2N_6,4H_3PO_4,4H_2O = 999.6.$

**Pharmacopoeias.** In *Chin.*

### Profile

Piperaquine phosphate is a 4-piperazinoquinoline derivative which has been studied in the treatment and prophylaxis of falciparum malaria. Combined treatment with dihydroartemisinin is also being investigated. A combination of piperaquine, dihydroartemisinin, and trimethoprim (Artecom) is available in some countries.

◊ References.


1. Denis MB, *et al.* Efficacy and safety of dihydroartemisinin-piperaquine (Artekin) in Cambodian children and adults with uncomplicated falciparum malaria. *Clin Infect Dis* 2002; **35:** 1469–76.
2. Karunajeewa H, *et al.* Safety evaluation of fixed combination piperaquine plus dihydroartemisinin (Artekin) in Cambodian children and adults with malaria. *Br J Clin Pharmacol* 2004; **57:** 93–9.
3. Hien TT, *et al.* Dihydroartemisinin-piperaquine against multi-drug-resistant Plasmodium falciparum malaria in Vietnam: randomised clinical trial. *Lancet* 2004; **363:** 18–22.


## Primaquine Phosphate *(BANM, rINNM)*

Difosfato de Primaquina; Fosfato de primaquina; Primachina Fosfato; Primachini Phosphas; Primaquine Diphosphate; Primaquini Diphosphas; Primaquinum Phosphoricum; SN-13,272. (*RS*)-8-(4-Amino-1-methylbutylamino)-6-methoxyquinoline diphosphate.

$C_{15}H_{21}N_3O,2H_3PO_4 = 455.3.$

*CAS — 90-34-6 (primaquine); 63-45-6 (primaquine phosphate).*

*ATC — P01BA03.*

**Pharmacopoeias.** In *Chin., Eur.* (see p.vi), *Int., US,* and *Viet.*

**Ph. Eur. 5.0** (Primaquine Diphosphate). An orange crystalline powder. Soluble in water; practically insoluble in alcohol. Protect from light.

**USP 27** (Primaquine Phosphate). An orange-red, odourless, crystalline powder. Soluble 1 in 15 of water; insoluble in chloroform and in ether. Its solutions are acid to litmus. Protect from light.

### Adverse Effects

Adverse effects with therapeutic doses of primaquine are usually minimal but abdominal pain and gastric distress are more common if taken on an empty stomach. Larger doses may cause nausea and vomiting. Methaemoglobinaemia may occur occasionally. Haemolytic anaemia can occur in persons with G6PD deficiency (see below). Other uncommon effects include mild anaemia and leucocytosis. Hypertension and cardiac arrhythmias have been reported on rare occasions. Primaquine may rarely produce leucopenia or agranulocytosis, usually following overdosage. Other effects associated with overdosage include gastrointestinal symptoms, haemolytic anaemia, and methaemoglobinaemia with cyanosis.

◊ A wide range of side-effects has been reported following the use of primaquine[1] but some, including pruritus and disturbances of visual accomodation, are considered to be inadequately documented or doubtfully attributed to the drug.

Acute intravascular haemolysis is the most serious toxic hazard of primaquine, especially in people with G6PD deficiency, other defects of the erythrocytic pentose phosphate pathway of glucose metabolism, or some types of haemoglobinopathy. In individuals with G6PD deficiency the severity of haemolysis is directly related to the degree of deficiency and to the quantity of primaquine administered. In patients with the African variant the standard course of primaquine generally produces a moderate and self-limiting anaemia, while in those with the Mediterranean and related Asian variants, haemolysis can result in progressive haemoglobinaemia and haemoglobinuria which can be fatal. Whenever possible, therapy with primaquine should be delayed until the acute stage of malaria has been brought under control by a blood schizontocide because of the risk of inducing haemolysis and compromising the gastrointestinal tolerance of therapy.


1. Clyde DF. Clinical problems associated with the use of primaquine as a tissue schizontocidal and gametocytocidal drug. *Bull WHO* 1981; **59:** 391–5.


### Precautions

Primaquine should be used cautiously in acutely ill patients with any serious systemic disease characterised by a tendency to granulocytopenia such as rheumatoid arthritis or lupus erythematosus. It should also be used with care in patients with G6PD deficiency. Primaquine should be withdrawn if signs of haemolysis or methaemoglobinaemia occur and the blood count should be monitored periodically.

**Pregnancy.** Radical cure of vivax or ovale malarias with primaquine should be delayed in pregnant women until after delivery.[1]


1. Panisko DM, Keystone JS. Treatment of malaria—1990. *Drugs* 1990; **39:** 160–89.


### Interactions

Primaquine should not be used with drugs liable to induce haemolysis or bone marrow depression. Theoretically, mepacrine may increase the plasma concentrations of primaquine resulting in a higher risk of toxicity, and it has been recommended that these drugs should not be used together.

**Antimalarials.** The pharmacokinetics of primaquine were not altered by *mefloquine* in healthy subjects,[1] although the effect of primaquine on mefloquine pharmacokinetics is uncertain (see under Mefloquine, p.455). In a study in patients with malaria, *quinine* reduced the plasma concentrations of primaquine, although the clinical importance of the interaction was unclear.[1]


1. Edwards G, *et al.* Interactions among primaquine, malaria infection and other antimalarials in Thai subjects. *Br J Clin Pharmacol* 1993; **35:** 193–8.


### Pharmacokinetics

Primaquine is readily absorbed from the gastrointestinal tract. Peak plasma concentrations occur about 1 to 2 hours after a dose is taken and then rapidly diminish with a reported elimination half-life of 3 to 6 hours. It is widely distributed into body tissues.

Primaquine is rapidly metabolised in the liver, its major metabolite being carboxyprimaquine, and little unchanged drug is excreted in the urine. Carboxyprimaquine accumulates in the plasma on repeated administration.

◊ References.


1. Fletcher KA, *et al.* Studies on the pharmacokinetics of primaquine. *Bull WHO* 1981; **59:** 407–12.
2. White NJ. Clinical pharmacokinetics of antimalarial drugs. *Clin Pharmacokinet* 1985; **10:** 187–215.
3. Mihaly GW, *et al.* Pharmacokinetics of primaquine in man, I: studies of the absolute bioavailability and effects of dose size. *Br J Clin Pharmacol* 1985; **19:** 745–50.
4. Ward SA, *et al.* Pharmacokinetics of primaquine in man, II: comparison of acute vs chronic dosage in Thai subjects. *Br J Clin Pharmacol* 1985; **19:** 751–5.
5. Bhatia SC, *et al.* Pharmacokinetics of primaquine in patients with P. vivax malaria. *Eur J Clin Pharmacol* 1986; **31:** 205–10.
6. Rønn A, Bygbjerg I. Unexpected high primaquine concentrations in acutely ill malaria patients. *Lancet* 1993; **341:** 305.


### Uses and Administration

Primaquine is an 8-aminoquinoline antimalarial that is effective as a tissue schizontocide against intrahepatic forms of all types of malaria parasite and is used to produce radical cure of vivax and ovale malarias.

Primaquine phosphate is given by mouth and doses may be expressed in terms of the base; primaquine phosphate 26.4 mg is approximately equivalent to 15 mg of primaquine base.

When used for radical cure of vivax and ovale malarias, a course of treatment with a blood schizontocide must be given first to kill any erythrocytic parasites. Primaquine phosphate is then given by mouth, usually in a dose equivalent to 15 mg of the base daily for 14 days but higher doses or longer courses may be required to overcome resistance in some strains of *P. vivax* (see below); WHO has advised that a treatment period of 21 days should be used to achieve radical cure in most of South-East Asia and the Pacific regions. A dose for children is 250 micrograms/kg daily for 14 days.

For patients with G6PD deficiency the use of 30 mg (children 500 to 750 micrograms/kg) once every 7 days for 8 weeks has been suggested to minimise haemolysis (but see Adverse Effects and Precautions, above).

Primaquine is also gametocytocidal and a single dose of 30 to 45 mg has been suggested to prevent transmission of falciparum malaria particularly in areas where there is potential for re-introduction of malaria.

Primaquine is also used with clindamycin in the treatment of *Pneumocystis carinii* pneumonia in AIDS patients.

**Malaria.** The overall treatment and prophylaxis of malaria and the place of primaquine in current recommendations are described on p.444.

Despite the generally successful use of primaquine for radical cure of benign malarias,[1,2] there has been a report[3] of a patient weighing 84 kg who had relapse of vivax malaria after treatment including primaquine 15 mg given daily for 21 days; no further symptoms occurred after a second course of 15 mg given daily for 3 months. It was suggested that a daily dose of 15 mg might be inadequate for patients weighing more than 50 kg and that patients with vivax malaria who have relapsed after the standard course of primaquine, and possibly those with vivax malaria acquired in South-East Asia or Melanesia, should receive a total dose of 6 mg/kg in daily doses of 15 to 22.5 mg. A report from Thailand,[4] where primaquine-resistant strains of *Plasmodium vivax* are increasing, showed that a dose of primaquine 22.5 mg daily for 14 days was safe and more effective in preventing relapses than 15 mg daily in patients with an average body-weight of about 51 kg. There have been several other reports of primaquine-resistant *P. vivax,*[5-8] and the suggestion has been made that higher doses of primaquine (15 mg twice daily for 14 days, to give a total dose of 6 mg/kg assuming a body-weight of 70 kg) should be considered wherever the vivax malaria was acquired.[8]

Variable responses to primaquine in the Amazonian region were attributed to considerable variation in the content of primaquine both between and within batches of tablets; primaquine content ranged from 19 to 168% of the labelled content.[9]

In the USA, the CDC have suggested the use of primaquine during the last 2 weeks of prophylaxis to prevent relapses due to *P. vivax* or *P. ovale* in persons returning from prolonged exposure in areas where relapsing malaria is endemic.[10]

Primaquine has also been tried for prophylaxis of falciparum and vivax malaria; use for a year produced effective cover and was well tolerated by Javanese men without G6PD deficiency.[11] It was also effective for prophylaxis in Colombian military personnel; it was noted that primaquine prophylaxis could be stopped 1 week after departing the endemic area.[12]


1. WHO. *WHO model prescribing information: drugs used in parasitic diseases.* 2nd ed. Geneva: WHO, 1995.
2. Molyneux M, Fox R. Diagnosis and treatment of malaria in Britain. *BMJ* 1993; **306:** 1175–80.
3. Luzzi GA, *et al.* Treatment of primaquine-resistant Plasmodium vivax malaria. *Lancet* 1992; **340:** 310.
4. Bunnag D, *et al.* High dose of primaquine in primaquine resistant vivax malaria. *Trans R Soc Trop Med Hyg* 1994; **88:** 218–19.
5. Collins WE, Jeffery GM. Primaquine resistance in Plasmodium vivax. *Am J Trop Med Hyg* 1996; **55:** 243–9.
6. Signorini L, *et al.* Short report: primaquine-tolerant Plasmodium vivax in an Italian traveler from Guatemala. *Am J Trop Med Hyg* 1996; **55:** 472–3.
7. Smoak BL, *et al.* Plasmodium vivax infections in US Army troops: failure of primaquine to prevent relapse in studies from Somalia. *Am J Trop Med Hyg* 1997; **56:** 231–4.
8. Doherty JF, *et al.* Treatment of Plasmodium vivax malaria—time for a change? *Trans R Soc Trop Med Hyg* 1997; **91:** 76.
9. Petralanda I. Quality of antimalarial drugs and resistance to Plasmodium vivax in Amazonian region. *Lancet* 1995; **345:** 1433.
10. CDC. Malaria. In: *The Yellow Book. Health Information for International Travel, 2003-2004.* Available at http://www.cdc.gov/travel/diseases/malaria/index.htm (accessed 19/04/04)
11. Fryauff DJ, *et al.* Randomised placebo-controlled trial of primaquine for prophylaxis of falciparum and vivax malaria. *Lancet* 1995; **346:** 1190–3.
12. Soto J, *et al.* Primaquine prophylaxis against malaria in nonimmune Colombian soldiers: efficacy and toxicity. *Ann Intern Med* 1998; **129:** 241–4.


**Pneumocystis carinii pneumonia.** Primaquine with clindamycin is used in the treatment of *Pneumocystis carinii* pneumonia as an alternative to co-trimoxazole or pentamidine (see p.389). Treatment has usually lasted 3 weeks, with primaquine being given by mouth in daily doses equivalent to 30 mg of the base, and clindamycin usually being given intravenously in doses of 600 mg four times daily or 300 to 450 mg four times daily by mouth.[1] The *British National Formulary* suggests clindamycin 600 mg by mouth every 6 hours with primaquine 15 mg daily by mouth for mild to moderate disease.

A randomised multicentre study[2] compared the use of a combination of primaquine (30 mg daily) and clindamycin (600 mg three times daily) with co-trimoxazole and with a combination of dapsone and trimethoprim in 181 AIDS patients who had confirmed mild to moderate *Pneumocystis carinii* pneumonia. Primaquine-clindamycin was as effective as the other two regimens, although the authors suggested that the combination might be best avoided in patients with severe myelosuppression.

Primaquine with clindamycin is not normally recommended for prophylaxis although there are reports of it being tried.[3]


1. Medical Letter on Drugs and Therapeutics. Drugs for parasitic infections (issued April 2002). Available at: http://www.medicalletter.com/freedocs/parasitic.pdf (accessed 19/04/04)
2. Safrin S, *et al.* Comparison of three regimens for treatment of mild to moderate Pneumocystis carinii pneumonia in patients with AIDS: a double-blind, randomized trial of oral trimethoprim-sulfamethoxazole, dapsone-trimethoprim, and clindamycin-primaquine. *Ann Intern Med* 1996; **124:** 792–802.
3. Kay R, DuBois RE. Clindamycin/primaquine therapy and secondary prophylaxis against Pneumocystis carinii pneumonia in patients with AIDS. *South Med J* 1990; **83:** 403–4.


### Preparations

***USP 27:*** Primaquine Phosphate Tablets.

**Proprietary Preparations** (details are given in Part 3)
***Austral.:*** Primacin; ***Braz.:*** Primakinder; ***India:*** Malirid; PMQ-INGA.

## Proguanil Hydrochloride *(BANM, rINNM)*

Bigumalum; Chloriguane Hydrochloride; Chloroguanide Hydrochloride; Hidrocloruro de proguanil; Proguanide Hydrochloride; Proguanili Hydrochloridum; RP-3359; SN-12,837. 1-(4-Chlorophenyl)-5-isopropylbiguanide hydrochloride.

$C_{11}H_{16}ClN_5,HCl = 290.2.$

*CAS — 500-92-5 (proguanil); 637-32-1 (proguanil hydrochloride).*

*ATC — P01BB01.*

**Pharmacopoeias.** In *Eur.* (see p.vi) and *Int.*

**Ph. Eur. 5.0** (Proguanil Hydrochloride). A white crystalline powder. Slightly soluble in water; sparingly soluble in dehydrated alcohol; practically insoluble in dichloromethane. Protect from light.

**Stability.** Although the Ph. Eur. 5.0 directs that proguanil hydrochloride should be protected from light, stability studies[1,2] suggest that it is a very stable compound with only small amounts of its major decomposition product 4-chloroaniline being formed during thermal and photochemical stress.


1. Owoyale JA, Elmarakby ZS. Effect of sunlight, ultraviolet irradiation and heat on proguanil. *Int J Pharmaceutics* 1989; **50:** 219–21.
2. Taylor RB, *et al.* A chemical stability study of proguanil hydrochloride. *Int J Pharmaceutics* 1990; **60:** 185–90.


### Adverse Effects and Precautions

Apart from mild gastric intolerance, diarrhoea, and some reports of aphthous ulceration there appear to be few adverse effects associated with usual doses of proguanil hydrochloride. There have been rare reports of hypersensitivity reactions including urticaria and angioedema. Haematological changes have been reported in patients with severe renal impairment. Overdosage may produce epigastric discomfort, vomiting, and renal irritation leading to haematuria.

Proguanil should be used with caution in patients with renal impairment; dosage should be reduced accordingly (see under Uses and Administration, below).

Proguanil may be taken during pregnancy, but UK authorities recommend that folate supplements (folic acid 5 mg daily) should also be given.

◊ Until 1985 proguanil was generally taken in a dose of 100 mg daily for malaria prophylaxis with few adverse effects. Although no serious adverse effects have been reported since the dose was increased to 200 mg daily, and it began to be used with chloroquine, there have been an increasing number of reports of reversible aphthous ulceration.[1] Chloroquine may exacerbate this effect.[2] There has also been a report of reversible alopecia in women and scaling of the skin in both men and women using proguanil.[3]

Megaloblastic anaemia and pancytopenia were associated with proguanil accumulation in 2 patients with renal failure receiving usual doses.[4]

Stevens-Johnson syndrome has been reported[5] in a patient taking proguanil with atovaquone.


1. Peto TEA. Toxicity of antimalarial drugs. *J R Soc Med* 1989; **82** (suppl 17): 30–4.
2. Drysdale SF, *et al.* Proguanil, chloroquine, and mouth ulcers. *Lancet* 1990; **335:** 164.
3. Hanson SN, *et al.* Hairloss and scaling with proguanil. *Lancet* 1989; **i:** 225.
4. Boots M, *et al.* Megaloblastic anemia and pancytopenia due to proguanil in patients with chronic renal failure. *Clin Nephrol* 1982; **18:** 106–8.
5. Emberger M, *et al.* Stevens-Johnson syndrome associated with Malarone antimalarial prophylaxis. Abstract: *Clin Infect Dis* 2003; **37:** 158. Full version: http://www.journals.uchicago.edu/CID/journal/issues/v37n1/30442/30442.html (accessed 19/04/04)


**Porphyria.** For a discussion of the problems of the use of antimalarials in patients with porphyria and a comment that proguanil may be safe for use in such patients, see under Precautions for Chloroquine, p.450.

### Interactions

**Fluvoxamine.** Fluvoxamine can virtually abolish[1] the metabolism of proguanil to its active metabolite cycloguanil via an inhibitory effect on the cytochrome P450 isoenzyme CYP2C19.


1. Jeppesen U, *et al.* The CYP2C19 catalyzed bioactivation of proguanil is abolished during fluvoxamine intake. *Eur J Clin Pharmacol* 1997; **52** (suppl): A134.


**Warfarin.** For a report of haematuria and high prothrombin ratio in a patient stabilised on warfarin who took proguanil for malaria prophylaxis, see p.1025.

### Pharmacokinetics

Proguanil is readily absorbed from the gastrointestinal tract after oral administration, peak plasma concentrations occurring within about 4 hours. Proguanil is metabolised in the liver to the active metabolite cycloguanil. Peak plasma concentrations of cycloguanil occur approximately 1 hour after those of the parent drug. The elimination half-lives of both proguanil and cycloguanil are about 20 hours. About 40 to 60% of proguanil is eliminated in the urine, of which 60% is unchanged and 30% cycloguanil. There is also some elimination via the faeces. Proguanil is distributed into breast milk in small amounts (which are not adequate to provide chemoprophylaxis for the infant).

◊ Early studies found proguanil to be well absorbed from the gastrointestinal tract with peak plasma concentrations occurring after about 4 hours.[1] In more recent studies, peak plasma concentrations of proguanil have been achieved within 2 to 4 hours.[2-4] Plasma protein binding for proguanil is 75%.[5] Proguanil is metabolised in the liver[3] to the active metabolite cycloguanil and to *p*-chlorophenylbiguanide which is inactive. Peak plasma concentrations of cycloguanil occur about 5.3 hours after administration of proguanil.[4] Unlike proguanil and *p*-chlorophenylbiguanide, cycloguanil is not concentrated in erythrocytes and thus concentrations of cycloguanil in plasma and whole blood are similar.[4] The elimination half-lives for proguanil and cycloguanil are about 20 hours.[3,4] A review of early studies states that 40 to 60% of a dose of proguanil is excreted in the urine, 60% of this as the unchanged drug, 30% as cycloguanil, and 8% as *p*-chlorophenylbiguanide.[1] About 10% of a dose is excreted in the faeces.[1] However, these values can vary greatly and wide interindividual variations in the ability to metabolise proguanil to cycloguanil have been reported.[3,6,7] Malaria prophylaxis with proguanil might be less effective in poor metabolisers although this has not been proved conclusively[8] and, anyway, other factors such as lack of protection against mosquitoes and sensitivity of the malaria parasite might be more important.[9]

Plasma concentrations of cycloguanil may be reduced in the third trimester of pregnancy.[10]


1. White NJ. Clinical pharmacokinetics of antimalarial drugs. *Clin Pharmacokinet* 1985; **10:** 187–215.
2. Kelly JA, *et al.* The kinetics of proguanil during prophylaxis. *Trans R Soc Trop Med Hyg* 1986; **80:** 338.
3. Watkins WM, *et al.* Variability in the metabolism of proguanil to the active metabolite cycloguanil in healthy Kenyan adults. *Trans R Soc Trop Med Hyg* 1990; **84:** 492–5.
4. Wattanagoon Y, *et al.* Single dose pharmacokinetics of proguanil and its metabolites in healthy subjects. *Br J Clin Pharmacol* 1987; **24:** 775–80.
5. Jaeger A, *et al.* Clinical features and management of poisoning due to antimalarial drugs. *Med Toxicol* 1987; **2:** 242–73.
6. Ward SA, *et al.* Inter-subject variability in the metabolism of proguanil to the active metabolite cycloguanil in man. *Br J Clin Pharmacol* 1989; **27:** 781–7.
7. Helsby NA, *et al.* The multiple dose pharmacokinetics of proguanil. *Br J Clin Pharmacol* 1993; **35:** 653–6.
8. Mberu EK, *et al.* Japanese poor metabolizers of proguanil do not have an increased risk of malaria chemoprophylaxis breakthrough. *Trans R Soc Trop Med Hyg* 1995; **89:** 658–9.
9. Skjelbo E, *et al.* Chloroguanide metabolism in relation to the efficacy in malaria prophylaxis and the S-mephenytoin oxidation in Tanzanians. *Clin Pharmacol Ther* 1996; **59:** 304–11.
10. Wangboonskul J, *et al.* Single dose pharmacokinetics of proguanil and its metabolites in pregnancy. *Eur J Clin Pharmacol* 1993; **44:** 247–51.


### Uses and Administration

Proguanil is a biguanide compound that has little antimalarial activity until metabolised in the body to the active antimalarial drug cycloguanil. Cycloguanil, like pyrimethamine, inhibits plasmodial dihydrofolate reductase and thus disrupts synthesis of nucleic acids in the parasite. Cycloguanil is active against pre-erythrocytic forms and is a slow-acting blood schizontocide. It also has some sporontocidal activity, rendering the gametocytes non-infective to the mosquito vector.

The value of proguanil is limited by the rapid development of resistance.

Proguanil is used as the hydrochloride for the chemoprophylaxis of malaria, in association with chloroquine or with atovaquone. The schizontocidal activity of cycloguanil on erythrocytic forms is too slow for cycloguanil or proguanil to be used alone for the treatment of malaria, but proguanil hydrochloride is given in combination with atovaquone for the treatment of uncomplicated falciparum malaria.

For prophylaxis of malaria in combination with chloroquine, the usual adult daily dose of proguanil hydrochloride is 200 mg taken after food. For prophylaxis in combination with atovaquone 250 mg, the daily dose of proguanil hydrochloride is 100 mg. It is generally recommended that chemoprophylaxis for travellers should start 1 week before exposure to malaria, but if this is not possible it can be started 1 to 2 days prior to travel. Administration should continue throughout exposure and for at least 4 weeks (1 week when proguanil is given with atovaquone) after leaving a malarious area.

In the treatment of uncomplicated falciparum malaria, adult doses are proguanil hydrochloride 400 mg together with atovaquone 1000 mg, each by mouth as a single dose for 3 consecutive days.

For children's doses in the prophylaxis and treatment of malaria, see below.

Cycloguanil was also formerly given by intramuscular injection as an oily suspension of the embonate.

◊ Reviews.


1. McKeage K, Scott LJ. Atovaquone/proguanil: a review of its use for the prophylaxis of Plasmodium falciparum malaria. *Drugs* 2003; **63:** 597–623.
2. Marra F, *et al.* Atovaquone-proguanil for prophylaxis and treatment of malaria. *Ann Pharmacother* 2003; **37:** 1266–75.


**Administration in children.** Dosage recommendations for proguanil with **chloroquine** for **malaria prophylaxis** in children have varied. A daily dose of proguanil hydrochloride 3 mg/kg has been recommended,[1,2] although UK malaria experts[1] have suggested the following prophylactic doses for children based on fractions of the adult dose of 200 mg daily:

- under 6.0 kg (0 to 12 weeks of age): one-eighth the adult dose
- 6 to 9.9 kg (3 to 11 months): one-quarter the adult dose
- 10 to 15.9 kg (1 year to 3 years 11 months): three-eighths the adult dose
- 16 to 24.9 kg (4 years to 7 years 11 months): half the adult dose
- 25 to 44.9 kg (8 years to 12 years 11 months): three-quarters the adult dose
- 45 kg and over (13 years or more): the adult dose

They noted that body-weight was a better guide to dosage than age for children over 6 months.

Children may be given proguanil with **atovaquone** for the **prophylaxis** of malaria in the following doses, based on the adult dose of 100 mg of proguanil hydrochloride daily:

- children weighing 11 to 20 kg: one-quarter the adult dose
- 21 to 30 kg: half the adult dose
- 31 to 40 kg: three-quarters the adult dose
- over 40 kg: the adult dose

Doses of proguanil with atovaquone for the **treatment** of malaria, based on the adult dose of 400 mg of proguanil hydrochloride daily, are:

- children weighing 5 to 8 kg: one-eighth the adult dose
- 9 to 10 kg: three-sixteenths the adult dose
- 11 to 20 kg: one-quarter the adult dose
- 21 to 30 kg: half the adult dose
- 31 to 40 kg: three-quarters the adult dose
- 40 kg and over: the adult dose

1. Bradley DJ, Bannister B. Guidelines for malaria prevention in travellers from the United Kingdom for 2001. *Commun Dis Public Health* 2001; **4:** 84–101. Also available at: http://www.hpa.org.uk/cdph/issues/CDPHVol4/no2/malaria_guidelinesp.pdf (accessed 16/04/04)
2. WHO. *International travel and health.* Geneva: WHO, 2003.

**Administration in renal impairment.** Proguanil is excreted by the kidneys and should be given in reduced dosage or avoided in patients with renal impairment. The following doses have been recommended based on creatinine clearance (CC):

- CC 20 to 59 mL/minute: 100 mg daily
- CC 10 to 19 mL/minute: 50 mg every other day
- CC less than 10 mL/minute: 50 mg once weekly

## Preparations

***BP 2003:*** Proguanil Tablets.

**Proprietary Preparations** (details are given in Part 3)
***Austral.:*** Paludrine; ***Austria:*** Paludrine; ***Belg.:*** Paludrine; ***Canad.:*** Paludrine†; ***Denm.:*** Paludrine; ***Fin.:*** Paludrine; ***Fr.:*** Paludrine; ***Ger.:*** Paludrine; ***India:*** Laveran; ***Irl.:*** Paludrine; ***Israel:*** Paludrin; ***Ital.:*** Paludrine; ***Malaysia:*** Paludrine; ***Neth.:*** Paludrine; ***Norw.:*** Paludrine; ***NZ:*** Paludrine†; ***Port.:*** Paludrine; ***S.Afr.:*** Paludrine; ***Singapore:*** Paludrine†; ***Swed.:*** Paludrine; ***Switz.:*** Paludrine; ***UK:*** Paludrine.

**Multi-ingredient:** ***Austral.:*** Malarone; ***Austria:*** Malarone; Promal; ***Belg.:*** Malarone; ***Braz.:*** Malarone†; ***Canad.:*** Malarone; ***Denm.:*** Malarone; ***Fr.:*** Malarone; Savarine; ***Ger.:*** Malarone; ***Norw.:*** Malarone; ***NZ:*** Malarone; ***S.Afr.:*** Daramal-Paludrine; ***Singapore:*** Malarone; ***Spain:*** Malarone; ***Swed.:*** Malarone; ***Switz.:*** Malarone; ***UK:*** Malarone; ***USA:*** Malarone.

# Pyrimethamine *(BAN, rINN)*

BW-50-63; Pirimetamina; Pyrimethaminum; RP-4753. 5-(4-Chlorophenyl)-6-ethylpyrimidine-2,4-diyldiamine.

$C_{12}H_{13}ClN_4$ = 248.7.

*CAS — 58-14-0.*

*ATC — P01BD01.*

**Pharmacopoeias.** In *Chin., Eur.* (see p.vi), *Int., Pol., US,* and *Viet.*

**Ph. Eur. 5.0** (Pyrimethamine). An almost white crystalline powder or colourless crystals. Practically insoluble in water; slightly soluble in alcohol. Protect from light.

**USP 27** (Pyrimethamine). A white, odourless, crystalline powder. Practically insoluble in water; soluble 1 in 200 of alcohol and 1 in 125 of chloroform; slightly soluble in acetone. Store in airtight containers. Protect from light.

## Adverse Effects and Treatment

Administration of pyrimethamine for prolonged periods, as used to be the case when it was *given alone* for the prophylaxis of malaria, can cause depression of haematopoiesis due to interference with folic acid metabolism. Skin rashes and hypersensitivity reactions also occurred.

Larger doses, such as those used in the treatment of toxoplasmosis, may cause gastrointestinal symptoms such as atrophic glossitis, abdominal pain, and vomiting; haematological effects such as megaloblastic anaemia, leucopenia, thrombocytopenia, and pancytopenia are also more likely to occur. CNS effects including headache, dizziness, and insomnia have also been reported.

Pulmonary eosinophilia has been reported in patients receiving pyrimethamine *with other antimalarials.* Severe and sometimes fatal reactions have occurred when pyrimethamine has been used with *sulfadoxine* (Fansidar), including erythema multiforme and the Stevens-Johnson syndrome, and toxic epidermal necrolysis; there have also been isolated reports of hepatotoxicity. Agranulocytosis occurs more frequently when pyrimethamine is used with *dapsone* (Maloprim) and fatalities have been reported.

Acute overdosage with pyrimethamine can cause gastrointestinal effects and CNS stimulation with vomiting, excitability, and convulsions. Tachycardia, respiratory depression, circulatory collapse, and death may follow. Treatment of overdosage is symptomatic.

**Adverse effects with dapsone.** Between 1972 and 1988, the UK Committee on Safety of Medicines received 76 reports of reactions that were attributed to the use of pyrimethamine with dapsone (Maloprim), of which 40 (53%) were considered to be serious including 6 deaths.[1] The incidence was estimated to be 1 in 9100 for serious reactions and 1 in 60 200 for fatalities. Serious blood disorders including agranulocytosis, granulocytopenia, or leucopenia occurred in 15 patients (estimated incidence of 1 in 20 000), five of whom died. The other death was in a patient with myocarditis. Three patients had cyanosis due to methaemoglobinaemia. Respiratory disorders such as pulmonary eosinophilia, flu-like syndrome, and dyspnoea occurred in 6 patients. In 4 patients skin disorders were the principal effect and included epidermal necrolysis, angioedema, and bullous eruptions. Hepatic disorders were also reported in 4 patients. Three women using pyrimethamine-dapsone during pregnancy delivered malformed babies, one of them being stillborn. Other effects in 4 patients included convulsions, exacerbated epilepsy, pancreatitis, or a generalised allergic reaction.

A review[2] of 21 cases of agranulocytosis associated with pyrimethamine-dapsone concluded that, although agranulocytosis can occur very rarely in patients taking pyrimethamine or dapsone alone, agranulocytosis due to the combination appears to be caused by an idiosyncratic reaction to dapsone exacerbated by pyrimethamine. Of the 18 individuals for whom dosage was certain, 12 had been taking one tablet of pyrimethamine-dapsone twice weekly, twice the recommended dose of one tablet once weekly. Of the 9 patients who died, 6 had been taking one tablet twice weekly and one patient had taken one tablet once weekly; the dosage was uncertain in the remaining patients. The time of onset of symptoms had been 7 to 9 weeks after starting therapy in 16 of 19 of the patients.

Some consider that pyrimethamine with dapsone may produce some degree of immunosuppression and render users more susceptible to common infections. A higher incidence of non-specific upper respiratory-tract infections occurred in military recruits receiving the combination than in those not receiving antimalarial prophylaxis.[3]

Pulmonary eosinophilia has also occurred in patients taking pyrimethamine with dapsone but, as there have also been similar reports of pulmonary toxicity in patients taking pyrimethamine with sulfadoxine (see below) or pyrimethamine with chloroquine, it has been suggested that pyrimethamine is probably the causative agent.[4]

1. Phillips-Howard PA, West LJ. Serious adverse drug reactions to pyrimethamine–sulphadoxine, pyrimethamine–dapsone and to amodiaquine in Britain. *J R Soc Med* 1990; **83:** 82–5.
2. Hutchinson DBA, *et al.* Agranulocytosis associated with Maloprim: review of cases. *Hum Toxicol* 1986; **5:** 221–7.
3. Lee PS, Lau EYL. Risk of acute non-specific upper respiratory tract infections in healthy men taking dapsone–pyrimethamine for prophylaxis against malaria. *BMJ* 1988; **296:** 893–5.
4. Davidson AC, *et al.* Pulmonary toxicity of malaria prophylaxis. *BMJ* 1988; **297:** 1240–1.

**Adverse effects with sulfonamides.** Severe and potentially fatal cutaneous reactions such as erythema multiforme, Stevens-Johnson syndrome, and toxic epidermal necrolysis have been associated with the combined use of pyrimethamine with sulfadoxine (Fansidar) for malaria prophylaxis. The reported incidence of these reactions has varied with surveys in the UK,[1] USA,[2] and Sweden[3] yielding similar results and a survey from Switzerland[4] finding a much lower incidence. The overall rate of serious reactions to pyrimethamine-sulfadoxine in the UK has been estimated to be 1 in 2100. The estimates for severe cutaneous reactions were 1 in 4900 in the UK, 1 in 5000 to 1 in 8000 in the USA, 1 in 10 000 in Sweden, and 1 in 150 000 in Switzerland, and the death rates were 1 in 11 100 in the UK, 1 in 11 000 to 1 in 25 000 in the USA, and 1 in 35 000 in Sweden; no fatalities were reported in Switzerland. Workers on the Swiss survey had suggested that the high incidence of cutaneous reactions reported in the USA might have been due to concurrent therapy with chloroquine but this has been disputed.[5] The authors of the UK survey[1] suggested that the lower incidence reported in Switzerland may have been due to the different methods used to estimate the amount of drug usage. Whether this toxicity is due to the combined use of pyrimethamine and sulfadoxine is unclear as the estimated frequency of fatal reactions associated with the use of sulfadoxine alone in Mozambique[6] was 1 in 50 000.

There have been isolated reports of other severe or life-threatening reactions associated with the use of pyrimethamine-sulfadoxine when used alone or with chloroquine, including hepatotoxicity[7-9] (estimated incidence of 1 in 11 100 in the UK[1]), fatal multisystem toxicity,[10] drug fever and photodermatitis,[11] agranulocytosis,[11] and erythroderma resembling Sézary syndrome.[12] Severe pulmonary reactions have also occurred[3,13] but, as similar reactions have also been reported when pyrimethamine has been used with other antimalarials, including dapsone, it has been suggested that pyrimethamine is the causative agent (see Adverse Effects with Dapsone, above). Hyperammonaemia and carnitine deficiency with deterioration in mental status has been reported in a patient receiving pyrimethamine and sulfadiazine for the treatment of toxoplasmosis.[14]

Severe megaloblastic anaemia in a patient receiving pyrimethamine and sulfadiazine for toxoplasmosis of the CNS[15] was treated by withdrawal of pyrimethamine and oral administration of folinic acid, together with a single platelet infusion.

For a comparison of the incidence of pruritus induced by various antimalarials including pyrimethamine with sulfadoxine, see Effects on the Skin under Chloroquine, p.449.

1. Phillips-Howard PA, West LJ. Serious adverse drug reactions to pyrimethamine–sulphadoxine, pyrimethamine–dapsone and to amodiaquine in Britain. *J R Soc Med* 1990; **83:** 82–5.
2. Miller KD, *et al.* Severe cutaneous reactions among American travelers using pyrimethamine–sulfadoxine (Fansidar®) for malaria prophylaxis. *Am J Trop Med Hyg* 1986; **35:** 451–8.
3. Hellgren U, *et al.* Adverse reactions to sulphadoxine–pyrimethamine in Swedish travellers: implications for prophylaxis. *BMJ* 1987; **295:** 365–6.
4. Steffen R, Somaini B. Severe cutaneous adverse reactions to sulfadoxine–pyrimethamine in Switzerland. *Lancet* 1986; **i:** 610.
5. Rombo L, *et al.* Does chloroquine contribute to the risk of serious adverse reactions to Fansidar? *Lancet* 1985; **ii:** 1298–9.
6. Hernborg A. Stevens-Johnson syndrome after mass prophylaxis with sulfadoxine for cholera in Mozambique. *Lancet* 1985; **ii:** 1072–3.
7. Lazar HP, *et al.* Fansidar and hepatic granulomas. *Ann Intern Med* 1985; **102:** 722.
8. Wejstal R, *et al.* Liver damage associated with Fansidar. *Lancet* 1986; **i:** 854–5.
9. Zitelli BJ, *et al.* Fatal hepatic necrosis due to pyrimethamine–sulfadoxine (Fansidar). *Ann Intern Med* 1987; **106:** 393–5.
10. Selby CD, *et al.* Fatal multisystemic toxicity associated with prophylaxis with pyrimethamine and sulfadoxine (Fansidar). *BMJ* 1985; **290:** 113–14.
11. Olsen VV, *et al.* Serious reactions during malaria prophylaxis with pyrimethamine–sulfadoxine. *Lancet* 1982; **ii:** 994.
12. Langtry JAA, *et al.* Erythroderma resembling Sézary syndrome after treatment with Fansidar and chloroquine. *BMJ* 1986; **292:** 1107–8.
13. Svanbom M, *et al.* Unusual pulmonary reaction during short term prophylaxis with pyrimethamine–sulfadoxine (Fansidar). *BMJ* 1984; **288:** 1876.
14. Sekas G, Harbhajan PS. Hyperammonemia and carnitine deficiency in a patient receiving sulfadiazine and pyrimethamine. *Am J Med* 1993; **95:** 112–13.
15. Chute JP, *et al.* Severe megaloblastic anemia complicating pyrimethamine therapy. *Ann Intern Med* 1995; **122:** 884–5.

**Overdosage.** Reports of overdosage with pyrimethamine in infants.

1. Akinyanju O, *et al.* Pyrimethamine poisoning. *BMJ* 1973; **4:** 147–8.
2. Elmalem J, *et al.* Les accidents graves lors de la prescription de pyriméthamine chez les nourrissons traités pour une toxoplasmose. *Therapie* 1985; **40:** 357–9.

## Precautions

Pyrimethamine may aggravate subclinical folic acid deficiency and it should not be given to patients with conditions associated with folate deficiency such as megaloblastic anaemia. Blood counts are required with prolonged treatment, and when large doses of pyrimethamine are used, as in the treatment of toxoplasmosis, blood counts should be checked twice weekly. Folinic acid, which does not interfere with the action of pyrimethamine against malaria or toxoplasmosis, has been given to prevent haematological toxicity due to pyrimethamine and its use is especially recommended if pyrimethamine is given during pregnancy. (Folic acid may be used as an alternative to folinic acid in malaria, but it interferes with the action of pyrimethamine against toxoplasmosis). Even if given with a folate supplement, some authorities consider pyrimethamine to be contra-indicated at least during the first trimester of pregnancy (see also under Pregnancy, below).

Pyrimethamine should be given with caution to patients with renal or hepatic impairment. When patients with convulsive disorders need to receive large doses, as in the treatment of toxoplasmosis, it is recommended that small starting doses should be used.

When pyrimethamine is used with sulfonamides or dapsone, the general precautions applicable to those drugs should also be observed (see under Sulfamethoxazole, p.261 and under Dapsone, p.203) and treatment should be discontinued immediately if any skin reactions, sore throat, or shortness of breath occurs.

**Breast feeding.** Pyrimethamine is distributed into breast milk[1] but as no adverse effects have been reported in breast-fed infants, the American Academy of Pediatrics considers breast feeding to be compatible with the use of pyrimethamine for malaria prophylaxis.[2] However, exposure of the infant to other folate antagonists should be avoided. The large doses of pyrimethamine used for treating toxoplasmosis may distribute into breast milk in sufficient quantities to interfere with folic acid metabolism in nursing infants.

1. Edstein MD, *et al.* Excretion of chloroquine, dapsone and pyrimethamine in human milk. *Br J Clin Pharmacol* 1986; **22:** 733–5.
2. American Academy of Pediatrics, Committee on Drugs. The transfer of drugs and other chemicals into human milk. *Pediatrics* 2001; **108:** 776–89. Correction. *ibid.*: 1029. Also available at: http://aappolicy.aappublications.org/cgi/content/full/pediatrics%3b108/3/776 (accessed 19/04/04)

**Porphyria.** For a discussion of the problems of the use of antimalarials in patients with porphyria and a comment that pyrimethamine is probably safe for use in such patients, see under Precautions for Chloroquine, p.450.

**Pregnancy.** There have been concerns over the use of pyrimethamine during pregnancy as it has been shown to be teratogenic in *animal* studies.[1] In one report, severe congenital defects in a stillborn infant were attributed to the use of pyrimethamine in early pregnancy,[2] but the association was considered to be questionable.[3] Other instances of congenital malformations with pyrimethamine and dapsone are given under Adverse Effects with Dapsone, above.

WHO considers that pyrimethamine combinations may be used after the first trimester of pregnancy in the treatment of toxoplasmosis,[4] and that pyrimethamine-sulfadoxine may be used for intermittent treatment in high-risk malaria-endemic regions.[5]

1. Anonymous. Pyrimethamine combinations in pregnancy. *Lancet* 1983; **ii:** 1005–7. Correction. *ibid.*; 1378.
2. Harpey J-P, *et al.* Teratogenicity of pyrimethamine. *Lancet* 1983; **ii:** 399.
3. Smithells RW, Sheppard S. Teratogenicity of Debendox and pyrimethamine. *Lancet* 1983; **ii:** 623–4.
4. WHO. *WHO model prescribing information: drugs used in parasitic diseases.* 2nd ed. Geneva: WHO, 1995.
5. WHO. WHO expert committee on malaria: twentieth report. *WHO Tech Rep Ser 892* 2000.

## Interactions

Use of pyrimethamine with other folate antagonists such as co-trimoxazole, trimethoprim, methotrexate, or phenytoin may exacerbate bone marrow depression.

**Lorazepam.** Signs of mild liver toxicity in 2 of 5 subjects who received lorazepam and pyrimethamine appeared to confirm earlier suspicions that concomitant administration of these drugs could cause hepatotoxicity. Both patients tolerated each drug when given separately.[1]

1. Briggs M, Briggs M. Pyrimethamine toxicity. *BMJ* 1974; **1:** 40.

**Zidovudine.** Studies *in vitro* and in *animals* suggest that zidovudine could reduce the effectiveness of pyrimethamine in the treatment of toxoplasmic encephalitis.[1] Furthermore, the dose of zidovudine may need to be altered if these drugs are used together as there has been a report that pyrimethamine with sulfadoxine (Fansidar) prolonged the serum half-life of zidovudine.[2]

1. Israelski DM, *et al.* Zidovudine antagonizes the action of pyrimethamine in experimental infection with Toxoplasma gondii. *Antimicrob Agents Chemother* 1989; **33:** 30–4.
2. Klein RS. Prophylaxis of opportunistic infections in individuals infected with HIV. *AIDS* 1989; **3** (suppl 1): S161–S173.

## Pharmacokinetics

Pyrimethamine is almost completely absorbed from the gastrointestinal tract and peak plasma concentrations of about 200 nanograms/mL are obtained 2 to 6 hours after administration of 25 mg orally. It is mainly concentrated in the kidneys, lungs, liver, and spleen and about 80 to 90% is bound to plasma proteins.

It is metabolised in the liver and slowly excreted via the kidney, the average half-life in plasma being about 4 days. Several metabolites have been detected in the urine. Pyrimethamine crosses the placenta. It is distributed into breast milk (see under Breast Feeding in Precautions, above).

◊ References.

1. White NJ. Clinical pharmacokinetics of antimalarial drugs. *Clin Pharmacokinet* 1985; **10:** 187–215.
2. Cook IF, *et al.* Race-linked differences in serum concentrations of dapsone, monoacetyldapsone and pyrimethamine during malaria prophylaxis. *Trans R Soc Trop Med Hyg* 1986; **80:** 897–901.
3. Weiss LM, *et al.* Pyrimethamine concentrations in serum and cerebrospinal fluid during treatment of acute toxoplasma encephalitis in patients with AIDS. *J Infect Dis* 1988; **157:** 580–3.
4. Hellgren U, *et al.* Plasma concentrations of sulfadoxine-pyrimethamine, mefloquine and its main metabolite after regular malaria prophylaxis for two years. *Trans R Soc Trop Med Hyg* 1991; **85:** 356–7.
5. Winstanley PA, *et al.* The disposition of oral and intramuscular pyrimethamine/sulphadoxine in Kenyan children with high parasitaemia but clinically non-severe falciparum malaria. *Br J Clin Pharmacol* 1992; **33:** 143–8.
6. Newton CRJC, *et al.* A single dose of intramuscular sulfadoxine-pyrimethamine as an adjunct to quinine in the treatment of severe malaria: pharmacokinetics and efficacy. *Trans R Soc Trop Med Hyg* 1993; **87:** 207–10.
7. Jacobson JM, *et al.* Pyrimethamine pharmacokinetics in human immunodeficiency virus-positive patients seropositive for Toxoplasma gondii. *Antimicrob Agents Chemother* 1996; **40:** 1360–5.
8. Klinker H, *et al.* Plasma pyrimethamine concentrations during long-term treatment for cerebral toxoplasmosis in patients with AIDS. *Antimicrob Agents Chemother* 1996; **40:** 1623–7.
9. Trenque T, *et al.* Human maternofoetal distribution of pyrimethamine-sulphadoxine. *Br J Clin Pharmacol* 1998; **45:** 179–80.

## Uses and Administration

Pyrimethamine is a diaminopyrimidine antimalarial used with a sulfonamide in the treatment of malaria and toxoplasmosis. Pyrimethamine with sulfadoxine has been tried in the treatment of actinomycetoma and for prophylaxis of *Pneumocystis carinii* pneumonia. Pyrimethamine alone or with sulfadoxine has also been tried in the treatment of isosporiasis.

Pyrimethamine exerts its antimalarial activity by inhibiting plasmodial dihydrofolate reductase, thus indirectly blocking the synthesis of nucleic acids in the malaria parasite. It is active against pre-erythrocytic forms and is also a slow-acting blood schizontocide. It also has some sporontocidal activity; it does not prevent the formation of gametocytes but renders them non-infective to the mosquito vector. It is mainly effective against *Plasmodium falciparum* but has some activity against *P. vivax*.

The development of plasmodial resistance has rendered obsolete the use of pyrimethamine on its own in malaria. Combinations of pyrimethamine with long-acting sulfonamides, such as sulfadoxine or sulfametopyrazine, are now used, although resistance has also developed to them.

For *treatment of chloroquine-resistant or multidrug-resistant falciparum malaria*, pyrimethamine is usually given with a long-acting sulfonamide, sometimes following a course of quinine, or with artesunate or amodiaquine. Pyrimethamine with sulfadoxine in a fixed dose ratio of 1 to 20 (Fansidar) is usually given by mouth. A single dose of pyrimethamine 75 mg with sulfadoxine 1.5 g is usually recommended. The dose should not be repeated for at least 7 days. Suggested doses for children are: 5 to 10 kg body-weight, 12.5 mg pyrimethamine and 250 mg sulfadoxine; 11 to 20 kg, 25 mg pyrimethamine and 500 mg sulfadoxine; 21 to 30 kg, 37.5 mg pyrimethamine and 750 mg sulfadoxine; 31 to 45 kg, 50 mg pyrimethamine and 1 g sulfadoxine. A combination of pyrimethamine with sulfametopyrazine is used similarly.

The combination of pyrimethamine with sulfadoxine has also been administered intramuscularly.

Pyrimethamine and pyrimethamine combinations are no longer recommended for *prophylaxis of malaria*. Combined preparations of pyrimethamine with sulfadoxine (Fansidar), and with dapsone in a fixed ratio of 1 to 8 (Maloprim), have been used in areas of chloroquine or multidrug resistance, although mefloquine is now preferred.

Pyrimethamine administered with a sulfonamide such as sulfadiazine is used in the *treatment of toxoplasmosis*. Alternatively, pyrimethamine may be given with clindamycin in AIDS patients with toxoplasmosis unable to tolerate a sulfonamide. For details of dosage regimens used, see below.

**Administration.** A formulation of pyrimethamine with sulfadoxine for intramuscular administration has been studied,[1-4] but its role in the treatment of falciparum malaria is not clear.

1. Harinasuta T, *et al.* Parenteral Fansidar® in falciparum malaria. *Trans R Soc Trop Med Hyg* 1988; **82:** 694.
2. Salako LA, *et al.* Parenteral sulphadoxine–pyrimethamine (Fansidar®): an effective and safe but under-used method of anti-malarial treatment. *Trans R Soc Trop Med Hyg* 1990; **84:** 641–3.
3. Simão F, *et al.* Comparison of intramuscular sulfadoxine-pyrimethamine and intramuscular quinine for the treatment of falciparum malaria in children. *Trans R Soc Trop Med Hyg* 1991; **85:** 341–4.
4. Newton CRJC, *et al.* A single dose of intramuscular sulfadoxine-pyrimethamine as an adjunct to quinine in the treatment of severe malaria: pharmacokinetics and efficacy. *Trans R Soc Trop Med Hyg* 1993; **87:** 207–10.

**Isosporiasis.** Isosporiasis (p.597) usually responds well to treatment with co-trimoxazole, but there is a high incidence of recurrence in immunocompromised patients, such as those with AIDS, and some form of maintenance therapy is generally required. Co-trimoxazole 960 mg given three times weekly or pyrimethamine 25 mg with sulfadoxine 500 mg given weekly were found to be equally effective maintenance regimens.[1] Pyrimethamine given alone in daily doses of 50 to 75 mg with folate therapy may be of use in the treatment of patients sensitive to sulfonamides.[2]

1. Pape JW, *et al.* Treatment and prophylaxis of Isospora belli infection in patients with the acquired immunodeficiency syndrome. *N Engl J Med* 1989; **320:** 1044–7.
2. Weiss LM, *et al.* Isospora belli infection: treatment with pyrimethamine. *Ann Intern Med* 1988; **109:** 474–5.

**Malaria.** The overall treatment and prophylaxis of malaria and the place of pyrimethamine-sulfadoxine (Fansidar) in current recommendations are discussed on p.444.

**Mycetoma.** For reference to the use of pyrimethamine as part of the treatment of actinomycetoma, see under Mycetoma, p.136.

**Pneumocystis carinii pneumonia.** For a mention of pyrimethamine in combination with dapsone or sulfadoxine for the prophylaxis of *Pneumocystis carinii* pneumonia, and a discussion of conventional prophylaxis and treatment, see p.389.

**Toxoplasmosis.** Pyrimethamine is given, usually in conjunction with sulfadiazine, in the treatment of toxoplasmosis (p.598). Folinic acid is also given to counteract the megaloblastic anaemia associated with these drugs. A suggested dosage regimen is pyrimethamine 50 to 200 mg daily with sulfadiazine 250 to 1000 mg every 6 hours for one or two days, then pyrimethamine 25 to 50 mg daily with sulfadiazine 125 to 500 mg every 6 hours for 2 to 4 weeks, or 4 to 6 weeks if the patient is immunocompromised. Treatment is ideally continued for several weeks after clinical cure. A suggested dose of pyrimethamine for children is 1 mg/kg daily for 1 to 3 days, then 0.5 mg/kg daily for 4 to 6 weeks, given with usual paediatric doses of sulfadiazine. Treatment may continue for 6 months to 1 year in infants with congenital toxoplasmosis.

Patients with AIDS may be given a loading dose of 100 to 200 mg pyrimethamine daily with sulfadiazine 500 to 1500 mg every 6 hours for one or two days, and then 50 to 100 mg pyrimethamine daily with the same dose of sulfadiazine for 3 to 6 weeks. Maintenance treatment for AIDS patients with pyrimethamine 25 to 50 mg daily and sulfadiazine 250 to 1000 mg every 6 hours may continue indefinitely. Pyrimethamine with clindamycin is an alternative in patients unable to tolerate a sulfonamide.

Other drugs tried in combination with pyrimethamine with promising results include azithromycin,[1] clarithromycin,[2] and doxycycline.[3,4]

Alternative regimens tried for long-term maintenance therapy in patients with AIDS have included pyrimethamine plus sulfadiazine given twice weekly[5,6] or pyrimethamine alone in doses of 25 mg or 50 mg daily or 50 mg three times weekly.[7-9] However, results from a study involving 396 patients suggested that the mortality rate was higher in those receiving pyrimethamine 25 mg three times weekly for primary prophylaxis than in those receiving placebo.[10] Pyrimethamine with dapsone given once a week can provide effective prophylaxis but was not well tolerated.[11] Pyrimethamine with sulfadoxine, also given once weekly, has produced promising results in bone-marrow transplant recipients.[12]

1. Saba J, *et al.* Pyrimethamine plus azithromycin for treatment of acute toxoplasmic encephalitis in patients with AIDS. *Eur J Clin Microbiol Infect Dis* 1993; **12:** 853–6.
2. Fernandez-Martin J, *et al.* Pyrimethamine-clarithromycin combination therapy of acute Toxoplasma encephalitis in patients with AIDS. *Antimicrob Agents Chemother* 1991; **35:** 2049–52.
3. Morris JT, Kelly JW. Effective treatment of cerebral toxoplasmosis with doxycycline. *Am J Med* 1992; **93:** 107–8.
4. Hagberg L, *et al.* Doxycycline and pyrimethamine for toxoplasmic encephalitis. *Scand J Infect Dis* 1993; **25:** 157–60.
5. Pedrol E, *et al.* Central nervous system toxoplasmosis in AIDS patients: efficacy of an intermittent maintenance therapy. *AIDS* 1990; **4:** 511–17.
6. Podzanczer D, *et al.* Twice-weekly maintenance therapy with sulfadiazine-pyrimethamine to prevent recurrent toxoplasmic encephalitis in patients with AIDS. *Ann Intern Med* 1995; **123:** 175–80.
7. Murphy K, *et al.* Pyrimethamine alone as long-term suppressive therapy in cerebral toxoplasmosis. *Am J Med* 1994; **96:** 95–6.
8. de Gans J, *et al.* Pyrimethamine alone as maintenance therapy for central nervous system toxoplasmosis in 38 patients with AIDS. *J Acquir Immune Defic Syndr Hum Retrovirol* 1992; **5:** 137–42.
9. Leport C, *et al.* Pyrimethamine for primary prophylaxis of toxoplasmic encephalitis in patients with human immunodeficiency virus infection: a double-blind, randomized trial. *J Infect Dis* 1996; **173:** 91–7.
10. Jacobson MA. *et al.* Primary prophylaxis with pyrimethamine for toxoplasmic encephalitis in patients with advanced human immunodeficiency virus disease: results of a randomized trial. *J Infect Dis* 1994; **169:** 384–94.
11. Opravil M, *et al.* Once-weekly administration of dapsone/pyrimethamine vs. aerosolized pentamidine as combined prophylaxis for Pneumocystis carinii pneumonia and toxoplasmic encephalitis in human immunodeficiency virus-infected patients. *Clin Infect Dis* 1995; **20:** 531–41.
12. Foot ABM, *et al.* Prophylaxis of toxoplasmosis infection with pyrimethamine/sulfadoxine (Fansidar) in bone marrow transplant recipients. *Bone Marrow Transplant* 1994; **14:** 241–5.

## Preparations

***BP 2003:*** Pyrimethamine Tablets;
***USP 27:*** Pyrimethamine Tablets; Sulfadoxine and Pyrimethamine Tablets.

**Proprietary Preparations** (details are given in Part 3)
***Arg.:*** Daraprim; ***Austral.:*** Daraprim; ***Austria:*** Daraprim; ***Belg.:*** Daraprim; ***Braz.:*** Daraprim†; Daraprin; ***Canad.:*** Daraprim; ***Chile:*** Daraprim; ***Fr.:*** Malocide; ***Ger.:*** Daraprim; ***Irl.:*** Daraprim; ***Israel:*** Daraprim; ***Mex.:*** Dar-

aprim; **Neth.:** Daraprim; **S.Afr.:** Daraprim; **Spain:** Daraprim; **Switz.:** Daraprim; **Thai.:** Daraprim; **UK:** Daraprim; **USA:** Daraprim.

**Multi-ingredient: Austral.:** Fansidar; **Belg.:** Fansidar†; Malastop; **Braz.:** Clopirim; Fansidar; Periodine Anti-Malarico†; **Canad.:** Fansidar; **Denm.:** Fansidar; **Fr.:** Fansidar; **India:** Laridox; Pyralfin; Rimodar; **Irl.:** Fansidar; Maloprim; **Israel:** Fansidar; **Ital.:** Metakelfin; **Malaysia:** Madomine; **S.Afr.:** Fansidar; Maloprim; **Singapore:** Madomine; **Swed.:** Fansidar†; **Switz.:** Fansidar; Fansimef; **Thai.:** Vivaxine; **UK:** Fansidar; Maloprim†; **USA:** Fansidar.

## Pyronaridine Phosphate

Malaridine Phosphate; Pironaridina, fosfato de. 7-Chloro-2-methoxy-10-[3,5-bis(pyrrolidinomethyl)-4-hydroxyanilino]benzo-[*b*]-1,5-naphthyridine phosphate.

$C_{29}H_{32}ClN_5O_2,4H_3PO_4 = 910.0.$

*CAS — 74847-35-1 (pyronaridine); 76748-86-2 (pyronaridine phosphate).*

**Pharmacopoeias.** In *Chin.*

### Profile

Pyronaridine is a naphthyridine derivative used in China in the treatment of vivax malaria and chloroquine-resistant falciparum malaria. Its use in Africa and in Thailand is also under investigation. Combination of pyronaridine with artesunate is also being investigated. Pyronaridine has been given as the phosphate by mouth or by intramuscular or intravenous injection.

◊ References.


1. Shao B-R. A review of antimalarial drug pyronaridine. *Chin Med J* 1990; **103:** 428–34.
2. Shao B-R, *et al.* A 5-year surveillance of sensitivity in vivo of Plasmodium falciparum to pyronaridine/sulfadoxine/pyrimethamine in Diaoluo area, Hainan province. *Southeast Asian J Trop Med Public Health* 1991; **22:** 65–7.
3. Chen C, *et al.* Studies on a new antimalarial compound: pyronaridine. *Trans R Soc Trop Med Hyg* 1992; **86:** 7–10.
4. Winstanley P. Pyronaridine: a promising drug for Africa? *Lancet* 1996; **347:** 2–3.
5. Ringwald P, *et al.* Randomised trial of pyronaridine versus chloroquine for acute uncomplicated falciparum malaria in Africa. *Lancet* 1996; **347:** 24–8.
6. Looareesuwan S, *et al.* Pyronaridine. *Lancet* 1996; **347:** 1189–90.
7. Anonymous. Pyronaridine: yet another promising antimalarial substance from China. *WHO Drug Inf* 1996; **10:** 9–10.
8. Looareesuwan S, *et al.* Clinical study of pyronaridine for the treatment of acute uncomplicated falciparum malaria in Thailand. *Am J Trop Med Hyg* 1996; **54:** 205–9.
9. Ringwald P, *et al.* Efficacy of oral pyronaridine for the treatment of acute uncomplicated falciparum malaria in African children. *Clin Infect Dis* 1998; **26:** 946–53.


# Quinine *(BAN)*

Chinina; Chininum; Quinina. (8*S*,9*R*)-6′-Methoxycinchonan-9-ol; (α*R*)-α-(6-Methoxy-4-quinolyl)-α-[(2*S*,4*S*,5*R*)-(5-vinylquinuclidin-2-yl)]methanol.

$C_{20}H_{24}N_2O_2 = 324.4.$

*CAS — 130-95-0 (anhydrous quinine).*

*ATC — P01BC01.*

**Description.** Quinine is the chief alkaloid of various species of *Cinchona* (Rubiaceae). It is an optical isomer of quinidine.

## Quinine Bisulfate

Chininum Bisulfuricum; Neutral Quinine Sulphate; Quinina, bisulfato de; Quinine Acid Sulphate; Quinine Bisulphate *(BANM)*; Quinini Bisulfas.

$C_{20}H_{24}N_2O_2,H_2SO_4,7H_2O = 548.6.$

*CAS — 549-56-4 (anhydrous quinine bisulfate).*

*ATC — P01BC01.*

**Pharmacopoeias.** In *Br., Int.,* and *Viet.*

**BP 2003** (Quinine Bisulphate). Colourless crystals or a white crystalline powder. It effloresces in dry air. Freely soluble in water; sparingly soluble in alcohol. A 1% solution in water has a pH of 2.8 to 3.4. Protect from light.

## Quinine Dihydrochloride *(BANM)*

Chinini Dihydrochloridum; Neutral Quinine Hydrochloride; Quinina, dihidrocloruro de; Quinine Acid Hydrochloride; Quinini Dihydrochloridum.

$C_{20}H_{24}N_2O_2,2HCl = 397.3.$

*CAS — 60-93-5.*

*ATC — P01BC01.*

**Pharmacopoeias.** In *Br., Chin.,* and *Int.*

*Viet.* includes the injection.

**BP 2003** (Quinine Dihydrochloride). A white or almost white powder. Very soluble in water; soluble in alcohol. A 3% solution in water has a pH of 2.0 to 3.0. Protect from light.

## Quinine Etabonate

Euquinina; Euquinine; Quinina, etilcarbonato de; Quinine Ethyl Carbonate.

$C_{23}H_{28}N_2O_4 = 396.5.$

*CAS — 83-75-0.*

*ATC — P01BC01.*

**Pharmacopoeias.** In *Jpn.*

## Quinine Hydrobromide *(BANM)*

Basic Quinine Hydrobromide; Chinini Bromidum; Quinina, hidrobromuro de; Quinine Monohydrobromide.

$C_{20}H_{24}N_2O_2,HBr,H_2O = 423.3.$

*CAS — 549-49-5 (anhydrous quinine hydrobromide).*

*ATC — P01BC01.*

**Pharmacopoeias.** In *Fr.*

## Quinine Hydrochloride *(BANM)*

Basic Quinine Hydrochloride; Chinini Hydrochloridum; Chininii Chloridum; Chininium Chloratum; Chininum Hydrochloricum; Quinina, hidrocloruro de; Quinine Monohydrochloride; Quinini Hydrochloridum.

$C_{20}H_{24}N_2O_2,HCl,2H_2O = 396.9.$

*CAS — 130-89-2 (anhydrous quinine hydrochloride); 6119-47-7 (quinine hydrochloride dihydrate).*

*ATC — P01BC01.*

**Pharmacopoeias.** In *Eur.* (see p.vi), *Int., Jpn, Pol.,* and *Viet.*

**Ph. Eur. 5.0** (Quinine Hydrochloride). Colourless, fine, silky needles, often grouped in clusters. Soluble in water; freely soluble in alcohol. A 1% solution in water has a pH of 6.0 to 6.8. Protect from light.

## Quinine Sulfate

Basic Quinine Sulphate; Chinini Sulfas; Chininum Sulfuricum; Quinina, sulfato de; Quinine Sulphate *(BANM)*; Quinini Sulfas.

$(C_{20}H_{24}N_2O_2)_2,H_2SO_4,2H_2O = 782.9.$

*CAS — 804-63-7 (anhydrous quinine sulfate); 6119-70-6 (quinine sulfate dihydrate).*

*ATC — P01BC01.*

**Pharmacopoeias.** In *Chin., Eur.* (see p.vi), *Int., Jpn, US,* and *Viet.*

**Ph. Eur. 5.0** (Quinine Sulphate). A white or almost white, crystalline powder or fine, colourless needles. Slightly soluble in water; sparingly soluble in boiling water and in alcohol. A 1% suspension in water has a pH of 5.7 to 6.6. Protect from light.

**USP 27** (Quinine Sulfate). It is the sulfate of an alkaloid obtained from the bark of species of *Cinchona*. White, odourless, fine needle-like crystals, usually lusterless, making a light and readily compressible mass. It darkens on exposure to light. Soluble 1 in 500 of water and 1 in 120 of alcohol; sparingly soluble in water at 100°; slightly soluble in chloroform; freely soluble in alcohol at 80° and in a mixture of 2 parts of chloroform and one part of dehydrated alcohol; very slightly soluble in ether; Its saturated solution in water is neutral or alkaline to litmus. Protect from light.

**Sorption.** For reference to loss of quinine sulfate from solutions during membrane filtration, see Chloroquine, p.448.

## Adverse Effects

Quinine or its salts given in usual therapeutic doses may give rise to a train of symptoms known as cinchonism, characterised in its mild form by tinnitus, impaired hearing, headache, nausea, and disturbed vision, with, in its more severe manifestations, vomiting, abdominal pain, diarrhoea, and vertigo.

Cinchonism may also occur after small doses in patients hypersensitive to quinine, but urticaria and flushing of the skin with intense pruritus are the most frequent reactions seen in these patients. Other effects include fever, skin rashes, and dyspnoea. Angioedema may also occur and asthma can be precipitated. Thrombocytopenia and other blood disorders have been reported. Thrombocytopenic purpura has been associated with quinine hypersensitivity. Haemoglobinuria occurs rarely.

Other adverse effects of quinine include hypoglycaemia, hypoprothrombinaemia, and renal failure.

The main symptoms of overdosage, which can be fatal, include gastrointestinal effects, oculotoxicity, CNS disturbances, and cardiotoxicity. Visual disturbances including sudden blindness are usually slowly reversible but there may be residual damage. Overdosage is discussed in detail below. Quinine can produce cardiovascular toxicity similar to that seen with quinidine including conduction disturbances, arrhythmias, anginal symptoms, and hypotension leading to cardiac arrest and circulatory failure. Severe or even fatal cardiovascular toxicity can result from rapid intravenous administration of quinine.

Large amounts of quinine can induce abortion; congenital malformations, particularly of the optic and auditory nerves, have been reported after failure to induce abortion with quinine. However, quinine should not be withheld from pregnant women with life-threatening malaria (see also under Pregnancy in Precautions, below).

Intramuscular injections of quinine can be irritant and have caused pain, focal necrosis, and abscess formation; tetanus has developed in some patients (see under Malaria in Uses and Administration, below).

**Effects on the blood.** Between 1966 and 1975 the Swedish Adverse Drug Reaction Committee received 43 reports of *thrombocytopenia* attributable to quinine or quinidine[1] and the Boston Collaborative Drug Surveillance Program had 11 similar reports in patients studied between 1972 and 1981.[2] The FDA in the USA subsequently received details of 2 fatalities due to quinine-induced thrombocytopenia.[3] Quinine-induced thrombocytopenia appears to be a hypersensitivity reaction and beverages containing quinine as a bitter in concentrations as low as 20 micrograms/mL have precipitated thrombocytopenic purpura in previously sensitised individuals.[4]

Although quinine can cause *haemolysis*, there is some doubt over the traditional view that irregular dosage with quinine predisposes patients with malaria to *blackwater fever*, a syndrome of severe haemolytic anaemia, haemoglobinuria, oliguria, and renal failure.[5] Some of the patients affected may have had G6PD deficiency.[5] Haemolytic-uraemic syndrome[6-8] and pancytopenia with coagulopathy and renal impairment[9,10] have also been associated with the use of quinine.

There have also been reports of *disseminated intravascular coagulation*, including one fatality, following the use of quinine by patients with quinine hypersensitivity.[11-13] In one case[13] the hypersensitivity reaction closely mimicked septic shock.

There have been isolated reports of *agranulocytosis* due to quinine.[14]


1. Böttiger LE, *et al.* Drug-induced blood dyscrasias. *Acta Med Scand* 1979; **205:** 457–61.
2. Danielson DA, *et al.* Drug-induced blood disorders. *JAMA* 1984; **252:** 3257–60.
3. Freiman JP. Fatal quinine-induced thrombocytopenia. *Ann Intern Med* 1990; **112:** 308–9.
4. Murray JA, *et al.* Bitter lemon purpura. *BMJ* 1979; **2:** 1551–2.
5. WHO. Severe and complicated malaria. 2nd ed. *Trans R Soc Trop Med Hyg* 1990; **84** (suppl 2): 1–65.
6. Hagley MT, *et al.* Hemolytic-uremic syndrome associated with ingestion of quinine. *Am J Nephrol* 1992; **12:** 192–5.
7. Gottschall JL, *et al.* Quinine-induced immune thrombocytopenia with hemolytic uremic syndrome: clinical and serological findings in nine patients and review of literature. *Am J Hematol* 1994; **47:** 283–9.
8. McDonald SP, *et al.* Quinine-induced hemolytic uremic syndrome. *Clin Nephrol* 1997; **47:** 397–400.
9. Maguire RB, *et al.* Recurrent pancytopenia, coagulopathy, and renal failure associated with multiple quinine-dependent antibodies. *Ann Intern Med* 1993; **119:** 215–17.
10. Schmitt SK, Tomford JW. Quinine-induced pancytopenia and coagulopathy. *Ann Intern Med* 1994; **120:** 90–1.
11. Spearing RL, *et al.* Quinine-induced disseminated intravascular coagulation. *Lancet* 1990; **336:** 1535–7.
12. Barr E, *et al.* Recurrent acute hypersensitivity to quinine. *BMJ* 1990; **301:** 323.
13. Schattner A. Quinine hypersensitivity simulating sepsis. *Am J Med* 1998; **104:** 488–90.
14. Sutherland R, *et al.* Quinine-induced agranulocytosis: toxic effect of quinine bisulphate on bone marrow cultures in vitro. *BMJ* 1977; **1:** 605–7.


**Effects on the ears.** Although ototoxicity such as tinnitus or deafness is known to be a possible adverse effect of quinine, reversible hearing loss may also occur. While one group of workers[1] found the reduction in auditory acuity to be greatest at higher frequencies, another group[2] have found that hearing loss was generally equal across the range of frequencies tested and appeared to be related to the plasma concentration of quinine.


1. Roche RJ, *et al.* Quinine induces reversible high-tone hearing loss. *Br J Clin Pharmacol* 1990; **29:** 780–2.
2. Karlsson KK, *et al.* Audiometry as a possible indicator of quinine plasma concentration during treatment of malaria. *Trans R Soc Trop Med Hyg* 1990; **84:** 765–7.


**Effects on the eyes.** Oculotoxicity following overdosage with quinine is well recognised (see below), but there has also been a report of blindness in two patients occurring during supposedly routine therapy.[1]


1. Waddell K. Blindness from quinine as an antimalarial. *Trans R Soc Trop Med Hyg* 1996; **90:** 331–2.


**Effects on glucose metabolism.** Hypoglycaemia is now recognised to be a frequent complication encountered in falciparum malaria and it is often associated with a poor prognosis. Children, pregnant women, and patients with severe disease appear to be particularly at risk. It is important to recognise that hypoglycaemia rather than cerebral malaria may be the cause of coma. Hypoglycaemia may also be induced by antimalarial therapy; first episodes of hypoglycaemia have been detected after patients received quinine[1-3] or quinidine[4] intravenously, although others have not found that quinine led to the development of hypoglycaemia.[5,6]

Quinine has also been reported to induce hypoglycaemia during treatment for leg cramps.[7]


1. White NJ, *et al.* Severe hypoglycemia and hyperinsulinemia in falciparum malaria. *N Engl J Med* 1983; **309:** 61–6.
2. Okitolonda W, *et al.* High incidence of hypoglycaemia in African patients treated with intravenous quinine for severe malaria. *BMJ* 1987; **295:** 716–18.
3. Looareesuwan S, *et al.* Quinine and severe falciparum malaria in late pregnancy. *Lancet* 1985; **ii:** 4–8.
4. Phillips RE, *et al.* Hypoglycaemia and antimalarial drugs: quinidine and release of insulin. *BMJ* 1986; **292:** 1319–21.

5. Taylor TE, *et al.* Blood glucose levels in Malawian children before and during the administration of intravenous quinine for severe falciparum malaria. *N Engl J Med* 1988; **319:** 1040–7.
6. Kawo NG, *et al.* The metabolic effects of quinine in children with severe and complicated Plasmodium falciparum malaria in Dar es Salaam. *Trans R Soc Trop Med Hyg* 1991; **85:** 711–13.
7. Limburg PJ, *et al.* Quinine-induced hypoglycemia. *Ann Intern Med* 1993; **119:** 218–19.


**Effects on the heart.** Cardiotoxicity following overdosage with quinine is well recognised, and prolongation of the QT interval has been noted with therapeutic doses. There has also been a report[1] of fatal ventricular fibrillation with QT prolongation in an elderly patient who received standard doses of quinine by slow intravenous infusion for falciparum malaria. It was noted that the patient had some prolongation of the QT interval before starting quinine and also that her free quinine concentrations were unusually high despite total quinine concentrations considered to be within the therapeutic range.


1. Bonington A, *et al.* Fatal quinine cardiotoxicity in the treatment of falciparum malaria. *Trans R Soc Trop Med Hyg* 1996; **90:** 305–7.


**Effects on the kidneys.** See Effects on the Blood, above.

**Effects on the liver.** Although hepatitis has been associated with quinidine therapy (see p.992), there appear to be few reports of hepatotoxicity due to quinine usage. Granulomatous hepatitis has been reported in 2 patients taking quinine,[1,2] but the diagnosis in the first of these cases was challenged as the histological findings were considered to be more indicative of non-specific reactive hepatitis.[3] Hepatotoxicity due to quinine hypersensitivity has been reported in another patient.[4] Symptoms of hepatotoxicity occurred within 24 hours in a further patient taking quinine for nocturnal leg cramps.[5]


1. Katz B, *et al.* Quinine-induced granulomatous hepatitis. *BMJ* 1983; **286:** 264–5.
2. Mathur S, *et al.* Quinine induced granulomatous hepatitis and vasculitis. *BMJ* 1990; **300:** 613.
3. Nirodi NS. Quinine induced granulomatous hepatitis. *BMJ* 1983; **286:** 647.
4. Punukollu RC, *et al.* Quinine hepatotoxicity: an underrecognized or rare phenomenon? *Arch Intern Med* 1990; **150:** 1112–13.
5. Farver DK, Lavin MN. Quinine-induced hepatotoxicity. *Ann Pharmacother* 1999; **33:** 32–4.


**Effects on the skin.** Urticaria, cutaneous flushing, various skin rashes, and pruritus are the commonest symptoms of hypersensitivity reactions to quinine.

Topical contact with quinine may cause contact as well as photocontact allergy, but quinine can also induce photosensitivity reactions following systemic administration.[1,2] Photosensitivity associated with quinine intake from excessive consumption of tonic water has been reported.[3] There have also been reports of eczematous dermatitis,[1] oedema and erythema,[4] and lichen planus.[4] Both phototoxic[4] and photoallergic[1] mechanisms have been suggested. Fatal cutaneous vasculitis related to quinine treatment for nocturnal cramps has been reported.[5]

For a comparison of the incidence of pruritus induced by various antimalarials, see under Chloroquine, p.449.


1. Ljunggren B, Sjövall P. Systemic quinine photosensitivity. *Arch Dermatol* 1986; **122:** 909–11.
2. Ljunggren B, *et al.* Systemic quinine photosensitivity with photoepicutaneous cross-reactivity to quinidine. *Contact Dermatitis* 1992; **26:** 1–4.
3. Wagner GH, *et al.* 'I'll have mine with a twist of lemon': quinine photosensitivity from excessive intake of tonic water. *Br J Dermatol* 1994; **131:** 734–5.
4. Ferguson J, *et al.* Quinine induced photosensitivity: clinical and experimental studies. *Br J Dermatol* 1987; **117:** 631–40.
5. Price EJ, *et al.* Quinine-induced cutaneous vasculitis. *Br J Clin Pract* 1992; **46:** 138–9.


**Hypersensitivity.** For reference to hypersensitivity reactions associated with quinine, see Effects on the Blood, Effects on the Liver, and Effects on the Skin, above.

**Overdosage.** Cinchonism may occur with therapeutic doses of quinine and symptoms include nausea, vomiting, tinnitus, deafness, headache, vasodilatation, and slightly disturbed vision. These symptoms may also occur in acute overdosage, but the visual disorders may be severe and there may be CNS disturbances and cardiotoxicity. A lethal dose or lethal plasma-quinine concentration has not been established but fatalities have been reported[1] in adults after doses of 2 to 8 g and in children after 1 g.

An analysis[2] of 165 cases of acute quinine poisoning revealed that: 21% had no symptoms, nausea with or without vomiting occurred in 47%, visual disturbances in 42%, tinnitus in 38%, other auditory disturbances in 23%, sinus tachycardia in 23%, and other ECG abnormalities in 8%. Mild impairment of consciousness was reported in 14% of the patients while 7 (4%) patients had deeper grades of coma. Of the 5 patients who died, 4 developed intractable ventricular arrhythmias and the fifth had a Jacksonian fit followed by cardiac arrest.

The effects of oculotoxicity may include blurred vision, defective colour perception, visual field constriction, and total blindness.[2,3] The onset of symptoms may vary from a few hours to a day or more after ingestion.[2,3] Suggested mechanisms for the oculotoxicity of quinine include an action on the retinal vasculature to produce ischaemia or a direct toxic effect on the retina.[1] Visual loss in one group of patients[3] was associated with plasma-quinine concentrations in excess of 10 micrograms/mL. However, in another group plasma-quinine concentrations were considered to be an imprecise guide to predicting visual disturbances.[2] The speed and degree of visual recovery varies. Of 70 patients with visual disturbances following quinine poisoning, 39 subsequently complained of a period of total blindness.[2] Permanent visual deficits remained in 19 of these but no patient had permanent bilateral blindness. All of the 31 patients who had had blurred vision recovered full visual acuity.

It is considered that the actions of quinine on the myocardium are similar to those of quinidine but that it is less potent.[1] Sinus tachycardia and minor ECG changes are the most common cardiovascular effects. Conduction abnormalities and ventricular dysrhythmias may occur with severe poisoning. Ventricular tachycardia is mostly associated with cardiogenic shock or circulatory collapse. Hypokalaemia may also occur.[1]


1. Jaeger A, *et al.* Clinical features and management of poisoning due to antimalarial drugs. *Med Toxicol* 1987; **2:** 242–73.
2. Boland ME, *et al.* Complications of quinine poisoning. *Lancet* 1985; **i:** 384–5.
3. Dyson EH, *et al.* Death and blindness due to overdose of quinine. *BMJ* 1985; **291:** 31–3.


## Treatment of Adverse Effects

In acute overdosage with quinine or its salts multiple doses of activated charcoal may be given to adults or children who present within one hour of ingesting more than the equivalent of 15 mg/kg of quinine base; gastric lavage may also be considered for use in adults. Other measures aimed at enhancing the elimination of quinine are largely ineffective. Treatment is mostly symptomatic with attention being given to maintaining blood pressure, respiration, and renal function, and to treating arrhythmias.

Vasodilators and stellate ganglion block have been used to prevent or reverse visual impairment but there is little evidence to support their use.

◊ It has been suggested that, as quinine has antimuscarinic effects, gastric emptying may be delayed and considerable amounts of drug might be removed from the stomach beyond the usual 4 hours.[1] Others consider that gastric lavage is of doubtful value as quinine is rapidly absorbed and vomiting has often occurred before admission.[2] However, studies in healthy subjects and poisoned patients suggest that oral administration of charcoal may increase the elimination of quinine.[3,4] Other methods of increasing elimination are probably ineffective. In a study involving 16 patients with quinine poisoning forced acid diuresis, haemodialysis, haemoperfusion, or plasma exchange were all found to be ineffective in increasing quinine elimination.[5]

Stellate ganglion block has been recommended to prevent or reverse retinal damage, the rationale being that quinine-induced oculotoxicity might arise from retinal arteriolar constriction. However, clinical studies have failed to find sufficient improvement to justify its use.[6,7] There has been a report of the intravenous administration of nitrates producing beneficial responses in 2 patients.[8]


1. Boland M, Volans G. ABC of poisoning: miscellaneous drugs. *BMJ* 1984; **289:** 1361–5.
2. Jaeger A, *et al.* Clinical features and management of poisoning due to antimalarial drugs. *Med Toxicol* 1987; **2:** 242–73.
3. Lockey D, Bateman DN. Effect of oral activated charcoal on quinine elimination. *Br J Clin Pharmacol* 1989; **27:** 92–4.
4. Prescott LF, *et al.* Treatment of quinine overdosage with repeated oral charcoal. *Br J Clin Pharmacol* 1989; **27:** 95–7.
5. Bateman DN, *et al.* Pharmacokinetics and clinical toxicity of quinine overdosage: lack of efficacy of techniques intended to enhance elimination. *Q J Med* 1985; **54:** 125–31.
6. Boland ME, *et al.* Complications of quinine poisoning. *Lancet* 1985; **i:** 384–5.
7. Dyson EH, *et al.* Quinine amblyopia: is current management appropriate? *J Toxicol Clin Toxicol* 1985–6; **23:** 571–8.
8. Moore D, *et al.* Research into quinine ocular toxicity. *Br J Ophthalmol* 1992; **76:** 703.


## Precautions

Quinine and its salts are contra-indicated in patients with a history of hypersensitivity to quinine or quinidine and in patients with tinnitus or optic neuritis. They should not be used in the presence of haemolysis. They should be used with caution in patients with atrial fibrillation, cardiac conduction defects, or heart block. Quinine should be avoided in patients with myasthenia gravis as it may aggravate their condition.

Pregnancy in a patient with malaria is not generally regarded as a contra-indication to the use of quinine.

As quinine has been implicated in precipitating blackwater fever it is generally contra-indicated in patients who have already suffered an attack. Quinine may also cause haemolysis in some types of G6PD deficiency and should be used with care.

It is important that when quinine is given intravenously it should be given by slow infusion and the patient observed closely for signs of cardiotoxicity. Blood-glucose concentrations should also be monitored. Problems that have been associated with intramuscular administration are discussed under Malaria in Uses and Administration, below.

**Breast feeding.** Although quinine is distributed into breast milk in small amounts,[1] the American Academy of Pediatrics considers that the use of quinine is probably compatible with breast feeding.[2]


1. Phillips RE, *et al.* Quinine pharmacokinetics and toxicity in pregnant and lactating women with falciparum malaria. *Br J Clin Pharmacol* 1986; **21:** 677–83.
2. American Academy of Pediatrics, Committee on Drugs. The transfer of drugs and other chemicals into human milk. *Pediatrics* 2001; **108:** 776–89. Correction. *ibid.*: 1029. Also available at: http://aappolicy.aappublications.org/cgi/content/full/pediatrics%3b108/3/776 (accessed 19/04/04)


**Liver disease.** See under Pharmacokinetics, below.

**Porphyria.** For a discussion of the problems of the use of antimalarials in patients with porphyria and a comment that quinine is considered to be safe for use in such patients, see under Precautions for Chloroquine, p.450.

**Pregnancy.** The use of quinine in large doses as an abortifacient in the past has led to concern over its use during pregnancy, but no evidence of an oxytocic effect was found when it was used to treat severe falciparum malaria in women in the third trimester of pregnancy.[1]

Congenital abnormalities including damage to the auditory and optic nerves have been seen, usually following attempted abortions, but WHO[2] considers quinine to be safe when used in normal therapeutic doses during pregnancy. Jitteriness attributed to quinine withdrawal has been reported in an infant whose mother had drunk large quantities of tonic water containing quinine during the last 17 weeks of pregnancy.[3]

As malaria is potentially serious during pregnancy and poses a threat to the mother and fetus, there appears to be little justification for withholding treatment in the absence of a suitable alternative. However, pregnant patients treated for malaria are at special risk from hypoglycaemia exacerbated or caused by quinine-induced hyperinsulinaemia (see under Effects on Glucose Metabolism in Adverse Effects, above) and should be managed appropriately.


1. Looareesuwan S, *et al.* Quinine and severe falciparum malaria in late pregnancy. *Lancet* 1985; **ii:** 4–8.
2. WHO. *WHO model prescribing information: drugs used in parasitic diseases.* 2nd ed. Geneva: WHO, 1995.
3. Evans ANW, *et al.* The ingestion by pregnant women of substances toxic to the foetus. *Practitioner* 1980; **224:** 315–19.


**Renal impairment.** See under Pharmacokinetics, below.

## Interactions

As quinine shares many of the actions of quinidine, interactions seen between quinidine and other drugs (see p.992) might also occur with quinine. Both have actions on skeletal muscle and may potentiate the effects of drugs with neuromuscular-blocking activity (see under Antiarrhythmics on p.1400). There is an increased risk of inducing ventricular arrhythmias if quinine is given with halofantrine (see p.452) or other arrhythmogenic drugs such as amiodarone, the antihistamines astemizole and terfenadine, cisapride, and the antipsychotic pimozide. There may be an increased risk of convulsions when quinine is administered with mefloquine.

**Amantadine.** For a report of quinine reducing renal clearance of amantadine, see p.1198.

**Anticoagulants.** Quinine can cause hypoprothrombinaemia and thereby enhance the effect of anticoagulants. In one report, reductions in *warfarin* dosage were necessary after ingestion of large amounts of tonic water containing quinine (see p.1025).

**Antimalarials.** Quinine and *chloroquine* may be antagonistic when used for falciparum malaria (see p.450). For a report of quinine reducing plasma concentrations of *primaquine*, see p.456.

**Ciclosporin.** For a report of quinine decreasing plasma concentrations of ciclosporin, see p.1355.

**Digoxin.** Quinidine has been reported to increase serum-digoxin concentrations (see p.896) and quinine has reduced total body clearance of digoxin (see p.897).

**Flecainide.** For a report of quinine inhibiting the metabolism of flecainide, see p.917.

**Histamine $H_2$-antagonists.** *Cimetidine* has been reported to reduce the clearance of quinine and prolong its elimination half-life in a study in healthy subjects; no significant effect was seen with *ranitidine*.[1]


1. Wanwimolruk S, *et al.* Effects of cimetidine and ranitidine on the pharmacokinetics of quinine. *Br J Clin Pharmacol* 1986; **22:** 346–50.


**Rifampicin.** Elimination of quinine has been reported to increase in patients also receiving rifampicin.[1]


1. Wanwimolruk S, *et al.* Marked enhancement by rifampicin and lack of effect of isoniazid on the elimination of quinine in man. *Br J Clin Pharmacol* 1995; **40:** 87–91.

**Tobacco smoking.** A single-dose study in healthy subjects has suggested that blood concentrations of quinine are lower in heavy smokers than in non-smokers, potentially impairing efficacy.[1]

1. Wanwimolruk S, *et al.* Cigarette smoking enhances the elimination of quinine. *Br J Clin Pharmacol* 1993; **36:** 610–14.

## Pharmacokinetics

The pharmacokinetics of quinine are altered significantly by malaria infection, the major effects being reductions in both its apparent volume of distribution and its clearance.

Quinine is rapidly and almost completely absorbed from the gastrointestinal tract and peak concentrations in the circulation are attained about 1 to 3 hours after oral administration of the sulfate or bisulfate. Plasma protein binding is about 70% in healthy subjects and rises to 90% or more in patients with malaria. Quinine is widely distributed throughout the body. Concentrations attained in the CSF of patients with cerebral malaria have been reported to be about 2 to 7% of those in the plasma.

Quinine is extensively metabolised in the liver and rapidly excreted mainly in the urine. Estimates of the proportion of unchanged quinine excreted in the urine vary from less than 5 to 20%. Excretion is increased in acid urine. The elimination half-life is about 11 hours in healthy subjects but may be prolonged in patients with malaria. Small amounts of quinine also appear in the bile and saliva.

Quinine crosses the placenta and is distributed into breast milk (see Breast Feeding, above).

◊ References.

1. White NJ. Clinical pharmacokinetics of antimalarial drugs. *Clin Pharmacokinet* 1985; **10:** 187–215.
2. Supanaranond W, *et al.* Disposition of oral quinine in acute falciparum malaria. *Eur J Clin Pharmacol* 1991; **40:** 49–52.
3. Wanwimolruk S, *et al.* Pharmacokinetics of quinine in young and elderly subjects. *Trans R Soc Trop Med Hyg* 1991; **85:** 714–17.
4. Dyer JR, *et al.* The pharmacokinetics and pharmacodynamics of quinine in the diabetic and non-diabetic elderly. *Br J Clin Pharmacol* 1994; **38:** 205–12.
5. Sowunmi A, Salako LA. Effect of dose size on the pharmacokinetics of orally administered quinine. *Eur J Clin Pharmacol* 1996; **49:** 383–6.
6. Krishna S, White NJ. Pharmacokinetics of quinine, chloroquine and amodiaquine: clinical implications. *Clin Pharmacokinet* 1996; **30:** 263–99.
7. Boele van Hensbroek M, *et al.* Quinine pharmacokinetics in young children with severe malaria. *Am J Trop Med Hyg* 1996; **54:** 237–42.
8. Zhang H, *et al.* Evidence for involvement of human CYP3A in the 3-hydroxylation of quinine. *Br J Clin Pharmacol* 1997; **43:** 245–52.
9. Viriyayudhakorn S, *et al.* Pharmacokinetics of quinine in obesity. *Trans R Soc Trop Med Hyg* 2000; **94:** 425–8.

**Administration in liver disease.** Reduced clearance of quinine and prolonged elimination half-life have been reported in patients with acute hepatitis B given a single intravenous dose.[1] The results suggested that quinine accumulation following multiple doses could be greater in patients with hepatitis, even once hepatic function had returned to normal. In another study[2] patients with moderate chronic liver disease were given quinine by mouth; the half-life was prolonged but total clearance was not affected.

1. Karbwang J, *et al.* The pharmacokinetics of quinine in patients with hepatitis. *Br J Clin Pharmacol* 1993; **35:** 444–6.
2. Auprayoon P, *et al.* Pharmacokinetics of quinine in chronic liver disease. *Br J Clin Pharmacol* 1995; **40:** 494–7.

**Administration in renal impairment.** As urinary clearance comprises only 20% of total clearance of quinine, it appears that high plasma concentrations reported in patients with severe falciparum malaria and acute renal failure may be related more to the severity of the malaria, and associated pharmacokinetic changes, rather than to any reduction in the glomerular filtration rate.[1] There were significant changes in the pharmacokinetics of quinine in 6 patients with chronic renal failure following a single oral dose.[2] The changes included a prolonged half-life, but there was no clear relationship between severity of renal failure and the degree of impairment of quinine clearance.

1. White NJ. Clinical pharmacokinetics of antimalarial drugs. *Clin Pharmacokinet* 1985; **10:** 187–215.
2. Rimchala P, *et al.* Pharmacokinetics of quinine in patients with chronic renal failure. *Eur J Clin Pharmacol* 1996; **49:** 497–501.

## Uses and Administration

Quinine is a cinchona alkaloid and a 4-methanolquinoline antimalarial that is a rapid-acting blood schizontocide with activity against *Plasmodium falciparum, P. vivax, P. ovale*, and *P. malariae*. It is active against the gametocytes of *P. malariae* and *P. vivax*, but not against mature gametocytes of *P. falciparum*. The precise mechanism of action of quinine is unclear but it may interfere with lysosome function or nucleic acid synthesis in the malaria parasite. Since it has no activity against exoerythrocytic forms, quinine does not produce a radical cure in vivax or ovale malarias. The increasing spread of resistance to chloroquine has been responsible for the re-emergence of quinine as an important drug in the treatment of falciparum malaria. Quinine is not generally used for malaria prophylaxis.

Quinine is also used to treat the protozoal infection babesiosis and for the relief of nocturnal leg cramps.

Quinine has mild analgesic and antipyretic properties and is sometimes included in preparations used for the symptomatic relief of the common cold and influenza; additional salts that have been used for this purpose include the camsilate and the gluconate.

Quinine is also used as a bitter and a flavour.

Quinine is given as a number of salts and 100 mg of anhydrous quinine is approximately equivalent to:

- 169 mg of quinine bisulfate
- 122 mg of quinine dihydrochloride
- 122 mg of quinine etabonate
- 130 mg of quinine hydrobromide
- 122 mg of quinine hydrochloride
- 121 mg of quinine sulfate

For the *treatment of malaria* quinine is given by mouth, usually as the sulfate, hydrochloride, or dihydrochloride, or parenterally as the dihydrochloride; quinine etabonate is sometimes used for oral administration because, unlike other quinine salts which are intensely bitter, it is tasteless. They all contain about the same amount of quinine and any of them can be used when the dose is cited in terms of "quinine salt"; this is not the case for the bisulfate, which contains a correspondingly smaller amount of quinine. Quinine formate is sometimes used for parenteral administration.

A course of treatment with quinine for falciparum malaria usually lasts 7 days and in uncomplicated infections treatment should preferably be given by the oral route. The usual oral dose is 600 mg of quinine salt given every 8 hours for 7 days. For children, a dose of 10 mg of quinine salt per kg body-weight given every 8 hours for 7 days is recommended.

In severe or complicated falciparum malaria, or when the patient is unable to take oral medication, quinine should be given parenterally by slow intravenous infusion, but this can be hazardous and patients generally need monitoring, particularly for signs of cardiotoxicity. Therapy should be changed to oral administration as soon as possible to complete the course. To obtain therapeutic concentrations rapidly with parenteral therapy, quinine is often given in an initial loading dose followed by maintenance doses. Recommended dosage regimens for intravenous administration include an initial loading dose of 20 mg of quinine dihydrochloride per kg (up to a maximum of 1.4 g) given over 4 hours with maintenance infusions being started 8 hours later, calculated from the start of the previous infusion. Alternatively, in intensive care units, an initial loading dose of 7 mg/kg may be given over 30 minutes followed immediately by the first of the maintenance infusions. Maintenance infusions consist of 10 mg/kg (up to a maximum of 700 mg) given over 4 hours every 8 hours. A loading dose should not be given if the patient has received quinine, quinidine, mefloquine, or halofantrine, during the previous 24 hours. If parenteral therapy is required for more than 48 hours the maintenance dose of quinine dihydrochloride should be reduced to 5 to 7 mg/kg. If intravenous infusion is not possible, quinine dihydrochloride has been given intramuscularly with doses, including the loading dose, the same as those used for intravenous administration; it should be diluted in sodium chloride 0.9% to a concentration of 60 to 100 mg of the dihydrochloride per mL, and the total dose divided between two administration sites, preferably each anterior thigh (not the buttock). However, intramuscular administration can be irritant and there have been concerns regarding its safety and efficacy (see under Malaria, below).

When used for the *relief of nocturnal leg cramps*, quinine is given at night in a dose of 200 to 300 mg by mouth of the sulfate or bisulfate. Quinine benzoate has also been used.

**Babesiosis.** Although there is no established specific treatment for babesiosis (p.595), a combination of quinine and clindamycin has been used for *Babesia microti* infections.[1-3] Suggested adult doses[3] are quinine 650 mg three times daily by mouth for 7 days, with clindamycin 1.2 g twice daily intravenously or 600 mg three times daily by mouth for 7 to 10 days. Children may be given quinine 25 mg/kg daily plus clindamycin 20 to 40 mg/kg daily, both by mouth in 3 divided doses and both for 7 days. Quinine with azithromycin was reported to be effective in a patient who had not responded to quinine with clindamycin.[4]

1. Wittner M, *et al.* Successful chemotherapy of transfusion babesiosis. *Ann Intern Med* 1982; **96:** 601–4.
2. Anonymous. Clindamycin and quinine treatment for Babesia microti infections. *MMWR* 1983; **32:** 65–6, 72.
3. Medical Letter on Drugs and Therapeutics. Drugs for parasitic infections (issued April 2002). Available at: http://www.medicalletter.com/freedocs/parasitic.pdf (accessed 26/01/04)
4. Shaio MF, Yang KD. Response of babesiosis to a combined regimen of quinine and azithromycin. *Trans R Soc Trop Med Hyg* 1997; **91:** 214–15.

**Flavouring.** The Joint FAO/WHO Expert Committee on Food Additives concluded that quinine levels in soft drinks of up to 100 mg/litre (as quinine base) were not of toxicological concern.[1] However, because of the possibility of hypersensitivity reactions in some individuals, the committee recommended that consumers be informed of the presence of quinine in food or beverages.

1. FAO/WHO. Evaluation of certain food additives and contaminants: forty-first report of the joint FAO/WHO expert committee on food additives. *WHO Tech Rep Ser 837* 1993.

**Malaria.** Quinine has an important role in the treatment of falciparum malaria (see p.444) being used where there is chloroquine or multidrug *Plasmodium falciparum* resistance,[1-4] and also (in view of the widespread problem of *P. falciparum* resistance) where the infective species is not known, or if the infection is mixed. Ideally treatment should be with one of the quinine salts given by mouth, with a dose of 600 mg of quinine salt for adults, or 10 mg/kg for children, every 8 hours for 7 days. However, to reduce quinine-related adverse effects and thereby improve compliance, a 3-day course of quinine salt combined with either 7 days of a tetracycline or a single dose of pyrimethamine-sulfadoxine (Fansidar) or clindamycin for 3 days may be considered in regions without quinine resistance. The dose of quinine salt applies to the hydrochloride, dihydrochloride, sulfate, and etabonate, but not to the bisulfate. Any quinine lost through vomiting within one hour after oral administration should be replaced by additional doses.[1]

The oral route may not provide effective treatment in severe infection and in such cases quinine should be given as the dihydrochloride by slow intravenous infusion, with the patient being observed closely, particularly for any signs of cardiotoxicity.[4] Loading doses of quinine are often used to obtain therapeutic blood concentrations as soon as possible in severely ill patients but they should not be given to patients who have received quinine, quinidine, mefloquine, or halofantrine, within the previous 24 hours.

WHO[4] recommends that an initial loading dose of quinine dihydrochloride 20 mg/kg [up to a maximum of 1.4 g] be given intravenously over 4 hours followed 8 hours after the start of the loading dose by maintenance infusions of 10 mg/kg given over 4 hours and repeated every 8 hours (sometimes the interval may be every 12 hours). Alternatively, in intensive care units, a loading dose of 7 mg/kg may be given by intravenous infusion over 30 minutes followed immediately by the first of the maintenance infusions. Patients are transferred to oral therapy as soon as possible, at a dose of 10 mg of quinine salt per kg every 8 hours, and treatment continued until a total of at least 7 days of therapy has been given. However, if patients still require parenteral therapy after 48 hours it has been suggested that maintenance doses should be reduced to 5 to 7 mg/kg. If intravenous formulations of quinine are unavailable quinidine may be used as an alternative; for further details, see under the Uses and Administration of Quinidine, p.993.

If facilities for administration by intravenous infusion, including monitoring, are not available WHO[4] recommends that quinine should be given by deep intramuscular injection. A loading dose of quinine dihydrochloride 20 mg/kg may be given by injection in divided sites followed by injections of 10 mg/kg every 8 hours; a dose interval of 12 hours has also been employed. Patients should be transferred to oral therapy as soon as possible. The use of the intramuscular route has been controversial because of concerns over safety and efficacy. However, some studies have demonstrated that it can safely be used in adults and children with severe infections.[5-8] Intramuscular injections of quinine can be irritant and have caused pain, focal necrosis, and abscess formation; fatal tetanus has developed in some patients.[9] It has been suggested that some such reactions may be related to the use of preparations formulated in urethane or other irritant substances. Diluted solutions of quinine dihydrochloride 60 mg/mL adjusted to neutral pH appear to be less painful than the usual undiluted preparation of 300 mg/mL.

If facilities do not exist to administer quinine parenterally then patients with severe malaria should receive quinine by mouth or nasogastric tube. Rectal administration has also been suggested.[10]

Quinine as formerly standardised used to contain a higher concentration of cinchona alkaloids and there might be synergy between mixtures of these alkaloids.[11] In practice no advantage has been demonstrated by such mixtures over quinine alone in the treatment of chloroquine-resistant falciparum malaria.[12]


1. WHO. *WHO model prescribing information: drugs used in parasitic diseases*. 2nd ed. Geneva: WHO, 1995.
2. Molyneux M, Fox R. Diagnosis and treatment of malaria in Britain. *BMJ* 1993; **306:** 1175–80.
3. Medical Letter on Drugs and Therapeutics. Drugs for parasitic infections (issued April 2002). Available at: http://www.medicalletter.com/freedocs/parasitic.pdf (accessed 19/04/04)
4. WHO. *Management of severe malaria: a practical handbook*. Geneva: WHO, 2000.
5. Wattanagoon Y, *et al.* Intramuscular loading dose of quinine for falciparum malaria: pharmacokinetics and toxicity. *BMJ* 1986; **293:** 11–13. Correction. *ibid.*; 362.
6. Mansor SM, *et al.* The safety and kinetics of intramuscular quinine in Malawian children with moderately severe falciparum malaria. *Trans R Soc Trop Med Hyg* 1990; **84:** 482–7.
7. Waller D, *et al.* The pharmacokinetic properties of intramuscular quinine in Gambian children with severe falciparum malaria. *Trans R Soc Trop Med Hyg* 1990; **84:** 488–91.
8. Schapira A, *et al.* Comparison of intramuscular and intravenous quinine for the treatment of severe and complicated malaria in children. *Trans R Soc Trop Med Hyg* 1993; **87:** 299–302.
9. Yen LM, *et al.* Role of quinine in the high mortality of intramuscular injection tetanus. *Lancet* 1994; **344:** 786–7.
10. Barennes H. Is intrarectal injectable quinine a safe alternative to intramuscular injectable quinine? *Trop Doct* 1994; **24:** 32–3.
11. Druilhe P, *et al.* Activity of a combination of three cinchona bark alkaloids against Plasmodium falciparum in vitro. *Antimicrob Agents Chemother* 1988; **32:** 250–4.
12. Bunnag D, *et al.* A combination of quinine, quinidine and cinchonine (LA 40221) in the treatment of chloroquine resistant falciparum malaria in Thailand: two double-blind trials. *Trans R Soc Trop Med Hyg* 1989; **83:** 66.


**Muscle spasm.** Quinine (usually as quinine sulfate or bisulfate) has traditionally been used for nocturnal cramps (p.1386) but there has been concern over its efficacy and potential for adverse effects, especially in the elderly. In the USA, for example, the FDA ruled that quinine products should no longer be used for the management of nocturnal cramps.[1,2] Meta-analyses[3,4] concluded that although quinine was effective in the treatment of nocturnal cramps in ambulatory patients the risk of serious adverse effects should be borne in mind. It was recommended that patients should be closely monitored while the efficacy of quinine is assessed over a period of at least 4 weeks. Some[5] have recommended that treatment be stopped every 3 months to see whether it is still needed.

Haemodialysis-induced cramp has been reported to respond to treatment with quinine.[6,7]


1. FDA. Drug products for the treatment and/or prevention of nocturnal leg muscle cramps for over-the-counter human use. *Fed Regist* 1994; **59:** 43234–52.
2. Nightingale SL. Quinine for nocturnal leg cramps. *ACP J Club* 1995; **123:** 86.
3. Man-Son-Hing M, Wells G. Meta-analysis of efficacy of quinine for treatment of nocturnal leg cramps in elderly people. *BMJ* 1995; **310:** 13–17.
4. Man-Son-Hing M, *et al.* Quinine for nocturnal leg cramps: a meta-analysis including unpublished data. *J Gen Intern Med* 1998; **13:** 600–606.
5. Anonymous. Quinine for nocturnal leg cramps? *Drug Ther Bull* 1996; **34:** 7–8.
6. Kaji DM, *et al.* Prevention of muscle cramps in haemodialysis patients by quinine sulphate. *Lancet* 1976; **ii:** 66–7.
7. Roca AO, *et al.* Dialysis leg cramps; efficacy of quinine versus vitamin E. *ASAIO J* 1992; **38:** M481–M485.


## Preparations

***BP 2003:*** Quinine Bisulphate Tablets; Quinine Dihydrochloride Intravenous Infusion; Quinine Sulphate Tablets;
***USP 27:*** Quinine Sulfate Capsules; Quinine Sulfate Tablets.

**Proprietary Preparations** (details are given in Part 3)
***Arg.:*** Circonyl; ***Austral.:*** Biquinate; Myoquin; Quinate; Quinbisul; Quinoctal; Quinsul; ***Braz.:*** Diclo†; Impalud†; Palukin; Paluquina; ***Denm.:*** Kinin; ***Fr.:*** Quinoforme; Surquina; ***Ger.:*** Limptar N; Sagittaproct†; ***India:*** Quininga; ***NZ:*** Q200; Q300; Quinoc†; ***Swed.:*** Kinin; ***Switz.:*** Circonyl N†; ***Thai.:*** Genin.

**Multi-ingredient:** ***Austria:*** Dilatol-Chinin; Iromin-Chinin-C; Limptar; Seltoc; Togal†; ***Belg.:*** Eugrippine†; Spasmosedine†; ***Braz.:*** Monotrean; Monotrean B6†; Paludil†; ***Fin.:*** Crampiton; Relapamil; ***Fr.:*** Arsiquinoformet; Dinacode; Hexaquine; Pholcones†; Quinimax; Quinisedine; Tussipax a l'Euquinine†; ***Ger.:*** Limptar; Togal; ***Irl.:*** Anadin; ***Ital.:*** Monotrean; ***Neth.:*** Aflukin C†; ***NZ:*** Nicobrevin; ***Port.:*** Broncosil; Bronquico†; Recto Bronco Tosse†; Rectopulmo Adultos; Transbronquina Rectal†; ***S.Afr.:*** Cetamine†; Ilvico; ***Spain:*** Brota Rectal Bals; ***UK:*** Nicobrevin; Ronpirin APCQ†.

## Tafenoquine *(BAN, rINN)*

Tafenoquina; WR-238605. (±)-8-[(4-Amino-1-methylbutyl)amino]-2,6-dimethoxy-4-methyl-5-[(α,α,α-trifluoro-*m*-tolyl)oxy]quinoline; (*RS*)-$N^4$-[2,6-Dimethoxy-4-methyl-5-(3-trifluoromethylphenoxy)quinolin-8-yl]pentane-1,4-diamine.

$C_{24}H_{28}F_3N_3O_3$ = 463.5.
*CAS — 106635-80-7.*

### Profile

Tafenoquine is an 8-aminoquinoline antimalarial. It acts as a tissue schizontocide and is under investigation as the succinate for the radical cure and prevention of relapse in vivax malaria. It may also have a role in the prophylaxis of falciparum malaria.

◊ References.


1. Walsh DS, *et al.* Randomized dose-ranging study of the safety and efficacy of WR 238605 (tafenoquine) in the prevention of relapse of Plasmodium vivax malaria in Thailand. *J Infect Dis* 1999; **180:** 1282–7.
2. Lell B, *et al.* Malaria chemoprophylaxis with tafenoquine: a randomised study. *Lancet* 2000; **355:** 2041–5.
3. Shanks GD, *et al.* A new primaquine analogue, tafenoquine (WR 238605), for prophylaxis against Plasmodium falciparum malaria. *Clin Infect Dis* 2001; **33:** 1968–74.
4. Nasveld P, *et al.* Comparison of tafenoquine (WR238605) and primaquine in the post-exposure (terminal) prophylaxis of vivax malaria in Australian Defence Force personnel. *Trans R Soc Trop Med Hyg* 2002; **96:** 683–4.
5. Hale BR, *et al.* A randomized, double-blind, placebo-controlled, dose-ranging trial of tafenoquine for weekly prophylaxis against Plasmodium falciparum. *Clin Infect Dis* 2003; **36:** 541–9.

# Antimigraine Drugs

Analgesic-induced headache, p.464
Cluster headache, p.464
Migraine, p.464
Post-dural puncture headache, p.465
Tension-type headache, p.465

This chapter reviews the management of headache, in particular migraine and cluster headache, and the drugs used mainly for their treatment. The mechanisms of head pain or headache are not fully understood but may involve neurovascular changes (as in migraine and cluster headache), muscle contraction (tension headache), nerve lesions (neuralgias), direct head injury, infection (meningitis), or referred pain (sinusitis, toothache, eye disorders). Headache is also an adverse effect of many drugs including, paradoxically, those used to treat it. The International Headache Society has published guidelines to aid the diagnosis of the various headache types. Patients may have more than one headache disorder simultaneously and require separate treatment for each.

◊ References.

1. Headache Classification Subcommittee of the International Headache Society. The international classification of headache disorders: 2nd edition. *Cephalalgia* 2004; **24** (suppl 1): 9–160. Also available at: http://216.25.100.131/ihscommon/guidelines/pdfs/ihc_II_main_no_print.pdf (accessed 01/06/04)

### Analgesic-induced headache

Overuse of analgesics and other drugs such as ergotamine or caffeine to treat headache can lead to dependence and paradoxical chronic daily headache in headache-prone patients; such headaches do not appear to occur when these drugs are used to treat other disorders.[1] Such analgesic-induced headaches, also referred to as rebound headaches or analgesic abuse headaches, are relieved by withdrawal of the offending drug, but the primary headache may still persist. Furthermore, abrupt discontinuation can exacerbate headache and produce other symptoms of withdrawal. This may then lead the patient to resume treatment to relieve the headache thereby setting up a vicious circle.

Analgesic-induced headache can be difficult to treat. Options for outpatient treatment include either gradual or abrupt withdrawal of the overused analgesic, sometimes together with substitution by a long-acting NSAID or intramuscular dihydroergotamine.[2,3] However, withdrawal symptoms may persist for up to 2 weeks and detoxification may require hospitalisation; intravenous metoclopramide and repetitive intravenous dihydroergotamine may be required to control nausea and vomiting and intractable headache, respectively. General advice on the prevention of analgesic-induced headache has included limiting the frequency of administration of analgesics and the avoidance of compound and opioid analgesics.[1,2]

1. Olesen J. Analgesic headache. *BMJ* 1995; **310:** 479–80.
2. Silberstein SD, Young WB. Analgesic rebound headache. *Drug Safety* 1995; **13:** 133–44.
3. Zed PJ, *et al.* Medication-induced headache: overview and systematic review of therapeutic approaches. *Ann Pharmacother* 1999; **33:** 61–72.

### Cluster headache

Cluster headache (migrainous neuralgia, histaminic cephalalgia, Horton's syndrome) is of unknown aetiology but may be neurovascular in origin.[1-3] Patients experience one or more short-lived attacks of intense unilateral head pain, usually at the same time of day (often at night). Restlessness during the attacks is characteristic. The period during which attacks occur is called a cluster period; it may last several weeks. In the typical episodic form of cluster headache, cluster periods are followed by periods of remission lasting for months or years but in the more rare chronic form, patients may have cluster periods lasting for more than a year, or with very short periods of remission in between. Substances such as alcohol or glyceryl trinitrate can precipitate headache attacks during cluster periods, but not during periods of remission. There is speculation that sleep disordered breathing[4] and increased body heat[5] may also trigger cluster headaches.

The **treatment** of individual acute attacks during a cluster period is difficult because the headache is short-lived and oral analgesics are unlikely to be absorbed fast enough to produce much benefit.[1,2] Inhalation of 100% oxygen is rapid and effective in aborting attacks, but because of practical difficulties other treatments such as inhaled ergotamine or subcutaneous sumatriptan are more likely to be used. Dihydroergotamine is also effective but generally requires administration by injection and is usually reserved for use in emergency settings. Intranasal instillation of lidocaine has been reported to be of some benefit but most patients do not obtain complete pain relief.[1,2]

Since individual attacks are difficult to treat it is probably more effective to manage cluster headache by **prophylaxis** once a cluster period has started. Ergotamine may be used for prevention in episodic cluster headache; it is given by mouth or rectally for limited periods of up to 2 weeks. It is often given for only 5 to 6 days in each week, which allows the patient to assess whether the cluster period has ended. Other drugs that have been used, either alone or with ergotamine, include verapamil, lithium carbonate, and prednisolone. Some consider verapamil to be the preventive therapy of choice.[1] Lithium may be particularly useful for the chronic form of the disorder. Methysergide, pizotifen, and valproate have also been tried.[1,2]

Chronic paroxysmal hemicrania is a rare variant of cluster headache in which patients experience numerous attacks every day for years. One of its features, which may be diagnostic, is its invariable response to indometacin.

1. Dodick DW, Capobianco DJ. Treatment and management of cluster headache. *Curr Pain Headache Rep* 2001; **5:** 83–91.
2. Ekbom K, Hardebo JE. Cluster headache: aetiology, diagnosis and management. *Drugs* 2002; **62:** 61–9.
3. Zakrzewska JM. Cluster headache: review of literature. *Br J Oral Maxillofac Surg* 2001; **39:** 103–13.
4. Chervin RD, *et al.* Sleep disordered breathing in patients with cluster headache. *Neurology* 2000; **54:** 2302–6.
5. Blau JN, Engel HO. A new cluster headache precipitant: increased body heat. *Lancet* 1999; **354:** 1001–2.

### Migraine

Migraine is characterised by recurrent attacks of headache which typically last 4 to 72 hours. Attacks persisting for longer than 72 hours are referred to as status migrainosus. The headache is usually a unilateral pulsating pain that is aggravated by movement and is usually of sufficient severity to disturb or prevent daily activities. It is frequently accompanied by nausea, vomiting, or other gastrointestinal disturbances and there may be photophobia and phonophobia. Migraine with aura (classic migraine) is characterised by an aura consisting of visual or sensory symptoms that lasts less than an hour. The headache usually follows the aura directly, or within 1 hour, but may begin simultaneously with the aura. In addition, aura can occur without headache. Migraine without aura (common migraine) is the more common form occurring in about 75% of patients with migraine. Premonitory symptoms may occur before a migraine attack (with or without aura). Familial hemiplegic migraine is a rare syndrome in which migraine with aura may be preceded or accompanied by aphasia, confusion, and hemiparesis. Basilar migraine is another rare form of migraine with aura in which there may be disturbances of the brain stem or occipital lobes accompanied by symptoms such as impairment of consciousness, vertigo, ataxia, dysarthria, and diplopia.

Migraine is described as a neurovascular headache. Traditionally, intracranial vasoconstriction was considered responsible for the aura and extracranial vasodilatation for the headache. However, it appears that vascular events may be secondary to neuropathic changes and the liberation of vasoactive substances including serotonin (5-HT), catecholamines, histamine, kinins, neuropeptides such as calcitonin gene-related peptide (CGRP), and prostaglandins.

There are several factors which may precipitate migraine attacks. These include anxiety, physical and emotional stress, a change in sleep pattern, bright lights, fasting, some foods, and menstruation. Menstrual migraine has no specific definition, but it is believed to occur around the time of menstruation and to be characterised by attacks without aura. Migraine may also be precipitated by drugs including combined oral contraceptives and oestrogens, and glyceryl trinitrate. The frequency of migraine attacks can be reduced if such precipitating factors can be identified and avoided. Quiet, darkness, and sleep can ease an attack, with sleep heralding recovery.

**Treatment**. There is evidence that therapy tailored to the severity of individual disease from the outset (stratified care) is preferable to beginning with simple analgesics and adjusting treatment subsequently according to response (step strategy).

Simple **analgesics** (paracetamol or aspirin and other NSAIDs) are effective if taken at the earliest signs of an attack. Weak opioid analgesics such as codeine are sometimes included in oral compound analgesic preparations, but many consider that opioids are best avoided, especially in patients who experience frequent headaches.

If the initial treatment of migraine is delayed, absorption of oral drugs may be compromised by development of gastric stasis and nausea and vomiting; **antiemetics** such as buclizine, cyclizine, and the **prokinetic** drugs metoclopramide and domperidone are often included in compound antimigraine preparations. Prokinetic drugs also have the advantage of promoting gastric emptying and normal peristalsis. Dispersible and effervescent analgesic preparations are preferable because of their more rapid absorption. If nausea and vomiting is prominent rectal administration may be necessary.

Attacks not responding to simple analgesics or NSAIDs may be treated with specific antimigraine drugs such as the selective serotonin ($5\text{-HT}_1$) agonists (e.g. sumatriptan) and the ergot derivatives ergotamine and dihydroergotamine; poor absorption and adverse effects limit the use of ergot derivatives and selective serotonin ($5\text{-HT}_1$) agonists are generally preferred.

Serotonin ($5\text{-HT}_1$) agonists are highly effective in relieving the pain and nausea of a migraine attack. There are a number of **triptans** available; patient characteristics and preferences vary in response to use and can sometimes be unpredictable. Some patients experience recurrence of the headache within 24 to 48 hours and often respond to a second dose. Finding the best triptan to suit the individual patient may involve trial and error. Triptans should not be used in patients with major risk factors for, or suffering from, cardiovascular disease. The main concern with all triptans is their potential for coronary vasoconstriction and no triptan appears to be safer than the others.

If **ergotamine** is used it should be given at the first warning of an attack; the earlier it is given, the more effective the treatment. Since its oral bioavailability is poor and may be reduced further during a migraine attack, ergotamine has sometimes been administered in sublingual or rectal preparations or by oral inhaler. Ergotamine can also exacerbate nausea and vomiting; metoclopramide or domperidone, or in severe cases the phenothiazines chlorpromazine or prochlorperazine, may be given. Dihydroergotamine may be of use if parenteral treatment is required; it can also be given intranasally but there is less experience with this route.

Patients who rapidly develop severe migraine may be given **parenteral** dihydroergotamine or sumatriptan. If there is no response to these drugs dopamine antagonists such as metoclopramide, chlorpromazine, or prochlorperazine given parenterally may be effective in relieving the pain of acute migraine attacks. Prolonged attacks (status migrainosus) may require intravenous administration of dihydroergotamine with metoclopramide.

**Other drugs** that may be given alone or in combination include prochlorperazine, chlorpromazine, corticosteroids, or pethidine. Lidocaine has been given intravenously for the emergency treatment of migraine; intranasal lidocaine has also been tried. The opioid agonist-antagonist butorphanol, administered by nasal spray, has been advocated, but its place in therapy, if any, remains to be established. Other drugs under investigation include botulinum A toxin and CGRP antagonists; intravenous valproic acid has also shown promise in aborting acute attacks.

**Prophylactic treatment** should be considered for patients in whom abortive measures are ineffective or migraine attacks occur frequently, or for those with less frequent but severe or prolonged attacks. Some recommend prophylaxis if attacks occur more often than once or twice a month. Prophylaxis can reduce the severity and/or frequency of attacks but does not eliminate them completely and patients still need additional abortive or symptomatic treatment. Drugs suggested for prophylaxis have a range of actions which reflects uncertainty over the pathogenesis of migraine. It is important to give prophylactic drugs for an adequate period before assessing their efficacy. Once an optimum effect has been achieved the need for continuing prophylaxis should be reviewed at intervals of about 3 to 6 months.

The main prophylactic drugs are **beta blockers**, **pizotifen**, tricyclic **antidepressants**, and **valproate**. Propranolol is considered by many to be the prophylactic drug of choice.

Lethargy appears to be the most common adverse effect. Other beta blockers reported to be effective are those that, like propranolol, possess no intrinsic sympathomimetic activity, which include atenolol, metoprolol, nadolol, and timolol. The potential for beta blockers to interact with some serotonin ($5-HT_1$) agonists and ergotamine should be borne in mind. Pizotifen, an antihistamine and serotonin antagonist, is one of the main alternatives to propranolol. Drowsiness and increased appetite with weight gain may be a problem, although these may be overcome to some extent by gradual increases in dose and administration at night. Tricyclic antidepressants, particularly amitriptyline, given in gradually increasing doses at night are useful for preventing migraine, especially in patients who also have depression or tension-type headache, although antimuscarinic side-effects may occur.

**Other drugs** have been used for the prophylaxis of migraine: of the drugs with calcium-channel blocking activity, flunarizine appears to be effective and verapamil may be useful, but evidence for the efficacy of other calcium-channel blockers such as diltiazem, nifedipine, or nimodipine is less convincing; NSAIDs may be worth trying. The use of methysergide, a potent serotonin antagonist, has declined because of serious side-effects, in particular retroperitoneal fibrosis. MAOIs such as phenelzine have been used occasionally but are best reserved for severe cases refractory to other forms of prophylactic treatment. Cyproheptadine, an antihistamine and serotonin antagonist, has been used for migraine prophylaxis, particularly in children. Other drugs used for the prophylaxis of migraine have included clonidine, cyclandelate, indoramin, and feverfew, and the ergot derivatives lisuride and metergoline. Positive results have been seen with riboflavin; magnesium (as the citrate) may also be of use. Other drugs still under investigation, which have shown potential for prevention of migraine attacks are: baclofen, botulinum A toxin, lisinopril, topiramate, and venlafaxine.

References.


1. Ferrari MD. Migraine. *Lancet* 1998; **351:** 1043–51.
2. Anonymous. Managing migraine. *Drug Ther Bull* 1998; **36:** 41–4.
3. Diener H-C, *et al.* A practical guide to the management and prevention of migraine. *Drugs* 1998; **56:** 811–24.
4. Bartleson JD. Treatment of migraine headaches. *Mayo Clin Proc* 1999; **74:** 702–8.
5. Tfelt-Hansen P, *et al.* Triptans in migraine: a comparative review of pharmacology, pharmacokinetics and efficacy. *Drugs* 2000; **60:** 1259–87.
6. Lipton RB, *et al.* Stratified care vs step care strategies for migraine: the Disability in Strategies of Care (DISC) study, a randomised trial. *JAMA* 2000; **284:** 2599–2605.
7. Ferrari MD, *et al.* Oral triptans (serotonin $5-HT_{1B/1D}$ agonists) in acute migraine treatment: a meta-analysis of 53 trials. *Lancet* 2001; **358:** 1668–75.
8. Rapaport AM, Tepper SJ. Triptans are all different. *Arch Neurol* 2001; **58:** 1479–80.
9. Anonymous. Drugs for migraine. In: *Drugs of choice from The Medical Letter.* 14th ed. New York: The Medical Letter, 2001: 131–7.
10. Jamieson DG. The safety of triptans in the treatment of patients with migraine. *Am J Med* 2002; **112:** 135–40.
11. Goadsby PJ, *et al.* Migraine—current understanding and treatment. *N Engl J Med* 2002; **346:** 257–70.
12. Cady R, Dodick DW. Diagnosis and treatment of migraine. *Mayo Clin Proc* 2002; **77:** 255–61.
13. Steiner TJ, Fontebasso M. Headache. *BMJ* 2002; **325:** 881–6.
14. Snow V, *et al.* Pharmacologic management of acute attacks of migraine and prevention of migraine headache. *Ann Intern Med* 2002; **137:** 840–9.
15. Silberstein SD. Migraine. *Lancet* 2004; **363:** 381–91.
16. Anonymous. Managing migraine in children. *Drug Ther Bull* 2004; **42:** 25–8.


### Post-dural puncture headache

For the management of headache associated with lumbar puncture or spinal anaesthesia, see Post-dural Puncture Headache under Local Anaesthetics, p.1368.

### Tension-type headache

Tension-type headaches, also referred to as muscle-contraction headaches, are probably the commonest form of headache. They are characterised by bilateral pain, which unlike migraine is continuous and non-pulsatile. The pain is often described by the patient as feeling like a tight band pressed around the head. Headaches of this type may be precipitated by many factors including psychosocial stress or muscular stress. Many patients also have associated symptoms of anxiety or depression. Also tension-type headaches and migraine frequently co-exist when they are often referred to as combination or mixed headaches. Some patients may only experience isolated acute attacks of tension-type headache (episodic tension-type headache), but others may develop chronic tension-type headache which is difficult to treat.

**Treatment** is aimed at removing the underlying causes where these can be identified. Simple massage may help if muscle contraction is a prominent component of the pain. Non-opioid analgesics, such as aspirin or other NSAIDs and paracetamol, may be tried for individual acute attacks of headache, but analgesic overuse must be avoided as this can lead to chronic headache resistant to other measures (see Analgesic-induced Headache, above). Opioids alone or in combination preparations with other analgesics should also be avoided. Hypnotics or sedatives have sometimes been used in combination preparations with analgesics in the management of tension-type headache that disrupts sleep but, because of the potential for abuse, they should be avoided in chronic headaches. Muscle relaxants appear to have little place in the management of tension-type headache; although some patients may respond results are generally disappointing. **Prophylaxis** is preferable to regular short-term use of analgesics in controlling chronic tension-type headache. Tricyclic antidepressants, particularly amitriptyline, are generally considered as first choice, although benefit is rarely complete. The mode of action is unclear and appears to be independent of any antidepressant action. In most cases, improvement is seen with low doses, but full antidepressant doses are necessary in the presence of underlying depression. Addition of a beta blocker such as propranolol may sometimes be of benefit for patients with some migraine features. Other drugs that have been tried include valproate and botulinum A toxin.

References.


1. Clough C. Non-migrainous headaches: classification and management. *BMJ* 1989; **299:** 70–2.
2. Olesen J, Schoenen J, eds. *Tension-type headache: classification, mechanisms, and treatment.* New York: Raven Press, 1993.
3. Silberstein SD. Tension-type and chronic daily headache. *Neurology* 1993; **43:** 1644–9.
4. Kumar KL, Cooney TG. Headaches. *Med Clin North Am* 1995; **79:** 261–86.
5. Anonymous. Management of tension-type headache. *Drug Ther Bull* 1999; **37:** 41–4.


## Almotriptan Malate *(BANM, USAN, rINNM)*

LAS-31416 (almotriptan); Malato de almotriptán; PNU-180638E (almotriptan malate). 1-[({3-[2-(Dimethylamino)ethyl]indol-5-yl}methyl)sulfonyl]pyrrolidine malate (1:1).

$C_{17}H_{25}N_3O_2S,C_4H_6O_5$ = 469.6.

*CAS — 154323-57-6 (almotriptan); 181183-52-8 (almotriptan malate).*

*ATC — N02CC05.*

### Adverse Effects and Precautions

As for Sumatriptan, p.471.

Almotriptan should not be used in patients with severe hepatic impairment since clearance is likely to be markedly impaired, and should be given with caution to patients with mild to moderate degrees of hepatic impairment. The dose of almotriptan should be reduced in patients with severe renal impairment.

Patients with hypersensitivity to sulfonamides may theoretically exhibit a similar reaction to almotriptan.

### Interactions

As for Sumatriptan, p.472.

### Pharmacokinetics

After oral doses, peak plasma-almotriptan concentrations are obtained in about 1 to 3 hours, with a bioavailability of about 70%. Protein binding is about 35%. Almotriptan is metabolised, primarily by monoamine oxidase type A to the inactive indole acetic acid derivative and to a lesser extent by cytochrome P450 isoenzymes CYP3A4 and CYP2D6 to the inactive gamma-aminobutyric acid derivative. More than 75% of an oral dose is excreted in the urine and the remainder in faeces. Approximately 40 to 50% of the dose in the urine and 5% in the faeces is excreted as unchanged drug. The plasma elimination half-life is about 3.5 hours in healthy subjects, increasing to about 7 hours in severe renal impairment.

Distribution into milk has been demonstrated in studies in *rats.*

### Uses and Administration

Almotriptan malate is a selective serotonin ($5-HT_1$) agonist with actions and uses similar to those of sumatriptan (p.473). It is used for the acute treatment of the headache phase of migraine attacks. It should not be used prophylactically. Almotriptan is given by mouth as the malate, and doses are expressed in terms of the base; almotriptan malate 8.75 mg is approximately equivalent to 6.25 mg of almotriptan.

The usual dose of almotriptan is 12.5 mg in the UK and 6.25 or 12.5 mg in the USA. If this is ineffective, a second dose should not be taken for the same attack. If the headache recurs within 24 hours, a second dose may be taken after an interval of at least 2 hours. No more than 2 doses should be taken in a 24-hour period. For doses in hepatic and renal impairment see below.

◊ References.


1. Holm KJ, Spencer CM. Almotriptan. *CNS Drugs* 1999; **11:** 159–64.
2. Keam SJ, *et al.* Almotriptan: a review of its use in migraine. *Drugs* 2002; **62:** 387–414.


**Administration in hepatic or renal impairment.** In patients with hepatic impairment or severe renal impairment, no more than 12.5 mg of almotriptan should be taken in 24 hours; a starting dose of 6.25 mg may be used. Almotriptan is contra-indicated in patients with severe hepatic disease.

**Migraine.** For comparison of the relative benefits of different triptans in migraine, see under Sumatriptan, p.473.

Further references.


1. Pascual J, *et al.* Consistent efficacy and tolerability of almotriptan in the acute treatment of multiple migraine attacks: results of a large, randomized, double-blind, placebo-controlled study. *Cephalalgia* 2000; **20:** 588–96.
2. Cabarrocas X, *et al.* Long-term efficacy and safety of oral almotriptan: interim analysis of a 1-year open study. *Headache* 2001; **41:** 57–62.
3. Balbisi EA. Efficacy and safety of almotriptan malate for migraine. *Am J Health-Syst Pharm* 2002; **59:** 2184–93.


### Preparations

**Proprietary Preparations** (details are given in Part 3)
**Belg.:** Almogran; **Denm.:** Almogran; **Fin.:** Almogran; **Fr.:** Almogran; **Ger.:** Almogran; **Irl.:** Almogran; **Ital.:** Almotrex; **Norw.:** Almogran; **Spain:** Almogran; **Swed.:** Almogran; **UK:** Almogran; **USA:** Axert.

## Alpiropride *(rINN)*

Alpiroprida. (±)-*N*-[(1-Allyl-2-pyrrolidinyl)methyl]-4-amino-5-(methylsulfamoyl)-*o*-anisamide.

$C_{17}H_{26}N_4O_4S$ = 382.5.

*CAS — 81982-32-3.*

### Profile

Alpiropride is a dopamine antagonist that has been given by mouth for the treatment and prophylaxis of migraine.

### Preparations

**Proprietary Preparations** (details are given in Part 3)
**Port.:** Rivistel.

## Dihydroergotamine *(BAN, rINN)*

Dihidroergotamina. (5′S,8R)-5′-Benzyl-9,10-dihydro-12′-hydroxy-2′-methyl-3′,6′,18-trioxoergotaman.

$C_{33}H_{37}N_5O_5$ = 583.7.

*CAS — 511-12-6.*

*ATC — N02CA01.*

## Dihydroergotamine Mesilate *(BANM, rINNM)*

Dihydroergotamine Mesylate *(USAN)*; Dihydroergotamine Methanesulphonate; Dihydroergotamini Mesilas; Mesilato de dihidroergotamina. (5′S,8R)-5′-Benzyl-9,10-dihydro-12′-hydroxy-2′-methyl-3′,6′,18-trioxoergotaman methanesulphonate.

$C_{33}H_{37}N_5O_5,CH_4O_3S$ = 679.8.

*CAS — 6190-39-2.*

*ATC — N02CA01.*

**Pharmacopoeias.** In *Eur.* (see p.vi), *Jpn, Pol.,* and *US.*

**Ph. Eur. 5.0** (Dihydroergotamine Mesilate). Colourless crystals or a white or almost white crystalline powder. Slightly soluble in water and in alcohol; sparingly soluble in methyl alcohol. A 0.1% solution in water has a pH of 4.4 to 5.4. Protect from light.

**USP 27** (Dihydroergotamine Mesylate). A white to slightly yellowish powder, or off-white to faintly red powder, having a faint odour. Soluble 1 in 125 of water, 1 in 90 of alcohol, 1 in 175 of chloroform, and 1 in 2600 of ether. pH of a 0.1% solution in water is between 4.4 and 5.4. Protect from light.

### Dihydroergotamine Tartrate *(BANM, rINNM)*

Dihydroergotamini Tartras; Tartrato de dihidroergotamina.

$(C_{33}H_{37}N_5O_5)_2,C_4H_6O_6$ = 1317.4.

*CAS — 5989-77-5.*

*ATC — N02CA01.*

**Pharmacopoeias.** In *Eur.* (see p.vi).

**Ph. Eur. 5.0** (Dihydroergotamine Tartrate). Colourless crystals or a white or almost white crystalline powder. Very slightly soluble in water; sparingly soluble in alcohol. A 0.1% suspension in water has a pH of 4.0 to 5.5. Protect from light.

## Adverse Effects and Treatment

As for Ergotamine Tartrate, p.467, although vasoconstriction may be less pronounced and the frequency of nausea and vomiting lower with dihydroergotamine mesilate than with ergotamine tartrate. Dihydroergotamine does not appear to produce physical dependence.

**Effects on the cardiovascular system.** There are conflicting reports on the risk of vasospasm in patients given dihydroergotamine with heparin for thromboembolism prophylaxis. Vasospastic or necrotic reactions have been reported on several occasions during such therapy.[1-4] In an Austrian study of 147 290 patients given drug prophylaxis for thromboembolism, complications attributable to ergotism were seen in 142 of 61 092 (0.23%) who received dihydroergotamine and heparin.[5] Others,[6] however, observed only 1 case of vasospasm in 5100 trauma patients (0.02%) given the combination. In 1989 the Swedish Adverse Drug Reactions Advisory Committee reported[7] that up to the end of September 1987 the manufacturer had received 201 reports of vasospastic reactions associated with the use of Orstanorm (dihydroergotamine + lidocaine) with heparin. Permanent damage occurred in 59% of these patients. Vasospastic reactions had occurred more frequently in patients who had undergone surgery for trauma and the prognosis for such patients was generally poorer than for others. Since the risk of permanent damage appeared to be related to treatment length the Committee recommended that this preparation should not be given for more than 7 days. The possibility of such reactions and the contra-indications of dihydroergotamine should be borne in mind when using this form of prophylaxis (see Venous Thromboembolism, under Uses, below).


1. van den Berg E, *et al.* Ergotism leading to threatened limb amputation or to death in two patients given heparin-dihydroergotamine prophylaxis. *Lancet* 1982; **i:** 955–6.
2. van den Berg E, *et al.* Vascular spasm during thromboembolism prophylaxis with heparin-dihydroergotamine. *Lancet* 1982; **ii:** 268–9.
3. Monreal M, *et al.* Skin and muscle necrosis during heparin-dihydroergotamine prophylaxis. *Lancet* 1984; **ii:** 820.
4. Kilroy RA, *et al.* Vascular spasm during heparin-dihydroergotamine prophylaxis. *Clin Pharm* 1987; **6:** 575–7.
5. Gatterer R. Ergotism as complication of thromboembolic prophylaxis with heparin and dihydroergotamine. *Lancet* 1986; **ii:** 638–9.
6. Schlag G, *et al.* Risk/benefit of heparin-dihydroergotamine thromboembolic prophylaxis. *Lancet* 1986; **ii:** 1465.
7. Swedish Adverse Drug Reaction Advisory Committee. Dihydroergotamine + lidocaine – vasospasm. *Bull Swed Adverse Drug React Advisory Committee* 1989; (54): 1.


**Fibrosis.** For reference to fibrosis associated with the administration of dihydroergotamine, see Methysergide Maleate, p.469.

## Precautions

As for Ergotamine Tartrate, p.467.

**Cardiovascular disorders.** For specific contra-indications and precautions in cardiovascular disorders, see under Ergotamine, p.468.

**Porphyria.** Dihydroergotamine has been associated with acute attacks of porphyria and is considered unsafe in porphyric patients.

## Interactions

See under ergotamine (p.468). Concurrent administration of other vasoconstrictive drugs, including supplementary antimigraine treatment with ergotamine or sumatriptan, should be avoided.

## Pharmacokinetics

Peak plasma-dihydroergotamine concentrations have been attained within about 1 to 2 hours after oral doses, about 30 minutes after intramuscular injection, about 15 to 45 minutes after subcutaneous injection, and about 45 to 55 minutes after administration by intranasal spray. However, the bioavailability of dihydroergotamine after oral administration is very low; values ranging from less than 0.1 to 1.5% have been reported. Although dihydroergotamine is incompletely absorbed from the gastrointestinal tract, the low bioavailability is considered to be determined primarily by extensive first-pass hepatic metabolism. It is 93% bound to plasma proteins.

Dihydroergotamine undergoes extensive metabolism, the major metabolite, 8′-β-hydroxydihydroergotamine, being pharmacologically active. Plasma concentrations of this metabolite are greater than those of dihydroergotamine. A further oxidation step produces 8′,10′-dihydroxydihydroergotamine which is also pharmacologically active. Other metabolites are also formed. Most of a dose is excreted as metabolites, mainly in the bile; 5 to 10% is excreted in the urine of which only trace amounts are of unchanged drug. The elimination of dihydroergotamine is biphasic; half-lives of about 1 to 2 hours and 22 to 32 hours have been reported for the 2 phases, respectively.

◊ References.


1. Bobik A, *et al.* Low oral bioavailability of dihydroergotamine and first-pass extraction in patients with orthostatic hypotension. *Clin Pharmacol Ther* 1981; **30:** 673–9.
2. Little PJ, *et al.* Bioavailability of dihydroergotamine in man. *Br J Clin Pharmacol* 1982; **13:** 785–90.
3. Lindblad B, *et al.* The pharmacokinetics of subcutaneous dihydroergotamine with and without a dextran 70 infusion. *Eur J Clin Pharmacol* 1983; **24:** 813–18.
4. Maurer G, Frick W. Elucidation of the structure and receptor binding studies of the major primary, metabolite of dihydroergotamine in man. *Eur J Clin Pharmacol* 1984; **26:** 463–70.
5. Müller-Schweinitzer E. Pharmacological actions of the main metabolites of dihydroergotamine. *Eur J Clin Pharmacol* 1984; **26:** 699–705.
6. Aellig WH, Rosenthaler J. Venoconstrictor effects of dihydroergotamine after intranasal and intramuscular administration. *Eur J Clin Pharmacol* 1986; **30:** 581–4.
7. de Marées H, *et al.* Relationship between the venoconstrictor activity of dihydroergotamine and its pharmacokinetics during acute and chronic oral dosing. *Eur J Clin Pharmacol* 1986; **30:** 685–9.
8. Humbert H, *et al.* Human pharmacokinetics of dihydroergotamine administered by nasal spray. *Clin Pharmacol Ther* 1996; **60:** 265–75.


## Uses and Administration

Dihydroergotamine is a semisynthetic ergot alkaloid that has weaker oxytocic and vasoconstrictor effects than ergotamine (p.468). Its activity as a 5-$HT_1$ agonist is believed to contribute to its antimigraine action. It is used in the treatment of migraine and cluster headache, and in the treatment of orthostatic hypotension. It has also been used for the prophylaxis of venous thromboembolism (see below).

Dihydroergotamine is commonly used as the mesilate by subcutaneous, intramuscular, or intravenous injection, although it may also be given as a nasal spray or by mouth.

For the treatment of migraine and to terminate an acute attack of cluster headache, dihydroergotamine mesilate is usually given by subcutaneous or intramuscular injection in doses of 1 mg repeated, if necessary, after 30 to 60 minutes up to a maximum daily dose of 3 mg. If a more rapid effect is desired it may be given intravenously in doses of 0.5 or 1 mg up to a maximum daily dose of 2 mg. The total weekly dose given by any route of injection should not exceed 6 mg. The usual nasal dose of dihydroergotamine mesilate for an acute attack of migraine is 0.5 mg sprayed into each nostril as a 0.4% solution followed after 15 minutes by an additional 0.5 mg in each nostril. A total intranasal dose of 2 mg per attack should not be exceeded. In the USA, the maximum dose in 24 hours is 3 mg and in a 7-day period is 4 mg, while maximum daily doses of up to 4 mg with a maximum dose of 12 mg in a 7-day period have been given in other countries. In some countries it is given by mouth; up to 10 mg daily has been given by mouth for the treatment of acute attacks of migraine. Lower oral doses have been given in some countries for migraine prophylaxis.

Dihydroergotamine mesilate has also been used alone or with etilefrine hydrochloride (p.914) in the treatment of orthostatic hypotension, in usual doses of up to 10 mg daily by mouth in divided doses. Doses of up to 40 to 60 mg have been used in some patients.

Dihydroergotamine tartrate has been used for indications similar to those of the mesilate.

**Analgesic-induced headache.** Dihydroergotamine may be used in the treatment of analgesic-induced headache (p.464), including symptoms of ergotamine withdrawal.

**Migraine and cluster headache.** Although sumatriptan is often the treatment of choice to abort acute attacks of migraine (p.464) that do not respond to simple analgesic preparations, parenteral dihydroergotamine is an alternative for patients who develop severe or refractory migraine.[1,2] Preparations for intranasal[3,4] administration are also available; in some countries, it is given orally. In a comparative study, relief of migraine was slower after subcutaneous dihydroergotamine than after subcutaneous sumatriptan, but headache recurred less often.[5] In another study, intranasal dihydroergotamine was not as effective as subcutaneous sumatriptan.[4]

Dihydroergotamine is also used in the treatment of cluster headache (p.464), usually in emergency settings, where it is given to abort individual headache attacks.


1. Scott AK. Dihydroergotamine: a review of its use in the treatment of migraine and other headaches. *Clin Neuropharmacol* 1992; **15:** 289–96.
2. Silberstein SD, Young WB. Safety and efficacy of ergotamine tartrate and dihydroergotamine in the treatment of migraine and status migrainosus. *Neurology* 1995; **45:** 577–84.
3. Ziegler D, *et al.* Dihydroergotamine nasal spray for the acute treatment of migraine. *Neurology* 1994; **44:** 447–53.
4. Touchon J, *et al.* A comparison of subcutaneous sumatriptan and dihydroergotamine nasal spray in the acute treatment of migraine. *Neurology* 1996; **47:** 361–5.
5. Winner P, *et al.* A double-blind study of subcutaneous dihydroergotamine vs subcutaneous sumatriptan in the treatment of acute migraine. *Arch Neurol* 1996; **53:** 180–4.


**Orthostatic hypotension.** Dihydroergotamine may be of use in patients with refractory orthostatic hypotension (p.1100). It is sometimes used in preparations with sympathomimetics such as etilefrine. After parenteral administration of dihydroergotamine, standing blood pressure is increased, but total peripheral resistance and supine blood pressure are also increased.[1] It does not prevent postprandial hypotension, presumably because it does not constrict the splanchnic veins, although administration with caffeine may overcome this problem. The main disadvantage of dihydroergotamine, however, is that it is ineffective, or at best weakly effective, when given by mouth although there has been some evidence that oral ergotamine tartrate may be of value.

Dihydroergotamine has been suggested for use in the prevention of hypotension associated with epidural anaesthesia,[2] the usual management of which is discussed under Treatment of Adverse Effects of Local Anaesthetics, p.1368. It has also been tried in the management of hypotension associated with haemodialysis.[3]


1. Anonymous. Management of orthostatic hypotension. *Lancet* 1987; **i:** 197–8.
2. Mattila M, *et al.* Dihydroergotamine in the prevention of hypotension associated with extradural anaesthesia. *Br J Anaesth* 1985; **57:** 976–82.
3. Milutinovic S. Dihydroergotamin in der Behandlung von Patienten mit symptomatischer Hypotonie während Dauerhämodialyse. *Arzneimittelforschung* 1987; **37:** 554–6.


**Venous thromboembolism.** Standard prophylaxis for surgical patients at high risk of venous thromboembolism is usually with heparin (p.839). Dihydroergotamine can reduce venous stasis by vasoconstriction of capacitance vessels and has enhanced postoperative prophylaxis when used in association with heparin.[1] Doses of dihydroergotamine mesilate 500 micrograms with heparin 5000 units, both given subcutaneously 2 hours before surgery, have been used. This regimen has then been given every 8 to 12 hours for 5 to 14 days depending on the risk of thrombosis. Some workers have investigated the use of dihydroergotamine with low-molecular-weight heparin fractions. Such a combination has been demonstrated to be of similar efficacy to dihydroergotamine with heparin[2,3] but might offer a more convenient dosing schedule. However, although dihydroergotamine might enhance the effect of heparin, a US National Institutes of Health consensus conference warned of the potential risk associated with its vasoconstrictive effects, and the contra-indications to its use.[4] In 1989 the Swedish Adverse Drug Reactions Advisory Committee recommended that dihydroergotamine with heparin should not be given for more than 7 days (see Effects on the Cardiovascular System, under Adverse Effects, above).


1. Lindblad B. Prophylaxis of postoperative thromboembolism with low dose heparin alone or in combination with dihydroergotamine: a review. *Acta Chir Scand* 1988; (suppl 543): 31–42.
2. Sasahara AA, *et al.* Low molecular weight heparin plus dihydroergotamine for prophylaxis of postoperative deep vein thrombosis. *Br J Surg* 1986; **73:** 697–700.
3. Haas S, *et al.* Prophylaxis of deep vein thrombosis in high risk patients undergoing total hip replacement with low molecular weight heparin plus dihydroergotamine. *Arzneimittelforschung* 1987; **37:** 839–43.
4. Consensus conference. Prevention of venous thrombosis and pulmonary embolism. *JAMA* 1986; **256:** 744–9.


## Preparations

***USP 27:*** Dihydroergotamine Mesylate Injection.

**Proprietary Preparations** (details are given in Part 3)

***Austral.:*** Dihydergot; ***Austria:*** Adhaegon; Detemes; Dihydergot; Divegal; Ergont; Ergovasan; Migranal; ***Belg.:*** Diergo; Dihydergot; Dystonal†; Ikaran†; ***Braz.:*** Dihydergot; ***Canad.:*** Migranal; ***Fin.:*** Orstanorm; ***Fr.:*** Ikaran; Seglor; Tamik; ***Ger.:*** Agit; Angionorm; Clavigrenin; DET MS; DET MS spezial; DHE; Dihydergot; Dihytamin; Endophleban†; Ergomimet; Ergont; ergotam; Tonopres†; Verladyn; ***Gr.:*** Dihydergot; Pervone; ***Hong Kong:*** Tamik; ***India:*** Dihydergot; Migranil; ***Ital.:*** Diidergot; Ikaran; Migranal; Seglor; ***Mex.:*** Dihydergot; ***Neth.:*** Dihydergot; ***Port.:*** Dihydergot; Seglor; ***S.Afr.:*** Dihydergot†; ***Spain:*** Dihydergot; Tenuatina†; ***Swed.:*** Migranal; Orstanorm; ***Switz.:*** Dihydergot; Ergotonine; Ikaran; ***Thai.:*** Poligot†; ***UK:*** Migranal†; ***USA:*** DHE; Migranal.

**Multi-ingredient:** ***Arg.:*** Parsel; Polper Vascular; ***Austria:*** Agilan; Defluina; Dihydergot; Effortil comp; Embolex; Hypodyn; Tonopan; Troparin compositum; Veno†; Venotop; Wallerox; ***Braz.:*** Cefalium; Cefaliv; Migraliv; Parcel; Tonopan; Vasofluina†; ***Chile:*** Migratapsin; Migrax; Parsel; ***Fr.:***

Diergospray; **Ger.:** Agit plus; Dihydergot plus; Effortil plus; Embolex NM; Ergo-Lonarid PD; Ergolefrin; Ergomimet plus; Optalidon special NOC; Venelbin†; **Mex.:** Parsel; Tonopan; **Spain:** Tonopan; **Switz.:** Dihydergot; Dihydergot plus; Effortil plus; Tonopan.

## Eletriptan Hydrobromide

*(BANM, USAN, rINNM)*

UK-116044-04. 3-{[(R)-1-Methyl-2-pyrrolidinyl]methyl}-5-[2-(phenylsulfonyl)ethyl]indole hydrobromide.

$C_{22}H_{26}N_2O_2S,HBr$ = 463.4.

*CAS — 143322-58-1 (eletriptan); 177834-92-3 (eletriptan hydrobromide).*

*ATC — N02CC06.*

### Adverse Effects and Precautions

As for Sumatriptan p.471.

Eletriptan should not be used in patients with severe hepatic or severe renal impairment. Blood pressure effects of eletriptan are increased in renal impairment and therefore the dose should be reduced in patients with mild to moderate renal impairment. No dosage adjustment is needed in mild or moderate hepatic impairment.

**Breast feeding.** Eletriptan is distributed into human breast milk and the manufacturer has suggested that infant exposure can be minimised by avoiding breast feeding for 24 hours after treatment.

### Interactions

As for Sumatriptan, p.472. Eletriptan should not be given with potent inhibitors of the cytochrome P450 isoenzyme CYP3A4 such as erythromycin and ketoconazole; increased plasma levels of eletriptan have been noted after such combinations.

### Pharmacokinetics

After oral doses eletriptan is rapidly and well absorbed (at least 81%) and has a bioavailability of about 50%. Peak plasma concentrations are attained within 1.5 hours. Eletriptan is about 85% protein bound. It is primarily metabolised by hepatic cytochrome P450 isoenzyme CYP3A4. Non-renal clearance accounts for about 90% of the elimination of eletriptan. A small amount is distributed into human breast milk.

◊ References.

1. Shah AK, *et al.* Pharmacokinetics and safety of oral eletriptan during different phases of the menstrual cycle in healthy volunteers. *J Clin Pharmacol* 2001; **41:** 1339–44.

### Uses and Administration

Eletriptan hydrobromide is a selective serotonin ($5\text{-}HT_1$) agonist with actions and uses similar to those of sumatriptan (p.473). It is used for acute treatment of the headache phase of migraine attacks. It should not be used prophylactically. Eletriptan is given by mouth as the hydrobromide, but doses are expressed in terms of the base; eletriptan hydrobromide 24.2 mg is approximately equivalent to 20 mg of eletriptan.

The usual dose is 40 mg; if this is ineffective a second dose should not be taken for the same attack. If the headache recurs within 24 hours a second dose may be taken after an interval of at least 2 hours. Doses of 80 mg may be used in subsequent attacks, but should not be repeated within a 24-hour period. For doses in hepatic and renal impairment, see below.

**Administration in hepatic impairment.** No dose adjustment for eletriptan is needed in patients with mild to moderate hepatic impairment. Eletriptan has not been studied in patients with severe hepatic impairment and therefore the manufacturers do not recommend its use.

**Administration in renal impairment.** In the UK, a dose of 20 mg of eletriptan is recommended in patients with mild to moderate renal impairment, increased if necessary to 40 mg. The maximum daily dose should not exceed 40 mg. Eletriptan should not be used in severe renal impairment.

**Migraine.** For comparison of the relative benefits of different triptans in migraine, see under Sumatriptan, p.473.

### Preparations

**Proprietary Preparations** (details are given in Part 3)

**Braz.:** Relpax†; **Denm.:** Relpax; **Fin.:** Relert; **Fr.:** Relepax; Relpax; **Israel:** Relert; **Ital.:** Relpax; **Mex.:** Relpax; **Norw.:** Relpax; **Spain:** Relert; Relpax; **Swed.:** Relpax; **Switz.:** Relpax; **UK:** Relpax; **USA:** Relpax.

## Ergotamine Tartrate *(BANM, rINNM)*

Ergotamini Tartras; Tartrato de ergotamina. (5′S)-12′-Hydroxy-2′-methyl-5′-benzylergotaman-3′,6′,18-trione tartrate; (5′S)-12′-Hydroxy-2′-methyl-3′,6′,18-trioxo-5-benzylergotaman (+)-tartrate.

$(C_{33}H_{35}N_5O_5)_2,C_4H_6O_6$ = 1313.4.

*CAS — 113-15-5 (ergotamine); 379-79-3 (ergotamine tartrate).*

*ATC — N02CA02.*

**Pharmacopoeias.** In *Chin., Eur.* (see p.vi), *Int., Jpn, Pol.,* and *US.*

**Ph. Eur. 5.0** (Ergotamine Tartrate). Slightly hygroscopic, colourless crystals or a white or almost white crystalline powder. It may contain 2 molecules of methanol of crystallisation. Slightly soluble in alcohol. Aqueous solutions slowly become cloudy owing to hydrolysis; this may be prevented by the addition of tartaric acid. A 0.25% suspension in water has a pH of 4.0 to 5.5. Store in airtight glass containers at a temperature of 2° to 8°. Protect from light.

**USP 27** (Ergotamine Tartrate). Colourless odourless crystals or a white or yellowish-white crystalline powder. Soluble 1 in about 3200 of water, but soluble 1 in about 500 of water in the presence of a slight excess of tartaric acid; soluble 1 in 500 of alcohol. Store at a temperature not exceeding 8°. Protect from light.

**Stability in solution.** References.

1. Kreilgård B, Kisbye J. Stability of ergotamine tartrate in aqueous solution. *Arch Pharm Chemi (Sci)* 1974; **2:** 1–13 and 38–49.

### Adverse Effects

The adverse effects of ergotamine may be attributed either to its effects on the CNS, or to vasoconstriction of blood vessels and possible thrombus formation.

After therapeutic doses nausea and vomiting commonly occur as a result of the direct emetogenic effect of ergotamine; some patients may also experience abdominal pain. Weakness and muscle pains in the extremities and numbness and tingling of the fingers and toes may occur. There may occasionally be localised oedema and itching in hypersensitive patients. Treatment should be stopped if symptoms of vasoconstriction develop. Susceptible patients, especially those with sepsis, liver disease, kidney disease, or occlusive peripheral vascular disease, may show signs of acute or chronic poisoning with normal doses of ergotamine.

Symptoms of acute overdosage include nausea, vomiting, diarrhoea, extreme thirst, coldness, tingling, and itching of the skin, a rapid and weak pulse, hypotension, shock, confusion, convulsions, and unconsciousness; fatalities have been reported. Further symptoms of peripheral vasoconstriction or of cardiovascular disturbances, as seen in chronic ergotamine poisoning, may also occur but may be delayed.

In chronic poisoning or ergotism, resulting from therapeutic overdosage or the use of ergotamine in susceptible patients, severe circulatory disturbances may develop. The extremities, especially the feet and legs, become numb, cold, tingling, and pale or cyanotic, with muscle pain; there may be no pulse in the affected limb. Eventually gangrene develops in the toes and sometimes the fingers. Anginal pain, tachycardia or bradycardia, and hypertension or hypotension have been reported. Myocardial infarction has occurred rarely. Pleural and peritoneal fibrosis may occur with excessive use and there have been rare cases of fibrosis of the cardiac valves. Chronic, intractable headache (rebound headache) may occur and is also a major withdrawal symptom following the development of ergotamine dependence (see under Precautions, below). Other adverse effects include confusion and convulsions. On rare occasions symptoms of vasoconstriction of blood vessels in the brain, eye, intestines, and kidneys occur. Anorectal ulceration, sometimes leading to rectal necrosis and stenosis or rectovaginal fistula, has been reported after excessive use of suppositories containing ergotamine.

**Effects on the cardiovascular system.** Reports of adverse cardiovascular effects associated with ergotamine, including mention of fatalities.

1. Joyce DA, Gubbay SS. Arterial complications of migraine treatment with methysergide and parenteral ergotamine. *BMJ* 1982; **285:** 260–1.
2. Corrocher R, *et al.* Multiple arterial stenoses in chronic ergot toxicity. *N Engl J Med* 1984; **310:** 261.
3. Fisher PE, *et al.* Ergotamine abuse and extra-hepatic portal hypertension. *Postgrad Med J* 1985; **61:** 461–3.
4. Deviere J, *et al.* Ischemic pancreatitis and hepatitis secondary to ergotamine poisoning. *J Clin Gastroenterol* 1987; **9:** 350–2.
5. Galer BS, *et al.* Myocardial ischemia related to ergot alkaloids: a case report and literature review. *Headache* 1991; **31:** 446–50.
6. Redfield MM, *et al.* Valve disease associated with ergot alkaloid use: echocardiographic and pathologic correlations. *Ann Intern Med* 1992; **117:** 50–2.
7. Lazarides MK, *et al.* Severe facial ischaemia caused by ergotism. *J Cardiovasc Surg* 1992; **33:** 383–5.
8. Hillis W, MacIntyre PD. Drug reactions: sumatriptan and chest pain. *Lancet* 1993; **341:** 1564–5. Correction. *ibid.*; **342:** 1310.

**Fibrosis.** For reference to fibrosis associated with the use of ergotamine tartrate, see Methysergide Maleate, p.469.

### Treatment of Adverse Effects

Treatment of acute poisoning with ergotamine is symptomatic. Following recent ingestion the stomach may be emptied by lavage; activated charcoal may be used to reduce absorption if ingestion has occurred within 1 hour. In chronic poisoning, withdrawal of ergotamine may be all that is required in some patients.

In both acute and chronic poisoning, attempts must be made to maintain an adequate circulation to the affected parts of the body in order to prevent the onset of gangrene. In severe arterial vasospasm vasodilators such as sodium nitroprusside by intravenous infusion have been given; heparin and dextran 40 have also been advocated to minimise the risk of thrombosis. Analgesics may be required for severe ischaemic pain.

◊ Sodium nitroprusside has been administered in severe ergotamine poisoning for its vasodilating and hypotensive actions; it should therefore be used with care if hypotension is a symptom of poisoning. It is usually given by intravenous infusion[1-4] although there have also been reports of intra-arterial infusion for ergotamine-induced ischaemia;[5,6] for details of precautions to be observed, see p.1001.

Many other drugs have been used in the treatment of circulatory disturbances induced by ergotamine. These include captopril by mouth[7] and alprostadil by intra-arterial infusion.[8,9]

For reference to the ergotamine withdrawal syndrome, see Dependence under Precautions, below.

1. Carliner NH, *et al.* Sodium nitroprusside treatment of ergotamine-induced peripheral ischemia. *JAMA* 1974; **277:** 308–9.
2. Andersen PK, *et al.* Sodium nitroprusside and epidural blockade in the treatment of ergotism. *N Engl J Med* 1977; **296:** 1271–3.
3. Eurin B, *et al.* Ergot and sodium nitroprusside. *N Engl J Med* 1978; **298:** 632–3.
4. Carr P. Self-induced myocardial infarction. *Postgrad Med J* 1981; **57:** 654–5.
5. O'Dell CW, *et al.* Sodium nitroprusside in the treatment of ergotism. *Radiology* 1977; **124:** 73–4.
6. Whitsett TL, *et al.* Nitroprusside reversal of ergotamine-induced ischemia. *Am Heart J* 1978; **96:** 700.
7. Zimran A, *et al.* Treatment with captopril for peripheral ischaemia induced by ergotamine. *BMJ* 1984; **288:** 364.
8. Levy JM, *et al.* Prostaglandin $E_1$ for alleviating symptoms of ergot intoxication: a case report. *Cardiovasc Intervent Radiol* 1984; **7:** 28–30.
9. Horstmann R, *et al.* Kritische Extremitätenischämie durch Ergotismus: Behandlung mit intraarterieller Prostaglandin-$E_1$-Infusion. *Dtsch Med Wochenschr* 1993; **118:** 1067–71.

### Precautions

Ergotamine tartrate is contra-indicated in patients with severe or uncontrolled hypertension, severe or persistent sepsis, peripheral vascular disease, ischaemic heart disease, temporal arteritis, hyperthyroidism, or hepatic or renal impairment. Ergotamine tartrate should be used with care in patients with anaemia. It is contra-indicated in pregnancy because of its oxytocic effect (see also below).

Patients should be warned to keep within the recommended dosage. Some symptoms of overdosage may mimic those of migraine. Numbness or tingling of the extremities generally indicates that ergotamine should be discontinued. Although ergotamine is used for limited periods in the prevention of episodic cluster headache, it should not be administered prophylactically in other circumstances, as prolonged use may give rise to gangrene. Dependence has occurred following regular use of ergotamine tartrate even if dosage recommendations are adhered to (see below).

**Breast feeding.** Although the American Academy of Pediatrics includes ergotamine among those drugs that may be given with caution to breast-feeding mothers,[1] it notes that maternal use in doses equivalent to those given for the treatment of migraine has been associated with vomiting, diarrhoea, and convulsions in nursing infants. The UK manufacturers recommend that ergotamine tartrate should be avoided during breast feeding; the distribution of unchanged drug and metabolites into breast milk presents a risk of ergotism in the infant and repeated doses of ergotamine may impair lactation.

1. American Academy of Pediatrics. The transfer of drugs and other chemicals into human milk. *Pediatrics* 2001; **108:** 776–89. Correction. *ibid.*; 1029. Also available at: http://aappolicy.aappublications.org/cgi/content/full/pediatrics%3b108/3/776 (accessed 01/06/04)

**Cardiovascular disorders.** In the USA, dihydroergotamine is contra-indicated in patients with ischaemic heart disease and other cardiovascular disorders such as hypertension, peripheral arterial disease, or coronary artery vasospasm and it is also recommended that it should not be given to those with a family history of ischaemic heart disease, to postmenopausal women or men aged over 40, or to those with other ischaemic risk factors such as hypertension, hypercholesterolaemia, smoking, or obesity, unless cardiovascular evaluation to exclude such disease has been carried out. Similar precautions and contra-indications, which resemble those that apply to serotonin ($5-HT_1$) agonists such as sumatriptan (p.472), may be applicable to other ergot derivatives used in migraine such as ergotamine.

In other countries, warnings concerning the use of ergot derivatives in patients with risk factors for myocardial ischaemia appear to be less stringent, although caution is clearly advisable.

**Dependence.** Dependence can develop insidiously when ergotamine tartrate is used for more than 2 days each week, even if total daily or weekly dosage recommendations are observed.[1] Individual reports indicate a state of addiction characterised by a predictable and irresistible pattern of drug usage, the development of tolerance to adverse effects, and a syndrome of withdrawal on discontinuing the drug. Ergotamine-dependent patients suffer from daily, or almost daily, migraine headaches, often referred to as 'analgesic-induced headaches' or 'rebound headaches', which are only alleviated by ergotamine. An intensifying headache in association with autonomic disturbances occurs within 24 to 48 hours of withdrawal of ergotamine and may continue for 72 hours or longer. As with other analgesic-induced headaches (p.464), supportive and symptomatic measures should be taken to treat the withdrawal syndrome.

1. Saper JR. Ergotamine dependency—a review. *Headache* 1987; **27:** 435–8.

**Porphyria.** Ergotamine tartrate has been associated with acute attacks of porphyria and is considered unsafe in porphyric patients.

**Pregnancy.** Ergotamine is contra-indicated in pregnancy because of its oxytocic effect. Accidental administration of ergotamine 2 mg in the form of a Cafergot suppository to a patient at 39 weeks of pregnancy caused uterine contractions and fetal tachycardia.[1] An emergency caesarean section was undertaken because of suspected placental abruption but no clear signs of retroplacental haemorrhage were found. The neonate recovered quickly after delivery and had developed normally during the next 10 years.

Jejunal atresia has been reported[2] in an infant born prematurely to a woman who had taken ergotamine tartrate 6 to 8 mg daily, as Cafergot tablets, throughout her pregnancy.

1. de Groot ANJA, *et al.* Ergotamine-induced fetal stress: review of side effects of ergot alkaloids during pregnancy. *Eur J Obstet Gynecol Reprod Biol* 1993; **51:** 73–7.
2. Graham JM, *et al.* Jejunal atresia associated with Cafergot ingestion during pregnancy. *Clin Pediatr (Phila)* 1983; **22:** 226–8.

## Interactions

The vasoconstrictor effects of ergotamine are enhanced by sympathomimetics such as adrenaline. There is also an increased risk of peripheral vasoconstriction during use of ergotamine with beta blockers.

Ergotamine is metabolised by the cytochrome P450 isoenzyme CYP3A4 and consequently it should not be given with potent inhibitors of this isoenzyme; elevated ergotamine concentrations sufficient to cause ergotism may occur with macrolide antibacterials such as erythromycin and clarithromycin, and HIV-protease inhibitors including indinavir and ritonavir.

Ergotamine should not be given until at least 6 hours after stopping a serotonin ($5-HT_1$) agonist such as sumatriptan, since there is an additional risk of prolonged vasospastic reactions (see also p.472). Conversely, a delay is advised before starting a serotonin agonist in patients who have been receiving ergotamine: sumatriptan, almotriptan, eletriptan, naratriptan, rizatriptan, or zolmitriptan should not be given until at least 24 hours after stopping the use of preparations containing ergotamine.

**Antibacterials.** Acute reactions ranging from minor ergotism[1] to severe vasospasm[2] have been reported in patients given *erythromycin* in addition to ergotamine. There is also a report of acute ergotism in 2 patients receiving ergotamine tartrate and *troleandomycin*.[3] The theoretical possibility exists that there may be a similar interaction with *azithromycin*. Ergotism has also been reported in patients receiving erythromycin[4] or troleandomycin[5] with dihydroergotamine.

1. Lagier G, *et al.* Un cas d'ergotisme mineur semblant en rapport avec une potentialisation de l'ergotamine par l'éthylsuccinate d'érythromycine. *Therapie* 1979; **34:** 515–21.
2. Ghali R, *et al.* Erythromycin-associated ergotamine intoxication: arteriographic and electrophysiologic analysis of a rare cause of severe ischemia of the lower extremities and associated ischemic neuropathy. *Ann Vasc Surg* 1993; **7:** 291–6.
3. Matthews NT, Havill JH. Ergotism with therapeutic doses of ergotamine tartrate. *N Z Med J* 1979; **89:** 476–7.
4. Leroy F, *et al.* Dihydroergotamine-erythromycin-induced ergotism. *Ann Intern Med* 1988; **109:** 249.
5. Franco A, *et al.* Ergotisme aigu par association dihydroergotamine-triacétyloléandomycine. *Nouv Presse Med* 1978; **7:** 205.

**Antidepressants.** There have been isolated case reports[1] of the serotonin syndrome (p.313) in patients receiving dihydroergotamine with *amitriptyline, imipramine, paroxetine,* or *sertraline.*

1. Mathew NT, *et al.* Serotonin syndrome complicating migraine pharmacotherapy. *Cephalalgia* 1996; **16:** 323–7.

**Antimigraine drugs.** Arterial occlusion has been reported[1] in 2 patients given *methysergide* with a high parenteral dosage of ergotamine for cluster headache; the combination should be avoided. Use of ergotamine as supplementary antimigraine medication in patients receiving *dihydroergotamine* is not recommended.

For reports of arterial vasoconstriction in patients taking *beta blockers* and antimigraine drugs, see below. See also above for a comment on the risk of vasospastic reactions with serotonin ($5-HT_1$) agonists such as *sumatriptan.*

1. Joyce DA, Gubbay SS. Arterial complications of migraine treatment with methysergide and parenteral ergotamine. *BMJ* 1982; **285:** 260–1.

**Antivirals.** Reports of ergotism in 5 patients who received ergotamine and combination antiviral treatment for HIV infection. It was suggested that the ergotism might have been caused by inhibition of ergotamine metabolism by *ritonavir* in 3 cases,[1-3] *indinavir* in one,[4] and *nelfinavir*[5] in the other.

The metabolism of ergot alkaloids may be inhibited by *efavirenz* (p.632).

1. Caballero-Granado FJ, *et al.* Ergotism related to concurrent administration of ergotamine tartrate and ritonavir in an AIDS patient. *Antimicrob Agents Chemother* 1997; **41:** 1207.
2. Montero A, *et al.* Leg ischemia in a patient receiving ritonavir and ergotamine. *Ann Intern Med* 1999; **130:** 329–30.
3. Liandet L, *et al.* Severe ergotism associated with interaction between ritonavir and ergotamine. *BMJ* 1999; **318:** 771.
4. Rosenthal E, *et al.* Ergotism related to concurrent administration of ergotamine tartrate and indinavir. *JAMA* 1999; **281:** 987.
5. Mortier E, *et al.* Ergotism related to interaction between nelfinavir and ergotamine. *Am J Med* 2001; **110:** 594.

**Beta blockers.** Peripheral vasoconstriction was reported in a patient with migraine after addition of *propranolol* to regular use of Cafergot (ergotamine and caffeine) suppositories twice daily.[1] This combination has been used without complication by others, who suggested that excessive dosage of ergotamine tartrate, rather than an interaction between ergotamine and propranolol, was responsible.[2] However, arterial vasoconstriction has been reported after concomitant use of methysergide and propranolol and of *oxprenolol* and ergotamine.[3] Such combinations should therefore be used with caution.

1. Baumrucker JF. Drug interaction—propranolol and Cafergot. *N Engl J Med* 1973; **288:** 916–17.
2. Diamond S. Propranolol and ergotamine tartrate. *N Engl J Med* 1973; **289:** 159.
3. Venter CP, *et al.* Severe peripheral ischaemia during concomitant use of beta blockers and ergot alkaloids. *BMJ* 1984; **289:** 288–9.

**Glyceryl trinitrate.** Glyceryl trinitrate has been reported to increase the oral bioavailability and plasma concentrations of dihydroergotamine in patients with orthostatic hypotension.[1]

1. Bobik A, *et al.* Low oral bioavailability of dihydroergotamine and first-pass extraction in patients with orthostatic hypotension. *Clin Pharmacol Ther* 1981; **30:** 673–9.

**Tacrolimus.** Ergotamine may inhibit the metabolism of tacrolimus (see p.1364).

## Pharmacokinetics

Absorption of ergotamine from the gastrointestinal tract after oral doses is poor and may be further decreased by the occurrence of gastric stasis during migraine attacks. Bioavailability is also diminished by a high first-pass hepatic metabolism. Ergotamine has been given rectally or by inhalation in an attempt to overcome these effects, with some improvement in absorption, but bioavailability is still of the order of 5% or less. Absorption of sublingual ergotamine is very poor. There is considerable interindividual variation in the bioavailability of ergotamine, regardless of the route of administration. Caffeine is sometimes included in oral and rectal preparations of ergotamine to improve the latter's absorption, although whether it does so is not clear. Drugs such as metoclopramide are sometimes given with the aim of alleviating gastric stasis and thus improve the absorption of ergotamine.

Ergotamine is metabolised extensively in the liver via the cytochrome P450 isoenzyme CYP3A4; the majority of metabolites are excreted in the bile. About 4% of a dose is excreted in the urine. Ergotamine or its metabolites have been detected in breast milk. Some of the metabolites are pharmacologically active. The elimination of ergotamine is biphasic; half-lives of about 2 hours and 21 hours have been reported for the 2 phases respectively.

◊ References.

1. Schmidt R, Fanchamps A. Effect of caffeine on intestinal absorption of ergotamine in man. *Eur J Clin Pharmacol* 1974; **7:** 213–16.
2. Eadie MJ. Ergotamine pharmacokinetics in man: an editorial. *Cephalalgia* 1983; **3:** 135–8.
3. Perrin VL. Clinical pharmacokinetics of ergotamine in migraine and cluster headache. *Clin Pharmacokinet* 1985; **10:** 334–52.

## Uses and Administration

Ergotamine is an alkaloid derived from ergot (p.1685). It has marked vasoconstrictor effects, and may have a partial agonist action at serotonin (5-HT) receptors; it also has a powerful oxytocic action on the uterus, although less so than ergometrine (p.1684). It is used in migraine and cluster headache, and has been tried in orthostatic hypotension.

Ergotamine is commonly used as the tartrate. It is usually given by mouth, but has also been given sublingually, rectally, and by oral inhalation. It was formerly given by subcutaneous or intramuscular injection. Caffeine is sometimes given with ergotamine tartrate with the intention of improving the latter's absorption, although whether it does so is not clear. Antiemetics such as cyclizine hydrochloride are sometimes included in combination preparations with ergotamine tartrate.

Ergotamine is used in migraine unresponsive to non-opioid analgesics. However, its adverse effects limit its use and prevent use for prophylaxis. It is most effective when given as early as possible in a migraine attack, preferably during the prodromal phase.

The usual dose is 1 to 2 mg of ergotamine tartrate by mouth, repeated, if necessary, half an hour later. Usually not more than 6 mg should be given in 24 hours, although some manufacturers recommend not more than 4 mg in 24 hours and others not more than 8 mg per attack. The recommended minimum interval between successive 24-hour courses is 4 days, and the total weekly dose is limited to a maximum of 12 mg, although some manufacturers recommend a lower weekly limit of 8 mg. It is also recommended that patients should receive no more than 2 courses per month. Similar doses may be given sublingually.

Ergotamine tartrate may also be given rectally as suppositories, especially if the oral route is not effective or not practicable. The rectal dose of ergotamine tartrate is 2 mg repeated, if necessary, one hour later. Usually, not more than 4 mg should be given in 24 hours and not more than 8 mg in one week with an interval of at least 4 days between successive 24-hour courses.

A more rapid onset of action may be achieved by oral inhalation. One dose containing 360 micrograms of ergotamine tartrate may be inhaled at the onset of the attack and repeated, if necessary, at 5-minute intervals. Not more than 6 inhalation doses should be taken in 24 hours and not more than 12 in one week, with an interval of at least 5 days between successive 24-hour courses.

Ergotamine is used in patients with cluster headache to treat individual attacks of headache but since such attacks are short-lived oral inhalation may be preferable to oral, sublingual, or rectal routes. Doses used are similar to those given to treat migraine. It has also been used to prevent headache attacks during cluster periods, when it is usually given daily in low doses for up to 2 weeks, either by mouth or rectally (see below).

**Migraine and cluster headache.** Ergotamine was formerly one of the main drugs used to treat acute attacks of migraine (p.464) unresponsive to non-opioid analgesics, but triptan serotonin ($5-HT_1$) agonists such as sumatriptan are now preferred. Since ergotamine may exacerbate the nausea and vomiting that commonly develops as a migraine attack progresses it is often necessary to give an antiemetic as well. Poor oral bioavailability may be reduced further during a migraine attack and ergotamine has sometimes been given sublingually, rectally, or by inhalation. Adverse effects limit the dose that can be used for an individual attack and prevent the long-term use that would be required for migraine prophylaxis.

Ergotamine may be used similarly in cluster headache (p.464) to treat individual headaches during a cluster period. Oral inhalation may be more effective than other routes. Ergotamine is also used in low doses given by mouth or rectally for limited periods of up to 2 weeks in the prophylaxis of cluster headache during a cluster period. Regimens that have been tried for such prophylaxis include 1 to 2 mg of ergotamine tartrate given 1 to 2 hours before an expected attack or 1 to 2 hours before bedtime for nocturnal attacks. The total maximum dose of ergotamine tartrate that may be given weekly for the prevention of cluster headache is less well established than for the treatment of migraine. Ergotamine is often given for only 5 to 6 days in each week, which allows the patient to assess whether the cluster period has ended.

References.


1. Silberstein SD, Young WB. Safety and efficacy of ergotamine tartrate and dihydroergotamine in the treatment of migraine and status migrainosus. *Neurology* 1995; **45:** 577–84.


**Orthostatic hypotension.** Ergotamine and dihydroergotamine might be of use in patients with refractory orthostatic hypotension (p.1100). Ergotamine is believed[1] to be less selective than dihydroergotamine (p.466) in its actions and affects both venous capacitance and peripheral resistance.[2,3] However, the oral bioavailability of ergotamine is greater[2] than that of dihydroergotamine and there have also been some reports of successful treatment with inhaled ergotamine.[3,4]


1. Anonymous. Management of orthostatic hypotension. *Lancet* 1987; **i:** 197–8.
2. Ahmad RAS, Watson RDS. Treatment of postural hypotension: a review. *Drugs* 1990; **39:** 74–85.
3. Tonkin AL, Wing LMH. Hypotension: assessment and management. *Med J Aust* 1990; **153:** 474–85.
4. Stumpf JL, Mitrzyk B. Management of orthostatic hypotension. *Am J Hosp Pharm* 1994; **51:** 648–60.


## Preparations

***BP 2003:*** Ergotamine Sublingual Tablets;
***USP 27:*** Ergotamine Tartrate and Caffeine Suppositories; Ergotamine Tartrate and Caffeine Tablets; Ergotamine Tartrate Inhalation Aerosol; Ergotamine Tartrate Injection; Ergotamine Tartrate Tablets.

**Proprietary Preparations** (details are given in Part 3)
***Austral.:*** Ergodryl Mono; ***Austria:*** Ergokapton; ***Braz.:*** Enxak†; Gynergene†; ***Canad.:*** Ergomar†; ***Chile:*** Jaquedryl; ***Ger.:*** ergo sanol spezial N; Ergo-Kranit mono; Migrexa; RubieNex mono†; ***Irl.:*** Lingraine†; ***Ital.:*** Ergotan; ***Thai.:*** Ergosia; Gynaemine; ***UK:*** Lingraine†; ***USA:*** Ergomar.

**Multi-ingredient:** ***Arg.:*** Cafergot; Cefalex; Ibu-Tetralgin; Ibumar Migra; Ibupirac Migra; Jaquedryl; Migra Dioxadol; Migra Dorixina; Migral; Migral Compositum; Migral II; Mikesan; Tetralgin; Tetralgin Novo; Zilactin-E; ***Austral.:*** Cafergot; Ergodryl; Migral†; ***Austria:*** Avamigran; Cafergot; Migril; Secokapton; Synkapton; ***Belg.:*** Cafergot; ***Braz.:*** Cafergot†; Migrane; Ormigrein; ***Canad.:*** Bellergal; Cafergot; Cafergot-PB; Ergodryl; Gravergol; Megral†; Wigraine†; ***Chile:*** Bellergal Retardado; Cafergot-PB; Cefalmin; Cinabel; Clonalgin Compuesto; Ergobelan; Ergonef; Fredol; Migra-Nefersil; Migragesic; Migranol; Migratam; Ultrimin; ***Denm.:*** Ergokoffin; Gynergen Comp; ***Fin.:*** Anervan; ***Fr.:*** Gynergene Cafeine; Migwell†; ***Ger.:*** Avamigran N; Cafergot N; Ergo-Kranit; Ergoffin; Migratan S; RubieNex spezial; ***Gr.:*** Cafergot; ***Hong Kong:*** Cafergot; Gravergol; Migril; ***India:*** Migranil; ***Irl.:*** Cafergot†; Migranat; Migril; ***Israel:*** Cafergot; Temigran; ***Ital.:*** Bellergil†; Cafergot; Virdex; ***Malaysia:*** Cafergot; ***Mex.:*** Cafergot; Ergocaf; Sydolil; Trinergot; ***Neth.:*** Cafergot; ***Norw.:*** Anervan; ***NZ:*** Cafergot; Ergodryl†; Migril†; ***Port.:*** Avamigran; Migretil; ***S.Afr.:*** Bellergal†; Cafergot; Cafergot-PB; Migril; ***Singapore:*** Cafergot; Migril†; ***Spain:*** Cafergot; Cafergot-PB; Distovagal†; Hemicraneal; Igril†; ***Swed.:*** Anervan; Cafergot; ***Switz.:*** Bellagotin; Bellergal†; Cafergot; Cafergot-PB; Ergosanol a la cafeine†; Ergosanol special a la cafeine†; Ergosanol special†; Migrexa†; Migril†; ***Thai.:*** Avamigran; Bellergal; Benera; Cafergot; Degran; Neuramizone; Poligot-CF; Polygot; ***UK:*** Cafergot; Migril; ***USA:*** Bel-Phen-Ergot S; Bellamine; Bellergal-S; Cafatine; Cafatine-PB; Cafergot; Cafetrate†; Ercaf; Folergot-DF; Phenerbel-S; Wigraine.

## Feverfew

Camomille (Grande); Matricaria; Tanaceti Parthenii Herba.

**Pharmacopoeias.** In *Eur.* (see p.vi). Also in *USNF* which describes additionally Powdered Feverfew.

**Ph. Eur. 5.0** (Feverfew). The dried, whole or fragmented aerial parts of *Tanacetum parthenium*. It contains not less than 0.2% of parthenolide ($C_{15}H_{20}O_3$ = 248.3), calculated with reference to the dried drug. It has a camphoraceous odour. Protect from light.

**USNF 22** (Feverfew). It consists of the dried leaves of *Tanacetum parthenium* (Asteraceae), collected when the plant is in flower. Store in a dry place. Protect from light.

### Adverse Effects and Precautions

Mouth ulceration and soreness have been reported following ingestion of feverfew, and may be due to sensitisation; if they occur feverfew should be discontinued. Contact dermatitis has been reported. Feverfew is reputed to have abortifacient properties and it is suggested that preparations should not be used in pregnancy.

**Effects on the blood.** There have been suggestions that feverfew may increase the risk of bleeding during surgery or in patients taking anticoagulants. However, although inhibition of platelet aggregation has been reported *in-vitro* or in *animals* a review[1] of clinical studies noted that feverfew did not appear to affect haematological safety parameters.


1. Pittler MH, *et al.* Feverfew for preventing migraine. Available in The Cochrane Library; Issue 2. Chichester: John Wiley; 2004.


### Interactions

It has been suggested that feverfew may enhance the effects of anticoagulants (but see Effects on the Blood, above).

### Uses and Administration

Feverfew is a traditional herbal remedy used in the prophylactic treatment of migraine. Its effects have been attributed to the plant's content of sesquiterpene lactones, notably parthenolide. A preparation of the dried leaf powder, which has been standardised to provide a minimum of 0.2% parthenolide, is available in some countries. Doses of 125 to 400 mg daily of the dried leaf powder have been recommended.

**Migraine.** Feverfew is a traditional herbal remedy used in the management of migraine (p.464).[1] Studies of standardised preparations of the freeze-dried powdered leaf have produced variable results in preventing or ameliorating migraine attacks,[2-4] and systematic reviews[5,6] suggest that its effectiveness in preventing migraine remains to be established.


1. Berry M. Feverfew. *Pharm J* 1994; **253:** 806–8.
2. Johnson ES, *et al.* Efficacy of feverfew as prophylactic treatment of migraine. *BMJ* 1985; **291:** 569–73.
3. Murphy JJ, *et al.* Randomised double-blind placebo controlled trial of feverfew in migraine prevention. *Lancet* 1988; **ii:** 189–92.
4. de Weerdt CJ, *et al.* Herbal medicines in migraine prevention: randomized double-blind placebo-controlled crossover trial of a feverfew preparation. *Phytomedicine* 1996; **3:** 225–30.
5. Vogler BK, *et al.* Feverfew as a preventive treatment for migraine: a systematic review. *Cephalalgia* 1998; **18:** 704–8.
6. Pittler MH, *et al.* Feverfew for preventing migraine. Available in The Cochrane Library; Issue 2. Chichester: John Wiley; 2004.


**Rheumatoid arthritis.** Feverfew has been used as a herbal medicine for the treatment of arthritis but although it has anti-inflammatory activity *in vitro*, a clinical trial[1] found it to be ineffective in rheumatoid arthritis.


1. Pattrick M, *et al.* Feverfew in rheumatoid arthritis: a double blind, placebo controlled study. *Ann Rheum Dis* 1989; **48:** 547–9.


### Preparations

**Proprietary Preparations** (details are given in Part 3)
***Austral.:*** Herbal Headache Relief†; ***Braz.:*** Tenliv; ***Canad.:*** Tanacet; ***UK:*** Tanacet.

**Multi-ingredient:** ***Austral.:*** Extralife Arthri-Care†; Extralife Migrai-Care†.

## Frovatriptan *(BAN, rINN)*

Frovatriptán; SB-209509AX (frovatriptan or frovatriptan succinate); VML-251 (frovatriptan or frovatriptan succinate). (6R)-5,6,7,8-Tetrahydro-6-methylaminocarbazole-3-carboxamide.

$C_{14}H_{17}N_3O$ = 243.3.
*CAS — 158747-02-5.*
*ATC — N02CC07.*

## Frovatriptan Succinate *(BANM, USAN, rINNM)*

SB-209509AX (frovatriptan or frovatriptan succinate); VML-251 (frovatriptan or frovatriptan succinate).

$C_{14}H_{17}N_3O,C_4H_6O_4,H_2O$ = 379.4.
*CAS — 158930-17-7.*
*ATC — N02CC07.*

### Profile

Frovatriptan is a serotonin (5-$HT_1$) agonist with actions similar to those of sumatriptan (p.471). It is used for the acute treatment of migraine attacks. It should not be used prophylactically or for the treatment of hemiplegic or basilar migraine. Frovatriptan is administered by mouth as the succinate although doses are expressed in terms of frovatriptan base; frovatriptan succinate 3.9 mg is approximately equivalent to 2.5 mg of frovatriptan base.

The recommended dose is 2.5 mg; if this is ineffective a second dose should not be taken for the same attack. If symptoms recur following an initial response, the dose may be repeated after an interval of at least 2 hours. The maximum dose of frovatriptan in 24 hours is 5 mg in the UK although, in the USA, a maximum daily dose of 7.5 mg is allowed.

◊ References.


1. Anonymous. Almotriptan (Axert) and frovatriptan (Frova) for migraine. *Med Lett Drugs Ther* 2002; **44:** 19–20.


### Preparations

**Proprietary Preparations** (details are given in Part 3)
***Irl.:*** Frovex; ***UK:*** Migard; ***USA:*** Frova.

## Iprazochrome *(rINN)*

3-Hydroxy-1-isopropyl-5,6-indolinedione 5-semicarbazone.

$C_{12}H_{16}N_4O_3$ = 264.3.
*CAS — 7248-21-7.*
*ATC — N02CX03.*

### Profile

Iprazochrome is a serotonin antagonist used in the prophylaxis of migraine (p.464) and in the management of diabetic retinopathy in usual doses of 2.5 to 5 mg three times daily.

### Preparations

**Proprietary Preparations** (details are given in Part 3)
***Ger.:*** Divascan.

## Methysergide *(BAN, USAN, rINN)*

1-Methyl-D-lysergic Acid Butanolamide. *N*-[1-(Hydroxymethyl)propyl]-1-methyl-D-lysergamide; 9,10-Didehydro-*N*-[1-(hydroxymethyl)propyl]-1,6-dimethylergoline-8β-carboxamide.

$C_{21}H_{27}N_3O_2$ = 353.5.
*CAS — 361-37-5.*
*ATC — N02CA04.*

## Methysergide Maleate *(BANM, rINNM)*

Maleato de metisergida.

$C_{21}H_{27}N_3O_2,C_4H_4O_4$ = 469.5.
*CAS — 129-49-7.*
*ATC — N02CA04.*

**Pharmacopoeias.** In *Br., Swiss,* and *US.*

**BP 2003** (Methysergide Maleate). A white or almost white crystalline powder which may have a yellow or pink tinge; odourless or almost odourless. Slightly soluble in water and in methyl alcohol; practically insoluble in chloroform and in ether. A 0.2% solution in water has a pH of 3.7 to 4.7. Store at a temperature of 2° to 8°. Protect from light.

**USP 27** (Methysergide Maleate). A white to yellowish-white or reddish-white, crystalline powder. Is odourless or has not more than a slight odour. Soluble 1 in 200 of water and 1 in 165 of alcohol; soluble 1 in 3400 of chloroform; practically insoluble in ether. pH of a 1 in 500 solution is between 3.7 and 4.7. Store in airtight containers at a temperature of 2° to 8°. Protect from light.

### Adverse Effects

Gastrointestinal effects such as nausea, vomiting, heartburn, and abdominal pain are common on initial treatment with methysergide maleate, as are dizziness and drowsiness. Other CNS effects reported include ataxia, insomnia, weakness, restlessness, lightheadedness, euphoria, and hallucinations. Peripheral or localised oedema, leg cramps, and weight gain have occurred and there have been occasional reports of skin rashes, loss of hair, joint and muscle pain, neutropenia, and eosinophilia. Orthostatic hypotension and tachycardia have been observed.

Arterial spasm has occurred in some patients with manifestations such as paraesthesia of the extremities and anginal pain, similar to those reported with ergotamine (p.467); if such symptoms occur methysergide should be withdrawn, although rebound headaches may be experienced if it is withdrawn suddenly. Vascular insufficiency of the lower limbs may represent arterial spasm or fibrotic changes. Retroperitoneal fibrosis, with obstruction of abdominal blood vessels and ureters, pleuropulmonary fibrosis, and fibrotic changes in heart valves have occurred in patients on long-term treatment. Methysergide must be withdrawn immediately if fibrosis occurs. Retroperitoneal fibrosis is usually reversible, but other fibrotic changes are less readily reversed.

**Fibrosis.** Fibrosis has been associated with the long-term use of methysergide maleate. In one early report[1] in 27 patients retroperitoneal fibrosis was attributed to daily administration of methysergide for periods of 9 to 54 months in doses ranging from 2 to 28 mg daily. There was partial or complete regression of fibrosis in 13 of the patients whose treatment was withdrawn. Improvement usually began within a few days, in some cases with the aid of prednisone. The other 14 patients were treated by surgery; those few who continued taking methysergide had difficult postoperative courses. Cardiac murmurs occurred in 7 patients, and regressed wholly or partially in 3 after therapy was stopped. Fibrotic changes affecting the aorta, heart valves, and pulmonary tissues occurred in a few of the patients. Others have reported the development of endocardial fibrosis indicated by cardiac murmurs in 48 patients receiving methysergide.[2] The murmurs gradually regressed in 27 when methysergide was discontinued. Retroperitoneal fibrosis was present in 9 patients and pleuropulmonary fibrosis in 2. A patient with fibrosis of the iliac vein has been described.[3]

A few cases of retroperitoneal fibrosis associated with ergotamine tartrate or dihydroergotamine have also been noted.[1] These 2 drugs have also been implicated in a few other cases of retroperitoneal fibrosis or other fibrotic disorders in patients taking high doses for long periods.[4-7]


1. Graham JR, *et al.* Fibrotic disorders associated with methysergide therapy for headache. *N Engl J Med* 1966; **274:** 359–68.
2. Bana DS, *et al.* Cardiac murmurs and endocardial fibrosis associated with methysergide therapy. *Am Heart J* 1974; **88:** 640–55.
3. Bucci JA, Manoharan A. Methysergide-induced retroperitoneal fibrosis: successful outcome and two new laboratory features. *Mayo Clin Proc* 1997; **72:** 1148–50.
4. Lepage-Savary D, Vallières A. Ergotamine as a possible cause of retroperitoneal fibrosis. *Clin Pharm* 1982; **1:** 179–80.
5. Robert M, *et al.* Fibrotic processes associated with long-term ergotamine therapy. *N Engl J Med* 1984; **311:** 601 and 602.
6. Damstrup L, Jensen TT. Retroperitoneal fibrosis after long-term daily use of ergotamine. *Int Urol Nephrol* 1986; **18:** 299–301.
7. Malaquin F, *et al.* Pleural and retroperitoneal fibrosis from dihydroergotamine. *N Engl J Med* 1989; **321:** 1760.


### Treatment of Adverse Effects

As for Ergotamine Tartrate, p.467. Methysergide maleate should be withdrawn immediately if fibrosis develops. Corticosteroids have been used to treat fibrosis, although surgery may be required.

### Precautions

As for Ergotamine Tartrate, p.467. In addition, methysergide maleate is contra-indicated in valvular heart disease, pulmonary and collagen diseases, diseases of the urinary tract, phlebitis and cellulitis of the lower extremities, and debilitated states. It should be used with caution in patients with peptic ulcer disease because it may increase gastric acidity. Patients should be closely supervised. Methysergide should not be given continuously for more than 6 months and should normally be withdrawn gradually (see Uses, below). However, it should be withdrawn immediately if symptoms of fibrosis or arterial spasm develop.

**Porphyria.** Methysergide is considered to be unsafe in patients with porphyria because it has been shown to be porphyrinogenic in *animals* or *in-vitro* systems.

### Interactions

Interactions involving those ergot alkaloids used primarily in the management of migraine are discussed under ergotamine (p.468). References specific to methysergide may be found there under the headings Antimigraine Drugs and Beta Blockers.

### Pharmacokinetics

Methysergide maleate is rapidly absorbed from the gastrointestinal tract with maximum plasma concentrations being obtained within about one hour of ingestion. Methysergide undergoes extensive first-pass hepatic metabolism to methylergometrine (p.1714). Methysergide is excreted in the urine as unchanged drug and metabolites.

◊ References.

1. Bredberg U, *et al.* Pharmacokinetics of methysergide and its metabolite methylergometrine in man. *Eur J Clin Pharmacol* 1986; **30:** 75–7.

### Uses and Administration

Methysergide maleate is a semisynthetic ergot alkaloid. It is a potent serotonin antagonist and, compared with ergotamine, has only feeble vasoconstrictor and oxytocic effects. It may be used prophylactically in the management of severe recurrent migraine (p.464) and in the prevention of headache attacks during cluster periods (p.464), although its use has declined because of adverse effects. It is ineffective in the treatment of acute attacks.

Methysergide is given by mouth as the maleate but doses are often expressed in terms of the base; 1.33 mg of methysergide maleate is approximately equivalent to 1 mg of methysergide. A usual dosage is 2 to 6 mg daily given in divided doses with meals. It is suggested that treatment should be started with 1 mg at bedtime and doses increased gradually over about 2 weeks; the minimum effective dose should be used. In the USA and some other countries doses are expressed in terms of the maleate, a usual dose of which is 4 to 8 mg daily. Careful and regular observation of the patient is essential because of the high incidence of adverse effects and it is recommended that treatment should only be carried out under hospital supervision. If treatment still proves to be ineffective after 3 weeks, further use is unlikely to be of benefit. Treatment should not be continued for more than 6 months, after which it should be gradually withdrawn over 2 or 3 weeks and then discontinued for at least a month for reassessment. Some consider that treatment courses should not exceed 3 months without a break.

Methysergide maleate has also been used to control diarrhoea associated with carcinoid syndrome (p.504) in high doses equivalent to 12 to 20 mg of methysergide daily.

As a serotonin antagonist, methysergide might be expected to help reverse the serotonin syndrome (p.313).

### Preparations

**BP 2003:** Methysergide Tablets;
**USP 27:** Methysergide Maleate Tablets.

**Proprietary Preparations** (details are given in Part 3)
**Austral.:** Deseril; **Belg.:** Deseril; **Braz.:** Deserila; **Canad.:** Sansert; **Fr.:** Desernil; **Ger.:** Deseril; **Irl.:** Deseril†; **Ital.:** Deserril†; **Neth.:** Deseril; **S.Afr.:** Deseril; **Switz.:** Deseril; **UK:** Deseril; **USA:** Sansert†.

## Naratriptan Hydrochloride

*(BANM, USAN, rINNM)*

GR-85548A; GR-85548X (naratriptan); Hidrocloruro de naratriptán. N-Methyl-3-(1-methyl-4-piperidyl)indole-5-ethanesulfonamide hydrochloride.

$C_{17}H_{25}N_3O_2S,HCl = 371.9.$

*CAS — 121679-13-8 (naratriptan); 121679-19-4 (naratriptan hydrochloride); 143388-64-1 (naratriptan hydrochloride).*

*ATC — N02CC02.*

**Pharmacopoeias.** In *US.*

**USP 27** (Naratriptan Hydrochloride). A white to pale yellow solid. Soluble in water. Store in airtight containers at a temperature not exceeding 30°.

### Adverse Effects and Precautions

As for Sumatriptan, p.471.

Naratriptan should not be used in patients with severe hepatic or renal impairment (creatinine clearance less than 15 mL/minute) and should be used with caution in mild or moderate renal or hepatic impairment. Patients with hypersensitivity to sulfonamides may theoretically exhibit a similar reaction to naratriptan.

**Analgesic-induced headache.** For a report of an association between naratriptan and analgesic-induced headache, see under Adverse Effects of Sumatriptan, p.471.

### Interactions

As for Sumatriptan, p.472.

### Pharmacokinetics

Following oral doses, peak plasma-naratriptan concentrations are observed at 2 to 3 hours, and bioavailability is reported to be 63% in men and 74% in women. Plasma protein binding is 29%. Naratriptan undergoes some hepatic metabolism by a wide range of cytochrome P450 isoenzymes. It is predominantly excreted in the urine with 50% of a dose being recovered as unchanged drug and 30% as inactive metabolites. The elimination half-life is 6 hours, and is significantly prolonged in patients with renal or hepatic impairment.

Distribution into milk has been demonstrated in studies in *rats.*

### Uses and Administration

Naratriptan is a selective serotonin (5-$HT_1$) agonist with actions and uses similar to those of sumatriptan (p.473). It is used for the acute treatment of migraine attacks, and should be administered as soon as possible after onset of migraine headache. It should not be used prophylactically. It is given by mouth as the hydrochloride, and doses are expressed in terms of the base; naratriptan hydrochloride 1.11 mg is approximately equivalent to 1 mg of naratriptan.

The recommended dose of naratriptan in the UK is 2.5 mg, and in the USA is 1 or 2.5 mg. If no response is obtained with the initial dose, a second dose should not be taken for the same attack. If symptoms recur following an initial response, the dose may be repeated after an interval of 4 hours, to a maximum of 5 mg in any 24-hour period. For doses in hepatic or renal impairment see below.

**Administration in hepatic or renal impairment.** Naratriptan is contra-indicated in patients with severe hepatic or severe renal impairment (creatinine clearance less than 15 mL/minute). In patients with mild to moderate hepatic or renal impairment, the recommended maximum dose in 24 hours is 2.5 mg and a lower starting dose should be considered.

**Migraine.** For comparison of the relative benefits of different triptans in migraine see under Sumatriptan, p.473.

Further references.

1. Klassen A, *et al.* Naratriptan is effective and well tolerated in the acute treatment of migraine: results of a double-blind, placebo-controlled, parallel-group study. *Headache* 1997; **37:** 640–5.
2. Mathew NT, *et al.* Naratriptan is effective and well tolerated in the acute treatment of migraine: results of a double-blind, placebo-controlled, crossover study. *Neurology* 1997; **49:** 1485–90.
3. Luciani R, *et al.* Prevention of migraine during prodrome with naratriptan. *Cephalalgia* 2000; **20:** 122–6.
4. Heywood J, *et al.* Tolerability and efficacy of naratriptan tablets in the acute treatment of migraine attacks for 1 year. *Cephalalgia* 2000; **20:** 470–4.

### Preparations

**USP 27:** Naratriptan Tablets.

**Proprietary Preparations** (details are given in Part 3)
**Arg.:** Naramig; **Austral.:** Naramig; **Austria:** Antimigrin; Naramig; **Belg.:** Naramig; **Braz.:** Naramig; **Canad.:** Amerge; **Chile:** Naramig; **Denm.:** Naragran; **Fin.:** Naramig; **Fr.:** Naramig; **Ger.:** Naramig; **Gr.:** Naramig; **Israel:** Naramig; **Mex.:** Naramig; **Neth.:** Naramig; **Norw.:** Naramig; **Port.:** Naramig; **S.Afr.:** Naramig; **Singapore:** Naramig; **Spain:** Colatan; Naramig; **Swed.:** Naramig; **Switz.:** Naramig; **Thai.:** Naramig; **UK:** Naramig; **USA:** Amerge.

## Oxetorone Fumarate *(USAN, rINNM)*

Fumarato de oxetorona; L-6257. 3-(6,12-Dihydrobenzofuro[3,2-c][1]benzoxepin-6-ylidene)-NN-dimethylpropylamine hydrogen fumarate.

$C_{21}H_{21}NO_2,C_4H_4O_4 = 435.5.$

*CAS — 26020-55-3 (oxetorone); 34522-46-8 (oxetorone fumarate).*

*ATC — N02CX06.*

### Profile

Oxetorone fumarate is an antihistamine and serotonin antagonist used in the treatment of migraine (p.464) and cluster headache (p.464) in doses of up to 180 mg daily by mouth. Oxetorone was reported to have induced hyperplastic changes in breast tissue and the uterine endometrium of *rodents.*

### Preparations

**Proprietary Preparations** (details are given in Part 3)
**Belg.:** Nocertone; **Fr.:** Nocertone.

## Pizotifen *(BAN, rINN)*

BC-105; Pizotifeno; Pizotyline *(USAN)*. 9,10-Dihydro-4-(1-methylpiperidin-4-ylidene)-4*H*-benzo[4,5]cyclohepta[1,2-*b*]thiophene.

$C_{19}H_{21}NS = 295.4.$

*CAS — 15574-96-6.*

*ATC — N02CX01.*

**Pharmacopoeias.** In *Chin.*

## Pizotifen Malate *(BANM, rINNM)*

Malato de pizotifeno; Pizotifen Hydrogen Malate; Pizotyline Malate.

$C_{19}H_{21}NS,C_4H_6O_5 = 429.5.$

*CAS — 5189-11-7.*

*ATC — N02CX01.*

**Pharmacopoeias.** In *Br.*

**BP 2003** (Pizotifen Malate). A white or slightly yellowish-white, odourless or almost odourless, crystalline powder. Very slightly soluble in water; slightly soluble in alcohol and in chloroform; sparingly soluble in methyl alcohol. Protect from light.

### Adverse Effects and Precautions

As for the sedating antihistamines in general, see p.419. Increased appetite and weight gain may occur with pizotifen. Drowsiness may be troublesome.

**Incidence of adverse effects.** Adverse effects were noted in 22 of 47 patients with severe migraine given pizotifen 1 to 2 mg daily.[1] These reactions included weight increase (15), muscle pain or cramps (3), heavy or restless legs (3), fluid retention (3), drowsiness (2), more frequent milder headaches (2), facial flushing (1), reduced libido (1), exacerbation of epilepsy (1), and dreaming (2). Adverse effects necessitating withdrawal occurred in 11 patients.

1. Peet KMS. Use of pizotifen in severe migraine: a long-term study. *Curr Med Res Opin* 1977; **5:** 192–9.

### Interactions

As for the sedating antihistamines in general, see p.421.

**Antihypertensives.** Following a report[1] of loss of blood pressure control when treatment with pizotifen was started in a patient receiving *debrisoquine* the manufacturer suggested that since pizotifen had a similar chemical structure to the tricyclic antidepressants it might antagonise the actions of adrenergic neurone blockers in a similar manner.

1. Bailey RR. Antagonism of debrisoquine sulphate by pizotifen (Sandomigran). *N Z Med J* 1976; **1:** 449.

### Pharmacokinetics

Pizotifen is well absorbed from the gastrointestinal tract, peak plasma concentrations occurring about 5 hours after a single oral dose. Over 90% is bound to plasma proteins. Pizotifen undergoes extensive metabolism. Over half of a dose is excreted in the urine, chiefly as metabolites; a significant proportion is excreted in the faeces. The primary metabolite of pizotifen (*N*-glucuronide conjugate) has a long elimination half-life of about 23 hours.

### Uses and Administration

Pizotifen is a sedating antihistamine (p.421) that has strong serotonin antagonist and weak antimuscarinic properties. It also antagonises the action of tryptamine. Pizotifen is used, usually as the malate, for the prophylaxis of migraine and for the prevention of headache attacks during cluster periods. It is not effective in treating an acute attack. Doses of pizotifen malate are expressed in terms of the equivalent amount of the base; pizotifen malate 1.45 mg is approximately equivalent to 1 mg of pizotifen.

The usual adult dose is 1.5 mg daily by mouth either in three divided doses or as a single dose at night. Gradual increase from an initial dose of 0.5 mg may help to avoid undue drowsiness. Doses in individual patients may vary from 0.5 mg up to a maximum of 4.5 mg daily. Not more than 3 mg should be given as a single dose. Up to 1.5 mg daily in divided doses (maximum single dose of 1 mg at night) has been recommended for children aged over 2 years.

Pizotifen hydrochloride has also been used in the management of migraine.

**Abdominal migraine.** Abdominal migraine is a recurrent disorder seen mainly in children and characterised by episodic midline abdominal pain lasting for up to 72 hours. The pain is severe enough to disrupt normal activities and may be associated with pallor, anorexia, nausea, and vomiting.[1] Sleep, and sometimes vomiting, terminate the attack.

Pizotifen was found to be effective for the prophylaxis of abdominal pain in children with abdominal migraine.[2] Prophylactic treatment with propranolol or cyproheptadine may also be of benefit.[3]


1. Headache Classification Subcommittee of the International Headache Society. The international classification of headache disorders: 2nd edition. *Cephalalgia* 2004; **24** (suppl 1): 9–160. Also available at: http://216.25.100.131/ihscommon/guidelines/pdfs/ihc_II_main_no_print.pdf (accessed 01/06/04)
2. Symon DNK, Russell G. Double blind placebo controlled trial of pizotifen syrup in the treatment of abdominal migraine. *Arch Dis Child* 1995; **72:** 48–50.
3. Worawattanakul M, *et al.* Abdominal migraine: prophylactic treatment and follow-up. *J Pediatr Gastroenterol Nutr* 1999; **28:** 37–40.


**Migraine and cluster headache.** Pizotifen is one of the main alternatives to propranolol for the prophylaxis of migraine (p.464). It has also been tried in the management of cluster headache (p.464) to prevent headache attacks during a cluster period.

References.


1. Bellavance AJ, Meloche JP. A comparative study of naproxen sodium, pizotyline and placebo in migraine prophylaxis. *Headache* 1990; **30:** 710–15.


### Preparations

***BP 2003:*** Pizotifen Tablets.

**Proprietary Preparations** (details are given in Part 3)
***Arg.:*** Sandomigran; ***Austral.:*** Sandomigran; ***Austria:*** Sandomigran†; ***Belg.:*** Sandomigran; ***Braz.:*** Sandomigran; ***Canad.:*** Sandomigran; ***Denm.:*** Sandomigrin; ***Fr.:*** Sanmigran; ***Ger.:*** Mosegor; Sandomigran†; ***Gr.:*** Mosegor; ***Hong Kong:*** Sandomigran; ***Irl.:*** Sanomigran; ***Israel:*** Sandomigran†; ***Ital.:*** Sandomigran; ***Malaysia:*** Sandomigran; ***Neth.:*** Sandomigran; ***NZ:*** Sandomigran; ***S.Afr.:*** Sandomigran; ***Spain:*** Mosegor; Sandomigran; ***Swed.:*** Sandomigrin; ***Switz.:*** Mosegor; ***Thai.:*** Anorsia; Mosegor; Moselar; Pizomed; Zofen; ***UK:*** Sanomigran.

## Rizatriptan Benzoate *(BANM, USAN, pINNM)*

Benzoato de rizatriptán; MK-462; MK-0462. 3-[2-(Dimethylamino)ethyl]-5-(1*H*-1,2,4-triazol-1-ylmethyl)indole monobenzoate; Dimethyl{2-[5-(1*H*-1,2,4-triazol-1-ylmethyl)indol-3-yl]ethyl}amine monobenzoate.

$C_{15}H_{19}N_5,C_7H_6O_2$ = 391.5.

*CAS — 144034-80-0 (rizatriptan); 145202-66-0 (rizatriptan benzoate).*

*ATC — N02CC04.*

### Adverse Effects and Precautions

As for Sumatriptan, p.471. Toxic epidermal necrolysis has also been reported with rizatriptan.

Rizatriptan should not be used in patients with severe hepatic or renal impairment and should be given with caution to patients with mild or moderate hepatic or renal impairment.

### Interactions

As for Sumatriptan, p.472. Propranolol increases plasma-rizatriptan concentrations and it is recommended that lower doses of rizatriptan should be used in patients receiving both drugs (see Uses and Administration, below).

### Pharmacokinetics

After oral doses, peak plasma-rizatriptan concentrations are obtained in about 1 to 1.5 hours or 1.6 to 2.5 hours depending on the formulation. Bioavailability is about 40 to 45%. Food may delay the time to peak-plasma concentrations of the tablet formulation by about 1 hour. Plasma protein binding is low (14%).

Rizatriptan is metabolised, primarily by monoamine oxidase type A to the inactive indole acetic acid derivative. The active metabolite *N*-monodesmethyl-rizatriptan is formed to a minor degree; other minor metabolites are also produced. About 14% of an oral dose is excreted in the urine as unchanged rizatriptan, 51% as the indole acetic acid metabolite, and 1% as *N*-monodesmethyl-rizatriptan. The plasma half-life is about 2 to 3 hours.

Distribution into milk has been demonstrated in *rats.*

◊ References.


1. Sciberras DG, *et al.* Initial human experience with MK-462 (rizatriptan): a novel 5-$HT_{1D}$ agonist. *Br J Clin Pharmacol* 1997; **43:** 49–54.
2. Lee Y, *et al.* Pharmacokinetics and tolerability of oral rizatriptan in healthy male and female volunteers. *Br J Clin Pharmacol* 1999; **47:** 373–8.
3. Goldberg MR, *et al.* Rizatriptan, a novel 5-$HT_{1B/1D}$ agonist for migraine: single- and multiple-dose tolerability and pharmacokinetics in healthy subjects. *J Clin Pharmacol* 2000; **40:** 74–83.


### Uses and Administration

Rizatriptan is a selective serotonin (5-$HT_1$) agonist with actions and uses similar to those of sumatriptan (p.473) but appears to have a faster onset of action. It is used for the acute treatment of the headache phase of migraine attacks. It should not be used prophylactically. Rizatriptan is given as the benzoate, and doses are expressed in terms of the base; rizatriptan benzoate 14.53 mg is approximately equivalent to 10 mg of rizatriptan.

The usual dose in the UK of rizatriptan is 10 mg by mouth. If this is ineffective, a second dose should not be taken for the same attack. If the headache recurs, a further dose of 10 mg may be taken after an interval of at least 2 hours. In the USA a dose of 5 or 10 mg is used. The recommended maximum dose in 24 hours is 20 mg in the UK and 30 mg in the USA. A reduced dose of 5 mg is recommended in patients also receiving propranolol, with the maximum in 24 hours reduced to 10 mg in the UK and 15 mg in the USA. It is also recommended that doses of the 2 drugs should be separated by at least 2 hours. For doses in hepatic or renal impairment, see below.

**Administration in hepatic or renal impairment.** In patients with mild to moderate hepatic or renal impairment, the dose of rizatriptan should be reduced to 5 mg. If the headache recurs, a further dose of 5 mg may be taken after an interval of at least 2 hours. The recommended maximum dose in 24 hours in these patients is 10 mg in the UK. Rizatriptan should not be used in patients with severe hepatic or severe renal impairment.

**Migraine.** For comparison of the relative benefits of different triptans in migraine, see under Sumatriptan, p.473.

Further references.


1. Dooley M, Faulds D. Rizatriptan: a review of its efficacy in the management of migraine. *Drugs* 1999; **58:** 699–723. Correction. *ibid.* 2000; **59:** 179.
2. Adelman JU, *et al.* Rizatriptan tablet versus wafer: patient preference. *Headache* 2000; **40:** 371–2.
3. Mathew NT, *et al.* Treatment of nonresponders to oral sumatriptan with zolmitriptan and rizatriptan: a comparative open trial. *Headache* 2000; **40:** 464–5.
4. Silberstein SD, *et al.* Rizatriptan in the treatment of menstrual migraine. *Obstet Gynecol* 2000; **96:** 237–42.
5. Wellington K, Plosker GL. Rizatriptan: an update of its use in the management of migraine. *Drugs* 2002; **62:** 1539–74.


### Preparations

**Proprietary Preparations** (details are given in Part 3)
***Arg.:*** Maxalt; ***Austria:*** Maxalt; Rizalief; ***Belg.:*** Maxalt; ***Braz.:*** Maxalt; ***Canad.:*** Maxalt; ***Chile:*** Maxalt; ***Denm.:*** Maxalt; ***Fin.:*** Maxalt; ***Ger.:*** Maxalt; ***Gr.:*** Maxalt; ***Israel:*** Rizalt; ***Ital.:*** Maxalt; Rizaliv; ***Mex.:*** Maxalt; ***Neth.:*** Maxalt; ***Norw.:*** Maxalt; ***NZ:*** Maxalt; ***Port.:*** Maxalt; ***S.Afr.:*** Maxalt; ***Spain:*** Maxalt; ***Swed.:*** Maxalt; ***Switz.:*** Maxalt; ***UK:*** Maxalt; ***USA:*** Maxalt.

## Sumatriptan Succinate

*(BANM, USAN, rINNM)*

GR-43175C; GR-43175X (sumatriptan); Succinato de sumatriptán; Sumatriptani Succinas. 3-(2-Dimethylaminoethyl)indol-5-yl-N-methylmethanesulphonamide succinate.

$C_{14}H_{21}N_3O_2S,C_4H_6O_4$ = 413.5.

*CAS — 103628-46-2 (sumatriptan); 103628-47-3 (sumatriptan hemisuccinate); 103628-48-4 (sumatriptan succinate).*

*ATC — N02CC01.*

**Pharmacopoeias.** In *Eur.* (see p.vi).

**Ph. Eur. 5.0** (Sumatriptan Succinate). A white or almost white powder. Freely soluble in water; practically insoluble in dichloromethane; sparingly soluble in methyl alcohol. A 1% solution in water has a pH of 4.5 to 5.3. Protect from light.

**Stability.** Oral liquid preparations of sumatriptan 5 mg/mL prepared from crushed sumatriptan succinate tablets in 3 different syrups were stable for at least 21 days when stored at 4° and protected from light.[1]


1. Fish DN, *et al.* Stability of sumatriptan succinate in extemporaneously prepared oral liquids. *Am J Health-Syst Pharm* 1997; **54:** 1619–22.


### Adverse Effects

The most commonly reported adverse effects of serotonin (5-$HT_1$) agonists such as sumatriptan include dizziness, flushing, weakness, drowsiness, and fatigue. Nausea and vomiting may occur. Pain or sensations of tingling, heaviness, heat, pressure, or tightness have also been commonly reported, can affect any part of the body including the throat and chest, and may be intense. These symptoms may be due to vasospasm, which on rare occasions has resulted in severe cardiovascular events including cardiac arrhythmias, myocardial ischaemia, or myocardial infarction. There have been isolated reports of associated cerebrovascular events in patients receiving sumatriptan. Transient increases in blood pressure may occur soon after treatment. Hypotension, bradycardia or tachycardia, and palpitations have been reported. Visual disturbances have also occurred.

Sumatriptan has occasionally been associated with minor disturbances in liver function. There have also been rare reports of seizures with sumatriptan. Hypersensitivity reactions ranging from skin rashes to, more rarely, anaphylaxis have occurred.

Transient pain at the injection site is common after subcutaneous sumatriptan administration; stinging, burning, erythema, bruising, and bleeding have also been reported. Irritation of the nasal mucosa and throat and epistaxis have been reported after intranasal sumatriptan administration.

**Incidence of adverse effects.** In a Dutch postmarketing survey[1] completed by 1187 patients who had taken sumatriptan the most common adverse reactions attributed to sumatriptan were paraesthesia (reported by 11.7% of patients), dizziness (8.1%), feeling of heaviness (8.0%), chest pain (7.9%), nausea and/or vomiting (7.3%), drowsiness/sedation (7.0%), flushing (5.1%), fatigue (4.6%), pressure in throat (3.3%), headache (3.1%), injection site reaction (3.0%), palpitations (2.8%), abdominal pain (2.6%), muscle pain (2.4%), and dyspnoea (2.2%).


1. Ottervanger JP, *et al.* Adverse reactions attributed to sumatriptan: a postmarketing study in general practice. *Eur J Clin Pharmacol* 1994; **47:** 305–9.


**Analgesic-induced headache.** Sumatriptan may have a similar risk of misuse to that associated with analgesics and ergotamine compounds in patients with analgesic-induced headache (p.464). There have been reports[1-3] of patients using one or more daily doses of sumatriptan to control migraine. Many of the patients had a history of abuse of other antimigraine drugs and were using sumatriptan to prevent recurrence of headache. Whether misuse of sumatriptan was due to addiction or rebound headache as seen with ergotamine, is unknown. A postmarketing study in 952 patients receiving sumatriptan found that 36 of the patients (4%) used sumatriptan daily or more than 10 times each week. This overuse was related to poor efficacy and not to rebound headache.[4] One study[5] and an anecdotal report[6] suggest that, rather than producing euphoria or other effects associated with drugs of abuse such as morphine, sumatriptan is more likely to be associated with dysphoria and apathetic sedation.

The development of analgesic-induced headache has also been reported with naratriptan and zolmitriptan.[7]


1. Osborne MJ, *et al.* Is there a problem with long term use of sumatriptan in acute migraine? *BMJ* 1994; **308:** 113.
2. Kaube H, *et al.* Sumatriptan. *BMJ* 1994; **308:** 1573–4.
3. Gaist D, *et al.* Misuse of sumatriptan. *Lancet* 1994; **344:** 1090.
4. Ottervanger JP, *et al.* Pattern of sumatriptan use and overuse in general practice. *Eur J Clin Pharmacol* 1996; **50:** 353–5.
5. Sullivan JT, *et al.* Psychoactivity and abuse potential of sumatriptan. *Clin Pharmacol Ther* 1992; **52:** 635–42.
6. Bakshi R, Yan-Go FL. Prolonged marijuana-like dysphoria after subcutaneous sumatriptan. *Ann Pharmacother* 1996; **30:** 683.
7. Limmroth V, *et al.* Headache after frequent use of serotonin agonists zolmitriptan and naratriptan. *Lancet* 1999; **353:** 378.


**Effects on the cardiovascular system.** About 10 months after sumatriptan injection had been made available commercially, the UK Committee on Safety of Medicines noted that it had received 34 reports of pain or tightness in the chest and 2 reports of myocardial ischaemia.[1] The Netherlands Centre for Monitoring of Adverse Reactions to Drugs reported about the same time that it had received 12 reports of chest or anginal pain mostly associated with oral sumatriptan.[2] A later postmarketing survey based on data from Dutch general practitioners identified chest pain in 1.3% of 1727 patients,[3] a figure considered to be lower than that seen in earlier studies, but in a subsequent questionnaire completed by 1187 of these patients 7.9% reported chest pain.[4] The Australian Adverse Drug Reactions Advisory Committee (ADRAC)[5] stated in December 1994 that it had received 114 reports of chest pain since sumatriptan had been marketed in mid 1992. Most patients had recovered quickly but 2 had died. The first developed a fatal myocardial infarction after coronary artery dissection but the causal relation between this and taking sumatriptan was unclear. The second patient who had hypertrophic obstructive cardiomyopathy developed ventricular fibrillation a few hours after the onset of chest pain and this led to fatal cardiac arrest.

One group of workers[6] who studied the effect of sumatriptan 16 mg given subcutaneously suggested that the symptoms of chest pain might be due to an effect of sumatriptan on oesophageal function, but others have argued against this suggestion.[7] ADRAC[5] considered that the reaction in the 28 reports of throat tightness they had received by December 1994 was a different reaction to that of chest pain, and probably resulted from changes in oesophageal motility.

Several reports have provided details of individual cases of the adverse cardiovascular effects of sumatriptan including arrhythmias (ventricular tachycardia,[8] ventricular fibrillation,[8] or atrial fibrillation[9]), acute myocardial infarction (sometimes in patients with no predisposing factors[10]),[10-14] and unstable angina.[15] Most of these reports concerned subcutaneous sumatriptan, but in one myocardial infarction occurred after oral use.[12]

A review[16] of published reports on chest pain as well as relevant data held by the UK manufacturer considered that the risk of myocardial ischaemia following vasoconstriction induced by sumatriptan was small. However, the contra-indications and cautions given under Precautions, below, should be observed. A recent study[17] of over 63 500 migraine patients in the UK General Practice Research Database failed to find an increased risk of cardiovascular death in those patients treated with serotonin agonists.

1. Committee on Safety of Medicines. Sumatriptan (Imigran) and chest pain. *Current Problems 34* 1992.
2. Stricker BHC. Coronary vasospasm and sumatriptan. *BMJ* 1992; **305:** 118.
3. Ottervanger JP, *et al.* Postmarketing study of cardiovascular adverse reactions associated with sumatriptan. *BMJ* 1993; **307:** 1185.
4. Ottervanger JP, *et al.* Adverse reactions attributed to sumatriptan: a postmarketing study in general practice. *Eur J Clin Pharmacol* 1994; **47:** 305–9.
5. Boyd IW, Rohan AP. Sumatriptan-induced chest pain. *Lancet* 1994; **344:** 1704–5.
6. Houghton LA, *et al.* Is chest pain after sumatriptan oesophageal in origin? *Lancet* 1994; **344:** 985–6.
7. Hood S, *et al.* Sumatriptan-induced chest pain. *Lancet* 1994; **344:** 1500–1.
8. Curtin T, *et al.* Cardiorespiratory distress after sumatriptan given by injection. *BMJ* 1992; **305:** 713–14.
9. Morgan DR, *et al.* Atrial fibrillation associated with sumatriptan. *BMJ* 2000; **321:** 275.
10. Ottervanger JP, *et al.* Transmural myocardial infarction with sumatriptan. *Lancet* 1993; **341:** 861–2.
11. Kelly KM. Cardiac arrest following use of sumatriptan. *Neurology* 1995; **45:** 1211–13.
12. O'Connor P, Gladstone P. Oral sumatriptan-associated transmural myocardial infarction. *Neurology* 1995; **45:** 2274–6.
13. Mueller L, *et al.* Vasospasm-induced myocardial infarction with sumatriptan. *Headache* 1996; **36:** 329–31.
14. Main ML *et al.* Cardiac arrest and myocardial infarction immediately after sumatriptan injection. *Ann Intern Med* 1998; **128:** 874.
15. Walton-Shirley M, *et al.* Unstable angina pectoris associated with Imitrex therapy. *Cathet Cardiovasc Diagn* 1995; **34:** 188.
16. Hillis WS, MacIntyre PD. Drug reactions: sumatriptan and chest pain. *Lancet* 1993; **341:** 1564–5. Correction. *ibid.*; **342:** 1310.
17. Hall GC, *et al.* Triptans in migraine: the risks of stroke, cardiovascular disease, and death in practice. *Neurology* 2004; **62:** 563–8.

**Effects on the cerebrovascular system.** Various adverse cerebrovascular effects have been reported after the use of subcutaneous sumatriptan including hemiparesis,[1] stroke,[2,3] and intracerebral haemorrhage.[4] However, a study[5] of over 63 500 migraine patients in the UK General Practice Research Database failed to find an increased risk of stroke in those patients treated with serotonin agonists.

1. Luman W, Gray RS. Adverse reactions associated with sumatriptan. *Lancet* 1993; **341:** 1091–2.
2. Cavazos J, *et al.* Sumatriptan-induced stroke in sagittal sinus thrombosis. *Lancet* 1994; **343:** 1105–6.
3. Meschia JF, *et al.* Reversible segmental cerebral arterial vasospasm and cerebral infarction: possible association with excessive use of sumatriptan and Midrin. *Arch Neurol* 1998; **55:** 712–14.
4. Edwards KR, *et al.* Intracerebral hemorrhage associated with sumatriptan. *Headache* 1995; **35:** 309.
5. Hall GC, *et al.* Triptans in migraine: the risks of stroke, cardiovascular disease, and death in practice. *Neurology* 2004; **62:** 563–8.

**Effects on the gastrointestinal tract.** Severe ischaemic colitis associated with sumatriptan use has been reported in 8 patients.[1] A further five episodes of mesenteric ischaemia occurred in 2 patients, each within hours of sumatriptan administration.[2] Three of these episodes in 1 patient were associated with doses of sumatriptan above the recommended daily maximum.

Oesophageal constriction or throat tightness has been reported in some patients taking sumatriptan and may be due to a direct effect on the oesophagus (see Effects on the Cardiovascular System, above).

1. Knudsen JF, *et al.* Ischemic colitis and sumatriptan use. *Arch Intern Med* 1998; **158:** 1946–8.
2. Liu JJ, Ardolf JC. Sumatriptan-associated mesenteric ischemia. *Ann Intern Med* 2000; **132:** 597.

**Effects on the respiratory system.** See Asthma under Precautions, below.

**Hypersensitivity.** Reactions to sumatriptan such as skin rashes and, more rarely, anaphylaxis have been noted by the manufacturer. Published reports include angioedema occurring in a patient 5 minutes after subcutaneous administration of sumatriptan,[1] and urticaria occurring 20 to 24 hours after oral or subcutaneous sumatriptan in another patient.[2]

1. Dachs R, Vitillo J. Angioedema associated with sumatriptan administration. *Am J Med* 1995; **99:** 684–5.
2. Pradalier A, *et al.* Delayed urticaria with sumatriptan. *Cephalalgia* 1996; **16:** 280–1.

## Precautions

Sumatriptan and other serotonin (5-$HT_1$) agonists should only be used where there is a clear diagnosis of migraine or cluster headache and care should be taken to exclude other potentially serious neurological conditions. They should not be used prophylactically and should not be administered to patients with basilar or hemiplegic migraine.

Serotonin (5-$HT_1$) agonists are contra-indicated in patients with uncontrolled hypertension, ischaemic heart disease (coronary artery disease), a history of myocardial infarction, coronary vasospasm (Prinzmetal's angina), peripheral vascular disease, or a previous cerebrovascular accident or transient ischaemic attack. Unrecognised cardiovascular disease should be excluded before the use of serotonin (5-$HT_1$) agonists in postmenopausal women, men over 40 years of age, and those with risk factors for ischaemic heart disease (see below). If chest pain and tightness occur during use, appropriate investigations should be performed. Sumatriptan injection should not be given intravenously because of the increased risk of producing coronary vasospasm.

Drowsiness may occur following treatment with serotonin (5-$HT_1$) agonists and patients thus affected should not drive or operate machinery.

Sumatriptan should be used with caution in patients with hepatic or renal impairment, and should generally be avoided if impairment is severe.

There have been rare reports of seizures following use of sumatriptan and it should therefore be used with caution in patients with a history of epilepsy or other conditions predisposing to seizures. Patients with hypersensitivity to sulfonamides may exhibit a similar reaction to sumatriptan.

**Asthma.** The manufacturers reviewed data from more than 75 clinical studies of sumatriptan involving 12 701 patients and reported[1] that the incidence of adverse events related to asthma did not differ between patients with or without asthma. Earlier there had been concern over the safety of sumatriptan in patients with asthma following 2 reports of bronchospasm and a report of a patient with asthma who died during a study of sumatriptan although the patient had not received sumatriptan in the month before her death.

1. Lloyd DK, Pilgrim AJ. The safety of sumatriptan in asthmatic migraineurs. *Cephalalgia* 1993; **13:** 201–4.

**Breast feeding.** No adverse effects have been observed in breast-feeding infants whose mothers were receiving sumatriptan, and the American Academy of Pediatrics considers that it is therefore usually compatible with breast feeding.[1] However, the manufacturers have suggested that infant exposure can be minimised by avoiding breast feeding for 24 hours after treatment.

The distribution of sumatriptan into breast milk following a 6-mg subcutaneous dose has been studied in 5 lactating mothers.[2] The mean total recovery of sumatriptan in breast milk was estimated to be 14.4 micrograms or 0.24% of the dose. It was calculated that on a weight adjusted basis an infant could receive a maximum of 3.5% of the maternal dose.

1. American Academy of Pediatrics. The transfer of drugs and other chemicals into human milk. *Pediatrics* 2001; **108:** 776–89. Correction. *ibid.*; 1029. Also available at: http://aappolicy.aappublications.org/cgi/content/full/pediatrics%3b108/3/776 (accessed 01/06/04)
2. Wojnar-Horton RE, *et al.* Distribution and excretion of sumatriptan in human milk. *Br J Clin Pharmacol* 1996; **41:** 217–21.

**Cardiovascular risk.** Patients with risk factors for ischaemic heart disease such as diabetes, hypertension, hypercholesterolaemia, obesity, and a strong family history of atheroma, as well as postmenopausal women, men over 40 years of age, and smokers should be given their first dose of sumatriptan under medical supervision.[1]

1. Hillis WS, MacIntyre PD. Drug reactions: sumatriptan and chest pain. *Lancet* 1993; **341:** 1564–5. Correction. *ibid.*; **342:** 1310.

**Cerebrovascular disorders.** A patient with a superior sagittal sinus thrombosis who presented with headache and was misdiagnosed as having migraine variant developed a cortical stroke within minutes of a second 6-mg subcutaneous injection of sumatriptan.[1] The importance of establishing a diagnosis of typical migraine or cluster headache before using sumatriptan was emphasised and caution given against its use in any patient who may have unstable cerebrovascular disease or raised intracranial pressure. Additionally, there was no clinical evidence that a second injection would relieve a headache when the initial injection had been ineffective.

1. Cavazos J, *et al.* Sumatriptan-induced stroke in sagittal sinus thrombosis. *Lancet* 1994; **343:** 1105–6.

## Interactions

Sumatriptan and other serotonin (5-$HT_1$) agonists should not be given with ergotamine or related compounds (including methysergide) since there is an increased risk of vasospastic reactions. In addition, a delay is advised before starting a serotonin (5-$HT_1$) agonist in patients who have been receiving ergotamine or related compounds: sumatriptan, almotriptan, eletriptan, naratriptan, rizatriptan, or zolmitriptan should not be given until at least 24 hours after stopping the use of preparations containing ergotamine. Conversely, ergotamine should not be given until 6 hours after stopping these drugs or at least 24 hours in the case of eletriptan. Serotonin (5-$HT_1$) agonists should not be given together.

It is recommended that sumatriptan or rizatriptan should not be used with, and for 2 weeks after stopping, an MAOI. Opinion varies on the concomitant use of zolmitriptan and inhibitors of monoamine oxidase type A such as moclobemide. In the UK the manufacturers recommend that the maximum dose of zolmitriptan should be reduced when used with inhibitors of monoamine oxidase type A whereas in the USA the manufacturers contra-indicate such combinations. There is a theoretical possibility that the use of serotonin (5-$HT_1$) agonists with SSRIs may increase the risk of serotonin syndrome, but see under Antidepressants, below.

◊ Oral sumatriptan appeared to delay gastric emptying and might affect the absorption of co-administered drugs, as judged by its delaying effect on paracetamol absorption in migraine patients.[1]

1. Rani PU, *et al.* Sumatriptan delays paracetamol absorption in migraine patients. *Clin Drug Invest* 1996; **11:** 300–304.

**Antidepressants.** Sumatriptan and rizatriptan are metabolised predominantly by monoamine oxidase type A and the manufacturers advise that patients taking *MAOIs*, including reversible selective type A inhibitors such as moclobemide, should not be given these serotonin (5-$HT_1$) agonists. Clearance of zolmitriptan was decreased after moclobemide; therefore, a reduced dose of zolmitriptan is advised if the drug is used with an inhibitor of monoamine oxidase type A. *SSRIs* such as fluoxetine may also interact with serotonin (5-$HT_1$) agonists with an increased risk of serotonin syndrome (p.313), and it has been suggested that *lithium* and sumatriptan may interact similarly. However, a review of the use of sumatriptan with MAOIs, SSRIs, or lithium found little evidence of an increased risk of serotonin syndrome.[1] It was concluded that most patients tolerate the combination of sumatriptan and an SSRI or lithium without incident. However, it was suggested that the use of sumatriptan with an MAOI should continue to be avoided until further data supporting safety becomes available. The manufacturers of zolmitriptan advise a reduction in dosage if it is given with fluvoxamine as the latter may inhibit zolmitriptan metabolism through its effects on the cytochrome P450 isoenzyme CYP1A2.

Increased serotonergic effects with increased incidence of adverse effects have been reported following the use of *hypericum* (St. John's Wort) with triptans.[2] Patients should be advised to stop taking hypericum if treatment with a serotonin (5-$HT_1$) agonist is necessary.

1. Gardner DM, Lynd LD. Sumatriptan contraindications and the serotonin syndrome. *Ann Pharmacother* 1998; **32:** 33–8.
2. Committee on Safety of Medicines/Medicines Control Agency. Reminder: St John's wort (Hypericum perforatum) interactions. *Current Problems* 2000; **26:** 6–7. Also available at: http://www.mca.gov.uk/ourwork/monitorsafequalmed/currentproblems/cpmay2000.pdf (accessed 01/06/04)

**Antimigraine drugs.** Although the efficacy and tolerability of subcutaneous sumatriptan in the acute treatment of migraine did not appear to be affected in patients already taking *dihydroergotamine* orally for migraine prophylaxis,[1] the bioavailability of oral dihydroergotamine is low and it could not be assumed that it was safe to use parenteral dihydroergotamine with sumatriptan.[2] The manufacturers of sumatriptan contra-indicate its use with *ergotamine* or other related compounds and also recommend that it should not be given until at least 24 hours after stopping ergotamine or related compounds (see above).

Acute myocardial infarction has been reported[3] in a premenopausal woman with controlled hypertension and no known coronary artery disease after subcutaneous use of sumatriptan within a few hours of taking *methysergide* by mouth.

1. Henry P, *et al.* Subcutaneous sumatriptan in the acute treatment of migraine in patients using dihydroergotamine as prophylaxis. *Headache* 1993; **33:** 432–5.
2. Campbell JK. [Editor's comment]. *Headache* 1993; **33:** 435.
3. Liston H, *et al.* The association of the combination of sumatriptan and methysergide in myocardial infarction in a premenopausal woman. *Arch Intern Med* 1999; **159:** 511–13.

**Antipsychotics.** For reference to a potential interaction between sumatriptan and *loxapine*, see Chlorpromazine, p.680.

## Pharmacokinetics

Sumatriptan is rapidly but incompletely absorbed when given orally and undergoes first-pass metabolism, resulting in a low absolute bioavailability of about 14%. Peak plasma concentrations following oral doses are achieved in about 2 hours. Bioavailability is much higher (96%) after subcutaneous doses with peak concentrations occurring within 25 minutes. Bioavailability after intranasal doses is 16% of that achieved subcutaneously, with peak concentrations occurring in 1 to 1.5 hours. Plasma protein binding is low at about 14 to 21%.

The elimination half-life of sumatriptan is about 2 hours. Sumatriptan is extensively metabolised in the liver predominantly by monoamine oxidase type A and is excreted mainly in the urine as the inactive indole acetic acid derivative and its glucuronide. Sumatriptan and its metabolites also appear in the faeces. Small amounts of sumatriptan are distributed into breast milk (see under Breast Feeding, above).

◊ Reviews.

1. Scott AK. Sumatriptan clinical pharmacokinetics. *Clin Pharmacokinet* 1994; **27:** 337–44.
2. Lacey LF, *et al.* Single dose pharmacokinetics of sumatriptan in healthy volunteers. *Eur J Clin Pharmacol* 1995; **47:** 543–8.

## Uses and Administration

Sumatriptan is a selective serotonin agonist which acts at 5-$HT_1$ receptors and produces vasoconstriction of cranial arteries. It is used for the acute treatment of migraine attacks and of cluster headache. It should not be used prophylactically. It may be given by mouth or subcutaneously as the succinate and intranasally as the base. Doses are expressed in terms of sumatriptan base; sumatriptan succinate 70 mg is approximately equivalent to 50 mg of sumatriptan.

For the acute treatment of **migraine** sumatriptan should be used as soon as possible after the onset of the headache phase, but efficacy is independent of the duration of the attack before starting treatment. If no response is obtained with the initial dose by any route, a second dose should not be given for the same attack.

The recommended dose by mouth in the UK is 50 mg, although some patients may require 100 mg. A clinical response can be expected after about 30 minutes. If there is a response but the migraine returns, further doses may be given provided that there is a minimum interval of 2 hours between doses and that not more than 300 mg is taken in any 24-hour period. In the USA a lower dose of 25 mg may be used, although some patients require 50 or 100 mg. This may be followed by a second dose of up to 100 mg if the headache returns or the patient has a partial response provided that the total daily dose does not exceed the recommended maximum of 200 mg. A minimum interval of 2 hours is recommended between doses. For oral doses in hepatic impairment, see below.

When used intranasally a clinical response can be expected in 15 minutes. In adults, the recommended dose of sumatriptan in the UK is 20 mg administered into one nostril; in the USA, the recommended dose is 5, 10, or 20 mg. If symptoms recur, a second dose may be given in the next 24 hours, at least 2 hours after the first dose. Not more than 40 mg should be used in a 24-hour period. Intranasal sumatriptan may also be given to adolescents aged 12 to below 18 years in a dose of 10 mg into one nostril; as with adults, the dose may be repeated if symptoms recur within 24 hours although not more than 20 mg should be taken within a 24-hour period.

Sumatriptan may be self-administered by subcutaneous injection in a single dose of 6 mg; a clinical response may be expected after 10 to 15 minutes. If symptoms recur, a second dose of 6 mg may be injected at least one hour after the first dose; not more than 12 mg should be given in a 24-hour period.

For the acute treatment of **cluster headache,** sumatriptan succinate is given by subcutaneous injection in similar doses to those used for migraine.

**Administration in hepatic impairment.** Sumatriptan should be used with caution in patients with hepatic impairment. A dose of up to 50 mg by mouth is considered suitable. It should not be given to patients with severe hepatic impairment.

**Migraine and cluster headache.** The use of sumatriptan and other triptans in the treatment of cluster headache (p.464) and migraine (p.464) has been reviewed.[1-7]

In **migraine** serotonin (5-$HT_1$) agonists are preferred to ergotamine for the treatment of acute attacks unresponsive to non-opioid analgesics.

There are several different triptans clinically available. In a meta-analysis of 53 trials (involving 24 089 patients) and a separate analysis of all direct comparative trials of 5 of the triptans and sumatriptan, all were found to be more effective than placebo.[5] At the marketed doses, all oral triptans (almotriptan, eletriptan, naratriptan, rizatriptan, sumatriptan, and zolmitriptan) were effective and well tolerated. Almotriptan, eletriptan, or rizatriptan were considered to provide the highest likelihood of consistent success. A review of the efficacy of the 5 triptans available in the USA also showed pain relief at 2 hours was comparable for all.[6] Almotriptan 12.5 mg offered high tolerability and good efficacy; eletriptan 80 mg provided high efficacy and low recurrence; and rizatriptan 10 mg was associated with consistent and rapid freedom from pain.[5] Frovatriptan was not included in the analyses, but publicly available data suggested lower efficacy. Only sumatriptan, though, has parenteral formulations and the 6-mg subcutaneous formulation is still the fastest and most effective acute treatment.[5]

About 21 to 57% of patients who initially respond to sumatriptan have a recurrence of their headache within 24 to 48 hours; this may be related in part to its short half-life. Such recurrences usually respond to a second dose[8,9] but if a first dose is ineffective subsequent doses for the same attack are of no benefit and should not be given. Sumatriptan is considered[10] to be effective when given at any time once the headache phase of migraine has started but giving it during migraine aura appears to be of little benefit since it does not affect the aura or prevent or delay the development of headache.[11] Repeated or long-term use does not appear to be associated with reduced efficacy.[12,13] For reports of an association between sumatriptan and analgesic-induced headache, see under Adverse Effects, above.

Sumatriptan's effectiveness appears to be maintained in menstrual migraine, a condition which is considered to be less responsive to treatment than nonmenstrual migraine.[14] Rizatriptan[15] has also been found to be effective in menstrual migraine.

Experience of use in children has been reported.[16] Results of a randomised, placebo-controlled study[17] in adolescents aged 12 to 17 years showed evidence of efficacy, tolerability, and safety in this age group; it was felt that the nasal spray might be particularly well suited for adolescent use.

Subcutaneous sumatriptan has also been shown to be effective in relieving acute attacks of headache in patients with **cluster headache**. In studies about 75% of patients have obtained relief within 15 minutes of a 6-mg subcutaneous injection;[18,19] the use of higher doses was found to be of no advantage. Long term efficacy appears to be maintained[20] but the significance of the transient increase in the frequency of attacks seen in some patients remains to be determined.[21] It does not appear to be effective for the prevention of headache during cluster periods.[22] Another triptan found to be effective in the treatment of episodic cluster headache is zolmitriptan.[23].

1. Fullerton T, Gengo FM. Sumatriptan: a selective 5-hydroxytryptamine receptor agonist for the acute treatment of migraine. *Ann Pharmacother* 1992; **26:** 800–8.
2. Hsu VD. Sumatriptan: a new drug for vascular headache. *Clin Pharm* 1992; **11:** 919–29.
3. Bateman DN. Sumatriptan. *Lancet* 1993; **341:** 221–4.
4. Perry CM, Markham A. Sumatriptan: an updated review of its use in migraine. *Drugs* 1998; **55:** 889–922.
5. Ferrari MD, *et al.* Oral triptans (serotonin 5-$HT_{1B/1D}$ agonists) in acute migraine treatment: a meta-analysis of 53 trials. *Lancet* 2001; **358:** 1668–75.
6. Jamieson DG. The safety of triptans in the treatment of patients with migraine. *Am J Med* 2002; **112:** 135–40.
7. Rapoport AM, Tepper SJ. Triptans are all different. *Arch Neurol* 2001; **58:** 1479–80.
8. Ferrari MD, *et al.* Oral sumatriptan: effect of a second dose, and incidence and treatment of headache recurrences. *Cephalalgia* 1994; **14:** 330–8.
9. Dahlöf C. Headache recurrence after subcutaneous sumatriptan and early treatment. *Lancet* 1992; **340:** 909.
10. Ferrari MD. Sumatriptan in the treatment of migraine. *Neurology* 1993; **43** (suppl 3): S43–S47.
11. Bates D, *et al.* Sumatriptan Aura Study Group. Subcutaneous sumatriptan during the migraine aura. *Neurology* 1994; **44:** 1587–92.
12. Cady RK, *et al.* Efficacy of subcutaneous sumatriptan in repeated episodes of migraine. *Neurology* 1993; **43:** 1363–8.
13. Tansey MJB, *et al.* Long-term experience with sumatriptan in treatment of migraine. *Eur Neurol* 1993; **33:** 310–15.
14. Solbach MP, Waymer RS. Treatment of menstruation-associated migraine headache with subcutaneous sumatriptan. *Obstet Gynecol* 1993; **82:** 769–72.
15. Silberstein SD, *et al.* Rizatriptan in the treatment of menstrual migraine. *Obstet Gynecol* 2000; **96:** 237–42.
16. Linder SL. Subcutaneous sumatriptan in the clinical setting: the first 50 consecutive patients with acute migraine in a pediatric neurology office practice. *Headache* 1996; **36:** 419–22.
17. Winner P, *et al.* A randomized, double-blind, placebo-controlled study of sumatriptan nasal spray in the treatment of acute migraine in adolescents. *Pediatrics* 2000; **106:** 989–997.
18. The Sumatriptan Cluster Headache Study Group. Treatment of acute cluster headache with sumatriptan. *N Engl J Med* 1991; **325:** 322–6.
19. Ekbom K, *et al.* Subcutaneous sumatriptan in the acute treatment of cluster headache: a dose comparison study. *Acta Neurol Scand* 1993; **88:** 63–9.
20. Ekbom K, *et al.* Cluster headache attacks treated for up to three months with subcutaneous sumatriptan (6 mg). *Cephalalgia* 1995; **15:** 230–6.
21. Hardebo JE. Subcutaneous sumatriptan in cluster headache: a time study of the effect on pain and autonomic symptoms. *Headache* 1993; **33:** 18–21.
22. Monstad I, *et al.* Preemptive oral treatment with sumatriptan during a cluster period. *Headache* 1995; **35:** 607–13.
23. Bahra A, *et al.* Oral zolmitriptan is effective in the acute treatment of cluster headache. *Neurology* 2000; **54:** 1832–39.

## Preparations

**Proprietary Preparations** (details are given in Part 3)

***Arg.:*** Imigran; Imitrex; Micranil; ***Austral.:*** Imigran; Suvalan; ***Austria:*** Imigran; ***Belg.:*** Imitrex; ***Braz.:*** Imigran; Migril†; Sumax; ***Canad.:*** Imitrex; ***Chile:*** Imigran; Liotrex; Somatran; ***Denm.:*** Imigran; ***Fin.:*** Imigran; ***Fr.:*** Imigrane; Imiject; ***Ger.:*** Imigran; ***Gr.:*** Imigran; ***Hong Kong:*** Imigran; ***India:*** Suminat; ***Irl.:*** Imigran; ***Israel:*** Imitrex; ***Ital.:*** Imigran; Sumigrene; ***Malaysia:*** Imigran; ***Mex.:*** Imigran; ***Neth.:*** Imigran; ***Norw.:*** Imigran; ***NZ:*** Imigran; ***Port.:*** Diletan; Imigran; ***S.Afr.:*** Imigran; ***Singapore:*** Imigran; ***Spain:*** Arcoiran; Dolmigral; Imigran; Novelian†; ***Swed.:*** Imigran; ***Switz.:*** Imigran; ***Thai.:*** Imigran; ***UK:*** Imigran; ***USA:*** Imitrex.

# Zolmitriptan *(BAN, USAN, rINN)*

311C90; Zolmitriptán. (S)-4-{3-[2-(Dimethylamino)ethyl]indol-5-ylmethyl}-1,3-oxazolidin-2-one.

$C_{16}H_{21}N_3O_2$ = 287.4.

*CAS — 139264-17-8.*

*ATC — N02CC03.*

## Adverse Effects and Precautions

As for Sumatriptan, p.471. Zolmitriptan should also be avoided in patients with Wolff-Parkinson-White syndrome or arrhythmias associated with accessory cardiac conduction pathways. It should be given with caution in patients with moderate to severe hepatic impairment.

**Analgesic-induced headache.** For a report of an association between zolmitriptan and analgesic-induced headache, see under Adverse Effects of Sumatriptan, p.471.

**Ischaemia.** A spinal cord lesion related to the use of zolmitriptan has been reported in a 50-year-old woman;[1] clinical features suggested that the lesion was an ischaemic infarct.

1. Vijayan N, Peacock JH. Spinal cord infarction during use of zolmitriptan: a case report. *Headache* 2000; **40:** 57–60.

## Interactions

As for Sumatriptan, p.472. It is recommended that the maximum dose of zolmitriptan in 24 hours should be reduced in patients receiving cimetidine (see under Uses and Administration, below). A similar reduction in zolmitriptan dosage is anticipated if it is given with drugs, such as fluvoxamine and ciprofloxacin, that inhibit the cytochrome P450 isoenzyme CYP1A2. Zolmitriptan should not be used within 12 hours of other serotonin (5-$HT_1$) agonists. Opinion varies on the use of zolmitriptan with inhibitors of monoamine oxidase type A such as moclobemide. In the UK the manufacturers recommend that the maximum dose of zolmitriptan should be reduced when used with inhibitors of monoamine oxidase type A (see under Uses and Administration, below), whereas in the USA the manufacturers contra-indicate such combinations.

◊ References.

1. Dixon R, *et al.* The metabolism of zolmitriptan: effects of an inducer and an inhibitor of cytochrome P450 on its pharmacokinetics in healthy volunteers. *Clin Drug Invest* 1998; **15:** 515–22.

**Beta blockers.** *Propranolol* increased plasma-zolmitriptan concentrations in a study in 12 healthy volunteers, but the changes were not thought to be clinically important, therefore dosage adjustment of zolmitriptan in patients taking propranolol for migraine prophylaxis was not considered necessary.[1]

1. Peck RW, *et al.* The interaction between propranolol and the novel antimigraine agent zolmitriptan (311C90). *Br J Clin Pharmacol* 1997; **44:** 595–9.

## Pharmacokinetics

The absolute bioavailability of zolmitriptan following oral doses is about 40 to 50%, and peak-plasma concentrations are achieved in about 1.5 to 3.5 hours depending on the formulation. Plasma protein binding is low (about 25%). Zolmitriptan undergoes hepatic metabolism, principally to the indole acetic acid, and also the *N*-oxide and *N*-desmethyl analogues. The *N*-desmethyl metabolite (183C91) was more active than the parent compound in *animal* studies, and would be expected to contribute to the therapeutic effect of zolmitriptan. The primary metabolism of zolmitriptan is mediated mainly by the cytochrome P450 isoenzyme CYP1A2 while monoamine oxidase type A is responsible for further metabolism of the *N*-desmethyl metabolite. Over 60% of a dose is excreted in the urine, mainly as the indole acetic acid, and about 30% appears in the faeces, mainly as unchanged drug. The elimination half-life is 2.5 to 3 hours, and is prolonged in patients with liver disease.

◊ References.

1. Seaber E, *et al.* The tolerability and pharmacokinetics of the novel antimigraine compound 311C90 in healthy male volunteers. *Br J Clin Pharmacol* 1996; **41:** 141–7.
2. Dixon R, *et al.* The pharmacokinetics and effects on blood pressure of multiple doses of the novel anti-migraine drug zolmitriptan (311C90) in healthy volunteers. *Br J Clin Pharmacol* 1997; **43:** 273–81.
3. Seaber E, *et al.* The absolute bioavailability and metabolic disposition of the novel antimigraine compound zolmitriptan (311C90). *Br J Clin Pharmacol* 1997; **43:** 579–87.
4. Peck RW, *et al.* The pharmacodynamics and pharmacokinetics of the $5HT_{1B/1D}$-agonist zolmitriptan in healthy young and elderly men and women. *Clin Pharmacol Ther* 1998; **63:** 342–53.
5. Seaber EJ, *et al.* The absolute bioavailability and effect of food on the pharmacokinetics of zolmitriptan in healthy volunteers. *Br J Clin Pharmacol* 1998; **46:** 433–9.
6. Dixon R, *et al.* A comparison of the pharmacokinetics and tolerability of the novel antimigraine compound zolmitriptan in adolescents and adults. *J Child Adolesc Psychopharmacol* 1999; **9:** 35–42.

## Uses and Administration

Zolmitriptan is a selective serotonin ($5-HT_1$) agonist with actions and uses similar to those of sumatriptan (p.473). It is used for the acute treatment of migraine attacks. Zolmitriptan should not be used prophylactically. It should be given as early as possible after the onset of migraine headache, but efficacy is independent of the duration of the attack before starting treatment.

The recommended dose in the UK is 2.5 mg by mouth. If symptoms persist or return within 24 hours, a second dose may be taken not less than 2 hours after the first dose. If a patient does not achieve satisfactory relief with a dose of 2.5 mg, subsequent attacks may be treated with doses of 5 mg. The maximum dose of zolmitriptan in 24 hours is 10 mg. Dose reductions are recommended in patients taking certain other drugs. The maximum dose of zolmitriptan in 24 hours should be 5 mg in those receiving cimetidine or an inhibitor of monoamine oxidase type A. A similar reduction is also recommended in those taking drugs, such as fluvoxamine and ciprofloxacin, that inhibit the cytochrome P450 isoenzyme CYP1A2.

Recommended doses in the USA are somewhat lower; the dose is 1.25 or 2.5 mg with a maximum dose of 10 mg in 24 hours.

In some countries, zolmitriptan is available as a nasal spray. When given intranasally the usual dose is 2.5 or 5 mg as a single dose into one nostril. If symptoms persist or return within 24 hours a second dose may be given after at least 2 hours, up to a maximum of 10 mg daily.

For dosage in hepatic or renal impairment see below.

**Administration in hepatic impairment.** A study[1] has indicated that while there is no need to reduce the size of the initial dose of zolmitriptan in patients with moderate or severe hepatic impairment, accumulation may occur with repeated doses in patients with severe hepatic impairment and their total daily dosage should be reduced.

A maximum oral dose of 5 mg in 24 hours is recommended by the manufacturers in the UK in patients with moderate to severe hepatic impairment. A dose of less than 2.5 mg is recommended in the USA.

1. Dixon R, *et al.* Effect of hepatic impairment on the pharmacokinetics of zolmitriptan. *J Clin Pharmacol* 1998; **38:** 694–701.

**Administration in renal impairment.** Although renal clearance of zolmitriptan and its metabolites was reduced in a study[1] in patients with moderate to severe renal impairment, the resulting effect was thought unlikely to be of clinical importance and adjustment of zolmitriptan dosage in patients with renal impairment was considered unnecessary.

1. Gillotin C, *et al.* No need to adjust the dose of 311C90 (zolmitriptan), a novel anti-migraine treatment in patients with renal failure not requiring dialysis. *Int J Clin Pharmacol Ther* 1997; **35:** 522–6.

**Migraine and cluster headache.** For comparison of the relative benefits of different triptans in migraine, see under Sumatriptan, p.473.

Further references.

1. Spencer CM, *et al.* Zolmitriptan: a review of its use in migraine. *Drugs* 1999; **58:** 347–74.
2. Bahra A, *et al.* Oral zolmitriptan is effective in the acute treatment of cluster headache. *Neurology* 2000; **54:** 1832–9.
3. Mathew NT, *et al.* Treatment of nonresponders to oral sumatriptan with zolmitriptan and rizatriptan: a comparative open trial. *Headache* 2000; **40:** 464–5.

## Preparations

**Proprietary Preparations** (details are given in Part 3)

***Arg.:*** Zomigon; ***Austral.:*** Zomig; ***Austria:*** Zomig; ***Belg.:*** Zomig; ***Braz.:*** Zomig; ***Canad.:*** Zomig; ***Denm.:*** Zomig; ***Fin.:*** Zomig; ***Fr.:*** Zomig; Zomigoro; ***Ger.:*** AscoTop; ***Gr.:*** Zomigon; ***Hong Kong:*** Zomig; ***Irl.:*** Zomig; ***Israel:*** Zomig; ***Ital.:*** Zomig; ***Mex.:*** Zomig; ***Neth.:*** Zomig; ***Norw.:*** Zomig; ***Port.:*** Zomig; ***S.Afr.:*** Zomig; ***Singapore:*** Zomig; ***Spain:*** Flezol; Zomig; ***Swed.:*** Zomig; ***Switz.:*** Zomig; ***Thai.:*** Zomig; ***UK:*** Zomig; ***USA:*** Zomig.

# Antimuscarinics

Anaesthesia, p.475
Biliary and renal colic, p.475
Cardiac disorders, p.475
Dystonias, p.475
Extrapyramidal disorders, p.475
Eye disorders, p.475
Gastrointestinal disorders, p.475
Hyperhidrosis, p.475
Micturition disorders, p.475
Nocturnal enuresis, p.475
Urinary incontinence and retention, p.476
Mydriasis and cycloplegia, p.476
Parkinsonism, p.476
Respiratory-tract disorders, p.476
Rhinitis, p.476
Vertigo, p.476

Antimuscarinic drugs are competitive inhibitors of the actions of acetylcholine at the muscarinic receptors of autonomic effector sites innervated by parasympathetic (cholinergic postganglionic) nerves; they are also inhibitors of the action of acetylcholine on smooth muscle lacking cholinergic innervation. They have been described as parasympatholytic, atropinic, atropine-like, and as anticholinergic, although the latter term should encompass compounds that also have antinicotinic actions.

Antimuscarinics can be classified as tertiary amine or quaternary ammonium compounds. The naturally occurring alkaloids such as atropine, hyoscine, and hyoscyamine are tertiary amines, that is they have a tertiary nitrogen atom; semisynthetic derivatives or synthetic antimuscarinics may be either tertiary (e.g. homatropine or trihexyphenidyl) or quaternary ammonium (e.g. homatropine methylbromide or ipratropium) compounds. At least 5 different pharmacologically identifiable types of **muscarinic receptor** ($M_1$, $M_2$, $M_3$, $M_4$, and $M_5$) have been described as have 5 different molecular forms ($m_1$, $m_2$, $m_3$, $m_4$, and $m_5$) of these receptors. While the traditional antimuscarinics appear to be relatively non-specific, newer compounds like pirenzepine and telenzepine have a selective action on the $M_1$ receptors within ganglia supplying cholinergic postganglionic nerves to the gastrointestinal tract. At therapeutic doses tertiary amine antimuscarinics have little effect on the actions of acetylcholine at nicotinic receptors. However, the quaternary ammonium antimuscarinics exhibit a greater degree of antinicotinic potency, and some of their side-effects at high doses are due to ganglionic blockade; excessively high doses may even produce neuromuscular block. There are also pharmacokinetic differences between tertiary amine and quaternary ammonium antimuscarinics. Quaternary ammonium compounds are less lipid soluble than tertiary amines; their gastrointestinal absorption is poor and they do not readily pass the blood-brain barrier or conjunctiva.

Antimuscarinics can produce a wide range of effects at therapeutic doses. The **peripheral** antimuscarinic effects that are produced as the dose increases are:

- decreased production of secretions from the salivary, bronchial, and sweat glands
- dilatation of the pupils (mydriasis) and paralysis of accommodation (cycloplegia)
- increased heart rate
- inhibition of micturition and reduction in gastrointestinal tone
- inhibition of gastric acid secretion

As for **central** effects, with the exception of hyoscine, which causes CNS depression at therapeutic doses, tertiary amines stimulate the medulla and higher cerebral centres producing mild central vagal excitation and respiratory stimulation. At toxic doses all tertiary amines, including hyoscine, cause stimulation of the CNS with restlessness, disorientation, hallucinations, and delirium. As the dose increases stimulation is followed by central depression and death from respiratory paralysis. Synthetic tertiary amines are less potent in their central effects than natural tertiary amines; quaternary ammonium compounds have negligible central effects.

These actions of antimuscarinics have led to their use in a variety of clinical conditions.

◊ References.

1. Goyal RK. Muscarinic receptor subtypes: physiology and clinical implications. *N Engl J Med* 1989; **321:** 1022–9.
2. Caulfield MP. Muscarinic receptors—characterization, coupling and function. *Pharmacol Ther* 1993; **58:** 319–79.
3. Caulfield MP, Birdsall NJM. International Union of Pharmacology. XVII. Classification of muscarinic acetylcholine receptors. *Pharmacol Rev* 1998; **50:** 279–90.

### Anaesthesia

Antimuscarinics, including *atropine, hyoscine,* and *glycopyrronium,* have been used pre-operatively to inhibit salivation and excessive secretions of the respiratory tract during anaesthesia (p.1296). This use is less important now that less irritating anaesthetics are used. Atropine and glycopyrronium are given to reduce intra-operative bradycardia and hypotension induced by drugs such as suxamethonium, halothane, or propofol, or following vagal stimulation. Glycopyrronium causes less tachycardia than atropine when given intravenously. When hyoscine is used as a premedicant it also provides some amnesia, sedation, and antiemesis but, unlike atropine, may cause bradycardia rather than tachycardia. Atropine or, preferably, glycopyrronium is also used before, or with, anticholinesterases such as neostigmine to prevent their muscarinic adverse effects (see p.1493).

### Biliary and renal colic

Antimuscarinics may relieve painful spasms of the biliary and genito-urinary systems and have been used in biliary or renal (ureteral) colic, although, as discussed on p.4, analgesics are normally used. However, an antispasmodic should be given with morphine and its derivatives in patients with biliary disorders to counteract painful spasms of the sphincter of Oddi which may be produced by the opioid. See Gastrointestinal Disorders (below) for reference to gastrointestinal spasm.

### Cardiac disorders

The cardiac uses of *atropine* are discussed on p.478.

### Dystonias

Antimuscarinics such as trihexyphenidyl have been used in the management of dystonias (p.1209). The high doses that may be required are tolerated much better by children and adolescents than by adults.

### Extrapyramidal disorders

See Dystonias (above) and Parkinsonism, including drug-induced extrapyramidal disorders (below).

### Eye disorders

See under Mydriasis and Cycloplegia (below).

### Gastrointestinal disorders

Antimuscarinics have been used to relieve **spasms** of the gastrointestinal tract in diverticular disease (p.1241), dyspepsia (p.1242), and irritable bowel syndrome (p.1244); they are no longer considered appropriate for use in infant colic (see Gastrointestinal Spasm, p.1242; see above for use in biliary and renal colic). Antimuscarinics have also been tried in an attempt to relax the smooth muscle in oesophageal spasm (see Oesophageal Motility Disorders, p.1246), although results are often disappointing. They should be avoided in patients with oesophageal reflux because of a tendency to relax the oesophageal sphincter.

Antimuscarinics (particularly selective antimuscarinics such as *pirenzepine*) have been used for their antisecretory effects in the treatment of **peptic ulcer disease** (p.1246), generally as adjuncts to other antiulcer drugs, but such therapy now plays a much reduced role in management.

*Hyoscine* is one of the principal drugs used to prevent **motion sickness** (see under Nausea and Vomiting, p.1245). It may be given by mouth for short-term protection or transdermally from controlled release systems for a prolonged duration of action.

### Hyperhidrosis

Antimuscarinics such as *diphemanil metilsulfate, glycopyrronium bromide,* and *hyoscine hydrobromide* have been applied topically as alternatives to aluminium salts in the treatment of hyperhidrosis (p.1136). Side-effects of antimuscarinics administered by mouth generally preclude their use by this route, although oral *propantheline* has been used successfully.

### Micturition disorders

Normal micturition (awareness of the need to void urine as a result of bladder filling, postponement of urination until convenient, and the ability to empty the bladder voluntarily) is controlled by the smooth detrusor muscle of the bladder (innervated predominantly by parasympathetic nerves) and the external sphincter (sympathetic innervation). During urination parasympathetic stimulation causes the detrusor muscle to contract while reduced sympathetic tone allows the external sphincter to relax. Micturition disorders can occur through local effects on the bladder or urethra or may result through disturbances of their nervous control. They include nocturnal enuresis, urinary incontinence, and urinary retention. The terms 'neurogenic bladder' and 'neuropathic bladder' are used loosely to describe any bladder dysfunction resulting from any neurological disturbance.

**Nocturnal enuresis.** Involuntary discharge of urine during sleep, termed nocturnal enuresis (bed-wetting), is a normal occurrence in young children, but may persist in up to 5% by the age of 10 years. Nocturnal enuresis is defined as primary if there has never been a period of dryness for more than 6 months, and secondary if the child was dry for such a period before the onset of bed-wetting. Nonpharmacological approaches to treatment include bladder retention training, motivational therapy, and behaviour modification or conditioning therapy using moisture-sensitive alarms. Drug therapy may initially produce a more rapid response, but training and the use of alarms has generally appeared to be more effective and to have a lower relapse rate. Although preparations are available to treat children as young as 5 years of age many consider drug therapy to be inappropriate for children under 7 years. Drug therapy is probably most useful for intermittent use on special occasions such as sleeping away from home or when added to treatment in children who fail to respond to nonpharmacological methods alone. The long-term use of drugs for enuresis is controversial.

Use of *desmopressin* at night can be effective in the short-term control of nocturnal enuresis and many now consider it to be the drug of choice in terms of safety. However, it should not be given when enuresis is due to polydipsia as desmopressin may provoke water intoxication and convulsions due to hyponatraemia.

Tricyclic antidepressants have also been used and of these most experience has been with *imipramine.* Their mechanism of action in nocturnal enuresis is unclear. It may be partly the result of their antimuscarinic and antispasmodic actions.

Antimuscarinics such as *oxybutynin* reduce uninhibited bladder contractions, but although they may be of benefit in diurnal enuresis they are rarely of benefit in nocturnal enuresis alone.

References.

1. Marcovitch H. Treating bed wetting. *BMJ* 1993; **306:** 536.
2. Rappaport L. The treatment of nocturnal enuresis—where are we now? *Pediatrics* 1993; **92:** 465–6.
3. Mark SD, Frank JD. Nocturnal enuresis. *Br J Urol* 1995; **75:** 427–34.
4. Monda JM, Husmann DA. Primary nocturnal enuresis: a comparison among observation, imipramine, desmopressin acetate and bed-wetting alarm systems. *J Urol (Baltimore)* 1995, **154:** 745–8.
5. Burke JR, *et al.* A comparison of amitriptyline, vasopressin and amitriptyline with vasopressin in nocturnal enuresis. *Pediatr Nephrol* 1995; **9:** 438–40.
6. Tietjen DN, Husmann DA. Nocturnal enuresis: a guide to evaluation and treatment. *Mayo Clin Proc* 1996; **71:** 857–62.
7. Owens RG, Karram MM. Comparative tolerability of drug therapies used to treat incontinence and enuresis. *Drug Safety* 1998; **19:** 123–39.
8. Evans JHC. Evidence based management of nocturnal enuresis. *BMJ* 2001; **323:** 1167–9. Correction. *ibid.* 2002; **324:** 98.
9. Glazener CMA, *et al.* Alarm interventions for nocturnal enuresis in children. Available in The Cochrane Library; Issue 1. Chichester: John Wiley; 2004.
10. Glazener CMA, Evans JHC. Desmopressin for nocturnal enuresis in children. Available in The Cochrane Library; Issue 1. Chichester: John Wiley; 2004.
11. Glazener CMA, *et al.* Drugs for nocturnal enuresis in children (other than desmopressin and tricyclics). Available in The Cochrane Library; Issue 1. Chichester: John Wiley; 2004.

12. Glazener CMA, *et al.* Tricyclic and related drugs for nocturnal enuresis in children. Available in The Cochrane Library; Issue 1. Chichester: John Wiley; 2004.
13. Anonymous. Management of bedwetting in children. *Drug Ther Bull* 2004; **42:** 33–7.

**Urinary incontinence and retention.** Urinary incontinence is defined as an involuntary loss of urine that is objectively demonstrable and a social or hygienic problem. Nocturnal enuresis in children is discussed above. Depending on the cause patients may have symptoms of urinary frequency, nocturia, urgency, dribbling, or dysuria. Classifications of incontinence vary but the main types include: stress incontinence, urge incontinence, and overflow incontinence (a consequence of urinary retention). The term functional incontinence is used when the patient's condition is due to impaired mobility or mental function. It is important to determine the type and, where possible, cause of urinary incontinence before attempting treatment. Urinary-tract infections, constipation, and benign prostatic hyperplasia may mimic or cause the symptoms of urinary incontinence and should be excluded.

**Stress incontinence** is the commonest form of incontinence in women. The patient usually has urethral sphincter incompetence and loss of urine is associated with increases in intra-abdominal pressure such as may occur on standing or coughing. Treatment may involve measures such as pelvic floor exercises, electrical stimulation, or biofeedback, and the use of devices such as vaginal cones; surgery; or drugs.

- Some consider that drug therapy has little part in the treatment of stress incontinence. Alpha-adrenoceptor agonists such as *ephedrine, phenylpropanolamine,* and *pseudoephedrine* have been used to increase tone in the muscles of the urethra and at the base of the bladder; they may prevent incontinence in certain stress situations, but long-term experience has been mostly disappointing. *Oestrogens* used with an alpha-adrenoceptor agonist such as phenylpropanolamine appear to be effective and may be of use for postmenopausal women with mild stress incontinence; unfortunately, addition of a progestogen (necessary in women with an intact uterus) might exacerbate the incontinence. The value of oestrogens used without an alpha-adrenoceptor agonist is less clear. The serotonin and noradrenaline reuptake inhibitor *duloxetine* has shown benefit in some studies in stress incontinence. Intra-urethral injections of *collagen* or *polytef* appear to be effective, but there are concerns over migration and granuloma formation with polytef.

In **urge incontinence**, also known as unstable bladder or detrusor instability, contractions of the detrusor muscle occur without warning and overcome urethral sphincter resistance, despite any attempt the patient might make to prevent it. Urge incontinence is the most common form of incontinence in the elderly and is often refractory to treatment. The cause is usually unknown and these cases are referred to as being due to **idiopathic detrusor instability.** When there is overt neurological disease, such as upper motor neurone lesions in spinal cord injury or multiple sclerosis, the term **detrusor hyperreflexia** is used. Reduction of excessive fluid intake and avoidance of drinks containing alcohol or caffeine may control mild symptoms of urge incontinence. Physiotherapy and behaviour therapy including bladder drill, biofeedback, hypnotherapy, acupuncture, and electrical stimulation may help.

- No drug treatment has been found to be universally effective. Drugs with antimuscarinic activity may inhibit unstable detrusor muscle contractions but the incidence of adverse effects can be high. As these drugs can increase bladder volume they should not be used in patients with urinary retention. The antimuscarinic *oxybutynin* also has direct smooth muscle relaxant properties and is considered by some to be the most useful drug, but adverse effects are common. *Tolterodine, trospium,* and *propiverine* have been introduced as alternatives to oxybutynin. *Flavoxate, propantheline,* and *emepronium* are now little used. *Tricyclic antidepressants* have also been used in urge incontinence because of their antimuscarinic activity but their main use has been in nocturnal enuresis and nocturia (see above). *Desmopressin* is also mainly used in nocturnal enuresis and nocturia. Evidence for *oestrogens* is inconclusive, but they may be useful as adjuncts in postmenopausal women with symptoms of urgency, frequency, and nocturia. Injection of *botulinum A toxin* into the detrusor muscle may be effective in the treatment of detrusor hyperreflexia that is resistant to antimuscarinics. Surgery is reserved for intractable cases.

Urge incontinence can also be due to abnormalities in bladder sensation; the causes of **sensory urgency** are often unknown but may be due to conditions such as urinary-tract infections or interstitial cystitis. Bladder retraining techniques and antimuscarinic therapy have been suggested when no underlying disorder can be identified.

Patients with **overflow incontinence** suffer from a continuous or frequent dribbling of urine as a consequence of an overdistended bladder produced by **urinary retention.** It may result from some form of urethral blockage or may be associated with drug treatment or conditions that reduce detrusor contractions or interfere with relaxation of the urethra. Overflow incontinence is uncommon in women and most patients are elderly men with urethral blockage due to benign prostatic hyperplasia (p.1555). However, urinary retention may also occur postpartum or postoperatively. Treatment depends on the underlying condition. Catheterisation is used to relieve acute painful urinary retention or when no cause can be found. Surgical procedures or dilatation are often used to correct any mechanical outflow obstruction.

- Alpha-adrenoceptor blocking drugs such as *alfuzosin, doxazosin, indoramin, prazosin, tamsulosin,* and *terazosin* may be given to patients waiting for surgery or to those unfit for surgery. They decrease outflow resistance and improve bladder emptying. Patients with detrusor hypotonicity have been given parasympathomimetics such as *bethanechol, carbachol,* and *distigmine* to increase detrusor muscle contractions but there have been doubts about their efficacy. Use of parasympathomimetics for postoperative urinary retention has been superseded by catheterisation.

References.

1. International Continence Society Standardization Committee. The standardization of terminology of lower urinary tract function. *Br J Obstet Gynaecol* 1990; **97** (suppl 6): 1–16.
2. Eckford SD, Keane DP. Management of detrusor instability. *Br J Hosp Med* 1993; **49:** 282–5.
3. Resnick NM. Urinary incontinence. *Lancet* 1995; **346:** 94–9.
4. Owens RG, Karram MM. Comparative tolerability of drug therapies used to treat incontinence and enuresis. *Drug Safety* 1998; **19:** 123–39.
5. Chutka DS, Takahashi PY. Urinary incontinence in the elderly: drug treatment options. *Drugs* 1998; **56:** 587–95.
6. Scientific Committee of the First International Consultation on Incontinence. Assessment and treatment of urinary incontinence. *Lancet* 2000; **355:** 2153–8.
7. Couture JA, Valiquette L. Urinary incontinence. *Ann Pharmacother* 2000; **34:** 646–55.
8. Thakar R, Stanton S. Management of urinary incontinence in women. *BMJ* 2000; **321:** 1326–31.
9. Haeusler G, *et al.* Drug therapy of urinary urge incontinence: a systematic review. *Obstet Gynecol* 2002; **100:** 1003–16.
10. Anonymous. Managing lower urinary tract symptoms in men. *Drug Ther Bull* 2003; **41:** 18–21.
11. Ouslander JG. Management of overactive bladder. *N Engl J Med* 2004; **350:** 786–99.
12. Holroyd-Leduc JM, Straus SE. Management of urinary incontinence in women: scientific review. *JAMA* 2004; **291:** 986–95.

### Mydriasis and cycloplegia

Drugs that dilate the pupil (mydriatics) and paralyse accommodation (cycloplegics) are used topically in the examination of the eye and other ophthalmic procedures, in the management of inflammatory conditions of the eye to treat or prevent the formation of adhesions between the lens and the iris (see Uveitis, p.1090), and in strabismus (p.1487).

Mydriasis requires paralysis of the pupillary constrictor muscles (which is how antimuscarinics act) or stimulation of the dilator muscles (which is how sympathomimetics act). Cycloplegia results from paralysis of the ciliary muscles (antimuscarinics, but not sympathomimetics, have this effect).

Antimuscarinics used in ophthalmology vary in onset and duration of action. *Atropine* can take up to 40 minutes or more to produce mydriasis, which persists for at least 7 days; it takes 1 to 3 hours to produce cycloplegia and 6 to 12 days for recovery of accommodation. *Hyoscine* has a shorter duration of action than atropine, although the effects may still persist for 3 to 7 days. For ophthalmic procedures, antimuscarinics such as *homatropine, cyclopentolate,* or *tropicamide,* with a more rapid onset and shorter duration of action than atropine, may be preferable. Recovery occurs up to 6 hours after tropicamide, and up to 24 hours after cyclopentolate; after homatropine it may take up to 3 days. Cycloplegia with homatropine may be incomplete, and particularly for young children (who are often resistant to the action of homatropine) cyclopentolate or atropine may be preferred.

The most common topical sympathomimetic is *phenylephrine,* but *hydroxyamfetamine* is also used in some countries. They are often used with an antimuscarinic to enhance mydriasis, especially in patients who might respond poorly to antimuscarinics alone, such as those with dark irides or diabetes, or those who are receiving prolonged miotic therapy. *Adrenaline* has been used for maintenance of mydriasis during ophthalmic surgery.

The local anaesthetic *cocaine* also has an independent mydriatic effect but because of concern over corneal toxicity it is now little used in ophthalmology.

Miosis (pupil constriction) resistant to conventional mydriatics often develops during ocular surgery, possibly due to the release of prostaglandins and other substances associated with trauma. *NSAIDs* are prostaglandin synthetase inhibitors and have been tried before ocular surgery to prevent or reduce intra-operative miosis. They do not possess intrinsic mydriatic properties.

### Parkinsonism

Antimuscarinics are used in Parkinson's disease (idiopathic or primary parkinsonism) and, particularly, drug-induced parkinsonism; they may be more suitable in younger rather than older patients. Those most commonly used are the tertiary amines, *trihexyphenidyl, benzatropine, orphenadrine,* and *procyclidine.* In Parkinson's disease (p.1196), antimuscarinics are generally used in the early stages when the condition is mild and tremor is the predominant symptom, as they provide little benefit in bradykinesia. They can also reduce the sialorrhoea experienced by patients with this disease but can aggravate other associated conditions such as constipation or dementia. Antimuscarinics may also be used later as adjuvant therapy to levodopa such as in patients with refractory tremor or dystonias.

Although antimuscarinics may provide relief from the extrapyramidal symptoms that occur as side-effects of antipsychotic therapy (see p.677), they do not relieve the symptoms of tardive dyskinesia and should be discontinued if it develops.

### Respiratory-tract disorders

The parasympathetic nervous system is involved in regulating bronchomotor tone; antimuscarinics have potent bronchodilatory activity and may be used in the management of bronchospasm. *Ipratropium* and *oxitropium* by inhalation are used in chronic bronchitis (p.779) and are at least as effective as beta$_2$ agonists. Ipratropium may produce additional bronchodilatation in severe acute asthma exacerbations (p.777) when life-threatening features are present or initial response to treatment with beta$_2$ agonists has been poor. In mild to moderate asthma, however, the addition of antimuscarinics has not been shown to add benefit to beta$_2$ agonist therapy.

*Atropine* and *glycopyrronium* have also been used.

### Rhinitis

The antimuscarinic drug ipratropium is used intranasally for the treatment of rhinitis (see p.787).

### Vertigo

Antihistamines are the mainstay of the treatment of vertigo (p.423), although the antimuscarinic drug *hyoscine* is effective in the prophylaxis and treatment of vertigo and nausea associated with vestibular disorders, such as Ménière's disease (p.422). See also motion sickness under Nausea and Vomiting (p.484).

## Atropine *(BAN)*

Atropina; Atropinum; (±)-Hyoscyamine. (1*R*,3*r*,5*S*,8*r*)-Tropan-3-yl (*RS*)-tropate.

$C_{17}H_{23}NO_3$ = 289.4.
*CAS — 51-55-8.*
*ATC — A03BA01; S01FA01.*

**Description.** Atropine is an alkaloid that may be obtained from solanaceous plants, or prepared by synthesis.

**Pharmacopoeias.** In *Eur.* (see p.vi) and *US.*

**Ph. Eur. 5.0** (Atropine). A white, crystalline powder or colourless crystals. Very slightly soluble in water; freely soluble in alcohol and in dichloromethane. Protect from light.

**USP 27** (Atropine). White crystals, usually needle-like, or white crystalline powder. Soluble 1 in 460 of water, 1 in 90 of water at 80°, 1 in 2 of alcohol, 1 in 1 of chloroform, and 1 in 25 of ether; soluble in glycerol. Its saturated solution in water is alkaline to phenolphthalein. Store in airtight containers. Protect from light.

## Atropine Methobromide *(BANM)*

Atropina, metilbromuro de; Atropine Methylbromide; Methylatropine Bromide; Methylatropini Bromidum; Methylatropinium Bromatum; Mydriasine. (1*R*,3*r*,5*S*)-8-Methyl-3-[(±)-tropoyloxy]tropanium bromide.

$C_{18}H_{26}BrNO_3$ = 384.3.
*CAS — 2870-71-5.*
*ATC — A03BA01.*

**Pharmacopoeias.** In *Eur.* (see p.vi).

**Ph. Eur. 5.0** (Methylatropine Bromide; Atropine Methobromide BP 2003). Colourless crystals or a white crystalline powder. Freely soluble in water; sparingly soluble in alcohol. Protect from light.

## Atropine Methonitrate *(BANM, rINN)*

Atrop. Methonit.; Atropini Methonitras; Methylatropine Nitrate *(USAN)*; Methylatropini Nitras; Metilnitrato de atropina.
(1*R*,3*r*,5*S*)-8-Methyl-3-[(±)-tropoyloxy]tropanium nitrate.
$C_{18}H_{26}N_2O_6$ = 366.4.
*CAS — 52-88-0.*
*ATC — A03BA01.*

**Pharmacopoeias.** In *Eur.* (see p.vi).

**Ph. Eur. 5.0** (Methylatropine Nitrate; Atropine Methonitrate BP 2003). A white, crystalline powder or colourless crystals. Freely soluble in water; soluble in alcohol. Protect from light.

**Stability.** Aqueous solutions of atropine methonitrate are unstable; stability is enhanced in acid solutions of pH below 6.

## Atropine Sulfate

Atrop. Sulph.; Atropina, sulfato de; Atropine Sulphate *(BANM)*; Atropini Sulfas.
$(C_{17}H_{23}NO_3)_2,H_2SO_4,H_2O$ = 694.8.
*CAS — 55-48-1 (anhydrous atropine sulfate); 5908-99-6 (atropine sulfate monohydrate).*
*ATC — A03BA01; S01FA01.*

NOTE. Compounded preparations of atropine sulfate may be represented by the following names:

- Co-phenotrope (*BAN*)—atropine sulfate 1 part and diphenoxylate hydrochloride 100 parts (w/w).

ATR is a code approved by the BP 2003 for use on single unit dose eye drops containing atropine sulfate where the individual container may be too small to bear all the appropriate labelling information.

**Pharmacopoeias.** In *Chin., Eur.* (see p.vi), *Int., Jpn, Pol., US,* and *Viet.*

**Ph. Eur. 5.0** (Atropine Sulphate). A white, crystalline powder or colourless crystals. Very soluble in water; freely soluble in alcohol. A 2% solution in water has a pH of 4.5 to 6.2. Protect from light.

**USP 27** (Atropine Sulfate). Odourless, colourless crystals or white crystalline powder. It effloresces in dry air. Soluble 1 in 0.5 of water, 1 in 2.5 of boiling water, 1 in 5 of alcohol, and 1 in 2.5 of glycerol. Store in airtight containers.

**Incompatibility.** Incompatibility between atropine sulfate and hydroxybenzoate preservatives has been observed,[1] resulting in a total loss of the atropine in 2 to 3 weeks.

1. Deeks T. Oral atropine sulphate mixtures. *Pharm J* 1983; **230:** 481.

## Adverse Effects

The pattern of adverse effects seen with atropine and other antimuscarinics can mostly be related to their pharmacological actions at muscarinic and, at high doses, nicotinic receptors (see p.475). These effects are dose-related and are usually reversible when therapy is discontinued. The **peripheral** side-effects of atropine and other antimuscarinics are a consequence of their inhibitory effect on muscarinic receptors within the autonomic nervous system. At therapeutic doses, adverse effects include dryness of the mouth with difficulty in swallowing and talking, thirst, reduced bronchial secretions, dilatation of the pupils (mydriasis) with loss of accommodation (cycloplegia) and photophobia, flushing and dryness of the skin, transient bradycardia followed by tachycardia, with palpitations and arrhythmias, and difficulty in micturition, as well as reduction in the tone and motility of the gastrointestinal tract leading to constipation. Some of the **central** side-effects of atropine and other tertiary antimuscarinics seen at toxic doses (see below) may also occur at therapeutic doses.

In **overdosage**, the peripheral effects become more pronounced and other symptoms such as hyperthermia, hypertension, increased respiratory rate, and nausea and vomiting may occur. A rash may appear on the face or upper trunk. Toxic doses also cause CNS stimulation marked by restlessness, confusion, excitement, ataxia, incoordination, paranoid and psychotic reactions, hallucinations and delirium, and occasionally seizures. However, in severe intoxication, central stimulation may give way to CNS depression, coma, circulatory and respiratory failure, and death.

There is considerable variation in susceptibility to atropine; recovery has occurred even after 1 g, whereas deaths have been reported from doses of 100 mg or less for adults and 10 mg for children.

Quaternary ammonium antimuscarinics, such as atropine methobromide or methonitrate and propantheline bromide, have some ganglion-blocking activity and high doses may cause orthostatic hypotension and impotence; in toxic doses non-depolarising neuromuscular block may be produced.

Systemic toxicity may be produced by the **local** instillation of antimuscarinic eye drops, particularly in children and in the elderly. Prolonged administration of atropine to the eye may lead to local irritation, hyperaemia, oedema, and conjunctivitis. An increase in intra-ocular pressure may occur, especially in patients with angle-closure glaucoma.

**Hypersensitivity** to atropine is not uncommon and may occur as conjunctivitis or a skin rash.

**Effects on body temperature.** Atropine can cause hyperthermia as a result of inhibition of sweating. This may be attenuated by atropine's ability to dilate cutaneous blood vessels. However, there has been a report of hypothermia in a 14-year-old feverish patient following intravenous administration of atropine.[1]

For reports of fatal heat stroke in patients receiving an antimuscarinic and an antipsychotic concomitantly, see under Interactions in Benzatropine, p.479.

1. Lacouture PG, *et al.* Acute hypothermia associated with atropine. *Am J Dis Child* 1983; **137:** 291–2.

**Effects on the eyes.** In addition to the expected ocular effects of atropine (see above) there have been instances of acute angle-closure glaucoma in patients receiving nebulised atropine.[1]

1. Berdy GJ, *et al.* Angle closure glaucoma precipitated by aerosolized atropine. *Arch Intern Med* 1991; **151:** 1658–60.

**Effects on the gastrointestinal tract.** A report of paralytic ileus in a 77-year-old man with Parkinson's disease who had been receiving atropine sulfate by mouth to control excess salivation.[1]

1. Beatson N. Atropine and paralytic ileus. *Postgrad Med J* 1982; **58:** 451–3.

**Effects on the heart.** Atropine sulfate to a total of 1 mg per 70 kg body-weight given intravenously to 79 patients before surgery produced arrhythmias in over 20% of patients but particularly frequently in the young.[1] Atrioventricular dissociation was the most common disturbance in adults and in children atrial rhythm disturbances were common. In another study[2] premedication including atropine or glycopyrronium given intramuscularly resulted in a significantly greater incidence of tachycardia during anaesthetic induction and intubation compared with controls who received no antimuscarinic drug. Patients who received glycopyrronium also had a higher incidence of tachycardia during surgery than the controls. No significant difference in bradycardia or extrasystoles was found in the atropine- or the glycopyrronium-treated patients. Atrial fibrillation has been reported in 2 elderly glaucoma patients following post-surgical application of atropine ointment or eye drops to the eye.[3]

1. Dauchot P, Gravenstein JS. Effects of atropine on the electrocardiogram in different age groups. *Clin Pharmacol Ther* 1971; **12:** 274–80.
2. Shipton EA, Roelofse JA. Effects on cardiac rhythm of premedication with atropine or glycopyrrolate. *S Afr Med J* 1984; **66:** 287–8.
3. Merli GJ, *et al.* Cardiac dysrhythmias associated with ophthalmic atropine. *Arch Intern Med* 1986; **146:** 45–7.

**Effects on mental function.** A study[1] in patients with Parkinson's disease and healthy control subjects suggested that although short-term memory was impaired in patients receiving long-term antimuscarinic therapy the effect was reversible on discontinuation.

See also under Trihexyphenidyl (p.490) and under Oxybutynin (p.486).

1. Van Herwaarden G, *et al.* Short-term memory in Parkinson's disease after withdrawal of long-term anticholinergic therapy. *Clin Neuropharmacol* 1993; **16:** 438–43.

**Hypersensitivity.** A report[1] of anaphylactic shock developing in a 38-year-old woman after an intravenous injection of atropine.

1. Aguilera L, *et al.* Anaphylactic reaction after atropine. *Anaesthesia* 1988; **43:** 955–7.

**Overdosage.** Reports of atropine poisoning or overdosage have included a respiratory therapist[1] who had given 10 atropine sulfate aerosol treatments in the preceding 24 hours and children who had taken overdoses of a preparation containing diphenoxylate and atropine.[2]

1. Larkin GL. Occupational atropine poisoning via aerosol. *Lancet* 1991; **337:** 917.
2. McCarron MM, *et al.* Diphenoxylate-atropine (Lomotil) overdose in children: an update (report of eight cases and review of the literature). *Pediatrics* 1991; **87:** 694–700.

## Treatment of Adverse Effects

If a patient presents within an hour of an overdose of atropine by mouth the stomach may be emptied or activated charcoal given to reduce absorption. Supportive therapy should be given as required.

Physostigmine has been tried for antimuscarinic poisoning (see p.1494) but such use can be hazardous and is not generally recommended. Diazepam may be given to control marked excitement and convulsions; phenothiazines should not be given as they may exacerbate antimuscarinic effects. Antiarrhythmics are not recommended if arrhythmias develop; hypoxia and acidosis should be corrected and sodium bicarbonate may be given even if acidosis is not present.

## Precautions

Atropine needs to be used with caution in children and the elderly (who may be more susceptible to its adverse effects). It is contra-indicated in patients with prostatic enlargement, in whom it may lead to urinary retention, and in those with paralytic ileus or pyloric stenosis. In patients with ulcerative colitis its use may lead to ileus or megacolon, and its effects on the lower oesophageal sphincter may exacerbate reflux. Caution is generally advisable in any patient with diarrhoea. It should not be given to patients with myasthenia gravis except to reduce adverse muscarinic effects of an anticholinesterase.

Atropine should not be given to patients with angle-closure glaucoma or with a narrow angle between the iris and the cornea, since it may raise intra-ocular pressure and precipitate an acute attack. Acute angle-closure glaucoma has been reported in patients receiving nebulised atropine. Some manufacturers recommend that atropine eye drops should not be used in infants aged less than 3 months due to the possible association between the induced cycloplegia and the development of amblyopia. Systemic reactions have followed the absorption of atropine from eye drops; overdosage is less likely if the eye ointment is used. In the event of blurred vision following topical administration of atropine to the eye patients should not drive or operate machinery. Systemic administration of antimuscarinics may also cause blurred vision, dizziness, and other effects that may impair a patient's ability to perform skilled tasks such as driving.

Because of the risk of provoking hyperthermia, atropine should not be given to patients, especially children, when the ambient temperature is high. It should also be used cautiously in patients with fever.

Atropine and other antimuscarinics need to be used with caution in conditions characterised by tachycardia such as thyrotoxicosis, heart failure, and in cardiac surgery, where they may further accelerate the heart rate. Care is required in patients with acute myocardial infarction, as ischaemia and infarction may be made worse, and in patients with hypertension.

Atropine may cause confusion, especially in the elderly. Reduced bronchial secretion caused by systemic administration of atropine may be associated with the formation of mucous plugs.

In the treatment of parkinsonism, increases in dosage and transfer to other forms of treatment should be gradual and antimuscarinic should not be withdrawn abruptly. Minor reactions may be controlled by reducing the dose until tolerance has developed.

Persons with Down's syndrome appear to have an increased susceptibility to some of the actions of atropine, whereas those with albinism may have a reduced susceptibility.

**Breast feeding.** No adverse effects have been observed in breast-feeding infants whose mothers were receiving atropine, and the American Academy of Pediatrics[1] considers that it is therefore usually compatible with breast feeding.

1. American Academy of Pediatrics. The transfer of drugs and other chemicals into human milk. *Pediatrics* 2001; **108:** 776–89. Correction. *ibid.*; 1029. Also available at: http://aappolicy.aappublications.org/cgi/content/full/pediatrics%3b108/3/776 (accessed 01/06/04)

## Interactions

The effects of atropine and other antimuscarinics may be enhanced by the concomitant use of other drugs with antimuscarinic properties, such as amantadine, some antihistamines, phenothiazine antipsychotics, and tricyclic antidepressants. Inhibition of drug-metabolising enzymes by MAOIs may possibly enhance the effects of antimuscarinics. The reduction in gastric motility caused by antimuscarinics may affect the absorption of other drugs. Antimuscarinics and parasympathomimetics may counteract each others effects.

## Pharmacokinetics

Atropine is readily absorbed from the gastrointestinal tract; it is also absorbed from mucous membranes, the eye, and to some extent through intact skin. It is rapidly cleared from the blood and is distributed throughout the body. It crosses the blood-brain barrier. It is incompletely metabolised in the liver and is excreted in the urine as unchanged drug and metabolites. A half-life of about 4 hours has been reported. Atropine crosses the placenta and traces appear in breast milk.

Quaternary ammonium salts of atropine, such as the methonitrate, are less readily absorbed after oral administration. They are highly ionised in body fluids and being poorly soluble in lipids they do not readily cross the blood-brain barrier.

**Pregnancy.** Studies of the pharmacokinetics of atropine in mother and fetus in late pregnancy[1-3] indicated that atropine rapidly crosses the placenta. However, whereas peak concentrations of atropine in fetal cord blood were reached about 5 minutes after intravenous administration, the maximum effect on fetal heart rate occurred after about 25 minutes.


1. Barrier G, *et al.* La pharmacocinétique de l'atropine chez la femme enceinte et le foetus en fin de grossesse. *Anesth Analg Reanim* 1976; **33:** 795–800.
2. Onnen I, *et al.* Placental transfer of atropine at the end of pregnancy. *Eur J Clin Pharmacol* 1979; **15:** 443–6.
3. Kanto J, *et al.* Placental transfer and pharmacokinetics of atropine after a single maternal intravenous and intramuscular administration. *Acta Anaesthesiol Scand* 1981; **25:** 85–8.


## Uses and Administration

Atropine is a tertiary amine antimuscarinic alkaloid with both central and peripheral actions (see p.475). It is usually given as the sulfate. It first stimulates and then depresses the CNS and has antispasmodic actions on smooth muscle and reduces secretions, especially salivary and bronchial secretions; it also reduces perspiration, but has little effect on biliary or pancreatic secretion. Atropine depresses the vagus and thereby increases the heart rate. When given orally atropine reduces smooth-muscle tone and diminishes gastric and intestinal motility but has little effect on gastric secretion in usual therapeutic doses. Quaternary ammonium derivatives, such as the methonitrate, have less effect on the CNS but strong ganglion-blocking activity.

Atropine has a variety of uses, including: in anaesthetic practice as a premedicant and to counteract the muscarinic effects of anticholinesterases such as neostigmine and other parasympathomimetics; as an antispasmodic in gastrointestinal disorders; as an adjunct to opioid analgesics for the symptomatic relief of biliary or renal colic; to treat bradycardia; to treat or prevent bronchospasm; and in the treatment of poisoning with mushrooms that contain muscarine and in organophosphorus pesticide poisoning. Atropine is used topically as a mydriatic and cycloplegic in ophthalmology.

See under headings below for details of dosage and administration of atropine and its derivatives in specific indications.

**Anaesthesia.** The role of antimuscarinics in anaesthesia is discussed on p.475.

Atropine has been given as a premedicant before general anaesthesia to diminish the risk of vagal inhibition of the heart and to reduce salivary and bronchial secretions. For premedication 300 to 600 micrograms of atropine sulfate may be given by subcutaneous or intramuscular injection, usually 30 to 60 minutes before anaesthesia. Alternatively 300 to 600 micrograms of atropine sulfate may be given intravenously immediately before induction of anaesthesia. The *British National Formulary* notes that atropine sulfate may also be given with up to 10 mg morphine sulfate by subcutaneous injection about an hour before anaesthesia. Suitable paediatric subcutaneous or intramuscular premedication doses of atropine sulfate are:

- children up to 3 kg in weight: 100 micrograms
- children 7 to 9 kg in weight: 200 micrograms
- children 12 to 16 kg in weight: 300 micrograms
- children over 20 kg in weight: the adult dose.

For intra-operative bradycardia the *British National Formulary* states that incremental doses of 100 micrograms may be given intravenously; larger doses may be used in emergencies.

To counteract the muscarinic effects of anticholinesterases when they are used to reverse the effects of competitive muscle relaxants (see Neostigmine, p.1493) adults are given atropine sulfate 0.6 to 1.2 mg by intravenous injection before or with the anticholinesterase. Neonates and infants may be given a dose of 20 micrograms/kg.

**Anoxic seizures.** A reflex anoxic seizure is a paroxysmal event triggered by a noxious stimulus which, by vagal stimulation, causes pronounced bradycardia or cardiac arrest and consequent relative cerebral ischaemia.[1] Certain features of the attack may lead to a misdiagnosis of epilepsy. To avoid confusion with epileptic seizures (p.349), reflex anoxic seizures have also been called white or type 2 breath holding attacks. Depending on the degree of vagal hypersensitivity or noxious stimulus, attacks may occur infrequently or several times a day.

Infants and young children are mainly affected, however, the condition usually resolves by early childhood. It is generally benign and children do not suffer cardiac or cerebral damage. Treatment is seldom necessary, but atropine has been advocated to prevent vagal hypersensitivity in those children with frequent, persistent attacks. As atropine may require frequent administration with an attendant risk of overdosage, transdermal hyoscine has been tried as an alternative.[2]


1. Appleton RE. Reflex anoxic seizures. *BMJ* 1993; **307:** 214–5.
2. Palm L, Blennow G. Transdermal anticholinergic treatment of reflex anoxic seizures. *Acta Paediatr Scand* 1985; **74:** 803–4.


**Biliary and renal colic.** Atropine has been used as an adjunct to opioid analgesics for symptomatic relief of biliary or renal colic (see p.475).

**Cardiac disorders.** Atropine depresses the vagus and thereby increases the heart rate. It is therefore used in a variety of disorders or circumstances in which bradyarrhythmias occur. It is frequently used in sudden onset bradyarrhythmias and although it may also be employed for the initial treatment of chronic arrhythmias (p.816), cardiac pacing is generally preferred for long-term control. Examples of acute use include the prevention and treatment of arrhythmias associated with anaesthesia (see above), the treatment of other drug-induced arrhythmias, and in cardiac arrest due to asystole or electromechanical dissociation (pulseless electrical activity—p.812). Atropine sulfate has been used in the management of bradycardia of acute myocardial infarction; however, caution is required, as atropine may exacerbate ischaemia or infarction in these patients.

International guidelines[1] for advanced life support in adults recommend doses of atropine sulfate in asystole and electromechanical dissociation, of 1 mg intravenously, repeated every 3 to 5 minutes to a total of 40 micrograms/kg. UK guidelines[2] for adults recommend a single dose of 3 mg intravenously or 6 mg via an endotracheal tube.

In **bradycardia**, atropine is given[1] in doses of 0.5 to 1 mg intravenously repeated every 3 to 5 minutes to a total dose of 40 micrograms/kg.

If an intravenous line cannot be established, atropine can be given via an endotracheal tube; 2 to 3 times the intravenous dose should be given, diluted in 10 mL of sterile water or sodium chloride 0.9%.


1. The American Heart Association in collaboration with the International Committee on Resuscitation (ILCOR). International guidelines 2000 for cardiopulmonary resuscitation and emergency cardiovascular care: a consensus on science. *Circulation* 2000; **102** (suppl I): I1–I384. Also published in *Resuscitation* 2000; **46:** 3–447.
2. Resuscitation Council (UK). Resuscitation Guidelines 2000. Available at: http://www.resus.org.uk/pages/guide.htm (accessed 01/06/04)


**Eye disorders.** Atropine is used to produce mydriasis and cycloplegia (p.476) for ophthalmic examination. One local application can take up to 40 minutes or more to produce mydriasis, which lasts for a week or more; marked paralysis of accommodation is obtained in 1 to 3 hours with recovery in 6 to 12 days. However, other antimuscarinics such as cyclopentolate, homatropine, or tropicamide may be preferred because they have a more rapid onset and shorter duration of action than atropine. Atropine is also used in the management of uveitis and iritis, and in strabismus. It is used in the treatment of iritis and uveitis to immobilise the ciliary muscle and iris and to prevent or break down adhesions. Because of its powerful cycloplegic action atropine is also used in the determination of refraction in children below the age of 6 and in children with convergent strabismus (p.1487).

In the treatment of **inflammatory eye disorders** such as uveitis or iritis (p.1090), the dose of atropine sulfate for adults is 1 or 2 drops of a 0.5 or 1% solution instilled into the eye(s) up to four times daily. The dose in children is 1 or 2 drops of a 0.5% solution (or one drop of a 1% solution) instilled up to three times daily. For **refraction** in adults the dose is one drop of a 1% solution of atropine sulfate; this may be instilled either twice daily for 1 or 2 days before the procedure or on a single occasion one hour before the procedure. In children the dose for refraction is 1 or 2 drops of a 0.5% solution (or one drop of a 1% solution) instilled twice daily for 1 to 3 days before the procedure, with a further dose given one hour before the procedure. An ophthalmic ointment of atropine sulfate 1% may be preferred for children under 5 years and particularly in infants under 3 months who are at increased risk of systemic effects with eye drops. Some manufacturers recommend that atropine sulfate should not be used in the eyes of children younger than 3 months due to a possible association between the cycloplegia produced and the development of amblyopia.

Atropine borate has also been used in ophthalmic preparations.

References.


1. Stolovitch C, *et al.* Atropine cycloplegia: how many instillations does one need? *J Pediatr Ophthalmol Strabismus* 1992; **29:** 175–6.
2. Foley-Nolan A, *et al.* Atropine penalisation versus occlusion as the primary treatment for amblyopia. *Br J Ophthalmol* 1997; **81:** 54–7.
3. Pediatric Eye Disease Investigator Group. A randomized trial of atropine vs. patching for treatment of moderate amblyopia in children. *Arch Ophthalmol* 2002; **120:** 268–78.


**Gastrointestinal disorders.** Antimuscarinics may be used in gastrointestinal disorders (see p.475) because of their marked inhibitory effect on gastrointestinal motility and their antisecretory effects. Atropine (as the sulfate or quaternary derivatives such as the methobromide or methonitrate) has been used to reduce smooth-muscle tone and diminish motility, but has little effect on gastric secretion at usual therapeutic doses (about 200 micrograms of atropine sulfate). It has been tried as an adjunct to the treatment of benign gastric and duodenal ulcers and the antispasmodic action of atropine has been used to facilitate radiological examination of the gut. Atropine sulfate has also been used in the treatment of irritable bowel syndrome. Atropine oxide hydrochloride is also used for gastrointestinal disorders.

**Poisoning.** Atropine is used in the management of overdosage or poisoning due to anticholinesterase compounds including organophosphorus pesticides,[1,2] chemical warfare nerve gases,[3] and parasympathomimetics such as neostigmine. It is also used to antagonise the effects of cholinomimetic substances in the treatment of overdosage with parasympathomimetics such as bethanechol, and in the treatment of poisoning with mushrooms that contain muscarine. Atropine blocks the action of these compounds at muscarinic receptors reversing bradycardia and decreasing tracheobronchial secretions, bronchoconstriction, intestinal secretions, and intestinal motility.

- In the treatment of poisoning with organophosphorus **pesticides** or chemical warfare **nerve gases** atropine sulfate may be given to adults in an initial dose of 2 mg or more intramuscularly or intravenously every 10 to 30 minutes until muscarinic effects disappear or signs of atropine toxicity are seen. In severe cases injections have been given as often as every 5 minutes in some centres. Continuous infusion has also been used.[4,5] A dose of at least 50 micrograms/kg has been suggested for children by some;[6] the *British National Formulary* includes a dose of 20 micrograms/kg given every 5 to 10 minutes.
- In moderate to severe poisoning a state of atropinisation is usually maintained for at least 2 days and continued for as long as symptoms are evident. In severely poisoned patients this may entail prolonged treatment.[7,8] As large amounts of atropine may be required it is important to use a preservative-free preparation to avoid the potential toxicity associated with administration of excess quantities of preservatives such as benzyl alcohol or chlorobutanol.
- Since atropine is ineffective against any nicotinic effects of these compounds a cholinesterase reactivator such as pralidoxime (p.1050) may be used as an adjunct.

The use of atropine in poisoning or overdosage with **other compounds** having muscarinic actions is similar to that for organophosphorus pesticides but the duration of treatment necessary is usually shorter. An initial dose of 0.6 to 1 mg given subcutaneously, intramuscularly, or intravenously and repeated every 2 hours may be adequate for overdosage with cholinomimetics such as bethanechol.


1. Singh S, *et al.* Is atropine alone sufficient in acute severe organophosphorus poisoning: experience of a North West Indian hospital. *Int J Clin Pharmacol Ther* 1995; **33:** 628–30.
2. Eddleston M, *et al.* Management of severe organophosphorus pesticide poisoning. *Crit Care* 2002; **6:** 259.
3. Anonymous. Treatment of nerve gas poisoning. *Med Lett Drugs Ther* 1995; **37:** 43–4.
4. Ram JS, *et al.* Continuous infusion of high doses of atropine in the management of organophosphorus compound poisoning. *J Assoc Physicians India* 1991; **39:** 190–3.
5. Sungur M, Güven M. Intensive care management of organophosphate insecticide poisoning. *Crit Care* 2001; **5:** 211–15.
6. Rotenberg JS, Newmark J. Nerve agent attacks on children: diagnosis and management. *Pediatrics* 2003; **112:** 648–58.
7. Golsousidis H, Kokkas V. Use of 19 590 mg of atropine during 24 days of treatment, after a case of unusually severe parathion poisoning. *Hum Toxicol* 1985; **4:** 339–40.
8. Afzaal S, *et al.* High dose atropine in organophosphorus poisoning. *Postgrad Med J* 1990; **66:** 70–1.


**Respiratory-tract disorders.** Although atropine is a potent bronchodilator its use in the management of reversible airways obstruction has largely been replaced by other antimuscarinics (see p.476). It is sometimes used in combination preparations with antihistamines and decongestants for the symptomatic relief of symptoms of the common cold.

References.


1. Sur S, *et al.* A random double-blind trial of the combination of nebulized atropine methylnitrate and albuterol in nocturnal asthma. *Ann Allergy* 1990; **65:** 384–8.
2. Vichyanond P, *et al.* Efficacy of atropine methylnitrate alone and in combination with albuterol in children with asthma. *Chest* 1990; **98:** 637–42.

## Preparations

***BP 2003:*** Atropine Eye Drops; Atropine Eye Ointment; Atropine Injection; Atropine Tablets; Morphine and Atropine Injection;
***USP 27:*** Atropine Sulfate Injection; Atropine Sulfate Ophthalmic Ointment; Atropine Sulfate Ophthalmic Solution; Atropine Sulfate Tablets; Diphenoxylate Hydrochloride and Atropine Sulfate Oral Solution; Diphenoxylate Hydrochloride and Atropine Sulfate Tablets.

**Proprietary Preparations** (details are given in Part 3)
***Arg.:*** Endotropina; Klonatropina; ***Austral.:*** Atropt; ***Belg.:*** Stellatropine; ***Braz.:*** Atropion; Sulfatina; ***Canad.:*** Atropisol; ***Fin.:*** Oftan Atropin; ***Fr.:*** Chibro-Atropine†; Genatropine†; ***Ger.:*** Atropinol; Dysurgal N; Noxenur S†; ***India:*** Bell Pino-Atrin; ***Israel:*** Atrospan; ***Ital.:*** Liotropina†; ***Malaysia:*** Atrop; ***Mex.:*** Atro Grin; Tropyn; ***NZ:*** Atropt; ***Port.:*** Atropocil; ***Switz.:*** Bellafit N; Skiatropine; ***USA:*** AtroPen; Atropisol†; Ocu-Tropine; Sal-Tropine.

**Multi-ingredient:** ***Arg.:*** Asmopul; Otorinazol; Saldeva; Trixol; Yanal; ***Austral.:*** Contac†; Donnagel; Donnalix; Donnatab; Neo-Diophen†; ***Austria:*** Causat; Dysurgal†; Ichtho-Bellol; Lactolavol; Myocardon; Noxenur†; Perphyllon†; ***Braz.:*** Enterotonus†; Espasmocron; Ormigrein; Sedabel; Tonaton; Vagostesyl; ***Canad.:*** Diban†; Donnatal†; ***Chile:*** Buton; Dipatropin; Dispasmol; Dolospam; Papatropin; ***Ger.:*** Angiocardyl N†; Causat B12 N†; Causat N†; Dilaudid-Atropin†; Ichtho-Bellol; Ichtho-Bellol compositum S; Mydrial-Atropin; ***Hong Kong:*** Virulex Forte; ***India:*** Atrisolon; Brovon; Pino-Cort; ***Israel:*** Patropin; Spasmalgin; ***Ital.:*** Cardiostenol; Deltamidrina; Genatrop; ***Mex.:*** Paliatil; Redotex NF; ***Port.:*** Cosmaxil; ***S.Afr.:*** Allertac†; Bellatard†; Colstat; Donnatal; Dyrosol†; Famucaps; Millerspas; Virobis; ***Spain:*** Abdominol; Laxo Vian†; Midriati; Rubia Paver†; Sulmetin Papaver; Sulmetin Papaverina; Tabletas Quimpe; ***Swed.:*** Dilaudid-Atropin; ***Switz.:*** Brosol†; Dilaudid-Atropin; Dolopyrine; Nardyl; Spasmosol; Viaggio†; ***Thai.:*** Alkamine; Alupep; Diolin†; Donnatal; Droximag; Stomac; ***UK:*** Actonorm; Brovon; Valonorm; ***USA:*** Accuhist LA; Antispasmodic Elixir; Antrocol†; Arco-Lase Plus†; Atrohist Plus†; Atropine and Demerol†; Atrosept; Barbidonna; Bellahist-D; Bellatal; Deconhist LA†; Dolsed; Donnatal†; Emergent-Ez; Hyosophen; MHP-A; Phenahist-TR†; Phenchlor SHA†; Prosed/DS; Ru-Tuss†; Stahist; Susano; Trac Tabs 2X; UAA; Uridon Modified; Urised; Uriseptic; Uritact.

*Used as an adjunct in:* ***Austral.:*** Lofenoxal; Lomotil; ***Belg.:*** Reasec†; ***Braz.:*** Colestase; Lomotil; ***Canad.:*** Lomotil; ***Denm.:*** Retardin†; ***Fr.:*** Diarsed; ***Ger.:*** Reasec†; ***Hong Kong:*** Dhamotil; Lomotil; ***India:*** Lomofen; Lomotil; ***Irl.:*** Lomotil; ***Ital.:*** Reasec†; ***Malaysia:*** Atrotil; Beamotil; Dhamotil; Lomotil; Setmotil; ***NZ:*** Diastop; Lomotil; ***Port.:*** Lomotil; ***S.Afr.:*** Eldox†; Lomotil; ***Singapore:*** Dhamotil; Erlotyl†; Lomotil; Remodil; ***Switz.:*** Reasec†; ***Thai.:*** Dilomil; Ditropine†; Lomotil; ***UAE:*** Intard; ***UK:*** Dymotil; Lomotil; Lotharin†; Tropergen†; ***USA:*** Enlon-Plus; Logen; Lomotil; Lonox; Motofen; Neostigmine Min-I-Mix.

---

# Belladonna

Belladona; Belladone; Deadly Nightshade; Tollkirschen.

*ATC — A03BA04.*

**Pharmacopoeias.** *Eur.* (see p.vi), *Pol.,* and *US* include a monograph for Belladonna Herb. *Chin.* includes Belladonna Herb. *Eur.* also includes Prepared Belladonna Leaf, Standardised Belladonna Leaf Tincture, and Standardised Belladonna Leaf Dry Extract.

*Jpn* includes only Belladonna Root.

**Ph. Eur. 5.0** (Belladonna Leaf; Belladonnae Folium; Belladonna Herb BP 2003). It consists of the dried leaf, or dried leaf and flowering, and occasionally fruit-bearing, tops of *Atropa belladonna*. It contains not less than 0.30% of total alkaloids, calculated as hyoscyamine. The alkaloids consist mainly of hyoscyamine together with smaller amounts of hyoscine. It has a slightly nauseous odour. Protect from light.

The BP 2003 directs that when Belladonna Herb, Belladonna Leaf, or Powdered Belladonna Herb is prescribed, Prepared Belladonna Herb shall be dispensed.

**Ph. Eur. 5.0** (Belladonna, Prepared; Belladonnae Pulvis Normatus; Prepared Belladonna Herb BP 2003). It is belladonna leaf powder adjusted to an alkaloidal content of 0.28 to 0.32% of total alkaloids, calculated as hyoscyamine. Store in airtight containers. Protect from light.

**USP 27** (Belladonna Leaf). It consists of the dried leaf and flowering or fruiting top of *Atropa belladonna* (Solanaceae). It yields not less than 0.35% of the alkaloids of belladonna leaf. When moistened, its odour is slight, somewhat tobacco-like. Avoid long exposure to direct sunlight. Protect powdered Belladonna Leaf from light.

**Stability in mixtures.** Atropine in belladonna preparations was unstable at alkaline pH and would quickly be degraded in mixtures with a pH above 7.[1] Such mixtures in the BPC 1973 included Aluminium Hydroxide and Belladonna Mixture, Cascara and Belladonna Mixture, and Magnesium Trisilicate and Belladonna Mixture.

1. *PSGB Lab Report P/71/9* 1971.

## Adverse Effects, Treatment, and Precautions

As for Atropine Sulfate, p.477.

## Interactions

As for antimuscarinics in general (see Atropine Sulfate, p.477).

## Uses and Administration

Belladonna has the actions of atropine (p.477). Belladonna herb and its preparations have been used for their antimuscarinic actions in a wide range of conditions, including the relief of gastrointestinal and urinary-tract disorders associated with smooth muscle spasm, but they are generally regarded as an outmoded form of treatment.

Belladonna liniments and plasters have been used as counter-irritants for the relief of pain but there is little evidence that they have a beneficial effect and side-effects have occurred.

Belladonna is used in homoeopathic medicine.

## Preparations

***Ph. Eur.:*** Belladonna Leaf Dry Extract, Standardised; Belladonna Leaf Tincture, Standardised;
***USP 27:*** Belladonna Extract; Belladonna Extract Tablets; Belladonna Tincture.

**Proprietary Preparations** (details are given in Part 3)
***Austral.:*** Atrobel; ***Austria:*** Bellanorm; ***Chile:*** Felaxen; ***Ger.:*** Belladonnysat Burger; Tremoforat.

**Multi-ingredient:** ***Arg.:*** Antipasmol; Cascara Sagrada Sanaplex; Dioxicolagol; Hepacur; Hepatodirectol; Opobyl; Passacanthine; Trixol; ***Austral.:*** Cold & Flu Tablets†; ***Austria:*** Asthma 23 D; Tampositorien mit Belladonna; ***Belg.:*** Baume Dalet†; Calmant Martou†; Colimax; Eucalyptine Pholcodine Le Brun; Folcodex†; Gastrofilm; Grains de Vals; Sanicolax†; Sirop Toux du Larynx†; Solucamphre†; ***Braz.:*** Acridin; Antispasmin†; Atroveran†; Atrovex†; Benzomel; Bismubell†; Bisuisan; Bromosedan†; Broncol; Bronquidex; Brontoss; Calminex Atleta; Calminex H; Cessatosse†; Colinex†; Cynarobil†; Cystex; Dorveran; Ductoveran; Efedronal†; Espasmolex†; Espasmosan Composto†; Espasmosan†; Etaverol†; Gastrobene; Gotas Hepaticas†; Gotas Nican; Gotas Preciosas†; Hemovirtu's Pomada†; Hepato-Flux†; Hepatobyl†; Hepavirmo†; Iodeto de Potassio; Neutracido†; Pilulas Ross; Pulmoiodo†; Pyelodion†; Regran†; Regulador Xavier n-1†; Regulador Xavier n-2†; Revulsan; Salicilato de Bismuto Composto; Solvobil; Teutoss; Tussifen; Tussucalman†; Xarope de Caraguata; Xarope Sao Joao; ***Canad.:*** Bellergal; Cafergot-PB; Rheumalan; Wigraine†; ***Chile:*** Bellergal Retardado; Belupan; Broncodeina; Cafergot-PB; Ergobelan; Fenokomp 39; Fenolftaleina Compuesta; Gotas Nican; Gruben; Ramistos; ***Denm.:*** Gynergen Comp; ***Fin.:*** Tannopon; ***Fr.:*** Bronpax†; Gastrosedyl†; Gelumaline; Humex; Mucinum†; Peter's Sirop†; Sirop Pectoral adulte†; Suppomaline; ***Ger.:*** Dalet Med Balsam; ***Hong Kong:*** Contac†; Rheogen†; ***India:*** Emantid; Molzyme; ***Israel:*** Laxative; Laxative Comp; ***Ital.:*** Antiemorroidali; Antispasmina Colica; Bellergil†; Farmospasmina†; Lassatina; Neo-Heparbil†; ***Mex.:*** Chofabol; ***Neth.:*** Abdijsiroop (Akker-Siroop)†; ***Port.:*** Anti-Gripe; Antispasmina Colica; Anucet; Calmo†; Codoforme†; Fluidin Antiasmatico†; Fluidin Infantil†; Lactucol†; Migretil; Servetinal; Vaporil; ***S.Afr.:*** Bellergal†; Cafergot-PB; ***Spain:*** Alofedina; Boldolaxin; Broncovital; Cafergot-PB; Carminativo Juventus; Crislaxo; Digestovital; Distovagal†; Dolokey; Laxante Bescansa Aloico; Medecitral†; Menabil Complex; Sin Mareo x 4; Tanagel; ***Switz.:*** Ajaka†; Aloinophen†; Bellagotin; Bellergal†; Bromocod N; Bronchalin†; Bronchofluid†; Cafergot-PB; Demo elixir pectoral N; Demo sirop contre la toux†; Dragees laxatives no 510†; Escotussin; Lysedil; Lysedil compositum†; Nican; Phol-Tux; Physiolax†; Phytolax†; Saintbois; Sirop pectoral DP2, DP3†; Spedro†; Tavolax†; Thymodrosin†; ***Thai.:*** Belacid; Bellergal; Benera; Contac†; Delta Charcoal; Diolin†; Neuramizone; ***UK:*** Enterosan†; Opazimes; ***USA:*** B & O Supprettes No. 15A; B & O Supprettes No. 16A; Bel-Phen-Ergot S; Bellamine; Bellergal-S; Butibel; Cafatine-PB; Folergot-DF; Phenerbel-S; Respa-ARM†.

---

# Benzatropine Mesilate *(BANM, rINNM)*

Benzatropine Methanesulfonate; Benztropine Mesylate; Mesilato de benzatropina. (1R,3r,5S)-3-Benzhydryloxytropane methanesulphonate.

$C_{21}H_{25}NO,CH_4O_3S$ = 403.5.

*CAS — 86-13-5 (benzatropine); 132-17-2 (benzatropine mesilate).*

*ATC — N04AC01.*

**Pharmacopoeias.** In *Br.* and *US.*

**BP 2003** (Benzatropine Mesilate). A white, odourless or almost odourless, crystalline powder. Very soluble in water; freely soluble in alcohol; practically insoluble in ether.

**USP 27** (Benztropine Mesylate). A white, slightly hygroscopic, crystalline powder. Very soluble in water; freely soluble in alcohol; very slightly soluble in ether. Store in airtight containers.

## Adverse Effects, Treatment, and Precautions

As for Atropine Sulfate, p.477. Drowsiness may be severe in some patients and patients so affected should not drive or operate machinery. Benzatropine may also produce severe mental disturbances and excitement.

**Abuse.** For mention of abuse of benzatropine see under Trihexyphenidyl Hydrochloride, p.490.

**Effects on the heart.** Paradoxical sinus bradycardia in a patient with depression and psychotic symptoms was attributed to benzatropine since it persisted despite modification to other treatment and resolved only when benzatropine was withdrawn.[1]

1. Voinov H, *et al.* Sinus bradycardia related to the use of benztropine mesylate. *Am J Psychiatry* 1992; **149:** 711.

## Interactions

As for antimuscarinics in general (see Atropine Sulfate, p.477).

**Antidepressants.** A report[1] of 5 patients who developed delirium while taking an antipsychotic, an SSRI, and benzatropine suggested that there might be an interaction between SSRIs and benzatropine.

1. Roth A, *et al.* Delirium associated with the combination of a neuroleptic, an SSRI, and benztropine. *J Clin Psychiatry* 1994; **55:** 492–5.

**Antipsychotics.** Fatal heat stroke after exposure to an ambient temperature of over 29° has been reported[1,2] in patients receiving benzatropine with antipsychotics. Paralytic ileus, sometimes fatal, has also been seen in patients taking benzatropine mesilate with antipsychotics.[3]

1. Stadnyk AN, Glezos JD. Drug-induced heat stroke. *Can Med Assoc J* 1983; **128:** 957–9.
2. Tyndel F, Labonté R. Drug-facilitated heat stroke. *Can Med Assoc J* 1983; **129:** 680.
3. Wade LC, Ellenor GL. Combination mesoridazine- and benztropine mesylate-induced paralytic ileus: two case reports. *Drug Intell Clin Pharm* 1980; **14:** 17–22.

## Uses and Administration

Benzatropine mesilate is a tertiary amine antimuscarinic with actions and uses similar to those of trihexyphenidyl (p.490); it also has antihistaminic properties.

Benzatropine is used for the symptomatic treatment of parkinsonism (p.476), including the alleviation of the extrapyramidal syndrome induced by drugs such as phenothiazines, but, like other antimuscarinics, is of no value against tardive dyskinesias.

Benzatropine mesilate is given by mouth or, if necessary, by intramuscular or intravenous injection.

In idiopathic parkinsonism benzatropine mesilate is usually given by mouth in an initial daily dose of 0.5 to 1 mg. Its actions are cumulative, and may not be manifest for several days after beginning therapy. Patients with post-encephalitic parkinsonism often tolerate an initial dose of 2 mg. The dose may be gradually increased by 500 micrograms every 5 to 6 days to a maximum of 6 mg daily until the optimum dose for each individual patient is reached. Maintenance therapy may be given as a single daily dose at bedtime or in divided doses 2 to 4 times daily.

In the management of drug-induced extrapyramidal disorders doses of 1 to 4 mg once or twice daily have been given orally or parenterally. Therapy may be withdrawn after one to two weeks to assess whether it is still necessary.

In an emergency, benzatropine mesilate may be injected intramuscularly or intravenously in a dose of 1 to 2 mg; intramuscular administration is reported to produce an effect as quickly as intravenous administration, so the latter is rarely necessary.

Benzatropine has also been given as the hydrochloride.

## Preparations

***BP 2003:*** Benzatropine Injection; Benzatropine Tablets;
***USP 27:*** Benztropine Mesylate Injection; Benztropine Mesylate Tablets.

**Proprietary Preparations** (details are given in Part 3)
***Austral.:*** Benztrop; Cogentin; ***Austria:*** BETE†; Cogentin; ***Canad.:*** Cogentin; ***Denm.:*** Cogentin; ***Ger.:*** Cogentinol†; ***Hong Kong:*** Cogentin; ***Irl.:*** Cogentin; ***Norw.:*** Cogentin; ***NZ:*** Cogentin; ***Port.:*** Cogentin; ***Swed.:*** Cogentin†; ***Thai.:*** Cogentin; Phatropine†; ***UK:*** Cogentin; ***USA:*** Cogentin.

---

# Biperiden *(BAN, rINN)*

Biperideno. 1-(Bicyclo[2.2.1]hept-5-en-2-yl)-1-phenyl-3-piperidinopropan-1-ol.

$C_{21}H_{29}NO$ = 311.5.

*CAS — 514-65-8.*

*ATC — N04AA02.*

**Pharmacopoeias.** In *Int.* and *US.*

**USP 27** (Biperiden). A white, practically odourless, crystalline powder. Practically insoluble in water; sparingly soluble in alcohol; freely soluble in chloroform. Protect from light.

## Biperiden Hydrochloride *(BANM, rINNM)*

Biperideni Hydrochloridum; Hidrocloruro de biperideno.

$C_{21}H_{29}NO,HCl$ = 347.9.

*CAS — 1235-82-1.*

*ATC — N04AA02.*

**Pharmacopoeias.** In *Eur.* (see p.vi), *Int., Jpn,* and *US.*

**Ph. Eur. 5.0** (Biperiden Hydrochloride). A white, crystalline powder. Slightly soluble in water and in alcohol; very slightly soluble in dichloromethane. A 0.2% solution in water has a pH of 5.0 to 6.5. Store in airtight containers. Protect from light.

**USP 27** (Biperiden Hydrochloride). A white, practically odourless, crystalline powder. Slightly soluble in water, in alcohol, in chloroform, and in ether; sparingly soluble in methyl alcohol. Protect from light.

## Biperiden Lactate *(BANM, rINNM)*

Lactato de biperideno.

$C_{21}H_{29}NO,C_3H_6O_3$ = 401.5.

*CAS — 7085-45-2.*

*ATC — N04AA02.*

**Pharmacopoeias.** *US* includes Biperiden Lactate Injection.

## Adverse Effects, Treatment, and Precautions

As for Atropine Sulfate, p.477.

Parenteral administration may be followed by slight transient hypotension. Biperiden may cause drowsiness and patients so affected should not drive or operate machinery.

**Abuse.** A report[1] of abuse of biperiden in psychiatric patients.

1. Pullen GP, *et al.* Anticholinergic drug abuse: a common problem? *BMJ* 1984; **289:** 612–13.

## Interactions

As for antimuscarinics in general (see Atropine Sulfate, p.477).

## Pharmacokinetics

Biperiden is readily absorbed from the gastrointestinal tract, but bioavailability is only about 30% suggesting that it undergoes extensive first-pass metabolism. Biperiden has an elimination half-life of about 20 hours.

◊ References.

1. Hollmann M, *et al.* Biperiden effects and plasma levels in volunteers. *Eur J Clin Pharmacol* 1984; **27:** 619–21.
2. Grimaldi R, *et al.* Pharmacokinetic and pharmacodynamic studies following the intravenous and oral administration of the antiparkinsonian drug biperiden to normal subjects. *Eur J Clin Pharmacol* 1986; **29:** 735–7.

## Uses and Administration

Biperiden is a tertiary amine antimuscarinic with actions and uses similar to those of trihexyphenidyl (p.490) but with more potent antinicotinic properties.

Biperiden is used in the symptomatic treatment of parkinsonism (p.476), including the alleviation of the extrapyramidal syndrome induced by drugs such as phenothiazines, but, like other antimuscarinics, is of no value against tardive dyskinesias.

Biperiden is administered by mouth as the hydrochloride and by injection as the lactate; doses are expressed in terms of the relevant salt. The initial dose by mouth for idiopathic parkinsonism is 2 mg of the hydrochloride three or four times daily increased according to the needs of the patient to a maximum of 16 mg daily. The dose for drug-induced extrapyramidal symptoms is 2 mg of the hydrochloride by mouth one to three times daily; alternatively, 2 mg of biperiden lactate may be given by intramuscular or slow intravenous injection and repeated every 30 minutes if needed up to a maximum of 4 doses in 24 hours.

## Preparations

***USP 27:*** Biperiden Hydrochloride Tablets; Biperiden Lactate Injection.

**Proprietary Preparations** (details are given in Part 3)

***Arg.:*** Akineton; Berofin; Darcipireno; ***Austral.:*** Akineton; ***Austria:*** Akineton; ***Belg.:*** Akineton; ***Braz.:*** Akineton; Cinetol; Parkinsol; ***Canad.:*** Akineton; ***Chile:*** Akineton; ***Denm.:*** Akineton; ***Fin.:*** Akineton; Ipsatol; ***Fr.:*** Akineton; ***Ger.:*** Akineton; Desiperiden†; Norakin N; ***Gr.:*** Akineton; ***India:*** Dyskinon; ***Irl.:*** Akineton; ***Israel:*** Dekinet; ***Ital.:*** Akineton; ***Mex.:*** Akineton; Kinex; Rolokent†; ***Neth.:*** Akineton; ***Norw.:*** Akineton; ***Port.:*** Akineton; ***S.Afr.:*** Akineton; ***Singapore:*** Akineton†; ***Spain:*** Akineton; ***Swed.:*** Akineton; ***Switz.:*** Akineton; ***Thai.:*** Akineton†; ***UK:*** Akineton†; ***USA:*** Akineton.

---

## Bornaprine Hydrochloride *(BANM, rINNM)*

Hidrocloruro de bornaprina. 3-Diethylaminopropyl 2-phenylbicyclo[2.2.1]heptane-2-carboxylate hydrochloride.

$C_{21}H_{31}NO_2,HCl = 365.9.$

*CAS — 20448-86-6 (bornaprine); 26908-91-8 (bornaprine hydrochloride).*

*ATC — N04AA11.*

### Profile

Bornaprine hydrochloride is a quaternary ammonium antimuscarinic with actions and uses similar to those of trihexyphenidyl (p.490). It is used in the symptomatic treatment of parkinsonism (p.476), but it is claimed to be mainly effective against tremor. It is given by mouth in initial doses of 2 mg daily gradually increased to 6 to 12 mg daily according to the response of the patient. It is also used in the treatment of hyperhidrosis (p.1136) in a dose of 4 to 8 mg daily.

### Preparations

**Proprietary Preparations** (details are given in Part 3)

***Austria:*** Sormodren; ***Ger.:*** Sormodren; ***Ital.:*** Sormodren; ***Mex.:*** Sormodren†.

---

## Butropium Bromide *(rINN)*

Bromuro de butropio. (−)-(1*R*,3*r*,5*S*)-8-(4-Butoxybenzyl)-3-[(*S*)-tropoyloxy]tropanium bromide.

$C_{28}H_{38}BrNO_4 = 532.5.$

*CAS — 29025-14-7.*

**Pharmacopoeias.** In *Jpn.*

### Profile

Butropium bromide is a quaternary ammonium antimuscarinic with peripheral effects similar to those of atropine (p.477). It has been used in the symptomatic treatment of visceral spasms in a dose of 30 mg daily in 3 divided doses.

### Preparations

**Proprietary Preparations** (details are given in Part 3)

***Hong Kong:*** Coliopan†; ***Jpn:*** Coliopan; ***Malaysia:*** Coliopan; ***Singapore:*** Coliopan.

---

## Buzepide Metiodide *(rINN)*

Diphexamide Iodomethylate; FI-6146; Metazepium Iodide; Metioduro de buzepida; R-661. 1-(3-Carbamoyl-3,3-diphenylpropyl)-1-methylperhydroazepinium iodide.

$C_{23}H_{31}IN_2O = 478.4.$

*CAS — 15351-05-0.*

### Profile

Buzepide metiodide is a quaternary ammonium antimuscarinic with peripheral effects similar to those of atropine (p.477). It has been given with other compounds for upper respiratory-tract disorders and in gastrointestinal disorders with smooth muscle spasm.

### Preparations

**Proprietary Preparations** (details are given in Part 3)

**Multi-ingredient:** ***Belg.:*** Denoral†; ***Fr.:*** Denoral†; Vesadol; ***Hong Kong:*** Denoral†; ***Ital.:*** Denoral.

---

## Ciclonium Bromide *(rINN)*

Asta-3746; Bromuro de ciclonio. Diethylmethyl{2-[(α-methyl-α-5-norbornen-2-ylbenzyl)oxy]ethyl}ammonium bromide.

$C_{22}H_{34}BrNO = 408.4.$

*CAS — 29546-59-6.*

### Profile

Ciclonium bromide is an antimuscarinic that has been used in the treatment of gastrointestinal and urinary-tract disorders.

### Preparations

**Proprietary Preparations** (details are given in Part 3)

***Thai.:*** Adamon.

**Multi-ingredient:** ***Arg.:*** Espasmo Motrax.

---

## Cimetropium Bromide *(rINN)*

Bromuro de cimetropio; DA-3177; Hyoscine-*N*-(cyclopropylmethyl) Bromide. 8-(Cyclopropylmethyl)-6β,7β-epoxy-3α-hydroxy-1αH,5αH-tropanium bromide, (−)-(*S*)-tropate.

$C_{21}H_{28}BrNO_4 = 438.4.$

*CAS — 51598-60-8.*

*ATC — A03BB05.*

### Profile

Cimetropium bromide is a quaternary ammonium antimuscarinic with peripheral effects similar to those of atropine (p.477). It has been used as an antispasmodic in the treatment of gastrointestinal disorders (p.475) in usual doses of 50 mg two or three times daily by mouth or by rectal suppository. It has also been given intramuscularly or intravenously in usual doses of 5 mg.

◊ References.

1. Dobrilla G, *et al.* Longterm treatment of irritable bowel syndrome with cimetropium bromide: a double blind placebo controlled clinical trial. *Gut* 1990; **31:** 355–8.
2. Marzio L, *et al.* Effect of cimetropium bromide on esophageal motility and transit in patients affected by primary achalasia. *Dig Dis Sci* 1994; **39:** 1389–94.
3. Savino F, *et al.* Cimetropium bromide in the treatment of crisis in infantile colic. *J Pediatr Gastroenterol Nutr* 2002; **34:** 417–9.

### Preparations

**Proprietary Preparations** (details are given in Part 3)

***Ital.:*** Alginor.

---

## Clidinium Bromide *(BAN, USAN, rINN)*

Bromuro de clidinio; Ro-2-3773. 3-Benziloyloxy-1-methylquinuclidinium bromide.

$C_{22}H_{26}BrNO_3 = 432.4.$

*CAS — 7020-55-5 (clidinium); 3485-62-9 (clidinium bromide).*

**Pharmacopoeias.** In *US.*

**USP 27** (Clidinium Bromide). A white or nearly white, practically odourless, crystalline powder. Soluble in water and in alcohol; slightly soluble in ether and in benzene. Store in airtight containers. Protect from light.

### Profile

Clidinium bromide is a quaternary ammonium antimuscarinic with peripheral effects similar to those of atropine (p.477). It has been used alone or more often with chlordiazepoxide in the symptomatic treatment of peptic ulcer disease and other gastrointestinal disorders.

### Preparations

***USP 27:*** Chlordiazepoxide Hydrochloride and Clidinium Bromide Capsules.

**Proprietary Preparations** (details are given in Part 3)

***USA:*** Quarzan†.

**Multi-ingredient:** ***Arg.:*** Librax; ***Belg.:*** Librax†; ***Canad.:*** Apo-Chlorax; Corium†; Librax; ***Chile:*** Gastrolen; Lerogin; Libraxin; Lironex; Sedogastrol; Tensoliv; ***Fin.:*** Librax; ***Fr.:*** Librax; ***Hong Kong:*** Bralix; Librax; Medocalum; ***India:*** Equirex; Normaxin; ***Israel:*** Librax†; Nirvaxal; ***Ital.:*** Librax; ***Malaysia:*** Apo-Chlorax; Liblan; ***Port.:*** Librax; ***S.Afr.:*** Librax; ***Singapore:*** Apo-Chlorax; Chlobax; Librax; Medocalum; ***Switz.:*** Librax; ***Thai.:*** Kenspa; Liblan†; Librax; Pobrax; Tumax; Zepobrax; ***USA:*** Clindex; Librax.

---

## Cyclodrine Hydrochloride

Ciclodrina, hidrocloruro de; GT-92. 2-Diethylaminoethyl 2-(1-hydroxycyclopentyl)-2-phenylacetate hydrochloride.

$C_{19}H_{29}NO_3,HCl = 355.9.$

*CAS — 52109-93-0 (cyclodrine); 78853-39-1 (cyclodrine hydrochloride).*

### Profile

Cyclodrine is an analogue of cyclopentolate (below). It has been used as the hydrochloride in eye drops to produce mydriasis and cycloplegia.

---

# Cyclopentolate Hydrochloride

*(BANM, rINNM)*

Cloridrato de Ciclopentolato; Cyclopentolati Hydrochloridum; Hidrocloruro de ciclopentolato. 2-Dimethylaminoethyl 2-(1-hydroxycyclopentyl)-2-phenylacetate hydrochloride.

$C_{17}H_{25}NO_3,HCl = 327.8.$

*CAS — 512-15-2 (cyclopentolate); 5870-29-1 (cyclopentolate hydrochloride).*

*ATC — S01FA04.*

NOTE. CYC is a code approved by the BP 2003 for use on single unit doses of eye drops containing cyclopentolate hydrochloride where the individual container may be too small to bear all the appropriate labelling information. PHNCYC is a similar code approved for eye drops containing phenylephrine hydrochloride and cyclopentolate hydrochloride.

**Pharmacopoeias.** In *Eur.* (see p.vi), *Jpn,* and *US.*

**Ph. Eur. 5.0** (Cyclopentolate Hydrochloride). A white, crystalline powder. Very soluble in water; freely soluble in alcohol. A 1% solution in water has a pH of 4.5 to 5.5.

**USP 27** (Cyclopentolate Hydrochloride). A white crystalline powder, which develops a characteristic odour on standing. Very soluble in water; freely soluble in alcohol; insoluble in ether. pH of a 1% solution in water is between 4.5 and 5.5. Store at a temperature not exceeding 8° in airtight containers.

## Adverse Effects, Treatment, and Precautions

As for Atropine Sulfate, p.477.

Eye drops of cyclopentolate hydrochloride may cause temporary irritation.

**Abuse.** A report[1] of abuse of cyclopentolate eye drops by 2 patients. One of the patients who had been instilling 200 to 400 drops of cyclopentolate into both eyes daily for about 4 months, presumably for its CNS effects, experienced intense nausea, vomiting, weakness, and tremors on withdrawal.

1. Sato EH, *et al.* Abuse of cyclopentolate hydrochloride (Cyclogyl) drops. *N Engl J Med* 1992; **326:** 1363–4.

**Hypersensitivity.** Two children developed hypersensitivity reactions shortly after the instillation of 1% cyclopentolate hydrochloride eye drops into each eye.[1] Both children initially had a facial rash but in one of them the rash later spread to include the arms and legs and was accompanied by mild breathlessness.

1. Jones LWJ, Hodes DT. Possible allergic reactions to cyclopentolate hydrochloride: case reports with literature review of uses and adverse reactions. *Ophthalmic Physiol Opt* 1991; **11:** 16–21.

**Systemic toxicity.** Ten of 66 patients who received one drop of 2% cyclopentolate eye drops in each eye developed systemic toxicity of mild to moderate severity; 9 of the 10 were female.[1] Toxic signs included physical weakness, nausea, lightheadedness, changes in emotional attitude, unprovoked weeping, and loss of equilibrium; tachycardia was always present but changes in blood pressure were insignificant. Spontaneous recovery occurred within 1 hour to several days.

As with atropine, it has been recommended that cyclopentolate eye drops should not be used during the first 3 months of life because of the possible association with development of amblyopia. Systemic toxicity has also been reported in neonates following ocular administration of cyclopentolate.[2]

A 4-year-old boy with cerebral palsy and paraplegia suffered tonic-clonic seizures, facial flushing, and tachycardia 70 minutes after one drop of a 1% cyclopentolate solution was instilled into each eye to dilate his pupils.[3] The child had no history of convulsions and had received 1% cyclopentolate eye drops on 2 previous occasions without incident.

1. Awan KJ. Adverse systemic reactions of topical cyclopentolate hydrochloride. *Ann Ophthalmol* 1976; **8:** 695–8.

2. Bauer CR, *et al.* Systemic cyclopentolate (Cyclogyl) toxicity in the newborn infant. *J Pediatr* 1973; **92:** 501–5.
3. Fitzgerald DA, *et al.* Seizures associated with 1% cyclopentolate eyedrops. *J Paediatr Child Health* 1990; **26:** 106–7.

### Interactions

As for antimuscarinics in general (see Atropine Sulfate, p.477).

### Uses and Administration

Cyclopentolate hydrochloride is a tertiary amine antimuscarinic with actions similar to those of atropine (p.477). It is used as eye drops to produce mydriasis and cycloplegia (p.476) for ophthalmic diagnostic procedures and also in the treatment of uveitis and iritis (p.1090). It acts more quickly than atropine and has a shorter duration of action; the maximum mydriatic effect is produced 30 to 60 minutes after instillation, and may persist for up to 24 hours; the maximum cycloplegic effect is produced within 25 to 75 minutes and accommodation recovers within 6 to 24 hours.

For diagnostic procedures, 1 drop of a 0.5% solution of cyclopentolate hydrochloride repeated after about 5 to 15 minutes is usually sufficient for adults. Higher strengths have been used. For children 1 or 2 drops of a 1% solution are instilled similarly, although some recommend that strengths greater than 0.5% should not be used in infants and that cyclopentolate should not be used at all during the first 3 months of life.

In the treatment of uveitis and iritis 1 or 2 drops of a 0.5% solution of cyclopentolate hydrochloride are instilled into the eye(s) up to four times daily.

Deeply pigmented eyes are more resistant to pupillary dilatation and may require the use of a 1% solution.

### Preparations

***BP 2003:*** Cyclopentolate Eye Drops;
***USP 27:*** Cyclopentolate Hydrochloride Ophthalmic Solution.

**Proprietary Preparations** (details are given in Part 3)
***Arg.:*** Ciclopenal; ***Austral.:*** Cyclogyl; ***Belg.:*** Cyclopentol; ***Braz.:*** Cicloplegico; ***Canad.:*** Cyclogyl; Diopentolate; ***Chile:*** Cyclogyl; ***Denm.:*** Cyclogyl; ***Fin.:*** Oftan Syklo; ***Fr.:*** Skiacol; ***Ger.:*** Zykolat-EDO; ***Gr.:*** Cyclogyl; ***Hong Kong:*** Cyclogyl; ***India:*** Bell Pentolate; Cyclogyl; ***Irl.:*** Mydrilate; ***Ital.:*** Ciclolux; ***Malaysia:*** Colircusi Cicloplejico; Cyclogyl; ***NZ:*** Cyclogyl; ***Port.:*** Cicloplegicedol; Midriodavi; ***S.Afr.:*** Cyclogyl; ***Singapore:*** Cyclogyl; ***Spain:*** Ciclople†; Cicloplejic†; Cicloplejico; ***Swed.:*** Cyclogyl; ***Switz.:*** Cyclogyl; ***Thai.:*** Cyclogyl; ***UK:*** Mydrilate; ***USA:*** Ak-Pentolate; Cyclogyl; Ocu-Pentolate; Pentolair.

**Multi-ingredient:** ***Malaysia:*** Cyclomydril; ***S.Afr.:*** Cyclomydril; ***Singapore:*** Cyclomydril; ***USA:*** Cyclomydril.

---

## Darifenacin *(BAN, rINN)*

Darifenacina; UK-88525. (S)-1-[2-(2,3-Dihydro-5-benzofuranyl)ethyl]-α,α-diphenyl-3-pyrrolidineacetamide.

$C_{28}H_{30}N_2O_2$ = 426.6.
*CAS — 133099-04-4 (darifenacin); 133099-07-7 (darifenacin hydrobromide).*

### Profile

Darifenacin is a selective $M_3$ antimuscarinic under investigation in the treatment of urinary incontinence. It is also being studied in irritable bowel syndrome.

◊ References.

1. Haab F, *et al.* Darifenacin, an M(3) selective receptor antagonist, is an effective and well-tolerated once-daily treatment for overactive bladder. *Eur Urol* 2004; **45:** 420–9.

---

## Dexetimide *(BAN, USAN, rINN)*

(S)-2-(1-Benzyl-4-piperidyl)-2-phenylglutarimide; (S)-3-Phenyl-1′-(phenylmethyl)-(3,4′-bipiperidine)-2,6-dione.

$C_{23}H_{26}N_2O_2$ = 362.5.
*CAS — 21888-98-2.*
*ATC — N04AA08.*

## Dexetimide Hydrochloride *(BANM, rINNM)*

Dexbenzetimide Hydrochloride; Hidrocloruro de dexetimida; R-16470.

$C_{23}H_{26}N_2O_2,HCl$ = 398.9.
*CAS — 21888-96-0.*
*ATC — N04AA08.*

### Profile

Dexetimide is a tertiary antimuscarinic with actions similar to those of trihexyphenidyl (p.490). It has been used to alleviate drug-induced extrapyramidal symptoms, but, like other antimuscarinics, it is of no value against tardive dyskinesias. Dexetimide is given as the hydrochloride although doses are expressed in terms of the base; dexetimide hydrochloride 1.1 mg is approximately equivalent to 1 mg of dexetimide. A usual dose is 0.5 to 1 mg once daily by mouth; it has also been given by intramuscular injection.

### Preparations

**Proprietary Preparations** (details are given in Part 3)
***Belg.:*** Tremblex; ***Neth.:*** Tremblex.

---

## Dicycloverine Hydrochloride

*(BANM, rINNM)*

Cloridrato de Diciclоverina; Dicyclomine Hydrochloride; Dicycloverini Hydrochloridum; Hidrocloruro de dicicloverina. 2-Diethylaminoethyl bicyclohexyl-1-carboxylate hydrochloride.

$C_{19}H_{35}NO_2,HCl$ = 345.9.
*CAS — 77-19-0 (dicycloverine); 67-92-5 (dicycloverine hydrochloride).*
*ATC — A03AA07.*

**Pharmacopoeias.** In *Eur.* (see p.vi) and *US.*

**Ph. Eur. 5.0** (Dicycloverine Hydrochloride). A white or almost white, crystalline powder. It shows polymorphism. Soluble in water; freely soluble in alcohol and in dichloromethane. A 1% solution in water has a pH of 5.0 to 5.5.

**USP 27** (Dicyclomine Hydrochloride). A fine white, practically odourless, crystalline powder. Soluble 1 in 13 of water, 1 in 5 of alcohol, 1 in 2 of chloroform and of glacial acetic acid, and 1 in 770 of ether. pH of a 1% solution in water is between 5.0 and 5.5.

### Adverse Effects, Treatment, and Precautions

As for Atropine Sulfate, p.477. Dicycloverine hydrochloride should not be given to infants younger than 6 months of age.

**Apnoea.** Reports of severe apnoea in infants aged 5 to 10 weeks associated with the administration of dicycloverine.

1. Williams J, Watkin-Jones R. Dicyclomine: worrying symptoms associated with its use in some small babies. *BMJ* 1984; **288:** 901.
2. Edwards PDL. Dicyclomine in babies. *BMJ* 1984; **288:** 1230.
3. Spoudeas H, Shribman S. Dicyclomine in babies. *BMJ* 1984; **288:** 1230.

**Pregnancy.** For a review of the risks to the fetus of antiemetic therapy during pregnancy, with particular reference to Debendox (Bendectin: dicycloverine with doxylamine and pyridoxine), see under Antihistamines on p.420.

### Interactions

As for antimuscarinics in general (see Atropine Sulfate, p.477).

### Uses and Administration

Dicycloverine hydrochloride is a tertiary amine antimuscarinic with effects similar to but weaker than those of atropine (p.477); it also has a direct antispasmodic action.

Dicycloverine is used in gastrointestinal spasm, particularly that associated with the irritable bowel syndrome. For adults, 10 to 20 mg of dicycloverine hydrochloride is given 3 times daily; in the USA, up to 40 mg four times daily has been recommended where adverse effects permit. Children aged 6 months to 2 years may be given 5 to 10 mg up to 3 or 4 times daily; doses are usually given 15 minutes before meals. Children aged 2 to 12 years may be given 10 mg three times daily.

Dicycloverine hydrochloride may be given intramuscularly in doses of 20 mg given 4 times daily to patients in whom oral therapy is temporarily impractical, but should not be used for longer than 1 to 2 days.

### Preparations

***BP 2003:*** Dicycloverine Oral Solution; Dicycloverine Tablets;
***USP 27:*** Dicyclomine Hydrochloride Capsules; Dicyclomine Hydrochloride Injection; Dicyclomine Hydrochloride Syrup; Dicyclomine Hydrochloride Tablets.

**Proprietary Preparations** (details are given in Part 3)
***Arg.:*** Babypasmil; ***Austral.:*** Merbentyl; ***Braz.:*** Bentyl; ***Canad.:*** Bentylol; Formulex; Lomine; ***India:*** Cyclominol; Cyclopam; Dysmen; Spasmo-Proxyvon; ***Irl.:*** Merbentyl; ***Israel:*** Notensyl; ***Mex.:*** Bentyl; Diclomin; Sediclon; ***NZ:*** Merbentyl; ***Port.:*** Optimal; ***S.Afr.:*** Clomin; Medicyclomine; Merbentyl; ***Thai.:*** Clomin†; Dicomin; ***UK:*** Merbentyl; ***USA:*** Antispas; Bentyl; Byclomine; Dibent; Or-Tyl.

**Multi-ingredient:** ***Arg.:*** Dafne; ***Braz.:*** Anacidron†; Gastricin†; Gastromag†; ***Canad.:*** Spasmo Nil†; ***Chile:*** Profisin; ***Hong Kong:*** Colimix; Crema-U†; Veragel; ***India:*** Colimex; Colirid; Cyclo-Meff; Cyclopam; Dysmen; Normaxin; Parvon-Spas; Spasmo-Proxyvon; Spasmo-Proxyvon Forte; ***Irl.:*** Kolanticon†; ***Ital.:*** Merankol Pastiglie; ***Malaysia:*** Colimix; Uphacol; ***Mex.:*** Alphalox-D; Farcolan; ***Port.:*** Nausefe; ***S.Afr.:*** Alkalite D; Alumite; Asic; Betaclomin; Co-Gel; Dynagastrin†; Gelumen; Kolantyl; Medigel; Microgel; Neutragel; Nu-Gel†; pH 550; Propan Gel-S; Remotrox; Spasmogel; ***Singapore:*** Colimix; Meclosil; Tocid†; Veragel DMS; ***Spain:*** Colchimax; Neocolan; ***Thai.:*** Berclomine; Biodan; Cymine; Difemic; Kremil-S; Mainnox; Med-Anspasmic; Veragel; ***UK:*** Diarrest†; Kolanticon.

---

## Diethazine Hydrochloride *(BANM, rINNM)*

Diethazinium Chloratum; Eazamine Hydrochloride; Hidrocloruro de dietazina; RP-2987. 10-(2-Diethylaminoethyl)phenothiazine hydrochloride.

$C_{18}H_{22}N_2S,HCl$ = 334.9.
*CAS — 60-91-3 (diethazine); 341-70-8 (diethazine hydrochloride).*

### Profile

Diethazine hydrochloride is an antimuscarinic with actions similar to those of profenamine hydrochloride (p.488), but it is more toxic and bone-marrow depression may occur. It has been used in the treatment of parkinsonism.

---

## Difemerine Hydrochloride *(rINNM)*

Hidrocloruro de difemerina; UP-57. 2-Dimethylamino-1,1-dimethylethyl benzilate hydrochloride.

$C_{20}H_{25}NO_3,HCl$ = 363.9.
*CAS — 80387-96-8 (difemerine); 70280-88-5 (difemerine hydrochloride).*
*ATC — A03AA09.*

### Profile

Difemerine hydrochloride is an antimuscarinic with effects similar to those of atropine (p.477) and was used in the symptomatic treatment of visceral spasms.

---

## Dihexyverine Hydrochloride *(USAN, rINNM)*

Dihexiverine Hydrochloride; Hidrocloruro de dihexiverina; JL-1078. 2-Piperidinoethyl bicyclohexyl-1-carboxylate hydrochloride.

$C_{20}H_{35}NO_2,HCl$ = 358.0.
*CAS — 561-77-3 (dihexyverine); 5588-25-0 (dihexyverine hydrochloride).*
*ATC — A03AA08.*

### Profile

Dihexyverine hydrochloride is an antimuscarinic with effects similar to those of atropine (p.477). It is given in the symptomatic treatment of gastrointestinal spasm in daily doses of 20 to 60 mg by mouth or 50 to 150 mg rectally. It has also been given in doses of 10 mg by intramuscular injection.

### Preparations

**Proprietary Preparations** (details are given in Part 3)
***Fr.:*** Spasmodex.

---

## Dimevamide *(rINN)*

Aminopentamide; Dimevamida. α-[2-(Dimethylamino)propyl]-α-phenylbenzeneacetamide.

$C_{19}H_{24}N_2O$ = 296.4.
*CAS — 60-46-8.*

## Dimevamide Sulfate *(rINNM)*

Aminopentamide Sulfate.

$C_{19}H_{24}N_2O,H_2SO_4$ = 394.5.

**Pharmacopoeias.** In *US* for veterinary use only.

### Profile

Dimevamide is a tertiary amine and has been used as an antimuscarinic.

### Preparations

**Proprietary Preparations** (details are given in Part 3)
**Multi-ingredient:** ***S.Afr.:*** Kantrexil.

---

## Diphemanil Metilsulfate *(BAN, rINN)*

Diphemanil Methylsulfate; Diphemanil Methylsulphate; Diphemethanil Methylsulphate; Metilsulfato de difemanilo; Vagophemanil Methylsulphate. 4-Benzhydrylidene-1,1-dimethylpiperidinium methylsulphate.

$C_{20}H_{24}N,CH_3SO_4$ = 389.5.
*CAS — 62-97-5.*
*ATC — A03AB15.*

### Profile

Diphemanil metilsulfate is a quaternary ammonium antimuscarinic with peripheral effects similar to those of atropine (p.477). It is used topically as a 2% cream or powder to treat hyperhidrosis (excessive sweating).

Diphemanil metilsulfate, given by mouth, has been investigated for the treatment of symptomatic bradycardia in infants.

◊ References.

1. Vidal AM, *et al.* Pharmacokinetics of diphemanil methylsulphate in healthy subjects. *Eur J Clin Pharmacol* 1992; **42:** 689–91.
2. Vidal AM, *et al.* Pharmacokinetics of diphemanil methylsulphate in infants. *Eur J Clin Pharmacol* 1993; **45:** 89–91.
3. Pariente-Khayat A, *et al.* Pharmacokinetics of diphemanil methylsulphate in neonates and in premature infants. *Eur J Clin Pharmacol* 1996; **50:** 429–30.

#### Preparations

**Proprietary Preparations** (details are given in Part 3)
***Austral.:*** Prantal; ***Chile:*** Nivelon; ***Ital.:*** Prantal; ***NZ:*** Prantal.

## Drofenine Hydrochloride *(pINNM)*

Hexahydroadiphenine Hydrochloride; Hidrocloruro de drofenina. 2-(Diethylamino)ethyl α-phenylcyclohexaneacetate hydrochloride.

$C_{20}H_{31}NO_2,HCl = 353.9.$

*CAS — 1679-76-1 (drofenine); 548-66-3 (drofenine hydrochloride).*

**Pharmacopoeias.** In *Swiss.*

#### Profile

Drofenine hydrochloride is an antimuscarinic available in preparations for the treatment of visceral spasms.

#### Preparations

**Proprietary Preparations** (details are given in Part 3)
**Multi-ingredient:** ***Arg.:*** Espasmo Cibalena; Espasmo Cibalena Fuerte; ***Austria:*** Spasmoplus; ***Belg.:*** Spasmo-Cibalgine†; Spasmoplus; ***Chile:*** Espasmo Cibalgina; Espasmo Cibalgina Compuesta; ***Ger.:*** Spasmo-Cibalgin compositum S†; Spasmo-Cibalgin S; ***Ital.:*** Spasmo-Cibalgina; ***Mex.:*** Espasmo Cibalgina; ***Switz.:*** Lunadon; Sonotryl†; Spasmo-Cibalgin; Spasmo-Cibalgin comp.

## Emepronium Bromide *(BAN, rINN)*

Bromuro de emepronio. Ethyldimethyl(1-methyl-3,3-diphenylpropyl)ammonium bromide.

$C_{20}H_{28}BrN = 362.3.$

*CAS — 27892-33-7 (emepronium); 3614-30-0 (emepronium bromide).*

*ATC — G04BD01.*

## Emepronium Carrageenate *(BAN)*

Emepronio, carragenato de.

*ATC — G04BD01.*

#### Adverse Effects, Treatment, and Precautions

As for Atropine Sulfate, p.477.

To avoid oesophageal ulceration, tablets of emepronium bromide should always be swallowed with an adequate volume of water, and patients should always be in the sitting or standing position while, and for 10 to 15 minutes after, taking the tablets. Emepronium is contra-indicated in patients with symptoms or signs of oesophageal obstruction or with pre-existing oesophagitis.

**Buccal and oesophageal ulceration.** Tablet-induced oesophageal damage is a widely recognised problem and is related to direct mucosal injury by the medication. Emepronium bromide has been frequently implicated in this type of mucosal injury, although it rarely results in stricture formation.[1]

1. McCord GS, Clouse RE. Pill-induced esophageal strictures: clinical features and risk factors for development. *Am J Med* 1990; **88:** 512–18.

#### Interactions

As for antimuscarinics in general (see Atropine Sulfate, p.477).

#### Pharmacokinetics

Emepronium is incompletely absorbed from the gastrointestinal tract and is mainly excreted unchanged in the urine and faeces. It does not readily cross the blood-brain barrier at therapeutic doses.

#### Uses and Administration

Emepronium is a quaternary ammonium antimuscarinic with peripheral effects similar to those of atropine (p.477). It is used mainly in the treatment of urinary frequency and incontinence (p.476). Emepronium is given by mouth as the carrageenate although doses are expressed in terms of the equivalent amount of the bromide; a usual dose is the equivalent of 200 mg three times daily. Emepronium as the bromide is also given by subcutaneous or intramuscular injection.

#### Preparations

**Proprietary Preparations** (details are given in Part 3)
***Austria:*** Cetiprin; ***Braz.:*** Cetiprin; ***Denm.:*** Cetiprin; ***Fin.:*** Cetiprin Novum; ***Ger.:*** Uro-Ripirin†; ***Hong Kong:*** Cetiprin Novum†; ***Irl.:*** Cetiprin†; ***Neth.:*** Cetiprin; ***Norw.:*** Cetiprin; ***NZ:*** Cetiprin†; ***Spain:*** Hexanium†; ***Swed.:*** Cetiprin; ***Switz.:*** Cetiprin†.

## Eucatropine Hydrochloride *(BANM, rINNM)*

Clorhidrato de Euftalmina; Eucatropinium Chloride; Hidrocloruro de eucatropina. 1,2,2,6-Tetramethyl-4-piperidyl mandelate hydrochloride.

$C_{17}H_{25}NO_3,HCl = 327.8.$

*CAS — 100-91-4 (eucatropine); 536-93-6 (eucatropine hydrochloride).*

**Pharmacopoeias.** In *US.*

**USP 27** (Eucatropine Hydrochloride). A white, odourless, granular powder. Very soluble in water; freely soluble in alcohol and in chloroform; insoluble in ether. Its solutions are neutral to litmus. Store in airtight containers. Protect from light.

#### Profile

Eucatropine hydrochloride is a tertiary amine antimuscarinic that has been used as a mydriatic. It has little or no effect on accommodation.

#### Preparations

**USP 27:** Eucatropine Hydrochloride Ophthalmic Solution.

## Fentonium Bromide *(rINN)*

Bromuro de fentonio; Fa-402; Fentonii Bromidum; Ketoscilium; *N*-(4-Phenylphenacyl)-1-hyoscyaminium Bromide; Z-326. (−)-(1*R*,3*r*,5*S*)-8-(4-Phenylphenacyl)-3-[(*S*)-tropoyloxy]tropanium bromide.

$C_{31}H_{34}BrNO_4 = 564.5.$

*CAS — 5868-06-4.*

*ATC — A03BB04.*

#### Profile

Fentonium bromide is a quaternary ammonium antimuscarinic with peripheral effects similar to those of atropine (p.477). It has been used to relieve visceral spasms.

#### Preparations

**Proprietary Preparations** (details are given in Part 3)
***Mex.:*** Ulcesium†.

## Flavoxate Hydrochloride *(BANM, USAN, rINNM)*

DW-61; Hidrocloruro de flavoxato; NSC-114649; Rec-7-0040. 2-Piperidinoethyl 3-methyl-4-oxo-2-phenyl-4*H*-chromene-8-carboxylate hydrochloride.

$C_{24}H_{25}NO_4,HCl = 427.9.$

*CAS — 15301-69-6 (flavoxate); 3717-88-2 (flavoxate hydrochloride).*

*ATC — G04BD02.*

**Pharmacopoeias.** In *Br.* and *Jpn.*

**BP 2003** (Flavoxate Hydrochloride). A white or almost white crystalline powder. Slightly soluble in water, in alcohol, and in dichloromethane. Protect from light.

#### Adverse Effects, Treatment, and Precautions

As for Atropine Sulfate, p.477. Ocular effects, including increased intra-ocular pressure, are occasionally troublesome. Other adverse effects include sedation or fatigue, vertigo, and hypersensitivity reactions. Leucopenia or eosinophilia has been reported rarely.

#### Interactions

As for antimuscarinics in general (see Atropine Sulfate, p.477).

#### Pharmacokinetics

Flavoxate is readily absorbed from the gastrointestinal tract and rapidly metabolised, about 50 to 60% of a dose being excreted in the urine within 24 hours as methyl flavone carboxylic acid.

#### Uses and Administration

Flavoxate hydrochloride is described as a smooth muscle relaxant but it also has antimuscarinic effects; it is a tertiary amine. It is used for the symptomatic relief of pain, urinary frequency, and incontinence associated with inflammatory disorders of the urinary tract. It is also used for the relief of vesico-urethral spasms resulting from instrumentation or surgery. A usual dose is 200 mg by mouth three times daily.

**Urinary incontinence.** Flavoxate is indicated mainly in the treatment of urge incontinence (p.476). Results of studies have sometimes been disappointing,[1-4] although side-effects are said to be less marked than those seen with other antimuscarinics such as oxybutynin.

1. Stanton SL. A comparison of emepronium bromide and flavoxate hydrochloride in the treatment of urinary incontinence. *J Urol (Baltimore)* 1973; **110:** 529–32.
2. Meyhoff HH, *et al.* Placebo—the drug of choice in female motor urge incontinence? *Br J Urol* 1983; **55:** 34–7.
3. Robinson JM, Brocklehurst JC. Emepronium bromide and flavoxate hydrochloride in the treatment of urinary incontinence associated with detrusor instability in elderly women. *Br J Urol* 1983; **55:** 371–6.
4. Chapple CR, *et al.* Double-blind, placebo-controlled, cross-over study of flavoxate in the treatment of idiopathic detrusor instability. *Br J Urol* 1990; **66:** 491–4.

#### Preparations

**BP 2003:** Flavoxate Tablets.

**Proprietary Preparations** (details are given in Part 3)
***Arg.:*** Bladuril; ***Austria:*** Urispas; ***Belg.:*** Urispas; ***Braz.:*** Genurin-S; ***Canad.:*** Urispas; ***Chile:*** Bladuril; ***Denm.:*** Urispadol; ***Fr.:*** Urispas; ***Ger.:*** Spasuret; ***Hong Kong:*** Genurin; Urispas; ***India:*** Urispas; ***Irl.:*** Urispas; ***Ital.:*** Genurin; ***Jpn:*** Bladderon; ***Malaysia:*** Urispas; ***Mex.:*** Bladuril; ***Neth.:*** Urispas; ***Port.:*** Urispas; ***S.Afr.:*** Urispas; ***Singapore:*** Cleanxate; Genurin; Urispas; ***Spain:*** Uronid; ***Switz.:*** Urispas; ***Thai.:*** Flavo-Spa; Flavorin; Spasdic; Spasuri; U-Spa; Uroxate; ***UK:*** Urispas; ***USA:*** Urispas.
**Multi-ingredient:** ***Arg.:*** Algio-Bladuril; ***Ital.:*** Cistalgan.

## Flutropium Bromide *(rINN)*

Ba-598BR; Bromuro de flutropio. (8*r*)-8-(2-Fluoroethyl)-3α-hydroxy-1α*H*,5α*H*-tropanium bromide benzilate.

$C_{24}H_{29}BrFNO_3 = 478.4.$

*CAS — 63516-07-4.*

#### Profile

Flutropium bromide is a quaternary ammonium antimuscarinic with peripheral effects similar to those of atropine (p.477). It has bronchodilator properties and has been tried in the treatment of respiratory-tract disorders.

## Glycopyrronium Bromide *(BAN, rINN)*

AHR-504; Bromuro de glicopirronio; Glycopyrrolate *(USAN)*. 3-(α-Cyclopentylmandeloyloxy)-1,1-dimethylpyrrolidinium bromide.

$C_{19}H_{28}BrNO_3 = 398.3.$

*CAS — 596-51-0.*

*ATC — A03AB02.*

**Pharmacopoeias.** In *US.*

**USP 27** (Glycopyrrolate). A white, odourless, crystalline powder. Soluble 1 in 4.2 of water, 1 in 30 of alcohol, 1 in 260 of chloroform, and 1 in 35 000 of ether. Store in airtight containers.

**Incompatibility.** Glycopyrronium bromide is incompatible with alkalis.

**Stability.** Investigation of the compatibility of glycopyrronium bromide with infusion solutions and additives showed that the stability of glycopyrronium bromide is questionable above a pH of 6, owing to ester hydrolysis.[1]

1. Ingallinera TS, *et al.* Compatibility of glycopyrrolate injection with commonly used infusion solutions and additives. *Am J Hosp Pharm* 1979; **36:** 508–10. Correction. *ibid.*; 745.

#### Adverse Effects, Treatment, and Precautions

As for Atropine Sulfate, p.477.

**Renal impairment.** A comparison[1] of the pharmacokinetics of intravenous glycopyrronium in 11 uraemic and 7 control patients indicated that the renal elimination of glycopyrronium is considerably prolonged in patients with uraemia. The mean amount of a dose excreted in the urine within 3 hours of administration was 0.7% in the uraemic patients and 50% in the control patients; 24-hour excretion was 7% and 65%, respectively. The authors concluded that repeated or large doses of glycopyrronium should be avoided or perhaps the drug should not be used in patients with uraemia.

1. Kirvelä M, *et al.* Pharmacokinetics of glycopyrronium in uraemic patients. *Br J Anaesth* 1993; **71:** 437–9.

#### Interactions

As for antimuscarinics in general (see Atropine Sulfate, p.477).

#### Pharmacokinetics

Glycopyrronium bromide is poorly absorbed from the gastrointestinal tract; about 10 to 25% has been stated to be absorbed after an oral dose. Glycopyrronium bromide penetrates the blood-brain barrier only poorly. Glycopyrronium is excreted in bile and urine.

◊ References.

1. Kaltiala E, *et al.* The fate of intravenous [³H]glycopyrrolate in man. *J Pharm Pharmacol* 1974; **26:** 352–4.
2. Ali-melkkilä TM, *et al.* Pharmacokinetics of IM glycopyrronium. *Br J Anaesth* 1990; **64:** 667–9.
3. Rautakorpi P, *et al.* Pharmacokinetics of glycopyrrolate in children. *J Clin Anesth* 1994; **6:** 217–20.

#### Uses and Administration

Glycopyrronium bromide is a quaternary ammonium antimuscarinic with peripheral effects similar to those of atropine (p.477). After intramuscular administration, onset of effects is within 15 to 30 minutes; vagal blocking effects last for 2 to 3 hours and antisialagogue effects persist for up to 7 hours. Following intravenous administration, onset of actions occurs within 1 minute.

Glycopyrronium bromide is used similarly to atropine in anaesthetic practice. It has also been used in the iontophoretic treatment of hyperhidrosis and as an adjunct in the treatment of peptic ulcer disease.

See under headings below for details of dosage and administration of glycopyrronium in specific indications.

**Anaesthesia.** Glycopyrronium bromide is given as a premedicant before general anaesthesia (see p.475) to diminish the risk of vagal inhibition of the heart and to reduce salivary and bronchial secretions. It is given in doses of 200 to 400 micrograms intravenously or intramuscularly before the induction of anaesthesia; alternatively, it may be given in a dose of 4 to 5 micrograms/kg to a maximum of 400 micrograms. If necessary, similar or lower doses may be given intravenously during the operation and repeated if required. A suggested dosage for premedication in children is 4 to 8 micrograms/kg intravenously or intramuscularly to a maximum of 200 micrograms.

Glycopyrronium bromide is given before or with anticholinesterases to counteract their muscarinic effects when they are used to reverse the effects of competitive muscle relaxants (see Neostigmine, p.1493). The dose is glycopyrronium bromide 200 micrograms intravenously per 1 mg of neostigmine (or per 5 mg of pyridostigmine); alternatively, it may be given in a dose of 10 to 15 micrograms/kg intravenously with neostigmine 50 micrograms/kg. A suggested dosage for children is 10 micrograms/kg intravenously with neostigmine 50 micrograms/kg. Glycopyrronium bromide can be administered mixed in the same syringe with the anticholinesterase, and it has been suggested that greater cardiovascular stability results from this method of administration.

**Gastrointestinal disorders.** Antimuscarinics, including glycopyrronium bromide, have a limited role in the treatment of gastrointestinal spasms and as an adjunct in the treatment of peptic ulcer disease (see p.475).

As an adjunct in the treatment of peptic ulcer disease the usual initial dose of glycopyrronium bromide is 3 to 6 mg daily by mouth in divided doses adjusted according to response to a maximum of 8 mg daily; a maintenance dose of 1 mg twice daily is often adequate. Doses of 100 to 200 micrograms have been given by intramuscular or intravenous injection.

**Hyperhidrosis.** Adverse effects generally preclude oral use of antimuscarinics for the management of hyperhidrosis (p.475), but some, such as glycopyrronium, have been applied topically as alternatives to aluminium salts.

In studies involving 22 patients with the Frey syndrome (localised flushing and sweating on eating) glycopyrronium bromide as 1 and 2% cream or roll-on solution gave good control of symptoms;[1] patients tended to prefer the roll-on lotion as it was easier to apply. Topical hyoscine as 0.25, 1, or 3% solution or cream also gave control of sweating, but was associated with a much higher incidence of side-effects. Patients with diabetic gustatory sweating have also noted a reduction in the frequency and severity of episodes after applying glycopyrronium 0.5% cream.[2]

Glycopyrronium bromide has also been used as a 0.05% solution in the iontophoretic treatment of hyperhidrosis.


1. Hays LL, *et al.* The Frey syndrome: a simple, effective treatment. *Otolaryngol Head Neck Surg* 1982; **90:** 419–25.
2. Shaw JE, *et al.* A randomised controlled trial of topical glycopyrrolate, the first specific treatment for diabetic gustatory sweating. *Diabetologia* 1997; **40:** 299–301.


**Palliative care.** Glycopyrronium bromide is used in palliative care as an alternative to hyoscine to reduce excessive respiratory secretions. A dose of 200 micrograms may be given subcutaneously or intramuscularly every 4 hours. Alternatively, a dose of 0.6 to 1.2 mg may be given by subcutaneous infusion over 24 hours.

**Respiratory-tract disorders.** Antimuscarinics have potent bronchodilatory activity and may be used in the management of reversible airways obstruction as discussed on p.476, although glycopyrronium is not one of the main ones used.

References.


1. Schroeckenstein DC, *et al.* Twelve-hour bronchodilation in asthma with a single aerosol dose of the anticholinergic compound glycopyrrolate. *J Allergy Clin Immunol* 1988; **82:** 115–19.
2. Gilman MJ, *et al.* Comparison of aerosolized glycopyrrolate and metaproterenol in acute asthma. *Chest* 1990; **98:** 1095–8.
3. Cydulka RK, Emerman CL. Effects of combined treatment with glycopyrrolate and albuterol in acute exacerbation of chronic obstructive pulmonary disease. *Ann Emerg Med* 1995; **25:** 470–3.


## Preparations

*USP 27:* Glycopyrrolate Injection; Glycopyrrolate Tablets.

**Proprietary Preparations** (details are given in Part 3)

***Arg.:*** Acpan; ***Austral.:*** Robinul; ***Austria:*** Robinul; ***Belg.:*** Robinul; ***Canad.:*** Robinul†; ***Denm.:*** Robinul; ***Fin.:*** Gastrodyn†; Robinul; ***Ger.:*** Robinul; ***Hong Kong:*** Robinul; ***Irl.:*** Robinul†; ***Neth.:*** Robinul†; ***Norw.:*** Robinul; ***NZ:*** Robinul; ***S.Afr.:*** Robinul; ***Swed.:*** Robinul; ***Switz.:*** Robinul†; ***UK:*** Robinul; ***USA:*** Robinul.

**Multi-ingredient:** ***Fin.:*** Gastrodyn comp.

*Used as an adjunct in:* ***Belg.:*** Robinul-Neostigmine; ***Denm.:*** Robinul-Neostigmin; ***Fin.:*** Glycostigmin; Robinul-Neostigmin; ***Irl.:*** Robinul-Neostigmine†; ***Norw.:*** Robinul-Neostigmin; ***Swed.:*** Robinul-Neostigmin; ***Switz.:*** Robinul-Neostigmine; ***UK:*** Robinul-Neostigmine.

## Homatropine *(BAN)*

Homatropina. (1*R*,3*r*,5*S*)-Tropan-3-yl (*RS*)-mandelate.
$C_{16}H_{21}NO_3$ = 275.3.
*CAS — 87-00-3.*
*ATC — S01FA05.*

## Homatropine Hydrobromide *(BANM)*

Homatr. Hydrobrom.; Homatropina, hidrobromuro de; Homatropini Hydrobromidum; Homatropinium Bromide; Homatropinum Bromatum; Omatropina Bromidrato; Oxtolyltropine Hydrobromide; Tropyl Mandelate Hydrobromide.
$C_{16}H_{21}NO_3,HBr$ = 356.3.
*CAS — 51-56-9.*
*ATC — S01FA05.*

NOTE. HOM is a code approved by the BP 2003 for use on single unit doses of eye drops containing homatropine hydrobromide where the individual container may be too small to bear all the appropriate labelling information.

**Pharmacopoeias.** In *Eur.* (see p.vi), *Int., Jpn, Pol.,* and *US.*

**Ph. Eur. 5.0** (Homatropine Hydrobromide). A white, crystalline powder or colourless crystals. Freely soluble in water; sparingly soluble in alcohol. A 5% solution in water has a pH of 5.0 to 6.5. Protect from light.

**USP 27** (Homatropine Hydrobromide). White crystals or a white crystalline powder. Soluble 1 in 6 of water, 1 in 40 of alcohol, and 1 in 420 of chloroform; insoluble in ether. pH of a 2% solution in water is between 5.7 and 7.0. Store in airtight containers. Protect from light.

## Homatropine Methylbromide *(BANM, rINN)*

Homatropine Methobromide; Homatropini Methylbromidum; Methylhomatropinium Bromatum; Methylhomatropinium Bromide; Metilbromuro de homatropina. (1*R*,3*r*,5*S*)-3-[(±)-Mandeloyloxy]-8-methyltropanium bromide.
$C_{16}H_{21}NO_3,CH_3Br$ = 370.3.
*CAS — 80-49-9.*

**Pharmacopoeias.** In *Eur.* (see p.vi), *Int.,* and *US.*

**Ph. Eur. 5.0** (Homatropine Methylbromide). A white, crystalline powder or colourless crystals. Freely soluble in water; soluble in alcohol. A 5% solution in water has a pH of 4.5 to 6.5. Protect from light.

**USP 27** (Homatropine Methylbromide). A white, odourless, powder that slowly darkens on exposure to light. Very soluble in water; freely soluble in alcohol and in acetone containing about 20% of water; practically insoluble in acetone and in ether. pH of a 1% solution in water is between 4.5 and 6.5. Store in airtight containers. Protect from light.

### Adverse Effects, Treatment, and Precautions

As for Atropine Sulfate, p.477.

**Ophthalmic use.** Antimuscarinic toxicity (including ataxia, restlessness, excitement, hallucinations) has been reported in children[1] and the elderly[2,3] following administration of homatropine eye drops.


1. Hoefnagel D. Toxic effects of atropine and homatropine eyedrops in children. *N Engl J Med* 1961; **264:** 168–71.
2. Reid D, Fulton JD. Tachycardia precipitated by topical homatropine. *BMJ* 1989; **299:** 795–6.
3. Tune LE, *et al.* Anticholinergic delirium caused by topical homatropine ophthalmologic solution: confirmation by anticholinergic radioreceptor assay in two cases. *J Neuropsychiatr Clin Neurosci* 1992; **4:** 195–7.


### Interactions

As for antimuscarinics in general (see Atropine Sulfate, p.477).

### Uses and Administration

Homatropine is a tertiary amine antimuscarinic with effects similar to those of atropine (p.477). It is used as the hydrobromide, also a tertiary amine, to produce mydriasis and cycloplegia (p.476); its actions are more rapid and of shorter duration than those of atropine, but it is less potent and has a relatively weak cycloplegic effect. In general, onset of action is between 30 and 60 minutes, and recovery within 1 to 3 days. Homatropine hydrobromide is generally used as a 1, 2, or 5% ophthalmic solution. For the determination of refraction, one or two drops may be instilled, repeated if necessary 5 to 10 minutes later. In the treatment of uveitis (p.1090), one or two drops may be instilled two or three times a day, or up to every 3 to 4 hours if required.

Homatropine has also been used as the quaternary ammonium methobromide derivative in the treatment of gastrointestinal spasm and as an adjunct in peptic ulcer disease.

## Preparations

*BP 2003:* Homatropine Eye Drops;
*USP 27:* Homatropine Hydrobromide Ophthalmic Solution; Homatropine Methylbromide Tablets.

**Proprietary Preparations** (details are given in Part 3)

***Arg.:*** Antiespasmodico; Dallapasmo; Espasmotropin; Paratropina; ***Braz.:*** Espasmofin†; Novatropina; ***Gr.:*** Nopar; ***Malaysia:*** Homa; ***Mex.:*** Homasedin; Homatropil†; Homo; Infafren Simple†; Pasmolit†; ***Port.:*** Homatrocil†; ***Spain:*** Coliriocilina Homatrop†; Homatrop.

**Multi-ingredient:** ***Arg.:*** Antispasmina; Asestor; Bellatotal; Bibol Leloup; Biliosan Compuesto; Carbogasol; Carbon Tabs; Colistop; Dimaval; Espasmo Ibupirac; Espasmofin; Factor AG Antiespasmodico; Hepatodirectol; Ibupirac Fem; Opoenterol; Paratropina Compuesta; Sumal; ***Braz.:*** Analgosedan†; Asmatiron†; Atapec; Belacodid; Calmazin†; Codeverin; Diapool†; Dipirol; Enterobion†; Enteropen†; Enterovit†; Espasmalgon; Espasmo Colic†; Espasmo Luftal; Espasmobel†; Etaverol†; Filinasma†; Flagass Baby; Glotil†; H-Sal†; Kaostase†; Linadin†; Marsonil†; Migrane; Naquinto†; Pasmalgin†; Plasmocolit†; Plenocedan†; Pulmoformil†; Sedalene; Somasedin†; Spasmotropin; Suspectim†; Tebasedan†; Tropinal; Vagoplex†; ***Chile:*** Codelasa; ***Hung.:*** Neotroparin; ***India:*** Dysfur-M; ***Mex.:*** Contefur; Coralzul; Dialgin; Facetin-D; Fuzotyl; Neoxil; Sultroquin; Tasakal; Threchop; Trilor; Yodozona; ***Port.:*** Fluidin Nocturno†; ***Spain:*** Cortenema; ***Thai.:*** Polyenzyme-I; ***USA:*** Gustase Plus†; Hycodan; Hydromet; Hydropane; Tussigon.

# Hyoscine *(BAN)*

Escopolamina; Scopolamine. (−)-(1*S*,3*s*,5*R*,6*R*,7*S*,8*s*)-6,7-Epoxy-3[(*S*)-tropoyloxy] tropane.
$C_{17}H_{21}NO_4$ = 303.4.
*CAS — 51-34-3.*
*ATC — A04AD01; N05CM05; S01FA02.*

## Hyoscine Butylbromide *(BANM)*

Butylscopolamine Bromide; *N*-Butylscopolammonium Bromide; Butylscopolamonii Bromidum; Escopolamina, butilbromuro de; Hyoscine-*N*-butyl Bromide; Hyoscini Butylbromidum; Scopolamine *N*-Butyl Bromide; Scopolamine Butylbromide; Scopolomini Butylbromidum. (−)-(1*S*,3*s*,5*R*,6*R*,7*S*,8*r*)-6,7-Epoxy-8-butyl-3-[(*S*)-tropoyloxy]tropanium bromide.
$C_{21}H_{30}BrNO_4$ = 440.4.
*CAS — 149-64-4.*

**Pharmacopoeias.** In *Chin., Eur.* (see p.vi), and *Jpn.*

**Ph. Eur. 5.0** (Hyoscine Butylbromide). A white or almost white, crystalline powder. Freely soluble in water and in dichloromethane; sparingly soluble in dehydrated alcohol. A 5% solution in water has a pH of 5.5 to 6.5.

## Hyoscine Hydrobromide *(BANM)*

Bromhidrato de Escopolamina; Escopolamina, hidrobromuro de; Hyoscini Hydrobromidum; Ioscina Bromidrato; Scopolamine Bromhydrate; Scopolamine Hydrobromide; Scopolamini Hydrobromidum. (−)-(1*S*,3*s*,5*R*,6*R*,7*S*)-6,7-Epoxytropan-3-yl (*S*)-tropate hydrobromide trihydrate.
$C_{17}H_{21}NO_4,HBr,3H_2O$ = 438.3.
*CAS — 114-49-8 (anhydrous hyoscine hydrobromide); 6533-68-2 (hyoscine hydrobromide trihydrate).*
*ATC — A04AD01; N05CM05; S01FA02.*

NOTE. HYO is a code approved by the BP 2003 for use on single unit doses of eye drops containing hyoscine hydrobromide where the individual container may be too small to bear all the appropriate labelling information.

**Pharmacopoeias.** In *Chin., Eur.* (see p.vi), *Jpn, Pol.,* and *US.*

**Ph. Eur. 5.0** (Hyoscine Hydrobromide). A white or almost white, efflorescent, crystalline powder or colourless crystals. Freely soluble in water; soluble in alcohol. A 5% solution in water has a pH of 4.0 to 5.5. Store in well-filled airtight containers of small capacity. Protect from light.

**USP 27** (Scopolamine Hydrobromide). Colourless or white crystals, or white granular powder. Is odourless and slightly efflorescent in dry air. Soluble 1 in 1.5 of water and 1 in 20 of alcohol; slightly soluble in chloroform; insoluble in ether. pH of a 5% solution in water is between 4.0 and 5.5. Store in airtight containers. Protect from light.

## Hyoscine Methobromide *(BAN)*

Epoxymethamine Bromide; Escopolamina, metilbromuro de; Hyoscine Methylbromide; Methscopolamine Bromide; Scopolamine Methobromide; Scopolamine Methylbromide. (−)-(1*S*,3*s*,5*R*,6*R*,7*S*)-6,7-Epoxy-8-methyl-3-[(*S*)-tropoyloxy]tropanium bromide.
$C_{18}H_{24}BrNO_4$ = 398.3.
*CAS — 155-41-9.*

## Hyoscine Methonitrate *(BANM)*

Escopolamina, metilnitrato de; Hyoscine Methylnitrate; Methscopolamine Nitrate; Methylhyoscini Nitras; Methylscopolamini Nitras; Scopolamine Methonitrate; Scopolamine Methylnitrate. (−)-(1*S*,3*s*,5*R*,6*R*,7*S*)-6,7-Epoxy-8-methyl-3-[(*S*)-tropoyloxy]tropanium nitrate.
$C_{18}H_{24}N_2O_7$ = 380.4.
*CAS — 6106-46-3.*

### Adverse Effects, Treatment, and Precautions

As for Atropine Sulfate, p.477. In contrast to atropine, hyoscine produces central depression at therapeutic doses and symptoms include drowsiness and fatigue. Toxic doses of hyoscine produce stimulation of the CNS in a similar manner to atropine. However, hyoscine does not stimulate the medullary centres and therefore does not produce the increases in respiration rate or blood pressure seen with atropine. Hyoscine may produce CNS stimulation rather than depression at therapeutic doses if used in the presence of pain without opioid analgesics; symptoms include excitement, restlessness, hallucinations, or delirium.

Patients who experience drowsiness should not drive or operate machinery. Caution has been advised in elderly patients and in patients with impaired metabolic, liver, or kidney function, as adverse CNS effects have been stated to be more likely in these patients. There have been rare reports of an increase in frequency of seizures in epileptic patients.

The quaternary derivatives, such as the butylbromide, methobromide, or methonitrate, do not readily cross the blood-brain barrier, so central effects are rare.

**Breast feeding.** The American Academy of Pediatrics[1] states that there have been no reports of any clinical effect on the infant associated with the use of hyoscine by breast-feeding mothers, and that therefore it may be considered to be usually compatible with breast feeding.

1. American Academy of Pediatrics. The transfer of drugs and other chemicals into human milk. *Pediatrics* 2001; **108:** 776–89. Correction. *ibid.*; 1029. Also available at: http://aappolicy.aappublications.org/cgi/content/full/pediatrics%3b108/3/776 (accessed 01/06/04)

**Effects on the eyes.** ANISOCORIA. Although bilateral mydriasis has occurred with the use of transdermal hyoscine, development of a unilateral fixed dilated pupil (anisocoria) may be due to contamination of a finger with hyoscine in applying the device, and then rubbing the eye.[1-4]

1. Chiaramonte JS. Cycloplegia from transdermal scopolamine. *N Engl J Med* 1982; **306:** 174.
2. Lepore FE. More on cycloplegia from transdermal scopolamine. *N Engl J Med* 1982; **307:** 824.
3. McCrary JA, Webb NR. Anisocoria from scopolamine patches. *JAMA* 1982; **248:** 353–4.
4. Bienia RA, *et al.* Scopolamine skin-disks and anisocoria. *Ann Intern Med* 1983; **99:** 572–3.

GLAUCOMA. A report[1] of 2 cases of angle-closure glaucoma precipitated by transdermal hyoscine.

1. Fraunfelder FT. Transdermal scopolamine precipitating narrow-angle glaucoma. *N Engl J Med* 1982; **307:** 1079.

STRABISMUS. Strabismus developed in a 4-year-old boy during treatment with transdermal hyoscine patches for drooling.[1] The strabismus resolved shortly after discontinuation of hyoscine.

1. Good WV, Crain LS. Esotropia in a child treated with a scopolamine patch for drooling. *Pediatrics* 1996; **97:** 126–7.

**Effects on mental function.** There have been reports of psychotic reactions associated with the transdermal administration of hyoscine.[1-4] Psychotic reactions have also occurred following instillation of hyoscine eye drops.[5]

1. Osterholm RK, Camoriano JK. Transdermal scopolamine psychosis. *JAMA* 1982; **247:** 3081.
2. Rodysill KJ, Warren JB. Transdermal scopolamine and toxic psychosis. *Ann Intern Med* 1983; **98:** 561.
3. MacEwan GW, *et al.* Psychosis due to transdermally administered scopolamine. *Can Med Assoc J* 1985; **133:** 431–2.
4. Rubner O, *et al.* Ungewöhnlicher Fall einer Psychose infolge einer Langzeiteinwirkung mit einem Skopolaminmembranpflaster: Paranoid-halluzinatorische und delirante Symptomatik. *Nervenarzt* 1997; **68:** 77–9.
5. Barker DB, Solomon DA. The potential for mental status changes associated with systemic absorption of anticholinergic ophthalmic medications: concerns for the elderly. *DICP Ann Pharmacother* 1990; **24:** 847–50.

**Effects on the skin.** Contact dermatitis occurred in 16 men being treated for seasickness with transdermal hyoscine for 6 weeks to 15 months.[1]

1. Gordon CR, *et al.* Allergic contact dermatitis caused by transdermal hyoscine. *BMJ* 1989; **298:** 1220–1.

**Porphyria.** Hyoscine butylbromide has been associated with acute attacks of porphyria and is considered unsafe in porphyric patients.

**Pregnancy.** A report[1] of hyoscine toxicity in a neonate born to a mother who had received a total of 1.8 mg of hyoscine in divided doses with pethidine and levorphanol prior to delivery. The neonate was lethargic, barrel chested, and had a heart rate of 200 beats per minute. Symptoms subsided following physostigmine 100 micrograms given intramuscularly.

1. Evens RP, Leopold JC. Scopolamine toxicity in a newborn. *Pediatrics* 1980; **66:** 329–30.

**Withdrawal.** Dizziness and nausea occurred three days after removal of a hyoscine transdermal delivery system. The patient had been using the transdermal patches to prevent seasickness during a 10-day cruise.[1]

1. Meyboom RHB. More on Transderm Scop patches. *N Engl J Med* 1984; **311:** 1377.

## Interactions

As for antimuscarinics in general (see Atropine Sulfate, p.477).

The sedative effect of hyoscine may be enhanced by alcohol or other CNS depressants.

## Pharmacokinetics

Hyoscine is readily absorbed from the gastrointestinal tract following oral doses of the hydrobromide. It is almost entirely metabolised, probably in the liver; only a small proportion of an oral dose has been reported to be excreted unchanged in the urine. It crosses the blood-brain barrier and has been stated to cross the placenta. Hyoscine is also well absorbed following application to the skin.

The quaternary derivatives, such as the butylbromide or methobromide, are poorly absorbed from the gastrointestinal tract and do not readily pass the blood-brain barrier.

◊ References.

1. Ebert U, *et al.* Pharmacokinetics and pharmacodynamics of scopolamine after subcutaneous administration. *J Clin Pharmacol* 1998; **38:** 720–6.

## Uses and Administration

Hyoscine is a tertiary amine antimuscarinic with central and peripheral actions (see p.475). It is a more powerful suppressant of salivation than atropine, and usually slows rather than increases heart rate, especially in low doses. Its central action differs from that of atropine in that it depresses the cerebral cortex and produces drowsiness and amnesia. Hyoscine hydrobromide is also a tertiary amine, whereas hyoscine butylbromide, hyoscine methobromide, and hyoscine methonitrate are quaternary ammonium derivatives.

Hyoscine and hyoscine hydrobromide are used in the management of motion sickness and other forms of nausea and vomiting; hyoscine hydrobromide is also given as a premedicant in anaesthesia, and to produce mydriasis and cycloplegia. Hyoscine butylbromide and other quaternary ammonium derivatives are used in conditions associated with visceral spasms. In addition, hyoscine methobromide has been employed as an adjunct in the treatment of peptic ulcer disease.

Other hyoscine salts or derivatives that have been used include hyoscine borate, hyoscine hydrochloride, and hyoscine oxide hydrobromide.

See under headings below for details of dosage and administration of hyoscine and its salts in specific indications.

**Anaesthesia.** The role of antimuscarinics, including hyoscine, in anaesthesia is discussed on p.475. For the use of hyoscine in the prevention of postoperative nausea and vomiting, see below. For premedication hyoscine hydrobromide is injected subcutaneously or intramuscularly in doses of 200 to 600 micrograms, usually with papaveretum about half to one hour before induction of general anaesthesia. In the UK, a dose of 15 micrograms/kg is licensed in children.

**Anoxic seizures.** For mention of the use of transdermal hyoscine as an alternative to atropine in the management of reflex anoxic seizures in children, see p.478.

**Biliary and renal colic.** Hyoscine has been used as an adjunct to opioid analgesics for symptomatic relief of biliary or renal colic (see p.475). See also Palliative Care, below.

**Cardiac disorders.** Although hyoscine is not one of the conventional therapies for heart failure (p.820) or myocardial infarction (p.828), low-dose transdermal hyoscine can increase cardiac vagal activity and thereby reduce the autonomic imbalance seen in patients with these conditions.[1-3]

1. Casadei B, *et al.* Low doses of scopolamine increase cardiac vagal tone in the acute phase of myocardial infarction. *Circulation* 1993; **88:** 353–7.
2. La Rovere MT, *et al.* Scopolamine improves autonomic balance in advanced congestive heart failure. *Circulation* 1994; **90:** 838–43.
3. Venkatesh G, *et al.* Double blind placebo controlled trial of short term transdermal scopolamine on heart rate variability in patients with chronic heart failure. *Heart* 1996; **76:** 137–43.

**Dysmenorrhoea.** Hyoscine as the butylbromide or hydrobromide has been used for its antispasmodic action in the treatment of dysmenorrhoea.

**Eye disorders.** Hyoscine hydrobromide is used in the eye for its mydriatic and cycloplegic actions (p.476) usually in a concentration of 0.25%. It has a faster onset and shorter duration of action than atropine although the effects may still persist for up to 3 to 7 days. It may be useful for patients who are hypersensitive to atropine.

**Gastrointestinal disorders.** Hyoscine has been used to relieve the pain of smooth muscle spasm associated with the gastrointestinal tract (p.475). In such conditions usual doses of 20 mg of hyoscine butylbromide are administered intramuscularly or intravenously, repeated after 30 minutes if necessary, up to a maximum of 100 mg daily; alternatively, 20 mg may be given by mouth four times daily. In irritable bowel syndrome the recommended starting dose by mouth is 10 mg three times daily which may be increased to 20 mg four times daily, if necessary. Children aged 6 to 12 years may be given 10 mg three times daily by mouth for gastrointestinal spasms. Hyoscine may also be useful as an antispasmodic in endoscopy and radiological procedures of the gastrointestinal tract.[1] Hyoscine has been used as an adjunct in the treatment of peptic ulcer disease. Its antiemetic effect is discussed under Nausea and Vomiting, below.

1. Goei R, *et al.* Use of antispasmodic drugs in double contrast barium enema examination: glucagon or Buscopan? *Clin Radiol* 1995: **50:** 553–7.

**Hyperhidrosis.** Adverse effects of antimuscarinics given orally generally preclude their use by this route for the management of hyperhidrosis (p.475), but some, such as hyoscine, have been applied topically as alternatives to aluminium salts. Hyoscine hydrobromide applied as a 3% cream was successful in reducing gustatory sweating, consisting of flushing and sweating over the right mandible during eating, in a patient who had previously undergone surgical excision of the right submandibular salivary gland.[1]

1. Bailey BMW, Pearce DE. Gustatory sweating following submandibular salivary gland removal. *Br Dent J* 1985; **158:** 17–18.

**Nausea and vomiting.** Hyoscine is an effective agent in the prevention of **motion sickness** and is one of the principal drugs used. It may be given by mouth for short-term protection or transdermally from controlled-release systems for a prolonged duration of action.

A usual dose of hyoscine hydrobromide by mouth is 300 micrograms taken 30 minutes before a journey, followed by 300 micrograms every 6 hours if required up to a maximum of 3 doses in 24 hours. Children aged 4 to 10 years may be given 75 to 150 micrograms and those over 10 years, 150 to 300 micrograms. Hyoscine is also given via a transdermal delivery system (Scopoderm, Transderm Scop) which is placed behind the ear and supplies 1 mg over 3 days. The patch may typically be used in adults and children aged 10 years and over and should be applied 5 to 6 hours before travelling or on the preceding evening and removed at the end of the journey.

An intranasal formulation of hyoscine hydrobromide has been investigated for the treatment and prevention of motion sickness.

Transdermal hyoscine has been used in adults and children for the prevention of **postoperative nausea and vomiting**.

Hyoscine hydrobromide has also been given by intravenous, subcutaneous, or intramuscular injection for its antiemetic effect in a usual dose of 300 to 600 micrograms.

The other drugs used in the management of motion sickness and postoperative nausea and vomiting are discussed on p.1245.

References.

1. Dahl E, *et al.* Transdermal scopolamine, oral meclizine, and placebo in motion sickness. *Clin Pharmacol Ther* 1984; **36:** 116–20.
2. Doyle E, *et al.* Prevention of postoperative nausea and vomiting with transdermal hyoscine in children using patient-controlled analgesia. *Br J Anaesth* 1994; **72:** 72–6.
3. Honkavaara P. Effect of transdermal hyoscine on nausea and vomiting during and after middle ear surgery under local anaesthesia. *Br J Anaesth* 1996; **76:** 49–53.

**Palliative care.** *Hyoscine hydrobromide* is used in palliative care to reduce excessive respiratory secretions. A dose of 400 to 600 micrograms may be given by subcutaneous injection every 4 to 8 hours. Alternatively 0.6 to 2.4 mg may be given over 24 hours by continuous subcutaneous infusion. Care should be taken to avoid the discomfort of a dry mouth. Hyoscine may also be given as a transdermal patch in some countries.

*Hyoscine butylbromide* is also used in palliative care in the treatment of bowel colic; however, it may not be adequate for the control of respiratory secretion. It is given as a subcutaneous infusion in a dose of 20 to 60 mg every 24 hours.

**Urinary incontinence.** Various antimuscarinics have been used in the management of urge incontinence (p.476) but the incidence of adverse effects can be high. Results of a small study[1] suggested that transdermal hyoscine might be of benefit in females with detrusor instability.

1. Muskat Y, *et al.* The use of scopolamine in the treatment of detrusor instability. *J Urol (Baltimore)* 1996; **156:** 1989–90.

**Vertigo.** Hyoscine has a long history of use in the management of vertigo, although other drugs are now preferred (p.423).

## Preparations

***BP 2003:*** Hyoscine Butylbromide Injection; Hyoscine Butylbromide Tablets; Hyoscine Eye Drops; Hyoscine Injection; Hyoscine Tablets;
***USP 27:*** Scopolamine Hydrobromide Injection; Scopolamine Hydrobromide Ophthalmic Ointment; Scopolamine Hydrobromide Ophthalmic Solution; Scopolamine Hydrobromide Tablets.

**Proprietary Preparations** (details are given in Part 3)
***Arg.:*** Buscapina; Cifespasmo; Colobolina; Luar-G; Pasmodina; Pasmovit; Rupe-N; ***Austral.:*** Buscopan; Kwells; Setacol; Travacalm HO; ***Austria:*** Buscopan; Scopoderm; ***Belg.:*** Aspasmine; Buscopan; ***Braz.:*** Algexin; Buscopan; Hiospan; Uni Hioscin; ***Canad.:*** Buscopan; Transderm-V; ***Chile:*** Buscapina; ***Denm.:*** Buscopan; Scopoderm; ***Fin.:*** Buscopan; Scopoderm; ***Fr.:*** Genoscopolamine†; Scoburen; Scopoderm TTS; ***Ger.:*** Boro-Scopol; BS-ratiopharm; Buscolysin; Buscopan; espa-butyl†; Scopoderm TTS; Spasman scop; Spasmowern; ***Gr.:*** Buscopan; ***Hong Kong:*** Buscopan; Busopin; Copan; Dhacopan; Holopon†; Hysopan; Scopoderm TTS; Vidaspan; ***India:*** Buscopan; ***Irl.:*** Buscopan; Kwells; ***Ital.:*** Buscopan; Transcop; ***Malaysia:*** Buscopan; Colospan; Dhacopan; Fucon; Hyomide; Spasmoliv; Vacopan; Vascopan; ***Mex.:*** Alpin†; Brolamina; Buscapina; Busina†; Busprina-S; Buticina†; Butiral; Cryopina; Espacil; Espasantral†; Grafin; Hiosinotil; Lemophar; Liliam; Selpiran-S; Tilosin†; ***Neth.:*** Buscopan; Scopoderm TTS; ***Norw.:*** Buscopan; Scopoderm; ***NZ:*** Buscopan; Scopoderm TTS; ***Port.:*** Buscopan; Vagotrope-S†; ***S.Afr.:*** Buscopan; Hyospasmol; Scopex; ***Singapore:*** Buscopan; Colospan; Dhacopan; Fucon; Hyomide; Scopoderm TTS†; Spasmoliv; Vacopan; ***Spain:*** Buscapina; Vorigeno; ***Swed.:*** Buscopan; Scopoderm; ***Switz.:*** Buscopan; Scopoderm TTS†; ***Thai.:*** Amcopan; Antispa; Bacotan; Buscono; Buscopan; Butyl; Cencopan; Eralga; Higan; Hy-Spa; Hybutyl; Hyosmed; Hyospan; Hyostan; Hyozin;

Hytic; Kanin; Scopas; Spascopan; Spasgone-H; Spatab; Vacopan; **UAE:** Scopinal; **UK:** Buscopan; Joy-Rides; Kwells; Scopoderm TTS; Travel Calm†; **USA:** Pamine; Scopace; Transderm Scop.

**Multi-ingredient: Arg.:** 6 Copin; Buscapina Compositum; Buscapina Compositum N; Cavodan; Cifespasmo Compuesto; Colobolina D; Dislembral; Espasmo Biotenk; Ibu-Buscapina; Lisalgil Compuesto; Luar-G Compositum; Novopasmil Compuesto; Rupe-N Compuesto; **Austral.:** Contac†; Donnagel; Donnalix; Donnatab; Travacalm; **Austria:** Asthma†; Buscopamol; Buscopan Compositum; Modiscop; **Belg.:** Buscopan Compositum; Spasma; **Braz.:** Analverin Composto; Analverin Plus; Binospan Composto; Bioscina Composta; Buscopan Composto; Buscopan Plus; Buscoveran Composto; Butilamin†; Disbuspan; Dorspan; Ductopan; Espasmodid Composto; Hiospan Composto; Inib-Dor†; Kindpasm; Neocopan; Sedabel; Sedobion†; Tropinal; Uzara†; Vagoplex†; Veratropan Composto; **Canad.:** Diban†; Donnatal†; **Chile:** Algion; Buscapina Compositum; Dolcopin; Kordinol Compuesto; Novalona; **Ger.:** Buscopan Plus; Oragallin S†; **Hong Kong:** Crema-U†; Unigan; Virulex Forte; **Irl.:** Feminax; **Ital.:** Buscopan Compositum; Spasmeridan; **Mex.:** Algosfar; Bipasmin Compuesto NF; Buscapina Compositum; Buscapina Compositum N; Busconet; Busepan; Busprina; Colepren; Donodol Compuesto; Escapin-N; Espacil Compuesto; Hiosinotil Compuesto; Ortran; Pasmodil; Pirobutil; Retodol Compositum; Selpiran; **Port.:** Buscopan Compositum N; **S.Afr.:** Allertac†; Bellatard†; Buscopan Compositum; Donnatal; Dyka-D†; Millerspas; Respinol; Respinol Compound; Scopex Co; Virobis; **Spain:** Buscapina Compositum; Midriati; Nolotil Compositum; Oragalin Espasmolitico; Psico Blocan; **Swed.:** Spasmofen; **Switz.:** Nardyl; Viaggio†; **Thai.:** Amcopan Plus; Buscopan Plus; Donnatal; Pacopan; Spasgone; Unigan; **UK:** Feminax; **USA:** Accuhist LA; AeroHist Plus; AeroKid; AH-chew; AlleRx; Antispasmodic Elixir; Atrohist Plus†; Barbidonna; Bellahist-D; Bellatal; Chlor-Mes D; CPM PSE MSC; CPM/PE/MSC; DA Chewable; DA II; Dallergy; Deconhist LA†; Dehistine; Donnatal†; DriHist; Dura-Vent/DA; Durahist; Ex-Histine; Extendryl; Hista-Vent DA; Histor-D Timecelles; Hyosophen; Mescolor; Murocoll-2; Norel DM; Omnihist LA; Pannaz; PCM; Phenahist-TR†; Phenchlor SHA†; Prehist D; PSE MSC; Rescon-MX; Ru-Tuss†; Stahist; Susano; Xiral.

## Hyoscyamine *(BAN)*

Hiosciamina; (−)-Hyoscyamine; *l*-Hyoscyamine. (−)-(1*R*,3*r*,5*S*)-Tropan-3-yl (*S*)-tropate.

$C_{17}H_{23}NO_3$ = 289.4.

*CAS — 101-31-5.*

*ATC — A03BA03.*

**Description.** Hyoscyamine is an alkaloid obtained from various solanaceous plants. It is the laevo-isomer of atropine into which it can be converted by heating or by the action of alkali.

**Pharmacopoeias.** In *US.*

**USP 27** (Hyoscyamine). A white crystalline powder. M.p. 106° to 109°. Slightly soluble in water and in benzene; freely soluble in alcohol, in chloroform, and in dilute acids; sparingly soluble in ether. Its solutions are alkaline to litmus. Store in airtight containers. Protect from light.

### Hyoscyamine Hydrobromide *(BANM)*

Bromidrato de Hiosciamina; Hiosciamina, hidrobromuro de; Hyoscyamine Bromhydrate.

$C_{17}H_{23}NO_3,HBr$ = 370.3.

*CAS — 306-03-6.*

*ATC — A03BA03.*

**Pharmacopoeias.** In *US.*

**USP 27** (Hyoscyamine Hydrobromide). White, odourless, crystals or crystalline powder. M.p. not less than 149°. Freely soluble in water; soluble 1 in 2.5 of alcohol, 1 in 1.7 of chloroform, and 1 in 2300 of ether. pH of a 5% solution in water is about 5.4. Store in airtight containers. Protect from light.

### Hyoscyamine Sulfate

Hiosciamina, sulfato de; Hyoscyamine Sulphate *(BANM)*; Hyoscyamini Sulfas; Hyoscyaminum Sulfuricum; Iosciamina Solfato.

$(C_{17}H_{23}NO_3)_2,H_2SO_4,2H_2O$ = 712.8.

*CAS — 620-61-1 (anhydrous hyoscyamine sulfate); 6835-16-1 (hyoscyamine sulfate dihydrate).*

*ATC — A03BA03.*

**Pharmacopoeias.** In *Eur.* (see p.vi) and *US.*

**Ph. Eur. 5.0** (Hyoscyamine Sulphate). A white or almost white, crystalline powder or colourless needles. Very soluble in water; sparingly soluble or soluble in alcohol. A 2% solution in water has a pH of 4.5 to 6.2. Store in airtight containers. Protect from light.

**USP 27** (Hyoscyamine Sulfate). White, odourless, crystals or crystalline powder. Soluble 1 in 0.5 of water and 1 in 5 of alcohol; practically insoluble in ether. pH of a 1% solution in water is about 5.3. Store in airtight containers. Protect from light.

### Adverse Effects, Treatment, and Precautions

As for Atropine Sulfate, p.477.

### Interactions

As for antimuscarinics in general (see Atropine Sulfate, p.477).

### Uses and Administration

Hyoscyamine is a tertiary amine antimuscarinic with the actions of atropine (which is racemic hyoscyamine, see p.477); hyoscyamine, the laevo-isomer, has about twice the potency of atropine since the dextro-isomer has only very weak antimuscarinic activity. Hyoscyamine is used mainly in the relief of conditions associated with visceral spasm. It has also been given for rhinitis and was formerly used in the treatment of parkinsonism.

Hyoscyamine is given in usual doses of 150 to 300 micrograms up to four times daily by mouth, but it is more usually employed as the sulfate; the hydrobromide is also used. Suggested doses of hyoscyamine sulfate are 125 to 250 micrograms by mouth or sublingually every four hours as needed, up to a maximum of 1.5 mg in 24 hours. Modified-release oral preparations of hyoscyamine sulfate are available in some countries; dosage is specific to a particular formulation. Hyoscyamine sulfate has also been given by injection.

### Preparations

***USP 27:*** Hyoscyamine Sulfate Elixir; Hyoscyamine Sulfate Injection; Hyoscyamine Sulfate Oral Solution; Hyoscyamine Sulfate Tablets; Hyoscyamine Tablets.

**Proprietary Preparations** (details are given in Part 3)
**Canad.:** Levsin; **Denm.:** Egazil; **Fin.:** Egazil; **Hong Kong:** Levsin; **Neth.:** Egacene†; **Norw.:** Egazil; **Swed.:** Egazil; **USA:** A-Spas; Anaspaz; Cystospaz; Cystospaz-M†; Donnamar; ED-SPAZ; Gastrosed; IB-Stat; Levbid; Levsin; Levsinex; Neosol; NuLev; Symax.

**Multi-ingredient: Austral.:** Contac†; Donnagel; Donnalix; Donnatab; **Austria:** Normensan†; **Braz.:** Analverin; Ormigrein; Tropinal; **Canad.:** Diban†; Donnatal†; **Ital.:** Antispasmina Colica; **S.Afr.:** Allertac†; Bellatard†; Donnatal; Millerspas; **Switz.:** Bronchalin†; Nardyl; Viaggio†; **Thai.:** Belloid†; Donnatal; **USA:** Accuhist LA; Antispasmodic Elixir; Arco-Lase Plus†; Atrohist Plus†; Atrosept; Barbidonna; Bellacane; Bellahist-D; Bellatal; Deconhist LA†; Dolsed; Donnatal†; Hyosophen; MHP-A; MSP-Blu; Phenahist-TR†; Phenchlor SHA†; Prosed/DS; Pyridium Plus; Ru-Tuss†; Stahist; Susano; Trac Tabs 2X; UAA; Urelief Plus; Urelle; Uretron; Uridon Modified; Urimar-T; Urimax; Urised; Uriseptic; Uritact; Uro Blue; Urogesic Blue; Utira.

## Hyoscyamus

Banotu; Beleño; Bilsenkraut; Giusquiamo; Henbane; Hyoscy.; Hyoscyami; Jusquiame; Jusquiame Noire; Meimendro.

**Pharmacopoeias.** *Chin.* specifies only the seeds.

### Profile

Hyoscyamus Leaf consists of the dried leaf, or the dried leaf and flowering, and occasionally fruit-bearing, tops of *Hyoscyamus niger.* The alkaloids consist mainly of hyoscyamine with varying amounts of hyoscine.

Hyoscyamus has peripheral and central effects similar to those of atropine (p.477); its preparations have been used mainly for the relief of visceral spasm. The fresh whole flowering plant (*Hyoscyamus niger*) has been used in herbal and homoeopathic medicine.

### Preparations

**Proprietary Preparations** (details are given in Part 3)
**Austria:** Kelosoft; **Switz.:** Kelosoft.

**Multi-ingredient: Arg.:** Hepacur; Trixol; **Belg.:** Sanicolax†; **Braz.:** Atroveran†; Atrovex†; Colinex†; Dorveran; Ductoveran; Espasmalgon; Espasmolex†; Expectolu†; Glicodin†; MM Expectorante; Sedatux; Subitan†; **Denm.:** Zink-Calmitol; **Fr.:** Asthmalgine†; Baume Dalet†; Creme Rap; Gastrosedyl†; Laccoderme a l'huile de cade; Thiosedal†; **Ger.:** Unguentum lymphaticum; **Spain:** Laxo Vian†; **Switz.:** Baby Liberol†; Gouttes contre la toux "S"; Keli-med; Kernosan Huile de Massage†; Liberol†; Sirop S contre la toux et la bronchite; **UK:** Onopordon Comp B.

## Isopropamide Iodide *(BAN, rINN)*

Ioduro de isopropamida. (3-Carbamoyl-3,3-diphenylpropyl)diisopropylmethylammonium iodide.

$C_{23}H_{33}IN_2O$ = 480.4.

*CAS — 7492-32-2 (isopropamide); 71-81-8 (isopropamide iodide).*

*ATC — A03AB09.*

**Pharmacopoeias.** In *US.*

**USP 27** (Isopropamide Iodide). A white to pale yellow crystalline powder. Soluble 1 in 50 of water, 1 in 10 of alcohol, and 1 in 5 of chloroform; very slightly soluble in ether and in benzene. Protect from light.

### Profile

Isopropamide iodide is a quaternary ammonium antimuscarinic with peripheral effects similar to those of atropine (p.477). It has been used as an adjunct in the treatment of peptic ulcer disease, in the relief of gastrointestinal and urinary-tract disorders associated with smooth muscle spasm, in rhinitis, and for the relief of symptoms of colds.

Isopropamide bromide has been used similarly.

### Preparations

***USP 27:*** Isopropamide Iodide Tablets.

**Proprietary Preparations** (details are given in Part 3)
**Belg.:** Priamide†.

**Multi-ingredient: Arg.:** Plidex; **Austria:** Vesalium†; **Belg.:** Vesalium†; **Braz.:** Descon AP†; Ornatrol; **Canad.:** Stelabid; **Fr.:** Enuretine†; **Hung.:** Bispan; Triospan; **Irl.:** Stelabid†; **Ital.:** Fluvaleas†; Raffreddoremed; Valtrax; **Mex.:** Stelabid; **Spain:** Ornade†.

## Mecloxamine Citrate *(rINNM)*

Citrato de mecloxamina. 2-[1-(4-Chlorophenyl)-1-phenylethoxy]-*N,N*-dimethyl-1-propanamine citrate.

$C_{19}H_{24}ClNO,C_6H_8O_7$ = 510.0.

*CAS — 5668-06-4 (mecloxamine); 56050-03-4 (mecloxamine citrate).*

### Profile

Mecloxamine citrate is reported to have antimuscarinic properties and has been used for its antiemetic action in antimigraine preparations.

### Preparations

**Proprietary Preparations** (details are given in Part 3)
**Multi-ingredient: Austria:** Avamigran.

## Mepenzolate Bromide *(BAN, rINN)*

Bromuro de mepenzolato; Mepenzolate Methylbromide; Mepenzolone Bromide. 3-Benziloyloxy-1,1-dimethylpiperidinium bromide.

$C_{21}H_{26}BrNO_3$ = 420.3.

*CAS — 25990-43-6 (mepenzolate); 76-90-4 (mepenzolate bromide).*

*ATC — A03AB12.*

**Pharmacopoeias.** In *Jpn.*

### Profile

Mepenzolate bromide is a quaternary ammonium antimuscarinic with peripheral actions similar to those of atropine (p.477). It has been used in the relief of gastrointestinal disorders associated with smooth muscle spasm and as an adjunct in the treatment of peptic ulcer disease. Up to 200 mg daily may be given in divided doses.

### Preparations

**Proprietary Preparations** (details are given in Part 3)
**Jpn:** Trancolon; **Swed.:** Cantil; **USA:** Cantil.

**Multi-ingredient: Jpn:** Trancolon P.

## Methanthelinium Bromide *(BAN, pINN)*

Bromuro de metantelinio; Dixamonum Bromidum; Methantheline Bromide; MTB-51; SC-2910. Diethylmethyl[2-(xanthen-9-ylcarbonyloxy)ethyl]ammonium bromide.

$C_{21}H_{26}BrNO_3$ = 420.3.

*CAS — 5818-17-7 (methanthelinium); 53-46-3 (methanthelinium bromide).*

*ATC — A03AB07.*

### Profile

Methanthelinium bromide is a quaternary ammonium antimuscarinic with peripheral effects similar to those of atropine (p.477). It has been used as an adjunct in the treatment of peptic ulcer disease, in gastrointestinal disorders associated with smooth muscle spasm, and in the management of urinary incontinence. A usual dose in gastrointestinal disorders is 50 mg by mouth three times daily.

### Preparations

**Proprietary Preparations** (details are given in Part 3)
**Ger.:** Vagantin; **USA:** Banthine†.

## Methylbenactyzium Bromide *(rINN)*

Benactyzine Methobromide; Bromuro de metilbenacticio. Diethyl(2-hydroxyethyl)methylammonium bromide benzilate.

$C_{21}H_{28}BrNO_3$ = 422.4.

*CAS — 3166-62-9.*

**Pharmacopoeias.** In *Jpn.*

### Profile

Methylbenactyzium bromide, a derivative of benactyzine (p.287), is an antimuscarinic with effects similar to those of atropine (p.477). It has been given by mouth for the treatment of gastrointestinal spasm and nocturnal enuresis.

### Preparations

**Proprietary Preparations** (details are given in Part 3)
**Multi-ingredient: Austria:** Anxiolit plus.

## Metixene Hydrochloride *(BANM, rINNM)*

Hidrocloruro de metixeno; Methixene Hydrochloride *(USAN)*; Methixene Hydrochloride Monohydrate; Metixeni Hydrochloridum; NSC-78194; SJ-1977. (*RS*)-9-(1-Methyl-3-piperidylmethyl)thioxanthene hydrochloride monohydrate.

$C_{20}H_{23}NS,HCl,H_2O$ = 363.9.

*CAS — 4969-02-2 (metixene); 1553-34-0 (anhydrous metixene hydrochloride); 7081-40-5 (metixene hydrochloride monohydrate).*

*ATC — N04AA03.*

**Pharmacopoeias.** In *Eur.* (see p.vi).

**Ph. Eur. 5.0** (Metixene Hydrochloride). A white or almost white, crystalline or fine crystalline powder. Soluble in water, in alcohol, and in dichloromethane. A 1.8% solution in water has a pH of 4.4 to 5.8. Protect from light.

**Profile**

Metixene hydrochloride is a tertiary antimuscarinic with actions similar to those of atropine (p.477); it also has antihistaminic and direct antispasmodic properties.

It is used for the symptomatic treatment of parkinsonism (p.476), including the alleviation of the extrapyramidal syndrome induced by other drugs such as phenothiazines, but, like other antimuscarinics, it is of no value against tardive dyskinesias. The usual dose by mouth of metixene hydrochloride is 2.5 mg three times daily initially, gradually increased according to the response of the patient to a total of 15 to 60 mg daily in divided doses.

Metixene hydrochloride has also been used in preparations to relieve gastrointestinal spasms.

**Preparations**

**Proprietary Preparations** (details are given in Part 3)
***Ger.:*** Metixen†; Tremarit; ***Ital.:*** Tremaril; ***Swed.:*** Tremoquil.

**Multi-ingredient:** ***Braz.:*** Dilubrin†; Espasmo Novozyme†; Flenalgin†; ***Port.:*** Espasmo Canulase; ***S.Afr.:*** Spasmo-Canulase; ***Switz.:*** Gillazyme plus†; Spasmo-Canulase.

## Metocinium Iodide *(pINN)*

(2-Hydroxyethyl)trimethylammonium iodide benzilate.
$C_{19}H_{24}INO_3$ = 441.3.
*CAS — 2424-71-7.*

**Profile**

Metocinium iodide is used as an antispasmodic.

## Octatropine Methylbromide *(BAN, rINN)*

Anisotropine Methobromide; Anisotropine Methylbromide *(USAN)*; Metilbromuro de octatropina. (1*R*,3*r*,5*S*)-8-Methyl-3-(2-propylvaleryloxy)tropanium bromide.
$C_{17}H_{32}BrNO_2$ = 362.3.
*CAS — 80-50-2.*

**Pharmacopoeias.** In *It.*

**Profile**

Octatropine methylbromide is a quaternary ammonium antimuscarinic with peripheral actions similar to those of atropine (p.477). It has been used as an adjunct in the treatment of peptic ulcer disease and to relieve visceral spasms.

**Preparations**

**Proprietary Preparations** (details are given in Part 3)
***Spain:*** Vapin†.

**Multi-ingredient:** ***Arg.:*** Espasmo Dioxadol; ***Chile:*** Bufacyl; Valpin; ***Ital.:*** Valpinax; ***Spain:*** Vapin Complex†.

# Orphenadrine Citrate *(BANM, rINNM)*

Citrato de orfenadrina; Mephenamine Citrate; Orphenadin Citrate; Orphenadrini Citras. (*RS*)-Dimethyl[2-(2-methylbenzhydryloxy)ethyl]amine dihydrogen citrate.
$C_{18}H_{23}NO,C_6H_8O_7$ = 461.5.
*CAS — 83-98-7 (orphenadrine); 4682-36-4 (orphenadrine citrate).*
*ATC — M03BC01.*

**Pharmacopoeias.** In *Eur.* (see p.vi) and *US.*

**Ph. Eur. 5.0** (Orphenadrine Citrate). A white or almost white crystalline powder. Sparingly soluble in water; slightly soluble in alcohol. Protect from light.

**USP 27** (Orphenadrine Citrate). A white, practically odourless, crystalline powder. Sparingly soluble in water; slightly soluble in alcohol; insoluble in chloroform, in ether, and in benzene. Store in airtight containers. Protect from light.

## Orphenadrine Hydrochloride *(BANM, rINNM)*

BS-5930; Hidrocloruro de orfenadrina; Mephenamine Hydrochloride; Orphenadin Hydrochloride; Orphenadrini Hydrochloridum. (*RS*)-Dimethyl[2-(2-methylbenzhydryloxy)ethyl]amine hydrochloride.
$C_{18}H_{23}NO,HCl$ = 305.8.
*CAS — 341-69-5.*
*ATC — N04AB02.*

**Pharmacopoeias.** In *Eur.* (see p.vi).

**Ph. Eur. 5.0** ( Orphenadrine Hydrochloride). A white or almost white crystalline powder. Freely soluble in water and in alcohol. Protect from light.

### Adverse Effects, Treatment, and Precautions

As for Atropine Sulfate, p.477. Orphenadrine may cause insomnia.

**Abuse.** A 23-year-old schizophrenic man, whose treatment included orphenadrine 100 mg three times daily, obtained illicit supplies and increased the dose for euphoric effect.[1] On one occasion he had an epileptic convulsion after a 600-mg dose.

See also under Trihexyphenidyl Hydrochloride, p.490.

1. Shariatmadari ME. Orphenadrine dependence. *BMJ* 1975; **3:** 486.

**Overdosage.** A report[1] of acute poisoning with orphenadrine following massive overdosage in a schizophrenic patient, who responded to intensive supportive treatment, including large doses of adrenaline, dopamine, and dobutamine to restore blood pressure following asystole. Between 1977 and 1980 twelve deaths due to orphenadrine were recorded by the UK National Poisons Unit.

1. Clarke B, *et al.* Acute poisoning with orphenadrine. *Lancet* 1985; **i:** 1386.

**Porphyria.** Orphenadrine has been associated with acute attacks of porphyria and is considered unsafe in porphyric patients.

### Interactions

As for antimuscarinics in general (see Atropine Sulfate, p.477).

**Chlorpromazine.** For the effect of orphenadrine on plasma concentrations of chlorpromazine, see under Antiparkinsonian Drugs, p.680.

**Dextropropoxyphene.** A suggested interaction between orphenadrine and dextropropoxyphene was open to question.[1,2]

1. Pearson RE, Salter FJ. Drug interaction? — orphenadrine with propoxyphene. *N Engl J Med* 1970; **282:** 1215.
2. Puckett WH, Visconti JA. Orphenadrine and propoxyphene (cont.). *N Engl J Med* 1970; **283:** 544.

### Pharmacokinetics

Orphenadrine is readily absorbed from the gastrointestinal tract and is almost completely metabolised to at least 8 metabolites. It is mainly excreted in the urine as metabolites and small amounts of unchanged drug.

**Half-life.** While the mean elimination half-life of orphenadrine in 5 healthy subjects given a single dose of the hydrochloride was found to be 15.5 hours, elimination half-lives of 30.5 and 40 hours were calculated in 2 patients who had received repeated oral administration.[1]

1. Labout JJM, *et al.* Difference between single and multiple dose pharmacokinetics of orphenadrine hydrochloride in man. *Eur J Clin Pharmacol* 1982; **21:** 343–50.

### Uses and Administration

Orphenadrine, which is a congener of diphenhydramine (p.431) without sharing its soporific effect, is a tertiary amine antimuscarinic with actions and uses similar to those of trihexyphenidyl (p.490). It also has weak antihistaminic and local anaesthetic properties.

Orphenadrine is used as the hydrochloride and the citrate; orphenadrine citrate 100 mg is approximately equivalent to 66 mg of orphenadrine hydrochloride.

Orphenadrine is used as the hydrochloride in the symptomatic treatment of **parkinsonism**, including the alleviation of the extrapyramidal syndrome induced by drugs such as phenothiazines, but, like other antimuscarinics, is of no value against tardive dyskinesias. The initial dose of orphenadrine hydrochloride is 150 mg daily in divided doses gradually increased by 50 mg every 2 or 3 days according to the response of the patient; the usual maintenance dose is in the range of 150 to 300 mg daily, but some patients may require a total of up to 400 mg daily. Orphenadrine hydrochloride has also been given intramuscularly.

Orphenadrine is also used as the citrate to relieve pain due to **skeletal muscle spasm**. It is given by mouth in a dose of 100 mg twice daily or by intramuscular or slow intravenous (over 5 minutes) injection in a dose of 60 mg which has been repeated every 12 hours.

Since the elderly are more susceptible to the adverse effects of antimuscarinics a dose at the lower end of the range is usually recommended.

**Hiccup.** Orphenadrine citrate has been used in some countries for the treatment of intractable hiccup. A protocol for the management of intractable hiccups may be found under Chlorpromazine, p.682.

**Muscle spasm.** References to the use of orphenadrine in the management of leg cramps and other painful conditions associated with skeletal muscle spasm.

1. Latta D, Turner E. An alternative to quinine in nocturnal leg cramps. *Curr Ther Res* 1989; **45:** 833–7.
2. Hunskaar S, Donnell D. Clinical and pharmacological review of the efficacy of orphenadrine and its combination with paracetamol in painful conditions. *J Int Med Res* 1991; **19:** 71–87.

### Preparations

***BP 2003:*** Orphenadrine Hydrochloride Tablets;
***USP 27:*** Orphenadrine Citrate Injection.

**Proprietary Preparations** (details are given in Part 3)
***Austral.:*** Norflex; ***Belg.:*** Disipal; Norflex†; ***Canad.:*** Disipal; Norflex; Orfenace†; ***Chile:*** Plenactol; ***Denm.:*** Disipal; Lysantin; Norflex; ***Fin.:*** Norflex; ***Ger.:*** Norflex; ***Gr.:*** Disipal; Norflex; ***India:*** Orphipal; ***Irl.:*** Disipal†; ***Israel:*** Flexin; ***Ital.:*** Disipal; ***Malaysia:*** Norflex; ***Mex.:*** Norflex; ***Norw.:*** Disipal; ***NZ:*** Disipal; Norflex; ***Port.:*** Norflex; ***S.Afr.:*** Disipal; Norflex; ***Singapore:*** Norflex†; ***Swed.:*** Disipal; Norflex; ***Switz.:*** Norflex†; ***Thai.:*** Norflex; Orfenal; ***UK:*** Biorphen; Disipal; ***USA:*** Banflex; Flexoject†; Flexon; Norflex.

**Multi-ingredient:** ***Arg.:*** Belmalen; Doloctaprin Plus; Flogodisten; Metaflex Plus; Mio Aldoron; Mio-Virobron; ***Austral.:*** Norgesic; ***Austria:*** Neodolpasse; Norgesic; ***Braz.:*** Algiflex†; Anapirol†; Banidor†; Dalgex; Dorflex; Doricin; Dorzone; Flexdor; Itaiflex†; Miorrelax; Nevralgex; Reciluго†; Relaflex†; Rielex; Sedalex; Theopirina; ***Canad.:*** Norgesic; ***Chile:*** Norgesic; ***Fin.:*** Dolan; Norgesic; ***Ger.:*** Norgesic N; ***Hong Kong:*** Norgesic; ***Irl.:*** Norgesic; ***Israel:*** Muscol; Norgesic; ***Malaysia:*** Anarex; Norgesic; ***Mex.:*** Norflex Plus; ***NZ:*** Norgesic†; ***Port.:*** Norgesic; ***S.Afr.:*** Besemax; Besenol; Norflex Co; ***Singapore:*** Anarex; Norgesic; Norphen; Orphenadol; ***Swed.:*** Norgesic; ***Switz.:*** Norgesic†; ***Thai.:*** Corilax; Dorpane; Med-Myolax; Medgesic; Muscol; Myodrine; Myoflex; Myopar†; Myosic; Neosec; Norgesic; Norgic; Norphen; Nurasic; Orflex; Orpar; Orphengesic; Poli-Relaxane; Polydol; Relar; Rena; ***UAE:*** Muscadol; ***USA:*** Norgesic; Orphengesic.

# Oxybutynin Hydrochloride

*(BANM, rINNM)*

5058; Hidrocloruro de oxibutinina; MJ-4309-1; Oxybutynin Chloride *(USAN)*; Oxybutynini Hydrochloridum. 4-Diethylaminobut-2-ynyl α-cyclohexylmandelate hydrochloride; 4-(Diethylamino)but-2-ynyl (*RS*)-2-cyclohexyl-2-hydroxy-2-phenylacetate hydrochloride.
$C_{22}H_{31}NO_3,HCl$ = 393.9.
*CAS — 5633-20-5 (oxybutynin); 1508-65-2 (oxybutynin hydrochloride).*
*ATC — G04BD04.*

**Pharmacopoeias.** In *Eur.* (see p.vi) and *US.*

**Ph. Eur. 5.0** (Oxybutynin Hydrochloride). A white or almost white, crystalline powder. Freely soluble in water and in alcohol; soluble in acetone; slightly soluble in cyclohexane. Protect from light.

**USP 27** (Oxybutynin Chloride). A white, practically odourless, crystalline powder. Freely soluble in water and in alcohol; soluble in acetone; very soluble in chloroform and in methyl alcohol; slightly soluble in ether; very slightly soluble in hexane.

### Adverse Effects, Treatment, and Precautions

As for Atropine Sulfate, p.477.

*Animal* studies have shown reproductive toxicity with high doses of oxybutynin, hence the recommendation that it should be avoided during pregnancy; caution should also be observed during breast feeding.

**Effects on body temperature.** A 76-year-old man taking oxybutynin hydrochloride 5 mg three times daily suffered heatstroke on a day when the ambient temperature was about 37°. He had had a similar febrile episode the previous summer while taking oxybutynin.[1]

1. Adubofour KO, *et al.* Oxybutynin-induced heatstroke in an elderly patient. *Ann Pharmacother* 1996; **30:** 144–7.

**Effects on the gastrointestinal tract.** Reflux oesophagitis has been reported[1] in a 36-year-old woman with cerebral palsy and hiatus hernia who had taken oxybutynin for 5 years to prevent urinary incontinence. Symptoms of gastro-oesophageal reflux resolved when oxybutynin was discontinued.

1. Lee M, Sharifi R. Oxybutynin-induced reflux esophagitis. *DICP Ann Pharmacother* 1990; **24:** 583–5.

**Effects on mental function.** Oxybutynin was associated with the development of acute confusional states in 4 patients with Parkinson's disease and some cognitive impairment.[1]

1. Donnellan CA, *et al.* Oxybutynin and cognitive dysfunction. *BMJ* 1997; **315:** 1363–4.

**Night terrors.** Night terrors have been reported in 5 patients taking oxybutynin.[1] Four of the patients were young children and the fifth was an elderly woman. Rechallenge was positive in 2 cases.

1. Valsecia ME, *et al.* New adverse effect of oxybutynin: "night terror". *Ann Pharmacother* 1998; **32:** 506.

**Overdosage.** A report[1] of a 34-year-old woman who ingested 100 mg of oxybutynin. The main symptoms were antimuscarinic effects and included drowsiness, hallucinations, dilatation of pupils, and urinary retention. Tachycardia resolved shortly after admission to hospital but ventricular ectopic beats and bigeminy persisted for over 24 hours. The patient recovered with symptomatic treatment.

1. Banerjee S, *et al.* Poisoning with oxybutynin. *Hum Exp Toxicol* 1991; **10:** 225–6.

**Porphyria.** Oxybutynin hydrochloride is considered to be unsafe in patients with porphyria because it has been shown to be porphyrinogenic in *animals* or *in-vitro* systems.

### Interactions

As for antimuscarinics in general (see Atropine Sulfate, p.477).

**Itraconazole.** Concomitant use of itraconazole and oxybutynin resulted in moderate increases of serum concentrations of the latter.[1] However, concentrations of the active metabolite of oxybutynin, *N*-desethyloxybutynin, were virtually unchanged and the interaction was considered to be of minor clinical significance.

1. Lukkari E, *et al.* Itraconazole moderately increases serum concentrations of oxybutynin but does not affect those of the active metabolite. *Eur J Clin Pharmacol* 1997; **52:** 403–6.

### Pharmacokinetics

Following oral administration of oxybutynin, peak plasma concentrations are reached within one hour. Oxybutynin is also absorbed following application to the skin. It undergoes extensive first-pass metabolism and systemic bioavailability has been reported to be only 6%. A half-life of 2 to 3 hours has been reported. *N*-desethyloxybutynin is an active metabolite. Oxybutynin has been detected in breast milk. Evidence suggests that it may cross the blood-brain barrier.

◊ References.

1. Douchamps J, *et al.* The pharmacokinetics of oxybutynin in man. *Eur J Clin Pharmacol* 1988; **35:** 515–20.
2. Pietzko A, *et al.* Influences of trospium chloride and oxybutynin on quantitative EEG in healthy volunteers. *Eur J Clin Pharmacol* 1994; **47:** 337–43.
3. Gupta SK, Sathyan G. Pharmacokinetics of an oral once-a-day controlled-release oxybutynin formulation compared with immediate-release oxybutynin. *J Clin Pharmacol* 1999; **39:** 289–96.
4. Appell RA, *et al.* Pharmacokinetics, metabolism, and saliva output during transdermal and extended-release oral oxybutynin administration in healthy subjects. *Mayo Clin Proc* 2003; **78:** 696–702.

### Uses and Administration

Oxybutynin hydrochloride is a tertiary amine antimuscarinic with actions similar to those of atropine (p.477); it also has direct effects on smooth muscle. It is used for the management of urinary frequency, urgency, and incontinence in neurogenic bladder disorders and in idiopathic detrusor instability and for nocturnal enuresis, as an adjunct to nonpharmacological therapy.

Usual doses of oxybutynin hydrochloride are 5 mg two or three times daily by mouth, increased to 5 mg four times daily if required. In elderly patients lower doses of 2.5 or 3 mg twice daily initially, increased to 5 mg twice daily if necessary, may be adequate. Modified-release preparations of oxybutynin hydrochloride are also available. The initial dose is 5 mg once daily, increased by 5 mg at weekly intervals if necessary, up to a maximum of 30 mg daily. Oxybutynin is also given via a transdermal delivery system that supplies 3.9 mg of oxybutynin daily. The patch should be applied to intact skin on the abdomen, hip, or buttocks and replaced every 3 to 4 days; re-application to the same site should be avoided for 7 days.

In children over 5 years, oxybutynin is used for neurogenic bladder disorders and nocturnal enuresis in an initial dose of 2.5 or 3 mg twice daily by mouth increased to 5 mg two or three times daily according to response. For nocturnal enuresis the last dose is usually given before bedtime. However, the *British National Formulary* considers that drug therapy for nocturnal enuresis is not appropriate in children under 7 years of age.

◊ Reviews.

1. Robinson TG, Castelden CM. Oxybutynin hydrochloride. *Prescribers' J* 1994; **34:** 27–30.

**Nocturnal enuresis.** Antimuscarinics such as oxybutynin reduce uninhibited bladder contractions but, although they may be of use in diurnal enuresis, they are rarely of benefit in nocturnal enuresis (p.475) alone. Oxybutynin did not appear to be effective in treating primary nocturnal enuresis in children with normal bladders.[1]

1. Lovering JS, *et al.* Oxybutynin efficacy in the treatment of primary enuresis. *Pediatrics* 1988; **82:** 104–6.

**Urinary incontinence.** In addition to its antimuscarinic effect, oxybutynin has a direct antispasmodic effect which also contributes to reducing the number of uninhibited bladder contractions in urge incontinence (see p.476). It is effective when given by mouth[1-4] or via a transdermal delivery system;[5-7] some consider oral oxybutynin to be the drug of choice.[8] However, frequent adverse effects particularly following oral administration may limit its use. Direct instillation of oxybutynin into the bladder has also been tried.[9,10]

Oxybutynin has also been studied in detrusor hyperreflexia[11] but, as most of these studies do not distinguish in their analyses between patients with neurogenic and non-neurogenic incontinence, its value remains to be determined. There is some evidence that doses up to 30 mg are well tolerated and effective in patients with neurogenic bladder.[12]

1. Riva D, Casolati E. Oxybutynin chloride in the treatment of female idiopathic bladder instability: results from double blind treatment. *Clin Exp Obstet Gynecol* 1984; **11:** 37–42.
2. Moore KH, *et al.* Oxybutynin hydrochloride (3 mg) in the treatment of women with idiopathic detrusor instability. *Br J Urol* 1990; **66:** 479–85.
3. Tapp AJS, *et al.* The treatment of detrusor instability in post-menopausal women with oxybutynin chloride: a double blind placebo controlled study. *Br J Obstet Gynaecol* 1990; **97:** 521–6.
4. Siddiqui MA, *et al.* Oxybutynin extended-release: a review of its use in the management of overactive bladder. *Drugs* 2004; **64:** 885–912.
5. Davila GW, *et al.* A short-term, multicenter, randomized double-blind dose titration study of the efficacy and anticholinergic side effects of transdermal compared to immediate release oral oxybutynin treatment of patients with urge urinary incontinence. *J Urol (Baltimore)* 2001; **166:** 140–5.
6. Dmochowski RR, *et al.* Efficacy and safety of transdermal oxybutynin in patients with urge and mixed urinary incontinence. *J Urol (Baltimore)* 2002; **168:** 580–6.
7. Dmochowski RR, *et al.* Comparative efficacy and safety of transdermal oxybutynin and oral tolterodine versus placebo in previously treated patients with urge and mixed urinary incontinence. *Urology* 2003; **62:** 237–42.
8. Yarker YE, *et al.* Oxybutynin: a review of its pharmacodynamic and pharmacokinetic properties, and its therapeutic use in detrusor instability. *Drugs Aging* 1995; **6:** 243–62.
9. Weese DL, *et al.* Intravesical oxybutynin chloride: experience with 42 patients. *Urology* 1993; **41:** 527–30.
10. Szollar SM, Lee SM. Intravesical oxybutynin for spinal cord injury patients. *Spinal Cord* 1996; **34:** 284–7.
11. Thüroff J, *et al.* Randomized, double-blind, multicenter trial on treatment of frequency, urgency and incontinence related to detrusor hyperactivity: oxybutynin versus propantheline versus placebo. *J Urol (Baltimore)* 1991; **145:** 813–17.
12. Bennett N, *et al.* Can higher doses of oxybutynin improve efficacy in neurogenic bladder? *J Urol (Baltimore)* 2004; **171:** 749–51.

### Preparations

***BP 2003:*** Oxybutynin Tablets;
***USP 27:*** Oxybutynin Chloride Syrup; Oxybutynin Chloride Tablets.

**Proprietary Preparations** (details are given in Part 3)
***Arg.:*** Delak; Ditropan; Oxitina; Oxyurin; Retebem; Urequin; ***Austral.:*** Ditropan; ***Austria:*** Cystrin; Detrusan; Ditropan; Oxybase; Oxybubene; ***Belg.:*** Ditropan; Driptane; ***Braz.:*** Frenurin; Incontinol; Retemic; ***Canad.:*** Ditropan; Nu-Oxybutyn; Oxybutyn; ***Chile:*** Odranal; Urazol; Uricont; ***Fin.:*** Cystrin; Ditropan; Oksibutin; Spasmoxyl; ***Fr.:*** Ditropan; Driptane; Zatur; ***Ger.:*** Cystonorm; Dridase; Oxyb; Oxybase; Oxybugamma; Oxybutin; Oxybuton; Oxymedin; Ryol; Spasyt; ***Gr.:*** Ditropan; ***Hong Kong:*** Ditropan; ***India:*** Oxyspas; ***Irl.:*** Cystrin; Ditropan; Renamel; ***Israel:*** Novitropan; Uricont; ***Ital.:*** Ditropan; ***Malaysia:*** Ditropan; ***Mex.:*** Nefryl; Tavor; ***Neth.:*** Dridase; ***NZ:*** Ditropan†; ***Port.:*** Ditropan; ***S.Afr.:*** Ditropan; Lenditro; Oxyspas; ***Singapore:*** Ditropan; ***Spain:*** Ditropan; Dresplan; ***Swed.:*** Ditropan; Oxybase; ***Switz.:*** Ditropan; ***Thai.:*** Diutropan; ***UK:*** Cystrin; Ditropan; Lyrinel XL; Promictuline†; ***USA:*** Ditropan; Oxytrol.

## Oxyphencyclimine Hydrochloride *(BANM, rINNM)*

Hidrocloruro de oxifenciclimina. 1,4,5,6-Tetrahydro-1-methylpyrimidin-2-ylmethyl α-cyclohexylmandelate hydrochloride.

$C_{20}H_{28}N_2O_3,HCl = 380.9.$

*CAS — 125-53-1 (oxyphencyclimine); 125-52-0 (oxyphencyclimine hydrochloride).*

*ATC — A03AA01.*

### Profile

Oxyphencyclimine hydrochloride is a tertiary amine antimuscarinic with effects similar to those of atropine (p.477). It has been used as an adjunct in the treatment of peptic ulcer disease and for the relief of smooth muscle spasms in gastrointestinal disorders.

### Preparations

**Proprietary Preparations** (details are given in Part 3)
***Hong Kong:*** Daricon; ***Thai.:*** Daricon; Med-Spastic; Oxyno; Proclimine.
**Multi-ingredient: *Hong Kong:*** Rudd-U.

## Oxyphenonium Bromide *(BAN, rINN)*

Bromuro de oxifenonio; Oxphenonii Bromidum; Oxyphenonium Bromatum. 2-(α-Cyclohexylmandeloyloxy)ethyldiethylmethylammonium bromide.

$C_{21}H_{34}BrNO_3 = 428.4.$

*CAS — 14214-84-7 (oxyphenonium); 50-10-2 (oxyphenonium bromide).*

*ATC — A03AB03.*

**Pharmacopoeias.** In *Pol.*

### Profile

Oxyphenonium bromide is a quaternary ammonium antimuscarinic with peripheral effects similar to those of atropine (p.477). It has been given by mouth to relieve visceral spasms.

### Preparations

**Proprietary Preparations** (details are given in Part 3)
***India:*** Antrenyl; ***S.Afr.:*** Spastrex.

## Parapenzolate Bromide *(USAN, rINN)*

Sch-3444. 4-Benziloyloxy-1,1-dimethylpiperidinium bromide.

$C_{21}H_{26}BrNO_3 = 420.3.$

*CAS — 5634-41-3.*

### Profile

Parapenzolate bromide is a quaternary ammonium antimuscarinic that has been used for the relief of visceral spasms.

### Preparations

**Proprietary Preparations** (details are given in Part 3)
**Multi-ingredient: *Chile:*** Tranvagal.

## Pargeverine Hydrochloride *(rINNM)*

Propinox Hydrochloride. 2-(Dimethylamino)ethyldiphenyl(2-propynyloxy)acetate hydrochloride.

$C_{21}H_{23}NO_3,HCl = 373.9.$

*CAS — 13479-13-5 (pargeverine); 2765-97-1 (pargeverine hydrochloride).*

### Profile

Pargeverine is reported to possess antimuscarinic and smooth-muscle relaxant properties and has been used in the treatment of gastrointestinal and smooth muscle spasm.

### Preparations

**Proprietary Preparations** (details are given in Part 3)
***Arg.:*** Nova Paratopina; Pasmosedan; Sertal; ***Braz.:*** Bipasmin†; Espasmo-Ped†; ***Chile:*** Bramedil; Pasmocalm; Viadil; ***Mex.:*** Bipasmin; Plidan; ***Port.:*** Vagopax.
**Multi-ingredient: *Arg.:*** Apasmo Compuesto; Binvex; Espasmo Dolex; Nova Paratropina Compositum; Pasmosedan Compuesto; Sertal Compuesto; ***Braz.:*** Bipasmin Composto†; ***Chile:*** Bramedil Compuesto; Scopanil; Viadil Compuesto; ***Mex.:*** Bipasmin Compuesto; Firac Plus; Plidan Compuesto.

## Phenamazide Hydrochloride

Fenamazida, hidrocloruro de; Phenamacide Hydrochloride. (±)-α-Aminobenzeneacetic acid 3-methylbutyl ester hydrochloride.

$C_{13}H_{19}NO_2,HCl = 257.8.$

*CAS — 84580-27-8 (phenamazide); 31031-74-0 (phenamazide hydrochloride).*

### Profile

Phenamazide is an antimuscarinic with actions similar to those of atropine (p.477). It has been used as the hydrochloride in the treatment of visceral spasms.

### Preparations

**Proprietary Preparations** (details are given in Part 3)
***Ger.:*** Aklonin†.

## Pipenzolate Bromide *(BAN, rINN)*

Bromuro de pipenzolato; Pipenzolate Methylbromide. 3-Benziloyloxy-1-ethyl-1-methylpiperidinium bromide.

$C_{22}H_{28}BrNO_3 = 434.4.$

*CAS — 13473-38-6 (pipenzolate); 125-51-9 (pipenzolate bromide).*

*ATC — A03AB14.*

### Profile

Pipenzolate bromide is a quaternary ammonium antimuscarinic with peripheral actions similar to those of atropine (p.477). It has been used as an adjunct in the treatment of gastrointestinal disorders characterised by smooth muscle spasm.

### Preparations

**Proprietary Preparations** (details are given in Part 3)
***Ger.:*** Ila-med m; ***Mex.:*** Expal; Poliptal†; Propedil†.
**Multi-ingredient: *Chile:*** Baldmin; Gasorbol; Sinpasmon; ***Mex.:*** Espasal; Finprob; ***S.Afr.:*** Pedrachol†.

## Piperidolate Hydrochloride *(BANM, rINNM)*

Hidrocloruro de piperidolato. 1-Ethyl-3-piperidyl diphenylacetate hydrochloride.

$C_{21}H_{25}NO_2,HCl = 359.9.$

*CAS — 82-98-4 (piperidolate); 129-77-1 (piperidolate hydrochloride).*

*ATC — A03AA30.*

### Profile

Piperidolate hydrochloride is a tertiary amine antimuscarinic with effects similar to those of atropine (p.477). It has been given in the symptomatic treatment of smooth muscle spasm associated with gastrointestinal disorders.

### Preparations

**Proprietary Preparations** (details are given in Part 3)
***Mex.:*** Dactil OB.
**Multi-ingredient: *Braz.:*** Dactil OB.

## Pipethanate Ethobromide *(rINNM)*

Ethylpipethanate Bromide; Etobromuro de pipetanato; Piperilate Ethobromide. 1-(2-Benziloyloxyethyl)-1-ethylpiperidinium bromide.

$C_{23}H_{30}BrNO_3 = 448.4.$

*CAS — 4546-39-8 (pipethanate); 23182-46-9 (pipethanate ethobromide).*

### Profile

Pipethanate ethobromide is an antimuscarinic with actions similar to those of atropine (p.477). It has been used in the symptomatic treatment of visceral spasms in doses by mouth of up to

160 mg daily in divided doses. Pipethanate ethobromide has also been given intramuscularly or intravenously in doses of 10 to 20 mg daily and rectally in doses of 60 or 120 mg daily.

### Preparations

**Proprietary Preparations** (details are given in Part 3)
***Chile:*** Nospasmin; ***Ital.:*** Panpurol†; Spalgin†; Spasmodene†; Spasmodil; ***Jpn:*** Panpurol; ***Thai.:*** Panpurol†.

**Multi-ingredient:** ***Chile:*** Nospasmin Compuesto.

## Pirenzepine Hydrochloride *(BANM, USAN, rINNM)*

Hidrocloruro de pirenzepina; LS-519 (pirenzepine); LS-519-Cl2; Pirenzepini Dihydrochloridum Monohydricum. 5,11-Dihydro-11-(4-methylpiperazin-1-ylacetyl)pyrido[2,3-*b*][1,4]benzodiazepin-6-one dihydrochloride monohydrate.

$C_{19}H_{21}N_5O_2,2HCl,H_2O$ = 442.3.

*CAS — 28797-61-7 (pirenzepine); 29868-97-1 (pirenzepine hydrochloride).*

*ATC — A02BX03.*

**Pharmacopoeias.** In *Eur.* (see p.vi).

**Ph. Eur. 5.0** (Pirenzepine Dihydrochloride Monohydrate; Pirenzepine Hydrochloride BP 2003). A white or yellowish crystalline powder. Freely soluble in water; very slightly soluble in dehydrated alcohol; practically insoluble in dichloromethane; slightly soluble in methyl alcohol. A 10% solution in water has a pH of 1.0 to 2.0. Protect from light.

### Adverse Effects and Precautions

Dry mouth and blurred vision have been reported but the risk of antimuscarinic effects (see Atropine Sulfate, p.477) may be reduced. Pirenzepine should be used with caution in patients with renal impairment, particularly those with end-stage renal failure.

**Effects on the blood.** Thrombocytopenia in one patient and agranulocytosis in another was probably associated with the administration of pirenzepine.[1]

1. Stricker BHC, *et al.* Blood disorders associated with pirenzepine. *BMJ* 1986; **293:** 1074.

### Interactions

As for antimuscarinics in general (see Atropine Sulfate, p.477).

### Pharmacokinetics

Pirenzepine is absorbed from the gastrointestinal tract but the bioavailability is reported to be only about 20 to 30% being decreased to about 10 to 20% when taken with food. Very little pirenzepine is metabolised. About 10% of an oral dose is excreted unchanged in the urine, the remainder being excreted in the faeces.

Pirenzepine has an elimination half-life of about 12 hours and is about 12% bound to plasma proteins. Diffusion across the blood-brain barrier is poor and only minimal amounts are stated to be present in breast milk.

◊ References.

1. Tanswell P, *et al.* Absolute bioavailability of pirenzepine in intensive care patients. *Eur J Clin Pharmacol* 1990; **38:** 265–8.

**Renal impairment.** The renal clearance and total plasma clearance of pirenzepine may be significantly reduced in patients with renal impairment,[1,2] with clearance decreasing proportionately with renal impairment. The half-life of pirenzepine is increased with reported values ranging from 14 to 20 hours.[1-3] Plasma concentrations of pirenzepine may be reduced by up to about 50% during haemodialysis.[2,3]

1. Krakamp B, *et al.* Steady-state intravenous pharmacokinetics of pirenzepine in patients with hepatic insufficiency and combined renal- and hepatic insufficiency. *Eur J Clin Pharmacol* 1989; **36:** 71–3.
2. Krakamp B, *et al.* Steady-state intravenous pharmacokinetics of pirenzepine in patients with differing degrees of renal dysfunction. *Eur J Clin Pharmacol* 1989; **36:** 75–8.
3. MacGregor T, *et al.* Oral pharmacokinetics of pirenzepine in patients with chronic renal insufficiency, failure, and maintenance haemodialysis. *Eur J Clin Pharmacol* 1990; **38:** 405–6.

### Uses and Administration

Pirenzepine is a selective $M_1$ tertiary amine antimuscarinic that displays a preferential action on the gastric mucosa thus causing a reduction in the secretion of gastric acid; it also reduces the secretion of pepsin. At therapeutic doses it has few other antimuscarinic actions.

Pirenzepine hydrochloride has been used in the management of peptic ulcer disease (p.475) in a usual dose of 50 mg two or three times daily by mouth for 4 to 6 weeks. It has also been given by slow intravenous injection in doses of up to 60 mg daily.

### Preparations

**Proprietary Preparations** (details are given in Part 3)
***Arg.:*** Droxol; ***Austria:*** Gastrozepin; ***Ger.:*** durapirenz†; Gastri-P†; Gastricur; Gastrozepin; Pirehexal†; Ulcoprotect; Ulcosafe†; Ulgescum†; ***Gr.:*** Gastrozepin; ***Israel:*** Ulcepin†; ***Ital.:*** Duogastral†; Frazim; Gastrol†; Gastropiren; Gastrosed†; Gastrozepin†; Ulcin†; Ulcopir†; ***Mex.:*** Gastropin†; ***Port.:*** Gastrozepina; ***Switz.:*** Gastrozepine†; piren-basan; ***Thai.:*** Cevanil.

**Multi-ingredient:** ***Arg.:*** Duo Vizerul.

## Platyphylline Acid Tartrate

Platyphylline Bitartrate; Platyphyllini Hydrotartras. 1,2-Dihydro-12-hydroxysenecionan-11,16-dione hydrogen tartrate.

$C_{18}H_{27}NO_5,C_4H_6O_6$ = 487.5.

*CAS — 480-78-4 (platyphylline); 1257-59-6 (platyphylline acid tartrate).*

### Profile

Platyphylline acid tartrate is a pyrrolizidine alkaloid occurring in *Senecio platyphyllus* and other *Senecio* spp. It has antimuscarinic actions and has been given with papaverine in antispasmodic preparations.

## Poldine Metilsulfate *(BAN, pINN)*

IS-499; McN-R-726-47; Metilsulfato de poldina; Poldine Methosulphate; Poldine Methylsulfate *(USAN)*; Poldine Methylsulphate. (*RS*)-2-Benziloyloxymethyl-1,1-dimethylpyrrolidinium methylsulphate.

$C_{21}H_{26}NO_3,CH_3O_4S$ = 451.5.

*CAS — 596-50-9 (poldine); 545-80-2 (poldine metilsulfate).*

*ATC — A03AB11.*

**Pharmacopoeias.** In *Br.*

**BP 2003** (Poldine Metilsulfate). A white odourless or almost odourless crystalline powder. Freely soluble in water; soluble in alcohol; slightly soluble in chloroform. A 1% solution in water has a pH of 5.0 to 7.0.

### Profile

Poldine metilsulfate is a quaternary ammonium antimuscarinic with peripheral actions similar to those of atropine (p.477) and has been used in the management of gastrointestinal disorders, including peptic ulcer disease.

### Preparations

***BP 2003:*** Poldine Tablets.

## Prifinium Bromide *(rINN)*

Bromuro de prifinio; PDB; Pyrodifenium Bromide. 3-Diphenylmethylene-1,1-diethyl-2-methylpyrrolidinium bromide.

$C_{22}H_{28}BrN$ = 386.4.

*CAS — 10236-81-4 (prifinium); 4630-95-9 (prifinium bromide).*

*ATC — A03AB18.*

### Profile

Prifinium bromide is a quaternary ammonium antimuscarinic with peripheral effects similar to those of atropine (p.477). It is structurally related to diphemanil metilsulfate (p.481).

Prifinium bromide is used to relieve visceral spasms. Oral doses usually range from 45 to 120 mg daily in divided doses; higher doses have sometimes been employed. It has also been given rectally in a dose of 60 mg three or four times daily, or by subcutaneous, intramuscular, or intravenous injection in a dose of 7.5 to 15 mg.

### Preparations

**Proprietary Preparations** (details are given in Part 3)
***Fr.:*** Riabal; ***Ital.:*** Riabal; ***Jpn:*** Padrin; ***Mex.:*** Anespas; ***Thai.:*** Riabal.

# Procyclidine Hydrochloride

*(BANM, rINNM)*

Hidrocloruro de prociclidina; Procyclidini Hydrochloridum. 1-Cyclohexyl-1-phenyl-3-(pyrrolidin-1-yl)propan-1-ol hydrochloride.

$C_{19}H_{29}NO,HCl$ = 323.9.

*CAS — 77-37-2 (procyclidine); 1508-76-5 (procyclidine hydrochloride).*

*ATC — N04AA04.*

**Pharmacopoeias.** In *Br.* and *US.*

**BP 2003** (Procyclidine Hydrochloride). A white, odourless or almost odourless, crystalline powder. Sparingly soluble in water; soluble in alcohol; practically insoluble in acetone and in ether. A 1% solution in water has a pH of 4.5 to 6.5.

**USP 27** (Procyclidine Hydrochloride). A white crystalline powder, having a moderate characteristic odour. Soluble 1 in 35 of water, 1 in 9 of alcohol, 1 in 6 of chloroform, and 1 in 11 000 of ether; insoluble in acetone. pH of a 1% solution in water is between 5.0 and 6.5. Store in a dry place in airtight containers. Protect from light.

## Adverse Effects, Treatment, and Precautions

As for Atropine Sulfate, p.477.

**Abuse.** Like other antimuscarinics (see also under Trihexyphenidyl Hydrochloride, p.490) procyclidine has been abused for its euphoriant effects.[1,2]

1. McGucken RB, *et al.* Teenage procyclidine abuse. *Lancet* 1985; **i:** 1514.
2. Dooris B, Reid C. Feigning dystonia to feed an unusual drug addiction. *J Accid Emerg Med* 2000; **17:** 311.

### Interactions

As for antimuscarinics in general (see Atropine Sulfate, p.477).

### Pharmacokinetics

Procyclidine hydrochloride is absorbed from the gastrointestinal tract and disappears rapidly from the tissues. Procyclidine given intravenously acts within 5 to 20 minutes and has a duration of effect of up to 4 hours.

◊ References.

1. Whiteman PD, *et al.* Pharmacokinetics and pharmacodynamics of procyclidine in man. *Eur J Clin Pharmacol* 1985; **28:** 73–8.

### Uses and Administration

Procyclidine hydrochloride is a tertiary amine antimuscarinic with actions and uses similar to those of trihexyphenidyl (p.490). It is used for the symptomatic treatment of parkinsonism (p.476), including the alleviation of the extrapyramidal syndrome induced by drugs such as phenothiazines, but, like other antimuscarinics, is of no value against tardive dyskinesias.

The initial dose of 2.5 mg three times daily by mouth may be increased gradually by 2.5 to 5 mg every 2 or 3 days (or daily if used for drug-induced extrapyramidal syndrome) until the optimum maintenance dose, usually 10 to 30 mg daily in 3 (or occasionally 4) divided doses, is reached; daily doses of up to 60 mg have occasionally been required. In emergency, 5 to 10 mg may be given by intravenous injection; higher doses have sometimes been used. The intramuscular route has also been employed: 5 to 10 mg may be given as a single injection, repeated if necessary after 20 minutes to a maximum of 20 mg daily. Parenteral doses are usually effective within 5 to 10 minutes but may need 30 minutes to produce relief.

### Preparations

***BP 2003:*** Procyclidine Injection; Procyclidine Tablets;
***USP 27:*** Procyclidine Hydrochloride Tablets.

**Proprietary Preparations** (details are given in Part 3)
***Austral.:*** Kemadrin†; ***Austria:*** Kemadrin; ***Belg.:*** Kemadrin; ***Canad.:*** Kemadrin; Procyclid; ***Denm.:*** Kemadrin; ***Ger.:*** Osnervan; ***India:*** Kemadrin; ***Irl.:*** Kemadrin; ***Israel:*** Kemadrin; ***Ital.:*** Kemadrin; ***Malaysia:*** Kemadrin; ***Neth.:*** Kemadrin†; ***NZ:*** Kemadrin; ***Spain:*** Kemadren; ***Swed.:*** Kemadrin†; ***Switz.:*** Kemadrin; ***UK:*** Arpicolin; Kemadrin; Muscinil; ***USA:*** Kemadrin.

## Profenamine Hydrochloride *(BANM, rINNM)*

Cloridrato de Profenamina; Ethopropazine Hydrochloride; Hidrocloruro de profenamina; Isothazine Hydrochloride; Profenamini Hydrochloridum; Prophenamini Chloridum. 10-(2-Diethylaminopropyl)phenothiazine hydrochloride.

$C_{19}H_{24}N_2S,HCl$ = 348.9.

*CAS — 522-00-9 (profenamine); 1094-08-2 (profenamine hydrochloride).*

*ATC — N04AA05.*

### Adverse Effects, Treatment, and Precautions

As for Atropine Sulfate, p.477.

Drowsiness and confusion are common in patients taking profenamine; patients so affected should not drive or operate machinery. Profenamine may also cause muscle cramps, paraesthesia, and a sense of heaviness in the limbs, epigastric discomfort, and nausea.

Profenamine is a phenothiazine derivative—for adverse effects associated with phenothiazines, see Chlorpromazine, p.675.

**Breast feeding.** Profenamine is distributed into the milk of lactating mothers.[1]

1. Rowan JJ. Excretion of drugs in milk. *Pharm J* 1976; **217:** 184–7.

### Interactions

As for antimuscarinics in general (see Atropine Sulfate, p.477).

### Uses and Administration

Profenamine hydrochloride is a phenothiazine derivative with antimuscarinic, adrenergic-blocking, antihistaminic, local anaesthetic and ganglion-blocking properties. It has been used in the symptomatic treatment of parkinsonism (p.476), including the alleviation of the extrapyramidal syndrome induced by drugs such as other phenothiazine compounds, but, like other compounds with antimuscarinic properties, is of no value against tardive dyskinesias. It has been used in a usual dose of 50 mg three times daily by mouth initially, gradually increased to up to 500 mg or more daily in divided doses, according to the response of the patient.

### Preparations

**Proprietary Preparations** (details are given in Part 3)
***Canad.:*** Parsitan.

## Propantheline Bromide *(BAN, rINN)*

Bromuro de propantelina; Propanthelini Bromidum. Di-isopropylmethyl[2-(xanthen-9-ylcarbonyloxy)ethyl]ammonium bromide.

$C_{23}H_{30}BrNO_3$ = 448.4.

*CAS — 298-50-0 (propantheline); 50-34-0 (propantheline bromide).*

*ATC — A03AB05.*

**Pharmacopoeias.** In *Chin., Eur.* (see p.vi), *Jpn*, and *US.*

**Ph. Eur. 5.0** (Propantheline Bromide). A white or yellowish-white, slightly hygroscopic powder. Very soluble in water, in alcohol, and in dichloromethane. Store in airtight containers.

**USP 27** (Propantheline Bromide). White or practically white, odourless, crystals. Very soluble in water, in alcohol, and in chloroform; practically insoluble in ether and in benzene.

### Adverse Effects, Treatment, and Precautions

As for Atropine Sulfate, p.477. Contact dermatitis has been reported following topical application of propantheline bromide.

**Buccal and oesophageal ulceration.** Severe buccal mucosal ulceration has been reported[1] in a 95-year-old woman as a result of retaining emepronium bromide tablets in her mouth, and recurred on administration of propantheline bromide tablets.

1. Huston GJ, *et al.* Anticholinergic drugs, buccal ulceration and mucosal potential difference. *Postgrad Med J* 1978; **54:** 331–2.

### Interactions

As for antimuscarinics in general (see Atropine Sulfate, p.477).

### Pharmacokinetics

Propantheline bromide is incompletely absorbed from the gastrointestinal tract and bioavailability is reported to be reduced by food; it is extensively metabolised in the small intestine before absorption. Propantheline is eliminated mainly in the urine as metabolites and less than 10% as unchanged drug. The duration of action is about 6 hours.

### Uses and Administration

Propantheline bromide is a quaternary ammonium antimuscarinic with peripheral effects similar to those of atropine (p.477). It has been used in the management of spasm of the gastrointestinal tract and as an adjunct in the treatment of peptic ulcer disease (p.475). The usual initial dose is 15 mg by mouth three times daily before meals and 30 mg at bedtime; doses of up to 120 mg daily may be needed in some patients. In elderly patients, doses of 7.5 mg three times daily may be sufficient.

Propantheline bromide has been used in the treatment of adult enuresis or urinary incontinence (p.476) in doses similar to those given above.

**Hyperhidrosis.** Some antimuscarinics, including propantheline, have been applied topically in the treatment of hyperhidrosis (p.475). Side-effects of antimuscarinics administered by mouth generally preclude their use by this route, although oral propantheline was used successfully to control excessive sweating in 2 patients with spinal cord injuries,[1] and it is sometimes used in palliative care to control night sweats. The *British National Formulary* notes that propantheline may be used for gustatory sweating in patients with diabetic neuropathy.

1. Canaday BR, Stanford RH. Propantheline bromide in the management of hyperhidrosis associated with spinal cord injury. *Ann Pharmacother* 1995; **29:** 489–92.

### Preparations

***BP 2003:*** Propantheline Tablets;
***USP 27:*** Propantheline Bromide Tablets.

**Proprietary Preparations** (details are given in Part 3)
***Austral.:*** Pro-Banthine; ***Belg.:*** Pro-Banthine†; ***Canad.:*** Pro-Banthine†; Propanthel; ***Denm.:*** Ercoril; Pro-Banthine†; ***India:*** Pro-Banthine; ***Irl.:*** Pro-Banthine†; ***Israel:*** Pro-Banthine†; ***Mex.:*** Bropantil†; Propantel†; ***NZ:*** Pro-Banthine; ***S.Afr.:*** Pro-Banthine; ***Swed.:*** Ercotina†; ***Switz.:*** Ercorax Roll-on†; Pro-Banthine†; ***UK:*** Pro-Banthine; ***USA:*** Pro-Banthine.
**Multi-ingredient:** ***Hong Kong:*** Crema-U†; ***Ital.:*** Lexil.

## Propiverine Hydrochloride *(BANM, rINNM)*

BUP-4 (propiverine); Hidrocloruro de propiverina. 1-Methyl-4-piperidyl diphenylpropoxyacetate hydrochloride.

$C_{23}H_{29}NO_3,HCl$ = 403.9.

*CAS — 60569-19-9 (propiverine); 54556-98-8 (propiverine hydrochloride).*

*ATC — G04BD06.*

### Adverse Effects, Treatment, and Precautions

As for Atropine Sulfate, p.477. Hypotension and drowsiness may also occur with propiverine. Propiverine is contra-indicated in patients with hepatic disorders (but see below) or severe renal impairment. Liver enzyme values should be monitored in patients receiving long-term therapy. Skeletal retardation has occurred in the offspring of *animals* given high doses of propiverine during pregnancy and therefore its use is not recommended during pregnancy.

### Interactions

As for antimuscarinics in general (see Atropine Sulfate, p.477). Hypotension may occur in patients treated with propiverine and isoniazid. Drowsiness may be enhanced by drugs with CNS-depressant properties.

### Pharmacokinetics

Propiverine is absorbed from the gastrointestinal tract and peak plasma concentrations are achieved about 2.3 hours after oral administration. It undergoes extensive first-pass metabolism and the average absolute bioavailability is reported to be about 41%. Plasma concentrations of the principal metabolite, the *N*-oxide, greatly exceed those of the parent compound. Protein binding is about 90% for propiverine and 60% for the *N*-oxide metabolite. Propiverine and its metabolites are excreted in the urine, bile, and faeces. The elimination half-life is about 20 hours.

◊ References.

1. Haustein KO, Huller G. On the pharmacokinetics and metabolism of propiverine in man. *Eur J Drug Metab Pharmacokinet* 1988; **13:** 81–90.

### Uses and Administration

Propiverine hydrochloride is a tertiary antimuscarinic with actions similar to those of atropine (p.477). It is used for the management of urinary frequency, urgency, and incontinence (p.476) in neurogenic bladder disorders and in idiopathic detrusor instability. Usual doses of propiverine hydrochloride are 15 mg two or three times daily by mouth, increased to 4 times daily if required. Some patients may respond to 15 mg once daily. A daily dose of 1 mg/kg should not be exceeded.

**Administration in hepatic impairment.** Although the manufacturers of propiverine do not recommend its use in patients with hepatic disorders, some[1] suggest that on pharmacokinetic grounds it may be given to those with mild to moderate hepatic impairment at recommended doses without increasing the risk of adverse effects.

1. Siepmann M, *et al.* Pharmacokinetics and safety of propiverine in patients with fatty liver disease. *Eur J Clin Pharmacol* 1998; **54:** 767–71.

### Preparations

**Proprietary Preparations** (details are given in Part 3)
***Ger.:*** Mictonetten; Mictonorm; ***UK:*** Detrunorm.

## Solifenacin Succinate *(USAN, rINNM)*

YM-905; YM-67905. (3*R*)-1-Azabicyclo[2.2.2]oct-3-yl (1*S*)-1-phenyl-3,4-dihydroisoquinoline-2(1*H*)-carboxylate compound with butanedioic acid (1:1).

$C_{23}H_{26}N_2O_2,C_4H_6O_4$ = 480.6.

*CAS — 242478-37-1 (solifenacin); 242478-38-2 (solifenacin succinate).*

*ATC — G04BD08.*

### Profile

Solifenacin succinate is a selective $M_3$-receptor antagonist that has been tried in the treatment of urinary incontinence.

◊ References.

1. Chapple CR, *et al.* Randomized, double-blind placebo- and tolterodine-controlled trial of the once-daily antimuscarinic agent solifenacin in patients with symptomatic overactive bladder. *BJU Int* 2004; **93:** 303–10.

## Stramonium

Datura; Estramonio; Inferno; Jamestown Weed; Jimson Weed; Stechapfel; Stramoine; Thornapple.

NOTE. The terms Datura, Datura Herb, and Datura Leaf have been applied to preparations of various species of the genus Datura including *Datura metel.*

**Pharmacopoeias.** *Eur.* (see p.vi) includes a monograph for Stramonium Leaf and Prepared Stramonium.

**Ph. Eur. 5.0** (Stramonium Leaf; Stramonii Folium). It consists of the dried leaf or the dried leaf, flowering tops and occasionally fruit-bearing tops of *Datura stramonium* and its varieties. It contains not less than 0.25% of total alkaloids, calculated as hyoscyamine. The alkaloids consist mainly of hyoscyamine with varying proportions of hyoscine. It has an unpleasant odour. Protect from light and moisture.

The BP 2003 directs that when stramonium leaf or powdered stramonium leaf is prescribed, prepared stramonium shall be dispensed.

**Ph. Eur. 5.0** (Stramonium, Prepared; Stramonii Pulvis Normatus). It is stramonium leaf powder adjusted to contain 0.23 to 0.27% of total alkaloids, calculated as hyoscyamine. Store in airtight containers. Protect from light.

### Adverse Effects, Treatment, and Precautions

As for Atropine Sulfate, p.477.

**Abuse.** Some reports[1-3] of poisoning following abuse of *Datura stramonium* or its preparations.

1. Gowdy JM. Stramonium intoxication: review of symptomatology in 212 cases. *JAMA* 1972; **221:** 585–7.
2. Shervette RE, *et al.* Jimson "Loco" weed abuse in adolescents. *Pediatrics* 1979; **63:** 520–3.
3. Anonymous. Jimson weed poisoning—Texas, New York, and California, 1994. *MMWR* 1995; **44:** 41–4.

**Effects on the eyes.** Anisocoria (unequal dilatation of the pupils) developed following accidental entry of a piece of jimson weed *(Datura stramonium)* into a patient's eye while gardening.[1]

1. Savitt DL, *et al.* Anisocoria from Jimsonweed. *JAMA* 1986; **255:** 1439–40.

### Uses and Administration

Stramonium has the actions of atropine (p.477). It has been given with other drugs in oral and rectal dosage forms for respiratory-tract disorders. It has also been smoked in cigarettes or burnt in powders and the fumes inhaled but the irritation produced by the fumes may aggravate bronchitis.

Stramonium has been used in homoeopathic medicine.

### Preparations

**Proprietary Preparations** (details are given in Part 3)
**Multi-ingredient:** ***Austral.:*** Potassium Iodide and Stramonium Compound†; ***Braz.:*** Asmatiron†; Expectol; Teutoss; Xarope de Eucalipto†; ***Spain:*** Balsamo Analgesic Karmel†.

## Tiemonium Iodide *(BAN, rINN)*

Ioduro de tiemonio; TE-114. 4-[3-Hydroxy-3-phenyl-3-(2-thienyl)propyl]-4-methylmorpholinium iodide.

$C_{18}H_{24}INO_2S$ = 445.4.

*CAS — 6252-92-2 (tiemonium); 144-12-7 (tiemonium iodide).*

*ATC — A03AB17.*

## Tiemonium Metilsulfate

Tiemonio, metilsulfato de; Tiemonium Methylsulphate. 4-[3-Hydroxy-3-phenyl-3-(2-thienyl)propyl]-4-methyl-morpholinium methylsulphate.

$C_{19}H_{27}NO_6S_2$ = 429.6.

*CAS — 6504-57-0.*

### Profile

Tiemonium iodide and tiemonium metilsulfate are quaternary ammonium antimuscarinics with peripheral effects similar to those of atropine (p.477) and are used in the relief of visceral spasms.

Tiemonium iodide is used in a usual dose of 100 mg twice daily by mouth. A dose of 5 mg has been given by intramuscular or slow intravenous injection.

Tiemonium metilsulfate is given in a dose of 100 to 300 mg daily in divided doses by mouth. A dose of 5 mg has been given three times daily by intramuscular or slow intravenous injection. Tiemonium metilsulfate has also been given as a rectal suppository in daily doses of 20 to 40 mg.

### Preparations

**Proprietary Preparations** (details are given in Part 3)
***Belg.:*** Visceralgine; ***Fr.:*** Visceralgine.
**Multi-ingredient:** ***Belg.:*** Asodal; Visceralgine Compositum†; ***Fr.:*** Colchimax; Visceralgine Forte.

## Timepidium Bromide *(rINN)*

Bromuro de timepidio; SA-504. 3-[Di-(2-thienyl)methylene]-5-methoxy-1,1-dimethylpiperidinium bromide monohydrate.

$C_{17}H_{22}BrNOS_2,H_2O$ = 418.4.

*CAS — 35035-05-3.*

*ATC — A03AB19.*

**Pharmacopoeias.** In *Jpn.*

### Profile

Timepidium bromide is a quaternary ammonium antimuscarinic with peripheral actions similar to those of atropine (p.477). It has been given for the symptomatic treatment of visceral spasms in usual doses of 30 mg three times daily by mouth. It has also been given by subcutaneous, intramuscular, and intravenous injection in a dose of 7.5 mg.

Urinary metabolites of timepidium may cause a reddish coloration of the urine.

### Preparations

**Proprietary Preparations** (details are given in Part 3)
***Jpn:*** Sesden; ***Singapore:*** Sesden.

## Tolterodine Tartrate *(BANM, USAN, rINNM)*

Kabi-2234 (tolterodine); PNU-200583E; Tartrato de tolterodina; Tolterodine L-Tartrate. (+)-(*R*)-2-{α-[2-(Diisopropylamino)ethyl]benzyl}-*p*-cresol tartrate.

$C_{22}H_{31}NO,C_4H_6O_6$ = 475.6.

*CAS — 124937-51-5 (tolterodine); 124937-52-6 (tolterodine tartrate).*

*ATC — G04BD07.*

## Adverse Effects, Treatment, and Precautions

As for Atropine Sulfate, p.477. Tolterodine should be used with caution in patients with hepatic or renal impairment. *Animal* studies have shown that high doses may cause fetal toxicity and it is recommended that tolterodine should be avoided during pregnancy.

◊ References.

1. Layton D, *et al.* Safety profile of tolterodine as used in general practice in England: results of prescription-event monitoring. *Drug Safety* 2001; **24:** 703–13.

## Interactions

As for antimuscarinics in general (see Atropine Sulfate, p.477).

There is a risk of interactions between tolterodine and other drugs metabolised by or inhibiting cytochrome P450 isoenzymes CYP2D6 (but see Antidepressants, below), or CYP3A4. The US manufacturers advise that the dose of tolterodine should not exceed 1 mg twice daily in patients receiving potent CYP3A4 inhibitors such as the macrolide antibiotics erythromycin or clarithromycin, and the antifungals ketoconazole, itraconazole, or miconazole; UK product information recommends against such combinations.

**Anticoagulants.** For reference to the effect of tolterodine on the activity of *warfarin*, see under Antimuscarinics, p.1025.

**Antidepressants.** The SSRI *fluoxetine* is a potent inhibitor of the cytochrome P450 isoenzyme CYP2D6 and use with tolterodine has resulted in more than a fourfold increase in the area-under-the-curve (AUC) of tolterodine, associated with an approximate 20% decrease in the AUC of its 5-hydroxymethyl metabolite.[1] However, since both are active these changes were thought likely to result in little clinical difference, and the manufacturers do not recommend a dose adjustment when tolterodine is given with fluoxetine.

1. Brynne N, *et al.* Fluoxetine inhibits the metabolism of tolterodine—pharmacokinetic implications and proposed clinical relevance. *Br J Clin Pharmacol* 1999; **48:** 553–63.

## Pharmacokinetics

Peak plasma concentrations of tolterodine occur 1 to 3 hours after a dose by mouth. Tolterodine is mainly metabolised by the cytochrome P450 isoenzyme CYP2D6 to the active 5-hydromethyl derivative (DD-01); in a minority of poor metabolisers tolterodine is metabolised by CYP3A4 isoenzymes to its inactive N-dealkylated derivative. Tolterodine is excreted primarily in the urine with about 17% appearing in the faeces; less than 1% of a dose is excreted as unchanged drug.

◊ References.

1. Brynne N, *et al.* Pharmacokinetics and pharmacodynamics of tolterodine in man: a new drug for the treatment of urinary bladder overactivity. *Int J Clin Pharmacol Ther* 1997; **35:** 287–95.
2. Brynne N, *et al.* Influence of CYP2D6 polymorphism on the pharmacokinetics and pharmacodynamics of tolterodine. *Clin Pharmacol Ther* 1998; **63:** 529–39.

## Uses and Administration

Tolterodine tartrate is a tertiary antimuscarinic with actions similar to those of atropine (p.477); it is claimed to have a greater selectivity for the muscarinic receptors of the bladder. Tolterodine is used in the management of urinary frequency, urgency, and incontinence in detrusor instability. Usual doses of tolterodine tartrate are 2 mg twice daily by mouth; modified-release preparations are given in a usual dose of 4 mg once daily. Doses of 1 mg twice daily (or 2 mg daily as a modified-release preparation) are recommended in patients experiencing troublesome adverse effects or receiving drugs that inhibit the cytochrome P450 isoenzyme CYP3A4 (see Interactions, above). See also below for doses in patients with hepatic or renal impairment.

**Administration in hepatic or renal impairment.** Doses of 1 mg of tolterodine tartrate twice daily by mouth (or 2 mg daily as a modified-release preparation) are recommended in patients with hepatic or severe renal impairment.

**Urinary incontinence.** Tolterodine is used as an alternative to oxybutynin in the treatment of urge incontinence (see p.476). Tolterodine is said to have fewer side-effects than oxybutynin.

References.

1. Hills CJ, *et al.* Tolterodine. *Drugs* 1998; **55:** 813–20.
2. Abrams P, *et al.* Tolterodine, a new antimuscarinic agent: as effective but better tolerated than oxybutynin in patients with an overactive bladder. *Br J Urol* 1998; **81:** 801–10.
3. Ruscin JM, Morgenstern NE. Tolterodine use for symptoms of overactive bladder. *Ann Pharmacother* 1999; **33:** 1073–82.
4. Abrams P. Evidence for the efficacy and safety of tolterodine in the treatment of overactive bladder. *Expert Opin Pharmacother* 2001; **2:** 1685–1701.
5. Jacquetin B, Wyndaele J. Tolterodine reduces the number of urge incontinence episodes in patients with an overactive bladder. *Eur J Obstet Gynecol Reprod Biol* 2001; **98:** 97–102.
6. Sussman D, Garely A. Treatment of overactive bladder with once-daily extended-release tolterodine or oxybutynin: the antimuscarinic clinical effectiveness trial (ACET). *Curr Med Res Opin* 2002; **18:** 177–84.

## Preparations

**Proprietary Preparations** (details are given in Part 3)

***Arg.:*** Breminal; Detrusitol; Toltem; Urginol; ***Austria:*** Detrusitol; ***Belg.:*** Detrusitol; ***Braz.:*** Detrusitol; ***Canad.:*** Detrol; ***Chile:*** Detrusitol; ***Denm.:*** Detrusitol; ***Fin.:*** Detrusitol; ***Fr.:*** Detrusitol; ***Ger.:*** Detrusitol; ***Gr.:*** Detrusitol; ***Hong Kong:*** Detrusitol; ***Irl.:*** Detrusitol; ***Israel:*** Detrusitol; ***Ital.:*** Detrusitol; ***Malaysia:*** Detrusitol; ***Mex.:*** Detrusitol; ***Neth.:*** Detrusitol; Detsel; ***Norw.:*** Detrusitol; ***NZ:*** Detrusitol; ***Port.:*** Detrusitol; ***S.Afr.:*** Detrusitol; ***Singapore:*** Detrusitol; ***Spain:*** Detrusitol; Urotrol; ***Swed.:*** Detrusitol; ***Switz.:*** Detrusitol; ***Thai.:*** Detrusitol; ***UK:*** Detrusitol; ***USA:*** Detrol.

## Tridihexethyl Chloride *(BAN)*

Tridihexetilo, cloruro de. (3-Cyclohexyl-3-hydroxy-3-phenylpropyl)triethylammonium chloride.

$C_{21}H_{36}ClNO$ = 354.0.

*CAS — 60-49-1 (tridihexethyl); 4310-35-4 (tridihexethyl chloride); 125-99-5 (tridihexethyl iodide).*

*ATC — A03AB08.*

NOTE. Tridihexethyl Iodide is *rINN*.

### Profile

Tridihexethyl chloride is a quaternary ammonium antimuscarinic with peripheral effects similar to those of atropine (p.477). It has been used as an adjunct in the treatment of peptic ulcer disease.

### Preparations

**Proprietary Preparations** (details are given in Part 3)

***USA:*** Pathilon†.

# Trihexyphenidyl Hydrochloride

*(BANM, rINNM)*

Benzhexol Hydrochloride; Cloridrato de Triexilfenidila; Cyclodolum; Hidrocloruro de trihexifenidilo; Trihexyphenidyli Hydrochloridum; Trihexyphenidylium Chloratum. 1-Cyclohexyl-1-phenyl-3-piperidinopropan-1-ol hydrochloride.

$C_{20}H_{31}NO,HCl$ = 337.9.

*CAS — 144-11-6 (trihexyphenidyl); 52-49-3 (trihexyphenidyl hydrochloride).*

*ATC — N04AA01.*

**Pharmacopoeias.** In *Chin., Eur.* (see p.vi), *Int., Jpn, Pol.*, and *US.*

**Ph. Eur. 5.0** (Trihexyphenidyl Hydrochloride). A white crystalline powder. Slightly soluble in water; sparingly soluble in alcohol and in dichloromethane. A 1% solution in water has a pH of 5.2 to 6.2.

**USP 27** (Trihexyphenidyl Hydrochloride). A white or slightly off-white, crystalline powder, having not more than a very faint odour. Slightly soluble in water; soluble in alcohol and in chloroform. Store in airtight containers.

## Adverse Effects, Treatment and Precautions

As for Atropine Sulfate, p.477. In some patients, such as those with arteriosclerosis or a history of drug idiosyncrasy, trihexyphenidyl may produce severe mental disturbances, excitement, nausea, and vomiting; such patients should be allowed to develop a tolerance by starting with a small initial dose and gradually increasing it until an effective level is reached.

**Abuse.** Trihexyphenidyl hydrochloride has been abused for its euphoric effect[1] especially by psychiatric patients.[2] Its abuse potential in schizophrenic patients has been questioned[3] and its unpleasant antimuscarinic effects tend to limit its repeated use,[4] but a small survey among psychiatric patients found that trihexyphenidyl was reported to be the antimuscarinic most frequently abused;[5] procyclidine, benzatropine, and orphenadrine (in decreasing order of frequency) were also misused.

1. Crawshaw JA, Mullen PE. A study of benzhexol abuse. *Br J Psychiatry* 1984; **145:** 300–3.
2. Pullen GP, *et al.* Anticholinergic drug abuse: a common problem? *BMJ* 1984; **289:** 612–13.
3. Goff DC, *et al.* A placebo-controlled trial of trihexyphenidyl in unmedicated patients with schizophrenia. *Am J Psychiatry* 1994; **151:** 429–31.
4. WHO. WHO expert committee on drug dependence: twenty-ninth report. *WHO Tech Rep Ser 856* 1995.
5. Buhrich N, *et al.* Misuse of anticholinergic drugs by people with serious mental illness. *Psychiatr Serv* 2000; **51:** 928–9.

**Effects on the heart.** Paradoxical sinus bradycardia developed in a schizophrenic patient after receiving trihexyphenidyl for extrapyramidal side-effects due to antipsychotic medication.[1] Normal sinus rhythm was restored after trihexyphenidyl was discontinued. The patient had previously received trihexyphenidyl and suffered bradycardia which at the time was attributed to haloperidol.

1. Blumensohn R, *et al.* Bradycardia due to trihexyphenidyl hydrochloride. *Drug Intell Clin Pharm* 1986; **20:** 786–7.

**Effects on mental function.** Trihexyphenidyl 2 mg by mouth significantly impaired memory function compared with placebo in a study in 13 elderly patients.[1] Impairment of memory has also been observed in patients with Parkinson's disease given antimuscarinics such as trihexyphenidyl.[2] However, impairment may be reversible on discontinuation of the antimuscarinic (see Atropine, p.477).

1. Potamianos G, Kellett JM. Anti-cholinergic drugs and memory: the effects of benzhexol on memory in a group of geriatric patients. *Br J Psychiatry* 1982; **140:** 470–2.
2. Sadeh M, *et al.* Effects of anticholinergic drugs on memory in Parkinson's disease. *Arch Neurol* 1982; **39:** 666–7.

**Overdosage.** A 34-year-old woman developed a toxic reaction with widely dilated pupils, dry skin, and visual hallucinations within 24 hours of taking about 300 mg of trihexyphenidyl hydrochloride with suicidal intent.[1] After 3 to 4 days the hallucinations were replaced by illusions; complete recovery occurred after a week, with no special treatment.

1. Ananth JV, *et al.* Toxic psychosis induced by benzhexol hydrochloride. *Can Med Assoc J* 1970; **103:** 771.

**Withdrawal.** A 61-year-old woman who had taken trihexyphenidyl 6 mg daily for a year for Parkinson's disease developed encephalopathy and miosis on two occasions when treatment was abruptly withdrawn.[1] Slowly tapered withdrawal avoided these effects.

1. Johkura K, *et al.* Trihexyphenidyl withdrawal encephalopathy. *Ann Neurol* 1997; **41:** 133–4.

## Interactions

As for antimuscarinics in general (see Atropine Sulfate, p.477).

**Chlorpromazine.** For the effect of trihexyphenidyl on plasma concentrations of chlorpromazine, see under Antiparkinsonian Drugs, p.680.

## Pharmacokinetics

Trihexyphenidyl hydrochloride is well absorbed from the gastrointestinal tract and has been stated to exert an effect within 1 hour of a dose by mouth.

**Half-life.** The reported half-life of trihexyphenidyl has varied according to the assay method used. Values reported when using radioreceptor and chromatographic techniques have ranged from about 1 to more than 24 hours[1] and from 10 to 29 hours,[2] respectively, but the sensitivity and specificity of these methods has been criticised.[3] With a more recently developed radio immunoassay it was found that following oral administration there was an initial elimination phase with an estimated half-life of 5.33 hours followed by a terminal elimination phase with an estimated half-life of 32.7 hours.

1. Burke RE, Fahn S. Pharmacokinetics of trihexyphenidyl after short-term and long-term administration to dystonic patients. *Ann Neurol* 1985; **18:** 35–40.
2. Garbarg S, *et al.* Comparaison pharmacoclinique de deux formes galéniques de trihexyphénidyle. *Encephale* 1983; **IX:** 167–74.
3. He H, *et al.* Development and application of a specific and sensitive radioimmunoassay for trihexyphenidyl to a pharmacokinetic study in humans. *J Pharm Sci* 1995; **84:** 561–7.

## Uses and Administration

Trihexyphenidyl hydrochloride is a tertiary amine antimuscarinic with actions similar to those of atropine (p.478). It also has a direct antispasmodic action on smooth muscle.

Trihexyphenidyl hydrochloride is employed in the symptomatic treatment of parkinsonism, including the alleviation of the extrapyramidal syndrome induced by drugs such as phenothiazines, but, like other antimuscarinics, is of no value against tardive dyskinesias. It has been used in the treatment of dystonias.

In idiopathic parkinsonism, trihexyphenidyl hydrochloride is given in 3 or 4 divided doses daily before or with food. The usual initial dose of 1 mg daily is gradually increased over a period of several days by increments of 2 mg to 6 to 10 mg daily according to the response of the patient; for advanced cases, 12 to 15 mg daily or even more may be needed. As a rule, postencephalitic patients tolerate and require the larger doses; elderly patients may require smaller doses.

Usual doses for drug-induced extrapyramidal symptoms lie within the range of 5 to 15 mg daily, although as little as 1 mg daily may be sufficient in some cases.

Antimuscarinic treatment of parkinsonism should never be terminated suddenly and it is usual when changing from one drug to another to withdraw one in small amounts while gradually increasing the dose of the other.

Trihexyphenidyl hydrochloride may be given with other drugs used for the relief of parkinsonism, such as levodopa, but the dose of each drug may need to be reduced.

**Extrapyramidal disorders.** Antimuscarinics such as trihexyphenidyl are used in the management of dystonias (p.1209) although only about half of all children and adolescents, and fewer adults (who tolerate antimuscarinics less well) show any response. Side-effects may be limited by starting with a low dose: one suggested regimen[1] starts with trihexyphenidyl 1 mg daily and rises up to 12 mg daily over the next 4 to 6 weeks; some patients may require up to 60 to 100 mg daily.

1. Jankovic J. Dystonia: medical therapy and botulinum toxin. *Adv Neurol* 2004; **94:** 275–86.

**Parkinsonism.** For the use of antimuscarinics, such as trihexyphenidyl, in the symptomatic treatment of parkinsonism, see p.476.

### Preparations

***BP 2003:*** Trihexyphenidyl Tablets;
***USP 27:*** Trihexyphenidyl Hydrochloride Elixir; Trihexyphenidyl Hydrochloride Extended-release Capsules; Trihexyphenidyl Hydrochloride Tablets.

**Proprietary Preparations** (details are given in Part 3)
***Arg.:*** Artane; ***Austral.:*** Artane; ***Austria:*** Artane; ***Belg.:*** Artane; ***Braz.:*** Artane; Triexidyl; ***Canad.:*** Apo-Trihex; Artane†; Novo-Hexidyl†; ***Chile:*** Artane; Tenvatil; Tonaril; ***Denm.:*** Peragit; ***Fin.:*** Artane†; ***Fr.:*** Artane; Parkinane; ***Ger.:*** Artane; Parkopan; ***Gr.:*** Artane; ***Hong Kong:*** Apo-Trihex; Artandyl; Artane; ***India:*** Pacitane; ***Irl.:*** Artane; ***Israel:*** Artane; Partane; Rodenal; ***Ital.:*** Artane; ***Malaysia:*** Aca; Apo-Trihex; Uphazhexol; ***Mex.:*** Artane; Hipokinon; Kexidil†; ***Neth.:*** Artane; ***Port.:*** Artane; ***S.Afr.:*** Artane†; ***Singapore:*** Apo-Trihex; B-Hex†; Beahexol; ***Spain:*** Artane; ***Swed.:*** Pargitan; ***Switz.:*** Artane†; ***Thai.:*** Aca; Acamed; Artane; Pozhexol; Tridyl; ***UK:*** Broflex; ***USA:*** Artane†; Trihexy.

**Multi-ingredient:** ***Ger.:*** Spasman; ***India:*** Sycot; Trinicalm Forte; Trinicalm Plus; ***Spain:*** Largatrex.

## Tropatepine Hydrochloride *(rINNM)*

Hidrocloruro de tropatepina; SD-1248-17. 3-(Dibenzo[*b*,*e*]thiepin-11(6*H*)-ylidene)tropane hydrochloride.
$C_{22}H_{23}NS,HCl = 370.0.$
*CAS — 27574-24-9 (tropatepine); 27574-25-0 (tropatepine hydrochloride).*
*ATC — N04AA12.*

### Profile

Tropatepine hydrochloride is an antimuscarinic with actions and uses similar to those of trihexyphenidyl (p.490). It is used in the management of parkinsonism, including the alleviation of extrapyramidal symptoms induced by drugs such as phenothiazines, but, like other antimuscarinics, it is of no value in tardive dyskinesias. Tropatepine hydrochloride is given in usual doses of 10 to 30 mg daily by mouth; it is also given intramuscularly or by slow intravenous injection in doses of 10 to 20 mg daily.

### Preparations

**Proprietary Preparations** (details are given in Part 3)
***Fr.:*** Lepticur.

## Tropicamide *(BAN, USAN, rINN)*

Bistropamide; Ro-1-7683; Tropicamida; Tropicamidum. *N*-Ethyl-*N*-(4-pyridylmethyl)tropamide; (2*RS*)-*N*-Ethyl-3-hydroxy-2-phenyl-*N*-(pyridin-4-ylmethyl)propanamide.
$C_{17}H_{20}N_2O_2 = 284.4.$
*CAS — 1508-75-4.*
*ATC — S01FA06.*

NOTE. TRO is a code approved by the BP 2003 for use on single unit doses of eye drops containing tropicamide where the individual container may be too small to bear all the appropriate labelling information.

**Pharmacopoeias.** In *Chin., Eur.* (see p.vi), *Int., Jpn,* and *US.*

**Ph. Eur. 5.0** (Tropicamide). A white or almost white, crystalline powder. M.p. 95° to 98°. Slightly soluble in water; freely soluble in alcohol and in dichloromethane. Protect from light.

**USP 27** (Tropicamide). A white or practically white crystalline powder, odourless or having not more than a slight odour. M.p. 96° to 100°. Slightly soluble in water; freely soluble in chloroform and in solutions of strong acids. Store in airtight containers. Protect from light.

### Adverse Effects, Treatment, and Precautions

As for Atropine Sulfate, p.477.

◊ References.

1. Vuori M-L, *et al.* Systemic absorption and anticholinergic activity of topically applied tropicamide. *J Ocul Pharmacol* 1994; **10:** 431–7.

### Interactions

As for antimuscarinics in general (see Atropine Sulfate, p.477).

### Uses and Administration

Tropicamide is a tertiary amine antimuscarinic with actions similar to those of atropine (p.477). It is used as eye drops to produce mydriasis and cycloplegia (p.476). It has a more rapid onset and a shorter duration of effect than atropine: mydriasis is produced within 20 to 40 minutes of instillation and usually lasts for about 6 hours; cycloplegia is maximal within about 30 minutes and is short-lasting, with complete recovery of accommodation normally within 6 hours. Tropicamide has been reported to be inadequate for cycloplegia in children.

To produce **mydriasis**, 1 or 2 drops of a 0.5% solution are instilled 15 to 20 minutes before examination of the eye. To produce **cycloplegia** 1 or 2 drops of a 1% solution are required, repeated after 5 minutes; a further drop may be necessary to prolong the effect after 20 to 30 minutes.

**Alzheimer's disease.** Tropicamide has been studied for use in the differential diagnosis of Alzheimer's disease (see Dementia, p.1484). Excessive pupil dilatation in response to tropicamide eye drops occurred in patients with signs and symptoms of Alzheimer's disease.[1] However, a double-blind placebo-controlled study[2] in similar patients and healthy subjects indicated that this was not a reliable diagnostic test for Alzheimer's disease.

1. Gómez-Tortosa E, *et al.* Pupil response to tropicamide in Alzheimer's disease and other neurodegenerative disorders. *Acta Neurol Scand* 1996; **94:** 104–9.
2. Graff-Radford NR, *et al.* Tropicamide eyedrops cannot be used for reliable diagnosis of Alzheimer's disease. *Mayo Clin Proc* 1997; **72:** 495–504.

### Preparations

***BP 2003:*** Tropicamide Eye Drops;
***USP 27:*** Tropicamide Ophthalmic Solution.

**Proprietary Preparations** (details are given in Part 3)
***Arg.:*** Midriaticum; Mydril; ***Austral.:*** Mydriacyl; ***Austria:*** Mydral; Mydriaticum; ***Belg.:*** Mydriaticum†; Tropicol†; ***Braz.:*** Mydriacyl; Tropinom; ***Canad.:*** Diotrope; Mydriacyl; ***Chile:*** Mydriacyl; ***Denm.:*** Mydriacyl; ***Fr.:*** Mydriaticum; ***Ger.:*** Mydriaticum; Mydrum; ***Gr.:*** Tropixal; ***Hong Kong:*** Mydriacyl; Mydriaticum; ***India:*** Tropico; ***Irl.:*** Mydriacil; ***Israel:*** Mydramide; ***Ital.:*** Tropimil; Visumidriatic; ***Malaysia:*** Mydriacyl; ***Mex.:*** Myriacyl; ***Norw.:*** Mydrian; ***NZ:*** Mydriacyl; ***Port.:*** Tropicil Top; ***S.Afr.:*** Mydriacyl; Mydriaticum; ***Singapore:*** Mydriacyl; ***Swed.:*** Mydriacyl; ***Switz.:*** Mydriaticum; ***Thai.:*** Mydriacyl; ***UK:*** Mydriacyl; ***USA:*** Mydral; Mydriacyl; Ocu-Tropic; Opticyl; Tropicacyl.

**Multi-ingredient:** ***Arg.:*** Fotorretin; ***Canad.:*** Diophenyl-T; ***Fr.:*** Mydriasert; ***Hong Kong:*** Mydrin-P; ***Ital.:*** Visumidriatic Antiflogistico†; Visumidriatic Fenilefrina; ***USA:*** Paremyd.

## Trospium Chloride *(BAN, USAN, rINN)*

Cloruro de trospio; IP-631. 3α-Benzilоyloxynortropane-8-spiro-1′-pyrrolidinium chloride.
$C_{25}H_{30}ClNO_3 = 428.0.$
*CAS — 10405-02-4.*
*ATC — A03AB20.*

### Adverse Effects, Treatment, and Precautions

As for Atropine Sulfate, p.477. Trospium should be used with caution in patients with hepatic or mild to moderate renal impairment, and avoided in those with severe renal impairment. *Animal* studies have shown that trospium crosses the placenta and is distributed into breast milk; the manufacturer therefore recommends that caution should be observed during pregnancy and breast feeding.

### Interactions

As for antimuscarinics in general (see Atropine Sulfate, p.477).

### Pharmacokinetics

Following oral administration of trospium chloride, peak plasma concentrations are reached at 4 to 6 hours. The bioavailability of trospium chloride is reduced by the simultaneous intake of food, especially with a high fat content. Trospium is excreted in the urine mainly as unchanged drug; about 10% appears as the spiroalcohol. The terminal elimination half-life has been reported to be between 10 and 20 hours. The mean half-life has been reported to be prolonged twofold in patients with severe renal impairment (creatinine clearance between 8 and 32 mL/minute). Trospium has been reported to cross the placenta and has been detected in the milk of *rats*.

◊ For reference to the bioavailability of trospium chloride after intravesical instillation, see below.

### Uses and Administration

Trospium chloride is a quaternary ammonium antimuscarinic with actions similar to those of atropine (p.477). It is used for the management of urinary frequency, urgency, and incontinence in detrusor instability or detrusor hyperreflexia. It has also been used as an antispasmodic.

Usual doses are 20 mg twice daily by mouth before meals on an empty stomach. Lower doses of 20 mg once daily may be warranted in patients aged 75 years and over. The need for continued treatment should be assessed at regular intervals of 3 to 6 months. For doses in renal impairment, see below.

It has also been given by intramuscular or slow intravenous injection, and rectally.

◊ References.

1. Madersbacher H, *et al.* Trospium chloride versus oxybutynin: a randomized, double-blind, multicentre trial in the treatment of detrusor hyper-reflexia. *Br J Urol* 1995; **75:** 452–6.
2. Walter P, *et al.* Bioavailability of trospium chloride after intravesical instillation in patients with neurogenic lower urinary tract dysfunction: a pilot study. *Neurourol Urodyn* 1999; **18:** 447–53.
3. Cardozo L, *et al.* Efficacy of trospium chloride in patients with detrusor instability: a placebo-controlled, randomized, double-blind, multicentre clinical trial. *BJU Int* 2000; **85:** 659–64.
4. Fusgen I, Hauri D. Trospium chloride: an effective option for medical treatment of bladder overactivity. *Int J Clin Pharmacol Ther* 2000; **38:** 223–34.

**Administration in renal impairment.** The UK manufacturer recommends that doses should be reduced to 20 mg daily or on alternate days in patients with a creatine clearance of 10 to 30 mL/minute.

### Preparations

**Proprietary Preparations** (details are given in Part 3)
***Arg.:*** Spasmex; ***Austria:*** Rekont; Spasmolyt; ***Chile:*** Spasmex; ***Denm.:*** Spasmo-Lyt; ***Fr.:*** Ceris; ***Ger.:*** Spasmex; Spasmo-Rhoival TC; Spasmo-Urgenin TC; Spasmolyt; Trospi; ***Irl.:*** Regurin; ***Ital.:*** Uraplex; ***Port.:*** Spasmoplex; ***Spain:*** Spasmosarto†; Uraplex; ***Switz.:*** Spasmo-Urgenine Neo; ***Thai.:*** Spasmo-Lyt; ***UK:*** Regurin; ***USA:*** Sanctura.

**Multi-ingredient:** ***Arg.:*** Keptan Compuesto; ***Austria:*** Spasmo-Urgenin; ***Port.:*** Spasmo-Urgenin; ***S.Afr.:*** Spasmo-Urgenin; ***Spain:*** Spasmo-Urgenin; ***Thai.:*** Spasmo-Urgenin.

## Valethamate Bromide

Valetamato, bromuro de. Diethylmethyl[2-(3-methyl-2-phenylvaleryloxy)ethyl]ammonium bromide.
$C_{19}H_{32}BrNO_2 = 386.4.$
*CAS — 16376-74-2 (valethamate); 90-22-2 (valethamate bromide).*

### Profile

Valethamate bromide is a quaternary ammonium antimuscarinic with peripheral effects similar to those of atropine (p.477). It has been given by mouth, by injection or rectally in the symptomatic treatment of visceral spasms.

### Preparations

**Proprietary Preparations** (details are given in Part 3)
***Ger.:*** Epidosin†; ***India:*** Epidosin.

## Xenytropium Bromide *(rINN)*

Bromuro de xenitropio; N-399. 8-(*p*-Phenylbenzyl)atropinium bromide.
$C_{30}H_{34}BrNO_3 = 536.5.$
*CAS — 511-55-7.*

### Profile

Xenytropium bromide is reported to have antimuscarinic properties; it has been given by mouth in preparations for the management of gastrointestinal disorders.

## Zamifenacin *(BAN, rINN)*

UK-76654-2 (zamifenacin fumarate); Zamifenacina. (*R*)-3-(Diphenylmethoxy)-1-[3,4-(methylenedioxy)phenetyl]piperidene.
$C_{27}H_{29}NO_3 = 415.5.$
*CAS — 127308-82-1 (zamifenacin); 127308-98-9 (zamifenacin fumarate).*

### Profile

Zamifenacin is an antimuscarinic with a selective action at $M_3$ receptors. It has been investigated for the treatment of irritable bowel syndrome and motion sickness.

◊ References.

1. Golding JF, Stott JRR. Comparison of the effects of a selective muscarinic receptor antagonist and hyoscine (scopolamine) on motion sickness, skin conductance and heart rate. *Br J Clin Pharmacol* 1997; **43:** 633–7.

# Antineoplastics

Adverse Effects, p.492
Treatment of Adverse Effects, p.495
Precautions, p.497
Interactions, p.498
Action, p.498
Resistance, p.498
Choice of Antineoplastic, p.499
Role of chemotherapy, p.499
Management of malignant disease, p.504
Carcinoid tumours and other secretory neoplasms, p.504
Gestational trophoblastic tumours, p.505
Histiocytic syndromes, p.505
Leukaemias, acute, p.505
Acute lymphoblastic leukaemia, p.506
Acute myeloid leukaemias, p.506
Leukaemias, chronic, p.507
Chronic lymphocytic leukaemia, p.507
Chronic myeloid leukaemia, p.507
Hairy-cell leukaemia, p.508
Myelodysplastic syndromes, p.508
Polycythaemia vera, p.508
Primary thrombocythaemia, p.509
Lymphomas, p.509
Hodgkin's disease, p.509
Non-Hodgkin's lymphomas, p.510
AIDS-related lymphomas, p.510
Burkitt's lymphoma, p.511
MALT lymphoma, p.511
Mycosis fungoides, p.511
Waldenström's macroglobulinaemia, p.511
Plasma cell neoplasms, p.511
Multiple myeloma, p.511
Malignant effusions, p.512
Malignant neoplasms of the bladder, p.512
Malignant neoplasms of the bone, p.513
Malignant neoplasms of the brain, p.513
Malignant neoplasms of the breast, p.514
Prophylaxis of breast cancer, p.515
Malignant neoplasms of the male breast, p.515
Malignant neoplasms of the cervix, p.515
Malignant neoplasms of the endometrium, p.516
Malignant neoplasms of the eye, p.516
Malignant neoplasms of the gastrointestinal tract, p.516
Malignant neoplasms of the head and neck, p.517
Malignant neoplasms of the kidney, p.518
Wilms' tumour, p.518
Malignant neoplasms of the liver, p.518
Malignant neoplasms of the lung, p.519
Malignant mesothelioma, p.520
Malignant neoplasms of the ovary, p.520
Malignant neoplasms of the pancreas, p.521
Malignant neoplasms of the prostate, p.521
Malignant neoplasms of the skin, p.522
Basal cell and squamous cell carcinoma, p.522
Melanoma, p.522
Malignant neoplasms of the testis, p.523
Malignant neoplasms of the thymus, p.523
Malignant neoplasms of the thyroid, p.523
Neuroblastoma, p.524
Retinoblastoma, p.524
Sarcomas, p.524
Bone sarcoma, p.524
Kaposi's sarcoma, p.524
Soft-tissue sarcoma, p.525

Antineoplastic drugs are used in the treatment of malignant neoplasms when surgery or radiotherapy is not possible or has proved ineffective, as an adjunct to surgery or radiotherapy, or, as in leukaemia, as the initial treatment. Therapy with antineoplastics is notably successful in a few malignant conditions and may be used to palliate symptoms and prolong life in others.

The two main groups of cytotoxic drugs used in the treatment of malignant disease are the alkylating agents and the antimetabolites. Nitrogen mustards, ethyleneimine compounds, and alkyl sulfonates are the main **alkylating agents**. Other compounds with an alkylating action are the various nitrosoureas. Cisplatin and dacarbazine appear to act similarly.

The **antimetabolites** may be subdivided into folic acid, purine, or pyrimidine antagonists.

Several natural products, or their derivatives, are used for their actions as **mitotic inhibitors**; they include the vinca alkaloids and the taxanes. Other drugs act as **topoisomerase inhibitors**, interfering with the coiling and uncoiling of DNA during replication. Drugs thought to act in this way include the podophyllotoxin derivatives such as etoposide, and camptothecin derivatives such as irinotecan and topotecan.

Some **antibiotics** also interfere with nucleic acids and are effective as antineoplastics.

Further described in this section are **other drugs** which act by various routes to affect the growth and proliferation of malignant cells. Some neoplasms express receptors to endogenous sex hormones, and various **hormone antagonists**, including, notably, the **aromatase inhibitors** are used in their management.

In recent years considerable interest has focused on immunological approaches to the treatment of malignant disease and a number of **monoclonal antibodies** have been, or are being, developed. The use of biological response modifiers such as interleukins continues to be the subject of investigation and attempts to develop vaccines against individual neoplasms also continue.

Glucocorticoids (see Corticosteroids, p.1073) are used with antineoplastics in the treatment of malignant disease, especially in acute leukaemias and lymphomas. Other agents used in antineoplastic therapy include sex hormones (p.1527) and radiopharmaceuticals (p.1522).

## Adverse Effects

The acute effects of antineoplastic drugs frequently include nausea and vomiting, often via a central mechanism, and sometimes extremely severe. In addition, many of these compounds are irritant or vesicant, and produce local pain, irritation, and inflammation at the administration site; extravasation may lead to ulceration and necrosis. Hypersensitivity reactions may also occur.

Many of the adverse effects of antineoplastics are an extension of their therapeutic action, which is not selective for malignant cells but affects all rapidly-dividing cells: antineoplastic therapy is made possible only by increased sensitivity or less effective recovery of malignant cells compared with normal cells, and administration is carefully controlled and timed, and, where possible, localised, to maximise the differences.

In consequence, adverse effects may be expected from most antineoplastics in tissues where normal cell division is fairly rapid, e.g. the bone marrow, lymphoreticular tissue, gastrointestinal mucosa, skin, and gonads, as well as in the fetus. The effects may not manifest for days or weeks, depending both on the drugs used and the rate of division in the tissue concerned, and may sometimes be cumulative. Perhaps the most common serious effect, and one which has frequently limited the doses that can be given, is bone-marrow depression. Because of their effects on the various types of white blood cell many antineoplastics also cause profound suppression of normal immunity, and patients may be at greatly increased risk of severe and disseminated infection.

The rapid destruction of large numbers of cells during antineoplastic therapy of certain highly sensitive tumours, and the consequent release of breakdown products, may also lead to problems with hyperuricaemia and acute renal failure due to uric acid nephropathy (the 'tumour lysis syndrome').

Additionally, some drugs may have specific toxicities which are not necessarily related to their therapeutic action, such as cardiotoxicity due to anthracycline antibiotics, nephrotoxicity with cisplatin, or the effects of bleomycin on the lung. Again these can be cumulative, and may limit the total lifetime dose that can be given.

In the very long term, patients who have undergone successful antineoplastic chemotherapy may develop secondary malignancies, suggesting that antineoplastics may themselves be carcinogenic. In addition, most are potentially mutagenic and teratogenic, and use in pregnancy, particularly in the first trimester, may lead to fetal abortion, stunting, or malformation.

**Carcinogenicity.** There is clear evidence that some antineoplastic drugs may themselves be carcinogenic, although it is difficult to control for the possible effects of primary disease, combination chemotherapy, and combined treatment with radiotherapy.[1]

Most convincingly associated with secondary malignancies are the various **alkylating agents**[2-4] including the nitrosoureas, and the topoisomerase II inhibitor **podophyllotoxin derivatives** such as etoposide and teniposide.[2,3,5] Leukaemias, particularly acute myeloid leukaemia, are the most common forms of secondary disease.[1-3] Leukaemia associated with alkylating agents usually occurs about 5 to 7 years after treatment, and is often preceded by a preleukaemic myelodysplasia.[2,3] The nitrosoureas are associated with a relatively high frequency of secondary leukaemia, and busulfan and melphalan are considered to be more leukaemogenic than cyclophosphamide.[3] Leukaemia associated with the podophyllotoxin derivatives has a shorter latency period of 2 to 3 years, with sudden onset and no myelodysplastic phase.[2,3] Solid tumours can also occur as secondary malignancies and include bladder cancer associated with cyclophosphamide used to treat non-Hodgkin's lymphoma,[4] and bone sarcomas, and breast and lung cancers following the use of various alkylating agents.[4,6]

There is little evidence of carcinogenicity associated with **antimetabolites** such as methotrexate, although it has been suggested that they may act as co-carcinogens.[7] Fludarabine therapy has been reported to be associated with the development of myelodysplasia and acute myeloid leukaemias,[8] although a review of the purine nucleoside analogues, cladribine and fludarabine, concluded that no significant increase in the risk of secondary malignancy had been demonstrated, but also that long-term follow-up of patients is needed.[9] Immunosuppression caused by antimetabolites including methotrexate, cladribine, and fludarabine, may also allow the development of Epstein-Barr virus-related lymphoma.[9,10] **Platinum derivatives** such as carboplatin and cisplatin have been found in large cohort studies[11,12] to have a dose-response relationship with the development of secondary leukaemia. Combinations that may also be associated with leukaemias include cisplatin with doxorubicin,[13] and other anthracycline-based regimens.[14] Another drug that has been associated with the development of secondary malignancies is **procarbazine**.[3,4,15,16]

Estimates of **risk** have varied very widely between studies, and have been calculated in various ways, making direct comparison impossible. Factors influencing the incidence of secondary malignancy include the use of combination chemotherapy regimens, combined treatment modalities, exposure to environmental carcinogens, predisposing genetic risk factors, ethnicity, age at time of treatment, gender, and spontaneous occurrence.[2,3]

The risk of secondary acute myeloid leukaemia appears to be associated primarily with the **cumulative dose** of antineoplastics.[2] Of patients at risk for secondary leukaemias, those with Hodgkin's disease have been most extensively studied. The cumulative 10-year incidence of secondary myeloid leukaemia has been reported to range from less than 1% up to 10%.[2,3] The highest risk is associated with the use of MOPP (chlormethine, vincristine, procarbazine, prednisone) and relative risk increases with cumulative dose of chlormethine.[2,3] Splenectomy or radiation of the spleen doubles the risk of leukaemia, as does being aged over 45 at the time of treatment.[2] Secondary solid tumours, such as lung cancer, in patients with Hodgkin's disease have also been attributed to the use of regimens such as MOPP.[4] The risk of secondary acute myeloid leukaemia, in patients treated with adjuvant chemotherapy for breast cancer, increases with cumulative doses of melphalan and cyclophosphamide, and high-dose regimens of doxorubicin with cyclophosphamide.[2,3] In patients treated for multiple myeloma, the increased risk of secondary leukaemia has been attributed to the prolonged use of melphalan.[2,3] Patients treated for testicular cancer appear to be at increased risk of secondary leukaemia associated with cumulative doses of podophyllotoxin derivatives (more than 2 g/m$^2$ etoposide), and the addition of high cisplatin doses may increase this risk.[2,3] Another review[17] of studies using etoposide or teniposide for various cancers found no relationship between the cumulative dose of these and secondary leukaemia, and suggested that other drugs used in treatment regimens had a greater effect on the development of secondary malignancy. There is growing evidence that the use of high-dose therapy with alkylating agents and/or anthracyclines, followed by autologous stem cell transplantation, is associated with an increased risk of secondary myelodysplasias and leukaemias, and a cumulative incidence of about 9% at 5 years.[2] However, it is unclear whether this is due to the high-dose therapy or to previous chemotherapy that has caused bone-marrow damage.[2,3]

Radiotherapy is an established cause of secondary malignancy. It remains unclear, however, to what extent the use of chemotherapy combined **with radiotherapy** could have an additive effect on the risk of secondary leukaemias, and how dose and treatment regimen influence this effect.[3] Similarly, the role of combined modality treatment in the development of secondary solid tumours has not been defined, even though the radiation-enhancing effect of some antineoplastics is known and used in chemoradiation regimens for this reason.[4]

In many cases the risk of secondary malignancy is far less than that of undertreating, or of failing to treat, the primary disease.[2,4] However, secondary malignancies may be more resistant to treatment and more aggressive than primary disease,[3,18] and the risk of inducing malignant neoplasia is certainly a consideration in the use of alkylating agents and podophyllotoxin derivatives to treat non-malignant disease,[3] and is an increasing challenge in the design of suitable treatment regimens for primary neoplastic disease.


1. Curtis RE, *et al.* Risk of leukemia associated with the first course of cancer treatment: an analysis of the surveillance, epidemiology, and end results program experience. *J Natl Cancer Inst* 1984; **72:** 531–44.
2. Kollmannsberger C, *et al.* Risk of secondary myeloid leukemia and myelodysplastic syndrome following standard-dose chemotherapy or high-dose chemotherapy with stem cell support in patients with potentially curable malignancies. *J Cancer Res Clin Oncol* 1998; **124:** 207–14.
3. Leone G, *et al.* Therapy related leukemias: susceptibility, prevention and treatment. *Leuk Lymphoma* 2001; **41:** 255–76.
4. Travis LB. Therapy-associated solid tumors. *Acta Oncol* 2002; **41:** 323–33.
5. Hawkins MM, *et al.* Epipodophyllotoxins, alkylating agents, and radiation and risk of secondary leukaemia after childhood cancer. *BMJ* 1992; **304:** 951–8.
6. Neglia JP, *et al.* Second malignant neoplasms in five-year survivors of childhood cancer: Childhood Cancer Survivor Study. *J Natl Cancer Inst* 2001; **93:** 618–29.
7. Zumtobel U, *et al.* Widespread cutaneous carcinomas associated with human papillomaviruses 5, 14 and 20 after introduction of methotrexate in two long-term PUVA-treated patients. *Dermatology* 2001; **202:** 127–30.
8. Micallef INM, *et al.* Therapy-related myelodysplasia and secondary acute myelogenous leukemia after high-dose therapy with autologous hematopoietic progenitor-cell support for lymphoid malignancies. *J Clin Oncol* 2000; **18:** 947–55.
9. Van Den Neste E, *et al.* Second primary tumors and immune phenomena after fludarabine or 2-chloro-2′-deoxyadenosine treatment. *Leuk Lymphoma* 2001; **40:** 541–50.
10. Kamel OW, *et al.* Brief report: reversible lymphomas associated with Epstein-Barr virus occurring during methotrexate therapy for rheumatoid arthritis and dermatomyositis. *N Engl J Med* 1993; **328:** 1317–21.
11. Travis LB, *et al.* Risk of leukemia after platinum-based chemotherapy for ovarian cancer. *N Engl J Med* 1999; **340:** 351–7.
12. Travis LB, *et al.* Treatment-associated leukemia following testicular cancer. *J Natl Cancer Inst* 2000; **92:** 1165–71.
13. Kaldor JM, *et al.* Leukemia following chemotherapy for ovarian cancer. *N Engl J Med* 1990; **322:** 1–6.
14. Levine MN, *et al.* Randomized trial of intensive cyclophosphamide, epirubicin, and fluorouracil chemotherapy compared with cyclophosphamide, methotrexate, and fluorouracil in premenopausal women with node-positive breast cancer. *J Clin Oncol* 1998; **16:** 2651–8.
15. Kaldor JM, *et al.* Leukemia following Hodgkin's disease. *N Engl J Med* 1990; **322:** 7–13.
16. Lee IP, Dixon RL. Mutagenicity, carcinogenicity and teratogenicity of procarbazine. *Mutat Res* 1978; **55:** 1–14.
17. Smith MA, *et al.* Secondary leukemia or myelodysplastic syndrome after treatment with epipodophyllotoxins. *J Clin Oncol* 1999; **17:** 569–77.
18. Neugut AI, *et al.* Poor survival of treatment-related acute nonlymphocytic leukemia. *JAMA* 1990; **264:** 1006–8.


EFFECTS ON CHROMOSOMES. Visible chromosome gaps, breaks, and structural rearrangements are found in blood lymphocytes from patients who have received substantial doses of combination chemotherapy, and the changes persist for years after the end of treatment. A more sensitive, if transient, measure of genetic damage is the increased rate of sister chromatid exchange (SCE) that occurs with even quite small doses of cytotoxic drugs.[1] Evidence from a study[2] in patients given chlorambucil suggests that as the dose increases so the capacity of the cells to cope with induced genetic damage is progressively exceeded, and thus SCE frequency reflects cumulative toxicity throughout the course of treatment.

In patients who develop acute myeloid leukaemia following alkylating agent therapy, the most common chromosomal losses involve deletions of chromosome 13, loss of the entire chromosomes 5 and 7, or deletions of part or the whole long arm of chromosomes 5 and 7. Molecular alterations of the suppressor gene p53 have also been found.[3] Balanced translocations, usually involving chromosomes 11 and 21, are associated with treatment using topoisomerase II inhibitors.[3,4]

See also under Effects on Reproductive Potential, below.


1. Anonymous. Drugs that can cause cancer. *Lancet* 1984; **i:** 261–2.
2. Palmer RG, *et al.* Chlorambucil-induced chromosome damage to human lymphocytes is dose-dependent and cumulative. *Lancet* 1984; **i:** 246–9.
3. Leone G, *et al.* Therapy related leukemias: susceptibility, prevention and treatment. *Leuk Lymphoma* 2001; **41:** 255–76.
4. Rowley JD, Olney HJ. International workshop on the relationship of prior therapy to balanced chromosome aberrations in therapy-related myelodysplastic syndromes and acute leukemia: overview report. *Genes Chromosomes Cancer* 2002; **33:** 331–45.


**Effects on the bladder.** Cyclophosphamide (p.540) and ifosfamide (p.561) are the antineoplastics most frequently associated with adverse effects on the bladder, but see also Busulfan, p.532, Chlorambucil, p.536, and Mitomycin, p.574.

**Effects on the blood.** BONE-MARROW DEPRESSION. Bone-marrow depression, or myelosuppression, is common to the majority of cytotoxic antineoplastics, and is probably the single most important dose-limiting adverse effect, although its significance has been somewhat reduced in recent years by improvements in supportive care, including the availability of colony-stimulating factors and the development of techniques such as peripheral blood stem cell transfusion.

The formation and development of blood cells takes place in the bone marrow. A common progenitor, the pluripotent stem cell, gives rise to 3 major cell lines from which red cells, white cells, and platelets are derived. All the cellular elements of blood may be affected by antineoplastic therapy, resulting in pancytopenia, but in many cases the toxicity appears to be greater for particular cell types. In addition, the different cell types have very different half-lives in the circulation. White blood cells and platelets tend to have the shortest half-lives in circulation. Hence the most usual manifestation of bone-marrow depression is leucopenia with a consequent increased risk of infection, and thrombocytopenia is also fairly common. Erythrocytes have the longest life (about 120 days) and anaemia is somewhat less frequent, and may be associated with megaloblastic changes in the bone marrow.

The onset, duration, and severity of bone-marrow depression vary considerably with different antineoplastics. Little or only relatively mild myelosuppression seems to occur with conventional regimens of bleomycin (p.530), mitotane (p.575), streptozocin (p.584), and vincristine (p.592). Megaloblastic anaemia occurring with hydroxycarbamide (p.559) may be treatable by blood transfusions, if necessary, without interrupting therapy.

Many of the alkylating agents are associated with severe and sometimes irreversible bone-marrow depression, particularly at high doses. Busulfan (p.532) and the nitrosoureas such as carmustine (p.535) pose a particular problem because the nadir of white-blood cell and platelet counts may not be reached for up to 6 weeks after a dose. These drugs affect both resting and actively cycling stem cells.

Many antimetabolites are also associated with myelosuppression and some such as cytarabine (p.543) may produce megaloblastic anaemia in addition to leucopenia and thrombocytopenia. Cytarabine has a biphasic effect on granulocytes, producing an initial nadir about 7 to 9 days after a dose, and a second and more severe one after 15 to 24 days. Unlike alkylating agents, antimetabolites affect actively proliferating, but not resting, stem cells. Cladribine (p.539) and fludarabine (p.553) produce a prolonged and profound lymphopenia.

Of the other drugs mitomycin (p.574) and procarbazine (p.581) in particular have both been associated with prolonged, delayed myelosuppression. Recovery from the bone-marrow toxicity of mitomycin may take months and about 25% of cases do not recover. Cisplatin (p.538) and anthracyclines such as doxorubicin (p.548) can cause severe myelosuppression, although other toxic effects may be more important in determining dose; myelosuppression is dose-limiting with carboplatin (p.534). Cisplatin-induced renal toxicity may lead to anaemia by decreasing erythropoietin production. Bone-marrow depression is also a significant adverse effect of vinblastine (p.591) vindesine, and vinorelbine, although the effects of vincristine on the bone marrow are much less marked, as mentioned above. Neutropenia is common with the camptothecin derivatives irinotecan (p.564) and topotecan (p.589) and can be dose-limiting. The monoclonal antibody alemtuzumab (p.526) and the conjugated antibody gemtuzumab ozogamicin (p.558) also produce severe and prolonged myelosuppression.

For further details, see under the individual monographs. For the management of bone-marrow depression, including discussion of the appropriate thresholds for treatment see under Treatment of Adverse Effects, below.

See also Effects on Immune Response, below.

**Effects on body-weight.** Although the effects of antineoplastics on the gastrointestinal tract (below) may lead to anorexia, malabsorption, and malnutrition, and hence to weight loss, antineoplastic therapy for breast cancer has also been associated with weight gain, sometimes dramatic.[1] Weight gain appeared to be more likely in premenopausal women, in those receiving multidrug regimens, and in those treated for longer periods of time. A study of premenopausal women found that reduced physical activity may be a contributing factor to the development of this form of weight gain.[2] Weight gain was also noted after long-term follow-up of paediatric leukaemia patients.[3,4]

Concurrent use of corticosteroids may also lead to weight gain.


1. Demark-Wahnefried W, *et al.* Why women gain weight with adjuvant chemotherapy for breast cancer. *J Clin Oncol* 1993; **11:** 1418–29.
2. Demark-Wahnefried W, *et al.* Changes in weight, body composition, and factors influencing energy balance among premenopausal breast cancer patients receiving adjuvant chemotherapy. *J Clin Oncol* 2001; **19:** 2381–9.
3. Birkebæk NH, Clausen N. Height and weight pattern up to 20 years after treatment for acute lymphoblastic leukaemia. *Arch Dis Child* 1998; **79:** 161–4.
4. Nysom K, *et al.* Degree of fatness after treatment for acute lymphoblastic leukaemia in childhood. *J Clin Endocrinol Metab* 1999; **84:** 4591–6.


**Effects on bones and joints.** Osteoporosis occurs as both an acute[1] and late complication of chemotherapy, but as multicomponent regimens are used and because the pathogenesis of osteoporosis is likely to be multifactorial, it is difficult to assess the impact of individual drugs.[2] However, chemotherapy that causes hypogonadism will decrease bone mineral density in the majority of patients.[2] This includes regimens for a variety of neoplasms, including breast, prostate and testicular cancers, lymphomas, and haematological malignancies. In particular, regimens containing cyclophosphamide, chlormethine, busulfan, or procarbazine may cause ovarian insufficiency and therefore have the potential to lead to osteoporosis in females. Males may be protected from the effects of pronounced hypogonadism, as the cells that produce testosterone only replicate slowly.[2]

In addition, several drugs may exert direct effects on the bone. Methotrexate has been found to increase bone resorption and inhibit bone formation to produce a massive uncoupling of bone turnover.[2] Other drugs, including doxorubicin, have been shown to be toxic to bone in *animals*.[2] High-dose conditioning regimens used for bone marrow transplantation may have a direct dose-dependent toxicity on bone marrow osteoprogenitor cells, contributing to osteopenia.[3]

Corticosteroids are believed to cause bone loss by decreasing osteoblast activity, an effect which may be alleviated by chlorambucil. Surprisingly, corticosteroids have not been implicated in bone loss for most chemotherapy regimens, perhaps because the duration of treatment is short.[2] Nevertheless, osteoporosis and fractures have occurred in young patients with acute lymphoblastic leukaemia, treated with regimens containing high total doses of corticosteroids.[4,5] However, the disease itself, other chemotherapy, and radiotherapy are also likely to be contributory factors in the development of osteopenia in these patients. Osteonecrosis has also been reported with high doses of corticosteroids used in the treatment of leukaemias and solid tumours in adults and children.[4,6,7] Adolescent patients may be at increased risk because their bones are in the process of maturation.[4,6]

A study in children with leukaemia has suggested that the effects of chemotherapy on gastrointestinal and renal handling of nutrients may lead to alterations in calcium and magnesium homoeostasis and hence to abnormal turnover of bone mineral.[8] Renal phosphate loss following damage to the renal tubule caused by ifosfamide can lead to osteomalacia.[2]


1. Arikoski P, *et al.* Reduced bone density at completion of chemotherapy for a malignancy. *Arch Dis Child* 1999; **80:** 143–8.
2. Pfeilschifter J, Diel IJ. Osteoporosis due to cancer treatment: pathogenesis and management. *J Clin Oncol* 2000; **18:** 1570–93.
3. Banfi A, *et al.* High-dose chemotherapy shows a dose-dependent toxicity to bone marrow osteoprogenitors: a mechanism for post-bone marrow transplantation osteopenia. *Cancer* 2001; **92:** 2419–28.
4. Strauss AJ, *et al.* Bony morbidity in children treated for acute lymphoblastic leukemia. *J Clin Oncol* 2001; **19:** 3066–72.
5. van der Sluis IM, *et al.* Altered bone mineral density and body composition, and increased fracture risk in childhood acute lymphoblastic leukemia. *J Pediatr* 2002; **141:** 204–10.
6. Mattano LA, *et al.* Osteonecrosis as a complication of treating acute lymphoblastic leukemia in children: a report from the Children's Cancer Group. *J Clin Oncol* 2000; **18:** 3262–72.
7. Winquist EW, *et al.* Nontraumatic osteonecrosis after chemotherapy for testicular cancer: a systematic review. *Am J Clin Oncol* 2001; **24:** 603–6.
8. Atkinson SA, *et al.* Mineral homeostasis and bone mass in children treated for acute lymphoblastic leukemia. *J Pediatr* 1989; **114:** 793–800.


**Effects on the cardiovascular system.** THROMBOEMBOLISM. Patients with cancer are at increased risk of thromboembolic disease, and thrombosis can be the earliest clinical sign of malignancy.[1] The risk of thromboembolism may be further increased by the use of antineoplastics. Deep-vein thrombosis and pulmonary embolism have been reported with a variety of chemotherapeutic regimens. Trials of patients with breast cancer have found that adjuvant chemotherapy can significantly increase the risk of venous thromboembolism.[2] An increase in venous thromboembolism, including CNS thromboses, has also been found with the use of asparaginase in the treatment of acute lymphoblastic leukaemia[2] (see also Effects on the Blood, under Asparaginase, p.528). Arterial thrombosis, including acute myocardial infarction, angina, stroke, and peripheral artery thrombosis, has also been reported with various regimens.[2] Mechanisms proposed for the possible role of antineoplastics in these effects include activation of coagulation, suppression of anticoagulant proteins and fibrinolysis, and a direct toxic effect on vascular endothelium.[1,2]

Several reports of arterial and venous thromboembolism have implicated combinations of bleomycin with cisplatin and another drug such as a vinca alkaloid or etoposide.[3-5] Such combinations, widely used for testicular cancer, have also been implicated in producing vasospastic reactions including angina[6] and Raynaud's syndrome,[7,8] although there is no evidence of a relationship between thromboembolism and vasospasm.[3]

In men with germ cell cancer there is some evidence that those with liver metastases, or receiving high-dose dexamethasone as antiemetic therapy, are at increased risk of thromboembolic complications.[9]

Treatment of venous thrombosis usually consists of the initiation of heparin therapy and long-term secondary prophylaxis with warfarin (or perhaps a low-molecular-weight heparin[10]), but patients with cancer may be at greater risk of recurrent thrombosis. Patients with arterial thrombosis may require heparin and warfarin, or anti-platelet therapy.[11]

Thromboembolic complications may also be associated with the indwelling catheters used to provide vascular access for antineoplastic therapy;[12] low-dose warfarin prophylaxis may reduce the risk.[13]

For a discussion of the cardiotoxicity of antineoplastics see Effects on the Heart, below.


1. Falanga A, Donati MB. Pathogenesis of thrombosis in patients with malignancy. *Int J Hematol* 2001; **73:** 137–44.
2. Lee AYY, Levine MN. The thrombophilic state induced by therapeutic agents in the cancer patient. *Semin Thromb Hemost* 1999; **25:** 137–45.
3. Cantwell BMJ, *et al.* Thromboembolic events during combination chemotherapy for germ cell malignancy. *Lancet* 1988; **ii:** 1086–7.
4. Hall MR, *et al.* Thromboembolic events during combination chemotherapy for germ cell malignancy. *Lancet* 1988; **ii:** 1259.
5. Garstin IWH, *et al.* Arterial thrombosis after treatment with bleomycin and cisplatin. *BMJ* 1990; **300:** 1018.
6. Rodriguez J, *et al.* Angina pectoris following cisplatin, etoposide, and bleomycin in a patient with advanced testicular cancer. *Ann Pharmacother* 1995; **29:** 138–9.
7. Vogelzang NJ, *et al.* Raynaud's phenomenon: a common toxicity after combination chemotherapy for testicular cancer. *Ann Intern Med* 1981; **95:** 288–92.
8. Pechère M, *et al.* Fingertip necrosis during chemotherapy with bleomycin, vincristine and methotrexate for HIV-related Kaposi's sarcoma. *Br J Dermatol* 1996; **134:** 378–9.
9. Weijl NI, *et al.* Thromboembolic events during chemotherapy for germ cell cancer: a cohort study and review of the literature. *J Clin Oncol* 2000; **18:** 2169–78.
10. Lee AYY, *et al.* Low-molecular-weight heparin versus a coumarin for the prevention of recurrent venous thromboembolism in patients with cancer. *N Engl J Med* 2003; **349:** 146–53.
11. Sutherland DE, *et al.* Thromboembolic complications of cancer: epidemiology, pathogenesis, diagnosis, and treatment. *Am J Hematol* 2003; **72:** 43–52.
12. Monreal M, Davant E. Thrombotic complications of central venous catheters in cancer patients. *Acta Haematol (Basel)* 2001; **106:** 69–72.
13. Bern MM, *et al.* Very low doses of warfarin can prevent thrombosis in central venous catheters: a randomized prospective trial. *Ann Intern Med* 1990; **112:** 423–8.


**Effects on electrolytes.** Fluid and electrolyte disturbances frequently occur in patients with cancer.[1] These can be caused by the disease process, or adverse effects of treatment such as surgery, chemotherapy, antibacterials and diuretics. Mechanisms of chemotherapy-induced electrolyte disturbances include loss of appetite, gastrointestinal electrolyte loss due to vomiting and diarrhoea, impaired intestinal absorption due to mucosal damage, direct nephrotoxicity causing renal electrolyte loss, and a syndrome of inappropriate antidiuretic hormone secretion or a condition resembling it. Hypoparathyroidism, which may be a complication of neck surgery, also affects electrolyte balance and is associated with hyperphosphataemia and hypocalcaemia. As well as the acute signs and symptoms of electrolyte disturbances, changes in electrolyte homoeostasis may result in abnormal bone turnover (see Effects on Bones and Joints, above). Release of the contents of cells destroyed by chemotherapy is well-known to be associated with hyperuricaemia, hyperphosphataemia, hyperkalaemia, and hypocalcaemia (see Tumour Lysis Syndrome, below).

Disturbances of electrolyte homoeostasis have been reported particularly with cisplatin (p.538), cyclophosphamide (p.541), ifosfamide (p.561), and vinblastine (p.591).


1. Kapoor M, Chan GZ. Fluid and electrolyte abnormalities. *Crit Care Clin* 2001; **17:** 503–29.


**Effects on the gastrointestinal tract.** Apart from anorexia, and nausea and vomiting (see below), many antineoplastics produce gastrointestinal disturbances. Mucosal inflammation (mucositis), notably as stomatitis and sometimes proctitis, is quite common, as are mucosal cellular changes, xerostomia, impaired absorption, and diarrhoea. In some cases gastrointestinal damage may progress to ulceration, haemorrhage, and perforation. Antimetabolites affecting pyrimidine metabolism, such as cytarabine (p.543) and fluorouracil (p.554), and the antifolates such as methotrexate (p.568), seem to be particularly associated with severe gastrointestinal effects, especially at high doses, but there appear to be few antineoplastics that do not cause some degree of gastrointestinal disturbance. Irinotecan (p.564) can produce both an initial transient diarrhoea related to cholinergic stimulation, and more severe prolonged diarrhoea with a delayed onset, which may be dose-limiting and potentially fatal. Use with radiotherapy may increase the toxicity of some drugs on the gastrointestinal tract. The neutropenia induced by many antineoplastic regimens may lead to secondary gastrointestinal effects, such as stomatitis and gastrointestinal inflammation, associated with infection.

CLOSTRIDIUM DIFFICILE INFECTION. Antineoplastic therapy has occasionally been associated with the development of *Clostridium difficile*-induced gastrointestinal disease, even in the absence of concomitant antibacterial therapy.[1] Most patients had received multiple drug regimens. Methotrexate, fluorouracil, cyclophosphamide, and doxorubicin have all been associated with a number of cases but this may simply reflect the frequency of their use. A retrospective analysis[2] of a group of patients treated for acute leukaemia or receiving bone marrow transplantation found that predictive variables for *C. difficile* diarrhoea included the use of low intensity chemotherapy, but speculated that patients receiving high intensity chemotherapy may be subjected to more strict isolation and infection control procedures, thereby reducing the risk of nosocomial transmission. Another review[3] of 875 courses of myelosuppressive chemotherapy found 61 episodes of *C. difficile* diarrhoea, and that in 36% of those episodes the patients had received high-dose cytarabine. In 35 of the 61 episodes, patients had also received prior intravenous antibacterials.

For discussion of the treatment of such disease, see Antibiotic-associated Colitis, p.128


1. Anand A, Glatt AE. Clostridium difficile infection associated with antineoplastic chemotherapy: a review. *Clin Infect Dis* 1993; **17:** 109–13.
2. Hornbuckle K, *et al.* Determination and validation of a predictive model for Clostridium difficile diarrhea in hospitalized oncology patients. *Ann Oncol* 1998; **9:** 307–11.
3. Gorschlüter M, *et al.* Clostridium difficile infection in patients with neutropenia. *Clin Infect Dis* 2001; **33:** 786–91.


MUCOSITIS. The suffering associated with oral mucositis is by far the worst part of treatment for many patients undergoing curative chemotherapy or bone marrow transplantation, and for those undergoing oral radiotherapy.[1,2] Apart from pain and dysphagia the ulcerated mucosa provides a portal of entry for infection; loss of weight and malnutrition may further impair immune function, and if symptoms are severe enough the treatment cycle may have to be interrupted. Before the patient starts any intensive chemotherapy or local or systemic radiotherapy the oral cavity must be assessed with a view to eliminating sources of infection and chronic irritation. For comment on the prophylaxis and treatment of mucositis, see under Treatment of Adverse Effects, below.


1. Calman FMB, Langdon J. Oral complications of cancer. *BMJ* 1991; **302:** 485–6.
2. Sonis ST. Mucositis as a biological process: a new hypothesis for the development of chemotherapy-induced stomatotoxicity. *Oral Oncol* 1998; **34:** 39–43.


NAUSEA AND VOMITING. Nausea and vomiting are common side-effects of antineoplastic therapy, and for many patients, represent a major drawback to treatment. Once experienced, anticipatory vomiting may occur at the sight of medical staff, or a needle. The problem may be severe enough in some cases to hinder or completely prevent further treatment.

Antineoplastic or cytotoxic drugs may induce vomiting by both a central action on the chemoreceptor trigger zone and a peripheral action on the gastrointestinal tract. Several neurotransmitters have been implicated over the years including acetylcholine, histamine, enkephalins, dopamine, and serotonin or 5-hydroxytryptamine (5-HT). The cerebral cortex is probably responsible for anticipatory vomiting. Antineoplastics may not all induce emesis by a common pathway, but 5-$HT_3$-receptor mechanisms are clearly important in the pathogenesis of *acute* cisplatin-associated vomiting. This was suspected when the antiemetic metoclopramide, a dopamine antagonist, was found to have serotonin (5-HT) antagonist activity at the high doses used against cisplatin emesis and confirmed when specific 5-$HT_3$ antagonists such as ondansetron proved to be effective. Different mechanisms are probably involved in *delayed* emesis since 5-$HT_3$ antagonists are less effective.

Some patients are more susceptible to emesis than others. The emetic potential of antineoplastics also varies in terms of severity and incidence, and may depend to some extent on the dose, route, and schedule of administration. Some combination therapy has resulted in a higher incidence of vomiting than would be expected from the constituents.

- Vomiting may be *very severe* with cisplatin, dacarbazine, dactinomycin, chlormethine, high-dose cyclophosphamide, and streptozocin, and occurs in most patients.
- *Moderate* vomiting is likely with the taxanes, doxorubicin, and more modest doses of cyclophosphamide, and high-dose methotrexate.
- Vinca alkaloids, fluorouracil, lower doses of methotrexate, chlorambucil, bleomycin, and etoposide have *low* emetogenic potential.

The *onset and duration* of vomiting also varies from drug to drug. With cisplatin the onset may be between 4 and 8 hours following a dose, while the duration may be up to 48 hours or occasionally even longer; a persistent feeling of nausea, and sometimes vomiting, lasting for several days may also occur. After chlormethine, vomiting may begin within a half to 2 hours, whereas after cyclophosphamide there may be a latent interval of 9 to 18 hours, but in both cases vomiting is generally less prolonged than with cisplatin. Acute emesis (that occurring within 24 hours) has generally been easier to control than delayed emesis (that occurring more than 24 hours after chemotherapy) or anticipatory emesis.

The management of chemotherapy-induced nausea and vomiting is discussed on p.1245.

**Effects on the heart.** The cardiotoxicity of antineoplastics has been reviewed.[1] Cardiotoxicity is the major dose-limiting toxicity with anthracyclines such as doxorubicin and daunorubicin, manifesting most seriously as drug-induced cardiomyopathy, which is frequently fatal, and for which no specific treatment exists. Some of the newer anthracycline analogues such as epirubicin or idarubicin were developed to be less toxic to the heart, although this has not always been easy to prove in controlled studies. Cardiotoxicity has also been associated with other antineoplastics, although less frequently. High-dose cyclophosphamide or ifosfamide may produce myocarditis, arrhythmias, and congestive heart failure, sometimes delayed by up to 2 weeks, while fluorouracil has been associated with angina pectoris and myocardial infarction, perhaps due to a combination of vasospastic effects and activation of coagulation. Amsacrine has been associated with arrhythmias, sometimes fatal. Occasional reports of cardiotoxicity associated with busulfan, carmustine, cisplatin, cytarabine, etoposide, mitomycin, paclitaxel, pentostatin, and vincristine also exist.

For a discussion of the thromboembolic events seen with antineoplastics see Effects on the Cardiovascular System, above.


1. Pai VB, Nahata MC. Cardiotoxicity of chemotherapeutic agents: incidence, treatment and prevention. *Drug Safety* 2000; **22:** 263–302.


**Effects on immune response.** Lymphocytes are produced by stem cells in the bone marrow and at other sites, including the thymus, and are involved in humoral and cell-mediated immunity. Most antineoplastics have a depressant effect on bone marrow (see Effects on the Blood, above) and many have immunosuppressant properties although the degree of suppression varies considerably and may depend on the dose and schedule used. Immunosuppression decreases the patient's resistance to infection and has been implicated in the development of malignancies. Response to vaccines may also be reduced, and there is a possibility of generalised infections with live viral vaccines (see Interactions, p.1606).

For a discussion on the effects of immunosuppressant therapy on the immune response and the infections associated with it, see Corticosteroids, p.1070.

**Effects on the kidneys.** Nephrotoxicity is well-recognised as an adverse effect of cisplatin (p.538), ifosfamide (p.561), and methotrexate (p.569), but renal toxicity may occur with other antineoplastics including the nitrosoureas, mitomycin (due to haemolytic-uraemic syndrome), azacitidine, gemcitabine, and pentostatin.[1]


1. Kintzel PE. Anticancer drug-induced kidney disorders: incidence, prevention and management. *Drug Safety* 2001; **24:** 19–38.


**Effects on the liver.** Occasional reports of hepatotoxicity exist for many antineoplastics including aminoglutethimide (p.526), busulfan (p.532), dacarbazine (p.544), dactinomycin (p.545), doxorubicin (p.548), floxuridine (p.553), flutamide (p.556), hydroxycarbamide (p.559), methotrexate (p.569), mitomycin (p.574), mitoxantrone (p.575), tamoxifen (p.585), and tioguanine (p.588). However, the relationship of the drug to the adverse effect is not always easy to establish.

An early but detailed review suggested that methotrexate, mercaptopurine, cytarabine, carmustine, streptozocin, asparaginase, and plicamycin could probably be classified as hepatotoxic. There was considered to be insufficient evidence to classify fluorouracil, cyclophosphamide, busulfan, dacarbazine, the anthracyclines, the vinca alkaloids, and the podophyllum derivatives as hepatotoxic, although this classification was not definitive.[1] Hepatic veno-occlusive disease has occurred following the use of high doses of chemotherapy for conditioning regimens before bone marrow transplantation.[2] Chemotherapy used in combination or with radiotherapy may also increase the risk of hepatotoxicity.[2] Liver toxicity may not be confined to patients: one report described 3 cases of liver damage in nurses working on an oncology ward.[3]


1. Ménard DB, *et al.* Antineoplastic agents and the liver. *Gastroenterology* 1980; **78:** 142–64.
2. King PD, Perry MC. Hepatotoxicity of chemotherapy. *Oncologist* 2001; **6:** 162–76.
3. Sotaniemi EA, *et al.* Liver damage in nurses handling cytostatic agents. *Acta Med Scand* 1983; **214:** 181–9.


**Effects on the lungs.** Lung injury leading to pulmonary fibrosis occurs in about 10% of all patients who receive bleomycin, being fatal in 1 to 2%. Clinically, the reaction usually presents several months after completion of therapy as non-productive cough and dyspnoea. The reaction is dose-related, being more likely at total doses over 400 000 international units (400 USP units), although it has occurred at much lower doses, and is more common in elderly patients. Injury may be exacerbated by the use of combination chemotherapy regimens and radiotherapy, and supplemental oxygen given even years after the use of bleomycin may precipitate pulmonary oedema.[1] Hypersensitivity pneumonitis, which is more amenable to treatment, has also been reported.[2]

Pulmonary damage has also been reported with an increasing number of antineoplastics apart from bleomycin.[1,3] Among the alkylating agents cyclophosphamide has been reported to produce lung injury in less than 1% of cases, although this may be increased where it is a component of combination regimens or given with radiotherapy. Busulfan may produce lung toxicity including insidious pulmonary fibrosis in as many as 4% of patients, usually developing several years after initiation of therapy, and with increased risk the longer that therapy lasts. A few reports exist of interstitial pneumonitis and fibrosis associated with chlorambucil and melphalan, but these appear to be extremely rare. The prognosis in patients with alkylating-agent-induced fibrosis is often poor, with mortality rates of 50% or more.

The antimetabolite methotrexate can produce symptoms similar to hypersensitivity pneumonitis in up to 7% of patients, sometimes with pleuritis and acute respiratory failure due to pulmonary oedema, but it is not clear whether a true hypersensitivity mechanism is involved, and symptoms are usually reversible even without stopping therapy. High-dose cytarabine has also been associated with pulmonary oedema.

Other antineoplastics known to be associated with pulmonary toxicity include mitomycin (usually in less than 10% of patients though the incidence may be much higher in combination regimens); the vinca alkaloids (generally in combination, and usually producing acute respiratory failure); chlorozotocin; procarbazine; and possibly teniposide. The nitrosoureas, and particularly carmustine, have also emerged as pulmonary toxins.

Carmustine has been associated with an insidious chronic pulmonary fibrosis, which in some early studies occurred in as many as 30% of patients and had a high mortality. Symptoms are associated particularly with cumulative doses in excess of about 1.4 g/m$^2$, although toxicity has occurred at cumulative doses as low as 240 mg/m$^2$. The onset of symptoms may be very delayed: some workers reported fibrosis occurring up to 17 years after treatment in patients who received carmustine as children.[4] Potentially life-threatening pneumonitis has occurred in patients receiving thoracic radiotherapy in association with gemcitabine (p.558).


1. Abid SH, *et al.* Radiation-induced and chemotherapy-induced pulmonary injury. *Curr Opin Oncol* 2001; **13:** 242–8.
2. Holoye PY, *et al.* Bleomycin hypersensitivity pneumonitis. *Ann Intern Med* 1978; **88:** 47–9.
3. Twohig KJ, Matthay RA. Pulmonary effects of cytotoxic agents other than bleomycin. *Clin Chest Med* 1990; **11:** 31–54.
4. O'Driscoll BR, *et al.* Active lung fibrosis up to 17 years after chemotherapy with carmustine (BCNU) in childhood. *N Engl J Med* 1990; **323:** 378–82.


**Effects on mental function.** Combination chemotherapy has been associated with psychiatric morbidity (anxiety, depression, behavioural changes) in both adults[1] and children.[2] It has been pointed out that patients receiving cancer chemotherapy inevitably suffer emotional distress, associated in part with the adverse effects of treatment. Patients should be fully informed of aims and likely outcomes of treatment, and adverse effects minimised, in order to keep emotional distress to a minimum.[3]

A number of individual antineoplastics have been associated with mental symptoms, including methotrexate (p.569), mitotane (p.575), and the vinca alkaloids (p.591). In many cases such symptoms can be attributed to direct central neurotoxicity (see also under Effects on the Nervous System, below).


1. Maguire GP, *et al.* Psychiatric morbidity and physical toxicity associated with adjuvant chemotherapy after mastectomy. *BMJ* 1980; **281:** 1179–80.
2. Dolgin MJ, *et al.* Behavioral distress in pediatric patients with cancer receiving chemotherapy. *Pediatrics* 1989; **84:** 103–10.
3. Brinkley D. Emotional distress during cancer chemotherapy. *BMJ* 1983; **286:** 663–4.


**Effects on the nervous system.** Neurotoxic effects have been reported for many antineoplastics, including altretamine (p.526), asparaginase (p.528), busulfan (p.532), carboplatin (p.534), carmustine (p.535), chlorambucil (p.536), chlormethine (p.537), cisplatin (p.538), cladribine (p.539), cytarabine (p.543), etanidazole (p.551), etoposide (p.551), fludarabine (p.553), fluorouracil (p.555), gemcitabine (p.558), hydroxycarbamide (p.559), ifosfamide (p.561), lomustine (p.565), methotrexate (p.569), mitotane (p.575), mitoxantrone (p.575), oxaliplatin (p.577), paclitaxel (p.577), pentostatin (p.579), procarbazine (p.581), tegafur (p.586), vinblastine (p.591), vincristine (p.592), and vindesine (p.593). In some cases these effects may be associated with particular routes such as the intrathecal. See under the individual monographs for further details. Radiotherapy can also cause damage to the nervous system so combination of the two modalities may lead to additive effects.

Reviews.


1. Verstappen CCP, *et al.* Neurotoxic complications of chemotherapy in patients with cancer: clinical signs and optimal management. *Drugs* 2003; **63:** 1549–63.


EFFECTS ON THE EARS. Several antineoplastics have been associated with ototoxicity,[1] including vincristine and vinblastine, but cisplatin in particular is associated with high-frequency hearing loss and tinnitus. In addition, agents such as the nitrogen mustards and bleomycin are potentially ototoxic.


1. Seligmann H, *et al.* Drug-induced tinnitus and other hearing disorders. *Drug Safety* 1996; **14:** 198–212.


**Effects on reproductive potential.** CHROMOSOMES. If patients are fertile after treatment with antineoplastics, no significant increase has been seen in fetal chromosome damage, fetal abnormality, or the miscarriage rate. A review[1] of reports of survivors of *childhood cancers* found that adverse pregnancy outcomes were limited to particular groups of survivors. Female survivors of Wilms' tumours who had been treated with abdominal radiation, with or without chemotherapy, appeared to be at increased risk of complications including miscarriage, low birth-weight neonates, and neonatal death. After treatment of childhood Hodgkin's disease using both radiotherapy and chemotherapy, female survivors and partners of male survivors might be at increased risk of miscarriage; however, treatment with radiotherapy or chemotherapy alone did not increase this risk. For other cancers, data was more limited, but suggested that the risk of adverse pregnancy outcomes was not increased in survivors.

Regarding the risk of congenital abnormalities in the offspring of survivors of childhood cancers, most studies have shown no excess of major or minor malformations.[1] There was also no evidence that the risk of cancer is increased in the offspring. However, because of the small numbers in many studies and heterogeneity regarding treatments used, it is possible that effects of individual drugs could have been masked. Long-term follow-up is needed as increasing numbers of children survive to adulthood following successful chemotherapy.

For *adult patients*, there is also a lack of evidence of adverse pregnancy outcomes and congenital abnormalities in offspring following chemotherapy. In a large series[2] of women treated with methotrexate, alone or in combination, for gestational trophoblastic tumours, there was no evidence of an increase in adverse outcomes or abnormalities, although women who had received three or more drugs in combination were less likely to have a live birth. A large case-control study carried out in Canada, and involving over 85 000 parents of children with congenital anomalies, also has failed to confirm a higher incidence of congenital abnormality in the offspring of patients treated with radiotherapy or alkylating agents.[3] However, despite these generally reassuring results, it has been suggested that women should delay conception for a year after cessation of chemotherapy to allow mature ova that might have been damaged to be eliminated.[4]

See also Effects on Chromosomes under Carcinogenicity, above.


1. Blatt J. Pregnancy outcome in long-term survivors of childhood cancer. *Med Pediatr Oncol* 1999; **33:** 29–33.
2. Rustin GJS, *et al.* Pregnancy after cytotoxic chemotherapy for gestational trophoblastic tumours. *BMJ* 1984; **288:** 103–6.
3. Dodds L, *et al.* Case-control study of congenital anomalies in children of cancer patients. *BMJ* 1993; **307:** 164–8.
4. Walden PAM, Bagshawe KD. Pregnancies after chemotherapy for gestational trophoblastic tumours. *Lancet* 1979; **ii:** 1241.


GONADS. The effects of cytotoxic drugs on the gonads have been reviewed.[1-3] In male patients, antineoplastic drugs may damage the seminiferous tubules, resulting in testicular atrophy with decreased sperm count and motility. Testosterone secretion may also be reduced after damage to Leydig cells. Chlorambucil, cyclophosphamide, chlormethine, busulfan, procarbazine, and the nitrosoureas have all been associated with testicular germ cell depletion. The total cumulative dose and the duration of treatment are important factors determining the degree of damage. Methotrexate, fluorouracil, and mercaptopurine appear less toxic than alkylating agents.

In women, cytotoxic drugs act on the ovary to produce loss of primordial follicles with failure of ovulation, oligomenorrhoea or amenorrhoea, and failure of endocrine function resulting in loss of libido and menopausal symptoms. As in men, reports of gonadal dysfunction are associated particularly with alkylating agents. The degree of damage and its reversibility depend partly on the drug and its dose but more on the age of the woman at the time of treatment, with older women (35 to 40 or over) being more sensitive, probably a reflection of the decrease in oocyte numbers with age. Ovarian suppression with oral contraceptives to protect the ovary from damage has been tried, but its effectiveness is not confirmed. Gonadotrophin-releasing hormone analogues are also under investigation for their potential protective effects.

Severe gonadal dysfunction in both men and women has been associated with combination chemotherapy regimens for Hodgkin's disease. Chlormethine and procarbazine are thought to be mainly responsible for the infertility produced. There is some evidence that the ABVD regimen (doxorubicin, bleomycin, vinblastine, and dacarbazine) results in less damage to gonadal cells than the MOPP regimen (chlormethine, vincristine, procarbazine, and prednisone). Prolonged gonadal dysfunction has also been seen in patients given combination chemotherapy for acute lymphoblastic leukaemia; girls appear to be at less risk than boys, especially if treated in the prepubertal period.


1. Goldman S, Johnson FL. Effects of chemotherapy and irradiation on the gonads. *Endocrinol Metab Clin North Am* 1993; **22:** 617–29.
2. Kovacs GT, Stern K. Reproductive aspects of cancer treatment: an update. *Med J Aust* 1999; **170:** 495–7.
3. Thomson AB, *et al.* Late reproductive sequelae following treatment of childhood cancer and options for fertility preservation. *Best Pract Res Clin Endocrinol Metab* 2002; **16:** 311–34.


SEXUAL FUNCTION. Loss of libido and decline in sexual performance seem to be relatively common in men receiving combination chemotherapy,[1,2] and may persist after chemotherapy has ended.[1] However, it may sometimes be difficult to distinguish the effects of chemotherapy from those of the disease and the patient's reaction to it: at least one study has shown that gonadal function is disturbed in patients with Hodgkin's disease before treatment.[2] Erectile dysfunction can also result from local damage caused by pelvic surgery or irradiation.[3] Evidence for decreased libido in women is harder to find, but failure of endocrine function after chemotherapy may lead to loss of libido and menopausal symptoms.[4]


1. Chapman RM, *et al.* Cyclical combination chemotherapy and gonadal function: retrospective study in males. *Lancet* 1979; **i:** 285–9.
2. Chapman RM, *et al.* Male gonadal dysfunction in Hodgkin's disease: a prospective study. *JAMA* 1981; **245:** 1323–8.
3. Costabile RA. Cancer and male sexual dysfunction. *Oncology (Huntingt)* 2000; **14:** 195–205.
4. Shalet SM. Effects of cancer chemotherapy on gonadal function of patients. *Cancer Treat Rev* 1980; **7:** 141–52.


**Effects on the skin and nails.** Alopecia occurs with many antineoplastics, and may be severe with anthracyclines such as doxorubicin, cyclophosphamide, ifosfamide, etoposide, or teniposide, the taxanes docetaxel and paclitaxel, and topotecan. The alkylating agents and some antibiotic antineoplastics are often associated with hyperpigmentation, most commonly of skin, although pigmentation of nails, hair, and teeth has occurred. Some drugs, such as the taxanes, cause dystrophic changes in the nails. Certain drugs may interact with UV light or x-ray radiation to enhance its effects on the skin and may cause radiation recall, photosensitivity, or, in the case of methotrexate, reactivation of UV light burns. Hypersensitivity to antineoplastics may produce cutaneous reactions including allergic rashes, angioedema, and pruritus. In addition to the above there may be local reactions to irritant and vesicant drugs following extravasation. Finally, certain drugs are associated with specific dermatological reactions: bleomycin may produce hyperkeratotic and sclerotic lesions, dactinomycin is associated with an erythematous papular or pustular rash mimicking septic emboli, fluorouracil may produce inflammation of solar keratoses, and plicamycin is associated with a distinctive flushing phenomenon. A palmar-plantar erythrodysesthesia syndrome has been seen with a number of antineoplastics (see below).

See also Local Toxicity, below. References may also be found under individual monographs.

PALMAR-PLANTAR ERYTHRODYSESTHESIA SYNDROME. Palmar-plantar erythrodysesthesia (PPE) associated with chemotherapy[1] usually presents as a tingling sensation in the palms and soles, which progresses in a few days to burning pain and well-defined swelling and erythema. In severe cases there is desquamation, ulceration, blistering, and severe pain. The reaction appears to be caused by a direct toxic effect and seems to be dose-dependent, affected by both peak drug concentration and total cumulative dose. The drugs most often associated with PPE are cytarabine (p.543), docetaxel (p.547), doxorubicin (p.548), and fluorouracil (p.555). It has also been reported for capecitabine (p.533), cisplatin (p.538), cyclophosphamide (p.541), and methotrexate (p.569). PPE is usually managed by reducing the drug dose, increasing the dosage interval, or withdrawing the drug, along with symptomatic treatment and wound care. Systemic corticosteroids and pyridoxine have been used in prophylaxis and treatment. Topical dimethyl sulfoxide has been used for PPE caused by liposomal doxorubicin.


1. Nagore E, *et al.* Antineoplastic therapy-induced palmar plantar erythrodysesthesia ('hand-foot') syndrome: incidence, recognition and management. *Am J Clin Dermatol* 2000; **1:** 225–34.


**Hyperuricaemia.** Overproduction of purines is a known complication of antineoplastic therapy and may result in hyperuricaemia (p.412). Hyperuricaemia is also an important part of the tumour lysis syndrome—see below.

**Local toxicity.** Local toxicity due to intravenous cancer chemotherapy may include local irritation, extravasation necrosis, and hypersensitivity.[1] Venous irritation, presenting as vasospasm and pain or endothelial chemical burn of the vessel, resulting in a painful, streaky, long-lasting sterile phlebitis, may be due to the drug, or, as with carmustine, due to the diluent (alcohol). Irritation and phlebitis have been reported particularly with fluorouracil, carmustine, bisantrene, vinorelbine, and chlormethine.

Up to 6% of patients treated with peripheral intravenous chemotherapy may experience extravasation, usually with pain, erythema, and swelling at the site of injection. Severe necrosis requiring surgical intervention may develop, particularly with antibiotic antineoplastics such as doxorubicin. For a discussion of extravasation and its management, including those drugs most commonly associated with problems, see Extravasation, p.496.

Local hypersensitivity reactions, usually self-limiting, may occur: it is important to distinguish such reactions from extravasation. In hypersensitivity reactions there is no swelling at the injection site, and pain is felt as a dull ache along the course of the vein, as opposed to the stinging commonly noted following extravasation.


1. Brigden ML, Barnett JB. Local toxicity of cancer chemotherapy—practical considerations. *Can J Hosp Pharm* 1986; **39:** 96–9.


**Tumour lysis syndrome.** The tumour lysis syndrome represents a biochemical disturbance following massive release of cellular breakdown products from tumour cells sensitive to therapy. The amount of breakdown products is sufficient to overwhelm normal excretory and metabolic mechanisms for their clearance, and the cardinal features of the syndrome are hyperkalaemia, hyperuricaemia, and hyperphosphataemia accompanied by hypocalcaemia. Clinical symptoms may include urate nephropathy or nephrocalcinosis leading to renal impairment, and cardiac arrhythmias associated with the potassium abnormalities. The syndrome is seen particularly when bulky chemosensitive disease is present, and may be more likely in patients with pre-existing renal impairment or hyperuricaemia. The most frequent cases are in patients with Burkitt's or lymphoblastic lymphoma, or an acute leukaemia. Of patients with solid tumours, reports have implicated those with germ-cell tumours, small-cell lung cancer, or neuroblastoma although, surprisingly, the syndrome has also been reported in patients with breast cancer, which is normally less rapidly responsive to chemotherapy.

References.


1. Kalemkerian GP, *et al.* Tumor lysis syndrome in small cell carcinoma and other solid tumors. *Am J Med* 1997; **103:** 363–7.
2. Jeha S. Tumor lysis syndrome. *Semin Hematol* 2001; **38** (suppl 10): 4–8.
3. Baeksgaard L, Sørensen JB. Acute tumor lysis syndrome in solid tumors–a case report and review of the literature. *Cancer Chemother Pharmacol* 2003; **51:** 187–92.


## Treatment of Adverse Effects

Intensive supportive care may be necessary to prevent or control the adverse effects of antineoplastic therapy. Antiemetic therapy should be given to reduce, and if possible prevent, nausea and vomiting, since once experienced it may become a conditioned response, and may not respond to antiemetics. Intensive oral care is desirable to minimise the effects of stomatitis, while corticosteroids, and if necessary nutritional supplements, may be of some help in patients with anorexia.

Techniques attempting to prevent the occurrence of alopecia have met with varying success (see below). Scalp tourniquets and local hypothermia have been used to minimise concentrations of antineoplastics in the scalp after intravenous injection. However, such methods may allow the development of a cancer-cell sanctuary and should not be used in patients with leukaemia or other conditions with circulating malignant cells.

Of particular importance is the management of bone-marrow depression. Colony-stimulating factors and epoetins can be used to promote the formation of replacement blood elements (see below). Active measures may be necessary to combat infection and bleeding. Transfusions of blood products may be required; granulocyte transfusions have been given for infections unresponsive to antibiotics, although their value is a matter of debate, while transfusion of blood platelets or use of growth factors such as oprelvekin (interleukin-11) may be of value in preventing thrombocytopenia-induced bleeding.

Extravasation of antineoplastics can pose serious problems. Infusion should be stopped immediately once extravasation is noticed and any drug remaining at the site aspirated if possible but the details of treatment are controversial (see below). If ulceration occurs plastic surgery may be required.

Hyperuricaemia secondary to tumour lysis in patients with leukaemias or lymphomas can be prevented by the addition of allopurinol or rasburicase to treatment schedules, and by adequate hydration and, if necessary, alkalinisation of the urine. Good hydration is also important to minimise the nephrotoxic effects of drugs such as cisplatin and methotrexate.

Specific treatments exist for the toxicity of certain antineoplastics (for example the use of calcium folinate to reduce methotrexate toxicity, or mesna to control the bladder toxicity of cyclophosphamide or ifosfamide). For further details of the treatment of specific adverse effects see under the individual monographs.

**Alopecia.** Attempts to prevent or reduce chemotherapy-induced alopecia have relied on either restriction of scalp blood flow with a tourniquet or the use of local hypothermia.[1] Both of these techniques have been based on the rationale that a temporary decrease in blood flow to the scalp will decrease the exposure of hair follicles to the antineoplastic. Therefore, most benefit would be expected for alopecia caused by drugs with a short half-life and for which both active drug and metabolites are rapidly cleared from the circulation.

Studies of scalp tourniquets carried out in the 1970s found head discomfort to be the main side-effect. They used different chemotherapy regimens, definitions for success, and tourniquet techniques, making conclusions difficult, and tourniquets were largely replaced by local hypothermia techniques.

Most studies of local hypothermia have attempted to prevent doxorubicin-induced alopecia. Again, chemotherapy regimens, devices used, and exposure times have varied between studies. Varying degrees of efficacy have been reported, but hypothermia has generally been of benefit, particularly with single-agent chemotherapy. The dose of chemotherapy may be relevant, with hypothermia being less effective at doxorubicin doses above 50 mg. Headache and cold intolerance may occur, but scalp hypothermia is generally well tolerated.

Despite the successes there is concern that this technique may provide a sanctuary for circulating malignant cells, with the potential risk of metastasis, and there are reports of scalp metastases following the use of hypothermia.[1,2] One reviewer suggests that the use of scalp hypothermia might therefore be restricted to patients receiving single-agent chemotherapy with a palliative intent, or those with solid tumours that rarely metastasise to the scalp.[1] The technique should probably be avoided in patients with leukaemias.[2]

In the USA commercial distribution of cooling caps designed to produce localised scalp hypothermia was halted by the FDA in 1990 because of concerns about their effectiveness and their potential to create sanctuary sites and interfere with drug distribution elsewhere in the head. However, they continue to be available in many countries.

For reference to the use of minoxidil to decrease the duration of alopecia following doxorubicin-containing chemotherapy, see p.961.

1. Dorr VJ. A practitioner's guide to cancer-related alopecia. *Semin Oncol* 1998; **25:** 562–70.
2. Forsberg SA. Scalp cooling therapy and cytotoxic treatment. *Lancet* 2001; **357:** 1134.

**Bone-marrow depression.** Bone-marrow depression in patients receiving chemotherapy may require a modification of the dose regimen in subsequent cycles, either by delaying or reducing doses, although it is recognised that this may sometimes reduce efficacy.

Licensed drug information for a number of myelosuppressive antineoplastics recommends that if neutropenia or thrombocytopenia occurs subsequent doses should be withheld until white cell counts have returned to 3000 to 3500 cells/mm$^3$ or more, and blood platelets to about 100 000 cells/mm$^3$. In practice, however, improved supportive care means that many expert centres routinely administer treatment at lower blood counts than these. The values at which it is acceptable to treat will be influenced by whether the regimen is likely to result in further significant falls, and whether the intent is curative (in which case maintaining treatment intensity is particularly important) or palliative (when avoiding toxicity becomes a prime consideration); local protocols may contain further guidance and should be consulted where available. However, it has been suggested[1] that with appropriate management treatment is usually possible at neutrophil counts of 1500 cells/mm$^3$ and platelet counts above 100 000 cells/mm$^3$.

For guidelines on the use of haematopoietic growth factors in the management of anaemia, neutropenia, and thrombocytopenia, see below.

1. Summerhayes M, Daniels S. *Practical chemotherapy: a multidisciplinary guide*. Oxford: Radcliffe Medical Press, 2003.

ANAEMIA. Chemotherapy-induced anaemia can be managed with transfusion of red cells (p.759) or treatment with epoetin (p.747),[1] and preliminary results suggest that epoetin may also potentiate the effects of colony-stimulating factors used to treat neutropenia.[2]

Guidelines for the use of epoetins have been issued jointly by the American Society of Clinical Oncology and the American Society of Hematology.[3] In the treatment of chemotherapy-induced anaemia, the use of epoetins can improve haemoglobin concentration and reduce the need for transfusion of red cells, but whether this improves symptoms and quality of life requires further study. The use of epoetins is recommended when haemoglobin has fallen to 10 g per 100 mL or less. For patients with a concentration between 10 and 12 g per 100 mL, the decision to use epoetins depends on clinical circumstances, and may be considered for patients at a higher risk of adverse effects related to anaemia, including elderly patients with limited cardiopulmonary reserve, or patients with underlying coronary artery disease and symptomatic angina.

1. Littlewood TJ. Management options for cancer therapy-related anaemia. *Drug Safety* 2002; **25:** 525–35.
2. Pierelli L, *et al.* Erythropoietin addition to granulocyte colony-stimulating factor abrogates life-threatening neutropenia and increases peripheral-blood progenitor-cell mobilization after epirubicin, paclitaxel, and cisplatin combination chemotherapy: results of a randomized comparison. *J Clin Oncol* 1999; **17:** 1288–95.
3. Rizzo JD, *et al.* Use of epoetin in patients with cancer: evidence-based clinical practice guidelines of the American Society of Clinical Oncology and the American Society of Hematology. *J Clin Oncol* 2002; **20:** 4083–4107. Also published in *Blood* 2002; **100:** 2303–20.

NEUTROPENIA. Use of granulocyte or granulocyte-macrophage colony-stimulating factors (G-CSF or GM-CSF), alone or with autologous bone marrow transplants or peripheral blood stem-cells, can markedly reduce the period of neutropenia after high-dose chemotherapy regimens (see Filgrastim, p.753, and Molgramostim, p.756).

The American Society of Clinical Oncology has issued detailed guidelines for the use of colony-stimulating factors (CSFs) in patients receiving chemotherapy.[1] These point out that in current practice infectious mortality resulting from febrile neutropenia is rare, and that the incidence with common chemotherapy regimens seldom exceeds 25 to 40% in previously untreated patients; however, episodes of febrile neutropenia prolong hospital stay, expose the patient to further interventions, and may result in delay or dose-reduction of further chemotherapy cycles. Unfortunately, although colony-stimulating factors can markedly reduce the incidence of febrile neutropenia, there was little evidence of improved clinical outcomes from the use of CSFs in most situations.

- Use of colony-stimulating factors for **primary prophylaxis** in previously untreated patients should not normally be considered except where bone-marrow compromise or comorbidity indicated a patient at high risk (and even here the evidence for improved clinical outcome was modest).
- There was no evidence of clinical benefit from the use of colony-stimulating factors in **secondary prophylaxis**. In patients with a previous episode of febrile neutropenia the usual option (except where it would compromise the chances of cure) was dose reduction of the chemotherapy regimen.
- For adjunctive **treatment** of episodes of neutropenia, it was recommended that CSFs should not be routinely used for patients who were *afebrile*; there was also strong and consistent evidence against routine use for uncomplicated fever and neutropenia in *febrile* patients. Use might be considered in high-risk patients with febrile neutropenia.
- Although CSFs could permit **increased dose-intensity** of chemotherapy, this was considered only justified within the context of a clinical trial, since increased dose-intensity had not been shown to improve survival or quality of life in most studies outside the haematological malignancies. Use in patients receiving combined **chemoradiotherapy** was not recommended.
- In patients with **haematological malignancies**, CSFs should be considered after induction chemotherapy in patients with acute myeloid leukaemias who were aged 55 or over, and after initial induction or postremission chemotherapy in patients with acute lymphoblastic leukaemia; a subset of patients with myelodysplastic syndrome might also benefit, but use in patients with refractory or relapsed myeloid leukaemia was not thought to be of benefit.
- CSFs were recommended as adjuncts to **progenitor cell transplantation** to help mobilise peripheral blood stem cells and to speed engraftment.
- Although the guidelines in adults were held to be generally applicable to **children**, it was recognised that there were differences of emphasis in practice and that CSFs tended to be used more often for prophylaxis in children than was recommended in adults, and less often for uncomplicated fever and neutropenia.

For details on the management of infections in neutropenic patients, see p.131.

1. Ozer H, *et al.* 2000 Update of recommendations for the use of hematopoietic colony-stimulating factors: evidence-based, clinical practice guidelines. *J Clin Oncol* 2000; **18:** 3558–85.

THROMBOCYTOPENIA. Chemotherapy-induced thrombocytopenia can be managed with transfusion of platelets (p.758). Recombinant thrombopoietin[1] (p.760), interleukin-3 (p.755), and interleukin-6 have been evaluated for their ability to increase platelet numbers *in vivo*. Interleukin-11 has also been studied and is now available as oprelvekin (p.757), which can reduce chemotherapy-induced thrombocytopenia.[2,3] Interleukin-1 (p.1701) and macrophage colony-stimulating factor (M-CSF) have also been investigated in the prevention or treatment of thrombocytopenia.

The American Society of Clinical Oncology has issued guidelines for the use of platelet transfusion.[4] They recommend that prophylactic platelet transfusion be administered for thrombocytopenia resulting from impaired bone-marrow function to reduce the risk of haemorrhage when the platelet count falls below a predefined threshold. This threshold will vary depending on the patient's diagnosis, clinical condition, and treatment modality. A threshold of 10 000 cells/mm$^3$ has been recommended for patients being treated for acute leukaemia, with haematopoietic stem cell transplantation, or for solid tumours. A higher threshold of 20 000 cells/mm$^3$ may need to be considered for patients with signs of haemorrhage, high fever, rapid fall of platelet count, coagulation abnormalities, patients receiving aggressive therapy for bladder tumours, or those with necrotic solid tumours who are at increased risk of bleeding from these sites.

1. Vadhan-Raj S, *et al.* Recombinant human thrombopoietin attenuates carboplatin-induced severe thrombocytopenia and the need for platelet transfusions in patients with gynecologic cancer. *Ann Intern Med* 2000; **132:** 364–8.
2. Gordon MS, *et al.* A phase I trial of recombinant human interleukin-11 (Neumega rhIL-11 growth factor) in women with breast cancer receiving chemotherapy. *Blood* 1996; **87:** 3615–24.
3. Isaacs C, *et al.* Randomized placebo-controlled study of recombinant human interleukin-11 to prevent chemotherapy-induced thrombocytopenia in patients with breast cancer receiving dose-intensive cyclophosphamide and doxorubicin. *J Clin Oncol* 1997; **15:** 3368–77.
4. Schiffer CA, *et al.* Platelet transfusion for patients with cancer: clinical practice guidelines of the American Society of Clinical Oncology. *J Clin Oncol* 2001; **19:** 1519–38.

**Extravasation.** Extravasation is the leakage of a drug into subcutaneous tissue during parenteral administration. Extravasation injuries can range from mild erythema to ulceration, and severe necrosis in some cases if not dealt with promptly. Antineoplastics vary in their propensity to cause extravasation injury:[1]

- *vesicant antineoplastics* cause pain, inflammation and blistering of the local skin, tissue death and necrosis; they include amsacrine, the anthracyclines (doxorubicin and its derivatives), carmustine, dacarbazine, dactinomycin, mitomycin, chlormethine, paclitaxel, plicamycin, streptozocin, and the vinca alkaloids
- *exfoliants* can cause inflammation and exfoliation, but are less likely to cause tissue death, and include cisplatin, docetaxel, mitoxantrone, oxaliplatin, and topotecan
- carboplatin, irinotecan, and the podophyllotoxin derivatives (etoposide and teniposide) are examples of *irritant* drugs which may cause inflammation and irritation, but rarely cause breakdown of tissue. Fluorouracil, methotrexate, and raltitrexed can cause mild to moderate inflammation of local tissue.

Measures to prevent the occurrence of extravasation include giving vesicant or irritant drugs via a central line, or peripherally via a recently sited cannula; vesicants are generally given by intravenous injection into a fast-running infusion. Glyceryl trinitrate patches applied distally to the cannula may be used to dilate veins where venous access is a problem. The site of administration should be regularly checked, and the patient asked to report any untoward sensations.

If extravasation should occur the infusion should be stopped immediately and as much as possible of the infiltrating drug removed by aspiration. Beyond this, however, the management of extravasation is not well standardised and there has been disagreement as to the most appropriate course; there is little data from controlled studies and much practice is based on anecdotal reports and individual experience. Intravenous and subcutaneous injection of a corticosteroid (usually hydrocortisone) has been suggested, although some consider it ineffective or possibly even disadvantageous. Topical application of a 1% hydrocortisone cream to inflamed skin has also been suggested, and antihistamines and, if necessary, analgesics, may be given by mouth. In most cases application of a cold dressing or ice pack is appropriate. However, following extravasation of the taxanes, vinca alkaloids, or cisplatin the use of warm packs with hyaluronidase to enhance uptake from the skin has been recommended; a similar procedure has been suggested for large volume extravasations of the podophyllotoxin derivatives.

The use of specific antidotes is a particularly contentious area, since few are clinically validated and some (such as the use of sodium bicarbonate 8.4% for anthracycline extravasations) may do more harm than good. Brief infiltration of a less concentrated (2.1%) sodium bicarbonate solution, followed after a few minutes by aspiration, is still, however, advocated by some in the management of extravasations of the anthracyclines, carmustine, and plicamycin. Better accepted in the management of anthracycline and mitomycin extravasation is the topical application of dimethyl sulfoxide about every 6 hours, sometimes alternated with hydrocortisone 1% cream. Sodium thiosulfate 3 or 4% has been used to infiltrate the site of extravasations of cisplatin, dactinomycin, or chlormethine.

The role of surgery is also important. It is unequivocally necessary in cases where other methods have failed to prevent evolving tissue damage, but there is some dispute as to the role of early surgery to remove drug-laden tissue and prevent the development of more serious ulceration and necrosis. Techniques of saline flushout and liposuction have been developed for removing drug and non-viable tissue while preserving overlying skin.

Some references to the management of extravasation are given below.[1-5]

1. Stanley A. Managing complications of chemotherapy administration. In: Allwood M, *et al.*, eds. *The Cytotoxics Handbook*. 4th ed. Oxford: Radcliffe Medical Press, 2002: 119–93.
2. Dorr RT. Antidotes to vesicant chemotherapy extravasations. *Blood Rev* 1990; **4:** 41–60.
3. Gault DT. Extravasation injuries. *Br J Plast Surg* 1993; **46:** 91–6.
4. Bertelli G. Prevention and management of extravasation of cytotoxic drugs. *Drug Safety* 1995; **12:** 245–55.
5. Kassner E. Evaluation and treatment of chemotherapy extravasation injuries. *J Pediatr Oncol Nurs* 2000; **17:** 135–48.

**Mucositis.** A number of drugs have been tried for the *prophylaxis* of mucositis caused by antineoplastic therapy, by modifying exposure of the oral mucosa to chemotherapy, modifying epithelial proliferation, or reducing the potential for infection and inflammatory complications of mucositis.[1] Some drugs showed limited evidence of benefit in small trials, including benzydamine, betacarotene, granulocyte-macrophage colony-stimulating factor, povidone-iodine, propantheline bromide, vitamin E, and tretinoin. There are conflicting reports of benefit from studies of sucralfate and chlorhexidine. Other options that have been tried with less success include aciclovir, allopurinol, dinoprostone, glutamine, misoprostol, pentoxifylline, and bacterial and fungal decontamination. A large systematic review[2] considered many of these but found that the only therapies with any significant benefit as prophylaxis for mucositis were local cooling with ice chips, granulocyte-macrophage colony-stimulating factor, and amifostine in patients treated with radiotherapy for head and neck cancer. There will be some overlap between measures for prophylaxis and treatment of mucositis, and another systematic review[3] of *treatment* strategies found that there was some evidence that topical allopurinol, intramuscular immunoglobulin, and human placental extract injection improved mucositis, but that the evidence was weak and unreliable. Given the number of variables involved in the development of mucositis it is unlikely that any one prophylactic or treatment regimen will prove suitable for all patients.

1. Knox JJ, *et al.* Chemotherapy-induced oral mucositis: prevention and management. *Drugs Aging* 2000; **17:** 257–67.
2. Clarkson JE, *et al.* Interventions for preventing oral mucositis for patients with cancer receiving treatment. Available in The Cochrane Library; Issue 2. Chichester: John Wiley; 2004.
3. Worthington HV, *et al.* Interventions for treating oral mucositis for patients with cancer receiving treatment. Available in The Cochrane Library; Issue 2. Chichester: John Wiley; 2004.

**Nausea and vomiting.** For a detailed discussion of the management of chemotherapy-induced nausea and vomiting, see p.1245.

## Precautions

In view of their severe toxicity and possible carcinogenicity these drugs should generally be reserved for severe or life-threatening disease, and it is widely suggested that their use and administration should be confined to experienced staff in specialised centres.

Immunosuppression and bone-marrow depression are features of many of these drugs and their use is associated with an increased risk of infections caused by pathogenic or opportunistic micro-organisms, and a reduced capacity to cope with them. Where possible, immunosuppressant drugs should not be given to patients with acute infections, and dosage reduction or withdrawal should be considered if infection develops, until the infection has been controlled. For cautions regarding the use of vaccines in patients receiving these drugs see Interactions, below. For discussion of the treatment of infections in immunosuppressed patients, see p.131. Special care is necessary in debilitated patients.

Blood counts and measurement of haemoglobin concentrations should be carried out routinely to help predict the onset of bone-marrow depression. Great caution is needed when the marrow is already depressed following radiotherapy or therapy with other antineoplastics, and modification of dosage regimens may be required. The blood count levels below which treatment is contra-indicated will vary depending on the regimen to be used and the therapeutic intent of that treatment (see Bone-Marrow Suppression, above); local protocols, including those for the use of colony-stimulating factors, should always be consulted.

Although positive evidence of teratogenicity in humans is not available for all antineoplastics, pregnancy should be avoided in women receiving them: in particular they should not be given, if possible, during the first trimester. Mothers receiving antineoplastic therapy should not breast feed. Because some regimens may result in permanent infertility, the storage of semen samples for male patients, and embryos for females before such therapy may be desirable.

Many antineoplastics are vesicant or irritant. Care must be taken to avoid extravasation since severe pain and tissue damage may ensue. They must be handled with great care and contact with skin and eyes avoided; they should not be inhaled. In many countries official or professional guidelines on precautions for the safe handling of cytotoxic drugs have been issued.

For precautions specific to particular drugs, see under the individual monographs.

**Administration in the elderly.** The use of antineoplastics in the elderly should take into consideration age-related physiological changes including decline in renal and hepatic function, reduced haematopoietic reserve, and reduced gastrointestinal and cardiac function. Other factors to consider are comorbid conditions and potential drug interactions with associated medications.[1,2] Neoplastic disorders in the elderly have been undertreated because of an impression that these diseases are less aggressive,[3] and the effects of chemotherapy more likely to be severe.[1-4] There is evidence, however, that healthy older patients can tolerate chemotherapy as well as younger patients.[1,2] However, there have been few studies of chemotherapy specifically in elderly patients,[3] and selection of a suitable dosage regimen is more difficult as a consequence, although there is increasing effort to address this lack of data.[2-4] Old people vary as much as any other group in their response to drugs, and the consensus is that they should not be excluded from any form of treatment on the grounds of age alone.

1. Kimmick GG, *et al.* Cancer chemotherapy in older adults: a tolerability perspective. *Drugs Aging* 1997; **10:** 34–49.
2. Lichtman SM, Skirvin JA. Pharmacology of antineoplastic agents in older cancer patients. *Oncology (Huntingt)* 2000; **14:** 1743–55.
3. Balducci L, Beghe' C. Cancer and age in the USA. *Crit Rev Oncol Hematol* 2001; **37:** 137–45.
4. Muss HB. Older age—not a barrier to cancer treatment. *N Engl J Med* 2001; **345:** 1128–9.

**Administration at home.** Outpatients taking oral antineoplastic therapy at home do not receive the same level of monitoring as inpatients, and should be cautioned to report any adverse effects, since such treatments may still produce severe toxicity.

**Contraception.** The *British National Formulary* recommends that intra-uterine devices for contraception be used with caution in patients with drug- or disease-induced immunosuppression, because of the risk of infection; such devices are contra-indicated in marked immunosuppression.

**Handling and disposal.** Many antineoplastics are potent and potentially highly toxic drugs that must be handled with due care. In many countries official or professional guidelines are available for the handling, reconstitution, and disposal of antineoplastics, and most centres or institutions in which these drugs are used will have individual handling policies based on these.[1]

Recommendations generally include:

- that these drugs be reconstituted by trained personnel;
- that reconstitution take place in designated areas, designed to protect personnel and the environment—for example, the use of safety cabinets;
- that protective clothing be worn, including gloves, eye protection, and masks if necessary (it should be noted that gloves may vary in their resistance to penetration, depending upon their thickness, the material of which they are made, and the drug in question[1,2]);
- that waste should be disposed of carefully in suitable separate containers, clearly labelled as to their contents (it should be noted that the patient's body fluids and excreta may contain appreciable amounts of antineoplastic agents and it has been suggested that they and materials such as bed linen contaminated with them should also be treated as hazardous waste[3,4]);
- that adequate procedures should be in place for accidental contamination due to spillages;
- that staff exposure to antineoplastic agents be recorded and monitored;
- that pregnant staff should avoid handling these drugs if possible.

1. Allwood M, *et al.* eds. *The Cytotoxics Handbook*. 4th ed. Oxford: Radcliffe Medical Press, 2002.
2. Connor TH. Permeability of nitrile rubber, latex, polyurethane, and neoprene gloves to 18 antineoplastic drugs. *Am J Health-Syst Pharm* 1999; **56:** 2450–3.
3. Harris J, Dodds LJ. Handling waste from patients receiving cytotoxic drugs. *Pharm J* 1985; **235:** 289–91.
4. Cass Y, Musgrave CF. Guidelines for the safe handling of excreta contaminated by cytotoxic agents. *Am J Hosp Pharm* 1992; **49:** 1957–8.

**Pregnancy.** Antineoplastics may be used during pregnancy for their immunosuppressant properties in auto-immune disease, and for the treatment of cancer, which can complicate 1 in 1000 pregnancies.[1,2] Although the use of potentially teratogenic drugs would normally be avoided during pregnancy, the risk to the mother of inadequate treatment may outweigh whatever risks exist of abnormality in the fetus.[1] The highest incidence of adverse effects appears to occur following exposure during the first trimester:[1,2] about 10 to 20% of fetuses exposed to cytotoxics during this period have major malformations, compared with 3% in the general population.[1] Anomalies may be found in the heart, neural tube, eye, ear, palate, haematopoietic system, and genital tract.[2] The risk of fetal malformations following exposure during the second and third trimesters is probably no higher than the background rate, but there may still be an increased risk of stillbirth, fetal growth restriction, premature birth, and maternal or fetal myelosuppression.[1,2] The delayed effects of antineoplastics on development have not been well-documented. Despite some small studies finding no abnormalities at follow-up assessments up to 19 years of age, premature birth and low birth-weight could contribute to retardation of growth, development, and intellect, and maternal antineoplastic therapy has been implicated in a case of childhood neuroblastoma and papillary thyroid cancer.[3] The highest risk of teratogenicity seems to be associated with alkylating agents and antimetabolites, in particular aminopterin, fluorouracil, and methotrexate.[1,2,4] The vinca alkaloids and doxorubicin may entail less risk,[2] although the former have produced malformations in *animals*.[1] Other drugs reported to be teratogenic or potentially teratogenic include busulfan,[1] chlorambucil,[1,4] chlormethine,[1] cyclophosphamide,[1,4] cytarabine,[1] mercaptopurine,[4] and the podophyllotoxin derivatives.[1]

There are no specific dosage recommendations for the use of antineoplastics during pregnancy, but physiological changes occurring in the mother can alter the pharmacokinetics of drugs.[1,2] This could potentially increase the toxicity of the antineoplastic, or decrease its efficacy.[2] Myelosuppressive chemotherapy should be avoided 3 weeks before the anticipated delivery so that the mother is neither neutropenic nor thrombocytopenic.[1,2] The timing of delivery is also critical for the neonate, as chemotherapy given shortly before delivery may not be eliminated through the placenta, prolonging exposure in the newborn.[1]

There has also been concern that long-term *occupational exposure* to antineoplastics might have an adverse effect on the fetus of pregnant health-care workers: a study in 650 Finnish nurses found that women who experienced fetal loss were more than twice as likely to have had first trimester exposure to antineoplastic drugs as women who successfully gave birth.[5] These results have been criticised on the grounds that such results are not generally seen in cancer patients,[6,7] who presumably are exposed to much higher doses of antineoplastics. However, similar results were seen in a cross-sectional analysis of 7094 pregnancies involving 2815 nursing and pharmacy staff.[8] Another study[9] has suggested that the rate of ectopic pregnancy may be increased in nurses occupationally exposed to antineoplastics, but the small number of ectopic pregnancies involved (15 in 734 pregnancies) means that the association with antineoplastics may be due to chance. A further, larger, case-control study[10] by the same investigators found no evidence of an increased rate of ectopic pregnancy, and suggested that occupational exposure to higher levels of antineoplastics in the past possibly explained the earlier findings. Again, such an effect does not appear to have been reported in women treated with antineoplastics.

See also Effects on Reproductive Potential, above.

1. Buekers TE, Lallas TA. Chemotherapy in pregnancy. *Obstet Gynecol Clin North Am* 1998; **25:** 323–9.
2. Falkenberry SS. Cancer in pregnancy. *Surg Oncol Clin N Am* 1998; **7:** 375–97.
3. Partridge AH, Garber JE. Long-term outcomes of children exposed to antineoplastic agents in utero. *Semin Oncol* 2000; **27:** 712–26.
4. Østensen M, Ramsey-Goldman R. Treatment of inflammatory rheumatic disorders in pregnancy: what are the safest treatment options? *Drug Safety* 1998; **19:** 389–410.
5. Selevan SG, *et al.* A study of occupational exposure to antineoplastic drugs and fetal loss in nurses. *N Engl J Med* 1985; **313:** 1173–8.
6. Kalter H. Antineoplastic drugs and spontaneous abortion in nurses. *N Engl J Med* 1986; **314:** 1048–9.

7. Mulvihill JJ, Stewart KR. Antineoplastic drugs and spontaneous abortion in nurses. *N Engl J Med* 1986; **314:** 1049.
8. Valanis B, *et al.* Occupational exposure to antineoplastic agents: self-reported miscarriages and stillbirths among nurses and pharmacists. *J Occup Environ Med* 1999; **41:** 632–8.
9. Saurel-Cubizolles MJ, *et al.* Ectopic pregnancy and occupational exposure to antineoplastic drugs. *Lancet* 1993; **341:** 1169–71.
10. Bouyer J, *et al.* Ectopic pregnancy and occupational exposure of hospital personnel. *Scand J Work Environ Health* 1998; **24:** 98–103.


## Interactions

Because of their effects on the gastrointestinal mucosa antineoplastics have the potential to interfere with the absorption of other drugs given by mouth. Antineoplastics that have an immunosuppressant effect may reduce the response to vaccines, and there is a possibility of generalised infection with live vaccines. Use with live vaccines should generally be avoided.

Many antineoplastics are inhibitors of certain isoenzymes of cytochrome P450 and some antineoplastics are also metabolised by these enzymes, and in consequence the possibility of interactions between antineoplastics, or between antineoplastics and concomitant medication, cannot be discounted.

Interactions affecting specific drugs are covered under the individual monographs.

◊ References.


1. Le Blanc GA, Waxman DJ. Interaction of anticancer drugs with hepatic monooxygenase enzymes. *Drug Metab Rev* 1989; **20:** 395–439.
2. Loadman PM, Bibby MC. Pharmacokinetic drug interactions with anticancer drugs. *Clin Pharmacokinet* 1994; **26:** 486–500.
3. Kivistö KT, *et al.* The role of human cytochrome P450 enzymes in the metabolism of anticancer agents: implications for drug interactions. *Br J Clin Pharmacol* 1995; **40:** 523–30.
4. McLeod HL. Clinically relevant drug-drug interactions in oncology. *Br J Clin Pharmacol* 1998; **45:** 539–44.


**Antiepileptics.** Retrospective review of outcomes in children treated for acute lymphoblastic leukaemia indicated that long-term antiepileptic therapy increased the clearance of several antileukaemic drugs and reduced the efficacy of therapy.[1]


1. Relling MV, *et al.* Adverse effect of anticonvulsants on efficacy of chemotherapy for acute lymphoblastic leukaemia. *Lancet* 2000; **356:** 285–90.


**Effects on other drugs.** Antineoplastics have been reported to affect a number of drugs including:

- digoxin (reduced absorption, see p.897)
- oral anticoagulants (increased or decreased effect, see Warfarin, p.1025)
- phenytoin (increased or decreased effect, see p.373)
- suxamethonium (prolonged effect, see p.1408)
- vaccines (decreased response, see p.1606).

## Action

Much of the development of cancer chemotherapy has been based on an understanding of the way in which tumour cells grow, and the way in which the drugs affect this growth.

After cell division the daughter cells enter a period of growth, **$G_1$**, which lasts for different lengths of time in different tissues. This is followed by a period of DNA synthesis, **S**, in which the amount of chromosomal material is doubled, then a postsynthetic, or premitotic, phase, **$G_2$**, then finally by mitotic cell division, **M**. As an alternative to re-entering the cycle, the products of cell division may enter a kinetically-dormant, nonproliferative stage, **$G_0$**, although it is not exactly clear what recruits such 'resting' cells back into the cell cycle.

The rate of cell division varies for different tumours; the doubling time for Burkitt's lymphoma and acute lymphoblastic leukaemia is less than 5 days, whereas the mean doubling time for seminoma is about 20 days, that for small-cell lung cancer about 50 days, and those for colon cancer and advanced breast cancer about 100 and 150 days respectively. The range of reported doubling times may also vary widely for a particular tumour type. The majority of common cancers increase very slowly in size in comparison with sensitive normal tissues, including those from which they derive, and the rate may decrease further in large tumours. This difference allows normal cells to recover more quickly than malignant ones from chemotherapy, and is the rationale behind current cyclic dosage schedules. The lethal body tumour burden is reached when the tumour cell mass approaches or exceeds $1 \times 10^{12}$ cells, equivalent to about 1 kg of tissue, and representing about 40 doublings.

Cell killing by cytotoxic agents is generally a first order process, so a given dose or course of antineoplastic kills a fixed percentage of tumour cells rather than a fixed number. Thus a drug that killed 99% of tumour cells would leave behind $10^{10}$ cells from a tumour containing $10^{12}$ cells, but only $10^2$ cells from one containing $10^4$, reinforcing the importance of treating malignant neoplasms as early as possible.

Cytotoxic drugs act to damage the reproductive integrity of cells. Some are active at a particular stage of the cell cycle. The antimetabolites all act at various points to interfere with DNA synthesis, as does hydroxycarbamide, and are thus active against cells in S phase, while the vinca alkaloids inhibit microtubular function and act on cells in phase M. Other drugs such as the alkylating agents, the anthracyclines, and cisplatin are not phase-specific, but since their actions are dependent at least in part on damaging DNA they are more effective against proliferating cells, particularly in S phase. It is now thought that many antineoplastics exert their ultimate effect by inducing cellular apoptosis (programmed cell death). Some drugs, such as bleomycin or vinblastine also have the property of arresting the cycle in a particular phase, and attempts have been made to synchronise tumour cell division in this way, to maximise the number of cells in a sensitive phase when a particular drug is used. However, in practice this approach has been less successful than early experimental results suggested.

Some drugs used in the treatment of neoplasms do not attack the tumour cells directly but are given in order to increase cell vulnerability to other modalities: these include radiosensitisers (which have proved of only limited benefit to date), and photosensitisers such as porfimer sodium, which are used in photodynamic therapy (PDT).

Apart from attacking cell division, increased understanding of the molecular biology of tumour cells has begun to open the possibility of other approaches to the treatment of malignant neoplasms. Some monoclonal antibodies are designed to bind to specific cell-surface proteins or receptors, enabling the immune system to recognise and attack tumour cells. Other areas of investigation include inducing tumour cells to differentiate into non-malignant forms, manipulation of cellular apoptosis and signal transduction, inhibiting the expression of abnormal growth factors, telomerases and other oncogene products (including the use of ribozymes or of 'antisense' compounds which inhibit oncogenic messenger RNA), control of tumour growth through inhibition of angiogenesis, and prevention or inhibition of metastasis. Gene therapy (p.1691) is another form of treatment under consideration. However, such approaches remain largely experimental.

◊ References to investigational modes of cancer therapy.


1. Gescher A, *et al.* Suppression of tumour development by substances derived from the diet—mechanisms and clinical implications. *Br J Clin Pharmacol* 1998; **45:** 1–12.
2. Sikic BI. New approaches in cancer treatment. *Ann Oncol* 1999; **10** (suppl 6): 149–53.
3. Knuth A, *et al.* Cancer immunotherapy in clinical oncology. *Cancer Chemother Pharmacol* 2000; **46** (suppl): S46–51.
4. Nelson AR, *et al.* Matrix metalloproteinases: biologic activity and clinical implications. *J Clin Oncol* 2000; **18:** 1135–49.
5. Diel IJ. Antitumour effects of bisphosphonates: first evidence and possible mechanisms. *Drugs* 2000; **59:** 391–9.
6. Noonberg SB, Benz CC. Tyrosine kinase inhibitors targeted to the epidermal growth factor receptor subfamily: role as anticancer agents. *Drugs* 2000; **59:** 753–67.
7. Vile RG, *et al.* Cancer gene therapy: hard lessons and new courses. *Gene Ther* 2000; **7:** 2–8.
8. Bodey B, *et al.* Failure of cancer vaccines: the significant limitations of this approach to immunotherapy. *Anticancer Res* 2000; **20:** 2665–76.
9. Green MC, *et al.* Monoclonal antibody therapy for solid tumors. *Cancer Treat Rev* 2000; **26:** 269–86.
10. Cox AD. Farnesyltransferase inhibitors: potential role in the treatment of cancer. *Drugs* 2001; **61:** 723–32.
11. Miller KD, *et al.* Redefining the target: chemotherapeutics as antiangiogenics. *J Clin Oncol* 2001; **19:** 1195–1206.
12. Kerbel RS. Clinical trials of antiangiogenic drugs: opportunities, problems, and assessment of initial results. *J Clin Oncol* 2001; **19** (suppl): 45s–51s.
13. Dermime S, *et al.* Cancer vaccines and immunotherapy. *Br Med Bull* 2002; **62:** 149–62.
14. Pirollo KF, *et al.* Antisense therapeutics: from theory to clinical practice. *Pharmacol Ther* 2003; **99:** 55–77.
15. Grunwald V, Hidalgo M. Developing inhibitors of the epidermal growth factor receptor for cancer treatment. *J Natl Cancer Inst* 2003; **95:** 851–67.
16. Dancey JE, Freidlin B. Targeting epidermal growth factor receptor—are we missing the mark? *Lancet* 2003; **362:** 62–4.
17. Kerbel RS. Antiangiogenic drugs and current strategies for the treatment of lung cancer. *Semin Oncol* 2004; **31** (suppl 1): 54–60.
18. Sattler M, *et al.* Therapeutic targeting of the receptor tyrosine kinase Met. *Cancer Treat Res* 2004; **119:** 121–38.


## Resistance

Resistance to antineoplastics is one of the greatest limitations to the use of chemotherapy in malignant disease. Resistance may be intrinsic to the tumour or may be acquired during chemotherapy, which effectively acts to select resistant cells from a heterogeneous population; the latter is one reason that relapses, or malignancies in heavily-pretreated patients, may be particularly difficult to treat.

The mechanisms of resistance in cancer cells are complex and imperfectly understood, but appear to include:

- hypoxia and imperfect drug penetration in the centre of large, solid tumours
- the small proportion of cells actively dividing and thus vulnerable to antineoplastics (particularly in slow-growing tumours)
- decreased cellular uptake or increased efflux of antineoplastic
- increased metabolic breakdown or decreased activation of antineoplastic
- increased expression of target enzymes
- metabolism via alternative biochemical pathways to those blocked by the antineoplastic
- more efficient repair of damaged DNA
- possibly the expression of genes which inhibit drug-induced apoptosis.

Several of these mechanisms may be in operation at one time. Much interest has been expressed in the potential use of drugs which can modulate or inhibit mechanisms of resistance, and in particular in compounds such as valspodar, verapamil, quinidine, and ciclosporin, which have the ability to block the action of p-glycoprotein, a membrane glycoprotein which acts as an efflux pump for a range of cytotoxic substances and which is responsible for the multi-drug resistant (MDR) phenotype. However, for sustained benefit it seems likely that several drugs would be required, each to overcome a different mechanism of resistance, and it would be necessary to ensure that toxicity of antineoplastics to normal cells was not also enhanced.

If the emergence of heritable resistant phenotypes is a natural part of tumour-cell biology (the Goldie-Coldman hypothesis) it implies that the larger and older the tumour, the more likely is resistance to occur. This would confirm the benefits of surgery and radiotherapy to shrink the primary tumour, and of starting chemotherapy as soon as possible after (a preferably early) diagnosis.

◊ Reviews of antineoplastic resistance.


1. Booser DJ, Hortobagyi GN. Anthracycline antibiotics in cancer therapy: focus on drug resistance. *Drugs* 1994; **47:** 223–58.
2. Ling V. P-Glycoprotein: its role in drug resistance. *Am J Med* 1995; **99** (suppl 6A): 31S–34S.
3. Kaye SB. Clinical drug resistance: the role of factors other than P-glycoprotein. *Am J Med* 1995; **99** (suppl 6A): 40S–44S.
4. Holmes J. Multidrug resistance as a cause of cytotoxic drug failure. *Pharm J* 1996; **257:** 294–6.
5. Dumontet C, Sikic BI. Mechanisms of action of and resistance to antitubulin agents: microtubule dynamics, drug transport, and cell death. *J Clin Oncol* 1999; **17:** 1061–70.
6. Sikic BI. Modulation of multidrug resistance: a paradigm for translational clinical research. *Oncology (Huntingt)* 1999; **13:** 183–7.


◊ Some drugs have been reported to partially abolish multidrug resistance to antineoplastics *in vitro*.[1,2] These include verapamil, its enantiomers and analogues such as Ro-11-2933; other calcium-channel blockers including prenylamine, diltiazem, nifedipine analogues such as nicardipine and bepridil; various phenothiazines and thioxanthenes including trifluoperazine and the *trans*-isomer of flupentixol; structural analogues of the anthracyclines and vinca alkaloids; progesterone and other steroid hormones, as well as, to some extent, anti-oestrogens such as tamoxifen; ciclosporin and various of its nonimmunosuppressive analogues (such as valspodar); and various miscellaneous agents including amiodarone, quinidine, propranolol, reserpine, yohimbine, dipyridamole, erythromycin, cefoperazone, and ceftriaxone.

However, despite reported effects on resistance *in vitro* clinical results may be less impressive: studies in which verapamil was added to therapy for small cell lung cancer[3] or multiple myeloma[4] failed to demonstrate any benefit, and second-generation P-glycoprotein inhibitors such as valspodar have shown unpredictable pharmacokinetic interactions with cytotoxics.[5] Nevertheless, there is ongoing development of P-glycoprotein inhibitors, and drugs such as tariquidar are undergoing clinical trials.[5]


1. Ford JM, Hait WN. Pharmacology of drugs that alter multidrug resistance in cancer. *Pharmacol Rev* 1990; **42:** 155–99.
2. Krishna R, Mayer LD. Multidrug resistance (MDR) in cancer: mechanisms, reversal using modulators of MDR and the role of MDR modulators in influencing the pharmacokinetics of anticancer drugs. *Eur J Pharm Sci* 2000; **11:** 265–83.
3. Milroy R, *et al.* A randomised clinical study of verapamil in addition to combination chemotherapy in small cell lung cancer. *Br J Cancer* 1993; **68:** 813–18.
4. Dalton WS, *et al.* A phase III randomized study of oral verapamil as a chemosensitizer to reverse drug resistance in patients with refractory myeloma: a Southwest Oncology Group Study. *Cancer* 1995; **75:** 815–20.
5. Thomas H, Coley HM. Overcoming multidrug resistance in cancer: an update on the clinical strategy of inhibiting P-glycoprotein. *Cancer Control* 2003; **10:** 159–65.


## Choice of Antineoplastic

The following section describes the treatment of some of the major malignant neoplasms, and in particular the role of combination chemotherapy with antineoplastics.

Table 1 (below) lists published initial doses for some well-known combination chemotherapy regimens. Doses may be modified (particularly in subsequent cycles) to allow for patient status and toxic effects, although in some cases this may be at the expense of efficacy. Regimens can also vary slightly between institutions, or may be modified as part of the ongoing evolution of cancer chemotherapy; such therapy should preferably take place only in expert centres. The same acronym has sometimes been used for regimens containing different drugs, or using the same drugs in different doses or in different ways, and the reader should consult the literature for further details.

### Role of chemotherapy

In 1999, in an update of a previous consultation document on cancer chemotherapy,[1] WHO listed those drugs it considered essential for the rational management of malignant neoplasms.

The list divides drugs into 3 categories [note: drugs in italics in this list were not in the previous 1994 list]:

- 17 essential drugs that are used to treat curable cancers or cancers for which the cost-benefit ratio clearly favours drug treatment (bleomycin, *chlorambucil,* cisplatin, cyclophosphamide, *cytarabine,* dactinomycin, daunorubicin, doxorubicin, etoposide, fluorouracil, mercaptopurine, methotrexate, prednisolone, procarbazine, tamoxifen, vinblastine, and vincristine)
- 12 drugs that may have advantages in certain clinical situations (*busulfan, carboplatin, flutamide,* folinic acid, *gonadorelin analogues, interferon alfa, melphalan, megestrol,* mitomycin, *mitoxantrone, paclitaxel, and vinorelbine*)
- 13 drugs judged as not essential for the effective delivery of cancer care (*aminoglutethimide, anastrozole, altretamine, carmustine,* dacarbazine, *docetaxel, epirubicin, gemcitabine, ifosfamide, irinotecan, lomustine, raltitrexed, and topotecan*).

WHO considers that for some tumours such as hepatocellular carcinoma and lung cancer the development of effective prevention programmes through hepatitis B immunisation and tobacco control is currently of greater priority than therapy.[1]

Despite the real benefits achieved in selected conditions, reassessment of the role and value of chemotherapy for malignant neoplasms has led a number of oncologists to express the view that it has not lived up to its promise. Braverman[2] suggested in 1991 that for many or most patients medical management should be confined to symptom management and enrolment in a hospice programme, with a considerable reduction in the prescription of antineoplastics and a confinement of studies to drugs with novel mechanisms of action, or refinement of regimens known to be effective, a view he subsequently re-iterated.[3] Similar views have been expressed by others during the 1980s and 90s, pointing out the failure of treatment for most common adult tumours,[4] and suggesting that widespread use of chemotherapy is not justified outside clinical trials or specialised centres.[5,6] Bailar and Smith, in a statistical review in 1986, suggested that the 'war against cancer' was being lost, and that concentration on prevention rather than treatment might produce more promising results.[7] Despite acknowledging some areas of progress, an update of this review including data up to the end of 1994 came to the same conclusion.[8] Others have also pointed out the failure to adequately address methods for cancer prevention.[9]

Such views have naturally provoked controversy, and others consider that developments in the use of adjuvant and intensive regimens, as well as the continuing development of new agents, are significant and should not be denigrated.[10-14] However, the frequent reference to the hoped-for benefits of a greatly-improved knowledge of the molecular biology of cancer, and in particular the use of biological response modifiers,[11,15] or gene therapy,[16] does seem to concede that present chemotherapeutic regimens could be improved. Whether dose intensification is one appropriate route for improvement is a matter of some debate,[17,18] and, so far, clear evidence of effectiveness has been reported only for certain leukaemias and lymphomas.[1]

It has been suggested that perhaps attempts to destroy cancer cells are based on a false analogy between oncology and microbiology, and that a more appropriate goal would be the restoration of mechanisms of cellular control, enabling the patient to live with their cancer. Understanding of malignancy as a process, involving complex interactions between the malignant cell and its environment, in which intervention may be feasible to restore regulation of cellular growth, offers a potentially useful approach to cancer treatment. Although such an approach remains largely theoretical at present,[9,19,20] some drugs currently available, such as imatinib and trastuzumab, offer glimpses of its potential.


1. Sikora K, *et al.* Essential drugs for cancer therapy: a World Health Organization consultation. *Ann Oncol* 1999; **10:** 385–90.
2. Braverman AS. Medical oncology in the 1990s. *Lancet* 1991; **337:** 901–2.
3. Braverman AS. Chemotherapeutic failure: resistance or insensitivity? *Ann Intern Med* 1993; **118:** 630–2.
4. Kearsley JH. Cytotoxic chemotherapy for common adult malignancies: the emperor's new clothes revisited? *BMJ* 1986; **293:** 871–6.
5. Milsted RAV, *et al.* Cancer chemotherapy—what have we achieved? *Lancet* 1980; **i:** 1343–6.
6. Mead GM. Chemotherapy for solid tumours: routine treatment not yet justified. *BMJ* 1995; **310:** 246–7.
7. Bailar JC, Smith EM. Progress against cancer? *N Engl J Med* 1986; **314:** 1226–32.
8. Bailar JC, Gornik HL. Cancer undefeated. *N Engl J Med* 1997; **336:** 1569–74.
9. Sporn MB. The war on cancer. *Lancet* 1996; **347:** 1377–81.
10. Tobias JS. Medical oncology in the 1990s. *Lancet* 1991; **337:** 1220.
11. Chabner BA, Rothenberg ML. Medical oncology in the 1990s. *Lancet* 1991; **338:** 576–7.
12. Chabner BA. Biological basis for cancer treatment. *Ann Intern Med* 1993; **118:** 633–7.
13. Cunningham D. Chemotherapy for solid tumours; important progress in treatment. *BMJ* 1995; **310:** 247–8.
14. Kramer BS, Klausner RD. Grappling with cancer—defeatism versus the reality of progress. *N Engl J Med* 1997; **337:** 931–4.
15. Malpas JS. Oncology. *Postgrad Med J* 1990; **66:** 80–93.
16. Lemoine NR, Sikora K. Interventional genetics and cancer treatment. *BMJ* 1993; **306:** 665–6.
17. Hryniuk W. Will increases in dose intensity improve outcome: pro. *Am J Med* 1995; **99** (suppl 6A): 69S–70S.
18. Souhami RL. Will increases in dose intensity improve outcome: con. *Am J Med* 1995; **99** (suppl 6A): 71S–76S.
19. Astrow AB. Rethinking cancer. *Lancet* 1994; **343:** 494–5.
20. Schipper H, *et al.* A new biological framework for cancer research. *Lancet* 1996; **348:** 1149–51.


**Table 1.** Common chemotherapy regimens for malignant disease.

| Regimen | Drugs and Administration | Cycle | Typically used for | References |
|---|---|---|---|---|
| ABCM | Doxorubicin 30 mg/m$^2$ iv day 1; carmustine 30 mg/m$^2$ iv day 1; cyclophosphamide 100 mg/m$^2$ oral days 22–25; and melphalan 6 mg/m$^2$ oral days 22–25. | 42 days | Multiple myeloma | 1 |
| ABVD | Doxorubicin 25 mg/m$^2$ iv days 1, 15; bleomycin 10 000 IU/m$^2$ iv$^{(b)}$ days 1, 15; vinblastine 6 mg/m$^2$ iv days 1, 15; and dacarbazine 375 mg/m$^2$ iv days 1, 15. | 28 days | Lymphomas | 2, 3 |
| AC | Doxorubicin 60 mg/m$^2$ iv day 1 and cyclophosphamide 600 mg/m$^2$ iv day 1. | 21 days (for 4 cycles; some studies used up to 8 cycles) | Breast cancer | 4–6 |
| AC + paclitaxel | As above, then followed by paclitaxel 175 mg/m$^2$ iv day 1. | 21 days (further 4 cycles) | Breast cancer | 7 |
| AC + trastuzumab | Doxorubicin 60 mg/m$^2$ iv day 1; cyclophosphamide 600 mg/m$^2$ iv day 1; and trastuzumab 4 mg/kg iv loading dose on day 1 then 2 mg/kg once each week. | 21 days (for 6 cycles) | Breast cancer (HER2 overexpressing) | 8 |
| ACE | Doxorubicin 45 mg/m$^2$ iv day 1; cyclophosphamide 1 g/m$^2$ iv day 1; and etoposide 50 mg/m$^2$ iv days 1–5. | 21 days | Small cell lung cancer | 9 |
| AT | Doxorubicin 60 mg/m$^2$ iv day 1 and paclitaxel 200 mg/m$^2$ iv day 1. | 21 days (for 4 cycles) | Breast cancer | 4 |
| Key to abbreviations: hrs – hours; im – intramuscular; iv – intravenous | | | | |

**Table 1.** Common chemotherapy regimens for malignant disease. *(continued)*

| Regimen | Drugs and Administration | Cycle | Typically used for | References |
|---|---|---|---|---|
| AT | Doxorubicin 50 mg/m$^2$ iv day 1 and docetaxel 75 mg/m$^2$ iv day 1. | 21 days (for up to 8 cycles) | Breast cancer (metastatic) | 5 |
| BEAM (Mini-BEAM) | Carmustine 60 mg/m$^2$ iv day 1; etoposide 75 mg/m$^2$ iv days 2–5; cytarabine 100 mg/m$^2$ twice daily iv days 2–5; and melphalan 30 mg/m$^2$ iv day 6. | usually 28 to 42 days | Lymphomas (salvage) | 10 |
| BEP | Bleomycin 30 000 IU iv[(b)] days 2, 9, 16; etoposide 100 mg/m$^2$ iv days 1–5; and cisplatin 20 mg/m$^2$ iv days 1–5. | 21 days (for 4 cycles) | Testicular cancer | 11 |
| CAF | Cyclophosphamide 500 mg/m$^2$ iv day 1; doxorubicin 50 mg/m$^2$ iv day 1; and fluorouracil 500 mg/m$^2$ iv day 1. | 21 days | Breast cancer | 12 |
| CAP | Cyclophosphamide 750 mg/m$^2$ iv day 1; doxorubicin 50 mg/m$^2$ iv day 1; and prednisone 40 mg/m$^2$ oral days 1–5. | 28 days | Chronic lymphocytic leukaemia | 13 |
| CAP | Cyclophosphamide 500 mg/m$^2$ iv day 1; doxorubicin 50 mg/m$^2$ iv day 1; and cisplatin 50 mg/m$^2$ iv day 1 (these doses are optimised from the original 600 mg/m$^2$, 45 mg/m$^2$, and 50 mg/m$^2$ respectively). | 21 days (for 6 cycles) | Ovarian cancer | 14, 15 |
| CAV | Cyclophosphamide 900 mg/m$^2$ iv day 1; doxorubicin 45 mg/m$^2$ iv day 1; and vincristine 2 mg iv day 1. | 21 days (for 6 cycles) | Small cell lung cancer | 16 |
| CHOP | Cyclophosphamide 750 mg/m$^2$ iv day 1; doxorubicin 50 mg/m$^2$ iv day 1; vincristine 1.4 mg/m$^2$ (max. 2mg) iv day 1; and prednisone 100 mg oral days 1–5. | 21 days (for 6 to 8 cycles) | Lymphomas, chronic lymphocytic leukaemia | 17, 18 |
| CMF | Cyclophosphamide 100 mg/m$^2$ oral days 1–14; methotrexate 40 mg/m$^2$ iv days 1, 8; and fluorouracil 600 mg/m$^2$ iv days 1, 8. | 28 days | Breast cancer | 6, 19 |
| CMF | Cyclophosphamide 600 mg/m$^2$ iv day 1; methotrexate 40 mg/m$^2$ iv day 1; and fluorouracil 600 mg/m$^2$ iv day 1. | 21 days | Breast cancer | 20 |
| CMF | Cyclophosphamide 750 mg/m$^2$ iv day 1; methotrexate 40 mg/m$^2$ iv days 1, 8; and fluorouracil 600 mg/m$^2$ iv days 1, 8. | 28 days | Breast cancer | 6 |
| CMV | Cisplatin 100 mg/m$^2$ iv day 2; methotrexate 30 mg/m$^2$ iv days 1, 8; and vinblastine 4 mg/m$^2$ iv days 1, 8. | 21 days | Bladder cancer | 21 |
| COP (CVP) | Cyclophosphamide 800 mg/m$^2$ iv day 1; vincristine 2 mg iv day 1; and prednisone 60 mg/m$^2$ oral days 1–5, then tapered over days 6–8. | 21 days (for 6 cycles) | Lymphomas (the original report of this regimen used a 14-day cycle) | 22 |
| CP | Cisplatin 100 mg/m$^2$ iv day 1 and cyclophosphamide 600 mg/m$^2$ iv day 1 *or* carboplatin 300 mg/m$^2$ iv day1 and cyclophosphamide 600 mg/m$^2$ iv day 1. | 28 days (for 6 cycles) | Ovarian cancer | 23 |
| CYVADIC | Cyclophosphamide 500 mg/m$^2$ iv day 1; vincristine 1.5 mg/m$^2$ iv[(a)] days 1, 5; doxorubicin 50 mg/m$^2$ iv day 1; and dacarbazine 250 mg/m$^2$ iv days 1–5. | 21 days | Sarcoma (alternative versions of this regimen using vincristine on day 1 only have also been reported) | 24 |
| Dartmouth regimen | Dacarbazine 220 mg/m$^2$ iv days 1–3, 22–24; cisplatin 25 mg/m$^2$ iv days 1–3, 22–24; carmustine 150 mg/m$^2$ iv day 1; and tamoxifen 10 mg oral twice daily. | 42 days | Melanoma (metastatic) | 25, 26 |
| DHAP | Dexamethasone 40 mg oral or iv days 1–4; cytarabine 2 g/m$^2$ iv over 3 hrs, repeated after 12 hrs, day 2; and cisplatin 100 mg/m$^2$ iv over 24 hrs, day 1. | 21–28 days | Lymphomas (salvage) | 27 |
| EAP | Etoposide 120 mg/m$^2$ iv days 4–6; doxorubicin 20 mg/m$^2$ iv days 1, 7; and cisplatin 40 mg/m$^2$ iv days 2, 8. | 21–28 days | Stomach cancer | 28, 29 |
| Key to abbreviations: hrs – hours; im – intramuscular; iv – intravenous | | | | |

**Table 1.** Common chemotherapy regimens for malignant disease. *(continued)*

| Regimen | Drugs and Administration | Cycle | Typically used for | References |
|---|---|---|---|---|
| EC | Etoposide 100 mg/m$^2$ iv days 1–3 and carboplatin 450 mg/m$^2$ iv day 1. | 28 days | Small cell lung cancer | 30 |
| EC | Etoposide 100 mg/m$^2$ iv days 1–3 and carboplatin 325 mg/m$^2$ iv day 1. | 21 days | Non-small cell lung cancer | 31 |
| ECF | Epirubicin 50 mg/m$^2$ iv day 1; cisplatin 60 mg/m$^2$ iv day 1; and fluorouracil 200 mg/m$^2$ daily continuous iv. | 21 days (for up to 8 cycles) | Stomach cancer | 32 |
| EDAP | Etoposide 100–200 mg/m$^2$ continuous iv, days 1–4; dexamethasone 40 mg oral or iv days 1–5; cytarabine 1 g/m$^2$ iv day 5; and cisplatin 20 mg/m$^2$ continuous iv, days 1–4. | 21–28 days | Multiple myeloma (salvage), lymphomas | 33 |
| EMA-CO (or EMA-EP) | Etoposide 100 mg/m$^2$ iv days 1, 2; methotrexate 300 mg/m$^2$ iv over 12 hrs, day 1; folinic acid 15 mg oral or im, twice daily for 4 doses, starting day 2; and dactinomycin 500 micrograms iv days 1, 2. *with* cyclophosphamide 600 mg/m$^2$ iv day 8 and vincristine 1 mg/m$^2$ iv[(a)] day 8. *or* etoposide 150 mg/m$^2$ iv day 8 and cisplatin 75 mg/m$^2$ iv day 8. | 14 days | Gestational trophoblastic tumours | 34 |
| EP (PE) | Etoposide 80 mg/m$^2$ iv days 1–3 and cisplatin 80 mg/m$^2$ iv day 1. | 21 days | Small cell lung cancer (standard dose – other versions exist) | 35 |
| EP (PE) | Etoposide 80 mg/m$^2$ iv days 1–5 and cisplatin 27 mg/m$^2$ iv days 1–5. | 21 days | Small cell lung cancer (high dose) | 35 |
| EP (PE) | Etoposide 100 mg/m$^2$ iv day 1, *then* 200 mg/m$^2$ oral days 2–4 and cisplatin 75 mg/m$^2$ iv day 1. | 21 days | Small cell lung cancer | 36 |
| EPOCH | Etoposide 50 mg/m$^2$ continuous iv days 1–4; vincristine 400 micrograms/m$^2$ continuous iv[(a)] days 1–4; doxorubicin 10 mg/m$^2$ continuous iv days 1–4; cyclophosphamide 750 mg/m$^2$ iv day 5; and prednisone 60 mg/m$^2$ oral days 1–5. | 21 days | Lymphomas (salvage) | 37 |
| ESHAP | Etoposide 40 mg/m$^2$ iv days 1–4; methylprednisolone 250–500mg iv days 1–5; cisplatin 25 mg/m$^2$ continuous iv days 1–4; and cytarabine 2 g/m$^2$ iv day 5. | 21–28 days (for up to 8 cycles) | Lymphomas (salvage) | 38 |
| FAM | Fluorouracil 600 mg/m$^2$ iv days 1, 8, 29, 36; doxorubicin 30 mg/m$^2$ iv days 1, 29; and mitomycin 10 mg/m$^2$ iv day 1. | 56 days | Stomach cancer, pancreatic cancer | 39–41 |
| FAMTX | Fluorouracil 1.5 g/m$^2$ iv day 1; doxorubicin 30 mg/m$^2$ iv day 15; methotrexate 1.5 g/m$^2$ iv day 1, 1 hour before fluorouracil; and folinic acid 15 mg/m$^2$ oral every 6 hrs for 3 days, starting 24 hrs after methotrexate. | 28 days | Stomach cancer | 29, 32 |
| 5FU/Folinic acid | Fluorouracil 370 mg/m$^2$ iv days 1–5 and folinic acid 200 mg/m$^2$ iv days 1–5. | 28–35 days | Colorectal cancer | 42 |
| 5FU/Folinic acid (Mayo regimen, Poon regimen) | Fluorouracil 425 mg/m$^2$ iv days 1–5 and folinic acid 20 mg/m$^2$ iv day 1–5. | 28–35 days | Stomach cancer, colorectal cancer | 42, 43 |
| 5FU/Folinic acid (de Gramont regimen) | Fluorouracil 400 mg/m$^2$ iv bolus then 600 mg/m$^2$ continuous iv infusion, days 1, 2 and folinic acid 200 mg/m$^2$ iv days 1, 2. | 14 days | Colorectal cancer | 44 |
| Gemcitabine + cisplatin | Gemcitabine 1 g/m$^2$ iv days 1, 8, 15 and cisplatin 70 mg/m$^2$ iv day 2. | 28 days | Bladder cancer (metastatic) | 45 |
| ICE (ICbE) | Ifosfamide 5 g/m$^2$ iv over 24hrs, day 1 (with mesna); carboplatin 400 mg/m$^2$ iv day 1; and etoposide 100 mg/m$^2$ iv days 1–3. | 28 days (for 6 cycles) | Small cell lung cancer | 46 |
| Irinotecan, folinic acid, and 5FU | Irinotecan 125 mg/m$^2$ iv; folinic acid 20 mg/m$^2$ iv; and fluorouracil 500 mg/m$^2$ iv all once a week for 4 weeks. | 42 days | Colorectal cancer | 47 |

Key to abbreviations: hrs – hours; im – intramuscular; iv – intravenous

**Table 1.** Common chemotherapy regimens for malignant disease. *(continued)*

| Regimen | Drugs and Administration | Cycle | Typically used for | References |
|---|---|---|---|---|
| Hyper-CVAD | *Course A:*<br>Cyclophosphamide 300 mg/m$^2$ iv every 12 hrs, days 1–3;<br>doxorubicin 50 mg/m$^2$ iv day 4;<br>vincristine 2 mg iv days 4, 11; and<br>dexamethasone 40 mg iv or oral, days 1–4, 11–14.<br><br>*CNS prophylaxis*<br>Methotrexate 12 mg intrathecal, day 2 and<br>cytarabine 100 mg intrathecal, day 8.<br><br>*Course B:*<br>Methotrexate 200 mg/m$^2$ iv over 2 hrs, then 800 mg/m$^2$ iv over 24 hrs, day 1;<br>folinic acid 15 mg iv every 6 hrs for 8 doses, from 24 hrs after methotrexate (increased to 50 mg iv every 6 hrs if methotrexate levels are high);<br>methylprednisolone 50 mg iv every 12 hrs, days 1–3; and<br>cytarabine 3 g/m$^2$ every 12 hrs, days 2, 3. | 4 cycles of A alternated with 4 cycles of B, given over as short a period as possible; the number of A cycles in which CNS prophylaxis is given varies with expected risk of CNS disease | Lymphomas, adult acute lymphoblastic leukaemia (some variants of this regimen exist, including the substitution of daunorubicin 60mg/m$^2$ for doxorubicin in course A, the omission of methylprednisolone and addition of oral bicarbonate in course B, and simplification of methotrexate and folinic acid dosing; mesna, which was given in course A of the original regimen, is usually omitted) | 48 |
| M2 | Vincristine 30 micrograms/kg iv[(a)] day 1;<br>carmustine 500 micrograms/kg iv day 1;<br>cyclophosphamide 10 mg/kg iv day 1;<br>melphalan 250 micrograms/kg oral days 1–4 *or* 100 micrograms/kg oral days 1–7 *or* 1–10; and<br>prednisone 1 mg/kg oral, days 1–7, then taper and discontinue by day 21 unless hypercalcaemia or bone disease persist. | 35 days | Multiple myeloma | 49 |
| MACOP-B | Methotrexate 400 mg/m$^2$ iv days 8, 36, 64 (as 100 mg/m$^2$ iv bolus, then 300 mg/m$^2$ iv over 4 hrs);<br>folinic acid 15 mg oral every 6 hrs for 6 doses, from 24 hrs after methotrexate;<br>doxorubicin 50 mg/m$^2$ iv days 1, 15, 29, 43, 57, 71;<br>cyclophosphamide 350 mg/m$^2$ iv days 1, 15, 29, 43, 57, 71;<br>vincristine 1.4 mg/m$^2$ iv[(a)] days 8, 22, 36, 50, 64, 78;<br>bleomycin 10 000 IU/m$^2$ iv[(b)] days 22, 50, 78; and<br>prednisone 75 mg oral, daily for 10 weeks then tapered over 15 days. | 12 weeks | Lymphomas | 50 |
| MIC | Mitomycin 6 mg/m$^2$ iv day 2;<br>ifosfamide 3 g/m$^2$ iv day 2; and<br>cisplatin 120 mg/m$^2$ iv day 1. | 21 days | Non-small cell lung cancer | 51 |
| MIC | Mitomycin 6 mg/m$^2$ iv day 1;<br>ifosfamide 3 g/m$^2$ iv day 1; and<br>cisplatin 50 mg/m$^2$ iv day 1. | 21 days | Non-small cell lung cancer | 52 |
| MOPP | Chlormethine 6 mg/m$^2$ iv days 1, 8;<br>vincristine 1.4 mg/m$^2$ (max. 2 mg), days 1, 8;<br>procarbazine 100 mg/m$^2$ oral days 1–14; and<br>prednisone 40 mg/m$^2$ oral days 1–14, cycles 1, 4. | 28 days (for 6 cycles) | Lymphomas, Hodgkin's disease | 3, 53 |
| M-VAC | Methotrexate 30 mg/m$^2$ iv days 1, 15, 22;<br>vinblastine 3 mg/m$^2$ iv days 2, 15, 22;<br>doxorubicin 30 mg/m$^2$ iv day 2; and<br>cisplatin 70 mg/m$^2$ iv day 2. | usually 28 days | Bladder cancer | 45, 54, 55 |
| MVP | Mitomycin 8 mg/m$^2$ iv day 1, cycles 1 and 2, day 15 cycle 3;<br>vinblastine 4 mg/m$^2$ iv day 1, cycle 1<br>2 mg/m$^2$ iv day 8, cycle 1<br>4.5 mg/m$^2$ iv days 15, 22, cycle 1<br>4.5 mg/m$^2$ iv days 1, 15, cycle 2 and later; and<br>cisplatin 120 mg/m$^2$ iv day 1 | 28 days | Non-small cell lung cancer (neoadjuvant) | 56 |
| MVP | Mitomycin 8 mg/m$^2$ iv day 1, cycles 1 and 2, day 15 cycle 3;<br>vindesine 3 mg/m$^2$ iv days 1, 8, 15, 22, day 1 of cycle 2, then every 2 weeks until the 15$^{th}$ week; and<br>cisplatin 120 mg/m$^2$ iv day 1, for 3 cycles. | 28 days | Non-small cell lung cancer (neoadjuvant) | 56, 57 |
| MVP | Mitomycin 8 mg/m$^2$ iv day 1, cycles 1 and 2, day 15 cycle 3;<br>vinorelbine 25 mg/m$^2$ iv once a week for 16 weeks; and<br>cisplatin 120 mg/m$^2$ iv day 1, for 3 cycles. | 28 days | Non-small cell lung cancer (neoadjuvant) | 57 |
| PAC | Cisplatin 50 mg/m$^2$ iv day 1;<br>doxorubicin 50 mg/m$^2$ iv day 1; and<br>cyclophosphamide 500 mg/m$^2$ iv day 1. | 21 days (for up to 8 cycles) | Thymoma | 58 |

Key to abbreviations: hrs – hours; im – intramuscular; iv – intravenous

**Table 1.** Common chemotherapy regimens for malignant disease. *(continued)*

| Regimen | Drugs and Administration | Cycle | Typically used for | References |
|---|---|---|---|---|
| Paclitaxel and carboplatin | Paclitaxel 175 mg/m$^2$ iv day 1 and carboplatin – adjust dose to AUC of 7.5 mg/mL/minute by Calvert formula, iv day 1. | 21 days (for 6 cycles) | Ovarian cancer | 59 |
| Paclitaxel and cisplatin | Paclitaxel 135 mg/m$^2$ continuous iv over 24 hrs, day 1 and cisplatin 75 mg/m$^2$ iv day 1. | 21 days (for 6 cycles) | Ovarian cancer | 60 |
| Paclitaxel (standard) and trastuzumab | Paclitaxel 175 mg/m$^2$ iv on day 1 and trastuzumab 4 mg/kg iv loading dose on day 1 then 2 mg/kg once each week. | 21 days | Breast cancer (HER2 overexpressing) | 8 |
| Paclitaxel (weekly) and trastuzumab | Paclitaxel 90 mg/m$^2$ iv on day 1 and trastuzumab 4 mg/kg iv loading dose on day 1 then 2 mg/kg once each week. | 7 days | Breast cancer (HER2 overexpressing) | 61 |
| PCV | Procarbazine 60 mg/m$^2$ oral days 8–21; lomustine 110 mg/m$^2$ oral day 1; and vincristine 1.4 mg/m$^2$ iv[(a)] days 8, 29. | 42–56 days | Gliomas (adjuvant) | 62 |
| PE | *See* EP | | | |
| ProMACE-CytaBOM | Prednisone 60 mg/m$^2$ oral days 1–14; doxorubicin 25 mg/m$^2$ iv day 1; cyclophosphamide 650 mg/m$^2$ iv day 1; etoposide 120 mg/m$^2$ iv day 1; cytarabine 300 mg/m$^2$ iv day 8; bleomycin 5000 IU/m$^2$ iv[(b)] day 8; vincristine 1.4 mg/m$^2$ iv[(a)] day 8; methotrexate 120 mg/m$^2$ iv day 8; and folinic acid 25 mg/m$^2$ oral every 6 hrs for 4 doses, from 24 hrs after methotrexate. | 21 days | Lymphomas | 63 |
| PVB | See VBP | | | |
| SMF | Streptozocin 1 g/m$^2$ iv days 1, 8, 29, 36; mitomycin 10 mg/m$^2$ iv day 1; and fluorouracil 600 mg/m$^2$ iv days 1, 8, 29, 36. | 56 days | Pancreatic cancer | 41 |
| Stanford V regimen | Doxorubicin 25 mg/m$^2$ iv days 1, 15; vinblastine 6 mg/m$^2$ iv days 1, 15; chlormethine 6 mg/m$^2$ iv day 1; vincristine 1.4 mg/m$^2$ iv (max 2mg) days 8, 22; bleomycin 5000 IU/m$^2$ iv[(b)] days 8, 22; etoposide 60 mg/m$^2$ iv days 15, 16; prednisone 40 mg/m$^2$ oral on alternate days for 10 weeks then tapered by 10 mg on alternate days. | 28 days (for 3 cycles) | Hodgkin's disease | 64 |
| VAD | Vincristine 400 micrograms iv days 1–4; doxorubicin 9 mg/m$^2$ iv days 1–4; and dexamethasone 40 mg oral days 1–4, 9–12, 17–20. | 28 days (usually for 4 cycles) | Multiple myeloma | 65 |
| VBAP | Vincristine 1 mg iv day 1; carmustine 30 mg/m$^2$ iv day 1; doxorubicin 30 mg/m$^2$ iv day 1; and prednisone 60 mg/m$^2$ oral or parenteral (may be rounded to 100 mg oral) days 1–4. | 21 or 28 days | Multiple myeloma | 66, 67 |
| VBP | Vinblastine 150 micrograms/kg iv days 1, 2; bleomycin 30 000 IU iv[(b)] days 2, 9, 16; and cisplatin 20 mg/m$^2$ iv days 1–5. | 21 days | Germ-cell (ovarian, testicular) cancer | 11 |
| VCMP | Vincristine 1 mg iv day 1; melphalan 9 mg/m$^2$ oral days 1–4; cyclophosphamide 500 mg/m$^2$ iv day 1; and prednisone 60 mg/m$^2$ oral or parenteral, days 1–4. | 28 days | Multiple myeloma | 67 |
| VeIP | Vinblastine 110 micrograms/kg iv days 1, 2; ifosfamide 1.2 g/m$^2$ iv days 1–5 (with mesna); and cisplatin 20 mg/m$^2$ iv days 1–5. | 21 days (for 4 cycles) | Germ-cell (especially testicular) cancer | 68 |
| VIP | Etoposide 75mg/m$^2$ iv days 1–5; ifosfamide 1.2 g/m$^2$ iv days 1–5 (with mesna); and cisplatin 20mg/m$^2$ iv days 1–5. | 21 days (for 4 cycles) | Germ-cell (especially testicular) cancer | 68 |
| Key to abbreviations: hrs – hours; im – intramuscular; iv – intravenous | | | | |

(a) Although not always reflected in the original papers it is now generally accepted that the total dose of vincristine should not exceed 2 mg, in order to minimise neurotoxicity

(b) Doses of bleomycin have been given in international units (IU) in this table, but doses in the original papers may be quoted in mg-potency or USP units. One mg-potency or one USP unit is equivalent to 1000 international units

**Table 1. References:**


1. MacLennan ICM, *et al.* Combined chemotherapy with ABCM versus melphalan for treatment of myelomatosis. *Lancet* 1992; **339:** 200–205.
2. Bonadonna G, Santoro A. ABVD chemotherapy in the treatment of Hodgkin's disease. *Cancer Treat Rev* 1982; **9:** 21–35.
3. Canellos GP, *et al.*. Chemotherapy of advanced Hodgkin's disease with MOPP, ABVD, or MOPP alternating with ABVD. *N Engl J Med* 1992; **327:** 1478–84.
4. Pouillart P, *et al.* Final results of a phase II randomized, parallel study of doxorubicin/cyclophosphamide (AC) and doxorubicin/Taxol® (paclitaxel) (AT) as neoadjuvant treatment of local-regional breast cancer. *Proc Am Soc Clin Oncol* 1999; **18:** 73.
5. Nabholtz J-M, *et al.* Docetaxel and doxorubicin compared with doxorubicin and cyclophosphamide as first-line chemotherapy for metastatic breast cancer: results of a randomized, multicenter, phase III trial. *J Clin Oncol* 2003; **21:** 968–75.
6. Fisher B, *et al.* Two months of doxorubicin-cyclophosphamide with and without interval reinduction therapy compared with 6 months of cyclophosphamide, methotrexate, and fluorouracil in positive-node breast cancer patients with tamoxifen-nonresponsive tumors: results from the National Surgical Adjuvant Breast and Bowel Project B-15. *J Clin Oncol.* 1990; **8:** 1483–96.
7. Henderson IC, *et al.* Improved outcomes from adding sequential paclitaxel but not from escalating doxorubicin dose in an adjuvant chemotherapy regimen for patients with node-positive primary breast cancer. *J Clin Oncol* 2003; **21:** 976–83.
8. Slamon DJ, *et al.* Use of chemotherapy plus a monoclonal antibody against HER2 for metastatic breast cancer that overexpresses HER2. *N Engl J Med* 2001; **344:** 783–92.
9. Aisner J, *et al.* Doxorubicin, cyclophosphamide and VP16-213 (ACE) in the treatment of small cell lung cancer. *Cancer Chemother Pharmacol* 1982; **7:** 187–93.
10. Colwill R, *et al.* Mini-BEAM as salvage therapy for relapsed or refractory Hodgkin's disease before intensive therapy and autologous bone marrow transplantation. *J Clin Oncol* 1995; **13:** 396–402.
11. Williams SD, *et al.* Treatment of disseminated germ-cell tumors with cisplatin, bleomycin, and either vinblastine or etoposide. *N Engl J Med* 1987; **316:** 1435–40.
12. Smalley RV, *et al.* A comparison of cyclophosphamide, adriamycin, 5-fluorouracil (CAF) and cyclophosphamide, methotrexate, 5-fluorouracil, vincristine, prednisone (CMFVP) in patients with metastatic breast cancer: a Southeastern Cancer Study Group project. *Cancer* 1977; **40:** 625–32.
13. The French Cooperative Group on Chronic Lymphocytic Leukemia. Comparison of fludarabine, cyclophosphamide/doxorubicin/prednisone, and cyclophosphamide/doxorubicin/vincristine/prednisone in advanced forms of chronic lymphocytic leukemia: preliminary results of a controlled clinical trial. *Semin Oncol* 1993; **20** (suppl 7): 21–3.
14. de Oliveira CF, *et al.* Randomized comparison of cyclophosphamide, doxorubicin and cisplatin (CAP) versus cyclophosphamide and doxorubicin (CA) for the treatment of advanced ovarian cancer (ADOVCA): a EORTC Gynecological Cancer Cooperative Group study. *Eur J Gynaecol Oncol* 1990; **11:** 323–30.
15. The ICON Collaborators. ICON2: randomised trial of single-agent carboplatin against three-drug combination of CAP (cyclophosphamide, doxorubicin, and cisplatin) in women with ovarian cancer. *Lancet* 1998; **352:** 1571–6.
16. Feld R, *et al.* Combined modality induction therapy without maintenance chemotherapy for small cell carcinoma of the lung. *J Clin Oncol* 1984; **2:** 294–304.
17. McKelvey EM, *et al.* Hydroxyldaunomycin (Adriamycin) combination chemotherapy in malignant lymphoma. *Cancer* 1976; **38:** 1484–93.
18. Fisher RI, *et al.* Comparison of a standard regimen (CHOP) with three intensive chemotherapy regimens for advanced non-Hodgkin's lymphoma. *N Engl J Med* 1993; **328:** 1002–6.
19. Bonadonna G, *et al.* Combination chemotherapy as an adjuvant treatment in operable breast cancer. *N Engl J Med* 1976; **294:** 405–10.
20. Weiss RB, *et al.* Adjuvant chemotherapy after conservative surgery plus irradiation versus modified radical mastectomy: analysis of drug dosing and toxicity. *Am J Med* 1987; **83:** 455–63.
21. Harker WG, *et al.* Cisplatin, methotrexate, and vinblastine (CMV): an effective chemotherapy regimen for metastatic transitional cell carcinoma of the urinary tract. A Northern California Oncology Group study. *J Clin Oncol* 1985; **3:** 1463–70.
22. Luce JK, *et al.* Combined cyclophosphamide, vincristine, and prednisone therapy of malignant lymphoma. *Cancer* 1971; **28:** 306–17.
23. Alberts DS, *et al.* Improved therapeutic index of carboplatin plus cyclophosphamide versus cisplatin plus cyclophosphamide: final report by the Southwest Oncology Group of a phase III randomized trial in stages III and IV ovarian cancer. *J Clin Oncol* 1992; **10:** 706–17.
24. Yap B-S, *et al.* Cyclophosphamide, vincristine, adriamycin, and DTIC (CYVADIC) combination chemotherapy for the treatment of advanced sarcomas. *Cancer Treat Rep* 1980; **64:** 93–8.
25. McClay EF, *et al.* Combination chemotherapy and hormonal therapy in the treatment of malignant melanoma. *Cancer Treat Rep* 1987; **71:** 465–9.
26. Chapman PB, *et al.* Phase III multicenter randomized trial of the Dartmouth regimen versus dacarbazine in patients with metastatic melanoma. *J Clin Oncol* 1999; **17:** 2745–51.
27. Velasquez WS, *et al.* Effective salvage therapy for lymphoma with cisplatin in combination with high-dose Ara-C and dexamethasone (DHAP). *Blood* 1988; **71:** 117–22.
28. Preusser P, *et al.* Phase II study with the combination etoposide, doxorubicin and cisplatin in advanced measurable gastric cancer. *J Clin Oncol* 1989; **7:** 1310–17.
29. Kelsen D, *et al.* FAMTX versus etoposide, doxorubicin, and cisplatin: a random assignment trial in gastric cancer. *J Clin Oncol* 1992; **10:** 541–8.
30. Viren M, *et al.* Carboplatin and etoposide in extensive small cell lung cancer. *Acta Oncol* 1994; **33:** 921–4.
31. Klastersky J, *et al.* A randomized study comparing cisplatin or carboplatin with etoposide in patients with advanced non-small-cell lung cancer: European Organization for Research and Treatment of Cancer Protocol 07861. *J Clin Oncol* 1990; **8:** 1556–62.
32. Waters JS, *et al.* Long-term survival after epirubicin, cisplatin and fluorouracil for gastric cancer: results of a randomized trial. *Br J Cancer* 1999; **80:** 269–72.
33. Barlogie B, *et al.* Etoposide, dexamethasone, cytarabine, and cisplatin in vincristine, doxorubicin, and dexamethasone-refractory myeloma. *J Clin Oncol* 1989; **7:** 1514–17.
34. Newlands ES, *et al.* Results with the EMA/CO (etoposide, methotrexate, actinomycin D, cyclophosphamide, vincristine) regimen in high risk gestational trophoblastic tumours, 1979 to 1989. *Br J Obstet Gynaecol* 1991; **98:** 550–7.
35. Ihde DC, *et al.* Prospective randomized comparison of high-dose and standard-dose etoposide and cisplatin chemotherapy in patients with extensive-stage small-cell lung cancer. *J Clin Oncol* 1994; **12:** 2022–34.
36. Sundstrøm S, *et al.* Cisplatin and etoposide regimen is superior to cyclophosphamide, epirubicin, and vincristine regimen in small-cell lung cancer: results from a randomized phase III trial with 5 years' follow-up. *J Clin Oncol* 2002; **20:** 4665–72.
37. Gutierrez M, *et al.* Role of a doxorubicin-containing regimen in relapsed and resistant lymphomas: an 8-year follow-up study of EPOCH. *J Clin Oncol* 2000; **18:** 3633–42.
38. Velasquez WS, *et al.* ESHAP—an effective chemotherapy regimen in refractory and relapsing lymphoma: a 4-year follow-up study. *J Clin Oncol* 1994; **12:** 1169–76.
39. Macdonald JS, *et al.* 5-Fluorouracil, doxorubicin and mitomycin (FAM) combination chemotherapy for advanced gastric cancer. *Ann Intern Med* 1980; **93:** 533–6.
40. Cullinan SA, *et al.* A comparison of three chemotherapeutic regimens in the treatment of advanced pancreatic and gastric carcinoma: fluorouracil vs fluorouracil and doxorubicin vs fluorouracil, doxorubicin, and mitomycin. *JAMA* 1985; **253:** 2061–7.
41. The Gastrointestinal Tumor Study Group. Phase II studies of drug combinations in advanced pancreatic carcinoma: fluorouracil plus doxorubicin plus mitomycin C and two regimens of streptozotocin plus mitomycin C plus fluorouracil. *J Clin Oncol* 1986; **4:** 1794–8.
42. Poon MA, *et al.* Biochemical modulation of fluorouracil: evidence of significant improvement of survival and quality of life in patients with advanced colorectal carcinoma. *J Clin Oncol* 1989; **7:** 1407–18.
43. Rubin J, *et al.* Phase II trials of 5-fluorouracil and leucovorin in patients with metastatic gastric or pancreatic carcinoma. *Cancer* 1996; **78:** 1888–91.
44. de Gramont A, *et al.* A review of GERCOD trials of bimonthly leucovorin plus 5-fluorouracil 48-h continuous infusion in advanced colorectal cancer: evolution of a regimen. *Eur J Cancer* 1998; **34:** 619–26.
45. von der Maase H, *et al.* Gemcitabine and cisplatin versus methotrexate, vinblastine, doxorubicin, and cisplatin in advanced or metastatic bladder cancer: results of a large, randomized, multinational, multicenter, phase III study. *J Clin Oncol* 2000; **17:** 3068–77.
46. Smith IE, *et al.* Carboplatin, etoposide, and ifosfamide as intensive chemotherapy for small-cell lung cancer. *J Clin Oncol* 1990; **8:** 899–905.
47. Saltz LB, *et al.* Irinotecan plus fluorouracil and leucovorin for metastatic colorectal cancer. *N Engl J Med* 2000; **343:** 905–14.
48. Kantarjian HM, *et al.* Results of treatment with hyper-CVAD, a dose-intensive regimen, in adult acute lymphocytic leukemia. *J Clin Oncol* 2000; **18:** 547–61.
49. Case DC, *et al.* Improved survival times in multiple myeloma treated with melphalan, prednisone, cyclophosphamide, vincristine and BCNU: M-2 protocol. *Am J Med* 1977; **63:** 897–903.
50. Klimo P, Connors JM. MACOP-B chemotherapy for the treatment of diffuse large-cell lymphoma. *Ann Intern Med* 1985; **102:** 596–602.
51. Crinò L, *et al.* Chemotherapy of advanced non-small-cell lung cancer: a comparison of three active regimens. A randomized trial of the Italian Oncology Group for Clinical Research. *Ann Oncol* 1995; **6:** 347–53.
52. Cullen MH, *et al.* Mitomycin, ifosfamide and cis-platin in non-small cell lung cancer: treatment good enough to compare. *Br J Cancer* 1988; **58:** 359–61.
53. DeVita VT, *et al.* Combination chemotherapy in the treatment of advanced Hodgkin's disease. *Ann Intern Med* 1970; **73:** 881–95.
54. Sternberg CN, *et al.* Preliminary results of M-VAC (methotrexate, vinblastine, doxorubicin and cisplatin) for transitional cell carcinoma of the urothelium. *J Urol (Baltimore)* 1985; **133:** 403–7.
55. Loehrer PJ, *et al.* A randomized comparison of cisplatin alone or in combination with methotrexate, vinblastine, and doxorubicin in patients with metastatic urothelial carcinoma: a cooperative group study. *J Clin Oncol* 1992; **10:** 1066–73.
56. Pisters KMW, *et al.* Pathologic complete response in advanced non-small-cell lung cancer following preoperative chemotherapy: implications for the design of future non-small-cell lung cancer combined modality trials. *J Clin Oncol* 1993; **11:** 1757–62.
57. Pérol M, *et al.* Multicenter randomized trial comparing cisplatin-mitomycin-vinorelbine versus cisplatin-mitomycin-vindesine in advanced non-small cell lung cancer. *Lung Cancer* 1996; **14:** 119–34.
58. Loehrer PJ, *et al.* Cisplatin plus doxorubicin plus cyclophosphamide in metastatic or recurrent thymoma: final results of an intergroup trial. *J Clin Oncol* 1994; **12:** 1164–8.
59. Coleman RL, *et al.* Carboplatin and short-infusion paclitaxel in high-risk and advanced-stage ovarian carcinoma. *Cancer J Sci Am* 1997; **3:** 246–53.
60. McGuire WP, *et al.* Cyclophosphamide and cisplatin compared with paclitaxel and cisplatin in patients with stage III and stage IV ovarian cancer. *N Engl J Med* 1996; **334:** 1–6.
61. Seidman AD, *et al.* Weekly trastuzumab and paclitaxel therapy for metastatic breast cancer with analysis of efficacy by HER2 immunophenotype and gene amplification. *J Clin Oncol* 2001; **19:** 2587–95.
62. Levin VA, *et al.* Superiority of post-radiotherapy adjuvant chemotherapy with CCNU, procarbazine, and vincristine (PCV) over BCNU for anaplastic gliomas: NCOG 6G61 final report. *Int J Radiat Oncol Biol Phys* 1990; **18:** 321–4.
63. Longo DL, *et al.* Superiority of ProMACE-CytaBOM over ProMACE-MOPP in the treatment of advanced diffuse aggressive lymphoma: results of a prospective randomized trial. *J Clin Oncol* 1991; **9:** 25–38.
64. Bartlett NL, *et al.* Brief chemotherapy, Stanford V, and adjuvant radiotherapy for bulky or advanced-stage Hodgkin's disease: a preliminary report. *J Clin Oncol* 1995; **13:** 1080–8.
65. Barlogie B, *et al.* Effective treatment of advanced multiple myeloma refractory to alkylating agents. *N Engl J Med* 1984; **310:** 1353–6.
66. Bonnet J, *et al.* Vincristine, BCNU, doxorubicin, and prednisone (VBAP) combination in the treatment of relapsing or resistant multiple myeloma: a Southwest Oncology Group study. *Cancer Treat Rep* 1982; **66:** 1267–71.
67. Bladé J, *et al.* Increased conventional chemotherapy does not improve survival in multiple myeloma: long-term results of two PETHEMA trials including 914 patients. *Hematol J* 2001; **2:** 272–8.
68. Loehrer PJ, *et al.* Salvage therapy in recurrent germ cell cancer: ifosfamide and cisplatin plus either vinblastine or etoposide. *Ann Intern Med* 1988; **109:** 540–6.


## Management of malignant disease

**Carcinoid tumours and other secretory neoplasms.** All neoplastic cells have some abnormalities of metabolism, and many secrete characteristic metabolic products. Where the substance secreted has hormonal or pharmacological properties profound clinical effects may result, particularly since secretion is generally unregulated by normal homoeostatic mechanisms. Examples of syndromes associated with such secretory neoplasms include acromegaly (p.1312), Cushing's syndrome (p.1313), hyperprolactinaemia (p.1315), and other endocrine disorders associated with pituitary adenomas; phaeochromocytoma (p.831); and carcinoid syndrome and the various syndromes associated with pancreatic endocrine tumours. Multiple endocrine neoplasia type 1 (MEN1) and type 2 (MEN2) are inherited conditions in which many tumours occur in often more than one endocrine organ; tumours in this disorder are often secretory.[1]

**Carcinoid syndrome.** Carcinoid tumours occur mainly in the gastrointestinal tract or lungs (bronchi), although they occasionally arise in other organs with a common embryological origin. Although they are relatively common, accounting for about 30% of all small bowel tumours, symptomatic carcinoid syndrome is rare, both because the tumours vary in their behaviour depending on their embryological origin and because the liver is capable of metabolising those tumour products which are secreted into the portal circulation; only if the carcinoid tumour secretes into the systemic circulation, notably after metastasis to the liver, do symptoms occur. Tumours of embryological fore-gut origin, usually found in the lung or stomach, predominantly secrete histamine or serotonin (5-HT); mid-gut tumours, with a usual primary site in the terminal ileum, are the most likely to metastasise and produce carcinoid syndrome, and predominantly secrete serotonin; hind-gut tumours, commonly benign, do not secrete active substances.

The characteristic symptoms of carcinoid syndrome include episodic flushing of the face and upper trunk (which may be provoked by alcohol, food, or stress), secretory diarrhoea, wheezing and dyspnoea, weight loss, pellagra, painful hepatomegaly, and right-sided valvular heart disease, which sometimes progresses to right heart failure and death.

The management of carcinoid tumours usually involves surgical resection, and this can be curative, particularly if the primary tumour has not metastasised.[2-4] Antineoplastic chemotherapy has limited benefit,[2] except perhaps in patients with atypical variants of carcinoid tumours.[3] There is some evidence that treatment with interferon alfa can stabilise the disease or occasionally produce tumour regression,[4] but adverse effects have limited its use.[3] Hepatic arterial embolisation to destroy the blood supply of hepatic metastases has produced symptomatic palliation, but its effects are temporary.[2,3] Results may be better in combination with systemic chemotherapy in selected patients.[5] Antineoplastics such as doxorubicin have also been given into the hepatic artery for treating hepatic metastases.[3]

For symptomatic relief of carcinoid syndrome somatostatin analogues such as octreotide or lanreotide are highly effective and are the treatment of choice.[2-4] The availability of depot intramuscular preparations has simplified treatment, removing the need for multiple daily subcutaneous injections. However, with prolonged use a few patients develop resistance even to the highest doses.[2] Octreotide is also used in the perioperative management of these patients to treat or prevent carcinoid crisis, when it may be given intravenously.[2,6] Other drugs that reduce the effects of serotonin that have been tried include cyproheptadine, ondansetron, ketanserin, and methysergide.[2]

Apart from such specific pharmacological therapies, antidiarrhoeals such as codeine and loperamide are sometimes helpful in controlling diarrhoea. Wheezing (bronchoconstriction) and heart failure are managed conventionally. Supplementation with nicotinamide is advisable to prevent pellagra. It is also important to avoid provocative factors such as stress, alcohol, and particular foods.[2]

**Pancreatic endocrine tumours**. Neoplasms of the pancreatic islet cells (pancreatic endocrine tumours) are uncommon compared with those of the exocrine pancreas (see Malignant Neoplasms of the Pancreas, p.521). Pancreatic endocrine tumours, whether benign or malignant, often secrete clinically significant amounts of hormone; the hormone secreted, and hence the resultant clinical syndrome, depends on which of the several types of hormone-secreting islet cells is the origin of the tumour (for example, insulinomas arise in islet beta cells).[7] Primary therapy for solitary pancreatic endocrine tumours is surgical resection; metastatic tumours may require a combination of symptomatic drug therapy, chemotherapy, radiotherapy, and surgical debulking. The most frequently used antineoplastic is streptozocin, either alone or combined with other drugs such as fluorouracil or doxorubicin.[7,8] Chlorozotocin is also active.[8] As with carcinoid tumours, hepatic metastases may be treated with hepatic artery embolisation.[4,5,7] Somatostatin analogues and interferon alfa may be used to control symptoms of pancreatic endocrine tumours.[4] Other therapies depend on the specific tumour type. In patients with **insulinoma** (tumours originating in the islet beta cells) excessive insulin secretion results in hypoglycaemia. Where surgical resection is not feasible or not successful diazoxide may be used to control hypoglycaemia. Beneficial results have also been achieved with octreotide. Intake of frequent small meals containing complex carbohydrates is also important.[7] Up to 90% of insulinomas are benign and do not metastasise. In **glucagonoma** the primary neoplasm derives from the alpha cell[7] and the clinical syndrome (a characteristic skin rash known as necrolytic migratory erythema, diabetes mellitus or glucose intolerance, weight loss, and anaemia) results from excessive glucagon secretion. Surgical resection is indicated for localised disease but 50 to 80% of cases have metastasised at presentation. Octreotide usually decreases glucagon secretion and improves symptoms. Another well characterised syndrome results from tumours which release vasoactive intestinal polypeptide (VIP). Such **vipomas** result in profound but intermittent secretory diarrhoea, with consequent hypokalaemia and acidosis;[7] the syndrome is sometimes known as pancreatic cholera. Metabolic imbalances should be corrected by fluid and electrolyte supplementation. Octreotide controls the secretory diarrhoea, and it may be useful for symptom control before surgery as well as for palliation in metastatic disease. About 80% of vipomas are malignant.[7]

Of the other pancreatic endocrine tumours **gastrinoma** is the commonest: it results in Zollinger-Ellison syndrome, the treatment of which is discussed on p.1247. Rarer tumours include **somatostatinoma** and **PPoma** (secreting pancreatic polypeptide).[7]


1. Brandi ML, *et al.* Guidelines for diagnosis and therapy of MEN type 1 and type 2. *J Clin Endocrinol Metab* 2001; **86:** 5658–71.
2. Caplin ME, *et al.* Carcinoid tumour. *Lancet* 1998; **352:** 799–805.
3. Kulke MH, Mayer RJ. Carcinoid tumors. *N Engl J Med* 1999; **340:** 858–68.
4. Öberg K. Advances in chemotherapy and biotherapy of endocrine tumours. *Curr Opin Oncol* 1998; **10:** 58–65.
5. Moertel CG, *et al.* The management of patients with advanced carcinoid tumors and islet cell carcinomas. *Ann Intern Med* 1994; **120:** 302–9.
6. Veall GRQ, *et al.* Review of the anaesthetic management of 21 patients undergoing laparotomy for carcinoid syndrome. *Br J Anaesth* 1994; **72:** 335–41.
7. Sharma V, Lynn JA. Rare tumours 1: the management of rare endocrine tumours of the pancreas. *CME Oncol* 1999; **1:** 85–92.
8. Moertel CG, *et al.* Streptozocin-doxorubicin, streptozocin-fluorouracil, or chlorozotocin in the treatment of advanced islet-cell carcinoma. *N Engl J Med* 1992; **326:** 519–23.


**Gestational trophoblastic tumours.** The gestational trophoblastic diseases arise from the trophoblast, the first tissue to differentiate in the early embryo: they are associated with conception and pregnancy and affect women of reproductive age. They may be divided into molar pregnancy (complete or partial hydatidiform mole), invasive mole (chorioadenoma destruens), choriocarcinoma, and placental site trophoblastic tumour. A persistent gestational trophoblastic tumour (invasive mole or choriocarcinoma) may develop in about 25% of women after evacuation of a complete molar pregnancy, and about 2 to 4% after a partial molar pregnancy.[1] Choriocarcinoma may also occur after normal delivery, abortion, or ectopic pregnancy.

All these tumours secrete human chorionic gonadotrophin (hCG), and measurement of the urinary or serum concentrations, which are generally proportional to the total tumour mass, is important in diagnosis of disease and monitoring of treatment.

The trophoblastic tumours vary in aggressiveness but some, such as choriocarcinoma, are highly invasive and rapidly fatal if untreated; however, appropriate treatment, based on the perceived risk category, can result in an excellent prognosis. Prognostic factors for increased risk include high titres of hCG, liver or brain metastases, and failure of previous single-agent chemotherapy as well as, perhaps, greater age. With current treatment, including local irradiation for metastases, virtually 100% of patients with localised disease should be cured, as are over 70% of patients with more advanced stages.

Prophylactic chemotherapy has been used in women considered at particular risk of persistent gestational trophoblastic tumour after evacuation of a complete molar pregnancy, but the practice is controversial.[1,2]

In patients who develop low- or moderate-risk choriocarcinoma or invasive mole, the treatment of choice is single-agent chemotherapy with methotrexate or dactinomycin.[1-4] The combination EMA-CO (etoposide, methotrexate, dactinomycin, cyclophosphamide, and vincristine) is the current preferred treatment in high-risk patients.[1,2,4,5] A combination of methotrexate, dactinomycin, and either cyclophosphamide or chlorambucil was the preferred combination in the past. In refractory disease, the salvage regimen EMA-EP uses etoposide and cisplatin in place of cyclophosphamide and vincristine in EMA-CO. Other regimens have used etoposide and cisplatin with either bleomycin or ifosfamide.[5]

Brain metastases are generally treated by local irradiation, given with chemotherapy. Liver metastases have been treated with irradiation, local chemoembolisation, or surgical resection.[2,5]

Patients with placental site trophoblastic tumour, which is relatively insensitive to chemotherapy, may be best treated by hysterectomy in the early stages.[1,2] In high-risk patients, a platinum-based regimen is preferred to EMA-CO.[4]


1. Berkowitz RS, Goldstein DP. Chorionic tumors. *N Engl J Med* 1996; **335:** 1740–8.
2. Shapter AP, McLellan R. Gestational trophoblastic disease. *Obstet Gynecol Clin North Am* 2001; **28:** 805–17.
3. Homesley HD. Single-agent therapy for nonmetastatic and low-risk gestational trophoblastic disease. *J Reprod Med* 1998; **43:** 69–74.
4. Newlands ES, *et al.* Recent advances in gestational trophoblastic disease. *Hematol Oncol Clin North Am* 1999; **13:** 225–44.
5. Lurain JR. Advances in management of high-risk gestational trophoblastic tumors. *J Reprod Med* 2002; **47:** 451–9.


**Histiocytic syndromes.** Histiocytic syndromes cover a broad range of proliferative disorders of histiocytes (macrophages and dendritic cells), for which the classification and diagnostic criteria are evolving.[1] Langerhans-cell histiocytosis (histiocytosis X) is one such disorder characterised by proliferation of CD1 positive Langerhans cells (a form of dendritic cell).[1] Terms that were formerly used for different clinical manifestations of Langerhans-cell histiocytosis include eosinophilic granuloma, Hand-Schüller-Christian disease, and Letterer-Siwe syndrome,[1-3] but these are now considered obsolete.[1] Langerhans-cell histiocytosis mainly presents in childhood, and is of uncertain aetiology: it is not clear whether it should be considered a malignancy.

The clinical presentation of Langerhans-cell histiocytosis is highly variable.[2-5] The classic feature is single or multiple bone lesions, and skin lesions may also occur (restricted disease).[3,5] The disorder may also involve visceral organs, ultimately causing dysfunction of the liver, lungs, or bone marrow (extensive or multisystem disease). Sequelae to the disease include diabetes insipidus, growth failure, and orthopaedic handicap.[3,4] The morbidity and prognosis depends upon the number of organ systems involved, and whether normal function of these organs is affected. Patients with restricted disease have a generally benign course, and single lesions often regress spontaneously. However, if a bone lesion does not resolve, or risks causing fracture or deformity before it resolves, or is causing disabling symptoms, it may be treated with curettage, intralesional corticosteroids, or radiotherapy.[3,5] Similarly, single skin lesions may be allowed to resolve without treatment or treated with methoxsalen plus UV light (PUVA) or topical chlormethine. Multiple bone lesions may be treated with single-agent chemotherapy.[5]

In more extensive disease the prognosis is not as good, mainly due to organ dysfunction.[3-5] Systemic chemotherapy has been widely used, because the disease tends to be progressive in these patients, but its degree of benefit is uncertain.[2-5] A comparative study in children with multisystem disease found treatment with vinblastine or etoposide for 6 months to be equally effective.[6] The overall response rate was 62%, but about half of the patients had switched to the alternate arm or other therapy during the drug treatment period. Half of those patients who became disease-free did have a reactivation, but these were generally milder than the original disease. Patients who failed to respond within the first 6 weeks of therapy were at increased risk for treatment failure. A randomised trial of combination chemotherapy has been started to study the effects of more intensive therapy in patients with a poor response to initial therapy. Systemic corticosteroids have also been used for recalcitrant skin disease or multisystem disease in children[7] and for pulmonary Langerhans-cell histiocytosis in adults.[8] In patients who have not responded to combination chemotherapy, a number of treatments may be considered including ciclosporin,[5] the nucleoside analogues cladribine or pentostatin,[9] thalidomide,[7] and bone marrow transplantation.[4,5] Anti-CD1 monoclonal antibodies[10] may offer improved therapeutic or diagnostic options in the future.


1. Favara BE, *et al.*. Contemporary classification of histiocytic disorders. The WHO Committee on Histiocytic/Reticulum Cell Proliferations and Reclassification Working Group of the Histiocyte Society. *Med Pediatr Oncol* 1997; **29:** 157–66.
2. Komp DM. Concepts in staging and clinical studies for treatment of Langerhans' cell histiocytosis. *Semin Oncol* 1991; **18:** 18–23.
3. Egeler RM, D'Angio GJ. Langerhans cell histiocytosis. *J Pediatr* 1995; **127:** 1–11.
4. The French Langerhans' Cell Histiocytosis Study Group. A multicentre retrospective survey of Langerhans' cell histiocytosis: 348 cases observed between 1983 and 1993. *Arch Dis Child* 1996; **75:** 17–24.
5. Ladisch S. Langerhans cell histiocytosis. *Curr Opin Hematol* 1998; **5:** 54–8.
6. Gadner H, *et al.* A randomized trial of treatment for multisystem Langerhans' cell histiocytosis. *J Pediatr* 2001; **138:** 728–34. Correction. *ibid.*; **139:** 170.
7. Chu T. Langerhans cell histiocytosis. *Australas J Dermatol* 2001; **42:** 237–42.
8. Vassallo R, *et al.* Pulmonary Langerhans'-cell histiocytosis. *N Engl J Med* 2000; **342:** 1969–78.
9. Weitzman S, *et al.* Nucleoside analogues in the therapy of Langerhans cell histiocytosis: a survey of members of the Histiocyte Society and review of the literature. *Med Pediatr Oncol* 1999; **33:** 476–81.
10. Kelly K, *et al.* CD1 antibody immunolocalisation in Langerhans' cell histiocytosis. *Lancet* 1993; **342:** 367–8.


**Leukaemias, acute.** The acute leukaemias are malignancies affecting haematopoietic precursor cells. They are relatively rare (about 1 to 3 cases per 100 000 of population), and of uncertain cause in the majority of cases, although radiation, carcinogenic substances, or oncogenic retroviruses have been implicated in some types, and certain individuals appear to have a genetic predisposition to these diseases.

Following the initiating event or events the progeny of the affected cell do not differentiate normally but proliferate in an uncontrolled fashion. The result is the accumulation in the blood and bone marrow of immature cell types (blasts) at the expense of normal functional blood cells.

The acute leukaemias may be broadly divided into **acute lymphoblastic leukaemia** (ALL), in which the neoplastic proliferation affects lymphoid cell lines, and the **acute myeloid leukaemias** (AML), variously known as acute myelogenous leukaemias or acute non-lymphoblastic leukaemias, which affect myeloid cell lines. These broad groups can be divided in various ways. ALL is subdivided by an immunophenotypic classification that distinguishes disease of B- and T-cell lineage; it was formerly divided morphologically into L1, L2, and L3 subtypes. For AML the French-American-British (FAB) classification has been widely used. This distinguishes, by lineage and estimated degree of differentiation:

- M0, undifferentiated AML
- M1, AML with minimal maturation
- M2, AML with maturation
- M3, acute promyelocytic leukaemia
- M4, acute myelomonocytic leukaemia
- M5, acute monocytic leukaemia
- M6, erythroid leukaemia
- M7, megakaryocytic leukaemia.

However, knowledge of the genotype, via cytogenetic or molecular analysis, is becoming increasingly important in the treatment of leukaemia. Consequently, a revised classification system has been proposed under the auspices of WHO, which uses a combination of morphology, immunophenotype, genetic, biological, and clinical features. In this classification,[1,2] AML is divided into 4 main groups:

- AML with recurrent cytogenic translocations
- AML with myelodysplasia-related features
- AML, therapy-related
- AML not otherwise specified.

In the WHO classification of lymphoid neoplasms, the Revised European-American Lymphoma (REAL) classification has been adopted, in which acute lymphoblastic leukaemias and lymphoblastic lymphomas are considered to be a single disease with different presentations.[1]

Acute leukaemia usually presents with fatigue, anaemia, infection (due to granulocytopenia), and easy bruisability or bleeding (mainly due to thrombocytopenia). Onset is usually rapid with ALL, although AML may be preceded by myelodysplasia lasting months or years. Bone pain, and enlargement of liver, spleen and lymph nodes due to infiltration of leukaemic cells may occur. Other organs may also be affected, and various metabolic disturbances, including hyperuricaemia, hyponatraemia, and hypokalaemia may be present.

If untreated the acute leukaemias are normally fatal, usually within months. However, these malignancies are among those in which medical treatment can make a substantial difference to life expectancy, and in some cases a permanent remission may be effected.


1. Harris NL, *et al.* World Health Organization classification of neoplastic diseases of the hematopoietic and lymphoid tissues: report of the clinical advisory committee meeting–Airlie House, Virginia, November 1997. *J Clin Oncol* 1999; **17:** 3835–49.
2. Vardiman JW, *et al.* The World Health Organization (WHO) classification of the myeloid neoplasms. *Blood* 2002; **100:** 2292–2302.


ACUTE LYMPHOBLASTIC LEUKAEMIA. With current chemotherapy regimens, long-term disease free survival can be achieved in 70 to 80% of children and 20 to 40% of adults with acute lymphoblastic leukaemia (ALL). While there is a lack of consensus on some prognostic factors, it is generally accepted that age less than 1 year or greater than 10 years, and high white cell count at the time of diagnosis indicate patients at higher risk of relapse. These factors probably reflect the presence of specific genotypes. The genotype with the worst prognosis is BCR-ABL t(9;22), which generates the Philadelphia chromosome; this occurs in 3 to 5 % of children and 25% of adults with ALL.

Standard treatment regimens for T-cell and precursor B-cell ALL generally consist of 2 to 3 years of therapy divided into several phases: a short induction phase; an intensification (consolidation) phase; therapy for prophylaxis of CNS disease, starting during the induction phase, and sometimes continuing for an extended period; and a prolonged continuation (maintenance) phase, sometimes including re-induction therapy.[1] Treatment for mature B-cell ALL (Burkitt cell leukaemia or lymphoma, see below) is different in terms of the drugs used, and the maintenance phase is not required.[1]

The aim of **induction therapy** is to induce complete remission, and a slow early response to this therapy has been reported to be an indicator of poor prognosis.[1] The level of minimal residual disease at completion of remission is an independent prognostic factor.[2]

Standard induction regimens include vincristine and a corticosteroid (prednisolone or prednisone, or dexamethasone), plus asparaginase in children and an anthracycline such as doxorubicin in adults. However, it is now accepted that better remission rates and more prolonged remissions can be achieved with more intensive induction therapy using 4 to 5 drugs—often vincristine, a corticosteroid, asparaginase, and an anthracycline, with or without cyclophosphamide.

The use of dexamethasone, rather than prednisolone, in the induction regimen appears to yield improved event-free survival and a lower incidence of CNS relapse,[3] and increasing its dose may result in a greater marrow blast response.[4] However, some have reported a higher incidence of fatal sepsis with the use of dexamethasone.[5] There is some suggestion that use of asparaginase derived from *Escherichia coli* may be associated with better event-free survival than that derived from *Erwinia chrysanthemi*,[6] and that pegaspargase may be more effective than asparaginase.[7]

For mature B-cell ALL, a 2- to 8-month intensive regimen of high-dose cyclophosphamide, high-dose methotrexate, and cytarabine is commonly used, sometimes with the addition of ifosfamide and/or etoposide.[1]

About 60% of children and 35% of adults who achieve an initial remission will subsequently relapse with meningeal involvement unless **CNS therapy** directed at the sanctuary sites in the meninges is undertaken. Effective prophylaxis can reduce the incidence of CNS relapse to around 2 to 5%.[1,3] Standard therapy consists of cranial irradiation and intrathecal methotrexate. However, concerns regarding the neurotoxicity of cranial irradiation and its ability to cause secondary brain tumours have led to the investigation of chemotherapy alone, particularly in children.[1,3,8] Regimens include intrathecal methotrexate combined with high-dose systemic methotrexate, and triple intrathecal chemotherapy with methotrexate, cytarabine and a corticosteroid. These regimens are started during induction therapy and continued intermittently for an extended period. Early intensification of triple intrathecal chemotherapy may be important in the prevention of CNS relapse, and successful CNS therapy may in turn prevent bone-marrow relapse.[9] Cranial irradiation may still be required in high-risk patients.[3]

**Intensification** (consolidation) therapy involves continuation of intensive chemotherapy regimens after the achievement of complete remission. Drugs used in intensification regimens include high-dose cytarabine, etoposide, teniposide, high-dose methotrexate, mercaptopurine, tioguanine, and the antineoplastics used in induction regimens; often 4- to 5-drug combinations are used. The UKALL Trial X showed that addition of intensification therapy at 5 and 20 weeks from the beginning of induction, (using cytarabine, etoposide, tioguanine, and daunorubicin), produced 5-year disease-free survival of 71% compared with 57% in those who received only maintenance therapy.[8] Benefit was seen even in children considered at low risk of treatment failure. Further intensification may benefit those children with a slow response to initial therapy and high-risk of relapse.[10] The value of intensification therapy in adults is less certain, but it appears to result in a longer duration of remission.[1]

**Continuation** (maintenance) therapy is generally given for some 2 to 3 years after remission;[1,8] three years rather than two years of maintenance therapy is associated with a lower risk of relapse but not a markedly different survival rate.[11] The standard combination of drugs consists of daily mercaptopurine, weekly methotrexate, and prednisolone and vincristine monthly. Many protocols provide for periods of **re-induction** therapy (repeating induction therapy) alternating with standard maintenance,[1] and such intensive therapy is associated with an absolute improvement of about 4% in long-term survival.[11] It has been suggested that individualisation of methotrexate dosage to take account of the patient's ability to clear the drug can improve the outcome.[12]

It is generally agreed that patients who maintain remission for 4 years after the end of maintenance therapy are at little risk of relapse and may be regarded as effectively cured.

Patients who relapse after stopping treatment can usually be brought to **second remission**, often by a repeat of their original induction therapy. However, if relapse occurs during treatment the prognosis is poor, and chemotherapy is unlikely to bring lasting benefit.

The role of **stem cell transplantation** (p.1344) in the treatment of ALL is a matter of some controversy. Bone marrow transplantation is associated with significant mortality and morbidity, and the relapse rate of ALL after transplantation is significant, with overall survival generally being similar to that for intensive chemotherapy in unselected patients. Consequently, allogeneic transplantation is usually reserved for patients who do not have a complete remission with induction therapy, and those who are in second remission after relapse.[1,13] Transplantation during first remission is considered for patients with Philadelphia-positive ALL, since these patients have a very poor prognosis[13,14] (although use of imatinib is under investigation). The lack of suitable HLA-matched family donors has led to the investigation of autologous purged marrow, or the use of marrow from mismatched family donors; however, generally neither of these options has proved more effective than chemotherapy.[14] The use of matched unrelated donors has shown some promise,[1,13] and the use of cord blood or peripheral blood stem cells is under investigation.


1. Pui C-H, Evans WE. Acute lymphoblastic leukemia. *N Engl J Med* 1998; **339:** 605–15.
2. Rubnitz JE, Pui C-H. Recent advances in the treatment and understanding of childhood acute lymphoblastic leukaemia. *Cancer Treat Rev* 2003; **29:** 31–44.
3. Pui C-H. Acute lymphoblastic leukemia in children. *Curr Opin Oncol* 2000; **12:** 3–12.
4. Schwartz CL, *et al.* Improved response with higher corticosteroid dose in children with acute lymphoblastic leukemia. *J Clin Oncol* 2001; **19:** 1040–6.
5. Hurwitz CA, *et al.* Substituting dexamethasone for prednisolone complicates remission induction in children with acute lymphoblastic leukemia. *Cancer* 2000; **88:** 1964–9.
6. Ronghe M, *et al.* Remission induction therapy for childhood acute lymphoblastic leukaemia: clinical and cellular pharmacology of vincristine, corticosteroids, L-asparaginase and anthracyclines. *Cancer Treat Rev* 2001; **27:** 327–37.
7. Avramis VI, *et al.* A randomized comparison of native Escherichia coli asparaginase and polyethylene glycol conjugated asparaginase for treatment of children with newly diagnosed standard-risk acute lymphoblastic leukemia: a Children's Cancer Group study. *Blood* 2002; **99:** 1986–94. Correction. *ibid.*; **100:** 1531.
8. Vora A. Acute lymphoblastic leukemia: optimizing treatment strategies in children. *Pediatr Drugs* 2002; **4:** 405–16.
9. Estlin EJ, *et al.* Consolidation therapy for childhood acute lymphoblastic leukaemia: clinical and cellular pharmacology of cytosine arabinoside, epipodophyllotoxins and cyclophosphamide. *Cancer Treat Rev* 2001; **27:** 339–50.
10. Nachman JB, *et al.* Augmented post-induction therapy for children with high-risk acute lymphoblastic leukemia and a slow response to initial therapy. *N Engl J Med* 1998; **338:** 1663–7.
11. Childhood ALL Collaborative Group. Duration and intensity of maintenance chemotherapy in acute lymphoblastic leukaemia: overview of 42 trials involving 12000 randomised children. *Lancet* 1996; **347:** 1783–8.
12. Evans WE, *et al.* Conventional compared with individualized chemotherapy for childhood acute lymphoblastic leukemia. *N Engl J Med* 1998; **338:** 499–505.
13. Finiewicz KJ, Larson RA. Dose-intensive therapy for adult acute lymphoblastic leukemia. *Semin Oncol* 1999; **26:** 6–20.
14. Aricò M, *et al.* Outcome of treatment in children with Philadelphia chromosome-positive acute lymphoblastic leukemia. *N Engl J Med* 2000; **342:** 998–1006.


ACUTE MYELOID LEUKAEMIAS. Treatment of acute myeloid leukaemias (AML) is problematic because normal stem-cell precursors are sensitive to the drugs used, and therapy aimed at myeloid leukaemic clones results in destruction of part of the normal stem-cell pool.

**Induction of remission** is usually possible with intensive chemotherapy. Complete remission has been stated to be achievable in up to 80% of younger patients and about 50% of older patients (who form the majority of those with AML), but patients suffer severe neutropenia during induction and remission rate is to some extent dependent upon the standard of supportive care. Remission rates are lower in those with adverse prognostic factors such as poor performance status, AML secondary to myelodysplasia or antineoplastics, high white cell count, features of multidrug resistance, and unfavourable cytogenetics.[1-3] Established regimens are based on cytarabine with the anthracycline daunorubicin.[1,2,4,5] Although idarubicin may be preferred to daunorubicin, especially in younger adult patients,[1,6] in children it is no more effective but may be associated with more toxicity.[7] Mitoxantrone is another alternative to daunorubicin,[1] and there is little evidence[2] that one anthracycline is better than another for induction protocols. Addition of etoposide or tioguanine to induction protocols of cytarabine and daunorubicin appears to be equally effective in younger adults and children,[8,9] but in older patients an induction regimen which added tioguanine was found to be more effective than one with etoposide.[10]

As in acute lymphoblastic leukaemia (see above) there is a trend towards the use of more intensive induction regimens.[5,9] Use of high-dose cytarabine compared with standard doses has been reported to improve the duration of first remission and disease-free survival, but overall survival and remission rates were not improved, and toxicity was greater at higher doses.[1,2] Neurotoxicity may be a problem in the elderly, and a combination of cytarabine with fludarabine may be an alternative in these patients.[3] Equally the timing of induction cycles may be important: intensive timing (where the second cycle was given 10 days after the first) has improved disease-free survival, despite more toxicity-related deaths, compared with the standard interval of 14 days or more.[11] Haematopoietic growth factors such as filgrastim and molgramostim may be used to accelerate recovery after induction regimens, although their role has not yet been clearly defined.[1-3]

Once remission is induced, **postremission therapy** is essential in preventing relapse.[1,4,5] Options include further chemotherapy, or allogeneic or autologous bone marrow transplantation (see Haematopoietic Stem Cell Transplantation, p.1344). Long-term survival of about 50% may be possible with these options when used in patients in first remission. However, which option to use is controversial.[5] The MRC AML10 Trial[12] demonstrated additional benefit from autologous bone marrow transplantation when used after intensive postremission chemotherapy, and it was suggested that while reserving transplantation for salvage therapy in children and patients with good-risk disease was appropriate, in older patients and those with standard risk it might be better to use the procedure in first remission. However, chemotherapy has continued to improve, and the most successful regimens use intensification or consolidation chemotherapy with high-dose cytarabine for up to 4 courses, and appear to be comparable to bone marrow transplantation in terms of survival.[13,14] Consequently, some advocate a policy of intensive postremission chemotherapy, reserving transplantation for subsequent relapse, particularly for patients with favourable cytogenetics.[15] Addition of gemtuzumab ozogamicin to therapy is under investigation.[16] Non-myeloablative chemotherapy with allogeneic transplantation is also being investigated as an alternative in older patients.[3,17]

Where possible, induction and postremission therapy is the treatment of choice in AML.[1,4] Low-dose **maintenance** chemotherapy (with cytarabine and tioguanine) may improve disease-free survival but not overall survival,[2] and prolonged maintenance therapy is generally considered unnecessary in patients with AML.[5,9] Where debility or concomitant medical conditions make intensive therapy impossible in the elderly, **palliative** treatment with oral hydroxycarbamide, tioguanine, or etoposide is often given, while idarubicin or low-dose subcutaneous cytarabine may also be of benefit.[3] Good results have been reported with a combination of idarubicin and etoposide in elderly patients.[3] Another option for elderly patients or those who are not able to receive chemotherapy is gemtuzumab ozogamicin.[3,17,18] The UK AML 14 study is investigating low-dose subcutaneous cytarabine, with or without gemtuzumab ozogamicin, in such patients.[19]

Acute promyelocytic leukaemia (APL) is a subtype of AML accounting for 10% of AML cases in adults. It is important to distinguish APL from other forms since, unlike other subtypes, standard therapy is tretinoin **differentiation** therapy. Although most patients with APL can achieve complete remission following treatment with tretinoin alone, remission durations are short and most patients relapse.[20] Induction therapy with tretinoin and chemotherapy (an anthracycline and cytarabine) improved event-free survival compared with chemotherapy alone, and has become routine in APL, although there is good evidence that cytarabine can be omitted.[20,21] Anthracycline-based consolidation therapy is mandatory, and, again, although most studies have included cytarabine, the role of high-dose cytarabine has been questioned.[20,21] Although maintenance therapy with tretinoin alone has been reported to be of benefit,[21,22] resistance has developed with continuous treatment,[23] and retinoic acid syndrome is a major toxicity.[20,21] Prolonged maintenance therapy (intermittent tretinoin plus continuous mercaptopurine and methotrexate for 2 years) also appears to reduce the rate of relapse in APL.[23] The synthetic retinoid, tamibarotene (AM-80), has been used to induce remission in patients who relapsed following successful remission induction with tretinoin.[24] Low doses of arsenic trioxide have also been effective in inducing complete remission in patients with APL who have relapsed,[21,25] although fatalities have been reported with its use.[20]

The efficacy of tretinoin appears to be achievable only because the characteristic chromosomal abnormalities in APL result in an abnormal retinoic acid receptor. The development of drugs that can effect differentiation in other forms of AML, and indeed in other neoplasms, seems likely to be a long and difficult task.

Other experimental therapies under investigation for AML include azacitidine, and imatinib.[9] The ciclosporin analogue valspodar, an inhibitor of multidrug resistance, has been investigated, but was associated with excessive early mortality.[26]


1. Löwenberg B, *et al.* Acute myeloid leukemia. *N Engl J Med* 1999; **341:** 1051–62. Correction. *ibid.*; 1484.
2. Tallman MS. Therapy of acute myeloid leukemia. *Cancer Control* 2001; **8:** 62–78.
3. Jackson GH, Taylor PRA. Acute myeloid leukaemia: optimising treatment in elderly patients. *Drugs Aging* 2002; **19:** 571–81.
4. Hiddemann W, *et al.* Management of acute myeloid leukemia in elderly patients. *J Clin Oncol* 1999; **17:** 3569–76.
5. Arceci RJ. Progress and controversies in the treatment of pediatric acute myelogenous leukemia. *Curr Opin Hematol* 2002; **9:** 353–60.
6. The AML Collaborative Group. A systematic collaborative overview of randomized trials comparing idarubicin with daunorubicin (or other anthracyclines) as induction therapy for acute myeloid leukaemia. *Br J Haematol* 1998; **103:** 100–109.
7. O'Brien TA, *et al.* Results of consecutive trials for children newly diagnosed with acute myeloid leukemia from the Australian and New Zealand Children's Cancer Study Group. *Blood* 2002; **100:** 2708–16.
8. Hann IM, *et al.* Randomized comparison of DAT versus ADE as induction chemotherapy in children and younger adults with acute myeloid leukemia: results of the Medical Research Council's 10th AML trial (MRC AML10). *Blood* 1997; **89:** 2311–18.
9. Loeb DM, Arceci RJ. What is the optimal therapy for childhood AML? *Oncology (Huntingt)* 2002; **16:** 1057–66.
10. Goldstone AH, *et al.* Attempts to improve treatment outcomes in acute myeloid leukemia (AML) in older patients: the results of the United Kingdom Medical Research Council AML11 trial. *Blood* 2001; **98:** 1302–11.
11. Woods WG, *et al.* Timed sequential therapy improves postremission outcome in acute myeloid leukemia: a report from the Children's Cancer Group. *Blood* 1996; **87:** 4979–89.
12. Burnett AK, *et al.* Randomised comparison of addition of autologous bone-marrow transplantation to intensive chemotherapy for acute myeloid leukaemia in first remission: results of MRC AML 10 trial. *Lancet* 1998; **351:** 700–8.
13. Mayer RJ, *et al.* Intensive postremission chemotherapy in adults with acute myeloid leukemia. *N Engl J Med* 1994; **331:** 896–903.
14. Cassileth PA, *et al.* Chemotherapy compared with autologous or allogeneic bone marrow transplantation in the management of acute myeloid leukemia in first remission. *N Engl J Med* 1998; **339:** 1649–56.
15. Edenfield WJ, Gore SD. Stage-specific application of allogeneic and autologous marrow transplantation in the management of acute myeloid leukemia. *Semin Oncol* 1999; **26:** 21–34.
16. Kell WJ, *et al.* A feasibility study of simultaneous administration of gemtuzumab ozogamicin with intensive chemotherapy in induction and consolidation in younger patients with acute myeloid leukemia. *Blood* 2003; **102:** 4277–83.
17. Stone RM. The difficult problem of acute myeloid leukemia in the older adult. *CA Cancer J Clin* 2002; **52:** 363–71.
18. Lang K, *et al.* Outcomes in patients treated with gemtuzumab ozogamicin for relapsed acute myelogenous leukemia. *Am J Health-Syst Pharm* 2002; **59:** 941–8.
19. Leukaemia Research Fund. AML14: Leukaemia Research Fund Acute Myeloid Leukaemia and High Risk MDS Trial 14. Available at: http://www.aml14.bham.ac.uk/trial/AmendmentJanuary2004/Protocol%20Jan%202004.pdf (accessed 29/06/04)
20. Tallman MS, *et al.* Acute promyelocytic leukemia: evolving therapeutic strategies. *Blood* 2002; **99:** 759–67.
21. Tallman MS, Nabhan C. Management of acute promyelocytic leukemia. *Curr Oncol Rep* 2002; **4:** 381–9.
22. Tallman MS, *et al.* All-trans retinoic acid in acute promyelocytic leukemia: long-term outcome and prognostic factor analysis from the North American Intergroup protocol. *Blood* 2002; **100:** 4298–4302.
23. Fenaux P, *et al.* A randomized comparison of all transretinoic acid (ATRA) followed by chemotherapy and ATRA plus chemotherapy and the role of maintenance therapy in newly diagnosed acute promyelocytic leukemia. *Blood* 1999; **94:** 1192–1200.
24. Tobita T, *et al.* Treatment with a new synthetic retinoid, Am80, of acute promyelocytic leukemia relapsed from complete remission induced by all-trans retinoic acid. *Blood* 1997; **90:** 967–73.
25. Soignet SL, *et al.* United States multicenter study of arsenic trioxide in relapsed acute promyelocytic leukemia. *J Clin Oncol* 2001; **19:** 3852–60.
26. Baer MR, *et al.* Phase 3 study of the multidrug resistance modulator PSC-833 in previously untreated patients 60 years of age and older with acute myeloid leukemia: Cancer and Leukemia Group B Study 9720. *Blood* 2002; **100:** 1224–32.


**Leukaemias, chronic.** The chronic leukaemias may be broadly divided into those in which the neoplastic proliferation affects lymphoid cell lines, and those affecting the myeloid cell lines.

Chronic leukaemias affecting the *lymphoid cell lines* include chronic lymphocytic leukaemia (CLL), which is B-cell in about 95% of cases and T-cell in about 5%, and hairy-cell leukaemia, which affects B-cells. The revised European-American lymphoma classification,[1] and a proposed WHO classification of haematologic malignancies,[2] consider lymphoid leukaemias and lymphomas of the same cell type to be one disease with different clinical presentations. Thus B-cell CLL is the same disease as B-cell small lymphocytic lymphoma.

Chronic neoplasms affecting the *myeloid cell lines* include the myeloproliferative disorders chronic myeloid leukaemia (CML), polycythaemia vera, and primary (essential) thrombocythaemia, and the myelodysplastic syndromes. All of these may undergo transformation to acute myeloid leukaemia.


1. Harris NL, *et al.* A revised European-American classification of lymphoid neoplasms: a proposal from the International Lymphoma Study Group. *Blood* 1994; **84:** 1361–92.
2. Harris NL, *et al.* World Health Organization classification of neoplastic diseases of the hematopoietic and lymphoid tissues: report of the clinical advisory committee meeting–Airlie House, Virginia, November 1997. *J Clin Oncol* 1999; **17:** 3835–49.


CHRONIC LYMPHOCYTIC LEUKAEMIA. Chronic lymphocytic leukaemia (CLL) typically occurs in people over 60 years of age, and accounts for about 30% of leukaemias in the West although it is rarer in the Far East. Stages of CLL are defined according to the American Rai system or the European Binet system, with both having prognostic value.[1-3] The clinical course is variable: low-risk patients (Rai stage O; Binet stage A) have a median survival of about 10 years, while high-risk patients (Rai stage III/IV; Binet stage C) have a median survival of about 1.5 years; median survival in the intermediate stages is about 6 years.[1,2]

In patients at low risk and those at intermediate risk with indolent disease cytotoxic chemotherapy is usually deferred until signs and symptoms of disease progression occur.[1,2,4] In these patient groups, trials of immediate versus deferred chemotherapy for early-stage CLL have shown no significant advantage, or disadvantage, for immediate chemotherapy in terms of 10-year survival.[5] Patients with high-risk or progressive disease are usually treated with immediate chemotherapy.

When therapy is required, it is essentially symptomatic and palliative. Continuous or intermittent chlorambucil has been most widely used, and is given for as long as the patient responds; response rates range from about 40 to 70%.[2,3] Although chlorambucil is often used with a corticosteroid (prednisone or prednisolone), there is some doubt as to whether this has a real advantage over chlorambucil alone.[1,2,4,5] Corticosteroid therapy is, however, the treatment of choice where patients present with cytopenias due to an immune mechanism.[1] Combination chemotherapy does not appear to offer any advantage over chlorambucil alone.[5] The most commonly used combinations are cyclophosphamide and prednisone or prednisolone plus either vincristine (COP or CVP) or doxorubicin (CAP), or both (CHOP).[1-3]

Once initial therapy has failed, the preferred second-line therapy is fludarabine.[1,2,4,6] Fludarabine has also been investigated as initial therapy, and while response rates have been found to be higher than with chlorambucil,[7] there appears to be no overall advantage in terms of survival.[1,2,8] Similarly, comparisons of fludarabine with CAP and CHOP found fludarabine gave better response rates in patients with advanced disease, but similar survival-times.[1,2] The combination of fludarabine and cyclophosphamide may be synergistic,[9] and has produced good overall response rates.[8] Cladribine may also be used for CLL refractory to alkylating agents. Compared with chlorambucil and prednisone, the combination of cladribine and prednisone gave higher response rates but increased toxicity, and overall survival was not statistically different.[10] Pentostatin[1] and bendamustine[2] have also been investigated. A combination of pentostatin and cyclophosphamide was well-tolerated and produced good overall response rates in a small group of patients refractory to fludarabine.[8]

In patients who fail treatment with conventional therapy, the monoclonal antibodies alemtuzumab and rituximab have produced encouraging results.[3,8,11,12] Various combinations of these antibodies with other drugs have been studied in CLL,[13] and the use of rituximab with fludarabine especially has shown marked clinical efficacy.[14] Other investigational drugs include oblimersen sodium and gomiliximab (IDEC-152).[13]

Patients may require supportive care for systemic complications of CLL. Hypogammaglobulinaemia is common, and the chief cause of infections. Normal immunoglobulin may reduce the infection rate in these patients but it is not clear that it improves survival.[15] If infection occurs broad spectrum antibacterials will be required. Colony-stimulating factors and erythropoietin may be useful for associated cytopenias.[4]

Recent results from patients given bone marrow transplants after chemoradiotherapy have suggested for the first time the possibility of cure in CLL, but this approach must still be considered experimental.[1,3,16]


1. Hamblin TJ. Achieving optimal outcomes in chronic lymphocytic leukaemia. *Drugs* 2001; **61:** 593–611.
2. Schriever F, Huhn D. New directions in the diagnosis and treatment of chronic lymphocytic leukaemia. *Drugs* 2003; **63:** 953–69.
3. Andritsos L, Khoury H. Chronic lymphocytic leukemia. *Curr Treat Options Oncol* 2002; **3:** 225–31.
4. Kalil N, Cheson BD. Chronic lymphocytic leukemia. *Oncologist* 1999; **4:** 352–69.
5. CLL Trialists' Collaborative Group. Chemotherapeutic options in chronic lymphocytic leukemia: a meta-analysis of the randomized trials. *J Natl Cancer Inst* 1999; **91:** 861–8.
6. National Institute for Clinical Excellence. Guidance on the use of fludarabine for B-cell chronic lymphocytic leukaemia (issued September 2001). Available at: http://www.nice.org.uk/pdf/NICEfludarab_E_29guidance.pdf (accessed 25/06/04)
7. Rai KR, *et al.* Fludarabine compared with chlorambucil as primary therapy for chronic lymphocytic leukemia. *N Engl J Med* 2000; **343:** 1750–7.
8. Weiss MA. Novel treatment strategies in chronic lymphocytic leukemia. *Curr Oncol Rep* 2001; **3:** 217–22.
9. O'Brien SM, *et al.* Results of the fludarabine and cyclophosphamide combination regimen in chronic lymphocytic leukemia. *J Clin Oncol* 2001; **19:** 1414–20.
10. Robak T, *et al.* Cladribine with prednisone versus chlorambucil with prednisone as first-line therapy in chronic lymphocytic leukemia: report of a prospective, randomized, multicenter trial. *Blood* 2000; **96:** 2723–9.
11. Keating MJ, *et al.* Therapeutic role of alemtuzumab (Campath-1H) in patients who have failed fludarabine: results of a large international study. *Blood* 2002; **99:** 3554–61.
12. O'Brien SM, *et al.* Rituximab dose-escalation trial in chronic lymphocytic leukemia. *J Clin Oncol* 2001; **19:** 2165–70.
13. Mavromatis B, Cheson BD. Monoclonal antibody therapy of chronic lymphocytic leukemia. *J Clin Oncol* 2003; **21:** 1874–81.
14. Byrd JC, *et al.* Randomized phase 2 study of fludarabine with concurrent versus sequential treatment with rituximab in symptomatic, untreated patients with B-cell chronic lymphocytic leukemia: results from Cancer and Leukemia Group B 9712 (CALGB 9712). *Blood* 2003; **101:** 6–14.
15. Morrison VA. The infectious complications of chronic lymphocytic leukemia. *Semin Oncol* 1998; **25:** 98–106.
16. Khouri IF, *et al.* Hematopoietic stem cell transplantation for chronic lymphocytic leukemia. *Curr Opin Hematol* 1998; **5:** 454–9.


CHRONIC MYELOID LEUKAEMIA. Chronic myeloid (myelogenous) or chronic granulocytic leukaemia (CML) is a rare disease, occurring usually in older patients, and representing about 15% of all adult leukaemias. It is associated in over 90% of cases with the presence in blood cells of an abnormal chromosome, the Philadelphia chromosome (Ph), which results from a reciprocal translocation between the long arms of chromosomes 9 and 22, with the fusion of the BCR gene and the ABL gene. The product of this gene, the protein BCR-ABL, is leukaemogenic. Ph-negative disease (atypical CML) carries a worse prognosis, and some classification systems consider it to be a separate disease.

During the **chronic phase**, which may last for several years, early allogeneic haematopoietic stem cell transplantation (HSCT) (p.1344) has the potential for cure of CML due to a graft-versus-leukaemia effect. Thus, in suitable patients (younger patients with HLA-matched sibling donors), allogeneic HSCT may be considered as first-line therapy.[1-3] The exact timing of the procedure after diagnosis is controversial;[4] however, there is evidence that it should be performed within 2 years.[2,4,5] Investigational procedures include matched unrelated HSCT, and purged autologous HSCT.[2,3] Options in patients who relapse following HSCT include a second transplant, the use of donor lymphocyte infusions, interferon alfa,[2] or imatinib.[3,6]

Imatinib, an inhibitor of the BCR-ABL protein tyrosine kinase, may also be considered for first-line therapy;[6,7] the International Randomized Study of Interferon and STI571 (IRIS), found imatinib to be superior to the combination of interferon alfa and low-dose cytarabine in newly diagnosed CML in chronic phase.[8] The current choice between transplantation and imatinib is a subject of much debate, and longer follow-up studies of imatinib are needed. Resistance may also be a problem.[9,10]

Interferon alfa has been used in those patients unsuitable for transplantation[2,11] since a number of randomised trials demonstrated that interferon alfa was associated with improved survival compared with busulfan or hydroxycarbamide,[12] the standard palliative therapy. Both busulfan and hydroxycarbamide produce haematological remissions in about 80 to 90% of patients, but do not affect disease progression or induce cytogenetic remissions.[1,2] Some 70 to 80% of patients treated with interferon experience a haematological response, and about 10 to 40% seem to undergo cytogenetic response, associated with more prolonged survival. The addition of low-dose cytarabine to interferon alfa has shown superior response rates, but increased toxicity, compared with interferon alfa alone.[4,11] Interferon, with or without cytarabine, may also be used if there is no response to, or relapse following, imatinib therapy.[6]

For initial management of symptoms, or to gain control of the white cell count, hydroxycarbamide or busulfan may be used.[4] Hydroxycarbamide is usually preferred,[6] as it is somewhat more effective, and better tolerated, than busulfan,[4,13] and use of the latter appears to adversely affect the outcome of allogeneic HSCT.[4,5] Investigational drugs in the chronic phase of CML include homoharringtonine, and a long-acting interferon, polyethylene glycol interferon.[2,4]

The onset of the subsequent **transformed phase** is unpredictable and may present as rapid onset of a blast cell crisis with the behaviour of an acute leukaemia, or a more gradual appearance of blast cells accompanied by gradual resistance to previous treatment (accelerated phase).[1,2] Transformation may produce lymphoblastic (25 to 33% of patients) or myeloblastic or undifferentiated cells (66 to 75% of patients), and the disease may then be treated as acute lymphoblastic or myeloid leukaemia, but cure, or even remission of long duration, is not generally possible with current chemotherapy regimens or allogeneic HSCT.[2,3,14] Patients with lymphoid blastic-phase disease have a better chance of response to chemotherapy (60%) than those with myeloid blastic-phase disease (20 to 30%).[2] High response rates and some prolonged responses have been seen in Ph-positive patients with myeloid blast crisis who were treated with imatinib.[3,14] However, relapse and resistance to imatinib are a problem,[3,9,10] and investigational strategies include combining imatinib with other therapies.[3] The outcome of HSCT is better when blast crisis has returned to chronic phase before transplantation, and imatinib may prove to be useful as a bridge to HSCT.[3] Other investigational drugs in the transformed phase include decitabine,[2-4,15] high-dose cladribine,[3] and farnesyl transferase inhibitors.[3,4]


1. Sawyers CL. Chronic myeloid leukemia. *N Engl J Med* 1999; **340:** 1330–40.
2. Faderl S, *et al.* Chronic myelogenous leukemia: biology and therapy. *Ann Intern Med* 1999; **131:** 207–19.
3. Schiffer CA, *et al.* Perspectives on the treatment of chronic phase and advanced phase CML and Philadelphia chromosome positive ALL. *Leukemia* 2003; **17:** 691–9.
4. Garcia-Manero G, *et al.* Current therapy of chronic myelogenous leukemia. *Intern Med* 2002; **41:** 254–64.
5. Silver RT, *et al.* An evidence-based analysis of the effect of busulfan, hydroxyurea, interferon, and allogeneic bone marrow transplantation in treating the chronic phase of chronic myeloid leukemia: developed for the American Society of Hematology. *Blood* 1999; **94:** 1517–36.
6. National Comprehensive Cancer Network. Clinical practice guidelines in oncology: chronic myelogenous leukemia (version 1.2004). Available at: http://www.nccn.org/professionals/physician_gls/PDF/cml.pdf (accessed 25/06/04)
7. National Institute for Clinical Excellence. Guidance on the use of imatinib for chronic myeloid leukaemia (October 2003). Available at: http://www.nice.org.uk/pdf/TA70_Imatinib_fullguidance.pdf (accessed 25/06/04)
8. O'Brien SG, *et al.* Imatinib compared with interferon and low-dose cytarabine for newly diagnosed chronic-phase chronic myeloid leukemia. *N Engl J Med* 2003; **348:** 994–1004.
9. Paterson SC, *et al.* Is there a cloud in the silver lining for imatinib? *Br J Cancer* 2003; **88:** 983–7.
10. Gambacorti-Passerini CB, *et al.* Molecular mechanisms of resistance to imatinib in Philadelphia-chromosome-positive leukaemias. *Lancet Oncol* 2003; **4:** 75–85.
11. Lindauer M, Fischer TH. Interferon-α combined with cytarabine in chronic myelogenous leukemia—clinical benefits. *Leuk Lymphoma* 2001; **41:** 523–33.
12. Chronic Myeloid Leukemia Trialists' Collaborative Group. Interferon alfa versus chemotherapy for chronic myeloid leukemia: a meta-analysis of seven randomized trials. *J Natl Cancer Inst* 1997; **89:** 1616–20.
13. Hehlmann R, *et al.* Randomized comparison of busulfan and hydroxyurea in chronic myelogenous leukemia: prolongation of survival by hydroxyurea. *Blood* 1993; **82:** 398–407.
14. Druker BJ, *et al.* Activity of a specific inhibitor of the BCR-ABL tyrosine kinase in the blast crisis of chronic myeloid leukemia and acute lymphoblastic leukemia with the Philadelphia chromosome. *N Engl J Med* 2001; **344:** 1038–42.
15. Sacchi S, *et al.* Chronic myelogenous leukemia in nonlymphoid blastic phase: analysis of the results of first salvage therapy with three different treatment approaches for 162 patients. *Cancer* 1999; **86:** 2632–41.


HAIRY-CELL LEUKAEMIA. Hairy-cell leukaemia is a rare, chronic, B-cell lymphoproliferative disorder marked by the presence of white blood cells with prominent cytoplasmic villi, pancytopenia, and splenomegaly. Many patients are asymptomatic and there is no clear advantage to early treatment before symptoms appear.[1-3] When treatment is required, splenectomy was formerly used as initial therapy, but response duration tended to be short. Interferon alfa-2a or -2b given for one year produces at least a partial response in most cases but patients have a tendency to relapse once therapy is discontinued,[1,2,4] although maintenance therapy with low-dose interferon alfa may prolong remission.[4]

Better results have been reported with the purine analogues cladribine and pentostatin, and these have now emerged as first-line treatments for this disease.[1,2,4] Durable complete remission rates of 50% or more are seen after relatively short courses of therapy.[4-7] Toxicity is generally acceptable.[4,6] They do not appear to show cross-resistance; cladribine has been used successfully in patients resistant to, or intolerant of, pentostatin, although it is not known whether the reverse is true.[2,4] For patients who relapse, re-treatment with initial therapy is advocated, although interferon alfa is an option in those patients relapsing after treatment with a purine analogue.[2] There are reports of remission following the use of rituximab in patients with refractory disease.[2,4,8] Other immunotherapy under investigation for hairy-cell leukaemia includes the recombinant immunotoxins LMB-2[9] and BL22.[10]


1. Tallman MS, *et al.* Treatment of hairy-cell leukemia: current views. *Semin Hematol* 1999; **36:** 155–63.
2. Mey U, *et al.* Advances in the treatment of hairy-cell leukaemia. *Lancet Oncol* 2003; **4:** 86–94.
3. Goodman GR, *et al.* Hairy cell leukemia: an update. *Curr Opin Hematol* 2003; **10:** 258–66.
4. Savoie L, Johnston JB. Hairy cell leukemia. *Curr Treat Options Oncol* 2001; **2:** 217–24.
5. Cheson BD, *et al.* Treatment of hairy cell leukemia with 2-chlorodeoxyadenosine via the group C protocol mechanism of the National Cancer Institute: a report of 979 patients. *J Clin Oncol* 1998; **16:** 3007–3015.
6. Flinn IW, *et al.* Long-term follow-up of remission duration, mortality, and second malignancies in hairy cell leukemia patients treated with pentostatin. *Blood* 2000; **96:** 2981–6.
7. Goodman GR, *et al.* Extended follow-up of patients with hairy cell leukemia after treatment with cladribine. *J Clin Oncol* 2003; **21:** 891–6.
8. Zinzani PL, *et al.* Efficacy of rituximab in hairy cell leukemia treatment. *J Clin Oncol* 2000; **18:** 3875–7.
9. Kreitman RJ, *et al.* Responses in refractory hairy cell leukemia to a recombinant immunotoxin. *Blood* 1999; **94:** 3340–8.
10. Kreitman RJ, *et al.* Efficacy of the anti-CD22 recombinant immunotoxin BL22 in chemotherapy-resistant hairy-cell leukemia. *N Engl J Med* 2001; **345:** 241–7.


MYELODYSPLASTIC SYNDROMES. Myelodysplastic syndromes are low-grade neoplasms of haematopoietic stem cells characterised by ineffective haematopoiesis that results in anaemia, neutropenia, or thrombocytopenia in various combinations. They have been described as smouldering leukaemia or preleukaemia, and transformation to acute myeloid leukaemia (AML) occurs in some patients. The clinical course of myelodysplastic syndromes is variable, and a precise individual determination of prognostic score is important in planning treatment.[1-3] In the few younger patients with suitable HLA-matched siblings, allogeneic bone marrow transplantation has curative potential.[1,2,4,5] Patients who are likely to have an indolent course are best treated conservatively with observation and supportive care (transfusions, antibacterials, or epoetins plus colony-stimulating factors).[1-5] The treatment of progressive or advanced myelodysplastic syndromes or those that have transformed to AML may involve intensive chemotherapy similar to that for AML (see p.506), but remission rates are lower.[1,2,4,5] However, many patients are elderly with poor performance status, and are unable to tolerate intensive chemotherapy. Low-intensity chemotherapy (low-dose cytarabine, azacitidine, or decitabine) may be tried in such patients,[3] but has had limited success.[2,4] A variety of antineoplastics and immunomodulating agents are being investigated for use in myelodysplastic syndromes, including amifostine,[2,5] antilymphocyte immunoglobulin,[2,6] arsenic trioxide,[5] azacitidine,[4,5,7] decitabine,[2,4] thalidomide,[2,5,8] and topotecan.[5] Attempts to induce cellular differentiation have generally been disappointing.[4]


1. Heaney ML, Golde DW. Myelodysplasia. *N Engl J Med* 1999; **340:** 1649–60.
2. Paquette RL. Diagnosis and management of aplastic anemia and myelodysplastic syndrome. *Oncology (Huntingt)* 2002; **16** (suppl): 153–61.
3. National Comprehensive Cancer Network. Clinical practice guidelines in oncology: myelodysplastic syndromes (version 1.2004). Available at: http://www.nccn.org/professionals/physician_gls/PDF/mds.pdf (accessed 25/06/04)
4. Steensma DP, Tefferi A. The myelodysplastic syndrome(s): a perspective and review highlighting current controversies. *Leuk Res* 2003; **27:** 95–120.
5. List AF. New approaches to the treatment of myelodysplasia. *Oncologist* 2002; **7** (suppl 1): 39–49.
6. Molldrem JJ, *et al.* Antithymocyte globulin for treatment of the bone marrow failure associated with myelodysplastic syndromes. *Ann Intern Med* 2002; **137:** 156–63.
7. Silverman LR, *et al.* Randomized controlled trial of azacitidine in patients with the myelodysplastic syndrome: a study of the Cancer and Leukemia Group B. *J Clin Oncol* 2002; **20:** 2429–40.
8. Zorat F, Pozzato G. Thalidomide in myelodysplastic syndromes. *Biomed Pharmacother* 2002; **56:** 20–30.


POLYCYTHAEMIA VERA. Polycythaemia vera (polycythaemia rubra vera) is a myeloproliferative disorder, apparently due to an abnormal stem cell clone, which results in increased red cell mass and packed cell volume, and is often associated with increases in white cell and platelet counts and splenomegaly. It is a disease of later life, with a median age at presentation of about 60 years. Patients may present with microvascular occlusion, marked by conditions such as erythromelalgia (burning pain and erythema of the hands and feet), paraesthesia, or migraine; and arterial or venous thrombosis (e.g. cerebrovascular accident, myocardial infarction, pulmonary embolism). The risk for thrombosis is highest in patients with a prior history of thrombosis and in those aged over 60 years. Other symptoms include pruritus, characteristically exacerbated by warmth, and hyperuricaemia. In up to 20% of patients the disease eventually enters a spent phase marked by fibrosis and marrow hypoplasia, and about 5% of patients have transformation to acute leukaemia (this is increased by some therapies). Median survival is in the region of 8 to 16 years.

The mainstay of treatment is periodic phlebotomy to maintain the haematocrit within normal values.[1-3] This may be all that is required in younger patients at low risk of thrombosis. In patients at high risk of thrombosis, including those who have a high phlebotomy requirement, some form of myelosuppressive therapy may be considered as a supplement to phlebotomy. Chlorambucil, which was formerly used for this purpose, has largely been discontinued because of a high incidence of leukaemia in patients so treated.[2,3] In patients with a life expectancy of less than 10 years, radioactive phosphorus-32 is probably appropriate, and produces good results with few immediate adverse effects.[1,2] However, like the alkylating agents it is associated with an increased risk of secondary malignancies.[3] In younger patients requiring myelosuppressive therapy hydroxycarbamide,[1,3] busulfan,[2,3] or in some countries pipobroman also,[2,4] have been preferred because they were considered to have lower risk of inducing leukaemia. However, there is some evidence[4,5] that they too may have leukaemogenic potential, especially when used in combination.[6] Non-cytotoxic therapies that have been shown to be effective include interferon alfa.[2,3,5,7] This may be preferred in younger patients requiring treatment.[1,2]

Symptoms resulting from microvascular occlusion can be controlled by the use of low-dose aspirin (less than about 80 mg/day).[1-3] Anagrelide, another antiplatelet agent, has also been tried in polycythaemia vera. Whether these antiplatelet agents can prevent thrombosis in early polycythaemia is being investigated,[2,8] but some[5] consider their routine use for this purpose to be unjustified.


1. Tefferi A. The Philadelphia chromosome negative chronic myeloproliferative disorders: a practical overview. *Mayo Clin Proc* 1998; **73:** 1177–84.

2. Tefferi A. Polycythemia vera: a comprehensive review and clinical recommendations. *Mayo Clin Proc* 2003; **78:** 174–94.
3. Solberg LA. Therapeutic options for essential thrombocythemia and polycythemia vera. *Semin Oncol* 2002; **29** (suppl 10): 10–15.
4. Najean Y, Rain JD. Treatment of polycythemia vera: the use of hydroxyurea and pipobroman in 292 patients under the age of 65 years. *Blood* 1997; **90:** 3370–7.
5. Spivak JL. The optimal management of polycythaemia vera. *Br J Haematol* 2002; **116:** 243–54.
6. Tefferi A, *et al.* A clinical update in polycythemia vera and essential thrombocythemia. *Am J Med* 2000; **109:** 141–9.
7. Lengfelder E, *et al.* Interferon α in the treatment of polycythemia vera. *Ann Hematol* 2000; **79:** 103–9.
8. Michiels JJ, *et al.*. Diagnosis and treatment of polycythemia vera and possible future study designs of the PVSG. *Leuk Lymphoma* 2000; **36:** 239–53.


PRIMARY THROMBOCYTHAEMIA. Primary thrombocythaemia (essential thrombocythaemia) is a rare myeloproliferative disorder in which abnormal platelet production results in elevated platelet counts. It occurs mainly during later life and unlike other myeloproliferative disorders, is associated with generally near-normal life expectancy.[1] However, microvascular occlusion marked by conditions such as erythromelalgia (burning pain and erythema of the hands and feet), paraesthesia, or migraine, and arterial or venous thrombosis (e.g. cerebrovascular accident, myocardial infarction, pulmonary embolism) may occur. The risk for thrombosis is highest in patients with a history of thrombosis and in those aged over 60 years. In less than 10% of patients the disease eventually enters a spent phase marked by fibrosis and marrow hypoplasia, or transforms to acute leukaemia.

Asymptomatic patients and those at low risk of thrombosis are generally not treated, but when to begin treatment is controversial.[1-3] Symptoms of microvascular occlusion can be controlled by low-dose aspirin (less than about 100 mg daily). In patients at risk of thrombosis, drugs that lower platelet counts are used, including cytotoxics.[1,2,4] Phosphorus-32 and alkylating agents such as busulfan are little used now because of their known potential to induce leukaemia.[4,5] Hydroxycarbamide can reduce thrombotic events,[4,6] and has tended to be preferred because it was thought to have lower risk of inducing leukaemia, but it too appears to have leukaemogenic potential.[4-8] Pipobroman may be substituted for hydroxycarbamide.[4,7] The increased risk of leukaemia from therapy is particularly relevant in younger patients, for whom non-cytotoxic drugs may be preferred. Non-cytotoxic therapies that have been shown to reduce platelet counts include anagrelide,[5,7] which is often substituted for hydroxycarbamide,[4,6] and interferon alfa,[4,7] which is the treatment of choice in pregnant women.[5,6]


1. Tefferi A. The Philadelphia chromosome negative chronic myeloproliferative disorders: a practical overview. *Mayo Clin Proc* 1998; **73:** 1177–84.
2. Bentley MA, *et al.* Essential thrombocythaemia. *Med J Aust* 1999; **171:** 210–13.
3. Tefferi A, *et al.* A clinical update in polycythemia vera and essential thrombocythemia. *Am J Med* 2000; **109:** 141–9.
4. Tefferi A, Murphy S. Current opinion in essential thrombocythemia: pathogenesis, diagnosis, and management. *Blood Rev* 2001; **15:** 121–31.
5. Andersson BS. Essential thrombocythemia: diagnosis and treatment, with special emphasis on the use of anagrelide. *Hematology* 2002; **7:** 173–7.
6. Solberg LA. Therapeutic options for essential thrombocythemia and polycythemia vera. *Semin Oncol* 2002; **29** (suppl 10): 10–15.
7. Briere J, Guilmin F. Management of patients with essential thrombocythemia: current concepts and perspectives. *Pathol Biol (Paris)* 2001; **49:** 178–83.
8. Finazzi G, Barbui T. Efficacy and safety of hydroxyurea in patients with essential thrombocythemia. *Pathol Biol (Paris)* 2001; **49:** 167–9.


**Lymphomas.** The malignant lymphomas are neoplastic disorders of the lymphoreticular cells. These cells are primarily located in the lymph nodes, but because of their wide distribution in the body lymphomas may arise in extranodal and extralymphatic tissues such as lung, gastrointestinal tract, and skin.

The term covers a heterogeneous group of diseases, comprising two main subgroups: Hodgkin's disease, and the non-Hodgkin's lymphomas (NHL). The cellular origin of Hodgkin's disease is uncertain; the NHL are monoclonal malignancies arising from B cells in about 80% of cases, with the remainder from cells of T lineage and from undifferentiated cells.

Management of patients with malignant lymphoma is largely determined by interpretation of histological features, and, especially for NHL by an allocation of subtype and grade. Various classification systems have been proposed for NHL of which the National Cancer Institute Working Formulation has been widely used.[1] Under the Working Formulation, NHL are divided into *low grade*, including small lymphocytic, follicular small cleaved cell, and follicular mixed small cleaved and large cell lymphoma; *intermediate grade*, including follicular large cell, diffuse large cell, diffuse small cleaved cell, and diffuse mixed types; and *high grade*, including large cell immunoblastic, lymphoblastic, and small non-cleaved cell (including Burkitt's) lymphomas. The International Lymphoma Study Group has proposed a revised European-American lymphoma (REAL) classification,[2] and this has subsequently also been published under the auspices of WHO.[3] It is based on a division into B-cell, T-cell and natural killer cell, and Hodgkin's neoplasms. In this classification, B-cell lymphomas include B-cell small lymphocytic lymphoma, MALT lymphoma, follicular lymphoma (35% of adult NHL, rare in children), diffuse large B-cell lymphoma (30% of adult NHL, 5% of NHL in children), and Burkitt's lymphoma (rare in adults; 30% of NHL in children) and Waldenström's macroglobulinaemia (lymphoplasmacytic lymphoma). Plasma-cell myeloma (multiple myeloma) is also a B-cell neoplasm. T-cell lymphomas include precursor T-cell lymphoblastic lymphoma (rare in adults; 45% of NHL in children) and mycosis fungoides; and Hodgkin's lymphoma is subdivided into nodular lymphocyte-predominant and classical (nodular sclerosis and mixed cellularity) forms.


1. Anonymous. Lymphoma classification—where now? *Lancet* 1992; **339:** 1084–5.
2. Harris NL, *et al.* A revised European-American classification of lymphoid neoplasms: a proposal from the International Lymphoma Study Group. *Blood* 1994; **84:** 1361–92.
3. Harris NL, *et al.* World Health Organization classification of neoplastic diseases of the hematopoietic and lymphoid tissues: report of the clinical advisory committee meeting–Airlie House, Virginia, November 1997. *J Clin Oncol* 1999; **17:** 3835–49.


HODGKIN'S DISEASE. Hodgkin's disease (Hodgkin's lymphoma) is characterised histologically by the presence of a particular type of giant cell, the Reed-Sternberg cell. It is more common in males than in females, and in the West is seen particularly in young adults and in the elderly, although the age distribution differs elsewhere.

It usually presents as painless enlargement of one or more lymph nodes, particularly in the neck or axillae. About a third of all patients also have constitutional symptoms of fever, weight loss, and night sweats, which carry adverse prognostic significance. In advanced disease, signs of organ infiltration may occur, as may infectious complications. The mass of the tumour may result in compression of vital organs.

Hodgkin's disease can be treated by radiotherapy or chemotherapy or both, and the choice of treatment depends on the volume and histological subtype of the tumour, the age of the patient, and, particularly, the stage of the disease.[1-3] The Ann Arbor classification (with Cotswold modifications) recognises 4 stages:

- Stage I, with involvement of a single lymph node region or extralymphatic site
- Stage II, in which spread is restricted to lymph nodes and sites on one side of the diaphragm only
- Stage III, involving spread on both sides of the diaphragm with possible splenic and extralymphatic involvement
- Stage IV, where the patient has diffuse or disseminated disease in one or more extralymphatic organs or tissues.

Stages are subclassified A or B according to the absence or presence respectively of the aforementioned constitutional symptoms. X indicates bulky disease and E the involvement of single extranodal sites. Survival rates following treatment for Hodgkin's disease are generally excellent, and there is increasing emphasis on better tailoring therapy to decrease early and late treatment-related morbidity while not compromising survival.[1,2] For prognostic and therapeutic considerations, patients are grouped into early stage favourable, early stage unfavourable or intermediate, and advanced stage disease.

In the treatment of early stage disease (stages I, II, and IIIA), radiotherapy alone was standard therapy for adult patients with limited disease, especially in those with good prognosis. However, there have been concerns about relapse rates and an increased risk of secondary malignancy after radiotherapy. Adjuvant chemotherapy (combined modality treatment) has been investigated in order to improve disease-free survival, reduce doses and volumes of radiotherapy, and avoid the need for surgical staging. A comprehensive meta-analysis of adjuvant chemotherapy in patients with early stage disease found a reduced risk of resistant or recurrent disease, but this did not translate to a significant improvement in 10-year survival.[4] A systematic review[5] came to the same conclusion. Most patients in the meta-analysis received the MOPP regimen (see below) and extended field radiotherapy, and some feel that the ABVD regimen (see below) and involved field radiotherapy may prove more effective in terms of toxicity and survival.[6] Combined modality treatment is now the preferred treatment for favourable early stage disease,[3,6-8] although the optimal chemotherapy regimen and radiation dose have yet to be determined. It is also generally accepted as the treatment of choice in those with unfavourable early stage disease, using the ABVD regimen.[3,6-8] Combined modality treatment is also preferred in children,[2,9] although evidence to support this is scanty.[10]

Chemotherapy alone is generally considered to be the treatment of choice in advanced disease (stages IIIB and IV), although the value of adding radiotherapy has still been debated. Meta-analyses or systematic reviews of combined modality therapy in advanced disease have found no survival benefit from additional radiotherapy, although it may have a role in initial bulky or residual disease.[5,11]

There are currently a number of 4-drug standard regimens available and the choice lies between one of these, alternating cycles of 2 different regimens, or a hybrid cycle that involves giving 7 or 8 drugs in the same course of treatment. However, the single most important factor governing the outcome of chemotherapy is thought to be dose intensity of the drugs given.

The earliest of the successful 4-drug regimens was combination chemotherapy with chlormethine, vincristine, procarbazine, and prednisone or prednisolone (MOPP). A number of MOPP-variant regimens exist which may be as effective and less toxic; these include substitution of chlorambucil or cyclophosphamide for chlormethine (LOPP or COPP, respectively), vinblastine for vincristine (MVPP), and both chlorambucil and vinblastine substituted in one regimen (ChlVPP). However, an alternative to the MOPP-based regimens, a non-cross resistant combination of doxorubicin, bleomycin, vinblastine, and dacarbazine (ABVD) was found to be as effective as MOPP with a reduced risk of inducing sterility or secondary leukaemia. Better results were later reported with ABVD alone, or with MOPP/ABVD, than with MOPP alone, and ABVD has become the basis of standard treatment for advanced stage Hodgkin's disease.[3,9,12]

More recent attempts to improve the results of ABVD or MOPP have centred on dose intensified hybrid regimens. The German Hodgkin's Lymphoma study group found improved results with a hybrid regimen of bleomycin, etoposide, doxorubicin, cyclophosphamide, vincristine, procarbazine, and prednisone (BEACOPP) compared with COPP/ABVD; overall survival was highest with an increased dose of BEACOPP, although toxicity was increased.[13] The Stanford V regimen (doxorubicin, vinblastine, chlormethine, vincristine, bleomycin, etoposide and prednisone, with consolidative radiotherapy) has also been used,[3] although a randomised study[14] comparing ABVD, Stanford V, and a MOPP-hybrid regimen found Stanford V to be inferior in terms of response and survival rates. Further comparative studies of ABVD versus BEACOPP or Stanford V are underway.[15]

Salvage treatment options for patients who relapse depend on the initial treatment and the interval between treatment and relapse. Patients who are candidates for salvage therapy can be divided into 4 groups:

- those initially treated with radiotherapy who have a recurrence, in whom standard chemotherapy regimens are effective
- those who never achieve complete remission with standard chemotherapy, in whom prognosis is very poor, and who are candidates for an intensive salvage chemotherapy regimen with autologous haematopoietic stem cell transplantation (HSCT)
- those whose original remission lasted for over a year, of whom some will respond to re-treatment with standard therapy, but in whom intensive salvage chemotherapy regimens with HSCT may be considered
- and those whose remission is short, less than one year, in whom standard chemotherapy may be used to reduce tumour volume before intensive salvage chemotherapy and HSCT.[8,16]

A common intensive salvage regimen consists of carmustine, etoposide, cytarabine, and melphalan (BEAM). Although intensive chemotherapy and HSCT is considered by some[8] to be the treatment of choice in relapsed patients, others[5] note that benefit on overall survival remains to be established.

Immunotherapies under investigation for Hodgkin's disease include the anti-CD20 monoclonal antibody rituximab,[6] and other monoclonal antibodies, some radiolabelled, to CD25 and CD30.[9] Gemcitabine is also being studied in refractory disease.[9]

1. Wolf J, *et al.* Issues in the treatment of Hodgkin's disease. *Curr Opin Oncol* 1998; **10:** 396–402.
2. Hudson MM, Donaldson SS. Treatment of pediatric Hodgkin's lymphoma. *Semin Hematol* 1999; **36:** 313–23.
3. National Comprehensive Cancer Network. Clinical practice guidelines in oncology: Hodgkin's disease (version 1.2003). Available at: http://www.nccn.org/professionals/physician_gls/PDF/hodgkins.pdf (accessed 27/05/04)
4. Specht L, *et al.* Influence of more extensive radiotherapy and adjuvant chemotherapy on long-term outcome of early-stage Hodgkin's disease: a meta-analysis of 23 randomized trials involving 3888 patients. *J Clin Oncol* 1998; **16:** 830–43.
5. Brandt L, *et al.* A systematic overview of chemotherapy effects in Hodgkin's disease. *Acta Oncol* 2001; **40:** 185–97.
6. Connors JM, *et al.* Hodgkin's lymphoma: basing the treatment on the evidence. *Hematology (Am Soc Hematol Educ Program)* 2001; **1:** 178–93.
7. Josting A, Diehl V. Early-stage Hodgkin's disease. *Curr Oncol Rep* 2001; **3:** 279–84.
8. Fung HC, Nademanee AP. Approach to Hodgkin's lymphoma in the new millennium. *Hematol Oncol* 2002; **20:** 1–15.
9. Yung L, Linch D. Hodgkin's lymphoma. *Lancet* 2003; **361:** 943–51.
10. Louw G, Pinkerton CR. Interventions for early stage Hodgkin's disease in children. Available in The Cochrane Library; Issue 2. Chichester: John Wiley; 2004.
11. Loeffler M, *et al.* Meta-analysis of chemotherapy versus combined modality treatment trials in Hodgkin's disease. *J Clin Oncol* 1998; **16:** 818–29.
12. Tesch H, *et al.* Treatment of advanced stage Hodgkin's disease. *Oncology* 2001; **60:** 101–9.
13. Diehl V, *et al.* Standard and increased-dose BEACOPP chemotherapy compared with COPP-ABVD for advanced Hodgkin's disease. *N Engl J Med* 2003; **348:** 2386–95.
14. Chisesi T, *et al.* ABVD versus Stanford V versus MEC in unfavourable Hodgkin's lymphoma: results of a randomised trial. *Ann Oncol* 2002; **13** (suppl 1): 102–6.
15. Hehn ST, Miller TP. What is the treatment of choice for advanced-stage Hodgkin's lymphoma: ABVD, Stanford V, or BEACOPP? *Curr Hematol Rep* 2004; **3:** 17–26.
16. Glossmann J-P, *et al.* New treatments for Hodgkin's disease. *Curr Treat Options Oncol* 2002; **3:** 283–90.

NON-HODGKIN'S LYMPHOMAS. The non-Hodgkin's lymphomas are a heterogeneous group of malignancies that vary considerably in their behaviour, prognosis, and management.[1] A variety of classifications have been used, grouping by grade (low, intermediate, or high) or cellular origin (B-cell or T-cell), and histology (see Lymphomas, above). The most recent WHO classification, while still separating B- and T-cell lymphoid neoplasms, does not group the non-Hodgkin's lymphomas into a distinct clinical framework.[2] The non-Hodgkin's lymphomas include Burkitt's lymphoma, MALT lymphoma, and mycosis fungoides, all of which are discussed separately.

The usual presentation of lymphomas is lymphadenopathy, which in low-grade lymphoma may develop insidiously over a long period. There may be constitutional symptoms of fever, night sweats, and weight loss. Extranodal involvement may occur, as may various symptoms due to organ compression by the tumour mass. Lymphomas of T-cell origin have a worse prognosis than B-cell lymphomas of the same type, and excess tumour bulk, involvement of bone marrow or gastrointestinal tract, and elevated serum-lactic dehydrogenase concentrations are also adverse prognostic factors. Staging is of somewhat less importance as a determinant of treatment and prognosis than in Hodgkin's disease.

About 40% of all lymphomas seen in North America and western Europe are *indolent* and of low grade; **follicular lymphoma** is the commonest form.[3] Indolent lymphomas are generally characterised as malignancies of small B lymphocytes,[4] and follicular large cell lymphomas should be treated as for diffuse large B-cell lymphoma (see below).[2] The approach to therapy of follicular lymphoma differs dramatically in patients with localised or disseminated (advanced) disease.[2] In the few patients with limited disease at presentation, radiotherapy is potentially curative,[1,2,5,6] with most patients achieving long-term freedom from disease, and low rates of relapse.[1] The addition of chemotherapy to radiotherapy does not convincingly prolong remission or improve overall survival.[6] Patients who do relapse after radiotherapy should be treated as those with more disseminated disease.[2] Even in more advanced disease, which is rarely curable,[1,2,5] follicular lymphoma may follow a fairly chronic course, with a median survival of 8 or more years[5] although transformation to more aggressive forms may occur.[1] Treatment in advanced disease has not been shown to affect survival, and a conservative approach of withholding treatment until symptoms require it is considered viable.[3-6] When treatment is required, single-agent therapy with chlorambucil or cyclophosphamide, sometimes with a corticosteroid such as prednisone in the initial stages, may be preferred.[4-6] Patients treated with combination chemotherapy tend to have remission earlier but the remissions do not last longer than those achieved more slowly with single-agent therapy,[1] and overall survival has not improved.[5,6] Nonetheless, because intensification of chemotherapy has improved response rates, combination therapy such as CHOP (cyclophosphamide, doxorubicin, vincristine, and prednisolone) has become widely used.[5] Some[4] consider this regimen too toxic for indolent lymphomas unless rapid tumour debulking is required. The use of interferon alfa with chemotherapy for first-line treatment has produced conflicting results. However, when interferon alfa was used with anthracycline-containing regimens, improvements in response rate and prolonged remission were reported;[4,5] prolonged survival has not been proven.[6] Interferon alfa as maintenance therapy appears to improve disease-free survival, but only if complete remission has been obtained with initial chemotherapy.[1,5] Results using the purine analogues, fludarabine and cladribine, for initial therapy have been promising, with high remission rates.[5]

Relapse of indolent lymphomas is generally inevitable. Although further remissions can be achieved with repeat of the initial alkylating agent, or an alternative alkylator, response rates and duration of remission tend to decrease.[6] Fludarabine and cladribine have shown responses in about half of those relapsing or refractory to initial chemotherapy.[5,6] Pentostatin has also been tried, with less response, but most studies were in patients refractory to the purine analogues, which show cross-resistance.[5] The anti-CD20 monoclonal antibody rituximab has shown response rates in relapsed disease similar to single-agent chemotherapy.[1,5] Radiolabelled monoclonal antibodies such as tositumomab and ibritumomab have shown promising results,[2] and, like rituximab, are under investigation in combination with chemotherapy,[4-7] although there may be practical difficulties to their use. High-dose chemotherapy followed by autologous[8,9] or allogeneic[10,11] haematopoietic stem cell transplantation (HSCT) may be an appropriate option for relapsed patients.[2,6] In those candidates considered for autologous HSCT, initial therapy should not be excessively myelotoxic, and in the case of allogeneic HSCT, nonmyeloablative approaches may be considered.[2]

Intermediate- to high-grade lymphomas, of which **diffuse large B-cell lymphoma** (DLCL) is the most common form,[2,12] are *aggressive*, and survival is measured in months in untreated patients. However, unlike indolent lymphomas, they are potentially curable with intensive therapy. DLCL occurs most commonly in patients aged 50 to 60 years, but also occurs in children. As with follicular lymphoma, approach to therapy differs in patients with localised or advanced disease.[2] Up to 20% of patients with aggressive lymphomas have localised disease at presentation, and combined modality treatment with a brief course of CHOP (see above) followed by involved field radiotherapy is the treatment of choice.[1,2,12-14] Combination chemotherapy is the treatment of choice in advanced aggressive lymphomas: cure can be achieved in about 35% of patients. Many of the regimens used have included the vinca alkaloids and doxorubicin with alkylating agents: CHOP and CVP (cyclophosphamide, vincristine, and prednisone) have been widely used.[3,12] More intensive second and third generation regimens such as MACOP-B (an intensive 12-week programme of cyclic methotrexate, doxorubicin, cyclophosphamide, vincristine, prednisone, and bleomycin), m-BACOD (with dexamethasone rather than prednisone), and ProMACE-CytaBOM (prednisone, doxorubicin, cyclophosphamide, etoposide, cytarabine, bleomycin, vincristine, and methotrexate), were then developed, and showed initial promising results. However, randomised studies failed to show any advantage for these second and third generation regimens over the less toxic and simpler CHOP regimen, and CHOP is once again considered the standard for care.[2,4,12,14] In a study in elderly patients, the addition of rituximab to CHOP increased complete response rate and prolonged survival, without significantly increasing toxicity,[15] and this combination has been recommended for first-line treatment in the UK.[16] High-dose chemotherapy with autologous HSCT has been tried for initial therapy in patients with diffuse aggressive non-Hodgkin's lymphoma, but remains investigational.[2,4,8,14]

Following relapse, patients are treated with salvage chemotherapy regimens such as DHAP (dexamethasone, cytarabine, and cisplatin), ICE (ifosfamide, carboplatin, etoposide), and ESHP or ESHAP (etoposide, methylprednisolone, cytarabine, cisplatin).[2,12] Patients are then evaluated for high-dose chemotherapy and autologous HSCT, which is considered the treatment of choice in suitable patients who respond to the salvage regimens.[1,2,12] In a randomised study, it was found to be superior to further courses of DHAP.[17] However, in disease resistant to salvage chemotherapy, its role has not been established,[12] and patients whose disease progresses are considered not likely to benefit from currently available standard therapy.[2]

High-grade lymphomas such as **precursor T-lymphoblastic lymphoma** (T-LBL) and Burkitt's lymphoma (see below) are *highly aggressive* and untreated patients survive only weeks. They occur principally in children and young adults, and are often widely disseminated with bone marrow, peripheral blood, and CNS involvement. In children with lymphoblastic lymphoma, good results have been seen with protocols based on those used for high-risk acute lymphoblastic leukaemia (see above), including the use of CNS prophylaxis.[18] It is unclear whether a similar approach would be beneficial in adults with lymphoblastic leukaemia: CHOP continues to be widely used, with generally poor results.[18] HSCT is an option in lymphoblastic lymphoma.[8]

1. Hauke RJ, Armitage JO. A new approach to non-Hodgkin's lymphoma. *Intern Med* 2000; **39:** 197–208.
2. National Comprehensive Cancer Network. Clinical practice guidelines in oncology: non-Hodgkin's lymphoma (version 1.2004). Available at: http://www.nccn.org/professionals/physician_gls/PDF/nhl.pdf (accessed 25/06/04)
3. Peterson BA. Current treatment of follicular low-grade lymphomas. *Semin Oncol* 1999; **26** (suppl 14): 2–11.
4. Fisher RI. Overview of non-Hodgkin's lymphoma: biology, staging, and treatment. *Semin Oncol* 2003; **30** (suppl 4): 3–9.
5. Reiser M, Diehl V. Current treatment of follicular non-Hodgkin's lymphoma. *Eur J Cancer* 2002; **38:** 1167–72.
6. Brandt L, *et al.* A systematic overview of chemotherapy effects in indolent non-Hodgkin's lymphoma. *Acta Oncol* 2001; **40:** 213–23.
7. McCune SL, *et al.* Monoclonal antibody therapy in the treatment of non-Hodgkin lymphoma. *JAMA* 2001; **286:** 1149–52.
8. Morrison VA, Peterson BA. High-dose therapy and transplantation in non-Hodgkin's lymphoma. *Semin Oncol* 1999; **26:** 84–98.
9. Brice P, *et al.* High-dose therapy with autologous stem-cell transplantation (ASCT) after first progression prolonged survival of follicular lymphoma patients included in the prospective GELF 86 protocol. *Ann Oncol* 2000; **11:** 1585–90.
10. van Besien K, *et al.* Allogeneic bone marrow transplantation for low-grade lymphoma. *Blood* 1998; **92:** 1832–6.
11. Khouri IF, *et al.* Nonablative allogeneic hematopoietic transplantation as adoptive immunotherapy for indolent lymphoma: low incidence of toxicity, acute graft-versus-host disease, and treatment-related mortality. *Blood* 2001; **98:** 3595–9.
12. Miller TP. Management of intermediate-grade lymphomas. *Oncology (Huntingt)* 1998; **12** (suppl 8): 35–9.
13. Miller TP, *et al.* Chemotherapy alone compared with chemotherapy plus radiotherapy for localized intermediate- and high-grade non-Hodgkin's lymphoma. *N Engl J Med* 1998; **339:** 21–6.
14. Godwin JE, Fisher RI. Diffuse large-cell lymphomas: a review of therapy. *Clin Lymphoma* 2001; **2:** 155–63.
15. Coiffier B, *et al.* CHOP chemotherapy plus rituximab compared with CHOP alone in elderly patients with diffuse large-B-cell lymphoma. *N Engl J Med* 2002; **346:** 235–42.
16. National Institute for Clinical Excellence. Rituximab for aggressive non-Hodgkin's lymphoma (September 2003). Available at: http://www.nice.org.uk/pdf/65_rituximab_nonhodgkins_fullguidance.pdf (accessed 25/06/04)
17. Philip T, *et al.* Autologous bone marrow transplantation as compared with salvage chemotherapy in relapses of chemotherapy-sensitive non-Hodgkin's lymphoma. *N Engl J Med* 1995; **333:** 1540–5.
18. Magrath IT. Management of high-grade lymphomas. *Oncology (Huntingt)* 1998; **12** (suppl 8): 40–8.

*AIDS-related lymphomas.* Non-Hodgkin's lymphoma is often a late complication of AIDS,[1] and its incidence in HIV-infected individuals is about 60 times greater than in the general population.[1-3] Histologically, it is usually diffuse large cell lymphoma (see above) or small non-cleaved lymphoma (Burkitt's lymphoma—see below).[1,2,4] About 50% of these are associated with the presence of Epstein-Barr virus. The other common HIV-associated lymphoma is primary CNS lymphoma, which is invariably associated with Epstein-Barr virus.[1,4] More recently primary effusion lymphoma or body cavity-based lymphoma has been identified,[1,2,4] which is associated with human herpes virus 8. The introduction of highly active antiretroviral therapy (HAART) for HIV infection (p.621) may reduce the risk of lymphomas by improving immune function,[2,4,5] but, conversely, may increase the incidence by allowing patients to survive long enough for lymphoma to develop.[1,2] The incidence of primary CNS lymphoma has decreased with the advent of HAART.[1,5] There is some evidence of tumour response when antiretroviral therapy is started in a patient who already has a lymphoma.[4]

A few patients with AIDS-related non-Hodgkin's lymphomas present with localised disease, and may benefit from radiotherapy, but most have disseminated disease, often extranodal, at presentation.[1,2,4] The common chemotherapy regimens used are similar to those used in non-HIV infected patients, combining cyclophosphamide, vincristine, doxorubicin, and corticosteroids (CHOP), and sometimes additional drugs such as bleomycin and methotrexate (m-BACOD).[1,3-5] However, although standard dose or even intensive chemotherapy regimens have been used successfully in selected patients, in general patients with AIDS tolerate chemotherapy poorly, and intensive regimens may even shorten their survival. A low-dose modification of m-BACOD has produced responses and survival comparable to standard dose m-BACOD,[6] and low-dose chemotherapy is likely to be preferred in patients with relatively poor immune function (CD4 cell count less than 200/mm$^3$).[3] Results of trials using cyclophosphamide, doxorubicin, and etoposide (CDE), sometimes with didanosine, have been promising.[1] A dose-adjusted regimen of etoposide, prednisone, vincristine, cyclophosphamide, and doxorubicin (EPOCH) has also been studied,[5] and is under investigation in combination with HAART.[1] The use of colony-stimulating factors with chemotherapy has reduced neutropenia and febrile episodes, but there has been no effect on remission rates or overall survival.[1] Most studies used granulocyte-macrophage colony-stimulating factor, but this may increase HIV-1 replication.[1] The prognosis for patients with poor immune status remains poor, and median survival remains only about 4 to 8 months.[3]

Primary CNS lymphoma has a very poor prognosis in patients with HIV infection, with a median survival of 3 months. Palliative radiotherapy is commonly used,[2,4] and may be combined with chemotherapy,[1,3] but it remains uncertain whether therapy improves survival.[5] Intrathecal cytarabine or methotrexate may be used to treat the meningitis associated with primary CNS lymphoma.[1]

1. Kersten MJ, Van Oers RHJ. Management of AIDS-related non-Hodgkin's lymphomas. *Drugs* 2001; **61:** 1301–15.
2. Tulpule A, Levine A. AIDS-related lymphoma. *Blood Rev* 1999; **13:** 147–50.
3. Mitsuyasu R. Oncological complications of human immunodeficiency virus disease and hematologic consequences of their treatment. *Clin Infect Dis* 1999; **29:** 35–43.
4. Hermans P. Opportunistic AIDS-associated malignancies in HIV-infected patients. *Biomed Pharmacother* 2000; **54:** 32–40.
5. Stebbing J, *et al.* The evidence-based treatment of AIDS-related non-Hodgkin's lymphoma. *Cancer Treat Rev* 2004; **30:** 249–53.
6. Kaplan LD, *et al.* Low-dose compared with standard-dose m-BACOD chemotherapy for non-Hodgkin's lymphoma associated with human immunodeficiency virus infection. *N Engl J Med* 1997; **336:** 1641–8.

*Burkitt's lymphoma.* Burkitt's lymphoma is a small non-cleaved cell lymphoma (SNCL) of B-cell origin, which is highly aggressive and is seen particularly in children; the rare cases in adults are most often associated with immunodeficiency such as AIDS. There is an endemic form occurring in equatorial Africa, which is associated with Epstein-Barr virus and commonly involves the jaws and other facial bones.

The primary mode of treatment for Burkitt's lymphoma is chemotherapy. Regimens are generally based on high-dose cyclophosphamide, in various combinations with high-dose methotrexate, high-dose cytarabine, vincristine, doxorubicin, etoposide, and prednisone or prednisolone. Ifosfamide may be substituted for cyclophosphamide.[1-3] Cytarabine and methotrexate may also be given intrathecally for CNS prophylaxis in advanced disease.[1] Although some groups have used an initial phase of low-intensity chemotherapy to reduce the risk of tumour lysis syndrome,[1] others[3] have shown that shorter duration, dose-intensive chemotherapy has resulted in improved survival.

In children complete remission is common and prognosis good: probability of long-term disease-free survival is usually greater than 80%.[3] Prognosis has been less good in adults, but with the increasing use of more intensive regimens similar to those used in children, is improving. About half of all adult cases are reported to be curable with intensive chemotherapy regimens.[2] It is possible that intensive regimens coupled with haematopoietic stem cell transplantation or monoclonal antibodies such as rituximab may improve results further.[2]

1. Magrath IT. Management of high-grade lymphomas. *Oncology (Huntingt)* 1998; **12** (suppl 8): 40–8.
2. Evens AM, Gordon LI. Burkitt's and Burkitt-like lymphoma. *Curr Treat Options Oncol* 2002; **3:** 291–305.
3. Cairo MS, *et al.* Burkitt's and Burkitt-like lymphoma in children and adolescents: a review of the Children's Cancer Group experience. *Br J Haematol* 2003; **120:** 660–70.

*MALT lymphoma.* Marginal zone B-cell lymphomas of mucosa-associated lymphoid tissue (MALT) occur most commonly in the stomach, but may also occur in the salivary gland, breast, thyroid, eye, or lung. They tend to be indolent and remain localised for long periods of time, but can transform to a more aggressive type.

Most gastric MALT lymphomas are associated with *Helicobacter pylori* infection.[1] The bacterium stimulates the formation of MALT in the stomach, which normally lacks organised lymphoid tissue, and there is evidence that it indirectly stimulates tumour growth. Eradication of *H. pylori* infection using antibacterial and antisecretory therapy, as described in Peptic Ulcer Disease, p.1246, has been shown to result in regression of gastric MALT lymphoma in a number of patients.[1-3] Increasing experience of the use of *H. pylori* eradication indicates that the lymphoma regression after eradication can take up to 14 months; eradication suppresses but does not necessarily eradicate the neoplastic clone; only lymphomas limited to the mucosa or submucosa regress after eradication; and that lymphoma can recur.[4] Thus, patients who are *H. pylori*-positive with early stage primary gastric MALT lymphomas may be treated solely with *H. pylori* eradication regimens and long-term endoscopic follow-up. The best treatment for patients without *H. pylori* infection, those whose tumours do not respond to eradication, and those with more advanced tumour stage at presentation remains to be established, but options include radiation, surgery, or chemotherapy.[1]

It has been suggested that screening for and eradication of *H. pylori* is worth investigating as a means of preventing gastric cancer.[5]

Non-gastrointestinal low-grade MALT lymphomas have been treated with surgery or radiation therapy if localised, and with single-agent or combination chemotherapy (similar to that used for other low-grade non-Hodgkin's lymphomas—see above) if advanced.[6]

1. Schechter NR, Yahalom J. Low-grade MALT lymphoma of the stomach: a review of treatment options. *Int J Radiat Oncol Biol Phys* 2000; **46:** 1093–1103.
2. Wotherspoon AC, *et al.* Regression of primary low-grade B-cell gastric lymphoma of mucosa-associated lymphoid tissue type after eradication of Helicobacter pylori. *Lancet* 1993; **342:** 575–7.
3. Wotherspoon AC, *et al.* Mucosa-associated lymphoid tissue lymphoma. *Curr Opin Hematol* 2002; **9:** 50–5.
4. Isaacson PG. Gastric MALT lymphoma: from concept to cure. *Ann Oncol* 1999; **10:** 637–45.
5. Peterson WL, *et al.* Helicobacter pylori-related disease. *Arch Intern Med* 2000; **160:** 1285–91.
6. Zinzani PL, *et al.* Nongastrointestinal low-grade mucosa-associated lymphoid tissue lymphoma: analysis of 75 patients. *J Clin Oncol* 1999; **17:** 1254–8.

*Mycosis fungoides.* Mycosis fungoides is the most common of the cutaneous T-cell lymphomas. It is considered to have 3 stages: a premycotic erythematous or patch phase, characterised by a pruritic rash resembling psoriasis, which may persist for years or even decades; an infiltrative or plaque phase, in which some patches become thickened, darker plaques with marked T-cell infiltration; and a tumour phase where lesions enlarge and ulcerate. Ultimately there may be visceral involvement or potentially fatal sepsis secondary to skin breakdown. A variant of mycosis fungoides presents as widespread pruritic erythroderma, accompanied by abnormal T-cells in the blood, and is known as the Sézary syndrome.

There are many therapeutic options for mycosis fungoides, but few have been evaluated in controlled trials. Treatment depends on disease stage and spread.[1-4] Patients with limited and slowly progressive *patch phase disease* have a good prognosis (median survival similar to age-matched controls) and may be managed with topical and local therapies. Topical therapies include emollients, corticosteroids, chlormethine, or carmustine. Phototherapy, using ultraviolet B light or a psoralen plus ultraviolet A light (PUVA), is a useful alternative when topical treatments are ineffective or not tolerated. Mycosis fungoides is very radiosensitive, and for clearly localised patches, or isolated patches that have failed to respond to other treatments, local x-ray or electron beam radiotherapy may be used.

The initial therapy for patients with widespread *patch/plaque phase disease* is also topical, using chlormethine or PUVA. Patients who fail to respond to a single drug may be treated with combinations such as chlormethine with either PUVA or electron beam therapy,[1] or PUVA with interferon alfa.[1,4] Total skin electron beam therapy may be used, but it may not be widely available and is usually only given once; it is generally used for thickened plaques or for disease that has not responded to other local therapies.

In the *tumour phase*, combination therapy as described above is often used. Systemic chemotherapy may be used for palliation in recalcitrant disease and advanced disease with extracutaneous involvement, but responses are often of short duration. Options include single-agent methotrexate, etoposide, or vinblastine; nucleoside analogues such as cladribine, fludarabine or pentostatin have also been tried.[1,3,4] Combination regimens include CHOP (cyclophosphamide, doxorubicin, vincristine, prednisone), CVP (CHOP without doxorubicin), or CAVE (cyclophosphamide, doxorubicin, vincristine, etoposide).[1]

Mycosis fungoides with erythrodermic features is treated similarly except that skin irradiation tends to be avoided or used in very low doses as it causes severe desquamation.[1] Extracorporeal photopheresis may be useful for disease with erythrodermic features.[1,4]

Newer therapies for persistent or recurrent mycosis fungoides include the interleukin-2 fusion toxin denileukin diftitox,[2,3] and bexarotene, a new retinoid analogue.[2,5-7]

1. Kim YH, Hoppe RT. Mycosis fungoides and the Sézary syndrome. *Semin Oncol* 1999; **26:** 276–89.
2. Duvic M, Cather JC. Emerging new therapies for cutaneous T-cell lymphoma. *Dermatol Clin* 2000; **18:** 147–56.
3. Siegel RS, *et al.* Primary cutaneous T-cell lymphoma: review and current concepts. *J Clin Oncol* 2000; **18:** 2908–25.
4. Whittaker SJ, *et al.* Joint British Association of Dermatologists and U.K. Cutaneous Lymphoma Group guidelines for the management of primary cutaneous T-cell lymphomas. *Br J Dermatol* 2003; **149:** 1095–1107.
5. Wong S-F. Oral bexarotene in the treatment of cutaneous T-cell lymphoma. *Ann Pharmacother* 2001; **35:** 1056–65.
6. Duvic M, *et al.* Bexarotene is effective and safe for treatment of refractory advanced-stage cutaneous T-cell lymphoma: multinational phase II-III trial results. *J Clin Oncol* 2001; **19:** 2456–71.
7. Heald P, *et al.* Topical bexarotene therapy for patients with refractory or persistent early-stage cutaneous T-cell lymphoma: results of the phase III clinical trial. *J Am Acad Dermatol* 2003; **49:** 801–15.

*Waldenström's macroglobulinaemia.* Waldenström's macroglobulinaemia (primary macroglobulinaemia) is a clinical syndrome associated with lymphoplasmacytic lymphoma in which the abnormal lymphocytes secrete a monoclonal serum paraprotein of immunoglobulin M type resulting in increased plasma viscosity. Patients are mainly elderly, and more often male. Although often asymptomatic, patients can present with weakness and fatigue, anaemia, hepatosplenomegaly, lymphadenopathy, or the hyperviscosity syndrome (characterised by oronasal bleeding, visual disturbances and retinal haemorrhage, neurological disturbances such as headache, vertigo, peripheral neuropathy, and hearing loss, and, rarely, heart failure).

Asymptomatic patients require no treatment and may remain stable for some years. Where treatment is required, it has usually been with chlorambucil (with or without prednisone) or, more recently, with cladribine or fludarabine.[1-4] Single-agent oral cyclophosphamide has also been used.[3,5] Rituximab is also recommended by some as a reasonable first choice, although patients should be closely monitored for symptoms of hyperviscosity;[6] plasmapheresis may be performed to reduce plasma viscosity.[3-6] Data on the use of rituximab are limited, and others consider its role has yet to be defined.[4,5]

When disease stabilises, treatment may be stopped and begun again on relapse, with either the same drug, or an alternative first-line agent.[3,6] Autologous haematopoietic stem cell transplantation (HSCT) may be considered for relapsed disease, although studies are limited and complete response rare;[3,4] it is recommended that exposure to alkylating agents or nucleoside analogues be limited if HSCT is considered.[5,6] Although there are few studies, combination chemotherapy does not appear to produce better responses than single-agent chlorambucil;[1,2,4] combination therapy with newer drugs remains investigational.[5,6] However, cyclophosphamide-containing regimens[6] are recommended in relapsed or refractory disease, if the re-use of a first-line drug is not feasible.

High-dose corticosteroids may be used to treat systemic vasculitis arising from deposition of paraproteins.[5,6] Splenectomy, although rarely indicated, may be used to manage painful splenomegaly and hypersplenic syndromes.[4-6] Small studies have reported benefit with thalidomide (with or without dexamethasone and/or clarithromycin),[3-6] high-dose dexamethasone,[6] or interferon alfa.[3,5,6]

1. Dimopoulos MA, *et al.* Waldenström's macroglobulinemia: clinical features, complications, and management. *J Clin Oncol* 2000; **18:** 214–26.
2. Gertz MA, *et al.* Waldenström's macroglobulinemia. *Oncologist* 2000; **5:** 63–7.
3. Johnson SA, *et al.* Waldenström's macroglobulinaemia. *Blood Rev* 2002; **16:** 175–84.
4. Desikan R, *et al.* Waldenström's macroglobulinaemia: current therapy and future approaches. *BioDrugs* 2002; **16:** 201–7.
5. Gertz MA. Waldenström's macroglobulinemia: a review of therapy. *Leuk Lymphoma* 2002; **43:** 1517–26.
6. Gertz MA, *et al.* Treatment recommendations in Waldenström's macroglobulinemia: consensus panel recommendations from the Second International Workshop on Waldenstrom's Macroglobulinemia. *Semin Oncol* 2003; **30:** 121–6.

PLASMA CELL NEOPLASMS. *Multiple myeloma.* Multiple myeloma (myelomatosis) is a lymphoproliferative disorder of B-cell origin, involving the development of an abnormal plasma-cell precursor. It occurs predominantly in the elderly, and accounts for only 1% or less of all malignancies. It is more common in black than in white patients and in men than in women.

The proliferation of the abnormal clone tends to suppress normal haematopoiesis, resulting in anaemia and immunosuppression, with an increased risk of serious infection. Perhaps the most characteristic complication, however, is skeletal destruction, apparently due to release of an osteoclast stimulating factor, resulting in osteoporosis, lytic lesions and fractures, and bone pain, as well as consequent hypercalcaemia. In addition, the plasma cells release large quantities of monoclonal immunoglobulins, known as paraproteins, which can produce a hyperviscosity syndrome and in some cases may interfere with platelet function. Renal failure of various causes and neurological problems due to compression are also common.

Multiple myeloma is not curable with presently-available treatment, and **therapy** is concerned with prolongation of survival and alleviation of symptoms.[1,2] Those patients with stable, indolent or smouldering myeloma, or benign monoclonal gammopathy, are followed carefully but not treated until overt progressive disease occurs. Early treatment may inhibit disease progression, but overall survival and response rates are not affected.[3] In patients with overt disease some form of haematopoietic stem cell **transplantation** may now be the treatment of choice.[4,5] If a syngeneic transplant (from an identical twin) is unavailable, high-dose chemotherapy combined with autologous peripheral blood stem cell (PBSC) transplantation improves response rate, event-free survival, and overall survival compared with standard chemotherapy. Evidence for these benefits is strongest for patients younger than 55 years old.[6] Although some[7] consider standard-dose chemotherapy to be the preferred initial treatment in patients older than 70 years, other reviews[4,5] have concluded that autologous PBSC transplantation is safe for the majority of patients older than 65 years, especially if they have good functional status and limited co-morbidity.

Patients may be treated with vincristine, doxorubicin, and dexamethasone (VAD) for 3 to 4 months prior to transplantation, although dexamethasone alone, or with thalidomide, has been suggested as alternative induction therapy.[5,7] Oral induction with cyclophosphamide, idarubicin, and dexamethasone has also been tried.[8] Peripheral stem cells are collected after administration of high-dose cyclophosphamide and granulocyte colony-stimulating factor.[4,7] Although some suggest the use of alkylating agents and interferon alfa after stem cell collection,[7] others do not recommend alkylator therapy before transplantation as it results in poor engraftment.[5,6] The standard conditioning regimen before transplantation is considered to be high-dose melphalan.[4,5,7] Total body irradiation is no longer recommended, as combined with lower dose melphalan, it resulted in higher toxicity and no significant survival benefit compared with high-dose melphalan alone.[4-6] Similarly, stem cells are not purged of contaminating myeloma cells as a randomised study[9] showed no benefit.

Where transplantation is infeasible or inappropriate, **chemotherapy** may be given to induce remission and prolong survival. The standard first-line regimen has long been a combination of oral melphalan and corticosteroids, usually prednisolone or prednisone.[1,5] This regimen produces an objective response in about half of all patients, and prolongs median survival to between 2 and 3 years.[1,5] The contribution of corticosteroids to the regimen has been controversial although a trend towards increased survival was noted[4] compared with melphalan alone, and high-dose dexamethasone given alone has been reported to be effective in producing remissions.[5] Cyclophosphamide is active,[4] and has been substituted for melphalan.[1] More intensive first-line combination regimens have also been used, particularly in younger, fitter patients. Examples include the ABCM regimen (doxorubicin, carmustine, cyclophosphamide, and melphalan), alternating combinations of VMCP (vincristine, melphalan, cyclophosphamide, and prednisone) with VBAP (vincristine, carmustine, doxorubicin, and prednisone), the VAD regimen (vincristine, doxorubicin, and dexamethasone), and the M2 or VBMCP protocol (vincristine, carmustine, melphalan, cyclophosphamide, and prednisolone).[1,5] However, although response rates are higher, meta-analysis[10] has not shown these combination regimens to be more effective than melphalan and prednisone in terms of survival. The use of interferon alfa as induction therapy is controversial, although a systematic review[4] found it improved progression-free survival.

**Maintenance** chemotherapy has not been shown convincingly to improve total duration of remissions or survival,[1] and although progression-free survival improved with interferon alfa treatment, overall survival benefit was considered to be minimal.[4] A study[11] found prednisone given on alternate days to be effective maintenance treatment in those patients responding to induction therapy.

In patients who fail to respond to initial treatment, or who subsequently **relapse**, various regimens have been tried. A systematic review found no particular regimen to be more effective than another.[4] Salvage regimens for progressive disease include VAD with the addition of cyclophosphamide, EDAP (etoposide, dexamethasone, cytarabine, and cisplatin), and high-dose cyclophosphamide.[1,2] About 60 to 70% of patients who relapse later than 6 months after stopping first-line therapy will respond to re-use of the initial regimen.[1] Thalidomide, with or without dexamethasone, has been shown to be effective in refractory myeloma.[2,4,12] Good responses have been reported with bortezomib[13] in relapsed, refractory myeloma, and there is some suggestion of an additive response with dexamethasone.

Although chemotherapy aimed at the myelomatous clone will produce symptomatic relief as disease is brought under control, **supportive and symptomatic care** is also important. Bisphosphonates such as clodronate, pamidronate, and zoledronic acid have been found to be effective in reducing skeletal complications,[14] and are recommended in those patients with bone disease.[2,15] Radiotherapy is used for impending fracture or impending spinal cord compression, and is often effective in relieving uncontrolled bone pain.[2,5] Erythropoietin therapy can improve anaemia and reduce the need for transfusion.[1,2,4,5,7] A high fluid intake is essential in patients with renal dysfunction or hypercalcaemia (for the appropriate management of the latter, see p.1218). Vigorous antibacterial treatment may be required if infection occurs (see Infections in Immunocompromised Patients, p.131) and plasma exchange may alleviate the hyperviscosity syndrome.[2,7]

Drugs under investigation for the treatment of multiple myeloma include oblimersen and various thalidomide analogues.


1. Huang Y-W, *et al.* Current drug therapy for multiple myeloma. *Drugs* 1999; **57:** 485–506.
2. National Comprehensive Cancer Network. Clinical practice guidelines in oncology: multiple myeloma (version 1.2004). Available at: http://www.nccn.org/professionals/physician_gls/PDF/myeloma.pdf (accessed 03/06/04)
3. He Y, *et al.* Early versus deferred treatment for early stage multiple myeloma. Available in The Cochrane Library; Issue 2. Chichester: John Wiley; 2004.
4. Kumar A, *et al.* Management of multiple myeloma: a systematic review and critical appraisal of published studies. *Lancet Oncol* 2003; **4:** 293–304.
5. Rajkumar SV, *et al.* Current therapy for multiple myeloma. *Mayo Clin Proc* 2002; **77:** 813–22.
6. Imrie K, *et al.* The role of high-dose chemotherapy and stem-cell transplantation in patients with multiple myeloma: a practice guideline of the Cancer Care Ontario Practice Guidelines Initiative. *Ann Intern Med* 2002; **136:** 619–29.
7. Kyle RA. Update on the treatment of multiple myeloma. *Oncologist* 2001; **6:** 119–24.
8. Spencer A, *et al.* Induction with oral chemotherapy (CID) followed by early autologous stem cell transplantation for de novo multiple myeloma patients. *Hematol J* 2004; **5:** 216–21.
9. Stewart AK, *et al.* Purging of autologous peripheral-blood stem cells using CD34 selection does not improve overall or progression-free survival after high-dose chemotherapy for multiple myeloma: results of a multicenter randomized controlled trial. *J Clin Oncol* 2001; **19:** 3771–9.
10. Myeloma Trialists' Collaborative Group. Combination chemotherapy versus melphalan plus prednisone as treatment for multiple myeloma: an overview of 6,633 patients from 27 randomized trials. *J Clin Oncol* 1998; **16:** 3832–42.
11. Berenson JR, *et al.* Maintenance therapy with alternate-day prednisone improves survival in multiple myeloma patients. *Blood* 2002; **99:** 3163–8.
12. Singhal S, *et al.* Antitumor activity of thalidomide in refractory multiple myeloma. *N Engl J Med* 1999; **341:** 1565–71.
13. Richardson PG, *et al.* A phase 2 study of bortezomib in relapsed, refractory myeloma. *N Engl J Med* 2003; **348:** 2609–17.
14. McCloskey EV, *et al.* The clinical and cost considerations of bisphosphonates in preventing bone complications in patients with metastatic breast cancer or multiple myeloma. *Drugs* 2001; **61:** 1253–74.
15. Berenson JR, *et al.* American Society of Clinical Oncology clinical practice guidelines: the role of bisphosphonates in multiple myeloma. *J Clin Oncol* 2002; **20:** 3719–36.


**Malignant effusions.** The amount of interstitial fluid is normally regulated by a complex equilibrium between capillary filtration, osmotic pressure, and physical hydrostatic or hydraulic forces. Malignant neoplasms can disturb this equilibrium by obstruction of capillary or lymphatic drainage as well as causing active exudation of additional fluid following metastatic implantation. Malignant effusions are associated most often with lung, breast, and ovarian malignancies and lymphomas. Symptoms vary, and the fluid build-up may be asymptomatic; both pleural and pericardial effusions can produce cough, pleuritic chest pain, and dyspnoea and pericardial effusions may progress to cardiac tamponade. Peritoneal effusions may lead to malignant ascites. The primary aim of treatment for malignant effusions is effective palliation of symptoms, and depends in part on the tumour type, patient performance status, and prognosis.[1-7] If the tumour is chemosensitive, systemic chemotherapy may resolve the effusion. Simple fluid drainage (thoracentesis or pericardiocentesis) will relieve symptoms until fluid build-up recurs, and in patients with very poor prognosis (life expectancy less than 1 month), may suffice for palliation.

In malignant ascites, paracentesis is usually necessary but spironolactone may be of benefit in some patients. In other patients with refractory tumours, fluid drainage followed by sclerotherapy is likely to be preferred. The principle involved is the instillation of an irritant agent into the pleural or pericardial cavity to promote inflammatory and fibrotic changes which result in the membranes adhering together and abolition of the space between the membranes in which fluid accumulates. In the case of pleural effusions, success of sclerotherapy is dependent on adequate fluid drainage beforehand and full re-expansion of the lung to bring the pleural surfaces together. Intrapleural thrombolytics such as streptokinase have been used to improve fluid drainage in cases of loculation of the effusion.[6,7]

Many drugs have been used for sclerotherapy, and the most common are a tetracycline (doxycycline or tetracycline), bleomycin, or talc. There are no clear data from large randomised studies to guide the choice between these three, and opinions on the preferred option differ.[1,4-7] Following drainage of the effusions the sclerosant is instilled in a small volume (20 to 50 mL) of liquid through the drainage tube. Talc may be also administered as a powder insufflation (rather than slurry), but this involves a surgical procedure under general anaesthesia. Sclerotherapy results in painful inflammation, and local anaesthetics or analgesics should be given. For patients who fail sclerotherapy, or for whom this is not considered suitable, there are various surgical options to manage effusions.[1-7]


1. Andrews CO, Gora ML. Pleural effusions: pathophysiology and management. *Ann Pharmacother* 1994; **28:** 894–903.
2. Vaitkus PT, *et al.* Treatment of malignant pericardial effusion. *JAMA* 1994; **272:** 59–64.
3. Shepherd FA. Malignant pericardial effusion. *Curr Opin Oncol* 1997; **9:** 170–4.
4. Light RW, Vargas FS. Pleural sclerosis for the treatment of pneumothorax and pleural effusion. *Lung* 1997; **175:** 213–23.
5. Grossi F, *et al.* Management of malignant pleural effusions. *Drugs* 1998; **55:** 47–58.
6. Erasmus JJ, Patz EF. Treatment of malignant pleural effusions. *Curr Opin Pulm Med* 1999; **5:** 250–5.
7. Antunes G, *et al.* BTS guidelines for the management of malignant pleural effusions. *Thorax* 2003; **58** (suppl 2): ii29–ii38.


**Malignant neoplasms of the bladder.** Cancer of the bladder is the fourth or fifth most common cancer in Europe and the USA, where over 90% of bladder cancers are transitional cell in type. About two-thirds of all cases occur in men, and the median age at diagnosis is 65 years. Known risk factors include smoking and exposure to aniline dyes. In countries where it is endemic, schistosomiasis is an important cause of squamous cell bladder cancer. Most patients present with haematuria; there may also be urinary frequency or dysuria.

Urothelial tumours fall into two major groups, superficial and invasive, which differ in prognosis and management.[1-4] About 70 to 80% of cases at presentation are superficial (non-muscle invasive), and 20 to 30% are invasive.

Of the *superficial* tumours, about 70% are low-grade transitional cell carcinomas confined to the mucosa (Ta), and have a low risk of progression to muscle invasive disease and a 50% chance of recurrence. Most of the remainder are higher-grade transitional cell carcinomas that have invaded the submucosa (T1), and a small percentage are high-grade carcinoma in situ (CIS). These high-grade tumours have a high risk of progression to muscle invasive disease, and a 50 to 90% chance of recurrence. The standard initial treatment for primary or recurrent superficial disease is surgery, in the form of transurethral resection. In an attempt to prolong remission and reduce the recurrence rate various antineoplastics have been instilled into the bladder after complete resection (prophylactic or adjuvant intravesical therapy). Effective agents include doxorubicin, epirubicin, mitomycin, and thiotepa. These have been shown to increase the disease-free interval, but not to reduce the risk of progression to invasive disease, nor to prolong survival.[5] Good results have also been reported with intravesical BCG,[6] and meta-analyses[7,8] have found it to produce lower recurrence rates than mitomycin. Currently, it is considered reasonable to use no adjuvant intravesical therapy in patients with primary resected low-grade tumours.[2,4] Adjuvant intravesical therapy with an antineoplastic (usually mitomycin) or BCG is recommended for patients with recurrent Ta tumours or primary higher grade T1, and BCG is generally preferred to antineoplastics in primary CIS.[2-4] Maintenance intravesical BCG therapy for CIS has been suggested.[4] Intravesical valrubicin is an alternative for CIS refractory to BCG, when surgery is contra-indicated. Other drugs under investigation for intravesical therapy include bropirimine and interferon alfa. Intravesical photodynamic therapy using porfimer sodium may be used as second-line therapy in recurring superficial disease, and 5-aminolevulinic acid is under investigation for both diagnosis and management. However, in recurrent or persistent superficial disease with high risk of progression, cystectomy is usually preferred.[2,4]

Management of *muscle-invasive* bladder cancer that has not yet metastasised is a matter of some controversy, but conventional therapy has revolved around radical surgery, radiotherapy, or a combination of the two. However, such conventional therapy offers a 5-year survival rate of only about 50%.[1] In consequence, alternatives that have been tried include systemic chemotherapy before or after cystectomy, or bladder-sparing options such as chemotherapy with radiotherapy.[4] The optimal regimen remains to be defined but regimens incorporating cisplatin and methotrexate, such as M-VAC (methotrexate, vinblastine, doxorubicin, and cisplatin), appear to be widely used. Such therapy has produced delays in recurrence of disease, but evidence for improved survival has been conflicting. For example, a large study comparing neoadjuvant therapy using CMV (cisplatin, methotrexate, and vinblastine) before cystectomy or radiotherapy, found this regimen to result in a higher response rate, but not to significantly prolong survival.[9] Although another study[10] has reported that neoadjuvant M-VAC provides a survival benefit over cystectomy alone, the strength of these results has been questioned.[11,12] A meta-analysis[13] that included both these studies concluded that neoadjuvant platinum-based combination chemotherapy did improve survival. However, the benefit was only modest, and there was no evidence of benefit for single-agent platinum therapy.

Patients with unresectable or *metastatic* disease, or who subsequently develop metastatic disease, are usually treated with systemic chemotherapy.[4] For patients with good prognosis, a combination regimen such as M-VAC or CMV may be used. Various combinations of gemcitabine or ifosfamide, paclitaxel, and cisplatin are under investigation,[4] and gemcitabine plus cisplatin has been shown to provide similar survival advantage to M-VAC with better tolerability: some now consider that it should be the preferred regimen in advanced disease.[14]


1. van der Meijden APM. Bladder cancer. *BMJ* 1998; **317:** 1366–9.
2. Otto T, *et al.* Therapy of superficial bladder carcinomas. *Urol Int* 1999; **63:** 32–9.
3. Smith JA, *et al.* The American Urological Association. Bladder Cancer Clinical Guidelines Panel summary report on the management of nonmuscle invasive bladder cancer (stages Ta, T1 and TIS). *J Urol (Baltimore)* 1999; **162:** 1697–1701.
4. National Comprehensive Cancer Network. Clinical practice guidelines in oncology: bladder cancer including upper tract tumors and transitional cell carcinoma of the prostate (version 1.2004). Available at: http://www.nccn.org/professionals/physician_gls/PDF/bladder.pdf (accessed 25/06/04)
5. Pawinski A, *et al.* A combined analysis of European Organization for Research and Treatment of Cancer, and Medical Research Council randomized clinical trials for the prophylactic treatment of stage TaT1 bladder cancer. *J Urol (Baltimore)* 1996; **156:** 1934–40.
6. Shelley MD, *et al.* Intravesical bacillus Calmette-Guerin in Ta and T1 bladder cancer. Available in The Cochrane Library; Issue 2. Chichester: John Wiley; 2004.
7. Böhle A, *et al.* Intravesical bacillus Calmette-Guerin versus mitomycin C for superficial bladder cancer: a formal meta-analysis of comparative studies on recurrence and toxicity. *J Urol (Baltimore)* 2003; **169:** 90–5.
8. Shelley MD, *et al.* Intravesical bacillus Calmette-Guerin versus mitomycin C for Ta and T1 bladder cancer. Available in The Cochrane Library; Issue 2. Chichester: John Wiley; 2004.
9. International Collaboration of Trialists. Neoadjuvant cisplatin, methotrexate, and vinblastine chemotherapy for muscle-invasive bladder cancer: a randomised controlled trial. *Lancet* 1999; **354:** 533–40. Correction. *ibid.*; 1650.
10. Grossman HB, *et al.* Neoadjuvant chemotherapy plus cystectomy compared with cystectomy alone for locally advanced bladder cancer. *N Engl J Med* 2003; **349:** 859–66. Correction. *ibid.*; 1880.
11. Sternberg CN, Parmar MKB. Neoadjuvant chemotherapy is not (yet) standard treatment for muscle-invasive bladder cancer. *J Clin Oncol* 2001; **19** (suppl): 21s–27s.
12. Dreicer R. Neoadjuvant chemotherapy for bladder cancer: current status. *Expert Opin Pharmacother* 2003; **4:** 853–8.
13. Advanced Bladder Cancer (ABC) Meta-analysis Collaboration. Neoadjuvant chemotherapy in invasive bladder cancer: a systematic review and meta-analysis. *Lancet* 2003; **361:** 1927–34.
14. von der Maase H, *et al.* Gemcitabine and cisplatin versus methotrexate, vinblastine, doxorubicin, and cisplatin in advanced or metastatic bladder cancer: results of a large, randomized, multinational, multicenter, phase III study. *J Clin Oncol* 2000; **17:** 3068–77.


**Malignant neoplasms of the bone.** Solid cancers frequently metastasise to the skeleton and metastatic bone disease is a common problem with cancers of the breast, prostate, and lung. Bone metastases are often responsible for cancer pain (the general management of which is discussed on p.5) and also result in immobility, bone fractures, bone-marrow failure, spinal cord compression, and hypercalcaemia.[1] The most common sites of metastasis are the spine, hip, and femur. Primary bone malignancies are rare, and are usually sarcomas (p.524). Multiple myeloma (p.511) also produces bone involvement.

Management of **bone metastases** is essentially palliative since cure is rarely possible.[1,2] External beam radiotherapy is the best treatment for localised metastatic bone pain, with responses occurring in over 70% of patients. Radiation delivered by bone seeking isotopes such as samarium-153 or strontium-89 is an alternative.[3,4] Bisphosphonates are of benefit in patients with severe bone pain that is too widespread for local use of radiotherapy and does not respond to other analgesics.[2,5]

Structural weakness secondary to extensive bone loss may require structural support.[1,2] Surgical fixation or stabilisation may be undertaken to treat or prevent fractures. Surgical excision and reconstruction with methylmethacrylate bone cement may also be required.

Bone metastases cause local osteolysis and various inhibitors of bone resorption have been tried, not only to correct hypercalcaemia of malignancy (p.1218), but also to relieve bone pain and reduce the risk of fractures. Several randomised trials in patients with metastatic bone disease from breast cancer or multiple myeloma have shown 25 to 50% reductions in skeletal events with the use of the bisphosphonates, clodronate or pamidronate.[2,6] Similar results have also been reported for zoledronate.[7] Various organisations have produced guidelines to suggest which patients are best treated with bisphosphonates.[2,8,9] The clearest evidence is in patients who already have lytic destruction of bone. There is much interest in the use of bisphosphonates to prevent the development of bone metastases. However, preliminary evidence of their efficacy is conflicting,[10] and further large controlled trials are considered warranted.[2,9]

Systemic antineoplastic therapy should also be given if the primary tumour is chemosensitive. Endocrine treatment is usually preferred for patients with breast and prostatic cancers, and can produce useful control of symptoms from bone metastases.[1,2] Patients who also have visceral metastases or who have hormone resistant tumours should probably be treated with cytotoxic antineoplastics.[2]


1. Aaron AD. The management of cancer metastatic to bone. *JAMA* 1994; **272:** 1206–9.
2. The Breast Specialty Group of the British Association of Surgical Oncology. The management of metastatic bone disease in the United Kingdom. *Eur J Surg Oncol* 1999; **25:** 3–23.
3. Nightengale B, *et al.* Strontium chloride Sr89 for treating pain from metastatic bone disease. *Am J Health-Syst Pharm* 1995; **52:** 2189–95.
4. McEwan AJB. Use of radionuclides for the palliation of bone metastases. *Semin Radiat Oncol* 2000; **10:** 103–114.
5. Wong R, Wiffen PJ. Bisphosphonates for the relief of pain secondary to bone metastases. Available in The Cochrane Library; Issue 2. Chichester: John Wiley; 2004.
6. Bloomfield DJ. Should bisphosphonates be part of the standard therapy of patients with multiple myeloma or bone metastases from other cancers? An evidence-based review. *J Clin Oncol* 1998; **16:** 1218–25.
7. Wellington K, Goa KL. Zoledronic acid: a review of its use in the management of bone metastases and hypercalcaemia of malignancy. *Drugs* 2003; **63:** 417–37.
8. Berenson JR, *et al.* American Society of Clinical Oncology clinical practice guidelines: the role of bisphosphonates in multiple myeloma. *J Clin Oncol* 2002; **20:** 3719–36.
9. Hillner BE, *et al.* American Society of Clinical Oncology 2003 update on the role of bisphosphonates and bone health issues in women with breast cancer. *J Clin Oncol* 2003; **21:** 4042–57. Correction. *ibid.* 2004; **22:** 1351.
10. Diel IJ, Mundy GR. Bisphosphonates in the adjuvant treatment of cancer: experimental evidence and first clinical results. *Br J Cancer* 2000; **82:** 1381–6.


**Malignant neoplasms of the brain.** Most primary brain malignancies are gliomas, such as astrocytoma and glioblastoma multiforme. The frequency and natural history of brain tumours differ between children and adults. Low-grade astrocytomas, and medulloblastomas are the commonest primary brain tumours in children and anaplastic astrocytomas and glioblastoma multiforme are the most common in adults. However, metastatic brain cancer is the most common cause of intracranial tumours in adults, being up to ten times more common than primary brain tumours. The cancers that most frequently metastasise to the brain are lung cancer, breast cancer, and melanoma. CNS involvement in patients with acute leukaemia (see Acute Lymphoblastic Leukaemia, p.506) or lymphoma (see Non-Hodgkin's Lymphomas, p.510) is also quite common.

The symptoms of primary and metastatic cranial neoplasms are those of local pressure and damage to the brain (such as focal seizures and visual field defects), of displacement of brain structures (like oculomotor paresis with tentorial herniation), and of raised intracranial pressure (such as impaired consciousness and papilloedema). The single most frequent symptom is headache, which is seen in about 60% of cases.

The mainstay of treatment for most primary brain tumours is surgery to relieve compression and cerebral oedema, establish diagnosis, and where feasible resect as much of the tumour as possible.[1-6] High-dose corticosteroids and computed tomography have reduced the morbidity of surgery, both for biopsy and excision. For benign tumours (such as pilocytic astrocytomas) resection may be curative; for malignant tumours (such as anaplastic astrocytomas, glioblastoma multiforme, and medulloblastomas) there is some evidence that extensive resection prolongs survival, but this may be biased by the selection of younger fitter patients for surgery. Adjuvant radiotherapy is widely used after surgical resection for malignant tumours in adults and children. Surgery alone or with radiotherapy is also used for single brain metastases.[7] For multiple brain metastases, most patients are treated with radiotherapy and corticosteroids. Radiosurgery is an investigational technique developed to reduce the radiation dose received by normal brain tissue. Radioactive implants (brachytherapy) are also being investigated.

The role of adjuvant chemotherapy for primary brain malignancies has been less certain, in part because of the difficulty in finding drugs that can cross the blood-brain barrier; the nitrosoureas such as carmustine and lomustine have been the drugs most frequently used, because of their lipid solubility. The PCV regimen, in which procarbazine, lomustine, and vincristine are given, is often preferred to single-agent nitrosoureas in the treatment of gliomas after surgical resection and radiation therapy.[2] The value of this regimen was called into question by a large randomised trial of adjuvant PCV plus radiotherapy versus radiotherapy alone in high-grade astrocytoma, in which PCV provided no additional survival benefit.[8] However, a meta-analysis including this and 11 smaller studies found that giving some form of adjuvant chemotherapy (usually based on nitrosoureas) modestly improves survival in adults with high-grade glioma.[9] Temozolomide is a newer alkylating agent that is given orally and is also being used for the treatment of recurrent gliomas.

In young children chemotherapy may be used as a stopgap measure to delay, or reduce the frequency of, radiotherapy, which can cause neurodevelopmental damage.[1,3] Studies in children under 3 years of age given combination chemotherapy regimens (often including cyclophosphamide, vincristine, cisplatin or carboplatin, and etoposide or methotrexate), after surgical resection of tumour found that radiotherapy could be safely delayed in most and that a few children might never require it.[3] Adjuvant chemotherapy (for example, vincristine and lomustine with or without cisplatin) has also been used to allow a reduction in radiation therapy in children aged between 3 and 10 years.[3] This chemotherapy regimen has also been used in children with poor-risk medulloblastoma.

Since present regimens for primary brain tumours are far from optimal, alternatives continue to be tried.[10] Newer antineoplastics include topoisomerase inhibitors such as irinotecan. Newer delivery techniques include implantation of biodegradable polymers impregnated with carmustine (which has been shown to improve survival in patients with malignant glioma), and the transient disruption of the blood-brain barrier to allow cytotoxics to cross. Other investigational treatments include thalidomide, lymphokine-activated killer cells, antisense oligonucleotides, and the use of gene therapy.[10,11] The most commonly investigated experimental technique for gene therapy involves the incorporation of the herpes simplex thymidine kinase gene into tumour cells via a retrovirus; such transduced tumour cells can then activate, and be killed by, the antiviral agent ganciclovir.[10]

The value of chemotherapy in cerebral metastatic disease remains to be defined:[7] the primary tumour may be intrinsically resistant to chemotherapy, or metastasis may develop despite treatment of the primary tumour, which will encourage the selection of resistant species. Furthermore, although the blood-brain barrier may not be completely intact in these patients, allowing some passage of antineoplastics into the brain, drug delivery of the less lipid-soluble drugs to cerebral metastases may not be sufficient, or sufficiently consistent, to produce a response. Nonetheless cerebral metastases of some chemosensitive primary tumours may respond to therapy.


1. Pollack IF. Brain tumors in children. *N Engl J Med* 1994; **331:** 1500–7.
2. Kaba SE, Kyritsis AP. Recognition and management of gliomas. *Drugs* 1997; **53:** 235–44.
3. Packer RJ. Childhood medulloblastoma: progress and future challenges. *Brain Dev* 1999; **21:** 75–81.
4. DeAngelis LM. Brain tumors. *N Engl J Med* 2001; **344:** 114–23.
5. Short SC, Brada M. The treatment of malignant cerebral tumours. *Hosp Med* 2000; **61:** 772–7.
6. Behin A, *et al.* Primary brain tumours in adults. *Lancet* 2003; **361:** 323–31.
7. Davey P. Brain metastases. *Curr Probl Cancer* 1999; **23:** 59–98.
8. Medical Research Council Brain Tumour Working Party. Randomized trial of procarbazine, lomustine, and vincristine in the adjuvant treatment of high-grade astrocytoma: a Medical Research Council Trial. *J Clin Oncol* 2001; **19:** 509–18.
9. Glioma Meta-analysis Trialists (GMT) Group. Chemotherapy for high-grade glioma. Available in The Cochrane Library; Issue 2. Chichester: John Wiley; 2004.
10. Avgeropoulos NG, Batchelor TT. New treatment strategies for malignant gliomas. *Oncologist* 1999; **4:** 209–24.
11. Jinnah HA, Friedmann T. Gene therapy and the brain. *Br Med Bull* 1995; **51:** 138–48.

**Malignant neoplasms of the breast.** Cancer of the breast is the most common malignant neoplasm in women. The disease is rare under the age of 25, and increases in incidence with age, although the rate of increase slows after the menopause. Risk factors include a family history (women with inherited BRCA1 or BRCA2 mutations are at higher risk), and reproductive hormonal factors such as early menarche, late menopause, nulliparity, and older age at birth of first child. Oral contraceptives and postmenopausal HRT are also associated with a small excess risk (see Carcinogenicity, Breast, on p.1528 and p.1536 respectively).

Ductal carcinoma in situ (DCIS) is a tumour localised to the breast ducts with no evidence of invasion. Invasive breast cancer can be divided into three main groups: early breast cancer (operable, primary, stage I/II); locally advanced disease (inoperable local, stage III); or advanced disease (metastatic; stage IV). Breast cancer is an extremely heterogeneous disorder, and the clinical course is consequently very variable; such factors as patient age and menopausal status, tumour size and grade, involvement of axillary lymph nodes or skin, and presence of hormone receptors within the tumour may be a guide to the extent and aggressiveness of disease, and hence have prognostic significance for treatment.[1-3]

Up to one-third of breast cancers detected by mammography screening are **ductal carcinomas in situ** (DCIS). The natural history of this cancer, which was rarely diagnosed before the use of mammography, is not fully understood, and there is controversy about its treatment.[4] Mastectomy was the standard treatment, but it is now felt that the majority of women with DCIS are candidates for breast conserving surgery. However, in contrast to invasive breast cancer, outcomes after mastectomy have not been directly compared with breast conserving surgery. There is good evidence that the use of radiotherapy after breast conserving surgery for DCIS reduces the risk of local recurrence and development of invasive disease. There is also evidence that the addition of tamoxifen further reduces the risk.[5] Currently there are no universally accepted prognostic factors for DCIS to allow tailoring of therapy to individual risk. Therefore decisions on therapy are based on the extent of the lesion, surgical margins, clinical judgement, and patient preference.[4]

In patients with **early disease** (stage I or II; a relatively small tumour with no or limited nodal involvement) the prognosis is fairly good. Primary treatment is surgical.[1,3] Breast conserving surgery followed by postoperative radiotherapy has been shown to have equivalent local recurrence rates and 10-year survival (about 60%) to mastectomy.[6] The use of postoperative radiotherapy after breast conserving surgery reduces local recurrence rates, but does not appear to affect overall survival.[6,7] Radiotherapy is not usually used after mastectomy, but there are some studies indicating that it may have additional benefits in patients at high risk of recurrence.[8,9]

Further adjuvant therapy with cytotoxic chemotherapy or hormonal manipulations such as tamoxifen and ovarian ablation by surgery, radiotherapy, or gonadorelin analogues has been given to try to eradicate the micrometastases which cause relapses. Overviews of a large number of trials by the Early Breast Cancer Trialists' Collaborative Group (EBCTCG) have confirmed the benefits of adjuvant therapy and attempted to determine which women derive most benefit and which regimens are most effective.[10-13] In these analyses, chemotherapy or hormonal therapy has been shown to have benefits in all women with early breast cancer, regardless of age and nodal status. However, the absolute benefits were greater in women with node-positive disease, and chemotherapy tended to have greater benefits in younger women. The analyses also indicate that the benefits of chemotherapy and tamoxifen are likely to be independent and probably additive. Adjuvant systemic therapy is now considered for all women with early breast cancer, except perhaps those with the lowest risk of recurrence.[1,3,14] The choice between adjuvant chemotherapy and hormonal therapy or a combination of both is less clear. Chemotherapy is preferred for both pre- and postmenopausal women with negative oestrogen receptor status.[1,3,14] For women at moderate or high risk of recurrence who are oestrogen-receptor positive, chemotherapy with tamoxifen may be used. For women at low risk of recurrence with oestrogen-receptor positive disease, tamoxifen with or without chemotherapy may be considered. Ovarian ablation by surgery or radiotherapy may be considered instead of chemotherapy in premenopausal women with oestrogen-receptor positive disease.[3,14] There is also growing evidence that a gonadorelin analogue, such as goserelin, can be used to suppress ovarian function.[14] Historically, the most common adjuvant *chemotherapy* regimen has been cyclophosphamide, methotrexate, and fluorouracil (CMF). Other suitable regimens include anthracycline-based combinations such as fluorouracil, doxorubicin, and cyclophosphamide (FAC or CAF), doxorubicin plus cyclophosphamide (AC), and AC followed by paclitaxel. Epirubicin is often used as an alternative to doxorubicin. Anthracycline regimens have been used particularly in women with node-positive disease.[3,14] The EBCTG analysis[11] found that 3 to 6 months of combination chemotherapy in women aged under 50 could produce reductions in risk of recurrence and of mortality of around 35% and 27% respectively. Moreover, the benefits were not confined to this age group: in older women chemotherapy reduced the risks of recurrence and death by about 20% and 8 to 14% (depending on age) respectively.[11] More prolonged chemotherapy had no greater benefit than treatment for 3 to 6 months, and there was some evidence that anthracycline-containing regimens produced more benefit than those without.[11]

The optimum sequencing of surgery, radiotherapy, and chemotherapy is being investigated. One study found that giving chemotherapy first followed by radiotherapy produced better overall results than the reverse order.[15] The use of neoadjuvant chemotherapy before surgery in locally advanced disease (see below) has led to its investigation in early disease. While studies have shown its use allows an increase in breast-conserving surgery, there is no clear evidence of an improvement in disease-free or overall survival.[16] Reducing dose intensity results in poorer survival, and this has led to the hypothesis that higher doses may offer more benefit, particularly in patients at high risk of recurrence. However, despite some positive reports of high-dose chemotherapy with stem-cell support, and the widespread use of such therapy, particularly in the USA, randomised trials have largely failed to show any benefit of high-dose over standard-dose therapy.[17]

In women with oestrogen-receptor positive tumours, the EBCTG analysis showed that 5 years of *hormonal therapy* with tamoxifen was associated with reductions in risk of disease recurrence and death of 50% and 28% respectively.[12] However, the effects of tamoxifen were small in women with oestrogen-receptor negative tumours,[12] and tamoxifen is no longer recommended in women with known oestrogen-receptor negative disease.[1,14] The optimum duration of tamoxifen remains to be determined, but more than 5 years' treatment does not appear to confer any additional benefits.[12,18,19] An EBCTG analysis has also shown that premenopausal women (but not postmenopausal women) also benefit from ovarian ablation by surgery or radiotherapy.[10,13] A number of studies are examining the role of neoadjuvant or adjuvant therapy using aromatase inhibitors, such as anastrozole or letrozole in postmenopausal women with early disease.[20] There is some early evidence that anastrozole is an effective adjuvant, but long-term follow-up is needed to adequately compare it with tamoxifen.[21] The use of letrozole after 5 years of tamoxifen therapy,[22] or switching to exemestane after 2 to 3 years of tamoxifen,[23] may improve disease-free survival, but again long-term safety and efficacy have not been studied.

In **locally advanced** breast cancer (stage III) the few patients for whom initial surgery is feasible may be treated as those with high-risk early breast cancer (see above). However, for most patients initial therapy is anthracycline-based neoadjuvant chemotherapy, which usually results in sufficient tumour shrinkage to allow surgical management. Radiotherapy and adjuvant chemotherapy are used after surgery, and tamoxifen is also added if the disease is oestrogen-receptor positive or unknown.[3]

The aims of therapy in **advanced disease** (stage IV) are palliation and prolongation of life; cure is generally not possible with current regimens,[1,3] and it is often appropriate to select therapy on the basis of its adverse effects, to achieve optimal risk/benefit ratios.[24] The choice of initial therapy is between hormonal treatment and combination chemotherapy. *Hormonal therapy* is likely to be favoured in patients with oestrogen-receptor positive tumours, postmenopausal status, long disease-free interval since primary treatment for early breast cancer, and disease limited to bone or soft tissues. *Chemotherapy* is preferred for oestrogen-receptor negative tumours and for aggressive disease, particularly where metastasis is to critical visceral sites such as the liver, or where there has been a short disease-free interval since treatment for early breast cancer. Chemotherapy is also used after failure of second- or third-line hormonal therapy. Tamoxifen is probably still the first option for hormonal therapy although results of comparative trials with aromatase inhibitors suggest that they are as effective or better.[20,25,26] It has been suggested that tamoxifen combined with a gonadorelin analogue is preferable in premenopausal women.[27] For patients who relapse during or after treatment with tamoxifen, selective aromatase inhibitors such as anastrozole or letrozole are the preferred second-line option in postmenopausal women, and ovarian ablation or suppression by surgery, radiotherapy, or gonadorelin analogue in premenopausal women. Other hormonal therapies that have been used include progestogens such as medroxyprogesterone or megestrol, androgens, and high-dose oestrogens. Fulvestrant, an oestrogen receptor downregulator, is another option for disease progression in postmenopausal women. Options for chemotherapy include CMF, FAC or related regimens, or a taxane. The prior use of adjuvant chemotherapy for early breast cancer is likely to influence the response to further treatment. In patients with CMF- or anthracycline-resistant disease the taxanes, paclitaxel and docetaxel, are favoured for second-line treatment, and vice versa. Other active agents include capecitabine, fluorouracil infusion, gemcitabine, and vinorelbine.[3] In cancers which overexpress HER2 (human epidermal growth factor receptor-2), the anti-HER2 monoclonal antibody trastuzumab may be added to paclitaxel therapy. Higher response rates have been achieved by intensive regimens, combined with autologous bone marrow transplants or stem cells in some studies. However, the results of randomised trials have been disappointing, with no improvement in survival with the use of stem-cell supported high-dose therapy in metastatic breast cancer.[17,28]

The use of bisphosphonates in women with bone metastases reduces bone pain and skeletal complications such as fracture, spinal cord compression, and hypercalcaemia (see Malignant Neoplasms of the Bone, above). Radiotherapy is also used for bone pain, and for the treatment of brain metastases (see Malignant Neoplasms of the Brain, above).


1. Hortobagyi GN. Treatment of breast cancer. *N Engl J Med* 1998; **339:** 974–84.
2. Buzdar AU, Hortobagyi GN. Breast cancer. *Cancer Chemother Biol Response Modif* 1999; **18:** 435–69.
3. National Comprehensive Cancer Network. Clinical practice guidelines in oncology: breast cancer (version 1.2004). Available at: http://www.nccn.org/professionals/physician_gls/PDF/breast.pdf (accessed 02/06/04)
4. Schwartz GF, *et al.* Consensus conference on the treatment of in situ ductal carcinoma of the breast, April 22-25, 1999. *Cancer* 2000; **88:** 946–54.
5. Fisher B, *et al.* Tamoxifen in treatment of intraductal breast cancer: National Surgical Adjuvant Breast and Bowel Project B-24 randomised controlled trial. *Lancet* 1999; **353:** 1993–2000.
6. Early Breast Cancer Trialists' Collaborative Group. Effects of radiotherapy and surgery in early breast cancer: an overview of the randomized trials. *N Engl J Med* 1995; **333:** 1444–55. Correction. *ibid.* 1996; **334:** 1003.
7. Early Breast Cancer Trialists' Collaborative Group. Favourable and unfavourable effects on long-term survival of radiotherapy for early breast cancer: an overview of the randomised trials. *Lancet* 2000; **355:** 1757–70.
8. Overgaard M, *et al.* Postoperative radiotherapy in high-risk premenopausal women with breast cancer who receive adjuvant chemotherapy. *N Engl J Med* 1997; **337:** 949–55.
9. Ragaz J, *et al.* Adjuvant radiotherapy and chemotherapy in node-positive premenopausal women with breast cancer. *N Engl J Med* 1997; **337:** 956–62.
10. Early Breast Cancer Trialists' Collaborative Group. Systematic treatment of early breast cancer by hormonal, cytotoxic, or immune therapy: 133 randomised trials involving 31 000 recurrences and 24 000 deaths among 75 000 women. *Lancet* 1992; **339:** 1–15 and 71–85.
11. Early Breast Cancer Trialists' Collaborative Group. Polychemotherapy for early breast cancer: an overview of the randomised trials. *Lancet* 1998; **352:** 930–42.
12. Early Breast Cancer Trialists' Collaborative Group. Tamoxifen for early breast cancer. Available in The Cochrane Library; Issue 2. Chichester: John Wiley; 2004.
13. Early Breast Cancer Trialists' Collaborative Group. Ovarian ablation for early breast cancer. Available in The Cochrane Library; Issue 2. Chichester: John Wiley; 2004.
14. Goldhirsch A, *et al.* Meeting highlights: international consensus panel on the treatment of primary breast cancer. *J Clin Oncol* 2001; **19:** 3817–27.
15. Recht A, *et al.* The sequencing of chemotherapy and radiation therapy after conservative surgery for early-stage breast cancer. *N Engl J Med* 1996; **334:** 1356–61.
16. Wolff AC, Davidson NE. Primary systemic therapy in operable breast cancer. *J Clin Oncol* 2000; **18:** 1558–69.
17. Bergh J. Where next with stem-cell-supported high-dose therapy for breast cancer. *Lancet* 2000; **355:** 944–5.
18. Stewart HJ, *et al.* Scottish adjuvant tamoxifen trial: a randomized study updated to 15 years. *J Natl Cancer Inst* 2001; **93:** 456–62.
19. Fisher B, *et al.* Five versus more than five years of tamoxifen for lymph node-negative breast cancer: updated findings from the National Surgical Adjuvant Breast and Bowel Project B-14 randomized trial. *J Natl Cancer Inst* 2001; **93:** 684–90.
20. Smith IE, Dowsett M. Aromatase inhibitors in breast cancer. *N Engl J Med* 2003; **348:** 2431–42.
21. The ATAC (Arimidex, Tamoxifen Alone or in Combination) Trialists' Group. Anastrozole alone or in combination with tamoxifen versus tamoxifen alone for adjuvant treatment of postmenopausal women with early breast cancer: first results of the ATAC randomised trial. *Lancet* 2002; **359:** 2131–9.

22. Goss PE, *et al.* A randomized trial of letrozole in postmenopausal women after five years of tamoxifen therapy for early-stage breast cancer. *N Engl J Med* 2003; **349:** 1793–1802.
23. Coombes RC, *et al.* A randomized trial of exemestane after two to three years of tamoxifen therapy in postmenopausal women with primary breast cancer. *N Engl J Med* 2004; **350:** 1081–92.
24. Fossati R, *et al.* Cytotoxic and hormonal treatment for metastatic breast cancer: a systematic review of published randomized trials involving 31510 women. *J Clin Oncol* 1998; **16:** 3439–60.
25. Bonneterre J, *et al.* Anastrozole is superior to tamoxifen as first-line therapy in hormone receptor positive advanced breast carcinoma. *Cancer* 2001; **92:** 2247–58.
26. Mouridsen H, *et al.* Superior efficacy of letrozole versus tamoxifen as first-line therapy for postmenopausal women with advanced breast cancer: results of a phase III study of the International Letrozole Breast Cancer Group. *J Clin Oncol* 2001; **19:** 2596–2606.
27. Klijn JGM, *et al.* Combined tamoxifen and luteinizing hormone-releasing hormone (LHRH) agonist versus LHRH agonist alone in premenopausal advanced breast cancer: a meta-analysis of four randomized trials. *J Clin Oncol* 2001; **19:** 343–53.
28. Lippman ME. High-dose chemotherapy plus autologous bone marrow transplantation for metastatic breast cancer. *N Engl J Med* 2000; **342:** 1119–20.

PROPHYLAXIS OF BREAST CANCER. The recognition of factors increasing the risk of breast cancer, and particularly the identification of specific genes that confer a high risk, has spurred the search for effective ways of preventing the disease. Current options, other than regular screening to detect the cancer at early stages, include surgery (prophylactic mastectomy and/or oophorectomy), drug therapy (below), and possibly some life-style modifications.[1] No option affords complete protection, and there are no clear data on the overall risks and benefits of each approach, but some recommendations for the management of hereditary breast cancer have been made.[2-5]

Treatment with tamoxifen as part of the adjuvant management of early breast cancer is associated with a reduced risk of developing cancer in the other breast (see above). In view of the difficulty of treating breast cancer once it develops this led to the suggestion that prophylactic tamoxifen might prevent the development of breast cancer in women at risk, and to trials to test this hypothesis. These studies were not without controversy, since the risk/benefit for tamoxifen use in healthy women differed from that in women with breast cancer. The first study to be reported was the US National Surgical Adjuvant Breast and Bowel Project (NSABP) P-1 trial,[6] which randomised 13 388 women to 5 years' treatment with tamoxifen or placebo. Participants were either aged 60 years or older, had a history of lobular carcinoma in situ, or had a 5-year predicted risk of developing breast cancer of greater than 1.66% (as assessed by number of first-degree relatives with breast cancer, number of previous breast biopsies, presence of atypical hyperplasia, and reproductive factors). In this study there was a highly significant 49% reduction in the occurrence of invasive breast cancer in women receiving tamoxifen (21.4 cancers prevented per 1000 women treated). The incidence of non-invasive breast cancer was reduced to a similar extent. Tamoxifen reduced the incidence of oestrogen-receptor positive, but not oestrogen-receptor negative, tumours. Adverse effects of tamoxifen included a modest increase in the risk of endometrial cancer and vascular events (stroke and pulmonary embolism). Preliminary results from 2 smaller randomised European trials did not confirm the benefit of tamoxifen in breast cancer prevention. The British trial[7] was in women with a first-degree family history of breast cancer, and their median age was younger than in the US trial. The Italian trial[8] was in hysterectomised women with no particular risk for breast cancer, and because of its size may not have been sufficiently powered to detect an effect of tamoxifen. The full follow-up[9] of 5 years' treatment in this study found no difference in breast cancer incidence between tamoxifen and placebo groups. A subgroup analysis of women at high risk of oestrogen-receptor positive breast cancer did find a protective effect from tamoxifen, and there was an apparent protective effect for women in this group who used HRT. However, this group was not identified at randomisation of the study and these results need to be confirmed. Initial results of a further placebo-controlled study (IBIS-I)[10] of women at increased risk of breast cancer found that during tamoxifen use for 5 years, the risk of all breast cancers was reduced by 32%. Like the NSABP P-1 trial, the reduction occurred in oestrogen-receptor positive tumours. Similar adverse effects were found with tamoxifen use, but there was also an unexpected increase in deaths from all causes in tamoxifen users. This may be associated with the excess in thromboembolic events reported, although statistical variability could not be ruled out. A retrospective analysis[11] of the NSABP P-1 data for women who had developed invasive breast cancer found that in carriers of the oncogene BRCA2, but not BRCA1 carriers, there was a reduction in breast cancer similar to the reduction in oestrogen-receptor positive cancer among all women in the study. The numbers available, however, were too small to be statistically significant, and it is therefore still not known if tamoxifen can reduce the risk of breast cancer in patients with these mutations. It is also unclear whether tamoxifen could improve overall survival or is merely delaying the development of breast cancer. Because the US trial was unblinded and all women were allowed to receive tamoxifen, it will not be possible to gain survival data from this trial. Long-term follow-up of large placebo-controlled trials is needed to provide answers to some of these questions. Until then, it is likely there will be continued disagreement on whether tamoxifen should be used for primary prevention, and if so, in whom, and for how long. Various groups have produced assessments of the prophylactic use of tamoxifen.[12-14]

Another anti-oestrogen, raloxifene, has reportedly shown a reduction in breast cancer risk while its effects on osteoporosis were being studied; further studies are ongoing.[14] The aromatase inhibitor, anastrozole, is also under investigation.

Other candidates for the prevention of breast cancer include plant oestrogens (phytoestrogens) such as those in soya. Epidemiological evidence suggests that diets high in these compounds may be protective. It was thought that retinoids might also be protective, but a secondary prevention trial of fenretinide failed to show any benefit.[15]

Various life-style modifications have the potential to reduce breast cancer risk based on epidemiological data. These include weight loss, increase in exercise, and dietary factors.[1] These may be proposed as part of an approach to a healthy life-style, but their real value in reducing breast cancer risk is unproven.

1. Chlebowski RT. Reducing the risk of breast cancer. *N Engl J Med* 2000; **343:** 191–8.
2. Burke W, *et al.* Recommendations for follow-up care of individuals with an inherited predisposition to cancer: BRCA1 and BRCA2. *JAMA* 1997; **277:** 997–1003.
3. Eisinger F, *et al.* Recommendations for medical management of hereditary breast and ovarian cancer: the French National Ad Hoc Committee. *Ann Oncol* 1998; **9:** 939–50.
4. Møller P, *et al.* Guidelines for follow-up of women at high risk for inherited breast cancer: consensus statement from the Biomed 2 Demonstration Programme on Inherited Breast Cancer. *Dis Markers* 1999; **15:** 207–11.
5. Eisen A, *et al.* Prophylactic surgery in women with a hereditary predisposition to breast and ovarian cancer. *J Clin Oncol* 2000; **18:** 1980–95.
6. Fisher B, *et al.* Tamoxifen for prevention of breast cancer: report of the National Surgical Adjuvant Breast and Bowel Project P-1 study. *J Natl Cancer Inst* 1998; **90:** 1371–88.
7. Powles T, *et al.* Interim analysis of the incidence of breast cancer in the Royal Marsden Hospital tamoxifen randomised chemoprevention trial. *Lancet* 1998; **352:** 98–101.
8. Veronesi U, *et al.* Prevention of breast cancer with tamoxifen: preliminary findings from the Italian randomised trial among hysterectomised women. *Lancet* 1998; **352:** 93–7.
9. Veronesi U, *et al.* Italian randomized trial among women with hysterectomy: tamoxifen and hormone-dependent breast cancer in high-risk women. *J Natl Cancer Inst* 2002; **95:** 160–5.
10. IBIS investigators. First results from the International Breast Cancer Intervention Study (IBIS-I): a randomised prevention trial. *Lancet* 2002; **360:** 817–24.
11. King M-C, *et al.* Tamoxifen and breast cancer incidence among women with inherited mutations in BRCA1 and BRCA2: National Surgical Adjuvant Breast and Bowel Project (NSABP-P1) Breast Cancer Prevention Trial. *JAMA* 2001; **286:** 2251–6.
12. American College of Obstetricians and Gynecologists. ACOG committee opinion; tamoxifen and the prevention of breast cancer in high-risk women. *Int J Gynecol Obstet* 2000; **68:** 73–5.
13. Anonymous. Pas de tamoxifène en prévention primaire du cancer du sein. *Rev Prescr* 1999; **19:** 775–8.
14. Chlebowski RT, *et al.* American Society of Clinical Oncology technology assessment of pharmacologic interventions for breast cancer risk reduction including tamoxifen, raloxifene, and aromatase inhibition. *J Clin Oncol* 2002; **20:** 3328–43.
15. Veronesi U, *et al.* Randomized trial of fenretinide to prevent second breast malignancy in women with early breast cancer. *J Natl Cancer Inst* 1999; **91:** 1847–56.

MALIGNANT NEOPLASMS OF THE MALE BREAST. Breast cancer can occur in men, although it has a much lower incidence than in women. Risk factors are not well understood, but it may sometimes be associated with abnormalities of sex hormone metabolism, including those acquired through liver disease or testicular trauma. In addition, the inherited mutation BRCA2, which is associated with an increased risk of breast cancer in women, also increases the risk of breast cancer in men. Breast cancer in men occurs at a slightly older median age than in women (60 to 70 years), and is more likely to be oestrogen-receptor positive. Survival by stage appears to be similar to that in women.

Treatment is similar to that for women.[1-4] Primary management is mastectomy and axillary lymph node dissection. Because of the rarity of the disease large controlled trials are lacking but studies in limited numbers of men and extrapolation from results in women suggest that adjuvant therapy should be considered on the same basis as for women. Radiotherapy may be used to reduce the rate of local recurrence in those considered at high risk. Adjuvant tamoxifen or chemotherapy may also be used, with tamoxifen being the most common. Chemotherapy is probably more appropriate in those with oestrogen-receptor negative tumours, locally advanced disease, or positive nodes. In advanced metastatic disease tamoxifen is generally the first choice treatment. Combination chemotherapy is reserved for unresponsive or relapsing disease; regimens that have been used include cyclophosphamide, methotrexate, and fluorouracil (CMF), cyclophosphamide, doxorubicin, and fluorouracil (CAF), or doxorubicin and vincristine. Hormonal ablation by adrenalectomy or orchidectomy is also effective, but has become less popular since the advent of tamoxifen.

1. Donegan WL, Redlich PN. Breast cancer in men. *Surg Clin North Am* 1996; **76:** 343–63.
2. Ravandi-Kashani F, Hayes TG. Male breast cancer: a review of the literature. *Eur J Cancer* 1998; **34:** 1341–7.
3. Jepson AS, Fentiman IS. Male breast cancer. *Int J Clin Pract* 1998; **52:** 571–6.
4. Giordano SH, *et al.* Breast cancer in men. *Ann Intern Med* 2002; **137:** 678–87.

**Malignant neoplasms of the cervix.** Cancer of the uterine cervix is one of the most common cancers in women, accounting for about 12% of all female malignancies. It is associated with vaginal intercourse and the presence of human papilloma virus; high-risk types of the virus (HPV-16 and 18) that produce proteins E6 and E7 inactivate host tumour suppressor proteins and thus encourage malignant transformation. Smoking and long-term use of oral contraceptives (p.1528) may also be risk factors. Widespread screening has meant that in many women the disease has been detected in the preinvasive or early stages, when the prognosis is excellent to good.

**Preinvasive cervical lesions** (cervical intraepithelial neoplasia; CIN) may resolve spontaneously if low-grade, and may be monitored by repeat screening.[1] High-grade CIN (cervical dysplasia) and cervical carcinoma in situ may progress to invasive carcinoma and are usually excised using diathermy or laser techniques. Conisation of the cervix (cone biopsy) may be used to rule out the presence of invasive disease. Investigational therapies include photodynamic therapy, and topical fluorouracil.

**Invasive cervical cancers** are mostly squamous cell in origin (80 to 90%), with 10 to 20% being adenocarcinoma. Invasive cervical cancers may be divided into early-stage (I and IIA), locally advanced (stages IIB to IVA), and metastatic (IVB). The earliest stage of invasive cervical cancer may be treated by conisation of the cervix (which maintains fertility) or simple hysterectomy.[1,2] Other early-stage cancers may be treated by surgery (radical hysterectomy) or by radiotherapy. Some patients treated with surgery may require adjuvant radiotherapy. Early-stage patients with poor prognostic factors have better survival if both chemotherapy and radiotherapy are given after surgery (adjuvant chemoradiotherapy).[2,3] Most regimens include cisplatin alone or combined with fluorouracil.[4,5] Hydroxycarbamide has also been used by some centres, but is less effective than cisplatin.[4] Patients with locally advanced cervical cancer are usually treated with primary chemoradiotherapy using cisplatin-based regimens.[2-5] The evidence for chemotherapy is stronger for stage IIB than for stages III/IVA. Neoadjuvant chemotherapy has been tried and although there is some indication that its use before surgery might be of benefit, no survival advantage has been shown; it does not appear to be beneficial before radiotherapy.[6] For local recurrence of disease, treatment options include radiotherapy if it has not already been used, more extensive surgery, or cisplatin-based chemoradiotherapy.[2,7] Treatment for metastatic disease consists of palliative radiotherapy or chemotherapy with cisplatin,[7] or chemoradiotherapy.[2] A combination of ifosfamide with cisplatin has been used but, despite improved response rates and progression-free survival, it is more toxic and has not improved overall survival. Bleomycin has also been used. Other drugs under investigation for locally advanced or recurrent disease, in combination with cisplatin, include gemcitabine, irinotecan, paclitaxel, and vinorelbine.[7] Human papilloma virus vaccines are under investigation for both therapeutic and prophylactic use.[8,9]

1. Miller AB, *et al.* Report on consensus conference on cervical cancer screening and management. *Int J Cancer* 2000; **86:** 440–7.
2. Waggoner SE. Cervical cancer. *Lancet* 2003; **361:** 2217–25.
3. Kim RY, *et al.* Advances in the treatment of gynecologic malignancies part 1: cancers of the cervix and vulva. *Oncology (Huntingt)* 2002; **16:** 1510–17, 1521.
4. Thomas GM. Concurrent chemotherapy and radiation for locally advanced cervical cancer: the new standard of care. *Semin Radiat Oncol* 2000; **10:** 44–50.
5. Green J, *et al.* Concomitant chemotherapy and radiation therapy for cancer of the uterine cervix. Available in The Cochrane Library; Issue 2. Chichester: John Wiley; 2004.
6. Moore DH. Neoadjuvant chemotherapy for cervical cancer. *Expert Opin Pharmacother* 2003; **4:** 859–67.

7. Friedlander M. Guidelines for the treatment of recurrent and metastatic cervical cancer. *Oncologist* 2002; **7:** 342–7.
8. Murakami M, *et al.* Human papillomavirus vaccines for cervical cancer. *J Immunother* 1999; **22:** 212–18.
9. Koutsky LA, *et al.* A controlled trial of a human papillomavirus type 16 vaccine. *N Engl J Med* 2002; **347:** 1645–51.


**Malignant neoplasms of the endometrium.** Cancer of the endometrium is a disease primarily of postmenopausal women, and is more common in developed than developing countries. Most of the risk factors for endometrial cancer are associated with increased oestrogen exposure. Factors resulting in increased endogenous exposure include obesity, anovulatory infertility, early menarche, and late menopause. Exogenous factors include use of oestrogens without progestogens for hormone replacement therapy (p.1537), and tamoxifen therapy (see Carcinogenicity, p.584). Postmenopausal vaginal bleeding is the most common sign of endometrial cancer, and allows the disease to be diagnosed at an early stage when the prognosis is good (80% of women have early stage disease at presentation). In menopausal or premenopausal women, diagnosis may be delayed because abnormal bleeding patterns may not be so obvious. Most endometrial cancers are adenocarcinomas. A small percentage are clear-cell or serous carcinomas, which are highly aggressive and have a poorer prognosis. Endometrial hyperplasia is generally regarded as a precancerous lesion; endometrial hyperplasia with cytological atypia, in particular, is associated with progression to adenocarcinoma.

Surgery is the primary therapy for endometrial cancers that are stage I to III;[1-4] oophorectomy is performed, as well as total abdominal hysterectomy, because of the significant incidence of ovarian metastases. No further treatment is required in women with stage I disease who are at low risk of recurrence. In those with stage I disease and a higher risk of recurrence, adjuvant brachytherapy or pelvic irradiation are used. In all other women, adjuvant radiotherapy is given, the field being tailored depending on the disease stage. Adjuvant progestogen therapy has not been shown to be effective.[5] There are a few studies of adjuvant chemotherapy in women at high risk of recurrence, but further data from randomised trials are required to assess its role.[6] For women with advanced disease (stage IV), systemic therapy with progestogens or cytotoxic chemotherapy can be considered, although response rates are only up to 30%.[1,3] Progestogens are likely to be preferred because of their better tolerability. Well-differentiated tumours, long disease-free interval, and positive hormone receptor status are factors that suggest increased response to progestogens. When progestogens are ineffective, chemotherapy may be tried. The drugs of choice are probably doxorubicin, cisplatin or carboplatin, and cyclophosphamide. Paclitaxel is also reported to have some activity. Investigational therapies include dactinomycin, gonadorelin analogues such as goserelin, and anastrozole.[3]


1. Rose PG. Endometrial carcinoma. *N Engl J Med* 1996; **335:** 640–9. Correction. *ibid.* 1997; **336:** 1335.
2. Semple D. Endometrial cancer. *Br J Hosp Med* 1997; **57:** 260–2.
3. Chen L-M, *et al.* Endometrial cancer: recent developments in evaluation and treatment. *Oncology (Huntingt)* 1999; **13:** 1665–70.
4. Southcott BM. Carcinoma of the endometrium. *Drugs* 2001; **61:** 1395–1405.
5. Martin-Hirsch PL, *et al.* Progestagens for endometrial cancer. Available in The Cochrane Library; Issue 2. Chichester: John Wiley; 2004.
6. Pustilnik T, Burke TW. Adjuvant chemotherapy for high-risk endometrial cancer. *Semin Radiat Oncol* 2000; **10:** 23–8.


**Malignant neoplasms of the eye.** Tumours of the orbit of the eye in adults are most commonly metastases from primary lesions elsewhere in the body, usually in the breast or lung, and local radiotherapy (external beam radiation or plaque radiotherapy) may be required for control of visual symptoms unresponsive to chemotherapeutic treatment of primary disease.[1]

Primary eye tumours are rare. In children, the most common intra-ocular tumour is retinoblastoma (see below), and the most common orbital tumour is rhabdomyosarcoma (see Soft-tissue Sarcomas, below). In adults, primary CNS lymphoma can originate in the eye (ocular lymphoma), and is treated with radiotherapy to the globe. However, the most common primary ocular cancer in adults is **intra-ocular melanoma** (posterior uveal melanoma), which accounts for 80% of all primary ocular cancers. Treatment options for small ocular melanomas include observation or local treatment (radiation, brachytherapy, cryotherapy, local resection, photocoagulation, or hyperthermia).[2,3] Large melanomas are treated by removal of the eye (enucleation). Treatment of medium-sized tumours is controversial, with some preferring treatments that preserve vision, and some enucleation. At present there are no good data to support the use of adjuvant chemotherapy. In the few patients with metastatic uveal melanoma, resection and intra-arterial chemotherapy or chemoembolisation may be used for isolated hepatic metastases.[2] Most of the combination chemotherapy regimens for palliative therapy have included dacarbazine.[2]

Ocular surface neoplasms (lesions of the conjunctival or corneal epithelium) are usually treated with local excision. Where surgery is not feasible, topical application of mitomycin (0.04%) or fluorouracil (1%) has been tried.[4]


1. Shields CL. Plaque radiotherapy for the management of uveal metastasis. *Curr Opin Ophthalmol* 1998; **9:** 31–7.
2. Wöll E, *et al.*. Uveal melanoma: natural history and treatment options for metastatic disease. *Melanoma Res* 1999; **9:** 575–81.
3. Char DH. Ocular melanoma. *Surg Clin North Am* 2003; **83:** 253–74.
4. Majmudar PA, Epstein RJ. Antimetabolites in ocular surface neoplasia. *Curr Opin Ophthalmol* 1998; **9:** 35–9.


**Malignant neoplasms of the gastrointestinal tract.** Considered as a whole (and excluding skin cancers, which are often poorly registered) the gastrointestinal tract is the most frequent site of malignancies worldwide, although the frequencies of the various types of gastrointestinal cancer vary greatly from country to country. Direct exposure to various environmental carcinogens is thought to play an important role in many of these cancers. Treatment may include surgery, radiotherapy, and chemotherapy, but the prognosis in most forms of gastrointestinal cancer is not encouraging.

**Oesophageal cancer** has perhaps the greatest variation in incidence between different geographical regions of any cancer, and is endemic in many parts of the world. The two major histological types are squamous cell carcinoma and adenocarcinoma. Squamous cell carcinoma is strongly associated with tobacco and alcohol use, and may occur as a second primary tumour in patients with tumours of the upper aerodigestive tract (see Malignant Neoplasms of the Head and Neck , below). Adenocarcinoma is more common in non-endemic regions, and is associated with Barrett's oesophagus (see Gastro-oesophageal Reflux Disease, p.1242). Oesophageal cancer usually develops as a growth or ulcerative lesion of the oesophagus with extensive infiltration of the mucosa and invasion of neighbouring structures. Lymphatic and blood-borne metastasis occurs at a relatively early stage. Symptoms of pain and dysphagia due to obstruction occur late and disease is usually well advanced at diagnosis.

Surgical resection is the preferred primary treatment in stage I oesophageal cancer. In general, in patients with localised disease, the choice is between surgery and primary chemoradiotherapy (with fluorouracil plus cisplatin), which appear to give equivalent results.[1,2] Because the overall 5-year survival rate in patients with operable tumours is only 5 to 20%, there has been great interest in adjuvant treatment (pre-operative or postoperative).[3,4] There is no clear evidence that pre-operative radiotherapy alone improves survival.[5] However, there is conflicting evidence on the value of chemoradiotherapy or chemotherapy used before surgery, with some trials showing improved survival, and others no additional benefit.[3] A randomised study[6] using cisplatin plus fluorouracil found an increase in median survival of about 3 months and improved 2-year survival rates. A systematic review[7] that included this study found that pre-operative chemotherapy appeared to improve survival, but this only became statistically significant after 5 years. This approach still requires continued evaluation in clinical trials.[2] In half to two-thirds of patients the disease is too advanced at presentation for anything but palliation. Those with poor performance status should be offered supportive care.[2] This may include brachytherapy, laser therapy, or photodynamic therapy with photosensitisers such as porfimer sodium to relieve obstruction. In those patients with good performance status, chemotherapy may offer some palliation of the disease. Standard options include cisplatin-based, fluorouracil-based, or taxane-based combinations.[2,4] Chemoradiotherapy may also be used.[4]

**Cancer of the stomach** is one of the most common cancers worldwide, with particularly high incidence in the Far East, Russia, and parts of Latin America, although the incidence is declining almost everywhere. Over 90% of malignant gastric neoplasms are adenocarcinomas. Less frequent gastric neoplasms include lymphomas (see MALT lymphoma, above) and carcinoid tumours (see above). Dietary factors, such as high consumption of salted or smoked foods, are thought to play a role in the development of gastric cancer. *Helicobacter pylori* infection, and resultant gastritis, plays a role in gastric lymphomas, and may also be a factor in gastric cancer. However, it is not yet known if elimination of *Helicobacter pylori* infection will prove useful in preventing the development of gastric cancer.[8]

Early disease is relatively asymptomatic or produces non-specific gastrointestinal symptoms such as dyspepsia. There is concern that the use of antisecretory drugs for these symptoms may delay the diagnosis of gastric cancer (see Gastric Carcinoma, under Omeprazole Precautions, p.1279). Gastric epithelial dysplasia is a premalignant condition, and warrants follow-up and possible surgical intervention. Similarly, persistent gastric ulcers may be malignant. More advanced disease may produce discomfort or pain, anaemia, weight loss, and anorexia; obstruction, haemorrhage, and perforation may develop. Extension to the liver and pancreas, and lymphatic and blood-borne (portal) metastases may occur. The overall prognosis is not good, and 5-year survival rates are only 5 to 10%.

Surgery is the mainstay of treatment for early disease,[4,9] and is all that is required for stage I. Survival rates are poorer in other stages of locoregional disease, and various adjuvant approaches have been tried. Gastric cancer is relatively chemoresistant; earlier meta-analyses[10,11] of postoperative chemotherapy failed to show a significant survival benefit, and although a more recent analysis[12] did find a small benefit, well-controlled trials are still needed to confirm this. Similarly adjuvant radiotherapy alone has not improved survival. More promising results have been obtained with combined chemoradiotherapy (most often with fluorouracil) after surgery.[13] Thus, some recommend the use of adjuvant chemoradiotherapy after resection in the case of positive margins.[9] In addition, this is also an option for the primary treatment of inoperable locoregional disease.[9] The use of neoadjuvant chemoradiotherapy is under investigation.[14]

Treatment for advanced disease is purely palliative, and options include supportive care with or without chemotherapy.[9,15,16] Supportive care includes the relief of luminal obstruction with, for example, photodynamic therapy. Chemotherapy may have substantial palliative effect and modest survival gains, and may be considered in those with good performance status. Fluorouracil alone produces responses in up to 20% of patients. Despite doubts about the superiority of combination chemotherapy over single agents, fluorouracil, doxorubicin, and mitomycin (FAM) has been widely used. Other combinations include the substitution of cisplatin or methotrexate for mitomycin (FAC and FAMTX, respectively) and the use of epirubicin instead of doxorubicin, (e.g. ECF—epirubicin, cisplatin, and fluorouracil). Investigational drugs include docetaxel, paclitaxel, gemcitabine, irinotecan, raltitrexed, and various oral agents such as etoposide, and fluorouracil derivatives. A study comparing FAMTX with fluorouracil plus cisplatin or a regimen of etoposide, fluorouracil and folinic acid found that all 3 had only modest clinical benefits.[17] There has been debate[18,19] about the possible superiority of ECF, and some[4] now recommend it as the preferred combination.

**Cancers of the colon and rectum** are very common in developed areas such as the USA and western Europe, but rare among African and Asian populations. Various genetic and dietary factors are thought to be related to development of the disease.[20] Inherited predisposition syndromes include familial adenomatous polyposis and hereditary non-polyposis colorectal cancer.[21] Most large bowel cancers arise within pre-existing intestinal polyps. Over 50% occur in the rectum and about 20% in the sigmoid colon. There may be direct invasion of neighbouring structures and metastatic spread to the lymph nodes, and to lungs, bone, and in particular, liver. Signs and symptoms include blood in the stools, altered bowel habit, anaemia, and weight loss; there may be local obstruction (depending on location) or perforation.

The first-line treatment for early-stage and locally-advanced disease (stages I to III; Dukes A to C) is surgery. Although complete surgical resection is possible in up to 80% of cases at the time of diagnosis, about 50% ultimately die of recurrent disease. Because of this, there has been much research in the use of adjuvant therapies. Local recurrence is more likely to occur with rectal cancers than colon cancers, since anatomical constraints make surgical removal of rectal tumours more difficult. Therefore, the use of local adjuvant (pre- or postoperative) radiotherapy has been extensively studied.[22]

Many consider the use of postoperative radiotherapy (combined with adjuvant chemotherapy) to be the standard of care in patients with rectal cancer.[22] A meta-analysis[23] has found that adjuvant radiotherapy reduced the risk of local recurrence; the risk of death from rectal cancer may have been reduced, particularly for pre-operative radiotherapy but there was little impact on overall survival. The dose of radiotherapy may be a significant factor in response, and further studies are needed to determine whether pre-operative radiotherapy really is more effective than postoperative.

Adjuvant chemotherapy, usually based on fluorouracil, is also widely used, both in rectal and colon cancer. In locally advanced colon and rectal cancer (Dukes C; stage III), the use of adjuvant systemic fluorouracil-based therapy has been shown to improve survival,[24-26] and is considered the standard of care.[27,28] The case for adjuvant therapy in stage II colon and rectal cancer is less clear,[29] no overall benefit has been shown,[28] and its use should preferably be within clinical trials.[27]

Fluorouracil is usually given with the biochemical modulator folinic acid (see also Administration under Fluorouracil, p.555) to increase its effect.[27] Continuing research suggests that fluorouracil combined with low-dose folinic acid may become the preferred regimen.[30] Fluorouracil is only effective against actively dividing cells, and there is some evidence that maximising the chances of exposure, by giving prolonged infusions, may improve the results of adjuvant therapy compared with bolus administration.

Newer antineoplastics such as oxaliplatin, irinotecan, and capecitabine, which have been used for palliative therapy, are also under investigation for adjuvant treatment.[27] Reports of improved survival with the adjuvant use of edrecolomab, a murine monoclonal antibody directed against an epithelial cell surface glycoprotein,[31,32] do not seem to have been borne out.[33] Another potential approach is the adjuvant use of intraportal chemotherapy directed at the liver, one of the commonest sites of metastasis for colon cancer. In a meta-analysis of 10 studies,[34] the reduction in hepatic metastases with intraportal vein chemotherapy given for about 1 week after surgery was not significant, although there was a trend towards increased 5-year survival. It was concluded that additional trial evidence was required.[34]

Palliative treatments for advanced colorectal cancer (stage IV; metastatic disease) include surgery, radiotherapy, and chemotherapy.[20,28,35] In patients with isolated hepatic metastases, these may be surgically resected, or intra-hepatic arterial chemotherapy may be considered (see Malignant Neoplasms of the Liver, below). In other patients with advanced colorectal cancer, palliative chemotherapy has resulted in modest survival benefits:[36] the combination of systemic fluorouracil with folinic acid has been recommended as standard chemotherapy for many years. There is evidence that the addition of folinic acid improves the efficacy of fluorouracil in this setting,[37] and that continuous infusion of fluorouracil is more effective than bolus administration.[38] Oral prodrug alternatives to parenteral fluorouracil have been investigated; capecitabine alone, or UFT (tegafur and uracil) combined with calcium folinate, can be used for first-line therapy in metastatic colorectal disease. A number of other drugs have been studied in advanced colorectal cancer[39] and may come to replace fluorouracil with folinic acid as standard therapy. Irinotecan combined with fluorouracil and folinic acid has been reported to increase response rate and survival compared with fluorouracil and folinic acid alone, and is now considered suitable for first-line therapy. Irinotecan monotherapy is used as second-line therapy after failure of fluorouracil, and has improved survival compared with supportive care. The platinum derivative oxaliplatin, used with fluorouracil and folinic acid, has also been reported to increase response rate and progression-free survival, and is another combination used for first-line therapy. Raltitrexed monotherapy is another option for the second-line treatment of advanced colorectal cancer when fluorouracil-based therapy is not tolerated or is inappropriate. Immunological therapies under investigation include monoclonal antibodies, and vaccination with autologous tumour cells or against tumour-associated antigens; gene therapy is another area of research.[40]

PROPHYLAXIS. Various drugs and dietary factors have been shown in epidemiological studies to be associated with a reduced risk of colorectal cancer, and some of these have been investigated in prospective randomised trials.[41] Aspirin and NSAIDs are the most widely studied. In short-term randomised trials, both sulindac and celecoxib have reduced the size and number of colonic polyps in patients with familial adenomatous polyposis. However, prophylactic surgical removal of the colon is still considered the standard of care for these patients.[41,42] Calcium supplementation has shown a moderate reduction in the formation of new adenomas in patients with a history of colorectal adenomas. Despite the epidemiological evidence for dietary fibre, a number of large randomised trials of fibre supplements or high-fibre diets have not found any reduction in the formation of new adenomas in patients with a history of colorectal adenomas. Antoxidant vitamins have also been investigated, but evidence for their benefit is conflicting (see Prophylaxis of Malignant Neoplasms, p.1420). Other potential chemopreventive agents on the basis of epidemiological evidence include folic acid, and menopausal HRT.[41]

An important component of the care of patients with inherited predisposition or other risk factors for colon cancer is regular screening.[42,43] Various screening methods are also under investigation for use in normal risk individuals.[44,45]

**Cancers of the anal canal** mucosa are most commonly squamous cell carcinomas. Risk factors include immunosuppression, genital human papillomavirus infection, and sexual activity. Combined chemotherapy and radiotherapy is the usual primary treatment.[46] Fluorouracil is commonly used, sometimes with mitomycin, and the combination of fluorouracil and cisplatin is being investigated. For patients who do not respond, or who subsequently relapse, surgical resection with the formation of a colostomy is preferred. There is no standard therapy for metastatic disease.[46]


1. Minsky BD. Carcinoma of the esophagus. Part 1: primary therapy. *Oncology (Huntingt)* 1999; **13:** 1225–32 and 1235–6.
2. National Comprehensive Cancer Network. Clinical practice guidelines in oncology: esophageal cancer (version 1.2004). Available at: http://www.nccn.org/professionals/physician_gls/PDF/esophageal.pdf (accessed 02/06/04)
3. Minsky BD. Carcinoma of the esophagus. Part 2: adjuvant therapy. *Oncology (Huntingt)* 1999; **13:** 1415–27.
4. Allum WH, *et al.* Guidelines for the management of oesophageal and gastric cancer. *Gut* 2002; **50** (suppl 5): v1–v23.
5. Arnott SJ, *et al.* Preoperative radiotherapy for esophageal carcinoma. Available in The Cochrane Library; Issue 2. Chichester: John Wiley; 2004.
6. Medical Research Council Oesophageal Cancer Working Party. Surgical resection with or without preoperative chemotherapy in oesophageal cancer: a randomised controlled trial. *Lancet* 2002; **359:** 1727–33.
7. Malthaner R, Fenlon D. Preoperative chemotherapy for resectable thoracic esophageal cancer. Available in The Cochrane Library; Issue 2. Chichester: John Wiley; 2004.
8. Scheiman JM, Cutler AF. Helicobacter pylori and gastric cancer. *Am J Med* 1999; **106:** 222–6.
9. National Comprehensive Cancer Network. Clinical practice guidelines in oncology: gastric cancer (version 1.2004). Available at: http://www.nccn.org/professionals/physician_gls/PDF/gastric.pdf (accessed 02/06/04)
10. Hermans J, *et al.* Adjuvant therapy after curative resection for gastric cancer: meta-analysis of randomised trials. *J Clin Oncol* 1993; **11:** 1441–7.
11. Earle CC, Maroun JA. Adjuvant chemotherapy after curative resection for gastric cancer in non-Asian patients: revisiting a meta-analysis of randomised trials. *Eur J Cancer* 1999; **35:** 1059–64.
12. Mari E, *et al.* Efficacy of adjuvant chemotherapy after curative resection for gastric cancer: a meta-analysis of published randomised trials. *Ann Oncol* 2000; **11:** 837–43.
13. Macdonald JS, *et al.* Chemoradiotherapy after surgery compared with surgery alone for adenocarcinoma of the stomach or gastroesophageal junction. *N Engl J Med* 2001; **345:** 725–30.
14. Sun W, Haller DG. Recent advances in the treatment of gastric cancer. *Drugs* 2001; **61:** 1545–51.
15. Fuchs CS, Mayer RJ. Gastric carcinoma. *N Engl J Med* 1995; **333:** 32–41.
16. Hendlisz A, Bleiberg H. Diagnosis and treatment of gastric cancer. *Drugs* 1995; **49:** 711–20.
17. Vanhoefer U, *et al.* Final results of a randomized phase III trial of sequential high-dose methotrexate, fluorouracil, and doxorubicin versus etoposide, leucovorin, and fluorouracil versus infusional fluorouracil and cisplatin in advanced gastric cancer: a trial of the European Organization for Research and Treatment of Cancer Gastrointestinal Tract Cancer Cooperative Group. *J Clin Oncol* 2000; **18:** 2648–57.
18. Ross PJ, *et al.* ECF in gastric cancer. *J Clin Oncol* 2000; **18:** 3874–5.
19. Ajani JA. Standard chemotherapy for gastric carcinoma: is it a myth? *J Clin Oncol* 2000; **18:** 4001–2.
20. Bodger K. Colorectal cancer. *J R Coll Physicians Lond* 2000; **34:** 197–201.
21. Midgley R, Kerr D. Colorectal cancer. *Lancet* 1999; **353:** 391–9.
22. Minsky BD. Adjuvant therapy of rectal cancer. *Semin Oncol* 1999; **26:** 540–4.
23. Colorectal Cancer Collaborative Group. Adjuvant radiotherapy for rectal cancer: a systematic overview of 8507 patients from 22 randomised trials. *Lancet* 2001; **358:** 1291–1304.
24. International Multicentre Pooled Analysis of Colon Cancer Trials (IMPACT) Investigators. Efficacy of adjuvant fluorouracil and folinic acid in colon cancer. *Lancet* 1995; **345:** 939–44.
25. Dube S, *et al.* Adjuvant chemotherapy in colorectal carcinoma: results of a meta-analysis. *Dis Colon Rectum* 1997; **40:** 35–41.
26. Midgley RSJ, Kerr DJ. Adjuvant therapy. *BMJ* 2000; **321:** 1208–11.
27. Moore HCF, Haller DG. Adjuvant therapy of colon cancer. *Semin Oncol* 1999; **26:** 545–55.
28. Scottish Intercollegiate Guidelines Network. Management of colorectal cancer: a national clinical guideline (March 2003). Available at: http://www.sign.ac.uk/pdf/sign67.pdf (accessed 25/06/04)
29. IMPACT B2 Investigators. Efficacy of adjuvant fluorouracil and folinic acid in B2 colon cancer. *J Clin Oncol* 1999; **17:** 1356–63.
30. QUASAR Collaborative Group. Comparison of fluorouracil with additional levamisole, higher-dose folinic acid, or both, as adjuvant chemotherapy for colorectal cancer: a randomised trial. *Lancet* 2000; **355:** 1588–96.
31. Riethmüller G, *et al.* Randomised trial of monoclonal antibody for adjuvant therapy of resected Dukes' C colorectal carcinoma. *Lancet* 1994; **343:** 1177–83.
32. Riethmüller G, *et al.* Monoclonal antibody therapy for resected Dukes' C colorectal cancer: seven-year outcome of a multicenter randomized trial. *J Clin Oncol* 1998; **16:** 1788–94.
33. Punt CJA, *et al.* Edrecolomab alone or in combination with fluorouracil and folinic acid in the adjuvant treatment of stage III colon cancer: a randomised study. *Lancet* 2002; **360:** 671–7.
34. Liver Infusion Meta-analysis Group. Portal vein chemotherapy for colorectal cancer: a meta-analysis of 4000 patients in 10 studies. *J Natl Cancer Inst* 1997; **89:** 497–505.
35. Napier MP, Ledermann JA. The management of advanced colorectal cancer. *CME Oncol* 2000; **2:** 31–6.
36. Best L, *et al.* Palliative chemotherapy for advanced or metastatic colorectal cancer. Available in The Cochrane Library; Issue 2. Chichester: John Wiley; 2004.
37. Advanced Colorectal Cancer Meta-analysis Project. Modulation of fluorouracil by leucovorin in patients with advanced colorectal cancer: evidence in terms of response rate. *J Clin Oncol* 1992; **10:** 896–903.
38. Meta-analysis Group in Cancer. Efficacy of intravenous continuous infusion of fluorouracil compared with bolus administration in advanced colorectal cancer. *J Clin Oncol* 1998; **16:** 301–308.
39. Anonymous. Chemotherapy for metastatic colorectal cancer. *Drug Ther Bull* 2002; **40:** 49–52.
40. Chung-Faye GA, Kerr DJ. Innovative treatment for colon cancer. *BMJ* 2000; **321:** 1397–9. Correction. *ibid.* 2001; **322:** 150.
41. Jänne PA, Mayer RJ. Chemoprevention of colorectal cancer. *N Engl J Med* 2000; **342:** 1960–8.
42. King JE, *et al.* Care of patients and their families with familial adenomatous polyposis. *Mayo Clin Proc* 2000; **75:** 57–67.
43. Cairns S, Scholefield JH, eds. Guidelines for colorectal cancer screening in high risk groups. *Gut* 2002; **51** (suppl 5): v1–v28.
44. Rhodes JM. Colorectal cancer screening in the UK: joint position statement by the British Society of Gastroenterology, the Royal College of Physicians, and the Association of Coloproctology of Great Britain and Ireland. *Gut* 2000; **46:** 746–8.
45. Pignone M, *et al.* Screening for colorectal cancer in adults at average risk: a summary of the evidence for the U.S. Preventive Services Task Force. *Ann Intern Med* 2002; **137:** 132–41.
46. Ryan DP, *et al.* Carcinoma of the anal canal. *N Engl J Med* 2000; **342:** 792–800.


**Malignant neoplasms of the head and neck.** Cancers of the head and neck are classically defined as those of the mucosal surfaces of the upper aerodigestive tract and include neoplasms of the oral cavity (accounting for 40%), pharynx (15%), and larynx (25%). The majority are squamous cell carcinomas, and the highest incidence is in men aged over 50 years. Overall, cancers of the head and neck account for about 5% of all malignant neoplasms in the West, but are the most common causes in other parts of the world. The major risk factor for these cancers is the use of tobacco (whether chewed, inhaled, or smoked). Alcohol acts synergistically with tobacco to increase the risk. Endemic nasopharyngeal cancer in parts of India, China, and North Africa is associated with Epstein-Barr virus and the consumption of salt-cured fish.

Premalignant lesions include leucoplakia and erythroplakia, and these can progress to invasive cancer. About one-third of cancers are diagnosed at early stages (I and II), and the rest are usually locally advanced (stage III and IVA). Although early-stage disease can be successfully treated, there is a high incidence of second primary cancers in the head and neck, lung, or oesophagus. Therefore, there is interest in the development of chemopreventive drugs to reduce this risk. Fewer than 30% of patients with locally advanced disease are cured.

Surgery or radiotherapy are the mainstays of treatment for early-stage cancers of the oral cavity and the oropharynx.[1-3] The choice is often debated, since both are equally effective, but have different complications. Radiotherapy is preferred for early-stage nasopharyngeal carcinoma, which is anatomically unresectable,[3,4] and for carcinoma of the larynx (vocal cords), to preserve the voice.[3]

Locally advanced disease is usually treated with combination therapy. Resectable disease is managed with surgery and adjuvant radiotherapy.[2,3] Chemotherapy with radiotherapy (either neoadjuvant chemotherapy or chemoradiotherapy) is used in patients with unresectable locally advanced tumours, and in resectable disease when the aim is to avoid the need for surgery and thereby allow organ preservation.[2,3,5] Some therefore recommend this as standard for cancers of the nasopharynx[3-5] and larynx.[3,5,6] A meta-analysis[7] showed only a small overall survival benefit (4%) for chemotherapy added to surgery and/or radiotherapy in locally advanced head and neck cancers. Further analysis by timing suggested that there was no significant benefit for adjuvant or neoadjuvant chemotherapy (except perhaps for neoadjuvant therapy with fluorouracil and a platinum compound), but that chemotherapy with radiotherapy (either concomitant or alternating) did offer significant benefits. Further studies have also shown overall survival benefit for chemoradiotherapy compared with radiotherapy alone.[2] Data from 3 trials of larynx preservation using neoadjuvant chemotherapy and radiotherapy in patients with locally advanced disease showed a non-significant negative effect in the chemotherapy arm.[7] The authors concluded that laryngeal preservation should remain investigational.[7]

Palliative chemotherapy is used in metastatic or recurrent disease.[3,5,6] Drugs used for single-agent treatment include methotrexate, cisplatin, carboplatin, fluorouracil, bleomycin, docetaxel, and paclitaxel. Combination regimens such as cisplatin and fluorouracil are commonly used and produce more responses, but no clear improvement in survival. The choice of best supportive care or single-agent or combination chemotherapy should be dictated by the patient's performance status, as the benefits of chemotherapy are limited.[3]

A local injection of cisplatin in a gel formulation containing adrenaline is under investigation in recurrent and refractory head and neck cancer.[8] Photodynamic therapy (p.581) using temoporfin is a more recent development for palliative management. Biological approaches being investigated include the monoclonal epidermal growth factor receptor antibody cetuximab, and various gene therapies. Chemoprevention is also under investigation (see Leucoplakia, p.531).


1. Zakrzewska JM. Oral cancer. *BMJ* 1999; **318:** 1051–4.
2. Sanderson RJ, Ironside JAD. Squamous cell carcinomas of the head and neck. *BMJ* 2002; **325:** 822–7.
3. National Comprehensive Cancer Network. Clinical practice guidelines in oncology: head and neck cancers (version 1.2004). Available at: http://www.nccn.org/professionals/physician_gls/PDF/head-and-neck.pdf (accessed 03/06/04)
4. Vokes EE, *et al.* Nasopharyngeal carcinoma. *Lancet* 1997; **350:** 1087–91.
5. Forastiere A, *et al.* Head and neck cancer. *N Engl J Med* 2001; **345:** 1890–1900. Correction. *ibid.* 2002; **346:** 788.
6. Catimel G. Head and neck cancer: guidelines for chemotherapy. *Drugs* 1996; **51:** 73–88.
7. Pignon JP, *et al.* Chemotherapy added to locoregional treatment for head and neck squamous-cell carcinoma: three meta-analyses of updated individual data. *Lancet* 2000; **355:** 949–55. Correction. *ibid.*; 1650.
8. Wenig BL, *et al.* The role of intratumoral therapy with cisplatin/epinephrine injectable gel in the management of advanced squamous cell carcinoma of the head and neck. *Arch Otolaryngol Head Neck Surg* 2002; **128:** 880–5.


**Malignant neoplasms of the kidney.** Cancer of the kidney is relatively uncommon. About 80% of such cancers in adults are renal cell carcinoma, with the remainder mostly cancer of the renal pelvis. The disease is about twice as common in men as in women. Risk factors include smoking, obesity, and phenacetin use. Disease is often clinically silent; there may however be haematuria, flank and back pain, and a palpable mass in the flank or abdomen. About 45% of patients have early-stage disease at presentation (I and II), 25% have locally advanced disease (stage III), and 30% metastatic disease (stage IV). The most common sites for metastases are the lung, liver, and bone, although unusual sites for metastases are a known feature of renal cancer.

Radical nephrectomy is the main treatment for early-stage disease although partial nephrectomy may be considered in some patients.[1,2] Minimally invasive procedures such as radiofrequency ablation and cryotherapy are under investigation for treatment of small tumours.[3] Radical nephrectomy is also used in selected patients with stage III disease. After radical nephrectomy 20 to 30% of patients with localised tumours will relapse, usually at distant sites.[2] This suggests that adjuvant therapy could be useful in reducing the risk of relapse.[1] However, radiotherapy is not beneficial, and no systemic therapy has been shown to reduce relapse (interferon alfa is not effective).[1,2] Standard care therefore remains close observation.[2]

In metastatic disease, nephrectomy may be considered in a few patients for palliation of symptoms. In addition, nephrectomy and surgical removal of solitary metastases may be appropriate in some patients.[2,4] In patients with minimal disease volume and good performance status, cytokine therapy with interleukin-2 or interferon alfa may be considered.[1,2] These cytokines have resulted in overall response rates of 10 to 20%, with a few long-term responses.[2,4,5] Meta-analysis has suggested a modest survival benefit for interferon alfa but the use of interleukin-2 has not been validated in appropriate comparative studies.[6] Two studies[7,8] of nephrectomy before interferon alfa therapy compared with interferon alone, in patients with good performance status, found that although overall response rates were similar there was a small survival benefit from nephrectomy. In other patients, supportive care remains the mainstay of therapy for metastatic disease.[2] Renal cell carcinoma is largely resistant to chemotherapy with currently available antineoplastics, and hormonal therapy with progestogens or anti-oestrogens has also had poor success.[1,5] The most extensively studied antineoplastics are vinblastine, fluorouracil, and floxuridine. However, reviews of up to 83 studies involving thousands of patients and over 70 different drugs found that only floxuridine and fluorouracil appeared to have even modest activity.[4,9] No antineoplastic can be considered standard in the treatment of metastatic disease.[5,10]

Investigational approaches include attempts to improve the response rates to interleukin-2 and interferon alfa by combining them, or adding antineoplastics or retinoids, but responses have been poor or toxicity significant.[4,5] There are also attempts to improve the tolerability of interleukin-2 by the use of continuous infusion, lower doses given by the subcutaneous route,[1,5] and inhalation.[5]

Because of the treatment resistance of renal cell carcinoma, there is an urgent need to develop innovative approaches. Various options in early phase development include radiolabelled monoclonal antibodies, allogeneic dendritic cell vaccines, and angiogenesis inhibitors.[1,11] Bevacizumab, a monoclonal antibody that binds to vascular endothelial growth factor (VEGF) and inhibits angiogenesis, has shown some promise in delaying progression of metastatic disease.[12] Regression of refractory metastatic disease after non-myeloablative allogeneic peripheral blood stem cell transplantation has been reported in a few patients.[13]


1. Vogelzang NJ, Stadler WM. Kidney cancer. *Lancet* 1998; **352:** 1691–6.
2. National Comprehensive Cancer Network. Clinical practice guidelines in oncology: kidney cancer (version 1.2004). Available at: http://www.nccn.org/professionals/physician_gls/PDF/kidney.pdf (accessed 03/06/04)
3. Reddan DN, *et al.* Management of small renal tumors: an overview. *Am J Med* 2001; **110:** 558–62.
4. Motzer RJ, Russo P. Systemic therapy for renal cell carcinoma. *J Urol (Baltimore)* 2000; **163:** 408–17.
5. Heinzer H, *et al.* Systemic chemotherapy and chemoimmunotherapy for metastatic renal cell cancer. *World J Urol* 2001; **19:** 111–19.
6. Coppin C, *et al.* Immunotherapy for advanced renal cell cancer. Available in The Cochrane Library; Issue 2. Chichester: John Wiley; 2004.
7. Mickisch GHJ, *et al.* Radical nephrectomy plus interferon-alfa-based immunotherapy compared with interferon alfa alone in metastatic renal-cell carcinoma: a randomised trial. *Lancet* 2001; **358:** 966–70.
8. Flanigan RC, *et al.* Nephrectomy followed by interferon alfa-2b compared with interferon alfa-2b alone for metastatic renal-cell cancer. *N Engl J Med* 2001; **345:** 1655–9.
9. Yagoda A, *et al.* Chemotherapy for advanced renal-cell carcinoma: 1983-1993. *Semin Oncol* 1995; **22:** 42–60.
10. Amato RJ. Chemotherapy for renal cell carcinoma. *Semin Oncol* 2000; **27:** 177–86.
11. Berg WJ, *et al.* Novel investigative approaches for advanced renal cell carcinoma. *Semin Oncol* 2000; **27:** 234–9.
12. Yang JC, *et al.* A randomized trial of bevacizumab, an anti-vascular endothelial growth factor antibody, for metastatic renal cancer. *N Engl J Med* 2003; **349:** 427–34.
13. Childs R, *et al.* Regression of metastatic renal-cell carcinoma after nonmyeloablative allogeneic peripheral-blood stem-cell transplantation. *N Engl J Med* 2000; **343:** 750–8.


WILMS' TUMOUR. In children most cases of renal tumours are due to Wilms' tumour (nephroblastoma). This is one of the most frequent solid tumours in childhood with a peak incidence between 1 and 5 years of age and accounting for about 6% of all childhood malignancies. The usual presentation is an asymptomatic abdominal mass; abdominal pain is less frequent and haematuria occurs only in about a quarter of patients. Metastasis in advanced disease is usually to the lungs and liver. Most primary tumours occur in one kidney, but some 5% involve both kidneys.

Unlike other forms of renal cancer Wilms' tumour responds well to chemotherapy. The basis of treatment is surgery, combined with chemotherapy, and if necessary radiotherapy. Management varies with disease stage and also varies between different study groups.[1-4] The US National Wilms' Tumour Study (NWTS) group and some other groups recommend initial surgery (nephrectomy) to confirm diagnosis and perform precise staging.[1,2] Others, including the European Société Internationale d'Oncologie Pédiatrique (SIOP), use neoadjuvant chemotherapy to reduce the tumour size and make surgery easier.[4] Overall survival for patients treated by either approach is very similar, being more than 90% for patients with favourable histology. The aim of the various study protocols has been to identify low-risk children who require less intensive therapy, and those with poor prognosis who require more intensive therapy or alternative investigative regimens.

Current SIOP neoadjuvant chemotherapy consists of 4 weeks of dactinomycin and vincristine for clinically localised disease, and 6 weeks of dactinomycin, vincristine, and epirubicin for metastatic disease.[3,4] Adjuvant chemotherapy regimens for disease with favourable histology are broadly similar between NWTS and SIOP.[2-4] In early disease, chemotherapy consists of vincristine combined with dactinomycin; in more advanced disease radiotherapy, and an anthracycline (doxorubicin or epirubicin) are added. Patients with unfavourable histology and stage I disease are treated the same as those with favourable histology early-stage disease.[3] Combination adjuvant chemotherapy regimens for patients with unfavourable histology and a poorer prognosis add drugs such as etoposide, carboplatin, and an alkylating agent (cyclophosphamide or ifosfamide), which may be combined with an anthracycline or vincristine; radiotherapy may also be used.[2-4] The duration of adjuvant chemotherapy is dependent on the disease stage. In children with recurrent disease, survival is usually poor: salvage rates of about 20 to 30% have been reported for those with favourable histology. A regimen of cyclophosphamide, carboplatin, and etoposide is being investigated.[3] Bilateral Wilms' tumour is not usually treated with primary bilateral nephrectomy because of the need to retain renal function. It may be biopsied to assess histology and stage and then treated with neoadjuvant chemotherapy.[2,3] Surgery is then performed, preserving as much of the kidneys as is possible. Survival has been reported to be comparable with that in other patients.[2] Because of these results, some have suggested the use of partial nephrectomy in patients with small unilateral tumours.[2]


1. Green DM, *et al.* The treatment of Wilms tumor: results of the National Wilms Tumor Studies. *Hematol Oncol Clin North Am* 1995; **9:** 1267–74.
2. Haase GM, Ritchey ML. Nephroblastoma. *Semin Pediatr Surg* 1997; **6:** 11–16.
3. Suryanarayan K, Marina N. Wilms' tumour: optimal treatment strategies. *Drugs* 1998; **56:** 597–605.
4. Graf N, *et al.* The role of preoperative chemotherapy in the management of Wilms' tumor: the SIOP studies. *Urol Clin North Am* 2000; **27:** 443–54.


**Malignant neoplasms of the liver.** Hepatocellular carcinoma (hepatoma) accounts for more than 90% of primary liver cancers. It is relatively uncommon in northern Europe and America but is the most common cancer among men in large parts of Africa and Asia. The incidence in men ranges from 2 to 8 times that in women. Chronic infection with hepatitis B or hepatitis C virus is by far the most important factor associated with development of liver cancer, although other risk factors include ingestion of foodstuffs contaminated with aflatoxins (see p.1648), alcoholic liver disease, haemochromatosis, and the long-term use of anabolic steroids (see under Testosterone, p.1570) and, rarely, combined oral contraceptives, (see p.1529). Over 70% of patients with hepatocellular carcinoma have cirrhosis of the liver.

Clinical manifestations of liver cancer include increasing obstructive jaundice, pain, malaise, and the presence of an epigastric mass; there may be metastasis to the lungs, kidney, bones, brain or other sites, or invasion of local structures.

Although diagnosis of *early disease* may be improved by screening at-risk groups, few patients have their tumours identified at a stage allowing prolongation of survival with surgical resection or liver transplantation.[1-3] **Liver transplantation** (p.1346) may be considered in those patients with very small tumours (stage I) and who have advanced cirrhosis and are therefore not suitable for surgical resection.[1,4] Patients with larger tumours or more advanced stages of disease are not candidates for transplantation because of the high rates of recurrence in the transplanted liver.[2,3] **Surgical resection** is considered in patients with no cirrhosis or mild liver impairment whose tumours are considered resectable (stages I to III). However, recurrence rates are high, and 5-year survival is only about 30%.[1,3,5]

As a result, **adjuvant** or **neoadjuvant chemotherapy** has been investigated in early-stage disease. Hepatocellular carcinoma is relatively resistant to chemotherapy, and a review of 8 studies concluded that none of the regimens of adjuvant or neoadjuvant therapy examined produced improvement in survival or disease-free survival.[6] However, a later review[7] of 21 studies found that chemotherapy injected into the hepatic artery after curative resection, usually with embolisation (see below), did improve survival and decrease recurrence. Neoadjuvant therapy may be considered to reduce tumour burden before transplantation[5] or to permit resection.[8] In patients who have small tumours and are not candidates for surgery or transplantation, percutaneous intratumoral alcohol injection is an option.[1,3-5,8] Other ablative therapies include radiofrequency ablation[4,5] and cryosurgery.[1,5]

Most patients present with *advanced stage* cancer and significant liver impairment. Options in unresectable disease include palliative medical treatments or supportive care.[1-3,5] **Systemic chemotherapy** has been tried, but has no standard role. Treatment with doxorubicin alone has been associated with a response rate of 3 to 30% and no increase in survival,[1,3,9] and this has not been bettered by combination chemotherapy. Doxorubicin has also been given by intra-arterial infusion into the hepatic artery, as have fluorouracil, floxuridine, and other drugs such as cisplatin and mitomycin.[1,3] Transcatheter arterial **chemo-em-**

**bolisation** combines intra-arterial chemotherapy with temporary occlusion of the artery (embolisation) using substances such as gelatine foam or iodised oil; this prolongs the duration of contact between drug and tumour, and attempts to induce tumour necrosis by ischaemia.[1,3,5] Although use of these techniques has given higher response rates than systemic therapy, there has been no evidence of an improvement in survival.[1-3,9] However, repeated chemo-embolisation was shown to improve survival compared with conservative treatment without chemotherapy in a study of selected patients with small unresectable tumours.[10] Systematic review[11] confirmed a survival benefit with chemo-embolisation, using doxorubicin or cisplatin, and suggested this method as standard therapy for selected patients with small unresectable tumours, and well-preserved liver function. **Other options** that have been tried include interferon alfa and tamoxifen.[1,3-5,9] Despite some initial positive data for tamoxifen, a large randomised clinical trial failed to show any survival benefit for therapy at conventional doses,[12] and meta-analysis[11] confirmed this. Adoptive immunotherapy, using activated T-cells cultured with interleukin-2 and a monoclonal anti-CD3 antibody, has been reported to lower recurrence after resection.[13] Trials of octreotide have produced conflicting results.[4]

In contrast to the poor response of hepatocellular carcinoma to therapy, better progress has been made in strategies for its **prevention**. Neonatal vaccination against hepatitis B has dramatically decreased the incidence of chronic infection in children in Taiwan, and reduced the incidence of hepatocellular carcinoma. This may be a more promising approach in areas where the disease is common.[2] There is evidence that interferon alfa may delay or prevent the development of hepatocellular carcinoma in cirrhotic patients with hepatitis C infection.[14] Chemoprevention may also be a useful approach after surgical resection: use of a synthetic retinoid, polyprenoic acid, was found to reduce the development of second primary tumours after resection.[15,16]

The liver is the most common site of *metastatic disease*.[17] For most malignancies the presence of liver metastases is indicative of generalised dissemination, but isolated metastatic liver disease is common in colorectal cancer (see Malignant Neoplasms of the Gastrointestinal Tract, above) and rarer cancers such as some neuroendocrine tumours (see Carcinoid Tumours, above). In contrast to disseminated disease, treatment of such isolated liver metastases can prolong survival. Surgical resection is the preferred treatment if feasible. Palliative or cytoreductive surgery is beneficial in hepatic metastases from neuroendocrine tumours because of their slow growth.[17] Combining resection with adjuvant hepatic arterial or systemic chemotherapy is under investigation for colorectal liver metastases. Unresectable colorectal liver metastases have been treated with systemic or hepatic intra-arterial chemotherapy, with modest survival benefits.[18]


1. Colleoni M, *et al.* Practical considerations in the treatment of hepatocellular carcinoma. *Drugs* 1998; **55:** 367–82.
2. Schafer DF, Sorrell MF. Hepatocellular carcinoma. *Lancet* 1999; **353:** 1253–7.
3. Badvie S. Hepatocellular carcinoma. *Postgrad Med J* 2000; **76:** 4–11.
4. Ryder SD. Guidelines for the diagnosis and treatment of hepatocellular carcinoma (HCC) in adults. *Gut* 2003; **52** (suppl): iii1–iii8. Also available at: http://www.bsg.org.uk/pdf_word_docs/hcc.pdf (accessed 28/06/04)
5. Yu AS, Keeffe EB. Management of hepatocellular carcinoma. *Rev Gastroenterol Disord* 2003; **3:** 8–24.
6. Chan ES-Y, *et al.* Neoadjuvant and adjuvant therapy for operable hepatocellular carcinoma. Available in The Cochrane Library; Issue 2. Chichester: John Wiley; 2004.
7. Mathurin P, *et al.* Meta-analysis: evaluation of adjuvant therapy after curative liver resection for hepatocellular carcinoma. *Aliment Pharmacol Ther* 2003; **17:** 1247–61.
8. Johnson PJ. Hepatocellular carcinoma: is current therapy really altering outcome? *Gut* 2002; **51:** 459–62.
9. Mathurin P, *et al.* Review article: overview of medical treatments in unresectable hepatocellular carcinoma-an impossible meta-analysis? *Aliment Pharmacol Ther* 1998; **12:** 111–126.
10. Llovet JM, *et al.* Arterial embolisation or chemoembolisation versus symptomatic treatment in patients with unresectable hepatocellular carcinoma: a randomised controlled trial. *Lancet* 2002; **359:** 1734–9.
11. Llovet JM, Bruix J. Systematic review of randomized trials for unresectable hepatocellular carcinoma: chemoembolization improves survival. *Hepatology* 2003; **37:** 429–42.
12. Cancer of the Liver Italian Programme Group. Tamoxifen in treatment of hepatocellular carcinoma: a randomised controlled trial. *Lancet* 1998; **352:** 17–20.
13. Takayama T, *et al.* Adoptive immunotherapy to lower postsurgical recurrence rates of hepatocellular carcinoma: a randomised trial. *Lancet* 2000; **356:** 802–7. Correction. *ibid.*; 1690.
14. Baffis V, *et al.* Use of interferon for prevention of hepatocellular carcinoma in cirrhotic patients with hepatitis B or hepatitis C virus infection. *Ann Intern Med* 1999; **131:** 696–701.
15. Muto Y, *et al.* Prevention of second primary tumors by an acyclic retinoid, polyprenoic acid, in patients with hepatocellular carcinoma. *N Engl J Med* 1996; **334:** 1561–7.
16. Muto Y, *et al.* Prevention of second primary tumors by an acyclic retinoid in patients with hepatocellular carcinoma. *N Engl J Med* 1999; **340:** 1046–7.
17. Choti MA, Bulkley GB. Management of hepatic metastases. *Liver Transpl Surg* 1999; **5:** 65–80.
18. Thirion P, *et al.* Survival impact of chemotherapy in patients with colorectal metastases confined to the liver: a re-analysis of 1458 non-operable patients randomised in 22 trials and 4 meta-analyses. *Ann Oncol* 1999; **10:** 1317–20.


**Malignant neoplasms of the lung.** Lung cancer is the most common non-skin cancer in the developed countries and the second most common overall worldwide. About 20 to 25% of all lung cancers are small cell lung cancers (SCLC) derived from endocrine cells in the bronchial mucosa; the remainder, comprising chiefly squamous cell carcinomas (40 to 45% of cases), adenocarcinoma (25 to 30%), and large-cell carcinoma (about 10%), are known collectively as non-small cell lung cancer (NSCLC). More than 80% of all lung cancers are associated with tobacco smoking, and there is also evidence that exposure to the cigarette smoke of others can increase the risk in non-smokers. Other risk factors may include occupational exposure to substances such as asbestos, and the effects of environmental toxins such as air pollutants.

Symptoms due to a lesion in a main bronchus (the most common site) include persistent cough, dyspnoea, haemoptysis, weight loss and sometimes chest pain. Metastatic spread is common, and may affect sites such as brain, liver, and bone. It occurs early with adenocarcinoma and SCLC, but late with squamous cell carcinoma.

Disease staging plays an important role in determining treatment. The management of SCLC differs significantly from that of non-small cell types.

The mainstay of treatment for **small cell lung cancer** is multi-drug chemotherapy.[1-4] Adjuvant thoracic radiotherapy is often used in patients with limited stage disease, and has been shown to improve survival.[5-7] The optimum scheduling of chemotherapy and radiotherapy is controversial, with some advocating early radiotherapy after chemotherapy,[1] and others radiotherapy concurrently with chemotherapy.[3,6] Surgical resection has been used in patients with limited stage disease, either alone or with other therapies, but it is not currently considered standard therapy.[1,3] Around 80% of patients with SCLC respond to primary therapy, with slightly better response in those with limited disease (confined to one hemithorax) than those with extensive disease. Despite these impressive responses, resistance and relapse almost always occur; the median survival is improved by treatment, but long-term survival is very poor: about 10 to 20% of patients with limited disease and 5% of those with extensive disease survive 2 years from the start of the treatment.

The most commonly used chemotherapy regimens for limited disease are etoposide and cisplatin (EP or PE), cyclophosphamide, doxorubicin, and vincristine (CAV), cyclophosphamide, doxorubicin, and etoposide (CAE or ACE), and ifosfamide, carboplatin, and etoposide (ICE).[1-3] Regimens containing cisplatin and etoposide are superior in limited-stage SCLC to regimens without these two drugs.[4] Various options for dose-intensification have been studied but there is no consistent evidence of improved survival, and such treatments remain investigational.[1,3,4] There is no role for maintenance chemotherapy in the treatment of SCLC.[4]

Similar combination regimens are used for extensive disease, but because of poor performance status, less aggressive treatments are sometimes used.[1,3] Oral etoposide was widely considered a useful palliative option, but the results of randomised controlled trials have shown slightly worse palliation of symptoms and reduced survival when compared with intravenous combination chemotherapy.[1,3,4] Paclitaxel and topotecan have been investigated, but have not proved better than standard EP therapy.[4,7] However, a recent phase III study[8] found a significant survival benefit over EP with the combination of irinotecan and cisplatin and further studies are underway.[4]

One of the most common sites for recurrence is the brain, and prophylactic cranial irradiation may be considered in an attempt to prevent this.[1-3] A recent meta-analysis[9] has confirmed that prophylactic cranial irradiation reduces the risk of brain recurrence and improves survival in patients in complete remission.

The value of chemotherapy in relapsed disease depends in part on the duration of remission before relapse, with greater responses the longer the remission.[3,7] Patients may be given the same initial therapy if they have received no treatment for 6 months or longer.[7] If cisplatin-based therapy was not used for initial treatment, it may be considered for second-line treatment.[3,7] Another option for second-line treatment is topotecan.[3,7] Palliative radiotherapy may also be given.[1,3]

Other drugs under investigation for the treatment of SCLC include vinorelbine and gemcitabine.[2-4]

In patients with **non-small cell lung cancer** presenting with tumour localised to the lung (generally stage I and II), the treatment of choice is surgery.[1,2,10] In patients with resectable disease who have medical contra-indications to surgery, radical radiotherapy is used with curative intent. More advanced disease is also treated with radiotherapy, although in disseminated disease this is purely palliative.[6] About 25 to 40% of patients resected for localised disease are still alive after 5 years, while 5-year survival is 4 to 8% in locally advanced disease and less than 1% in disseminated disease. Because of these poor results there has been great interest in the role of adjuvant therapies. In early-stage disease, use of radiotherapy after complete resection has been shown to result in worse survival than surgery alone,[11] and is not recommended.[1,2] Conversely, some recommend[1,10] that postoperative radiotherapy be considered if there is residual disease after surgery, although there is a lack of good evidence for a reduction in local recurrence in this setting. Chemotherapy has also been investigated as an adjuvant to surgery and/or radiotherapy. There is some evidence that cisplatin-based postoperative therapy improves survival, but that alkylating agent-based therapy decreases survival.[12] Recent results of a large international trial suggest that 5-year survival and disease-free survival were significantly increased in patients randomised to receive adjuvant chemotherapy compared with those receiving surgery alone. Chemotherapy consisted of 3 to 4 cycles of cisplatin combined with etoposide or a vinca alkaloid (vinblastine, vindesine, or vinorelbine).[13] In patients with unresectable locally advanced disease (stage IIIB), the use of cisplatin-based chemotherapy either before or concurrently with radiotherapy has resulted in a modest increase in survival according to the findings of a number of meta-analyses[12,14,15] and subsequent clinical trials.[6,16-18] Various combinations have been used including cisplatin plus etoposide, cisplatin plus vinblastine or vindesine or vinorelbine, carboplatin plus paclitaxel, and mitomycin, ifosfamide, plus cisplatin. The issue of dosage and sequencing is under investigation;[6] nonetheless concurrent chemotherapy with radiotherapy (chemoradiotherapy) is considered by some to be superior to sequential therapy.[6,18] Chemoradiotherapy followed by surgery (trimodality therapy) is also under investigation.[18] Recent results[13] suggest that this approach of chemotherapy, radiation, and surgery may improve progression-free survival when compared with chemotherapy and radiation alone.

Chemotherapy may also be used for advanced metastatic disease (stage IV), which is detected in 40 to 50% of patients at presentation. Various meta-analyses have shown a modest improvement in survival and symptom control in patients receiving chemotherapy compared with those receiving best supportive care.[12,19,20] The use of cisplatin-based chemotherapy resulted in an increase in median survival of 6 weeks, and an increase in 1-year survival of 10%.[12] To date no particular regimen has been identified as superior.[21] Regimens include cisplatin combined with either gemcitabine, irinotecan, vinorelbine, docetaxel, or paclitaxel,[22] or triple regimens such as mitomycin, vinblastine, and cisplatin (MVP) or mitomycin, ifosfamide, and cisplatin (MIC).[17] In the UK, gemcitabine, paclitaxel, or vinorelbine are recommended for first-line treatment, combined with platinum-based chemotherapy where tolerated with the choice of drug depending on patient characteristics, adverse effects, and institutional and individual preferences.[23] Drugs that have shown benefit in patients failing initial therapy include docetaxel,[2] gefitinib,[22] gemcitabine,[2] and pemetrexed.[13]

Photodynamic therapy, with porfimer sodium, may be considered for the palliative treatment of bronchial obstruction. Photodynamic therapy may also be used as an alternative to surgery in patients with very early-stage (in situ) endobronchial NSCLC.[24]

Despite the recent advances in chemotherapy for NSCLC, the median survival for this disease remains poor, and there is a need to identify alternative approaches to treatment. Those in preclinical development include gene therapy with the tumour suppressor gene p53 (which is abnormal in up to 75% of patients), monoclonal antibodies against epidermal growth factors, and angiogenesis inhibitors. Drugs under investigation include trastuzumab[25] and erlotinib.[18,25]

Given the poor prognosis of lung cancers, and the high incidence of secondary primaries in patients curatively treated for early-stage disease, there has been great interest in **prophylaxis.** The most important factor in primary and secondary prevention is cessation of tobacco smoking, for which a number of interventions may be tried (see Smoking Cessation, p.1721). Diets rich in fruit and vegetables have been associated with a lower incidence of malignant disease, and have prompted the investigation of antioxidant vitamins. However, primary prevention studies in those at risk of lung cancer have failed to show any benefit for vitamin supplements, and in the case of betacarotene, an increase in lung cancer was seen in those most at risk (see Prophylaxis of Malignant Neoplasms, p.1420). Other drugs under investigation are retinoids and NSAIDs.[26]

While a meta-analysis[27] concluded that screening of patients with chest radiography or sputum cytology was ineffective, the Early Lung Cancer Action Project found that computed tomography improves the likelihood of detection of nodules suggestive of lung cancer in high-risk patients.[28] Since most of those cancers detected were at an early stage, resection was possible, and it is theorised that this technique may reduce mortality,[25] although it remains investigational.

**Metastatic lung disease.** The lung is the second most frequent site for metastatic disease, occurring in about 30% of cancer patients. Surgical resection may be used to treat pulmonary metastases when there are no effective systemic therapies, no extrapulmonary metastases, the pulmonary metastasis is completely resectable, and the patient is able to undergo surgery.[29] Specific cancers for which surgical resection of pulmonary metastases is considered include soft-tissue sarcoma, osteosarcoma, and sometimes breast cancer.


1. The Royal College of Radiologists Clinical Oncology Information Network. Guidelines on the non-surgical management of lung cancer. *Clin Oncol* 1999; **11:** S1–S53.
2. Hoffman PC, *et al.* Lung cancer. *Lancet* 2000; **355:** 479–85.
3. Adjei AA, *et al.* Current guidelines for the management of small cell lung cancer. *Mayo Clin Proc* 1999; **74:** 809–16.
4. Sandler AB. Chemotherapy for small cell lung cancer. *Semin Oncol* 2003; **30:** 9–25.
5. Pignon JP, *et al.* A meta-analysis of thoracic radiotherapy for small cell lung cancer. *N Engl J Med* 1992; **327:** 1618–24.
6. Price A. Lung cancer 5: state of the art radiotherapy for lung cancer. *Thorax* 2003; **58:** 447–52.
7. Okuno SH, Jett JR. Small cell lung cancer: current therapy and promising new regimens. *Oncologist* 2002; **7:** 234–8.
8. Noda K, *et al.* Irinotecan plus cisplatin compared with etoposide plus cisplatin for extensive small-cell lung cancer. *N Engl J Med* 2002; **346:** 85–91.
9. The Prophylactic Cranial Irradiation Overview Collaborative Group. Cranial irradiation for preventing brain metastases of small cell lung cancer in patients in complete remission. Available in The Cochrane Library; Issue 2. Chichester: John Wiley; 2004.
10. Bastin KT, Curley R. Non-small-cell lung carcinoma: current and future therapeutic management. *Drugs* 1995; **49:** 362–75.
11. PORT Meta-analysis Trialists Group. Postoperative radiotherapy in non-small-cell lung cancer: systematic review and meta-analysis of individual patient data from nine randomised controlled trials. *Lancet* 1998; **352:** 257–63.
12. Non-small Cell Lung Cancer Collaborative Group. Chemotherapy for non-small cell lung cancer. Available in The Cochrane Library; Issue 2. Chichester: John Wiley; 2004.
13. McCarthy M. Scientists report progress against non-small cell lung cancer. *Lancet* 2003; **361:** 2055.
14. Pritchard RS, Anthony SP. Chemotherapy plus radiotherapy compared with radiotherapy alone in the treatment of locally advanced, unresectable, non-small-cell lung cancer: a meta-analysis. *Ann Intern Med* 1996; **125:** 723–9. Correction. *ibid.* 1997; **126:** 670.
15. Marino P, *et al.* Randomized trials of radiotherapy alone versus combined chemotherapy and radiotherapy in stages IIIa and IIIb nonsmall cell lung cancer. *Cancer* 1995; **76:** 593–601.
16. Movsas B. Innovative treatment strategies in locally advanced and/or unresectable non-small cell lung cancer. *Cancer Control* 2000; **7:** 25–34.
17. Cullen M. Lung cancer 4: chemotherapy for non-small cell lung cancer: the end of the beginning. *Thorax* 2003; **58:** 352–6.
18. Edelman MJ. Neoadjuvant chemotherapy and chemoradiotherapy for non-small cell lung cancer: current status and future prospects. *Expert Opin Pharmacother* 2003; **4:** 843–52.
19. Souquet PJ, *et al.* Polychemotherapy in advanced non small cell lung cancer: a meta-analysis. *Lancet* 1993; **342:** 19–21.
20. Lilenbaum RC, *et al.* Single agent versus combination chemotherapy in patients with advanced nonsmall cell lung carcinoma: a meta-analysis of response, toxicity, and survival. *Cancer* 1998; **82:** 116–26.
21. Schiller JH, *et al.* Comparison of four chemotherapy regimens for advanced non-small-cell lung cancer. *N Engl J Med* 2002; **346:** 92–8.
22. Pfister DG, *et al.* American Society of Clinical Oncology treatment of unresectable non—small-cell lung cancer guideline: update 2003. *J Clin Oncol* 2004; **22:** 330–53.
23. National Institute for Clinical Excellence. Guidance on the use of docetaxel, paclitaxel, gemcitabine and vinorelbine for the treatment of non-small cell lung cancer (issued June 2001, reviewed May 2003). Available at: http://www.nice.org.uk/pdf/lungcancerguidance.pdf (accessed 28/06/04)
24. Sheski FD, Mathur PN. Endoscopic treatment of early-stage lung cancer. *Cancer Control* 2000; **7:** 35–44.
25. Carney DN. Lung cancer—time to move on from chemotherapy. *N Engl J Med* 2002; **346:** 126–8.
26. Goodman GE. Lung cancer 1: prevention of lung cancer. *Thorax* 2002; **57:** 994–9.
27. Manser RL, *et al.* Screening for lung cancer. Available in The Cochrane Library; Issue 2. Chichester: John Wiley; 2004.
28. Henschke CI, *et al.* Early Lung Cancer Action Project: overall design and findings from baseline screening. *Lancet* 1999; **354:** 99–105.
29. Downey RJ. Surgical treatment of pulmonary metastases. *Surg Oncol Clin N Am* 1999; **8:** 341–54.


MALIGNANT MESOTHELIOMA. Malignant mesothelioma is a relatively rare tumour of the lining of the lung, yet its incidence is increasing. Occupational exposure to asbestos is the causative factor in most cases, with a mean latent interval of about 40 years between first exposure and death. Typical clinical manifestations include chest pain or dyspnoea or both. Neurological entrapment and pericardial involvement may occur. The disease is progressive, and median survival is poor. Histologically, disease may be epithelioid, sarcomatoid, or a mixture of the two. The epithelioid type is the most common, and may be confused with adenocarcinoma (see non-small cell lung cancer, above). In patients with small epithelioid tumours, radical surgery may be considered, but otherwise is seldom appropriate. Pleurodesis is usually the treatment of choice in the management of pleural effusions associated with mesothelioma; pleurectomy is an alternative. Palliative radiotherapy may be effective for pain relief.[1]

Responses to single-agent chemotherapy have been in the region of 10 to 20%. Doxorubicin, epirubicin, mitomycin, cyclophosphamide, ifosfamide, cisplatin, and carboplatin have all been tried.[1,2] Irinotecan, topotecan, gemcitabine, vinorelbine, docetaxel, and paclitaxel have also been investigated.[2] Combination chemotherapy, mostly with doxorubicin- or cisplatin-based regimens, have not shown any survival advantage over single-agent therapy.[2] However, encouraging results have been obtained in a large phase 3 study using pemetrexed and cisplatin, and some suggest this combination should be standard first-line therapy.[2,3] Other regimens, including vinorelbine compared with mitomycin, vinblastine, and cisplatin (MVP),[3] and raltitrexed with oxaliplatin[2] are being investigated.


1. British Thoracic Society Standards of Care Committee. Statement on malignant mesothelioma in the United Kingdom. *Thorax* 2001; **56:** 250–65. Correction. *ibid.*; 820.
2. Tomek S, *et al.* Chemotherapy for malignant pleural mesothelioma: past results and recent developments. *Br J Cancer* 2003; **88:** 167–74.
3. Steele JPC. The new front line treatment for malignant pleural mesothelioma? *Thorax* 2003; **58:** 96–7.


**Malignant neoplasms of the ovary.** Ovarian cancers account for about 5% of all malignancies in women. The most common form (90% of cases) is **epithelial ovarian cancer**, which ranks as fourth in the leading causes of cancer deaths in women. The lethality of this disease is related to the absence of symptoms in the majority of women during its early stages: in about three-quarters of all patients disease is advanced at diagnosis and has spread to the peritoneum or beyond. It is predominantly a disease of older women, the median age at diagnosis being 61 years. The risk of epithelial ovarian cancer appears to be related to the number of ovulatory cycles a women has in her lifetime, thus nulliparity increases the risk, whereas multiparity, breast feeding, and combined oral contraceptives (p.1529) decrease the risk. Other risk factors are a family history (particularly when associated with the BRCA1 gene), and possibly fertility drugs (see Clomifene, p.1542), perineal talc use (p.1159), and menopausal HRT (p.1538).

The primary treatment for epithelial ovarian cancer in the majority of patients is surgical removal of womb, ovaries and fallopian tubes, and omentum, together with debulking of any remaining gross disease.[1-3] The use of adjuvant chemotherapy depends on disease stage.

The minority of patients who have localised disease at diagnosis have a good prognosis. Patients with well differentiated early disease (stage IA) have a 5-year disease-free survival of at least 90%; adjuvant therapy has not been shown to improve survival in this group,[4] and conservative fertility-sparing surgery is possible at this stage in women of child-bearing age.[2,3] In those subgroups with poorly differentiated or more extensive localised disease (stage IC and II) postoperative platinum-based chemotherapy has been reported to improve both recurrence-free and overall survival at 5 years,[5] and is usually considered appropriate.[2,3] Adjuvant intraperitoneal phosphorus-32 and oral melphalan have also been used.

Prognosis is less good in patients with advanced disease (stage III and IV), who presently form the majority at diagnosis. Patients with extra-pelvic disease or positive nodes who have only minimal residual disease after surgery have a 5-year survival rate of less than 30% but in patients with distant metastases or suboptimal debulking there is a less than 10% chance of long-term survival. Many adjuvant regimens have been tried in advanced ovarian cancer, often based on platinum derivatives, alkylating agents, and sometimes also anthracyclines. Cisplatin or carboplatin with cyclophosphamide (CP) and sometimes doxorubicin (CAP) have been widely used. In 1991, a meta-analysis[6] failed to reach any definite conclusions about the relative benefits of differing chemotherapeutic regimens, but did suggest that immediate treatment was better than delaying until relapse, that platinum-based regimens were probably better than those without a platinum derivative, that combination regimens were better than single-agent platinum where the doses were equivalent, and that carboplatin was as effective as cisplatin. A subsequent updated analysis[7] by the same group reached similar conclusions. Two similar analyses in 1991 and 1992 suggested that regimens of cisplatin, doxorubicin, and cyclophosphamide offered a survival advantage over cisplatin with cyclophosphamide alone.[8,9] Subsequent to these analyses, a large randomised study (ICON2) was instigated to compare carboplatin alone with cyclophosphamide, doxorubicin and cisplatin. This study[10] found no difference in progression-free or overall survival (median 33 months) between the 2 treatment arms, and single-agent carboplatin was less toxic. In the early 1990's, the finding of significant activity for paclitaxel in ovarian cancer led to various studies incorporating this drug. Two studies[11,12] comparing cisplatin plus cyclophosphamide with cisplatin plus paclitaxel found improved overall survival for the paclitaxel-containing arm (median 38 and 36 months versus 24 and 26 months). Substitution of carboplatin for cisplatin resulted in similar overall survival,[13] and subsequently a number of reviews and guidelines have recommended paclitaxel plus cisplatin or carboplatin as the first-line adjuvant treatment of ovarian cancer.[1-3] Conversely, another study[14] found cisplatin alone (100 mg/m$^2$) to be no different to cisplatin (75 mg/m$^2$) plus paclitaxel (135 mg/m$^2$) in terms of overall survival (median 30 versus 26 months) and progression-free survival, although cisplatin alone was poorly tolerated. This study also contained a single-agent paclitaxel arm (200 mg/m$^2$), which had poorer progression-free survival, but similar overall survival (26 months) to the other arms. Results of a further study (ICON3)[15] also failed to demonstrate an improvement in progression-free or overall survival for carboplatin plus paclitaxel (median 17 and 36 months) compared with carboplatin alone or cisplatin-based CAP (median 16 and 35 months); single-agent carboplatin had a more favourable toxicity profile. Subsequent guidelines[16] have recommended that platinum-based therapy alone or with paclitaxel are both reasonable options for first-line adjuvant therapy.

Investigational therapies in the adjuvant setting include interval surgical debulking in those with suboptimal debulking at primary surgery,[3] and intraperitoneal chemotherapy in those with minimal residual disease after primary surgery.[3,13]

In patients with recurrent disease, the choice of therapy depends on the time since initial therapy and the drugs used.[3,17] Relapse occurring more than 6 months after initial therapy is potentially platinum-sensitive and may be re-treated with the initial therapy. In patients who are potentially not sensitive to platinum derivatives, paclitaxel may be used if it was not used previously. Combining paclitaxel with platinum chemotherapy may further improve survival in patients who are platinum-sensitive.[18] Other drugs with second-line activity include topotecan,[19] liposomal doxorubicin,[20] and altretamine. Investigational agents include gemcitabine, oral etoposide, ifosfamide, and tamoxifen,[17] and the monoclonal antibodies oregovomab and pemtumomab. Some success has been reported using high-dose chemotherapy followed by autologous stem cell transplantation.[21]

PROPHYLAXIS. The identification of genes conferring an inherited predisposition to ovarian cancer, and the difficulty in identifying the disease and its poor prognosis has led to increased interest in prevention. Oral contraceptives are known to be protective in the general population, but there is conflicting evidence as to whether they are protective in carriers of the BRCA1 gene.[22,23] Prophylactic oophorectomy may be considered in women with BRCA1 mutations after child-bearing or at age 35 years.[24,25] The risk/benefit ratio of this procedure is not known, and a few women who undergo this procedure subsequently develop a primary peritoneal cancer.

**Ovarian germ-cell cancers** account for less than 3% of ovarian cancers and typically occur in women aged 20 to 30 years. Unlike epithelial ovarian cancer, most patients present with early disease, and even in advanced disease, combination chemotherapy can be curative.[26] Conservative fertility-sparing surgery is the primary therapy. Adjuvant chemotherapy is used except in those with stage I disease able to undergo frequent follow-up. Commonly used regimens are similar to those used in male germ-cell tumours such as bleomycin, etoposide, and cisplatin (BEP) or vinblastine, bleomycin, and cisplatin (VBP).[26]


1. Society of Gynecologic Oncologists. Practice guidelines: ovarian cancer. *Oncology (Huntingt)* 1998; **12:** 129–33.
2. American College of Obstetricians and Gynecologists. ACOG educational bulletin: ovarian cancer. *Int J Gynaecol Obstet* 1998; **63:** 301–10.
3. Gibbs DD, Gore ME. Pursuit of optimum outcomes in ovarian cancer: methodological approaches to therapy. *Drugs* 2001; **61:** 1103–20.
4. Young RC. Early-stage ovarian cancer: to treat or not to treat. *J Natl Cancer Inst* 2003; **95:** 94–5.
5. International Collaborative Ovarian Neoplasm 1 (ICON1) and European Organisation for Research and Treatment of Cancer Collaborators-Adjuvant ChemoTherapy in Ovarian Neoplasm (EORTC-ACTION). International collaborative ovarian neoplasm trial 1 and adjuvant chemotherapy in ovarian neoplasm trial: two parallel randomized phase III trials of adjuvant chemotherapy in patients with early-stage ovarian carcinoma. *J Natl Cancer Inst* 2003; **95:** 105–12.
6. Advanced Ovarian Cancer Trialists Group. Chemotherapy in advanced ovarian cancer: an overview of randomised clinical trials. *BMJ* 1991; **303:** 884–93.
7. Advanced Ovarian Cancer Trialists Group. Chemotherapy for advanced ovarian cancer. Available in The Cochrane Library; Issue 2. Chichester: John Wiley; 2004.
8. Fanning J, *et al.* Meta-analysis of cisplatin, doxorubicin, and cyclophosphamide versus cisplatin and cyclophosphamide chemotherapy of ovarian carcinoma. *Obstet Gynecol* 1992; **80:** 954–60.
9. Ovarian Cancer Meta-analysis Project. Cyclophosphamide plus cisplatin versus cyclophosphamide, doxorubicin, and cisplatin chemotherapy of ovarian carcinoma: a meta-analysis. *J Clin Oncol* 1991; **9:** 1668–74.
10. The ICON Collaborators. ICON2: randomised trial of single-agent carboplatin against three-drug combination of CAP (cyclophosphamide, doxorubicin, and cisplatin) in women with ovarian cancer. *Lancet* 1998; **352:** 1571–76.
11. McGuire WP, *et al.* Cyclophosphamide and cisplatin compared with paclitaxel and cisplatin in patients with stage III and stage IV ovarian cancer. *N Engl J Med* 1996; **334:** 1–6.
12. Piccart MJ, *et al.* Randomized intergroup trial of cisplatin-paclitaxel versus cisplatin-cyclophosphamide in women with advanced epithelial ovarian cancer: three-year results. *J Natl Cancer Inst* 2000; **92:** 699–708.
13. Herrin VE, Thigpen JT. Chemotherapy for ovarian cancer: current concepts. *Semin Surg Oncol* 1999; **17:** 181–8.
14. Muggia FM, *et al.* Phase III randomized study of cisplatin versus paclitaxel versus cisplatin and paclitaxel in patients with suboptimal stage III or IV ovarian cancer: a Gynecologic Oncology Group study. *J Clin Oncol* 2000; **18:** 106–115.
15. The International Collaborative Ovarian Neoplasms (ICON) Group. Paclitaxel plus carboplatin versus standard chemotherapy with either single-agent carboplatin or cyclophosphamide, doxorubicin, and cisplatin in women with ovarian cancer: the ICON3 randomised trial. *Lancet* 2002; **360:** 505–15. Correction. *ibid.* 2003; **361:** 706.
16. National Institute for Clinical Excellence. Guidance on the use of paclitaxel in the treatment of ovarian cancer (issued January 2003). Available at: http://www.nice.org.uk/pdf/55_Paclitaxel_ovarianreviewfullguidance.pdf (accessed 28/06/04)
17. Markman M, Bookman MA. Second-line treatment of ovarian cancer. *Oncologist* 2000; **5:** 26–35.
18. The ICON and AGO collaborators. Paclitaxel plus platinum-based chemotherapy versus conventional platinum-based chemotherapy in women with relapsed ovarian cancer: the ICON4/AGO-OVAR-2.2 trial. *Lancet* 2003; **361:** 2099–2106.
19. National Institute for Clinical Excellence. Guidance on the use of topotecan for the treatment of advanced ovarian cancer (issued August 2001). Available at: http://www.nice.org.uk/pdf/topotecanguidance.pdf (accessed 28/06/04)
20. National Institute for Clinical Excellence. Guidance on the use of pegylated liposomal doxorubicin hydrochloride (PLDH) for the treatment of advanced ovarian cancer (issued July 2002). Available at: http://www.nice.org.uk/pdf/Fullguidance-PDF-ovariancancer.pdf (accessed 28/06/04)
21. Stiff PJ, *et al.* High-dose chemotherapy and autologous stem-cell transplantation for ovarian cancer: an autologous blood and marrow transplant registry report. *Ann Intern Med* 2000; **133:** 504–15.
22. Narod SA, *et al.* Oral contraceptives and the risk of hereditary ovarian cancer. *N Engl J Med* 1998; **339:** 424–8.
23. Modan B, *et al.* Parity, oral contraceptives, and the risk of ovarian cancer among carriers and noncarriers of a BRCA1 or BRCA2 mutation. *N Engl J Med* 2001; **345:** 235–40.
24. Burke W, *et al.* Recommendations for follow-up care of individuals with an inherited predisposition to cancer: BRCA1 and BRCA2. *JAMA* 1997; **277:** 997–1003.
25. Eisinger F, *et al.* Recommendations for medical management of hereditary breast and ovarian cancer: the French National Ad Hoc Committee. *Ann Oncol* 1998; **9:** 939–50.
26. Bridgewater JA, Rustin GJS. Management of non-epithelial ovarian tumours. *Oncology* 1999; **57:** 89–98.


**Malignant neoplasms of the pancreas.** Pancreatic adenocarcinoma (cancer of the exocrine pancreas) accounts for about 95% of pancreatic tumours. A very small percentage of pancreatic tumours arise in the endocrine pancreas, and have different clinical features and treatment (see under Carcinoid Tumours and Other Secretory Neoplasms, above). Although rare below the age of 30 the incidence of pancreatic adenocarcinoma rises steadily with age; overall, it accounts for about 3% of all cancers, but is the fifth leading cause of cancer deaths. Pancreatic adenocarcinoma is ductal in origin and metastasises early to the lymph nodes, and by the time of diagnosis more than half of all patients have liver metastases, more than a quarter have peritoneal seeding, and a third have invasion of the duodenum causing ulceration. The most frequent symptom at presentation in patients with cancer of the pancreatic head is jaundice, often with other symptoms indicative of obstruction of the bile duct. In lesions of the body and tail of the pancreas severe and relentless pain may develop. Diabetes mellitus is a manifestation of the disease, but there is also some evidence that it may be a predisposing factor. About 30% of pancreatic cancers are probably due to tobacco smoking.

Pancreatic adenocarcinoma has a very poor prognosis because of its usually advanced stage at diagnosis and lack of effective therapies.[1-3] Apart from a small number of patients with resectable carcinoma of the head of the pancreas, in whom radical surgery results in a 5-year survival of about 10 to 20% most patients with pancreatic adenocarcinoma will be dead within 1 year. Adjuvant therapy with irradiation and fluorouracil has been used in those with resectable disease,[1-3] based on early evidence[4] that it optimised the chance for long-term survival. However, a systematic review[5] concluded that there was no convincing evidence of benefit from adjuvant chemotherapy, with or without radiotherapy. The preliminary results of a further large randomised study[6] also suggest that there is no benefit from adjuvant fluorouracil-based chemoradiotherapy but that there may be a survival benefit from chemotherapy alone. In patients with symptomatic localised unresectable disease, palliative radiotherapy alone or combined with chemotherapy may be used. There is interest in neoadjuvant chemoradiotherapy to improve resectability rates in locally advanced disease, but this remains investigational.[2,4] In patients with advanced (metastatic) disease, supportive care alone remains appropriate. Palliative chemotherapy may be considered, but benefits are modest (pancreatic adenocarcinoma is a chemoresistant tumour).[1-3,5,7] Single-agent fluorouracil has been most extensively used. Combination regimens, such as FAM (fluorouracil, doxorubicin, mitomycin) SMF (streptozocin, mitomycin, fluorouracil), and FAP (fluorouracil, doxorubicin, cisplatin), have not proved more effective than fluorouracil alone.[2,5] More recently, gemcitabine improved survival over fluorouracil by 5 weeks but with more adverse events.[8] It may be used instead of fluorouracil, and is being studied in a number of combination regimens.[7] Rubitecan is one of many other antineoplastics under investigation for advanced pancreatic cancer,[7] and various other therapies being investigated include somatostatin analogues, other hormonal strategies, and biological therapies.[9] A preliminary study suggested that flutamide (an anti-androgen) might be beneficial[10] but flutamide with gemcitabine proved of no more benefit than gemcitabine alone.[11]


1. Rosewicz S, Wiedenmann B. Pancreatic carcinoma. *Lancet* 1997; **349:** 485–9.
2. Sporn JR. Practical recommendations for the management of adenocarcinoma of the pancreas. *Drugs* 1999; **57:** 69–79.
3. DiMagno EP, *et al.* American Gastroenterological Association medical position statement: epidemiology, diagnosis, and treatment of pancreatic ductal adenocarcinoma. *Gastroenterology* 1999; **117:** 1463–84.
4. Ghaneh P, *et al.* Adjuvant therapy for pancreatic cancer. *World J Surg* 1999; **23:** 937–45.
5. Permert J, *et al.* A systematic overview of chemotherapy effects in pancreatic cancer. *Acta Oncol* 2001; **40:** 361–70.
6. Neoptolemos JP, *et al.* Adjuvant chemoradiotherapy and chemotherapy in resectable pancreatic cancer: a randomised controlled trial. *Lancet* 2001; **358:** 1576–85.
7. El Kamar FG, *et al.* Metastatic pancreatic cancer: emerging strategies in chemotherapy and palliative care. *Oncologist* 2003; **8:** 18–34.
8. Burris HA, *et al.* Improvements in survival and clinical benefit with gemcitabine as first-line therapy for patients with advanced pancreas cancer: a randomized trial. *J Clin Oncol* 1997; **15:** 2403–13.
9. Rosenberg L. Pancreatic cancer: a review of emerging therapies. *Drugs* 2000; **59:** 1071–89.
10. Greenway BA. Effect of flutamide on survival in patients with pancreatic cancer: results of a prospective, randomised, double blind, placebo controlled trial. *BMJ* 1998; **316:** 1935–8.
11. Corrie P, *et al.* Phase II study to evaluate combining gemcitabine with flutamide in advanced pancreatic cancer patients. *Br J Cancer* 2002; **87:** 716–19.


**Malignant neoplasms of the prostate.** Prostatic cancer is the most commonly diagnosed non-skin malignancy in men in the western world, and the second most common cause of cancer deaths in men: about one in 6 men can be expected to develop clinically evident carcinoma of the prostate during his lifetime. The incidence rises steadily with age. More than 95% of all prostate cancer is adenocarcinoma, which begins as a hard mass in the peripheral portion of the gland and infiltrates surrounding tissues slowly. Metastasis may occur in advanced disease, notably to bone. Presenting symptoms of advanced disease are usually those of urinary outflow obstruction, or pelvic or back pain due to bone metastases. However, as a result of the slow rate of tumour growth and usually advanced age at diagnosis, many patients die of other illnesses without having suffered significant disability from the cancer.

Controversy exists regarding all aspects of the management of prostate cancer, from screening to the best treatment for each stage of the disease. Much of this is because of the lack of clear data to guide treatment decisions. Factors that guide treatment decisions include the extent (stage) of the tumour, tumour grade (Gleason score), the patient's life expectancy (based on age and comorbid conditions), and patient preference.[1-4]

There is great controversy over the value of **screening** for early disease by detection of prostate specific antigen (PSA), and other tests, because of the uncertainties regarding interpretation of the test results, and controversy over the management of asymptomatic early localised disease.[5-7] Screening studies are currently underway.

In patients with **localised disease**, detected incidentally or by screening, the choices are radical prostatectomy, radical external beam radiotherapy, brachytherapy, or deferred treatment (watchful waiting). There is currently no evidence to suggest one form of therapy is more effective than another, except perhaps for poorly differentiated tumours, which have a faster rate of progression and may benefit from earlier therapy.[4] Because of the lack of differences in efficacy, treatment morbidity and patient preferences are particularly important. Adverse effects of surgery include impotence and incontinence, and for radiotherapy, radiation proctitis, impotence and incontinence, and these complications may be severe in up to 5% of patients.[4] In medically fit patients with a life expectancy of 10 years or more many clinicians would consider radical prostatectomy or radiotherapy with curative intent,[1,4,8] although it should be noted that these patients are the ones for whom treatment complications are likely to have the most impact on quality of life.[4] In men with a life expectancy of less than 10 years and with low-grade tumours, there is a definite role for deferring treatment.[1,4,8] Interstitial implantation of radioisotopes (brachytherapy) is an alternative to external beam radiotherapy; a more localised dose is possible but inadequate dose distribution can occur and some patients may also need adjuvant external beam radiotherapy.[8] Cryosurgery, and ultrasound or radiofrequency interstitial tumour ablation are other options for localised disease, but are less well investigated.[8] In patients who undergo radical surgery and who are found to have positive margins, adjuvant radiotherapy or hormonal therapy may be used. Neoadjuvant hormonal therapy has been used before radiotherapy, but its role in early disease remains to be established. Hormonal therapy has also been used alone when there is a risk of disease progression but local therapy is not deemed necessary.[8]

For patients with **locally advanced disease**, options include radiotherapy with or without neoadjuvant or adjuvant hormonal therapy, hormonal treatment alone, or, in those who are asymptomatic, deferred treatment.[1,4,9] Although radiotherapy alone produces good local control, most patients eventually develop metastatic disease. There is increasing evidence that the use of hormonal therapy before or after radiotherapy improves disease-free and overall survival.[9,10] Deferred treatment was less effective than immediate treatment in one study,[11] but the form of follow-up for deferred treatment was not regulated. In patients for whom deferred treatment is considered, close surveillance is required. Surgery alone is rarely used in locally advanced disease[1] but there is some evidence to suggest that adjuvant hormonal therapy may delay disease progression, and neoadjuvant hormonal therapy is under investigation.[9]

PSA may be used to monitor the efficacy of therapy and detect biochemical relapse, but the interpretation of the test and when to instigate further treatment in patients with no clinical evidence of disease is controversial.[9,12]

For patients with **metastatic disease** cure is not possible and therapy is aimed at prolonging survival and palliating symptoms. The basis of therapy is hormonal manipulation: about 80% of patients will respond to such therapy, but resistance eventually develops. The first choice is between orchidectomy or a gonadorelin analogue, which have been shown to be equally effective.[4,13]

An alternative to orchidectomy or gonadorelin analogues is the use of an anti-androgen (such as flutamide, nilutamide, or bicalutamide) alone. However, there is some evidence that these may be less effective and cause more treatment withdrawals (due to gastrointestinal intolerance),[13] although they may have less adverse effect on libido. Although historically oestrogens such as diethylstilbestrol have been used in patients with prostate cancer they are now less favoured because of their cardiovascular adverse effects.

The combined use of anti-androgens such as flutamide with ablation of testicular androgen production (by surgery or gonadorelin analogues) has the advantage of blocking the effects of adrenal androgen production as well (maximal or complete androgen blockade). An early meta-analysis[14] seemed to indicate that this approach did not produce a better survival rate compared with conventional castration, and an update of this meta-analysis[15] confirmed that any survival advantage from maximum androgen blockade using nonsteroidal anti-androgens was likely to be in the region of 3%.

In patients who relapse after or during hormonal therapy, second-line hormonal therapy may be tried, although responses are variable. Drugs that have been used include aminoglutethimide, high-dose bicalutamide, corticosteroids, ketoconazole, and megestrol.[12] Some patients treated with anti-androgens experience a paradoxical response to withdrawal of the drug, but it is not possible to predict which patients will respond. Gonadorelin analogue therapy must be continued, to maintain testosterone suppression.[16]

Chemotherapy for recurrent hormone-refractory prostate cancer is still undergoing clinical trials and has no routine place in therapy. Some patients with soft-tissue disease may benefit from an anthracycline.[4] Mitoxantrone has a palliative benefit and improves quality of life, but does not prolong survival. Single-agent taxane therapy has shown some promise, and docetaxel plus prednisone may improve survival. Combinations of estramustine with docetaxel, etoposide, vinblastine, or vinorelbine have also shown favourable results.[12,17]

Preliminary results have indicated that a herbal combination preparation, PC-SPES, may have beneficial effects in both androgen-dependent and androgen-independent disease. It has been used widely as a complementary medicine, but there have been reports of adverse cardiovascular effects and contamination with diethylstilbestrol and warfarin, resulting in the withdrawal of this product from most markets.[18] Although suramin originally showed promise, later results were less favourable, and it appears its development has been discontinued. Bone metastases are usually treated with palliative radiotherapy (see p.513). Bone-targeted therapy with strontium-89 has been tried,[17,19] and gene therapy is under investigation.[20] Prostate cancer growth is thought to be stimulated by endothelin-1, a small peptide that acts at endothelin-A receptors; atrasentan is an endothelin-A receptor antagonist under investigation, and early studies have shown improvements in time to disease progression and markers of bone metastases.[17]

Because of the difficulties involved in managing prostate cancer there has been interest in the concept of disease **prophylaxis**. One small study of finasteride in men at high risk of prostate cancer showed little evidence to support such use.[21] In healthy men, a large controlled trial[22] found that seven years of finasteride prophylaxis reduced the incidence of prostate cancer by about 25% compared with placebo, but this benefit was offset by an increased risk of high-grade tumours associated with finasteride. There is preliminary evidence that selenium (see p.1444) or vitamin E (see p.1420) supplementation may reduce the risk of prostate cancer, and a large randomised study is underway to further investigate this.


1. Frydenberg M, *et al.* Prostate cancer diagnosis and management. *Lancet* 1997; **349:** 1681–7.
2. Rosenthal MA. Management of metastatic prostate cancer. *Med J Aust* 1998; **169:** 46–50.
3. Moffat LEF. Therapeutic choices in prostate cancer. *Prescribers' J* 1999; **39:** 16–23.
4. The Royal College of Radiologists' Clinical Oncology Information Network and British Association of Urological Surgeons. Guidelines on the management of prostate cancer. *Clin Oncol* 1999; **11:** S53–S88.
5. US Preventive Services Task Force. Screening for prostate cancer: recommendation and rationale. *Ann Intern Med* 2002; **137:** 915–6.
6. Harris R, Lohr KN. Screening for prostate cancer: an update of the evidence for the US Preventive Services Task Force. *Ann Intern Med* 2002; **137:** 917–29.
7. Frankel S, *et al.* Screening for prostate cancer. *Lancet* 2003; **361:** 1122–8.
8. Jani AB, Hellman S. Early prostate cancer: clinical decision-making. *Lancet* 2003; **361:** 1045–53.
9. Boccon-Gibod L, *et al.* Management of locally advanced prostate cancer: a European consensus. *Int J Clin Pract* 2003; **57:** 187–94.
10. Vicini FA, *et al.* The role of androgen deprivation in the definitive management of clinically localized prostate cancer treated with radiation therapy. *Int J Radiat Oncol Biol Phys* 1999; **43:** 707–13.
11. Medical Research Council Prostate Cancer Working Party Investigators Group. Immediate versus deferred treatment for advanced prostatic cancer: initial results of the Medical Research Council Trial. *Br J Urol* 1997; **79:** 235–46.
12. Harris KA, Reese DM. Treatment options in hormone-refractory prostate cancer: current and future approaches. *Drugs* 2001; **61:** 2177–92.
13. Seidenfeld J, *et al.* Single-therapy androgen suppression in men with advanced prostate cancer: a systematic review and meta-analysis. *Ann Intern Med* 2000; **132:** 566–77.
14. Prostate Cancer Trialists' Collaborative Group. Maximum androgen blockade in advanced prostate cancer: an overview of 22 randomised trials with 3283 deaths in 5710 patients. *Lancet* 1995; **346:** 265–9.
15. Prostate Cancer Trialists' Collaborative Group. Maximum androgen blockade in advanced prostate cancer: an overview of the randomised trials. *Lancet* 2000; **355:** 1491–8.
16. Paul R, Breul J. Antiandrogen withdrawal syndrome associated with prostate cancer therapies: incidence and clinical significance. *Drug Safety* 2000; **23:** 381–90.
17. Rosenbaum E, Carducci MA. Pharmacotherapy of hormone refractory prostate cancer: new developments and challenges. *Expert Opin Pharmacother* 2003; **4:** 875–87.
18. de Lemos ML. Herbal supplement PC-Spes for prostate cancer. *Ann Pharmacother* 2002; **36:** 921–6.
19. Tu S-M, *et al.* Bone-targeted therapy for advanced androgen-independent carcinoma of the prostate: a randomised phase II trial. *Lancet* 2001; **357:** 336–41. Correction. *ibid.*; 1210.
20. Harrington KJ, *et al.* Gene therapy for prostate cancer: current status and future prospects. *J Urol (Baltimore)* 2001; **166:** 1220–33.
21. Cote RJ, *et al.* The effect of finasteride on the prostate gland in men with elevated serum prostate-specific antigen levels. *Br J Cancer* 1998; **78:** 413–18.
22. Thompson IM, *et al.* The influence of finasteride on the development of prostate cancer. *N Engl J Med* 2003; **349:** 215–24.


**Malignant neoplasms of the skin.** Basal cell carcinoma is the most common form of skin cancer, accounting for about 80% of cases. The second most common skin cancer is squamous cell carcinoma. These 2 types of carcinoma (collectively referred to as nonmelanoma skin cancers) are the most common malignancies among white populations, but because many are not recorded the exact incidence is uncertain and they are often omitted from calculations of the relative frequency of malignancy. A small but increasing proportion of all skin cancers are melanomas, arising from melanocytes (pigment cells). Other cancers that manifest in the skin include cutaneous T-cell lymphomas (see Mycosis Fungoides, above) and Kaposi's sarcoma (see below).

Nonmelanoma and melanoma skin cancers are related to solar radiation, and the incidence is greatest in those regions where light-skinned populations live closest to the equator. Individuals at particular risk include those with fair skin, blue eyes, red hair, a tendency to freckle, and to burn rather than tan. Use of methoxsalen with ultraviolet light (PUVA) has also been associated with an increased incidence of skin cancers (see p.1152). Other risk factors for nonmelanoma skin cancers include various inherited disorders such as xeroderma pigmentosum and albinism. Immunosuppressive therapy, as used after solid organ transplantation, is associated with a very large increase in risk of squamous cell carcinoma.

PROPHYLAXIS. Although nonmelanoma and melanoma skin cancers are related to solar radiation, and measures to reduce sun exposure are therefore advocated for prophylaxis, the relationship appears to differ between the types.

- Squamous cell carcinoma and its precursor lesions are clearly linked to cumulative chronic sun exposure.[1,2] These lesions are more common on frequently exposed skin (head, neck, and back of hands), and are more common in individuals with outdoor occupations. In addition, there is evidence that regular sunscreen use can reduce the incidence of new actinic keratoses and increase remission of existing lesions,[3] and reduce incident squamous cell carcinomas.[4]
- Although basal cell carcinomas are also common on sun-exposed skin (head and neck), it appears that they may be more related to a history of severe sunburns, particularly in childhood and adolescence, rather than to cumulative sun exposure.[1] In 1 study,[4] there was no difference in incidence of basal cell carcinomas between sunscreen users and non-users.
- Cutaneous melanoma is more common on skin exposed to the sun occasionally (particularly the legs in women, and the back in men), and appears to be more common in indoor than outdoor workers. This suggests that intermittent sun exposure may be more risky than regular exposure for this cancer.[1,2,5] In addition, preliminary evidence suggests that spending more time in the sun could offset any protective effect of sunscreens.[5]

In addition to sun protection measures, chemoprevention has been investigated as a means of reducing the incidence of squamous and basal cell cancers, particularly in those most at risk. Retinoids such as acitretin, etretinate, and isotretinoin have been shown to reduce the incidence of new squamous cell carcinomas in individuals with xeroderma pigmentosum, and in renal transplant recipients.[6] Conversely, neither betacarotene (p.1420) nor selenium (p.1444) has reduced the incidence of squamous or basal cell carcinomas in patients previously treated for these disorders. There is some evidence that a low-fat diet may reduce the incidence of actinic keratosis in patients with a history of nonmelanoma skin cancer.[7]


1. Anonymous. Do sunscreens prevent skin cancer? *Drug Ther Bull* 1998; **36:** 49–51.
2. Bruce AJ, Brodland DG. Overview of skin cancer detection and prevention for the primary care physician. *Mayo Clin Proc* 2000; **75:** 491–500.
3. Thompson SC, *et al.* Reduction of solar keratoses by regular sunscreen use. *N Engl J Med* 1993; **329:** 1147–51.
4. Green A, *et al.* Daily sunscreen application and betacarotene supplementation in prevention of basal-cell and squamous-cell carcinomas of the skin: a randomised controlled trial. *Lancet* 1999; **354:** 723–9.
5. Finkel E. Sorting the hype from the facts in melanoma. *Lancet* 1998; **351:** 1866.
6. DiGiovanna JJ. Retinoid chemoprevention in patients at high risk for skin cancer. *Med Pediatr Oncol* 2001; **36:** 564–7.
7. Black HS, *et al.* Effect of a low-fat diet on the incidence of actinic keratosis. *N Engl J Med* 1994; **330:** 1272–5.


BASAL CELL AND SQUAMOUS CELL CARCINOMA. The great majority of skin cancers are basal cell carcinomas, which are completely curable if diagnosed early and treated appropriately. Although they rarely metastasise, they have a tendency to be locally destructive. The remainder are mainly squamous cell carcinomas, which, although curable when treated early, have a greater risk of metastatic spread. Common precursor lesions for squamous cell carcinoma are actinic keratosis (solar keratosis) and Bowen's disease (squamous cell carcinoma in situ).

- Treatments for **actinic keratosis** and **Bowen's disease** include cryosurgery, curettage, excision, laser treatment, photodynamic therapy (see Porfimer Sodium, p.581) using 5-aminolevulinic acid or methyl aminolevulinate, and topical fluorouracil.[1-3] Topical diclofenac or topical imiquimod may be used for actinic keratosis.[2,3] The choice of treatment depends on the site and size of the lesion, evidence for efficacy, ease of application, and availability.[1]
- Treatment options for superficial low-risk **basal cell carcinomas** include curettage and electrodessication or cryosurgery.[4,5] Topical fluorouracil may be used for superficial lesions in some instances, as is photodynamic therapy using methyl aminolevulinate. Imiquimod is under investigation.
- For superficial tumours at high-risk sites, and for most **squamous cell carcinomas**, excision with postoperatively determined margins or Mohs' micrographic surgery (tumour margins examined during the procedure) is more appropriate.[4-6] Radiotherapy is an alternative in patients at risk of surgical complications or where surgery would be difficult or extensive.

The prognosis with appropriate treatment is good, with 5-year disease free survival of over 90%. However, about 50% of patients will subsequently develop another skin cancer, and regular monitoring to detect this as early as possible is desirable.[5] In addition, patients should be educated about sun protection measures, and chemoprevention with retinoids may be appropriate for some high-risk patients (see Prophylaxis, in Malignant Neoplasms of the Skin, above).


1. Cox NH, *et al.* Guidelines for management of Bowen's disease. *Br J Dermatol* 1999; **141:** 633–41.
2. Anonymous. New treatments for actinic keratoses. *Med Lett Drugs Ther* 2002; **44:** 57–8.
3. Anonymous. Managing solar keratoses. *Drug Ther Bull* 2002; **40:** 33–5.
4. Telfer NR, *et al.* Guidelines for the management of basal cell carcinoma. *Br J Dermatol* 1999; **141:** 415–23.
5. Martinez J-C, Otley CC. The management of melanoma and nonmelanoma skin cancer: a review for the primary care physician. *Mayo Clin Proc* 2001; **76:** 1253–65.
6. Alam M, Ratner D. Cutaneous squamous-cell carcinoma. *N Engl J Med* 2001; **344:** 975–83.


MELANOMA. Although cutaneous melanoma is rare it is the most aggressive skin cancer, accounting for the majority of all skin cancer deaths. Melanoma may arise in apparently normal skin or from an existing naevus. Early signs of a naevus that may indicate development of a melanoma are change in size, shape, or colour. Other signs include itching, ulceration, and bleeding. The most common site in women is the legs, and in men the back. For a discussion of sun protection measures in the prevention of melanoma, see Prophylaxis, in Malignant Neoplasms of the Skin, above.

Surgical resection is the mainstay of curative treatment for melanomas, and the margins of excision are determined by tumour depth.[1,2] Patients with thin tumours (less than 1 mm) can be treated with wide local excision only; patients with intermediate (1 to 4 mm) or thick (more than 4 mm) melanoma are at high risk for nodal disease, and lymph node dissection may also be performed following positive node biopsy. Because of the high risk of recurrence after surgery in the latter group, there is great interest in adjuvant therapies. The most common adjuvant treatment is interferon alfa, which is the subject of ongoing clinical trials. Of the studies reported so far, high-dose interferon has shown a clinical benefit in terms of relapse-free survival, but the effect on overall survival is less clear.[3-6] Isolated limb perfusion with melphalan has been used as adjuvant therapy, but a review of four randomised trials failed to show any survival benefit for this compared with surgery alone.[7] Similarly, systemic chemotherapy has not proved useful in the adjuvant setting.[8] Various melanoma vaccines (e.g. GM2 ganglioside, autologous melanoma-associated antigens) are being investigated for adjuvant use,[9] but high-dose interferon alfa has been shown to produce greater clinical benefit than vaccination with GM2.[5] Isolated recurrences are treated with surgical resection.

For patients who present with metastatic melanoma the 5-year survival rate is poor.[8] There is no evidence to show that any systemic treatments are better than best supportive care in these patients.[10] Because of this, surgery is still considered an option, and a few patients may survive long term after resection of isolated metastases. Chemotherapy has been tried,[11] and dacarbazine, with a response rate of about 20%, is the most common single agent. However, the response duration is usually only 4 to 6 months, and complete responses are rare. The orally active analogue temozolomide produces similar responses,[12] and is an alternative. Nitrosoureas (such as carmustine, lomustine, and semustine) have response rates around 15% as single agents.[11] Fotemustine appears to be more active, particularly in the treatment of brain metastases. Other drugs with a response rate of about 15% include cisplatin, vinblastine, vindesine, docetaxel, and paclitaxel; response duration has generally been poor.

Combination regimens have been used, such as CVD (cisplatin, a vinca alkaloid, and dacarbazine). Tamoxifen has also been added to regimens, on the hypothesis that melanoma is oestrogen-dependent; an example is the CDBT or Dartmouth regimen (cisplatin, dacarbazine, carmustine, and tamoxifen). However, a randomised study found that this regimen was no more effective than dacarbazine alone,[13] and there is a lack of evidence that tamoxifen potentiates the action of cytotoxics in melanoma.[11]

Cytokines such as interferon alfa and interleukin-2 have similar activity to chemotherapy in metastatic melanoma.[11] Cytotoxic chemotherapy has been given with these cytokines and there have been some reports of improved response rates, but large controlled studies are needed to confirm a benefit. Melanoma vaccines are also being investigated in metastatic or recurrent disease,[9] as is gene therapy, and antiangiogenic agents such as thalidomide.[11]


1. Australian Cancer Network/National Health and Medical Research Council. The management of cutaneous melanoma. Available at: http://www.nhmrc.gov.au/publications/pdf/cp68.pdf (accessed 28/06/04)
2. Martinez J-C, Otley CC. The management of melanoma and nonmelanoma skin cancer: a review for the primary care physician. *Mayo Clin Proc* 2001; **76:** 1253–65.
3. Hancock BW, *et al.* Adjuvant interferon-alpha in malignant melanoma: current status. *Cancer Treat Rev* 2000; **26:** 81–9.
4. Kirkwood JM, *et al.* High- and low-dose interferon alfa-2b in high-risk melanoma: first analysis of intergroup trial E1690/S9111/C9190. *J Clin Oncol* 2000; **18:** 2444–58.
5. Kirkwood JM, *et al.* High-dose interferon alfa-2b significantly prolongs relapse-free and overall survival compared with the GM2-KLH/QS-21 vaccine in patients with resected stage IIB-III melanoma: results of intergroup trial E1694/S9512/C509801. *J Clin Oncol* 2001; **19:** 2370–80.
6. Sabel MS, Sondak VK. Is there a role for adjuvant high-dose interferon-α-2b in the management of melanoma? *Drugs* 2003; **63:** 1053–58.
7. Lens MB, Dawes M. Isolated limb perfusion with melphalan in the treatment of malignant melanoma of the extremities: a systematic review of randomised controlled trials. *Lancet Oncol* 2003; **4:** 359–64.
8. Jackson DP, Patel PM. The current place of systemic therapy in the treatment of malignant melanoma. *CME Oncology* 1998; **1:** 4–8.
9. Brinckerhoff LH, *et al.* Melanoma vaccines. *Curr Opin Oncol* 2000; **12:** 163–73.
10. Crosby T, *et al.* Systemic treatments for metastatic cutaneous melanoma. Available in The Cochrane Library; Issue 2. Chichester: John Wiley; 2004.
11. Bajetta E, *et al.* Metastatic melanoma: chemotherapy. *Semin Oncol* 2002; **29:** 427–45.
12. Middleton MR, *et al.* Randomized phase III study of temozolomide versus dacarbazine in the treatment of patients with advanced metastatic malignant melanoma. *J Clin Oncol* 2000; **18:** 158–66.
13. Chapman PB, *et al.* Phase III multicenter randomized trial of the Dartmouth regimen versus dacarbazine in patients with metastatic melanoma. *J Clin Oncol* 1999; **17:** 2745–51.


**Malignant neoplasms of the testis.** Testicular cancer only accounts for about 1% of all male malignancies but it is the most common cancer in young men. Patients with a history of cryptorchidism are at increased risk. About 95% of testicular tumours arise in germ cells, and 40% or so of these are pure seminomas. The remainder are collectively known as nonseminomatous germ cell tumours (NSGCT) in the WHO classification, and are commonly of mixed cell types with or without a seminoma component. Nonseminomatous tumours have been referred to as teratomas in the British classification system, but this term has a more specific meaning in the WHO classification.[1]

Metastasis first occurs to the lymph nodes, then, in advanced disease, to distant sites such as lung, liver, brain, and bones. The leading symptom is a hard, painless swelling of the testis, but once metastasis occurs the patient may present with back pain (due to enlargement of retroperitoneal lymph nodes), cough, dyspnoea, gynaecomastia due to chorionic gonadotrophin production, or weight loss.

Surgical removal of the testis (orchidectomy) when diagnosis is confirmed is fundamental to the treatment of all types of testicular cancer, but further therapy depends upon the disease type and stage.[1-3]

In patients with **nonseminomatous** disease with the tumour confined to the testis (stage I), options for post-orchidectomy management include surveillance or a short course of adjuvant chemotherapy. With surveillance, about 20 to 30% of patients will relapse and are subsequently treated with curative chemotherapy. Surveillance is thus not appropriate for patients who are unable to undergo regular follow-up, or who have prognostic factors suggesting a high risk of relapse such as vascular or lymphatic invasion. In the UK, these patients would be treated with adjuvant chemotherapy with 2 cycles of BEP (bleomycin, etoposide, and cisplatin), which will prevent relapse in the vast majority of cases.[1] In the USA, retroperitoneal lymph-node dissection may be carried out to further stage the disease before making a decision regarding surveillance or adjuvant chemotherapy.[3] If resected nodes are clear, patients undergo surveillance, but if they involve tumour (stage II) the decision to give adjuvant chemotherapy is based on the degree of nodal involvement and the ability of the patient to undergo regular follow-up.[3]

Where metastasis to the lymph nodes (stage II) or beyond (stage III) has occurred, standard postorchidectomy therapy is now combination chemotherapy with BEP,[1,3] which has largely replaced the effective but more toxic PVB regimen (cisplatin, vinblastine, and bleomycin).[2,4] Based on serum markers and the presence or absence of non-pulmonary visceral metastases, patients with metastatic disease can be categorised into good, intermediate, and poor-risk groups, with 5-year survival rates of 91%, 79%, and 48%, respectively.[3] Consequently, there has been interest in minimising the treatment in patients with good prognosis in order to reduce long-term morbidity. In such patients, 3 cycles of BEP,[1,3] or 4 cycles of cisplatin and etoposide, may be adequate.[2,3] The substitution of carboplatin for cisplatin has resulted in a 10% lower relapse-free survival, and slightly reduced overall survival, and is not usually recommended,[2] although some have reported good results with such a regimen in children.[5] There is evidence that overall survival is improved by increased dose-intensity of etoposide and perhaps bleomycin.[6] Standard management for patients with intermediate- or poor-risk disease is 4 cycles of BEP.[1,3] However, less than 50% of poor-risk patients achieve a durable response and they may be offered more intensive chemotherapy such as accelerated therapy, dose escalation with use of haematopoietic growth factors, or high-dose chemotherapy with stem cell support, with the aim of improving responses. So far, those intensive treatments evaluated in randomised clinical trials have not proved more effective than BEP, and have often been more toxic.[2] Various trials are ongoing.[2] Secondary resection of residual tumour after chemotherapy is commonly undertaken.[1-3]

Patients who fail, or who relapse after, standard chemotherapy have a poor prognosis, with an overall survival of only 20 to 25%.[2,3] Common salvage regimens include cisplatin, ifosfamide, and etoposide or vinblastine. High-dose chemotherapy with stem cell support may also be considered.[1-3] Newer drugs with activity in relapsed disease include paclitaxel and gemcitabine.[1,2]

**Seminoma** is extremely sensitive to radiation, and adjuvant radiotherapy is the treatment of choice after orchidectomy in limited disease (stage I) and disease with low tumour burden (stages IIA and IIB).[1-3] About three-quarters of patients have stage I disease at diagnosis and cure rates are between 95 and 100%. However, seminoma also responds very well to chemotherapy and adjuvant single-agent carboplatin is currently being compared with adjuvant radiotherapy for stage I disease,[1,2] and chemotherapy is being used in some patients with stage IIB disease.[1] Patients with stages IIC to III seminoma have a relapse rate of over 35% after adjuvant radiotherapy, and adjuvant chemotherapy is preferred.[1-3] Standard regimens are BEP (3 cycles for good prognosis patients and 4 cycles for others[3]), or cisplatin with etoposide,[1] which produce survival rates of approximately 90%.[2] Salvage regimens for relapsed or unresponsive seminoma are similar to those used for nonseminomatous disease.[3]


1. Clinical Oncology Information Network and Scottish Intercollegiate Guidelines Network. Guidelines on the management of adult testicular germ cell tumours. *Clin Oncol* 2000; **12:** S173–S210. Also available at: http://www.rcr.ac.uk/upload/TestisGuidelines2000.pdf (accessed 28/06/04)
2. Hartmann JT, *et al.* Diagnosis and treatment of patients with testicular germ cell cancer. *Drugs* 1999; **58:** 257–81.
3. National Comprehensive Cancer Network. Clinical practice guidelines in oncology: testicular cancer (version 1.2004). Available at: http://www.nccn.org/professionals/physician_gls/PDF/testicular.pdf (accessed 03/06/04)
4. Culine S, Droz J-P. Comparative tolerability of chemotherapy regimens for germ cell cancer. *Drug Safety* 2000; **22:** 373–88.
5. Mann JR, *et al.* The United Kingdom Children's Cancer Study Group's second germ cell tumor study: carboplatin, etoposide, and bleomycin are effective treatment for children with malignant extracranial germ cell tumours, with acceptable toxicity. *J Clin Oncol* 2000; **18:** 3809–18.
6. Toner GC, *et al.* Comparison of two standard chemotherapy regimens for good-prognosis germ-cell tumours: a randomised trial. *Lancet* 2001; **357:** 739–45.


**Malignant neoplasms of the thymus.** Thymomas are tumours of the mediastinum, arising from thymic tissue. They are rare, and most commonly present in patients between 40 and 60 years of age. Thymoma originates from the epithelium of the thymus but may also contain a lymphocyte component, which is probably not neoplastic. Up to 50% of patients are asymptomatic, and others have local symptoms such as cough, chest pain, dyspnoea, and obstruction of the vena cava; paraneoplastic syndromes such as myasthenia gravis, red cell aplasia, and hypogammaglobulinaemia may also develop.

Thymomas may be classified as non-invasive (encapsulated, stage I), invasive (localised, stage II; extensive, stage III and IVa), and metastatic (IVb). The majority of patients present with non-invasive disease, and can be treated solely by surgical resection with low recurrence rates and long-term survival approaching 100%.[1-3] Patients with invasive disease have a higher risk of recurrence, even if the tumour is completely resected, and they are usually treated with adjuvant radiotherapy.[1-3]

In patients with unresectable invasive disease, radiotherapy alone has been used, but high recurrence rates are seen.[1] There is increasing interest in combined modality approaches to improve survival in this group.[1-3] For example, radiotherapy followed by chemotherapy may be used, and neoadjuvant chemotherapy followed by surgical resection then adjuvant radiotherapy with or without further chemotherapy is being investigated. Chemotherapy regimens used in this approach are similar to those used in metastatic disease.

The role of therapies in recurrent or metastatic disease is not well established because of its rarity.[1-3] Various case series and phase II trials have shown that the tumour is chemosensitive. The demonstration that cisplatin had activity against thymoma has led to much interest in cisplatin-containing regimens such as cisplatin, doxorubicin, and cyclophosphamide (PAC), and the same drugs with addition of vincristine.[1-3] Ifosfamide is also active as a single agent against thymoma, and has been given with cisplatin and etoposide.[1,3] A combination of carboplatin and paclitaxel is under investigation.[3] Interleukin-2 has not proved beneficial.[1,3] There is some evidence that thymomas possess somatostatin receptors, and there have been a few reports of the benefit of octreotide.[1,3]


1. Thomas CR, *et al.* Thymoma: state of the art. *J Clin Oncol* 1999; **17:** 2280–9.
2. Johnson SB, *et al.* Thymoma: update for the new millenium. *Oncologist* 2001; **6:** 239–46.
3. Schmidt-Wolf IGH, *et al.* Malignant thymoma: current status of classification and multimodality treatment. *Ann Hematol* 2003; **82:** 69–76.


**Malignant neoplasms of the thyroid.** Thyroid cancer accounts for only about 1% of all malignancies. The incidence is reportedly higher in women than men, in patients who received irradiation of the thyroid during childhood, and in populations where goitre is endemic. The natural history varies with the cell type and degree of differentiation. Well-differentiated papillary or follicular tumours (which constitute about 70% and 15% of cases, respectively) are very slow to grow and metastasise, sometimes persisting for years with little change in size and extent, although they may prove more aggressive in children. In contrast medullary carcinomas (5 to 10% of cases), which develop from the cells responsible for calcitonin secretion, and undifferentiated (anaplastic) tumours (5%)

metastasise early and follow a much more rapid and aggressive course. About 25% of medullary cancers are hereditary, including those due to multiple endocrine neoplasia type 2.

The well-differentiated types usually present as a thyroid nodule, although most nodules are not malignant, while with anaplastic tumours there is usually bulky disease and often difficulty in breathing due to encroachment on the tracheal lumen.

In patients with **well-differentiated tumours** total or partial thyroidectomy is the treatment of choice.[1-3] This may be followed by a course of iodine-131 to destroy any residual tumour, although in low-risk patients the prognosis after surgery alone is so favourable that iodine-131 is not usually recommended.[1-3] Levothyroxine treatment should be given to all patients to suppress thyroid stimulating hormone (TSH) production, and must be continued for life.[1-4] Ten-year survival of up to 75% in patients with follicular tumours and up to 90% with papillary tumours has been seen.[4] Disease recurrence is commonly treated with further surgery and ablative iodine-131 therapy.[1,2]

In patients with **medullary cancers** total thyroidectomy and neck dissection are indicated, followed by levothyroxine treatment.[2,3] Ten-year survival of 60 to 70% has been reported.[4,5] Adjuvant external beam radiotherapy may be used in patients at high risk of regional recurrence[3] but routine use has not shown any survival benefit.[2] Prophylactic thyroidectomy may be considered in patients with a hereditary predisposition to medullary cancer.[3,5] Resection may relieve symptoms in patients with **anaplastic tumours**, but cure is impossible and treatment is purely palliative, with survival measured in months.[3,4,6] Neither medullary[5] nor anaplastic tumours[4] are sensitive to iodine-131. External radiation therapy is commonly used.[2,3,6] Chemotherapy has been tried in anaplastic thyroid cancer, as well as in unresponsive disease of other cell types, with limited benefit. Drugs tried, often in combination regimens, include cisplatin, cyclophosphamide, bleomycin, dacarbazine, doxorubicin, fluorouracil, paclitaxel, and vincristine.[4-6]

1. Schlumberger MJ. Papillary and follicular thyroid carcinoma. *N Engl J Med* 1998; **338:** 297–306.
2. British Thyroid Association and Royal College of Physicians. Guidelines for the management of thyroid cancer in adults (March 2002). Available at: http://www.british-thyroid-association.org/complete%20guidelines.pdf (accessed 28/06/04)
3. Sherman SI. Thyroid carcinoma. *Lancet* 2003; **361:** 501–11.
4. O'Doherty MJ, Coakley AJ. Drug therapy alternatives in the treatment of thyroid cancer. *Drugs* 1998; **55:** 801–12.
5. Heshmati HM, *et al.* Advances and controversies in the diagnosis and management of medullary thyroid carcinoma. *Am J Med* 1997; **103:** 60–69.
6. Ain KB. Anaplastic thyroid carcinoma: a therapeutic challenge. *Semin Surg Oncol* 1999; **16:** 64–9.

**Neuroblastoma.** Neuroblastoma accounts for about 7% of all childhood malignancies overall but is probably the most frequent neoplasm in the first year of life. Three-quarters of all cases present before the age of 5 years. The tumour is derived from cells of the neural crest, and may occur anywhere within the sympathetic nervous system, notably the sympathetic ganglia and the adrenal medulla. It is characterised by a diversity of clinical behaviour ranging from spontaneous remission to rapid metastatic progression and death. Sites of metastasis include lymph nodes, bone marrow, liver, and skin. Adverse prognostic factors include age over 1 year at diagnosis, stage IV (distant metastases), and amplification of the oncogene MYCN.

Progress in the treatment of neuroblastoma over the last 20 years has increased 10-year survival to about 60% overall, although in patients with disseminated disease the gains have been modest.[1] In those with localised disease (stage I or II) surgical resection alone is appropriate, with good long-term survival prospects. In addition, asymptomatic infants less than one year of age with localised tumours and limited dissemination (stage IV special) usually experience a high rate of tumour regression, and can be considered for surgical resection then close observation.[1] Low-dose chemotherapy generally arrests tumour progression should this occur. In those with localised but unresectable disease (stage II and III), subtotal surgical resection may be followed by standard-dose chemotherapy.[1] Chemotherapy regimens include cyclophosphamide and doxorubicin, sometimes with vincristine for good prognosis patients, and with the addition of cisplatin and etoposide (or teniposide) for poorer prognosis patients. Further surgery may be undertaken, with further chemotherapy and/or radiotherapy used in those with residual disease.[1] Disseminated disease (stage IV) and tumours with adverse prognostic features such as MYCN amplification are often more resistant to chemotherapy, and more intensive therapy is used.[1,2] Surgery and radiation therapy may also be combined with chemotherapy. Regimens used for remission induction include cyclophosphamide, doxorubicin, cisplatin, etoposide or teniposide, and vincristine. Another option is cisplatin, etoposide, and vindesine alternating with vincristine, dacarbazine, ifosfamide, and doxorubicin.[1] After remission induction, consolidation with myeloablative chemotherapy and autologous stem cell or bone marrow rescue may be used. Maintenance therapy with oral cyclophosphamide is being investigated. Isotretinoin, fenretinide, and monoclonal antibodies are also being investigated for their ability to maintain remissions after chemotherapy.[1,3] Targeted radiation, using iodine-131-labelled *m*-iodobenzylguanidine, which is actively taken up by cells synthesising catecholamines, may be used for scanning, and is also being investigated for treatment.[4]

1. Berthold F, Hero B. Neuroblastoma: current drug therapy recommendations as part of the total treatment approach. *Drugs* 2000; **59:** 1261–77.
2. Katzenstein HM, Cohn SL. Advances in the diagnosis and treatment of neuroblastoma. *Curr Opin Oncol* 1998; **10:** 43–51.
3. Reynolds CP, *et al.* Retinoid therapy of high-risk neuroblastoma. *Cancer Lett* 2003; **197:** 185–92.
4. Meller S. Targeted radiotherapy for neuroblastoma. *Arch Dis Child* 1997; **77:** 389–91.

**Retinoblastoma.** Retinoblastoma is the most common eye tumour in children and accounts for about 3% of all childhood malignancies (for other malignant neoplasms of the eye, see above). In 60 to 70% of cases the tumour is sporadic and non-hereditary, producing a unilateral, unifocal lesion. In the remaining 30 to 40% of cases there is an abnormal tumour suppressor gene (RB1) inherited: these tumours are typically bilateral and are sometimes associated with an intracranial neuroblastic tumour (trilateral retinoblastoma or pinealoblastoma). In addition, patients with the hereditary form are at very high risk of secondary primary malignancies, particularly osteosarcoma and soft tissue sarcomas. The most common manifestations of retinoblastoma are leukocoria (white pupil), strabismus (squint) and nystagmus. Retinoblastoma is confined to the eye(s) (intra-ocular) at presentation in about 80% of patients, although the majority have extensive disease within the eye. Nevertheless, 5-year disease-free survival after treatment in these patients is greater than 90%. The remainder of patients with extra-ocular disease in the tissues around the eye or with metastatic spread to the CNS and beyond, have a poor 5-year survival of less than 10% despite treatment.

The aim of treatment for intra-ocular retinoblastoma is to cure the disease, and to preserve as much vision as possible.[1-5] In patients with unilateral tumours, enucleation (removal of the eye) is the standard primary treatment when there is no expectation of useful vision (e.g. extensive disease within the eye). In bilateral retinoblastoma, standard treatment was enucleation of the advanced eye and external beam radiation therapy in the less advanced eye. However, there is increasing use of therapies to preserve the eye and to reduce the use of external radiotherapy which further increases the risk of secondary malignancies.[2-4] These include local treatments such as cryotherapy, thermotherapy, and plaque radiotherapy. Intravenous neoadjuvant chemotherapy may be given to reduce tumour size before use of these local treatments (chemoreduction); regimens usually include carboplatin, etoposide (or teniposide), and vincristine.[2-4] Ciclosporin has also been included to overcome the multidrug resistance gene, P-glycoprotein.[3]

Patients who undergo enucleation and who are found to have optic nerve involvement (micrometastatic retinoblastoma) are at high risk of recurrence. Although there is no consensus on further treatment, these patients are often treated with adjuvant chemotherapy (cyclophosphamide, doxorubicin, and vincristine) and radiotherapy.[3]

Patients with orbital extension may be treated with enucleation, radiotherapy, and intensive chemotherapy.[3] Regimens typically include cyclophosphamide, doxorubicin, and vincristine, and may include carboplatin and etoposide. Intrathecal methotrexate and cranial irradiation may be added for CNS involvement or trilateral retinoblastoma. Metastatic disease may be treated similarly, but although combination chemotherapy may produce a response it is rarely curative in such advanced disease. High-dose chemotherapy with autologous stem cell rescue has been tried in metastatic disease, but it has not been effective for disease involving the CNS.[4]

1. Zucker JM, *et al.* Retinoblastoma. *Eur J Cancer* 1998; **34:** 1045–9.
2. Shields CL, Shields JA. Recent developments in the management of retinoblastoma. *J Pediatr Ophthalmol Strabismus* 1999; **36:** 8–18.
3. Finger PT, *et al.* Chemotherapy for retinoblastoma: a current topic. *Drugs* 1999; **58:** 983–96.
4. De Potter P. Current treatment of retinoblastoma. *Curr Opin Ophthalmol* 2002; **13:** 331–6.
5. Deegan WF. Emerging strategies for the treatment of retinoblastoma. *Curr Opin Ophthalmol* 2003; **14:** 291–5.

**Sarcomas.** The sarcomas are tumours arising from mesodermal cells which form the bone and connective tissue (as opposed to carcinomas, which arise from ectodermal and endodermal cells, and leukaemias and lymphomas which arise from the bone marrow and immune system). Sarcomas are uncommon, and vary considerably in their sites, presentation, and prognosis. The primary malignancies of bone include osteosarcoma and Ewing's sarcoma, which most often occur in older children and adolescents, and chondrosarcoma which is most common in later life. Soft tissue sarcomas include those of fibrous tissue (fibrosarcoma), skeletal muscle (rhabdomyosarcoma), smooth muscle (leiomyosarcoma), adipose tissue (liposarcoma), and blood vessels (a group which includes Kaposi's sarcoma).

BONE SARCOMA. The commonest primary malignant tumour of bone is **osteosarcoma** (osteogenic sarcoma) which accounts for about 3 to 4% of all childhood malignancies. It is composed of malignant osteoblasts which form an osteoid matrix within which new bone formation may occur. Most osteosarcomas are aggressive high-grade malignancies which destroy overlying cortical bone and invade adjacent soft tissue, as well as spreading along the medulla. Metastasis, almost exclusively via the vascular system to the lungs and other distant sites, is usual and occurs early.

The primary therapy is surgery, with an increasing trend to more conservative, limb-sparing operations rather than amputation. Adjuvant chemotherapy is an important component of therapy, however, as metastasis of the tumour is common.[1,2] The most widely used combination is doxorubicin and cisplatin, sometimes with high-dose methotrexate and folinic acid rescue. Ifosfamide and cyclophosphamide are also used.[1-3] Chemotherapy is often started before surgery to attack micrometastases, shrink the primary tumour and enable evaluation of the tumour response.[3] Aggressive treatment regimens can result in long-term relapse-free survival rates of 70%, although patients with overt metastatic disease at presentation have a poorer prognosis.[3]

Like osteosarcoma, **Ewing's sarcoma** is seen mainly in adolescents and older children. It is a round cell tumour that most commonly arises in the pelvis or the long bones of the limbs. There may be diffuse erosion of the bone and marked periosteal reaction. It spreads through the medullary cavity, and metastases to lung and other bones are common.

Unlike most bone sarcomas this is highly radiosensitive, so radiotherapy is frequently used to control local disease. The role of surgery has been controversial, but as adjuvant chemotherapy has increased survival to over 50%, limb-sparing surgery is gaining popularity.[2] The majority of patients will have micrometastatic disease, and therefore adjuvant chemotherapy remains essential.[3] In the USA, good results have been achieved with a combination of etoposide and ifosfamide added to intermittent high-dose vincristine, doxorubicin or dactinomycin or both, and cyclophosphamide.[1-4] These aggressive treatment regimens are not without risk; a significant proportion of successfully treated patients develop secondary cancers, such as radiation-induced sarcomas or treatment-related leukaemias, as well as anthracycline-induced cardiomyopathy.[1] Although multimodal therapy has improved survival, the prognosis for patients with overt metastatic disease remains poor; survival has been estimated to be only 20 to 30%.[3] Myeloablative therapy followed by stem cell transplantation has met with limited success in patients with metastatic disease at diagnosis.[1]

Chemotherapy appears to have little place in the treatment of other bone sarcomas such as **chondrosarcoma** or **osteoclastoma**; it has been used in high-grade **fibrosarcomas** and in **histiocytoma** but its value is uncertain.

1. Arndt CAS, Crist WM. Common musculoskeletal tumors of childhood and adolescence. *N Engl J Med* 1999; **341:** 342–52.
2. Yaw KM. Pediatric bone tumors. *Semin Surg Oncol* 1999; **16:** 173–83.
3. Russell EC, *et al.* Lymphomas and bone marrow tumors: clinical presentation, management, and potential late effects of current treatment strategies. *Adolesc Med* 1999; **10:** 419–35.
4. Grier HE, *et al.* Addition of ifosfamide and etoposide to standard chemotherapy for Ewing's sarcoma and primitive neuroectodermal tumor of bone. *N Engl J Med* 2003; **348:** 694–701.

KAPOSI'S SARCOMA. Kaposi's sarcoma is a tumour of endothelial or spindle cell origin. In its classical form it manifests as red or violet cutaneous lesions of the limbs in elderly men, usually of Jewish or Mediterranean ancestry. An endemic form is also seen in certain areas of Africa.[1] Lesions may eventually affect the whole of the skin, upper airways, gastrointestinal tract, lungs, and lymph nodes, but in general disease is only very slowly progressive, and may require no treatment. Patients receiving immunosuppressive therapy may be at greater risk of developing Kaposi's sarcoma, particularly if they are from ethnic groups that are susceptible to the classic or endemic forms of the disease.[1] In recent years an epidemic form of the disease has appeared in patients with disease due to HIV infection (p.621). HIV-associated Kaposi's sarcoma is more aggressive, with a greater tendency to disseminated and metastatic disease.

A novel herpesvirus (human herpesvirus 8, HHV8) has been implicated in the pathogenesis of Kaposi's sarcoma. HHV8 induces changes in endothelial cells that make them more susceptible to inflammatory cytokines and angiogenesis.[2] Some antivirals, such as cidofovir and to a lesser extent foscarnet and ganciclovir, have shown activity against HHV8 *in vitro*, but they have not been equally successful in treating Kaposi's sarcoma *in vivo*. Treatment with highly active antiretroviral therapy has greatly reduced the occurrence of Kaposi's sarcoma in AIDS patients, and may cause regression of milder forms of the disease, but this is thought to be due to improvements in immune function rather than a direct effect on Kaposi's sarcoma.[3] The development of Kaposi's sarcoma is likely to be multifactorial, and as infection with HHV8 alone does not produce disease, and the replication of HHV8 in sarcoma cells is low, antiviral therapy alone is unlikely to be sufficient to control symptoms.[3]

Patients with classic or endemic Kaposi's sarcoma are often treated with surgery or radiotherapy of individual lesions.[1] Extensive or recurrent disease may be treated with vinca alkaloids, bleomycin, doxorubicin, and dacarbazine, alone or in combination.[1] Etoposide and interferon alfa have also been tried.[1] Patients with immunosuppression-associated Kaposi's sarcoma may receive similar treatment to those with the classic form, or preferably by alteration of the immunosuppressive regimen if this can be done without graft loss.[1]

The epidemic form of Kaposi's sarcoma is associated with HIV infection, and seen particularly in homosexual patients. In the early stages, highly active antiretroviral therapy may resolve the immunosuppression and therefore control Kaposi's sarcoma, but the response is unpredictable, so specific therapy is often needed.[1] Localised disease may be managed with cryotherapy or radiotherapy, but intralesional vinblastine, interferon alfa, and topical alitretinoin are also used.[2,4] Photodynamic therapy is under investigation.

Systemic chemotherapy is generally reserved for patients with more extensive disease or mucosal or visceral involvement. In patients with a CD4 cell count of 200 cells/microlitre or above, treatment with interferon alfa, in combination with zidovudine, has been advocated by some, but systemic chemotherapy is the treatment of choice.[1-3] The main combination regimens use a vinca alkaloid and bleomycin, with or without doxorubicin.[2,3] Liposomal formulations of doxorubicin and daunorubicin have produced response rates of 40-85%, and may be less toxic than conventional chemotherapy;[2-4] many now consider a liposomal anthracycline the drug of choice in extensive disease.[1,2] Paclitaxel is also used as a single agent in advanced disease.[2-4] Some response has also been reported for oral etoposide.[1]

Control of Kaposi's sarcoma has been reported in a few patients given high-dose intramuscular chorionic gonadotrophin, but tumour regression ceased and regrowth occurred when dosage was reduced or withdrawn.[5] Further reports of intralesional or systemic administration have included partial remissions and disease stabilisation, as well as no effect or disease progression. The reasons for these contradictory results are unclear, but they may be due to variability in chorionic gonadotrophin preparations, which contain a mixture of biological contaminants. A cytotoxic ribonuclease and the degradation product of the β-hCG subunit have been proposed as active contaminants against Kaposi's sarcoma, but other contaminants may stimulate the tumour.[6] Other lines of investigation include the use of sulfated polysaccharide peptidoglycans, various other inhibitors of angiogenesis including thalidomide, and the retinoids.[1,4]


1. Antman K, Chang Y. Kaposi's sarcoma. *N Engl J Med* 2000; **342:** 1027–38.
2. Mitsuyasu RT. Update on the pathogenesis and treatment of Kaposi sarcoma. *Curr Opin Oncol* 2000; **12:** 174–80.
3. Hermans P. Opportunistic AIDS-associated malignancies in HIV-infected patients. *Biomed Pharmacother* 2000; **54:** 32–40.
4. Dezube BJ, *et al.* Management of AIDS-related Kaposi sarcoma: advances in target discovery and treatment. *AIDS Read* 2004; **14:** 236–8, 243–4, 251–3.
5. Harris PJ. Treatment of Kaposi's sarcoma and other manifestations of AIDS with human chorionic gonadotropin. *Lancet* 1995; **346:** 118–19.
6. Simonart T, *et al.* Treatment of Kaposi's sarcoma with human chorionic gonadotropin. *Dermatology* 2002; **204:** 330–3.


SOFT-TISSUE SARCOMA. Soft-tissue sarcomas are a group of malignant tumours that originate from mesenchymal stem cells. **Rhabdomyosarcoma** is the commonest soft-tissue sarcoma in childhood, and is thought to arise from progenitor cells for skeletal muscle found throughout the body. The most frequent sites are the head and neck, genito-urinary tract, and extremities. The tumour spreads at an early stage into adjacent tissues and regional lymph nodes, and about 20% of patients have metastatic disease at diagnosis, most frequently in the lungs.

Effective treatment of soft-tissue sarcoma, particularly rhabdomyosarcoma, requires a combination of surgery, radiotherapy, and chemotherapy. Complete surgical excision is to be preferred, but where this is impossible wide-field irradiation should be given. Adjuvant chemotherapy is frequently used to control micrometastatic disease and has increased recurrence-free survival.[1-3] Most regimens use doxorubicin, with various combinations of ifosfamide, etoposide, cisplatin, dactinomycin, dacarbazine, cyclophosphamide, and vincristine.[1,4] Although doxorubicin and ifosfamide are considered to be the most active drugs, there is no consensus on the optimal drug regimen or dose.[1,2] For palliative treatment in advanced soft-tissue sarcoma, a systematic review[5] concluded that combination chemotherapy did not significantly increase survival rates compared with single-agent doxorubicin.

Dose-intensified combination regimens, with colony-stimulating factor support, have been investigated as adjuvant therapy[6] and in advanced disease;[7] although both these studies found a delay in disease progression, a beneficial effect on overall survival was only found in the former. Response to topotecan has been reported in a study of metastatic rhabdomyosarcoma,[8] and trabectedin is a novel antineoplastic under investigation for advanced soft-tissue sarcomas. Tasonermin and melphalan can be used together for isolated limb perfusion of unresectable soft-tissue sarcomas, but severe toxicity may limit use of this regimen.


1. Bishop JM, Lorigan P. Systemic therapy of soft tissue sarcomas. *CME Oncol* 1999; **1:** 81–4.
2. Sarcoma Meta-analysis Collaboration (SMAC). Adjuvant chemotherapy for localised resectable soft tissue sarcoma in adults. Available in The Cochrane Library; Issue 2. Chichester: John Wiley; 2004.
3. Pellitteri PK, *et al.* Management of sarcomas of the head and neck in adults. *Oral Oncol* 2003; **39:** 2–12.
4. Seynaeve C, Verweij J. High-dose chemotherapy in adult sarcomas: no standard yet. *Semin Oncol* 1999; **26:** 119–33.
5. Bramwell VHC, *et al.* Doxorubicin-based chemotherapy for the palliative treatment of adult patients with locally advanced or metastatic soft tissue sarcoma. Available in The Cochrane Library; Issue 2. Chichester: John Wiley; 2004.
6. Frustaci S, *et al.* Adjuvant chemotherapy for adult soft tissue sarcomas of the extremities and girdles: results of the Italian randomized cooperative trial. *J Clin Oncol* 2001; **19:** 1238–47.
7. Le Cesne A, *et al.* Randomized phase III study comparing conventional-dose doxorubicin plus ifosfamide versus high-dose doxorubicin plus ifosfamide plus recombinant human granulocyte-macrophage colony-stimulating factor in advanced soft tissue sarcomas: a trial of the European Organization for Research and Treatment of Cancer/Soft Tissue and Bone Sarcoma Group. *J Clin Oncol* 2000; **18:** 2676–84.
8. Pappo AS, *et al.* Up-front window trial of topotecan in previously untreated children and adolescents with metastatic rhabdomyosarcoma: an intergroup rhabdomyosarcoma study. *J Clin Oncol* 2001; **19:** 213–19.


---

## Aclarubicin *(BAN, USAN, rINN)*

Aclacinomycin A; NSC-208734. Methyl (1*R*,2*R*,4*S*)-4-(*O*-{2,6-dideoxy-4-*O*-[(2*R*,6*S*)-tetrahydro-6-methyl-5-oxopyran-2-yl]-α-L-*lyxo*-hexopyranosyl}-(1→4)-2,3,6-trideoxy-3-dimethylamino-L-*lyxo*-hexopyranosyloxy)-2-ethyl-1,2,3,4,6,11-hexahydro-2,5,7-trihydroxy-6,11-dioxonaphthacene-1-carboxylate.

$C_{42}H_{53}NO_{15}$ = 811.9.

*CAS — 57576-44-0.*

*ATC — L01DB04.*

**Description.** Aclarubicin is an anthracycline antineoplastic antibiotic isolated from *Streptomyces galilaeus*.

## Aclarubicin Hydrochloride *(BANM, rINNM)*

Hidrocloruro de aclarubicina.

$C_{42}H_{53}NO_{15},HCl$ = 848.3.

*CAS — 75443-99-1.*

*ATC — L01DB04.*

**Pharmacopoeias.** In *Jpn.*

**Stability.** In a study of the stability of anthracycline antineoplastic agents in 4 infusion fluids—glucose 5%, sodium chloride 0.9%, lactated Ringer's injection, and a commercial infusion fluid—stability appeared to be partly related to pH; aclarubicin was most stable in sodium chloride injection, with a pH of 6.2, and any increase or decrease in pH appeared to affect stability adversely.[1]


1. Poochikian GK, *et al.* Stability of anthracycline antitumor agents in four infusion fluids. *Am J Hosp Pharm* 1981; **38:** 483–6.


### Adverse Effects, Treatment, and Precautions

As for Doxorubicin Hydrochloride, p.548. Alopecia and cardiotoxicity may be less pronounced than with doxorubicin, and extravasation of aclarubicin causes less local tissue inflammation. Bone-marrow depression is dose-limiting, with platelet counts reaching a nadir 1 to 2 weeks after administration, while leucopenia is greatest after 2 to 3 weeks; recovery generally occurs within 4 weeks. Myelosuppression may be particularly severe in patients who have received mitomycin or a nitrosourea.

◊ An early review[1] noted that a strikingly high incidence of ECG changes had been observed with aclarubicin, but that although acute cardiotoxicity occurred, the chronic cardiomyopathy classically associated with the anthracyclines (see p.548) appeared to be rare. Alopecia was also rare, although gastrointestinal disturbances and mucositis were as common or more common than with doxorubicin.


1. Warrell RP. Aclacinomycin A: clinical development of a novel anthracycline antibiotic in the haematological cancers. *Drugs Exp Clin Res* 1986; **12:** 275–82.


### Pharmacokinetics

Aclarubicin is rapidly distributed into tissues after intravenous injection. Clearance is triphasic, with a terminal elimination half-life of about 3 hours; the principal active metabolite has a terminal half-life of about 13 hours. Aclarubicin is extensively metabolised and only about 1% of the total dose is eliminated unchanged. It is excreted in urine, chiefly as metabolites; some is also eliminated in bile.

### Uses and Administration

Aclarubicin is an anthracycline antibiotic with antineoplastic actions similar to those of the other anthracyclines (see Doxorubicin Hydrochloride, p.549), although it inhibits RNA synthesis more strongly than DNA synthesis. It is used as the hydrochloride in the treatment of malignant blood disorders, such as acute myeloid leukaemia (p.506). Aclarubicin hydrochloride 104 mg is approximately equivalent to 100 mg of aclarubicin. The usual initial dose as a single agent is the equivalent of 175 to 300 mg/m² of aclarubicin, given divided over 3 to 7 consecutive days, by intravenous infusion over 30 to 60 minutes. Where appropriate and tolerated, maintenance doses of the equivalent of 25 to 100 mg/m² may be given as a single infusion every 3 to 4 weeks. The total dose that can be given over the patient's lifetime depends upon cardiological status but most patients have not received more than 400 mg/m². Dosages may need to be reduced when given as part of a combination regimen.

◊ An early review of studies in patients with relapsed acute myeloid leukaemia confirmed the activity of aclarubicin, with reported complete remission rates of the order of 12 to 24%.[1] Doses varied from 10 to 30 mg/m² daily to higher doses of 75 to 120 mg/m² for 2 to 4 days; in general a total dose of about 300 mg/m² appeared to be necessary to induce remission. Less information was available concerning activity in acute lymphoblastic leukaemia, but response rates were lower than those in acute myeloid leukaemia. Results in the malignant lymphomas were generally disappointing.

Longer-term follow-up has confirmed that remission rates and survival are similar for induction regimens in acute myeloid leukaemia using either aclarubicin or daunorubicin.[2,3]


1. Warrell RP. Aclacinomycin A: clinical development of a novel anthracycline antibiotic in the haematological cancers. *Drugs Exp Clin Res* 1986; **12:** 275–82.
2. de Nully Brown P, *et al.* Long-term survival and development of secondary malignancies in patients with acute myeloid leukemia treated with aclarubicin or daunorubicin plus cytosine arabinoside followed by intensive consolidation chemotherapy in a Danish national phase III trial. *Leukemia* 1997; **11:** 37–41.
3. Öberg G, *et al.* Long-term follow-up of patients ≥60 yr old with acute myeloid leukaemia treated with intensive chemotherapy. *Eur J Haematol* 2002; **68:** 376–81.


### Preparations

**Proprietary Preparations** (details are given in Part 3)
***Ger.:*** Aclaplastin†; ***UK:*** Aclacin†.

---

## AE-941

### Profile

AE-941 is an angiogenesis inhibitor derived from shark cartilage extract. It is under investigation for the treatment of various malignant neoplasms, particularly non-small cell lung cancer. It is also being investigated for the treatment of psoriasis.

◊ References.


1. Sauder DN, *et al.* Neovastat (AE-941), an inhibitor of angiogenesis: randomized phase I/II clinical trial results in patients with plaque psoriasis. *J Am Acad Dermatol* 2002; **47:** 535–41.
2. Gingras D, *et al.* Neovastat—a novel antiangiogenic drug for cancer therapy. *Anticancer Drugs* 2003; **14:** 91–6.

## Alemtuzumab (BAN, rINN)

Campath-1; Campath-1H.
CAS — 216503-57-0.
ATC — L01XC04.

### Adverse Effects and Precautions

For general discussions, see Antineoplastics, p.492 and p.497.

Alemtuzumab commonly causes neutropenia, thrombocytopenia, anaemia, or pancytopenia. It has been associated with severe and prolonged myelosuppression and fatalities have occurred. Auto-immune thrombocytopenia and haemolytic anaemia have been reported less commonly. Single doses greater than 30 mg, or cumulative weekly doses greater than 90 mg should not be used, because of the increased incidence of pancytopenia. Complete blood and platelet counts should be measured weekly during alemtuzumab therapy, and more frequently if anaemia, neutropenia, or thrombocytopenia occur; treatment should be discontinued if severe myelosuppression or evidence of haematological toxicity are seen.

Alemtuzumab commonly causes infusion-related reactions due to an acute cytokine release syndrome. The reaction usually includes mild to moderate rigors, fever, nausea and vomiting, hypotension, rash, urticaria, pruritus, shortness of breath, headache, and diarrhoea. More serious reactions have occurred, including bronchospasm, syncope, pulmonary infiltrates, acute respiratory distress syndrome, respiratory arrest, myocardial infarction, and cardiac arrest. These reactions are most common at the start of therapy: the dose must be increased gradually when beginning treatment, or if it is interrupted for 7 days or more. Pre-medication with an oral or intravenous corticosteroid, oral antihistamine, and paracetamol should also be used, particularly before the first dose, and with dose increases. If acute infusion reactions persist, the infusion time may be extended to 8 hours from the time of reconstitution.

Other adverse effects include fatigue, arthralgia, myalgia, back pain, chest pain, hypertension, and tachycardia. Opportunistic infections are common, and antimicrobial prophylaxis is recommended.

Alemtuzumab is contra-indicated for patients with active systemic infection, or underlying immunodeficiency.

### Uses and Administration

Alemtuzumab is a humanised derivative of campath-1G, a rat monoclonal antibody to the CD52 antigen found on lymphocytes. Alemtuzumab is used in the treatment of B-cell chronic lymphocytic leukaemia (p.507) resistant to conventional chemotherapy. The dose of alemtuzumab must be increased gradually to avoid infusion-related reactions (see above). Alemtuzumab should be filtered via a 5 micron filter prior to dilution in 100 mL sodium chloride 0.9% or glucose 5%. The initial dose is 3 mg daily, given as an intravenous infusion over 2 hours (it may be increased up to 8 hours in some patients, see above). When this dose is tolerated, the dose is gradually increased until 10 mg daily can be tolerated. The maintenance dose of 30 mg can then be started; this dose escalation usually takes 3 to 7 days. A maximum maintenance dose of 30 mg given three times per week on alternate days can then be used for up to 12 weeks. The dose should be modified according to haematological toxicity.

Alemtuzumab has been tried in patients with lymphomas and lymphoproliferative disorders, and has also been investigated for the prevention of graft-versus-host disease. It has been tried with variable results in auto-immune disorders including vasculitis and rheumatoid arthritis, and multiple sclerosis. Subcutaneous alemtuzumab has been investigated.

◊ References.


1. Coles AJ, *et al.* Pulsed monoclonal antibody treatment and autoimmune thyroid disease in multiple sclerosis. *Lancet* 1999; **354:** 1691–5.
2. Dick AD, *et al.* Campath-1H therapy in refractory ocular inflammatory disease. *Br J Ophthalmol* 2000; **84:** 107–9.
3. Ferrajoli A, *et al.* Alemtuzumab: a novel monoclonal antibody. *Expert Opin Biol Ther* 2001; **1:** 1059–65.
4. Hale G, *et al.* CAMPATH-1 antibodies in stem-cell transplantation. *Cytotherapy* 2001; **3:** 145–64.
5. Marsh JC, Gordon-Smith EC. CAMPATH-1H in the treatment of autoimmune cytopenias. *Cytotherapy* 2001; **3:** 189–95.
6. Rebello P, *et al.* Pharmacokinetics of CAMPATH-1H in BMT patients. *Cytotherapy* 2001; **3:** 261–7.
7. Keating MJ, *et al.* Therapeutic role of alemtuzumab (Campath-1H) in patients who have failed fludarabine: results of a large international study. *Blood* 2002; **99:** 3554–61.
8. Osterborg A, *et al.* Clinical effects of alemtuzumab (Campath-1H) in B-cell chronic lymphocytic leukemia. *Med Oncol* 2002; **19** (suppl): S21–S26.
9. Dearden CE, *et al.* Alemtuzumab in T-cell malignancies. *Med Oncol* 2002; **19** (suppl): S27–S32.
10. Kennedy B, Hillmen P. Immunological effects and safe administration of alemtuzumab (MabCampath) in advanced B-cLL. *Med Oncol* 2002; **19** (suppl): S49–S55.
11. Lundin J, *et al.* Phase II trial of subcutaneous anti-CD52 monoclonal antibody alemtuzumab (Campath-1H) as first-line treatment for patients with B-cell chronic lymphocytic leukemia (B-CLL). *Blood* 2002; **100:** 768–73.
12. Hale G, *et al.* Alemtuzumab (Campath-1H) for treatment of lymphoid malignancies in the age of nonmyeloablative conditioning? *Bone Marrow Transplant* 2002; **30:** 797–804.
13. Frampton JE, Wagstaff AJ. Alemtuzumab. *Drugs* 2003; **63:** 1229–43.


### Preparations

**Proprietary Preparations** (details are given in Part 3)
***Denm.:*** MabCampath; ***Fin.:*** MabCampath; ***Fr.:*** MabCampath; ***Ger.:*** MabCampath; ***Irl.:*** MabCampath; ***Ital.:*** MabCampath; ***Port.:*** MabCampath; ***Spain:*** MabCampath; ***Swed.:*** MabCampath; ***UK:*** MabCampath; ***USA:*** Campath.

## Alitretinoin (BAN, USAN, rINN)

AGN-192013; Alitretinoína; ALRT-1057; LG-100057; LGD-1057; NSC-659772; 9-*cis*-Retinoic Acid. (2*E*,4*E*,6*Z*,8*E*)-3,7-Dimethyl-9-(2,6,6-trimethyl-1-cyclohexen-1-yl)-2,4,6,8-nonatetraenoic acid.
$C_{20}H_{28}O_2$ = 300.4.
CAS — 5300-03-8.
ATC — L01XX22.

### Profile

Alitretinoin is a retinoid related to tretinoin (p.1161). It is used topically, as a 0.1% gel, in the management of AIDS-related Kaposi's sarcoma (p.524). It is applied directly to the lesions twice daily, increasing to up to 4 times daily if tolerated. Local skin toxicity may occur, in particular erythema and oedema, and in some patients this may be dose-limiting. An oral formulation of alitretinoin is under investigation for the treatment of various malignant neoplasms.

◊ References.


1. Walmsley S, *et al.* Treatment of AIDS-related cutaneous Kaposi's sarcoma with topical alitretinoin (9-cis-retinoic acid) gel. *J Acquir Immune Defic Syndr* 1999; **22:** 235–46.
2. Cheer SM, Foster RH. Alitretinoin. *Am J Clin Dermatol* 2000; **1:** 307–14.
3. Bodsworth NJ, *et al.* Phase III vehicle-controlled, multi-centered study of topical alitretinoin gel 0.1% in cutaneous AIDS-related Kaposi's sarcoma. *Am J Clin Dermatol* 2001; **2:** 77–87.
4. Miles SA, *et al.* Antitumor activity of oral 9-cis-retinoic acid in HIV-associated Kaposi's sarcoma. *AIDS* 2002; **16:** 421–9.
5. Kurie JM, *et al.* Treatment of former smokers with 9-cis-retinoic acid reverses loss of retinoic acid receptor-beta expression in the bronchial epithelium: results from a randomized placebo-controlled trial. *J Natl Cancer Inst* 2003; **95:** 206–14.


### Preparations

**Proprietary Preparations** (details are given in Part 3)
***Canad.:*** Panretin†; ***Fr.:*** Panretin; ***USA:*** Panretin.

## Altretamine (BAN, USAN, rINN)

Altretamina; Hexamethylmelamine; HMM; NSC-13875; WR-95704. 2,4,6-Tris(dimethylamino)-1,3,5-triazine; $N^2,N^2,N^4,N^4,N^6,N^6$-Hexamethyl-1,3,5-triazine-2,4,6-triamine.
$C_9H_{18}N_6$ = 210.3.
CAS — 645-05-6.
ATC — L01XX03.

**Pharmacopoeias.** In *Chin.* and *US.*

**USP 27** (Altretamine). A white crystalline powder. Insoluble in water; soluble in chloroform. Store in airtight containers.

### Adverse Effects, Treatment, and Precautions

For a general outline see Antineoplastics, p.492, p.495, and p.497.

Bone-marrow depression is usually moderate, manifesting as leucopenia, thrombocytopenia, and anaemia, and may require dosage reduction; blood counts should be monitored regularly. Nausea and vomiting are common and usually moderate although they may be dose-limiting. Prolonged or high-dose therapy may be associated with neurotoxicity, both peripheral (neuropathies) and central (ataxia, depression, confusion, drowsiness, and hallucinations); neurological examination should be performed regularly and administration interrupted or the dose reduced as appropriate. Renal toxicity may also be dose-limiting. Other rare adverse effects include rashes, alopecia, and hepatic toxicity.

**Handling.** Altretamine is irritant; avoid contact with skin and mucous membranes.

### Interactions

For a general outline of antineoplastic drug interactions, see p.498. Pyridoxine appears to reduce the activity of altretamine.

**Antidepressants.** Severe and potentially life-threatening orthostatic hypotension developed in 3 patients who received *amitriptyline* or *imipramine* with altretamine and in a fourth patient who took *phenelzine* and altretamine concurrently.[1] One patient was able to tolerate a combination of the antineoplastic with *nortriptyline.*


1. Bruckner HW, Schleifer SJ. Orthostatic hypotension as a complication of hexamethylmelamine antidepressant interaction. *Cancer Treat Rep* 1983; **67:** 516.


### Pharmacokinetics

Altretamine is well absorbed from the gastrointestinal tract after oral doses, but is rapidly demethylated in the liver producing variation in plasma-altretamine concentrations. The principal metabolites are pentamethylmelamine and tetramethylmelamine, which are excreted in urine. The elimination half-life has been reported to be 4 to 10 hours.

◊ References.


1. Damia G, D'Incalci M. Clinical pharmacokinetics of altretamine. *Clin Pharmacokinet* 1995; **28:** 439–48.


### Uses and Administration

Altretamine is an antineoplastic agent structurally similar to the alkylating agent tretamine (triethylenemelamine) although its mode of action may be different. It is given by mouth and is licensed for use as a single agent in the palliative treatment of ovarian carcinoma (p.520). Altretamine has also been tried in lung cancer. The usual dose as a single agent in ovarian cancer is 260 mg/m$^2$ daily in four divided doses, for 14 or 21 consecutive days out of a 28-day cycle. Up to 12 cycles may be given. Therapy should be interrupted for at least 14 days, and subsequently restarted at a lower dose of 200 mg/m$^2$ daily, if the white cell count falls below 2000 cells/mm$^3$ or the platelet count below 75 000 cells/mm$^3$ or if neurotoxic or intolerable gastrointestinal symptoms occur. Lower doses are also used in combination regimens.

◊ Reviews.


1. Hansen LA, Hughes TE. Altretamine. *DICP Ann Pharmacother* 1991; **25:** 146–52.
2. Lee CR, Faulds D. Altretamine: a review of its pharmacodynamic and pharmacokinetic properties, and therapeutic potential in cancer chemotherapy. *Drugs* 1995; **49:** 932–53.
3. Manetta A, *et al.* Hexamethylmelamine as a single second-line agent in ovarian cancer: follow-up report and review of the literature. *Gynecol Oncol* 1997; **66:** 20–6.


### Preparations

***USP 27:*** Altretamine Capsules.

**Proprietary Preparations** (details are given in Part 3)
***Austral.:*** Hexalen; ***Canad.:*** Hexalen†; ***Fr.:*** Hexastat†; ***Hong Kong:*** Hexastat†; ***Israel:*** Hexalen†; ***Ital.:*** Hexastat†; ***Norw.:*** Hexalen; Hexastat†; ***NZ:*** Hexalen; ***Spain:*** Hexinawas†; ***Swed.:*** Hexalen; ***UK:*** Hexalen†; ***USA:*** Hexalen.

## Aminoglutethimide (BAN, rINN)

Aminoglutetimida; Ba-16038. 2-(4-Aminophenyl)-2-ethylglutarimide; 3-(4-Aminophenyl)-3-ethylpiperidine-2,6-dione.
$C_{13}H_{16}N_2O_2$ = 232.3.
CAS — 125-84-8.
ATC — L02BG01.

**Pharmacopoeias.** In *Chin., Eur.* (see p.vi), and *US.*

**Ph. Eur. 5.0** (Aminoglutethimide). A white or slightly yellow, crystalline powder. Practically insoluble in water; freely soluble in acetone; soluble in methyl alcohol.

**USP 27** (Aminoglutethimide). A white or creamy-white, fine, crystalline powder. Very slightly soluble in water; readily soluble in most organic solvents. It forms water-soluble salts with strong acids. The pH of a 0.1% solution in dilute methyl alcohol (1 in 20) is between 6.2 and 7.3.

### Adverse Effects

The most frequent adverse effects reported with aminoglutethimide include drowsiness, lethargy, and skin rashes (sometimes with fever); these generally diminish after the first 6 weeks of therapy. Dizziness and nausea occasionally occur. Leucopenia, thrombocytopenia, agranulocytosis, or severe pancytopenia have occurred rarely. Adrenal insufficiency may rarely occur, and there have been reports of other endocrine disturbances including hypothyroidism, and virilisation. Other rare effects include ataxia, headache, depression, gastrointestinal disturbances, hypercholesterolaemia, and orthostatic hypotension.

Overdosage may lead to CNS depression and impairment of consciousness, electrolyte disturbances, and respiratory depression.

**Effects on the liver.** Aminoglutethimide has been associated with reports of cholestatic jaundice, accompanied by rash[1,2] and fever,[2] and probably due to an idiosyncratic hypersensitivity reaction.[1] It has been suggested that liver function tests should be carried out in patients receiving aminoglutethimide who develop fever and eruptions.[2]


1. Gerber SB, Miller KB. Cholestatic jaundice and aminoglutethimide. *Ann Intern Med* 1982; **97:** 138.
2. Perrault DJ, Domovitch E. Aminoglutethimide and cholestasis. *Ann Intern Med* 1984; **100:** 160.


**Effects on the lungs.** Pulmonary infiltrates in a patient who developed progressive dyspnoea on commencing therapy with aminoglutethimide were found to be due to diffuse alveolar damage and haemorrhage; thrombocytopenia was present but prothrombin and bleeding times were normal. The patient's gas exchange and chest radiographs improved on discontinuation of aminoglutethimide and institution of corticosteroid therapy.[1]

Blood and pulmonary eosinophilia, which resolved on cessation of aminoglutethimide therapy, has also been reported.[2]

1. Rodman DM, *et al.* Aminoglutethimide, alveolar damage, and hemorrhage. *Ann Intern Med* 1986; **105:** 633.
2. Bell SC, Anderson EG. Pulmonary eosinophilia associated with aminoglutethimide. *Aust N Z J Med* 1998; **28:** 670–1.

**Lupus.** Systemic lupus erythematosus occurred in a patient who received aminoglutethimide, and resolved when the drug was withdrawn.[1] In another report, however, a patient with a lupus-like syndrome experienced a reduction in disease activity when tamoxifen therapy was changed to aminoglutethimide.[2]

1. McCraken M, *et al.* Systemic lupus erythematosus induced by aminoglutethimide. *BMJ* 1980; **281:** 1254.
2. Etherington J, *et al.* Effect of aminoglutethimide on the activity of a case of a connective tissue disorder with features of systemic lupus erythematosus. *Lupus* 1993; **2:** 387.

### Precautions

Aminoglutethimide inhibits adrenal steroid production so supplementary glucocorticoid therapy with hydrocortisone must normally be given, although supplementation may not be necessary in patients with Cushing's syndrome. Some patients also require a mineralocorticoid. It has been suggested that aminoglutethimide should be temporarily withdrawn in patients who undergo shock or trauma, or develop intercurrent infection.

Blood pressure, blood counts, and serum electrolytes should be regularly monitored during aminoglutethimide therapy and periodic monitoring of liver and thyroid function is recommended.

Aminoglutethimide should not be given during pregnancy as pseudohermaphroditism may occur in the fetus.

Aminoglutethimide frequently causes drowsiness: patients so affected should not drive or operate machinery.

**Porphyria.** Aminoglutethimide has been associated with acute attacks of porphyria and is considered unsafe in porphyric patients.

### Interactions

The rate of metabolism of some drugs is increased by aminoglutethimide; patients also taking warfarin or other coumarin anticoagulants, theophylline, tamoxifen, medroxyprogesterone, or oral hypoglycaemics, may require increased dosages of these drugs. The metabolism of dexamethasone is also accelerated, which limits its value for corticosteroid supplementation in patients receiving aminoglutethimide. Use with diuretics may lead to hyponatraemia, while alcohol may potentiate the central effects of aminoglutethimide.

◊ See also references to aminoglutethimide's interactions with *digitoxin* (p.894), *theophylline* (p.802), *progestogens* (p.1567), *tamoxifen* (p.585), and *anticoagulants* (under Warfarin, p.1025).

### Pharmacokinetics

Aminoglutethimide is well absorbed after oral doses, with peak plasma concentrations occurring after 1 to 4 hours. It is metabolised in the liver, primarily to *N*-hydroxylaminoglutethimide and *N*-acetylaminoglutethimide, and appears to induce its own metabolism. The half-life, which is reported to be about 13 hours after a single dose, is decreased to around 9 hours after about 2 weeks of continuous therapy. Aminoglutethimide is excreted in urine, about half a dose being excreted unchanged and the remainder as metabolites. Only about 20 to 25% of a dose is bound to plasma protein.

**Half-life.** A pharmacokinetic study of aminoglutethimide in 17 patients demonstrated that the plasma half-life had a mean value of 15.5 hours after single doses but fell to 8.9 hours during multiple-dose therapy.[1] This marked reduction could largely be attributed to a decrease in the volume of distribution; auto-induction of metabolism might be of less importance in decreasing half-life than had been previously suggested.

1. Lønning PE, *et al.* Single-dose and steady-state pharmacokinetics of aminoglutethimide. *Clin Pharmacokinet* 1985; **10:** 353–64.

### Uses and Administration

Aminoglutethimide is an analogue of glutethimide (p.701) and was formerly used for its weak anticonvulsant properties. Aminoglutethimide blocks the production of adrenal steroids and acts as an aromatase inhibitor to block the conversion of androgens to oestrogens (the major source of oestrogens in women without ovarian function). It has been used in the treatment of metastatic breast cancer (p.514) in postmenopausal or oophorectomised women, in doses of 250 mg up to four times daily by mouth. Aminoglutethimide has also been used in similar doses as palliative treatment in men with advanced prostatic cancer (p.521). Replacement therapy with a corticosteroid must also be given, usually hydrocortisone 20 to 30 mg daily in divided doses (see Adrenocortical Insufficiency, p.1075 for a description of corticosteroid replacement therapy).

Aminoglutethimide is used in similar or higher doses in the treatment of Cushing's syndrome (p.1313); up to 2 g daily may be needed. Corticosteroid supplementation may not be required in these patients.

The *dextro*-isomer of aminoglutethimide, dexaminoglutethimide has also been investigated.

### Preparations

***BP 2003:*** Aminoglutethimide Tablets;
***USP 27:*** Aminoglutethimide Tablets.

**Proprietary Preparations** (details are given in Part 3)
***Arg.:*** Orimeten; ***Austral.:*** Cytadren; ***Austria:*** Orimeten; ***Belg.:*** Orimeten; ***Braz.:*** Orimeten; ***Chile:*** Orimeten; ***Fr.:*** Orimetene; ***Ger.:*** Orimeten; Rodazol†; ***Hong Kong:*** Orimetene; ***Irl.:*** Orimeten†; ***Israel:*** Orimetene†; ***Ital.:*** Orimeten; ***Malaysia:*** Orimetene; ***Neth.:*** Orimeten; ***NZ:*** Cytadren; ***S.Afr.:*** Orimeten; ***Spain:*** Orimeten; ***Swed.:*** Orimeten†; ***Switz.:*** Orimetene; ***UK:*** Orimeten; ***USA:*** Cytadren.

## 5-Aminolevulinic Acid

ALA; 5-ALA; δ-Aminolaevulinic Acid; 5-Aminolaevulinic Acid; 5-Aminolevulínico, ácido. 5-Amino-4-oxopentanoic acid.

$C_5H_9NO_3$ = 131.1.
*CAS — 106-60-5.*
*ATC — L01XD04.*

### Aminolevulinic Acid Hydrochloride *(USAN)*

Aminolaevulinic Acid Hydrochloride. 5-Aminolevulinic acid hydrochloride.

$C_5H_9NO_3$, HCl = 167.6.
*CAS — 5451-09-2.*
*ATC — L01XD04.*

### Methyl Aminolevulinate Hydrochloride *(USAN)*

Methyl Aminolaevulinate Hydrochloride; P-1202. Methyl 5-amino-4-oxopentanoate hydrochloride.

$C_6H_{11}NO_3$,HCl = 181.6.
*CAS — 79416-27-6.*
*ATC — L01XD03.*

### Adverse Effects and Precautions

The mechanism of action of topical 5-aminolevulinic acid or its derivatives generally results in local phototoxicity, manifest as a localised burning or stinging sensation, erythema, oedema, pruritus, crusting, or pain. Ulceration, suppuration, blistering, erosion, or changes in skin pigmentation are common. Symptoms are usually mild to moderate, and transient. Skin infections may occur.

During treatment, patients should be advised to avoid sunlight or prolonged exposure to bright light.

**Porphyria.** 5-Aminolevulinic acid and its derivatives are considered to be unsafe in patients with porphyria.

### Interactions

**Hypericum.** A patient given oral aminolevulinic acid experienced a pronounced phototoxic reaction 6 hours later, consisting of an erythematous rash and swelling of the face, neck, and hands. She was also taking hypericum. Although both drugs have been associated with photosensitivity, the authors suggested a synergistic effect had occurred. Tests *in vitro* appeared to confirm this.[1]

1. Ladner DP, *et al.* Synergistic toxicity of δ-aminolaevulinic acid-induced protoporphyrin IX used for photodiagnosis and hypericum extract, a herbal antidepressant. *Br J Dermatol* 2001; **144:** 916–8.

### Uses and Administration

5-Aminolevulinic acid is a naturally occurring haem precursor that is metabolised in the body to protoporphyrin IX, a photosensitiser, and then to haem. It has been formulated for topical use in the photodynamic treatment (p.581) of actinic keratoses and basal cell carcinoma (see p.522). Aminolevulinic acid hydrochloride is applied topically as a 20% solution in the treatment of non-hyperkeratotic actinic keratoses of the face or scalp. This is followed, 14 to 18 hours later, by illumination with blue wavelength light sufficient to supply a dose of 10 J/cm$^2$. Treatment may be repeated once after 8 weeks if necessary.

Methyl aminolevulinate hydrochloride is a derivative of 5-aminolevulinic acid that is applied topically for the treatment of basal cell carcinoma and actinic keratoses of the face or scalp. A cream containing the equivalent of 16% methyl aminolevulinate is applied to the lesions and covered with an occlusive dressing. After 3 hours, the lesions are exposed to red wavelength light in a dose of 75 J/cm$^2$. Treatment is repeated one week later, and again after 3 months if necessary.

Patients should avoid sunlight or bright light sources for at least 40 hours after application.

◊ References to use in actinic keratoses and skin cancers.

1. Ormrod D, Jarvis B. Topical aminolevulinic acid HCl photodynamic therapy. *Am J Clin Dermatol* 2000; **1:** 133–9.
2. Jeffes EW, *et al.* Photodynamic therapy of actinic keratoses with topical aminolevulinic acid hydrochloride and fluorescent blue light. *J Am Acad Dermatol* 2001; **45:** 96–104.
3. Morton CA, *et al.* Guidelines for topical photodynamic therapy: report of a workshop of the British Photodermatology Group. *Br J Dermatol* 2002; **146:** 552–67.
4. Szeimies RM, *et al.* Photodynamic therapy using topical methyl 5-aminolevulinate compared with cryotherapy for actinic keratosis: a prospective, randomized study. *J Am Acad Dermatol* 2002; **47:** 258–62.
5. Pariser DM, *et al.* Photodynamic therapy with topical methyl aminolevulinate for actinic keratosis: results of a prospective randomized multicenter trial. *J Am Acad Dermatol* 2003; **48:** 227–32.
6. Marmur ES, *et al.* A review of laser and photodynamic therapy for the treatment of nonmelanoma skin cancer. *Dermatol Surg* 2004; **30:** 264–71.

◊ 5-Aminolevulinic acid has been used topically in the photodynamic therapy of skin conditions such as psoriasis, recalcitrant viral warts, acne vulgaris, and cutaneous T-cell lymphoma.[1] An intravesical solution has been instilled for the detection[2] and management[3] of superficial bladder cancer. A topical application of 5-aminolevulinic acid 3% has been tried in the treatment of cervical intraepithelial neoplasia, with poor response.[4]

Photodynamic therapy using *oral* 5-aminolevulinic acid as the photosensitiser, at doses of 30 or 60 mg/kg, has been used to treat Barrett's oesophagus.[5,6] It is also under investigation for the photodynamic detection and treatment of brain tumours.[7]

1. Ibbotson SH. Topical 5-aminolaevulinic acid photodynamic therapy for the treatment of skin conditions other than non-melanoma skin cancer. *Br J Dermatol* 2002; **146:** 178–88.
2. Zaak D, *et al.* Role of 5-aminolevulinic acid in the detection of urothelial premalignant lesions. *Cancer* 2002; **95:** 1234–8. Correction. *ibid.*; 2580.
3. Kriegmair M, *et al.* Early clinical experience with 5-aminolevulinic acid for the photodynamic therapy of superficial bladder cancer. *Br J Urol* 1996; **77:** 667–71.
4. Barnett AA, *et al.* A randomised, double-blind, placebo-controlled trial of photodynamic therapy using 5-aminolaevulinic acid for the treatment of cervical intraepithelial neoplasia. *Int J Cancer* 2003; **103:** 829–32.
5. Ackroyd R, *et al.* Photodynamic therapy for dysplastic Barrett's oesophagus: a prospective, double blind, randomised, placebo controlled trial. *Gut* 2000; **47:** 612–17.
6. Barr H. Barrett's esophagus: treatment with 5-aminolevulinic acid photodynamic therapy. *Gastrointest Endosc Clin N Am* 2000; **10:** 421–37.
7. Friesen SA, *et al.* 5-Aminolevulinic acid-based photodynamic detection and therapy of brain tumors (review). *Int J Oncol* 2002; **21:** 577–82.

### Preparations

**Proprietary Preparations** (details are given in Part 3)
***Swed.:*** Metvix; ***UK:*** Metvix; Porphin; ***USA:*** Levulan Kerastick.

## Amrubicin *(rINN)*

SM-5887. (+)-(7*S*,9*S*)-9-Acetyl-9-amino-7-[(2-deoxy-β-D-*erythro*-pentopyranosyl)oxy]-7,8,9,10-tetrahydro-6,11-dihydroxy-5,12-naphthacenedione.

$C_{25}H_{25}NO_9$ = 483.5.
*CAS — 110267-81-7.*

### Profile

Amrubicin is a synthetic anthracycline derivative related to compounds such as doxorubicin (p.547). It is under investigation as an antineoplastic in the treatment of lung cancers, superficial bladder cancers, and lymphomas.

## Amsacrine *(BAN, USAN, pINN)*

Acridinyl Anisidide; *m*-AMSA; Amsacrina; CI-880; NSC-249992. 4′-(Acridin-9-ylamino)methanesulphon-*m*-anisidide.

$C_{21}H_{19}N_3O_3S$ = 393.5.
*CAS — 51264-14-3.*
*ATC — L01XX01.*

**Incompatibility.** Amsacrine is incompatible with sodium chloride 0.9% injection and with other chloride-containing solutions,[1,2] apparently because of the poor solubility of the hydrochloride salt in aqueous solution.[2] Amsacrine reacts with certain plastics.[1]

1. D'Arcy PF. Reactions and interactions in handling anticancer drugs. *Drug Intell Clin Pharm* 1983; **17:** 532–8.
2. Trissel LA, *et al.* Visual compatibility of amsacrine with selected drugs during simulated Y-site injection. *Am J Hosp Pharm* 1990; **47:** 2525–8.

### Adverse Effects, Treatment, and Precautions

For a general outline see Antineoplastics, p.492, p.495, and p.497.

Bone-marrow depression is usually dose-limiting and may be severe. The nadir of the white cell count has been reported at about 12 days after treatment, with recovery usually by the 25th day. Pancytopenia and haemorrhage may occur. Nausea and vomiting (mild to moderate), stomatitis (mild to life-threatening), rashes, and alopecia may occur. Grand mal seizures, renal dysfunction, hepatotoxicity, and cardiotoxicity, have been reported. Amsacrine is irritant: there may be phlebitis and local tissue necrosis particularly with administration of high concentrations.

Amsacrine should be given with caution to patients with liver or kidney disease, who may require dosage adjustments.

### Interactions

For a general outline of antineoplastic drug interactions, see p.498. Use with diuretics or nephrotoxic drugs such as the aminoglycosides may theoretically increase the risk of cardiotoxicity with amsacrine by precipitating hypokalaemia.

#### Pharmacokinetics

Amsacrine is poorly absorbed after oral doses. When given intravenously it has a reported terminal half-life of about 5 to 8 hours. It is metabolised in the liver and excreted primarily in the bile, mostly as metabolites. It is reported to be about 98% protein bound.

#### Uses and Administration

Amsacrine is an antineoplastic agent that appears to act by intercalation with DNA and inhibition of nucleic acid synthesis. It may also exert an action on cell membranes. Cells in $G_2$ or S phases may be most sensitive to its actions.

It is used for the induction and maintenance of remission in adult acute leukaemias, particularly acute myeloid leukaemia.

Amsacrine is prepared as a solution in lactic acid and dimethylacetamide, and is given, diluted in glucose 5%, by intravenous infusion over 60 to 90 minutes.

For the induction of remission, amsacrine may be given at a dose of 90 mg/m$^2$ daily for 5 to 8 days, depending on clinical response. Courses may be repeated at 2- to 4-week intervals according to response, and the dose may be increased to 120 mg/m$^2$ daily in subsequent courses if tolerated. Maintenance doses of 150 mg/m$^2$ as a single dose or divided over 3 consecutive days have been given every 3 to 4 weeks, adjusted if necessary according to response.

Complete blood counts should be performed regularly, and cardiac, liver, kidney, and CNS function should be monitored.

Doses should be reduced in patients with hepatic or renal impairment (see below).

**Administration in hepatic impairment.** In moderate to severe hepatic impairment, dosage of amsacrine may need to be reduced by up to 50%. Some manufacturers recommend an initial reduction of 20 to 30%, to a dose between 60 and 75 mg/m$^2$ per day.

**Administration in renal impairment.** In moderate to severe renal impairment, dosage of amsacrine may need to be reduced by up to 50%. Some manufacturers recommend an initial reduction of 20 to 30%, to a dose between 60 and 75 mg/m$^2$ per day.

#### Preparations

**Proprietary Preparations** (details are given in Part 3)
***Austral.:*** Amsidyl; ***Belg.:*** Amsidine; ***Canad.:*** Amsa P-D; ***Denm.:*** Amekrin; ***Fin.:*** Amekrin; ***Fr.:*** Amsidine†; ***Ger.:*** Amsidyl; ***Irl.:*** Amsidine; ***Neth.:*** Amsidine; ***Norw.:*** Amekrin†; ***NZ:*** Amsidyl†; ***Swed.:*** Amekrin; ***Switz.:*** Amsidyl; ***UK:*** Amsidine.

## Anastrozole *(BAN, USAN, rINN)*

Anastrozol; ICI-D1033; ZD-1033. 2,2′-Dimethyl-2,2′-[5-(1*H*-1,2,4-triazol-1-ylmethyl)-1,3-phenylene]bis(propiononitrile); α,α,α′,α′-Tetramethyl-5-(1*H*-1,2,4-triazol-1-ylmethyl)-*m*-benzenediacetonitrile.
$C_{17}H_{19}N_5$ = 293.4.
*CAS — 120511-73-1.*
*ATC — L02BG03.*

### Adverse Effects and Precautions

The most frequent adverse effects are gastrointestinal disturbances including anorexia, nausea and vomiting, and diarrhoea; asthenia; hot flushes; dizziness; drowsiness; headache; and rash. Other reported effects include hair thinning, vaginal dryness or bleeding, oedema, dyspnoea, myalgia and arthralgia, bone fractures, fever, weight gain, leucopenia, and a flu-like syndrome. Abnormalities in liver enzyme values, thromboembolism, and increases in total cholesterol, have occurred in some patients receiving anastrozole. Very rare cases of erythema multiforme and Stevens-Johnson syndrome have occurred.

The use of anastrozole is contra-indicated in premenopausal women (particularly in pregnancy).

**Effects on the musculoskeletal system.** In a series of 77 postmenopausal women treated with anastrozole for metastatic breast cancer, 12 complained of joint pains within 2 months of beginning therapy. Based on this experience and the incidence of arthralgia reported during clinical trials, the authors estimated that arthralgia occurs in 10 to 15% of patients treated with anastrozole, possibly as a result of the very low oestrogen concentrations achieved.[1]

1. Donnellan PP, *et al.* Aromatase inhibitors and arthralgia. *J Clin Oncol* 2001; **19:** 2767.

### Pharmacokinetics

Anastrozole is rapidly and almost completely absorbed from the gastrointestinal tract after oral doses, with peak plasma concentrations within about 2 hours. Food decreases the rate of absorption, though this is not considered clinically significant. Anastrozole is 40% bound to plasma proteins. It is metabolised in the liver, and excreted in urine, chiefly as metabolites. The terminal elimination half-life is about 50 hours, and steady-state concentrations are achieved after about 7 days in patients receiving once-daily doses.

### Uses and Administration

Anastrozole is a potent and selective nonsteroidal inhibitor of the aromatase (oestrogen synthetase) system, which converts adrenal androgens to oestrogens in peripheral tissue. It is used in the treatment of advanced or locally advanced breast cancer, and as adjuvant treatment in early breast cancer (p.514), in postmenopausal women in a dose of 1 mg daily by mouth. Responses are unlikely in patients with oestrogen receptor-negative disease. Adjuvant therapy may be continued for up to 5 years, although the optimum duration is uncertain.

◊ References.

1. Anonymous. Anastrozole for metastatic breast cancer. *Med Lett Drugs Ther* 1996; **38:** 61–2.
2. Buzdar A, *et al.* Anastrozole, a potent and selective aromatase inhibitor, versus megestrol acetate in postmenopausal women with advanced breast cancer: results of overview analysis of two phase III trials. *J Clin Oncol* 1996; **14:** 2000–11.
3. Bonneterre J, *et al.* Anastrozole versus tamoxifen as first-line therapy for advanced breast cancer in 668 postmenopausal women: results of the Tamoxifen or Arimidex Randomized Group Efficacy and Tolerability study. *J Clin Oncol* 2000; **18:** 3748–57.
4. Nabholtz JM, *et al.* Anastrozole is superior to tamoxifen as first-line therapy for advanced breast cancer in postmenopausal women: results of a North American multicenter randomized trial. *J Clin Oncol* 2000; **18:** 3758–67.
5. The ATAC (Arimidex, Tamoxifen Alone or in Combination) trialists' group. Anastrozole alone or in combination with tamoxifen versus tamoxifen alone for adjuvant treatment of postmenopausal women with early breast cancer: first results of the ATAC randomised trial. *Lancet* 2002; **359:** 2131–9.
6. Wellington K, Faulds DM. Anastrozole in early breast cancer. *Drugs* 2002; **62:** 2483–90.
7. Baum M, *et al.* Anastrozole alone or in combination with tamoxifen versus tamoxifen alone for adjuvant treatment of postmenopausal women with early-stage breast cancer: results of the ATAC (Arimidex, Tamoxifen Alone or in Combination) trial efficacy and safety update analyses. *Cancer* 2003; **98:** 1802–10.

**Gynaecomastia.** Anastrozole is reported[1] to be under investigation for the treatment of gynaecomastia (p.1546).

1. Gruntmanis U, Braunstein GD. Treatment of gynecomastia. *Curr Opin Investig Drugs* 2001; **2:** 643–9.

### Preparations

**Proprietary Preparations** (details are given in Part 3)
***Arg.:*** Arimidex; Asiolex; Distalene; Gondonar; Lezole; Pantestone; Trozolite; ***Austral.:*** Arimidex; ***Austria:*** Arimidex; ***Belg.:*** Arimidex; ***Braz.:*** Arimidex; ***Canad.:*** Arimidex; ***Chile:*** Arimidex; Trozolet; ***Denm.:*** Arimidex; ***Fin.:*** Arimidex; ***Fr.:*** Arimidex; ***Ger.:*** Arimidex; ***Gr.:*** Arimidex; ***Hong Kong:*** Arimidex; ***Irl.:*** Arimidex; ***Israel:*** Arimidex; ***Ital.:*** Arimidex; ***Malaysia:*** Arimidex; ***Mex.:*** Arimidex; ***Neth.:*** Arimidex; ***Norw.:*** Arimidex; ***NZ:*** Arimidex; ***Port.:*** Arimidex; ***S.Afr.:*** Arimidex; ***Singapore:*** Arimidex; ***Spain:*** Arimidex; ***Swed.:*** Arimidex; ***Switz.:*** Arimidex; ***Thai.:*** Arimidex; ***UK:*** Arimidex; ***USA:*** Arimidex.

## Antineoplaston A10

3-Phenylacetylamino-2,6-piperidinedione.
$C_{13}H_{14}N_2O_3$ = 246.3.

#### Profile

Antineoplaston A10, one of a group of peptide derivatives isolated from blood and urine, has been investigated for the treatment of breast cancer and other malignant neoplasms although its value has been questioned (see below).

◊ A critical review of the antineoplastons.[1] Most work has been done with antineoplaston A10, which is insoluble in aqueous solutions, and its derivatives antineoplaston AS2.5 (phenylacetylglutamine), and antineoplaston AS2.1 (a 4:1 mixture of phenylacetic acid and phenylacetylglutamine), which have not been independently shown to be active against cancer. Nonetheless, later references[2,3] suggest that interest in the antineoplastons continues.

1. Green S. Antineoplastons: an unproved cancer therapy. *JAMA* 1992; **267:** 2924–8.
2. Buckner JC, *et al.* Phase II study of antineoplastons A10 (NSC 648539) and AS2-1 (NSC 620261) in patients with recurrent glioma. *Mayo Clin Proc* 1999; **74:** 137–45.
3. Badria F, *et al.* Immune modulatory potentials of antineoplaston A-10 in breast cancer patients. *Cancer Lett* 2000; **157:** 57–63.

## AP-12009

TGF-β2 antisense oligonucleotide; Transforming growth factor-β2-specific phosphorothioate antisense oligodeoxynucleotide.

#### Profile

AP-12009 is an antisense oligonucleotide that specifically suppresses the production of transforming growth factor-beta-2, an immunosuppressive protein produced by tumour cells. It is under investigation for the treatment of high-grade glioma (p.513).

## Asparaginase *(USAN)*

Asparaginasa; L-Asparaginase; L-Asparagine Amidohydrolase; MK-965; NSC-109229; Re-82-TAD-15.
*CAS — 9015-68-3.*
*ATC — L01XX02.*

NOTE. Colaspase and crisantaspase are *BAN* for asparaginase obtained from cultures of *Escherichia coli* and *Erwinia chrysanthemi* (*E. carotovora*) respectively.

**Pharmacopoeias.** In *Chin.*

**Incompatibility.** Asparaginase is incompatible with rubber. The manufacturers recommend that it should not be mixed with other drugs.

**Storage.** Asparaginase should be stored at 2° to 8° (see also Stability, below).

### Pegaspargase *(USAN, rINN)*

PEG-L-asparaginase; Pegaspargasa. A conjugate of colaspase with a polyethylene glycol of molecular weight 5000; Monomethoxypolyethylene glycol succinimidyl L-asparaginase.
*CAS — 130167-69-0.*
*ATC — L01XX24.*

**Stability.** Although asparaginase was routinely kept under refrigeration,[1] information from a manufacturer (Merck Sharp & Dohme) indicated that it would remain stable for 48 hours at 15° to 30°. The manufacturer of pegaspargase states it should not be used if stored at room temperature for more than 48 hours.

1. Vogenberg FR, Souney PF. Stability guidelines for routinely refrigerated drug products. *Am J Hosp Pharm* 1983; **40:** 101–2.

**Storage.** Pegaspargase should be stored at 2° to 8°.

### Units

One unit of asparaginase splits 1 micromole of ammonia from L-asparagine in 1 minute under standard conditions.

### Adverse Effects

Asparaginase is a protein and may produce anaphylaxis and other hypersensitivity reactions including fever, rashes, and bronchospasm; there does not appear to be cross-sensitivity between asparaginase derived from *Escherichia coli* and that from *Erwinia chrysanthemi.* Hypersensitivity to pegaspargase is less common, but about 30% of patients hypersensitive to the native enzyme experience hypersensitivity to pegaspargase treatment.

Liver function abnormalities occur in many patients, and there may be decreased blood concentrations of fibrinogen and clotting factors, alterations in blood lipids and cholesterol, and hypoalbuminaemia. Hyperammonaemia, due to the production of ammonia from asparagine, may occur. Uraemia, and occasionally renal failure, have been reported. Pancreatitis may occur and may be fatal: there may also be hyperglycaemia due to decreased insulin production, and death from ketoacidosis has occurred.

Gastrointestinal disturbances, including nausea and vomiting, and CNS disturbances, including drowsiness, depression, coma, hallucinations, and a Parkinson-like syndrome, have also been reported. Transient bone-marrow depression has occurred rarely, as has marked leucopenia.

**Effects on the blood.** Central thrombosis or intracranial haemorrhage as well as peripheral thrombosis and haemorrhage have been reported following asparaginase therapy.[1-4] Although the precise mechanism for this effect remains unclear, asparaginase appears to deplete certain clotting factors as well as antithrombin III, plasminogen, and fibrinogen.[4] These decreases may be dependent on the formulation and resultant asparaginase activity of preparations,[5] and there is some suggestion that *Erwinia chrysanthemi* asparaginase may affect coagulation factors less severely than that of *Escherichia coli* origin.[6] A multicentre, retrospective survey[3] of paediatric patients with acute lymphoblastic leukaemia found that concurrent use of corticosteroids and *E. coli* asparaginase may be an additional risk factor for thromboembolic events.

1. Priest JR, *et al.* A syndrome of thrombosis and hemorrhage complicating L-asparaginase therapy for childhood acute lymphoblastic leukemia. *J Pediatr* 1982; **100:** 984–9.
2. Ott N, *et al.* Sequelae of thrombotic or hemorrhagic complications following L-asparaginase therapy for childhood lymphoblastic leukemia. *Am J Pediatr Hematol Oncol* 1988; **10:** 191–5.
3. Sutor AH, *et al.* Bleeding and thrombosis in children with acute lymphoblastic leukemia, treated according to the ALL-BFM-90 protocol. *Klin Padiatr* 1999; **211:** 201–4.
4. Alberts SR, *et al.* Thrombosis related to the use of L-asparaginase in adults with acute lymphoblastic leukemia: a need to consider coagulation monitoring and clotting factor replacement. *Leuk Lymphoma* 1999; **32:** 489–96.

5. Nowak-Göttl U, *et al.* Influence of two different Escherichia coli asparaginase preparations on fibrinolytic proteins in childhood ALL. *Haematologica* 1996; **81:** 127–31.
6. Carlsson H, *et al.* Effects of Erwinia-asparaginase on the coagulation system. *Eur J Haematol* 1995; **55:** 289–93.

### Precautions

Asparaginase is contra-indicated in patients with pancreatitis, and should be avoided in pregnancy. It should be given cautiously to patients with hepatic impairment. Facilities for the management of anaphylaxis (see p.855) should be available during treatment. Some manufacturers recommend an intradermal test dose at the start of asparaginase treatment to check for hypersensitivity, as described under Uses, below, although such tests may not always be predictive. Re-treatment with asparaginase may be associated with an increased risk of allergic reactions. Serum amylase concentrations should be monitored regularly as should blood glucose concentrations. Asparaginase has been reported to interfere with tests of thyroid function by transient reduction of concentrations of thyroxine-binding globulin.

### Interactions

If asparaginase is given before, rather than after, methotrexate the activity of the latter may be reduced (see below). Vincristine neurotoxicity may possibly be increased by use with intravenous asparaginase (see p.593).

**Methotrexate.** Asparaginase inhibits protein synthesis and cell replication, and therefore may interfere with the action of drugs such as methotrexate that require cell replication for their antineoplastic effect.[1] It has been suggested that a 24-hour interval between methotrexate and a subsequent dose of asparaginase permits at least an additive therapeutic effect.[2]

1. Jolivet J, *et al.* Prevention of methotrexate cytotoxicity by asparaginase inhibition of methotrexate polyglutamate formation. *Cancer Res* 1985; **45:** 217–20.
2. Capizzi RL. Asparaginase-methotrexate in combination chemotherapy: schedule-dependent differential effects on normal versus neoplastic cells. *Cancer Treat Rep* 1981; **65** (suppl 4): 115–21.

### Pharmacokinetics

Following intravenous injection the plasma half-life of the native enzyme has varied from about 8 to 30 hours; half-lives of up to 49 hours may be seen after intramuscular dosage. The mean half-life of pegaspargase is reported to be between 6 and 14 days. Asparaginase is found in the lymph at about 20% of the concentration in plasma. There is virtually no diffusion into the CSF. Little is excreted in the urine.

### Uses and Administration

Asparaginase is an enzyme which acts by breaking down the amino acid L-asparagine to aspartic acid and ammonia. It interferes with the growth of those malignant cells which, unlike most healthy cells, are unable to synthesise L-asparagine for their metabolism, but resistance to its action develops fairly rapidly. Its action is reportedly specific for the $G_1$ phase of the cell cycle.

Asparaginase is used mainly for the induction of remissions in acute lymphoblastic leukaemia (p.506). Regimens vary but it may be given intravenously in a dose of 1000 units/kg daily for 10 days following treatment with vincristine and prednisone or prednisolone, or intramuscularly in a dose of 6000 units/$m^2$ given every third day for 9 doses during treatment with vincristine and prednisone or prednisolone. Alternatively, in patients hypersensitive to the native enzyme it may be given as pegaspargase, in doses of 2500 units/$m^2$ every 14 days, preferably by intramuscular injection although the intravenous route may also be used. In patients with a body-surface less than 0.6 $m^2$ a dose of 82.5 units/kg of pegaspargase, given every 14 days, has been recommended.

Asparaginase is not generally used alone as an induction agent but doses of 200 units/kg daily have been given intravenously for 28 days to adults and children. If pegaspargase is used alone doses are the same as for combination regimens. Children appear to tolerate asparaginase better than adults.

Although not entirely reliable, an intradermal test dose of about 2 units has been recommended in the USA, to test for hypersensitivity, before treatment with asparaginase or where more than a week has elapsed between doses. Desensitisation has been advocated if no alternative antineoplastic treatment is available. The incidence of hypersensitivity is lower in patients given pegaspargase, and a test dose is not advocated.

When administered intravenously a solution of asparaginase in Water for Injections or sodium chloride 0.9% should be given over not less than 30 minutes through a running infusion of sodium chloride 0.9% or glucose 5%. When given intramuscularly no more than 2 mL of a solution in sodium chloride 0.9% should be injected at a single site.

◊ References.

1. Muller HJ, Boos J. Use of L-asparaginase in childhood ALL. *Crit Rev Oncol Hematol* 1998; **28:** 97–113.
2. Asselin BL. The three asparaginases: comparative pharmacology and optimal use in childhood leukemia. *Adv Exp Med Biol* 1999; **457:** 621–9.
3. Abshire TC, *et al.* Weekly polyethylene glycol conjugated L-asparaginase compared with biweekly dosing produces superior induction remission rates in childhood relapsed acute lymphoblastic leukemia: a Pediatric Oncology Group study. *Blood* 2000; **96:** 1709–15.

### Preparations

**Proprietary Preparations** (details are given in Part 3)
***Arg.:*** Kidrolase; L-Asp; ***Austral.:*** Leunase; ***Belg.:*** Paronal; ***Braz.:*** Elspar; ***Canad.:*** Kidrolase; Oncaspar; ***Denm.:*** Erwinase; ***Fin.:*** Erwinase; ***Fr.:*** Kidrolase; ***Ger.:*** Erwinase; Oncaspar; ***Gr.:*** Erwinase; ***Hong Kong:*** Elspar; Leunase; ***India:*** Leunase; ***Irl.:*** Erwinase; ***Israel:*** Kidrolase; ***Ital.:*** Crasnitin†; ***Jpn:*** Leunase; ***Malaysia:*** Erwinase; Leunase; ***Mex.:*** Leunase; Serasa†; ***NZ:*** Erwinase; Leunase; ***S.Afr.:*** Laspar; ***Singapore:*** Erwinase; Leunase; ***Swed.:*** Erwinase; ***Thai.:*** Erwinase; Leunase; ***UK:*** Erwinase; ***USA:*** Elspar; Oncaspar.

---

## Azacitidine *(USAN, rINN)*

Azacitidina; 5-Azacytidine; Ladakamycin; NSC-102816; U-18496. 4-Amino-1-β-D-ribofuranosyl-1,3,5-triazin-2(1*H*)-one.

$C_8H_{12}N_4O_5$ = 244.2.

*CAS — 320-67-2.*

### Profile

Azacitidine is an antimetabolite antineoplastic with general properties similar to those of cytarabine (p.543). It also inhibits cellular pyrimidine synthesis. It has been used in the treatment of acute myeloid leukaemia (p.506). Azacitidine is used in myelodysplastic syndromes (p.508) in a dose of 75 mg/$m^2$ subcutaneously daily for 7 days, in 4-week cycles. If there is no benefit after 2 cycles, and no toxicity other than nausea and vomiting has occurred, the dose may be increased to 100 mg/$m^2$ daily. Treatment for at least 4 cycles is usually needed.

Azacitidine causes anaemia, neutropenia, and thrombocytopenia, and complete blood counts should be monitored. It also commonly causes erythema at the injection site, fever, and gastrointestinal disturbances including nausea and vomiting, diarrhoea or constipation. Azacitidine is contra-indicated in patients with advanced hepatic malignancies, because of rare reports of progressive hepatic coma and death in such patents. It should be used with caution in renal impairment (see below).

◊ References.

1. Silverman LR, *et al.* Randomized controlled trial of azacitidine in patients with the myelodysplastic syndrome: a study of the cancer and leukemia group B. *J Clin Oncol* 2002; **20:** 2429–40.
2. Kornblith AB, *et al.* Impact of azacytidine on the quality of life of patients with myelodysplastic syndrome treated in a randomized phase III trial: a Cancer and Leukemia Group B study. *J Clin Oncol* 2002; **20:** 2441–52.

**Administration in renal impairment.** Adverse renal effects of azacitidine include abnormalities in renal-function tests, renal tubular acidosis, and renal failure. The manufacturers recommend that if serum-bicarbonate concentrations fall to below 20 mEq/litre, the dose of azacitidine should be halved for the next course. If there are rises in serum concentrations of urea or creatinine, the next cycle of azacitidine should be delayed until these return to normal or baseline, and the dose should be halved.

### Preparations

**Proprietary Preparations** (details are given in Part 3)
***USA:*** Vidaza.

---

## Batimastat *(BAN, USAN, rINN)*

BB-94. (2*S*,3*R*)-5-Methyl-3-{[(α*S*)-α-(methylcarbamoyl)phenethyl]carbamoyl}-2-[(2-thienylthio)methyl]hexanohydroxamic acid; (2*S*,3*R*)-*N*[1]-Hydroxy-3-isobutyl-*N*[4]-[(*S*)-α-(methylcarbamoyl)phenethyl]-2-(2-thienylthiomethyl)succinamide.

$C_{23}H_{31}N_3O_4S_2$ = 477.6.

*CAS — 130370-60-4.*

### Profile

Batimastat is an inhibitor of matrix metalloproteinases, enzymes which are thought to play a role in the metastasis of cancer cells. It has been investigated in a variety of malignant disorders but development was subsequently abandoned. Preliminary studies of a batimastat-releasing stent for the reduction of restenosis after coronary angioplasty failed to show any benefit.

---

## Bendamustine Hydrochloride *(rINNM)*

IMET-3393. 5-[Bis(2-chloroethyl)amino]-1-methyl-2-benzimidazolebutyric acid hydrochloride.

$C_{16}H_{21}Cl_2N_3O_2$, HCl = 394.7.

*CAS — 16506-27-7 (bendamustine); 3543-75-7 (bendamustine hydrochloride).*

### Profile

Bendamustine is an antineoplastic alkylating agent. It is given intravenously as the hydrochloride in lymphomas, including Hodgkin's disease, chronic lymphocytic leukaemia, multiple myeloma, and breast cancer.

◊ References.

1. Barman Balfour JA, Goa KL. Bendamustine. *Drugs* 2001; **61:** 631–8.

### Preparations

**Proprietary Preparations** (details are given in Part 3)
***Ger.:*** Ribomustin.

---

## Bevacizumab *(rINN)*

*CAS — 216974-75-3.*

### Profile

Bevacizumab is a recombinant humanised monoclonal antibody that binds to vascular endothelial growth factor (VEGF), thereby inhibiting the angiogenesis that occurs during tumour growth. Bevacizumab is used with fluorouracil-based chemotherapy in the treatment of metastatic colorectal cancer (p.516); a dose of 5 mg/kg once every 14 days is given in a solution of 100 mL of sodium chloride 0.9%. The first dose should be given as an intravenous infusion over 90 minutes; if this is well tolerated the second dose should be given over 60 minutes, and if this is well tolerated then subsequent doses may be given over 30 minutes.

Bevacizumab may impair wound healing; therapy should be stopped at least several weeks before elective surgery, and should not be restarted until the surgical incision is fully healed. It should be stopped permanently in patients who develop gastrointestinal perforation, wound dehiscence needing medical intervention, serious bleeding, nephrotic syndrome, or hypertensive crisis. Bevacizumab may cause congestive heart failure.

### Preparations

**Proprietary Preparations** (details are given in Part 3)
***USA:*** Avastin.

---

## Bexarotene *(BAN, USAN, rINN)*

Bexaroteno; LG-100069; LGD-1069. *p*-[1-(5,6,7,8-Tetrahydro-3,5,5,8,8-pentamethyl-2-naphthyl)vinyl]benzoic acid.

$C_{24}H_{28}O_2$ = 348.5.

*CAS — 153559-49-0.*
*ATC — L01XX25.*

### Adverse Effects and Precautions

The main adverse effects noted after oral therapy with bexarotene include hyperlipidaemia, hypothyroidism, leucopenia, headache, oedema, altered liver function, rash, and pruritus. Exfoliative dermatitis, alopecia, and skin disorders may occur. Other common adverse effects include anaemia, insomnia, dizziness, eye or ear disorders, gastrointestinal disturbances, arthralgia, and myalgia. Acute pancreatitis has been associated with hypertriglyceridaemia, and patients with risk factors for pancreatitis should generally not be given bexarotene. If triglyceride concentrations rise during therapy, dose reductions are recommended, and lipid-lowering therapy may be instituted (with the exception of gemfibrozil, see below). The most common adverse events associated with topical therapy are rash, pruritus, and pain. Bexarotene capsules and gel should not be used during pregnancy because of the risk of fetal malformation.

### Interactions

**Gemfibrozil.** Gemfibrozil inhibits clearance of bexarotene, resulting in extremely high triglyceride levels and pancreatitis.[1]

1. Talpur R, *et al.* Optimizing bexarotene therapy for cutaneous T-cell lymphoma. *J Am Acad Dermatol* 2002; **47:** 672–84.

### Uses and Administration

Bexarotene is an agonist at the retinoid X receptor, which is involved in the regulation of cell differentiation and proliferation. It is used in the treatment of cutaneous T-cell lymphoma (see Mycosis Fungoides, p.511), in a usual dose of 300 mg/$m^2$ daily by mouth, adjusted according to toxicity. For the topical treatment of refractory disease a 1% gel may be applied on alternate days for the first week, gradually increased to up to 4 times daily, depending on tolerance.

◊ References.

1. Anonymous. Bexarotene (Targretin) for cutaneous T-cell lymphoma. *Med Lett Drugs Ther* 2000; **42:** 31–2.
2. Lowe MN, Plosker GL. Bexarotene. *Am J Clin Dermatol* 2000; **1:** 245–50.

3. Duvic M, *et al.* Bexarotene is effective and safe for treatment of refractory advanced-stage cutaneous T-cell lymphoma: multinational phase II-III trial results. *J Clin Oncol* 2001; **19:** 2456–71.
4. Wong S-F. Oral bexarotene in the treatment of cutaneous T-cell lymphoma. *Ann Pharmacother* 2001; **35:** 1056–65.
5. Heald P, *et al.* Topical bexarotene therapy for patients with refractory or persistent early-stage cutaneous T-cell lymphoma: results of the phase III clinical trial. *J Am Acad Dermatol* 2003; **49:** 801–15.

### Preparations

**Proprietary Preparations** (details are given in Part 3)
***Irl.:*** Targretin; ***Spain:*** Targretin; ***UK:*** Targretin; ***USA:*** Targretin.

## Bicalutamide *(BAN, USAN, rINN)*

Bicalutamida; ICI-176334. (*RS*)-4′-Cyano-α′,α′,α′-trifluoro-3-(4-fluorophenylsulphonyl)-2-hydroxy-2-methylpropiono-*m*-toluidide.

$C_{18}H_{14}F_4N_2O_4S$ = 430.4.
*CAS — 90357-06-5.*
*ATC — L02BB03.*

### Adverse Effects and Precautions

As for Flutamide, p.556.

Cardiovascular effects including angina, heart failure, arrhythmias, and ECG changes have been reported rarely. Interstitial pneumonitis and pulmonary fibrosis have also been reported rarely.

**Effects on the gastrointestinal tract.** There is some evidence that bicalutamide is associated with a lower incidence of diarrhoea than flutamide.[1]

1. Schellhammer P, *et al.* A controlled trial of bicalutamide versus flutamide, each in combination with luteinizing hormone-releasing hormone analogue therapy, in patients with advanced prostate cancer. *Urology* 1995; **45:** 745–52.

### Interactions

Bicalutamide inhibits various cytochrome P450 isoenzymes, particularly CYP3A4, *in vitro*, and the manufacturer recommends that terfenadine, astemizole, and cisapride should not be given with bicalutamide, and that other drugs with a narrow therapeutic index that are metabolised by cytochrome P450 isoenzymes should be used with caution.

### Pharmacokinetics

Bicalutamide is well absorbed after oral doses. It undergoes extensive metabolism in the liver, the active *R*-enantiomer predominantly by oxidation, the inactive *S*-enantiomer primarily by glucuronidation. It is excreted as metabolites in urine and faeces. The half-life of the *R*-enantiomer is about 6 to 7 days, and may be prolonged still further in severe hepatic impairment. The *S*-enantiomer is cleared more rapidly. Bicalutamide is about 96% bound to plasma proteins.

### Uses and Administration

Bicalutamide is a nonsteroidal anti-androgen with actions and uses similar to those of flutamide (p.557). It is used by mouth in the treatment of prostatic cancer (p.521). When used with a gonadorelin analogue in the palliative treatment of advanced prostatic cancer the usual dose is 50 mg daily. In the UK treatment is started at least 3 days before commencing the gonadorelin analogue to suppress any flare reaction, but in the USA treatment is started at the same time. A similar dose is used with surgical castration, starting on the same day as surgery.

Bicalutamide in a dose of 150 mg daily may be given as monotherapy or adjuvant therapy to surgery or radiotherapy in men with locally advanced disease. It has been used as monotherapy in localised disease, but there is some evidence to suggest that in men without high risk of disease progression, who would otherwise be managed with watchful waiting, the immediate use of bicalutamide may increase the risk of death.

◊ References.

1. Schellhammer P, *et al.* A controlled trial of bicalutamide versus flutamide, each in combination with luteinizing hormone-releasing hormone analogue therapy, in patients with advanced prostate cancer. *Urology* 1995; **45:** 745–52.
2. Anonymous. Bicalutamide for prostate cancer. *Med Lett Drugs Ther* 1996; **38:** 56–7.
3. Schellhammer PF, *et al.* Clinical benefits of bicalutamide compared with flutamide in combined androgen blockade for patients with advanced prostatic carcinoma: final report of a double-blind, randomized, multicenter trial. *Urology* 1997; **50:** 330–6.
4. Iversen P, *et al.* Casodex (bicalutamide) 150-mg monotherapy compared with castration in patients with previously untreated nonmetastatic prostate cancer: results from two multicenter randomized trials at a median follow-up of 4 years. *Urology* 1998; **51:** 389–96.
5. Goa KL, Spencer CM. Bicalutamide in advanced prostate cancer: a review. *Drugs Aging* 1998; **12:** 401–22.
6. Tyrrell CJ, *et al.* A randomised comparison of 'Casodex' (bicalutamide) 150 mg monotherapy versus castration in the treatment of metastatic and locally advanced prostate cancer. *Eur Urol* 1998; **33:** 447–56.
7. Wirth M, *et al.* Bicalutamide (Casodex) 150 mg as immediate therapy in patients with localized or locally advanced prostate cancer significantly reduces the risk of disease progression. *Urology* 2001; **58:** 146–51.
8. Carswell CI, Figgitt DP. Bicalutamide in early-stage prostate cancer. *Drugs* 2002; **62:** 2471–9.

### Preparations

**Proprietary Preparations** (details are given in Part 3)
***Arg.:*** Androxinon; Bicaprost; Bidrostat; Bosconar; Casodex; Gepeprostin; Imda; Liberprost; Raffolutil; ***Austral.:*** Cosudex; ***Austria:*** Casodex; ***Belg.:*** Casodex; ***Braz.:*** Casodex; ***Canad.:*** Casodex; ***Chile:*** Casodex; Lutamidal; ***Denm.:*** Casodex; ***Fin.:*** Casodex; ***Fr.:*** Casodex; ***Ger.:*** Casodex; ***Gr.:*** Casodex; ***Hong Kong:*** Casodex; ***Irl.:*** Casodex; ***Israel:*** Casodex; ***Ital.:*** Casodex; ***Malaysia:*** Casodex; ***Mex.:*** Casodex; ***Neth.:*** Casodex; ***Norw.:*** Casodex; ***NZ:*** Cosudex; ***Port.:*** Casodex; ***S.Afr.:*** Casodex; ***Singapore:*** Casodex; ***Spain:*** Casodex; ***Swed.:*** Casodex; ***Switz.:*** Casodex; ***Thai.:*** Casodex; ***UK:*** Casodex; ***USA:*** Casodex.

## Bisantrene Hydrochloride *(USAN, rINNM)*

ADAH; ADCA; CL-216942; Hidrocloruro de bisantreno; NSC-337766; Orange Crush. 9,10-Anthracenedicarboxaldehyde bis-(2-imidazolin-2-ylhydrazone) dihydrochloride.

$C_{22}H_{22}N_8,2HCl$ = 471.4.
*CAS — 78186-34-2 (bisantrene); 71439-68-4 (bisantrene hydrochloride).*

### Profile

Bisantrene is a cell-cycle non-specific antineoplastic agent that is believed to act by intercalation with DNA. It has been used as the hydrochloride in the treatment of acute myeloid leukaemias relapsed or refractory to other therapy.

## Bleomycin Sulfate *(USAN, pINNM)*

Bleomycin Sulphate *(BANM)*; Bleomycini Sulfas; Sulfato de bleomicina.

*CAS — 11056-06-7 (bleomycin); 67763-87-5 (bleomycin hydrochloride); 9041-93-4 (bleomycin sulfate).*
*ATC — L01DC01.*

**Pharmacopoeias.** In *Eur.* (see p.vi), *Int., Jpn,* and *US.*
*Int.* and *Jpn* also include Bleomycin Hydrochloride. *Chin.* includes Bleomycin A5 Hydrochloride for Injection.

**Ph. Eur. 5.0** (Bleomycin Sulphate). The sulfate of a mixture of glycopeptides obtained by the growth of *Streptomyces verticillus* or by any other means; the two principal components of the mixture are $N^1$-[3-(dimethylsulphonio)propyl]bleomycinamide (bleomycin $A_2$) and $N^1$-4-(guanidobutyl)bleomycinamide (bleomycin $B_2$). A white or yellowish-white, very hygroscopic powder. It loses not more than 3% of its weight when dried. Very soluble in water; slightly soluble in dehydrated alcohol; practically insoluble in acetone. A 0.5% solution in water has a pH of 4.5 to 6.0. Store in airtight containers at a temperature of 2° to 8°.

**USP 27** (Bleomycin Sulfate). The sulfate salt of a mixture of basic cytotoxic glycopeptides, produced by the growth of *Streptomyces verticillus* or produced by other means. It has a potency of not less than 1.5 units and not more than 2.0 units/mg. It contains between 55 and 70% of bleomycin $A_2$ and between 25 and 32% of bleomycin $B_2$; the content of bleomycin $B_4$ is not more than 1%. The combined percentage of bleomycin $A_2$ and $B_2$ is not less than 90%. A cream-coloured, amorphous powder. It loses not more than 6% of its weight when dried. Very soluble in water. A solution in water containing 10 units/mL has a pH of 4.5 to 6.0. Store in airtight containers.

**Incompatibility.** A loss of bleomycin activity was reported when bleomycin sulfate solutions were mixed with solutions of carbenicillin, cefazolin or cefalotin sodium, nafcillin sodium, benzylpenicillin sodium, methotrexate, mitomycin, hydrocortisone sodium succinate, aminophylline, ascorbic acid, or terbutaline.[1] The interactions of bleomycin have been summarised as the chelation of divalent and trivalent cations (especially copper), inactivation by compounds containing sulfhydryl groups, and precipitation by hydrophobic anions; solutions of bleomycin should not be mixed with solutions of essential amino acids, riboflavin, dexamethasone, or furosemide.[2]

1. Dorr RT, *et al.* Bleomycin compatibility with selected intravenous medications. *J Med* 1982; **13:** 121–30.
2. D'Arcy PF. Reactions and interactions in handling anticancer drugs. *Drug Intell Clin Pharm* 1983; **17:** 532–8.

**Stability.** The UK manufacturers of bleomycin sulfate state that it should be protected from light.

Bleomycin sulfate solutions appear to be equally stable in plastic or glass,[1,2] despite some earlier studies suggesting loss of potency in plastic.[3,4] There is some evidence[5] that bleomycin is more stable in sodium chloride 0.9% than glucose 5%, and sodium chloride 0.9% is the diluent recommended by the manufacturer.

1. De Vroe C, *et al.* A study on the stability of three antineoplastic drugs and on their sorption by iv delivery systems and end-line filters. *Int J Pharmaceutics* 1990; **65:** 49–56.
2. Stajich GV, *et al.* In vitro evaluation of bleomycin-induced cell lethality from plastic and glass containers. *DICP Ann Pharmacother* 1991; **25:** 14–16.
3. Benvenuto JA, *et al.* Stability and compatibility of antitumor agents in glass and plastic containers. *Am J Hosp Pharm* 1981; **38:** 1914–18.
4. Adams J, *et al.* Instability of bleomycin in plastic containers. *Am J Hosp Pharm* 1982; **39:** 1636.
5. Koberda M, *et al.* Stability of bleomycin sulfate reconstituted in 5% dextrose injection or 0.9% sodium chloride injection stored in glass vials or polyvinyl chloride containers. *Am J Hosp Pharm* 1990; **47:** 2528–9.

### Units

8910 units of bleomycin complex $A_2/B_2$ are contained in 5 mg of bleomycin complex in one ampoule of the first International Reference Preparation (1980). The Ph. Eur. 5.0 specifies a potency of not less than 1500 international units per mg, calculated with reference to the dried substance. These units differ from those used by the USP: Bleomycin Sulfate (USP 27) contains 1.5 to 2.0 units of bleomycin in each mg. A change in the labelling of preparations in the UK, from units equivalent to those of the USP to international units in line with the Ph. Eur., resulted in an apparent but artefactual increase in UK doses by a factor of 1000.

In some countries doses were *formerly* described in terms of mg-potency, where 1 mg-potency corresponded to 1 unit. In the original preparation 1 mg-potency was equivalent to 1 mg-weight but improvements in purification of the product led to a situation in which ampoules labelled as containing 15 mg (i.e. 15 units) contained far fewer mg-weight of bleomycin.

### Adverse Effects and Treatment

For a general outline see Antineoplastics, p.492 and p.495.

The most frequent side-effects with bleomycin involve the skin and mucous membranes and include rash, erythema, pruritus, vesiculation, hyperkeratosis, nail changes, alopecia, hyperpigmentation, striae, and stomatitis. Fever is also common, and acute anaphylactoid reactions with hyperpyrexia and cardiorespiratory collapse have been reported in about 1% of patients with lymphoma. There is little depression of the bone marrow. Local reactions and thrombophlebitis may occur at the site of parenteral administration.

The most serious delayed effect is pulmonary toxicity; interstitial pneumonitis occurs in about 10% of patients and progresses to fibrosis and death in about 1% of patients treated with bleomycin (see also Effects on the Lungs, p.494). Pulmonary toxicity is more likely in elderly patients and those given total doses greater than 400 000 international units (400 USP units). It is also more likely in patients who have had previous radiotherapy to the chest. For the suggestion that pulmonary toxicity may be potentiated by cisplatin or colony-stimulating factors, see under Interactions, below.

**Effects on the nails.** Permanent nail loss and nail loss followed by regrowth with dystrophy have been reported following intralesional injection of bleomycin for periungual warts.[1-3] In 2 cases this was preceded by blistering and ulceration,[1] or swelling, severe pain, and a burning sensation.[2] All 3 patients had received injections on one or two previous occasions when 2 patients had reported only mild pain.[1,3] One patient also developed Raynaud's phenomenon in one finger.[1]

1. Czarnecki D. Bleomycin and periungual warts. *Med J Aust* 1984; **141:** 40.
2. Miller RAW. Nail dystrophy following intralesional injections of bleomycin for a periungual wart. *Arch Dermatol* 1984; **120:** 963–4.
3. Urbina González F, *et al.* Cutaneous toxicity of intralesional bleomycin administration in the treatment of periungual warts. *Arch Dermatol* 1986; **122:** 974–5.

**Effects on the vascular system.** Although thromboembolic disorders and Raynaud's syndrome have been associated with use of bleomycin in combination regimens, particularly with cisplatin and the vinca alkaloids or etoposide (see Effects on the Cardiovascular System, p.493) there is some evidence for an association of Raynaud's syndrome with the use of bleomycin alone.[1,2]

There have also been cases of Raynaud's phenomenon reported after intralesional injection of bleomycin for treatment of warts on the hands and feet.[3-6] See also Effects on the Nails, above.

1. Sundstrup B. Raynaud's phenomenon after bleomycin treatment. *Med J Aust* 1978; **2:** 266.

2. Adoue D, Arlet P. Bleomycin and Raynaud's phenomenon. *Ann Intern Med* 1984; **100:** 770.
3. Epstein E. Intralesional bleomycin and Raynaud's phenomenon. *J Am Acad Dermatol* 1991; **24:** 785–6.
4. Gregg LJ. Intralesional bleomycin and Raynaud's phenomenon. *J Am Acad Dermatol* 1992; **26:** 279–80.
5. de Pablo P, *et al.* Raynaud's phenomenon and intralesional bleomycin. *Acta Derm Venereol (Stockh)* 1992; **72:** 465.
6. Vanhooteghem O, *et al.* Raynaud phenomenon after treatment of verruca vulgaris of the sole with intralesional injection of bleomycin. *Pediatr Dermatol* 2001; **18:** 249–51.

## Precautions

For reference to the precautions necessary with antineoplastics, see p.497.

Bleomycin should be used with caution in the elderly, in patients with renal impairment or pulmonary infection or pre-existing impairment of pulmonary function, and in those who have received radiotherapy, particularly to the thorax. Patients should undergo regular chest X-rays. If these show infiltrates, or if basal lung crepitations occur, bleomycin should be stopped.

In view of the risk of an anaphylactoid reaction it has been suggested that patients with lymphomas should receive two test doses of 2000 international units (2 USP units) or less initially.

**AIDS.** Cutaneous adverse effects occurred in 12 of 50 patients being treated with bleomycin for AIDS-associated Kaposi's sarcoma and increased in severity until bleomycin was withdrawn.[1] Bleomycin should be stopped in people with AIDS if cutaneous side-effects are seen, and rechallenge should be avoided. However, the incidence of side-effects did not appear to be higher in these patients than in cancer patients, and patients with AIDS seem to be less sensitive to bleomycin than to antibacterials such as co-trimoxazole and penicillins.

1. Caumes E, *et al.* Cutaneous side-effects of bleomycin in AIDS patients with Kaposi's sarcoma. *Lancet* 1990; **336:** 1593.

**Diving.** Since the partial pressure of oxygen in the inspired air of a scuba diver increases with increasing depth, a theoretical possibility exists of a toxic [pulmonary] reaction to oxygen in bleomycin-treated patients who subsequently go diving, and such a risk would increase with the depth and duration of each dive.[1]

1. Zanetti CL. Scuba diving and bleomycin therapy. *JAMA* 1990; **264:** 2869.

**Handling and disposal.** *Urine* produced for up to 72 hours after a dose of bleomycin should be handled wearing protective clothing.[1]

1. Harris J, Dodds LJ. Handling waste from patients receiving cytotoxic drugs. *Pharm J* 1985; **235:** 289–91.

## Interactions

For a general outline of antineoplastic drug interactions, see p.498. There may be an increased risk of pulmonary toxicity in patients given bleomycin who receive oxygen, for example as part of a general anaesthetic procedure; a reduction in inspired oxygen concentration is recommended.

**Cisplatin.** Enhanced pulmonary toxicity, in some cases fatal, has been reported in patients given bleomycin and cisplatin,[1-4] presumably because cisplatin-induced renal impairment led to a decrease in bleomycin elimination. It seems reasonable to assume that similar interactions might occur if bleomycin were given with other nephrotoxic agents. It has been suggested that apart from a decrease in bleomycin dosage if nephrotoxicity occurs with such a combination, administration of bleomycin by constant infusion rather than intermittent bolus might be less toxic.[1,5]

1. Bennett WM, *et al.* Fatal pulmonary bleomycin toxicity in cisplatin-induced acute renal failure. *Cancer Treat Rep* 1980; **64:** 921–4.
2. van Barneveld PWC, *et al.* Influence of platinum-induced renal toxicity on bleomycin-induced pulmonary toxicity in patients with disseminated testicular carcinoma. *Oncology* 1984; **41:** 4–7.
3. Brodsky A, *et al.* Stevens-Johnson syndrome, respiratory distress and acute renal failure due to synergic bleomycin-cisplatin toxicity. *J Clin Pharmacol* 1989; **29:** 821–3.
4. Sleijfer S, *et al.* Enhanced effects of bleomycin on pulmonary function disturbances in patients with decreased renal function due to cisplatin. *Eur J Cancer* 1996; **32A:** 550–2.
5. Chisholm RA, *et al.* Bleomycin lung: the effect of different chemotherapeutic regimens. *Cancer Chemother Pharmacol* 1992; **30:** 158–60.

**Colony-stimulating factors.** An increased incidence of pulmonary toxicity has been reported in patients receiving bleomycin as part of the ABVD regimen (with doxorubicin, vinblastine, and dacarbazine) who were given granulocyte colony-stimulating factor to alleviate neutropenia.[1] Another case of rapidly developing and fatal pneumonitis in a patient given BEP (bleomycin, etoposide, and cisplatin) with granulocyte colony-stimulating factor has been reported.[2] However, analysis of two randomised controlled trials failed to show increased pulmonary toxicity when granulocyte colony-stimulating factor was added to bleomycin therapy.[3,4]

1. Matthews JH. Pulmonary toxicity of ABVD chemotherapy and G-CSF in Hodgkin's disease: possible synergy. *Lancet* 1993; **342:** 988.
2. Dirix LY, *et al.* Pulmonary toxicity and bleomycin. *Lancet* 1994; **344:** 56.
3. Bastion Y, *et al.* Possible toxicity with the association of G-CSF and bleomycin. *Lancet* 1994; **343:** 1221–2.
4. Bastion Y, Coiffier B. Pulmonary toxicity of bleomycin: is G-CSF a risk factor? *Lancet* 1994; **344:** 474.

## Pharmacokinetics

Bleomycin is thought to be poorly absorbed from the gastrointestinal tract. After parenteral doses some 60 to 70% of a dose has been reported to be excreted in urine as active drug. Enzymic degradation of bleomycin occurs, primarily in plasma, the liver and other organs, and to a much lesser extent in skin and lungs. Elimination is biphasic: mean initial and terminal half-lives of 0.5 and 4 hours respectively have been reported after an intravenous bolus. Elimination may be more prolonged after intravenous infusion and mean half-lives of 1.3 and 9 hours respectively have been reported. Bleomycin does not cross the blood-brain barrier but appears to cross the placenta.

◊ References.

1. Broughton A, *et al.* Clinical pharmacology of bleomycin following intravenous infusion as determined by radioimmunoassay. *Cancer* 1977; **40:** 2772–8.
2. Alberts DS, *et al.* Bleomycin pharmacokinetics in man I: intravenous administration. *Cancer Chemother Pharmacol* 1978; **1:** 177–81.
3. Yee GC, *et al.* Bleomycin disposition in children with cancer. *Clin Pharmacol Ther* 1983; **33:** 668–73.

## Uses and Administration

Bleomycin is an antineoplastic antibiotic which binds to DNA and causes strand scissions, and is probably most effective in the $G_2$ and M phases of the cell cycle. It is widely used to treat malignant disease; particularly squamous cell carcinomas, including those of the cervix and external genitalia, oesophagus, skin, and head and neck; Hodgkin's disease and other lymphomas; malignant neoplasms of the testis, and malignant effusions. It has also been tried in other malignancies, including carcinoma of the bladder, lung, and thyroid, and some sarcomas, including Kaposi's sarcoma.

Bleomycin is often used with other antineoplastics, notably with doxorubicin, vinblastine, and dacarbazine (ABVD) for Hodgkin's disease, and with etoposide and cisplatin (BEP) in testicular tumours. Bleomycin is given as the sulfate by either the intramuscular, intravenous, or subcutaneous route. It may also be given intra-arterially or instilled intrapleurally or intraperitoneally. If intramuscular injections are painful they may be given in a 1% solution of lidocaine.

- *Doses are calculated in terms of the base, and are given in* ***units****, but the units used for preparations in the UK, which were formerly equivalent to those of the USP, are now international units equivalent to those of the Ph. Eur. (see Units, above). Since 1000 international units is equivalent to 1 USP unit, UK doses now appear to be 1000 times greater than those previously in use, or than those in use in the USA, and care is recommended in evaluating the literature.*

In the UK the licensed dose as a single agent for **squamous cell** or **testicular tumours** is 15 000 international units (15 USP units) three times a week, or 30 000 international units twice a week, by intramuscular or intravenous injection, although in practice treatment of malignancy will generally be with combination regimens. This may be repeated, at usual intervals of 3 to 4 weeks, up to a total cumulative dose of 500 000 international units. The dose and total cumulative dose should be reduced in those over 60 years of age (see below). Doses should be adjusted according to tolerance, and may need to be adjusted as part of combination chemotherapy. Continuous intravenous infusion at a rate of 15 000 international units per 24 hours for up to 10 days or 30 000 international units per 24 hours for up to 5 days may also be used. In patients with **lymphoma** a dose of 15 000 international units once or twice weekly by intramuscular injection has been suggested, to a total dose of 225 000 international units. Again, dosage should be reduced in older patients and in combination regimens if necessary. In the treatment of **malignant effusions** a solution of 60 000 international units in 100 mL of sodium chloride 0.9% may be instilled into the affected serous cavity. Treatment may be repeated as necessary up to a total cumulative dose of 500 000 international units depending on the patient's age. Local anaesthetics or analgesics are given concomitantly.

In the USA licensed doses for **lymphomas** as well as **squamous cell** and **testicular** neoplasms are 250 to 500 international units/kg (0.25 to 0.5 USP units/kg), or 10 000 to 20 000 international units/m$^2$ (10 to 20 USP units/m$^2$), given once or twice weekly. In view of the risk of an anaphylactoid reaction it has been suggested that patients with lymphomas should receive two test doses of 2000 international units (2 USP units) or less initially. In patients with Hodgkin's disease, once a 50% response has been achieved it may be maintained with 1000 international units (1 USP unit) of bleomycin daily, or 5000 international units (5 USP units) weekly.

In the UK, manufacturers suggest that a **total dose** of 500 000 international units (500 USP units) should not be exceeded. Total cumulative dose should not exceed 300 000 international units in those aged 60 to 69 years, 200 000 international units in those 70 to 79, and 100 000 international units in those 80 and over; the weekly dose should be no more than 30 000 and 15 000 international units respectively in the latter 2 groups. In the USA the recommended maximum total dose is 400 000 international units (400 USP units); it is generally agreed that patients receiving 400 000 international units or more are at increased risk of pulmonary toxicity (see Adverse Effects, above).

Dosage should be reduced in patients with renal impairment (see below).

Bleomycin hydrochloride has also been given parenterally for malignant neoplasms, and bleomycin sulfate has been applied topically for the local treatment of skin tumours.

**Administration.** For the suggestion that giving bleomycin by intravenous infusion rather than bolus injection in combination regimens may result in reduced pulmonary toxicity, see Interactions, Cisplatin, above.

**Administration in renal impairment.** A significant portion of a dose of bleomycin is excreted largely unchanged in the urine, and dose reduction should be considered in patients with renal impairment. Firm guidelines for dose adjustment have not been established but manufacturers' suggestions include dose reductions of 40 to 75% for patients with a creatinine clearance of 40 mL/minute or less, or a 50% dose reduction when the serum creatinine concentration is between 20 and 40 micrograms/mL and further reduction for serum creatinine above this.

**Leucoplakia.** Leucoplakia is used to describe a white patch or plaque in the mouth which cannot be otherwise characterised. Such lesions are of concern because they may be pre-malignant, and patients with evidence of dysplasia may be at higher risk of transformation (see also Malignant Neoplasms of the Head and Neck, p.517). Leucoplakia must be distinguished from other conditions such as candidiasis, lichen planus, and oral hairy leucoplakia which is associated with HIV infection.[1]

Leucoplakia is often associated with tobacco smoking, and smoking cessation can result in regression.[1] Where active treatment is desirable, small and easily accessible lesions can be removed surgically or by laser therapy, although they may recur.[1] For extensive patches or those in which surgery would be difficult, the treatments described include topical bleomycin 1%, dissolved in dimethyl sulfoxide and applied for 5 minutes daily for 14 consecutive days. In a group of 19 patients with dysplastic leucoplakia, improvement in the appearance of lesions and histological evidence of remission of the dysplasia occurred in the majority of patients. Sustained effects were also found on long-term follow-up for up to 10 years.[2]

There have been reports of partial or complete remission of leucoplakia in studies of vitamin A or betacarotene given orally long-term,[3-5] but lesions have recurred when supplementation was stopped.[4] Topical treatment with retinoids such as tretinoin or isotretinoin has also been tried, with similar results to those of oral vitamin A and retinoid treatments.[6,7] A small open study has also suggested that topical calcipotriol may be effective.[8]

A systematic review of treatments for leucoplakia found that there were few controlled trials reported, and that although these treatments might be effective in the resolution of lesions, the rate of relapse was high, and there was no evidence that they prevent malignant transformation.[9]

1. Scully C, Porter S. ABC of oral health: swellings and red, white, and pigmented lesions. *BMJ* 2000; **321:** 225–8.

2. Epstein JB, *et al.* Topical bleomycin for the treatment of dysplastic oral leukoplakia. *Cancer* 1998; **83:** 629–34.
3. Issing WJ, *et al.* Long-term follow-up of larynx leukoplakia under treatment with retinyl palmitate. *Head Neck* 1996; **18:** 560–5.
4. Sankaranarayanan R, *et al.* Chemoprevention of oral leukoplakia with vitamin A and beta carotene: an assessment. *Oral Oncol* 1997; **33:** 231–6.
5. Garewal HS, *et al.* β-Carotene produces sustained remissions in patients with oral leukoplakia: results of a multicenter prospective trial. *Arch Otolaryngol Head Neck Surg* 1999; **125:** 1305–10.
6. Epstein JB, Gorsky M. Topical application of vitamin A to oral leukoplakia: a clinical case series. *Cancer* 1999; **86:** 921–7.
7. Gorsky M, Epstein JB. The effect of retinoids on premalignant oral lesions: focus on topical therapy. *Cancer* 2002; **95:** 1258–64.
8. Femiano F, *et al.* Oral leukoplakia: open trial of topical therapy with calcipotriol compared with tretinoin. *Int J Oral Maxillofac Surg* 2001; **30:** 402–6.
9. Lodi G, *et al.* Interventions for treating oral leukoplakia. Available in The Cochrane Library; Issue 2. Chichester: John Wiley; 2004.


**Malignant effusions.** Bleomycin is used for the sclerotherapy of malignant pleural and pericardial effusions (p.512).

**Malignant neoplasms.** Bleomycin is employed in regimens for the management of Hodgkin's disease and non-Hodgkin's lymphomas (see p.509, p.510, and p.510), and for germ-cell tumours of the ovary and testis (see p.520, and p.523), as well as for some other malignancies including those of the head and neck, (p.517), and Kaposi's sarcoma (p.524).

**Pneumothorax.** In a patient with AIDS and *Pneumocystis carinii* pneumonia who developed pneumothorax, instillation of bleomycin into each pleural cavity was successful in resolving the pneumothorax after tetracycline sclerotherapy failed to do so.[1]


1. Hnatiuk OW, *et al.* Bleomycin sclerotherapy for bilateral pneumothoraces in a patient with AIDS. *Ann Intern Med* 1990; **113:** 988–90.


**Warts.** A number of studies have examined the local use of bleomycin sulfate to treat severe or resistant warts (p.1139) of the common, plane, plantar, eponychial, and mosaic types, usually by intralesional injection.[1-3] At the doses used, adverse effects, other than pain at the injection site,[1-3] do not seem to be common; however, nail dystrophy and Raynaud's phenomenon have been reported (see under Effects on the Nails and Effects on the Vascular System, under Adverse Effects, above). Bleomycin has also been applied as a pressure-sensitive adhesive tape,[4] and various techniques for the improvement of intralesional administration have been investigated.[5-7]


1. Shumack PH, Haddock MJ. Bleomycin: an effective treatment for warts. *Australas J Dermatol* 1979; **20:** 41–2.
2. Bunney MH, *et al.* The treatment of resistant warts with intralesional bleomycin: a controlled clinical trial. *Br J Dermatol* 1984; **111:** 197–207.
3. Munkvad M, *et al.* Locally injected bleomycin in the treatment of warts. *Dermatologica* 1983; **167:** 86–9.
4. Takigawa M, *et al.* Treatment of viral warts with pressure-sensitive adhesive tape containing bleomycin sulfate. *Arch Dermatol* 1985; **121:** 1108.
5. Munn SE, *et al.* A new method of intralesional bleomycin therapy in the treatment of recalcitrant warts. *Br J Dermatol* 1996; **135:** 969–71.
6. van der Velden EM, *et al.* Dermatography with bleomycin as a new treatment for verrucae vulgaris. *Int J Dermatol* 1997; **36:** 145–50.
7. Pollock B, Sheehan-Dare R. Pulsed dye laser and intralesional bleomycin for treatment of resistant viol [sic] hand warts. *Lasers Surg Med* 2002; **30:** 135–40.


## Preparations

***BP 2003:*** Bleomycin Injection;
***USP 27:*** Bleomycin for Injection.

**Proprietary Preparations** (details are given in Part 3)
***Arg.:*** Bileco; Bleocris; Blocamicina; ***Austral.:*** Blenamax; Blenoxane; ***Braz.:*** Blenoxane; Bonar; Tecnomicina; ***Canad.:*** Blenoxane; ***Chile:*** Blexit; Nikableomicina; ***Ger.:*** Bleo-cell; ***Gr.:*** Bleocin; ***India:*** Bleocin; ***Jpn:*** Bleo-S; Bleocin; ***Mex.:*** Blanoxan; Bleolem; ***NZ:*** Blenoxane; ***Port.:*** Blio; ***S.Afr.:*** Blenoxane; ***Thai.:*** Bleolem; ***UK:*** Bleo; ***USA:*** Blenoxane.

## Bortezomib *(USAN, rINN)*

LDP-341; PS-341. *N*-((1*S*)-1-Benzyl-2-{[(1*R*)-1-(dihydroxyboranyl)-3-methylbutyl]amino}-2-oxoethyl)pyrazinecarboxamide.
$C_{19}H_{25}BN_4O_4$ = 384.2.
*CAS — 179324-69-7.*
*ATC — L01XX32.*

### Profile

Bortezomib is an inhibitor of proteasomes, which are enzyme complexes in cells responsible for breaking down regulatory proteins of the cell cycle. Such inhibition disrupts tumour cell turnover and induces apoptosis. It is used for the treatment of relapsed refractory multiple myeloma in doses of 1.3 mg/m², given intravenously on days 1, 4, 8 and 11 of a 21-day cycle. Common adverse effects of bortezomib include asthenia, gastrointestinal disturbances, peripheral neuropathy, fever, thrombocytopenia, and anaemia. Orthostatic hypotension and pneumonia have been reported.

◊ References.


1. Richardson PG, *et al.* A phase 2 study of bortezomib in relapsed, refractory myeloma. *N Engl J Med* 2003; **348:** 2609–17.
2. Stanford BL, Zondor SD. Bortezomib treatment for multiple myeloma. *Ann Pharmacother* 2003; **37:** 1825–30.


## Preparations

**Proprietary Preparations** (details are given in Part 3)
***UK:*** Velcade; ***USA:*** Velcade.

## Bropirimine *(BAN, USAN, rINN)*

ABPP; Bropirimina; U-54461; U-54461S. 2-Amino-5-bromo-6-phenyl-4(3*H*)-pyrimidinone.
$C_{10}H_8BrN_3O$ = 266.1.
*CAS — 56741-95-8.*

### Profile

Bropirimine is reported to have immunomodulatory actions, possibly due to the induction of interferons. It has been investigated in the management of carcinoma in situ of the bladder (p.512).

## Broxuridine *(rINN)*

Bromodeoxyuridine; Broxuridina; BUDR; NSC-38297. 5-Bromo-2′-deoxyuridine; 5-Bromo-1-(2-deoxy-β-D-ribofuranosyl)pyrimidine-2,4(1*H*,3*H*)-dione.
$C_9H_{11}BrN_2O_5$ = 307.1.
*CAS — 59-14-3.*

### Profile

Broxuridine is a thymidine analogue which acts as a radiosensitiser to enhance the effects of radiotherapy. It is also reported to possess antiviral activity. A related compound brivudine (p.629) is used as an antiviral.

Broxuridine has been given by intra-arterial infusion, with radiotherapy and other antineoplastic agents, in the treatment of tumours of the brain, head, and neck. It has also been used diagnostically.

◊ References.


1. Freese A, *et al.* The application of 5-bromodeoxyuridine in the management of CNS tumors. *J Neurooncol* 1994; **20:** 81–95.
2. Phillips TL, *et al.* Results of a randomized comparison of radiotherapy and bromodeoxyuridine with radiotherapy alone for brain metastases: report of RTOG trial 89-05. *Int J Radiat Oncol Biol Phys* 1995; **33:** 339–48.
3. Prados MD, *et al.* Influence of bromodeoxyuridine radiosensitization on malignant glioma patient survival: a retrospective comparison of survival data from the Northern California Oncology Group (NCOG) and Radiation Therapy Oncology Group trials (RTOG) for glioblastoma multiforme and anaplastic astrocytoma. *Int J Radiat Oncol Biol Phys* 1998; **40:** 653–9.
4. Prados MD, *et al.* Phase III randomized study of radiotherapy plus procarbazine, lomustine, and vincristine with or without BUdR for treatment of anaplastic astrocytoma: final report of RTOG 9404. *Int J Radiat Oncol Biol Phys* 2004; **58:** 1147–52.


# Busulfan *(BAN, rINN)*

Bussulfam; Busulfano; Busulfanum; Busulphan; CB-2041; GT-41; Myelosan; NSC-750; WR-19508. Tetramethylene di(methanesulphonate); Butane-1,4-diol di(methanesulphonate).
$C_6H_{14}O_6S_2$ = 246.3.
*CAS — 55-98-1.*
*ATC — L01AB01.*

**Pharmacopoeias.** In *Chin., Eur.* (see p.vi), *Int., Jpn, Pol.*, and *US.*

**Ph. Eur. 5.0** (Busulfan). A white or almost white, crystalline powder. Very slightly soluble in water and in alcohol; freely soluble in acetone and in acetonitrile. Store in airtight containers. Protect from light.

**USP 27** (Busulfan). A white, crystalline powder. Very slightly soluble in water; slightly soluble in alcohol; soluble 1 in 45 of acetone. Store in airtight containers.

## Adverse Effects and Treatment

For a general outline see Antineoplastics, p.492 and p.495.

The major side-effect of busulfan with standard doses is bone-marrow depression, manifest as leucopenia, thrombocytopenia, and sometimes, anaemia. The nadir of the granulocyte count usually occurs after about 10 to 30 days with recovery occurring over up to 5 months, but busulfan has sometimes caused irreversible or extremely-prolonged bone-marrow depression.

Hyperpigmentation is common, and in a few cases after long-term therapy may be part of a syndrome simulating Addison's disease.

Rarely, progressive interstitial pulmonary fibrosis, known as 'busulfan lung', can occur on prolonged treatment. Gastrointestinal disturbances are rare at usual therapeutic doses but may be dose-limiting where high doses are given before bone marrow transplantation. Other rare adverse effects include dry skin and other skin reactions, liver damage, gynaecomastia, cataract formation, and, at high doses, CNS effects including convulsions.

Busulfan may result in impaired fertility and gonadal function. As with other alkylating agents, it is potentially carcinogenic, mutagenic, and teratogenic.

**Effects on the bladder.** Haemorrhagic cystitis occurred in a patient who had received prolonged therapy with busulfan.[1] High-dose busulfan used in conditioning regimens for haematopoietic stem cell transplantation may increase the risk of late-onset haemorrhagic cystitis.[2,3]


1. Pode D, *et al.* Busulfan-induced hemorrhagic cystitis. *J Urol (Baltimore)* 1983; **130:** 347–8.
2. Kondo M, *et al.* Late-onset hemorrhagic cystitis after hematopoietic stem cell transplantation in children. *Bone Marrow Transplant* 1998; **22:** 995–8.
3. Leung AYH, *et al.* Clinicopathological features and risk factors of clinically overt haemorrhagic cystitis complicating bone marrow transplantation. *Bone Marrow Transplant* 2002; **29:** 509–13.


**Effects on the liver.** Jaundice in the terminal phase of chronic myeloid leukaemia in a 31-year-old man was attributed to busulfan which had been taken for 6 years.[1] Busulfan toxicity involving the liver was also reported in a patient who had taken busulfan for 54 months,[2] while hepatitis possibly associated with busulfan therapy has also been described.[3] Dose-dependent veno-occlusive disease has been reported in 20 to 40% of patients receiving high-dose busulfan before bone marrow transplantation.[4]


1. Underwood JCE, *et al.* Jaundice after treatment of leukaemia with busulphan. *BMJ* 1971; **1:** 556–7.
2. Foadi MD, *et al.* Portal hypertension in a patient with chronic myeloid leukaemia. *Postgrad Med J* 1977; **53:** 267–9.
3. Morris L, Guthrie T. Busulfan-induced hepatitis. *Am J Gastroenterol* 1988; **83:** 682–3.
4. Hassan M. The role of busulfan in bone marrow transplantation. *Med Oncol* 1999; **16:** 166–76.


**Effects on the nervous system.** High-dose busulfan, used in conditioning regimens for bone marrow transplantation, has been associated with the development of convulsions,[1-4] both generalised[1,3,4] and myoclonic.[2,4] As a result, the use of prophylactic antiepileptic therapy has been suggested as a component of such regimens.[1,3,4] However, some do not consider the routine use of prophylactic antiepileptics justified,[5] and the potential for phenytoin to increase the metabolism of busulfan, thereby possibly decreasing its myeloablative efficacy, has been pointed out.[6] In addition, phenytoin plasma concentrations have been found to be subtherapeutic in patients who developed convulsions despite a standard prophylactic dose,[4] and the regimen was subsequently adjusted to take account of plasma concentrations. Clobazam has been suggested as an alternative to phenytoin for prophylaxis of busulfan-induced seizures.[7] The UK manufacturer GlaxoSmithKline recommends the use of prophylactic anticonvulsants, and prefers a benzodiazepine to phenytoin. However, other manufacturers suggest use with phenytoin; Orphan Medical in the USA state that the recommended dose of their parenteral product is based on the concurrent use of phenytoin, and that if other anticonvulsants are used a 15% increase in plasma-busulfan may be expected, with increased risk of toxicity.


1. Marcus RE, Goldman JM. Convulsions due to high-dose busulphan. *Lancet* 1984; **ii:** 1463.
2. Martell RW, *et al.* High-dose busulfan and myoclonic epilepsy. *Ann Intern Med* 1987; **106:** 173.
3. Sureda A, *et al.* High-dose busulfan and seizures. *Ann Intern Med* 1989; **111:** 543–4.
4. Grigg AP, *et al.* Busulphan and phenytoin. *Ann Intern Med* 1989; **111:** 1049–50. Correction. *ibid.*; **112:** 313.
5. Hugh-Jones K, Shaw PJ. No convulsions in children on high-dose busulphan. *Lancet* 1985; **i:** 220.
6. Fitzsimmons WE, *et al.* Anticonvulsants and busulfan. *Ann Intern Med* 1990; **112:** 552–3.
7. Schwarer AP, *et al.* Clobazam for seizure prophylaxis during busulfan chemotherapy. *Lancet* 1995; **346:** 1238.


**Effects on the skin.** For the effect of radiotherapy in activating skin lesions in busulfan-treated patients, see under Precautions, below.

## Precautions

For reference to the precautions necessary with antineoplastics, see p.497. Careful attention should be given to monitoring blood counts during therapy. These should initially be monitored at least weekly during standard dose therapy. With high dose therapy blood counts should be monitored daily, as should liver function. Prophylactic anticonvulsants should be used during high dose therapy (see Effects on the Nervous System, above).

Busulfan should be stopped if lung toxicity develops. In patients with possible lung toxicity, the use of oxygen may accentuate this; if anaesthesia is required the concentration of oxygen should be minimised.

**Handling.** Busulfan is irritant; avoid contact with skin and mucous membranes.

**Porphyria.** Busulfan is considered to be unsafe in patients with porphyria because it has been shown to be porphyrinogenic in *animals*.

**Radiotherapy.** Severe cutaneous reactions occurred in patients given radiotherapy at least 30 days after combined chemotherapy with high-dose busulfan.[1]

It is possible that subsequent radiotherapy could augment subclinical lung injury caused by busulfan.

1. Vassal G, *et al.* Radiosensitisation after busulphan. *Lancet* 1987; **i:** 571.

## Interactions

For a general outline of antineoplastic drug interactions, see p.498. Phenytoin increases the clearance of busulfan (see Effects on the Nervous System, above).

**Antifungals.** Giving *itraconazole* with busulfan resulted in a decrease in the clearance of busulfan; *fluconazole* had no such effect.[1] Busulfan doses may need to be decreased if itraconazole is also given.

1. Buggia I, *et al.* Itraconazole can increase systemic exposure to busulfan in patients given bone marrow transplantation. *Anticancer Res* 1996; **16:** 2083–8.

**Antineoplastics.** When *tioguanine* was given with busulfan for chronic myeloid leukaemia, a number of cases of hepatic nodular regenerative hyperplasia, with abnormal liver function tests, portal hypertension, and oesophageal varices were noted. There were no cases in patients treated with busulfan alone, and the mechanism of this possible interaction is unclear.[1,2]

1. Key NS, *et al.* Oesophageal varices associated with busulfan-thioguanine combination therapy for chronic myeloid leukaemia. *Lancet* 1987; **ii:** 1050–2.
2. Shepherd PCA, *et al.* Thioguanine used in maintenance therapy of chronic myeloid leukaemia causes non-cirrhotic portal hypertension. *Br J Haematol* 1991; **79:** 185–92.

**Antiprotozoals.** In a study[1] of patients who received high-dose busulfan as part of a myeloablative regimen before stem cell transplantation, the use of *metronidazole* significantly increased plasma concentrations of busulfan and the degree of associated toxicity, including elevation of liver function tests, veno-occlusive disease, and mucositis.

1. Nilsson C, *et al.* The effect of metronidazole on busulfan pharmacokinetics in patients undergoing hematopoietic stem cell transplantation. *Bone Marrow Transplant* 2003; **31:** 429–35.

**Interferons.** For reports of severe cytopenia in patients receiving busulfan and *interferon alfa*, see p.642.

## Pharmacokinetics

Busulfan is readily absorbed from the gastrointestinal tract and rapidly disappears from the blood with a half-life of 2 to 3 hours. It is extensively metabolised, and excreted in the urine almost entirely as sulfur-containing metabolites. It crosses the blood-brain barrier.

◊ In a study of the pharmacokinetics of high-dose busulfan in 5 patients receiving 1 mg/kg by mouth every six hours for 4 days, the mean elimination half-life decreased from about 3.4 hours after the first dose to about 2.3 hours after the final dose, suggesting that busulfan may induce its own metabolism.[1]

1. Hassan M, *et al.* Pharmacokinetic and metabolic studies of high-dose busulphan in adults. *Eur J Clin Pharmacol* 1989; **36:** 525–30.

## Uses and Administration

Busulfan is an antineoplastic with a cell-cycle non-specific alkylating action unlike that of the nitrogen mustards, and having a selective depressant action on bone marrow. In small doses, it depresses granulocytopoiesis and to a lesser extent thrombocytopoiesis but has little effect on lymphocytes. With larger doses, severe bone-marrow depression eventually ensues.

Because of its selective action, busulfan has been used in the palliative treatment of chronic myeloid leukaemia (p.507). It provides symptomatic relief with a reduction in spleen size and a general feeling of well-being. The fall in leucocyte count is usually accompanied by a rise in the haemoglobin concentration. Permanent remission is not induced and resistance to its beneficial effects gradually develops.

Busulfan may be used in patients with polycythaemia vera (p.508) and in some patients with myelofibrosis and primary thrombocythaemia (p.509). It is also used at high doses as part of a conditioning regimen to prepare patients for bone marrow transplantation, a procedure discussed on p.1344 under Haematopoietic Stem Cell Transplantation.

The licensed initial dosage of busulfan in **chronic myeloid leukaemia** is 60 micrograms/kg daily by mouth, with a usual maximum single daily dose of 4 mg. This is continued until the white cell count has fallen to between 15 000 and 25 000 cells/mm$^3$ (typically 12 to 20 weeks). It should be stopped earlier if the platelet count falls below 100 000 cells/mm$^3$. Higher doses may be given if the response after 3 weeks is inadequate but this increases the risk of irreversible damage to the bone marrow and calls for special vigilance. Complete blood counts should be made at least every week and the trends followed closely; if haemorrhagic tendencies occur or there is a steep fall in the white cell count indicating severe bone-marrow depression, busulfan should be withdrawn until marrow function has returned.

Once an initial remission has been attained treatment is stopped and not resumed until the white cell count returns to 50 000 cells/mm$^3$. If this occurs within 3 months continuous maintenance treatment with a usual dose of 0.5 to 2 mg daily may be given.

In patients with **polycythaemia vera** the usual dose is 4 to 6 mg daily by mouth, continued for 4 to 6 weeks with careful monitoring of blood counts. Further courses are given when relapse occurs, or alternatively maintenance therapy may be given at half the dose required for induction. Doses of 2 to 4 mg daily have been given for **essential thrombocythaemia** or myelofibrosis.

In conditioning regimens for **bone marrow transplantation** busulfan has been given in usual doses of 3.5 to 4 mg/kg daily in divided doses for 4 days by mouth (total dose 14 to 16 mg/kg), with cyclophosphamide, for ablation of the recipient's bone marrow. When given by intravenous infusion in a regimen with phenytoin (see Effects on the Nervous System, above), a recommended dose is 3.2 mg/kg ideal body-weight daily for 4 days (total dose 12.8 mg/kg); actual body-weight is used for the calculation if it is less than the ideal weight. The daily dose is given as 4 infusions of 800 micrograms/kg at intervals of 6 hours; each dose should be diluted in sodium chloride 0.9% or glucose 5% to a final concentration of about 500 micrograms/mL, and given over 2 hours through a central venous catheter using an infusion pump.

◊ References.

1. Buggia I, *et al.* Busulfan. *Ann Pharmacother* 1994; **28:** 1055–62.

## Preparations

***BP 2003:*** Busulfan Tablets;
***USP 27:*** Busulfan Tablets.

**Proprietary Preparations** (details are given in Part 3)
***Arg.:*** Myleran; ***Austral.:*** Myleran; ***Austria:*** Myleran; ***Belg.:*** Myleran; ***Braz.:*** Mielucin†; Myleran; ***Canad.:*** Busulfex; Myleran; ***Chile:*** Myleran; ***Fr.:*** Myleran; ***Ger.:*** Myleran; ***Gr.:*** Myleran; ***Hong Kong:*** Myleran; ***India:*** Myleran; ***Irl.:*** Myleran; ***Israel:*** Busulfex; Myleran; ***Ital.:*** Misulban†; Myleran; ***Malaysia:*** Myleran; ***Mex.:*** Myleran; ***Neth.:*** Myleran; ***Norw.:*** Myleran†; ***NZ:*** Myleran; ***Port.:*** Myleran; ***S.Afr.:*** Myleran; ***Singapore:*** Myleran; ***Swed.:*** Myleran; ***Switz.:*** Myleran; ***Thai.:*** Myleran; ***UK:*** Busilvex; Myleran; ***USA:*** Busulfex; Myleran.

# Capecitabine *(BAN, USAN, rINN)*

Capecitabina; Ro-09-1978/000. Pentyl 1-(5-deoxy-β-D-ribofuranosyl)-5-fluoro-1,2-dihydro-2-oxo-4-pyrimidinecarbamate.
$C_{15}H_{22}FN_3O_6$ = 359.4.
*CAS — 154361-50-9; 158798-73-3.*
*ATC — L01BC06.*

## Adverse Effects and Precautions

As for Fluorouracil, p.554. Diarrhoea, nausea and vomiting, stomatitis, palmar-plantar erythrodysesthesia syndrome (erythema and desquamation of hands and feet), dermatitis, cardiotoxicity, and bone-marrow depression have all been reported. Hyperbilirubinaemia has occurred. Doses should be reduced in patients with moderate renal impairment and capecitabine is contra-indicated in those with severe impairment.

**Effects on the eyes.** A report of severe ocular irritation with corneal deposits and impaired visual acuity in 2 patients who received capecitabine.[1] Symptoms resolved within several weeks of discontinuing the drug.

1. Walkhom B, *et al.* Severe ocular irritation and corneal deposits associated with capecitabine use. *N Engl J Med* 2000; **343:** 740–1.

## Interactions

As for Fluorouracil, p.555. Altered coagulation parameters and bleeding have occurred in patients on warfarin given capecitabine. Increased phenytoin plasma concentrations and symptoms of toxicity during use with capecitabine have been reported.

## Pharmacokinetics

Capecitabine is readily absorbed from the gastrointestinal tract, with peak plasma concentrations occurring at about 1.5 hours. Food reduces the rate and extent of absorption. Capecitabine is hydrolysed in the liver to 5′-deoxy-5-fluorocytidine, which is then converted to 5′-deoxy-5-fluorouridine and subsequently to 5-fluorouracil in body tissues. 5-Fluorouracil is further metabolised, as discussed on p.555.

◊ References.

1. Reigner B, *et al.* Effect of food on the pharmacokinetics of capecitabine and its metabolites following oral administration in cancer patients. *Clin Cancer Res* 1998; **4:** 941–8.
2. Reigner B, *et al.* Clinical pharmacokinetics of capecitabine. *Clin Pharmacokinet* 2001; **40:** 85–104.

## Uses and Administration

Capecitabine is a prodrug that is converted to fluorouracil (p.555) in body tissues. It is given by mouth for the treatment of metastatic colorectal cancer (p.516) and locally advanced or metastatic breast cancer (p.514). The recommended daily dose is 2.5 g/m$^2$ in 2 divided doses about 12 hours apart with food; doses are given for 2 weeks, followed by a 1-week rest period. Doses should be modified in subsequent cycles according to toxicity. Capecitabine doses should be reduced in patients with renal impairment (see below).

Capecitabine is also under investigation in the treatment of other malignancies.

◊ References.

1. Blum JL, *et al.* Multicenter phase II study of capecitabine in paclitaxel-refractory metastatic breast cancer. *J Clin Oncol* 1999; **17:** 485–93.
2. Van Cutsem E, *et al.* Capecitabine, an oral fluoropyrimidine carbamate with substantial activity in advanced colorectal cancer: results of a randomized phase II study. *J Clin Oncol* 2000; **18:** 1337–45.
3. Hoff PM, *et al.* Comparison of oral capecitabine versus intravenous fluorouracil plus leucovorin as first-line treatment in 605 patients with metastatic colorectal cancer: results of a randomized phase III study. *J Clin Oncol* 2001; **19:** 2282–92.
4. Van Cutsem E, *et al.* Oral capecitabine compared with intravenous fluorouracil plus leucovorin in patients with metastatic colorectal cancer: results of a large phase III study. *J Clin Oncol* 2001; **19:** 4097–4106.
5. McGavin JK, Goa KL. Capecitabine: a review of its use in the treatment of advanced or metastatic colorectal cancer. *Drugs* 2001; **61:** 2309–26.
6. Talbot DC, *et al.* Randomised, phase II trial comparing oral capecitabine (Xeloda) with paclitaxel in patients with metastatic/advanced breast cancer pretreated with anthracyclines. *Br J Cancer* 2002; **86:** 1367–72.
7. O'Shaughnessy J, *et al.* Superior survival with capecitabine plus docetaxel combination therapy in anthracycline-pretreated patients with advanced breast cancer: phase III trial results. *J Clin Oncol* 2002; **20:** 2812–23.
8. Wagstaff AJ, *et al.* Capecitabine: a review of its pharmacology and therapeutic efficacy in the management of advanced breast cancer. *Drugs* 2003; **63:** 217–36.
9. Van Cutsem E, *et al.* Oral capecitabine vs intravenous 5-fluorouracil and leucovorin: integrated efficacy data and novel analyses from two large, randomised, phase III trials. *Br J Cancer* 2004; **90:** 1190–7.

**Administration in renal impairment.** Renal impairment increases systemic exposure to 5′-deoxy-5-fluorouridine, a metabolite of capecitabine. An increase in the severity of adverse effects appears to correlate with decreased renal function and increased exposure to this metabolite.[1]

In patients with renal impairment (creatinine clearance 30 to 50 mL/minute) initial doses of capecitabine should be reduced to 1.875 g/m$^2$ daily. Capecitabine is contra-indicated in patients with more severe renal impairment.

1. Poole C, *et al.* Effect of renal impairment on the pharmacokinetics and tolerability of capecitabine (Xeloda) in cancer patients. *Cancer Chemother Pharmacol* 2002; **49:** 225–34.

## Preparations

**Proprietary Preparations** (details are given in Part 3)
***Arg.:*** Apecitab; Xeloda; ***Austral.:*** Xeloda; ***Belg.:*** Xeloda; ***Braz.:*** Xeloda; ***Canad.:*** Xeloda; ***Chile:*** Xeloda; ***Denm.:*** Xeloda; ***Fin.:*** Xeloda; ***Fr.:*** Xeloda; ***Ger.:*** Xeloda; ***Gr.:*** Xeloda; ***Hong Kong:*** Xeloda; ***Irl.:*** Xeloda; ***Israel:*** Xeloda; ***Ital.:*** Xeloda; ***Mex.:*** Xeloda; ***Norw.:*** Xeloda; ***NZ:*** Xeloda; ***Port.:*** Xeloda; ***S.Afr.:*** Xeloda; ***Singapore:*** Xeloda; ***Spain:*** Xeloda; ***Swed.:*** Xeloda; ***Switz.:*** Xeloda; ***Thai.:*** Xeloda; ***UK:*** Xeloda; ***USA:*** Xeloda.

# Carboplatin *(BAN, USAN, rINN)*

Carboplatino; Carboplatinum; CBDCA; JM-8; NSC-241240. *cis*-Diammine(cyclobutane-1,1-dicarboxylato)platinum.
$C_6H_{12}N_2O_4Pt$ = 371.2.
*CAS — 41575-94-4.*
*ATC — L01XA02.*

**Pharmacopoeias.** In *Chin., Eur.* (see p.vi), and *US.*

**Ph. Eur. 5.0** (Carboplatin). A colourless, crystalline powder. Sparingly soluble in water; very slightly soluble in alcohol and in acetone. Protect from light.

**USP 27** (Carboplatin). A 1% solution in water has a pH of 5.0 to 7.0. Store in airtight containers. Protect from light.

**Incompatibility.** Carboplatin reacts with aluminium causing loss of potency and precipitate formation. Needles, syringes, catheters or administration sets that contain aluminium should not be used for preparation or administration of carboplatin.

**Stability.** About 5% of the initial carboplatin concentration was lost over 24 hours when solutions were diluted in sodium chloride 0.9% and stored at 25°; lesser degrees of degradation were seen at lower sodium chloride concentrations, but carboplatin was apparently stable over this period if diluted with glucose 5%.[1] The authors suggested that chloride-containing infusion solutions are not suitable for carboplatin, not only because of the loss of active drug but because of the possibility that conversion to cisplatin may be occurring, with a risk of increased toxicity.[1] This has been contested by the manufacturers (*Bristol-Myers, USA*), who found that only 0.5% or 0.7%, depending on formulation, of a carboplatin solution in sodium chloride 0.9%, had been converted to cisplatin after 24 hours.[2] However, the total degradation of carboplatin was not measured. In another study, the authors calculated the time to 5% degradation of carboplatin at 25° as 29.2 hours in sodium chloride 0.9% compared with 52.7 hours in water.[3] They concluded that carboplatin should not be diluted in sodium chloride 0.9% when intended for continuous infusion over a prolonged period.[3] Carboplatin in glucose 5% was reported to be stable for 7 days at 25° in PVC bags when protected from light.[4]

1. Cheung Y-W, *et al.* Stability of cisplatin, iproplatin, carboplatin, and tetraplatin in commonly used intravenous solutions. *Am J Hosp Pharm* 1987; **44:** 124–30.
2. Perrone RK, *et al.* Extent of cisplatin formation in carboplatin admixtures. *Am J Hosp Pharm* 1989; **46:** 258–9.
3. Allsopp MA, *et al.* The degradation of carboplatin in aqueous solutions containing chloride or other selected nucleophiles. *Int J Pharmaceutics* 1991; **69:** 197–210.
4. Diaz Amador F, *et al.* Stability of carboplatin in polyvinyl chloride bags. *Am J Health-Syst Pharm* 1998; **55:** 602, 604.

## Adverse Effects, Treatment, and Precautions

As for Cisplatin, p.538; nephrotoxicity and gastrointestinal toxicity are less severe than with cisplatin and reversible myelosuppression is the dose-limiting toxicity; platelet counts reach a nadir between 14 and 21 days after a dose, with recovery within 35 days, but recovery from leucopenia may be slower. Myelosuppression may be more severe and prolonged in patients with impaired renal function. Carboplatin should therefore be given at reduced doses to these patients and should be avoided if creatinine clearance is 20 mL/minute or less. Weekly blood counts and regular renal and hepatic function tests are recommended in all patients during therapy. Neurological function including assessment of hearing should also be monitored.

**Incidence of adverse effects.** Analysis by the manufacturers of the adverse effects of carboplatin, in studies involving 710 patients.[1] Myelosuppression was the dose-limiting toxicity: leucopenia occurred in 55% of the evaluable patients. Leucopenia and thrombocytopenia result in symptomatic events such as infection or bleeding in a minority of patients. Anaemia was frequent (59%) and required transfusional support in about one-fifth of the patients. Nephrotoxicity and serum electrolyte loss were much less of a problem; no high-volume fluid hydration or electrolyte supplementation was given during treatment. Vomiting occurred in about half the patients, and a further 25% had nausea without vomiting. Peripheral neurotoxicity was reported in 6% of evaluable patients and clinical ototoxicity occurred in only 8 cases (about 1%), but see also Effects on the Ears, below. Increases in liver enzyme values have also been reported, as well as, more rarely, alopecia, skin rash, a flu-like syndrome, and local effects at the injection site.

1. Canetta R, *et al.* Carboplatin: the clinical spectrum to date. *Cancer Treat Rev* 1985; **12** (suppl A): 125–36.

**Effects on the ears.** Carboplatin is less ototoxic than cisplatin, but ototoxicity is still common with carboplatin when used in high doses, for example, as part of conditioning regimens for bone marrow transplantation.[1,2] There was some evidence that sodium thiosulfate reduced carboplatin-induced hearing loss, when carboplatin was used for CNS malignancy.[3,4]

1. Freilich RJ, *et al.* Hearing loss in children with brain tumors treated with cisplatin and carboplatin-based high-dose chemotherapy with autologous bone marrow rescue. *Med Pediatr Oncol* 1996; **26:** 95–100.
2. Parsons SK, *et al.* Severe ototoxicity following carboplatin-containing conditioning regimen for autologous marrow transplantation for neuroblastoma. *Bone Marrow Transplant* 1998; **22:** 669–74.
3. Neuwelt EA, *et al.* First evidence of otoprotection against carboplatin-induced hearing loss with a two-compartment system in patients with central nervous system malignancy using sodium thiosulfate. *J Pharmacol Exp Ther* 1998; **286:** 77–84.
4. Doolittle ND, *et al.* Delayed sodium thiosulfate as an otoprotectant against carboplatin-induced hearing loss in patients with malignant brain tumors. *Clin Cancer Res* 2001; **7:** 493–500.

**Effects on the eyes.** Cortical blindness developed in 2 patients with impaired renal function receiving high-dose carboplatin;[1] although 10 cases of visual disturbances in patients receiving carboplatin had been reported to the manufacturers, none of these had sudden blindness and it was thought that the effect represented CNS toxicity in the presence of poor renal excretion. It was concluded that it was unwise to give high-dose carboplatin to patients whose glomerular filtration rate is less than 50 mL/minute.

1. O'Brien MER, *et al.* Blindness associated with high-dose carboplatin. *Lancet* 1992; **339:** 558.

**Effects on the kidneys.** Although carboplatin is reported to be much less nephrotoxic than cisplatin it is not devoid of adverse effects on the kidney. Salt wasting nephropathy (similar to that seen with cisplatin),[1] and decreased creatinine clearance[2] and glomerular filtration rate[3] have occurred, as has acute renal failure in 2 patients given intraperitoneal carboplatin[4] (although these patients had been heavily pretreated with cisplatin). It has been suggested that renal toxicity may be more likely at cumulative carboplatin doses of about 750 mg/m$^2$ or more,[3] and there is some evidence to suggest that intensive hydration may ameliorate nephrotoxic effects.[2]

1. Welborn J, *et al.* Renal salt wasting and carboplatinum. *Ann Intern Med* 1988; **108:** 640.
2. Reed E, Jacob J. Carboplatin and renal dysfunction. *Ann Intern Med* 1989; **110:** 409.
3. Smit EF, *et al.* Carboplatin and renal function. *Ann Intern Med* 1989; **110:** 1034.
4. McDonald BR, *et al.* Acute renal failure associated with the use of intraperitoneal carboplatin: a report of two cases and review of the literature. *Am J Med* 1991; **90:** 386–91.

**Hypersensitivity.** In one series, 12% of 205 patients treated with carboplatin developed a hypersensitivity reaction after a median of 8 courses of platinum therapy.[1] Symptoms were at least moderately severe in half of the patients. Reactions to cisplatin would be anticipated in patients who have been previously sensitised to carboplatin—for 1 such case see p.538. In another study,[2] patients receiving more than 7 courses of carboplatin therapy were given a skin test before each course in an attempt to identify patients at risk for hypersensitivity reactions. The test consisted of 0.02 mL of an undiluted aliquot of their planned infusion, injected intradermally 1 hour before administration. A negative skin test was found to accurately predict the absence of a hypersensitivity reaction. In a further extended report[3] by the same group, the skin test had been given about 30 minutes before carboplatin doses in 126 women who had already received at least 6 courses of a platinum-based regimen for a gynaecological cancer. Following 668 negative skin tests, a hypersensitivity reaction developed on 10 occasions (in 7 patients), giving a false-negative rate of 1.5%. None of the reactions were severe. Of the 39 patients who had a positive skin test, 7 elected to receive the dose of carboplatin; 6 of these developed a hypersensitivity reaction but none were severe.

The use of a desensitisation regimen has been successful in a small number of patients.[4]

1. Markman M, *et al.* Clinical features of hypersensitivity reactions to carboplatin. *J Clin Oncol* 1999; **17:** 1141–5.
2. Zanotti KM, *et al.* Carboplatin skin testing: a skin-testing protocol for predicting hypersensitivity to carboplatin chemotherapy. *J Clin Oncol* 2001; **19:** 3126–9.
3. Markman M, *et al.* Expanded experience with an intradermal skin test to predict for the presence or absence of carboplatin hypersensitivity. *J Clin Oncol* 2003; **21:** 4611–14.
4. Markman M, *et al.* Initial experience with a novel desensitization strategy for carboplatin-associated hypersensitivity reactions: carboplatin-hypersensitivity reactions. *J Cancer Res Clin Oncol* 2004; **130:** 25–8.

## Interactions

As for Cisplatin, p.539.

## Pharmacokinetics

Intravenous carboplatin exhibits a biphasic elimination and is excreted primarily in the urine, about 70% of a dose being excreted within 24 hours, almost all unchanged. The terminal half-life of intact carboplatin is reported to be about 1.5 to 6 hours. Platinum from carboplatin slowly becomes protein bound, and is subsequently excreted with a half-life of 5 days or more.

◊ References.

1. van der Vijgh WJF. Clinical pharmacokinetics of carboplatin. *Clin Pharmacokinet* 1991; **21:** 242–61.

## Uses and Administration

Carboplatin is an analogue of cisplatin with similar actions and uses (see p.539). It is used in the treatment of advanced ovarian cancers and of small-cell lung cancer, both alone and combined with other antineoplastics. It has also been tried as an alternative to cisplatin in other solid tumours (see below).

Carboplatin is given by intravenous infusion over 15 minutes to 1 hour. In the UK an initial dose of 400 mg/m$^2$ is licensed for use as a single agent in previously untreated patients with normal renal function, reduced by 20 to 25% (300 to 320 mg/m$^2$) in patients who have previously been treated with myelosuppressive therapy or who have poor performance status. In the USA an initial dose of 360 mg/m$^2$ is licensed as a single agent in previously treated patients with recurrent disease, and an initial dose of 300 mg/m$^2$ when used with cyclophosphamide in previously untreated patients.

Dosage adjustments are necessary in patients with renal impairment (see below) and when carboplatin is given as part of a combination regimen. The dose in mg may be calculated using the Calvert formula as described under Administration, below. Subsequent doses should be adjusted according to the nadir of the white cell and platelet counts (see also Bone-marrow Depression, p.496), and should not be given more frequently than every 4 weeks.

**Administration.** Pharmacokinetic studies by Calvert and colleagues[1] have indicated that the dose of carboplatin to produce a desired area under the concentration-time curve (AUC) could be calculated, based on the patient's glomerular filtration rate (GFR), as:

$$\text{Dose in mg} = \text{target AUC} \times (\text{GFR} + 25)$$

It should be noted that the resultant dose is given in mg and not in mg/m$^2$. This formula was found to be useful in patients with higher than normal as well as reduced GFR. Suggested target AUCs were 5 mg/mL per minute in previously treated patients and 7 mg/mL per minute in those who had not previously received chemotherapy. In combination therapy the appropriate AUC value depended on the other drugs used: an AUC of 4.5 mg/mL per minute gave acceptable results when carboplatin was combined with bleomycin and etoposide for testicular teratoma.

However, determination of GFR may be a problem: clearance of technetium-99m-labelled diethylenetriamine penta-acetic acid (DTPA) or chromium-51-labelled edetic acid is more accurate than 24-hour creatinine clearance, with the first of these more convenient than the second.[2] (It has been suggested that creatinine clearance should not be used to estimate GFR for the Calvert equation.[3]) Nonetheless, radioisotopic determination of GFR is still an elaborate procedure, and may be less accurate in children than adults.[4] Chatelut and colleagues have proposed formulae for determining clearance of carboplatin in both adults[5] and children.[4]

It has been suggested that the Calvert and Chatelut formulae are not sufficiently accurate for use in children, or in adults with very severe renal impairment. Bayesian methods are the technique of choice where serum carboplatin concentrations can be monitored.[3] However, a study in children showed that dosage based on determination of the GFR results in more consistent carboplatin exposure than administration based on body-surface area.[6]

1. Calvert AH, *et al.* Carboplatin dosage: prospective evaluation of a simple formula based on renal function. *J Clin Oncol* 1989; **7:** 1748–56.
2. Millward MJ, *et al.* Carboplatin dosing based on measurement of renal function—experience at the Peter MacCallum Cancer Institute. *Aust N Z J Med* 1996; **26:** 372–9.
3. Duffull SB, Robinson BA. Clinical pharmacokinetics and dose optimisation of carboplatin. *Clin Pharmacokinet* 1997; **33:** 161–83.
4. Chatelut E, *et al.* Population pharmacokinetics of carboplatin in children. *Clin Pharmacol Ther* 1996; **59:** 436–43.
5. Chatelut E, *et al.* Prediction of carboplatin clearance from standard morphological and biological patient characteristics. *J Natl Cancer Inst* 1995; **87:** 573–80.
6. Thomas H, *et al.* Prospective validation of renal-function-based carboplatin dosing in children with cancer: a United Kingdom Children's Cancer Study Group Trial. *J Clin Oncol* 2000; **18:** 3614–21.

**Administration in renal impairment.** The initial dose of carboplatin is usually determined using a formula (see Administration, above). If this approach is not adopted, the UK manufacturers recommend that carboplatin be given at a dose of 250 mg/m$^2$ if creatinine clearance is between 20 and 39 mL/minute, and that patients with a creatinine clearance of 40 mL/minute or more be given the standard dose of 400 mg/m$^2$. However, in the USA, the manufacturers recommend a dose of 200 mg/m$^2$ for patients with a creatinine clearance of between 16 and 40 mL/minute, and a dose of 250 mg/m$^2$ for those with a creatinine clearance of between 41 and 59 mL/minute.

**Malignant neoplasms.** A preliminary review[1] of carboplatin, concluded that it was active in ovarian cancer (p.520), with similar responses to those seen with cisplatin; its activity in small-cell lung cancer (p.519), seminoma, and squamous cell carcinomas of the head and neck seemed likely to be comparable, whereas results in gastrointestinal and breast cancers, lymphomas and leukaemias, melanoma, mesothelioma, renal carcinoma, and sarcoma were, generally unimpressive. A subsequent review[2] suggested that in testicular cancer, where there was a prospect of cure, cisplatin, which appeared to give better results in some studies should be preferred. However, in ovarian cancer, where treatment was largely palliative, carboplatin had the advantage of being better tolerated. A further review[3] of randomised studies concurred that carboplatin was equivalent to cisplatin in suboptimally debulked ovarian cancer and extensive-stage small-cell lung cancer, and was inferior to cisplatin in testicular cancer. It was also concluded that carboplatin was inferior to cisplatin in head and neck and oesophageal cancers. There was insufficient comparative evidence for other cancers for which cisplatin has a role.

1. Wagstaff AJ, *et al.* Carboplatin: a preliminary review of its pharmacodynamic and pharmacokinetic properties and therapeutic efficacy in the treatment of cancer. *Drugs* 1989; **37:** 162–90.
2. Anonymous. Cisplatin or carboplatin for ovarian and testicular cancer? *Drug Ther Bull* 1994; **32:** 62–3.
3. Go RS, Adjei AA. Review of the comparative pharmacology and clinical activity of cisplatin and carboplatin. *J Clin Oncol* 1999; **17:** 409–22.

## Preparations

***BP 2003:*** Carboplatin Injection;
***USP 27:*** Carboplatin for Injection.

**Proprietary Preparations** (details are given in Part 3)
***Arg.:*** Carboplat; Carboxtie; Omilipis; Paraplatin; ***Austria:*** Carbosol; Paraplatin; ***Belg.:*** Paraplatin; ***Braz.:*** B-Platin; Biocarbo; Oncocarb; Paraplatin; Platamine; Platicarb; Tecnocarb; ***Canad.:*** Paraplatin; ***Chile:*** Blastocarb; ***Denm.:*** Carbosin†; Paraplatin; ***Fin.:*** Carbosin; Paraplatin; ***Fr.:*** Paraplatine; ***Ger.:*** Carboplat; Neocarbo; Ribocarbo; ***Gr.:*** Carbosin; Emorzim; Megaplatin; Paraplatin; ***Hong Kong:*** Paraplatin; ***India:*** Kemocarb; ***Irl.:*** Paraplatin; ***Israel:*** Paraplatin; ***Ital.:*** Paraplatin; ***Malaysia:*** Paraplatin; ***Mex.:*** Blastocarb; Boplatex; Carboplat; Carbotec†; Displata†; Ifacap; Novoplat†; Paraplatin; ***Neth.:*** Paraplatin; ***Norw.:*** Carbosin; Paraplatin; ***NZ:*** Carbosin; Paraplatin; ***Port.:*** Nealorin†; Novoplatinum; Paraplatin; ***S.Afr.:*** Carbosin; Paraplatin; ***Singapore:*** Paraplatin; ***Spain:*** Ercar; Nealorin; Paraplatin; Platinwas; ***Swed.:*** Paraplatin; ***Switz.:*** Paraplatin; ***Thai.:*** Carbosin; Kemocarb; Paraplatin; ***UK:*** Paraplatin; ***USA:*** Paraplatin.

---

## Carboquone *(rINN)*

Carbazilquinone; Carbocuona. 2,5-Bis(aziridin-1-yl)-3-(2-hydroxy-1-methoxyethyl)-6-methyl-*p*-benzoquinone carbamate.
$C_{15}H_{19}N_3O_5$ = 321.3.
*CAS — 24279-91-2.*
*ATC — L01AC03.*

### Profile

Carboquone is an alkylating agent that has been used in the treatment of a variety of malignant neoplasms including those of the lung, stomach, and ovary; it has also been used in lymphomas and in chronic myeloid leukaemia. It has been given by the intravenous or intra-arterial route, or by mouth.

---

## Carmofur *(rINN)*

HCFU. 5-Fluoro-*N*-hexyl-3,4-dihydro-2,4-dioxo-1-(2*H*)-pyrimidinecarboxamide; 1-Hexylcarbamoyl-5-fluorouracil; .
$C_{11}H_{16}FN_3O_3$ = 257.3.
*CAS — 61422-45-5.*
*ATC — L01BC04.*

**Pharmacopoeias.** In *Jpn.*

### Profile

Carmofur is an orally active derivative of fluorouracil (p.554) and has similar actions. It is used in the adjuvant treatment of colorectal cancer, and has been used in breast and ovarian cancers. Carmofur has been associated with the development of neurological disorders including leukoencephalopathy.

◊ References.

1. Yamada T, *et al.* Leukoencephalopathy following treatment with carmofur: a case report and review of the Japanese literature. *Asia Oceania J Obstet Gynaecol* 1989; **15:** 161–8.
2. Sakamoto J, *et al.* An individual patient data meta-analysis of long supported adjuvant chemotherapy with oral carmofur in patients with curatively resected colorectal cancer. *Oncol Rep* 2001; **8:** 697–703.
3. Nakamura T, *et al.* Optimal duration of oral adjuvant chemotherapy with Carmofur in the colorectal cancer patients: the Kansai Carmofur Study Group trial III. *Int J Oncol* 2001; **19:** 291–8.
4. Tominaga T, *et al.* Postoperative chemoendocrine therapy for women with node-positive stage II breast cancer with combined cyclophosphamide, tamoxifen, and 1-hexylcarbamoyl-5-fluorouracil. *Eur J Surg* 2001; **167:** 598–604.
5. Iwagaki H, *et al.* Post-operative adjuvant chemotherapy for colorectal cancer with 5-fluorouracil (5-FU) infusion combined with 1-hexylcarbamoyl-5-fluorouracil (HCFU) oral administration after curative resection. *Anticancer Res* 2001; **21:** 4163–8.

### Preparations

**Proprietary Preparations** (details are given in Part 3)
***Fin.:*** Mirafur.

---

# Carmustine *(BAN, USAN, rINN)*

BCNU; BiCNU; Carmustina; Carmustinum; NSC-409962; WR-139021. 1,3-Bis(2-chloroethyl)-1-nitrosourea.
$C_5H_9Cl_2N_3O_2$ = 214.0.
*CAS — 154-93-8.*
*ATC — L01AD01.*

**Pharmacopoeias.** In *Chin.* and *Eur.* (see p.vi).

**Ph. Eur. 5.0** (Carmustine). A yellowish, granular powder. Very slightly soluble in water; freely soluble in dehydrated alcohol; very soluble in dichloromethane. It melts at about 31° with decomposition. Store at a temperature of 2° to 8° in airtight containers. Protect from light.

**Stability.** The manufacturers state that, when reconstituted, resulting carmustine solutions (undiluted or further diluted in sodium chloride 0.9% or glucose 5%) are stable for 8 hours at room temperature, or 24 hours at 2° to 8°, when protected from light. There is some evidence that carmustine interacts with plastic giving sets and containers, and the manufacturers recommend the use of polyethylene or glass.

A study has indicated that diluted solutions of carmustine undergo increased degradation in the presence of sodium bicarbonate, with only 73% of the original concentration of carmustine remaining after 90 minutes, much of the loss being in the first 15 minutes.[1]

1. Colvin M, *et al.* Stability of carmustine in the presence of sodium bicarbonate. *Am J Hosp Pharm* 1980; **37:** 677–8.

## Adverse Effects and Treatment

For a general outline see Antineoplastics, p.492 and p.495. Delayed and cumulative bone-marrow depression is the most frequent and serious side-effect of intravenous carmustine. Platelets and leucocytes are mainly affected, with platelet nadirs occurring at 4 to 5 weeks after administration and leucocyte nadirs at 5 to 6 weeks after administration; although thrombocytopenia is usually more severe, leucopenia may also be dose-limiting. Other side-effects include pulmonary fibrosis (mainly but not exclusively at high cumulative doses—see also Effects on the Lungs, p.494), renal and hepatic damage, and optic neuritis. Nausea and vomiting, beginning up to 2 hours after a dose, is common but can be reduced by prophylactic antiemetic therapy. Venous irritation may follow intravenous injection and transient hyperpigmentation has been noted after contact of a solution with the skin. Flushing of the skin and suffusion of the conjunctiva may occur following rapid intravenous infusion.

Convulsions, cerebral oedema, and various neurological symptoms have been reported in patients given carmustine-containing polymer implants; abnormalities of wound healing at the site of implantation, and an increased incidence of intracranial infection have also been reported.

As with other alkylating agents, carmustine is potentially carcinogenic, mutagenic, and teratogenic.

**Effects on the eyes.** Ocular toxicity has been reported in patients receiving carmustine,[1,2] and seems to be more likely when given into the carotid artery,[1,2] although it was also seen with high-dose intravenous therapy. There is some evidence that the alcohol diluent used to prepare carmustine solutions may contribute to the retinopathy.[2]

1. Shingleton BJ, *et al.* Ocular toxicity associated with high-dose carmustine. *Arch Ophthalmol* 1982; **100:** 1766–72.
2. Greenberg HS, *et al.* Intra-arterial BCNU chemotherapy for treatment of malignant gliomas of the central nervous system. *J Neurosurg* 1984; **61:** 423–9.

**Extravasation.** For mention of the use of sodium bicarbonate as a specific antidote following carmustine extravasation, see under Treatment of Adverse Effects of Antineoplastics, p.496.

## Precautions

For reference to the precautions necessary with antineoplastics, see p.497. Carmustine should be used with extreme caution in children, who are at particular risk of severe delayed pulmonary toxicity. It should also be used with caution in patients with reduced lung function. Lung function should be monitored before and frequently during therapy. Blood counts should be monitored weekly during therapy, and for at least 6 weeks after the last dose. Renal and hepatic function should also be monitored periodically.

**Handling and disposal.** Carmustine has been shown to permeate latex, PVC, and rubber gloves, the degree of permeation tending to increase with time,[1-3] up to an equilibrium value.[2] The permeation rate appears not to depend solely on glove thickness and material, and may be different for different gloves made from the same material.[2] The time for initial penetration was reported to vary between 4.7 and 66.0 minutes in one study,[2] and gloves could be chosen accordingly depending on the anticipated length of exposure. Double-gloving, particularly with thicker PVC[1] or ethylmethacrylate[3] gloves, may offer some additional protection.

1. Connor TH, *et al.* Permeability of latex and polyvinyl chloride gloves to carmustine. *Am J Hosp Pharm* 1984; **41:** 676–9.
2. Thomas PH, Fenton-May V. Protection offered by various gloves to carmustine exposure. *Pharm J* 1987; **238:** 775–7.
3. Mellström GA, *et al.* Barrier effect of gloves against cytostatic drugs. *Curr Probl Dermatol* 1996; **25:** 163–9.

## Interactions

For a general outline of antineoplastic drug interactions, see p.498.

**Cimetidine.** Reductions in white cell counts and platelet counts well below those normally attributed to treatment with carmustine alone were seen in 6 of 8 patients receiving their first course of carmustine and steroids with cimetidine given prophylactically,[1] and in 9 patients in a further study.[2] Cimetidine was also reported to exacerbate the neutropenia and leucopenia in a patient receiving lomustine.[3]

1. Selker RG, *et al.* Bone-marrow depression with cimetidine plus carmustine. *N Engl J Med* 1978; **299:** 834.
2. Volkin RL, *et al.* Potentiation of carmustine-cranial irradiation-induced myelosuppression by cimetidine. *Arch Intern Med* 1982; **142:** 243–5.
3. Hess WA, Kornblith PL. Combination of lomustine and cimetidine in the treatment of a patient with malignant glioblastoma: a case report. *Cancer Treat Rep* 1985; **69:** 733.

## Pharmacokinetics

Intravenous carmustine is rapidly metabolised, and no intact drug is detectable after 15 minutes; metabolites have a much longer half-life and are presumed to be responsible for its activity. It is primarily excreted in the urine; some is also excreted as carbon dioxide, via the lungs. Carmustine readily crosses the blood-brain barrier, appearing in CSF in substantial concentrations almost immediately after intravenous injection.

## Uses and Administration

Carmustine is a cell-cycle phase non-specific antineoplastic belonging to the nitrosourea group of compounds, which are considered to function as alkylating agents. It is believed to alkylate DNA and RNA, and may also inhibit enzymatic processes by carbamoylation of amino acids in proteins. It is used in the treatment of brain tumours, and in combination chemotherapy for multiple myeloma, and may be given as second-line therapy in Hodgkin's disease, and some other malignancies (see below).

Carmustine is licensed for use as a single agent either as a single dose of 150 to 200 mg/m² or divided into doses of 75 to 100 mg/m² given on 2 successive days. Doses are given by intravenous infusion over 1 to 2 hours in sodium chloride 0.9% or glucose 5%. Lower doses are usually given in combination therapy, except for conditioning before stem-cell transplantation. Doses may be repeated every 6 weeks provided that blood counts have returned to acceptable levels. Subsequent doses must be adjusted according to the haematological response (see also Bone-marrow Depression, p.496).

Polymer implants containing carmustine have been developed for implantation into the brain in the localised treatment of malignant glioma. Each implant contains 7.7 mg of carmustine: up to 8 such implants are inserted into the cavity left by surgical removal of the tumour.

**Administration.** In a multicentre study[1] in patients with recurrent malignant glioma, biodegradable poly(carboxyphenoxypropane/sebacic acid)anhydride polymer (BIODEL) wafers containing carmustine 7.7 mg or placebo were implanted into the brain after tumour resection to a maximum dose of 8 wafers. The effects of treatment favoured the carmustine implant; 59 of 112 patients given placebo implants were dead at 6 months, compared with 44 of 110 given carmustine implants, with a median survival of 23 and 31 weeks, respectively. A subsequent small cohort study[2] failed to find a clear survival benefit associated with wafer implantation in recurrent glioma, and reported a higher rate of complications including seizures, cerebral oedema, CSF leaks, sepsis, and wound infections. The limitations of this small study were acknowledged by the authors, and a review[3] that included these studies concluded that despite limited data, carmustine wafers do provide some survival benefit.

1. Brem H, *et al.* Placebo-controlled trial of safety and efficacy of intraoperative controlled delivery by biodegradable polymers of chemotherapy for recurrent gliomas. *Lancet* 1995; **345:** 1008–12.
2. Subach BR, *et al.* Morbidity and survival after 1,3-bis(2-chloroethyl)-1-nitrosourea wafer implantation for recurrent glioblastoma: a retrospective case-matched cohort series. *Neurosurgery* 1999; **45:** 17–23.
3. Engelhard HH. The role of interstitial BCNU chemotherapy in the treatment of malignant glioma. *Surg Neurol* 2000; **53:** 458–64.

**Amyloidosis.** For mention of chemotherapy with epirubicin, cyclophosphamide, and carmustine to suppress amyloidosis after cardiac transplantation, see p.567.

**Malignant neoplasms.** Carmustine has been used in chemotherapeutic regimens for a number of malignancies. Because of its ability to pass the blood-brain barrier it has been extensively used in malignant neoplasms of the brain, the management of which is discussed further on p.513. Other conditions in which it has been employed, include malignant melanoma (p.522), Hodgkin's disease (p.509), and multiple myeloma (p.511).

**Mycosis fungoides.** Topical application of carmustine has been used successfully[1-4] in early mycosis fungoides (p.511). Erythema and telangiectasia were the most frequent side-effects.

1. Zackheim HS, *et al.* Topical carmustine (BCNU) for mycosis fungoides and related disorders: a 10-year experience. *J Am Acad Dermatol* 1983; **9:** 363–74.
2. Zackheim HS, *et al.* Topical carmustine (BCNU) for cutaneous T cell lymphoma: a 15-year experience in 143 patients. *J Am Acad Dermatol* 1990; **22:** 802–10.
3. Zackheim HS. Topical carmustine (BCNU) for patch/plaque mycosis fungoides. *Semin Dermatol* 1994; **13:** 202–6.
4. Heald PW, Glusac EJ. Unilesional cutaneous T-cell lymphoma: clinical features, therapy, and follow-up of 10 patients with a treatment-responsive mycosis fungoides variant. *J Am Acad Dermatol* 2000; **42:** 283–5.

## Preparations

**Proprietary Preparations** (details are given in Part 3)
***Arg.:*** BiCNU; ***Austral.:*** BiCNU; Gliadel; ***Austria:*** Carmubris; ***Belg.:*** Nitrumon; ***Braz.:*** Becenun; Gliadel†; ***Canad.:*** BiCNU; Gliadel†; ***Chile:*** BiCNU; Gliadel; ***Denm.:*** Becenun†; ***Fr.:*** BiCNU; Gliadel†; ***Ger.:*** Carmubris; ***Gr.:*** Nitrumon; ***Hong Kong:*** BiCNU; ***Irl.:*** BiCNU; ***Israel:*** BiCNU; Gliadel; ***Malaysia:*** BiCNU; ***Mex.:*** BiCNU; ***Norw.:*** Becenun†; ***NZ:*** BiCNU; Gliadel†; ***Port.:*** Gliadel†; ***S.Afr.:*** BiCNU; ***Singapore:*** BiCNU; Gliadel†; ***Spain:*** Nitroureant†; ***Swed.:*** Becenun†; ***Thai.:*** BiCNU†; ***UK:*** BiCNU; Gliadel; ***USA:*** BiCNU; Gliadel.

## Cetuximab *(USAN, rINN)*

C-225.
*CAS — 205923-56-4.*

### Profile

Cetuximab is a monoclonal antibody that binds to the epidermal growth factor receptor (EGFR). It is used alone or with irinotecan in the treatment of EGFR-expressing metastatic colorectal cancer (p.516). It is also under investigation for the treatment of cancer of the head and neck, and other solid tumours. In colorectal cancer, cetuximab 400 mg/m$^2$ is given as a loading dose by intravenous infusion over 2 hours. This is followed by once weekly maintenance doses of 250 mg/m$^2$ given over 1 hour. A low-protein-binding 0.22-micrometre in-line filter and infusion or syringe pump should be used.

Adverse effects associated with cetuximab include acneform rash, asthenia, and gastrointestinal disturbances. Infusion reactions suggestive of a cytokine release syndrome can occur, usually with the first dose. Mild reactions include chills, fever, and dyspnoea; severe reactions include bronchospasm, urticaria, and hypotension, and fatalities have occurred. Pre-medication with a histamine $H_1$-receptor antagonist is recommended. Interstitial lung disease and pneumonitis have been reported rarely. Cetuximab doses should be halved in patients who have experienced a mild to moderate infusion reaction, and permanently discontinued if a severe reaction has occurred. When a severe acneform rash has occurred, the next dose should be delayed by 1 to 2 weeks. After the first occurrence, the full maintenance dose may be given if there has been improvement in the rash; after a second occurrence the next dose should be delayed and reduced to 200 mg/m$^2$; after a third occurrence the next dose should be delayed and reduced to 150 mg/m$^2$. If there is no improvement in the rash when therapy has been delayed, or if the rash has occurred 4 times, cetuximab should be stopped.

◊ Reviews.

1. Reynolds NA, Wagstaff AJ. Cetuximab: in the treatment of metastatic colorectal cancer. *Drugs* 2004; **64:** 109–18.

### Preparations

**Proprietary Preparations** (details are given in Part 3)
***USA:*** Erbitux.

# Chlorambucil *(BAN, rINN)*

CB-1348; Chlorambucilum; Chloraminophene; Chlorbutinum; Clorambucilo; NSC-3088; WR-139013. 4-[4-Bis(2-chloroethyl)aminophenyl]butyric acid.
$C_{14}H_{19}Cl_2NO_2$ = 304.2.
*CAS — 305-03-3.*
*ATC — L01AA02.*

**Pharmacopoeias.** In *Chin., Eur.* (see p.vi), *Int., Pol.,* and *US.*

**Ph. Eur. 5.0** (Chlorambucil). A white, crystalline powder. Practically insoluble in water; freely soluble in alcohol and in acetone. Protect from light.

**USP 27** (Chlorambucil). An off-white, slightly granular powder. M.p. 65° to 69°. Very slightly soluble in water; soluble 1 in 2 of acetone; soluble in dilute alkali. Store in airtight containers. Protect from light.

**Storage.** The manufacturers recommend that tablets of chlorambucil should be stored at 2° to 8° and kept dry.

## Adverse Effects and Treatment

For a general outline see Antineoplastics, p.492 and p.495.

A reversible progressive lymphocytopenia tends to develop during treatment with chlorambucil. Neutropenia may continue to develop up to 10 days after the last dose. Irreversible bone-marrow depression can occur particularly when the total dosage for the course approaches 6.5 mg/kg.

Other reported adverse effects include gastrointestinal disturbances, hepatotoxicity, skin rashes (rarely Stevens-Johnson syndrome or toxic epidermal necrolysis), peripheral neuropathy, and central neurotoxicity, including seizures. Interstitial pneumonia and pulmonary fibrosis have occurred; the latter is usually reversible but fatalities have been recorded. Chlorambucil in high doses may produce azoospermia and amenorrhoea; sterility has developed particularly when chlorambucil has been given to boys at or before puberty.

Overdosage may result in pancytopenia and in neurotoxicity, including agitation, ataxia, and grand mal seizures.

Like other alkylating agents, chlorambucil is potentially mutagenic, teratogenic, and carcinogenic, and an increased incidence of acute leukaemias and other secondary malignancies has been reported in patients who have received the drug.

**Effects on the bladder.** Chlorambucil-induced cystitis was reported in a 73-year-old woman given 2 mg daily for over 2 years for the treatment of lymphocytic lymphoma.[1]

1. Daoud D, *et al.* Sterile cystitis associated with chlorambucil. *Drug Intell Clin Pharm* 1977; **11:** 491.

**Effects on the eyes.** Visual impairment and optic atrophy in a patient who had been receiving chlorambucil for five years to control non-Hodgkin's lymphoma were thought to be due to the drug,[1] although ocular effects are extremely rare with chlorambucil.

1. Yiannakis PH, Larner AJ. Visual failure and optic atrophy associated with chlorambucil therapy. *BMJ* 1993; **306:** 109.

**Effects on the nervous system.** There have been a small number of reports of seizures in patients given chlorambucil. A review[1] of these suggested that in adults, patients with a history of seizures, or those given high doses of chlorambucil may be at increased risk. The reports in children consisted mainly of patients being treated for nephrotic syndrome, possibly because the condition may alter the pharmacokinetics of chlorambucil.

1. Salloum E, *et al.* Chlorambucil-induced seizures. *Cancer* 1997; **79:** 1009–13.

## Precautions

For reference to the precautions necessary with antineoplastics, see p.497. Chlorambucil should not be administered, or should be given with great care and at reduced doses, for at least 4 weeks after treatment with radiotherapy or other antineoplastics unless only low doses of radiation have been given to parts remote from the bone marrow and the neutrophil and platelet counts are not depressed. The dose should be reduced if there is lymphocytic involvement of the bone marrow or if it is hypoplastic. Chlorambucil should be given with care to patients with impaired renal function; the manufacturers state that consideration should also be given to dose reduction in patients with gross hepatic dysfunction. Children with nephrotic syndrome, patients receiving high-dose pulse therapy with chlorambucil, and those with a history of seizures, may be at increased risk of seizures. Regular blood counts are required during therapy.

**Handling and disposal.** Chlorambucil is irritant; avoid contact with skin and mucous membranes.

*Urine* produced for up to 48 hours after a dose of chlorambucil should be handled wearing protective clothing.[1]

1. Harris J, Dodds LJ. Handling waste from patients receiving cytotoxic drugs. *Pharm J* 1985; **235:** 289–91.

**Porphyria.** Chlorambucil is considered to be unsafe in patients with porphyria because it has been shown to be porphyrinogenic in *animals.*

## Interactions

For a general outline of antineoplastic drug interactions, see p.498.

## Pharmacokinetics

Chlorambucil is rapidly and almost completely absorbed from the gastrointestinal tract following oral doses and is reported to have a terminal half-life in plasma of about 1.5 hours. It is extensively metabolised in the liver, primarily to active phenylacetic acid mustard, which has a slightly longer plasma half-life of about 1.8 to 2.5 hours, and which like chlorambucil also undergoes some spontaneous degradation to further derivatives. Chlorambucil and its metabolites are extensively protein bound. It is excreted in the urine almost entirely as metabolites with less than 1% unchanged.

## Uses and Administration

Chlorambucil is an antineoplastic derived from chlormethine (p.537) and has a similar mode of action. It acts on lymphocytes and to a lesser extent on neutrophils and platelets. Chlorambucil is most valuable in those conditions associated with the proliferation of white blood cells, especially lymphocytes, and is used in the treatment of chronic lymphocytic leukaemia and lymphomas, including Hodgkin's disease. It is also used in Waldenström's macroglobulinaemia and has been given in gestational trophoblastic tumours. Although formerly widely used in the management of polycythaemia vera it has largely been superseded.

Chlorambucil also has immunosuppressant properties and has been given in various auto-immune disorders including amyloidosis, Behçet's syndrome, glomerular kidney disease, primary biliary cirrhosis, polymyositis, rheumatoid arthritis, and sarcoidosis.

The use of chlorambucil in these disorders is discussed further elsewhere, as indicated by the cross-references given below.

Chlorambucil is better tolerated than chlormethine hydrochloride and serious bone-marrow toxicity is not usually a problem with normal doses. When used as a single-agent antineoplastic for chronic lymphocytic leukaemia and lymphomas, chlorambucil is licensed for use by mouth in usual initial doses of 100 to 200 micrograms/kg daily (usually 4 to 10 mg once daily), for 3 to 8 weeks. A dose of 100 micrograms/kg daily may be adequate for the treatment of non-Hodgkin's lymphoma; 150 micrograms/kg daily until the total leukocyte count falls below 10 000 cells/mm$^3$ may be used in chronic lymphocytic leukaemia; and in Hodgkin's disease, 200 micrograms/kg daily is usually required. Lower doses may be given as part of a combination regimen. If lymphocytic infiltration of the bone marrow is present or if the bone marrow is hypoplastic, the daily dose should not exceed 100 micrograms/kg. Alternatively, high-dose chlorambucil may be given intermittently. For example, in chronic lymphocytic leukaemia it may be given in an initial single dose of 400 micrograms/kg increased by 100 micrograms/kg at each 2- or 4-week dose interval until control of lymphocytosis is achieved or toxicity occurs.

Once a remission has been established the patient may receive continuous maintenance with 30 to 100 micrograms/kg daily. However, short intermittent courses appear to be safer and are generally preferred for maintenance.

In patients with Waldenström's macroglobulinaemia chlorambucil is licensed in an initial dose of 6 to 12 mg daily by mouth until leucopenia develops. Maintenance therapy with doses of 2 to 8 mg daily may then be given indefinitely.

Total and differential white cell counts and haemoglobin and platelet examinations are recommended each week during treatment with chlorambucil.

**Amyloidosis.** Chlorambucil may be of use in preserving kidney function and improving survival in patients with amyloidosis secondary to rheumatic disease,[1-4] the management of which is discussed in more detail on p.567.

1. Berglund K, *et al.* Alkylating cytostatic treatment in renal amyloidosis secondary to rheumatic disease. *Ann Rheum Dis* 1987; **46:** 757–62.
2. Berglund K, *et al.* Results, principles and pitfalls in the management of renal AA-amyloidosis; a 10-21 year followup of 16 patients with rheumatic disease treated with alkylating cytostatics. *J Rheumatol* 1993; **20:** 2051–7.
3. David J, *et al.* Amyloidosis in juvenile chronic arthritis: a morbidity and mortality study. *Clin Exp Rheumatol* 1993; **11:** 85–90.
4. Savolainen HA. Chlorambucil in severe juvenile chronic arthritis: longterm followup with special reference to amyloidosis. *J Rheumatol* 1999; **26:** 898–903.

**Blood disorders, non-malignant.** Chlorambucil may produce a response in cold auto-immune haemolytic anaemia (p.733).

**Connective tissue and muscular disorders.** Chlorambucil has been used as a corticosteroid-sparing agent in patients with Behçet's syndrome (p.1076). It has occasionally been tried in polymyositis (p.1086). In both these conditions, the potential benefits must be weighed against the possibility of toxicity.

**Kidney disorders, non-malignant.** Chlorambucil has been used in some forms of glomerular kidney disease (p.1080). In minimal change nephropathy, in which cytotoxics are reserved for the most severe cases because of fears about toxicity, cyclophosphamide is generally preferred to chlorambucil because it is perceived as entailing somewhat less risk, but chlorambucil has been used with corticosteroids in patients with membranous nephropathy.[1-3]

1. Ponticelli C, *et al.* Methylprednisolone plus chlorambucil as compared with methylprednisolone alone for the treatment of idiopathic membranous nephropathy. *N Engl J Med* 1992; **327:** 599–603.
2. Reichert LJM, *et al.* Preserving renal function in patients with membranous nephropathy: daily oral chlorambucil compared with intermittent monthly pulses of cyclophosphamide. *Ann Intern Med* 1994; **121:** 328–33.
3. Ponticelli C, *et al.* A 10-year follow-up of a randomized study with methylprednisolone and chlorambucil in membranous nephropathy. *Kidney Int* 1995; **48:** 1600–4.

**Liver disorders, non-malignant.** No treatment has proven unequivocally successful in the management of primary biliary cirrhosis (p.1761). Chlorambucil is one of a number of drugs for which reports of benefit exist.[1]

1. Hoofnagle JH, *et al.* Randomized trial of chlorambucil for primary biliary cirrhosis. *Gastroenterology* 1986; **91:** 1327–34.

**Malignant neoplasms.** Chlorambucil is used in the management of a number of haematological malignancies including chronic lymphocytic leukaemia (p.507), Hodgkin's disease (p.509), indolent low-grade non-Hodgkin's lymphomas (p.510), and Waldenström's macroglobulinaemia (p.511). It was formerly used in polycythaemia vera (p.508) but is now largely superseded.

**Ocular disorders, non-malignant.** Chlorambucil is one of the immunosuppressants that may be considered for patients with uveitis (p.1090) unresponsive to corticosteroids in tolerable doses.[1-3]

1. Mudun AB, *et al.* Short-term chlorambucil for refractory uveitis in Behcet's disease. *Ocul Immunol Inflamm* 2001; **9:** 219–29.
2. Miserocchi E, *et al.* Efficacy and safety of chlorambucil in intractable noninfectious uveitis. *Ophthalmology* 2002; **109:** 137–42.
3. Goldstein DA, *et al.* Long-term follow-up of patients treated with short-term high-dose chlorambucil for sight-threatening ocular inflammation. *Ophthalmology* 2002; **109:** 370–7.

**Rheumatoid arthritis.** Chlorambucil has been used for its immunosuppressant properties in a few patients with severe rheumatoid arthritis (p.9), especially with vasculitis, who have failed to respond to other drugs. However, the use of cytotoxic immunosuppressants other than methotrexate is considered debatable.

**Sarcoidosis.** Where drug therapy is required for sarcoidosis (p.1087), corticosteroids are the usual treatment. Chlorambucil is one of a number of cytotoxic immunosuppressants that have been tried, with variable results, as a second-line therapy.

## Preparations

***BP 2003:*** Chlorambucil Tablets;
***USP 27:*** Chlorambucil Tablets.

**Proprietary Preparations** (details are given in Part 3)
***Arg.:*** Leukeran; ***Austral.:*** Leukeran; ***Austria:*** Leukeran; ***Belg.:*** Leukeran; ***Braz.:*** Leukeran; ***Canad.:*** Leukeran; ***Chile:*** Leukeran; ***Denm.:*** Leukeran; ***Fin.:*** Leukeran; ***Ger.:*** Leukeran; ***Gr.:*** Leukeran; ***Hong Kong:*** Leukeran; ***India:*** Leukeran; ***Irl.:*** Leukeran; ***Israel:*** Leukeran; ***Ital.:*** Leukeran; Linfolysin†; ***Malaysia:*** Leukeran; ***Mex.:*** Leukeran; ***Mon.:*** Chloraminophene; ***Neth.:*** Leukeran; ***Norw.:*** Leukeran; ***NZ:*** Leukeran; ***Port.:*** Leukeran; ***S.Afr.:*** Leukeran; ***Singapore:*** Leukeran; ***Spain:*** Leukeran; ***Swed.:*** Leukeran; ***Switz.:*** Leukeran; ***Thai.:*** Leukeran; ***UK:*** Leukeran; ***USA:*** Leukeran†.

# Chlormethine Hydrochloride

*(BANM, rINNM)*

Chlorethazine Hydrochloride; Hidrocloruro de clormetina; HN2 (chlormethine); Mechlorethamine Hydrochloride; Mustine Hydrochloride; Nitrogen Mustard (chlormethine); NSC-762; WR-147650. Bis(2-chloroethyl)methylamine hydrochloride; 2,2′-Dichloro-*N*-methyldiethylamine hydrochloride.

$C_5H_{11}Cl_2N,HCl = 192.5.$

*CAS — 51-75-2 (chlormethine); 55-86-7 (chlormethine hydrochloride).*

*ATC — L01AA05.*

**Pharmacopoeias.** In *Br., Chin., Int.,* and *US.*

**BP 2003** (Chlormethine Hydrochloride). A white or almost white, hygroscopic, vesicant, crystalline powder or mass. Very soluble in water. Store at a temperature of 8° to 15°.

**USP 27** (Mechlorethamine Hydrochloride). A white, hygroscopic, crystalline powder. A 0.2% solution in water has a pH of 3.0 to 5.0. Store in airtight containers. Protect from light.

**Stability.** Solutions of chlormethine hydrochloride lose their activity very rapidly, particularly at neutral or alkaline pH.

A study[1] using an assay specific for chlormethine found that a 0.1% solution in Water for Injections or sodium chloride 0.9% injection underwent a loss of approximately 10% when stored for 6 hours at room temperature, and of approximately 4 to 6% when stored for the same period at 4°; similar results were obtained whether the solution was stored in glass vials or plastic syringes. Solutions in 500 mL of sodium chloride or glucose 5% injection and stored in PVC infusion bags were still less stable, with 15% and 10% degradation respectively after 6 hours at room temperature.

Chlormethine hydrochloride has been used in extemporaneous ointment preparations in the treatment of mycosis fungoides.[2] One formulation of chlormethine hydrochloride, dissolved in acetone and worked into white soft paraffin, was reported[3] to be stable for at least 84 days when stored at 4°, and for at least 40 days at 37°.

1. Kirk B. Stability of reconstituted Mustine Injection BP during storage. *Br J Parenter Ther* 1986; **7:** 86–92.
2. Price NM, *et al.* Ointment-based mechlorethamine treatment for mycosis fungoides. *Cancer* 1983; **52:** 2214–19.
3. Cummings J, *et al.* The long term stability of mechlorethamine hydrochloride (nitrogen mustard) ointment measured by HPLC. *J Pharm Pharmacol* 1993; **45:** 6–9.

## Adverse Effects, Treatment, and Precautions

For general discussions see Antineoplastics, p.492, p.495, and p.497.

Chlormethine hydrochloride is extremely toxic and its use is invariably accompanied by side-effects. Severe nausea and vomiting may commence within an hour of injection of the drug and last for some hours; antiemetics should be given before treatment. It causes varying degrees of bone-marrow depression depending on the dose. In heavily pretreated patients, or when the total dose for a single course exceeds 400 micrograms/kg, there is a risk of severe and possibly fatal depression with anaemia, lymphocytopenia, granulocytopenia, and thrombocytopenia with consequent haemorrhage. Depression of lymphocytes may be apparent within 24 hours of a dose and maximum suppression of granulocytes and platelets occurs within 7 to 21 days; haematological recovery may be adequate after 4 weeks.

Tinnitus, vertigo, deafness, headache, drowsiness, and other neurological symptoms have been reported, as have episodes of jaundice. Skin reactions to chlormethine hydrochloride include maculopapular rashes. There is a high incidence of hypersensitivity when topical preparations are used.

Chlormethine hydrochloride has a powerful vesicant action on the skin and mucous membranes and great care must be taken to avoid contact with the eyes. Thrombophlebitis is a potential hazard of chlormethine particularly if it is not sufficiently diluted. Extravasation of the injection causes severe irritation and even sloughing. If extravasation occurs during injection, the manufacturers suggest that the involved area should be infiltrated with an isotonic 4% solution of sodium thiosulfate, followed by the application of an ice compress intermittently for 6 to 12 hours, although the role of specific antidotes in antineoplastic extravasation is somewhat contentious (see p.496).

Chlormethine hydrochloride may produce temporary or permanent inhibition of fertility. There is some evidence of mutagenicity, teratogenicity, and carcinogenicity.

**Effects on the nervous system.** Severe immediate neurotoxicity developed[1] in 14 of 21 evaluable patients who underwent bone marrow transplantation after preparation with cytotoxic regimens including chlormethine 0.3 to 2 mg/kg. Symptoms, which developed a median of 4 days after treatment, included headache, hallucinations, confusion, convulsions, paraplegia, and tremor. Symptoms resolved in most, although in some they had not done so before their death. However, of the 13 patients who survived more than 60 days, 6, all of whom had earlier recovered from acute toxicity, developed a delayed neurotoxicity, beginning a median of 169 days after the first chlormethine injection and characterised by symptoms including confusion, somnolence, personality change, dementia, focal motor seizures, and hydrocephalus. Patients older than 21 years, those who had received CNS irradiation, and those treated concomitantly with other cytotoxic agents were at increased risk of neurotoxicity.

1. Sullivan KM, *et al.* Immediate and delayed neurotoxicity after mechlorethamine preparation for bone marrow transplantation. *Ann Intern Med* 1982; **97:** 182–9.

**Handling and disposal.** Chlormethine hydrochloride is a strong vesicant; avoid contact with skin and mucous membranes.

The manufacturers state that *unused injection* solutions of chlormethine hydrochloride may be neutralised by mixing with an equal volume of a solution containing sodium thiosulfate 5% and sodium bicarbonate 5% and allowing to stand for 45 minutes. Equipment used in the preparation and administration of such solutions may be treated similarly. Alternatively a solution containing sodium carbonate 2.5% or sodium hydroxide in a mixture of industrial methylated spirit and water has been suggested for the decontamination of equipment.

*Urine* produced for up to 48 hours after a dose of chlormethine should be handled wearing protective clothing.[1]

1. Harris J, Dodds LJ. Handling waste from patients receiving cytotoxic drugs. *Pharm J* 1985; **235:** 289–91.

## Pharmacokinetics

On intravenous injection, chlormethine is rapidly converted to a reactive ethyleneimmonium ion. It usually disappears from the blood in a few minutes. A very small proportion is excreted unchanged in the urine.

## Uses and Administration

Chlormethine belongs to the group of antineoplastic drugs described as alkylating agents. It also possesses weak immunosuppressant properties.

Chlormethine hydrochloride is used in the treatment of advanced Hodgkin's disease (p.509), historically in conjunction with a vinca alkaloid, procarbazine, and prednisone or prednisolone (the MOPP regimen). Chlormethine has also been tried in non-Hodgkin's lymphomas, notably mycosis fungoides (p.511), and some other malignancies including chronic leukaemias, tumours of the breast, ovary, and lung, and in polycythaemia vera. Chlormethine has been used in the management of malignant effusions but is not the agent of choice.

In the MOPP regimen chlormethine hydrochloride has been given in doses of 6 mg/m$^2$. However, when licensed for use as a single agent, the usual dose of chlormethine hydrochloride is 400 micrograms/kg, preferably as a single dose, although it may be divided into 2 or 4 equal doses on successive days. It is given by intravenous injection in a strength of 1 mg/mL in Water for Injections or sodium chloride 0.9%. Injection over 2 minutes into the tubing of a fast running intravenous infusion of sodium chloride 0.9% or glucose 5% may reduce the incidence of thrombophlebitis and the risk of extravasation.

The response should be assessed by the trend of the blood counts. Treatment with chlormethine may be repeated when the bone-marrow function has recovered.

Intracavitary injections of 200 to 400 micrograms/kg have been given in the treatment of malignant, especially pleural, effusions. In mycosis fungoides with extensive skin involvement, very dilute solutions of chlormethine (e.g. 200 micrograms/mL) have been applied topically.

**Histiocytic syndromes.** Dilute solutions of chlormethine (200 micrograms/mL) have been applied topically for the cutaneous symptoms of Langerhans-cell histiocytosis (p.505).[1,2] Such therapy was reported to effectively clear skin lesions in most patients, and be well tolerated. However, although no malignant skin disease developed during the follow-up of one group of children, the long-term effects of topical chlormethine are of concern in young patients.[2]

1. Sheehan MP, *et al.* Topical nitrogen mustard: an effective treatment for cutaneous Langerhans cell histiocytosis. *J Pediatr* 1991; **119:** 317–21.
2. Hoeger PH, *et al.* Long term follow up of topical mustine treatment for cutaneous Langerhans cell histiocytosis. *Arch Dis Child* 2000; **82:** 483–7.

**Mycosis fungoides.** Chlormethine is used topically in the management of mycosis fungoides (p.511). A retrospective cohort analysis[1] of 203 patients treated with chlormethine found a partial response rate of 33% and a complete response rate of 50%. The median time to achieve complete response was 12 months and the time to relapse was also 12 months. Mild disease of limited skin involvement responded better than generalised patch/plaque disease, and more patients with mild disease obtained long-term remission. Maintenance therapy was used in some patients, but on cessation the relapse rate was similar to patients who did not receive maintenance therapy. Treatment had usually been applied as either an aqueous solution or an ointment containing chlormethine 100 to 200 micrograms/mL.

1. Kim YH, *et al.* Topical nitrogen mustard in the management of mycosis fungoides: update of the Stanford experience. *Arch Dermatol* 2003; **139:** 165–73.

## Preparations

***BP 2003:*** Chlormethine Injection;
***USP 27:*** Mechlorethamine Hydrochloride for Injection.

**Proprietary Preparations** (details are given in Part 3)
***Braz.:*** Onco-Cloramin†; ***Canad.:*** Mustargen; ***Fr.:*** Caryolysine†; ***Gr.:*** Caryolysine; ***Israel:*** Mustargen; ***Switz.:*** Mustargen; ***USA:*** Mustargen.

## Chlorozotocin

Clorozotocina; DCNU; NSC-178248. 2-[3-(2-Chloroethyl)-3-nitrosoureido]-2-deoxy-D-glucopyranose.

$C_9H_{16}ClN_3O_7$ = 313.7.

*CAS — 54749-90-5.*

### Profile

Chlorozotocin is an analogue of the antineoplastic streptozocin (p.584) but has been reported to have little diabetogenic effect. It has been tried as an antineoplastic, notably in pancreatic endocrine tumours (p.504). Renal toxicity has occurred.

◊ References.


1. Baker JJ, *et al.* Renal-failure anemia and nitrosourea therapy. *N Engl J Med* 1979; **301:** 662.
2. Bukowski RM, *et al.* Phase II trial of chlorozotocin and fluorouracil in islet cell carcinoma: a Southwest Oncology Group study. *J Clin Oncol* 1992; **10:** 1914–8.


## Cisplatin *(BAN, USAN, rINN)*

CDDP; Cisplatina; Cisplatino; Cisplatinum; Cis-platinum; DDP; *cis*-DDP; NSC-119875; Peyrone's Salt; Platinum Diamminodichloride. *cis*-Diamminedichloroplatinum.

$(NH_3)_2.PtCl_2$ = 300.0.

*CAS — 15663-27-1.*

*ATC — L01XA01.*

**Pharmacopoeias.** In *Chin., Eur.* (see p.vi), *Int.*, and *US.*

**Ph. Eur. 5.0** (Cisplatin). A yellow powder or yellow or orange-yellow crystals. Slightly soluble in water; practically insoluble in alcohol; sparingly soluble in dimethylformamide. A 0.1% solution in sodium chloride 0.9% has a pH of 4.5 to 6.0 immediately after preparation. Store in airtight containers. Protect from light.

**USP 27** (Cisplatin). Store in airtight containers. Protect from light.

**Incompatibility.** Cisplatin is rapidly degraded in the presence of bisulfite or metabisulfite,[1,2] and admixture with preparations containing these as preservatives may result in loss of activity.[2] Sodium bicarbonate may also increase the loss of cisplatin from solution, and in some cases may cause precipitation.[3] The stability of cisplatin when mixed with fluorouracil is reported to be limited, with 10% loss of cisplatin in 1.2 to 1.5 hours.[4] Mixtures with etoposide[5] in sodium chloride 0.9% injection formed a precipitate if mannitol and potassium chloride were present as additives, but not when the diluent was glucose 5% with sodium chloride 0.45%. Turbidity has been reported[6] within 4 hours of mixing 0.1% solutions of cisplatin and thiotepa in glucose 5%. Cisplatin exhibits variable incompatibility with paclitaxel, depending on the paclitaxel concentration and the temperature.[7]

Cisplatin reacts with aluminium causing loss of potency and precipitate formation. Needles, syringes, catheters or administration sets that contain aluminium should not be used for preparation or administration of cisplatin.


1. Hussain AA, *et al.* Reaction of cis-platinum with sodium bisulfite. *J Pharm Sci* 1980; **69:** 364–5.
2. Garren KW, Repta AJ. Incompatibility of cisplatin and Reglan Injectable. *Int J Pharmaceutics* 1985; **24:** 91–9.
3. Hincal AA, *et al.* Cis-platin stability in aqueous parenteral vehicles. *J Parenter Drug Assoc* 1979; **33:** 107–16.
4. Stewart CF, Fleming RA. Compatibility of cisplatin and fluorouracil in 0.9% sodium chloride injection. *Am J Hosp Pharm* 1990; **47:** 1373–7.
5. Stewart CF, Hampton EM. Stability of cisplatin and etoposide in intravenous admixtures. *Am J Hosp Pharm* 1989; **46:** 1400–4.
6. Trissel LA, Martinez JF. Compatibility of thiotepa (lyophilized) with selected drugs during simulated Y-site administration. *Am J Health-Syst Pharm* 1996; **53:** 1041–5.
7. Zhang Y, *et al.* Compatibility and stability of paclitaxel combined with cisplatin and with carboplatin in infusion solutions. *Ann Pharmacother* 1997; **31:** 1465–70.


**Stability.** Decomposition of cisplatin in aqueous solutions is primarily due to reversible substitution of water for chloride, and its stability is enhanced in sodium chloride solutions because of the excess of chloride ions available.[1,2] A solution in sodium chloride 0.9% injection has been reported to lose 3% of the drug in less than one hour and to remain stable at this equilibrium value for 24 hours at room temperature.[1] Stability is decreased if exposed to intense light, but the effect of normal lighting conditions is apparently smaller.[1,2] It has been recommended that admixtures of cisplatin with mannitol and magnesium sulfate (in glucose 5% with sodium chloride 0.45%) stored at room temperature in PVC bags should be used within 48 hours, but may be stored for 4 days at 4° or frozen and stored at −15° for up to 30 days.[3] However, solutions containing 600 micrograms/mL or more of cisplatin precipitate out when refrigerated and are slow to redissolve.[1]


1. Greene RF, *et al.* Stability of cisplatin in aqueous solution. *Am J Hosp Pharm* 1979; **36:** 38–43.
2. Hincal AA, *et al.* Cis-platin stability in aqueous parenteral vehicles. *J Parenter Drug Assoc* 1979; **33:** 107–16.
3. LaFollette JM, *et al.* Stability of cisplatin admixtures in polyvinyl chloride bags. *Am J Hosp Pharm* 1985; **42:** 2652.


### Adverse Effects and Treatment

For a general outline see Antineoplastics, p.492 and p.495.

Severe nausea and vomiting occur in most patients during treatment with cisplatin; nausea may persist for up to a week.

Serious toxic effects on the kidneys, bone marrow, and ears have been reported in up to about one third of patients given a single dose of cisplatin; the effects are generally dose-related and cumulative.

Damage to the renal tubules may be evident during the second week after a dose of cisplatin and renal function must return to normal before further cisplatin is given. Adequate hydration, and use of osmotic diuretics such as mannitol to increase urine volume and thus decrease the urinary concentration of platinum, can reduce the incidence of nephrotoxicity. Electrolyte disturbances, particularly hypomagnesaemia and hypocalcaemia, may occur, possibly as a result of renal tubular damage. Hyperuricaemia is also seen.

Bone-marrow depression may be severe with higher doses of cisplatin. Nadirs in platelet and leucocyte counts occur between days 18 and 23 and most patients recover by day 39; anaemia is commonly seen and may be partly related to decreased production of erythropoietin following renal damage.

Ototoxicity may be more severe in children. It can manifest as tinnitus, loss of hearing in the high frequency range, and occasionally deafness or vestibular toxicity. Other neurological effects reported include peripheral neuropathies, loss of taste, and seizures. Ocular toxicities include optic neuritis, papilloedema, and cerebral blindness.

Anaphylactoid reactions and cardiac abnormalities have occurred.

Platinum derivatives are potentially mutagenic and teratogenic, and there is some evidence they may be associated with the development of secondary leukaemias—see p.492.

**Effects on the blood.** Cisplatin-induced anaemia appears to be disproportionate to the effects on other blood cells, and to correlate with renal tubular dysfunction.[1] It may therefore be due to an erythropoietin deficiency state resulting from cisplatin-induced renal tubular damage. Haemolysis has also been reported.[2]


1. Wood PA, Hrushesky WJ. Cisplatin-associated anemia: an erythropoietin deficiency syndrome *J Clin Invest* 1995; **95:** 1650–9.
2. Rothmann SA, Weick JK. Cisplatin toxicity for erythroid precursors. *N Engl J Med* 1981; **304:** 360.


THROMBOEMBOLISM. For discussion of thromboembolic events possibly associated with cisplatin-containing chemotherapy regimens see Effects on the Cardiovascular System, p.493.

**Effects on electrolytes.** Renal-magnesium wasting and, less commonly, symptomatic hypomagnesaemia occurs with cisplatin therapy.[1,2] Adding magnesium to the pre- and posthydration fluids has been suggested.[2] When hypocalcaemia is also present, tetany may result,[1,3] although this has responded to electrolyte infusion without the need to interrupt chemotherapy.[1] Cisplatin therapy may also be associated with significant hypokalaemia[1] and hyponatraemia.[4,5]

See also Effects on the Kidneys, below.


1. Winkler CF, *et al.* Cisplatin and renal magnesium wasting. *Ann Intern Med* 1979; **91:** 502.
2. Lajer H, Daugaard G. Cisplatin and hypomagnesemia. *Cancer Treat Rev* 1999; **25:** 47–58.
3. Stuart-Harris R, *et al.* Tetany associated with cis-platin. *Lancet* 1980; **ii:** 1303.
4. Hutchison FN, *et al.* Renal salt wasting in patients treated with cisplatin. *Ann Intern Med* 1988; **108:** 21–5.
5. Mariette X, *et al.* Cisplatin and hyponatremia. *Ann Intern Med* 1988; **108:** 770–1.


**Effects on the kidneys.** Nephrotoxicity is a well established adverse effect of cisplatin, may be dose-limiting, and can manifest as acute or chronic renal failure, polyuria, or chronic hypomagnesaemia.[1] The mechanism appears to involve primarily damage to the proximal renal tubule; selective magnesium loss may be due to a specific membrane or transport system abnormality. Sulfhydryl metabolism and oxidative stress play a role in toxicity, and measures that reduce glutathione depletion and scavenge intracellular free oxygen radicals have been tried in an attempt to modulate nephrotoxicity.[1-3] However, the primary measures for reducing renal damage have been aggressive hydration with chloride-containing solutions, and the use of mannitol (see also Prophylaxis, below). It has been suggested that cisplatin may mobilise lead accumulated in bone and cause temporary accumulation in the kidney, with concomitant toxicity,[4] but this has been vigorously disputed.[5-7]

See also under Effects on Electrolytes, above.


1. Anand AJ, Bashey B. Newer insights into cisplatin nephrotoxicity. *Ann Pharmacother* 1993; **27:** 1519–25.
2. Meyer KB, Madias NE. Cisplatin nephrotoxicity. *Miner Electrolyte Metab* 1994; **20:** 201–13.
3. Kuhlmann MK, *et al.* Insights into potential cellular mechanisms of cisplatin nephrotoxicity and their clinical application. *Nephrol Dial Transplant* 1997; **12:** 2478–80.
4. El-Sharkawi AM, *et al.* Unexpected mobilisation of lead during cisplatin chemotherapy. *Lancet* 1986; **ii:** 249–50.
5. Tothill P, *et al.* Is lead mobilised by cisplatin? *Lancet* 1989; **ii:** 333.
6. Tothill P, *et al.* Mobilisation of lead by cisplatin. *Lancet* 1989; **ii:** 1342.
7. Hainsworth IR, Morgan WD. Plasma lead and cisplatin. *Lancet* 1989; **ii:** 624.


PROPHYLAXIS. Hydration with 1 to 2 litres of fluid before treatment, and infusion of cisplatin in a further 2 litres of infusion fluid containing an osmotic diuretic such as mannitol reduces the nephrotoxicity of cisplatin, but does not abolish it. Maintaining adequate hydration and urinary output post-treatment is also important. Administering cisplatin over 6 to 8 hours rather than 1 to 2 hours may also decrease renal toxicity.

Sulfur-containing nucleophiles can inactivate cisplatin, and have therefore been investigated for their chemoprotective potential. Amifostine is a prodrug which is selectively activated by normal tissue, and has been shown to protect normal tissue (principally the kidney) against the cytotoxicity of cisplatin without affecting antitumour activity (for references, see p.1032). Glutathione (p.1040) is a similar agent, which may be selectively taken up by kidney and neural tissue. Sodium thiosulfate (p.1053) does not show selective activation or uptake, and its use is therefore limited to situations where cisplatin is given locally (e.g. intraperitoneal[1]) or directly (e.g. intra-arterial).


1. Howell SB, *et al.* Intraperitoneal cisplatin with systemic thiosulfate protection. *Ann Intern Med* 1982; **97:** 845–51.


**Effects on the nervous system.** The features of cisplatin-induced peripheral neuropathy are consistent with damage predominantly to sensory fibres, with numbness, tingling, and decreased vibratory sensation and deep tendon reflexes, progressing in severe cases to disabling sensory ataxia.[1] The toxicity is dose-dependent, with symptoms usually appearing in patients who have received cumulative doses of 300 to 600 mg/m², although individuals vary in susceptibility. Neuropathy is reversible but recovery may take a year or more. The pathophysiology is unknown. Peripheral neuropathy can be a dose-limiting toxicity for cisplatin and agents such as Org-2766 (a corticotropin analogue) and amifostine (p.1031) have been investigated for their potential in protecting peripheral nerves.[1-3] Glutathione is also under investigation for the prevention of neurotoxicity (see p.1040). Autonomic neuropathy, with, in some cases, consequent orthostatic hypotension, has also been described following treatment with cisplatin-containing regimens.[4] Apart from ototoxicity, cisplatin has also been associated with central neurotoxicity, including focal encephalopathy, seizures, aphasia, confusion, agitation, and cortical blindness.[5-7] It has been suggested that the mechanism of focal encephalopathy may be vascular,[5] although this is uncertain.


1. Mollman JE. Cisplatin neurotoxicity. *N Engl J Med* 1990; **322:** 126–7.
2. Alberts DS, Noel JK. Cisplatin-associated neurotoxicity: can it be prevented? *Anticancer Drugs* 1995; **6:** 369–83.
3. Cavaletti G, *et al.* Neuroprotectant drugs in cisplatin neurotoxicity. *Anticancer Res* 1996; **16:** 3149–59.
4. Richardson P, Cantwell BMJ. Autonomic neuropathy after cisplatin based chemotherapy. *BMJ* 1990; **300:** 1466–7.
5. Lindeman G, *et al.* Cisplatin neurotoxicity. *N Engl J Med* 1990; **323:** 64–5.
6. Philip PA, *et al.* Convulsions and transient cortical blindness after cisplatin. *BMJ* 1991; **302:** 416.
7. Higa GM, *et al.* Severe, disabling neurologic toxicity following cisplatin retreatment. *Ann Pharmacother* 1995; **29:** 134–7.


**Extravasation.** For discussion of the management of extravasation, including mention of the potential use of sodium thiosulfate in cisplatin extravasation, see under Treatment of the Adverse Effects of Antineoplastics, p.496.

**Hypersensitivity.** Anaphylactoid reactions to intravenous cisplatin generally appear within a few minutes of administration and have manifested as facial oedema, wheezing, tachycardia, and hypotension.[1] A high incidence of anaphylactoid reaction has also been seen following intravesical instillation in patients with bladder cancer,[2] but intraperitoneal or intrapleural administration does not seem to be associated with an enhanced risk of hypersensitivity,[3] although anaphylactoid reactions have occurred when cisplatin is given intraperitoneally.[4] Anaphylactoid symptoms and ischaemia of the hands accompanied severe exfoliative dermatitis in one patient on the second cycle of cisplatin-based chemotherapy;[5] she had earlier experienced exfoliative dermatitis associated with carboplatin. Palmar-plantar erythrodysesthesia (p.495) has also occurred.[6]


1. Von Hoff DD, *et al.* Allergic reactions to cis platinum. *Lancet* 1976; **i:** 90.
2. Denis L. Anaphylactic reactions to repeated intravesical instillation with cisplatin. *Lancet* 1983; **i:** 1378–9.
3. Markman M. No increase in allergic reactions with intracavitary administration of cisplatin. *Lancet* 1984; **ii:** 1164.
4. Hebert ME, *et al.* Anaphylactoid reactions with intraperitoneal cisplatin. *Ann Pharmacother* 1995; **29:** 260–3.
5. Lee TC, *et al.* Severe exfoliative dermatitis associated with hand ischemia during cisplatin therapy. *Mayo Clin Proc* 1994; **69:** 80–2.
6. Vakalis D, *et al.* Acral erythema induced by chemotherapy with cisplatin. *Br J Dermatol* 1998; **139:** 750–1.


**Nausea and vomiting.** For discussion of the management of chemotherapy-induced nausea and vomiting, see under Nausea and Vomiting, p.1245.

### Precautions

For reference to the precautions necessary with antineoplastics, see p.497. Cisplatin is generally contra-indicated in patients with renal or hearing impairment, or bone-marrow depression. Renal and neurological function and hearing should be monitored during treatment, and regular blood counts performed. Electrolytes should be measured before starting therapy, and before each subsequent course. Adequate hydration and urinary output must be maintained before, and for 24 hours after, a dose.

**Breast feeding.** Platinum concentrations in a patient receiving cisplatin were 0.9 micrograms/mL in breast milk and 0.8 micrograms/mL in plasma.[1] Although most of the platinum in breast milk is probably protein-bound the authors considered that a mother should not breast feed while receiving cisplatin chemotherapy. However, in another report,[2] cisplatin was undetectable in breast milk and the American Academy of Pediatrics[3] considers its use to be compatible with breast feeding.

1. de Vries EGE, *et al.* Excretion of platinum into breast milk. *Lancet* 1989; **i:** 497. Correction. *ibid.*; 798.
2. Egan PC, *et al.* Doxorubicin and cisplatin excretion into human milk. *Cancer Treat Rep* 1985; **69:** 1387–9.
3. American Academy of Pediatrics. The transfer of drugs and other chemicals into human milk. *Pediatrics* 2001; **108:** 776–89. Correction. *ibid.*; 1029. Also available at: http://aappolicy.aappublications.org/cgi/content/full/pediatrics%3b108/3/776 (accessed 29/06/04)

**Handling and disposal.** Methods for the destruction of *cisplatin wastes* by reduction with zinc powder under acidic conditions or by reaction with ditiocarb sodium have been described.[1] Residue produced by the degradation of cisplatin by either method showed no mutagenicity *in vitro*.

*Urine* produced for up to 7 days after a dose of cisplatin should be handled wearing protective clothing.[2]

1. Castegnaro M, *et al.*, eds. Laboratory decontamination and destruction of carcinogens in laboratory wastes: some antineoplastic agents. *IARC Scientific Publications 73*. Lyon: WHO/International Agency for Research on Cancer, 1985.
2. Harris J, Dodds LJ. Handling waste from patients receiving cytotoxic drugs. *Pharm J* 1985; **235:** 289–91.

**Radiotherapy.** Enhanced ototoxicity has been reported in patients given cisplatin for brain tumours who had also received cranial irradiation.[1,2]

1. Granowetter L, *et al.* Enhanced cis-platinum neurotoxicity in pediatric patients with brain tumors. *J Neurooncol* 1983; **1:** 293–7.
2. Mahoney DH, *et al.* Ototoxicity with cisplatin therapy. *J Pediatr* 1983; **103:** 1006.

### Interactions

For a general outline of antineoplastic drug interactions, see p.498. Use with other myelosuppressive, nephrotoxic or ototoxic drugs may exacerbate the adverse effects of cisplatin. The effects of cisplatin on renal function may also affect the pharmacokinetics of other drugs excreted by the renal route.

**Antibacterials.** Although the use of cisplatin with other nephrotoxic or ototoxic drugs requires great caution, there is some evidence that *aminoglycosides* can be used in patients who have recently received cisplatin if appropriate supportive care is available.[1]

1. Cooper BW, *et al.* Renal dysfunction during high-dose cisplatin therapy and autologous hematopoietic stem cell transplantation: effect of aminoglycoside therapy. *Am J Med* 1993; **94:** 497–504.

**Antineoplastics.** The ototoxicity of cisplatin was reportedly enhanced by *ifosfamide*,[1] a drug that is not ototoxic when given alone, although it does have nephrotoxic potential, making reports of increased nephrotoxicity in patients who have received both unsurprising.[2,3]

For a report of increased toxicity with *etoposide*, see p.552. Cisplatin may reduce the clearance of *paclitaxel*, see p.578.

1. Meyer WH, *et al.* Ifosfamide and exacerbation of cisplatin-induced hearing loss. *Lancet* 1993; **341:** 754–5.
2. Rossi R, Ehrich JHH. Partial and complete de Toni-Debré-Fanconi syndrome after ifosfamide chemotherapy of childhood malignancy. *Eur J Clin Pharmacol* 1993; **44** (suppl 1): S43–S45.
3. Martinez F, *et al.* Ifosfamide nephrotoxicity: deleterious effect of previous cisplatin administration. *Lancet* 1996; **348:** 1100–1.

**Cardiovascular drugs.** A patient whose renal function was unaffected by cisplatin alone developed nephrotoxicity when given cisplatin and antihypertensive therapy with *furosemide, hydralazine, diazoxide,* and *propranolol*.[1] Previous results in *animals* suggest that furosemide may aggravate cisplatin nephrotoxicity, while the other antihypertensives might have contributed to a transient fall in renal-blood flow with resultant increased renal-tubular cisplatin concentration.

1. Markman M, Trump DL. Nephrotoxicity with cisplatin and antihypertensive medications. *Ann Intern Med* 1982; **96:** 257.

**Gastrointestinal drugs.** For mention of 2 retrospective studies, one showing a decreased area under the plasma-concentration time curve of high-dose cisplatin with *ondansetron* and the other an increase, see p.541.

### Pharmacokinetics

After intravenous doses cisplatin disappears from the plasma in a biphasic manner and half-lives of 25 to 49 minutes and 3 to 4 days have been reported for total platinum. More than 90% of the platinum from a dose is protein bound within 2 to 4 hours; only the unbound fraction has significant antineoplastic activity. Cisplatin is concentrated in the liver, kidneys, and large and small intestines. Penetration into the CNS appears to be poor. Excretion is mainly in the urine but is incomplete and prolonged: up to about 50% of a dose has been reported to be excreted in urine over 5 days, and platinum may be detected in tissue for several months afterwards. The unbound fraction, which is more rapidly cleared, may be actively secreted by the renal tubules. Cisplatin is well-absorbed on intraperitoneal use. Cisplatin may be distributed into breast milk (see Breast Feeding, above).

### Uses and Administration

The antineoplastic cisplatin is a platinum-containing complex which may act similarly to the alkylating agents. Its antineoplastic actions are cell-cycle non-specific and are dependent upon its *cis* configuration; they appear to be related to its hydrolysis in the body to form reactive aquated species. Although it causes immunosuppression, stimulation of the host immune response against the tumour has been suggested as contributing to cisplatin's antineoplastic action.

Cisplatin is of value in the treatment of metastatic tumours of the testis, usually as a major component of combination chemotherapy regimens, and particularly with bleomycin and etoposide (BEP). It is also used in metastatic ovarian tumours, lung cancer, and advanced bladder cancer, and has been reported to be active against a wide range of other solid tumours, as indicated by the cross references given below.

Cisplatin is given by intravenous infusion in sodium chloride 0.9% or sodium chloride and glucose. It is usually given as a single dose of 50 to 120 mg/m$^2$ every 3 to 4 weeks in the treatment of ovarian and bladder cancers. Lower doses are generally used for combination chemotherapy regimens than for single agent therapy. A dose of 20 mg/m$^2$ daily for 5 days every 3 to 4 weeks has been employed in combination chemotherapy of testicular tumours; this dose is also used for single agent therapy.

The manufacturers recommend that cisplatin is given in 2 litres of chloride-containing infusion fluid over at least 1 to 2 hours, and that an infusion time of 6 to 8 hours may further reduce the toxicity. In practice, volumes of less than 2 litres have been used in expert centres.

To aid diuresis and protect the kidneys, 37.5 g of mannitol (e.g. 375 mL of mannitol 10%) is usually added to the infusion or is infused separately immediately before cisplatin. In order to begin diuresis the patient is usually hydrated by the infusion of 1 to 2 litres of a suitable fluid over several hours before giving cisplatin. Adequate hydration must also be maintained for up to 24 hours after a dose. Renal, haematological, auditory, and neurological function should be monitored during therapy, and dosage adjusted accordingly.

Cisplatin has also been given by the intra-arterial and intraperitoneal routes, and by instillation into the bladder. It is being investigated as a liposomal formulation, and as a collagen-based injectable gel containing cisplatin and adrenaline (MPI-5010) to localise the effect.

Various analogues of cisplatin have been developed or investigated including those with fewer adverse effects (e.g. carboplatin, p.533; nedaplatin, p.576), an altered spectrum of activity (oxaliplatin, p.577), or activity following oral administration (satraplatin, p.583).

**Administration.** Various adjustments to the administration of cisplatin have been suggested in an attempt to improve effectiveness while reducing toxicity.

Hydration before and after a dose of cisplatin, together with the use of mannitol to promote diuresis, is now standard (see Uses and Administration, above). Higher doses of cisplatin (up to 200 mg/m$^2$ per treatment cycle) have been successfully given by infusion in hypertonic sodium chloride, accompanied by intensive hydration.[1,2] However, while such a regimen may limit nephrotoxicity, other toxic effects, such as peripheral neuropathy, are not prevented;[1-4] myelosuppression may be less if the total dose is given in 2 divided doses rather than divided over 5 days.[2]

Toxicity has been reported to be reduced when cisplatin was given by continuous intra-arterial[5] or intravenous[6] infusion. It has also been suggested that giving cisplatin in the evening rather than the morning results in less damage to renal function, apparently because of circadian variations in urine production.[7] However, another study[8] found that morning, rather than evening, administration of cisplatin resulted in less renal damage. Noting the inconsistency with previous reports, the authors concluded that use of a prolonged hydration protocol and concomitant furosemide might have been responsible for these results (see also under Interactions, above). It was also found that morning administration of cisplatin may be more emetogenic than evening administration, although the use of prophylactic ondansetron prior to cisplatin diminished this apparent circadian effect on vomiting.

A suggested alternative way to increase the platinum dose without producing incapacitating toxicity has been the combination of cisplatin and carboplatin.[9]

Various drugs have been investigated to reduce toxicity, including amifostine, glutathione, and thiosulfate, as discussed under Effects on the Kidneys, and Effects on the Nervous System, above.

1. Ozols RF, *et al.* High-dose cisplatin in hypertonic saline. *Ann Intern Med* 1984; **100:** 19–24.
2. Gandara DR, *et al.* Cisplatin dose intensity in non-small cell lung cancer: phase II results of a day 1 and day 8 high-dose regimen. *J Natl Cancer Inst* 1989; **81:** 790–4.
3. Bagley CM, *et al.* High-dose cisplatin therapy for cancer of the ovary: neurotoxicity. *Ann Intern Med* 1985; **102:** 719.
4. Ozols RF, Young RC. High-dose cisplatin therapy for cancer of the ovary: neurotoxicity. *Ann Intern Med* 1985; **102:** 719.
5. Jacobs SC, *et al.* Intraarterial cisplatin infusion in the management of transitional cell carcinoma of the bladder. *Cancer* 1989; **64:** 388–91.
6. Salem P, *et al.* Cis-diamminedichloroplatinum (II) by 5-day continuous infusion: a new dose schedule with minimal toxicity. *Cancer* 1984; **53:** 837–40.
7. Hrushesky WJM, *et al.* Circadian time dependence of cisplatin urinary kinetics. *Clin Pharmacol Ther* 1982; **32:** 330–9.
8. Kobayashi M, *et al.* Cisplatin-induced vomiting depends on circadian timing. *Chronobiol Int* 2001; **18:** 851–63.
9. Piccart MJ, *et al.* Cisplatin combined with carboplatin: a new way of intensification of platinum dose in the treatment of advanced ovarian cancer. *J Natl Cancer Inst* 1990; **82:** 703–7.

**Malignant neoplasms.** Cisplatin is used in the management of many solid malignancies, notably those of the bladder, cervix, lung, ovary, and testis, as discussed on p.512, p.515, p.519, p.520, and p.523 respectively. Other malignancies where cisplatin may be employed, as discussed in the introduction to this chapter, include non-Hodgkin's lymphomas (p.510), tumours of brain (p.513), endometrium (p.516), upper gastrointestinal tract (p.516), head and neck (p.517), and thymus (p.523), neuroblastoma (p.524), and sarcoma of bone and soft tissue (p.524 and p.525).

### Preparations

***BP 2003:*** Cisplatin Injection;
***USP 27:*** Cisplatin for Injection.

**Proprietary Preparations** (details are given in Part 3)
***Arg.:*** Elvecis; Platamine; Platino II; Platinol; Sicatem; ***Austria:*** Abiplatin; Cishexal; Platiblastin; Platinol; Platosin; ***Belg.:*** Platinol; Platistine; ***Braz.:*** Astaplatin; Bioplatino; C-Platin; Cisplatex; Cisplatyl†; Platiran; Platistine; Tecnoplatin; Unistin; ***Canad.:*** Platinol†; ***Chile:*** Blastolem; ***Denm.:*** Citosin†; Lederplatin; Platinol; ***Fin.:*** Platinol; ***Fr.:*** Cisplatyl; ***Ger.:*** Cis-Gry; Platiblastin†; Platinex; ***Gr.:*** Cisplatyl; Platamine; Platinol; Platosin; ***India:*** Kemoplat; ***Israel:*** Abiplatin; Cisplatyl†; Platinex†; Platinol†; Platosin†; ***Ital.:*** Citoplatino; Platamine; Platinex; Pronto Platamine; ***Malaysia:*** Platosin; ***Mex.:*** Blastolem; Niyaplat†; Noveldexis; Plastistil†; Platinol; Seroplatin†; Tecnoplatin†; Tisplal†; ***Neth.:*** Platinol†; ***Norw.:*** Platinol; Platistin; ***NZ:*** Platamine†; ***Port.:*** Faulplatin; ***S.Afr.:*** Abiplatin; Platamine†; Platosin; ***Spain:*** Neoplatin; Placis; Platistil; ***Swed.:*** Platinol; ***Switz.:*** Platiblastin-S; Platinol; ***Thai.:*** Abiplatin; Kemoplat; Platinol; Platosin; ***UK:*** Platinex; ***USA:*** Platinol.

---

## Cladribine *(BAN, USAN, rINN)*

2-Chlorodeoxyadenosine; Cladribina; RWJ-26251; RWJ-26251-000. 2-Chloro-2′-deoxyadenosine.

$C_{10}H_{12}ClN_5O_3$ = 285.7.

*CAS — 4291-63-8.*

*ATC — L01BB04.*

**Stability.** Cladribine shows increased degradation in glucose 5%, therefore this diluent should not be used. Cladribine in sodium chloride 0.9% is stable for at least 24 hours at room temperature and ambient lighting in PVC infusion containers.

The manufacturers recommend that cladribine should be stored at 2° to 8° and protected from light.

### Adverse Effects and Treatment

For a general outline see Antineoplastics, p.492 and p.495.

Cladribine produces severe myelosuppression, with neutropenia, anaemia, and thrombocytopenia. Transfusion of blood products may be required. Prolonged CD4 lymphopenia with a nadir at 4 to 6 months also occurs. Prolonged bone-marrow hypocellularity may occur, although it is not clear if this is due to the drug or underlying disease. Haemolytic anaemia has also been reported.

Other adverse effects include fever, fatigue, malaise, mild nausea and gastrointestinal disturbances, rashes, pruritus, purpura, headache, dizziness, cough, dyspnoea, oedema, tachycardia, arthralgia, and myalgia.

Very high doses of cladribine have been associated with severe renal and nervous system toxicity as well as myelosuppression. Severe neurotoxicity is rare at currently recommended doses, but confusion, neuropathy, ataxia, insomnia, and somnolence have occurred.

**Carcinogenicity.** As with some other antimetabolites (see p.492), Epstein-Barr virus-related lymphoma has been reported after cladribine therapy.[1]

1. Niesvizky R, *et al.* Epstein-Barr virus-associated lymphoma after treatment of macroglobulinemia with cladribine. *N Engl J Med* 1999; **341:** 55.

## Precautions

For the precautions necessary with antineoplastics, see p.497. Careful haematological monitoring is recommended, especially during the first 4 to 8 weeks of therapy. Renal and hepatic function should also be monitored.

## Pharmacokinetics

Plasma-cladribine concentrations are reported to decline multi-exponentially after intravenous infusion, with terminal half-lives ranging from 3 to 22 hours. Cladribine is extensively distributed and penetrates into the CNS. It is about 20% bound to plasma proteins. Cladribine is phosphorylated within cells by deoxycytidine kinase to form cytotoxic nucleotides.

◊ References.

1. Liliemark J. The clinical pharmacokinetics of cladribine. *Clin Pharmacokinet* 1997; **32:** 120–31.

## Uses and Administration

Cladribine is a chlorinated purine nucleoside analogue that inhibits DNA synthesis and repair, particularly in lymphocytes and monocytes. It is used as an antimetabolite antineoplastic for the treatment of lymphoid malignancies including hairy-cell leukaemia (p.508) and chronic lymphocytic leukaemia (p.507). It has been tried in indolent low-grade non-Hodgkin's lymphomas (p.510), histiocytic syndromes (p.505), and in Waldenström's macroglobulinaemia (p.511).

The recommended dose of cladribine in hairy-cell leukaemia is a single course of 90 micrograms/kg (3.6 mg/m$^2$) daily for 7 days by continuous intravenous infusion. If the patient does not respond to the initial course, they are unlikely to respond to further doses. Cladribine has also been given subcutaneously in a dose of 140 micrograms/kg (5.6 mg/m$^2$) daily for 5 consecutive days.

For the treatment of chronic lymphocytic leukaemia the recommended dose is 120 micrograms/kg (4.8 mg/m$^2$) daily for 5 consecutive days of a 28-day cycle; the infusion is given over 2 hours. Response should be determined every 2 cycles, and once maximum response has occurred a further 2 cycles of treatment are recommended, up to a maximum of 6 cycles. Patients who do not respond with a lymphocyte reduction of 50% or more after 2 cycles should not receive further therapy. Cladribine has also been given subcutaneously in a dose of 100 micrograms/kg (4 mg/m$^2$) daily for 5 consecutive days.

The use of cladribine by mouth in chronic lymphocytic leukaemia is under investigation.

Cladribine has also been tried in the management of multiple sclerosis (see below).

◊ Reviews.

1. Beutler E. Cladribine (2-chlorodeoxyadenosine). *Lancet* 1992; **340:** 952–6.
2. Bryson HM, Sorkin EM. Cladribine: a review of its pharmacodynamic and pharmacokinetic properties and therapeutic potential in haematological malignancies. *Drugs* 1993; **46:** 872–94.
3. Baltz JK, Montello MJ. Cladribine for the treatment of hematologic malignancies. *Clin Pharm* 1993; **12:** 805–13.
4. Saven A, Piro LD. 2-Chlorodeoxyadenosine: a newer purine analog active in the treatment of indolent lymphoid malignancies. *Ann Intern Med* 1994; **120:** 784–91.

**Multiple sclerosis.** Cladribine has shown some evidence of benefit in multiple sclerosis (p.646) but it is not clear whether it improves attack rate or disease progression.

References.

1. Sipe JC, *et al.* Cladribine in treatment of chronic progressive multiple sclerosis. *Lancet* 1994; **344:** 9–13.
2. Romine JS, *et al.* A double-blind, placebo-controlled, randomized trial of cladribine in relapsing-remitting multiple sclerosis. *Proc Assoc Am Physicians* 1999; **111:** 35–44.
3. Rice GPA, *et al.* Cladribine and progressive MS: clinical and MRI outcomes of a multicenter controlled trial. *Neurology* 2000; **54:** 1145–55.

## Preparations

**Proprietary Preparations** (details are given in Part 3)
***Arg.:*** Intocel; Leustat; ***Austral.:*** Leustatin; ***Austria:*** Leustatin; ***Braz.:*** Leustatin; ***Canad.:*** Leustatin; ***Denm.:*** Leustatin; ***Fin.:*** Leustatin; ***Fr.:*** Leustatine; ***Ger.:*** Leustatin; ***Gr.:*** Leustatin; ***Hong Kong:*** Leustatin; ***Israel:*** Leustatin; Litak; ***Ital.:*** Leustatin; ***Neth.:*** Leustatin; ***Norw.:*** Leustatin; ***NZ:*** Leustatin; ***S.Afr.:*** Leustatin; ***Spain:*** Leustatin; ***Swed.:*** Leustatin; ***Switz.:*** Leustatin; Litak; ***Thai.:*** Leustatin; ***UK:*** Leustat; ***USA:*** Leustatin.

---

## Clofarabine *(USAN, pINN)*

2-Chloro-9-(2-deoxy-2-fluoro-β-D-arabinofuranosyl)-9*H*-purin-6-amine.

$C_{10}H_{11}ClFN_5O_3$ = 303.7.
*CAS — 123318-82-1.*

### Profile

Clofarabine, a purine nucleoside analogue, is an antimetabolite antineoplastic under investigation for the treatment of leukaemias.

---

## Corynebacterium parvum

*C. parvum*; NSC-220537; *Propionibacterium acnes.*

### Profile

Inactivated *Corynebacterium parvum* has been used in the treatment of malignant effusions, and has been tried as an adjuvant to cancer chemotherapy for its immunostimulant properties. It has also been used in the treatment of musculoskeletal and joint disorders.

Fever and pain have occurred after intracavitary injection. There have been reports of nephrotoxicity following intravenous use.

### Preparations

**Proprietary Preparations** (details are given in Part 3)
***Braz.:*** Corymunum†; Imunoparvum†; ***Ger.:*** Arthrokehlan A.

---

## Crisnatol Mesilate *(rINNM)*

BW-A770U (crisnatol); BW-A770U (crisnatol mesilate); Crisnatol Mesylate *(USAN)*; Mesilato de crisnatol.
*CAS — 96389-68-3 (crisnatol); 96389-69-4 (crisnatol mesilate).*

### Profile

Crisnatol is reported to act as a topoisomerase inhibitor and an intercalator of DNA. It has been investigated for its antineoplastic properties, notably for malignant neoplasms of the brain.

---

## Cyclophosphamide *(BAN, rINN)*

B-518; Ciclofosfamida; Cyclophosphamidum; Cyclophosphanum; NSC-26271; WR-138719. 2-[Bis(2-chloroethyl)amino]perhydro-1,3,2-oxazaphosphorinan 2-oxide monohydrate.

$C_7H_{15}Cl_2N_2O_2P,H_2O$ = 279.1.
*CAS — 6055-19-2 (cyclophosphamide monohydrate); 50-18-0 (anhydrous cyclophosphamide).*
*ATC — L01AA01.*

**Pharmacopoeias.** In *Chin., Eur.* (see p.vi), *Int., Jpn, Pol.,* and *US.*

**Ph. Eur. 5.0** (Cyclophosphamide). A white or almost white, crystalline powder. Soluble in water; freely soluble in alcohol. A freshly prepared 2% solution in water has a pH of 4.0 to 6.0.

**USP 27** (Cyclophosphamide). A white, crystalline powder. It liquefies upon loss of its water of crystallisation. Soluble in water and in alcohol. A 1% solution in water has a pH of 3.9 to 7.1 when determined 30 minutes after preparation. Store in airtight containers at 2° to 30°.

### Adverse Effects and Treatment

For a general outline see Antineoplastics, p.492 and p.495. The major dose-limiting effect is myelosuppression. After single doses the nadir of the white cell count may occur in around 1 to 2 weeks with full recovery usually in 3 to 4 weeks. Thrombocytopenia and anaemia may occur but tend to be less common and less severe.

Haemorrhagic cystitis may develop after high or prolonged dosage, and can be life-threatening. Adequate hydration to maintain urine output at 100 mL/hour and use of mesna (see p.1041) are generally recommended in an attempt to reduce urotoxicity. If mesna is used, frequent emptying of the bladder should be avoided. Doses of cyclophosphamide should be given early in the day.

Alopecia occurs in about 20% of patients given low doses and in practically all patients given high doses. Hair loss starts after 3 weeks of treatment but regrowth is usually evident after 3 months, even with continued treatment. Hyperpigmentation of skin, especially that of the palms and soles, and of the nails, has been reported.

Nausea and vomiting commonly occur, and may be reduced by prophylactic antiemetics. Mucositis may also occur.

Other adverse effects include a syndrome resembling inappropriate secretion of antidiuretic hormone (which may require diuretic therapy), disturbances of carbohydrate metabolism, gonadal suppression (common and occasionally resulting in sterility), interstitial pulmonary fibrosis, and, especially at high doses, cardiotoxicity.

Cyclophosphamide, in common with other alkylating agents, has carcinogenic, mutagenic, and teratogenic potential and secondary malignancies have occurred in patients given previous antineoplastic therapy including cyclophosphamide—see p.492.

**Effects on the bladder.** *Sterile haemorrhagic cystitis* can occur following high-dose infusions of cyclophosphamide or after prolonged low-dose oral administration.[1,2] It is believed to be secondary to renal excretion of alkylating metabolites, particularly the acrolein metabolite, that cause sloughing, thinning, and inflammation of the bladder wall. Damage ranges from minor bleeding to diffuse necrotic ulceration, and can lead to anaemia, constriction of the bladder, bladder perforation, and death.[2] Symptoms may be delayed, and have been reported to occur up to 6 months after discontinuation of the drug.[3] An increased incidence of cystitis when patients on a high-dose cyclophosphamide regimen were transferred from one brand to another has been reported,[4] apparently because one was labelled in terms of the anhydrous substance and one as the monohydrate, resulting in a 6.4% difference in the content of active substance.[5]

Measures used to prevent haemorrhagic cystitis include intravenous hydration with diuresis, frequent voiding, or bladder catheterisation with irrigation, to increase urine output and dilute the excreted metabolites. Mesna may be used as a uroprotectant to reduce exposure to the metabolites.[2] If bleeding occurs, intravesical treatments that have been used include irrigation with sodium chloride 0.9%,[2] alum instillation, which has an astringent effect,[2] or prostaglandins such as alprostadil, carboprost, or dinoprostone.[2,6-9] Silver nitrate, formaldehyde, or phenol instillations have been used but are painful and patients require anaesthesia.[2] There is limited information to suggest that conjugated oestrogens given orally or intravenously may be effective.[2,10] Nonpharmacological techniques are reserved for refractory cases and include arterial embolisation or surgery.[2]

In addition to the shorter term effects, cyclophosphamide has been reported to be associated with the development of *bladder carcinoma*.[1,11-14] A history of cyclophosphamide-induced cystitis may be associated with an increased risk of bladder carcinoma[1,11] but some studies have not found a link,[13] and bladder malignancies can develop in patients who have not experienced cystitis while receiving cyclophosphamide.[12] For a discussion of the carcinogenic effects of antineoplastics, including cyclophosphamide, see p.492.

1. Talar-Williams C, *et al.* Cyclophosphamide-induced cystitis and bladder cancer in patients with Wegener granulomatosis. *Ann Intern Med* 1996; **124:** 477–84.
2. West NJ. Prevention and treatment of hemorrhagic cystitis. *Pharmacotherapy* 1997; **17:** 696–706.
3. Armstrong B, *et al.* Delayed cystitis due to cyclophosphamide. *N Engl J Med* 1979; **300:** 45.
4. Shaw IC, *et al.* Difference in bioactivity between two preparations of cyclophosphamide. *Lancet* 1983; **i:** 709.
5. Hilgard P, *et al.* Bioactivity of cyclophosphamide preparations. *Lancet* 1983; **i:** 1436.
6. Mohiuddin J, *et al.* Treatment of cyclophosphamide-induced cystitis with prostaglandin $E_2$. *Ann Intern Med* 1984; **101:** 142.
7. Miller LJ, *et al.* Treatment of cyclophosphamide-induced hemorrhagic cystitis with prostaglandins. *Ann Pharmacother* 1994; **28:** 590–4.
8. Ippoliti C, *et al.* Intravesicular carboprost for the treatment of hemorrhagic cystitis after marrow transplantation. *Urology* 1995; **46:** 811–15.
9. Laszlo D, *et al.* Prostaglandin E2 bladder instillation for the treatment of hemorrhagic cystitis after allogeneic bone marrow transplantation. *Haematologica* 1995; **80:** 421–5.
10. Ordemann R, *et al.* Encouraging results in the treatment of haemorrhagic cystitis with estrogen – report of 10 cases and review of the literature. *Bone Marrow Transplant* 2000; **25:** 981–5.
11. Wall RL, Clausen KP. Carcinoma of the urinary bladder in patients receiving cyclophosphamide. *N Engl J Med* 1975; **293:** 271–3.
12. Plotz PH, *et al.* Bladder complications in patients receiving cyclophosphamide for systemic lupus erythematosus or rheumatoid arthritis. *Ann Intern Med* 1979; **91:** 221–3.

13. Pedersen-Bjergaard J, *et al.* Carcinoma of the urinary bladder after treatment with cyclophosphamide for non-Hodgkin's lymphoma. *N Engl J Med* 1988; **318:** 1028–32.
14. Travis LB, *et al.* Bladder cancer after chemotherapy for non-Hodgkin's lymphoma. *N Engl J Med* 1989; **321:** 544–5.

**Effects on the blood.** Amifostine has been reported to protect against the myelosuppressive effects of cyclophosphamide, and may be used to reduce neutropenia-related infection associated with the combination of cyclophosphamide and cisplatin (see p.1031).

**Effects on carbohydrate metabolism.** Acute onset type 1 diabetes occurred in a patient treated with cyclophosphamide, doxorubicin, vincristine and prednisone (CHOP), and was thought to be due to the cyclophosphamide.[1]

1. Atlan-Gepner C, *et al.* A cyclophosphamide-induced autoimmune diabetes. *Lancet* 1998; **352:** 373–4.

**Effects on electrolytes.** Water intoxication has been reported with cyclophosphamide,[1-4] usually in high doses (30 to 50 mg/kg or more) although symptoms have been reported after a dose of 20 mg/kg in a patient with renal disease,[3] and in another patient with systemic lupus erythematosus but apparently normal renal function who received 10 mg/kg.[4] One case of severe hyponatraemia leading to convulsions and death has been reported.[5] Symptoms resemble the syndrome of inappropriate antidiuretic hormone secretion (SIADH)[5] but plasma concentrations of antidiuretic hormone do not appear to be raised in these patients.[3]

1. DeFronzo RA, *et al.* Water intoxication in man after cyclophosphamide therapy: time course and relation to drug activation. *Ann Intern Med* 1973; **78:** 861–9.
2. Green TP, Mirkin BL. Prevention of cyclophosphamide-induced antidiuresis by furosemide infusion. *Clin Pharmacol Ther* 1981; **29:** 634–42.
3. Bressler RB, Huston DP. Water intoxication following moderate-dose intravenous cyclophosphamide. *Arch Intern Med* 1985; **145:** 548–9.
4. McCarron MO, *et al.* Water intoxication after low dose cyclophosphamide. *BMJ* 1995; **311:** 292.
5. Harlow PJ, *et al.* A fatal case of inappropriate ADH secretion induced by cyclophosphamide therapy. *Cancer* 1979; **44:** 896–8.

**Effects on the eyes.** Recurrent transient myopia, apparently due to increased hydration of the lens of the eye, was induced by an intravenous bolus of cyclophosphamide in an adolescent with systemic lupus erythematosus.[1]

1. Arranz JA, *et al.* Cyclophosphamide-induced myopia. *Ann Intern Med* 1992; **116:** 92–3.

**Effects on reproductive potential.** Severe gonadal failure with transient or permanent azoospermia is common in men treated with cyclophosphamide. Suppression of germ-cell function with intramuscular testosterone in 5 men during cyclophosphamide therapy for nephrotic syndrome was associated with a more rapid return of spermatogenesis compared with 10 patients who did not receive the androgen.[1]

1. Masala A, *et al.* Use of testosterone to prevent cyclophosphamide-induced azoospermia. *Ann Intern Med* 1997; **126:** 292–5.

**Effects on the skin.** An erythematous pruritic rash, similar to the palmar-plantar erythrodysesthesia syndrome (p.495) but occurring on the dorsal surfaces of the hands and feet, occurred 6 days after the first high dose of cyclophosphamide in a patient being prepared for bone marrow transplantation.[1] Previous cyclophosphamide-containing chemotherapy did not produce this reaction. The symptoms improved somewhat on treatment with triamcinolone ointment, and subsequently desquamation of the hands occurred with decreased purplish discoloration and oedema of the feet. There has also been a report of 2 patients who developed Stevens-Johnson syndrome, with some features suggestive of overlapping toxic epidermal necrolysis.[2]

1. Matsuyama JR, Kwok KK. A variant of the chemotherapy-associated erythrodysesthesia syndrome related to high-dose cyclophosphamide. *DICP Ann Pharmacother* 1989; **23:** 776–9.
2. Assier-Bonnet H, *et al.* Stevens-Johnson syndrome induced by cyclophosphamide: report of two cases. *Br J Dermatol* 1996; **135:** 864–6.

**Hypersensitivity.** Occasional anaphylaxis has been reported with cyclophosphamide;[1] analysis of data by the Boston Collaborative Drug Surveillance Program detected only one allergic skin reaction among 210 patients given cyclophosphamide, resulting in a calculated incidence of 4.8 reactions per 1000 recipients.[2]

1. Jones JB, *et al.* Cyclophosphamide anaphylaxis. *DICP Ann Pharmacother* 1989; **23:** 88–9.
2. Bigby M, *et al.* Drug-induced cutaneous reactions: a report from the Boston Collaborative Drug Surveillance Program on 15 438 consecutive inpatients, 1975 to 1982. *JAMA* 1986; **256:** 3358–63.

## Precautions

For reference to the precautions necessary with antineoplastics, see p.497.

Cyclophosphamide should not be given to patients with bone-marrow aplasia, acute infection, or drug- or radiation-induced urothelial toxicity. It should be given with care to those with diabetes mellitus. Care is also needed in elderly or debilitated patients, or those with renal or hepatic impairment or who have undergone adrenalectomy. Liberal fluid intake and frequent micturition are advised to reduce the risk of cystitis but care must be taken to avoid water retention and intoxication. Urine should be examined regularly for red cells, which may precede haemorrhagic cystitis. The haematological profile should be monitored regularly. The use of cyclophosphamide in pregnancy should be avoided where possible.

**Breast feeding.** Cyclophosphamide has been detected in breast milk,[1] and there are reports of neutropenia,[2] and leucopenia and thrombocytopenia,[3] in infants who have been breast fed by women receiving cyclophosphamide. The American Academy of Pediatrics considers[4] that cyclophosphamide may interfere with cellular metabolism, causing neutropenia and possibly immune suppression in the infant, and has unknown effects on growth, and an association with carcinogenesis.

1. Wiernik PH, Duncan JH. Cyclophosphamide in human milk. *Lancet* 1971; **1:** 912.
2. Amato D, Niblett JS. Neutropenia from cyclophosphamide in breast milk. *Med J Aust* 1977; **1:** 383–4.
3. Durodola JI. Administration of cyclophosphamide during late pregnancy and early lactation: a case report. *J Natl Med Assoc* 1979; **71:** 165–6.
4. American Academy of Pediatrics. The transfer of drugs and other chemicals into human milk. *Pediatrics* 2001; **108:** 776–89. Correction. *ibid.*; 1029. Also available at: http://aappolicy.aappublications.org/cgi/content/full/pediatrics%3b108/3/776 (accessed 29/06/04)

**Handling and disposal.** *Residues* of cyclophosphamide or ifosfamide destroyed using alkaline hydrolysis in the presence of dimethylformamide showed no mutagenicity *in vitro*.[1] An alternative method, involving refluxing of cyclophosphamide with hydrochloric acid, neutralising, and then reacting with sodium thiosulfate, was effective for the degradation of cyclophosphamide, but residues from ifosfamide were still highly mutagenic *in vitro* and this second method should therefore not be used to degrade ifosfamide.

*Urine and faeces* produced for up to 72 hours and 5 days respectively after an oral dose of cyclophosphamide should be handled wearing protective clothing.[2] As cyclophosphamide was present in sweat and saliva, protective clothing was advised for 72 hours after a dose when bathing the patient or carrying out oral procedures.

1. Castegnaro M, *et al.*, eds. Laboratory decontamination and destruction of carcinogens in laboratory wastes: some antineoplastic agents. *IARC Scientific Publications 73*. Lyon: WHO/International Agency for Research on Cancer, 1985.
2. Harris J, Dodds LJ. Handling waste from patients receiving cytotoxic drugs. *Pharm J* 1985; **235:** 289–91.

**Porphyria.** Cyclophosphamide is considered to be unsafe in patients with porphyria because it has been shown to be porphyrinogenic in *animals*.

## Interactions

For a general outline of antineoplastic drug interactions, see p.498. Since cyclophosphamide must undergo hepatic metabolism before it is active, interactions are possible with drugs that inhibit or stimulate the mixed function oxidase enzymes responsible. There may be an increased risk of cardiotoxicity in patients who have also received doxorubicin or other cardiotoxic drugs.

**Allopurinol.** Although the Boston Collaborative Drug Surveillance Program reported an increased incidence of bone-marrow depression in patients who received allopurinol with cyclophosphamide than in those receiving cyclophosphamide without allopurinol (15 of 26 compared with only 6 of 32),[1] a subsequent study in patients receiving combination chemotherapy, including cyclophosphamide, for lymphomas failed to find any difference in the nadirs of the platelet and white blood cell counts in cycles in which allopurinol was given.[2] Although allopurinol pretreatment resulted in a longer cyclophosphamide half-life in 4 of 26 patients given cyclophosphamide urinary excretion of cyclophosphamide was unchanged.[3] A longer cyclophosphamide half-life was also seen in a study in children who had received allopurinol.[4]

1. Boston Collaborative Drug Surveillance Program. Allopurinol and cytotoxic drugs: interaction in relation to bone marrow depression. *JAMA* 1974; **227:** 1036–40.
2. Stolbach L, *et al.* Evaluation of bone marrow toxic reaction in patients treated with allopurinol. *JAMA* 1982; **247:** 334–6.
3. Bagley CM, *et al.* Clinical pharmacology of cyclophosphamide. *Cancer Res* 1973; **33:** 226–33.
4. Yule SM, *et al.* Cyclophosphamide pharmacokinetics in children. *Br J Clin Pharmacol* 1996; **41:** 13–19.

**Antibacterials.** *Chloramphenicol* given before cyclophosphamide prolonged the mean cyclophosphamide serum half-life from 7.5 to 11.5 hours and reduced the peak activity in all of 5 subjects.[1] Giving *sulfaphenazole* before cyclophosphamide significantly inhibited the rate of biotransformation of cyclophosphamide in 2 of 7 subjects and enhanced it in 2; it remained unchanged in 3.

1. Faber OK, *et al.* The effect of chloramphenicol and sulphaphenazole on the biotransformation of cyclophosphamide in man. *Br J Clin Pharmacol* 1975; **2:** 281–5.

**Anticoagulants.** For reference to the interaction of cyclophosphamide with *warfarin*, see p.1025.

**Barbiturates.** Although patients receiving cyclophosphamide developed higher peak plasma concentrations of active cyclophosphamide metabolites when given enzyme-inducing agents such as barbiturates, the active metabolites also disappeared rapidly.[1]

1. Bagley CM, *et al.* Clinical pharmacology of cyclophosphamide. *Cancer Res* 1973; **33:** 226–33.

**Chlorpromazine.** The half-life of cyclophosphamide was approximately 200% greater in 2 children also taking chlorpromazine than in children not receiving the phenothiazine.[1]

1. Yule SM, *et al.* Cyclophosphamide pharmacokinetics in children. *Br J Clin Pharmacol* 1996; **41:** 13–19.

**Colony-stimulating factors.** Fatal respiratory insufficiency associated with alveolar fibrosis developed in an infant given cyclophosphamide and doxorubicin followed by *filgrastim*.[1] Since pulmonary toxicity with cyclophosphamide is normally associated with high cumulative doses it was suggested that in this case the effects might have been exacerbated by the granulocyte colony-stimulating factor. (The pulmonary toxicity of bleomycin has also been suggested to be exacerbated by colony-stimulating factors, as discussed on p.531).

1. van Woensel JBM, *et al.* Acute respiratory insufficiency during doxorubicin, cyclophosphamide, and G-CSF therapy. *Lancet* 1994; **344:** 759–60.

**Corticosteroids.** Single doses of *prednisone* have been found to inhibit the activation of cyclophosphamide but after longer-term treatment the rate of activation has increased.[1] A study in children found that pretreatment with *dexamethasone* was associated with increased clearance of cyclophosphamide and a decrease in its half-life relative to children who had not received the corticosteroid.[2]

1. Faber OK, Mouridsen HT. Cyclophosphamide activation and corticosteroids. *N Engl J Med* 1974; **291:** 211.
2. Yule SM, *et al.* Cyclophosphamide pharmacokinetics in children. *Br J Clin Pharmacol* 1996; **41:** 13–19.

**Gastrointestinal drugs.** In a retrospective study in patients receiving high-dose cyclophosphamide, cisplatin, and carmustine,[1] the area under the plasma-concentration time curve (AUC) for cyclophosphamide (measured as the parent compound) was 17% lower when *ondansetron* rather than prochlorperazine was added to the antiemetic regimen. In addition, the AUC for cisplatin was 10% higher with the ondansetron regimen. In a similar study,[2] the AUCs for both cyclophosphamide and cisplatin were lower in patients receiving an antiemetic regimen including ondansetron rather than prochlorperazine. The authors of both studies noted that the relevance of these findings to toxicity and antitumour effect of the antineoplastics remained to be determined.

1. Gilbert CJ, *et al.* Pharmacokinetic interaction between ondansetron and cyclophosphamide during high-dose chemotherapy for breast cancer. *Cancer Chemother Pharmacol* 1998; **42:** 497–503.
2. Cagnoni PJ, *et al.* Modification of the pharmacokinetics of high-dose cyclophosphamide and cisplatin by antiemetics. *Bone Marrow Transplant* 1999; **24:** 1–4.

**NSAIDs.** Acute life-threatening water intoxication was reported in a patient given low-dose cyclophosphamide with *indometacin*.[1] The patient had previously received treatment with cyclophosphamide (for multiple myeloma) without significant adverse effect.

1. Webberley MJ, Murray JA. Life-threatening acute hyponatraemia induced by low dose cyclophosphamide and indomethacin. *Postgrad Med J* 1989; **65:** 950–2.

**Suxamethonium.** For reference to a possible interaction between cyclophosphamide and suxamethonium, see under Suxamethonium Chloride, p.1408.

## Pharmacokinetics

After oral doses, cyclophosphamide is well absorbed from the gastrointestinal tract with a bioavailability greater than 75%. It is widely distributed in the tissues and crosses the blood-brain barrier. It undergoes activation by the mixed function oxidase systems in the liver. The initial metabolites are 4-hydroxycyclophosphamide and its acyclic tautomer, aldophosphamide, which both undergo further metabolism; aldophosphamide may undergo non-enzymatic conversion to active phosphoramide mustard. Acrolein is also produced and may be responsible for bladder toxicity. Cyclophosphamide is excreted principally in urine, as metabolites and some unchanged drug. It crosses the placenta, and is found in breast milk.

◊ Reviews.

1. Moore MJ. Clinical pharmacokinetics of cyclophosphamide. *Clin Pharmacokinet* 1991; **20:** 194–208.
2. Boddy AV, Yule SM. Metabolism and pharmacokinetics of oxazaphosphorines. *Clin Pharmacokinet* 2000; **38:** 291–304.

**Absorption.** Cyclophosphamide was detected in the urine of 5 patients following application to intact skin, demonstrating that cyclophosphamide can be absorbed via this route.[1] Absorption continued after the site of application had been cleaned, suggesting that cyclophosphamide had penetrated subcutaneous lipid and was slowly released to the circulation from this depot. Cyclophosphamide was also identified in the urine of 2 oncology nurses but appeared more quickly than in patients, suggesting a faster route of absorption, perhaps by inhalation of aerosols generated during dissolution of the drug.

1. Hirst M, *et al.* Occupational exposure to cyclophosphamide. *Lancet* 1984; **i:** 186–8.

## Uses and Administration

Cyclophosphamide is an antineoplastic that is converted in the body to active alkylating metabolites with properties similar to those of chlormethine (p.537). It also possesses marked immunosuppressant properties.

Cyclophosphamide is widely used, often in combination with other agents, in the treatment of malignant diseases as indicated by the cross-references below. It is given for Burkitt's and other non-Hodgkin's lymphomas, multiple myeloma, and mycosis fungoides. It is also used in gestational trophoblastic tumours and malignancies of the brain, breast, endometrium, lung, and ovary; in childhood malignancies such as neuroblastoma, retinoblastoma, Wilms' tumour; and in sarcomas and some leukaemias.

The immunosuppressant properties of cyclophosphamide have been used in organ and tissue transplantation. It has also been used in the management of disorders thought to have an auto-immune component including amyloidosis, Behçet's syndrome, glomerular kidney disease, idiopathic thrombocytopenic purpura, aplastic anaemia, cryptogenic fibrosing alveolitis, polymyositis, scleroderma, systemic lupus erythematosus, and vasculitic syndromes including the Churg-Strauss syndrome, polyarteritis nodosa, and Wegener's granulomatosis, as indicated by the cross references below.

Cyclophosphamide is usually given by mouth or intravenous injection.

In the BP 2003 the content of Cyclophosphamide Injection is expressed in terms of the equivalent amount of anhydrous cyclophosphamide whereas the content of Cyclophosphamide Tablets is given in terms of the monohydrate; the USP 27 expresses content in terms of anhydrous cyclophosphamide for both injection and tablets. Confusion has arisen when patients were changed from a preparation in which the content was expressed as the monohydrate to one in which it was expressed as the anhydrous substance (see Effects on the Bladder, above). 53.45 mg of cyclophosphamide monohydrate is equivalent to 50 mg of anhydrous cyclophosphamide. *Doses below are given in terms of anhydrous cyclophosphamide.*

The dosage given may vary considerably depending on the disease being treated, the condition of the patient including the state of the bone marrow, and use with radiotherapy or other chemotherapy. The white cell count is usually used to guide the dose.

In the UK an example of a licensed *low-dose* regimen is cyclophosphamide 2 to 6 mg/kg weekly as a single intravenous dose or in divided doses by mouth; a *moderate-dose* regimen might be 10 to 15 mg/kg weekly as a single intravenous dose. An example of a *high-dose* regimen is 20 to 40 mg/kg as a single intravenous dose every 10 to 20 days, although higher doses have been used. Alternative regimens include 100 to 300 mg daily in divided doses by mouth, 80 to 300 mg/m$^2$ daily as a single intravenous dose, 300 to 600 mg/m$^2$ weekly as a single intravenous dose, and 600 to 1500 mg/m$^2$ as a single intravenous dose or short infusion at 10 to 20 day intervals. The use of mesna is generally recommended with single doses of cyclophosphamide over 2 g, but one manufacturer suggests its use with doses as low as 10 mg/kg.

In the USA, an initial dose of 40 to 50 mg/kg has been licensed for single agent therapy of malignancy, given intravenously in divided doses over 2 to 5 days although in practice treatment of malignancy will generally be with combination regimens. Other intravenous regimens include 3 to 5 mg/kg twice weekly or 10 to 15 mg/kg every 7 to 10 days. Alternatively, 1 to 5 mg/kg daily has been given orally.

A daily oral dose of 2 to 3 mg/kg has been used in children with minimal change nephropathy leading to the nephrotic syndrome, in whom corticosteroids have been unsuccessful.

In patients who are to undergo bone marrow transplantation very high doses of cyclophosphamide such as 60 mg/kg daily for 2 days may be given as part of the conditioning regimen.

Cyclophosphamide has also been given intramuscularly, intraperitoneally, and intrapleurally, as well as intra-arterially, and by local perfusion (but passage through the liver is required for its activation—see Pharmacokinetics, above). A liquid preparation of cyclophosphamide for oral use may be prepared using the powder for injection.

Regular blood counts are essential during therapy with cyclophosphamide and treatment should be withdrawn or delayed if leucopenia or thrombocytopenia becomes severe (see also Bone-marrow Depression, p.496). Patients should be adequately hydrated and urine output maintained.

**Amyloidosis.** Although there is no unequivocally effective treatment for amyloidosis (p.567), cyclophosphamide may reduce the decline in renal function and prolong survival;[1-3] it has also been used with epirubicin and carmustine to suppress the disease in a patient who had undergone heart transplantation for cardiac amyloid.[4]

1. Berglund K, *et al.* Alkylating cytostatic treatment in renal amyloidosis secondary to rheumatic disease. *Ann Rheum Dis* 1987; **46:** 757–62.
2. Berglund K, *et al.* Results, principles and pitfalls in the management of renal AA-amyloidosis; a 10-21 year followup of 16 patients with rheumatic disease treated with alkylating cytostatics. *J Rheumatol* 1993; **20:** 2051–7.
3. Chevrel G, *et al.* Renal type AA amyloidosis associated with rheumatoid arthritis: a cohort study showing improved survival on treatment with pulse cyclophosphamide. *Rheumatology (Oxford)* 2001; **40:** 821–5.
4. Hall R, *et al.* Cardiac transplantation for AL amyloidosis. *BMJ* 1994; **309:** 1135–7.

**Blood disorders, non-malignant.** Cyclophosphamide has been used in patients with idiopathic thrombocytopenic purpura (p.1082), but cytotoxic immunosuppressants tend to be a treatment of last resort. Responses generally occur within 8 weeks.[1] In patients with refractory life-threatening disease, high-dose cyclophosphamide[1] may be tried. Combination chemotherapy including cyclophosphamide has also produced responses in a few patients.[2]

Cyclophosphamide is commonly used in preparation for bone marrow transplantation in patients with aplastic anaemia (p.732), and complete remission has also been reported with high-dose cyclophosphamide alone.[3] However, a randomised trial[4] of high-dose cyclophosphamide plus ciclosporin compared with conventional immunosuppression was stopped early when a higher mortality was observed in those receiving cyclophosphamide. Further follow-up[5] also found that relapse rates were no different.

1. McMillan R. Therapy for adults with refractory chronic immune thrombocytopenic purpura. *Ann Intern Med* 1997; **126:** 307–14.
2. Figueroa M, *et al.* Combination chemotherapy in refractory immune thrombocytopenic purpura. *N Engl J Med* 1993; **328:** 1226–9.
3. Brodsky RA, *et al.* Durable treatment-free remission after high-dose cyclophosphamide therapy for previously untreated severe aplastic anemia. *Ann Intern Med* 2001; **135:** 477–83.
4. Tisdale JF, *et al.* High-dose cyclophosphamide in severe aplastic anaemia: a randomised trial. *Lancet* 2000; **356:** 1554–9.
5. Tisdale JF, *et al.* Late complications following treatment for severe aplastic anemia (SAA) with high-dose cyclophosphamide (Cy): follow-up of a randomized trial. *Blood* 2002; **100:** 4668–70.

**Cogan's syndrome.** For reference to the use of cyclophosphamide in combination with corticosteroids for Cogan's syndrome, see p.1078.

**Connective tissue and muscular disorders.** Cyclophosphamide is one of a number of immunosuppressants that have been tried for disease control in Behçet's syndrome (p.1076); such agents may permit a reduction in the use of corticosteroids, although they carry their own risks of toxicity. In polymyositis (p.1086) cyclophosphamide may have a role where there is lung disease; the role of immunosuppressants other than azathioprine or methotrexate is poorly defined. In patients with systemic lupus erythematosus (p.1088), cyclophosphamide has been used with some success for severe disease or disease refractory to corticosteroids alone, and appears to be more effective than corticosteroids for lupus nephritis.

**Kidney disorders, non-malignant.** Cyclophosphamide is used with corticosteroids in the treatment of a number of forms of glomerular kidney disease (p.1080). In minimal change nephropathy, cyclophosphamide 2 to 3 mg/kg daily for 8 weeks may be added to a course of corticosteroid therapy in relapsing disease;[1] addition of cyclophosphamide to corticosteroid therapy also improves the prospect of remission in focal glomerulosclerosis. Oral cyclophosphamide helps to stabilise progressive disease in patients with membranous nephropathy[2] although intermittent intravenous pulses are reported to be ineffective.[3] Such treatment is usually reserved for those whose disease is severe and progressive enough to justify it. Cyclophosphamide has been given with methylprednisolone for rapidly progressive glomerulonephritis,[4] and has been used as part of the aggressive management of renal lesions in Goodpasture's syndrome.

1. Durkan A, *et al.* Non-corticosteroid treatment for nephrotic syndrome in children. Available in The Cochrane Library; Issue 2. Chichester: John Wiley; 2004.
2. Falk RJ, *et al.* Treatment of progressive membranous glomerulopathy: a randomized trial comparing cyclophosphamide and corticosteroids with corticosteroids alone. *Ann Intern Med* 1992; **116:** 438–45.
3. Reichert LJM, *et al.* Preserving renal function in patients with membranous nephropathy: daily oral chlorambucil compared with intermittent monthly pulses of cyclophosphamide. *Ann Intern Med* 1994; **121:** 328–33.
4. Bruns FJ, *et al.* Long-term follow-up of aggressively treated idiopathic rapidly progressive glomerulonephritis. *Am J Med* 1989; **86:** 400–6.

**Liver disorders, non-malignant.** For mention of the use of cyclophosphamide in auto-immune hepatitis inadequately controlled by corticosteroids and azathioprine see Chronic Active Hepatitis, p.1078.

**Lung disorders, non-malignant.** Cyclophosphamide may be useful with corticosteroids in patients with cryptogenic fibrosing alveolitis, as mentioned under Diffuse Parenchymal Lung Disease, p.1079.

**Malignant neoplasms.** Cyclophosphamide is one of the most widely used drugs for the chemotherapy of malignancy, and mention of its role may be found in the discussions of the management of gestational trophoblastic tumours (p.505); the non-Hodgkin's lymphomas, including AIDS-related lymphoma, Burkitt's lymphoma, and mycosis fungoides (p.510, p.510, p.511, p.511); malignancies of the brain (p.513), breast (p.514), endometrium (p.516), lung (p.519), ovary (p.520) and thymus (p.523); multiple myeloma (p.511); Wilms' tumour, neuroblastoma, and retinoblastoma (p.518, p.524, and p.524 respectively); and sarcomas of bone (p.524) and rhabdomyosarcoma (p.525). Cyclophosphamide is also used in the management of acute lymphoblastic leukaemia (p.506) and chronic lymphocytic leukaemia (p.507).

**Neuromuscular disorders.** Cyclophosphamide has been tried in myasthenia gravis (p.1486) in patients who require immunosuppressants but are intolerant of or unresponsive to corticosteroids and azathioprine. Cyclophosphamide has also been tried in various regimens for the management of multiple sclerosis (p.646), but the reported benefits have generally been slight and outweighed by toxicity, such that it is usually reserved for patients with severe disease resistant to standard therapies.

References.

1. De Feo LG, *et al.* Use of intravenous pulsed cyclophosphamide in severe, generalized myasthenia gravis. *Muscle Nerve* 2002; **26:** 31–6.
2. Drachman DB, *et al.* Treatment of refractory myasthenia: "rebooting" with high-dose cyclophosphamide. *Ann Neurol* 2003; **53:** 29–34.
3. Portaccio E, *et al.* Safety and tolerability of cyclophosphamide 'pulses' in multiple sclerosis: a prospective study in a clinical cohort. *Multiple Sclerosis* 2003; **9:** 446–50.
4. Zephir H, *et al.* Treatment of progressive forms of multiple sclerosis by cyclophosphamide: a cohort study of 490 patients. *J Neurol Sci* 2004; **218:** 73–7.
5. La Mantia L, *et al.* Cyclophosphamide for multiple sclerosis. Available in The Cochrane Library; Issue 2. Chichester: John Wiley; 2004.

**Ocular disorders, non-malignant.** Immunosuppressive agents, including cyclophosphamide, have been used in scleritis and uveitis (see p.1088 and p.1090) unresponsive to corticosteroids in tolerable doses.

**Organ and tissue transplantation.** Cyclophosphamide is used in high doses, usually with busulfan or irradiation, in conditioning regimens for bone marrow transplantation (see Haematopoietic Stem Cell Transplantation, p.1344). It has been tried as part of immunosuppressant regimens following transplantation of heart grafts (p.1345).

**Paraquat poisoning.** For reference to the use of cyclophosphamide in paraquat poisoning, see p.1508.

**Pemphigus and pemphigoid.** Corticosteroids are the main treatment for blistering in pemphigus and pemphigoid (p.1137). Immunosuppressive therapy, including cyclophosphamide,[1,2] has been used in combination with corticosteroids to permit a reduction in corticosteroid dosage. Cyclophosphamide with a corticosteroid is also reported to be of value in ocular cicatricial pemphigoid,[3] although treatment may not completely prevent cicatrisation. However, it has been suggested that evidence for the corticosteroid-sparing effect is lacking and that immunosuppressants should be reserved for patients who cannot tolerate corticosteroids or in whom they are contra-indicated.[4]

1. Pandya AG, Sontheimer RD. Treatment of pemphigus vulgaris with pulse intravenous cyclophosphamide. *Arch Dermatol* 1992; **128:** 1626–30.
2. Itoh T, *et al.* Successful treatment of bullous pemphigoid with pulsed intravenous cyclophosphamide. *Br J Dermatol* 1996; **134:** 931–3.
3. Elder MJ, *et al.* Role of cyclophosphamide and high dose steroid in ocular cicatricial pemphigoid. *Br J Ophthalmol* 1995; **79:** 264–6.
4. Bystryn J-C, Steinman NM. The adjuvant therapy of pemphigus: an update. *Arch Dermatol* 1996; **132:** 203–12.

**Rheumatoid arthritis.** Cyclophosphamide has been used as a disease-modifying antirheumatic drug in rheumatoid arthritis (p.9), usually in patients with severe disease unresponsive to other drugs; its severe toxicity limits its usefulness.[1] It is of most value in controlling antibody-mediated systemic complications of the disease such as vasculitis[2] through inhibition of B-cell function.

1. Suarez-Almazor ME, *et al.* Cyclophosphamide for treating rheumatoid arthritis. Available in The Cochrane Library; Issue 2. Chichester: John Wiley; 2004.
2. Choy E, Kingsley G. How do second-line agents work? *Br Med Bull* 1995; **51:** 472–92.

**Sarcoidosis.** Where drug therapy is required for sarcoidosis (p.1087), corticosteroids are the usual treatment. Cyclophosphamide is one of a number of cytotoxic immunosuppressants that have been tried, with variable results, as a second-line therapy; its use has been limited by toxicity.

**Scleroderma.** As discussed on p.1348 the role of drug treatment for scleroderma is not well determined, but cyclophosphamide may be useful combined with a corticosteroid for patients with lung involvement.

**Vasculitic syndromes.** Treatment of the systemic vasculitides has revolved around the use of corticosteroids and cyclophosphamide. The benefits are uncertain in polyarteritis nodosa (p.1085) and Takayasu's arteritis (p.1089), but the benefits of combined therapy are generally accepted in Churg-Strauss syndrome (p.1078) and microscopic polyangiitis (p.1085), and cyclophosphamide is the mainstay of effective treatment of Wegener's granulomatosis (p.1090). A number of regimens are in use; in particular intermittent high-dose intravenous ('pulsed') use is being evaluated in comparison with continuous therapy.[1]

1. Richmond R, *et al.* Optimisation of cyclophosphamide therapy in systemic vasculitis. *Clin Pharmacokinet* 1998; **34:** 79–90.

## Preparations

***BP 2003:*** Cyclophosphamide Injection; Cyclophosphamide Tablets;
***USP 27:*** Cyclophosphamide for Injection; Cyclophosphamide Tablets.

**Proprietary Preparations** (details are given in Part 3)
***Arg.:*** Endoxan; Genoxal; ***Austral.:*** Cycloblastin; Endoxan; ***Austria:*** Endoxan; ***Belg.:*** Cycloblastine†; Endoxan; ***Braz.:*** Ciclosmida†; Cyclan; Enduxan†; Genuxal; ***Canad.:*** Cytoxan; Procytox; ***Chile:*** Endoxan; Ledoxina; ***Denm.:*** Carloxan; Sendoxan; ***Fin.:*** Sendoxan; ***Fr.:*** Endoxan; ***Ger.:*** Cyclo-cell†; Cyclostin; Endoxan; ***Gr.:*** Endoxan; ***Hong Kong:*** Endoxan; ***India:*** Cycloxan; Endoxan; ***Irl.:*** Endoxana; ***Israel:*** Cytophosphan; Cytoxan; Endoxan; ***Ital.:*** Endoxan; ***Malaysia:*** Endoxan; ***Mex.:*** Fosfaseron†; Genoxal; Ledoxina; ***Neth.:*** Endoxan; ***Norw.:*** Sendoxan; ***NZ:*** Cycloblastin; Cytoxan; Endoxan; ***Port.:*** Endoxan; ***S.Afr.:*** Cycloblastin; Endoxan; ***Singapore:*** Alkyloxan†; Endoxan; ***Spain:*** Cicloxal†; Genoxal; ***Swed.:*** Sendoxan; ***Switz.:*** Endoxan; ***Thai.:*** Endoxan; Endoxana†; ***UK:*** Endoxana; ***USA:*** Cytoxan; Neosar.

# Cytarabine *(BAN, USAN, rINN)*

Arabinosylcytosine; Ara-C; Citarabina; Cytarabinum; Cytosine Arabinoside; NSC-63878 (cytarabine hydrochloride); U-19920; U-19920A (cytarabine hydrochloride); WR-28453. 1-β-D-Arabinofuranosylcytosine; 4-Amino-1-β-D-arabinofuranosylpyrimidin-2(1*H*)-one.

$C_9H_{13}N_3O_5$ = 243.2.

*CAS — 147-94-4 (cytarabine); 69-74-9 (cytarabine hydrochloride).*

*ATC — L01BC01.*

**Pharmacopoeias.** In *Eur.* (see p.vi), *Int., Jpn, Pol.,* and *US. Chin.* includes the hydrochloride.

**Ph. Eur. 5.0** (Cytarabine). A white or almost white, crystalline powder. Freely soluble in water; very slightly soluble in alcohol and in dichloromethane. Store in airtight containers. Protect from light.

**USP 27** (Cytarabine). An odourless, white to off-white, crystalline powder. Freely soluble in water; slightly soluble in alcohol and in chloroform. Protect from light.

**Incompatibility.** Although cytarabine has been stated in the literature to be incompatible with solutions of fluorouracil[1,2] and methotrexate[2] some studies have reported it to be stable for some hours when mixed with the latter.[3]

1. McRae MP, King JC. Compatibility of antineoplastic, antibiotic and corticosteroid drugs in intravenous admixtures. *Am J Hosp Pharm* 1976; **33:** 1010–13.
2. D'Arcy PF. Reactions and interactions in handling anticancer drugs. *Drug Intell Clin Pharm* 1983; **17:** 532–8.
3. Cheung Y-W, *et al.* Stability of cytarabine, methotrexate sodium, and hydrocortisone sodium succinate admixtures. *Am J Hosp Pharm* 1984; **41:** 1802–6.

## Adverse Effects, Treatment, and Precautions

For general discussions see Antineoplastics, p.492, p.495, and p.497.

The major dose-limiting adverse effect of cytarabine is bone-marrow depression, manifest as leucopenia (particularly granulocytopenia), thrombocytopenia, and anaemia, sometimes with striking megaloblastic changes. Myelosuppression appears to be more evident after continuous infusions. Leucopenia is biphasic, with a nadir at 7 to 9 days after a dose and another, more severe, at 15 to 24 days. The nadir of the platelet count occurs at about 12 to 15 days. Recovery generally occurs in a further 10 days.

Gastrointestinal disturbances may occur: nausea and vomiting may be more severe when doses are given rapidly (but other adverse effects are reported to be worse when the drug is given by infusion). Other adverse effects reported include hepatic dysfunction, renal dysfunction, neurotoxicity, bleeding complications, rashes, oral and anal ulceration, gastrointestinal haemorrhage, oesophagitis, and conjunctivitis. A syndrome of bone and muscle pain, fever, malaise, conjunctivitis, and rash, sometimes described as flu-like, has been reported 6 to 12 hours after cytarabine administration, which may be treated or prevented with corticosteroid therapy. Anaphylactoid reactions and pancreatitis have occurred rarely. There may be local pain, cellulitis, and thrombophlebitis at the site of injection.

Intrathecal administration of the liposomal cytarabine formulation commonly causes chemical arachnoiditis manifesting as neck stiffness or pain, nausea, vomiting, headache, and fever. Dexamethasone should be used prophylactically to reduce the incidence and severity of this complication. Other rare adverse effects include encephalopathy, and focal seizures. Intrathecal administration of conventional cytarabine formulations has rarely been associated with severe spinal cord toxicity, necrotising encephalopathy, blindness, and other neurotoxicities. If used intrathecally, preservative-free diluents must be used.

High-dose therapy has been associated with particularly severe gastrointestinal and CNS effects, including severe ulceration of the gastrointestinal tract, pneumatosis cystoides leading to peritonitis, necrotising colitis and bowel necrosis, peripheral neuropathy, and cerebral and cerebellar dysfunction, with personality changes, somnolence, and coma. There may also be corneal toxicity leading to punctate keratitis and haemorrhagic conjunctivitis, sepsis, liver abscess, severe skin rash leading to desquamation, alopecia, and cardiac disorders including pericarditis and fatal cardiomyopathy. Pulmonary oedema, sometimes fatal, has occurred.

Cytarabine is teratogenic in *animals* (but see Pregnancy, below).

In addition to frequent white blood cell and platelet counts, blood-uric acid should be monitored because of the risk of hyperuricaemia secondary to lysis of neoplastic cells, and renal and hepatic function should be periodically assessed. Cytarabine should be given with care to patients with impaired liver function; dosage reduction may be necessary.

◊ The toxicity of cytarabine has been reviewed.[1] The principal toxicity of standard dosage regimens is myelosuppression but bleeding complications and gastrointestinal toxicity are also major problems at standard doses. With the high-dose regimens neurological toxicity may be dose-limiting: severe and sometimes irreversible symptoms have been seen in some 6 to 10% of patients receiving a cumulative dose of 36 g/m$^2$. Ocular toxicity may occur in up to 80% of patients at the highest doses. Since cytarabine toxicity is largely dose-related, low-dose cytarabine is generally well tolerated, even in elderly patients (who are more susceptible): its only significant toxicity is myelosuppression.

1. Stentoft J. The toxicity of cytarabine. *Drug Safety* 1990; **5:** 7–27.

**Effects on the nervous system.** Although paraplegia has been reported with intrathecal cytarabine[1] (see also under Benzyl Alcohol, p.1170) and peripheral neuropathy has occurred in a patient who had received only conventional intravenous doses,[2] the majority of cases of neurotoxicity associated with cytarabine appear to be in patients given high-dose regimens.[3-7] Although some cases have manifested as demyelinating peripheral neuropathy,[3,4] including a syndrome of painful legs and involuntary movements in the toes which showed some response to carbamazepine,[3] most studies have reported in particular a syndrome of cerebellar toxicity,[5-8] with symptoms such as dysarthria, nystagmus, and ataxia. Toxicity appears to be dose-related: in one series[5] CNS toxicity occurred in none of 12 patients given total doses of up to 24 g/m$^2$ of cytarabine, 3 of 19 receiving 36 g/m$^2$, and 1 of 12 given 48 g/m$^2$, none of which were life-threatening or irreversible, whereas 4 of 6 given 54 g/m$^2$ (as 4.5 g/m$^2$ every 12 hours for 12 doses) developed neurotoxicity, which was fatal in one and irreversible in another. However, persistent, severe cerebellar toxicity has also been reported in a patient who had received a total dose of only 36 g/m$^2$ (as 3 g/m$^2$ every 12 hours).[8] There is some evidence[6] that patients aged over 50, and those who have recently received conventional-dose cytarabine[7] may be at increased risk. Intracranial hypertension (pseudotumor cerebri) has occurred rarely.[9]

1. Saleh MN, *et al.* Intrathecal cytosine arabinoside-induced acute, rapidly reversible paralysis. *Am J Med* 1989; **86:** 729–30.
2. Russell JA, Powles RL. Neuropathy due to cytosine arabinoside. *BMJ* 1974; **4:** 652–3.
3. Malapert D, Degos JD. Jambes douloureuses et orteils instables: neuropathie induite par la cytarabine. *Rev Neurol (Paris)* 1989; **145:** 869–71.
4. Openshaw H, *et al.* Acute polyneuropathy after high dose cytosine arabinoside in patients with leukemia. *Cancer* 1996; **78:** 1899–1905.
5. Lazarus HM, *et al.* Central nervous system toxicity of high-dose systemic cytosine arabinoside. *Cancer* 1981; **48:** 2577–82.
6. Graves T, Hooks MA. Drug-induced toxicities associated with high-dose cytosine arabinoside infusions. *Pharmacotherapy* 1989; **9:** 23–8.
7. Barnett MJ, *et al.* Neurotoxicity of high-dose cytosine arabinoside. *Prog Exp Tumor Res* 1985; **29:** 177–82.
8. Dworkin LA, *et al.* Cerebellar toxicity following high-dose cytosine arabinoside. *J Clin Oncol* 1985; **3:** 613–16.
9. Fort JA, Smith LD. Pseudotumor cerebri secondary to intermediate-dose cytarabine HCl. *Ann Pharmacother* 1999; **33:** 576–8.

**Effects on the skin.** A syndrome of pain and erythema of the palms and soles, progressing to bullae and desquamation, has been seen in patients receiving intermediate- or high-dose cytarabine.[1-3] The syndrome is similar to the palmar-plantar erythrodysesthesia syndrome (p.495) reported in patients receiving chemotherapy not including cytarabine,[4] although some considered the two forms of toxicity distinct.[5] Cutaneous small vessel necrotising vasculitis has been reported after high-dose therapy with cytarabine.[6]

1. Baer MR, *et al.* Palmar-plantar erythrodysesthesia and cytarabine. *Ann Intern Med* 1985; **102:** 556.
2. Peters WG, Willemze R. Palmar-plantar skin changes and cytarabine. *Ann Intern Med* 1985; **103:** 805.
3. Calista D, Landi C. Cytarabine-induced acral erythema: a localized form of toxic epidermal necrolysis? *J Eur Acad Dermatol Venereol* 1998; **10:** 274–5.
4. Lokich JJ, Moore C. Chemotherapy-associated palmar-plantar erythrodysesthesia syndrome. *Ann Intern Med* 1984; **101:** 798–800.
5. Vogelzang NJ, Ratain MJ. Cancer chemotherapy and skin changes. *Ann Intern Med* 1985; **103:** 303–4.
6. Ahmed I, *et al.* Cytosine arabinoside-induced vasculitis. *Mayo Clin Proc* 1998; **73:** 239–42.

**Pregnancy.** Although there has been a report of limb and ear deformities in the infant of a woman given cytarabine at the estimated time of conception and 4 to 8 weeks later,[1] no congenital abnormalities were noted in 17 infants, 5 therapeutic abortions, and one still-birth (following pre-eclamptic toxaemia) resulting from over 20 known cases in which cytarabine was given during pregnancy.[2]

1. Wagner VM, *et al.* Congenital abnormalities in baby born to cytarabine treated mother. *Lancet* 1980; **ii:** 98–9.
2. Morgenstern G. Cytarabine in pregnancy. *Lancet* 1980; **ii:** 259.

## Interactions

For a general outline of antineoplastic drug interactions, see p.498.

**Antifungals.** Cytarabine has been reported to inhibit the action of *flucytosine*—see p.400.

**Antineoplastics.** Acute pancreatitis has been reported in patients given cytarabine who had previously received *asparaginase* therapy.[1] Subclinical damage to the pancreas by asparaginase may have rendered it susceptible to cytarabine.

For a report of hepatic dysfunction in patients who had received cytarabine and *daunorubicin* see under Daunorubicin Hydrochloride, p.546.

Giving cytarabine after *fludarabine* is reported to result in a five-fold increase in intracellular cytarabine concentrations in leukaemic cells,[2] producing improved clinical response rates.

1. Altman AJ, *et al.* Acute pancreatitis in association with cytosine arabinoside therapy. *Cancer* 1982; **49:** 1384–6.
2. Avramis VI, *et al.* Pharmacokinetic and pharmacodynamic studies of fludarabine and cytosine arabinoside administered as loading boluses followed by continuous infusions after a phase I/II study in pediatric patients with relapsed leukemias. *Clin Cancer Res* 1998; **4:** 45–52.

## Pharmacokinetics

Cytarabine is not effective by mouth due to rapid deamination in the gastrointestinal tract; less than 20% of an oral dose is absorbed. After intravenous injection it disappears rapidly from the plasma with an initial half-life of about 10 minutes; the terminal elimination half-life ranges from 1 to 3 hours. It is converted by phosphorylation to an active form which is rapidly deaminated, mainly in the liver and the kidneys, to inactive 1-β-D-arabinofuranosyluracil (uracil arabinoside, ara-U). The majority of an intravenous dose is excreted in the urine within 24 hours, mostly as the inactive metabolite with about 10% as unchanged cytarabine.

There is only moderate diffusion of cytarabine across the blood-brain barrier following intravenous injection, but, because of low deaminase activity in the CSF, concentrations achieved after continuous intravenous infusion or intrathecal injection are maintained for longer in the CSF than are those in plasma, with a terminal elimination half-life of 3.5 hours. After intrathecal administration of the liposomal formulation, a terminal elimination half-life of 100 to 263 hours was seen. Cytarabine also crosses the placenta.

◊ References.


1. Slevin ML, *et al.* The pharmacokinetics of subcutaneous cytosine arabinoside in patients with acute myelogenous leukaemia. *Br J Clin Pharmacol* 1981; **12:** 507–10.
2. DeAngelis LM, *et al.* Pharmacokinetics of ara-C and ara-U in plasma and CSF after high-dose administration of cytosine arabinoside. *Cancer Chemother Pharmacol* 1992; **29:** 173–7.
3. Hamada A, *et al.* Clinical pharmacokinetics of cytarabine formulations. *Clin Pharmacokinet* 2002; **41:** 705–18.


## Uses and Administration

Cytarabine, a pyrimidine nucleoside analogue, is an antimetabolite antineoplastic which inhibits the synthesis of deoxyribonucleic acid. Its actions are specific for the S phase of the cell cycle. It also has antiviral and immunosuppressant properties. Cytarabine is one of the mainstays of the treatment of acute myeloid leukaemias, together with an anthracycline, (see p.506), and is used for the prophylaxis of meningeal leukaemia, as well as in regimens for consolidation, in patients with acute lymphoblastic leukaemia (p.506). It has also been investigated in the blast crisis of chronic myeloid leukaemia (p.507) and the myelodysplasias (p.508) (see also Administration, below). It may also be used in salvage regimens for Hodgkin's disease (p.509), as part of the complex regimens sometimes employed in aggressive intermediate- and high-grade non-Hodgkin's lymphomas (p.510), and for meningeal lymphoma.

Cytarabine is usually given by the intravenous route. Higher doses can be tolerated when given by rapid injection rather than slow infusion, because of the rapid clearance of cytarabine, but there is little evidence of clinical advantage either way. Cytarabine may be given by the intrathecal route for leukaemic or lymphomatous meningitis.

For the induction of remission in adults and children with acute leukaemias a wide variety of dosage regimens have been used: 100 mg/m$^2$ twice daily by rapid intravenous injection, or 100 mg/m$^2$ daily by continuous intravenous infusion, have often been employed. These doses are generally given for 5 to 10 days, depending on therapeutic response and toxicity. Children reportedly tolerate high doses better than adults.

For maintenance 1 to 1.5 mg/kg once or twice weekly have been given intravenously or subcutaneously; other regimens have been used.

In the treatment of refractory disease high-dose regimens have been employed, with cytarabine given in doses of up to 3 g/m$^2$ every 12 hours for up to 6 days. These doses should be given by intravenous infusion over at least 1 hour.

In leukaemic meningitis cytarabine has been given intrathecally, often in a dose of 10 to 30 mg/m$^2$ every 2 to 4 days; it has also been used prophylactically. A liposomal formulation is available in some countries for intrathecal administration and permits less frequent dosing because of its longer duration of action. The recommended dose for lymphomatous meningitis is 50 mg intrathecally every 2 weeks for 5 doses then every 4 weeks for 5 doses.

White cell and platelet counts should be determined regularly during treatment with cytarabine and therapy should be stopped immediately if the count falls rapidly or to low values (see also Bone-marrow Depression, p.496).

Cytarabine ocfosfate is an orally active prodrug of cytarabine under investigation in chronic myeloid leukaemia.

**Administration.** INTRATHECAL. Intrathecal administration of the liposomal formulation of cytarabine results in prolonged drug exposure when compared with intrathecal administration of the conventional formulation (see Pharmacokinetics, above). In a randomised study,[1] the liposomal formulation administered once every 2 weeks gave a higher response rate and improved Karnofsky score compared with the conventional formulation administered twice a week in patients with lymphomatous meningitis secondary to lymphoma.


1. Glantz MJ, *et al.* Randomized trial of a slow-release versus a standard formulation of cytarabine for the intrathecal treatment of lymphomatous meningitis. *J Clin Oncol* 1999; **17:** 3110–16.


LOW-DOSE THERAPY. Because of initial suggestions that low doses of cytarabine might induce differentiation and maturation of leukaemic cells, low-dose therapy (usually 5 to 10 mg/m$^2$ twice daily) has been tried in patients with myelodysplastic syndrome and acute myeloid leukaemia.[1] The UK AML14 study is examining low-dose subcutaneous cytarabine (20 mg twice daily for 10 days every 28 to 42 days, with or without gemtuzumab ozogamicin), for the non-intensive treatment of acute myeloid leukaemia or myelodysplasia in elderly patients.[2] Although complete remission may occur in about 20% of patients with myelodysplastic syndromes a similar proportion succumb to treatment-related mortality, and remissions do not appear to be particularly long-lasting. Bone-marrow suppression may be marked even at these doses.[1]


1. Aul C, Gattermann N. The role of low-dose chemotherapy in myelodysplastic syndrome. *Leuk Res* 1992; **16:** 207–15.
2. Leukaemia Research Fund. AML14: Leukaemia Research Fund Acute Myeloid Leukaemia and High Risk MDS Trial 14. Available at: http://www.aml14.bham.ac.uk/trial/AmendmentJanuary2004/Protocol%20Jan%202004.pdf (accessed 29/06/04)


**Leukoencephalopathy.** There are anecdotal reports[1-3] of marked improvement in patients with progressive multifocal leukoencephalopathy secondary to AIDS or chemotherapy-induced immunosuppression following intravenous or intrathecal cytarabine. However, a randomised multicentre study[4] has indicated that cytarabine was ineffective and has no role in this condition (see also Infections in Immunocompromised Patients, p.624). Another group[5] have suggested that even intrathecal administration may not provide adequate delivery of cytarabine to target cells, and a trial of delivering the drug directly into the brain under pressure is underway.


1. O'Riordan T, *et al.* Progressive multifocal leukoencephalopathy-remission with cytarabine. *J Infect* 1990; **20:** 51–4.
2. Portegies P, *et al.* Response to cytarabine in progressive multifocal leucoencephalopathy in AIDS. *Lancet* 1991; **337:** 680–1.
3. Nicoli F, *et al.* Efficacy of cytarabine in progressive multifocal leucoencephalopathy in AIDS. *Lancet* 1992; **339:** 306.
4. Hall CD, *et al.* Failure of cytarabine in progressive multifocal leukoencephalopathy associated with human immunodeficiency virus infection. *N Engl J Med* 1998; **338:** 1345–51.
5. Levy RM, *et al.* Convection-enhanced intraparenchymal delivery (CEID) of cytosine arabinoside (AraC) for the treatment of HIV-related progressive multifocal leukoencephalopathy (PML). *J Neurovirol* 2001; **7:** 382–5.


## Preparations

***BP 2003:*** Cytarabine Injection;
***USP 27:*** Cytarabine for Injection.

**Proprietary Preparations** (details are given in Part 3)
***Arg.:*** Aracytin; Citagenin; ***Austral.:*** Cytosar-U†; ***Austria:*** Alexan; Cytosar; ***Belg.:*** Cytosar; ***Braz.:*** Alexan†; Aracytin; Citab; Tabine; ***Canad.:*** Cytosar; DepoCyt; ***Chile:*** Alexan; Aracytin; Laracit; ***Denm.:*** Arabine; Cytosar; ***Fin.:*** Arabine; ***Fr.:*** Aracytine; Cytarbel†; ***Ger.:*** Alexan; ARA-cell; Udicil; ***Gr.:*** Aracytin; ***Hong Kong:*** Alexan; Cytosar; ***India:*** Cytarine; ***Irl.:*** Cytosar; ***Israel:*** Alexan; Cytosar; ***Ital.:*** Aracytin; Erpalfa; ***Jpn:*** Cylocide; ***Malaysia:*** Cytosar-U; ***Mex.:*** Alexan; Ifarab; Laracit; Medsara; Novutrax; Serotabir†; ***Neth.:*** Cytosar; ***Norw.:*** Cytosar; ***NZ:*** Cytosar-U†; ***Port.:*** Alexan; Citaloxan; Cytosar; ***S.Afr.:*** Alexan; Cytosar; ***Singapore:*** Alexan; Cytosar; ***Swed.:*** Alexan†; Arabine; Cytosar; ***Switz.:*** Alexan†; Cytosar; ***Thai.:*** Alexan; Cytarine; Cytosar; ***UK:*** Cytosar†; DepoCyte; ***USA:*** Cytosar-U; DepoCyt.

---

# Dacarbazine *(BAN, USAN, rINN)*

Dacarbazina; Dacarbazinum; DIC; DTIC; Imidazole Carboxamide; NSC-45388; WR-139007. 5-(3,3-Dimethyltriazeno)imidazole-4-carboxamide.

$C_6H_{10}N_6O$ = 182.2.

*CAS — 4342-03-4.*

*ATC — L01AX04.*

**Pharmacopoeias.** In *Br., Int.,* and *US.*

**BP 2003** (Dacarbazine). A colourless or pale yellow, crystalline powder. Slightly soluble in water and in alcohol. Store at 2° to 8°. Protect from light.

**USP 27** (Dacarbazine). Store in airtight containers at 2° to 8°. Protect from light.

**Incompatibility.** Dacarbazine has been reported to be incompatible with hydrocortisone sodium succinate but not with the sodium phosphate.[1] It has been reported to be incompatible with heparin,[2] although only with concentrated dacarbazine solutions (25 mg/mL).


1. Dorr RT. Incompatibilities with parenteral anticancer drugs. *Am J Intravenous Ther* 1979; **6:** 42–52.
2. Nelson RW, *et al.* Visual incompatibility of dacarbazine and heparin. *Am J Hosp Pharm* 1987; **44:** 2028.


**Stability.** References to the photodegradation of dacarbazine solution.[1-4] Dacarbazine is more sensitive to direct sunlight than to artificial lighting or diffuse daylight.


1. Stevens MFG, Peatey L. Photodegradation of solutions of the antitumour drug DTIC. *J Pharm Pharmacol* 1978; **30** (suppl): 47P.
2. Horton JK, Stevens MFG. Search for drug interactions between the antitumour agent DTIC and other cytotoxic agents. *J Pharm Pharmacol* 1979; **31** (suppl): 64P.
3. Kirk B. The evaluation of a light-protecting giving set. *Intensive Therapy Clin Monit* 1987; **8:** 78–86.
4. El Aatmani M, *et al.* Stability of dacarbazine in amber glass vials and polyvinyl chloride bags. *Am J Health-Syst Pharm* 2002; **59:** 1351–6.


## Adverse Effects, Treatment, and Precautions

For general discussions see Antineoplastics, p.492, p.495, and p.497.

Leucopenia and thrombocytopenia with dacarbazine, although usually moderate, may be severe. The nadir of the white cell count usually occurs 21 to 25 days after a dose. Anorexia, nausea, and vomiting occur in more than 90% of patients initially but tolerance may develop after repeated doses. Less frequent adverse effects include diarrhoea, skin reactions, alopecia, a flu-like syndrome, facial flushing and paraesthesia, headache, blurred vision, seizures, and rare but potentially fatal hepatotoxicity. There may be local pain at the injection site; extravasation produces pain and tissue damage. Anaphylaxis has occurred occasionally.

Dacarbazine should be used with caution in hepatic and renal impairment, and consideration given to reducing the dose. Haematological monitoring is required during therapy. Dacarbazine is potentially carcinogenic, mutagenic, and teratogenic.

**Effects on the liver.** Dacarbazine has been associated with fatal hepatic vascular toxicity, caused by thrombosis of the hepatic veins, necrosis, and extensive haemorrhage.[1] As the reaction usually occurs during the second course of dacarbazine it is thought to be immune mediated, and early corticosteroid treatment has been tried with a few reported cases of patient survival.[2] Other adverse hepatic effects have included[3] necrosis without inflammation, granulomatous hepatitis, and acute toxic hepatitis during the first course of dacarbazine. Morphological studies have suggested that dacarbazine may exert a toxic effect on the microfilamentous cytoskeleton of the hepatocytes.[3]


1. Ceci G, *et al.* Fatal hepatic vascular toxicity of DTIC: is it really a rare event? *Cancer* 1988; **61:** 1988–91.
2. Herishanu Y, *et al.* The role of glucocorticoids in the treatment of fulminant hepatitis induced by dacarbazine. *Anticancer Drugs* 2002; **13:** 177–9.
3. Dancygier H, *et al.* Dacarbazine (DTIC)-induced human liver injury. *Gut* 1982; **23:** A447.


**Handling.** Dacarbazine is irritant; avoid contact with skin and mucous membranes.

## Interactions

For a general outline of antineoplastic drug interactions, see p.498.

**Levodopa.** For a report of dacarbazine reducing the effects of levodopa, see Antineoplastics, p.1208.

## Pharmacokinetics

Dacarbazine is poorly absorbed from the gastrointestinal tract. On intravenous injection it is rapidly distributed with an initial plasma half-life of about 20 minutes; the terminal half-life is reported to be about 5 hours. The volume of distribution is larger than body water content, suggesting localisation in some body tissues, probably mainly the liver. Only about 5% is bound to plasma protein. It crosses the blood-brain barrier to a limited extent with concentrations in CSF about 14% of those in plasma. Dacarbazine is extensively metabolised in the liver by the cytochrome P450 isoenzyme system to its active metabolite 5-(3-methyl-1-triazeno)imidazole-4-carboxamide (MTIC), which spontaneously decomposes to the major metabolite 5-aminoimidazole-4-carboxamide (AIC). About half of a dose is excreted unchanged in the urine by tubular secretion.

## Uses and Administration

Dacarbazine is a cell-cycle non-specific antineoplastic that is thought to function as an alkylating agent after it has been activated in the liver. Dacarbazine is used mainly in the treatment of metastatic malignant melanoma (p.522). It is also given to patients with Hodgkin's disease (p.509), notably with doxorubicin, bleomycin, and vinblastine (ABVD), and may be given in neuroblastoma (p.524), and in the treatment of soft-tissue sarcoma (p.525), Kaposi's sarcoma (p.524), and other tumours.

Dacarbazine is given by the intravenous route. Injections may be given over one to two minutes. The reconstituted solution can be further diluted with up to 300 mL of glucose 5% or sodium chloride 0.9% and given by infusion over 15 to 30 minutes.

Dacarbazine is licensed for use as a single agent for metastatic melanoma in doses of 2 to 4.5 mg/kg daily for 10 days, repeated at intervals of 4 weeks, or 200 to 250 mg/m$^2$ daily for 5 days, repeated at intervals of 3 weeks. It can also be given in a dose of 850 mg/m$^2$ by intravenous infusion at 3-week intervals. In the treatment of Hodgkin's disease doses of 150 mg/m$^2$ daily for 5 days repeated every 4 weeks, or 375 mg/m$^2$ every 15 days have been given with other agents.

### Preparations

**BP 2003:** Dacarbazine Injection;
**USP 27:** Dacarbazine for Injection.

**Proprietary Preparations** (details are given in Part 3)
**Arg.:** Deticene; Oncocarbil; **Austral.:** DTIC; **Austria:** DTIC-Dome; **Belg.:** DTIC-Dome†; **Braz.:** Dacarb; Dacarbaziba†; **Canad.:** DTIC; **Fin.:** Dacatic; **Fr.:** Deticene; **Ger.:** Detimedac; DTIC†; **Gr.:** Deticene; **Hong Kong:** Deticene†; **India:** DTIC; **Irl.:** DTIC-Dome†; **Israel:** Deticene; **Ital.:** Deticene; **Malaysia:** DTI; **Mex.:** Asercit†; Deticene; Detilem; Ifadac; **Neth.:** Deticene; **NZ:** DTIC-Dome; **Port.:** Deticene; Fauldetic; **S.Afr.:** DTIC-Dome; **Spain:** DTIC-Dome†; **Swed.:** DTIC; **Switz.:** DTIC; **UK:** DTIC-Dome; **USA:** DTIC-Dome.

## Dactinomycin *(BAN, USAN, rINN)*

Actinomycin $C_1$; Actinomycin D; Dactinomicina; Meractinomycin; NSC-3053. $N^{2.1},N^{2'.1'}$-(2-Amino-4,6-dimethyl-3-oxo-3*H*-phenoxazine-1,9-diyldicarbonyl)bis[threonyl-D-valylprolyl(*N*-methylglycyl)(*N*-methylvaline) 1.5–3.1-lactone].

$C_{62}H_{86}N_{12}O_{16}$ = 1255.4.

*CAS — 50-76-0.*

*ATC — L01DA01.*

**Description.** Dactinomycin is an antineoplastic antibiotic produced by *Streptomyces parvulus* and other species of *Streptomyces*.

Cactinomycin (actinomycin C; HBF-386; NSC-18268) is a mixture of dactinomycin (actinomycin D) (10%), actinomycin $C_2$ (45%), and actinomycin $C_3$ (45%) produced by *Streptomyces chrysomallus*.

**Pharmacopoeias.** In *Chin., Int., Jpn, Pol.,* and *US.*

**USP 27** (Dactinomycin). A bright red, somewhat hygroscopic, crystalline powder, affected by light and heat. It has a potency of not less than 950 and not more than 1030 micrograms/mg, calculated on the dried basis. Soluble in water at 10° and slightly soluble in water at 37°; freely soluble in alcohol; very slightly soluble in ether. Store at a temperature not exceeding 40° in airtight containers. Protect from light.

**Adsorption.** Dactinomycin binds to cellulose ester filters,[1] and such filtration should be avoided.[2] Although it has been suggested that significant amounts of drug may be adsorbed to glass or plastic,[3] dactinomycin is reportedly compatible with glass and PVC infusion containers,[4] and administration into the tubing of a fast-running intravenous infusion is recommended—see Uses and Administration, below.

1. Kanke M, *et al.* Binding of selected drugs to a "treated" inline filter. *Am J Hosp Pharm* 1983; **40:** 1323–8.
2. D'Arcy PF. Reactions and interactions in handling anticancer drugs. *Drug Intell Clin Pharm* 1983; **17:** 532–8.
3. Rapp RP, *et al.* Guidelines for the administration of commonly-used intravenous drugs—1984 update. *Drug Intell Clin Pharm* 1984; **18:** 218–32.
4. Benvenuto JA, *et al.* Stability and compatibility of antitumor agents in glass and plastic containers. *Am J Hosp Pharm* 1981; **38:** 1914–18.

### Adverse Effects, Treatment, and Precautions

For general discussions see Antineoplastics, p.492, p.495, and p.497.

Apart from nausea and vomiting adverse effects are often delayed, beginning 2 to 4 days after the completion of a course of treatment and reaching a maximum after 1 to 2 weeks. Fatalities have occurred. Bone-marrow depression and gastrointestinal effects (particularly stomatitis and diarrhoea) may prove dose-limiting. Bone-marrow depression is apparent 1 to 7 days after therapy and may be manifest first as thrombocytopenia; the nadir of the platelet and white cell counts usually occurs within 14 to 21 days, with recovery in 21 to 25 days. Other adverse effects include oral and gastrointestinal effects such as cheilitis, oesophagitis, gastrointestinal ulceration, and proctitis; fever, malaise, hypocalcaemia, erythema, myalgia, alopecia, pneumonitis, and kidney and liver abnormalities. Anaphylactoid reactions have occurred. Dactinomycin is very irritant and extravasation results in severe tissue damage.

The effects of radiotherapy are enhanced by dactinomycin and severe reactions may follow the concomitant use of high doses. Erythema and pigmentation of the skin may occur in areas previously irradiated. An increase in incidence of second primary tumours has been seen in patients treated with radiation and dactinomycin.

Dactinomycin should not be given to patients with varicella or herpes zoster, as severe and even fatal systemic disease may occur. Its use is best avoided in infants under 1 year as they are reported to be highly susceptible to the toxicity of dactinomycin. Blood counts and renal and hepatic function should be monitored frequently.

**Effects on the liver.** Although doses below about 50 micrograms/kg or 1.5 mg/m$^2$ do not seem to be associated with an unacceptable degree of hepatotoxicity,[1] giving dactinomycin as a single dose of 60 micrograms/kg (about 1.8 mg/m$^2$) every 3 weeks to children with Wilms' tumour was associated with a high incidence of severe hepatotoxicity;[2] reduction of the dose to 45 micrograms/kg every 3 weeks reduced this incidence to levels comparable with a standard regimen of 15 micrograms/kg daily for 5 successive days.[3] Others have not seen such a high incidence of hepatotoxicity with doses of 60 micrograms/kg (despite some raised liver enzyme values), but in this case the high dose was given only every 6 weeks.[4] In general, dactinomycin should be given with caution to children with a history of antecedent liver damage, including abdominal irradiation or recent halothane anaesthesia.[1]

Reversible veno-occlusive disease in particular has been found in children with Wilms' tumour who have received dactinomycin and vincristine. One study[5] found age of less than 1 year to be a risk factor. A literature review[6] noted a significant predominance of veno-occlusive disease in right-sided Wilms' tumour, possibly because the tumour mass could interfere with blood flow in the hepatic veins, which might make the liver more susceptible to the effects of dactinomycin.

1. Pritchard J, *et al.* Hepatotoxicity of actinomycin-D. *Lancet* 1989; **i:** 168.
2. D'Angio GJ. Hepatotoxicity with actinomycin D. *Lancet* 1987; **ii:** 104.
3. D'Angio GJ. Hepatotoxicity and actinomycin D. *Lancet* 1990; **335:** 1290.
4. de Camargo B. Hepatotoxicity and actinomycin D. *Lancet* 1990; **335:** 1290.
5. Bisogno G, *et al.* Veno-occlusive disease of the liver in children treated for Wilms tumor. *Med Pediatr Oncol* 1997; **29:** 245–51.
6. Tornesello A, *et al.* Veno-occlusive disease of the liver in right-sided Wilms' tumours. *Eur J Cancer* 1998; **34:** 1220–3.

**Handling.** Dactinomycin is irritant; avoid contact with skin and mucous membranes.

### Interactions

For a general outline of antineoplastic drug interactions, see p.498.

### Pharmacokinetics

Intravenous doses of dactinomycin are rapidly distributed with high concentrations in bone marrow and nucleated cells. It undergoes only minimal metabolism and is slowly excreted in urine and bile. The terminal plasma half-life is reported to be about 36 hours. It does not cross the blood-brain barrier but is thought to cross the placenta.

### Uses and Administration

Dactinomycin is a highly toxic antibiotic with antineoplastic properties. It inhibits the proliferation of cells in a cell-cycle non-specific way by forming a stable complex with DNA and interfering with DNA-dependent RNA synthesis. It may enhance the cytotoxic effects of radiotherapy (see also Adverse Effects, above). Dactinomycin also has immunosuppressant properties.

It has been used, usually with other drugs or radiotherapy, in the treatment of Wilms' tumour (p.518), gestational trophoblastic tumours (p.505), nonseminomatous testicular cancer (p.523), and sarcomas such as rhabdomyosarcoma (p.525) and Ewing's sarcoma (p.524).

In the treatment of Wilms' tumour, childhood rhabdomyosarcoma, or Ewing's sarcoma, a dose of 15 micrograms/kg daily for 5 days has been used in combination regimens. In adults, gestational trophoblastic tumours have been treated with 12 micrograms/kg daily for 5 days as a single agent, or 500 micrograms on days 1 and 2 of combination regimens. Metastatic nonseminomatous testicular cancer has been treated with 1 mg/m$^2$ on day 1 of combination regimens. The dose intensity for adults or children should not exceed 15 micrograms/kg or 400 to 600 micrograms/m$^2$ daily for 5 days per 2-week cycle, and lower doses may need to be used in some chemotherapy combinations or with radiotherapy. Localised administration using a regional perfusion technique has permitted the use of higher doses, 50 micrograms/kg being suggested for an isolated lower extremity or pelvis and 35 micrograms/kg for an upper extremity.

Great care must be taken to avoid extravasation and administration should, for preference, be into the tubing of a fast-running intravenous infusion. Platelet and white cell counts should be performed frequently to detect bone-marrow depression; if either count shows a marked decrease the drug should be withheld until recovery occurs, which may take up to 3 weeks (see also Bone-marrow Depression, p.496).

### Preparations

**USP 27:** Dactinomycin for Injection.

**Proprietary Preparations** (details are given in Part 3)
**Arg.:** Cosmegen; **Austral.:** Cosmegen; **Austria:** Cosmegen; **Belg.:** Lyovac Cosmegen; **Braz.:** Bioact-D†; Cosmegen; **Canad.:** Cosmegen; **Fin.:** Cosmegen; **Ger.:** Lyovac Cosmegen; **Gr.:** Cosmegen; **Hong Kong:** Cosmegen; **India:** Dacmozen; **Irl.:** Cosmegen; **Ital.:** Cosmegen; **Malaysia:** Cosmegen; **Mex.:** Ac-De; **Neth.:** Lyovac Cosmegen; **Norw.:** Cosmegen; **NZ:** Cosmegen; **S.Afr.:** Cosmegen†; **Swed.:** Cosmegen; **Switz.:** Cosmegen; **Thai.:** Cosmegen; **UK:** Cosmegen; **USA:** Cosmegen.

## Daunorubicin Hydrochloride

*(BANM, USAN, rINNM)*

Cloridrato de Daunorrubicina; Daunomycin Hydrochloride; Daunorubicini Hydrochloridum; FI-6339 (daunorubicin); Hidrocloruro de daunorubicina; NDC-0082-4155; NSC-82151; RP-13057 (daunorubicin); Rubidomycin Hydrochloride. (1*S*,3*S*)-3-Acetyl-1,2,3,4,6,11-hexahydro-3,5,12-trihydroxy-10-methoxy-6,11-dioxonaphthacen-1-yl 3-amino-2,3,6-trideoxy-α-L-*lyxo*-pyranoside hydrochloride; (8*S*-*cis*)-8-Acetyl-10-[(3-amino-2,3,6-trideoxy-α-L-*lyxo*-hexopyranosyl)]oxy-7,8,9,10-tetrahydro-6,8,-11-trihydroxy-1-methoxy-5,12-naphthacenedione hydrochloride.

$C_{27}H_{29}NO_{10}$,HCl = 564.0.

*CAS — 20830-81-3 (daunorubicin); 23541-50-6 (daunorubicin hydrochloride).*

*ATC — L01DB02.*

NOTE. Daunorubicin citrate is used in the preparation of liposomal preparations (see Uses and Administration, below).

**Pharmacopoeias.** In *Eur.* (see p.vi), *Jpn,* and *US.*

**Ph. Eur. 5.0** (Daunorubicin Hydrochloride). The hydrochloride of a substance produced by certain strains of *Streptomyces coeruleorubidus* or *S. peucetius* or obtained by any other means. It is manufactured by methods designed to minimise or eliminate the presence of histamine. An orange-red, hygroscopic, crystalline powder. It contains between 95 and 102% of the hydrochloride (anhydrous and solvent-free basis). Freely soluble in water and in methyl alcohol; slightly soluble in alcohol; practically insoluble in acetone. A 0.5% solution in water has a pH of 4.5 to 6.5. Store in airtight containers. Protect from light.

**USP 27** (Daunorubicin Hydrochloride). An orange-red, hygroscopic, crystalline powder. It has a potency equivalent to not less than 842 and not more than 1030 micrograms of the base per mg. Freely soluble in water and in methyl alcohol; slightly soluble in alcohol; practically insoluble in acetone; very slightly soluble in chloroform. A 0.5% solution in water has a pH of 4.5 to 6.5. Store at a temperature not exceeding 40° in airtight containers. Protect from light.

**Incompatibility.** Daunorubicin is incompatible with heparin sodium,[1] and has also been reported to be incompatible with a solution of dexamethasone sodium phosphate.

1. D'Arcy PF. Reactions and interactions in handling anticancer drugs. *Drug Intell Clin Pharm* 1983; **17:** 532–8.

**Stability.** In a study[1] of the stability of anthracycline antineoplastic agents in 4 infusion fluids (glucose 5%, sodium chloride 0.9%, lactated Ringer's injection, and a commercial infusion fluid) daunorubicin hydrochloride was stable in all 4, the percentage remaining after 24 hours being 98.5%, 97.4%, 94.7%, and 95.4% respectively. Stability appeared to be partly related to pH; daunorubicin was more stable as the pH of the mixture became more acidic, with the best stability in glucose 5% with a pH of 4.5. Although daunorubicin solutions are degraded by light, the effect is reported not to be significant at concentrations of 500 micrograms/mL or above; however, below this concentration precautions should be taken to protect solutions from light, and storage should be in polyethylene or polypropylene containers to minimise adsorptive losses.[2] It has been suggested that formulation with the food colouring Scarlet GN, which absorbs light over the same spectral region as daunorubicin, would stabilise daunorubicin solutions to light.[3]

Liposomal daunorubicin should be diluted with glucose 5% solution as aggregation of the liposomes may result with sodium chloride. In addition, the manufacturers advise that liposomal daunorubicin not be mixed with substances containing benzyl alcohol or other detergent-like molecules, which can lead to premature rupture of the liposomes.

1. Poochikian GK, *et al.* Stability of anthracycline antitumor agents in four infusion fluids. *Am J Hosp Pharm* 1981; **38:** 483–6.
2. Wood MJ, *et al.* Photodegradation of doxorubicin, daunorubicin and epirubicin measured by high-performance liquid chromatography. *J Clin Pharm Ther* 1990; **15:** 291–300.
3. Thoma K, Klimek R. Photostabilization of drugs in dosage forms without protection from packaging materials. *Int J Pharmaceutics* 1991; **67:** 169–75.

## Adverse Effects, Treatment, and Precautions

As for Doxorubicin Hydrochloride, p.548 and p.548.

Cardiotoxicity is more likely when the total cumulative dose of daunorubicin exceeds 550 mg/m$^2$ in adults, 300 mg/m$^2$ in children, or in children aged under 2 years, 10 mg/kg. The manufacturers of liposomal daunorubicin recommend determining ventricular ejection fraction after cumulative doses of 320 mg/m$^2$, and every 160 mg/m$^2$ thereafter. Daunorubicin should be used in reduced doses in hepatic and renal impairment.

*Liposomal formulations* of daunorubicin may be associated with a reduced potential for local tissue necrosis although current clinical experience is limited and such toxicity remains a possibility. An acute syndrome of back pain, flushing, and chest tightness may occur during infusion, but generally resolves on slowing or temporarily discontinuing the infusion.

**Effects on the heart.** For a discussion of the cardiotoxicity of anthracyclines, and its management, see Effects on the Heart, under Doxorubicin Hydrochloride, p.548.

**Effects on the skin and nails.** For reports of hyperpigmentation in patients given daunorubicin, see under Doxorubicin Hydrochloride, p.548.

**Handling and disposal.** Daunorubicin hydrochloride is irritant; avoid contact with skin and mucous membranes.

For a method for the destruction of daunorubicin in wastes see under Doxorubicin Hydrochloride, p.549.

## Interactions

As for Doxorubicin Hydrochloride, p.549.

**Antineoplastics.** Hepatic dysfunction was reported[1] in 13 patients who had received daunorubicin 180 to 450 mg/m$^2$. Ten of them had also received *tioguanine* or *cytarabine*, or a combination of these. The authors also noted that other studies had suggested that the related drug doxorubicin might enhance the hepatotoxicity of *mercaptopurine*, and thought that a similar interaction could occur between daunorubicin and tioguanine.

1. Penta JS, *et al.* Hepatotoxicity of combination chemotherapy for acute myelocytic leukemia. *Ann Intern Med* 1977; **87:** 247–8.

## Pharmacokinetics

After intravenous injection, daunorubicin is rapidly distributed into body tissues, particularly the liver, lungs, kidneys, spleen, and heart with an initial distribution half-life of about 45 minutes. It is rapidly metabolised in the liver, and is excreted in bile and urine as unchanged drug and metabolites. The major metabolite, daunorubicinol, has antineoplastic activity. Up to 25% of a dose is excreted in urine in an active form over several days (the terminal plasma elimination half-lives of daunorubicin and its major metabolite are reported to be 18.5 and 26.7 hours respectively); an estimated 40% is excreted in bile. Daunorubicin does not appear to cross the blood-brain barrier, but crosses the placenta.

The pharmacokinetics of liposomal doxorubicin are significantly different from those of the conventional drug formulation, with a decreased uptake by normal tissues (although tumour neovasculature is reported to have increased permeability to the liposomes), and a terminal half-life of 4 to 5 hours.

## Uses and Administration

Daunorubicin is an antineoplastic anthracycline antibiotic with actions similar to those of doxorubicin (p.549), to which it is closely related. It is used with other antineoplastics to induce remissions in acute leukaemias. Daunorubicin is given in combination regimens for acute lymphoblastic leukaemia (see p.506) and acute myeloid leukaemias (see p.506). It has also been tried in some other malignancies. A liposomal formulation of daunorubicin has been developed for use in the management of Kaposi's sarcoma in patients with AIDS (see also p.524).

Daunorubicin is usually given as the hydrochloride, but doses are expressed in terms of the base. Daunorubicin hydrochloride 21.4 mg is approximately equivalent to 20 mg daunorubicin.

In combination treatment regimens for adult acute leukaemia, the usual dose is 30 to 45 mg/m$^2$ daily on days 1 to 3 of the first course, and days 1 and 2 of subsequent courses. Daunorubicin is given as a solution in sodium chloride 0.9% into a fast-running infusion of sodium chloride or glucose. Courses may be repeated after 3 to 6 weeks. A dose of 25 mg/m$^2$ has been given intravenously once a week, in combination regimens, to children with acute lymphoblastic leukaemia. For children less than 2 years of age, or less than 0.5 m$^2$, a dose of 1 mg/kg has been used instead.

The total cumulative dose in adults should not exceed 550 mg/m$^2$; in patients who have received radiotherapy to the chest it may be advisable to limit the total dose to about 400 mg/m$^2$. Lower limits apply in children: a total cumulative dose of no more than 300 mg/m$^2$, or in children aged under 2 years 10 mg/kg, is recommended. Dosage should be reduced in patients with impaired hepatic or renal function (see below), and elderly patients with inadequate bone marrow reserves.

In the treatment of Kaposi's sarcoma, liposomal daunorubicin is given intravenously every 2 weeks starting with a dose of 40 mg/m$^2$, and continued for as long as disease control can be maintained. It is diluted with glucose 5% (sodium chloride 0.9% should not be used) to a concentration between 0.2 and 1 mg/mL, and given over 30 to 60 minutes.

Blood counts should be determined frequently during treatment as daunorubicin has a potent effect on bone-marrow function (see also Bone-marrow Depression, p.496). Cardiac function should be monitored at regular intervals to detect signs of cardiotoxicity.

**Administration in hepatic impairment.** Doses of daunorubicin should be reduced in hepatic impairment. Some manufacturers recommend that patients with serum-bilirubin concentrations of 12 to 30 micrograms/mL should receive 75% of the usual dose, and those with concentrations greater than 30 micrograms/mL should be given 50% of the usual dose.

**Administration in renal impairment.** Doses of daunorubicin should be reduced in renal impairment. Some manufacturers recommend that patients with serum-creatinine concentrations of 105 to 265 micromoles/litre should receive 75% of the usual dose, and those with concentrations greater than 265 micromoles/litre should be given 50% of the usual dose.

## Preparations

*USP 27:* Daunorubicin Hydrochloride for Injection.

**Proprietary Preparations** (details are given in Part 3)
***Arg.:*** Daunoblastina; Maxidauno; ***Austral.:*** DaunoXome; ***Austria:*** Daunoblastin; DaunoXome; ***Belg.:*** Cerubidine; DaunoXome†; ***Braz.:*** Daunoblastina; Daunocin; DaunoXome†; ***Canad.:*** Cerubidine; ***Chile:*** Daurocina; ***Denm.:*** Cerubidin; DaunoXome; ***Fin.:*** DaunoXome; ***Fr.:*** Cerubidine; DaunoXome; ***Ger.:*** Daunoblastin; DaunoXome; ***Gr.:*** DaunoXome; ***Hong Kong:*** Daunoblastina; ***Irl.:*** Cerubidin; DaunoXome; ***Israel:*** Cerubidine; ***Ital.:*** Daunoblastina; DaunoXome; ***Mex.:*** Rubilem; ***Neth.:*** Cerubidine; DaunoXome; ***Norw.:*** Cerubidin; ***NZ:*** Cerubidine†; ***Port.:*** Daunoblastina; ***S.Afr.:*** Cerubidin; Daunoblastin; ***Singapore:*** Daunoblastina; ***Spain:*** Daunoblastina; DaunoXome; ***Swed.:*** Cerubidin; DaunoXome; ***Switz.:*** Cerubidine; DaunoXome; ***UK:*** Cerubidin†; DaunoXome; ***USA:*** Cerubidine; DaunoXome.

# Decitabine *(BAN, USAN, rINN)*

5-Aza-2′-deoxycytidine; DAC; Decitabina; NSC-127716. 4-Amino-1-(2-deoxy-β-D-*erythro*-pentofuranosyl)-1,3,5-triazin-2(1*H*)-one.

$C_8H_{12}N_4O_4$ = 228.2.
*CAS — 2353-33-5.*

## Profile

Decitabine is an antineoplastic antimetabolite structurally related to cytarabine (p.543). It is reported to cause DNA hypomethylation by the inhibition of DNA methyltransferase, which has the potential to alter gene expression (re-activate silent genes) and limit disease progression and resistance. It is under investigation in the treatment of myelodysplastic syndromes (p.508), chronic myeloid leukaemia (p.507), and some solid tumours. It is also reported to increase fetal haemoglobin in patients with sickle-cell disease (p.734).

◊ References.

1. Momparler RL, *et al.* Pilot phase I-II study on 5-aza-2′-deoxycytidine (decitabine) in patients with metastatic lung cancer. *Anticancer Drugs* 1997; **8:** 358–68.
2. Kantarjian HM, *et al.* Results of decitabine therapy in the accelerated and blastic phases of chronic myelogenous leukemia. *Leukemia* 1997; **11:** 1617–20.
3. Sacchi S, *et al.* Chronic myelogenous leukemia in nonlymphoid blastic phase: analysis of the results of first salvage therapy with three different treatment approaches for 162 patients. *Cancer* 1999; **86:** 2632–41.
4. Wijermans P, *et al.* Low-dose 5-aza-2′-deoxycytidine, a DNA hypomethylating agent, for the treatment of high-risk myelodysplastic syndrome: a multicenter phase II study in elderly patients. *J Clin Oncol* 2000; **18:** 956–62.
5. Koshy M, *et al.* 2-Deoxy 5-azacytidine and fetal hemoglobin induction in sickle cell anemia. *Blood* 2000; **96:** 2379–84.
6. Lübbert M, *et al.* Cytogenetic responses in high-risk myelodysplastic syndrome following low-dose treatment with the DNA methylation inhibitor 5-aza-2′-deoxycytidine. *Br J Haematol* 2001; **114:** 349–57.
7. DeSimone J, *et al.* Maintenance of elevated fetal hemoglobin levels by decitabine during dose interval treatment of sickle cell anemia. *Blood* 2002; **99:** 3905–8.
8. Kantarjian HM, *et al.* Results of decitabine (5-aza-2′deoxycytidine) therapy in 130 patients with chronic myelogenous leukemia. *Cancer* 2003; **98:** 522–8.
9. Issa JP, *et al.* Phase 1 study of low-dose prolonged exposure schedules of the hypomethylating agent 5-aza-2′-deoxycytidine (decitabine) in hematopoietic malignancies. *Blood* 2004; **103:** 1635–40.

# Denileukin Diftitox *(USAN, rINN)*

$DAB_{389}IL2$; Denileucina diftitox; Denileukin Difitox *(BAN)*; LY-335348.
*CAS — 173146-27-5.*
*ATC — L01XX29.*

## Adverse Effects and Precautions

Denileukin diftitox can cause an acute hypersensitivity reaction within 24 hours of infusion with symptoms reminiscent of a cytokine release syndrome. Anaphylaxis and death have also been reported. A more delayed flu-like syndrome may also occur up to several days after infusion. Vascular leak syndrome, characterised by hypotension, oedema, or hypoalbuminaemia, may also be delayed. Gastrointestinal disturbances, chills, fever, and asthenia are common. Other adverse effects include rash, predisposition to cutaneous infections, and thrombotic events.

## Uses and Administration

Denileukin diftitox is a recombinant interleukin fusion toxin comprised of interleukin-2 linked to the A and B fragments of diphtheria toxin. It is given by intravenous infusion for the management of persistent or recurrent cutaneous T-cell lymphoma (see Mycosis Fungoides, p.511), in patients whose malignant cells express the CD25 interleukin-2 receptor. The concentration of denileukin diftitox must be at least 15 micrograms/mL during all steps in the preparation of the solution for infusion. The recommended dose is 9 or 18 micrograms/kg daily, given over 15 minutes or more, for 5 consecutive days every 3 weeks.

◊ References.

1. Olsen E, *et al.* Pivotal phase III trial of two dose levels of denileukin diftitox for the treatment of cutaneous T-cell lymphoma. *J Clin Oncol* 2001; **19:** 376–88.
2. Martin A, *et al.* A multicenter dose-escalation trial with denileukin diftitox (ONTAK, DAB(389)IL-2) in patients with severe psoriasis. *J Am Acad Dermatol* 2001; **45:** 871–81.
3. Talpur R, *et al.* Treatment of refractory peripheral T-cell lymphoma with denileukin diftitox (ONTAK). *Leuk Lymphoma* 2002; **43:** 121–6.
4. Frankel AE, *et al.* A phase II study of DT fusion protein denileukin diftitox in patients with fludarabine-refractory chronic lymphocytic leukemia. *Clin Cancer Res* 2003; **9:** 3555–61.

## Preparations

**Proprietary Preparations** (details are given in Part 3)
***USA:*** Ontak.

# Diaziquone *(USAN, rINN)*

Aziridinylbenzoquinone; AZQ; CI-904; Diazicuona; NSC-182986. Diethyl 2,5-bis-(1-aziridinyl)-3,6-dioxo-1,4-cyclohexadiene-1,4-dicarbamate.

$C_{16}H_{20}N_4O_6$ = 364.4.
*CAS — 57998-68-2.*

## Profile

Diaziquone has been investigated as an antineoplastic in the treatment of malignant brain tumours and acute myeloid leukaemia. It is thought to act as an alkylating agent. Adverse effects include bone-marrow suppression, manifesting chiefly as leucopenia and thrombocytopenia, gastrointestinal disturbances, and alopecia. Anaphylactoid reactions have occurred.

# Didemnin B

Didemnina B; NSC-325319.

$C_{57}H_{89}N_7O_{15}$ = 1112.4.
*CAS — 77327-05-0.*

## Profile

The didemnins are biologically active peptides extracted from a marine sea squirt of the genus *Trididemnum*. They possess antineoplastic and antiviral properties; didemnin B is reported to be more active than didemnin A or didemnin C and has been investigated as an antineoplastic, although results have not generally been favourable. Nausea and vomiting are dose-limiting; myelosuppression, cardiac and renal toxicity, liver dysfunction, other gastrointestinal disturbances, myalgia, fatigue, and phlebitis may occur. Hypersensitivity reactions, possibly due to the polyethoxylated castor oil vehicle, are common.

## Docetaxel *(BAN, USAN, rINN)*

NSC-628503; RP-56976. (2*R*,3*S*)-*N*-Carboxy-3-phenylisoserine, *N*-*tert*-butyl ester, 13-ester with 5β-20-epoxy-1,2α,4,7β,10β,13α-hexahydroxytax-11-en-9-one 4-acetate 2-benzoate; *tert*-Butyl {(1*S*,2*S*)-2-[(2*S*,5*R*,7*S*,10*R*,13*S*)-4-acetoxy-2-benzoyloxy-1,7,10-trihydroxy-9-oxo-5,20-epoxytax-11-en-13-yloxycarbonyl]-2-hydroxy-1-phenylethyl}carbamate.

$C_{43}H_{53}NO_{14}$ = 807.9.

*CAS — 114977-28-5 (anhydrous docetaxel); 148408-66-6 (docetaxel trihydrate).*

*ATC — L01CD02.*

### Adverse Effects, Treatment, and Precautions

As for Paclitaxel, p.577. Anaemia and skin reactions are common and may be severe. Fluid retention, resulting in oedema, ascites, pleural and pericardial effusion, and weight gain, is also common, and may be cumulative; premedication with a corticosteroid can reduce fluid retention as well as the severity of hypersensitivity reactions.

Docetaxel should not be used in patients hypersensitive to polysorbate 80, which is contained in the formulation. Patients with hepatic impairment show increased sensitivity to toxic effects of docetaxel, and should be given the drug with great care and in reduced doses, if at all.

**Effects on the eyes.** Excessive tear formation severe enough to interfere with reading and driving has been reported in patients given docetaxel. Canalicular stenosis has been described as the mechanism for this effect, and docetaxel has been measured in tear fluid suggesting that irritation of the ocular surface and fibrosis of the tear drainage ducts may be caused by direct contact with docetaxel.[1] In a report of 36 patients receiving docetaxel-containing regimens for metastatic breast cancer, the effect developed in 14 of 18 patients receiving docetaxel weekly compared with only 2 of 18 on a 3-weekly regimen. The onset ranged from 4 to 16 weeks and the mean cumulative dose of docetaxel was found to be higher in those patients who developed stenosis.[2] Management of this adverse effect includes probing and irrigation of the lachrymal ducts and canalicular silicone tubing placement, or surgery followed by tube placement. The condition is generally reversible and tubing can be removed 4 to 6 weeks after cessation of docetaxel therapy.[3]

Very rare cases of transient visual disturbances such as flashing lights and scotomata have occurred during docetaxel infusion, and in association with hypersensitivity reactions. For reference to a report of glaucoma possibly related to docetaxel, see Paclitaxel, p.578.

1. Esmaeli B, *et al.* Docetaxel secretion in tears: association with lacrimal drainage obstruction. *Arch Ophthalmol* 2002; **120:** 1180–2.
2. Esmaeli B, *et al.* Canalicular stenosis secondary to weekly versus every-3-weeks docetaxel in patients with metastatic breast cancer. *Ophthalmology* 2002; **109:** 1188–91.
3. Ahmadi MA, Esmaeli B. Surgical treatment of canalicular stenosis in patients receiving docetaxel weekly. *Arch Ophthalmol* 2001; **119:** 1802–4.

**Effects on the gastrointestinal tract.** Ischaemic colitis has occurred in women treated with docetaxel, some of whom also received vinorelbine, which may have exacerbated this complication.[1,2]

1. Ibrahim NK, *et al.* Colitis associated with docetaxel-based chemotherapy in patients with metastatic breast cancer. *Lancet* 2000; **355:** 281–3.
2. de Matteis A, *et al.* Intestinal side-effects of docetaxel/vinorelbine combination. *Lancet* 2000; **355:** 1098–9.

**Effects on the musculoskeletal system.** For reference to a case of docetaxel-induced myalgia successfully treated with gabapentin, see Paclitaxel, p.578.

**Effects on the skin and nails.** Palmar-plantar erythrodysesthesia syndrome (p.495) has been reported with the use of docetaxel.[1] For reference to reports of adverse effects on the nails following the use of docetaxel, see Paclitaxel, p.578.

1. Eich D, *et al.* Acral erythrodysesthesia syndrome caused by intravenous infusion of docetaxel in breast cancer. *Am J Clin Oncol* 2002; **25:** 599–602.

### Interactions

For a general outline of antineoplastic drug interactions, see p.498.

◊ Docetaxel is metabolised by cytochrome P450 isoenzyme CYP3A, and theoretically has the potential to interact with other drugs that are inhibitors or inducers of this enzyme.[1]

1. Royer I, *et al.* Metabolism of docetaxel by human cytochromes P450: interactions with paclitaxel and other antineoplastic drugs. *Cancer Res* 1996; **56:** 58–65.

**Antineoplastics.** The clearance of a dose of docetaxel was markedly reduced[1] when it was given after 4 days' treatment with *topotecan*, rather than on day 1; this resulted in worsened neutropenia.

1. Zamboni WC, *et al.* Pharmacokinetic and pharmacodynamic study of the combination of docetaxel and topotecan in patients with solid tumors. *J Clin Oncol* 2000; **18:** 3288–94.

### Pharmacokinetics

On intravenous dosage docetaxel is rapidly distributed to body tissues. Docetaxel is more than 95% bound to plasma proteins. It is extensively metabolised via hepatic cytochrome P450 isoenzyme CYP3A and excreted chiefly in the faeces as metabolites. Only about 6% of a dose is excreted in urine. The terminal elimination half-life is about 11 hours. Clearance is reduced in hepatic impairment.

◊ References.

1. Bruno R, *et al.* Pharmacokinetic and pharmacodynamic properties of docetaxel: results of phase I and phase II trials. *Am J Health-Syst Pharm* 1997; **54** (suppl 2): S16–S19.
2. Clarke SJ, Rivory LP. Clinical pharmacokinetics of docetaxel. *Clin Pharmacokinet* 1999; **36:** 99–114.

### Uses and Administration

Docetaxel is a semisynthetic taxane similar to paclitaxel (see p.578). It is manufactured from a taxane precursor derived from the needles of the European yew tree *Taxus baccata*. Docetaxel is used for locally advanced or metastatic breast cancer (p.514) and non-small cell lung cancer (p.519). It may be used in hormone-refractory metastatic prostate cancer (p.521), and is being investigated in various other malignant neoplasms including the palliative treatment of cancers of the head and neck.

Docetaxel is given by intravenous infusion in glucose 5% or sodium chloride 0.9% at a concentration not exceeding 0.74 mg/mL. Infusion is normally over 1 hour. The licensed dose for docetaxel as a single agent in the treatment of breast cancer after failure of previous chemotherapy is 60 to 100 $mg/m^2$ once every 3 weeks; a dose of 75 $mg/m^2$ is given in first-line combination therapy. The dose for non-small cell lung cancer is 75 $mg/m^2$ once every 3 weeks, for both first-line combination therapy and monotherapy after failure of previous chemotherapy. Premedication with an oral corticosteroid for 3 days starting 1 day before docetaxel is recommended.

For prostate cancer, the dose of docetaxel is 75 $mg/m^2$ once every 3 weeks, with prednisone 5 mg orally twice daily given continuously. The use of prednisone reduces the need for a premedication corticosteroid, which may be given for just the 12 hours before docetaxel.

Regular blood counts are required, and dosage in subsequent courses should be reduced in patients who experience severe or febrile neutropenia (see also Bone-marrow Depression, p.496), or severe cutaneous reactions or peripheral neuropathy. The dose of docetaxel should be reduced in hepatic impairment, see below.

◊ References. For references to taxanes as a class, see Paclitaxel, p.578.

1. Anonymous. Docetaxel (Taxotere) for advanced breast cancer. *Med Lett Drugs Ther* 1996; **38:** 87–8.
2. Leahy M, Howell A. Docetaxel. *Br J Hosp Med* 1997; **57:** 141–4.
3. Tankanow RM. Docetaxel: a taxoid for the treatment of metastatic breast cancer. *Am J Health-Syst Pharm* 1998; **55:** 1777–91.
4. Figgitt DP, Wiseman LR. Docetaxel: an update of its use in advanced breast cancer. *Drugs* 2000; **59:** 621–51.
5. Shepherd FA, *et al.* Prospective randomized trial of docetaxel versus best supportive care in patients with non-small-cell lung cancer previously treated with platinum-based chemotherapy. *J Clin Oncol* 2000; **18:** 2095–2103.

**Administration.** Docetaxel has been investigated as a low-dose weekly infusion, in patient groups such as the elderly, those with poor performance status, or refractory disease.[1-3]

1. Hainsworth JD, *et al.* Weekly docetaxel in the treatment of elderly patients with advanced breast cancer: a Minnie Pearl Cancer Research Network phase II trial. *J Clin Oncol* 2001; **19:** 3500–5.
2. Mekhail T, *et al.* Phase I trial of weekly docetaxel and gemcitabine in patients with refractory malignancies. *Cancer* 2003; **97:** 170–8.
3. Petrioli R, *et al.* Weekly low-dose docetaxel in advanced non-small cell lung cancer previously treated with two chemotherapy regimens. *Lung Cancer* 2003; **39:** 85–9.

**Administration in hepatic impairment.** The UK manufacturers recommend that doses of docetaxel monotherapy should be reduced from 100 $mg/m^2$ to 75 $mg/m^2$ in moderate hepatic impairment, and hepatic function should be monitored; use should be avoided if possible in severe hepatic impairment. The US manufacturers contra-indicate the use of docetaxel in hepatic impairment.

### Preparations

**Proprietary Preparations** (details are given in Part 3)

***Arg.:*** Asodocel; Dolectran; Donataxel; Doxetal; Doxmil; Neocel; Plustaxano; Taxotere; Texot; Trazoteva; Trixotene; ***Austral.:*** Taxotere; ***Austria:*** Taxotere; ***Belg.:*** Taxotere; ***Braz.:*** Taxotere; ***Canad.:*** Taxotere; ***Denm.:*** Taxotere; ***Fin.:*** Taxotere; ***Fr.:*** Taxotere; ***Ger.:*** Taxotere; ***Gr.:*** Taxotere; ***Hong Kong:*** Taxotere; ***India:*** Daxotel; ***Irl.:*** Taxotere; ***Israel:*** Taxotere; ***Ital.:*** Taxotere; ***Jpn:*** Taxotere; ***Malaysia:*** Taxotere; ***Mex.:*** Taxotere; ***Neth.:*** Taxotere; ***Norw.:*** Taxotere; ***NZ:*** Taxotere; ***Port.:*** Taxotere; ***S.Afr.:*** Taxotere; ***Singapore:*** Taxotere; ***Spain:*** Taxotere; ***Swed.:*** Taxotere; ***Switz.:*** Taxotere; ***Thai.:*** Daxotel; Taxotere; ***UK:*** Taxotere; ***USA:*** Taxotere.

## Doxifluridine *(rINN)*

5′-Deoxy-5-fluorouridine; 5-DFUR; Doxifluridina; FUDR; Ro-21-9738.

$C_9H_{11}FN_2O_5$ = 246.2.

*CAS — 3094-09-5.*

### Profile

Doxifluridine is an antineoplastic that probably acts through its conversion in the body to fluorouracil (p.554). It is given orally in the management of malignant neoplasms of the breast (p.514) and gastrointestinal tract (p.516), and of other solid tumours, in doses of 0.8 to 1.2 g daily in divided doses. It has also been given by the intravenous route.

**Pharmacokinetics.** Doxifluridine is metabolised to fluorouracil and 5,6-dihydrofluorouracil. It is orally active with a bioavailability of 34 to 47%.

References.

1. Sommadossi J-P, *et al.* Kinetics and metabolism of a new fluoropyrimidine, 5′-deoxy-5-fluorouridine, in humans. *Cancer Res* 1983; **43:** 930–3.
2. Van Der Heyden SAM, *et al.* Pharmacokinetics and bioavailability of oral 5′-deoxy-5-fluorouridine in cancer patients. *Br J Clin Pharmacol* 1999; **47:** 351–6.

### Preparations

**Proprietary Preparations** (details are given in Part 3)

***Jpn:*** Furtulon.

## Doxorubicin *(BAN, USAN, rINN)*

Adriamycin; FI-106; 3-Hydroxyacetyldaunorubicin; 14-Hydroxydaunomycin. 8-Hydroxyacetyl (8*S*,10*S*)-10-[(3-amino-2,3,6-trideoxy-α-L-*lyxo*-hexopyranosyl)oxy]-6,8,11-trihydroxy-1-methoxy-7,8,9,10-tetrahydronaphthacene-5,12-dione.

$C_{27}H_{29}NO_{11}$ = 543.5.

*CAS — 23214-92-8.*

*ATC — L01DB01.*

NOTE. In many countries the name Adriamycin is a trademark.

## Doxorubicin Hydrochloride *(BANM, rINNM)*

Cloridrato de Doxorrubicina; Doxorubicini Hydrochloridum; Hidrocloruro de doxorubicina; NSC-123127.

$C_{27}H_{29}NO_{11}$,HCl = 580.0.

*CAS — 25316-40-9.*

*ATC — L01DB01.*

NOTE. Doxorubicin citrate complex is a constituent of some liposomal products (see Uses and Administration, below).

**Pharmacopoeias.** In *Eur.* (see p.vi), *Int., Jpn, Pol.*, and *US.*

**Ph. Eur. 5.0** (Doxorubicin Hydrochloride). The hydrochloride of a substance isolated from certain strains of *Streptomyces coeruleorubidus* or *S. peucetius* or obtained by any other means. It contains between 98 and 102% of the hydrochloride, calculated on the anhydrous substance. An orange-red, hygroscopic, crystalline powder. Soluble in water; slightly soluble in methyl alcohol. A 0.5% solution in water has a pH of 4.0 to 5.5. Store in airtight containers.

**USP 27** (Doxorubicin Hydrochloride). A red-orange, hygroscopic, crystalline powder. It contains not less than 98% and not more than 102% of $C_{27}H_{29}NO_{11}$,HCl, calculated on the anhydrous, solvent-free basis. Soluble in water, in sodium chloride 0.9%, and in methyl alcohol; practically insoluble in chloroform, in ether, and in other organic solvents. A 0.5% solution in water has a pH of 4.0 to 5.5. Store in airtight containers.

**Incompatibility.** Admixture of doxorubicin hydrochloride with cefalotin sodium, dexamethasone, diazepam, or hydrocortisone sodium succinate is reported to result in immediate precipitation;[1] similarly precipitation has occurred when doxorubicin hydrochloride was mixed with furosemide or heparin sodium.[2] A mixture of fluorouracil or aminophylline with doxorubicin hydrochloride is reported to darken in colour from red to purple, indicating degradation of doxorubicin.[1] For mention of the compatibility of doxorubicin with paclitaxel, see p.577.

Liposomal doxorubicin differs in its incompatibilities from conventional formulations: whereas the latter are reportedly incompatible with allopurinol, cefepime, and ganciclovir, there was no visual evidence of this with the liposomal formulation. However, it was incompatible with a number of drug solutions including amphotericin B, docetaxel, gallium nitrate, hydroxyzine hydrochloride, metoclopramide hydrochloride, miconazole, mitoxantrone hydrochloride, morphine sulfate and some other opioids, paclitaxel, sodium bicarbonate, and some antibacterials.[3]


1. Dorr RT. Incompatibilities with parenteral anticancer drugs. *Am J Intravenous Ther* 1979; **6:** 42–52.
2. Cohen MH, *et al.* Drug precipitation within IV tubing: a potential hazard of chemotherapy administration. *Cancer Treat Rep* 1985; **69:** 1325–6.
3. Trissel LA, *et al.* Compatibility of doxorubicin hydrochloride liposome injection with selected other drugs during simulated Y-site administration. *Am J Health-Syst Pharm* 1997; **54:** 2708–13.


**Stability.** Although sensitive to light at low concentrations, doxorubicin is not subject to significant photodegradation at clinical concentrations and special precautions to protect solutions from light during administration do not appear to be necessary.[1,2] Solutions in sodium chloride solution 0.9% were reported[3] to be stable for 24 days when stored in PVC minibags at 25° and for even longer if stored in minibags or polypropylene syringes at 4°. Stability in solution seems to be partly related to pH, with doxorubicin becoming more stable[3-5] at acid pH. A fall in pH of the solution also significantly decreases the loss of doxorubicin by adsorption and precipitation onto the surface of a positively-charged in-line filter.[6]

Some liposomal doxorubicin formulations should be diluted only with glucose 5%. If not used immediately, they may be stored for 24 hours at 2° to 8°.


1. Tavoloni N, *et al.* Photolytic degradation of adriamycin. *J Pharm Pharmacol* 1980; **32:** 860–2.
2. Wood MJ, *et al.* Photodegradation of doxorubicin, daunorubicin and epirubicin measured by high-performance liquid chromatography. *J Clin Pharm Ther* 1990; **15:** 291–300.
3. Wood MJ, *et al.* Stability of doxorubicin, daunorubicin and epirubicin in plastic syringes and minibags. *J Clin Pharm Ther* 1990; **15:** 279–89.
4. Poochikian GK, *et al.* Stability of anthracycline antitumor agents in four infusion fluids. *Am J Hosp Pharm* 1981; **38:** 483–6.
5. Beijnen JH, *et al.* Stability of anthracycline antitumour agents in infusion fluids. *J Parenter Sci Technol* 1985; **39:** 220–2.
6. Francomb MM, *et al.* Effect of pH on the adsorption of cytotoxic drugs to a 96 hour intravenous filter. *Pharm J* 1991; **247:** R26.


## Adverse Effects and Treatment

For general discussions see Antineoplastics, p.492 and p.495.

Doxorubicin and other anthracyclines cause pronounced bone-marrow depression, which may be dose-limiting. White cell count reaches a nadir 10 to 15 days after a dose and usually recovers by about 21 days.

The anthracyclines may produce cardiac toxicity, both as an acute, usually transient disturbance of cardiac function marked by ECG abnormalities and, sometimes, arrhythmias; and as a delayed, sometimes fatal, irreversible congestive heart failure, which may occur suddenly. Severe cardiotoxicity is more likely in adults receiving total cumulative doses of doxorubicin greater than 450 to 550 mg/m², and may occur months or even years after administration.

Gastrointestinal disturbances include moderate or sometimes severe nausea and vomiting; stomatitis and oesophagitis may progress to ulceration. More rarely, facial flushing, conjunctivitis, and lachrymation may occur. Alopecia occurs in the majority of patients. The urine may be coloured red. Occasional hypersensitivity reactions may occur. Hyperuricaemia may occur due to tumour lysis syndrome.

Doxorubicin and other anthracyclines are very irritant and thrombophlebitis and streaking of the skin over the vein used for injection has been reported; extravasation is serious and may produce extensive local necrosis and ulceration. Intravesical instillation can cause bladder and urethral irritation, haematuria, and haemorrhagic cystitis.

Combination therapy including doxorubicin has rarely been associated with secondary acute myeloid leukaemia (see also Carcinogenicity, p.492).

Formulations of liposomal doxorubicin may be associated with a reduced potential for local tissue necrosis, and possibly a reduced incidence of cardiotoxicity, although current clinical experience is limited, and such toxicity remains a possibility. Conversely, palmar-plantar erythrodysesthesia (p.495) appears to be more common, and may be dose-limiting. In addition, an acute pseudo-allergic reaction may be seen on initial infusion, but generally resolves on slowing or temporarily stopping the infusion.

**Effects on the heart.** Cardiotoxicity has been a major factor in limiting the use of the anthracyclines, doxorubicin and daunorubicin.[1-5] Toxicity is essentially of 2 kinds: acute, usually reversible ECG changes, including a wide range of arrhythmias, and a delayed, usually irreversible dose-related cardiomyopathy, resulting in congestive heart failure.[3-5] The latter may be further subdivided into chronic effects, occurring up to about a year after administration, and late-onset toxicity occurring years after treatment.[4] Delayed toxicity may be fatal in as many as 60% of patients who develop it.[2]

The single most important determinant of cardiac toxicity appears to be *cumulative dose*, with the risk of toxicity becoming ever greater at cumulative doxorubicin doses of 550 mg/m² or more,[2] and daunorubicin doses of 600 mg/m² or more.[1] However, patients vary widely in sensitivity,[4] and these values represent relatively arbitrary choices on a continuum of risk: there is no single safe dose.[2] Even at doses which produce no symptoms, subclinical myocardial damage may occur, and in children this may result in diminished cardiac reserve and heart disease in later life.[3,6,7] The *dosage schedule* also appears to be important; relatively high single doses on an infrequent schedule (presumably resulting in higher peak concentrations) appear to be more cardiotoxic than lower, weekly doses, or continuous infusion.[2,3,5,8-10] Cardiotoxicity is also reported to be more likely in *children and elderly* patients, and in those who have received prior *radiotherapy* to the chest.[1-5] There is reason to believe that previous *cardiovascular disease* may also increase the risk,[2-4] although such patients are commonly excluded from studies of anthracycline therapy.[2] *Females* may be at greater risk than males.[11] Use with cyclophosphamide, trastuzumab, or *other antineoplastics* with cardiotoxic potential may increase the likelihood of cardiomyopathy.

The late development of cardiac toxicity is a source of some concern: although in one study the mean time to development of symptoms was 33 days after administration, with a range of 0 to 231 days,[2] several reports have indicated that late cardiac failure may occur up to 18 years after anthracycline therapy.[4,12,13]

PREVENTION. Given that doxorubicin-induced cardiac failure has been reported to occur in between 0.4 and 9% of all recipients, and that the fatality rate is high, much effort has gone into ways of predicting and preventing anthracycline-induced cardiotoxicity. Although ECG changes are commonly monitored, most of the changes are not predictive of cardiomyopathy and severe cardiac toxicity can occur without ECG changes. However, a persistent reduction in the voltage of the QRS wave is generally indicative of the need to perform further tests. Non-invasive cardiac monitoring, by means of echocardiography or radionuclide angiography, is useful in predicting the development of cardiomyopathy, but may give normal results until damage is quite advanced; sensitivity may be improved with exercise stress tests.[3-5] Endomyocardial biopsy is the most sensitive indicator of cardiomyopathy, but it is invasive and not widely available. The Childrens Cancer Study Group[14] has issued guidelines for monitoring using ECG, echocardiography, and radionuclide angiocardiography in patients receiving anthracyclines. The role of such techniques in predicting late-onset cardiotoxicity remains to be clarified.[4] There is some preliminary evidence to suggest that concentrations of cardiac troponins and natriuretic peptides could be used as predictive markers of myocardial damage.[15]

Dexrazoxane (p.1036) has shown some protective effect against the cardiotoxicity of doxorubicin and other anthracyclines, and is used to reduce cardiomyopathy in women receiving doxorubicin for metastatic breast cancer.

Alteration of the dosage schedule to weekly rather than three-weekly dosage, or the use of continuous infusion, has also been advocated as a way of reducing doxorubicin cardiotoxicity,[8-10] as has administration of anthracyclines formulated in liposomes.[4]

Several anthracycline derivatives have been developed with the aim of reducing the inherent cardiotoxicity of this class of compounds, including aclarubicin (p.525), epirubicin (p.550), and mitoxantrone (p.575). However, although this strategy has met with some success, almost all these compounds exhibit some degree of cardiotoxicity.

TREATMENT. The result of treatment for such cardiotoxicity has generally been poor. Options have included digoxin, diuretics, low-salt diet, and bed rest. However, beta blockers may be useful, and results in patients with epirubicin-induced cardiotoxicity[16] have indicated that treatment with an ACE inhibitor can improve cardiac function and survival. Study is underway to determine whether ACE inhibitors can also prevent the initial toxicity if given immediately after an anthracycline.[17] Heart transplantation has been used.[5]


1. Von Hoff DD, *et al.* Daunomycin-induced cardiotoxicity in children and adults: a review of 110 cases. *Am J Med* 1977; **62:** 200–8.
2. Von Hoff DD, *et al.* Risk factors for doxorubicin-induced congestive heart failure. *Ann Intern Med* 1979; **91:** 710–17.
3. Hale JP, Lewis IJ. Anthracyclines: cardiotoxicity and its prevention. *Arch Dis Child* 1994; **71:** 457–62.
4. Shan K, *et al.* Anthracycline-induced cardiotoxicity. *Ann Intern Med* 1996; **125:** 47–58.
5. Singal PK, Iliskovic N. Doxorubicin-induced cardiomyopathy. *N Engl J Med* 1998; **339:** 900–905.
6. Yeung ST, *et al.* Functional myocardial impairment in children treated with anthracyclines for cancer. *Lancet* 1991; **337:** 816–18.
7. Lipschultz SE, *et al.* Late cardiac effects of doxorubicin therapy for acute lymphoblastic leukemia in childhood. *N Engl J Med* 1991; **324:** 808–15.
8. Legha SS, *et al.* Reduction of doxorubicin cardiotoxicity by prolonged continuous intravenous infusion. *Ann Intern Med* 1982; **96:** 133–9.
9. Torti FM, *et al.* Reduced cardiotoxicity of doxorubicin delivered on a weekly schedule: assessment by endomyocardial biopsy. *Ann Intern Med* 1983; **99:** 745–9.
10. Lum BL, *et al.* Doxorubicin: alteration of dose scheduling as a means of reducing cardiotoxicity. *Drug Intell Clin Pharm* 1985; **19:** 259–64.
11. Lipshultz SE, *et al.* Female sex and higher drug dose as risk factors for late cardiotoxic effects of doxorubicin therapy for childhood cancer. *N Engl J Med* 1995; **332:** 1738–43.
12. Goorin AM, *et al.* Initial congestive heart failure, six to ten years after doxorubicin chemotherapy for childhood cancer. *J Pediatr* 1990; **116:** 144–7.
13. Steinherz LJ, *et al.* Cardiac toxicity 4 to 20 years after completing anthracycline therapy. *JAMA* 1991; **266:** 1672–7.
14. Steinherz LJ, *et al.* Guidelines for cardiac monitoring of children during and after anthracycline therapy: report of the Cardiology Committee of the Childrens Cancer Study Group. *Pediatrics* 1992; **89:** 942–9.
15. Sparano JA, *et al.* Predicting cancer therapy-induced cardiotoxicity: the role of troponins and other markers. *Drug Safety* 2002; **25:** 301–11.
16. Jensen BV, *et al.* Treatment with angiotensin-converting-enzyme inhibitor for epirubicin-induced dilated cardiomyopathy. *Lancet* 1996; **347:** 297–9.
17. Jensen BV, *et al.* Angiotensin-converting enzyme inhibitor for epirubicin-induced dilated cardiomyopathy. *Lancet* 1996; **347:** 1485.


**Effects on the liver.** Hepatitis and non-specific hepatocellular damage has been reported in patients receiving doxorubicin as part of combination therapy.[1] A characteristic hepatotoxicity can also be produced by the combination of radiotherapy with doxorubicin.[2]


1. Avilés A, *et al.* Hepatic injury during doxorubicin therapy. *Arch Pathol Lab Med* 1984; **108:** 912–13.
2. Price LA. Surviving malignant disease: medical and oncological aspects. *Br J Hosp Med* 1983; **30:** 8–12.


**Effects on the skin and nails.** Hyperpigmentation has occurred in patients who have received daunorubicin, doxorubicin, or idarubicin.[1-6] Reports described pigmentation of the skin and transverse hyperpigmented bands of the nails. Effects on the skin resolved over several weeks, and bands on the nails moved with normal nail growth. Dark-skinned patients appear to be more susceptible to this adverse effect. Biopsy has found an increase in melanin granules in the affected tissues. An unusual blue-grey pigmentation of the face was reported in a patient who received doxorubicin.[7]

For specific reference to treatment of alopecia caused by doxorubicin, and for extravasation, see p.496.


1. Kelly TM, *et al.* Hyperpigmentation with daunorubicin therapy. *Arch Dermatol* 1984; **120:** 262–3.
2. Kumar L, Kochupillai V. Doxorubicin induced hyperpigmentation. *N Z Med J* 1990; **103:** 165.
3. Curran CF. Doxorubicin-associated hyperpigmentation. *N Z Med J* 1990; **103:** 517.
4. Anderson LL, *et al.* Cutaneous pigmentation after daunorubicin chemotherapy. *J Am Acad Dermatol* 1992; **26:** 255–6.
5. Borecky DJ, *et al.* Idarubicin-induced pigmentary changes of the nails. *Cutis* 1997; **59:** 203–4.
6. Kroumpouzos G, *et al.* Generalized hyperpigmentation with daunorubicin chemotherapy. *J Am Acad Dermatol* 2002; **46** (suppl): S1–S3.
7. Konohana A. Blue-gray pigmentation in a patient receiving doxorubicin. *J Dermatol* 1992; **19:** 250–2.


## Precautions

For a general discussion see Antineoplastics, p.497.

Doxorubicin and other anthracyclines are generally contra-indicated in patients with heart disease. The total cumulative dose should be limited, and cardiac function should be monitored during treatment (see Effects on the Heart, above). Blood counts should be monitored and doses should not be repeated while there is bone-marrow depression or ulceration of the mouth. Doxorubicin should be given with great care in reduced doses to patients with hepatic impairment; dosage reduction may also be necessary in children and the elderly. Extravasation results in severe tissue damage and doxorubicin and other anthracyclines should not be given by intramuscular or subcutaneous injection. The adverse effects of irradiation may be enhanced by doxorubicin and skin reactions previously induced by radiotherapy may recur; the maximum cumulative dose should be reduced to no more than 400 mg/m² in patients who have received radiotherapy to the chest or heart. Different liposomal formulations may not be interchangeable with conventional formulations, or with each other.

**Breast feeding.** Doxorubicin and its metabolites have been detected in breast milk.[1] The American Academy of Pediatrics considers[2] that doxorubicin is concentrated in breast milk, that it may possibly cause immune suppression in the infant, has unknown effects on growth, and an association with carcinogenesis.

1. Egan PC, *et al.* Doxorubicin and cisplatin excretion into human milk. *Cancer Treat Rep* 1985; **69:** 1387–9.
2. American Academy of Pediatrics. The transfer of drugs and other chemicals into human milk. *Pediatrics* 2001; **108:** 776–89. Correction. *ibid.*; 1029. Also available at: http://aappolicy.aappublications.org/cgi/content/full/pediatrics%3b108/3/776 (accessed 29/06/04)

**Handling and disposal.** Doxorubicin hydrochloride is irritant; avoid contact with skin and mucous membranes.

A method for the destruction of doxorubicin or daunorubicin *wastes* using sulfuric acid and potassium permanganate.[1] Residues produced by degradation of daunorubicin by this method showed no mutagenicity *in vitro*; some mutagenicity was seen with high concentrations of residues from doxorubicin.

*Urine and faeces* produced for up to 7 days after a dose of doxorubicin should be handled wearing protective clothing.[2]

1. Castegnaro M, *et al.*, eds. Laboratory decontamination and destruction of carcinogens in laboratory wastes; some antineoplastic agents. *IARC Scientific Publications 73*. Lyon: WHO/International Agency for Research on Cancer, 1985.
2. Harris J, Dodds LJ. Handling waste from patients receiving cytotoxic drugs. *Pharm J* 1985; **235:** 289–91.

**Pregnancy.** Although doxorubicin has been reported to be undetectable in amniotic fluid[1,2] it has been found in fetal tissue (liver, kidney, and lungs) at concentrations several times those in maternal plasma,[2] indicating that it does pass the placenta. The effect of anthracyclines on the outcome of 160 pregnancies has been analysed.[3] Most women had received combination chemotherapy that included doxorubicin or daunorubicin, for haematological malignancies or breast cancer. Most outcomes (73%) were normal. There were 5 malformations, most often associated with regimens that also included antimetabolites or alkylating agents; the malformations were highly variable. Fetal toxicity was associated with chemotherapy use for solid tumours during the first trimester, and the risk of severe fetal toxicity was significantly increased with doxorubicin doses above 70 mg/m$^2$ per cycle. Fetal cardiac toxicity occurred in 2 cases and was associated with anthracycline use during the second and third trimesters. It has been suggested that the use of epirubicin may reduce the risk of fetal myocardiopathy. Fetal death was more frequent in women with acute leukaemia; it was associated with disease progression and the authors recommended that chemotherapy should not be postponed.

1. Roboz J, *et al.* Does doxorubicin cross the placenta? *Lancet* 1979; **ii:** 1382–3.
2. D'Incalci M, *et al.* Transplacental passage of doxorubicin. *Lancet* 1983; **i:** 75.
3. Germann N, *et al.* Anthracyclines during pregnancy: embryo-fetal outcome in 160 patients. *Ann Oncol* 2004; **15:** 146–50.

## Interactions

For a general outline of antineoplastic drug interactions, see p.498. The cumulative dose of doxorubicin should be reduced in patients who have received other cardiotoxic drugs such as daunorubicin or cyclophosphamide. Doxorubicin is reported to inhibit the intracellular activation of stavudine and hence its antiviral effect.

**Antibacterials.** Hypersensitivity reactions to doxorubicin or daunorubicin have been reported in 2 patients with recent exposure to *clindamycin*, one of whom had exhibited hypersensitivity to that antibiotic.[1] The possibility of cross-sensitivity between anthracyclines and clindamycin should be considered.

1. Arena FP, Sherlock S. Doxorubicin hypersensitivity and clindamycin. *Ann Intern Med* 1990; **112:** 150.

**Antineoplastics.** Giving doxorubicin with or after agents, such as *streptozocin*[1] or *methotrexate*,[2] that can impair hepatic function, has resulted in increased doxorubicin toxicity, possibly due to reduced hepatic clearance. A high incidence of cardiotoxicity (manifest as congestive heart failure) has been reported in patients who received doxorubicin with *paclitaxel* (which also has cardiotoxic effects).[3] Any interaction may be schedule dependent.[4] Similarly an increased incidence of cardiotoxicity has been seen when *trastuzumab* was given with or after anthracyclines (see Effects on the Heart under Trastuzumab, p.589).

*Valspodar* inhibits P-glycoprotein, and a pharmacokinetic study[5] found that it decreased clearance of doxorubicin and prolonged the terminal half-life, increasing exposure to doxorubicin and myelosuppressive effects. The authors suggested that the dose of doxorubicin might need to be reduced by about 60%.

For a suggestion that doxorubicin might enhance the hepatotoxicity of *mercaptopurine*, see under Daunorubicin Hydrochloride, p.546.

1. Anonymous. Two drugs may not be better than one. *JAMA* 1976; **236:** 913.
2. Robertson JH, *et al.* Toxicity of doxorubicin and methotrexate in osteogenic sarcoma. *BMJ* 1976; **1:** 23.
3. Gianni L, *et al.* Paclitaxel by 3-hour infusion in combination with bolus doxorubicin in women with untreated metastatic breast cancer: high antitumor efficacy and cardiac effects in a dose-finding and sequence-finding study. *J Clin Oncol* 1995; **13:** 2688–99.
4. Danesi R, *et al.* Pharmacokinetic optimisation of treatment schedules for anthracyclines and paclitaxel in patients with cancer. *Clin Pharmacokinet* 1999; **37:** 195–211.
5. Advani R, *et al.* A phase I trial of doxorubicin, paclitaxel, and valspodar (PSC 833), a modulator of multidrug resistance. *Clin Cancer Res* 2001; **7:** 1221–9.

**Immunosuppressants.** Increased plasma-doxorubicin concentrations and myelotoxicity have occurred when *ciclosporin* was used to modulate tumour resistance.[1] Severe neurological toxicity occurred in another patient given doxorubicin after long-term ciclosporin therapy.[2] It has been suggested that the use of ciclosporin or its analogues (see above for the effect of valspodar) to modulate doxorubicin resistance should be undertaken with caution.[3]

1. Rushing DA, *et al.* The effects of cyclosporine on the pharmacokinetics of doxorubicin in patients with small cell lung cancer. *Cancer* 1994; **74:** 834–41.
2. Barbui T, *et al.* Neurological symptoms and coma associated with doxorubicin administration during chronic cyclosporin therapy. *Lancet* 1992; **339:** 1421.
3. Beck WT, Kuttesch JF. Neurological symptoms associated with cyclosporin plus doxorubicin. *Lancet* 1992; **340:** 496.

**Thalidomide.** In a comparison of two treatment regimens for multiple myeloma (thalidomide, dexamethasone, cisplatin, cyclophosphamide, and etoposide, with or without doxorubicin), there was an increased risk of deep-vein thrombosis in those patients who received the combination that included doxorubicin.[1] The authors cited a previous study[2] in which the addition of thalidomide to an antineoplastic regimen increased the risk of deep-vein thrombosis, and concluded that patients with multiple myeloma treated with the combination of doxorubicin and thalidomide are at increased risk.

1. Zangari M, *et al.* Thrombogenic activity of doxorubicin in myeloma patients receiving thalidomide: implications for therapy. *Blood* 2002; **100:** 1168–71.
2. Zangari M, *et al.* Increased risk of deep-vein thrombosis in patients with multiple myeloma receiving thalidomide and chemotherapy. *Blood* 2001; **98:** 1614–15.

## Pharmacokinetics

Following intravenous injection, doxorubicin is rapidly cleared from the blood, and distributed into tissues including lungs, liver, heart, spleen, and kidneys. It undergoes rapid metabolism in the liver to metabolites including the active metabolite doxorubicinol (adriamycinol). About 40 to 50% of a dose is stated to be excreted in bile within 7 days, of which about half is as unchanged drug. Only about 5% of a dose is excreted in urine within 5 days. It does not cross the blood-brain barrier but may cross the placenta and is distributed into breast milk. The disappearance of doxorubicin from the blood is triphasic: mean half-lives are 12 minutes, 3.3 hours and about 30 hours.

The pharmacokinetics of liposomal formulations are somewhat different from the conventional drug. The use of macrogols in the surface layer of the liposomes (pegylation) reduces removal of liposomes by macrophages. This results in prolonged circulation in the plasma, with relatively little tissue distribution, but tumour neovasculature is reported to permit penetration of liposomes into tumour tissue. Pharmacokinetics are reported to be biphasic with mean half-lives of 5 hours and 55 to 75 hours respectively. A non-pegylated liposomal formulation also exists and is reported to produce higher peak plasma concentrations of total doxorubicin than conventional formulations, but lower free (not liposome-encapsulated) concentrations. Clearance is reduced, and peak plasma concentrations of doxorubicinol delayed.

◊ References.

1. Speth PAJ, *et al.* Clinical pharmacokinetics of doxorubicin. *Clin Pharmacokinet* 1988; **15:** 15–31.
2. Rushing DA, *et al.* The disposition of doxorubicin on repeated dosing. *J Clin Pharmacol* 1993; **33:** 698–702.
3. Piscitelli SC, *et al.* Pharmacokinetics and pharmacodynamics of doxorubicin in patients with small cell lung cancer. *Clin Pharmacol Ther* 1993; **53:** 555–61.
4. Amantea MA, *et al.* Population pharmacokinetics and pharmacodynamics of pegylated-liposomal doxorubicin in patients with AIDS-related Kaposi's sarcoma. *Clin Pharmacol Ther* 1997; **61:** 301–11.
5. Danesi R, *et al.* Pharmacokinetic-pharmacodynamic relationships of the anthracycline anticancer drugs. *Clin Pharmacokinet* 2002; **41:** 431–44.
6. Swenson CE, *et al.* Pharmacokinetics of doxorubicin administered i.v. as Myocet (TLC D-99; liposome-encapsulated doxorubicin citrate) compared with conventional doxorubicin when given in combination with cyclophosphamide in patients with metastatic breast cancer. *Anticancer Drugs* 2003; **14:** 239–46.
7. Gabizon A, *et al.* Pharmacokinetics of pegylated liposomal doxorubicin : review of animal and human studies. *Clin Pharmacokinet* 2003 **42:** 419–36.

## Uses and Administration

Doxorubicin is an anthracycline antineoplastic antibiotic which may act by forming a stable complex with DNA and interfering with the synthesis of nucleic acids. It is a cell-cycle non-specific agent but is most active against cells in S phase. It also has actions on cell membranes, and antibacterial and immunosuppressant properties. It is an effective antineoplastic against a wide range of tumours as indicated by the cross-references given below. Doxorubicin is used, often in association with other antineoplastics, in the treatment of Hodgkin's disease, non-Hodgkin's lymphomas, bone and soft-tissue sarcomas, neuroblastoma, Wilms' tumour, and malignant neoplasms of the bladder, breast, lung, ovary, and thyroid. It has also been used in a wide variety of other tumours. Liposomal doxorubicin is used in the management of Kaposi's sarcoma in patients with AIDS and metastatic breast and ovarian cancers.

Doxorubicin hydrochloride is given by intravenous injection of a solution in sodium chloride 0.9% into a fast-running infusion of sodium chloride 0.9% or glucose 5% over 3 minutes or more. When used as a single agent, the dose is 60 to 75 mg/m$^2$, or 1.2 to 2.4 mg/kg, once every 3 weeks. Alternatively, doses of 20 to 25 mg/m$^2$ have been given daily for 3 days every 3 weeks, although dividing the dose in this way may increase the incidence of mucositis. A regimen of 20 mg/m$^2$ as a single weekly dose may be used, and is reported to be associated with a lower incidence of cardiotoxicity.

Doses may need to be reduced if doxorubicin is given with other antineoplastics: a dose of 30 to 40 mg/m$^2$ every 3 weeks has been suggested. Doses should also be reduced in patients with liver dysfunction (see below).

The maximum total dose should not exceed 450 to 550 mg/m$^2$; in patients who have received radiotherapy to the chest, or other cardiotoxic drugs, it may be advisable to further limit the total dose.

In the management of AIDS-related Kaposi's sarcoma pegylated liposomal doxorubicin hydrochloride is given in a dose of 20 mg/m$^2$ infused over 30 minutes once every 2 to 3 weeks. For the treatment of breast and ovarian cancers, the suggested dose of this liposomal formulation is 50 mg/m$^2$ infused over 1 hour once every 4 weeks. In these three conditions, treatment should be continued for as long as the patient responds satisfactorily and tolerates treatment. The pegylated liposomal formulation should be diluted only with glucose 5%.

A non-pegylated liposomal formulation is also available and contains a doxorubicin citrate complex prepared with the aid of doxorubicin hydrochloride. It is given in the treatment of metastatic breast cancer in doses equivalent to doxorubicin hydrochloride 60 to 75 mg/m$^2$ every 3 weeks, with cyclophosphamide. Doses are given by intravenous infusion over 1 hour, diluted in sodium chloride 0.9% or glucose 5%.

Blood counts should be made routinely during treatment with doxorubicin (see also Bone-marrow Depression, p.496) and cardiac function should be monitored at regular intervals for early signs of cardiotoxicity.

Doxorubicin hydrochloride has also been instilled into the bladder in the local treatment of malignant neoplasms. For this purpose 50 mL of a 1 mg/mL solution may be instilled into the bladder for one hour once a month. Doxorubicin has been given intra-arterially.

A formulation of doxorubicin with carbon/iron carrier particles (MTC-DOX) is under investigation as magnetically targeted treatment for hepatocellular carcinoma, using an external magnet to keep the drug at the tumour site.

◊ Reviews and studies of liposomal formulations.

1. Working PK, Dayan AD. CPMP Preclinical Expert Report: Caelyx (Stealth liposomal doxorubicin HCL). *Hum Exp Toxicol* 1996; **15:** 752–85.
2. Batist G, *et al.* Reduced cardiotoxicity and preserved antitumor efficacy of liposome-encapsulated doxorubicin and cyclophosphamide compared with conventional doxorubicin and cyclophosphamide in a randomized, multicenter trial of metastatic breast cancer. *J Clin Oncol* 2001; **19:** 1444–54.

3. Gordon AN, *et al.* Recurrent epithelial ovarian carcinoma: a randomized phase III study of pegylated liposomal doxorubicin versus topotecan. *J Clin Oncol* 2001; **19:** 3312–22.
4. Sharpe M, *et al.* Polyethylene glycol-liposomal doxorubicin: a review of its use in the management of solid and haematological malignancies and AIDS-related Kaposi's sarcoma. *Drugs* 2002; **62:** 2089–2126.
5. Harris L, *et al.* Liposome-encapsulated doxorubicin compared with conventional doxorubicin in a randomized multicenter trial as first-line therapy of metastatic breast carcinoma. *Cancer* 2002; **94:** 25–36.

**Administration in hepatic impairment.** Doses of doxorubicin should be adjusted as follows in patients with liver dysfunction:

- moderate impairment (serum-bilirubin concentrations of 12 to 30 micrograms/mL), half the normal dose
- severe impairment (serum-bilirubin greater than 30 micrograms/mL), quarter of the usual dose

**Amyloidosis.** For mention of the use of doxorubicin in patients with amyloidosis (and of the increased risk this may carry in cardiac amyloidosis) see p.567.

**Malignant neoplasms.** Doxorubicin plays a major role in combination regimens for chemotherapy of solid malignancies; it is often employed for tumours of the breast and lung (see p.514 and p.519) and for Wilms' tumour and neuroblastoma or retinoblastoma in children (see p.518, p.524, and p.524) but has been used for malignancies of the bladder (p.512); for various gynaecological cancers including those of the endometrium, and ovary (see p.516, and p.520); for cancer of the liver, stomach, and pancreas (p.518, p.516, p.521); and for neoplasms of prostate, and thymus (p.521 and p.523). It is also used in the treatment of sarcomas of bone and soft-tissue (see p.524 and p.525) and liposomal doxorubicin is used in patients with Kaposi's sarcoma (see p.524).

In addition, doxorubicin is a component of the ABVD regimen used to treat Hodgkin's disease (see p.509) and is part of the CHOP regimen used for non-Hodgkin's lymphoma (p.510). Doxorubicin is also used in Burkitt's lymphoma (p.511), mycosis fungoides (p.511), and the lymphomas associated with AIDS (see p.510). It has been employed in acute lymphoblastic leukaemia (p.506), in chronic lymphocytic leukaemia as part of the CHOP regimen (though with uncertain benefit—see p.507), and in multiple myeloma (p.511).

## Preparations

***BP 2003:*** Doxorubicin Injection;
***USP 27:*** Doxorubicin Hydrochloride for Injection; Doxorubicin Hydrochloride Injection.

**Proprietary Preparations** (details are given in Part 3)
***Arg.:*** Adriblastina; Caelyx; Colhidrol; Dicladox; Doxocris; Doxorbin; Doxtie; Flavicina; Nagun; Ranxas; Roxorin; ***Austral.:*** Caelyx; Doxorubin†; ***Austria:*** Adriblastin; Caelyx; Doxolem; Doxorubin; ***Belg.:*** Adriblastina; Caelyx; ***Braz.:*** Adriblastina; Biorrub; Caelyx†; Doxolem; Neoxane; Rubex; ***Canad.:*** Caelyx; ***Chile:*** Adriblastina; Caelyx; Daxotel; ***Denm.:*** Caelyx; Doxorubin†; ***Fin.:*** Caelyx; ***Fr.:*** Adriblastine; Caelyx; Myocet; ***Ger.:*** Adriblastin; Adrimedac; Caelyx; DOXO-cell; Myocet; Ribodoxo-L; ***Gr.:*** Adriblastina; Caelyx; ***Hong Kong:*** Caelyx; ***India:*** Adrim; ***Irl.:*** Caelyx; Myocet; ***Israel:*** Adriblastina; Caelyx; ***Ital.:*** Adriblastina; Caelyx; Myocet; ***Malaysia:*** Caelyx; Doxorubin; ***Mex.:*** Adriblastina; Caelyx; Doxolem; Doxotec†; Ifadox; ***Neth.:*** Adriblastina; Caelyx; ***Norw.:*** Caelyx; ***NZ:*** Doxorubin; ***Port.:*** Adriblastina; Caelyx†; Fauldoxo; Myocet; ***S.Afr.:*** Adriblastina†; Caelyx; ***Singapore:*** Caelyx; Doxorubin; ***Spain:*** Caelyx; Farmiblastina; Myocet; ***Swed.:*** Caelyx; ***Switz.:*** Adriblastin; Caelyx; ***Thai.:*** Adriblastina; Adrim; Caelyx; Doxolem; Doxorubin; ***UK:*** Caelyx; Myocet; ***USA:*** Doxil; Rubex.

---

## Droloxifene *(USAN, rINN)*

Droloxifeno; 3-Hydroxytamoxifen; K-21060E. *(E)*-α-{*p*-[2-(Dimethylamino)ethoxy]phenyl}-α′-ethyl-3-stilbenol.
$C_{26}H_{29}NO_2$ = 387.5.
*CAS — 82413-20-5.*

### Profile

Droloxifene is a selective oestrogen receptor modulator related to tamoxifen (p.584) and with similar general properties. It has been investigated in the hormonal treatment and prophylaxis of breast cancer and is under study for osteoporosis.

---

## Edatrexate *(USAN, rINN)*

CGP-30694; Edatrexato. *N*-(*p*-{1-[(2,4-Diamino-6-pteridinyl)-methyl]propyl}benzoyl)-L-glutamic acid.
$C_{22}H_{25}N_7O_5$ = 467.5.
*CAS — 80576-83-6.*

### Profile

Edatrexate is an analogue of methotrexate (p.568) and has similar general properties. It is under investigation as an antineoplastic in the treatment of various malignant neoplasms. Mucositis may be dose limiting.

◊ References.

1. Schornagel JH, *et al.* Randomized phase III trial of edatrexate versus methotrexate in patients with metastatic and/or recurrent squamous cell carcinoma of the head and neck: a European Organization for Research and Treatment of Cancer Head and Neck Cancer Cooperative Group study. *J Clin Oncol* 1995; **13:** 1649–55.
2. Dreicer R, *et al.* A phase II trial of edatrexate in patients with advanced renal cell carcinoma: an Eastern Cooperative Oncology Group study. *Am J Clin Oncol* 1997; **20:** 251–3.
3. D'Andrea G, *et al.* Phase I study of escalating doses of edatrexate in combination with paclitaxel in patients with metastatic breast cancer. *Clin Cancer Res* 1999; **5:** 275–9.
4. Kindler HL, *et al.* Edatrexate (10-ethyl-deaza-aminopterin) (NSC 626715) with or without leucovorin rescue for malignant mesothelioma: sequential phase II trials by the cancer and leukemia group B. *Cancer* 1999; **86:** 1985–91.
5. Laurie SA, *et al.* Phase I and pharmacological study of two schedules of the antifolate edatrexate in combination with cisplatin. *Clin Cancer Res* 2001; **7:** 501–9.
6. Colon-Otero G, *et al.* A phase II trial of edatrexate, vinblastine, adriamycin, cisplatin, and filgrastim (EVAC/G-CSF) in patients with non-small-cell carcinoma of the lungs: a North Central Cancer Treatment Group Trial. *Am J Clin Oncol* 2001; **24:** 551–5.
7. Kuriakose P, *et al.* Phase I trial of edatrexate in advanced breast and other cancers. *Cancer Invest* 2002; **20:** 473–9.

---

## Edrecolomab *(USAN, rINN)*

17-1A Antibody; C1; Monoclonal Antibody 17-1A.
*CAS — 156586-89-9.*
*ATC — L01XC01.*

### Profile

Edrecolomab is a monoclonal antibody of murine origin directed at epithelial cell surface glycoproteins that has been used as adjuvant therapy following surgery in patients with colorectal cancer (p.516), although reports of improved survival do not seem to have been borne out. It has been given by intravenous infusion over 2 hours, in an initial dose of 500 mg, followed by 4 further doses of 100 mg at monthly intervals. The drug is of murine origin and most patients develop antibodies following administration. Hypersensitivity reactions, including anaphylactic reactions, have occurred.

It has also been tried for other malignant neoplasms including pancreatic cancer and advanced breast cancer.

◊ References.

1. Riethmüller G, *et al.* Randomised trial of monoclonal antibody for adjuvant therapy of resected Dukes' C colorectal carcinoma. *Lancet* 1994; **343:** 1177–83.
2. Riethmüller G, *et al.* Monoclonal antibody therapy for resected Dukes' C colorectal cancer: seven-year outcome of a multicenter randomized trial. *J Clin Oncol* 1998; **16:** 1788–94.
3. Adkins JC, Spencer CM. Edrecolomab (monoclonal antibody 17-1A). *Drugs* 1998; **56:** 619–26.
4. Punt CJA, *et al.* Edrecolomab alone or in combination with fluorouracil and folinic acid in the adjuvant treatment of stage III colon cancer: a randomised study. *Lancet* 2002; **360:** 671–7.

### Preparations

**Proprietary Preparations** (details are given in Part 3)
***Ger.:*** Panorex†.

---

## Eniluracil *(BAN, USAN, rINN)*

776C85; Eniluracilo. 5-Ethynyluracil.
$C_6H_4N_2O_2$ = 136.1.
*CAS — 59989-18-3.*

### Profile

Eniluracil inactivates the enzyme dihydropyrimidine dehydrogenase, which plays an important role in fluorouracil metabolism. Eniluracil increases the bioavailability of fluorouracil, particularly when the latter is given by mouth. It has been investigated as an adjunct to fluorouracil therapy in the treatment of colorectal, breast, and pancreatic cancer.

---

## Enocitabine *(rINN)*

Behenoyl Cytarabine; Behenoylcytosine Arabinoside; BH-AC; Enocitabina; NSC-239336. *N*-(1-β-D-Arabinofuranosyl-1,2-dihydro-2-oxo-4-pyrimidinyl)docosanamide.
$C_{31}H_{55}N_3O_6$ = 565.8.
*CAS — 55726-47-1.*

### Profile

Enocitabine is an antineoplastic that is converted in the body to cytarabine (p.543). It has been used similarly in the treatment of acute leukaemias.

---

# Epirubicin Hydrochloride

*(BANM, USAN, rINNM)*

4′-Epiadriamycin Hydrochloride; 4′-Epidoxorubicin Hydrochloride; Epirubicini Hydrochloridum; Hidrocloruro de epirubicina; IMI-28; Pidorubicin Hydrochloride. (8*S*,10*S*)-10-(3-Amino-2,3,6-trideoxy-α-L-*arabino*-hexopyranosyloxy)-8-glycolloyl-7,8,9,10-tetrahydro-6,8,11-trihydroxy-1-methoxynaphthacene-5,12-dione hydrochloride.
$C_{27}H_{29}NO_{11}$,HCl = 580.0.
*CAS — 56420-45-2 (epirubicin); 56390-09-1 (epirubicin hydrochloride).*
*ATC — L01DB03.*

**Pharmacopoeias.** In *Eur.* (see p.vi) and *Jpn.*

**Ph. Eur. 5.0** (Epirubicin Hydrochloride). A substance obtained by chemical transformation of a substance produced by certain strains of *Streptomyces peucetius*. An orange-red powder. Soluble in water and in methyl alcohol; slightly soluble in dehydrated alcohol; practically insoluble in acetone. A 0.5% solution in water has a pH of 4.0 to 5.5. Store at 2° to 8° in airtight containers. Protect from light.

**Incompatibility.** The manufacturers state that epirubicin hydrochloride is incompatible with heparin or fluorouracil, resulting in precipitation, and that it is hydrolysed in alkaline solutions.

**Stability.** Epirubicin was not subject to significant photodegradation at clinical concentrations,[1,2] and special precautions to protect solutions from light during administration do not appear to be necessary. However, photodegradation may be significant at lower concentrations (below 500 micrograms/mL).[1]

1. Wood MJ, *et al.* Photodegradation of doxorubicin, daunorubicin and epirubicin measured by high-performance liquid chromatography. *J Clin Pharm Ther* 1990; **15:** 291–300.
2. Pujol M, *et al.* Stability study of epirubicin in NaCl 0.9% injection. *Ann Pharmacother* 1997; **31:** 992–5.

## Adverse Effects, Treatment, and Precautions

As for Doxorubicin Hydrochloride, p.548. Cardiotoxicity and myelotoxicity may be less than with doxorubicin. Cardiotoxicity is more likely when the cumulative dose exceeds 0.9 to 1 g/m$^2$.

**Effects on the heart.** For further discussion of the cardiotoxicity of anthracyclines, see under Adverse Effects of Doxorubicin, p.548.

## Interactions

As for Doxorubicin Hydrochloride, p.549.

**Antineoplastics.** Increased exposure to epirubicin, and a consequent increase in myelotoxicity, has been reported in patients given epirubicin immediately after *paclitaxel*, compared with patients who received epirubicin before paclitaxel.[1] Similar interactions have been seen when paclitaxel was given before other anthracyclines.[2] These and other studies[3,4] have suggested that paclitaxel given in this way is associated with a reduced conversion of epirubicin to the less myelotoxic metabolite, epirubicinol, although the interaction is complex, and may involve both disposition and pharmacodynamics.

1. Venturini M, *et al.* Sequence effect of epirubicin and paclitaxel treatment on pharmacokinetics and toxicity. *J Clin Oncol* 2000; **18:** 2116–25.
2. Danesi R, *et al.* Pharmacokinetic optimisation of treatment schedules for anthracyclines and paclitaxel in patients with cancer. *Clin Pharmacokinet* 1999; **37:** 195–211.
3. Grasselli G, *et al.* Clinical and pharmacologic study of the epirubicin and paclitaxel combination in women with metastatic breast cancer. *J Clin Oncol* 2001; **19:** 2222–31.
4. Danesi R, *et al.* Pharmacokinetics and pharmacodynamics of combination chemotherapy with paclitaxel and epirubicin in breast cancer patients. *Br J Clin Pharmacol* 2002; **53:** 508–18.

**Cimetidine.** Cimetidine increased the formation of the active metabolite of epirubicin in a study in 8 patients; there was also a substantial increase in systemic exposure to unchanged epirubicin.[1] The mechanisms and potential clinical significance of the interaction were unclear.

1. Murray LS, *et al.* The effect of cimetidine on the pharmacokinetics of epirubicin in patients with advanced breast cancer: preliminary evidence of a potentially common drug interaction. *Clin Oncol* 1998; **10:** 35–8.

## Pharmacokinetics

After intravenous doses epirubicin is rapidly and extensively distributed into body tissues, and undergoes metabolism in the liver, with the formation of epirubicinol (13-hydroxyepirubicin) and appreciable amounts of glucuronide derivatives. Epirubicin is eliminated mainly in bile, with a terminal plasma elimination half-life of about 30 to 40 hours. About 10% of a dose is recovered in urine within 48 hours. Epirubicin does not cross the blood-brain barrier.

◊ References.

1. Morris RG, *et al.* Disposition of epirubicin and metabolites with repeated courses to cancer patients. *Eur J Clin Pharmacol* 1991; **40:** 481–7.
2. Robert J. Clinical pharmacokinetics of epirubicin. *Clin Pharmacokinet* 1994; **26:** 428–38.

## Uses and Administration

Epirubicin is an anthracycline antibiotic with antineoplastic actions similar to those of doxorubicin (p.549). It is used, alone or in combination with other antineoplastics, in acute leukaemias, lymphomas, multiple myeloma, and in solid tumours including Wilms' tumour (p.518), cancer of the bladder (p.512), breast (p.514), and gastrointestinal tract (p.516).

Epirubicin hydrochloride is given by intravenous injection of a solution in sodium chloride 0.9% or Water for Injections into a fast-running infusion of sodium chloride 0.9% or glucose 5% over 3 to 5 minutes, or by infusion over up to 30 minutes. It is given as a single agent in usual doses of 60 to 90 mg/m² as a single dose every 3 weeks; this dose may be divided over 2 or 3 days if desired. A regimen of 12.5 to 25 mg/m² once a week has also been tried in palliative care. High-dose regimens, of 120 mg/m² or more every 3 weeks, or 45 mg/m² for 3 consecutive days every 3 weeks have been used.

Doses may need to be reduced if epirubicin is given with other antineoplastics. Doses should also be reduced in patients with liver impairment (see below) and in those whose bone-marrow function is impaired by age or previous chemotherapy or radiotherapy.

A total cumulative dose of 0.9 to 1 g/m² should not generally be exceeded, because of the risk of cardiotoxicity.

Epirubicin has also been given by intravesical instillation in the local treatment of bladder cancer. Instillation of 50 mg weekly as a 0.1% solution (in sodium chloride 0.9% or sterile water) for 8 weeks has been suggested, reduced to 30 mg in 50 mL weekly if chemical cystitis develops; for carcinoma in-situ, the dose may be increased, if tolerated, to 80 mg in 50 mL weekly. For the prophylaxis of recurrence in patients who have undergone transurethral resection, 50 mg weekly for 4 weeks, followed by 50 mg instilled once a month for 11 months is the suggested regimen. The solution should be retained in the bladder for 1 hour.

Blood counts should be made routinely during treatment with epirubicin (see also Bone-marrow Depression, p.496) and cardiac function should be carefully monitored. Liver function should be assessed before and if possible during therapy.

◊ References.

1. Plosker GL, Faulds D. Epirubicin: a review of its pharmacodynamic and pharmacokinetic properties, and therapeutic use in cancer chemotherapy. *Drugs* 1993; **45:** 788–856.
2. Coukell AJ, Faulds D. Epirubicin: an updated review of its pharmacodynamic and pharmacokinetic properties and therapeutic efficacy in the management of breast cancer. *Drugs* 1997; **53:** 453–82.

**Administration in hepatic impairment.** Doses of epirubicin should be halved in patients with moderate liver dysfunction (serum bilirubin concentrations of 12 to 30 micrograms/mL), while those with severe liver impairment (serum bilirubin greater than 30 micrograms/mL) should be given a quarter of the usual dose.

**Amyloidosis.** For reference to a regimen including epirubicin used to control disease in a patient with amyloidosis, see p.567.

### Preparations

**Proprietary Preparations** (details are given in Part 3)
***Arg.:*** Crisabon; Cuatroepi; Epidoxo; Epifil; Epikebir; EPR; Farmorubicin; Robanul; Rubifarm; ***Austral.:*** Pharmorubicin; ***Austria:*** Farmorubicin; ***Belg.:*** Farmorubicine; ***Braz.:*** Farmorubicina; Rubina; ***Canad.:*** Pharmorubicin; ***Chile:*** Farmorrubicina; ***Denm.:*** Farmorubicin; ***Fin.:*** Farmorubicin; ***Fr.:*** Farmorubicine; ***Ger.:*** Epi-Cell; Farmorubicin; ***Gr.:*** Farmorubicin; ***Hong Kong:*** Pharmorubicin; ***Irl.:*** Pharmorubicin; ***Israel:*** Farmorubicin; ***Ital.:*** Farmorubicina; ***Malaysia:*** Pharmorubicin; ***Mex.:*** Epilem; Farmorubicin; ***Neth.:*** Farmorubicine; ***Norw.:*** Farmorubicin; ***NZ:*** Pharmorubicin; ***Port.:*** Farmorubicina; ***S.Afr.:*** Farmorubicin; ***Singapore:*** Pharmorubicin; ***Spain:*** Farmorubicina; ***Swed.:*** Farmorubicin; ***Switz.:*** Farmorubicin; ***Thai.:*** Epilem; Farmorubicin; ***UK:*** Pharmorubicin; ***USA:*** Ellence.

---

## Epratuzumab *(rINN)*

*CAS — 205923-57-5.*

### Profile

Epratuzumab is a humanised anti-CD22 monoclonal antibody under investigation, alone or conjugated with yttrium-90, for the treatment of non-Hodgkin's lymphoma.

---

## Estramustine Sodium Phosphate *(BANM, rINNM)*

Estramustine Phosphate Sodium *(USAN)*; Fosfato sódico de estramustina; NSC-89199 (estramustine phosphate); Ro-21-8837/001; Ro-22-2296/000 (estramustine). Estra-1,3,5(10)-triene-3,17β-diol 3-[bis(2-chloroethyl)carbamate] 17-(disodium phosphate); Disodium 3-[bis(2-chloroethyl)-carbamoyloxy]estra-1,3,5(10)-trien-17β-yl orthophosphate.

$C_{23}H_{30}Cl_2NNa_2O_6P$ = 564.3.

*CAS — 2998-57-4 (estramustine); 4891-15-0 (estramustine phosphate); 52205-73-9 (estramustine sodium phosphate).*

*ATC — L01XX11.*

**Pharmacopoeias.** In *Br.*

**BP 2003** (Estramustine Sodium Phosphate). A white or almost white powder. Freely soluble in water and in methyl alcohol; very slightly soluble in dehydrated alcohol and in chloroform. A 0.5% solution in water has a pH of 8.5 to 10.0. Protect from light.

### Adverse Effects, Treatment, and Precautions

Oestrogenic side-effects are fairly common, and may include gynaecomastia, fluid retention, and cardiovascular effects. Gastrointestinal disturbances, hepatic dysfunction, loss of libido, hypersensitivity reactions, and occasionally leucopenia and thrombocytopenia may occur. Estramustine is contra-indicated in patients with peptic ulceration and severe hepatic or cardiovascular disease. Diabetes mellitus may be exacerbated, and it should be given with care to patients with disorders such as congestive heart failure, epilepsy, hypertension, migraine, and renal impairment which may be adversely affected by additional fluid retention. Care is also required in patients with conditions predisposing to hypercalcaemia, and serum calcium should be monitored in hypercalcaemic patients.

**Porphyria.** Estramustine has been associated with acute attacks of porphyria and is considered unsafe in porphyric patients.

### Interactions

Estramustine sodium phosphate should not be given with milk products or products high in calcium, which may interfere with its absorption. Hypersensitivity reactions including angioedema have occurred rarely in patients given estramustine who were also receiving an ACE inhibitor.

### Pharmacokinetics

Up to 75% of a dose of estramustine sodium phosphate is absorbed from the gastrointestinal tract and rapidly dephosphorylated. Estramustine is found in the body mainly as its oxidised isomer estromustine; both forms accumulate in the prostate. Some hydrolysis of the carbamate linkage occurs in the liver, releasing estradiol, estrone, and the normustine group. Estramustine and estromustine have plasma half-lives of 10 to 20 hours, and are excreted with their metabolites mainly in the faeces.

### Uses and Administration

Estramustine is a combination of estradiol and normustine and has weaker oestrogenic activity than estradiol and weaker antineoplastic activity than most other alkylating agents. Estramustine phosphate is given by mouth as the disodium salt. Doses are calculated in terms of estramustine phosphate; 108 mg of estramustine sodium phosphate is approximately equivalent to 100 mg of estramustine phosphate. Estramustine phosphate with meglumine has been given by intravenous injection.

Estramustine sodium phosphate is licensed for use in the treatment of advanced prostatic carcinoma (p.521). An estramustine phosphate dose of about 14 mg/kg daily in divided doses is used. The usual initial dose is 560 to 840 mg daily, which may be adjusted to between 140 mg and 1.4 g daily according to the response and gastrointestinal tolerance. It should be given not less than 1 hour before or 2 hours after meals.

◊ References.

1. Bergenheim AT, Henriksson R. Pharmacokinetics and pharmacodynamics of estramustine phosphate. *Clin Pharmacokinet* 1998; **34:** 163–72.
2. Sangrajrang S, *et al.* Estramustine resistance. *Gen Pharmacol* 1999; **33:** 107–13.
3. Kreis W, Budman D. Daily oral estramustine and intermittent intravenous docetaxel (Taxotere) as chemotherapeutic treatment for metastatic, hormone-refractory prostate cancer. *Semin Oncol* 1999; **26** (suppl 17): 34–8.
4. Kitamura T. Necessity of re-evaluation of estramustine phosphate sodium (EMP) as a treatment option for first-line monotherapy in advanced prostate cancer. *Int J Urol* 2001; **8:** 33–6.
5. Hamilton A, Muggia F. Estramustine potentiates taxane in prostate and refractory breast cancers. *Oncology (Huntingt)* 2001; **15** (suppl 7): 40–3.
6. Kitamura T, *et al.* EMP combination chemotherapy and low-dose monotherapy in advanced prostate cancer. *Expert Rev Anticancer Ther* 2002; **2:** 59–71.

### Preparations

***BP 2003:*** Estramustine Phosphate Capsules.

**Proprietary Preparations** (details are given in Part 3)
***Arg.:*** Amsupros; Estracyt; ***Austral.:*** Estracyt†; ***Austria:*** Estracyt; ***Belg.:*** Estracyt; ***Braz.:*** Estracyt†; ***Canad.:*** Emcyt; ***Chile:*** Estracyt; ***Denm.:*** Estracyt; ***Fin.:*** Estracyt; ***Fr.:*** Estracyt; ***Ger.:*** cellmustin; Estracyt; Multosin; Prostamustin; ***Gr.:*** Estracyt; ***Hong Kong:*** Estracyt; ***Irl.:*** Estracyt; ***Israel:*** Estracyt; ***Ital.:*** Estracyt; ***Jpn:*** Estracyt; ***Malaysia:*** Estracyt; ***Mex.:*** Emcyt; ***Neth.:*** Estracyt; ***Norw.:*** Estracyt; ***Port.:*** Estracyt; ***S.Afr.:*** Estracyt; ***Singapore:*** Estracyt; ***Spain:*** Estracyt; ***Swed.:*** Estracyt; ***Switz.:*** Estracyt; ***UK:*** Estracyt; ***USA:*** Emcyt.

---

## Etanidazole *(USAN, rINN)*

Etanidazol; NSC-301467; SR-2508. N-(2-Hydroxyethyl)-2-nitroimidazole-1-acetamide.

$C_7H_{10}N_4O_4$ = 214.2.

*CAS — 22668-01-5.*

### Profile

Etanidazole is a radiosensitiser structurally related to metronidazole, and which is under investigation as an adjunct to radiotherapy in the treatment of cancer. Peripheral neuropathy may be dose-limiting.

◊ References.

1. Lee DJ, *et al.* Results of an RTOG phase III trial (RTOG 85-27) comparing radiotherapy plus etanidazole with radiotherapy alone for locally advanced head and neck carcinomas. *Int J Radiat Oncol Biol Phys* 1995; **32:** 567–76.
2. Eschwege F, *et al.* Results of a European randomized trial of etanidazole combined with radiotherapy in head and neck carcinomas. *Int J Radiat Oncol Biol Phys* 1997; **39:** 275–81.

---

## Etoposide *(BAN, USAN, rINN)*

EPEG; Etopósido; Etoposidum; NSC-141540; VP-16; VP-16-213. 4′-Demethylepipodophyllotoxin 9-[4,6-O-(R)-ethylidene-β-D-glucopyranoside]; (5S,5aR,8aS,9R)-9-(4,6-O-Ethylidene-β-D-glucopyranosyloxy)-5,8,8a,9-tetrahydro-5-(4-hydroxy-3,5-dimethoxyphenyl)-isobenzofuro[5,6-f][1,3]benzodioxol-6(5aH)-one.

$C_{29}H_{32}O_{13}$ = 588.6.

*CAS — 33419-42-0.*

*ATC — L01CB01.*

NOTE. The trivial name epipodophyllotoxin has occasionally been used incorrectly for this derivative.

**Pharmacopoeias.** In *Eur.* (see p.vi), *Int.*, and *US.*

**Ph. Eur. 5.0** (Etoposide). A white or almost white, crystalline powder. Practically insoluble in water; slightly soluble in alcohol and in dichloromethane; sparingly soluble in methyl alcohol. Store in airtight containers.

**USP 27** (Etoposide). A fine, white to off-white, crystalline powder. Very slightly soluble in water; slightly soluble in alcohol, in chloroform, in dichloromethane, and in ethyl acetate; sparingly soluble in methyl alcohol. Store in airtight containers. Protect from light.

## Etoposide Phosphate *(USAN)*

BMY-40481. {5R-[5α,5aβ,8aα,9β(R*)]}-5-[3,5-Dimethoxy-4-(phosphonooxy)phenyl]-9-[(4,6-O-ethylidene-β-D-glucopyranosyl)oxy]-5,8,8a,9-tetrahydrofuro-[3′,4′:6,7]naphtho[2,3-d]-1,3-dioxol-6(5aH)-one; 4′-Demethylepipodophyllotoxin 9-(4,6-O-ethylidene-β-D-glucopyranoside) 4′-(dihydrogen phosphate).

$C_{29}H_{33}O_{16}P$ = 668.5.

*CAS — 117091-64-2.*

*ATC — L01CB01.*

**Incompatibility.** For reference to precipitation when mannitol or potassium chloride was added to mixtures of etoposide and cisplatin in sodium chloride injection, see Cisplatin, p.538.

### Adverse Effects, Treatment, and Precautions

For general discussions see Antineoplastics, p.492, p.495, and p.497.

The dose-limiting toxicity with etoposide is myelosuppression, predominantly manifesting as leucopenia, but also thrombocytopenia, and sometimes anaemia. The nadir of the granulocyte count usually occurs 7 to 14 days after a dose, with recovery by about 21 days. Nausea and vomiting are common; there may also be anorexia, diarrhoea, and stomatitis. Gastrointestinal toxicity may be more common after oral administration. Reversible alopecia may occur in about two-thirds of all patients. Peripheral or central neuropathies, including transient cortical blindness, have been reported rarely, as have hypersensitivity or anaphylactoid reactions, apnoea, fever, rashes and skin pigmentation, pruritus, and dysphagia. Disturbances of liver function have been reported, mainly at high doses. There have been occasional reports of cardiotoxicity. Local irritation and thrombophlebitis may occur at the site of injection. Care should be taken to avoid extravasation although tissue damage (possibly associated with the vehicle) is rare.

Rapid intravenous doses may cause hypotension; etoposide should be given by infusion over at least 30 minutes. Etoposide should not be given to patients with severe hepatic impairment nor by intracavitary administration.

Some adverse effects associated with intravenous etoposide may be due to the formulation of the vehicle.

There is evidence that etoposide may be associated with the development of secondary leukaemias—see Carcinogenicity, p.492.

**Breast feeding.** Some licensed information states that it is not known whether etoposide is excreted into breast milk. However, in breast milk samples from a woman given consolidation therapy, including etoposide,[1] for acute promyelocytic leukaemia, etoposide concentrations were maximal just after a dose, but decreased rapidly to undetectable levels within 24 hours on each of three days. She started to breast feed her baby 3 weeks after the completion of therapy, and no abnormalities were observed in the infant up to 16 months of age.

1. Azuno Y, *et al.* Mitoxantrone and etoposide in breast milk. *Am J Hematol* 1995; **48:** 131–2.

**Effects on the nervous system.** A report of an acute dystonic reaction in a child given etoposide as part of a combined maintenance regimen for acute lymphoblastic leukaemia;[1] the patient had been receiving the same regimen uneventfully for over a year but symptoms (which responded to diphenhydramine) recurred on rechallenge with etoposide.

1. Ascher DP, Delaney RA. Acute dystonia from etoposide. *Drug Intell Clin Pharm* 1988; **22:** 41–2.

**Handling and disposal.** *Urine and faeces* produced for up to 4 and 7 days respectively after a dose of etoposide should be handled wearing protective clothing.[1]

1. Harris J, Dodds LJ. Handling waste from patients receiving cytotoxic drugs. *Pharm J* 1985; **235:** 289–91.

**Hypersensitivity.** Hypersensitivity reactions to intravenous etoposide are characterised by one or more of: hypotension, bronchospasm, flushing, exanthema, dyspnoea, fever, chills, tachycardia, tightness in the chest, cyanosis, and hypertension. Although originally stated to be rare, some investigators[1] have reported an incidence of up to about 50%, particularly in younger patients. The mechanism is uncertain, but a literature review[1] supported the hypothesis that it might not be antibody-mediated, as reducing the rate of infusion may prevent reactions, as may reducing etoposide concentration in the infusion solution. However, an immunogenic mechanism cannot be excluded as hypersensitivity appears to have been reported less frequently with the oral formulation, which unlike the infusion does not contain polysorbate 80. In addition, there are reports[2,3] of successful administration of etoposide phosphate formulations, not containing polysorbate 80, after hypersensitivity reactions to etoposide, suggesting that the solvent may be responsible.

1. Hoetelmans RMW, *et al.* Hypersensitivity reactions to etoposide. *Ann Pharmacother* 1996; **30:** 367–71.
2. Bernstein BJ, Troner MB. Successful rechallenge with etoposide phosphate after an acute hypersensitivity reaction to etoposide. *Pharmacotherapy* 1999; **19:** 989–91.
3. Siderov J, *et al.* Safe administration of etoposide phosphate after hypersensitivity reaction to intravenous etoposide. *Br J Cancer* 2002; **86:** 12–13.

## Interactions

For a general outline of antineoplastic drug interactions, see p.498.

**Antineoplastics.** Giving etoposide 2 days after a dose of *cisplatin* was associated with a marked decrease in etoposide clearance and more toxicity, compared with the same dose given 21 days after a dose of cisplatin, in a study involving 17 children.[1] There was no evidence of a persistent decrease in etoposide clearance associated with the cumulative dose of cisplatin, however. In a randomised, crossover trial,[2] cisplatin or *carboplatin* were given alternately during 2 courses of etoposide. Although increases in the area under the concentration-time curve of etoposide were seen in the second course, effects were modest and, given the pharmacokinetic variability seen with etoposide, the authors considered any clinical impact to be small.

1. Relling MV, *et al.* Etoposide pharmacokinetics and pharmacodynamics after acute and chronic exposure to cisplatin. *Clin Pharmacol Ther* 1994; **56:** 503–11.
2. Thomas HD, *et al.* Randomized cross-over clinical trial to study potential pharmacokinetic interactions between cisplatin or carboplatin and etoposide. *Br J Clin Pharmacol* 2002; **53:** 83–91.

**Ciclosporin.** High-dose ciclosporin therapy was found to increase the exposure to etoposide by 80%, and to reduce etoposide clearance by 38%. Leucopenia was increased. Etoposide doses should be halved when the drug is given with high-dose ciclosporin.[1] In a study[2] of children who received etoposide and mitoxantrone for acute myeloid leukaemia, the addition of ciclosporin with a 40% reduction in the doses of the antineoplastics still resulted in a 71% reduction in the clearance of etoposide, and a 42% reduction for mitoxantrone. However, there was wide interpatient variability, and the rates of stomatitis and infection were similar between the groups, with or without ciclosporin.

1. Lum BL, *et al.* Alteration of etoposide pharmacokinetics and pharmacodynamics by cyclosporine in a phase I trial to modulate drug resistance. *J Clin Oncol* 1992; **10:** 1635–42.
2. Lacayo NJ, *et al.* Pharmacokinetic interactions of cyclosporine with etoposide and mitoxantrone in children with acute myeloid leukemia. *Leukemia* 2002; **16:** 920–7.

**Grapefruit juice.** In a randomised crossover study[1] of 6 patients, grapefruit juice appeared to reduce the oral bioavailability of etoposide. Initially the authors had expected the opposite since etoposide is demethylated by cytochrome P450 isoenzyme CYP3A4. Although no definite conclusions could be made due to the small number of patients studied, a possible mechanism might have been alteration of P-glycoprotein mediated transport.

1. Reif S, *et al.* Effect of grapefruit juice intake on etoposide bioavailability. *Eur J Clin Pharmacol* 2002; **58:** 491–4.

## Pharmacokinetics

After doses by mouth absorption is variable, but on average about 50% of the dose of etoposide is absorbed. The pharmacokinetics of etoposide are subject to considerable interindividual variation. It is rapidly distributed, and concentrations in plasma fall in a biphasic manner, with a terminal half-life of 4 to 11 hours. Etoposide is about 94% bound to plasma protein. It is metabolised by the cytochrome P450 isoenzyme CYP3A4. Etoposide is excreted in urine and faeces as unchanged drug and metabolites: about 45% of a dose is reported to be excreted in urine over 72 hours. It crosses the blood-brain barrier poorly; concentrations in CSF are 1 to 10% of those in plasma. It is distributed into breast milk (see above).

**Metabolism.** Studies *in vitro* suggested that metabolic activation of etoposide by oxidation into the *O*-quinone derivative might play an essential role in its activity against DNA.[1]

1. van Maanen JMS, *et al.* Metabolic activation of anti-tumour agent VP 16-213. *Hum Toxicol* 1986; **5:** 136.

## Uses and Administration

Etoposide is a semisynthetic derivative of podophyllotoxin with antineoplastic properties; it interferes with the function of topoisomerase II thus inhibiting DNA synthesis, and is most active against cells in the late S and $G_2$ phases of the cell cycle.

It is used, usually in combination with other antineoplastics, in the treatment of tumours of the testis, and cancers of the lung. It has also been tried in other solid tumours including those of the brain, gastrointestinal tract, ovary, and thymus, and some childhood neoplasms; in lymphomas and acute leukaemias, and in the treatment of Kaposi's sarcoma associated with AIDS. These uses are discussed further under Choice of Antineoplastic, as indicated by the cross-references given below.

It is given by slow intravenous infusion over at least 30 minutes, as a solution in sodium chloride 0.9% or glucose 5% injection. In the UK the manufacturers recommend that the concentration of the infusion should not exceed 250 micrograms/mL, to avoid the risk of the drug crystallising out of solution, but in the USA an upper limit of 400 micrograms/mL is regarded as acceptable. Etoposide phosphate, a prodrug with improved solubility in water, has been developed. 113.6 mg of etoposide phosphate is equivalent to 100 mg of etoposide. Intravenous doses are calculated in terms of etoposide, and are identical to those of the base, but it may be given in concentrations up to the equivalent of etoposide 20 mg/mL. Etoposide phosphate solutions may be infused over 5 minutes to 3.5 hours.

The usual intravenous dose is 50 to 120 mg/m$^2$ of etoposide daily for 5 days. Somewhat lower doses have been suggested in lung cancer. Alternatively, 100 mg/m$^2$ has been given on alternate days to a total of 300 mg/m$^2$. The usual oral dose of etoposide is 100 to 240 mg/m$^2$ daily for 5 consecutive days. Courses may be repeated after 3 to 4 weeks. Doses should be reduced in renal impairment (see below).

**Administration in renal impairment.** Some manufacturers of etoposide or etoposide phosphate recommend that patients with a creatinine clearance of between 15 and 50 mL/minute be given 75% of the recommended dose. No recommendations are given for those patients having a creatinine clearance of below 15 mL/minute, although one manufacturer suggests that further dose reduction in these patients be considered.

**Blood disorders, non-malignant.** For reference to the use of combination chemotherapy, including etoposide, in a few patients with refractory idiopathic thrombocytopenic purpura, see p.1082.

**Histiocytic syndromes.** Systemic chemotherapy is often tried in patients with extensive Langerhans-cell histiocytosis (p.505), although its value is uncertain. Etoposide is one of the drugs widely used for this purpose.

**Hypereosinophilic syndrome.** Etoposide has been reported to produce clinical responses in patients with the hypereosinophilic syndrome.[1]

1. Bourrat E, *et al.* Etoposide for treating the hypereosinophilic syndrome. *Ann Intern Med* 1994; **121:** 899–900.

**Malignant neoplasms.** Etoposide has been used for a variety of solid tumours: in particular it is part of curative regimens used in the treatment of testicular cancer and germ-cell tumours of the ovary (see p.523 and p.520), and is used with cisplatin and other drugs in the treatment of lung cancer (p.519). Other solid neoplasms in which it is sometimes employed include those of the brain (p.513), stomach (p.516), and thymus (p.523), as well as in neuroblastoma (p.524), Wilms' tumour (p.518), retinoblastoma (p.524), and rhabdomyosarcoma (p.525); it has also formed part of systemic regimens for bone sarcomas (p.524), disseminated Kaposi's sarcoma (see p.524), and gestational trophoblastic tumours (p.505). Etoposide is used in regimens for Hodgkin's disease (see p.509); it is also sometimes used in aggressive intermediate- and high-grade non-Hodgkin's lymphomas (p.510), and may produce short-term responses in mycosis fungoides (p.511). It is also used in Burkitt's lymphoma (p.511). Etoposide may have benefits when added to induction protocols for acute myeloid leukaemia (p.506), and when used as part of intensification therapy in acute lymphoblastic leukaemia (p.506). It has formed part of salvage regimens in multiple myeloma (p.511).

**Vasculitic syndromes.** For mention of the use of etoposide to induce remission in patients with Wegener's granulomatosis resistant to standard therapy with cyclophosphamide and corticosteroids, see p.1090.

## Preparations

***BP 2003:*** Etoposide Capsules; Etoposide Intravenous Infusion;
***USP 27:*** Etoposide Capsules; Etoposide Injection.

**Proprietary Preparations** (details are given in Part 3)
***Arg.:*** Citodox; Etocris; Etopofos; Euvaxon; Labimion; Neoplaxol; Optasid; Percas; Vepesid; VP-Gen; ***Austral.:*** Etopophos; Vepesid; ***Austria:*** Abiposid†; Etopofos; Exitop†; Vepesid; ***Belg.:*** Etopophos; Vepesid; ***Braz.:*** Eposido; Etopos; Etopul; Etosin; Eunades; Nexvep; Vepesid; ***Canad.:*** Vepesid; ***Chile:*** Epsidox; Lastet; ***Denm.:*** Eposid†; Etopofos; Vepesid; ***Fin.:*** Eposin; Etopofos; Exitop; Vepesid; ***Fr.:*** Celltop; Etopophos; Vepeside; ***Ger.:*** ETO CS; Eto-Gry; Etomedac; Etopophos; Exitop; Onkoposid; Riboposid; Vepesid; ***Gr.:*** Vepesid; ***Hong Kong:*** Vepesid; ***India:*** Etosid; Lastet; ***Irl.:*** Etopophos; Vepesid; ***Israel:*** Etopophos; Vepesid; ***Ital.:*** Lastet; Vepesid; ***Jpn:*** Lastet; ***Malaysia:*** Eposin; Vepesid; ***Mex.:*** Etopos; Kenazol; Lastet; Seroposide†; Vepesid; VP-Tec†; ***Neth.:*** Etopophos†; Vepesid; ***Norw.:*** Eposin; Etopofos; Vepesid; ***NZ:*** Etopophos; Vepesid; ***Port.:*** Lastet†; Vepesid; ***S.Afr.:*** Eposin; Etopophos; Vepesid; ***Singapore:*** Vepesid; ***Spain:*** Eposin; Lastet; Vepesid; ***Swed.:*** Eposin; Etopofos; Exitop; Vepesid; ***Switz.:*** Etopophos; Vepesid; ***Thai.:*** Eposin; Fytosid; Vepesid; ***UK:*** Eposin; Etopophos; Vepesid; ***USA:*** Etopophos; Toposar; Vepesid.

# Exemestane *(BAN, USAN, rINN)*

Exemestano; FCE-24304. 6-Methyleneandrosta-1,4-diene-3,17-dione.

$C_{20}H_{24}O_2$ = 296.4.
*CAS — 107868-30-4.*
*ATC — L02BG06.*

## Adverse Effects and Precautions

The most frequently reported adverse effects for exemestane are gastrointestinal disturbances, hot flushes, sweating, fatigue, and dizziness. Other reported effects include headache, insomnia, depression, skin rashes, alopecia, and peripheral and leg oedema. Thrombocytopenia and leucopenia have been reported occasionally.

The use of exemestane is contra-indicated in premenopausal women (particularly in pregnancy).

## Pharmacokinetics

Exemestane is rapidly absorbed from the gastrointestinal tract. Its bioavailability is limited by first-pass metabolism, but is increased when taken with food. Exemestane is widely distributed, and is extensively bound to plasma proteins. It is cleared from the circulation mainly by metabolism; metabolites are excreted in the urine and faeces, and less than 1% of a dose is excreted unchanged in the urine. Exemestane has a terminal elimination half-life of about 24 hours.

## Uses and Administration

Exemestane is a selective inhibitor of the aromatase (oestrogen synthase) system, similar to formestane (p.557). It is used in the treatment of advanced breast cancer (p.514), in postmenopausal women who are no longer responsive to anti-oestrogen therapy. The recommended dose is 25 mg daily by mouth, preferably after a meal.

◊ References.

1. Clemett D, Lamb HM. Exemestane: a review of its use in postmenopausal women with advanced breast cancer. *Drugs* 2000; **59:** 1279–96.
2. Kaufmann M, *et al.* Exemestane is superior to megestrol acetate after tamoxifen failure in postmenopausal women with advanced breast cancer: results of a phase III randomized double-blind trial. *J Clin Oncol* 2000; **18:** 1399–1411.
3. Lønning PE, *et al.* Activity of exemestane in metastatic breast cancer after failure of nonsteroidal aromatase inhibitors: a phase II trial. *J Clin Oncol* 2000; **18:** 2234–44.
4. Coombes RC, *et al.* A randomized trial of exemestane after two to three years of tamoxifen therapy in postmenopausal women with primary breast cancer. *N Engl J Med* 2004; **350:** 1081–92.

## Preparations

**Proprietary Preparations** (details are given in Part 3)
***Arg.:*** Aromasin; ***Austral.:*** Aromasin; ***Austria:*** Aromasin; ***Belg.:*** Aromasin; ***Braz.:*** Aromasin; ***Canad.:*** Aromasin; ***Chile:*** Aromasin; ***Denm.:*** Aromasin; ***Fin.:*** Aromasin; ***Fr.:*** Aromasine; ***Ger.:*** Aromasin; ***Gr.:*** Aromacin; ***Hong Kong:*** Aromasin; ***Irl.:*** Aromasin; ***Israel:*** Aromasin; ***Ital.:*** Aromasin; ***Neth.:*** Aromasin; ***Norw.:*** Aromasin; ***Port.:*** Aromasin; ***Singapore:*** Aromasin; ***Spain:*** Aromasil; ***Swed.:*** Aromasin; ***Switz.:*** Aromasin; ***Thai.:*** Aromasin; ***UK:*** Aromasin; ***USA:*** Aromasin.

# Exisulind *(rINN)*

FGN-1; Sulindac Sulfone. 5-Fluoro-2-methyl-1-[(*Z*)-*p*-(methylsulfonyl)benzylidene]indene-3-acetic acid.

$C_{20}H_{17}FO_4S$ = 372.4.
*CAS — 59973-80-7.*

## Profile

Exisulind is a sulfone metabolite of sulindac (p.91) that is reported to induce apoptosis in cancerous and precancerous cells. It has been studied for the treatment of familial adenomatous polyposis, with variable results. It is also being investigated for the prevention and treatment of malignant neoplasms, including those of the breast, prostate, and lung.

◊ References.


1. Stoner GD, *et al.* Sulindac sulfone induced regression of rectal polyps in patients with familial adenomatous polyposis. *Adv Exp Med Biol* 1999; **470:** 45–53.
2. van Stolk R, *et al.* Phase I trial of exisulind (sulindac sulfone, FGN-1) as a chemopreventive agent in patients with familial adenomatous polyposis. *Clin Cancer Res* 2000; **6:** 78–89.
3. Goluboff ET, *et al.* Safety and efficacy of exisulind for treatment of recurrent prostate cancer after radical prostatectomy. *J Urol (Baltimore)* 2001; **166:** 882–6.
4. Goluboff ET. Exisulind, a selective apoptotic antineoplastic drug. *Expert Opin Invest Drugs* 2001; **10:** 1875–82.
5. Pusztai L, *et al.* Phase I and II study of exisulind in combination with capecitabine in patients with metastatic breast cancer. *J Clin Oncol* 2003; **21:** 3454–61.


## Fadrozole Hydrochloride *(USAN, rINNM)*

CGS-16949 (fadrozole); CGS-16949A; Hidrocloruro de fadrozol. (±)-*p*-(5,6,7,8-Tetrahydroimidazo[1,5-*a*]pyridin-5-yl)benzonitrile monohydrochloride.

$C_{14}H_{13}N_3HCl = 259.7$.

*CAS — 102676-47-1 (fadrozole); 102676-96-0 (fadrozole hydrochloride).*

### Profile

Fadrozole hydrochloride is a selective nonsteroidal inhibitor of the aromatase (oestrogen synthetase) system, similar to anastrozole (p.528). It is used for the treatment of breast cancer. It has been given in doses of 1 mg twice daily by mouth.

◊ References.


1. Buzdar AU, *et al.* Fadrozole HCl (CGS-16949A) versus megestrol acetate treatment of postmenopausal patients with metastatic breast carcinoma: results of two randomized double blind controlled multiinstitutional trials. *Cancer* 1996; **77:** 2503–13.
2. Miller AA, *et al.* Fadrozole hydrochloride in postmenopausal patients with metastatic breast carcinoma. *Cancer* 1996; **78:** 789–93.
3. Falkson CI, Falkson HC. A randomised study of CGS 16949A (fadrozole) versus tamoxifen in previously untreated postmenopausal patients with metastatic breast cancer. *Ann Oncol* 1996; **7:** 465–9.
4. Thurlimann B, *et al.* First-line fadrozole HCl (CGS 16949A) versus tamoxifen in postmenopausal women with advanced breast cancer: prospective randomised trial of the Swiss Group for Clinical Cancer Research SAKK 20/88. *Ann Oncol* 1996; **7:** 471–9.


## Fenretinide *(USAN, rINN)*

Fenretinida; 4-HPR; 4-Hydroxyphenylretinamide; McN-R-1967. *all-trans*-4′-Hydroxyretinanilide.

$C_{26}H_{33}NO_2 = 391.5$.

*CAS — 65646-68-6.*

### Profile

Fenretinide is a retinoid derivative that is given by mouth and is being studied in the management of breast and prostate cancer and some other malignancies. It has also been tried in oral lichen planus and leucoplakia. Fenretinide has been investigated in the treatment of psoriasis, but was associated with unacceptable adverse effects such as night blindness and severe toxic erythema.

◊ Fenretinide has been studied for the treatment of breast cancer and cutaneous malignancies but early results were disappointing and night blindness and mucocutaneous effects have been associated with this use.[1] Fenretinide has been investigated for the prevention of breast cancer (p.515), but a large randomised study of secondary prevention failed to show any benefit.[2] A follow-up of the same study[3] found that patients receiving fenretinide had a lower incidence of ovarian carcinoma during the 5-year treatment period, but that this apparently protective effect disappeared after treatment was discontinued. Combinations of tamoxifen and fenretinide, given intermittently (for treatment or prevention), have been reported to be well tolerated.[4,5]


1. Modiano MR, *et al.* Phase II study of fenretinide (N-[4-hydroxyphenyl]retinamide) in advanced breast cancer and melanoma. *Invest New Drugs* 1990; **8:** 317–19.
2. Veronesi U, *et al.* Randomized trial of fenretinide to prevent second breast malignancy in women with early breast cancer. *J Natl Cancer Inst* 1999; **91:** 1847–56.
3. De Palo G, *et al.* Effect of fenretinide on ovarian carcinoma occurrence. *Gynecol Oncol* 2002; **86:** 24–7.
4. Cobleigh MA, *et al.* Phase I/II trial of tamoxifen with or without fenretinide, an analog of vitamin A, in women with metastatic breast cancer. *J Clin Oncol* 1993; **11:** 474–7.
5. Conley B, *et al.* Pilot trial of the safety, tolerability, and retinoid levels of N-(4-hydroxyphenyl) retinamide in combination with tamoxifen in patients at high risk for developing invasive breast cancer. *J Clin Oncol* 2000; **18:** 275–83.


## Floxuridine *(USAN, rINN)*

Floxuridina; 5-Fluorouracil Deoxyriboside; FUDR; NSC-27640; WR-138720. 2′-Deoxy-5-fluorouridine; 5-Fluoro-2′-deoxyuridine; 1-(2-Deoxy-β-D-ribofuranosyl)-5-fluoropyrimidine-2,4(1*H*,3*H*)-dione.

$C_9H_{11}FN_2O_5 = 246.2$.

*CAS — 50-91-9.*

**Pharmacopoeias.** In *US.*

**USP 27** (Floxuridine). Store in airtight containers. Protect from light.

### Adverse Effects, Treatment, and Precautions

As for Fluorouracil, p.554. Adverse reactions following intra-arterial infusion commonly include local reactions, thromboembolic complications, and infection or bleeding at the catheter site, or blockage of the catheter. Erythema, stomatitis, and gastrointestinal disturbances are relatively common. There have also been signs of liver dysfunction.

**Effects on the liver.** Serious biliary toxicity has been reported in over half of all patients receiving hepatic arterial infusions of floxuridine, usually manifesting as sclerosing cholangitis or acalculous cholecystitis;[1] as a result some surgeons routinely remove the gallbladder at the time of infusion pump implantation.[2] Extrahepatic biliary stenosis with jaundice and cholestasis has also been described;[3] the authors suggest that this could lead to intrahepatic biliary damage from bile stasis and infection, recurrent cholangitis, and biliary sclerosis. Floxuridine infusions have also been associated with a case of fatal progressive cirrhosis of the liver in the absence of overt cholestasis.[4]


1. Sherlock S. The spectrum of hepatotoxicity due to drugs. *Lancet* 1986; **ii:** 440–4.
2. Anonymous. An implanted infusion pump for chemotherapy of liver metastases. *Med Lett Drugs Ther* 1984; **26:** 89–90.
3. Aldrighetti L, *et al.* Extrahepatic biliary stenoses after hepatic arterial infusion (HAI) of floxuridine (FUdR) for liver metastases from colorectal cancer. *Hepatogastroenterology* 2001; **48:** 1302–7.
4. Pettavel J, *et al.* Fatal liver cirrhosis associated with long-term arterial infusion of floxuridine. *Lancet* 1986; **ii:** 1162–3.


### Interactions

As for Fluorouracil, p.555.

### Pharmacokinetics

Floxuridine is poorly absorbed from the gastrointestinal tract and it is usually given by injection. Floxuridine is metabolised mainly in the liver to fluorouracil following rapid injection. When given by slow intra-arterial infusion, more of the drug is metabolised to floxuridine monophosphate (F-dUMP). It is excreted as carbon dioxide via the lungs; some is excreted, as unchanged drug and metabolites, in urine. Floxuridine crosses the blood-brain barrier to some extent and is found in CSF.

### Uses and Administration

Floxuridine is an antineoplastic which acts as an antimetabolite, either by conversion to fluorouracil (after rapid injection), or, when given by slow intra-arterial infusion, partly via floxuridine monophosphate (F-dUMP), which produces greater inhibition of DNA synthesis.

Floxuridine is used in the palliative treatment of hepatic metastases of colorectal cancer—see Malignant Neoplasms of the Liver, p.518. It has been tried in some other solid neoplasms. Doses of 100 to 600 micrograms/kg daily are given by continuous hepatic arterial infusion, usually with the aid of an infusion pump, until toxicity occurs.

White cell and platelet counts should be carried out regularly during therapy and treatment should be stopped if the white cell count falls rapidly or if the white cell or platelet count falls below acceptable levels (see also Bone-marrow Depression, p.496), or if major adverse effects occur.

◊ References.


1. Fordy C, *et al.* Hepatic arterial floxuridine as second-line treatment for systemic fluorouracil-resistant colorectal liver metastases. *Br J Cancer* 1998; **78:** 1058–60.
2. Kemeny N, *et al.* Hepatic arterial infusion of chemotherapy after resection of hepatic metastases from colorectal cancer. *N Engl J Med* 1999; **341:** 2039–48.
3. Lorenz M, Muller HH. Randomized, multicenter trial of fluorouracil plus leucovorin administered either via hepatic arterial or intravenous infusion versus fluorodeoxyuridine administered via hepatic arterial infusion in patients with nonresectable liver metastases from colorectal carcinoma. *J Clin Oncol* 2000; **18:** 243–54.
4. Fiorentini G, *et al.* Locoregional therapy for liver metastases from colorectal cancer: the possibilities of intraarterial chemotherapy, and new hepatic-directed modalities. *Hepatogastroenterology* 2001; **48:** 305–12.


### Preparations

***USP 27:*** Floxuridine for Injection.

**Proprietary Preparations** (details are given in Part 3)
***Singapore:*** FUDR†; ***USA:*** FUDR.

## Fludarabine Phosphate *(BAN, USAN, rINNM)*

2-F-ara-AMP; Fludarabine Monophosphate; 2-Fluoro-ara-AMP; Fosfato de fludarabina; NSC-312887. 9-β-D-Arabinofuranosyl-2-fluoroadenine 5′-dihydrogenphosphate.

$C_{10}H_{13}FN_5O_7P = 365.2$.

*CAS — 21679-14-1 (fludarabine); 75607-67-9 (fludarabine phosphate).*

*ATC — L01BB05.*

**Pharmacopoeias.** In *US.*

**USP 27** (Fludarabine Phosphate). A white to off-white, hygroscopic, crystalline powder. Slightly soluble in water and in 0.1M hydrochloric acid; practically insoluble in dehydrated alcohol; freely soluble in dimethylformamide. Store at 2° to 8°. Protect from light.

### Adverse Effects, Treatment, and Precautions

For general discussions see Antineoplastics, p.492, p.495, and p.497.

Bone-marrow suppression from fludarabine is dose-limiting, manifesting as neutropenia, thrombocytopenia, and anaemia; the nadir of the white cell and platelet counts usually occurs after about 13 to 16 days. Myelosuppression can be severe and cumulative; prolonged lymphopenia with concomitant risk of opportunistic infections may occur.

Other adverse effects include fever, chills, cough, dyspnoea, pneumonia, gastrointestinal disturbances, stomatitis, oedema, the tumour lysis syndrome, skin rashes, haemolytic anaemia, haemorrhagic cystitis, and neurological disturbances including peripheral neuropathy, agitation, confusion, visual disturbances, and coma. High doses have been associated with progressive encephalopathy, blindness, and death.

Dosage should be reduced in renal impairment and fludarabine should not be given if creatinine clearance is less than 30 mL/minute (see below). It should also be avoided in patients with decompensated haemolytic anaemia.

**Carcinogenicity.** A study in patients with chronic lymphocytic leukaemia who were treated with fludarabine found that there was no significantly increased risk of secondary malignancy following therapy, despite the immunosuppressive properties of this drug.[1] A review[2] of this and other studies concluded that no significant increase in the risk of secondary malignancy has been demonstrated, but also that long-term follow-up of patients treated with fludarabine is needed.


1. Cheson BD, *et al.* Second malignancies as a consequence of nucleoside analog therapy for chronic lymphoid leukaemias. *J Clin Oncol* 1999; **17:** 2454–60.
2. Van Den Neste E, *et al.* Second primary tumors and immune phenomena after fludarabine or 2-chloro-2′-deoxyadenosine treatment. *Leuk Lymphoma* 2001; **40:** 541–50.


**Effects on the lungs.** Pulmonary toxicity manifest as dyspnoea, fever, hypoxaemia, and radiographic evidence of interstitial and alveolar infiltrates was diagnosed in 9 patients of a cohort of 105 treated with fludarabine.[1] Lung biopsies were performed in 6 patients and showed diffuse chronic interstitial inflammation and fibrosis. Patients with chronic lymphocytic leukaemia appeared to be at greater risk of developing this complication than those with non-Hodgkin's lymphoma.


1. Helman DL, *et al.* Fludarabine-related pulmonary toxicity: a distinct clinical entity in chronic lymphoproliferative syndromes. *Chest* 2002; **122:** 785–90.


**Effects on the nervous system.** High doses (of the order of 100 mg/m$^2$ daily intravenously) of fludarabine are associated with severe, life-threatening neurotoxicity. However, a few cases of progressive multifocal leukoencephalopathy have also been reported in patients who had received fludarabine in usual doses.[1-4] The prolonged immunosuppression caused by fludarabine might increase the risk of developing this fatal demyelinating disease, which is caused by opportunistic JC virus infection.


1. Zabernigg A, *et al.* Late-onset fatal neurological toxicity of fludarabine. *Lancet* 1994; **344:** 1780.
2. Gonzalez H, *et al.* Progressive multifocal leukoencephalitis (PML) in three patients treated with standard-dose fludarabine (FAMP). *Hematol Cell Ther* 1999; **41:** 183–6.
3. Cid J, *et al.* Progressive multifocal leukoencephalopathy following oral fludarabine treatment of chronic lymphocytic leukemia. *Ann Hematol* 2000; **79:** 392–5.
4. Vidarsson B, *et al.* Progressive multifocal leukoencephalopathy after fludarabine therapy for low-grade lymphoproliferative disease. *Am J Hematol* 2002; **70:** 51–4.


**Graft-versus-host disease.** Transfusion-associated graft-versus-host disease has been reported following administration of blood products in patients treated with fludarabine.[1] Fludarabine-treated patients should receive irradiated red cells and platelets (to inactivate any viable T-cells) if they require a transfusion.


1. Williamson LM, *et al.* Fludarabine treatment and transfusion-associated graft-versus-host disease. *Lancet* 1996; **348:** 472–3.


**Infection.** A review[1] of patients treated with fludarabine-containing regimens showed that therapy was associated with a variety of serious infections including listeriosis, *Pneumocystis carinii* pneumonia, mycobacterial infections, and opportunistic fungal and viral infections. The risk was exacerbated by previous or concomitant corticosteroid therapy. Prophylactic therapy with co-trimoxazole, triazole antifungals, aciclovir, and colony-stimulating factors was recommended in at-risk patients. A high incidence of herpesvirus infections was also found in another review[2] of patients treated with fludarabine. In another study,[3] combination therapy using chlorambucil and fludarabine resulted in more infections than when either was used alone, but single-agent fludarabine was associated with more major infections and herpesvirus infections than chlorambucil alone. The frequency of serious infection has also been reported[4] to be increased in patients after their conditions became refractory to fludarabine and they were being treated with conventional chemotherapy.

For reports of progressive multifocal leukoencephalopathy caused by opportunistic JC virus infection, see Effects on the Nervous System, above.


1. Anaissie EJ, *et al.* Infections in patients with chronic lymphocytic leukemia treated with fludarabine. *Ann Intern Med* 1998; **129:** 559–66.
2. Byrd JC, *et al.* Herpes virus infections occur frequently following treatment with fludarabine: results of a prospective natural history study. *Br J Haematol* 1999; **105:** 445–7.
3. Morrison VA, *et al.* Impact of therapy with chlorambucil, fludarabine, or fludarabine plus chlorambucil on infections in patients with chronic lymphocytic leukemia: Intergroup Study Cancer and Leukemia Group B 9011. *J Clin Oncol* 2001; **19:** 3611–21.
4. Perkins JG, *et al.* Frequency and type of serious infections in fludarabine-refractory B-cell chronic lymphocytic leukemia and small lymphocytic lymphoma: implications for clinical trials in this patient population. *Cancer* 2002; **94:** 2033–9.


## Interactions

Increased pulmonary toxicity, including fatalities, has been reported in patients given fludarabine with pentostatin. Cytarabine may reduce the metabolic activation of fludarabine but use together results in increased intracellular concentrations of cytarabine—see p.543. The therapeutic efficacy of fludarabine may also be reduced by dipyridamole and other inhibitors of adenosine uptake.

**Aminoglycosides.** Severe ototoxicity occurred when a short course of *gentamicin* was given to a patient who had recently completed a course of fludarabine.[1]


1. O'Brien RK, Sparling TG. Gentamicin and fludarabine ototoxicity. *Ann Pharmacother* 1995; **29:** 200–1.


**Corticosteroids.** For a suggestion that use of fludarabine with corticosteroids may increase the risk of infection, see above.

## Pharmacokinetics

Intravenous fludarabine phosphate is rapidly dephosphorylated to fludarabine which is taken up by lymphocytes and rephosphorylated to the active triphosphate nucleotide. Peak intracellular concentrations of fludarabine triphosphate are seen about 4 hours after a dose. Fludarabine has a bioavailability of about 50 to 65% after doses of the phosphate by mouth.

Clearance of fludarabine from the plasma is triphasic with a terminal half-life of about 20 hours. Elimination is mostly via renal excretion: 60% of a dose is excreted in the urine. The pharmacokinetics of fludarabine exhibit considerable interindividual variation.

◊ References.


1. Johnson SA. Clinical pharmacokinetics of nucleoside analogues: focus on haematological malignancies. *Clin Pharmacokinet* 2000; **39:** 5–26.
2. Gandhi V, Plunkett W. Cellular and clinical pharmacology of fludarabine. *Clin Pharmacokinet* 2002; **41:** 93–103.


## Uses and Administration

Fludarabine is a fluorinated nucleotide analogue of the antiviral vidarabine (p.657); it acts as a purine antagonist antimetabolite. It is used for its antineoplastic properties in the treatment of chronic lymphocytic leukaemia. Fludarabine phosphate is given by bolus injection or by intravenous infusion over 30 minutes in a usual dose of 25 mg/m$^2$ daily for 5 consecutive days. Alternatively it may be given by mouth in a dose of 40 mg/m$^2$ daily for 5 consecutive days. Courses may be repeated every 28 days, usually for up to 6 cycles.

Haematological function should be monitored regularly; the dosage may need to be reduced, or further courses delayed, if blood counts indicate severe or persistent myelosuppression (see also Bone-marrow Depression, p.496). Doses should be reduced in renal impairment (see below).

◊ General references.


1. Adkins JC, *et al.* Fludarabine: an update of its pharmacology and use in the treatment of haematological malignancies. *Drugs* 1997; **53:** 1005–37.
2. Plosker GL, Figgitt DP. Oral fludarabine. *Drugs* 2003; **63:** 2317–23.


**Administration in renal impairment.** Doses of fludarabine phosphate should be reduced by up to 50% in patients with mild to moderate renal impairment (creatinine clearance between 30 and 70 mL/minute); the drug should not be given in more severe renal impairment.

**Malignant neoplasms.** Fludarabine is the preferred second-line therapy for chronic lymphocytic leukaemia once initial alkylating agent therapy fails,[1] and may also be used for initial therapy (see p.507). It has also been tried in other malignancies. Listed below are some references to the use of fludarabine phosphate for the treatment of chronic lymphocytic leukaemia,[2,3] and its potential activity against a variety of other malignancies, including indolent low-grade non-Hodgkin's lymphoma[4] (p.510), mycosis fungoides,[5] heavy chain disease,[6] prolymphocytic leukaemia,[7,8] hairy cell leukaemia,[9] and Waldenström's macroglobulinaemia.[10,11]


1. National Institute for Clinical Excellence. Guidance on the use of fludarabine for B-cell chronic lymphocytic leukaemia (issued September 2001). Available at: http://www.nice.org.uk/pdf/NICEfludarab_E_29guidance.pdf (accessed 29/06/04)
2. Keating MJ, *et al.* Clinical experience with fludarabine in leukaemia. *Drugs* 1994; **47** (suppl 6): 39–49.
3. French Cooperative Group on CLL, *et al.* Multicentre prospective randomised trial of fludarabine versus cyclophosphamide, doxorubicin, and prednisone (CAP) for treatment of advanced-stage chronic lymphocytic leukaemia. *Lancet* 1996; **347:** 1432–8.
4. Hiddemann W, Pott-Hoeck C. Fludarabine in the management of malignant lymphomas. *Drugs* 1994; **47** (suppl 6): 50–6.
5. Scarisbrick JJ, *et al.* A trial of fludarabine and cyclophosphamide combination chemotherapy in the treatment of advanced refractory primary cutaneous T-cell lymphoma. *Br J Dermatol* 2001; **144:** 1010–15.
6. Agrawal S, *et al.* First report of fludarabine in gamma-heavy chain disease. *Br J Haematol* 1994; **88:** 653–5.
7. Smith OP, Mehta AB. Fludarabine monophosphate for prolymphocytic leukaemia. *Lancet* 1990; **336:** 820.
8. Kantarjian HM, *et al.* Efficacy of fludarabine, a new adenine nucleoside analogue, in patients with prolymphocytic leukemia and the prolymphocytoid variant of chronic lymphocytic leukemia. *Am J Med* 1991; **90:** 223–8.
9. Kantarjian HM, *et al.* Fludarabine therapy in hairy cell leukemia. *Cancer* 1991; **67:** 1291–3.
10. Dhodapkar MV, *et al.* Prognostic factors and response to fludarabine therapy in patients with Waldenström macroglobulinemia: results of United States intergroup trial (Southwest Oncology Group S9003). *Blood* 2001; **98:** 41–8.
11. Leblond V, *et al.* Multicenter, randomized comparative trial of fludarabine and the combination of cyclophosphamide-doxorubicin-prednisone in 92 patients with Waldenström macroglobulinemia in first relapse or with primary refractory disease. *Blood* 2001; **98:** 2640–4.


## Preparations

*USP 27:* Fludarabine Phosphate for Injection.

**Proprietary Preparations** (details are given in Part 3)
***Arg.:*** Fludara; Forclina; ***Austral.:*** Fludara; ***Austria:*** Fludara; ***Belg.:*** Fludara; ***Braz.:*** Fludara; ***Canad.:*** Fludara; ***Chile:*** Fludara; ***Denm.:*** Fludara; ***Fin.:*** Fludara; ***Fr.:*** Fludara; ***Ger.:*** Fludara; ***Gr.:*** Fludara; ***Hong Kong:*** Fludara; ***Irl.:*** Fludara; ***Israel:*** Fludara; ***Ital.:*** Fludara; ***Malaysia:*** Fludara; ***Mex.:*** Fludara; ***Neth.:*** Fludara; ***Norw.:*** Fludara; ***NZ:*** Fludara; ***Port.:*** Fludara; ***S.Afr.:*** Fludara; ***Singapore:*** Fludara; ***Spain:*** Beneflur; ***Swed.:*** Fludara; ***Switz.:*** Fludara; ***Thai.:*** Fludara; ***UK:*** Fludara; ***USA:*** Fludara.

# Fluorouracil *(BAN, USAN, rINN)*

5-Fluoracil; Fluorouracilo; Fluorouracilum; 5-FU; NSC-19893; Ro-2-9757; WR-69596. 5-Fluoropyrimidine-2,4(1*H*,3*H*)-dione.

$C_4H_3FN_2O_2$ = 130.1.

*CAS — 51-21-8.*

*ATC — L01BC02.*

**Pharmacopoeias.** In *Chin., Eur.* (see p.vi), *Int., Jpn, Pol.,* and *US.*

**Ph. Eur. 5.0** (Fluorouracil). A white or almost white, crystalline powder. Sparingly soluble in water; slightly soluble in alcohol. A 1% solution in water has a pH of 4.5 to 5.0. Protect from light.

**USP 27** (Fluorouracil). A white to practically white, practically odourless, crystalline powder. Sparingly soluble in water; slightly soluble in alcohol; practically insoluble in chloroform and in ether. Store in airtight containers. Protect from light.

**Incompatibility.** Preparations of fluorouracil are alkaline, and compatibility problems may be expected with acidic drugs and preparations, or those which are unstable in the presence of alkali. Fluorouracil is reported to be incompatible with cytarabine,[1] diazepam,[2] doxorubicin[2] (and presumably other anthracyclines that are unstable at alkaline pH), and calcium folinate.[3] Although fluorouracil has been stated to be incompatible with methotrexate[1] a study of the long-term stability of an admixture of the 2 drugs in sodium chloride 0.9% injection suggests otherwise.[4]


1. McRae MP, King JC. Compatibility of antineoplastic, antibiotic and corticosteroid drugs in intravenous admixtures. *Am J Hosp Pharm* 1976; **33:** 1010–13.
2. Dorr RT. Incompatibilities with parenteral anticancer drugs. *Am J Intravenous Ther* 1979; **6:** 42–52.
3. Trissel LA, *et al.* Incompatibility of fluorouracil with leucovorin calcium or levoleucovorin calcium. *Am J Health-Syst Pharm* 1995; **52:** 710–15.
4. Vincké BJ, *et al.* Extended stability of 5-fluorouracil and methotrexate solutions in PVC containers. *Int J Pharmaceutics* 1989; **54:** 181–9.


**Stability.** Despite one report[1] that fluorouracil had limited stability when dissolved in glucose 5% at room temperature (10% loss from solution in 43 hours when stored in PVC and in only 7 hours when stored in glass), others[2] found such a solution to be stable for at least 16 weeks when stored in PVC at 5°. When stored at room temperature in PVC, solutions of fluorouracil may lose water by evaporation, which slowly increases their concentration.[2,3] Results of a study of fluorouracil and methotrexate admixtures in sodium chloride 0.9% suggest that extended stability (up to 13 weeks) is possible in this diluent at 5° in PVC bags.[3] Commercial solutions of fluorouracil for injection have been reported to be stable for 7 days at 37° in a portable infusion pump, although at 25° one brand showed evidence of precipitation.[4] Fluorouracil solutions may be incompatible with synthetic elastomers: microscopic precipitation has been reported as soon as 4 hours after placement into polyisoprene reservoirs of elastomeric infusers and in polypropylene syringes with an elastomeric joint.[5] Some have questioned the validity of this finding.[6,7]


1. Benvenuto JA, *et al.* Stability and compatibility of antitumor agents in glass and plastic containers. *Am J Hosp Pharm* 1981; **38:** 1914–18.
2. Quebbeman EJ, *et al.* Stability of fluorouracil in plastic containers used for continuous infusion at home. *Am J Hosp Pharm* 1984; **41:** 1153–6.
3. Vincké B, *et al.* Extended stability of 5-fluorouracil and methotrexate solutions in PVC containers. *Int J Pharmaceutics* 1989; **54:** 181–9.
4. Stiles ML, *et al.* Stability of fluorouracil administered through four portable infusion pumps. *Am J Hosp Pharm* 1989; **46:** 2036–40.
5. Corbrion V, *et al.* Precipitation of fluorouracil in elastomeric infusers with a polyisoprene reservoir and in polypropylene syringes with an elastomeric joint. *Am J Health-Syst Pharm* 1997; **54:** 1845–8.
6. Trissel LA. Fluorouracil precipitate. *Am J Health-Syst Pharm* 1998; **55:** 1314–15.
7. Allwood MC. Fluorouracil precipitate. *Am J Health-Syst Pharm* 1998; **55;** 1315–16.


## Adverse Effects and Treatment

For general discussions see Antineoplastics, p.492 and p.495.

The main adverse effects of fluorouracil are on the bone marrow and the gastrointestinal tract, and may be dose-limiting. Toxicity is schedule dependent: reducing the rate of injection to a slow infusion is associated with less haematological toxicity but does not decrease gastrointestinal toxicity. With protracted continuous infusion in particular, the palmar-plantar erythrodysesthesia syndrome (erythema and painful desquamation of the hands and feet) may occur. Gastrointestinal toxicity may be exacerbated if fluorouracil is given with folinic acid.

Leucopenia, thrombocytopenia, stomatitis, gastrointestinal ulceration and bleeding, diarrhoea, or haemorrhage from any site, are signs that treatment should be stopped. The nadir of the white cell count may occur from 7 to 20 days after a dose, and counts usually return to normal after about 30 days. Thrombocytopenia is usually at a maximum 7 to 17 days after a dose. Anaemia may also occur. Nausea and vomiting, rashes, and alopecia are common. Ocular irritation, central neurotoxicity (notably cerebellar ataxia), and myocardial ischaemia have occurred.

Local inflammatory and photosensitivity reactions have occurred following topical use. Dermatitis and, rarely, erythema multiforme have been reported.

**Effects on the eyes.** Systemic fluorouracil therapy has been associated with various types of ocular toxicity including several cases of excessive lachrymation and watering of the eyes,[1] in one patient associated with symptoms suggesting fibrosis of the tear duct,[1] and possibly representing local irritation due to the presence of fluorouracil in tear fluid[2] although symptoms have not always resolved on discontinuing the drug.[1] More seriously a case of bilateral total corneal epithelial erosion has been described.[3] Optic neuropathy, culminating in near blindness, has also occurred in a patient receiving fluorouracil as part of a combination regimen.[4] Severe ulceration and corneal abscess with hypopyon has followed local injection of fluorouracil into the eye in a diabetic patient with idiopathic band keratopathy.[5]


1. Haidak DJ, *et al.* Tear-duct fibrosis (dacryostenosis) due to 5-fluorouracil. *Ann Intern Med* 1978; **88:** 657.
2. Christophidis N, *et al.* Lacrimation and 5-fluorouracil. *Ann Intern Med* 1978; **89:** 574.
3. Hirsh A, *et al.* Bilateral total corneal epithelial erosion as a side effect of cytotoxic therapy. *Br J Ophthalmol* 1990; **74:** 638.
4. Adams JW, *et al.* Recurrent acute toxic optic neuropathy secondary to 5-FU. *Cancer Treat Rep* 1984; **68:** 565–6.
5. Hickey-Dwyer M, Wishart PK. Serious corneal complication of 5-fluorouracil. *Br J Ophthalmol* 1993; **77:** 250–1.


**Effects on the heart.** Life-threatening cardiotoxicity (arrhythmias, ventricular tachycardia, and cardiac arrest, secondary to transmural ischaemia) has been reported to occur in 0.55% of patients given fluorouracil,[1] although the incidence of angina and less severe cardiotoxicity associated with coronary artery spasm may be higher.[1-3] Possible risk factors include pre-existing heart disease or mediastinal radiotherapy and administration by prolonged infusion, but symptoms can also occur in patients without these risk factors.[2-4] Therefore, at present, it is not possible to reliably predict patients at risk.[5]


1. Keefe DL, *et al.* Clinical cardiotoxicity of 5-fluorouracil. *J Clin Pharmacol* 1993; **33:** 1060–70.
2. McLachlan SA, *et al.* The spectrum of 5-fluorouracil cardiotoxicity. *Med J Aust* 1994; **161:** 207–9.
3. Anand AJ. Fluorouracil cardiotoxicity. *Ann Pharmacother* 1994; **28:** 374–8.
4. Hannaford R. Sudden death associated with 5-fluorouracil. *Med J Aust* 1994; **161:** 225.
5. Becker K, *et al.* Cardiotoxicity of the antiproliferative compound fluorouracil. *Drugs* 1999; **57:** 475–84.

**Effects on the nervous system.** Central neurotoxicity, including cerebellar ataxia, confusion, disorientation, and emotional lability is reported to occur rarely in patients receiving fluorouracil, although the incidence may be increased with high-dose or intensive regimens. Patients with disorders of pyrimidine metabolism may be at increased risk of neurotoxicity.[1-3] It has also been suggested that fluorouracil may produce neurotoxicity by causing thiamine deficiency, and that thiamine may be used to treat it.[4]

1. Tuchman M, *et al.* Familial pyrimidinemia and pyrimidinuria associated with severe fluorouracil toxicity. *N Engl J Med* 1985; **313:** 245–9.
2. Stéphan F, *et al.* Depressed hepatic dihydropyrimidine dehydrogenase activity and fluorouracil-related toxicities. *Am J Med* 1995; **99:** 685–8.
3. Takimoto C, *et al.* Reversible 5-fluorouracil-associated encephalopathy in a dihydropyrimidine dehydrogenase (DPD) deficient patient. *Clin Pharmacol Ther* 1996; **59:** 161.
4. Pirzada NA, *et al.* Fluorouracil-induced neurotoxicity. *Ann Pharmacother* 2000; **34:** 35–8.

**Effects on the skin.** In addition to reports of fluorouracil-associated dermatitis and photosensitivity a syndrome of erythema, pain, and desquamation of the skin of palms and soles has been reported[1-4] (the palmar-plantar erythrodysesthesia syndrome, p.495). Although particularly associated with continuous infusion[1,2] the syndrome may also occur following bolus doses.[3,4] Symptoms generally respond to stopping the drug, but addition of oral pyridoxine to chemotherapy regimens has been reported to prevent or resolve symptoms,[5] as has application of a nicotine patch in one patient.[6]

Rash and confusion developing in an elderly man with malabsorption and poor nutritional intake who received fluorouracil for a biliary-tract tumour were diagnosed as pellagra.[7] Symptoms responded to nicotinic acid therapy.

1. Lokich JJ, Moore C. Chemotherapy-associated palmar-plantar erythrodysesthesia syndrome. *Ann Intern Med* 1984; **101:** 798–800.
2. Feldman LD, Ajani JA. Fluorouracil-associated dermatitis of the hands and feet. *JAMA* 1985; **254:** 3479.
3. Atkins JN. Fluorouracil and the palmar-plantar erythrodysesthesia syndrome. *Ann Intern Med* 1985; **102:** 419.
4. Curran CF, Luce JK. Fluorouracil and palmar-plantar erythrodysesthesia. *Ann Intern Med* 1989; **111:** 858.
5. Vukelja SJ, *et al.* Pyridoxine for the palmar-plantar erythrodysesthesia syndrome. *Ann Intern Med* 1989; **111:** 688–9.
6. Kingsley EC. 5-Fluorouracil dermatitis prophylaxis with a nicotine patch. *Ann Intern Med* 1994; **120:** 813.
7. Stevens HP, *et al.* Pellagra secondary to 5-fluorouracil. *Br J Dermatol* 1993; **128:** 578–80.

## Precautions

For general discussions see Antineoplastics, p.497.

Fluorouracil should be given with care to weak or malnourished patients, to those with a history of heart disease, or to those with hepatic or renal insufficiency. Patients with a history of high-dose pelvic irradiation or treatment with alkylating agents, and those with widespread metastases to the bone marrow should also be treated with extreme caution. Blood cell counts should be determined frequently during therapy.

Topical fluorouracil should not be used on mucous membranes. There is a possibility of increased absorption if used excessively or on ulcerated or inflamed skin. Occlusive dressings may increase inflammatory actions. Exposure to sunlight during treatment should be avoided. Creams are preferably applied using a non-metal applicator or gloved hand; if bare fingertips are used the hands must be washed immediately afterwards.

**Handling and disposal.** Fluorouracil is irritant; avoid contact with skin and mucous membranes.

*Urine and faeces* produced for up to 48 hours and 5 days respectively after an oral dose of fluorouracil should be handled wearing protective clothing.[1]

1. Harris J, Dodds LJ. Handling waste from patients receiving cytotoxic drugs. *Pharm J* 1985; **235:** 289–91.

**Metabolic disorders.** For reference to increased neurotoxicity in patients with a defect of pyrimidine metabolism given fluorouracil, see under Effects on the Nervous System, above.

## Interactions

For a general discussion of antineoplastic drug interactions, see p.498. The actions of fluorouracil may be modified by other drugs including allopurinol, cimetidine, folinic acid, methotrexate, and metronidazole (see also under Administration, below).

**Antineoplastics.** *Oxaliplatin*, which is given with fluorouracil and folinic acid in the treatment of colorectal cancer, reduced fluorouracil clearance in a study[1] of 29 patients with colorectal cancer. The effect was delayed and prolonged, lasting about 15 days, and an increase in toxicity correlated with raised fluorouracil concentrations. The mechanism of this interaction is unclear.

For reference to the effect of fluorouracil on the action of *paclitaxel*, see Antineoplastics, p.578. For the increased risk of haemolytic-uraemic syndrome that may be seen if fluorouracil is used with *mitomycin*, see Effects on the Kidneys, p.574.

1. Boisdron-Celle M, *et al.* Influence of oxaliplatin on 5-fluorouracil plasma clearance and clinical consequences. *Cancer Chemother Pharmacol* 2002; **49:** 235–43.

**Antiprotozoals.** *Metronidazole* increased the toxicity of fluorouracil in patients with colorectal cancer, apparently by reducing the clearance of the antineoplastic. No enhanced antineoplastic effect was seen with the combination *in vitro*.[1]

1. Bardakji Z, *et al.* 5-Fluorouracil–metronidazole combination therapy in metastatic colorectal cancer. *Cancer Chemother Pharmacol* 1986; **18:** 140–4.

**Antivirals.** Giving *interferon alfa-2b* with fluorouracil has produced a marked increase in the initial plasma concentration of fluorouracil and a decrease in fluorouracil clearance.[1]

Severe leucopenia, fatal in some cases, has been reported in patients given fluorouracil or fluorouracil prodrugs (such as tegafur) with *sorivudine*.[2,3] A metabolite of sorivudine appears to inhibit dihydropyrimidine dehydrogenase, the primary enzyme responsible for the inactivation of fluorouracil.[3]

1. Czejka MJ, *et al.* Clinical pharmacokinetics of 5-fluorouracil: influence of the biomodulating agents interferon, dipyridamole and folic acid alone and in combination. *Arzneimittelforschung* 1993; **43:** 387–90.
2. Yawata M. Deaths due to drug interaction. *Lancet* 1993; **342:** 1166.
3. Diasio RB. Sorivudine and 5-fluorouracil; a clinically significant drug-drug interaction due to inhibition of dihydropyrimidine dehydrogenase. *Br J Clin Pharmacol* 1998; **46:** 1–4.

**Gastrointestinal drugs.** Pretreatment with *cimetidine* for 4 weeks led to increased plasma concentrations of fluorouracil after intravenous and oral doses in 6 patients.[1] The effect was probably due to a combination of hepatic enzyme inhibition and reduced hepatic blood flow. No such effect was seen following single doses of cimetidine in 5 patients or pretreatment for just 1 week in 6. Care is required in patients taking both drugs simultaneously.

1. Harvey VJ, *et al.* The influence of cimetidine on the pharmacokinetics of 5-fluorouracil. *Br J Clin Pharmacol* 1984; **18:** 421–30.

## Pharmacokinetics

Absorption of fluorouracil from the gastrointestinal tract is unpredictable and fluorouracil is usually given intravenously. Little is absorbed when fluorouracil is applied to healthy skin.

After intravenous injection fluorouracil is cleared rapidly from plasma with a mean half-life of about 16 minutes. It is distributed throughout body tissues and fluids including crossing the blood-brain barrier to appear in the CSF, and disappears from the plasma within about 3 hours. Within the target cell fluorouracil is converted to 5-fluorouridine monophosphate and floxuridine monophosphate (5-fluorodeoxyuridine monophosphate), the former undergoing conversion to the triphosphate which can be incorporated into RNA while the latter inhibits thymidylate synthetase. About 15% of an intravenous dose is excreted unchanged in the urine within 6 hours. The remainder is inactivated primarily in the liver and is catabolised via dihydropyrimidine dehydrogenase similarly to endogenous uracil. A large amount is excreted as respiratory carbon dioxide; urea and other metabolites are also produced.

**Chronopharmacology.** The plasma concentrations of fluorouracil during continuous intravenous infusion are reported to undergo circadian variations of as much as 50% of the mean, peak concentrations occurring in the middle of the night.[1] The variation may be due to a circadian variation in the activity of the enzyme dihydropyrimidine dehydrogenase in blood,[2] but striking interpatient variations in peak concentrations of fluorouracil and peak enzyme activity suggest that any adjustment of infusion times would need to be individualised.[2] It has been suggested that pharmacokinetic monitoring should be investigated as a means of individualizing fluorouracil doses with the aim of improving efficacy and reducing toxicity.[3]

1. Petit E, *et al.* Circadian rhythm-varying plasma concentration of 5-fluorouracil during a five-day continuous venous infusion at a constant rate in cancer patients. *Cancer Res* 1988; **48:** 1676–9.
2. Harris BE, *et al.* Relationship between dihydropyrimidine dehydrogenase activity and plasma 5-fluorouracil levels with evidence for circadian variation of enzyme activity and plasma drug levels in cancer patients receiving 5-fluorouracil by protracted continuous infusion. *Cancer Res* 1990; **50:** 197–201.
3. Young AM, *et al.* Can pharmacokinetic monitoring improve clinical use of fluorouracil. *Clin Pharmacokinet* 1999; **36:** 391–8.

## Uses and Administration

Fluorouracil, an analogue of the pyrimidine uracil, is an antineoplastic that acts as an antimetabolite. After intracellular conversion to the active deoxynucleotide it interferes with the synthesis of DNA by blocking the conversion of deoxyuridylic acid to thymidylic acid by the cellular enzyme thymidylate synthetase. It can also interfere with RNA synthesis.

Fluorouracil is used alone or in combination in the adjuvant and palliative treatment of gastrointestinal cancer. In this setting it may be combined with folinic acid (see Administration, below). Fluorouracil is often used with cyclophosphamide and methotrexate or doxorubicin in the adjuvant treatment of breast cancer. It may also be used in the palliation of other malignant neoplasms such as those of the head and neck, liver, and pancreas. In addition, it may be used topically for treating malignant or premalignant lesions of the skin. Its use in these malignancies is further discussed under Choice of Antineoplastic as indicated by the cross-references given below.

A wide range of dosage regimens has been used. Although it is most often given in combination regimens for the treatment of malignancy many of the licensed dosage regimens relate to single-agent use. Such licensed regimens include:

- by *intravenous injection*, usual doses of 12 mg/kg daily (to a maximum of 0.8 to 1 g daily) for 3 or 4 days. If there is no evidence of toxicity, this may be followed after 1 day by 6 mg/kg on alternate days for 3 or 4 further doses. An alternative schedule is to give 15 mg/kg intravenously once a week throughout the course. The course may be repeated after 4 to 6 weeks or maintenance doses of 5 to 15 mg/kg to a maximum of 1 g may be given weekly.
- by *intravenous infusion*, usual doses of 15 mg/kg daily (to a maximum of 1 g daily) being infused in 500 mL of sodium chloride 0.9% or glucose 5% over 4 hours and repeated on successive days until toxicity occurs or a total of 12 to 15 g has been given. *Continuous infusion* may also be used. The course may be repeated after 4 to 6 weeks.
- by continuous *intra-arterial infusion*, in doses of 5 to 7.5 mg/kg daily (regional perfusion).
- by *mouth*, although the parenteral route is generally preferred a dose of 15 mg/kg, to a maximum of 1 g in one day, has been given once weekly for maintenance.

A variety of regimens have also been used in combination with folinic acid. One suggested regimen is 200 mg/m$^2$ of folinic acid (as calcium folinate) by slow intravenous injection followed immediately by an intravenous bolus of fluorouracil 370 mg/m$^2$; the treatment is given daily for 5 consecutive days, and may be repeated after 21 to 28 days. Lower doses of folinic acid (20 mg/m$^2$) followed by fluorouracil 425 mg/m$^2$ for 5 consecutive days, repeated every 4 to 5 weeks (the Mayo regimen) has also been used. A third, widely-used protocol (the de Gramont regimen) employs an initial dose of 200 mg/m$^2$ of folinic acid, followed by fluorouracil 400 mg/m$^2$ as an initial intravenous bolus injection and then 600 mg/m$^2$ by continuous intravenous infusion. This dosage is given for 2 consecutive days every 2 weeks.

The white cell count should be determined frequently during treatment with fluorouracil and therapy stopped immediately if the count falls rapidly or if the white cell or platelet count falls below acceptable levels (see also Bone-marrow Depression, p.496) or if severe adverse effects occur. Doses should be reduced by up to half in patients with poor nutritional status, impaired bone-marrow, hepatic, or renal function, and within 30 days of major surgery.

Fluorouracil is used topically in the treatment of solar (actinic) keratoses and other superficial tumours and premalignant conditions of the skin including Bowen's disease and superficial basal cell carcinomas. For actinic keratosis it is usually applied as a 0.5 to 5% cream or as a 1 to 5% solution in propylene glycol once or twice daily for 2 to 4 weeks; the higher strength may be applied for at least 3 to 6 weeks for superficial basal cell carcinomas.

**Administration.** Modulation of fluorouracil by other drugs has been tried in an effort to enhance its effects, particularly in the treatment of colorectal cancer (p.516).

*Folinic acid* has been extensively used to modulate the effects of fluorouracil, and has become the agent of choice. Various regimens have been used, modifying the fluorouracil schedule (continuous infusion versus bolus), folinic acid dose (low-dose versus high-dose) and the regimen frequency (monthly, bimonthly, or weekly). Despite numerous studies, the optimum regimen in terms of efficacy and tolerability has yet to be determined. In the adjuvant setting, a recent large-scale randomised trial[1] found no difference in efficacy between low-dose and high-dose folinic acid when added to fluorouracil given either once weekly for 30 doses, or for 5 consecutive days per month over 6 months. Fluorouracil and low-dose folinic acid may therefore become the preferred regimen in the adjuvant setting. In the palliation of advanced disease, meta-analyses have revealed the value of the addition of folinic acid to fluorouracil,[2] and the use of infusions rather than bolus fluorouracil,[3] in terms of response rates. However, the data for low-dose folinic acid versus high-dose are less clear.[4] In 1 randomised trial,[5] a bimonthly infusion regimen of fluorouracil plus high-dose folinic acid (the de Gramont regimen[6]) was more effective than a monthly bolus regimen of fluorouracil plus low-dose folinic acid. Further studies comparing the effect of high- and low-dose folinic acid added to the same schedule of continuous infusion fluorouracil are required.

*Interferon alfa* also appears to modify the actions of fluorouracil (see also under Interactions, above), and has been investigated in combination with fluorouracil and folinic acid. Although some early results were promising, recent randomised controlled trials have failed to show any benefit for the addition of interferon alfa to fluorouracil or fluorouracil plus folinic acid.[7] It is not clear whether interferon beta will prove of any greater benefit.

Based on the results of early adjuvant trials, *levamisole* was used as standard therapy to modulate fluorouracil, particularly in the USA. However, more recent trials indicate that levamisole is no more effective than placebo when added to fluorouracil,[1] or to fluorouracil plus folinic acid.[8]

*Methotrexate* has also been used to modulate fluorouracil. Meta-analysis of several studies of fluorouracil preceded by methotrexate found that the combination doubled the response rate to fluorouracil in metastatic colorectal cancer and produced some survival benefits.[9] (Combination in the reverse order, i.e. methotrexate preceded by fluorouracil, may reduce methotrexate toxicity—see under Treatment of Adverse Effects, p.570.)


1. QUASAR Collaborative Group. Comparison of fluorouracil with additional levamisole, higher-dose folinic acid, or both, as adjuvant chemotherapy for colorectal cancer: a randomised trial. *Lancet* 2000; **355:** 1588–96.
2. Advanced Colorectal Cancer Meta-analysis Project. Modulation of fluorouracil by leucovorin in patients with advanced colorectal cancer: evidence in terms of response rate. *J Clin Oncol* 1992; **10:** 896–903.
3. Meta-analysis Group in Cancer. Efficacy of intravenous continuous infusion of fluorouracil compared with bolus administration in advanced colorectal cancer. *J Clin Oncol* 1998; **16:** 301–8.
4. Rustum YM, *et al.* Rationale for treatment design: biochemical modulation of 5-fluorouracil by leucovorin. *Cancer J Sci Am* 1998; **4:** 12–18.
5. de Gramont A, *et al.* Randomized trial comparing monthly low-dose leucovorin and fluorouracil bolus with bimonthly high-dose leucovorin and fluorouracil bolus plus continuous infusion for advanced colorectal cancer: a French Intergroup study. *J Clin Oncol* 1997; **15:** 808–15.
6. de Gramont A, *et al.* A review of GERCOD trials of bimonthly leucovorin plus 5-fluorouracil 48-h continuous infusion in advanced colorectal cancer: evolution of a regimen. *Eur J Cancer* 1998; **34:** 619–26.
7. Makower D, Wadler S. Interferons as biomodulators of fluoropyrimidines in the treatment of colorectal cancer. *Semin Oncol* 1999; **26:** 663–71.
8. Wolmark N, *et al.* Clinical trial to assess the relative efficacy of fluorouracil and leucovorin, fluorouracil and levamisole, and fluorouracil, leucovorin, and levamisole in patients with Dukes' B and C carcinoma of the colon: results from National Surgical Adjuvant Breast and Bowel Project C-04. *J Clin Oncol* 1999; **17:** 3553–9.
9. Advanced Colorectal Cancer Meta-analysis Project. Meta-analysis of randomized trials testing the biochemical modulation of fluorouracil by methotrexate in metastatic colorectal cancer. *J Clin Oncol* 1994; **12:** 960–9.


**Darier's disease.** Two patients with resistant Darier's disease (p.1134) receiving long-term oral retinoid therapy responded to treatment with topical fluorouracil applied as a 1% cream once daily.[1] There was complete clearance of skin lesions after 3 weeks of treatment.


1. Knulst AC, *et al.* Topical 5-fluorouracil in the treatment of Darier's disease. *Br J Dermatol* 1995; **133:** 463–6.


**Glaucoma.** A regimen of subconjunctival injections of fluorouracil is effective in improving the outcome of glaucoma filtering surgery[1-3] in selected patients when used as an adjunct to prevent the formation of scar tissue (see p.1485). However, in view of the increased risk of late-onset conjunctival wound leaks caution has been suggested in its use in eyes with a good prognosis.[3] Although one study[4] found that fluorouracil improved the success rate of combined glaucoma filtering surgery and cataract surgery earlier studies had failed to demonstrate any advantage.[5,6] A systematic review[7] of these and 2 other studies concluded that fluorouracil reduced the risk of surgical failure of trabeculectomy in eyes at high risk of failure, and in those undergoing surgery for the first time, but noted that the methodological quality of the studies was not high, and that this practice has largely been superseded by the use of intra-operative mitomycin.

Intra-operative topical application of fluorouracil has been tried as an alternative to subconjunctival injection with conflicting results.[8-10]


1. Ophir A, Ticho U. A randomized study of trabeculectomy and subconjunctival administration of fluorouracil in primary glaucomas. *Arch Ophthalmol* 1992; **110:** 1072–5.
2. Goldenfeld M, *et al.* 5-Fluorouracil in initial trabeculectomy: a prospective, randomized, multicenter study. *Ophthalmology* 1994; **101:** 1024–9.
3. The Fluorouracil Filtering Surgery Study Group. Five-year follow-up of the Fluorouracil Filtering Surgery Study. *Am J Ophthalmol* 1996; **121:** 349–66.
4. Gandolfi SA, Vecchi M. 5-Fluorouracil in combined trabeculectomy and clear-cornea phacoemulsification with posterior chamber intraocular lens implantation: a one-year randomized, controlled clinical trial. *Ophthalmology* 1997; **104:** 181–6.
5. Wong PC, *et al.* 5-Fluorouracil after primary combined filtration surgery. *Am J Ophthalmol* 1994; **117:** 149–54.
6. O'Grady JM, *et al.* Trabeculectomy, phacoemulsification, and posterior chamber lens implantation with and without 5-fluorouracil. *Am J Ophthalmol* 1993; **116:** 594–9.
7. Wormald R, *et al.* Post-operative 5-fluorouracil for glaucoma surgery. Available in The Cochrane Library; Issue 2. Chichester: John Wiley; 2004.
8. Egbert PR, *et al.* A prospective trial of intraoperative fluorouracil during trabeculectomy in a black population. *Am J Ophthalmol* 1993; **116:** 612–16.
9. Lachkar Y, *et al.* Trabeculectomy with intraoperative sponge 5-fluorouracil in Afro-Caribbeans. *Br J Ophthalmol* 1997; **81:** 555–8.
10. Yorston D, Khaw PT. A randomised trial of the effect of intra-operative 5-FU on the outcome of trabeculectomy in east Africa. *Br J Ophthalmol* 2001; **85:** 1028–30.


**Malignant neoplasms.** Fluorouracil plays an important role in the adjuvant treatment of gastrointestinal cancer, as discussed on p.516, and is widely used in adjuvant regimens for early breast cancer (p.514). It may also be employed in the management of a wide variety of other malignancies including pancreatic endocrine tumours (p.504), cancers of the cervix (p.515) and head and neck (p.517), liver metastases (p.518), and tumours of the exocrine pancreas (p.521). It is reported to have only modest activity in neoplasms of the kidney (p.518). In addition, it is sometimes applied topically as part of the management of malignant or pre-malignant lesions of the skin (p.522), or surface neoplasia of the eye (p.516).

**Toxoplasmosis.** For mention of the use of fluorouracil with clindamycin to treat cerebral toxoplasmosis, see p.598.

**Warts.** Fluorouracil has been used, as a 1% or, more usually, a 5% cream or solution in the treatment of genital warts (condylomata acuminata).[1-3] It has been tried as an adjuvant to laser therapy in severe papillomavirus-associated vulvar disease,[4] with variable results, and in men with subclinical or clinically apparent penile lesions.[5] A preparation of fluorouracil 3% in a collagen gel basis, together with adrenaline as a local vasoconstrictor, has been tried by injection into genital warts.[6] For a discussion of the various agents, including cytotoxics such as fluorouracil employed to produce destruction of warts, see p.1139.


1. Kling AR. Genital warts—therapy. *Semin Dermatol* 1992; **11:** 247–55.
2. Stone KM. Human papillomavirus infection and genital warts: update on epidemiology and treatment. *Clin Infect Dis* 1995; **20** (suppl 1): S91–7.
3. Beutner KR, Ferenczy A. Therapeutic approaches to genital warts. *Am J Med* 1997; **102:** 28–37.
4. Reid R, *et al.* Superficial laser vulvectomy IV: extended laser vaporization and adjunctive 5-fluorouracil therapy of human papillomavirus-associated vulvar disease. *Obstet Gynecol* 1990; **76:** 439–48.
5. Bergman A, Nalick R. Genital human papillomavirus infection in men: diagnosis and treatment with a laser and 5-fluorouracil. *J Reprod Med* 1991; **36:** 363–6.
6. Swinehart JM, *et al.* Intralesional fluorouracil/epinephrine injectable gel for treatment of condylomata acuminata: a phase 3 clinical study. *Arch Dermatol* 1997; **133:** 67–73.


## Preparations

***BP 2003:*** Fluorouracil Cream; Fluorouracil Injection;
***USP 27:*** Fluorouracil Cream; Fluorouracil Injection; Fluorouracil Topical Solution.

**Proprietary Preparations** (details are given in Part 3)
***Arg.:*** Cinco-Fu; Efudix; Ifocid; Oncofu; ***Austral.:*** Efudix; Fluoroplex†; ***Belg.:*** Efudix†; Fluroblastine; ***Braz.:*** Killit; Utoral; ***Canad.:*** Adrucil; Efudex; Fluoroplex†; ***Denm.:*** Flurablastin; ***Fin.:*** Flurablastin; ***Fr.:*** Efudix; ***Ger.:*** Actino-Hermal†; Efudix; Fluroblastin†; O-fluor; Onkofluor; Ribofluor; ***Hong Kong:*** Efudix; ***India:*** Fivefluro; Fluracil; ***Irl.:*** Efudix; ***Israel:*** Efudix; Fluracedyl†; ***Ital.:*** Efudix; ***Mex.:*** Efudix; Fiverocil†; Flurox; Ifacil; Rhonuracil†; ***Neth.:*** Efudix; ***Norw.:*** Flurablastin; Fluracedyl†; ***NZ:*** Efudix; ***Port.:*** Cinkef-U; ***S.Afr.:*** Efudix; Fluroblastin; ***Singapore:*** Efudix; ***Spain:*** Efudix; ***Swed.:*** Flurablastin; Fluracedyl; ***Switz.:*** Efudix; ***Thai.:*** Efudix†; Fivoflu; Fluracedyl; ***UK:*** Efudix; ***USA:*** Adrucil; Carac; Efudex; Fluoroplex.

**Multi-ingredient:** ***Braz.:*** Efurix; ***Ger.:*** Verrumal; ***Hong Kong:*** Verrumal; ***Israel:*** Verrumal; Verucid; ***Malaysia:*** Verrumal; ***Port.:*** Verrucare; Verrumal; ***Singapore:*** Verrumal; ***Switz.:*** Verrumal; ***Thai.:*** Verrumal.

# Flutamide *(BAN, USAN, rINN)*

Flutamida; Flutamidum; Sch-13521. α′,α′,α′-Trifluoro-4′-nitroisobutyro-*m*-toluidide; α,α,α-Trifluoro-2-methyl-4′-nitro-*m*-propionotoluidide.

$C_{11}H_{11}F_3N_2O_3$ = 276.2.
*CAS — 13311-84-7.*
*ATC — L02BB01.*

**Pharmacopoeias.** In *Eur.* (see p.vi) and *US.*

**Ph. Eur. 5.0** (Flutamide). A pale yellow, crystalline powder. Practically insoluble in water; freely soluble in alcohol and in acetone. Protect from light.

**USP 27** (Flutamide). A pale yellow, crystalline powder. Practically insoluble in water, in liquid paraffin, and in petroleum spirit; freely soluble in acetone, in ethyl acetate, and in methyl alcohol; soluble in chloroform and in ether. Store in airtight containers. Protect from light.

## Adverse Effects and Precautions

The most frequently reported adverse effects with flutamide are hot flushes and reversible gynaecomastia or breast tenderness, sometimes accompanied by galactorrhoea. Nausea, vomiting, diarrhoea, increased appetite, anorexia, and sleep disturbances may occur. There have been reports of skin reactions, including epidermal necrolysis, and of liver damage, sometimes fatal. Other adverse effects reported in patients receiving flutamide include anaemias, haemolysis, headache, dizziness, malaise, blurred vision, anxiety, depression, decreased libido, impotence, and hypertension. Discoloration of the urine to amber or yellow-green can be caused by the presence of flutamide and/or its metabolites.

Flutamide should be used with care in patients with cardiovascular disease because of the possibility of fluid retention. It should also be used with caution in patients with hepatic impairment and is contra-indicated in those with severe impairment. Regular liver function testing is recommended in all patients: therapy should be discontinued or dosage reduced if there is evidence of hepatotoxicity.

**Effects on the blood.** A report[1] of methaemoglobinaemia in an elderly man was attributed to flutamide. A study[2] of 45 patients receiving flutamide found no cases of methaemoglobinaemia, but the authors noted a further three published case reports.


1. Schott AM, *et al.* Flutamide-induced methemoglobinemia. *DICP Ann Pharmacother* 1991; **25:** 600–1.
2. Schulz M, *et al.* Lack of methemoglobinemia with flutamide. *Ann Pharmacother* 2001; **35:** 21–5.


**Effects on the liver.** Hepatitis occurred in a 79-year-old man receiving flutamide 750 mg daily as sole therapy following a prostatectomy,[1] but a subsequent study[2] in 1091 patients receiving flutamide 250 mg three times daily as part of a regimen for prostate cancer found marked signs of liver damage only in 4, of whom only 2 had clinical evidence of liver toxicity. In the USA, the FDA had received reports of 46 patients with hepatotoxicity associated with flutamide up to December 1994. Of these patients, 20 died from progressive liver disease.[3] Further cases have continued to be reported.[4,5]


1. Hart W, Stricker BHC. Flutamide and hepatitis. *Ann Intern Med* 1989; **110:** 943–4.
2. Gomez J-L, *et al.* Incidence of liver toxicity associated with the use of flutamide in prostate cancer patients. *Am J Med* 1992; **92:** 465–70.
3. Wysowski DK, Fourcroy JL. Flutamide hepatotoxicity. *J Urol (Baltimore)* 1996; **155:** 209–12. Correction *ibid:* 396.
4. Garcia Cortes M, *et al.* Flutamide-induced hepatotoxicity: report of a case series. *Rev Esp Enferm Dig* 2001; **93:** 423–32. Correction. *ibid.*; 634.
5. Lubbert C, *et al.* Ikterus und schwere Leberfunktionsstorung bei der hormonablativen Behandlung des Prostatakarzinoms. *Internist (Berl)* 2004; **45:** 333–40.


**Effects on the lungs.** In a review[1] of 78 cases of pneumonitis reported to the FDA between 1998 and 2000 that were associated with bicalutamide, flutamide, or nilutamide, it was found that 14 patients had died of respiratory failure. It was estimated that the incidence of pneumonitis was highest for nilutamide (0.77%), but lower for flutamide (0.04%) and bicalutamide (0.01%).


1. Bennett CL, *et al.* Pneumonitis associated with nonsteroidal antiandrogens: presumptive evidence of a class effect. *Ann Intern Med* 2002; **137:** 625.


**Effects on the skin.** A report of photosensitivity reactions in 2 patients receiving flutamide.[1]


1. Fujimoto M, *et al.* Photosensitive dermatitis induced by flutamide. *Br J Dermatol* 1996; **135:** 496–7.


## Interactions

Flutamide may increase the effect of warfarin, see Antineoplastics, p.1025.

## Pharmacokinetics

Flutamide is reported to be rapidly and completely absorbed from the gastrointestinal tract with peak plasma concentrations occurring 1 hour after a dose. It is rapidly and extensively metabolised; the major metabolite (2-hydroxyflutamide) possesses anti-androgenic properties. The half-life of the metabolite is about 6 hours. Both flutamide and 2-hydroxyflutamide are more than 90% bound to plasma proteins. Excretion is predominantly in the urine with only minor amounts appearing in the faeces.

◊ References.


1. Radwanski E, *et al.* Single and multiple dose pharmacokinetic evaluation of flutamide in normal geriatric volunteers. *J Clin Pharmacol* 1989; **29:** 554–8.

### Uses and Administration

Flutamide is a nonsteroidal compound with anti-androgenic properties which appears to act by inhibiting the uptake and/or binding of androgens in target tissues. It is used, usually with gonadorelin analogues, in the palliative treatment of prostatic carcinoma (p.521). The usual dose by mouth is 250 mg three times daily. When used in combination therapy the UK manufacturers recommend that flutamide treatment should be started at least 3 days before the gonadorelin analogue to suppress any 'flare' reaction; however, in the USA the manufacturers recommend beginning treatment with both agents simultaneously for optimum effect.

**Congenital adrenal hyperplasia.** For mention of the use of flutamide with testolactone to block androgenic effects in congenital adrenal hyperplasia, see p.1078.

**Hirsutism.** Anti-androgens (usually cyproterone or spironolactone) are widely used for the drug treatment of hirsutism (p.1545). Flutamide has no particular advantage in this context;[1,2] one study has found flutamide to be more effective than spironolactone in inhibiting hirsutism,[3] but others found them to be of similar efficacy,[4,5] and the risk of hepatotoxicity with flutamide is a problem.[2] Nonetheless, flutamide has continued to be investigated.[6-8]

1. Rittmaster RS. Hyperandrogenism—what is normal? *N Engl J Med* 1992; **327:** 194–6.
2. Rittmaster RS. Hirsutism. *Lancet* 1997; **349:** 191–5.
3. Cusan L, *et al.* Comparison of flutamide and spironolactone in the treatment of hirsutism: a randomized controlled trial. *Fertil Steril* 1994; **61:** 281–7.
4. Erenus M, *et al.* Comparison of the efficacy of spironolactone versus flutamide in the treatment of hirsutism. *Fertil Steril* 1994; **61:** 613–6.
5. Moghetti P, *et al.* Comparison of spironolactone, flutamide, and finasteride efficacy in the treatment of hirsutism: a randomized, double blind, placebo-controlled trial. *J Clin Endocrinol Metab* 2000; **85:** 89–94.
6. Muderris II, *et al.* Treatment of hirsutism with lowest-dose flutamide (62.5 mg/day). *Gynecol Endocrinol* 2000; **14:** 38–41.
7. Venturoli S, *et al.* Low-dose flutamide (125 mg/day) as maintenance therapy in the treatment of hirsutism. *Horm Res* 2001; **56:** 25–31.
8. Gambineri A, *et al.* Effect of flutamide and metformin administered alone or in combination in dieting obese women with polycystic ovary syndrome. *Clin Endocrinol (Oxf)* 2004; **60:** 241–9.

**Malignant neoplasms.** Androgen blockade, which may include the use of flutamide, is used in the management of metastatic hormone-responsive prostate cancer (p.521); once the cancer begins to progress despite such therapy, discontinuation of flutamide occasionally produces paradoxical disease regression. Promising preliminary results have also followed the use of flutamide in patients with adenocarcinoma of the pancreas (p.521).

### Preparations

***USP 27:*** Flutamide Capsules.

**Proprietary Preparations** (details are given in Part 3)
***Arg.:*** Asoflut; Dedile; Eulexin; Flutaplex; Flutax; Flutepan; Flutrax; FTDA; Olter; ***Austral.:*** Eulexin; Flutamin; Fugerel; ***Austria:*** Afluta; Androbloc; Flutabene; Flutastad; Fugerel; ***Belg.:*** Eulexin; Flutaplex†; ***Braz.:*** Biomida; Eulexin; Tecnoflut; ***Canad.:*** Euflex; ***Chile:*** Androdor; Drogenil; Etaconil; Flulem; ***Denm.:*** Eulexin; Fluprosin; Flutacan; Flutaplex†; Profamid; ***Fin.:*** Eulexin; Profamid; ***Fr.:*** Eulexine; Prostadirex; ***Ger.:*** Apimid; Flumid; Fluta; Flutamex†; Fugerel; Prostica; Prostogenat; Testac†; Testotard; ***Gr.:*** Elbat; Flucinom; Palistop; Tremexal; ***Hong Kong:*** Flutan; Fugerel; ***India:*** Prostamid; ***Irl.:*** Drogenil; ***Israel:*** Eulexin; ***Ital.:*** Drogenil; Eulexin; Fluprost; Virflutam; ***Malaysia:*** Flutan; Flutaplex; Fugerel; ***Mex.:*** Eulexin; Fluken; Flulem; Tafenil; ***Neth.:*** Drogenil; Eulexin; ***Norw.:*** Eulexin; ***NZ:*** Eulexin†; Flutamin; Flutol; ***Port.:*** Draxon†; Eulexin; ***S.Afr.:*** Eulexin; Flutaplex; ***Singapore:*** Fugerel†; ***Spain:*** Eulexin; Flutandrona; Flutaplex; Grisetin; Oncosal; Prostacur; ***Swed.:*** Eulexin; Flutacan; ***Switz.:*** Flucinome; ***Thai.:*** Flutan; Fugerel; ***UK:*** Chimax; Drogenil; ***USA:*** Eulexin.

## Formestane *(BAN, rINN)*

CGP-32349; Formestano; 4-Hydroxyandrostenedione; 4-OHA; 4-OHAD. 4-Hydroxyandrost-4-ene-3,17-dione.

$C_{19}H_{26}O_3$ = 302.4.
*CAS — 566-48-3.*
*ATC — L02BG02.*

### Adverse Effects, Treatment, and Precautions

The most frequent adverse effects of formestane are local irritation and pain at the site of injection. Patients may experience hot flushes due to oestrogen deprivation. Other occasional or rare adverse effects include rashes and pruritus, alopecia or hypertrichosis, drowsiness, dizziness, emotional lability, oedema of the leg, thrombophlebitis, vaginal spotting or bleeding, gastrointestinal disturbances, pelvic or muscle cramps, arthralgia, exacerbation of bone pain, and a vasovagal reaction. Hypersensitivity reactions to the drug or the formulation have occurred.

Care should be taken to avoid intravascular injection. Injection into or near the sciatic nerve may result in pain and nerve trauma. Caution is required if patients drive or operate machinery.

**Effects on carbohydrate metabolism.** Recurrent hypoglycaemic episodes developed in a diabetic patient previously well maintained on gliclazide following addition of formestane to treatment for metastatic breast cancer.[1] Episodic hypoglycaemia continued following dosage reduction, and eventually withdrawal, of gliclazide, suggesting that the effect was not simply an interaction with the sulfonylurea.

1. Brankin E, *et al.* Hypoglycaemia associated with formestane treatment. *BMJ* 1997; **314:** 869.

### Pharmacokinetics

Intramuscular formestane is reported to form a depot which slowly releases active drug into the systemic circulation; maximum plasma concentrations occur about 30 to 48 hours after a single dose and then decline fairly rapidly over 2 to 4 days before declining more slowly, with an apparent elimination half-life of 5 to 6 days. The systemic uptake has been estimated at 20 to 25% of the dose in 14 days. Formestane is about 85% bound to plasma protein in the circulation. It is metabolised by conjugation to the inactive glucuronide: less than 1% of the dose is excreted in urine unchanged.

### Uses and Administration

Formestane is an inhibitor of the aromatase (oestrogen synthetase) system which is responsible for the production of oestrogens from androgens. It is used for its anti-oestrogenic properties in the endocrine treatment of advanced breast cancer in postmenopausal women (p.514).

It is given by intramuscular injection, as an aqueous suspension, in doses of 250 mg every 2 weeks. Injections should be given into each buttock alternately.

◊ Reviews.

1. Wiseman LR, McTavish D. Formestane: a review of its pharmacodynamic and pharmacokinetic properties and therapeutic potential in the management of breast cancer and prostatic cancer. *Drugs* 1993; **45:** 66–84.
2. Anonymous. Formestane for advanced breast cancer in postmenopausal women. *Drug Ther Bull* 1993; **31:** 85–7.

### Preparations

**Proprietary Preparations** (details are given in Part 3)
***Arg.:*** Lentaron; ***Austria:*** Lentaron; ***Belg.:*** Lentaron†; ***Braz.:*** Lentaron; ***Chile:*** Lentaron; ***Denm.:*** Lentaron; ***Fr.:*** Lentaron†; ***Ger.:*** Lentaron; ***Gr.:*** Lentaron; ***Hong Kong:*** Lentaron; ***Irl.:*** Lentaron†; ***Israel:*** Lentaron†; ***Ital.:*** Lentaron; ***Malaysia:*** Lentaron; ***Neth.:*** Lentaron; ***Port.:*** Lentaron†; ***S.Afr.:*** Lentare; ***Spain:*** Lentaron; ***Switz.:*** Lentaron†; ***UK:*** Lentaron†.

## Fotemustine *(BAN, rINN)*

Fotemustina; S-10036. (±)-Diethyl {1-[3-(2-chloroethyl)-3-nitrosoureido]ethyl}phosphonate.

$C_9H_{19}ClN_3O_5P$ = 315.7.
*CAS — 92118-27-9.*
*ATC — L01AD05.*

### Profile

Fotemustine is a nitrosourea derivative and alkylating agent with actions similar to those of carmustine (p.535). It is used in the treatment of disseminated malignant melanoma, particularly where cerebral metastases are present (p.522) and has been tried in primary malignancies of the brain (p.513). When used as a single agent it is licensed for intravenous or intra-arterial infusion in usual doses of 100 mg/m$^2$ weekly for 3 weeks to induce remission, followed after 4 to 5 weeks, if blood counts permit, by maintenance dosage with 100 mg/m$^2$ every 3 weeks. Intravenous infusions are given over 1 hour and intra-arterial infusions over 4 hours. Liver function should be monitored regularly during induction treatment. Regular blood counts should be taken and dosage should be reduced or withheld if white cell or platelet counts are below acceptable levels (see also Bone-marrow Depression, p.496). Bone-marrow suppression may be delayed, with the nadir of the white cell counts 5 or 6 weeks after administration. Solutions for infusion must be freshly prepared and protected from light.

◊ References.

1. Pujol JL, *et al.* Phase II study of nitrosourea fotemustine as single-drug chemotherapy in poor-prognosis non-small-cell lung cancer. *Br J Cancer* 1994; **69:** 1136–40.
2. Kleeberg UR, *et al.* Palliative therapy of melanoma patients with fotemustine: inverse relationship between tumour load and treatment effectiveness. A multicentre phase II trial of the EORTC-Melanoma Cooperative Group (MCG). *Melanoma Res* 1995; **5:** 195–200.
3. Rougier P, *et al.* Fotemustine in patients with advanced gastric cancer, a phase II trial from the EORTC-GITCCG. *Eur J Cancer* 1996; **32A:** 1432–3.
4. Pontes L, *et al.* Isolated limb perfusion with fotemustine after chemosensitization with dacarbazine in melanoma. *Melanoma Res* 1997; **7:** 417–9.
5. Mohr P, *et al.* Combined treatment of stage IV melanoma patients with amifostine and fotemustine—a pilot study. *Melanoma Res* 1998; **8:** 166–9.
6. Marzolini C, *et al.* Pharmacokinetics of temozolomide in association with fotemustine in malignant melanoma and malignant glioma patients: comparison of oral, intravenous, and hepatic intra-arterial administration. *Cancer Chemother Pharmacol* 1998; **42:** 433–40.
7. Ulrich J, *et al.* Management of cerebral metastases from malignant melanoma: results of a combined, simultaneous treatment with fotemustine and irradiation. *J Neurooncol* 1999; **43:** 173–8.
8. Terheyden P, *et al.* Sequential interferon-alpha2b, interleukin-2 and fotemustine for patients with metastatic melanoma. *Melanoma Res* 2000; **10:** 475–82.
9. Frenay M, *et al.* Up-front chemotherapy with fotemustine (F) / cisplatin (CDDP) / etoposide (VP16) regimen in the treatment of 33 non-removable glioblastomas. *Eur J Cancer* 2000; **36:** 1026–31.
10. Mornex F, *et al.* A prospective randomized multicentre phase III trial of fotemustine plus whole brain irradiation versus fotemustine alone in cerebral metastases of malignant melanoma. *Melanoma Res* 2003; **13:** 97–103.
11. Aapro MS, *et al.* Phase II study of fotemustine in patients with advanced ovarian carcinoma: a trial of the EORTC Gynecological Cancer Group. *Eur J Cancer* 2003; **39:** 1141–13.
12. Fazeny-Dorner B, *et al.* Second-line chemotherapy with dacarbazine and fotemustine in nitrosourea-pretreated patients with recurrent glioblastoma multiforme. *Anticancer Drugs* 2003; **14:** 437–42.
13. Avril MF, *et al.* Fotemustine compared with dacarbazine in patients with disseminated malignant melanoma: a phase III study. *J Clin Oncol* 2004; **22:** 1118–25.

### Preparations

**Proprietary Preparations** (details are given in Part 3)
***Arg.:*** Muforan; ***Austral.:*** Muphoran; ***Austria:*** Muphoran; ***Braz.:*** Muphoran; ***Fr.:*** Muphoran; ***Gr.:*** Muphoran; ***Hong Kong:*** Muphoran†; ***Israel:*** Muphoran; ***Ital.:*** Muphoran; ***Spain:*** Mustoforan.

## Fulvestrant *(BAN, USAN, rINN)*

ICI-182780; ZD-9238. 7α-[9-(4,4,5,5,5-Pentafluoropentylsulfinyl)nonyl]estra-1,3,5(10)-triene-3,17β-diol.

$C_{32}H_{47}F_5O_3S$ = 606.8.
*CAS — 129453-61-8.*
*ATC — L02BA03.*

### Adverse Effects and Precautions

The most commonly reported adverse effects of fulvestrant are nausea, vomiting, constipation, diarrhoea, abdominal pain, headache, back pain, hot flushes, and pharyngitis. Injection site reactions can occur.

### Pharmacokinetics

Fulvestrant is highly bound to plasma proteins. It is metabolised primarily in the liver to a number of metabolites, some of which have oestrogen antagonist activity, and is excreted in the faeces. Following intramuscular injection fulvestrant has a half-life of about 40 days.

### Uses and Administration

Fulvestrant is an oestrogen antagonist that downregulates the oestrogen receptor and is used for the treatment of oestrogen-receptor positive, locally advanced or metastatic breast cancer in postmenopausal women (p.514). The recommended dose is 250 mg, administered intramuscularly at monthly intervals.

◊ References.

1. Howell A, *et al.* ICI 182,780 (Faslodex): development of a novel, pure antioestrogen. *Cancer* 2000; **89:** 817–25.
2. Curran M, Wiseman L. Fulvestrant. *Drugs* 2001; **61:** 807–13.
3. Cheung KL, Robertson JF. Fulvestrant. *Expert Opin Invest Drugs* 2002; **11:** 303–8.
4. Wardley AM. Fulvestrant: a review of its development, pre-clinical and clinical data. *Int J Clin Pract* 2002; **56:** 305–9.
5. Osborne CK, *et al.* Double-blind, randomized trial comparing the efficacy and tolerability of fulvestrant versus anastrozole in postmenopausal women with advanced breast cancer progressing on prior endocrine therapy: results of a North American trial. *J Clin Oncol* 2002; **20:** 3386–95.
6. Howell A, *et al.* Fulvestrant, formerly ICI 182,780, is as effective as anastrozole in postmenopausal women with advanced breast cancer progressing after prior endocrine treatment. *J Clin Oncol* 2002; **20:** 3396–3403.
7. Bross PF, *et al.* Fulvestrant in postmenopausal women with advanced breast cancer. *Clin Cancer Res* 2003; **9:** 4309–17.
8. Howell A, *et al.* Comparison of fulvestrant versus tamoxifen for the treatment of advanced breast cancer in postmenopausal women previously untreated with endocrine therapy: a multinational, double-blind, randomized trial. *J Clin Oncol* 2004; **22:** 1605–13.

### Preparations

**Proprietary Preparations** (details are given in Part 3)
***UK:*** Faslodex; ***USA:*** Faslodex.

## Gefitinib *(BAN, USAN, rINN)*

ZD-1839. N-(3-Chloro-4-fluorophenyl)-7-methoxy-6-[3-(morpholin-4-yl)propoxy]quinazolin-4-amine.

$C_{22}H_{24}ClFN_4O_3$ = 446.9.
*CAS — 184475-35-2.*
*ATC — L01XX31.*

### Profile

Gefitinib is a selective inhibitor of the tyrosine kinase activity of the epidermal growth factor receptor. It blocks signal transduction pathways implicated in the growth of tumour cells. It is used for the management of advanced or metastatic non-small cell lung cancer (p.519) unresponsive to other therapy; the usual dose is 250 mg daily by mouth. Adverse effects include rashes and diarrhoea. There have been reports of severe diffuse parenchymal lung disease, including fatalities. It is under investigation in the management of other solid tumours.

◊ References.


1. Culy CR, Faulds D. Gefitinib. *Drugs* 2002; **62:** 2237–48.
2. Inoue A, *et al.* Severe acute interstitial pneumonia and gefitinib. *Lancet* 2003; **361:** 137–9.
3. Kris MG, *et al.* Efficacy of gefitinib, an inhibitor of the epidermal growth factor receptor tyrosine kinase, in symptomatic patients with non–small cell lung cancer: a randomized trial. *JAMA* 2003; **290:** 2149–58.
4. Liu CY, Seen S. Gefitinib therapy for advanced non–small-cell lung cancer. *Ann Pharmacother* 2003; **37:** 1644–53.
5. Cersosimo RJ. Gefitinib: a new antineoplastic for advanced non-small-cell lung cancer. *Am J Health-Syst Pharm* 2004; **61:** 889–98.
6. Giaccone G, *et al.* Gefitinib in combination with gemcitabine and cisplatin in advanced non-small-cell lung cancer: a phase III trial—INTACT 1. *J Clin Oncol* 2004; **22:** 777–84.
7. Herbst RS, *et al.* Gefitinib in combination with paclitaxel and carboplatin in advanced non-small-cell lung cancer: a phase III trial—INTACT 2. *J Clin Oncol* 2004; **22:** 785–94.


### Preparations

**Proprietary Preparations** (details are given in Part 3)
***UK:*** Iressa; ***USA:*** Iressa.

## Gemcitabine Hydrochloride

*(BANM, USAN, rINNM)*

Hidrocloruro de gemcitabina; LY-188011 (gemcitabine). 4-Amino-1-(2-deoxy-2,2-difluoro-β-D-ribofuranosyl)pyrimidin-2(1*H*)-one hydrochloride; 2′-Deoxy-2′,2′-difluorocytidine hydrochloride.

$C_9H_{11}F_2N_3O_4,HCl = 299.7.$

*CAS — 95058-81-4 (gemcitabine); 122111-03-9 (gemcitabine hydrochloride).*

*ATC — L01BC05.*

**Pharmacopoeias.** In *US.*

**USP 27** (Gemcitabine Hydrochloride). A white to off-white solid. Soluble in water; practically insoluble in alcohol and in polar organic solvents; slightly soluble in methyl alcohol. pH of a 1% solution in water is between 2.0 and 3.0. Store in airtight containers.

**Incompatibility.** Gemcitabine hydrochloride was reported to be physically incompatible with aciclovir sodium, amphotericin B, cefoperazone sodium, cefotaxime sodium, furosemide, ganciclovir sodium, imipenem with cilastatin sodium, irinotecan, methotrexate sodium, methylprednisolone sodium succinate, mezlocillin sodium, mitomycin, piperacillin sodium, piperacillin sodium with tazobactam, and prochlorperazine edisilate during simulated Y-site administration.[1]

1. Trissel LA, *et al.* Compatibility of gemcitabine hydrochloride with 107 selected drugs during simulated Y-site injection. *J Am Pharm Assoc* 1999; **39:** 514–18.

### Adverse Effects, Treatment, and Precautions

As for Cytarabine, p.543; myelotoxicity is, however, reported to be modest even at high doses, although rashes and flu-like symptoms are relatively common. Oedema, dyspnoea, and alopecia are also commonly reported. Pulmonary oedema has been reported infrequently and there are rare cases of hypotension. Gemcitabine may produce somnolence: patients so affected should not drive or operate machinery. Severe toxicity, in the form of potentially life-threatening oesophagitis and pneumonitis has been seen in patients given radical radiotherapy to the thorax concurrently with gemcitabine. It should be used with caution in patients with impaired renal or hepatic function. Haemolytic-uraemic syndrome has been reported and has led to irreversible renal failure; gemcitabine should be stopped at the first signs of microangiopathic haemolytic anaemia.

**Effects on the nervous system.** A report of autonomic neuropathy associated with gemcitabine therapy.[1] Symptoms resolved 4 weeks after stopping therapy.

1. Dormann AJ, *et al.* Gemcitabine-associated autonomic neuropathy. *Lancet* 1998; **351:** 644.

### Interactions

**Antineoplastics.** In a study[1] of 14 patients with lung cancer, the use of *paclitaxel* before gemcitabine caused a decrease in the systemic clearance, volume of distribution, and interpatient pharmacokinetic variability of gemcitabine. This resulted in plasma concentrations of gemcitabine slightly higher than the desired range. However, there was no apparent relationship between pharmacokinetic changes and toxicity, and the clinical significance of this possible interaction is unclear.

1. Shord SS, *et al.* Gemcitabine pharmacokinetics and interaction with paclitaxel in patients with advanced non-small-cell lung cancer. *Cancer Chemother Pharmacol* 2003; **51:** 328–36.

### Pharmacokinetics

After intravenous doses gemcitabine is rapidly cleared from the blood and metabolised by cytidine deaminase in the liver, kidney, blood, and other tissues. Clearance is approximately 25% lower in women than in men. Almost all of the dose is excreted in urine as 2′-deoxy-2′,2′-difluorouridine (dFdU), only about 1% being found in the faeces. Intracellular metabolism produces mono-, di-, and triphosphate metabolites, the latter two active. The half-life of gemcitabine ranges from 42 to 94 minutes depending on age and gender. The intracellular half-life of the triphosphate is stated to range from 0.7 to 12 hours.

◊ References.


1. Johnson SA. Clinical pharmacokinetics of nucleoside analogues: focus on haematological malignancies. *Clin Pharmacokinet* 2000; **39:** 5–26.


### Uses and Administration

Gemcitabine is an analogue of cytarabine (p.543) that is metabolised intracellularly to active diphosphate and triphosphate nucleosides, which inhibit DNA synthesis and induce apoptosis. It is primarily active against cells in S phase. It is given in the management of solid tumours including those of the bladder, breast, lung, and pancreas (see p.512, p.514, p.519, and p.521, respectively). It is also being tried in cancers of the cervix and ovary.

Gemcitabine is given intravenously as the hydrochloride. Doses are calculated in terms of the base; gemcitabine hydrochloride 1.14 g is approximately equivalent to 1 g of gemcitabine. Doses are reconstituted in sodium chloride 0.9%. The concentration of the infusion solution should not exceed the equivalent of gemcitabine 40 mg/mL.

The recommended initial dose is the equivalent of gemcitabine 1 $g/m^2$, by infusion over 30 minutes, subsequently adjusted according to response and toxicity.

In the treatment of pancreatic cancer, an initial course of up to 7 such doses at weekly intervals may be given, followed after a one-week recovery period by a regimen of infusions once weekly for 3 consecutive weeks out of 4.

In the treatment of non-small cell lung cancer and bladder cancer, gemcitabine is usually given with cisplatin. The recommended dose of gemcitabine above is given once weekly for 3 weeks, followed by a one-week rest period. Alternatively the equivalent of gemcitabine 1.25 $g/m^2$ may be given on days 1 and 8 of a 21-day cycle to patients with lung cancer. Doses are adjusted according to toxicity.

In breast cancer, gemcitabine is usually given with a taxane such as paclitaxel. A dose of gemcitabine 1.25 $g/m^2$ is given on days 1 and 8 of a 21-day cycle, and adjusted according to toxicity.

◊ References.


1. Michael M, Moore M. Clinical experience with gemcitabine in pancreatic carcinoma. *Oncology (Huntingt)* 1997; **11:** 1615–22.
2. Hui YF, Reitz J. Gemcitabine: a cytidine analogue active against solid tumors. *Am J Health-Syst Pharm* 1997; **54:** 162–70.
3. Noble S, Goa KL. Gemcitabine: a review of its pharmacology and clinical potential in non-small cell lung cancer and pancreatic cancer. *Drugs* 1997; **54:** 447–72.
4. Rosell R, *et al.* The activity of gemcitabine plus cisplatin in randomized trials in untreated patients with advanced non-small cell lung cancer. *Semin Oncol* 1998; **25:** (suppl 9): 27–34.
5. Thomas A, Steward WP. Gemcitabine: a major advance? *Ann Oncol* 1998; **9:** 1265–7.
6. Stadler WM. Gemcitabine doublets in advanced urothelial cancer. *Semin Oncol* 2002; **29** (suppl 3): 15–19.
7. Hussain M, *et al.* Novel gemcitabine-containing triplets in the management of urothelial cancer. *Semin Oncol* 2002; **29** (suppl 3): 20–4.
8. Hochster HS. Newer approaches to gemcitabine-based therapy of pancreatic cancer: fixed-dose-rate infusion and novel agents. *Int J Radiat Oncol Biol Phys* 2003; **56** (suppl): 24–30.
9. Yardley DA. Gemcitabine and taxanes as a new standard of care in breast cancer. *Clin Breast Cancer* 2004; **4** (suppl 3): S107–S112.


### Preparations

***USP 27:*** Gemcitabine for Injection.

**Proprietary Preparations** (details are given in Part 3)
***Arg.:*** Abine; Antoril; Gemtro; ***Austral.:*** Gemzar; ***Austria:*** Gemzar; ***Belg.:*** Gemzar; ***Braz.:*** Gemzar; ***Canad.:*** Gemzar; ***Chile:*** Gemzar; ***Denm.:*** Gemzar; ***Fin.:*** Gemzar; ***Fr.:*** Gemzar; ***Ger.:*** Gemzar; ***Gr.:*** Gemzar; ***Hong Kong:*** Gemzar; ***India:*** Gemcite; ***Irl.:*** Gemzar; ***Israel:*** Gemzar; ***Ital.:*** Gemzar; ***Malaysia:*** Gemzar; ***Mex.:*** Gemzar; ***Neth.:*** Gemzar; ***Norw.:*** Gemzar; ***NZ:*** Gemzar; ***Port.:*** Gemzar; ***S.Afr.:*** Gemzar; ***Singapore:*** Gemzar; ***Spain:*** Gemzar; ***Swed.:*** Gemzar; ***Switz.:*** Gemzar; ***Thai.:*** Gemzar; ***UK:*** Gemzar; ***USA:*** Gemzar.

## Gemtuzumab Ozogamicin *(USAN, rINN)*

CDP-771; CMA-676; Gemtuzumab ozogamicina; Gemtuzumab Zogamicin; WAY-CMA-676.

*CAS — 220578-59-6.*

*ATC — L01XC05.*

### Adverse Effects and Precautions

For general discussions see Antineoplastics, p.492 and p.497.

Myelosuppression is common with gemtuzumab ozogamicin, and thrombocytopenia may be prolonged. Infusion-related reactions characteristic of a cytokine release syndrome (including fever, chills, dyspnoea, and hypotension) and hypersensitivity may occur; prophylactic use of an antihistamine and paracetamol is recommended. Pulmonary sequelae may be fatal. Hepatotoxicity, including severe veno-occlusive disease, has also been reported. Electrolyte imbalances, especially hypokalaemia and hypomagnesaemia, and gastrointestinal disturbances may occur. Blood and platelet counts, electrolytes, and liver function tests should be regularly monitored.

### Uses and Administration

Gemtuzumab ozogamicin is a recombinant humanised monoclonal antibody conjugated with calicheamicin, a cytotoxic antibiotic. The antibody binds specifically to the CD33 antigen, which is expressed on leukaemic myeloblasts but not normal haematopoietic stem cells. Gemtuzumab ozogamicin is licensed for the second-line treatment of CD33-positive acute myeloid leukaemia (p.506) in elderly patients who are unable to tolerate conventional chemotherapy. It is given in 100 mL of sodium chloride 0.9% via an in-line 1.2 micron filter. The licensed dose is 9 $mg/m^2$ given by intravenous infusion over 2 hours, repeated once after 14 days. Lower doses are under investigation as part of combined induction or consolidation regimens.

◊ References.


1. McGavin JK, Spencer CM. Gemtuzumab ozogamicin. *Drugs* 2001; **61:** 1317–22.
2. Dowell JA, *et al.* Pharmacokinetics of gemtuzumab ozogamicin, an antibody-targeted chemotherapy agent for the treatment of patients with acute myeloid leukemia in first relapse. *J Clin Pharmacol* 2001; **41:** 1206–14.
3. Sievers EL, *et al.* Efficacy and safety of gemtuzumab ozogamicin in patients with CD33-positive acute myeloid leukemia in first relapse. *J Clin Oncol* 2001; **19:** 3244–54.
4. Sievers EL, Linenberger M. Mylotarg: antibody-targeted chemotherapy comes of age. *Curr Opin Oncol* 2001; **13:** 522–7.
5. Larson RA, *et al.* Antibody-targeted chemotherapy of older patients with acute myeloid leukemia in first relapse using Mylotarg (gemtuzumab ozogamicin). *Leukemia* 2002; **16:** 1627–36.
6. Leukaemia Research Fund. AML14: Leukaemia Research Fund Acute Myeloid Leukaemia and High Risk MDS Trial 14. Available at: http://www.aml14.bham.ac.uk/trial/AmendmentJanuary2004/Protocol%20Jan%202004.pdf (accessed 30/06/04)
7. Medical Research Council. AML15: Medical Research Council Working Parties on Leukaemia in Adults and Children Acute Myeloid Leukaemia Trial 15. Available at: http://www.aml15.bham.ac.uk/trial/ApplyingForLRECApproval/AML15%20Amendment%20January%202004/AML15ProtocolVersion2Jan2004FINAL.pdf (accessed 30/06/04)


### Preparations

**Proprietary Preparations** (details are given in Part 3)
***Arg.:*** Mylotarg; ***USA:*** Mylotarg.

## Homoharringtonine

Homoharringtonina; NSC-141633. Cephalotaxine 2-(methoxycarbonylmethyl)-2,6-dihydroxy-5-methylheptanoate.

$C_{29}H_{39}NO_9 = 545.6.$

**Pharmacopoeias.** In *Chin.*

### Profile

Homoharringtonine is an alkaloid derived from the tree *Cephalotaxus harringtonia*, and related species. It is thought to act at the ribosome to inhibit protein synthesis and is most active against cells in stage $G_1$. It has been tried as an antineoplastic in the treatment of acute myeloid leukaemias (p.506) and other neoplastic disorders. Some benefit has also been seen in chronic myeloid leukaemia (p.507).

The related compounds harringtonine, isoharringtonine, and deoxyharringtonine have also been investigated.

Reported adverse effects of homoharringtonine include severe hypotension, cardiac arrhythmias, myelosuppression, gastrointestinal disturbances, alopecia, rashes, and hyperglycaemia.

◊ References.


1. Feldman E, *et al.* Homoharringtonine is safe and effective for patients with acute myelogenous leukemia. *Leukemia* 1992; **6:** 1185–8.
2. Feldman EJ, *et al.* Homoharringtonine in patients with myelodysplastic syndrome (MDS) and MDS evolving to acute myeloid leukemia. *Leukemia* 1996; **10:** 40–2.
3. Kantarjian HM, *et al.* Homoharringtonine and low-dose cytarabine in the management of late chronic-phase chronic myelogenous leukemia. *J Clin Oncol* 2000; **18:** 3513–21.
4. Kantarjian HM, *et al.* Homoharringtonine: history, current research, and future direction. *Cancer* 2001; **92:** 1591–1605.
5. O'Brien S, *et al.* Simultaneous homoharringtonine and interferon-alpha in the treatment of patients with chronic-phase chronic myelogenous leukemia. *Cancer* 2002; **94:** 2024–32.

6. Tang J, *et al.* A homoharringtonine-based regimen for childhood acute myelogenous leukemia. *Med Pediatr Oncol* 2003; **41:** 70–2.
7. O'Brien S, *et al.* Results of triple therapy with interferon-alpha, cytarabine, and homoharringtonine, and the impact of adding imatinib to the treatment sequence in patients with Philadelphia chromosome-positive chronic myelogenous leukemia in early chronic phase. *Cancer* 2003; **98:** 888–93.

# Hydroxycarbamide *(BAN, rINN)*

Hidroxicarbamida; Hydroxycarbamidum; Hydroxyurea *(USAN)*; NSC-32065; SQ-1089; WR-83799.

$NH_2.CO.NHOH = 76.05.$

*CAS — 127-07-1.*

*ATC — L01XX05.*

**Pharmacopoeias.** In *Chin., Eur.* (see p.vi), and *US.*

**Ph. Eur. 5.0** (Hydroxycarbamide). A white or almost white, hygroscopic, crystalline powder. It exhibits polymorphism. Freely soluble in water; practically insoluble in alcohol. Store in airtight containers. Protect from light.

**USP 27** (Hydroxyurea). A white to off-white powder. It is somewhat hygroscopic and decomposes in the presence of moisture. Freely soluble in water and in hot alcohol. Store in airtight containers in a dry atmosphere.

## Adverse Effects, Treatment, and Precautions

For general discussions see Antineoplastics, p.492, p.495, and p.497.

Bone-marrow suppression, including megaloblastic changes, is the main adverse effect of hydroxycarbamide. The erythema caused by irradiation may be exacerbated. Other side-effects reported have included gastrointestinal disturbances, impairment of renal function, pulmonary oedema, dermatological reactions, alopecia, and neurological reactions such as headache, dizziness, drowsiness, disorientation, hallucinations, and convulsions. There are rare reports of acute pulmonary reactions consisting of pulmonary infiltrates or fibrosis, dyspnoea and fever.

Pre-existing anaemia should be corrected before beginning therapy with hydroxycarbamide and the haemoglobin concentration, white cell and platelet counts, and hepatic and renal function should be determined repeatedly during treatment. Treatment should be interrupted if the white cell or platelet count fall below acceptable levels (see also Bone-marrow Depression, p.496). If anaemia occurs when hydroxycarbamide is used as an antineoplastic, it may be corrected by transfusions of whole blood without stopping therapy. If anaemia (haemoglobin less than 4.5 g per 100 mL, or reticulocyte count less than 80 000 cells/$mm^3$ when haemoglobin is less than 9 g per 100 mL) occurs when the drug is used for sickle-cell disease, therapy should be interrupted. Megaloblastic changes are usually self-limiting.

Hydroxycarbamide should be used with caution in patients with impaired renal function. The elderly may be more sensitive to its adverse effects.

**Breast feeding.** Hydroxycarbamide is excreted into human breast milk. In milk samples from a woman given 500 mg three times daily, the mean concentration of the drug was found to be about 6 mg/L. It was estimated that, had the infant been breast-fed, it would have received about 3 to 4 mg daily. Although this amount appears to be low, women are advised not to breast feed their infants while taking hydroxycarbamide.[1]

1. Sylvester RK, *et al.* Excretion of hydroxyurea into milk. *Cancer* 1987; **60:** 2177–8.

**Carcinogenicity.** Secondary leukaemias have occurred in patients receiving hydroxycarbamide for myeloproliferative disorders, although the extent to which this is due to the treatment or the underlying disorder is unknown.

Skin cancers have also been associated with its use. These are often multiple and include both squamous cell and basal cell carcinomas.

References.

1. Liozon E, *et al.* Is treatment with hydroxyurea leukemogenic in patients with essential thrombocythemia? An analysis of three new cases of leukaemic transformation and review of the literature. *Hematol Cell Ther* 1997; **39:** 11–18.
2. Pearson TC, *et al.* Leukemic transformation in polycythemia vera. *Blood* 1998; **92:** 1837–8.
3. De Simone C, *et al.* Multiple squamous cell carcinomas of the skin during long-term treatment with hydroxyurea. *Eur J Dermatol* 1998; **8:** 114–15.
4. Best PJM, Petitt RM. Multiple skin cancers associated with hydroxyurea therapy. *Mayo Clin Proc* 1998; **73:** 961–3.

**Effects on the liver.** Fever and hepatitis have been reported[1,2] in patients receiving hydroxycarbamide. Symptoms recurred when patients were rechallenged with the drug.

1. Heddle R, Calvert AF. Hydroxyurea induced hepatitis. *Med J Aust* 1980; **1:** 121.
2. Westerman DA, *et al.* Hydroxyurea-induced fever and hepatitis. *Aust N Z J Med* 1998; **28:** 657–9.

**Effects on the skin and nails.** Reports of skin reactions with hydroxycarbamide include hyperpigmentation of the skin,[1] and of nails (melanonychia).[2]

Hydroxycarbamide therapy has been associated with scaly erythematous skin lesions often resembling those of dermatomyositis.[1,3,4] Such lesions usually occur after several years of treatment and the course is usually benign. However, withdrawal of the drug is usually necessary for healing or improvement, in which case resolution may take several months.[1,4] Hydroxycarbamide may also cause painful leg ulcers, often on the malleoli, which may require treatment discontinuation.[1,5,6] Leg ulcers often co-exist with dermatomyositis-like eruptions and may be caused by the same mechanism.[7] Although mechanical injury may have a role in malleolar ulceration,[5] histologically, perivascular lymphocytic infiltration without vasculitis occurs in both early dermatomyositis-like lesions[1] and in leg ulcers.[5,8]

Skin cancers have also occurred, see Carcinogenicity above.

1. Vassallo C, *et al.* Muco-cutaneous changes during long-term therapy with hydroxyurea in chronic myeloid leukaemia. *Clin Exp Dermatol* 2001; **26:** 141–8.
2. Aste N, *et al.* Nail pigmentation caused by hydroxyurea: report of 9 cases. *J Am Acad Dermatol* 2002; **47:** 146–7.
3. Senet P, *et al.* Hydroxyurea-induced dermatomyositis-like eruption. *Br J Dermatol* 1995; **133:** 455–9.
4. Daoud MS, *et al.*. Hydroxyurea dermopathy: a unique lichenoid eruption complicating long-term therapy with hydroxyurea. *J Am Acad Dermatol* 1997; **36:** 178–82.
5. Best PJ, *et al.* Hydroxyurea-induced leg ulceration in 14 patients. *Ann Intern Med* 1998; **128:** 29–32.
6. Chaine B, *et al.* Cutaneous adverse reactions to hydroxyurea in patients with sickle cell disease. *Arch Dermatol* 2001; **137:** 467–70.
7. Suehiro M, *et al.* Hydroxyurea dermopathy with a dermatomyositis-like eruption and a large leg ulcer. *Br J Dermatol* 1998; **139:** 748–9.
8. Tarumoto T, *et al.* A case of bilateral heel ulcers associated with hydroxyurea therapy for chronic myelogenous leukemia. *Jpn J Clin Oncol* 2000; **30:** 159–62.

**Handling and disposal.** *Urine* produced for up to 48 hours after a dose of hydroxycarbamide should be handled wearing protective clothing.[1]

1. Harris J, Dodds LJ. Handling waste from patients receiving cytotoxic drugs. *Pharm J* 1985; **235:** 289–91.

## Interactions

For a general discussion of antineoplastic drug interactions, see p.498.

## Pharmacokinetics

Hydroxycarbamide is readily absorbed from the gastrointestinal tract and distributed throughout the body. Peak plasma concentrations are reached within 2 hours. Up to 50% of a dose is metabolised by the liver; hydroxycarbamide is excreted in urine as metabolites and unchanged drug. Some is excreted as carbon dioxide via the lungs. About 80% of a dose is reported to be excreted in the urine within 12 hours. Hydroxycarbamide crosses the blood-brain barrier and the placenta, and is distributed into breast milk.

◊ References.

1. Gwilt PR, Tracewell WG. Pharmacokinetics and pharmacodynamics of hydroxyurea. *Clin Pharmacokinet* 1998; **34:** 347–58.

## Uses and Administration

Hydroxycarbamide is an antineoplastic that may cause inhibition of DNA synthesis by acting as a ribonucleotide reductase inhibitor. It is S-phase specific. Hydroxycarbamide is used in the treatment of chronic myeloid leukaemia, and may be used in the myeloproliferative disorders polycythaemia vera and primary (essential) thrombocythaemia. It has also been tried, often combined with radiotherapy, in some solid malignancies (see Malignant Neoplasms, below). Hydroxycarbamide has also been found to be of benefit in the haemoglobinopathies, particularly in sickle-cell disease (see below).

In the treatment of chronic myeloid leukaemia and solid tumours, hydroxycarbamide is given by mouth, typically in a single dose of 20 to 30 mg/kg daily or in a single dose of 80 mg/kg every third day. If a beneficial effect is evident after 6 weeks, therapy may be continued indefinitely. Doses of 15 mg/kg daily, adjusted according to response, are used in polycythaemia vera and primary thrombocythaemia. In sickle-cell disease initial doses of 15 mg/kg daily are suggested, increased if necessary by 5 mg/kg daily every 12 weeks according to response and blood counts, up to a maximum of 35 mg/kg daily.

Blood counts and hepatic and renal function should be monitored during therapy; treatment may need to be interrupted if leucopenia or thrombocytopenia occur (see Adverse Effects, Treatment, and Precautions, above).

**Haemoglobinopathies.** Hydroxycarbamide is considered a promising treatment for the haemoglobinopathies. It can stimulate fetal haemoglobin production, which in turn can reduce haemoglobin polymerisation and the numbers of deformed, dense, and damaged erythrocytes.[1] In adult patients with **sickle-cell disease** (p.734), a randomised controlled study produced evidence that initial doses of 15 mg/kg daily, adjusted according to response and tolerance to up to 35 mg/kg daily, reduced the rate of sickle-cell crisis compared with placebo.[2] An observational follow-up study[3] of this group found that patients taking hydroxycarbamide for frequent sickle-cell episodes appeared to have reduced mortality. A report in 2 adults has suggested that it might reverse splenic dysfunction.[4]

Despite some concerns about giving a potential carcinogen to children, preliminary studies in paediatric populations have also reported evidence of benefit in terms of decreased hospitalisation[5,6] and sickle-cell crisis.[6,7] Hydroxycarbamide may be an alternative to blood transfusions in children who have had a stroke.[6,8] Although a small trial[9] has suggested benefit in paediatric patients in terms of splenic preservation, long-term prevention of organ damage remains to be established.[10,11]

It has been suggested that use of the drug with erythropoietin might enhance the production of fetal haemoglobin, but results from studies of the combination have been conflicting.[12,13]

There appear to have been few studies of hydroxycarbamide specifically in **thalassaemia** (p.735). Initial doses of 8.2 to 10.3 mg/kg daily by mouth, increased until toxicity occurred did produce increases in fetal haemoglobin in 3 patients, but these were not sustained.[14] Conversely, sustained responses have been seen in other studies.[15-17] Use with sodium phenylbutyrate has produced conflicting results.[18-20]

1. Halsey C, Roberts IAG. The role of hydroxyurea in sickle cell disease. *Br J Haematol* 2003; **120:** 177–86.
2. Charache S, *et al.* Effect of hydroxyurea on the frequency of painful crises in sickle cell anemia. *N Engl J Med* 1995; **332:** 1317–22.
3. Steinberg MH, *et al.* Effect of hydroxyurea on mortality and morbidity in adult sickle cell anemia: risks and benefits up to 9 years of treatment. *JAMA* 2003; **289:** 1645–51.
4. Claster S, Vichinsky E. First report of reversal of organ dysfunction in sickle cell anemia by the use of hydroxyurea: splenic regeneration. *Blood* 1996; **88:** 1951–3.
5. Scott JP, *et al.* Hydroxyurea therapy in children severely affected with sickle cell disease. *J Pediatr* 1996; **128:** 820–8.
6. Ferster A, *et al.* Five years of experience with hydroxyurea in children and young adults with sickle cell disease. *Blood* 2001; **97:** 3628–32.
7. Jayabose S, *et al.* Clinical and hematologic effects of hydroxyurea in children with sickle cell anemia. *J Pediatr* 1996; **129:** 559–65.
8. Ware RE, *et al.* Hydroxyurea as an alternative to blood transfusions for the prevention of recurrent stroke in children with sickle cell disease. *Blood* 1999; **94:** 3022–6.
9. Wang WC, *et al.* A two-year pilot trial of hydroxyurea in very young children with sickle-cell anemia. *J Pediatr* 2001; **139:** 790–6.
10. Powars DR. Hydroxyurea in very young children with sickle cell anemia is not a cure-all. *J Pediatr* 2001; **139:** 763–4.
11. Kinney TR, *et al.* Safety of hydroxyurea in children with sickle cell anemia: results of the HUG-KIDS study, a phase I/II trial. *Blood* 1999; **94:** 1550–4.
12. Goldberg MA, *et al.* Treatment of sickle cell anemia with hydroxyurea and erythropoietin. *N Engl J Med* 1990; **323:** 366–72.
13. Rodgers GP, *et al.* Augmentation by erythropoietin of the fetal-hemoglobin response to hydroxyurea in sickle-cell disease. *N Engl J Med* 1993; **328:** 73–80.
14. Hajjar FM, Pearson HA. Pharmacologic treatment of thalassemia intermedia with hydroxyurea. *J Pediatr* 1994; **125:** 490–2.
15. Loukopoulos D, *et al.* Hydroxyurea therapy in thalassemia. *Ann N Y Acad Sci* 1998; **30:** 120–8.
16. Rigano P, *et al.* Clinical and hematological responses to hydroxyurea in Sicilian patients with Hb S/β-thalassemia. *Hemoglobin* 2001; **25:** 9–17.
17. Loukopoulos D, *et al.* Reduction of the clinical severity of sickle cell/β-thalassemia with hydroxyurea: the experience of a single center in Greece. *Blood Cells Mol Dis* 2000; **26:** 453–66.
18. Olivieri NF, *et al.* Treatment of thalassaemia major with phenylbutyrate and hydroxyurea. *Lancet* 1997; **350:** 491–2.
19. Hoppe C, *et al.* Hydroxyurea and sodium phenylbutyrate therapy in thalassemia intermedia. *Am J Hematol* 1999; **62:** 221–7.
20. Dover GJ. Hemoglobin switching protocols in thalassemia. *Ann N Y Acad Sci* 1998; **850:** 80–6.

**HIV infection and AIDS.** Unlike most drugs used to treat HIV, which target viral enzymes, hydroxycarbamide inhibits ribonucleotide reductase, a host cellular enzyme that is less prone to mutation and subsequent development of resistance.[1] The drug acts synergistically with didanosine (p.630). Of 25 HIV-positive patients given didanosine 200 mg twice daily with hydroxycarbamide 15 mg/kg daily in 2 divided doses, all showed a drop in viral load and an increase in CD4+ lymphocyte count.[2] Viraemia was not detectable in 13 of 24 patients evaluated at 6 months and 10 of 20 patients evaluated at 1 year. In 2 of these patients who subsequently received no antiviral treatments for 1 year there was no viral rebound, although some proviral DNA was detected.[3] In another study in 6 patients, didanosine 200 mg twice daily with hydroxycarbamide 250 mg four times daily (suggested to be a better regimen because of the short half-life of the antineoplastic) produced a sharp decrease in viraemia, which was maintained for up to 72 weeks.[4] A rebound occurred in 1 patient on interrupting treatment but viral replication was again suppressed when treatment was restarted.

Combinations with didanosine and other HIV drugs have also been tried.[1] A controlled trial[5] of hydroxycarbamide, didanosine, and stavudine indicated significantly enhanced activity when the antivirals were used with the antineoplastic rather than placebo. However, in a long-term follow-up[6] there was a high withdrawal rate amongst patients receiving this combination, due to virological failure and adverse effects such as peripheral neuropathy and fatigue. Another study[7] (ACTG 5025) was terminated due to the high risk of toxicity, including fatal pancreatitis, in patients receiving the hydroxycarbamide regimens. The authors noted that the use of a higher daily dosage of 1200 mg of hydroxycarbamide (rather than the usual 1000 mg daily) and increased exposure to didanosine (itself associated with pancreatitis) may have contributed to toxicity. An analysis of 2613 patients[8] determined that the use of hydroxycarbamide with didanosine, or didanosine and stavudine, resulted in a fourfold increase in the risk for development of pancreatitis, compared to didanosine alone. In a study of patients who had failed protease-inhibitor based regimens,[9] the addition of the antineoplastic to reverse transcriptase inhibitor-based therapy significantly improved virologic response. Despite an increased incidence of adverse events associated with its use, hydroxycarbamide was considered to be a valuable alternative in these patients. A small randomised study[10] of patients with chronic HIV infection given structured treatment interruptions with cycles of highly active antiretroviral therapy (HAART) or HAART and hydroxycarbamide found that use of the latter decreased viral load. For further discussion of the management of HIV infection and AIDS, see p.621.

1. Gibbs MA, Sorensen SJ. Hydroxyurea in the treatment of HIV-1. *Ann Pharmacother* 2000; **34:** 89–93.
2. Vila J, *et al.* 1-year follow-up of the use of hydroxycarbamide and didanosine in HIV infection. *Lancet* 1996; **848:** 203–4.
3. Vila J, *et al.* Absence of viral rebound after treatment of HIV-infected patients with didanosine and hydroxycarbamide. *Lancet* 1997; **350:** 635–6.
4. Lori F, *et al.* Long-term suppression of HIV-1 by hydroxyurea and didanosine. *JAMA* 1997; **277:** 1437–8.
5. Rutschmann OT, *et al.* A placebo-controlled trial of didanosine plus stavudine, with and without hydroxyurea, for HIV infection. *AIDS* 1998; **12:** F71–7.
6. Rutschmann OT, *et al.* Long-term hydroxyurea in combination with didanosine and stavudine for the treatment of HIV-1 infection. *AIDS* 2000; **14:** 2145–51.
7. Havlir DV, *et al.* Effects of treatment intensification with hydroxyurea in HIV-infected patients with virologic suppression. *AIDS* 2001; **15:** 1379–88.
8. Moore RD, *et al.* Incidence of pancreatitis in HIV-infected patients receiving nucleoside reverse transcriptase inhibitor drugs. *AIDS* 2001; **15:** 617–20.
9. Lafeuillade A, *et al.* The HYDILE trial: efficacy and tolerance of a quadruple combination of reverse transcriptase inhibitors versus the same regimen plus hydroxyurea or hydroxyurea and interleukin-2 in HIV-infected patients failing protease inhibitor-based combinations. *HIV Clin Trials* 2002; **3:** 263–71.
10. García F, *et al.* A cytostatic drug improves control of HIV-1 replication during structured treatment interruptions: a randomized study. *AIDS* 2003; **17:** 43–51.

**Malignant neoplasms.** Hydroxycarbamide is used in the treatment of chronic myeloid leukaemia (p.507), and may be used in the myeloproliferative disorders polycythaemia vera (p.508) and primary (essential) thrombocythaemia (p.509). Hydroxycarbamide has been tried, often with radiotherapy, in some solid malignancies such as tumours of the cervix (p.515), head and neck (p.517), and ovary (p.520).

**Psoriasis.** An immunosuppressant (usually methotrexate or ciclosporin) may be useful in patients with severe refractory psoriasis (p.1137). Hydroxycarbamide has also been tried, although experience is limited.[1,2]

1. Layton AM, *et al.* Hydroxyurea in the management of therapy resistant psoriasis. *Br J Dermatol* 1989; **121:** 647–53.
2. Smith CH, *et al.*. Use of hydroxyurea in psoriasis. *Clin Exp Dermatol* 1999; **24:** 2–6.

### Preparations

***BP 2003:*** Hydroxycarbamide Capsules;
***USP 27:*** Hydroxyurea Capsules.

**Proprietary Preparations** (details are given in Part 3)
***Arg.:*** Dacrodil; Droxiurea; Hydrea; ***Austral.:*** Hydrea; ***Austria:*** Litalir; ***Belg.:*** Hydrea; ***Braz.:*** Hydrea; Hydrine; ***Canad.:*** Hydrea; ***Chile:*** Hydrea; ***Denm.:*** Hydrea; ***Fin.:*** Hydrea; ***Fr.:*** Hydrea; ***Ger.:*** Litalir; Syrea; ***Gr.:*** Medroxyurea; ***Hong Kong:*** Hydrea; ***India:*** Neodrea; ***Irl.:*** Hydrea; ***Israel:*** Hydrea; ***Ital.:*** Onco-Carbide; ***Malaysia:*** Hydrea; ***Mex.:*** Hydrea; Oxeron†; ***Neth.:*** Hydrea; ***NZ:*** Hydrea; ***Port.:*** Hydrea; ***S.Afr.:*** Hydrea; ***Singapore:*** Hydrea; ***Spain:*** Hydrea; ***Swed.:*** Hydrea; ***Switz.:*** Litalir; ***Thai.:*** Hydrea; ***UK:*** Hydrea; ***USA:*** Droxia; Hydrea; Mylocel.

## Ibritumomab Tiuxetan *(BAN, USAN, rINN)*

IDEC-129; IDEC-Y2B8.

*CAS — 206181-63-7.*

### Adverse Effects and Precautions

For general discussions, see Antineoplastics, p.492 and p.497.

Myelosuppression is common after administration of ibritumomab tiuxetan, and may be prolonged. Thrombocytopenia resulting in fatal haemorrhage has occurred. Infections, and hypersensitivity reactions manifest as bronchospasm and angioedema, may also be severe. As ibritumomab tiuxetan is given with rituximab, severe infusion reactions due to the cytokine release syndrome may occur (see under Rituximab, p.582). Gastrointestinal disturbances are common.

Complete blood and platelet counts should be monitored weekly, or more frequently if cytopenia is present, until haematological recovery. Ibritumomab tiuxetan should not be administered to patients with extensive marrow involvement, impaired bone marrow reserve, or platelet or neutrophil counts below acceptable levels (see also Bone-marrow Depression, p.496). Care should be taken during and after radiolabelling with indium-111 or yttrium-90 to minimise radiation exposure.

### Uses and Administration

Ibritumomab is a murine monoclonal antibody to CD20 antigen, which is conjugated with tiuxetan to provide a chelation site for radioactive isotopes. Radiolabelled ibritumomab tiuxetan is used in the treatment of relapsed or refractory, low-grade, follicular, or transformed B-cell non-Hodgkin's lymphoma (p.510). Patients are pretreated with a low dose of rituximab (p.582). In the USA this is followed by slow intravenous injection of ibritumomab tiuxetan chelated with indium-111 (p.1523) for imaging to confirm that biodistribution of tumour cells is acceptable. A second rituximab treatment is given 7 to 9 days after the first, followed by ibritumomab tiuxetan chelated with yttrium-90 (p.1526) for radio-immunotherapy.

◊ References.

1. Witzig TE, *et al.* Phase I/II trial of IDEC-Y2B8 radioimmunotherapy for treatment of relapsed or refractory CD20+ B-cell non-Hodgkin's lymphoma. *J Clin Oncol* 1999; **17:** 3793–3803.
2. Wiseman GA, *et al.* Biodistribution and dosimetry results from a phase III prospectively randomized controlled trial of Zevalin radioimmunotherapy for low-grade, follicular, or transformed B-cell non-Hodgkin's lymphoma. *Crit Rev Oncol Hematol* 2001; **39:** 181–94.
3. Wagner HN, *et al.* Administration guidelines for radioimmunotherapy of non-Hodgkin's lymphoma with $^{90}$Y-labeled anti-CD20 monoclonal antibody. *J Nucl Med* 2002; **43:** 267–72.
4. Witzig TE, *et al.* Randomized controlled trial of yttrium-90-labeled ibritumomab tiuxetan radioimmunotherapy versus rituximab immunotherapy for patients with relapsed or refractory low-grade, follicular, or transformed B-cell non-Hodgkin's lymphoma. *J Clin Oncol* 2002; **20:** 2453–63.
5. Witzig TE, *et al.* Treatment with ibritumomab tiuxetan radioimmunotherapy in patients with rituximab-refractory follicular non-Hodgkin's lymphoma. *J Clin Oncol* 2002; **20:** 3262–9.
6. Ansell SM, *et al.* Subsequent chemotherapy regimens are well tolerated after radioimmunotherapy with yttrium-90 ibritumomab tiuxetan for non-Hodgkin's lymphoma. *J Clin Oncol* 2002; **20:** 3885–90.

### Preparations

**Proprietary Preparations** (details are given in Part 3)
***UK:*** Zevalin; ***USA:*** Zevalin.

## Idarubicin Hydrochloride

*(BANM, USAN, rINNM)*

4-Demethoxydaunorubicin Hydrochloride; Hidrocloruro de idarubicina; IMI-30; NSC-256439 (idarubicin). (7*S*,9*S*)-9-Acetyl-7-(3-amino-2,3,6-trideoxy-α-L-*lyxo*-hexopyranosyloxy)-7,8,9,10-tetrahydro-6,9,11-trihydroxynaphthacene-5,12-dione hydrochloride.

$C_{26}H_{27}NO_9,HCl = 534.0.$

*CAS — 58957-92-9 (idarubicin); 57852-57-0 (idarubicin hydrochloride).*

*ATC — L01DB06.*

**Pharmacopoeias.** In *Jpn* and *US.*

**USP 27** (Idarubicin Hydrochloride). A red-orange to red-brown powder. Slightly soluble in water; insoluble in acetone and in solvent ether; soluble in methyl alcohol. A 0.5% solution in water has a pH between 5.0 and 6.5. Store in airtight containers.

**Incompatibility.** The manufacturers state that precipitation occurs when idarubicin hydrochloride is mixed with heparin, and that it will degrade in alkaline solution.

### Adverse Effects, Treatment, and Precautions

As for Doxorubicin Hydrochloride, p.548. Raised liver enzymes and bilirubin occur in about 20 to 30% of patients. Severe enterocolitis with perforation has been reported rarely. A cumulative total dose limit of 400 mg/m² has been recommended for oral therapy, although it has been suggested that idarubicin may be associated with less cardiotoxicity than doxorubicin. Idarubicin should be given with caution, and in reduced doses, to patients with renal or hepatic impairment.

**Effects on the skin and nails.** For a report of transverse hyperpigmented bands of the nails in a patient who received idarubicin, see under Doxorubicin Hydrochloride, p.548.

### Pharmacokinetics

On intravenous dosage idarubicin is rapidly distributed into body tissues and extensively tissue bound, with a volume of distribution which may be in excess of 2000 litres. It is extensively metabolised, both in the liver and extrahepatically; the principal metabolite, idarubicinol (13-dihydroidarubicin) has equal antineoplastic activity. Peak concentrations of idarubicin and idarubicinol in bone marrow and nucleated blood cells are 400 (idarubicin) and 200 (idarubicinol) times greater than those in plasma; cellular concentrations of drug and metabolite decline with apparent terminal half-lives of 15 and 72 hours respectively, whereas plasma half-lives are reported to be 20 to 22 hours and about 45 hours respectively. Idarubicin is excreted in bile, and to a lesser extent in urine, as unchanged drug and metabolites.

Idarubicin is also absorbed orally, but estimates of its oral bioavailability vary from about 20 to 50%.

◊ References.

1. Robert J. Clinical pharmacokinetics of idarubicin. *Clin Pharmacokinet* 1993; **24:** 275–88.

### Uses and Administration

Idarubicin is an anthracycline antibiotic with antineoplastic actions similar to those of doxorubicin (p.549). It is used as the hydrochloride, alone or in combination with other drugs, for the induction of remission in patients with acute myeloid leukaemias (p.506). It is also used as a second-line treatment in acute lymphoblastic leukaemia (p.506), and advanced breast cancer (p.514). It has been tried in multiple myeloma (p.511) and non-Hodgkin's lymphoma (p.510).

Idarubicin hydrochloride is given by intravenous injection (reconstituted with Water for Injections) into a fast-running infusion of sodium chloride 0.9% or glucose 5% over 5 to 15 minutes. The suggested dose in adult acute myeloid leukaemia is 12 mg/m² daily for 3 days, with cytarabine. A similar dose, as a single agent, has been given in acute lymphoblastic leukaemia. An alternative dosage schedule in acute myeloid leukaemia is 8 mg/m² given daily for 5 days, either alone or in combination therapy. In children with acute lymphoblastic leukaemia a dose of 10 mg/m² daily for 3 days as a single agent has been suggested. When the intravenous route cannot be used, idarubicin hydrochloride may be given by mouth. A suggested dose in adult acute myeloid leukaemia as a single agent is 30 mg/m² daily for 3 days; 15 to 30 mg/m² daily may be given for 3 days when used with other drugs.

In patients with refractory breast cancer idarubicin hydrochloride has been given by mouth in doses of 45 mg/m², as a single dose or divided over 3 consecutive days; the treatment may be repeated every 3 or 4 weeks depending on the haematological recovery.

Blood counts should be performed frequently in patients receiving idarubicin, and monitoring of cardiac, hepatic, and renal function is recommended. Doses should be reduced in patients with hepatic or renal impairment (for further information on the former, see below). In patients who receive a second course of idarubicin dosage should be reduced by 25% if severe mucositis developed with the first course.

◊ The actions and uses of idarubicin have been reviewed.[1] A study in leukaemia cells *in vitro* suggested that idarubicin was more active than a conventional anthracycline, daunorubicin, against cells with the multidrug resistance (MDR) phenotype.[2] A collaborative overview of randomised trials for acute myeloid leukaemia found that idarubicin-based therapy achieved better remission rates and overall survival than daunorubicin-based regimens.[3]

1. Cersosimo RJ. Idarubicin: an anthracycline antineoplastic agent. *Clin Pharm* 1992; **11:** 152–67.
2. Berman E, McBride M. Comparative cellular pharmacology of daunorubicin and idarubicin in human multidrug-resistant leukaemia cells. *Blood* 1992; **79:** 3267–73.
3. AML Collaborative Group. A systematic collaborative overview of randomised trials comparing idarubicin with daunorubicin (or other anthracyclines) as induction therapy for acute myeloid leukaemia. *Br J Haematol* 1998; **103:** 100–9.

**Administration in hepatic impairment.** UK licensing information for idarubicin hydrochloride recommends that a dose reduction be considered in patients with hepatic impairment. Although no specific doses are suggested, it is noted that a 50% reduction in dosage has been employed with some other anthracyclines in patients with acute leukaemias whose bilirubin levels were between 12 and 20 micrograms/mL, and that in studies in breast cancer a 50% dosage reduction with idarubicin has sometimes been employed in those whose bilirubin rose to 20 to 30 micrograms/mL, with withdrawal if levels rose above this. However, in other studies idarubicin was not used if bilirubin values were above 20 micrograms/mL.

In the USA, similar cautions apply but licensing information only suggests that idarubicin should be withheld if bilirubin levels exceed 50 micrograms/mL.

## Preparations

*USP 27:* Idarubicin Hydrochloride for Injection.

**Proprietary Preparations** (details are given in Part 3)
***Arg.:*** Idarrux; Zavedos; ***Austral.:*** Zavedos; ***Austria:*** Zavedos; ***Belg.:*** Zavedos; ***Braz.:*** Zavedos; ***Canad.:*** Idamycin; ***Chile:*** Zavedos; ***Denm.:*** Zavedos; ***Fin.:*** Zavedos; ***Fr.:*** Zavedos; ***Ger.:*** Zavedos; ***Gr.:*** Zavedos; ***Hong Kong:*** Zavedos; ***Irl.:*** Zavedos; ***Israel:*** Zavedos; ***Ital.:*** Zavedos; ***Malaysia:*** Zavedos; ***Mex.:*** Idamycin; Idaralem; ***Neth.:*** Zavedos; ***Norw.:*** Zavedos; ***NZ:*** Zavedos; ***Port.:*** Zavedos; ***S.Afr.:*** Zavedos; ***Singapore:*** Zavedos; ***Spain:*** Zavedos; ***Swed.:*** Zavedos; ***Switz.:*** Zavedos; ***Thai.:*** Zavedos; ***UK:*** Zavedos; ***USA:*** Idamycin.

# Ifosfamide *(BAN, USAN, rINN)*

Ifosfamida; Ifosfamidum; Iphosphamide; Isophosphamide; MJF-9325; NSC-109724; Z-4942. 3-(2-Chloroethyl)-2-(2-chloroethylamino)perhydro-1,3,2-oxazaphosphorinane 2-oxide.

$C_7H_{15}Cl_2N_2O_2P$ = 261.1.

*CAS — 3778-73-2.*

*ATC — L01AA06.*

**Pharmacopoeias.** In *Eur.* (see p.vi) and *US.*

**Ph. Eur. 5.0** (Ifosfamide). A white or almost white, hygroscopic, fine crystalline powder. Soluble in water; freely soluble in dichloromethane. Store in airtight containers.

**USP 27** (Ifosfamide). A white, crystalline powder. M.p. about 40°. Freely soluble in water; very soluble in alcohol, in methyl alcohol, in isopropyl alcohol, in dichloromethane, and in ethyl acetate; very slightly soluble in hexanes. A 10% solution in water has a pH of between 4.0 and 7.0. Store in airtight containers at a temperature not exceeding 25°.

**Incompatibility.** Ifosfamide appears to be compatible when mixed in solution with mesna.[1,2] However, ifosfamide appears to be incompatible with benzyl alcohol used as a preservative in Water for Injections: solutions made up with water preserved in this way became turbid, with the formation of aqueous and oily phases, at concentrations of ifosfamide greater than 60 mg/mL.[3]

1. Shaw IC, Rose JWP. Infusion of ifosphamide plus mesna. *Lancet* 1984; **i:** 1353–4.
2. Rowland CG, *et al.* Infusion of ifosfamide plus mesna. *Lancet* 1984; **ii:** 468.
3. Behme RJ, *et al.* Incompatibility of ifosfamide with benzyl-alcohol-preserved bacteriostatic water for injection. *Am J Hosp Pharm* 1988; **45:** 627–8.

**Stability.** Ifosfamide undergoes a reversible chemical re-arrangement in aqueous solution, which is sensitive to changes in pH.[1] The ratio of these compounds to one another in biological fluids may have a bearing on the toxicity and efficacy of ifosfamide.

1. Küpfer A, *et al.* Intramolecular rearrangement of ifosfamide in aqueous solutions. *Lancet* 1990; **335:** 1461.

## Adverse Effects, Treatment, and Precautions

As for Cyclophosphamide, p.540. Toxic effects on the urinary tract may be more severe with ifosfamide and may involve the kidneys as well as the bladder. CNS side-effects have been reported, especially confusion, drowsiness, depressive psychosis, hallucinations, and rarely, seizures.

**Effects on the heart.** Severe myocardial depression, with heart failure and ventricular arrhythmias, has been reported in patients receiving high-dose ifosfamide.[1] Symptoms were reversible with appropriate treatment in most cases although one patient died of cardiogenic shock.

1. Quezado ZMN, *et al.* High-dose ifosfamide is associated with severe, reversible cardiac dysfunction. *Ann Intern Med* 1993; **118:** 31–6.

**Effects on the kidneys.** In addition to its effects on the bladder ifosfamide may be associated with serious nephrotoxicity. Both proximal and distal tubular damage,[1,2] and to a lesser extent glomerular effects,[2] are seen, and the Fanconi syndrome (with development of hypophosphataemic rickets in a number of children),[2-6] and nephrogenic diabetes insipidus[1,6] may result. Progressive chronic renal failure after high-dose ifosfamide has been described.[7] Life-threatening hypokalaemia possibly due to a renal lesion has also occurred.[8] Results in *rats* suggest that generation of toxic metabolites within the kidney itself may be responsible, and that repairable renal damage occurs after the first dose, which is aggravated by repeated toxic insults.[9] This is in agreement with clinical results, since although renal damage has been seen after a single dose, perhaps representing an idiosyncratic reaction,[10,11] most cases have been in children receiving relatively high doses long-term. Renal damage appears to persist after withdrawal of ifosfamide in these patients and may be largely irreversible.[12]

A combination of younger age and high cumulative doses of ifosfamide was found to convey the highest risk of toxicity, but concomitant use of cisplatin may also increase the risk.[13] The maximum safe dose of ifosfamide remains controversial.[13-15] It has been suggested that cumulative doses of ifosfamide of 100 g/m² or more should be avoided in children in an attempt to reduce the incidence of nephrotoxicity,[14] although subsequent reviews have suggested that lower cumulative doses may be toxic, especially in younger children.[13,15]

1. Skinner R, *et al.* Nephrotoxicity after ifosfamide. *Arch Dis Child* 1990; **65:** 732–8.
2. Burk CD, *et al.* Ifosfamide-induced renal tubular dysfunction and rickets in children with Wilms tumor. *J Pediatr* 1990; **117:** 331–5.
3. Skinner R, *et al.* Hypophosphataemic rickets after ifosfamide treatment in children. *BMJ* 1989; **298:** 1560–1.
4. Newbury-Ecob RA, Barbor PRH. Hypophosphataemic rickets after ifosfamide treatment. *BMJ* 1989; **299:** 258.
5. Newbury-Ecob RA, *et al.* Ifosfamide-induced Fanconi syndrome. *Lancet* 1989; **i:** 1328.
6. Skinner R, *et al.* Nephrotoxicity of ifosfamide in children. *Lancet* 1989; **ii:** 159.
7. Krämer A, *et al.* Progressive renal failure in two breast cancer patients after high-dose ifosfamide. *Lancet* 1994; **334:** 1569.
8. Husband DJ, Watkin SW. Fatal hypokalaemia associated with ifosfamide/mesna chemotherapy. *Lancet* 1988; **i:** 1116.
9. Graham MI, *et al.* A proposed mechanism for isophosphamide-induced kidney toxicity. *Hum Toxicol* 1985; **4:** 545–6.
10. Heney D, *et al.* Acute ifosfamide-induced tubular toxicity. *Lancet* 1989; **ii:** 103–4.
11. Devalck C, *et al.* Acute ifosfamide-induced proximal tubular toxic reaction. *J Pediatr* 1991; **118:** 325–6.
12. Heney D, *et al.* Progressive renal toxicity due to ifosfamide. *Arch Dis Child* 1991; **66:** 966–70.
13. Loebstein R, *et al.* Risk factors for long-term outcome of ifosfamide-induced nephrotoxicity in children. *J Clin Pharmacol* 1999; **39:** 454–61.
14. Skinner R, *et al.* Risk factors for ifosfamide nephrotoxicity in children. *Lancet* 1996; **348:** 578–80.
15. Loebstein R, Koren G. Ifosfamide-induced nephrotoxicity in children: critical review of predictive risk factors. *Pediatrics* 1998; **101:** 1067. Full version: http://pediatrics.aappublications.org/cgi/content/full/101/6/e8 (accessed 30/06/04)

**Effects on the nervous system.** Use of ifosfamide (with mesna for urothelial protection) may be associated with the development of severe encephalopathy, with EEG abnormalities, disorientation, hallucinations, catatonia, and coma; occasionally CNS depression has led to circulatory collapse and death.[1,2] The effect has been suggested to be due to a metabolite, perhaps chloroacetaldehyde,[3] a hypothesis with which the increased incidence of encephalopathy after oral rather than intravenous doses may agree.[4,5] Others suggest that the dechloroethylated metabolites may contribute, and in particular the *R*-enantiomer of 3-dechloroethyl-ifosfamide which is a metabolite of *S*-ifosfamide.[6] There is some uncertainty about the contributory role of mesna, if any: encephalopathy has not been seen when mesna is given with cyclophosphamide,[7] and has been seen when ifosfamide is given alone,[5] but an exacerbatory role for mesna cannot be ruled out,[8] perhaps via its chelating properties.[1,7] A nomogram has been proposed to identify patients at greatest risk of toxicity,[9,10] such as those with renal or hepatic impairment,[9] although doubts have been raised as to its general applicability,[11] and it has also been suggested that the drug be given by continuous infusion over several days where possible, since this route has by far the lowest incidence of encephalopathy (7%, versus 26% with intravenous bolus and 43% with oral doses).[4] Care may also be required when giving other antineoplastics to patients who have experienced encephalopathy after ifosfamide, since a case of encephalopathy following bleomycin (not normally associated with neurotoxicity) has been reported in such a patient.[12]

There are a few reports of the use of methylthioninium chloride effectively preventing or reversing signs of encephalopathy.[13] A number of mechanisms have been proposed for this observation.

1. Meanwell CA, *et al.* Encephalopathy associated with ifosphamide/mesna therapy. *Lancet* 1985; **i:** 406–7.
2. Cantwell BMJ, Harris AL. Ifosfamide/mesna and encephalopathy. *Lancet* 1985; **i:** 752.
3. Goren MP, *et al.* Dechloroethylation of ifosfamide and neurotoxicity. *Lancet* 1986; **ii:** 1219–20.
4. Cerny T, *et al.* Ifosfamide by continuous infusion to prevent encephalopathy. *Lancet* 1990; **335:** 175.
5. Lewis LD, Meanwell CA. Ifosfamide pharmacokinetics and neurotoxicity. *Lancet* 1990; **335:** 175–6.
6. Wainer IW, *et al.* Ifosfamide stereoselective dichloroethylation [sic] and neurotoxicity. *Lancet* 1994; **343:** 982–3.
7. Osborne RJ, Slevin ML. Ifosfamide, mesna, and encephalopathy. *Lancet* 1985; **i:** 1398–9.
8. Pinkerton R, *et al.* Ifosfamide, mesna, and encephalopathy. *Lancet* 1985; **i:** 1399.
9. Meanwell CA, *et al.* Avoiding ifosfamide/mesna encephalopathy. *Lancet* 1986; **ii:** 406.
10. Perren TJ, *et al.* Encephalopathy with rapid infusion ifosfamide/mesna. *Lancet* 1987; **i:** 390–1.
11. McCallum AK. Ifosfamide/mesna encephalopathy. *Lancet* 1987; **i:** 987. Correction. *ibid.*; 1048.
12. Atherton P, *et al.* Drug-induced encephalopathy after previous ifosfamide treatment. *Lancet* 1988; **ii:** 1084.
13. Pelgrims J, *et al.* Methylene blue in the treatment and prevention of ifosfamide-induced encephalopathy: report of 12 cases and a review of the literature. *Br J Cancer* 2000; **82:** 291–4.

**Handling and disposal.** A study[1] found that ifosfamide 8% solution penetrated all of 4 brands of latex glove and one PVC glove, although the diffusion rate was 4 or more times slower than through cadaver skin. Permeation was greater through the PVC glove than the latex gloves, partly due to its lesser thickness, although permeation was not dependent on thickness alone and varied between gloves of the same brand as well as between brands. They recommended that latex gloves of a suitable brand should be worn when handling ifosfamide, and changed at least every 2 hours. For reference to a method for the destruction of ifosfamide waste, see under Cyclophosphamide, p.541.

1. Corlett SA, *et al.* Permeation of ifosfamide through gloves and cadaver skin. *Pharm J* 1991; **247:** R39.

## Interactions

As for Cyclophosphamide, p.541. For a general outline of antineoplastic drug interactions, see p.498.

◊ For reference to the effects of ifosfamide on oral anticoagulants, see under Warfarin Sodium, p.1025. For a report of the enhancement of cisplatin-induced ototoxicity and nephrotoxicity, see under Cisplatin, p.539.

## Pharmacokinetics

Ifosfamide is normally given intravenously, although it is well absorbed from the gastrointestinal tract. The pharmacokinetics of ifosfamide are reported to exhibit considerable interindividual variation. It is a prodrug that is extensively metabolised, chiefly by the cytochrome P450 isoenzyme system in the liver, to a variety of active and inactive metabolites; there is some evidence that metabolism is saturated at very high doses. Although the manufacturers state that a mean terminal elimination half-life of about 15 hours has been reported following a single high-dose intravenous bolus, most studies at lower doses appear to have recorded elimination half-lives of about 4 to 8 hours. Following repeated doses (fractionated therapy) there is a decrease in the elimination half-life, apparently due to autoinduction of metabolism. Ifosfamide is distributed into the CSF. It is excreted largely in urine, as unchanged drug and metabolites.

◊ General references.

1. Wagner T. Ifosfamide clinical pharmacokinetics. *Clin Pharmacokinet* 1994; **26:** 439–56.
2. Boddy AV, Yule SM. Metabolism and pharmacokinetics of oxazaphosphorines. *Clin Pharmacokinet* 2000; **38:** 291–304.
3. Kerbusch T, *et al.* Clinical pharmacokinetics and pharmacodynamics of ifosfamide and its metabolites. *Clin Pharmacokinet* 2001; **40:** 41–62.

◊ In a study[1] in 20 patients receiving intravenous ifosfamide over 3 or 5 days, the median elimination half-life of ifosfamide was 3.85 hours in patients under 60 years of age compared with 6.03 hours in those over age 60; this difference appeared to be due to an increased volume of distribution in the older age group. The autoinduction of metabolism typically seen with multiple doses of ifosfamide was not affected by age. The increased clearance seen over time during a 5-day cycle of ifosfamide treatment[2] was not sustained over the 21 days between cycles, but was reproducible and of similar magnitude in the subsequent cycle.

In another study[3] the half-life of the *S*-enantiomer of ifosfamide was found to be 5.98 hours after an intravenous bolus of the racemate, compared with 7.12 hours for the *R*-enantiomer.

1. Lind MJ, *et al.* The effect of age on the pharmacokinetics of ifosfamide. *Br J Clin Pharmacol* 1990; **30:** 140–3.
2. Lewis LD. A study of 5 day fractionated ifosfamide pharmacokinetics in consecutive treatment cycles. *Br J Clin Pharmacol* 1996; **42:** 179–86.
3. Corlett SA, *et al.* Pharmacokinetics of ifosfamide and its enantiomers following a single 1h intravenous infusion of the racemate in patients with small cell lung carcinoma. *Br J Clin Pharmacol* 1995; **39:** 452–5.

## Uses and Administration

Ifosfamide is an alkylating agent with properties similar to those of cyclophosphamide (p.542), of which it is a congener. It is used in the treatment of a variety of solid tumours including those of the cervix, lung, ovary, testis, and thymus, as well as in sarcoma and in the treatment of lymphomas. For further mention of these uses see the cross-references given below.

Ifosfamide is given intravenously, either by injection as a solution diluted to less than 4%, or by infusion. Licensed dosage regimens include a total dose of 8 to 12 g/m² divided over 3 to 5 days, with the course repeated at 2 to 4 week intervals; a total dose of 6 g/m² divided over 5 days, repeated every 3 weeks; and doses of 5 to 6 g/m², to a maximum of 10 g, given as a single 24-hour infusion, repeated at 3 to 4 week intervals. The interval between courses also depends on the blood count (see also Bone-marrow Depression, p.496). Oral ifosfamide has also been studied but is associated with neurotoxicity (see Effects on the Nervous System, above).

Ifosfamide should be given with mesna (below), and adequate hydration should be maintained, to avoid urological toxicity; fluid intake should not be less than 2 litres daily.

**Administration.** Mesna (p.1041) can combine with urotoxic ifosfamide metabolites in the kidney to form stable and non-toxic compounds. It is therefore given prophylactically with ifosfamide. It has a shorter half-life than ifosfamide so repeated doses are needed to provide adequate protection of the bladder. A common schedule uses intravenous mesna at 60% of the ifosfamide dose, divided into 3 doses given with, or 15 minutes before, ifosfamide, then 4 and 8 hours after ifosfamide.[1] Mesna may also be given orally, but higher doses are required.

1. Siu LL, Moore MJ. Use of mesna to prevent ifosfamide-induced urotoxicity. *Support Care Cancer* 1998; **6:** 144–54.

**Malignant neoplasms.** Ifosfamide may be used as an alternative to cyclophosphamide in lymphomas such as Burkitt's lymphoma (p.511). It is also used in a variety of solid neoplasms, including in palliative regimens for advanced cervical cancer (p.515); in the treatment of lung cancer (p.519); in ovarian cancer (p.520) and second-line and salvage regimens for testicular cancer (p.523); in thymoma (p.523); in adjuvant therapy for bone sarcomas (p.524) and rhabdomyosarcoma (p.525).

## Preparations

***USP 27:*** Ifosfamide for Injection.

**Proprietary Preparations** (details are given in Part 3)
***Arg.:*** Asoifos; Cuantil; Duvaxan; Fentul; Holoxan; Ifocris; Ifosmixan; IFX; ***Austral.:*** Holoxan; ***Austria:*** Holoxan; ***Belg.:*** Holoxan; ***Braz.:*** Holoxane; Ifos†; ***Canad.:*** Ifex; ***Chile:*** Holoxan; Ifolem; ***Denm.:*** Holoxan; ***Fin.:*** Holoxan; ***Fr.:*** Holoxan; ***Ger.:*** Holoxan; IFO-cell; ***Gr.:*** Holoxan; ***Hong Kong:*** Holoxan; ***Irl.:*** Mitoxana; ***Israel:*** Ifoxan; ***Ital.:*** Holoxan; ***Malaysia:*** Holoxan; ***Mex.:*** Holoxan†; Ifolem; Ifomida; Ifoxan; Seromida†; ***Neth.:*** Holoxan; ***Norw.:*** Holoxan; ***NZ:*** Holoxan; ***Port.:*** Holoxan; ***S.Afr.:*** Holoxan; ***Singapore:*** Holoxan; ***Spain:*** Tronoxal; ***Swed.:*** Holoxan; ***Switz.:*** Holoxan; ***Thai.:*** Holoxan; ***UK:*** Mitoxana; ***USA:*** Ifex.

**Multi-ingredient:** ***India:*** Holoxan Uromitexan.

## Imatinib Mesilate *(BANM, rINNM)*

CGP-57-148B; Imatinib Mesylate *(USAN)*; Mesilato de imatinib; STI-571. α-(4-Methyl-1-piperazinyl)-3′-{[4-(3-pyridyl)-2-pyrimidinyl]amino}-p-tolu-p-toluidide methanesulfonate.

$C_{29}H_{31}N_7O,CH_4O_3S = 589.7$.

*CAS — 152459-95-5 (imatinib); 220127-57-1 (imatinib mesilate).*

*ATC — L01XX28.*

### Adverse Effects and Precautions

The most common adverse effects of imatinib mesilate include gastrointestinal disturbances, superficial oedema, myalgia, muscle cramps, rashes, and headache. Myelosuppression, manifest as neutropenia, thrombocytopenia, or anaemia, occurs more frequently in leukaemic patients, and may be associated with the underlying disease. Gastrointestinal bleeding, however, occurs more frequently in those patients treated for stromal tumours. Severe fluid retention can occur, which may result in pleural and pericardial effusion, pulmonary oedema, and ascites. Some fatalities have been reported, and treatment may need to be stopped if there is unexpected, rapid weight gain. Elderly patients and those with a history of cardiac disease may be at increased risk. There are reports, including fatalities, of cerebral oedema, increased intracranial pressure and papilloedema. Hepatotoxicity may occur.

Imatinib mesilate should be taken with food and a large glass of water to minimise gastrointestinal irritation. Complete blood counts and liver function should be monitored regularly.

**Effects on the skin and hair.** There are reports of acute generalised exanthematous pustulosis in patients receiving imatinib.[1,2] The authors noted that severe skin reactions had been reported in some other patients receiving the drug, and speculated that the effect might be dose-dependent and related to its pharmacological action. In subsequent reports[3-5] of cutaneous adverse effects, this dose-dependency has also been observed, with effects especially at doses of 600 mg daily and above. Epidermal necrolysis occurred in a patient who underwent stem cell transplantation after treatment with imatinib.[6] The authors suggested that prolonged inhibition of platelet-derived growth factor by imatinib may have impaired the repair of skin damage caused by the conditioning therapy. Repigmentation of grey hair has also been reported.[7]

1. Brouard M, Saurat J-H. Cutaneous reactions to STI571. *N Engl J Med* 2001; **345:** 618–19.
2. Schwarz M, *et al.* Imatinib-induced acute generalized exanthematous pustulosis (AGEP) in two patients with chronic myeloid leukemia. *Eur J Haematol* 2002; **69:** 254–6.
3. Valeyrie L, *et al.* Adverse cutaneous reactions to imatinib (STI571) in Philadelphia chromosome-positive leukemias: a prospective study of 54 patients. *J Am Acad Dermatol* 2003; **48:** 201–6.
4. Drummond A, *et al.* A spectrum of skin reactions caused by the tyrosine kinase inhibitor imatinib mesylate (STI 571, Glivec®). *Br J Haematol* 2003; **120:** 911–13.
5. Ugurel S, *et al.* Dose-dependent severe cutaneous reactions to imatinib. *Br J Cancer* 2003; **88:** 1157–9.
6. Schaich M, *et al.* Severe epidermal necrolysis after treatment with imatinib and consecutive allogeneic hematopoietic stem cell transplantation. *Ann Hematol* 2003; **82:** 303–4.
7. Etienne G, *et al.* Imatinib mesylate and gray hair. *N Engl J Med* 2002; **347:** 446.

**Effects on the spleen.** There are isolated reports of splenic rupture in patients receiving imatinib mesilate.[1]

1. Elliott MA, *et al.* Adverse events after imatinib mesylate therapy. *N Engl J Med* 2002; **346:** 712–13.

### Interactions

Imatinib mesilate is metabolised by the cytochrome P450 isoenzyme CYP3A4, and drugs that inhibit this enzyme system, such as azole antifungals and macrolide antibacterials, may increase blood concentrations of imatinib. Equally, inducers of this enzyme system (such as carbamazepine, dexamethasone, hypericum, phenobarbital, phenytoin, and rifampicin) may reduce blood concentrations of imatinib.

*In vitro* studies have indicated that imatinib itself inhibits the cytochrome P450 isoenzymes CYP3A4, CYP2C9, and CYP2D6, and may increase blood concentrations of drugs that are substrates of these enzymes.

### Pharmacokinetics

Imatinib mesilate is well absorbed after oral doses with peak blood concentrations occurring after 2 to 4 hours. The mean bioavailability is about 98%. Imatinib is reported to be about 95% bound to plasma proteins. Plasma elimination half-lives of imatinib and its major active metabolite, the *N*-demethylated piperazine derivative, are about 18 and 40 hours respectively. The major enzyme responsible for the metabolism of imatinib is cytochrome P450 isoenzyme CYP3A4; isoenzymes CYP1A2, CYP2D6, CYP2C9, and CYP2C19 also play a minor role. About 81% of a dose is eliminated within 7 days in the faeces (68%) and urine (13%). It is excreted mostly as metabolites, with only 25% as unchanged drug (20% faeces, 5% urine).

### Uses and Administration

Imatinib mesilate is a tyrosine kinase inhibitor that inhibits the BCR-ABL tyrosine kinase created by the Philadelphia chromosome abnormality in chronic myeloid leukaemia (p.507). It also inhibits the tyrosine kinase for platelet-derived growth factor and stem cell factor, c-kit (CD117), which is overexpressed in gastrointestinal stromal tumours. Imatinib is given as the mesilate but doses are expressed as the base. Imatinib mesilate 119.5 mg is approximately equivalent to 100 mg of imatinib.

In the treatment of chronic myeloid leukaemia, patients in chronic phase may be given the equivalent of 400 mg of the base daily by mouth, increased to 600 mg daily if required. Patients in blast crisis or accelerated phase are given 600 mg daily, increased to 400 mg twice daily if necessary. Children over 3 years may be given 260 mg/m² daily (to a maximum of 400 mg) in chronic phase, and 340 mg/m² daily (maximum 600 mg) in advanced phase.

In the treatment of unresectable or metastatic malignant gastrointestinal stromal tumours, doses of 400 or 600 mg daily are recommended.

Doses should be taken with food, and accompanied by plenty of water, to minimise gastric irritation. Dose adjustments may be necessary if myelosuppression or hepatotoxicity occurs; blood counts and liver function should be regularly monitored.

◊ References.

1. Druker BJ, *et al.* Efficacy and safety of a specific inhibitor of the BCR-ABL tyrosine kinase in chronic myeloid leukemia. *N Engl J Med* 2001; **344:** 1031–7.
2. Druker BJ, *et al.* Activity of a specific inhibitor of the BCR-ABL tyrosine kinase in the blast crisis of chronic myeloid leukemia and acute lymphoblastic leukemia with the Philadelphia chromosome. *N Engl J Med* 2001; **344:** 1038–42.
3. Joensuu H, *et al.* Effect of the tyrosine kinase inhibitor STI571 in a patient with a metastatic gastrointestinal stromal tumor. *N Engl J Med* 2001; **344:** 1052–6.
4. van Oosterom AT, *et al.* Safety and efficacy of imatinib (STI571) in metastatic gastrointestinal stromal tumours: a phase I study. *Lancet* 2001; **358:** 1421–3.
5. Savage DG, Antman KH. Imatinib mesylate—a new oral targeted therapy. *N Engl J Med* 2002; **346:** 683–93.
6. Kantarjian H, *et al.* Hematologic and cytogenetic responses to imatinib mesylate in chronic myelogenous leukemia. *N Engl J Med* 2002; **346:** 645–52. Correction. *ibid.* 1923.
7. Demetri GD, *et al.* Efficacy and safety of imatinib mesylate in advanced gastrointestinal stromal tumors. *N Engl J Med* 2002; **347:** 472–80.
8. Kantarjian HM, *et al.* Imatinib mesylate therapy in newly diagnosed patients with Philadelphia chromosome-positive chronic myelogenous leukemia: high incidence of early complete and major cytogenetic responses. *Blood* 2003; **101:** 97–100.
9. Kantarjian HM, *et al.* Dose escalation of imatinib mesylate can overcome resistance to standard-dose therapy in patients with chronic myelogenous leukemia. *Blood* 2003; **101:** 473–5.
10. Peggs K, Mackinnon S. Imatinib mesylate—the new gold standard for treatment of chronic myeloid leukemia. *N Engl J Med* 2003; **348:** 1048–50.
11. Deininger MW, *et al.* Practical management of patients with chronic myeloid leukemia receiving imatinib. *J Clin Oncol* 2003; **21:** 1637–47.
12. Croom KF, Perry CM. Imatinib mesylate: in the treatment of gastrointestinal stromal tumours. *Drugs* 2003; **63:** 513–22.
13. Druker BJ. Imatinib mesylate in the treatment of chronic myeloid leukaemia. *Expert Opin Pharmacother* 2003; **4:** 963–71.
14. O'Brien SG, Deininger MWN. Imatinib in patients with newly diagnosed chronic-phase chronic myeloid leukemia. *Semin Hematol* 2003; **40** (suppl 2): 26–30.

### Preparations

**Proprietary Preparations** (details are given in Part 3)
***Austral.:*** Glivec; ***Braz.:*** Glivec; ***Chile:*** Glivec; ***Denm.:*** Glivec; ***Fin.:*** Glivec; ***Fr.:*** Glivec; ***Irl.:*** Glivec; ***Israel:*** Glivec; ***Ital.:*** Glivec; ***Malaysia:*** Glivec; ***Norw.:*** Glivec; ***NZ:*** Glivec; ***Port.:*** Glivec; ***S.Afr.:*** Gleevec; ***Spain:*** Glivec; ***Switz.:*** Glivec; ***Thai.:*** Glivec; ***UK:*** Glivec; ***USA:*** Gleevec.

## Interleukin-2

BG-8301 (teceleukin); Epidermal Thymocyte Activating Factor; ETAF; IL-2; Interleucina 2; T-cell Growth Factor.

**Description.** Interleukin-2 is a naturally-occurring 133-amino-acid glycoprotein with a molecular weight of about 15 000. It is available from natural sources or as a product of recombinant DNA technology (rIL-2).

In addition to aldesleukin (below) modified forms of interleukin-2 produced by recombinant DNA technology have included celmoleukin and teceleukin.

## Aldesleukin *(BAN, USAN, rINN)*

Aldesleukina; Des-alanyl-1, Serine-125 Human Interleukin-2; Recombinant Interleukin-2; 125-L-Serine-2–133-interleukin 2 (human reduced).

*CAS — 110942-02-4.*

*ATC — L03AC01.*

**Description.** Aldesleukin (modified human recombinant interleukin-2) is produced by recombinant DNA technology using an *Escherichia coli* strain containing an analogue of the human interleukin-2 gene. It differs from native interleukin-2 in that it is not glycosylated, it has no N-terminal alanine, and it has serine substituted for cysteine at position 125.

**Incompatibility.** Aldesleukin 33 800 units/mL in glucose 5% lost significant biological activity when mixed with a variety of other drugs including ganciclovir sodium, lorazepam, pentamidine isetionate, prochlorperazine edisilate, and promethazine hydrochloride.[1] However, the incompatibility was not detectable by spectrophotometric methods and only lorazepam was visually incompatible, suggesting that these methods may be invalid for assessing the compatibility of proteins.

1. Alex S, *et al.* Compatibility and activity of aldesleukin (recombinant interleukin-2) in presence of selected drugs during simulated Y-site administration: evaluation of three methods. *Am J Health-Syst Pharm* 1995; **52:** 2423–6.

**Stability.** Aldesleukin lost 75 to 100% of activity when reconstituted with glucose 5% or sodium chloride 0.9% in a plastic syringe and administered over 24 hours with a syringe driver.[1,2] Loss of activity was not seen if aldesleukin was reconstituted with water alone[2] or with the addition of albumin.[1,2] It was suggested that loss of activity could be suspected because of lack of toxicity,[1,2] and that the lack of toxicity in some published studies could be due to this.[1,3] However, the authors of these studies indicated that they had reconstituted aldesleukin with albumin.[4,5] Reconstitution with low concentrations of albumin has been advocated to avoid bioavailability problems,[1,4,6] but is not recommended for currently licensed preparations

For short intravenous infusion, the US manufacturer indicates that dilution outside of a specified range (below 30 micrograms/mL and above 70 micrograms/mL) results in increased variability in drug delivery.

Dilution of aldesleukin preparations with sodium chloride 0.9% is not recommended because increased aggregation occurs.

1. Miles DW, *et al.* Reconstitution of interleukin 2 with albumin for infusion. *Lancet* 1990; **335:** 1602–3.
2. Vlasveld LT, *et al.* Reconstitution of interleukin-2. *Lancet* 1990; **336:** 446.
3. Miles DW, *et al.* Toxicity and reconstitution of recombinant interleukin-2 with albumin. *Lancet* 1991; **338:** 1464.
4. Franks CR. Reconstitution of interleukin-2. *Lancet* 1990; **336:** 445–6.
5. Hamblin T. Reconstitution of interleukin-2 with albumin for infusion. *Lancet* 1990; **336:** 251.
6. Lamers CHJ, *et al.* Bioavailability of interleukin-2 after reconstitution with albumin. *Lancet* 1992; **340:** 241.

### Units

100 units of human interleukin-2 are contained in one ampoule of the first International Standard Preparation (1987). The activity of interleukin-2 has also been expressed in Nutley and Cetus units: 100 international units is reportedly equivalent to about 83.3 Nutley units and to about 16.7 Cetus units. According to the manufacturers, 18 million international units of aldesleukin are equivalent to 1.1 mg of protein.

### Adverse Effects and Treatment

Toxicity is related to dose and route and is often severe; fatalities have been recorded. Decreased vascular resistance and increased capillary permeability (the 'capillary leak syndrome') is common in patients given aldesleukin, and results in hypotension, reduced organ perfusion, and oedema. The incidence and severity of this syndrome is lower after subcutaneous than intravenous dosage. Fluid replacement may be necessary to treat the resultant hypovolaemia and dopamine or other pressor agents may be needed to help maintain organ perfusion. Capillary leak syndrome may also be associated with cardiac effects including tachycardia, angina, myocardial infarction; respiratory effects such as dyspnoea, pulmonary oedema, and respiratory failure; renal abnormalities including uraemia and oliguria or anuria; mental status changes including irritability, depression, confusion, and drowsiness. Therapy should be stopped if patients develop severe lethargy or somnolence, as continuing may result in coma. Raised liver enzymes, gastrointestinal disturbances, fever and flu-like symptoms (malaise, rigors, chills, arthralgia, and myalgia), rashes, pruritus, anaemia, leucopenia, and thrombocytopenia, are also relatively common. Paracetamol (but not NSAIDs, see Effects on the Kidneys, below) may be used prophylactically for fever. Pethidine may be used to control rigors. Antiemetics and antidiarrhoeals may also be required. Antihistamines may benefit some patients with pruritic rash. Injection site reactions are common after subcutaneous doses; necrosis has occurred. Aldesleukin therapy is associated with impaired neutrophil function, and an increased risk of bacterial infections, including sepsis and bacterial endocarditis (see below); this has been reported mainly after intravenous use, and antibacterial prophylaxis may be necessary.

◊ References.


1. Sundin DJ, Wolin MJ. Toxicity management in patients receiving low-dose aldesleukin therapy. *Ann Pharmacother* 1998; **32:** 1344–52.
2. Schwartzentruber DJ. Guidelines for the safe administration of high-dose interleukin-2. *J Immunother* 2001; **24:** 287–93.
3. Dutcher J, *et al.* Kidney cancer: the Cytokine Working Group experience (1986-2001): part II: management of IL-2 toxicity and studies with other cytokines. *Med Oncol* 2001; **18:** 209–19.
4. Schwartz RN, *et al.* Managing toxicities of high-dose interleukin-2. *Oncology (Huntingt)* 2002; **16** (suppl 13): 11–20.


**Bacterial infections.** The incidence of sepsis and bacteraemia is increased in patients receiving interleukin-2 via intravenous catheters,[1,2] and possibly subcutaneously,[3] although others have not found this to be the case.[4,5] The increased incidence of nonopportunistic bacterial infection may be a particular problem in patients with AIDS who are treated with interleukin-2.[6] The mechanism is uncertain, but may be related to impairment of neutrophil function by the cytokine.[7]


1. Snydman DR, *et al.* Nosocomial sepsis associated with interleukin-2. *Ann Intern Med* 1990; **112:** 102–7.
2. Shiloni E, *et al.* Interleukin-2 therapy, central venous catheters, and nosocomial sepsis. *Ann Intern Med* 1990; **112:** 882–3.
3. Jones AL, *et al.* Infectious complications of subcutaneous interleukin-2 and interferon-alpha. *Lancet* 1992; **339:** 181–2.
4. Buter J, *et al.* Infection after subcutaneous interleukin-2. *Lancet* 1992; **339:** 552.
5. Schomburg AG, *et al.* Cytokines and infection in cancer patients. *Lancet* 1992; **339:** 1061.
6. Murphy PM, *et al.* Marked disparity in incidence of bacterial infections in patients with the acquired immunodeficiency syndrome receiving interleukin-2 or interferon-γ. *Ann Intern Med* 1988; **108:** 36–41.
7. Klempner MS, *et al.* An acquired chemotactic defect in neutrophils from patients receiving interleukin-2 immunotherapy. *N Engl J Med* 1990; **322:** 959–65.


**Effects on endocrine function.** It has been suggested that patients with adrenal metastases may be particularly susceptible to adrenal haemorrhage and consequent failure during interleukin therapy.[1] Results also suggested that lack of endogenous steroid production may increase the risk of early severe interleukin-2 toxicity.[1]

Effects on thyroid function have also been reported, with the development of hypothyroidism[2-4] and goitre.[3]


1. VanderMolen LA, *et al.* Adrenal insufficiency and interleukin-2 therapy. *Ann Intern Med* 1989; **111:** 185.
2. Atkins MB, *et al.* Hypothyroidism after treatment with interleukin-2 and lymphokine-activated killer cells. *N Engl J Med* 1988; **318:** 1557–63.
3. van Liessum PA, *et al.* Hypothyroidism and goitre during interleukin-2 therapy without LAK cells. *Lancet* 1989; **i:** 224.
4. Sauter NP, *et al.* Transient thyrotoxicosis and persistent hypothyroidism due to acute autoimmune thyroiditis after interleukin-2 and interferon-α therapy for metastatic carcinoma: a case report. *Am J Med* 1992; **92:** 441–4.


**Effects on the kidneys.** Intravenous aldesleukin therapy was associated with varying degrees of acute renal dysfunction in almost all of 99 adult patients.[1] The clinical syndrome of hypotension, oliguria, fluid retention, and associated azotaemia with intense tubular avidity for filtered sodium all support prerenal acute renal failure as the cause of renal dysfunction. However, renal function values returned to baseline levels within 7 days in 62% of patients and in 95% by 30 days. Patients with elevated pretreatment serum-creatinine values, particularly those aged over 60 years, and those who had previously undergone a nephrectomy, were at risk of more severe and prolonged changes in renal function, and might be particularly vulnerable to the use of indometacin for associated fever and chills, which could potentiate renal impairment through its effects on intrarenal prostaglandin production. Similar effects were noted in a study[2] of 15 children given continuous infusion of aldesleukin. A further study[3] of the renal haemodynamic effects of aldesleukin infusion found it to have a specific renal vasoconstrictor effect; changes in renal prostaglandin synthesis contributed to the decreased renal blood flow.


1. Belldegrun A, *et al.* Effects of interleukin-2 on renal function in patients receiving immunotherapy for advanced cancer. *Ann Intern Med* 1987; **106:** 817–22.
2. Cochat P, *et al.* Renal effects of continuous infusion of recombinant interleukin-2 in children. *Pediatr Nephrol* 1991; **5:** 33–7.
3. Geertsen PF, *et al.* Renal haemodynamics, sodium and water reabsorption during continuous intravenous infusion of recombinant interleukin-2. *Clin Sci* 1998; **95:** 73–81.


## Precautions

Aldesleukin should be given with great care, if at all, to patients with pre-existing cardiac or pulmonary disease, and those with severe renal or hepatic impairment. It should be avoided in patients with CNS metastases or seizure disorders.

Risk factors for toxicity and poor response include Eastern Co-operative Oncology Group performance status of 1 or greater, 2 or more metastatic sites, and a period of less than 24 months between diagnosis of primary tumour and consideration for aldesleukin therapy. The manufacturer in the UK considers that aldesleukin should not be used to treat metastatic renal cell carcinoma in patients with all three of these risk factors.

Aldesleukin may exacerbate auto-immune diseases, and should be used with caution in patients with these conditions. Bacterial infections should be adequately treated before beginning therapy. Aldesleukin may exacerbate effusions from serosal surfaces, and these should generally be treated before aldesleukin therapy.

Vital signs, blood counts, renal and hepatic function, serum electrolytes, and pulmonary and cardiac function should be monitored before starting treatment and then regularly during therapy.

**Activity.** For mention of the loss of activity when aldesleukin was given by continuous infusion without albumin, see Stability above.

**Inflammatory bowel disease.** Two patients with a history of Crohn's disease had a recurrence of the condition when given aldesleukin. It was suggested that interleukin-2 should be contraindicated in such patients.[1]


1. Sparano JA, *et al.* Symptomatic exacerbation of Crohn disease after treatment with high-dose interleukin-2. *Ann Intern Med* 1993; **118:** 617–18.


**Psoriasis.** Exacerbations of psoriasis developed in 3 patients during therapy with aldesleukin alone or with lymphokine-activated killer cells. The psoriatic symptoms remitted with topical therapy.[1]


1. Lee RE, *et al.* Interleukin 2 and psoriasis. *Arch Dermatol* 1988; **124:** 1811–15.


## Interactions

Corticosteroids (which reduce some of the adverse effects of interleukin-2) may also reduce its antineoplastic properties: use together should generally be avoided. The use of iodinated contrast media after aldesleukin therapy may result in symptoms resembling the immediate adverse effects of aldesleukin. Although most events were reported to occur within 2 to 4 weeks of the last dose of aldesleukin, some occurred several months afterward.

**Antivirals.** For the effect of interleukin-2 on plasma concentrations of *indinavir*, see p.639.

**NSAIDs.** NSAIDs are effective in preventing or reducing fever and myalgia caused by interleukin-2. However, there is concern that they could exacerbate renal toxicity (see also Effects on the Kidneys, above). Use of *indometacin* in patients receiving interleukin-2 led to more severe weight gain, oliguria, and azotaemia in 1 study.[1] However, *ibuprofen* was used successfully to reduce interleukin-2 toxicity in another study.[2]


1. Sosman JA, *et al.* Repetitive weekly cycles of interleukin-2 II: clinical and immunologic effects of dose, schedule, and addition of indomethacin. *J Natl Cancer Inst* 1988; **80:** 1451–61.
2. Eberlein TJ, *et al.* Ibuprofen causes reduced toxic effects of interleukin 2 administration in patients with metastatic cancer. *Arch Surg* 1989; **124:** 542–7.


## Pharmacokinetics

After intravenous bolus, the serum distribution and elimination half-lives of aldesleukin are 13 and 85 minutes, respectively. After subcutaneous doses, the absorption half-life is 45 minutes and the elimination half-life is 5.3 hours, while bioavailability ranges between 35 and 47%.

Aldesleukin is metabolised to amino acids by the kidneys.

◊ References.


1. Anderson PM, Sorenson MA. Effects of route and formulation on clinical pharmacokinetics of interleukin-2. *Clin Pharmacokinet* 1994; **27:** 19–31.
2. Piscitelli SC, *et al.* Pharmacokinetics and pharmacodynamics of subcutaneous interleukin-2 in HIV-infected patients. *Pharmacotherapy* 1996; **16:** 754–9.
3. Kirchner GI, *et al.* Pharmacokinetics of recombinant human interleukin-2 in advanced renal cell carcinoma patients following subcutaneous application. *Br J Clin Pharmacol* 1998; **46:** 5–10.


## Uses and Administration

Interleukin-2 is a lymphokine which stimulates the proliferation of T-lymphocytes and thus amplifies immune response to an antigen; it also has actions on B-lymphocytes, and induces the production of interferon-γ and the activation of natural killer cells. Interleukin-2 is used in the immunotherapy of metastatic renal cell carcinoma in selected patients (see p.518). It is also used in melanoma (p.522), and has been tried in non-Hodgkin's lymphoma and acute myeloid leukaemia.

Interleukin-2 is usually given by intravenous infusion or subcutaneous injection of one of its recombinant forms, such as aldesleukin.

A variety of dosage regimens have been tried. In the UK, the recommended dose of aldesleukin for metastatic renal cell carcinoma is 18 million units given subcutaneously once daily for 5 days, followed by 2 days rest for the first week. For the next 3 weeks, 18 million units are then given on days 1 and 2 of each week, and 9 million units on days 3 to 5 of each week, followed by 2 days rest. This 4-week cycle may be repeated after an interval of 1 week. Doses may be delayed or reduced if the regimen is not tolerated.

Aldesleukin was formerly given by intravenous infusion, in similar doses, but this is no longer advocated in the UK. However, in the USA, aldesleukin is given by intravenous infusion for metastatic renal cell carcinoma or melanoma. The recommended dose is an infusion of 600 000 units/kg over 15 minutes, every 8 hours for up to 14 doses. This 5-day cycle is repeated after 9 days. Further courses may be given at intervals of at least 7 weeks in patients who respond. Doses should be withheld for toxicity.

Aldesleukin given by inhalation is being investigated in the treatment of renal cell carcinoma.

Interleukin-2 has also been given in adoptive immunotherapy with lymphokine-activated killer (LAK) cells or tumour-infiltrating lymphocytes (TIL), which are harvested from the patient, activated *ex vivo,* and then re-infused.

Interleukin-2 is also being tried in patients with HIV infection and AIDS in an attempt to restore immune response (see below) and has been given in some other infections or immune diseases.

Other interleukins are under investigation (see also Interleukin-1, p.1701). Conjugates of interleukin-2 with macrogol (PEG-IL2; pegaldesleukin) have also been investigated and liposome-encapsulated interleukin-2 has also been investigated for the treatment of renal, brain and CNS tumours.

◊ Reviews.


1. Noble S, Goa K. Aldesleukin (recombinant interleukin-2): a review of its pharmacological properties, clinical efficacy and tolerability in patients with metastatic melanoma. *BioDrugs* 1997; **7:** 394–422.
2. Atkins MB, *et al.* High-dose recombinant interleukin 2 therapy for patients with metastatic melanoma: analysis of 270 patients treated between 1985 and 1993. *J Clin Oncol* 1999; **17:** 2105–16.
3. Malaguarnera M, *et al.* Use of interleukin-2 in advanced renal carcinoma: meta-analysis and review of the literature. *Eur J Clin Pharmacol* 2001; **57:** 267–73.
4. Atkins MB, *et al.* Kidney cancer: the Cytokine Working Group experience (1986-2001): part I: IL-2-based clinical trials. *Med Oncol* 2001; **18:** 197–207.


**HIV infection and AIDS.** The immunodeficiency of HIV infection and AIDS (p.621) has been associated with a defect in interleukin-2 production. Interleukin-2 stimulates the proliferation of lymphocytes and activates natural killer cells and a number of studies have therefore examined the potential benefits of adding interleukin-2 to the treatment of patients with HIV infection.[1] Following earlier pilot studies, trials of antiretroviral therapy plus interleukin-2 have shown it to produce a much greater increase in CD4 cell counts than antiretroviral therapy alone,[2-6] even where therapy included highly active antiretroviral therapy (HAART). Given the efficacy of current therapies demonstrating additional benefits on survival or disease progression is difficult, although some studies have been undertaken.[1] In the interim, a pooled analysis[7] of earlier results showed a non-significant trend towards improved clinical outcome.

Although teceleukin has been tried[2] most studies of interleukin-2 therapy in HIV have used aldesleukin. Doses and routes have varied: in general doses seem to have ranged from 6 to 18 million units daily by intravenous infusion, or 3 to 30 million units daily subcutaneously, given in most cases for a 5-day cycle every 8 weeks. Subcutaneous dosage appears to be as effective as intravenous,[3,8] is more convenient,[3] and may be less toxic.[9] There is evidence that 5-day dose cycles of 3, 4.5 or

7.5 million units twice daily by subcutaneous injection are effective,[4,5,8,10,11] whereas cycles with a lower dose of 1.5 million units twice daily are not.[4,10] However, others have reported benefit from a dose as low as 3 million units daily in combination with HAART in patients with advanced disease.[12] Continuous low-dose daily therapy appears to accelerate the normalisation of T-cell and natural killer cell concentrations over the course of several months.[9]

Adverse effects are common, particularly at higher doses and with intravenous infusion rather than subcutaneous use.[6,9] However, concerns about a potential stimulant effect on viral replication with a consequent increase in viral load do not seem to have been borne out.[3-6,8] Some studies have reported reduced viral loads in interleukin-treated patients,[5,13] including decreases in hepatitis C viral load in those HIV patients co-infected with hepatitis C.[8,14]

The macrogol conjugate of interleukin-2, PEG-IL2, has also been investigated in this context, but results have been disappointing, since it appears markedly less effective than aldesleukin in stimulating CD4 counts.[3,15]

1. Pau AK, Tavel JA. Therapeutic use of interleukin-2 in HIV-infected patients. *Curr Opin Pharmacol* 2002; **2:** 433–9.
2. Bartlett JA, *et al.* Coadministration of zidovudine and interleukin-2 increases absolute CD4 cells in subjects with Walter Reed stage 2 human immunodeficiency virus infection: results of ACTG protocol 042. *J Infect Dis* 1998; **178:** 1170–3.
3. Levy Y, *et al.* Comparison of subcutaneous and intravenous interleukin-2 in asymptomatic HIV-1 infection: a randomised controlled trial. *Lancet* 1999; **353:** 1923–9.
4. Losso MH, *et al.* A randomized, controlled, phase II trial comparing escalating doses of subcutaneous interleukin-2 plus antiretrovirals versus antiretrovirals alone in human immunodeficiency virus-infected patients with CD4+ cell counts ≥350/mm³. *J Infect Dis* 2000; **181:** 1614–21. Correction. *ibid.*; 2122.
5. Davey RT, *et al.* Immunologic and virologic effects of subcutaneous interleukin 2 in combination with antiretroviral therapy: a randomized controlled trial. *JAMA* 2000; **284:** 183–9.
6. Piscitelli SC, *et al.* A risk-benefit assessment of interleukin-2 as an adjunct to antiviral therapy in HIV infection. *Drug Safety* 2000; **22:** 19–31.
7. Emery S, *et al.* Pooled analysis of 3 randomized, controlled trials of interleukin-2 therapy in adult human immunodeficiency virus type 1 disease. *J Infect Dis* 2000; **182:** 428–34.
8. Tambussi G, *et al.* Efficacy of low-dose intermittent subcutaneous interleukin (IL)–2 in antiviral drug–experienced human immunodeficiency virus–infected persons with detectable virus load: a controlled study of 3 IL-2 regimens with antiviral drug therapy. *J Infect Dis* 2001; **183:** 1476–84.
9. Smith KA. Low-dose daily interleukin-2 immunotherapy: accelerating immune restoration and expanding HIV-specific T-cell immunity without toxicity. *AIDS* 2001; **15** (suppl 2): S28–S35.
10. Davey RT, *et al.* A randomized trial of high- versus low-dose subcutaneous interleukin-2 outpatient therapy for early human immunodeficiency virus type 1 infection. *J Infect Dis* 1999; **179:** 849–58.
11. David D, *et al.* Rapid effect of interleukin-2 therapy in human immunodeficiency virus–infected patients whose CD4 cell counts increase only slightly in response to combined antiretroviral treatment. *J Infect Dis* 2001; **183:** 730–5.
12. Arnó A, *et al.* Efficacy of low-dose subcutaneous interleukin-2 to treat advanced human immunodeficiency virus type 1 in persons with ≤250/microlitre CD4 T cells and undetectable plasma virus load. *J Infect Dis* 1999; **180:** 56–60.
13. Lafeuillade A, *et al.* Pilot study of a combination of highly active antiretroviral therapy and cytokines to induce HIV-1 remission. *J Acquir Immune Defic Syndr* 2001; **26:** 44–55.
14. Schlaak JF, *et al.* Sustained suppression of HCV replication and inflammatory activity after interleukin-2 therapy in patients with HIV/hepatitis C virus coinfection. *J Acquir Immune Defic Syndr* 2002; **29:** 145–8.
15. Carr A, *et al.* Outpatient continuous intravenous interleukin-2 or subcutaneous, polyethylene glycol-modified interleukin-2 in human immunodeficiency virus-infected patients: a randomized, controlled, multicenter study. *J Infect Dis* 1998; **178:** 992–9.

### Preparations

**Proprietary Preparations** (details are given in Part 3)
***Arg.:*** Ilgen; Proleukin; ***Austral.:*** Proleukin; ***Austria:*** Proleukin; ***Belg.:*** Proleukin; ***Braz.:*** Proleukin; ***Canad.:*** Proleukin; ***Denm.:*** Proleukin; ***Fr.:*** Macrolin†; Proleukin; ***Ger.:*** Proleukin; ***Gr.:*** Proleukin; ***Hong Kong:*** Proleukin; ***Israel:*** Proleukin; ***Ital.:*** Proleukin; ***Mex.:*** Proleukin; ***Neth.:*** Proleukin; ***NZ:*** Proleukin; ***Port.:*** Proleukin†; ***Singapore:*** Proleukin; ***Spain:*** Proleukin; ***Switz.:*** Proleukin; ***UK:*** Proleukin; ***USA:*** Proleukin.

## Irinotecan Hydrochloride

*(BANM, USAN, rINNM)*

CPT-11 (irinotecan); Hidrocloruro de irinotecán; U-101440E.
(+)-7-Ethyl-10-hydroxycamptothecine 10-[1,4′-bipiperidine]-1′-carboxylate hydrochloride trihydrate; (*S*)-4,11-Diethyl-3,4,-12,14-tetrahydro-4-hydroxy-3,14-dioxo-1*H*-pyrano[3′,4′:6′,7′]-indolizino[1,2-*b*]quinolin-9-yl [1,4′-dipiperidine]-1′-carboxylate hydrochloride trihydrate.
$C_{33}H_{38}N_4O_6,HCl,3H_2O = 677.2.$
*CAS — 97682-44-5 (irinotecan); 136572-09-3 (irinotecan hydrochloride trihydrate).*
*ATC — L01XX19.*

### Adverse Effects, Treatment, and Precautions

For general discussions, see Antineoplastics, p.492, p.495, and p.497. Neutropenia and diarrhoea may be dose-limiting in patients receiving irinotecan. The nadir of the white cell count usually occurs about 8 days after a dose, with recovery by about day 22. Anaemia also occurs and, less commonly, thrombocytopenia. Gastrointestinal disturbances are common: acute diarrhoea, occurring within 24 hours of administration, may be part of a cholinergic syndrome which can also include sweating, hypersalivation, abdominal cramps, lachrymation, and miosis. These symptoms can be controlled with atropine. However a more severe, prolonged diarrhoea may occur, beginning more than 24 hours after a dose, and can be life-threatening; prompt management with high-dose loperamide and fluid replacement is required (see below), and irinotecan treatment should be interrupted and any further doses reduced. Other adverse effects include nausea and vomiting, weakness, alopecia, and skin reactions. Hypertension has occurred rarely during or after infusion, and there are rare reports of hypersensitivity reactions, interstitial pneumonia, and pneumonitis, in patients who have received irinotecan.

Irinotecan should not be given to patients with inflammatory bowel disease. The risk of diarrhoea may be increased in the elderly and in patients who have received radiotherapy to the abdomen or pelvis. Blood counts should be monitored weekly and liver function tests should be regularly performed.

Severe toxicity resulting in an increased number of deaths has been reported from the combination of irinotecan with fluorouracil and folinic acid (see under Interactions, below).

**Effects on the gastrointestinal system.** Acute diarrhoea occurring as part of a cholinergic syndrome is rarely severe. The syndrome is usually treated or prevented with atropine, but pretreatment with hyoscine butylbromide has also been tried.[1] In contrast, delayed diarrhoea can be dose-limiting or even fatal in some patients. Standard treatment involves fluid and electrolyte replacement and a high-dose loperamide regimen consisting of 4 mg loperamide immediately after the first loose stool, then 2 mg every 2 hours until 12 hours after the last liquid stool. The high-dose therapy should not be given for more than 48 hours and should never be given prophylactically. Specific recommendations[2] state that if the diarrhoea persists for more than 24 hours despite loperamide therapy, patients should also take an oral fluoroquinolone for 7 days. If the diarrhoea persists for more than 48 hours, patients should be hospitalised for parenteral hydration. Other treatments have been tried,[3-7] including acetorphan,[3] budesonide,[4] glutamine,[5] and octreotide.[7] A small study[8] found that a regimen of thalidomide with irinotecan had a striking lack of gastrointestinal adverse effects such as diarrhoea and nausea.

1. Zampa G, Magnolfi E. Premedication for irinotecan. *J Clin Oncol* 2000; **18:** 237.
2. Rothenberg ML, *et al.* Mortality associated with irinotecan plus bolus fluorouracil/leucovorin: summary findings of an independent panel. *J Clin Oncol* 2001; **19:** 3801–7.
3. Saliba F, *et al.* Pathophysiology and therapy of irinotecan-induced delayed-onset diarrhea in patients with advanced colorectal cancer: a prospective assessment. *J Clin Oncol* 1998; **16:** 2745–51.
4. Lenfers BHM, *et al.* Substantial activity of budesonide in patients with irinotecan (CPT-11) and 5-fluorouracil induced diarrhea and failure of loperamide treatment. *Ann Oncol* 1999; **10:** 1251–3.
5. Savarese D, *et al.* Glutamine for irinotecan diarrhea. *J Clin Oncol* 2000; **18:** 450–1.
6. Ychou M, *et al.* Randomized comparison of prophylactic antidiarrheal treatment versus no prophylactic antidiarrheal treatment in patients receiving CPT-11 (irinotecan) for advanced 5-FU-resistant colorectal cancer: an open-label multicenter phase II study. *Am J Clin Oncol* 2000; **23:** 143–8.
7. Pro B, *et al.* Therapeutic response to octreotide in patients with refractory CPT-11 induced diarrhea. *Invest New Drugs* 2001; **19:** 341–3.
8. Govindarajan R, *et al.* Effect of thalidomide on gastrointestinal toxic effects of irinotecan. *Lancet* 2000; **356:** 566–7.

### Interactions

**Antidepressants.** In a small, crossover study[1] of cancer patients, use of *hypericum* during irinotecan therapy was found to decrease plasma concentrations of SN-38, the active metabolite of irinotecan. Myelosuppression was also reduced with this combination. The interaction is thought to be due to the induction of the cytochrome P450 isoenzyme CYP3A4 by hypericum.

1. Mathijssen RHJ, *et al.* Effects of St. John's Wort on irinotecan metabolism. *J Natl Cancer Inst* 2002; **94:** 1247–9.

**Antineoplastics.** Although previously reported to be effective, and not associated with excessive toxicity,[1] a regimen of irinotecan with bolus *fluorouracil* and folinic acid was found to be associated with an excess of early deaths in 2 further studies, which were consequently terminated.[2] Deaths were associated with a variety of events including dehydration (due to diarrhoea, nausea, and vomiting), neutropenia, and sepsis. It has been suggested that use of irinotecan with fluorouracil by continuous infusion might be better tolerated,[3,4] and a small study[5] found that the sequence of administration may be important. Irinotecan followed by an infusion of fluorouracil over 48 hours, was associated with less dose-limiting toxicity, and higher maximum tolerated doses, than fluorouracil infusion followed by irinotecan.

1. Saltz LB, *et al.* Irinotecan plus fluorouracil and leucovorin for metastatic colorectal cancer. *N Engl J Med* 2000; **343:** 905–14.
2. Sargent DJ, *et al.* Recommendation for caution with irinotecan, fluorouracil, and leucovorin for colorectal cancer. *N Engl J Med* 2001; **345:** 144–5.
3. Ledermann JA, *et al.* Recommendation for caution with irinotecan, fluorouracil, and leucovorin for colorectal cancer. *N Engl J Med* 2001; **345:** 145–6.
4. Van Cutsem E, *et al.* Toxicity of irinotecan in patients with colorectal cancer. *N Engl J Med* 2001; **345:** 1351–2.
5. Falcone A, *et al.* Sequence effect of irinotecan and fluorouracil treatment on pharmacokinetics and toxicity in chemotherapy-naive metastatic colorectal cancer patients. *J Clin Oncol* 2001; **19:** 3456–62.

### Pharmacokinetics

After intravenous doses irinotecan is metabolised by carboxylesterase in body tissues to active SN-38 (7-ethyl-10-hydroxycamptothecin). Irinotecan exhibits biphasic or triphasic pharmacokinetics, with a terminal half-life of about 14 hours. Only about 20% of a dose is excreted in urine within 24 hours.

◊ References.

1. Chabot GG. Clinical pharmacokinetics of irinotecan. *Clin Pharmacokinet* 1997; **33:** 245–59.
2. Rivory LP. Metabolism of CPT-11: impact on activity. *Ann N Y Acad Sci* 2000; **922:** 205–15.
3. Mathijssen RH, *et al.* Clinical pharmacokinetics and metabolism of irinotecan (CPT-11). *Clin Cancer Res* 2001; **7:** 2182–94.

### Uses and Administration

Irinotecan is a derivative of the alkaloid camptothecin, obtained from the shrub *Camptotheca acuminata*. The camptothecin derivatives are inhibitors of the enzyme topoisomerase I which thus interfere with the coiling and uncoiling of DNA during replication and prevent nucleic acid synthesis. This action is specific for S phase.

Irinotecan is used, alone or with fluorouracil, in the treatment of metastatic colorectal cancer (p.516). It has been tried in the management of other solid tumours including those of the lung (p.519).

It is given as the hydrochloride, by intravenous infusion, in at least 250 mL of glucose 5%, or sodium chloride 0.9%. In the treatment of refractory colorectal malignancies one suggested single-agent dose regimen is irinotecan hydrochloride 125 mg/m² infused over 90 minutes once a week for 4 weeks, followed by a 2-week rest period. Additional courses may be given if required, with doses modified according to toxicity. Another regimen requires an initial dose of 350 mg/m² over 30 to 90 minutes repeated every 3 weeks and adjusted according to toxicity.

Irinotecan hydrochloride may also be given as part of a regimen with fluorouracil and folinic acid in the first-line treatment of metastatic colorectal cancer. The irinotecan component of the course is given at a dose of 180 mg/m² over 30 to 90 minutes every 2 weeks for 3 doses; alternatively, 125 mg/m² may be given weekly for 4 doses. (For reference to toxicity from such regimens see under Interactions, above.)

◊ References.

1. Douillard JY, *et al.* Irinotecan combined with fluorouracil compared with fluorouracil alone as first-line treatment for metastatic colorectal cancer: a multicentre randomised trial. *Lancet* 2000; **355:** 1041–7. Correction. *ibid.*; 1372.
2. Saltz LB, *et al.* Irinotecan plus fluorouracil and leucovorin for metastatic colorectal cancer. *N Engl J Med* 2000; **343:** 905–14.
3. Rothenberg ML. Irinotecan (CPT-11): recent developments and future directions—colorectal cancer and beyond. *Oncologist* 2001; **6:** 66–80.
4. Saltz LB, *et al.* Irinotecan plus fluorouracil/leucovorin for metastatic colorectal cancer: a new survival standard. *Oncologist* 2001; **6:** 81–91.
5. Cunningham D, *et al.* Optimizing the use of irinotecan in colorectal cancer. *Oncologist* 2001; **6** (suppl 4): 17–23.
6. Vanhoefer U, *et al.* Irinotecan in the treatment of colorectal cancer: clinical overview. *J Clin Oncol* 2001; **19:** 1501–18.
7. Douillard JY, *et al.* Update on European adjuvant trials with irinotecan for colorectal cancer. *Oncology (Huntingt)* 2002; **16** (suppl 3): 13–15.
8. Pizzolato JF, Saltz LB. The camptothecins. *Lancet* 2003; **361:** 2235–42.

### Preparations

**Proprietary Preparations** (details are given in Part 3)
***Arg.:*** Biotecan; Camptosar; CPT; Efixano; Irenax; Irinogen; Itoxaril; Kebirtecan; Pipetecan; Satigene; Sibudan; Trinotecan; Winol; ***Austral.:*** Camptosar; ***Austria:*** Campto; ***Belg.:*** Campto; ***Braz.:*** Camptosar; Tecnotecan; ***Canad.:*** Camptosar; ***Chile:*** Camptosar; ***Denm.:*** Campto; ***Fin.:*** Campto; ***Fr.:*** Campto; ***Ger.:*** Campto; ***Gr.:*** Campto; ***Hong Kong:*** Camp-

to; **India:** Irinotel; **Irl.:** Campto; **Israel:** Campto; **Ital.:** Campto; **Malaysia:** Campto; **Mex.:** Camptosar; **Neth.:** Campto; **Norw.:** Campto; **NZ:** Camptosar; **Port.:** Campto; **S.Afr.:** Campto; **Singapore:** Campto; **Spain:** Campto; **Swed.:** Campto; **Switz.:** Campto; **Thai.:** Campto; **UK:** Campto; **USA:** Camptosar.

## Letrozole *(BAN, USAN, rINN)*

CGS-20267; Letrozol. 4,4′-(1H-1,2,4-Triazol-1-ylmethylene)-dibenzonitrile.

$C_{17}H_{11}N_5$ = 285.3.
*CAS — 112809-51-5.*
*ATC — L02BG04.*

**Pharmacopoeias.** In *US.*

**USP 27** (Letrozole). A white to yellowish, crystalline powder. Practically insoluble in water; slightly soluble in alcohol; freely soluble in dichloromethane. Store in airtight containers.

### Adverse Effects and Precautions

As for Anastrozole, p.528.

### Interactions

**Tamoxifen.** In a study[1] of postmenopausal women with breast cancer, the addition of tamoxifen reduced letrozole plasma concentrations by a mean of about 38%, but the effect of letrozole on hormone concentrations was unchanged. The mechanism and possible clinical effect of this interaction are unknown.

1. Dowsett M, *et al.* Impact of tamoxifen on the pharmacokinetics and endocrine effects of the aromatase inhibitor letrozole in postmenopausal women with breast cancer. *Clin Cancer Res* 1999; **5:** 2338–43.

### Pharmacokinetics

Letrozole is rapidly and completely absorbed from the gastrointestinal tract. About 60% of letrozole in the circulation is bound to plasma protein, mainly albumin. Most of an oral dose is slowly metabolised to an inactive carbinol metabolite, which is then excreted as the glucuronide in the urine. Letrozole has a terminal elimination half-life of about 2 days.

### Uses and Administration

Letrozole is a selective nonsteroidal inhibitor of the aromatase (oestrogen synthetase) system, similar to anastrozole (p.528). It is used in the treatment of advanced or locally advanced breast cancer (p.514) in postmenopausal women. It may also be given as neoadjuvant (pre-operative) therapy to those with localised hormone-receptor positive disease, to allow subsequent breast-conserving surgery. The usual dose is 2.5 mg daily by mouth.

◊ References.

1. Lamb HM, Adkins JC. Letrozole: a review of its use in postmenopausal women with advanced breast cancer. *Drugs* 1998; **56:** 1125–40.
2. Dombernowsky P, *et al.* Letrozole, a new oral aromatase inhibitor for advanced breast cancer: double-blind randomized trial showing a dose effect and improved efficacy and tolerability compared with megestrol acetate. *J Clin Oncol* 1998; **16:** 453–61.
3. Gershanovich M, *et al.* Letrozole, a new oral aromatase inhibitor: randomised trial comparing 2.5 mg daily, 0.5 mg daily and aminoglutethimide in postmenopausal women with advanced breast cancer. *Ann Oncol* 1998; **9:** 639–45.
4. Chaudri HA, Trunet PF. Letrozole: updated duration of response. *J Clin Oncol* 1999; **17:** 3859–60.
5. Mouridsen H, *et al.* Superior efficacy of letrozole versus tamoxifen as first-line therapy for postmenopausal women with advanced breast cancer: results of a phase III study of the International Letrozole Breast Cancer Group. *J Clin Oncol* 2001; **19:** 2596–2606.
6. Buzdar A, *et al.* Phase III, multicenter, double-blind, randomized study of letrozole, an aromatase inhibitor, for advanced breast cancer versus megestrol acetate. *J Clin Oncol* 2001; **19:** 3357–66.
7. Ellis MJ, *et al.* Letrozole is more effective neoadjuvant endocrine therapy than tamoxifen for ErbB-1- and/or ErbB-2-positive, estrogen receptor-positive primary breast cancer: evidence from a phase III randomized trial. *J Clin Oncol* 2001; **19:** 3808–16.
8. Goss PE, *et al.* A randomized trial of letrozole in postmenopausal women after five years of tamoxifen therapy for early-stage breast cancer. *N Engl J Med* 2003; **349:** 1793–1802.

### Preparations

***USP 27:*** Letrozole Tablets.

**Proprietary Preparations** (details are given in Part 3)
**Arg.:** Cendalon; Fecinole; Femara; **Austral.:** Femara; **Austria:** Femara; **Belg.:** Femara; **Braz.:** Femara; **Canad.:** Femara; **Chile:** Femara; **Denm.:** Femar; **Fin.:** Femar; **Fr.:** Femara; **Ger.:** Femara; **Gr.:** Femara; **Hong Kong:** Femara; **Irl.:** Femara; **Israel:** Femara; **Ital.:** Femara; **Malaysia:** Femara; **Mex.:** Femara; **Neth.:** Femara; **Norw.:** Femar; **NZ:** Femara; **Port.:** Femara; **S.Afr.:** Femara; **Singapore:** Femara†; **Spain:** Femara; **Swed.:** Femar; **Switz.:** Femara; **Thai.:** Femara; **UK:** Femara; **USA:** Femara.

## Lobaplatin *(rINN)*

D-19466; Lobaplatino. *cis*-[*trans*-1,2-Cyclobutanebis(methylamine)][(*S*)-lactato-*O*¹,*O*²]platinum.

$C_9H_{18}N_2O_3Pt$ = 397.3.
*CAS — 135558-11-1.*

### Profile

Lobaplatin is an analogue of cisplatin (p.538) that has been investigated for its antineoplastic properties. Thrombocytopenia is reported to be dose-limiting. It may be active against some cancer cells resistant to cisplatin or carboplatin.

◊ References.

1. Manegold C, *et al.* Lobaplatin (D-19466) in patients with advanced non-small-cell lung cancer: a trial of the association for medical oncology (AIO) phase II study group. *Onkologie* 1996; **19:** 248–51.
2. Fiebig HH, *et al.* Phase II clinical trial of lobaplatin (D-19466) in pretreated patients with small-cell lung cancer. *Onkologie* 1996; **19:** 328–32.
3. Sternberg CN, *et al.* Lobaplatin in advanced urothelial tract tumors. *Ann Oncol* 1997; **8:** 695–6.
4. Welink J, *et al.* Pharmacokinetics and pharmacodynamics of lobaplatin (D-19466) in patients with advanced solid tumors, including patients with impaired renal or liver function. *Clin Cancer Res* 1999; **5:** 2349–58.
5. McKeage MJ. Lobaplatin: a new antitumour platinum drug. *Expert Opin Invest Drugs* 2001; **10:** 119–28.

## Lomustine *(BAN, USAN, rINN)*

CCNU; Lomustina; Lomustinum; NSC-79037; RB-1509; WR-139017. 1-(2-Chloroethyl)-3-cyclohexyl-1-nitrosourea.

$C_9H_{16}ClN_3O_2$ = 233.7.
*CAS — 13010-47-4.*
*ATC — L01AD02.*

**Pharmacopoeias.** In *Chin., Eur.* (see p.vi), and *Pol.*

**Ph. Eur. 5.0** (Lomustine). A yellow, crystalline powder. Practically insoluble in water; soluble in alcohol; freely soluble in acetone and in dichloromethane. Protect from light.

### Adverse Effects, Treatment, and Precautions

As for Carmustine, p.535. Neurological reactions such as confusion and lethargy have been reported.

**Handling and disposal.** A method for the destruction of lomustine *waste* by reaction with hydrobromic acid in glacial acetic acid has been described.[1] The residue produced by the degradation of lomustine by this method showed no mutagenicity. This method is not suitable for the degradation of carmustine or semustine.

1. Castegnaro M, *et al.*, eds. Laboratory decontamination and destruction of carcinogens in laboratory wastes: some antineoplastic agents. *IARC Scientific Publications 73.* Lyon: WHO/International Agency for Research on Cancer, 1985.

**Overdosage.** A patient who inadvertently received 200 mg of lomustine for 7 days instead of a single 200-mg dose developed pancytopenia and subsequent multiorgan dysfunction including liver dysfunction, abdominal pain, pulmonary toxicity with tachypnoea and hypoxaemia, and CNS toxicity leading to confusion and disorientation.[1] Although the white cell count recovered other signs of toxicity did not and the patient developed fever and hypotension and died 59 days after the initial dose of lomustine. In another case of accidental overdose, a 30-year old female received a cumulative dose of 28 mg/kg over 7 days.[2] Severe myelosuppression developed soon after the overdose and lasted for 50 days. The patient was treated with granulocyte colony-stimulating factor and antibiotic cover, norethisterone (to prevent menstruation), and acetylcysteine (to protect against organ toxicity). Gastrointestinal necrosis occurred, and liver enzymes remained elevated even after recovery from the overdose, but the patient survived and her tumour regressed without further chemotherapy.

1. Trent KC, *et al.* Multiorgan failure associated with lomustine overdose. *Ann Pharmacother* 1995; **29:** 384–6.
2. Abele M, *et al.* CCNU overdose during PCV chemotherapy for anaplastic astrocytoma. *J Neurol* 1998; **245:** 236–8.

### Interactions

For a general outline of antineoplastic drug interactions, see p.498.

**Cimetidine.** For a report of a possible interaction between lomustine and cimetidine, see under Carmustine, p.535.

**Theophylline.** Leucopenia and thrombocytopenia in a 45-year-old woman were believed to have been secondary to an interaction between theophylline and lomustine.[1]

1. Zeltzer PM, Feig SA. Theophylline-induced lomustine toxicity. *Lancet* 1979; **ii:** 960–1.

### Pharmacokinetics

Lomustine is absorbed from the gastrointestinal tract and is rapidly metabolised, with peak plasma concentrations of metabolites occurring within 4 hours of a dose by mouth. Metabolites have a prolonged plasma half-life reported to range from 16 to 48 hours. Active metabolites readily cross the blood-brain barrier and appear in the CSF in concentrations higher than those in plasma. About half a dose is excreted as metabolites in the urine within 24 hours and about 75% is excreted within 4 days.

### Uses and Administration

Lomustine is a nitrosourea with actions and uses similar to those of carmustine (p.535). It has been used in the treatment of brain tumours (p.513) and resistant or relapsed Hodgkin's disease and other lymphomas (p.509), and also lung cancer (p.519), malignant melanoma (p.522), and various solid tumours.

When given as a single agent, lomustine is licensed for use by mouth in adults and children as a single dose of 120 to 130 mg/m²; division of the dose over 3 consecutive days may reduce gastrointestinal effects. A dose of 100 mg/m² should be given to patients with compromised bone-marrow function. Doses are also generally reduced when lomustine is given as part of a combination regimen. Providing blood counts have returned to acceptable levels, doses may be repeated every 6 to 8 weeks, and should be adjusted according to the haematological response (see also Bone-marrow Depression, p.496).

### Preparations

***BP 2003:*** Lomustine Capsules.

**Proprietary Preparations** (details are given in Part 3)
**Arg.:** CeeNU; **Austral.:** CeeNU; **Belg.:** Cecenu†; **Braz.:** Citostal; **Canad.:** CeeNU; **Chile:** CeeNU; **Fr.:** Belustine†; **Ger.:** Cecenu; **Hong Kong:** Belustine†; CeeNU; **Israel:** CeeNU; **Ital.:** Belustine†; **Malaysia:** CeeNU; **Mex.:** CeeNU; **NZ:** CeeNU; **S.Afr.:** CeeNU†; **Singapore:** CeeNU; **Spain:** Belustine†; **Switz.:** Prava; **Thai.:** CeeNU†; **UK:** CCNU; **USA:** CeeNU.

## Lonidamine *(BAN, rINN)*

AF-1890; Diclondazolic Acid; Lonidamina. 1-(2,4-Dichlorobenzyl)indazole-3-carboxylic acid.

$C_{15}H_{10}Cl_2N_2O_2$ = 321.2.
*CAS — 50264-69-2.*
*ATC — L01XX07.*

### Profile

Lonidamine is an antineoplastic that is thought to act by inhibiting mitochondrial function in tumour cells. It may be given by mouth in the treatment of various solid neoplasms, including those of the lung, breast, prostate, and brain, in usual doses of 450 to 900 mg daily, in 3 divided doses. Myalgia is common, and may be dose-limiting. Other adverse effects include testicular pain, auditory dysfunction, gastrointestinal disturbances, drowsiness, weakness, and conjunctivitis with photophobia, but it is reported to lack myelosuppressive effects and not to cause stomatitis or alopecia.

◊ References.

1. De Marinis F, *et al.* The role of vindesine and lonidamine in the treatment of elderly patients with advanced non-small cell lung cancer: a phase III randomized FONICAP trial. *Tumori* 1999; **85:** 177–82.
2. Pacini P, *et al.* FEC (5-fluorouracil, epidoxorubicin and cyclophosphamide) versus EM (epidoxorubicin and mitomycin-C) with or without lonidamine as first-line treatment for advanced breast cancer: a multicentric randomised study. Final results. *Eur J Cancer* 2000; **36:** 966–75.
3. Berruti A, *et al.* Time to progression in metastatic breast cancer patients treated with epirubicin is not improved by the addition of either cisplatin or lonidamine: final results of a phase III study with a factorial design. *J Clin Oncol* 2002; **20:** 4150–9.
4. Papaldo P, *et al.* Addition of either lonidamine or granulocyte colony-stimulating factor does not improve survival in early breast cancer patients treated with high-dose epirubicin and cyclophosphamide. *J Clin Oncol* 2003; **21:** 3462–8.

### Preparations

**Proprietary Preparations** (details are given in Part 3)
**Ital.:** Doridamina.

## Mafosfamide *(rINN)*

Mafosfamida. (±)-2-({2-[Bis(2-chloroethyl)amino]tetrahydro-2H-1,3,2-oxazaphosphorin-4-yl}thio)ethanesulphonic acid *P-cis* oxide.

$C_9H_{19}Cl_2N_2O_5PS_2$ = 401.3.
*CAS — 88859-04-5.*

### Profile

Mafosfamide is a derivative of cyclophosphamide (p.540) that has been used to treat bone marrow for transplantation. It is also under investigation in the treatment of neoplastic meningitis.

## Marimastat *(BAN, USAN, rINN)*

BB-2516. (2S,3R)-3-{(S)-[2,2-Dimethyl-1-(methylcarbamoyl)propyl]carbamoyl}-2-hydroxy-5-methylhexanohydroxamic acid.

$C_{15}H_{29}N_3O_5$ = 331.4.
*CAS — 154039-60-8.*

### Profile

Like batimastat (p.529) marimastat is an inhibitor of matrix metalloproteinases, enzymes which are thought to play a role in the metastasis of cancer cells. It has been investigated by mouth in various malignant disorders.

◊ References.
1. Bramhall SR, *et al.* Marimastat as first-line therapy for patients with unresectable pancreatic cancer: a randomized trial. *J Clin Oncol* 2001; **19:** 3447–55.
2. Bramhall SR, *et al.* A double-blind placebo-controlled, randomised study comparing gemcitabine and marimastat with gemcitabine and placebo as first line therapy in patients with advanced pancreatic cancer. *Br J Cancer* 2002; **87:** 161–7.
3. Miller KD, *et al.* A randomized phase II trial of adjuvant marimastat in patients with early-stage breast cancer. *Ann Oncol* 2002; **13:** 1220–4.
4. Quirt I, *et al.* Phase II study of marimastat (BB-2516) in malignant melanoma: a clinical and tumor biopsy study of the National Cancer Institute of Canada Clinical Trials Group. *Invest New Drugs* 2002; **20:** 431–7.
5. Shepherd FA, *et al.* Prospective, randomized, double-blind, placebo-controlled trial of marimastat after response to first-line chemotherapy in patients with small-cell lung cancer: a trial of the National Cancer Institute of Canada-Clinical Trials Group and the European Organization for Research and Treatment of Cancer. *J Clin Oncol* 2002; **20:** 4434–9.
6. Groves MD, *et al.* Phase II trial of temozolomide plus the matrix metalloproteinase inhibitor, marimastat, in recurrent and progressive glioblastoma multiforme. *J Clin Oncol* 2002; **20:** 1383–8.
7. Larson DA, *et al.* Phase II study of high central dose Gamma Knife radiosurgery and marimastat in patients with recurrent malignant glioma. *Int J Radiat Oncol Biol Phys* 2002; **54:** 1397–1404.
8. King J, *et al.* Randomised double blind placebo control study of adjuvant treatment with the metalloproteinase inhibitor, marimastat in patients with inoperable colorectal hepatic metastases: significant survival advantage in patients with musculoskeletal side-effects. *Anticancer Res* 2003; **23:** 639–45.

## Masoprocol *(USAN, rINN)*

CHX-10; CHX-100; Mesonordihydroguaiaretic Acid; *meso*-NDGA. *meso*-4,4′-(2,3-Dimethyltetramethylene)dipyrocatechol.

$C_{18}H_{22}O_4$ = 302.4.

*CAS — 27686-84-6.*

*ATC — L01XX10.*

### Profile

Masoprocol is a 5-lipoxygenase inhibitor isolated from the chaparral or creosote bush, *Larrea tridentata* (p.1670). It is reported to have antineoplastic activity. It has been used in the topical treatment of actinic (solar) keratoses. Local irritation and contact dermatitis have occurred.

## Melphalan *(BAN, USAN, rINN)*

CB-3025; Melfalán; NSC-8806 (melphalan hydrochloride); PAM; Phenylalanine Mustard; Phenylalanine Nitrogen Mustard; L-Sarcolysine; WR-19813. 4-Bis(2-chloroethyl)amino-L-phenylalanine.

$C_{13}H_{18}Cl_2N_2O_2$ = 305.2.

*CAS — 148-82-3 (melphalan); 3223-07-2 (melphalan hydrochloride).*

*ATC — L01AA03.*

NOTE. Merphalan (CB-3007; NSC-14210; sarcolysine) is the racemic form of melphalan; Medphalan (CB-3026; NSC-35051) is the D-isomer of melphalan.

**Pharmacopoeias.** In *Br., Jpn,* and *US.*

**BP 2003** (Melphalan). A white or almost white, odourless or almost odourless, powder. It loses not more than 7% of its weight on drying. Practically insoluble in water, in chloroform, and in ether; slightly soluble in methyl alcohol; dissolves in dilute mineral acids. Store at a temperature not exceeding 25°. Protect from light.

**USP 27** (Melphalan). An off-white to buff powder with a faint odour. Practically insoluble in water, in chloroform, and in ether; slightly soluble in alcohol and in methyl alcohol; soluble in dilute mineral acids. Store in airtight, glass containers. Protect from light.

**Stability.** A study of the stability of melphalan 40 and 400 micrograms/mL in infusion fluids reported that the time for a 10% loss of drug at 20° in sodium chloride 0.9% injection was 4.5 hours, compared with 2.9 hours in lactated Ringer's injection, which has a considerably lower chloride ion content, and only 1.5 hours in glucose 5% injection.[1] At 25° the corresponding figures were 2.4, 1.5, and 0.6 hours, and at 37° they were 0.6, 0.4, and 0.3 hours. It was concluded that melphalan is sufficiently stable at 20° in sodium chloride injection to permit infusion, but that increased temperature and decreased chloride ion concentration were associated with faster degradation rates.[1] Another study recommended that solutions of melphalan be handled at temperatures above 5° for the minimum time but found that a solution containing 20 micrograms/mL in sodium chloride 0.9% could be stored for at least 6 months at −20° without significant deterioration.[2] A more recent study, while recommending storage at 4° from preparation of the admixture until the infusion began, considered that administration at a room temperature of 20° or below, and use of hypertonic (3%) saline as a diluent, would be sufficient to allow prolonged infusion.[3] The practicalities of such a procedure were not addressed.

1. Tabibi SE, Cradock JC. Stability of melphalan in infusion fluids. *Am J Hosp Pharm* 1984; **41:** 1380–2.
2. Bosanquet AG. Stability of melphalan solutions during preparation and storage. *J Pharm Sci* 1985; **74:** 348–51.
3. Pinguet F, *et al.* Effect of sodium chloride concentration and temperature on melphalan stability during storage and use. *Am J Hosp Pharm* 1994; **51:** 2701–4.

### Adverse Effects and Treatment

For general discussions see Antineoplastics, p.492 and p.495.

The onset of neutropenia and thrombocytopenia is variable; the nadir of bone-marrow depression usually occurs at 2 to 3 weeks after starting treatment with melphalan, with recovery after 4 to 5 weeks.

Skin rashes and hypersensitivity reactions, including anaphylaxis, may occur. Cardiac arrest has been reported in association with such effects. Gastrointestinal disturbances may sometimes occur, particularly at high doses where diarrhoea, vomiting, and stomatitis may become dose-limiting. Haemolytic anaemia, vasculitis, pulmonary fibrosis, and hepatic disorders including hepatitis and jaundice have been reported. Suppression of ovarian function is common in premenopausal women; temporary or permanent sterility may occur in male patients. Extravasation of melphalan injection can cause skin ulceration and necrosis. As with other alkylating agents, melphalan also has carcinogenic, mutagenic, and teratogenic potential.

**Overdosage.** A 12-month old child given melphalan 140 mg intravenously (a tenfold overdose) developed pronounced lymphopenia within 24 hours but had no other significant adverse effects until the seventh day, when neutropenia, thrombocytopenia, oral ulceration, and diarrhoea developed.[1] Bone marrow recovered within 40 days. Treatment was by vigorous hyperalimentation and close surveillance during this period and the patient subsequently remained well 9 months afterwards, without complications. Cases of intravenous melphalan overdose have also been reported in adults,[2] resulting in bone-marrow depression, haemorrhagic diarrhoea, and electrolyte disturbances. Bone-marrow depression has also been reported following cumulative oral doses of 360 mg over 3 weeks,[3] and 560 mg over 2 weeks.[4] Filgrastim was used in one of these cases to stimulate bone-marrow recovery.[4]

1. Coates TD. Survival from melphalan overdose. *Lancet* 1984; **ii:** 1048.
2. Jost LM. Überdosierung von Melphalan (Alkeran®): Symptome und Behandlung: eine Übersicht. *Onkologie* 1990; **13:** 96–101.
3. Grimes DJ, *et al.* Complete remission of paraproteinaemia and neuropathy following iatrogenic oral melphalan overdose. *Br J Haematol* 1993; **83:** 675–7.
4. Jirillo A, *et al.* Accidental overdose of melphalan per os in a 69-year-old woman treated for advanced endometrial carcinoma. *Tumori* 1998; **84:** 611.

### Precautions

For general discussions see Antineoplastics, p.497.

Care is required in patients with impaired renal function.

**Handling and disposal.** *Urine and faeces* produced for up to 48 hours and 7 days respectively after a dose of melphalan by mouth should be handled wearing protective clothing.[1]

1. Harris J, Dodds LJ. Handling waste from patients receiving cytotoxic drugs. *Pharm J* 1985; **235:** 289–91.

### Interactions

Use of nalidixic acid with high-dose intravenous melphalan in children has resulted in fatal haemorrhagic enterocolitis.

**Ciclosporin.** For reference to enhanced toxicity when melphalan was given with ciclosporin, see under Ciclosporin, p.1355.

**Food.** The bioavailability of oral melphalan is significantly reduced, by up to 45%, by food. Some recommend that melphalan should not be taken with food, and that if dosage is switched from after to before food patients should be monitored for increased toxicity.[1]

1. Nathan C, Betmouni R. Melphalan: avoid with food. *Pharm J* 1996; **257:** 264.

**Interferons.** The fever induced by interferon alfa resulted in a reduction in the area under the plasma concentration-time curve for melphalan in a study of 10 patients, although the peak plasma concentration and time to peak concentration were not affected.[1] The effect was thought to represent increased chemical reactivity of melphalan at the elevated temperature.

1. Ehrsson H, *et al.* Oral melphalan pharmacokinetics: influence of interferon-induced fever. *Clin Pharmacol Ther* 1990; **47:** 86–90.

### Pharmacokinetics

Absorption of melphalan from the gastrointestinal tract is variable; the mean bioavailability is reported to be 56% but it may range from 25 to 89%. Absorption is reduced by the presence of food (see above). Following absorption it is rapidly distributed throughout body water with a volume of distribution of about 0.5 litres/kg, and has been reported to be inactivated mainly by spontaneous hydrolysis. About 60 to 90% is bound to plasma proteins, mainly albumin. The terminal plasma half-life of melphalan has been reported to be of the order of 30 to 150 minutes. Melphalan is excreted in the urine, about 10% as unchanged drug.

### Uses and Administration

Melphalan is an antineoplastic that acts as a bifunctional alkylating agent. It is used mainly in the treatment of multiple myeloma. Melphalan has also been given to patients with carcinoma of the breast and ovary, neuroblastoma, Hodgkin's disease, and in polycythaemia vera, and has been given by intra-arterial regional perfusion for malignant melanoma and soft-tissue sarcomas. See also the cross-references given below. Melphalan is also used in the treatment of amyloidosis, see below.

Melphalan is usually given by mouth as a single daily dose or in divided doses; it is also given intravenously as the hydrochloride. Doses are calculated in terms of the base; 1.12 mg of melphalan hydrochloride is equivalent to 1 mg of melphalan. Frequent blood counts are essential and dosage should be adjusted according to haematological response. Therapy should be interrupted if the platelet or white cell count fall below acceptable levels (see also Bone-marrow Depression, p.496). It should be given with great caution if the neutrophil count has recently been depressed by chemotherapy or radiotherapy.

Numerous conventional-dose regimens have been tried for the treatment of multiple myeloma and there is still uncertainty as to the best schedule. Licensed **oral** dosage regimens include: 150 micrograms/kg daily in divided doses for 4 to 7 days; or 250 micrograms/kg daily for 4 days; or 6 mg daily for 2 to 3 weeks. Melphalan is usually combined with corticosteroids. Courses are followed by a rest period of up to 6 weeks to allow recovery of haematological function and are then repeated, or maintenance therapy may be instituted, usually with a daily dose of 1 to 3 mg, or up to 50 micrograms/kg. For optimum effect, therapy is usually adjusted to produce a moderate leucopenia, with white cell counts in the range 3000 to 3500 cells/$mm^3$.

In the treatment of breast cancer, licensed doses are 150 micrograms/kg daily or 6 mg/$m^2$ daily for 5 days, repeated every 6 weeks. Doses of 200 micrograms/kg daily for 5 days every 4 to 8 weeks have been given to patients with ovarian carcinoma.

In patients with polycythaemia vera, doses of 6 to 10 mg daily for 5 to 7 days, and then 2 to 4 mg daily, have been used for remission induction; a dose of 2 to 6 mg weekly has been used for maintenance.

Melphalan is also given **intravenously**; a single dose of 1 mg/kg, repeated in 4 weeks if the platelet and neutrophil counts permit, has been licensed in ovarian adenocarcinoma. It may be infused in sodium chloride 0.9% or injected into the tubing of a fast-running drip; when given by infusion the time from reconstitution of the solution to completion of infusion should not exceed 1.5 hours and prolonged infusions should be carried out with several batches of solution, each freshly prepared. In multiple myeloma, the licensed dose for use as a single agent is an intravenous dose of 400 micrograms/kg or 16 mg/$m^2$, infused over 15 to 20 minutes; the first 4 doses may be given at 2-week intervals, but further doses should be given at 4-week intervals depending on toxicity.

**High-dose** melphalan has been given intravenously in some malignancies: doses of 100 to 240 mg/$m^2$ have been licensed in neuroblastoma, and 100 to 200 mg/$m^2$ in multiple myeloma, generally followed by autologous stem cell rescue, which becomes essential where doses exceed 140 mg/$m^2$. High doses should be given through a central venous catheter.

Melphalan may be given by **local arterial perfusion** in the management of melanoma and soft-tissue sarcomas. A typical dosage range for upper extremity perfusions is 0.6 to 1 mg/kg, whereas for lower extremity perfusions doses of 0.8 to 1.5 mg/kg (in melanoma) or 1 to 1.4 mg/kg (in sarcoma) are typically used.

The dose of melphalan should be reduced in patients with **renal impairment** (see below).

**Administration in renal impairment.** The initial dose of intravenous melphalan should be reduced by about 50% in patients with renal impairment and dosage reduction should be considered when giving it by mouth. High-dose regimens are not recommended in patients with moderate to severe renal impairment.

**Amyloidosis.** Amyloidosis refers to a group of conditions characterised by accumulation of a waxy proteinaceous infiltrate within body tissues. Various forms are known,[1,2] including:

- primary or AL amyloidosis, in which the amyloid is derived from immunoglobulin light chains
- ATTR amyloidosis (a familial form), in which amyloid is derived from transthyretin
- AA amyloidosis, which is most often secondary to chronic inflammation, such as that associated with rheumatoid arthritis, tuberculosis, or familial Mediterranean fever (p.416)

Symptoms vary, depending on where the amyloid is deposited. The organs most commonly affected are the heart and kidneys. Renal amyloidosis can present as proteinuria, leading to nephrotic syndrome and renal failure. While renal disease is common in the AA and AL forms, it is less prevalent in ATTR amyloidosis, which commonly presents with neuropathy. Cardiac involvement, rare in AA amyloidosis, is variable in the ATTR form, and common in the AL form; it manifests as restrictive cardiomyopathy, leading to congestive heart failure. Painful peripheral sensory neuropathy and carpal tunnel syndrome also occur frequently. Amyloid deposition in the gastrointestinal tract can lead to malabsorption. Hepatomegaly is common. Macroglossia, due to deposition of amyloid in the tongue, occurs only in the AL form.[1,2]

Management depends to some extent upon the type of amyloidosis involved, and the site, but no drug or combination of drugs is unequivocally effective. Colchicine is extremely effective at preventing renal deterioration in patients with familial Mediterranean fever, but is not considered to be of benefit in other forms of amyloidosis.[1] Melphalan plus prednisone is the standard therapy, and has been shown to increase median survival in primary amyloidosis patients. Melphalan, prednisone, and colchicine was found to be more effective than colchicine alone in the treatment of AL amyloidosis,[3] but a later trial[4] found no benefit in adding colchicine to the standard therapy. Addition of multiple alkylating agents such as vincristine, carmustine, and cyclophosphamide to the standard therapy[5] did not improve survival or response. Alternatively, cycles of vincristine, doxorubicin, and dexamethasone may be effective, but patients with cardiac amyloidosis may be at increased risk of anthracycline toxicity.[6] High-dose intravenous melphalan with autologous haematopoietic stem cell transplantation may result in complete remission of primary amyloidosis,[7,8] and some[1] consider it the treatment of choice. While this may improve renal disease,[7] the therapy remains very toxic, and patient selection on the basis of limited organ disease and no significant cardiac involvement, may reduce morbidity and mortality.[8] High-dose dexamethasone has also been tried for the treatment of amyloidosis, although its value is controversial, as has local application or oral administration of dimethyl sulfoxide, and 4′-iodo-4′-deoxydoxorubicin has been investigated.[1,6]

Symptomatic management is also important. Care must be taken to avoid digitalis toxicity when cardiac amyloid is present, as well as to avoid salt and water depletion through injudicious use of diuretics. Calcium-channel blockers and beta blockers should be avoided.[1] Renal transplantation may be considered in end-stage renal failure due to amyloidosis, but unless amyloid production has been stopped disease is likely to recur in the new kidney. Cardiac transplantation, and subsequent chemotherapy with epirubicin, carmustine, and cyclophosphamide to suppress the underlying disease and control amyloid deposition in the graft has also been described.[9] Liver transplantation is the definitive therapy for patients with ATTR amyloidosis.[1,10] Because amyloid deposits contain a plasma glycoprotein serum amyloid P component (SAP) that contributes to the stability of the deposits, and thus contributes to the pathogenesis of amyloidosis, future therapeutic approaches include the targeting of SAP to deplete it from the tissues and clear it from the plasma. Ro-63-8695(CPHPC) is being investigated.[11]


1. Khan MF, Falk RH. Amyloidosis. *Postgrad Med J* 2001; **77:** 686–93.
2. Falk RH, Skinner M. The systemic amyloidoses: an overview. *Adv Intern Med* 2000; **45:** 107–37.
3. Skinner M, *et al.* Treatment of 100 patients with primary amyloidosis: a randomized trial of melphalan, prednisone, and colchicine versus colchicine only. *Am J Med* 1996; **100:** 290–8.
4. Kyle RA, *et al.* A trial of three regimens for primary amyloidosis: colchicine alone, melphalan and prednisone, and melphalan, prednisone, and colchicine. *N Engl J Med* 1997; **336:** 1202–7.
5. Gertz MA, *et al.* Prospective randomized trial of melphalan and prednisone versus vincristine, carmustine, melphalan, cyclophosphamide, and prednisone in the treatment of primary systemic amyloidosis. *J Clin Oncol* 1999; **17:** 262–7.
6. Sezer O, *et al.* New therapeutic approaches in primary systemic AL amyloidosis. *Ann Hematol* 2000; **79:** 1–6.
7. Dember LM, *et al.* Effect of dose-intensive intravenous melphalan and autologous blood stem-cell transplantation on AL amyloidosis-associated renal disease. *Ann Intern Med* 2001; **134:** 746–53.
8. Comenzo RL, Gertz MA. Autologous stem cell transplantation for primary systemic amyloidosis. *Blood* 2002; **99:** 4276–82.
9. Hall R, *et al.* Cardiac transplantation for AL amyloidosis. *BMJ* 1994; **309:** 1135–7.
10. Suhr OB, *et al.* Liver transplantation for hereditary transthyretin amyloidosis. *Liver Transpl* 2000; **6:** 263–76.
11. Pepys MB, *et al.* Targeted pharmacological depletion of serum amyloid P component for treatment of human amyloidosis. *Nature* 2002; **417:** 254–9.


**Bone disorders, non-malignant.** Fibrogenesis imperfecta ossium is a rare progressive bone disease in which disorders of bone collagen and mineralisation, and subsequent abnormal bone structure, result in bone pain and fractures. A patient responded to treatment with melphalan 10 mg and prednisolone 20 or 30 mg daily, in 7-day courses every 2 months.[1,2] Another showed some improvement with intermittent 5-day courses of melphalan 10 mg daily and prednisolone 40 mg daily.[3] However, melphalan alone was reported to be ineffective in two other patients; both experienced bone-marrow depression.[3,4]


1. Stamp TCB, *et al.* Fibrogenesis imperfecta ossium: remission with melphalan. *Lancet* 1985; **i:** 582–3.
2. Ralphs JR, *et al.* Ultrastructural features of the osteoid of patients with fibrogenesis imperfecta ossium. *Bone* 1989; **10:** 243–9.
3. Carr AJ, *et al.* Fibrogenesis imperfecta ossium. *J Bone Joint Surg Br* 1995; **77:** 820–9.
4. Lafage-Proust M-H, *et al.* Fibrogenesis imperfecta ossium: ineffectiveness of melphalan. *Calcif Tissue Int* 1996; **59:** 240–4.


**Malignant neoplasms.** The important role played by melphalan in the management of multiple myeloma is discussed on p.511. Melphalan is also used as part of salvage regimens for relapsed Hodgkin's disease (see p.509), in ovarian cancer (p.520), and for local perfusion of melanoma (p.522).

## Preparations

***BP 2003:*** Melphalan Injection; Melphalan Tablets;
***USP 27:*** Melphalan Tablets.

**Proprietary Preparations** (details are given in Part 3)
***Arg.:*** Alkerana; ***Austral.:*** Alkeran; ***Austria:*** Alkeran; ***Belg.:*** Alkeran; ***Braz.:*** Alkeran; ***Canad.:*** Alkeran; ***Chile:*** Alkeran; ***Denm.:*** Alkeran; ***Fin.:*** Alkeran; ***Fr.:*** Alkeran; ***Ger.:*** Alkeran; ***Gr.:*** Alkeran; ***Hong Kong:*** Alkeran; ***India:*** Alkeran; ***Irl.:*** Alkeran; ***Israel:*** Alkeran; ***Ital.:*** Alkeran; ***Malaysia:*** Alkeran; ***Mex.:*** Alkeran; ***Neth.:*** Alkeran; ***Norw.:*** Alkeran; ***NZ:*** Alkeran; ***Port.:*** Alkeran; ***S.Afr.:*** Alkeran; ***Singapore:*** Alkeran; ***Swed.:*** Alkeran; ***Switz.:*** Alkeran; ***Thai.:*** Alkeran; ***UK:*** Alkeran; ***USA:*** Alkeran.

# Mercaptopurine *(BAN, rINN)*

Mercaptopurina; Mercaptopurinum; NSC-755; 6MP; Purinethiol; WR-2785. 6-Mercaptopurine monohydrate; Purine-6-thiol monohydrate; 1,7-Dihydro-6*H*-purine-6-thione monohydrate.

$C_5H_4N_4S,H_2O$ = 170.2.

*CAS — 50-44-2 (anhydrous mercaptopurine); 6112-76-1 (mercaptopurine monohydrate).*

*ATC — L01BB02.*

**Pharmacopoeias.** In *Chin., Eur.* (see p.vi), *Jpn, Pol.,* and *US.*

**Ph. Eur. 5.0** (Mercaptopurine). A yellow, crystalline powder. Practically insoluble in water; slightly soluble in alcohol; dissolves in solutions of alkali hydroxides. Protect from light.

**USP 27** (Mercaptopurine). A yellow, odourless or practically odourless, crystalline powder. Insoluble in water, in acetone, and in ether; soluble in hot alcohol and in dilute alkali solutions; slightly soluble in 2N sulfuric acid.

## Adverse Effects, Treatment, and Precautions

For general discussions see Antineoplastics, p.492, p.495, and p.497.

Bone-marrow depression with mercaptopurine, manifesting as leucopenia, thrombocytopenia, and anaemia, may be delayed; hypoplasia may occur. Mercaptopurine is less toxic to the gastrointestinal tract than the folic acid antagonists or fluorouracil but gastrointestinal disturbances may occur. Hepatotoxicity has been reported, with cholestatic jaundice and necrosis, sometimes fatal. Gastrointestinal and hepatic toxicity are reported to be more frequent in adults than in children, and are more likely at higher doses. Crystalluria with haematuria has been observed rarely as have skin disorders including hyperpigmentation. Fever may occur.

Mercaptopurine is potentially carcinogenic and mutagenic; an increased incidence of abortion has occurred in women given mercaptopurine during the first trimester of pregnancy.

Mercaptopurine should be used with care in patients with impaired hepatic or renal function. Hepatic function should be monitored periodically.

**Effects on the blood.** Measurement of the activity of thiopurine methyltransferase or the concentration of its substrate, tioguanine nucleotide, has been suggested as a way of predicting those individuals likely to experience severe myelotoxicity with mercaptopurine and related drugs (see Azathioprine, p.1349).

**Effects on the pancreas.** Pancreatitis occurred in 13 of 396 patients given mercaptopurine for inflammatory bowel disease.[1] Symptoms resolved on withdrawal but recurred in 7 who were re-challenged with mercaptopurine or azathioprine. Acute pancreatitis has also been reported in 2 children given mercaptopurine during maintenance chemotherapy for acute lymphoblastic leukaemia.[2] They had also suffered pancreatitis from asparaginase during earlier therapy, and the authors suggested that subclinical damage to the pancreas by asparaginase may have been exacerbated by mercaptopurine, but also noted that most patients who develop asparaginase-induced pancreatitis receive mercaptopurine without developing this complication.


1. Present DH, *et al.* 6-Mercaptopurine in the management of inflammatory bowel disease: short- and long-term toxicity. *Ann Intern Med* 1989; **111:** 641–9.
2. Willert JR, *et al.* Recurrent mercaptopurine-induced acute pancreatitis: a rare complication of chemotherapy for acute lymphoblastic leukemia in children. *Med Pediatr Oncol* 2002; **38:** 73–4.


**Handling and disposal.** A method for the destruction of mercaptopurine or tioguanine in *wastes* by oxidation with potassium permanganate in sulfuric acid.[1] Residues produced by this method had no mutagenic activity. *Urine and faeces* produced for up to 48 hours and 5 days, respectively after a dose of mercaptopurine should be handled wearing protective clothing.[2]


1. Castegnaro M, *et al.,* eds. Laboratory decontamination and destruction of carcinogens in laboratory wastes: some antineoplastic agents. *IARC Scientific Publications 73.* Lyon: WHO/International Agency for Research on Cancer, 1985.
2. Harris J, Dodds LJ. Handling waste from patients receiving cytotoxic drugs. *Pharm J* 1985; **235:** 289–91.


**Porphyria.** Mercaptopurine has been associated with acute attacks of porphyria and is considered unsafe in porphyric patients.

## Interactions

Mercaptopurine should be given with particular caution with other hepatotoxic drugs. Its effects are enhanced by allopurinol and the dose of mercaptopurine should be reduced to one-third to one-quarter of the usual dose when allopurinol is also given.

**Allopurinol.** Mercaptopurine plasma concentrations were markedly increased by allopurinol when mercaptopurine was given by mouth but not when it was given intravenously.[1] The results appear to indicate that allopurinol inhibits the first-pass metabolism of mercaptopurine.


1. Zimm S, *et al.* Inhibition of first-pass metabolism in cancer chemotherapy: interaction of 6-mercaptopurine and allopurinol. *Clin Pharmacol Ther* 1983; **34:** 810–17.


**Anticoagulants.** For reference to mercaptopurine diminishing the activity of *warfarin,* see p.1025.

**Antineoplastics.** For a suggestion that *doxorubicin* might enhance the hepatotoxicity of mercaptopurine, see under Daunorubicin Hydrochloride, p.546.

Giving mercaptopurine with low-dose *methotrexate* by mouth resulted in an increase in mean peak plasma concentrations of mercaptopurine of 26% compared with use of the same dose of mercaptopurine alone in a study in 14 patients with acute lymphoblastic leukaemia.[1] The effect was probably due to inhibition of the first-pass metabolism of mercaptopurine by methotrexate, which is a potent inhibitor of xanthine oxidase. In another study[2] of 10 children with acute lymphoblastic leukaemia, high-dose intravenous methotrexate (2 or 5 g/m²) increased the peak plasma concentrations of mercaptopurine by 108 and 121% respectively. However, the clinical effect of this pharmacokinetic interaction is probably only minor because of the low, and highly variable, mercaptopurine bioavailability and the lack of correlation between mercaptopurine plasma concentrations and effect.[3] Mercaptopurine and methotrexate have been widely used in combination chemotherapy regimens for acute lymphoblastic leukaemia for their synergistic pharmacodynamic interaction.


1. Balis FM, *et al.* The effect of methotrexate on the bioavailability of oral 6-mercaptopurine. *Clin Pharmacol Ther* 1987; **41:** 384–7.
2. Innocenti F, *et al.* Clinical and experimental pharmacokinetic interaction between 6-mercaptopurine and methotrexate. *Cancer Chemother Pharmacol* 1996; **37:** 409–14.
3. Giverhaug T, *et al.* The interaction of 6-mercaptopurine (6-MP) and methotrexate (MTX). *Gen Pharmacol* 1999; **33:** 341–6.


**Gastrointestinal drugs.** The enzyme thiopurine methyltransferase was inhibited *in vitro* by *sulfasalazine* and *mesalazine,* raising the possibility of an interaction in patients treated simultaneously with an aminosalicylate and a thiopurine such as mercaptopurine or azathioprine.[1] Myelotoxicity has been reported in a patient receiving mercaptopurine concomitantly with *olsalazine.*[2] Similarly, severe pancytopenia has occurred in a 13-year-old boy when azathioprine was added to mesalazine therapy.[3] In a study[4] of 34 patients with Crohn's disease in which *balsalazide,* mesalazine, or sulfasalazine was added to established azathioprine or mercaptopurine therapy, there was a high frequency of mild leucopenia in patients who received mesalazine or sulfasalazine, and whole blood concentrations of tioguanine nucleotide were found to be increased, probably due to thiopurine methyltransferase inhibition. These effects were not statistically significant in patients receiving balsalazide.

1. Szumlanski C, Weinshilboum RM. Sulfasalazine inhibition of thiopurine methyltransferase: possible mechanism for interaction with 6-mercaptopurine and azathioprine. *Br J Clin Pharmacol* 1995; **39:** 456–9.
2. Lewis LD, *et al.* Olsalazine and 6-mercaptopurine-related bone marrow suppression: a possible drug-drug interaction. *Clin Pharmacol Ther* 1997; **62:** 464–75.
3. Chouragui JP, *et al.* Azathioprine toxicity in a child with ulcerative colitis: interaction with mesalazine. *Gastroenterology* 1996; **110** (suppl): A883.
4. Lowry PW, *et al.* Leucopenia resulting from a drug interaction between azathioprine or 6-mercaptopurine and mesalamine, sulphasalazine, or balsalazide. *Gut* 2001; **49:** 656–64.

## Pharmacokinetics

Mercaptopurine is variably and incompletely absorbed from the gastrointestinal tract; about 50% of an oral dose has been reported to be absorbed, but the absolute bioavailability is somewhat lower, probably due to gastrointestinal or first-pass metabolism, and is also subject to wide interindividual variation. Once absorbed it is widely distributed throughout body water and tissues. Plasma half-lives ranging from about 20 to 90 minutes have been reported after intravenous injection and the drug is not found in plasma after about 8 hours but this is of limited significance since mercaptopurine is activated intracellularly by conversion to nucleotide derivatives which persist for much longer. It is rapidly and extensively metabolised in the liver, by methylation and oxidation as well as by the formation of inorganic sulfates. Considerable amounts are oxidised to thiouric acid by the enzyme xanthine oxidase. It is excreted in urine as metabolites and some unchanged drug; about half an oral dose has been recovered in 24 hours. A small proportion is excreted over several weeks.

Mercaptopurine crosses the blood-brain barrier to some extent and is found in the CSF, but only in subtherapeutic concentrations.

**Therapeutic drug monitoring.** For a discussion of therapeutic drug monitoring for mercaptopurine, see under Azathioprine, p.1349.

## Uses and Administration

Mercaptopurine is an antineoplastic that acts as an antimetabolite. It is an analogue of the natural purines hypoxanthine and adenine. After the intracellular conversion of mercaptopurine to active nucleotides, including thioinosinic acid, it appears to exhibit a variety of actions including interfering with nucleic acid synthesis. It also has immunosuppressant properties. Its actions are specific for cells in S phase.

Mercaptopurine is used, usually with other agents, in the treatment of leukaemia. It induces remissions in acute lymphoblastic and myeloid leukaemias (p.506 and p.506, respectively) but other agents are generally preferred and mercaptopurine is chiefly employed in maintenance programmes, commonly in association with methotrexate. It may also be effective in chronic myeloid leukaemia (p.507). There is cross-resistance between mercaptopurine and tioguanine (p.588).

Mercaptopurine has been used for its immunosuppressant properties in the treatment of various auto-immune disorders such as inflammatory bowel disease but has been largely replaced by azathioprine.

Mercaptopurine is given by mouth. The usual initial antineoplastic dose for children and adults is 2.5 mg/kg or 50 to 75 mg/m² daily but dosage varies according to individual response and tolerance. If there is no clinical improvement and no evidence of white-cell depression after 4 weeks, the dose may be cautiously increased up to 5 mg/kg daily. In maintenance schedules the dose may vary from 1.5 to 2.5 mg/kg daily. Blood counts should be taken at least once a week and if there is a steep fall in the white cell count or severe bone-marrow depression the drug should be withdrawn immediately. Therapy may be resumed carefully if the white cell count remains constant for 2 or 3 days or rises.

It has been used intravenously as mercaptopurine sodium. Thioinosine (mercaptopurine riboside) has also been used.

**Administration.** There is evidence[1] that the maintenance dosage of mercaptopurine should be tailored individually to achieve an appropriate systemic exposure in children with acute lymphoblastic leukaemia (although this would involve determining mercaptopurine pharmacokinetics in each child). Improvements in survival since 1980 may be associated with changes in the prescribing of mercaptopurine which have resulted in greater cumulative doses being given;[2] some children may have been under-treated in the past because of variations in the pharmacokinetics of mercaptopurine (particularly boys, who tolerate mercaptopurine better than girls,[3] but who have a poorer prognosis).[2] The concentration of tioguanine nucleotide metabolites in the erythrocytes has been shown to be directly related to the risk of relapse in children with acute lymphoblastic leukaemia.[4] Thiopurine methyltransferase activity (which results in methylation and inactivation of mercaptopurine rather than the formation of active nucleotides) may play a substantial role in this variation,[5] but titration of the dose of mercaptopurine until myelotoxicity occurs may prevent the problem:[2] despite gaps in therapy caused by more frequent drug withdrawal, it appears to result in greater accumulation of tioguanine nucleotides in the cells.[6]

1. Koren G, *et al.* Systemic exposure to mercaptopurine as a prognostic factor in acute lymphocytic leukemia in children. *N Engl J Med* 1990; **323:** 17–21.
2. Hale JP, Lilleyman JS. Importance of 6-mercaptopurine dose in lymphoblastic leukaemia. *Arch Dis Child* 1991; **66:** 462–6.
3. Lilleyman JS, *et al.* Childhood lymphoblastic leukaemia: sex difference in 6-mercaptopurine utilization. *Br J Cancer* 1984; **49:** 703–7.
4. Lilleyman JS, Lennard L. Mercaptopurine metabolism and risk of relapse in childhood lymphoblastic leukaemia. *Lancet* 1994; **343:** 1188–90.
5. Lennard L, *et al.* Genetic variation in response to 6-mercaptopurine for childhood acute lymphoblastic leukaemia. *Lancet* 1990; **336:** 225–9.
6. Lennard L, *et al.* Mercaptopurine in childhood leukaemia: the effects of dose escalation on thioguanine nucleotide metabolites. *Br J Clin Pharmacol* 1996; **42:** 525–7.

**Inflammatory bowel disease.** Mercaptopurine has been reported to be of benefit in ulcerative colitis[1,2] and Crohn's disease,[3-5] although azathioprine has generally been preferred (see p.1350). The *British National Formulary* considers that in resistant or frequently relapsing cases mercaptopurine 1 to 1.5 mg/kg given daily may be of use.

1. Adler DJ, Korelitz BI. The therapeutic efficacy of 6-mercaptopurine in refractory ulcerative colitis. *Am J Gastroenterol* 1990; **85:** 717–22.
2. George J, *et al.* The long-term outcome of ulcerative colitis treated with 6-mercaptopurine. *Am J Gastroenterol* 1996; **91:** 1711–14.
3. Present DH, *et al.* Treatment of Crohn's disease with 6-mercaptopurine: a long-term randomized, double-blind study. *N Engl J Med* 1980; **302:** 981–7.
4. Sandborn W, *et al.* Azathioprine or 6-mercaptopurine for induction of remission in Crohn's disease. Available in The Cochrane Library; Issue 2. Chichester: John Wiley; 2004.
5. Markowitz J, *et al.* A multicenter trial of 6-mercaptopurine and prednisone in children with newly diagnosed Crohn's disease. *Gastroenterology* 2000; **119:** 895–902.

**Polymyositis.** Mercaptopurine has been tried in a few patients with polymyositis but has not been formally assessed.

## Preparations

***BP 2003:*** Mercaptopurine Tablets;
***USP 27:*** Mercaptopurine Tablets.

**Proprietary Preparations** (details are given in Part 3)
***Arg.:*** Puri-Nethol; Varimer; ***Austral.:*** Puri-Nethol; ***Austria:*** Puri-Nethol; ***Belg.:*** Puri-Nethol; ***Braz.:*** Mercaptina†; Puri-Nethol; ***Canad.:*** Puri-Nethol; ***Chile:*** Puri-Nethol; ***Fr.:*** Puri-Nethol; ***Ger.:*** Mercap†; Puri-Nethol; ***Hong Kong:*** Puri-Nethol; ***India:*** Puri-Nethol; ***Irl.:*** Puri-Nethol; ***Israel:*** Puri-Nethol; ***Ital.:*** Ismipur†; Puri-Nethol; ***Mex.:*** Flocofil†; Puri-Nethol; ***Neth.:*** Puri-Nethol; ***Norw.:*** Puri-Nethol; ***NZ:*** Puri-Nethol; ***S.Afr.:*** Puri-Nethol; ***Singapore:*** Puri-Nethol; ***Swed.:*** Puri-Nethol; ***Switz.:*** Puri-Nethol; ***Thai.:*** Puri-Nethol; ***UK:*** Puri-Nethol; ***USA:*** Puri-Nethol.

# Methotrexate *(BAN, USAN, rINN)*

Amethopterin; 4-Amino-4-deoxy-10-methylpteroyl-L-glutamic Acid; 4-Amino-10-methylfolic Acid; CL-14377; α-Methopterin; Methotrexatum; Metotrexato; MTX; NSC-740; WR-19039. N-{4-[(2,4-Diamino-6-pteridinylmethyl)methylamino]benzoyl}-L-glutamic acid.

$C_{20}H_{22}N_8O_5$ = 454.4.
*CAS — 59-05-2.*
*ATC — L01BA01; L04AX03.*

**Pharmacopoeias.** In *Chin., Eur.* (see p.vi), *Int., Jpn,* and *US.*
**Ph. Eur. 5.0** (Methotrexate). It contains between 98 and 102% of $C_{20}H_{22}N_8O_5$, calculated with reference to the anhydrous substance. A yellow or orange, hygroscopic, crystalline powder. It contains not more than 13% of water. Practically insoluble in water, in alcohol, and in dichloromethane; dissolves in dilute solutions of mineral acids and of alkali hydroxides and carbonates. Store in airtight containers. Protect from light.
**USP 27** (Methotrexate). It is a mixture of 4-amino-10-methylfolic acid and closely related substances; it contains not less than 98% and not more than 102% of $C_{20}H_{22}N_8O_5$, calculated on the anhydrous basis. A yellow or orange-brown crystalline powder. It contains not more than 12% of water. Practically insoluble in water, in alcohol, in chloroform, and in ether; freely soluble in dilute solutions of alkali hydroxides and carbonates; slightly soluble in 6N hydrochloric acid. Store in airtight containers. Protect from light.

## Methotrexate Sodium *(BANM, rINNM)*

Methotrexate Disodium; Metotrexate sodium.
$C_{20}H_{20}N_8Na_2O_5$ = 498.4.
*CAS — 7413-34-5 (methotrexate disodium); 15475-56-6 (methotrexate sodium, xNa).*
*ATC — L01BA01; L04AX03.*

**Incompatibility.** Methotrexate sodium has been reported to be incompatible with cytarabine, fluorouracil, and prednisolone sodium phosphate;[1] however, another study suggests it is compatible with fluorouracil.[2] Furthermore a mixture of methotrexate sodium with cytarabine and hydrocortisone sodium succinate in various infusion fluids has been reported to be visually compatible for at least 8 hours at 25°, although precipitation did occur on storage for several days.[3]

1. McRae MP, King JC. Compatibility of antineoplastic, antibiotic and corticosteroid drugs in intravenous admixtures. *Am J Hosp Pharm* 1976; **33:** 1010–13.
2. Vincké BJ, *et al.* Extended stability of 5-fluorouracil and methotrexate solutions in PVC containers. *Int J Pharmaceutics* 1989; **54:** 181–9.
3. Cheung Y-W, *et al.* Stability of cytarabine, methotrexate sodium, and hydrocortisone sodium succinate admixtures. *Am J Hosp Pharm* 1984; **41:** 1802–6.

**Stability to light.** Methotrexate undergoes photodegradation when stored in the light in diluted solutions, although undiluted commercial preparations are reported to show negligible photodegradation.[1] The bicarbonate ion catalyses this reaction and such admixtures should be avoided if possible, although they may be stable in light for 12 hours. Storage of solutions diluted in sodium chloride 0.9% injection in PVC bags was reported to protect against photodegradation although the length of the study was only 4 hours.[2] Photodegradation can take place under normal lighting, but is more rapid in direct sunlight, with about 11% drug loss from a 1 mg/mL solution after 7 hours; storage under normal lighting resulted in little change in drug concentration over 24 hours with a decrease of up to 12% by 48 hours.[3] Loss was greatest from unprotected polybutadiene tubing, with almost 80% drug loss in 48 hours.

1. Chatterji DC, Gallelli JF. Thermal and photolytic decomposition of methotrexate in aqueous solutions. *J Pharm Sci* 1978; **67:** 526–31.
2. Dyvik O, *et al.* Methotrexate in infusion solutions—a stability test for the hospital pharmacy. *J Clin Hosp Pharm* 1986; **11:** 343–8.
3. McElnay JC, *et al.* Stability of methotrexate and vinblastine in burette administration sets. *Int J Pharmaceutics* 1988; **47:** 239–47.

## Adverse Effects

For general discussions see Antineoplastics, p.492.

The most common dose-related toxic effects of methotrexate are on the bone marrow and gastrointestinal tract. Bone-marrow depression can occur abruptly, and leucopenia, thrombocytopenia, and anaemia may all occur. The nadir of the platelet and white-blood cell counts is usually around 5 to 10 days after a bolus dose, with recovery between about 14 to 28 days, but some sources suggest that leucocytes may exhibit an early fall and rise, followed by a second nadir and recovery, within this period. Ulceration of the mouth and gastrointestinal disturbances are also early signs of toxicity: stomatitis and diarrhoea during treatment indicate that it may need to be interrupted, otherwise haemorrhagic enteritis, intestinal perforation, and death may follow.

Methotrexate is associated with liver damage, both acute (notably after high doses) and, more seriously, chronic (generally after long-term use). Hepatic fibrosis and cirrhosis may develop without obvious signs of hepatotoxicity, and have led to eventual death.

Other adverse effects include renal failure and tubular necrosis following high doses, pulmonary reactions including life-threatening interstitial lung disease, skin reactions (sometimes severe), alopecia, and ocular irritation. Neurotoxicity may be seen: leukoencephalopathy, paresis, demyelination are associated particularly with intrathecal use and are more likely when cranial irradiation is also given. Intrathecal administration may also produce arachnoiditis, an acute syndrome of headache, nuchal rigidity, back pain, and fever. Other rarer reactions may include megaloblastic anaemia, osteoporosis, precipitation of diabetes, arthralgias, necrosis of soft tissue and bone, and anaphylaxis.

Methotrexate may cause defective oogenesis and spermatogenesis, and fertility may be impaired (this may be reversible). Like other folate inhibitors it is teratogenic, and it has been associated with fetal deaths. Lymphomas (generally reversible on withdrawal of treatment) have occasionally been reported with methotrexate therapy, although the association has been questioned (see Carcinogenicity, below).

**Carcinogenicity.** There are reports of lymphomas associated with low-dose methotrexate therapy for rheumatic disorders,[1-3] which in some cases have been associated with concomitant Epstein-Barr virus infection.[2] Transitional cell bladder cancer has also been associated with such therapy.[4] However, a retrospective analysis involving 16 263 patients with rheumatoid arthritis found no evidence of a relationship between the use of methotrexate as an antirheumatic and the development of haematological malignancy.[5] Nonetheless, the spontaneous remission of lymphoma after withdrawal of methotrexate in some patients seems to support an association[6] A later prospective study[7] of all new cases of lymphoma, detected over 3 years in patients treated with methotrexate for rheumatoid arthritis, also found a higher incidence of Hodgkin's disease compared with the general population. The carcinogenic risk with antimetabolites such as methotrexate has generally been considered less than with alkylating agents (p.492).


1. Zimmer-Galler I, Lie JT. Choroidal infiltrates as the initial manifestation of lymphoma in rheumatoid arthritis after treatment with low-dose methotrexate. *Mayo Clin Proc* 1994; **69:** 258–61.
2. Kamel OW, *et al.* Brief report: reversible lymphomas associated with Epstein-Barr virus occurring during methotrexate therapy for rheumatoid arthritis and dermatomyositis. *N Engl J Med* 1993; **328:** 1317–21.
3. Viraben R, *et al.* Reversible cutaneous lymphoma occurring during methotrexate therapy. *Br J Dermatol* 1996; **135:** 116–18.
4. Millard RJ, McCredie S. Bladder cancer in patients on low-dose methotrexate and corticosteroids. *Lancet* 1994; **343:** 1222–3.
5. Moder KG, *et al.* Hematologic malignancies and the use of methotrexate in rheumatoid arthritis: a retrospective study. *Am J Med* 1995; **99:** 276–81.
6. Georgescu L, Paget SA. Lymphoma in patients with rheumatoid arthritis: what is the evidence of a link with methotrexate? *Drug Safety* 1999; **20:** 475–87.
7. Mariette X, *et al.* Lymphomas in rheumatoid arthritis patients treated with methotrexate: a 3-year prospective study in France. *Blood* 2002; **99:** 3909–15.


**Effects on the blood.** Although serious and sometimes fatal blood dyscrasias are a well-known consequence of high-dose methotrexate therapy the UK Committee on Safety of Medicines[1] stated in September 1997 that it was also aware of 83 reports of blood dyscrasias associated with low-dose methotrexate used to treat psoriasis or rheumatoid arthritis; there were 36 fatalities. Many of the cases had contributing factors such as advanced age, renal impairment, or concomitant use of interacting drugs.


1. Committee on Safety Medicines/Medicines Control Agency. Blood dyscrasias and other ADRs with low-dose methotrexate. *Current Problems* 1997; **23:** 12. Also available at: http://medicines.mhra.gov.uk/ourwork/monitorsafequalmed/currentproblems/page1.htm (accessed 30/06/04)


MEGALOBLASTIC ANAEMIA. Megaloblastic anaemia, usually with marked macrocytosis, has been reported in mainly elderly patients receiving long-term weekly methotrexate therapy.[1-3] It has been suggested that therapy should be withdrawn if the mean corpuscular volume exceeds 106 femtolitres.[1] Symptoms appear to be associated with folate depletion by methotrexate,[2,4,5] probably due to increased excretion,[6] and in one case megaloblastic anaemia developed following embarkation on a weight-reducing diet poor in folate.[4] Folate supplementation, conversely, may permit continuation of methotrexate therapy with resolution of the anaemia.[5]


1. Dodd HJ, *et al.* Megaloblastic anaemia in psoriatic patients treated with methotrexate. *Br J Dermatol* 1985; **112:** 630.
2. Dahl MGC. Folate depletion in psoriatics on methotrexate. *Br J Dermatol* 1984; **111** (suppl 26): 18.
3. Casserly CM, *et al.* Severe megaloblastic anemia in a patient receiving low-dose methotrexate for psoriasis. *J Am Acad Dermatol* 1993; **29:** 477–80.
4. Fulton RA. Megaloblastic anaemia and methotrexate treatment. *Br J Dermatol* 1986; **114:** 267–8.
5. Oxholm A, Thomsen K. Megaloblastic anaemia and methotrexate treatment. *Br J Dermatol* 1986; **114:** 268–9.
6. Duhra P, *et al.* Intestinal folate absorption in methotrexate treated psoriatic patients. *Br J Dermatol* 1988; **119:** 327–32.


**Effects on the kidneys.** High-dose methotrexate therapy can result in supersaturation of the urine with methotrexate and its metabolites leading to crystal formation.[1] These crystals can cause intrarenal obstruction and are a factor in the development of acute renal failure. Risk factors for crystal formation are acid urine, volume depletion, and renal impairment. Adequate hydration, and urinary alkalinisation with sodium bicarbonate or acetazolamide play an important role in minimising nephrotoxicity in high-dose methotrexate regimens.


1. Perazella MA. Crystal-induced acute renal failure. *Am J Med* 1999; **106:** 459–65.


**Effects on the liver.** Methotrexate is well established as a cause of hepatotoxicity including periportal fibrosis when given in relatively high doses as an antineoplastic, and it has become clear that its long-term use in lower doses for disorders such as psoriasis and rheumatoid arthritis can also be associated with liver toxicity.[1] There has been some difficulty in these patients in distinguishing the effects of the drug from the effects of the disease, but there is good evidence that the risk is increased in patients given doses on a daily rather than a weekly regimen, and in those with a high alcohol intake.[1] Pre-existing liver disease, obesity (especially if associated with diabetes mellitus), renal impairment, and increasing total cumulative dose may also increase the risk of hepatotoxicity.[1] A lower incidence of hepatotoxicity in patients with rheumatoid arthritis (compared with older studies in patients with psoriasis) may be due to improved dosage regimens and greater awareness of the risks.[1]

In order to minimise the risks of serious liver damage various guidelines and recommendations have been issued for the use of methotrexate in psoriasis and rheumatoid arthritis, and the appropriate monitoring.

- For patients with *psoriasis*, US guidelines[2] recommend a liver biopsy at the beginning of treatment and after each cumulative dose of 1 to 1.5 g, together with monitoring of alanine aminotransferase (ALT), aspartate aminotransferase (AST), alkaline phosphatase, bilirubin, and albumin. Practice in the UK has been similar, although recommendations on biopsy are less firm.[3] The need to repeat routine liver biopsies has been questioned.[4]
- In patients with *rheumatoid arthritis* US guidelines[5] suggest an initial biopsy only in patients with a history of excessive alcohol consumption, persistently abnormal AST values or chronic hepatitis B or C infection. All patients should undergo monitoring of liver enzyme values (AST and ALT) and albumin every 4 to 8 weeks, and a biopsy should be performed if 5 of 9 or 6 of 12 measurements of AST are elevated in a 12-month interval; if liver changes are moderate to severe, methotrexate should be discontinued.

The UK Committee on Safety of Medicines advised in 1997 that liver-function tests (together with blood count and renal-function testing) should be performed before beginning long-term low-dose methotrexate therapy and repeated weekly until therapy was stabilised, and thereafter every 2 to 3 months.[6]


1. West SG, *et al.* Methotrexate hepatotoxicity. *Rheum Dis Clin North Am* 1997; **23:** 883–915.
2. Roenigk HH, *et al.* Methotrexate in psoriasis: revised guidelines. *J Am Acad Dermatol* 1988; **19:** 145–6.
3. Research Unit of the Royal College of Physicians of London, *et al.* Guidelines for management of patients with psoriasis. *BMJ* 1991; **303:** 829–35.
4. Boffa MJ, *et al.* Sequential liver biopsies during long-term methotrexate treatment for psoriasis: a reappraisal. *Br J Dermatol* 1995; **133:** 774–8.
5. Kremer JM, *et al.* Methotrexate for rheumatoid arthritis: suggested guidelines for monitoring liver toxicity. *Arthritis Rheum* 1994; **37:** 316–28.
6. Committee on Safety of Medicines/Medicines Control Agency. Blood dyscrasias and other ADRs with low-dose methotrexate. *Current Problems* 1997; **23:** 12. Also available at: http://medicines.mhra.gov.uk/ourwork/monitorsafequalmed/currentproblems/page1.htm (accessed 30/06/04)


**Effects on the lungs.** A review[1] of over 120 reports of methotrexate pneumonitis found that onset usually occurred during treatment, presenting as dyspnoea, cough, and fever. Examination often found tachypnoea and crackles, eosinophilia, reduced pulmonary function, interstitial and alveolar infiltrates on chest radiography, and interstitial inflammation and fibrosis. The majority of cases were managed with cessation of methotrexate with or without corticosteroid therapy; most patients improved, but there were 16 deaths caused by respiratory disease. Methotrexate was restarted in 16 patients, and pneumonitis recurred in 4 of these.

A multicentre case-control study[2] which examined 29 cases of methotrexate-induced lung injury among rheumatoid arthritis patients reported a number of risk factors. These included age over 60 years, pleuropulmonary disease (or to a lesser extent other extra-articular disease), previous use of other disease-modifying antirheumatic drugs, and low serum-albumin; an association with smoking, nonsedentary occupations, and diabetes mellitus was also noted.


1. Imokawa S, *et al.* Methotrexate pneumonitis: review of the literature and histopathological findings in nine patients. *Eur Respir J* 2000; **15:** 373–81.
2. Alarcón GS, *et al.* Risk factors for methotrexate-induced lung injury in patients with rheumatoid arthritis: a multicenter, case-control study. *Ann Intern Med* 1997; **127:** 356–64.


**Effects on mental function.** Children who had received intrathecal methotrexate with cranial irradiation for the prophylaxis of CNS leukaemia, had a significant intellectual deficit compared with their siblings.[1] There was no corresponding significant reduction in IQ in a group of children who had received systemic chemotherapy and radiotherapy when compared with their sibling controls. The results suggest that intrathecal methotrexate and cranial irradiation cause intellectual problems, particularly on the higher, more complex and integrated intellectual functions, and that the repercussions are greater in younger children. Subsequent results in these patients indicated that although the lowering of IQ had persisted, it had not progressed since the original study.[2] A further study confirmed the adverse neurological effects of leukaemia treatment, and its effects on IQ, and did not find a reduced radiation dose to be any less toxic.[3] Neurotoxicity appeared to be greater when systemic therapy with intramuscular rather than oral methotrexate was given with CNS prophylaxis. A study[4] of children who underwent surgery, chemotherapy, and craniospinal radiotherapy for medulloblastoma also found that those patients who received intrathecal methotrexate had significantly worse cognitive deficits than those who did not, and all patients performed worse than a control group of cousins and siblings.

In a small study[5] of children treated for leukaemia with chemotherapy that included intrathecal methotrexate, but without irradiation, there were lower cognitive scores in some measures compared with a group of healthy controls, but overall no major cognitive impairment was found.

A study in 20 patients receiving intermittent oral methotrexate for psoriasis found no evidence of psychological impairment.[6]


1. Twaddle V, *et al.* Intellectual function after treatment for leukaemia or solid tumours. *Arch Dis Child* 1983; **58:** 949–52.
2. Twaddle V, *et al.* Intellect after malignancy. *Arch Dis Child* 1986; **61:** 700–2.
3. Chessells JM, *et al.* Neurotoxicity in lymphoblastic leukaemia: comparison of oral and intramuscular methotrexate and two doses of radiation. *Arch Dis Child* 1990; **65:** 416–22.
4. Riva D, *et al.* Intrathecal methotrexate affects cognitive function in children with medulloblastoma. *Neurology* 2002; **59:** 48–53.
5. Kingma A, *et al.* No major cognitive impairment in young children with acute lymphoblastic leukemia using chemotherapy only: a prospective longitudinal study. *J Pediatr Hematol Oncol* 2002; **24:** 106–14.
6. Duller P, van de Kerkhof PCM. The impact of methotrexate on psycho-organic functioning. *Br J Dermatol* 1985; **113:** 503–4.


**Effects on the nervous system.** Methotrexate has a cumulative toxic effect on the nervous system, and generalised and focal neurotoxic reactions are associated with intrathecal and high-dose intravenous use.[1] An immediate, usually transient, effect occurring within a day of high intravenous doses can cause nausea and vomiting, headache, somnolence, lethargy, confusion, disorientation, seizures, and increased intracranial pressure. Reversible acute meningitis can follow intrathecal use, with similar results. Spinal cord myelopathy resulting in transient or permanent paraplegia has also followed intrathecal methotrexate use, especially if other neurotoxic treatments have also been used. A subacute form of toxic reaction can occur up to several weeks after treatment. It is usually transient and characterised by seizures, varying degrees of paresis, aphasia, anaesthesia, blurred vision, and pseudobulbar palsy. A more delayed syndrome occurs weeks to months after treatment and is of variable severity, but can progress to lethargy, seizures, spasticity, paresis, drooling, and dementia. This condition is characterised by leukoencephalopathy and chronic calcification of brain tissue. It is dose-related, and more severe if the patient has also received radiotherapy.

See also Effects on Mental Function, above.


1. Shuper A, *et al.* Methotrexate treatment protocols and the central nervous system: significant cure with significant neurotoxicity. *J Child Neurol* 2000; **15:** 573–80.


**Effects on the skin.** There are rare reports[1,2] of painful erythema of the hands and feet, particularly the fingertips, with progression to blistering and desquamation (palmar-plantar erythrodysesthesia syndrome, p.495) after the use of high-dose intravenous methotrexate. Purpuric skin lesions due to vasculitis have occurred following both high-dose[3] and low-dose[4,5] methotrexate. Accelerated rheumatoid nodulosis has been reported[6,7] after the use of methotrexate in patients with rheumatoid arthritis. Erosion of psoriatic plaques, accompanied by pain and erythema, has been seen[8,9] following the use of low-dose methotrexate therapy; blistering and necrosis consistent with toxic epidermal necrolysis has occurred.[8] Possible exacerbation of a photosensitivity reaction to ciprofloxacin has been described,[10] and reactivation of sunburn has also been reported[11] in a number of cases where methotrexate was given within 2 to 5 days following the initial sunburn.


1. Doyle LA, *et al.* Erythema and desquamation after high-dose methotrexate. *Ann Intern Med* 1983; **98:** 611–12.
2. Millot F, *et al.* Acral erythema in children receiving high-dose methotrexate. *Pediatr Dermatol* 1999; **16:** 398–400.
3. Navarro M, *et al.* Leukocytoclastic vasculitis after high-dose methotrexate. *Ann Intern Med* 1986; **105:** 471–2.
4. Marks CR, *et al.* Small-vessel vasculitis and methotrexate. *Ann Intern Med* 1984; **100:** 916.
5. Torner O, *et al.* Methotrexate related cutaneous vasculitis. *Clin Rheumatol* 1997; **16:** 108–9.
6. Williams FM, *et al.* Accelerated cutaneous nodulosis during methotrexate therapy in a patient with rheumatoid arthritis. *J Am Acad Dermatol* 1998; **39:** 359–62.
7. Filosa G, *et al.* Accelerated nodulosis during methotrexate therapy for refractory rheumatoid arthritis: a case report. *Adv Exp Med Biol* 1999; **455:** 521–4.
8. Reed KM, Sober AJ. Methotrexate-induced necrolysis. *J Am Acad Dermatol* 1983; **8:** 677–9.
9. Pearce HP, Wilson BB. Erosion of psoriatic plaques: an early sign of methotrexate toxicity. *J Am Acad Dermatol* 1996; **35:** 835–8.
10. Nedorost ST, *et al.* Drug-induced photosensitivity reaction. *Arch Dermatol* 1989; **125:** 433–4.
11. Khan AJ, *et al.* Methotrexate and the photodermatitis reactivation reaction: a case report and review of the literature. *Cutis* 2000; **66:** 379–82.


**Hypersensitivity.** There are rare reports of anaphylactic reactions in patients given methotrexate. Reactions have usually occurred in patients who had previous exposure to methotrexate, but there are also reports of reaction during initial exposure to high-dose intravenous therapy.[1] Serious reactions have also been described following low-dose intravenous[2] and intrathecal[3] administration. See also under Effects on the Lungs, above.


1. Alkins SA, *et al.* Anaphylactoid reactions to methotrexate. *Cancer* 1996; **77:** 2123–6.
2. Cohn JR, *et al.* Systemic anaphylaxis from low dose methotrexate. *Ann Allergy* 1993; **70:** 384–5.
3. Devecioğlu Ö, *et al.* Systemic near-fatal anaphylactic reaction after intrathecal methotrexate administration. *Med Pediatr Oncol* 2000; **34:** 151–2.

**Treatment of Adverse Effects**

For general guidelines, see p.495.

Folinic acid neutralises the immediate toxic effects of methotrexate on the bone marrow. It is given as sodium or calcium folinate by mouth, intramuscularly, by intravenous bolus injection, or by infusion. When overdosage is suspected the dose of folinate should be at least as high as that of methotrexate and should be given as soon as possible; further doses are given as required preferably based on serum-methotrexate concentrations. Folinate should be continued until serum-methotrexate concentrations fall below 0.05 to 0.1 micromol/litre, which may necessitate prolonged treatment in patients with delayed elimination. Other dosage regimens, given intramuscularly or by mouth, may be appropriate for more modest toxicity associated with conventional doses of methotrexate. For details, see under Folinic Acid, p.1431. Following intrathecal overdose, the drainage of 30 mL of CSF within 15 minutes removes about 95% of methotrexate; but methotrexate rapidly enters the systemic circulation and folinic acid treatment should be based on serum-methotrexate concentrations.

Folinic acid is usually given in association with high-dose methotrexate regimens to prevent damage to normal tissue ('folinic acid rescue') and this is discussed in Uses and Administration, below.

An adequate flow of alkaline urine should be maintained following high doses of methotrexate to prevent precipitation of methotrexate or its metabolites in the renal tubules; in addition to adequate hydration, the use of acetazolamide or sodium bicarbonate is recommended.

**Folinic acid.** A discussion of the selection of the appropriate route for folinic acid rescue.[1] The general objective is to give folinic acid (as folinate) at doses that maintain plasma concentrations of reduced folates at a level equivalent to or greater than the plasma-methotrexate concentration. In any clinical situation suggesting impaired gastrointestinal function calcium folinate should be given by injection. Although absorption of intramuscular doses is relatively complete and rapid the intravenous route is usually preferable for other reasons, such as a reduced risk of bleeding at injection sites. In the absence of impaired gastrointestinal function, and where there are no concomitant risk factors for methotrexate toxicity, the oral route may be used provided that methotrexate concentrations are expected to be less than 1 micromol/litre. For very high dose methotrexate regimens it is generally appropriate to begin folinic acid rescue intravenously to ensure adequate initial therapy, but the majority of the dosage regimen can generally be given orally.

1. Rodman JH, Crom WR. Selecting an administration route for leucovorin rescue. *Clin Pharm* 1989; **8:** 617, 621.

**Other drugs.** Pretreatment with fluorouracil is reported to reduce the toxicity of subsequent methotrexate doses to a degree sufficient to permit high-dose methotrexate without the need for folinic acid rescue.[1] Methotrexate has also been given before fluorouracil to modulate its activity (see Administration, in Fluorouracil, p.555).

The acute neurotoxic effects of methotrexate have been reported to be relieved by intravenous aminophylline or oral theophylline in some children.[2]

For reference to the ineffectiveness of diltiazem in preventing the nephrotoxicity due to high-dose methotrexate, see Kidney Disorders, under Diltiazem p.902.

For evidence that colestyramine might decrease serum-methotrexate concentrations, see Interactions, below.

1. White RM. 5-Fluorouracil modulates the toxicity of high dose methotrexate. *J Clin Pharmacol* 1995; **35:** 1156–65.
2. Bernini JC, *et al.* Aminophylline for methotrexate-induced neurotoxicity. *Lancet* 1995; **345:** 544–7.

## Precautions

For general discussions see p.497.

Methotrexate should be used with great care in patients with bone-marrow, hepatic, or renal impairment. It should also be used cautiously in ulcerative disorders of the gastrointestinal tract, and in the elderly and the very young. Pleural or ascitic effusions may act as a depot for methotrexate and produce enhanced toxicity, and should be drained before treatment.

Regular monitoring of haematological, renal, and hepatic function, and gastrointestinal toxicity is advisable. Treatment should be interrupted if myelosuppression, diarrhoea, or stomatitis occur. Dyspnoea or cough may be a sign of pulmonary toxicity and patients should be advised to contact their doctor if they develop these symptoms. Treatment should be withdrawn and the patient investigated to exclude infection. If methotrexate-induced lung disease is suspected corticosteroid therapy may be initiated but treatment with methotrexate should not be restarted. Patients or their carers should report any symptoms or signs suggestive of infection, especially sore throat.

In patients receiving **low-dose methotrexate for psoriasis or rheumatoid arthritis** full blood counts and renal and liver function tests should be performed before starting treatment and repeated regularly thereafter (for discussion of guidelines for monitoring in these patients see Effects on the Liver, above). Treatment should be interrupted if myelosuppression, stomatitis, or any abnormality of liver function is detected. Methotrexate should not be used to treat rheumatoid arthritis or psoriasis in patients with alcoholism, liver disease or persistent abnormal liver function tests, or in those with significant renal impairment, immunodeficiency, or blood disorders. A test dose has been recommended.

With **high-dose regimens**, serum concentrations of methotrexate should be monitored. Maintenance of an adequate flow of alkaline urine is essential (see Treatment of Adverse Effects, above).

Methotrexate is a potent teratogen and should be avoided in **pregnancy**. Some manufacturers advise that conception should be avoided for at least 6 months after therapy but others consider 3 months adequate.

**Blood products.** Enhanced toxicity was seen in 2 of 14 patients receiving methotrexate by 24-hour infusion when packed red cells were transfused immediately after the methotrexate infusion.[1] Erythrocytes act as reservoirs for methotrexate and probably resulted in the prolonged high serum-methotrexate concentrations seen in these patients. Great care should be exercised whenever packed red blood cells and methotrexate are given concurrently.

1. Yap AKL, *et al.* Methotrexate toxicity coincident with packed red cell transfusions. *Lancet* 1986; **ii:** 641.

**Breast feeding.** Methotrexate has been detected in breast milk in low concentrations.[1] The American Academy of Pediatrics considers[2] that methotrexate may interfere with cellular metabolism, causing neutropenia and possibly immune suppression in the nursing infant, and has unknown effects on growth, and an association with carcinogenesis.

1. Johns DG, *et al.* Secretion of methotrexate into human milk. *Am J Obstet Gynecol* 1972; **112:** 978–80.
2. American Academy of Pediatrics. The transfer of drugs and other chemicals into human milk. *Pediatrics* 2001; **108:** 776–89. Correction. *ibid.*; 1029. Also available at: http://aappolicy.aappublications.org/cgi/content/full/pediatrics%3b108/3/776 (accessed 30/06/04)

**Handling and disposal.** Care should be taken to avoid inhalation of methotrexate or contact with skin and mucous membranes. It may cause irritation of the eyes.

Methods have been published for the oxidative destruction of methotrexate *wastes* using potassium permanganate and sulfuric acid, aqueous alkaline potassium permanganate, or sodium hypochlorite.[1] The first method may also be used for dichloromethotrexate. Residues produced by the degradation of methotrexate by these methods showed no mutagenicity *in vitro*.

*Urine and faeces* produced for up to 72 hours and 7 days respectively after a dose of methotrexate should be handled wearing protective clothing.[2]

1. Castegnaro M, *et al.* eds. Laboratory decontamination and destruction of carcinogens in laboratory wastes: some antineoplastic agents. *IARC Scientific Publications 73*. Lyon: WHO/International Agency for Research on Cancer, 1985.
2. Harris J, Dodds LJ. Handling waste from patients receiving cytotoxic drugs. *Pharm J* 1985; **235:** 289–91.

**Hepatitis.** Reactivation of hepatitis B infection, with the development of hepatocellular necrosis and fulminant hepatic failure requiring liver transplantation, developed on discontinuation of low-dose methotrexate therapy in a patient with rheumatoid arthritis who was also an asymptomatic chronic hepatitis B carrier.[1] It was suggested that all patients being considered for low-dose methotrexate therapy should be screened for the presence of serum HBsAg before beginning therapy.

1. Flowers MA, *et al.* Fulminant hepatitis as a consequence of reactivation of hepatitis B virus infection after discontinuation of low-dose methotrexate therapy. *Ann Intern Med* 1990; **112:** 381–2.

**Porphyria.** Methotrexate is considered to be unsafe in patients with porphyria because it has been shown to be porphyrinogenic in *animals*.

**PUVA.** Of a total of 94 patients with psoriasis and 38 with mycosis fungoides treated with PUVA therapy (methoxsalen and ultraviolet light) 2 psoriatics who received concomitant methotrexate and PUVA therapy developed skin cancers.[1] It was suggested that the combination of methotrexate and PUVA may be synergistic in inducing cutaneous malignancy. However, in a cohort study[2] of patients with severe psoriasis, exposure to methotrexate for at least 4 years was associated with an increase in risk of squamous cell carcinoma but not basal cell carcinoma, and no interaction was found between methotrexate and PUVA.

1. Fitzsimons CP, *et al.* Synergistic carcinogenic potential of methotrexate and PUVA in psoriasis. *Lancet* 1983; **i:** 235–6.
2. Stern RS, Laird N. The carcinogenic risk of treatments for severe psoriasis. *Cancer* 1994; **73:** 2759–64.

**Radiation.** Analysis of neutrophil counts for 18 months in children with acute lymphoblastic leukaemia showed that methotrexate-induced neutropenia was significantly greater in patients given CNS irradiation and was considered to have contributed to 3 of 5 deaths during remission.[1]

For the effect of cranial irradiation and intrathecal methotrexate on intellectual development, see Effects on Mental Function, above.

1. Report to the Medical Research Council of the Working Party on Leukaemia in Childhood. Analysis of treatment in childhood leukaemia: I—predisposition to methotrexate-induced neutropenia after craniospinal irradiation. *BMJ* 1975; **3:** 563–6.

## Interactions

For a general outline of antineoplastic drug interactions, see p.498. The effects of methotrexate may be enhanced by drugs that decrease its renal excretion, such as NSAIDs and salicylates, probenecid, and some penicillins. Fatal toxicity has occurred in patients given NSAIDs concurrently with methotrexate (see below). Severe toxicity has occurred rarely when co-trimoxazole or trimethoprim was given with methotrexate. Use with other myelotoxic, hepatotoxic, or nephrotoxic agents may increase the risk of toxicity. Folic acid and its derivatives may decrease the effectiveness of methotrexate, although they are often used together to reduce methotrexate toxicity (see Treatment of Adverse Effects, above).

Animal studies suggested methotrexate toxicity may be increased by chloramphenicol, para-aminobenzoic acid, and hypoglycaemics, but there does not appear to be any evidence of this clinically.

**Antibacterials.** The oral *aminoglycosides* neomycin[1] and paromomycin[2] have been reported to reduce the gastrointestinal absorption of methotrexate. Various *penicillins* have been reported to markedly decrease the clearance of methotrexate given intravenously for treatment of neoplasms,[3-6] although *ceftazidime* may not.[4] There have also been a few reports of penicillins possibly exacerbating the toxicity of low-dose methotrexate in patients being treated for psoriasis or rheumatoid arthritis, but a small study found that although flucloxacillin decreased methotrexate clearance slightly, this was not clinically significant.[7] Methotrexate toxicity has been reported in a patient receiving low-dose methotrexate following a course of *tetracycline*.[8] In a patient receiving high-dose methotrexate, giving *doxycycline* before the eleventh cycle was believed to be responsible for an exacerbation of methotrexate toxicity, with raised plasma concentrations and reduced clearance of methotrexate.[9] The *sulfonamides* such as sulfafurazole and sulfamethoxazole may displace methotrexate from binding sites[10] and reduce renal clearance.[11] Megaloblastic pancytopenia has been reported on a number of occasions when methotrexate was given with *co-trimoxazole*[12-14] or *trimethoprim*;[13,15,16] possible mechanisms involved include an additive antifolate effect, in addition to the effect of the sulfamethoxazole component in the case of co-trimoxazole.

1. Shen DD, Azarnoff DL. Clinical pharmacokinetics of methotrexate. *Clin Pharmacokinet* 1978; **3:** 1–13.
2. Cohen MH, *et al.* Effect of oral prophylactic broad spectrum nonabsorbable antibiotics on the gastrointestinal absorption of nutrients and methotrexate in small cell bronchogenic carcinoma patients. *Cancer* 1976; **38:** 1556.
3. Bloom EJ, *et al.* Delayed clearance (CL) of methotrexate (MTX) associated with antibiotics and antiinflammatory agents. *Clin Res* 1986; **34:** 560A.
4. Yamamoto K, *et al.* Delayed elimination of methotrexate associated with piperacillin administration. *Ann Pharmacother* 1997; **31:** 1261–2.
5. Dean R, *et al.* Possible methotrexate-mezlocillin interaction. *Am J Pediatr Hematol Oncol* 1992; **14:** 88–9.
6. Ronchera CL, *et al.* Pharmacokinetic interaction between high-dose methotrexate and amoxycillin. *Ther Drug Monit* 1993; **15:** 375–9.
7. Herrick AL, *et al.* Lack of interaction between flucloxacillin and methotrexate in patients with rheumatoid arthritis. *Br J Clin Pharmacol* 1996; **41:** 223–7.
8. Turck M. Successful psoriasis treatment then sudden 'cytotoxicity'. *Hosp Pract* 1984; **19:** 175–6.
9. Tortajada-Ituren JJ, *et al.* High-dose methotrexate—doxycycline interaction. *Ann Pharmacother* 1999; **33:** 804–8.
10. Liegler DG, *et al.* The effect of organic acids on renal clearance of methotrexate in man. *Clin Pharmacol Ther* 1969; **10:** 849–57.
11. Ferrazzini G, *et al.* Interaction between trimethoprim-sulfamethoxazole and methotrexate in children with leukemia. *J Pediatr* 1990; **117:** 823–6.
12. Liddle BJ, Marsden JR. Drug interactions with methotrexate. *Br J Dermatol* 1989; **120:** 582–3.
13. Jeurissen ME, *et al.* Pancytopenia and methotrexate with trimethoprim-sulfamethoxazole. *Ann Intern Med* 1989; **111:** 261.
14. Groenendal H, Rampen FHJ. Methotrexate and trimethoprim-sulphamethoxazole—a potentially hazardous combination. *Clin Exp Dermatol* 1990; **15:** 358–60.

15. Steuer A, Gumpel JM. Methotrexate and trimethoprim: a fatal interaction. *Br J Rheumatol* 1998; **37:** 105–6.
16. Govert JA, *et al.* Pancytopenia from using trimethoprim and methotrexate. *Ann Intern Med* 1992; **117:** 877–8.

**Antiepileptics.** For mention of the reduction in serum-*valproate* concentration produced by methotrexate see p.382.

**Antineoplastics.** Enhanced methotrexate toxicity might be expected with nephrotoxic agents (such as *cisplatin*) that can reduce methotrexate excretion by impairing renal function. Sequential use of methotrexate and *fluorouracil* may result in synergistic enhancement of effect (see Administration, in Fluorouracil, p.555), and equally, fluorouracil before methotrexate may reduce its toxicity (see under Treatment of Adverse Effects, above), but if *asparaginase* (p.529) is given before methotrexate the cytotoxic effect of methotrexate may be reduced.

Methotrexate may increase the bioavailability of *mercaptopurine* by interference with first-pass metabolism (see p.567).

**Colestyramine.** Serum-methotrexate concentrations were markedly reduced in 3 patients given colestyramine to treat methotrexate toxicity.[1,2] Colestyramine appears to bind methotrexate and reduce its enterohepatic recirculation.

1. Erttmann R, Landbeck G. Effect of oral cholestyramine on the elimination of high-dose methotrexate. *J Cancer Res Clin Oncol* 1985; **110:** 48–50.
2. Shinozaki T, *et al.* Successful rescue by oral cholestyramine of a patient with methotrexate nephrotoxicity: nonrenal excretion of serum methotrexate. *Med Pediatr Oncol* 2000; **34:** 226–8.

**Gastrointestinal drugs.** Elevated serum concentrations of methotrexate were reported when it was given to 2 patients also receiving *omeprazole*.[1,2] The effect was not seen with subsequent cycles of methotrexate therapy once omeprazole had been discontinued. In another case[3] however, raised methotrexate concentrations were thought to be due to an interaction with omeprazole, but were identical during a second cycle after omeprazole had been withdrawn. Severe generalised myalgia and bone pain were reported in a patient who received methotrexate and *pantoprazole*.[4] The same reaction occurred on rechallenge with the combination, but not with methotrexate alone. Although methotrexate concentrations were unchanged, concentrations of the metabolite 7-hydroxymethotrexate were raised suggesting an interaction with its renal elimination.

1. Reid T, *et al.* Impact of omeprazole on the plasma clearance of methotrexate. *Cancer Chemother Pharmacol* 1993; **33:** 82–4.
2. Beorlegui B, *et al.* Potential interaction between methotrexate and omeprazole. *Ann Pharmacother* 2000; **34:** 1024–7.
3. Whelan J, *et al.* Omeprazole does not alter plasma methotrexate clearance. *Cancer Chemother Pharmacol* 1999; **44:** 88–9.
4. Tröger U, *et al.* Severe myalgia from an interaction between treatments with pantoprazole and methotrexate. *BMJ* 2002; **324:** 1497.

**Immunosuppressants.** For reports of enhanced toxicity with *ciclosporin* in patients who have received methotrexate see p.1355.

**Nitrous oxide.** Severe unpredictable myelosuppression and stomatitis have been attributed to the use of nitrous oxide anaesthesia in patients receiving methotrexate, potentiating the effects of methotrexate on folate metabolism.[1] The effect could be reduced by the use of folinic acid rescue.

1. Goldhirsch A, *et al.* Methotrexate/nitrous-oxide toxic interaction in perioperative chemotherapy for early breast cancer. *Lancet* 1987; **ii:** 151.

**NSAIDs.** Severe, and in some cases fatal, aggravation of methotrexate toxicity has been reported when it was given with various NSAIDs including *aspirin* and other *salicylates*,[1,2] *azapropazone*,[3] *diclofenac*,[4] *indometacin*,[4,5] and *ketoprofen*.[6] The mechanism is uncertain but may include both displacement of methotrexate from protein-binding sites or an effect of NSAIDs on the kidney resulting in reduced methotrexate excretion.[6,7] *Naproxen* has been reported not to affect the pharmacokinetics of methotrexate,[8] but a fatal interaction has nonetheless been reported.[9] Despite the risks, some commentators have pointed out that methotrexate and NSAIDs are frequently used together in the treatment of rheumatoid arthritis,[10,11] and that provided this is done with caution, in low doses, and patients are appropriately monitored and cautioned to avoid additional 'over-the-counter' analgesics, such combinations need not be contra-indicated. A study in patients receiving low-dose methotrexate for rheumatoid arthritis suggested that *flurbiprofen*, *ketoprofen*, or *piroxicam* did not influence methotrexate clearance.[12] A case of methotrexate toxicity has nevertheless been described[13] in an elderly woman when flurbiprofen was added to low-dose methotrexate therapy.

Manufacturers of methotrexate generally contra-indicate the use of NSAIDs with high-dose methotrexate.

1. Baker H. Intermittent high dose oral methotrexate therapy in psoriasis. *Br J Dermatol* 1970; **82:** 65–9.
2. Zuik M, Mandel MA. Methotrexate-salicylate interaction: a clinical and experimental study. *Surg Forum* 1975; **26:** 567–9.
3. Daly HM, *et al.* Methotrexate toxicity precipitated by azapropazone. *Br J Dermatol* 1986; **114:** 733–5.
4. Gabrielli A, *et al.* Methotrexate and nonsteroidal anti-inflammatory drugs. *BMJ* 1987; **294:** 776.
5. Maiche AG. Acute renal failure due to concomitant action of methotrexate and indomethacin. *Lancet* 1986; **i:** 1390.
6. Thyss A, *et al.* Clinical and pharmacokinetic evidence of a life-threatening interaction between methotrexate and ketoprofen. *Lancet* 1986; **i:** 256–8.
7. Furst DE, *et al.* Effect of aspirin and sulindac on methotrexate clearance. *J Pharm Sci* 1990; **79:** 782–6.
8. Stewart CF, *et al.* Coadministration of naproxen and low-dose methotrexate in patients with rheumatoid arthritis. *Clin Pharmacol Ther* 1990; **47:** 540–6.
9. Singh RR, *et al.* Fatal interaction between methotrexate and naproxen. *Lancet* 1986; **i:** 1390.
10. Tully M. NSAIDs. *Pharm J* 1991; **247:** 746.
11. Zachariae H. Methotrexate and nonsteroidal anti-inflammatory drugs. *Br J Dermatol* 1992; **126:** 95.
12. Tracy TS, *et al.* Methotrexate disposition following concomitant administration of ketoprofen, piroxicam and flurbiprofen in patients with rheumatoid arthritis. *Br J Clin Pharmacol* 1994; **37:** 453–6.
13. Frenia ML, Long KS. Methotrexate and nonsteroidal antiinflammatory drug interactions. *Ann Pharmacother* 1992; **26:** 234–7.

**Probenecid.** Probenecid can produce two- to fourfold increases in serum-methotrexate concentrations,[1-3] presumably by inhibiting renal excretion of methotrexate. Although probenecid has been shown to reduce protein binding of methotrexate,[4] usual doses of probenecid are unlikely to significantly affect methotrexate elimination by this mechanism. A woman receiving low-dose weekly methotrexate for rheumatoid arthritis developed severe pancytopenia when probenecid was given for asymptomatic hyperuricaemia.[5]

1. Aherne GW, *et al.* Prolongation and enhancement of serum methotrexate concentrations by probenecid. *BMJ* 1978; **1:** 1097–9.
2. Howell SB, *et al.* Effect of probenecid on cerebrospinal fluid methotrexate kinetics. *Clin Pharmacol Ther* 1979; **26:** 641–6.
3. Lilly MB, Omura GA. Clinical pharmacology of oral intermediate-dose methotrexate with or without probenecid. *Cancer Chemother Pharmacol* 1985; **15:** 220–2.
4. Paxton JW. Interaction of probenecid with the protein binding of methotrexate. *Pharmacology* 1984; **28:** 86–9.
5. Basin KS, *et al.* Severe pancytopenia in a patient taking low dose methotrexate and probenecid. *J Rheumatol* 1991; **18:** 609–10.

**Retinoids.** An increased risk of hepatotoxicity has been reported when methotrexate and *etretinate* are given together,[1] possibly due to increased plasma concentrations of methotrexate.[2,3]

1. Zachariae H. Dangers of methotrexate/etretinate combination therapy. *Lancet* 1988; **i:** 422.
2. Harrison PV, *et al.* Methotrexate and retinoids in combination for psoriasis. *Lancet* 1987; **ii:** 512.
3. Larsen FG, *et al.* Interaction of etretinate with methotrexate pharmacokinetics in psoriatic patients. *J Clin Pharmacol* 1990; **30:** 802–7.

## Pharmacokinetics

When given in low doses, methotrexate is rapidly absorbed from the gastrointestinal tract, but higher doses are less well absorbed. It is also rapidly and completely absorbed after intramuscular doses. Peak serum concentrations are achieved in 1 to 2 hours after an oral dose, and 30 to 60 minutes after an intramuscular one.

Methotrexate is distributed to tissues and extracellular fluid with a steady-state volume of distribution of 0.4 to 0.8 litres/kg; it penetrates ascitic fluid and effusions, which may act as a depot and thus enhance toxicity. Clearance from plasma is reported to be triphasic, with a terminal elimination half-life of between 3 and 10 hours after doses less than 30 mg/m$^2$ or 8 to 15 hours after high-dose parenteral therapy. It is about 50% bound to plasma protein. Methotrexate enters the cells in part by an active transport mechanism and is bound as polyglutamate conjugates: bound drug may remain in the body for several months, particularly in the liver. Only small or insignificant amounts cross the blood-brain barrier and enter the CSF after oral or parenteral doses although this may be increased by giving higher doses; however, after intrathecal doses there is significant passage into the systemic circulation.

Methotrexate has been detected in very small amounts in saliva and breast milk. It crosses the placenta.

Methotrexate does not appear to undergo significant metabolism at low doses; following high-dose therapy the 7-hydroxy metabolite has been detected. Methotrexate may be partly metabolised by the intestinal flora after oral doses. It is excreted primarily in the urine, by glomerular filtration and active tubular secretion. Small amounts are excreted in bile and found in faeces; there is some evidence for enterohepatic recirculation.

Considerable interindividual variation exists in the pharmacokinetics of methotrexate: those patients in whom clearance is delayed are at increased risk of toxicity.

◊ References.

1. Shen DD, Azarnoff DL. Clinical pharmacokinetics of methotrexate. *Clin Pharmacokinet* 1978; **3:** 1–13.
2. Balis FM, *et al.* Clinical pharmacokinetics of commonly used anticancer drugs. *Clin Pharmacokinet* 1983; **8:** 202–32.
3. Wang Y-M, Fujimoto T. Clinical pharmacokinetics of methotrexate in children. *Clin Pharmacokinet* 1984; **9:** 335–48.
4. Witter FR. Clinical pharmacokinetics in the treatment of rheumatoid arthritis in pregnancy. *Clin Pharmacokinet* 1993; **25:** 444–9.
5. Bannwarth B, *et al.* Clinical pharmacokinetics of low-dose pulse methotrexate in rheumatoid arthritis. *Clin Pharmacokinet* 1996; **30:** 194–210.
6. Chládek J, *et al.* Pharmacokinetics and pharmacodynamics of low-dose methotrexate in the treatment of psoriasis. *Br J Clin Pharmacol* 2002; **54:** 147–56.
7. Grim J, *et al.* Pharmacokinetics and pharmacodynamics of methotrexate in non-neoplastic diseases. *Clin Pharmacokinet* 2003; **42:** 139–51.

## Uses and Administration

Methotrexate is an antineoplastic which acts as an antimetabolite of folic acid. It also has immunosuppressant properties. Within the cell, folic acid is reduced to dihydrofolic and then tetrahydrofolic acid. Methotrexate competitively inhibits the enzyme dihydrofolate reductase and prevents the formation of tetrahydrofolate which is necessary for purine and pyrimidine synthesis and consequently the formation of DNA and RNA. It is most active against cells in the S phase of the cell cycle. Folinic acid (the 5-formyl derivative of tetrahydrofolic acid) has been given after high doses to bypass the block in tetrahydrofolate production in normal cells and prevent the adverse effects of methotrexate. A suggested schedule for *folinic acid rescue* is described under Folinic Acid, p.1431. (See also under Treatment of Adverse Effects, above). Methotrexate, in very high doses, followed by folinic acid rescue, is used in treating some malignant diseases.

Methotrexate is used in the management of acute lymphoblastic leukaemia. It is seldom used for the induction of remission but is employed in maintenance programmes and in the prophylaxis and treatment of meningeal leukaemia. It may be used for Burkitt's and other non-Hodgkin's lymphomas. In the solid neoplasms it is an important part of curative regimens for choriocarcinoma and other gestational trophoblastic tumours, and for the adjuvant therapy of osteosarcoma and breast cancer. It may also be used in malignant neoplasms of the bladder and head and neck, and a variety of other neoplasms, as indicated by the cross references given below.

Methotrexate is of value in the treatment of psoriasis but because of the risks associated with this use, it should only be given when the disease is severe and has not responded to other forms of treatment. It is used widely as a disease-modifying antirheumatic drug in rheumatoid arthritis. Methotrexate may be used to prevent graft-versus-host disease after bone marrow transplantation and may be used as a cytotoxic immunosuppressant and corticosteroid-sparing agent in a variety of non-malignant diseases.

Methotrexate has a role in the management of ectopic pregnancy (see below).

Methotrexate may be given by mouth as the base or the sodium salt, or by injection as the sodium salt. Doses are calculated in terms of methotrexate. Methotrexate sodium 16.5 mg is approximately equivalent to 15 mg of methotrexate. The doses and regimens used vary enormously, and may need to be adjusted according to bone marrow or other toxicity (see also under Bone-marrow Depression, p.496). Doses larger than 100 mg are usually given partly or wholly by intravenous infusion over not more than 24 hours.

A common dose for maintenance therapy of acute lymphoblastic leukaemia is 15 mg/m$^2$ once or twice weekly, by mouth or intramuscularly, with other agents such as mercaptopurine. Alternatively, 2.5 mg/kg may be given intravenously every 14 days. Meningeal leukaemia may be treated by the intrathecal injection of 12 mg/m$^2$ (maximum 15 mg) once weekly for 2 to 3 weeks, then once monthly; an alternative is 200 to 500 micrograms/kg at intervals of 2 to 5 days until the cell count of the CSF returns to normal. Another regimen has been recommended for children based on age, with children under the age of 1 year receiving 6 mg, 8 mg for those 1 year of age, 10 mg in 2-year-olds, and 12 mg in those 3 years of age or older. Intrathecal doses have also sometimes been given prophylactically to patients with lymphoblastic leukaemia in association with intrathecal cytarabine and hydrocortisone. Methotrexate in intravenous doses of about 500 mg/m$^2$, followed by folinic acid rescue, may also produce effective concentrations in the CSF and has been used for meningeal leukaemia.

Choriocarcinoma has been treated with doses of 15 to 30 mg daily by mouth or intramuscularly for 5 days repeated after an interval of 1 week or more, for 3 to 5 courses. Alternatively 0.25 to 1 mg/kg up to a maximum of 60 mg has been given intramuscularly every 48 hours for 4 doses, followed by folinic acid rescue, and repeated at intervals of 7 days for 4 or more courses. Combination chemotherapy may be necessary in patients with metastases.

Doses of 10 to 60 mg/m$^2$ are employed intravenously in the treatment of breast cancer, often with cyclophosphamide and fluorouracil.

In advanced lymphosarcoma doses of 0.625 to 2.5 mg/kg daily have been suggested with other antineoplastics. Alternatively, higher doses of up to 30 mg/kg have been given intravenously, followed by folinic acid rescue. For Burkitt's lymphoma 10 to 25 mg of methotrexate has been given daily by mouth for 4 to 8 days, repeated after an interval of 7 to 10 days, while patients with mycosis fungoides may be given 2.5 to 10 mg daily by mouth to induce remission; alternatively 50 mg may be given weekly as a single dose or two divided doses, by intramuscular injection.

Very high doses, in the range 12 to 15 g/m$^2$ have been given by intravenous infusion, followed by folinic acid, as part of combined adjuvant therapy in patients with osteosarcoma. High-dose regimens have been tried in a variety of other malignancies, including carcinoma of the lung and of the head and neck.

Single weekly doses of 10 to 25 mg may be given by mouth or by intramuscular or intravenous injection in the treatment of psoriasis and adjusted by response. Other, more frequent, regimens have been used but a weekly dosage regimen appears to be less hepatotoxic than a daily one. In the treatment of rheumatoid arthritis doses of 7.5 mg by mouth once weekly are used, adjusted by response and not exceeding 20 mg/week.

It is essential that blood counts and tests of renal and liver function should be made before, during, and after each course of treatment with methotrexate (see Precautions, above).

**Asthma.** Various immunosuppressants, including methotrexate, have been tried for their anti-inflammatory and corticosteroid-sparing properties in chronic asthma (p.777), but because of fears about toxicity are largely reserved for certain patients dependent upon systemic corticosteroids. Results of individual studies with methotrexate have been conflicting, but it appears that some patients may benefit from the corticosteroid-sparing effects of methotrexate.[1,2] However, other reviewers considered that the reduction in corticosteroid dose was insufficient to offset the adverse effects of methotrexate.[3] Methotrexate therapy must be given for at least 3 months for an adequate assessment of efficacy.


1. Shulimzon TR, Shiner RJ. A risk-benefit assessment of methotrexate in corticosteroid-dependent asthma. *Drug Safety* 1996; **15:** 283–90.
2. Marin MG. Low-dose methotrexate spares steroid usage in steroid-dependent asthmatic patients: a meta-analysis. *Chest* 1997; **112:** 29–33.
3. Davies H, *et al.* Methotrexate as a steroid sparing agent for asthma in adults. Available in The Cochrane Library; Issue 2. Chichester: John Wiley; 2004.


**Connective tissue and muscular disorders.** Reports in a limited number of patients indicate that methotrexate given once weekly in low to moderate doses may be of benefit in patients with systemic lupus erythematosus (p.1088), with benefit reported particularly for joint and mucocutaneous symptoms.[1]

Methotrexate therapy has been investigated for its potential corticosteroid-sparing properties in polymyalgia rheumatica (p.1086). Different regimens have been tried and although one study[2] reported benefit, others[3,4] found no evidence of clinical efficacy or a corticosteroid-sparing effect.

Methotrexate is widely employed in rheumatoid arthritis (see below) and in polymyositis (p.1086), and has been tried in Cogan's syndrome (p.1078).


1. Sato EI. Methotrexate therapy in systemic lupus erythematosus. *Lupus* 2001; **10:** 162–4.
2. Ferraccioli G, *et al.* Methotrexate in polymyalgia rheumatica: preliminary results of an open, randomized study. *J Rheumatol* 1996; **23:** 624–8.
3. Feinberg HL, *et al.* The use of methotrexate in polymyalgia rheumatica. *J Rheumatol* 1996; **23:** 1550–2.
4. van der Veen MJ, *et al.* Can methotrexate be used as a steroid sparing agent in the treatment of polymyalgia rheumatica and giant cell arteritis? *Ann Rheum Dis* 1996; **55:** 218–23.


**Ectopic pregnancy.** Ectopic pregnancy occurs when the fertilised ovum implants outside the uterus, usually in the fallopian tube itself (tubal pregnancy). The problem is increasingly encountered in some developed countries such as the USA, due in part to improved diagnostic techniques.[1] Although ectopic pregnancies may spontaneously abort early, without clinical sequelae, the potential adverse effects are serious, ranging from pelvic pain and bleeding at 5 to 6 weeks of gestation (indistinguishable from spontaneous abortion), to potentially fatal intra-abdominal haemorrhage later in the course of an otherwise asymptomatic pregnancy.

Laparoscopic surgery remains the standard treatment.[1-3] In some countries non-surgical methods are increasing in popularity because of earlier diagnosis.[4] Perhaps the most experience of the latter has been with methotrexate. Management with intramuscular methotrexate may be appropriate for selected women with small unruptured tubal pregnancies who are haemodynamically stable, have low serum-chorionic gonadotrophin concentrations, and lack contra-indications to methotrexate use.[2-6] Surgery is preferred where there is cardiac activity in the conceptus, since a living embryo increases resistance to methotrexate.[5,6] Two regimens of intramuscular methotrexate have been described. A multiple-dose regimen of 1 mg/kg on 4 alternate days, with folinic acid rescue,[1] has similar efficacy to surgery.[3] A single dose of 50 mg/m$^2$ can be used instead[4] but systematic reviews have indicated that it has a higher failure rate than surgery[3,7] and about 20% of patients will require more than one cycle of treatment.[4] The addition of an oral dose of mifepristone to single-dose methotrexate has been investigated[8,9] and may reduce treatment failure rates.

Methotrexate has been given by local injection directly into the ectopic (salpingocentesis). Doses of 1 mg/kg or 50 mg have been used[10] but this technique is significantly less successful than surgery.[3] Systemic methotrexate (with folinic acid rescue) has also been reported to be effective in resolving persistent ectopic pregnancy unsuccessfully treated with surgery.

The role of other agents in the management of ectopic pregnancy is less well established. Local instillation of glucose 50% by salpingocentesis has also been used in the treatment of ectopic pregnancy,[10,11] but one study was discontinued because of a higher failure rate with glucose treatment compared with local methotrexate.[12]


1. Pisarska MD, *et al.* Ectopic pregnancy. *Lancet* 1998; **351:** 1115–20.
2. Tay JI, *et al.* Ectopic pregnancy. *BMJ* 2000; **320:** 916–9. Correction. *ibid.*; **321:** 424.
3. Hajenius PJ, *et al.* Interventions for tubal ectopic pregnancy. Available in The Cochrane Library; Issue 2. Chichester: John Wiley; 2004.
4. Lipscomb GH, *et al.* Nonsurgical treatment of ectopic pregnancy. *N Engl J Med* 2000; **343:** 1325–9.
5. Lipscomb GH, *et al.* Predictors of success of methotrexate treatment in women with tubal ectopic pregnancies. *N Engl J Med* 1999; **341:** 1974–8.
6. American College of Obstetricians and Gynecologists. ACOG practice bulletin: medical management of tubal pregnancy. Number 3, December 1998. *Int J Gynecol Obstet* 1999; **65:** 97–103.
7. Parker J, *et al.* A systematic review of single-dose intramuscular methotrexate for the treatment of ectopic pregnancy. *Aust N Z J Obstet Gynaecol* 1998; **38:** 145–50.
8. Gazvani MR, *et al.* Mifepristone in combination with methotrexate for the medical treatment of tubal pregnancy: a randomized, controlled trial. *Hum Reprod* 1998; **13:** 1987–90.
9. Perdu M, *et al.* Treating ectopic pregnancy with the combination of mifepristone and methotrexate: a phase II nonrandomized study. *Am J Obstet Gynecol* 1998; **179:** 640–3.
10. Natofsky JG, *et al.* Ultrasound-guided injection of ectopic pregnancy. *Clin Obstet Gynecol* 1999; **42:** 39–47.
11. Lang PFJ, *et al.* Laparoscopic instillation of hyperosmolar glucose vs. expectant management of tubal pregnancies with serum hCG≤2500 mIU/mL. *Acta Obstet Gynecol Scand* 1997; **76:** 797–800.
12. Sadan O, *et al.* Methotrexate versus hyperosmolar glucose in the treatment of extrauterine pregnancy. *Arch Gynecol Obstet* 2001; **265:** 82–4.


**Inflammatory bowel disease.** Methotrexate (given intramuscularly once weekly in a dose of 25 mg) was reported to improve symptoms and reduce corticosteroid requirements in a large controlled study in patients with chronic active Crohn's disease.[1] Those patients who were in remission after 16 weeks of methotrexate treatment were entered into a further placebo-controlled trial[2] of methotrexate 15 mg weekly by intramuscular injection. During 40 weeks of follow-up, a higher proportion of patients receiving methotrexate remained in remission, and had fewer relapses. Smaller studies have also reported modest benefit for oral methotrexate 12.5 to 22.5 mg/week in chronic active disease.[3,4] Subcutaneous methotrexate has also been used.[5] A review[6] concluded that low-dose methotrexate could be recommended for induction of remission and for its corticosteroid-sparing effect in refractory and corticosteroid-dependent Crohn's disease, although the precise indications, dose, and route for its use were still unclear. The value of methotrexate in ulcerative colitis is also uncertain, although benefits have been seen in some patients.[5,7] However, one study in active ulcerative colitis found no significant differences between oral methotrexate 12.5 mg/week and placebo.[8] For a discussion of inflammatory bowel disease, see p.1243.


1. Feagan BG, *et al.* Methotrexate for the treatment of Crohn's disease. *N Engl J Med* 1995; **332:** 292–7.
2. Feagan BG, *et al.* A comparison of methotrexate with placebo for the maintenance of remission in Crohn's disease. *N Engl J Med* 2000; **342:** 1627–32.
3. Oren R, *et al.* Methotrexate in chronic active Crohn's disease: a double-blind, randomized, Israeli multicenter trial. *Am J Gastroenterol* 1997; **92:** 2203–9.
4. Arora S, *et al.* Methotrexate in Crohn's disease: results of a randomized, double-blind, placebo-controlled trial. *Hepatogastroenterology* 1999; **46:** 1724–9.
5. Egan LJ, *et al.* A randomized dose-response and pharmacokinetic study of methotrexate for refractory inflammatory Crohn's disease and ulcerative colitis. *Aliment Pharmacol Ther* 1999; **13:** 1597–1604.
6. Egan LJ, Sandborn WJ. Methotrexate for inflammatory bowel disease: pharmacology and preliminary results. *Mayo Clin Proc* 1996; **71:** 69–80.
7. Kozarek RA. Methotrexate for refractory Crohn's disease: preliminary answers to definitive questions. *Mayo Clin Proc* 1996; **71:** 104–5.
8. Oren R, *et al.* Methotrexate in chronic active ulcerative colitis: a double-blind, randomized, Israeli multicenter trial. *Gastroenterology* 1996; **110:** 1416–21.


**Malignant neoplasms.** Methotrexate is extensively used in the management of malignant disease. In acute lymphoblastic leukaemia it is used for maintenance therapy, and intrathecally for prophylaxis of CNS relapse, as discussed on p.506, while it also forms part of a number of regimens used for Burkitt's and other aggressive, intermediate- to high-grade non-Hodgkin's lymphomas (see p.511 and p.510), including mycosis fungoides (p.511) and those associated with AIDS (p.510). In the solid neoplasms it is an important part of curative regimens for gestational trophoblastic tumours (p.505), the adjuvant therapy of osteosarcoma (p.524) and is used in regimens for tumours of the bladder (p.512), brain (p.513), breast (p.514), gastrointestinal tract (p.516), and head and neck (p.517).

**Multiple sclerosis.** Results suggest that methotrexate 7.5 mg by mouth weekly may be of benefit[1] in slowing the progression of multiple sclerosis (p.646). Although the results of studies of immunosuppressant therapy in this condition have tended to be disappointing, it has been pointed out that benefit was assessed differently in the methotrexate study,[2] which may have a bearing on its more favourable conclusions.


1. Goodkin DE, *et al.* Low-dose (7.5 mg) oral methotrexate reduces the rate of progression in chronic progressive multiple sclerosis. *Ann Neurol* 1995; **37:** 30–40.
2. Whitaker JN, *et al.* Clinical outcomes and documentation of partial beneficial effects of immunotherapy for multiple sclerosis. *Ann Neurol* 1995; **37:** 5–6.


**Myasthenia gravis.** Methotrexate has been tried in the management of myasthenia gravis (p.1486) in patients who require immunosuppression but are intolerant of or unresponsive to corticosteroids and azathioprine.

**Organ and tissue transplantation.** For reference to the use of methotrexate (usually with ciclosporin) in bone marrow transplantation, see Haematopoietic Stem Cell Transplantation, p.1344.

**Primary biliary cirrhosis.** Like other drugs used for primary biliary cirrhosis (p.1761) methotrexate has been associated with biochemical improvement but evidence of clinical and in particular histological improvement is harder to demonstrate, and the toxicity of immunosuppressants such as methotrexate is problematic.

**Psoriatic arthritis.** Methotrexate may be useful for severe or progressive cases of psoriatic arthritis (see under Spondyloarthropathies, p.11) when the arthritis is not controlled by physical therapy and NSAIDs, although toxicity may limit long-term use in some patients.

**Rheumatoid arthritis.** Therapy of rheumatoid arthritis (p.9) is conventionally begun with an analgesic and an NSAID for symptomatic relief, to which a disease-modifying antirheumatic drug (DMARD) is subsequently added in an attempt to retard the disease process. It is now clear that irreversible joint damage commonly occurs in early disease and rheumatologists now generally add the DMARD shortly after rheumatoid arthritis has been diagnosed. Methotrexate or sulfasalazine tend to be the most widely used of such DMARDs.[1] Systematic review has confirmed that methotrexate has significant benefit in the short-term treatment of the disease.[2] Methotrexate has also been tried with ciclosporin, hydroxychloroquine and sulfasalazine, leflunomide, etanercept, and infliximab. Studies have shown improved responses to these combinations compared with methotrexate alone, but long-term efficacy and safety has not been studied.[3]

Methotrexate may be of benefit in juvenile idiopathic arthritis (p.9).[4-6]

Methotrexate may also be of value in the management of associated uveitis (p.1090).


1. Anonymous. Modifying disease in rheumatoid arthritis. *Drug Ther Bull* 1998; **36:** 3–6.
2. Suarez-Almazor ME, *et al.* Methotrexate for treating rheumatoid arthritis. Available in The Cochrane Library; Issue 2. Chichester: John Wiley; 2004.
3. Kremer JM. Rational use of new and existing disease-modifying agents in rheumatoid arthritis. *Ann Intern Med* 2001; **134:** 695–706.
4. Ravelli A, *et al.* Radiologic progression in patients with juvenile chronic arthritis treated with methotrexate. *J Pediatr* 1998; **133:** 262–5.
5. Takken T, *et al.* Methotrexate for treating juvenile idiopathic arthritis. Available in The Cochrane Library; Issue 2. Chichester: John Wiley; 2004.
6. Ramanan AV, *et al.* Use of methotrexate in juvenile idiopathic arthritis. *Arch Dis Child* 2003; **88:** 197–200.

**Sarcoidosis.** Where therapy is required for sarcoidosis (p.1087) corticosteroids are the first choice of drug; methotrexate is one of the preferred second-line immunosuppressants.

References.


1. Webster GF, *et al.* Methotrexate therapy in cutaneous sarcoidosis. *Ann Intern Med* 1989; **111:** 538–9.
2. Soriano FG, *et al.* Neurosarcoidosis: therapeutic success with methotrexate. *Postgrad Med J* 1990; **66:** 142–3.
3. Lower EE, Baughman RP. Prolonged use of methotrexate for sarcoidosis. *Arch Intern Med* 1995; **155:** 846–51.
4. Baughman RP, Lower EE. A clinical approach to the use of methotrexate for sarcoidosis. *Thorax* 1999; **54:** 742–6.


**Scleroderma.** There is some evidence of benefit with methotrexate in patients with scleroderma (p.1348), particularly for cutaneous symptoms, although not all studies have demonstrated clear value.

References.


1. van den Hoogen FH, *et al.* Comparison of methotrexate with placebo in the treatment of systemic sclerosis: a 24 week randomized double-blind trial, followed by a 24 week observational trial. *Br J Rheumatol* 1996; **35:** 364–72.
2. Seyger MMB, *et al.* Low-dose methotrexate in the treatment of widespread morphea. *J Am Acad Dermatol* 1998; **39:** 220–5.
3. Uziel Y, *et al.* Methotrexate and corticosteroid therapy for pediatric localized scleroderma. *J Pediatr* 2000; **136:** 91–5.
4. Pope JE, *et al.* A randomized, controlled trial of methotrexate versus placebo in early diffuse scleroderma. *Arthritis Rheum* 2001; **44:** 1351–8.


**Skin disorders, non-malignant.** Methotrexate is widely used in the treatment of severe refractory psoriasis. As discussed on p.1137 the aim of such therapy is to bring the disease under control, enabling a return to other therapy. For use in psoriatic arthritis see above. Methotrexate is also used in conjunction with corticosteroids in the management of pemphigus and pemphigoid (p.1137) but its value has been questioned.[1]


1. Carson PJ, *et al.* Influence of treatment on the clinical course of pemphigus vulgaris. *J Am Acad Dermatol* 1996; **34:** 645–52.


**Termination of pregnancy.** Methotrexate has been investigated as an alternative to mifepristone for use with misoprostol for the termination of pregnancy (p.1512). Intramuscular methotrexate followed 3 days later by intravaginal misoprostol was more effective than misoprostol alone for termination at 56 days or less;[1] the combination was reported to be less successful after 57 to 63 days' gestation.[2] Later studies[3,4] however found the combination to be safe and effective in terminating pregnancies up to 63 days' gestation; in these the misoprostol was administered up to 7 days after the methotrexate. Oral methotrexate is also effective.[5-7]

For the role of methotrexate in the management of ectopic pregnancy, see above.


1. Creinin MD, Vittinghoff E. Methotrexate and misoprostol vs misoprostol alone for early abortion: a randomized controlled trial. *JAMA* 1994; **272:** 1190–5.
2. Creinin MD. Methotrexate and misoprostol for abortion at 57-63 days gestation. *Contraception* 1994; **50:** 511–15.
3. Hausknecht RU. Methotrexate and misoprostol to terminate early pregnancy. *N Engl J Med* 1995; **333:** 537–40.
4. Creinin MD, *et al.* A randomized trial comparing misoprostol three and seven days after methotrexate for early abortion. *Am J Obstet Gynecol* 1995; **173:** 1578–84.
5. Creinin MD. Oral methotrexate and vaginal misoprostol for early abortion. *Contraception* 1996; **54:** 15–18.
6. Creinin MD, *et al.* Medical abortion with oral methotrexate and vaginal misoprostol. *Obstet Gynecol* 1997; **90:** 611–16.
7. Carbonell JLL, *et al.* Oral methotrexate and vaginal misoprostol for early abortion. *Contraception* 1998; **57:** 83–8.


**Vasculitic syndromes.** In giant cell arteritis (p.1080), improved clinical response and a corticosteroid-sparing effect have been reported with the addition of methotrexate to corticosteroid therapy,[1] but other studies using different designs and dosages[2,3] have failed to find any benefit. For the use of methotrexate in Takayasu's arteritis and Wegener's granulomatosis see p.1089 and p.1090, respectively.


1. Jover JA, *et al.* Combined treatment of giant-cell arteritis with methotrexate and prednisone: a randomized, double-blind, placebo-controlled trial. *Ann Intern Med* 2001; **134:** 106–14.
2. Spiera RF, *et al.* A prospective, double-blind, randomized, placebo controlled trial of methotrexate in the treatment of giant cell arteritis (GCA). *Clin Exp Rheumatol* 2001; **19:** 495–501.
3. Hoffman GS, *et al.* A multicenter, randomized, double-blind, placebo-controlled trial of adjuvant methotrexate treatment for giant cell arteritis. *Arthritis Rheum* 2002; **46:** 1309–18.


## Preparations

***BP 2003:*** Methotrexate Injection; Methotrexate Tablets;
***USP 27:*** Methotrexate for Injection; Methotrexate Injection; Methotrexate Tablets.

**Proprietary Preparations** (details are given in Part 3)
***Arg.:*** Artrait; Ervemin; Xantromid; ***Austral.:*** Ledertrexate; Methoblastin; ***Austria:*** Abitrexate; Emthexate; ***Belg.:*** Ledertrexate; Methoblastine†; ***Braz.:*** Biometrox; Emthexate; Metrexato; Metrotex†; Miantrex; Unitrexate; ***Canad.:*** Rheumatrex†; ***Chile:*** Trixilem; ***Denm.:*** Emthexate; ***Fin.:*** Emthexat; Trexan; ***Fr.:*** Ledertrexate; Novatrex; ***Ger.:*** Farmitrexat; Lantarel; Metex; MTX; O-trexat; ***Gr.:*** Emthexate; ***India:*** Biotrexate; Neotrexate; ***Israel:*** Abitrexate; Emthexate†; ***Malaysia:*** Emthexate; ***Mex.:*** Ifamet; Ledertrexate; Medsatrexate; Methoblastin†; Rhodamer†; Texate†; Trexeron†; Trixilem; Xaken†; ***Neth.:*** Ledertrexate; ***Norw.:*** Emthexat; ***NZ:*** Emthexate†; Ledertrexate; Methoblastin; ***Port.:*** Fauldexato; ***S.Afr.:*** Abitrexate; Emthexate; Methoblastin†; ***Singapore:*** Emthexate†; MTX†; ***Spain:*** Emthexate; ***Swed.:*** Emthexat; ***Thai.:*** Abitrexate; Emthexate; Trixilem; ***UK:*** Maxtrex; ***USA:*** Rheumatrex; Trexall.

## Miltefosine *(BAN, rINN)*

D-18506; HDPC; Hexadecylphosphocholine; Miltefosina. [2-(Trimethylammonio)ethyl][hexadecyloxyphosphonate].

$C_{21}H_{46}NO_4P$ = 407.6.
*CAS — 58066-85-6.*
*ATC — L01XX09.*

### Profile

Miltefosine is a phospholipid derivative which is structurally related to the phospholipid components of the cell membrane and is thought to exert its antineoplastic actions by disruption of cell-membrane function. A 6% solution is applied once or twice daily as a topical antineoplastic agent for skin metastases of breast cancer. Miltefosine has also been tried by mouth for various malignant neoplasms and is used for the treatment of visceral leishmaniasis.

**Leishmaniasis.** Miltefosine, given by mouth in doses of 50 to 150 mg daily, or approximately 2.5 mg/kg daily, for 28 days, appears to be of benefit[1-6] in the treatment of visceral leishmaniasis (p.597), and has been licensed for this purpose in India. It is also under investigation in New World cutaneous leishmaniasis.[7]


1. Sundar S, *et al.* Trial of oral miltefosine for visceral leishmaniasis. *Lancet* 1998; **352:** 1821–3.
2. Jha TK, *et al.* Miltefosine, an oral agent, for the treatment of Indian visceral leishmaniasis. *N Engl J Med* 1999; **341:** 1795–1800.
3. Thakur CP, *et al.* Miltefosine in a case of visceral leishmaniasis with HIV co-infection; and rising incidence of this disease in India. *Trans R Soc Trop Med Hyg* 2000; **94:** 696–7.
4. Sundar S, *et al.* Short-course of oral miltefosine for treatment of visceral leishmaniasis. *Clin Infect Dis* 2001; **31:** 1110–13.
5. Sundar S, *et al.* Oral miltefosine for Indian visceral leishmaniasis. *N Engl J Med* 2002; **347:** 1739–46.
6. Bhattacharya SK, *et al.* Efficacy and tolerability of miltefosine for childhood visceral leishmaniasis in India. *Clin Infect Dis* 2004; **38:** 217–21.
7. Soto J, *et al.* Miltefosine for new world cutaneous leishmaniasis. *Clin Infect Dis* 2004; **38:** 1266–72.


**Malignant neoplasms.** References to the use of topical miltefosine in breast cancer.


1. Terwogt JM, *et al.* Phase II trial of topically applied miltefosine solution in patients with skin-metastasized breast cancer. *Br J Cancer* 1999; **79:** 1158–61.
2. Smorenburg CH, *et al.* Phase II study of miltefosine 6% solution as topical treatment of skin metastases in breast cancer patients. *Anticancer Drugs* 2000; **11:** 825–8.
3. Leonard R, *et al.* Randomized, double-blind, placebo-controlled, multicenter trial of 6% miltefosine solution, a topical chemotherapy in cutaneous metastases from breast cancer. *J Clin Oncol* 2001; **19:** 4150–9.


## Preparations

**Proprietary Preparations** (details are given in Part 3)
***Arg.:*** Mitex; ***Austria:*** Miltex; ***Braz.:*** Miltex; ***Chile:*** Miltex; ***Fin.:*** Miltex; ***Fr.:*** Miltex; ***Ger.:*** Miltex; ***Israel:*** Miltex; ***Singapore:*** Miltex; ***Spain:*** Miltex; ***Swed.:*** Miltex; ***UK:*** Miltex.

## Mitobronitol *(BAN, rINN)*

DBM; Dibromomannitol; NSC-94100; R-54; WR-220057. 1,6-Dibromo-1,6-dideoxy-D-mannitol.

$C_6H_{12}Br_2O_4$ = 308.0.
*CAS — 488-41-5.*
*ATC — L01AX01.*

**Pharmacopoeias.** In *Br.*

**BP 2003** (Mitobronitol). A white or almost white crystalline solid. Slightly soluble in water, in alcohol, and in acetone; practically insoluble in chloroform. Protect from light.

### Profile

Mitobronitol is an antineoplastic which appears to act as an alkylating agent, perhaps by epoxide formation. It has been used in the management of thrombocythaemia, both primary, and secondary to chronic myeloid leukaemia or polycythaemia vera.

The usual dose is 250 mg daily by mouth until the platelet count falls to acceptable levels. Intermittent dosage has been given for maintenance therapy, adjusted according to the blood count. Frequent examination of the blood should be performed during treatment.

Mitobronitol is well absorbed from the gastrointestinal tract and is excreted through the liver into the bile, with reabsorption from the small intestine. It is eliminated as unchanged drug and some bromine-containing metabolites in the urine over several days.

**Carcinogenicity.** Long-term follow-up of a cooperative study[1] involving 350 patients with polycythaemia vera and treated with mitobronitol was thought to indicate that mitobronitol was less likely than phosphorus-32 or busulfan to induce acute myeloid leukaemia.

For a discussion of the usual management of polycythaemia vera, see p.508.


1. Kelemen E, *et al.* Decreasing risk of leukaemia during prolonged follow-up after mitobronitol therapy for polycythaemia vera. *Lancet* 1987; **ii:** 625.


## Preparations

***BP 2003:*** Mitobronitol Tablets.

**Proprietary Preparations** (details are given in Part 3)
***Austria:*** Myelobromol; ***UK:*** Myelobromol.

## Mitoguazone Dihydrochloride *(rINNM)*

Dihidrocloruro de mitoguazona; Methyl-GAG; Methylglyoxal Bis-guanylhydrazone (mitoguazone); MGBG; NSC-32946. 1,1′-[(Methylethanediylidene)dinitrilo]diguanidine dihydrochloride.

$C_5H_{12}N_8,2HCl$ = 257.1.
*CAS — 459-86-9 (mitoguazone); 7059-23-6 (mitoguazone dihydrochloride).*
*ATC — L01XX16.*

### Profile

Mitoguazone is an antineoplastic which may exert its cytotoxic effects by its ability to inhibit polyamine biosynthesis. It has been tried as the dihydrochloride monohydrate or the acetate, in the treatment of leukaemias, lymphomas, and some solid tumours.

Mitoguazone may produce hypoglycaemia and should be given dissolved in glucose-containing infusion fluids; sugar may be taken by mouth if hypoglycaemia develops during infusion. Granulocytopenia and thrombocytopenia are generally mild and reversible on stopping treatment. Gastrointestinal effects frequently occur.

## Mitolactol *(rINN)*

DBD; Dibromodulcitol; NSC-104800; WR-138743. 1,6-Dibromo-1,6-dideoxy-D-galactitol.

$C_6H_{12}Br_2O_4$ = 308.0.
*CAS — 10318-26-0.*

### Profile

Mitolactol is an antineoplastic which may act by alkylation, probably as epoxide metabolites including dianhydrogalactitol. It has been given by mouth in the treatment of metastatic breast and cervical carcinoma, although other drugs are usually preferred, and has also been tried in other malignant neoplasms, notably those of the brain.

In addition to myelosuppression, which is usually dose-limiting, and manifests chiefly as leucopenia and thrombocytopenia, adverse effects include gastrointestinal disturbances, skin rashes, grey pigmentation of the skin, transient disturbances of hepatic function, elevated blood-urea nitrogen (BUN), and hypersensitivity reactions. Blood counts should be taken regularly during treatment and mitolactol withdrawn if bone-marrow depression occurs.

## Mitomycin *(BAN, USAN, rINN)*

Mitomicina; Mitomycin C; Mitomycine C; Mitomycinum; NSC-26980. 6-Amino-1,1a,2,8,8a,8b-hexahydro-8-hydroxymethyl-8a-methoxy-5-methylazirino[2′,3′:3,4]pyrrolo[1,2-*a*]indole-4,7-dione carbamate; (1*S*,2*S*,9*S*,9a*R*)-7-Amino-2,3,5,8,9,9a-hexahydro-9a-methoxy-6-methyl-5,8-dioxo-1,2-epimino-1-*H*-pyrrolo[1,2-*a*]indol-9-ylmethyl carbamate.

$C_{15}H_{18}N_4O_5$ = 334.3.
*CAS — 50-07-7.*
*ATC — L01DC03.*

**Description.** Mitomycin is an antineoplastic antibiotic produced by the growth of *Streptomyces caespitosus.*

**Pharmacopoeias.** In *Chin., Eur.* (see p.vi), *Jpn,* and *US.*

**Ph. Eur. 5.0** (Mitomycin). A substance produced by a strain of *Streptomyces caespitosus.* Blue-violet crystals or crystalline powder. Slightly soluble in water and in acetone; freely soluble in dimethylacetamide; sparingly soluble in methyl alcohol. A 0.1% solution in water has a pH of 5.5 to 7.5. Protect from light.

**USP 27** (Mitomycin). A blue-violet crystalline powder. It has a potency of not less than 970 micrograms/mg. Slightly soluble in water; soluble in acetone, in butyl acetate, in cyclohexanone, and in methyl alcohol. A 0.5% suspension in water has a pH of 6.0 to 7.5. Store in airtight containers at a temperature of 25°, excursions permitted between 15° and 30°. Protect from light.

**Incompatibility.** Mitomycin may be incompatible with drugs that are acid in solution—for a report of incompatibility with topotecan, see p.589.

**Stability.** Mitomycin undergoes degradation in acid solution,[1] and two studies[2,3] suggested that mitomycin was much less stable in glucose 5% injection than in sodium chloride 0.9%. These findings were queried by a manufacturer (*Bristol, USA*) whose own results suggested[4] that mitomycin was stable for 48 hours in glucose injection 5% at 25°, and it is uncertain whether different manufacturers' formulations differ in stability, or, as has been suggested, that an unsuitable assay was used by the manufacturer to measure stability.[5]


1. Beijnen JH, Underberg WJM. Degradation of mitomycin C in acidic solution. *Int J Pharmaceutics* 1985; **24:** 219–29.
2. Benvenuto JA, *et al.* Stability and compatibility of antitumour agents in glass and plastic containers. *Am J Hosp Pharm* 1981; **38:** 1914–18.
3. Quebbeman EJ, *et al.* Stability of mitomycin admixtures. *Am J Hosp Pharm* 1985; **42:** 1750–4.
4. Keller JH. Stability of mitomycin admixtures. *Am J Hosp Pharm* 1986; **43:** 59,64.
5. Quebbeman EJ, Hoffman NE. Stability of mitomycin admixtures. *Am J Hosp Pharm* 1986; **43:** 64.

### Adverse Effects, Treatment, and Precautions

For general discussions see Antineoplastics, p.492, p.495, and p.497.

The main adverse effect of mitomycin is delayed cumulative bone-marrow suppression. Profound leucopenia and thrombocytopenia occurs after about 4 weeks with recovery in about 8 to 10 weeks after a dose. Blood counts may not recover in about one-quarter of patients. Other serious adverse effects include renal damage and pulmonary reactions; a potentially fatal haemolytic-uraemic syndrome has been reported in some patients. The US manufacturer states that the degree of renal impairment does not appear to be related to dose or duration of therapy but some in the UK consider that the incidence of renal toxicity is greatly increased if the total cumulative dose exceeds 120 mg (see also Effects on the Kidneys, below). Gastrointestinal toxicity, dermatitis, alopecia, fever, malaise, and rarely cardiotoxicity may also occur. Local tissue necrosis, ulceration, and cellulitis may occur following extravasation.

Mitomycin is contra-indicated in patients with impaired renal function or coagulation disorders. Renal function should be tested before beginning treatment and after each course.

**Effects on the bladder.** Intravesical instillation of mitomycin after resection of superficial bladder tumours has led to the development of indolent asymptomatic ulcers at the resection site which may persist for months, and must be distinguished from persistent infiltrating bladder cancer.[1,2] Persistent ulceration, inflammation, necrosis, and pain has also occurred, possibly because of mitomycin extravasation at the resection site.[3] There are also a few reports[4] of eosinophilic cystitis, in which eosinophilic infiltration of the mucosa and muscle were accompanied by oedema, inflammation, muscle necrosis and fibrosis. Severe bladder contracture is a rare, and often irreversible, complication of intravesical mitomycin;[5] urinary diversion may be required in cases of intolerable urinary frequency.[6] Formation of papillary-like calcifications at the resection site,[7] and calcification of the bladder wall have also been described after the use of mitomycin for superficial transitional cell carcinoma of the bladder.

See also under Effects on the Skin, below.

1. Richards B, Tolley D. Benign ulcers after bladder instillation of mitomycin C. *Lancet* 1986; **i:** 45.
2. Hetherington JW, Whelan P. Persistent ulcers after bladder instillation of mitomycin C. *Lancet* 1986; **i:** 324.
3. Cliff AM, *et al.* Perivesical inflammation after early mitomycin C instillation. *BJU Int* 2000; **85:** 556–7.
4. Ülker V, *et al.* Eosinophilic cystitis induced by mitomycin-C. *Int Urol Nephrol* 1996; **28:** 755–9.
5. Punga-Maole ML, *et al.* Rétraction vésicale, complication de la chimioprophylaxie du cancer vésical superficiel par mitomycine C endovésicale: a propos d'un cas et revue de la littérature. *Prog Urol* 1995; **5:** 580–5.
6. Wajsman Z, *et al.* Severely contracted bladder following intravesical mitomycin C therapy. *J Urol (Baltimore)* 1983; **130:** 340–1.
7. Fiore AA, *et al.* Papillary-like bladder calcifications following intravesical mitomycin C: a case report. *Minerva Urol Nefrol* 1993; **45:** 171–3.

**Effects on the eye.** Early complications following the topical use of mitomycin with glaucoma filtering surgery (see Glaucoma, below) include hypotony, shallow anterior chamber, cataract formation, choroidal effusions, hypotonous maculopathy, and suprachoroidal haemorrhage.[1] Late complications include bleb leak, blebitis, and endophthalmitis.[2] Complications following the topical use of mitomycin with or following pterygium surgery (see Pterygium, below) commonly include irritation and photophobia. Other effects include delayed epithelial healing, avascularity of the sclera and cornea, scleral calcification and ulceration, necrotising scleritis, corneal or scleral perforation, iridocyclitis, cataract formation, glaucoma, and symblepharon.[1] Some of these effects may be severe and sight-threatening, and require further surgery.[3]

1. Hardten DR, Samuelson TW. Ocular toxicity of mitomycin-C. *Int Ophthalmol Clin* 1999; **39:** 79–90.
2. DeBry PW, *et al.* Incidence of late-onset bleb-related complications following trabeculectomy with mitomycin. *Arch Ophthalmol* 2002; **120:** 297–300.
3. Rubinfeld RS, *et al.* Serious complications of topical mitomycin C after pterygium surgery. *Ophthalmology* 1992; **99:** 1647–54.

**Effects on the kidneys.** A syndrome of thrombotic microangiopathy resembling the haemolytic-uraemic syndrome has been seen in patients receiving mitomycin, either alone[1] or more frequently combined with other drugs, particularly fluorouracil[2] or tamoxifen.[3,4] The syndrome is characterised by haemolytic anaemia, thrombocytopenia, and progressive renal failure, and may be accompanied by hypertension, pulmonary oedema, and neurological effects including confusion, headache, and seizures.[1,2] Onset is usually delayed, sometimes occurring several months after the end of a course of mitomycin.[1,2] There is some uncertainty as to whether mitomycin dose is significant, but one study[1] found that all of 25 cases they reported had received total doses of 70 mg or more, and another[2] reported that 74 of 83 cases had received 60 mg or more. Symptoms may be exacerbated by blood transfusions.[2] The use of erythropoietin allowed the cessation of blood transfusion, with subsequent haematological improvement and slower progression of chronic renal failure in one case report.[5] Plasma exchange has been suggested as possibly helpful,[1] although only a minority of patients may benefit from this treatment.[2] Captopril therapy may also be useful.[6]

1. Cordonnier D, *et al.* La néphrotoxicité de la mitomycine C (à propos de 25 observations): résultats d'une enquête multicentrique organisée par la société de néphrologie. *Nephrologie* 1985; **6:** 19–26.
2. Lesesne JB, *et al.* Cancer-associated hemolytic-uremic syndrome: analysis of 85 cases from a national registry. *J Clin Oncol* 1989; **7:** 781–9.
3. Montes A, *et al.* A toxic interaction between mitomycin C and tamoxifen causing the haemolytic uraemic syndrome. *Eur J Cancer* 1993; **29A:** 1854–7.
4. Ellis PA, *et al.* Haemolytic uraemic syndrome in a patient with lung cancer: further evidence for a toxic interaction between mitomycin-C and tamoxifen. *Clin Oncol (R Coll Radiol)* 1996; **8:** 402–3.
5. Catalano C, *et al.* Erythropoietin is beneficial in mitomycin-induced hemolytic-uremic syndrome. *Nephron* 2002; **91:** 324–6.
6. Schiebe ME, *et al.* Mitomycin C-related hemolytic uremic syndrome in cancer patients. *Anticancer Drugs* 1998; **9:** 433–5.

**Effects on the liver.** Hepatic veno-occlusive disease developed in 6 of 29 patients given intensive mitomycin therapy and autologous bone marrow transplantation.[1] The effect was manifest as abdominal pain, hepatomegaly, and ascites, and liver failure was progressive and fatal in 3. A further patient, who had no symptoms, was found to have veno-occlusive disease at post mortem.

1. Lazarus HM, *et al.* Veno-occlusive disease of the liver after high-dose mitomycin C therapy and autologous bone marrow transplantation. *Cancer* 1982; **49:** 1789–95.

**Effects on respiratory function.** Mitomycin-induced pulmonary toxicity has been reviewed.[1,2] There have been reports of toxicity at total dosages as low as 20 mg/m$^2$ of mitomycin,[2] although others report[1] that the average cumulative dose associated with toxicity is 78 mg. Premedication with corticosteroids may reduce the incidence of lung toxicity.[2]

See also Effects on the Lungs, p.494. For reference to the respiratory effects of mitomycin in combination with a vinca alkaloid see Interactions, Antineoplastics, under Vinblastine Sulfate, p.592.

1. Linette DC, *et al.* Mitomycin-induced pulmonary toxicity: case report and review of the literature. *Ann Pharmacother* 1992; **26:** 481–4.
2. Okuno SH, Frytak S. Mitomycin lung toxicity: acute and chronic phases. *Am J Clin Oncol* 1997; **20:** 282–4.

**Effects on the skin.** Severe eczema of the hands and feet and generalised rash have been reported in patients receiving intravesical mitomycin.[1,2] These symptoms appear to be due to a delayed hypersensitivity (type IV) reaction,[1,2] which is probably also responsible for the bladder irritation and cystitis that may follow intravesical mitomycin[1] (see above). Leucocytoclastic vasculitis caused by an immune-complex mediated (type III) reaction and presenting as purpuric papules has also been described.[2]

1. Colver GB, *et al.* Dermatitis due to intravesical mitomycin C: a delayed-type hypersensitivity reaction? *Br J Dermatol* 1990; **122:** 217–24.
2. Kunkeler L, *et al.* Type III and type IV hypersensitivity reactions due to mitomycin C. *Contact Dermatitis* 2000; **42:** 74–6.

### Interactions

For a general outline of antineoplastic drug interactions, see p.498.

**Antineoplastics.** Cardiotoxicity developed in 14 of 91 patients who received mitomycin therapy as second-line treatment for breast cancer after the failure of *doxorubicin*-containing regimens, compared with 3 of 89 similar patients whose second-line treatment did not include mitomycin.[1]

For reports of acute bronchospasm following injection of a *vinca alkaloid* in patients pretreated with mitomycin see Vinblastine Sulfate, p.592. For the increased risk of haemolytic-uraemic syndrome that may occur if mitomycin is given with *fluorouracil* or *tamoxifen* see under Effects on the Kidneys, above.

1. Buzdar AU, *et al.* Adriamycin and mitomycin C: possible synergistic cardiotoxicity. *Cancer Treat Rep* 1978; **62:** 1005–8.

### Pharmacokinetics

Mitomycin disappears rapidly from the blood after intravenous injection with an initial (distribution) half-life of 17 minutes. It is widely distributed but does not appear to cross the blood-brain barrier. Mitomycin is metabolised mainly but not exclusively in the liver. The terminal half-life is about 50 minutes. Following normal doses about 10% of a dose is excreted unchanged in the urine; small amounts are also present in bile and faeces. With increasing doses metabolic pathways are saturated, and more drug is excreted unchanged in the urine.

### Uses and Administration

Mitomycin is a highly toxic antibiotic with antineoplastic properties. It acts as an alkylating agent after activation *in vivo* and suppresses the synthesis of nucleic acids. It is a cell-cycle non-specific agent, but is most active in the late $G_1$ and early S phases.

Mitomycin is used, with other antineoplastic agents, in the treatment of many solid tumours including those of the bladder, breast, cervix, eye, liver, lung, stomach, and prostate as indicated by the cross-references given below. Mitomycin has been tried in various other neoplasms including those of the gastrointestinal tract, head and neck, pancreas, in melanoma, sarcomas, and in leukaemias.

Various dosage regimens have been tried. An initial dose of 10 to 20 mg/m$^2$ intravenously has been given; subsequent doses may be repeated at intervals of 6 to 8 weeks if blood counts permit, and should be reduced according to the previous haematological response. Another suggested regimen is 2 mg/m$^2$ daily for 5 days, repeated after 2 days. Other regimens may be used, particularly in combination.

Doses are adjusted according to the effect on bone marrow and treatment should not be repeated until the leucocyte and platelet counts are above acceptable levels (see also Bone-marrow Depression, p.496). The drug should not be given again if the nadir of the leucocyte count is below 2000 cells/mm$^3$. Dosage may need to be reduced when used in combination with other antineoplastics.

Mitomycin is also used as a bladder instillation: 10 to 40 mg is instilled one to three times a week for a total of 20 doses in the treatment of superficial bladder tumours. For the prevention of recurrent bladder tumours 20 mg may be instilled every 2 weeks, or 40 mg monthly or 3-monthly. Alternatively 4 to 10 mg may be instilled one to three times a week. These doses are usually given in 10 to 40 mL of water for injection. The solution should be retained in the bladder for at least 1 hour.

Mitomycin has been given by the intra-arterial route in the treatment of liver tumours, sometimes as an infusion of microcapsules designed to produce localised embolisation.

**Glaucoma.** Mitomycin, like fluorouracil, is effective in improving the outcome of glaucoma filtering surgery in selected patients when used as an adjunct to prevent the formation of scar tissue (see p.1485). Fluorouracil is usually administered as a regimen of multiple injections but mitomycin given as a single intra-operative topical application in usual concentrations ranging from 0.2 to 0.5 mg/mL appears to be of similar efficacy.[1,2] A systematic review of 11 studies concluded that intra-operative mitomycin reduced the chances of failure in high-risk patients, and in those having their first trabeculectomy.[3] However it was noted that the nature of the data might have led to overestimation of the effect and that there was some evidence of an increased risk of cataract with mitomycin. Late hypotony is also a problem.[4] For other potential complications see Effects on the Eye, above.

1. Skuta GL, *et al.* Intraoperative mitomycin versus postoperative 5-fluorouracil in high-risk glaucoma filtering surgery. *Ophthalmology* 1992; **99:** 438–44.
2. Katz GJ, *et al.* Mitomycin C versus 5-fluorouracil in high-risk glaucoma filtering surgery: extended follow-up. *Ophthalmology* 1995; **102:** 1263–9.
3. Wilkins M, *et al.* Intra-operative mitomycin C for glaucoma surgery. Available in The Cochrane Library. Issue 2. Chichester: John Wiley; 2004.
4. Bindlish R, *et al.* Efficacy and safety of mitomycin-C in primary trabeculectomy: five-year follow-up. *Ophthalmology* 2002; **109:** 1336–42.

**Malignant neoplasms.** Mitomycin is used in the prevention of recurrent bladder cancer (p.512), in the palliative therapy of advanced breast cancer (p.514), in malignancies of the cervix (p.515), eye (p.516), gastrointestinal tract (p.516), liver (p.518), non-small cell lung cancer (p.519), and has been tried in advanced prostatic cancer (see p.521).

**Pterygium.** Pterygium is a degenerative condition of subconjunctival tissues that results in a vascularised overgrowth of the conjunctiva and cornea. It is cosmetically unappealing but does not usually require treatment. However, if it affects the pupillary area it can be treated surgically. Pterygium often recurs after removal and methods used to prevent recurrence include radiotherapy or the topical application of mitomycin or thiotepa.[1]

Thiotepa has been applied postoperatively as 0.05% eye drops for several weeks, but pterygium may still recur[2] and adverse effects include conjunctival injection, granuloma, hypertrophic conjunctiva, and black deposits in the conjunctival fornix.[1] Depigmentation of the eyelids may also be a problem, so patients should avoid direct sunlight during thiotepa use.[1]

Mitomycin has been applied topically to the surgical site, or given as eye drops postoperatively.[1] The optimal intra-operative exposure time and concentration are uncertain: concentrations of 0.02 or 0.04% have been applied for up to 5 minutes,[1,3] and low-dose treatment with mitomycin 0.02% for 30 seconds has been reported to be effective with few complications.[4] Postoperative treatment has generally been given as 0.02, 0.04, or 0.1% eye drops for up to 2 weeks, but the higher concentrations and longer treatment periods have been associated with more adverse effects,[1] some of which may be severe and sight-threatening (see also Effects on the Eye, above). Comparisons of intra-operative with postoperative use suggest that pterygium recurrence rates are similar.[1,5]

A range of β-irradiation doses and fractionation methods have been used. Long-term complications include posterior subcapsular changes of the lens, atrophy and ulceration of the sclera, and scleral necrosis leading to endophthalmitis.[1] In one retrospective study,[6] intra-operative administration of 0.04% mitomycin was found to be more effective than β-irradiation in preventing recurrence after surgery. In another study,[7] postoperative mitomycin 0.02% for one week was less effective than radiation therapy.

1. Hoffman RS, Power WJ. Current options in pterygium management. *Int Ophthalmol Clin* 1999; **39:** 15–26.
2. Chapman-Smith JS. Pterygium treatment with triethylene thiophosphoramide. *Aust N Z J Ophthalmol* 1992; **20:** 129–31.
3. Anduze AL. Pterygium surgery with mitomycin-C: ten-year results. *Ophthalmic Surg Lasers* 2001; **32:** 341–5.
4. Cheng H-C, *et al.* Low-dose intraoperative mitomycin C as chemoadjuvant for pterygium surgery. *Cornea* 2001; **20:** 24–9.
5. Oguz H, *et al.* Intraoperative application versus postoperative mitomycin C eye drops in pterygium surgery. *Acta Ophthalmol Scand* 1999; **77:** 147–50.
6. Amano S, *et al.* Comparative study of intraoperative mitomycin C and β irradiation in pterygium surgery. *Br J Ophthalmol* 2000; **84:** 618–21.
7. Şimşek T, *et al.* Comparative efficacy of β-irradiation and mitomycin-C in primary and recurrent pterygium. *Eur J Ophthalmol* 2001; **11:** 126–32.

### Preparations

***USP 27:*** Mitomycin for Injection.

**Proprietary Preparations** (details are given in Part 3)
***Arg.:*** Asomutan; Crisofimina; Datisan; Maximiton; Mitocyna; Mitokebir; Mitonovag; Mitotie; Oncotaxina; Sintemicina; Vetio; ***Braz.:*** Mitocin; ***Canad.:*** Mutamycin; ***Chile:*** Metomit; ***Fin.:*** Mitostat; Mutamycin; ***Fr.:*** Ametycine; ***Ger.:*** Ametycine; Mito-medac; ***Mex.:*** Ifamit; Mitocin-C; Mitolem; Mixandex; ***Norw.:*** Mutamycin; ***Swed.:*** Mutamycin; ***Switz.:*** Mutamycine; ***USA:*** Mitozytrex; Mutamycin.

## Mitotane *(USAN, rINN)*

CB-313; *o,p'*DDD; Mitotano; NSC-38721; WR-13045. 1,1-Dichloro-2-(2-chlorophenyl)-2-(4-chlorophenyl)ethane.

$C_{14}H_{10}Cl_4$ = 320.0.
*CAS — 53-19-0.*
*ATC — L01XX23.*

**Pharmacopoeias.** In *US.*

**USP 27** (Mitotane). A white crystalline powder with a slight aromatic odour. M.p. is between 75° and 81°. Practically insoluble in water; soluble in alcohol, in ether, in petroleum spirit, and in fixed oils and fats. Store in airtight containers. Protect from light.

### Adverse Effects

Almost all patients given mitotane experience anorexia, nausea and vomiting, and sometimes diarrhoea, and about 40% suffer some central toxicity with dizziness, vertigo, sedation, lethargy, and depression. Permanent brain damage may develop with prolonged dosage. Ocular side-effects may occur including blurred vision, diplopia, lenticular opacities, and retinopathy. Other side-effects include hypersensitivity reactions, haematuria, albuminuria, skin rashes, fever, myalgia, haemorrhagic cystitis, flushing, hypertension, and orthostatic hypotension.

### Precautions

Mitotane inhibits the adrenal cortex and adrenocortical insufficiency may develop during treatment; corticosteroid therapy is often required. In trauma or shock the drug should be temporarily withdrawn and corticosteroids should be given systemically. Mitotane should be given with care to patients with liver disease. Before mitotane therapy is begun, all possible tumour tissue from large metastases should be surgically removed, in order to minimise possible infarction or haemorrhage in the tumour. Patients should not drive or operate machinery. Behavioural and neurological assessments should be carried out regularly in patients who have been receiving treatment for 2 years or more.

### Interactions

Mitotane may induce hepatic microsomal enzymes and enhance the metabolism of some other drugs, including coumarin anticoagulants.

**Spironolactone.** Mitotane in a dose of up to 3 g daily in a 65-year-old patient with Cushing's syndrome appeared to be ineffective and did not produce the usual side-effects associated with mitotane while the patient was also receiving spironolactone.[1]

1. Wortsman J, Soler NG. Mitotane: spironolactone antagonism in Cushing's syndrome. *JAMA* 1977; **238:** 2527.

### Pharmacokinetics

Up to 40% of a dose of mitotane is absorbed from the gastrointestinal tract. After daily doses of 5 to 15 g, concentrations in the blood of 7 to 90 micrograms/mL of unchanged drug and 29 to 54 micrograms/mL of metabolite have been reported. Mitotane has been detected in the blood 6 to 9 weeks after stopping treatment. It is widely distributed and appears to be stored mainly in fatty tissues. It is metabolised in the liver and other tissues and excreted as metabolites in urine and bile. From 10 to 25% of a dose has been recovered in the urine as a water-soluble metabolite.

**Therapeutic drug monitoring.** Monitoring of mitotane and its major metabolite *o,p'*-DDE in 2 patients receiving mitotane in low doses for Cushing's disease demonstrated that there is a prolonged lag time in the plasma concentration changes in response to alterations in dosage,[1] presumably because of the lipophilicity of both compounds which leads to accumulation in adipose tissue. A study[2] in adrenal carcinoma found that mitotane is preferentially distributed into the very-low-density lipoprotein (VLDL) fraction of the serum of patients with hypertriglyceridaemia, whereas under normolipidaemic conditions, it is bound to high-density lipoproteins and albumin. Because VLDL is not incorporated into the human adrenal cells, mitotane's lipophilicity has implications for treatment and monitoring in patients with hypertriglyceridaemia. In some studies[3,4] tumour responses were seen only in those patients achieving a serum concentration of mitotane above 14 micrograms/mL, and a small prospective study[5] found that therapeutic concentrations (defined as between 14 and 20 micrograms/mL) could be reached by sustained low doses (1 to 3 g daily), thus limiting side-effects.

1. Benecke R, *et al.* Plasma level monitoring of mitotane (o,p'-DDD) and its metabolite (o,p'-DDE) during long-term treatment of Cushing's disease with low doses. *Eur J Clin Pharmacol* 1991; **41:** 259–61.
2. Gebhardt DOE, *et al.* The distribution of *o,p'*-DDD (mitotane) among serum lipoproteins in normo- and hypertriglyceridemia. *Cancer Chemother Pharmacol* 1992; **29:** 331–4.
3. Haak HR, *et al.* Optimal treatment of adrenocortical carcinoma with mitotane: results in a consecutive series of 96 patients. *Br J Cancer* 1994; **69:** 947–51.
4. Baudin E, *et al.* Impact of monitoring plasma 1,1-dichlorodiphenildichloroethane (o,p'DDD) levels on the treatment of patients with adrenocortical carcinoma. *Cancer* 2001; **92:** 1385–92.
5. Terzolo M, *et al.* Low-dose monitored mitotane treatment achieves the therapeutic range with manageable side effects in patients with adrenocortical cancer. *J Clin Endocrinol Metab* 2000; **85:** 2234–8.

### Uses and Administration

Mitotane is an antineoplastic with a selective inhibitory action on adrenal cortex activity. It may also modify peripheral steroid metabolism. It is given in the treatment of inoperable adrenocortical tumours and has also been used in patients with Cushing's syndrome (p.1313).

The usual initial dosage is 2 to 6 g daily by mouth in 3 or 4 divided doses, adjusted to the maximum tolerated dose which may range from 2 to 16 g daily.

◊ A retrospective study involving 105 patients with adrenocortical carcinoma found the prognosis to be generally poor with a 5-year survival of 22% among 88 patients followed up.[1] Surgical resection was the treatment of choice; mitotane treatment had no effect on survival although 8 patients had transient tumour regression and it was of some benefit in controlling adrenal hypersecretion. However, others have previously reported improved survival in patients with adrenocortical carcinoma in whom mitotane serum concentrations were above 14 micrograms/mL, and some[2] have suggested that the poor results with mitotane in the retrospective study may have been due to low serum-mitotane concentrations (see Therapeutic Drug Monitoring, above). A further study[3] found mitotane to be of benefit only in patients with adrenocortical carcinoma undergoing palliative surgery, but of no additional benefit as an adjuvant therapy for survival amongst patients receiving curative surgical resection. A review[4] concluded that, although mitotane is recommended for patients with unresectable tumours, only about 35% of tumours respond.

1. Luton J-P, *et al.* Clinical features of adrenocortical carcinoma, prognostic factors, and the effect of mitotane therapy. *N Engl J Med* 1990; **322:** 1195–1201.
2. Haak HR, *et al.* Mitotane therapy of adrenocortical carcinoma. *N Engl J Med* 1990; **323:** 758.
3. Icard P, *et al.* Adrenocortical carcinomas: surgical trends and results of a 253-patient series from the French Association of Endocrine Surgeons study group. *World J Surg* 2001; **25:** 891–7.
4. Wooten MD, King DK. Adrenal cortical carcinoma: epidemiology and treatment with mitotane and a review of the literature. *Cancer* 1993; **72:** 3145–55.

### Preparations

***USP 27:*** Mitotane Tablets.

**Proprietary Preparations** (details are given in Part 3)
***Braz.:*** Lisodren; ***Canad.:*** Lysodren; ***Gr.:*** Lysodren; ***USA:*** Lysodren.

## Mitoxantrone Hydrochloride

*(BANM, USAN, rINNM)*

CL-232315; DHAD; Dihydroxyanthracenedione Dihydrochloride; Hidrocloruro de mitoxantrona; Mitoxantroni Hydrochloridum; Mitozantrone Hydrochloride; NSC-301739. 1,4-Dihydroxy-5,8-bis[2-(2-hydroxyethylamino)ethylamino]anthraquinone dihydrochloride.

$C_{22}H_{28}N_4O_6,2HCl$ = 517.4.
*CAS — 65271-80-9 (mitoxantrone); 70476-82-3 (mitoxantrone hydrochloride).*
*ATC — L01DB07.*

**Pharmacopoeias.** In *Chin., Eur.* (see p.vi), and *US.*

**Ph. Eur. 5.0** (Mitoxantrone Hydrochloride). A dark-blue, electrostatic, hygroscopic powder. Sparingly soluble in water; practically insoluble in acetone; slightly soluble in methyl alcohol. Store in airtight containers.

**USP 27** (Mitoxantrone Hydrochloride). A dark-blue powder. Sparingly soluble in water; practically insoluble in acetone, in acetonitrile, and in chloroform; slightly soluble in methyl alcohol. Store in airtight containers.

### Adverse Effects, Treatment, and Precautions

As for Doxorubicin Hydrochloride, p.548. Mitoxantrone is reported to be better tolerated than doxorubicin. The nadir of the white cell count usually occurs about 10 days after a dose, with recovery by day 21. Elevation in liver enzyme values may occur; there are occasional reports of severe hepatic impairment in patients with leukaemia, in whom doses are generally higher and adverse effects of mitoxantrone may be more frequent and severe.

Transient blue-green coloration of the urine, and occasionally the sclerae, may occur. Tissue necrosis is rare following extravasation.

Severe neurotoxicity has resulted from erroneous intrathecal administration; local or regional neuropathy has followed intra-arterial injection. Care is required in patients with pre-existing heart disease, or who have had prior anthracycline treatment or radiotherapy to the chest, as they are at increased risk of cardiotoxicity; regular examinations of cardiac function should be performed in such patients and in those who receive a total cumulative dose of mitoxantrone in excess of 160 mg/m$^2$. Care is also required in patients with hepatic impairment. Regular blood counts should be performed during treatment.

**Alopecia.** Two patients receiving therapy with mitoxantrone developed selective alopecia of white but not of dark hair.[1]

1. Arlin ZA, *et al.* Selective alopecia with mitoxantrone. *N Engl J Med* 1984; **310:** 1464.

**Breast feeding.** Mitoxantrone was detected in the breast milk of a woman with acute promyelocytic leukaemia in remission who was given consolidation chemotherapy that included mitoxantrone 6 mg/m$^2$ on days 1 to 3. A concentration of 120 nanograms/mL was measured just after the third dose and a concentration of 18 nanograms/mL was still measurable 28 days after treatment. Although she breast fed her neonate from 3 weeks after the completion of the course of treatment and no adverse effects were observed, the authors recommended that women treated with mitoxantrone should be advised not to breast feed.[1]

1. Azuno Y, *et al.* Mitoxantrone and etoposide in breast milk. *Am J Hematol* 1995; **48:** 131–2.

**Effects on the heart.** Data from over 4000 patients treated with mitoxantrone included 172 reports of cardiac events, including 42 cases of congestive heart failure and 66 of decreased ejection fraction.[1] Prior treatment with an anthracycline increased the risk, and congestive heart failure seemed to be more likely in patients exposed to a cumulative mitoxantrone dose of 160 mg/m$^2$ or 100 mg/m$^2$ in those who had already received anthracyclines. In a further 78 patients,[2] clinical heart failure developed in 2 after cumulative doses of 174 and 243 mg/m$^2$. Four of 9 other patients who received mitoxantrone in doses above 100 mg/m$^2$ showed signs of cardiotoxicity, and a further patient who had previously received doxorubicin 313 mg/m$^2$ had a fall in stress ejection fraction after only 47 mg/m$^2$ of mitoxantrone. However, sinus bradycardia has also been reported[3] in 2 previously untreated patients after commencing continuous infusions of mitoxantrone 10 mg/m$^2$. For information on the cardiotoxicity of anthracyclines, to which mitoxantrone is structurally related, see under Adverse Effects and Treatment of Doxorubicin Hydrochloride, p.548.

1. Crossley RJ. Clinical safety and tolerance of mitoxantrone. *Semin Oncol* 1984; **11:** (suppl 1): 54–8.
2. Stuart-Harris R, *et al.* Cardiotoxicity associated with mitoxantrone. *Lancet* 1984; **ii:** 219–20.
3. Benekli M, *et al.* Mitoxantrone-induced bradycardia. *Ann Intern Med* 1997; **126:** 409.

**Handling and disposal.** *Urine and faeces* produced for up to 7 days after a dose of mitoxantrone should be handled wearing protective clothing.[1]

1. Harris J, Dodds LJ. Handling waste from patients receiving cytotoxic drugs. *Pharm J* 1985; **235:** 289–91.

**Hypersensitivity.** In a report of 3 patients, allergic-type reactions to mitoxantrone included vasculitis, facial oedema and skin rashes, and in one, breathlessness, tachypnoea, cyanosis, and unrecordable pulse and blood pressure.[1] Allergic reactions to the drug appear to be rare.

1. Taylor WB, *et al.* Allergic reactions to mitoxantrone. *Lancet* 1986; **i:** 1439.

## Interactions

For a report of the effect of ciclosporin in patients receiving mitoxantrone and etoposide, see p.552.

## Pharmacokinetics

After intravenous doses mitoxantrone is rapidly and extensively distributed to body tissues, and slowly excreted in urine and bile as unchanged drug and metabolites. The elimination half-life is reported to range from 5 to 18 days. Between 6 and 11% of a dose has been recovered from urine, and 13 to 25% in faeces, within 5 days. It does not appear to cross the blood-brain barrier, but it is distributed into breast milk.

◊ References.

1. Ehninger G, *et al.* Pharmacokinetics and metabolism of mitoxantrone: a review. *Clin Pharmacokinet* 1990; **18:** 365–80.

## Uses and Administration

Mitoxantrone is an antineoplastic structurally related to doxorubicin (p.547). Its mode of action has not been fully established but it inhibits topoisomerase II and causes DNA strand breakage, as well as intercalating with DNA. It is cell-cycle non-specific but is most active against cells in the late S phase.

It is used in the treatment of metastatic breast cancer (p.514), and of non-Hodgkin's lymphomas (p.510), alone or in combination with other agents. It may also be given to treat adult acute myeloid leukaemias (p.506), and has been used in patients with hormone-refractory prostate cancer (p.521). Mitoxantrone has also been used in the treatment of ovarian and liver cancer.

In addition, mitoxantrone is used in the management of secondary progressive or relapsing multiple sclerosis (see below), to reduce neurological disability or the frequency of relapses.

Mitoxantrone is given as the hydrochloride, but doses are expressed in terms of the base; 1.2 mg of the hydrochloride is approximately equivalent to 1 mg of mitoxantrone. In the treatment of breast cancer, prostate cancer, and lymphomas, a dose equivalent to mitoxantrone 14 mg/m² is given initially, then repeated every 3 weeks. It is diluted to at least 50 mL in sodium chloride 0.9% or glucose 5% and injected over at least 3 minutes into a freely-running intravenous infusion of either. Subsequent doses may be adjusted according to the degree of myelosuppression produced. Initial dosage may need to be reduced to 12 mg/m² in debilitated patients or those who have had previous chemotherapy. Doses should also probably be reduced when mitoxantrone is given as part of a combination regimen: an initial dose of 10 to 12 mg/m² has been suggested.

In the treatment of patients with acute myeloid leukaemia a dose of 12 mg/m² daily for 5 days may be given to induce remission; alternatively a similar dose may be given for 3 days in association with cytarabine.

Cardiac examinations are recommended in all patients who receive a cumulative dose of mitoxantrone greater than 160 mg/m². Regular blood counts should be performed during treatment and courses should not be repeated until blood counts have recovered (see also Bone-marrow Depression, p.496).

In the management of multiple sclerosis, the recommended dose is the equivalent of mitoxantrone 12 mg/m² by intravenous infusion over 5 to 15 minutes. This dose may be given once every 3 months initially provided that neutrophil counts are above 1500 cells/mm³ and that left ventricular ejection fraction (LVEF) is greater than 50%. Blood counts should be monitored before each dose. LVEF should be evaluated before beginning mitoxantrone therapy and before all doses in patients who have received a cumulative dose in excess of 100 mg/m²; a total cumulative lifetime dose in excess of 140 mg/m² should be avoided. LVEF should also be measured if signs or symptoms of heart failure develop.

◊ References.

1. Faulds D, *et al.* Mitoxantrone: a review of its pharmacodynamic and pharmacokinetic properties, and therapeutic potential in the chemotherapy of cancer. *Drugs* 1991; **41:** 400–49.

**Multiple sclerosis.** Mitoxantrone has produced clinical benefit[1-3] in terms of reduced relapse rate and a slowing of disease progression in patients with multiple sclerosis (p.646). It has been given intravenously in doses of 5 or 12 mg/m² every 3 months, or 8 mg/m² every month. Benefit has also been demonstrated in combination with corticosteroids,[4] although the combination was not compared with mitoxantrone alone. However, cardiotoxicity limits the dose that can be given.[5]

1. Millefiorini E, *et al.* Randomized placebo-controlled trial of mitoxantrone in relapsing-remitting multiple sclerosis: 24-month clinical and MRI outcome. *J Neurol* 1997; **244:** 153–9.
2. van de Wyngaert FA, *et al.* A double-blind clinical trial of mitoxantrone versus methylprednisolone in relapsing, secondary progressive multiple sclerosis. *Acta Neurol Belg* 2001; **101:** 210–16.
3. Hartung H-P, *et al.* Mitoxantrone in progressive multiple sclerosis: a placebo-controlled, double-blind, randomised, multicentre trial. *Lancet* 2002; **360:** 2018–25.
4. Edan G, *et al.* Therapeutic effect of mitoxantrone combined with methylprednisolone in multiple sclerosis: a randomised multicentre study of active disease using MRI and clinical criteria. *J Neurol Neurosurg Psychiatry* 1997; **62:** 112–118.
5. Ghalie RG, *et al.* Cardiac adverse effects associated with mitoxantrone (Novantrone) therapy in patients with MS. *Neurology* 2002; **59:** 909–13.

## Preparations

***BP 2003:*** Mitoxantrone Intravenous Infusion;
***USP 27:*** Mitoxantrone Injection.

**Proprietary Preparations** (details are given in Part 3)
***Arg.:*** Batinel; Micraleve; Mitoxgen; Mitoxmar; ***Austral.:*** Novantrone; Onkotrone; ***Austria:*** Novantron; ***Belg.:*** Novantrone; ***Braz.:*** Misostol; Mitoxal; Novantrone†; ***Canad.:*** Novantrone; ***Chile:*** Neotalem; ***Denm.:*** Novantrone; ***Fin.:*** Novantrone; ***Fr.:*** Novantrone; ***Ger.:*** Novantron; Onkotrone; ***Gr.:*** Genefadrone; Novantrone; ***Hong Kong:*** Novantrone; ***India:*** Oncotron; ***Irl.:*** Novantrone; ***Israel:*** Novantrone; ***Ital.:*** Novantrone; ***Malaysia:*** Novantrone; ***Mex.:*** Formyxan; Mitroxone†; Neotalem; Novantrone†; Serotron†; ***Neth.:*** Novantrone; ***Norw.:*** Novantrone; ***NZ:*** Novantrone; ***Port.:*** Novantrone†; ***S.Afr.:*** Novantrone; ***Singapore:*** Novantrone; ***Spain:*** Novantrone; Pralifan; ***Swed.:*** Novantrone; ***Switz.:*** Novantron; ***Thai.:*** Novantrone; ***UK:*** Novantrone; Onkotrone; ***USA:*** Novantrone.

---

# Multialchilpeptide

Multialquilpéptido.
*CAS — 9076-25-9.*

## Profile

Multialchilpeptide is a complex of metamelfalan, an analogue of melphalan (p.566) with peptides. It has been used in the treatment of malignant neoplasms of the blood and lymphatic systems.

## Preparations

**Proprietary Preparations** (details are given in Part 3)
***Ital.:*** Peptichemio†.

---

# Nedaplatin *(rINN)*

Nedaplatino. *cis*-Diammine(glycolato-O$^1$,O$^2$)platinum.
$C_2H_8N_2O_3Pt$ = 303.2.
*CAS — 95734-82-0.*

## Profile

Nedaplatin is a platinum derivative with general properties similar to those of cisplatin (p.538) although it may be associated with less nephrotoxicity. It is used in the treatment of a variety of malignant neoplasms. It is given by intravenous infusion over 1 hour or more, dissolved in at least 300 mL of an appropriate infusion solution, in doses of 80 to 100 mg/m². Administration should be followed by infusion of at least 1 litre of fluid to ensure adequate hydration and reduce the risk of renal damage.

◊ References.

1. Adachi S, *et al.* A pilot study of nedaplatin and etoposide for recurrent gynecological malignancies. *Oncol Rep* 1998; **5:** 881–4.
2. Ito K, *et al.* A dose-finding study of nedaplatin and cyclophosphamide for patients with gynecological malignancies. *Jpn J Clin Oncol* 1999; **29:** 299–302.
3. Yoshioka T, *et al.* A new combination chemotherapy with cis-diammine-glycolatoplatinum (Nedaplatin) and 5-fluorouracil for advanced esophageal cancers. *Intern Med* 1999; **38:** 844–8.
4. Adachi S, *et al.* Intravenous nedaplatin and intraarterial cisplatin with transcatheter arterial embolization for patients with locally advanced uterine cervical cancer. *Int J Clin Pharmacol Res* 2001; **21:** 105–10.

## Preparations

**Proprietary Preparations** (details are given in Part 3)
***Jpn:*** Aqupla.

---

# Nilutamide *(BAN, USAN, rINN)*

Nilutamida; RU-23908. 5,5-Dimethyl-3-(α,α,α-trifluoro-4-nitro-*m*-tolyl)-imidazolidine-2,4-dione.
$C_{12}H_{10}F_3N_3O_4$ = 317.2.
*CAS — 63612-50-0.*
*ATC — L02BB02.*

## Adverse Effects and Precautions

As for Flutamide, p.556. Interstitial pneumonitis has occurred in patients receiving nilutamide, and the drug is contra-indicated in those with severe respiratory insufficiency.

**Effects on the eyes.** Reversible visual disturbances, particularly delayed dark adaptation, have been associated with nilutamide.[1,2] Although some consider such visual disturbances to be mild and generally well tolerated,[3] others suggest that these, together with alcohol intolerance and, more seriously, effects on the lung, mean that other nonsteroidal anti-androgens should be preferred.[4]

1. Harnois C, *et al.* Ocular toxicity of Anandron in patients treated for prostatic cancer. *Br J Ophthalmol* 1986; **70:** 471–3.
2. Brisset JM, *et al.* Ocular toxicity of Anandron. *Br J Ophthalmol* 1987; **71:** 639.
3. Dijkman GA, *et al.* Comment: clinical experiences of visual disturbances with nilutamide. *Ann Pharmacother* 1997; **31:** 1550–1.
4. Dole EJ, Holdsworth MT. Comment: clinical experiences of visual disturbances with nilutamide. *Ann Pharmacother* 1997; **31:** 1551–2.

## Interactions

Patients receiving nilutamide may exhibit intolerance to alcohol.

## Pharmacokinetics

Nilutamide is rapidly and completely absorbed from the gastrointestinal tract. It is extensively metabolised although it may inhibit its own metabolism to some extent after multiple doses. About 60% of an oral dose of nilutamide is eliminated in the urine and less than 10% in the faeces, with an elimination half-life of 41 to 49 hours.

## Uses and Administration

Nilutamide is a nonsteroidal anti-androgen that is used similarly to flutamide (p.557) in the treatment of prostatic carcinoma (p.521). It is given by mouth in a dose of 300 mg daily, usually starting on the same day that the patient undergoes orchidectomy or receives treatment with a gonadorelin analogue. Dosage may be reduced to 150 mg daily after 1 month.

◊ References.

1. Dole EJ, Holdsworth MT. Nilutamide: an antiandrogen for the treatment of prostate cancer. *Ann Pharmacother* 1997; **31:** 65–75.
2. Desai A, *et al.* Nilutamide: possible utility as a second-line hormonal agent. *Urology* 2001; **58:** 1016–20.
3. Kassouf W, *et al.* Nilutamide as second line hormone therapy for prostate cancer after androgen ablation fails. *J Urol (Baltimore)* 2003; **169:** 1742–4.

## Preparations

**Proprietary Preparations** (details are given in Part 3)
***Arg.:*** Anandron; ***Austral.:*** Anandron; ***Braz.:*** Anandron; ***Canad.:*** Anandron; ***Denm.:*** Anandron†; ***Fin.:*** Anandron†; ***Fr.:*** Anandron; ***Gr.:*** Anandron; ***Mex.:*** Anandron; ***Neth.:*** Anandron; ***Norw.:*** Anandron†; ***Port.:*** Anandron; ***Swed.:*** Anandron; ***USA:*** Nilandron.

---

# Nimustine Hydrochloride *(rINNM)*

ACNU; Hidrocloruro de nimustina; NSC-245382; Pimustine Hydrochloride. 3-[(4-Amino-2-methylpyrimidin-5-yl)methyl]-1-(2-chloroethyl)-1-nitrosourea hydrochloride.
$C_9H_{13}ClN_6O_2,HCl$ = 309.2.
*CAS — 42471-28-3 (nimustine); 55661-38-6 (nimustine hydrochloride).*
*ATC — L01AD06.*

## Profile

Nimustine is a nitrosourea antineoplastic with actions and uses similar to those of carmustine (p.535). It is licensed for use in the treatment of brain tumours, brain metastases from lung cancers, and colorectal cancer. Nimustine hydrochloride is given in doses of 2 to 3 mg/kg or 90 to 100 mg/m² as a single dose by slow intravenous injection, repeated at intervals of 4 to 6 weeks depending on haematological response. It may also be given intra-arterially. Solutions for injection must be freshly prepared and protected from light.

◊ References.

1. Anders K, *et al.* Accelerated radiotherapy with concomitant ACNU/Ara-C for the treatment of malignant glioma. *J Neurooncol* 2000; **48:** 63–73.
2. Kochii M, *et al.* Randomized comparison of intra-arterial versus intravenous infusion of ACNU for newly diagnosed patients with glioblastoma. *J Neurooncol* 2000; **49:** 63–70.
3. Silvani A, *et al.* Intra-arterial ACNU and carboplatin versus intravenous chemotherapy with cisplatin and BCNU in newly diagnosed patients with glioblastoma. *Neurol Sci* 2002; **23:** 219–24.
4. Weller M, *et al.* Neuro-Oncology Working Group 01 trial of nimustine plus teniposide versus nimustine plus cytarabine chemotherapy in addition to involved-field radiotherapy in the first-line treatment of malignant glioma. *J Clin Oncol* 2003; **21:** 3276–84.

## Preparations

**Proprietary Preparations** (details are given in Part 3)
***Ger.:*** ACNU; ***Jpn:*** Nidran; ***Neth.:*** ACNU; ***Switz.:*** ACNU.

---

# Nolatrexed *(rINN)*

AG-337 (nolatrexed dihydrochloride). 2-Amino-6-methyl-5-(4-pyridylthio)-4(3*H*)-quinazolinone.
$C_{14}H_{12}N_4OS$ = 284.3.
*CAS — 147149-76-6 (nolatrexed); 152946-68-4 (nolatrexed dihydrochloride).*

## Profile

Nolatrexed is, like raltitrexed (p.582), a selective inhibitor of thymidylate synthase. It is under investigation as an antimetabolite antineoplastic for the treatment of hepatocellular carcinoma.

◊ References.


1. Hughes AN, *et al.* Phase I studies with the nonclassical antifolate nolatrexed dihydrochloride (AG337, Thymitaq) administered orally for 5 days. *Clin Cancer Res* 1999; **5:** 111–8.
2. Stuart K, *et al.* A phase II trial of nolatrexed dihydrochloride in patients with advanced hepatocellular carcinoma. *Cancer* 1999; **86:** 410–4.
3. Jodrell DI, *et al.* A phase I study of the lipophilic thymidylate synthase inhibitor Thymitaq (nolatrexed dihydrochloride) given by 10-day oral administration. *Br J Cancer* 1999; **79:** 915–20.
4. Mok TS, *et al.* A multi-centre randomized phase II study of nolatrexed versus doxorubicin in treatment of Chinese patients with advanced hepatocellular carcinoma. *Cancer Chemother Pharmacol* 1999; **44:** 307–11.
5. Hughes AN, *et al.* Clinical pharmacokinetic and in vitro combination studies of nolatrexed dihydrochloride (AG337, Thymitaq) and paclitaxel. *Br J Cancer* 2000; **82:** 1519–27.
6. Estlin EJ, *et al.* A phase I study of nolatrexed dihydrochloride in children with advanced cancer. *Br J Cancer* 2001; **84:** 11–18.
7. Pivot X, *et al.* Result of two randomized trials comparing nolatrexed (Thymitaq) versus methotrexate in patients with recurrent head and neck cancer. *Ann Oncol* 2001; **12:** 1595–9.


## Oblimersen Sodium *(USAN, rINNM)*

G-3139.

$C_{172}H_{204}N_{62}$-$Na_{17}O_{91}P_{17}S_{17}$ = 6058.3.

*CAS — 190977-41-4.*

### Profile

Oblimersen sodium is an antisense oligonucleotide that blocks the production of BCL-2, a mitochondrial protein that prevents apoptosis. It is under investigation for the treatment of leukaemias and multiple myeloma.

◊ References.


1. Frankel SR. Oblimersen sodium (G3139 Bcl-2 antisense oligonucleotide) therapy in Waldenstrom's macroglobulinemia: a targeted approach to enhance apoptosis. *Semin Oncol* 2003; **30:** 300–304.


## Oregovomab *(USAN, rINN)*

MAb-B43.13.

*CAS — 213327-37-8.*

### Profile

Oregovomab is a murine monoclonal antibody that binds to CA-125, an antigen that is overexpressed in the majority of ovarian cancer patients, and stimulates an immune response to the tumour cells. It is under investigation for the treatment of ovarian cancer.

## Oxaliplatin *(BAN, USAN, rINN)*

JM-83; NSC-266046; *l*-OHP; Oxaliplatino; Oxaliplatinum; RP-54780; SR-96669. [(1*R*,2*R*)-1,2-Cyclohexanediamine-*N*,*N'*]-[oxalato(2-)-*O*,*O'*]platinum.

$C_8H_{14}N_2O_4Pt$ = 397.3.

*CAS — 61825-94-3.*

*ATC — L01XA03.*

**Pharmacopoeias.** In *Eur.* (see p.vi).

**Ph. Eur. 5.0** (Oxaliplatin). A white or almost white, crystalline powder. Slightly soluble in water; practically insoluble in dehydrated alcohol; very slightly soluble in methyl alcohol.

**Incompatibility.** The manufacturers state that oxaliplatin should not be mixed with chloride-containing solutions (including sodium chloride) or alkaline drugs or solutions. They also recommend that the infusion line be flushed with glucose 5% prior to any administration of concomitant medication. Oxaliplatin may degrade on contact with aluminium.

### Adverse Effects and Precautions

The adverse affects of oxaliplatin are similar to those of cisplatin (p.538) but nausea and vomiting, nephrotoxicity, and myelosuppression, seem to be less marked. Raised liver enzyme values may occur. Neurotoxicity can be dose-limiting. Peripheral neuropathy occurs in 85 to 95% of patients given oxaliplatin; pain, functional impairment, and loss of tendon reflexes may develop. Pulmonary fibrosis, potentially fatal, has also been reported. Extravasation of oxaliplatin can cause local pain and inflammation; complications may sometimes be severe, including necrosis.

Neurological examinations should be carried out at regular intervals during treatment and the dose should be reduced if symptoms are prolonged or severe. Regular blood counts should be performed during treatment and courses should not be repeated until blood counts have recovered (see also Bone-marrow Depression, p.496). Oxaliplatin should not be given to patients with pre-existing sensory neuropathies or myelosuppression, nor to those with severe renal impairment. Renal function and toxicity should be carefully monitored in those with more moderate degrees of renal impairment.

**Effects on the nervous system.** Neurological toxicity is the principal dose-limiting adverse effect with oxaliplatin. The toxicity is biphasic:

- acute paraesthesias or dysaesthesias of the extremities, triggered or exacerbated by cold, are seen in 85 to 95% of patients within hours of infusion, but are normally mild and resolve within hours or days. Some patients also experience distressing laryngopharyngeal symptoms, such as difficulty in breathing or swallowing.
- with increasing cumulative dose, peripheral sensory symptoms increase in duration and intensity. Symptoms are sometimes associated with pain and cramps, and may progress to functional impairment (loss of fine sensorimotor coordination). Dosage reduction may be required, but in clinical practice the onset of functional impairment often occurs after the maximum response to therapy has been attained. Cumulative neurotoxicity is reversible in most cases, and about 80% of patients exhibit symptom regression within 4 to 6 months.

The incidence of neurotoxicity may be higher when oxaliplatin is given with fluorouracil. There is some evidence that more prolonged infusion of oxaliplatin can reduce acute toxicity, particularly laryngopharyngeal symptoms. Antiepileptics such as carbamazepine (see Neuropathic Pain, p.358) or gabapentin have been investigated in the management of oxaliplatin-induced neurotoxicity and glutathione has been tried for prevention.

References.


1. Extra JM, *et al.* Pharmacokinetics and safety profile of oxaliplatin. *Semin Oncol* 1998; **25** (suppl 5): 13–22.
2. Culy CR, *et al.* Oxaliplatin: a review of its pharmacological properties and clinical efficacy in metastatic colorectal cancer and its potential in other malignancies. *Drugs* 2000; **60:** 895–924.
3. Cassidy J, Misset J-L. Oxaliplatin-related side effects: characteristics and management. *Semin Oncol* 2002; **29** (suppl 15): 11–20.


### Interactions

For reference to the effect of oxaliplatin on fluorouracil, see Antineoplastics, p.555.

### Pharmacokinetics

After intravenous doses, oxaliplatin is widely distributed throughout the body. It binds irreversibly to red blood cells, which can prolong the half-life of the drug. The mean terminal half-life has been variously stated to be 273 hours and 391 hours.

Oxaliplatin is extensively metabolised to both inactive and active compounds and is predominantly excreted in the urine.

◊ References.


1. Lévi F, *et al.* Oxaliplatin: pharmacokinetics and chronopharmacological aspects. *Clin Pharmacokinet* 2000; **38:** 1–21.
2. Graham MA, *et al.* Clinical pharmacokinetics of oxaliplatin: a critical review. *Clin Cancer Res* 2000; **6:** 1205–18.


### Uses and Administration

Oxaliplatin is a platinum-containing complex similar to cisplatin (see p.538). It is given with fluorouracil and folinic acid in the treatment of metastatic colorectal cancer (p.516). The recommended dose is 85 $mg/m^2$ by intravenous infusion over 2 to 6 hours, dissolved in 250 to 500 mL of glucose 5%. The dose may be repeated at intervals of 2 weeks if toxicity permits, reduced according to tolerance. Following persistent neurotoxicity or recovery from severe adverse effects the manufacturers recommend an initial reduction to 65 $mg/m^2$. Oxaliplatin should always be administered before fluoropyrimidines.

Oxaliplatin is under investigation for the treatment of ovarian cancer.

◊ References.


1. Piccart MJ, *et al.* Oxaliplatin or paclitaxel in patients with platinum-pretreated advanced ovarian cancer: a randomized phase II study of the European Organization for Research and Treatment of Cancer Gynecology Group. *J Clin Oncol* 2000; **18:** 1193–1202.
2. Culy CR, *et al.* Oxaliplatin: a review of its pharmacological properties and clinical efficacy in metastatic colorectal cancer and its potential in other malignancies. *Drugs* 2000; **60:** 895–924.
3. Monnet I, *et al.* Oxaliplatin plus vinorelbine in advanced non-small-cell lung cancer: final results of a multicenter phase II study. *Ann Oncol* 2002; **13:** 103–7.
4. Dieras V, *et al.* Multicentre phase II study of oxaliplatin as a single-agent in cisplatin/carboplatin +/− taxane-pretreated ovarian cancer patients. *Ann Oncol* 2002; **13:** 258–66.
5. Schmoll HJ. The role of oxaliplatin in the treatment of advanced metastatic colorectal cancer: prospects and future directions. *Semin Oncol* 2002; **29** (suppl 15): 34–9.
6. Louvet C, *et al.* Phase II study of oxaliplatin, fluorouracil, and folinic acid in locally advanced or metastatic gastric cancer patients. *J Clin Oncol* 2002; **20:** 4543–8.
7. Simpson D, *et al.* Oxaliplatin: a review of its use in combination therapy for advanced metastatic colorectal cancer. *Drugs* 2003; **63:** 2127–56.


### Preparations

**Proprietary Preparations** (details are given in Part 3)

***Arg.:*** Crisapla; Dabenzol; Dacplat; Kebir; Metaplatin; Mitog; O-Plat; Oxaltie; Platenk; Platinostyl; Plusplatin; Uxalun; Xaliplat; ***Austral.:*** Eloxatin; ***Belg.:*** Eloxatin; ***Braz.:*** Eloxatin; O-Plat; ***Chile:*** O-Plat; ***Fr.:*** Eloxatine; ***Ger.:*** Eloxatin; ***Hong Kong:*** Eloxatin; ***Ital.:*** Eloxatin; ***Malaysia:*** Eloxatin; ***Mex.:*** Eloxatin; ***Neth.:*** Eloxatin; ***Singapore:*** Eloxatin; ***Spain:*** Eloxatin; ***Swed.:*** Eloxatin; ***Switz.:*** Eloxatine; ***Thai.:*** Eloxatin; ***UK:*** Eloxatin; ***USA:*** Eloxatin.

## Paclitaxel *(BAN, USAN, rINN)*

BMS-181339-01; NSC-125973; Taxol; Taxol A. (2*S*,5*R*,7*S*,-10*R*,13*S*)-10,20-Bis(acetoxy)-2-benzoyloxy-1,7-dihydroxy-9-oxo-5,20-epoxytax-11-en-13-yl (3*S*)-3-benzoylamino-3-phenyl-D-lactate.

$C_{47}H_{51}NO_{14}$ = 853.9.

*CAS — 33069-62-4.*

*ATC — L01CD01.*

NOTE. Paclitaxel was formerly referred to as taxol, but the use of this name is now limited, as Taxol is a trademark.

**Pharmacopoeias.** In *US.*

**USP 27** (Paclitaxel). A white to off-white powder. Insoluble in water; soluble in alcohol. Store in airtight containers at a temperature between 20° and 25°. Protect from light.

**Incompatibility.** The vehicle for paclitaxel injection, which contains alcohol and polyethoxylated castor oil, was found to leach the plasticiser diethylhexyl phthalate from some plastic administration sets.[1,2] Consequently, the manufacturer recommends the use of non-PVC containers and administration sets.

Paclitaxel was found to be compatible with doxorubicin for at least 24 hours, but microcrystalline precipitation of paclitaxel occurred after 3 to 5 days.[3] For mention of the incompatibility of paclitaxel and cisplatin see p.538.


1. Trissel LA, *et al.* Compatibility of paclitaxel injection vehicle with intravenous administration and extension sets. *Am J Hosp Pharm* 1994; **51:** 2804–10.
2. Mazzo DJ, *et al.* Compatibility of docetaxel and paclitaxel in intravenous solutions with polyvinyl chloride infusion materials. *Am J Health-Syst Pharm* 1997; **54:** 566–9.
3. Trissel LA, *et al.* Compatibility and stability of paclitaxel combined with doxorubicin hydrochloride in infusion solutions. *Ann Pharmacother* 1998; **32:** 1013–6.


### Adverse Effects, Treatment, and Precautions

For a general outline see Antineoplastics, p.492, p.495, and p.497.

Paclitaxel produces severe dose-limiting bone marrow depression, the nadir of the white cell count usually occurring after about 11 days, with recovery usually by day 15 to 21 after a dose. Myelosuppression may be less frequent and less severe when infusions are given over 3 rather than 24 hours.

Peripheral neuropathy may also be severe, and occasionally dose-limiting. Hypersensitivity reactions, with flushing, rash, dyspnoea, hypotension, chest pain, and angioedema may occur, and all patients should receive initial premedication with corticosteroids, antihistamines, and histamine $H_2$-antagonists. Other adverse effects include alopecia, arthralgia and myalgia, gastrointestinal disturbances, mucositis, bradycardia and ECG changes, nail dystrophies, and elevation of liver enzyme values. Extravasation may result in tissue damage. Rare adverse events include hypertension, severe thrombotic events, myocardial infarction, severe cardiac conduction abnormalities, seizures, neuroencephalopathy, paralytic ileus, optic nerve disturbances, severe skin reactions, hepatic necrosis, and hepatic encephalopathy.

Paclitaxel is not recommended in patients with severely impaired hepatic function. The drug is formulated in polyethoxylated castor oil and should be avoided in patients hypersensitive to this substance. The formulation also contains alcohol, the CNS effects of which should be considered. Blood counts should be monitored frequently. Continuous cardiac monitoring should be performed in patients who have experienced previous significant conduction abnormalities while receiving paclitaxel.

**Alcohol intoxication.** Acute alcohol intoxication resulting from high-dose paclitaxel infusion has been reported;[1] it was calculated that the dose used (348 mg/m$^2$) supplied 50 mL of alcohol, or the equivalent of about 3 drinks (half a bottle of wine).

1. Wilson DB, *et al.* Paclitaxel formulation as a cause of ethanol intoxication. *Ann Pharmacother* 1997; **31:** 873–5.

**Effects on the eyes.** Optic neuritis has occurred with paclitaxel. There is a report of glaucoma possibly related to the use of docetaxel and paclitaxel in a patient also receiving corticosteroids.[1]

1. Fabre-Guillevin E, *et al.* Taxane-induced glaucoma. *Lancet* 1999; **354:** 1181–2.

**Effects on the heart.** Infusion of paclitaxel has been associated with sinus bradycardia, atrial arrhythmias, ventricular tachycardia, heart block, myocardial infarction, and sudden death.[1,2] Symptoms of heart failure have been reported.[3] In another report sudden death 7 days after paclitaxel treatment raised the question of whether paclitaxel might have had a delayed effect.[4] There is some evidence of cellular damage to the myocardium of a patient with paclitaxel-associated cardiac symptoms.[3] The manufacturers note that severe cardiovascular events have been observed more frequently following the use of paclitaxel in patients with non-small cell lung cancer than in those with breast or ovarian carcinoma.

1. Rowinsky EK, *et al.* Cardiac disturbances during the administration of taxol. *J Clin Oncol* 1991; **9:** 1704–12.
2. Arbuck SG, *et al.* A reassessment of cardiac toxicity associated with Taxol. *J Natl Cancer Inst Monogr* 1993; **15:** 117–30.
3. Jekunen A, *et al.* Paclitaxel-induced myocardial damage detected by electron microscopy. *Lancet* 1994; **343:** 727–8.
4. Alagaratnam TT. Sudden death 7 days after paclitaxel infusion for breast cancer. *Lancet* 1993; **342:** 1232–3.

**Effects on the musculoskeletal system.** Myalgia induced by paclitaxel and docetaxel was successfully treated with gabapentin in 2 patients.[1]

1. van Deventer H, Bernard S. Use of gabapentin to treat taxane-induced myalgias. *J Clin Oncol* 1999; **17:** 434–5.

**Effects on the respiratory system.** Acute bilateral interstitial pneumonitis has been reported rarely in patients receiving paclitaxel, despite premedication with corticosteroids and histamine antagonists.[1] Symptoms resolved on treatment with parenteral corticosteroids.

1. Khan A, *et al.* Paclitaxel-induced acute bilateral pneumonitis. *Ann Pharmacother* 1997; **31:** 1471–4.

**Effects on the skin and nails.** Nail changes, noted as pigmentation or discoloration of the nail-bed, may occur with paclitaxel. Onycholysis (separation of the nail from the nail-bed) has also been reported.[1] Discoloration and onycholysis can also occur following docetaxel use, and there are reports of subungual hyperkeratosis and haemorrhage.[2-4]

1. Flory SM, *et al.* Onycholysis associated with weekly administration of paclitaxel. *Ann Pharmacother* 1999; **33:** 584–5.
2. Wasner G, *et al.* Clinical picture: nail changes secondary to docetaxel. *Lancet* 2001; **357:** 910.
3. Pavithran K, Doval DC. Nail changes due to docetaxel. *Br J Dermatol* 2002; **146:** 709–10.
4. Leonard GD, Zujewski JA. Docetaxel-related skin, nail, and vascular toxicity. *Ann Pharmacother* 2003; **37:** 148.

**Hypersensitivity.** Despite premedication with corticosteroids, antihistamines, and $H_2$-antagonists, hypersensitivity reactions occur frequently in patients given paclitaxel; up to about 40% of patients may experience a mild reaction and about 2% a severe reaction. Although the manufacturers consider further use to be contra-indicated following a severe reaction, strategies for continuation of treatment and desensitisation have been described.[1]

1. Markman M, *et al.* Paclitaxel-associated hypersensitivity reactions: experience of the gynecologic oncology program of the Cleveland Clinic Cancer Center. *J Clin Oncol* 2000; **18:** 102–5.

**Pregnancy.** Paclitaxel has been shown to be fetotoxic in *animal* studies, but although the use of potentially teratogenic drugs would normally be avoided during pregnancy, the risk to the mother of inadequate treatment may outweigh whatever risks exist of abnormality in the fetus. Paclitaxel has been used in the treatment of a patient who presented at 27 weeks' gestation with ovarian cancer. She underwent cytoreductive surgery followed by adjuvant chemotherapy consisting of 3 cycles of paclitaxel and cisplatin given every 3 weeks. A healthy child was delivered by caesarean section at 37 weeks, and showed normal growth and development at 30 months of age.[1]

1. Sood AK, *et al.* Paclitaxel and platinum chemotherapy for ovarian carcinoma during pregnancy. *Gynecol Oncol* 2001; **83:** 599–600.

## Interactions

For a general outline of antineoplastic drug interactions, see p.498. Pretreatment with cisplatin may reduce the clearance of paclitaxel, resulting in increased toxicity, and when both drugs are given, paclitaxel should be given first.

**Antineoplastics.** For reference to enhanced cardiotoxicity when paclitaxel was given in association with *doxorubicin*, see p.549. For the pharmacokinetic changes reported when paclitaxel was given with *gemcitabine*, see p.558.

Pretreatment with *fluorouracil* has been reported to inhibit paclitaxel's cytotoxic action, possibly by preventing tumour cells from entering the $G_2$-M phases of the cell cycle.[1] The effect also occurred when the 2 drugs were given simultaneously, suggesting that combination therapy might not be appropriate.

*Valspodar* inhibits P-glycoprotein, and a pharmacokinetic study[2] found that it decreased clearance of paclitaxel and prolonged the terminal half-life, increasing exposure to paclitaxel and myelosuppressive effects. The authors suggested that the dose of paclitaxel may need to be reduced by about 60%.

1. Johnson KR, *et al.* 5-Fluorouracil interferes with paclitaxel cytotoxicity against human solid tumor cells. *Clin Cancer Res* 1997; **3:** 1739–45.
2. Advani R, *et al.* A phase I trial of doxorubicin, paclitaxel, and valspodar (PSC 833), a modulator of multidrug resistance. *Clin Cancer Res* 2001; **7:** 1221–9.

**Immunosuppressants.** *Ciclosporin* increased the oral absorption of paclitaxel, possibly by inhibiting the multidrug transporter P-glycoprotein in the gastrointestinal tract.[1]

For the effects of *valspodar* (an analogue of ciclosporin) on paclitaxel, see above.

1. Meerum Terwogt JM, *et al.* Co-administration of cyclosporin enables oral therapy with paclitaxel. *Lancet* 1998; **352:** 285. Correction. *ibid.*; 824.

## Pharmacokinetics

Intravenous paclitaxel exhibits a biphasic decline in plasma concentrations, with a mean terminal half-life of anywhere between about 3 and 50 hours. The pharmacokinetics are non-linear. The steady-state volume of distribution is reported to range from 200 to 700 litres/m$^2$, indicating extensive extravascular distribution, tissue binding, or both. Paclitaxel is 89% or more bound to plasma protein *in vitro*. The elimination of paclitaxel has not been fully elucidated; only about 1 to 12% of a dose is reported to be excreted in urine, as unchanged drug, indicating extensive non-renal clearance. Paclitaxel is metabolised in the liver, with the major metabolic pathway apparently mediated by the cytochrome P450 isoenzyme CYP2C8, although CYP3A4 may play a minor role. Metabolites are excreted in the faeces via the bile, the primary metabolite being 6α-hydroxypaclitaxel.

◊ References.

1. Sonnichsen DS, Relling MV. Clinical pharmacokinetics of paclitaxel. *Clin Pharmacokinet* 1994; **27:** 256–69.
2. Walle T, *et al.* Taxol metabolism and disposition in cancer patients. *Drug Metab Dispos* 1995; **23:** 506–12.
3. Sonnichsen DS, *et al.* Variability in human cytochrome P450 paclitaxel metabolism. *J Pharmacol Exp Ther* 1995; **275:** 566–75.
4. Henningsson A, *et al.* Mechanism-based pharmacokinetic model for paclitaxel. *J Clin Oncol* 2001; **19:** 4065–73.

## Uses and Administration

Paclitaxel is a taxane originally derived from the bark of the Pacific yew tree *Taxus brevifolia* (Taxaceae), and now obtained semisynthetically from a taxane precursor derived from the needles of the European yew, *Taxus baccata*. Its antineoplastic action arises from its induction of microtubule formation and stabilisation of microtubules, thereby disrupting normal cell division in the $G_2$ and M phases of the cell cycle.

Paclitaxel is used for the primary treatment of advanced ovarian cancer (p.520) with cisplatin or carboplatin, and for secondary treatment. In the treatment of breast cancer (p.514) paclitaxel is used for primary adjuvant therapy, and as second-line treatment in advanced disease, usually after failure of anthracycline-based therapy; in patients with metastatic disease who overexpress HER2 (human epidermal growth receptor 2) it may be used with trastuzumab as initial therapy. Paclitaxel is used with cisplatin or carboplatin, for the primary treatment of advanced non-small cell lung cancer (p.519). It may be used for the second-line treatment of AIDS-related Kaposi's sarcoma (p.524), and has been tried in a variety of other neoplasms including cancers of the head and neck, and relapsed germ-cell tumours.

The recommended dose for the primary treatment of **ovarian cancer** is 135 mg/m$^2$ infused over 24 hours, followed by cisplatin, and repeated at 3-week intervals. Alternatively 175 mg/m$^2$ may be infused over 3 hours, followed by cisplatin, every 3 weeks. For the secondary treatment of ovarian cancer, the suggested dose as a single agent is 135 or 175 mg/m$^2$ infused over 3 hours once every 3 weeks.

A dose of 175 mg/m$^2$ infused over 3 hours once every 3 weeks is recommended for the treatment of **breast cancer**; for adjuvant therapy 4 such courses may be given sequentially after an anthracycline-based regimen. In **non-small cell lung cancer**, the recommended dose is 135 mg/m$^2$ over 24 hours or 175 mg/m$^2$ over 3 hours, followed by cisplatin, and repeated at 3-week intervals.

A dose of 135 mg/m$^2$ over 3 hours once every 3 weeks has been suggested for AIDS-related **Kaposi's sarcoma**. Alternatively, 100 mg/m$^2$ over 3 hours every 2 weeks may be given, especially in patients with poor performance status.

Regular blood counts should be performed, and dosage should not be repeated until the neutrophil and platelet counts are at acceptable levels; the neutrophil count should be above 1000 cells/mm$^3$ in patients with AIDS (see also Bone-marrow Depression, p.496). The dose should be reduced by 20% in subsequent courses in patients who experience severe neutropenia or peripheral neuropathy. Patients should be pretreated with corticosteroids, antihistamines, and histamine $H_2$-antagonists. The dose of paclitaxel may need to be reduced in patients with hepatic impairment (see below).

Various formulations are in development to avoid the use of polyethoxylated castor oil and improve the efficacy and safety of paclitaxel, including an albumin-based formulation, paclitaxel linked to docosahexaenoic acid or biodegradable polymers, an injectable emulsion, micellar and liposomal formulations, and an oral dosage form.

Paclitaxel-releasing stents may be used to reduce restenosis after coronary artery stent placement.

◊ References to paclitaxel, and to taxanes as a class.

1. Rowinsky EK, *et al.* Taxol: the first of the taxanes, an important new class of antitumor agents. *Semin Oncol* 1992; **19:** 646–62.
2. Gelmon K. The taxoids: paclitaxel and docetaxel. *Lancet* 1994; **344:** 1267–72.
3. Long HJ. Paclitaxel (Taxol): a novel anticancer chemotherapeutic drug. *Mayo Clin Proc* 1994: **69:** 341–5.
4. Spencer CM, Faulds D. Paclitaxel: a review of its pharmacodynamic and pharmacokinetic properties and therapeutic potential in the treatment of cancer. *Drugs* 1994; **48:** 794–847.
5. Rowinsky EK, Donehower RC. Paclitaxel (Taxol). *N Engl J Med* 1995; **332:** 1004–14. Correction. *ibid.*; **333:** 75.
6. Anonymous. Paclitaxel and docetaxel in breast and ovarian cancer. *Drug Ther Bull* 1997; **35:** 43–6.
7. Eisenhauer EA, Vermorken JB. The taxoids: comparative clinical pharmacology and therapeutic potential. *Drugs* 1998; **55:** 5–30.
8. Crown J, O'Leary M. The taxanes: an update. *Lancet* 2000; **355:** 1176–8.
9. Michaud LB, *et al.* Risks and benefits of taxanes in breast and ovarian cancer. *Drug Safety* 2000; **23:** 401–28.

**Administration.** Although many of the original studies of paclitaxel employed a 24-hour infusion regimen, the use of *3-hour infusions* has subsequently become widespread. A systematic review[1] noted that although it was difficult to compare efficacy in studies of unlike malignancies there was no conclusive evidence of a difference in effectiveness with differing length of infusion; however, there were differences in the adverse effect profile, neutropenia being much less marked with the shorter infusion, although neurotoxic effects were reduced with 24-hour administration.

There has also been considerable interest in evaluating the use of paclitaxel in reduced-dose *weekly* schedules.[2-10] Various dosage regimens have been tried: most have found that doses of between 50 and about 100 mg/m$^2$ weekly, usually by infusion over 1 hour rather than a conventional 3-hour infusion, can be given with relatively modest toxicity. Although higher doses have been tried, neurotoxicity and myelosuppression become problematic and tend to limit dose intensity. A number of studies have addressed the combination of weekly paclitaxel with other antineoplastics, for example with trastuzumab in breast cancer, estramustine in prostate cancer, and in combination with platinum compounds or gemcitabine in other solid tumours such as those of the ovary or lung. Weekly paclitaxel is also under investigation in combination with radiotherapy in the management of lung cancer and glioblastoma multiforme.

1. Williams C, *et al.* Short versus long duration infusions of paclitaxel for any advanced adenocarcinoma. Available in The Cochrane Library, Issue 2. Chichester: John Wiley; 2004.
2. Seidman AD, *et al.* Dose-dense therapy with weekly 1-hour paclitaxel infusions in the treatment of metastatic breast cancer. *J Clin Oncol* 1998; **16:** 3353–61.
3. Fountzilas G, *et al.* Radiation and concomitant weekly administration of paclitaxel in patients with glioblastoma multiforme: a phase II study. *J Neurooncol* 1999; **45:** 159–65.
4. Markman M. Weekly paclitaxel in the management of ovarian cancer. *Semin Oncol* 2000; **27** (suppl 7): 37–40.
5. De Pas T, *et al.* Phase I and pharmacologic study of weekly gemcitabine and paclitaxel in chemo-naive patients with advanced non-small-cell lung cancer. *Ann Oncol* 2000; **11:** 821–7.
6. Langer CJ, *et al.* Paclitaxel by 1-h infusion in combination with carboplatin in advanced non-small cell lung carcinoma (NSCLC). *Eur J Cancer* 2000; **36:** 183–93.
7. Akerley W. Recent developments in weekly paclitaxel therapy in lung cancer. *Curr Oncol Rep* 2001; **3:** 165–9.

8. Haas N, *et al.* Phase I trial of weekly paclitaxel plus oral estramustine phosphate in patients with hormone-refractory prostate cancer. *Urology* 2001; **58:** 59–64.
9. Seidman AD, *et al.* Weekly trastuzumab and paclitaxel therapy for metastatic breast cancer with analysis of efficacy by HER2 immunophenotype and gene amplification. *J Clin Oncol* 2001; **19:** 2587–95.
10. Kouroussis C, *et al.* A dose-finding study of the weekly administration of paclitaxel in patients with advanced solid tumors. *Am J Clin Oncol* 2001; **24:** 404–7.


**Administration in hepatic impairment.** The manufacturers in the USA have made recommendations for initial dosage adjustment of some paclitaxel regimens in patients with hepatic impairment, according to transaminase and bilirubin concentrations. They suggest paclitaxel should not be given if transaminase values are more than 10 times normal upper limits, or if bilirubin is more than 75 micrograms/mL or 5 times the normal upper limit.

**Reperfusion and revascularisation procedures.** In a study compared with bare metal stents,[1] paclitaxel-releasing stents reduced the risk of restenosis and the need for repeat revascularisation procedures (p.834), although the follow-up rates of death from cardiac causes or myocardial infarction were not significantly reduced at 9 months.


1. Stone GW, *et al.* A polymer-based, paclitaxel-eluting stent in patients with coronary artery disease. *N Engl J Med* 2004; **350:** 221–31.


## Preparations

***USP 27:*** Paclitaxel Injection.

**Proprietary Preparations** (details are given in Part 3)

***Arg.:*** Asotax; Clitaxel; Dalys; Drifen; Paclikebir; Pacliteva; Paklitaxfil; Panataxel; Tarvexol; Taxocris; Taxol; Taycovit; ***Austral.:*** Anzatax; Taxol; ***Austria:*** Taxol; ***Belg.:*** Taxol; ***Braz.:*** Biopaxel; Paclitax; Parexel; Paxel; Taclipaxol; Taxol; ***Canad.:*** Taxol; ***Chile:*** Britaxol; Praxel; Taxodiol; ***Denm.:*** Taxol; ***Fin.:*** Taxol; ***Fr.:*** Taxol; ***Ger.:*** Taxol; ***Gr.:*** Taxol; ***Hong Kong:*** Anzatax; Taxol; ***India:*** Intaxel; ***Irl.:*** Taxol; ***Israel:*** Biotax; Medixel; Taxol; ***Ital.:*** Taxol; ***Jpn:*** Taxol; ***Malaysia:*** Anzatax; Taxol; ***Mex.:*** Asotax; BrisTaxol; Ifaxol; Praxel; ***Neth.:*** Taxol; ***Norw.:*** Taxol; ***NZ:*** Taxol; ***Port.:*** Taxol; ***S.Afr.:*** Taxol; Yewtaxan†; ***Singapore:*** Anzatax; Taxol; ***Spain:*** Taxol; ***Swed.:*** Taxol; ***Switz.:*** Taxol; ***Thai.:*** Anzatax; Intaxel; Taxol; ***UK:*** Paxene; Taxol; ***USA:*** Onxol; Taxol.

## Peldesine *(USAN, pINN)*

BCX-34; Peldesina; Peldésine. 2-Amino-3,5-dihydro-7-(3-pyridylmethyl)-4*H*-pyrrolo[3,2-*d*]pyrimidin-4-one.

$C_{12}H_{11}N_5O = 241.2.$

*CAS — 133432-71-0.*

### Profile

Peldesine is an inhibitor of the enzyme purine nucleoside phosphorylase and is reported to suppress T-cell proliferation. It has been investigated in the management of cutaneous T-cell lymphomas, and has also been tried topically in psoriasis and some T-cell mediated eye disorders.

## Pemetrexed Disodium *(BANM, USAN, rINNM)*

LY-231514; MTA; Multi-targeted Antifolate; Pemetrexed disódico. Disodium *N*-{*p*-[2-(2-amino-4,7-dihydro-4-oxo-1*H*-pyrrolo[2,3-*d*]pyrimidin-5-yl)ethyl]benzoyl}-L-glutamate.

$C_{20}H_{19}N_5Na_2O_6 = 471.4.$

*CAS — 137281-23-3 (pemetrexed); 150399-23-8 (pemetrexed disodium).*

NOTE. In practice, pemetrexed is given as the disodium heptahydrate ($C_{20}H_{19}N_5Na_2O_6,7H_2O = 597.5$).

### Profile

Pemetrexed is primarily a thymidylate synthase inhibitor like raltitrexed (p.582), but it also inhibits other folate-dependent enzymes involved in purine synthesis. It is used with cisplatin in the treatment of unresectable malignant pleural mesothelioma (p.520). Pemetrexed is given as the disodium heptahydrate but doses are expressed in terms of the base: pemetrexed disodium heptahydrate 1.4 g is approximately equivalent to pemetrexed 1 g.

In malignant mesothelioma, a dose of pemetrexed 500 mg/m² is given by intravenous infusion over 10 minutes. The dose may be repeated in 21-day cycles, and doses should be adjusted according to toxicity. Cisplatin is given 30 minutes after the end of pemetrexed infusion.

Pemetrexed is associated with dose-limiting myelosuppression, including neutropenia, anaemia, and thrombocytopenia. It may also cause gastrointestinal disturbances, stomatitis, pharyngitis, dyspnoea, chest pain, and rash. Complete blood cell counts should be monitored, and folate and vitamin $B_{12}$ are given as prophylaxis against haematological and gastrointestinal toxicity during pemetrexed therapy. Pre-treatment with a corticosteroid, such as oral dexamethasone, reduces the incidence and severity of skin reactions.

Pemetrexed is under investigation as an antifolate antimetabolite in the treatment of lung, colon, pancreatic, breast, and head and neck cancer.

◊ References.


1. Miller KD, *et al.* Phase II study of the multitargeted antifolate LY231514 (ALIMTA, MTA, pemetrexed disodium) in patients with advanced pancreatic cancer. *Ann Oncol* 2000; **11:** 101–3.
2. John W, *et al.* Activity of multitargeted antifolate (pemetrexed disodium, LY231514) in patients with advanced colorectal carcinoma: results from a phase II study. *Cancer* 2000; **88:** 1807–13.
3. Manegold C, *et al.* Front-line treatment of advanced non-small-cell lung cancer with MTA (LY231514, pemetrexed disodium, ALIMTA) and cisplatin: a multicenter phase II trial. *Ann Oncol* 2000; **11:** 435–40.
4. Miles DW, *et al.* A phase II study of pemetrexed disodium (LY231514) in patients with locally recurrent or metastatic breast cancer. *Eur J Cancer* 2001; **37:** 1366–71.
5. Shepherd FA, *et al.* Phase II study of pemetrexed disodium, a multitargeted antifolate, and cisplatin as first-line therapy in patients with advanced nonsmall cell lung carcinoma: a study of the National Cancer Institute of Canada Clinical Trials Group. *Cancer* 2001; **92:** 595–600.
6. Pivot X, *et al.* Pemetrexed disodium in recurrent locally advanced or metastatic squamous cell carcinoma of the head and neck. *Br J Cancer* 2001; **85:** 649–55.
7. Clarke SJ, *et al.* Phase II trial of pemetrexed disodium (ALIMTA, LY231514) in chemotherapy-naive patients with advanced non-small-cell lung cancer. *Ann Oncol* 2002; **13:** 737–41.
8. Hughes A, *et al.* Phase I clinical and pharmacokinetic study of pemetrexed and carboplatin in patients with malignant pleural mesothelioma. *J Clin Oncol* 2002; **20:** 3533–44.
9. Vogelzang NJ, *et al.* Phase III study of pemetrexed in combination with cisplatin versus cisplatin alone in patients with malignant pleural mesothelioma. *J Clin Oncol* 2003; **21:** 2636–44.
10. Hanna N, *et al.* Randomized phase III trial of pemetrexed versus docetaxel in patients with non-small-cell lung cancer previously treated with chemotherapy. *J Clin Oncol* 2004; **22:** 1589–97.


## Pemtumomab

### Profile

Pemtumomab is a radiolabelled monoclonal antibody of murine origin that binds to muc-1, an epithelial cell surface protein on tumour cells. It has been investigated for the treatment of various cancers, including ovarian and gastric cancers, but results have been disappointing.

## Pentostatin *(BAN, USAN, rINN)*

CI-825; Covidarabine; Co-vidarabine; Deoxycoformycin; 2′-Deoxycoformycin; NSC-218321; PD-81565; Pentostatina. (*R*)-3-(2-Deoxy-β-D-*erythro*-pentofuranosyl)-3,6,7,8-tetrahydroimidazo[4,5-*d*][1,3]diazepin-8-ol; 1,2-Dideoxy-1-[(*R*)-3,6,7,8-tetrahydro-8-hydroxyimidazo[4,5-*d*][1,3]diazepin-3-yl]-D-*erythro*-pentofuranose.

$C_{11}H_{16}N_4O_4 = 268.3.$

*CAS — 53910-25-1.*

*ATC — L01XX08.*

### Adverse Effects and Precautions

The most common adverse effects in patients receiving pentostatin include myelosuppression (and in particular suppression of CD4+ lymphocyte subset), headache, abdominal pain, fever and chills, gastrointestinal disturbances (notably diarrhoea and nausea and vomiting), hypersensitivity reactions, and hepatotoxicity. Central neurotoxicity may be manifest as tiredness, anxiety, depression, sleep disturbances, and paraesthesias: treatment should be withheld or discontinued in such patients. Impaired renal function and pulmonary toxicity (cough, dyspnoea, and pneumonia) may occur. Severe toxicity in early studies, affecting mainly the CNS, kidneys, liver, and lungs, was associated with the use of doses higher than those currently recommended and produced some fatalities.

Other adverse effects reported with pentostatin include dry skin and rashes (sometimes severe and worsening with continued treatment), pruritus, conjunctivitis, alopecia, arthralgia and myalgia, peripheral oedema, thrombophlebitis, and cardiovascular disorders including arrhythmias, angina pectoris, and heart failure.

Pentostatin should not be given to patients with impaired renal function, or in active infection. It is teratogenic in *animals* and potentially genotoxic: it is therefore contra-indicated in pregnancy and men receiving pentostatin should not father children for 6 months after therapy.

### Interactions

Pentostatin should not be given with fludarabine, as the combination may result in enhanced pulmonary toxicity. A similar increase in toxicity is expected when pentostatin is used with vidarabine.

Use of pentostatin with carmustine, etoposide and high-dose cyclophosphamide, has produced acute pulmonary oedema and hypotension, leading to death. Pentostatin should therefore not be given with high-dose cyclophosphamide.

**Allopurinol.** Fatal acute necrotising arteritis developed in a patient given pentostatin and allopurinol.[1] Although the hypersensitivity vasculitis may have been due to allopurinol alone there is circumstantial evidence to suggest that pentostatin may predispose patients to drug hypersensitivity and it may be wise to avoid this combination, and to observe pentostatin-treated patients closely for allergic manifestations.


1. Steinmetz JC, *et al.* Hypersensitivity vasculitis associated with 2-deoxycoformycin and allopurinol therapy. *Am J Med* 1989; **86:** 498–9.


### Pharmacokinetics

Following intravenous injection, pentostatin has an elimination half-life of about 6 hours. Approximately 90% of a dose is excreted in the urine as unchanged drug and metabolites. Pentostatin crosses the blood-brain barrier and can be measured in the CSF.

### Uses and Administration

Pentostatin is a potent inhibitor of the enzyme adenosine deaminase that probably exerts its cytotoxic actions through the interruption of normal purine metabolism and DNA synthesis. Lymphocytes are particularly sensitive to its actions.

Pentostatin is used as a single agent in the treatment of hairy-cell leukaemia (p.508), in usual doses of 4 mg/m² every other week. The dose is given as an intravenous bolus injection, or as an infusion over 20 to 30 minutes. Hydration with 500 mL to 1 litre of glucose 5% in sodium chloride 0.18 or 0.9%, or equivalent, is recommended before administration; a further 500 mL of the hydration solution should be infused once the drug has been given.

Pentostatin has been tried in cutaneous T-cell lymphomas (see Mycosis Fungoides, p.511) and histiocytic syndromes (p.505). It is also under investigation in some other lymphoid malignancies, including chronic lymphocytic leukaemia (p.507) and non-Hodgkin's lymphomas (p.510) and for the management of chronic graft-versus-host disease following haematopoietic stem cell transplantation (p.1344).

◊ References.


1. Brogden RN, Sorkin EM. Pentostatin: a review of its pharmacodynamic and pharmacokinetic properties, and therapeutic potential in lymphoproliferative disorders. *Drugs* 1993; **46:** 652–77.
2. Ho AD, *et al.* Pentostatin in T-cell malignancies—a phase II trial of the EORTC. *Ann Oncol* 1999; **10:** 1493–8.
3. Grever MR, *et al.* Pentostatin in the treatment of hairy-cell leukemia. *Best Pract Res Clin Haematol* 2003; **16:** 91–9.
4. Drapkin R, *et al.* Results of a phase II multicenter trial of pentostatin and rituximab in patients with low grade B-cell non-Hodgkin's lymphoma: an effective and minimally toxic regimen. *Clin Lymphoma* 2003; **4:** 169–75.
5. Tsimberidou AM, *et al.* Phase II study of pentostatin in advanced T-cell lymphoid malignancies: update of an MD Anderson Cancer Center series. *Cancer* 2004; **100:** 342–9.
6. Tsiara SN, *et al.* Treatment of resistant/relapsing chronic lymphocytic leukemia with a combination regimen containing deoxycoformycin and rituximab. *Acta Haematol (Basel)* 2004; **111:** 185–8.


## Preparations

**Proprietary Preparations** (details are given in Part 3)

***Canad.:*** Nipent; ***Fr.:*** Nipent; ***Ger.:*** Nipent; ***Gr.:*** Nipent; ***Ital.:*** Nipent; ***Port.:*** Nipent†; ***Spain:*** Nipent†; ***UK:*** Nipent; ***USA:*** Nipent.

## Peplomycin Sulfate *(USAN, rINNM)*

NK-631; Pepleomycin Sulphate; Peplomycin Sulphate; Sulfato de peplomicina. $N^1$-{3-[(*S*)-(α-Methylbenzyl)amino]propyl}bleomycinamide sulphate.

$C_{61}H_{88}N_{18}O_{21}S_2,H_2SO_4 = 1571.7.$

*CAS — 68247-85-8 (peplomycin); 70384-29-1 (peplomycin sulfate).*

**Pharmacopoeias.** In *Jpn.*

### Profile

Peplomycin is an antineoplastic derived from bleomycin (see p.530) and with similar properties. It has been given as the sulfate in the treatment of a variety of malignant neoplasms, including tumours of the head and neck, lung, prostate, and skin.

## Pipobroman (USAN, pINN)

A-8103; NSC-25154; Pipobromán. 1,4-Bis(3-bromopropionyl)piperazine.

$C_{10}H_{16}Br_2N_2O_2$ = 356.1.
*CAS — 54-91-1.*
*ATC — L01AX02.*

### Profile

Pipobroman is an antineoplastic which appears to act by alkylation. It may be used in the treatment of polycythaemia vera (p.508), in patients requiring myelosuppressive therapy, and in refractory chronic myeloid leukaemia (p.507).

The usual dose initially is 1 mg/kg by mouth daily, increased to 3 mg/kg, if necessary, according to the patient's response. Maintenance dosage is 100 to 200 micrograms/kg daily for polycythaemia vera.

The principal adverse effect is moderate bone-marrow depression, which may be delayed 4 weeks or more from initiation of treatment. Anaemia may be marked at higher doses and is usually accompanied by leucopenia. Thrombocytopenia and haemolysis have occurred. In the initial stages of treatment, white cell and platelet counts should be determined on alternate days and complete blood counts once or twice weekly. Doses should be discontinued if the white cell or platelet counts fall below acceptable levels (see also Bone-marrow Depression, p.496).

### Preparations

**Proprietary Preparations** (details are given in Part 3)
**Fr.:** Vercyte; **Ital.:** Vercite.

## Pirarubicin (rINN)

1609RB; Pirarubicina; Tepirubicin; THP-ADM; THP-doxorubicin. (8S,10S)-10-{[3-Amino-2,3,6-trideoxy-4-O-(2R-tetrahydro-2H-pyran-2-yl)-α-L-*lyxo*-hexopyranosyl]oxy}-8-glycoloyl-7,8,9,10-tetrahydro-6,8,11-trihydroxy-1-methoxy-5,12-naphthacenedione.

$C_{32}H_{37}NO_{12}$ = 627.6.
*CAS — 72496-41-4.*
*ATC — L01DB08.*

**Pharmacopoeias.** In *Jpn.*

### Profile

Pirarubicin is an antineoplastic anthracycline antibiotic that is a structural analogue of doxorubicin (p.547), and has similar properties. It is used in the management of breast cancer and has also been tried in other solid neoplasms, acute leukaemias and lymphomas.

Pirarubicin is formulated as the hydrochloride but doses are in terms of the base. A usual dose of 25 to 50 mg/$m^2$ every 3 to 4 weeks has been recommended in breast cancer, according to response, but other dosage regimens have been used. Doses may be given by intravenous injection over 5 to 10 minutes into a rapidly-flowing intravenous infusion of glucose 5%. Patients should undergo regular blood counts and monitoring of cardiac function: at cumulative doses above 600 mg/$m^2$ ventricular ejection fraction should be checked before each course. Pirarubicin has also been given by the intra-arterial and intravesical routes.

### Preparations

**Proprietary Preparations** (details are given in Part 3)
**Fr.:** Theprubicine.

## Piritrexim Isetionate (rINNM)

BW-301U (piritrexim); Isetionato de piritrexima; NSC-351521; Piritrexim Isethionate (USAN). 2,4-Diamino-6-(2,5-dimethoxybenzyl)-5-methylpyrido[2,3-*d*]pyrimidine mono(2-hydroxyethanesulphonate).

$C_{17}H_{19}N_5O_2,C_2H_6O_4S$ = 451.5.
*CAS — 72732-56-0 (piritrexim); 79483-69-5 (piritrexim isetionate).*

### Profile

Piritrexim is a folate antagonist with general properties similar to those of methotrexate (p.568) and that has been tried by mouth for its antineoplastic properties, and has also been used (as the isetionate) for the treatment of opportunistic infections in immunosuppressed patients. Myelosuppression, gastrointestinal disturbances, and hepatotoxicity have been reported.

Piritrexim isetionate has also been investigated for severe psoriasis.

◊ References.

1. Feun LG, *et al.* Phase II trial of piritrexim in metastatic melanoma using intermittent, low-dose administration. *J Clin Oncol* 1991; **9:** 464–7.
2. Feun LG, *et al.* Phase II trial of piritrexim and DTIC using an alternating dose schedule in metastatic melanoma. *Am J Clin Oncol* 1995; **18:** 488–90.
3. Khorsand M, *et al.* Phase II trial of oral piritrexim in advanced, previously treated transitional cell cancer of bladder. *Invest New Drugs* 1997; **15:** 157–63.

## Plicamycin (BAN, USAN, rINN)

A-2371; Aureolic Acid; Mithramycin; NSC-24559; PA-144; Plicamicina.

$C_{52}H_{76}O_{24}$ = 1085.1.
*CAS — 18378-89-7.*
*ATC — L01DC02.*

**Description.** Plicamycin is an antineoplastic antibiotic produced by the growth of *Streptomyces argillaceus, S. plicatus* and *S. tanashiensis*.

**Pharmacopoeias.** In *US.*

**USP 27** (Plicamycin). A yellow, odourless, hygroscopic, crystalline powder, with a potency of not less than 900 micrograms/mg, calculated on the dry basis. It loses not more than 8% of its weight when dried. Slightly soluble in water and in methyl alcohol; very slightly soluble in alcohol; freely soluble in ethyl acetate. A 0.05% solution in water has a pH of 4.5 to 5.5. Store at 2° to 8° in airtight containers. Protect from light.

**Adsorption.** Plicamycin is bound to cellulose filters used for in-line filtration of intravenous infusions,[1] with more drug likely to be lost from glucose than from sodium chloride injection at the low concentrations of drug used in therapy.

1. Butler LD, *et al.* Effect of inline filtration on the potency of low-dose drugs. *Am J Hosp Pharm* 1980; **37:** 935–41.

**Incompatibility.** Plicamycin readily chelates divalent cations, especially iron. Admixture with trace element solutions should be avoided.[1]

1. D'Arcy PF. Reactions and interactions in handling anticancer drugs. *Drug Intell Clin Pharm* 1983; **17:** 532–8.

### Adverse Effects, Treatment, and Precautions

For general discussions see Antineoplastics, p.492, p.495, and p.497.

The major adverse effect of plicamycin is a dose-related bleeding syndrome, manifest initially as epistaxis, which may progress to haematemesis and potentially fatal haemorrhage. Effects on clotting factors in the blood are thought to contribute to this syndrome. Severe thrombocytopenia may also occur due to bone-marrow depression. Leucopenia is relatively uncommon.

Gastrointestinal effects are common during treatment with plicamycin. Other side-effects include fever, malaise, drowsiness, lethargy and weakness, headache, depression, skin rashes, facial flushing, and reduced serum concentrations of calcium, phosphorus, and potassium. There may also be reversible impairment of renal and hepatic function.

Extravasation of plicamycin solutions may cause local irritation, cellulitis, and phlebitis. Application of moderate heat to the site of extravasation may aid dispersal of plicamycin and minimise discomfort and local irritation.

Plicamycin should only be given with great care to patients with hepatic or renal impairment. It should not be given to patients with thrombocytopenia or depressed bone-marrow function, coagulation disorders, or increased susceptibility to bleeding for any cause.

**Administration rate.** Although it is recommended that plicamycin is given as an intravenous infusion over 4 to 6 hours, on the grounds that more rapid administration is associated with increased severity of gastrointestinal toxicity, a search of the literature failed to find any evidence of improved tolerance or enhanced efficacy with infusion rather than bolus injection of plicamycin.[1]

1. Mutch RS, *et al.* Plicamycin: bolus or infusion? *DICP Ann Pharmacother* 1990; **24:** 885–6.

**Effects on the kidneys.** A report of reversible oliguria and deterioration of renal function occurring on 2 occasions in a patient given single doses of plicamycin.[1]

1. Benedetti RG, *et al.* Nephrotoxicity following single dose mithramycin therapy. *Am J Nephrol* 1983; **3:** 277–8.

**Effects on the skin.** Toxic epidermal necrolysis occurring in a 22-year-old man was attributed to treatment with plicamycin.[1]

1. Purpora D, *et al.* Toxic epidermal necrolysis after mithramycin. *N Engl J Med* 1978; **299:** 1412.

**Local toxicity.** Disodium edetate has been suggested as an antidote to local toxicity following extravasation of plicamycin.[1] However, there is a suggestion that the classification of plicamycin as a vesicant is inappropriate.[2]

1. MacCara ME. Extravasation: a hazard of intravenous therapy. *Drug Intell Clin Pharm* 1983; **17:** 713–17.
2. Loughner JE, Olek C. Comment; plicamycin infusion. *DICP Ann Pharmacother* 1991; **25:** 215.

### Uses and Administration

Plicamycin is a highly toxic antibiotic with antineoplastic and hypocalcaemic properties. It may act by complexing with DNA in the presence of divalent cations and inhibiting synthesis of ribonucleic acid. Lowering of serum calcium concentrations has been suggested to result from antagonism of the effects of vitamin D and parathyroid hormone on osteoclasts.

Plicamycin has been used in the symptomatic management of hypercalcaemia and hypercalciuria associated with malignancy if it cannot be managed by other means (see below). The usual dose is 25 micrograms/kg daily by slow intravenous infusion over 4 to 6 hours in a litre of glucose 5% or sodium chloride 0.9%, for 3 or 4 days if necessary. Further courses may be given at intervals of a week or more if required.

Plicamycin has also been used in the treatment of malignant neoplasms of the testis not susceptible to surgery or radiotherapy; however, other agents are preferred (p.523).

Blood counts, bleeding time, prothrombin time, and hepatic and renal function should be determined frequently during treatment and for several days after, and treatment stopped if there is any sudden change.

**Administration.** The manufacturers recommend that plicamycin be given by infusion rather than bolus injection, as this is reportedly associated with fewer and less severe gastrointestinal adverse effects. For a suggestion that this distinction is unjustified, see under Adverse Effects, above.

**Hypercalcaemia.** Where treatment is required for hypercalcaemia it is aimed at increasing urinary excretion of calcium and maintaining adequate hydration. Drugs that inhibit bone resorption may also be employed if hypercalcaemia is severe, particularly when it is associated with malignancy (see p.1218). Although plicamycin is effective, it is highly toxic, and the bisphosphonates and calcitonins are generally preferred.

**Paget's disease of bone.** Plicamycin remains a second- or third-line drug in the therapy of Paget's disease of bone (p.764), reserved for patients refractory to other treatment. Nonetheless, occasional successes are reported: one patient with refractory Paget's disease had apparent cure of her symptoms after treatment with plicamycin 25 micrograms/kg daily for 15 doses, followed by 1500 micrograms weekly for about 2 months and every 2 weeks for 6 weeks.[1] She had remained asymptomatic for 18 years after treatment. However, similar regimens have been used in other patients without this degree of success.[1] Another patient, who was refractory to calcitonin and pamidronate therapy, showed a considerable improvement in pain relief and biochemical parameters when treated with 30 micrograms/kg plicamycin daily for 3 days.[2]

1. Ryan WG, *et al.* Apparent cure of Paget's disease of bone. *Am J Med* 1990; **89:** 825–6.
2. Wimalawansa SJ. Dramatic response to plicamycin in a patient with severe Paget's disease refractory to calcitonin and pamidronate. *Semin Arthritis Rheum* 1994; **23:** 267.

### Preparations

**USP 27:** Plicamycin for Injection.

**Proprietary Preparations** (details are given in Part 3)
**Fr.:** Mithracine†; **Gr.:** Mithracin; **Norw.:** Mithracin†; **USA:** Mithracin†.

## Porfimer Sodium (BAN, USAN, rINN)

CL-184116; Dihaematoporphyrin Ether; Porfímero sódico.
*CAS — 87806-31-3.*
*ATC — L01XD01.*

### Adverse Effects and Precautions

Photosensitivity occurs in all patients treated with porfimer sodium. This effect is likely to be prolonged, and patients should avoid sunlight or bright indoor light for at least 30 days. However, exposure to ambient indoor light is encouraged, as it allows gradual inactivation of any remaining drug. Other reported adverse effects include local inflammation, chest pain, respiratory insufficiency or distress (including dyspnoea), abdominal pain, dysphagia, constipation, nausea and vomiting, fever, tachycardia and atrial fibrillation, pleural effusion, mucositis, and anaemia due to tumour bleeding. Pneumonia and bronchitis may occur. Anxiety and insomnia have also been reported. Photodynamic therapy with porfimer sodium is contra-indicated in patients with severe hepatic impairment, oesophageal fistulae, erosion of major blood vessels, or severe acute respiratory distress. Sufficient time should be allowed between photodynamic therapy and radiotherapy to allow inflammatory reactions from either treatment to subside.

**Porphyria.** The use of porfimer sodium is contra-indicated in patients with porphyria.

### Interactions

Use of porfimer sodium with other drugs causing photosensitivity should be avoided as the reaction may be increased.

### Pharmacokinetics

Porfimer sodium is distributed and eliminated slowly after intravenous injection, with plasma elimination half-life reported to be between 11 and 28 days. *In vitro* studies indicate that plasma protein binding is about 90%. Excretion occurs primarily via the faeces.

### Uses and Administration

Porfimer sodium is a haematoporphyrin derivative that reportedly accumulates in malignant tissue on injection. It is then activated by laser light to release oxygen radicals within malignant cells, producing cytotoxicity. Porfimer sodium is used as a photosensitiser in the photodynamic therapy of non-small cell lung cancer (p.519), oesophageal cancer (p.516), and superficial bladder cancer (p.512). It is also used for the treatment of dysplasia associated with Barrett's oesophagus (see Gastro-oesophageal Reflux Disease, p.1242), and has been investigated in various other neoplasms, including tumours of the gastrointestinal tract and cervix.

Porfimer sodium should be reconstituted with glucose 5% to a final concentration of 2.5 mg/mL. It is given by slow intravenous injection at a dose of 2 mg/kg. This is followed, 40 to 50 hours later, by activation using a laser tuned to a wavelength of 630 nanometres and delivered to the area of the tumour using a fibre optic guide. Residual tumour may subsequently be debrided surgically. A second laser treatment may be given 96 to 120 hours after the original injection. A maximum of 3 courses of photodynamic therapy may be used, with each injection separated by a minimum of 30 days for oesophageal and endobronchial tumours, and a minimum of 90 days for dysplasia in Barrett's oesophagus. However, in the treatment of superficial bladder cancer, only one dose of drug and light is administered due to an increased risk of bladder contracture, and no surgical debridement is performed.

**Photodynamic therapy.** Photodynamic therapy probably has the greatest potential of the various forms of light-activated treatment.[1] Photosensitising drugs are given intravenously, orally, or topically, and are selectively retained by tumour cells. When exposed to the correct wavelength of light the drug produces toxic oxygen radicals that destroy cell membranes and thereby kill the tumour cells. Vascular damage and immune-mediated injury may also occur.[2,3] Tumour cells must have an adequate supply of oxygen to be sensitive to photodynamic therapy,[2] and as light penetration is usually limited, early or superficial malignant lesions respond best to therapy.[1,2] Photodynamic therapy has been tried in skin, gastrointestinal, head and neck, bladder, gynaecological, pulmonary, and various intraperitoneal malignancies[2-8] It is also used for the treatment of Barrett's oesophagus.[9,10] There is also an interesting report of cytotoxicity against leukaemic cells *in vitro* when exposure to porfimer sodium was combined with ultrasound.[5]

The main adverse effect of photosensitisers such as porfimer is photosensitivity lasting 4 to 8 weeks; patients should be advised to avoid sunlight during this period and therapy is best delayed until the darker winter months if possible.[1] Newer photosensitisers are being developed to show increased tissue penetration and less prolonged photosensitivity.[2] The natural haem precursor 5-aminolevulinic acid (p.527) has the advantage that photosensitivity lasts only a few hours.


1. Bown SG. New techniques in laser therapy. *BMJ* 1998; **316:** 754–7.
2. Hsi RA, *et al.* Photodynamic therapy in the treatment of cancer: current state of the art. *Drugs* 1999; **57:** 725–34.
3. Ost D, *et al.* Photodynamic therapy in lung cancer. *Oncology* 2000; **14:** 379–86.
4. Wilson JHP, *et al.* Photodynamic therapy for gastrointestinal tumors. *Scand J Gastroenterol* 1991; **26** (suppl 188): 20–5.
5. Tachibana K, *et al.* Eliminating adult T-cell leukaemia cells with ultrasound. *Lancet* 1997; **349:** 325.
6. Walther MM. The role of photodynamic therapy in the treatment of recurrent superficial bladder cancer. *Urol Clin North Am* 2000; **27:** 163–70.
7. Metz JM, Friedberg JS. Endobronchial photodynamic therapy for the treatment of lung cancer. *Chest Surg Clin North Am* 2001; **11:** 829–39.
8. Biel MA. Photodynamic therapy in head and neck cancer. *Curr Oncol Rep* 2002; **4:** 87–96.
9. Wolfsen HC, *et al.* Photodynamic therapy for dysplastic Barrett esophagus and early esophageal adenocarcinoma. *Mayo Clin Proc* 2002; **77:** 1176–81.
10. Kelty CJ, *et al.* Photodynamic therapy for Barrett's esophagus: a review. *Dis Esophagus* 2002; **15:** 137–44.


### Preparations

**Proprietary Preparations** (details are given in Part 3)
***Canad.:*** Photofrin; ***Ger.:*** Photofrin; ***Israel:*** Photofrin; ***UK:*** Photofrin†; ***USA:*** Photofrin.

## Porfiromycin *(BAN, USAN)*

Methyl Mitomycin; NSC-56410; Porfiromicina; U-14743. 6-Amino-1,1a,2,8,8a,8b-hexahydro-8-(hydroxymethyl)-8a-methoxy-1,5-dimethylazirino[2′,3′:3,4]pyrrolo[1,2-*a*]indole-4,7-dione carbamate ester.

$C_{16}H_{20}N_4O_5$ = 348.4.
*CAS — 801-52-5.*

### Profile

Porfiromycin is an antibiotic antineoplastic structurally related to mitomycin (p.573). It is being studied as a radiosensitiser in the management of malignant neoplasms of the head and neck.

◊ References.


1. Haffty BG, *et al.* Bioreductive alkylating agent porfiromycin in combination with radiation therapy for the management of squamous cell carcinoma of the head and neck. *Radiat Oncol Invest* 1997; **5:** 235–45.


## Prednimustine *(USAN, rINN)*

Leo-1031; NSC-134087; Prednimustina. 11β,17,21-Trihydroxypregna-1,4-diene-3,20-dione 21-(4-{4-[bis(2-chloroethyl)amino]phenyl}butyrate).

$C_{35}H_{45}Cl_2NO_6$ = 646.6.
*CAS — 29069-24-7.*
*ATC — L01AA08.*

### Profile

Prednimustine is the prednisolone ester of chlorambucil, (p.536) and has been given by mouth in the treatment of various malignant diseases.

## Procarbazine Hydrochloride

*(BANM, USAN, rINNM)*

Hidrocloruro de procarbazina; Ibenzmethyzin Hydrochloride; NSC-77213; Ro-4-6467/1. *N*-Isopropyl-α-(2-methylhydrazino)-*p*-toluamide hydrochloride.

$C_{12}H_{19}N_3O,HCl$ = 257.8.
*CAS — 671-16-9 (procarbazine); 366-70-1 (procarbazine hydrochloride).*
*ATC — L01XB01.*

**Pharmacopoeias.** In *Chin., Int., Jpn,* and *US.*
**USP 27** (Procarbazine Hydrochloride). Store in airtight containers. Protect from light.

### Adverse Effects, Treatment, and Precautions

For general discussions see Antineoplastics, p.492, p.495, and p.497.

The most common adverse effects associated with procarbazine are gastrointestinal disturbances such as anorexia, nausea and vomiting (although patients may soon become tolerant), and bone-marrow depression. Leucopenia and thrombocytopenia may be delayed with a nadir at about 4 weeks after a dose, and recovery usually within 6 weeks. Anaemia, haemolysis, and bleeding tendencies have been reported.

Neurotoxicity is also common, with central effects such as somnolence, depression, nervousness or confusion, headache, hallucinations, and dizziness, and peripheral neuropathies including paraesthesias and decreased reflexes. Lethargy, ataxia, and sleep disorders have also occurred, and tremors, convulsions, and coma have been reported.

Other side-effects reported include fever and myalgia, pulmonary fibrosis or pneumonitis, haematuria, urinary frequency, skin reactions including dermatitis, pruritus, and hyperpigmentation, tachycardia, orthostatic hypotension, ocular defects, infertility, and hepatic impairment.

Procarbazine is a carcinogen, mutagen, and teratogen.

Procarbazine should be used with caution in patients with hepatic or renal impairment, and is contra-indicated if impairment is severe. The haematological status of the patient should be determined at least every 3 or 4 days and hepatic and renal function determined weekly. Care is also advisable in patients with phaeochromocytoma, epilepsy, or cardiovascular or cerebrovascular disease. Treatment should be interrupted if allergic skin reactions occur.

**Handling and disposal.** *Urine* produced for up to 48 hours after a dose of procarbazine should be handled wearing protective clothing.[1]


1. Harris J, Dodds LJ. Handling waste from patients receiving cytotoxic drugs. *Pharm J* 1985; **235:** 289–91.


### Interactions

For a general outline of antineoplastic drug interactions, see p.498. Procarbazine is a weak MAOI and the possibility of reactions with other drugs and food, although very rare, must be borne in mind—for details of MAOI reactions see p.314. Procarbazine may enhance the sedative effects of other CNS depressants. A disulfiram-like reaction has been reported with alcohol and the effects of antihypertensive agents may be enhanced.

**Antiepileptics.** Use with enzyme-inducing antiepileptics is associated with an increased risk of hypersensitivity reactions to procarbazine, possibly through a reactive intermediate generated by induction of the cytochrome P450 isoenzyme CYP3A subfamily.[1] Non-enzyme-inducing antiepileptics might be more appropriate in patients with brain tumours in whom procarbazine therapy is anticipated.


1. Lehmann DF, *et al.* Anticonvulsant usage is associated with an increased risk of procarbazine hypersensitivity reactions in patients with brain tumors. *Clin Pharmacol Ther* 1997; **62:** 225–9.


### Pharmacokinetics

Procarbazine is readily absorbed from the gastrointestinal tract. It crosses the blood-brain barrier and diffuses into the CSF. A plasma half-life of about 10 minutes has been reported. Procarbazine is rapidly metabolised (mainly in liver and kidneys) and only about 5% is excreted unchanged in the urine. The remainder is oxidised to *N*-isopropylterephthalamic acid and excreted in the urine, up to about 70% of a dose being excreted in 24 hours. Some of the drug is excreted as carbon dioxide and methane via the lungs. During oxidative breakdown in the body hydrogen peroxide is formed which may account for some of the drug's actions.

### Uses and Administration

Procarbazine hydrochloride is a methylhydrazine derivative whose antineoplastic effect, although not fully understood, may resemble that of the alkylating agents; it appears to inhibit protein and nucleic acid synthesis and suppress mitosis. It does not exhibit cross-resistance with other cytotoxic drugs.

Its main use is the treatment of Hodgkin's disease (p.509) when it is usually given with other drugs, as in the MOPP regimen (with chlormethine, vincristine, and prednisone) and its variants. Procarbazine has also been used in the treatment of other lymphomas (p.510) and in some other malignant neoplasms including tumours of the brain (p.513).

Doses of procarbazine hydrochloride are calculated in terms of procarbazine; procarbazine hydrochloride 116 mg is approximately equivalent to 100 mg of procarbazine. In many of the combination regimens it has been given by mouth to adults and children in doses of the equivalent of procarbazine 100 mg/m$^2$ on days 1 to 14 of each 4- or 6-week cycle. If used as a single agent in adults a dose equivalent to 50 mg of procarbazine daily, increased by 50 mg daily to 250 to 300 mg daily in divided doses has been suggested in the UK, while in the USA the recommended regimen is 2 to 4 mg/kg daily for the first week, subsequently increased to 4 to 6 mg/kg, doses being given to the nearest 50 mg. These doses are continued until maximum response is achieved or leucopenia, thrombocytopenia, or other signs of toxicity ensue. Maintenance doses are usually 50 to 150 mg, or 1 to 2 mg/kg, daily, until a cumulative dose of at least 6 g has been given. In children, initial daily doses of the equivalent of 50 mg/m$^2$ have been suggested (some sources simply suggest a dose of 50 mg), increased to 100 mg/m$^2$ and then adjusted according to response.

**Blood disorders, non-malignant.** Chemotherapy with regimens including procarbazine has been used in a few patients with refractory idiopathic thrombocytopenic purpura (p.1082), and has produced prolonged remission although in most cases of the disease such aggressive therapy is difficult to justify.

### Preparations

***USP 27:*** Procarbazine Hydrochloride Capsules.

**Proprietary Preparations** (details are given in Part 3)
***Austral.:*** Natulan; ***Belg.:*** Natulan†; ***Braz.:*** Natulanar†; ***Canad.:*** Natulan; ***Fr.:*** Natulan; ***Ger.:*** Natulan; ***Gr.:*** Natulan; ***Israel:*** Natulan†; ***Ital.:*** Natulan; ***Mex.:*** Natulan†; ***Neth.:*** Natulan; ***NZ:*** Natulan; ***S.Afr.:*** Natulan†; ***Spain:*** Natulan; ***Switz.:*** Natulan†; ***USA:*** Matulane.

## Raltitrexed *(BAN, USAN, rINN)*

D-1694; ICI-D1694; ZD-1694. *N*-{5-[3,4-Dihydro-2-methyl-4-oxoquinazolin-6-ylmethyl(methyl)amino]-2-thenoyl}-L-glutamic acid.

$C_{21}H_{22}N_4O_6S$ = 458.5.
*CAS — 112887-68-0.*
*ATC — L01BA03.*

### Adverse Effects, Treatment, and Precautions

Raltitrexed produces bone marrow depression, usually mild to moderate, with leucopenia, anaemia, and, less frequently, thrombocytopenia. The nadir of the white cell count usually occurs 7 to 14 days after a dose, with recovery by the third week. Gastrointestinal toxicity is also common, with nausea and vomiting, diarrhoea, and anorexia: mucositis may occur. Reversible increases in liver enzyme values have occurred. Other adverse effects include weakness and malaise, fever, pain, headache, skin rashes, arthralgia, muscle cramps, weight loss, peripheral oedema, alopecia, taste disturbance, and conjunctivitis. The use of folinic acid 25 mg/m² every 6 hours intravenously has been suggested by the manufacturer in patients who develop very severe toxicity.

Raltitrexed should be given with care to patients with hepatic impairment and should be avoided if impairment is severe. It should also be avoided in severe renal impairment and be given in reduced doses in moderate impairment. Care is also advisable in debilitated or elderly patients.

Raltitrexed is teratogenic; pregnancy should be avoided while either partner is receiving the drug and for at least 6 months after treatment. It may impair male fertility.

**Toxicity.** A large multicentre study comparing raltitrexed with fluorouracil plus folinic acid was suspended in 1999 due to an excess of deaths in the raltitrexed arm.[1] This decision has led to some controversy,[1-3] as in 11 of the 17 deaths in patients taking raltitrexed there was evidence that the dose had not been correctly adjusted to take account of renal function. In addition, and further confusing the issue, the incidence of reported serious adverse effects was lower in raltitrexed-treated patients than in controls. A further study[4] reported an increased rate of raltitrexed-related deaths compared with fluorouracil-based regimens. Almost all of the 18 deaths were caused by gastrointestinal and haematological toxicity, and in 3 of these the dose of raltitrexed had not been adjusted for toxicity.

1. Anonymous. Drug-company decision to end cancer trial. *Lancet* 1999; **354:** 1045.
2. Ford HER, Cunningham D. Safety of raltitrexed. *Lancet* 1999; **354:** 1824–5.
3. Kerr D. Safety of raltitrexed. *Lancet* 1999; **354:** 1825.
4. Maughan TS, *et al.* Comparison of survival, palliation, and quality of life with three chemotherapy regimens in metastatic colorectal cancer: a multicentre randomised trial. *Lancet* 2002; **359:** 1555–63.

### Interactions

Raltitrexed should not be given with folic or folinic acid which may impair its cytotoxic action. (For the deliberate use of folinic acid to counteract the effects of raltitrexed in patients with severe toxicity, see above.)

### Pharmacokinetics

After intravenous doses raltitrexed exhibits triphasic pharmacokinetics, with an initial rapid decline from peak plasma concentrations followed by a slow terminal elimination phase. Raltitrexed is actively transported into cells and metabolised to active polyglutamate forms. The remainder of a dose is excreted unchanged, about 50% of a dose appearing in the urine, and about 15% in the faeces. The terminal elimination half-life is stated to be about 8 days. Clearance is markedly reduced in renal impairment.

◊ References.

1. Clarke SJ, *et al.* Clinical and preclinical pharmacokinetics of raltitrexed. *Clin Pharmacokinet* 2000; **39:** 429–43.

### Uses and Administration

Raltitrexed is a folate analogue that is a potent and specific inhibitor of the enzyme thymidylate synthase, which is involved in the synthesis of DNA. It is used in the treatment of advanced colorectal cancer (p.516) and has also been tried in breast cancer (p.514) and other solid neoplasms.

The recommended initial dose of raltitrexed in patients with normal renal function is 3 mg/m² given by intravenous infusion over 15 minutes. Subsequent doses, which should be reduced by up to 50% depending on the severity of initial toxicity, may be given at intervals of 3 weeks provided toxicity has resolved.

A full blood count should be performed before each dose and treatment withheld if the white cell or platelet counts are below acceptable levels (see also Bone-marrow Depression, p.496). Hepatic and renal function should also be tested. It is essential that doses be adjusted in renal impairment (see below).

◊ References.

1. Gunasekara NS, Faulds D. Raltitrexed: a review of its pharmacological properties and clinical efficacy in the management of advanced colorectal cancer. *Drugs* 1998; **55:** 423–35.
2. Cunningham D, *et al.* Efficacy, tolerability and management of raltitrexed (Tomudex) monotherapy in patients with advanced colorectal cancer: a review of phase II/III trials. *Eur J Cancer* 2002; **38:** 478–86.
3. Scheithauer W, *et al.* Randomized multicenter phase II trial of oxaliplatin plus irinotecan versus raltitrexed as first-line treatment in advanced colorectal cancer. *J Clin Oncol* 2002; **20:** 165–72.
4. Feliu J, *et al.* Raltitrexed in the treatment of elderly patients with advanced colorectal cancer: an active and low toxicity regimen. *Eur J Cancer* 2002; **38:** 1204–11.
5. Comella P, *et al.* Oxaliplatin plus raltitrexed and leucovorin-modulated 5-fluorouracil i.v. bolus: a salvage regimen for colorectal cancer patients. *Br J Cancer* 2002; **86:** 1871–5.
6. Maughan TS, *et al.* Comparison of survival, palliation, and quality of life with three chemotherapy regimens in metastatic colorectal cancer: a multicentre randomised trial. *Lancet* 2002; **359:** 1555–63.

**Administration in renal impairment.** It is essential that doses of raltitrexed be adjusted in renal impairment (creatinine clearance less than 65 mL/minute) as fatalities have been associated with the failure to make such adjustments (see under Adverse Effects, above). The dosage interval should be increased from 3 to 4 weeks and the dose adjusted on the basis of creatinine clearance (CC) as follows:

- CC of 55 to 65 mL/minute, 2.25 mg/m²
- CC of 25 to 54 mL/minute, 1.5 mg/m² (in some countries, adjustment of the dose to a percentage of the full dose equivalent to the value of the CC in mL/minute is suggested in this group, e.g. reduction to 30% in those with a CC of 30 mL/minute, or 40% if CC is 40 mL/minute)
- CC less than 25 mL/minute, treatment contra-indicated

### Preparations

**Proprietary Preparations** (details are given in Part 3)
***Arg.:*** Tomudex; ***Austral.:*** Tomudex; ***Austria:*** Tomudex; ***Belg.:*** Tomudex; ***Braz.:*** Tomudex; ***Canad.:*** Tomudex; ***Fin.:*** Tomudex; ***Fr.:*** Tomudex; ***Hong Kong:*** Tomudex; ***Irl.:*** Tomudex; ***Ital.:*** Tomudex; ***Mex.:*** Tomudex; ***Neth.:*** Tomudex; ***Norw.:*** Tomudex; ***Port.:*** Tomudex; ***S.Afr.:*** Tomudex; ***Singapore:*** Tomudex; ***Spain:*** Tomudex; ***Switz.:*** Tomudex; ***UK:*** Tomudex.

## Ranimustine *(rINN)*

MCNU; NSC-0270516; Ranimustina; Ranomustine. Methyl 6-[3-(2-chloroethyl)-3-nitrosoureido]-6-deoxy-α-D-glucopyranoside.

$C_{10}H_{18}ClN_3O_7$ = 327.7.
*CAS — 58994-96-0.*
*ATC — L01AD07.*

### Profile

Ranimustine is a nitrosourea derivative with general properties similar to those of carmustine (p.535). It is used intravenously in the treatment of malignant neoplasms in usual doses of 50 to 90 mg/m² every 6 to 8 weeks according to haematological response.

◊ References.

1. Wada M, *et al.* Induction therapy consisting of alternating cycles of ranimustine, vincristine, melphalan, dexamethasone and interferon alpha (ROAD-IN) and a randomized comparison of interferon alpha maintenance in multiple myeloma: a co-operative study in Japan. *Br J Haematol* 2000; **109:** 805–14.
2. Hatano N, *et al.* Efficacy of post operative adjuvant therapy with human interferon beta, MCNU and radiation (IMR) for malignant glioma: comparison among three protocols. *Acta Neurochir (Wien)* 2000; **142:** 633–8.
3. Wakabayashi T, *et al.* Initial and maintenance combination treatment with interferon-beta, MCNU (ranimustine), and radiotherapy for patients with previously untreated malignant glioma. *J Neurooncol* 2000; **49:** 57–62.
4. Mizuno H, *et al.* Superior efficacy of MMCP regimen compared with VMCP and MMPP regimens in the treatment of multiple myeloma. *Intern Med* 2002; **41:** 290–4.
5. Takenaka T, *et al.* Phase III study of ranimustine, cyclophosphamide, vincristine, melphalan, and prednisolone (MCNU-COP/MP) versus modified COP/MP in multiple myeloma: a Japan clinical oncology group study, JCOG 9301. *Int J Hematol* 2004; **79:** 165–73.

### Preparations

**Proprietary Preparations** (details are given in Part 3)
***Jpn:*** Cymerin.

## Ranpirnase *(USAN, rINN)*

P-30 Protein; Ranpirnasa.
*CAS — 196488-72-9.*

NOTE. P-30 protein has been incorrectly stated to contain ergotamine.

### Profile

Ranpirnase is a ribonuclease reported to have antineoplastic properties. It is under investigation in the treatment of malignant mesothelioma. Ranpirnase has also been investigated in the management of a variety of solid tumours. It is also reported to have activity *in vitro* against HIV.

## Razoxane *(BAN, rINN)*

ICI-59118; ICRF-159; NSC-129943; Razoxano. (±)-4,4′-Propylenebis(piperazine-2,6-dione).

$C_{11}H_{16}N_4O_4$ = 268.3.
*CAS — 21416-87-5.*

### Profile

Razoxane is an antineoplastic with inhibitory activity during the pre-mitotic and early mitotic phases of cell growth ($G_2$-M). It enhances the effects of radiotherapy. It has been used in association with radiotherapy in the treatment of sarcomas, including Kaposi's sarcoma. Razoxane has also been tried in other malignant diseases including acute leukaemias and non-Hodgkin's lymphomas. However, it is no longer widely used. Razoxane was formerly used in psoriasis, but its carcinogenic properties militate against such use, as discussed below.

In the treatment of sarcomas it has generally been given by mouth in doses of 125 mg twice daily; higher doses have been given in the management of acute leukaemias and Kaposi's sarcoma. The peripheral blood count should be monitored during treatment.

The principal adverse effects of razoxane include bone-marrow depression, gastrointestinal disturbances, skin reactions, and alopecia. It may enhance the adverse effects of radiotherapy. Razoxane therapy has been associated with the development of secondary malignancies: it is contra-indicated in the treatment of non-malignant conditions.

Dexrazoxane (p.1036) is the (+)-enantiomer of razoxane. It is used to reduce anthracycline-induced cardiotoxicity.

**Malignant neoplasms.** References to the use of razoxane in association with radiotherapy.

1. Rhomberg W, *et al.* Radiotherapy vs radiotherapy and razoxane in the treatment of soft tissue sarcomas: final results of a randomized study. *Int J Radiat Oncol Biol Phys* 1996; **36:** 1077–84.
2. Rhomberg W, *et al.* A small prospective study of chordomas treated with radiotherapy and razoxane. *Strahlenther Onkol* 2003; **179:** 249–53.

**Skin disorders, non-malignant.** Razoxane was formerly used in the systemic treatment of psoriasis, and has been found to be extremely effective, with an initial response rate of 97% overall. It was found to be of use in all forms of cutaneous psoriasis and psoriatic arthropathy.[1] However, the development of acute myeloid leukaemias and other malignancies in patients given razoxane[2-5] has led to its being contra-indicated in non-malignant conditions.

For a discussion of psoriasis and its management, see p.1137.

1. Horton JJ, Wells RS. Razoxane: a review of 6 years' therapy in psoriasis. *Br J Dermatol* 1983; **109:** 669–73.
2. Horton JJ, *et al.* Epitheliomas in patients receiving razoxane therapy for psoriasis. *Br J Dermatol* 1983; **109:** 675–8.
3. Lakhani S, *et al.* Razoxane and leukaemia. *Lancet* 1984; **ii:** 288–9.
4. Caffrey EA, *et al.* Acute myeloid leukaemia after treatment with razoxane. *Br J Dermatol* 1985; **113:** 131–4.
5. Zuiable AG, *et al.* Razoxane and T-cell lymphoma. *Br J Dermatol* 1989; **121:** 149.

## Rituximab *(BAN, USAN, rINN)*

IDEC-102; IDEC-C2B8.
*CAS — 174722-31-7.*
*ATC — L01XC02.*

### Adverse Effects, Treatment, and Precautions

For general discussions see Antineoplastics, p.492, p.495, and p.497.

Infusion of rituximab has been associated with a cytokine release syndrome of fever and rigors, usually within 2 hours of beginning therapy (see also below). Other reported symptoms include pruritus and rashes, dyspnoea, bronchospasm, angioedema, transient hypotension, and flushing. Severe cases may be associated with tumour lysis syndrome, respiratory failure, and death. Thrombocytopenia, neutropenia, leucopenia, and anaemia have occurred in a few patients, as have exacerbation of angina pectoris and heart failure. Hypersensitivity reactions manifest similarly to the cytokine release syndrome, but usually occur within minutes of starting infusion. Mucocutaneous reactions, some fatal, and including Stevens-Johnson syndrome or toxic epidermal necrolysis have also occurred.

Patients with an extensive tumour burden, pulmonary tumour infiltration or pulmonary insufficiency may be at increased risk of severe reactions and should be treated with caution and possibly a decreased initial infusion rate. Therapy should be interrupted in patients who develop severe symptoms and only resumed, at half the previous rate, once all signs and symptoms have resolved. Premedication with analgesics, antihistamines, and possibly corticosteroids is recommended in all patients before receiving rituximab. Complete blood and platelet counts should be monitored regularly.

**Infusion-related reactions.** By November 1998 there had been 74 cases of serious infusion-related reactions to rituximab reported worldwide, with 8 fatal cases.[1] An estimated 12 000 to 14 000 patients had been treated.

The reaction usually occurs within the first 2 hours of infusion and the underlying mechanism is believed to be a severe cytokine release syndrome, with some elements of tumour lysis syndrome.[1-3] In one series of cases tumour necrosis factor-α and interleukin-6 levels were found to peak 90 minutes after the onset of the infusion, and these elevated cytokine levels coincided with infusion-related symptoms.[2] The reaction is usually most marked after the first infusion and subsequent infusions are usually tolerated, emphasising that this is not a true hypersensitivity reaction.[4]

Patients with a high tumour burden (lesions over 10 cm in diameter or more than 500 000 circulating malignant cells/mm$^3$), a history of pulmonary infiltration or insufficiency, or underlying cardiac disease are believed to be at greater risk of severe reactions.[1,2,4] The UK Committee on Safety of Medicines recommends that premedication with an analgesic and an antihistamine should always be given before rituximab, and corticosteroids should be considered.[1] However, serious or fatal reactions have occurred despite such premedication.[3,4] Alternative infusion schedules and/or combination therapy with chemotherapeutic drugs may be required to decrease the tumour burden before rituximab therapy.[2,4]

1. Committee on Safety of Medicines/Medicines Control Agency. Rituximab (MabThera): serious infusion-related adverse reactions. *Current Problems* 1999; **25:** 2–3. Also available at: http://www.mca.gov.uk/ourwork/monitorsafequalmed/currentproblems/volume25feb.htm (accessed 30/06/04)
2. Winkler U, *et al.* Cytokine-release syndrome in patients with B-cell chronic lymphocytic leukaemia and high lymphocyte counts after treatment with an anti-CD20 monoclonal antibody (rituximab, IDEC-C2B8). *Blood* 1999; **94:** 2217–24.
3. Lim L-C, *et al.* Fatal cytokine release syndrome with chimeric anti-CD20 monoclonal antibody rituximab in a 71-year-old patient with chronic lymphocytic leukaemia. *J Clin Oncol* 1999; **17:** 1962–3.
4. Byrd JC, *et al.* Rituximab therapy in hematologic malignancy patients with circulating blood tumor cells: association with increased infusion-related side effects and rapid blood tumor clearance. *J Clin Oncol* 1999; **17:** 791–5.

**Pregnancy.** Giving 4 cycles of rituximab (with doxorubicin, vincristine, and prednisolone) to a pregnant woman with lymphoma, from 21 weeks' gestation until delivery at 35 weeks, resulted in no adverse effects to either the mother or the infant.[1] However, since human immunoglobulin G (IgG) crosses the placenta, and rituximab has an IgG component, the manufacturers advise against its use during pregnancy, as it may potentially cause B-cell depletion in the fetus; women of child-bearing potential should use effective contraceptive methods during treatment and for up to 12 months following therapy.

1. Herold M, *et al.* Efficacy and safety of a combined rituximab chemotherapy during pregnancy. *J Clin Oncol* 2001; **19:** 3439.

### Pharmacokinetics

Serum concentration and half-life of rituximab are reported to be proportional to dose, but show considerable interindividual variation. Mean serum half-life after intravenous infusion of 375 mg/m$^2$ was about 76 hours after an initial infusion and about 205 hours after 3 further infusions at weekly intervals. Serum concentrations are negatively correlated with tumour burden and the number of circulating B-cells. Rituximab is bound to B lymphocytes, and is detectable in the body for 3 to 6 months after treatment.

### Uses and Administration

Rituximab is a chimeric monoclonal antibody to CD20 antigen used as monotherapy in the treatment of indolent low-grade non-Hodgkin's lymphoma, and in combination with CHOP chemotherapy (cyclophosphamide, doxorubicin, vincristine, and prednisone) for CD20-positive diffuse large B-cell non-Hodgkin's lymphoma (p.510). Rituximab also forms part of the combination regimen employing ibritumomab tiuxetan (p.560). Rituximab is given diluted in sodium chloride 0.9% or glucose 5%, to a final concentration of between 1 and 4 mg/mL. Recommended doses are 375 mg/m$^2$ by intravenous infusion once weekly, for 4 doses. The first infusion is given initially at a rate of 50 mg/hour; subsequently this may be increased in increments of 50 mg/hour every 30 minutes to a maximum of 400 mg/hour, if well tolerated. Subsequent doses may be begun at a rate of 100 mg/hour, and incremented to a maximum of 400 mg/hour.

Rituximab is also under investigation for the treatment of a number of other conditions in which B cells are implicated, including chronic lymphocytic leukaemia (p.507), idiopathic thrombocytopenic purpura, and rheumatoid arthritis.

◊ References.

1. Wood AM. Rituximab: an innovative therapy for non-Hodgkin's lymphoma. *Am J Health-Syst Pharm* 2001; **58:** 215–32.
2. Coiffier B, *et al.* CHOP chemotherapy plus rituximab compared with CHOP alone in elderly patients with diffuse large-B-cell lymphoma. *N Engl J Med* 2002; **346:** 235–42.
3. Hainsworth JD, *et al.* Rituximab as first-line and maintenance therapy for patients with indolent non-Hodgkin's lymphoma. *J Clin Oncol* 2002; **20:** 4261–7.
4. Plosker GL, Figgitt DP. Rituximab: a review of its use in non-Hodgkin's lymphoma and chronic lymphocytic leukaemia. *Drugs* 2003; **63:** 803–43.
5. National Institute for Clinical Excellence. Rituximab for aggressive non-Hodgkin's lymphoma (issued September 2003). Available at: http://www.nice.org.uk/pdf/65_rituximab_nonhodgkins_fullguidance.pdf (accessed 30/06/04)

### Preparations

**Proprietary Preparations** (details are given in Part 3)
***Arg.:*** Mabthera; ***Austral.:*** Mabthera; ***Austria:*** Mabthera; ***Belg.:*** Mabthera; ***Braz.:*** Mabthera; ***Canad.:*** Rituxan; ***Chile:*** Mabthera; ***Denm.:*** Mabthera; ***Fin.:*** Mabthera; ***Fr.:*** Mabthera; ***Ger.:*** Mabthera; ***Gr.:*** Mabthera; ***Hong Kong:*** Mabthera; ***Irl.:*** Mabthera; ***Israel:*** Mabthera; ***Ital.:*** Mabthera; ***Mex.:*** Mabthera; ***Neth.:*** Mabthera; ***Norw.:*** Mabthera; ***NZ:*** Mabthera; ***Port.:*** Mabthera; ***S.Afr.:*** Mabthera; ***Singapore:*** Mabthera; ***Spain:*** Mabthera; ***Swed.:*** Mabthera; ***Switz.:*** Mabthera; ***Thai.:*** Mabthera; ***UK:*** Mabthera; ***USA:*** Rituxan.

---

## Roquinimex *(USAN, rINN)*

FCF-89; LS-2616. 1,2-Dihydro-4-hydroxy-*N*,1-dimethyl-2-oxo-3-quinolinecarboxanilide.
$C_{18}H_{16}N_2O_3$ = 308.3.
*CAS — 84088-42-6.*
*ATC — L03AX02.*

### Profile

Roquinimex is an immunomodulator which is reported to stimulate various immune functions including macrophage cytotoxicity. It has been investigated for its potential against various malignant neoplasms including as adjuvant therapy following bone marrow transplantation in acute leukaemia, to prolong the time to relapse. Roquinimex has also been investigated in various immune and auto-immune disorders including multiple sclerosis. However serious cardiovascular toxicity following roquinimex therapy has led to several trials being terminated.

◊ References.

1. Coutant R, *et al.* Low dose linomide in type I juvenile diabetes of recent onset: a randomised placebo-controlled double blind trial. *Diabetologia* 1998; **41:** 1040–6.
2. Simonsson B, *et al.* Roquinimex (Linomide) vs placebo in AML after autologous bone marrow transplantation. *Bone Marrow Transplant* 2000; **25:** 1121–7.
3. Tan IL, *et al.* Linomide in the treatment of multiple sclerosis: MRI results from prematurely terminated phase-III trials. *Multiple Sclerosis* 2000; **6:** 99–104.
4. Noseworthy JH, *et al.* Linomide in relapsing and secondary progressive MS. Part 1: trial design and clinical results. *Neurology* 2000; **54:** 1726–33.

---

## Rubitecan *(USAN, rINN)*

9-NC; 9-Nitrocamptothecin; RFS-2000; Rubitecán. 9-Nitro-20(*S*)-camptothecin.
$C_{20}H_{15}N_3O_6$ = 393.3.
*CAS — 91421-42-0.*

### Profile

Like irinotecan (p.564), rubitecan is a topoisomerase I inhibitor related to camptothecin. It is under investigation for its antineoplastic properties particularly in the treatment of pancreatic cancer.

---

## Satraplatin *(USAN, rINN)*

BMS-182751; BMY-45594; JM-216; Satraplatino. (*OC*-6-43)-Bis(acetato)amminedichloro(cyclohexylamine)platinum.
$C_{10}H_{22}Cl_2N_2O_4Pt$ = 500.3.
*CAS — 129580-63-8.*

### Profile

Satraplatin is an analogue of cisplatin (p.538) with generally similar properties, but which is well absorbed following oral administration. It is under investigation for its antineoplastic properties.

◊ References.

1. Fokkema E, *et al.* Phase II study of oral platinum drug JM216 as first-line treatment in patients with small-cell lung cancer. *J Clin Oncol* 1999; **17:** 3822–7.
2. Kelland LR. An update on satraplatin: the first orally available platinum anticancer drug. *Expert Opin Invest Drugs* 2000; **9:** 1373–82.
3. Jones S, *et al.* Phase I study of JM-216 (an oral platinum analogue) in combination with paclitaxel in patients with advanced malignancies. *Invest New Drugs* 2002; **20:** 55–61.

---

## Semustine *(USAN, rINN)*

Methyl Lomustine; Methyl-CCNU; NSC-95441; Semustina; WR-220076. 1-(2-Chloroethyl)-3-(4-methylcyclohexyl)-1-nitrosourea.
$C_{10}H_{18}ClN_3O_2$ = 247.7.
*CAS — 13909-09-6.*
*ATC — L01AD03.*

**Pharmacopoeias.** In *Chin.*

### Adverse Effects, Treatment, and Precautions

As for Carmustine, p.535.

**Effects on the kidneys.** Nephrotoxicity has been reported in patients receiving high cumulative doses of semustine. Severe renal damage was reported in 6 of 17 children given semustine after radiotherapy for brain tumours; all 6 children had received a total dose above 1.5 g/m$^2$ in contrast to those not so affected, who had received lower doses.[1] A decrease in kidney size was seen in 2 patients who had received lower cumulative doses. There had been no evidence during treatment that patients were losing renal function. Similarly others have reported an increased risk of renal abnormalities in patients given a cumulative dose of 1.4 g/m$^2$ or more.[2] Some 25% of patients given higher doses were so affected, while those given lower doses were not. Overall, however, the problem may not be particularly frequent: in one study it was considered that only 4 of 857 patients treated with semustine over 6 years might have had delayed renal insufficiency possibly related to semustine.[3]

1. Harmon WE, *et al.* Chronic renal failure in children treated with methyl-CCNU. *N Engl J Med* 1979; **300:** 1200–3.
2. Micetich KC, *et al.* Nephrotoxicity of semustine (methyl-CCNU) in patients with malignant melanoma receiving adjuvant chemotherapy. *Am J Med* 1981; **71:** 967–72.
3. Nichols WC, Moertel CG. Nephrotoxicity of methyl-CCNU. *N Engl J Med* 1979; **301:** 1181.

### Pharmacokinetics

Semustine is well absorbed from the gastrointestinal tract following oral doses, and is rapidly metabolised. The metabolites are reported to possess prolonged plasma half-lives, and cross the blood-brain barrier into the CSF. It is excreted in urine as metabolites: up to 60% of a dose is excreted in this way within 48 hours. Small amounts may be excreted in faeces and via the lungs as carbon dioxide.

### Uses and Administration

Semustine is a nitrosourea with actions and uses similar to those of carmustine (p.535) and lomustine (p.565).

---

## Seocalcitol *(BAN, rINN)*

EB-1089. (5*Z*,7*E*,22*E*,24*E*)-24a,26a,27a-Trihomo-9,10-secocholesta-5,7,10(19),22,24-pentaene-1α,3β,25-triol.
$C_{30}H_{46}O_3$ = 454.7.
*CAS — 134404-52-7.*

### Profile

Seocalcitol is a vitamin D analogue under investigation for the treatment of hepatocellular carcinoma.

---

## Sizofiran *(rINN)*

Schizophyllan; Sizofirán. Poly[3→(*O*-β-D-glucopyranosyl-(1→3)-*O*-[β-D-glucopyranosyl-(1→6)]-*O*-β-D-glucopyranosyl-(1→3)-*O*-β-D-glucopyranosyl)→1].
$(C_{24}H_{40}O_{20})_n$.
*CAS — 9050-67-3.*

### Profile

Sizofiran is a polysaccharide obtained from cultures of the basidiomycete fungus *Schizophyllum commune*. It is reported to have antineoplastic and immunomodulating activity and is given with radiotherapy in malignant neoplasms of the cervix (p.515). It is given by intramuscular injection in usual doses of 40 mg weekly. It has also been tried with chemotherapy or radiotherapy in other malignant neoplasms. Hypersensitivity reactions, including anaphylactoid shock, may occur.

◊ References.

1. Fujimoto S, *et al.* Clinical outcome of postoperative adjuvant immunochemotherapy with sizofiran for patients with resectable gastric cancer: a randomised controlled study. *Eur J Cancer* 1991; **27:** 1114–18.
2. Shimizu Y, *et al.* Augmenting effect of sizofiran on the immunofunction of regional lymph nodes in cervical cancer. *Cancer* 1992; **69:** 1188–94.
3. Kano Y, *et al.* Effect of sizofiran on regional lymph nodes in patients with head and neck cancer. *Biotherapy* 1996; **9:** 257–62.

### Preparations

**Proprietary Preparations** (details are given in Part 3)
***Jpn:*** Sonifilan.

---

## Sobuzoxane *(rINN)*

MST-16; Sobuzoxano. 4,4′-Ethylenebis[1-(hydroxymethyl)-2,6-piperazinedione] bis(isobutyl carbonate).
$C_{22}H_{34}N_4O_{10}$ = 514.5.
*CAS — 98631-95-9.*

### Profile

Sobuzoxane is an orally active inhibitor of topoisomerase II that has been used for its antineoplastic properties in the treatment of non-Hodgkin's lymphomas and adult T-cell leukaemia/lymphoma. Adverse effects include myelosuppression, bleeding tendency, renal and hepatic dysfunction, gastrointestinal disturbances, alopecia, headache, and fever.

## Streptozocin *(USAN, rINN)*

Estreptozocina; NSC-85998; Streptozotocin; U-9889. 2-Deoxy-2-(3-methyl-3-nitrosoureido)-D-glucopyranose.

$C_8H_{15}N_3O_7$ = 265.2.

*CAS — 18883-66-4.*

*ATC — L01AD04.*

**Storage.** The manufacturers recommend that the freeze-dried streptozocin preparation be stored at 2° to 8° and protected from light.

### Adverse Effects, Treatment, and Precautions

For general discussions see Antineoplastics, p.492, p.495, and p.497.

Cumulative nephrotoxicity is common with streptozocin and may be severe and irreversible. Intra-arterial administration may be associated with increased risk of nephrotoxicity.

Other adverse effects include severe nausea and vomiting and alterations in liver function or occasionally severe hepatotoxicity. Myelosuppression may occur but is rarely severe. Streptozocin may affect glucose metabolism. A diabetogenic effect has been reported; hypoglycaemia attributed to the release of insulin from damaged cells has also occurred.

Streptozocin is irritant to tissues and extravasation may lead to local ulceration and necrosis.

Streptozocin should be used with extreme care in patients with pre-existing renal impairment.

**Handling and disposal.** Methods for the destruction of streptozocin *waste* by reaction with hydrobromic acid in glacial acetic acid or by oxidation with a solution of potassium permanganate in sulfuric acid.[1] Residues produced by either method were free of mutagenic activity.

1. Castegnaro M, *et al.*, eds. Laboratory decontamination and destruction of carcinogens in laboratory wastes: some antineoplastic agents. *IARC Scientific Publications 73.* Lyon: WHO/International Agency for Research on Cancer, 1985.

### Interactions

Streptozocin should not be given in association with other potentially nephrotoxic drugs. For increased doxorubicin toxicity when given with streptozocin see p.549.

**Phenytoin.** It has been suggested that because phenytoin appeared to protect the beta cells of the pancreas from the cytotoxic effects of streptozocin, its use with streptozocin should be avoided in patients being treated for pancreatic tumours.[1]

1. Koranyi L, Gero L. Influence of diphenylhydantoin on the effect of streptozotocin. *BMJ* 1979; **1:** 127.

### Pharmacokinetics

After intravenous doses streptozocin is rapidly cleared from the blood and distributed to body tissues, particularly the liver, kidneys, intestines, and pancreas. It is extensively metabolised, mainly in the liver and perhaps the kidney, and excreted principally in the urine as metabolites and a small amount of unchanged drug. Approximately 60 to 70% of an intravenous dose is excreted in urine within 24 hours. Some is also excreted via the lungs. Streptozocin itself does not cross the blood-brain barrier but its metabolites are found in the CSF.

### Uses and Administration

Streptozocin is an antibiotic antineoplastic belonging to the nitrosoureas (see Carmustine, p.535) and is used, alone or in combination with other antineoplastics, mainly in the treatment of pancreatic endocrine (islet-cell) tumours (p.504). It has been tried in other tumours including exocrine pancreatic cancer and prostate cancer. It is licensed for intravenous injection or infusion in doses of 1 g/m$^2$ weekly, increased if necessary after 2 weeks to up to 1.5 g/m$^2$. Alternatively doses of 500 mg/m$^2$ may be given daily for 5 days and repeated every 6 weeks.

Streptozocin has also been given by intra-arterial infusion (but see Adverse Effects above).

Full blood counts, and renal and hepatic function tests should be performed routinely during treatment; doses should be reduced or treatment withdrawn if renal toxicity occurs.

### Preparations

**Proprietary Preparations** (details are given in Part 3)
***Canad.:*** Zanosar; ***Fr.:*** Zanosar; ***Gr.:*** Zanosar; ***Israel:*** Zanosar; ***USA:*** Zanosar.

---

## Tamoxifen Citrate *(BANM, USAN, rINNM)*

Citrato de tamoxifeno; ICI-46474; Tamoxifeni Citras. (Z)-2-[4-(1,2-Diphenylbut-1-enyl)phenoxy]ethyldimethylamine citrate.

$C_{26}H_{29}NO,C_6H_8O_7$ = 563.6.

*CAS — 10540-29-1 (tamoxifen); 54965-24-1 (tamoxifen citrate).*

*ATC — L02BA01.*

**Pharmacopoeias.** In *Chin., Eur.* (see p.vi), *Int.*, and *US.*

**Ph. Eur. 5.0** (Tamoxifen Citrate). A white or almost white, polymorphic, crystalline powder. Slightly soluble in water and in acetone; soluble in methyl alcohol.

**USP 27** (Tamoxifen Citrate). A white, fine, crystalline powder. Very slightly soluble in water, in alcohol, in acetone, and in chloroform; soluble in methyl alcohol. Protect from light.

### Adverse Effects

The most frequent adverse effects of tamoxifen are hot flushes. Other adverse effects include fluid retention, nausea, gastrointestinal intolerance, vaginal bleeding or discharge, pruritus vulvae, rashes, dry skin, and alopecia. There have also been reports of dizziness, headache, depression, confusion, fatigue, and muscle cramps. There may be an increased tendency to thromboembolism, and pulmonary embolism has occurred. Tumour pain and flare may be a sign of response, but hypercalcaemia, sometimes severe, has developed in patients with bony metastases. Transient thrombocytopenia and leucopenia have been reported. Blurred vision and loss of visual acuity, corneal opacities, retinopathies, and cataracts have occurred rarely. Tamoxifen has been associated with increased liver enzymes, and rarely with cholestasis and hepatitis. Hypertriglyceridaemia has occurred. Uterine fibroids and endometrial changes including hyperplasia and polyps may occur, and an increased incidence of endometrial carcinoma, and rarely uterine sarcoma, has been reported. Suppression of menstruation may occur in premenopausal women and cystic ovarian swellings have occasionally occurred. Very rare cases of interstitial pneumonitis have been reported.

**Carcinogenicity.** Tamoxifen has a stimulant effect on the endometrium (probably by acting as a partial oestrogen agonist) and its use has been associated with the development of endometrial polyps[1] and endometriosis,[2] and an increased risk of endometrial cancer.[3-5] The risk, which increases with duration of therapy, is generally agreed to be modest, and the clinical benefit in women with breast cancer outweighs any increased risk of endometrial neoplasm.[6-9] Women taking tamoxifen to prevent breast cancer have been estimated to have a 2.53-fold greater risk of developing endometrial carcinoma than untreated women.[10] The risk may increase with more prolonged use and a case-control study has reported that long-term (over 2 years) users may have a worse prognosis if endometrial cancer develops, due to less favourable history and stage.[11] It has been recommended that women with breast cancer taking tamoxifen should be given annual gynaecological examinations, and any unusual symptoms, including abnormal bleeding or spotting should be investigated promptly.[12] Women taking tamoxifen for prophylaxis of breast cancer should be monitored carefully for endometrial hyperplasia. If atypical hyperplasia develops, tamoxifen should be discontinued while the condition is treated and a hysterectomy should be considered before tamoxifen is re-started.[12] However, up to 39% of postmenopausal women taking tamoxifen show endometrial changes and as these seldom progress to cancer, the value of routine endometrial biopsies has been questioned.[7,8,12,13] Transvaginal ultrasonography has been used as a noninvasive method of endometrial screening, but has a high rate of false-positive results.[14] It has been suggested that colour doppler ultrasonography, which distinguishes vascularised lesions such as polyps and carcinomas from avascular atrophic lesions, may be a useful alternative.[15] There is some evidence that a levonorgestrel-releasing intra-uterine device can protect against the uterine changes induced by tamoxifen.[16]

Although rare, there is an increase in the risk of uterine sarcoma in women receiving tamoxifen. Between 1978, when tamoxifen was first marketed in the USA, and April 2001, the FDA was aware of 43 cases in women who had been receiving tamoxifen; there had also been reports in 116 women in other countries.[17] Although less than the expected rate in this population, this was considered to be due to underreporting.

Tamoxifen has been shown to form DNA adducts in *rat* livers, and there has been speculation that it may cause liver cancer in humans. However, there is considerable interspecies variation in the metabolism of tamoxifen and several large-scale clinical trials did not find an increase in liver carcinogenicity in humans.[9] There is also little evidence of an increased relative risk of other secondary malignancies such as gastrointestinal or ovarian cancers.[9]

1. Corley D, *et al.* Postmenopausal bleeding from unusual endometrial polyps in women on chronic tamoxifen therapy. *Obstet Gynecol* 1992; **79:** 111–16.
2. Cano A, *et al.* Tamoxifen and the uterus and endometrium. *Lancet* 1989, **i:** 376.
3. Fornander T, *et al.* Adjuvant tamoxifen in early breast cancer: occurrence of new primary cancers. *Lancet* 1989; **i:** 117–20.
4. Gusberg SB. Tamoxifen for breast cancer: associated endometrial cancer. *Cancer* 1990; **65:** 1463–4.
5. van Leeuwen FE, *et al.* Risk of endometrial cancer after tamoxifen treatment of breast cancer. *Lancet* 1994; **343:** 448–52.
6. Baum M, *et al.* Endometrial cancer during tamoxifen treatment. *Lancet* 1994; **343:** 1291.
7. Bissett D, *et al.* Gynaecological monitoring during tamoxifen therapy. *Lancet* 1994; **344:** 1244.
8. Neven P, Vergote I. Should tamoxifen users be screened for endometrial lesions? *Lancet* 1998; **351:** 155–7.
9. Stearns V, Gelmann EP. Does tamoxifen cause cancer in humans? *J Clin Oncol* 1998; **16:** 779–92.
10. Fisher B, *et al.* Tamoxifen for prevention of breast cancer: report of the National Surgical Adjuvant Breast and Bowel Project P-1 Study. *J Natl Cancer Inst* 1998; **90:** 1371–88.
11. Bergman L, *et al.* Risk and prognosis of endometrial cancer after tamoxifen for breast cancer. *Lancet* 2000; **356:** 881–7.
12. American College of Obstetrics and Gynaecologists. ACOG Committee Opinion: tamoxifen and endometrial cancer. *Int J Gynaecol Obstet* 1996; **53:** 197–9.
13. Barakat RR, *et al.* Effect of adjuvant tamoxifen on the endometrium in women with breast cancer: a prospective study using office endometrial biopsy. *J Clin Oncol* 2000; **18:** 3459–63.
14. Gerber B, *et al.* Effects of adjuvant tamoxifen on the endometrium in postmenopausal women with breast cancer: a prospective long-term study using transvaginal ultrasound. *J Clin Oncol* 2000; **18:** 3464–70.
15. Aleem FA, Predanic M. Endometrial changes in patients on tamoxifen. *Lancet* 1995; **346:** 1292–3.
16. Gardner FJE, *et al.* Endometrial protection from tamoxifen-stimulated changes by a levonorgestrel-releasing intrauterine system: a randomised controlled trial. *Lancet* 2000; **356:** 1711–17.
17. Wysowski DK, *et al.* Uterine sarcoma associated with tamoxifen use. *N Engl J Med* 2002; **346:** 1832–3.

**Effects on the blood.** Pancytopenia developed shortly after beginning tamoxifen therapy in an elderly woman, and persisted for some years;[1] the patient eventually developed very severe leucopenia and died of infection.

1. Miké V, *et al.* Fatal neutropenia associated with long-term tamoxifen therapy. *Lancet* 1994; **344:** 541–2.

**Effects on blood lipids.** Tamoxifen has been reported to have a generally favourable effect on serum lipid profiles.[1] However, some cases of increased serum triglycerides in women with pre-existing hypertriglyceridaemia have been reported. Pancreatitis has also resulted. It has been suggested that tamoxifen should be used with caution in patients with hypertriglyceridaemia.[2,3]

1. Love RR, *et al.* Effects of tamoxifen on cardiovascular risk factors in postmenopausal women. *Ann Intern Med* 1991; **115:** 860–4.
2. Kanel KT, *et al.* Delayed severe hypertriglyceridaemia from tamoxifen. *N Engl J Med* 1997; **337:** 281.
3. Colls BM, George PM. Severe hypertriglyceridaemia and hypercholesterolaemia associated with tamoxifen use. *Clin Oncol* 1998; **10:** 270–1.

**Effects on the cardiovascular system.** ISCHAEMIC HEART DISEASE. For discussion of whether the effects of tamoxifen on lipid profiles can alter the incidence of ischaemic heart disease, see Cardiovascular Disorders under Uses and Administration, below.

STROKE. An excess risk of stroke was seen in tamoxifen compared with placebo recipients (5 cases versus 1) in a study of adjuvant tamoxifen.[1] A non-statistically significant increase in stroke was seen in a study on the use of tamoxifen for breast cancer prevention (0.5 excess cases per 1000 women per year).[2]

1. Dignam JJ, Fisher B. Occurrence of stroke with tamoxifen in NSABP B-24. *Lancet* 2000; **355:** 848–9.
2. Fisher B, *et al.* Tamoxifen for prevention of breast cancer: report of the National Surgical Adjuvant Breast and Bowel Project P-1 study. *J Natl Cancer Inst* 1998; **90:** 1371–88.

THROMBOEMBOLISM. A case control study,[1] involving 25 cases of deep-vein thrombosis or pulmonary embolism among more than 10 000 women with breast cancer, suggested that current use of tamoxifen was associated with an estimated relative risk of developing idiopathic venous thromboembolism of 7.1 (95% confidence interval 1.5 to 33). Past use of tamoxifen was not associated with a materially increased risk. In a randomised placebo-controlled study, there was an increase in pulmonary emboli in women receiving tamoxifen for cancer prevention (excess of 0.46 cases per 1000 women per year).[2] The fatality rate from pulmonary emboli in tamoxifen recipients was about 17%. In this study, there was also a trend towards more deep-vein thrombosis in tamoxifen recipients. In another controlled study[3] of breast cancer prevention, tamoxifen approximately doubled the risk of developing a major thromboembolic event such as pulmonary embolism, deep-vein thrombosis, or retinal thrombosis.

1. Meier CR, Jick H. Tamoxifen and risk of idiopathic venous thromboembolism. *Br J Clin Pharmacol* 1998; **45:** 608–12.
2. Fisher B, *et al.* Tamoxifen for prevention of breast cancer: report of the National Surgical Adjuvant Breast and Bowel Project P-1 study. *J Natl Cancer Inst* 1998; **90:** 1371–88.
3. Duggan C, *et al.* Inherited and acquired risk factors for venous thromboembolic disease among women taking tamoxifen to prevent breast cancer. *J Clin Oncol* 2003; **21:** 3588–93.

**Effects on the eyes.** Tamoxifen has been reported to be associated with decreased visual acuity, corneal opacities and cataract, and retinopathy. The latter is sometimes progressive although in most cases it has shown improvement once the drug was discontinued.[1] A prospective study in 63 patients receiving tamoxifen 20 mg daily found evidence of decreased visual acuity, macular oedema, and retinal opacities in 4, occurring after 10 to 35 months of therapy.[2] A small excess risk of developing cataracts (3.1 extra per year per 1000 women) and of requiring cataract surgery (1.7 per year per 1000 women) was found in women receiving tamoxifen for up to 5 years to reduce the risk of breast cancer when compared with women receiving placebo.[3] Studies *in vitro* have suggested that cataract formation may be due to inhibition of chloride channels in the lens by tamoxifen or its hydroxy metabolite.[4]

1. Mihm LM, Barton TL. Tamoxifen-induced ocular toxicity. *Ann Pharmacother* 1994; **28:** 740–2.
2. Pavlidis NA, *et al.* Clear evidence that long-term, low-dose tamoxifen treatment can induce ocular toxicity. *Cancer* 1992; **69:** 2961–4.

3. Fisher B, *et al.* Tamoxifen for prevention of breast cancer: report of the National Surgical Adjuvant Breast and Bowel Project P-1 study. *J Natl Cancer Inst* 1998; **90:** 1371–88.
4. Zhang JJ, *et al.* Tamoxifen blocks chloride channels: a possible mechanism for cataract formation. *J Clin Invest* 1994; **94:** 1690–7.

**Effects on the genito-urinary system.** Persistent nocturnal priapism was reported in a man receiving tamoxifen 20 mg daily.[1] Symptoms abated within 24 hours of withdrawing the drug. Impotence has been reported in men receiving tamoxifen, and has been attributed to a paradoxical oestrogenic effect.[2]

1. Fernando IN, Tobias JS. Priapism in patient on tamoxifen. *Lancet* 1989; **i:** 436.
2. Collinson MP, *et al.* Two case reports of tamoxifen as a cause of impotence in male subjects with carcinoma of the breast. *Breast* 1993; **2:** 48–9.

**Effects on the liver.** Cholestasis and increased liver enzyme values have been reported following use of tamoxifen in a 75-year-old patient.[1] Enzyme activity rose again on rechallenge with tamoxifen. Fatal hepatocellular necrosis and agranulocytosis, possibly exacerbated by continuing to take the drug once jaundice developed, has also been reported;[2] the authors noted that 4 cases of hepatic failure (3 fatal) and 5 cases of hepatitis (1 fatal) had been reported to the UK Committee on Safety of Medicines. Patients taking tamoxifen may also develop steatohepatitis,[3-6] which must be distinguished from alcohol-induced liver disease. Steatohepatitis is reversible on withdrawal of tamoxifen.[3,5,6] Bezafibrate has been tried to prevent progression of steatohepatitis and permit continued use of tamoxifen.[7]

For a report of peliosis hepatis and liver haemorrhage in a patient receiving tamoxifen and warfarin, see under Interactions, below.

For reference to the development of liver cancer in *animals* given tamoxifen, see Carcinogenicity, above.

1. Blackburn AM, *et al.* Tamoxifen and liver damage. *BMJ* 1984; **289:** 288.
2. Ching CK, *et al.* Tamoxifen-associated hepatocellular damage and agranulocytosis. *Lancet* 1992; **339:** 940.
3. Pratt DS, *et al.* Tamoxifen-induced steatohepatitis. *Ann Intern Med* 1995; **123:** 236.
4. Van Hoof M, *et al.* Tamoxifen-induced steatohepatitis. *Ann Intern Med* 1996; **124:** 855–6.
5. Ogawa Y, *et al.* Tamoxifen-induced fatty liver in patients with breast cancer. *Lancet* 1998; **351:** 725.
6. Oien KA, *et al.* Cirrhosis with steatohepatitis after adjuvant tamoxifen. *Lancet* 1999; **353:** 36–7.
7. Saibara T, *et al.* Bezafibrate for tamoxifen-induced non-alcoholic steatohepatitis. *Lancet* 1999; **353:** 1802.

**Effects on the ovaries.** Ovarian cysts are relatively common as an adverse effect in women receiving adjuvant tamoxifen: a study[1] in 95 such women reported the development of ovarian cysts in 6 of 16 (37.5%) who were premenopausal and in 5 of 79 postmenopausal women (6.3%). In 2 of the premenopausal women the cysts were complex. Two women underwent laparotomy for persistent cysts that were found to be benign, and 1 for leiomyoma; the cysts in the other 8 women resolved after withdrawal of tamoxifen. A study of 142 breast cancer patients receiving tamoxifen found ovarian cysts in 24 patients after treatment. Cyst development was more common in pre-menopausal women, patients with high oestrogen levels, and patients who did not receive high-dose chemotherapy.[2] There is a little evidence that tamoxifen increases the risk of ovarian cancer (see Carcinogenicity, above).

1. Shushan A, *et al.* Ovarian cysts in premenopausal and postmenopausal tamoxifen-treated women with breast cancer. *Am J Obstet Gynecol* 1996; **174:** 141–4.
2. Mourits MJE, *et al.* Ovarian cysts in women receiving tamoxifen for breast cancer. *Br J Cancer* 1999; **79:** 1761–64.

**Effects on the skin and hair.** Purpuric leucocytoclastic vasculitis has been reported in a patient receiving tamoxifen.[1] Withdrawal of the drug resulted in complete clearance of the lesions within 2 weeks; on re-introduction purpura developed again within a few days. The results suggest that tamoxifen can produce immune-mediated vascular damage.

In another report a patient with white hair developed darkening and repigmentation of the hair after about 2½ years of tamoxifen therapy.[2] Alopecia has also been reported in women receiving tamoxifen,[3,4] and in older patients the follicle may not recover.[3]

1. Drago F, *et al.* Tamoxifen and purpuric vasculitis. *Ann Intern Med* 1990; **112:** 965–6.
2. Hampson JP, *et al.* Tamoxifen-induced hair colour change. *Br J Dermatol* 1995; **132:** 483–4.
3. Gateley CA, Bundred NJ. Alopecia and breast disease. *BMJ* 1997; **314:** 481.
4. Ayoub J-PM, *et al.* Tamoxifen-induced female androgenetic alopecia in a patient with breast cancer. *Ann Intern Med* 1997; **126:** 745–6.

## Precautions

All patients being considered for treatment with tamoxifen should be assessed for any increased risk of thromboembolism. Tamoxifen should not be used for treatment of infertility or the prophylaxis of breast cancer in women with a history of thromboembolic events. When used to treat breast cancer in such women, the risks and benefits should be considered; in some patients, especially those receiving cytotoxic drugs, prophylactic anticoagulation may be justified. Care is also needed during or immediately after major surgery or prolonged immobility; all patients should receive thrombosis prophylactic measures. For patients being treated for infertility tamoxifen should be stopped at least 6 weeks before surgery or long-term immobility and only restarted when the patient is fully mobile. Patients should be made aware of the symptoms of thromboembolism and advised to report sudden breathlessness or any pain in the calf of one leg. Tamoxifen should be withdrawn immediately in any patient developing thromboembolism and anti-thrombosis measures initiated. Treatment should not usually be restarted for infertility therapy but the resumed use of tamoxifen with prophylactic anticoagulation may be justified in selected patients with breast cancer.

Women treated with tamoxifen should have routine gynaecological monitoring, and any abnormal symptoms such as menstrual irregularities, abnormal vaginal bleeding or discharge, or pelvic pain should be investigated (see also under Carcinogenicity, above). Periodic complete blood counts and liver function tests have been suggested.

**Breast feeding.** Tamoxifen was shown to inhibit lactation in 60 puerperal women.[1] The manufacturers recommend that it should not be given to lactating women.

1. Masala A, *et al.* Inhibition of lactation and inhibition of prolactin release after mechanical breast stimulation in puerperal women given tamoxifen or placebo. *Br J Obstet Gynaecol* 1978; **85:** 134–7.

**Porphyria.** Tamoxifen has been associated with acute attacks of porphyria and is considered unsafe in porphyric patients.

**Pregnancy.** Tamoxifen is contra-indicated in pregnancy. Ambiguous genitalia have been reported in an infant exposed to tamoxifen *in utero*, although no causal link was demonstrated.[1] Another infant was born with Goldenhar's syndrome (oculoauriculovertebral dysplasia) following exposure to tamoxifen throughout a 26-week pregnancy.[2] The mother had also taken cocaine and marijuana during the first 6 weeks of pregnancy, and a bone scan using technetium Tc99m medronate had been performed. The US manufacturer of tamoxifen (Zeneca USA) was aware of 50 pregnancies in patients taking tamoxifen, resulting in 19 normal births, 8 terminations, 13 unknown outcomes and 10 infants with fetal or neonatal abnormalities.[2]

Tamoxifen has also been used to stimulate ovulation in women with luteal phase dysfunction. In one study tamoxifen was given to 40 women, resulting in 14 pregnancies. Although 9 infants were born with no congenital abnormalities, there were 5 spontaneous abortions, which the authors felt was unacceptably high.[3] Another study, using lower doses of tamoxifen (in some cases sequentially with clomifene), reported 32 pregnancies and only 3 spontaneous abortions in 65 treated patients.[4]

1. Tewari K, *et al.* Ambiguous genitalia in infant exposed to tamoxifen in utero. *Lancet* 1997; **350:** 183.
2. Cullins SL, *et al.* Goldenhar's syndrome associated with tamoxifen given to the mother during gestation. *JAMA* 1994; **271:** 1905–6.
3. Ruiz-Velasco V, *et al.* Chemical inducers of ovulation: comparative results. *Int J Fertil* 1979; **24:** 61–64.
4. Wu CH. Less miscarriage in pregnancy following tamoxifen treatment of infertile patients with luteal phase dysfunction as compared to clomiphene treatment. *Early Pregnancy* 1997; **3:** 301–5.

**Radiotherapy.** There are reports of radiation recall, with erythema at the site of previous radiotherapy, in patients receiving tamoxifen.[1,2]

1. Parry BR. Radiation recall induced by tamoxifen. *Lancet* 1992; **340:** 49.
2. Extermann M, *et al.* Radiation recall in a patient with breast cancer treated for tuberculosis. *Eur J Clin Pharmacol* 1995; **48:** 77–8.

## Interactions

There is a risk of increased anticoagulant effect if tamoxifen is given with coumarin anticoagulants. Conversely, use with cytotoxic drugs may increase the risk of thromboembolic events; prophylactic anticoagulation should be considered. Tamoxifen increases the dopaminergic effect of bromocriptine.

**Allopurinol.** For reference to exacerbation of hepatotoxicity when tamoxifen was given with allopurinol, see under Allopurinol, p.413.

**Antibacterials.** *Rifampicin* was found to decrease plasma concentrations of tamoxifen in 10 healthy subjects. This was thought to be due to induction of cytochrome P450 isoenzyme CYP3A4 by rifampicin.[1]

1. Kivistö KT, *et al.* Tamoxifen and toremifene concentrations in plasma are greatly decreased by rifampin. *Clin Pharmacol Ther* 1998; **64:** 648–54.

**Anticoagulants.** A potentially life-threatening interaction between tamoxifen and *warfarin*, with marked prolongation of prothrombin times, haematuria, and haematoma, has been reported in a number of cases.[1-3] It has been suggested that in addition to enhancement of the effects of warfarin, competition for the same metabolic enzyme systems might reduce the activity of tamoxifen against tumours,[2] but such a suggestion remains speculative.

Peliosis hepatis and fatal liver haemorrhage have been reported in a patient who was receiving tamoxifen with warfarin and a liothyronine-levothyroxine preparation.[4]

1. Lodwick R, *et al.* Life threatening interaction between tamoxifen and warfarin. *BMJ* 1987; **295:** 1141.
2. Tenni P, *et al.* Life threatening interaction between tamoxifen and warfarin. *BMJ* 1989; **298:** 93.
3. Ritchie LD, Grant SMT. Tamoxifen-warfarin interaction: the Aberdeen hospitals drug file. *BMJ* 1989; **298:** 1253.
4. Loomus GN, *et al.* A case of peliosis hepatis in association with tamoxifen therapy. *Am J Clin Pathol* 1983; **80:** 881–3.

**Antineoplastics.** *Aminoglutethimide* reduces serum tamoxifen concentrations, possibly by increasing its metabolism.[1] For mention of an increased risk of haemolytic-uraemic syndrome in patients who received therapy with tamoxifen and *mitomycin* see Effects on the Kidneys, under Mitomycin, p.574. Tamoxifen is reported to reduce plasma concentrations of *letrozole*, see p.565.

1. Lien EA, *et al.* Decreased serum concentrations of tamoxifen and its metabolites induced by aminoglutethimide. *Cancer Res* 1990; **50:** 5851–7.

**Immunosuppressants.** For the results of a study *in vitro* suggesting that tamoxifen might inhibit the metabolism of *tacrolimus*, see under Interactions of Tacrolimus, p.1364.

**Neuromuscular blockers.** For reference to prolonged neuromuscular blockade in a patient given *atracurium* while receiving tamoxifen, see p.1400.

## Pharmacokinetics

Peak plasma concentrations of tamoxifen occur 4 to 7 hours after an oral dose. It is extensively protein bound. Plasma clearance is reported to be biphasic and the terminal half-life may be up to 7 days. It is extensively metabolised, the major serum metabolite being *N*-desmethyltamoxifen; the half-life of this metabolite at steady state is about 14 days. Several of the metabolites are stated to have similar pharmacological activity to the parent compound. Tamoxifen is excreted slowly in the faeces, mainly as conjugates. Small amounts are excreted in urine. Tamoxifen appears to undergo enterohepatic circulation.

## Uses and Administration

Tamoxifen is an oestrogen antagonist with actions similar to those of clomifene citrate (see p.1543). It may also inhibit the production or release of cellular growth factors and induce apoptosis. It is used in the adjuvant endocrine therapy of early breast cancer, in the palliative treatment of advanced disease, and for prophylaxis in women at increased risk. It has been tried in some other malignancies including tumours of the ovary and in malignant melanoma. Tamoxifen is also used to stimulate ovulation in women with anovulatory infertility. See also the cross-references below.

Tamoxifen is given by mouth as the citrate but doses are calculated in terms of the base; tamoxifen citrate 15.2 mg is approximately equivalent to 10 mg of tamoxifen. In the treatment of breast cancer, usual doses are tamoxifen 20 mg daily, in 2 divided doses or as a single daily dose. Doses of up to 40 mg daily may be given but no additional benefit has been demonstrated. Adjuvant therapy is normally continued for up to 5 years, although the optimum duration is still uncertain (p.514). To reduce breast cancer incidence in women at high risk of the disease, the licensed dose of tamoxifen is 20 mg daily for 5 years.

In the treatment of anovulatory infertility the usual dose is tamoxifen 20 mg daily on days 2 to 5 of the menstrual cycle, increased if necessary in subsequent cycles up to 80 mg daily. In women with irregular menstruation the initial course may be begun on any day, and a second course begun at a higher dose after 45 days if there has been no response. If the patient responds with menstruation, subsequent courses may begin on day 2 of the cycle.

◊ Reviews.

1. Osborne CK. Tamoxifen in the treatment of breast cancer. *N Engl J Med* 1998; **339:** 1609–18.
2. Mitlak BH, Cohen FJ. Selective estrogen receptor modulators: a look ahead. *Drugs* 1999; **57:** 653–63.

**Breast disorders, non-malignant.** GYNAECOMASTIA. Tamoxifen, usually in doses of 10 mg twice daily, has been reported to be effective[1-4] in relieving pain and swelling in men or pubertal boys with gynaecomastia (p.1546). Tamoxifen has been recommended as a drug of choice in patients requiring drug therapy, given for 3 months to see if a response occurs.[5]

1. Jefferys DB. Painful gynaecomastia treated with tamoxifen. *BMJ* 1979; **1:** 1119–20.
2. Hooper PD. Puberty gynaecomastia. *J R Coll Gen Pract* 1985; **35:** 142.
3. McDermott MT, *et al.* Tamoxifen therapy for painful idiopathic gynecomastia. *South Med J* 1990; **83:** 1283–5.
4. Ting AC, *et al.* Comparison of tamoxifen with danazol in the management of idiopathic gynecomastia. *Am Surg* 2000; **66:** 38–40.
5. Braunstein GD. Gynecomastia. *N Engl J Med* 1993; **328:** 490–5.


MASTALGIA. Tamoxifen 20 mg daily has been shown to be effective in patients with both cyclic and non-cyclic mastalgia,[1] and improvement has also been reported at a lower dose of 10 mg daily.[2] However, there is concern about the use of tamoxifen in otherwise healthy premenopausal women,[3-5] particularly since many patients relapse on withdrawal,[2] and it has been recommended[6,7] that tamoxifen be reserved for patients who fail to respond to other drugs (see p.1546).


1. Fentiman IS, *et al.* Double-blind controlled trial of tamoxifen therapy for mastalgia. *Lancet* 1986; **i:** 287–8.
2. Fentiman IS, *et al.* Studies of tamoxifen in women with mastalgia. *Br J Clin Pract* 1989; **43** (suppl 68): 34–6.
3. Anonymous. Tamoxifen for benign breast disease. *Lancet* 1986; **i:** 305.
4. Smallwood JA, Taylor I. Tamoxifen for mastalgia. *Lancet* 1986; **i:** 680–1.
5. Fentiman IS, *et al.* Tamoxifen for mastalgia. *Lancet* 1986; **i:** 681.
6. Gateley CA, Mansel RE. Management of the painful and nodular breast. *Br Med Bull* 1991; **47:** 284–94.
7. Anonymous. Cyclical breast pain: what works and what doesn't. *Drug Ther Bull* 1992; **30:** 1–3.


**Cardiovascular disorders.** Tamoxifen has been reported to have a generally favourable effect on lipid profiles (see Effects on Blood Lipids, under Adverse Effects, above) suggesting it may have cardiovascular benefits. A cohort study of adjuvant tamoxifen found that the drug reduced the incidence of myocardial infarction,[1] and a randomised study of the same therapy also showed a trend towards a decrease in mortality from coronary heart disease.[2] However, in a much larger breast cancer prevention trial, tamoxifen did not reduce the risk of, and mortality from, ischaemic heart disease, neither of which differed between placebo and tamoxifen recipients.[3,4] This lack of difference was independent of pre-existing cardiovascular disease.[4]


1. McDonald CC, *et al.* Scottish Cancer Trials Breast Group. Cardiac and vascular morbidity in women receiving adjuvant tamoxifen for breast cancer in a randomised trial. *BMJ* 1995; **311:** 977–80.
2. Costantino JP, *et al.* Coronary heart disease mortality and adjuvant tamoxifen therapy. *J Natl Cancer Inst* 1997; **89:** 776–82.
3. Fisher B, *et al.* Tamoxifen for prevention of breast cancer: report of the National Surgical Adjuvant Breast and Bowel Project P-1 study. *J Natl Cancer Inst* 1998; **90:** 1371–88.
4. Reis SE, *et al.* Cardiovascular effects of tamoxifen in women with and without heart disease: breast cancer prevention trial. *J Natl Cancer Inst* 2001; **93:** 16–21.


**Disorders related to the menstrual cycle.** Apart from cyclic mastalgia (see above) tamoxifen has been used in a number of cases in which disorders were linked to the hormonal changes of the menstrual cycle, including menorrhagia due to myometrial hypertrophy,[1] an auto-immune dermatitis due to post-ovulatory rises in serum progesterone,[2,3] and premenstrual migraine.[4] However, tamoxifen was thought to be a cause of recurrent migraines in another patient, because of its action at oestrogen receptors.[5]


1. Fraser IS. Menorrhagia due to myometrial hypertrophy: treatment with tamoxifen. *Obstet Gynecol* 1987; **70:** 505–6.
2. Wojnarowska F, *et al.* Progesterone-induced erythema multiforme. *J R Soc Med* 1985; **78:** 407–8.
3. Stephens CJM, *et al.* Autoimmune progesterone dermatitis responding to tamoxifen. *Br J Dermatol* 1989; **121:** 135–7.
4. O'Dea JPK, Davis EH. Tamoxifen in the treatment of menstrual migraine. *Neurology* 1990; **40:** 1470–1.
5. Mathew P, Fung F. Recapitulation of menstrual migraine with tamoxifen. *Lancet* 1999; **353:** 467–8.


**Infertility.** Tamoxifen is reported to be as effective as clomifene in the treatment of anovulatory infertility (p.1316) in women,[1,2] and may be useful in women in whom abnormal cervical mucus acts as a barrier to spermatozoa.[3] In infertile men, however, results are reportedly contradictory, with some studies reporting increase in sperm density and improved pregnancy rates while others failed to demonstrate any effect.[4] A systematic review, originally published in 1996, of 5 trials in men with oligo/asthenospermia showed that although anti-oestrogen therapy improved serum testosterone concentrations, there was no increase in the overall pregnancy rate.[5]


1. Messinis IE, Nillius SJ. Comparison between tamoxifen and clomiphene for induction of ovulation. *Acta Obstet Gynecol Scand* 1982; **61:** 377–9.
2. Boostanfar R, *et al.* A prospective randomized trial comparing clomiphene citrate with tamoxifen citrate for ovulation induction. *Fertil Steril* 2001; **75:** 1024–6.
3. Roumen FJME, *et al.* Treatment of infertile women with a deficient postcoital test with two antiestrogens: clomiphene and tamoxifen. *Fertil Steril* 1984; **41:** 237–43.
4. Howards SS. Treatment of male infertility. *N Engl J Med* 1995; 312–17.
5. Vandekerckhove P, *et al.* Clomiphene or tamoxifen for idiopathic oligo/asthenospermia,. Available in The Cochrane Library; Issue 3. Oxford: Update Software; 2002.


**Malignant neoplasms.** For reference to the use of tamoxifen in malignant neoplasms of breast, ovary, and in cutaneous melanoma, see p.514, p.520, and p.522. The most common use of tamoxifen is for the endocrine therapy of oestrogen-receptor positive early or advanced breast cancer, where there seems to be a clear benefit. How long such therapy should be continued, however, remains uncertain although recent results suggest that continuing therapy beyond 5 years may not increase the overall benefit. Extension of tamoxifen use to the attempted prophylaxis of breast cancer has proved controversial (see p.515). Nonetheless, evidence that tamoxifen can reduce short-term incidence of breast cancer in some women at increased risk has been seen, and tamoxifen has been approved for such use in the USA.

Despite some positive data, tamoxifen does not appear to be effective in the treatment of hepatocellular carcinoma (see p.518).

**Osteoporosis.** Tamoxifen has been reported to have favourable effects on bone mass,[1-3] but any general role in the prevention of osteoporosis (p.763) seems unlikely given concerns about the carcinogenicity of tamoxifen. The effects are reported to be comparable in magnitude to those of calcium supplementation, and less than those of oestrogens (see also p.1541) or bisphosphonates. It has been suggested that such an effect on bone would provide an additional benefit in women receiving tamoxifen for the prophylaxis of breast cancer,[4] although others dispute the benefits.[5]


1. Love RR, *et al.* Effects of tamoxifen on bone mineral density in postmenopausal women with breast cancer. *N Engl J Med* 1992; **326:** 852–6.
2. Love RR, *et al.* Effect of tamoxifen on lumbar spine bone mineral density in postmenopausal women after 5 years. *Arch Intern Med* 1994; **154:** 2585–8.
3. Grey AB, *et al.* The effect of the antiestrogen tamoxifen on bone mineral density in normal late postmenopausal women. *Am J Med* 1995; **99:** 636–41.
4. Powles TJ. The case for clinical trials of tamoxifen for prevention of breast cancer. *Lancet* 1992; **340:** 1145–7.
5. Fugh-Berman A, Epstein S. Tamoxifen: disease prevention or disease substitution? *Lancet* 1992; **340:** 1143–5.


## Preparations

***BP 2003:*** Tamoxifen Tablets;
***USP 27:*** Tamoxifen Citrate Tablets.

**Proprietary Preparations** (details are given in Part 3)
***Arg.:*** Crisafeno; Diemon; Farmifeno; Ginarsan; Nolvadex; Rolap; Tamofen; Tamoxis; Taxfeno; Trimetrox; ***Austral.:*** Estroxyn†; Genox; Kessar†; Nolvadex; Tamosin; Tamoxen; ***Austria:*** Ebefen; Kessar; Nolvadex; Tamax; Tamofen; Tamoplex; ***Belg.:*** Nolvadex; Tamizam; ***Braz.:*** Bioxifeno; Kessar; Nolvadex; Tamofen†; Tamooex; Tamoplex; Tamox; Tamoxin; Taxofen; Tecnotax; ***Canad.:*** Apo-Tamox; Nolvadex; Tamofen; Tamone†; ***Chile:*** Kessar; Nolvadex; Tamolem; Taxus; ***Denm.:*** Tamofen; ***Fin.:*** Nolvadex; Tadex; Tamexin; Tamofen; ***Fr.:*** Kessar; Nolvadex; Oncotam; Tamofene; ***Ger.:*** duratamoxifen†; Jenoxifen; Kessar; Nolvadex; Nourytam; Tamobeta†; Tamofen†; Tamokadin; Tamopham; Tamox; Tamoxasta; Tamoxigenat†; Tamoximerck; Tamoxistad; Zemide; ***Gr.:*** Adifen; Defarol; Kessar; Nolvadex; Puretam; Tamoplex; Zymoplex; ***Hong Kong:*** Apo-Tamox; Nolvadex; Tamifen; Tamofen†; Zitazonium; ***India:*** Mamofen; Nolvadex; ***Irl.:*** Clonoxifen†; Nolgen; Nolvadex; Tamofen; Tamox; ***Israel:*** Nolvadex; Tamofen; Tamoplex†; Tamoxen; Tamoxi; ***Ital.:*** Kessar; Ledertam; Nolvadex; Nomafen; Tamoxene; Virtamox; ***Malaysia:*** Genox; Nolvadex; Novofen; Tamoplex; Zitazonium; ***Mex.:*** Bilem; Cryoxifeno; Kessar; Nolvadex; Ralsifen-X; Tamofen†; Tamoxan†; Taxus; Tecnofen†; ***Neth.:*** Nolvadex; ***Norw.:*** Nolvadex; Tamofen†; ***NZ:*** Genox; Nolvadex; Tamofen; ***Port.:*** Nolvadex; Tamoxan; ***S.Afr.:*** Kessar; Nephedan; Nolvadex; Tamoplex; ***Singapore:*** Apo-Tamox; Nolvadex; Tamofen; Tamoplex†; ***Spain:*** Nolvadex; Oxeprax†; Sinmaren; ***Swed.:*** Nolvadex; Tamaxin†; ***Switz.:*** Kessar; Nolvadex; Tamec; ***Thai.:*** Nolvadex; Novofen; Tamofen; Tamoplex; Tuosomin; Zitazonium; ***UAE:*** Tamophar; ***UK:*** Emblon†; Nolvadex; Oestrifen†; Soltamox; Tamofen†; ***USA:*** Nolvadex.

---

## Tegafur *(BAN, USAN, rINN)*

FT-207; Ftorafur; MJF-12264; NSC-148958; WR-220066. 5-Fluoro-1-(tetrahydro-2-furyl)uracil; 5-Fluoro-1-(tetrahydro-2-furyl)pyrimidine-2,4(1*H*,3*H*)-dione.

$C_8H_9FN_2O_3 = 200.2.$
*CAS — 17902-23-7.*
*ATC — L01BC03.*

**Pharmacopoeias.** In *Chin.* and *Jpn.*

### Adverse Effects, Treatment, and Precautions

As for Fluorouracil, p.554.

Bone-marrow depression may be less severe with tegafur but gastrointestinal toxicity is often dose-limiting and central neurotoxicity is more common. Peripheral oedema and dyspnoea occur commonly. Increases in liver function test values are common and there are reports of fatal fulminant hepatitis. Liver function should be monitored in patients with hepatic impairment given tegafur; it should not be given in severe hepatic impairment.

### Interactions

Tegafur should not be used with drugs that inhibit dihydropyrimidine dehydrogenase; fatalities have occurred in patients given tegafur and sorivudine (see Antivirals under Interactions of Fluorouracil, p.555).

### Pharmacokinetics

Tegafur is well absorbed from the gastrointestinal tract after oral administration. Following an intravenous dose it is reported to have a prolonged plasma half-life of 6 to 16 hours. Tegafur appears to be slowly metabolised in the liver to fluorouracil (p.555), and some intracellular conversion to fluorouracil may also occur. It crosses the blood-brain barrier and is found in the CSF.

### Uses and Administration

Tegafur is considered to be an orally active prodrug of fluorouracil (p.555). It has been used in the management of a variety of malignant neoplasms including those of the breast, gallbladder, gastrointestinal tract, head and neck, liver, and pancreas. Tegafur has been given by mouth in doses up to 1 g/m$^2$ daily. It is often given with uracil (UFT). Tegafur 300 mg/m$^2$ daily, with uracil 672 mg/m$^2$ daily, may be given in 3 divided doses by mouth, together with calcium folinate, in the management of metastatic colorectal cancer. Doses are given for a cycle of 28 days, followed by 7 days without treatment. The drugs should be taken 1 hour before or after meals, and doses modified according to toxicity. Doses of tegafur 1 to 3 g/m$^2$ daily for 5 days have been given intravenously.

**Administration.** Tegafur is an orally active prodrug of fluorouracil. Although it has been given as a single agent, it is more commonly used with drugs that modify its bioavailability and toxicity.[1] These include drugs such as uracil and gimestat (5-chlorodihydropyrimidine, CDHP) which can increase fluorouracil concentrations by inhibition of dihydropyrimidine dehydrogenase, the enzyme responsible for its further catabolism,[1-3] and oxonic acid (otastat), which inhibits another enzyme, orotate pyrimidine phosphoribosyl transferase, thought to play a role in the gastrointestinal toxicity of fluorouracil and its prodrugs.[2]

UFT consists of tegafur and uracil in the optimal molar ratio 1:4.[1] It is available for the treatment of colorectal cancer (p.516)—for doses, see above. A preliminary analysis of a large trial comparing oral UFT and calcium folinate therapy with intravenous fluorouracil and calcium folinate found both regimens to be well tolerated with similar levels of toxicity.[4]

S-1 (TS-1, *Taiho Jpn*) is a combination of tegafur, gimestat and the potassium salt of oxonic acid in the molar ratio 10:4:10. It has been tried in gastric and colorectal cancers,[2,3,5] and initial results have suggested comparable activity to fluorouracil and calcium folinate in induction regimens, but the incidence of diarrhoea and stomatitis was reduced.


1. Adjei AA. A review of the pharmacology and clinical activity of new chemotherapy agents for the treatment of colorectal cancer. *Br J Clin Pharmacol* 1999; **48:** 265–77.
2. Sakata Y, *et al.* Late phase II study of novel oral fluoropyrimidine anticancer drug S-1 (1 M tegafur-0.4 M gimestat-1 M otastat potassium) in advanced gastric cancer patients. *Eur J Cancer* 1998; **34:** 1715–20.
3. Sugimachi K, *et al.* An early phase II study of oral S-1, a newly developed 5-fluorouracil derivative for advanced and recurrent gastrointestinal cancers. *Oncology* 1999; **57:** 202–10.
4. Smith R, *et al.* UFT plus calcium folinate vs 5-FU plus calcium folinate in colon cancer. *Oncology (Huntingt)* 1999; **13** (suppl 3): 44–7.
5. Osugi H, *et al.* Oral fluoropyrimidine anticancer drug TS-1 for gastric cancer patients with peritoneal dissemination. *Oncol Rep* 2002; **9:** 811–15.


## Preparations

**Proprietary Preparations** (details are given in Part 3)
***Austria:*** Ftoralon; ***Hong Kong:*** Ftoral†; Futraful†; ***Israel:*** Ftoral; ***Ital.:*** Citofur; ***Spain:*** Utefos.

**Multi-ingredient:** ***Arg.:*** Asofurtal; UFT; ***Austria:*** UFT; ***Belg.:*** UFT; ***Braz.:*** UFT; ***Denm.:*** Uftoral; ***Fr.:*** UFT; ***Ger.:*** UFT; ***Hong Kong:*** UFT; ***Israel:*** UFT; ***Ital.:*** UFT; ***Jpn:*** UFT; ***Malaysia:*** UFT; ***Mex.:*** UFT; ***Norw.:*** UFT; ***Port.:*** UFT; ***S.Afr.:*** UFT; ***Singapore:*** UFT; ***Spain:*** UFT; ***Swed.:*** UFT; ***Thai.:*** UFT; ***UK:*** Uftoral.

---

## Temoporfin *(BAN, USAN, rINN)*

EF-9; mTHPC; Temoporfina; *meso*-Tetrahydroxyphenylchlorin; *meta*-Tetrahydroxyphenylchlorin. 3,3′,3″,3‴-(7,8-Dihydroporphyrin-5,10,15,20-tetrayl)tetraphenol; 7,8-Dihydro-5,10,15,20-tetrakis(3-hydroxyphenyl)porphyrin.

$C_{44}H_{32}N_4O_4 = 680.7.$
*CAS — 122341-38-2.*

### Profile

Temoporfin is a porphyrin derivative used palliatively as a photosensitiser in the photodynamic therapy (p.581) of head and neck cancers (p.517). It is also under investigation in the treatment of various other malignant neoplasms. Temoporfin is given by slow intravenous injection over at least 6 minutes, at a dose of 150 micrograms/kg. This is followed 96 hours later by activation using a laser tuned to a wavelength of 652 nanometres for about 200 seconds, sufficient to supply a dose of 20 J/cm$^2$. Treatment may be repeated once after 4 weeks if necessary. Adverse effects of temoporfin include photosensitivity, local inflammatory reactions, and gastrointestinal disturbances. Patients should be advised to avoid direct sunlight or bright indoor light for 15 days, and to protect the injection site from light for at least 3 months if extravasation has occurred.

**Porphyria.** The use of temoporfin is contra-indicated in patients with porphyria.

**Use.** References.


1. Kubler AC, *et al.* Photodynamic therapy of primary nonmelanomatous skin tumours of the head and neck. *Lasers Surg Med* 1999; **25:** 60–8.
2. Baas P, *et al.* Photodynamic therapy with *meta*-tetrahydroxyphenylchlorin for basal cell carcinoma: a phase I/II study. *Br J Dermatol* 2001; **145:** 75–8.
3. Kubler AC, *et al.* Treatment of squamous cell carcinoma of the lip using Foscan-mediated photodynamic therapy. *Int J Oral Maxillofac Surg* 2001; **30:** 504–9.
4. Javaid B, *et al.* Photodynamic therapy (PDT) for oesophageal dysplasia and early carcinoma with mTHPC (m-tetrahydroxyphenyl chlorin): a preliminary study. *Lasers Med Sci* 2002; **17:** 51–6.
5. Friedberg JS, *et al.* A phase I study of Foscan-mediated photodynamic therapy and surgery in patients with mesothelioma. *Ann Thorac Surg* 2003; **75:** 952–9.

## Preparations

**Proprietary Preparations** (details are given in Part 3)
*UK:* Foscan.

## Temozolomide (BAN, USAN, rINN)

CCRG-81045; M&B-39831; NSC-362856; Sch-52365; Temozolomida. 3,4-Dihydro-3-methyl-4-oxoimidazo[5,1-*d*][1,2,3,5]-tetrazine-8-carboxamide.

$C_6H_6N_6O_2$ = 194.2.
*CAS — 85622-93-1.*
*ATC — L01AX03.*

### Adverse Effects, Treatment, and Precautions

For general discussions see Antineoplastics, p.492, p.495, and p.497. Myelosuppression is dose-limiting. The nadir of cell counts usually occurs 21 to 28 days after treatment, with recovery within the next 1 to 2 weeks. Patients over 70 years of age are thought to be more susceptible to severe myelosuppression. Other common adverse effects include gastrointestinal disturbances, headache, rashes, fever, and somnolence. Asthenia, dizziness, malaise, pain, pruritus, and paraesthesia have also been reported. Hypersensitivity reactions, including anaphylaxis, and erythema multiforme have been reported rarely. Temozolomide has carcinogenic, mutagenic, and teratogenic potential.

### Pharmacokinetics

Temozolomide is rapidly and completely absorbed from the gastrointestinal tract, with peak plasma concentrations occurring 0.5 to 1.5 hours after a dose. Food reduces the rate and extent of absorption. It readily crosses the blood-brain barrier and can be detected in the CSF. The plasma elimination half-life is 1.8 hours. Temozolomide undergoes spontaneous hydrolysis to its active metabolite 5-(3-methyl-1-triazeno)imidazole-4-carboxamide (MTIC), which is then further hydrolysed to active and inactive compounds. It is largely eliminated by the kidneys, about 5 to 10% as unchanged drug.

### Uses and Administration

Temozolomide is a prodrug that is converted to MTIC (see Pharmacokinetics, above), the active metabolite of dacarbazine (p.544). MTIC acts as an alkylating agent. Temozolomide is given by mouth and is licensed for the treatment of malignant gliomas such as glioblastoma multiforme and anaplastic astrocytoma, and malignant melanoma (below).

The usual dose for malignant gliomas in adults and children over 3 years of age is 200 mg/m$^2$ daily by mouth for 5 days, repeated every 28 days. In patients who have received previous courses of chemotherapy the dose should be reduced to 150 mg/m$^2$ for the first cycle of therapy, but may be increased for subsequent courses if there is no haematological toxicity. A dose of 200 mg/m$^2$ daily for 5 days every 28 days is also used for metastatic malignant melanoma.

**Malignant neoplasms.** Temozolomide has been studied[1-7] particularly in the management of malignant neoplasms of the brain (p.513). In the UK, patients with recurrent progressive malignant glioma who have failed first-line chemotherapy treatment with other agents (either because of lack of efficacy or because of side-effects) may be considered for treatment with temozolomide.[8]


1. Newlands ES, *et al.* Temozolomide: a review of its discovery, chemical properties, pre-clinical development and clinical trials. *Cancer Treat Rev* 1997; **23:** 35–61.
2. Bower M, *et al.* Multicentre CRC phase II trial of temozolomide in recurrent or progressive high-grade glioma. *Cancer Chemother Pharmacol* 1997; **40:** 484–8.
3. Estlin EJ, *et al.* Phase I study of temozolomide in paediatric patients with advanced cancer. *Br J Cancer* 1998; **78:** 652–61.
4. Yung WKA, *et al.* Multicenter phase II trial of temozolomide in patients with anaplastic astrocytoma or anaplastic oligoastrocytoma at first relapse. *J Clin Oncol* 1999; **17:** 2762–71.
5. Yung WK, *et al.* A phase II study of temozolomide vs procarbazine in patients with glioblastoma multiforme at first relapse. *Br J Cancer* 2000; **83:** 588–93.
6. Brada M, *et al.* Multicenter phase II trial of temozolomide in patients with glioblastoma multiforme at first relapse. *Ann Oncol* 2001; **12:** 259–66.
7. Dinnes J, *et al.* A rapid and systematic review of the effectiveness of temozolomide for the treatment of recurrent malignant glioma. *Br J Cancer* 2002; **86:** 501–5.
8. National Institute for Clinical Excellence. Guidance on the use of temozolomide for the treatment of recurrent malignant glioma (brain cancer) (issued April 2001). Available at: http://www.nice.org.uk/pdf/temozolomideguidance.pdf (accessed 30/06/04)


MELANOMA. Temozolomide has been studied[1,2] as a treatment for advanced metastatic melanoma (p.522). A phase III trial compared the overall survival-time in 305 patients treated with either oral temozolomide or intravenous dacarbazine in standard doses for up to 12 cycles of therapy. Temozolomide was found to be at least equivalent to dacarbazine in these patients, and there were no major differences in adverse effects.[2] However, median survival-times were short in both groups (7.7 months and 6.4 months respectively).


1. Bleehen NM, *et al.* Cancer research campaign phase II trial of temozolomide in metastatic melanoma. *J Clin Oncol* 1995; **13:** 910–13.
2. Middleton MR, *et al.* Randomized phase III study of temozolomide versus dacarbazine in the treatment of patients with advanced metastatic malignant melanoma. *J Clin Oncol* 2000; **18:** 158–66.


### Preparations

**Proprietary Preparations** (details are given in Part 3)
*Arg.:* Temodal; *Austral.:* Temodal; *Austria:* Temodal; *Belg.:* Temodal; *Braz.:* Temodal; *Canad.:* Temodal; *Chile:* Temodal; *Denm.:* Temodal; *Fin.:* Temodal; *Fr.:* Temodal; *Ger.:* Temodal; *Gr.:* Temodal; *Hong Kong:* Temodal; *Irl.:* Temodal; *Israel:* Temodal; *Ital.:* Temodal; *Mex.:* Temodal; *Neth.:* Temodal; *Norw.:* Temodal; *NZ:* Temodal; *Port.:* Temodal†; *S.Afr.:* Temoxol; *Singapore:* Temodal; *Spain:* Temodal; *Swed.:* Temodal; *Switz.:* Temodal; *Thai.:* Temodal; *UK:* Temodal; *USA:* Temodar.

## Teniposide (BAN, USAN, rINN)

ETP; NSC-122819; Tenipósido; VM-26. (5S,5aR,8aS,9R)-5,8,8a,9-Tetrahydro-5-(4-hydroxy-3,5-dimethoxyphenyl)-9-(4,6-*O*-thenylidene-β-D-glucopyranosyloxy)isobenzofuro[5,6-*f*][1,3]benzodioxol-6(5a*H*)-one.

$C_{32}H_{32}O_{13}S$ = 656.7.
*CAS — 29767-20-2.*
*ATC — L01CB02.*

**Stability.** Precipitation occurred repeatedly in preparations for infusion containing teniposide 200 micrograms/mL in either glucose 5% or sodium chloride 0.9% injection, although previously such preparations had been used uneventfully.[1] Dilution of teniposide solutions to 100 micrograms/mL or less reduced the frequency of the problem, which could not be attributed to a change in formulation and remained unexplained.


1. Strong DK, Morris LA. Precipitation of teniposide during infusion. *Am J Hosp Pharm* 1990; **47:** 512,518.


### Adverse Effects, Treatment, and Precautions

As for Etoposide, p.551. There is some evidence that teniposide may be a more potent mutagen and carcinogen than etoposide.

**Hypersensitivity.** The development of haemolytic anaemia and acute renal failure with tubular necrosis has been reported in a patient who developed an antibody to teniposide.[1] As with etoposide (p.552) hypersensitivity or infusion reactions occur, sometimes with the first dose, and may be severe;[2,3] the frequency may be as high as 13% in neuroblastoma patients.[2] Although it has been suggested that hypersensitivity reactions might be due to the polyethoxylated castor oil in the injection vehicle,[2] studies *in vitro* suggest that it is the drug rather than the vehicle that is responsible.[3]


1. Habibi B, *et al.* Immune hemolytic anemia and renal failure due to teniposide. *N Engl J Med* 1982; **306:** 1091–3.
2. Siddall SJ, *et al.* Anaphylactic reactions to teniposide. *Lancet* 1989; **i:** 394.
3. Carstensen H, *et al.* Teniposide-induced hypersensitivity reactions in children. *Lancet* 1989; **ii:** 55.


### Interactions

For a general outline of antineoplastic drug interactions, see p.498.

**Antiepileptics.** Clearance of teniposide was markedly increased by *phenytoin* or *phenobarbital*; the resultant decrease in systemic exposure to the antineoplastic might reduce its efficacy, and increased dosage would be needed in patients receiving anticonvulsants to guarantee equivalent exposure.[1]


1. Baker DK, *et al.* Increased teniposide clearance with concomitant anticonvulsant therapy. *J Clin Oncol* 1992; **10:** 311–15.


**Ciclosporin.** Use of ciclosporin with teniposide has been reported[1] to produce a decrease in the clearance of the latter, with increased terminal half-life, peak plasma concentrations, and toxicity.


1. Toffoli G, *et al.* Cyclosporin A as a multidrug-resistant modulator in patients with renal cell carcinoma treated with teniposide. *Br J Cancer* 1997; **75:** 715–21.


### Uses and Administration

Teniposide is an antineoplastic agent with general properties similar to those of etoposide (p.551). It has been given alone or with other antineoplastic agents in the treatment of refractory acute lymphoblastic leukaemia (p.506). Teniposide has been tried in various solid tumours including neuroblastoma (p.524), and retinoblastoma (p.524).

A variety of dosage regimens have been used, ranging from 30 mg/m$^2$ every 5 days, to 180 mg/m$^2$ weekly, as a single agent. Doses of 165 mg/m$^2$ twice weekly for 8 or 9 doses with cytarabine, or up to 250 mg/m$^2$ weekly for 4 to 8 weeks with vincristine and prednisone have been given in the treatment of refractory acute lymphoblastic leukaemia. Teniposide is given by slow intravenous infusion over at least 30 to 60 minutes, as a solution of up to 1 mg/mL in sodium chloride 0.9% injection or glucose 5% injection.

### Preparations

**Proprietary Preparations** (details are given in Part 3)
*Arg.:* Vumon; *Austral.:* Vumon; *Austria:* Vumon; *Belg.:* Vumon; *Braz.:* Vumon; *Canad.:* Vumon; *Chile:* Vumon; *Denm.:* Vumon†; *Fr.:* Vehem†; *Ger.:* VM 26; *Gr.:* Vumon; *Hong Kong:* Vumon; *Israel:* Vumon; *Ital.:* Vumon; *Malaysia:* Vumon; *Mex.:* Vumon; *Neth.:* Vumon; *NZ:* Vumon; *Port.:* Vumon; *S.Afr.:* Vumon; *Singapore:* Vumon; *Spain:* Vumon; *Swed.:* Vumon†; *USA:* Vumon.

## Tesmilifene Hydrochloride (USAN, rINNM)

BMS-217380-01; BMY-33419; DPPE. 2-[(α-Phenyl-*p*-tolyl)oxy]-triethylamine hydrochloride; *N,N*-Diethyl-2-[4-(phenylmethyl)-phenoxy]-ethanamine hydrochloride.

$C_{19}H_{25}NO,HCl$ = 319.9.
*CAS — 98774-23-3 (tesmilifene); 92981-78-7 (tesmilifene hydrochloride).*

### Profile

Tesmilifene hydrochloride is an intracellular histamine antagonist that appears to augment the antineoplastic activity of drugs such as the anthracyclines and taxanes. It is under investigation for the treatment of various cancers, including metastatic breast cancer, and hormone-refractory cancer of the prostate.

## Testolactone (USAN, rINN)

1-Dehydrotestololactone; NSC-23759; SQ-9538; Testolactona. D-Homo-17a-oxaandrosta-1,4-diene-3,17-dione.

$C_{19}H_{24}O_3$ = 300.4.
*CAS — 968-93-4.*

**Pharmacopoeias.** In *US.*

**USP 27** (Testolactone). A white to off-white, practically odourless, crystalline powder. Soluble 1 in 4050 of water; soluble in alcohol and in chloroform; slightly soluble in benzyl alcohol; insoluble in ether and in petroleum spirit. Store in airtight containers.

### Profile

Testolactone is a derivative of testosterone (see p.1569). It is reported to be an aromatase inhibitor that reduces peripheral oestrogen synthesis but has no significant androgenic activity. It has been used in the palliative treatment of advanced breast cancer in postmenopausal women (p.514).

The usual dose is 250 mg four times daily by mouth.

It should not be given to men with breast cancer.

Peripheral neuropathies have occurred in patients receiving testolactone; gastrointestinal disturbances, pain or oedema of the extremities, hypertension, rashes, and glossitis have also been reported.

**Congenital adrenal hyperplasia.** For mention of the use of testolactone with flutamide to block androgenic effects in congenital adrenal hyperplasia, see p.1078.

**Precocious puberty.** Encouraging results have been reported using testolactone in the treatment of 5 girls with precocious puberty (p.1318) due to the McCune-Albright syndrome.[1] Testolactone is an aromatase inhibitor and blocks the synthesis of oestrogens from androgens. Long-term therapy (for up to 5 years) was associated with continued benefit in many patients; however, signs of puberty were not always completely suppressed, in some cases perhaps because of difficulties in maintaining the dosage regimen.[2] Encouraging results were also obtained using testolactone with spironolactone in the treatment of familial precocious puberty in boys, although neither agent was successful when used alone.[3] Again, signs of a diminished response to longer-term therapy have occurred; in this case control was restored by addition of a gonadorelin analogue.[4] Another study[5] in 10 boys who were treated for at least 6 years with spironolactone and testolactone, with deslorelin added at the onset of secondary central precocious puberty, found normalisation in growth rate and bone maturation, and improvements in predicted adult height.


1. Feuillan PP, *et al.* Treatment of precocious puberty in the McCune-Albright syndrome with the aromatase inhibitor testolactone. *N Engl J Med* 1986; **315:** 1115–19.
2. Feuillan PP, *et al.* Long term testolactone therapy for precocious puberty in girls with the McCune-Albright syndrome. *J Clin Endocrinol Metab* 1993; **77:** 647–51.
3. Laue L, *et al.* Treatment of familial male precocious puberty with spironolactone and testolactone. *N Engl J Med* 1989; **320:** 496–502.
4. Laue L, *et al.* Treatment of familial male precocious puberty with spironolactone, testolactone, and deslorelin. *J Clin Endocrinol Metab* 1993; **76:** 151–5.
5. Leschek EW, *et al.* Six-year results of spironolactone and testolactone treatment of familial male-limited precocious puberty with addition of deslorelin after central puberty onset. *J Clin Endocrinol Metab* 1999; **84:** 175–8.


### Preparations

*USP 27:* Testolactone Tablets.

**Proprietary Preparations** (details are given in Part 3)
*Chile:* Teslac; *Ger.:* Fludestrin; *USA:* Teslac.

**Thiotepa** *(BAN, rINN)*

NSC-6396; TESPA; Thiophosphamide; Tiotepa; Triethylenethiophosphoramide; TSPA; WR-45312. Phosphorothioic tri(ethyleneamide); Tris(aziridin-1-yl)phosphine sulphide.

$C_6H_{12}N_3PS$ = 189.2.

*CAS — 52-24-4.*

*ATC — L01AC01.*

**Pharmacopoeias.** In *Br., Chin., Fr., Jpn,* and *US.*

**BP 2003** (Thiotepa). Fine white, odourless or almost odourless, crystalline flakes. M.p. 52° to 57°. Freely soluble in water, in alcohol, and in chloroform. Store at 2° to 8°. At higher temperatures it polymerises and becomes inactive.

**USP 27** (Thiotepa). Fine white, crystalline flakes, having a faint odour. M.p. 52° to 57°. Soluble 1 in 13 of water, 1 in about 8 of alcohol, 1 in about 2 of chloroform, and 1 in about 4 of ether. Store at 2° to 8° in airtight containers. Protect from light.

**Incompatibility.** Lyophilised thiotepa 1 mg/mL in glucose 5% was incompatible when mixed with solutions of cisplatin or minocycline hydrochloride.[1]

1. Trissel LA, Martinez JF. Compatibility of thiotepa (lyophilized) with selected drugs during simulated Y-site administration. *Am J Health-Syst Pharm* 1996; **53:** 1041–5.

**Stability.** A solution of a lyophilised thiotepa preparation 0.5 mg/mL in glucose 5% was considered to be stable (less than 10% loss of thiotepa) for 8 hours at both 4° and 23°.[1] After 24 hours losses ranged between about 10 and 17%. A higher thiotepa concentration (5 mg/mL) was stable for 3 days at 23° and 14 days at 4°. Another study found that solutions containing 1 or 3 mg/mL of thiotepa in sodium chloride 0.9% were stable for 24 hours at 25° and 48 hours at 8°, but solutions containing 0.5% thiotepa needed to be used immediately.[2]

1. Xu QA, *et al.* Stability of thiotepa (lyophilized) in 5% dextrose injection at 4 and 23°C. *Am J Health-Syst Pharm* 1996; **53:** 2728–30.
2. Murray KM, *et al.* Stability of thiotepa (lyophilized) in 0.9% sodium chloride injection. *Am J Health-Syst Pharm* 1997; **54:** 2588–91.

### Adverse Effects, Treatment, and Precautions

For general discussions, see Antineoplastics, p.492, p.495, and p.497.

Bone-marrow depression may be delayed; the nadir of white cell and platelet counts may occur up to 30 days after therapy has been discontinued. Bone-marrow depression has been reported after intravesical as well as parenteral use, and has occasionally been prolonged or fatal.

Gastrointestinal disturbances, fatigue, weakness, headache and dizziness, hypersensitivity reactions, blurred vision and conjunctivitis may occur. Amenorrhoea and impaired fertility have also been reported. Local irritation, and rarely frank chemical or haemorrhagic cystitis may follow intravesical instillation. Depigmentation of periorbital skin has occurred following the use of thiotepa eye drops. As with other alkylating agents, thiotepa is potentially mutagenic, teratogenic, and carcinogenic.

Thiotepa should be given with extreme care, if at all, to patients with pre-existing impairment of hepatic, renal, or bone-marrow function.

### Pharmacokinetics

The absorption of thiotepa from the gastrointestinal tract is incomplete and unreliable; variable absorption also occurs from intramuscular injection sites. Absorption through serous membranes such as the bladder and pleura occurs to some extent. After intravenous doses it is rapidly cleared from plasma, with an elimination half-life of about 2.4 hours. It is extensively metabolised: triethylenephosphoramide (TEPA), the primary metabolite, and some of the other metabolites have cytotoxic activity and are eliminated more slowly than the parent compound. It is excreted in the urine: less than 2% of a dose is reported to be present as unchanged drug or its primary metabolite.

### Uses and Administration

Thiotepa is an ethyleneimine compound whose antineoplastic effect is related to its alkylating action. It has generally been replaced by cyclophosphamide (p.542) or other drugs. It is not a vesicant and may be given by all parenteral routes, as well as directly into tumour masses.

Instillations of thiotepa may be used in the adjuvant treatment of superficial tumours of the bladder (p.512) and in the control of malignant effusions (p.512). It has been given parenterally in the palliative treatment of various solid tumours, including those of breast and ovary (p.514 and p.520). It has also been given intrathecally to patients with malignant meningeal disease, and has been used, in the form of eye drops, as an adjunct to the surgical removal of pterygium, to prevent recurrence (see p.574).

Thiotepa is given in a variety of dosage schedules. In general, initial doses to suit the individual patient are followed by maintenance doses given at intervals of 1 to 4 weeks. Blood counts are recommended before and during therapy and should continue for at least 3 weeks after stopping. Thiotepa should not be given if the white cell or platelet counts fall below acceptable levels (see also Bone-marrow Depression, p.496) and treatment should be stopped if the white cell count falls rapidly. Dosage should be reduced in patients with lesser degrees of leucopenia.

In the treatment of bladder cancer thiotepa in doses up to 60 mg may be instilled in 30 to 60 mL of sterile water or sodium chloride 0.9% into the bladder of a patient previously dehydrated for 8 to 12 hours, and retained if possible for 2 hours. The instillation may be repeated weekly for up to 4 weeks. Similar instillations have been given at intervals of 1 to 2 weeks, for up to 8 instillations in the prophylaxis of recurrence after surgical removal of bladder cancer. Single doses of 90 mg in 100 mL of sterile water have also been used prophylactically. For malignant effusions, doses of up to 60 mg of thiotepa in 20 to 60 mL of sterile water may be instilled after aspiration; in the USA the licensed dose is 600 to 800 micrograms/kg, a dose similar to that suggested for injection directly into tumours. Thiotepa for local use may be mixed with solutions of procaine and adrenaline.

Intramuscular and intravenous dosage regimens vary considerably; several regimens have used courses of 15 mg daily for 4 days. In the USA a licensed dose is 300 to 400 micrograms/kg given at 1- to 4-week intervals. A solution containing 1 mg/mL in sterile water has been tried intrathecally in doses of up to 10 mg given on alternate days, for up to 4 doses.

Thiotepa 0.05% in sterile Ringer's solution has been instilled as eye drops every 3 hours for up to 6 weeks following surgical removal of pterygium in order to reduce the likelihood of recurrence.

A dose of 60 mg weekly has been instilled into the urethra for the treatment of condylomata acuminata (genital warts). Topical application of thiotepa has also been used for condylomata.

### Preparations

***BP 2003:*** Thiotepa Injection;
***USP 27:*** Thiotepa for Injection.

**Proprietary Preparations** (details are given in Part 3)
***Belg.:*** Ledertepa†; ***Braz.:*** Onco Tiotepa†; ***Gr.:*** Ledertepa; ***Ital.:*** Thioplex; ***Neth.:*** Ledertepa; ***Spain:*** Onco Tiotepa; ***USA:*** Thioplex.

## Tioguanine *(BAN, rINN)*

NSC-752; 6-TG; Thioguanine *(USAN)*; 6-Thioguanine; Tioguanina; WR-1141. 2-Aminopurine-6(1*H*)-thione; 2-Amino-6-mercaptopurine; 2-Aminopurine-6-thiol.

$C_5H_5N_5S$ = 167.2.

*CAS — 154-42-7 (anhydrous tioguanine); 5580-03-0 (tioguanine hemihydrate).*

*ATC — L01BB03.*

**Pharmacopoeias.** In *Br., Chin.,* and *US.*

**BP 2003** (Tioguanine). A pale yellow, odourless or almost odourless, crystalline powder. Practically insoluble in water, in alcohol, and in chloroform; dissolves in dilute solutions of alkali hydroxides.

**USP 27** (Thioguanine). It is anhydrous or contains one-half molecule of water of hydration. A pale yellow, odourless or practically odourless, crystalline powder. Insoluble in water and in chloroform; soluble 1 in 7700 of alcohol; freely soluble in dilute solutions of alkali hydroxides. Store in airtight containers.

### Adverse Effects, Treatment, and Precautions

As for Mercaptopurine, p.567.

In some patients, gastrointestinal reactions are reported to be less frequent than with mercaptopurine.

**Effects on the blood.** For the view that it may be possible to predict those individuals likely to experience severe bone-marrow depression with tioguanine based on measurement of the activity of thiopurine methyltransferase or the concentration of tioguanine nucleotide, see under Azathioprine, p.1349.

**Effects on the liver.** There have been occasional reports of hepatic veno-occlusive disease attributed to tioguanine.[1-4]

1. Gill RA, *et al.* Hepatic veno-occlusive disease caused by 6-thioguanine. *Ann Intern Med* 1982; **96:** 58–60.
2. Krivoy N, *et al.* Reversible hepatic veno-occlusive disease and 6-thioguanine. *Ann Intern Med* 1982; **96:** 788.
3. Kao NL, Rosenblate HJ. 6-Thioguanine therapy for psoriasis causing toxic hepatic venoocclusive disease. *J Am Acad Dermatol* 1993; **28:** 1017–18.
4. Romagosa R, *et al.* Treatment of psoriasis with 6-thioguanine and hepatic venoocclusive disease. *J Am Acad Dermatol* 2002; **47:** 970–2.

**Handling and disposal.** For reference to a method for the destruction of tioguanine in wastes, see Mercaptopurine, p.567.

### Interactions

Unlike mercaptopurine (p.567), normal doses of tioguanine may be used with allopurinol.

A number of cases of portal hypertension with hepatic nodular regenerative hyperplasia have been reported in patients who received tioguanine with busulfan (see p.533).

It has been suggested that daunorubicin might enhance the hepatotoxicity of tioguanine (see p.546).

### Pharmacokinetics

Tioguanine is incompletely and variably absorbed from the gastrointestinal tract; on average about 30% of a dose is absorbed after oral doses. It is rapidly activated in the body by intracellular conversion to its nucleotide, thioguanylic acid and its thioguanosine phosphate derivatives. With repeated doses increasing amounts of the nucleotide are incorporated into DNA. Very little unchanged tioguanine has been detected circulating in the blood but the half-life of the nucleotide in the tissues is prolonged. Tioguanine is inactivated primarily by methylation to aminomethylthiopurine; small amounts are deaminated to thioxanthine, and may go on to be oxidised by xanthine oxidase to thiouric acid, but inactivation is essentially independent of xanthine oxidase and is not affected by inhibition of the enzyme.

It is excreted in the urine almost entirely as metabolites; only negligible amounts of tioguanine have been detected. Tioguanine does not appear to cross the blood-brain barrier to a significant extent; very little is found in CSF after normal clinical doses. It crosses the placenta.

### Uses and Administration

Tioguanine is an analogue of the naturally occurring purine, guanine, and is an antineoplastic with actions and uses similar to those of mercaptopurine (p.568). It appears to cause fewer gastrointestinal reactions but cross-resistance exists so that patients who do not respond to one are unlikely to respond to the other.

Tioguanine may be given by mouth, usually with cytarabine and an anthracycline, in the induction and maintenance of remissions in acute myeloid leukaemia (p.506), but there is some uncertainty about its value. It has also been used in other malignancies including acute lymphoblastic leukaemia (p.506) and chronic myeloid leukaemia.

Doses up to 200 mg/m$^2$ daily have been given for 5 to 20 days as part of a combined induction regimen; similar doses have been used in children as well as lower doses of 60 to 75 mg/m$^2$. For maintenance therapy, intermittent or continuous daily doses of up to 200 mg/m$^2$ have been used in both adults and children. A dose of 2 mg/kg daily increased after 4 weeks, if there is no response or toxicity allows, to 3 mg/kg daily may be given to adults and children in those rare cases when single agent therapy is considered appropriate.

Blood counts should be made frequently, particularly during induction and when tioguanine is given with other antineoplastic agents. Therapy should be withdrawn at the first sign of severe bone-marrow depression.

Tioguanine has been given intravenously as the sodium salt.

**Psoriasis.** A report of the use of tioguanine, in doses ranging from 20 mg twice weekly to 120 mg daily, in the management of patients with refractory psoriasis.[1] Dramatic improvement occurred in 14 of 18 patients, but a further 2 were unable to tolerate the drug. Myelosuppression was the principal toxic effect and it was suggested that thiopurine methyltransferase activity could be measured as a basis to determine initial dosage and the risk of toxicity. For the conventional management of psoriasis see p.1137.

1. Mason C, Krueger GG. Thioguanine for refractory psoriasis. *J Am Acad Dermatol* 2001; **44:** 67–72.

### Preparations

***BP 2003:*** Tioguanine Tablets;
***USP 27:*** Thioguanine Tablets.

**Proprietary Preparations** (details are given in Part 3)
***Arg.:*** Lanvis; ***Austral.:*** Lanvis; ***Belg.:*** Lanvis; ***Braz.:*** Lanvis; ***Canad.:*** Lanvis; ***Chile:*** Lanvis; ***Fr.:*** Lanvis; ***Gr.:*** Lanvis; Tioguanina; ***Hong Kong:*** Lanvis; ***Irl.:*** Lanvis; ***Israel:*** Lanvis; ***Malaysia:*** Lanvis; ***Neth.:*** Lanvis; ***NZ:*** Lanvis; ***S.Afr.:*** Lanvis; ***Singapore:*** Lanvis; ***Swed.:*** Lanvis; ***Switz.:*** Lanvis; ***Thai.:*** Lanvis; ***UK:*** Lanvis; ***USA:*** Tabloid.

## Tirapazamine *(USAN, rINN)*

SR-4233; Tirapazamina; Win-59075. 3-Amino-1,2,4-benzotriazine 1,4-dioxide.

$C_7H_6N_4O_2$ = 178.1.

*CAS — 27314-97-2.*

### Profile

Tirapazamine is reported to be reduced in hypoxic cells to an active anion that causes DNA strand breaks. It sensitises hypoxic tumour cells to the cytotoxic activity of other drugs. It is under investigation for its cytotoxic actions, alone or in combination with cisplatin or radiotherapy. Adverse effects reported with tirapazamine include nausea and vomiting, diarrhoea, skin rashes, muscle cramps and fatigue; myelosuppression is said to be rare.

◊ References.

1. Von Pawel J, *et al.* Tirapazamine plus cisplatin versus cisplatin in advanced non-small-cell lung cancer: a report of the international CATAPULT I study group. *J Clin Oncol* 2000; **18:** 1351–9.
2. Gandara DR, *et al.* Tirapazamine: prototype for a novel class of therapeutic agents targeting tumor hypoxia. *Semin Oncol* 2002; **29** (suppl 4): 102–9.

## Topotecan Hydrochloride

*(BANM, USAN, pINNM)*

Hidrocloruro de topotecán; SKF-104864A; SKFS-104864-A. (*S*)-10-Dimethylaminomethyl-4-ethyl-4,9-dihydroxy-1*H*-pyrano-[3′,4′:6,7]indolizino[1,2*b*]quinoline-3,14(4*H*,12*H*)-dione hydrochloride.

$C_{23}H_{23}N_3O_5,HCl = 457.9.$

*CAS — 123948-87-8 (topotecan); 119413-54-6 (topotecan hydrochloride).*

*ATC — L01XX17.*

**Incompatibility.** Topotecan hydrochloride was found to degrade to 88.7% of its original concentration over 4 hours when mixed with ticarcillin sodium or potassium clavulanate. It was also found to be incompatible with dexamethasone sodium phosphate and fluorouracil.[1] When mixed with mitomycin solution an immediate colour change took place and concentrations of mitomycin fell by 15 to 20% over 4 hours. The pH of the mixtures remained constant at 3.3 to 3.5.

1. Mayron D, Gennaro AR. Stability and compatibility of topotecan hydrochloride with selected drugs. *Am J Health-Syst Pharm* 1999; **56:** 875–81.

### Adverse Effects and Precautions

For general discussions, see Antineoplastics, p.492 and p.497. Neutropenia is common and is usually dose-limiting. The nadir of white cell count usually occurs about 9 to 12 days after a dose. Thrombocytopenia and anaemia are less frequent. Gastrointestinal disturbances are also common. Other adverse effects include fatigue and weakness, alopecia, malaise, and hyperbilirubinaemia.

Topotecan should be avoided in patients with pre-existing bone-marrow depression, and the manufacturers suggest that it should not be given in severe renal or hepatic impairment. Blood counts should be monitored regularly. Topotecan has been reported to produce fetal death and malformations in *animals*.

### Interactions

For a report of topotecan reducing the clearance of docetaxel, see Antineoplastics, p.547.

### Pharmacokinetics

Topotecan is widely distributed after intravenous doses. It undergoes reversible hydrolysis of the lactone ring to the inactive hydroxy acid form; only small amounts are demethylated in the liver. A significant proportion of a dose is excreted in urine. Topotecan has a terminal half-life of 2 to 3 hours.

◊ References.

1. Herben VMM, *et al.* Clinical pharmacokinetics of topotecan. *Clin Pharmacokinet* 1996; **31:** 85–102.

### Uses and Administration

Like irinotecan (p.564), topotecan is a semisynthetic derivative of the alkaloid camptothecin that exerts its antineoplastic activity by inhibition of topoisomerase I. It is used in the treatment of metastatic carcinoma of the ovary refractory to other therapy (see p.520) and in small cell lung cancer (p.519) refractory to standard therapy. Topotecan is also under investigation in the management of myelodysplastic syndromes.

Topotecan is given as the hydrochloride but doses are calculated in terms of the base. Topotecan hydrochloride 1.09 mg is approximately equivalent to 1 mg of topotecan. The recommended initial dose is the equivalent of topotecan 1.5 mg/m², given by intravenous infusion over 30 minutes, on days 1 to 5 of a 21-day course. A minimum of 4 courses should be given, provided that blood counts and haemoglobin have recovered adequately (see also Bone-marrow Depression, p.496).

If severe neutropenia occurs in any course the dose in the subsequent courses may be reduced by 0.25 mg/m², or a granulocyte colony-stimulating factor may be given from day 6 of the course once topotecan dosage is complete. If severe toxicity recurs once the dose has been reduced to 1 mg/m² withdrawal of topotecan may be required. Dosage should also be reduced after severe thrombocytopenia and in patients with renal impairment (see below).

Oral formulations of topotecan are under investigation.

◊ Reviews.

1. Cersosimo RJ. Topotecan: a new topoisomerase I inhibiting antineoplastic agent. *Ann Pharmacother* 1998; **32:** 1334–43.
2. Estey EH. Topotecan for myelodysplastic syndromes. *Oncology (Huntingt)* 1998; **12:** 81–6.
3. Huang CH, Treat J. New advances in lung cancer chemotherapy: topotecan and the role of topoisomerase I inhibitors. *Oncology* 2001; **61** (suppl 1): 14–24.
4. Schiller JH. Future role of topotecan in the treatment of lung cancer. *Oncology* 2001; **61** (suppl 1): 55–9.
5. Herzog TJ. Update on the role of topotecan in the treatment of recurrent ovarian cancer. *Oncologist* 2002; **7** (suppl 5): 3–10.
6. Coleman RL. Emerging role of topotecan in front-line treatment of carcinoma of the ovary. *Oncologist* 2002; **7** (suppl 5): 46–55.

**Administration in renal impairment.** The initial dose of intravenous topotecan should be halved to 0.75 mg/m² in patients with a creatinine clearance of between 20 and 39 mL/minute.

### Preparations

**Proprietary Preparations** (details are given in Part 3)
***Arg.:*** Asotecan; Hycamtin; Potekam; Tisogen; Topestin; Topokebir; Topotag; TPT; ***Austral.:*** Hycamtin; ***Austria:*** Hycamtin; ***Belg.:*** Hycamtin; ***Braz.:*** Hycamtin; ***Canad.:*** Hycamtin; ***Chile:*** Hycamtin; ***Denm.:*** Hycamtin; ***Fin.:*** Hycamtin; ***Fr.:*** Hycamtin; ***Ger.:*** Hycamtin; ***Gr.:*** Hycamtin; ***Hong Kong:*** Hycamtin; ***India:*** Topotel; ***Irl.:*** Hycamtin; ***Israel:*** Hycamtin; ***Ital.:*** Hycamtin; ***Neth.:*** Hycamtin; ***Norw.:*** Hycamtin; ***Port.:*** Hycamtin; ***S.Afr.:*** Hycamtin; ***Singapore:*** Hycamtin; ***Spain:*** Hycamtin; ***Swed.:*** Hycamtin; ***Switz.:*** Hycamtin; ***Thai.:*** Hycamtin; ***UK:*** Hycamtin; ***USA:*** Hycamtin.

## Toremifene Citrate *(BANM, USAN, rINNM)*

FC-1157a. 2-{*p*-[(*Z*)-4-Chloro-1,2-diphenyl-1-butenyl]phenoxy}-*N*,*N*-dimethylethylamine citrate.

$C_{26}H_{28}ClNO,C_6H_8O_7 = 598.1.$

*CAS — 89778-26-7 (toremifene); 89778-27-8 (toremifene citrate).*

*ATC — L02BA02.*

### Adverse Effects and Precautions

As for Tamoxifen Citrate, p.584.

Use of toremifene is contra-indicated in patients with pre-existing endometrial hyperplasia, or in those with severe thromboembolic disease or severe hepatic impairment. Toremifene must be used with caution in patients with uncompensated heart failure or severe angina.

### Interactions

Toremifene is metabolised by cytochrome P450 isoenzyme CYP3A4, and potent enzyme-inducing drugs such as phenytoin, phenobarbital and carbamazepine, might be expected to increase toremifene metabolism, thereby lowering the serum concentration. Conversely, azole antifungals and macrolide antibiotics may inhibit toremifene metabolism by inhibiting the isoenzyme.

Use with drugs that decrease renal calcium excretion, such as thiazide diuretics, may increase the incidence of hypercalcaemia.

**Antibacterials.** *Rifampicin* was found to decrease plasma concentrations of toremifene in 9 volunteers. This was thought to be due to induction of cytochrome P450 isoenzyme CYP3A4 by rifampicin.[1]

1. Kivistö KT, *et al.* Tamoxifen and toremifene concentrations in plasma are greatly decreased by rifampin. *Clin Pharmacol Ther* 1998; **64:** 648–54.

### Pharmacokinetics

Toremifene citrate is well absorbed from the gastrointestinal tract, reaching peak plasma concentrations of toremifene within 3 hours. It is extensively bound to plasma proteins, mainly albumin. Toremifene is metabolised principally by the cytochrome P450 isoenzyme CYP3A4; some metabolites are reported to be active. It undergoes enterohepatic circulation and is eliminated mainly in the faeces as metabolites, with an elimination half-life of about 5 days. About 10% is excreted in the urine.

◊ Reviews.

1. Taras TL, *et al.* Clinical pharmacokinetics of toremifene. *Clin Pharmacokinet* 2000; **39:** 327–34.

### Uses and Administration

Toremifene is an anti-oestrogen with properties similar to those of tamoxifen (p.585), and is used similarly in the treatment of advanced breast cancer (p.514) in postmenopausal women. It is also being investigated as an adjuvant for the treatment of lung tumours.

Toremifene is given by mouth as the citrate, but doses are calculated in terms of the base; 88.4 mg of toremifene citrate is approximately equivalent to 60 mg of toremifene. A dose of toremifene 60 mg daily is used.

◊ References.

1. Wiseman LR, Goa KL. Toremifene: a review of its pharmacological properties and clinical efficacy in the management of advanced breast cancer. *Drugs* 1997; **54:** 141–60.
2. Anonymous. Toremifene and letrozole for advanced breast cancer. *Med Lett Drugs Ther* 1998; **40:** 43–5.
3. Holli K. Adjuvant trials of toremifene vs tamoxifen: the European experience. *Oncology (Huntingt)* 1998; **12** (suppl 5): 23–7.
4. Holli K, *et al.* Safety and efficacy results of a randomized trial comparing adjuvant toremifene and tamoxifen in postmenopausal patients with node-positive breast cancer. *J Clin Oncol* 2000; **18:** 3487–94.

### Preparations

**Proprietary Preparations** (details are given in Part 3)
***Arg.:*** Fareston; ***Austral.:*** Fareston; ***Austria:*** Fareston; ***Belg.:*** Fareston; ***Braz.:*** Fareston†; ***Denm.:*** Fareston†; ***Fin.:*** Fareston; ***Fr.:*** Fareston; ***Ger.:*** Fareston; ***Gr.:*** Fareston; ***Irl.:*** Fareston; ***Ital.:*** Fareston; ***Mex.:*** Fareston; ***Neth.:*** Fareston†; ***NZ:*** Fareston; ***Port.:*** Fareston; ***S.Afr.:*** Fareston; ***Spain:*** Fareston; ***Swed.:*** Fareston; ***Switz.:*** Fareston; ***Thai.:*** Fareston; ***UK:*** Fareston; ***USA:*** Fareston.

## Tositumomab *(rINN)*

B-1.

*CAS — 192391-48-3.*

*ATC — V10XA53.*

### Profile

Tositumomab is an anti-B1 monoclonal antibody that is directed against the CD20 antigen found on the surface of B lymphocytes. It is radiolabelled with iodine-131 (p.1524) for the treatment of follicular non-Hodgkin's lymphoma (p.510), in patients with CD20-positive disease refractory to rituximab and who have relapsed following chemotherapy.

Infusion reactions suggestive of a cytokine release syndrome, and other hypersensitivity reactions including anaphylaxis, have been reported. Prolonged and severe neutropenia, thrombocytopenia, and anaemia occur commonly. Other adverse effects include nausea, vomiting, diarrhoea, and abdominal pain, pleural effusion, and increased susceptibility to infection.

### Preparations

**Proprietary Preparations** (details are given in Part 3)
***USA:*** Bexxar.

## Trabectedin *(USAN, rINN)*

Ecteinascidin-743; ET-743; NSC-648766. (1′*R*,6*R*,6a*R*,7*R*,13*S*,14*S*,16*R*)-6′,8,14-Trihydroxy-7′,9-dimethoxy-4,10,23-trimethyl-19-oxo-3′,4′,6,7,12,13,14,16-octahydrospiro[6,16-(epithiopropanooxymethano)-7,13-imino-6a*H*-1,3-dioxolo[7,8]isoquino-[3,2-*b*][3]benzazocine-20,1′(2′*H*)-isoquinolin]-5-yl acetate.

$C_{39}H_{43}N_3O_{11}S = 761.8.$

*CAS — 114899-77-3.*

*ATC — L01CX01.*

### Profile

Trabectedin is a novel DNA-binding agent derived from the marine tunicate, *Ecteinascidia turbinata*. It is under investigation for the treatment of advanced soft-tissue sarcomas and ovarian cancer.

◊ References.

1. Cvetkovic RS, *et al.* ET-743. *Drugs* 2002; **62:** 1185–92.
2. van Kesteren C, *et al.* Yondelis (trabectedin, ET-743): the development of an anticancer agent of marine origin. *Anticancer Drugs* 2003; **14:** 487–502.
3. D'Incalci M, Jimeno J. Preclinical and clinical results with the natural marine product ET-743. *Expert Opin Invest Drugs* 2003; **12:** 1843–53.

## Trastuzumab *(BAN, rINN)*

HER-2 Monoclonal Antibody; rhuMAb HER2.

*CAS — 180288-69-1.*

*ATC — L01XC03.*

### Adverse Effects, Treatment, and Precautions

For general discussions see Antineoplastics, p.492, p.495 and p.497.

Trastuzumab has been associated with fatal hypersensitivity reactions, infusion reactions characteristic of a cytokine release syndrome, and pulmonary events including acute respiratory distress syndrome. These usually occur after the first dose of trastuzumab and are more common in patients with reduced lung function. Use of trastuzumab is contra-indicated in patients with severe dyspnoea at rest. Cardiac dysfunction and congestive heart failure may also occur and left ventricular function should be monitored before and during therapy. The risk of cardiotoxicity is increased if trastuzumab is given with anthracyclines or cyclophosphamide (see below).

There is an increase in incidence of leucopenia, thrombocytopenia, and anaemia when trastuzumab is given with chemotherapy, but it infrequently causes myelosuppression when used alone. Diarrhoea occurs in about 25% of patients given trastuzumab. Other common adverse effects include chills, fever, headache, arthralgia, myalgia, and rashes.

**Effects on the heart.** Cardiac events related to the administration of trastuzumab include asymptomatic decreases in left ventricular ejection fraction, tachycardia, palpitations, dyspnoea, and chest pain. Congestive heart failure may develop.[1]

In a pivotal comparative trial,[2] an increased incidence of cardiac adverse events prompted a retrospective analysis. This independent review identified cardiac dysfunction in 27% of patients receiving trastuzumab, an anthracycline, and cyclophosphamide, compared with only 8% receiving an anthracycline and cyclophosphamide. In patients given trastuzumab and paclitaxel, 13% developed cardiac dysfunction compared with 1% of patients given paclitaxel alone, although all these patients had previously received an anthracycline. The incidence of severe dysfunction was highest in those patients receiving trastuzumab, an anthracycline, and cyclophosphamide.

Further analysis[3] of this trial and 6 other studies found that, in a total of 1219 patients, 10 heart-related deaths had been reported, and that 9 of these were patients who had received trastuzumab. However, the risk of developing cardiotoxicity was less when trastuzumab was given alone than with concomitant anthracycline therapy. Advanced age was found to be a significant risk factor, whereas giving trastuzumab and the anthracycline at different times appeared to decrease the rate of cardiotoxicity.

The manufacturers of trastuzumab warn that patients who have previously received anthracyclines may also be at increased risk of cardiotoxicity with trastuzumab treatment. Furthermore, because the half-life of trastuzumab is approximately 28.5 days, trastuzumab may persist in the circulation for up to 24 weeks, and patients receiving anthracyclines after stopping trastuzumab may still be at increased risk of cardiotoxicity. If anthracyclines are used, the patient's cardiac function should be carefully monitored. Patients with pre-existing cardiovascular disease should also be treated with caution. However, the majority of patients who develop congestive heart failure improve with standard treatment, including the use of ACE inhibitors, beta blockers, cardiac glycosides and diuretics.[1]

The pathogenesis of the cardiotoxicity associated with trastuzumab is under investigation. A small study[4] showed specific uptake of a pretreatment tracer dose of radiolabelled trastuzumab into the myocardium of patients who subsequently developed cardiac adverse events.

1. Keefe DL. Trastuzumab-associated cardiotoxicity. *Cancer* 2002; **95:** 1592–1600.
2. Slamon DJ, *et al.* Use of chemotherapy plus a monoclonal antibody against HER2 for metastatic breast cancer that overexpresses HER2. *N Engl J Med* 2001; **344:** 783–92.
3. Seidman A, *et al.* Cardiac dysfunction in the trastuzumab clinical trials experience. *J Clin Oncol* 2002; **20:** 1215–21.
4. Behr TM, *et al.* Trastuzumab and breast cancer. *N Engl J Med* 2001; **345:** 995–6.

## Uses and Administration

Trastuzumab is a humanised monoclonal antibody directed against a cell surface protein produced by the human epidermal growth factor receptor 2 (HER2) gene. HER2 protein is overexpressed in about one-third of all breast cancers. Trastuzumab is used in the treatment of metastatic breast cancer (p.514) with such characteristics. The recommended dose, alone or with paclitaxel, is 4 mg/kg initially, by intravenous infusion in 250 mL of sodium chloride 0.9% over 90 minutes. This may be followed by 2 mg/kg over 30 minutes at weekly intervals.

HER2 may also be overexpressed in other epithelial cancers, and trastuzumab is under investigation for use in non-small cell lung cancer, bladder, and ovarian malignancies.

◊ References.

1. Cobleigh MA, *et al.* Multinational study of the efficacy and safety of humanized anti-HER2 monoclonal antibody in women who have HER2-overexpressing metastatic breast cancer that has progressed after chemotherapy for metastatic disease. *J Clin Oncol* 1999; **17:** 2639–48.
2. Treish L, *et al.* Pharmacology and therapeutic use of trastuzumab in breast cancer. *Am J Health-Syst Pharm* 2000; **57:** 2063–79.
3. Agus DB, *et al.* HER-2/neu as a therapeutic target in non-small cell lung cancer, prostate cancer, and ovarian cancer. *Semin Oncol* 2000; **27** (suppl 11): 53–63.
4. Seidman AD, *et al.* Weekly trastuzumab and paclitaxel therapy for metastatic breast cancer with analysis of efficacy by HER2 immunophenotype and gene amplification. *J Clin Oncol* 2001; **19:** 2587–95.
5. Eiermann W, *et al.* Trastuzumab combined with chemotherapy for the treatment of HER2-positive metastatic breast cancer: pivotal trial data. *Ann Oncol* 2001; **12** (suppl 1): S57–S62.
6. Slamon DJ, *et al.* Use of chemotherapy plus a monoclonal antibody against HER2 for metastatic breast cancer that overexpresses HER2. *N Engl J Med* 2001; **344:** 783–92.
7. McKeage K, Perry CM. Trastuzumab: a review of its use in the treatment of metastatic breast cancer overexpressing HER2. *Drugs* 2002; **62:** 209–43.
8. Bookman MA, *et al.* Evaluation of monoclonal humanized anti-HER2 antibody, trastuzumab, in patients with recurrent or refractory ovarian or primary peritoneal carcinoma with overexpression of HER2: a phase II trial of the Gynecologic Oncology Group. *J Clin Oncol* 2003; **21:** 283–90.
9. Spigel DR, Burstein HJ. Trastuzumab regimens for HER2-overexpressing metastatic breast cancer. *Clin Breast Cancer* 2003; **4:** 329–37.
10. Ferrone M, Motl SE. Trastuzumab for the treatment of non-small-cell lung cancer. *Ann Pharmacother* 2003; **37:** 1904–8.
11. Hirsch FR, Langer CJ. The role of HER2/neu expression and trastuzumab in non-small cell lung cancer. *Semin Oncol* 2004; **31** (suppl 1): 75–82.

## Preparations

**Proprietary Preparations** (details are given in Part 3)
***Arg.:*** Herceptin; ***Austral.:*** Herceptin; ***Belg.:*** Herceptin; ***Braz.:*** Herceptin; ***Canad.:*** Herceptin; ***Chile:*** Herceptin; ***Denm.:*** Herceptin; ***Fin.:*** Herceptin; ***Fr.:*** Herceptin; ***Ger.:*** Herceptin; ***Gr.:*** Herceptin; ***Irl.:*** Herceptin; ***Israel:*** Herceptin; ***Ital.:*** Herceptin; ***Mex.:*** Herceptin; ***Norw.:*** Herceptin; ***NZ:*** Herceptin; ***Port.:*** Herceptin; ***S.Afr.:*** Herceptin; ***Singapore:*** Herceptin; ***Spain:*** Herceptin; ***Swed.:*** Herceptin; ***Switz.:*** Herceptin; ***Thai.:*** Herceptin; ***UK:*** Herceptin; ***USA:*** Herceptin.

## Treosulfan *(BAN, rINN)*

Dihydroxybusulphan; NSC-39069; Treosulfano. L-Threitol 1,4-dimethanesulphonate.

$C_6H_{14}O_8S_2$ = 278.3.
*CAS — 299-75-2.*
*ATC — L01AB02.*

### Profile

Treosulfan is an antineoplastic agent related to busulfan (p.532), which is reported to act by alkylation after conversion *in vivo* to epoxide compounds. It is used palliatively or as an adjunct to surgery mainly in the treatment of ovarian cancer (p.520).

Treosulfan 1 g daily is licensed for use by mouth in 4 divided doses for 2 or 4 weeks followed by the same period without treatment. Alternatively 1.5 g daily in 3 divided doses may be given for 1 week, followed by 3 weeks without therapy. The cycle is then repeated, the dose being adjusted if necessary according to the effect on bone marrow. Doses of 3 to 8 g/m² may instead be given intravenously every 1 to 3 weeks. Doses larger than 3 g/m² should be given by infusion at a rate of 3 g/m² every 5 to 10 minutes. Doses up to 1.5 g/m² have been given intraperitoneally. Lower doses should be used if treatment with other antineoplastic drugs or radiotherapy is being given.

Regular blood counts should be made and treatment should be interrupted if the white cell or platelet counts fall below acceptable levels (see also Bone-marrow Depression, p.496). Because bone-marrow depression may be cumulative the interval between blood counts should be reduced after the second course of treatment with treosulfan.

### Preparations

**Proprietary Preparations** (details are given in Part 3)
***Ger.:*** Ovastat.

## Trofosfamide *(rINN)*

A-4828; NSC-109723; Trilophosphamide; Trofosfamida; Trophosphamide; Z-4828. 3-(2-Chloroethyl)-2-[bis(2-chloroethyl)amino]tetrahydro-2*H*-1,3,2-oxazaphosphorine-2-oxide.

$C_9H_{18}Cl_3N_2O_2P$ = 323.6.
*CAS — 22089-22-1.*
*ATC — L01AA07.*

### Profile

Trofosfamide is a derivative of cyclophosphamide (p.540) and has the same general properties. It is used in the treatment of a variety of malignant disorders in usual initial doses of 300 to 400 mg daily by mouth. Doses of 50 to 150 mg daily have been given for maintenance therapy.

### Preparations

**Proprietary Preparations** (details are given in Part 3)
***Austria:*** Ixoten; ***Ger.:*** Ixoten; ***Spain:*** Genoxal Trofosfamida.

## Tumour Necrosis Factor

Factor de necrosis tumoral; TNF.

## Tasonermin *(BAN, rINN)*

Tasonermina; TNFα-1a.

$C_{778}H_{1225}N_{215}O_{231}S_2$ = 17350.5.
*CAS — 94948-59-1.*
*ATC — L03AX11.*

### Profile

Tumour necrosis factor is a cytokine of which 2 forms have been identified with similar biological properties: TNFα or cachectin, which is produced predominantly by macrophages, and TNFβ or lymphotoxin, which is produced by lymphocytes. Various recombinant forms of TNFα, both human and mouse, are available: the names sonermin and sertenef have been used for such products.

The antitumour effects of tumour necrosis factor *in vitro* and in *animals* have prompted investigation of recombinant TNFα in the treatment of cancer either alone or in combination with other cytokines such as interleukin-2 or the interferons. Tasonermin is a recombinant TNFα used in combination with melphalan (p.566) for soft tissue sarcomas. It is administered by mild hyperthermic isolated limb perfusion at a total dose of 3 mg for upper limbs and 4 mg for lower limbs. Leakage of tasonermin into the systemic circulation should not exceed 10%, as severe toxicity may occur. Local adverse effects include skin reactions, oedema, and pain; less commonly, vascular thrombosis, onycholysis, or severe tissue damage have occurred. Systemic effects include fever, chills, nausea and vomiting, arrhythmias, hepatotoxicity, and infections. Shock or hypotension, neurological disorders, thrombocytopenia, leucopenia, acute renal failure, and hypersensitivity reactions have all been reported.

◊ References.

1. van Der Veen AH, *et al.* An overview on the use of TNF-alpha: our experience with regional administration and developments towards new opportunities for systemic application. *Anticancer Res* 2000; **20:** 3467–74.
2. Libutti SK, *et al.* Technique and results of hyperthermic isolated hepatic perfusion with tumor necrosis factor and melphalan for the treatment of unresectable hepatic malignancies. *J Am Coll Surg* 2000; **191:** 519–30.
3. Lejeune FJ, *et al.* Limb salvage by neoadjuvant isolated perfusion with TNFα and melphalan for non-resectable soft tissue sarcoma of the extremities. *Eur J Surg Oncol* 2000; **26:** 669–78.
4. Eggermont AM, ten Hagen TL. Tumor necrosis factor-based isolated limb perfusion for soft tissue sarcoma and melanoma: ten years of successful antivascular therapy. *Curr Oncol Rep* 2003; **5:** 79–80.
5. ten Hagen TL, Eggermont AM. Solid tumor therapy: manipulation of the vasculature with TNF. *Technol Cancer Res Treat* 2003; **2:** 195–203.
6. Noorda EM, *et al.* Isolated limb perfusion with tumor necrosis factor-alpha and melphalan for patients with unresectable soft tissue sarcoma of the extremities. *Cancer* 2003; **98:** 1483–90.
7. Corti A. Strategies for improving the anti-neoplastic activity of TNF by tumor targeting. *Methods Mol Med* 2004; **98:** 247–64.

**Units.** The first International Standard for human tumour necrosis factor α, which contained 40 000 international units/ampoule, was considered unsuitable for the assay of recombinant *mouse* tumour necrosis factor α, for human tumour necrosis factor β, or for preparations of tumour necrosis factor α of modified structure.[1]

The first Reference Reagent for tumour necrosis factor β had an assigned potency of 150 000 units/ampoule.[2]

1. WHO. WHO expert committee on biological standardization: forty-second report. *WHO Tech Rep Ser 822* 1992.
2. WHO. WHO expert committee on biological standardization: forty-seventh report. *WHO Tech Rep Ser 878* 1998.

### Preparations

**Proprietary Preparations** (details are given in Part 3)
***Belg.:*** Beromun; ***Gr.:*** Beromun; ***Ital.:*** Beromun; ***Neth.:*** Beromun†; ***Spain:*** Beromun; ***Swed.:*** Beromun.

## Ubenimex *(rINN)*

NK-421; NSC-265489. (−)-*N*-[(2*S*,3*R*)-3-Amino-2-hydroxy-4-phenylbutyryl]-L-leucine.

$C_{16}H_{24}N_2O_4$ = 308.4.
*CAS — 58970-76-6.*

### Profile

Ubenimex is a peptide derived from *Streptomyces olivoreticuli.* It is reported to have antineoplastic and immunostimulant properties. It has been used in the adjuvant treatment of acute myeloid leukaemia and is under investigation for the treatment of lung cancer. Adverse effects include gastrointestinal and hepatic function disturbances, skin rashes, headache, and paraesthesias.

◊ References.

1. Ichinose Y, *et al.* Randomized double-blind placebo-controlled trial of bestatin in patients with resected stage I squamous-cell lung carcinoma. *J Natl Cancer Inst* 2003; **95:** 605–10.

## Valrubicin *(USAN, rINN)*

AD-32; NSC-246131; *N*-Trifluoroacetyladriamycin-14-valerate; *N*-Trifluoroacetyldoxorubicin-14-valerate; Valrubicina. (8*S*,10*S*)-8-Glycoloyl-7,8,9,10-tetrahydro-6,8,11-trihydroxy-1-methoxy-10-{[2,3,6-trideoxy-3-(2,2,2-trifluoroacetamido)-α-L-*lyxo*-hexopyranosyl]oxy}-5,12-naphthacenedione 8²-valerate.

$C_{34}H_{36}F_3NO_{13}$ = 723.6.
*CAS — 56124-62-0.*
*ATC — L01DB09.*

**Pharmacopoeias.** In *US.*

**USP 27** (Valrubicin). An orange to orange-red crystalline powder. Very slightly soluble in water, in hexane, and in petroleum spirit; soluble in dehydrated alcohol, in acetone, in dichloromethane, and in methyl alcohol. Store in airtight containers. Protect from light.

### Adverse Effects, Treatment, and Precautions

Increased urinary frequency and urgency, dysuria, bladder spasm and pain may follow intravesical use of valrubicin due to local irritation of the bladder, and usually resolve within 1 to 7 days of treatment. Gross haematuria has occurred rarely but should be distinguished from drug-induced red coloration of the urine. Abdominal pain and nausea may occur.

Myelosuppression similar to that seen with other anthracyclines (see Adverse Effects of Doxorubicin Hydrochloride, p.548) is possible if significant systemic exposure occurs. Therefore valrubicin should not be given to patients with a perforated bladder or compromised bladder mucosa.

Because of the risk of metastasis, cystectomy should be reconsidered for patients with carcinoma *in situ* who do not respond completely to valrubicin treatment after three months.

### Pharmacokinetics

On intravesical use valrubicin penetrates the bladder wall but systemic absorption is low in patients who have an intact bladder mucosa. The drug is almost entirely excreted by voiding after the installation period.

### Uses and Administration

Valrubicin is a semisynthetic analogue of the anthracycline doxorubicin (p.547). It is used for carcinoma *in situ* of the bladder (p.512) refractory to BCG vaccine, when surgery is contra-indicated, although only about 20% of such patients exhibit a complete response. The recommended dose is 800 mg given intravesically once a week for 6 weeks, as 75 mL of a solution diluted with sodium chloride 0.9%. The solution should be retained for 2 hours if possible before voiding.

◊ References.

1. Steinberg G, *et al.* Efficacy and safety of valrubicin for the treatment of Bacillus Calmette-Guerin refractory carcinoma in situ of the bladder. *J Urol (Baltimore)* 2000; **163:** 761–7.
2. Kuznetsov DD, *et al.* Intravesical valrubicin in the treatment of carcinoma in situ of the bladder. *Expert Opin Pharmacother* 2001; **2:** 1009–13.

### Preparations

***USP 27:*** Valrubicin Intravesical Solution.

**Proprietary Preparations** (details are given in Part 3)
***Canad.:*** Valtaxin; ***Israel:*** Valstar; ***USA:*** Valstar.

---

## Valspodar *(BAN, USAN, rINN)*

PSC-833; SDZ-PSC-833. Cyclo{[(2*S*,4*R*,6*E*)-4-methyl-2-(methylamino)-3-oxo-6-octenoyl]-L-valyl-*N*-methylglycyl-*N*-methyl-L-leucyl-L-valyl-*N*-methyl-L-leucyl-L-alanyl-D-alanyl-*N*-methyl-L-leucyl-*N*-methyl-L-leucyl-*N*-methyl-L-valyl}.

$C_{63}H_{111}N_{11}O_{12}$ = 1214.6.
*CAS — 121584-18-7.*

### Profile

Valspodar is an analogue of ciclosporin (p.1351). It inhibits P-glycoprotein, which is associated with multidrug resistance. Valspodar is being investigated in various neoplasms to restore sensitivity of resistant tumour cells to anticancer drugs.

Valspodar inhibits the cytochrome P450 isoenzyme CYP3A4, and may reduce the metabolism and clearance of other drugs.

◊ References.

1. Advani, R, *et al.* Treatment of poor prognosis AML patients using PSC833 (valspodar) plus mitoxantrone, etoposide, and cytarabine (PSC-MEC). *Adv Exp Med Biol* 1999; **457:** 47–56.
2. Sparreboom A, Nooter K. Does P-glycoprotein play a role in anticancer drug pharmacokinetics? *Drug Resist Updat* 2000; **3:** 357–63.
3. Kang MH, *et al.* The P-glycoprotein antagonist PSC 833 increases the plasma concentrations of 6α-hydroxypaclitaxel, a major metabolite of paclitaxel. *Clin Cancer Res* 2001; **7:** 1610–17.
4. Fracasso PM, *et al.* Phase II study of paclitaxel and valspodar (PSC 833) in refractory ovarian carcinoma: a gynecologic oncology group study. *J Clin Oncol* 2001; **19:** 2975–82.
5. Baekelandt M, *et al.* Phase I/II trial of the multidrug-resistance modulator valspodar combined with cisplatin and doxorubicin in refractory ovarian cancer. *J Clin Oncol* 2001; **19:** 2983–93.
6. Baer MR, *et al.* Phase 3 study of the multidrug resistance modulator PSC-833 in previously untreated patients 60 years of age and older with acute myeloid leukemia: Cancer and Leukemia Group B Study 9720. *Blood* 2002; **100:** 1224–32.
7. Ma MK, *et al.* Pharmacokinetic study of infusional valspodar. *J Clin Pharmacol* 2002; **42:** 412–18.

---

## Verteporfin *(BAN, USAN, rINN)*

Benzoporphyrin Derivative; BPD; CL-318952; Verteporfina. *trans*-18-Ethenyl-4,4a-dihydro-3,4-bis(methoxycarbonyl)-4a,8,14,19-tetramethyl-23*H*,25*H*-benzo[*b*]porphine-9,13-dipropanoic acid monomethyl ester.

$C_{41}H_{42}N_4O_8$ = 718.8.
*CAS — 129497-78-5.*
*ATC — L01XD02.*

**Pharmacopoeias.** In *US.*

**USP 27** (Verteporfin). Store at a temperature between −25° and −10° in airtight containers.

### Adverse Effects and Precautions

Photosensitivity will occur in all patients treated with verteporfin and patients should not be exposed to direct sunlight for 2 to 5 days after treatment. However, exposure to ambient indoor light is encouraged, as it allows gradual inactivation of any remaining drug. Headaches, injection site reactions, and visual disturbances occur frequently. Extravasation at the injection site may be severe and may require interruption of therapy. Patients who experience a severe decrease in vision should not be re-treated until their vision recovers. Other reported adverse effects include hypersensitivity, infusion-related pain (primarily presenting as back pain), chest pain, gastrointestinal disturbances, atrial fibrillation, hypertension, decreased hearing, and anaemia. Verteporfin should be used with care in patients with hepatic impairment.

**Porphyria.** The use of verteporfin is contra-indicated in patients with porphyria.

### Interactions

Use of verteporfin with other drugs causing photosensitivity should be avoided as the reaction may be increased.

### Pharmacokinetics

After intravenous doses, elimination of verteporfin is bi-exponential, with a terminal plasma elimination half-life of about 5 to 6 hours. Protein binding is about 90%. It is metabolised in the liver. It is excreted in faeces via the bile, mostly as unchanged drug, with less than 1% of a dose recovered in the urine.

◊ References.

1. Houle J-M, Strong A. Clinical pharmacokinetics of verteporfin. *J Clin Pharmacol* 2002; **42:** 547–57.

### Uses and Administration

Verteporfin is a photosensitiser used in the photodynamic therapy (see Porfimer Sodium, p.581) of age-related macular degeneration. Following intravenous administration verteporfin accumulates preferentially in the endothelial cells of actively growing blood vessels, including those in the choroid. When activated by laser light it produces local vascular occlusion and this inhibits neovascularisation and reduces the decline in visual acuity. It is given by intravenous infusion over 10 minutes at a dose of 6 mg/m$^2$. This is followed 15 minutes after the start of the infusion by activation using a laser tuned to a wavelength of 689 nanometres and delivered to the eye via a fibre optic device and a slit lamp, together with a suitable contact lens. The recommended light dose is 50 J/cm$^2$, given over 83 seconds. Therapy may be repeated every 3 months for recurrent choroidal neovascular leakage. Verteporfin has also been investigated in the photodynamic therapy of a variety of other disorders including malignant neoplasms.

◊ References.

1. Treatment of age-related macular degeneration with photodynamic therapy (TAP) Study Group. Photodynamic therapy of subfoveal choroidal neovascularization in age-related macular degeneration with verteporfin: one-year results of 2 randomized clinical trials—TAP report 1. *Arch Ophthalmol* 1999; **117:** 1329–45.
2. Soubrane G, Bressler NM. Treatment of subfoveal choroidal neovascularisation in age related macular degeneration: focus on clinical application of verteporfin photodynamic therapy. *Br J Ophthalmol* 2001; **85:** 483–95.
3. Messmer KJ, Abel SR. Verteporfin for age-related macular degeneration. *Ann Pharmacother* 2001; **35:** 1593–8.
4. Blumenkranz MS, *et al.* Verteporfin therapy for subfoveal choroidal neovascularization in age-related macular degeneration: three-year results of an open-label extension of 2 randomized clinical trials—TAP report no. 5. *Arch Ophthalmol* 2002; **120:** 1307–14.
5. Blinder KJ, *et al.* Verteporfin therapy of subfoveal choroidal neovascularization in pathologic myopia: 2-year results of a randomized clinical trial—VIP report no. 3. *Ophthalmology* 2003; **110:** 667–73.
6. Keam SJ, *et al.* Verteporfin: a review of its use in the management of subfoveal choroidal neovascularisation. *Drugs* 2003; **63:** 2521–54.
7. National Institute for Clinical Excellence. Guidance on the use of photodynamic therapy for age-related macular degeneration (September 2003). Available at: http://www.nice.org.uk/pdf/68_PDTGuidance.pdf (accessed 10/06/04)

### Preparations

***USP 27:*** Verteporfin for Injection.

**Proprietary Preparations** (details are given in Part 3)
***Arg.:*** Visudyne; ***Austral.:*** Visudyne; ***Braz.:*** Visudyne; ***Canad.:*** Visudyne; ***Chile:*** Visudyne; ***Denm.:*** Visudyne; ***Fin.:*** Visudyne; ***Fr.:*** Visudyne; ***Ger.:*** Visudyne; ***Gr.:*** Visudyne; ***Hong Kong:*** Visudyne; ***Israel:*** Visudyne; ***Ital.:*** Visudyne; ***Norw.:*** Visudyne; ***NZ:*** Visudyne; ***Singapore:*** Visudyne; ***Spain:*** Visudyne; ***Swed.:*** Visudyne; ***Switz.:*** Visudyne; ***Thai.:*** Visudyne; ***UK:*** Visudyne; ***USA:*** Visudyne.

---

## Vinblastine Sulfate *(USAN, rINNM)*

29060-LE; NSC-49842; Sulfato de Vimblastina; Sulfato de vinblastina; Vinblastine Sulphate *(BANM)*; Vinblastini Sulfas; Vincaleukoblastine Sulphate; VLB (vinblastine).

$C_{46}H_{58}N_4O_9,H_2SO_4$ = 909.1.
*CAS — 865-21-4 (vinblastine); 143-67-9 (vinblastine sulfate).*
*ATC — L01CA01.*

**Description.** Vinblastine sulfate is the sulfate of an alkaloid, vincaleukoblastine, extracted from *Catharanthus roseus* (*Vinca rosea*) (Apocynaceae).

**Pharmacopoeias.** In *Chin., Eur.* (see p.vi), *Int., Jpn, Pol., US* and *Viet.*

**Ph. Eur. 5.0** (Vinblastine Sulphate). A white or slightly yellowish, very hygroscopic, crystalline powder. It loses not more than 15% of its weight on drying. Freely soluble in water; practically insoluble in alcohol. A 0.15% solution in water has a pH of 3.5 to 5.0. Store at a temperature not exceeding −20° in airtight glass containers. Protect from light.

**USP 27** (Vinblastine Sulfate). A white or slightly yellow, odourless, hygroscopic, amorphous or crystalline powder. It loses not more than 15% of its weight on drying. Freely soluble in water. A 0.15% solution in water has a pH of 3.5 to 5.0. Store at a temperature between −25° and −10° in airtight containers. Protect from light.

**Stability.** Between about 5 and 20% of active drug was lost from solution when a solution of vinblastine sulfate 3 micrograms/mL in glucose 5% injection was stored for 48 hours in a range of intravenous burette giving sets, the highest loss being from cellulose propionate sets and the lowest from one made from methacrylate butadiene styrene.[1] Similarly, storage in PVC tubing led to a 42 to 44% loss from solution whereas only about 6% was lost over the 48 hours in polybutadiene tubing. The losses appeared to be due to drug sorption, and were therefore greater from the tubing which had a greater surface-area-to-volume ratio than the burettes.

1. McElnay JC, *et al.* Stability of methotrexate and vinblastine in burette administration sets. *Int J Pharmaceutics* 1988; **47:** 239–47.

### Adverse Effects, Treatment, and Precautions

For general discussions, see Antineoplastics, p.492, p.495, and p.497.

Bone-marrow depression, especially leucopenia, is the most common adverse effect with vinblastine and tends to be dose-limiting. Maximum depression occurs 5 to 10 days after a dose with recovery in a further 7 to 14 days. Leucopenia may be more severe in patients with cachexia or extensive skin ulceration: vinblastine should not be used in elderly patients with these conditions. Stomatitis and gastrointestinal bleeding may occur; nausea and vomiting respond to treatment with antiemetics.

The vinca alkaloids can produce central and peripheral (including autonomic) neurotoxicity, although these effects are less frequent with vinblastine. Symptoms include malaise, weakness, headache, depression, paraesthesia and numbness, loss of deep tendon reflexes, peripheral neuropathies, constipation and adynamic ileus, jaw pain, and convulsions. Damage to the eighth cranial nerve may result in vestibular and auditory toxicity leading to dizziness, nystagmus, vertigo, and partial or total deafness. A routine prophylactic regimen against constipation is recommended in patients receiving high doses of vinblastine. Overdosage has caused permanent damage to the CNS. Intrathecal use of the vinca alkaloids is contra-indicated because of the likelihood of fatal neurotoxicity (see Administration Error, below).

Other reported effects include skin reactions, alopecia, ischaemic cardiac toxicity, hypertension, dyspnoea and bronchospasm, and bone and tumour pain. A syndrome of inappropriate secretion of antidiuretic hormone has occurred at high doses, and may be relieved by fluid restriction and, if necessary, a suitable diuretic.

Vinblastine is irritant to the skin and mucous membranes and extravasation may cause necrosis, cellulitis, and sloughing. The application of warmth and local injection of hyaluronidase may be of benefit in relieving the effects of extravasation. By analogy with its use in the management of vincristine overdosage (see p.592), folinic acid has been suggested for use in overdosage with vinblastine.

Vinblastine should not be injected into an extremity with impaired circulation because of an increased risk of thrombosis. It should be given with caution and at reduced dosage to patients with hepatic impairment (see under Uses, below).

**Administration error.** *Intrathecal administration of vinca alkaloids, including vinblastine, results in ascending paralysis and death.* For reference to the successful treatment of inadvertent intrathecal administration of vincristine, and UK guidelines on dilution of vinca alkaloids to avoid intrathecal use, see p.592.

**Handling and disposal.** A method for the destruction of vincristine or vinblastine *wastes* using sulfuric acid and potassium permanganate.[1] Residues produced by degradation of either drug by this method showed no mutagenicity *in vitro.*

*Urine and faeces* produced for up to 4 and 7 days respectively after a dose of vinblastine should be handled wearing protective clothing.[2]

1. Castegnaro M, *et al.*, eds. Laboratory decontamination and destruction of carcinogens in laboratory wastes: some antineoplastic agents. *IARC Scientific Publications 73* Lyon: WHO/International Agency for Research on Cancer, 1985.
2. Harris J, Dodds LJ. Handling waste from patients receiving cytotoxic drugs. *Pharm J* 1985; **235:** 289–91.

**Porphyria.** Vinblastine is considered to be unsafe in patients with porphyria because it has been shown to be porphyrinogenic in *in-vitro* systems, although there is conflicting evidence of porphyrinogenicity.

### Interactions

For a general outline of antineoplastic drug interactions, see p.498. Use with drugs that inhibit cytochromes of the CYP3A subfamily may result in decreased metabolism of vinblastine and increased toxicity. For a report of the possible contribution of vinblastine to reduced plasma concentrations of phenytoin, see p.373.

**Analgesics.** A report of enhanced hepatotoxicity in patients treated with interferon alfa and vinblastine who were given *paracetamol.*[1]

1. Kellokumpu-Lehtinen P, *et al.* Hepatotoxicity of paracetamol in combination with interferon and vinblastine. *Lancet* 1989; **i:** 1143.

**Antibacterials.** There is a report of severe vinblastine toxicity in 3 patients who received vinblastine and ciclosporin with *erythromycin.*[1] Adverse effects resolved on stopping erythromycin and recurred in 1 patient who was rechallenged with erythromycin.

1. Tobe SW, *et al.* Vinblastine and erythromycin: an unrecognised serious drug interaction. *Cancer Chemother Pharmacol* 1995; **35:** 188–90.

**Antineoplastics.** Acute bronchospastic reactions following injection of a vinca alkaloid have been reported, usually in patients who have also received *mitomycin*,[1] and presenting as acute respiratory distress, cyanosis, and dyspnoea, often with the development of pulmonary infiltrates and pneumonitis.[2,3] A number of fatalities due to respiratory complications have occurred. For reports of vascular toxicity and Raynauds syndrome associated with the use of vinca alkaloids with *bleomycin* and other drugs, see Effects on the Cardiovascular System, p.493.

1. Dyke RW. Acute bronchospasm after a vinca alkaloid in patients previously treated with mitomycin. *N Engl J Med* 1984; **310:** 389.
2. Konits PH, *et al.* Possible pulmonary toxicity secondary to vinblastine. *Cancer* 1982; **50:** 2771–4.
3. Ozols RF, *et al.* MVP (mitomycin, vinblastine, and progesterone): a second-line regimen in ovarian cancer with a high incidence of pulmonary toxicity. *Cancer Treat Rep* 1983; **67:** 721–2.

**Interferons.** Severe myelosuppression has occurred in patients receiving relatively high doses of vinblastine with interferon alfa-n1.

## Pharmacokinetics

Vinblastine is not reliably absorbed from the gastrointestinal tract. After intravenous use it is rapidly cleared from the blood and distributed to tissues; it is reported to be concentrated in blood platelets. It is extensively protein bound. Vinblastine is metabolised in the liver, by cytochrome P450 isoenzymes of the CYP3A subfamily, to an active metabolite desacetylvinblastine, and is excreted in faeces via the bile, and in urine; some is excreted as unchanged drug. The terminal half-life is reported to be about 25 hours. It does not cross the blood-brain barrier in significant amounts.

## Uses and Administration

Vinblastine sulfate is an antineoplastic agent that apparently acts by binding to the microtubular proteins of the spindle and arresting mitosis at the metaphase; it is thus specific for the M phase of the cell cycle. It also interferes with glutamate metabolism and possibly nucleic acid synthesis, and has some immunosuppressant activity. Significant cross-resistance with vincristine has not been reported although pleiotropic resistance may occur.

Vinblastine sulfate is used, usually with other antineoplastics, in the treatment of Hodgkin's disease and other lymphomas, for some inoperable malignant neoplasms including those of the breast, bladder, and kidney, and in non-small cell lung cancer, choriocarcinoma, and Kaposi's sarcoma; vinblastine has also been employed in the management of Langerhans-cell histiocytosis. It was formerly used with bleomycin and cisplatin (PVB) for testicular cancer, but other regimens are now preferred. The management of these conditions is discussed under Choice of Antineoplastic, as indicated by the cross-references given below.

Vinblastine sulfate may be given by intravenous injection as a solution containing 1 mg/mL in sodium chloride 0.9%. However, UK guidelines recommend that for patients over the age of 10 years, solutions of vinblastine should generally be diluted to a volume of at least 20 mL to avoid inadvertent intrathecal use; higher concentrations can be used for children under 10 years of age. Care should be taken to avoid extravasation and the intravenous injection may be given into a freely running infusion of sodium chloride injection if preferred. The usual dose is about 6 mg/m$^2$, not more often than every 7 days, although doses starting at 3.7 mg/m$^2$ and increasing to 18.5 mg/m$^2$ have been given as a single agent. If a maintenance dose is required, it may be given every 7 days provided white cell counts permit (see below), and should be one decrement smaller than the maximum dose that the patient is able to tolerate without serious leucopenia occurring.

Children may be given vinblastine sulfate in a usual maximum weekly dose of 7.5 mg/m$^2$. Doses of up to 12.5 mg/m$^2$ per week as a single agent have been given.

White cell counts should be made before each injection and some US sources suggest a repeat dose should never be given unless the count has risen to at least 4000 cells/mm$^3$ (but see also Bone-marrow Depression, p.496). A dosage reduction is advised in patients with hepatic impairment (see below).

**Administration in hepatic impairment.** The manufacturers recommend that the dose of vinblastine be reduced by 50% in patients having a serum bilirubin value above 3 mg/100 mL.

**Blood disorders, non-malignant.** The vinca alkaloids vinblastine and vincristine have been used experimentally in the treatment of various auto-immune blood disorders such as idiopathic thrombocytopenic purpura, and auto-immune haemolytic anaemia (p.1082 and p.733 respectively). There are also reports of the haemolytic-uraemic syndrome/thrombotic thrombocytopenic purpura responding to treatment with intravenous injection of vincristine.[1-3] For further details on the treatment of thrombotic microangiopathies, see p.758. Vincristine has been given with normal immunoglobulin in the management of a patient with life-threatening thrombocytopenia due to sarcoidosis.[4] Vincristine has also been used for life-threatening haemangioma (p.1081).

1. Gutterman LA, *et al.* The hemolytic-uremic syndrome: recovery after treatment with vincristine. *Ann Intern Med* 1983; **98:** 612–13.
2. Ferrara F, *et al.* Vincristine as salvage treatment for refractory thrombotic thrombocytopenic purpura. *Ann Hematol* 1999; **78:** 521–3.
3. Ferrara F, *et al.* Vincristine as treatment for recurrent episodes of thrombotic thrombocytopenic purpura. *Ann Hematol* 2002; **81:** 7–10.
4. Larner AJ. Life threatening thrombocytopenia in sarcoidosis. *BMJ* 1990; **300:** 317–19.

**Histiocytic syndromes.** The value of systemic chemotherapy in patients with Langerhans-cell histiocytosis (p.505) is uncertain; however, it is certainly widely used in extensive disease, vinblastine being one of the drugs often employed.[1,2]

1. The French Langerhans' Cell Histiocytosis Study Group. A multicentre retrospective survey of Langerhans' cell histiocytosis: 348 cases observed between 1983 and 1993. *Arch Dis Child* 1996; **75:** 17–24.
2. Gadner H, *et al.* A randomized trial of treatment for multisystem Langerhans' cell histiocytosis. *J Pediatr* 2001; **138:** 728–34. Correction. *ibid.*; **139:** 170.

**Malignant neoplasms.** Vinblastine plays an important role in the ABVD regimen in patients with Hodgkin's disease (p.509). It also formed part of the effective, if toxic, PVB regimen used to treat germ cell (ovarian or testicular) cancer, p.520 and p.523 respectively, although other regimens tend now to be preferred. The vinca alkaloids are also active in gestational trophoblastic tumours (p.505), and vinblastine is also used in the therapy of invasive bladder cancer (p.512); it may be used in the adjuvant or palliative treatment of non-small-cell lung cancer (p.519) and in the palliative care of advanced breast cancer (p.514) and mycosis fungoides (p.511). It has been used in malignancies of the kidney (p.518). Vinca alkaloids are also used to treat Kaposi's sarcoma (p.524).

## Preparations

***BP 2003:*** Vinblastine Injection;
***USP 27:*** Vinblastine Sulfate for Injection.

**Proprietary Preparations** (details are given in Part 3)
***Arg.:*** Blastovin; Velbe; Xintoprost; ***Austral.:*** Velbe; ***Austria:*** Velbe; ***Belg.:*** Velbe; ***Braz.:*** Velban; ***Canad.:*** Velbe†; ***Chile:*** Lemblastine; Velbe; ***Denm.:*** Velbe; ***Fin.:*** Velbe; ***Fr.:*** Velbe; ***Ger.:*** Cellblastin; Velbe; ***Gr.:*** Velbe; ***Hong Kong:*** Velbe; ***India:*** Cytoblastin; ***Israel:*** Blastovin; Velbe†; ***Ital.:*** Velbe; ***Mex.:*** Ifabla; Lemblastine; Serovin†; Velbe; ***Neth.:*** Velbe; ***Norw.:*** Velbe; ***Port.:*** Solblastin; Velbe; ***S.Afr.:*** Periblastine†; ***Swed.:*** Velbe; ***Switz.:*** Velbe; ***UK:*** Velbe; ***USA:*** Velban.

---

# Vincristine Sulfate *(USAN, rINNM)*

Compound 37231; Leurocristine Sulphate; NSC-67574; 22-Oxovincaleukoblastine Sulphate; Sulfato de vincristina; Sulfato de Vincristina; Vincristine Sulphate *(BANM)*; Vincristini Sulfas.

$C_{46}H_{56}N_4O_{10},H_2SO_4$ = 923.0.

*CAS — 57-22-7 (vincristine); 2068-78-2 (vincristine sulfate).*

*ATC — L01CA02.*

**Description.** Vincristine sulfate is the sulfate of an alkaloid, 22-oxovincaleukoblastine, obtained from *Catharanthus roseus* (*Vinca rosea*) (Apocynaceae).

**Pharmacopoeias.** In *Chin., Eur.* (see p.vi), *Int., Jpn, Pol., US,* and *Viet.*

**Ph. Eur. 5.0** (Vincristine Sulphate). A white or slightly yellowish, very hygroscopic, crystalline powder. It loses not more than 12% of its weight on drying. Freely soluble in water; slightly soluble in alcohol. A 0.1% solution in water has a pH of 3.5 to 4.5. Store at a temperature not exceeding −20° in airtight glass containers. Protect from light.

**USP 27** (Vincristine Sulfate). A white to slightly yellow, odourless, hygroscopic, amorphous or crystalline powder. It loses not more than 12% of its weight on drying. Freely soluble in water; slightly soluble in alcohol; soluble in methyl alcohol. A 0.1% solution in water has a pH of 3.5 to 4.5. Store at a temperature between −25° and −20° in airtight containers. Protect from light.

## Adverse Effects, Treatment, and Precautions

As for Vinblastine Sulfate, p.591.

Bone-marrow depression occurs less commonly than with vinblastine but neurological and neuromuscular effects are more severe with vincristine and are dose-limiting. Walking may be impaired and the neurological effects may not be reversed for several months after the drug is discontinued. Convulsions, often with hypertension, have occurred. Constipation is common and there may be abdominal pain. Urinary disturbances have occurred and alopecia is frequent.

Folinic acid has been given for the treatment of overdosage: suggested doses are as much as 100 mg of folinic acid intravenously every 3 hours for 24 hours, then every 6 hours for at least 48 hours. However, this is unlikely to be of benefit in reversing neuromuscular toxicity. For mention of the use of glutamic acid in managing the usually fatal consequences of inadvertent intrathecal administration, see below.

Because severe constipation and impaction of faeces often occur with vincristine, laxatives or enemas may be necessary to ensure regular bowel function. Vincristine should be given with caution to patients with pre-existing neuromuscular disease and is contra-indicated in patients with the demyelinating form of Charcot-Marie-Tooth syndrome (see under Effects on the Nervous System, below). Doses may need to be adjusted in patients with hepatic impairment. Care should also be taken in elderly patients, who may be more susceptible to neurotoxicity.

**Administration error.** *Inadvertent intrathecal administration of vincristine results in ascending paralysis and death.*[1,2] However, in one case[1] treatment immediately following the error, and consisting of removal of contaminated spinal fluid and flushing with lactated Ringer's solution and fresh frozen plasma diluted in lactated Ringer's solution, plus intravenous and oral glutamic acid, was reported successful in stabilising neurological dysfunction and preventing death. The role of glutamic acid in this case is uncertain, but a study involving 84 patients found that glutamic acid 1.5 g daily given by mouth in divided doses during a 6-week induction chemotherapy course decreased vincristine-induced neurotoxicity.[3] One manufacturer (Lilly) has stated that folinic acid and pyridoxine intravenously have also been used, but that, like glutamic acid, their roles in the reduction of neurotoxicity remain unclear.

While early recognition and immediate treatment with cerebrospinal fluid drainage and exchange may improve survival,[4] fatalities still occur despite these measures.[4,5] Recommendations[2,5] have been made in order to prevent further errors occurring, including restrictions on the prescription, administration, and storage of intrathecal drugs. In the UK, recommendations state that vinca alkaloids for intravenous use in adults or children over 10 years should be diluted to a maximum concentration of 100 micrograms/mL (vincristine) or a volume of at least 20 mL (vinblastine, vindesine, or vinorelbine) and labelled with a clear warning of the consequences of use by other routes. Higher concentrations may be used in children under 10 years, and in certain specialised centres.[2]

1. Dyke RW. Treatment of inadvertent intrathecal injection of vincristine. *N Engl J Med* 1989; **321:** 1270–1.
2. Department of Health. Updated national guidance on the safe administration of intrathecal chemotherapy (HSC 2003/010, 2 October 2003). Available at: http://www.dh.gov.uk/assetRoot/04/06/43/17/04064317.pdf (accessed 01/07/04)
3. Jackson DV, *et al.* Amelioration of vincristine neurotoxicity by glutamic acid. *Am J Med* 1988; **84:** 1016–22.
4. Alcaraz A, *et al.* Intrathecal vincristine: fatal myeloencephalopathy despite cerebrospinal fluid perfusion. *J Toxicol Clin Toxicol* 2002; **40:** 557–61.
5. Fernandez CV, *et al.* Intrathecal vincristine: an analysis of reasons for recurrent fatal chemotherapeutic error with recommendations for prevention. *J Pediatr Hematol Oncol* 1998; **20:** 587–90.

**Effects on the nervous system.** In its most typical form, vincristine neurotoxicity[1] manifests as a mixed sensorimotor neuropathy of the distal type. The earliest symptoms are sensory changes in the form of paraesthesias, accompanied by impairment and ultimately loss of deep tendon reflexes. In more severe forms, impairment of motor function occurs with wrist drop and foot drop, ataxia and gait abnormalities, and occasionally progressive quadriparesis.

In contrast to these peripheral neuropathies which are usually associated with long-term usage there may be short-term autonomic neuropathy resulting in constipation and occasionally ileus, abdominal pain, atony of the urinary bladder (which may lead to urinary retention), orthostatic hypotension, and rarely, impotence. There may be effects on the cranial nerves, resulting in ptosis, hoarseness (due to laryngeal nerve paralysis), or optic neuropathies. Effects on the CNS are rare, probably in part because of poor penetration into CSF, but include excessive release of antidiuretic hormone and consequent hyponatraemia.

Hallucinations have occurred[2] and effects on the special senses have been reported: both bilateral optic atrophy and blindness,[3] and profound neurological deafness (which was largely reversible on drug withdrawal)[4] have occurred. Convulsions associated with hypertension are another feature of vincristine toxicity.[5]

Toxicity is related to both the cumulative and the individual dose.[1] It usually begins in adults after receiving a total of 5 to 6 mg, and is significant by the time a cumulative dose of 15 to 20 mg is reached. If individual doses are low (less than 2 mg) or intervals between doses are longer than the usual week, patients can tolerate higher cumulative doses. Children tolerate vincristine better than adults, but the elderly are particularly prone to neurotoxicity. Patients with existing neurological disorders such as poliomyelitis or the Charcot-Marie-Tooth syndrome may be at increased risk of neurotoxicity.[6-9] It has been suggested that increased neurotoxicity may be associated with the use of ready-to-use solutions rather than reconstituted lyophilised preparations but this has not been proved.[10-14]

There is no good treatment for the effects of vincristine on the nervous system: symptoms are largely reversible once administration is interrupted, and should be managed with appropriate symptomatic care.[1] However, there is some suggestion that glutamic acid may be of benefit in treating neurotoxicity—see Administration Error, above. For the use of dinoprost to alleviate ileus induced by vinca alkaloids, see p.1515.


1. Legha SS. Vincristine neurotoxicity: pathophysiology and management. *Med Toxicol* 1986; **1:** 421–7.
2. Holland JF, *et al.* Vincristine treatment of advanced cancer: a cooperative study of 392 cases. *Cancer Res* 1973; **33:** 1258–64.
3. Awidi AS. Blindness and vincristine. *Ann Intern Med* 1980; **93:** 781.
4. Yousif H, *et al.* Partially reversible nerve deafness due to vincristine. *Postgrad Med J* 1990; **66:** 688–9.
5. Ito S, *et al.* Seizures and hypertension complicating vincristine therapy in children. *Clin Pharmacol Ther* 1995; **57:** 208.
6. Hogan-Dann CM, *et al.* Polyneuropathy following vincristine therapy in two patients with Charcot-Marie-Tooth syndrome. *JAMA* 1984; **252:** 2862–3.
7. Miller BR. Neurotoxicity and vincristine. *JAMA* 1985; **253:** 2045.
8. Chauncey TR, *et al.* Vincristine neurotoxicity. *JAMA* 1985; **254:** 507.
9. Griffiths JD, *et al.* Vincristine neurotoxicity in Charcot-Marie-Tooth syndrome. *Med J Aust* 1985; **143:** 305–6.
10. Arnold AM, *et al.* Acute vincristine neurotoxicity. *Lancet* 1985; **i:** 346.
11. Jalihal S, Roebuck N. Acute vincristine neurotoxicity. *Lancet* 1985; **i:** 637.
12. Davies CE, *et al.* Acute vincristine neurotoxicity. *Lancet* 1985; **i:** 637–8.
13. Warrier RP, Ducos R. Acute vincristine neurotoxicity. *Lancet* 1985; **i:** 980.
14. Gennery BA. Vincristine neurotoxicity. *Lancet* 1985; **ii:** 385.


**Handling and disposal.** For a method for the destruction of vincristine *wastes*, see under Vinblastine Sulfate, p.591.

*Urine and faeces* produced for up to 4 and 7 days respectively after a dose of vincristine should be handled wearing protective clothing.[1]


1. Harris J, Dodds LJ. Handling waste from patients receiving cytotoxic drugs. *Pharm J* 1985; **235:** 289–91.


**Porphyria.** Vincristine is considered to be unsafe in patients with porphyria because it has been shown to be porphyrinogenic in *in-vitro* systems, although there is conflicting evidence of porphyrinogenicity.

## Interactions

For a general outline of antineoplastic drug interactions, see p.498. Use of vincristine with drugs that inhibit cytochromes of the CYP3A subfamily may result in decreased metabolism of vincristine and increased toxicity. If vincristine is used with asparaginase it should be given 12 to 24 hours before the enzyme: giving asparaginase with or before vincristine may reduce vincristine clearance and increase toxicity. For reports of vascular toxicity and Raynaud's syndrome associated with the use of vinca alkaloids with bleomycin and other drugs see Effects on the Cardiovascular System, p.493.

**Antibacterials.** Severe neurotoxicity has occurred when *isoniazid* was added to the regimen of a patient receiving vincristine.[1]


1. Carrión C, *et al.* Possible vincristine-isoniazid interaction. *Ann Pharmacother* 1995; **29:** 201.


**Antiepileptics.** A pharmacokinetic study showed that systemic clearance of vincristine was 63% higher when it was given with *phenytoin* or *carbamazepine*, two inducers of the cytochrome P450 isoenzyme CYP3A4. The clinical significance of this finding is unknown.[1]


1. Villikka K, *et al.* Cytochrome P450-inducing antiepileptics increase the clearance of vincristine in patients with brain tumours. *Clin Pharmacol Ther* 1999; **66:** 589–93.


**Antifungals.** Toxicity has been reported to be increased in children who received *itraconazole* with or without nifedipine during treatment involving vincristine.[1-4] Itraconazole is presumed to potentiate the toxicity of vincristine either by inhibition of cytochrome P450 isoenzymes, thus reducing the clearance of vincristine,[1-4] or by inhibiting the P-glycoprotein efflux pump,[2,3] and increasing intracellular concentrations of vincristine. Nifedipine also decreases the clearance of vincristine, by similar mechanisms,[1,3,4] and can theoretically further potentiate toxicity.


1. Murphy JA, *et al.* Vincristine toxicity in five children with acute lymphoblastic leukaemia. *Lancet* 1995; **346:** 443.
2. Jeng MR, Feusner J. Itraconazole-enhanced vincristine neurotoxicity in a child with acute lymphoblastic leukemia. *Pediatr Hematol Oncol* 2001; **18:** 137–42.
3. Sathiapalan RK, El-Solh H. Enhanced vincristine neurotoxicity from drug interactions: case report and review of literature. *Pediatr Hematol Oncol* 2001; **18:** 543–6.
4. Kamaluddin M, *et al.* Potentiation of vincristine toxicity by itraconazole in children with lymphoid malignancies. *Acta Paediatr* 2001; **90:** 1204–7.


**Nifedipine.** Vincristine toxicity may be potentiated by nifedipine, see Antifungals, above.

## Pharmacokinetics

Vincristine is not reliably absorbed from the gastrointestinal tract. After intravenous injection it disappears rapidly from the blood. It is extensively protein bound and is reported to be concentrated in blood platelets. It is metabolised in the liver and excreted primarily in the bile; about 70 to 80% of a dose is found in faeces, as unchanged drug and metabolites, while 10 to 20% appears in the urine. The terminal half-life is reported to be about 85 hours but may range from about 19 to 155 hours. Vincristine does not appear to cross the blood-brain barrier in significant amounts.

## Uses and Administration

Vincristine is an antineoplastic agent that may act similarly to vinblastine (above) by arresting mitosis at the metaphase. Significant cross-resistance with vinblastine has not been reported although pleiotropic resistance may occur.

Vincristine sulfate is used principally in combination chemotherapy regimens for acute leukaemia and Hodgkin's disease and other lymphomas, including Burkitt's lymphoma. It may also be used in the treatment of Wilms' tumour, myeloma, neuroblastoma, in sarcomas including Kaposi's sarcoma and rhabdomyosarcoma and in tumours of the brain, breast, head and neck, and lung, among others. It has also been given in idiopathic thrombocytopenic purpura refractory to other agents. See also the cross-references given below.

Vincristine sulfate is given by intravenous injection. It has been given as a solution containing 1 mg/mL. However, UK guidelines recommend that for patients over the age of 10 years, solutions of vincristine should generally be diluted to a maximum concentration of 100 micrograms/mL and to a volume of at least 10 mL, to avoid inadvertent intrathecal use; higher concentrations can be used for children under 10 years of age. Care should be taken to avoid extravasation and the injection may be given into a freely-running intravenous infusion of sodium chloride injection if preferred.

In acute leukaemia the usual once-weekly dose of vincristine sulfate for induction of remission in children is 2 mg/m$^2$, or an initial dose of 50 micrograms/kg in those weighing 10 kg or less. Adults may be given about 1.4 mg/m$^2$ or 25 to 75 micrograms/kg weekly; a maximum weekly dose of 2 mg has been suggested (but see Administration, below). For other malignancies 25 micrograms/kg may be given weekly and reduced to 5 to 10 micrograms/kg for maintenance.

Blood counts should be carried out before giving each dose. A dose reduction is recommended in patients with hepatic impairment (see below).

A liposomal formulation of vincristine is under investigation.

**Action.** Results *in vitro* suggested[1] a selective action of vincristine against lymphocytes of patients with chronic lymphocytic leukaemia; lymphocytes of healthy subjects were not so affected. A further study[2] confirmed these findings, and also found marked variation in vincristine susceptibility among individual chronic lymphocytic leukaemic cells. This suggests that vincristine may have effects other than arrest of mitosis.


1. Vilpo J, Vilpo L. Selective toxicity of vincristine against chronic lymphocytic leukaemia in vitro. *Lancet* 1996; **347:** 1491–2.
2. Vilpo JA, *et al.* Selective toxicity of vincristine against chronic lymphocytic leukemia cells in vitro. *Eur J Haematol* 2000; **65:** 370–8.


**Administration.** Although a maximum single dose of 2 mg is recommended for vincristine sulfate to reduce neurotoxicity, a review[1] has suggested that this guideline is overly rigid, since it does not take into account interindividual variations in pharmacokinetics and susceptibility to toxicity, which may be considerable. Furthermore the authors considered the evidence for effectiveness of this dosage limitation to be equivocal. They suggested beginning therapy at 1.4 mg/m$^2$ and adjusting subsequent doses according to toxicity.

For UK recommendations on dilution of intravenous vinca alkaloids see Administration Error, under Adverse Effects, above.


1. McCune JS, Lindley C. Appropriateness of maximum-dose guidelines for vincristine. *Am J Health-Syst Pharm* 1997; **54:** 1755–8.


**Administration in hepatic impairment.** The manufacturers recommend that the dose of vincristine be reduced by 50% in patients having a serum bilirubin value above 3 mg/100 mL.

**Amyloidosis.** For mention of regimens including vincristine used in the management of amyloidosis, see p.567.

**Blood disorders, non-malignant.** Vincristine may be employed in the treatment of various auto-immune blood disorders, see under Vinblastine, p.592.

**Malignant neoplasms.** Vincristine is widely used in the treatment of malignant neoplasms. It is a fundamental part of potentially curative regimens for acute lymphoblastic leukaemia, Hodgkin's disease and aggressive non-Hodgkins lymphomas (see p.506, p.509 and p.510). It has also been used in chronic lymphocytic leukaemia (p.507) and in other non-Hodgkin's lymphomas including AIDS-related lymphoma (p.510), Burkitt's lymphoma (p.511) and mycosis fungoides (p.511). Other haematological malignancies in which it may be tried include multiple myeloma (p.511). Among the solid neoplasms, vincristine is used in regimens to treat gestational trophoblastic tumours (p.505), tumours of the brain (p.513), head and neck (p.517), Wilms' tumour (p.518), small-cell lung cancer (p.519), and thymoma (p.523). It is also employed in regimens for neuroblastoma (p.524), retinoblastoma (p.524), and some sarcomas including sarcomas of bone, Kaposi's sarcoma, and rhabdomyosarcoma (see p.524, p.524, and p.525).

## Preparations

***BP 2003:*** Vincristine Injection;
***USP 27:*** Vincristine Sulfate for Injection; Vincristine Sulfate Injection.

**Proprietary Preparations** (details are given in Part 3)
***Arg.:*** Vinces; ***Austral.:*** Oncovin; ***Austria:*** Oncovin; ***Belg.:*** Oncovin; ***Braz.:*** Biocrist; Oncovin; Tecnocris; Vincizina; Vincristex; Vinracine; ***Canad.:*** Oncovin†; ***Chile:*** Citomid; Oncovin; ***Denm.:*** Oncovin; ***Fin.:*** Oncovin; Vincrin†; ***Fr.:*** Oncovin; ***Ger.:*** Cellcristin; Farmistin; Onkocristin; ***Gr.:*** Oncovin; ***India:*** Cytocristin; Neocristin; ***Irl.:*** Oncovin†; ***Israel:*** Oncovin†; ***Malaysia:*** Vinracine; ***Mex.:*** Citomid; Filcrin†; Ifavin; Oncovin; Vincasar†; Vintec†; ***Neth.:*** Oncovin†; ***Norw.:*** Oncovin; ***NZ:*** Oncovin†; ***Port.:*** Faulcris; Oncovin; ***S.Afr.:*** Oncovin; Pericristine†; ***Spain:*** Vincrisul; ***Swed.:*** Oncovin; ***Switz.:*** Oncovin; ***UK:*** Oncovin; ***USA:*** Oncovin; Vincasar PFS.

# Vindesine Sulfate *(USAN, rINNM)*

Compound 112531 (vindesine); Desacetyl Vinblastine Amide Sulfate; LY-099094; NSC-245467 (vindesine or vindesine sulfate); Sulfato de vindesina; Vindesine Sulphate *(BANM)*; Vindesini Sulfas. 3-Carbamoyl-4-O-deacetyl-3-de(methoxycarbonyl)vincaleukoblastine sulfate.

$C_{43}H_{55}N_5O_7,H_2SO_4$ = 852.0.
*CAS — 53643-48-4 (vindesine); 59917-39-4 (vindesine sulfate).*
*ATC — L01CA03.*

**Pharmacopoeias.** In *Eur.* (see p.vi).

**Ph. Eur. 5.0** (Vindesine Sulphate). A white or almost white, hygroscopic, amorphous substance. Freely soluble in water and in methyl alcohol; practically insoluble in cyclohexane. The pH of a 0.5% solution in water is 3.5 to 5.5. Store in airtight polypropylene containers with a polypropylene cap, at a temperature not exceeding −50°.

## Adverse Effects, Treatment, and Precautions

As for Vinblastine Sulfate, p.591.

The main dose-limiting effect of vindesine is granulocytopenia, with the nadir of the white cell count usually occurring 3 to 5 days after a dose and recovery after a further 4 to 5 days. Although neurotoxicity occurs it may be less severe than that seen with vincristine (see p.592). Alopecia is the most common side-effect.

Folinic acid has been suggested for the treatment of overdosage by analogy with vincristine.

Vindesine should not be given by the intrathecal route, as this may produce fatal toxicity. Care should be taken if acute abdominal pain occurs: further doses may result in paralytic ileus.

**Administration error.** *Inadvertent intrathecal administration of vinca alkaloids results in ascending paralysis and death.* In a 10-year-old child accidentally given an intrathecal injection of vindesine, treatment with folinic acid and dexamethasone produced transient recovery but symptoms subsequently recurred and the patient died of progressive ascending paralysis.[1] The CNS showed changes at necropsy similar to those seen following intrathecal administration of vincristine. For reference to the successful treatment of inadvertent intrathecal administration of vincristine, and UK recommendations on dilution of vinca alkaloids to avoid intrathecal use, see p.592.


1. Robbins G. Accidental intrathecal injection of vindesine. *BMJ* 1985; **291:** 1094.


## Interactions

As for Vinblastine Sulfate, p.591.

### Pharmacokinetics

The pharmacokinetics of vindesine are similar to those of the other vinca alkaloids. After intravenous doses elimination from the blood is triphasic; the drug is rapidly distributed to body tissues. The terminal half-life is reported to be about 20 hours. It is metabolised primarily in the liver and excreted in bile and urine.

### Uses and Administration

Vindesine sulfate is an antineoplastic agent derived from vinblastine (see p.591); like the other vinca alkaloids it causes mitotic arrest in metaphase by binding to microtubular protein. It is used in the treatment of refractory acute lymphoblastic or chronic myeloid leukaemias, and malignant melanoma. It has also been tried in malignant neoplasms of the breast, and lung. See also the cross references given below.

Vindesine sulfate is given weekly by intravenous injection. It may be given as a solution containing 1 mg/mL in sodium chloride injection 0.9%. However, UK guidelines recommend that for patients over the age of 10 years, solutions of vindesine should generally be diluted to a volume of at least 20 mL to avoid inadvertent intrathecal use; higher concentrations can be used for children under 10 years of age. Care should be taken to avoid extravasation and it may be given into a fast-running infusion of sodium chloride, glucose 5%, or glucose-saline injection. The usual starting dose for adults is 3 mg/m$^2$ which may be raised by increments of 500 micrograms/m$^2$ weekly providing that the granulocyte and platelet counts do not fall below acceptable levels (see also Bone-marrow Depression, p.496), and acute abdominal pain is not experienced; weekly doses are usually between 3 and 4 mg/m$^2$. Children may be given 4 mg/m$^2$ initially, with weekly doses usually ranging between 4 and 5 mg/m$^2$. An alternative regimen for children with leukaemia is 2 mg/m$^2$ daily for 2 consecutive days, repeated after an interval of 5 to 7 days. Blood counts should be made before each injection. It may be necessary to reduce initial doses in patients with significantly impaired hepatic function.

**Malignant neoplasms.** Vindesine has been tried in refractory metastatic melanoma (p.522), childhood acute lymphoblastic leukaemia (p.506), chronic myeloid leukaemia in blastic crisis (p.507), and neuroblastoma (p.524). It is also under investigation in lung cancer, particularly non-small cell lung cancer (p.519) and responses have been reported in advanced breast cancer (p.514).

### Preparations

***BP 2003:*** Vindesine Injection.

**Proprietary Preparations** (details are given in Part 3)
***Arg.:*** Eldisine; ***Austral.:*** Eldisine; ***Austria:*** Eldisin; ***Belg.:*** Eldisine; ***Canad.:*** Eldisine†; ***Fin.:*** Eldisine; ***Fr.:*** Eldisine; ***Ger.:*** Eldisine; ***Gr.:*** Gesidine; ***Hong Kong:*** Eldisine†; ***Irl.:*** Eldisine; ***Ital.:*** Eldisine; ***Neth.:*** Eldisine; ***Port.:*** Gesidine; ***S.Afr.:*** Eldisine; ***Spain:*** Enison; ***Swed.:*** Eldisine; ***Switz.:*** Eldisine; ***UK:*** Eldisine.

---

## Vinorelbine Tartrate *(BANM, USAN, rINNM)*

5′-Nor-anhydrovinblastine Tartrate; Tartrato de vinorelbina; Vinorelbine Ditartrate; Vinorelbini Tartras. 3′,4′-Didehydro-4′-deoxy-8′-norvincaleukoblastine ditartrate.

$C_{45}H_{54}N_4O_8,2C_4H_6O_6$ = 1079.1.

*CAS — 71486-22-1 (vinorelbine); 125317-39-7 (vinorelbine tartrate).*

*ATC — L01CA04.*

**Pharmacopoeias.** In *Eur.* (see p.vi) and *US.*

**Ph. Eur. 5.0** (Vinorelbine Tartrate). A white or almost white, hygroscopic powder. Freely soluble in water and in methyl alcohol; practically insoluble in hexane. A 1.4% solution in water has a pH of 3.3 to 3.8. Store under an inert gas at a temperature not exceeding −15°. Protect from light.

**USP 27** (Vinorelbine Tartrate). A white to yellow or light brown amorphous powder. Freely soluble in water. pH of a 1% solution in water is between 3.3 and 3.8. Store at a temperature between −25° and −10° in airtight containers. Protect from light.

### Adverse Effects and Precautions

As for Vinblastine Sulfate, p.591. The main dose-limiting effect of vinorelbine is granulocytopenia. The nadir of the granulocyte count occurs 5 to 10 days after a dose, with recovery usually after a further 7 to 14 days. The drug should be discontinued if moderate or severe neurotoxicity develops. Local pain and thrombophlebitis may be seen with repeated injection of vinorelbine. Gastrointestinal effects such as nausea and vomiting are common with the oral formulation.

**Administration error.** *Inadvertent intrathecal administration of vinca alkaloids results in ascending paralysis and death.* For reference to the successful treatment of inadvertent intrathecal administration of vincristine, and UK recommendations on dilution of vinca alkaloids to avoid intrathecal use, see p.592.

**Effects on the gastrointestinal tract.** For reference to a report of vinorelbine possibly exacerbating ischaemic colitis in patients receiving docetaxel, see p.547.

### Interactions

As for Vinblastine Sulfate, p.591.

### Pharmacokinetics

As with the other vinca alkaloids, vinorelbine exhibits triphasic pharmacokinetics after intravenous injection, and has a terminal half-life of between about 28 and 44 hours. It is rapidly absorbed from the gastrointestinal tract with peak plasma concentrations achieved between 1.5 and 3 hours after oral doses. It is metabolised in the liver; deacetylvinorelbine has antineoplastic activity. Vinorelbine and its metabolites are excreted primarily in faeces via the bile but also in urine.

◊ References.

1. Levêque D, Jehl F. Clinical pharmacokinetics of vinorelbine. *Clin Pharmacokinet* 1996; **31:** 184–97.
2. Marty M, *et al.* Oral vinorelbine pharmacokinetics and absolute bioavailability study in patients with solid tumors. *Ann Oncol* 2001; **12:** 1643–9.
3. Bugat R, *et al.* The effects of food on the pharmacokinetic profile of oral vinorelbine. *Cancer Chemother Pharmacol* 2002; **50:** 285–90.
4. Variol P, *et al.* A simultaneous oral/intravenous population pharmacokinetic model for vinorelbine. *Eur J Clin Pharmacol* 2002; **58:** 467–76.

### Uses and Administration

Vinorelbine is a semisynthetic derivative of vinblastine (p.592) with similar general properties. It is used as the tartrate in the treatment of advanced breast cancer and non-small cell lung cancers (see p.514 and p.519 respectively), and has been tried in other malignancies including lymphomas and tumours of ovary and prostate.

Vinorelbine is given as the tartrate but doses are calculated in terms of vinorelbine: vinorelbine tartrate 1.385 mg is approximately equivalent to 1 mg of vinorelbine. It may be given by intravenous injection over 5 to 10 minutes, as a solution containing the equivalent of vinorelbine 1.5 to 3 mg/mL in glucose 5% or sodium chloride 0.9% injection, directly or into a freely-running intravenous infusion. However, UK guidelines recommend that for patients over the age of 10 years, solutions of vinorelbine should generally be diluted to a volume of at least 20 mL to avoid inadvertent intrathecal use; higher concentrations can be used for children under 10 years of age. It may also be given by intravenous infusion over 20 to 30 minutes after dilution in 125 mL of glucose 5% or sodium chloride 0.9%. The usual initial dose is the equivalent of vinorelbine 25 to 30 mg/m$^2$ weekly. In the UK, the manufacturers recommend that if the neutrophil count falls below 2000 cells/mm$^3$ subsequent doses should be delayed until recovery. In the USA it is suggested that subsequent doses should be halved if granulocyte counts fall to between 1000 and 1500 cells/mm$^3$; treatment should be interrupted if counts are below 1000 cells/mm$^3$ and discontinued if granulocytopenia persists for more than 2 weeks (see also Bone-marrow Depression, p.496). Doses should also be reduced in hepatic impairment and in patients with massive liver metastases (but see also below).

In the treatment of non-small cell lung cancer, vinorelbine is also given orally at a dose of 60 mg/m$^2$ once weekly for 3 weeks. Subsequent doses may be increased to 80 mg/m$^2$, unless the neutrophil count falls below 500 cells/mm$^3$, or to between 500 and 1000 cells/mm$^3$ on two separate occasions.

◊ References.

1. Gregory RK, Smith IE. Vinorelbine—a clinical review. *Br J Cancer* 2000; **82:** 1907–13.
2. Sarris AH, *et al.* Infusional vinorelbine in relapsed or refractory lymphomas. *Leuk Lymphoma* 2000; **39:** 291–9.
3. Sorensen P, *et al.* Phase II study of vinorelbine in the treatment of platinum-resistant ovarian carcinoma. *Gynecol Oncol* 2001; **81:** 58–62.
4. Oudard S, *et al.* Phase II study of vinorelbine in patients with androgen-independent prostate cancer. *Ann Oncol* 2001; **12:** 847–52.
5. Domenech GH, Vogel CL. A review of vinorelbine in the treatment of breast cancer. *Clin Breast Cancer* 2001; **2:** 113–28.
6. Aapro MS, *et al.* Developments in cytotoxic chemotherapy: advances in treatment utilising vinorelbine. *Crit Rev Oncol Hematol* 2001; **40:** 251–63.
7. Gridelli C, De Vivo R. Vinorelbine in the treatment of non-small cell lung cancer. *Curr Med Chem* 2002; **9:** 879–91.
8. Freyer G, *et al.* Phase II study of oral vinorelbine in first-line advanced breast cancer chemotherapy. *J Clin Oncol* 2003; **21:** 35–40.

**Administration in hepatic impairment.** Clearance of vinorelbine was markedly reduced in patients with diffuse liver metastases and hence severely altered hepatic function: a 50% dose reduction was probably appropriate in such patients even if hyperbilirubinaemia was not marked.[1] However, reduced doses were not necessary in patients with moderate liver involvement in whom liver function, as measured by lidocaine metabolism, was not markedly reduced. The manufacturers in the UK suggest that the intravenous dose be reduced by one-third in patients with massive liver metastases (more than 75% of liver volume replaced by tumour cells).

In the USA, the manufacturers recommend that the intravenous dose of vinorelbine be reduced by 50% in patients with bilirubin values of 2.1 to 3 mg/100 mL and by 75% in those with bilirubin greater than 3 mg/100 mL.

1. Robieux I, *et al.* Pharmacokinetics of vinorelbine in patients with liver metastases. *Clin Pharmacol Ther* 1996; **59:** 32–40.

### Preparations

**Proprietary Preparations** (details are given in Part 3)
***Arg.:*** Filcrin; Navelbine; Neocitec; Sulcoline; Vilbine; Vilne; Vinarine; Vinorgen; ***Austral.:*** Navelbine; ***Austria:*** Navelbine; ***Belg.:*** Navelbine; ***Braz.:*** Navelbine; Norelbin; ***Canad.:*** Navelbine; ***Chile:*** Navelbine; ***Denm.:*** Navelbine; ***Fin.:*** Navelbine; ***Fr.:*** Navelbine; ***Ger.:*** Navelbine; ***Gr.:*** Navelbine; ***Hong Kong:*** Navelbine; ***India:*** Vinelbine; ***Israel:*** Navelbine; ***Ital.:*** Navelbine; ***Malaysia:*** Navelbine; ***Mex.:*** Navelbine; ***Norw.:*** Navelbine; ***NZ:*** Navelbine; ***Port.:*** Navelbine; ***S.Afr.:*** Navelbine; ***Singapore:*** Navelbine; ***Spain:*** Biovelbin†; Navelbine; ***Swed.:*** Navelbine; ***Switz.:*** Navelbine; ***Thai.:*** Navelbine; ***UK:*** Navelbine; ***USA:*** Navelbine.

---

## Vorozole *(BAN, USAN, rINN)*

R-83842; Vorozol. (+)-6-[4-Chloro-α-(1,2,4-triazol-1-yl)benzyl]-1-methyl-1*H*-benzotriazole.

$C_{16}H_{13}ClN_6$ = 324.8.

*CAS — 129731-10-8.*

*ATC — L02BG05.*

### Profile

Vorozole is a selective nonsteroidal inhibitor of the aromatase (oestrogen synthetase) system. It has been investigated in the treatment of breast cancer.

◊ References.

1. Goss PE, *et al.* Phase II study of vorozole (R83842), a new aromatase inhibitor, in postmenopausal women with advanced breast cancer in progression on tamoxifen. *Clin Cancer Res* 1995; **1:** 287–94.
2. Paridaens R, *et al.* Vorozole (Rivizor): an active and well tolerated new aromatase inhibitor for the treatment of advanced breast cancer patients with prior tamoxifen exposure. *Anticancer Drugs* 1998; **9:** 29–35.
3. Goss PE, *et al.* Randomized phase III trial comparing the new potent and selective third-generation aromatase inhibitor vorozole with megestrol acetate in postmenopausal advanced breast cancer patients. *J Clin Oncol* 1999; **17:** 52–63.
4. Harper-Wynne CL, *et al.* Comparison of the systemic and intratumoral effects of tamoxifen and the aromatase inhibitor vorozole in postmenopausal patients with primary breast cancer. *J Clin Oncol* 2002; **20:** 1026–35.

---

## Zinostatin *(USAN, rINN)*

Neocarzinostatin; NSC-69856; NSC-157365; Zinostatina.

*CAS — 9014-02-2.*

**Description.** Zinostatin is an antineoplastic antibiotic obtained from *Streptomyces carzinostaticus*.

**Pharmacopoeias.** *Jpn* includes zinostatin stimalamer.

### Profile

Zinostatin is an antibiotic with antineoplastic activity and has been used in the treatment of malignant neoplasms.

Zinostatin stimalamer (SMANCS), a conjugate of zinostatin with a styrene-maleic acid polymer, is used for the treatment of liver cancer.

---

## Zorubicin Hydrochloride *(USAN, rINNM)*

Hidrocloruro de zorubicina; NSC-164011; RP-22050 (zorubicin). Benzoic acid (2*S*-*cis*)-{1-[4-(3-amino-2,3,6-trideoxy-α-L-*lyxo*-hexopyranosyloxy)-1,2,3,4,6,11-hexahydro-2,5,12-trihydroxy-7-methoxy-6,11-dioxonaphthacen-2-yl]ethylidene}hydrazide hydrochloride.

$C_{34}H_{35}N_3O_{10},HCl$ = 682.1.

*CAS — 54083-22-6 (zorubicin); 36508-71-1 (zorubicin hydrochloride).*

*ATC — L01DB05.*

### Profile

Zorubicin is an anthracycline antibiotic with antineoplastic actions similar to those of doxorubicin (see p.547). It has been used as the hydrochloride in the treatment of acute leukaemias.

# Antiprotozoals


Amoebic infections, p.595
Acanthamoeba infections, p.595
Acanthamoeba keratitis, p.595
Disseminated acanthamoeba infection, p.595
Amoebiasis, p.595
Naegleria infections, p.595
Primary amoebic meningoencephalitis, p.595
Babesiosis, p.595
Balantidiasis, p.596
Blastocystis hominis infection, p.596
Coccidiosis, p.596
Cryptosporidiosis, p.596
Cyclosporiasis, p.596
Gastro-enteritis, p.596
Giardiasis, p.596
Infections in immunocompromised patients, p.597
Isosporiasis, p.597
Leishmaniasis, p.597
Malaria, p.598
Microsporidiosis, p.598
Pneumocystis carinii pneumonia, p.598
Toxoplasmosis, p.598
Trichomoniasis, p.599
African trypanosomiasis, p.599
American trypanosomiasis, p.600


The drugs described in this chapter are those used primarily in the treatment of parasitic protozoal infections. In addition to their use as antiprotozoals, metronidazole and related nitroimidazole derivatives are also important in the treatment of anaerobic bacterial infections. Some veterinary antiprotozoal drugs are included. Drugs used in the treatment of malaria are described in the Antimalarials chapter; some of these are also used in other protozoal infections.

The principal antiprotozoal drugs are listed in Table 1, below.

**Table 1.** Classification of principal antiprotozoals.

| | |
|---|---|
| *Antimony compounds* | *Nitrofurans* |
| Meglumine antimonate | Furazolidone |
| Sodium stibogluconate | Nifuratel |
| | Nifurtimox |
| *Aromatic diamidines* | *5-Nitroimidazoles* |
| Pentamidine | Metronidazole |
| *Arsenicals, pentavalent* | Nimorazole |
| Acetarsol | Ornidazole |
| Tryparsamide | Secnidazole |
| | Tinidazole |
| *Arsenicals, trivalent* | |
| Melarsoprol | *Miscellaneous* |
| | Atovaquone |
| *Dichloroacetamides* | Benznidazole |
| Diloxanide | Dehydroemetine |
| *Halogenated hydroxyquinolines* | Eflornithine |
| Diiodohydroxyquinoline | Mepacrine |
| | Paromomycin |
| | Suramin |

## Choice of Antiprotozoal

Protozoal infections occur throughout the world and are a major cause of morbidity and mortality in some regions. The choice of treatment for the principal protozoal diseases in humans is discussed below.

### Amoebic infections

The most common amoebic infection of man is amoebiasis caused by infection with the protozoan parasite *Entamoeba histolytica* and related species. Free-living amoebae can also cause disease in man, though these infections are rare. Infection with *Naegleria fowleri* results in primary amoebic meningoencephalitis, while infection with *Acanthamoeba* species or leptomyxid amoebae leads to granulomatous amoebic encephalitis. *Acanthamoeba* is also a cause of keratitis.

**Acanthamoeba infections.** ACANTHAMOEBA KERATITIS. *Acanthamoeba* keratitis is usually associated with the wearing of soft contact lenses. It is treated by prompt topical antiamoebic therapy,[1-3] although an optimum regimen has yet to be determined. Surgery may be needed in severe cases. The antiseptic propamidine isetionate applied topically is a mainstay of treatment, and has been used in various combinations with aminoglycosides such as neomycin or a neomycin-polymyxin-gramicidin preparation, and/or a biguanide (usually polihexanide but chlorhexidine has also been used). Systemic itraconazole or ketoconazole with topical miconazole have also been tried with some success. Clotrimazole has also been used successfully. Hexamidine isetionate has been suggested as an alternative to propamidine isetionate.

*Acanthamoeba* keratitis in contact lens wearers should be preventable by good lens hygiene (see Contact Lens Care, p.1164).


1. Illingworth CD, *et al.* Acanthamoeba keratitis: risk factors and outcome. *Br J Ophthalmol* 1995; **79:** 1078–82.
2. Elder MJ, Dart JKG. Chemotherapy for acanthamoeba keratitis. *Lancet* 1995; **345:** 791–2.
3. Lindquist TD. Treatment of Acanthamoeba keratitis. *Cornea* 1998; **17:** 11–16.


DISSEMINATED ACANTHAMOEBA INFECTION. Granulomatous amoebic encephalitis is caused by infection with free-living amoebae, usually *Acanthamoeba* spp. or sometimes leptomyxid amoebae. It is an opportunistic infection occurring mainly in debilitated or immunocompromised individuals. The protozoa spread to the CNS from pulmonary or skin lesions and produce focal neurological deficits that progress over days or weeks to a diffuse meningoencephalitis. The infection is usually fatal and most cases have been diagnosed postmortem so little is known about effective treatments.

Clinical responses to chemotherapy have been reported in a few patients[1-3] with disseminated infection but no evidence of CNS involvement. Disseminated *Acanthamoeba* infection in an immunocompromised patient was successfully treated with intravenous pentamidine followed by maintenance therapy with oral itraconazole.[1] Skin lesions were treated topically with chlorhexidine and ketoconazole. Clinical improvement of disseminated acanthamoebiasis in a patient with AIDS followed treatment with intravenous pentamidine and oral flucytosine; an infant with HIV infection was treated with fluconazole, flucytosine, and sulfadiazine.[2] A lung transplant patient with disseminated acanthamoebiasis was also successfully treated with pentamidine, flucytosine, and azithromycin, together with topical chlorhexidine and ketoconazole.[3]


1. Slater CA, *et al.* Brief report: successful treatment of disseminated Acanthamoeba infection in an immunocompromised patient. *N Engl J Med* 1994; **331:** 85–7.
2. Murakawa GJ, *et al.* Disseminated Acanthamoeba in patients with AIDS: a report of five cases and a review of the literature. *Arch Dermatol* 1995; **131:** 1291–6.
3. Oliva S, *et al.* Successful treatment of widely disseminated acanthamoebiasis. *South Med J* 1999; **92:** 55–7.


**Amoebiasis.** The term amoebiasis is generally applied to infections with obligate parasitic species of amoeba, principally *Entamoeba histolytica*.[1,2] Other parasitic species which occasionally cause human infections include *E. polecki* (primarily a parasite of pigs and reported mainly in Papua New Guinea) and *Dientamoeba fragilis* (often found in association with the helminth *Enterobius vermicularis* and now thought to be a trichomonad).

Transmission of *E. histolytica* is by the faeco-oral route and infection results from the ingestion of cysts, usually in contaminated food and drink. The cysts transform to trophozoites in the intestines and reproduction occurs by fission of the trophozoites. Further cysts develop and are excreted in the faeces. Amoebiasis occurs throughout the world. It is more prevalent and severe in the tropics and subtropics, but is more closely related to sanitation and socio-economic status than to climate. Colonisation with *E. histolytica* can result in asymptomatic infection, but in other cases the trophozoites invade the wall of the large intestine causing ulceration and may migrate to other tissues, especially the liver, where they continue to divide and destroy tissue. Factors increasing susceptibility to tissue invasion include malnutrition, immunosuppression, and pregnancy.

Symptomatic amoebiasis may be classified as intestinal or extra-intestinal amoebiasis. Intestinal amoebiasis comprises two main states, amoebic dysentery and non-dysenteric amoebic colitis; amoeboma, a localised form of intestinal amoebiasis, and amoebic appendicitis may also occur. Hepatic amoebiasis, the most common form of extra-intestinal amoebic disease, may present as acute non-suppurative disease or as amoebic liver abscess. Amoebic infection is a less common cause of liver abscess than bacterial infection. Amoebiasis may also involve the skin, genito-urinary tract, or organs such as the lungs and brain.

Drugs used in the **treatment** of amoebiasis may be classified according to their site of action as follows:

- *luminal amoebicides* acting principally in the bowel lumen.
  Diloxanide furoate is widely used as the luminal amoebicide of choice, although clefamide, etofamide, and teclozan are also effective.[3] Paromomycin and diiodohydroxyquinoline have also been used[1,2,4] although most oral preparations of halogenated hydroxyquinolines have been withdrawn because of the association between clioquinol and subacute myelo-opticoneuropathy
- *tissue* or *systemic amoebicides* acting principally in the intestinal wall and liver. These have included the alkaloid emetine, its synthetic derivative dehydroemetine, and the antimalarial chloroquine which acts principally in the liver
- *mixed amoebicides* acting at all sites of infection, that is within the intestinal lumen and in the intestinal wall and other tissues. These have included metronidazole and other 5-nitroimidazole derivatives. However, because of their rapid absorption from the gastrointestinal tract, the nitroimidazoles are less effective against parasites in the lumen

In non-endemic areas, patients with asymptomatic intestinal amoebiasis (cyst passers) are generally treated with a luminal amoebicide. The choice of drug is influenced by availability; diloxanide furoate is generally used in the UK while diiodohydroxyquinoline or paromomycin are used in the USA.[5] Standard treatment for invasive amoebiasis (amoebic dysentery; hepatic amoebiasis) is metronidazole, ornidazole, or tinidazole, followed by a luminal amoebicide to eradicate any surviving organisms from the lumen of the large intestine and prevent relapse. The majority of patients with amoebic liver abscess defervesce after 3 to 4 days of treatment with metronidazole. Addition of chloroquine is an option in patients who do not respond;[4] WHO recommends that hepatic abscesses should be lanced by needle aspiration.[3] In severe cases of amoebic dysentery tetracycline given in combination with a systemic amoebicide lessens the risk of superinfection, intestinal perforation, and peritonitis.

In acute diarrhoea of any aetiology the priority is to maintain hydration by prevention or treatment of fluid and electrolyte depletion, especially in infants and the elderly. Oral rehydration therapy is discussed under Diarrhoea on p.1241.

Drugs suggested for the treatment of *Dientamoeba fragilis* infections include diiodohydroxyquinoline, metronidazole, paromomycin, or tetracycline.[5] Metronidazole has been suggested for *E. polecki* infections.[5]


1. Stanley SL. Amoebiasis. *Lancet* 2003; **361:** 1025–34.
2. Haque R, *et al.* Amebiasis. *N Engl J Med* 2003; **348:** 1565–73.
3. WHO. *WHO model formulary.* Geneva: WHO, 2004.
4. Petri WA, Singh U. Diagnosis and management of amebiasis. *Clin Infect Dis* 1999; **29:** 1117–25.
5. Medical Letter on Drugs and Therapeutics. Drugs for parasitic infections (issued April 2002). Available at: http://www.medicalletter.com/freedocs/parasitic.pdf (accessed 02/06/04)


**Naegleria infections.** PRIMARY AMOEBIC MENINGOENCEPHALITIS. Primary amoebic meningoencephalitis is usually caused by the free-living amoeba *Naegleria fowleri*. It occurs mainly in healthy children and young adults and is usually associated with swimming in warm fresh water. The protozoa invade the CNS directly through the nasal mucosa to produce a meningoencephalitis that is usually rapidly fatal. Few cases of successful treatment have been reported, and have generally involved intravenous, and usually intrathecal, amphotericin B;[1-3] some patients were also given oral rifampicin.


1. Anderson K, Jamieson A. Primary amoebic meningoencephalitis. *Lancet* 1972; **i:** 902–3.
2. Seidel JS, *et al.* Successful treatment of primary amebic meningoencephalitis. *N Engl J Med* 1982; **306:** 346–8.
3. Brown RL. Successful treatment of primary amebic meningoencephalitis. *Arch Intern Med* 1991; **151:** 1201–2.


### Babesiosis

Babesiosis (piroplasmosis) is a rare infection caused by protozoa of the *Babesia* spp., which are transmitted to man by the bite of infected *Ixodes* ticks. Transmission by blood transfusion has also been reported. Infections in North America are commonly due to *B. microti* and, although often asymptomatic, may produce prolonged severe illness with fever and haemolytic anaemia, particularly in patients who are asplenic, elderly, debilitated, or immunocompromised. Co-infection with *B. microti* and *Borrelia burgdorferi* (Lyme disease) has resulted in more severe symptoms. In Europe, infections are principally caused by *B. divergens* or *B. bovis* and have only been described in asplenic persons, in most of whom the infection was rapidly fatal. Clinical features include severe haemolytic anaemia, jaundice, and renal failure.

There is no established specific treatment for babesiosis. For serious infections, supportive therapies include blood transfusion and haemodialysis. Exchange transfusions have been used to reduce parasitaemia. Clindamycin with quinine has been used[1-3] for the treatment of *B. microti* infections. A prospective randomised study[4] in 58 patients has suggested that azithromycin with atovaquone may be as effective as clindamycin and quinine. Azithromycin with quinine has been reported to be effective in 2 patients who had not responded to quinine plus clindamycin.[5,6] In *B. divergens* infections, treatment is complicated by the rapid progression of the disease. Antiprotozoal and antimalarial drugs have been tried with limited success, although pentamidine with co-trimoxazole was successful in a patient,[7] and a marked reduction in parasite load was seen in a patient treated with pentamidine plus exchange transfusions.[8] Pentamidine has also been reported to produce clinical improvement in patients with *B. microti* infection,[9] but the efficacy and safety of pentamidine in this self-limiting disease has been questioned.[10]


1. Wittner M, *et al.* Successful chemotherapy of transfusion babesiosis. *Ann Intern Med* 1982; **96:** 601–4.
2. Gorenflot A, *et al.* Human babesiosis. *Ann Trop Med Parasitol* 1998; **92:** 489–501.
3. Medical Letter on Drugs and Therapeutics. Drugs for parasitic infections (issued April 2002). Available at: http://www.medicalletter.com/freedocs/parasitic.pdf (accessed 02/06/04)
4. Krause PJ, *et al.* Atovaquone and azithromycin for the treatment of babesiosis. *N Engl J Med* 2000; **343:** 1454–8.
5. Shaio MF, Yang KD. Response of babesiosis to a combined regimen of quinine and azithromycin. *Trans R Soc Trop Med Hyg* 1997; **91:** 214–15.
6. Shih C-M, Wang C-C. Ability of azithromycin in combination with quinine for the elimination of babesial infection in humans. *Am J Trop Med Hyg* 1998; **59:** 509–12.
7. Raoult D, *et al.* Babesiosis, pentamidine, and cotrimoxazole. *Ann Intern Med* 1987; **107:** 944.
8. Clarke CS, *et al.* Babesiosis: under-reporting or case-clustering? *Postgrad Med J* 1989; **65:** 591–3.
9. Francioli PB, *et al.* Response of babesiosis to pentamidine therapy. *Ann Intern Med* 1981; **94:** 326–30.
10. Teutsch SM, Juranek DD. Babesiosis. *Ann Intern Med* 1981; **95:** 241.


## Balantidiasis

Infection with the ciliate protozoan *Balantidium coli* results from the ingestion of cysts, the commonest sources of which are pigs. Water-borne epidemics of balantidiasis have been reported. Most infections are asymptomatic and the organism lives in the large intestine as a luminal commensal, but those with symptomatic infections have diarrhoea. Colonic ulceration resulting in a severe dysenteric syndrome resembling amoebic dysentery may occur in some individuals, especially if malnourished. Treatment is with tetracycline; metronidazole or diiodohydroxyquinoline are alternatives.[1]


1. Medical Letter on Drugs and Therapeutics. Drugs for parasitic infections (issued April 2002). Available at: http://www.medicalletter.com/freedocs/parasitic.pdf (accessed 02/06/04)


## Blastocystis hominis infection

There is controversy over whether the protozoan parasite *Blastocystis hominis* is a pathogen or a harmless commensal of the intestinal tract. It has increasingly been reported both in immunocompetent and immunocompromised subjects,[1] with transmission probably by the faeco-oral route. Diarrhoea and other gastrointestinal symptoms have been ascribed to the organism.

Treatment with standard antiprotozoals, especially metronidazole, has had variable success; metronidazole resistance may occur.[2] Diiodohydroxyquinoline may also be effective.[3] Co-trimoxazole was reported to have eliminated *B. hominis* from the stools of all but one of 47 otherwise healthy subjects with diarrhoea in one study,[4] and similarly in 36 of 38 children, and 14 of 15 adults, in another.[5]


1. Anonymous. Blastocystis hominis: commensal or pathogen? *Lancet* 1991; **337:** 521–2.
2. Haresh K, *et al.* Isolate resistance of Blastocystis hominis to metronidazole. *Trop Med Int Health* 1999; **4:** 274–7.
3. Stenzel DJ, Boreham PFL. Blastocystis hominis revisited. *Clin Microbiol Rev* 1996; **9:** 563–84.
4. Schwartz E, Houston R. Effect of co-trimoxazole on stool recovery of Blastocystis hominis. *Lancet* 1992; **339:** 428–9.
5. Ok UZ, *et al.* Effect of trimethoprim-sulfamethaxazole [sic] in Blastocystis hominis infection. *Am J Gastroenterol* 1999; **94:** 3245–7.


## Coccidiosis

Coccidiosis is a term sometimes applied to infections with protozoa of the order *Eucoccidiorida.* The predominant coccidian infections in man are caused by *Cryptosporidium* (below), *Cyclospora cayetanensis* (below), *Isospora* (below), *Plasmodium* (see Malaria, p.444), and *Toxoplasma* (below). Coccidian protozoa, primarily *Eimeria,* cause economically important infections in domesticated animals.

## Cryptosporidiosis

Cryptosporidiosis is a gastrointestinal infection caused by species of the coccidian protozoan parasite *Cryptosporidium.* It has a worldwide distribution and occurs in many animal species as well as in man. Infection is acquired through ingestion, and perhaps inhalation, of oocysts. Infection in immunocompetent individuals usually causes a self-limiting diarrhoea lasting up to 2 weeks. In immunocompromised patients there may be profuse and persistent diarrhoea, profound weight loss, and severe abdominal pain, and the infection may be life-threatening. Cryptosporidiosis is a cause of diarrhoea in patients with AIDS. Other sites of infection include the respiratory and biliary tracts.

There is currently no consistently effective specific therapy[1] and priority should be given to maintaining hydration by prevention or treatment of fluid and electrolyte depletion, especially in infants and the elderly. Oral rehydration therapy is discussed under Diarrhoea on p.1241. In patients with AIDS the best treatment is improvement of immune function with highly active antiretroviral therapy, but where this is not possible therapy with an antimicrobial and an antidiarrhoeal drug continues to be standard.[1] Paromomycin,[2-9] azithromycin,[10,11] and nitazoxanide[12-14] are widely used, although benefits are at best moderate.[1] Therapy with paromomycin plus azithromycin has produced some beneficial responses in patients with AIDS-related cryptosporidiosis.[15] Other treatments reported to have produced benefit include hyperimmune bovine colostrum,[16-20] eflornithine,[21] normal immunoglobulin with high cryptosporidium antibody titres,[22] or letrazuril,[23,24] but again the numbers of patients involved are small. Responses to spiramycin have not been consistent.[25-27] Beneficial responses to octreotide have been reported in a few cases,[28,29] but a study in patients with refractory AIDS-related diarrhoea suggested that response was better in patients without identifiable pathogens.[30]

Clarithromycin and rifabutin may be useful for disease prophylaxis,[31] although the efficacy of clarithromycin has been questioned.[32]


1. Chen X-M, *et al.* Cryptosporidiosis. *N Engl J Med* 2002; **346:** 1723–31.
2. Clezy K, *et al.* Paromomycin for the treatment of cryptosporidial diarrhoea in AIDS patients. *AIDS* 1991; **5:** 1146–7.
3. Armitage K, *et al.* Treatment of cryptosporidiosis with paromomycin: a report of five cases. *Arch Intern Med* 1992; **152:** 2497–9.
4. Danziger LH, *et al.* Treatment of cryptosporidial diarrhea in an AIDS patient with paromomycin. *Ann Pharmacother* 1993; **27:** 1460–2.
5. Fichtenbaum CJ, *et al.* Use of paromomycin for treatment of cryptosporidiosis in patients with AIDS. *Clin Infect Dis* 1993; **16:** 298–300.
6. White AC, *et al.* Paromomycin for cryptosporidiosis in AIDS: a prospective, double-blind trial. *J Infect Dis* 1994; **170:** 419–24.
7. Bissuel F, *et al.* Paromomycin: an effective treatment for cryptosporidial diarrhea in patients with AIDS. *Clin Infect Dis* 1994; **18:** 447–9.
8. Mohri H, *et al.* Case report: inhalation therapy of paromomycin is effective for respiratory infection and hypoxia by Cryptosporidium with AIDS. *Am J Med Sci* 1995; **309:** 60–2.
9. Flanigan TP, *et al.* Prospective trial of paromomycin for cryptosporidiosis in AIDS. *Am J Med* 1996; **100:** 370–2.
10. Vargas SL, *et al.* Azithromycin for treatment of severe Cryptosporidium diarrhea in two children with cancer. *J Pediatr* 1993; **123:** 154–6.
11. Bessette RE, Amsden GW. Treatment of non-HIV cryptosporidial diarrhea with azithromycin. *Ann Pharmacother* 1995; **29:** 991–3.
12. Rossignol J-F, *et al.* A double-'blind' placebo-controlled study of nitazoxanide in the treatment of cryptosporidial diarrhoea in AIDS patients in Mexico. *Trans R Soc Trop Med Hyg* 1998; **92:** 663–6.
13. Rossignol J-FA, *et al.* Treatment of diarrhea caused by Cryptosporidium parvum: a prospective randomized, double-blind, placebo-controlled study of nitazoxanide. *J Infect Dis* 2001; **184:** 103–6.
14. Amadi B, *et al.* Effect of nitazoxanide on morbidity and mortality in Zambian children with cryptosporidiosis: a randomised controlled trial. *Lancet* 2002; **360:** 1375–80.
15. Smith NH, *et al.* Combination drug therapy for cryptosporidiosis in AIDS. *J Infect Dis* 1998; **178:** 900–903.
16. Tzipori S, *et al.* Remission of diarrhoea due to cryptosporidiosis in an immunodeficient child treated with hyperimmune bovine colostrum. *BMJ* 1986; **293:** 1276–7.
17. Tzipori S, *et al.* Chronic cryptosporidial diarrhoea and hyperimmune cow colostrum. *Lancet* 1987; **ii:** 344–5.
18. Nord J, *et al.* Treatment with bovine hyperimmune colostrum of cryptosporidial diarrhea in AIDS patients. *AIDS* 1990; **4:** 581–4.
19. Shield J, *et al.* Bovine colostrum immunoglobulin concentrate for cryptosporidiosis in AIDS. *Arch Dis Child* 1993; **69:** 451–3.
20. Greenberg PD, Cello JP. Treatment of severe diarrhea caused by Cryptosporidium parvum with oral bovine immunoglobulin concentrate in patients with AIDS. *J Acquir Immune Defic Syndr Hum Retrovirol* 1996; **13:** 348–54.
21. Rolston KVI, *et al.* Intestinal crytosporidiosis treated with eflornithine: a prospective study among patients with AIDS. *J Acquir Immune Defic Syndr* 1989; **2:** 426–30.
22. Borowitz SM, Saulsbury FT. Treatment of chronic cryptosporidial infection with orally administered human serum immune globulin. *J Pediatr* 1991; **119:** 593–5.
23. Harris M, *et al.* A phase I study of letrazuril in AIDS-related cryptosporidiosis. *AIDS* 1994; **8:** 1109–13.
24. Loeb M, *et al.* Treatment with letrazuril of refractory cryptosporidial diarrhea complicating AIDS. *J Acquir Immune Defic Syndr Hum Retrovirol* 1995; **10:** 48–53.
25. Portnoy D, *et al.* Treatment of intestinal cryptosporidiosis with spiramycin. *Ann Intern Med* 1984; **101:** 202–4.
26. Moskovitz BL, *et al.* Spiramycin therapy for cryptosporidial diarrhoea in immunocompromised patients. *J Antimicrob Chemother* 1988; **22** (suppl B): 189–91.
27. Wittenberg DF, *et al.* Spiramycin is not effective in treating cryptosporidium diarrhea in infants: results of a double-blind randomized trial. *J Infect Dis* 1989; **159:** 131–2.
28. Cook DJ, *et al.* Somatostatin treatment for cryptosporidial diarrhea in a patient with the acquired immunodeficiency syndrome (AIDS). *Ann Intern Med* 1988; **108:** 708–9.
29. Clotet B, *et al.* Efficacy of the somatostatin analogue (SMS-201-995), Sandostatin, for cryptosporidial diarrhoea in patients with AIDS. *AIDS* 1989; **3:** 857–8.
30. Cello JP, *et al.* Effect of octreotide on refractory AIDS-associated diarrhea: a prospective, multicenter clinical trial. *Ann Intern Med* 1991; **115:** 705–10.
31. Holmberg SD, *et al.* Possible effectiveness of clarithromycin and rifabutin for cryptosporidiosis chemoprophylaxis in HIV disease. *JAMA* 1998; **279:** 384–6.
32. Fichtenbaum CJ, *et al.* Rifabutin but not clarithromycin prevents cryptosporidiosis in persons with advanced HIV infection. *AIDS* 2000; **14:** 2889–93.


## Cyclosporiasis

An organism originally described as cyanobacterium-like or coccidian-like bodies, but now identified as the coccidian protozoan *Cyclospora cayetanensis,* has been reported to be a cause of diarrhoea in both immunocompromised and immunocompetent patients. Infection results from ingestion of spores or oocysts in contaminated food or water. In immunocompetent patients, infection may be asymptomatic or cause a self-limiting diarrhoeal illness. Immunocompromised patients may develop severe or persistent symptoms. Beneficial responses have been reported with co-trimoxazole.[1-3] Ciprofloxacin may be an alternative in those unable to tolerate co-trimoxazole, although it is somewhat less effective.[3]


1. Pape JW, *et al.* Cyclospora infection in adults infected with HIV: clinical manifestations, treatment, and prophylaxis. *Ann Intern Med* 1994; **121:** 654–7.
2. Hoge CW, *et al.* Placebo-controlled trial of co-trimoxazole for cyclospora infections among travellers and foreign residents in Nepal. *Lancet* 1995; **345:** 691–3. Correction. *ibid.;* 1060.
3. Verdier R-I, *et al.* Trimethoprim-sulfamethoxazole compared with ciprofloxacin for treatment and prophylaxis of Isospora belli and Cyclospora cayetanensis infection in HIV-infected patients: a randomized, controlled trial. *Ann Intern Med* 2000; **132:** 885–8.


## Gastro-enteritis

Although bacteria and viruses are responsible for many cases of infective diarrhoea, protozoal infections are also a cause of diarrhoea, which can be severe (especially in immunocompromised patients, including those with AIDS). In acute diarrhoea of any aetiology the priority is to maintain hydration by prevention or treatment of fluid and electrolyte depletion, especially in infants and the elderly. Oral rehydration therapy is discussed under Diarrhoea on p.1241. Specific therapy with antiprotozoals may also be necessary to control enteric protozoal infections. For the management of the protozoal infections that are generally associated with diarrhoea, see under Amoebiasis (above), Balantidiasis (above), *Blastocystis hominis* infections (above), Cryptosporidiosis (above), Cyclosporiasis (above), Giardiasis (below), Isosporiasis (below), and Microsporidiosis (below).

References.


1. Goodgame RW. Diagnosis and treatment of gastrointestinal protozoal infections. *Curr Opin Infect Dis* 1996; **9:** 346–52.
2. Okhuysen PC. Traveler's diarrhea due to intestinal protozoa. *Clin Infect Dis* 2001; **33:** 110–14.


## Giardiasis

Infection with *Giardia intestinalis* (*G. lamblia*; *Lamblia intestinalis*) occurs throughout the world and is one of the commonest intestinal protozoal infections. Infection is acquired by oral ingestion of *Giardia* cysts, and transmission may be person-to-person or from contaminated drinking water or foodstuffs. Infected patients may have acute or chronic diarrhoea or they may be asymptomatic. In acute diarrhoea of any aetiology the priority is to maintain hydration by prevention or treatment of fluid and electrolyte depletion, especially in infants and the elderly. Oral rehydration therapy is discussed under Diarrhoea on p.1241.

Treatment is with metronidazole or another nitroimidazole derivative such as tinidazole.[1] Albendazole, furazolidone, mebendazole, and mepacrine have all also been used but some of them may be less well tolerated than the nitroimidazoles. Nitazoxanide has also been reported to be effective.[2-4] Paromomycin has been suggested;[5] although it is less effective than other drugs, it is not absorbed systemically and may be a useful alternative during pregnancy. Treatment may sometimes need to be repeated, possibly due to resistance,[6,7] and drug combinations such as metronidazole with mepacrine[6,8] have been reported to be of value in these cases.


1. Zaat JOM, *et al.* Drugs for treating giardiasis. Available in The Cochrane Library; Issue 2. Chichester: John Wiley; 2004.
2. Rossignol J-F, *et al.* Treatment of diarrhea caused by Giardia intestinalis and Entamoeba histolytica or E. dispar: a randomized, double-blind, placebo-controlled study of nitazoxanide. *J Infect Dis* 2001; **184:** 381–4.
3. Abboud P, *et al.* Successful treatment of metronidazole- and albendazole-resistant giardiasis with nitazoxanide in a patient with acquired immunodeficiency syndrome. *Clin Infect Dis* 2001; **32:** 1792–4.
4. Ortiz JJ, *et al.* Randomized clinical study of nitazoxanide compared to metronidazole in the treatment of symptomatic giardiasis in children from Northern Peru. *Aliment Pharmacol Ther* 2001; **15:** 1409–15.
5. Medical Letter on Drugs and Therapeutics. Drugs for parasitic infections (Issued April 2002). Available at: http://www.medicalletter.com/freedocs/parasitic.pdf (accessed 02/06/04)
6. Farthing MJG. Giardia comes of age: progress in epidemiology, immunology and chemotherapy. *J Antimicrob Chemother* 1992; **30:** 563–6.
7. Boreham PFL. Giardiasis and its control. *Pharm J* 1991; **247:** 271–4.
8. Nash TE, *et al.* Treatment of patients with refractory giardiasis. *Clin Infect Dis* 2001; **33:** 22–8.


### Infections in immunocompromised patients

Patients with a defective immune system are at particular risk of infection. Primary immune deficiency is rare, whereas secondary deficiency is more common: immunosuppressive therapy, cancer and its treatment, HIV infection, and splenectomy may all cause neutropenia and impaired humoral and cellular immunity in varying degrees. The risk of infection is linked to the duration and severity of neutropenia. Most protozoal infections present in a more severe form in immunocompromised patients than in immunocompetent patients. Those of particular concern in patients with HIV infection include Cryptosporidiosis (above), Isosporiasis (below), Leishmaniasis (below), Microsporidiosis (below), and Toxoplasmosis (below).

References.


1. Sharpstone D, Gazzard B. Gastrointestinal manifestations of HIV infection. *Lancet* 1996; **348:** 378–83.
2. Centers for Disease Control and Prevention. Guidelines for preventing opportunistic infections among HIV-infected persons—2002: recommendations of the US Public Health Service and the Infectious Diseases Society of America. *MMWR* 2002; **51** (RR-8): 1–52. Also available at: http://www.cdc.gov/mmwr/PDF/rr/rr5108.pdf (accessed 02/06/04)


### Isosporiasis

Isosporiasis is a coccidian protozoal infection of the gastrointestinal tract caused by *Isospora belli*. Oocysts are excreted in faeces and infection is acquired when sporulated oocysts are ingested. In immunocompetent individuals the infection is usually mild and self-limiting but in immunocompromised patients there may be severe, chronic gastroenteritis. Treatment is usually with co-trimoxazole.[1-3] Ciprofloxacin may be an alternative in those unable to tolerate co-trimoxazole, although it is somewhat less effective.[3] Pyrimethamine has been used successfully in individual patients with sulfonamide sensitivity.[4] In acute diarrhoea of any aetiology the priority is to maintain hydration by prevention or treatment of fluid and electrolyte depletion, especially in infants and the elderly. Oral rehydration therapy is discussed under Diarrhoea on p.1241.

Recurrence of infection is common and long-term suppressive treatment with either co-trimoxazole or pyrimethamine plus sulfadoxine has been recommended.[5]


1. WHO. *WHO model prescribing information: drugs used in parasitic diseases.* 2nd ed. Geneva: WHO, 1995.
2. Medical Letter on Drugs and Therapeutics. Drugs for parasitic infections (issued April 2002). Available at: http://www.medicalletter.com/freedocs/parasitic.pdf (accessed 02/06/04)
3. Verdier R-I, *et al.* Trimethoprim-sulfamethoxazole compared with ciprofloxacin for treatment and prophylaxis of Isospora belli and Cyclospora cayetanensis infection in HIV-infected patients: a randomized, controlled trial. *Ann Intern Med* 2000; **132:** 885–8.
4. Weiss LM, *et al.* Isospora belli infection: treatment with pyrimethamine. *Ann Intern Med* 1988; **109:** 474–5.
5. Pape JW, *et al.* Treatment and prophylaxis of Isospora belli infection in patients with the acquired immunodeficiency syndrome. *N Engl J Med* 1989; **320:** 1044–7.


### Leishmaniasis

Leishmaniasis is caused by parasitic protozoa of the genus *Leishmania*. It occurs throughout Africa, the Middle East, Central Asia, and the Mediterranean (Old World leishmaniasis), and throughout Central and South America (New World leishmaniasis). In endemic areas there is generally a reservoir of disease in a mammalian host, often dogs or rodents. The usual vectors are sandflies of the genus *Phlebotomus* in the Old World and *Lutzomyia* in the New World. Leishmaniasis can be categorised as cutaneous, mucosal, and visceral and ranges from self-limiting, localised, cutaneous ulcers to widely disseminated progressive disease and involvement of the reticuloendothelial system. Incubation periods can be prolonged, with clinical features not appearing until several months or even years after the primary infection.

In endemic areas an integrated approach to controlling leishmaniasis involves case detection and treatment of patients, vector and animal reservoir control, environmental management to reduce suitable vector habitats, and personal protection against sandfly bites including the use of insect repellents and bednets.[1] Strategies aimed at controlling malaria are believed to have reduced leishmaniasis transmission dramatically.[1]

**Visceral leishmaniasis** of the Old World is mainly caused by *L. donovani* and *L. infantum* and of the New World by *L. chagasi*. The onset of the disease is gradual in residents of an endemic area but may present as an acute illness in non-immune visitors to the region. Many infections result in sub-clinical or self-limiting disease. Fever, malaise, shivering or chills, weight loss, anorexia, and discomfort in the left hypochondrium are common; there is often non-tender splenomegaly with or without hepatomegaly, wasting, pallor of mucous membranes, anaemia, leucopenia, and lymphadenopathy. Continued deterioration can lead to potentially fatal secondary infection. Darkening of the skin of the face, hands, feet, and abdomen is common in endemic visceral leishmaniasis in India (kala-azar = black sickness). Rare complications can include severe acute haemolytic anaemia, acute renal damage, and severe mucosal haemorrhage. In recent years, visceral leishmaniasis has emerged as an opportunistic infection in patients with HIV or other conditions associated with reduced immunity, in whom it is particularly difficult to treat.

A small percentage of patients develop post-kala-azar dermal leishmaniasis following recovery from visceral leishmaniasis and such patients represent a human reservoir for the disease.

The pentavalent antimonials meglumine antimonate and sodium stibogluconate are the traditional first-line drugs for the treatment of visceral leishmaniasis.[1-3] Patients relapsing after the initial course of treatment may be given a further course, but there is growing evidence that responsiveness to the antimonials is declining. Resistance to antimonials is widespread in parts of India.[3] Miltefosine has been shown to be effective[4-6] and has recently been introduced in India for treatment. Four regimens have been suggested for the first-line treatment of visceral leishmaniasis due to *L. infantum* in Mediterranean countries.[7] They are:

- pentavalent antimonials
- pentavalent antimonials plus allopurinol
- liposomal amphotericin B
- paromomycin alone or in combination with pentavalent antimonials

These regimens have also been evaluated in other regions and in patients with HIV infection.[8-14] Amphotericin B has been tried successfully as a second-line drug in drug-resistant infections[15-18] and increasingly as a useful alternative first-line drug.[2,3,19,20] Lipid complex and other non-conventional forms of amphotericin B are better tolerated than conventional amphotericin B, and are likely to be preferred when the toxicity and duration of therapy with conventional forms would compromise patient compliance.[2] Pentamidine has also been used as a second-line drug but its usefulness as alternative first-line therapy is doubtful[21] given its toxicity, increasing failure rates, and slow disease response. Nevertheless it has been tried as an adjunct to meglumine antimonate for first-line therapy[22] and alone for long-term secondary prophylaxis in patients with HIV infection.[23] Beneficial responses to ketoconazole have been reported in some patients[24,25] but unfavourable reports have also appeared.[26,27] Another line of investigation is to boost the immune response to the parasite by adding interferon gamma to conventional treatment, although results have been variable.[28-31]

**Cutaneous leishmaniasis** is caused by various species of *Leishmania* and a wide variety of clinical presentations is possible. A 'classical' lesion starts as a nodule at the site of inoculation. A crust develops centrally which may fall away exposing an ulcer which heals gradually. Satellite nodules at the edge of the lesion are common. Cutaneous leishmaniasis of the Old World is normally caused by *L. tropica*, *L. major*, or *L. aethiopica*, although cutaneous lesions due to *L. infantum* have been reported. New World cutaneous leishmaniasis (American cutaneous leishmaniasis) is caused by numerous species and subspecies of *Leishmania* including *L. braziliensis*, *L. mexicana*, *L. panamensis*, and *L. peruviana*. In general, New World forms tend to be more severe and longer lasting than Old World forms. The disease ranges from single, self-healing lesions which are troublesome and unsightly but not a threat to life, to multiple, deep, and destructive ulcers which cause considerable disfigurement and disability.

Diffuse cutaneous leishmaniasis occurs occasionally following infection with *L. aethiopica* or members of the *L. mexicana* complex and involves dissemination of the disease from the original site of infection to distant skin sites, typically the face and exterior surfaces of the limbs. The lesions resemble lepromatous leprosy, do not heal spontaneously, and are resistant to treatment.

Another variant is leishmaniasis recidivans which is a lupoid or tuberculoid form. This chronic disease often occurs as slowly progressive, destructive and disfiguring lesions on the face which are very resistant to most forms of therapy.

There is no established treatment for cutaneous leishmaniasis.[3] The decision to treat depends upon the site and extent of the lesions and the likelihood of dissemination. Small lesions, particularly in Old World cutaneous leishmaniasis, may be left untreated if they are not troublesome to the patient. Treatment for disfiguring or potentially disabling lesions may be local or systemic. Systemic treatment is required where there is a risk that the infecting organism may be one causing mucocutaneous leishmaniasis (see below) or where there is evidence of lymphatic spread or extensive local involvement.

WHO[1] suggested that early noninflamed nodular lesions due to *L. tropica*, *L. major*, *L. mexicana*, *L. panamensis*, or *L. peruviana* might be treated with intralesional injections of mepacrine, sodium stibogluconate, or meglumine antimonate, or removed by surgery and curettage. Benefit has been reported with this therapy.[3,32,33] However, local infiltration of drugs can be difficult as well as painful. Surgical curettage may promote dissemination of the parasite.[34] Other local treatments include cryotherapy or, alternatively, application of heat to bring the temperature of the lesion to about 40° which may aid healing.[35] Topical treatment with paromomycin sulfate 15% plus methylbenzethonium chloride 5 or 12% has produced promising responses;[36-39] paromomycin 12 to 15% with urea 10% was better tolerated.[40] However, not all studies have shown benefit.[41,42]

Systemic treatment is similar to that of visceral leishmaniasis[1,3,43,44] (see above). Topical paromomycin plus systemic meglumine antimonate was initially found to be promising in patients with New World infections,[45] but a subsequent randomised, controlled trial[46] found that application of paromomycin sulfate 15%/methylbenzethonium chloride 12% did not augment the clinical response to parenteral meglumine antimonate. Cutaneous leishmaniasis due to *L. aethiopica*, including diffuse cutaneous leishmaniasis, does not generally respond to antimonials[1] although responses to antimonials in combination with paromomycin have been reported.[47] It may also be treated with pentamidine.[1,3]

Other drugs tried in cutaneous leishmaniasis have included fluconazole,[48] itraconazole,[49-52] and ketoconazole.[39,53-56] Variable responses to allopurinol have been reported in patients with New World infections.[57-59] Dapsone was reported to be effective in a study in patients in India[60] but not in Colombia.[61] Among the non-specific therapies tried in cutaneous leishmaniasis, topical application of the nitric oxide donor *S*-nitroso-*N*-acetylpenicillamine (SNAP)[62] and intralesional injection of hypertonic sodium chloride solution[63] have produced beneficial responses. Immunomodulation using leishmania antigens mixed with BCG,[64,65] or interferon gamma,[66,67] has produced encouraging results.

While there has been some work on vaccines against cutaneous leishmaniasis much more needs to be done. However, leishmanisation (deliberate infection with *L. major*) has been used as a last resort in some countries when other measures have failed.

**Mucocutaneous leishmaniasis** of the New World (espundia) is caused by *L. braziliensis* or *L. panamensis*. In mucocutaneous leishmaniasis the primary lesions do not heal spontaneously. Metastatic spread to the mucosa may occur during the presence of the primary lesion or up to 30 years later. The nasal mucosa is always affected. Ulceration and erosion progressively destroy the soft tissue and cartilage of the oronasal/pharyngeal cavity. Mutilation is severe and secondary bacterial infection is frequent and can be fatal.

Mucocutaneous leishmaniasis responds poorly to treatment and relapses are common. Initial treatment is with pentavalent antimony;[3] failure to respond is an indication to use amphotericin B or pentamidine. Nifurtimox may be effective in some cases of mucocutaneous leishmaniasis.[1] Treatment with corticosteroids may be needed to control severe inflammation. Mucosal disease in Old World leishmaniasis is much less common than visceral or cutaneous forms, but treatment with antimony compounds or ketoconazole has been described.[68]

1. WHO. Control of the leishmaniases. *WHO Tech Rep Ser 793* 1990.
2. Berman JD. Human leishmaniasis: clinical, diagnostic, and chemotherapeutic developments in the last 10 years. *Clin Infect Dis* 1997; **24:** 684–703.
3. Herwaldt BL. Leishmaniasis. *Lancet* 1999; **354:** 1191–9.
4. Jha TK, *et al.* Miltefosine, an oral agent, for the treatment of Indian visceral leishmaniasis. *N Engl J Med* 1999; **341:** 1795–1800.
5. Sundar S, *et al.* Short-course of oral miltefosine for treatment of visceral leishmaniasis. *Clin Infect Dis* 2001; **31:** 1110–13.
6. Sundar S, *et al.* Oral miltefosine for Indian visceral leishmaniasis. *N Engl J Med* 2002; **347:** 1739–46.
7. Gradoni L, *et al.* Treatment of Mediterranean visceral leishmaniasis. *Bull WHO* 1995; **73:** 191–7.
8. Laguna F, *et al.* Assessment of allopurinol plus meglumine antimoniate in the treatment of visceral leishmaniasis in patients infected with HIV. *J Infect* 1994; **28:** 255–9.
9. Mishra M, *et al.* Amphotericin versus sodium stibogluconate in first-line treatment of Indian Kala-azar. *Lancet* 1994; **344:** 1599–1600.
10. Dietze R, *et al.* Treatment of kala-azar in Brazil with Amphocil (amphotericin B cholesterol dispersion) for 5 days. *Trans R Soc Trop Med Hyg* 1995; **89:** 309–11.
11. Russo R, *et al.* Visceral leishmaniasis in HIV infected patients: treatment with high dose liposomal amphotericin B (AmBisome). *J Infect* 1996; **32:** 133–7.
12. Sundar S, *et al.* Short-course, low-dose amphotericin B lipid complex therapy for visceral leishmaniasis unresponsive to antimony. *Ann Intern Med* 1997; **127:** 133–7.
13. Jha TK, *et al.* Randomised controlled trial of aminosidine (paromomycin) v sodium stibogluconate for treating visceral leishmaniasis in North Bihar, India. *BMJ* 1998; **316:** 1200–5.
14. Thakur CP, *et al.* A prospective randomized, comparative, open-label trial of the safety and efficacy of paromomycin (aminosidine) plus sodium stibogluconate versus sodium stibogluconate alone for the treatment of visceral leishmaniasis. *Trans R Soc Trop Med Hyg* 2000; **94:** 429–31.
15. Davidson RN, *et al.* Liposomal amphotericin B in drug-resistant visceral leishmaniasis. *Lancet* 1991; **337:** 1061–2.
16. Mishra M, *et al.* Amphotericin versus pentamidine in antimony-unresponsive kala-azar. *Lancet* 1992; **340:** 1256–7.
17. Jha TK, *et al.* Use of amphotericin B in drug-resistant cases of visceral leishmaniasis in North Bihar, India. *Am J Trop Med Hyg* 1995; **52:** 536–8.
18. Sundar S, Murray HW. Cure of antimony-unresponsive Indian visceral leishmaniasis with amphotericin B lipid complex. *J Infect Dis* 1996; **173:** 762–5.
19. Sundar S, *et al.* Treatment of Indian visceral leishmaniasis with single or daily infusions of low dose liposomal amphotericin B: randomised trial. *BMJ* 2001; **323:** 419–22.
20. Thakur CP, *et al.* Amphotericin B deoxycholate treatment of visceral leishmaniasis with newer modes of administration and precautions: a study of 938 cases. *Trans R Soc Trop Med Hyg* 1999; **93:** 319–23.
21. Baily GG, Nandy A. Visceral leishmaniasis: more prevalent and more problematic. *J Infect* 1994; **29:** 241–7.
22. Özsoylu S. Treatment of kala azar. *Lancet* 1996; **347:** 1701.
23. Pérez-Molina JA, *et al.* Pentamidine isethionate as secondary prophylaxis against visceral leishmaniasis in HIV-positive patients. *AIDS* 1996; **10:** 237–8.
24. Wali JP, *et al.* Ketoconazole in the treatment of antimony- and pentamidine-resistant kala-azar. *J Infect Dis* 1992; **166:** 215–16.
25. Kuyucu N, *et al.* Successful treatment of visceral leishmaniasis with allopurinol plus ketoconazole in an infant who developed pancreatitis caused by meglumine antimoniate. *Pediatr Infect Dis J* 2001; **20:** 455–7.
26. Sundar S, *et al.* Ketoconazole in visceral leishmaniasis. *Lancet* 1990; **336:** 1582–3.
27. Wali JP, *et al.* Efficacy of sodium antimony gluconate and ketoconazole in the treatment of kala-azar—a comparative study. *J Commun Dis* 1997; **29:** 73–83.
28. Badaro R, *et al.* Treatment of visceral leishmaniasis with pentavalent antimony and interferon gamma. *N Engl J Med* 1990; **322:** 16–21.
29. Sundar S, *et al.* Successful treatment of refractory visceral leishmaniasis in India using antimony plus interferon-γ. *J Infect Dis* 1994; **170:** 659–62.
30. Sundar S, *et al.* Immunochemotherapy for a systemic intracellular infection: accelerated response using interferon-γ in visceral leishmaniasis. *J Infect Dis* 1995; **171:** 992–6.
31. Sundar S, *et al.* Response to interferon-γ plus pentavalent antimony in Indian visceral leishmaniasis. *J Infect Dis* 1997; **176:** 1117–19.
32. Alkhawajah AM, *et al.* Treatment of cutaneous leishmaniasis with antimony: intramuscular versus intralesional administration. *Ann Trop Med Parasitol* 1997; **91:** 899–905.
33. Aste N, *et al.* Intralesional treatment of cutaneous leishmaniasis with meglumine antimoniate. *Br J Dermatol* 1998; **138:** 370–1.
34. Moss JT, Wilson JP. Current treatment recommendations for leishmaniasis. *Ann Pharmacother* 1992; **26:** 1452–5.
35. Navin TR, *et al.* Placebo-controlled clinical trial of meglumine antimonate (Glucantime) vs localized controlled heat in the treatment of cutaneous leishmaniasis in Guatemala. *Am J Trop Med Hyg* 1990; **42:** 43–50.
36. El-On J, *et al.* Topical treatment of Old World cutaneous leishmaniasis caused by Leishmania major: a double-blind control study. *J Am Acad Dermatol* 1992; **27:** 227–31.
37. Krause G, Kroeger A. Topical treatment of American cutaneous leishmaniasis with paromomycin and methylbenzethonium chloride: a clinical study under field conditions in Ecuador. *Trans R Soc Trop Med Hyg* 1994; **88:** 92–4.
38. Arana BA, *et al.* Randomized, controlled, double-blind trial of topical treatment of cutaneous leishmaniasis with paromomycin plus methylbenzethonium chloride ointment in Guatemala. *Am J Trop Med Hyg* 2001; **65:** 466–70.
39. Ozgoztasi O, Baydar I. A randomized clinical trial of topical paromomycin versus oral ketoconazole for treating cutaneous leishmaniasis in Turkey. *Int J Dermatol* 1997; **36:** 61–3.
40. Bryceson ADM, *et al.* Treatment of Old World cutaneous leishmaniasis with aminosidine ointment: results of an open study in London. *Trans R Soc Trop Med Hyg* 1994; **88:** 226–8.
41. Ben Salah A, *et al.* A randomized, placebo-controlled trial in Tunisia treating cutaneous leishmaniasis with paromomycin ointment. *Am J Trop Med Hyg* 1995; **53:** 162–6.
42. Asilian A, *et al.* A randomized, placebo-controlled trial of a two week regimen of aminosidine (paromomycin) ointment for treatment of cutaneous leishmaniasis in Iran. *Am J Trop Med Hyg* 1995; **53:** 648–51.
43. Soto J, *et al.* Limited efficacy of injectable aminosidine as single-agent therapy for Colombian cutaneous leishmaniasis. *Trans R Soc Trop Med Hyg* 1994; **88:** 695–8.
44. Hepburn NC, *et al.* Aminosidine (paromomycin) versus sodium stibogluconate for the treatment of American cutaneous leishmaniasis. *Trans R Soc Trop Med Hyg* 1994; **88:** 700–3.
45. Soto J, *et al.* Successful treatment of New World cutaneous leishmaniasis with a combination of topical paromomycin/methylbenzethonium chloride and injectable meglumine antimonate. *Clin Infect Dis* 1995; **20:** 47–51.
46. Soto J, *et al.* Topical paromomycin/methylbenzethonium chloride plus parenteral meglumine antimonate as treatment for American cutaneous leishmaniasis: controlled study. *Clin Infect Dis* 1998; **26:** 56–8.
47. Teklemariam S, *et al.* Aminosidine and its combination with sodium stibogluconate in the treatment of diffuse cutaneous leishmaniasis caused by Leishmania aethiopica. *Trans R Soc Trop Med Hyg* 1994; **88:** 334–9.
48. Alrajhi AA, *et al.* Fluconazole for the treatment of cutaneous leishmaniasis caused by Leishmania major. *N Engl J Med* 2002; **346:** 891–5.
49. Albanese G, *et al.* Cutaneous leishmaniasis: treatment with itraconazole. *Arch Dermatol* 1989; **125:** 1540–2.
50. Pialoux G, *et al.* Cutaneous leishmaniasis in an AIDS patient: cure with itraconazole. *J Infect Dis* 1990; **162:** 1221–2.
51. Akuffo H, *et al.* The use of itraconazole in the treatment of leishmaniasis caused by Leishmania aethiopica. *Trans R Soc Trop Med Hyg* 1990; **84:** 532–4.
52. Dogra J, Saxena VN. Itraconazole and leishmaniasis: a randomised double-blind trial in cutaneous disease. *Int J Parasitol* 1996; **26:** 1413–15.
53. Dedet J-P, *et al.* Failure to cure Leishmania braziliensis guyanensis cutaneous leishmaniasis with oral ketoconazole. *Trans R Soc Trop Med Hyg* 1986; **80:** 176.
54. Weinrauch L, *et al.* Ketoconazole in cutaneous leishmaniasis. *Br J Dermatol* 1987; **117:** 666–7.
55. Saenz RE, *et al.* Efficacy of ketoconazole against Leishmania braziliensis panamensis cutaneous leishmaniasis. *Am J Med* 1990; **89:** 147–55.
56. Navin TR, *et al.* Placebo-controlled clinical trial of sodium stibogluconate (Pentostam) versus ketoconazole for treating cutaneous leishmaniasis in Guatemala. *J Infect Dis* 1992; **165:** 528–34.
57. Martinez S, Marr JJ. Allopurinol in the treatment of American cutaneous leishmaniasis. *N Engl J Med* 1992; **326:** 741–4.
58. Velez I, *et al.* Inefficacy of allopurinol as monotherapy for Colombian cutaneous leishmaniasis: a randomized, controlled trial. *Ann Intern Med* 1997; **126:** 232–6.
59. Martinez S, *et al.* Treatment of cutaneous leishmaniasis with allopurinol and stibogluconate. *Clin Infect Dis* 1997; **24:** 165–9.
60. Dogra J. A double-blind study on the efficacy of oral dapsone in cutaneous leishmaniasis. *Trans R Soc Trop Med Hyg* 1991; **85:** 212–13.
61. Osorio LE, *et al.* Treatment of cutaneous leishmaniasis in Colombia with dapsone. *Lancet* 1998; **351:** 498–9.
62. López-Jaramillo P, *et al.* Treatment of cutaneous leishmaniasis with nitric-oxide donor. *Lancet* 1998; **351:** 1176–7.
63. Sharquie KE. A new intralesional therapy of cutaneous leishmaniasis with hypertonic sodium chloride solution. *J Dermatol* 1995; **22:** 732–7.
64. Convit J, *et al.* Immunotherapy of localized, intermediate, and diffuse forms of American cutaneous leishmaniasis. *J Infect Dis* 1989; **160:** 104–15.
65. Sharifi I, *et al.* Randomised vaccine trial of single dose of killed Leishmania major plus BCG against anthroponotic cutaneous leishmaniasis in Bam, Iran. *Lancet* 1998; **351:** 1540–3.
66. Harms G, *et al.* A randomized trial comparing a pentavalent antimonial drug and recombinant interferon-γ in the local treatment of cutaneous leishmaniasis. *Trans R Soc Trop Med Hyg* 1991; **85:** 214–16.
67. Falcoff E, *et al.* Clinical healing of antimony-resistant cutaneous or mucocutaneous leishmaniasis following the combined administration of interferon-γ and pentavalent antimonial compounds. *Trans R Soc Trop Med Hyg* 1994; **88:** 95–7.
68. El-Hassan AM, Zijlstra EE. Leishmaniasis in Sudan 2: Mucosal leishmaniasis. *Trans R Soc Trop Med Hyg* 2001; **95** (suppl 1): S19–S26.

## Malaria

For a discussion of malaria, its prophylaxis and treatment, see p.444.

## Microsporidiosis

Microsporidia are obligate intracellular spore-forming protozoal parasites. They were primarily regarded as a cause of disease in nonhuman species but some, including *Encephalitozoon*, *Enterocytozoon*, *Pleistophora*, and *Trachipleistophora* spp. and *Brachiola vesicularum* and *Vittaforma corneae (Nosema corneum)*, are now recognised as human pathogens. Transmission is believed to be predominantly faeco-oral although inhalation and direct inoculation also occur. Infections usually occur only in immunocompromised patients. Small bowel infection with *Enterocytozoon bieneusi* has been reported in AIDS patients as a cause of chronic diarrhoea and weight loss. Other manifestations of microsporidiosis in AIDS include keratoconjunctivitis, respiratory-tract infections, renal and urinary-tract infections, peritonitis, cholangitis, granulomatous hepatitis, and disseminated myositis.

There is no established treatment.[1] Beneficial responses have been reported with albendazole[2-6] and atovaquone.[7] Metronidazole has been reported to produce a transient symptomatic response in some patients[8] but not in those with severe diarrhoea.[9] There has also been a report of a patient treated successfully with nitazoxanide.[10] Fumagillin appears effective in the treatment of infection due to *E. bieneusi*.[11]

Topical treatment of keratoconjunctivitis has been disappointing, although there are reports of individual patients responding to topical propamidine isetionate,[12] topical fumagillin,[13,14] oral albendazole,[15] oral albendazole plus topical fumagillin,[16] or oral itraconazole plus topical antibacterials.[17]

1. Conteas CN, *et al.* Therapy for human gastrointestinal microsporidiosis. *Am J Trop Med Hyg* 2000; **63:** 121–7.
2. Blanshard C, *et al.* Treatment of intestinal microsporidiosis with albendazole in patients with AIDS. *AIDS* 1992; **6:** 311–13.
3. Dieterich DT, *et al.* Treatment with albendazole for intestinal disease due to Enterocytozoon bieneusi in patients with AIDS. *J Infect Dis* 1994; **169:** 178–82.
4. Franzen C, *et al.* Intestinal microsporidiosis with Septata intestinalis in a patient with AIDS—response to albendazole. *J Infect* 1995; **31:** 237–9.
5. Dore GJ, *et al.* Disseminated microsporidiosis due to Septata intestinalis in nine patients infected with the human immunodeficiency virus: response to therapy with albendazole. *Clin Infect Dis* 1995; **21:** 70–6.
6. Molina J-M, *et al.* Albendazole for treatment and prophylaxis of microsporidiosis due to Encephalitozoon intestinalis in patients with AIDS: a randomized double-blind controlled trial. *J Infect Dis* 1998; **177:** 1373–7.
7. Anwar-Bruni DM, *et al.* Atovaquone is effective treatment for the symptoms of gastrointestinal microsporidiosis in HIV-1-infected patients. *AIDS* 1996; **10:** 619–23.
8. Schattenkerk JKME, *et al.* Clinical significance of small-intestinal microsporidiosis in HIV-1-infected individuals. *Lancet* 1991; **337:** 895–8.
9. Blanshard C, Gazzard BG. Microsporidiosis in HIV-1-infected individuals. *Lancet* 1991; **337:** 1488–9.
10. Bicart-See A, *et al.* Successful treatment with nitazoxanide of Enterocytozoon bieneusi microsporidiosis in a patient with AIDS. *Antimicrob Agents Chemother* 2000; **44:** 167–8.
11. Molina J-M, *et al.* Fumagillin treatment of intestinal microsporidiosis. *N Engl J Med* 2002; **346:** 1963–9.
12. Metcalfe TW, *et al.* Microsporidial keratoconjunctivitis in a patient with AIDS. *Br J Ophthalmol* 1992; **76:** 177–8.
13. Diesenhouse MC, *et al.* Treatment of microsporidial keratoconjunctivitis with topical fumagillin. *Am J Ophthalmol* 1993; **115:** 293–8.
14. Garvey MJ, *et al.* Topical fumagillin in the treatment of microsporidial keratoconjunctivitis in AIDS. *Ann Pharmacother* 1995; **29:** 872–4.
15. Silverstein BE, *et al.* Microsporidial keratoconjunctivitis in a patient without human immunodeficiency virus infection. *Am J Ophthalmol* 1997; **124:** 395–6.
16. Theng J, *et al.* Microsporidial keratoconjunctivitis in a healthy contact lens wearer without human immunodeficiency virus infection. *Ophthalmology* 2001; **108:** 976–8.
17. Yee RW, *et al.* Resolution of microsporidial epithelial keratopathy in a patient with AIDS. *Ophthalmology* 1991; **98:** 196–201.

## Pneumocystis carinii pneumonia

Although *Pneumocystis carinii* has been classified as a protozoan, current evidence suggests that it is probably a fungus. For the management of *Pneumocystis carinii* pneumonia, see p.389.

## Toxoplasmosis

Toxoplasmosis is a zoonosis with a worldwide distribution caused by the protozoan parasite *Toxoplasma gondii*. There is a high incidence of *Toxoplasma* antibody, an indication of previous infection, in the general population, although infection will have been diagnosed in few individuals. Sexual reproduction of *T. gondii* occurs in the gastrointestinal tract of cats. Soil becomes contaminated from excretion of oocysts in cat faeces. Other animals, such as pigs and sheep, may become infected by ingestion of these oocysts and act as intermediate hosts. In man, infection is acquired through contact with infected cat faeces or contaminated soil, or from eating raw or undercooked meat from infected animals. Ingested oocysts rapidly transform into trophozoites which multiply in tissue macrophages. The intracellular trophozoites disseminate in the bloodstream and lymphatic system to reach the brain, heart, and lungs. As immunity develops the trophozoites form latent cystic aggregates (bradyzoites), mainly in the brain, heart, and skeletal muscle, and these are subject to reactivation throughout the life of the host.

Toxoplasma infection in immunocompetent individuals is usually asymptomatic and if symptomatic infection does occur it is usually self-limiting. Very rarely myocarditis or encephalitis may occur. Patients with impaired immunity may develop serious complications such as encephalitis, chorioretinitis, myocarditis, and pneumonitis. Toxoplasmic encephalitis is the most common presentation in patients with AIDS.

Congenital toxoplasmosis is not a problem in women who have *Toxoplasma* antibody before conception, but primary toxoplasmosis during early pregnancy is serious because of the risk of transplacental transmission which may result in fetal death or congenital toxoplasmosis. Primary infection during later pregnancy can also result in congenital infection, although this often only becomes symptomatic later in life. The sequelae in live-born infants with signs of infection are generally severe and include a potentially fatal syndrome in which hydrocephalus, hepatosplenomegaly with jaundice, mental retardation, and chorioretinitis may occur. Congenital disease that becomes clinically evident later in life is usually less severe, but often results in ocular or neurological impairment. Infection in the pregnant woman is usually asymptomatic and antenatal screening programmes have been set up in some countries for the diagnosis of acute infections during pregnancy. However, the value and practicality of such schemes has been debated.[1-5] Ocular toxoplasmosis causes chorioretinitis and is often a result of congenital infection; patients may be asymptomatic until later in life.

**Treatment.** Toxoplasmosis in immunocompetent patients is not usually treated unless symptoms are severe. Currently there is no drug active against the cystic form, so any treatment is directed against the acute forms of the disease. Active toxoplasmosis in immunocompromised patients requires prompt treatment. Toxoplasmosis is normally treated with pyrimethamine together with sulfadiazine.[6] Folinic acid should also be given during treatment to counteract the megaloblastic anaemia associated with these drugs. Treatment is ideally continued for several weeks after clinical cure. Indefinite, usually lifelong, maintenance therapy should be given to AIDS patients. Clindamycin plus pyrimethamine has been used as an alternative in patients unable to take the sulfonamide.[7-10] Other approaches for such patients are to give pyrimethamine alone[6] or to carry out sulfadiazine desensitisation.[11] Other drug regimens which have produced encouraging results in small numbers of AIDS patients with encephalitis include pyrimethamine with clarithromycin,[12] pyrimethamine with doxycycline,[13] atovaquone,[14,15] clindamycin with fluorouracil,[16] clarithromycin with minocycline,[17] co-trimoxazole,[18] and azithromycin with pyrimethamine.[19] Atovaquone has also been studied for long-term suppressive therapy.[15,20]

Pyrimethamine should not be used to treat primary toxoplasmosis during the first trimester of **pregnancy** in immunocompetent patients.[6] Spiramycin has been used throughout the first trimester but, although it reduces the risk of congenital transmission, it does not readily penetrate the cerebrospinal space and does not prevent toxoplasmic encephalitis in immunocompromised women. After the first trimester pyrimethamine may be given with sulfadiazine and folinic acid and, when there is evidence of placental or fetal infection, this treatment may be alternated with courses of spiramycin until term. In **neonates** without overt disease, but born to mothers known to have become infected during pregnancy, pyrimethamine together with sulfadiazine and folinic acid are given for the first 4 weeks with further courses of treatment if the infants are subsequently shown to be infected.[6] Some workers have suggested treatment for one year initially.[5,21] Alternate courses of pyrimethamine-sulfadiazine with spiramycin have been suggested as a means of reducing the risk of bone marrow suppression and have produced good results when given throughout the first year of life. Severely infected neonates are given daily pyrimethamine-sulfadiazine for 6 months after which alternating monthly courses of pyrimethamine-sulfadiazine and spiramycin for at least a further 6 months have been used.[6] A corticosteroid, usually prednisolone, is added for active chorioretinitis or CNS involvement.[6]

In immunocompetent individuals, **ocular toxoplasmosis** is a self-limiting disease and requires no treatment, unless visual acuity is threatened or there is a large retinal lesion with marked vitritis.[22-24] All immunocompromised patients should be treated and prolonged treatment is necessary to prevent recrudescence. The best drug regimen is unknown. The most commonly used regimens are pyrimethamine with sulfadiazine or pyrimethamine with clindamycin (which is concentrated in the choroid). Benefit has been reported from clindamycin with corticosteroids,[25] although corticosteroids should never be used alone since fulminant cases may occur. Spiramycin is not indicated for ocular toxoplasmosis.

**Prophylaxis.** Primary prophylaxis against *T. gondii* infection has been investigated in AIDS patients and recipients of organ transplants. Clindamycin[26] alone was found to be too toxic. While some studies have suggested that pyrimethamine[26-29] alone may be of value, increased mortality risk has been reported[30] and a controlled study has shown no benefit.[31] Co-trimoxazole, in regimens designed for *Pneumocystis carinii* pneumonia prophylaxis, appears to provide effective primary prophylaxis for toxoplasma encephalitis.[32,33] Alternatively, pyrimethamine plus dapsone may be effective[32,34] but in one study was not tolerated by 30% of patients.[35] Pyrimethamine plus sulfadoxine has also been used, with promising results.[36]

Secondary prophylaxis, or chronic maintenance therapy, should be given after treatment of toxoplasmic encephalitis in patients with HIV infection. Pyrimethamine with sulfadiazine plus folinic acid may be used; clindamycin may be substituted for sulfadiazine in patients unable to tolerate sulfa drugs.[32]

It may be possible to discontinue primary and secondary prophylaxis in patients with HIV infection who obtain a sustained response to highly active antiretroviral therapy with at least partial recovery of immune function.[32]


1. Anonymous. Antenatal screening for toxoplasmosis in the UK. *Lancet* 1990; **336:** 346–8. Correction. *ibid.*: 576.
2. Jeannel D, *et al.* What is known about the prevention of congenital toxoplasmosis? *Lancet* 1990; **336:** 359–61.
3. Ho-Yen DO, *et al.* Congenital toxoplasmosis and TORCH. *Lancet* 1990; **336:** 624.
4. Desmonts G. Preventing congenital toxoplasmosis. *Lancet* 1990; **336:** 1017–18.
5. Guerina NG, *et al.* Neonatal serologic screening and early treatment for congenital Toxoplasma gondii infection. *N Engl J Med* 1994; **330:** 1858–63.
6. WHO. *WHO model prescribing information: drugs used in parasitic diseases.* 2nd ed. Geneva: WHO, 1995.
7. Remington JS, Vildé JL. Clindamycin for toxoplasma encephalitis in AIDS. *Lancet* 1991; **338:** 1142–3.
8. Luft BJ, *et al.* Toxoplasmic encephalitis in patients with the acquired immunodeficiency syndrome. *N Engl J Med* 1993; **329:** 995–1000.
9. Dannemann B, *et al.* Treatment of toxoplasmic encephalitis in patients with AIDS: a randomized trial comparing pyrimethamine plus clindamycin to pyrimethamine plus sulfadiazine. *Ann Intern Med* 1992; **116:** 33–43.
10. Katlama C, *et al.* Pyrimethamine-clindamycin vs pyrimethamine-sulfadiazine as acute and long-term therapy for toxoplasmic encephalitis in patients with AIDS. *Clin Infect Dis* 1996; **22:** 268–75.
11. Tenant-Flowers M, *et al.* Sulphadiazine desensitization in patients with AIDS and cerebral toxoplasmosis. *AIDS* 1991; **5:** 311–15.
12. Fernandez-Martin J, *et al.* Pyrimethamine-clarithromycin combination for therapy of acute Toxoplasma encephalitis in patients with AIDS. *Antimicrob Agents Chemother* 1991; **35:** 2049–52.
13. Hagberg L, *et al.* Doxycycline and pyrimethamine for toxoplasmic encephalitis. *Scand J Infect Dis* 1993; **25:** 157–60.
14. Kovacs JA, *et al.* Efficacy of atovaquone in treatment of toxoplasmosis in patients with AIDS. *Lancet* 1992; **340:** 637–8.
15. Torres RA, *et al.* Atovaquone for salvage treatment and suppression of toxoplasmic encephalitis in patients with AIDS. *Clin Infect Dis* 1997; **24:** 422–9.
16. Dhiver C, *et al.* 5-Fluoro-uracil–clindamycin for treatment of cerebral toxoplasmosis. *AIDS* 1993; **7:** 143–4.
17. Lacassin F, *et al.* Clarithromycin-minocycline combination as salvage therapy for toxoplasmosis in patients infected with human immunodeficiency virus. *Antimicrob Agents Chemother* 1995; **39:** 276–7.
18. Torre D, *et al.* Randomized trial of trimethoprim-sulfamethoxazole versus pyrimethamine-sulfadiazine for therapy of toxoplasmic encephalitis in patients with AIDS. *Antimicrob Agents Chemother* 1998; **42:** 1346–9.
19. Saba J, *et al.* Pyrimethamine plus azithromycin for treatment of acute toxoplasmic encephalitis in patients with AIDS. *Eur J Clin Microbiol Infect Dis* 1993; **12:** 853–6.
20. Katlama C, *et al.* Atovaquone as long-term suppressive therapy for toxoplasmic encephalitis in patients with AIDS and multiple drug intolerance. *AIDS* 1996; **10:** 1107–12.
21. Roizen N, *et al.* Neurologic and developmental outcome in treated congenital toxoplasmosis. *Pediatrics* 1995; **95:** 11–20.
22. Rothova A. Ocular involvement in toxoplasmosis. *Br J Ophthalmol* 1993; **77:** 371–7.
23. Nussenblatt RB, Belfort R. Ocular toxoplasmosis: an old disease revisited. *JAMA* 1994; **271:** 304–7. Correction. *ibid.*; **272:** 356.
24. Hay J, Dutton GN. Toxoplasma and the eye. *BMJ* 1995; **310:** 1021–2.
25. Djurković-Djaković O, *et al.* Short-term effects of the clindamycin-steroid regimen in the treatment of ocular toxoplasmosis. *J Chemother* 1995; **7** (suppl 4): 199–201.
26. Jacobson MA, *et al.* Toxicity of clindamycin as prophylaxis for AIDS-associated toxoplasmic encephalitis. *Lancet* 1992; **339:** 333–4.
27. Wreghitt TG, *et al.* Efficacy of pyrimethamine for the prevention of donor-acquired Toxoplasma gondii infection in heart and heart-lung transplant recipients. *Transpl Int* 1992; **5:** 197–200.
28. Murphy K, *et al.* Pyrimethamine alone as long-term suppressive therapy in cerebral toxoplasmosis. *Am J Med* 1994; **96:** 95–6.
29. Klinker H, *et al.* Pyrimethamine alone as prophylaxis for cerebral toxoplasmosis in patients with advanced HIV infection. *Infection* 1996; **24:** 324–7.
30. Jacobson MA, *et al.* Primary prophylaxis with pyrimethamine for toxoplasmic encephalitis in patients with advanced human immunodeficiency virus disease: results of a randomized trial. *J Infect Dis* 1994; **169:** 384–94.
31. Leport C, *et al.* Pyrimethamine for primary prophylaxis of toxoplasmic encephalitis in patients with human immunodeficiency virus infection: a double-blind, randomized trial. *J Infect Dis* 1996; **173:** 91–7.
32. Centers for Disease Control and Prevention. Guidelines for preventing opportunistic infections among HIV-infected persons—2002: recommendations of the US Public Health Service and the Infectious Diseases Society of America. *MMWR* 2002; **51** (RR-8): 1–52. Also available at: http://www.cdc.gov/mmwr/PDF/rr/rr5108.pdf (accessed 02/06/04)
33. Bucher HC, *et al.* Meta-analysis of prophylactic treatments against Pneumocystis carinii pneumonia and toxoplasma encephalitis in HIV-infected patients. *J Acquir Immune Defic Syndr Hum Retrovirol* 1997; **15:** 104–14.
34. Podzamczer D, *et al.* Intermittent trimethoprim-sulfamethoxazole compared with dapsone-pyrimethamine for the simultaneous primary prophylaxis of Pneumocystis pneumonia and toxoplasmosis in patients infected with HIV. *Ann Intern Med* 1995; **122:** 755–61.
35. Opravil M, *et al.* Once-weekly administration of dapsone/pyrimethamine vs aerosolized pentamidine as combined prophylaxis for Pneumocystis carinii pneumonia and toxoplasmic encephalitis in human immunodeficiency virus-infected patients. *Clin Infect Dis* 1995; **20:** 531–41.
36. Schürmann D, *et al.* Twice-weekly pyrimethamine-sulfadoxine effectively prevents Pneumocystis carinii pneumonia and toxoplasmic encephalitis in patients with AIDS. *J Infect* 2001; **42:** 8–15.


## Trichomoniasis

Trichomoniasis is caused by invasion of the genito-urinary tract with the protozoan *Trichomonas vaginalis*. Transmission is primarily sexual. Trichomoniasis is a common cause of vaginitis and vaginal discharge; some infected women are asymptomatic but should still be treated to prevent sexual transmission and symptomatic infection. Men are usually asymptomatic, although they may experience urethritis.

Treatment is usually with a nitroimidazole such as metronidazole when a single oral dose can be effective.[1-5] Sexual partners should be treated concomitantly. The incidence of treatment failures appears to be increasing and some at least have been due to metronidazole resistance. Patients who do not respond to single-dose treatment may be given a more intensive course of metronidazole for 5 to 7 days. Tinidazole has been widely used as an alternative to metronidazole, and may be effective in cases of metronidazole resistance.[6] A patient with metronidazole- and tinidazole-resistant infection was successfully treated with paromomycin.[7] Local application of paromomycin has also been tried in a small number of patients with moderate success.[8] Clotrimazole, given intravaginally, has been suggested[1] for symptomatic relief during pregnancy, especially during the first trimester when metronidazole therapy is not recommended. However, clotrimazole is curative in only about 20% of patients and definitive treatment may be required later in pregnancy.


1. WHO. *WHO model prescribing information: drugs used in sexually transmitted diseases and HIV infection.* Geneva: WHO, 1995.
2. Clinical Effectiveness Group (Association for Genitourinary Medicine and the Medical Society for the Study of Venereal Diseases). 2001 National guideline on the management of Trichomonas vaginalis. Available at: http://www.bashh.org.guidelines/2002/tv%200601.PDF (accessed 02/06/04)
3. WHO. *Guidelines for the management of sexually transmitted infections.* Geneva: WHO, 2003. Also available at: http://whqlibdoc.who.int/publications/2003/9241546263.pdf (accessed 13/05/04)
4. Forna F, Gülmezoglu AM. Interventions for treating trichomoniasis in women. Available in The Cochrane Library; Issue 2. Chichester: John Wiley; 2004.
5. Centers for Disease Control. Sexually transmitted diseases treatment guidelines 2002. *MMWR* 2002; **51** (RR-6): 1–80. Also available at: http://www.cdc.gov/mmwr/PDF/rr/rr5106.pdf (accessed 02/06/04)
6. Sobel JD, *et al.* Tinidazole therapy for metronidazole-resistant vaginal trichomoniasis. *Clin Infect Dis* 2001; **33:** 1341–6.
7. Nyirjesy P, *et al.* Paromomycin for nitroimidazole-resistant trichomonosis. *Lancet* 1995; **346:** 1110.
8. Nyirjesy P, *et al.* Difficult-to-treat trichomoniasis: results with paromomycin cream. *Clin Infect Dis* 1998; **26:** 986–8.


## African trypanosomiasis

African trypanosomiasis (sleeping sickness) is caused by subspecies of the protozoan *Trypanosoma brucei*, transmitted by the bite of infected tsetse flies (*Glossina* spp.). Gambian or West African sleeping sickness is caused by *T. brucei gambiense*, carried by riverine tsetse flies, and Rhodesian or East African sleeping sickness is caused by *T. brucei rhodesiense*, carried by savannah tsetse flies. Infection can follow blood transfusion and congenital trypanosomiasis has also occurred.

Although it has proven impractical to eliminate trypanosomiasis from endemic areas, the intensity of transmission can be reduced by detection and treatment of cases and vector control, including insecticide spraying of breeding sites and the use of insecticide-impregnated traps and screens.[1,2] Control of infection in domestic animals may also be beneficial.[1]

Trypanosomiasis can be divided into the early haematolymphatic stage (infection of the bloodstream and lymph nodes), with lymphadenopathy, pruritus, fever, headache, and muscle and joint pain, and the late or meningoencephalitic stage (infection of the CNS) which is marked by signs including sleep disturbances, confusion, incoordination, psychiatric disorders, and eventual deterioration of consciousness.[1-3] Trypanosomiasis due to *T. b. gambiense* develops slowly over several months or even years and the disease stages are relatively distinct. Infection with *T. b. rhodesiense* is more acute with a rapid onset of symptoms and indistinct disease stages and, if left untreated, will usually lead to death in a matter of weeks or months.

The **haematolymphatic** phase of African trypanosomiasis is treated with suramin or pentamidine.[1-3] Pentamidine may be used for treatment of *T. b. gambiense* infections, but increasing resistance makes it unsuitable for *T. b. rhodesiense* infections; suramin is used for *T. b. rhodesiense* infections and for *T. b. gambiense* infections which are resistant to pentamidine. Giving both pentamidine and suramin for *T. b. gambiense* infections has not been shown to reduce the incidence of relapse.[4] Eflornithine can also be effective in this phase of infection caused by *T. b. gambiense*; it is not very effective on its own against *T. b. rhodesiense*.[2]

Suramin and pentamidine penetrate the blood-brain barrier poorly and are only used in the **meningoencephalitic** stage as adjuncts before starting treatment with melarsoprol or eflornithine. Melarsoprol, which is effective against both *T. b. gambiense* and *T. b. rhodesiense*, is usually only given to treat the meningoencephalitic stage of the infection because it may produce potentially fatal encephalopathy. However, protection against this toxicity may be provided by prophylaxis with prednisolone.[5,6] Patients with *T. b. gambiense* infection may be treated more safely with eflornithine than melarsoprol on its own. Combination therapy with melarsoprol and eflornithine was reported to be effective in a patient who had not responded to either drug alone.[7] Eflornithine given in combination with suramin produced disappointing results in 6 patients with *T. b. rhodesiense*.[8]

Nifurtimox[1,9,10] is an alternative treatment to melarsoprol for relapse of *T. b. gambiense* infection.

There is no established effective alternative treatment for melarsoprol-resistant *T. b. rhodesiense*, although suramin given in combination with high-dose metronidazole was successful in a patient.[11]

Patients should be seen every 6 months for a follow-up period of at least 2 years, to ascertain if treatment has been successful.


1. WHO. Control and surveillance of African trypanosomiasis. *WHO Tech Rep Ser 881* 1998.
2. WHO. *WHO model prescribing information: drugs used in parasitic diseases.* 2nd ed. Geneva: WHO, 1995.
3. Stich A, *et al.* Human African trypanosomiasis. *BMJ* 2002; **325:** 203–6.
4. Pépin J, Khonde N. Relapses following treatment of early-stage Trypanosoma brucei gambiense sleeping sickness with a combination of pentamidine and suramin. *Trans R Soc Trop Med Hyg* 1996; **90:** 183–6.
5. Pepin J, *et al.* Trial of prednisolone for prevention of melarsoprol-induced encephalopathy in gambiense sleeping sickness. *Lancet* 1989; **i:** 1246–50.
6. Pepin J, *et al.* Risk factors for encephalopathy and mortality during melarsoprol treatment of Trypanosoma brucei gambiense sleeping sickness. *Trans R Soc Trop Med Hyg* 1995; **89:** 92–7.
7. Simarro PP, Asumu PN. Gambian trypanosomiasis and synergism between melarsoprol and eflornithine: first case report. *Trans R Soc Trop Med Hyg* 1996; **90:** 315.
8. Clerinx J, *et al.* Treatment of late stage rhodesiense trypanosomiasis using suramin and eflornithine: report of six cases. *Trans R Soc Trop Med Hyg* 1998; **92:** 449–50.
9. Pepin J, *et al.* An open clinical trial of nifurtimox for arseno-resistant Trypanosoma brucei gambiense sleeping sickness in central Zaire. *Trans R Soc Trop Med Hyg* 1989; **83:** 514–17.
10. Pepin J, *et al.* High-dose nifurtimox for arseno-resistant Trypanosoma brucei gambiense sleeping sickness: an open trial in central Zaire. *Trans R Soc Trop Med Hyg* 1992; **86:** 254–6.
11. Foulkes JR. Metronidazole and suramin combination in the treatment of arsenical refractory rhodesian sleeping sickness—a case study. *Trans R Soc Trop Med Hyg* 1996; **90:** 422.


### American trypanosomiasis

American trypanosomiasis (Chagas' disease) is caused by *Trypanosoma cruzi*, carried by reduviid or triatomine bugs which feed on human blood.[1] Infected bugs defecate on the human host while feeding and metacyclic trypanosomes are shed and enter the host via skin abrasions or by direct penetration of mucous membranes such as the conjunctiva. Transmission by blood transfusion has been a large problem. Congenital infection can also occur. Control measures include case detection and treatment, vector control by insecticide applications within domestic buildings, and screening of blood donors.[1]

Infection with *T. cruzi* is found throughout South and Central America and has been recorded in Mexico and Texas; there have also been reports of transfusion-induced infection in northern USA and Canada. Three phases of the disease are recognised. In the early acute phase of infection parasites are present in the blood; this phase may be asymptomatic or there may be a swelling or chagoma at the site of infection, allergic reactions, and more rarely acute heart failure or meningoencephalitis. The acute phase may be fatal in children, but patients usually survive to enter an indeterminate phase, in which infection may be present in tissue for years without clinical manifestations. Classical features of the final chronic phase are cardiomyopathy, megacolon, and mega-oesophagus. Parasitaemia falls to undetectable levels after the acute phase.

Available treatment is generally unsatisfactory but, despite their toxicity, nifurtimox or benznidazole are of value especially in the acute phase; it is not certain whether trypanocidal treatment during the indeterminate phase can prevent the development of chronic disease although favourable results were obtained in a small study in children given benznidazole.[2] Although it is generally felt that there is no benefit from treatment in the chronic phase, treatment during the early chronic phase was reported to be beneficial,[3] and long-term follow-up of patients who had received benznidazole showed a reduction in cardiac complications and parasitaemia.[4] Symptomatic treatment is often given, particularly in the chronic stage for cardiac and gastrointestinal lesions.

The efficacy of treatment varies from country to country and may be linked to variations in the sensitivity of different strains of *T. cruzi*. Treatment is said to be successful when both parasitaemia and serological tests become negative and remain so for at least one year after the end of treatment.

Allopurinol and allopurinol riboside are under investigation for the treatment of American trypanosomiasis since they have shown trypanocidal activity. Allopurinol has been reported to be as effective as nifurtimox or benznidazole in reducing parasitaemia during the indeterminate phase and to be better tolerated.[5] Combined allopurinol and itraconazole has produced beneficial responses in patients with chronic disease.[6]

In areas where the proportion of seropositive blood donors is high, emergency blood supplies positive for *T. cruzi* have been made safe by the addition of methylrosanilinium chloride. It has been suggested that the risk of transmission to transplant recipients can be reduced considerably by nifurtimox or benznidazole treatment of the donor for 2 weeks before transplantation, and of the recipient for 2 weeks after transplantation. In laboratory workers at risk of an infection after an accident, treatment with benznidazole for 10 days should be started immediately.


1. WHO. Control of Chagas disease: second report of the WHO expert committee. *WHO Tech Rep Ser 905* 2002.
2. Sosa Estani S, *et al.* Efficacy of chemotherapy with benznidazole in children in the indeterminate phase of Chagas' disease. *Am J Trop Med Hyg* 1998; **59:** 526–9.
3. de Andrade ALSS, *et al.* Randomised trial of efficacy of benznidazole in treatment of early Trypanosoma cruzi infection. *Lancet* 1996; **348:** 1407–13.
4. Viotti R, *et al.* Treatment of chronic Chagas' disease with benznidazole: clinical and serologic evolution of patients with long-term follow-up. *Am Heart J* 1994; **127:** 151–62.
5. Gallerano RH, *et al.* Therapeutic efficacy of allopurinol in patients with chronic Chagas' disease. *Am J Trop Med Hyg* 1990; **43:** 159–66.
6. Apt W, *et al.* Treatment of chronic Chagas' disease with itraconazole and allopurinol. *Am J Trop Med Hyg* 1998; **59:** 133–8.


## Acetarsol *(BAN, rINN)*

Acetaminohydroxyphenylarsonsäure; Acetarsone; Acetphenarsinum; Osarsolum. 3-Acetamido-4-hydroxyphenylarsonic acid.

$C_8H_{10}AsNO_5$ = 275.1.

*CAS — 97-44-9.*

*ATC — A07AX02; G01AB01; P01CD02.*

### Profile

Acetarsol, a pentavalent organic arsenical derivative, was formerly given orally in the treatment of intestinal amoebiasis and vaginally in the treatment of trichomoniasis, but the use of pentavalent arsenical compounds has been abandoned in favour of more effective and less toxic drugs. For the adverse effects of arsenic and their treatment, see Arsenic Trioxide, p.1657.

Acetarsol suppositories were once tried in the treatment of proctitis. Acetarsol lithium and acetarsol sodium have been included in some preparations for minor mouth infections.

### Preparations

**Proprietary Preparations** (details are given in Part 3)
***Ital.:*** Gynoplix Theraplix†.

**Multi-ingredient: *Belg.:*** Sulfaryl†; ***Ital.:*** Sanogyl Bianco†.

## Amprolium Hydrochloride *(BANM, rINNM)*

Hidrocloruro de amprolio. 1-(4-Amino-2-propylpyrimidin-5-ylmethyl)-2-methylpyridinium chloride hydrochloride.

$C_{14}H_{19}ClN_4,HCl$ = 315.2.

*CAS — 121-25-5 (amprolium); 137-88-2 (amprolium hydrochloride).*

**Pharmacopoeias.** In *Fr.* and *US* for veterinary use only. Also in *BP(Vet).*

**BP(Vet) 2003** (Amprolium Hydrochloride). A white or almost white, odourless or almost odourless powder. Freely soluble in water; slightly soluble in alcohol; practically insoluble in chloroform; very slightly soluble in ether.

**USP 27** (Amprolium). A white to light yellow powder. Freely soluble in water, in alcohol, in dimethylformamide and in methyl alcohol; sparingly soluble in dehydrated alcohol; practically insoluble in acetone, in butyl alcohol, and in isopropyl alcohol.

### Profile

Amprolium hydrochloride is an antiprotozoal used in veterinary practice, alone or with other drugs such as ethopabate, for the control of coccidiosis in pigeons and in poultry.

# Pentavalent Antimony Compounds

Compuestos de antimonio pentavalente.

## Meglumine Antimonate

Antimoniato de meglumina; Antimony Meglumine; Meglumine Antimoniate; Protostib; RP-2168. 1-Deoxy-1-methylamino-D-glucitol antimonate.

$C_7H_{18}NO_8Sb$ = 366.0.

*CAS — 133-51-7.*

*ATC — P01CB01.*

## Sodium Stibogluconate *(BAN, rINN)*

Estibogluconato de sodio; Sod. Stibogluc.; Sodium Antimony Gluconate; Stibogluconat-Natrium.

*CAS — 16037-91-5.*

*ATC — P01CB02.*

**Description.** A pentavalent antimony compound of indefinite composition. It has been represented by the formula $C_6H_9Na_2O_9Sb$ but usually there are less than 2 atoms of Na for each atom of Sb. Solutions may be sterilised by autoclaving.

**Pharmacopoeias.** In *Br., Chin., Int.,* and *It.*

**BP 2003** (Sodium Stibogluconate). It is mainly the disodium salt of μ-oxy-bis[gluconato(3-)$O^2,O^3,O^4$-hydroxo-antimony]. It contains not less than 30.0% and not more than 34.0% of antimony(V), calculated with reference to the dried and methanol-free substance. It is a colourless, odourless or almost odourless, mostly amorphous powder. Very soluble in water; practically insoluble in alcohol and in ether. A solution in water containing 10% of pentavalent antimony has a pH of 5.0 to 5.6 after autoclaving.

## Adverse Effects, Treatment, and Precautions

As for Trivalent Antimony Compounds, p.103.

Adverse effects are generally less frequent and less severe with the pentavalent antimony compounds sodium stibogluconate and meglumine antimonate than with trivalent compounds such as antimony sodium tartrate. Nevertheless, similar precautions should be observed, especially in patients on high-dose therapy.

Intramuscular injections of sodium stibogluconate can be painful and intravenous use has been associated with thrombophlebitis.

◊ Common side-effects of pentavalent antimony are anorexia, vomiting, nausea, malaise, arthralgia and myalgia, headache, lethargy, and pancreatitis. ECG changes are dose-dependent and most commonly include T-wave inversion and prolonged QT interval. Renal damage is a rarely reported toxic effect. Pentavalent antimony is usually well tolerated. Serious side-effects when they occur usually involve the liver or the heart when it is prudent to interrupt the course temporarily.

References.


1. WHO. Control of the leishmaniases. *WHO Tech Rep Ser 793* 1990.
2. Aronson NE, *et al.* Safety and efficacy of intravenous sodium stibogluconate in the treatment of leishmaniasis: recent US military experience. *Clin Infect Dis* 1998; **27:** 1457–64.


**Breast feeding.** The amount of antimony distributed into the breast milk of a patient given sodium stibogluconate was considered not to constitute a hazard and oral absorption was not detected in an *animal* study.[1] The American Academy of Pediatrics also considers that the use of antimony is usually compatible with breast feeding.[2] Others, however, have felt that more safety evaluation was required before antimony could be considered completely safe during breast feeding.[3]


1. Berman JD, *et al.* Concentration of Pentostam in human breast milk. *Trans R Soc Trop Med Hyg* 1989; **83:** 784–5.

2. American Academy of Pediatrics. The transfer of drugs and other chemicals into human milk. *Pediatrics* 2001; **108:** 776–89. Correction. *ibid.*; 1029. Also available at: http://aappolicy.aappublications.org/cgi/content/full/pediatrics%3b108/3/776 (accessed 02/06/04)
3. Verschoyle RD. Comment. *Trop Dis Bull* 1990; **87:** 919.

**Effects on the blood.** Although thrombocytopenia is associated with leishmaniasis, there are case reports of it also being associated with sodium stibogluconate.[1,2]

1. Braconier JH, Miörner H. Recurrent episodes of thrombocytopenia during treatment with sodium stibogluconate. *J Antimicrob Chemother* 1993; **31:** 187–8.
2. Hepburn NC. Thrombocytopenia complicating sodium stibogluconate therapy for cutaneous leishmaniasis. *Trans R Soc Trop Med Hyg* 1993; **87:** 691.

**Effects on the heart.** The ECG was monitored during 65 courses of treatment with sodium stibogluconate in 59 Kenyan patients with leishmaniasis.[1] ECG abnormalities developed during 35 treatment courses. They were qualitatively similar to those previously described during treatment with trivalent antimonial drugs, but occurred less frequently and later during the course of treatment. The most common abnormality was inversion and/or decreased amplitude of T waves. Incidence was related to total daily dose and duration of treatment. One patient died suddenly during the 4th week of treatment with antimony 60 mg/kg daily. Other deaths probably related to cardiac toxicity have been reported in patients receiving 60 mg/kg daily[2] and 30 mg/kg daily.[3] Guidelines[1] for monitoring during treatment with sodium stibogluconate recommend that ECGs be obtained every 3 to 4 days in patients receiving antimony 20 mg/kg daily for more than 20 days or a higher dose for more than 10 days. If Stokes-Adams attacks or ventricular tachyarrhythmias develop, sodium stibogluconate should be stopped and appropriate treatment given.

1. Chulay JD, *et al.* Electrocardiographic changes during treatment of leishmaniasis with pentavalent antimony (sodium stibogluconate). *Am J Trop Med Hyg* 1985; **34:** 702–9.
2. Bryceson ADM, *et al.* Visceral leishmaniasis unresponsive to antimonial drugs II: response to high dosage sodium stibogluconate or prolonged treatment with pentamidine. *Trans R Soc Trop Med Hyg* 1985; **79:** 705–14.
3. Thakur CP. Harmful effect of high stibogluconate treatment of kala-azar in India. *Trans R Soc Trop Med Hyg* 1986; **80:** 672–3.

**Effects on the kidneys.** Sodium stibogluconate given for 10 days to 16 young men with cutaneous leishmaniasis had no apparent adverse effect on glomerular or tubular renal function.[1] However, evidence of renal tubular dysfunction has been reported in patients with mucocutaneous leishmaniasis given meglumine antimonate or sodium stibogluconate for 30 days or more[2] and acute renal failure has occurred in patients both with,[3] and without,[4] pre-existing renal impairment, the latter resulting in death.

1. Joliffe DS. Nephrotoxicity of pentavalent antimonials. *Lancet* 1985; **i:** 584.
2. Veiga JPR, *et al.* Renal tubular dysfunction in patients with mucocutaneous leishmaniasis treated with pentavalent antimonials. *Lancet* 1983; **ii:** 569.
3. Balzan M, Fenech F. Acute renal failure in visceral leishmaniasis treated with sodium stibogluconate. *Trans R Soc Trop Med Hyg* 1992; **86:** 515–16.
4. Rodrigues MLO, *et al.* Nephrotoxicity attributed to meglumine antimoniate (Glucantime) in the treatment of generalized cutaneous leishmaniasis. *Rev Inst Med Trop Sao Paulo* 1999; **41:** 33–7.

**Effects on the liver.** WHO has reported that when serious side-effects occur with sodium stibogluconate they usually involve the liver or the heart.[1] There have been reports of disturbed liver function[2,3] in patients given sodium stibogluconate, although there has also been a report[4] that signs of altered liver function, which may be a feature of visceral leishmaniasis, improved during treatment with sodium stibogluconate.

1. WHO. Control of the leishmaniases. *WHO Tech Rep Ser 793* 1990.
2. Ballou WR, *et al.* Safety and efficacy of high-dose sodium stibogluconate therapy of American cutaneous leishmaniasis. *Lancet* 1987; **ii:** 13–16.
3. Hepburn NC, *et al.* Hepatotoxicity of sodium stibogluconate in leishmaniasis. *Lancet* 1993; **342:** 238–9.
4. Misbahuddin M, *et al.* Stibogluconate for leishmaniasis. *Lancet* 1993; **342:** 804.

**Effects on the musculoskeletal system.** Arthralgia is common with pentavalent antimony compounds. It is usually dose-dependent[1] but a patient has been described who experienced symptoms early in treatment.[2] Palindromic arthropathy with effusion was associated with sodium stibogluconate treatment in another patient.[3]

1. Ballou WR, *et al.* Safety and efficacy of high-dose sodium stibogluconate therapy of American cutaneous leishmaniasis. *Lancet* 1987; **ii:** 13–16.
2. Castro C, *et al.* Severe arthralgia, not related to dose, associated with pentavalent antimonial therapy for mucosal leishmaniasis. *Trans R Soc Trop Med Hyg* 1990; **84:** 362.
3. Donovan KL, *et al.* Pancreatitis and palindromic arthropathy with effusions associated with sodium stibogluconate treatment in a renal transplant recipient. *J Infect* 1990; **21:** 107–10.

**Effects on the nervous system.** Peripheral neuropathy developed in a patient about 8 days after starting therapy with sodium stibogluconate.[1] The symptoms were generally reversible when treatment was stopped (after 17 days), although there was some slight persistent hypoaesthesia in the toes. An interaction with a single dose of amitriptyline, taken on the second day of stibogluconate therapy, seemed unlikely but could not be ruled out.

1. Brummitt CF, *et al.* Reversible peripheral neuropathy associated with sodium stibogluconate therapy for American cutaneous leishmaniasis. *Clin Infect Dis* 1996; **22:** 878–9.

**Effects on the pancreas.** Pancreatitis has been associated with sodium stibogluconate treatment.[1-3] Withdrawing treatment usually resulted in resolution of pancreatitis.

1. Donovan KL, *et al.* Pancreatitis and palindromic arthropathy with effusions associated with sodium stibogluconate treatment in a renal transplant recipient. *J Infect* 1990; **21:** 107–10.
2. Gasser RA, *et al.* Pancreatitis induced by pentavalent antimonial agents during treatment of leishmaniasis. *Clin Infect Dis* 1994; **18:** 83–90.
3. Domingo P, *et al.* Treatment of Indian kala-azar with pentavalent antimony. *Lancet* 1995; **345:** 584–5.

## Pharmacokinetics

The pentavalent antimony compounds are poorly absorbed from the gastrointestinal tract. After intravenous doses an initial distribution phase is followed by biexponential elimination by the kidneys. The elimination half-life of the initial phase is about 1.7 hours and that of the slow terminal phase is about 33 hours. The corresponding half-lives after intramuscular doses are reported to be 2 hours and 766 hours respectively. The slow elimination phase may reflect reduction to trivalent antimony. Accumulation occurs on daily use and maximum tissue concentrations may not be reached for 7 days or more. Antimony has been detected in breast milk (see Breast Feeding, above).

◊ References.

1. Rees PH, *et al.* Renal clearance of pentavalent antimony (sodium stibogluconate). *Lancet* 1980; **ii:** 226–9.
2. Chulay JD, *et al.* Pharmacokinetics of antimony during treatment of visceral leishmaniasis with sodium stibogluconate or meglumine antimoniate. *Trans R Soc Trop Med Hyg* 1988; **82:** 69–72.
3. Al Jaser M, *et al.* Pharmacokinetics of antimony in patients treated with sodium stibogluconate for cutaneous leishmaniasis. *Pharm Res* 1995; **12:** 113–16.

## Uses and Administration

Pentavalent antimony, as sodium stibogluconate or meglumine antimonate, is used as first-line treatment for all forms of leishmaniasis except *Leishmania aethiopica* infections.

For systemic use, sodium stibogluconate is given by intramuscular or intravenous injection as a solution containing the equivalent of 100 mg of pentavalent antimony per mL. Intramuscular injection is generally preferable. Intravenous injections must be administered very slowly (over at least 5 minutes) and preferably through a fine needle to avoid thrombophlebitis; as with trivalent antimony compounds, they should be stopped immediately if coughing, vomiting, or substernal pain occurs. Meglumine antimonate is given by deep intramuscular injection as a solution containing the equivalent of 85 mg of pentavalent antimony per mL. Doses are expressed in terms of the equivalent amount of pentavalent antimony.

Local variations exist in treatment schedules but WHO recommends the following regimens:

- In **visceral leishmaniasis**, initial treatment is based on daily injection of pentavalent antimony 20 mg/kg to a maximum of 850 mg (but see below) for at least 20 days. The length of treatment varies from one endemic area to another, but is continued until no parasites are detected in consecutive splenic aspirates taken at 14-day intervals. Patients who relapse are re-treated at the same dose
- Early non-inflamed lesions of **cutaneous leishmaniasis** due to all forms of *Leishmania* except *L. aethiopica*, *L. amazonensis*, and *L. braziliensis* may be treated by infiltration with intralesional injections of 1 to 3 mL of sodium stibogluconate or meglumine antimonate (approximately 100 to 300 mg of pentavalent antimony), repeated once or twice if necessary at intervals of 1 to 2 days. Systemic therapy with pentavalent antimony 10 to 20 mg/kg daily is given if the lesions are more severe and continued until a few days after clinical and parasitological cure is achieved.

  Cutaneous leishmaniasis due to *L. aethiopica* is not responsive to antimonials at conventional doses. In cutaneous leishmaniasis due to *L. braziliensis*, prolonged systemic treatment with pentavalent antimony 20 mg/kg daily for a minimum of 4 weeks is indicated. Similar doses are required for **diffuse cutaneous leishmaniasis** due to *L. amazonensis* and are continued for several months after clinical improvement occurs. Relapses should be expected until immunity develops.
- In **mucocutaneous leishmaniasis**, daily doses of pentavalent antimony 20 mg/kg are given for a minimum of 4 weeks; if the response is poor, 10 to 15 mg/kg may be given every 12 hours. Relapses are well known and have generally been associated with inadequate or interrupted treatment; they are treated with the same drug given for at least twice as long as the original treatment. Only when that fails should alternative treatment be given.

**Leishmaniasis.** The main treatment for leishmaniasis (p.597) is a pentavalent antimony compound such as sodium stibogluconate. Higher doses of antimony compounds than those recommended by WHO (see above) have been tried in order to overcome the unresponsiveness of leishmaniasis to therapy. In the USA, the use of 20 mg/kg daily of pentavalent antimony has been recommended, without restriction to an 850-mg maximum daily dose.[1,2] At 20 mg/kg daily the most common adverse effects are musculoskeletal disorders, elevated liver enzyme values, and T-wave changes on the ECG, and the CDC recommends that the ECG, blood chemistry, and blood count should be monitored throughout therapy if resources permit.[1] Severe cardiotoxicity is rare at this dose but fatal cardiac toxicity has been reported with doses of up to 60 mg/kg daily (see under Effects on the Heart, above). Drug-resistant strains of *Leishmania infantum* have been associated with unresponsiveness to treatment with meglumine antimonate.[3] It was suggested[4] that the use of suboptimal doses may be increasing the prevalence of drug-resistant strains of the parasite. However, low doses of antimony compounds (5 mg/kg daily for 30 days) have produced long-term cure in patients with cutaneous *L. braziliensis* infection followed for up to 10 years.[5]

INTRALESIONAL ADMINISTRATION. Intralesional infiltration of 3 doses of sodium stibogluconate on alternate days or once weekly was more effective than daily treatment in a study of 96 patients in Saudi Arabia.[6] Local infiltration of meglumine antimonate in usual doses of 150 to 900 mg (maximum 1500 mg) once each week for up to 6 weeks produced microbiological and clinical cures in all of 45 patients in Italy with cutaneous leishmaniasis.[7]

1. Herwaldt BL, Berman JD. Recommendations for treating leishmaniasis with sodium stibogluconate (Pentostam) and review of pertinent clinical studies. *Am J Trop Med Hyg* 1992; **46:** 296–306.
2. Medical Letter on Drugs and Therapeutics. Drugs for parasitic infections (issued April 2002). Available at: http://www.medicalletter.com/freedocs/parasitic.pdf (accessed 03/06/04)
3. Faraut-Gambarelli F, *et al.* In vitro and in vivo resistance of Leishmania infantum to meglumine antimoniate: a study of 37 strains collected from patients with visceral leishmaniasis. *Antimicrob Agents Chemother* 1997; **41:** 827–30.
4. Grogl M, *et al.* Drug resistance in leishmaniasis: its implication in systemic chemotherapy of cutaneous and mucocutaneous disease. *Am J Trop Med Hyg* 1992; **47:** 117–26.
5. Oliveira-Neto MP, *et al.* A low-dose antimony treatment in 159 patients with American cutaneous leishmaniasis: extensive follow-up studies (up to 10 years). *Am J Trop Med Hyg* 1997; **57:** 651–5.
6. Tallab TM, *et al.* Cutaneous leishmaniasis: schedules for intralesional treatment with sodium stibogluconate. *Int J Dermatol* 1996; **35:** 594–7.
7. Aste N, *et al.* Intralesional treatment of cutaneous leishmaniasis with meglumine antimoniate. *Br J Dermatol* 1998; **138:** 370–1.

## Preparations

***BP 2003:*** Sodium Stibogluconate Injection.

**Proprietary Preparations** (details are given in Part 3)
***Braz.:*** Glucantime; ***Fr.:*** Glucantime; ***Israel:*** Pentostam; ***Ital.:*** Glucantim; ***Spain:*** Glucantime; ***UK:*** Pentostam.

# Atovaquone *(BAN, USAN, rINN)*

Atovacuona; BW-A566C; BW-566C; BW-566C80; 566C; 566C80. 2-[*trans*-4-(4-Chlorophenyl)cyclohexyl]-3-hydroxy-1,4-naphthoquinone.

$C_{22}H_{19}O_3Cl$ = 366.8.

*CAS — 95233-18-4.*

*ATC — P01AX06.*

**Pharmacopoeias.** In *US.*

**USP 27** (Atovaquone). A yellow powder. Insoluble in water; slightly soluble in alcohol, in butanediol, in ethyl acetate, in glycerol, in octanol, and in macrogol 200; sparingly soluble in acetone, in di-*n*butyl adipate, in dimethyl sulfoxide, and in macrogol 400; soluble in chloroform; freely soluble in *N*-methyl-2-pyrrolidone and in tetrahydrofuran; very slightly soluble in 0.1N sodium hydroxide. Store in airtight containers. Protect from light.

### Adverse Effects and Precautions

Adverse reactions to atovaquone include skin rashes, headache, fever, insomnia, and gastrointestinal effects such as nausea, diarrhoea, and vomiting. Raised liver enzyme values, hyponatraemia, and haematological disturbances such as anaemia and neutropenia may occur occasionally. Atovaquone should be avoided in patients with gastrointestinal disorders that may limit absorption of the drug.

**Effects on the skin.** Stevens-Johnson syndrome has been reported[1] in a patient taking atovaquone with proguanil.

1. Emberger M, *et al.* Stevens-Johnson syndrome associated with Malarone antimalarial prophylaxis. Abstract: *Clin Infect Dis* 2003; **37:** 158. Full version: http://www.journals.uchicago.edu/CID/journal/issues/v37n1/30442/30442.html (accessed 03/06/04)

### Interactions

Use of atovaquone with either metoclopramide, tetracycline, or rifampicin (and possibly also rifabutin) may result in decreases in plasma-atovaquone concentrations. Other drugs which have produced small reductions in plasma-atovaquone concentrations include aciclovir, antidiarrhoeals, benzodiazepines, cephalosporins, laxatives, opioids, and paracetamol.

Atovaquone is reported to decrease the metabolism of zidovudine resulting in moderate increases in zidovudine plasma concentrations. A decrease in trough concentrations of indinavir, and in the area under the indinavir time-concentration curve has been reported when atovaquone was also given. Small decreases in the plasma concentrations of co-trimoxazole have been noted in patients taking atovaquone. There is a theoretical possibility that atovaquone could displace other highly protein-bound drugs from plasma-protein binding sites.

### Pharmacokinetics

Atovaquone is poorly absorbed from the gastrointestinal tract after oral doses; bioavailability is especially poor in patients with AIDS. Bioavailability from commercial oral liquid formulations is better than from tablets and can be further improved if taken with food, particularly meals with a high fat content. Atovaquone is more than 99% bound to plasma proteins and has a long plasma half-life of 2 to 3 days, thought to be due to enterohepatic recycling. It is excreted almost exclusively in faeces as unchanged drug.

◊ References.

1. Hughes WT, *et al.* Safety and pharmacokinetics of 566C80, a hydroxynaphthoquinone with anti-Pneumocystis carinii activity: a phase I study in human immunodeficiency virus (HIV)-infected men. *J Infect Dis* 1991; **163:** 843–8.
2. Rolan PE, *et al.* Examination of some factors responsible for a food-induced increase in absorption of atovaquone. *Br J Clin Pharmacol* 1994; **37:** 13–20.
3. Dixon R, *et al.* Single-dose and steady-state pharmacokinetics of a novel microfluidized suspension of atovaquone in human immunodeficiency virus-seropositive patients. *Antimicrob Agents Chemother* 1996; **40:** 556–60.
4. Hussein Z, *et al.* Population pharmacokinetics of atovaquone in patients with acute malaria caused by Plasmodium falciparum. *Clin Pharmacol Ther* 1997; **61:** 518–30.
5. Rolan PE, *et al.* Disposition of atovaquone in humans. *Antimicrob Agents Chemother* 1997; **41:** 1319–21.

### Uses and Administration

Atovaquone is a hydroxynaphthoquinone antiprotozoal that is also active against the fungus *Pneumocystis carinii.* It is used in the treatment and prophylaxis of *Pneumocystis carinii* pneumonia in patients unable to tolerate co-trimoxazole, and with proguanil in the treatment and prophylaxis of malaria.

In the treatment of mild to moderate *Pneumocystis carinii* pneumonia, atovaquone is given by mouth in a dose of 750 mg with food three times daily as tablets, or twice daily as a suspension, for 21 days. For prophylaxis 1500 mg is given once daily with food.

In the treatment of uncomplicated falciparum malaria, atovaquone is given in a single daily dose of 1 g with proguanil hydrochloride 400 mg, as a combined preparation, for 3 days.

For prophylaxis of falciparum malaria, atovaquone 250 mg is given once daily in combination with proguanil 100 mg. Prophylaxis should commence 1 to 2 days before travel to the malarious area, continue daily throughout exposure, and for 7 days after leaving the area.

For both treatment and prophylaxis of malaria, children weighing 11 to 20 kg may be given one-quarter the adult dose, those weighing 21 to 30 kg may be given half the adult dose, and those weighing 31 to 40 kg may be given three-quarters the adult dose.

◊ Reviews.

1. Haile LG, Flaherty JF. Atovaquone: a review. *Ann Pharmacother* 1993; **27:** 1488–94.
2. Artymowicz RJ, James VE. Atovaquone: a new antipneumocystis agent. *Clin Pharm* 1993; **12:** 563–70.
3. Spencer CM, Goa KL. Atovaquone: a review of its pharmacological properties and therapeutic efficacy in opportunistic infections. *Drugs* 1995; **50:** 176–96.
4. Baggish AL, Hill DR. Antiparasitic agent atovaquone. *Antimicrob Agents Chemother* 2002; **46:** 1163–73.
5. McKeage K, Scott LJ. Atovaquone/proguanil: a review of its use for the prophylaxis of Plasmodium falciparum malaria. *Drugs* 2003; **63:** 597–623.
6. Marra F, *et al.* Atovaquone-proguanil for prophylaxis and treatment of malaria. *Ann Pharmacother* 2003; **37:** 1266–75.

**Babesiosis.** In a prospective, randomised study[1] involving 58 patients with babesiosis (p.595), atovaquone with azithromycin was found to be equivalent in efficacy to, and associated with fewer adverse effects than, standard therapy with quinine and clindamycin.

1. Krause PJ, *et al.* Atovaquone and azithromycin for the treatment of babesiosis. *N Engl J Med* 2000; **343:** 1454–8.

**Malaria.** Atovaquone with proguanil (Malarone) is used in the treatment and prophylaxis of uncomplicated malaria caused by *Plasmodium falciparum* (see p.444).

Atovaquone, a blood schizontocide, is associated with an unacceptably high rate of recrudescence when used alone[1,2] for *treatment* but is more successful in malaria when used with proguanil,[2,3] including that produced by multidrug-resistant strains.[4] Use of the combination to treat *P. ovale* and *P. malariae* malarias has also been studied.[5] Atovaquone with proguanil followed by primaquine may also be effective for the treatment of *P. vivax* malaria.[6]

Atovaquone with proguanil has also been found to be useful for *prophylaxis* of falciparum malaria in both children[7] and adults[8] in endemic areas. It may also be used for prophylaxis in non-immune travellers[9] and appears to be well tolerated.[10]

1. Chiodini PL, *et al.* Evaluation of atovaquone in the treatment of patients with uncomplicated Plasmodium falciparum malaria. *J Antimicrob Chemother* 1995; **36;** 1073–5.
2. Looareesuwan S, *et al.* Clinical studies of atovaquone, alone or in combination with other antimalarial drugs, for treatment of acute uncomplicated malaria in Thailand. *Am J Trop Med Hyg* 1996; **54:** 62–6.
3. Radloff PD, *et al.* Atovaquone and proguanil for Plasmodium falciparum malaria. *Lancet* 1996; **347:** 1511–14.
4. Sabchareon A, *et al.* Efficacy and pharmacokinetics of atovaquone and proguanil in children with multidrug-resistant Plasmodium falciparum malaria. *Trans R Soc Trop Med Hyg* 1998; **92:** 201–6.
5. Radloff PD, *et al.* Atovaquone plus proguanil is an effective treatment for Plasmodium ovale and P. malariae malaria. *Trans R Soc Trop Med Hyg* 1996; **90:** 682.
6. Looareesuwan S, *et al.* Atovaquone and proguanil hydrochloride followed by primaquine for treatment of plasmodium vivax malaria in Thailand. *Trans R Soc Trop Med Hyg* 1999; **93:** 637–40.
7. Lell B, *et al.* Randomised placebo-controlled study of atovaquone plus proguanil for malaria prophylaxis in children. *Lancet* 1998; **351:** 709–13.
8. Shanks GD, *et al.* Efficacy and safety of atovaquone/proguanil as suppressive prophylaxis for Plasmodium falciparum malaria. *Clin Infect Dis* 1998; **27:** 494–9.
9. Overbosch D, *et al.* Atovaquone-proguanil versus mefloquine for malaria prophylaxis in nonimmune travelers: results from a randomized, double-blind study. *Clin Infect Dis* 2001; **33:** 1015–21.
10. Høgh B, *et al.* Atovaquone-proguanil versus chloroquine-proguanil for malaria prophylaxis in non-immune travellers: a randomised, double-blind study. *Lancet* 2000; **356:** 1888–94.

**Microsporidiosis.** There is no established effective treatment for microsporidiosis (p.598). Beneficial responses were reported with atovaquone in a preliminary study.[1]

1. Anwar-Bruni DM, *et al.* Atovaquone is effective treatment for the symptoms of gastrointestinal microsporidiosis in HIV-1-infected patients. *AIDS* 1996; **10:** 619–23.

**Pneumocystis carinii pneumonia.** Atovaquone is one alternative to co-trimoxazole or pentamidine for the treatment of mild to moderate *Pneumocystis carinii* pneumonia (p.389). In open studies, a clinical response to atovaquone was reported in 78% of patients with mild to moderate disease and in 56% of patients with severe disease who were intolerant of, or who failed to respond to, both co-trimoxazole and pentamidine.[1] Comparative studies have shown atovaquone to be less effective than co-trimoxazole[2] and probably less effective than pentamidine,[3,4] but to produce fewer treatment-limiting adverse effects than either. For primary or secondary *prophylaxis,* atovaquone was as effective as dapsone[5] or inhaled pentamidine[6] in studies in patients intolerant of co-trimoxazole.

1. White A, *et al.* Clinical experience with atovaquone on a treatment investigational new drug protocol for Pneumocystis carinii pneumonia. *J Acquir Immune Defic Syndr Hum Retrovirol* 1995; **9:** 280–5.
2. Hughes W, *et al.* Comparison of atovaquone (566C80) with trimethoprim-sulfamethoxazole to treat Pneumocystis carinii pneumonia in patients with AIDS. *N Engl J Med* 1993; **328:** 1521–7.
3. Dohn MN, *et al.* Oral atovaquone compared with intravenous pentamidine for Pneumocystis carinii pneumonia in patients with AIDS. *Ann Intern Med* 1994; **121:** 174–80.
4. Lederman MM, van der Horst C. Atovaquone for Pneumocystis carinii pneumonia. *Ann Intern Med* 1995; **122:** 314.
5. El-Sadr WM, *et al.* Atovaquone compared with dapsone for the prevention of Pneumocystis carinii pneumonia in patients with HIV infection who cannot tolerate trimethoprim, sulfonamides, or both. *N Engl J Med* 1998; **339:** 1889–95.
6. Chan C, *et al.* Atovaquone suspension compared with aerosolized pentamidine for prevention of Pneumocystis carinii pneumonia in human immunodeficiency virus-infected subjects intolerant of trimethoprim or sulfonamides. *J Infect Dis* 1999; **180:** 369–76.

**Toxoplasmosis.** Atovaquone, either alone or with pyrimethamine or sulfadiazine, has produced encouraging results for treatment[1-3] or long-term suppression[2-4] of toxoplasmosis (p.598) in patients with AIDS.

1. Kovacs JA, *et al.* Efficacy of atovaquone in treatment of toxoplasmosis in patients with AIDS. *Lancet* 1992; **340:** 637–8.
2. Torres RA, *et al.* Atovaquone for salvage treatment and suppression of toxoplasmic encephalitis in patients with AIDS. *Clin Infect Dis* 1997; **24:** 422–9.
3. Chirgwin K, *et al.* Randomized phase II trial of atovaquone with pyrimethamine or sulfadiazine for treatment of toxoplasmic encephalitis in patients with acquired immunodeficiency syndrome: ACTG 237/ANRS 039 Study. *Clin Infect Dis* 2002; **34:** 1243–50.
4. Katlama C, *et al.* Atovaquone as long-term suppressive therapy for toxoplasmic encephalitis in patients with AIDS and multiple drug intolerance. *AIDS* 1996; **10:** 1107–12.

### Preparations

***USP 27:*** Atovaquone Oral Suspension.

**Proprietary Preparations** (details are given in Part 3)
***Austral.:*** Wellvone; ***Austria:*** Wellvone; ***Belg.:*** Wellvone; ***Canad.:*** Mepron; ***Denm.:*** Wellvone†; ***Fr.:*** Wellvone; ***Ger.:*** Wellvone; ***Gr.:*** Wellvone; ***Ital.:*** Wellvone; ***Neth.:*** Wellvone; ***S.Afr.:*** Wellvone; ***Spain:*** Wellvone†; ***Swed.:*** Wellvone; ***Switz.:*** Wellvone; ***UK:*** Wellvone; ***USA:*** Mepron.

**Multi-ingredient:** ***Austral.:*** Malarone; ***Austria:*** Malarone; Promal; ***Belg.:*** Malarone; ***Braz.:*** Malarone†; ***Canad.:*** Malarone; ***Denm.:*** Malarone; ***Fr.:*** Malarone; ***Ger.:*** Malarone; ***Norw.:*** Malarone; ***NZ:*** Malarone; ***Singapore:*** Malarone; ***Spain:*** Malarone; ***Swed.:*** Malarone; ***Switz.:*** Malarone; ***UK:*** Malarone; ***USA:*** Malarone.

---

## Azanidazole *(BAN, USAN, rINN)*

Azanidazol; F-4. 4-[(*E*)-2-(1-Methyl-5-nitroimidazol-2-yl)vinyl]pyrimidin-2-ylamine.
$C_{10}H_{10}N_6O_2$ = 246.2.
*CAS — 62973-76-6.*
*ATC — G01AF13; P01AB04.*

### Profile

Azanidazole is a 5-nitroimidazole derivative similar to metronidazole (p.607) and is used in the treatment of trichomoniasis in usual doses of 200 mg twice daily by mouth or 250 mg once daily intravaginally.

### Preparations

**Proprietary Preparations** (details are given in Part 3)
***Ital.:*** Triclose.

---

## Benznidazole *(rINN)*

Benznidazol; Benznidazolum; Ro-7-1051. *N*-Benzyl-2-(2-nitroimidazol-1-yl)acetamide.
$C_{12}H_{12}N_4O_3$ = 260.2.
*CAS — 22994-85-0.*
*ATC — P01CA02.*

**Pharmacopoeias.** In *Int.*

### Adverse Effects

Nausea, vomiting, abdominal pain, peripheral neuropathy, blood dyscrasias, and severe skin reactions have been reported with benznidazole.

◊ A study[1] involving 20 patients with chronic American trypanosomiasis given benznidazole 5 mg/kg daily had to be stopped because of the high incidence of skin rashes and neurological symptoms.

1. Apt W, *et al.* Clinical trial of benznidazole and an immunopotentiator against Chagas disease in Chile. *Trans R Soc Trop Med Hyg* 1986; **80:** 1010.

### Pharmacokinetics

Benznidazole is absorbed from the gastrointestinal tract after oral doses.

◊ References.

1. Raaflaub J, Ziegler WH. Single-dose pharmacokinetics of the trypanosomicide benznidazole in man. *Arzneimittelforschung* 1979; **29:** 1611–14.

### Uses and Administration

Benznidazole is a 2-nitroimidazole derivative with antiprotozoal activity. It is of value in the treatment of American trypanosomiasis (Chagas' disease) due to infection with *Trypanosoma cruzi,* especially during the early acute stage of the disease.

Benznidazole has been given by mouth in a dose of 5 to 7 mg/kg daily in two divided doses usually for 60 days (but see below). Children have been given 10 mg/kg daily in two divided doses.

**American trypanosomiasis.** Available treatment for American trypanosomiasis (p.600) is generally unsatisfactory, but benznidazole is of value especially in the acute phase. WHO[1] recommends that benznidazole should be given for 60 days but some in the USA[2] suggest courses of 30 to 90 days. Although treatment is usually confined to the acute phase of the disease, therapy during the early chronic phase was reported to be beneficial,[3] and long-term follow-up in patients who had received benznidazole has shown a reduction in cardiac complications and parasitaemia.[4]

1. WHO. Control of Chagas disease: second report of the WHO expert committee. *WHO Tech Rep Ser 905* 2002.
2. Medical Letter on Drugs and Therapeutics. Drugs for parasitic infections (issued April 2002). Available at: http://www.medicalletter.com/freedocs/parasitic.pdf (accessed 03/06/04)
3. de Andrade ALSS, *et al.* Randomised trial of efficacy of benznidazole in treatment of early Trypanosoma cruzi infection. *Lancet* 1996; **348:** 1407–13.
4. Viotti R, *et al.* Treatment of chronic Chagas' disease with benznidazole: clinical and serologic evolution of patients with long-term follow-up. *Am Heart J* 1994; **127:** 151–62.

## Preparations

**Proprietary Preparations** (details are given in Part 3)
***Arg.:*** Radanil; ***Braz.:*** Rochagan; ***Ecuad.:*** Ragonil.

## Buparvaquone *(BAN, rINN)*

Buparvacuona; BW-720C. *trans*-2-(4-*tert*-butylcyclohexylmethyl)-3-hydroxy-1,4-naphthoquinone.
$C_{21}H_{26}O_3$ = 326.4.
*CAS — 88426-33-9.*

### Profile

Buparvaquone is an antiprotozoal used in veterinary practice for the treatment of theileriosis in cattle.

## Carnidazole *(BAN, USAN, pINN)*

Carnidazol; R-25831; R-28096 (carnidazole hydrochloride). *O*-Methyl [2-(2-methyl-5-nitroimidazol-1-yl)ethyl]thiocarbamate.
$C_8H_{12}N_4O_3S$ = 244.3.
*CAS — 42116-76-7.*

### Profile

Carnidazole is a 5-nitroimidazole derivative similar to metronidazole. It is used in veterinary practice for the control of trichomoniasis in pigeons.

## Clazuril *(BAN, USAN, rINN)*

Clazurilo; Clazurilum; R-62690. (±)-[2-Chloro-4-(4,5-dihydro-3,5-dioxo-*as*-triazin-2(3*H*)-yl)phenyl]-(*p*-chlorophenyl)acetonitrile.
$C_{17}H_{10}Cl_2N_4O_2$ = 373.2.
*CAS — 101831-36-1.*

**Pharmacopoeias.** In *Eur.* (see p.vi) for veterinary use only.
**Ph. Eur. 5.0** (Clazuril for Veterinary Use). A white or light yellow powder. Practically insoluble in water; slightly soluble in alcohol and in dichloromethane; freely soluble in dimethylformamide. Protect from light.

### Profile

Clazuril is an antiprotozoal used in veterinary practice for the control of coccidiosis in pigeons.

## Clefamide *(BAN, rINN)*

Chlorphenoxamide. 2,2-Dichloro-*N*-(2-hydroxyethyl)-*N*-[4-(4-nitrophenoxy)benzyl]acetamide.
$C_{17}H_{16}Cl_2N_2O_5$ = 399.2.
*CAS — 3576-64-5.*
*ATC — P01AC02.*

### Profile

Clefamide is an antiprotozoal that has been used as a luminal amoebicide in the treatment of *Entamoeba histolytica* infections.

## Clopidol *(BAN, USAN, rINN)*

Clopindol; Meticlorpindol. 3,5-Dichloro-2,6-dimethylpyridin-4-ol.
$C_7H_7Cl_2NO$ = 192.0.
*CAS — 2971-90-6.*

### Profile

Clopidol is an antiprotozoal used in veterinary practice for the prevention of coccidiosis in poultry and rabbits either alone or in combination with methyl benzoquate (p.607).

## Decoquinate *(BAN, USAN, rINN)*

Decoquinato; HC-1528; M&B-15497. Ethyl 6-decyloxy-7-ethoxy-4-hydroxyquinoline-3-carboxylate.
$C_{24}H_{35}NO_5$ = 417.5.
*CAS — 18507-89-6.*

**Pharmacopoeias.** In *US* for veterinary use only. Also in *BP(Vet).*
**BP(Vet) 2003** (Decoquinate). A cream to buff-coloured, odourless or almost odourless, microcrystalline powder. Insoluble in water; practically insoluble in alcohol; very slightly soluble in chloroform and in ether.
**USP 27** (Decoquinate). Store in airtight containers.

### Profile

Decoquinate is an antiprotozoal used in veterinary practice for the control of coccidiosis in calves, sheep, and chickens. It is also used for toxoplasmosis in sheep.

## Dehydroemetine Hydrochloride *(BANM, rINNM)*

BT-436; 2,3-Dehydroemetine Hydrochloride; DHE; Hidrocloruro de deshidroemetina; Ro-1-9334. 2,3-Didehydro-6′,7′,10,11-tetramethoxyemetan dihydrochloride; 3-Ethyl-1,6,7,11b-tetrahydro-9,10-dimethoxy-2-(1,2,3,4-tetrahydro-6,7-dimethoxy-1-isoquinolylmethyl)-4*H*-benzo[*a*]quinolizine dihydrochloride.
$C_{29}H_{38}N_2O_4,2HCl$ = 551.5.
*CAS — 4914-30-1 (dehydroemetine); 2228-39-9 (dehydroemetine hydrochloride).*

NOTE. The name DHE has been used to denote a preparation of dihydroergotamine mesilate.

**Pharmacopoeias.** In *Int.*

### Profile

Dehydroemetine, a synthetic derivative of emetine (p.604), is a tissue amoebicide with similar actions and uses, although probably of a lower toxicity.

Dehydroemetine should be avoided in patients with cardiac, renal, or neuromuscular disease and patients should be monitored for cardiac toxicity during treatment.

When used in the treatment of amoebiasis (p.595), dehydroemetine hydrochloride is given by intramuscular injection in a dose of 1 mg/kg daily (maximum daily dose of 60 mg), generally for up to 4 to 6 days, but for no more than 5 days in children. A dose of 0.5 mg/kg has been suggested for elderly or severely ill patients. At least 6 weeks should elapse before treatment is repeated. Following treatment with dehydroemetine, all patients should receive a luminal amoebicide to eliminate organisms from the colon. Patients with hepatic amoebiasis may be given supplementary treatment with chloroquine.

**Liver fluke infections.** Dehydroemetine has been given[1] in the treatment of the liver fluke infection fascioliasis (see p.99).

1. Farid Z, *et al.* Treatment of acute toxaemic fascioliasis. *Trans R Soc Trop Med Hyg* 1988; **82:** 299.

## Diaveridine *(BAN, USAN, rINN)*

BW-49-210; Diaveridina; NSC-408735. 5-Veratrylpyrimidine-2,4-diyldiamine.
$C_{13}H_{16}N_4O_2$ = 260.3.
*CAS — 5355-16-8.*

**Pharmacopoeias.** In *Fr.* for veterinary use.

### Profile

Diaveridine is an antiprotozoal used in veterinary practice for the control of coccidiosis in poultry.

## Diclazuril *(BAN, USAN, rINN)*

Diclazurilo; Diclazurilum; R-64433. (±)-4-Chlorophenyl[2,6-dichloro-4-(2,3,4,5-tetrahydro-3,5-dioxo-1,2,4-triazin-2-yl)phenyl]acetonitrile.
$C_{17}H_9Cl_3N_4O_2$ = 407.6.
*CAS — 101831-37-2.*

**Pharmacopoeias.** In *Eur.* (see p.vi) for veterinary use only.
**Ph. Eur. 5.0** (Diclazuril for Veterinary Use). A white or light yellow powder. Practically insoluble in water, in alcohol, and in dichloromethane; sparingly soluble in dimethylformamide. Protect from light.

### Profile

Diclazuril is an antiprotozoal that has been tried in AIDS patients for the management of diarrhoea associated with protozoal infection. It is used in veterinary practice for the control of coccidiosis in lambs and poultry.

◊ References.

1. Kayembe K, *et al.* Diclazuril for Isospora belli infections in AIDS. *Lancet* 1989; **i:** 1397.
2. Connolly GM, *et al.* Diclazuril in the treatment of severe cryptosporidial diarrhoea in AIDS patients. *AIDS* 1990; **4:** 700–701.
3. Menichetti F, *et al.* Diclazuril for cryptosporidiosis in AIDS. *Am J Med* 1991; **90:** 271–2.
4. Limson-Pobre RNR, *et al.* Use of diclazuril for the treatment of isosporiasis in patients with AIDS. *Clin Infect Dis* 1995; **20:** 201–2.

## Diiodohydroxyquinoline *(rINN)*

Diiodohidroxiquinoleína; Diiodohydroxyquin; Di-iodohydroxyquinoline *(BAN)*; Di-iodoxychinolinum; Diiodoxyquinoléine; Iodoquinol *(USAN)*. 5,7-Di-iodoquinolin-8-ol.
$C_9H_5I_2NO$ = 397.0.
*CAS — 83-73-8.*
*ATC — G01AC01.*

**Pharmacopoeias.** In *US.*
**USP 27** (Iodoquinol). A light yellowish to tan, microcrystalline powder, not readily wetted in water, odourless or has a faint odour. Practically insoluble in water; sparingly soluble in alcohol and in ether.

### Adverse Effects

Major concerns have been expressed about the safety of the halogenated hydroxyquinolines since the recognition of severe neurotoxicity with clioquinol (p.196). In Japan, the epidemic development of subacute myelo-opticoneuropathy (SMON) in the 1960s was associated with the ingestion of normal or high doses of clioquinol for prolonged periods and the sale of clioquinol and related hydroxyquinolines was subsequently banned there. Symptoms of subacute myelo-opticoneuropathy are principally those of peripheral neuropathy, including optic atrophy, and myelopathy. Abdominal pain and diarrhoea often precede neurological symptoms such as paraesthesias in the legs, progressing to paraplegia in some patients, and loss of visual acuity sometimes leading to blindness. Cerebral disturbances, including confusion and retrograde amnesia, have also been reported. Although many patients improved when clioquinol was withdrawn, others had residual disability.

It was suggested that the Japanese epidemic might have been due to genetic susceptibility, but a few cases of subacute myelo-opticoneuropathy associated with clioquinol or related hydroxyquinoline derivatives, including broxyquinoline and diiodohydroxyquinoline, have been reported elsewhere.

Diiodohydroxyquinoline has also been associated with gastrointestinal effects such as abdominal cramps, nausea, and diarrhoea. Adverse effects which may be attributable to the iodine content of diiodohydroxyquinoline include pruritus ani, skin eruptions, and enlargement of the thyroid gland. Fever, chills, headache, and vertigo have also occurred.

### Precautions

Diiodohydroxyquinoline is contra-indicated in patients known to be hypersensitive to iodine or halogenated hydroxyquinolines and in those with hepatic or renal impairment. It should be used with caution in thyroid disease and may interfere with determinations of protein-bound iodine in tests for thyroid function for up to 6 months after therapy. Its use is best avoided in patients with neurological disorders. Long-term use should be avoided.

**Children.** The Committee on Drugs of the American Academy of Pediatrics[1] considered that there was a potential risk of toxicity to infants and children from clioquinol and diiodohydroxyquinoline applied topically. Since alternative effective preparations are available for dermatitis, the Committee recommended that products containing either of these compounds should not be used.

WHO considers that the use of halogenated hydroxyquinolines for the treatment of acute diarrhoea or amoebiasis in children cannot be justified.[2] There is no evidence of their efficacy in acute diarrhoea and they have been associated with severe neurological effects. On the rare occasions when a luminal amoebicide is required, other less toxic and more effective agents are available.

1. Kauffman RE, *et al.* Clioquinol (iodochlorhydroxyquin, Vioform) and iodoquinol (diiodohydroxyquin): blindness and neuropathy. *Pediatrics* 1990; **86:** 797–8.
2. WHO. The rational use of drugs in the management of acute diarrhoea in children. Geneva: WHO, 1990.

### Pharmacokinetics

Diiodohydroxyquinoline is poorly absorbed from the gastrointestinal tract. Concern has been expressed about possible absorption following application to the skin (see Children, under Precautions, above).

### Uses and Administration

Diiodohydroxyquinoline, a halogenated hydroxyquinoline, is a luminal amoebicide acting principally in the bowel lumen and is used in the treatment of intestinal amoebiasis, although a less toxic amoebicide such as diloxanide furoate is usually preferred; children should not be treated with diiodohydroxyquinoline (see Precautions, above). It is given alone in the treatment of asymptomatic cyst passers and with an amoebicide that acts in the tissues, such as metronidazole, in patients with invasive amoebiasis (p.595). The usual dosage in the treatment of amoebiasis is 630 or 650 mg three times daily by mouth for 20 days.

Diiodohydroxyquinoline has also been given in the treatment of *Dientamoeba fragilis* infections, in balantidiasis (p.596) as an alternative to tetracycline, and in *Blastocystis hominis* infections (p.596).

Diiodohydroxyquinoline was formerly used in the treatment of acrodermatitis enteropathica; it is reported to act by enhancing zinc absorption and has now been superseded by oral zinc therapy.

Diiodohydroxyquinoline is claimed to have some antibacterial and antifungal activity and has been used topically (but see under Precautions, above).

### Preparations

**USP 27:** Iodoquinol Tablets.

**Proprietary Preparations** (details are given in Part 3)

**Canad.:** Diodoquin; **Mex.:** Amabagyl†; Antidifar; Carsuquin; Depofin; Diameb†; Diodolina†; Diodoquin; Diyomex†; Diyosul†; Diyowil†; Drioquilen†; Entero-Diyod; Entodiba; Flanoquin†; Versamiv; Yopin†; **Thai.:** Dysetrin†; **USA:** Sebaquin; Yodoxin.

**Multi-ingredient: Arg.:** Hipoglos Cicatrizante; Plusderm; **Austral.:** Floraquin†; **Braz.:** Dexacloran†; **Chile:** Kordinol Compuesto; **Mex.:** Amebyl; Coralzul; Decadron con Nistatina; Dialgin; Facetin-D; Farmeban; Flagenase 400; Flagosil; Metodine; Metrodiyod; Norecil; Threchop; **S.Afr.:** Vagarsol; Viocort; Viodor; **Thai.:** Coccila; Diolin†; Disento; Floraquin†; Gynecon; Gynoco; Gynova; Gyracon; Mediocin; Nystin; Quinradon-N; Quinradon†; Vagicin; **USA:** Vytone.

## Diloxanide Furoate *(BANM, rINNM)*

Furoato de diloxanida. 4-(*N*-Methyl-2,2-dichloroacetamido)phenyl 2-furoate.

$C_{14}H_{11}Cl_2NO_4$ = 328.1.

*CAS — 579-38-4 (diloxanide); 3736-81-0 (diloxanide furoate).*

*ATC — P01AC01.*

**Pharmacopoeias.** In *Br., Int.,* and *US.*

**BP 2003** (Diloxanide Furoate). A white or almost white, odourless or almost odourless, crystalline powder. Very slightly soluble in water; slightly soluble in alcohol and in ether; freely soluble in chloroform. Protect from light.

**USP 27** (Diloxanide Furoate). A white or almost white, crystalline powder. Very slightly soluble in water; slightly soluble in alcohol and in ether; freely soluble in chloroform. Store in airtight containers. Protect from light.

### Adverse Effects

Flatulence is the most common adverse effect during treatment with diloxanide furoate. Vomiting, pruritus, and urticaria may occasionally occur.

### Pharmacokinetics

Diloxanide furoate is hydrolysed before absorption from the gastrointestinal tract. The resulting diloxanide is readily absorbed and excreted mainly in the urine as the glucuronide; less than 10% of a dose appears in the faeces.

### Uses and Administration

Diloxanide furoate, a dichloroacetamide derivative, is a luminal amoebicide acting principally in the bowel lumen and is used in the treatment of intestinal amoebiasis (p.595). It is given alone in the treatment of asymptomatic cyst passers and with an amoebicide that acts in the tissues, such as metronidazole, in patients with invasive amoebiasis.

Diloxanide furoate is given by mouth in a dosage of 500 mg three times daily for 10 days; children weighing more than 25 kg may be given 20 mg/kg daily, in divided doses, for 10 days. The course of treatment may be repeated if necessary.

### Preparations

**BP 2003:** Diloxanide Tablets.

**Proprietary Preparations** (details are given in Part 3)

**Irl.:** Furamide†; **Switz.:** Furamid†; **UK:** Furamide†.

**Multi-ingredient: India:** Dyrade-M; Entamizole; Entrolate; Qugyl; Tinidafyl Plus; Wotinex.

## Dimetridazole *(BAN, pINN)*

Dimetridazol. 1,2-Dimethyl-5-nitroimidazole.

$C_5H_7N_3O_2$ = 141.1.

*CAS — 551-92-8.*

**Pharmacopoeias.** In *Fr.* for veterinary use. Also in *BP(Vet).*

**BP(Vet) 2003** (Dimetridazole). An almost white to brownish-yellow, odourless or almost odourless powder which darkens on exposure to light. Slightly soluble in water; sparingly soluble in alcohol; freely soluble in chloroform; slightly soluble in ether. Protect from light.

### Profile

Dimetridazole is a 5-nitroimidazole derivative similar to metronidazole. It is used in veterinary practice for the control of various protozoal infections in birds, fish, and reptiles. It is also used for swine dysentery.

## Diminazene Aceturate *(BANM, rINNM)*

Aceturato de diminazeno. 1,3-Bis(4-amidinophenyl)triazene bis(*N*-acetylglycinate).

$C_{22}H_{29}N_9O_6$ = 515.5.

*CAS — 536-71-0 (diminazene); 908-54-3 (diminazene aceturate).*

NOTE. Diminazene aceturate is often referred to by its veterinary proprietary name Berenil.

### Profile

Diminazene aceturate, an aromatic diamidine derivative related to pentamidine, is an antiprotozoal that has been used in veterinary practice in the treatment of trypanosomiasis and babesiosis. It has also been tried in human infections.

## Dinitolmide *(BAN, rINN)*

Dinitolmida; Dinitrotoluamide; Methyldinitrobenzamide. 3,5-Dinitro-o-toluamide.

$C_8H_7N_3O_5$ = 225.2.

*CAS — 148-01-6.*

**Pharmacopoeias.** In *BP(Vet).*

**BP(Vet) 2003** (Dinitolmide). A cream-coloured to light tan-coloured odourless or almost odourless powder. Practically insoluble in water; slightly soluble in alcohol, in chloroform, and in ether; soluble in acetone.

### Profile

Dinitolmide is an antiprotozoal used in veterinary practice for the prevention of coccidiosis in poultry.

## Eflornithine Hydrochloride

*(BANM, USAN, rINNM)*

DFMO; α-Difluoromethylornithine Hydrochloride; Hidrocloruro de eflornitina; MDL-71782; MDL-71782A; RMI-71782. 2-(Difluoromethyl)-DL-ornithine monohydrochloride monohydrate.

$C_6H_{12}F_2N_2O_2,HCl,H_2O$ = 236.6.

*CAS — 67037-37-0 (eflornithine); 96020-91-6 (eflornithine hydrochloride).*

*ATC — D11AX16; P01CX03.*

### Adverse Effects and Precautions

Myelosuppression may lead to anaemia, leucopenia, and thrombocytopenia. Some patients have experienced hearing loss and alopecia. Gastrointestinal disturbances, especially diarrhoea, may occur. Seizures have occurred in about 8% of patients given eflornithine but they may have been related to the disease rather than treatment.

Dosage should be reduced in patients with renal impairment.

Skin irritation, such as erythema or a stinging or burning sensation, has been reported following topical application of eflornithine.

**Effects on the ears.** A study in 58 patients[1] receiving eflornithine alone or with interferon alfa for the treatment of metastatic melanoma found that hearing loss was related to the cumulative dose of eflornithine and was worse in patients with pre-existing hearing deficit.

1. Croghan MK, *et al.* Dose-related α-difluoromethylornithine ototoxicity. *Am J Clin Oncol* 1991; **14:** 331–5.

**Effects on the heart.** Fatal cardiac arrest occurred in an AIDS patient with *Pneumocystis carinii* pneumonia during the intravenous infusion of eflornithine 100 mg/kg over 1 hour.[1] Sudden death after infusion of eflornithine had occurred in several other critically ill patients with AIDS.

1. Barbarash RA, *et al.* Alpha-difluoromethylornithine infusion and cardiac arrest. *Ann Intern Med* 1986; **105:** 141–2.

### Pharmacokinetics

Eflornithine hydrochloride is absorbed from the gastrointestinal tract. After intravenous doses about 80% is excreted unchanged in the urine in 24 hours. The terminal elimination half-life is about 3 hours. It is distributed to the CSF.

Less than 1% of a dose is absorbed following topical application.

◊ References.

1. Haegele KD, *et al.* Kinetics of α-difluoromethylornithine: an irreversible inhibitor of ornithine decarboxylase. *Clin Pharmacol Ther* 1981; **30:** 210–17.
2. Milord F, *et al.* Eflornithine concentrations in serum and cerebrospinal fluid of 63 patients treated for Trypanosoma brucei gambiense sleeping sickness. *Trans R Soc Trop Med Hyg* 1993; **87:** 473–7.
3. Malhotra B, *et al.* Percutaneous absorption and pharmacokinetics of eflornithine HCl 13.9% cream in women with unwanted facial hair. *J Clin Pharmacol* 2001; **41:** 972–8.

### Uses and Administration

Eflornithine is an antiprotozoal that acts as an irreversible inhibitor of ornithine decarboxylase, the rate-limiting enzyme in polyamine biosynthesis; trypanosomes are more susceptible to the effects of eflornithine than are humans, probably because of their slower turnover of this enzyme.

Eflornithine is used in African trypanosomiasis due to *Trypanosoma brucei gambiense*. It is effective in the early and, more importantly, in the late stage of the disease (when there is CNS involvement).

In the treatment of African trypanosomiasis, eflornithine hydrochloride is given by intravenous infusion. The dose is 100 mg/kg every 6 hours for at least 14 days. Each dose should be administered over a period of at least 45 minutes. Dosage should be reduced in patients with impaired renal function. It has also been given by mouth, in some instances following intravenous therapy, but diarrhoea can be troublesome with this route.

Eflornithine hydrochloride is also applied topically as a 13.9% cream twice daily for the reduction of unwanted facial hair in women.

**Cryptosporidiosis.** Eflornithine has been tried in the treatment of cryptosporidiosis (p.596) in AIDS patients.[1]

1. Rolston KVI, *et al.* Intestinal cryptosporidiosis treated with eflornithine: a prospective study among patients with AIDS. *J Acquir Immune Defic Syndr* 1989; **2:** 426–30.

**Hirsutism.** Topical eflornithine hydrochloride applied twice daily as a 13.9% cream is effective in reducing the growth of unwanted facial hair in females (see Hirsutism, p.1545), although it must be used indefinitely to prevent regrowth.[1] Its action is thought to be due to the irreversible inhibition of ornithine decarboxylase in hair follicles.

1. Barman Balfour JA, McClellan K. Topical eflornithine. *Am J Clin Dermatol* 2001; **2:** 197–201.

**Malignant neoplasms.** Eflornithine has antimetabolic activity and is being studied as a potential chemopreventive agent in patients at high risk of a variety of malignant diseases, including cancer of the bladder, breast, cervix, colon, oesophagus, prostate, and skin.[1]

1. Meyskens FL, Gerner EW. Development of difluoromethylornithine (DFMO) as a chemoprevention agent. *Clin Cancer Res* 1999; **5:** 945–51.

**African trypanosomiasis.** Eflornithine is effective in the treatment of *Trypanosoma brucei gambiense* infections (p.599), and is particularly valuable in providing an alternative to melarsoprol in meningoencephalitic disease. Eflornithine 100 mg/kg intravenously every 6 hours for 7 days, rather than the standard 14 days, produced long-term responses in 42 of 47 patients who had relapsed after other treatment regimens.[1] Similar positive results in relapsing cases were obtained with a short 7-day course in a multicentre randomised controlled study,[2] although this short course was inferior to the 14-day course for new cases, in whom it could not be recommended. A patient who had relapsed after treatment with melarsoprol and eflornithine given singly was cured when the drugs were given together.[3] Eflornithine is not effective when given alone in *T. b. rhodesiense* infections, and early reports of its use with suramin were not encouraging.[4]

1. Khonde N, *et al.* A seven days course of eflornithine for relapsing Trypanosoma brucei gambiense sleeping sickness. *Trans R Soc Trop Med Hyg* 1997; **91:** 212–13.
2. Pepin J, *et al.* Short-course eflornithine in Gambian trypanosomiasis: a multicentre randomized controlled trial. *Bull WHO* 2000; **78:** 1284–95.
3. Simarro PP, Asumu PN. Gambian trypanosomiasis and synergism between melarsoprol and eflornithine: first case report. *Trans R Soc Trop Med Hyg* 1996; **90:** 315.
4. Clerinx J, *et al.* Treatment of late stage rhodesiense trypanosomiasis using suramin and eflornithine: report of six cases. *Trans R Soc Trop Med Hyg* 1998; **92:** 449–50.

### Preparations

**Proprietary Preparations** (details are given in Part 3)

**USA:** Ornidyl; Vaniqa.

## Emetine Hydrochloride *(BANM)*

Cloridrato de Emetina; Emet. Hydrochlor.; Emetina, hidrocloruro de; Emetine Dihydrochloride; Emetine Hydrochloride Heptahydrate; Emetini Chloridum; Emetini Hydrochloridum Heptahydricum; Ipecine Hydrochloride; Methylcephaëline Hydrochloride. 6′,7′,10,11-Tetramethoxyemetan dihydrochloride heptahydrate; (2*S*,3*R*,11b*S*)-3-Ethyl-1,3,4,6,7,11b-hexahydro-9,10-dimethoxy-2-[(1*R*)-1,2,3,4-tetrahydro-6,7-dimethoxy-1-isoquinolylmethyl]-2*H*-benzo[*a*]quinolizine dihydrochloride heptahydrate.

$C_{29}H_{40}N_2O_4,2HCl,7H_2O$ = 679.7.

*CAS — 483-18-1 (emetine); 316-42-7 (anhydrous emetine hydrochloride); 7083-71-8 (emetine hydrochloride, hydrate); 79300-08-6 (emetine hydrochloride, heptahydrate).*

*ATC — P01AX02.*

**Pharmacopoeias.** In *Chin., Eur.* (see p.vi), and *Viet.*

*Eur.* also has a monograph for Emetine Hydrochloride Pentahydrate; *Int.* permits the heptahydrate or pentahydrate in the same monograph. *US* has a monograph for the anhydrous salt.

**Ph. Eur. 5.0** (Emetine Hydrochloride Heptahydrate; Emetine Hydrochloride BP 2003). A white or slightly yellow crystalline powder. Freely soluble in water and in alcohol. A 2% solution in water has a pH of 4.0 to 6.0. Protect from light.

**Ph. Eur. 5.0** (Emetine Hydrochloride Pentahydrate ). A white or slightly yellow crystalline powder. Freely soluble in water and in alcohol. A 2% solution in water has a pH of 4.0 to 6.0. Protect from light.

**USP 27** (Emetine Hydrochloride). The hydrochloride of an alkaloid obtained from ipecacuanha, or prepared by methylation of cephaëline, or prepared synthetically. Anhydrous emetine hydrochloride is a white or slightly yellowish, odourless, crystalline powder. Freely soluble in water and in alcohol. Store in airtight containers at a temperature of 25°, excursions permitted between 15° and 30°. Protect from light.

## Adverse Effects

Emetine hydrochloride is commonly associated with aching, tenderness, stiffness, and weakness of the muscles in the area of the injection site; there may be necrosis and abscess formation. After injection, diarrhoea and nausea and vomiting, sometimes with dizziness and headache, are common. There may be generalised muscle weakness and muscular pain, especially in the neck and limbs, and, more rarely, mild sensory disturbances. Eczematous, urticarial, and purpuric skin lesions have been reported.

Cardiovascular effects are considered the most serious and include precordial pain, dyspnoea, tachycardia, and hypotension. Changes in the ECG, particularly flattening or inversion of the T-wave and prolongation of the QT interval, occur in many patients. Emetine accumulates in the body and large doses or prolonged use may cause lesions of the heart, gastrointestinal tract, kidneys, liver, and skeletal muscle. Severe acute degenerative myocarditis may occur and may give rise to sudden cardiac failure and death. In some patients cardiotoxic effects have appeared after the completion of treatment with therapeutic doses.

Emetine hydrochloride is very irritant and contact with mucous membranes should be avoided.

## Precautions

Emetine is contra-indicated in cardiac, renal, or neuromuscular disease. Its use should be avoided during pregnancy and it should not be given to children, except in severe amoebic dysentery unresponsive to other drugs. It should be used with great caution in old or debilitated patients. Patients receiving emetine should be closely supervised; ECG monitoring is advisable during treatment.

## Pharmacokinetics

After injection emetine hydrochloride is concentrated in the liver, and to some extent in kidney, lung, and spleen. Excretion is slow and detectable amounts may persist in urine 40 to 60 days after treatment has been discontinued.

## Uses and Administration

Emetine, an alkaloid of ipecacuanha (p.1122), is a tissue amoebicide acting principally in the bowel wall and in the liver. It has been given by deep subcutaneous or intramuscular injection in the treatment of severe invasive amoebiasis (p.595), including hepatic amoebiasis in patients who do not respond to metronidazole, although dehydroemetine has tended to replace it. Emetine was formerly given by mouth as emetine and bismuth iodide.

Emetine has also been included in combination preparations for the symptomatic relief of cough.

## Preparations

**USP 27:** Emetine Hydrochloride Injection.

**Proprietary Preparations** (details are given in Part 3)

**Multi-ingredient:** ***Austria:*** Spirbon; ***Canad.:*** Cophylac†; ***Switz.:*** Ipeca; Sano Tuss.

# Ethopabate *(BAN)*

Etopabato. Methyl 4-acetamido-2-ethoxybenzoate.

$C_{12}H_{15}NO_4$ = 237.3.

*CAS — 59-06-3.*

**Pharmacopoeias.** In *US* for veterinary use only. Also in *BP(Vet).*

**BP(Vet) 2003** (Ethopabate). A white or pinkish-white powder. Very slightly soluble in water; sparingly soluble in alcohol; soluble in chloroform and in methyl alcohol; slightly soluble in ether.

**USP 27** (Ethopabate). A white or pinkish-white, odourless or practically odourless, powder. Very slightly soluble in water; soluble in dehydrated alcohol, in acetone, in methyl alcohol, and in acetonitrile; slightly soluble in ether; sparingly soluble in dichloromethane, in dioxan, in ethyl acetate, and in isopropyl alcohol. Protect from light.

## Profile

Ethopabate is an antiprotozoal used in veterinary practice with other drugs, such as amprolium, for the control of coccidiosis in poultry.

# Etofamide *(rINN)*

Ethychlordiphene; Etofamida; K-430. 2,2-Dichloro-N-(2-ethoxyethyl)-N-[4-(4-nitrophenoxy)benzyl]acetamide.

$C_{19}H_{20}Cl_2N_2O_5$ = 427.3.

*CAS — 25287-60-9.*

*ATC — P01AC03.*

## Profile

Etofamide, a dichloroacetamide derivative, is a luminal amoebicide with actions and uses similar to those of diloxanide furoate (p.604).

## Preparations

**Proprietary Preparations** (details are given in Part 3)

***Braz.:*** Kitnos; ***Mex.:*** Kitnos.

# Fumagillin *(BAN)*

Fumagilina. 4-(1,2-Epoxy-1,6-dimethylhex-4-enyl)-5-methoxy-1-oxaspiro[2.5]oct-6-yl hydrogen deca-2,4,6,8-tetraenedioate.

$C_{26}H_{34}O_7$ = 458.5.

*CAS — 23110-15-8.*

## Profile

Fumagillin is an alicyclic antibiotic produced by certain strains of *Aspergillus fumigatus*. It has activity against Microsporidia and is used in veterinary practice to control *Nosema apis* infection in honeybees. It has also been tried in humans in the topical treatment of microsporidial keratoconjunctivitis and for the treatment of intestinal microsporidiosis due to *Enterocytozoon bieneusi* in patients with HIV infection. It was formerly given by mouth in the treatment of intestinal amoebiasis, but produced an unacceptably high frequency of adverse effects. Analogues of fumagillin have been investigated for effects on angiogenesis in solid tumours.

**Microsporidiosis.** As discussed on p.598, topical treatment of microsporidial keratoconjunctivitis has been disappointing. There have been several reports of successful treatment in individual patients using fumagillin topically,[1-3] usually as a solution of bicyclohexylammonium fumagillin containing the equivalent of 70 micrograms of fumagillin per mL.

Oral fumagillin in a dose of 20 mg three times daily has been effective in the treatment of diarrhoea due to intestinal microsporidial infection with *Enterocytozoon bieneusi* in patients with HIV infection.[4-7]


1. Rosberger DF, *et al.* Successful treatment of microsporidial keratoconjunctivitis with topical fumagillin in a patient with AIDS. *Cornea* 1993; **12:** 261–5.
2. Diesenhouse MC, *et al.* Treatment of microsporidial keratoconjunctivitis with topical fumagillin. *Am J Ophthalmol* 1993; **115:** 293–8.
3. Garvey MJ, *et al.* Topical fumagillin in the treatment of microsporidial keratoconjunctivitis in AIDS. *Ann Pharmacother* 1995; **29:** 872–4.
4. Molina J-M, *et al.* Potential efficacy of fumagillin in intestinal microsporidiosis due to Enterocytozoon bieneusi in patients with HIV infection: results of a drug screening study. *AIDS* 1997; **11:** 1603–10.
5. Molina J-M, *et al.* Trial of oral fumagillin for the treatment of intestinal microsporidiosis in patients with HIV infection. *AIDS* 2000; **14:** 1341–8.
6. Molina J-M, *et al.* Fumagillin treatment of intestinal microsporidiosis. *N Engl J Med* 2002; **346:** 1963–9.
7. Medical Letter on Drugs and Therapeutics. Drugs for parasitic infections (issued April 2002). Available at: http://www.medicalletter.com/freedocs/parasitic.pdf (accessed 03/06/04)


# Furazolidone *(BAN, rINN)*

Furazolidona; Nifurazolidonum. 3-(5-Nitrofurfurylideneamino)-2-oxazolidone.

$C_8H_7N_3O_5$ = 225.2.

*CAS — 67-45-8.*

*ATC — G01AX06.*

**Pharmacopoeias.** In *Br., Fr.,* and *US.*

**BP 2003** (Furazolidone). A yellow odourless or almost odourless crystalline powder. Very slightly soluble in water and in alcohol; slightly soluble in chloroform; practically insoluble in ether. The filtrate from a 1% suspension in water has a pH of 4.5 to 7.0. Protect from light.

**USP 27** (Furazolidone). A yellow, odourless, crystalline powder. Practically insoluble in water, in alcohol, and in carbon tetrachloride. Store in airtight containers. Protect from light and avoid exposure to direct sunlight.

## Adverse Effects

The most common adverse effects of furazolidone involve the gastrointestinal tract and include nausea and vomiting. Dizziness, drowsiness, headache, and a general malaise have also been reported.

Allergic reactions, most commonly skin reactions such as rashes or angioedema, may occur. There have been instances of acute pulmonary reactions, similar to those seen with the structurally related drug nitrofurantoin, and of hepatotoxicity. Agranulocytosis has been reported rarely. Haemolytic anaemia may occur in patients with G6PD deficiency given furazolidone.

Darkening of the urine has been attributed to the presence of metabolites.

## Precautions

Furazolidone should be used with caution in those with G6PD deficiency because of the risk of haemolytic anaemia. It should not be given to infants under 1 month of age since their enzyme systems are immature.

## Interactions

A disulfiram-like reaction has been reported in patients taking alcohol while on furazolidone therapy; alcohol should be avoided during, and for a short period after, treatment with furazolidone.

Furazolidone is an MAOI and the cautions advised for these drugs regarding use with other drugs, especially indirect-acting sympathomimetic amines, and the consumption of food and drink containing tyramine, should be observed (see Phenelzine Sulfate, p.314). However, there appear to be no reports of hypertensive crises in patients receiving furazolidone and it has been suggested that, since furazolidone inhibits monoamine oxidase gradually over several days, the risks are small if treatment is limited to a 5-day course. Toxic psychosis has been reported in a patient receiving furazolidone and amitriptyline (see Antiprotozoals, under Interactions of Amitriptyline, p.284).

## Pharmacokinetics

Although furazolidone has been considered to be largely unabsorbed when given orally, the occurrence of systemic adverse effects and coloured metabolites in the urine suggest that this may not be the case. Rapid and extensive metabolism, possibly in the intestine, has been proposed.

## Uses and Administration

Furazolidone is a nitrofuran derivative with antiprotozoal and antibacterial activity. It is active against the protozoan *Giardia intestinalis* (*Giardia lamblia*) and against a range of enteric bacteria *in vitro*, including staphylococci, enterococci, *Escherichia coli, Salmonella* spp., *Shigella* spp., and *Vibrio cholerae*. Furazolidone is bactericidal and appears to act by interfering with bacterial enzyme systems. Resistance is reported to be limited. It is used in the treatment of giardiasis (p.596) and cholera (p.128). It has been suggested for other bacterial gastrointestinal infections, but antibacterial therapy is regarded as unnecessary in mild and self-limiting gastro-enteritis (see p.127).

Furazolidone is given by mouth in a dose of 100 mg four times daily; children may be given 1.25 mg/kg four times daily. It is usually given for 2 to 5 days, but may be given for up to 7 days in some patients, or for up to 10 days for giardiasis.

**Peptic ulcer disease.** Furazolidone is not one of the main antibacterials used in *Helicobacter pylori* eradication regimens for peptic ulceration (p.1246), but there are some studies suggesting its efficacy.[1-8]


1. Segura AM, *et al.* Furazolidone, amoxycillin, bismuth triple therapy for Helicobacter pylori infection. *Aliment Pharmacol Ther* 1997; **11:** 529–32.
2. Xiao S-D, *et al.* High cure rate of Helicobacter pylori infection using tripotassium dicitrato bismuthate, furazolidone and clarithromycin triple therapy for 1 week. *Aliment Pharmacol Ther* 1999; **13:** 311–15.
3. Liu W-Z, *et al.* Furazolidone-containing short-term triple therapies are effective in the treatment of Helicobacter pylori infection. *Aliment Pharmacol Ther* 1999; **13:** 317–22.
4. Dani R, *et al.* Omeprazole, clarithromycin and furazolidone for the eradication of Helicobacter pylori in patients with duodenal ulcer. *Aliment Pharmacol Ther* 1999; **13:** 1647–52.
5. Graham DY, *et al.* Furazolidone combination therapies for Helicobacter pylori infection in the United States. *Aliment Pharmacol Ther* 2000; **14:** 211–15.
6. Liu W-Z, *et al.* A new quadruple therapy for Helicobacter pylori using tripotassium dicitrato bismuthate, furazolidone, josamycin and famotidine. *Aliment Pharmacol Ther* 2000; **14:** 1519–22.
7. Fakheri H, *et al.* Clarithromycin vs furazolidone in quadruple therapy regimens for the treatment of Helicobacter pylori in a population with a high metronidazole resistance rate. *Aliment Pharmacol Ther* 2001; **15:** 411–16.
8. Lu H, *et al.* One-week regimens containing ranitidine bismuth citrate, furazolidone and either amoxicillin or tetracycline effectively eradicate Helicobacter pylori: a multicentre, randomized, double-blind study. *Aliment Pharmacol Ther* 2001; **15:** 1975–9.


## Preparations

**USP 27:** Furazolidone Oral Suspension; Furazolidone Tablets.

**Proprietary Preparations** (details are given in Part 3)

***Arg.:*** Giardil; ***Braz.:*** Enterolidon†; Giarcid; Giarlam; Neo Furasil; ***Chile:*** Furoxona; ***Ger.:*** Nifuran; ***India:*** Furoxone; ***Ital.:*** Furoxone†; ***Mex.:*** Exofur; Furoxona; Fuxol†; Novafur†; Salmocide; Seformant†; ***Thai.:*** Furasian; Furion; ***USA:*** Furoxone.

**Multi-ingredient:** ***Arg.:*** Endomicina; ***Braz.:*** Atapec; Colestase; Enterobion†; Furazolin†; Lisoquinol†; Magnostase†; Plasmocolit†; Suspectim†; Tratocolit†; ***Chile:*** Furazolidona; ***India:*** Dysfur-M; Emantid; Flagyl-F; Kaltin MF; Lomofen; Metrogyl-F; ***Ital.:*** Ginecofuran†; ***Mex.:*** Caopecfar; Colfur; Contefur; Coralzul; Dialgin; Dibapec Compuesto; Fuzotyl; Neo-Kap; Optazol; Solfurol; Threchop; Trilor; Yodozona; ***Spain:*** Desinvag; ***Thai.:*** Attafur†; Coccila; Di-Su-Frone; Difuran; Diolin†; Disento; Disento PF; Furasian; Furopectin; Med-Kafuzone; Mediocin.

# Halofuginone Hydrobromide *(BANM, USAN, rINNM)*

Hidrobromuro de halofuginona; RU-19110. (±)-*trans*-7-Bromo-6-chloro-3-[3-(3-hydroxy-2-piperidyl)acetonyl]quinazolin-4(3*H*)-one hydrobromide.

$C_{16}H_{17}BrClN_3O_3,HBr$ = 495.6.

*CAS — 55837-20-2 (halofuginone); 64924-67-0 (halofuginone hydrobromide).*

## Profile

Halofuginone is an antiprotozoal used as the hydrobromide in veterinary practice for the prevention of coccidiosis in poultry and for the control of cryptosporidiosis in calves. It is also under investigation for use in neoplastic disease in humans and in the treatment of scleroderma.

## Imidocarb Dipropionate *(BANM, rINNM)*

4A65 (imidocarb hydrochloride); Dipropionato de imidocarbo. 1,3-Bis[3-(2-imidazolin-2-yl)phenyl]urea dipropionate; 3,3′-Di-2-imidazolin-2-ylcarbanilide dipropionate.

$C_{19}H_{20}N_6O,2C_3H_6O_2$ = 496.6.

*CAS — 27885-92-3 (imidocarb); 55750-06-6 (imidocarb dipropionate); 5318-76-3 (imidocarb hydrochloride).*

NOTE. Imidocarb Hydrochloride is *USAN*.

### Profile

Imidocarb has antiprotozoal and antibacterial activity and is used as the dipropionate in veterinary practice in the treatment of babesiosis and anaplasmosis in cattle. Imidocarb hydrochloride has also been used.

## Isometamidium Chloride *(BAN, rINN)*

Cloruro de isometamidio; Isometamidium. 8-[3-(*m*-Amidinophenyl)-2-triazeno]3-amino-5-ethyl-6-phenylphenanthridinium chloride.

$C_{28}H_{26}ClN_7$ = 496.0.

*CAS — 34301-55-8.*

### Profile

Isometamidium is an antiprotozoal used as the chloride in veterinary practice for the control of trypanosomiasis.

## Lasalocid *(BAN, USAN, rINN)*

Ro-02-2985. 6-[(3*R*,4*S*,5*S*,7*R*)-7-{(2*S*,3*S*,5*S*)-5-Ethyl-5-[(2*R*,5*R*,6*S*)-5-ethyltetrahydro-5-hydroxy-6-methyl-2*H*-pyran-2-y]tetrahydro-3-methyl-2-fury l}4-hydroxy-3,5-dimethyl-6-oxononyl]-2-hydroxy-*m*-toluic acid.

$C_{34}H_{54}O_8$ = 590.8.

*CAS — 11054-70-9; 25999-31-9.*

## Lasalocid Sodium *(BANM, rINNM)*

Lasalocid sódico.

$C_{34}H_{53}NaO_8$ = 612.8.

*CAS — 25999-20-6.*

### Profile

Lasalocid, an antibiotic produced by *Streptomyces lasaliensis*, is an antiprotozoal used as the sodium salt in veterinary practice for the prevention of coccidiosis in birds.

## Letrazuril *(rINN)*

Letrazurilo. (±)-[2,6-Dichloro-4-(4,5-dihydro-3,5-dioxo-*as*-triazin-2(3*H*)-yl)phenyl](*p*-fluorophenyl)acetonitrile.

$C_{17}H_9Cl_2FN_4O_2$ = 391.2.

*CAS — 103337-74-2.*

### Profile

Letrazuril is an antiprotozoal that has been investigated in the treatment of cryptosporidiosis (p.596) in patients with AIDS.

## Maduramicin *(BAN, USAN, rINN)*

CL-273703; Maduramicin Ammonium; Maduramicina. Ammonium (2*R*,3*S*,4*S*,5*R*,6*S*)-tetrahydro-2-hydroxy-6-{(*R*)-1-[(2*S*,5*R*,7*S*,8*R*,9*S*)-9-hydroxy-2,8-dimethyl-2-{(2*S*,2′*R*,3′*S*,5*R*,5′*R*)-octahydro-2-methyl-3′-[(2*R*,4*S*,5*S*,6*S*)-tetrahydro-4,5-dimethoxy-6-methyl-2*H*-pyran-2-yl]oxy}-5′-[(2*S*,3*S*,5*R*,6*S*)-tetrahydro-6-hydroxy-3,5,6-trimethyl-2*H*-pyran-2-yl](2,2′-bifuran-5-yl)-1,6-dioxaspiro[4.5]dec-7-yl]ethyl}-4,5-dimethoxy-3-methyl-2*H*-pyran-2-acetate.

$C_{47}H_{80}O_{17},NH_3$ = 934.2.

*CAS — 84878-61-5.*

NOTE. The name maduramicin has also been used to denote the acid.

### Profile

Maduramicin is an antiprotozoal used in veterinary practice for the prevention of coccidiosis in poultry.

# Melarsoprol *(BAN, rINN)*

Mel B; Melarsen Oxide-BAL; RP-3854. 2-[4-(4,6-Diamino-1,3,5-triazin-2-ylamino)phenyl]-1,3,2-dithiarsolan-4-ylmethanol.

$C_{12}H_{15}AsN_6OS_2$ = 398.3.

*CAS — 494-79-1.*

*ATC — P01CD01.*

### Adverse Effects and Treatment

Adverse effects are common and may be severe during the treatment of African trypanosomiasis with melarsoprol. It may be difficult to distinguish between effects of the disease, Jarisch-Herxheimer reactions resulting from the trypanocidal activity of melarsoprol, and adverse effects due to the drugs arsenic content or to hypersensitivity. For the adverse effects of arsenic and their treatment, see Arsenic Trioxide, p.1657.

A severe febrile reaction may occur after the first injection of melarsoprol, especially in patients with large numbers of trypanosomes in their blood. It is therefore common practice to give two or three injections of suramin or pentamidine before starting melarsoprol therapy.

The greatest risk is from reactive encephalopathy which occurs in about 10% of patients treated with melarsoprol and is usually seen between the end of the first 3- or 4-day course of injections and the start of the second course. Some have attributed it to a toxic effect of melarsoprol and others to a Jarisch-Herxheimer reaction resulting from the release of antigen from trypanosomes killed in the brain; a combination of drug toxicity and host immune responses may be responsible. Encephalopathy may be sudden in onset or develop slowly. Symptoms include fever, headache, tremor, slurring of speech, convulsions, and coma; death has occurred in up to 5% of patients treated with melarsoprol. Less commonly, haemorrhagic encephalopathy may occur. The prophylactic use of corticosteroids has been suggested during treatment courses of melarsoprol (see African Trypanosomiasis, below). Treatment of reactive encephalopathy has included the use of corticosteroids, hypertonic solutions to combat cerebral oedema, anticonvulsants such as diazepam, and subcutaneous adrenaline; dimercaprol has been given on the assumption that encephalopathy resulted from arsenic poisoning, but has not generally been of benefit.

Hypersensitivity reactions to melarsoprol may occur during the second and subsequent courses of treatment. Desensitisation with gradually increasing doses of melarsoprol has been attempted; corticosteroids may help to control symptoms during this procedure. Some authorities consider that the use of small doses of melarsoprol may increase the risk of resistance.

Melarsoprol injection is very irritant and extravasation during intravenous use should be avoided. Vomiting and abdominal colic may occur if it is injected too rapidly. Other adverse effects reported include agranulocytosis, hypertension, peripheral neuropathy, proteinuria, severe diarrhoea, myocardial damage, exfoliative dermatitis, and hepatic disturbances.

◊ References.

1. Pepin J, *et al.* Trial of prednisolone for prevention of melarsoprol-induced encephalopathy in gambiense sleeping sickness. *Lancet* 1989; **i:** 1246–50.
2. Pepin J, Milord F. African trypanosomiasis and drug-induced encephalopathy: risk factors and pathogenesis. *Trans R Soc Trop Med Hyg* 1991; **85:** 222–4.
3. Pepin J, *et al.* Risk factors for encephalopathy and mortality during melarsoprol treatment of Trypanosoma brucei gambiense sleeping sickness. *Trans R Soc Trop Med Hyg* 1995; **89:** 92–7.

### Precautions

Use of melarsoprol in febrile patients has been associated with an increased incidence of reactive encephalopathy, and therefore it should not be given during epidemics of influenza. Intercurrent infections such as malaria and pneumonia should be treated before melarsoprol is used. Severe haemolytic reactions have been reported in patients with G6PD deficiency. It may precipitate erythema nodosum when given to patients with leprosy.

Patients should be in hospital when they are treated with melarsoprol and dosage decided after taking into account their general condition.

Treatment of pregnant women with trypanosomiasis should be deferred until after delivery. Pregnant women with meningoencephalitis may be treated with pentamidine (*Trypanosoma brucei gambiense*) or suramin (*T. b. rhodesiense*).

### Pharmacokinetics

Melarsoprol is reported to be unreliably absorbed if given by mouth and is usually given by intravenous injection. A small amount penetrates into the CSF where it has a local trypanocidal action. It is rapidly metabolised and excreted in the faeces and urine so any prophylactic effect is short-lived.

### Uses and Administration

Melarsoprol, a trivalent arsenical derivative, is a trypanocide which appears to act by inhibiting trypanosomal pyruvate kinase. It is effective in the treatment of all stages of African trypanosomiasis due to *Trypanosoma brucei gambiense* or *T. brucei rhodesiense*, but because of its toxicity its use is usually reserved for stages of the disease involving the CNS. Resistance has been reported to develop.

Patients undergoing therapy with melarsoprol should be treated in hospital. Melarsoprol is administered by intravenous injection as a 3.6% solution in propylene glycol. The injection should be given slowly, care being taken to prevent leakage into the surrounding tissues, and the patient should remain supine and fasting for several hours after the injection.

Treatment protocols vary, but in general melarsoprol is given in low doses initially, especially in children and debilitated patients, increased gradually to the maximum daily dose of 3.6 mg/kg. Doses are given daily for 3 or 4 days and the course repeated 2 or 3 times with an interval of 7 to 10 days between courses. Since massive destruction of parasites resulting in a Jarisch-Herxheimer reaction is particularly dangerous during treatment with melarsoprol, several doses of suramin or pentamidine may be given to induce the reaction before melarsoprol is started.

Melarsonyl potassium is a water-soluble derivative of melarsoprol which was formerly used as an alternative to melarsoprol but was probably more toxic and less effective.

**African trypanosomiasis.** Melarsoprol, which is effective against both *Trypanosoma brucei gambiense* and *T. b. rhodesiense*, is usually only given to treat the meningoencephalitic stage of African trypanosomiasis (p.599) because it may produce potentially fatal encephalopathy. However, protection against this toxicity may be provided by prophylaxis with prednisolone.[1,2] Therapy with melarsoprol and eflornithine was reported to be effective in a patient who had not responded to either drug alone.[3] A comparative study[4] in 500 patients with second-stage infection with *T. b. gambiense* found that a more concise dosage regimen of melarsoprol 2.2 mg/kg daily, as a single course over 10 days, was similar in efficacy to standard regimens of 1.2 to 3.6 mg/kg daily for 3 or 4 days repeated twice over a 26-day period with 7-day intervals between series, although there was no difference between the regimens in the incidence of associated encephalopathy.

1. Pepin J, *et al.* Trial of prednisolone for prevention of melarsoprol-induced encephalopathy in gambiense sleeping sickness. *Lancet* 1989; **i:** 1246–50.
2. Pepin J, *et al.* Risk factors for encephalopathy and mortality during melarsoprol treatment of Trypanosoma brucei gambiense sleeping sickness. *Trans R Soc Trop Med Hyg* 1995; **89:** 92–7.
3. Simarro PP, Asumu PN. Gambian trypanosomiasis and synergism between melarsoprol and eflornithine: first case report. *Trans R Soc Trop Med Hyg* 1996; **90:** 315.
4. Burri C, *et al.* Efficacy of new, concise schedule for melarsoprol in treatment of sleeping sickness caused by Trypanosoma brucei gambiense: a randomised trial. *Lancet* 2000; **355:** 1419–25.

## Mepacrine Hydrochloride *(BANM, rINNM)*

Acrichinum; Acrinamine; Antimalarinae Chlorhydras; Chinacrina; Hidrocloruro de mepacrina; Mepacrini Hydrochloridum; Quinacrine Hydrochloride. 6-Chloro-9-(4-diethylamino-1-methylbutylamino)-2-methoxyacridine dihydrochloride dihydrate.

$C_{23}H_{30}ClN_3O,2HCl,2H_2O$ = 508.9.

*CAS — 83-89-6 (mepacrine); 69-05-6 (anhydrous mepacrine dihydrochloride); 6151-30-0 (mepacrine dihydrochloride dihydrate).*

*ATC — P01AX05.*

### Adverse Effects

The most common adverse effects associated with mepacrine are dizziness, headache, and gastrointestinal disturbances such as nausea and vomiting. Reversible yellow discoloration of the skin, conjunctiva, and urine may occur during long-term use or after large doses; blue/black discoloration of the palate and discoloration of the nails have also been reported. Doses such as those used in the treatment of giardiasis may occasionally cause transient acute toxic psychosis and CNS stimulation. Convulsions have been reported at high doses. Ocular toxicity similar to that seen with chloroquine (p.448) and chronic dermatoses, including severe exfoliative dermatitis and lichenoid eruptions, have also occurred after prolonged use of mepacrine. Hepatotoxicity and aplastic anaemia occur rarely.

**Effects on the nervous system.** Two patients had convulsions a few hours after mepacrine hydrochloride 400 mg was given intrapleurally for malignant effusions. One developed status epilepticus and died and the other was successfully treated with anticonvulsants.[1]

1. Borda I, Krant M. Convulsions following intrapleural administration of quinacrine hydrochloride. *JAMA* 1967; **201:** 1049–50.

### Precautions

Mepacrine should be used with caution in elderly patients or patients with a history of psychosis, or in the presence of hepatic disease. Mepacrine can cause exacerbation of psoriasis and should be avoided in psoriatic patients.

**Porphyria.** Mepacrine should be used with caution in patients with porphyria.

### Interactions

Mepacrine has been reported to produce a mild disulfiram-like reaction (see p.1681) when taken with alcohol.

Theoretically, mepacrine may increase the plasma concentrations of primaquine resulting in a higher risk of toxicity, and it has been recommended that these drugs should not be used together.

### Pharmacokinetics

Mepacrine is readily absorbed from the gastrointestinal tract and widely distributed throughout the body. It accumulates in body tissues, particularly the liver, and is liberated slowly. It is excreted slowly mainly in the urine, and is still detectable in the urine after 2 months. Mepacrine crosses the placenta.

**Intrapleural administration.** Peak plasma concentrations of mepacrine far above those associated with CNS effects were rapidly attained in 3 of 4 patients following intrapleural instillation of a solution of mepacrine hydrochloride and remained at these levels for several hours.[1]

1. Björkman S, *et al.* Pharmacokinetics of quinacrine after intrapleural instillation in rabbits and man. *J Pharm Pharmacol* 1989; **41:** 160–73.

### Uses and Administration

Mepacrine is a 9-aminoacridine antiprotozoal used as the hydrochloride mainly as an alternative to the nitroimidazoles in the treatment of giardiasis (p.596).

In giardiasis, mepacrine hydrochloride is given by mouth in doses of 100 mg three times daily after food for 5 to 7 days. A dose for children is 2 mg/kg given three times daily (maximum 300 mg daily).

Mepacrine hydrochloride may also be used, alone or with hydroxychloroquine, for the treatment of discoid and subcutaneous lupus erythematosus. It has also been used locally in the treatment of some forms of cutaneous leishmaniasis, as a sterilisation technique for contraception, and in the management of malignant effusions. It was formerly used to treat malaria.

The mesilate was also formerly used.

Mepacrine is under investigation for the treatment of variant Creutzfeldt-Jakob Disease.

**Contraception.** Sterilisation with intra-uterine mepacrine has been attempted as an irreversible method of contraception (p.1535). It produces occlusion of the fallopian tube and has been reported to be an effective nonsurgical means of female sterilisation.[1] There has been speculation about the risk of cancer from this technique but there appeared to be no evidence to confirm such a risk.[2,3] However, the method remains controversial and a full evaluation of its safety and efficacy has been recommended.[4] The Indian government has banned the use of mepacrine for sterilisation.

1. Hieu DT, *et al.* 31 781 Cases of non-surgical female sterilisation with quinacrine pellets in Vietnam. *Lancet* 1993; **342:** 213–17.
2. Anonymous. Death of a study: WHO, what, and why. *Lancet* 1994; **343:** 987–8.
3. Hieu DT. Quinacrine method of family planning. *Lancet* 1994; **343:** 1040.
4. Benagiano G. Sterilisation by quinacrine. *Lancet* 1994; **344:** 689.

**Leishmaniasis.** Mepacrine has been suggested for intralesional injection in the treatment of early noninflamed nodular lesions of cutaneous leishmaniasis (p.597) due to *Leishmania tropica, L. major, L. mexicana, L. panamensis*, or *L. peruviana.*[1] The suggested course of treatment was 3 intralesional injections of a 5% solution of mepacrine given at intervals of 3 to 5 days. However, local infiltration of drugs can be difficult and painful.

1. WHO. Control of the leishmaniases. *WHO Tech Rep Ser 793* 1990.

**Sclerotherapy.** Intrapleural instillations of mepacrine hydrochloride or mesilate have been used as sclerosants in the management of malignant pleural effusions (p.512) and recurrent pneumothorax but the treatment is associated with pain and a high frequency of toxic effects.

### Preparations

**Proprietary Preparations** (details are given in Part 3)
***India:*** Maladin.
**Multi-ingredient:** ***Austria:*** Acrisuxin†; ***Switz.:*** Acrisuxin†.

## Methyl Benzoquate *(BAN)*

Nequinate *(USAN, pINN)*; AY-20385; ICI-55052; Nequinato. Methyl 7-benzyloxy-6-butyl-1,4-dihydro-4-oxoquinoline-3-carboxylate.
$C_{22}H_{23}NO_4$ = 365.4.
*CAS — 13997-19-8.*

### Profile

Methyl benzoquate is an antiprotozoal used in veterinary practice with clopidol (p.603) for the prevention of coccidiosis in poultry.

## Metronidazole *(BAN, USAN, rINN)*

Bayer-5360; Metronidazol; Metronidazolum; NSC-50364; RP-8823; SC-10295. 2-(2-Methyl-5-nitroimidazol-1-yl)ethanol.
$C_6H_9N_3O_3$ = 171.2.
*CAS — 443-48-1.*
*ATC — A01AB17; D06BX01; G01AF01; J01XD01; P01AB01.*

**Pharmacopoeias.** In *Chin., Eur.* (see p.vi), *Int., Jpn, Pol., US,* and *Viet.*

**Ph. Eur. 5.0** (Metronidazole). A white or yellowish, crystalline powder. Slightly soluble in water, in alcohol, in acetone, and in dichloromethane. Protect from light.

**USP 27** (Metronidazole). White to pale yellow, odourless crystals or crystalline powder. It darkens on exposure to light. Sparingly soluble in water and in alcohol; slightly soluble in chloroform and in ether. Store at a temperature of 25°, excursions permitted between 15° and 30°. Protect from light.

**Incompatibility.** See below.

## Metronidazole Benzoate *(BAN)*

Benzoato de metronidazol; Benzoyl Metronidazole; Metronidazoli Benzoas; RP-9712. 2-(2-Methyl-5-nitroimidazol-1-yl)ethyl benzoate.
$C_{13}H_{13}N_3O_4$ = 275.3.
*CAS — 13182-89-3.*
*ATC — A01AB17; D06BX01; G01AF01; J01XD01; P01AB01.*

**Pharmacopoeias.** In *Eur.* (see p.vi), *Int.*, and *US.*

**Ph. Eur. 5.0** (Metronidazole Benzoate). White or slightly yellowish, crystalline powder or flakes. Practically insoluble in water; slightly soluble in alcohol; soluble in acetone; freely soluble in dichloromethane. Protect from light.

**USP 27** (Metronidazole Benzoate). A white to slightly yellow, crystalline powder. Practically insoluble in water; slightly soluble in alcohol; soluble in acetone; freely soluble in dichloromethane; very slightly soluble in solvent ether. Store at a temperature of 25°, excursions permitted between 15° and 30°. Protect from light.

## Metronidazole Hydrochloride *(BANM, USAN)*

Metronidazol, hidrocloruro de; SC-32642.
$C_6H_9N_3O_3,HCl$ = 207.6.
*CAS — 69198-10-3.*
*ATC — A01AB17; D06BX01; G01AF01; J01XD01; P01AB01.*

**Incompatibility.** Solutions of metronidazole hydrochloride have a low pH, usually of less than 2.0, before dilution and neutralisation for intravenous use. These undiluted solutions react with aluminium in equipment such as needles to produce red-dish-brown discoloration, and a precipitate has been reported with ready-to-use preparations of metronidazole hydrochloride, although this occurred after contact for 6 hours or more.[1,2]

Several studies have assessed the compatibility of antibacterial injections and other drugs when added to metronidazole solution for intravenous infusion.[3-7] Results have varied according to the criteria applied and the preparations and conditions used. Physical incompatibilities due to the low pH of metronidazole injections appear to be more of a problem than chemical incompatibility. Regardless of these studies, it is generally recommended that other drugs should not be added to intravenous solutions of metronidazole or its hydrochloride. Specific information on the compatibility of individual formulations may be found in the manufacturers' literature.

1. Schell KH, Copeland JR. Metronidazole hydrochloride-aluminum interaction. *Am J Hosp Pharm* 1985; **42:** 1040, 1042.
2. Struthers BJ, Parr RJ. Clarifying the metronidazole hydrochloride-aluminum interaction. *Am J Hosp Pharm* 1985; **42:** 2660.
3. Bisaillon S, Sarrazin R. Compatibility of several antibiotics or hydrocortisone when added to metronidazole solution for intravenous infusion. *J Parenter Sci Technol* 1983; **37:** 129–32.
4. Gupta VD, Stewart KR. Chemical stabilities of hydrocortisone sodium succinate and several antibiotics when mixed with metronidazole injection for intravenous infusion. *J Parenter Sci Technol* 1985; **39:** 145–8.
5. Gupta VD, *et al.* Chemical stabilities of cefamandole nafate and metronidazole when mixed together for intravenous infusion. *J Clin Hosp Pharm* 1985; **10:** 379–83.
6. Barnes AR. Chemical stabilities of cefuroxime sodium and metronidazole in an admixture for intravenous infusion. *J Clin Pharm Ther* 1990; **15:** 187–96.
7. Nahata MC, *et al.* Stability of metronidazole and ceftizoxime sodium in ready-to-use metronidazole bags stored at 4 and 25° C. *Am J Health-Syst Pharm* 1996; **53:** 1046–8.

### Adverse Effects

The adverse effects of metronidazole are generally dose-related. The most common are gastrointestinal disturbances, especially nausea and an unpleasant metallic taste. Vomiting, and diarrhoea or constipation may also occur. A furred tongue, glossitis, and stomatitis may be associated with an overgrowth of *Candida*. There have been rare reports of antibiotic-associated colitis associated with metronidazole, although it is also used in the treatment of this condition.

Weakness, dizziness, ataxia, headache, drowsiness, insomnia, and changes in mood or mental state such as depression or confusion have also been reported. Peripheral neuropathy, usually presenting as numbness or tingling in the extremities, and epileptiform seizures have been associated with high doses of metronidazole or prolonged treatment.

Temporary moderate leucopenia and thrombocytopenia may occur in some patients receiving metronidazole. Skin rashes, urticaria, and pruritus occur occasionally and erythema multiforme, angioedema, and anaphylaxis have been reported rarely. Other side-effects include urethral discomfort and darkening of the urine. Raised liver enzyme values, cholestatic hepatitis, and jaundice have occasionally been reported. Thrombophlebitis may follow the intravenous administration of metronidazole.

Studies have shown metronidazole to be mutagenic in bacteria and carcinogenic in some *animals*.

**Carcinogenicity and mutagenicity.** Metronidazole is mutagenic in bacterial assays, and its hydroxy metabolite even more so, but studies of mammalian cells *in vitro* and *in vivo* have not consistently demonstrated a mutagenic effect. Similarly, there is no uniformity in the limited data concerning genotoxicity in humans,[1] and although metronidazole has been classified as a carcinogen in *animals*, the evidence of human carcinogenicity is ambiguous. There was no appreciable increase in the incidence of cancer in a retrospective study of 771 patients given metronidazole for vaginal trichomoniasis,[2] nor in another similar study of 2460 patients.[3] The first study[2] did show an excess of cases of lung cancer, although all 4 were in women who were smokers. Subsequent follow-up[4] to 1984, covering a period of 15 to 25 years, still showed an excess of lung cancer cases even after allowing for smoking status. However, this follow-up also continued to show no significant increase overall in cancer-related morbidity or mortality. Follow-up[5] of the patients from the second study for 11 to 15 years to 1984 also showed no increase in the overall incidence of cancers nor did it confirm any increase in lung cancer.

Risks to the fetus are discussed under Pregnancy in Precautions, below.

1. Bendesky A, *et al.* Is metronidazole carcinogenic? *Mutat Res* 2002; **511:** 133–44.
2. Beard CM, *et al.* Lack of evidence for cancer due to use of metronidazole. *N Engl J Med* 1979; **301:** 519–22.
3. Friedman GD. Cancer after metronidazole. *N Engl J Med* 1980; **302:** 519.
4. Beard CM, *et al.* Cancer after exposure to metronidazole. *Mayo Clin Proc* 1988; **63:** 147–53.
5. Friedman GD, Selby JV. Metronidazole and cancer. *JAMA* 1989; **261:** 866.

**Effects on the blood.** Adverse haematological effects associated with metronidazole therapy include a report of bone marrow aplasia, with leucopenia and markedly reduced erythropoiesis and granulopoiesis,[1] aplastic anaemia,[2] and the haemolytic-uraemic syndrome.[3]

1. White CM, *et al.* Bone marrow aplasia associated with metronidazole. *BMJ* 1980; **280:** 647.
2. Raman R, *et al.* Metronidazole induced aplastic anaemia. *Clinician* 1982; **46:** 464–8.
3. Powell HR, *et al.* Haemolytic-uraemic syndrome after treatment with metronidazole. *Med J Aust* 1988; **149:** 222–3.

**Effects on the ears.** A review of reports of ototoxicity notified to the Australian Adverse Drug Reactions Advisory Committee revealed a number of cases of deafness associated with the use of metronidazole.[1]

1. Anonymous. Drug-induced ototoxicity. *WHO Drug Inf* 1991; **5:** 12.

**Effects on the eyes.** Myopia which developed in a patient after 11 days of oral metronidazole for trichomoniasis had resolved 4 days after withdrawal of treatment, but recurred when she resumed treatment.[1]

Retrobulbar or optic neuritis was reported in 7 patients receiving metronidazole.[2] Dosage varied from 0.75 to 1 g daily by mouth and duration of treatment from 7 days to a year. Abnormalities included defects in colour vision, decreased vision, and scotomas. Vision improved following withdrawal of metronidazole, although there was a residual deficit in 2 patients.

1. Grinbaum A, *et al.* Transient myopia following metronidazole treatment for Trichomonas vaginalis. *JAMA* 1992; **267:** 511–12.
2. Putnam D, *et al.* Metronidazole and optic neuritis. *Am J Ophthalmol* 1991; **112:** 737.

**Effects on the gastrointestinal tract.** ANTIBIOTIC-ASSOCIATED COLITIS. Reports of pseudomembranous colitis associated with the administration of metronidazole.


1. Thomson G, *et al.* Pseudomembranous colitis after treatment with metronidazole. *BMJ* 1981; **282:** 864–5.
2. Daly JJ, Chowdary KVS. Pseudomembranous colitis secondary to metronidazole. *Dig Dis Sci* 1983; **28:** 573–4.


**Effects on the liver.** Severely elevated liver enzyme values, consistent with a drug-induced hepatitis, occurred in a patient given metronidazole hydrochloride 500 mg every 6 hours intravenously for 4 days. He was also receiving cefapirin sodium and tobramycin sulfate.[1] A case of reversible hepatotoxicity caused by an overdose of metronidazole 12.5 g has also been reported.[2]


1. Appleby DH, Vogtland HD. Suspected metronidazole toxicity. *Clin Pharm* 1983; **2:** 373–4.
2. Lam S, Bank S. Hepatotoxicity caused by metronidazole overdose. *Ann Intern Med* 1995; **122:** 803.


**Effects on the nervous system.** CONVULSIONS. Reports of convulsions associated with metronidazole therapy (usually in high doses or in patients with renal impairment).


1. Halloran TJ. Convulsions associated with high cumulative doses of metronidazole. *Drug Intell Clin Pharm* 1982; **16:** 409.
2. Wienbren M, *et al.* Convulsions and encephalopathy in a patient with leukemia after treatment with metronidazole. *J Clin Pathol* 1985; **38:** 1076.
3. Ferroir JP, *et al.* Polynévrite, crises convulsives et syndrome cérébelleux, complications d'un traitement par le métronidazole. *Presse Med* 1985; **14:** 2108.
4. Moulin B, *et al.* Risque neurotoxique du métronidazole (MN) au cours de l'insuffisance rénale sévère. *Ann Med Interne (Paris)* 1988; **139:** 369.
5. Sopena B, *et al.* Convulsiones inducidas por la asociación de metronidazol y cloroquina. *Med Clin (Barc)* 1990; **95:** 675.
6. Beloosesky Y, *et al.* Convulsions induced by metronidazole treatment for Clostridium difficile-associated disease in chronic renal failure. *Am J Med Sci* 2000; **319:** 338–9.


EFFECTS ON MENTAL FUNCTION. Although metronidazole is sometimes used to reduce colonic flora in the treatment of hepatic encephalopathy, impaired metabolism of metronidazole in such patients can result in elevated plasma concentrations and consequent toxicity. Psychosis and manic behaviour were reported in one such patient during treatment for hepatic encephalopathy with metronidazole and lactulose, although plasma-metronidazole concentrations were not found to be raised (24 micrograms/mL).[1] Symptoms resolved when metronidazole was discontinued. Acute psychosis has also been reported in a patient following a 5-day course of intravenous metronidazole 1 g daily for a gynaecological disorder.[2]


1. Uhl MD, Riely CA. Metronidazole in treating portosystemic encephalopathy. *Ann Intern Med* 1996; **124:** 455.
2. Schreiber W, Spernal J. Metronidazole-induced psychotic disorder. *Am J Psychiatry* 1997; **154:** 1170–1.


PERIPHERAL NEUROPATHY. Peripheral neuropathy has been reported in patients receiving prolonged treatment with metronidazole.[1-4] Stopping metronidazole or lowering the dose usually results in complete resolution or improvement of the neuropathy but in some patients it may persist despite these measures. For reports of retrobulbar or optic neuritis associated with metronidazole, see Effects on the Eyes, above.


1. Duffy LF, *et al.* Peripheral neuropathy in Crohn's disease patients treated with metronidazole. *Gastroenterology* 1985; **88:** 681–4.
2. Boyce EG, *et al.* Persistent metronidazole-induced peripheral neuropathy. *DICP Ann Pharmacother* 1990; **24:** 19–21.
3. Learned-Coughlin S. Peripheral neuropathy induced by metronidazole. *Ann Pharmacother* 1994; **28:** 536.
4. Dreger LM, *et al.* Intermittent-dose metronidazole-induced peripheral neuropathy. *Ann Pharmacother* 1998; **32:** 267–8.


**Effects on the pancreas.** A small number of cases of acute pancreatitis associated with metronidazole, in some cases recurrent on rechallenge, have been reported.[1-3] No cases were found in a retrospective study of about 6500 patients who had received metronidazole.[4]


1. Plotnick BH, *et al.* Metronidazole-induced pancreatitis. *Ann Intern Med* 1985; **103:** 891–2.
2. Sanford KA, *et al.* Metronidazole-associated pancreatitis. *Ann Intern Med* 1988; **109:** 756–7.
3. Sura ME, *et al.* Metronidazole-associated pancreatitis. *Ann Pharmacother* 2000; **34:** 1152–5.
4. Friedman G, Selby JV. How often does metronidazole induce pancreatitis? *Gastroenterology* 1990; **98:** 1702–3.


**Gynaecomastia.** Gynaecomastia occurred in a 36-year-old man with ulcerative colitis after taking metronidazole for about a month.[1]


1. Fagan TC, *et al.* Metronidazole-induced gynecomastia. *JAMA* 1985; **254:** 3217.


**Hypersensitivity.** A hypersensitivity reaction with chills, fever, generalised erythema, and a maculopapular rash developed after a single dose of metronidazole in a patient who had previously developed a rash during treatment with intravaginal metronidazole.[1]


1. Knowles S, *et al.* Metronidazole hypersensitivity. *Ann Pharmacother* 1994; **28:** 325–6.


## Precautions

Peripheral neuropathy, transient epileptiform seizures, and leucopenia have sometimes been associated with prolonged or intensive treatment with metronidazole (see Adverse Effects, above). Clinical and laboratory monitoring is advised in patients receiving metronidazole for more than 10 days. Doses should be reduced in patients with severe hepatic impairment.

It is suggested that the use of metronidazole should be avoided during pregnancy, and this caution applies especially to use during the first trimester and to the use of high-dose regimens (see also below).

Patients are advised not to drink alcoholic beverages while taking metronidazole (see Interactions, below).

**Breast feeding.** Metronidazole is distributed into breast milk giving it a bitter taste which may impair feeding.[1] The American Academy of Pediatrics considers that although the effects of metronidazole on breast-fed infants are unknown they may be of concern. It recommends that breast feeding should be discontinued for 12 to 24 hours when single-dose therapy is used;[2] no specific recommendations are given for long-term treatment.


1. Rubin PC. Prescribing in pregnancy: general principles. *BMJ* 1986; **293:** 1415–17.
2. American Academy of Pediatrics. The transfer of drugs and other chemicals into human milk. *Pediatrics* 2001; **108:** 776–89. Correction. *ibid.*; 1029. Also available at: http://aappolicy.aappublications.org/cgi/content/full/pediatrics%3b108/3/776 (accessed 03/02/04)


**Pregnancy.** Metronidazole is mutagenic in bacteria and carcinogenic in *rodents*. It readily crosses the placenta achieving similar concentrations in the placental cord and maternal plasma and its use in pregnancy is controversial. Meta-analyses of studies involving the use of metronidazole in the first trimester of pregnancy[1,2] concluded that there did not appear to be an increased risk of teratogenicity. However, in the USA the manufacturer considers metronidazole to be contra-indicated during the first trimester in patients with trichomoniasis; use for trichomoniasis during the second and third trimesters may be acceptable. For other indications the risks and benefits of treatment with metronidazole should be weighed carefully, especially in the first trimester.


1. Burtin P, *et al.* Safety of metronidazole in pregnancy: a meta-analysis. *Am J Obstet Gynecol* 1995; **172:** 525–9.
2. Caro-Patón T, *et al.* Is metronidazole teratogenic? A meta-analysis. *Br J Clin Pharmacol* 1997; **44:** 179–82.


## Interactions

When given with alcohol, metronidazole may provoke a disulfiram-like reaction in some patients. Acute psychoses or confusion have been associated with the use of metronidazole and disulfiram together.

Metronidazole is reported to impair the metabolism or excretion of several drugs including warfarin (p.1026), phenytoin (p.373), lithium (p.303), ciclosporin, and fluorouracil (p.555), with the consequent potential for an increased incidence of adverse effects. There is some evidence that phenytoin might accelerate the metabolism of metronidazole. Plasma concentrations of metronidazole are decreased by phenobarbital, with a consequent reduction in the effectiveness of metronidazole. Cimetidine has increased plasma concentrations of metronidazole and might increase the risk of neurological side-effects. For references to some of these interactions, see below.

For incompatibilities between metronidazole and other drugs in solutions for injection, see above.

**Alcohol.** Metronidazole may provoke a disulfiram-like reaction in some individuals when given with alcohol; reactions have occurred after the use of preparations formulated with alcohol, including injections, as well as after drinking alcohol.[1] Acute psychosis or confusional state was reported in 6 of 29 alcoholic patients who were also receiving disulfiram.[2] However, an analysis of published reports[3] and a study in volunteers[4] both found that there was no convincing evidence of a disulfiram-like reaction between metronidazole and alcohol although caution was still advised.


1. Edwards DL, *et al.* Disulfiram-like reaction associated with intravenous trimethoprim-sulfamethoxazole and metronidazole. *Clin Pharm* 1986; **5:** 999–1000.
2. Rothstein E, Clancy DD. Toxicity of disulfiram combined with metronidazole. *N Engl J Med* 1969; **280:** 1006–7.
3. Williams CS, Woodcock KR. Do ethanol and metronidazole interact to produce a disulfiram-like reaction? *Ann Pharmacother* 2000; **34:** 255–7.
4. Visapää J-P, *et al.* Lack of disulfiram-like reaction with metronidazole and ethanol. *Ann Pharmacother* 2002; **36:** 971–4.


**Antineoplastics.** For reference to the effect of metronidazole on busulfan, see p.533.

**Carbamazepine.** For a report of a possible interaction between metronidazole and carbamazepine, see p.356.

**Cimetidine.** In a study in 6 healthy volunteers metronidazole plasma concentrations were increased by twice-daily administration of cimetidine. The effect was presumed to be due to inhibition of cytochrome P450 isoenzymes responsible for metronidazole metabolism.[1] However, cimetidine was not found to affect the pharmacokinetics of metronidazole in a study in patients with Crohn's disease[2] nor in a single-dose study in healthy subjects.[3]


1. Gugler R, Jansen JC. Interaction between cimetidine and metronidazole. *N Engl J Med* 1983; **309:** 1518–19.
2. Eradiri O, *et al.* Interaction of metronidazole with cimetidine and phenobarbital in Crohn's disease. *Clin Pharmacol Ther* 1987; **41:** 235.
3. Loft S, *et al.* Lack of effect of cimetidine on the pharmacokinetics and metabolism of a single oral dose of metronidazole. *Eur J Clin Pharmacol* 1988; **35:** 65–8.


**Disulfiram.** For a report of acute psychosis or confusional state following metronidazole treatment in alcoholic patients receiving disulfiram, see under Alcohol, above.

**Omeprazole.** Although concentrations in plasma and saliva of metronidazole and its hydroxy metabolite were unaffected by omeprazole in healthy volunteers, those in gastric juice were substantially lowered, possibly as a result of a reduction in transfer from the plasma.[1] However, this may be of limited clinical significance during treatment of *Helicobacter pylori* infections.


1. Jessa MJ, *et al.* The effect of omeprazole on the pharmacokinetics of metronidazole and hydroxymetronidazole in human plasma, saliva and gastric juice. *Br J Clin Pharmacol* 1997; **44:** 245–53.


**Phenobarbital.** An increase in the rate of metabolism of metronidazole, resulting in treatment failure, was reported in a patient receiving phenobarbital.[1] In a retrospective survey of patients who had not responded to treatment with metronidazole, 80% were found to be receiving long-term phenobarbital therapy.[2] Subsequently it was found that up to three times the usual dose was required to produce a parasitological cure of giardiasis in such patients.


1. Mead PB, *et al.* Possible alteration of metronidazole metabolism by phenobarbital. *N Engl J Med* 1982; **306:** 1490.
2. Gupte S. Phenobarbital and metabolism of metronidazole. *N Engl J Med* 1983; **308:** 529.


**Phenytoin.** In addition to conflicting reports on the effects of metronidazole on the metabolism of phenytoin (p.373), increased metabolism of metronidazole was reported in a patient during treatment with phenytoin.[1]


1. Wheeler LA, *et al.* Use of high-pressure liquid chromatography to determine plasma levels of metronidazole and metabolites after intravenous administration. *Antimicrob Agents Chemother* 1978; **13:** 205–9.


## Antimicrobial Action

Metronidazole is active against several protozoa including *Balantidium coli*, *Blastocystis hominis*, *Entamoeba histolytica*, *Giardia intestinalis* (*Giardia lamblia*), and *Trichomonas vaginalis*. Most obligate anaerobic bacteria, including *Bacteroides* and *Clostridium* spp., are sensitive *in vitro* to metronidazole. It is bactericidal. It also has activity against the facultative anaerobes *Gardnerella vaginalis* and *Helicobacter pylori* and against some spirochaetes. Resistance to metronidazole has been reported and cross-resistance to other nitroimidazoles, such as tinidazole, may occur.

◊ Metronidazole has well-established bactericidal activity against obligate anaerobic bacteria *in vitro*, including the Gram-negative organisms *Bacteroides fragilis* and other *Bacteroides* spp., *Fusobacterium* spp., and *Veillonella* spp., and the Gram-positive organisms *Clostridium difficile, Cl. perfringens,* and other *Clostridium* spp., *Eubacterium* spp., *Peptococcus* spp., and *Peptostreptococcus* spp.; *Propionibacterium* and *Actinomyces* spp. are often resistant.[1-6] It also has activity against the facultative anaerobe *Gardnerella vaginalis*, although its bactericidal effect is reported to be much slower than against obligate anaerobes,[7] against some strains of *Campylobacter* spp. including *C. fetus* subsp. *jejuni*,[8,9] and against *Helicobacter pylori*.[10,11]

The oxidative metabolites of metronidazole also have antibacterial activity; the hydroxy metabolite has been reported to be consistently more active than metronidazole against strains of *G. vaginalis*.[12,13]

The mode of action of metronidazole is not entirely clear, but is thought to involve reduction by bacterial 'nitroreductases' to an unstable intermediate which interacts with DNA, effectively preventing further replication.[14] A number of factors affect the sensitivity of micro-organisms to metronidazole *in vitro*. Anaerobic conditions are important for optimal activity. Interactions between micro-organisms and metronidazole have been described, including inhibition of *Escherichia coli* by metronidazole in the presence of *B. fragilis* and enhancement of the rate of killing of *B. fragilis* by metronidazole in the presence of *E. coli*.

Resistance to metronidazole has developed in sensitive species. Although no resistance among the *B. fragilis* group was observed over several years,[15,16] there have been occasional reports of resistance in this group[17-22] and in other *Bacteroides* spp.[23-25] now known as *Prevotella* spp. Nitroimidazole resistance in *Helicobacter pylori* has been increasing and may be associated with reduced response rates to anti-*Helicobacter* therapy for peptic ulcer disease in some populations (see Peptic Ulcer Disease under Uses, below).


1. Wüst J. Susceptibility of anaerobic bacteria to metronidazole, ornidazole, and tinidazole and routine susceptibility testing by standardized methods. *Antimicrob Agents Chemother* 1977; **11:** 631–7.

2. Dubreuil L, *et al.* Susceptibility of anaerobic bacteria from several French hospitals to three major antibiotics. *Antimicrob Agents Chemother* 1984; **25:** 764–6.
3. Hill GB, Ayers OM. Antimicrobial susceptibilities of anaerobic bacteria isolated from female genital tract infections. *Antimicrob Agents Chemother* 1985; **27:** 324–31.
4. Chow AW, *et al.* In vitro susceptibility of Clostridium difficile to new β-lactam and quinolone antibiotics. *Antimicrob Agents Chemother* 1985; **28:** 842–4.
5. Brazier JS, *et al.* Antibiotic susceptibility of clinical isolates of clostridia. *J Antimicrob Chemother* 1985; **15:** 181–5.
6. Van der Auwera P, *et al.* Comparative serum bactericidal activity against test anaerobes in volunteers receiving imipenem, clindamycin, latamoxef and metronidazole. *J Antimicrob Chemother* 1987; **19:** 205–10.
7. Ralph ED, Amatnieks YE. Metronidazole in treatment against Haemophilus vaginalis (Corynebacterium vaginale). *Antimicrob Agents Chemother* 1980; **18:** 101–4.
8. Hof H, *et al.* Comparative in vitro activities of niridazole and metronidazole against anaerobic and microaerophilic bacteria. *Antimicrob Agents Chemother* 1982; **22:** 332–3.
9. Freydière AM, *et al.* In vitro susceptibilities of 40 Campylobacter fetus subsp jejuni strains to niridazole and metronidazole. *Antimicrob Agents Chemother* 1984; **25:** 145–6.
10. Marshall BJ, *et al.* Pyloric campylobacter infection and gastroduodenal disease. *Med J Aust* 1985; **142:** 439–44.
11. Howden A, *et al.* In-vitro sensitivity of Campylobacter pyloridis to furazolidone. *Lancet* 1986; **ii:** 1035.
12. Ralph ED, Amatnieks YE. Relative susceptibilities of Gardnerella vaginalis (Haemophilus vaginalis), Neisseria gonorrhoeae, and Bacteroides fragilis to metronidazole and its two major metabolites. *Sex Transm Dis* 1980; **7:** 157–60.
13. Shanker S, Munro R. Sensitivity of Gardnerella vaginalis to metabolites of metronidazole and tinidazole. *Lancet* 1982; **i:** 167.
14. Ingham HR, *et al.* Interactions between micro-organisms and metronidazole. *J Antimicrob Chemother* 1982; **10:** 84–7.
15. Tally FP, *et al.* Susceptibility of the Bacteroides fragilis group in the United States in 1981. *Antimicrob Agents Chemother* 1983; **23:** 536–40.
16. Tally FP, *et al.* Nationwide study of the susceptibility of the Bacteroides fragilis group in the United States. *Antimicrob Agents Chemother* 1985; **28:** 675–7.
17. Ingham HR, *et al.* Bacteroides fragilis resistance to metronidazole after long-term therapy. *Lancet* 1978; **i:** 214.
18. Eme A, *et al.* Bacteroides fragilis resistant to metronidazole. *J Antimicrob Chemother* 1983; **12:** 523–5.
19. Lamothe F, *et al.* Bacteroides fragilis resistant to both metronidazole and imipenem. *J Antimicrob Chemother* 1986; **18:** 642–3.
20. Brogan O, *et al.* Bacteroides fragilis resistant to metronidazole, clindamycin and cefoxitin. *J Antimicrob Chemother* 1989; **23:** 660–2.
21. Hickey MM, *et al.* Metronidazole resistant Bacteroides fragilis infection of a prosthetic hip joint. *J Infect* 1990; **20:** 129–33.
22. Turner P, *et al.* Simultaneous resistance to metronidazole, co-amoxiclav, and imipenem in clinical isolate of Bacteroides fragilis. *Lancet* 1995; **345:** 1275–7.
23. Sprott MS, *et al.* Metronidazole-resistant anaerobes. *Lancet* 1983; **i:** 1220.
24. McWalter PW, Baird DR. Metronidazole-resistant anaerobes. *Lancet* 1983; **i:** 1220.
25. Sprott MS, Kearns AM. Metronidazole-resistant Bacteroides melaninogenicus. *J Antimicrob Chemother* 1988; **22:** 951–2.

## Pharmacokinetics

Metronidazole is readily and almost completely absorbed after oral doses. Peak plasma concentrations of about 6 and 12 micrograms/mL are achieved, usually within 1 to 2 hours, after single doses of 250 and 500 mg respectively. Some accumulation occurs and consequently there are higher concentrations when multiple doses are given. Absorption may be delayed, but is not reduced overall by food. Metronidazole benzoate given by mouth is hydrolysed in the gastrointestinal tract to release metronidazole, which in turn is then absorbed.

Peak steady-state plasma concentrations of about 25 micrograms/mL with trough concentrations of about 18 micrograms/mL have been reported in patients given an intravenous loading dose of 15 mg/kg followed by 7.5 mg/kg every 6 hours. The bioavailability of metronidazole from rectal suppositories is 60 to 80%; peak plasma concentrations are half those achieved with equivalent oral doses and effective concentrations occur after about 5 to 12 hours. Absorption from vaginal pessaries is poor with a reported bioavailability of about 20 to 25%; absorption is gradual producing peak plasma concentrations of about 2 micrograms/mL following a dose of 500 mg. An intravaginal gel formulation providing a dose of 37.5 mg metronidazole produced peak plasma concentrations of 0.3 micrograms/mL at 8 hours, with a bioavailability of 56%.

Metronidazole is widely distributed. It appears in most body tissues and fluids including bile, bone, breast milk, cerebral abscesses, CSF, liver and liver abscesses, saliva, seminal fluid, and vaginal secretions, and achieves concentrations similar to those in plasma. It also crosses the placenta and rapidly enters the fetal circulation. No more than 20% is bound to plasma proteins.

Metronidazole is metabolised in the liver by side-chain oxidation and glucuronide formation. The principal oxidative metabolites are 1-(2-hydroxyethyl)-2-hydroxymethyl-5-nitroimidazole (the hydroxy metabolite), which has antibacterial activity and is detected in plasma and urine, and 2-methyl-5-nitroimidazole-1-acetic acid (the acid metabolite), which has virtually no antibacterial activity and is often not detected in plasma, but is excreted in urine. Small amounts of reduced metabolites, acetamide and *N*-(2-hydroxyethyl)oxamic acid (HOA), have also been detected in urine and are probably formed by the intestinal flora.

The elimination half-life of metronidazole is about 8 hours; that of the hydroxy metabolite is slightly longer. The half-life of metronidazole is reported to be longer in neonates and in patients with severe hepatic impairment; that of the hydroxy metabolite is prolonged in patients with substantial renal impairment.

The majority of a dose of metronidazole is excreted in the urine, mainly as metabolites; a small amount appears in the faeces.

◊ References.

1. Cunningham FE, *et al.* Pharmacokinetics of intravaginal metronidazole gel. *J Clin Pharmacol* 1994; **34:** 1060–5.
2. Lamp KC, *et al.* Pharmacokinetics and pharmacodynamics of the nitroimidazole antimicrobials. *Clin Pharmacokinet* 1999; **36:** 353–73.

**Hepatic impairment.** There have been differing results from pharmacokinetic studies of the elimination of metronidazole in patients with hepatic impairment. No marked difference was reported[1] between patients with cirrhosis or hepatosplenic schistosomiasis given a single 500-mg oral dose of metronidazole when compared with healthy subjects; this suggested that, in the absence of renal impairment, dosage adjustment was not needed in patients with hepatic impairment. However, others found[2] that elimination of metronidazole, given intravenously, was considerably impaired in a study of 10 patients with alcoholic liver disease or chronic active hepatitis, 7 of whom also had reduced creatinine clearance. Responding to the comment[3] that these differing results were probably due to impaired renal elimination, the authors suggested[4] that impaired elimination of metronidazole was due to impaired hepatic metabolism rather than decreased renal clearance; other studies have shown metronidazole clearance to be normal in renal impairment. They nevertheless agreed that reduction in the dosage of metronidazole is required only when hepatic function is very poor, particularly when renal function is impaired. A study in 10 severely ill patients with or without impaired hepatic and/or renal function[5] also suggested that hepatic function is a very important determinant of metronidazole elimination.

1. Daneshmend TK, *et al.* Disposition of oral metronidazole in hepatic cirrhosis and in hepatosplenic schistosomiasis. *Gut* 1982; **23:** 807–13.
2. Farrell G, *et al.* Impaired elimination of metronidazole in decompensated chronic liver disease. *BMJ* 1983; **287:** 1845.
3. Daneshmend TK, Roberts CJC. Impaired elimination of metronidazole in decompensated chronic liver disease. *BMJ* 1984; **288:** 405.
4. Farrell G, *et al.* Impaired elimination of metronidazole in decompensated chronic liver disease. *BMJ* 1984, **288:** 1009.
5. Ljungberg B, *et al.* Metronidazole: pharmacokinetic observations in severely ill patients. *J Antimicrob Chemother* 1984; **14:** 275–83.

**Infants and children.** A single intravenous dose of 15 mg/kg has been suggested for neonates[1] which would produce therapeutic concentrations of metronidazole for around 24 hours in term neonates and 48 hours in preterm neonates. Renal and hepatic function is incompletely developed in newborn infants and consequently the elimination half-life of metronidazole is prolonged and has been reported to range from 25 to 109 hours.[1] Elimination half-life is inversely proportional to gestational age[1,2] and as the infant matures half-life is reduced to values closer to those in adults.[1,3]

1. Jager-Roman E, *et al.* Pharmacokinetics and tissue distribution of metronidazole in the newborn infant. *J Pediatr* 1982; **100:** 651–4.
2. Hall P, *et al.* Intravenous metronidazole in the newborn. *Arch Dis Child* 1983; **58:** 529–31.
3. Amon I, *et al.* Disposition kinetics of metronidazole in children. *Eur J Clin Pharmacol* 1983; **24:** 113–19.

**Renal impairment.** Pharmacokinetic studies have indicated that doses of metronidazole need not be altered in patients with renal impairment,[1] although adjustments might be required in patients undergoing haemodialysis, since metronidazole and its hydroxy metabolite are efficiently cleared and extensively removed in such patients.[2] However, in another study[3] the amount of metronidazole and its hydroxy metabolite cleared was found to depend on the type of dialysis membrane used; the authors concluded that dosage supplementation may be needed only for seriously ill patients undergoing haemodialysis with a membrane having high metronidazole clearance.

Routine adjustment of dosage was not considered necessary in patients undergoing peritoneal dialysis.[4] However, the potential for metabolites to accumulate was noted in patients on continuous ambulatory peritoneal dialysis[5] and it was suggested that dosage reduction may be necessary if excessive concentrations of metabolites are found to be toxic.

1. Houghton GW, *et al.* Pharmacokinetics of metronidazole in patients with varying degrees of renal failure. *Br J Clin Pharmacol* 1985; **19:** 203–9.
2. Somogyi A, *et al.* Disposition and removal of metronidazole in patients undergoing haemodialysis. *Eur J Clin Pharmacol* 1983; **25:** 683–7.
3. Lau AH, *et al.* Hemodialysis clearance of metronidazole and its metabolites. *Antimicrob Agents Chemother* 1986; **29:** 235–8.
4. Cassey JG, *et al.* Pharmacokinetics of metronidazole in patients undergoing peritoneal dialysis. *Antimicrob Agents Chemother* 1983; **24:** 950–1.
5. Guay DR, *et al.* Pharmacokinetics of metronidazole in patients undergoing continuous ambulatory peritoneal dialysis. *Antimicrob Agents Chemother* 1984; **25:** 306–10.

## Uses and Administration

Metronidazole is a 5-nitroimidazole derivative with activity against anaerobic bacteria and protozoa (see Antimicrobial Action, above); it also has a radiosensitising effect on hypoxic tumour cells. Its mechanism of action is thought to involve interference with DNA by a metabolite in which the nitro group of metronidazole has been reduced.

Metronidazole is used in the treatment of susceptible protozoal infections such as amoebiasis, balantidiasis, *Blastocystis hominis* infections, giardiasis, and trichomoniasis; it has also been tried in leishmaniasis and microsporidiosis. For details of these infections and their treatment see under Choice of Antiprotozoal, p.595. Metronidazole is also used in the treatment and prophylaxis of anaerobic bacterial infections. Specific bacterial infections treated with metronidazole include bacterial vaginosis, acute necrotising ulcerative gingivitis, pelvic inflammatory disease, tetanus, and antibiotic-associated colitis. For details of these infections and their treatment see under Choice of Antibacterial, p.120.

Metronidazole is used to eradicate *Helicobacter pylori* in peptic ulcer disease (in combination with other antimicrobials, and either bismuth compounds or proton pump inhibitors) and in the management of malodorous tumours and ulcers where there is anaerobic infection. It is also used in the treatment of rosacea and of dracunculiasis (guinea-worm infection) and has been given in the treatment of perianal Crohn's disease and hepatic encephalopathy. It has also been tried as an adjunct to the radiotherapy of malignant neoplasms. See also below for these miscellaneous uses.

ADMINISTRATION AND DOSAGE. Metronidazole is given by mouth in tablets or, as metronidazole benzoate, in oral suspension; the tablets are taken with or after food and the suspension at least 1 hour before food. Metronidazole is also given rectally in suppositories, applied topically as a cream or gel, or given by intravenous infusion of metronidazole or metronidazole hydrochloride. Doses are expressed in terms of metronidazole base.

In **amoebiasis**, metronidazole acts as an amoebicide at all sites of infection with *Entamoeba histolytica*. Because of its rapid absorption it is probably less effective against parasites in the bowel lumen and is therefore used with a luminal amoebicide such as diloxanide furoate or diiodohydroxyquinoline in the treatment of invasive amoebiasis. Metronidazole is given in doses of 400 to 800 mg three times daily by mouth for 5 to 10 days. Children aged 1 to 3 years may be given one-quarter, those aged 3 to 7 years one-third, and those aged 7 to 10 years one-half the total adult daily dose; alternatively 35 to 50 mg/kg daily in divided doses has been used. An alternative adult dose is 1.5 to 2.5 g as a single daily dose for 2 or 3 days.

In **balantidiasis** and ***Blastocystis hominis* infection**, metronidazole has been given in doses similar to those used in amoebiasis.

In **giardiasis**, the usual dose of metronidazole is 2 g once daily by mouth for 3 successive days, or 400 mg three times daily for 5 days, or 500 mg twice daily for 7 to 10 days. Dosage for children is proportional, as for amoebiasis (above). An alternative schedule for children is 15 mg/kg daily in divided doses.

In **trichomoniasis**, metronidazole is given by mouth either as a single 2-g dose, as a 2-day course of 800 mg in the morning and 1.2 g in the evening, or as a 7-day course of 600 mg to 1 g daily in two or three divided doses. Sexual partners should also be treated. If treatment needs to be repeated, an interval of 4 to 6 weeks between courses has been recommended. Vaginal preparations containing metronidazole are available for the treatment of vaginal trichomoniasis in some countries. Children with trichomoniasis may be given a 7-day course of metronidazole by mouth as follows: 1 to 3 years, 50 mg three times daily; 3 to 7 years, 100 mg twice daily, and 7 to 10 years, 100 mg three times daily. An alternative children's dose is 15 mg/kg daily in divided doses for 7 days.

**Bacterial vaginosis** is treated similarly to vaginal trichomoniasis with which it may co-exist; metronidazole is usually given by mouth as a single 2-g dose or as a 5 to 7-day course of 400 or 500 mg twice daily. Alternatively it may be applied locally as 5 g of a 0.75% gel once or twice daily for 5 days.

In **acute necrotising ulcerative gingivitis**, metronidazole 200 mg three times daily is given by mouth for 3 days; similar doses are used in acute dental infections. A 25% dental gel has also been used as an adjunct to the treatment of chronic periodontal infections.

For the treatment of most **anaerobic bacterial infections**, metronidazole is given by mouth in an initial dose of 800 mg followed by 400 mg every 8 hours, usually for about 7 days. A regimen of 500 mg every 8 hours is alternatively used. When oral therapy is precluded metronidazole may be given intravenously, 500 mg being infused as 100 mL of a 5 mg/mL solution at a rate of 5 mL/minute every 8 hours, or rectally as a 1-g suppository every 8 hours for 3 days, then every 12 hours; oral therapy should be substituted as soon as possible. Suppositories may be unsuitable for beginning therapy in serious infections because of the slower absorption of metronidazole. Children may be given 7.5 mg/kg every 8 hours by mouth or by intravenous infusion; recommended rectal doses for children, to be given every 8 hours for 3 days, then every 12 hours thereafter, are: for those aged under 1 year, 125 mg; 1 to 5 years, 250 mg; 5 to 10 years, 500 mg. In the USA recommended adult doses of metronidazole are 7.5 mg/kg every 6 hours by mouth or 15 mg/kg by intravenous infusion followed by 7.5 mg/kg every 6 hours, doses being infused over 1 hour; by either route a total dose of 4 g in 24 hours should not be exceeded. In mixed anaerobic and aerobic infections metronidazole is given with the appropriate antibacterials.

For the **prevention of postoperative anaerobic bacterial infections**, especially in patients undergoing abdominal or gynaecological surgery, metronidazole is given orally, intravenously, or rectally in doses similar to those used for treatment, usually together with a beta-lactam or an aminoglycoside antibacterial. Various schedules have been employed. In the UK, licensed doses for adults are:

- by mouth, 400 mg every 8 hours in the 24 hours before surgery followed postoperatively by intravenous or rectal administration until oral therapy is possible
- by intravenous infusion, 500 mg shortly before operation and repeated every 8 hours, oral doses of 200 or 400 mg every 8 hours being substituted as soon as possible
- by rectum, 1 g every 8 hours starting 2 hours before surgery.

The *British National Formulary*, however, recommends that oral doses should be started only 2 hours before the operation and that the number of doses for all administration routes be limited to a total of four. In the USA the recommended schedule for adults undergoing colorectal surgery is metronidazole 15 mg/kg by intravenous infusion over 30 to 60 minutes, completed about 1 hour before surgery, followed by two further intravenous doses of 7.5 mg/kg infused at 6 and 12 hours after the initial dose.

In **peptic ulcer disease**, metronidazole is used in combination therapy to eradicate *Helicobacter pylori*. Typical regimens include metronidazole plus another antibacterial (clarithromycin or amoxicillin) given with either a proton pump inhibitor (omeprazole or lansoprazole) or with ranitidine bismuth citrate. The usual dose of metronidazole is 400 mg twice daily except when given with omeprazole and amoxicillin, when metronidazole 400 mg three times daily is used. Treatment is continued for 1 week.

For **leg ulcers** and **pressure sores** infected with anaerobic bacteria, metronidazole 400 mg may be given three times daily by mouth for 7 days. Metronidazole is also applied topically as a 0.75% or 0.8% gel to reduce the odour associated with anaerobic infection in **fungating tumours**.

In the treatment of **rosacea** metronidazole is given by mouth or applied topically.

**Administration in hepatic impairment.** Since metronidazole is mainly metabolised by hepatic oxidation, accumulation of metronidazole and its metabolites is likely in patients with severely impaired hepatic function. Metronidazole should therefore be administered with caution and at reduced doses to patients with severe hepatic impairment, and especially hepatic encephalopathy when adverse affects of metronidazole can add to the symptoms of the disease. One-third of the usual daily dose may be administered once daily in these patients. For patients with lesser degrees of hepatic impairment, pharmacokinetic studies have not produced consistent results (see under Pharmacokinetics, above) and no recommendations about dosage reduction have been made by the manufacturers.

**Administration in renal impairment.** The elimination of metronidazole is largely unchanged in patients with renal impairment, although metabolites may accumulate in patients with end-stage renal disease on dialysis (see under Pharmacokinetics, above). Dosage reductions are therefore not usually recommended for patients with renal impairment although, since both metronidazole and its metabolites are removed by haemodialysis, doses need to be given immediately after haemodialysis.

**Dracunculiasis.** Metronidazole may be beneficial in the management of dracunculiasis (p.98). It provides symptomatic relief and is also thought to weaken the anchorage of the worms within subcutaneous tissue, thus allowing them to be removed more quickly.

Metronidazole has been given in a variety of regimens, including doses of 400 mg three times daily for 5 days,[1] 40 mg/kg daily in three divided doses (to a maximum daily dose of 2.4 g) for 3 days,[2] and 400 mg daily for 10 to 20 days.[3] WHO recommends 25 mg/kg daily for 10 days;[4] in the USA, a dose of 250 mg three times daily for 10 days has also been recommended.[5]

1. Padonu KO. A controlled trial of metronidazole in the treatment of dracontiasis in Nigeria. *Am J Trop Med Hyg* 1973; **22:** 42–4.
2. Kale OO. A controlled field trial of the treatment of dracontiasis with metronidazole and niridazole. *Ann Trop Med Parasitol* 1974; **68:** 91–5.
3. Muller R. Guinea worm disease: epidemiology, control, and treatment. *Bull WHO* 1979; **57:** 683–9.
4. WHO. *WHO model prescribing information: drugs used in parasitic diseases.* 2nd ed. Geneva: WHO, 1995.
5. Medical Letter on Drugs and Therapeutics. Drugs for parasitic infections (issued April 2002). Available at: http://www.medicalletter.com/freedocs/parasitic.pdf (accessed 03/06/04)

**Hepatic encephalopathy.** The treatment of hepatic encephalopathy is discussed on p.1243. It includes the use of an antimicrobial such as metronidazole to reduce the intestinal flora.

**Inflammatory bowel disease.** Metronidazole is used in the treatment of perineal Crohn's disease (see Inflammatory Bowel Disease, p.1243) and may also be used in colonic Crohn's disease, when it has been tried with ciprofloxacin. It has also proved effective for the prevention of postsurgical recurrence. Duration of therapy is usually limited to 3 months.

References.

1. Bernstein LH, *et al.* Healing of perineal Crohn's disease with metronidazole. *Gastroenterology* 1980; **79:** 357–65.
2. Brandt LJ, *et al.* Metronidazole therapy for perineal Crohn's disease: a follow-up study. *Gastroenterology* 1982; **83:** 383–7.
3. Ursing B, *et al.* A comparative study of metronidazole and sulfasalazine for active Crohn's disease: the cooperative Crohn's disease study in Sweden. *Gastroenterology* 1982; **83:** 550–62.
4. Sutherland L, *et al.* Double blind, placebo controlled trial of metronidazole in Crohn's disease. *Gut* 1991; **32:** 1071–5.
5. Rutgeerts P, *et al.* Controlled trial of metronidazole treatment for prevention of Crohn's recurrence after ileal resection. *Gastroenterology* 1995; **108:** 1617–21.
6. Prantera C, *et al.* An antibiotic regimen for the treatment of active Crohn's disease: a randomized, controlled clinical trial of metronidazole plus ciprofloxacin. *Am J Gastroenterol* 1996; **91:** 328–32.

**Metabolic disorders.** There are case reports of children with excesses of methylmalonic[1,2] and propionic[3] acid in their blood or urine showing clinical improvement when given metronidazole which reduced the excretion of faecal propionate and urinary methylmalonate. Metronidazole is considered to act through its antimicrobial effect on gut anaerobes that are involved in propionate production; such propionate cannot be handled by these children who are deficient in the relevant enzyme.

1. Bain MD, *et al.* Contribution of gut bacterial metabolism to human metabolic disease. *Lancet* 1988; **i:** 1078–9.
2. Koletzko B, *et al.* Antibiotic therapy for improvement of metabolic control in methylmalonic aciduria. *J Pediatr* 1990; **117:** 99–101.
3. Mellon AF, *et al.* Effect of oral antibiotics on intestinal production of propionic acid. *Arch Dis Child* 2000; **82:** 169–72.

**Mouth disorders and infections.** Ciclosporin-induced gingival hyperplasia resolved in 4 patients following treatment with metronidazole.[1]

Metronidazole is considered to be effective for the treatment of acute necrotising ulcerative gingivitis and is an alternative to penicillin in other dental infections (see Mouth Infections, p.136).

1. Wong W, *et al.* Resolution of cyclosporin-induced gingival hypertrophy with metronidazole. *Lancet* 1994; **343:** 986.

**Peptic ulcer disease.** The use of metronidazole is well established in regimens for eradicating *Helicobacter pylori* (see Peptic Ulcer Disease, p.1246). However, the emergence of metronidazole-resistant strains of *H. pylori* has been associated with an increased rate of treatment failures with some regimens.[1-4] Difficulties arise in assessing metronidazole resistance and in correlating *in-vitro* results with clinical response.[5] In populations in which the incidence of resistance is high, it may become necessary to use alternative regimens,[6] although some clinicians report that regimens containing metronidazole continue to produce adequate response rates.[7]

1. Buckley MJM, *et al.* Metronidazole resistance reduces efficacy of triple therapy and leads to secondary clarithromycin resistance. *Dig Dis Sci* 1997; **42:** 2111–15.
2. Lerang F, *et al.* Highly effective twice-daily triple therapies for Helicobacter pylori infection and peptic ulcer disease: does in vitro metronidazole resistance have any clinical relevance? *Am J Gastroenterol* 1997; **92:** 248–53.
3. Misiewicz JJ, *et al.* One week triple therapy for Helicobacter pylori: a multicentre comparative study. *Gut* 1997; **41:** 735–9.
4. van Zanten SV, *et al.* Adding once-daily omeprazole 20 mg to metronidazole/amoxicillin treatment for Helicobacter pylori gastritis: a randomized, double-blind trial showing the importance of metronidazole resistance. *Am J Gastroenterol* 1998; **93:** 5–10.
5. Goddard AF, Logan RPH. Antimicrobial resistance and Helicobacter pylori. *J Antimicrob Chemother* 1996; **37:** 639–43.
6. Fennerty MB. Should we abandon metronidazole containing Helicobacter pylori treatment regimens? The clinical relevance of metronidazole resistance. *Am J Gastroenterol* 1998; **93:** 2–3.
7. Walt RP. Metronidazole-resistant H pylori—of questionable clinical importance. *Lancet* 1996; **348:** 489–90.

**Skin disorders.** Metronidazole may be effective in the management of malodorous anaerobic skin infections associated with ulceration (p.146), including *pressure sores* and *fungating tumours*. Both the oral and topical routes have been employed but the evidence in favour of its use is largely anecdotal as few randomised controlled trials have yet been performed.[1]

Several studies have indicated that metronidazole by mouth or applied topically is effective in the treatment of *rosacea* (p.1138). Metronidazole 200 mg twice daily by mouth was more effective than placebo[2] and as effective as oral oxytetracycline.[3] Similarly, topical preparations (for example, 0.75% cream, gel, or lotion or 1% cream) have been found to be better than placebo and as effective as oral oxytetracycline.[4,5]

1. Clark J. Metronidazole gel in managing malodorous fungating wounds. *Br J Nurs* 2002 **11** (suppl): S54–S60.
2. Pye RJ, Burton JL. Treatment of rosacea by metronidazole. *Lancet* 1976; **i:** 1211–12.
3. Saihan EM, Burton JL. A double-blind trial of metronidazole versus oxytetracycline therapy for rosacea. *Br J Dermatol* 1980; **102:** 443–5.
4. McClellan KJ, Noble S. Topical metronidazole: a review of its use in rosacea. *Am J Clin Dermatol* 2000; **1:** 191–9.
5. Dahl MV, *et al.* Once-daily topical metronidazole cream formulations in the treatment of the papules and pustules of rosacea. *J Am Acad Dermatol* 2001; **45:** 723–30.

**Surgical infection.** Metronidazole and related nitroimidazoles are used in surgical infection prophylaxis (p.147) to reduce the rate of wound infection.

HAEMORRHOIDECTOMY. Prophylactic metronidazole reduced pain following haemorrhoidectomy in a small study.[1]

1. Carapeti EA, *et al.* Double-blind randomised controlled trial of effect of metronidazole on pain after day-case haemorrhoidectomy. *Lancet* 1998; **351:** 169–72.

**African trypanosomiasis.** Although there is no established alternative treatment for *Trypanosoma brucei rhodesiense* infections that are resistant to melarsoprol (see p.599), metronidazole and suramin were effective in 1 patient.[1]

1. Foulkes JR. Metronidazole and suramin combination in the treatment of arsenical refractory rhodesian sleeping sickness—a case study. *Trans R Soc Trop Med Hyg* 1996; **90:** 422.

## Preparations

***BP 2003:*** Metronidazole Gel; Metronidazole Intravenous Infusion; Metronidazole Oral Suspension; Metronidazole Suppositories; Metronidazole Tablets;

***USP 27:*** Metronidazole Gel; Metronidazole Injection; Metronidazole Tablets.

**Proprietary Preparations** (details are given in Part 3)

***Arg.:*** Bexon; Epaq; Etronil; Flagyl; Format; Ginkan; Metral; Nalox; Noritate; Padet; Repligen; Rozex; Tricofin; Trimstat; ***Austral.:*** Flagyl; Metrogyl; Metronide; Rozex; ***Austria:*** Acsacea; Anaerobex; Ariline; Elyzol; Flagyl†; Oecozol†; Rozex; Trichex; ***Belg.:*** Anaeromet; Flagyl; Pharmaflex; Rozex; ***Braz.:*** Astergyl; Canderme; Dalzolston; Flagyl; Flanizol; Ginovagin†; Helmizol; Metrodax; Metronib†; Metronide†; Metronil; Metronix; Metroval; Metrozol†; Minegyl; Neo Metrodazol; Rozex; ***Canad.:*** Flagyl; Metrocream; Metrogel; NidaGel; Noritate; Novo-Nidazol; Trikacide†; **Chile:** Deprocid; Flagyl; Geloderm; Medazol Gel; Metrocream; Metrogel; Metropast; Noritate; **Denm.:** Elyzol; Flagyl; Metrogel; Rozex; Zidoval; **Fin.:** Elyzol; Flagyl; Rozex; Trikozol; **Fr.:** Elyzol; Flagyl; Rosiced; Rozacreme; Rozagel; Rozex; **Ger.:** Arilin; Clont; Elyzol; Flagyl; Fossyol; Infectoclont; Metrogel; Metronid-Puren; Metronimerck; Metronour; Metront; Ulcolind Metro†; Vagimid; **Gr.:** Colpocin-T; Emedal; Flagyl; Gnostol; Metrogyl; Robaz; **Hong Kong:** Elyzol; Flagyl; Gynoplix; Metole; Metrogyl; Metrozine†; Noritate; Protogyl†; Rozex; Trizele†; Unigo; **India:** Aristogyl; Flagyl; Metrogyl; Monizole; Unimezol; **Irl.:** Anabact; Elyzol†; Flagyl; Metrogel†; Metronide; Metrotop; Rozex; **Israel:** Elyzol; Flagyl; Metrogyl; Noritate; Rozex; Venogyl; Zadstat†; Zidoval; **Ital.:** Deflamon; Elyzol; Flagyl; Pernyzol†; Rosased; Rozex; Vagilen; **Malaysia:** Flagyl; Frotin; Protogyl; Ranigyl; Rozex; Setrozole; **Mex.:** Ameblin; Amiyodazol†; Antral†; Biomona; Biotazol; Cryozol†; Dasmetrol†; Dasolin†; Dualizol; Elyzol; Epaq; Fagizol†; Fartricon; Flagenase; Flagenol; Flaginazol†; Flagyl; Flamin; Fresenizol; Fusanidazol†; Hemestal; Juaflor†; Labitrix†; Lagylan†; Lamblit; Medazol; Medizol; Meredazol†; Metricom†; Metrizol; Metrocream; Metrogel; Metronil†; Metroson; Mibazol†; Niacel†; Nidazolem†; Nidralon; Nidrozol; Nitromidager†; Ortrizol; Otrozol; Planizol; Proflag†; Promibasol; Prozolin; Retofar†; Samonil; Selegil; Servizol; Solumidazol; Valpar; Vatrix-S†; Vertisal; **Neth.:** Flagyl; Metrogel; Rozex; **Norw.:** Elyzol; Flagyl; Rozex; Zidoval; **NZ:** Flagyl; Rozex; Trichozole; **Port.:** Dumozol; Flagyl; Metroderme; Rodermil; **S.Afr.:** Acuzole†; Ambral†; Bemetrazole; Berazole†; Dynametron†; Flagyl; Medamet; Metagyl; Metazol; Metrazole; Metrostat; Narobic; Rozex; Trichazole; Zagyl†; Zobacide; **Singapore:** Anabact†; Elyzol†; Fladex; Flagyl; Metrozole; MND; Nizole; Protogyl†; Rozex; Servizol†; **Spain:** Amotein; Flagyl; Rozex; Tricowas B; **Swed.:** Elyzol; Flagyl; Rozex; Zidoval; **Switz.:** Arilin; Elyzol; Flagyl; Perilox; Rivozol; Rosalox; Rozex; Servizol†; **Thai.:** Anabact†; Asiazole; Biogyl; Elyzol; Flagyl; Klion†; Klont†; Med-Tricocide; Medazyl; Mefiron; Menisole; Mepagyl; Mesolex; Metrazole; Metrocide; Metrogyl; Metrolex; Milanidazole; Servizol†; Tricomed; Unimezol†; Vagil; Vagyl; **UAE:** Negazole; **UK:** Acea; Anabact; Elyzol†; Flagyl; Metrogel; Metrolyl; Metrosa; Metrotop; Metrozol; Noritate; Norzol; Rozex; Vaginyl; Zadstat†; Zidoval; Zyomet; **USA:** Flagyl; Metro†; Metrocream; Metrogel; Metrogel Vaginal; Noritate; Protostat.

**Multi-ingredient: Arg.:** Bexon; Ciprocort; Estilomicin; Farm-X Duo; Farm-X Ginecologico; Flagystatin; Ginal Cent; Ginkan; Linfol; Naxo TV; Vagicural Plus; **Austral.:** Helidac†; Losec Helicopak†; Somac-MA†; **Austria:** Helicocin; **Braz.:** Bio-Vagin; Colpanist†; Colpatrin; Colpist; Colpistar; Colpistatin; Donnagel; Flagyl Nistatina; Fungimax; Ginestatin; Minegyl C/Nistatina; Nistazol; Periodontil; Profargil†; Tricolpex; Trisdazol†; Vagi Biotic†; Vagimax; **Canad.:** Flagystatin; Losec 1-2-3 M; **Fin.:** Flagyl Comp; Helipak A; Helipak T; Losec Helira; **Fr.:** Birodogyl; Rodogyl; **India:** Dyrade-M; Dysfur-M; Entamizole; Flagyl-F; Kaltin MF; Metrogyl-F; Qugyl; **Irl.:** Flagyl Compak†; **Ital.:** Meclon; **Mex.:** Amebyl; Flagenase 400; Flagosil; Flagystatin V; Flamin 400†; Madecassol C; Metodine; Metrodiyod; Metrofur; Norecil; Promibasol-Plus; Rodogyl; Vagitrol-V; **NZ:** Helicosec†; **Singapore:** Flagystatin; Neo-Penotran; **Spain:** Blastoestimulina; Rhodogil; **UK:** Flagyl Compak†; HeliMet; **USA:** Helidac.

## Monensin (BAN, USAN, rINN)

Lilly-67314. 4-{2-[2-Ethyl-3′-methyl-5′-(tetrahydro-6-hydroxy-6-hydroxymethyl-3,5-dimethylpyran-2-yl)perhydro-2,2′-bifuran-5-yl]-9-hydroxy-2,8-dimethyl-1,6-dioxaspiro[4.5]dec-7-yl}3-methoxy-2-methylpentanoic acid.

$C_{36}H_{62}O_{11}$ = 670.9.

*CAS — 17090-79-8.*

**Pharmacopoeias.** In *US* for veterinary use only.

**USP 27** (Monensin). A mixture of antibiotic substances produced by *Streptomyces cinnamonensis*.

## Monensin Sodium (BANM, rINNM)

Monensina sódica.

$C_{36}H_{61}NaO_{11}$ = 692.9.

*CAS — 22373-78-0.*

**Pharmacopoeias.** In *US* for veterinary use only.

**USP 27** (Monensin Sodium). An off-white to tan crystalline powder. Slightly soluble in water; soluble in chloroform and in methyl alcohol; practically insoluble in petroleum spirit. Avoid moisture and excessive heat.

### Profile

Monensin is an antiprotozoal used as the sodium salt in veterinary practice for the prevention of coccidiosis in poultry and as a growth promotor for cattle.

## Narasin (BAN, USAN, rINN)

Compound 79891; Lilly-79891; Narasina. 2-(6-{5-[2-(5-Ethyltetrahydro-5-hydroxy-6-methylpyran-2-yl)-15-hydroxy-2,10,12-trimethyl-1,6,8-trioxadispiro[4.1.5.3]pentadec-13-en-9-yl]-2-hydroxy-1,3-dimethyl-4-oxoheptyl}tetrahydro-3,5-dimethylpyran-2-yl)butyric acid.

$C_{43}H_{72}O_{11}$ = 765.0.

*CAS — 55134-13-9.*

**Pharmacopoeias.** In *US* for veterinary use only.

**USP 27** (Narasin Granular). It contains narasin mixed with suitable carriers and inactive ingredients prepared in a granular form that is free-flowing and free of aggregates. Narasin is a white to off-white crystalline powder. Soluble in water and in methyl alcohol.

### Profile

Narasin, an antibiotic produced by *Streptomyces aureofaciens*, is an antiprotozoal used in veterinary practice for the prevention of coccidiosis in chickens.

## Nicarbazin (BAN)

Nicarbazina. An equimolecular complex of 1,3-bis(4-nitrophenyl)urea ($C_{13}H_{10}N_4O_5$) and 4,6-dimethylpyrimidin-2-ol ($C_6H_8N_2O$).

$C_{19}H_{18}N_6O_6$ = 426.4.

*CAS — 330-95-0.*

### Profile

Nicarbazin is an antiprotozoal used in veterinary practice for the prevention of coccidiosis in poultry.

## Nifuratel (BAN, USAN, rINN)

Methylmercadone. 5-Methylthiomethyl-3-(5-nitrofurfurylideneamino)-2-oxazolidone.

$C_{10}H_{11}N_3O_5S$ = 285.3.

*CAS — 4936-47-4.*

*ATC — G01AX05.*

### Adverse Effects

Adverse effects associated with nifuratel include gastrointestinal disturbances, peripheral neuropathy, and thrombocytopenic purpura. Allergic reactions, hepatotoxicity, blood dyscrasias, and pulmonary reactions similar to those seen with the structurally related drug nitrofurantoin have been reported rarely. Haemolytic anaemia may occur in patients with G6PD deficiency given nifuratel.

**Hypersensitivity.** There have been several reports of contact dermatitis associated with nifuratel, including a report after only one application of nifuratel ointment in a man whose wife was undergoing treatment with nifuratel vaginal pessaries.[1]

1. Bedello PG, *et al.* Contact dermatitis from nifuratel. *Contact Dermatitis* 1983; **9:** 166.

### Precautions

Nifuratel should not be given to patients with renal impairment, neuropathies, or G6PD deficiency.

### Interactions

A disulfiram-like reaction may occur in patients taking alcohol while on nifuratel therapy.

### Pharmacokinetics

When taken by mouth nifuratel is absorbed from the gastrointestinal tract. A metabolite, with activity against bacteria but not against trichomonads, is excreted in the urine.

### Uses and Administration

Nifuratel is a nitrofuran derivative with a broad antimicrobial spectrum. It is active against the protozoan *Trichomonas vaginalis* and has an antibacterial spectrum similar to that of nitrofurantoin and some antifungal activity against *Candida albicans*. Although other drugs are preferred, nifuratel has been used to treat susceptible infections of the genito-urinary tract in doses of 200 to 400 mg three times daily by mouth. It has also been given vaginally.

### Preparations

**Proprietary Preparations** (details are given in Part 3)

**Austria:** Macmiror; **Ger.:** Inimur; **Hong Kong:** Macmiror†; **Ital.:** Macmiror; **Mex.:** Macmiror; **Spain:** Macmiror†; **Switz.:** Macmiror†.

**Multi-ingredient: Hong Kong:** Macmiror Complex†; **Ital.:** Macmiror Complex; **Mex.:** Macmiror Complex V; **Port.:** Dafnegil; **Switz.:** Dafnegil†.

## Nifursol (BAN, USAN, pINN)

3,5-Dinitro-2′-(5-nitrofurfurylidene)salicylohydrazide.

$C_{12}H_7N_5O_9$ = 365.2.

*CAS — 16915-70-1.*

### Profile

Nifursol is an antiprotozoal used in veterinary practice for the prevention of blackhead (histomoniasis) in poultry.

## Nifurtimox (BAN, rINN)

Bayer-2502. Tetrahydro-3-methyl-4-(5-nitrofurfurylideneamino)-1,4-thiazine 1,1-dioxide.

$C_{10}H_{13}N_3O_5S$ = 287.3.

*CAS — 23256-30-6.*

*ATC — P01CC01.*

**Pharmacopoeias.** In *Fr.* and *Int.*

### Adverse Effects

Adverse effects are common with nifurtimox and include gastrointestinal effects such as anorexia with loss of weight, abdominal pain, nausea and vomiting, and effects on the nervous system, especially peripheral neuropathy. Psychoses, CNS excitement, insomnia, drowsiness, headache, myalgia, arthralgia, dizziness, and convulsions have also been reported. Skin rashes and other allergic reactions may occur.

**Mutagenicity.** An increase in chromosomal aberrations has been observed in children given nifurtimox.[1]

1. Gorla NB, *et al.* Thirteenfold increase of chromosomal aberrations non-randomly distributed in chagasic children treated with nifurtimox. *Mutat Res* 1989; **224:** 263–7.

### Pharmacokinetics

Nifurtimox is well absorbed and rapidly metabolised after doses by mouth.

◊ References.

1. Paulas C, *et al.* Pharmacokinetics of a nitrofuran compound, nifurtimox, in healthy volunteers. *Int J Clin Pharmacol Ther Toxicol* 1989; **27:** 454–7.
2. Gonzalez-Martin G, *et al.* The pharmacokinetics of nifurtimox in chronic renal failure. *Eur J Clin Pharmacol* 1992; **42:** 671–3.

### Uses and Administration

Nifurtimox is a nitrofuran derivative with antiprotozoal activity. It is of value in the treatment of American trypanosomiasis (Chagas' disease) due to infection by *Trypanosoma cruzi*, especially the early acute stage of the disease. In African trypanosomiasis it has some activity against *T. brucei gambiense*, the organism responsible for West African sleeping sickness.

Nifurtimox is given orally in divided doses. It is better tolerated by children than by adults. Treatment for American trypanosomiasis is given for 60 to 120 days (but see below). Doses for adults are 8 to 10 mg/kg daily. Doses for children are: aged 1 to 10 years, 15 to 20 mg/kg daily for 90 days; aged 11 to 16 years, 12.5 to 15 mg/kg daily for 90 days.

**Leishmaniasis.** Mucocutaneous leishmaniasis of the New World (p.597) is usually treated with pentavalent antimony or, in those who do not respond, with amphotericin B or pentamidine. However, nifurtimox 10 mg/kg daily for a minimum of 4 weeks has been shown to be effective in cases of mucocutaneous leishmaniasis in Colombia and Brazil. Despite this, toxic effects with nifurtimox are common and its role as a second-line drug or with pentavalent antimony has not been established.[1]

1. WHO. Control of the leishmaniases. *WHO Tech Rep Ser 793,* 1990.

**African trypanosomiasis.** Nifurtimox has been tried as an alternative to melarsoprol or eflornithine in the meningoencephalitic stage of *Trypanosoma brucei gambiense* infection (p.599), but higher doses than those used in American trypanosomiasis are necessary. A good initial response was achieved[1] in 25 patients with nifurtimox 15 mg/kg daily for 60 days, but 3 patients relapsed while still receiving nifurtimox and a further 12 of 19 patients who were followed up relapsed subsequently. An attempt[2] to improve the response by increasing the daily dose even higher to 30 mg/kg for 30 days resulted in substantial toxicity and only a modest improvement in results, with 9 of 25 patients relapsing.

1. Pepin J, *et al.* An open clinical trial of nifurtimox for arseno-resistant Trypanosoma brucei gambiense sleeping sickness in central Zaire. *Trans R Soc Trop Med Hyg* 1989; **83:** 514–17.
2. Pépin J, *et al.* High-dose nifurtimox for arseno-resistant Trypanosoma brucei gambiense sleeping sickness: an open trial in central Zaire. *Trans R Soc Trop Med Hyg* 1992; **86:** 254–6.

**American trypanosomiasis.** The treatment of American trypanosomiasis (p.600) is generally unsatisfactory, but nifurtimox is of value especially in the acute phase. However, there has been controversy over its ability to cure completely, that is to eradicate all parasites, in chronic disease.[1] Doses recommended by WHO[2-4] are 8 to 10 mg/kg daily in three divided doses for adults, and 15 to 20 mg/kg daily in four divided doses for children. WHO recommends that nifurtimox should be given for 60 or 90 days.[2-4] Some in the USA[5] suggest a 90- to 120-day regimen for adults but nifurtimox is not well tolerated and the experience of other workers[1] suggests that few patients may complete the full course.

1. Gutteridge WE. Existing chemotherapy and its limitations. *Br Med Bull* 1985; **41:** 162–8.
2. WHO. *WHO model prescribing information: drugs used in parasitic diseases.* 2nd ed. Geneva: WHO, 1995.
3. WHO. Control of Chagas disease: second report of the WHO expert committee. *WHO Tech Rep Ser 905* 2002.
4. WHO. *WHO model formulary.* Geneva: WHO, 2004.
5. Medical Letter on Drugs and Therapeutics. Drugs for parasitic infections (issued April 2002). Available at: http://www.medicalletter.com/freedocs/parasitic.pdf (accessed 03/06/04)

## Nimorazole (BAN, rINN)

Nimorazol; Nitrimidazine. 4-[2-(5-Nitroimidazol-1-yl)ethyl]morpholine.

$C_9H_{14}N_4O_3$ = 226.2.

*CAS — 6506-37-2.*

*ATC — P01AB06.*

**Pharmacopoeias.** In *It.*

### Adverse Effects and Precautions

As for Metronidazole, p.607.

### Pharmacokinetics

Nimorazole is readily absorbed from the gastrointestinal tract. Peak blood concentrations are achieved within 2 hours, and high concentrations are reported to occur in salivary and vaginal secretions. Trichomonicidal urinary concentrations may persist for up to 48 hours after a dose. It is excreted in the urine together with 2 active metabolites. Unchanged drug and metabolites also appear in breast milk.

### Uses and Administration

Nimorazole is a 5-nitroimidazole derivative. It has antimicrobial actions and uses similar to those of metronidazole (p.609).

In the treatment of trichomoniasis, the usual dose of nimorazole is 2 g by mouth as a single dose with a main meal. It may alternatively be given in a dose of 1 g every 12 hours for three doses, or 250 mg three times daily for 5 to 7 days. Sexual partners should also be treated. In giardiasis or amoebiasis, nimorazole 500 mg to 1 g is given twice daily, usually for 5 to 7 days; a dose for children is 15 to 30 mg/kg daily in divided doses.

Nimorazole may also be used in the treatment of acute ulcerative gingivitis in a dose of 500 mg twice daily for 2 days.

### Preparations

**Proprietary Preparations** (details are given in Part 3)
***Arg.:*** Naxogin; Vagarne; ***Austria:*** Naxogin; ***Belg.:*** Naxogin; ***Braz.:*** Naxogin; ***Chile:*** Naxogin; ***Fr.:*** Naxogyn†; ***Ger.:*** Esclama; ***Hong Kong:*** Naxogin†; ***Mex.:*** Naxogil†; ***Thai.:*** Naxogin†.

**Multi-ingredient:** ***Arg.:*** Vagarne; ***Braz.:*** Floregin Composto†; Floregin†; Naxogin Composto; ***Chile:*** Naxogin Compositum; Naxogin Dos.

## Nitazoxanide *(BAN, USAN, rINN)*

Nitazoxanida; PH-5776. *N*-(5-Nitro-2-thiazolyl)salicylamide acetate.

$C_{12}H_9N_3O_5S = 307.3.$
*CAS — 55981-09-4.*

### Adverse Effects

The most common adverse effects associated with nitazoxanide are abdominal pain and diarrhoea. Nausea and vomiting, flatulence, and increased appetite have also been reported. Headache may occur. Other reported adverse effects include fever, malaise, pruritus, sweating, dizziness, and rhinitis. Discoloration of urine and of the eyes has been reported rarely. Increased creatinine and liver enzyme values have been noted.

### Uses and Administration

Nitazoxanide is used in the treatment of cryptosporidiosis and of giardiasis in children aged 1 to 11 years. It is given with food as an oral suspension for 3 days, in doses of 100 mg twice daily in children aged 1 to 3 years, and 200 mg twice daily in those aged 4 to 11 years. A tablet formulation for use in adults is also under development. Nitazoxanide has also been tried in a number of other protozoal and helminth infections, in particular in immunocompromised patients, including those with AIDS or HIV infection.

◊ References.


1. Doumbo O, *et al.* Nitazoxanide in the treatment of cryptosporidial diarrhea and other intestinal parasitic infections associated with acquired immunodeficiency syndrome in tropical Africa. *Am J Trop Med Hyg* 1997; **56:** 637–9.
2. Romero Cabello R, *et al.* Nitazoxanide for the treatment of intestinal protozoan and helminthic infections in Mexico. *Trans R Soc Trop Med Hyg* 1997; **91:** 701–3.
3. Rossignol J-F, *et al.* Successful treatment of human fascioliosis with nitazoxanide. *Trans R Soc Trop Med Hyg* 1998; **92:** 103–4.
4. Abaza H, *et al.* Nitazoxanide in the treatment of patients with intestinal protozoan and helminthic infections: a report on 546 patients in Egypt. *Curr Ther Res* 1998; **59:** 116–21.
5. Rossignol J-F, *et al.* A double-'blind' placebo-controlled study of nitazoxanide in the treatment of cryptosporidial diarrhoea in AIDS patients in Mexico. *Trans R Soc Trop Med Hyg* 1998; **92:** 663–6.
6. Megraud F, *et al.* Nitazoxanide, a potential drug for eradication of Helicobacter pylori with no cross-resistance to metronidazole. *Antimicrob Agents Chemother* 1998; **42:** 2836–40.
7. Bicart-See A, *et al.* Successful treatment with nitazoxanide of Enterocytozoon bieneusi microsporidiosis in a patient with AIDS. *Antimicrob Agents Chemother* 2000; **44:** 167–8.
8. Abboud P, *et al.* Successful treatment of metronidazole- and albendazole-resistant giardiasis with nitazoxanide in a patient with acquired immunodeficiency syndrome. *Clin Infect Dis* 2001; **32:** 1792–1794.
9. Rossignol J-FA, *et al.* Treatment of diarrhea caused by Cryptosporidium parvum: a prospective randomized, double-blind, placebo-controlled study of nitazoxanide. *J Infect Dis* 2001; **184:** 103–6.
10. Rossignol J-F, *et al.* Treatment of diarrhea caused by Giardia intestinalis and Entamoeba histolytica or E dispar: a randomized, double-blind, placebo-controlled study of nitazoxanide. *J Infect Dis* 2001; **184:** 381–4.
11. Ortiz JJ, *et al.* Randomized clinical study of nitazoxanide compared to metronidazole in the treatment of symptomatic giardiasis in children from Northern Peru. *Aliment Pharmacol Ther* 2001; **15:** 1409–15.
12. Ortiz JJ, *et al.* Comparative clinical studies of nitazoxanide, albendazole and praziquantel in the treatment of ascariasis, trichuriasis and hymenolepiasis in children from Peru. *Trans R Soc Trop Med Hyg* 2002; **96:** 193–6.
13. Amadi B, *et al.*. Effect of nitazoxanide on morbidity and mortality in Zambian children with cryptosporidiosis: a randomised controlled trial. *Lancet* 2002; **360:** 1375–80.
14. Anonymous. Nitazoxanide (Alinia)—a new anti-protozoal agent. *Med Lett Drugs Ther* 2003; **45:** 29–31.


### Preparations

**Proprietary Preparations** (details are given in Part 3)
***Arg.:*** Heliton; ***Braz.:*** Heliton†; ***Mex.:*** Daxon; ***USA:*** Alinia.

**Multi-ingredient:** ***Mex.:*** Heliton.

## Ornidazole *(USAN, rINN)*

Ornidazol; Ro-7-0207. 1-Chloro-3-(2-methyl-5-nitroimidazol-1-yl)propan-2-ol.

$C_7H_{10}ClN_3O_3 = 219.6.$
*CAS — 16773-42-5.*
*ATC — G01AF06; J01XD03; P01AB03.*

### Adverse Effects and Precautions

As for Metronidazole, p.607.

### Pharmacokinetics

Ornidazole is readily absorbed from the gastrointestinal tract and peak plasma concentrations are reached within 3 hours. After repeated oral doses of 500 mg every 12 hours, steady-state peak and trough concentrations are 14 and 6 micrograms/mL respectively.

The plasma elimination half-life of ornidazole is 12 to 14 hours. Less than 15% is bound to plasma proteins. It is widely distributed in body tissues and fluids, including the CSF.

Ornidazole is metabolised in the liver and is excreted in the urine, mainly as conjugates and metabolites, and to a lesser extent in the faeces. Biliary excretion may be important in the elimination of ornidazole and its metabolites.

◊ References.


1. Schwartz DE, Jeunet F. Comparative pharmacokinetic studies of ornidazole and metronidazole in man. *Chemotherapy* 1976; **22:** 19–29.
2. Matheson I, *et al.* Plasma levels after a single oral dose of 1.5 g ornidazole. *Br J Vener Dis* 1977; **53:** 236–9.
3. Schwartz DE, *et al.* Metabolic studies of ornidazole in the rat, in the dog and in man. *Xenobiotica* 1979; **9:** 571–81.
4. Turcant A, *et al.* Pharmacokinetics of ornidazole in neonates and infants after a single intravenous infusion. *Eur J Clin Pharmacol* 1987; **32:** 111–13.
5. Martin C, *et al.* Pharmacokinetics and tissue penetration of a single dose of ornidazole (1,000 milligrams intravenously) for antibiotic prophylaxis in colorectal surgery. *Antimicrob Agents Chemother* 1990; **34:** 1921–4.
6. Bourget P, *et al.* Disposition of ornidazole and its metabolites during pregnancy. *J Antimicrob Chemother* 1995; **35:** 691–6.


**Hepatic impairment.** The elimination of ornidazole after a single intravenous dose of 500 mg was impaired in 10 patients with severe liver cirrhosis when compared with 10 healthy subjects; mean half-lives were 21.9 hours and 14.1 hours respectively.[1] These results suggested that the interval between doses of ornidazole should be doubled in patients with marked hepatic impairment. The need for dose adjustment was confirmed in further studies of patients with other forms of liver disease.[2,3]


1. Taburet AM, *et al.* Pharmacokinetics of ornidazole in patients with severe liver cirrhosis. *Clin Pharmacol Ther* 1986; **40:** 359–64.
2. Bourget P, *et al.* Ornidazole pharmacokinetics in several hepatic diseases. *J Pharmacol Clin* 1988; **7:** 25–32.
3. Taburet AM, *et al.* Pharmacokinetics of ornidazole in patients with acute viral hepatitis, alcoholic cirrhosis, and extrahepatic cholestasis. *Clin Pharmacol Ther* 1989; **45:** 373–9.


**Renal impairment.** The half-life of intravenous ornidazole was not prolonged in a study in patients with advanced chronic renal failure, including those on continuous ambulatory peritoneal dialysis, although total plasma clearance was halved; modification of the usual dosage is not necessary in such patients. However, the drug was removed by haemodialysis and ornidazole should be given after the dialysis session rather than before.[1] In another study[2] the systemic availability and total body clearance of ornidazole were unaffected in chronic renal failure; it was considered that an additional dose should be given before haemodialysis to compensate for removal during that procedure.


1. Merdjan H, *et al.* Pharmacokinetics of ornidazole in patients with renal insufficiency; influence of haemodialysis and peritoneal dialysis. *Br J Clin Pharmacol* 1985; **19:** 211–17.
2. Horber FF, *et al.* High haemodialysis clearance of ornidazole in the presence of a negligible renal clearance. *Eur J Clin Pharmacol* 1989; **36:** 389–93.


### Uses and Administration

Ornidazole is a 5-nitroimidazole derivative. It has the antimicrobial actions of metronidazole and is used similarly (see p.609) in the treatment of susceptible protozoal infections and also in the treatment and prophylaxis of anaerobic bacterial infections.

It is given by mouth after food, or intravenously. Intravenous solutions of ornidazole should be diluted to 5 mg or less per mL and 100 or 200 mL infused over 15 to 30 minutes. It has also been given by vaginal pessary.

In **amoebiasis**, 500 mg of ornidazole is given twice daily by mouth for 5 to 10 days; children are given 25 mg/kg as a single daily dose for 5 to 10 days. Patients with amoebic dysentery may be given 1.5 g as a single daily dose for 3 days; the children's dose is 40 mg/kg daily. In severe amoebic dysentery and amoebic liver abscess, ornidazole may be given by intravenous infusion in a dose of 0.5 to 1 g initially, followed by 500 mg every 12 hours for 3 to 6 days; the children's dose is 20 to 30 mg/kg daily.

In **giardiasis**, 1 or 1.5 g of ornidazole is given by mouth as a single daily dose for 1 or 2 days; the children's dose is 30 or 40 mg/kg daily.

In **trichomoniasis**, a single dose of 1.5 g is given by mouth; alternatively, a 5-day course of ornidazole 500 mg twice daily by mouth may be used. Sexual partners should be treated concomitantly. The children's dose is 25 mg/kg as a single dose by mouth.

For the treatment of **anaerobic bacterial infections,** ornidazole is given by intravenous infusion in an initial dose of 0.5 to 1 g, followed by 1 g daily as a single dose or in two divided doses for 5 to 10 days; oral therapy with 500 mg every 12 hours should be substituted as soon as possible. Children may be given 10 mg/kg intravenously every 12 hours for 5 to 10 days.

For the prevention of postoperative anaerobic bacterial infections, 1 g is given by intravenous infusion about 30 minutes before surgery.

**Administration in hepatic impairment.** In view of the prolonged half-life and reduced clearance of ornidazole reported in patients with hepatic dysfunction (see above), the interval between doses should be doubled in patients with severe hepatic impairment.

**Administration in renal impairment.** The elimination of ornidazole is reported to be largely unaltered in patients with impaired renal function (see under Pharmacokinetics, above). Dosage adjustment is therefore usually unnecessary, although patients receiving haemodialysis should be given a supplemental dose equivalent to one-half of the usual dose before dialysis.

### Preparations

**Proprietary Preparations** (details are given in Part 3)
***Arg.:*** Mebaxol; ***Belg.:*** Tiberal; ***Chile:*** Invigan; ***Fr.:*** Tiberal; ***Gr.:*** Betiral; ***India:*** Oniz; ***Israel:*** Tiberal†; ***Ital.:*** Tiberal†; ***Mex.:*** Danubial; Tiberal†; ***NZ:*** Tiberal; ***Spain:*** Tinerol; ***Switz.:*** Tiberal.

## Paromomycin Sulfate *(rINNM)*

Aminosidin Sulphate; Aminosidine Sulphate; Catenulin Sulphate; Crestomycin Sulphate; Estomycin Sulphate; Hydroxymycin Sulphate; Monomycin A Sulphate; Neomycin E Sulphate; Paromomycin Sulphate *(BANM)*; Paucimycin Sulphate; Sulfato de paromomicina. *O*-2,6-Diamino-2,6-dideoxy-β-L-idopyranosyl-(1→3)-*O*-β-D-ribofuranosyl-(1→5)-*O*-[2-amino-2-deoxy-α-D-glucopyranosyl-(1→4)]-2-deoxystreptamine sulphate.

$C_{23}H_{45}N_5O_{14},xH_2SO_4.$
*CAS — 59-04-1 (paromomycin); 7542-37-2 (paromomycin); 1263-89-4 (paromomycin sulfate).*
*ATC — A07AA06.*

**Pharmacopoeias.** In *Chin., Int., It.,* and *US.*

**USP 27** (Paromomycin Sulfate). The sulfate salt of an antibiotic substance produced by the growth of *Streptomyces rimosus* var. *paromomycinus*, or a mixture of two or more such salts.
A creamy-white to light yellow, odourless or practically odourless, very hygroscopic powder. It loses not more than 5% of its weight on drying. Very soluble in water; insoluble in alcohol, in chloroform, and in ether. pH of a 3% solution in water is between 5.0 and 7.5. Store in airtight containers.

### Adverse Effects, Treatment, and Precautions

As for Neomycin, p.235.

**Effects on the pancreas.** Pancreatitis was associated with use of paromomycin during treatment of cryptosporidiosis in a patient with HIV infection.[1]


1. Tan WW, *et al.* Paromomycin-associated pancreatitis in HIV-related cryptosporidiosis. *Ann Pharmacother* 1995; **29:** 22–4.


### Interactions

As for Neomycin, p.235.

## Antimicrobial Action

Paromomycin is active against various protozoa including *Leishmania* spp., *Entamoeba histolytica*, and *Cryptosporidium* spp. In addition, it has an antibacterial spectrum similar to that of neomycin (p.235). There is cross-resistance between paromomycin and kanamycin, framycetin, neomycin, and streptomycin.

Paromomycin also has anthelmintic properties against tapeworms.

**Antimycobacterial activity.** References.


1. Kanyok TP, *et al.* Activity of aminosidine (paromomycin) for Mycobacterium tuberculosis and Mycobacterium avium. *J Antimicrob Chemother* 1994; **33:** 323–7.
2. Piersimoni C, *et al.* Bacteriostatic and bactericidal activities of paromomycin against Mycobacterium avium complex isolates. *J Antimicrob Chemother* 1994; **34:** 421–4.
3. Kanyok TP, *et al.* In vivo activity of paromomycin against susceptible and multidrug-resistant Mycobacterium tuberculosis and M. avium complex strains. *Antimicrob Agents Chemother* 1994; **38:** 170–3.


## Pharmacokinetics

Paromomycin is poorly absorbed from the gastrointestinal tract and most of the dose is eliminated unchanged in the faeces.

**Parenteral administration.** References.


1. Kanyok TP, *et al.* Pharmacokinetics of intramuscularly administered aminosidine in healthy subjects. *Antimicrob Agents Chemother* 1997; **41:** 982–6.


## Uses and Administration

Paromomycin is an aminoglycoside antibiotic that has been given by mouth in the treatment of intestinal protozoal infections, including amoebiasis, cryptosporidiosis, and giardiasis. It has also been tried parenterally for visceral, and topically for cutaneous, leishmaniasis. For details of these infections and their treatment, see under Choice of Antiprotozoal, p.595. It has been used in the treatment of tapeworm infection, but it is not the treatment of choice. Like neomycin (p.235), it has been used in the suppression of intestinal flora both pre-operatively and in the management of hepatic encephalopathy.

Paromomycin is given as the sulfate although doses are expressed in terms of the base. In intestinal amoebiasis, the dose for both adults and children is the equivalent of paromomycin 25 to 35 mg/kg daily by mouth in 3 divided doses with meals for 5 to 10 days. Similar doses have been tried in cryptosporidiosis.

In taeniasis and other tapeworm infections, a dose of 4 g is given by mouth as a single dose or in divided doses over the course of one hour.

For hepatic coma, 4 g is given daily by mouth in divided doses at regular intervals for 5 to 6 days.

**Leishmaniasis.** Topical treatment with paromomycin 15% plus methylbenzethonium chloride 5 or 12% has produced promising results[1-3] in *cutaneous leishmaniasis* (p.597); paromomycin 12 to 15% with urea 10% was better tolerated.[4] However, benefit has not been seen in all studies.[5,6] Treatment with topical paromomycin plus systemic meglumine antimonate was initially promising in patients with New World cutaneous leishmaniasis;[7] however, a subsequent study[8] found no clear advantage over treatment with meglumine antimonate alone. Good responses to parenteral paromomycin 14 mg/kg daily, in combination with sodium stibogluconate 10 mg/kg daily, in cases of *diffuse cutaneous leishmaniasis* have also been reported.[9]

Paromomycin has also been used intramuscularly, either alone[10] or with sodium stibogluconate,[11] in the treatment of *visceral leishmaniasis* in an area of India with increasing resistance to pentavalent antimony compounds. The authors of one study[10] found paromomycin 16 or 20 mg/kg daily for 21 days to be significantly more effective than sodium stibogluconate 20 mg/kg daily for 30 days and suggested that paromomycin be considered as first-line treatment for visceral leishmaniasis in this region.


1. El-On J, *et al.* Topical treatment of Old World cutaneous leishmaniasis caused by Leishmania major: a double-blind control study. *J Am Acad Dermatol* 1992; **27:** 227–31.
2. Krause G, Kroeger A. Topical treatment of American cutaneous leishmaniasis with paromomycin and methylbenzethonium chloride: a clinical study under field conditions in Ecuador. *Trans R Soc Trop Med Hyg* 1994; **88:** 92–4.
3. Arana BA, *et al.* Randomized, controlled, double-blind trial of topical treatment of cutaneous leishmaniasis with paromomycin plus methylbenzethonium chloride ointment in Guatemala. *Am J Trop Med Hyg* 2001; **65:** 466–70.
4. Bryceson ADM, *et al.* Treatment of Old World cutaneous leishmaniasis with aminosidine ointment: results of an open study in London. *Trans R Soc Trop Med Hyg* 1994; **88:** 226–8.
5. Ben Salah A, *et al.* A randomized, placebo-controlled trial in Tunisia treating cutaneous leishmaniasis with paromomycin ointment. *Am J Trop Med Hyg* 1995; **53:** 162–6.
6. Asilian A, *et al.* A randomized, placebo-controlled trial of a two week regimen of aminosidine (paromomycin) ointment for treatment of cutaneous leishmaniasis in Iran. *Am J Trop Med Hyg* 1995; **53:** 648–51.
7. Soto J, *et al.* Successful treatment of New World cutaneous leishmaniasis with a combination of topical paromomycin/methylbenzethonium chloride and injectable meglumine antimonate. *Clin Infect Dis* 1995; **20:** 47–51.
8. Soto J, *et al.* Topical paromomycin/methylbenzethonium chloride plus parenteral meglumine antimonate as treatment for American cutaneous leishmaniasis: controlled study. *Clin Infect Dis* 1998; **26:** 56–8.
9. Teklemariam S, *et al.* Aminosidine and its combination with sodium stibogluconate in the treatment of diffuse cutaneous leishmaniasis caused by Leishmania aethiopica. *Trans R Soc Trop Med Hyg* 1994; **88:** 334–9.
10. Jha TK, *et al.* Randomised controlled trial of aminosidine (paromomycin) v sodium stibogluconate for treating visceral leishmaniasis in North Bihar, India. *BMJ* 1998; **316:** 1200–5.
11. Thakur CP, *et al.* A prospective randomized, comparative, open-label trial of the safety and efficacy of paromomycin (aminosidine) plus sodium stibogluconate versus sodium stibogluconate alone for the treatment of visceral leishmaniasis. *Trans R Soc Trop Med Hyg* 2000; **94:** 429–31.


**Trichomoniasis.** Local application of a paromomycin cream has been tried in a small number of patients with metronidazole-resistant vaginal trichomoniasis (p.599) with moderate success.[1]


1. Nyirjesy P, *et al.* Difficult-to-treat trichomoniasis: results with paromomycin cream. *Clin Infect Dis* 1998; **26:** 986–8.


## Preparations

***USP 27:*** Paromomycin Sulfate Capsules; Paromomycin Sulfate Syrup.

**Proprietary Preparations** (details are given in Part 3)
***Austria:*** Humatin; ***Belg.:*** Gabbroral; ***Canad.:*** Humatin; ***Ger.:*** Humatin; ***Hong Kong:*** Gabbromicina†; ***Ital.:*** Gabbroral; Humatin; Kaman; ***Spain:*** Humatin; ***Switz.:*** Humatin; ***USA:*** Humatin.

**Multi-ingredient:** ***Braz.:*** Leshcutan†; ***Israel:*** Leshcutan.

# Pentamidine Isetionate *(BANM, rINNM)*

Isetionato de pentamidina; M&B-800; Pentamidine Diisetionate; Pentamidine Isethionate; Pentamidini Diisetionas; Pentamidini Isethionas. 4,4′-(Pentamethylenedioxy)dibenzamidine bis(2-hydroxyethanesulphonate).

$C_{19}H_{24}N_4O_2,2C_2H_6O_4S = 592.7.$

*CAS — 100-33-4 (pentamidine); 140-64-7 (pentamidine isetionate).*

*ATC — P01CX01.*

**Pharmacopoeias.** In *Eur.* (see p.vi) and *Int.*

**Ph. Eur. 5.0** (Pentamidine Diisetionate; Pentamidine Isetionate BP 2003). A white or almost white powder or colourless crystals; it is hygroscopic. Freely soluble in water; sparingly soluble in alcohol; practically insoluble in dichloromethane. A 5% solution in water has a pH of 4.5 to 6.5. Store in airtight containers.

**Incompatibility.** Immediate precipitation was observed when a solution of pentamidine isetionate 3 mg/mL in glucose 5% was mixed with each of 5 cephalosporin and 1 cephamycin injections.[1]

Pentamidine isetionate is reported to be incompatible with foscarnet


1. Lewis JD, El-Gendy A. Cephalosporin-pentamidine isethionate incompatibilities. *Am J Health-Syst Pharm* 1996; **53:** 1461–2.


# Pentamidine Mesilate *(BANM, rINNM)*

Mesilato de pentamidina; Pentamidine Dimethylsulphonate; Pentamidine Mesylate; Pentamidine Methanesulphonate; RP-2512. Pentamidine dimethanesulphonate.

$C_{19}H_{24}N_4O_2,2CH_3SO_3H = 532.6.$

*CAS — 6823-79-6.*

**Pharmacopoeias.** In *Int.*

## Adverse Effects

Pentamidine is a toxic drug and adverse effects are frequent and sometimes severe when given parenterally; fatalities have been reported. Renal impairment is common, usually manifesting as mild and reversible raised blood urea nitrogen and serum creatinine concentrations, but acute renal failure can occur. Raised liver enzyme values and haematological disturbances such as leucopenia, anaemia, and occasionally thrombocytopenia, may develop. Hypoglycaemia, sometimes followed by hyperglycaemia and type 1 diabetes mellitus, is well documented; there have been occasional reports of acute pancreatitis.

The rapid intravenous injection of pentamidine has resulted in sudden hypotension and immediate reactions such as dizziness, headache, vomiting, breathlessness, tachycardia, and fainting. Hypotension may also occur when pentamidine is given intramuscularly or by slow intravenous infusion. Intramuscular pentamidine often causes pain, swelling, sterile abscess formation, and tissue necrosis at the site of injection. Similar damage can follow extravasation during intravenous administration.

Other adverse effects reported include hypocalcaemia, hyperkalaemia, skin rashes, the Stevens-Johnson syndrome, fever, flushing, gastrointestinal effects such as nausea, vomiting, and taste disturbances, confusion, hallucinations, and cardiac arrhythmias.

Pentamidine is not as toxic when administered by inhalation for the prophylaxis of *Pneumocystis carinii* pneumonia. The commonest adverse effects with this route are cough and bronchoconstriction and may be controlled by a bronchodilator. Inhalation may leave a bitter taste. Pneumothorax has been reported, but may be associated with the disease. There have been rare reports of adverse effects such as those observed when pentamidine is given by injection.

**Incidence of adverse effects.** Adverse effects were observed in 46.8% of 404 patients given pentamidine parenterally for the treatment of *Pneumocystis carinii* pneumonia, according to an analysis from the CDC in the USA.[1] The reactions included impaired renal function (23.5% of patients), abnormal liver function (9.6%), hypoglycaemia (6.2%), haematological disturbances (4.2%), skin rashes (1.5%), and hypocalcaemia (1.2%). Local reactions at injection sites such as pain and abscess occurred in 18.3% and immediate side-effects such as hypotension in 9.6%. Retrospective studies[2-4] suggest that adverse reactions occur more commonly in patients with AIDS.

An evaluation of pentamidine in the treatment of 82 patients with visceral leishmaniasis further illustrates its toxicity.[5] Cardiotoxicity (tachycardia, hypotension, and ECG changes of non-specific myocarditis), occurred in about 23% of patients. No hypoglycaemic reaction was noted, but 4 patients developed diabetes mellitus and 3 of them were found to be insulin-dependent. Other adverse reactions included gastrointestinal effects (anorexia, nausea, vomiting, abdominal pain, or diarrhoea) in about 78%, CNS effects (headache associated with flushing, delirium, or sensory disturbances resembling pins and needles) in about 24%, mild reversible albuminuria in about 7%, and allergic manifestations (generalised urticaria, itching, and conjunctival congestion) in about 5%. One patient had severe anaphylaxis.


1. Walzer PD, *et al.* Pneumocystis carinii pneumonia in the United States: epidemiologic, diagnostic and clinical features. *Ann Intern Med* 1974; **80:** 83–93.
2. Lachaal M, Venuto RC. Nephrotoxicity and hyperkalemia in patients with acquired immunodeficiency syndrome treated with pentamidine. *Am J Med* 1989; **87:** 260–3.
3. Briceland LL, Bailie GR. Pentamidine-associated nephrotoxicity and hyperkalemia in patients with AIDS. *DICP Ann Pharmacother* 1991; **25:** 1171–4.
4. O'Brien JG, *et al.* A 5-year retrospective review of adverse drug reactions and their risk factors in human immunodeficiency virus-infected patients who were receiving intravenous pentamidine therapy for Pneumocystis carinii pneumonia. *Clin Infect Dis* 1997; **24:** 854–9.
5. Jha TK. Evaluation of diamidine compound (pentamidine isethionate) in the treatment of resistant cases of kala-azar occurring in North Bihar, India. *Trans R Soc Trop Med Hyg* 1983; **77:** 167–70.


**Effects on carbohydrate metabolism.** As reported, above, pentamidine can have a range of effects on carbohydrate metabolism. Four patients receiving pentamidine for *Pneumocystis carinii* pneumonia developed severe fasting hypoglycaemia followed later by hyperglycaemia and type 1 diabetes mellitus.[1] It has been suggested that pentamidine has a toxic effect on the β-cells of the pancreatic islets and can induce an early cytolytic release of insulin and hypoglycaemia, followed by β-cell destruction, insulin deficiency, and diabetes mellitus.[1,2] AIDS patients appear to be highly susceptible and have a higher incidence of hypoglycaemia due to pentamidine.[3] The action on the pancreas has led to fatal acute *pancreatitis*;[4-6] fatal hypoglycaemia has also been reported.[7] These reports[1-5,7] involved pentamidine given by injection; pancreatitis[8,9] and diabetes mellitus[10,11] have also been reported in patients given pentamidine by aerosol inhalation.


1. Bouchard P, *et al.* Diabetes mellitus following pentamidine-induced hypoglycemia in humans. *Diabetes* 1982; **31:** 40–5.
2. Osei K, *et al.* Diabetogenic effect of pentamidine: in vitro and in vivo studies in a patient with malignant insulinoma. *Am J Med* 1984; **77:** 41–6.
3. Stahl-Bayliss CM, *et al.* Pentamidine-induced hypoglycemia in patients with the acquired immune deficiency syndrome. *Clin Pharmacol Ther* 1986; **39:** 271–5.
4. Salmeron S, *et al.* Pentamidine and pancreatitis. *Ann Intern Med* 1986; **105:** 140–1.
5. Zuger A, *et al.* Pentamidine-associated fatal acute pancreatitis. *JAMA* 1986; **256:** 2383–5.
6. Sauleda J, *et al.* Probable pentamidine-induced acute pancreatitis. *Ann Pharmacother* 1994; **28:** 52–3.
7. Sattler FR, Waskin H. Pentamidine and fatal hypoglycemia. *Ann Intern Med* 1987; **107:** 789–90.
8. Herer B, *et al.* Pancreatitis associated with pentamidine by aerosol. *BMJ* 1989; **298:** 605.
9. Hart CC. Aerosolized pentamidine and pancreatitis. *Ann Intern Med* 1989; **111:** 691.
10. Fisch A. Diabetes mellitus in a patient with AIDS after treatment with pentamidine aerosol. *BMJ* 1990; **301:** 875.
11. Chen JP, *et al.* Diabetes after aerosolized pentamidine. *Ann Intern Med* 1991; **114:** 913–14.


**Effects on the cardiovascular system.** *Hypotension* is a problem with intravenous pentamidine, but can be reduced by infusing the dose over 60 minutes, when the incidence of hypotension appears to be similar to that with the intramuscular route.[1,2] Intravenous pentamidine has also been associated with *torsade de pointes*.[3-5]


1. Navin TR, Fontaine RE. Intravenous versus intramuscular administration of pentamidine. *N Engl J Med* 1984; **311:** 1701.
2. Helmick CG, Green JK. Pentamidine-associated hypotension and route of administration. *Ann Intern Med* 1985; **103:** 480.
3. Harel Y, *et al.* Pentamidine-induced torsade de pointes. *Pediatr Infect Dis J* 1993; **12:** 692–4.
4. Miller HC. Cardiac arrest after intravenous pentamidine in an infant. *Pediatr Infect Dis J* 1993; **12:** 694–6.
5. Zanetti LAF, Oliphant CM. Pentamidine-induced torsade de pointes. *Ann Pharmacother* 1994; **28:** 282–3.


**Effects on the kidneys.** In an analysis[1] of the adverse effects of parenteral pentamidine (see also above), *nephrotoxicity* was often the most serious adverse reaction, although it was impossible to attribute it solely to pentamidine. Severe renal impairment occurred in 15 of 404 patients and contributed materially to 12 of 14 ensuing deaths. However, elevation of blood urea nitrogen was usually relatively mild and reversible in those patients who had normal pretreatment renal function and had received no other nephrotoxic agents. In two studies in patients with AIDS,[2,3] severe nephrotoxicity (increase in serum creatinine concentration of 0.5 mg per 100 mL) was reported in about 40% of patients. Analysis of risk factors suggested that the development of adverse reactions to parenteral pentamidine is correlated with the total dose received and the duration of treatment,[2,3] but not with the initial degree of renal function.[2] It has been observed that renal toxicity is more common when pentamidine is given intramuscularly, rather than intravenously, to AIDS patients with diarrhoea, suggesting that fluid status might have an important role.[4] There have been instances of renal failure occurring when pentamidine is inhaled as an aerosol for its local effect.[5,6]


1. Walzer PD, *et al.* Pneumocystis carinii pneumonia in the United States: epidemiologic, diagnostic and clinical features. *Ann Intern Med* 1974; **80:** 83–93.
2. Briceland LL, Bailie GR. Pentamidine-associated nephrotoxicity and hyperkalemia in patients with AIDS. *DICP Ann Pharmacother* 1991; **25:** 1171–4.
3. O'Brien JG, *et al.* A 5-year retrospective review of adverse drug reactions and their risk factors in human immunodeficiency virus-infected patients who were receiving intravenous pentamidine therapy for Pneumocystis carinii pneumonia. *Clin Infect Dis* 1997; **24:** 854–9.
4. Stehr-Green JK, Helmick CG. Pentamidine and renal toxicity. *N Engl J Med* 1985; **313:** 694–5.
5. Miller RF, *et al.* Acute renal failure after nebulised pentamidine. *Lancet* 1989; **i:** 1271–2.
6. Chapelon C, *et al.* Renal insufficiency with nebulised pentamidine. *Lancet* 1989; **ii:** 1045–6.


**Effects on the respiratory system.** Although inhaled pentamidine has produced reactions that are normally associated with the parenteral route, the main problem following inhalation is bronchoconstriction;[1] it can be prevented by prior use of a bronchodilator. Acute eosinophilic pneumonia associated with nebulised pentamidine administration has been reported in a patient.[2] Concern has also been expressed at the risks to those who are with the patient at the time of inhalation and are exposed to nebulised pentamidine.[3-5]


1. Smith DE, *et al.* Reversible bronchoconstriction with nebulised pentamidine. *Lancet* 1988; **ii:** 905.
2. Dupon M, *et al.* Acute eosinophilic pneumonia induced by inhaled pentamidine isethionate. *BMJ* 1993; **306:** 109.
3. McDiarmid MA, Jacobson-Kram D. Aerosolised pentamidine and public health. *Lancet* 1989; **ii:** 863–4.
4. Thomas SHL, *et al.* Aerosolised pentamidine. *Lancet* 1989; **ii:** 1284.
5. Smaldone GC, *et al.* Detection of inhaled pentamidine in health care workers. *N Engl J Med* 1991; **325:** 891–2.


## Precautions

Pentamidine should be used under close supervision and great care is necessary if it is used in patients suffering from any condition likely to be exacerbated by its adverse effects. The CSF should be checked for signs of CNS involvement before giving pentamidine for trypanosomiasis, since it is unlikely to be effective in such cases. Patients should remain supine during administration and their blood pressure should be monitored. Kidney and liver function, blood-glucose concentrations, blood and platelet counts, and other parameters indicative of developing toxicity, such as serum-calcium concentrations and the ECG, should also be assessed regularly during courses of treatment with pentamidine.

Patients with a history of asthma or smoking may be at increased risk of cough and bronchospasm during inhalation of nebulised pentamidine. Symptoms may be controlled by giving a bronchodilator before pentamidine. Pentamidine solution should not be mixed with other drugs nor should a bronchodilator be given in the same nebuliser. Extrapulmonary *P. carinii* infections may occur in patients receiving nebulised pentamidine and should be considered in patients with unexplained signs and symptoms. Precautions should be taken to minimise atmospheric pollution with pentamidine during nebulisation and to minimise exposure of medical personnel to pentamidine.

## Interactions

Use of pentamidine with other nephrotoxic drugs such as amphotericin B or foscarnet should preferably be avoided. Extreme caution is also necessary if pentamidine is given with other drugs, such as foscarnet, that can cause hypocalcaemia. There is an increased risk of ventricular arrhythmias if pentamidine is given with drugs which prolong the QT interval such as amiodarone, levacetylmethadol, or terfenadine. There may be an increased risk of pancreatitis when intravenous pentamidine is used with didanosine or zalcitabine and such combinations should be avoided.

## Pharmacokinetics

After intravenous doses of the isetionate, pentamidine is rapidly distributed to body tissues and this is followed by a prolonged elimination phase. Elimination half-lives of 6 hours following intravenous infusion and 9 hours following intramuscular injection have been cited, but probably represent an intermediate value, and terminal elimination half-lives of between several days and weeks have been reported. During repeated dosing accumulation is believed to occur, particularly in the liver and kidneys, and only small concentrations of pentamidine are found in the urine.

Distribution to the lung is relatively poor following administration by injection. Systemic absorption after inhalation is reported to result in peak plasma concentrations of 5 to 10% of those after parenteral administration, and there have been a few reports of systemic adverse effects. Particle or droplet size appears to be important in achieving adequate pulmonary distribution.

◊ References.


1. O'Doherty MJ, *et al.* Differences in relative efficiency of nebulisers for pentamidine administration. *Lancet* 1988; **ii:** 1283–6.
2. Simonds AK, *et al.* Aerosolised pentamidine. *Lancet* 1989; **i:** 221–2.
3. Baskin MI, *et al.* Regional deposition of aerosolized pentamidine: effects of body position and breathing pattern. *Ann Intern Med* 1990; **113:** 677–83.
4. Bronner U, *et al.* Pentamidine concentrations in plasma, whole blood and cerebrospinal fluid during treatment of Trypanosoma gambiense in Côte d'Ivoire. *Trans R Soc Trop Med Hyg* 1991; **85:** 608–11.
5. Lidman C, *et al.* Plasma pentamidine concentrations vary between individuals with Pneumocystis carinii pneumonia and the drug is actively secreted by the kidney. *J Antimicrob Chemother* 1994; **33:** 803–10.
6. Bronner U, *et al.* Pharmacokinetics and adverse reactions after a single dose of pentamidine in patients with Trypanosoma gambiense sleeping sickness. *Br J Clin Pharmacol* 1995; **39:** 289–95.
7. Conte JE, Golden JA. Intrapulmonary and systemic pharmacokinetics of aerosolized pentamidine used for prophylaxis of Pneumocystis carinii pneumonia in patients infected with the human immunodeficiency virus. *J Clin Pharmacol* 1995; **35:** 1166–73.


**Renal impairment.** In a study[1] of patients with normal renal function or on haemodialysis, renal clearance of pentamidine during the 24 hours after intravenous use was 2.1% of the plasma clearance in those with normal renal function, suggesting that pentamidine elimination would be largely unaffected by renal impairment. In those with end-stage renal disease on haemodialysis the terminal elimination half-life after a single dose was prolonged to about 75 hours, compared with 30 hours in the patients with normal renal function, but the volumes of distribution and area under the concentration-time curve were not significantly different. In patients with normal or mildly impaired renal function who had received between 12 and 21 doses, the terminal elimination half-life after the final dose was about 12 days and pentamidine was still detectable in the plasma after 6 weeks. There was evidence of accumulation of pentamidine during repeated daily dosing.


1. Conte JE. Pharmacokinetics of intravenous pentamidine in patients with normal renal function or receiving hemodialysis. *J Infect Dis* 1991; **163:** 169–75.


## Uses and Administration

Pentamidine, an aromatic diamidine derivative, is an antiprotozoal used in the treatment of the early stages of African trypanosomiasis, especially *Trypanosoma brucei gambiense* infections, and in some forms of leishmaniasis. It is also used in the treatment and prophylaxis of *Pneumocystis carinii* pneumonia. It may act by several mechanisms, including interference with protozoal DNA and folate transformation and by inhibition of RNA and protein synthesis.

Pentamidine has been given as the isetionate or mesilate salt, but the isetionate is the only form now available in most countries. There is considerable confusion in the literature regarding the dosage of pentamidine since it is often not clear whether doses are being expressed in terms of pentamidine base, the isetionate salt, or the mesilate salt. In general it would appear that when the isetionate is used doses are expressed in terms of pentamidine isetionate, whereas when the mesilate is used doses are expressed in terms of pentamidine base. Pentamidine isetionate 4 mg/kg is approximately equivalent to pentamidine base 2.3 mg/kg; pentamidine mesilate 3.6 mg/kg is approximately equivalent to pentamidine base 2.3 mg/kg.

Pentamidine isetionate is given by deep intramuscular injection or by slow intravenous infusion over at least 60 minutes; direct intravenous injection must be avoided. Patients should be lying down. The mesilate has usually been given intramuscularly.

In the treatment of early **African trypanosomiasis** due to *T. b. gambiense*, pentamidine isetionate 4 mg/kg may be given daily or on alternate days by intramuscular injection or intravenous infusion to a total of 7 to 10 doses. Pentamidine is not effective in trypanosomiasis with CNS involvement, but 2 doses of pentamidine may be given in late-stage *T. b. gambiense* infection before starting treatment with melarsoprol or eflornithine.

In the treatment of visceral **leishmaniasis**, and of mucocutaneous leishmaniasis due to *Leishmania braziliensis* or *L. aethiopica* that have not responded to antimonials, pentamidine isetionate 4 mg/kg may be given, preferably intramuscularly three times weekly, for 5 to 25 weeks or longer. An alternative regimen in visceral leishmaniasis is to give 3 to 4 mg/kg on alternate days to a maximum of 10 injections; the course may need to be repeated. In cutaneous leishmaniasis due to *L. aethiopica* or *L. guyanensis*, pentamidine isetionate 3 to 4 mg/kg may be given, preferably intramuscularly once or twice weekly, until the condition resolves. A weekly dose of 3 to 4 mg/kg is also used for diffuse cutaneous leishmaniasis due to *L. aethiopica* and should be continued for at least 4 months after parasites are no longer detectable on skin smears.

In the treatment of ***Pneumocystis carinii*** pneumonia, pentamidine isetionate 4 mg/kg is given once daily for 14 days or longer, by intramuscular injection or preferably slow intravenous infusion. Pentamidine isetionate is given by inhalation through a nebuliser to prevent *P. carinii* pneumonia in HIV-positive patients in a dose of 300 mg once every 4 weeks; in those who cannot tolerate this dose 150 mg every 2 weeks may be used. It has also occasionally been used by this route for treating mild to moderate *P. carinii* infection in a dose of 600 mg daily for 3 weeks. Nebuliser design can affect the droplet size delivered and hence the amount of pentamidine reaching sites of action within the lungs. The optimal particle size is 1 to 2μ m. Precautions should be taken to minimise atmospheric pollution with pentamidine during nebulisation and to minimise exposure of medical personnel to the drug.

**Administration in renal impairment.** Since renal clearance accounts for only a small proportion of pentamidine elimination, dosage adjustment is not generally considered necessary for mild to moderate degrees of renal impairment. The UK manufacturer recommends dosage reductions in patients with *P. carinii* pneumonia who have a creatinine clearance of less than 10 mL/minute. In patients with life-threatening disease the recommended dose of 4 mg/kg daily should be given for 7 to 10 days and then on alternate days for the remainder of the 14-dose course. In less severe disease the suggested dose is 4 mg/kg on alternate days for 14 doses.

**Amoebic infections.** ACANTHAMOEBA INFECTIONS. Pentamidine was used to treat disseminated *Acanthamoeba* infection (p.595) without evidence of CNS involvement in 2 immunocompromised patients.[1,2] It is unlikely that pentamidine would be effective in infections involving the CNS.


1. Slater CA, *et al.* Brief report: successful treatment of disseminated Acanthamoeba infection in an immunocompromised patient. *N Engl J Med* 1994; **331:** 85–7.
2. Murakawa GJ, *et al.* Disseminated Acanthamoeba in patients with AIDS: a report of five cases and a review of the literature. *Arch Dermatol* 1995; **131:** 1291–6.

**Babesiosis.** Pentamidine has been tried for babesiosis (p.595), but while some patients showed clinical improvements,[1-3] the value of pentamidine in this infection was considered to be doubtful.[4]


1. Francioli PB, *et al.* Response of babesiosis to pentamidine therapy. *Ann Intern Med* 1981; **94:** 326–30.
2. Raoult D, *et al.* Babesiosis, pentamidine, and cotrimoxazole. *Ann Intern Med* 1987; **107:** 944.
3. Clarke CS, *et al.* Babesiosis: under-reporting or case-clustering? *Postgrad Med J* 1989; **65:** 591–3.
4. Teutsch SM, Juranek DD. Babesiosis. *Ann Intern Med* 1981; **95:** 241.


**Leishmaniasis.** Pentamidine has been used in the treatment of visceral leishmaniasis (p.597) both alone and with antimonials in patients who have failed to respond to antimonials alone.[1,2] It has also been tried for long-term secondary prophylaxis in patients with HIV infection.[3] Cutaneous leishmaniasis due to *L. guyanensis* is usually treated with pentamidine to reduce the risk of dissemination;[1] beneficial results in patients infected with *L. infantum, L. major*, or *L. tropica* have also been reported.[4] Lesions due to *L. aethiopica* may also respond to pentamidine, but can be left to heal spontaneously since the risk of diffuse cutaneous involvement is small.[1] Diffuse cutaneous or mucocutaneous disease which is unresponsive to antimonials may respond to pentamidine, especially when due to *L. aethiopica*.[1]


1. WHO. *WHO model prescribing information: drugs used in parasitic diseases.* 2nd ed. Geneva: WHO, 1995.
2. Baily GG, Nandy A. Visceral leishmaniasis: more prevalent and more problematic. *J Infect* 1994; **29:** 241–7.
3. Pérez-Molina JA, *et al.* Pentamidine isethionate as secondary prophylaxis against visceral leishmaniasis in HIV-positive patients. *AIDS* 1996; **10:** 237–8.
4. Hellier I, *et al.* Treatment of Old World cutaneous leishmaniasis by pentamidine isethionate: an open study of 11 patients. *Dermatology* 2000; **200:** 120–3.


**Pneumocystis carinii pneumonia.** In the treatment of *Pneumocystis carinii* pneumonia (p.389) intravenous pentamidine is generally reserved for patients who do not respond to, or cannot tolerate, co-trimoxazole.[1,2] Co-trimoxazole with pentamidine is no more effective than pentamidine alone in these patients and is potentially more toxic than either drug.[3] Inhaled pentamidine has occasionally been suggested for mild to moderate infection, but is now generally only used for prophylaxis. However, patients receiving inhaled pentamidine may be prone to extrapulmonary *Pneumocystis* infections.[4,5]

In both primary and secondary prophylaxis of *P. carinii* pneumonia in immunocompromised patients, co-trimoxazole has been preferred to inhaled pentamidine. Comparative studies have shown that, in the short term, inhaled pentamidine has been less effective than co-trimoxazole[6,7] and no more effective than the other common prophylactic drug, dapsone.[8,9] In addition, both co-trimoxazole and dapsone (given with pyrimethamine) also provide protection against toxoplasmosis and extrapulmonary *P. carinii* infections. However, inhaled pentamidine is better tolerated than either of the alternatives, and studies have suggested that in the long term the efficacy of the three drugs is comparable,[10,11] at least in patients with CD4+ T lymphocyte counts of more than 100 cells/microlitre. Increasing the dose of pentamidine from 300 mg every four weeks to 300 mg every two weeks[12,13] or 600 mg every week[14] may improve efficacy further.


1. Anonymous. Prevention and treatment of Pneumocystis carinii pneumonia in patients infected with HIV. *Drug Ther Bull* 1994; **32:** 12–15.
2. Medical Letter on Drugs and Therapeutics. Drugs for parasitic infections (issued April 2002). Available at: http://www.medicalletter.com/freedocs/parasitic.pdf (accessed 03/06/04)
3. PCP Therapy Project Group. Assessment of therapy for Pneumocystis carinii pneumonia. *Am J Med* 1984; **76:** 501–8.
4. Witt K, *et al.* Dissemination of Pneumocystis carinii in patients with AIDS. *Scand J Infect Dis* 1991; **23:** 691–5.
5. Sha BE, *et al.* Pneumocystis carinii choroiditis in patients with AIDS: clinical features, response to therapy, and outcome. *J Acquir Immune Defic Syndr Hum Retrovirol* 1992; **5:** 1051–8.
6. Schneider MME, *et al.* A controlled trial of aerosolized pentamidine or trimethoprim-sulfamethoxazole as primary prophylaxis against Pneumocystis carinii pneumonia in patients with human immunodeficiency virus infection. *N Engl J Med* 1992; **327:** 1836–41.
7. Hardy WD, *et al.* A controlled trial of trimethoprim-sulfamethoxazole or aerosolized pentamidine for secondary prophylaxis of Pneumocystis carinii pneumonia in patients with the acquired immunodeficiency syndrome. *N Engl J Med* 1992; **327:** 1842–8.
8. Girard P-M, *et al.* Dapsone-pyrimethamine compared with aerosolized pentamidine as primary prophylaxis against Pneumocystis carinii pneumonia and toxoplasmosis in HIV infection. *N Engl J Med* 1993; **328:** 1514–20.
9. Torres RA, *et al.* Randomized trial of dapsone and aerosolized pentamidine for the prophylaxis of Pneumocystis carinii pneumonia and toxoplasmic encephalitis. *Am J Med* 1993; **95:** 573–83.
10. Bozzette SA, *et al.* A randomized trial of three antipneumocystis agents in patients with advanced human immunodeficiency virus infection. *N Engl J Med* 1995; **332:** 693–9.
11. Rizzardi GP, *et al.* Risks and benefits of aerosolized pentamidine and cotrimoxazole in primary prophylaxis of Pneumocystis carinii pneumonia in HIV-1-infected patients: a two-year Italian multicentric randomized controlled trial. *J Infect* 1996; **32:** 123–31.
12. Kronawitter U, *et al.* Low incidence of Pneumocystis carinii pneumonia in HIV patients receiving 300 mg pentamidine aerosol every 2 weeks. *Clin Invest* 1992; **70:** 1089–91.
13. Rizzardi GP, *et al.* Better efficacy of twice-monthly than monthly aerosolised pentamidine for secondary prophylaxis of Pneumocystis carinii pneumonia in patients with AIDS: an Italian multicentric randomised controlled trial. *J Infect* 1995; **31:** 99–105.
14. Ong ELC, *et al.* Efficacy and effects on pulmonary function tests of weekly 600 mg aerosol pentamidine as prophylaxis against Pneumocystis carinii pneumonia. *Infection* 1992; **20:** 136–9.


**African trypanosomiasis.** Pentamidine is used for the haematolymphatic phase of African trypanosomiasis caused by *Trypanosoma brucei gambiense* (p.599), and as an adjunct to other treatment for the meningoencephalitic stage of the infection.[1] It is reported to be less effective against *T. b. rhodesiense* and in some areas resistance of *T. b. gambiense* to pentamidine is increasing.[2] Pentamidine has been used with suramin for *T. b. gambiense* infections but this has not been shown to be clinically superior to pentamidine alone.[3]


1. WHO. Control and surveillance of African trypanosomiasis: report of a WHO expert committee. *WHO Tech Rep Ser 881* 1998.
2. WHO. *WHO model prescribing information: drugs used in parasitic diseases.* 2nd ed. Geneva: WHO, 1995.
3. Pépin J, Khonde N. Relapses following treatment of early-stage Trypanosoma brucei gambiense sleeping sickness with a combination of pentamidine and suramin. *Trans R Soc Trop Med Hyg* 1996; **90:** 183–6.


### Preparations

***BP 2003:*** Pentamidine Injection.

**Proprietary Preparations** (details are given in Part 3)
***Austria:*** Pentacarinat; ***Belg.:*** Pentacarinat; ***Braz.:*** Pentacarinat; ***Canad.:*** Pentacarinat; ***Denm.:*** Pentacarinat; ***Fin.:*** Pentacarinat; ***Fr.:*** Pentacarinat; ***Ger.:*** Pentacarinat; ***Gr.:*** Pentacarinat; ***Irl.:*** Pentacarinat; ***Israel:*** Pentacarinat; ***Ital.:*** Pentacarinat; Pneumopent†; ***Mex.:*** Pentam†; ***Neth.:*** Pentacarinat; ***Norw.:*** Pentacarinat†; ***NZ:*** Pentacarinat; ***Port.:*** Pentacarinat; Pentamina; ***S.Afr.:*** Pentacarinat†; ***Spain:*** Pentacarinat; ***Swed.:*** Pentacarinat; ***Switz.:*** Pentacarinat; ***Thai.:*** Pentacarinat; ***UK:*** Pentacarinat; ***USA:*** NebuPent; Pentacarinat; Pentam.

## Quinfamide *(USAN, rINN)*

Win-40014. 1-(Dichloroacetyl)-1,2,3,4-tetrahydroquinolin-6-ol 2-furoic acid ester.

$C_{16}H_{13}Cl_2NO_4$ = 354.2.
*CAS — 62265-68-3.*

### Profile

Quinfamide is a luminal amoebicide. It is given by mouth for intestinal amoebiasis in a dose of 300 mg, either as a single dose or as three divided doses over 24 hours.

### Preparations

**Proprietary Preparations** (details are given in Part 3)
***Mex.:*** Amefin; Amefur; Amenox; Celemin; Falacid; Luminovag; Protosin; Quinfamex†; Quocel.

## Robenidine Hydrochloride *(BANM, USAN, rINNM)*

CL-78116; Hidrocloruro de robenidina; Robenzidene Hydrochloride. 1,3-Bis(4-chlorobenzylideneamino)guanidine hydrochloride.

$C_{15}H_{13}Cl_2N_5,HCl$ = 370.7.
*CAS — 25875-51-8 (robenidine); 25875-50-7 (robenidine hydrochloride).*

### Profile

Robenidine is an antiprotozoal used as the hydrochloride in veterinary practice for the prevention of coccidiosis in poultry and rabbits.

## Ronidazole *(BAN, USAN, pINN)*

Ronidazol. (1-Methyl-5-nitroimidazol-2-yl)methyl carbamate.

$C_6H_8N_4O_4$ = 200.2.
*CAS — 7681-76-7.*

**Pharmacopoeias.** In *BP(Vet).*

**BP(Vet) 2003** (Ronidazole). A white to yellowish-brown, odourless or almost odourless powder. Slightly soluble in water, in alcohol, and in chloroform; very slightly soluble in ether. Protect from light.

### Profile

Ronidazole is a 5-nitroimidazole antiprotozoal that is used in veterinary practice for the control of trichomoniasis in cage birds and pigeons. It has also been added to turkey feeding stuffs and has been used for the control of swine dysentery.

## Salinomycin Sodium *(BANM, rINNM)*

AHR-3096 (salinomycin); K-364 (salinomycin); K-748364A (salinomycin); Salinomicina sódica. Sodium (2R)-2-{(2R,5S,6R)-6-[(1S,2S,3S,5R)-5-{(2S,5S,7R,9S,10S,12R,15R)-2-[(2R,5R,6S)-5-ethyltetrahydro-5-hydroxy-6-methylpyran-2-yl]-15-hydroxy-2,10,12-trimethyl-1,6,8-trioxadispiro[4.1.5.3]pentadec-13-en-9-yl}-2-hydroxy-1,3-dimethyl-4-oxoheptyl]tetrahydro-5-methylpyran-2-yl}butyrate.

$C_{42}H_{69}NaO_{11}$ = 773.0.
*CAS — 53003-10-4 (salinomycin); 55721-31-8 (salinomycin sodium).*

### Profile

Salinomycin, an antibiotic produced by *Streptomyces albus*, is an antiprotozoal used as the sodium salt in veterinary practice for the prevention of coccidiosis in poultry and as a growth promotor in pigs.

## Secnidazole *(BAN, rINN)*

PM-185184; 14539-RP; RP-14539; Secnidazol. 1-(2-Methyl-5-nitroimidazol-1-yl)propan-2-ol.

$C_7H_{11}N_3O_3$ = 185.2.
*CAS — 3366-95-8.*
*ATC — P01AB07.*

### Profile

Secnidazole is a 5-nitroimidazole derivative with properties similar to those of metronidazole (p.607), apart from a much longer plasma half-life of 20 hours or more. It is used in the treatment of amoebiasis, giardiasis, and trichomoniasis.

Secnidazole is given by mouth, usually as a single dose of 2 g in adults or 30 mg/kg in children. In invasive (hepatic) amoebiasis a dose of 1.5 g daily is given in single or divided doses for 5 days; children may be given 30 mg/kg daily.

◊ References.


1. Gillis JC, Wiseman LR. Secnidazole: a review of its antimicrobial activity, pharmacokinetic properties and therapeutic use in the management of protozoal infections and bacterial vaginosis. *Drugs* 1996; **51:** 621–38.


### Preparations

**Proprietary Preparations** (details are given in Part 3)
***Arg.:*** Flagentyl; ***Braz.:*** Deprozol; Neodazol; Secni-Plus; Secnid†; Secnidal; Secnidalin; Secnizol; Tecnid; ***Fr.:*** Flagentyl†; Secnol; ***India:*** Noameba-DS; Secnil; ***Mex.:*** Minovag; Sabima; Secnidal; ***Port.:*** Flagentyl.
**Multi-ingredient: *Arg.:*** Gynerium; ***Mex.:*** Sporasec.

## Semduramicin *(BAN, USAN, rINN)*

Semduramicina; UK-61689; UK-61689-2 (semduramicin sodium). (2R,3S,4S,5R,6S)-Tetrahydro-2,4-dihydroxy-6-{(R)-1-[(2S,5R,7S,8R,9S)-9-hydroxy-2,8-dimethyl-2-{(2S,2′R,3′S,5′R)-octahydro-2-methyl-5′-[(2S,3S,5R,6S)-tetrahydro-6-hydroxy-3,5,6-trimethyl-2H-pyran-2-yl]-3′-[(2S, 5S, 6R)-tetrahydro-5-methoxy-6-methyl-2H-pyran-2-yloxy]-2,2′-bifuran-5-yl}-1,6-dioxaspiro[4.5]dec-7-yl]ethyl}-5-methoxy-3-methyl-2H-pyran-2-ylacetic acid.

$C_{45}H_{76}O_{16}$ = 873.1.
*CAS — 113378-31-7 (semduramicin); 119068-77-8 (semduramicin sodium).*

### Profile

Semduramicin is an antiprotozoal used in veterinary practice for the prevention of coccidiosis in poultry. It is also used as the sodium salt.

# Suramin Sodium

Antrypol; Bayer-205; CI-1003; Fourneau-309; Naganinum; Naganol; Suramin Hexasodium *(USAN)*; Suramina sódica. The symmetrical 3″-urea of the sodium salt of 8-(3-benzamido-4-methylbenzamido)naphthalene-1,3,5-trisulphonic acid; Hexasodium 8,8′-{carbonylbis[imino-3,1-phenylenecarbonylimino(4-methyl-3,1-phenylene)carbonylimino]}bis(1,3,5-naphthalenetrisulfonate).

$C_{51}H_{34}N_6Na_6O_{23}S_6$ = 1429.2.
*CAS — 145-63-1 (suramin); 129-46-4 (suramin sodium).*
*ATC — P01CX02.*

**Pharmacopoeias.** In *Fr., Int.*, and *It.*

## Adverse Effects

An immediate and potentially fatal reaction, with nausea, vomiting, shock, seizures, and loss of consciousness, may follow the injection of suramin sodium in some patients and thus it is usual practice to give a small test dose before starting treatment.

Abdominal pain, mouth ulceration, and skin reactions such as urticaria and pruritus may occur. The risk of hypersensitivity reactions is reported to be greater when onchocerciasis is present.

Other adverse effects include paraesthesia, hyperaesthesia of the palms and soles, skin eruptions, blood dyscrasias, fever, polyuria, increased thirst, raised liver enzyme values, fatigue, and effects on the eye including photophobia and lachrymation. Proteinuria is common; haematuria and casts in the urine may also occur. There have been occasional reports of adrenal insufficiency.

**Effects on the blood.** Thrombocytopenia has been reported in patients receiving suramin, generally during treatment for AIDS or cancer.[1-4] An immune-mediated mechanism has been proposed[3] although there is evidence that multiple mechanisms may be involved.[4] Other adverse effects on the blood include neutropenia,[1,5] anaemia,[1] deterioration of pre-existing lymphocytopenia,[5] and fatal myelosuppression.[5] Agranulocytosis and haemolytic anaemia have occurred rarely.

1. Levine AM, *et al.* Suramin antiviral therapy in the acquired immunodeficiency syndrome. *Ann Intern Med* 1986; **105:** 32–7.
2. Arlt W, *et al.* Suramin in adrenocortical cancer: limited efficacy and serious toxicity. *Clin Endocrinol (Oxf)* 1994; **41:** 299–307.
3. Seidman AD, *et al.* Immune-mediated thrombocytopenia secondary to suramin. *Cancer* 1993; **71:** 851–4.
4. Tisdale JF, *et al.* Severe thrombocytopenia in patients treated with suramin: evidence for an immune mechanism in one. *Am J Hematol* 1996; **51:** 152–7.
5. Rosen PJ, *et al.* Suramin in hormone-refractory metastatic prostate cancer: a drug with limited efficacy. *J Clin Oncol* 1996; **14:** 1626–36.

**Effects on the eyes.** Late effects on the eyes associated with suramin include photophobia, lachrymation, and palpebral oedema. Keratopathy characterised by corneal deposits has been reported in patients receiving suramin. In a study of 114 patients receiving suramin for prostatic cancer, 13 developed corneal deposits similar to those reported with chloroquine therapy after 34 to 98 days of therapy.[1] Symptoms in 10 of the 13 included lachrymation and foreign body sensation. The remaining 3 patients were asymptomatic. Shifts in refractive error were also found. Keratopathy has also been reported in patients with AIDS receiving suramin.[2] In patients treated with suramin for ocular onchocerciasis, the incidence of optic atrophy was higher after 3 years than in untreated patients.[3] A prolonged inflammatory response to dying microfilariae in the optic nerve might be responsible, although a direct toxic or allergic effect could not be ruled out.

1. Hemady RK, *et al.* Ocular symptoms and signs associated with suramin sodium treatment for metastatic cancer of the prostate. *Am J Ophthalmol* 1996; **121:** 291–6.
2. Teich SA, *et al.* Toxic keratopathy associated with suramin therapy. *N Engl J Med* 1986; **314:** 1455–6.
3. Thylefors B, Rolland A. The risk of optic atrophy following suramin treatment of ocular onchocerciasis. *Bull WHO* 1979; **57:** 479–80.

**Effects on the kidneys.** In addition to the proteinuria commonly seen during suramin therapy, there have been reports of individual cases of renal glycosuria[1] and of acute renal dysfunction.[2]

1. Awadzi K, *et al.* The chemotherapy of onchocerciasis XVIII: aspects of treatment with suramin. *Trop Med Parasitol* 1995; **46:** 19–26.
2. Figg WD, *et al.* Acute renal toxicity associated with suramin in the treatment of prostate cancer. *Cancer* 1994; **74:** 1612–14.

**Effects on the nervous system.** Neurological disorders reported in patients receiving suramin include paraesthesia and polyneuropathy. Severe polyneuropathy with generalised flaccid paralysis has generally been associated with serum-suramin concentrations greater than 350 micrograms/mL,[1,2] but motor neuropathy was reported in 8 patients with serum concentrations of 275 micrograms/mL.[3]

1. La Rocca RV, *et al.* Suramin-induced polyneuropathy. *Neurology* 1990; **40:** 954–60.
2. Arlt W, *et al.* Suramin in adrenocortical cancer: limited efficacy and serious toxicity. *Clin Endocrinol (Oxf)* 1994; **41:** 299–307.
3. Bitton RJ, *et al.* Pharmacologic variables associated with the development of neurologic toxicity in patients treated with suramin. *J Clin Oncol* 1995; **13:** 2223–9.

**Effects on the skin.** Pruritus and urticaria may occur as hypersensitivity reactions to suramin. Late skin reactions include erythematous maculopapular rashes.[1] Severe reactions including erythema multiforme,[2] exfoliative dermatitis, and fatal toxic epidermal necrolysis[3,4] have been reported.

1. O'Donnell BP, *et al.* Suramin-induced skin reactions. *Arch Dermatol* 1992; **128:** 75–9.
2. Katz SK, *et al.* Erythema multiforme induced by suramin. *J Am Acad Dermatol* 1995; **32:** 292–3.
3. May E, Allolio B. Fatal toxic epidermal necrolysis during suramin therapy. *Eur J Cancer* 1991; **27:** 1338.
4. Falkson G, Rapoport BL. Lethal toxic epidermal necrolysis during suramin treatment. *Eur J Cancer* 1992; **28A:** 1294.

## Precautions

Suramin sodium should be used under close supervision, and the general condition of patients improved as far as possible before treatment starts. Patients who have a severe reaction to the first dose should never receive suramin again. It should not be used in elderly or infirm patients or in the presence of severe hepatic or renal disease. The urine should be tested before treatment starts and weekly during treatment; dosage should be reduced if moderate proteinuria develops and stopped if it becomes severe or if casts appear in the urine.

**Pregnancy.** Suramin has been reported to be teratogenic in *mice* but not in *rats*.[1] WHO[2] recommends that when necessary suramin should be used in pregnant women with *T. b. rhodesiense* trypanosomiasis, even those with meningoencephalitic disease, because melarsoprol is contra-indicated; in onchocerciasis, suramin treatment should be delayed until after delivery.

1. Mercier-Parot L, Tuchmann-Duplessis H. Action abortive et tératogène d'un trypanocide, la suramine. *C R Soc Biol* 1973; **167:** 1518–22.
2. WHO. *WHO model prescribing information: drugs used in parasitic diseases.* 2nd ed. Geneva: WHO, 1995.

## Pharmacokinetics

After intravenous injection, suramin becomes bound to plasma proteins and plasma concentrations over 100 micrograms/mL are maintained for several weeks. Unbound suramin is excreted in the urine. Penetration of suramin into the CSF appears to be poor.

◊ The clinical pharmacokinetics of suramin were studied in 4 patients with AIDS given 6.2 g intravenously over 5 weeks.[1] Suramin accumulated during treatment and plasma concentrations exceeded 100 micrograms/mL for several weeks. After the last dose the terminal half-life of suramin ranged from 44 to 54 days. At least 99.7% was bound to plasma proteins. Renal clearance accounted for most of the elimination of suramin from the body. There appeared to be little or no metabolism of suramin.

In another study,[2] ten male patients with onchocerciasis received weekly infusions of suramin for 6 weeks, according to the dose regimen recommended by WHO (see below). In these patients the median elimination half-life was about 92 days, and in each case, the maximum plasma concentration remained below 300 micrograms/mL.

1. Collins JM, *et al.* Clinical pharmacokinetics of suramin in patients with HTLV-III/LAV infection. *J Clin Pharmacol* 1986; **26:** 22–6.
2. Chijioke CP, *et al.* Clinical pharmacokinetics of suramin in patients with onchocerciasis. *Eur J Clin Pharmacol* 1998; **54:** 249–51.

## Uses and Administration

Suramin is a trypanocide used in the treatment of African trypanosomiasis and as an anthelmintic in the treatment of onchocerciasis.

Suramin is given as suramin sodium by slow intravenous injection, usually as a 10% solution. Because of the danger of severe reactions it is advisable to give a test dose before initiating treatment.

In African trypanosomiasis suramin is used mainly for the early (haematolymphatic) stages of *Trypanosoma brucei rhodesiense* infection; pentamidine may be preferred for early-stage treatment of *T. b. gambiense* infection. Suramin is not used as sole therapy for late-stage infections with CNS involvement. Early-stage trypanosomiasis may be treated with a dose of 5 mg/kg of suramin on day 1, 10 mg/kg on day 3, then 20 mg/kg on days 5, 11, 17, 23, and 30. Another schedule consists of 5 doses of 1 g given over 3 weeks following a test dose of 100 to 200 mg. In late-stage trypanosomiasis injections of suramin are often given before starting treatment with melarsoprol; 5 and 10 mg/kg are given on days 1 and 3 respectively, and in some regimens 20 mg/kg is also given on day 5.

For doses used in onchocerciasis see below.

**Malignant neoplasms.** Suramin is reported to have antineoplastic activity and has been studied in a number of malignant neoplasms, in particular hormone-resistant prostatic cancer (p.521). However, its clinical usefulness is hindered by dose-limiting toxicity and problems in developing a simple dose schedule.

References.

1. Stein CA, *et al.* Suramin: an anticancer drug with a unique mechanism of action. *J Clin Oncol* 1989; **7:** 499–508.
2. Kilbourn RG. Suramin: new therapeutic concepts for an old drug. *Cancer Bull* 1991; **43:** 265–7.
3. Rapoport BL, *et al.* Suramin in combination with mitomycin C in hormone-resistant prostate cancer: a phase II clinical study. *Ann Oncol* 1993; **4:** 567–73.
4. Woll PJ, *et al.* Suramin for breast and prostate cancer: a pilot study of intermittent short infusions without adaptive controls. *Ann Oncol* 1994; **5:** 597–600.
5. Arlt W, *et al.* Suramin in adrenocortical cancer: limited efficacy and serious toxicity. *Clin Endocrinol (Oxf)* 1994; **41:** 299–307.
6. Eisenberger MA, Reyno LM. Suramin. *Cancer Treat Rev* 1994; **20:** 259–73.
7. Rosen PJ, *et al.* Suramin in hormone-refractory metastatic prostate cancer: a drug with limited efficacy. *J Clin Oncol* 1996; **14:** 1626–36.
8. Small EJ, *et al.* Suramin therapy for patients with symptomatic hormone-refractory prostate cancer: results of a randomized phase III trial comparing suramin plus hydrocortisone to placebo plus hydrocortisone. *J Clin Oncol* 2000; **18:** 1440–50.

**Onchocerciasis.** Although suramin is the only drug in clinical use for onchocerciasis that is effective against adult worms, its use is restricted because of the frequency of associated complications and its intrinsic toxicity. Treatment of onchocerciasis (p.100) is currently based on continuous suppression of microfilariae by regular use of ivermectin. WHO[1] advises that suramin should only be considered for the curative treatment of individuals in areas without transmission of onchocerciasis and of individuals leaving an endemic area, and for severe hyperreactive onchodermatitis where symptoms are not adequately controlled with ivermectin. WHO[2,3] also recommends that it should not be used to treat onchocerciasis in the elderly or infirm, in patients with severe liver or renal disease, in children aged less than 10 years, in totally blind patients (unless they require relief from intensely itchy lesions), in light to moderately infected people with no symptoms and whose eyes are not at risk, or in pregnant women (who should be treated after delivery).

A total dose of 66.7 mg/kg in six incremental weekly doses is recommended.[1-3] The first (test) dose of suramin sodium 3.3 mg/kg should be given very cautiously by slow intravenous injection; this is followed at weekly intervals by incremental doses of 6.7 mg/kg, 10.0 mg/kg, 13.3 mg/kg, 16.7 mg/kg and 16.7 mg/kg.[3]

1. WHO. Onchocerciasis and its control: report of a WHO expert committee. *WHO Tech Rep Ser 852* 1995.
2. WHO. *WHO model prescribing information: drugs used in parasitic diseases.* 2nd ed. Geneva: WHO, 1995.
3. WHO. *WHO model formulary.* Geneva: WHO, 2004.

**African trypanosomiasis.** Suramin is used in the treatment of the early haematolymphatic phase of African trypanosomiasis (p.599) caused by *Trypanosoma brucei rhodesiense* and for *T. b. gambiense* infections which are resistant to pentamidine.[1] In some regions, suramin is used with pentamidine for *T. b. gambiense* infections but it has not been shown to be clinically superior to pentamidine alone.[2] Although suramin does not reach sufficient concentrations in the CSF to produce a cure in the meningoencephalitic phase, it is used to reduce the number of trypanosomes in the blood and lymph before treatment with melarsoprol.[1] Case reports have suggested that suramin with metronidazole[3] or eflornithine[4] could be useful in *T. b. rhodesiense* infections, although response to suramin plus eflornithine was disappointing in a study involving 6 patients.[5]

1. WHO. *WHO model prescribing information: drugs used in parasitic diseases.* 2nd ed. Geneva: WHO, 1995.
2. Pépin J, Khonde N. Relapses following treatment of early-stage Trypanosoma brucei gambiense sleeping sickness with a combination of pentamidine and suramin. *Trans R Soc Trop Med Hyg* 1996; **90:** 183–6.
3. Foulkes JR. Metronidazole and suramin combination in the treatment of arsenical refractory rhodesian sleeping sickness—a case study. *Trans R Soc Trop Med Hyg* 1996; **90:** 422.
4. Taelman H, *et al.* Combination treatment with suramin and eflornithine in late stage rhodesian trypanosomiasis: case report. *Trans R Soc Trop Med Hyg* 1996; **90:** 572–3.
5. Clerinx J, *et al.* Treatment of late stage rhodesiense trypanosomiasis using suramin and eflornithine: report of six cases. *Trans R Soc Trop Med Hyg* 1998; **92:** 449–50.

## Preparations

**Proprietary Preparations** (details are given in Part 3)
**Ger.:** Germanin.

---

# Teclozan *(USAN, rINN)*

NSC-107433; Teclozán; Win-13146. *NN'*-*p*-Phenylenedimethylenebis[2,2-dichloro-*N*-(2-ethoxyethyl)acetamide].

$C_{20}H_{28}Cl_4N_2O_4$ = 502.3.
*CAS — 5560-78-1.*
*ATC — P01AC04.*

## Profile

Teclozan, a dichloroacetamide derivative, is a luminal amoebicide with actions and uses similar to those of diloxanide furoate (p.604). It has been given by mouth in the treatment of intestinal amoebiasis.

## Preparations

**Proprietary Preparations** (details are given in Part 3)
**Braz.:** Falmonox.

---

# Tenonitrozole *(rINN)*

TC-109; Tenonitrozol; Thenitrazole. *N*-(5-Nitrothiazol-2-yl)thiophene-2-carboxamide.

$C_8H_5N_3O_3S_2$ = 255.3.
*CAS — 3810-35-3.*
*ATC — P01AX08.*

## Profile

Tenonitrozole is an antiprotozoal given in the treatment of trichomoniasis (p.599). It is given by mouth in a dose of 250 mg twice daily with meals, for 4 days.

## Preparations

**Proprietary Preparations** (details are given in Part 3)
**Fr.:** Atrican.

---

# Ternidazole *(rINN)*

Ternidazol. 2-Methyl-5-nitroimidazole-1-propanol.

$C_7H_{11}N_3O_3$ = 185.2.
*CAS — 1077-93-6.*

## Profile

Ternidazole is a 5-nitroimidazole antiprotozoal with properties similar to those of metronidazole (p.607). It has been an ingredient of preparations used for the treatment of vaginitis.

### Preparations

**Proprietary Preparations** (details are given in Part 3)
**Multi-ingredient:** ***Fr.:*** Tergynan†.

## Tilbroquinol *(pINN)*

7-Bromo-5-methylquinolin-8-ol.
$C_{10}H_8BrNO$ = 238.1.
*CAS — 7175-09-9.*
*ATC — P01AA05.*

### Profile

Tilbroquinol is a halogenated hydroxyquinoline antiprotozoal with properties similar to those of diiodohydroxyquinoline (p.603). It has been used with tiliquinol (below) in the treatment of intestinal infections including amoebiasis but less toxic drugs are preferred.

**Adverse effects.** A report of neurotoxicity, considered to be subacute myelo-opticoneuropathy, in a patient who had taken tilbroquinol together with tiliquinol for 4 years.[1] Hepatotoxicity has also been reported[2] with this combination.

1. Soffer M, *et al.* Oxyquinoline toxicity. *Lancet* 1983; **i:** 709.
2. Caroli-Bosc F-X, *et al.* Hépatite aiguë due à l'association de tiliquinol et tilbroquinol (Intétrix). *Gastroenterol Clin Biol* 1996; **20:** 605–6.

### Preparations

**Proprietary Preparations** (details are given in Part 3)
***Fr.:*** Intetrix P†.
**Multi-ingredient:** ***Fr.:*** Intetrix.

## Tiliquinol *(rINN)*

5-Methylquinolin-8-ol.
$C_{10}H_9NO$ = 159.2.
*CAS — 5541-67-3.*

### Profile

Tiliquinol has been used with tilbroquinol (above) in the treatment of intestinal infections including amoebiasis but less toxic drugs are preferred.

### Preparations

**Proprietary Preparations** (details are given in Part 3)
**Multi-ingredient:** ***Fr.:*** Intetrix.

## Tinidazole *(BAN, USAN, rINN)*

CP-12574; Tinidazol; Tinidazolum. 1-[2-(Ethylsulphonyl)ethyl]-2-methyl-5-nitroimidazole.
$C_8H_{13}N_3O_4S$ = 247.3.
*CAS — 19387-91-8.*
*ATC — J01XD02; P01AB02.*

**Pharmacopoeias.** In *Chin., Eur.* (see p.vi), *Jpn, Pol.,* and *US.*

**Ph. Eur. 5.0** (Tinidazole). An almost white or pale yellow, crystalline powder. Practically insoluble in water; soluble in acetone and in dichloromethane; sparingly soluble in methyl alcohol. Protect from light.

**USP 27** (Tinidazole). An almost white or pale yellow crystalline powder. Practically insoluble in water; soluble in acetone and in dichloromethane; sparingly soluble in methyl alcohol. Store in airtight containers. Protect from light.

### Adverse Effects and Precautions

As for Metronidazole, p.607.

**Breast feeding.** The American Academy of Pediatrics[1] considers that the use of tinidazole by mothers during breast feeding may be of concern, since it is mutagenic *in vitro.* Following single-dose therapy, breast feeding may be discontinued for 12 to 24 hours to allow excretion of the dose.

1. American Academy of Pediatrics. The transfer of drugs and other chemicals into human milk. *Pediatrics* 2001; **108:** 776–89. Correction. *ibid.*; 1029. Also available at: http://aappolicy.aappublications.org/cgi/content/full/pediatrics%3b108/3/776 (accessed 03/06/04)

**Porphyria.** Tinidazole is considered to be unsafe in patients with porphyria because it has been shown to be porphyrinogenic in *in-vitro* systems.

**Shock.** An acute severe toxic reaction, considered not to be allergic, occurred in a healthy subject shortly after the intravenous infusion of tinidazole 1.6 g over 80 minutes.[1] He fainted for about 10 seconds and low blood pressure, nausea, and tiredness persisted for several hours. Spasms in the left arm were also experienced but no generalised convulsions.

1. Aase S, *et al.* Severe toxic reaction to tinidazole. *Eur J Clin Pharmacol* 1983; **24:** 425–7.

### Interactions

Tinidazole may, like metronidazole (p.608), produce a disulfiram-like reaction with alcohol.

### Pharmacokinetics

The pharmacokinetics of tinidazole resemble those of metronidazole although the half-life is longer.

Tinidazole is rapidly and almost completely absorbed after oral doses and, typically, a peak plasma concentration of about 40 micrograms/mL is achieved 2 hours after a single 2-g dose, falling to about 10 micrograms/mL at 24 hours and 2.5 micrograms/mL at 48 hours; concentrations above 8 micrograms/mL are maintained by daily maintenance doses of 1 g. Comparable concentrations are achieved with equivalent intravenous doses. The plasma elimination half-life of tinidazole is 12 to 14 hours.

Tinidazole is widely distributed and concentrations similar to those in plasma have been achieved in bile, breast milk, CSF, saliva, and a variety of body tissues; it crosses the placenta readily. Only 12% is reported to be bound to plasma proteins. An active hydroxy metabolite has been identified.

Unchanged drug and metabolites are excreted in the urine and, to a lesser extent, in the faeces.

◊ References.

1. Wood BA, *et al.* The pharmacokinetics, metabolism and tissue distribution of tinidazole. *J Antimicrob Chemother* 1982; **10** (suppl A): 43–57.
2. Karhunen M. Placental transfer of metronidazole and tinidazole in early human pregnancy after a single infusion. *Br J Clin Pharmacol* 1984; **18:** 254–7.
3. Evaldson GR, *et al.* Tinidazole milk excretion and pharmacokinetics in lactating women. *Br J Clin Pharmacol* 1985; **19:** 503–7.
4. Wood SG, *et al.* Pharmacokinetics and metabolism of $^{14}$C-tinidazole in humans. *J Antimicrob Chemother* 1986; **17:** 801–9.

**Renal impairment.** Single-dose studies indicate that the pharmacokinetics of tinidazole in patients with chronic renal failure are not significantly different from those in healthy subjects and that no modification of tinidazole dosage is necessary. However, tinidazole is rapidly removed by haemodialysis.[1,2]

1. Flouvat BL, *et al.* Pharmacokinetics of tinidazole in chronic renal failure and in patients on haemodialysis. *Br J Clin Pharmacol* 1983; **15:** 735–41.
2. Robson RA, *et al.* Tinidazole pharmacokinetics in severe renal failure. *Clin Pharmacokinet* 1984; **9:** 88–94.

### Uses and Administration

Tinidazole is a 5-nitroimidazole derivative. It has the antimicrobial actions of metronidazole and is used similarly (see p.609) in the treatment of susceptible protozoal infections and in the treatment and prophylaxis of anaerobic bacterial infections. It has also been used in regimens for the eradication of *Helicobacter pylori* in peptic ulcer disease.

Tinidazole is usually given as a single daily dose by mouth with or after food; it is also given by intravenous infusion and as vaginal pessaries.

In invasive **amoebiasis**, tinidazole is usually given with a luminal amoebicide. In intestinal amoebiasis, a single daily dose of 2 g is given by mouth for 2 or 3 days; in hepatic amoebiasis, 1.5 to 2 g as a single daily dose may be given for 3 days or occasionally up to 6 days. Children are given 50 to 60 mg/kg daily for 3 or 5 days respectively.

A single dose of tinidazole 2 g is given by mouth in the treatment of **giardiasis, trichomoniasis**, and acute necrotising **ulcerative gingivitis**; 50 to 75 mg/kg as a single dose is given to children with giardiasis or trichomoniasis. It may sometimes be necessary to repeat this dose once. In trichomoniasis, sexual partners should also be treated.

In **bacterial vaginosis**, a single 2-g dose of tinidazole is usually given by mouth, although higher cure rates have been achieved with a 2-g dose on 2 successive days.

For the treatment of most **anaerobic bacterial infections**, tinidazole is given by mouth, usually for 5 or 6 days, in an initial dose of 2 g followed on subsequent days by 1 g daily or 500 mg twice daily. If oral therapy is not possible, tinidazole may be given intravenously, 800 mg being infused as 400 mL of a 2 mg/mL solution at a rate of 10 mL/minute; this initial dose is followed by 800 mg daily or 400 mg twice daily until oral therapy can be substituted. For the *prevention* of postoperative anaerobic bacterial infections, 2 g is given by mouth about 12 hours before surgery. Alternatively 1.6 g is given as a single intravenous infusion before surgery.

In regimens for the treatment of **peptic ulcer disease**, tinidazole 500 mg twice daily has been given with clarithromycin and omeprazole for 7 days.

**Administration in renal impairment.** The elimination of tinidazole is largely unchanged in patients with impaired renal function (see under Pharmacokinetics, above) and dosage adjustment is not generally considered necessary. However tinidazole is removed by haemodialysis, and patients may need additional doses to compensate.

### Preparations

**Proprietary Preparations** (details are given in Part 3)
***Arg.:*** Fasigyn; Gynormal; Ladylen Duo; ***Austral.:*** Fasigyn; Simplotan; ***Belg.:*** Fasigyn; ***Braz.:*** Amplium; Fa-Cyl; Fasigyn; Ginosutin; Pletil; Tinoral; Trinizol; ***Chile:*** Fasigyn; Triconidazol; Troxxil; ***Fr.:*** Fasigyne; ***Ger.:*** Simplotan; Sorquetan†; ***Gr.:*** Fasigyn; ***Hong Kong:*** Fasigyn; ***India:*** Amebamagma; Enidazol; Fasigyn; Tinidafyl; Zil; ***Israel:*** Fasigyn; Protocide; ***Ital.:*** Fasigin; Trimonase; ***Malaysia:*** Fasigyn; ***Mex.:*** Amebysol; Ametricid; Estovyn-T; Fasigyn; Induken; Triseptil; ***Neth.:*** Fasigyn; ***NZ:*** Dyzole; ***Port.:*** Fasigyn; ***S.Afr.:*** Fasigyn; ***Singapore:*** Fasigyn; ***Spain:*** Tricolam; ***Swed.:*** Fasigyn; ***Switz.:*** Fasigyne; ***Thai.:*** Asiazole-TN; Fasigyn; Funida; Idazole; Sporinex; Tinazole; Tini; Tonid; Trichonas; Tricogyn; Tricozone; Trigyn; ***UK:*** Fasigyn.
**Multi-ingredient:** ***Arg.:*** Aduar; Fasigyn Nistatina; Gynormal; Ladylen; Mebutar Compuesto; Tru Compuesto; ***Braz.:*** Amplium-G; Cartrax; Colpolase; Duozol; Facyl M; Ginec; Gino Pletil; Ginometrim Oral; Ginometrim†; Ginosutin M; Gynomax; Poliginax; Seczol; Takil; Trinizol M; ***Chile:*** Doxifen; Famidal; Famidal Ad; Ginecopast; Ginedazol Dual; Mizonase; ***India:*** Candizole-T; Entrolate; Tinidafyl Plus; Wotinex; ***Ital.:*** Fasigin N; ***Mex.:*** Fasigyn VT; Mebeciclol.

## Toltrazuril *(BAN, USAN, rINN)*

Bay-Vi-9142; Toltrazurilo. 1-Methyl-3-(4-{*p*-[(trifluoromethyl)thio]phenoxy}-*m*-tolyl)-s-triazine-2,4,6(1*H*,3*H*,5*H*)-trione.
$C_{18}H_{14}F_3N_3O_4S$ = 425.4.
*CAS — 69004-03-1.*

### Profile

Toltrazuril is an antiprotozoal used in veterinary practice for the treatment of coccidiosis in poultry and piglets, and for the treatment of isosporiasis in piglets.

## Tryparsamide *(rINN)*

Glyphenarsine; Triparsamida; Tryparsam.; Tryparsone. Sodium hydrogen 4-(carbamoylmethylamino)phenylarsonate hemihydrate.
$C_8H_{10}AsN_2NaO_4,\frac{1}{2}H_2O$ = 305.1.
*CAS — 554-72-3 (anhydrous tryparsamide); 6159-29-1 (tryparsamide hemihydrate).*

### Profile

Tryparsamide, a pentavalent arsenical compound, is a trypanocide which penetrates into the CSF and has been used with suramin in the treatment of late-stage African trypanosomiasis due to *Trypanosoma brucei gambiense*, as an alternative to melarsoprol or eflornithine (see p.599). However, because of its toxicity, especially the risk of blindness resulting from damage to the optic nerve, melarsoprol or eflornithine are preferred.

For the adverse effects of arsenic and their treatment, see Arsenic Trioxide, p.1657. Like melarsoprol, tryparsamide can cause encephalopathy.

# Antivirals

Common cold, p.618
Encephalitis, p.618
Gastro-enteritis, p.618
Haemorrhagic fevers, p.618
Hantavirus pulmonary syndrome, p.618
Hepatitis, p.618
Herpesvirus infections, p.619
Cytomegalovirus infections, p.619
Epstein-Barr virus infections, p.620
Herpes simplex infections, p.620
Herpesvirus simiae infections, p.621
Varicella-zoster infections, p.621
HIV infection and AIDS, p.621
HIV-associated infections, p.623
HIV-associated malignancies, p.623
HIV-associated neurological complications, p.623
HIV-associated wasting and diarrhoea, p.623
HIV infection prophylaxis, p.623
Infections in immunocompromised patients, p.624
Influenza, p.624
Measles, p.624
Respiratory syncytial virus infection, p.625
SARS, p.625
Warts, p.625

The drugs described in this chapter are used in the treatment of viral infections; they may also be used to provide protection, usually for a brief period only, against infection. Treatment has to be started early in the infection for the drug to be effective and inhibit the replicating virus. There is little evidence that these compounds affect latent or nonreplicating viruses. They do not provide an alternative to available immunisation for the long-term prophylaxis of infection—for details of such treatment see the chapter on Vaccines, p.1605.

## Choice of Antiviral

Antiviral drugs are effective for the treatment and prophylaxis of a range of viral infections as described below. Non-specific symptomatic and supportive treatments are also important in the management of viral infections. Those viral infections not amenable to antiviral drug therapy include mumps, poliomyelitis, rabies, and rubella.

### Common cold

A cold is usually a mild, self-limiting respiratory infection with a range of viruses, the rhinoviruses and coronaviruses being most frequently involved. Symptoms include nasal discharge and obstruction, sneezing, sore throat, and cough; there is little or no fever. Occasionally there may be concurrent or subsequent bacterial infection of the upper respiratory tract.

The variety of causative agents makes vaccination an unlikely prospect. Not only are there different groups of viruses, but within the rhinoviruses, for example, there are many different serotypes.

Treatment of the common cold is symptomatic, using analgesics, cough suppressants, and decongestants but symptoms usually last for about a week whether or not treatment is taken. Antibacterial[1] and antiviral[2] therapy has consistently failed to show any benefit and antibacterials are indicated only if there is secondary bacterial infection. Very large doses of ascorbic acid have been widely used to prevent and treat colds but a systematic review[3] has concluded that, although there has been evidence of benefit in published studies, it has generally been modest, and that long-term supplementation with vitamin C does not appear to prevent colds; there may be a slight reduction in duration of cold symptoms when it is used therapeutically. Other drugs[4] tried have included mast-cell stabilisers, interferon alfa-2b, and zinc lozenges. Intranasal interferons, tried for prophylaxis or treatment, have not fulfilled their early promise. Results of trials of zinc treatment have been inconclusive.[5] Similarly, there is insufficient evidence to support the use of Echinacea for treatment or prevention of colds.[6] A soluble recombinant intercellular adhesion molecule 1 (ICAM-1), tremacamra, is under investigation. Pleconaril has also been investigated.

1. Arroll B, Kenealy T. Antibiotics for the common cold and acute purulent rhinitis. Available in The Cochrane Library; Issue 1. Chichester: John Wiley; 2004.
2. Jefferson TO, Tyrrell D. Antivirals for the common cold. Available in The Cochrane Library; Issue 1. Chichester: John Wiley; 2004.
3. Douglas RM, *et al.* Vitamin C for preventing and treating the common cold. Available in The Cochrane Library; Issue 1. Chichester: John Wiley; 2004.
4. Mossad SB. Treatment of the common cold. *BMJ* 1998; **317:** 33–6.
5. Marshall I. Zinc for the common cold. Available in The Cochrane Library; Issue 1. Chichester: John Wiley; 2004.
6. Melchart D, *et al.* Echinacea for preventing and treating the common cold. Available in The Cochrane Library; Issue 1. Chichester: John Wiley; 2004.

### Encephalitis

Viral infections that can produce encephalitis[1] include Epstein-Barr virus infections, herpes simplex infections, HIV infection, influenza, Lassa fever, measles, mumps, rubella, and varicella-zoster infections; the specific treatment of these infections, if any, is described under the appropriate heading. However, there is also a group of viruses known as encephalitis viruses that cause infections in which encephalitis is a major clinical feature.

They include:

- alphaviruses (previously arbovirus Group A) including Eastern, Western, and Venezuelan equine viruses transmitted by mosquitoes
- bunyaviruses including California encephalitis virus and La Crosse virus both transmitted by mosquitoes
- flaviviruses (previously arbovirus Group B) including Japanese encephalitis virus, St Louis encephalitis virus, Murray Valley encephalitis virus, Rocio virus, and West Nile virus all transmitted by mosquitoes and the tick-borne viruses of this group, louping ill virus, Powassan virus, and the Eastern and Western subtype viruses
- paramyxoviruses including Nipah virus and Hendra virus, the reservoir for both of which is bats, but which are transmitted to humans via close contact with secondary hosts such as pigs and horses

Encephalitis virus infections usually present with fever, headache, nausea, vomiting, and neck rigidity. Some infections progress to produce confusion, convulsions, coma, and sometimes death. Patients who recover may be left with some permanent neurological damage. There is generally no specific treatment for encephalitis virus infections and patients must be managed with vigorous supportive care. Control of mosquito and tick populations in endemic areas and minimising contact with these vectors are important means of preventing infections. Japanese encephalitis vaccine and tick-borne encephalitis vaccine are available for active immunisation of individuals at risk of infection and tick-borne encephalitis immunoglobulins are available in some countries for passive immunisation against infection.

1. Whitley RJ, Gnann JW. Viral encephalitis: familiar infections and emerging pathogens. *Lancet* 2002; **359:** 507–14.

### Gastro-enteritis

Viral infections are an important cause of diarrhoea, especially in children and immunocompromised patients. Those causing diarrhoea and other gastrointestinal symptoms include adenovirus, astrovirus, calicivirus, rotavirus, Norwalk virus, and related small round structured virus infections. Cytomegalovirus is an important cause of diarrhoea in AIDS (see HIV-associated Wasting and Diarrhoea, below). Rotavirus infection is recognised as the commonest cause of endemic acute diarrhoea in childhood, and is associated with severe vomiting and fever. In acute diarrhoea of any aetiology the priority is to maintain hydration by prevention or treatment of fluid and electrolyte depletion, especially in infants and the elderly (see p.1241). Antivirals are not used in the management of viral diarrhoeas. Several rotavirus vaccines are under development.

### Haemorrhagic fevers

Viruses causing haemorrhagic fever form a diverse group from several viral families. They are usually transmitted via mosquitoes, ticks, or rodents.

The more important viruses responsible for haemorrhagic fevers in man include:

- alphaviruses (previously arbovirus Group A) causing Chikungunya, transmitted by mosquitoes
- arenaviruses causing Argentinian haemorrhagic fever, Bolivian haemorrhagic fever, and Lassa fever and transmitted by rodents
- Bunyaviridae causing Crimean Congo haemorrhagic fever, haemorrhagic fever with renal syndrome, and Rift Valley fever and transmitted by ticks, rodents and insectivores, and mosquitoes, respectively
- the filoviruses Ebola virus and Marburg virus
- flaviviruses (previously arbovirus Group B) causing dengue fever and yellow fever transmitted by mosquitoes, and Kyasanur forest fever and Omsk haemorrhagic fever transmitted by ticks

As suggested by the name, fever and haemorrhage of varying severity are characteristics of these infections. Chills, headache, malaise, myalgia, and nausea usually occur and sometimes flushing and rashes. Severe vomiting, diarrhoea, and shock may occur in advanced infections. There is often some degree of renal or hepatic impairment and occasionally CNS involvement.

While ribavirin has been reported to reduce mortality in patients with Lassa fever, haemorrhagic fever with renal syndrome, and possibly Crimean Congo haemorrhagic fever, there is generally no specific antiviral treatment for haemorrhagic fever and patients must be managed symptomatically. Control of vector populations and prevention of vector contact have an important role to play (see p.1500). Guidelines for the prevention, control, and treatment of dengue and yellow fevers have been produced by WHO[1,2] and related organisations.[3] National guidelines exist in some countries.[4]

Rift Valley fever vaccines and yellow fever vaccines are available for active immunisation of individuals at risk of infection; dengue fever vaccines and haemorrhagic fever with renal syndrome vaccines are under development. Crimean Congo haemorrhagic fever immunoglobulins are available in some countries for passive immunisation against the disease.

1. Vainio J, Cutts F. *Yellow fever.* Geneva: WHO, 1998. Also available at: http://www.who.int/vaccines-documents/DocsPDF/www9842.pdf (accessed 11/03/04)
2. WHO. *Prevention and control of dengue and dengue haemorrhagic fever: comprehensive guidelines.* New Delhi: WHO, 1999.
3. Pan American Health Organization. *Dengue and dengue hemorrhagic fever in the Americas: Guidelines for prevention and control.* Washington, DC: PAHO, 1994.
4. Advisory Committee on Dangerous Pathogens. *Management and control of viral haemorrhagic fevers.* London: HMSO, 1996.

### Hantavirus pulmonary syndrome

A number of hantaviruses related to the virus causing haemorrhagic fever with renal syndrome (see above) have been identified as the probable cause of an acute, severe respiratory illness which has been named hantavirus pulmonary syndrome. Its main symptoms are fever, myalgia, headache, and cough rapidly progressing to respiratory failure; the mortality rate may be about 50% and death is usually due to non-cardiogenic pulmonary oedema and acute respiratory distress syndrome. The virus is transmitted by rodents and the syndrome has mainly been described in the USA.

Treatment is primarily symptomatic including respiratory and circulatory support with the early use of cardiac inotropes being particularly important. Intravenous ribavirin has been tried but preliminary data have not indicated improved mortality. Guidelines for the management of hantavirus pulmonary syndrome have been produced in the USA.[1]

1. Pan American Health Organization. *Hantavirus in the Americas: guidelines for diagnosis, treatment, prevention and control.* Washington, DC: PAHO, 1999.

### Hepatitis

Viral hepatitis refers to infection of the liver caused by a group of hepatitis viruses. Those so far identified are designated A, B, C, D, E, and G. Other viruses such as Epstein-Barr virus and yellow fever virus may be secondary causes of hepatitis and it may also be caused by nonviral infections, many drugs and chemicals, and alcoholism.

Hepatitis viruses are endemic worldwide. Hepatitis A and E are spread via the faecal-oral route. Hepatitis B, C, and D, and probably also G are transmitted in blood and blood products and by sexual contact. Hepatitis B may also be transmitted by contact with infectious body fluids. Hepatitis C probably accounts for most cases of blood-transmitted hepatitis. Hepatitis D only occurs in the presence of hepatitis B since it requires multiplication of the hepatitis B virus for its own replication.

Acute viral hepatitis results in inflammation of the liver and hepatocellular necrosis, but clinical presentation varies widely from subclinical asymptomatic illness to fulminant hepatic failure. Initial symptoms may include malaise, weakness, anorexia, nausea, vomiting, fever, and abdominal pain, followed after 3 to 10 days by jaundice. In some cases the condition may progress to fulminant hepatitis with hepatic encephalopathy, coma, and death. In patients who survive, recovery usually takes a few months but some will have residual liver damage. Some patients infected with the B, C, or D virus may develop chronic hepatitis, which may lead to hepatocellular carcinoma or cirrhosis.

Active immunisation of individuals at risk of infection is possible for hepatitis A and B with specific vaccines, or passive immunisation can be achieved using immunoglobulins.

The management of uncomplicated acute viral hepatitis is largely symptomatic. However, there is some evidence[1,2] that treatment with *interferon* might prevent the progression of acute hepatitis C to the chronic stage, and meta-analyses[3,4] also suggest that it can promote more rapid resolution of viraemia and normalisation of aminotransferase. Additionally, improvements in liver function were reported in 4 patients with fulminant hepatitis A following treatment with interferon beta.[5]

Chronic viral hepatitis has usually been treated with interferon alfa. Guidelines and other recommendations have been issued in the UK and USA for the management of hepatitis C.[6-8] Prolonged therapy for between 4 (hepatitis B) and 12 months (hepatitis C or D) is necessary, although long-term remission of disease is achieved in less than half of patients treated. Relapse is common and, in patients with hepatitis C especially, may be expected in half of responding patients on cessation of treatment. Response rates may be determined by the level of viraemia and the genotype. In view of these difficulties, a number of other antiviral and immunomodulating drugs have been used or investigated. In hepatitis B, responses to interferon alfa may be improved by pretreatment with prednisone[9,10] or prednisolone.[11,12] Studies[13] have shown that once-weekly peginterferon alfa, a formulation of interferon alfa with monomethoxy polyethylene glycol, is more effective than interferon alfa given three times weekly in patients with chronic hepatitis C, including those with cirrhosis or extensive fibrosis.[14] *Ribavirin*, a nucleoside analogue, has also been shown to have some activity against hepatitis C, although biochemical improvements are generally not sustained once treatment is stopped.[15,16] However, the use of ribavirin with interferon alfa (or beta[17]) is more effective than either drug alone with sustained responses having been recorded and many now consider combination therapy to be the treatment of first choice.[7,18,19] A meta-analysis[20] and a systematic review[19] of randomised studies have concluded that combination therapy is also more effective for chronic hepatitis C in patients who had failed to respond to interferon alone or to any other previous treatment. Recent studies[21,22] have suggested that combination therapy with peginterferon alfa and ribavirin may be more effective and better tolerated than interferon alfa plus ribavirin, and a review[23] of the use of peginterferon alfa with ribavirin has also concluded that this combination was superior to interferon alfa plus ribavirin or to peginterferon alfa alone.

Several other nucleoside analogues are active against hepatitis B virus, the most widely used being *lamivudine*. It has been extensively studied and has produced promising responses, although relapse rates tend to be high after withdrawal.[24-28] There is also a suggestion that lamivudine might prevent recurrence of hepatitis B infection in patients with chronic hepatitis B who undergo liver transplantation.[29] Encouraging results have also been obtained in hepatitis B with *adefovir*.[30,31]

*Other drugs* that have been tried as adjuncts to conventional therapy include thymosin $\alpha_1$.[32,33]


1. Omata M, *et al.* Resolution of acute hepatitis C after therapy with natural beta interferon. *Lancet* 1991; **338:** 914–15.
2. Jaeckel E, *et al.* Treatment of acute hepatitis C with interferon alfa-2b. *N Engl J Med* 2001; **345:** 1452–7.
3. Cammà C, *et al.* Interferon as treatment for acute hepatitis C: a meta-analysis. *Dig Dis Sci* 1996; **41:** 1248–55.
4. Quin JW. Interferon therapy for acute hepatitis C viral infection—a review by meta-analysis. *Aust N Z J Med* 1997; **27:** 611–18.
5. Yoshiba M, *et al.* Interferon for hepatitis A. *Lancet* 1994; **343:** 288–9.
6. Centers for Disease Control. Recommendations for prevention and control of hepatitis C virus (HCV) infection and HCV-related chronic disease. *MMWR* 1998; **47** (RR-19): 1–39. Also available at: http://www.cdc.gov/mmwr/PDF/rr/rr4719.pdf (accessed 15/04/04)
7. Booth JCL, *et al.*, Royal College of Physicians of London and the British Society of Gastroenterology. Clinical guidelines on the management of hepatitis C. *Gut* 2001; **49** (suppl 1): i1–i21.
8. National Institutes of Health Consensus Development Conference Statement. Management of hepatitis C: 2002. Available at: http://consensus.nih.gov/cons/116/091202116cdc_statement.htm (accessed 10/03/04) Revisions available at: http://consensus.nih.gov/cons/116/revisions.htm (accessed 10/03/04)
9. Perrillo RP, *et al.* A randomized, controlled trial of interferon alfa-2b alone and after prednisone withdrawal for the treatment of chronic hepatitis B. *N Engl J Med* 1990; **323:** 295–301.
10. Fevery J, *et al.* Efficacy of interferon alfa-2b with or without prednisone withdrawal in the treatment of chronic viral hepatitis B: a prospective double-blind Belgian-Dutch study. *J Hepatol* 1990; **11:** S108–S112.
11. Krogsgaard K, *et al.* Prednisolone withdrawal therapy enhances the effect of human lymphoblastoid interferon in chronic hepatitis B. *J Hepatol* 1996; **25:** 803–13.
12. Lin S-M, *et al.* Long-term beneficial effect of interferon therapy in patients with chronic hepatitis B virus infection. *Hepatology* 1999; **29:** 971–5.
13. Zeuzem S, *et al.* Peginterferon alfa-2a in patients with chronic hepatitis C. *N Engl J Med* 2000; **343:** 1666–72.
14. Heathcote EJ, *et al.* Peginterferon alfa-2a in patients with chronic hepatitis C and cirrhosis. *N Engl J Med* 2000; **343:** 1673–80.
15. Reichard O, *et al.* Ribavirin treatment for chronic hepatitis C. *Lancet* 1991; **337:** 1058–61.
16. Di Bisceglie AM, *et al.* Ribavirin as therapy for chronic hepatitis C: a randomized, double-blind, placebo-controlled trial. *Ann Intern Med* 1995; **123:** 897–903.
17. Kakumu S, *et al.* A pilot study of ribavirin and interferon beta for the treatment of chronic hepatitis C. *Gastroenterology* 1993; **105:** 507–12.
18. Scott LJ, Perry CM. Interferon-α-2b plus ribavirin: a review of its use in the management of chronic hepatitis C. *Drugs* 2002; **62:** 507–56.
19. Kjaergard LL, *et al.* Ribavirin with or without alpha interferon for chronic hepatitis C. Available in The Cochrane Library; Issue 1. Chichester: John Wiley; 2004.
20. Cummings KJ, *et al.* Interferon and ribavirin vs interferon alone in the re-treatment of chronic hepatitis C previously nonresponsive to interferon: a meta-analysis of randomized trials. *JAMA* 2001; **285:** 193–9.
21. Manns MP, *et al.* Peginterferon alfa-2b plus ribavirin compared with interferon alfa-2b plus ribavirin for initial treatment of chronic hepatitis C: a randomised trial. *Lancet* 2001; **358:** 958–65.
22. Fried MW, *et al.* Peginterferon alfa-2a plus ribavirin for chronic hepatitis C virus infection. *N Engl J Med* 2002; **347:** 975–82.
23. Keating GM, Curran MP. Peginterferon-α-2a (40kD) plus ribavirin: a review of its use in the management of chronic hepatitis C. *Drugs* 2003; **63:** 701–30.
24. Benhamou Y, *et al.* Efficacy of lamivudine on replication of hepatitis B virus in HIV-infected patients. *Lancet* 1995; **345:** 396–7.
25. Dienstag JL, *et al.* A preliminary trial of lamivudine for chronic hepatitis B infection. *N Engl J Med* 1995; **333:** 1657–61.
26. Lai C-L, *et al.* A one-year trial of lamivudine for chronic hepatitis B. *N Engl J Med* 1998; **339:** 61–8.
27. Dienstag JL, *et al.* Lamivudine as initial treatment for chronic hepatitis B in the United States. *N Engl J Med* 1999; **341:** 1256–63.
28. Jonas MM, *et al.* Clinical trial of lamivudine in children with chronic hepatitis B. *N Engl J Med* 2002; **346:** 1706–13. Correction. *ibid.*; **347:** 955.
29. Perrillo RP, *et al.* A multicenter United States-Canadian trial to assess lamivudine monotherapy before and after liver transplantation for chronic hepatitis B. *Hepatology* 2001; 33: 424–32.
30. Hadziyannis SJ, *et al.* Adefovir dipivoxil for the treatment of hepatitis B e antigen-negative chronic hepatitis B. *N Engl J Med* 2003; **348:** 800–7. Correction. *ibid.*: 1192.
31. Marcellin P, *et al.* Adefovir dipivoxil for the treatment of hepatitis B e antigen-positive chronic hepatitis B. *N Engl J Med* 2003; **348:** 808–16. Correction. *ibid.*: 1192.
32. Sherman KE, *et al.* Hepatitis C RNA response to combined therapy with thymosin alpha-1 and interferon. *Hepatology* 1994; **20:** 207A.
33. Chien R-N, *et al.* Efficacy of thymosin α-1 in patients with chronic hepatitis B: a randomized, controlled trial. *Hepatology* 1998; **27:** 1383–7.


## Herpesvirus infections

Established herpesvirus pathogens discussed below include cytomegalovirus, Epstein-Barr virus, Herpesvirus simiae, herpes simplex virus, and varicella-zoster virus. Herpesviruses 6, 7, and 8 have also emerged as potential pathogens and have been associated with a variety of disorders including childhood febrile illnesses, various malignancies including Kaposi's sarcoma (p.524), and multiple sclerosis (p.646).

**Cytomegalovirus infections.** Cytomegaloviruses are members of the herpesvirus group, and are widely distributed in many animal species. Infection may occur through intra-uterine or perinatal transmission, by oral contact with the saliva of infected individuals, or by sexual transmission. Transmission by blood transfusion or by transplantation of infected tissue can also occur. After infection, viral DNA becomes incorporated into the host cells and persists for the life of the individual with occasional reactivation when infectious virions appear in the saliva and urine.

Most congenitally infected infants are asymptomatic, but some infants may present with intra-uterine growth retardation, jaundice, hepatosplenomegaly, encephalitis, and thrombocytopenia. Acquired infections generally do not cause clinical symptoms, although they may occasionally present as infectious mononucleosis, lymphocytosis, or lymphadenopathy. The virus is a common cause of infection in the immunocompromised, particularly transplant recipients and patients with AIDS, when it commonly presents as cytomegalovirus retinitis or enteritis and is a major cause of morbidity and mortality.

Specific **treatment** for cytomegalovirus infection is usually only given to immunocompromised patients, in whom the infection is often complicated by extensive tissue damage leading to target organ failure and secondary opportunistic infections. Relapses are likely to occur after treatment is stopped due to the latent nature of cytomegaloviruses. *Ganciclovir* is used in the treatment of severe cytomegalovirus infections in transplant recipients and patients with AIDS. However, ganciclovir may cause neutropenia and many AIDS patients receiving zidovudine cannot tolerate the combined haematological toxicity of these two drugs, hence the use of colony-stimulating factors to treat or prevent ganciclovir-induced neutropenia. Although less experience has been gained with *foscarnet*, it appears to be an alternative to ganciclovir with similar efficacy. It does not produce myelosuppression, but nephrotoxicity and electrolyte disturbances are common. The two drugs given in combination may be more effective than monotherapy with either. Other approaches to treatment have involved the use of ganciclovir with *cytomegalovirus immunoglobulins* or *normal immunoglobulins*.

Cytomegalovirus retinitis is usually treated intravenously with ganciclovir or foscarnet.[1] This route has the advantage that extra-retinal and bilateral infections are also reduced. In AIDS patients, the initial induction treatment is generally followed by lifelong maintenance therapy, since ganciclovir and foscarnet both suppress rather than eliminate the virus. However, some workers consider that maintenance therapy may be discontinued in patients who have received highly active antiretroviral therapy (HAART) and have had a sufficient resultant increase in their CD4+ count.[2-4] Oral ganciclovir is reported to be an effective and more convenient alternative to intravenous maintenance in selected patients. The oral prodrug of ganciclovir, valganciclovir, may be used for either induction or maintenance treatment as an alternative to intravenous administration.[5] Despite maintenance treatment, recurrence is considered to be almost inevitable, although it usually responds to an increase in dosage. Foscarnet therapy has been associated with improved survival in AIDS patients, although it is often tolerated less well than ganciclovir and the need for long-term intravenous administration poses practical problems.

*Cidofovir* is another alternative for the treatment of cytomegalovirus retinitis, and has the advantage of intermittent administration. However, long-term treatment may be limited by toxicity.

For patients unable to tolerate systemic therapy, use of a modified-release intravitreal ganciclovir insert may be beneficial, although the risk of increased bilateral and extra-ocular infection is not affected. Adjunctive treatment with oral ganciclovir has been tried to overcome this.[6] Ganciclovir with foscarnet, each given by intravitreal injection, has been reported to be effective.[7] Intravitreal injection of the antisense oligonucleotide *fomivirsen* has also been used. Intra-ocular injection of cidofovir, foscarnet, or ganciclovir is now rarely used because of the high incidence of associated complications.

Guidelines for the treatment of cytomegalovirus infections have been produced by the International AIDS Society—USA.[8]

US guidelines[9] for the **prevention** of opportunistic infections, including cytomegalovirus infection, in HIV-infected patients emphasise the importance of teaching patients to recognise early symptoms of cytomegalovirus retinitis. Ophthalmic screening is also sometimes used.

Primary prophylaxis of cytomegalovirus infection in high-risk patients, particularly transplant recipients, has been reported using intravenous *ganciclovir*,[10-12] *foscarnet*,[13] *valaciclovir*,[14] and *cytomegalovirus immunoglobulins*.[15] Oral ganciclovir may be useful for prophylaxis or pre-emptive therapy in selected transplant patients.[16-18] Conflicting results have been reported from studies of the efficacy of oral ganciclovir for primary prophylaxis in patients with HIV infection,[19,20] but it is recommended in the US guidelines.[9]

*Aciclovir*, with[21] or without[22,23] cytomegalovirus immunoglobulins, has been successful in preventing infection in some transplant patients, but failure of prophylaxis has been reported,[24-26] and comparison of aciclovir with ganciclovir for prophylaxis in liver transplant recipients has found ganciclovir to be the more effective drug.[27,28] The US guidelines[9] consider aciclovir and valaciclovir to be unsuitable for prophylaxis in patients with HIV infection, although preliminary studies suggest that valaciclovir may be effective in these patients.[29] The efficacy of prophylaxis also varies with the organ transplanted.[30]

*Cytomegalovirus vaccines* are currently in development.


1. Jacobson MA. Treatment of cytomegalovirus retinitis in patients with the acquired immunodeficiency syndrome. *N Engl J Med* 1997; **337:** 105–14.
2. Whitcup SM. Cytomegalovirus retinitis in the era of highly active antiretroviral therapy. *JAMA* 2000; **283:** 653–7.
3. Jouan M, *et al.* Discontinuation of maintenance therapy for cytomegalovirus retinitis in HIV-infected patients receiving highly active antiretroviral therapy. *AIDS* 2001; **15:** 23–31.

4. Curi ALL, *et al.* Suspension of anticytomegalovirus maintenance therapy following immune recovery due to highly active antiretroviral therapy. *Br J Ophthalmol* 2001; **85:** 471–3.
5. Martin DF, *et al.* A controlled trial of valganciclovir as induction therapy for cytomegalovirus retinitis. *N Engl J Med* 2002; **346:** 1119–26. Correction. *ibid.*; **347:** 862.
6. Martin DF, *et al.* Oral ganciclovir for patients with cytomegalovirus retinitis treated with a ganciclovir implant. *N Engl J Med* 1999; **340:** 1063–70.
7. Velez G, *et al.* High-dose intravitreal ganciclovir and foscarnet for cytomegalovirus retinitis. *Am J Ophthalmol* 2001; **131:** 396–7.
8. Whitley RJ, *et al.* Guidelines for the treatment of cytomegalovirus diseases in patients with AIDS in the era of potent antiretroviral therapy: recommendation of an international panel. *Arch Intern Med* 1998; **158:** 957–69.
9. Centers for Disease Control and Prevention. Guidelines for preventing opportunistic infections among HIV-infected persons—2002: recommendations of the US Public Health Service and the Infectious Diseases Society of America. *MMWR* 2002; **51** (RR-8): 1–52. Also available at: http://www.cdc.gov/mmwr/PDF/rr/rr5108.pdf (accessed 10/03/04)
10. Goodrich JM, *et al.* Ganciclovir prophylaxis to prevent cytomegalovirus disease after allogeneic marrow transplant. *Ann Intern Med* 1993; **118:** 173–8.
11. Winston DJ, *et al.* Ganciclovir prophylaxis of cytomegalovirus infection and disease in allogeneic bone marrow transplant recipients. *Ann Intern Med* 1993; **118:** 179–84.
12. Hibberd PL, *et al.* Preemptive ganciclovir therapy to prevent cytomegalovirus disease in cytomegalovirus antibody-positive renal transplant recipients: a randomized controlled trial. *Ann Intern Med* 1995; **123:** 18–26.
13. Ippoliti C, *et al.* Foscarnet for prevention of cytomegalovirus infection in allogeneic marrow transplant recipients unable to receive ganciclovir. *Bone Marrow Transplant* 1997; **20:** 491–5.
14. Lowance D, *et al.* Valacyclovir for the prevention of cytomegalovirus disease after renal transplantation. *N Engl J Med* 1999; **340:** 1462–70.
15. Wittes JT, *et al.* Meta-analysis of CMVIG studies for the prevention and treatment of CMV infection in transplant patients. *Transplant Proc* 1996; **28** (suppl 2): 17–24.
16. Goodrich J, Khardori N. Cytomegalovirus: the taming of the beast? *Lancet* 1997; **350:** 1718–19.
17. Singh N. Preemptive therapy versus universal prophylaxis with ganciclovir for cytomegalovirus in solid organ transplant recipients. *Clin Infect Dis* 2001; **32:** 742–51.
18. Paya CV, *et al.* Preemptive use of oral ganciclovir to prevent cytomegalovirus infection in liver transplant patients: a randomized, placebo-controlled trial. *J Infect Dis* 2002; **185:** 854–60.
19. McCarthy M. Oral ganciclovir fails to prevent CMV in HIV trial. *Lancet* 1995; **346:** 895.
20. Spector SA, *et al.* Oral ganciclovir for the prevention of cytomegalovirus disease in persons with AIDS. *N Engl J Med* 1996; **334:** 1491–7.
21. Eisenmann D, *et al.* Prevention of cytomegalovirus disease in heart transplant recipients by prophylaxis with cytomegalovirus hyperimmune globulin plus oral acyclovir. *Transplant Proc* 1990; **22:** 2322–3.
22. Balfour HH, *et al.* A randomized, placebo-controlled trial of oral acyclovir for the prevention of cytomegalovirus disease in recipients of renal allografts. *N Engl J Med* 1989; **320:** 1381–7.
23. Prentice HG, *et al.* Impact of long-term acyclovir on cytomegalovirus infection and survival after allogeneic bone marrow transplantation. *Lancet* 1994; **343:** 749–53.
24. Bailey TC, *et al.* Failure of high-dose oral acyclovir with or without immune globulin to prevent primary cytomegalovirus disease in recipients of solid organ transplants. *Am J Med* 1993; **95:** 273–8.
25. Singh N, *et al.* High-dose acyclovir compared with short-course pre-emptive ganciclovir therapy to prevent cytomegalovirus disease in liver transplant recipients: a randomized trial. *Ann Intern Med* 1994; **120:** 375–81.
26. Boeckh M, *et al.* Failure of high-dose acyclovir to prevent cytomegalovirus disease after autologous marrow transplantation. *J Infect Dis* 1995; **172:** 939–43.
27. Winston DJ, *et al.* Randomised comparison of ganciclovir and high-dose acyclovir for long-term cytomegalovirus prophylaxis in liver-transplant recipients. *Lancet* 1995; **346:** 69–74.
28. Winston DJ, Busuttil RW. Randomized controlled trial of oral ganciclovir versus oral acyclovir after induction with intravenous ganciclovir for long-term prophylaxis of cytomegalovirus disease in cytomegalovirus-seropositive liver transplant recipients. *Transplantation* 2003; **75:** 229–33.
29. Feinberg JE, *et al.* A randomized, double-blind trial of valaciclovir prophylaxis for cytomegalovirus disease in patients with advanced human immunodeficiency virus infection. *J Infect Dis* 1998; **177:** 48–56.
30. Griffiths PD. Prophylaxis against CMV infection in transplant patients. *J Antimicrob Chemother* 1997; **39:** 299–301.

**Epstein-Barr virus infections.** Epstein-Barr virus (EBV) is a DNA virus of the herpesvirus group occurring worldwide. Following primary exposure the individual becomes a lifelong carrier of EBV, but associated disease only occurs if the normal immune mechanisms are compromised and the virus can be reactivated. EBV is the causative agent in infectious mononucleosis and is associated with several diseases including Burkitt's lymphoma, nasopharyngeal carcinoma, chronic interstitial pneumonitis in infants with AIDS, and oral hairy leucoplakia in AIDS patients. It may also be associated with Hodgkin's disease and with amyloidosis.

Infectious mononucleosis (glandular fever) is an acute, self-limiting, lymphoproliferative infection occurring mainly in adolescents and young adults, transmission usually being via close oral contact. Symptoms may last for several weeks and include sore throat, swelling of the neck, fever, sweating, chills, and anorexia. Lymphadenopathy and splenomegaly usually occur and some patients may experience hepatomegaly and jaundice. Most patients recover uneventfully with only supportive treatment, although they may continue to be easily exhausted for some time. Complications may occur in a few patients and can be fatal. They include meningitis, encephalitis, seizures, hepatic necrosis, splenic rupture, haemolytic and aplastic anaemia, agranulocytosis, and thrombocytopenia. Very rarely the illness may become chronic, with symptoms persisting for years, and may result in death from lymphomatous disease.

There is no specific treatment for EBV infections. Aciclovir,[1,2] ganciclovir,[3,4] and interferons[1,5-7] are some of the drugs that have been reported to produce some clinical or immunological improvement, but this is usually reversible on stopping treatment. Corticosteroids may be useful in severe, prolonged, or complicated infections, although concern has been expressed that they might impair immunity and increase the risk of EBV-related tumours in later years.[8] Concurrent throat infection with streptococci should not be treated with amoxicillin or ampicillin since they may cause a maculopapular rash in patients with infectious mononucleosis.

1. Drago F, *et al.* Epstein-Barr virus-related primary cutaneous amyloidosis: successful treatment with acyclovir and interferon-alpha. *Br J Dermatol* 1996; **134:** 170–4.
2. Torre D, Tambini R. Acyclovir for treatment of infectious mononucleosis: a meta-analysis. *Scand J Infect Dis* 1999; **31:** 543–7.
3. Ishida Y, *et al.* Ganciclovir for chronic active Epstein-Barr virus infection. *Lancet* 1993; **341:** 560–1.
4. Pirsch JD, *et al.* Treatment of severe Epstein-Barr virus-induced lymphoproliferative syndrome with ganciclovir: two cases after solid organ transplantation. *Am J Med* 1989; **86:** 241–4.
5. Cheeseman SH, *et al.* Epstein-Barr virus infection in renal transplant recipients: effects of antithymocyte globulin and interferon. *Ann Intern Med* 1980; **93:** 39–42.
6. Fujisaki T, *et al.* Gamma-interferon for severe chronic active Epstein-Barr virus. *Ann Intern Med* 1993; **118:** 474–5.
7. Sakai Y, *et al.* Interferon-α therapy for chronic active Epstein-Barr virus infection: potential effect on the development of T-lymphoproliferative disease. *J Pediatr Hematol Oncol* 1998; **20:** 342–6.
8. Sheagren JN. Corticosteroids for treatment of mononucleosis and aphthous stomatitis. *JAMA* 1986; **256:** 1051.

**Herpes simplex infections.** Herpes simplex virus (HSV, herpesvirus hominis) is distributed worldwide and is most often classified[1] into serotypes HSV-1 and HSV-2. Transmission is by direct contact with infected secretions, with HSV-1 being associated primarily with oral and ocular transmission and HSV-2 primarily with genital transmission. Symptomatic disease normally affects the skin or mucous membranes, when HSV replicates in the epithelium with subsequent lysis of infected cells and local inflammation to produce characteristic painful lesions. Viraemia occurs rarely, except in immunocompromised individuals in whom disseminated disease can develop.

HSV becomes latent within sensory nerve ganglia from where it can be reactivated by various triggers such as stress, bacterial infection, fever, irradiation (including sunlight), or menstruation. Reactivation leads to a prodromal period before the lesions emerge.

Primary infections are usually in the perioral, ocular, or genital areas, but infection may occur at any skin site if the skin is damaged or if the patient is immunocompromised. Anorectal lesions including herpes proctitis are especially prevalent in homosexual men with AIDS. Most primary HSV-1 infections are asymptomatic but may occasionally present as acute gingivostomatitis and pharyngitis. Infections commonly recur as *herpes labialis*, also known as fever blisters or cold sores. *Ocular herpes* is also generally caused by HSV-1, and infections range in severity from superficial conjunctivitis or dendritic keratitis to sight-threatening diseases of the inner eye such as iridocyclitis or herpetic disciform keratitis. *Genital herpes* is usually caused by HSV-2 and tends to be a more severe condition than other herpes simplex infections, especially in women. *Herpes encephalitis* and *neonatal herpes* are rare, but occasionally fatal, complications of herpes simplex infections.

**Management.** The most widely used antiviral for herpes simplex infections is aciclovir. In clinical practice, treatment of primary herpes simplex infections, while relieving symptoms and reducing the duration of viral shedding, does not prevent recurrences. Antiviral therapy is generally more effective for primary infections than for recurrences, and should be given as early as possible during the course of an active infection, preferably within 3 days of the onset of symptoms. Aciclovir may be administered topically, orally, or intravenously depending on the severity and nature of the infection. Resistance to aciclovir is emerging, mainly in immunocompromised patients.

Assessment of antivirals with improved bioavailability or pharmacokinetic profiles that allow less frequent dosing and antivirals that are effective against aciclovir-resistant strains is continuing. Such drugs include the nucleoside analogues valaciclovir and cidofovir, and the immunomodulators interferon alfa and imiquimod. Herpes simplex vaccines have also been tried but with generally disappointing results.

- **Herpes labialis** is a self-limiting disorder that rarely requires antiviral therapy but if used it should be started early in the prodromal phase. Topical preparations of antivirals, including aciclovir, penciclovir, and tromantadine, are used but there is conflicting evidence regarding their efficacy. Docosanol may be a further alternative. Oral aciclovir may suppress frequently recurrent herpes labialis,[2] and protect those at high risk of recurrence. Oral valaciclovir has also been reported to be effective for suppression of recurrences and may provide the convenience of single-day treatment.[3] However, for the majority of patients careful hygiene and, if necessary, symptomatic treatment with analgesics and the use of antiseptics such as povidone-iodine to reduce secondary infection will suffice; sunscreens may reduce the frequency of recurrences.
- **Ocular herpes simplex infections** usually require treatment with a suitable antiviral. Aciclovir is commonly applied as an ointment.[1] Trifluridine[1] and vidarabine are alternatives. Ganciclovir gel might be as effective as aciclovir.[4] The use of topical corticosteroids alone is contra-indicated for most forms of ocular herpes as they can increase disease severity, but a combination of a corticosteroid with an antiviral, such as prednisolone with aciclovir[5] or trifluridine[6] may be useful. Long-term treatment with oral aciclovir has been found to reduce the rate of recurrence of ocular herpes simplex disease.[7] Patients with intra-ocular infections require systemic treatment, usually with aciclovir. However, the addition of oral aciclovir to topical therapy with trifluridine and a corticosteroid was reported to be of no benefit in patients with stromal keratitis.[8] A systematic review[9] has concluded that using an antiviral nucleoside with interferon appears to speed healing in patients with epithelial keratitis.
- **Genital herpes** is usually treated with systemic aciclovir; alternatives are famciclovir and valaciclovir.[10-12] Topical aciclovir has been used but it is less effective. As with other herpes simplex infections, therapy of the initial infection appears to have no effect on subsequent recurrences. In patients experiencing a recognisable prodrome, a 5-day course of oral aciclovir, famciclovir, or valaciclovir initiated by the patient may abort the recurrence or reduce its severity.[10-12] In patients who do not experience a prodrome or those with frequent recurrences, continuous suppressive therapy with aciclovir, famciclovir, or valaciclovir should be considered.[10-12] There is a risk of *neonatal herpes* in the infants of mothers with genital herpes infection. Prophylactic administration of aciclovir to the mother during late pregnancy is not routinely recommended[10] but may be indicated in HIV-infected mothers if recurrence is frequent.[13] Infants with evidence of neonatal herpes infection should be given systemic aciclovir.[10,12]
- **Severe or disseminated herpes simplex infections**, particularly those occurring in immunocompromised patients, usually require intravenous therapy. Aciclovir is used most commonly,[1] with foscarnet or cidofovir as alternatives for infections resistant to aciclovir. Immunocompromised patients with frequent or disabling recurrences may benefit from prophylactic oral aciclovir or famciclovir administration.[13]

1. Whitley RJ, Roizman B. Herpes simplex virus infections. *Lancet* 2001; **357:** 1513–18.
2. Worrall G. Acyclovir in recurrent herpes labialis. *BMJ* 1996; **312:** 6.
3. Spruance SL, *et al.* High-dose, short-duration, early valacyclovir therapy for episodic treatment of cold sores: results of two randomized, placebo-controlled, multicenter studies. *Antimicrob Agents Chemother* 2003; **47:** 1072–80.
4. Hoh HB, *et al.* Randomised trial of ganciclovir and acyclovir in the treatment of herpes simplex dendritic keratitis: a multicentre study. *Br J Ophthalmol* 1996; **80:** 140–3.
5. Collum LMT, *et al.* Acyclovir (Zovirax) in herpetic disciform keratitis. *Br J Ophthalmol* 1983; **67:** 115–18.
6. Wilhelmus KR, *et al.* Herpetic eye disease study: a controlled trial of topical corticosteroids for herpes simplex stromal keratitis. *Ophthalmology* 1994; **101:** 1883–96.
7. Herpetic Eye Disease Study Group. Acyclovir for the prevention of recurrent herpes simplex virus eye disease. *N Engl J Med* 1998; **339:** 300–6.
8. Barron BA, *et al.* Herpetic eye disease study: a controlled trial of oral acyclovir for herpes simplex stromal keratitis. *Ophthalmology* 1994; **101:** 1871–82.
9. Wilhelmus KR. Interventions for herpes simplex virus epithelial keratitis. Available in The Cochrane Library; Issue 1. Chichester: John Wiley; 2004.
10. Centers for Disease Control. Sexually transmitted diseases treatment guidelines 2002. *MMWR* 2002; **51** (RR-6): 1–80. Also available at: http://www.cdc.gov/mmwr/PDF/rr/rr5106.pdf (accessed 10/03/04)

11. Clinical Effectiveness Group (Association for Genitourinary Medicine and the Medical Society for the Study of Venereal Diseases). 2001 National guideline for the management of genital herpes. Available at: http://www.bashh.org/guidelines/2002/hsv%2006%2001.PDF (accessed 10/03/04)
12. WHO. *Guidelines for the management of sexually transmitted infections*. Geneva: WHO, 2003 Also available at: http://whqlibdoc.who.int/publications/2003/9241546263.pdf (accessed 26/04/04)
13. Centers for Disease Control and Prevention. Guidelines for preventing opportunistic infections among HIV-infected persons—2002: recommendations of the US Public Health Service and the Infectious Diseases Society of America. *MMWR* 2002; **51** (RR-8): 1–52. Also available at: http://www.cdc.gov/mmwr/PDF/rr/rr5108.pdf (accessed 10/03/04)

**Herpesvirus simiae infections.** Herpesvirus simiae (monkey B virus, herpes B virus) is a herpesvirus that usually infects macaque monkeys, but may rarely be transmitted to man by laboratory accidents or bites or scratches from infected monkeys.

Initially there may be vesicles at the site of the bite or scratch. As the infection progresses there is increasing neurological involvement that can lead to encephalitis, coma, and death.

Aciclovir is recommended[1] for the treatment of symptomatic or culture-confirmed infection. It should be started intravenously for symptomatic infections or orally for those that are asymptomatic but culture-positive. Intravenous use should be followed by oral therapy. An alternative is ganciclovir given similarly. Prophylactic use of antivirals is not recommended, although empirical therapy with aciclovir may be considered if there is clear evidence of viral shedding by the monkey.

1. Holmes GP, *et al.* Guidelines for the prevention and treatment of B-virus infections in exposed persons. *Clin Infect Dis* 1995; **20:** 421–39.

**Varicella-zoster infections.** Varicella-zoster virus (VZV) is a herpesvirus which causes chickenpox (varicella) and herpes zoster (zoster, shingles). The virus is easily transmitted, particularly by close contact with infected individuals.

Primary infection usually results in *chickenpox*, which presents with a characteristic generalised vesicular eruption, fever, and malaise. Chickenpox is commonly a benign disease of childhood of short duration. It can occur in adults when it can be severe, and is potentially fatal in immunocompromised patients: complications include secondary bacterial skin infections, pneumonia, and neurological disorders such as encephalitis and cerebral ataxia. Reye's syndrome, which is principally associated with viral infections in childhood, may also be a cause of encephalopathy in patients with chickenpox. Infection during early pregnancy may result rarely in fetal varicella syndrome while infection during late pregnancy may cause neonatal varicella after delivery.

Patients who recover from primary infections with varicella-zoster have lifelong immunity against chickenpox. However, a permanent latent infection of sensory nerve ganglia is established, and reactivation produces herpes zoster.

*Herpes zoster* is characterised by painful vesicular eruptions localised to a single dermatome of skin, and sometimes preceded by a prodromal phase with fever, malaise, and headache. Involvement of the trigeminal nerve can lead to sight-threatening ophthalmic herpes zoster. As with chickenpox, herpes zoster is more serious in immunocompromised patients and may be severe, prolonged, or disseminated. Chronic pain that persists after the rash has healed is termed postherpetic neuralgia (p.7) and occurs in about 10% of patients who have had herpes zoster.

Management of **chickenpox** in otherwise healthy patients is usually symptomatic using antipyretics, analgesics, and antipruritics. Antibacterials may be required for secondary infections. The value of antivirals in the treatment of chickenpox in such patients has been questioned, and their use is not recommended for the treatment of uncomplicated chickenpox in otherwise healthy children.[1] However, oral aciclovir has been reported to reduce the duration and severity of symptoms when administered within 24 hours of onset of symptoms,[2] but may not reduce the incidence of chickenpox-associated complications. It may be useful in immunocompromised patients or those who have developed complications. Intravenous therapy may be necessary in severe chickenpox. Recommendations for the use of aciclovir in children,[1] adults,[3] and during pregnancy[4] have been developed.

Transmission of chickenpox to household contacts is not prevented by administration of aciclovir to the primary case but there is evidence to suggest that transmission can be suppressed by giving aciclovir to susceptible contacts during the incubation period.[5,6] Although the need for such prophylaxis has been questioned, especially in otherwise healthy children,[7] prophylaxis or early treatment may be useful for household contacts in whom the infection might prove to be more severe.[1,8,9]

Varicella-zoster immunoglobulins are used for the prevention of chickenpox in patients at high risk of developing complications, such as the immunocompromised, neonates, and in susceptible pregnant women following significant exposure. There have been reports of severe chickenpox occurring in patients undergoing corticosteroid therapy and in the UK administration of varicella-zoster immunoglobulins is recommended in persons exposed to the virus who have received therapeutic doses of corticosteroids within the previous 3 months[10] (see also under Precautions for Corticosteroids, p.1072). Varicella-zoster vaccines are available in some countries.

The place of antivirals in the treatment of **herpes zoster** is well established and guidelines on management have been produced.[11] Antiviral treatment can reduce the severity and duration of acute pain, minimise complications and propagation of the rash, and reduce viral shedding.[11] Aciclovir may be given orally or intravenously, depending upon the severity of the infection. Oral famciclovir or valaciclovir are alternatives. Treatment should be started within 72 hours of the onset of the rash and is usually continued for 7 to 10 days. Amantadine has also been used in the acute phase. Nothing appears to be gained from extending the treatment period or from adding systemic corticosteroids,[12] which are best avoided anyway in patients with acute infection since they can increase the risk of viral dissemination.[13] Immunocompromised patients or others at high risk of severe or disseminated varicella-zoster infections should receive intravenous aciclovir. Combined therapy with aciclovir and vidarabine may be considered in the severely immunocompromised.[13] Foscarnet may be of value in aciclovir-resistant varicella-zoster infections[14-16] although treatment failures have been reported.[17] Sorivudine has been reported to be more effective than aciclovir[18] in HIV-infected patients and has produced benefit in immunocompromised patients with recurrent cutaneously disseminated varicella-zoster infection refractory to aciclovir and to foscarnet.[19] Brivudine has displayed comparable efficacy to that of aciclovir.[20]

*Ophthalmic herpes zoster* may be treated with topical aciclovir, although concurrent treatment with systemic aciclovir may be needed for optimum results.[13,21] Oral famciclovir may have similar efficacy to oral aciclovir.[22] However, a study in 20 patients with AIDS suggested that ganciclovir given either alone or with foscarnet was more effective than aciclovir in terms of preserving long-term visual acuity.[23] Topical corticosteroids are usually avoided during the acute phase of the infection, but may be needed if there is a substantial inflammatory component.

There has been controversy over the use of oral aciclovir to *prevent* postherpetic neuralgia and ocular complications. A meta-analysis suggested that treatment of herpes zoster with oral aciclovir within 72 hours of the onset of rash could reduce the incidence of residual pain at 6 months by 46% in immunocompetent adults.[24] A more recent analysis[25] considered that there was only marginal evidence that aciclovir decreased the incidence of postherpetic neuralgia and that there was no reduction in incidence with either famciclovir or valaciclovir. It is, however, generally agreed that antivirals do reduce the duration of postherpetic neuralgia.[25]

1. Tarlow MJ, Walters S. Chickenpox in childhood: a review prepared for the UK Advisory Group on Chickenpox on behalf of the British Society for the Study of Infection. *J Infect* 1998; **36** (suppl 1): 39–47.
2. Klassen TP, *et al.* Acyclovir for treating varicella in otherwise healthy children and adolescents. Available in The Cochrane Library; Issue 1. Chichester: John Wiley; 2004.
3. Wilkins EGL, *et al.* Management of chickenpox in the adult: a review prepared for the UK Advisory Group on Chickenpox on behalf of the British Society for the Study of Infection. *J Infect* 1998; **36** (suppl 1): 49–58.
4. Nathwani D, *et al.* Varicella infections in pregnancy and the newborn: a review prepared for the UK Advisory Group on Chickenpox on behalf of the British Society for the Study of Infection. *J Infect* 1998; **36** (suppl 1): 59–71.
5. Asano Y, *et al.* Postexposure prophylaxis of varicella in family contact by oral acyclovir. *Pediatrics* 1993; **92:** 219–22.
6. Suga S, *et al.* Effect of oral acyclovir against primary and secondary viraemia in incubation period of varicella. *Arch Dis Child* 1993; **69:** 639–42.
7. Conway SP. Effect of oral acyclovir against primary and secondary viraemia in incubation period of varicella: commentary. *Arch Dis Child* 1993; **69:** 642–3.
8. Ogilvie MM. Antiviral prophylaxis and treatment in chickenpox: a review prepared for the UK Advisory Group on Chickenpox on behalf of the British Society for the Study of Infection. *J Infect* 1998; **36:** (suppl 1): 31–8.
9. Lin TY, *et al.* Oral acyclovir prophylaxis of varicella after intimate contact. *Pediatr Infect Dis J* 1997; **16:** 1162–5.
10. Department of Health. *Immunisation against infectious disease* 1996: "The Green Book". Available at: http://www.dh.gov.uk/PublicationsAndStatistics/Publications/PublicationsPolicyAndGuidance/PublicationsPolicyAndGuidanceArticle/fs/en?CONTENT_ID=4072977&chk=87uz6M (accessed 26/02/04)
11. BSSI Working Group. Guidelines for the management of shingles: report of a working group of the British Society for the Study of Infection (BSSI). *J Infect* 1995; **30:** 193–200.
12. Wood MJ, *et al.* A randomized trial of acyclovir for 7 days or 21 days with and without prednisolone for treatment of acute herpes zoster. *N Engl J Med* 1994; **330:** 896–900.
13. Nikkels AF, Piérard GE. Recognition and treatment of shingles. *Drugs* 1994; **48:** 528–48.
14. Safrin S, *et al.* Foscarnet therapy in five patients with AIDS and acyclovir-resistant varicella-zoster virus infection. *Ann Intern Med* 1991; **115:** 19–21.
15. Smith KJ, *et al.* Acyclovir-resistant varicella zoster responsive to foscarnet. *Arch Dermatol* 1991; **127:** 1069–71.
16. Breton G, *et al.* Acyclovir-resistant herpes zoster in human immunodeficiency virus-infected patients: results of foscarnet therapy. *Clin Infect Dis* 1998; **27:** 1525–7.
17. Bendel AE, *et al.* Failure of foscarnet in disseminated herpes zoster. *Lancet* 1993; **341:** 1342.
18. Gnann JW, *et al.* Sorivudine versus acyclovir for treatment of dermatomal herpes zoster in human immunodeficiency virus-infected patients: results from a randomized, controlled clinical trial. *Antimicrob Agents Chemother* 1998; **42:** 1139–45.
19. Burdge DR, *et al.* Sorivudine (BV-ara-U) for the treatment of complicated refractory varicella zoster virus infection in HIV-infected patients. *AIDS* 1995; **9:** 810–12.
20. Wutzler P, *et al.* Oral brivudin vs intravenous acyclovir in the treatment of herpes zoster in immunocompromised patients: a randomized double-blind trial. *J Med Virol* 1995; **46:** 252–7.
21. Anonymous. Treatment of ocular herpes zoster. *Lancet* 1991; **338:** 1244–5.
22. Tyring S, *et al.* Famciclovir for ophthalmic zoster: a randomised aciclovir controlled study. *Br J Ophthalmol* 2001; **85:** 576–81.
23. Moorthy RS, *et al.* Management of varicella zoster virus retinitis in AIDS. *Br J Ophthalmol* 1997; **81:** 189–94.
24. Jackson JL, *et al.* The effect of treating herpes zoster with oral acyclovir in preventing postherpetic neuralgia: a meta-analysis. *Arch Intern Med* 1997; **157:** 909–12.
25. Alper BS, Lewis PR. Does treatment of acute herpes zoster prevent or shorten postherpetic neuralgia? *J Fam Pract* 2000; **49:** 255–64.

## HIV infection and AIDS

The causative agent of AIDS (acquired immunodeficiency syndrome) is the human immunodeficiency virus (HIV; previously known as HTLV-III or LAV), a retrovirus transmitted by sexual contact, blood and blood products, the use of contaminated needles, or from mother to fetus. Two subtypes of HIV have been identified. The most common is HIV-1, which occurs worldwide. HIV-2 is found mainly in Africa and is associated with a slower progression to AIDS than HIV-1.

HIV has a high affinity for the CD4 receptor on T lymphocytes and its major effect on the immune system is a progressive depletion of CD4+ T lymphocytes.[1] Although there is no rigid pattern in progression from HIV infection to AIDS, a typical course is as follows. Infection is followed by development of anti-HIV antibodies (seroconversion). During seroconversion the patient may remain asymptomatic or have transient symptoms including rash, sore throat, and lymphadenopathy. Despite the antibodies the infection progresses over a period of months to several years to persistent generalised lymphadenopathy (lymphadenopathy syndrome) or to a more serious collection of symptoms, sometimes known as AIDS-related complex (ARC), and including fatigue, weight loss, recurrent fever, diarrhoea, and persistent infections. AIDS is characterised by severe impairment of the immune system leading to the development of secondary infections, particularly *Pneumocystis carinii* pneumonia, *Toxoplasma* encephalitis, oropharyngeal and oesophageal candidiasis, cryptococcal meningitis, cytomegalovirus retinitis, and tuberculosis, or to secondary neoplasms such as Kaposi's sarcoma, primary CNS lymphomas, invasive cervical cancer, and non-Hodgkin's lymphoma. Other complications are numerous and may include dementia and thrombocytopenia. Series of articles in *Lancet* 1996, *Med J Aust* 1995/96, and *J Antimicrob Chemother* 1996[2] have discussed various aspects of HIV infection and the associated disorders.

The revised definition of AIDS by the US Centers for Disease Control[1] (as all HIV-infected patients with a CD4+ T lymphocyte count of less than 200/microlitre or less than 14% of the total lymphocyte count) has not generally been adopted outside the USA.[3] Measurement of both the CD4+ T lymphocyte count and HIV RNA may be a more accurate surrogate marker for clinical outcome and is increasingly used to assess prognosis before starting treatment and to monitor progress of the disease during treatment.[4] WHO has produced guidelines[5,6] for the diagnosis and treatment of HIV infection and related disorders in resource-limited settings and has declared[6] the aim of having 3 million people taking antiretrovirals in the developing world by the end of 2005.

In general, HIV infections eventually result in AIDS, which is invariably fatal. However, in a small proportion of patients the immune system stabilises after an initial decline in CD4+ count despite continued HIV infection.[7]

Cases of clearance of HIV infection in neonates infected prenatally have been reported.[8] Variation in the genes for recently identified coreceptors necessary for HIV infection may be involved[9] and may offer new therapeutic targets.

**Treatment**. The following discussion relates to the use of antiretrovirals in HIV infection and AIDS. The treatment of secondary and opportunistic infections and other complications is covered under the relevant sections, below.

Treatment strategies for HIV infection have been changing rapidly with the advent of new antiretroviral drugs and improved timing of treatment and guidelines for the treatment of HIV infection published in the USA[10,11,51] and in the UK[12] are frequently updated. Until recently monotherapy with zidovudine (or an alternative nucleoside reverse transcriptase inhibitor) was most commonly used, but combination therapy is now considered essential. There is still debate over whether to start treatment early in the course of the infection or to delay until the disease progresses.[10,13-15] However, in view of the adverse effects of current treatment regimens, in the USA treatment is often deferred to a later stage in the disease process than was formerly recommended.[10] Treatment during the acute infection has also been advocated,[16] but a more conservative approach is often adopted in view of the lack of evidence of long-term benefits.[10]

The main drugs used in combination therapy are nucleoside reverse transcriptase inhibitors (such as zidovudine, abacavir, didanosine, lamivudine, stavudine, and zalcitabine), HIV-protease inhibitors (such as amprenavir, atazanavir, fosamprenavir, indinavir, lopinavir, nelfinavir, ritonavir, and saquinavir), and non-nucleoside reverse transcriptase inhibitors (such as delavirdine, efavirenz, and nevirapine). Those that inhibit reverse transcriptase act by preventing the spread of the virus to uninfected cells. HIV-protease inhibitors act at a late stage of viral replication, preventing the maturation of the viral particle to an infective form. The HIV-fusion inhibitor enfuvirtide may herald a new class of drugs and acts by blocking fusion of HIV with cells, thereby blocking entry. Many other drugs have been investigated, including transactivator gene (tat) inhibitors, integrase inhibitors, TIBO derivatives, and recombinant soluble CD4 (rs CD4). There are also strategies involving linking toxins to a CD4 carrier. Therapies aimed at modifying the immune response to HIV include the use of interleukin-2 (see p.563), normal immunoglobulins (see p.1629), and hyperimmune plasma products; a number of vaccines are also being developed. The response to interferon therapy has generally been disappointing (see p.644). Gene therapies, antisense oligonucleotides, modified chemokines, and ribozymes have also been investigated.

**Monotherapy** with zidovudine was generally considered to produce an improvement, albeit short-lived, in the incidence of opportunistic infections and in mortality in patients with ARC or AIDS (there might also be an improvement in some of the other features of AIDS such as dementia)[17,18] and early studies produced promising results. For example, a placebo-controlled study[19] was terminated prematurely when the results at up to 24 weeks showed a significantly reduced mortality rate and incidence of opportunistic infections in the zidovudine group. Unfortunately, subsequent studies showed that the benefits in AIDS and ARC patients were limited to the first few months of treatment.[20] It was also shown that while the death rate was reduced during the first year of zidovudine treatment,[21] after 2 years there was no difference between patients who did or did not receive zidovudine; beyond 2 years the death rate was higher in the zidovudine group.

Similarly, expectations that giving zidovudine monotherapy to patients in the early stages of HIV infection before symptoms developed might delay progression and reduce the mortality rate were not fulfilled. Various studies in asymptomatic or mildly symptomatic patients showed that zidovudine started early could delay progression to ARC or AIDS within a follow-up period of about 2 years.[22-25] However, with the exception of the European-Australian Collaborative Group study[26] (which reported continued benefits at up to 3 years), the delay in disease progression was found to be transitory,[27,28] and in general no improvements in survival rates were seen.[24,27,28] In addition, adverse effects of zidovudine may counterbalance any improvements in quality of life to be gained from a prolonged disease-free period.[29] Nevertheless, the successful reduction of vertical transmission from mother to child with zidovudine therapy (see under HIV Infection Prophylaxis, below) and findings that zidovudine given early in the primary infection might delay disease progression[30] did suggest that early antiretroviral treatment may be beneficial. The failure of monotherapy with antiretrovirals to produce sustained clinical benefits including improved survival is due, at least in part, to the selection of drug-resistant variants of HIV. Resistance develops rapidly during monotherapy and cross-resistance is reported between related drugs.

**Combination therapy** with antiretroviral drugs given early in the infection (a strategy analogous to the treatment of tuberculosis and other infectious diseases) aims to improve efficacy, minimise toxicity, and delay drug resistance. Results from the Delta study[31] and the US AIDS Clinical Trial Group 175 (ACTG 175) study,[32] showing combination therapy to be more effective than monotherapy in antiretroviral-naive patients, have led to profound changes in clinical practice. Both studies showed substantial reductions in mortality at 30 months in antiretroviral-naive patients treated with zidovudine plus either didanosine or zalcitabine compared with those receiving zidovudine alone. Combinations of three antiretrovirals, typically two nucleoside reverse transcriptase inhibitors plus either an HIV-protease inhibitor or a non-nucleoside reverse transcriptase inhibitor, referred to as **highly active antiretroviral therapy** or **HAART**, have produced reductions in viral loads, often to levels below the limits of detection, and have been associated with sustained improvements in disease progression. It appears that it is necessary to suppress viral replication to this extent in order to inhibit the emergence of resistant variants and consequent disease progression.[33] The decline in CD4+ count has been arrested or reversed in patients on HAART therapy, even in the absence of profound suppression of viraemia,[34] and there is some evidence that immune function may be partially restored in the long term.[35] Declining morbidity and mortality among patients with HIV infection have been attributed to the introduction of more effective treatment regimens.[36-40] Systematic review and meta-analysis has concluded that triple therapy regimens are superior to dual therapy or monotherapy.[41] Quadruple therapy regimens may be of further benefit but this requires further study.[41]

Although HAART regimens are generally most effective in antiretroviral-naive patients, good responses can also be achieved in patients who have received previous treatment.[42] When a new regimen is started, drugs should be started simultaneously rather than sequentially.[43] Ideally, drug regimens should be changed entirely to drugs that have not been taken previously, or at least two drugs of a triple-drug regimen should be changed.

Despite the ability of HAART regimens to maintain the viral loads at undetectable levels, clinical experience shows that viral load rapidly returns to pretreatment levels once treatment is stopped. The reason for this appears to be the persistence of the virus in a latent state or in compartments not accessible to antiretrovirals. At present it has not been possible to stop treatment in the majority of patients. Although intermittent therapy may eventually be possible,[44] there is currently no evidence to support its use.[45-47] The continued effectiveness of any HAART regimen is dependent on compliance with treatment, since lapses in compliance can rapidly lead to the emergence of HIV variants resistant to one or more of the drugs being used and consequent disease progression. However, compliance is difficult to maintain due to the complexity of many regimens and to poor tolerability and long-term adverse effects of the drugs used. In addition, the cost of treatment is high and access to effective treatment in developing countries with high burdens of disease is of particular concern.[6] There has been some interest in the use of hydroxycarbamide with conventional antiretrovirals[48] and this may result in the development of regimens that are particularly useful in developing countries. Approaches being tried to overcome compliance problems include: the use of simplified dosage regimens using combined products or utilising pharmacokinetic interactions to reduce doses or extend the dosing interval; the investigation of simplified maintenance regimens (although preliminary results were disappointing[49]); activating latent HIV-1 with immunostimulant treatment (for example interleukins, colony-stimulating factors, or antibodies to CD3) thereby making it susceptible to antiretrovirals;[50] and the development of new drugs with novel modes of action.


1. Anonymous. 1993 Revised classification system for HIV infection and expanded surveillance case definition for AIDS among adolescents and adults. *JAMA* 1993; **269:** 729–80.
2. Various. HIV infection. *J Antimicrob Chemother* 1996; **37** (suppl B): 1–198.
3. Ancelle Park RA. European AIDS definition. *Lancet* 1992; **339:** 671.
4. Saag MS. Use of HIV viral load in clinical practice: back to the future. *Ann Intern Med* 1997; **126:** 983–5.
5. WHO. *Global programme on AIDS: guidelines for the clinical management of HIV infection in adults.* Geneva: WHO, 1991.
6. WHO. Scaling up antiretroviral therapy in resource-limited settings: guidelines for a public health approach. Available at: http://www.who.int/hiv/pub/prev_care/en/ScalingUp_E.pdf (accessed 10/03/04)
7. Cao Y, *et al.* Virologic and immunologic characterization of long-term survivors of human immunodeficiency virus type 1 infection. *N Engl J Med* 1995; **332:** 201–8.
8. Bryson YJ, *et al.* Clearance of HIV infection in a perinatally infected infant. *N Engl J Med* 1995; **332:** 833–8.
9. Bradbury J. HIV-1-resistant individuals may lack HIV-1 coreceptor. *Lancet* 1996; **348:** 463. Correction. *ibid.*; 626.
10. Department of Health and Human Services. Guidelines for the use of antiretroviral agents in HIV-1-infected adults and adolescents. Available at: http://www.aidsinfo.nih.gov/guidelines/ (accessed 10/03/04)
11. National Resource Center at the François-Xavier Bagnoud Center, Health Resources and Services Administration, National Institutes of Health. Guidelines for the use of antiretroviral agents in pediatric HIV infection. Available at: http://www.aidsinfo.nih.gov/guidelines/ (accessed 10/03/04)
12. BHIVA Writing Committee. British HIV Association (BHIVA) guidelines for the treatment of HIV-infected adults with antiretroviral therapy. Available at: http://www.bhiva.org/pdf/2003/guides/BHIVA_2003_Guidelines.pdf (accessed 10/03/04)
13. Walker BD, Basgoz N. Treat HIV-1 infection like other infections—treat it. *JAMA* 1998; **280:** 91–3.
14. Burman WJ, *et al.* The case for conservative management of early HIV disease. *JAMA* 1998; **280:** 93–5.
15. Levy JA. Caution: should we be treating HIV infection early? *Lancet* 1998; **352:** 982–3.
16. Kahn JO, Walker BD. Acute human immunodeficiency virus type 1 infection. *N Engl J Med* 1998; **339:** 33–9.
17. Portegies P, *et al.* Declining incidence of AIDS dementia complex after introduction of zidovudine treatment. *BMJ* 1989; **299:** 819–21. Correction. *ibid.*; 1141.
18. Schmitt FA, *et al.* Neuropsychological outcome of zidovudine (AZT) treatment of patients with AIDS and AIDS-related complex. *N Engl J Med* 1988; **319:** 1573–8.
19. Fischl MA, *et al.* The efficacy of azidothymidine (AZT) in the treatment of patients with AIDS and AIDS-related complex: a double-blind, placebo-controlled trial. *N Engl J Med* 1987; **317:** 185–91.
20. Dournon E, *et al.* Effects of zidovudine in 365 consecutive patients with AIDS or AIDS-related complex. *Lancet* 1988; **ii:** 1297–1302.
21. Lundgren JD, *et al.* Comparison of long-term prognosis of patients with AIDS treated and not treated with zidovudine. *JAMA* 1994; **271:** 1088–92.
22. Fischl MA, *et al.* The safety and efficacy of zidovudine (AZT) in the treatment of subjects with mildly symptomatic human immunodeficiency virus type 1 (HIV) infection: a double-blind, placebo-controlled trial. *Ann Intern Med* 1990; **112:** 727–37.
23. Volberding PA, *et al.* Zidovudine in asymptomatic human immunodeficiency virus infection: a controlled trial in persons with fewer than 500 CD4-positive cells per cubic millimeter. *N Engl J Med* 1990; **322:** 941–9.
24. Hamilton JD, *et al.* A controlled trial of early versus late treatment with zidovudine in symptomatic human immunodeficiency virus infection. *N Engl J Med* 1992; **326:** 437–43.
25. Graham NMH, *et al.* The effects on survival of early treatment of human immunodeficiency virus infection. *N Engl J Med* 1992; **326:** 1037–42.
26. Cooper DA, *et al.* Zidovudine in persons with asymptomatic HIV infection and CD4+ cell counts greater than 400 per cubic millimeter. *N Engl J Med* 1993; **329:** 297–303.
27. Concorde Coordinating Committee. Concorde: MRC/ANRS randomised double-blind controlled trial of immediate and deferred zidovudine in symptom-free HIV infection. *Lancet* 1994; **343:** 871–81.
28. Volberding PA, *et al.* The duration of zidovudine benefit in persons with asymptomatic HIV infection: prolonged evaluation of protocol 019 of the AIDS clinical trials group. *JAMA* 1994; **272:** 437–42.
29. Lenderking WR, *et al.* Evaluation of the quality of life associated with zidovudine treatment in asymptomatic human immunodeficiency virus infection. *N Engl J Med* 1994; **330:** 738–43.
30. Kinloch-de Loës S, *et al.* A controlled trial of zidovudine in primary human immunodeficiency virus infection. *N Engl J Med* 1995; **333:** 408–13.
31. Delta Coordinating Committee. Delta: a randomised double-blind controlled trial comparing combination of zidovudine plus didanosine or zalcitabine with zidovudine alone in HIV-infected individuals. *Lancet* 1996; **348:** 283–91.
32. Hammer SM, *et al.* A trial comparing nucleoside monotherapy with combination therapy in HIV-infected adults with CD4 cell counts from 200 to 500 per cubic millimeter. *N Engl J Med* 1996; **335:** 1081–90.
33. Raboud JM, *et al.* Suppression of plasma viral load below 20 copies/mL is required to achieve a long-term response to therapy. *AIDS* 1998; **12:** 1619–24.
34. Kaufmann D, *et al.* CD4-cell count in HIV-1-infected individuals remaining viraemic with highly active antiretroviral therapy (HAART). *Lancet* 1998; **351:** 723–4.
35. Graham BS. Infection with HIV-1. *BMJ* 1998; **317:** 1297–1301.
36. Palella FJ, *et al.* Declining morbidity and mortality among patients with advanced human immunodeficiency virus infection. *N Engl J Med* 1998; **338:** 853–60.
37. Detels R, *et al.* Effectiveness of potent antiretroviral therapy on time to AIDS and death in men with known HIV infection duration. *JAMA* 1998; **280:** 1497–1503.
38. Mocroft A, *et al.* Changing patterns of mortality across Europe in patients infected with HIV-1. *Lancet* 1998; **352:** 1725–30.
39. Gortmaker SL, *et al.* Effect of combination therapy including protease inhibitors on mortality among children and adolescents infected with HIV-1. *N Engl J Med* 2001; **345:** 1522–8.
40. Mocroft A, *et al.* Decline in the AIDS and death rates in the EuroSIDA study: an observational study. *Lancet* 2003; **362:** 22–9.
41. Jordan R, *et al.* Systematic review and meta-analysis of evidence for increasing numbers of drugs in antiretroviral combination therapy. *BMJ* 2002; **324:** 757–60.
42. Ledergerber B, *et al.* Clinical progression and virological failure on highly active antiretroviral therapy in HIV-1 patients: a prospective cohort study. *Lancet* 1999; **353:** 863–8.
43. Gulick RM, *et al.* Simultaneous vs sequential initiation of therapy with indinavir, zidovudine, and lamivudine for HIV-1 infection: 100-week follow-up. *JAMA* 1998; **280:** 35–41.
44. Youle M. Is interruption of HIV therapy always harmful? *J Antimicrob Chemother* 2000; **45:** 137–8.

45. Lori F, *et al.* Structured treatment interruptions as a potential alternative therapeutic regimen for HIV-infected patients: a review of recent clinical data and future prospects. *J Antimicrob Chemother* 2002; **50:** 155–60.
46. Gulick RM. Structured treatment interruption in patients infected with HIV: a new approach to therapy? *Drugs* 2002; **62:** 245–53.
47. Lawrence J, *et al.* Structured treatment interruption in patients with multidrug-resistant human immunodeficiency virus. *N Engl J Med* 2003; **349:** 837–46.
48. Lisziewicz J, *et al.* Hydroxyurea in the treatment of HIV infection: clinical efficacy and safety concerns. *Drug Safety* 2003; **26:** 605–24.
49. Cooper DA, Emery S. Therapeutic strategies for HIV infection—time to think hard. *N Engl J Med* 1998; **339:** 1319–21.
50. Morris K. HAART and host: balancing the response to HIV-1. *Lancet* 1998; **352:** 1686.
51. Yeni PG, et al. Treatment for adult HIV infection: 2004 recommendations of the International AIDS Society—USA panel. *JAMA* 2004; **292:** 251–65. Also available at: http://www.iasusa.org/pub/arv_2004.pdf (accessed 29/07/04)

**HIV-associated infections.** Patients with HIV infection and AIDS are at special risk of other infections because of their impaired cell-mediated immunity. The successful management of such patients depends as much on the prophylaxis and treatment of secondary and opportunistic infections as on the antiretroviral therapy aimed at the primary infection. There is growing concern that infections such as herpesviruses[1] and tuberculosis[2] may promote HIV replication and thereby accelerate the development of immunodeficiency. Some infections have particular significance in AIDS and are regarded as disease-defining events in patients testing positive for HIV.[3] They are: oesophageal candidiasis (p.386), cryptococcal meningitis (p.387), severe or recurrent pneumonia (p.141), and tuberculosis (p.150). Other common AIDS-related infections include mucosal candidiasis (p.386), coccidioidomycosis (p.387), cryptococcosis (p.387), herpesvirus infections (p.619), histoplasmosis (p.388), disseminated *Mycobacterium avium* complex infections (p.137), *Pneumocystis carinii* pneumonia (p.389), syphilis (p.148), and toxoplasmosis (p.598). Cytomegalovirus retinitis (p.619) is a common cause of blindness. Cryptosporidiosis (p.596) and microsporidiosis (p.598) have been identified as common causes of diarrhoea (see also below). Papovavirus infection can cause progressive multifocal leukoencephalopathy (see Infections in Immunocompromised Patients, p.624).

Recommendations for both treatment[4,5] and infection prophylaxis in AIDS patients who have not previously contracted an opportunistic infection (primary prophylaxis) and following treatment of an infection (secondary prophylaxis) have been published.[6,7] Improvements in opportunistic infections have been reported in patients receiving combination antiretroviral therapy containing HIV-protease inhibitors.[8] Recovery of immune function in patients responding to intensive antiretroviral combination therapy may be sufficient to protect against some opportunistic infections.[9]

1. Wood MJ. Antivirals in the context of HIV disease. *J Antimicrob Chemother* 1996; **37** (suppl B): 97–112.
2. Goletti D, *et al.* Effect of Mycobacterium tuberculosis on HIV replication: role of immune activation. *J Immunol* 1996; **157:** 1271–8.
3. Harries AD, Maher D. *TB/HIV: a clinical manual.* Geneva: WHO, 1996.
4. British Society for Antimicrobial Chemotherapy Working Party. Antifungal chemotherapy in patients with acquired immunodeficiency syndrome. *Lancet* 1992; **340:** 648–51.
5. American Thoracic Society. Fungal infection in HIV-infected persons. *Am J Respir Crit Care Med* 1995; **152:** 816–22.
6. Mijch AM, Quin J. Recommendations for antimicrobial prophylaxis in HIV. *Med J Aust* 1996; **164:** 551.
7. Centers for Disease Control and Prevention. Guidelines for preventing opportunistic infections among HIV-infected persons—2002: recommendations of the US Public Health Service and the Infectious Diseases Society of America. *MMWR* 2002; **51**(RR-8): 1–52. Also available at http://www.cdc.gov/mmwr/PDF/rr/rr5108.pdf (accessed 10/03/04)
8. Carr A, *et al.* Treatment of HIV-1-associated microsporidiosis and cryptosporidiosis with combination antiretroviral therapy. *Lancet* 1998; **351:** 256–61.
9. Powderly WG, *et al.* Recovery of the immune system with antiretroviral therapy: the end of opportunism? *JAMA* 1998; **280:** 72–7.

**HIV-associated malignancies.** There is an increased incidence of some malignancies in patients with the long-term immunodeficiency related to HIV infection. The malignancies most frequently associated with HIV infection are Kaposi's sarcoma (p.524), and non-Hodgkin's lymphoma and primary CNS lymphoma (see AIDS-related Lymphomas, p.510). In addition, invasive cervical cancer (p.515) may occur in a particularly aggressive form and this and Kaposi's sarcoma are classified as AIDS-defining events in patients testing positive for HIV. Other malignancies that may be associated with AIDS include Hodgkin's lymphoma (p.509) and, in some patient populations, tumours of the anus and rectum (see Malignant Neoplasms of the Gastrointestinal Tract p.516). Tumours may regress or the range of malignancies may change in patients responding to intensive antiretroviral combination therapy.

**HIV-associated neurological complications.** Neurological complications of HIV infection can arise from opportunistic infections of the CNS, auto-immune disorders, HIV infection of the CNS, malignancies, and metabolic or drug toxicities.

- **AIDS dementia complex** (HIV-1-associated cognitive/motor complex) and related transient neurological deficits occur mainly in patients with late HIV infection and severe immunodepression. It is thought to be due to HIV infection of the brain and there is evidence to suggest that antiretroviral therapy may have both prophylactic and therapeutic benefits. While most studies have used high-dose zidovudine, anecdotal reports suggest that intensive antiretroviral combination therapy may also be beneficial.
- **HIV headache** is not well understood and occurs in late HIV infections. Headache can also be a symptom of meningitis.
- **Neuropathies** may result from auto-immune mechanisms (for example idiopathic demyelinating neuropathies), cytomegalovirus infection, or HIV infection. One of the commonest is distal predominantly sensory polyneuropathy seen in the late stages of the disease. Effective antiretroviral combination therapy has produced improvement of neuropathies in some patients although toxicity caused by some antiretrovirals can produce similar symptoms.
- **Progressive multifocal leukoencephalopathy** due to papovavirus infection is discussed under Infections in Immunocompromised Patients, p.624.

References.

1. Melton ST, *et al.* Pharmacotherapy of HIV dementia. *Ann Pharmacother* 1997; **31:** 457–73.
2. Skolnick AA. Protease inhibitors may reverse AIDS dementia. *JAMA* 1998; **279:** 419.
3. Gendelman HE, *et al.* Suppression of inflammatory neurotoxins by highly active antiretroviral therapy in human immunodeficiency virus-associated dementia. *J Infect Dis* 1998; **178:** 1000–1007.
4. Markus R, Brew BJ. HIV-1 peripheral neuropathy and combination antiretroviral therapy. *Lancet* 1998; **352:** 1906–7.
5. Simpson DM. Human immunodeficiency virus-associated dementia: review of pathogenesis, prophylaxis, and treatment studies of zidovudine therapy. *Clin Infect Dis* 1999; **29:** 19–34.
6. Wulff EA, *et al.* HIV-associated peripheral neuropathy: epidemiology, pathophysiology and treatment. *Drugs* 2000; **59:** 1251–60.

**HIV-associated wasting and diarrhoea.** Diarrhoea and the wasting syndrome (with weight loss and cachexia) are major contributors to the morbidity and mortality of late HIV infection and AIDS, particularly in Africa where the syndrome has been termed 'slim disease'. Although the pathology is poorly understood, opportunistic infections, principally with Microsporidia and Cryptosporidia, cytomegalovirus, and *Mycobacterium avium-intracellulare*, are the most common causes of diarrhoea, while histopathological changes in the small bowel mucosa may also contribute. Malnutrition is thought to be a more likely cause of wasting than increased resting energy expenditure although nutritional supplementation is not consistently effective. Management of diarrhoea relies primarily on rehydration, antidiarrhoeal drugs, and antimicrobial treatment. If no causative pathogen is identified, elimination of common bacterial pathogens by empirical treatment with a fluoroquinolone such as ciprofloxacin has been suggested. Albendazole has also produced beneficial responses when given empirically. Details of specific management of the common infections are on p.596 (Cryptosporidiosis), p.619 (Cytomegalovirus Infections), p.598 (Microsporidiosis), and p.137 (Opportunistic Mycobacterial Infections). Other common microbial causes of diarrhoea are dealt with under Gastro-enteritis on p.127 (bacterial), p.596 (protozoal), and p.618 (viral). The use of antidiarrhoeals and rehydration techniques is discussed under Diarrhoea, p.1241. Antisecretory drugs such as octreotide have been tried with some success but are unlikely to have a wide role in the treatment of HIV-associated diarrhoea. Recombinant growth hormone has been suggested for cachectic patients who do not respond to nutritional supplementation. Other drugs tried in cachexia include megestrol and dronabinol (as appetite stimulants), the growth hormone mediator mecasermin, testosterone, and drugs that decrease cytokine production including pentoxifylline and thalidomide.

References.

1. Von Roenn JH. Management of HIV-related bodyweight loss. *Drugs* 1994; **47:** 774–83.
2. Weinroth SE, *et al.* Wasting syndrome in AIDS: pathophysiologic mechanisms and therapeutic approaches. *Infect Agents Dis* 1995; **4:** 76–94.
3. Corcoran C, Grinspoon S. Treatments for wasting in patients with the acquired immunodeficiency syndrome. *N Engl J Med* 1999; **340:** 1740–50. Correction. *ibid.*; **341:** 776.
4. Nemechek PM, *et al.* Treatment guidelines for HIV-associated wasting. *Mayo Clin Proc* 2000; **75:** 386–94.
5. Grinspoon S, Mulligan K. Weight loss and wasting in patients infected with human immunodeficiency virus. *Clin Infect Dis* 2003; **36** (suppl 2): S69–S78.

## HIV infection prophylaxis

Despite remaining uncertainties over the efficacy and toxicity of prophylactic antiretroviral regimens following accidental exposure to HIV, they are becoming more widely accepted, particularly after **occupational exposure**.[1] Zidovudine has been commonly used, and has been reported[2] to reduce seroconversion after percutaneous exposure by 79%, but there are case reports of seroconversion,[3-6] including some where zidovudine was given within an hour of exposure.[5,6] The risk of seroconversion is estimated at about 0.3 to 0.4% following percutaneous contamination with HIV-infected blood[4,7,8] and considerably less for accidents involving contamination of intact skin or mucous membranes.[7,8] In view of short-term and potential long-term toxicity of antiretrovirals, chemoprophylaxis should only be offered to high-risk cases.[9] If chemoprophylaxis is given it should preferably be started as soon as possible after the accident. In the UK,[10] guidelines recommend that prophylaxis with a combination of zidovudine 300 mg twice daily (or 250 mg twice daily), lamivudine 150 mg twice daily, and nelfinavir 1250 mg twice daily (or 750 mg three times daily) should be offered for 4 weeks following occupational percutaneous, mucous membrane, or broken skin site exposure to high-risk body fluids or tissues known to be, or strongly suspected of being, infected with HIV. Other HIV-protease inhibitors considered suitable alternatives to nelfinavir include lopinavir-ritonavir, saquinavir, and amprenavir. Guidelines in the USA[7] recommend a basic two-drug regimen of zidovudine 600 mg daily in two or three divided doses plus lamivudine 150 mg twice daily when there is a recognised risk of transmission; alternative basic regimens are lamivudine as above plus stavudine 40 mg twice daily (30 mg twice daily in those weighing less than 60 kg), or didanosine 400 mg daily (125 mg twice daily in those weighing less than 60 kg) plus stavudine as above. An expanded regimen is recommended when there is an increased risk of transmission, consisting of one of the basic regimens above with the addition of one of indinavir 800 mg every 8 hours, or nelfinavir 750 mg three times daily or 1250 mg twice daily, or efavirenz 600 mg once daily at bedtime, or abacavir 300 mg twice daily. They also recommend that such treatment should continue for 4 weeks, if tolerated. Serious adverse effects have been reported following the use of regimens containing nevirapine[11] and US guidelines state that it should not be used for postexposure prophylaxis.[7]

Hygienic measures and behavioural changes are the most effective methods of **reducing the spread of HIV infection in the general population**. These include needle exchange schemes for intravenous drug abusers and the promotion of safe-sex practices. Guidelines have been published in the USA[12] for the management of non-occupational exposure to HIV amongst the general population. There is some evidence that heterosexual transmission may be inhibited if the infected partner is receiving zidovudine.[13] However, transmission is only reduced by about 50% and zidovudine treatment does not obviate the need for behavioural changes to reduce the risk of transmission. Prophylaxis following sexual exposure similar to that following occupational exposure has also been proposed,[14] although the disadvantages of antiretroviral prophylaxis in this setting may outweigh the advantages.[12,15] Vaccination against HIV infection is being investigated, but it is not clear yet if this is a feasible approach.

Measures aimed at **reducing vertical transmission** from mothers with HIV infection to their infants include perinatal chemotherapy and discouraging breast feeding. The Pediatric AIDS Clinical Trial Group protocol 076 (ACTG 076) study[16] of zidovudine therapy during pregnancy, labour, and given to the infant postpartum was stopped prematurely when good preliminary results were observed. Further analysis[17] of the results of ACTG 076 showed that the risk of vertical transmission was reduced regardless of the maternal viral load or CD4+ count. The protocol, which involved starting oral zidovudine at 14 to 34 weeks' gestation, giving the mother an intravenous dose at birth, and administering zidovudine to the infant for 6 weeks, has been widely adopted in the USA.[18] However, short-course oral therapy comprising less frequent doses given from 36 weeks' gestation, oral doses during labour and without treatment of the infant has also been shown to cut transmission,[19-21] and may be more appropriate for use in developing countries. Combination therapy with antiretrovirals has been investigated for prevention of vertical transmission; in one study in France,[22] lamivudine given from 32 weeks' gestation and to the infant for 6 weeks, in addition to the ACTG 076 zidovudine regimen, was effective in reducing vertical transmission, but severe adverse effects occurred and resistance to lamivudine emerged and it was concluded that the role of combination therapy was unclear. A further study in Africa[23] comparing short-course combination regimens found that zidovudine and lamivudine started at 36 weeks' gestation then given during labour and for 1 week to the mother and neonate resulted in a greater reduction in transmission than the same combination given without the prepartum component, although both regimens were effective; the combination had no efficacy when given during labour alone. Moreover, the benefits from the first two regimens diminished considerably after 18 months of follow-up.[23] There is also evidence that prophylactic zidovudine begun as late as the first 48 hours of life may still be of benefit in reducing vertical transmission.[24] Nevirapine given in single doses to the mother before delivery and to the neonate has also been shown to reduce transmission in breast-feeding women who were not receiving antiretroviral therapy,[25] but did not demonstrate additional benefit in reducing transmission in women who were receiving antiretrovirals but who were not breast feeding.[26] Another study[27] in sub-Saharan Africa involving HIV-positive women who were not tested or counselled during pregnancy but who did breast feed has suggested that treatment of the neonate only with a single oral dose of nevirapine as soon as possible after birth together with oral zidovudine for 7 days may offer greater protection against vertical transmission than nevirapine alone. Maternal vitamin A deficiency has been identified as a risk factor for vertical transmission in Africa (see p.1453). Nutritional intervention and vaginal cleansing during labour could reduce vertical transmission in regions where zidovudine therapy is not readily available.

**Other measures** necessary to minimise the transmission of infection include the rigorous selection of blood donors, microbiological screening of the blood, and, where possible, heat treatment of blood products.


1. Henderson DK. Postexposure chemoprophylaxis for occupational exposures to the human immunodeficiency virus. *JAMA* 1999; **281:** 931–6.
2. Centers for Disease Control. Case-control study of HIV seroconversion in health-care workers after percutaneous exposure to HIV-infected blood—France, United Kingdom, and United States, January 1988–August 1994. *MMWR* 1995; **44:** 929–33.
3. Looke DFM, Grove DI. Failed prophylactic zidovudine after needlestick injury. *Lancet* 1990; **335:** 1280.
4. Tokars JI, *et al.* Surveillance of HIV infection and zidovudine use among health care workers after occupational exposure to HIV-infected blood. *Ann Intern Med* 1993; **118:** 913–19.
5. Lange JMA, *et al.* Failure of zidovudine prophylaxis after accidental exposure to HIV-1. *N Engl J Med* 1990; **322:** 1375–7.
6. Anonymous. HIV seroconversion after occupational exposure despite early prophylactic zidovudine therapy. *Lancet* 1993; **341:** 1077–8.
7. Centers for Disease Control and Prevention. Updated US Public Health Service guidelines for the management of occupational exposures to HBV, HCV, and HIV and recommendations for postexposure prophylaxis. *MMWR* 2001; **50** (RR-11): 1–52. Also available at: http://www.cdc.gov/mmwr/PDF/rr/rr5011.pdf (accessed 10/03/04)
8. Jeffries DJ. Zidovudine after occupational exposure to HIV. *BMJ* 1991; **302:** 1349–51.
9. Easterbrook P, Ippolito G. Prophylaxis after occupational exposure to HIV. *BMJ* 1997; **315:** 557–8.
10. UK Department of Health. HIV post-exposure prophylaxis: guidance from the UK Chief Medical Officers' Expert Advisory Group on AIDS. London: Department of Health, February 2004. Available at: http://www.advisorybodies.doh.gov.uk/eaga/prophylaxisguidancefeb04.pdf (accessed 10/03/04)
11. Centers for Disease Control. Serious adverse events attributed to nevirapine regimens for postexposure prophylaxis after HIV exposure—worldwide, 1997-2000. *MMWR* 2001; **49:** 1153–6.
12. Centers for Disease Control. Management of possible sexual, injecting-drug-use, or other nonoccupational exposure to HIV, including considerations related to antiretroviral therapy: Public Health Service statement. *MMWR* 1998; **47** (RR-17): 1–14. Also available at: http://www.cdc.gov/mmwr/PDF/rr/rr4717.pdf (accessed 10/03/04)
13. Musicco M, *et al.* Antiretroviral treatment of men infected with human immunodeficiency virus type 1 reduces the incidence of heterosexual transmission. *Arch Intern Med* 1994; **154:** 1971–6.
14. Katz MH, Gerberding JL. The care of persons with recent sexual exposure to HIV. *Ann Intern Med* 1998; **128:** 306–12.
15. Lurie P, *et al.* Postexposure prophylaxis after nonoccupational HIV exposure: clinical, ethical, and policy considerations. *JAMA* 1998; **280:** 1769–73.
16. Connor EM, *et al.* Reduction of maternal-infant transmission of human immunodeficiency virus type 1 with zidovudine treatment. *N Engl J Med* 1994; **331:** 1173–80.
17. Sperling RS, *et al.* Maternal viral load, zidovudine treatment, and the risk of transmission of human immunodeficiency virus type 1 from mother to infant. *N Engl J Med* 1996; **335:** 1621–9.
18. Perinatal HIV Guidelines Working Group. Public Health Service Task Force recommendations for use of antiretroviral drugs in pregnant HIV-1-infected women for maternal health and interventions to reduce perinatal HIV-1 transmission in the United States. Available at: http://www.aidsinfo.nih.gov/guidelines/ (accessed 10/03/04)
19. Shaffer N, *et al.* Short-course zidovudine for perinatal HIV-1 transmission in Bangkok, Thailand: a randomised controlled trial. *Lancet* 1999; **353:** 773–80.
20. Wiktor SZ, *et al.* Short-course oral zidovudine for prevention of mother-to-child transmission of HIV-1 in Abidjan, Côte d'Ivoire: a randomised trial. *Lancet* 1999; **353:** 781–5.
21. Dabis F, *et al.* 6-Month efficacy, tolerance, and acceptability of a short regimen of oral zidovudine to reduce vertical transmission of HIV in breastfed children in Côte d'Ivoire and Burkina Faso: a double-blind placebo-controlled multicentre trial. *Lancet* 1999; **353:** 786–92.
22. Mandelbrot L, *et al.* Lamivudine-zidovudine combination for prevention of maternal-infant transmission of HIV-1. *JAMA* 2001; **285:** 2083–93.
23. The Petra Study Team. Efficacy of three short-course regimens of zidovudine and lamivudine in preventing early and late transmission of HIV-1 from mother to child in Tanzania, South Africa, and Uganda (Petra study): a randomised, double-blind, placebo-controlled trial. *Lancet* 2002; **359:** 1178–86.
24. Wade NA, *et al.* Abbreviated regimens of zidovudine prophylaxis and perinatal transmission of the human immunodeficiency virus. *N Engl J Med* 1998; **339:** 1409–14.
25. Guay LA, *et al.* Intrapartum and neonatal single-dose nevirapine compared with zidovudine for prevention of mother-to-child transmission of HIV-1 in Kampala, Uganda: HIVNET 012 randomised trial. *Lancet* 1999; **354:** 795–802.
26. Dorenbaum A, *et al.* Two-dose intrapartum/newborn nevirapine and standard antiretroviral therapy to reduce perinatal HIV transmission: a randomized trial. *JAMA* 2002; **288:** 189–98.
27. Taha TE, *et al.* Short postexposure prophylaxis in newborn babies to reduce mother-to-child transmission of HIV-1: NVAZ randomised clinical trial. *Lancet* 2003; **362:** 1171–7.


## Infections in immunocompromised patients

Most viral infections present in a more severe form in immunocompromised patients than in immunocompetent patients. Among the viral infections that may be a particular problem in immunocompromised patients are hepatitis, herpesvirus infections (including cytomegalovirus and Epstein-Barr virus infections), measles, and respiratory syncytial virus infections. For further information and treatment of these infections, see under the individual diseases. For secondary infections occurring in HIV-infected patients, see p.623.

Persistent infection with human **parvovirus B19** can cause red cell aplasia with resultant anaemia, particularly in immunocompromised patients; treatment with immunoglobulin has been reported to be successful.

Infection with a papovavirus (JC virus)[1,2] can cause **progressive multifocal leukoencephalopathy**. Although no treatment has been consistently successful,[1] prolonged survival has been reported in patients receiving interferon alfa[3] and in those receiving highly active antiretroviral therapy (HAART).[4-6] Cidofovir may be of benefit in patients unresponsive to HAART.[7,8]


1. Brink NS, Miller RF. Clinical presentation, diagnosis and therapy of progressive multifocal leukoencephalopathy. *J Infect* 1996; **32:** 97–102.
2. Greenlee JE. Progressive multifocal leukoencephalopathy—progress made and lessons relearned. *N Engl J Med* 1998; **338:** 1378–80.
3. Huang SS, *et al.* Survival prolongation in HIV-associated progressive multifocal leukoencephalopathy treated with alpha-interferon: an observational study. *J Neurovirol* 1998; **4:** 324–32.
4. Albrecht H, *et al.* Highly active antiretroviral therapy significantly improves the prognosis of patients with HIV-associated progressive multifocal leukoencephalopathy. *AIDS* 1998; **12:** 1149–54.
5. Elliot B, *et al.* 2.5 Year remission of AIDS-associated progressive multifocal leukoencephalopathy with combined antiretroviral therapy. *Lancet* 1997; **349:** 850.
6. Domingo P, *et al.* Remission of progressive multifocal leucoencephalopathy after antiretroviral therapy. *Lancet* 1997; **349:** 1554–5.
7. Segarra-Newnham M, Vodolo KM. Use of cidofovir in progressive multifocal leukoencephalopathy. *Ann Pharmacother* 2001; **35:** 741–4.
8. Razonable RR, *et al.* Cidofovir treatment of progressive multifocal leukoencephalopathy in a patient receiving highly active antiretroviral therapy. *Mayo Clin Proc* 2001; **76:** 1171–5.


## Influenza

Influenza is caused by RNA viruses of the family Orthomyxoviridae. Three types of influenza virus, A, B, and C, have been classified. Type A causes most infections in man; type B causes a similar though possibly milder infection than type A; type C causes only a mild infection. Epidemic influenza is usually caused by the type A influenza virus. Outbreaks of influenza due to the type A virus occur in most years while those due to the type B virus tend to occur at intervals of several years. Influenza viruses, especially influenza A, are antigenically labile with the principal surface antigens, haemagglutinin and neuraminidase, undergoing antigenic changes. Major changes (antigenic shifts) in these surface antigens of the influenza A virus occur periodically and are responsible for the emergence of the subtypes of virus which may cause pandemic influenza; more minor changes (antigenic drift) occur more frequently and are responsible for the annual epidemic outbreaks of influenza.

Influenza is transmitted from person to person in respiratory droplets. Infection with influenza A or B virus typically causes fever, chills, headache, malaise, myalgia, dry cough, nasal obstruction, and a dry or sore throat. Such infections are usually acute but self-limiting. Complications can occur though, and include primary viral pneumonia, secondary bacterial pneumonia, croup, exacerbation of asthma or chronic bronchitis, myositis, Reye's syndrome, and the toxic shock syndrome. Patients at high risk of complications include the elderly and those with heart and chronic chest disease.

Treatment of influenza is largely symptomatic and supportive. Amantadine and rimantadine have both been shown to reduce the duration of influenza A symptoms when given within 48 hours of the onset of symptoms and may be given to high-risk patients. Treatment and prophylaxis failures may be due to the rapid emergence of drug-resistant viruses. Oseltamivir and zanamivir, which inhibit viral neuraminidase, are active against both influenza A and B viruses. Response to ribavirin has generally been disappointing.

The most effective means of preventing influenza is with influenza vaccine adjusted to take account of current antigenic drifts and shifts and to provide protection against both influenza A and B. Amantadine and rimantadine are also effective at preventing influenza A but are not a substitute for vaccination unless the vaccine is contra-indicated. Prophylaxis with amantadine or rimantadine should be considered in addition to vaccination in individuals such as the immunocompromised whose antibody response to the vaccine is likely to be incomplete, in persons vaccinated after an influenza outbreak has begun, and in residents and carers in institutions to prevent or abort outbreaks of influenza. To be fully effective chemoprophylaxis must be started as early as possible and be taken each day for the duration of influenza activity or until an adequate antibody response to vaccination has occurred. Neuraminidase inhibitors may also be useful for prophylaxis.

References.


1. Couch RB. Prevention and treatment of influenza. *N Engl J Med* 2000; **343:** 1778–87.
2. Jefferson T, *et al.* Neuraminidase inhibitors for preventing and treating influenza in healthy adults. Available in The Cochrane Library; Issue 1. Chichester: John Wiley; 2004.
3. Nicholson KG, *et al.* Influenza. *Lancet* 2003; **362:** 1733–45.
4. Matheson NJ, *et al.* Neuraminidase inhibitors for preventing and treating influenza in children. Available in The Cochrane Library; Issue 1. Chichester: John Wiley; 2004.
5. Jefferson TO, *et al.* Amantadine and rimantadine for preventing and treating influenza A in adults. Available in The Cochrane Library; Issue 1. Chichester: John Wiley; 2004.


## Measles

Measles is caused by an RNA virus of the family Paramyxoviridae. It is a highly contagious disease spread by direct contact with respiratory secretions of infected persons, allowing the virus to invade the upper respiratory tract, nose, and possibly the conjunctivae. During the prodromal phase patients usually experience malaise, fever, conjunctivitis, cough, rhinitis, congestion, and later Koplik's spots on the buccal mucosa. An erythematous, maculopapular rash then develops starting on the face and spreading over the trunk and limbs. Immunocompromised patients are at special risk of respiratory and central complications. Recovery usually takes place during the week following the rash's appearance. However, potentially fatal complications may develop, especially in immunocompromised patients. There may be respiratory complications, including giant cell pneumonia and bacterial and viral superinfections, and central complications including acute encephalitis, a progressive subacute encephalitis, and the more slowly progressive subacute sclerosing panencephalitis (SSPE) that may develop several years after the original measles infection.

Measles usually requires only symptomatic and supportive treatment.[1] Administration of vitamin A supplements to prevent complications from measles is well established in children in developing countries and may be beneficial in children in developed countries (see p.1453). The use of prophylactic antibacterials remains controversial but has not been supported by clinical trials.[2-4] There appears to be no good evidence for antivirals being effective in the complications of measles.

Measles can be prevented by active immunisation with measles vaccine, and measles immunoglobulins may be used for passive immunisation against measles. Normal immunoglobulins may be used to prevent, or possibly modify, an attack of measles in those at risk of developing severe or fatal disease such as immunocompromised patients.

1. Hussey G. Managing measles. *BMJ* 1997; **314:** 316–17.
2. Shann F. Meta-analysis of trials of prophylactic antibiotics for children with measles: inadequate evidence. *BMJ* 1997; **314:** 334–7.
3. Duke T, Mgone CS. Measles: not just another viral exanthem. *Lancet* 2003; **361:** 763–73.
4. Shann F, *et al.* Antibiotics for preventing pneumonia in children with measles. Available in The Cochrane Library; Issue 1. Chichester: John Wiley; 2004.

### Respiratory syncytial virus infection

Respiratory syncytial virus (RSV) is an RNA virus of the family Paramyxoviridae. RSV infection is generally confined to the respiratory tract; it commonly occurs in young children, and is also increasingly recognised as a common infection in the elderly. Acquired immunity is incomplete and of short duration and therefore re-infection is common. In young children, the infection generally spreads to the lower respiratory-tract and may cause bronchiolitis and pneumonia, which can be life-threatening. In older children and adults, infection occurs as an upper respiratory-tract illness or tracheobronchitis. Severe or complicated infection is more common in children with underlying cardiac or pulmonary disease and in immunocompromised patients.

The management of RSV infection is largely supportive.[1-4] Supplementary oxygen is useful in patients with bronchiolitis. Measures to limit the spread of infection in hospitals and institutions through attention to good hygiene and control of cross-infection are important. Ribavirin administered by aerosol has been shown to have beneficial effects in infants with lower respiratory-tract RSV infection, but trials lack sufficient power to provide reliable estimates of the effects and further study is needed.[5] Ribavirin has been less frequently used in the UK than in the USA and some[1] suggest its use be restricted to patients with RSV and cystic fibrosis, severe immunodeficiency, congenital heart disease and pulmonary hypertension, and patients with bronchopulmonary dysplasia and dependence on supplementary oxygen. Similarly, bronchodilators have been reported to be more commonly used for RSV bronchiolitis in the USA than in the UK.[1] The difference in clinical management could result from differences in diagnostic criteria for bronchiolitis.[1,6] It has also been considered that the evidence of efficacy of bronchodilators in bronchiolitis is uncertain.[7] Corticosteroids are deemed to be of no value.[1,2,8-10]

Respiratory syncytial virus immunoglobulin or a human monoclonal antibody to RSV, palivizumab, is recommended in the USA for prophylaxis in infants and children at high risk of severe RSV infections.[11] RSV immunoglobulin has not, however, been found to be effective in the treatment of RSV infections.[12]

Vaccines to prevent RSV infection are currently under development.

1. Rakshi K, Couriel JM. Management of acute bronchiolitis. *Arch Dis Child* 1994; **71:** 463–9.
2. Everard ML. Bronchiolitis: origins and optimal management. *Drugs* 1995; **49:** 885–96.
3. Rodriguez WJ. Management strategies for respiratory syncytial virus infections in infants. *J Pediatr* 1999; **135:** S45–S50.
4. Simoes EAF. Respiratory syncytial virus infection. *Lancet* 1999; **354:** 847–52.
5. Randolph AG, Wang EEL. Ribavirin for respiratory syncytial virus infection of the lower respiratory tract. Available in The Cochrane Library; Issue 1. Chichester: John Wiley; 2004.
6. Everard ML. Acute bronchiolitis—a perennial problem. *Lancet* 1996; **348:** 279–80.
7. Kellner JD, *et al.* Bronchodilators for bronchiolitis. Available in The Cochrane Library; Issue 1. Chichester: John Wiley; 2004.
8. Isaacs D. Bronchiolitis. *BMJ* 1995; **310:** 4–5.
9. Roosevelt G, *et al.* Dexamethasone in bronchiolitis: a randomised controlled trial. *Lancet* 1996; **348:** 292–5.
10. Cade A, *et al.* Randomised placebo controlled trial of nebulised corticosteroids in acute respiratory syncytial viral bronchiolitis. *Arch Dis Child* 2000; **82:** 126–30.
11. Committee on Infectious Diseases and Committee on Fetus and Newborn, American Academy of Pediatrics. Revised indications for the use of palivizumab and respiratory syncytial virus immune globulin intravenous for the prevention of respiratory syncytial virus infections. *Pediatrics* 2003; **112:** 1442–6. Also available at: http://www.aap.org/policy/rsv-tr9-12-03.pdf (accessed 10/03/04)
12. Rodriguez WJ, *et al.* Respiratory syncytial virus (RSV) immune globulin intravenous therapy for RSV lower respiratory tract infection in infants and young children at high risk for severe RSV infections. *Pediatrics* 1997; **99:** 454–61.

### SARS

Severe acute respiratory syndrome (SARS) is a respiratory illness thought to be caused by a novel virus that may be related to a coronavirus, although its precise aetiology is poorly understood. SARS has presented primarily in previously healthy adults although there have been some cases reported in children. The incubation period for SARS is usually 2 to 7 days, after which the disease manifests initially in the form of fever associated with dry cough or dyspnoea and may progress to hypoxia; up to about 20% of patients require mechanical ventilation and the fatality rate is thought to be around 3%. Optimal treatment of SARS is not known. Treatment regimens have included the use of antibacterials, typically clarithromycin or levofloxacin, to presumptively treat known bacterial causes of atypical pneumonia. Antiviral drugs including ribavirin and oseltamivir have also been tried. Corticosteroids have been tried orally or intravenously in combination with ribavirin.[1,2] Guidelines for the surveillance and management of SARS have been developed by WHO.[3]

1. So LK-Y, *et al.* Development of a standard treatment protocol for severe acute respiratory syndrome. *Lancet* 2003; **361:** 1615–17.
2. Peiris JSM, *et al.* The severe acute respiratory syndrome. *N Engl J Med* 2003; **349:** 2431–41.
3. WHO. Alert, verification and public health management of SARS in the post-outbreak period. Available at: http://www.who.int/csr/sars/postoutbreak/en/ (accessed 10/03/04)

### Warts

Warts are caused by human papillomaviruses. The lesions present in several different forms and can affect any skin site although the hands, feet, and anogenital areas are most frequently affected. Anogenital warts are known as condylomata acuminata. Treatment generally relies on some form of local tissue destruction and is described on p.1139. Interferons have also been used (see p.645).

---

## Abacavir *(BAN, rINN)*

{(1*S*,4*R*)-4-[2-Amino-6-(cyclopropylamino)-9*H*-purin-9-yl]cyclopent-2-enyl}methanol.

$C_{14}H_{18}N_6O$ = 286.3.

*CAS — 136470-78-5.*

*ATC — J05AF06.*

NOTE. The code 1592U89 has been applied to abacavir but is more properly reserved for abacavir sulfate.

### Abacavir Succinate *(BANM, USAN, rINNM)*

Succinato de abacavir.

$C_{14}H_{18}N_6O,C_4H_6O_4$ = 404.4.

*CAS — 168146-84-7.*

*ATC — J05AF06.*

NOTE. The code 1592U89 has been applied to abacavir succinate but is more properly reserved for abacavir sulfate.

### Abacavir Sulfate *(USAN, rINNM)*

Abacavir Sulphate *(BANM)*; Sulfato de abacavir; 1592U89.

$(C_{14}H_{18}N_6O)_2,H_2SO_4$ = 670.7.

*CAS — 188062-50-2.*

*ATC — J05AF06.*

NOTE. The code 1592U89 and its abbreviated form, 1592, have also been applied to abacavir and abacavir succinate.

### Adverse Effects

Severe hypersensitivity reactions, sometimes fatal, have occurred in about 4% of patients receiving abacavir, especially (but not exclusively) during the first 6 weeks of treatment, or during intermittent therapy. Symptoms of hypersensitivity commonly include fever, rash, cough, dyspnoea, lethargy, malaise, headache, myalgia, and gastrointestinal disturbances, particularly nausea and vomiting, diarrhoea, and abdominal pain. Anaphylaxis has occurred. Caution is needed as hypersensitivity may be misdiagnosed as influenza, respiratory disease, or gastroenteritis. Erythema multiforme, Stevens-Johnson syndrome, and toxic epidermal necrolysis have occurred rarely. Other adverse effects associated with abacavir include pancreatitis and elevated blood glucose and triglyceride concentrations. There may be raised liver enzyme values. Lactic acidosis, sometimes fatal and usually associated with severe hepatomegaly and steatosis, has been reported in patients receiving nucleoside reverse transcriptase inhibitors (see Zidovudine, p.658).

**Effects on the skin.** Stevens-Johnson syndrome occurring in a patient receiving antiretroviral therapy with abacavir, lamivudine, and zidovudine was considered to be probably associated with abacavir.[1] Resolution occurred upon discontinuation of antiretroviral therapy and the condition did not recur upon rechallenge with an alternative regimen also containing lamivudine and zidovudine.

1. Bossi P, *et al.* Stevens-Johnson syndrome associated with abacavir therapy. *Clin Infect Dis* 2002; **35:** 902.

**Hypersensitivity.** A review of hypersensitivity associated with abacavir.[1]

1. Hewitt RG. Abacavir hypersensitivity reaction. *Clin Infect Dis* 2002; **34:** 1137–42.

### Precautions

Abacavir should be discontinued immediately if symptoms associated with hypersensitivity occur and should *never be recommenced* in patients who have stopped therapy due to a hypersensitivity reaction. Patients should be closely monitored for signs of hypersensitivity during the first 2 months of treatment, although hypersensitivity reactions can occur at any time. Patients restarting therapy after an interruption are at particular risk even if they have not previously shown symptoms of hypersensitivity. Since intermittent therapy may increase the risk of hypersensitivity developing, patients should be advised of the importance of regular dosing.

Abacavir should not be used in patients with moderate to severe hepatic impairment, and should be used with caution in those with lesser degrees of impairment and those with risk factors for liver disease; for dose reductions to be employed in those with mild hepatic impairment, see Administration in Hepatic Impairment under Uses and Administration, below. Treatment should be discontinued if liver function deteriorates rapidly or if hepatomegaly or unexplained metabolic acidosis develop.

Abacavir should be avoided in patients with end-stage renal disease.

### Interactions

Administration of abacavir with alcohol may result in decreased elimination of abacavir and consequent increases in the area under the plasma concentration-time curve.

**Alcohol.** References.

1. McDowell JA, *et al.* Pharmacokinetic interaction of abacavir (1592U89) and ethanol in human immunodeficiency virus-infected adults. *Antimicrob Agents Chemother* 2000; **44:** 1686–90.

### Antiviral Action

Abacavir is converted intracellularly in stages to carbovir triphosphate, which halts the DNA synthesis of retroviruses, including HIV, through competitive inhibition of reverse transcriptase and incorporation into viral DNA.

◊ References.

1. Faletto MB, *et al.* Unique intracellular activation of the potent anti-human immunodeficiency virus agent 1592U89. *Antimicrob Agents Chemother* 1997; **41:** 1099–1107.

### Pharmacokinetics

Abacavir is rapidly absorbed following oral administration with a bioavailability of about 80%. Absorption is delayed slightly by food but the extent is unaffected. Abacavir crosses the blood-brain barrier. It is about 50% bound to plasma proteins. The elimination half-life is about 1.5 hours following a single dose. Abacavir undergoes intracellular metabolism to the active antiviral metabolite carbovir triphosphate. Elimination is via hepatic metabolism primarily by alcohol dehydrogenase and by glucuronidation and the metabolites are excreted mainly in the urine. There is no significant metabolism by hepatic cytochrome P450 isoenzymes.

◊ References.

1. Kumar PN, *et al.* Safety and pharmacokinetics of abacavir (1592U89) following oral administration of escalating single doses in human immunodeficiency virus type 1-infected adults. *Antimicrob Agents Chemother* 1999; **43:** 603–8.
2. Hughes W, *et al.* Safety and single-dose pharmacokinetics of abacavir (1592U89) in human immunodeficiency virus type 1-infected children. *Antimicrob Agents Chemother* 1999; **43:** 609–15.
3. McDowell JA, *et al.* Multiple-dose pharmacokinetics and pharmacodynamics of abacavir alone and in combination with zidovudine in human immunodeficiency virus-infected adults. *Antimicrob Agents Chemother* 2000; **44:** 2061–7.
4. Izzedine H, *et al.* Pharmacokinetics of abacavir in HIV-1-infected patients with impaired renal function. *Nephron* 2001; **89:** 62–7.

### Uses and Administration

Abacavir is a nucleoside reverse transcriptase inhibitor with antiretroviral activity against HIV. It is given by mouth as the sulfate with other antiretrovirals for combination therapy of HIV infection (p.621). Doses are expressed in terms of the base. 1.17 g of abacavir sulfate is approximately equivalent to 1 g of abacavir. The adult dose is 300 mg twice daily. The dose for children over 3 months of age is 8 mg/kg twice daily up to a maximum of 600 mg daily. Doses should be reduced in patients with hepatic impairment (see below).

◊ Reviews.

1. Hervey PS, Perry CM. Abacavir: a review of its clinical potential in patients with HIV infection. *Drugs* 2000; **60:** 447–79.

**Administration in hepatic impairment.** Abacavir should not be used in patients with moderate to severe hepatic impairment, although reduced doses of 200 mg twice daily may be given to patients with mild impairment.

### Preparations

**Proprietary Preparations** (details are given in Part 3)
***Arg.:*** Ziagenavir; ***Austral.:*** Ziagen; ***Belg.:*** Ziagen; ***Braz.:*** Ziagenavir; ***Canad.:*** Ziagen; ***Chile:*** Ziagen; ***Denm.:*** Ziagen; ***Fin.:*** Ziagen; ***Fr.:*** Ziagen; ***Ger.:*** Ziagen; ***Gr.:*** Ziagen; ***Hong Kong:*** Ziagen; ***Irl.:*** Ziagen; ***Israel:*** Ziagen; ***Ital.:*** Ziagen; ***Mex.:*** Ziagenavir; ***Norw.:*** Ziagen; ***NZ:*** Ziagen; ***Port.:*** Ziagen; ***S.Afr.:*** Ziagen; ***Singapore:*** Ziagen; ***Spain:*** Ziagen; ***Swed.:*** Ziagen; ***Switz.:*** Ziagen; ***Thai.:*** Ziagenavir; ***UK:*** Ziagen; ***USA:*** Ziagen.

**Multi-ingredient:** ***Arg.:*** Tricivir; ***Austral.:*** Trizivir; ***Belg.:*** Trizivir; ***Chile:*** Tricivir; ***Denm.:*** Trizivir; ***Fin.:*** Trizivir; ***Fr.:*** Trizivir; ***Ger.:*** Trizivir; ***Irl.:*** Trizivir; ***Israel:*** Trizivir; ***Ital.:*** Trizivir; ***Norw.:*** Trizivir; ***Port.:*** Trizivir; ***Singapore:*** Trizivir; ***Spain:*** Trizivir; ***Swed.:*** Trizivir; ***Switz.:*** Trizivir; ***UK:*** Trizivir; ***USA:*** Trizivir.

## Aciclovir *(BAN, rINN)*

Aciclovirum; Acycloguanosine; Acyclovir *(USAN)*; BW-248U. 9-[(2-Hydroxyethoxy)methyl]guanine; 2-Amino-1,9-dihydro-9-(2-hydroxyethoxymethyl)-6*H*-purin-6-one.

$C_8H_{11}N_5O_3$ = 225.2.

*CAS — 59277-89-3.*

*ATC — D06BB03; J05AB01; S01AD03.*

**Pharmacopoeias.** In *Chin.*, *Eur.* (see p.vi), and *US.*

**Ph. Eur. 5.0** (Aciclovir). A white to almost white crystalline powder. Slightly soluble in water; very slightly soluble in alcohol; freely soluble in dimethyl sulfoxide; soluble in dilute solutions of alkali hydroxides and mineral acids.

**USP 27** (Acyclovir). A white to off-white crystalline powder. Slightly soluble in water; insoluble in alcohol; soluble in dilute hydrochloric acid. Store in airtight containers at a temperature of 15° to 25°. Protect from light and moisture.

### Aciclovir Sodium *(BANM, rINNM)*

Aciclovir sódico; Acyclovir Sodium *(USAN)*.

$C_8H_{10}N_5NaO_3$ = 247.2.

*CAS — 69657-51-8.*

*ATC — D06BB03; J05AB01; S01AD03.*

**Incompatibility.** Aciclovir is reported to be incompatible with foscarnet.

**Stability.** References.

1. Zhang Y, *et al.* Stability of acyclovir sodium 1, 7, and 10 mg/mL in 5% dextrose injection and 0.9% sodium chloride injection. *Am J Health-Syst Pharm* 1998; **55:** 574–7.

### Adverse Effects

Aciclovir is generally well tolerated. When administered intravenously as aciclovir sodium it may cause local reactions at the injection site with inflammation and phlebitis; these reactions may be associated with extravasation that leads rarely to ulceration.

Renal impairment may be associated with systemic use of aciclovir in some patients; it is usually reversible and is reported to respond to hydration and/or dosage reduction or withdrawal, but may progress to acute renal failure. The risk of renal toxicity is increased by conditions favouring deposition of aciclovir crystals in the tubules such as when the patient is poorly hydrated, has existing renal impairment, or when the drug is given at a high dosage or by rapid or bolus injection. Some patients receiving systemic aciclovir may experience transient increases in blood concentrations of urea and creatinine although this is more acute with intravenous administration.

Occasional adverse effects following systemic administration include increased serum bilirubin and liver enzymes, haematological changes, skin rashes (including erythema multiforme, Stevens-Johnson syndrome, and toxic epidermal necrolysis), fever, headache, dizziness, and gastrointestinal effects such as nausea, vomiting, and diarrhoea. Anaphylaxis has been reported. Hepatitis and jaundice have been reported rarely. Neurological effects including lethargy, somnolence, confusion, hallucinations, agitation, tremors, psychosis, convulsions, and coma have been reported in a small number of patients, particularly in those receiving intravenous aciclovir and with predisposing factors such as renal impairment; these effects may be more marked in older patients. Thrombotic thrombocytopenic purpura and haemolytic uraemic syndrome, sometimes resulting in death, have occurred in immunocompromised patients receiving high parenteral doses of aciclovir. Accelerated diffuse hair loss has also been reported.

Topical application of aciclovir, especially to genital lesions, may sometimes produce transient stinging, burning, itching, or erythema. Eye ointments may occasionally produce transient stinging, superficial punctate keratopathy, blepharitis, or conjunctivitis.

**Effects on the blood.** There has been no evidence of bone-marrow toxicity in patients given aciclovir following bone marrow transplantation.[1,2] However, megaloblastic haematopoiesis has been observed in the bone marrow of 3 patients given aciclovir for suspected or proven herpes simplex encephalitis.[3] There has also been a report of inhibition of human peripheral blood lymphocytes in samples taken from healthy subjects given aciclovir.[4]

1. Serota FT, *et al.* Acyclovir treatment of herpes zoster infections: use in children undergoing bone marrow transplantation. *JAMA* 1982; **247:** 2132–5.
2. Gluckman E, *et al.* Oral acyclovir prophylactic treatment of herpes simplex infection after bone marrow transplantation. *J Antimicrob Chemother* 1983; **12** (suppl B): 161–7.
3. Amos RJ, Amess JAL. Megaloblastic haemopoiesis due to acyclovir. *Lancet* 1983; **i:** 242–3.
4. Tauris P, *et al.* Evaluation of the acyclovir-induced modulation of the plaque-forming cell response of human peripheral blood lymphocytes. *J Antimicrob Chemother* 1984; **13:** 71–7.

**Effects on the kidneys.** Transient renal impairment occurred in 2 adequately hydrated patients following aciclovir 10 mg/kg infused over 1 hour every 8 hours.[1] In another patient[2] severe acute renal failure occurred following administration of aciclovir 5 mg/kg over 90 minutes daily for 2 days. This reaction did not appear to be related to dosage or manner of administration, but may have been idiosyncratic or immunological.[2] Acute renal failure (with no evidence of crystals) and coma developed in 2 elderly patients receiving high dose oral therapy (800 mg five times daily) with aciclovir.[3,4]

1. Harrington MG, *et al.* Renal impairment and acyclovir. *Lancet* 1981; **ii:** 1281.
2. Giustina A, *et al.* Low-dose acyclovir and acute renal failure. *Ann Intern Med* 1988; **108:** 312.
3. Eck P, *et al.* Acute renal failure and coma after a high dose of oral acyclovir. *N Engl J Med* 1991; **325:** 1178.
4. Johnson GL, *et al.* Acute renal failure and neurotoxicity following oral acyclovir. *Ann Pharmacother* 1994; **28:** 460–3.

**Effects on the nervous system.** Of 143 patients given aciclovir by intravenous infusion in doses ranging from 0.75 to 3.6 g/m² daily for the treatment of herpesvirus infections following bone marrow transplantation, 6 developed reversible neurological symptoms including tremor, agitation, nausea, lethargy, mild disorientation, autonomic instability, hemiparaesthesia, and slurred speech.[1] EEGs were diffusely abnormal in all 6. Symptoms improved in all patients on withdrawing aciclovir; reinstituting aciclovir in 2 produced a recurrence of symptoms. Concomitant therapy included irradiation and methotrexate intrathecally for all 6, interferon alfa for 3, and ciclosporin for 1. There are individual case reports of neurological and, less frequently, psychiatric adverse effects in patients given intravenous aciclovir.[2-8] Neurological toxicity following oral aciclovir was possibly associated with elevated plasma concentrations in patients with end-stage renal disease.[9,10] The association between plasma-aciclovir concentrations and neurotoxicity has been difficult to establish because of a delay of 24 to 48 hours in the development of symptoms following a concentration peak.[11]

1. Wade JC, Meyers JD. Neurologic symptoms associated with parenteral acyclovir treatment after marrow transplantation. *Ann Intern Med* 1983; **98:** 921–5.
2. Vartian CV, Shlaes DM. Intravenous acyclovir and neurologic effects. *Ann Intern Med* 1983; **99:** 568.
3. Auwerx J, *et al.* Acyclovir and neurologic manifestations. *Ann Intern Med* 1983; **99:** 882–3.
4. Cohen SMZ, *et al.* Severe but reversible neurotoxicity from acyclovir. *Ann Intern Med* 1984; **100:** 920.
5. Tomson CR, *et al.* Psychiatric side-effects of acyclovir in patients with chronic renal failure. *Lancet* 1985; **ii:** 385–6.
6. Bataille P, *et al.* Psychiatric side-effects with acyclovir. *Lancet* 1985; **ii:** 724.
7. Sirota P, *et al.* Major depression with psychotic features associated with acyclovir therapy. *Drug Intell Clin Pharm* 1988; **22:** 306–8.
8. Revankar SG, *et al.* Delirium associated with acyclovir treatment in a patient with renal failure. *Clin Infect Dis* 1995; **21:** 435–6.
9. Swan SK, Bennett WM. Oral acyclovir and neurotoxicity. *Ann Intern Med* 1989; **111:** 188.
10. Mataix AL, *et al.* Oral acyclovir and neurologic adverse effects in endstage renal disease. *Ann Pharmacother* 1994; **28:** 961–2.
11. Haefeli WE, *et al.* Acyclovir-induced neurotoxicity: concentration-side effect relationship in acyclovir overdose. *Am J Med* 1993; **94:** 212–15.

**Effects on the skin.** A report of vesicular lesions associated with intravenous administration of aciclovir in a patient thought to have herpes simplex encephalitis.[1] Careful evaluation is necessary to differentiate the reaction from herpetic lesions.

1. Buck ML, *et al.* Vesicular eruptions following acyclovir administration. *Ann Pharmacother* 1993; **27:** 1458–9.

**Vasculitis.** Aciclovir has been associated with vasculitis. In one patient[1] it was one of many drugs given that may have caused a necrotising vasculitis. In another report an immunocompromised child with chickenpox given aciclovir by infusion developed a vasculitic rash which diminished on withdrawal of the drug.[2]

1. von Schulthess GK, Sauter C. Acyclovir and herpes zoster. *N Engl J Med* 1981; **305:** 1349.
2. Platt MPW, Eden OB. Vasculitis in association with chickenpox treatment in childhood acute lymphoblastic leukaemia. *Lancet* 1982; **ii:** 763–4.

### Precautions

Aciclovir should be used with caution in patients with renal impairment and doses should be adjusted according to creatinine clearance (see Administration in Renal Impairment, under Uses and Administration, below). Parenteral administration should be by slow intravenous infusion over one hour to avoid precipitation of aciclovir in the kidney; rapid or bolus injection should be avoided and adequate hydration maintained. The risk of renal impairment is increased by use with other nephrotoxic drugs. Intravenous aciclovir should also be used with caution in patients with underlying neurological abnormalities, with significant hypoxia, or with serious hepatic or electrolyte abnormalities.

**Breast feeding.** Aciclovir is distributed into breast milk[1-4] and in some instances higher concentrations are obtained than in maternal serum.[1-3] The manufacturers report that a maternal dose of 200 mg five times daily by mouth could expose a suckling infant to 300 micrograms/kg daily and advise caution when treating nursing mothers with aciclovir. However, no adverse effects have been observed in breast-fed infants whose mothers were receiving aciclovir, and the American Academy of Pediatrics considers[5] that it is therefore usually compatible with breast feeding.

1. Lau RJ, *et al.* Unexpected accumulation of acyclovir in breast milk with estimation of infant exposure. *Obstet Gynecol* 1987; **69:** 468–71.
2. Meyer LJ, *et al.* Acyclovir in human breast milk. *Am J Obstet Gynecol* 1988; **158:** 586–8.
3. Bork K, Benes P. Concentration and kinetic studies of intravenous acyclovir in serum and breast milk of a patient with eczema herpeticum. *J Am Acad Dermatol* 1995; **32:** 1053–5.
4. Taddio A, *et al.* Acyclovir excretion in human breast milk. *Ann Pharmacother* 1994; **28:** 585–7.
5. American Academy of Pediatrics. The transfer of drugs and other chemicals into human milk. *Pediatrics* 2001; **108:** 776–89. Correction. *ibid.*; 1029. Also available at: http://aappolicy.aappublications.org/cgi/content/full/pediatrics%3b108/3/776 (accessed 10/03/04)

**Pregnancy.** The incidence of congenital abnormality and spontaneous fetal loss did not appear to be greater among 312 cases of prenatal exposure to aciclovir than among the general population, and this data was supported by evidence from 145 further retrospective reports.[1]

1. Andrews EB, *et al.* Acyclovir in Pregnancy Registry: six years' experience. *Obstet Gynecol* 1992; **79:** 7–13.

**Sodium content.** Each g of aciclovir sodium represents 4.05 mmol of sodium.

### Interactions

Probenecid is reported to block the renal clearance of aciclovir. The risk of renal impairment is increased by use with other nephrotoxic drugs.

**Antivirals.** Combined therapy with *zidovudine* and aciclovir is not generally associated with additional toxicity.[1] However, there is a report[2] of a patient who had overwhelming fatigue when given aciclovir and zidovudine together; no such effect occurred when each drug was given alone.

The manufacturer of *interferon alfa-n1* has reported progressive renal failure in patients also given aciclovir.

1. Tartaglione TA, *et al.* Pharmacokinetic evaluations of low- and high-dose zidovudine plus high-dose acyclovir in patients with symptomatic human immunodeficiency virus infection. *Antimicrob Agents Chemother* 1991; **35:** 2225–31.
2. Bach MC. Possible drug interaction during therapy with azidothymidine and acyclovir for AIDS. *N Engl J Med* 1987; **316:** 547.

**Xanthines.** For reference to evidence that aciclovir inhibits *theophylline* metabolism, resulting in accumulation, see p.802.

### Antiviral Action

Aciclovir is active against herpes simplex virus type 1 and type 2 and against varicella-zoster virus. This activity is due to intracellular conversion of aciclovir by viral thymidine kinase to the monophosphate with subsequent conversion by cellular enzymes to the diphosphate and the active triphosphate. This active form inhibits viral DNA synthesis and replication by inhibiting the herpesvirus DNA polymerase enzyme as well as being incorporated into viral DNA. This process is highly selective for infected cells. Studies in *animals* and *in vitro* show various sensitivities but demonstrate that these viruses are inhibited by concentrations of aciclovir that are readily achieved clinically. Herpes simplex virus type 1 appears to be the most susceptible, then type 2, followed by varicella-zoster virus.

The Epstein-Barr virus and cytomegalovirus are also susceptible to aciclovir to a lesser extent. However, for cytomegalovirus it does not appear to be activated by thymidine kinase and may act via a different mechanism. Epstein-Barr virus may have reduced thymidine kinase activity but its DNA polymerase is very sensitive to inhibition by aciclovir triphosphate, which may account for the partial activity.

Aciclovir has no activity against latent viruses, but there is some evidence that it inhibits latent herpes simplex virus at an early stage of reactivation.

## Resistance

Herpes simplex virus develops resistance to aciclovir *in vitro* and *in vivo* by selection of mutants deficient in thymidine kinase. Other mechanisms of resistance include altered substrate specificity of thymidine kinase and reduced sensitivity of viral DNA polymerase. Resistance has also been reported with varicella-zoster virus, probably by similar mechanisms.

Although occasional treatment failures have been reported, resistance has not yet emerged as a major problem in treating herpes simplex infections. However, resistant viruses are more likely to be a problem in patients with a suppressed immune response; AIDS patients may be particularly prone to aciclovir-resistant mucocutaneous herpes simplex virus infections.

Viruses resistant to aciclovir because of absence of thymidine kinase may be cross-resistant to other antivirals phosphorylated by this enzyme, such as brivudine, idoxuridine, and ganciclovir. Viruses resistant because of altered substrate specificity of thymidine kinase may display cross-resistance to brivudine; those with altered DNA polymerase sensitivity may be resistant to brivudine and vidarabine. However, those viruses with altered enzyme specificity or sensitivity tend to have variable cross-resistance patterns and may be relatively susceptible to the aforementioned antivirals.

◊ References.

1. Christophers J, *et al.* Survey of resistance of herpes simplex virus to acyclovir in Northwest England. *Antimicrob Agents Chemother* 1998; **42:** 868–72.

## Pharmacokinetics

The intravenous infusion of aciclovir as the sodium salt produces plasma-aciclovir concentrations that demonstrate a biphasic pattern. The infusion over 1 hour of a dose equivalent to 5 mg of aciclovir per kg in adults produces therapeutic steady-state plasma concentrations similar to those achieved following doses of 250 mg/m² in children over 1 year and doses of 10 mg/kg in neonates of up to 3 months of age.

Aciclovir is excreted through the kidney by both glomerular filtration and tubular secretion. The terminal or beta-phase half-life is reported to be about 2 to 3 hours for adults without renal impairment. In chronic renal failure, this value is increased and may be up to 19.5 hours in anuric patients. During haemodialysis the half-life has been reported to be reduced to 5.7 hours, with 60% of a dose of aciclovir being removed. Most of a dose by intravenous infusion is excreted unchanged with only up to 14% appearing in the urine as the inactive metabolite 9-carboxymethoxymethylguanine. Faecal excretion may account for about 2% of a dose. There is wide distribution, including into the CSF where concentrations achieved are about 50% of those achieved in plasma. Protein binding is reported to range from 9 to 33%.

Probenecid increases the half-life and the area under the plasma concentration-time curve of aciclovir.

About 15 to 30% of a dose of aciclovir given by mouth is considered to be absorbed from the gastrointestinal tract. Orally active prodrugs such as valaciclovir (p.656) have been developed to overcome this poor absorption.

Aciclovir crosses the placenta and is distributed into breast milk in concentrations about 3 times higher than those in maternal serum.

Absorption of aciclovir is usually slight following topical application to intact skin, although it may be increased by changes in formulation. Aciclovir is absorbed following application of a 3% ointment to the eye giving a relatively high concentration in the aqueous humour but negligible amounts in the blood.

◊ Reviews.

1. de Miranda P, Blum MR. Pharmacokinetics of acyclovir after intravenous and oral administration. *J Antimicrob Chemother* 1983; **12** (suppl B): 29–37.
2. Laskin OL. Clinical pharmacokinetics of acyclovir. *Clin Pharmacokinet* 1983; **8:** 187–201.
3. Wagstaff AJ, *et al.* Aciclovir: a reappraisal of its antiviral activity, pharmacokinetic properties and therapeutic efficacy. *Drugs* 1994; **47:** 153–205.

**Distribution.** References to the pharmacokinetics of aciclovir and its distribution into the eye[1] and the CSF.[2,3]

1. Hung SO, *et al.* Pharmacokinetics of oral acyclovir (Zovirax) in the eye. *Br J Ophthalmol* 1984; **68:** 192–5.
2. Lycke J, *et al.* Acyclovir concentrations in serum and cerebrospinal fluid at steady state. *J Antimicrob Chemother* 1989; **24:** 947–54.
3. Chavanet P, *et al.* Meningeal diffusion of high doses of acyclovir given with probenecid. *J Antimicrob Chemother* 1990; **26:** 294–5.

## Uses and Administration

Aciclovir is a synthetic purine nucleoside analogue structurally related to guanine. It is used mainly for the treatment of viral infections due to herpes simplex virus (types 1 and 2) and varicella-zoster virus (herpes zoster and chickenpox).

Herpes simplex infections, including herpes keratitis, herpes labialis, and genital herpes, respond to aciclovir by the intravenous, oral, or topical route, given as soon as possible after symptoms appear. Both initial and recurrent infections can be successfully treated. Prolonged treatment can reduce the incidence of recurrence which is particularly important in immunocompromised patients. However, when prolonged treatment is withdrawn, infections may recur.

Aciclovir also improves the healing of herpes zoster lesions and reduces acute pain when given intravenously or by mouth; use to prevent postherpetic neuralgia is controversial (see p.7). Beneficial effects may be more marked in immunocompromised patients.

ADMINISTRATION AND DOSAGE. Aciclovir is administered by *intravenous infusion* as the sodium salt over 1 hour. Doses are expressed in terms of the base. Aciclovir sodium 1.1 g is approximately equivalent to 1 g of aciclovir. Solutions for infusion are usually prepared to give a concentration of 25 or 50 mg of aciclovir per mL; this must then be further diluted in a suitable infusion fluid such as water for injections or sodium chloride 0.9% to a final concentration not greater than about 5 mg/mL (0.5%). Alternatively, a solution containing 25 mg/mL may be given by injection using a controlled-rate infusion pump, over 1 hour.

For herpes simplex infections in the immunocompromised, and for severe initial genital herpes, or varicella-zoster infections in immunocompetent patients, the dose by the intravenous route is 5 mg/kg given every 8 hours, and recommended periods of treatment range from 5 to 7 days. A similar dose may be used for prophylaxis of herpes simplex infections in immunocompromised patients. A higher dose of 10 mg/kg every 8 hours is given in the treatment of herpes simplex encephalitis. This higher dose is also given in varicella-zoster infections in immunocompromised patients. Herpes simplex encephalitis usually requires treatment for 10 days.

*Oral doses* of aciclovir vary according to indication. For treatment of primary herpes simplex infections, including genital herpes, the usual oral dose is 200 mg five times daily (usually every 4 hours while awake) for 5 to 10 days. Severely immunocompromised patients or those with impaired absorption may be given 400 mg five times daily for 5 days. For suppression of recurrent herpes simplex in immunocompetent patients, the oral dose is 800 mg daily in two to four divided doses; dosage reduction to 400 to 600 mg daily can be tried. Higher doses of 1 g daily have also been used. Therapy should be interrupted every 6 to 12 months for reassessment of the condition. For prophylaxis of herpes simplex in immunocompromised patients, the dose is 200 to 400 mg four times daily. Chronic suppressive treatment is not suitable for mild or infrequent recurrences of herpes simplex. In such cases episodic treatment of recurrences may be more beneficial; a dose of 200 mg five times daily for 5 days has been recommended, preferably initiated during the prodromal period. The usual oral dose of aciclovir for treatment of chickenpox is 800 mg four or five times daily for 5 to 7 days; for herpes zoster 800 mg five times daily may be given for 7 to 10 days.

In herpes simplex infections of the skin, including genital herpes and herpes labialis, *topical treatment* with an ointment or cream containing aciclovir 5% may be applied 5 or 6 times daily for periods of 5 to 10 days. In herpes simplex keratitis a 3% eye ointment may be applied 5 times daily until 3 days after healing.

Doses should be reduced in *renal impairment* (see below).

*Children's doses.* In children, the 8-hourly intravenous dose is best calculated by body-surface using 250 mg/m² for herpes simplex and varicella-zoster infections in immunocompetent patients and 500 mg/m² for herpes simplex encephalitis and varicella-zoster infection in the immunocompromised. A suggested 8-hourly dose for infants and neonates is 10 mg/kg; treatment for neonatal herpes usually continues for 10 days. In the treatment of herpes simplex infections, and in the prophylaxis of herpes simplex infections in the immunocompromised, oral doses of aciclovir for children aged 2 years and over are as for adults. Children aged under 2 years are given half the adult dose. In the treatment of chickenpox, children over 2 years of age may be given 20 mg/kg, up to a maximum of 800 mg, four times daily for 5 days. Alternatively, children aged 6 years and over may be given 800 mg four times daily, those aged 2 to 5 years may be given 400 mg four times daily, and those aged under 2 years may be given 200 mg four times daily.

◊ Reviews.

1. Wagstaff AJ, *et al.* Aciclovir: a reappraisal of its antiviral activity, pharmacokinetic properties and therapeutic efficacy. *Drugs* 1994; **47:** 153–205.
2. Welsby PD. Acyclovir: is the honeymoon coming to an end? *J Infect* 1994; **28:** 121–9.
3. Leflore S, *et al.* A risk-benefit evaluation of aciclovir for the treatment and prophylaxis of herpes simplex virus infections. *Drug Safety* 2000; **23:** 131–42.

**Administration in renal impairment.** Doses of aciclovir should be reduced in renal impairment according to creatinine clearance (CC) and the manufacturers have given the following guidance:

*intravenous* administration:

- CC between 25 and 50 mL/minute: the interval between infusions may be increased to 12 hours
- CC 10 to 25 mL/minute: the interval between infusions may be increased to 24 hours
- CC less than 10 mL/minute: patients on *peritoneal dialysis* should receive half the usual appropriate dose given once every 24 hours; patients on *haemodialysis* should receive half the usual dose every 24 hours plus an extra half-dose following haemodialysis

*oral* administration:

- CC less than 10 mL/minute: *herpes simplex infections*: 200 mg every 12 hours; *varicella-zoster infections*: 800 mg every 12 hours
- CC between 10 and 25 mL/minute: *varicella-zoster infections*: 800 mg three times daily every 8 hours

**Erythema multiforme.** For patients with recurrent erythema multiforme (p.1135) associated with herpes simplex infection a 5-day course of oral aciclovir at the start of the infection has been proposed to prevent the subsequent skin lesions.[1] If this fails, a 6-month course of oral aciclovir has been found to be of benefit,[2] even if the association with herpes is not obvious. It should be noted, however, that erythema multiforme may occur as an adverse effect of systemic aciclovir.

1. Schofield JK, *et al.* Recurrent erythema multiforme: clinical features and treatment in a large series of patients. *Br J Dermatol* 1993; **128:** 542–5.
2. Tatnall FM, *et al.* A double-blind, placebo-controlled trial of continuous acyclovir therapy in recurrent erythema multiforme. *Br J Dermatol* 1995; **132:** 267–70.

## Preparations

***BP 2003:*** Aciclovir Cream; Aciclovir Eye Ointment; Aciclovir Intravenous Infusion; Aciclovir Oral Suspension; Aciclovir Tablets; Dispersible Aciclovir Tablets;

***USP 27:*** Acyclovir Capsules; Acyclovir for Injection; Acyclovir Ointment; Acyclovir Oral Suspension; Acyclovir Tablets.

**Proprietary Preparations** (details are given in Part 3)
***Arg.:*** Acerpes; Aciclo; Lisovyr; Poviral; Xiclovir; Zovirax; ***Austral.:*** Acihexal; Acyclo-V; Chemists Own Cold Sore; Lovir; Zolaten; Zovirax; Zyclir; ***Austria:*** Acic; Aciclobene; Aciclostad; Aciclotyrol; Activir; Exviral; Farocid; Fibral; Herpomed; Nycovir; Simplex-Fieberblasen; Stadovir; ViroMed; Xorox; Zovirax; ***Belg.:*** Zovirax; ***Braz.:*** Aciclomed; Aciclor†; Aciveral; Anclomax; Antivirax; Aviral; Ciclavix; Ciclocris; Clovir; Exavir; Ezopen; Heclivir; Herpesil; Uni Vir; Zovirax; Zoylex; ***Canad.:*** Avirax; Zovirax; ***Chile:*** Eurovir; Lisovyr; Oftavir; Vironida; Zovirax; ***Denm.:*** Aciclodan; Avirox; Geavir; Orivir; Zoviplus†; Zovir; ***Fin.:*** Aclovir; Acyclostad; Acyrax; Geavir; Herpolips; Zovirax; ***Fr.:*** Activir; Kendix; Zovirax; ***Ger.:*** Acerpes; Aci-Sanorania†; Acic; Acic-Ophtal; Aciclobeta; Aciclostad; Acivir; Dynexan Herpescreme; Herpetad; Herpofug†; Herpotern†; Herpoviric†; Mapox; Supraviran; Virax; Virupos; Viruseen; Virzin; Zoliparin; Zovirax; ***Gr.:*** Abduce; Cargosil; Cevinolon; Clovirax; Cyclovir; Cycloviran; Etasisen; Hagevir; Helposol; Herzkur; Pulibex; Uniplex; Verpir; Virusteril; Xorox; Zidovimm; Zovirax; ***Hong Kong:*** Acilax; Acyvir; Avorax; Cusiviral; Cyclorax; Cyclovax; Entir; Medovir; Synclovir; Vidaclovir; Wariviron; Zevin; Zoral; Zovirax; ***India:*** Acivir; Cyclovir; Herpex; Zovirax; ***Irl.:*** Clonorax†; Soothelip; Viralief; Zovirax; ***Israel:*** Acivir; Cyclomed; Supra-Vir; Viroxy; Zovirax; ***Ital.:*** Aciclin; ACY; Acyvir; Alovir; Amodivyr; Avirase; Avix; Avyclor; Avyplus; Avysal; Cevirin; Citivir; Cycloviran; Dravyr; Efriviral; Esavir; Fuviron; Herpesnil†; Iliaclor; Immunovir; Ipaviran; Ipsovir; Neclovir; Neviran; Rexan; Riduvir; Sanavir; Sifiviral; Voraclor; Zovirax; ***Malaysia:*** Avorax; Cusiviral; Cyclovax; Declovir; Hepirax; Lovir; Medovir; Virest; Virless; Zevin; Zoral; Zorax; Zovirax; ***Mex.:*** Acifur; Akevir†; Avirex-T; Cicloferon; Ciclor†; Epsin; Exaliver; Filivir†; Herpilem; Isavir; Laciken; Maclov; Opthavir; Soviclor; Virazone†; Zetavir; Ziverone; Zovirax; ***Neth.:*** Previum†; Zovirax; ***Norw.:*** Geavir†; Zovirax; ***NZ:*** Acicvir; Lovir; Viraban; Zolaten; Zovirax; ***Port.:*** Aciclosina; Cicloviral; Divicil; Faulviral; Hermixsofex; Hermocil; Zov800; Zovirax; ***S.Afr.:*** Acitop; Activir; Cyclivex; Lovire; Zovirax; ***Singapore:*** Avorax; Bearax; Cusiviral; Danovir; Dravyr; Entir; Erlvirax; Lovir; Medovir; Vacrax; Virest; Virless; Zoral; Zorax; Zovirax; ***Spain:*** Aciclostad; Cusiviral†; Maynar; Milavir; Virbelte†; Virherpes; Virmen; Viruderm; Zovirax; ***Swed.:*** Geavir; Zovirax; ***Switz.:*** Acerpes; Aviral; Helvevir; Virucalm; Zovirax; ***Thai.:*** ACV; Acyvir; Clinovir; Clovin; Clovira; Colsor; Cyclorax; Entir; Herpenon; Lermex; Medovir†; Norum; Ranvir; Vermis; Vilerm; Viraxy; Virogon; Virolan; Viromed; Viropox; Vivir; Zevin; Zocovin; Zovirax; ***UAE:*** Lovrak; ***UK:*** Clearsore; Herpetad; Soothelip; Virasorb; Virovir; Zovirax; ***USA:*** Zovirax.

---

## Adefovir *(BAN, USAN, rINN)*

GS-0393; PMEA. {[2-(6-Amino-9*H*-purin-9-yl)ethoxy]methyl}phosphonic acid; 9-[2-(Phosphonomethoxy)ethyl]adenine.
$C_8H_{12}N_5O_4P$ = 273.2.
*CAS — 106941-25-7.*
*ATC — J05AF08.*

### Adefovir Dipivoxil *(BANM, USAN, rINNM)*

Dipivoxilo de adefovir; GS-0840; Piv2PMEA; *Bis*(POM)PMEA. 9-[2-({Bis[(pivaloyloxy)methoxy]phosphinyl}methoxy)ethyl]adenine.
$C_{20}H_{32}N_5O_8P$ = 501.5.
*CAS — 142340-99-6.*
*ATC — J05AF08.*

### Adverse Effects

The most common adverse effects reported from adefovir have been gastrointestinal effects including nausea, flatulence, diarrhoea, dyspepsia, and abdominal pain. Other common adverse effects are headache and asthenia. There have also been reports of pruritus, skin rashes, and respiratory effects including increased cough, pharyngitis, and sinusitis. Increases in serum-creatinine concentrations may occur and there have been instances of renal impairment and acute renal failure. Raised liver enzyme concentrations may occur and exacerbation of hepatitis has been reported after cessation of treatment with adefovir.

Lactic acidosis, usually associated with severe hepatomegaly and steatosis, has been associated with treatment with nucleoside reverse transcriptase inhibitors (see Zidovudine, p.658).

### Precautions

Treatment with adefovir should be discontinued if there is a rapid increase in aminotransferase concentrations, progressive hepatomegaly or steatosis, or metabolic or lactic acidosis of unknown aetiology. Adefovir should be given with caution to patients with hepatomegaly or other risk factors for liver disease. Careful differentiation should be made between patients whose liver enzyme concentrations become elevated due to response to treatment and those in whom it is indicative of toxicity. Exacerbation of hepatitis has been reported after cessation of treatment with adefovir and patients who discontinue treatment should be monitored closely for an appropriate period. Patients receiving adefovir should be monitored every 3 months for signs of deteriorating renal function; particular care should be exercised in patients with a creatinine clearance of less than 50 mL/minute, who may require dosage modification (see below), and in those receiving other drugs that may affect renal function.

### Interactions

Caution should be exercised when adefovir is given with other drugs eliminated by active tubular secretion as competition for the elimination pathway may increase the serum concentrations of either drug. Care is required when adefovir is given with other drugs with the potential for nephrotoxicity.

### Antiviral Action

Adefovir is converted intracellularly in stages to the diphosphate. This diphosphate halts the DNA synthesis of hepatitis B virus through competitive inhibition of reverse transcriptase and incorporation into viral DNA.

### Pharmacokinetics

Following oral administration adefovir dipivoxil is rapidly converted to adefovir. Peak plasma concentrations of adefovir are reported after about 0.6 to 4 hours. Bioavailability is reported to be 59% after a single dose. Absorption is delayed but not reduced by administration with food. Adefovir is widely distributed to body tissues, particularly into the kidneys, liver, and intestines. Less than 4% is bound to plasma or serum proteins. Adefovir is excreted renally by glomerular filtration and active tubular secretion; the terminal elimination half-life is reported to be about 7 hours. Adefovir is partially removed by haemodialysis.

### Uses and Administration

Adefovir is a nucleotide reverse transcriptase inhibitor, structurally related to adenine, with antiviral activity against hepatitis B virus and HIV. It is given by mouth as the prodrug adefovir dipivoxil for the treatment of chronic hepatitis B in adults with decompensated liver disease, or with compensated liver disease with evidence of active viral replication, persistently raised serum alanine aminotransferase concentrations, and histological evidence of active liver inflammation and fibrosis. The usual dose of adefovir dipivoxil is 10 mg once daily. For details of dosage modification in patients with renal impairment, see below.

Adefovir dipivoxil has also been investigated for the treatment of HIV infection.

◊ References.


1. Noble S, Goa KL. Adefovir dipivoxil. *Drugs* 1999; **58:** 479–87.
2. Kahn J, *et al.* Efficacy and safety of adefovir dipivoxil with antiretroviral therapy: a randomized controlled trial. *JAMA* 1999; **282:** 2305–12.
3. Walsh KM, *et al.* Successful treatment with adefovir dipivoxil in a patient with fibrosing cholestatic hepatitis and lamivudine resistant hepatitis B virus. *Gut* 2001; **49:** 436–40.
4. Benhamou Y, *et al.* Safety and efficacy of adefovir dipivoxil in patients co-infected with HIV-1 and lamivudine-resistant hepatitis B virus: an open-label pilot study. *Lancet* 2001; **358:** 718–23.
5. Hadziyannis SJ, *et al.* Adefovir dipivoxil for the treatment of hepatitis B e antigen-negative chronic hepatitis B. *N Engl J Med* 2003; **348:** 800–7. Correction. *ibid.*: 1192.
6. Marcellin P, *et al.* Adefovir dipivoxil for the treatment of hepatitis B e antigen-positive chronic hepatitis B. *N Engl J Med* 2003; **348:** 808–16. Correction. *ibid.*: 1192.


**Administration in renal impairment.** The dosage of adefovir dipivoxil should be reduced in patients with renal impairment. The dosing interval should be modified according to the creatinine clearance (CC) of the patient:

- CC 50 mL or more per minute: usual once-daily dosage
- CC 20 to 49 mL/minute: every 48 hours
- CC 10 to 19 mL/minute: every 72 hours
- haemodialysis patients: every 7 days following dialysis or after a cumulative total of 12 hours of dialysis

### Preparations

**Proprietary Preparations** (details are given in Part 3)
***UK:*** Hepsera; ***USA:*** Hepsera.

**Multi-ingredient:** ***Fr.:*** Hepsera.

---

## Amprenavir *(BAN, USAN, rINN)*

KVX-478; VX-478; 141W94. (3*S*)-Tetrahydro-3-furyl{(*S*)-α-[(1*R*)-1-hydroxy-2-($N^1$-isobutylsulfanilamido)ethyl]phenethyl}carbamate.
$C_{25}H_{35}N_3O_6S$ = 505.6.
*CAS — 161814-49-9.*
*ATC — J05AE05.*

### Adverse Effects and Precautions

As for HIV-protease inhibitors in general (see Indinavir Sulfate, p.638). A possible association with Stevens-Johnson syndrome has been reported with amprenavir. Mild to moderate rashes usually resolve within 2 weeks but treatment with amprenavir should be permanently discontinued in patients who develop skin rashes with associated systemic or allergic symptoms or mucosal involvement.

Depressive or mood disorders have occurred.

Amprenavir is a sulfonamide and should be used with caution in patients known to be allergic to sulfonamides. The oral solution and capsule formulations (*Agenerase, GlaxoSmithKline*) also provide high daily doses of vitamin E (see p.1465); the oral solution has a high content of propylene glycol, present as an excipient, and appropriate precautions should be taken.

### Interactions

Interactions involving HIV-protease inhibitors are discussed under Indinavir Sulfate, p.639. Amprenavir is reported to be both a substrate for, and inhibitor of, the cytochrome P450 isoenzyme CYP3A4 and may thus interact with drugs that are metabolised by, or which inhibit, this isoenzyme.

### Antiviral Action

As for HIV-protease inhibitors in general (see Indinavir Sulfate, p.639). Mechanisms of resistance to amprenavir may differ sufficiently from those of other HIV-protease inhibitors to reduce the occurrence of cross-resistance between amprenavir and some other HIV-protease inhibitors.

### Pharmacokinetics

Amprenavir is absorbed from the gastrointestinal tract following oral administration. Absorption is impaired by ingestion with a high-fat meal. Bioavailability is about 14% lower from the oral solution formulation than from the capsule formulation (*Agenerase, GlaxoSmithKline*). Peak plasma concentrations are attained 1 to 2 hours after a single dose. It is about 90% bound to plasma proteins. Amprenavir is metabolised by hepatic cytochrome P450 isoenzyme CYP3A4. It is excreted mainly in the faeces as metabolites. The plasma elimination half-life is 7.1 to 10.6 hours.

◊ References.


1. Sadler BM, Stein DS. Clinical pharmacology and pharmacokinetics of amprenavir. *Ann Pharmacother* 2002; **36:** 102–18.


### Uses and Administration

Amprenavir is a protease inhibitor with antiviral activity against HIV. It is used with other antiretrovirals for combination therapy of HIV infection (p.621).

Amprenavir is given by mouth as capsules or an oral solution but the bioavailability of these formulations (*Agenerase, GlaxoSmithKline*) differ and their doses are not interchangeable. The *capsules* are given in an adult dose of 1.2 g twice daily (or 600 mg twice daily if given in combination with ritonavir) and the *oral solution* is given in a dose of 17 mg/kg three times daily (maximum daily dose 2.8 g).

Children aged 4 to 12 years and patients under 50 kg body-weight may be given 20 mg/kg twice daily or 15 mg/kg three times daily to a maximum daily dose of 2.4 g as *capsules*, or 22.5 mg/kg twice daily or 17 mg/kg three times daily as *oral solution* (maximum daily dose 2.8 g).

Doses should be reduced in patients with moderate to severe hepatic impairment.

Amprenavir is also used in the form of the prodrug fosamprenavir (see p.634), which may aid compliance by reducing adverse effects and increasing flexibility of dosing.

◊ Reviews.


1. Noble S, Goa KL. Amprenavir: a review of its clinical potential in patients with HIV infection. *Drugs* 2000; **60:** 1383–1410.


### Preparations

**Proprietary Preparations** (details are given in Part 3)
***Arg.:*** Agenerase; ***Austral.:*** Agenerase; ***Belg.:*** Agenerase; ***Braz.:*** Agenerase; ***Canad.:*** Agenerase; ***Chile:*** Agenerase; ***Denm.:*** Agenerase; ***Fin.:***

Agenerase; **Fr.:** Agenerase; **Ger.:** Agenerase; **Gr.:** Agenerase; **Israel:** Agenerase; **Ital.:** Agenerase; **Mex.:** Agenerase; **Norw.:** Agenerase; **NZ:** Agenerase; **Port.:** Agenerase; **Spain:** Agenerase; **Swed.:** Agenerase; **Switz.:** Agenerase; **UK:** Agenerase; **USA:** Agenerase.

## Atazanavir Sulfate *(USAN, rINNM)*

Atazanavir Sulphate *(BANM)*; BMS-232632-05; BMS-232632 (atazanavir). Dimethyl (3*S*,8*S*,9*S*,12*S*)-9-Benzyl-3,12-di-*tert*-butyl-8-hydroxy-4,11-dioxo-6-(*p*-2-pyridylbenzyl)-2,5,6,10,13-pentaazatetradecanedioate sulfate (1:1).

$C_{38}H_{52}N_6O_7,H_2SO_4$ = 802.9.

*CAS — 198904-31-3 (atazanavir); 229975-97-7 (atazanavir sulfate).*

### Adverse Effects and Precautions

As for HIV-protease inhibitors in general (see Indinavir Sulfate, p.638). It has been suggested that atazanavir may not adversely affect the lipid profile to the extent seen with other HIV-protease inhibitors. Atazanavir may prolong the PR interval on the ECG and asymptomatic first-degree atrioventricular block has been reported in some patients; caution should be exercised in patients with pre-existing cardiac conduction disorders.

### Interactions

Interactions involving HIV-protease inhibitors are discussed under Indinavir Sulfate, p.639. Caution should be exercised when atazanavir is given with drugs known to prolong the PR interval on the ECG.

### Antiviral Action

As for HIV-protease inhibitors in general (see Indinavir Sulfate, p.639).

### Pharmacokinetics

Atazanavir is absorbed from the gastrointestinal tract following oral administration with peak plasma concentrations occurring after 2 to 2.5 hours. Bioavailability is enhanced by administration with food. Atazanavir is reported to be 86% bound to serum proteins. It is distributed into semen and into the CSF. Atazanavir is extensively metabolised, mainly by oxidation by cytochrome P450 isoenzyme CYP3A; the metabolites appear to be inactive. Atazanavir is predominantly excreted in faeces, mainly as metabolites, and to a smaller extent in the urine. The terminal elimination half-life is reported to be about 7 hours.

### Uses and Administration

Atazanavir is a protease inhibitor with antiviral activity against HIV. It is used with other antiretrovirals for combination therapy of HIV infection (p.621).

Atazanavir is given with food by mouth as the sulfate, but doses are expressed in terms of atazanavir; 228 mg of atazanavir sulfate is approximately equivalent to 200 mg atazanavir. The usual adult dose is 400 mg once daily. Alternatively, it is given in a dose of 300 mg once daily with ritonavir 100 mg once daily, which acts as a pharmacokinetic enhancer.

For details of reduced dosage of atazanavir to be used in patients with moderate hepatic impairment, see below.

◊ Reviews.


1. Goldsmith DR, Perry CM. Atazanavir. *Drugs* 2003; **63:** 1679–93.


**Administration in hepatic impairment.** Atazanavir should not be used in patients with severe hepatic impairment. A reduced dose of 300 mg once daily should be used in patients with moderate impairment.

### Preparations

**Proprietary Preparations** (details are given in Part 3)
**UK:** Reyataz; **USA:** Reyataz.

## Atevirdine Mesilate *(rINNM)*

Atevirdine Mesylate *(USAN)*; U-87201 (atevirdine); U-87201E. 1-[3-(Ethylamino)-2-pyridyl]-4-[(5-methoxyindol-2-yl)carbonyl]piperazine monomethanesulfonate.

$C_{21}H_{25}N_5O_2,CH_4O_3S$ = 475.6.

*CAS — 136816-75-6 (atevirdine); 138540-32-6 (atevirdine mesilate).*

### Profile

Atevirdine is a non-nucleoside reverse transcriptase inhibitor that was formerly investigated for the treatment of HIV infection, but development was discontinued.

## Brivudine *(rINN)*

Brivudina; BVDU. (*E*)-5-(2-Bromovinyl)-2′-deoxyuridine.

$C_{11}H_{13}BrN_2O_5$ = 333.1.

*CAS — 69304-47-8.*

### Profile

Brivudine is a nucleoside analogue effective *in vitro* against herpes simplex virus type 1 and varicella-zoster virus; other viruses including herpes simplex virus type 2 have been reported to be sensitive, but only at relatively high concentrations. The activity appears to be due, at least in part, to selective phosphorylation of brivudine by viral deoxythymidine kinase in preference to cellular kinases. There is the possibility of cross-resistance developing between brivudine and aciclovir because of some similar features in their mode of action (see p.627).

Brivudine is given by mouth in the treatment of herpes zoster (p.621) in a dose of 125 mg daily for 7 days. It has also been given orally for herpes simplex infection and has been used topically.

◊ References.


1. Wutzler P, *et al.* Oral brivudin vs intravenous acyclovir in the treatment of herpes zoster in immunocompromised patients: a randomized double-blind trial. *J Med Virol* 1995; **46:** 252–7.
2. Wassilew SW, *et al.* Oral brivudin in comparison with acyclovir for improved therapy of herpes zoster in immunocompetent patients: results of a randomized, double-blind, multicentered study. *Antiviral Res* 2003; **59:** 49–56.
3. Wassilew SW, *et al.* Oral brivudin in comparison with acyclovir for herpes zoster: a survey study on postherpetic neuralgia. *Antiviral Res* 2003; **59:** 57–60.


### Preparations

**Proprietary Preparations** (details are given in Part 3)
**Ger.:** Helpin†; Zostex.

## Cidofovir *(BAN, USAN, rINN)*

GS-504; GS-0504; HPMPC. {[(*S*)-2-(4-Amino-2-oxo-1(2*H*)-pyrimidinyl)-1-(hydroxymethyl)ethoxy]methyl}phosphonic acid; 1-[(*S*)-3-Hydroxy-2-(phosphonomethoxy)propyl]-cytosine.

$C_8H_{14}N_3O_6P$ = 279.2.

*CAS — 113852-37-2 (anhydrous cidofovir); 149394-66-1 (cidofovir dihydrate).*

*ATC — J05AB12.*

### Adverse Effects

The most serious dose-limiting adverse effect of cidofovir is nephrotoxicity, the incidence and severity of which can be reduced by administration with probenecid and by ensuring adequate hydration. There have been instances of acute renal failure occurring after only 1 or 2 doses, and some fatalities. Low plasma-bicarbonate concentrations and metabolic acidosis, sometimes associated with proximal tubule injury and renal wasting syndrome (including Fanconi's syndrome) or with liver dysfunction and pancreatitis, have been reported. Reversible neutropenia has also occurred. Other adverse effects include nausea and vomiting, fever, asthenia, skin rash, dyspnoea, alopecia, and ocular hypotony (decreased intra-ocular pressure). Iritis or uveitis has been reported.

Cidofovir is carcinogenic and embryotoxic in *animals* and may have the potential to cause male infertility; for further details see Precautions, below.

**Effects on the eyes.** Ocular adverse effects associated with intravenous administration of cidofovir include iritis,[1] uveitis,[2] and ocular hypotony. While development of ocular hypotony is considered to warrant withdrawal of cidofovir,[2] uveitis or iritis alone may respond to topical corticosteroids and cycloplegics thus allowing antiviral therapy to be continued; no response or worsening of symptoms would necessitate discontinuation of cidofovir.


1. Tseng AL, *et al.* Iritis associated with intravenous cidofovir. *Ann Pharmacother* 1999; **33:** 167–71.
2. Ambati J, *et al.* Anterior uveitis associated with intravenous cidofovir use in patients with cytomegalovirus retinitis. *Br J Ophthalmol* 1999; **83:** 1153–8.


**Effects on the kidneys.** Dose-related nephrotoxicity is the most severe adverse effect of cidofovir and severe proteinuria has been reported in 13% of patients. There have been instances of acute renal failure occurring after only 1 or 2 doses, and some fatalities. Fanconi's syndrome associated with renal tubular damage has been reported in 2% of patients and, in one such patient, occurred on the third injection of cidofovir and resulted in irreversible renal impairment.[1] A case of nephrogenic diabetes insipidus occurring without premonitory laboratory abnormalities has also been reported in a patient given cidofovir.[2]


1. Vittecoq D, *et al.* Fanconi syndrome associated with cidofovir therapy. *Antimicrob Agents Chemother* 1997; **41:** 1846.
2. Schliefer K, *et al.* Nephrogenic diabetes insipidus in a patient taking cidofovir. *Lancet* 1997; **350:** 413–14. Correction. *ibid.*; 1558.


### Precautions

Cidofovir is contra-indicated in patients with renal impairment. Renal function should be measured before each dose. In the UK it is recommended that treatment should be interrupted or discontinued if renal function deteriorates, but in the USA reduction of the dosage is permitted for increases in serum creatinine up to 400 micrograms/dL above baseline. Patients should receive oral probenecid and intravenous hydration with each dose of cidofovir. Neutrophil counts should also be monitored and regular ophthalmological follow-up is recommended. Patients with diabetes mellitus are at increased risk of ocular hypotony.

Cidofovir is carcinogenic and embryotoxic in *animals*. Cidofovir should not be administered during pregnancy and both sexes should use effective methods of contraception during treatment; in addition, effective contraception should be used, for 1 month by women and for 3 months by men, after the end of treatment. There is also a possibility that cidofovir may cause male infertility.

Cidofovir should be given intravenously only; direct intra-ocular injection has been associated with significant ocular hypotony and visual impairment and is contra-indicated.

### Interactions

Additive nephrotoxicity may occur if cidofovir is given with other nephrotoxic drugs such as aminoglycosides, amphotericin B, foscarnet, intravenous pentamidine, vancomycin, or NSAIDs. Potentially nephrotoxic drugs should be discontinued at least 7 days before starting cidofovir. Probenecid, which is given with cidofovir, may alter the clearance of other drugs given concomitantly (see Interactions under Probenecid, p.417).

Patients with cytomegalovirus retinitis are at increased risk of adverse inflammatory effects if cidofovir is given within 2 to 4 weeks of intravitreal fomivirsen.

### Antiviral Action

Cidofovir undergoes intracellular phosphorylation by cellular kinases to the antiviral metabolite, cidofovir diphosphate, which acts as a competitive inhibitor of viral DNA polymerase. It is active against a range of herpesviruses including cytomegalovirus, and, since its activity is not reliant on viral enzymes, may retain activity against some aciclovir- and foscarnet-resistant viruses. Cross-resistance with ganciclovir is common.

◊ References.


1. Cherrington JM, *et al.* In vitro antiviral susceptibilities of isolates from cytomegalovirus retinitis patients receiving first- or second-line cidofovir therapy: relationship to clinical outcome. *J Infect Dis* 1998; **178:** 1821–5.
2. Jabs DA, *et al.* Incidence of foscarnet resistance and cidofovir resistance in patients treated for cytomegalovirus retinitis. *Antimicrob Agents Chemother* 1998; **42:** 2240–4.


### Pharmacokinetics

Following intravenous administration of cidofovir, serum concentrations decline with a reported terminal half-life of about 2.2 hours (the intracellular half-life of the active diphosphate may be up to 65 hours). Cidofovir is eliminated mainly by renal excretion, both by glomerular filtration and tubular secretion. About 80 to 100% of a dose is recovered unchanged from the urine within 24 hours. Administration with probenecid may reduce the excretion of cidofovir to some extent by blocking tubular secretion, although 70 to 85% has still been reported to be excreted unchanged in the urine within 24 hours.

◊ References.


1. Cundy KC. Clinical pharmacokinetics of the antiviral nucleotide analogues cidofovir and adefovir. *Clin Pharmacokinet* 1999; **36:** 127–43.
2. Brody SR, *et al.* Pharmacokinetics of cidofovir in renal insufficiency and in continuous ambulatory peritoneal dialysis or high-flux hemodialysis. *Clin Pharmacol Ther* 1999; **65:** 21–8.

### Uses and Administration

Cidofovir is a nucleoside analogue that is active against herpesviruses. It is used in the treatment of cytomegalovirus retinitis (p.619) in patients with AIDS, and is being investigated for herpes simplex and other viral infections.

In the treatment of cytomegalovirus retinitis, cidofovir is given in a dose of 5 mg/kg by intravenous infusion over 1 hour once a week for 2 consecutive weeks, then once every 2 weeks for maintenance. Probenecid 2 g is given by mouth 3 hours before each dose of cidofovir and further 1-g doses of probenecid at 2 and 8 hours after completion of the infusion. To ensure adequate hydration, 1 litre of sodium chloride 0.9% is administered by intravenous infusion over 1 to 2 hours immediately before each infusion of cidofovir; if the additional fluid load can be tolerated, a further 1 litre of sodium chloride 0.9% may be infused over 1 to 3 hours, starting at the same time as (or immediately after) the cidofovir infusion. For details of modified use of cidofovir in patients with renal impairment, see below.

Cidofovir has also been given experimentally by intravitreal injection but the commercially available formulation is unsuitable for use by this route and the manufacturers advise against it (see Precautions, above).

An orally active prodrug of cidofovir known as cyclic-HPMPC (GS-930) is under investigation.

◊ Reviews.

1. Lea AP, Bryson HM. Cidofovir. *Drugs* 1996; **52:** 225–30.
2. Kendle JB, Fan-Havard P. Cidofovir in the treatment of cytomegaloviral disease. *Ann Pharmacother* 1998; **32:** 1181–92.
3. Plosker GL, Noble S. Cidofovir: a review of its use in cytomegalovirus retinitis in patients with AIDS. *Drugs* 1999; **58:** 325–45.

**Administration in renal impairment.** Cidofovir is contra-indicated in patients with pre-existing renal impairment (serum creatinine more than 1.5 mg/dL) and should be interrupted or discontinued if serum creatinine increases by more than 500 micrograms/dL during therapy; in the USA, a reduction in the maintenance dose from 5 to 3 mg/kg is permitted for increases of serum creatinine of up to 300 to 400 micrograms/dL above baseline.

**Viral infections.** In addition to its use in cytomegalovirus retinitis, cidofovir has been studied in herpes simplex infections,[1-6] papillomavirus infections,[7-10] molluscum contagiosum,[11,12] and progressive multifocal leukoencephalopathy.[13,14]

1. Snoeck R, *et al.* A new topical treatment for resistant herpes simplex infections. *N Engl J Med* 1993; **329:** 968–9.
2. Lalezari JP, *et al.* Treatment with intravenous (S)-1-[3-hydroxy-2-(phosphonylmethoxy)propyl]-cytosine of acyclovir-resistant mucocutaneous infection with herpes simplex virus in a patient with AIDS. *J Infect Dis* 1994; **170:** 570–2.
3. Lalezari J, *et al.* A randomized, double-blind, placebo-controlled trial of cidofovir gel for the treatment of acyclovir-unresponsive mucocutaneous herpes simplex virus infection in patients with AIDS. *J Infect Dis* 1997; **176:** 892–8.
4. Sacks SL, *et al.* A multicenter phase I/II dose escalation study of single-dose cidofovir gel for treatment of recurrent genital herpes. *Antimicrob Agents Chemother* 1998; **42:** 2996–9.
5. Bryant P, *et al.* Successful treatment of foscarnet-resistant herpes simplex stomatitis with intravenous cidofovir in a child. *Pediatr Infect Dis J* 2001; **20:** 1083–6.
6. Kopp T, *et al.* Successful treatment of an aciclovir-resistant herpes simplex type 2 infection with cidofovir in an AIDS patient. *Br J Dermatol* 2002; **147:** 134–8.
7. Snoeck R, *et al.* Treatment of anogenital papillomavirus infections with an acyclic nucleoside phosphonate analogue. *N Engl J Med* 1995; **333:** 943–4.
8. Davis MDP, *et al.* Large plantar wart caused by human papillomavirus-66 and resolution by topical cidofovir therapy. *J Am Acad Dermatol* 2000; **43:** 340–3.
9. Descamps V, *et al.* Topical cidofovir for bowenoid papulosis in an HIV-infected patient. *Br J Dermatol* 2001; **144:** 642–3.
10. Snoeck R, *et al.* Phase II double-blind, placebo-controlled study of the safety and efficacy of cidofovir topical gel for the treatment of patients with human papillomavirus infection. *Clin Infect Dis* 2001; **33:** 597–602.
11. Davies EG, *et al.* Topical cidofovir for severe molluscum contagiosum. *Lancet* 1999; **353:** 2042.
12. Toro JR, *et al.* Topical cidofovir: a novel treatment for recalcitrant molluscum contagiosum in children infected with human immunodeficiency virus 1. *Arch Dermatol* 2000; **136:** 983–5.
13. Segarra-Newnham M, Vodolo KM. Use of cidofovir in progressive multifocal leukoencephalopathy. *Ann Pharmacother* 2001; **35:** 741–4.
14. Razonable RR, *et al.* Cidofovir treatment of progressive multifocal leukoencephalopathy in a patient receiving highly active antiretroviral therapy. *Mayo Clin Proc* 2001; **76:** 1171–5.

### Preparations

**Proprietary Preparations** (details are given in Part 3)

***Austral.:*** Vistide; ***Austria:*** Vistide; ***Belg.:*** Vistide; ***Braz.:*** Vistide†; ***Fr.:*** Vistide; ***Ger.:*** Vistide; ***Ital.:*** Vistide; ***Port.:*** Vistide; ***Spain:*** Vistide; ***Switz.:*** Vistide; ***UK:*** Vistide; ***USA:*** Vistide.

## Delavirdine Mesilate *(rINNM)*

Delavirdine Mesylate *(USAN)*; Mesilato de delavirdina; U-90152S.
1-[3-(Isopropylamino)-2-pyridyl]-4-[(5-methanesulfonamidoindol-2-yl)carbonyl]-piperazine monomethanesulfonate.
$C_{22}H_{28}N_6O_3S,CH_4O_3S = 552.7$.
*CAS — 136817-59-9 (delavirdine); 147221-93-0 (delavirdine mesilate).*
*ATC — J05AG02.*

### Adverse Effects

The most common adverse effect of delavirdine is skin rash, usually occurring within the first 3 weeks of starting therapy and resolving in 3 to 14 days. Severe skin reactions, including erythema multiforme and Stevens-Johnson syndrome, have occurred. Additional adverse effects may include nausea and vomiting, diarrhoea, headache, asthenia, and increased liver enzyme values.

### Precautions

Delavirdine should be discontinued if a severe skin rash develops or if a rash is accompanied by fever, blistering, oral lesions, conjunctivitis, swelling, or muscle or joint aches. Delavirdine should be used with caution in patients with hepatic impairment.

### Interactions

Similarly to the HIV-protease inhibitors (see Indinavir Sulfate, p.639), delavirdine is metabolised mainly by cytochrome P450 isoenzymes of the CYP3A family. Consequently it may compete with other drugs metabolised by this system, potentially resulting in toxic concentrations; co-administration of amfetamines, the non-sedating antihistamines astemizole and terfenadine, antiarrhythmics, the benzodiazepines alprazolam, midazolam, and triazolam, calcium-channel blockers, cisapride, ergot alkaloids, pimozide, sildenafil, and statins may be particularly hazardous. Alternatively, enzyme inducers such as rifabutin, rifampicin, hypericum, and the antiepileptics carbamazepine, phenobarbital, and phenytoin, may decrease plasma concentrations of delavirdine. The absorption of delavirdine is reduced by drugs that raise gastric pH such as antacids and histamine $H_2$-antagonists.

**Antibacterials.** Plasma concentrations of *dapsone* and *rifabutin* may be increased by delavirdine; *rifabutin* and *rifampicin*[1] may reduce delavirdine plasma concentrations and the use of either of these drugs with delavirdine is not recommended. Plasma concentrations of both delavirdine and *clarithromycin* may be increased by concurrent administration although this may not be clinically significant.

1. Borin MT, *et al.* Pharmacokinetic study of the interaction between rifampin and delavirdine mesylate. *Clin Pharmacol Ther* 1997; **61:** 544–53.

**Antidepressants.** Plasma concentrations of delavirdine may be increased by *fluoxetine*.

**Antifungals.** Plasma concentrations of delavirdine may be increased by *ketoconazole*.

**Antivirals.** Administration of delavirdine with *didanosine* may result in reduced plasma concentrations of both drugs[1] and they should be given at least 1 hour apart; plasma concentrations of HIV-protease inhibitors including *indinavir* and *saquinavir* may be increased by delavirdine (see Antivirals, under Interactions of Indinavir, p.639) and liver function should be monitored in patients receiving delavirdine and saquinavir.

1. Morse GD, *et al.* Single-dose pharmacokinetics of delavirdine mesylate and didanosine in patients with human immunodeficiency virus infection. *Antimicrob Agents Chemother* 1997; **41:** 169–74.

### Antiviral Action

Delavirdine acts by non-competitive inhibition of HIV-1 reverse transcriptase.

Resistance to delavirdine and emergence of cross-resistance to other non-nucleoside reverse transcriptase inhibitors has been seen.

### Pharmacokinetics

Delavirdine is rapidly absorbed following oral administration, peak plasma concentrations occurring after about 1 hour. It is about 98% bound to plasma proteins. Delavirdine is extensively metabolised by hepatic microsomal enzymes, principally by cytochrome P450 isoenzymes of the CYP3A family, to several inactive metabolites. Plasma half-life following the usual dosage has ranged from 2 to 11 hours. Delavirdine is excreted as metabolites in the urine and faeces. Less than 5% is excreted in the urine unchanged.

◊ Reviews.

1. Tran JQ, *et al.* Delavirdine: clinical pharmacokinetics and drug interactions. *Clin Pharmacokinet* 2001; **40:** 207–26.

**Bioavailability.** The manufacturers report that bioavailability of delavirdine tablets is about 85% of that from an oral solution following a single dose and that the bioavailability increases by about 20% if the tablets are dispersed in water before use.

### Uses and Administration

Delavirdine is a non-nucleoside reverse transcriptase inhibitor with activity against HIV-1. Viral resistance emerges rapidly when delavirdine is used alone, and it is therefore used with other antiretrovirals for combination therapy of HIV infection (p.621).

Delavirdine is given by mouth as the mesilate in a usual dose of 400 mg three times daily. Some tablet formulations may be dispersed in water before administration in order to increase bioavailability (see above).

◊ Reviews.

1. Scott LJ, Perry CM. Delavirdine: a review of its use in HIV infection. *Drugs* 2000; **60:** 1411–44.

### Preparations

**Proprietary Preparations** (details are given in Part 3)

***Austral.:*** Rescriptor; ***Braz.:*** Rescriptor†; ***Canad.:*** Rescriptor; ***Mex.:*** Rescriptor; ***USA:*** Rescriptor.

## Didanosine *(BAN, USAN, rINN)*

BMY-40900; DDI; ddI; ddIno; Didanosina; Dideoxyinosine; NSC-612049. 2′,3′-Dideoxyinosine.
$C_{10}H_{12}N_4O_3 = 236.2$.
*CAS — 69655-05-6.*
*ATC — J05AF02.*

### Adverse Effects

The most common serious adverse effects of didanosine are peripheral neuropathy and potentially fatal pancreatitis. Abnormal liver function tests may occur and hepatitis or fatal hepatic failure has been reported rarely. Retinal depigmentation and optic neuritis have been reported in patients receiving high doses of didanosine. Other adverse effects include nausea, vomiting, and abdominal pain (which may also be symptoms of pancreatitis), diarrhoea, headache, hyperglycaemia, fatigue, myalgia, rash, parotid gland enlargement, alopecia, rhabdomyolysis, hypersensitivity reactions including anaphylaxis, and hyperuricaemia. Lactic acidosis, usually associated with severe hepatomegaly and steatosis, has been reported in patients receiving nucleoside reverse transcriptase inhibitors (see Zidovudine, p.658).

**Effects on the blood.** In general, haematological abnormalities are less common in patients taking didanosine than in those taking zidovudine. However, there have been reports of thrombocytopenia associated with didanosine.[1-3]

1. Butler KM, *et al.* Dideoxyinosine in children with symptomatic human immunodeficiency virus infection. *N Engl J Med* 1991; **324:** 137–44.
2. Lor E, Liu YQ. Didanosine-associated eosinophilia with acute thrombocytopenia. *Ann Pharmacother* 1993; **27:** 23–5.
3. Herranz P, *et al.* Cutaneous vasculitis associated with didanosine. *Lancet* 1994; **344:** 680.

**Effects on the eyes.** Retinal lesions with atrophy of the retinal pigment epithelium at the periphery of the retina was reported in 4 children receiving didanosine doses of 270 to 540 mg/m$^2$ daily.[1]

1. Whitcup SM, *et al.* Retinal lesions in children treated with dideoxyinosine. *N Engl J Med* 1992; **326:** 1226–7.

**Effects on glucose metabolism.** Hyperglycaemia, glucose intolerance, diabetes mellitus, and hyperosmolar nonketotic diabetic syndrome have been associated with didanosine.[1-3] The effect may be dose-related, and has been reported[4] in patients who subsequently developed pancreatitis (see Effects on the Pancreas, below). The manufacturer also reports cases of hypoglycaemia in patients taking didanosine.

1. Munshi MN, *et al.* Hyperosmolar nonketotic diabetic syndrome following treatment of human immunodeficiency virus infection with didanosine. *Diabetes Care* 1994; **17:** 316–17.
2. Jablonowski H, *et al.* A dose comparison study of didanosine in patients with very advanced HIV infection who are intolerant to or clinically deteriorate on zidovudine. *AIDS* 1995; **9:** 463–9.
3. Nguyen B-Y, *et al.* Five-year follow-up of a phase I study of didanosine in patients with advanced human immunodeficiency virus infection. *J Infect Dis* 1995; **171:** 1180–9.
4. Albrecht H, *et al.* Didanosine-induced disorders of glucose tolerance. *Ann Intern Med* 1993; **119:** 1050.

**Effects on the liver.** Fatal fulminant hepatic failure was reported[1] in a patient receiving didanosine. A further 14 cases had been noted by the manufacturer, and elevated liver enzymes have been recorded during clinical studies.[2-5]

1. Lai KK, *et al.* Fulminant hepatic failure associated with 2′,3′-dideoxyinosine (ddI). *Ann Intern Med* 1991; **115:** 283–4.
2. Dolin R, *et al.* Zidovudine compared with didanosine in patients with advanced HIV type 1 infection and little or no experience with zidovudine. *Arch Intern Med* 1995; **155:** 961–74.
3. Jablonowski H, *et al.* A dose comparison study of didanosine in patients with very advanced HIV infection who are intolerant to or clinically deteriorate on zidovudine. *AIDS* 1995; **9:** 463–9.
4. Alpha International Coordinating Committee. The Alpha trial: European/Australian randomized double-blind trial of two doses of didanosine in zidovudine-intolerant patients with symptomatic HIV disease. *AIDS* 1996; **10:** 867–80.
5. Gatell JM, *et al.* Switching from zidovudine to didanosine in patients with symptomatic HIV infection and disease progression. *J Acquir Immune Defic Syndr Hum Retrovirol* 1996; **12:** 249–58.

**Effects on mental state.** Recurrent mania associated with didanosine treatment has been reported in a patient.[1]

1. Brouillette MJ, *et al.* Didanosine-induced mania in HIV infection. *Am J Psychiatry* 1994; **151:** 1839–40.

**Effects on metabolism.** Hyperuricaemia has been reported to be a common adverse effect during clinical studies of didanosine.[1,2] Hypokalaemia occurred during didanosine therapy in 3 patients, 2 of whom had diarrhoea.[3] There has also been a report of hypertriglyceridaemia occurring on 2 occasions in a patient given didanosine;[4] it was suggested that this hyperlipidaemic effect might be a possible aetiological factor in the development of pancreatitis. For effects on glucose metabolism, see above.

1. Cooley TP, *et al.* Once-daily administration of 2′,3′-dideoxyinosine (ddI) in patients with the acquired immunodeficiency syndrome or AIDS-related complex: results of a phase I trial. *N Engl J Med* 1990; **322:** 1340–5.
2. Montaner JSG, *et al.* Didanosine compared with continued zidovudine therapy for HIV-infected patients with 200 to 500 CD4 cells/mm³: a double-blind, randomized, controlled trial. *Ann Intern Med* 1995; **123:** 561–71.
3. Katlama C, *et al.* Dideoxyinosine-associated hypokalaemia. *Lancet* 1991; **337:** 183.
4. Tal A, Dall L. Didanosine-induced hypertriglyceridemia. *Am J Med* 1993; **95:** 247.

**Effects on the mouth.** Xerostomia (dry mouth) may be a troublesome effect in patients receiving didanosine.[1,2]

1. Dodd CL, *et al.* Xerostomia associated with didanosine. *Lancet* 1992; **340:** 790.
2. Valentine C, *et al.* Xerostomia associated with didanosine. *Lancet* 1992; **340:** 1542.

**Effects on the nervous system.** Peripheral neuropathy is a well recognised adverse effect of didanosine and has been the subject of a review.[1]

1. Moyle GJ, Sadler M. Peripheral neuropathy with nucleoside antiretrovirals: risk factors, incidence and management. *Drug Safety* 1998; **19:** 481–94.

**Effects on the pancreas.** Pancreatitis is recognised as being the most serious adverse effect of didanosine and can be fatal.[1-3] It appears to be dose-related, occurring in up to 13% of patients receiving 750 mg of didanosine daily.[2,4] Pancreatitis can resolve if didanosine is withdrawn[5] and cautious reintroduction of didanosine has been possible in some patients.[6] Raised amylase concentrations[3] and glucose intolerance (see above) have been reported in patients who subsequently developed pancreatitis.

1. Bouvet E, *et al.* Fatal case of 2′,3′-dideoxyinosine-associated pancreatitis. *Lancet* 1990; **336:** 1515.
2. Kahn JO, *et al.* A controlled trial comparing continued zidovudine with didanosine in human immunodeficiency virus infection. *N Engl J Med* 1992; **327:** 581–7.
3. Dolin R, *et al.* Zidovudine compared with didanosine in patients with advanced HIV-type 1 infection and little or no previous experience with zidovudine. *Arch Intern Med* 1995; **155:** 961–74.
4. Jablonowski H, *et al.* A dose comparison study of didanosine in patients with very advanced HIV infection who are intolerant to or clinically deteriorate on zidovudine. *AIDS* 1995; **9:** 463–9.
5. Nguyen B-Y, *et al.* Five-year follow-up of a phase I study of didanosine in patients with advanced human immunodeficiency virus infection. *J Infect Dis* 1995; **171:** 1180–9.
6. Butler KM, *et al.* Pancreatitis in human immunodeficiency virus-infected children receiving dideoxyinosine. *Pediatrics* 1993; **91:** 747–51.

**Effects on the skin.** Didanosine has been implicated in a case of Stevens-Johnson syndrome[1] and of cutaneous vasculitis.[2]

1. Parneix-Spake A, *et al.* Didanosine as probable cause of Stevens-Johnson syndrome. *Lancet* 1992; **340:** 857–8.
2. Herranz P, *et al.* Cutaneous vasculitis associated with didanosine. *Lancet* 1994; **344:** 680.

## Precautions

Patients with a history of pancreatitis and those with increased triglyceride concentrations should be observed carefully for signs of pancreatitis and treatment with didanosine interrupted in all patients with raised serum amylase or lipase or other signs of possible pancreatitis, until it has been excluded. Use with other drugs likely to cause pancreatitis or peripheral neuropathy (see Interactions, below) should be avoided if possible.

It may be necessary to interrupt didanosine treatment in patients who develop peripheral neuropathy; on recovery from peripheral neuropathy a reduced dose may be tolerated. Treatment should also be interrupted if uric acid concentrations are elevated.

Didanosine should be used with caution in patients with renal or hepatic impairment, and dosage reduction may be necessary. Regular checks of liver function are recommended. If liver function deteriorates during treatment then didanosine should be withdrawn. Treatment with didanosine may be associated with lactic acidosis and should be discontinued if there is a rapid increase in aminotransferase concentrations, progressive hepatomegaly, steatosis, or metabolic or lactic acidosis of unknown aetiology. Didanosine should be given with caution to patients with hepatomegaly or other risk factors for liver disease.

Children should be monitored for retinal lesions and didanosine withdrawn if they occur. Monitoring should also be considered in adults.

## Interactions

Use of didanosine with other drugs known to cause pancreatitis (for example intravenous pentamidine) or with drugs that may cause peripheral neuropathy (for example metronidazole, isoniazid, and vincristine) should be avoided. If co-administration is unavoidable, patients should be monitored carefully for these adverse effects.

An increase in the area under the plasma concentration-time curve for didanosine has been reported when allopurinol is given concurrently.

Plasma concentrations of didanosine may be reduced by methadone.

Since didanosine is generally taken with an antacid (often included in the formulation), drugs that could be affected by an increased gastric pH (for example HIV-protease inhibitors, ketoconazole, fluoroquinolone antibacterials, and dapsone) should be given at least 2 hours before didanosine. Didanosine preparations containing magnesium or aluminium antacids should not be given with tetracyclines.

See also below for interactions with antivirals.

**Antidiabetics.** Fatal lactic acidosis has been reported[1] in a patient who received *metformin* together with didanosine, stavudine, and tenofovir.

1. Worth L, *et al.* A cautionary tale: fatal lactic acidosis complicating nucleoside analogue and metformin therapy. *Clin Infect Dis* 2003; **37:** 315–16.

**Antivirals.** Plasma concentrations of didanosine are approximately doubled when *ganciclovir* is given concurrently.[1-3]

Changes in the pharmacokinetics of didanosine and *zidovudine* have occurred when these drugs are given together, but results of studies have not been consistent, and the effects have generally been of limited clinical significance. For further details, see under Interactions in Zidovudine, p.660. *Tenofovir* has been reported to significantly increase plasma concentrations of didanosine,[4] and may increase the risk of pancreatitis associated with didanosine.[5] There has also been a report of acute renal failure and fatal lactic acidosis when tenofovir was added to a regimen containing didanosine.[6]

Concurrent administration of didanosine and *delavirdine* resulted in reductions in the area under the concentration-time curve for both drugs in a single-dose study.[7] The manufacturer of delavirdine recommends that administration of these two drugs should be separated by at least 1 hour.

Absorption of some *HIV-protease inhibitors* may be reduced by the antacids in didanosine formulations and doses should be separated by at least 2 hours (see p.639).

1. Griffy KG. Pharmacokinetics of oral ganciclovir capsules in HIV-infected persons. *AIDS* 1996; **10** (suppl 4): S3–S6.
2. Jung D, *et al.* Effect of high-dose oral ganciclovir on didanosine disposition in human immunodeficiency virus (HIV)-positive patients. *J Clin Pharmacol* 1998; **38:** 1057–62.
3. Cimoch PJ, *et al.* Pharmacokinetics of oral ganciclovir alone and in combination with zidovudine, didanosine, and probenecid in HIV-infected subjects. *J Acquir Immune Defic Syndr Hum Retrovirol* 1998; **17:** 227–34.
4. Pecora Fulco P, Kirian MA. Effect of tenofovir on didanosine absorption in patients with HIV. *Ann Pharmacother* 2003; **37:** 1325–8.
5. Blanchard JN, *et al.* Pancreatitis with didanosine and tenofovir disoproxil fumarate. *Clin Infect Dis* 2003; **37:** e57–e62. Correction. *ibid.*: 995. [title of paper corrected]
6. Murphy MD, *et al.* Fatal lactic acidosis and acute renal failure after addition of tenofovir to an antiretroviral regimen containing didanosine. *Clin Infect Dis* 2003; **36:** 1082–5.
7. Morse GD, *et al.* Single-dose pharmacokinetics of delavirdine mesylate and didanosine in patients with human immunodeficiency virus infection. *Antimicrob Agents Chemother* 1997; **41:** 169–74.

## Antiviral Action

Didanosine is converted intracellularly to its active form dideoxyadenosine triphosphate. This triphosphate halts the DNA synthesis of retroviruses, including HIV, through competitive inhibition of reverse transcriptase and incorporation into viral DNA.

Didanosine-resistant strains of HIV emerge during didanosine therapy. Cross-resistance to other nucleoside reverse transcriptase inhibitors has been recognised.

**Resistance.** Evidence for the development of didanosine-resistant HIV was reported in 36 of 64 patients with advanced HIV infection within 24 weeks of switching from zidovudine to didanosine monotherapy.[1] Patients with the didanosine resistance mutation for HIV reverse transcriptase showed a greater decline in CD4+ T cell count and increase in viral burden than those without.

Multiple-drug resistant mutations have been identified in patients receiving long-term antiretroviral therapy with combinations containing didanosine.[2]

1. Kozal MJ, *et al.* Didanosine resistance in HIV-infected patients switched from zidovudine to didanosine monotherapy. *Ann Intern Med* 1994; **121:** 263–8.
2. Kavlick MF, *et al.* Emergence of multi-dideoxynucleoside-resistant human immunodeficiency virus type 1 variants, viral sequence variation, and disease progression in patients receiving antiretroviral chemotherapy. *J Infect Dis* 1998; **98:** 1506–13.

## Pharmacokinetics

Didanosine is rapidly hydrolysed in the acid medium of the stomach and is therefore given by mouth with pH buffers or antacids. Bioavailability is reported to range from 20 to 40% depending on the formulation used; the bioavailability is substantially reduced by administration with or after food. Maximum plasma concentrations are achieved about 1 hour after oral administration. Binding to plasma proteins is reported to be less than 5%. Didanosine has been reported not to cross the blood brain barrier.

Didanosine is metabolised intracellularly to the active antiviral metabolite dideoxyadenosine triphosphate. The plasma elimination half-life is reported to be about 1.5 hours. Renal clearance is by glomerular filtration and active tubular secretion; about 20% of an oral dose is recovered in the urine. Didanosine is partially cleared by haemodialysis but not by peritoneal dialysis.

◊ References.

1. Balis FM, *et al.* Clinical pharmacology of 2′,3′-dideoxyinosine in human immunodeficiency virus-infected children. *J Infect Dis* 1992; **165:** 99–104.
2. Morse GD, *et al.* Comparative pharmacokinetics of antiviral nucleoside analogues. *Clin Pharmacokinet* 1993; **24:** 101–23.
3. Mueller BU, *et al.* Clinical and pharmacokinetic evaluation of long-term therapy with didanosine in children with HIV infection. *Pediatrics* 1994; **94:** 724–31.
4. Knupp CA, *et al.* Disposition of didanosine in HIV-seropositive patients with normal renal function or chronic renal failure: influence of hemodialysis and continuous ambulatory peritoneal dialysis. *Clin Pharmacol Ther* 1996; **60:** 535–42.
5. Wintergerst U, *et al.* Lack of absorption of didanosine after rectal administration in human immunodeficiency virus-infected patients. *Antimicrob Agents Chemother* 1999; **43:** 699–701.
6. Abreu T, *et al.* Bioavailability of once- and twice-daily regimens of didanosine in human immunodeficiency virus-infected children. *Antimicrob Agents Chemother* 2000; **44:** 1375–6.

**Pregnancy.** Fetal blood concentrations of 14 and 19% of the maternal serum-didanosine concentrations have been reported.[1] There is evidence of extensive metabolism in the placenta.[2]

1. Pons JC, *et al.* Fetoplacental passage of 2′,3′-dideoxyinosine. *Lancet* 1991; **337:** 732.
2. Dancis J, *et al.* Transfer and metabolism of dideoxyinosine by the perfused human placenta. *J Acquir Immune Defic Syndr* 1993; **6:** 2–6.

## Uses and Administration

Didanosine is a nucleoside reverse transcriptase inhibitor structurally related to inosine with activity against retroviruses including HIV. It is used in the treatment of HIV infection, usually with other antiretrovirals as part of combination therapy.

Didanosine is given by mouth, usually as buffered chewable/dispersible tablets, or enteric-coated capsules, or oral solution. The tablets have a bioavailability 20 to 25% greater than that of the solution. Doses should be taken at least 30 minutes before, or 2 hours after, a meal. The total daily dose may be given as either a single dose or as two divided doses, the choice being dependent upon both the formulation and the strength used. Doses for adults are: greater than 60 kg body-weight, 400 mg (tablets or capsules) or 500 mg (oral solution) daily; under 60 kg, 250 mg (tablets or capsules) or 334 mg (oral solution) daily.

Children's doses are determined by body-surface: in the UK, children over 3 months of age (or over 6 years with enteric-coated capsules) may be given 240 mg/m² daily, or 180 mg/m² daily when didanosine is given in combination with zidovudine. In the USA, infants aged 2 weeks to 8 months may be given a dose of 100 mg/m² twice daily and children aged 8 months or over 120 mg/m² twice daily.

Dosage reduction may be necessary in patients with renal (see below) or hepatic impairment.

◊ Reviews.

1. Shelton MJ, *et al.* Didanosine. *Ann Pharmacother* 1992; **26:** 660–70.
2. Lipsky JJ. Zalcitabine and didanosine. *Lancet* 1993; **341:** 30–2.
3. Perry CM, Noble S. Didanosine: an updated review of its use in HIV infection. *Drugs* 1999; **58:** 1099–1135.

**Administration in renal impairment.** Dosage of didanosine should be reduced in patients with renal impairment. The following doses are recommended by the manufacturer based on the patient's creatinine clearance (CC):

Adults greater than 60 kg:

- CC more than 60 mL/minute: usual adult doses
- CC 30 to 59 mL/minute: 200 mg daily as a single dose or in two equally divided doses (tablets); 100 mg twice daily (oral solution)
- CC 10 to 29 mL/minute: 150 mg once daily (tablets); 167 mg once daily (oral solution)
- CC less than 10 mL/minute: 100 mg once daily (tablets or oral solution)

Adults less than 60 kg:

- CC more than 60 mL/minute: usual adult doses
- CC 30 to 59 mL/minute: 150 mg daily as a single dose or in two equally divided doses (tablets); 100 mg twice daily (oral solution)
- CC 10 to 29 mL/minute: 100 mg once daily (tablets or oral solution)
- CC less than 10 mL/minute: 75 mg once daily (tablets); 100 mg once daily (oral solution)

### Preparations

**Proprietary Preparations** (details are given in Part 3)
***Arg.:*** Aso DDI; Bandotan; Dibistic; Megavir; Ronvir; Videx; ***Austral.:*** Videx; ***Austria:*** Videx; ***Belg.:*** Videx; ***Braz.:*** Videx; ***Canad.:*** Videx; ***Chile:*** Videx; ***Denm.:*** Videx; ***Fin.:*** Videx; ***Fr.:*** Videx; ***Ger.:*** Videx; ***Gr.:*** Videx; ***Hong Kong:*** Videx; ***Irl.:*** Videx; ***Israel:*** Videx; ***Ital.:*** Videx; ***Malaysia:*** Videx; ***Mex.:*** Videx; ***Neth.:*** Videx; ***Norw.:*** Videx; ***NZ:*** Videx; ***Port.:*** Videx; ***S.Afr.:*** Videx; ***Singapore:*** Videx; ***Spain:*** Videx; ***Swed.:*** Videx; ***Switz.:*** Videx; ***Thai.:*** Videx; ***UK:*** Videx; ***USA:*** Videx.

## Docosanol *(USAN)*

Behenyl Alcohol; *n*-Docosanol; Docosyl Alcohol; IK-2. 1-Docosanol.

$C_{22}H_{46}O$ = 326.6.
*CAS — 661-19-8.*
*ATC — D06BB11.*

### Profile

Docosanol is an antiviral used topically five times daily as a 10% cream in the treatment of recurrent herpes labialis (p.620). Docosanol acts by inhibiting fusion between the cell plasma membrane and the herpes simplex virus, thereby preventing viral entry into cells and subsequent viral replication. It is also under investigation for genital herpes.

◊ References.

1. Habbema L, *et al.* n-Docosanol 10% cream in the treatment of recurrent herpes labialis: a randomised, double-blind, placebo-controlled study. *Acta Derm Venereol* 1996; **76:** 479–81.
2. Sacks SL, *et al.* Clinical efficacy of topical docosanol 10% cream for herpes simplex labialis: a multicenter, randomized, placebo-controlled trial. *J Am Acad Dermatol* 2001; **45:** 222–30.

### Preparations

**Proprietary Preparations** (details are given in Part 3)
***USA:*** Abreva.

## Edoxudine *(USAN, rINN)*

Edoxudina; EDU; Ethyl Deoxyuridine; EUDR; ORF-15817; RWJ-15817. 2′-Deoxy-5-ethyluridine.

$C_{11}H_{16}N_2O_5$ = 256.3.
*CAS — 15176-29-1.*
*ATC — D06BB09.*

### Profile

Edoxudine is an antiviral used topically as a 1.2% gel in the treatment of mucocutaneous herpes simplex infections (p.620); it has also been used as a 3% cream and as a 0.3% ophthalmic preparation.

### Preparations

**Proprietary Preparations** (details are given in Part 3)
***Canad.:*** Virostat†; ***Switz.:*** Edurid.

## Efavirenz *(BAN, rINN)*

5B706; DMP-266; L-743; L-743726. (*S*)-6-Chloro-4-(cyclopropylethynyl)-1,4-dihydro-4-(trifluoromethyl)-2*H*-3,1-benzoxazin-2-one.

$C_{14}H_9ClF_3NO_2$ = 315.7.
*CAS — 154598-52-4.*
*ATC — J05AG03.*

### Adverse Effects

The most common adverse effects associated with efavirenz are skin rashes and CNS disturbances. Mild rashes may resolve on continued treatment, but severe forms may occur and erythema multiforme and Stevens-Johnson syndrome have been reported occasionally. CNS symptoms include dizziness, headache, insomnia or somnolence, impaired concentration, abnormal dreaming, and convulsions. Symptoms resembling psychoses and severe acute depression have also been reported. Other adverse effects include nausea and vomiting, diarrhoea, fatigue, and pancreatitis. Raised liver enzyme values have occurred, particularly in patients with viral hepatitis. Raised serum-cholesterol and -triglyceride concentrations have been reported.

### Precautions

Efavirenz is contra-indicated in patients with severe hepatic impairment, and should be used with caution, and liver enzymes values monitored, in patients with mild to moderate liver disease. Caution should be exercised in patients with a history of seizures or psychiatric disorders. Efavirenz should be discontinued if a severe skin rash, associated with blistering, desquamation, mucosal involvement, or fever, develops. Monitoring of plasma-cholesterol concentrations may be considered during efavirenz treatment.

False-positive results in some urinary cannabinoid tests have been reported in subjects receiving efavirenz.

Efavirenz has been associated with carcinogenicity and teratogenicity in *animals*.

### Interactions

Similarly to the HIV-protease inhibitors (see Indinavir Sulfate, p.639), efavirenz is metabolised mainly by cytochrome P450 isoenzymes including CYP3A4. Consequently, it may compete with other drugs metabolised by this system, potentially resulting in mutually increased plasma concentrations and toxicity. Enzyme inducers may decrease plasma concentrations of efavirenz; efavirenz itself acts as an enzyme inducer and can reduce plasma concentrations of other drugs. Inhibition of some P450 isoenzymes has also been demonstrated *in vitro*.

Efavirenz can inhibit the metabolism of astemizole, terfenadine, cisapride, the benzodiazepines midazolam and triazolam, and ergot alkaloids, resulting in serious adverse effects and such combinations should be avoided.

**Antibacterials.** Plasma concentrations of efavirenz may be reduced by *rifampicin* and may necessitate an increase in the dose of efavirenz. A similar interaction might occur with *rifabutin*. Use of efavirenz with *clarithromycin* has resulted in a decrease in the plasma concentration of clarithromycin and an increase in its active hydroxy metabolite. The combination has been associated with a high incidence of skin rashes.

**Antivirals.** For the effect of efavirenz on *HIV-protease inhibitors*, see p.639.

**Grapefruit.** The metabolism of efavirenz may be inhibited by concomitant ingestion of grapefruit juice.

**Hormonal contraceptives.** For the effect of efavirenz on *ethinylestradiol* concentrations, see p.1534.

### Antiviral Action

Efavirenz acts by non-competitive inhibition of HIV-1 reverse transcriptase.

Resistance to efavirenz and emergence of cross-resistance to other non-nucleoside reverse transcriptase inhibitors has been seen.

### Pharmacokinetics

Efavirenz is absorbed following oral administration with peak plasma concentrations being achieved about 5 hours after the dose. Steady-state plasma concentrations are reached in 6 to 7 days following multiple dosing. Bioavailability is increased following a high-fat meal. Efavirenz is more than 99% bound to plasma proteins and is distributed into the CSF. It is metabolised principally by hepatic cytochrome P450 isoenzymes CYP3A4 and CYP2B6. Efavirenz acts as an enzyme inducer and induces its own metabolism resulting in a terminal half-life of 40 to 55 hours after multiple doses compared with 52 to 76 hours after a single dose. About 14 to 34% of a dose is excreted in the urine as metabolites, and 16 to 61% in the faeces.

### Uses and Administration

Efavirenz is a non-nucleoside reverse transcriptase inhibitor with activity against HIV. It is used with other antiretrovirals for combination therapy of HIV infection (p.621).

Efavirenz is administered by mouth as capsules or tablets in an adult dose of 600 mg once daily; alternatively, it may be given as an oral solution in an adult dose of 720 mg once daily. Dosing at bedtime is recommended during the first 2 to 4 weeks of therapy to improve tolerability. Doses (as capsules) for children over the age of 3 years are based on body-weight: children weighing 13 to 14 kg are given 200 mg once daily; those weighing 15 to 19 kg, 250 mg once daily; those weighing 20 to 24 kg, 300 mg once daily; those weighing 25 to 32.4 kg, 350 mg once daily; those weighing 32.5 to 39 kg, 400 mg once daily; and those weighing 40 kg or more, 600 mg once daily. Bioavailability of efavirenz from the oral solution is less than that from the capsule and so proportionately higher doses are used; the dose ranges, which are again calculated in terms of body-weight, also depend on the age range.

◊ References.

1. Adkins JC, Noble S. Efavirenz. *Drugs* 1998; **56:** 1055–64.
2. Gazzard BG. Efavirenz in the management of HIV infection. *Int J Clin Pract* 1999; **53:** 60–4.

### Preparations

**Proprietary Preparations** (details are given in Part 3)
***Arg.:*** Filginase; Stocrin; ***Austral.:*** Stocrin; ***Belg.:*** Stocrin; ***Braz.:*** Stocrin; ***Canad.:*** Sustiva; ***Chile:*** Stocrin; ***Denm.:*** Stocrin; ***Fin.:*** Stocrin; ***Fr.:*** Sustiva; ***Ger.:*** Sustiva; ***Gr.:*** Stocrin; ***Hong Kong:*** Stocrin; ***India:*** Efavir; ***Irl.:*** Sustiva; ***Israel:*** Stocrin; ***Ital.:*** Sustiva; ***Malaysia:*** Stocrin; ***Mex.:*** Stocrin; ***Neth.:*** Stocrin; ***Norw.:*** Stocrin; ***NZ:*** Stocrin; ***Port.:*** Stocrin; ***S.Afr.:*** Stocrin; ***Singapore:*** Stocrin; ***Spain:*** Sustiva; ***Swed.:*** Stocrin; ***Switz.:*** Stocrin; ***Thai.:*** Stocrin; ***UK:*** Sustiva; ***USA:*** Sustiva.

## Emtricitabine *(USAN, rINN)*

BW-524W91; Emtricitabina; FTC; (–)-FTC; FTC-(–). 5-Fluoro-1-[(2*R*,5*S*)-2-(hydroxymethyl)-1,3-oxathiolan-5-yl]cytosine.

$C_8H_{10}FN_3O_3S$ = 247.2.
*CAS — 143491-57-0.*
*ATC — J05AF09.*

### Adverse Effects

The most common adverse effects reported from the use of emtricitabine have been headache, diarrhoea, nausea and vomiting, and rashes. Abdominal pain and dyspepsia may occur and raised serum amylase and lipase concentrations have been reported. Skin discoloration may occur, manifested as hyperpigmentation of the palms and soles, but it is generally mild. Other adverse effects reported have included peripheral neuropathy, asthenia, dizziness, sleep disturbances, and depression. Elevation of creatine kinase concentration is common and arthralgia and myalgia have been reported. Raised liver enzyme concentrations and hyperbilirubinaemia may also occur during treatment. There have also been reports of hypertriglyceridaemia, hyperglycaemia, neutropenia, and anaemia.

Lactic acidosis, usually associated with severe hepatomegaly and steatosis, has been associated with treatment with nucleoside reverse transcriptase inhibitors (see Zidovudine, p.658).

### Precautions

Treatment with emtricitabine should be discontinued if

there is a rapid increase in aminotransferase concentrations, progressive hepatomegaly or steatosis, or metabolic or lactic acidosis of unknown aetiology. Emtricitabine should be given with caution to patients with hepatomegaly or other risk factors for liver disease. In particular, extreme caution should be exercised in patients with co-existing hepatitis B infection; it is recommended that all patients should be tested for the presence of hepatitis B infection before treatment is initiated, and that patients co-infected with HIV and hepatitis B should be monitored for several months after stopping treatment with emtricitabine for signs of exacerbations of hepatitis. Emtricitabine should be used with caution and doses reduced in patients with renal impairment.

## Interactions

Caution should be exercised when emtricitabine is given with other drugs eliminated by active tubular secretion as competition for the elimination pathway may increase the serum concentrations of either drug.

## Antiviral Action

Emtricitabine is converted intracellularly in stages to the triphosphate. This triphosphate halts the DNA synthesis of HIV through competitive inhibition of reverse transcriptase. Emtricitabine-resistant strains of HIV have been identified and cross-resistance to other nucleoside reverse transcriptase inhibitors may occur.

## Pharmacokinetics

Emtricitabine is rapidly and extensively absorbed from the gastrointestinal tract following oral administration, with peak plasma concentrations occurring after 1 to 2 hours. Bioavailability is reported to be 93% following administration of the capsules. Binding to plasma proteins is reported to be less than 4%. The plasma elimination half-life is about 10 hours. Emtricitabine is metabolised to a limited degree, but is excreted largely unchanged in the urine and to a lesser extent in the faeces. It is partially removed by haemodialysis.

## Uses and Administration

Emtricitabine is a nucleoside reverse transcriptase inhibitor related to cytosine with antiretroviral activity against HIV. It is also active against hepatitis B virus. It is used with other antiretrovirals for combination therapy of HIV infection. Emtricitabine is given once daily by mouth as capsules in a usual adult dose of 200 mg. Children weighing at least 33 kg may be given adult doses.

For details of reduced doses of emtricitabine to be used in patients with renal impairment, see below.

◊ Reviews.

1. Bang LM, Scott LJ. Emtricitabine: an antiretroviral agent for HIV infection. *Drugs* 2003; **63:** 2413–24.

**Administration in renal impairment.** Doses of emtricitabine should be reduced in patients with renal impairment, according to the patient's creatinine clearance (CC):

- CC at least 50 mL/minute: usual adult doses (as capsules)
- CC 30 to 49 mL/minute: 200 mg every 48 hours
- CC 15 to 29 mL/minute: 200 mg every 72 hours
- CC less than 15 mL/minute: 200 mg every 96 hours

## Preparations

**Proprietary Preparations** (details are given in Part 3)
**UK:** Emtriva; **USA:** Emtriva.

# Enfuvirtide *(BAN, USAN, rINN)*

DP-178; Enfuvirtida; Pentafuside; T-20.

$C_{204}H_{301}N_{51}O_{64}$ = 4491.9.

*CAS — 159519-65-0.*

## Adverse Effects

The most common adverse effects associated with enfuvirtide are local injection site reactions with resultant pain, erythema, induration, or nodules and cysts. These reactions have been reported to occur in 98% of patients, but have only necessitated discontinuation of therapy in a small minority. Other common adverse effects include nausea, diarrhoea, constipation, abdominal pain, anorexia, taste disturbance, and fatigue. An increased incidence of some bacterial infections, in particular of pneumonia, has occurred in patients receiving enfuvirtide. Hypersensitivity reactions have occurred in about 1% of patients. Pancreatitis has occurred. Eosinophilia has been reported. Other adverse effects have included insomnia, headache, dizziness, depression, anxiety, peripheral neuropathy, myalgia, arthralgia, sweating, conjunctivitis, and cough.

## Precautions

Enfuvirtide should be discontinued immediately and should not be restarted in patients who develop signs of a systemic hypersensitivity reaction. An increased incidence of some bacterial infections, in particular of pneumonia, has been observed and patients receiving enfuvirtide should be closely monitored for signs of pneumonia. Enfuvirtide should be used with caution in patients with hepatic impairment and in those with moderate to severe renal impairment.

## Antiviral Action

Enfuvirtide is an HIV fusion inhibitor that interferes with entry of HIV into cells by binding to the gp41 subunit of the viral envelope glycoprotein, thereby inhibiting fusion of viral and cellular membranes. Strains of HIV with reduced susceptibility to enfuvirtide have been isolated in patients receiving it but, owing to the different mode of action of enfuvirtide and the fact that it does not require intracellular activation for its activity, cross-resistance with other antiretrovirals may occur less frequently.

## Pharmacokinetics

Enfuvirtide is absorbed following subcutaneous injection with a reported mean absolute bioavailability of 84%. It is 92% bound to plasma proteins. Enfuvirtide is a peptide and is metabolised by hydrolysis; it does not appear to interact with cytochrome P450 isoenzymes. The elimination half-life is reported to be 3.8 hours following subcutaneous administration, although elimination pathways have yet to be identified.

## Uses and Administration

Enfuvirtide is a synthetic 36-amino acid peptide that blocks HIV cell fusion and viral entry. It is used with other antiretrovirals for combination therapy of HIV infection. Enfuvirtide is given by subcutaneous injection into the upper arm, anterior thigh, or abdomen in a usual adult dose of 90 mg twice daily. Each injection should be given at a different site from the preceding one.

◊ References.

1. Lalezari JP, *et al.* Enfuvirtide, an HIV-1 fusion inhibitor, for drug-resistant HIV infection in North and South America. *N Engl J Med* 2003; **348:** 2175–85. Correction. *ibid.*; **349:** 1100.
2. Duffalo ML, James CW. Enfuvirtide: a novel agent for the treatment of HIV-1 infection. *Ann Pharmacother* 2003; **37:** 1448–56.
3. Cervia JS, Smith MA. Enfuvirtide (T-20): a novel human immunodeficiency virus type 1 fusion inhibitor. *Clin Infect Dis* 2003; **37:** 1102–6.
4. Dando TM, Perry CM. Enfuvirtide. *Drugs* 2003; **63:** 2755–66.

## Preparations

**Proprietary Preparations** (details are given in Part 3)
**Fr.:** Fuzeon; **UK:** Fuzeon; **USA:** Fuzeon.

# Famciclovir *(BAN, USAN, rINN)*

AV-42810; BRL-42810. 2[2-(2-Amino-9*H*-purin-9-yl)ethyl]trimethylene diacetate.

$C_{14}H_{19}N_5O_4$ = 321.3.

*CAS — 104227-87-4.*

*ATC — J05AB09; S01AD07.*

## Adverse Effects and Precautions

The most common adverse effects of famciclovir are headache and nausea. Other adverse effects include vomiting, dizziness, skin rash, confusion, and hallucinations. In addition, abdominal pain and fever have been reported in immunocompromised patients receiving famciclovir.

Dosage should be reduced in patients with renal impairment (see below) Acute renal failure has been reported in patients with renal impairment receiving inappropriately high doses of famciclovir.

◊ References.

1. Saltzman R, *et al.* Safety of famciclovir in patients with herpes zoster and genital herpes. *Antimicrob Agents Chemother* 1994; **38:** 2454–7.

## Interactions

As for Penciclovir, p.651.

## Antiviral Action

As for Penciclovir, p.651.

## Pharmacokinetics

Famciclovir is rapidly absorbed following oral administration. Absorption is delayed but not reduced by administration with food. Famciclovir is rapidly converted to penciclovir (see p.651), peak plasma concentrations occurring within about 1 hour of administration, and virtually no famciclovir is detectable in the plasma or urine. Bioavailability of penciclovir is reported to be 77%. Famciclovir is principally excreted in the urine (partly by renal tubular secretion) as penciclovir and its 6-deoxy precursor; elimination is reduced in patients with renal impairment.

◊ References.

1. Pue MA, Benet LZ. Pharmacokinetics of famciclovir in man. *Antiviral Chem Chemother* 1993; **4** (suppl 1): 47–55.
2. Boike SC, *et al.* Pharmacokinetics of famciclovir in subjects with varying degrees of renal impairment. *Clin Pharmacol Ther* 1994; **55:** 418–26.
3. Boike SC, *et al.* Pharmacokinetics of famciclovir in subjects with chronic hepatic disease. *J Clin Pharmacol* 1994; **34:** 1199–1207.
4. Gill KS, Wood MJ. The clinical pharmacokinetics of famciclovir. *Clin Pharmacokinet* 1996; **31:** 1–8.

## Uses and Administration

Famciclovir is a prodrug of the antiviral penciclovir (p.651). It is given by mouth in the treatment of herpes zoster (see Varicella-zoster Infections, p.621) and genital and mucocutaneous herpes (see Herpes Simplex Infections, p.620).

For herpes zoster, famciclovir is given in a dose of 250 mg three times daily, or 750 mg once daily, for 7 days (in the USA the recommended dose is 500 mg three times daily for 7 days); immunocompromised patients are given 500 mg three times daily for 10 days.

For first episodes of genital herpes, famciclovir is given in a dose of 250 mg three times daily for 5 days; immunocompromised patients are given 500 mg twice daily for 7 days. For acute treatment of recurrent episodes of genital herpes, 125 mg is given twice daily for 5 days; immunocompromised patients are given 500 mg twice daily for 7 days. For suppression of recurrent episodes of genital herpes, 250 mg is given twice daily; HIV patients may be given 500 mg twice daily. Such suppressive treatment is interrupted every 6 to 12 months to observe possible changes in the natural history of the disease.

For acute treatment of recurrent mucocutaneous herpes in HIV-infected patients, 500 mg is given twice daily for 7 days.

Doses of famciclovir should be reduced in patients with renal impairment (see below).

◊ Reviews.

1. Perry CM, Wagstaff AJ. Famciclovir: a review of its pharmacological properties and therapeutic efficacy in herpesvirus infections. *Drugs* 1995; **50:** 396–415.

**Administration in renal impairment.** Doses of famciclovir need to be reduced in patients with renal impairment. The UK manufacturer recommends the following doses based on creatinine clearance (CC):

Immunocompetent patients:

- Herpes zoster or an initial episode of genital herpes
  - CC 30 to 59 mL/minute: 250 mg twice daily
  - CC 10 to 29 mL/minute: 250 mg once daily
- Acute recurrent genital herpes, treatment
  - CC 30 to 59 mL/minute: no dosage adjustment necessary
  - CC 10 to 29 mL/minute: 125 mg once daily
- Recurrent genital herpes, suppression
  - CC over 30 mL/minute: 250 mg twice daily
  - CC 10 to 29 mL/minute: 125 mg twice daily

Immunocompromised patients:

- Herpes zoster
  - CC over 40 mL/minute: 500 mg three times daily
  - CC 30 to 39 mL/minute: 250 mg three times daily

- CC 10 to 29 mL/minute: 125 mg three times daily

Herpes simplex infections
- CC over 40 mL/minute: 500 mg twice daily
- CC 30 to 39 mL/minute: 250 mg twice daily
- CC 10 to 29 mL/minute: 125 mg twice daily

Patients on haemodialysis should be given doses of famciclovir immediately following dialysis.

## Preparations

**Proprietary Preparations** (details are given in Part 3)
***Arg.:*** Zosvir; ***Austral.:*** Famvir; ***Austria:*** Famvir; ***Belg.:*** Famvir; ***Braz.:*** Famvir; Fanclomax; Penvir; ***Canad.:*** Famvir; ***Denm.:*** Famvir; ***Fin.:*** Famvir; ***Fr.:*** Oravir; ***Ger.:*** Famvir; ***Gr.:*** Famvir; ***Hong Kong:*** Famvir; ***Irl.:*** Famvir; ***Israel:*** Famvir; ***Ital.:*** Famvir; ***Neth.:*** Famvir; ***NZ:*** Famvir†; ***S.Afr.:*** Famvir; ***Singapore:*** Famvir; ***Spain:*** Ancivin; Famvir; ***Swed.:*** Famvir; ***Switz.:*** Famvir; ***Thai.:*** Famvir; ***UK:*** Famvir; ***USA:*** Famvir.

# Fomivirsen Sodium *(BANM, USAN, rINNM)*

Fomivirseno sódico; Isis-2922.
$C_{204}H_{243}N_{63}Na_{20}O_{114}P_{20}S_{20}$ = 7122.0.
*CAS — 144245-52-3 (fomivirsen); 160369-77-7 (fomivirsen sodium).*
*ATC — S01AD08.*

## Adverse Effects and Precautions

Adverse effects following intra-ocular administration of fomivirsen are confined to the treated eye. They include intra-ocular inflammation, transient increases in intra-ocular pressure, retinal detachment and oedema, and visual abnormalities. Other adverse effects associated with the intravitreal injection procedure include vitreal haemorrhage, endophthalmitis, uveitis, and cataract formation.

Patients should be monitored during treatment for changes in intra-ocular pressure and visual field and for extra-ocular cytomegalovirus disease or disease in the contralateral eye.

## Interactions

In order to reduce the risk of inflammation, intra-ocular administration of fomivirsen is not recommended within 2 to 4 weeks of cidofovir treatment.

## Antiviral Action

Fomivirsen is an antisense oligonucleotide that inhibits human cytomegalovirus replication. It is active against strains of cytomegalovirus resistant to ganciclovir, foscarnet, and cidofovir. Resistance to fomivirsen has been induced *in vitro*, but cross-resistance to antivirals with other modes of action is unlikely.

## Uses and Administration

Fomivirsen is an antisense oligonucleotide that is used as the sodium salt for the local treatment of cytomegalovirus retinitis (p.619) in patients with AIDS. For newly diagnosed disease, a dose of 165 micrograms may be given by intravitreal injection into the affected eye once each week for 3 weeks, then on alternate weeks thereafter. For previously treated disease, 330 micrograms may be injected into the affected eye; this dose is then repeated once after 2 weeks and then once every 4 weeks thereafter.

◊ Reviews.

1. Perry CM, Barman Balfour JA. Fomivirsen. *Drugs* 1999; **57:** 375–80.
2. Geary RS, *et al.* Fomivirsen: clinical pharmacology and potential drug interactions. *Clin Pharmacokinet* 2002; **41:** 255–60.

## Preparations

**Proprietary Preparations** (details are given in Part 3)
***Braz.:*** Vitravene†; ***Denm.:*** Vitravene†; ***Fin.:*** Vitravene†; ***Fr.:*** Vitravene†; ***Ger.:*** Vitravene†; ***Irl.:*** Vitravene†; ***Ital.:*** Vitravene†; ***Swed.:*** Vitravene†; ***Switz.:*** Vitravene; ***UK:*** Vitravene†; ***USA:*** Vitravene.

# Fosamprenavir Calcium *(USAN, rINNM)*

GW-433908G. (3S)-Tetrahydro-3-furyl {(αS)-α-[(1R)-1-hydroxy-2-($N^1$-isobutylsulfanilamido)ethyl]phenethyl}carbamate calcium phosphate (1:1).
$C_{25}H_{36}CaN_3O_9PS$ = 625.7.
*CAS — 226700-79-4 (fosamprenavir); 226700-81-8 (fosamprenavir calcium).*

## Adverse Effects and Precautions

As for Amprenavir, p.628.

## Interactions

Interactions involving HIV-protease inhibitors are discussed under Indinavir Sulfate, p.639. Drugs interacting with amprenavir (p.628) might reasonably also be expected to interact with fosamprenavir.

## Antiviral Action

As for HIV-protease inhibitors in general (see Indinavir Sulfate, p.639). Fosamprenavir itself has little or no antiviral activity but is converted *in vivo* to the active drug amprenavir (p.628).

## Pharmacokinetics

Following oral administration, fosamprenavir is rapidly hydrolysed to amprenavir in the gastrointestinal epithelium as it is absorbed. Peak plasma concentrations of amprenavir are attained 1.5 to 4 hours after administration of fosamprenavir. Fosamprenavir may be given with or without food. For details of the pharmacokinetics of amprenavir, see p.628.

## Uses and Administration

Fosamprenavir is a prodrug of amprenavir, which is a protease inhibitor with antiviral activity against HIV. Fosamprenavir is used with other antiretrovirals for combination therapy of HIV infection (p.621).

Fosamprenavir may be given with or without food. It is given by mouth as the calcium salt, but doses are expressed in terms of the base. Fosamprenavir calcium 748 mg is approximately equivalent to 700 mg of fosamprenavir or to 600 mg of amprenavir. The usual adult dose is 1.4 g twice daily in antiretroviral-naive patients. Doses should be reduced in patients with mild or moderate hepatic impairment (see below). A lower dose of 1.4 g once daily is used when fosamprenavir is given with ritonavir 200 mg once daily; similarly fosamprenavir is given in a dose of 700 mg twice daily when given with ritonavir 100 mg twice daily. The twice daily regimen with ritonavir twice daily is preferred in protease inhibitor-experienced patients.

**Administration in hepatic impairment.** Fosamprenavir should not be used in patients with severe hepatic impairment. A reduced dose of 700 mg twice daily may be used in patients with mild or moderate impairment who are not receiving ritonavir.

## Preparations

**Proprietary Preparations** (details are given in Part 3)
***USA:*** Lexiva.

# Foscarnet Sodium *(BAN, USAN, rINN)*

A-29622; EHB-776 (anhydrous and hexahydrate); Foscarnet sódico; Foscarnetum Natricum Hexahydricum; Phosphonoformate Trisodium; Phosphonoformate Trisodium. Trisodium phosphonatoformate hexahydrate.
$CNa_3O_5P,6H_2O$ = 300.0.
*CAS — 63585-09-1 (foscarnet sodium); 34156-56-4 (foscarnet sodium hexahydrate).*
*ATC — J05AD01.*

**Pharmacopoeias.** In *Eur.* (see p.vi).

**Ph. Eur. 5.0** (Foscarnet Sodium Hexahydrate; Foscarnet Sodium BP 2003). A white or almost white crystalline powder. Soluble in water; practically insoluble in alcohol. A 2% solution in water has a pH of 9.0 to 11.0. Protect from light.

**Incompatibility.** Foscarnet sodium has been found to be visually incompatible with a number of commonly used injectable drugs and the manufacturer also lists incompatibilities with glucose 30% solutions and solutions containing calcium. It is therefore recommended that foscarnet should not be infused via an intravenous line with any other drug.

References.

1. Lor E, Takagi J. Visual compatibility of foscarnet with other injectable drugs. *Am J Hosp Pharm* 1990; **47:** 157–9.
2. Baltz JK, *et al.* Visual compatibility of foscarnet with other injectable drugs during simulated Y-site administration. *Am J Hosp Pharm* 1990; **47:** 2075–7.

## Adverse Effects and Treatment

The most serious common adverse effect of foscarnet sodium is renal impairment, which may be severe. Anaemia may be common and granulocytopenia and thrombocytopenia have been reported. Foscarnet sodium may cause hypocalcaemia and other electrolyte disturbances. Some patients may experience convulsions. Excretion of high concentrations in the urine can cause local irritation and genital ulceration. Other adverse effects reported include nausea, vomiting, diarrhoea, malaise, fatigue, fever, headache, dizziness, paraesthesia, tremor, mood disturbances, rash, abnormal liver function tests, blood pressure and ECG changes, and isolated reports of pancreatitis. Intravenous injection may cause phlebitis at the site of injection.

In cases of overdosage it is important to maintain hydration. Foscarnet elimination may be increased by haemodialysis.

**Effects on the CNS.** Convulsions may occur in up to 10% of AIDS patients receiving foscarnet and have been reported following overdoses. Contributing factors include underlying CNS pathology (HIV-related encephalopathy or other infections) and foscarnet-related electrolyte disturbances. However, seizures have been reported in patients without apparent risk factors.[1]

1. Lor E, Liu YQ. Neurologic sequelae associated with foscarnet therapy. *Ann Pharmacother* 1994; **28:** 1035–7.

**Effects on electrolyte balance.** Foscarnet chelates divalent metal ions and acute hypocalcaemia has been reported to occur in about 15% of patients receiving foscarnet. Other electrolyte disturbances include hypokalaemia and hypomagnesaemia (each in about 15%), hypophosphataemia (8%), and hyperphosphataemia (6%). The incidence of electrolyte disturbances is higher in patients receiving hydration. Hypocalcaemia may cause paraesthesias and, together with hypomagnesaemia and hypokalaemia, may predispose to seizures and cardiovascular disturbances.

**Effects on the kidneys.** The most serious common adverse effect of foscarnet sodium is nephrotoxicity. Clinically significant increases in serum-creatinine concentrations occur in about 30% of patients, and the incidence of nephrotoxicity tends to increase with increasing dose[1] and with duration of therapy.[2] Foscarnet sodium is excreted unchanged in the urine and tubulo-interstitial lesions and deposition of crystals in the glomerular capillary lumen have been implicated.[3] Acute renal failure has occurred and haemodialysis has been reported to have reduced plasma-foscarnet concentrations.[4] The risk of nephrotoxicity can be minimised by ensuring adequate hydration, the use of intermittent dosing schedules,[5] and by adjusting the dose according to serum-creatinine concentrations. Nephrogenic diabetes insipidus and renal tubular acidosis associated with foscarnet have been reported.[6-8]

1. Jacobson MA, *et al.* A dose-ranging study of daily maintenance intravenous foscarnet therapy for cytomegalovirus retinitis in AIDS. *J Infect Dis* 1993; **168:** 444–8.
2. Gaub J, *et al.* The effect of foscarnet (phosphonoformate) on human immunodeficiency virus isolation, T-cell subsets and lymphocyte function in AIDS patients. *AIDS* 1987; **1:** 27–33.
3. Beaufils H, *et al.* Foscarnet and crystals in glomerular capillary lumens. *Lancet* 1990; **336:** 755.
4. Deray G, *et al.* Foscarnet-induced acute renal failure and effectiveness of haemodialysis. *Lancet* 1987; **ii:** 216.
5. Deray G, *et al.* Prevention of foscarnet nephrotoxicity. *Ann Intern Med* 1990; **113:** 332.
6. Farese RV, *et al.* Nephrogenic diabetes insipidus associated with foscarnet treatment of cytomegalovirus retinitis. *Ann Intern Med* 1990; **112:** 955–6.
7. Conn J, *et al.* Nephrogenic diabetes insipidus associated with foscarnet—a case report. *J Antimicrob Chemother* 1996; **37:** 1180–1.
8. Navarro JF, *et al.* Nephrogenic diabetes insipidus and renal tubular acidosis secondary to foscarnet therapy. *Am J Kidney Dis* 1996; **27:** 431–4.

**Effects on the skin and mucous membranes.** A generalised pruritic macular rash was reported in a patient receiving foscarnet which subsided after the drug was withdrawn.[1]

There have been several reports of genital ulceration,[2-7] possibly related to local toxicity arising from high concentrations of foscarnet in the urine. Oral ulceration has occurred, usually in patients also presenting with genital ulceration during foscarnet treatment.[3-5] Uvular and oesophageal ulcerations have also been reported.[4,8]

1. Green ST, *et al.* Generalised cutaneous rash associated with foscarnet usage in AIDS. *J Infect* 1990; **21:** 227–8.
2. Van Der Pijl JW, *et al.* Foscarnet and penile ulceration. *Lancet* 1990; **335:** 286.
3. Gilquin J, *et al.* Genital and oral erosions induced by foscarnet. *Lancet* 1990; **335:** 287.
4. Féguex S, *et al.* Penile ulcerations with foscarnet. *Lancet* 1990; **335:** 547.
5. Moyle G, *et al.* Penile ulcerations with foscarnet. *Lancet* 1990; **335:** 547–8.
6. Lacey HB, *et al.* Vulval ulceration associated with foscarnet. *Genitourin Med* 1992; **68:** 182.
7. Caumes E, *et al.* Foscarnet-induced vulvar erosion. *J Am Acad Dermatol* 1993; **28:** 799.
8. Saint-Marc T, *et al.* Uvula and oesophageal ulcerations with foscarnet. *Lancet* 1992; **340:** 970–1.

## Precautions

Foscarnet sodium should be used with caution in renal impairment and doses should be reduced if serum creatinine is raised. Serum-creatinine concentrations should be measured on alternate days throughout induction treatment; monitoring may be weekly during maintenance therapy. An adequate state of hydration must be maintained during therapy to prevent renal toxicity. Electrolytes, especially calcium and magnesium, should also be monitored and deficiencies corrected before and during foscarnet therapy.

**Electrolyte content.** Each g of foscarnet sodium represents about 15.6 mmol of sodium and about 5.2 mmol of phosphate.

## Interactions

Foscarnet should not be given with other nephrotoxic drugs such as aminoglycosides, amphotericin B, and ciclosporin, or with other drugs that can affect serum-calcium concentrations. Intravenous pentamidine can produce both of these effects and severe additive toxicity may result from its use in combination with foscarnet.

**Ciprofloxacin.** Tonic-clonic seizures associated with foscarnet administration in 2 patients receiving multiple antimicrobial drugs were thought to have been exacerbated by the concurrent administration of ciprofloxacin.[1]

1. Fan-Havard P, *et al.* Concurrent use of foscarnet and ciprofloxacin may increase the propensity for seizures. *Ann Pharmacother* 1994; **28:** 869–72.

## Antiviral Action

Foscarnet inhibits replication of human herpesviruses including cytomegalovirus, herpes simplex virus types 1 and 2, herpesvirus 6, Epstein-Barr virus, and varicella-zoster virus. Activity is also reported against hepatitis B virus and HIV. Foscarnet acts by inhibition of virus-specific DNA polymerases and reverse transcriptases: unlike the nucleoside reverse transcriptase inhibitors and ganciclovir, foscarnet does not require intracellular conversion to an active triphosphate.

◊ References.

1. Balfour HH, *et al.* Effect of foscarnet on quantities of cytomegalovirus and human immunodeficiency virus in blood of persons with AIDS. *Antimicrob Agents Chemother* 1996; **40:** 2721–6.
2. Jabs DA, *et al.* Incidence of foscarnet resistance and cidofovir resistance in patients treated for cytomegalovirus retinitis. *Antimicrob Agents Chemother* 1998; **42:** 2240–4.

## Pharmacokinetics

The pharmacokinetics of foscarnet are complicated by the high incidence of renal impairment during therapy and by the deposition and subsequent gradual release of foscarnet from bone. Thus the estimation of half-life depends upon the duration of foscarnet therapy and the duration of the observation period. The plasma half-life in patients with normal renal function is in the order of 2 to 4 hours, but terminal half-lives in excess of 100 hours have been reported. Plasma protein binding is about 14 to 17%. Foscarnet crosses the blood-brain barrier in variable amounts; CSF concentrations ranging from zero to more than three times the plasma concentration have been reported. Foscarnet is mostly excreted unchanged in the urine.

◊ In 13 HIV-infected male patients with lymphadenopathy or AIDS-related complex[1] foscarnet [sodium] by continuous intravenous infusion (0.14 to 0.19 mg/kg per minute) produced plasma-foscarnet concentrations of about 100 to 500 nanomol/mL. There appeared to be a link between the degree of adverse effects experienced and plasma-foscarnet concentrations above 350 nanomol/mL. Foscarnet was excreted mainly via the kidneys. It was thought that up to 20% of the cumulative intravenous dose may have been deposited in bone 7 days after the end of infusion.

Penetration of foscarnet into the CSF is very variable and in 5 patients[1] CSF concentrations of foscarnet were found to be 13 to 68% of those in the plasma. Subsequent studies showed that CSF concentrations of foscarnet would be virostatic in the majority of patients,[2] attaining a mean concentration of about 25% of plasma concentration following a single infusion[2,3] and 66% under steady state conditions.[3] CSF concentrations ranged from 0 to 340%[2] and 5 to 72%[3] of those in plasma. A correlation between the amount of foscarnet in the CSF and the inflammation of the meninges was found in one of the studies,[2] and with the HIV infection stage in another,[3] but neither reported a correlation with plasma concentration.

Evidence from a study of the effects of probenecid on foscarnet excretion[4] suggested that renal excretion was via glomerular filtration and not tubular excretion.

1. Sjövall J, *et al.* Pharmacokinetics of foscarnet and distribution to cerebrospinal fluid after intravenous infusion in patients with human immunodeficiency virus infection. *Antimicrob Agents Chemother* 1989; **33:** 1023–31.
2. Raffi F, *et al.* Penetration of foscarnet into cerebrospinal fluid of AIDS patients. *Antimicrob Agents Chemother* 1993; **37:** 1777–80.
3. Hengge UR, *et al.* Foscarnet penetrates the blood-brain barrier: rationale for therapy of cytomegalovirus encephalitis. *Antimicrob Agents Chemother* 1993; **37:** 1010–14.
4. Noormohamed FH, *et al.* Renal excretion and pharmacokinetics of foscarnet in HIV sero-positive patients: effect of probenecid pretreatment. *Br J Clin Pharmacol* 1997; **43:** 112–15.

## Uses and Administration

Foscarnet is a non-nucleoside pyrophosphate analogue active against herpesviruses. It is used as the trisodium salt mainly for the treatment of cytomegalovirus retinitis in AIDS patients and for aciclovir-resistant mucocutaneous herpes simplex virus infections in immunocompromised patients.

Foscarnet is given by intravenous infusion. A solution containing foscarnet sodium 24 mg/mL may be administered via a central vein or diluted with glucose 5% or sodium chloride 0.9% to a concentration of 12 mg/mL and administered via a peripheral vein. Hydration with 0.5 to 1 litre of sodium chloride 0.9% or glucose 5% is recommended with each infusion to reduce renal toxicity.

For the treatment of cytomegalovirus retinitis in adults with normal renal function, the usual dose is 60 mg/kg infused over at least 1 hour every 8 hours, or 90 mg/kg infused over 1½ to 2 hours every 12 hours, for 2 to 3 weeks; this should then be followed by maintenance therapy with 60 mg/kg daily, increasing to 90 to 120 mg/kg daily infused over 2 hours if tolerated.

For the treatment of aciclovir-resistant mucocutaneous herpes simplex virus infections in adults with normal renal function, a dose of 40 mg/kg, infused over at least 1 hour every 8 or 12 hours is given for 2 to 3 weeks or until lesions have healed.

Doses of foscarnet should be reduced in patients with renal impairment (see below).

◊ Reviews.

1. Chrisp P, Clissold SP. Foscarnet: a review of its antiviral activity, pharmacokinetic properties and therapeutic use in immunocompromised patients with cytomegalovirus retinitis. *Drugs* 1991; **41:** 104–29.
2. Wagstaff AJ, Bryson HM. Foscarnet: a reappraisal of its antiviral activity, pharmacokinetic properties and therapeutic use in immunocompromised patients with viral infections. *Drugs* 1994; **48:** 199–226.

**Administration in renal impairment.** For patients with renal impairment, the UK manufacturers of foscarnet sodium consider the following doses, based on creatinine clearance (CC), to be equivalent to the 60 mg/kg dose given to patients with normal renal function for the treatment of cytomegalovirus retinitis:

- CC more than 1.6 mL/kg per minute: 60 mg/kg
- CC 1.6 to 1.4 mL/kg per minute: 55 mg/kg
- CC 1.4 to 1.2 mL/kg per minute: 49 mg/kg
- CC 1.2 to 1.0 mL/kg per minute: 42 mg/kg
- CC 1.0 to 0.8 mL/kg per minute: 35 mg/kg
- CC 0.8 to 0.6 mL/kg per minute: 28 mg/kg
- CC 0.6 to 0.4 mL/kg per minute: 21 mg/kg
- CC of less than 0.4 mL/kg per minute: use not recommended

The UK manufacturers also suggest similar proportional reductions of the dose of 40 mg/kg used to treat aciclovir-resistant mucocutaneous herpes simplex infections in patients with normal renal function.

The US manufacturers recommend modification of doses by extending the dose interval in patients with more severe renal impairment, although the total daily doses are reduced proportionally similarly to those in the UK.

**Cytomegalovirus infections.** Foscarnet is used in the treatment of severe cytomegalovirus infections (p.619) in immunocompromised patients. It has been particularly useful instead of ganciclovir in patients with AIDS who require concurrent zidovudine therapy but are unable to tolerate ganciclovir (because of haematological toxicity) and appears to possess similar efficacy (see also under Ganciclovir, p.637). For patients unable to tolerate systemic therapy foscarnet has been tried as an intravitreal injection as an alternative to intravitreal inserts of ganciclovir. Beneficial responses have been reported with intravitreal injections of foscarnet 1.2 mg every 48 hours for 4 doses[1] or 2.4 mg every 72 hours for 6 doses, then once weekly thereafter.[2] Combined treatment with foscarnet and ganciclovir each given intravitreally has also been reported to be effective.[3]

Foscarnet has also been investigated for primary prophylaxis of cytomegalovirus infection in bone marrow transplant recipients at high risk of infection.[4]

1. Lieberman RM, *et al.* Efficacy of intravitreal foscarnet in a patient with AIDS. *N Engl J Med* 1994; **330:** 868–9.
2. Diaz-Llopis M, *et al.* High dose intravitreal foscarnet in the treatment of cytomegalovirus retinitis in AIDS. *Br J Ophthalmol* 1994; **78:** 120–4.
3. Velez G, *et al.* High-dose intravitreal ganciclovir and foscarnet for cytomegalovirus retinitis. *Am J Ophthalmol* 2001; **131:** 396–7.
4. Ippoliti C, *et al.* Foscarnet for prevention of cytomegalovirus infection in allogeneic marrow transplant recipients unable to receive ganciclovir. *Bone Marrow Transplant* 1997; **20:** 491–5.

**Herpes simplex infections.** Although foscarnet is effective in the treatment of herpes simplex infections it is usually reserved for severe mucocutaneous infections, particularly in immunocompromised patients who have failed to respond to aciclovir (see p.620). Topical treatment with a 1% foscarnet cream has also been investigated.[1]

1. Javaly K, *et al.* Treatment of mucocutaneous herpes simplex virus infections unresponsive to acyclovir with topical foscarnet cream in AIDS patients: a phase I/II study. *J Acquir Immune Defic Syndr* 1999; **21:** 301–6.

**Varicella-zoster infections.** Although topical or systemic aciclovir is the usual treatment for ophthalmic herpes zoster (p.621), a study in 20 patients with AIDS suggested that ganciclovir alone or in combination with foscarnet was more effective than aciclovir in terms of preservation of long-term visual acuity.[1] In another study,[2] 10 of 13 HIV-infected patients with aciclovir-resistant herpes zoster had complete healing in response to intravenous foscarnet, although 5 of these 10 experienced relapse within 5 days of cessation of foscarnet therapy. It was suggested that previous treatment with foscarnet in 2 of the 3 patients who experienced treatment failure may have resulted in foscarnet-resistant strains.

1. Moorthy RS, *et al.* Management of varicella zoster virus retinitis in AIDS. *Br J Ophthalmol* 1997; **81:** 189–94.
2. Breton G, *et al.* Acyclovir-resistant herpes zoster in human immunodeficiency virus-infected patients: results of foscarnet therapy. *Clin Infect Dis* 1998; **27:** 1525–7.

## Preparations

***BP 2003:*** Foscarnet Intravenous Infusion.

**Proprietary Preparations** (details are given in Part 3)

***Austral.:*** Foscavir; ***Austria:*** Foscavir; ***Belg.:*** Foscavir; ***Braz.:*** Foscavir; ***Denm.:*** Foscovir†; ***Fin.:*** Foscavir†; ***Fr.:*** Foscavir; ***Ger.:*** Foscavir; Triapten; ***Gr.:*** Foscavir; ***Hong Kong:*** Foscavir†; ***Israel:*** Foscavir; ***Ital.:*** Foscavir; Virudin†; ***Jpn:*** Foscavir; ***Neth.:*** Foscavir; ***Norw.:*** Foscavir; ***Port.:*** Foscavir; ***Spain:*** Foscavir; ***Swed.:*** Foscavir; ***Switz.:*** Foscavir; ***Thai.:*** Foscavir†; ***UK:*** Foscavir; ***USA:*** Foscavir.

# Ganciclovir *(BAN, USAN, rINN)*

BIOLF-62; BN-B759V; BW-759; BWB-759U; BW-759U; DHPG; Dihydroxypropoxymethylguanine; 9-(1,3-Dihydroxy-2-propoxymethyl)guanine; 2′-NDG; 2′-Nor-2′-deoxyguanosine; RS-21592. 9-[2-Hydroxy-1-(hydroxymethyl)ethoxymethyl]guanine.

$C_9H_{13}N_5O_4$ = 255.2.

*CAS — 82410-32-0.*

*ATC — J05AB06; S01AD09.*

**Pharmacopoeias.** In *US.*

**USP 27** (Ganciclovir). A white to off-white crystalline powder. Store at a temperature of 25°, excursions permitted between 15° and 30°.

## Ganciclovir Sodium *(BANM, USAN, rINNM)*

Ganciclovir sódico.

$C_9H_{12}N_5NaO_4$ = 277.2.

*CAS — 107910-75-8.*

*ATC — J05AB06; S01AD09.*

**Incompatibility.** Ganciclovir is reported to be incompatible with foscarnet.

**Stability.** Ganciclovir sodium solution in sodium chloride 0.9% was found[1] to be stable when stored in polypropylene infusion-pump syringes for 12 hours at 25° and for 10 days at 4°. Little variation was found in ganciclovir concentration following storage of a 2% solution at room temperature, 5°, and −8° for 10 to 24 days.[2]

1. Mulye NV, *et al.* Stability of ganciclovir sodium in an infusion-pump syringe. *Am J Hosp Pharm* 1994; **51:** 1348–9.
2. Morlet N, *et al.* High dose intravitreal ganciclovir for CMV retinitis: a shelf life and cost comparison study. *Br J Ophthalmol* 1995; **79:** 753–5.

## Adverse Effects and Treatment

The most common adverse effects of intravenous ganciclovir are haematological and include neutropenia and thrombocytopenia; anaemia also occurs. Neutropenia affects up to 40% of patients receiving ganciclovir intravenously, most commonly starting in the first or second week of ganciclovir treatment. It is usually reversible but may be prolonged or irreversible and can lead to potentially fatal infections. AIDS patients may be at a greater risk of neutropenia than other immunosuppressed patients. Thrombocytopenia occurs in about 20% of patients given ganciclovir intravenously. Those with iatrogenic immunosuppression may be more at risk of developing thrombocytopenia than AIDS patients. Other adverse effects occurring in patients given intravenous ganciclovir include fever, rash, and abnormal liver function tests. Irritation or phlebitis may occur at the site of injection due to the high pH. Less frequent adverse effects reported have included cardiovascular, CNS, gastrointestinal, metabolic, musculoskeletal, respiratory, urogenital, and cutaneous symptoms, and increased serum-creatinine and blood-urea nitrogen concentrations.

The most frequent adverse effects associated with orally administered ganciclovir include neutropenia, thrombocytopenia, anaemia, gastrointestinal disturbances, asthenia, headache, rash, pruritus, fever, abnormal liver function tests, pain, and infection.

Local adverse effects have been associated with the insertion of ocular implants containing ganciclovir.

*Animal* studies have suggested that there may be a risk of adverse testicular effects with temporary or permanent inhibition of spermatogenesis. Female fertility may also be affected. Such studies also suggest that ganciclovir is a potential mutagen, teratogen, and carcinogen.

Haemodialysis and hydration may be useful in reducing plasma concentrations of ganciclovir. Haematological adverse effects may be reversed in some patients by stopping treatment or reducing dosage; blood cell counts should return to normal within 3 to 7 days.

Colony-stimulating factors have been given with ganciclovir to limit its haematological toxicity.

**Effects on the blood.** Ganciclovir-induced neutropenia was successfully treated in a patient with cytomegalovirus retinitis and bone-marrow suppression by intravenous administration of *molgramostim* 5 micrograms/kg.[1] In a multicentre, randomised placebo-controlled trial[2] in 69 AIDS patients with cytomegalovirus infection who developed neutropenia from ganciclovir therapy, *lenograstim* given in a dose of 50 micrograms/m$^2$ subcutaneously yielded similarly positive results.

1. Russo CL, *et al.* Treatment of neutropenia associated with dyskeratosis congenita with granulocyte-macrophage colony-stimulating factor. *Lancet* 1990; **336:** 751–2.
2. Dubreuil-Lemaire M-L, *et al.* Lenograstim for the treatment of neutropenia in patients receiving ganciclovir for cytomegalovirus infection: a randomised, placebo-controlled trial in AIDS patients. *Eur J Haematol* 2000; **65:** 337–43.

**Effects on mental function.** Psychosis was associated with ganciclovir administration in a patient on 2 occasions.[1]

1. Hansen BA, *et al.* Ganciclovir-induced psychosis. *N Engl J Med* 1996; **335:** 1397.

## Precautions

Ganciclovir should be used with caution in patients with renal impairment and doses should be adjusted according to the serum-creatinine concentration (see Administration in Renal Impairment under Uses and Administration, below). It should not be given by rapid or bolus injection and adequate hydration should be maintained during intravenous infusion. It should be given with caution to patients with low blood counts or with a history of cytopenic reactions to drugs. Monitoring of white blood cell and platelet counts should be performed every 2 days or daily during the first 14 days of intravenous therapy and once weekly thereafter; ganciclovir should be withdrawn if the neutrophil count falls below 500 cells/microlitre or the platelet count falls below 25 000 cells/microlitre. Patients receiving oral ganciclovir should also be monitored regularly.

Ganciclovir is contra-indicated in pregnancy; contraception is recommended during ganciclovir treatment and, additionally for men, for 90 days thereafter. Adverse effects have been observed in the offspring of lactating animals.

Because of the risk of carcinogenicity and the high pH of the solution, contact with the skin and eyes should be avoided during the reconstitution of ganciclovir sodium injection.

**Sodium content.** Each g of ganciclovir sodium represents about 2.8 mmol of sodium.

## Interactions

Zidovudine given with ganciclovir may have an additive neutropenic effect and should not be given during intravenous ganciclovir induction therapy, although it has been given with caution during oral maintenance therapy. Probenecid and other drugs that inhibit renal tubular secretion and resorption may reduce the renal clearance of ganciclovir, and so increase its serum concentrations. Administration of intravenous ganciclovir with oral mycophenolate mofetil may result in increased plasma concentrations of both drugs due to competition for renal tubular secretion. Drugs that inhibit rapid cell division such as myelosuppressants may have additive toxic effects if given with ganciclovir. Convulsions have been reported when ganciclovir was given with imipenem and cilastatin.

**Antivirals.** An additive neutropenic effect may occur if ganciclovir is given with *zidovudine* (see Zidovudine, p.660), and there are reports of increased plasma concentrations of *didanosine* when given with ganciclovir (see p.631). There has also been a report[1] of decreased blood concentrations of ganciclovir when didanosine (200 mg every 12 hours) was given 2 hours before ganciclovir (1 g every 8 hours orally) but not when the two drugs were given at the same time. However, a later study[2] using twice the dose of ganciclovir found no effect irrespective of whether ganciclovir was administered 2 hours before or 2 hours after didanosine. The UK manufacturer also reports that decreased blood concentrations of ganciclovir have occurred when it is given orally 2 hours before didanosine.

When ganciclovir was given with *zalcitabine*, a 22% increase in the area under the concentration-time curve for ganciclovir was noted although it was believed that this did not necessitate any dosage modification.[3] No pharmacokinetic changes were reported when ganciclovir was given with *stavudine*.[3]

1. Cimoch PJ, *et al.* Pharmacokinetics of oral ganciclovir alone and in combination with zidovudine, didanosine, and probenecid in HIV-infected subjects. *J Acquir Immune Defic Syndr Hum Retrovirol* 1998; **17;** 227–34.
2. Jung D, *et al.* Effect of high-dose oral ganciclovir on didanosine disposition in human immunodeficiency virus (HIV)-positive patients. *J Clin Pharmacol* 1998; **38:** 1057–62.
3. Jung D, *et al.* The pharmacokinetics and safety profile of oral ganciclovir combined with zalcitabine or stavudine in asymptomatic HIV- and CMV-seropositive patients. *J Clin Pharmacol* 1999; **39:** 505–12.

**Ciclosporin.** Reversible acute unilateral or bilateral eye movement disorders typical of sixth cranial nerve palsies[1] occurred in 4 patients who received ciclosporin and ganciclovir following bone marrow transplantation.

1. Openshaw H, *et al.* Eye movement disorders in bone marrow transplant patients on cyclosporin and ganciclovir. *Bone Marrow Transpl* 1997; **19:** 503–5.

## Antiviral Action

Ganciclovir inhibits replication of human herpesviruses *in vivo* and *in vitro*. It is active against cytomegalovirus, herpes simplex virus types 1 and 2, Epstein-Barr virus, varicella-zoster virus, and herpesvirus 6. This activity is due to intracellular conversion of ganciclovir by viral thymidine kinase (in herpes simplex and varicella-zoster infected cells) or possibly by cellular deoxyguanosine kinase (in Epstein-Barr infected cells) to ganciclovir monophosphate with subsequent cellular conversion to the diphosphate and the active triphosphate. Ganciclovir triphosphate inhibits viral DNA synthesis by inhibiting the viral DNA polymerase enzyme as well as being incorporated into the viral DNA. This process is selective for infected cells; the concentration of ganciclovir triphosphate may be up to a hundredfold higher in cytomegalovirus-infected cells than in uninfected cells.

Ganciclovir has a similar spectrum of activity to aciclovir, herpes simplex virus types 1 and 2 being the most susceptible of the herpesviruses. However, cytomegalovirus is much more susceptible to ganciclovir than aciclovir.

## Resistance

Resistance to ganciclovir has been demonstrated *in vitro* in herpes simplex viruses, varicella-zoster virus, and cytomegalovirus. Possible mechanisms of resistance include a reduction in the phosphorylation of ganciclovir to the active form and reduced sensitivity of viral DNA polymerase. Resistance has been reported in cytomegalovirus strains isolated from patients receiving ganciclovir for prolonged periods and in those with an initially high viral load. It has also been observed in AIDS patients with cytomegalovirus retinitis who have never previously received the drug. Cross-resistance with cidofovir is common.

◊ The development of cytomegalovirus resistance to ganciclovir may be a factor in disease progression in patients receiving prolonged therapy with ganciclovir and the incidence of resistance is reported to increase with duration of therapy.[1] A ganciclovir-resistant isolate of cytomegalovirus has been detected in about 30% of 95 patients after 9 months of treatment and correlated with development of dissemination of infection to the contralateral eye.[2]

Ganciclovir-resistant cytomegalovirus has been reported[3] to be an important cause of late morbidity in seronegative patients who received cytomegalovirus-seropositive organ transplants; in one study,[4] 5 of 67 seronegative recipients developed ganciclovir-resistant cytomegalovirus disease compared with none of 173 seropositive subjects.

1. Drew WL. Cytomegalovirus resistance to antiviral therapies. *Am J Health-Syst Pharm* 1996; **53** (suppl 2): S17–S23.
2. Jabs DA, *et al.* Cytomegalovirus retinitis and viral resistance: ganciclovir resistance. *J Infect Dis* 1998; **177:** 770–3.
3. Limaye AP. Ganciclovir-resistant cytomegalovirus in organ transplant recipients. *Clin Infect Dis* 2002; **35:** 866–72.
4. Limaye AP, *et al.* Emergence of ganciclovir-resistant cytomegalovirus disease among recipients of solid-organ transplants. *Lancet* 2000; **356:** 645–9.

## Pharmacokinetics

Ganciclovir is poorly absorbed from the gastrointestinal tract following oral administration and there is minimal systemic absorption after intravitreal injection. Bioavailability of oral ganciclovir is about 5%, and is increased by intake with food to 6 to 9%. Following intravenous administration as ganciclovir sodium it is widely distributed to body tissues and fluids including intra-ocular fluid and CSF. Binding to plasma proteins is reported to be 1 to 2%. Ganciclovir is excreted unchanged in the urine mainly by glomerular filtration and also active tubular secretion. The half-life is about 2.5 to 4.5 hours in patients with normal renal function following intravenous administration and about 4 to 5.7 hours after oral administration. In patients with renal impairment, the renal clearance decreases and the half-life increases; a half-life of 28.5 hours has been reported when the serum-creatinine concentration was greater than 398 micromol/litre.

Haemodialysis has been reported to reduce plasma-ganciclovir concentrations by about 50%.

◊ References.

1. Arevalo JF, *et al.* Intravitreous and plasma concentrations of ganciclovir and foscarnet after intravenous therapy in patients with AIDS and cytomegalovirus retinitis. *J Infect Dis* 1995; **172:** 951–6.
2. Morlet N, *et al.* High dose intravitreal ganciclovir injection provides a prolonged therapeutic intraocular concentration. *Br J Ophthalmol* 1996; **80:** 214–16.
3. Lavelle J, *et al.* Effect of food on the relative bioavailability of oral ganciclovir. *J Clin Pharmacol* 1996; **36:** 238–41.
4. Zhou X-J, *et al.* Population pharmacokinetics of ganciclovir in newborns with congenital cytomegalovirus infection. *Antimicrob Agents Chemother* 1996; **40:** 2202–5.
5. Giffy KG. Pharmacokinetics of oral ganciclovir capsules in HIV-infected persons. *AIDS* 1996; **10** (suppl 4): S3–S6.
6. Jung D, *et al.* Steady-state relative bioavailability of three oral ganciclovir dosage regimens delivering 6,000 mg/day in patients with human immunodeficiency virus. *J Clin Pharmacol* 1998; **38:** 1021–4.
7. Jung D, *et al.* Absolute bioavailability and dose proportionality of oral ganciclovir after ascending multiple doses in human immunodeficiency virus (HIV)-positive patients. *J Clin Pharmacol* 1998; **38:** 1122–8.
8. Jung D, *et al.* Effect of food on high-dose oral ganciclovir disposition in HIV-positive subjects. *J Clin Pharmacol* 1999; **39:** 161–5.
9. Snell GI, *et al.* Pharmacokinetic assessment of oral ganciclovir in lung transplant recipients with cystic fibrosis. *J Antimicrob Chemother* 2000; **45:** 511–16.

## Uses and Administration

Ganciclovir is a synthetic nucleoside analogue of guanine closely related to aciclovir, but has greater activity against cytomegalovirus. It is used for the treatment and suppression of life-threatening or sight-threatening cytomegalovirus infections in immunocompromised patients, including those with AIDS and those with iatrogenic immunosuppression associated with organ transplantation or chemotherapy of neoplastic disease. It has also been used for superficial ocular herpes simplex infections.

Ganciclovir is administered by intravenous infusion as the sodium salt but doses are expressed in terms of ganciclovir; 54.3 mg of ganciclovir sodium is approximately equivalent to 50 mg of ganciclovir. Solutions for infusion are usually prepared to give a concentration of 50 mg of ganciclovir per mL, then further diluted to contain not more than 10 mg/mL. An intravenous solution is given over 1 hour. Ganciclovir may alternatively be given by mouth.

In **cytomegalovirus infections**, the usual *initial* dose for *treatment* is 5 mg/kg by intravenous infusion every 12 hours for 14 to 21 days. This induction period may be followed by *maintenance* therapy to prevent recurrence or progression of the disease. The usual maintenance dosage is 5 mg/kg by intravenous infusion as a single daily dose for 7 days each week or 6 mg/kg daily for 5 days each week. If retinitis recurs or progresses a further induction course of ganciclovir may be given. AIDS patients who have received initial treatment with intravenous ganciclovir, and who have stable cytomegalovirus retinitis following at least 3 weeks of intravenous therapy, may be given ganciclovir by mouth in a dose of 3 g daily in 3 or 6 divided doses, with food.

For *prevention* of cytomegalovirus infection in immunocompromised patients, specifically those receiving immunosuppressive therapy following organ transplantation, ganciclovir may be given in an *initial* dose of 5 mg/kg by intravenous infusion every 12 hours for 7 to 14 days, followed by intravenous *maintenance* therapy as above. Ganciclovir prophylaxis may be given orally in a dose of 1 g three times daily with food to immunocompromised patients including those with advanced HIV infection.

Doses of ganciclovir should be reduced in renal impairment (see below).

Intravitreal implants providing controlled release of ganciclovir are available for those patients with cytomegalovirus retinitis who are unable to tolerate systemic therapy; the implants are designed to release ganciclovir over a period of 5 to 8 months.

Ganciclovir is used as a topical ophthalmic 0.15% gel for the treatment of superficial ocular **herpes simplex infections**.

◊ General references.


1. Faulds D, Heel RC. Ganciclovir: a review of its antiviral activity, pharmacokinetic properties and therapeutic efficacy in cytomegalovirus infections. *Drugs* 1990; **39:** 597–638.
2. Markham A, Faulds D. Ganciclovir: an update of its therapeutic use in cytomegalovirus infection. *Drugs* 1994; **48:** 455–84.
3. Crumpacker CS. Ganciclovir. *N Engl J Med* 1996; **335:** 721–9.
4. McGavin JK, Goa KL. Ganciclovir: an update of its use in the prevention of cytomegalovirus infection and disease in transplant recipients. *Drugs* 2001; **61:** 1153–83.


**Administration in renal impairment.** Doses of ganciclovir should be reduced in renal impairment. This may be done by reducing the dose and/or increasing the dosage interval according to creatinine clearance (CC). The following doses have been recommended by the manufacturers:

*intravenous* administration:

- CC 70 mL/minute or more: 5 mg/kg every 12 hours for induction, followed by 5 mg/kg every 24 hours for maintenance
- CC 50 to 69 mL/minute: 2.5 mg/kg every 12 hours for induction, 2.5 mg/kg every 24 hours for maintenance
- CC 25 to 49 mL/minute: 2.5 mg/kg every 24 hours for induction, 1.25 mg/kg every 24 hours for maintenance
- CC 10 to 24 mL/minute: 1.25 mg/kg every 24 hours for induction, 0.625 mg/kg every 24 hours for maintenance
- dialysis patients, on days when dialysis is performed 1.25 mg/kg for induction, or 0.625 mg/kg for maintenance, in each case given shortly after the end of dialysis (in the USA, a maximum of 3 doses each week is recommended)

*oral* administration:

- CC of 70 mL/minute or more: 3000 mg daily in 3 or 6 divided doses
- CC 50 to 69 mL/minute: 1500 mg daily
- CC 25 to 49 mL/minute: 1000 mg daily
- CC 10 to 24 mL/minute: 500 mg daily
- CC less than 10 mL/minute: 500 mg three times a week, following haemodialysis.

**Cytomegalovirus infections.** Ganciclovir is used in both the treatment and prophylaxis of cytomegalovirus infections (p.619) in immunocompromised patients.

As with other herpesvirus infections, antiviral treatment tends to be suppressive rather than curative, and long-term maintenance therapy is necessary. Treatment in patients with AIDS is complicated by the additive haematological toxicity of ganciclovir and zidovudine. Clinical studies comparing ganciclovir with foscarnet for AIDS-related cytomegalovirus retinopathy have shown higher mortality rates in patients receiving ganciclovir than in those receiving foscarnet,[1,2] leading to the suggestion that foscarnet may possess intrinsic antiretroviral activity. However, an alternative explanation is that fewer patients receiving ganciclovir could tolerate full doses of zidovudine and were thus receiving suboptimal therapy. If it is possible to overcome the drug-induced neutropenia by giving colony-stimulating factors (thus enabling the use of full therapeutic doses of zidovudine), ganciclovir may remain the preferred treatment for cytomegalovirus retinitis, since foscarnet is less well tolerated. The use of ganciclovir with cytomegalovirus immunoglobulins[3,4] or normal immunoglobulins,[5] or with foscarnet[6,7] has been reported to improve both efficacy and tolerance. An alternative is the use of intravitreal controlled-release ganciclovir implants[8-10] to avoid systemic adverse effects. Intravitreal ganciclovir in combination with intravitreal foscarnet has been reported to be effective.[11] Another development has been the introduction of oral preparations of ganciclovir for maintenance therapy. Oral ganciclovir may be a useful adjunct to prevent systemic infection in patients treated with the intravitreal implants.[12] The use of oral ganciclovir in high doses has been investigated;[13] daily doses of up to 6 g have been reported to be of benefit, although a conclusive comparison with standard intravenous doses could not be made. Cytomegalovirus infections at other sites in AIDS patients, including gastrointestinal and pulmonary infections, respond less well to ganciclovir than does retinitis.

Ganciclovir is also valuable for prophylaxis and early treatment of cytomegalovirus infections in transplant recipients.[7,14-20] For established infections, ganciclovir is reported to be more effective in solid organ transplant recipients than in bone marrow transplant recipients. Ganciclovir has also been tried for prevention of cytomegalovirus infection in patients with AIDS, although results are conflicting.[21,22]

Treatment of congenital infections has a generally poor outcome. Prolonged treatment periods may improve the response, but the safety of extended treatment with ganciclovir in this age group has not been fully evaluated and there is a need for further randomised controlled studies.[23] There is some recent evidence[24] that a 6-week treatment course started in neonates with clinically apparent disease affecting the CNS prevents hearing deterioration at 6 months and may also prevent deterioration at or beyond 1 year of age.


1. Studies of Ocular Complications of AIDS Research Group, in Collaboration with the AIDS Clinical Trials Group. Mortality in patients with the acquired immunodeficiency syndrome treated with either foscarnet or ganciclovir for cytomegalovirus retinitis. *N Engl J Med* 1992; **326:** 213–20.
2. Polis MA, *et al.* Increased survival of a cohort of patients with acquired immunodeficiency syndrome and cytomegalovirus retinitis who received sodium phosphonoformate (foscarnet). *Am J Med* 1993; **94:** 175–80.
3. D'Alessandro AM, *et al.* Successful treatment of severe cytomegalovirus infections with ganciclovir and CMV hyperimmune globulin in liver transplant recipients. *Transplant Proc* 1989; **21:** 3560–1.
4. Salmela K, *et al.* Ganciclovir in the treatment of severe cytomegalovirus disease in liver transplant patients. *Transplant Proc* 1990; **22:** 238–40.
5. Emanuel D, *et al.* Cytomegalovirus pneumonia after bone marrow transplantation successfully treated with the combination of ganciclovir and high-dose intravenous immune globulin. *Ann Intern Med* 1988; **109:** 777–82.
6. Studies of Ocular Complications of AIDS Research Group, in Collaboration with the AIDS Clinical Trials Group. Combination foscarnet and ganciclovir therapy vs monotherapy for the treatment of relapsed cytomegalovirus retinitis in patients with AIDS: the Cytomegalovirus Retreatment Trial. *Arch Ophthalmol* 1996; **114:** 23–33.
7. Mylonakis E, *et al.* Combination antiviral therapy for ganciclovir-resistant cytomegalovirus infection in solid-organ transplant recipients. *Clin Infect Dis* 2002; **34:** 1337–41.
8. Anand R, *et al.* Control of cytomegalovirus retinitis using sustained release of intraocular gancyclovir. *Arch Ophthalmol* 1993; **111:** 223–7.
9. Martin DF, *et al.* Treatment of cytomegalovirus retinitis with an intraocular sustained-release ganciclovir implant: a randomized controlled clinical trial. *Arch Ophthalmol* 1994; **112:** 1531–9.
10. Musch DC, *et al.* Treatment of cytomegalovirus retinitis with a sustained-release ganciclovir implant. *N Engl J Med* 1997; **337:** 83–90.
11. Velez G, *et al.* High-dose intravitreal ganciclovir and foscarnet for cytomegalovirus retinitis. *Am J Ophthalmol* 2001; **131:** 396–7.
12. Martin DF, *et al.* Oral ganciclovir for patients with cytomegalovirus retinitis treated with a ganciclovir implant. *N Engl J Med* 1999; **340:** 1063–70.
13. Lalezari JP, *et al.* High dose oral ganciclovir treatment for cytomegalovirus retinitis. *J Clin Virol* 2002; **24:** 67–77.
14. Goodrich JM, *et al.* Ganciclovir prophylaxis to prevent cytomegalovirus disease after allogeneic marrow transplant. *Ann Intern Med* 1993; **118:** 173–8.
15. Winston DJ, *et al.* Ganciclovir prophylaxis of cytomegalovirus infection and disease in allogeneic bone marrow transplant recipients. *Ann Intern Med* 1993; **118:** 179–84.
16. Hibberd PL, *et al.* Preemptive ganciclovir therapy to prevent cytomegalovirus disease in cytomegalovirus antibody-positive renal transplant recipients: a randomized controlled trial. *Ann Intern Med* 1995; **123:** 18–26.
17. Winston DJ, *et al.* Randomised comparison of ganciclovir and high-dose acyclovir for long-term cytomegalovirus prophylaxis in liver-transplant recipients. *Lancet* 1995; **346:** 69–74.
18. Gane E, *et al.* Randomised trial of efficacy and safety of oral ganciclovir in the prevention of cytomegalovirus disease in liver-transplant recipients. *Lancet* 1997; **350:** 1729–33.
19. Singh N. Preemptive therapy versus universal prophylaxis with ganciclovir for cytomegalovirus in solid organ transplant recipients. *Clin Infect Dis* 2001; **32:** 742–51.
20. Paya CV, *et al.* Preemptive use of oral ganciclovir to prevent cytomegalovirus infection in liver transplant patients: a randomized, placebo-controlled trial. *J Infect Dis* 2002; **185:** 854–60.
21. McCarthy M. Oral ganciclovir fails to prevent CMV in HIV trial. *Lancet* 1995; **346:** 895.
22. Spector SA, *et al.* Oral ganciclovir for the prevention of cytomegalovirus disease in persons with AIDS. *N Engl J Med* 1996; **334:** 1491–7.
23. Michaels MG, *et al.* Treatment of children with congenital cytomegalovirus infection with ganciclovir. *Pediatr Infect Dis J* 2003; **22:** 504–8.
24. Kimberlin DW, *et al.* Effect of ganciclovir therapy on hearing in symptomatic congenital cytomegalovirus disease involving the central nervous system: a randomized, controlled trial. *J Pediatr* 2003; **143:** 16–25.


**Epstein-Barr virus infections.** There have been anecdotal reports[1,2] of some improvement in patients with Epstein-Barr virus (EBV) infection given ganciclovir, although no antiviral therapy is entirely satisfactory (p.620).


1. Pirsch JD, *et al.* Treatment of severe Epstein-Barr virus-induced lymphoproliferative syndrome with ganciclovir: two cases after solid organ transplantation. *Am J Med* 1989; **86:** 241–4.
2. Ishida Y, *et al.* Ganciclovir for chronic active Epstein-Barr virus infection. *Lancet* 1993; **341:** 560–1.


**Herpesvirus infections.** In patients with herpes simplex keratitis, ganciclovir 0.15% gel was reported to be as effective as aciclovir 3% ointment,[1] the drug most commonly used in this infection (see Ocular Herpes Simplex Infections, p.620).

Ganciclovir was also reported to produce beneficial responses in AIDS patients with ocular varicella zoster infections.[2]


1. Hoh HB, *et al.* Randomised trial of ganciclovir and acyclovir in the treatment of herpes simplex dendritic keratitis: a multicentre study. *Br J Ophthalmol* 1996; **80:** 140–3.
2. Moorthy RS, *et al.* Management of varicella zoster virus retinitis in AIDS. *Br J Ophthalmol* 1997; **81:** 189–94.


### Preparations

**USP 27:** Ganciclovir for Injection.

**Proprietary Preparations** (details are given in Part 3)

***Arg.:*** Ciganclor; Cymevene; Cytovene; Gasmilen; Grinevel; Virgan; ***Austral.:*** Cymevene; Vitrasert; ***Austria:*** Cymevene; ***Belg.:*** Cymevene; ***Braz.:*** Cymevene; Ganvirt†; Ganvirax; ***Canad.:*** Cytovene; ***Chile:*** Cymevene; ***Denm.:*** Cymevene; ***Fin.:*** Cymevene; ***Fr.:*** Cymevan; Virgan; ***Ger.:*** Cymeven; ***Gr.:*** Cymevene; ***Hong Kong:*** Cymevene; ***Irl.:*** Cymevene; ***Israel:*** Cymevene; ***Ital.:*** Citovirax; Cymevene; ***Mex.:*** Cymevene; ***Neth.:*** Cymevene; ***Norw.:*** Cymevene; ***NZ:*** Cymevene; ***Port.:*** Cymevene; ***S.Afr.:*** Cymevene; ***Singapore:*** Cymevene; ***Spain:*** Cymevene; ***Swed.:*** Cymevene; ***Switz.:*** Cymevene; ***Thai.:*** Cymevene; ***UK:*** Cymevene; Virgan; Vitrasert†; ***USA:*** Cytovene; Vitrasert.

## Ibacitabine *(rINN)*

Ibacitabina; Iododesoxycytidine. 2′-Deoxy-5-iodocytidine.

$C_9H_{12}IN_3O_4$ = 353.1.

*CAS — 611-53-0.*

*ATC — D06BB08.*

### Profile

Ibacitabine is an antiviral used topically as a 1% gel in the treatment of herpes labialis (p.620).

### Preparations

**Proprietary Preparations** (details are given in Part 3)

***Fr.:*** Cuterpes; ***Hong Kong:*** Cuterpes†; ***Ital.:*** Herpes-Gel†.

## Idoxuridine *(BAN, USAN, rINN)*

Allergan 211; GF-I115; Idoxuridina; Idoxuridinum; IDU; 5-IDUR; 5-IUDR; NSC-39661; SKF-14287. 2′-Deoxy-5-iodouridine.

$C_9H_{11}IN_2O_5$ = 354.1.

*CAS — 54-42-2.*

*ATC — D06BB01; J05AB02; S01AD01.*

**Pharmacopoeias.** In *Chin., Eur.* (see p.vi), *Int., Jpn,* and *US.*

**Ph. Eur. 5.0** (Idoxuridine). A white or almost white crystalline powder. M.p. about 180°, with decomposition. Slightly soluble in water and in alcohol; dissolves in dilute solutions of alkali hydroxides. A 0.1% solution in water has a pH of 5.5 to 6.5. Protect from light.

**USP 27** (Idoxuridine). A white, practically odourless, crystalline powder. Slightly soluble in water and in alcohol; practically insoluble in chloroform and in ether. Store in airtight containers. Protect from light.

**Stability.** Iodine vapour is liberated on heating idoxuridine. It has been reported that some decomposition products such as iodouracil are more toxic than idoxuridine and reduce its antiviral activity.

### Adverse Effects

Adverse effects that occur occasionally when idoxuridine is applied to the eyes include irritation, pain, stinging, conjunctivitis, oedema and inflammation of the eye or eyelids, photophobia, pruritus, and rarely, occlusion of the lachrymal duct. Hypersensitivity reactions may occur rarely. Prolonged use may damage the cornea. Taste disturbance may occur.

Idoxuridine applied to the skin may produce irritation, stinging, and hypersensitivity reactions. Excessive application of topical idoxuridine to the eyes or skin may cause punctate defects in the cornea or skin maceration.

Adverse effects after intravenous administration of idoxuridine have included bone-marrow depression and liver damage.

Idoxuridine is a potential carcinogen and teratogen.

**Carcinogenicity.** Squamous carcinoma in a patient was associated with topical idoxuridine treatment.[1] Reference is made to an earlier similar case.


1. Koppang HS, Aas E. Squamous carcinoma induced by topical idoxuridine therapy? *Br J Dermatol* 1983; **108:** 501–3.


### Precautions

Idoxuridine should be used with caution in conditions where there is deep ulceration involving the stromal layers of the cornea, as delayed healing has resulted in corneal perforation. Prolonged topical use should be avoided.

The potential teratogenicity of idoxuridine should be taken into account when treating pregnant patients or patients likely to become pregnant. Corticosteroids should be applied with caution in patients also receiving idoxuridine as they may accelerate the spread of viral infection. Preparations containing boric acid should not be applied to the eye in patients also receiving ocular preparations of idoxuridine as irritation ensues.

### Antiviral Action

Following intracellular phosphorylation to the triphosphate, idoxuridine is incorporated into viral DNA instead of thymidine so inhibiting replication of the virus. Idoxuridine is also incorporated into mammalian DNA. Idoxuridine is active against herpes simplex and varicella zoster viruses. It has also been shown to inhibit vaccinia virus, cytomegalovirus, and adenovirus.

Resistance to idoxuridine occurs *in vitro* and *in vivo*.

### Pharmacokinetics

Penetration of idoxuridine into the cornea and skin is reported to be poor. Following systemic administration idoxuridine is rapidly metabolised to iodouracil, uracil, and iodide, which are excreted in the urine.

### Uses and Administration

Idoxuridine is a pyrimidine nucleoside structurally related to thymidine. It has been used topically in the treatment of herpes simplex keratitis and cutaneous forms of herpes simplex (p.620) and herpes zoster (p.621), but has generally been superseded by other antivirals.

In the treatment of herpes simplex keratitis, idoxuridine has been applied as a 0.1% ophthalmic solution.

Idoxuridine 5% in dimethyl sulfoxide (to aid absorption) can be painted onto the lesions of cutaneous herpes simplex and herpes zoster four times daily for 4 days.

### Preparations

***BP 2003:*** Idoxuridine Eye Drops;
***USP 27:*** Idoxuridine Ophthalmic Ointment; Idoxuridine Ophthalmic Solution.

**Proprietary Preparations** (details are given in Part 3)
***Arg.:*** Idulea; ***Austral.:*** Herplex-D†; Stoxil; ***Belg.:*** Virexen; ***Braz.:*** Herpesine; ***Canad.:*** Herplex; ***Fr.:*** Iduviran†; ***Ger.:*** Iducutit†; Ophtal†; Virunguent; Zostrum; ***Hong Kong:*** Herpidu†; Herplex†; Oftalmolosa Cusi Virucida†; Stoxil†; ***India:*** Ridinox; ***Irl.:*** Zostrum; ***Israel:*** Virusan; ***Ital.:*** Iducher; Iduridin†; Idustatin; ***Malaysia:*** Virunguent; ***Mex.:*** Idina; ***Norw.:*** Iduridin†; ***NZ:*** Virasolve; ***Port.:*** Virexen; Virunguent; ***Singapore:*** Stoxil†; Virunguent; ***Spain:*** Antizona†; Virexen; ***Switz.:*** Iderpes; Virexen†; Virunguent; ***Thai.:*** Herpidu†; ***UK:*** Herpid.

**Multi-ingredient:** ***Austral.:*** Virasolve; ***Ger.:*** Virunguent P; ***Hong Kong:*** Virasolve; ***Ital.:*** Iducol†; Idustatin†.

## Imiquimod *(BAN, USAN, rINN)*

R-837; S-26308. 4-Amino-1-isobutyl-1*H*-imidazo[4,5-*c*]quinoline.

$C_{14}H_{16}N_4$ = 240.3.
*CAS — 99011-02-6.*
*ATC — D06BB10.*

### Adverse Effects

Adverse effects following topical application of imiquimod include local skin erosion, erythema, excoriation, flaking, and oedema. There have been reports of localised hypopigmentation and hyperpigmentation. Skin reactions away from the site of application have been reported. Systemic effects following topical application include headache, flu-like symptoms, and myalgia.

Hypotension has occurred after repeated ingestion.

### Uses and Administration

Imiquimod is an immune response modifier used topically in the treatment of external genital and perianal warts. It is applied as a 5% cream three times each week for up to 16 weeks and is left on the skin for 6 to 10 hours.

Imiquimod is being investigated for the treatment of basal cell and squamous cell carcinoma.

◊ Reviews.


1. Perry CM, Lamb HM. Topical imiquimod: a review of its use in genital warts. *Drugs* 1999; **58:** 375–90.
2. Tyring S, *et al.* Imiquimod; an international update on therapeutic uses in dermatology. *Int J Dermatol* 2002; **41:** 810–16.
3. Garland SM. Imiquimod. *Curr Opin Infect Dis* 2003; **16:** 85–9.


**Basal cell and squamous cell carcinoma.** Imiquimod is under investigation and has been found to be of benefit in the treatment of actinic keratosis,[1,2] Bowen's disease,[3] and basal cell carcinoma.[4-10]


1. Stockfleth E, *et al.* Successful treatment of actinic keratosis with imiquimod cream 5%: a report of six cases. *Br J Dermatol* 2001; **144:** 1050–3.
2. Persaud AN, *et al.* Clinical effect of imiquimod 5% cream in the treatment of actinic keratosis. *J Am Acad Dermatol* 2002; **47:** 553–6.
3. Mackenzie-Wood A, *et al.* Imiquimod 5% cream in the treatment of Bowen's disease. *J Am Acad Dermatol* 2001; **44:** 462–70.
4. Beutner KR, *et al.* Therapeutic response of basal cell carcinoma to the immune response modifier imiquimod 5% cream. *J Am Acad Dermatol* 1999; **41:** 1002–7.
5. Marks R, *et al.* Imiquimod 5% cream in the treatment of superficial basal cell carcinoma: results of a multicenter 6-week dose-response trial. *J Am Acad Dermatol* 2001; **44:** 807–13.
6. Chen TM, *et al.* Treatment of a large superficial basal cell carcinoma with 5% imiquimod: a case report and review of the literature. *Dermatol Surg* 2002; **28:** 344–6.
7. Drehs MM, *et al.* Successful treatment of multiple superficial basal cell carcinomas with topical imiquimod: case report and review of the literature. *Dermatol Surg* 2002; **28:** 427–9.
8. Geisse JK, *et al.* Imiquimod 5% cream for the treatment of superficial basal cell carcinoma: a double-blind, randomized, vehicle-controlled study. *J Am Acad Dermatol* 2002; **47:** 390–8.
9. Sterry W, *et al.* Imiquimod 5% cream for the treatment of superficial and nodular basal cell carcinoma: randomized studies comparing low-frequency dosing with and without occlusion. *Br J Dermatol* 2002; **147:** 1227–36.
10. Stockfleth E, *et al.* Successful treatment of basal cell carcinomas in a nevoid basal cell carcinoma syndrome with topical 5% imiquimod. *Eur J Dermatol* 2002; **12:** 569–72.


### Preparations

**Proprietary Preparations** (details are given in Part 3)
***Arg.:*** Aldara; ***Austral.:*** Aldara; ***Belg.:*** Aldara; ***Canad.:*** Aldara; ***Chile:*** Aldara; ***Denm.:*** Aldara; ***Fin.:*** Aldara; ***Fr.:*** Aldara; ***Ger.:*** Aldara; ***Gr.:*** Aldara; ***Hong Kong:*** Aldara; ***Irl.:*** Aldara; ***Israel:*** Aldara; ***Ital.:*** Aldara; ***Malaysia:*** Aldara; ***Mex.:*** Aldara; ***Neth.:*** Aldara; ***Norw.:*** Aldara; ***NZ:*** Aldara; ***S.Afr.:*** Aldara; ***Singapore:*** Aldara; ***Spain:*** Aldara; ***Swed.:*** Aldara; ***Switz.:*** Aldara; ***Thai.:*** Aldara; ***UK:*** Aldara; ***USA:*** Aldara.

## Indinavir Sulfate *(USAN, pINNM)*

Indinavir Sulphate *(BANM)*; L-735524; MK-639; MK-0639; Sulfato de indinavir. (αR,γS,2S)-α-Benzyl-2-(*tert*-butylcarbamoyl)-γ-hydroxy-*N*-[(1S,2R)-2-hydroxy-1-indanyl]-4-(3-pyridylmethyl)-1-piperazinevaleramide sulfate (1:1).

$C_{36}H_{47}N_5O_4,H_2SO_4$ = 711.9.
*CAS — 150378-17-9 (indinavir); 157810-81-6 (indinavir sulfate).*
*ATC — J05AE02.*

### Adverse Effects

The general spectrum of adverse effects associated with indinavir and other HIV-protease inhibitors commonly includes nausea, vomiting, and diarrhoea (which can be severe enough to cause dehydration with its potential for adverse renal effects). Other side-effects reported include taste disturbances, abdominal pain, anorexia, increased appetite, flatulence, asthenia, fatigue, sleep disturbances, headache, dizziness, paraesthesia, hypoaesthesia, myalgia, arthralgia, alopecia, pruritus, and renal insufficiency. Myositis and rhabdomyolysis have occurred. Skin rashes occur commonly and may occasionally be severe; a possible association with Stevens-Johnson syndrome and erythema multiforme has been reported for several HIV-protease inhibitors.

Lipodystrophy (redistribution of peripheral subcutaneous fat to the shoulders and abdomen) may occur.

Hyperglycaemia and an association with the onset or exacerbation of diabetes mellitus has also occurred in patients receiving HIV-protease inhibitors.

Hypersensitivity reactions, including vasculitis and sometimes anaphylaxis, have been associated with several HIV-protease inhibitors including indinavir.

Effects on the blood associated with indinavir and other HIV-protease inhibitors are, notably, anaemia including acute haemolytic anaemia, thrombocytopenia, and, generally, reduced neutrophil counts. Abnormal laboratory test results associated with HIV-protease inhibitors have included raised liver enzymes and bilirubin (jaundice and hepatitis have occurred), raised creatine phosphokinase, and raised blood lipids (with rare cases of pancreatitis).

Nephrolithiasis, often with flank pain and occurring with or without haematuria, has been associated with indinavir. It is often resolved by withdrawal for 1 to 3 days and administration of fluids, but interstitial nephritis and acute renal failure have been reported.

There have been reports of ingrowing toenails and paronychia of the great toes associated with indinavir. Additional side-effects reported with indinavir include acid regurgitation, dyspepsia, dry mouth, dysuria, dry skin, and hyperpigmentation.

◊ Reviews.


1. Moyle GJ, Gazzard BG. A risk-benefit assessment of HIV protease inhibitors. *Drug Safety* 1999; **20:** 299–321.


**Effects on carbohydrate and lipid metabolism.** HIV-protease inhibitors have been associated with a lipodystrophy syndrome characterised by peripheral fat wasting, central adiposity and the so called 'buffalo hump', hyperlipidaemia, and insulin resistance.[1]

A survey of 113 HIV-infected patients receiving HIV-protease inhibitors found lipodystrophy in 83% (severe in 11%) and impaired glucose tolerance in 23% (including diabetes mellitus in 7%) after a mean of 21 months of therapy.[2]

A systematic review[3] of published material has concluded that use of protease inhibitors is associated with increased concentrations of total cholesterol, triglycerides, and low-density lipoprotein; that use is often associated with morphological signs of cardiovascular disease such as increased carotid intima thickness or atherosclerotic lesions; and that there is some evidence of an increased risk of myocardial infarction. Comparison of the effect of specific protease inhibitors showed that ritonavir was consistently associated with elevated lipids and that, although some studies showed that saquinavir was associated with elevated lipids, it was to a lesser degree than other drugs. Guidelines[4] have been published outlining the management, including drug therapy, of antiretroviral-induced lipid disorders in HIV-infected patients.

Impaired glucose tolerance has been linked to reduction in insulin sensitivity[5] and has responded to treatment with sulfonylureas or insulin.[6]


1. Carr A, *et al.* Pathogenesis of HIV-1-protease inhibitor-associated peripheral lipodystrophy, hyperlipidaemia, and insulin resistance. *Lancet* 1998; **351:** 1881–3.
2. Carr A, *et al.* Diagnosis, prediction, and natural course of HIV-1 protease-inhibitor-associated lipodystrophy, hyperlipidaemia, and diabetes mellitus: a cohort study. *Lancet* 1999; **353:** 2093–9.
3. Rhew DC, *et al.* Association between protease inhibitor use and increased cardiovascular risk in patients infected with human immunodeficiency virus: a systematic review. *Clin Infect Dis* 2003; **37:** 959–72.
4. Dubé MP, *et al.* Guidelines for the evaluation and management of dyslipidemia in human immunodeficiency virus (HIV)-infected adults receiving antiretroviral therapy: recommendations of the HIV Medicine Association of the Infectious Disease Society of America and the Adult AIDS Clinical Trials Group. *Clin Infect Dis* 2003; **37:** 613–27.
5. Walli R, *et al.* Impaired glucose tolerance and protease inhibitors. *Ann Intern Med* 1998; **129:** 837–8.
6. Dubé MP, *et al.* Protease inhibitor-associated hyperglycaemia. *Lancet* 1997; **350:** 713–14.


**Effects on the cardiovascular system.** For adverse effects of HIV-protease inhibitors on carbohydrate and lipid metabolism that increase the risk of coronary vascular disease, see above.

**Effects on the kidneys.** Nephrolithiasis has been reported in about 10% of patients receiving indinavir, and the incidence may be higher in patients with haemophilia or hepatitis C infection.[1] Both asymptomatic[2] and symptomatic[3,4] crystalluria have been reported in patients receiving indinavir, with symptomatic urinary-tract disease in 8%. Indinavir has been identified as the major constituent of both urinary crystals[2] and calculi.[5] In addition there have been reports of acute interstitial nephritis associated with indinavir[6] and deterioration of renal function associated with both indinavir[7] and ritonavir.[8,9] Renal atrophy was associated with long-term treatment with indinavir.[10,11]


1. Brodie SB, *et al.* Variation in incidence of indinavir-associated nephrolithiasis among HIV-positive patients. *AIDS* 1998; **12:** 2433–7.
2. Kopp JB, *et al.* Crystalluria and urinary tract abnormalities associated with indinavir. *Ann Intern Med* 1997; **127:** 119–25.
3. Hachey DM, *et al.* Indinavir crystalluria in an HIV-positive man. *Ann Pharmacother* 2000; **34:** 403.
4. Famularo G, *et al.* Symptomatic crystalluria associated with indinavir. *Ann Pharmacother* 2000; **34:** 1414–18.
5. Daudon M, *et al.* Urinary stones in HIV-1-positive patients treated with indinavir. *Lancet* 1997; **349:** 1294–5.
6. Marroni M, *et al.* Acute interstitial nephritis secondary to the administration of indinavir. *Ann Pharmacother* 1998; **32:** 843–4.
7. Boubaker K, *et al.* Changes in renal function associated with indinavir. *AIDS* 1998; **12:** F249–F254.
8. Duong M, *et al.* Renal failure after treatment with ritonavir. *Lancet* 1996; **348:** 693–4.
9. Chugh S, *et al.* Ritonavir and renal failure. *N Engl J Med* 1997; **336:** 138.
10. Hanabusa H, *et al.* Renal atrophy associated with long-term treatment with indinavir. *N Engl J Med* 1999; **340:** 392–3.
11. Cattelan AM, *et al.* Severe hypertension and renal atrophy associated with indinavir. *Clin Infect Dis* 2000; **30:** 619–21.


**Effects on the liver.** The use of indinavir with other antiretroviral drugs has been associated with the development of severe hepatitis.[1,2]

Hepatic failure was attributed to ritonavir in a patient receiving combination therapy for AIDS.[3]


1. Bräu N, *et al.* Severe hepatitis in three AIDS patients treated with indinavir. *Lancet* 1997; **349:** 924–5.
2. Matsuda J, *et al.* Severe hepatitis in patients with AIDS and haemophilia B treated with indinavir. *Lancet* 1997; **350:** 364.
3. Picard O, *et al.* Hepatotoxicity associated with ritonavir. *Ann Intern Med* 1998; **129:** 670–1.


**Effects on the menstrual cycle.** Irregular, prolonged, or heavy menstruation[1] in 4 patients receiving ritonavir subsequently returned to normal in the 3 who were transferred to a different HIV-protease inhibitor.


1. Nielsen H. Hypermenorrhoea associated with ritonavir. *Lancet* 1999; **353:** 811–12.


**Effects on mental state.** Acute paranoid reactions occurred on two occasions in a patient receiving saquinavir.[1]


1. Finlayson JA, Laing RBS. Acute paranoid reaction to saquinavir. *Am J Health-Syst Pharm* 1998; **55:** 2016–17.


**Effects on the pancreas.** Pancreatitis was associated with use of ritonavir with saquinavir in 1 patient,[1] and with ritonavir (other drugs unspecified) in 2 others,[2] and was believed to be secondary to hyperlipidaemia (see Effects on Carbohydrate and Lipid Metabolism, above).


1. McBride M, *et al.* Lipid lowering therapy in patients with HIV infection. *Lancet* 1998; **352:** 1782–3.
2. Di Perri G, *et al.* HIV-protease inhibitors. *N Engl J Med* 1998; **339:** 773–4.


**Effects on sexual function.** Sexual dysfunction has been reported in patients given combination therapy with HIV-protease inhibitors and reverse transcriptase inhibitors.[1,2]


1. Martínez E, *et al.* Sexual dysfunction with protease inhibitors. *Lancet* 1999; **353:** 810–11.
2. Colebunders R, *et al.* Sexual dysfunction with protease inhibitors. *Lancet* 1999; **353:** 1802.


**Effects on the skin.** Skin rashes have been reported in about 20% of patients receiving indinavir and in 3 to 5% of patients receiving nelfinavir or saquinavir. Rash is described as a frequent adverse effect of ritonavir. In patients taking indinavir who reported rashes,[1] the rash commonly appeared within 2 weeks of starting treatment, was frequently accompanied by pruritus, and was usually self-limiting, commonly resolving within 4 weeks.

Paronychia and pyogenic granuloma of the great toes has been reported in patients receiving indinavir.[2]

1. Gajewski LK, *et al.* Characterization of rash with indinavir in a national patient cohort. *Ann Pharmacother* 1999; **33:** 17–21.
2. Bouscarat F, *et al.* Paronychia and pyogenic granuloma of the great toes in patients treated with indinavir. *N Engl J Med* 1998; **338:** 1776–7.

## Precautions

Indinavir and similar HIV-protease inhibitors are primarily metabolised in the liver and therefore caution and possible dosage reduction are required in hepatic impairment; deterioration in hepatic function has been reported in patients with pre-existing hepatitis or hepatic impairment receiving HIV-protease inhibitors, and where the hepatic impairment is severe they should be avoided.

Although renal excretion is a relatively minor route of elimination, adequate hydration is recommended to reduce the risk of nephrolithiasis; monitoring is advised in the presence of renal impairment. Treatment may need to be temporarily interrupted or discontinued completely in patients developing nephrolithiasis.

Patients receiving HIV-protease inhibitors should be monitored for signs of lipodystrophy. Caution is needed in diabetic patients since HIV-protease inhibitors have been associated with hyperglycaemia and the onset or exacerbation of diabetes mellitus. Caution is also needed in patients with haemophilia who may experience increased bleeding. Treatment with HIV-protease inhibitors may need to be discontinued should acute haemolytic anaemia occur.

**Mycobacterial infections.** Patients with a previously unsuspected *Mycobacterium avium* complex infection experienced a severe febrile syndrome with inflammatory lymphadenitis after starting indinavir treatment.[1] The reaction resolved with appropriate antimycobacterial therapy.

1. Race EM, *et al.* Focal mycobacterial lymphadenitis following initiation of protease-inhibitor therapy in patients with advanced HIV-1 disease. *Lancet* 1998; **351:** 252–5.

**Pregnancy.** A retrospective survey[1] involving 89 women who received HIV-protease inhibitors during pregnancy indicated that these antivirals appeared generally safe.

1. Morris AB, *et al.* Multicenter review of protease inhibitors in 89 pregnancies. *J Acquir Immune Defic Syndr* 2000; **25:** 306–11.

## Interactions

Indinavir and similar HIV-protease inhibitors are metabolised principally by cytochrome P450 isoenzymes of the CYP3A family. They consequently compete for the same metabolic pathways with a wide range of drugs that are metabolised similarly, often resulting in mutually increased plasma concentrations. The extent of such interactions depends on a number of factors, including the affinity of the relevant HIV-protease inhibitor for the various cytochrome P450 isoenzymes; in the case of indinavir, CYP3A4 is reported to be the only P450 isoenzyme that plays a major role. Where significant competition for metabolism does occur, the margin between therapeutic and toxic concentrations has a major role in determining the severity of the interaction. Thus, concurrent administration of a drug with a narrow therapeutic window, such as cisapride or terfenadine, is contra-indicated, whereas a drug with a wider therapeutic window, such as erythromycin, may only require dosage reduction at its highest dose level.

Conversely, a drug that is a significant inducer of microsomal enzymes, particularly isoenzymes of the CYP3A family, may reduce plasma concentrations of HIV-protease inhibitors. A potent enzyme inducer, such as rifampicin, may reduce the plasma concentration of an HIV-protease inhibitor to a subtherapeutic level and therefore its concurrent use is contra-indicated. Other well known enzyme inducers, such as carbamazepine, phenobarbital, and phenytoin, also possibly reduce the plasma concentrations of HIV-protease inhibitors.

In turn, HIV-protease inhibitors may themselves induce metabolism and may reduce plasma concentrations of other drugs, such as theophylline and hormonal contraceptives.

The principal interactions that have been reported as a risk for one or more of the various HIV-protease inhibitors are listed below.

◊ References to interactions associated with HIV-protease inhibitors.

1. Eagling VA, *et al.* Differential inhibition of cytochrome P450 isoforms by the protease inhibitors, ritonavir, saquinavir and indinavir. *Br J Clin Pharmacol* 1997; **44:** 190–4.
2. von Moltke LL, *et al.* Protease inhibitors as inhibitors of human cytochromes P450: high risk associated with ritonavir. *J Clin Pharmacol* 1998; **38:** 106–11.
3. Malaty LI, Kuper JJ. Drug interactions of HIV protease inhibitors. *Drug Safety* 1999; **20:** 147–69.

**Amfetamines.** For mention of interactions, including a fatal serotonergic reaction, with *methylenedioxymethamfetamine* (Ecstasy) in patients receiving ritonavir, see p.1590.

**Analgesics.** Ritonavir and possibly other HIV-protease inhibitors produce complex and potentially serious interactions with some opioids (see p.73). Interactions between ritonavir and *dextropropoxyphene* (p.29) or *pethidine* (p.81) are considered to be especially hazardous. Lopinavir-ritonavir, nelfinavir, and ritonavir may reduce plasma concentrations of *methadone* (see p.58).

Use of ritonavir with *piroxicam* can result in potentially toxic concentrations of piroxicam (see p.84).

**Antiarrhythmics.** Use of HIV-protease inhibitors with the antiarrhythmics *amiodarone, flecainide, propafenone*, or *quinidine* may result in potentially toxic plasma concentrations of these drugs with an increased risk of ventricular arrhythmias.

**Antibacterials.** Plasma concentrations of HIV-protease inhibitors may be reduced to subtherapeutic levels by *rifabutin* or *rifampicin*. In addition, plasma concentrations of rifabutin may be increased, with a consequent risk of uveitis. In general, HIV-protease inhibitors should not be used with rifampicin (p.251) and dosage modifications may be necessary if used with rifabutin; further information is given in Rifabutin under Interactions, p.249 and Uses, Tuberculosis and HIV Infection, p.250.

HIV-protease inhibitors may inhibit the metabolism of *clarithromycin* (p.192) and possibly other macrolides.

**Antidepressants.** HIV-protease inhibitors may inhibit the metabolism of *desipramine* and other tricyclic antidepressants (p.284) and *fluoxetine* (p.296).

Plasma concentrations of HIV-protease inhibitors may be reduced by *Hypericum* (*St John's Wort*) as a result of induction of cytochrome P450; concomitant use should be avoided.[1]

1. Piscitelli SC, *et al.* Indinavir concentrations and St John's wort. *Lancet* 2000; **355:** 547–8. Correction. *ibid.* 2001; **357:** 1210.

**Antiepileptics.** Reduced plasma concentrations of HIV-protease inhibitors may be anticipated if the enzyme inducers *carbamazepine, phenobarbital*, or *phenytoin* are given concurrently. Nelfinavir has been reported to reduce the plasma concentration of phenytoin (p.374). In addition, carbamazepine concentrations have been reported to be increased by ritonavir (p.356).

**Antifungals.** Plasma concentrations of HIV-protease inhibitors may be increased by azole antifungals. The manufacturers recommend that the dose of indinavir should be reduced to 600 mg every 8 hours when given with *itraconazole* 200 mg twice daily. A dose reduction is not considered necessary by the UK manufacturer when indinavir is given with *ketoconazole*, but the US manufacturer recommends a reduction to indinavir 600 mg every 8 hours.

Conversely, plasma concentrations of ketoconazole are increased by ritonavir.

**Antihistamines.** HIV-protease inhibitors inhibit the metabolism of non-sedating antihistamines such as *terfenadine* resulting in increased plasma concentrations of these drugs and an increased risk of serious ventricular arrhythmias. Such combinations should be avoided.

**Antipsychotics.** Ritonavir and possibly other HIV-protease inhibitors may increase plasma concentrations of *clozapine* (but see p.688), *pimozide* (p.715), and *sertindole* (p.722) resulting in increased toxicity. Concomitant use should be avoided. Plasma concentrations of *thioridazine* may also be increased when given with some HIV-protease inhibitors.

**Antivirals.** HIV-protease inhibitors can inhibit metabolism of other drugs from the same class and increases in adverse effects have in particular resulted from use of *saquinavir* with *ritonavir*. However, there have been suggestions that judicious administration of two of these drugs could be utilised to simplify dosage regimens and thereby improve compliance.[1] An increase in the plasma concentrations of both *indinavir* and *nelfinavir* may occur when they are co-administered; a similar effect may be seen with concurrent use of *amprenavir* with ritonavir, of nelfinavir with saquinavir, or of nelfinavir with ritonavir. Ritonavir also appears to increase indinavir and saquinavir plasma concentrations, and indinavir to increase saquinavir concentrations when given concomitantly.

Plasma concentrations of indinavir[2] and saquinavir may be reduced by *nevirapine*; the manufacturers of indinavir recommend a dose increase of indinavir to 1 g every 8 hours be considered.

Plasma concentrations of indinavir[3] and saquinavir may be increased by *delavirdine*; the manufacturers of indinavir recommend a dose reduction of indinavir to 400 to 600 mg every 8 hours in patients receiving delavirdine and the manufacturers of saquinavir recommend that liver function should be monitored if saquinavir is given with delavirdine.

Plasma concentrations of amprenavir, indinavir, *lopinavir*, and saquinavir are decreased when given with *efavirenz*. Increased doses of indinavir to 1 g every 8 hours are recommended when it is given with efavirenz, but the use of saquinavir with efavirenz is not recommended unless saquinavir concentrations are increased by the addition of other antiretrovirals such as ritonavir. The use of efavirenz with ritonavir is associated with an increased frequency of adverse effects, presumably due to competitive inhibition of metabolism, and the manufacturer recommends that liver enzymes should be monitored in patients receiving this combination. Plasma concentrations of nelfinavir are increased when given with efavirenz, but the combination is usually well tolerated at standard doses.

Although there is no direct interaction between HIV-protease inhibitors and *didanosine*, the buffer included in the didanosine formulation can impair the absorption of indinavir; doses of nelfinavir or ritonavir, both of which should be given with food, should also be separated by at least 1 hour from didanosine doses, which should be given on an empty stomach.

Use of lopinavir with *tenofovir* may result in decreased plasma concentrations of lopinavir but increased plasma concentrations of tenofovir.

For a report of reduced area under the plasma concentration-time curve for *zidovudine* in patients receiving ritonavir, see p.660.

1. Hsu A, *et al.* Pharmacokinetic interaction between ritonavir and indinavir in healthy volunteers. *Antimicrob Agents Chemother* 1998; **42:** 2784–91.
2. Murphy RL, *et al.* Antiviral effect and pharmacokinetic interaction between nevirapine and indinavir in persons infected with human immunodeficiency virus type 1. *J Infect Dis* 1999; **179:** 1116–23.
3. Ferry JJ, *et al.* Pharmacokinetic drug-drug interaction study of delavirdine and indinavir in healthy subjects. *J Acquir Immune Defic Syndr Hum Retrovirol* 1998; **18:** 252–9.

**Benzodiazepines.** For the effect of HIV-protease inhibitors on benzodiazepines, see Diazepam, p.693.

**Ciclosporin.** Mutual increases in the area under the plasma concentration-time curves for saquinavir and ciclosporin were reported in a kidney transplant recipient.[1] The resultant adverse effects subsided when doses of both drugs were reduced by half. Similar interactions with other HIV-protease inhibitors are possible.

1. Brinkman K, *et al.* Pharmacokinetic interaction between saquinavir and cyclosporine. *Ann Intern Med* 1998; **129:** 914–15.

**Cisapride.** For the effect of HIV-protease inhibitors on cisapride, see p.1260.

**Corticosteroids.** Corticosteroids, in particular *dexamethasone*, may induce the metabolism of HIV-protease inhibitors resulting in reduced plasma concentrations. For the effect of ritonavir on plasma concentrations of *fluticasone*, see p.1072

**Ergot alkaloids.** For reports of ergotism in patients receiving HIV-protease inhibitors and ergot alkaloids, see Ergotamine, p.468.

**Grapefruit.** The area under the plasma concentration-time curve for saquinavir was increased by 50% when taken with grapefruit juice;[1] however, the manufacturers do not recommend any adjustment of dosage of saquinavir.

1. Kupferschmidt HHT, *et al.* Grapefruit juice enhances the bioavailability of the HIV protease inhibitor saquinavir in men. *Br J Clin Pharmacol* 1998; **45:** 355–9.

**Hormonal contraceptives.** For the effect of HIV-protease inhibitors on hormonal contraceptives, see p.1534.

**Interleukin-2.** Plasma concentrations of indinavir were increased[1] during concurrent administration of interleukin-2.

1. Piscitelli SC, *et al.* Alteration in indinavir clearance during interleukin-2 infusions in patients infected with the human immunodeficiency virus. *Pharmacotherapy* 1998; **18:** 1212–16.

**Phenylpropanolamine.** For a possible interaction between phenylpropanolamine and antiretrovirals including indinavir, see Stavudine, p.654.

**Sildenafil.** For the effect of HIV-protease inhibitors on sildenafil, including a report of fatal myocardial infarction following sildenafil in a patient receiving ritonavir and saquinavir, see p.1744.

**Statins.** HIV-protease inhibitors may inhibit the metabolism of statins metabolised by CYP3A4 isoenzymes resulting in an increased risk of myopathy. Although some statins may be used in certain circumstances to manage HIV-protease inhibitor-induced lipid disorders, the use of indinavir with lovastatin or simvastatin should be avoided, and it should be given with caution in patients receiving atorvastatin or cerivastatin.

**Tacrolimus.** HIV-protease inhibitors may inhibit the metabolism of tacrolimus (see Antivirals, p.1365).

**Theophylline.** For a potential effect of ritonavir on theophylline, see p.802.

**Warfarin.** For the effect of HIV-protease inhibitors on warfarin, see p.1026.

## Antiviral Action

Indinavir and similar HIV-protease inhibitors are antiretrovirals that act by binding reversibly to HIV-protease thereby preventing cleavage of the viral precursor polyproteins. This results in the formation of immature viral particles incapable of infecting other cells. Viral resistance develops rapidly when HIV-protease inhibitors are given alone and therefore they are used in combination with other antiretrovirals. Cross-resistance between HIV-protease inhibitors may occur, but cross-resistance between HIV-protease inhibitors and reverse transcriptase inhibitors is considered unlikely.

**Resistance.** References.

1. Boden D, Markowitz M. Resistance to human immunodeficiency virus type 1 protease inhibitors. *Antimicrob Agents Chemother* 1998; **42:** 2775–83.

## Pharmacokinetics

Indinavir is rapidly absorbed following oral administration producing peak plasma concentrations in 0.8 hours. Bioavailability is about 65% following a single dose. Absorption is reduced by administration with a meal high in calories, fat, and protein but is less affected by a light meal. At doses up to 1 g, increases in plasma concentration are proportionately greater than increases in dose. Plasma protein binding is about 60%. Indinavir is reported to cross the blood-brain barrier. It undergoes oxidative metabolism by cytochrome P450 isoenzyme CYP3A4 and glucuronidation. The elimination half-life is 1.8 hours. Less than 20% of the absorbed dose is excreted in the urine, about half of this as unchanged drug. The remainder is excreted in the faeces.

◊ References.

1. Ståhle L, *et al.* Indinavir in cerebrospinal fluid of HIV-1-infected patients. *Lancet* 1997; **350:** 1823.
2. Bernard L, *et al.* Indinavir concentrations in hair from patients receiving highly active antiretroviral therapy. *Lancet* 1998; **352:** 1757–8.
3. Wintergerst U, *et al.* Use of saliva specimens for monitoring indinavir therapy in human immunodeficiency virus-infected patients. *Antimicrob Agents Chemother* 2000; **44:** 2572–4.
4. Haas DW, *et al.* Steady-state pharmacokinetics of indinavir in cerebrospinal fluid and plasma among adults with human immunodeficiency virus type 1 infection. *Clin Pharmacol Ther* 2000; **68:** 367–74.
5. Burger DM, *et al.* Pharmacokinetics of the protease inhibitor indinavir in human immunodeficiency virus type 1-infected children. *Antimicrob Agents Chemother* 2001; **45:** 701–5.

## Uses and Administration

Indinavir is a protease inhibitor with antiviral activity against HIV. It is used with nucleoside reverse transcriptase inhibitors for combination therapy of HIV infection (p.621).

Indinavir is given by mouth as the sulfate, but doses are expressed in terms of the base. 116 mg of indinavir sulfate is approximately equivalent to 100 mg of indinavir. It is given in a usual adult dose of 800 mg every 8 hours. It should be given either an hour before or two hours after meals, or with a light, low-fat meal. Adequate hydration should be maintained. Treatment may have to be interrupted if acute episodes of nephrolithiasis occur. Children over 4 years of age may be given 500 mg/m$^2$ every 8 hours, the dose not to exceed the adult dose.

For details of reduced dosage to be used in patients with hepatic impairment, see below, or for those receiving azole antifungals or other antivirals, see above.

Indinavir has also been recommended as part of the chemoprophylactic regimen with zidovudine and lamivudine in patients at high risk of HIV infection following occupational percutaneous exposure (see p.623).

**Administration in hepatic impairment.** A reduction in the dose of indinavir to 600 mg every 8 hours is recommended for patients with mild to moderate hepatic insufficiency due to cirrhosis.

**HIV infection and AIDS.** Reviews on the use of indinavir and other HIV-protease inhibitors.

1. Deeks SG, *et al.* HIV-1 protease inhibitors: a review for clinicians. *JAMA* 1997; **277:** 145–53.
2. Flexner C. HIV-protease inhibitors. *N Engl J Med* 1998; **338:** 1281–92.
3. Plosker GL, Noble S. Indinavir: a review of its use in the management of HIV infection. *Drugs* 1999; **58:** 1165–1203.

**Other viral infections.** Infection with human herpesvirus-8 (a virus associated with an increased risk of developing Kaposi's sarcoma) resolved in a patient when indinavir was added to combination therapy for HIV infection.[1] Regression of progressive multifocal leukoencephalopathy (the result of a papovavirus infection of the CNS) has been reported in 2 patients receiving combination antiretroviral therapy including indinavir for HIV infection.[2,3]

1. Rizzieri DA, *et al.* Clearance of HHV-8 from peripheral blood mononuclear cells with a protease inhibitor. *Lancet* 1997; **349:** 775–6.
2. Elliot B, *et al.* 2.5 Year remission of AIDS-associated progressive multifocal leukoencephalopathy with combined antiretroviral therapy. *Lancet* 1997; **349:** 850.
3. Domingo P, *et al.* Remission of progressive multifocal leucoencephalopathy after antiretroviral therapy. *Lancet* 1997; **349:** 1554–5.

## Preparations

**Proprietary Preparations** (details are given in Part 3)
***Arg.:*** Avural; Crixivan; Elvenavir; Forli; Indilea; Inhibisam; ***Austral.:*** Crixivan; ***Austria:*** Crixivan; ***Belg.:*** Crixivan; ***Braz.:*** Crixivan; Dinavir†; Indinax; ***Canad.:*** Crixivan; ***Chile:*** Crixivan; ***Denm.:*** Crixivan; ***Fin.:*** Crixivan; ***Fr.:*** Crixivan; ***Ger.:*** Crixivan; ***Gr.:*** Crixivan; ***Hong Kong:*** Crixivan; ***Irl.:*** Crixivan; ***Israel:*** Crixivan; ***Ital.:*** Crixivan; ***Jpn:*** Crixivan; ***Malaysia:*** Crixivan; ***Mex.:*** Crixivan; ***Neth.:*** Crixivan; ***Norw.:*** Crixivan; ***NZ:*** Crixivan; ***Port.:*** Crixivan; ***S.Afr.:*** Crixivan; ***Singapore:*** Crixivan; ***Spain:*** Crixivan; ***Swed.:*** Crixivan; ***Switz.:*** Crixivan; ***Thai.:*** Crixivan; ***UK:*** Crixivan; ***USA:*** Crixivan.

# Inosine Pranobex *(BAN, rINNM)*

Inosiplex; Isoprinosine; Methisoprinol; Metisoprinol; NP-113; NPT-10381. Inosine 2-hydroxypropyldimethylammonium 4-acetamidobenzoate (1:3).

$C_{10}H_{12}N_4O_5{:}C_{14}H_{22}N_2O_4$ (1:3) = 1115.2.

*CAS — 36703-88-5.*

*ATC — J05AX05.*

NOTE. Inosine pranobex has sometimes been expressed as inosine with dimepranol (*pINN*) ((±)-1-(dimethylamino)-2-propanol) and acedoben (*pINN*) (*p*-acetamidobenzoic acid).
Dimepranol Acedoben is *USAN.*

## Adverse Effects and Precautions

Some patients have experienced transient nausea and vomiting. Metabolism of the inosine content of inosine pranobex leads to increased serum and urine concentrations of uric acid; caution is therefore recommended in treating patients with renal impairment, gout, or hyperuricaemia.

## Antiviral Action

Inosine pranobex appears to owe its activity in viral infections more to its capacity to modify or stimulate cell-mediated immune processes than to a direct action on the virus.

## Pharmacokinetics

Inosine pranobex is reported to be rapidly absorbed after oral administration. It is also rapidly metabolised with a plasma half-life of 50 minutes, the inosine portion of the complex yielding uric acid; the other components undergo oxidation and glucuronidation. The metabolites are excreted in the urine.

◊ References.

1. Nielsen P, Beckett AH. The metabolism and excretion in man of NN-dimethylamino-isopropanol and p-acetamido-benzoic acid after administration of isoprinosine. *J Pharm Pharmacol* 1981; **33:** 549–50.

## Uses and Administration

Inosine pranobex has been used in the treatment of various viral infections, including herpes simplex, genital warts, and subacute sclerosing panencephalitis, although other treatments or measures are preferred. The dose in mucocutaneous herpes simplex is 1 g four times daily by mouth for 7 to 14 days. A dose of 1 g three times daily is given for 14 to 28 days as an adjunct to standard topical treatment for genital warts. In subacute sclerosing panencephalitis, the dose is 50 to 100 mg/kg daily in divided doses given every 4 hours.

◊ Reviews.

1. Campoli-Richards DM, *et al.* Inosine pranobex: a preliminary review of its pharmacodynamic and pharmacokinetic properties, and therapeutic efficacy. *Drugs* 1986; **32:** 383–424.

**Subacute sclerosing panencephalitis.** Inosine pranobex has been tried in the treatment of subacute sclerosing panencephalitis, a complication of measles (p.624), but the results of clinical studies have been equivocal.[1-8] Some success has been reported when inosine pranobex has been given with interferons and other antivirals.[9-12]

1. Streletz LJ, Cracco J. The effect of isoprinosine in subacute sclerosing panencephalitis (SSPE). *Ann Neurol* 1977; **1:** 183–4.
2. Huttenlocher PR, Mattson RH. Isoprinosine in subacute sclerosing panencephalitis. *Neurology* 1979; **29:** 763–71.
3. Silverberg R, *et al.* Inosiplex in the treatment of subacute sclerosing panencephalitis. *Arch Neurol* 1979; **36:** 374–5.
4. Haddad FS, Risk WS. Isoprinosine treatment in 18 patients with subacute sclerosing panencephalitis: a controlled study. *Ann Neurol* 1980; **7:** 185–8.
5. Jones CE, *et al.* Inosiplex therapy in subacute sclerosing panencephalitis: a multicentre, non-randomised study in 98 patients. *Lancet* 1982; **i:** 1034–7.
6. Anonymous. Inosiplex: antiviral, immunomodulator, or neither? *Lancet* 1982; **i:** 1052–4.
7. DuRant RH, *et al.* The influence of inosiplex treatment on the neurological disability of patients with subacute sclerosing panencephalitis. *J Pediatr* 1982; **101:** 288–93.
8. DuRant RH, Dyken PR. The effect of inosiplex on the survival of subacute sclerosing panencephalitis. *Neurology* 1983; **33:** 1053–5.
9. Anlar B, *et al.* β-Interferon plus inosiplex in the treatment of subacute sclerosing panencephalitis. *J Child Neurol* 1998; **13:** 557–9.
10. Gokcil Z, *et al.* α-Interferon and isoprinosine in adult-onset subacute sclerosing panencephalitis. *J Neurol Sci* 1999; **162:** 62–4.
11. Solomon T, *et al.* Treatment of subacute sclerosing panencephalitis with interferon-α, ribavirin, and inosiplex. *J Child Neurol* 2002; **17:** 703–5.
12. Aydin ÖF, *et al.* Combined treatment with subcutaneous interferon-α, oral isoprinosine, and lamivudine for subacute sclerosing panencephalitis. *J Child Neurol* 2003; **18:** 104–8.

## Preparations

**Proprietary Preparations** (details are given in Part 3)
***Belg.:*** Isoprinosine; ***Canad.:*** Imunovir; ***Chile:*** Isoprinosine; ***Fr.:*** Isoprinosine; ***Ger.:*** delimmun; Isoprinosine; ***Gr.:*** Isoprinosine; ***Irl.:*** Imunovir; Isoprinosine; ***Ital.:*** Avirin; Farviran; Isoprinosina†; Metivirol†; Stimuzim†; Viract†; Viralin†; Virustop; Viruxan; ***Mex.:*** Isoprinosine; Pranosine; ***NZ:*** Imunovir; ***Port.:*** Isovir; ***Singapore:*** Imin; ***Spain:*** Bodaril†; ***UK:*** Imunovir.

# Interferon Alfa *(BAN, rINN)*

IFN-α; Interferon-α; Interferón alfa; Ro-22-8181 (interferon alfa-2a); Sch-30500 (interferon alfa-2b).

*CAS — 74899-72-2 (interferon alfa); 76543-88-9 (interferon alfa-2a); 99210-65-8 (interferon alfa-2b); 118390-30-0 (interferon alfacon-1); 198153-51-4 (peginterferon alfa-2a); 215647-85-1 (peginterferon alfa-2b).*

*ATC — L03AB01 (natural); L03AB04 (2a); L03AB05 (2b); L03AB06 (n1); L03AB09 (alfacon-1); L03AB10 (peginterferon alfa-2b); L03AB11 (peginterferon alfa-2a).*

NOTE. Interferon alfa was previously known as leucocyte interferon or lymphoblastoid interferon.
Interferon alfa-2a, alfa-2b, alfa-n1, and alfa-n3 are *USAN.*
Interferon alfacon-1 (*BAN, USAN, rINN*) is a recombinant non-naturally occurring alfa interferon. Peginterferon alfa-2a (*BAN, USAN, rINN*) and peginterferon alfa-2b (*BAN, rINN*) are interferons pegylated by conjugation with macrogols.

**Pharmacopoeias.** *Chin.* includes Lyophilized Recombinant Human Interferon α-2a. *Eur.* (see p.vi) includes Interferon Alfa-2 Concentrated Solution.

**Ph. Eur. 5.0** (Interferon Alfa-2 Concentrated Solution; Interferoni Alfa-2 Solutio Concentrata). It is produced by a method based on recombinant DNA technology using bacteria as host cells. It is a clear, colourless or slightly yellowish liquid. Store in airtight containers at a temperature of −20° or below. Protect from light.

**Nomenclature.** Interferon alfa may be derived from leucocytes or lymphoblasts as well as through recombinant DNA technology. Sub-species of the human alfa gene may produce interferon alfa with protein variants or a mixture of proteins. The protein variants may be designated by a number (as in interferon alfa-2) which may be further qualified by a letter to indicate the amino-acid sequences at positions 23 and 34. Interferon alfa-2a has lysine at 23 and histidine at 34, interferon alfa-2b has arginine at 23 and histidine at 34, and interferon alfa-2c has arginine at both positions. In the case of a mixture of proteins an alphanumeric designation is given (as in interferon alfa-n1). Interferon alfacon-1 varies from interferon alfa-2 in 20 of 166 amino acids.

The name may be further elaborated on the label by approved sets of initials in parentheses to indicate the method of production: (rbe) indicates production from bacteria (*Escherichia coli*) genetically modified by recombinant DNA technology; (lns) indicates production from cultured lymphoblasts from the Namalwa cell line that have been stimulated by a Sendai virus; (bls) indicates production from leucocytes from human blood that have been stimulated by a Sendai virus.

References.

1. Finter NB. The naming of cats—and alpha-interferons. *Lancet* 1996; **348:** 348–9.

## Adverse Effects and Treatment

Most reports of the adverse effects of interferons have involved interferon alfa, but limited clinical experience suggests that interferons beta and gamma have similar adverse effects.

Interferons produce influenza-like symptoms with fever, chills, fatigue, headache, malaise, myalgia, and arthralgia. These symptoms tend to be dose-related, are most likely to occur at the start of treatment, and mostly respond to paracetamol (but for a possible interaction with paracetamol, see Interactions, below).

Other adverse effects include nausea, vomiting, diarrhoea, anorexia with weight loss, bone marrow depression, alopecia, rash, taste alteration and, rarely, epistaxis, cough, and pharyngitis. There may be signs of altered liver function and hepatitis has been reported. Renal failure and the nephrotic syndrome have occurred. Severe hypersensitivity reactions including anaphylaxis and bronchospasm have been reported rarely. Cardiovascular effects include hypotension or hypertension, arrhythmias, oedema, myocardial infarction, and stroke. High doses may cause electrolyte disturbances including decreased calcium concentrations. Hyperglycaemia and thyroid dysfunction have been reported as have pulmonary oedema and pneumonitis. EEG abnormalities and neurological symptoms including ataxia, paraesthesia, somnolence, dizziness, confusion, and rarely, convulsions and coma have been reported. Depression, anxiety, depersonalisation, or emotional lability may be severe. Visual disturbances and, rarely, ischaemic retinopathy may occur. Menstrual irregularities have been reported, particularly with interferon beta.

Subcutaneous injection may produce a reaction at the injection site. The reaction is reported frequently with interferon beta, which can produce severe reactions including local necrosis.

Nasal administration may produce mucosal irritation and damage.

◊ Reviews.


1. Vial T, Descotes J. Clinical toxicity of the interferons. *Drug Safety* 1994; **10:** 115–50.
2. Pardo M, *et al.* Risks and benefits of interferon-α in the treatment of hepatitis. *Drug Safety* 1995; **13:** 304–16.
3. Kirkwood JM, *et al.* Mechanisms and management of toxicities associated with high-dose interferon alfa-2b therapy. *J Clin Oncol* 2002; **20:** 3703–18.


**Auto-immune disorders.** For exacerbation or development of auto-immune disorders in patients receiving interferon, see under Precautions, below.

**Effects on the blood.** Restoration of bone-marrow function following marrow transplantation was delayed in 3 patients given a human interferon alfa preparation.[1] Laboratory results showed an inhibition of granulocyte colony growth by human leucocyte interferon alfa. It was considered that interferon alfa was contra-indicated in patients with severe bone-marrow insufficiency and should not be given to marrow transplant patients before the graft was fully functional. However, in another 5 patients recombinant interferon alfa did not affect bone-marrow transplants, although 3 patients experienced fever and chills, 4 experienced more than a 60% reduction in absolute peripheral granulocyte counts, and 4 had a 37 to 80% reduction in absolute platelet counts.[2] Lymphocytes were increased in all patients; blood counts returned to normal when interferon therapy stopped. Interferon alfa produced a decline in CD4+ T-lymphocytes resulting in opportunistic infections in 2 HIV-positive patients being treated for chronic hepatitis C.[3]

Other haematological effects reported to be associated with interferon alfa include immune haemolytic anaemia[4] and immune thrombocytopenia.[5,6] Haemorrhage occurred in a patient with immune thrombocytopenic purpura treated with interferon alfa,[7] and it was thought prudent to use interferons with caution, if at all, in this condition.[6,7] Bleeding associated with induction of factor VIII inhibitor has been reported in a patient receiving interferon alfa to enhance hydroxycarbamide therapy for chronic myeloid leukaemia.[8] Thrombosis associated with interferon alfa has also been reported.[9]


1. Nissen C, *et al.* Toxicity of human leucocyte interferon preparations in human bone-marrow cultures. *Lancet* 1977; **i:** 203–4.
2. Winston DJ, *et al.* Safety and tolerance of recombinant leukocyte A interferon in bone marrow transplant recipients. *Antimicrob Agents Chemother* 1983; **23:** 846–51.
3. Pesce A, *et al.* Opportunistic infections and CD4 lymphocytopenia with interferon treatment in HIV-1 infected patients. *Lancet* 1993; **341:** 1597.
4. Akard LP, *et al.* Alpha-interferon and immune hemolytic anemia. *Ann Intern Med* 1986; **105:** 306.
5. McLaughlin P, *et al.* Immune thrombocytopenia following α-interferon therapy in patients with cancer. *JAMA* 1985; **254:** 1353–4.
6. Färkkilä M, Iivanainen M. Thrombocytopenia and interferon. *BMJ* 1988; **296:** 642.
7. Matthey F, *et al.* Bleeding in immune thrombocytopenic purpura after alpha-interferon. *Lancet* 1990; **335:** 471–2.
8. English KE, *et al.* Acquired factor VIII inhibitor in a patient with chronic myelogenous leukaemia receiving interferon-alfa therapy. *Ann Pharmacother* 2000; **34:** 737–9.
9. Durand JM, *et al.* Thrombosis and recombinant interferon-α. *Am J Med* 1993; **95:** 115.


**Effects on the cardiovascular system.** There have been reports of cardiomyopathy[1-4] and of Raynaud's syndrome[5-10] associated with interferon alfa therapy.


1. Deyton LR, *et al.* Reversible cardiac dysfunction associated with interferon alfa therapy in AIDS patients with Kaposi's sarcoma. *N Engl J Med* 1989; **321:** 1246–9.
2. Sonnenblick M, *et al.* Reversible cardiomyopathy induced by interferon. *BMJ* 1990; **300:** 1174–5.
3. Angulo MP, *et al.* Reversible cardiomyopathy secondary to α-interferon in an infant. *Pediatr Cardiol* 1999; **20:** 293–4.
4. Kuwata A, *et al.* A case of reversible dilated cardiomyopathy after α-interferon therapy in a patient with renal cell carcinoma. *Am J Med Sci* 2002; **324:** 331–4.
5. Roy V, Newland AC. Raynaud's phenomenon and cryoglobulinaemia associated with the use of recombinant human alpha-interferon. *Lancet* 1988; **i:** 944–5.
6. Bachmeyer C, *et al.* Raynaud's phenomenon and digital necrosis induced by interferon-alpha. *Br J Dermatol* 1996; **135:** 481–3.
7. Linden D. Severe Raynaud's phenomenon associated with interferon-β treatment for multiple sclerosis. *Lancet* 1998; **352:** 878–9.
8. Kruit WH, *et al.* Interferon-α induced Raynaud's syndrome. *Ann Oncol* 2000; **11:** 1501–2.
9. Schapira D, *et al.* Interferon-induced Raynaud's syndrome. *Semin Arthritis Rheum* 2002; **32:** 157–62.
10. Iorio R, *et al.* Severe Raynaud's phenomenon with chronic hepatitis C disease treated with interferon. *Pediatr Infect Dis J* 2003; **22:** 195–7.


**Effects on the endocrine system.** Both hypothyroidism[1,2] and hyperthyroidism[2,3] have been associated with interferon alfa therapy. Recombinant interferon gamma was reported not to affect thyroid function.[4] The development of type 1 diabetes has been associated with interferon alfa therapy.[5-8] Exacerbation of existing type 2 diabetes has also been reported.[9,10] Reversible hypopituitarism has been reported in patients receiving interferon alfa.[11,12]


1. Fentiman IS, *et al.* Primary hypothyroidism associated with interferon therapy of breast cancer. *Lancet* 1985; **i:** 1166.
2. Burman P, *et al.* Autoimmune thyroid disease in interferon-treated patients. *Lancet* 1985; **ii:** 100–1.
3. Schultz M, *et al.* Induction of hyperthyroidism by interferon-α-2b. *Lancet* 1989; **i:** 1452.
4. Bhakri H, *et al.* Recombinant gamma interferon and autoimmune thyroid disease. *Lancet* 1985; **ii:** 457.
5. Fabris P, *et al.* Development of type 1 diabetes mellitus during interferon alfa therapy for chronic HCV hepatitis. *Lancet* 1992; **340:** 548.
6. Guerci A-P, *et al.* Onset of insulin-dependent diabetes mellitus after interferon-alfa therapy for hairy cell leukaemia. *Lancet* 1994; **343:** 1167–8.
7. Gori A, *et al.* Reversible diabetes in patient with AIDS-related Kaposi's sarcoma treated with interferon α-2a. *Lancet* 1995; **345:** 1438–9.
8. Murakami M, *et al.* Diabetes mellitus and interferon-α therapy. *Ann Intern Med* 1995; **123:** 318.
9. Campbell S, *et al.* Rapidly reversible increase in insulin requirement with interferon. *BMJ* 1996; **313:** 92.
10. Lopes EPA, *et al.* Exacerbation of type 2 diabetes mellitus during interferon-alfa therapy for chronic hepatitis B. *Lancet* 1994; **343:** 244. Correction. *ibid.*: 680.
11. Sakane N, *et al.* Reversible hypopituitarism after interferon-alfa therapy. *Lancet* 1995; **345:** 1305.
12. Concha LB, *et al.* Interferon-induced hypopituitarism. *Am J Med* 2003; **114:** 161–3.


**Effects on the eyes.** Reports of interferon-associated retinopathy have been reviewed.[1]

In a study of 43 patients with chronic hepatitis receiving interferon alfa, retinopathy developed in 11 of 37 non-diabetic patients and in 3 of 6 diabetic patients after about 8 to 10 weeks of therapy.[2] None of the patients had had retinopathy before treatment; the condition was reversible in the non-diabetic patients on cessation of therapy. Visual acuity remained unchanged. Subconjunctival haemorrhage occurred in a further 3 of the non-diabetic patients. Severe irreversible loss of vision has been reported in a non-diabetic patient receiving interferon alfa.[3]

Pain in one eyeball leading to exophthalmos and complete visual loss has been reported in a patient receiving interferon alfa;[4] despite withdrawal of interferon and instigation of antibacterial and corticosteroid treatment, the eyeball subsequently ruptured necessitating ophthalmectomy.


1. Hayasaka S, *et al.* Interferon associated retinopathy. *Br J Ophthalmol* 1998; **82:** 323–5.
2. Hayasaka S, *et al.* Retinopathy and subconjunctival haemorrhage in patients with chronic viral hepatitis receiving interferon alfa. *Br J Ophthalmol* 1995; **79:** 150–2.
3. Lohmann CP, *et al.* Severe loss of vision during adjuvant interferon alfa-2b treatment for malignant melanoma. *Lancet* 1999; **353:** 1326.
4. Yamada H, *et al.* Acute onset of ocular complications with interferon. *Lancet* 1994; **343:** 914.


**Effects on the gastrointestinal tract.** There have been reports[1-3] of the onset of coeliac disease during treatment of hepatitis C with interferon alfa, in some cases in combination with ribavirin. Symptoms generally resolved after interferon was discontinued and a gluten-free diet instituted.


1. Bardella MT, *et al.* Celiac disease during interferon treatment. *Ann Intern Med* 1999; **131:** 157–8.
2. Cammarota G, *et al.* Onset of coeliac disease during treatment with interferon for chronic hepatitis C. *Lancet* 2000; **356:** 1494–5.
3. Bourlière M, *et al.* Onset of coeliac disease and interferon treatment. *Lancet* 2001; **357:** 803–4.


**Effects on the hair.** A report of marked greying of the hair in a patient beginning after 5 months of treatment with interferon alfa for metastatic malignant melanoma; on completion of interferon therapy the hair regrowth returned to its normal colour.[1] Marked straightening of scalp and body hair has been reported in 2 patients following combined treatment with interferon alfa-2b or peginterferon alfa-2b and ribavirin for chronic hepatitis C.[2] In the first patient, there was also diffuse thinning of scalp hair, change in hair texture, increased greying of the hair, and eyebrow lengthening; the original curly hair began to regrow 6 months after discontinuation of treatment, but the hair abnormalities recurred on rechallenge despite switching from interferon alfa-2b to peginterferon alfa-2b. In the second patient, treatment with peginterferon alfa-2b and ribavirin was associated with straightening of scalp hair, eyebrow hair, and pubic hair.[2] Lengthening and thickening of eyelashes has also been reported in association with interferon alfa therapy.[3,4]

Reversible mild to moderate alopecia has been reported by the manufacturers.


1. Fleming CJ, MacKie RM. Alpha interferon-induced hair discolouration. *Br J Dermatol* 1996; **135:** 337–8.
2. Bessis D, *et al.* Straight hair associated with interferon-alfa plus ribavirin in hepatitis C infection. *Br J Dermatol* 2002; **147:** 392–3.
3. Hernández-Núñez A, *et al.* Trichomegaly following treatment with interferon alpha-2b. *Lancet* 2002; **359:** 1107.
4. Dikici B, *et al.* Interferon alpha and hypertrichosis of eyelashes. *Pediatr Infect Dis J* 2002; **21:** 448–9.


**Effects on hearing.** Sensorineural hearing loss was reported in 18 of 49 patients and tinnitus in 14 of 49 patients receiving interferons.[1] The effects were more common in those receiving interferon beta than in those receiving interferon alfa, and resolved in all patients on discontinuation of therapy.


1. Kanda Y, *et al.* Sudden hearing loss associated with interferon. *Lancet* 1994; **343:** 1134–5.


**Effects on the kidneys.** In a double-blind parallel-group study all of 8 renal transplant patients given, in addition to routine immunosuppression, high doses of recombinant interferon alfa (36 million units intramuscularly three times a week for 6 weeks followed by twice weekly for a further 6 weeks) had early rejection episodes which were corticosteroid-resistant; 3 also had transient nephrotic syndrome.[1] All of 8 control patients, given human albumin and saline solution, also had early rejection episodes but only one was corticosteroid-resistant. These adverse effects on the transplant contrasted with the absence of adverse effects on kidney transplants reported by other workers[2] who gave lower doses of leucocyte interferon alfa for the prophylaxis of cytomegalovirus infections. There have been a number of other reports of nephrotic syndrome associated with interferon alfa;[3-6] in one patient this was secondary to membranoproliferative glomerulonephritis.[5] Nephrotic syndrome has also occurred following interferon beta administration.[7]


1. Kramer P, *et al.* Recombinant leucocyte interferon A induces steroid-resistant acute vascular rejection episodes in renal transplant recipients. *Lancet* 1984; **i:** 989–90.
2. Hirsch MS, *et al.* Effects of interferon-alpha on cytomegalovirus reactivation syndromes in renal-transplant recipients. *N Engl J Med* 1983; **308:** 1489–93.
3. Averbuch SD, *et al.* Acute interstitial nephritis with the nephrotic syndrome following recombinant leukocyte A interferon therapy for mycosis fungoides. *N Engl J Med* 1984; **310:** 32–5.
4. Selby P, *et al.* Nephrotic syndrome during treatment with interferon. *BMJ* 1985; **290:** 1180.
5. Herrman J, Gabriel F. Membranoproliferative glomerulonephritis in a patient with hairy-cell leukemia treated with alpha-II interferon. *N Engl J Med* 1987; **316:** 112–13.
6. Endo M, *et al.* Appearance of nephrotic syndrome following interferon-α therapy in a patient with hepatitis B virus and hepatitis C virus coinfection. *Am J Nephrol* 1998; **18:** 439–43.
7. Nakao K, *et al.* Minimal change nephrotic syndrome developing during postoperative interferon-beta therapy for malignant melanoma. *Nephron* 2002; **90:** 498–500.


**Effects on lipids.** Reversible hypertriglyceridaemia has been associated with interferon alfa treatment for chronic hepatitis C.[1] Gemfibrozil reduced the hypertriglyceridaemia but lipid concentrations did not return to baseline values and interferon treatment had to be withdrawn. Reversible hypertriglyceridaemia has also occurred in patients given interferon alfa for malignant melanoma.[2]


1. Graessle D, *et al.* Alpha-interferon and reversible hypertriglyceridemia. *Ann Intern Med* 1993; **118:** 316–17.
2. Junghans V, Rünger TM. Hypertriglyceridaemia following adjuvant interferon-α treatment in two patients with malignant melanoma. *Br J Dermatol* 1999; **140:** 183–4.


**Effects on the liver.** Therapy with interferon alfa has been associated with cases of fatal liver failure,[1,2] sometimes in association with chronic hepatitis B and/or C infection.[3,4]


1. Durand JM, *et al.* Liver failure due to recombinant alpha interferon. *Lancet* 1991; **338:** 1268–9.
2. Wandl UB, *et al.* Liver failure due to recombinant alpha interferon for chronic myelogenous leukaemia. *Lancet* 1992; **339:** 123–4.
3. Marcellin P, *et al.* Fatal exacerbation of chronic hepatitis B induced by recombinant alpha-interferon. *Lancet* 1991; **338:** 828.
4. Janssen HLA, *et al.* Fatal hepatic decompensation associated with interferon alfa. *BMJ* 1993; **306:** 107–8.


**Effects on the nervous system and mental state.** Neurological effects, reported in 10 women with advanced breast cancer treated for up to 12 weeks with recombinant interferon alfa in doses of 20 million units daily or 50 million units three times weekly, included abnormal EEG patterns in all 10 patients, profound lethargy and somnolence in 6, confusion and dysphasia in 5, paraesthesia in 2, and an upper motor-neurone lesion of the legs in one.[1] These effects resolved when interferon alfa was withdrawn and all patients tolerated its reintroduction at a lower dose. Reversible EEG abnormalities were observed in a further 11 patients given interferon alfa in doses of 100 million units/m² daily for 7 days by continuous intravenous infusion,[2] in 3 patients given 5 to 10 million units/m² three times weekly by subcutaneous injection,[3] and in another patient given 4 million units/m² daily for 6 weeks.[4] Other adverse neurological effects reported with interferon alfa include delusions and hallucinations,[5] neuropsychiatric changes,[6] neuralgic amyotrophy and polyradiculopathy,[7] seizures,[8-10] spastic diplegia (in infants),[11] and severe neuropathy.[12] Mania attributed to interferon-induced hypothyroidism has been described.[13] Some of these effects were observed with doses as low as 1.5 million units[8] or 3 million units daily.[6]

Psychiatric effects including depression and suicidal ideation have been associated with interferon alfa.[14-16] Preliminary findings suggest that patients who develop depression may have higher pretreatment depression scores in psychometric tests,[17] although a prospective study of 50 patients receiving interferon alfa found that patients with pre-existing mood or anxiety disorders were no more likely than controls to interrupt therapy.[18]

SSRIs have been used successfully to both treat patients with interferon-associated depression, thus allowing therapy to be continued,[19,20] and to prevent its occurrence via pretreatment.[21]


1. Smedley H, *et al.* Neurological effects of recombinant human interferon. *BMJ* 1983; **286:** 262–4.
2. Rohatiner AZS, *et al.* Central nervous system toxicity of interferon. *Br J Cancer* 1983; **47:** 419–22.
3. Suter CC, *et al.* Electroencephalographic abnormalities in interferon encephalopathy: a preliminary report. *Mayo Clin Proc* 1984; **59:** 847–50.
4. Honigsberger L, *et al.* Neurological effects of recombinant human interferon. *BMJ* 1983; **286:** 719.
5. Tamam L, *et al.* Psychosis associated with interferon alfa therapy for chronic hepatitis B. *Ann Pharmacother* 2003; **37:** 384–7.
6. Adams F, *et al.* Neuropsychiatric manifestations of human leukocyte interferon therapy in patients with cancer. *JAMA* 1984; **252:** 938–41.
7. Bernsen PLJA, *et al.* Neuralgic amyotrophy and polyradiculopathy during interferon therapy. *Lancet* 1985; **i:** 50.
8. Janssen HLA, *et al.* Seizures associated with low-dose α-interferon. *Lancet* 1990; **336:** 1580.
9. Brouwers PJ, *et al.* Photosensitive seizures associated with interferon alpha-2a. *Ann Pharmacother* 1999; **33:** 113–14.
10. Ameen M, Russell-Jones R. Seizures associated with interferon-α treatment of cutaneous malignancies. *Br J Dermatol* 1999; **141:** 386–7.
11. Barlow CF, *et al.* Spastic diplegia as a complication of interferon alfa-2a treatment of hemangiomas of infancy. *J Pediatr* 1998; **132:** 527–30.
12. Gastineau DA, *et al.* Severe neuropathy associated with low-dose recombinant interferon-alpha. *Am J Med* 1989; **87:** 116.
13. Kingsley D. Interferon-alpha induced 'tertiary mania'. *Hosp Med* 1999; **60:** 381–2.
14. Janssen HLA, *et al.* Suicide associated with alfa-interferon therapy for chronic viral hepatitis. *J Hepatol* 1994; **21:** 241–3.
15. Renault PF, *et al.* Psychiatric complications of long-term interferon alfa therapy. *Arch Intern Med* 1987; **147:** 1577–80.
16. Adverse Drug Reactions Advisory Committee (ADRAC). Depression with interferon. *Aust Adverse Drug React Bull* 1999; **18:** 6.
17. Capuron L, Ravaud A. Prediction of the depressive effects of interferon alfa therapy by the patient's initial affective state. *N Engl J Med* 1999; **340:** 1370.
18. Parinate CM, *et al.* Treatment with interferon-α in patients with chronic hepatitis and mood or anxiety disorders. *Lancet* 1999; **354:** 131–2.
19. Levenson JL, Fallon HJ. Fluoxetine treatment of depression caused by interferon-α. *Am J Gastroenterol* 1993; **88:** 760–1.
20. Schramm TM, *et al.* Sertraline treatment of interferon-alfa-induced depressive disorder. *Med J Aust* 2000; **173:** 359–61.
21. Musselman DL, *et al.* Paroxetine for the prevention of depression induced by high-dose interferon alfa. *N Engl J Med* 2001; **344:** 961–6.


**Effects on the oral mucosa.** Painful oral ulcers, necessitating withdrawal of interferon alfa therapy, have occurred in a patient treated for chronic hepatitis.[1] Oropharyngeal lichen planus was associated with interferon alfa in another patient.[2]


1. Qaseem T, *et al.* A case report of painful oral ulcerations associated with the use of alpha interferon in a patient with chronic hepatitis due to non-A non-B non-C virus. *Mil Med* 1993; **158:** 126–7.
2. Kütting B, *et al.* Oropharyngeal lichen planus associated with interferon-α treatment for mycosis fungoides: a rare side-effect in the therapy of cutaneous lymphomas. *Br J Dermatol* 1997; **137:** 836–7.


**Effects on the respiratory system.** Treatment with interferon alfa resulted in severe exacerbation of mild asthma in 2 patients with hepatitis C.[1]


1. Bini EJ, Weinshel EH. Severe exacerbation of asthma: a new side effect of interferon-α in patients with asthma and chronic hepatitis C. *Mayo Clin Proc* 1999; **74:** 367–70.


**Effects on skeletal muscle.** Myalgia is one of the influenza-like symptoms frequently associated with interferons. Rhabdomyolysis has occurred and in one case proved fatal when associated with multiple organ failure in a patient receiving high-dose interferon alfa.[1]


1. Reinhold U, *et al.* Fatal rhabdomyolysis and multiple organ failure associated with adjuvant high-dose interferon alfa in malignant melanoma. *Lancet* 1997; **349:** 540–1.


**Effects on the skin.** Exacerbation or development of psoriasis was reported in patients given recombinant interferon alfa.[1,2] However, no such effect was seen in 7 patients given interferon gamma.[3] Exacerbation of lichen planus has also been reported[4] during interferon alfa treatment (see also Effects on the Oral Mucosa, above). Cutaneous vascular lesions with punctate telangiectasias were noted in 18 of 44 patients treated with interferon alfa-2a; lesions did not appear at the injection site.[5] Severe necrotising cutaneous lesions were reported at injection sites in a patient receiving recombinant interferon beta-1b; the lesions healed when interferon alfa-n3 was substituted.[6] However, cutaneous necrosis has also been associated with interferon alfa[7,8] and peginterferon alfa.[9] Fatal paraneoplastic pemphigus developed in a patient receiving interferon alfa-2a.[10] Cutaneous sarcoidosis has also been reported.[11] Hyperpigmentation of the skin and tongue has been described[12] in 2 dark-skinned patients during treatment with interferon alfa and ribavirin.


1. Quesada JR, Gutterman JU. Psoriasis and alpha-interferon. *Lancet* 1986; **i:** 1466–8.
2. Funk J, *et al.* Psoriasis induced by interferon-α. *Br J Dermatol* 1991; **125:** 463–5.
3. Schulze H-J, Mahrle G. Gamma interferon and psoriasis. *Lancet* 1986; **ii:** 926–7.
4. Protzer U, *et al.* Exacerbation of lichen planus during interferon alfa-2a therapy for chronic active hepatitis C. *Gastroenterology* 1993; **104:** 903–5.
5. Dreno B, *et al.* Alpha-interferon therapy and cutaneous vascular lesions. *Ann Intern Med* 1989; **111:** 95–6.
6. Sheremata WA, *et al.* Severe necrotizing cutaneous lesions complicating treatment with interferon beta-1b. *N Engl J Med* 1995; **332:** 1584.
7. Shinohara K. More on interferon-induced cutaneous necrosis. *N Engl J Med* 1995; **333:** 1222.
8. Sasseville D, *et al.* Interferon-induced cutaneous necrosis. *J Cutan Med Surg* 1999; **3:** 320–3.
9. Bessis D, *et al.* Necrotizing cutaneous lesions complicating treatment with pegylated-interferon alfa in an HIV-infected patient. *Eur J Dermatol* 2002; **12:** 99–102.
10. Kirsner RS, *et al.* Treatment with alpha interferon associated with the development of paraneoplastic pemphigus. *Br J Dermatol* 1995; **132:** 474–8.
11. Eberlein-König B, *et al.* Cutaneous sarcoid foreign body granulomas developing in sites of previous skin injury after systemic interferon-alpha treatment for chronic hepatitis C. *Br J Dermatol* 1999; **140:** 370–2.
12. Willems M, *et al.* Hyperpigmentation during interferon-alpha therapy for chronic hepatitis C virus infection. *Br J Dermatol* 2003; **149:** 390–4.


**Shock.** Fatal non-cardiogenic shock occurred following the third dose of interferon alfa-2b in a patient with malignant melanoma.[1] There were similarities to a fatal reaction reported in another patient with malignant melanoma (see under Effects on Skeletal Muscle, above).


1. Carson JJ, *et al.* Fatality and interferon α for malignant melanoma. *Lancet* 1998; **352:** 1443–4.


## Precautions

Interferons should be used with caution or avoided altogether in patients with depression or psychiatric disorders, epilepsy or other CNS diseases, renal or hepatic impairment, cardiac disorders, myelosuppression, poorly controlled thyroid dysfunction, pulmonary disease, diabetes mellitus, auto-immune diseases, coagulation disorders, or a history of these conditions. Patients with psoriasis or sarcoidosis have been reported to experience exacerbations during interferon alfa therapy.

Blood counts should be monitored, particularly in patients at high risk of myelosuppression (for example those with haematological malignancies). Assessment of cardiac function is advised before treatment is started. Patients receiving interferons who experience visual disturbances should receive an eye examination. A baseline ocular examination is recommended prior to treatment, and periodic eye examinations should be performed throughout treatment in patients predisposed to retinopathy, such as those with diabetes mellitus or hypertension. Hepatic and renal function should be monitored during treatment with interferons. Interferon alfa should be discontinued in patients with chronic hepatitis who develop liver decompensation. Patients should receive adequate fluids to maintain hydration during treatment with interferon alfa.

Interferons may affect the ability to drive or operate machinery.

Antibodies may develop to exogenous interferon that reduce its activity.

**Asthma.** For a report of severe exacerbation of asthma in patients receiving interferon alfa, see Effects on the Respiratory System, above.

**Auto-immune disorders.** A number of disorders thought to have an auto-immune component have developed or been exacerbated during therapy with interferon alfa, including diabetes mellitus,[1] auto-immune hepatitis,[2,3] multiple sclerosis,[4,5] rheumatoid arthritis,[6] systemic lupus erythematosus,[7] and thyroid disease.[8]

For mention of a possible association between interferons and the occurrence of coeliac disease, see Effects on the Gastrointestinal Tract under Adverse Effects, above.


1. Fabris P, *et al.* Development of type 1 diabetes mellitus during interferon alfa therapy for chronic HCV hepatitis. *Lancet* 1992; **340:** 548.
2. Vento S, *et al.* Hazards of interferon therapy for HBV-seronegative chronic hepatitis. *Lancet* 1989; **ii:** 926.
3. Papo T, *et al.* Autoimmune chronic hepatitis exacerbated by alpha-interferon. *Ann Intern Med* 1992; **116:** 51–3.
4. Larrey D, *et al.* Exacerbation of multiple sclerosis after the administration of recombinant human interferon alfa. *JAMA* 1989; **261:** 2065.
5. Coyle JT. Multiple sclerosis and human interferon alfa. *JAMA* 1989; **262:** 2684.
6. Chazerain P, *et al.* Rheumatoid arthritis-like disease after alpha-interferon therapy. *Ann Intern Med* 1992; **116:** 427.
7. Tolaymat A, *et al.* Systemic lupus erythematosus in a child receiving long-term interferon therapy. *J Pediatr* 1992; **120:** 429–32.
8. Fernandez-Soto L, *et al.* Increased risk of autoimmune thyroid disease in hepatitis C vs hepatitis B before, during, and after discontinuing interferon therapy. *Arch Intern Med* 1998; **158:** 1445–8.


**Breast feeding.** The American Academy of Pediatrics[1] states that there have been no reports of any clinical effect on the infant associated with the use of interferon alfa by breast-feeding mothers, and that therefore it may be considered to be usually compatible with breast feeding. It has been suggested that interferons are too large in molecular weight to transfer into breast milk in clinically relevant amounts.[2]


1. American Academy of Pediatrics. The transfer of drugs and other chemicals into human milk. *Pediatrics* 2001; **108:** 776–89. Correction. *ibid.*; 1029. Also available at: http://aappolicy.aappublications.org/cgi/content/full/pediatrics%3b108/3/776 (accessed 10/03/04)
2. Kumar AR, *et al.* Transfer of interferon alfa into human breast milk. *J Hum Lact* 2000; **16:** 226–8.


**Psychiatric disorders.** For comment on the incidence of adverse effects in patients with pre-existing mood or anxiety disorders, see Effects on the Nervous System and Mental State, above.

## Interactions

Interactions involving interferons have not been fully evaluated, but it is known that they can inhibit hepatic oxidative metabolism via cytochrome P450 enzymes and thus caution should be exercised during use with drugs metabolised in this way. Drugs likely to exacerbate the effects of interferons, such as those with myelosuppressant activity, should also be used with caution.

**ACE inhibitors.** For a report of possible synergistic haematological toxicity in patients receiving interferon alfa and ACE inhibitors, see p.845.

**Anticoagulants.** For reference to potentiation of *acenocoumarol* or *warfarin* necessitating dosage reduction in patients also receiving interferon alfa, see p.1026.

**Antineoplastics.** The manufacturer of interferon alfa-n1 has reported occasional cases of severe cytopenia with or without bone marrow aplasia in patients with chronic myeloid leukaemia who received interferon alfa-n1 immediately following *busulfan*. Caution has been advised if busulfan or *hydroxycarbamide* are reintroduced in combination with interferon alfa-n1. Severe myelosuppression has been reported in patients receiving interferon alfa-n1 with relatively high doses of *vinblastine*.

For reduction in the area under the plasma concentration-time curve for *melphalan* in patients receiving interferon alfa, see p.566.

**Antivirals.** The manufacturer of interferon alfa-n1 has reported progressive renal failure in patients receiving interferon alfa-n1 and high doses of *aciclovir*.

For a report of synergistic bone-marrow toxicity with interferon alfa and *zidovudine*, see p.660.

**Paracetamol.** Three patients experienced increases in liver enzyme values when given paracetamol 1 g two or three times daily on three days each week to coincide with the days of administration of interferon alfa; vinblastine was also given every third week.[1] Paracetamol has also been found to enhance the antiviral effect of interferon alfa in healthy subjects.[2]


1. Kellokumpu-Lehtinen P, *et al.* Hepatotoxicity of paracetamol in combination with interferon and vinblastine. *Lancet* 1989; **i:** 1143.
2. Hendrix CW, *et al.* Modulation of α-interferon's antiviral and clinical effects by aspirin, acetaminophen, and prednisone in healthy volunteers. *Antiviral Res* 1995; **28:** 121–31.


**Theophylline.** For reference to reduced clearance of theophylline in patients receiving interferon alfa, see p.802.

## Antiviral Action

Interferons are produced by virus-infected cells and confer protection on uninfected cells of the same species. They affect many cell functions demonstrating, in addition to their antiviral activity, antiproliferative and immunoregulatory properties; interferon gamma in particular is a potent macrophage-stimulating factor. These activities are considered to be interrelated. Following binding of interferons to a specific cell-surface protein, several enzyme systems appear to be activated to block viral and possibly cellular RNA development.

Studies have shown interferons to have benefit in infections with hepatitis B virus, hepatitis C virus, herpes simplex viruses, varicella-zoster virus, cytomegalovirus, rhinoviruses, and papillomaviruses.

## Pharmacokinetics

Interferons are not absorbed from the gastrointestinal tract. More than 80% of a subcutaneous or intramuscular dose of interferon alfa is absorbed. Following intramuscular injection, interferon alfa produced by recombinant techniques or from cultured leucocytes produce similar plasma concentrations, usually reaching a peak within 4 to 8 hours. Half-lives of about 3 to 8 hours have been reported. Intravenous administration produces more rapid distribution and elimination with a half-life of 2 to 3 hours. Interferon alfa does not readily cross the blood-brain barrier. Interferon alfa undergoes renal catabolism and negligible amounts of interferons are excreted in the urine.

Pegylation reduces the rate of absorption and excretion of interferon.

## Uses and Administration

The interferons have a range of activities. In addition to their action against viruses they are active against malignant neoplasms and have an immunomodulating effect. Several alfa interferons are available: interferon alfa-2a (rbe), interferon alfa-2b (rbe), alfa-n1 (lns), alfa-n3 (bls), alfacon-1 (rbe), and the pegylated interferons peginterferon alfa-2a (rbe) and peginterferon alfa-2b (rbe).

Alfa interferons are used in chronic hepatitis B (alfa-2a, alfa-2b, and alfa-n1) and chronic hepatitis C (alfa-2a and its pegylated form, alfa-2b and its pegylated form, alfa-n1, and alfacon-1); in several malignant neoplasms including AIDS-related Kaposi's sarcoma (alfa-2a and alfa-2b), hairy-cell leukaemia (alfa-2a, alfa-2b, and alfa-n1), chronic myeloid leukaemia (alfa-2a, alfa-2b, and alfa-n1), follicular lymphoma (alfa-2a and alfa-2b), cutaneous T-cell lymphoma (alfa-2a), carcinoid tumours (alfa-2b), melanoma (alfa-2a and alfa-2b), myeloma (alfa-2b), and renal cell carcinoma (alfa-2a); and in condylomata acuminata (alfa-2b and alfa-n3).

ADMINISTRATION AND DOSAGE. Dosage regimens for alfa interferons are as follows:

- **Chronic active hepatitis B.** *Interferon alfa-2a* is given in a dose of 2.5 to 5 million units/m$^2$ three times weekly by subcutaneous injection for 4 to 6 months. *Interferon alfa-2b* is given in a dose of 5 to 10 million units three times weekly for 4 to 6 months, or 5 million units daily for 16 weeks, by subcutaneous or intramuscular injection. *Interferon alfa-n1* is given either in doses of 10 to 15 million units (to a maximum of 7.5 million units/m$^2$) three times weekly for 12 weeks, or 5 to 10 million units (to a maximum of 5 million units/m$^2$) three times weekly for up to 6 months, by subcutaneous or intramuscular injection. An initial escalating dosing schedule, usually over 5 days, may improve tolerance.
- **Chronic hepatitis C.** *Interferon alfa-2a* is given in a dose of 3 to 4.5 million units three times weekly by subcutaneous or intramuscular injection for 6 months when it is used with ribavirin. In patients unable to tolerate ribavirin, interferon alfa-2a monotherapy is given either in an initial dose of 3 to 6 million units three times weekly for 6 months followed by 3 million units three times weekly for an additional 6 months, or in a dose of 3 million units three times weekly for 12 months, by subcutaneous or intramuscular injection. *Peginterferon alfa-2a* is given in a dose of 180 micrograms once weekly subcutaneously, in combination with ribavirin or as monotherapy, for up to 48 weeks. *Interferon alfa-2b* is given in a dose of 3 million units three times weekly for 6 to 12 months in combination with ribavirin or, when given as monotherapy, for 12 to 18 months, or for up to 24 months, by subcutaneous or intramuscular injection. *Peginterferon alfa-2b* is given subcutaneously in a dose of 1.5 micrograms/kg once weekly for 6 to 12 months in combination with ribavirin, or in a dose of 0.5 or 1 microgram/kg once weekly for 6 to 12 months when given as monotherapy. *Interferon alfa-n1* is given in a dose of 3 or 5 million units three times weekly for 48 weeks by subcutaneous or intramuscular injection. *Interferon alfacon-1* is given in a dose of 9 micrograms three times weekly by subcutaneous injection for 24 weeks followed by 15 micrograms three times weekly for up to 48 weeks if necessary.
- **AIDS-related Kaposi's sarcoma.** *Interferon alfa-2a* is usually given in an escalating dose of 3 million units daily for 3 days, 9 million units daily for 3 days, 18 million units daily for 3 days, and 36 million units daily, if tolerated, on days 10 to 84, by subcutaneous or intramuscular injection; thereafter the maximum tolerated dose (up to 36 million units) may be given three times weekly. *Interferon alfa-2b* is given in a dose of 30 million units/m$^2$ three times weekly, by subcutaneous or intramuscular injection.
- **Hairy-cell leukaemia.** *Interferon alfa-2a* is given in an initial dose of 3 million units daily for 16 to 24 weeks, then the same dose three times weekly, by subcutaneous or intramuscular injection. Treatment has continued for up to 20 months. *Interferon alfa-2b* is given in a dose of 2 million units/m$^2$ three times weekly by subcutaneous or intramuscular injection for up to 6 months or more. *Interferon alfa-n1* is given in an initial dose of 3 million units daily by subcutaneous or intramuscular injection, commonly for 12 to 16 weeks, then the same dose three times weekly thereafter. Alternative doses of 2 million units/m$^2$ or 0.2 million units/m$^2$ of interferon alfa-n1 have also been tried. Treatment may continue for 6 months or more.
- **Chronic myeloid leukaemia.** *Interferon alfa-2a* is given by subcutaneous or intramuscular injection in an escalating dose of 3 million units daily for 3 days, 6 million units daily for 3 days, and 9 million units daily thereafter. Patients showing a response after 12 weeks should continue treatment until a complete haematological response is achieved or for a maximum of 18 months; those who achieve a complete haematological response should continue on 9 million units daily (or a minimum of 9 million units three times weekly) in order to achieve a cytogenetic response. *Interferon alfa-2b* is given in a dose of 4 to 5 million units/m$^2$ daily by subcutaneous injection, continuing at the maximum tolerated dose to maintain remission (usually 4 to 10 million units/m$^2$ daily). *Interferon alfa-n1* is given, once the white blood cell count has been controlled by cytotoxic chemotherapy, in a dose of 3 million units daily for three weeks by subcutaneous injection. The dose is then adjusted to maintain a suitable leucocyte count (typically about 20 million units/week). Doses of 3 or 6 million units (occasionally 9 million units) daily have been used to achieve initial control of the white blood cell count.
- **Follicular lymphoma.** *Interferon alfa-2a* is given as an adjunct to chemotherapy in a dose of 6 million units/m$^2$ daily by subcutaneous or intramuscular injection on days 22 to 26 of each 28-day chemotherapy cycle. *Interferon alfa-2b* is given as an adjunct to chemotherapy in a dose of 5 million units three times weekly by subcutaneous injection for 18 months.
- **Cutaneous T-cell lymphoma.** *Interferon alfa-2a* is given by subcutaneous or intramuscular injection in an escalating dose of 3 million units daily for 3 days, then 9 million units daily for 3 days, and then 18 million units daily to complete 12 weeks of treatment. The maximum tolerated dose (up to 18 million units) is then given three times weekly for a minimum of 12 months in responding patients.
- **Carcinoid tumours.** *Interferon alfa-2b* is given in a dose of 3 to 9 million units (usually 5 million units) three times weekly by subcutaneous injection. In advanced disease, 5 million units may be given daily.
- **Melanoma.** *Interferon alfa-2a* is given in a dose of 3 million units three times weekly by subcutaneous or intramuscular injection for 18 months. Treatment should start no later than 6 weeks after surgery. *Interferon alfa-2b* is given in an initial dose of 20 million units/m$^2$ daily on 5 days each week for 4 weeks by intravenous infusion over 20 minutes, and then for maintenance 10 million units/m$^2$ three times weekly by subcutaneous injection for 48 weeks.
- **Multiple myeloma.** *Interferon alfa-2b* is given as maintenance treatment following chemotherapy induction at a dose of 3 million units/m$^2$ three times weekly by subcutaneous injection.
- **Renal cell carcinoma.** *Interferon alfa-2a* is given as an adjunct to cytotoxic chemotherapy in an escalating dose of 3 million units three times weekly for one week, then 9 million units three times weekly for one week, then 18 million units three times weekly thereafter for 3 to 12 months, by subcutaneous or intramuscular injection.
- **Condylomata acuminata.** *Interferon alfa-2b* is given in a dose of 1 million units injected into each lesion three times weekly for 3 weeks, and repeated after 12 to 16 weeks if necessary. No more than 5 lesions should be treated in each treatment course, but courses for additional lesions may run sequentially. *Interferon alfa-n3* is given in a dose of 0.25 million units per lesion twice weekly for up to 8 weeks, to a maximum of 2.5 million units in each session.

See below for further details of these as well as some other uses of alfa interferons.

◊ General reviews of interferons.


1. Baron S, *et al.* The interferons: mechanisms of action and clinical applications. *JAMA* 1991; **266:** 1375–83.
2. Finter NB, *et al.* The use of interferon-α in virus infections. *Drugs* 1991; **42:** 749–65.
3. Volz MA, Kirkpatrick CH. Interferons 1992: how much of the promise has been realised? *Drugs* 1992; **43:** 285–94.
4. Dorr RT. Interferon-α malignant and viral diseases: a review. *Drugs* 1993; **45:** 177–211.
5. Haria M, Benfield P. Interferon-α-2a: a review of its pharmacological properties and therapeutic use in the management of viral hepatitis. *Drugs* 1995; **50:** 873–96.


**Age-related macular degeneration.** In age-related macular degeneration (senile macular degeneration), a common cause of visual impairment in the elderly, there is a gradual and progressive deterioration of central vision usually affecting both eyes. Although some encouraging results[1-4] have been obtained with systemic interferon alfa-2a or alfa-2b for the treatment of choroidal neovascularisation considered unsuitable for laser therapy, adverse effects have been common and often severe and a randomised study in 481 patients showed no benefit after treatment for one year.[5]


1. Gillies MC, *et al.* Treatment of choroidal neovascularisation in age-related macular degeneration with interferon alfa-2a and alfa-2b. *Br J Ophthalmol* 1993; **77:** 759–65.
2. Kirkpatrick JNP, *et al.* Clinical experience with interferon alfa-2a for exudative age-related macular degeneration. *Br J Ophthalmol* 1993; **77:** 766–70.
3. Poliner LS, *et al.* Interferon alpha-2a for subfoveal neovascularization in age-related macular degeneration. *Ophthalmology* 1993; **100:** 1417–24.
4. Engler C, *et al.* Interferon alfa-2a modifies the course of subfoveal and juxtafoveal choroidal neovascularisation. *Br J Ophthalmol* 1994; **78:** 749–53.
5. Pharmacological Therapy for Macular Degeneration Study Group. Interferon alfa-2a in ineffective for patients with choroidal neovascularization secondary to age-related macular degeneration: results of a prospective randomized placebo-controlled clinical trial. *Arch Ophthalmol* 1997; **115:** 865–72.


**Angiomatous disease.** Encouraging responses were reported in 4 of 5 children treated with interferon alfa-2a for various angiomatous diseases.[1] Regression of haemangioma size by more than 50% was achieved in 11 of 18 infants and children given interferon alfa-2a for 1 to 5 months,[2] and in 11 of 19 children treated for at least 4 months.[3] Interferon alfa-2b has also been found to cause regression of haemangioma in 27 of 38 children treated for at least 6 months.[4] In addition, there have been reports of the successful use of interferon alfa-2b to treat infantile giant cell angioblastoma[5] and pelvic metastases of adult haemangioendothelioma of the liver.[6]

The use of interferons as anti-angiogenic agents has been reviewed.[7]


1. White CW, *et al.* Treatment of childhood angiomatous diseases with recombinant interferon alfa-2a. *J Pediatr* 1991; **118:** 59–66.
2. Deb G, *et al.* Treatment of hemangiomas of infants and babies with interferon alfa-2a: preliminary results. *Int J Pediatr Hematol/Oncol* 1996; **3:** 109–13.
3. Greinwald JH, *et al.* An update on the treatment of hemangiomas in children with interferon alfa-2a. *Arch Otolaryngol Head Neck Surg* 1999; **125:** 21–7.
4. Garmendía G, *et al.* Regression of infancy hemangiomas with recombinant IFN-α 2b. *J Interferon Cytokine Res* 2001; **21:** 31–8.
5. Marler JJ, *et al.* Successful antiangiogenic therapy of giant cell angioblastoma with interferon alfa 2b: report of 2 cases. *Pediatrics* 2002; **109:** e37. Also available at: http://pediatrics.aappublications.org/cgi/content/full/109/2/e37 (accessed 10/03/04)
6. Kayler LK, *et al.* Epithelioid hemangioendothelioma of the liver disseminated to the peritoneum treated with liver transplantation and interferon alpha-2B. *Transplantation* 2002; **74:** 128–30.
7. Lindner DJ. Interferons as antiangiogenic agents. *Curr Oncol Rep* 2002; **4:** 510–14.


**Behçet's syndrome.** Behçet's syndrome (p.1076) is usually managed with corticosteroids. Among many other drugs that have been tried, interferon alfa-2b was reported to produce beneficial responses in 3 patients with refractory ocular symptoms.[1] Encouraging results have also been obtained with interferon alfa-2a.[2,3]


1. Feron EJ, *et al.* Interferon-α2b for refractory ocular Behçet's disease. *Lancet* 1994; **343:** 1428.
2. Alpsoy E, *et al.* Interferon alfa-2a in the treatment of Behçet disease: a randomized placebo-controlled and double-blind study. *Arch Dermatol* 2002; **138:** 467–71.
3. Kötter I, *et al.* Human recombinant interferon alfa-2a for the treatment of Behçet's disease with sight threatening posterior or panuveitis. *Br J Ophthalmol* 2003; **87:** 423–31.


**Blood disorders.** Interferon alfa may be used in the management of the myeloproliferative disorders *primary (essential) thrombocythaemia*[1] (p.509) and *polycythaemia vera*[1,2] (p.508). A study in patients with a variety of chronic myeloproliferative disorders suggested that interferon alfa-2b could also be useful in the management of *myeloid metaplasia*.[3]

Paradoxically, interferon alfa has also been used with some success in patients with *thrombocytopenia* associated with hepatitis C[4-6] and with HIV infection[7] (see also HIV Infection and AIDS, below).

In addition to case reports of interferon alfa producing improvements in patients with idiopathic *hypereosinophilic syndrome*[8-10] who had not responded to corticosteroids or hydroxycarbamide, studies have also shown beneficial responses to interferon alfa alone[11] and in combination with corticosteroids or hydroxycarbamide.[12,13]

See also under Malignant Neoplasms, below.


1. Elliott MA, Tefferi A. Interferon-alpha therapy in polycythemia vera and essential thrombocythemia. *Semin Thromb Hemost* 1997; **23:** 463–72.
2. Lengfelder E, *et al.*. Interferon alpha in the treatment of polycythemia vera. *Ann Hematol* 2000; **79:** 103–9.
3. Gilbert HS. Long term treatment of myeloproliferative disease with interferon-α-2b: feasibility and efficacy. *Cancer* 1998; **83:** 1205–13.
4. Uygun A, *et al.* Interferon treatment for thrombocytopenia associated with chronic HCV infection. *Int J Clin Pract* 2000; **54:** 683–4.
5. Rajan S, Liebman HA. Treatment of hepatitis C related thrombocytopenia with interferon alpha. *Am J Hematol* 2001; **68:** 202–9.
6. Benci A, *et al.* Thrombocytopenia in patients with HCV-positive chronic hepatitis: efficacy of leucocyte interferon-α treatment. *Int J Clin Pract* 2003; **57:** 17–19.
7. Marroni M, *et al.* Interferon-α is effective in the treatment of HIV-1-related, severe, zidovudine-resistant thrombocytopenia. *Ann Intern Med* 1994; **121:** 423–9.
8. Zielinski RM, Lawrence WD. Interferon-α for the hypereosinophilic syndrome. *Ann Intern Med* 1990; **113:** 716–18.

9. Busch FW, *et al.* Alpha-interferon for the hypereosinophilic syndrome. *Ann Intern Med* 1991; **114:** 338–9.
10. Yoon T-Y, *et al.* Complete remission of hypereosinophilic syndrome after interferon-α therapy: report of a case and literature review. *J Dermatol* 2000; **27:** 110–15.
11. Butterfield JH, Gleich GJ. Interferon-α treatment of six patients with the idiopathic hypereosinophilic syndrome. *Ann Intern Med* 1994; **121:** 648–53.
12. Coutant G, *et al.* Traitement des syndromes hyperéosinophiliques à expression myeloproliferative par l'association hydroxyurée-interféron alpha. *Ann Med Interne (Paris)* 1993; **144:** 243–50.
13. Baratta L, *et al.* Favorable response to high-dose interferon-alpha in idiopathic hypereosinophilic syndrome with restrictive cardiomyopathy: case report and literature review. *Angiology* 2002; **53:** 465–70.


**Churg-Strauss syndrome.** For a report that interferon alfa may be beneficial in Churg-Strauss syndrome, see p.1078.

**Hepatitis.** Interferon alfa is the main drug used in the treatment of chronic viral hepatitis (p.618). Interferon beta has also been used. Although the response and relapse rates following treatment of chronic hepatitis with interferons have been disappointing, prolonging treatment with higher doses (if tolerated) may be beneficial.[1-3] However, in an interim analysis of a study of 29 patients with AIDS and chronic hepatitis C, escalating doses of interferon alfa did not improve response rates.[4] A meta-analysis[5] suggested that treatment with interferon alfa 3 million units three times weekly for at least 12 months had the best risk:benefit ratio for patients with chronic hepatitis C. Once-weekly peginterferon alfa has been shown to be more effective than interferon alfa given three times weekly in patients with chronic hepatitis C,[6,7] including those with cirrhosis or extensive fibrosis.[8] The use of ribavirin with interferon alfa or interferon beta[9] for the treatment of chronic hepatitis C is more effective than either drug alone with sustained responses having been recorded, and many now consider combination therapy to be the treatment of first choice.[10-14] A meta-analysis[15] and a systematic review[14] of randomised studies have concluded that combination therapy is also more effective for chronic hepatitis C in patients who had failed to respond to interferon alone or to any other previous treatment. Recent studies[16,17] have suggested that combination therapy with peginterferon alfa and ribavirin may be more effective and better tolerated than interferon alfa plus ribavirin, and a review[18] of the use of peginterferon alfa with ribavirin has also concluded that this combination was superior to interferon alfa plus ribavirin or to peginterferon alfa alone.

In hepatitis B, responses to interferon alfa can be improved by pre-treatment with corticosteroids.[19-21]

Evidence of improved long-term outcomes following treatment is accumulating. Long-term follow-up of patients has demonstrated a lower incidence of hepatocellular carcinoma in patients who had received interferons than in untreated patients.[22-26] Risk reduction is apparently greatest in patients with chronic hepatitis C and without hepatitis B infection.[26]

Interferon alfa can produce benefit in some patients with chronic hepatitis D[27] or hepatitis G.[28]

Although antivirals are generally not required in uncomplicated acute hepatitis, treatment with interferons has been shown to produce more rapid resolution of viraemia[5,29,30] and may decrease the risk of chronic hepatitis developing.[31,32] Improvements in liver function were reported in 4 patients with fulminant hepatitis A treated with interferon beta.[33]


1. Reichard O, *et al.* Two-year biochemical, virological, and histological follow-up in patients with chronic hepatitis C responding in a sustained fashion to interferon alfa-2b treatment. *Hepatology* 1995; **21:** 918–22.
2. Poynard T, *et al.* A comparison of three interferon alfa-2b regimens for the long-term treatment of chronic non-A, non-B hepatitis. *N Engl J Med* 1995; **332:** 1457–62.
3. Degos F, *et al.* Reinforced regimen of interferon alfa-2a reduces the incidence of cirrhosis in patients with chronic hepatitis C: a multicentre randomised trial. *J Hepatol* 1998; **29:** 224–32.
4. Soriano V, *et al.* A pilot study on the efficacy of escalating dosage of alpha-interferon for chronic hepatitis C in HIV-infected patients. *J Infect* 1997; **35:** 225–30.
5. Poynard T, *et al.* Meta-analysis of interferon randomized trials in the treatment of viral hepatitis C: effects of dose and duration. *Hepatology* 1996; **24:** 778–89.
6. Zeuzem S, *et al.* Peginterferon alfa-2a in patients with chronic hepatitis C. *N Engl J Med* 2000; **343:** 1666–72.
7. Perry CM, Jarvis B. Peginterferon-α-2a (40 kD): a review of its use in the management of chronic hepatitis C. *Drugs* 2001; **61:** 2263–88.
8. Heathcote EJ, *et al.* Peginterferon alfa-2a in patients with chronic hepatitis C and cirrhosis. *N Engl J Med* 2000; **343:** 1673–80.
9. Kakumu S, *et al.* A pilot study of ribavirin and interferon beta for the treatment of chronic hepatitis C. *Gastroenterology* 1993; **105:** 507–12.
10. Poynard T, *et al.* Randomised trial of interferon α2b plus ribavirin for 48 weeks or for 24 weeks versus interferon α2b plus placebo for 48 weeks for treatment of chronic infection with hepatitis C virus. *Lancet* 1998; **352:** 1426–32.
11. Davis GL, *et al.* Interferon alfa-2b alone or in combination with ribavirin for the treatment of relapse of chronic hepatitis C. *N Engl J Med* 1998; **339:** 1493–9.
12. McHutchison JG, *et al.* Interferon alfa-2b alone or in combination with ribavirin as initial treatment for chronic hepatitis C. *N Engl J Med* 1998; **339:** 1485–92.
13. Scott LJ, Perry CM. Interferon-α-2b plus ribavirin: a review of its use in the management of chronic hepatitis C. *Drugs* 2002; **62:** 507–56.
14. Kjaergard LL, *et al.* Ribavirin with or without alpha interferon for chronic hepatitis C. Available in The Cochrane Library; Issue 1. Chichester: John Wiley; 2004.
15. Cummings KJ, *et al.* Interferon and ribavirin vs interferon alone in the re-treatment of chronic hepatitis C previously nonresponsive to interferon: a meta-analysis of randomized trials. *JAMA* 2001; **285:** 193–9.
16. Manns MP, *et al.* Peginterferon alfa-2b plus ribavirin compared with interferon alfa-2b plus ribavirin for initial treatment of chronic hepatitis C: a randomised trial. *Lancet* 2001; **358:** 958–65.
17. Fried MW, *et al.* Peginterferon alfa-2a plus ribavirin for chronic hepatitis C virus infection. *N Engl J Med* 2002; **347:** 975–82.
18. Keating GM, Curran MP. Peginterferon-α-2a (40kD) plus ribavirin: a review of its use in the management of chronic hepatitis C. *Drugs* 2003; **63:** 701–30.
19. Perrillo RP, *et al.* A randomized, controlled trial of interferon alfa-2b alone and after prednisone withdrawal for the treatment of chronic hepatitis B. *N Engl J Med* 1990; **323:** 295–301.
20. Fevery J, *et al.* Efficacy of interferon alfa-2b with or without prednisone withdrawal in the treatment for chronic viral hepatitis B: a prospective double-blind Belgian-Dutch study. *J Hepatol* 1990; **11:** S108–S112.
21. Krogsgaard K, *et al.* Prednisolone withdrawal therapy enhances the effect of human lymphoblastoid interferon in chronic hepatitis B. *J Hepatol* 1996; **25:** 803–13.
22. Nishiguchi S, *et al.* Randomised trial of effects of interferon-α on incidence of hepatocellular carcinoma in chronic active hepatitis C with cirrhosis. *Lancet* 1995; **346:** 1051–5.
23. Kuwana K, *et al.* Risk factors and the effect of interferon therapy in the development of hepatocellular carcinoma: a multivariate analysis in 343 patients. *J Gastroenterol Hepatol* 1997; **12:** 149–55.
24. Imai Y, *et al.* Relation of interferon therapy and hepatocellular carcinoma in patients with chronic hepatitis C. *Ann Intern Med* 1998; **129:** 94–9.
25. Lin S-M, *et al.* Long-term beneficial effect of interferon therapy in patients with chronic hepatitis B virus infection. *Hepatol* 1999; **29:** 971–5.
26. International Interferon-α Heptocellular Carcinoma Study Group. Effect of interferon-α on progression of cirrhosis to hepatocellular carcinoma: a retrospective cohort study. *Lancet* 1998; **351:** 1535–9.
27. Farci P, *et al.* Treatment of chronic hepatitis D with interferon alfa-2a. *N Engl J Med* 1994; **330:** 88–94.
28. Tanaka E, *et al.* Effect of hepatitis G virus infection on chronic hepatitis C. *Ann Intern Med* 1996; **125:** 740–3.
29. Cammà C, *et al.* Interferon as treatment for acute hepatitis C: a meta-analysis. *Dig Dis Sci* 1996; **41:** 1248–55.
30. Quin JW. Interferon therapy for acute hepatitis C viral infection—a review by meta-analysis. *Aust N Z J Med* 1997; **27:** 611–18.
31. Omata M, *et al.* Resolution of acute hepatitis C after therapy with natural beta interferon. *Lancet* 1991; **338:** 914–15.
32. Jaeckel E, *et al.* Treatment of acute hepatitis C with interferon alfa-2b. *N Engl J Med* 2001; **345:** 1452–7.
33. Yoshiba M, *et al.* Interferon for hepatitis A. *Lancet* 1994; **343:** 288–9.


**Herpes simplex infections.** Although herpes simplex infections are commonly treated with aciclovir (see p.620), beneficial responses to interferon alfa, administered topically[1-5] or subcutaneously,[6] have been reported in genital herpes and, in combination with trifluridine[7,8] or brivudine,[9] in herpes keratitis. A systematic review[10] of interventions for herpes simplex epithelial keratitis found that interferon monotherapy had a slightly beneficial effect on dendritic epithelial keratitis, but no more than that of other antivirals and concluded that the combination of an antiviral nucleoside and interferon seemed to speed healing.

Similarly, there are case reports of improvement in herpes labialis with topical interferon alfa with trifluridine in 3 patients resistant to aciclovir, 2 of whom were also resistant to foscarnet.[11] In a comparative study[12] intramuscular interferon alfa was not superior to topical aciclovir either in treating first-episode genital herpes or in altering the frequency of recurrences. Topical application of interferon beta has also been tried in a small number of patients for the treatment of labial and genital herpes[13] and in one study,[14] it did reduce the rate of recurrence of genital herpes.


1. Friedman-Kien AE, *et al.* Treatment of recurrent genital herpes with topical alpha interferon gel combined with nonoxynol 9. *J Am Acad Dermatol* 1986; **15:** 989–94.
2. Sacks SL, *et al.* Randomized, double-blind, placebo-controlled, patient-initiated study of topical high- and low-dose interferon-α with nonoxynol-9 in the treatment of recurrent genital herpes. *J Infect Dis* 1990; **161:** 692–8.
3. Shupack J, *et al.* Topical alpha-interferon in recurrent genital herpes simplex infection. *Dermatologica* 1990; **181:** 134–8.
4. Syed TA, *et al.* Human leukocyte interferon-alpha in cream for the management of genital herpes in Asian women: a placebo-controlled, double-blind study. *J Mol Med* 1995; **73:** 141–4.
5. Syed TA, *et al.* Human leukocyte interferon-alpha in cream for the treatment of genital herpes in Asian males: a placebo-controlled, double-blind study. *Dermatology* 1995; **191:** 32–5.
6. Cardamakis E, *et al.* Treatment of recurrent genital herpes with interferon alpha-2α. *Gynecol Obstet Invest* 1998; **46:** 54–7.
7. de Koning EWJ, *et al.* Combination therapy for dendritic keratitis with human leucocyte interferon and trifluorothymidine. *Br J Ophthalmol* 1982; **66:** 509–12.
8. Sundmacher R, *et al.* Combination therapy for dendritic keratitis: high-titer α-interferon and trifluridine. *Arch Ophthalmol* 1984; **102:** 554–5.
9. van Bijsterveld OP, *et al.* Bromovinyldeoxyuridine and interferon treatment in ulcerative herpetic keratitis: a double masked study. *Br J Ophthalmol* 1989; **73:** 604–7.
10. Wilhelmus KR. Interventions for herpes simplex virus epithelial keratitis. Available in The Cochrane Library; Issue 1. Chichester: John Wiley; 2004.
11. Birch CJ, *et al.* Clinical effects and in vitro studies of trifluorothymidine combined with interferon-α for treatment of drug-resistant and -sensitive herpes simplex virus infections. *J Infect Dis* 1992; **166:** 108–12.
12. Levin MJ, *et al.* Comparison of intramuscular recombinant alpha interferon (rIFN-2A) with topical acyclovir for the treatment of first-episode herpes genitalis and prevention of recurrences. *Antimicrob Agents Chemother* 1989; **33:** 649–52.
13. Glezerman M, *et al.* Placebo-controlled trial of topical interferon in labial and genital herpes. *Lancet* 1988; **i:** 150–2.
14. Ophir J, *et al.* Effect of topical interferon-β on recurrence rates in genital herpes: a double-blind, placebo-controlled, randomized study. *J Interferon Cytokine Res* 1995; **15:** 625–31.


**HIV infection and AIDS.** The effects of interferons on the progression of AIDS (p.621) have been mixed.[1-6] Combinations of interferon alfa with antiretroviral reverse transcriptase inhibitors have produced variable responses,[7-12] with some investigators reporting enhanced[7,11] or synergistic[9] antiretroviral effects, though often at doses associated with a high incidence of adverse effects.

Interferons have been tried with some success in the management of Kaposi's sarcoma and mycobacterial infections in patients with AIDS (see below and under Interferon Gamma, p.648).

Benefit has been reported with interferon alfa in patients with HIV-associated thrombocytopenia,[13] although interferons have been reported to induce immune thrombocytopenia, and there has been a report of bleeding in a patient with idiopathic thrombocytopenic purpura (see Effects on the Blood under Adverse Effects, above).


1. Puppo F, *et al.* Low doses of alpha-interferon for the treatment of AIDS-related syndromes: a preliminary study. *Int J Immunother* 1988; **4:** 165–8.
2. Brook MG, *et al.* Anti-HIV effects of alpha-interferon. *Lancet* 1989; **i:** 42.
3. Ellis ME, *et al.* An open study of interferon in HIV-antibody-positive men. *AIDS* 1989; **3:** 851–3.
4. Lane HC, *et al.* Interferon-α in patients with asymptomatic human immunodeficiency virus (HIV) infection: a randomized placebo-controlled trial. *Ann Intern Med* 1990; **112:** 805–11.
5. Frissen PHJ, *et al.* High-dose interferon-α2a exerts potent activity against human immunodeficiency virus type 1 not associated with antitumor activity in subjects with Kaposi's sarcoma. *J Infect Dis* 1997; **176:** 811–14.
6. Katabira ET, *et al.* Lack of efficacy of low dose oral interferon alfa in symptomatic HIV-1 infection: a randomised, double blind, placebo controlled trial. *Sex Transm Infect* 1998; **74:** 265–70.
7. Berglund O, *et al.* Combined treatment of symptomatic human immunodeficiency virus type 1 infection with native interferon-α and zidovudine. *J Infect Dis* 1991; **163:** 710–15.
8. Bissuel F, *et al.* Tolerance of a triple combination therapy with zidovudine, didanosine and interferon-α in seven HIV-infected patients. *AIDS* 1995; **9:** 1285.
9. Mildvan D, *et al.* Synergy, activity and tolerability of zidovudine and interferon-alpha in patients with symptomatic HIV-1 infection: ACTG 068. *Antivir Ther* 1996; **1:** 77–88.
10. Kovacs JA, *et al.* Combination therapy with didanosine and interferon-α in human immunodeficiency virus-infected patients: results of a phase I/II trial. *J Infect Dis* 1996; **173:** 840–8.
11. Fischl MA, *et al.* Safety and antiviral activity of combination therapy with zidovudine, zalcitabine, and two doses of interferon-$α_{2a}$ in patients with HIV: AIDS Clinical Trials Group Study 197. *J Acquir Immune Defic Syndr Hum Retrovirol* 1997; **16:** 247–53.
12. Krown SE, *et al.* Phase II, randomized, open-label, community-based trial to compare the safety and activity of combination therapy with recombinant interferon-α2b and zidovudine versus zidovudine alone in patients with asymptomatic to mildly symptomatic HIV infection. *J Acquir Immune Defic Syndr Hum Retrovirol* 1999; **20:** 245–54.
13. Marroni M, *et al.* Interferon-α is effective in the treatment of HIV-1-related, severe, zidovudine-resistant thrombocytopenia. *Ann Intern Med* 1994; **121:** 423–9.


PROGRESSIVE MULTIFOCAL LEUKOENCEPHALOPATHY. Beneficial responses were reported in patients with HIV-associated progressive multifocal leucoencephalopathy following treatment with interferon alfa.[1] However, in a retrospective analysis[2] of the relative value of highly active antiretroviral therapy (HAART) and interferon alfa in the treatment of progressive multifocal leucoencephalopathy, prolonged survival associated with interferon alfa was found to be not independent of the effects of HAART and it was concluded that interferon alfa provided no additional benefit.


1. Huang SS, *et al.* Survival prolongation in HIV-associated progressive multifocal leukoencephalopathy treated with alpha-interferon: an observational study. *J Neurovirol* 1998; **4:** 324–32.
2. Geschwind MD, *et al.* The relative contributions of HAART and alpha-interferon for therapy of progressive multifocal leukoencephalopathy in AIDS. *J Neurovirol* 2001; **7:** 353–7.


**Inflammatory bowel disease.** Interferon alfa is one of many drugs that have been tried in inflammatory bowel disease (p.1243). A study[1] found that clinical remission was achieved in 26 of 28 patients with ulcerative colitis after 6 to 12 months of treatment with interferon alfa-2a. Partial remission was reported in 2 of 5 patients with Crohn's disease[2] who received interferon alfa, but in another study in 12 patients[3] interferon alfa was of no benefit. Interferon beta has also been investigated and found to be of benefit for the treatment of ulcerative colitis unresponsive to corticosteroids.[4]


1. Sümer N, Palabiyikoğlu M. Induction of remission by interferon-α in patients with chronic active ulcerative colitis. *Eur J Gastroenterol Hepatol* 1995; **7:** 597–602.
2. Davidsen B, *et al.* Tolerability of interferon alpha-2b, a possible new treatment of active Crohn's disease. *Aliment Pharmacol Ther* 1995; **9:** 75–9.
3. Gasché C, *et al.* Prospective evaluation of interferon-α in treatment of chronic active Crohn's disease. *Dig Dis Sci* 1995; **40:** 800–4.
4. Musch E, *et al.* Induction and maintenance of clinical remission by interferon-β in patients with steroid-refractory active ulcerative colitis—an open long-term pilot trial. *Aliment Pharmacol Ther* 2002; **16:** 1233–9.


**Kaposi's sarcoma.** The various treatments used for Kaposi's sarcoma are discussed on p.524. Interferon alfa has been used in AIDS-related Kaposi's sarcoma[1-9] and in patients with the classical, nonepidemic form.[10-13] There have been several small studies of interferon alfa in patients with immunodeficiency- or AIDS-related Kaposi's sarcoma.[1-3] Results have been mixed. A review[8] concluded that the best responses to interferon alfa were achieved in asymptomatic patients with relatively high CD4+ T lymphocyte counts (200 cells/microlitre or better) and no prior opportunistic infections. However, the adverse effects which occur at the doses required limit the tolerability of long-term administration.

Interferons have also been tried in AIDS-related Kaposi's sarcoma in combination with other drugs including antineoplastics (with disappointing results)[9] and zidovudine (complete or partial tumour response and/or evidence of antiviral effects in some patients).[4-7] Low doses of interferons in combination with nucleoside reverse transcriptase inhibitors have been used for AIDS-associated Kaposi's sarcoma;[9] efficacy and toxicity of these combinations have been reported to be dose-related.[14,15]


1. de Wit R, *et al.* Clinical and virological effects of high-dose recombinant interferon-α in disseminated AIDS-related Kaposi's sarcoma. *Lancet* 1988; **ii:** 1214–17.
2. Lane HC, *et al.* Anti-retroviral effects of interferon-α in AIDS-associated Kaposi's sarcoma. *Lancet* 1988; **ii:** 1218–22.
3. Sulis E, *et al.* Interferon administered intralesionally in skin and oral cavity lesions in heterosexual drug addicted patients with AIDS-related Kaposi's sarcoma. *Eur J Cancer Clin Oncol* 1989; **25:** 759–61.
4. Kovacs JA, *et al.* Combined zidovudine and interferon-α therapy in patients with Kaposi sarcoma and the acquired immunodeficiency syndrome (AIDS). *Ann Intern Med* 1989; **111:** 280–7.
5. Brockmeyer NH, *et al.* Regression of Kaposi's sarcoma and improvement of performance status by a combined interferon β and zidovudine therapy in AIDS patients. *J Invest Dermatol* 1989; **92:** 776.
6. Edlin BR, *et al.* Interferon-alpha plus zidovudine in HIV infection. *Lancet* 1989; **i:** 156.
7. Krown SE, *et al.* Interferon-α with zidovudine: safety, tolerance, and clinical and virologic effects in patients with Kaposi sarcoma associated with the acquired immunodeficiency syndrome (AIDS). *Ann Intern Med* 1990; **112:** 812–21.
8. Krown SE. Interferon and other biologic agents for the treatment of Kaposi's sarcoma. *Hematol Oncol Clin North Am* 1991; **5:** 311–22.
9. Northfelt DW. Treatment of Kaposi's sarcoma: current guidelines and future perspectives. *Drugs* 1994; **48:** 569–82.
10. Killeen RB, Marsh RD. α-Interferon for Kaposi's sarcoma in HIV-negative, non-homosexual man. *Lancet* 1991; **337:** 309–10.
11. Trattner A, *et al.* The therapeutic effect of intralesional interferon in classical Kaposi's sarcoma. *Br J Dermatol* 1993; **129:** 590–3.
12. Shimizu S, *et al.* Classic (non-AIDS-related) Kaposi's sarcoma in a Japanese patient, successfully treated with alpha-2b-interferon. *Br J Dermatol* 1995; **133:** 332–4.
13. Deichmann M, *et al.* Non-human immunodeficiency virus Kaposi's sarcoma can be effectively treated with low-dose interferon-α despite the persistence of herpesvirus-8. *Br J Dermatol* 1998; **139:** 1052–4.
14. Shepherd FA, *et al.* Prospective randomized trial of two dose levels of interferon alfa with zidovudine for the treatment of Kaposi's sarcoma associated with human immunodeficiency virus infection: a Canadian HIV Clinical Trials Network study. *J Clin Oncol* 1998; **16:** 1736–42.
15. Krown SE, *et al.* Efficacy of low-dose interferon with antiretroviral therapy in Kaposi's sarcoma: a randomized phase II AIDS clinical trials group study. *J Interferon Cytokine Res* 2002; **22:** 295–303.


**Malignant neoplasms.** Many reports have been published on the effects of interferons on various neoplasms; most have involved interferon alfa.

Interferons have become established in the treatment of a few malignant disorders, notably hairy-cell leukaemia (but see p.508), Kaposi's sarcoma (see above), and chronic myeloid leukaemia (p.507).[1-6] Alfa interferons may improve the duration of remission in multiple myeloma,[7-10] but not necessarily survival.[8,11] Combination therapy including interferons has also been used in indolent low-grade non-Hodgkin's lymphoma (p.510) and interferon alfa has been used alone to maintain remission. In renal cell carcinoma (p.518) response to interferon alfa in combination with interleukin-2 has been promising, but toxicity high;[12,13] interferon alfa alone produces very modest benefit.[14] Beneficial responses have also been reported in a number of other neoplasms including melanoma (p.522); carcinoid tumours[15,16] (p.504); myelodysplasia; cutaneous T cell lymphomas including mycosis fungoides (p.511); and in meningioma.[17] Interferons have been administered locally as an adjunct to surgery for superficial bladder tumours[18] and intralesionally in basal cell carcinoma[19-21] and also for keloid scars.[22,23] Combination of interferon alfa with fluorouracil has been tried in inoperable colorectal cancer but does not appear to be more beneficial than fluorouracil alone.[24] Interferon alfa in combination with zidovudine has produced encouraging results in adult T-cell leukaemia-lymphoma.[25]


1. The Italian Cooperative Study Group on Chronic Myeloid Leukemia. Interferon alfa-2a as compared with conventional chemotherapy for the treatment of chronic myeloid leukemia. *N Engl J Med* 1994; **330:** 820–5.
2. Schofield JR, *et al.* Low doses of interferon-α are as effective as higher doses in inducing remissions and prolonging survival in chronic myeloid leukemia. *Ann Intern Med* 1994; **121:** 736–44.
3. Allan NC, *et al.* UK Medical Research Council randomised, multicentre trial of interferon-αnl for chronic myeloid leukaemia: improved survival irrespective of cytogenetic response. *Lancet* 1995; **345:** 1392–7.
4. Kantarjian HM, *et al.* Prolonged survival in chronic myelogenous leukemia after cytogenetic response to interferon-α therapy. *Ann Intern Med* 1995; **122:** 254–61.
5. Talpaz M, Kantarjian H. Low-dose interferon-α in chronic myeloid leukemia. *Ann Intern Med* 1995; **122:** 728.
6. Mahon F-X, *et al.* Response to IFNα in myelogenous leukaemia. *Lancet* 1996; **347:** 57–8.
7. Mandelli F, *et al.* Maintenance treatment with recombinant interferon alfa-2b in patients with multiple myeloma responding to conventional induction chemotherapy. *N Engl J Med* 1990; **322:** 1430–4.
8. Nordic Myeloma Study Group. Interferon-α2b added to melphalan-prednisone for initial and maintenance therapy in multiple myeloma: a randomized, controlled trial. *Ann Intern Med* 1996; **124:** 212–22.
9. Fritz E, Ludwig H. Interferon-α treatment in multiple myeloma: meta-analysis of 30 randomised trials among 3948 patients. *Ann Oncol* 2000; **11:** 1427–36.
10. Myeloma Trialists' Collaborative Group. Interferon as therapy for multiple myeloma: an individual patient data overview of 24 randomized trials and 4012 patients. *Br J Haematol* 2001; **113:** 1020–34.
11. Österborg A, *et al.* Natural interferon-α in combination with melphalan/prednisone versus melphalan/prednisone in the treatment of multiple myeloma stages II and III: a randomized study from the myeloma group of central Sweden. *Blood* 1993; **81:** 1428–34.
12. Besana C, *et al.* Treatment of advanced renal cell cancer with sequential intravenous recombinant interleukin-2 and subcutaneous α-interferon. *Eur J Cancer* 1994; **30A** 1292–8.
13. Négrier S, *et al.* Intensive regimen of cytokines with interleukin-2 and interferon alfa-2b in selected patients with metastatic renal carcinoma. *J Immunother* 1995; **17:** 62–8.
14. Medical Research Council Renal Cancer Collaborators. Interferon-α and survival in metastatic renal carcinoma: early results of a randomised controlled study. *Lancet* 1999; **353:** 14–17.
15. Öberg K, *et al.* Treatment of malignant carcinoid tumors: a randomized controlled study of streptozocin plus 5-FU and human leukocyte interferon. *Eur J Cancer Clin Oncol* 1989; **25:** 1475–9.
16. Kölby L, *et al.* Randomized clinical trial of the effect of interferon α on survival in patients with disseminated midgut carcinoid tumours. *Br J Surg* 2003; **90:** 687–93.
17. Wöber-Bingöl Ç, *et al.* Interferon-alfa-2b for meningioma. *Lancet* 1995; **345:** 331.
18. Brown DH, *et al.* Interferons and bladder cancer. *Urol Clin North Am* 2000; **27:** 171–8.
19. Pizarro A, Fonseca E. Treatment of basal cell carcinoma with intralesional interferon alpha-2b: evaluation of efficacy with emphasis on tumours located on "H" zone on face. *Eur J Dermatol* 1994; **4:** 287–90.
20. LeGrice P, *et al.* Treatment of basal cell carcinoma with intralesional interferon alpha-2A. *N Z Med J* 1995; **108:** 206–7.
21. Kowalzick L, *et al.* Intralesional recombinant interferon beta-1a in the treatment of basal cell carcinoma: results of an open-label multicentre study. *Eur J Dermatol* 2002; **12:** 558–61.
22. Granstein RD, *et al.* A controlled trial of intralesional recombinant interferon-γ in the treatment of keloidal scarring. *Arch Dermatol* 1990; **126:** 1295–1302.
23. Larrabee WF, *et al.* Intralesional interferon gamma treatment for keloids and hypertrophic scars. *Arch Otolaryngol Head Neck Surg* 1990; **116:** 1159–62.
24. Thirion P, *et al.* Alpha-interferon does not increase the efficacy of 5-fluorouracil in advanced colorectal cancer: Meta-analysis Group in Cancer. *Br J Cancer* 2001; **84:** 611–20.
25. Gill PS, *et al.* Treatment of adult T-cell leukemia-lymphoma with a combination of interferon alfa and zidovudine. *N Engl J Med* 1995; **332:** 1744–8.


**Mycobacterial infections.** For the use of interferon alfa in mycobacterial infections, see Interferon Gamma, p.648.

**Skin disorders.** For the use of interferon alfa in skin disorders associated with raised IgE concentrations, see Interferon Gamma, p.648.

**Warts.** Various interferons have been tried by various routes in the treatment of anogenital warts (condylomata acuminata) (p.1139).

*Intralesional* injection has been used to ensure relatively high concentrations of interferon in the wart but the occurrence of systemic adverse effects demonstrates that there is absorption from this site. Complete responses were reported[1] in 36% of patients receiving intralesional interferon alfa-2b compared with 17% receiving placebo, and a corresponding overall reduction in the affected area of 62.4% compared with 1.2% respectively. However, follow-up was not sufficiently long to comment on relapse rates. Another study[2] found similar responses using interferons alfa-2b, alfa-n1, or beta in patients with refractory warts, with complete responses in 47% of patients receiving intralesional interferons compared with 22% of patients receiving placebo. A study[3] evaluating two different doses of intralesional interferon beta given three times weekly for three weeks reported complete responses in 63% of lesions injected with 1 million units compared with 38% of lesions injected with 33 000 units. Good responses have also been reported in patients with both refractory and recurrent warts treated with intralesional interferon alfa-n3.[4] Relapses were delayed and fewer warts recurred in patients who had received interferon rather than placebo. Intralesional interferon alfa-2b given in combination with podophyllum was more effective that podophyllum alone,[5] although about 66% of patients in each group subsequently relapsed.

*Topical* application of interferon alfa has also been reported to be more effective than podophyllotoxin.[6,7] Interferon beta has also been applied topically following removal of warts surgically.[8]

Theoretically, *systemic* administration should have advantages in controlling subclinical infections and reducing relapses. However, responses to subcutaneous interferon alfa have generally been disappointing[9-11] although responses comparable with cauterisation and a reduction in relapse rates with either subcutaneous or intramuscular interferon alfa-2b have been obtained.[12] Information on the use of systemic interferons as an adjunct to conventional therapy is scarce but a study in 97 patients[13] with recurrent warts found no difference in either response or relapse rates in patients receiving cryotherapy with subcutaneous interferon alfa or cryotherapy alone. A study comparing subcutaneous interferon alfa, beta, and gamma in combination with cryotherapy found no significant difference in response rate, although patients receiving interferon beta or gamma developed new warts at a lower frequency.[14]


1. Eron LJ, *et al.* Interferon therapy for condylomata acuminata. *N Engl J Med* 1986; **315:** 1059–64.
2. Reichman RC, *et al.* Treatment of condyloma acuminatum with three different interferons administered intralesionally: a double-blind, placebo-controlled trial. *Ann Intern Med* 1988; **108:** 675–9.
3. Monsonego J, *et al.* Randomised double-blind trial of recombinant interferon-beta for condyloma acuminatum. *Genitourin Med* 1996; **72:** 111–14.
4. Friedman-Kien AE, *et al.* Natural interferon alfa for treatment of condylomata acuminata. *JAMA* 1988; **259:** 533–8.
5. Douglas JM, *et al.* A randomized trial of combination therapy with intralesional interferon $\alpha_{2b}$ and podophyllin versus podophyllin alone for the therapy of anogenital warts. *J Infect Dis* 1990; **162:** 52–9.
6. Syed TA, *et al.* Human leukocyte interferon-alpha versus podophyllotoxin in cream for the treatment of genital warts in males: a placebo-controlled, double-blind, comparative study. *Dermatology* 1995; **191:** 129–32.
7. Syed TA, *et al.* Management of genital warts in women with human leukocyte interferon-α vs podophyllotoxin in cream: a placebo-controlled, double-blind, comparative study. *J Mol Med* 1995; **73:** 255–8.
8. Gross G, *et al.* Recombinant interferon beta gel as an adjuvant in the treatment of recurrent genital warts: results of a placebo-controlled double-blind study in 120 patients. *Dermatology* 1998; **196:** 330–4.
9. Reichman RC, *et al.* Treatment of condyloma acuminatum with three different interferon-α preparations administered parenterally: a double-blind, placebo-controlled trial. *J Infect Dis* 1990; **162:** 1270–6.
10. Condylomata International Collaborative Study Group. Recurrent condylomata acuminata treated with recombinant interferon alfa-2a: a multicenter double-blind placebo-controlled clinical trial. *JAMA* 1991; **265:** 2684–7.
11. Condylomata International Collaborative Study Group. Recurrent condylomata acuminata treated with recombinant interferon alpha-2a: a multicenter double-blind placebo-controlled clinical trial. *Acta Derm Venereol (Stockh)* 1993; **73:** 223–6.
12. Panici PB, *et al.* Randomized clinical trial comparing systemic interferon with diathermocoagulation in primary multiple and widespread anogenital condyloma. *Obstet Gynecol* 1989; **74:** 393–7.
13. Eron LJ, *et al.* Recurrence of condylomata acuminata following cryotherapy is not prevented by systemically administered interferon. *Genitourin Med* 1993; **69:** 91–3.
14. Bonnez W, *et al.* A randomized, double-blind, placebo-controlled trial of systemically administered interferon-α, -β, or -γ in combination with cryotherapy for the treatment of condyloma acuminatum. *J Infect Dis* 1995; **171:** 1081–9.


## Preparations

**Proprietary Preparations** (details are given in Part 3)

***Arg.:*** Avirostat; Bioferon; INF; Infostat; Inmutag; Intron A; Intron A Peg; Roferon-A; ***Austral.:*** Intron A; PegIntron; Roferon-A; ***Austria:*** Berofor†; IntronA; Roferon-A; Wellferon†; ***Belg.:*** Infergen; Introna; PegIntron; Roferon-A; ***Braz.:*** Beferon; Blauferon; Inter IF†; Intron A; Pegasys; PegIntron; Roferon-A; Wellferon†; ***Canad.:*** Infergen; Intron A; PegIntron; Roferon-A; Wellferon†; ***Chile:*** Intermax-Alpha; Intron A; Introna; Pegasys; PegIntron; Roferon-A; ***Denm.:*** Introna; PegIntron; Roceron-A; ***Fin.:*** Finnferon-Alpha; Introna; PegIntron; Roferon-A; Wellferon†; ***Fr.:*** Infergen; Introna; Laroferon†; Pegasys; Roferon-A; Viraferon; ViraferonPeg; ***Ger.:*** Cellferon†; Inferax; Introna; PegIntron; Roferon-A; ***Gr.:*** Infergen; Intron A; PegIntron; Roferon-A; ***Hong Kong:*** Intron A; PegIntron; Roferon-A; Wellferon†; ***India:*** Roferon-A; ***Irl.:*** Introna; Pegasys; PegIntron; Roferon-A; ViraferonPeg; ***Israel:*** Intron A; PegIntron; Roferon-A; Wellferon†; ***Ital.:*** Alfaferone; Alfater; Biaferone; Cilferon-A; Haimaferone; Humoferon; Infergen; Introna; Isiferone; PegIntron; Roferon-A; Wellferon; ***Jpn:*** OIF; Roferon-A; Sumiferon; ***Malaysia:*** Intron A; ***Mex.:*** Alferon; Altemol; Intron A; Lemeron; Roferon-A; Urifron; Viraferon; Wellferon†; ***Neth.:*** Infergen; Intron A; PegIntron; Roferon-A; ***Norw.:*** IntronA; PegIntron; Roceron; ***NZ:*** Intron A; Pegasys; Roferon-A; Wellferon†; ***Port.:*** Intron A; Pegasys; PegIntron; Roferon-A; ***S.Afr.:*** Intron A; Roferon-A; ***Singapore:*** Intron A; Roferon-A; Wellferon†; ***Spain:*** Intron A; PegIntron; Roferon-A; Viraferon†; Wellferon†; ***Swed.:*** Introna; Multiferon; PegIntron; Roferon-A; Wellferon†; ***Switz.:*** Intron A; Pegasys; Roferon-A; Wellferon†; ***Thai.:*** Bioferon; Introna; Roferon-A; Wellferon; ***UK:*** Introna; Pegasys; PegIntron; Roferon-A; Viraferon; ViraferonPeg; ***USA:*** Alferon N; Infergen; Intron A; Pegasys; PegIntron; Roferon-A; Wellferon†.

**Multi-ingredient:** ***Arg.:*** Bioferon Hepakit; Rebetron; ***Austral.:*** Pegatron; Rebetron; ***Canad.:*** Rebetron; ***Mex.:*** Hepatron C; ***S.Afr.:*** Rebetron; ***Switz.:*** Intron A/Rebetol; ***USA:*** Rebetron.

---

# Interferon Beta *(BAN, rINN)*

IFN-β; Interferon-β; Interferón beta; SH-Y-579A (interferon beta-1b).

*CAS — 74899-71-1 (interferon beta); 145258-61-3 (interferon beta-1a); 145155-23-3 (interferon beta-1b); 90598-63-3 (interferon beta-1b).*

*ATC — L03AB02 (natural); L03AB07 (1a); L03AB08 (1b).*

NOTE. Interferon beta was previously known as fibroblast interferon.

Interferon beta-1a and Interferon beta-1b are both *USAN.*

**Nomenclature.** Interferon beta may be derived from fibroblasts as well as through recombinant DNA technology. Sub-species of the human beta gene produce interferon beta with protein variants designated by a number (as in interferon beta-1). Interferon beta-1 is further qualified by a letter to indicate the amino-acid sequences at positions 1 and 17, and to indicate whether or not glycosylation is present. Interferon beta-1a has methionine at position 1 and cysteine at 17 and is glycosylated at position 80. Interferon beta-1b has serine at position 17 and is not glycosylated.

The name may be further elaborated on the label by approved sets of initials in parentheses to indicate the method of production: (rch) indicates production from genetically engineered Chinese hamster ovary cells; (rbe) indicates production from bacteria (*Escherichia coli*) genetically modified by recombinant DNA technology.

## Adverse Effects

As for interferons in general (see Interferon Alfa, p.640).

Severe local reactions at injection sites, including tissue necrosis, have been reported. Menstrual irregularities have been associated with interferon beta administration. Syncope and muscle hypertonia have been reported, usually early in a course of treatment.

◊ Reviews.

1. Bayas A, Rieckmann P. Managing the adverse effects of interferon-beta therapy in multiple sclerosis. *Drug Safety* 2000; **22:** 149–59.

**Auto-immune disorders.** Subacute cutaneous lupus erythematosus has been reported in a patient following administration of interferon beta.[1]

1. Nousari HC, *et al.* Subacute cutaneous lupus erythematosus associated with interferon beta-1a. *Lancet* 1998; **352:** 1825–6.

**Effects on the cardiovascular system.** Severe Raynaud's syndrome developed in a patient during treatment with interferon beta.[1] Symptoms subsided once interferon beta was stopped.

1. Linden D. Severe Raynaud's phenomenon associated with interferon-β treatment for multiple sclerosis. *Lancet* 1998; **352:** 878–9.

**Effects on hearing.** For a report of sensorineural hearing loss in patients receiving interferon beta, see Interferon Alfa, p.641.

**Effects on the liver.** Hepatotoxicity, sometimes severe and in rare cases fatal, has been reported with interferons and its association specifically with the use of interferon-beta-1a in multiple sclerosis patients has been reviewed.[1]

1. Francis GS, *et al.* Hepatic reactions during treatment of multiple sclerosis with interferon-β-1a: incidence and clinical significance. *Drug Safety* 2003; **26:** 815–27.

**Effects on the skin.** For a report of severe necrotising cutaneous lesions at injection sites in a patient receiving interferon beta, see Interferon Alfa, p.642. See also Auto-immune Disorders, above for a report of cutaneous lupus erythematosus associated with interferon beta.

## Precautions

As for interferons in general (see Interferon Alfa, p.642).

Interferon beta in high doses is fetotoxic and abortifacient in *primates* and should be avoided during pregnancy.

## Interactions

As for interferons in general (see Interferon Alfa, p.642).

## Antiviral Action

As for interferons in general (see Interferon Alfa, p.642).

## Pharmacokinetics

Interferons are not absorbed from the gastrointestinal tract. About 50% of a subcutaneous or intramuscular dose of interferon beta is absorbed. For some formulations of interferon beta-1a, bioavailability and area under the plasma concentration-time curves are equivalent for subcutaneous and intramuscular administration, but for others, intramuscular administration produces higher values than subcutaneous administration. Peak serum concentrations of interferon beta-1a have been reported to be reached 3 hours after subcutaneous injection and between 5 and 15 hours after intramuscular injection, and those for beta-1b have been reported to be reached 1 to 8 hours after subcutaneous injection. The elimination half-life for interferon beta-1a is about 10 hours.

## Uses and Administration

Interferon beta has antiviral and immunomodulating activities. It is mainly used in the management of multiple sclerosis, although its mode of action is unclear.

**Interferon beta-1a** is given in relapsing-remitting multiple sclerosis in a dose dependent upon the formulation used:

- *Avonex* (Biogen) is given in a dose of 6 million units (30 micrograms) once weekly by intramuscular injection.
- *Rebif* (Serono) is given in an escalating dose over 4 weeks, to 12 million units (44 micrograms) three times weekly by subcutaneous injection, or to 6 million units (22 micrograms) three times weekly by subcutaneous injection in patients unable to tolerate the higher dose.

*Avonex* is also indicated for the treatment of patients who have experienced a single demyelinating event with an active inflammatory process if it is sufficiently severe to warrant intravenous corticosteroids.

**Interferon beta-1b** is given in both relapsing-remitting and in secondary progressive multiple sclerosis in a dose of 8 million units (250 micrograms) on alternate days by subcutaneous injection.

◊ Reviews.

1. Goodkin DE. Interferon beta-1b. *Lancet* 1994; **344:** 1057–60.

**Guillain-Barré syndrome.** Rapid improvement in motor function was reported during administration of interferon beta-1a in a patient with Guillain-Barré syndrome associated with *Campylobacter jejuni* infection.[1] However, the relative contributions of interferon therapy and a course of plasma exchange which immediately preceded it could not be assessed.[2]

1. Créange A, *et al.* Treatment of Guillain-Barré syndrome with interferon-β. *Lancet* 1998; **352:** 368.
2. Sawaya RA. Interferon beta for Guillain-Barré syndrome. *Lancet* 1998; **352:** 1550–1.

**Hepatitis.** For mention of the use of interferon beta in chronic hepatitis, see Interferon Alfa, p.644. See also Effects on the Liver, under Adverse Effects, above.

**Herpes simplex infections.** For a report of the use of interferon beta in small numbers of patients for the treatment of labial and genital herpes, see Interferon Alfa, p.644.

**Multiple sclerosis.** Multiple sclerosis (MS) is characterised by patches of demyelination that can be scattered throughout the white matter of the CNS, but are usually localised in the brain stem, periventricular areas, the optic nerve, and the cervical spinal cord. The cause is unknown but may have an immunological basis. Symptoms may vary according to the areas affected but typically include weakness, paraesthesias, vision loss, incoordination, and bladder dysfunction. Most patients improve to some degree after the initial attack but the course and severity of the disease are unpredictable. The disease is classified according to the clinical course. In many patients the disease follows a relapsing-remitting course in which there are recurrent exacerbations followed by clinical improvement and relatively long periods of remission. The patients may subsequently develop progressive neurological deterioration, categorised as secondary progressive disease. About 10% of patients have gradual continuous deterioration, classified as primary progressive disease. In a few patients the disease is described as progressive relapsing when there is little or no improvement after each exacerbation and disability slowly increases.

The evaluation of therapy for any disease such as MS that has spontaneous remissions is difficult[1-5] and, until relatively recently, there has been little convincing evidence that any treatment affects the outcome of the disease. Despite the increasing use of disease-modifying treatment, **symptomatic treatment** aimed at the management of spasticity, pain, fatigue, and bladder dysfunction remains important. Baclofen, dantrolene, diazepam, and tizanidine are the usual drugs given for spasticity (see p.1386). There is also some evidence to suggest that cannabis and individual cannabinoids, including synthetic cannabinoids such as nabilone, may improve spasticity.[6] Patients with MS can suffer from a number of different types of pain, including pain from spasticity, and therapy must be individualised for each specific pain syndrome (see Choice of Analgesic, p.2). Pain, spasms, and spasticity have responded to gabapentin in preliminary studies.[7-12] A review has noted, however, that the absolute and comparative efficacy and tolerability of anti-spasticity drugs is poorly documented.[13] Paraesthesia and dysaesthesia, which can be common, may respond to tricyclic antidepressants or antiepileptics. Amantadine may alleviate fatigue associated with MS. Treatment of bladder dysfunction may include an alpha blocker such as phenoxybenzamine and appropriate parasympathomimetic or antimuscarinic therapy to control bladder contractions (see Urinary Incontinence and Retention, p.476). Fampridine and 3,4-diaminopyridine have been reported to produce beneficial symptomatic responses such as improvement in walking, dexterity, and vision, possibly as a result of potassium-channel blocking activity but a systematic review[14] was unable to come to a conclusion about safety and efficacy, noting that publication bias posed a problem in this area.

A wide range of drugs with immunological actions has been tried in the **treatment** of MS itself with the aim of improving recovery from acute attacks, preventing or decreasing the number of relapses, and halting the progressive stage of the disease.

*Corticosteroids* are used for their immunomodulatory and anti-inflammatory effects in acute relapses. Corticosteroid therapy reduces the duration of the relapse and accelerates recovery, but it is not known whether it alters the course of the disease in the long term.[15] Methylprednisolone has superseded corticotropin and prednisolone as the drug of choice. Methylprednisolone is usually given intravenously in high doses (typically 1 g daily) for 3 to 5 days, sometimes followed by a tapering dose of oral prednisolone. Doses of up to 2 g daily have been tried.[16] In patients with acute optic neuritis (frequently the first manifestation of multiple sclerosis), methylprednisolone delayed the onset of other symptoms of multiple sclerosis,[17] although the effect was not sustained beyond 2 years.[18] Beneficial responses have also been reported with oral methylprednisolone at doses including 500 mg once daily for 5 days followed by a tapering dose over 10 days[19] and 48 mg once daily for 7 days followed by a tapering dose over 14 days.[20]

In patients with primary progressive disease, the benefits of short-course methylprednisolone lasted no longer than 3 months[21] although, in patients with secondary progressive disease, a preliminary study has suggested that progression may be delayed by intermittent high-dose methylprednisolone therapy.[22]

*Interferon beta* has become established for treatment of relapsing-remitting disease in selected patients, and is also used in secondary progressive disease. Many early studies using interferons were conducted before the immunomodulating effects of interferons were understood, but they did demonstrate that natural interferon beta could reduce exacerbations by inhibiting interferon gamma which in itself appeared to act as a disease activator. Natural interferon alfa alone was found to produce little or no benefit.[23] Subsequent studies in patients with relapsing-remitting disease have used recombinant interferon beta and patients treated with interferon *beta-1b* have obtained a reduction in the rate and severity of exacerbations;[24,25] there was also evidence from magnetic resonance imaging[26] of reduced disease activity and burden. Encouraging results have also been obtained with interferon beta-1b in patients with secondary progressive disease.[27] Similar results in relapsing-remitting disease have been obtained with interferon *beta-1a*;[28-30] although there has been some suggestion that some interferon beta-1a products might be more effective than others,[31] this remains a matter of controversy. A prospective, randomised, multicentre study[32] comparing the different frequencies of dosing with interferon beta-1a and beta-1b has concluded that high-dose interferon beta-1b given on alternate days is more effective in relapsing-remitting disease than once-weekly interferon beta-1a. No effect has been demonstrated on disability progression from use of interferon beta-1a in secondary progressive disease.[33] There may be some benefit from interferon beta in patients presenting with a first demyelinating event, or other manifestation of early disease, in terms of subsequent development of definitive disease.[34,35] However, the effect of interferon beta on the progression of disability remains to be determined. Concern has been expressed over the detection of neutralising antibodies against interferon in up to 46% of patients.[36-38]

Results of studies with *glatiramer* have shown that it can reduce the number of relapses and may produce some improvements in neurological disability. These benefits are produced in a different way from those gained with interferon beta leading to expectations of possible treatment with both drugs.

Guidelines[39] have been produced by the Association of British Neurologists for the use of interferon beta and of glatiramer in selected patients, although a systematic review[40] did not support the routine use of glatiramer.

Intermittent intravenous *normal immunoglobulins* might also be able to reduce the frequency of exacerbations and slow disease progression without producing troublesome adverse effects.[41]

Although some studies have shown modest benefits with *immunosuppressants*, the general conclusions of large controlled studies have tended to be that any slight benefits of existing therapies with immunosuppressants such as azathioprine, ciclosporin, or cyclophosphamide are outweighed by the toxicity of the doses required to have an effect.[42-48] However, it has been pointed out that in terms of relapse reduction azathioprine appeared to be as effective as newer treatments such as interferon beta.[49] Studies with cladribine suggested that it might provide some benefit at well-tolerated doses,[50,51] and low-dose methotrexate might also slow progression of chronic disease and provide a relatively non-toxic treatment option.[52] Mitoxantrone has also been studied[53-55] but its use may be limited by dose-related cardiotoxicity. Benefit has been reported with *roquinimex* (but see p.583).

*Other immunological approaches* evaluated have included the use of monoclonal antibodies such as CD4 antibodies, altered peptide ligands from myelin basic protein, and T-cell vaccination.[56] Combined total lymphoid irradiation with low-dose corticosteroid therapy has also been investigated and may slow progression of disease.[57]

A review of the relationship between *dietary fat* and MS concluded that the role of lipids remained to be proven.[58] Some studies found a reduction of severity and duration of relapse in patients taking linoleic acid supplements (as sunflower oil)[59] while another reported benefit in patients who limited their intake of dietary saturated fatty acids and supplemented their diet with polyunsaturated fatty acids.[60] Despite a lack of firm evidence many patients with MS practice dietary modification and take supplements of omega-6 group polyunsaturated acids, sunflower oil, evening primrose oil, fish oils, and omega-3 fatty acids.[58]

The use of *hyperbaric oxygen* therapy in MS was a matter of debate for many years. Some workers reported benefit, especially in bladder and bowel function or in cerebellar function whereas others were unable to substantiate any useful long-term effect and reviews have concluded that there is no convincing evidence that hyperbaric oxygen therapy is successful.[61,62]

1. Weinstock-Guttman B, Jacobs LD. What is new in the treatment of multiple sclerosis? *Drugs* 2000; **59:** 401–10.
2. Pender MP. Multiple sclerosis. *Med J Aust* 2000; **172:** 556–62.

3. Polman CH, Vitdehaag BMJ. Drug treatment of multiple sclerosis. *BMJ* 2000; **321:** 490–4.
4. Noseworthy JH, *et al.* Multiple sclerosis. *N Engl J Med* 2000; **343:** 938–52.
5. Compston A, Coles A. Multiple sclerosis. *Lancet* 2002; **359:** 1221–31. Correction. *ibid.*; **360:** 648.
6. Martyn CN, *et al.* Nabilone in the treatment of multiple sclerosis. *Lancet* 1995; **345:** 579.
7. Mueller ME, *et al.* Gabapentin for relief of upper motor neuron symptoms in multiple sclerosis. *Arch Phys Med Rehabil* 1997; **78:** 521–4.
8. Samkoff LM, *et al.* Amelioration of refractory dysesthetic limb pain in multiple sclerosis by gabapentin. *Neurology* 1997; **49:** 304–5.
9. Solaro C, *et al.* An open-label trial of gabapentin treatment of paroxysmal symptoms in multiple sclerosis patients. *Neurology* 1998; **51:** 609–11.
10. Dunevsky A, Perel AB. Gabapentin for relief of spasticity associated with multiple sclerosis. *Am J Phys Med Rehabil* 1998; **77:** 451–4.
11. Cutter NC, *et al.* Gabapentin effect on spasticity in multiple sclerosis: a placebo-controlled, randomized trial. *Arch Phys Med Rehabil* 2000; **81:** 164–9.
12. Solaro C, *et al.* Gabapentin is effective in treating nocturnal painful spasms in multiple sclerosis. *Multiple Sclerosis* 2000; **6:** 192–3.
13. Shakespeare DT, *et al.* Anti-spasticity agents for multiple sclerosis. Available in The Cochrane Library; Issue 1. Chichester: John Wiley; 2004.
14. Solari A, *et al.* Aminopyridines for symptomatic treatment in multiple sclerosis. Available in The Cochrane Library; Issue 1. Chichester: John Wiley; 2004.
15. Filippini G, *et al.* Corticosteroids or ACTH for acute exacerbations in multiple sclerosis. Available in The Cochrane Library; Issue 1. Chichester: John Wiley; 2004.
16. Oliveri RL, *et al.* Randomized trial comparing two different high doses of methylprednisolone in MS: a clinical and MRI study. *Neurology* 1998; **50:** 1833–6.
17. Beck RW, *et al.* The effect of corticosteroids for acute optic neuritis on the subsequent development of multiple sclerosis. *N Engl J Med* 1993; **329:** 1764–9.
18. Beck RW, *et al.* The optic neuritis treatment trial: three-year follow-up results. *Arch Ophthalmol* 1995; **113:** 136–7.
19. Sellebjerg F, *et al.* Double-blind, randomized, placebo-controlled study of oral, high-dose methylprednisolone in attacks of MS. *Neurology* 1998; **51:** 529–34.
20. Barnes D, *et al.* Randomised trial of oral and intravenous methylprednisolone in acute relapses of multiple sclerosis. *Lancet* 1997; **349:** 902–6.
21. Cazzato G, *et al.* Double-blind, placebo-controlled, randomized, crossover trial of high-dose methylprednisolone in patients with chronic progressive form of multiple sclerosis. *Eur Neurol* 1995; **35:** 193–8.
22. Goodkin DE, *et al.* A phase II study of IV methylprednisolone in secondary-progressive multiple sclerosis. *Neurology* 1998; **51:** 239–45.
23. Panitch HS. Interferons in multiple sclerosis: a review of the evidence. *Drugs* 1992; **44:** 946–62.
24. The IFNB Multiple Sclerosis Study Group. Interferon beta-1b is effective in relapsing-remitting multiple sclerosis I: clinical results of a multicenter, randomized, double-blind, placebo-controlled trial. *Neurology* 1993; **43:** 655–61.
25. The IFNB Multiple Sclerosis Study Group and the University of British Columbia MS/MRI Analysis Group. Interferon beta-1b in the treatment of multiple sclerosis: final outcome of the randomised controlled trial. *Neurology* 1995; **45:** 1277–85.
26. Paty DW, *et al.* Interferon beta-1b is effective in relapsing-remitting multiple sclerosis II: MRI analysis results of a multicenter, randomized, double-blind, placebo-controlled trial. *Neurology* 1993; **43:** 662–7.
27. European Study Group on Interferon β-1b in Secondary Progressive MS. Placebo-controlled multicentre randomised trial of interferon β-1b in secondary progressive multiple sclerosis. *Lancet* 1998; **352:** 1491–7.
28. Jacobs LD, *et al.* Intramuscular interferon beta-1a for disease progression in relapsing multiple sclerosis. *Ann Neurol* 1996; **39:** 285–94.
29. Rudick RA, *et al.* Impact of interferon beta-1a on neurologic disability in relapsing multiple sclerosis. *Neurology* 1997; **49:** 358–63.
30. PRISMS Study Group. Randomised double-blind placebo-controlled study of interferon β-1a in relapsing/remitting multiple sclerosis. *Lancet* 1998; **352:** 1498–1504.
31. Panitch H, *et al.* Randomized, comparative study of interferon β-1a treatment regimens in MS: the EVIDENCE trial. *Neurology* 2002; **59:** 1496–1506.
32. Durelli L, *et al.* Every-other-day interferon beta-1b versus once-weekly interferon beta-1a for multiple sclerosis: results of a 2-year prospective randomised multicentre study (INCOMIN). *Lancet* 2002; **359:** 1453–60.
33. Secondary Progressive Efficacy Clinical Trial of Recombinant Interferon-beta-1a in MS (SPECTRIMS) Study Group. Randomized controlled trial of interferon- beta-1a in secondary progressive MS: clinical results. *Neurology* 2001; **56:** 1496–1504.
34. Jacobs LD, *et al.* Intramuscular interferon beta-1a therapy initiated during a first demyelinating event in multiple sclerosis. *N Engl J Med* 2000; **343:** 898–904.
35. Comi G, *et al.* Effect of early interferon treatment on conversion to definite multiple sclerosis: a randomised study. *Lancet* 2001; **357:** 1576–82.
36. Paty DW, *et al.* Guidelines for physicians with patients on IFNB-1b: the use of an assay for neutralizing antibodies (NAB). *Neurology* 1996; **47:** 865–6.
37. IFNB Multiple Sclerosis Study Group, University of British Columbia MS/MRI Analysis Group. Neutralizing antibodies during treatment of multiple sclerosis with interferon beta-1b: experience during the first three years. *Neurology* 1996; **47:** 889–94.
38. Sorensen PS, *et al.* Clinical importance of neutralising antibodies against interferon beta in patients with relapsing-remitting multiple sclerosis. *Lancet* 2003; **362:** 1184–91. Correction. *ibid.* 2004; **363:** 402.
39. Association of British Neurologists. Guidelines for the use of beta interferons and glatiramer acetate in multiple sclerosis: January 2001. Available at: http://www.theabn.org/downloads/msdoc.pdf (accessed 15/08/03)
40. Munari L, *et al.* Therapy with glatiramer acetate for multiple sclerosis. Available in The Cochrane Library; Issue 1. Chichester: John Wiley; 2004.
41. Gray OM, *et al.* Intravenous immunoglobulins for multiple sclerosis. Available in The Cochrane Library; Issue 1. Chichester: John Wiley; 2004.
42. British and Dutch Multiple Sclerosis Azathioprine Trial Group. Double-masked trial of azathioprine in multiple sclerosis. *Lancet* 1988; **ii:** 179–83.
43. Ellison GW, *et al.* A placebo-controlled, randomized, double-masked, variable dosage, clinical trial of azathioprine with and without methylprednisolone in multiple sclerosis. *Neurology* 1989; **39:** 1018–26.
44. Rudge P, *et al.* Randomised double blind controlled trial of cyclosporin in multiple sclerosis. *J Neurol Neurosurg Psychiatry* 1989; **52:** 559–65.
45. The Multiple Sclerosis Study Group. Efficacy and toxicity of cyclosporine in chronic progressive multiple sclerosis: a randomized, double-blinded, placebo-controlled clinical trial. *Ann Neurol* 1990; **27:** 591–605.
46. The Canadian Cooperative Multiple Sclerosis Study Group. The Canadian cooperative trial of cyclophosphamide and plasma exchange in progressive multiple sclerosis. *Lancet* 1991; **337:** 441–6.
47. La Mantia L, *et al.* Cyclophosphamide for multiple sclerosis. Available in The Cochrane Library; Issue 3. Chichester: John Wiley; 2003.
48. Yudkin PL, *et al.* Overview of azathioprine treatment in multiple sclerosis. *Lancet* 1991; **338:** 1051–5.
49. Palace J, Rothwell P. New treatments and azathioprine in multiple sclerosis. *Lancet* 1997; **350:** 261.
50. Sipe JC, *et al.* Cladribine in treatment of chronic progressive multiple sclerosis. *Lancet* 1994; **344:** 9–13.
51. Romine JS, *et al.* A double-blind, placebo-controlled, randomized trial of cladribine in relapsing-remitting multiple sclerosis. *Proc Assoc Am Physicians* 1999; **111:** 35–44.
52. Goodkin DE, *et al.* Low-dose (7.5 mg) oral methotrexate reduces the rate of progression in chronic progressive multiple sclerosis. *Ann Neurol* 1995; **37:** 30–40.
53. Gonsette RE. Mitoxantrone immunotherapy in multiple sclerosis. *Multiple Sclerosis* 1996; **1:** 329–32.
54. Millefiorini E, *et al.* Randomized placebo-controlled trial of mitoxantrone in relapsing-remitting multiple sclerosis: 24-month clinical and MRI outcome. *J Neurol* 1997; **244:** 153–9.
55. Hartung H-P, *et al.* Mitoxantrone in progressive multiple sclerosis: a placebo-controlled, double-blind, randomised, multicentre trial. *Lancet* 2002; **360:** 2018–25.
56. Medaer R, *et al.* Depletion of myelin-basic-protein autoreactive T cells by T-cell vaccination: pilot trial in multiple sclerosis. *Lancet* 1995; **346:** 807–8.
57. Cook SD, *et al.* Combination total lymphoid irradiation and low-dose corticosteroid therapy for progressive multiple sclerosis. *Acta Neurol Scand* 1995; **91:** 22–7.
58. Anonymous. Lipids and multiple sclerosis. *Lancet* 1990; **336:** 25–6.
59. Millar JHD, *et al.* Double-blind trial of linoleate supplementation of the diet in multiple sclerosis. *BMJ* 1973; **1:** 765–8.
60. Swank RL, Dugan BB. Effect of low saturated fat diet in early and late cases of multiple sclerosis. *Lancet* 1990; **336:** 37–9.
61. Webb HE. Multiple sclerosis: therapeutic pessimism. *BMJ* 1992; **304:** 1260–1.
62. Bennett M, Heard R. Hyperbaric oxygen therapy for multiple sclerosis. Available in The Cochrane Library; Issue 1. Chichester: John Wiley; 2004.


**Rheumatoid arthritis.** Preliminary studies suggest that interferon beta may have a beneficial effect on rheumatoid arthritis,[1] the conventional management of which is described on p.9.


1. van Holten J, *et al.* Interferon-β for treatment of rheumatoid arthritis? *Arthritis Res* 2002; **4:** 346–52.


**Warts.** For the use of interferon beta in the management of warts, see Interferon Alfa, p.645.

## Preparations

**Proprietary Preparations** (details are given in Part 3)

***Arg.:*** Avonex; Betaferon; Rebif; ***Austral.:*** Avonex; Betaferon; Rebif; ***Austria:*** Avonex; Betaferon; Rebif; ***Belg.:*** Avonex; Betaferon; ***Braz.:*** Avonex; Betaferon; Fronet†; Rebif; ***Canad.:*** Avonex; Betaseron; Rebif; ***Chile:*** Avonex; ***Denm.:*** Avonex; Betaferon; Rebif; ***Fin.:*** Avonex; Betaferon; Rebif; ***Fr.:*** Avonex; Betaferon; Rebif; ***Ger.:*** Avonex; Betaferon; Fiblaferon; Rebif; ***Gr.:*** Avonex; Betaferon; Rebif; ***Hong Kong:*** Rebif; ***Irl.:*** Avonex; Betaferon; Rebif; ***Israel:*** Avonex; Betaferon; Rebif; ***Ital.:*** Avonex; Betaferon; Betron R; Fronet†; Naferon†; Rebif; Serobif; ***Jpn:*** Feron; ***Malaysia:*** Betaferon; Rebif; ***Mex.:*** Avonex; Betaferon; Rebif; ***Neth.:*** Avonex; Betaferon; Rebif; ***Norw.:*** Avonex; Betaferon; Rebif; ***NZ:*** Avonex; Betaferon; ***Port.:*** Avonex†; Betaferon; Rebif; ***S.Afr.:*** Avonex; Betaferon; Rebif; ***Singapore:*** Betaferon; Rebif; ***Spain:*** Avonex; Betaferon; Fronet†; Rebif; ***Swed.:*** Avonex; Betaferon; Rebif; ***Switz.:*** Avonex; Betaferon; Rebif; ***Thai.:*** Rebif; ***UK:*** Avonex; Betaferon; Rebif; ***USA:*** Avonex; Betaseron; Rebif.

# Interferon Gamma *(BAN, rINN)*

IFN-γ; Interferon-γ; Interferón gamma.

*CAS — 98059-18-8 (interferon gamma-1a); 98059-61-1 (interferon gamma-1b).*

*ATC — L03AB03.*

NOTE. Interferon gamma was previously known as immune interferon.

Interferon gamma-1b is *USAN* and was previously known as interferon gamma-2a.

**Pharmacopoeias.** *Eur.* (see p.vi) includes Interferon Gamma-1b Concentrated Solution.

**Ph. Eur. 5.0** (Interferon Gamma-1b Concentrated Solution; Interferoni Gamma-1b Solutio Concentrata). It is a solution of the *N*-terminal methionyl form of interferon gamma. It is produced by a method based on recombinant DNA technology using bacteria as host cells. It is a clear, colourless or slightly yellowish liquid. The pH of the solution is 4.5 to 5.5. Store in airtight containers at a temperature of −70°. Protect from light.

**Nomenclature.** Interferon gamma may be derived from immunologically stimulated T-lymphocytes (hence its former name of immune interferon) as well as through recombinant DNA technology. Similarly to interferon alfa, protein variants of interferon gamma are designated by a number and further qualified by a letter to indicate the amino-acid sequences at terminal positions 1 and 139. Interferon gamma-1a has at position 1 hydrogen, cysteine, tyrosine, and cysteine and at position 139 arginine, alanine, serine, glutamine, and a hydroxyl group. Interferon gamma-1b, formerly known as interferon gamma-2a, has at position 1 hydrogen and methionine and at position 139 a hydroxyl group. Interferon gamma derived through recombinant DNA technology is labelled (rbe).

## Adverse Effects

As for interferons in general (see Interferon Alfa, p.640)

## Precautions

As for interferons in general (see Interferon Alfa, p.642).

## Interactions

As for interferons in general (see Interferon Alfa, p.642).

## Antiviral Action

Interferons are produced by virus-infected cells and confer protection on uninfected cells of the same species. They affect many cell functions demonstrating, in addition to their antiviral activity, antiproliferative and immunomodulating properties. Interferon gamma in particular is a potent macrophage-stimulating factor.

## Pharmacokinetics

Interferons are not absorbed from the gastrointestinal tract. Peak plasma concentrations of interferon gamma-1b occur about 4 hours after intramuscular injection and about 7 hours after subcutaneous injection. Half-lives of 38 minutes (intravenous administration), 2.9 hours (intramuscular administration), and 5.9 hours (subcutaneous administration) have been reported.

## Uses and Administration

Interferon gamma has antiviral and immunomodulating effects. Interferon gamma-1b is used for its action as a macrophage-stimulating factor as an adjunct to antimicrobial therapy in chronic granulomatous disease. It is also used to delay time to disease progression in patients with severe malignant osteopetrosis.

Interferon gamma-1b is given in a dose of 50 micrograms/m$^2$ body-surface (1 million units/m$^2$) three times weekly by subcutaneous injection. Patients with a body-surface less than 0.5 m$^2$ should receive 1.5 micrograms/kg body-weight three times weekly.

Interferon gamma-1b is also under investigation for the treatment of cryptogenic fibrosing alveolitis (see below).

Interferon gamma-n1 has also been used.

◊ Reviews.


1. Todd PA, Goa KL. Interferon gamma-1b: a review of its pharmacology and therapeutic potential in chronic granulomatous disease. *Drugs* 1992; **43:** 111–22.


**Bacterial infections.** In addition to its use to control infections in chronic granulomatous disease, interferon gamma was used with some success as an adjunct to antibacterials in a patient with Whipple's disease[1] but was of no benefit in a study in burn-related infections.[2] For the conventional management of these infections, see Whipple's Disease, p.153 and Skin Infections, p.146.


1. Schneider T, *et al.* Treatment of refractory Whipple disease with interferon-γ. *Ann Intern Med* 1998; **129:** 875–7.
2. Wasserman D, *et al.* Interferon-γ in the prevention of severe burn-related infections: a European phase III multicenter trial. *Crit Care Med* 1998; **26:** 434–9.


**Cryptogenic fibrosing alveolitis.** In a preliminary study[1] in patients with cryptogenic fibrosing alveolitis who had not responded to treatment with corticosteroids or to other immunosuppressive therapy, lung capacity increased in 9 patients treated with interferon gamma-1b in combination with prednisolone for 12 months, but deteriorated in 9 who were treated with prednisolone alone for the same period. The study was, however, criticised for its methodology and the statistical significance of its findings questioned.[2] A later study[3] involving 330 patients with cryptogenic fibrosing alveolitis did not find interferon gamma 1-b to be of benefit.


1. Ziesche R, *et al.* A preliminary study of long-term treatment with interferon gamma-1b and low-dose prednisolone in patients with idiopathic pulmonary fibrosis. *N Engl J Med* 1999; **341:** 1264–9.

2. King TE. Interferon gamma-1b for the treatment of idiopathic pulmonary fibrosis. *N Engl J Med* 2000; **342:** 974–5.
3. Raghu G, *et al.* A placebo-controlled trial of interferon gamma-1b in patients with idiopathic pulmonary fibrosis. *N Engl J Med* 2004; **350:** 125–33.

**Leishmaniasis.** Interferon gamma has been tried both systemically and locally as an adjunct to standard treatment of leishmaniasis (p.597) with encouraging results. A review[1] of the use of interferon gamma in non-viral infections concluded that interferon gamma was effective when combined with antimony compounds for treatment failures in visceral leishmaniasis and could enhance the response to initial therapy in untreated patients. However, the response to adjunctive interferon gamma was limited in patients with a high degree of resistance to antimony compounds.[2] For cutaneous infections, intralesional interferon gamma has been shown to be effective[3] but less so than intralesional antimony compounds.[4] Subcutaneous administration of interferon gamma with antimony given intravenously was no more effective than antimony alone when administered as a short course over 10 days.[5] However, encouraging responses have been reported in patients who have failed to respond to antimony compounds alone.[6]

1. Murray HW. Interferon-gamma and host antimicrobial defense: current and future clinical applications. *Am J Med* 1994; **97:** 459–67.
2. Sundar S, *et al.* Response to interferon-γ plus pentavalent antimony in Indian visceral leishmaniasis. *J Infect Dis* 1997; **176:** 1117–19.
3. Harms G, *et al.* Effects of intradermal gamma-interferon in cutaneous leishmaniasis. *Lancet* 1989; **i:** 1287–92.
4. Harms G, *et al.* A randomized trial comparing a pentavalent antimonial drug and recombinant interferon-γ in the local treatment of cutaneous leishmaniasis. *Trans R Soc Trop Med Hyg* 1991; **85:** 214–16.
5. Arana BA, *et al.* Efficacy of a short course (10 days) of high-dose meglumine antimonate with or without interferon-γ in treating cutaneous leishmaniasis in Guatemala. *Clin Infect Dis* 1994; **18:** 381–4.
6. Falcoff E, *et al.* Clinical healing of antimony-resistant cutaneous or mucocutaneous leishmaniasis following the combined administration of interferon-γ and pentavalent antimonial compounds. *Trans R Soc Trop Med Hyg* 1994; **88:** 95–7.

**Mycobacterial infections.** Interferon alfa has been tried as an adjunct to conventional therapy in *multibacillary leprosy.*[1] Experience with interferons for *opportunistic mycobacterial infections* in patients with AIDS is limited. Interferon gamma given with antimycobacterials produced beneficial responses in 3 patients with *Mycobacterium avium* complex infections, but produced no response or only a transient response in 3 others who received interferon gamma alone.[2,3]

Beneficial responses have also been reported following use of interferon alfa[4] or gamma[5] as an adjunct to antimycobacterial therapy in HIV-negative patients with mycobacterial infections unresponsive to conventional therapy.

Inhaled interferon alfa[6] or gamma[7] may be a useful adjunct to conventional antimycobacterial treatment for *pulmonary tuberculosis.*

For discussion of these infections and their standard treatment, see Leprosy, p.133, Opportunistic Mycobacterial Infections, p.137, and Tuberculosis, p.150.

1. Ganapati R, *et al.* A multicenter study of recombinant interferon-alpha2b in the treatment of multibacillary leprosy. *Int J Lepr* 1997; **65:** 495–7.
2. Squires KE, *et al.* Interferon-γ and Mycobacterium avium-intracellulare infection. *J Infect Dis* 1989; **159:** 599–600.
3. Squires KE, *et al.* Interferon-γ treatment for Mycobacterium avium-intracellulare complex bacillemia in patients with AIDS. *J Infect Dis* 1992; **166:** 686–7.
4. Maziarz RT, *et al.* Reversal of infection with Mycobacterium avium intracellulare by treatment with alpha-interferon in a patient with hairy cell leukemia. *Ann Intern Med* 1988; **109:** 292–4.
5. Holland SM, *et al.* Treatment of refractory disseminated nontuberculous mycobacterial infection with interferon gamma: a preliminary report. *N Engl J Med* 1994; **330:** 1348–55.
6. Giosuè S, *et al.* Effects of aerosolized interferon-α in patients with pulmonary tuberculosis. *Am J Respir Crit Care Med* 1998; **158:** 1156–62.
7. Condos R, *et al.* Treatment of multidrug-resistant pulmonary tuberculosis with interferon-γ via aerosol. *Lancet* 1997; **349:** 1513–15.

**Osteopetrosis.** Interferon gamma has been tried in the treatment of malignant osteopetrosis (p.1085). A study[1] in 14 patients found that interferon gamma-1b increased bone resorption. In 11 who received this treatment for 18 months there was stabilisation or improvement in clinical condition and a reduction in the frequency of serious infection.

1. Key LL, *et al.* Long-term treatment of osteopetrosis with recombinant human interferon gamma. *N Engl J Med* 1995; **332:** 1594–9.

**Skin disorders.** Interferons have been tried in skin disorders in which IgE levels are raised. Subcutaneous interferon gamma improved *eczema* and reduced serum-IgE concentration in one patient, but the condition gradually returned within a week of stopping treatment.[1] In two studies[2,3] subcutaneous interferon gamma given to patients with severe atopic dermatitis and raised serum-IgE concentrations resulted in improvement of the skin condition; IgE concentrations were reduced in one study[2] but remained high in the other.[3] Subcutaneous interferon alfa, however, was unsuccessful in 2 patients with very severe atopic dermatitis; serum-IgE concentrations and severity of the skin condition remained unaffected.[4] Interferon alfa has been tried in subacute *cutaneous lupus erythematosus*[5,6] and *discoid lupus erythematosus.*[6] Although marked improvement generally occurred, the condition tended to recur within several weeks of stopping treatment. For discussion of the conventional treatment of eczema, see p.1135 and of lupus erythematosus, see Systemic Lupus Erythematosus, p.1088.

There have been reports[7,8] of the successful use of interferon alfa to control the symptoms of *urticaria* associated with mastocytosis (p.797).

Interferons have also been proposed for antifibrotic therapy in the management of diffuse *scleroderma* (see p.1348). A multicentre study of interferon gamma in scleroderma[9] found that cutaneous symptoms might be improved but that treatment was associated with an unacceptable incidence of adverse effects. Interferon gamma has also been tried in *eosinophilic pustular folliculitis.*[10]

Interferons have also been used for the treatment of warts (see under Interferon Alfa, p.645).

1. Souillet G, *et al.* Alpha-interferon treatment of patient with hyper IgE syndrome. *Lancet* 1989; **i:** 1384.
2. Reinhold U, *et al.* Recombinant interferon-γ in severe atopic dermatitis. *Lancet* 1990; **335:** 1282.
3. Boguniewicz M, *et al.* Recombinant gamma interferon in treatment of patients with atopic dermatitis and elevated IgE levels. *Am J Med* 1990; **88:** 365–70.
4. MacKie RM. Interferon-α for atopic dermatitis. *Lancet* 1990; **335:** 1282–3.
5. Nicolas J-F, Thivolet J. Interferon alfa therapy in severe unresponsive subacute cutaneous lupus erythematosus. *N Engl J Med* 1989; **321:** 1550–1.
6. Thivolet J, *et al.* Recombinant interferon α2a is effective in the treatment of discoid and subacute cutaneous lupus erythematosus. *Br J Dermatol* 1990; **122:** 405–9.
7. Kolde G, *et al.* Treatment of urticaria pigmentosa using interferon alpha. *Br J Dermatol* 1995; **133:** 91–4.
8. Lippert U, Henz BM. Long-term effect of interferon alpha treatment in mastocytosis. *Br J Dermatol* 1996; **134:** 1164–5.
9. Polisson RP, *et al.* A multicenter trial of recombinant human interferon gamma in patients with systemic sclerosis: effects on cutaneous fibrosis and interleukin 2 receptor levels. *J Rheumatol* 1996; **23:** 654–8.
10. Fushimi M, *et al.* Eosinophilic pustular folliculitis effectively treated with recombinant interferon-γ: suppression of mRNA expression of interleukin 5 in peripheral blood mononuclear cells. *Br J Dermatol* 1996; **134:** 766–72.

## Preparations

**Proprietary Preparations** (details are given in Part 3)
***Arg.:*** Imufor; ***Austral.:*** Imukin; ***Austria:*** Imufor; Imukin; ***Belg.:*** Immukine; ***Denm.:*** Imukin; ***Fin.:*** Imukin; ***Fr.:*** Imukin; ***Ger.:*** Imukin; ***Gr.:*** Imukin; ***Hong Kong:*** Immukin; ***Irl.:*** Immukin; ***Ital.:*** Gammakine; Imukin; ***Jpn:*** Ogamma; ***Neth.:*** Immukine; ***Norw.:*** Imukin; ***NZ:*** Imukin; ***Port.:*** Imukin; ***Spain:*** Imukin; ***Swed.:*** Imukin; ***Switz.:*** Imukin; ***UK:*** Immukin; ***USA:*** Actimmune.

# Lamivudine *(BAN, USAN, rINN)*

3TC; (−)-2′-Deoxy-3′-thiacytidine; GR-109714X; Lamivudina. (−)-1-[(2R,5S)-2-(Hydroxymethyl)-1,3-oxathiolan-5-yl]cytosine.
$C_8H_{11}N_3O_3S = 229.3.$
*CAS — 131086-21-0; 134678-17-4.*
*ATC — J05AF05.*

**Pharmacopoeias.** In *US.*

**USP 27** ( Lamivudine). A white to off-white solid. Soluble in water. Protect from light.

## Adverse Effects

Adverse effects commonly associated with lamivudine include abdominal pain, nausea, vomiting, diarrhoea, headache, fever, rash, alopecia, malaise, insomnia, cough, nasal symptoms, arthralgia, musculoskeletal pain, and peripheral neuropathy. There have been rare instances of rhabdomyolysis. Pancreatitis has been reported rarely. Neutropenia and anaemia (usually when given in combination with zidovudine), thrombocytopenia, and increases in liver enzymes and rare cases of hepatitis have occurred. Lactic acidosis, usually associated with severe hepatomegaly and steatosis, has been reported during treatment with nucleoside reverse transcriptase inhibitors (see Zidovudine, p.658).

**Effects on the blood.** Although anaemia associated with lamivudine usually occurs when it is used in combination with zidovudine, there has been a report[1] of severe anaemia in a 62-year-old HIV-infected man who received lamivudine in the absence of zidovudine.

1. Weitzel T, *et al.* Severe anaemia as a newly recognized side-effect caused by lamivudine. *AIDS* 1999; **13:** 2309–11.

**Effects on the hair.** Hair loss was associated with lamivudine treatment in 5 patients.[1]

1. Fong IW. Hair loss associated with lamivudine. *Lancet* 1994; **344:** 1702.

**Effects on the nails.** Paronychia was reported in 12 HIV-infected patients receiving lamivudine.[1] In a further report, 6 patients developed paronychia while receiving lamivudine in combination with indinavir.[2]

1. Zerboni R, *et al.* Lamivudine-induced paronychia. *Lancet* 1998; **351:** 1256.
2. Tosti A, *et al.* Paronychia associated with antiretroviral therapy. *Br J Dermatol* 1999; **140:** 1165–8.

**Effects on the nervous system.** Exacerbation of peripheral neuropathy has been reported in a patient following substitution of lamivudine for zalcitabine.[1]

1. Cupler EJ, Dalakas MC. Exacerbation of peripheral neuropathy by lamivudine. *Lancet* 1995; **345:** 460–1.

**Hypersensitivity.** Angioedema, urticaria, and anaphylactoid reaction occurred in a patient 30 minutes after receiving the first dose of lamivudine.[1]

1. Kainer MA, Mijch A. Anaphylactoid reaction, angioedema, and urticaria associated with lamivudine. *Lancet* 1996; **348:** 1519.

## Precautions

Lamivudine therapy should be stopped in patients who develop abdominal pain, nausea, or vomiting or with abnormal biochemical test results until pancreatitis has been excluded.

Treatment with lamivudine may be associated with lactic acidosis and should be discontinued if there is a rapid increase in aminotransferase concentrations, progressive hepatomegaly, or metabolic or lactic acidosis of unknown aetiology. Lamivudine should be used with caution in patients with hepatomegaly or other risk factors for hepatic disease. In patients with chronic hepatitis B, there is a risk of rebound hepatitis when lamivudine is discontinued, and liver function should be monitored in such patients. The possibility of HIV infection should be excluded before beginning lamivudine therapy for hepatitis B, since the lower doses used to treat the latter may permit the development of lamivudine-resistant strains of HIV.

Dosage reduction may be necessary in patients with impaired renal function (see below).

## Interactions

The renal excretion of lamivudine may be inhibited by concomitant administration of other drugs mainly eliminated by active renal secretion, for example trimethoprim. Usual prophylactic doses of trimethoprim are unlikely to necessitate reductions in lamivudine dosage unless the patient has renal impairment, but the co-administration of lamivudine with the high therapeutic doses of trimethoprim (as co-trimoxazole) used in *Pneumocystis carinii* pneumonia and toxoplasmosis should be avoided. Although there is usually no clinically significant interaction with zidovudine, severe anaemia has occasionally been reported in patients receiving lamivudine and zidovudine in combination (see Zidovudine, Interactions, p.660). Lamivudine may antagonise the antiviral action of zalcitabine and the two drugs should not be used in combination.

**Microbiological interactions.** The intracellular phosphorylation of lamivudine was increased by the addition of *hydroxycarbamide* in an *in-vitro* study.[1]

Modest increases in *zidovudine* plasma concentrations may occur on concurrent administration of lamivudine, but are not usually clinically significant.

1. Palmer S, Cox S. Increased activation of the combination of 3′-azido-3′-deoxythymidine and 2′-deoxy-3′-thiacytidine in the presence of hydroxyurea. *Antimicrob Agents Chemother* 1997; **41:** 460–4.

**Phenylpropanolamine.** For a possible interaction between phenylpropanolamine and antiretrovirals, see Stavudine, p.654.

## Antiviral Action

Lamivudine is converted intracellularly in stages to the triphosphate. This triphosphate halts the DNA synthesis of retroviruses, including HIV, through competitive inhibition of reverse transcriptase and incorporation into viral DNA. Lamivudine is also active against hepatitis B virus. Resistance to lamivudine has been reported in isolates of HIV and hepatitis B virus.

## Pharmacokinetics

Lamivudine is rapidly absorbed following oral administration and peak plasma concentrations are achieved in about 1 hour. Absorption is delayed, but not reduced, by ingestion with food. Bioavailability is between 80 and 87%. Binding to plasma protein is reported to be up to 36%. Lamivudine crosses the blood-brain barrier with a ratio of CSF to serum concentrations of about 0.12. It crosses the placenta and is distributed into breast milk.

Lamivudine is metabolised intracellularly to the active antiviral triphosphate. Hepatic metabolism is low and it is cleared mainly unchanged by active renal excretion. An elimination half-life of 5 to 7 hours has been reported following a single dose.

◊ References.

1. Mueller BU, *et al.* Serum and cerebrospinal fluid pharmacokinetics of intravenous and oral lamivudine in human immunodeficiency virus-infected children. *Antimicrob Agents Chemother* 1998; **42:** 3187–92.
2. Johnson MA, *et al.* Clinical pharmacokinetics of lamivudine. *Clin Pharmacokinet* 1999; **36:** 41–66.
3. Bruno R, *et al.* Comparison of the plasma pharmacokinetics of lamivudine during twice and once daily administration in patients with HIV. *Clin Pharmacokinet* 2001; **40:** 695–700.

## Uses and Administration

Lamivudine is a nucleoside reverse transcriptase inhibitor structurally related to cytosine with activity against retroviruses including HIV. It is used, usually with other antiretrovirals, for combination therapy of HIV infection. It is also used for the treatment of chronic hepatitis B.

For HIV infection, the dose of lamivudine for adults is 300 mg by mouth daily as a single dose or in two divided doses. A dose for children aged between 3 months and 12 years is 4 mg/kg twice daily to a maximum daily dose of 300 mg.

For chronic hepatitis B, the adult dose is 100 mg once daily by mouth. A dose for children aged over 2 years is 3 mg/kg once daily to a maximum daily dose of 100 mg. In patients with concomitant HIV and hepatitis B infection the dosage regimen appropriate for HIV should be used.

Reduction of dosage is recommended for patients with renal impairment (see below).

**Administration in renal impairment.** Dosage of lamivudine should be reduced in patients with moderate to severe renal impairment (creatinine clearance (CC) below 50 mL/minute).

*adults*: HIV infection:

- CC 30 to 49 mL/minute: 150 mg for the first dose then 150 mg once daily
- CC 15 to 29 mL/minute: 150 mg for the first dose then 100 mg once daily
- CC 5 to 14 mL/minute: 150 mg for the first dose then 50 mg once daily
- CC less than 5 mL/minute: 50 mg for the first dose then 25 mg once daily
- dialysis patients: not recommended

*adults*: chronic hepatitis B infection:

- CC 30 to 49 mL/minute: 100 mg for the first dose then 50 mg once daily
- CC 15 to 29 mL/minute: 100 mg for the first dose then 25 mg once daily
- CC 5 to 14 mL/minute: 35 mg for the first dose then 15 mg once daily
- CC less than 5 mL/minute: 35 mg for the first dose then 10 mg once daily
- haemodialysis patients: no further dose adjustment other than in accordance with CC is required
- peritoneal dialysis patients: not recommended

*children*:

- doses should be reduced according to CC by the same proportions as in adults.

**Hepatitis.** Lamivudine is one of the more promising antivirals being used as an alternative to interferon alfa in the treatment of chronic hepatitis B (p.618).[1-3] In a preliminary study, lamivudine 100 or 300 mg daily reduced hepatitis B virus DNA to low or undetectable levels.[4] In a 1-year double-blind study involving about 350 patients with chronic hepatitis B, lamivudine 100 mg daily was associated with substantial histological improvement in many patients; a dose of 25 mg daily was less effective.[5] Relapses have been reported once treatment with lamivudine is stopped, and a case of reactivation of hepatitis B infection has been observed.[6] Lamivudine may also be effective in preventing re-infection with hepatitis B in patients who have received liver transplants,[7,8] and beneficial responses have been seen in transplant patients with acute hepatitis B infection treated with lamivudine 100 mg daily for prolonged periods.[9]

1. Dienstag JL, *et al.* Lamivudine as initial treatment for chronic hepatitis B in the United States. *N Engl J Med* 1999; **341:** 1256–63.
2. Hagmeyer KO, Pan Y-Y. Role of lamivudine in the treatment of chronic hepatitis B virus infection. *Ann Pharmacother* 1999; **33:** 1104–12.
3. Jonas MM, *et al.* Clinical trial of lamivudine in children with chronic hepatitis B. *N Engl J Med* 2002; **346:** 1706–13. Correction. *ibid.*; **347:** 955.
4. Dienstag JL, *et al.* A preliminary trial of lamivudine for chronic hepatitis B infection. *N Engl J Med* 1995; **333:** 1657–61.
5. Lai C-L, *et al.* A one-year trial of lamivudine for chronic hepatitis B. *N Engl J Med* 1998; **339:** 61–8.
6. Honkoop P, *et al.* Hepatitis B reactivation after lamivudine. *Lancet* 1995; **346:** 1156–7.
7. Grellier L, *et al.* Lamivudine prophylaxis against reinfection in liver transplantation for hepatitis B cirrhosis. *Lancet* 1996; **348:** 1212–15. Correction. *ibid.* 1997; **349:** 364.
8. Perrillo RP, *et al.* A multicenter United States-Canadian trial to assess lamivudine monotherapy before and after liver transplantation for chronic hepatitis B. *Hepatology* 2001; **33:** 424–32.
9. Andreone P, *et al.* Lamivudine treatment for acute hepatitis B after liver transplantation. *J Hepatol* 1998; **29:** 985–9.

**HIV infection and AIDS.** Lamivudine is a potent inhibitor of HIV-1 and HIV-2 *in vitro*, including variants resistant to zidovudine.[1] Resistance emerges rapidly when lamivudine is given alone to patients with HIV infections,[2] although sustained responses have been reported despite the emergence of resistance.[3] Combination therapy with lamivudine delays, and may even reverse, the emergence of zidovudine resistance and produces a sustained synergistic antiretroviral effect,[4] but HIV strains resistant to both lamivudine and zidovudine may arise.[5] As discussed on p.621, combination therapy, typically with two nucleoside reverse transcriptase inhibitors and either a non-nucleoside reverse transcriptase inhibitor or an HIV-protease inhibitor, is standard therapy for HIV infection. Treatment with lamivudine plus zidovudine has produced better responses than either drug alone in antiretroviral-naive patients,[6,7] and has produced additional responses in antiretroviral-experienced patients,[8,9] with little additional toxicity. The addition of lamivudine to existing antiretroviral therapy was reported to slow the progression of the disease and improve survival,[10] and treatment with lamivudine, indinavir, and nevirapine produced beneficial responses in patients who had previously failed on combined nucleoside analogue therapy.[11] Clinically useful CNS concentrations of lamivudine were achieved in patients with HIV infection given combination therapy with lamivudine and zidovudine or stavudine.[12]

Lamivudine is also used in prophylactic regimens following occupational exposure to HIV infection (see p.623) and has been tried for reducing vertical transmission from mother to neonate.[13,14]

1. Anonymous. Lamivudine: impressive benefits in combination with zidovudine. *WHO Drug Inf* 1996; **10:** 5–7.
2. Wainberg MA, *et al.* Development of HIV-1 resistance to (−)2′-deoxy-3′-thiacytidine in patients with AIDS or advanced AIDS-related complex. *AIDS* 1995; **9:** 351–7.
3. Ingrand D, *et al.* Phase I/II study of 3TC (lamivudine) in HIV-positive, asymptomatic or mild AIDS-related complex patients: sustained reduction in viral markers. *AIDS* 1995; **9:** 1323–9.
4. Larder BA, *et al.* Potential mechanism for sustained antiretroviral efficacy of AZT-3TC combination therapy. *Science* 1995; **269:** 696–9.
5. Miller V, *et al.* Dual resistance to zidovudine and lamivudine in patients treated with zidovudine-lamivudine combination therapy: association with therapeutic failure. *J Infect Dis* 1998; **177:** 1521–32.
6. Eron JJ, *et al.* Treatment with lamivudine, zidovudine, or both in HIV-positive patients with 200 to 500 CD4+ cells per cubic millimeter. *N Engl J Med* 1995; **333:** 1662–9.
7. Katlama C, *et al.* Safety and efficacy of lamivudine-zidovudine combination therapy in antiretroviral-naive patients: a randomized controlled comparison with zidovudine monotherapy. *JAMA* 1996; **276:** 118–25.
8. Staszewski S, *et al.* Safety and efficacy of lamivudine-zidovudine combination therapy in zidovudine-experienced patients: a randomized controlled comparison with zidovudine monotherapy. *JAMA* 1996; **276:** 111–17.
9. Bartlett JA, *et al.* Lamivudine plus zidovudine compared with zalcitabine plus zidovudine in patients with HIV infection: a randomized, double-blind, placebo-controlled trial. *Ann Intern Med* 1996; **125:** 161–72.
10. CAESAR Coordinating Committee. Randomised trial of addition of lamivudine or lamivudine plus loviride to zidovudine-containing regimens for patients with HIV-1 infection: the CAESAR trial. *Lancet* 1997; **349:** 1413–21.
11. Harris M, *et al.* A pilot study of nevirapine, indinavir, and lamivudine among patients with advanced human immunodeficiency virus disease who have had failure of combination nucleoside therapy. *J Infect Dis* 1998; **177:** 1514–20.
12. Foudraine NA, *et al.* Cerebrospinal-fluid HIV-1 RNA and drug concentrations after treatment with lamivudine plus zidovudine or stavudine. *Lancet* 1998; **351:** 1547–51.
13. Mandelbrot L, *et al.* Lamivudine-zidovudine combination for prevention of maternal-infant transmission of HIV-1. *JAMA* 2001; **285:** 2083–93.
14. The Petra Study Team. Efficacy of three short-course regimens of zidovudine and lamivudine in preventing early and late transmission of HIV-1 from mother to child in Tanzania, South Africa, and Uganda (Petra study): a randomised, double-blind, placebo-controlled trial. *Lancet* 2002; **359:** 1178–86.

## Preparations

**Proprietary Preparations** (details are given in Part 3)

***Arg.:*** 3TC; Birvac; Ganvirel; Hivirux; Imunoxa; Kess; Lamilea; Oralmuv; Ultraviral; Vuclodir; Zeffix; ***Austral.:*** 3TC; Zeffix; ***Austria:*** Epivir; ***Belg.:*** Epivir; Zeffix; ***Braz.:*** Epivir; Lamiden†; Vudirax; Zeffix; ***Canad.:*** 3TC; Heptovir; ***Chile:*** 3TC/Epivir; ***Denm.:*** Epivir; Zeffix; ***Fin.:*** Epivir; Zeffix; ***Fr.:*** Epivir; Zeffix; ***Ger.:*** Epivir; Zeffix; ***Gr.:*** Epivir; Zeffix; ***Hong Kong:*** 3TC; Zeffix; ***India:*** Ladiwin; Lamidac; ***Irl.:*** Epivir; Zeffix; ***Israel:*** Epivir; Zeffix; ***Ital.:*** Epivir; Zeffix; ***Jpn:*** Epivir; ***Malaysia:*** 3TC; Zeffix; ***Mex.:*** 3TC; ***Neth.:*** Epivir; ***Norw.:*** Epivir; ***NZ:*** 3TC; Zeffix; ***Port.:*** Epivir; Zeffix; ***S.Afr.:*** 3TC; ***Singapore:*** Epivir; Zeffix; ***Spain:*** Epivir; Zeffix; ***Swed.:*** Epivir; Zeffix; ***Switz.:*** 3TC; Zeffix; ***Thai.:*** Epivir; Zeffix; ***UK:*** Epivir; Zeffix; ***USA:*** Epivir.

**Multi-ingredient:** ***Arg.:*** 3TC Complex; 3TC/AZT; Ganvirel Duo; Hivirux Complex; Imunoxa Complex; Kess Complex; Muvidina; Tricivir; Ultraviral Duo; Zetavudin; ***Austral.:*** Combivir; Trizivir; ***Austria:*** Combivir; ***Belg.:*** Combivir; Trizivir; ***Braz.:*** Biovir; Combivir†; Duovir; Zidolam; ***Canad.:*** Combivir; ***Chile:*** Combivir; Tricivir; ***Denm.:*** Combivir; Trizivir; ***Fin.:*** Combivir; Trizivir; ***Fr.:*** Combivir; Trizivir; ***Ger.:*** Combivir; Trizivir; ***Gr.:*** Combivir; ***Hong Kong:*** Combivir; ***India:*** Duovir; Lamuzid; ***Irl.:*** Combivir; Trizivir; ***Israel:*** Combivir; Trizivir; ***Ital.:*** Combivir; Trizivir; ***Malaysia:*** Combivir; ***Mex.:*** Combivir; ***Neth.:*** Combivir; ***Norw.:*** Combivir; Trizivir; ***NZ:*** Combivir; ***Port.:*** Combivir; Trizivir; ***S.Afr.:*** Combivir; Retrovir/3TC Post-HIV Exposure; ***Singapore:*** Combivir; Trizivir; ***Spain:*** Combivir; Trizivir; ***Swed.:*** Combivir; Trizivir; ***Switz.:*** Combivir; Trizivir; ***Thai.:*** Combid; ***UK:*** Combivir; Trizivir; ***USA:*** Combivir; Trizivir.

## Lobucavir *(USAN, rINN)*

BMS-180194; SQ-34514. 9-[(1*R*,2*R*,3*S*)-2,3-Bis(hydroxymethyl)cyclobutyl]guanine.

$C_{11}H_{15}N_5O_3$ = 265.3.

*CAS — 127759-89-1.*

### Profile

Lobucavir is a nucleoside analogue with antiviral activity that has been studied for the treatment of herpesvirus and hepatitis B infections. Clinical studies were suspended in 1999 following observation of possible carcinogenicity in *rodents*.

## Lopinavir *(BAN, USAN, rINN)*

A-157378.0; ABT-378. (α*S*)-Tetrahydro-*N*-((α*S*)-α-{(2*S*,3*S*)-2-hydroxy-4-phenyl-3-[2-(2,6-xylyloxy)acetamido]butyl}phenethyl)-α-isopropyl-2-oxo-1(2*H*)-pyrimidineacetamide.

$C_{37}H_{48}N_4O_5$ = 628.8.

*CAS — 192725-17-0.*

*ATC — J05AE06.*

### Adverse Effects and Precautions

As for HIV-protease inhibitors in general (see Indinavir Sulfate, p.638). Lopinavir has been associated with increases in serum cholesterol and triglycerides, and cases of pancreatitis have been reported. It should be discontinued if symptoms of pancreatitis occur.

The oral solution (*Kaletra, Abbott*) has a high content of alcohol and propylene glycol, present as excipients, and appropriate precautions should be taken.

### Interactions

Interactions involving HIV-protease inhibitors are discussed under Indinavir Sulfate, p.639.

### Antiviral Action

As for HIV-protease inhibitors in general (see Indinavir Sulfate, p.639).

### Uses and Administration

Lopinavir is a protease inhibitor with antiviral activity against HIV. It is used with other antiretrovirals for combination therapy of HIV infection (p.621). It is given with low-dose ritonavir, which acts as a pharmacokinetic enhancer. The dose in adults is lopinavir 400 mg (with ritonavir 100 mg) twice daily with food. Children over 2 years of age may be given lopinavir 230 mg (with ritonavir 57.5 mg) per $m^2$ twice daily, up to a maximum of lopinavir 400 mg twice daily.

◊ Reviews.

1. Hurst M, Faulds D. Lopinavir. *Drugs* 2000; **60:** 1371–9.
2. Cvetkovic RS, Goa KL. Lopinavir/ritonavir: a review of its use in the management of HIV infection. *Drugs* 2003; **63:** 769–802.

### Preparations

**Proprietary Preparations** (details are given in Part 3)

**Multi-ingredient:** ***Arg.:*** Kaletra; ***Austral.:*** Kaletra; ***Belg.:*** Kaletra; ***Braz.:*** Kaletra; ***Canad.:*** Kaletra; ***Chile:*** Kaletra; ***Denm.:*** Kaletra; ***Fin.:*** Kaletra; ***Fr.:*** Kaletra; ***Ger.:*** Kaletra; ***Gr.:*** Kaletra; ***Hong Kong:*** Kaletra; ***Israel:*** Kaletra; ***Ital.:*** Kaletra; ***Norw.:*** Kaletra; ***NZ:*** Kaletra; ***Port.:*** Kaletra; ***Spain:*** Kaletra; ***Swed.:*** Kaletra; ***Switz.:*** Kaletra; ***Thai.:*** Kaletra; ***UK:*** Kaletra; ***USA:*** Kaletra.

## Moroxydine Hydrochloride *(BANM, rINNM)*

Abitilguanide Hydrochloride; ABOB; Hidrocloruro de moroxidina. 1-(Morpholinoformimidoyl)guanidine hydrochloride.

$C_6H_{13}N_5O,HCl$ = 207.7.

*CAS — 3731-59-7 (moroxydine); 3160-91-6 (moroxydine hydrochloride).*

*ATC — J05AX01.*

### Profile

Moroxydine hydrochloride has been given by mouth in the treatment of herpes simplex and varicella-zoster infections. It has also been used topically. It is included as an ingredient in preparations for the treatment of cold and influenza symptoms.

### Preparations

**Proprietary Preparations** (details are given in Part 3)

***Hong Kong:*** Virustat†.

**Multi-ingredient:** ***Hong Kong:*** Virulex Forte; ***Mex.:*** Amgrip; Clorfriol; Cortigrin; Flepin X-3; Friral; Singril; Singrilen; ***S.Afr.:*** Corenza C; Virobis.

## Nelfinavir Mesilate *(BANM, rINNM)*

AG-1343 (nelfinavir or nelfinavir mesilate); Mesilato de nelfinavir; Nelfinavir Mesylate *(USAN)*. 3S[2(2S*,3S*),3α,4aβ,8aβ]-N-(1,1-Dimethylethyl)decahydro-2-[2-hydroxy-3-[(3-hydroxy-2-methylbenzoyl)amino]-4-(phenylthio)butyl-3-isoquinolinecarboxamide monomethanesulphonate; (3S,4aS,8aS)-N-tert-Butyldecahydro-2-[(2R,3R)-3-(3-hydroxy-o-toluamido)-2-hydroxy-4-(phenylthio)butyl]isoquinoline-3-carboxamide monomethanesulphonate.

$C_{32}H_{45}N_3O_4S,CH_4O_3S = 663.9.$

*CAS — 159989-64-7 (nelfinavir); 159989-65-8 (nelfinavir mesilate).*

*ATC — J05AE04.*

NOTE. Nelfinavir should not be confused with nevirapine (p.650).

### Adverse Effects and Precautions

As for HIV-protease inhibitors in general (see Indinavir Sulfate, p.638).

### Interactions

Interactions involving HIV-protease inhibitors are discussed under Indinavir Sulfate, p.639. Nelfinavir is reported to be metabolised in part by cytochrome P450 isoenzymes of the CYP3A family and to be unlikely to inhibit other cytochrome P450 isoforms at therapeutic concentrations.

### Antiviral Action

As for HIV-protease inhibitors in general (see Indinavir Sulfate, p.639). Mechanisms of resistance to nelfinavir may differ sufficiently from those to other HIV-protease inhibitors to reduce the occurrence of cross-resistance between nelfinavir and other HIV-protease inhibitors.

**Resistance.** References.

1. Patick AK, *et al.* Genotypic and phenotypic characterization of human immunodeficiency virus type 1 variants isolated from patients treated with the protease inhibitor nelfinavir. *Antimicrob Agents Chemother* 1998; **42:** 2637–44.

### Pharmacokinetics

Nelfinavir is absorbed from the gastrointestinal tract and peak plasma concentrations occur in 2 to 4 hours. Absorption is enhanced by administration with food. Nelfinavir is extensively bound to plasma proteins (more than 98%). It is distributed into breast milk. Nelfinavir is metabolised by oxidation by cytochrome P450 isoenzymes including CYP3A. The major oxidative metabolite has *in-vitro* antiviral activity equal to that of nelfinavir. The terminal half-life is 3.5 to 5 hours. Nelfinavir is excreted in the faeces mainly as metabolites. Only about 1 to 2% is excreted in the urine.

### Uses and Administration

Nelfinavir is a protease inhibitor with antiviral activity against HIV. It is used with nucleoside reverse transcriptase inhibitors for combination therapy of HIV infection (p.621).

Nelfinavir is given by mouth as the mesilate, but doses are expressed in terms of the base. Nelfinavir mesilate 292 mg is approximately equivalent to 250 mg of nelfinavir. Nelfinavir is available as tablets and oral powder. The oral powder should not be taken with acidic foods or drinks as this may result in a bitter taste. Nelfinavir is given in an adult dose of 1.25 g twice daily or 0.75 g three times daily with food. Children aged 3 to 13 years may be given 50 to 55 mg/kg twice daily or 25 to 30 mg/kg three times daily.

◊ Reviews.

1. Pai VB, Nahata MC. Nelfinavir mesylate: a protease inhibitor. *Ann Pharmacother* 1999; **33:** 325–39.
2. Bardsley-Elliot A, Plosker GL. Nelfinavir: an update on its use in HIV infection. *Drugs* 2000; **59:** 581–620.

### Preparations

**Proprietary Preparations** (details are given in Part 3)

**Arg.:** Filosfil; Nalvir; Nelfilea; Viracept; **Austral.:** Viracept; **Austria:** Viracept; **Belg.:** Viracept; **Braz.:** Nelfir†; Viracept; **Canad.:** Viracept; **Chile:** Viracept; **Denm.:** Viracept; **Fin.:** Viracept; **Fr.:** Viracept; **Ger.:** Viracept; **Gr.:** Viracept; **Irl.:** Viracept; **Israel:** Viracept; **Ital.:** Viracept; **Jpn:** Viracept; **Mex.:** Viracept; **Neth.:** Viracept; **Norw.:** Viracept; **NZ:** Viracept; **Port.:** Viracept; **S.Afr.:** Viracept; **Singapore:** Viracept; **Spain:** Viracept; **Swed.:** Viracept; **Switz.:** Viracept; **Thai.:** Viracept; **UK:** Viracept; **USA:** Viracept.

## Nevirapine *(BAN, USAN, rINN)*

BI-RG-587; BIRG-0587; Nevirapina. 11-Cyclopropyl-5,11-dihydro-4-methyl-6H-dipyrido[3,2-b:2′,3′-e]-[1,4]diazepin-6-one.

$C_{15}H_{14}N_4O = 266.3.$

*CAS — 129618-40-2.*

*ATC — J05AG01.*

NOTE. Nevirapine should not be confused with nelfinavir (p.650).

### Adverse Effects

The most common adverse effect of nevirapine is skin rash, usually occurring within the first 6 weeks of starting therapy. Severe and life-threatening skin reactions (with some fatalities) have occurred, including Stevens-Johnson syndrome and, more rarely, toxic epidermal necrolysis. Hypersensitivity reactions including angioedema, urticaria, and anaphylaxis have been reported. Rashes may occur alone or in the context of hypersensitivity reactions when they may be accompanied by other symptoms such as fever, arthralgia, myalgia, lymphadenopathy, eosinophilia, granulocytopenia, or renal dysfunction. Severe hepatotoxicity, including hepatitis and hepatic necrosis, occasionally fatal, has occurred and may be more prevalent in women. Other common adverse effects include nausea, vomiting, diarrhoea, abdominal pain, fatigue, drowsiness, and headache.

**Effects on the liver.** References.

1. Cattelan AM, *et al.* Severe hepatic failure related to nevirapine treatment. *Clin Infect Dis* 1999; **29:** 455–6.
2. Clarke S, *et al.* Late onset hepatitis and prolonged deterioration in hepatic function associated with nevirapine therapy. *Int J STD AIDS* 2000; **11:** 336–7.
3. Prakash M, *et al.* Jaundice and hepatocellular damage associated with nevirapine therapy. *Am J Gastroenterol* 2001; **96:** 1571–4.
4. Martinez E, *et al.* Hepatotoxicity in HIV-1-infected patients receiving nevirapine-containing antiretroviral therapy. *AIDS* 2001; **15:** 1261–8.
5. Committee on Safety of Medicines/Medicines Control Agency. Nevirapine (Viramune): serious adverse reactions when used in HIV post exposure prophylaxis. *Current Problems* 2001; **27:** 13. Also available at: http://www.mca.gov.uk/ourwork/monitorsafequalmed/currentproblems/cpaug2001.pdf (accessed 13/03/04)
6. Gonzalez de Requena D, *et al.* Liver toxicity caused by nevirapine. *AIDS* 2002; **16:** 290–1.
7. De Maat MM, *et al.* Hepatotoxicity following nevirapine-containing regimens in HIV-1-infected individuals. *Pharmacol Res* 2002; **46:** 295–300.

**Effects on the skin.** References.

1. Warren KJ, *et al.* Nevirapine-associated Stevens-Johnson syndrome. *Lancet* 1998; **351:** 567.
2. Barner A, Myers M. Nevirapine and rashes. *Lancet* 1998; **351:** 1133.
3. Wetterwald E, *et al.* Nevirapine-induced overlap Stevens-Johnson syndrome/toxic epidermal necrolysis. *Br J Dermatol* 1999; **140:** 980–2.
4. Committee on Safety of Medicines/Medicines Control Agency. Nevirapine (Viramune): serious adverse reactions when used in HIV post exposure prophylaxis. *Current Problems* 2001; **27:** 13. Also available at: http://www.mca.gov.uk/ourwork/monitorsafequalmed/currentproblems/cpaug2001.pdf (accessed 13/03/04)

### Precautions

Nevirapine should be used with extreme caution in patients with mild to moderate hepatic impairment; it is contra-indicated in those with severe hepatic impairment. Women and patients with higher CD4+ cell counts are at increased risk of hepatotoxicity. Liver function should be monitored every 2 weeks during the first 2 months of treatment, again at 3 months, and every 3 to 6 months thereafter. Treatment should be interrupted if moderate or severe abnormalities occur; nevirapine may be restarted at the initial dose if liver function returns to normal, but should be permanently discontinued if abnormalities recur or if abnormal liver function is accompanied by symptoms suggestive of a hypersensitivity reaction.

Nevirapine should also be used with caution in patients with renal impairment.

Patients receiving nevirapine should be closely monitored for adverse skin reactions and hepatotoxicity during the first 18 weeks of treatment. Nevirapine should be permanently discontinued if a severe skin rash develops or if a rash is accompanied by fever, blistering, oral lesions, conjunctivitis, swelling, muscle or joint aches, or general malaise. Dose escalation should not be attempted in patients developing any rash during the first 14 days of treatment until the rash has resolved. Patients or their carers should be counselled on how to recognise hypersensitivity reactions and instructed to seek immediate medical attention if they occur.

### Interactions

Similarly to the HIV-protease inhibitors (see Indinavir Sulfate, p.639), nevirapine is metabolised mainly by cytochrome P450 isoenzymes of the CYP3A family. Consequently it may compete with other drugs metabolised by this system, possibly resulting in mutually increased plasma concentrations. Alternatively, enzyme inducers may decrease plasma concentrations of nevirapine; nevirapine itself acts as a mild to moderate enzyme inducer and may thus reduce plasma concentrations of other drugs.

**Antibacterials.** Plasma concentrations of nevirapine may be decreased by *rifabutin* and *rifampicin*, probably as a result of enzyme induction.

**Antifungals.** Use of nevirapine and *ketoconazole* may result in reduction in the plasma concentration of ketoconazole and increase in that of nevirapine. The manufacturers recommend that this combination should be avoided. Use of nevirapine with *fluconazole* may increase bioavailability of nevirapine and caution is required when the drugs are used together.

**Antivirals.** For the effect of nevirapine on *indinavir* and *saquinavir*, see p.639.

**Hormonal contraceptives.** The manufacturers suggest that nevirapine may decrease the plasma concentrations of hormonal contraceptives. Although the clinical significance of this potential interaction is unknown they advise the use of alternative contraceptive methods.

**Methadone.** Nevirapine may induce the metabolism of methadone (p.58) resulting in reduced plasma-methadone concentrations.

### Antiviral Action

Nevirapine acts by non-competitive inhibition of HIV-1 reverse transcriptase.

Resistance to nevirapine and emergence of cross-resistance to other non-nucleoside reverse transcriptase inhibitors has been seen.

### Pharmacokinetics

Nevirapine is readily absorbed following oral administration and absorption is not affected by food. Bioavailability is greater than 90%. Peak plasma concentrations occur 4 hours after a single dose. Nevirapine is about 60% bound to plasma proteins. Concentrations in the CSF are about 45% of those in plasma. Nevirapine crosses the placenta and is distributed into breast milk. It is extensively metabolised by hepatic microsomal enzymes, principally by cytochrome P450 isoenzymes of the CYP3A family. Autoinduction of these enzymes results in a 1.5- to 2-fold increase in apparent oral clearance after 2 to 4 weeks' administration of usual doses, and a decrease in terminal half-life from 45 hours to 25 to 30 hours over the same period. In children, half-life at steady state varies with age, being 32 hours in children less than 1 year of age, 21 hours in children aged 1 to 4 years, 18 hours in children aged 4 to 8 years, and 28 hours in children over 8 years. Apparent clearance, adjusted for body-weight, also varies with age, that in children under 8 years being about twice that in adults. Nevirapine is mainly excreted in the urine as glucuronide conjugates of the hydroxylated metabolites.

◊ References.

1. Mirochnick M, *et al.* Nevirapine: pharmacokinetic considerations in children and pregnant women. *Clin Pharmacokinet* 2000; **39:** 281–93.

### Uses and Administration

Nevirapine is a non-nucleoside reverse transcriptase inhibitor with activity against HIV-1. It is used in the treatment of HIV infection (p.621). Viral resistance emerges rapidly when nevirapine is used alone, and it is used in combination with other antiretrovirals.

Nevirapine is given by mouth in an adult dose of 200 mg once daily for the first 14 days, then increased to 200 mg twice daily provided that no rash is present (see Precautions, above). Children aged 2 months to 8 years may be given 4 mg/kg once daily for 14 days and then, if no rash is present, 7 mg/kg twice daily; those aged 8 to 16 years may be given 4 mg/kg once daily for

14 days then 4 mg/kg twice daily thereafter. A total dose of 400 mg daily should not be exceeded.

If treatment is interrupted for more than 7 days, it should be reintroduced using the lower dose for the first 14 days as for new treatment.

◊ References.


1. Floridia M, *et al.* A randomized, double-blind trial on the use of a triple combination including nevirapine, a nonnucleoside reverse transcriptase HIV inhibitor, in antiretroviral-naive patients with advanced disease. *J Acquir Immune Defic Syndr Hum Retrovirol* 1999; **20:** 11–19.
2. Guay LA, *et al.* Intrapartum and neonatal single-dose nevirapine compared with zidovudine for prevention of mother-to-child transmission of HIV-1 in Kampala, Uganda: HIVNET 012 randomised trial. *Lancet* 1999; **354:** 795–802.
3. Bardsley-Elliot A, Perry CM. Nevirapine: a review of its use in the prevention and treatment of paediatric HIV infection. *Paediatr Drugs* 2000; **2:** 373–407.
4. Dorenbaum A, *et al.* Two-dose intrapartum/newborn nevirapine and standard antiretroviral therapy to reduce perinatal HIV transmission: a randomized trial. *JAMA* 2002; **288:** 189–98.
5. Moodley D, *et al.* A multicenter randomized controlled trial of nevirapine versus a combination of zidovudine and lamivudine to reduce intrapartum and early postpartum mother-to-child transmission of human immunodeficiency virus type 1. *J Infect Dis* 2003; **187:** 725–35.
6. Taha TE, *et al.* Short postexposure prophylaxis in newborn babies to reduce mother-to-child transmission of HIV-1: NVAZ randomised clinical trial. *Lancet* 2003; **362:** 1171–7.


## Preparations

**Proprietary Preparations** (details are given in Part 3)
***Arg.:*** Filide; Nerapin; Neviralea; Protease; Ritvir; Viramune; ***Austral.:*** Viramune; ***Austria:*** Viramune; ***Belg.:*** Viramune; ***Braz.:*** Viramune†; ***Canad.:*** Viramune; ***Chile:*** Viramune; ***Denm.:*** Viramune; ***Fin.:*** Viramune; ***Fr.:*** Viramune; ***Ger.:*** Viramune; ***Gr.:*** Viramune; ***Hong Kong:*** Viramune; ***India:*** Nevimune; ***Irl.:*** Viramune; ***Israel:*** Viramune; ***Ital.:*** Viramune; ***Jpn:*** Viramune; ***Malaysia:*** Viramune; ***Mex.:*** Viramune; ***Neth.:*** Viramune; ***Norw.:*** Viramune; ***NZ:*** Viramune; ***Port.:*** Viramune; ***S.Afr.:*** Viramune; ***Singapore:*** Viramune; ***Spain:*** Viramune; ***Swed.:*** Viramune; ***Switz.:*** Viramune; ***Thai.:*** Viramune; ***UK:*** Viramune; ***USA:*** Viramune.

# Oseltamivir Phosphate *(USAN, rINNM)*

Fosfato de oseltamivir; GS-4104/002; Ro-64-0796/002. Ethyl (3R,4R,5S)-4-acetamido-5-amino-3-(1-ethylpropoxy)-1-cyclohexene-1-carboxylate phosphate (1:1).

$C_{16}H_{28}N_2O_4,H_3PO_4$ = 410.4.

*CAS — 196618-13-0 (oseltamivir); 204255-11-8 (oseltamivir phosphate).*

*ATC — J05AH02.*

## Adverse Effects

The most commonly reported adverse effects associated with oseltamivir are nausea and vomiting, abdominal pain, bronchitis, insomnia, and vertigo. Diarrhoea, dizziness, headache, cough, and fatigue may occur, but many adverse effects may be difficult to distinguish from the symptoms of influenza. Other adverse effects occurring less commonly have included unstable angina, anaemia, pseudomembranous colitis, pneumonia, pyrexia, and peritonsillar abscess. There have been occasional reports of skin rash and, rarely, elevated liver enzymes and hepatitis.

## Precautions

Oseltamivir is not recommended in patients with severe renal impairment and it should be given with caution and dosage should be reduced in patients with moderate renal impairment (see Administration in Renal Impairment, below).

## Pharmacokinetics

Oseltamivir is readily absorbed from the gastrointestinal tract following oral administration and is extensively metabolised in the liver to the active entity, oseltamivir carboxylate. At least 75% of an oral dose reaches the systemic circulation as the carboxylate. Binding to plasma proteins is about 3% for the carboxylate and 42% for the parent drug. Oseltamivir has a plasma half-life of 1 to 3 hours. The carboxylate is not metabolised further and is eliminated in the urine.

## Uses and Administration

Oseltamivir is an oral prodrug of oseltamivir carboxylate, an inhibitor of the enzyme neuraminidase (sialidase), which has a role in the infectivity and replication of influenza A and B viruses. It is used for the treatment and prevention of influenza A and B.

For treatment, oseltamivir is given as the phosphate, but doses are expressed in terms of the base. Oseltamivir phosphate 98.5 mg is approximately equivalent to 75 mg of oseltamivir. The usual adult dose is 75 mg twice daily for 5 days, beginning as soon as possible (within 48 hours) after the onset of symptoms.

For the prevention of influenza, the adult dose is 75 mg once daily for at least 7 days for postexposure prophylaxis and for up to 6 weeks during an epidemic; therapy should begin within 48 hours of exposure.

Doses in children over 1 year for the treatment of influenza are, according to body-weight: over 40 kg, the adult dose; 23 to 40 kg, 60 mg twice daily; 15 to 23 kg, 45 mg twice daily; less than 15 kg, 30 mg twice daily.

Dosage should be reduced in patients with moderate renal impairment (see below).

◊ Reviews.


1. Gubareva LV, *et al.* Influenza virus neuraminidase inhibitors. *Lancet* 2000; **355:** 827–35.
2. McClellan K, Perry CM. Oseltamivir: a review of its use in influenza. *Drugs* 2001; **61:** 263–83.
3. Jefferson T, *et al.* Neuraminidase inhibitors for preventing and treating influenza in healthy adults. Available in The Cochrane Library; Issue 1. Chichester: John Wiley; 2004.
4. Matheson NJ, *et al.* Neuraminidase inhibitors for preventing and treating influenza in children. Available in The Cochrane Library; Issue 1. Chichester: John Wiley; 2004.
5. Cooper NJ, *et al.* Effectiveness of neuraminidase inhibitors in treatment and prevention of influenza A and B: systematic review and meta-analyses of randomised controlled trials. *BMJ* 2003; **326:** 1235–9.


**Administration in renal impairment.** Dosage of oseltamivir should be reduced in patients with moderate renal impairment, according to creatinine clearance (CC):

- CC 10 to 30 mL/minute: *treatment of influenza*: 75 mg once daily or 30 mg twice daily; *prevention*: 75 mg on alternate days or 30 mg daily
- CC less than 10 mL/minute: not recommended

## Preparations

**Proprietary Preparations** (details are given in Part 3)
***Arg.:*** Tamiflu; ***Austral.:*** Tamiflu; ***Braz.:*** Tamiflu; ***Canad.:*** Tamiflu; ***Chile:*** Tamiflu; ***Fr.:*** Tamiflu; ***Hong Kong:*** Tamiflu; ***Irl.:*** Tamiflu; ***Israel:*** Tamiflu; ***Jpn:*** Tamiflu; ***NZ:*** Tamiflu; ***Port.:*** Tamiflu; ***Singapore:*** Tamiflu; ***Switz.:*** Tamiflu; ***UK:*** Tamiflu; ***USA:*** Tamiflu.

# Penciclovir *(BAN, USAN, rINN)*

BRL-39123 (penciclovir); BRL-39123-D (penciclovir sodium). 9-[4-Hydroxy-3-(hydroxymethyl)butyl]guanine.

$C_{10}H_{15}N_5O_3$ = 253.3.

*CAS — 39809-25-1 (penciclovir); 97845-62-0 (penciclovir sodium).*

*ATC — D06BB06; J05AB13.*

## Adverse Effects and Precautions

Penciclovir applied topically may cause transient stinging, burning, and numbness.

For adverse effects of penciclovir following systemic administration of famciclovir, see p.633.

## Interactions

Plasma concentrations of penciclovir may be increased in patients receiving *probenecid* with the prodrug famciclovir.

## Antiviral Action

Penciclovir has antiviral activity similar to that of aciclovir (p.626). It is active *in vitro* and *in vivo* against herpes simplex virus types 1 and 2 and against varicella-zoster virus. This activity is due to intracellular conversion by virus-induced thymidine kinase into penciclovir triphosphate, which inhibits replication of viral DNA and persists in infected cells for more than 12 hours. It also has activity against Epstein-Barr virus and hepatitis B virus.

◊ References.


1. Vere-Hodge RA. Famciclovir and penciclovir: the mode of action of famciclovir including its conversion to penciclovir. *Antiviral Chem Chemother* 1993; **4:** 67–84.
2. Boyd MR, *et al.* Penciclovir: a review of its spectrum of activity, selectivity, and cross-resistance pattern. *Antiviral Chem Chemother* 1993; **4** (suppl 1): 3–11.
3. Bacon TH, Boyd MR. Activity of penciclovir against Epstein-Barr virus. *Antimicrob Agents Chemother* 1995; **39:** 1599–1602.


## Pharmacokinetics

Penciclovir is poorly absorbed from the gastrointestinal tract. For systemic use it is usually given orally as the prodrug famciclovir, which is rapidly converted to penciclovir, producing peak plasma concentrations proportional to the dose (over the range 125 to 750 mg) after 45 minutes to 1 hour. The plasma elimination half-life is about 2 hours. The intracellular half-life of the active triphosphate metabolite is longer. Penciclovir is less than 20% bound to plasma proteins. Penciclovir is mainly excreted unchanged in the urine.

## Uses and Administration

Penciclovir is a nucleoside analogue structurally related to guanine, which is active against herpesviruses. It is applied topically as a 1% cream every 2 hours during waking hours for 4 days in the treatment of herpes labialis (see Herpes Simplex Infections, p.620).

For systemic use, penciclovir is administered by mouth as the prodrug famciclovir (see p.633). Intravenous administration of penciclovir has been investigated.

◊ References.


1. Spruance SL, *et al.* Penciclovir cream for the treatment of herpes simplex labialis: a randomized, multicenter, double-blind, placebo-controlled trial. *JAMA* 1997; **277:** 1374–9.
2. Lazarus HM, *et al.* Intravenous penciclovir for treatment of herpes simplex infections in immunocompromised patients: results of a multicenter, acyclovir-controlled trial. *Antimicrob Agents Chemother* 1999; **43:** 1192–7.
3. Boon R, *et al.* Penciclovir cream for the treatment of sunlight-induced herpes simplex labialis: a randomized, double-blind, placebo-controlled trial. *Clin Ther* 2000; **22:** 76–90.
4. Raborn GW, *et al.* Effective treatment of herpes simplex labialis with penciclovir cream: combined results of two trials. *J Am Dent Assoc* 2002; **133:** 303–9.
5. Lin L, *et al.* Topical application of penciclovir cream for the treatment of herpes simplex facialis/labialis: a randomized, double-blind, multicentre, aciclovir-controlled trial. *J Dermatol Treat* 2002; **13:** 67–72.


## Preparations

**Proprietary Preparations** (details are given in Part 3)
***Austral.:*** Vectavir; ***Austria:*** Famvir; Vectavir; ***Belg.:*** Vectavir; ***Braz.:*** Famvir; ***Denm.:*** Vectavir; ***Fin.:*** Vectavir; ***Fr.:*** Denavir†; ***Ger.:*** Vectavir; ***Gr.:*** Vectavir; ***Hong Kong:*** Vectavir; ***Israel:*** Vectavir; ***Ital.:*** Vectavir; ***Neth.:*** Famvir; ***Norw.:*** Vectavir; ***NZ:*** Vectavir; ***Spain:*** Vectavir; ***Swed.:*** Vectavir; ***Switz.:*** Famvir; ***UK:*** Vectavir; ***USA:*** Denavir.

# Peptide T

D-Ala-peptide-T-amide; Péptido T.

## Profile

Peptide T is an octapeptide segment of the envelope glycoprotein of HIV. It has been investigated for the treatment of HIV infection and HIV-associated neurological disorders. Peptide T has also been tried in the treatment of psoriasis.

# Pleconaril *(USAN, rINN)*

Pleconarilo; VP-63843; Win-63843. 3-{4-[3-(3-Methyl-5-isoxazolyl)propoxy]-3,5-xylyl}-5-(trifluoromethyl)-1,2,4-oxadizole.

$C_{18}H_{18}F_3N_3O_3$ = 381.3.

*CAS — 153168-05-9.*

*ATC — J05AX06.*

## Profile

Pleconaril is an oral antiviral with activity against a range of picornaviruses. It is under investigation for the treatment of viral meningitis, upper respiratory-tract viral infections including the common cold, and other enteroviral infections.

◊ References.


1. Nowak-Wegrzyn A, *et al.* Successful treatment of enterovirus infection with the use of pleconaril in 2 infants with severe combined immunodeficiency. *Clin Infect Dis* 2001; **32:** E13–E14.
2. Rotbart HA, Webster AD. Treatment of potentially life-threatening enterovirus infections with pleconaril. *Clin Infect Dis* 2001; **32:** 228–35.
3. Aradottir E, *et al.* Severe neonatal enteroviral hepatitis treated with pleconaril. *Pediatr Infect Dis J* 2001; **20:** 457–9.
4. Starlin R, *et al.* Acute flaccid paralysis syndrome associated with echovirus 19, managed with pleconaril and intravenous immunoglobulin. *Clin Infect Dis* 2001; **33:** 730–2.
5. Hayden FG, *et al.* Oral pleconaril treatment of picornavirus-associated viral respiratory illness in adults: efficacy and tolerability in phase II clinical trials. *Antivir Ther* 2002; **7:** 53–65.
6. Abzug MJ, *et al.* Double blind placebo-controlled trial of pleconaril in infants with enterovirus meningitis. *Pediatr Infect Dis J* 2003; **22:** 335–41.
7. Hayden FG, *et al.* Efficacy and safety of oral pleconaril for treatment of colds due to picornaviruses in adults: results of 2 double-blind, randomized, placebo-controlled trials. *Clin Infect Dis* 2003; **36:** 1523–32.


# Poly I.poly C12U

Poli(I)²poli($C_{12}$U); Poly(I):poly($C_{12}$,U).

## Profile

Poly I.poly C12U is a synthetic mismatched polymer of double-stranded RNA with antiviral and immunomodulatory activity. It is under investigation in the treatment of HIV infection, and also in renal cell carcinoma, chronic fatigue syndrome, invasive melanoma, and hepatitis B and C.

For a reference to the enhancement by poly I.poly C12U of zidovudine's anti-HIV activity *in vitro*, see Microbiological Interactions under Antiviral Action of Zidovudine, p.660.

## Propagermanium (rINN)

Propagermanio. A polymer obtained from 3-(trihydroxygermyl)propionic acid.

$(C_3H_5GeO_{3.5})_n$.

### Profile

Propagermanium is an immunomodulator that has been used in chronic hepatitis B infections. Acute exacerbation of hepatitis, including some fatalities, has been reported in patients receiving propagermanium.

◊ References.


1. Hirayama C, *et al.* Propagermanium: a nonspecific immune modulator for chronic hepatitis B. *J Gastroenterol* 2003; **38:** 525–32.


## Resiquimod (rINN)

R-848; S-28463; VML-600. 4-Amino-2-(ethoxymethyl)-α,α-dimethyl-1*H*-imidazo[4,5-*c*]quinoline-1-ethanol.

$C_{17}H_{22}N_4O_2$ = 314.4.

*CAS — 144875-48-9.*

### Profile

Resiquimod is an immune response modifier that has been investigated for the topical treatment of genital herpes.

◊ References.


1. Spruance SL, *et al.* Application of a topical immune response modifier, resiquimod gel, to modify the recurrence rate of recurrent genital herpes: a pilot study. *J Infect Dis* 2001; **184:** 196–200.


## Ribavirin (BAN, USAN, rINN)

ICN-1229; Ribavirina; Ribavirinum; Tribavirin. 1-β-D-Ribofuranosyl-1*H*-1,2,4-triazole-3-carboxamide.

$C_8H_{12}N_4O_5$ = 244.2.

*CAS — 36791-04-5.*

*ATC — J05AB04.*

**Pharmacopoeias.** In *Chin., Eur.* (see p.vi), and *US.*

**Ph. Eur. 5.0** (Ribavirin). A white or almost white crystalline powder. It exhibits polymorphism. Freely soluble in water; slightly soluble in alcohol; slightly soluble or very slightly soluble in dichloromethane. A 2% solution in water has a pH of 4.0 to 6.5. Protect from light.

**USP 27** (Ribavirin). A white crystalline powder. Freely soluble in water; slightly soluble in dehydrated alcohol. Store in airtight containers.

### Adverse Effects

When given *by inhalation*, ribavirin has sometimes led to deterioration in pulmonary function, bacterial pneumonia, and pneumothorax, to cardiovascular effects (including a fall in blood pressure and cardiac arrest), and, rarely, to anaemia and reticulocytosis. Conjunctivitis and skin rash have also occurred. Precipitation of inhaled ribavirin and consequent accumulation of fluid has occurred in the tubing of ventilating equipment.

Patients receiving ribavirin *by mouth* have experienced haemolytic anaemia, sometimes with associated increased serum concentrations of bilirubin and uric acid. A wide range of other adverse effects may occur as a result of the use of ribavirin with interferon alfa (see under Adverse Effects in Interferon Alfa, p.640).

### Precautions

SPECIFIC CAUTIONS FOR ORAL TREATMENT. Ribavirin should not be given orally to patients with pre-existing medical conditions that could be exacerbated by ribavirin-induced haemolysis, including unstable cardiac disease or haemoglobinopathies (thalassaemia or sickle-cell anaemia). Blood cell counts and chemistry should be measured at the start of treatment, after 2 and 4 weeks of treatment, and periodically thereafter. Patients with renal impairment and a creatinine clearance of less than 50 mL/minute should not receive oral ribavirin. It should be avoided in patients with severe hepatic impairment or decompensated cirrhosis of the liver. The potential for development of gout should be considered in predisposed patients.

Ribavirin has been reported to be teratogenic in *animals* and is contra-indicated in pregnancy or in those who may become pregnant. Pregnancy should also be avoided in partners of male patients taking ribavirin orally. Effective contraception should be used, and monthly pregnancy tests conducted, during treatment and for 6 months after the end of treatment in women and for 6 to 7 months after the end of treatment in men. Male patients whose partners are pregnant should use a condom to minimise vaginal exposure to ribavirin.

SPECIFIC CAUTIONS FOR INHALED TREATMENT. Standard supportive respiratory and fluid management should be maintained during aerosol treatment with ribavirin and electrolytes should be monitored closely. Administration equipment should be monitored for precipitation of ribavirin. Precautions should be taken to minimise atmospheric pollution with ribavirin during aerosol administration. Pregnant women and those planning pregnancy should avoid exposure to the aerosol.

**Contact lenses.** Report of damage to a nurse's soft contact lenses following intermittent occupational exposure to ribavirin over a period of 1 month.[1]


1. Diamond SA, Dupuis LL. Contact lens damage due to ribavirin exposure. *DICP Ann Pharmacother* 1989; **23:** 428–9.


### Interactions

**Anticoagulants.** For reference to the effect of ribavirin on the activity of *warfarin*, see under Antivirals, p.1026.

### Antiviral Action

Ribavirin inhibits a wide variety of viruses *in vitro* and in *animal* models. However, this activity has not necessarily correlated with activity against human infections. Ribavirin is phosphorylated but its mode of action is still unclear; it may act at several sites, including cellular enzymes, to interfere with viral nucleic acid synthesis. The mono- and triphosphate derivatives are believed to be responsible for its antiviral activity. Susceptible DNA viruses include herpesviruses, adenoviruses, and poxviruses. Susceptible RNA viruses include Lassa virus, members of the bunyaviridae group, influenza, parainfluenza, measles, mumps, and respiratory syncytial viruses, and (HIV).

**Microbiological interactions.** Ribavirin and *zidovudine* inhibited each others' antiviral activity *in vitro*.[1]


1. Vogt MW, *et al.* Ribavirin antagonizes the effect of azidothymidine on HIV replication. *Science* 1987; **235:** 1376–9.


### Pharmacokinetics

Ribavirin is rapidly absorbed following oral administration and peak plasma concentrations have been reported within 1 to 2 hours. Bioavailability following oral administration is about 45 to 65% as a result of first-pass metabolism. Steady state plasma concentrations are achieved after about 4 weeks with twice-daily oral doses. Ribavirin is also absorbed from the respiratory tract following inhalation. Ribavirin crosses the blood-brain barrier and, at steady state, concentrations in the CSF are 70% or more of those in the plasma. Accumulation occurs in red blood cells and ribavirin is detectable in sperm. Ribavirin undergoes phosphorylation by cellular enzymes to the mono-, di-, and triphosphate derivatives. Distribution and elimination is triphasic. The β-phase half-life is about 2 hours, and the terminal elimination half-life is reported to be 20 to 50 hours depending on the sampling time. Ribavirin is mainly excreted in the urine as unchanged drug and metabolites. Insignificant amounts of the drug are removed by haemodialysis. Ribavirin is still detectable in the plasma for up to 4 weeks after cessation of therapy.

◊ References.


1. Crumpacker C, *et al.* Ribavirin enters cerebrospinal fluid. *Lancet* 1986; **ii:** 45–6.
2. Laskin OL, *et al.* Ribavirin disposition in high-risk patients for acquired immunodeficiency syndrome. *Clin Pharmacol Ther* 1987; **41:** 546–55.
3. Roberts RB, *et al.* Ribavirin pharmacodynamics in high-risk patients for acquired immunodeficiency syndrome. *Clin Pharmacol Ther* 1987; **42:** 365–73.
4. Paroni R, *et al.* Pharmacokinetics of ribavirin and urinary excretion of the major metabolite 1,2,4-triazole-3-carboxamide in normal volunteers. *Int J Clin Pharmacol Ther Toxicol* 1989; **27:** 302–7.
5. Kramer TH, *et al.* Hemodialysis clearance of intravenously administered ribavirin. *Antimicrob Agents Chemother* 1990; **34:** 489–90.
6. Connor E, *et al.* Safety, tolerance, and pharmacokinetics of systemic ribavirin in children with human immunodeficiency virus infection. *Antimicrob Agents Chemother* 1993; **37:** 532–9.
7. Glue P, *et al.* The single dose pharmacokinetics of ribavirin in subjects with chronic liver disease. *Br J Clin Pharmacol* 2000; **49:** 417–21.


### Uses and Administration

Ribavirin is a synthetic nucleoside analogue structurally related to guanine. It is administered by aerosol in the treatment of respiratory syncytial virus infections (p.625); this route appears to give better results than the oral route although its efficacy by any route is questionable. It is used orally in combination with interferon alfa-2a or alfa-2b (or peginterferon alfa-2a or alfa-2b) in the treatment of chronic hepatitis C (p.618). Ribavirin has been tried in haemorrhagic fever with renal syndrome and in other types of haemorrhagic fever including Lassa fever.

Preparations of ribavirin are available for aerosol administration to infants and children with *severe respiratory syncytial virus infection* via a small particle aerosol generator. Solutions containing 20 mg/mL are used; 300 mL, representing 6 g of ribavirin, is delivered over a 12-to 18-hour period by aerosol at an average concentration of 190 micrograms/litre of air. Treatment is given for 3 to 7 days.

For the treatment of *chronic hepatitis C*, ribavirin is given daily by mouth in doses determined according to body-weight. In the UK, the dose of ribavirin in combination with interferon alfa-2b or peginterferon alfa-2b is 400 mg twice daily, in the morning and evening, for patients up to 65 kg; 400 mg in the morning and 600 mg in the evening for those between 65 and 85 kg; and 600 mg twice daily, in the morning and evening, for those over 85 kg. In combination with interferon alfa-2a or peginterferon alfa-2a, the UK dose is as in the USA regardless of the interferon used, namely 400 mg (in patients up to 75 kg) or 600 mg (in patients over 75 kg) in the morning, and 600 mg in the evening (regardless of body-weight). Children's doses in the USA are: 200 mg both in the morning and in the evening for those of body-weight 25 to 36 kg; 200 mg in the morning and 400 mg in the evening for those weighing 37 to 49 kg; and 400 mg both in the morning and evening for those weighing 50 to 61 kg. Treatment is continued for 6 to 12 months. Dose reductions of ribavirin may be necessary in patients who develop low haemoglobin concentrations.

**Encephalitis.** A beneficial response to ribavirin was reported in a child with severe La Crosse encephalitis.[1] Ribavirin was given intravenously in a dose of 25 mg/kg over the first 24 hours and then reduced to 15 mg/kg daily for a further 9 days.


1. McJunkin JE, *et al.* Treatment of severe La Crosse encephalitis with intravenous ribavirin following diagnosis by brain biopsy. *Pediatrics* 1997; **99:** 261–7.


**Haemorrhagic fevers.** The treatment of haemorrhagic fevers (p.618) is primarily symptomatic. However, ribavirin has been reported to reduce mortality in patients with Lassa fever,[1] haemorrhagic fever with renal syndrome,[2] and possibly Crimean-Congo haemorrhagic fever[3,4] and Bolivian haemorrhagic fever.[5] Ribavirin has also been tried in the related hantavirus pulmonary syndrome,[6,7] but preliminary results did not indicate an improvement in mortality.[8]

For treatment of *Lassa fever*, ribavirin has been given intravenously in a dose of 2 g initially, then 1 g every 6 hours for 4 days, then 500 mg every 8 hours for 6 days.[1] Treatment is most effective if instituted within 6 days of the onset of fever. Experience has shown that rigors may occur if the drug is given as a bolus injection, but that this can be overcome by giving it as an infusion over 30 minutes.[9] For prophylaxis, a dose of ribavirin 600 mg by mouth 4 times daily for 10 days has been suggested for adults,[10] although this was considered to be excessive by other commentators[11] who suggested that oral doses of 1 g daily (following an intravenous loading dose for those in whom the start of prophylaxis is delayed) might be suitable.


1. McCormick JB, *et al.* Lassa fever: effective therapy with ribavirin. *N Engl J Med* 1986; **314:** 20–6.
2. Huggins JW, *et al.* Prospective, double-blind, concurrent, placebo-controlled clinical trial of intravenous ribavirin therapy of hemorrhagic fever with renal syndrome. *J Infect Dis* 1991; **164:** 1119–27.
3. Fisher-Hoch SP, *et al.* Crimean Congo-haemorrhagic fever treated with oral ribavirin. *Lancet* 1995; **346:** 472–5.
4. Mardani M, *et al.* The efficacy of oral ribavirin in the treatment of crimean-congo hemorrhagic fever in Iran. *Clin Infect Dis* 2003; **36:** 1613–18.
5. Kilgore PE, *et al.* Treatment of Bolivian hemorrhagic fever with intravenous ribavirin. *Clin Infect Dis* 1997; **24:** 718–22.
6. Anonymous. Hantavirus pulmonary syndrome—northeastern United States, 1994. *JAMA* 1994; **272:** 997–8.
7. Prochoda K, *et al.* Hantavirus-associated acute respiratory failure. *N Engl J Med* 1993; **329:** 1744.
8. Khan AS, *et al.* Hantavirus pulmonary syndrome. *Lancet* 1996; **347:** 739–41.
9. Fisher-Hoch SP, *et al.* Unexpected adverse reactions during a clinical trial in rural West Africa. *Antiviral Res* 1992; **19:** 139–47.
10. Holmes GP, *et al.* Lassa fever in the United States: investigation of a case and new guidelines for management. *N Engl J Med* 1990; **323:** 1120–23.
11. Johnson KM, Monath TP. Imported Lassa fever—reexamining the algorithms. *N Engl J Med* 1990; **323:** 1139–41.

## Preparations

**BP 2003:** Ribavirin Nebuliser Solution;
**USP 27:** Ribavirin for Inhalation Solution.

**Proprietary Preparations** (details are given in Part 3)
**Austral.:** Virazide; **Austria:** Rebetol; **Belg.:** Rebetol; Virazole†; **Braz.:** Rebetol; Ribav; Ribaviron C; Viramid; Virazole; **Canad.:** Virazole; **Chile:** Rebetol; **Denm.:** Rebetol; **Fin.:** Rebetol; **Fr.:** Rebetol; **Ger.:** Rebetol; Virazole; **Gr.:** Rebetol; **Hong Kong:** Rebetol; Virazole; **India:** Ribavin; **Irl.:** Rebetol; **Israel:** Rebetol; **Ital.:** Rebetol; **Malaysia:** Rebetol; **Mex.:** Desiken; Vilona; Virazide; **Neth.:** Rebetol; Virazole; **Norw.:** Rebetol; **NZ:** Copegus; **Port.:** Copegus; Rebetol; **Singapore:** Rebetol; Virazole; **Spain:** Rebetol; Virazid†; Virazole; **Swed.:** Rebetol; Virazole; **Thai.:** Rebetol; **UK:** Copegus; Rebetol; Virazole; **USA:** Copegus; Virazole.

**Multi-ingredient: Arg.:** Bioferon Hepakit; Rebetron; **Austral.:** Pegatron; Rebetron; **Canad.:** Rebetron; **Mex.:** Hepatron C; **S.Afr.:** Rebetron; **Switz.:** Intron A/Rebetol; **USA:** Rebetron.

# Rimantadine Hydrochloride *(BANM, USAN, rINNM)*

EXP-126; Hidrocloruro de rimantadina. (*RS*)-1-(Adamantan-1-yl)ethylamine hydrochloride; α-Methyl-1-adamantanemethylamine hydrochloride.

$C_{12}H_{21}N,HCl = 215.8.$
*CAS — 13392-28-4 (rimantadine); 1501-84-4 (rimantadine hydrochloride).*
*ATC — J05AC02.*

**Pharmacopoeias.** In *US.*

**USP 27** (Rimantadine Hydrochloride). Store at a temperature of 15° to 30°.

## Adverse Effects and Precautions

The incidence and severity of adverse effects associated with rimantadine appear to be low. Those reported include gastrointestinal disturbances such as nausea, vomiting, and anorexia and CNS effects such as headache, insomnia, nervousness, dizziness, and concentration difficulties. It should be given with caution to patients with epilepsy. Doses are reduced in severe renal or hepatic impairment; reduced doses are also used in the elderly .

◊ A review[1] of clinical studies in healthy subjects concluded that rimantadine and amantadine were equally effective for prevention and treatment of influenza A, but rimantadine was significantly better tolerated than amantadine at usual doses.

In a study to evaluate the safety of long-term rimantadine hydrochloride for elderly, chronically ill individuals during an influenza A epidemic,[2] a significantly greater proportion of patients taking rimantadine developed anxiety and/or nausea compared with those taking placebo. There was also a significantly greater number of days in which anxiety, nausea, confusion, depression, or vomiting were reported. Most of these side-effects lasted less than 9 days and were seldom severe except in 2 patients who withdrew from the study because of insomnia, anxiety, or both and a third who suffered a generalised convulsion. In a larger study[3] the incidence of these symptoms was similar in treatment and placebo groups.

Observations of seizures in 2 patients receiving influenza prophylaxis with rimantadine hydrochloride emphasised that chronically ill and elderly patients prone to seizures (especially those who may have had antiepileptic therapy withdrawn) may be at risk of developing seizures.[4] A precautionary measure of reducing the rimantadine hydrochloride dosage to 100 mg daily together with temporary re-introduction of antiepileptics was suggested.


1. Jefferson TO, *et al.* Amantadine and rimantadine for preventing and treating influenza A in adults. Available in The Cochrane Library; Issue 1. Chichester: John Wiley; 2004.
2. Patriarca PA, *et al.* Safety of prolonged administration of rimantadine hydrochloride in the prophylaxis of influenza A virus infections in nursing homes. *Antimicrob Agents Chemother* 1984; **26:** 101–3.
3. Monto AS, *et al.* Safety and efficacy of long-term use of rimantadine for prophylaxis of type A influenza in nursing homes. *Antimicrob Agents Chemother* 1995; **39:** 2224–8.
4. Bentley DW, *et al.* Rimantadine and seizures. *Ann Intern Med* 1989; **110:** 323–4.


## Antiviral Action

Rimantadine inhibits influenza A viruses, probably at an early stage of replication, but its mechanism of action is not fully understood.

Resistance to rimantadine can be induced in influenza A virus *in vitro* and *in vivo* although resistance in clinical isolates is reported to occur infrequently. Transmission of rimantadine-resistant influenza A virus has been found among household contacts, and young children treated for established influenza A infection may excrete resistant virus within a week of beginning treatment.

◊ References to rimantadine resistance in influenza A virus.


1. Hall CB, *et al.* Children with influenza A infection: treatment with rimantadine. *Pediatrics* 1987; **80:** 275–82.
2. Belshe RB, *et al.* Genetic basis of resistance to rimantadine emerging during treatment of influenza virus infection. *J Virol* 1988; **62:** 1508–12.
3. Belshe RB, *et al.* Resistance of influenza A virus to amantadine and rimantadine: results of one decade of surveillance. *J Infect Dis* 1989; **159:** 430–5.
4. Hayden FG, *et al.* Emergence and apparent transmission of rimantadine-resistant influenza A virus in families. *N Engl J Med* 1989; **321:** 1696–1702.
5. Ziegler T, *et al.* Low incidence of rimantadine resistance in field isolates of influenza A viruses. *J Infect Dis* 1999; **180:** 935–9.


## Pharmacokinetics

Rimantadine hydrochloride is well, but slowly, absorbed from the gastrointestinal tract. Maximum plasma concentrations are reached about 6 hours after administration. It has a long plasma half-life; reported figures range from 24 to 36 hours. Protein binding of rimantadine is about 40%. The elimination half-life following a single dose is 13 to 65 hours in healthy subjects. It is extensively metabolised with less than 25% of a dose being excreted unchanged in the urine; about 75% is excreted as hydroxylated metabolites over 72 hours. In severe renal or hepatic impairment the half-life approximately doubles, necessitating a dosage reduction.

## Uses and Administration

Rimantadine hydrochloride is used similarly to amantadine hydrochloride (p.1197) in the prophylaxis and treatment of influenza A infections (p.624). It is given in usual adult doses of 200 mg daily by mouth in divided doses. Children may be given 5 mg/kg daily, up to a maximum of 150 mg. In elderly patients the usual daily dose is 100 mg. A dosage reduction is also necessary in patients with severe renal or severe hepatic impairment (see below).

◊ Reviews.


1. Jefferson TO, *et al.* Amantadine and rimantadine for preventing and treating influenza A in adults. Available in The Cochrane Library; Issue 1. Chichester: John Wiley; 2004.


**Administration in hepatic or renal impairment.** The usual oral dose of rimantadine in patients with severe renal or severe hepatic impairment is 100 mg daily.

## Preparations

**USP 27:** Rimantadine Hydrochloride Tablets.

**Proprietary Preparations** (details are given in Part 3)
**Arg.:** Germic; Oclovir; **Israel:** Flumadine; **USA:** Flumadine.

# Ritonavir *(BAN, USAN, rINN)*

A-84538; Abbott-84538; ABJ-538. 5-Thiazolylmethyl {(αS)-α-[(1*S*,3*S*)-1-hydroxy-3-((2*S*)-2-{3-[(2-isopropyl-4-thiazolyl)methyl]-3-methylureido}-3-methylbutyramido)-4-phenylbutyl]phenethyl}carbamate; *N*[1]-[(1*S*,3*S*,4*S*)-1-Benzyl-3-hydroxy-5-phenyl-4-(1,3-thiazol-5-ylmethoxycarbonylamino)pentyl]-*N*[2]-{[(2-isopropyl-1,3-thiazol-4-yl)methyl](methyl)carbamoyl}-L-valinamide.

$C_{37}H_{48}N_6O_5S_2 = 720.9.$
*CAS — 155213-67-5.*
*ATC — J05AE03.*

## Adverse Effects and Precautions

As for HIV-protease inhibitors in general (see Indinavir Sulfate, p.638). Vasodilatation has been commonly associated with ritonavir, and syncope and orthostatic hypotension have been reported. Pancreatitis has occurred in patients receiving ritonavir, and has been associated with hypertriglyceridaemia. Additional adverse effects reported with ritonavir include dyspepsia, dry mouth, ulceration of the oral mucosa, throat irritation and cough, hyperaesthesia, seizures, anxiety, sweating, and fever. Allergic reactions, rarely anaphylaxis, have been associated with ritonavir. There may be increases in uric acid concentrations and decreased free and total thyroxine concentrations. Neutrophil counts may be reduced or increased.

Ritonavir treatment should be discontinued in patients developing pancreatitis.

## Interactions

Interactions involving HIV-protease inhibitors are discussed under Indinavir Sulfate, p.639. Ritonavir is reported to have a high affinity for several cytochrome P450 isoenzymes with the following ranked order:

$$CYP3A > CYP2D6 > CYP2C9$$

Oral liquid formulations of ritonavir currently contain alcohol and concurrent administration with disulfiram or metronidazole should be avoided.

## Antiviral Action

As for HIV-protease inhibitors in general (see Indinavir Sulfate, p.639).

## Pharmacokinetics

Ritonavir is absorbed following oral administration and peak plasma concentrations occur in about 2 to 4 hours. Absorption is enhanced when ritonavir is taken with food, and is dose-related. Protein binding is reported to be about 98% and penetration into the CNS is minimal. Ritonavir is extensively metabolised in the liver principally by cytochrome P450 isoenzymes CYP3A and CYP2D6. The major metabolite has antiviral activity, but concentrations in plasma are low. Ritonavir is mainly excreted in the faeces, with a half-life of 3 to 5 hours.

◊ References.


1. Hsu A, *et al.* Multiple-dose pharmacokinetics of ritonavir in human immunodeficiency virus-infected subjects. *Antimicrob Agents Chemother* 1997; **41:** 898–905.
2. Hsu A, *et al.* Ritonavir: clinical pharmacokinetics and interactions with other anti-HIV agents. *Clin Pharmacokinet* 1998; **35:** 275–91.


## Uses and Administration

Ritonavir is a protease inhibitor with antiviral activity against HIV (see Antiviral Action, under Indinavir, p.639). It is used with other antiretrovirals for combination therapy of HIV infection (p.621).

Ritonavir is given by mouth in an adult dose of 600 mg twice daily with food. In order to minimise nausea, ritonavir may be started at a dose of 300 mg twice daily and gradually increased over a period of up to 14 days by 100 mg twice daily to a total of 600 mg twice daily. Children over the age of 2 years may be given an initial dose of 250 mg/m$^2$ twice daily increasing by 50 mg/m$^2$ twice daily at 2- or 3-day intervals up to 350 to 400 mg/m$^2$ twice daily, but not exceeding a total dose of 600 mg twice daily.

Ritonavir in doses of 100 mg twice daily is also used with some other HIV-protease inhibitors as a pharmacokinetic enhancer.

◊ Reviews.


1. Lea AP, Faulds D. Ritonavir. *Drugs* 1996; **52:** 541–6.
2. Cooper CL, *et al.* A review of low-dose ritonavir in protease inhibitor combination therapy. *Clin Infect Dis* 2003; **36:** 1585–92.


**Administration.** Adjusting the dosage regimen for ritonavir from 600 mg twice daily to 300 mg every 6 hours improved tolerability in 2 patients who would otherwise have discontinued the drug.[1]


1. Merry C, *et al.* Improved tolerability of ritonavir derived from pharmacokinetic principles. *Br J Clin Pharmacol* 1996; **42:** 787.


**Molluscum contagiosum.** Intractable molluscum contagiosum, a viral skin infection, resolved when a patient was given ritonavir for treatment of HIV infection.[1]


1. Hicks CB, *et al.* Resolution of intractable molluscum contagiosum in a human immunodeficiency virus-infected patient after institution of antiretroviral therapy with ritonavir. *Clin Infect Dis* 1997; **24:** 1023–5.


## Preparations

**Proprietary Preparations** (details are given in Part 3)
**Austral.:** Norvir; **Belg.:** Norvir; **Canad.:** Norvir; **Chile:** Norvir; **Denm.:** Norvir; **Fin.:** Norvir; **Fr.:** Norvir; **Ger.:** Norvir; **Gr.:** Norvir; **Hong Kong:** Norvir; **Irl.:** Norvir; **Israel:** Norvir; **Ital.:** Norvir; **Jpn:** Norvir; **Malaysia:** Norvir; **Mex.:** Norvir; **Neth.:** Norvir; **Norw.:** Norvir; **NZ:** Norvir; **Port.:** Norvir†; **S.Afr.:** Norvir; **Spain:** Norvir; **Swed.:** Norvir; **Switz.:** Norvir; **Thai.:** Norvir; **UK:** Norvir; **USA:** Norvir.

**Multi-ingredient: Arg.:** Kaletra; **Austral.:** Kaletra; **Belg.:** Kaletra; **Braz.:** Kaletra; **Canad.:** Kaletra; **Chile:** Kaletra; **Denm.:** Kaletra; **Fin.:** Kaletra; **Fr.:** Kaletra; **Ger.:** Kaletra; **Gr.:** Kaletra; **Hong Kong:** Kaletra; **Israel:** Kaletra; **Ital.:** Kaletra; **Norw.:** Kaletra; **NZ:** Kaletra; **Port.:** Kaletra; **Spain:** Kaletra; **Swed.:** Kaletra; **Switz.:** Kaletra; **Thai.:** Kaletra; **UK:** Kaletra; **USA:** Kaletra.

# Saquinavir *(BAN, USAN, rINN)*

Ro-31-8959. *N*[1]-{(1*S*,2*R*)-1-Benzyl-3-[(3*S*,4a*S*,8a*S*)-3-(*tert*-butylcarbamoyl)perhydroisoquinolin-2-yl]-2-hydroxypropyl}-*N*[2]-(2-quinolylcarbonyl)-L-aspartamide; (*S*)-*N*-[(α*S*)-α-{(1*R*)-2-[(3*S*,4a*S*,8a*S*)-3-(*tert*-Butylcarbamoyl)octahydro-2(1*H*)-isoquinolyl]-1-hydroxyethyl}phenethyl]-2-quinaldamidosuccinamide.

$C_{38}H_{50}N_6O_5 = 670.8.$
*CAS — 127779-20-8.*
*ATC — J05AE01.*

## Saquinavir Mesilate *(BANM, rINNM)*

Mesilato de saquinavir; Ro-31-8959/003; Saquinavir Mesylate (*USAN*). Saquinavir methanesulfonate.

$C_{38}H_{50}N_6O_5,CH_4O_3S = 766.9.$
*CAS — 149845-06-7.*
*ATC — J05AE01.*

**Pharmacopoeias.** In *US.*

**USP 27** (Saquinavir Mesylate). Store in airtight containers.

## Adverse Effects and Precautions

As for HIV-protease inhibitors in general (see Indinavir Sulfate, p.638). Stevens-Johnson syndrome, nephrolithiasis, and pancreatitis (in some cases fatal) have been associated with saquinavir. Additional adverse effects reported with saquinavir include ulceration of the oral mucosa, verruca, depression, seizures, and peripheral neuropathy. Allergic reactions have been associated with saquinavir. Acute haemolytic anaemia has occurred.

Bioavailability of some formulations of saquinavir is reported to be low owing to a combination of incomplete absorption and extensive first-pass metabolism; saquinavir may therefore be particularly susceptible to malabsorption (e.g. in the presence of diarrhoea).

### Interactions

Interactions involving HIV-protease inhibitors are discussed under Indinavir Sulfate, p.639.

Saquinavir is reported to be metabolised by the cytochrome P450 system, with the specific isoenzyme CYP3A4 responsible for more than 90% of the hepatic metabolism.

### Antiviral Action

As for HIV-protease inhibitors in general (see Indinavir Sulfate, p.639). HIV isolates resistant to saquinavir are reported to show cross-resistance to at least one other HIV-protease inhibitor in most patients.

### Pharmacokinetics

Saquinavir is absorbed to a limited extent (about 30%) following oral administration of the mesilate and undergoes extensive first-pass hepatic metabolism, resulting in a bioavailability of 4% when taken with food. Bioavailability is greater from a soft gelatin capsule formulation of saquinavir base in a suitable vehicle (*Fortovase, Roche*) than from the hard capsule formulation (*Invirase, Roche*). Bioavailability is substantially less when saquinavir is taken in the fasting state. Plasma concentrations are reported to be higher in HIV-infected patients than in healthy subjects. Saquinavir is about 98% bound to plasma proteins and extensively distributed into the tissues, although CSF concentrations are reported to be negligible. It is rapidly metabolised by the cytochrome P450 system (specifically the isoenzyme CYP3A4) to a number of inactive monohydroxylated and dihydroxylated compounds. It is excreted predominantly in the faeces with a reported terminal elimination half-life of 13.2 hours.

◊ References.


1. Regazzi MB, *et al.* Pharmacokinetic variability and strategy for therapeutic drug monitoring of saquinavir (SQV) in HIV-1 infected individuals. *Br J Clin Pharmacol* 1999; **47:** 379–82.
2. Grub S, *et al.* Pharmacokinetics and pharmacodynamics of saquinavir in pediatric patients with human immunodeficiency virus infection. *Clin Pharmacol Ther* 2002; **71:** 122–30.


### Uses and Administration

Saquinavir is a protease inhibitor with antiviral activity against HIV (see Antiviral Action, under Indinavir, p.639). It is used with other antiretrovirals for combination therapy of HIV infection (p.621).

Saquinavir is given by mouth as the mesilate (*Invirase, Roche*), but doses are expressed in terms of the base. 229 mg of saquinavir mesilate is approximately equivalent to 200 mg of saquinavir. The adult dose is 1 g twice daily given with ritonavir 100 mg twice daily, in combination with other antiretrovirals. Despite the greater bioavailability of saquinavir base formulated as soft gelatin capsules, this formulation (*Fortovase, Roche*) is also given in doses of 1 g twice daily with ritonavir and other antiretrovirals. It may be given in doses of 1.2 g three times daily after meals without ritonavir but with other antiretrovirals.

◊ Reviews.


1. Noble S, Faulds D. Saquinavir: a review of its pharmacology and clinical potential in the management of HIV infection. *Drugs* 1996; **52:** 93–112.
2. Moyle G. Saquinavir in the management of HIV infection. *Br J Hosp Med* 1997; **57:** 560–4.
3. Vella S, Floridia M. Saquinavir: clinical pharmacology and efficacy. *Clin Pharmacokinet* 1998; **34:** 189–201.
4. Figgitt DP, Plosker GL. Saquinavir soft-gel capsule: an updated review of its use in the management of HIV infection. *Drugs* 2000; **60:** 481–516.
5. Plosker GL, Scott LJ. Saquinavir: a review of its use in boosted regimens for treating HIV infection. *Drugs* 2003; **63:** 1299–1324.


#### Preparations

***USP 27:*** Saquinavir Capsules.

**Proprietary Preparations** (details are given in Part 3)
***Arg.:*** Fortovase; ***Austral.:*** Fortovase; Invirase; ***Austria:*** Fortovase; Invirase; ***Belg.:*** Fortovase; Invirase; ***Braz.:*** Fortovase; Invirase; ***Canad.:*** Fortovase; Invirase; ***Chile:*** Fortovase; ***Denm.:*** Fortovase; Invirase; ***Fin.:*** Fortovase; Invirase; ***Fr.:*** Fortovase; Invirase; ***Ger.:*** Fortovase; Invirase; ***Gr.:*** Fortovase; Invirase; ***Hong Kong:*** Fortovase; Invirase; ***Irl.:*** Fortovase; Invirase; ***Israel:*** Fortovase; Invirase; ***Ital.:*** Fortovase; Invirase; ***Jpn:*** Invirase; ***Mex.:*** Fortovase; Invirase†; ***Neth.:*** Fortovase; Invirase; ***Norw.:*** Fortovase; Invirase†; ***NZ:*** Fortovase; Invirase; ***Port.:*** Fortovase; Invirase†; ***S.Afr.:*** Fortovase; Invirase; ***Singapore:*** Invirase†; ***Spain:*** Fortovase; Invirase; ***Swed.:*** Fortovase; Invirase; ***Switz.:*** Fortovase; Invirase; ***Thai.:*** Fortovase; Invirase†; ***UK:*** Fortovase; Invirase; ***USA:*** Fortovase; Invirase.

## Sorivudine *(BAN, USAN, rINN)*

Bravavir; Bromovinylarauracil; Brovavir; BV-araU; BVAU; Sorivudina; SQ-32756; YN-72. (*E*)-1-β-D-Arabinofuranosyl-5-(2-bromovinyl)uracil.

$C_{11}H_{13}BrN_2O_6$ = 349.1.
*CAS — 77181-69-2.*

#### Profile

Sorivudine is a synthetic thymidine derivative with antiviral activity against varicella-zoster virus. It has been investigated for the treatment of herpes zoster but has been withdrawn from the market in Japan following deaths in patients receiving fluorouracil concomitantly.

◊ References.


1. Yawata M. Deaths due to drug interaction. *Lancet* 1993; **342:** 1166.
2. Diasio RB. Sorivudine and 5-fluorouracil: a clinically significant drug-drug interaction due to inhibition of dihydropyrimidine dehydrogenase. *Br J Clin Pharmacol* 1998; **46:** 1–4.


## Stavudine *(BAN, USAN, pINN)*

BMY-27857; d4T; Estavudina. 1-(2,3-Dideoxy-β-D-*glycero*-pent-2-enofuranosyl)thymine.

$C_{10}H_{12}N_2O_4$ = 224.2.
*CAS — 3056-17-5.*
*ATC — J05AF04.*

### Adverse Effects

Stavudine produces dose-related peripheral neuropathy. Raised liver enzyme concentrations and, rarely, hepatitis or hepatic failure may also occur during treatment. Pancreatitis has been reported and fatalities have occurred.

Other adverse effects noted in patients taking stavudine have included asthenia, chest pain, hypersensitivity reactions, and a flu-like syndrome; dizziness, headache, and insomnia; abdominal pain, anorexia, constipation, diarrhoea, nausea, and vomiting; neutropenia and thrombocytopenia; arthralgia and myalgia; mood changes; dyspnoea; pruritus and rashes; and lymphadenopathy and neoplasms.

Lactic acidosis, usually associated with severe hepatomegaly and steatosis, has been associated with treatment with nucleoside reverse transcriptase inhibitors (see Zidovudine, p.658).

There have been reports of motor weakness associated with stavudine, occurring particularly in association with lactic acidosis.

**Effects on the nervous system.** Peripheral neuropathy is a well recognised adverse effect of stavudine and has been the subject of a review.[1]


1. Moyle GJ, Sadler M. Peripheral neuropathy with nucleoside antiretrovirals: risk factors, incidence and management. *Drug Safety* 1998; **19:** 481–94.


**Gynaecomastia.** Bilateral gynaecomastia was associated with stavudine use in a patient with HIV infection who was also receiving lamivudine and co-trimoxazole.[1] Symptoms resolved when stavudine was discontinued. Four further cases of gynaecomastia were reported in HIV-infected patients receiving highly active antiretroviral therapy regimens all involving stavudine.[2]


1. Melbourne KM, *et al.* Gynecomastia with stavudine treatment in an HIV-positive patient. *Ann Pharmacother* 1998; **32:** 1108.
2. Manfredi R, *et al.* Gynecomastia associated with highly active antiretroviral therapy. *Ann Pharmacother* 2001; **35:** 438–9.


### Precautions

Stavudine should be used with caution in patients with a history of peripheral neuropathy and treatment suspended if peripheral neuropathy develops; if symptoms resolve on withdrawal, stavudine may be resumed at half the previous dose. Treatment with stavudine may be associated with lactic acidosis and should be discontinued if there is a rapid increase in aminotransferase concentrations, progressive hepatomegaly or steatosis, or metabolic or lactic acidosis of unknown aetiology. Stavudine should be given with caution to patients with hepatomegaly or other risk factors for liver disease. Patients with a history of pancreatitis should also be observed carefully for signs of pancreatitis during treatment with stavudine. Concomitant use of other drugs likely to cause peripheral neuropathy or pancreatitis should be avoided if possible. Stavudine should be used with caution and doses reduced in patients with renal impairment.

### Interactions

The intracellular activation of stavudine and hence its antiviral effect may be inhibited by zidovudine, doxorubicin, and ribavirin.

Use of stavudine with other drugs known to cause pancreatitis or peripheral neuropathy should be avoided if possible.

**Antidiabetics.** Fatal lactic acidosis has been reported[1] in a patient who received *metformin* together with didanosine, stavudine, and tenofovir.


1. Worth L, *et al.* A cautionary tale: fatal lactic acidosis complicating nucleoside analogue and metformin therapy. *Clin Infect Dis* 2003; **37:** 315–16.


**Antivirals.** References to *in-vivo* antagonism of the antiretroviral effect of stavudine when used with *zidovudine*.[1]


1. Havlir DV, *et al.* In vivo antagonism with zidovudine plus stavudine combination therapy. *J Infect Dis* 2000; **182:** 321–5.


**Phenylpropanolamine.** Hypertensive crisis associated with use of phenylpropanolamine and clemastine occurred in a patient receiving HIV prophylaxis with indinavir, lamivudine, and stavudine.[1] The most likely cause was an interaction between phenylpropanolamine and stavudine, although interactions with the other antiretrovirals could not be ruled out.


1. Khurana V, *et al.* Hypertensive crisis secondary to phenylpropanolamine interacting with triple-drug therapy for HIV prophylaxis. *Am J Med* 1999; **106:** 118–19.


### Antiviral Action

Stavudine is converted intracellularly in stages to the triphosphate. This triphosphate halts the DNA synthesis of retroviruses, including HIV, through competitive inhibition of reverse transcriptase and incorporation into viral DNA. Stavudine-resistant strains of HIV have been identified and cross-resistance to other nucleoside reverse transcriptase inhibitors may occur.

### Pharmacokinetics

Stavudine is absorbed rapidly following oral administration producing peak plasma concentrations within 1 hour and with a reported bioavailability of about 86%. Administration with food delays but does not reduce absorption. Stavudine crosses the blood-brain barrier producing a CSF to plasma ratio of about 0.4 after 4 hours. Binding to plasma proteins is negligible. Stavudine is metabolised intracellularly to the active antiviral triphosphate. The elimination half-life is reported to be about 1 to 1.5 hours following single or multiple doses. The intracellular half-life of stavudine triphosphate has been estimated to be 3.5 hours *in vitro*. About 40% of a dose is excreted in the urine by active tubular secretion and glomerular filtration. Stavudine is removed by haemodialysis.

◊ References.


1. Rana KZ, Dudley MN. Clinical pharmacokinetics of stavudine. *Clin Pharmacokinet* 1997; **33:** 276–84.
2. Kaul S, *et al.* Effect of food on bioavailability of stavudine in subjects with human immunodeficiency virus infection. *Antimicrob Agents Chemother* 1998; **42:** 2295–8.
3. Grasela DM, *et al.* Pharmacokinetics of single-dose oral stavudine in subjects with renal impairment and in subjects requiring hemodialysis. *Antimicrob Agents Chemother* 2000; **44:** 2149–53.


### Uses and Administration

Stavudine is a nucleoside reverse transcriptase inhibitor related to thymidine with activity against retroviruses including HIV. It is used in the treatment of HIV infection, usually in combination with other antiretrovirals. However, use with zidovudine is not recommended (see Interactions, above). Usual adult doses of stavudine are 40 mg every 12 hours by mouth for patients weighing 60 kg or more or 30 mg every 12 hours for patients weighing less than 60 kg. The dose in children over 3 months of age and weighing less than 30 kg is 1 mg/kg every 12 hours; children weighing more than 30 kg are given the adult dose.

For details of reduced doses of stavudine to be used in patients with renal impairment, see below.

Stavudine is also available in some countries as an extended-release preparation suitable for once-daily administration in adults in a dose of 100 mg daily (in those weighing 60 kg or more) or 75 mg daily (in those weighing less than 60 kg).

◊ Reviews.


1. Hurst M, Noble S. Stavudine: an update of its use in the treatment of HIV infection. *Drugs* 1999; **58:** 919–49.
2. Cheer SM, Goa KL. Stavudine once daily. *Drugs* 2002; **62:** 2667–74.


**Administration in renal impairment.** Dosage reduction according to creatinine clearance (CC) is recommended for patients receiving stavudine who have renal impairment:

- CC 26 to 50 mL/minute: 20 mg every 12 hours (those weighing 60 kg or more) or 15 mg every 12 hours (those weighing less than 60 kg)
- CC below 25 mL/minute: 20 mg every 24 hours (those weighing 60 kg or more) or 15 mg every 24 hours (those weighing less than 60 kg)

### Preparations

**Proprietary Preparations** (details are given in Part 3)
***Arg.:*** Birac; Lion; Revixil; Stamar; Stelea; STV; Tonavir; Zerit; ***Austral.:*** Zerit; ***Austria:*** Zerit; ***Belg.:*** Zerit; ***Braz.:*** Zeritavir; ***Canad.:*** Zerit; ***Chile:*** Zerit; ***Denm.:*** Zerit; ***Fin.:*** Zerit; ***Fr.:*** Zerit; ***Ger.:*** Zerit; ***Gr.:*** Zerit; ***Hong Kong:*** Zerit; ***India:*** Stavir; ***Irl.:*** Zerit; ***Israel:*** Zerit; ***Ital.:*** Zerit; ***Jpn:*** Zerit; ***Malaysia:*** Zerit; ***Mex.:*** Zerit; ***Neth.:*** Zerit; ***Norw.:*** Zerit; ***NZ:*** Zerit; ***Port.:*** Zerit; ***S.Afr.:*** Zerit; ***Singapore:*** Zerit; ***Spain:*** Zerit; ***Swed.:*** Zerit; ***Switz.:*** Zerit; ***Thai.:*** Zerit; ***UK:*** Zerit; ***USA:*** Zerit.

## Tenofovir *(BAN, USAN, rINN)*

GS-1278; PMPA; (R)-PMPA. 9-[(R)-2-(Phosphonomethoxy)propyl]adenine monohydrate; {[(R)-2-(6-Amino-9H-purin-9-yl)-1-methylethoxy]methyl}phosphonic acid monohydrate.

$C_9H_{14}N_5O_4P,H_2O$ = 305.2.

*CAS — 147127-20-6 (anhydrous tenofovir); 206184-49-8 (tenofovir monohydrate).*

## Tenofovir Disoproxil Fumarate *(BANM, USAN, rINNM)*

Fumarato de disoproxilo de tenofovir; GS-4331/05. 9-{(R)-2-[(Bis{[(isopropoxycarbonyl)oxy]methoxy}phosphinyl)methoxy]propyl}adenine fumarate (1:1).

$C_{19}H_{30}N_5O_{10}P,C_4H_4O_4$ = 635.5.

*CAS — 202138-50-9.*

*ATC — J05AF07.*

### Adverse Effects

The most common adverse effects reported from the use of tenofovir disoproxil fumarate are mild gastrointestinal effects, particularly diarrhoea, nausea and vomiting, abdominal pain, flatulence, dyspepsia, and anorexia. Serum-amylase concentrations may be raised and pancreatitis has been reported. Hypophosphataemia occurs commonly. Skin rashes may occur. Other adverse effects occurring commonly include peripheral neuropathy, headache, dizziness, insomnia, depression, asthenia, sweating, and myalgia. There have also been reports of raised liver enzymes, hypertriglyceridaemia, hyperglycaemia, and neutropenia. There have also been reports of renal impairment, acute renal failure, and effects on the renal proximal tubules, including Fanconi syndrome.

Lactic acidosis, usually associated with severe hepatomegaly and steatosis, has been associated with treatment with nucleoside reverse transcriptase inhibitors (see Zidovudine, p.658).

### Precautions

Treatment with tenofovir disoproxil fumarate should be discontinued if there is a rapid increase in aminotransferase concentrations, progressive hepatomegaly or steatosis, or metabolic or lactic acidosis of unknown aetiology. It should be given with caution to patients with hepatomegaly or other risk factors for liver disease. In particular, extreme caution should be exercised in patients with co-existing hepatitis C infection who are receiving treatment with interferon alfa and ribavirin.

Tenofovir should be used with caution, and doses modified, in patients with renal impairment. Monitoring of renal function and serum phosphates is recommended before treatment with tenofovir disoproxil fumarate and every 4 weeks during therapy; in patients with a history of renal impairment, consideration should be given to more frequent monitoring. If serum phosphate concentrations fall markedly or if creatinine clearance is below 50 mL/minute, renal function should be evaluated within a week, and consideration given to interruption of treatment. Tenofovir disoproxil fumarate may be associated with reduction in bone density and patients should be observed for evidence of bone abnormalities.

### Interactions

Use of tenofovir disoproxil fumarate with other drugs eliminated by active tubular secretion is not recommended; if such use is unavoidable, renal function should be monitored weekly. For reference to the effects of concomitant use of tenofovir with didanosine, see p.631.

**Antidiabetics.** Fatal lactic acidosis has been reported[1] in a patient who received *metformin* together with didanosine, stavudine, and tenofovir.


1. Worth L, *et al.* A cautionary tale: fatal lactic acidosis complicating nucleoside analogue and metformin therapy. *Clin Infect Dis* 2003; **37:** 315–16.


### Antiviral Action

Tenofovir is converted intracellularly to the diphosphate. This diphosphate halts the DNA synthesis of HIV through competitive inhibition of reverse transcriptase and incorporation into viral DNA. Tenofovir-resistant strains of HIV have been identified and cross-resistance to other reverse transcriptase inhibitors may occur.

### Pharmacokinetics

Tenofovir disoproxil fumarate is rapidly absorbed and converted to tenofovir following oral administration, with peak plasma concentrations occurring after 1 to 2 hours. Bioavailability in fasting patients is reported to be 25%, but this is enhanced when tenofovir disoproxil fumarate is taken with a high fat meal. Tenofovir is widely distributed into body tissues, particularly the kidneys and liver. Binding to plasma proteins is reported to be less than 1% and that to serum proteins about 7%. The terminal elimination half-life of tenofovir is 12 to 18 hours. Tenofovir is excreted mainly in the urine by both active tubular secretion and glomerular filtration. It is removed by haemodialysis.

### Uses and Administration

Tenofovir is a nucleotide reverse transcriptase inhibitor used, in combination with other antiretrovirals, for the treatment of HIV infection. It is given by mouth as the disoproxil fumarate ester. Tenofovir disoproxil fumarate 300 mg is equivalent to 245 mg of tenofovir disoproxil and to 136 mg of tenofovir. The usual dose is 300 mg of the disoproxil fumarate ester once daily with food. The base has been given intravenously.

For details of modified doses of tenofovir disoproxil fumarate to be used in patients with renal impairment, see below.

◊ Reviews.


1. Grim SA, Romanelli F. Tenofovir disoproxil fumarate. *Ann Pharmacother* 2003; **37:** 849–59.
2. Chapman TM, *et al.* Tenofovir disoproxil fumarate. *Drugs* 2003; **63:** 1597–1608.
3. Gallant JE, Deresinski S. Tenofovir disoproxil fumarate. *Clin Infect Dis* 2003; **37:** 944–50.


**Administration in renal impairment.** Doses of tenofovir disoproxil fumarate should be modified by adjustment of the dosing interval in patients with renal impairment according to their creatinine clearance (CC):

- CC 50 mL or more per minute: usual once-daily dosage
- CC 30 to 49 mL/minute: every 48 hours
- CC 10 to 29 mL/minute: every 72 to 96 hours
- haemodialysis patients: a dose every 7 days or after a cumulative total of 12 hours of dialysis

### Preparations

**Proprietary Preparations** (details are given in Part 3)
***Austral.:*** Viread; ***Canad.:*** Viread; ***Fr.:*** Viread; ***Irl.:*** Viread; ***Spain:*** Viread; ***UK:*** Viread; ***USA:*** Viread.

## Tipranavir *(rINN)*

PNU-140690; U-140690. 3′-{(1R)-1-[(6R)-5,6-Dihydro-4-hydroxy-2-oxo-6-phenethyl-6-propyl-2H-pyran-3-yl]propyl}-5-(trifluoromethyl)-2-pyridinesulfonanilide.

$C_{31}H_{33}F_3N_2O_5S$ = 602.7.

*CAS — 174484-41-4 (tipranavir); 191150-83-1 (tipranavir disodium).*

NOTE. Tipranavir Disodium is *USAN*.

### Profile

Tipranavir is an HIV-protease inhibitor under investigation for the treatment, in combination with other antiretrovirals, of HIV infection.

◊ Reviews.


1. Plosker GL, Figgitt DP. Tipranavir. *Drugs* 2003; **63:** 1611–18.


## Tremacamra *(USAN, rINN)*

BIRR-004; 1–453-Glycoprotein ICAM-1 (human reduced). 1-453-Glycoprotein ICAM-1 (human reduced).

*CAS — 155576-45-7.*

### Profile

Tremacamra is a recombinant soluble intercellular adhesion molecule 1 (ICAM-1) under investigation for the treatment of the common cold.

◊ References.


1. Turner RB, *et al.* Efficacy of tremacamra, a soluble intercellular adhesion molecule 1, for experimental rhinovirus infection: a randomized clinical trial. *JAMA* 1999; **281:** 1797–1804.


## Trichosanthin

Compound Q; GLQ-223 (a purified form of trichosanthin); Tricosantina.

*CAS — 60318-52-7 (trichosanthins); 116899-30-0 (Trichosanthes kirilowii); 160185-58-0 (Trichosanthes kirilowii root); 120947-28-6 (GLQ-223).*

### Profile

Trichosanthin is a polypeptide extracted from the tuber of the Chinese cucumber, *Trichosanthes kirilowii* (Cucurbitaceae). It is under investigation in the treatment of HIV infection and is used in China as an abortifacient.

**HIV infection and AIDS.** Trichosanthin has been given to patients with AIDS, AIDS-related complex, or HIV infection.[1,2] It has generally been given by intravenous injection. In one study[1] it was also given by intramuscular injection but that route was abandoned due to the occurrence of pain and necrosis at the injection site. A common adverse effect on intravenous administration was a flu-like syndrome with headache, myalgias, fever, and arthralgia and was generally mild to moderate,[3] although neurological effects progressing to coma with fatalities have been reported.[1,2] Improvements in surrogate markers for HIV infection have been reported including increases in CD4+ T lymphocyte counts in patients with moderate disease[3] and in patients failing to respond to reverse transcriptase inhibitors.[4]


1. Byers VS, *et al.* A phase I/II study of trichosanthin treatment of HIV disease. *AIDS* 1990; **4:** 1189–96.
2. Kahn JO, *et al.* The safety and pharmacokinetics of GLQ223 in subjects with AIDS and AIDS-related complex: a phase I study. *AIDS* 1990; **4:** 1197–1204.
3. Kahn JO, *et al.* Safety, activity, and pharmacokinetics of GLQ223 in patients with AIDS and AIDS-related complex. *Antimicrob Agents Chemother* 1994; **38:** 260–7.
4. Byers VS, *et al.* A phase II study of effect of addition of trichosanthin to zidovudine in patients with HIV disease and failing antiretroviral agents. *AIDS Res Hum Retroviruses* 1994; **10:** 413–20.


## Trifluridine *(USAN, rINN)*

$F_3T$; $F_3TDR$; NSC-75520; Trifluorothymidine; Trifluridina. ααα-Trifluorothymidine; 2′-Deoxy-5-trifluoromethyluridine.

$C_{10}H_{11}F_3N_2O_5$ = 296.2.

*CAS — 70-00-8.*

*ATC — S01AD02.*

**Pharmacopoeias.** In *US.*

**USP 27** (Trifluridine). A white, odourless powder, appearing under the microscope as rod-like crystals. Store in airtight containers. Protect from light.

### Adverse Effects

Adverse effects occurring after the use of trifluridine in the eyes are similar to those for idoxuridine (p.637) but have been reported to occur less frequently.

◊ References.


1. Udell IJ. Trifluridine-associated conjunctival cicatrization. *Am J Ophthalmol* 1985; **99:** 363–4.


### Antiviral Action

Trifluridine acts similarly to idoxuridine to interfere with viral DNA synthesis following phosphorylation. It is reported to be active against herpes simplex viruses, some adenoviruses, vaccinia viruses, and cytomegalovirus. Like idoxuridine it is incorporated into mammalian DNA.

### Pharmacokinetics

Trifluridine is absorbed through the cornea following ocular administration and penetration may be increased in the presence of damage or inflammation. Systemic absorption does not appear to follow ocular administration.

### Uses and Administration

Trifluridine is a pyrimidine nucleoside structurally related to thymidine. It is used in the treatment of primary keratoconjunctivitis and recurrent epithelial keratitis due to herpes simplex viruses. One drop of a 1% ophthalmic solution is instilled into the eye every 2 hours up to a maximum of 9 times daily until complete re-epithelialisation has occurred. Treatment is then reduced to one drop every 4 hours to a minimum of 5 drops daily for a further 7 days.

◊ Reviews.

1. Heidelberger C, King DH. Trifluorothymidine. *Pharmacol Ther* 1979; **6:** 427–42.
2. Carmine AA, *et al.* Trifluridine: a review of its antiviral activity and therapeutic use in the topical treatment of viral eye infections. *Drugs* 1982; **23:** 329–53.

### Preparations

**Proprietary Preparations** (details are given in Part 3)
***Belg.:*** TFT Ophtiole†; ***Braz.:*** Zost†; ***Canad.:*** Viroptic†; ***Fr.:*** Triherpine†; Virophta; ***Ger.:*** TFT†; Triflumann; ***Gr.:*** Thilol; ***Hong Kong:*** Bephen†; Triherpine; ***Ital.:*** Triherpine; ***Neth.:*** TFT Ophtiole; ***Port.:*** Adrocil; Viridin; ***S.Afr.:*** TFT; ***Spain:*** Viromidin; ***Switz.:*** Triherpine; ***Thai.:*** Triherpine; ***USA:*** Viroptic.

## Tromantadine Hydrochloride *(rINNM)*

D-41; Hidrocloruro de tromantadina. N-1-Adamantyl-2-(2-dimethylaminoethoxy)acetamide hydrochloride; 2-(2-Dimethylaminoethoxy)-N-(tricyclo[3.3.1.1$^{3,7}$]dec-1-yl)acetamide hydrochloride.

$C_{16}H_{28}N_2O_2,HCl = 316.9.$

*CAS — 53783-83-8 (tromantadine); 41544-24-5 (tromantadine hydrochloride).*

*ATC — D06BB02; J05AC03.*

### Profile

Tromantadine hydrochloride is a derivative of amantadine (p.1197) used for its antiviral activity. It is applied topically at a concentration of 1% in the treatment of herpes simplex infections of the skin and mucous membranes and of herpes zoster.

Contact dermatitis has been reported following the topical use of tromantadine hydrochloride.

**Effects on the skin.** References to contact dermatitis associated with the use of tromantadine.

1. Fanta D, Mischer P. Contact dermatitis from tromantadine hydrochloride. *Contact Dermatitis* 1976; **2:** 282–4.
2. Lembo G, *et al.* Allergic dermatitis from Viruserol ointment probably due to tromantadine hydrochloride. *Contact Dermatitis* 1984; **10:** 317.
3. Jauregui I, *et al.* Allergic contact dermatitis from tromantadine. *J Investig Allergol Clin Immunol* 1997; **7:** 260–1.

### Preparations

**Proprietary Preparations** (details are given in Part 3)
***Austria:*** Viru-Merz; ***Belg.:*** Viru-Merz; ***Braz.:*** Herpex; ***Chile:*** Viru-Merz; ***Denm.:*** Viru-Merz†; ***Ger.:*** Viru-Merz; ***Gr.:*** Viru-Merz Serol; ***Hong Kong:*** Viru-Merz; ***Israel:*** Viru-Merz; ***Ital.:*** Viruserol; ***Malaysia:*** Viru-Merz; ***Mex.:*** Viru-Serol; ***Neth.:*** Viru-Merz; ***Port.:*** Viru-Merz; ***Singapore:*** Viru-Merz; ***Spain:*** Viru-Serol; ***Switz.:*** Viru-Merz Serol.

## Valaciclovir Hydrochloride

*(BANM, rINNM)*

Hidrocloruro de valaciclovir; 256U87 (valaciclovir); Valacyclovir Hydrochloride *(USAN)*. L-Valine, ester with 9-[(2-hydroxyethoxy)methyl]guanine hydrochloride.

$C_{13}H_{20}N_6O_4,HCl = 360.8.$

*CAS — 124832-26-4 (valaciclovir); 124832-27-5 (valaciclovir hydrochloride);.*

*ATC — J05AB11.*

### Adverse Effects and Precautions

As for Aciclovir, p.626.

### Interactions

As for Aciclovir, p.626.

### Antiviral Action

As for Aciclovir, p.626.

### Pharmacokinetics

Valaciclovir is readily absorbed from the gastrointestinal tract following oral administration, and is rapidly converted to aciclovir and valine by first-pass intestinal or hepatic metabolism. The bioavailability of aciclovir following valaciclovir administration is reported to be 54% and peak plasma concentrations of aciclovir are achieved after 1.5 hours. Valaciclovir is eliminated principally as aciclovir and its metabolite 9-carboxymethoxymethylguanine (see p.627); less than 1% of a dose of valaciclovir is excreted unchanged in the urine.

◊ References.

1. Steingrimsdottir H, *et al.* Bioavailability of aciclovir after oral administration of aciclovir and its prodrug valaciclovir to patients with leukopenia after chemotherapy. *Antimicrob Agents Chemother* 2000; **44:** 207–9.
2. Höglund M, *et al.* Comparable aciclovir exposures produced by oral valaciclovir and intravenous aciclovir in immunocompromised cancer patients. *J Antimicrob Chemother* 2001; **47:** 855–61.
3. Bras AP, *et al.* Comparative bioavailability of acyclovir from oral valacyclovir and acyclovir in patients treated for recurrent genital herpes simplex virus infection. *Can J Clin Pharmacol* 2001; **8:** 207–11.
4. Nadal D, *et al.* An investigation of the steady-state pharmacokinetics of oral valacyclovir in immunocompromised children. *J Infect Dis* 2002; **186** (suppl 1): S123–S130.

### Uses and Administration

Valaciclovir is a prodrug of the antiviral aciclovir (p.627). It is used in the treatment of herpes zoster (p.621) and herpes simplex infections (p.620) of the skin and mucous membranes, including genital herpes. Treatment should be started as soon as symptoms occur. It is also used for the prophylaxis of cytomegalovirus infection following renal transplantation. Valaciclovir is given by mouth as the hydrochloride; doses are expressed in terms of the base. Valaciclovir hydrochloride 1.11 g is approximately equivalent to 1 g of valaciclovir.

For herpes zoster, the dose is 1 g three times daily for 7 days. For treatment of herpes simplex infections, 500 mg is given twice daily for 5 days (3 days in the USA) for recurrent episodes or for up to 10 days for a first episode; in the USA, the recommended dose for a first episode of genital herpes is 1 g twice daily for 10 days. For the suppression of herpes simplex infection, a dose of 500 mg daily as a single dose or in two divided doses, is recommended; in the USA, a dose of 1 g daily as a single dose is recommended for suppression of recurrent genital herpes. A dose of 500 mg twice daily may be used in immunocompromised patients. For the treatment of herpes labialis, a dose of 4 g in two divided doses 12 hours apart is recommended. A dose of 2 g four times daily is recommended for prophylaxis of cytomegalovirus infection in renal transplant recipients; prophylaxis should begin within 72 hours and is usually continued for 90 days.

Doses of valaciclovir may need to be reduced in patients with renal impairment (see Administration in Renal Impairment, below).

◊ References.

1. Ormrod D, *et al.* Valaciclovir: a review of its long term utility in the management of genital herpes simplex virus and cytomegalovirus infections. *Drugs* 2000; **59:** 839–63.
2. Ormrod D, Goa K. Valaciclovir: a review of its use in the management of herpes zoster. *Drugs* 2000; **59:** 1317–40.
3. Baker DA. Valacyclovir in the treatment of genital herpes and herpes zoster. *Expert Opin Pharmacother* 2002; **3:** 51–8.
4. Tyring SK, *et al.* Valacyclovir for herpes simplex virus infection: long-term safety and sustained efficacy after 20 years' experience with acyclovir. *J Infect Dis* 2002; **186** (suppl 1): S40–S46.
5. Corey L, *et al.* Once-daily valacyclovir to reduce the risk of transmission of genital herpes. *N Engl J Med* 2004; **350:** 11–20.

**Administration in renal impairment.** Doses of valaciclovir may need to be reduced in patients with renal impairment. The following dosage reductions are suggested by the UK manufacturer according to creatinine clearance (CC):

*herpes zoster:*
- CC 15 to 30 mL/minute: 1 g twice daily
- CC less than 15 mL/minute: 1 g daily
- patients on haemodialysis: 1 g daily after haemodialysis

*herpes simplex infections:*
- CC 15 to 30 mL/minute: no modification
- CC less than 15 mL/minute: 500 mg daily
- patients on haemodialysis: 500 mg daily after haemodialysis

*suppression of herpes simplex:*
- CC below 15 mL/minute: *immunocompetent patients*: 250 mg once daily; *immunocompromised patients*: 500 mg once daily
- patients on haemodialysis: *immunocompetent patients*: 250 mg once daily after haemodialysis; *immunocompromised patients*: 500 mg once daily after haemodialysis

*prophylaxis of cytomegalovirus:*
- CC 50 to 74 mL/minute: 1.5 g four times daily
- CC 25 to 49 mL/minute: 1.5 g three times daily
- CC 10 to 24 mL/minute: 1.5 g twice daily
- CC less than 10 mL/minute: 1.5 g once daily
- patients on haemodialysis: 1.5 g once daily after haemodialysis

### Preparations

**Proprietary Preparations** (details are given in Part 3)
***Arg.:*** Valtrex; Viranet; ***Austral.:*** Valtrex; ***Austria:*** Valtrex; ***Belg.:*** Zelitrex; ***Braz.:*** Valtrex; ***Canad.:*** Valtrex; ***Chile:*** Pervioral; Vadiral; Valtrex; Virmax; ***Denm.:*** Zelitrex; ***Fin.:*** Valavir; Valtrex; ***Fr.:*** Zelitrex; ***Ger.:*** Valtrex; ***Gr.:*** Valtrex; ***Hong Kong:*** Valtrex; ***Irl.:*** Valtrex; ***Israel:*** Valtrex; ***Ital.:*** Talavir; Zelitrex; ***Malaysia:*** Valtrex; ***Mex.:*** Rapivir; ***Neth.:*** Zelitrex; ***Norw.:*** Valtrex; ***Port.:*** Valavir; Valtrex; ***S.Afr.:*** Zelitrex; ***Singapore:*** Valtrex; ***Spain:*** Valherpes; Valpridol†; Valtrex; Virval; ***Swed.:*** Valtrex; ***Switz.:*** Valtrex; ***Thai.:*** Valtrex; ***UK:*** Valtrex; ***USA:*** Valtrex.

## Valganciclovir Hydrochloride

*(BANM, USAN, rINNM)*

Hidrocloruro de valganciclovir; Ro-107-9070/194; RS-079070-194. L-Valine, ester with 9-{[2-hydroxy-1-(hydroxymethyl)-ethoxy]methyl} guanine hydrochloride.

$C_{14}H_{22}N_6O_5,HCl = 390.8.$

*CAS — 175865-60-8 (valganciclovir); 175865-59-5 (valganciclovir hydrochloride).*

*ATC — J05AB14.*

**Stability.** References.

1. Anaizi NH, *et al.* Stability of valganciclovir in an extemporaneously compounded oral liquid. *Am J Health-Syst Pharm* 2002; **59:** 1267–70.
2. Henkin CC, *et al.* Stability of valganciclovir in extemporaneously compounded liquid formulations. *Am J Health-Syst Pharm* 2003; **60:** 687–90.

### Adverse Effects, Treatment, and Precautions

As for Ganciclovir, p.635.

### Interactions

As for Ganciclovir, p.636.

### Antiviral Action

As for Ganciclovir, p.636.

### Pharmacokinetics

Valganciclovir is well absorbed from the gastrointestinal tract following oral administration and is rapidly converted to ganciclovir by first-pass intestinal or hepatic metabolism. The bioavailability of ganciclovir following valganciclovir administration is reported to be about 60% and peak plasma concentrations of ganciclovir are achieved between 1 and 3 hours after administration. Valganciclovir is eliminated in the urine as ganciclovir (see p.636).

◊ References.

1. Brown F, *et al.* Pharmacokinetics of valganciclovir and ganciclovir following multiple oral dosages of valganciclovir in HIV- and CMV-seropositive volunteers. *Clin Pharmacokinet* 1999; **37:** 167–76.
2. Jung D, Dorr A. Single-dose pharmacokinetics of valganciclovir in HIV- and CMV-seropositive subjects. *J Clin Pharmacol* 1999; **39:** 800–4.
3. Pescovitz MD, *et al.* Valganciclovir results in improved oral absorption of ganciclovir in liver transplant recipients. *Antimicrob Agents Chemother* 2000; **44:** 2811–15.

### Uses and Administration

Valganciclovir is a prodrug of the antiviral ganciclovir (p.636) that is used for the treatment of cytomegalovirus retinitis in patients with AIDS, and for the prevention of cytomegalovirus disease in heart, kidney, or kidney-pancreas transplant recipients who have received an organ from a cytomegalovirus-positive donor.

Valganciclovir is given by mouth with food as the hydrochloride; doses are expressed in terms of the base. Valganciclovir hydrochloride 1.1 g is approximately equivalent of 1 g of valganciclovir.

For induction in patients with active cytomegalovirus retinitis, the dose is 900 mg twice daily for 21 days. For maintenance following induction, or in patients with inactive cytomegalovirus retinitis, the dose is 900 mg daily. Patients whose retinitis deteriorates during maintenance may repeat induction but the possibility of viral resistance should be considered. For prevention of cytomegalovirus disease in organ transplant recipients, the dose is 900 mg daily starting within 10 days and continuing until 100 days after transplantation. Doses of valganciclovir may need to be reduced in renal impairment (see Administration in Renal Impairment, below).

◊ Reviews.

1. Curran M, Noble S. Valganciclovir. *Drugs* 2001; **61:** 1145–50.
2. Cocohoba JM, McNicholl IR. Valganciclovir: an advance in cytomegalovirus therapeutics. *Ann Pharmacother* 2002: **36:** 1075–9.

**Administration in renal impairment.** Doses of valganciclovir in patients with renal impairment may need to be reduced according to creatinine clearance (CC):

- CC 40 to 59 mL/minute: 450 mg twice daily for induction and 450 mg daily for maintenance
- CC 25 to 39 mL/minute: 450 mg daily for induction and 450 mg every two days for maintenance
- CC 10 to 24 mL/minute: 450 mg every two days for induction and 450 mg twice weekly for maintenance
- haemodialysis patients: not recommended

### Preparations

**Proprietary Preparations** (details are given in Part 3)
***Austral.:*** Valcyte; ***Fr.:*** Rovalcyte; ***Irl.:*** Valcyte; ***NZ:*** Valcyte; ***UK:*** Valcyte; ***USA:*** Valcyte.

## Vidarabine *(BAN, USAN, rINN)*

Adenine Arabinoside; Ara-A; CI-673; Vidarabina. 9-β-D-Arabinofuranosyladenine monohydrate.

$C_{10}H_{13}N_5O_4,H_2O = 285.3$.
*CAS — 5536-17-4 (anhydrous vidarabine); 24356-66-9 (vidarabine monohydrate).*
*ATC — J05AB03; S01AD06.*

**Pharmacopoeias.** In *US.*

**USP 27** (Vidarabine). A white to off-white powder. Very slightly soluble in water; slightly soluble in dimethylformamide. Store in airtight containers.

## Vidarabine Phosphate *(BANM, USAN, rINNM)*

Ara-AMP; Arabinosyladenine Monophosphate; CI-808; Fosfato de vidarabina; Vidarabine 5′-Monophosphate. 9-β-D-Arabinofuranosyladenine 5′-(dihydrogen phosphate).

$C_{10}H_{14}N_5O_7P = 347.2$.
*CAS — 29984-33-6.*
*ATC — J05AB03; S01AD06.*

## Vidarabine Sodium Phosphate *(BANM, USAN, rINNM)*

CI-808 Sodium. 9-β-D-Arabinofuranosyladenine 5′-(dihydrogen phosphate) disodium.

$C_{10}H_{12}N_5Na_2O_7P = 391.2$.
*CAS — 71002-10-3.*
*ATC — J05AB03; S01AD06.*

### Adverse Effects

Adverse effects that may occur when vidarabine is applied to the eyes include irritation, pain, superficial punctate keratitis, photophobia, lachrymation, and occlusion of the lachrymal duct.

### Pharmacokinetics

Systemic absorption does not occur following application of vidarabine to the eye; trace amounts of its principal metabolite hypoxanthine arabinoside (arabinosyl hypoxanthine), and vidarabine, if the cornea is damaged, may be found in the aqueous humour.

### Uses and Administration

Vidarabine is a purine nucleoside obtained from *Streptomyces antibioticus*. It has been used in the treatment of herpes simplex and varicella-zoster infections, although aciclovir and related drugs are generally preferred.

Vidarabine has been administered topically in the treatment of herpes simplex keratitis and keratoconjunctivitis as a 3% ophthalmic ointment, applied 5 times daily every 3 hours until corneal re-epithelialisation has occurred, then twice daily for a further 7 days to prevent recurrence.

Vidarabine has also been used as the sodium phosphate as a 10% gel for the treatment of genital herpes, applied four times daily at four-hourly intervals for 7 days.

Vidarabine was formerly used intravenously in the treatment of severe and disseminated herpes simplex infections and herpes zoster but aciclovir is preferred.

### Preparations

***USP 27:*** Vidarabine Ophthalmic Ointment.

**Proprietary Preparations** (details are given in Part 3)
***Austral.:*** Vira-A†; ***Fr.:*** Vira-MP†; ***NZ:*** Vira-A†; ***USA:*** Vira-A†.

# Zalcitabine *(BAN, USAN, rINN)*

DDC; ddC; ddCyd; Dideoxycytidine; NSC-606170; Ro-24-2027; Ro-24-2027/000; Zalcitabina. 2′,3′-Dideoxycytidine.

$C_9H_{13}N_3O_3 = 211.2$.
*CAS — 7481-89-2.*
*ATC — J05AF03.*

**Pharmacopoeias.** In *US.*

**USP 27** (Zalcitabine). A white to off-white, crystalline powder. Soluble in water and in methyl alcohol; sparingly soluble in alcohol, in acetonitrile, in chloroform, and in dichloromethane; slightly soluble in cyclohexane. Store in airtight containers. Protect from light.

### Adverse Effects

The most serious adverse effects of zalcitabine are peripheral neuropathy, which can affect up to one-third of patients, and pancreatitis which is rare, affecting up to about 1% of patients, but which can be fatal. Other severe adverse effects include oral and oesophageal ulceration, hypersensitivity reactions including anaphylaxis, cardiomyopathy and heart failure, lactic acidosis and severe hepatomegaly with steatosis (both potentially life-threatening), and hepatic failure.

Other adverse effects noted in patients taking zalcitabine have included asthenia, chest pain, fatigue, and fever; dizziness, headache, and insomnia; abdominal pain, anorexia, constipation, diarrhoea, dysphagia, nausea, and vomiting; anaemia, leucopenia, neutropenia, and thrombocytopenia; raised liver enzyme values; arthralgia and myalgia; mood changes; dyspnoea and pharyngitis; alopecia, pruritus, and rashes; hearing and visual disturbances; hyperuricaemia; and renal disorders.

**Effects on the nervous system.** Reviews of peripheral neuropathy associated with the use of zalcitabine.

1. Moyle GJ, Sadler M. Peripheral neuropathy with nucleoside antiretrovirals: risk factors, incidence and management. *Drug Safety* 1998; **19:** 481–94.
2. Carey P. Peripheral neuropathy: zalcitabine reassessed. *Int J STD AIDS* 2000; **11:** 417–23.

### Precautions

Zalcitabine should be interrupted or discontinued if peripheral neuropathy develops. Neuropathy is usually slowly reversible if treatment is stopped promptly but may be irreversible if treatment is continued after symptoms develop. Zalcitabine should be avoided in patients who already have peripheral neuropathy. It should be used with caution in patients at risk of developing peripheral neuropathy (especially those with a low CD4+ cell count) and in those receiving other drugs that may cause it (see Interactions, below).

Treatment should be interrupted in patients who develop abdominal pain, nausea, or vomiting or with abnormal biochemical test results until pancreatitis has been excluded. Zalcitabine should be discontinued permanently if pancreatitis develops. Patients with a history of pancreatitis or of raised serum amylase should be monitored closely. Zalcitabine should not be used with other drugs known to cause pancreatitis (see Interactions, below).

Zalcitabine should be used with caution in patients with hepatic impairment and treatment interrupted or discontinued if hepatic function deteriorates or there are signs of hepatic damage or lactic acidosis. It should be used with caution in patients with renal impairment, and dosage reductions may be necessary. It should also be used with caution in patients with cardiomyopathy or heart failure.

Complete blood count and biochemical tests should be carried out before treatment starts and at regular intervals throughout therapy.

**Handling.** Exposure of the skin to zalcitabine and inhalation of zalcitabine powder should be avoided.

### Interactions

Zalcitabine should not be used with other drugs known to cause pancreatitis (for example intravenous pentamidine). Caution is necessary when zalcitabine is given with other drugs that may cause peripheral neuropathy, such as other nucleoside reverse transcriptase inhibitors, chloramphenicol, dapsone, ethionamide, isoniazid (the clearance of which may also be affected—see p.223), metronidazole, nitrofurantoin, ribavirin, and vincristine. Use of zalcitabine with didanosine is not recommended.

The absorption of zalcitabine is reduced by about 25% when given with aluminium- or magnesium-containing antacids.

Cimetidine, probenecid, or trimethoprim can reduce the renal excretion of zalcitabine, resulting in elevated plasma concentrations. Renal excretion of zalcitabine may also be reduced by amphotericin B, aminoglycosides, or foscarnet, potentially increasing its toxicity.

The antiviral action of zalcitabine may be antagonised by lamivudine and the two drugs should not be used together.

### Antiviral Action

Zalcitabine is converted intracellularly in stages to the triphosphate. This triphosphate halts the DNA synthesis of retroviruses, including HIV, through competitive inhibition of reverse transcriptase and incorporation into viral DNA.

The emergence of zalcitabine-resistant strains of HIV has been reported.

◊ References.

1. Jeffries DJ. The antiviral activity of dideoxycytidine. *J Antimicrob Chemother* 1989; **23** (suppl A): 29–34.

### Pharmacokinetics

Zalcitabine is absorbed from the gastrointestinal tract with a bioavailability of greater than 80%. The rate of absorption is reduced by administration with food. Peak plasma concentrations in the fasting state are achieved within about 1 hour. Zalcitabine crosses the blood-brain barrier producing CSF concentrations ranging from 9 to 37% of those in plasma. Binding to plasma proteins is negligible. The plasma elimination half-life is about 2 hours.

Zalcitabine is metabolised intracellularly to the active antiviral triphosphate. It does not appear to undergo any substantial hepatic metabolism and is excreted mainly in the urine, in part by active tubular secretion.

◊ References.

1. Morse GD, *et al.* Comparative pharmacokinetics of antiviral nucleoside analogues. *Clin Pharmacokinet* 1993; **24:** 101–23.
2. Devineni D, Gallo JM. Zalcitabine: clinical pharmacokinetics and efficacy. *Clin Pharmacokinet* 1995; **28:** 351–60.
3. Chadwick EG, *et al.* Phase I evaluation of zalcitabine administered to human immunodeficiency virus-infected children. *J Infect Dis* 1995; **172:** 1475–9.
4. Bazunga M, *et al.* The effects of renal impairment on the pharmacokinetics of zalcitabine. *J Clin Pharmacol* 1998; **38:** 28–33.

### Uses and Administration

Zalcitabine is a nucleoside reverse transcriptase inhibitor derived from cytidine with activity against retroviruses including HIV. It is used in the treatment of HIV infection, usually in combination with other antiretrovirals.

Zalcitabine is given by mouth in a dose of 750 micrograms every 8 hours. Doses should be reduced in patients with renal impairment (see below).

◊ Reviews.

1. Whittington R, Brodgen RN. Zalcitabine: a review of its pharmacology and clinical potential in acquired immunodeficiency syndrome (AIDS). *Drugs* 1992; **44:** 656–83.
2. Lipsky JJ. Zalcitabine and didanosine. *Lancet* 1993; **341:** 30–2.
3. Shelton MJ, *et al.* Zalcitabine. *Ann Pharmacother* 1993; **27:** 480–9.
4. Adkins JC, *et al.* Zalcitabine: an update of its pharmacodynamic and pharmacokinetic properties and clinical efficacy in the management of HIV infection. *Drugs* 1997; **53:** 1054–80.

**Administration in renal impairment.** Doses of zalcitabine should be reduced for patients with renal impairment according to creatinine clearance (CC):

- CC 10 to 40 mL/minute: 750 micrograms every 12 hours
- CC less than 10 mL/minute: 750 micrograms every 24 hours

**HIV infection and AIDS.** Zalcitabine has been used as an alternative antiretroviral to treat HIV infection in patients intolerant of or unresponsive to zidovudine, although it has not been shown to have any great advantage over zidovudine in patients with advanced disease[1,2] and may be less well tolerated.[3]

Zalcitabine is now generally used with other antiretrovirals, usually another nucleoside reverse transcriptase inhibitor and either an HIV-protease inhibitor or a non-nucleoside reverse transcriptase inhibitor. Combination therapy with zalcitabine and zidovudine was superior to zidovudine alone in delaying disease progression and in prolonging life in patients who had not previously received antiretroviral therapy.[4,5] Combination therapy has been less successful in patients who have previously received zidovudine than in zidovudine-naive patients,[6] and zalcitabine with zidovudine was reported to be less effective than combinations of zidovudine with didanosine[4,5] or lamivudine.[7] Use of zalcitabine and saquinavir, with or without zidovudine, has shown favourable responses.[8-10]

For a general discussion on the management of HIV infection and AIDS, see p.621.


1. Fischl MA, *et al.* Zalcitabine compared with zidovudine in patients with advanced HIV-1 infection who received previous zidovudine therapy. *Ann Intern Med* 1993; **118:** 762–9.
2. Fischl MA, *et al.* Combination and monotherapy with zidovudine and zalcitabine in patients with advanced HIV disease. *Ann Intern Med* 1995; **122:** 24–32.
3. Bozzette SA, *et al.* Health status and function with zidovudine or zalcitabine as initial therapy for AIDS: a randomized controlled trial. *JAMA* 1995; **273:** 295–301.
4. Delta Coordinating Committee. Delta: a randomised double-blind controlled trial comparing combinations of zidovudine plus didanosine or zalcitabine with zidovudine alone in HIV-infected individuals. *Lancet* 1996; **348:** 283–91.
5. Hammer SM, *et al.* A trial comparing nucleoside monotherapy with combination therapy in HIV-infected adults with CD4 cell counts from 200 to 500 per cubic millimeter. *N Engl J Med* 1996; **335:** 1081–90.
6. Saravolatz LD, *et al.* Zidovudine alone or in combination with didanosine or zalcitabine in HIV-infected patients with the acquired immunodeficiency syndrome or fewer than 200 CD4 cells per cubic millimeter. *N Engl J Med* 1996; **335:** 1099–1106.
7. Bartlett JA, *et al.* Lamivudine plus zidovudine compared with zalcitabine plus zidovudine in patients with HIV infection: a randomized, double-blind, placebo-controlled trial. *Ann Intern Med* 1996; **125:** 161–72.
8. Collier AC, *et al.* Treatment of human immunodeficiency virus infection with saquinavir, zidovudine, and zalcitabine. *N Engl J Med* 1996; **334:** 1011–17.
9. Revicki DA, *et al.* Quality of life outcomes of combination zalcitabine-zidovudine, saquinavir-zidovudine, and saquinavir-zalcitabine-zidovudine therapy for HIV-infected adults with CD4 cell counts between 50 and 350 per cubic millimeter. *AIDS* 1999; **13:** 851–8.
10. Revicki DA, *et al.* Quality of life outcomes of saquinavir, zalcitabine and combination saquinavir plus zalcitabine therapy for adults with advanced HIV infection with CD4 counts between 50 and 300 cells/mm³. *Antivir Ther* 1999; **4:** 35–44.


## Preparations

***USP 27:*** Zalcitabine Tablets.

**Proprietary Preparations** (details are given in Part 3)
***Arg.:*** Hivid; Inxibir; ***Austral.:*** Hivid; ***Austria:*** Hivid; ***Belg.:*** Hivid; ***Braz.:*** Citavir†; Hivid; ***Canad.:*** Hivid; ***Chile:*** Hivid; ***Denm.:*** Hivid; ***Fin.:*** Hivid; ***Fr.:*** Hivid; ***Ger.:*** Hivid; ***Gr.:*** Hivid; ***Hong Kong:*** Hivid; ***Irl.:*** Hivid; ***Israel:*** Hivid; ***Ital.:*** Hivid; ***Jpn:*** Hivid; ***Mex.:*** Hivid; ***Neth.:*** Hivid; ***Norw.:*** Hivid†; ***NZ:*** Hivid†; ***Port.:*** Hivid; ***S.Afr.:*** Hivid; ***Singapore:*** Hivid; ***Spain:*** Hivid; ***Swed.:*** Hivid; ***Switz.:*** Hivid; ***Thai.:*** Hivid; ***UK:*** Hivid; ***USA:*** Hivid.

---

# Zanamivir *(BAN, USAN, rINN)*

GG-167; GR-121167X; 4-Guanidino-2,4-dideoxy-2,3-dehydro-*N*-acetylneuraminic Acid. 5-Acetamido-2,6-anhydro-3,4,5-trideoxy-4-guanidino-D-*glycero*-D-*galacto*-non-2-enonic acid.

$C_{12}H_{20}N_4O_7$ = 332.3.

*CAS — 139110-80-8.*

*ATC — J05AH01.*

## Adverse Effects

Inhaled zanamivir has generally been well tolerated. Acute bronchospasm or decline in respiratory function, with some fatalities, has been reported rarely in patients with a history of respiratory disease and very rarely in those with no such history. Other effects that have been noted include nasal symptoms, headache, gastrointestinal symptoms, cough, and bronchitis, but they may be difficult to distinguish from the symptoms of influenza. There have also been rare reports of hypersensitivity reactions, including oropharyngeal oedema and severe skin rashes, in association with zanamivir.

◊ Reviews.


1. Freund B, *et al.* Zanamivir: a review of clinical safety. *Drug Safety* 1999; **21:** 267–81.
2. Gravenstein S, *et al.* Zanamivir: a review of clinical safety in individuals at high risk of developing influenza-related complications. *Drug Safety* 2001; **24:** 1113–25.


## Precautions

Zanamivir should be used with caution in patients with chronic respiratory diseases as they may be at increased risk of bronchospasm; if zanamivir use is considered appropriate, patients with asthma or chronic obstructive pulmonary disease should have a fast-acting bronchodilator available during treatment. Patients on maintenance therapy with inhaled bronchodilators should administer the bronchodilator before zanamivir. Patients experiencing bronchospasm should be advised to discontinue zanamivir and seek medical attention.

## Antiviral Action

Zanamivir inhibits the viral surface enzyme neuraminidase (sialidase) which is essential for the release of newly formed viral particles from infected cells, and may facilitate access of virus through mucus to the cell surface. Zanamivir is active against influenza A and B virus replication.

**Resistance.** References.


1. Gubareva LV, *et al.* Evidence for zanamivir resistance in an immunocompromised child infected with influenza B virus. *J Infect Dis* 1998; **178:** 1257–62.
2. McKimm-Breschkin JL. Resistance of influenza viruses to neuraminidase inhibitors—a review. *Antiviral Res* 2000; **47:** 1–17.


## Pharmacokinetics

Zanamivir is poorly absorbed following oral administration with a bioavailability of about 2%. About 10 to 20% of the inhaled dose is absorbed producing peak serum concentrations at about 1 to 2 hours. The remainder is deposited in the oropharynx and eliminated via the gastrointestinal tract. The absorbed portion is excreted unchanged in the urine with a serum half-life of 2.6 to 5 hours.

◊ References.


1. Aoki FY, Hayden FG (eds.). The pharmacokinetics of zanamivir: a new inhaled antiviral for influenza. *Clin Pharmacokinet* 1999; **36** (suppl 1): 1–58.


## Uses and Administration

Zanamivir is a neuraminidase inhibitor used for the treatment of influenza A and B (p.624). It is administered by inhalation in a dose of 10 mg twice daily for 5 days, starting as soon as possible (within 48 hours) after the onset of symptoms.

Zanamivir is also under investigation for prophylaxis of influenza.

◊ Reviews.


1. Gubareva LV, *et al.* Influenza virus neuraminidase inhibitors. *Lancet* 2000; **355:** 827–35.
2. Cheer SM, Wagstaff AJ. Zanamivir: an update of its use in influenza. *Drugs* 2002; **62:** 71–106.
3. Jefferson T, *et al.* Neuraminidase inhibitors for preventing and treating influenza in healthy adults. Available in The Cochrane Library; Issue 1. Chichester: John Wiley; 2004.
4. Matheson NJ, *et al.* Neuraminidase inhibitors for preventing and treating influenza in children. Available in The Cochrane Library; Issue 1. Chichester: John Wiley; 2004.
5. Fleming DM. Zanamivir in the treatment of influenza. *Expert Opin Pharmacother* 2003; **4:** 799–805.
6. Cooper NJ, *et al.* Effectiveness of neuraminidase inhibitors in treatment and prevention of influenza A and B: systematic review and meta-analyses of randomised controlled trials. *BMJ* 2003; **326:** 1235–9.


**Influenza prophylaxis.** Randomised, placebo-controlled studies in healthy subjects[1] have shown intranasal zanamivir to be well tolerated and effective for prophylaxis of experimental influenza A. Early use (within 32 hours of inoculation with the virus) reduced the occurrence of fever, peak viral titres, and the duration of viral shedding by 3 days.[1] Delayed use (beginning 50 hours after inoculation) produced rapid decline in viral titres and subsequent reduction of the duration of viral shedding by 1 day, but had no effect on symptoms.[1] Zanamivir has been reported to be effective for prophylaxis in household contacts of patients with suspected influenza.[2]


1. Hayden FG, *et al.* Safety and efficacy of the neuraminidase inhibitor GG167 in experimental human influenza. *JAMA* 1996; **275:** 295–9.
2. Monto AS, *et al.* Zanamivir prophylaxis: an effective strategy for the prevention of influenza types A and B within households. *J Infect Dis* 2002; **186:** 1582–8.


## Preparations

**Proprietary Preparations** (details are given in Part 3)
***Arg.:*** Relenza; ***Austral.:*** Relenza; ***Austria:*** Relenza; ***Belg.:*** Relenza; ***Braz.:*** Relenza†; ***Canad.:*** Relenza; ***Chile:*** Relenza; ***Denm.:*** Relenza; ***Fin.:*** Relenza; ***Fr.:*** Relenza; ***Ger.:*** Relenza; ***Gr.:*** Relenza; ***Hong Kong:*** Relenza; ***Irl.:*** Relenza; ***Israel:*** Relenza; ***Ital.:*** Relenza; ***Mex.:*** Relenza; ***Neth.:*** Relenza; ***Norw.:*** Relenza; ***NZ:*** Relenza; ***Port.:*** Relenza; ***S.Afr.:*** Relenza; ***Singapore:*** Relenza†; ***Spain:*** Relenza; ***Swed.:*** Relenza; ***Switz.:*** Relenza; ***UK:*** Relenza; ***USA:*** Relenza.

---

# Zidovudine *(BAN, USAN, rINN)*

Azidodeoxythymidine; Azidothymidine; AZT; BW-A509U; BW-509U; Compound-S; Zidovudina; Zidovudinum. 3′-Azido-3′-deoxythymidine.

$C_{10}H_{13}N_5O_4$ = 267.2.

*CAS — 30516-87-1.*

*ATC — J05AF01.*

NOTE. The abbreviation AZT has also been used for azathioprine.

**Pharmacopoeias.** In *Eur.* (see p.vi), *Pol.*, and *US.*

**Ph. Eur. 5.0** (Zidovudine). A white to brownish powder. It shows polymorphism. Sparingly soluble in water; soluble in dehydrated alcohol. Protect from light.

**USP 27** (Zidovudine). A white to yellowish powder. Exhibits polymorphism. Sparingly soluble in water; soluble in alcohol. Store in airtight containers at a temperature of 25°, excursions permitted between 15° and 30°. Protect from light.

## Adverse Effects

The commonest serious adverse effects reported with zidovudine are anaemia and leucopenia, mainly neutropenia, occurring within a few weeks of starting treatment. This haematological toxicity occurs most commonly in those with pre-existing haematological abnormalities and is usually reversed by interrupting treatment or reducing dosage but it can be severe enough to require blood transfusion.

Other reported adverse effects include asthenia, fever, malaise, dizziness, headache, insomnia, myalgia, myopathy, paraesthesia, dyspnoea, cough, abdominal pain, anorexia, dyspepsia, taste disturbance, diarrhoea, nausea, vomiting, and rashes. Lactic acidosis and severe hepatomegaly with steatosis have been reported as rare, but potentially fatal, occurrences in patients taking zidovudine. Pancreatitis, convulsions, and pigmentation of nails, skin, and oral mucosa have occurred.

Zidovudine is reported to be carcinogenic in *rodents*.

◊ Adverse effects with zidovudine tend to be dose-related and reversible. In more advanced disease, the risk of zidovudine toxicity is greater.

Some references to the incidence and range of adverse effects are given below.


1. Richman DD, *et al.* The toxicity of azidothymidine (AZT) in the treatment of patients with AIDS and AIDS-related complex: a double-blind, placebo-controlled trial. *N Engl J Med* 1987; **317:** 192–7.
2. Gelmon K, *et al.* Nature, time course and dose dependence of zidovudine-related side effects: results from the Multicenter Canadian Azidothymidine Trial. *AIDS* 1989; **3:** 555–61.
3. Fischl MA, *et al.* The safety and efficacy of zidovudine (AZT) in the treatment of subjects with mildly symptomatic human immunodeficiency virus type 1 (HIV) infection: a double-blind, placebo-controlled trial. *Ann Intern Med* 1990; **112:** 727–37.
4. McKinney RE, *et al.* Safety and tolerance of intermittent intravenous and oral zidovudine therapy in human immunodeficiency virus-infected pediatric patients. *J Pediatr* 1990; **116:** 640–7.
5. Koch MA, *et al.* Toxic effects of zidovudine in asymptomatic human immunodeficiency-virus-infected individuals with CD4+ cell counts of 0.5x10⁹/L or less: detailed and updated results from protocol 019 of the AIDS Clinical Trials Group. *Arch Intern Med* 1992; **152:** 2286–92.


**Effects on the blood.** Adverse haematological effects reported with zidovudine may be severe and include anaemia with erythroid aplasia or hypoplasia, and neutropenia.[1-5] Although these effects may be reversed by withdrawal,[5] they may persist for weeks afterwards[2,3] and blood transfusions may be required in some patients.[1-4] A study indicated that zidovudine-induced neutropenia only significantly increased the risk of bacterial infection in patients whose polymorphonuclear cell count fell below 500/microlitre.[6] The effects of zidovudine on the platelet count are considered to be complex, but patients with thrombocytopenia appeared not to be at risk during treatment.[7]

Recombinant erythropoietin has been used in an attempt to reduce blood-transfusion requirements in zidovudine-induced anaemia,[8,9] although the proportion of patients who derive benefit may be limited and some have reported it to have no effect.[10] Similarly granulocyte-macrophage colony-stimulating factor has been reported to improve the neutrophil count in some but not all patients.[11]


1. Forester G. Profound cytopenia secondary to azidothymidine. *N Engl J Med* 1987; **317:** 772.
2. Gill PS, *et al.* Azidothymidine associated with bone marrow failure in the acquired immunodeficiency syndrome (AIDS). *Ann Intern Med* 1987; **107:** 502–5.
3. Mir N, Costello C. Zidovudine and bone marrow. *Lancet* 1988; **ii:** 1195–6.
4. Walker RE, *et al.* Anemia and erythropoiesis in patients with the acquired immunodeficiency syndrome (AIDS) and Kaposi sarcoma treated with zidovudine. *Ann Intern Med* 1988; **108:** 372–6.
5. Cohen H, *et al.* Reversible zidovudine-induced pure red-cell aplasia. *AIDS* 1989; **3:** 177–8.
6. Shaunak S, Bartlett JA. Zidovudine-induced neutropenia: are we too cautious? *Lancet* 1989; **ii:** 91–2.
7. Flegg PJ, *et al.* Effect of zidovudine on platelet count. *BMJ* 1989; **298:** 1074–5.
8. Fischl M, *et al.* Recombinant human erythropoietin for patients with AIDS treated with zidovudine. *N Engl J Med* 1990; **322:** 1488–93.
9. Henry DH, *et al.* Recombinant human erythropoietin in the treatment of anemia associated with human immunodeficiency virus (HIV) infection and zidovudine therapy: overview of four clinical trials. *Ann Intern Med* 1992; **117:** 739–48.
10. Shepp DH, *et al.* Erythropoietin for zidovudine-induced anemia. *N Engl J Med* 1990; **323:** 1069–70.
11. Hewitt RG, *et al.* Pharmacokinetics and pharmacodynamics of granulocyte-macrophage colony-stimulating factor and zidovudine in patients with AIDS and severe AIDS-related complex. *Antimicrob Agents Chemother* 1993; **37:** 512–22.


**Effects on the CNS.** Reports of adverse effects on the CNS associated with zidovudine include mania,[1,2] seizures[3,4] (following an overdose in one patient[5]), psychogenic panic,[6] and Wernicke's encephalopathy,[7] mostly involving one or two patients in each case. CNS toxicity, thought to be zidovudine-related, contributed to the death of an AIDS patient.[8]

For reports of neurological symptoms associated with mitochondrial dysfunction in infants whose mothers received perinatal zidovudine, see Effects on Mitochondria, below.

1. Maxwell S, *et al.* Manic syndrome associated with zidovudine treatment. *JAMA* 1988; **259:** 3406–7.
2. Wright JM, *et al.* Zidovudine-related mania. *Med J Aust* 1989; **150:** 339–40.
3. Harris PJ, Caceres CA. Azidothymidine in the treatment of AIDS. *N Engl J Med* 1988; **318:** 250.
4. D'Silva M, *et al.* Seizure associated with zidovudine. *Lancet* 1995; **346:** 452.
5. Routy JP, *et al.* Seizure after zidovudine overdose. *Lancet* 1989; **i:** 384–5.
6. Levitt AJ, Lippert GP. Psychogenic panic after zidovudine therapy—the therapeutic benefit of an N of 1 trial. *Can Med Assoc J* 1990; **142:** 341–2.
7. Davtyan DG, Vinters HV. Wernicke's encephalopathy in AIDS patient treated with zidovudine. *Lancet* 1987; **i:** 919–20.
8. Hagler DN, Frame PT. Azidothymidine neurotoxicity. *Lancet* 1986; **ii:** 1392–3.


**Effects on the liver.** The development of acute cholestatic hepatitis necessitated the withdrawal of zidovudine in a patient who was later unable to tolerate its re-institution.[1] Zidovudine also had to be withdrawn in 3 patients after abnormal liver-function values occurred;[2] it was reinstated in 2 patients without further liver changes. Reversible increases in liver enzymes and rashes were also reported in 2 patients receiving prophylaxis with zidovudine and zalcitabine following exposure to HIV.[3] There has been a report of iron deposition in the liver of patients receiving blood transfusions for zidovudine-related anaemia.[4]

Fatal hepatic dysfunction associated with steatosis in the liver was reported in 6 patients with HIV infection, who were either receiving zidovudine or had previously done so.[5] Five of these 6 patients also developed metabolic acidosis. Cases of fatal lactic acidosis and hepatic failure or steatosis have been reported in patients receiving zidovudine and other nucleoside analogues.[6,7]


1. Dubin G, Braffman MN. Zidovudine-induced hepatotoxicity. *Ann Intern Med* 1989; **110:** 85–6.
2. Melamed AJ, *et al.* Possible zidovudine-induced hepatotoxicity. *JAMA* 1987; **258:** 2063.
3. Henry K, *et al.* Hepatotoxicity and rash associated with zidovudine and zalcitabine chemoprophylaxis. *Ann Intern Med* 1996; **124:** 855.
4. Lindley R, *et al.* Iron deposition in liver in zidovudine-related transfusion-dependent anaemia. *Lancet* 1989; **ii:** 681.
5. Freiman JP, *et al.* Hepatomegaly with severe steatosis in HIV-seropositive patients. *AIDS* 1993; **7:** 379–85.
6. Sundar K, *et al.* Zidovudine-induced fatal lactic acidosis and hepatic failure in patients with acquired immunodeficiency syndrome: report of two patients and review of the literature. *Crit Care Med* 1997; **25:** 1425–30. Correction. *ibid.*: 1762.
7. Acosta BS, Grimsley EW. Zidovudine-associated type B lactic acidosis and hepatic steatosis in an HIV-infected patient. *South Med J* 1999; **92:** 421–3.


**Effects on the metabolism.** Lactic acidosis, sometimes in association with myopathy or hepatotoxicity (see above) and in some instances fatal, has been reported following zidovudine treatment.[1-6] However, lactic acidosis with no apparent cause[7] has also been reported in 7 patients with HIV infection: 4 patients were receiving zidovudine, 1 ganciclovir, and 1 clofazimine. The disorder in these patients resembled Reye's syndrome and it was not clear whether the acidosis was induced by zidovudine or the HIV infection.

Lactic acidosis associated with nucleoside reverse transcriptase inhibitors responded to treatment with riboflavin in 4 patients.[8,9]


1. Olano JP, *et al.* Massive hepatic steatosis and lactic acidosis in a patient with AIDS who was receiving zidovudine. *Clin Infect Dis* 1995; **21:** 973–6.
2. Sundar K, *et al.* Zidovudine-induced fatal lactic acidosis and hepatic failure in patients with acquired immunodeficiency syndrome: report of two patients and review of the literature. *Crit Care Med* 1997; **25:** 1425–30. Correction. *ibid.*: 1762.
3. Scalfaro P, *et al.* Severe transient neonatal lactic acidosis during prophylactic zidovudine treatment. *Intensive Care Med* 1998; **24:** 247–50.
4. Chariot P, *et al.* Zidovudine-induced mitochondrial disorder with massive liver steatosis, myopathy, lactic acidosis, and mitochondrial DNA depletion. *J Hepatol* 1999; **30:** 156–60.
5. Acosta BS, Grimsley EW. Zidovudine-associated type B lactic acidosis and hepatic steatosis in an HIV-infected patient. *South Med J* 1999; **92:** 421–3.
6. Roy P-M, *et al.* Severe lactic acidosis induced by nucleoside analogues in an HIV-infected man. *Ann Emerg Med* 1999; **34:** 282–4.
7. Chattha G, *et al.* Lactic acidosis complicating the acquired immunodeficiency syndrome. *Ann Intern Med* 1993; **118:** 37–9.
8. Fouty B, *et al.* Riboflavin to treat nucleoside analogue-induced lactic acidosis. *Lancet* 1998; **352:** 291–2.
9. Luzzati R, *et al.* Riboflavine and severe lactic acidosis. *Lancet* 1999; **353:** 901–2.


**Effects on mitochondria.** Concern has been expressed[1] over the effects of nucleoside reverse transcriptase inhibitors on mitochondria following reports in France[2] of mitochondrial dysfunction in 8 infants whose mothers had received zidovudine alone, or with lamivudine, to prevent vertical transmission of HIV infection during pregnancy. The effects manifested themselves as severe demyelinating neurological disorder in 2 of the 8, both of whom died after about one year of life. Three other infants experienced seizures, 1 with severe cardiomyopathy and 1 with spastic diplegia, while the remaining 3 were asymptomatic. None were infected with HIV. A study[3] involving echocardiograms performed from birth to 5 years of age in 382 infants without HIV infection (36 with zidovudine exposure) and 58 infants with HIV infection (12 with zidovudine exposure), all of whom were born to HIV-infected women, found, however, that there was no evidence of abnormality in left ventricular structure or function associated with perinatal zidovudine. While it was considered that further assessment of this toxicity was required, it was emphasised that current recommendations for zidovudine monotherapy during pregnancy should be maintained.[1,2]


1. Committee on Safety of Medicines. Antiretroviral drugs in pregnancy and mitochondrial cytopathy in infants. *Current Problems* 1999; **25:** 15. Also available at: http://www.mca.gov.uk/ourwork/monitorsafequalmed/currentproblems/volume25nov.htm (accessed 13/03/04)
2. Blanche S, *et al.* Persistent mitochondrial dysfunction and perinatal exposure to antiretroviral nucleoside analogues. *Lancet* 1999; **354:** 1084–9.
3. Lipshultz SE, *et al.* Absence of cardiac toxicity of zidovudine in infants. *N Engl J Med* 2000; **343:** 759–66.


**Effects on the musculoskeletal system.** Myalgia and other adverse effects on the muscle can occur in patients taking zidovudine, although it has sometimes been difficult to determine whether the effects were caused by the drug or by the underlying HIV infection.[1-4] Zidovudine-induced myopathy has been considered to be a distinct condition characterised by the presence of abnormal mitochondria in muscle-biopsy specimens;[2] this view is supported by the fact that the myopathy readily responds to the withdrawal of zidovudine or to treatment with corticosteroids or other anti-inflammatory drugs.[1-3] For further discussion of the effects of zidovudine on mitochondria, see above.

Arthralgia involving the knees, elbows, ankles, and wrists has been reported in a patient receiving zidovudine.[5]


1. Gertner E, *et al.* Zidovudine-associated myopathy. *Am J Med* 1989; **86:** 814–18.
2. Dalakas MC, *et al.* Mitochondrial myopathy caused by long-term zidovudine therapy. *N Engl J Med* 1990; **322:** 1098–1105.
3. Till M, MacDonell KB. Myopathy with human immunodeficiency virus type 1 (HIV-1) infection: HIV-1 or zidovudine? *Ann Intern Med* 1990; **113:** 492–4.
4. Simpson DM, *et al.* Myopathies associated with human immunodeficiency virus and zidovudine: can their effects be distinguished? *Neurology* 1993; **43:** 971–6.
5. Murphy D, *et al.* Zidovudine related arthropathy. *BMJ* 1994; **309:** 97.


**Effects on the nails.** Bluish or brownish discoloration of fingernails and/or toenails has been reported in a number of patients receiving zidovudine.[1-5] Dark-skinned patients appear to be most commonly affected.[2,4] Occasionally the abnormal pigmentation also involves the skin.[3,5] It has been pointed out that discoloration of nails has occurred in HIV-infected patients without exposure to zidovudine.[6]


1. Furth PA, Kazakis AM. Nail pigmentation changes associated with azidothymidine (zidovudine). *N Engl J Med* 1987; **107:** 350.
2. Vaiopoulos G, *et al.* Nail pigmentation and azidothymidine. *Ann Intern Med* 1988; **108:** 777.
3. Merenich JA, *et al.* Azidothymidine-induced hyperpigmentation mimicking primary adrenal insufficiency. *Am J Med* 1989; **86:** 469–70.
4. Don PC, *et al.* Nail dyschromia associated with zidovudine. *Ann Intern Med* 1990; **112:** 145–6.
5. Bendick C, *et al.* Azidothymidine-induced hyperpigmentation of skin and nails. *Arch Dermatol* 1989; **125:** 1285–6.
6. Chandrasekar PH. Nail discoloration and human immunodeficiency virus infection. *Am J Med* 1989; **86:** 506–7.


## Precautions

Zidovudine should be used with care in patients with anaemia or bone-marrow suppression. The incidence of neutropenia is greater in patients with low vitamin $B_{12}$ concentrations. Dosage adjustments may be necessary and it has been recommended that it should not be used if the neutrophil count or haemoglobin value is abnormally low. Care is also required in the elderly and in patients with reduced renal or hepatic function who may require reductions in dose. Patients with risk factors for liver disease should be monitored during treatment. Particular care may be necessary in obese patients and in women. Patients with hepatitis receiving interferon alfa and ribavirin may be at special risk. Zidovudine treatment should be stopped if there is symptomatic hyperlactataemia and metabolic or lactic acidosis, progressive hepatomegaly, or a rapid increase in aminotransferase concentrations. It should not be given to neonates with hyperbilirubinaemia requiring treatment other than phototherapy or with markedly increased aminotransferase concentrations.

Because of the haematological toxicity of zidovudine it is recommended that, in patients with advanced symptomatic HIV disease taking oral zidovudine, blood tests should be carried out at least every 2 weeks for the first 3 months of treatment and at least monthly thereafter; blood tests should be performed at least every week in those receiving intravenous zidovudine. In patients with early HIV infection blood tests may be performed less frequently (e.g. every 1 to 3 months).

**Interference with laboratory tests.** Raised urinary thymine concentrations in neonates, due to maternal zidovudine treatment, could produce erroneous results in screening tests for inborn errors of metabolism.[1]


1. Sewell AC. Zidovudine and confusion in urinary metabolic screening. *Lancet* 1998; **352:** 1227.


**Pregnancy.** Administration of zidovudine to pregnant women with HIV infection from 14 weeks of gestation until delivery, and subsequently to the neonate, has been shown to reduce vertical transmission of the infection (see Uses and Administration, below). However, studies have shown that zidovudine can be fetotoxic in *animals* when given early in pregnancy, and the long-term consequences for the infant are as yet unknown although no adverse effects were seen in a group of infants followed for up to 5.6 years.[1] The manufacturer therefore recommends that zidovudine should not generally be administered before 14 weeks of gestation.


1. Culnane M, *et al.* Lack of long-term effects of in utero exposure to zidovudine among uninfected children born to HIV-infected women. *JAMA* 1999; **281:** 151–7.


## Interactions

Care should be taken during concomitant therapy with zidovudine and drugs that are myelosuppressive or nephrotoxic. Drugs that undergo glucuronidation may delay the metabolism of zidovudine but few of these appear to produce clinically important increases in zidovudine plasma concentrations. Increased toxicity and decreased antiretroviral activity has been reported when zidovudine is given with some other antiviral drugs, and pharmacokinetic interactions have been reported with a number of anti-infective drugs used commonly in patients with HIV infection.

**Analgesics.** There may be an increased risk of haematotoxicity during use of zidovudine with *NSAIDs*.

Decreased zidovudine clearance[1] and increased area under the zidovudine plasma concentration-time curve[2] has been observed in patients receiving *methadone*.

Severe hepatotoxicity has occurred after use of *paracetamol* in a patient taking zidovudine and co-trimoxazole.[3] However, neither short-term[4] nor long-term[5] studies (the latter also in an individual patient) have shown any alteration of zidovudine elimination in patients taking zidovudine and paracetamol.


1. Burger DM, *et al.* Pharmacokinetic variability of zidovudine in HIV-infected individuals: subgroup analysis and drug interactions. *AIDS* 1994; **8:** 1683–9.
2. Schwartz EL, *et al.* Pharmacokinetic interactions of zidovudine and methadone in intravenous drug-using patients with HIV infection. *J Acquir Immune Defic Syndr* 1992; **5:** 619–26.
3. Shriner K, Goetz MB. Severe hepatotoxicity in a patient receiving both acetaminophen and zidovudine. *Am J Med* 1992; **93:** 94–6.
4. Sattler FR, *et al.* Acetaminophen does not impair clearance of zidovudine. *Ann Intern Med* 1991; **114:** 937–40.
5. Burger DM, *et al.* Pharmacokinetics of zidovudine and acetaminophen in a patient on chronic acetaminophen therapy. *Ann Pharmacother* 1994; **28:** 327–30.


**Antibacterials.** Studies have indicated that the absorption of zidovudine could be reduced by *clarithromycin*.[1] The manufacturers of clarithromycin recommend giving zidovudine and clarithromycin 1 to 2 hours apart since this has been shown to have no overall effect on the bioavailability of zidovudine.[2] Administration of *rifampicin* to patients taking zidovudine has been reported to reduce the area under the plasma concentration-time curve of zidovudine, probably by inducing glucuronidation and amination. The manufacturers of zidovudine have warned that this may result in a partial, or total, loss of efficacy of the drug.[3,4] *Rifabutin* has not been shown to have a marked effect on zidovudine clearance.[5] *Trimethoprim* has been reported[6,7] to decrease the renal clearance of zidovudine by up to 60% with a consequent increase in plasma concentrations, although it was only thought likely to be of clinical significance in patients with hepatic impairment.[7]

For a report of reduced *pyrazinamide* concentrations in patients receiving zidovudine, see p.247.


1. Polis MA, *et al.* Clarithromycin lowers plasma zidovudine levels in persons with human immunodeficiency virus infection. *Antimicrob Agents Chemother* 1997; **41:** 1709–14.
2. Vance E, *et al.* Pharmacokinetics of clarithromycin and zidovudine in patients with AIDS. *Antimicrob Agents Chemother* 1995; **39:** 1355–60.
3. Burger DM, *et al.* Pharmacokinetic interaction between rifampin and zidovudine. *Antimicrob Agents Chemother* 1993; **37:** 1426–31.
4. Gallicano KD, *et al.* Induction of zidovudine glucuronidation and amination pathways by rifampicin in HIV-infected patients. *Br J Clin Pharmacol* 1999; **48:** 168–79.
5. Gallicano K, *et al.* Effect of rifabutin on the pharmacokinetics of zidovudine in patients infected with human immunodeficiency virus. *Clin Infect Dis* 1995; **21:** 1008–11.
6. Chatton JY, *et al.* Trimethoprim, alone or in combination with sulphamethoxazole, decreases the renal excretion of zidovudine and its glucuronide. *Br J Clin Pharmacol* 1992; **34:** 551–4.
7. Lee BL, *et al.* Zidovudine, trimethoprim, and dapsone pharmacokinetic interactions in patients with human immunodeficiency virus infection. *Antimicrob Agents Chemother* 1996; **40:** 1231–6.


**Antiepileptics.** Administration of *valproic acid* to 6 patients receiving zidovudine produced increases in plasma-zidovudine concentrations and the area under the plasma concentration-time curve.[1] The evidence suggested that this was due to reduced glucuronidation of zidovudine. Zidovudine may possibly reduce or increase plasma concentrations of *phenytoin*.


1. Lertora JJL, *et al.* Pharmacokinetic interaction between zidovudine and valproic acid in patients infected with human immunodeficiency virus. *Clin Pharmacol Ther* 1994; **56:** 272–8.

**Antifungals.** Administration of *fluconazole* with zidovudine produced higher serum-zidovudine concentrations, increases in the area under the serum concentration-time curve and prolonged terminal half-life compared with zidovudine alone in a study in 12 patients.[1] Studies *in vitro* suggested that fluconazole could inhibit the glucuronidation of zidovudine; inhibition was also seen with *amphotericin B*, *ketoconazole*, and *miconazole*, but not with *flucytosine* or *itraconazole*.[2]

1. Sahai J, *et al.* Effect of fluconazole on zidovudine pharmacokinetics in patients infected with human immunodeficiency virus. *J Infect Dis* 1994; **169:** 103–7.
2. Sampol E, *et al.* Comparative effects of antifungal agents on zidovudine glucuronidation by human liver microsomes. *Br J Clin Pharmacol* 1995; **40:** 83–6.

**Antivirals.** Studies *in vitro* have shown that *ribavirin* and zidovudine inhibit each other's activity and the manufacturer recommends that this combination should be avoided. The manufacturer also recommends that the use of zidovudine with *stavudine* be avoided since similar antagonism has been shown *in vivo*.[1] *Interferon alfa* and zidovudine had a synergistic cytotoxicity to bone-marrow progenitor cells.[2] Severe haematological toxicity occurred when zidovudine was added to *ganciclovir* therapy in AIDS patients with cytomegalovirus retinitis, necessitating substantial dosage reductions or withdrawal of zidovudine in the majority of patients;[3,4] this additive toxicity with ganciclovir may be one reason why patients receiving zidovudine and ganciclovir do less well than those receiving zidovudine and foscarnet. Combined therapy with zidovudine and *aciclovir* is not generally associated with additional toxicity[5] but severe fatigue and lethargy were reported in a patient receiving aciclovir with zidovudine; this did not occur when either drug was given alone.[6] Evidence of a pharmacokinetic interaction between zidovudine and *didanosine* has been conflicting, with reports of no effect,[7] increased,[8] and decreased[9] plasma concentrations of zidovudine. Small reductions in didanosine plasma concentrations have been reported in patients also receiving zidovudine.[10] However, all changes have generally been small and are likely to be of limited clinical significance. Exposure to zidovudine (as measured by peak plasma concentrations and area under the concentration-time curve) was reduced in HIV patients given *ritonavir* concomitantly, whereas the pharmacokinetics of ritonavir were not affected by zidovudine;[11] the clinical relevance of this was not known. Modest increases in plasma-zidovudine concentrations occur on use with *lamivudine*. Although this interaction is usually clinically insignificant, profound anaemia has been reported rarely in patients receiving this combination.[12,13]

For the enhanced *in-vitro* antiviral activity of zidovudine in combination with other antivirals, see Microbiological Interactions under Antiviral Action, below.

1. Havlir DV, *et al.* In vivo antagonism with zidovudine plus stavudine combination therapy. *J Infect Dis* 2000; **182:** 321–5.
2. Berman E, *et al.* Synergistic cytotoxic effect of azidothymidine and recombinant interferon alpha on normal human bone marrow progenitor cells. *Blood* 1989; **74:** 1281–6.
3. Millar AB, *et al.* Treatment of cytomegalovirus retinitis with zidovudine and ganciclovir in patients with AIDS: outcome and toxicity. *Genitourin Med* 1990; **66:** 156–8.
4. Hochster H, *et al.* Toxicity of combined ganciclovir and zidovudine for cytomegalovirus disease associated with AIDS: an AIDS Clinical Trials Group study. *Ann Intern Med* 1990; **113:** 111–17.
5. Tartaglione TA, *et al.* Pharmacokinetic evaluations of low- and high-dose zidovudine plus high-dose acyclovir in patients with symptomatic human immunodeficiency virus infection. *Antimicrob Agents Chemother* 1991; **35:** 2225–31.
6. Bach MC. Possible drug interaction during therapy with azidothymidine and acyclovir for AIDS. *N Engl J Med* 1987; **316:** 547.
7. Collier AC, *et al.* Combination therapy with zidovudine and didanosine compared with zidovudine alone in HIV-1 infection. *Ann Intern Med* 1993; **119:** 786–93.
8. Barry M, *et al.* Pharmacokinetics of zidovudine and dideoxyinosine alone and in combination in patients with the acquired immunodeficiency syndrome. *Br J Clin Pharmacol* 1994; **37:** 421–6.
9. Burger DM, *et al.* Pharmacokinetic interaction study of zidovudine and didanosine. *J Drug Dev* 1994; **6:** 187–94.
10. Gibb D, *et al.* Pharmacokinetics of zidovudine and dideoxyinosine alone and in combination in children with HIV infection. *Br J Clin Pharmacol* 1995; **39:** 527–30.
11. Cato A, *et al.* Multidose pharmacokinetics of ritonavir and zidovudine in human immunodeficiency virus-infected patients. *Antimicrob Agents Chemother* 1998; **42:** 1788–93.
12. Hester EK, Peacock JE. Profound and unanticipated anemia with lamivudine-zidovudine combination therapy in zidovudine-experienced patients with HIV infection. *AIDS* 1998; **12:** 439–40.
13. Tseng A, *et al.* Precipitous declines in hemoglobin levels associated with combination zidovudine and lamivudine therapy. *Clin Infect Dis* 1998; **27:** 908–9.

**Atovaquone.** Use of atovaquone with zidovudine produced moderate increases in the zidovudine plasma concentration and area under the plasma concentration-time curve, probably by inhibition of glucuronidation.[1]

1. Lee BL, *et al.* Atovaquone inhibits the glucuronidation and increases the plasma concentrations of zidovudine. *Clin Pharmacol Ther* 1996; **59:** 14–21.

**Probenecid.** Use of probenecid with zidovudine results in increased plasma concentrations and area under the plasma concentration-time curve of zidovudine, probably due to inhibition of glucuronidation;[1] tubular secretion of the glucuronide metabolite is also reduced. A high incidence of adverse effects has been reported in some patients receiving this combination.[2]

1. de Miranda P, *et al.* Alteration of zidovudine pharmacokinetics by probenecid in patients with AIDS or AIDS-related complex. *Clin Pharmacol Ther* 1989; **46:** 494–500.
2. Petty BG, *et al.* Zidovudine with probenecid: a warning. *Lancet* 1990; **335:** 1044–5.

## Antiviral Action

Zidovudine is converted intracellularly in stages to the triphosphate via thymidine kinase and other kinases. This triphosphate halts the DNA synthesis of retroviruses, including HIV, through competitive inhibition of reverse transcriptase and incorporation into viral DNA. It has also been shown to possess activity against Epstein-Barr virus and Gram-negative bacteria *in vitro*.

Zidovudine-resistant strains of HIV emerge rapidly during zidovudine therapy and are responsible for the lack of benefit with long-term monotherapy. Cross-resistance to other nucleoside reverse transcriptase inhibitors has been recognised.

**Microbiological interactions.** The anti-HIV activity of zidovudine has been enhanced *in vitro* by a number of drugs including dextran sulfate,[1] granulocyte-macrophage colony-stimulating factor,[2,3] hydroxycarbamide,[4] foscarnet,[5,6] poly I.poly C12U,[7] carbovir,[8] castanospermine,[9] zalcitabine,[10] and didanosine.[11] Antiviral synergy was demonstrated against HIV *in vitro* with a combination of zidovudine, soluble CD4, and interferon alfa.[12] Interferon alfa also enhanced the activity of zidovudine in cells acutely and persistently infected with HIV.[13] Zidovudine blocked the HIV replication-enhancing effect of tumour necrosis factor.[14]

For a report of zidovudine and ribavirin mutually inhibiting each other's antiviral activity *in vitro*, and reports of increased toxicity of some antiviral combinations, see Antivirals, under Interactions, above.

1. Ueno R, Kuno S. Dextran sulphate, a potent anti-HIV agent in vitro having synergism with zidovudine. *Lancet* 1987; **i:** 1379.
2. Hammer SM, Gillis JM. Synergistic activity of granulocyte-macrophage colony-stimulating factor and 3′-azido-3′-deoxythymidine against human immunodeficiency virus in vitro. *Antimicrob Agents Chemother* 1987; **31:** 1046–50.
3. Perno C-F, *et al.* Replication of human immunodeficiency virus in monocytes: granulocyte/macrophage colony-stimulating factor (GM-CSF) potentiates viral production yet enhances the antiviral effect mediated by 3′-azido-2′3′-dideoxythymidine (AZT) and other dideoxynucleoside congeners of thymidine. *J Exp Med* 1989; **169:** 933–51.
4. Palmer S, Cox S. Increased activity of the combination of 3′-azido-3′-deoxythymidine and 2′-deoxy-3′-thiacytidine in the presence of hydroxyurea. *Antimicrob Agents Chemother* 1997; **41:** 460–4.
5. Eriksson BFH, Schinazi RF. Combinations of 3′-azido-3′-deoxythymidine (zidovudine) and phosphonoformate (foscarnet) against human immunodeficiency virus type 1 and cytomegalovirus replication in vitro. *Antimicrob Agents Chemother* 1989; **33:** 663–9.
6. Koshida R, *et al.* Inhibition of human immunodeficiency virus in vitro by combination of 3′-azido-3′-deoxythymidine and foscarnet. *Antimicrob Agents Chemother* 1989; **33:** 778–80.
7. Mitchell WM, *et al.* Mismatched double-stranded RNA (ampligen) reduces concentration of zidovudine (azidothymidine) required for in-vitro inhibition of human immunodeficiency virus. *Lancet* 1987; **i:** 890–2.
8. Smith MS, *et al.* Evaluation of synergy between carbovir and 3′-azido-2′3′-deoxythymidine for inhibition of human immunodeficiency virus type 1. *Antimicrob Agents Chemother* 1993; **37:** 144–7.
9. Johnson VA, *et al.* Synergistic inhibition of human immunodeficiency virus type 1 and type 2 replication in vitro by castanospermine and 3′-azido-3′-deoxythymidine. *Antimicrob Agents Chemother* 1989; **33:** 53–7.
10. Spector SA, *et al.* Human immunodeficiency virus inhibition is prolonged by 3′-azido-3′-deoxythymidine alternating with 2′,3′-dideoxycytidine compared with 3′-azido-3′-deoxythymidine alone. *Antimicrob Agents Chemother* 1989; **33:** 920–3.
11. Dornsife RE, *et al.* Anti-human immunodeficiency virus synergism by zidovudine (3′-azidothymidine) and didanosine (dideoxyinosine) contrasts with their additive inhibition of normal human marrow progenitor cells. *Antimicrob Agents Chemother* 1991; **35:** 322–8.
12. Johnson VA, *et al.* Three-drug synergistic inhibition of HIV-1 replication in vitro by zidovudine, recombinant soluble CD4, and recombinant interferon-alpha A. *J Infect Dis* 1990; **161:** 1059–67.
13. Pincus SH, Wehrly K. AZT demonstrates anti-HIV-1 activity in persistently infected cell lines: implications for combination chemotherapy and immunotherapy. *J Infect Dis* 1990; **162:** 1233–8.
14. Michihiko S, *et al.* Augmentation of in-vitro HIV replication in peripheral blood mononuclear cells of AIDS and ARC patients by tumour necrosis factor. *Lancet* 1989; **i:** 1206–7.

**Resistance.** The emergence of zidovudine-resistant HIV strains in patients receiving long-term therapy with zidovudine has been recognised since 1989.[1,2] The emergence of drug resistance is associated with the duration[3] of treatment with zidovudine, but not the dose,[4] and is attributed to a high frequency of mutations in the HIV reverse transcriptase gene.[3,5] Development of high-level resistance to zidovudine in patients with advanced HIV infection is associated with rapid disease progression and death.[6] Primary infection with zidovudine-resistant HIV strains has been recorded,[7] as has zidovudine resistance in patients receiving other nucleoside reverse transcriptase inhibitors,[8,9] although it is possible that these patients had unrecorded exposure to zidovudine.[8] Cross-resistance with other reverse transcriptase inhibitors has been recorded and, although the use of zidovudine in combination with lamivudine has been reported to delay or reverse the emergence of some mutations conferring zidovudine resistance, dual resistance to zidovudine and lamivudine has occurred.[10] Analysis of the Delta trial[11] found no delay in the emergence of zidovudine resistance when used in combinations with didanosine or zalcitabine, although circulating concentrations of resistant virus were lower during combination therapy and antiviral activity was apparently not impaired. Nevertheless, it could be anticipated that the use of zidovudine in combination with other antiretrovirals, and particularly the highly active regimens which suppress viral replication to a high degree, could delay the emergence of resistance. The clinical response of patients with previous exposure to a number of regimens could be compromised by the presence of multidrug resistance.[12,13]

1. Larder BA, *et al.* HIV with reduced sensitivity to zidovudine (AZT) isolated during prolonged therapy. *Science* 1989; **243:** 1731–4.
2. Rooke R, *et al.* Isolation of drug-resistant variants of HIV-1 from patients on long-term zidovudine therapy. *AIDS* 1989; **3:** 411–15.
3. Japour AJ, *et al.* Prevalence and clinical significance of zidovudine resistance mutations in human immunodeficiency virus isolated from patients after long-term zidovudine treatment. *J Infect Dis* 1995; **171:** 1172–9.
4. Richman DD, *et al.* Effect of stage of disease and drug dose on zidovudine susceptibilities of isolates of human immunodeficiency virus. *J Acquir Immune Defic Syndr* 1990; **3:** 743–6.
5. Loveday C, *et al.* HIV-1 RNA serum-load and resistant viral genotypes during early zidovudine therapy. *Lancet* 1995; **345:** 820–4.
6. D'Aquila RT, *et al.* Zidovudine resistance and HIV-1 disease progression during antiretroviral therapy. *Ann Intern Med* 1995; **122:** 401–8.
7. Erice A, *et al.* Brief report: primary infection with zidovudine-resistant human immunodeficiency virus type 1. *N Engl J Med* 1993; **328:** 1163–5.
8. Lin P-F, *et al.* Genotypic and phenotypic analysis of human immunodeficiency virus type 1 isolates from patients on prolonged stavudine therapy. *J Infect Dis* 1994; **170:** 1157–64.
9. Demeter LM, *et al.* Development of zidovudine resistance mutations in patients receiving prolonged didanosine monotherapy. *J Infect Dis* 1995; **172:** 1480–5.
10. Miller V, *et al.* Dual resistance to zidovudine and lamivudine in patients treated with zidovudine-lamivudine combination therapy: association with therapy failure. *J Infect Dis* 1998; **177:** 1521–32.
11. Brun-Vézinet F, *et al.* HIV-1 viral load, phenotype, and resistance in a subset of drug-naive participants from the Delta trial. *Lancet* 1997; **350:** 983–90.
12. Kavlick MF, *et al.* Emergence of multi-dideoxynucleoside-resistant human immunodeficiency virus type 1 variants, viral sequence variation, and disease progression in patients receiving antiretroviral chemotherapy. *J Infect Dis* 1998; **177:** 1506–13.
13. Shafer RW, *et al.* Multiple concurrent reverse transcriptase and protease mutations and multidrug resistance of HIV-1 isolates from heavily treated patients. *Ann Intern Med* 1998; **128:** 906–11.

## Pharmacokinetics

Zidovudine is rapidly absorbed from the gastrointestinal tract and undergoes first-pass hepatic metabolism with a bioavailability of about 60 to 70%. Peak plasma concentrations occur after about 1 hour. Absorption is delayed by administration with food, but bioavailability is probably unaffected. Zidovudine crosses the blood-brain barrier producing CSF to plasma ratios of about 0.5. It crosses the placenta and is distributed into breast milk. It has been detected in semen. Plasma protein binding is reported to be 34 to 38%. The plasma half-life is about 1 hour.

Zidovudine is metabolised intracellularly to the antiviral triphosphate. It is also metabolised in the liver, mainly to the inactive glucuronide, and is excreted in the urine as unchanged drug and metabolite.

◊ Reviews.

1. Acosta EP, *et al.* Clinical pharmacokinetics of zidovudine: an update. *Clin Pharmacokinet* 1996; **30:** 251–62.

**Neonates.** The pharmacokinetics of zidovudine in infants more than 14 days old are reported to be similar to those in adults. Following maternal administration the half-life of zidovudine in 7 neonates has been reported to be extended to a mean of 13 hours.[1] In infants receiving zidovudine, those under 14 days of age had lower total clearance, longer terminal half-life (about 3 hours), and higher bioavailability than older infants.[2] Zidovudine clearance was low and the half-life prolonged to about 7 hours in premature infants.[3]

1. O'Sullivan MJ, *et al.* The pharmacokinetics and safety of zidovudine in the third trimester of pregnancy for women infected with human immunodeficiency virus and their infants: phase 1 Acquired Immunodeficiency Syndrome Clinical Trials Group Study (protocol 082). *Am J Obstet Gynecol* 1993; **168:** 1510–16.
2. Boucher FD, *et al.* Phase 1 evaluation of zidovudine administered to infants exposed at birth to the human immunodeficiency virus. *J Pediatr* 1993; **122:** 137–44.
3. Mirochnick M, *et al.* Zidovudine pharmacokinetics in premature infants exposed to human immunodeficiency virus. *Antimicrob Agents Chemother* 1998; **42:** 808–12.

**Pregnancy.** In a study in 3 pregnant women with HIV infection,[1] the area under the concentration-time curve for zidovudine was reduced and the clearance of an oral dose increased during pregnancy when compared with up to 4 weeks postpartum. These results differed from those reported from another study which reported no differences during or after pregnancy.[2] This latter study, however, used values obtained no later than 48 hours postpartum for comparison, at which time it is unlikely that physiological functions would have returned to the nonpregnant state. Zidovudine and its glucuronide metabolite cross the placenta reaching concentrations in the fetal blood similar to those in maternal blood.[3,4] However, concentrations of zidovudine in the fetal CNS have been reported to be below those required to exert an anti-HIV effect.[5]


1. Watts DH, *et al.* Pharmacokinetic disposition of zidovudine during pregnancy. *J Infect Dis* 1991; **163:** 226–32.
2. O'Sullivan MJ, *et al.* The pharmacokinetics and safety of zidovudine in the third trimester of pregnancy for women infected with human immunodeficiency virus and their infants: phase 1 Acquired Immunodeficiency Syndrome Clinical Trials Group Study (protocol 082). *Am J Obstet Gynecol* 1993; **168:** 1510–16.
3. Gillet JY, *et al.* Fetoplacental passage of zidovudine. *Lancet* 1989; **ii:** 269–70.
4. Chavanet P, *et al.* Perinatal pharmacokinetics of zidovudine. *N Engl J Med* 1989; **321:** 1548–9.
5. Lyman WD, *et al.* Zidovudine concentrations in human fetal tissue: implications for perinatal AIDS. *Lancet* 1990; **335:** 1280–1.


## Uses and Administration

Zidovudine is a nucleoside reverse transcriptase inhibitor structurally related to thymidine. It has activity against retroviruses including HIV and is used in the management of HIV infection. Zidovudine is given in combination with other antiretrovirals to symptomatic and selected asymptomatic patients. It is used alone to prevent vertical transmission from mother to infant.

Zidovudine is given by mouth to *adults* in doses of 500 to 600 mg daily in divided doses. Higher doses may be required for neurological disease. Zidovudine may be given by intravenous infusion of a solution containing 2 to 4 mg/mL over 1 hour for short-term management of patients unable to take it by mouth. The adult dose is 1 to 2 mg/kg every 4 hours (equivalent to an oral dose of 1.5 to 3 mg/kg every 4 hours).

The oral dose for *children* over 3 months of age is 360 to 480 mg/m$^2$ daily in 3 or 4 divided doses, although doses of up to 720 mg/m$^2$ daily (180 mg/m$^2$ every 6 hours) are used and may be necessary for neurological disease. The dose should not exceed 200 mg every 6 hours. Intravenous doses of 80 to 160 mg/m$^2$ have been given every 6 hours. An intravenous dose of 120 mg/m$^2$ every 6 hours is approximately equivalent to an oral dose of 180 mg/m$^2$ every 6 hours.

For the *prevention of maternal-fetal HIV transmission*, zidovudine may be given after the fourteenth week of pregnancy until the beginning of labour in a dose of 100 mg five times daily by mouth. During labour and delivery, zidovudine is given by intravenous infusion in a dose of 2 mg/kg over 1 hour, then 1 mg/kg per hour until the umbilical cord is clamped. When a caesarean section is planned the intravenous infusion is started 4 hours before the operation. The newborn infant is given 2 mg/kg orally every 6 hours starting within 12 hours after birth and continuing for 6 weeks. Short-course regimens are being assessed (see HIV Infection Prophylaxis, below). Neonates unable to receive oral doses are given 1.5 mg/kg by intravenous infusion over 30 minutes every 6 hours.

Blood tests should be carried out regularly as described under Precautions, above. If the white cell count or haemoglobin level fall, the dose should be reduced or, alternatively, treatment interrupted briefly, until there is evidence of recovery. Treatment should be discontinued if toxicity is severe and cautiously reintroduced once the bone marrow has recovered. Dosage adjustments may also be necessary in patients with renal or hepatic impairment.

**Administration and dosage.** A number of studies have been performed to determine the optimal dosage regimen of zidovudine and as a result there has been a general trend to use lower doses for both prophylaxis and treatment of HIV infection and AIDS. Doses studied in patients with AIDS have ranged from 400 to 1500 mg daily in a variety of divided-dose regimens.[1,2] These studies found that low-dose regimens were as effective as higher doses in terms of prolongation of survival and were better tolerated. Similar results were found in patients with AIDS-related complex[3] and asymptomatic HIV infection,[4] and it was concluded that doses above 400 to 600 mg daily[5,6] offered no clinical advantage.


1. Fischl MA, *et al.* A randomized controlled trial of a reduced daily dose of zidovudine in patients with the acquired immunodeficiency syndrome. *N Engl J Med* 1990; **323:** 1009–14.
2. Nordic Medical Research Councils' HIV Therapy Group. Double blind dose-response study of zidovudine in AIDS and advanced HIV infection. *BMJ* 1992; **304:** 13–17.
3. Collier AC, *et al.* A pilot study of low-dose zidovudine in human immunodeficiency virus infection. *N Engl J Med* 1990; **323:** 1015–21.
4. Volberding PA, *et al.* Zidovudine in asymptomatic human immunodeficiency virus infection: a controlled trial in persons with fewer than 500 CD4-positive cells per cubic millimeter. *N Engl J Med* 1990; **322:** 941–9.
5. Gøtzshe PC. Zidovudine dosage. *BMJ* 1993; **307:** 682–3.
6. McLeod GX, Hammer SM. Zidovudine: five years later. *Ann Intern Med* 1992; **117:** 487–501.


**HIV infection and AIDS.** As discussed on p.621, the use of antiretroviral drugs in HIV infection has changed following studies that indicated that combination therapy could improve response. Monotherapy with zidovudine reduced the incidence of opportunistic infections and mortality in patients with AIDS or ARC. Benefit might also be seen in other features of AIDS such as dementia (see HIV-associated Neurological Complications, below). Unfortunately such benefit was found to be transient[1-4] and treatment during the early stages of HIV infection, while delaying disease progression,[5-10] failed to produce improvements in long-term outcome or the quality of life;[7,10-12] in addition there were concerns about resistance.[13,14]

Therapy with a combination of zidovudine and other antiretroviral drugs might improve efficacy, minimise toxicity, and delay drug resistance. Results from the Delta study[15] and the US AIDS Clinical Trial Group 175 (ACTG 175) study[16] showed combination therapy to be more effective than monotherapy in antiretroviral-naive patients and have led to profound changes in clinical practice. Both studies showed substantial reductions in mortality at 30 months in antiretroviral-naive patients treated with zidovudine plus either didanosine or zalcitabine compared with those receiving zidovudine alone. Triple therapy with zidovudine combined with another nucleoside reverse transcriptase inhibitor and either an HIV-protease inhibitor or a non-nucleoside reverse transcriptase inhibitor (HAART regimens) have been found to reduce viral loads more effectively than monotherapy or two-drug combination therapy and such regimens are currently regarded as standard.


1. Fischl MA, *et al.* The efficacy of azidothymidine (AZT) in the treatment of patients with AIDS and AIDS-related complex: a double-blind, placebo-controlled trial. *N Engl J Med* 1987; **317:** 185–91.
2. Dournon E, *et al.* Effects of zidovudine in 365 consecutive patients with AIDS or AIDS-related complex. *Lancet* 1988; **ii:** 1297–1302.
3. Lundgren JD, *et al.* Comparison of long-term prognosis of patients with AIDS treated and not treated with zidovudine. *JAMA* 1994; **271:** 1088–92.
4. Kinloch-de Loës S, Perneger TV. Primary HIV infection: follow-up of patients initially randomized to zidovudine or placebo. *J Infect* 1997; **35:** 111–16.
5. Fischl MA, *et al.* The safety and efficacy of zidovudine (AZT) in the treatment of subjects with mildly symptomatic human immunodeficiency virus type 1 (HIV) infection: a double-blind, placebo-controlled trial. *Ann Intern Med* 1990; **112:** 727–37.
6. Volberding PA, *et al.* Zidovudine in asymptomatic human immunodeficiency virus infection: a controlled trial in persons with fewer than 500 CD4-positive cells per cubic millimeter. *N Engl J Med* 1990; **322:** 941–9.
7. Hamilton JD, *et al.* A controlled trial of early versus late treatment with zidovudine in symptomatic human immunodeficiency virus infection. *N Engl J Med* 1992; **326:** 437–43.
8. Graham NMH, *et al.* The effects on survival of early treatment of human immunodeficiency virus infection. *N Engl J Med* 1992; **326:** 1037–42.
9. Cooper DA, *et al.* Zidovudine in persons with asymptomatic HIV infection and CD4+ cell counts greater than 400 per cubic millimeter. *N Engl J Med* 1993; **329:** 297–303.
10. Concorde Coordinating Committee. Concorde: MRC/ANRS randomised double-blind controlled trial of immediate and deferred zidovudine in symptom-free HIV infection. *Lancet* 1994; **343:** 871–81.
11. Volberding PA, *et al.* The duration of zidovudine benefit in persons with asymptomatic HIV infection: prolonged evaluation of protocol 019 of the AIDS clinical trials group. *JAMA* 1994; **272:** 437–42.
12. Lenderking WR, *et al.* Evaluation of the quality of life associated with zidovudine treatment in asymptomatic human immunodeficiency virus infection *N Engl J Med* 1994; **330:** 738–43.
13. Ogino MT, *et al.* Development and significance of zidovudine resistance in children infected with human immunodeficiency virus. *J Pediatr* 1993; **123:** 1–8.
14. Husson RN, *et al.* High-level resistance to zidovudine but not to zalcitabine or didanosine in human immunodeficiency virus from children receiving antiretroviral therapy. *J Pediatr* 1993; **123:** 9–16.
15. Delta Coordinating Committee. Delta: a randomised double-blind controlled trial comparing combinations of zidovudine plus didanosine or zalcitabine with zidovudine alone in HIV-infected individuals. *Lancet* 1996; **348:** 283–91.
16. Hammer SM, *et al.* A trial comparing nucleoside monotherapy with combination therapy in HIV-infected adults with CD4 cell counts from 200 to 500 per cubic millimeter. *N Engl J Med* 1996; **335:** 1081–90.


**HIV-associated malignancies.** As discussed on p.524, zidovudine in combination with interferons has been advocated for the management of Kaposi's sarcoma in HIV-infected patients with a CD4+ count of 200 cells/microlitre or above.[1-5] Benefit has also been seen in patients with lower CD4+ counts.[6,7]

In patients with AIDS-associated non-Hodgkin's lymphoma, zidovudine in combination with interferon alfa[8] and with methotrexate[9] has been reported to produce beneficial responses in small numbers of patients.


1. Brockmeyer NH, *et al.* Regression of Kaposi's sarcoma and improvement of performance status by a combined interferon β and zidovudine therapy in AIDS patients. *J Invest Dermatol* 1989; **92:** 776.
2. Edlin BR, *et al.* Interferon-alpha plus zidovudine in HIV infection. *Lancet* 1989; **i:** 156.
3. Kovacs JA, *et al.* Combined zidovudine and interferon-α therapy in patients with Kaposi sarcoma and the acquired immunodeficiency syndrome (AIDS). *Ann Intern Med* 1989; **111:** 280–7.
4. Krown SE, *et al.* Interferon-α with zidovudine: safety, tolerance, and clinical and virologic effects in patients with Kaposi sarcoma associated with the acquired immunodeficiency syndrome (AIDS). *Ann Intern Med* 1990; **112:** 812–21.
5. Northfelt DW. Treatment of Kaposi's sarcoma: current guidelines and future perspectives. *Drugs* 1994; **48:** 569–82.
6. Fischl MA, *et al.* A phase II study of recombinant human interferon-$\alpha_{2a}$ and zidovudine in patients with AIDS-related Kaposi's sarcoma. *J Acquir Immune Defic Syndr Hum Retrovirol* 1996; **11:** 379–84.
7. Shepherd FA, *et al.* Prospective randomized trial of two dose levels of interferon alfa with zidovudine for the treatment of Kaposi's sarcoma associated with human immunodeficiency virus infection: a Canadian HIV Clinical Trials Network study. *J Clin Oncol* 1998; **16:** 1736–42.
8. Harrington WJ, *et al.* Azothymidine and interferon-α are active in AIDS-associated small non-cleaved cell lymphoma but not large-cell lymphoma. *Lancet* 1996; **348:** 833.
9. Tosi P, *et al.* 3′-Azido-3′-deoxythymidine + methotrexate as a novel antineoplastic combination in the treatment of human immunodeficiency virus-related non-Hodgkin's lymphomas. *Blood* 1997; **89:** 419–25.


**HIV-associated neurological complications.** Dementia is one of the complications associated with HIV infection and AIDS[1] (see p.623). In a retrospective study of AIDS patients it was noted that the incidence of dementia fell after the institution of zidovudine therapy.[2] Despite criticisms of this study,[3] others have also noted an improvement in dementia and other AIDS-related neurological disorders with zidovudine.[4-8] The improvement was sustained for up to 18 months in one patient.[4] Zidovudine given intrathecally for AIDS-related dementia produced improvement in 3 patients, with minimal toxicity,[9] but no improvement was observed in a further patient given zidovudine intrathecally and intravenously.[10]


1. Simpson DM. Human immunodeficiency virus-associated dementia: review of pathogenesis, prophylaxis, and treatment studies of zidovudine therapy. *Clin Infect Dis* 1999; **29:** 19–34.
2. Portegies P, *et al.* Declining incidence of AIDS dementia complex after introduction of zidovudine treatment. *BMJ* 1989; **299:** 819–21. Correction. *ibid.*; 1141.
3. Morriss R, House A. Zidovudine in AIDS dementia complex. *BMJ* 1989; **299:** 1218.
4. Yarchoan R, *et al.* Long-term administration of 3′-azido-2′,3′-dideoxythymidine to patients with AIDS-related neurological disease. *Ann Neurol* 1988; **23** (suppl): S82–7.
5. Schmitt FA, *et al.* Neuropsychological outcome of zidovudine (AZT) treatment of patients with AIDS and AIDS-related complex. *N Engl J Med* 1988; **319:** 1573–8.
6. Conway B, *et al.* Human immunodeficiency virus-associated progressive multifocal leukoencephalopathy: apparent response to 3′-azido-3′-deoxythymidine. *Rev Infect Dis* 1990; **12:** 479–82.
7. Chiesi A, *et al.* Epidemiology of AIDS dementia complex in Europe. *J Acquir Immune Defic Syndr Hum Retrovirol* 1996; **11:** 39–44.
8. Evers S, *et al.* Impact of antiretroviral treatment on AIDS dementia: a longitudinal prospective event-related potential study. *J Acquir Immune Defic Syndr Hum Retrovirol* 1998; **17:** 143–8.
9. Routy JP, *et al.* Intrathecal zidovudine for AIDS dementia. *Lancet* 1990; **336:** 248.
10. Lucht F, *et al.* Intrathecal zidovudine for AIDS dementia. *Lancet* 1990; **336:** 813.


**HIV infection prophylaxis.** Antiretroviral drugs are becoming more widely accepted for chemoprophylaxis after *occupational exposure* to HIV infection. Zidovudine is commonly used in combination with other antiretroviral drugs after exposure with a risk of infection (see p.623).

Zidovudine monotherapy has been shown to be of value in *reducing vertical transmission* from mother to infant.[1,2] A typical dosage regimen is given under Uses and Administration, above, but the effectiveness of shorter courses is being assessed in developing countries. Short-course regimens have typically involved starting zidovudine 300 mg twice daily by mouth at 36 to 38 weeks' gestation, and giving, during labour, either 300 mg every 3 hours[3,4] or 500 or 600 mg as a single dose.[5] In the latter study, treatment was continued for a further week postpartum,[5] but no treatment was given to the infants in any of these studies. Although the reductions in transmission rates were lower than those achieved with the high-dose regimen, they were nevertheless regarded as useful in the populations studied.[6] Abbreviated regimens, even begun as late as the first 48 hours of life, do seem still to be of benefit.[7] Combination therapy with zidovudine and other antiretrovirals has been investigated for prevention of vertical transmission; in one study in France,[8] lamivudine, given from 32 weeks' gestation, in addition to the standard zidovudine regimen was effective, but severe adverse effects occurred and resistance to lamivudine emerged. A further study in Africa[9] comparing short-course combination regimens found that zidovudine and lamivudine started at 36 weeks' gestation then given during labour and for 1 week to the mother and neonate resulted in a greater reduction in transmission than the same combination given without the prepartum component, although both regimens were effective; the combination had no efficacy when given during labour alone. Moreover, the benefits from the first two regimens diminished considerably after 18 months of follow-up.[9] Another study[10] in sub-Saharan Africa involving HIV-positive women who were not tested or counselled during pregnancy but who did breast feed has suggested that treatment of the neonate only with oral zidovudine for 7 days together with a single oral dose of nevirapine as soon as possible after birth may offer greater protection against vertical transmission than nevirapine alone.

1. Connor EM, *et al.* Reduction of maternal-infant transmission of human immunodeficiency virus type 1 with zidovudine treatment. *N Engl J Med* 1994; **331:** 1173–80.
2. Sperling RS, *et al.* Maternal viral load, zidovudine treatment, and the risk of transmission of human immunodeficiency virus type 1 from mother to infant. *N Engl J Med* 1996; **335:** 1621–9.
3. Shaffer N, *et al.* Short-course zidovudine for perinatal HIV-1 transmission in Bangkok, Thailand: a randomised controlled trial. *Lancet* 1999; **353:** 773–80.
4. Wiktor SZ, *et al.* Short-course oral zidovudine for prevention of mother-to-child transmission of HIV-1 in Abidjan, Côte d'Ivoire: a randomised trial. *Lancet* 1999; **353:** 781–5.
5. Dabis F, *et al.* 6-Month efficacy, tolerance, and acceptability of a short regimen of oral zidovudine to reduce vertical transmission of HIV in breastfed children in Côte d'Ivoire and Burkina Faso: a double-blind placebo-controlled multicentre trial. *Lancet* 1999; **353:** 786–92.
6. Mofenson LM. Short-course zidovudine for prevention of perinatal infection. *Lancet* 1999; **353:** 766–7.
7. Wade NA, *et al.* Abbreviated regimens of zidovudine prophylaxis and perinatal transmission of the human immunodeficiency virus. *N Engl J Med* 1998; **339:** 1409–14.
8. Mandelbrot L, *et al.* Lamivudine-zidovudine combination for prevention of maternal-infant transmission of HIV-1. *JAMA* 2001; **285:** 2083–93.
9. The Petra Study Team. Efficacy of three short-course regimens of zidovudine and lamivudine in preventing early and late transmission of HIV-1 from mother to child in Tanzania, South Africa, and Uganda (Petra study): a randomised, double-blind, placebo-controlled trial. *Lancet* 2002; **359:** 1178–86.
10. Taha TE, *et al.* Short postexposure prophylaxis in newborn babies to reduce mother-to-child transmission of HIV-1: NVAZ randomised clinical trial. *Lancet* 2003; **362:** 1171–7.

## Preparations

***USP 27:*** Zidovudine Capsules; Zidovudine Injection; Zidovudine Oral Solution; Zidovudine Tablets.

**Proprietary Preparations** (details are given in Part 3)
***Arg.:*** Azoazol; Azotine; Crisazet; Enper; Exovir; Iduvo; Retrovir; Zetrotax; ***Austral.:*** Retrovir; ***Austria:*** Retrovir; ***Belg.:*** Retrovir; ***Braz.:*** Produvir; Retrovir; Revirax; Virozid; Virustat†; Zidix†; Zidovir; Zidovusan; ***Canad.:*** Novo-AZT; Retrovir; ***Chile:*** Retrovir; ***Denm.:*** Retrovir; ***Fin.:*** Retrovir; ***Fr.:*** Retrovir; ***Ger.:*** Retrovir; ***Gr.:*** Retrovir; ***Hong Kong:*** Retrovir; ***India:*** Retrovir; Zidovir; Zydowin; ***Irl.:*** Retrovir; ***Israel:*** Retrovir; ***Ital.:*** Retrovir; ***Malaysia:*** Retrovir; ***Mex.:*** Azetavir; Dipedyne†; Isadol†; Novavir†; Prandox; Retrovir; Serovidina†; Zidovir†; ***Neth.:*** Retrovir; ***Norw.:*** Retrovir; ***NZ:*** Retrovir; ***Port.:*** Retrovir; ***S.Afr.:*** Retrovir; ***Singapore:*** Retrovir; ***Spain:*** Retrovir; ***Swed.:*** Retrovir; ***Switz.:*** Retrovir; ***Thai.:*** Retrovir; T-ZA†; T.O.Vir; Zidis; ***UK:*** Retrovir; ***USA:*** Retrovir.

**Multi-ingredient:** ***Arg.:*** 3TC Complex; 3TC/AZT; Ganvirel Duo; Hivirux Complex; Imunoxa Complex; Kess Complex; Muvidina; Tricivir; Ultraviral Duo; Zetavudin; ***Austral.:*** Combivir; Trizivir; ***Austria:*** Combivir; ***Belg.:*** Combivir; Trizivir; ***Braz.:*** Biovir; Combivir†; Duovir; Zidolam; ***Canad.:*** Combivir; ***Chile:*** Combivir; Tricivir; ***Denm.:*** Combivir; Trizivir; ***Fin.:*** Combivir; Trizivir; ***Fr.:*** Combivir; Trizivir; ***Ger.:*** Combivir; Trizivir; ***Gr.:*** Combivir; ***Hong Kong:*** Combivir; ***India:*** Duovir; Lamuzid; ***Irl.:*** Combivir; Trizivir; ***Israel:*** Combivir; Trizivir; ***Ital.:*** Combivir; Trizivir; ***Malaysia:*** Combivir; ***Mex.:*** Combivir; ***Neth.:*** Combivir; ***Norw.:*** Combivir; Trizivir; ***NZ:*** Combivir; ***Port.:*** Combivir; Trizivir; ***S.Afr.:*** Combivir; Retrovir/3TC Post-HIV Exposure; ***Singapore:*** Combivir; Trizivir; ***Spain:*** Combivir; Trizivir; ***Swed.:*** Combivir; Trizivir; ***Switz.:*** Combivir; Trizivir; ***Thai.:*** Combid; ***UK:*** Combivir; Trizivir; ***USA:*** Combivir; Trizivir.

# Anxiolytic Sedatives Hypnotics and Antipsychotics

Anxiety disorders, p.663
Obsessive-compulsive disorder, p.663
Panic attacks, p.663
Phobic disorders, p.663
Post-traumatic stress disorder, p.664
Extrapyramidal disorders, p.664
Ballism, p.664
Chorea, p.664
Tics, p.664
Hypochondriasis, p.664
Psychoses, p.665
Disturbed behaviour, p.665
Mania, p.665
Schizophrenia, p.665
Sedation, p.666
Dental sedation, p.666
Endoscopy, p.666
Intensive care, p.666
Sleep disorders, p.667
Insomnia, p.667
Parasomnias, p.667

The drugs in this chapter include:

- anxiolytic sedatives, formerly called minor tranquillisers, which have been used in the management of anxiety disorders
- drugs used to produce sleep (hypnotics)
- drugs used in the treatment of psychoses (antipsychotics, formerly called major tranquillisers). The term neuroleptic is sometimes used to describe those antipsychotics that have effects on the extrapyramidal system.

The difference in action between anxiolytics and hypnotics is mainly one of degree and the same drug or group of drugs can have both effects, larger doses being necessary to produce a state of sleep.

The benzodiazepines (typified by Diazepam, p.690) replaced the barbiturates (typified by Amobarbital, p.670) and related sedatives as the major group of drugs used as anxiolytics and hypnotics. Some benzodiazepines are also used for their muscle relaxant and anticonvulsant properties. Newer anxiolytics include buspirone (p.672), a drug that affects serotonin neurotransmission.

The classical antipsychotics (typified by Chlorpromazine, p.675) include the butyrophenones, the diphenylbutylpiperidines, the indole derivatives, the phenothiazines, and the thioxanthenes. Some newer antipsychotics such as clozapine (p.685), risperidone (p.719), olanzapine (p.710), quetiapine (p.718), and amisulpride (p.669) are often referred to as atypical antipsychotics because of their reduced tendency to cause the extrapyramidal effects typical of classical antipsychotics.

◊ General references.

1. WHO. Evaluation of methods for the treatment of mental disorders. *WHO Tech Rep Ser 812* 1991.

## Anxiety disorders

Anxiety is an emotional condition characterised by feelings such as apprehension and fear accompanied by physical symptoms such as tachycardia, increased respiration, sweating, and tremor. It can be a normal emotion but when it is severe and disabling it becomes pathological.

Anxiety disorders are difficult to define and various classifications exist:

- in **acute stress disorder** anxiety is associated with a recent extremely stressful event such as bereavement, and is likely to resolve within a few weeks
- in **generalised anxiety disorders** there is persistent pervasive anxiety usually lasting 6 months or more. Symptoms include fatigue and disturbed sleep, motor tension, autonomic hyperactivity, irritability, and loss of concentration.

The first step in the **management** of anxiety that cannot be attributed to an underlying disease is the use of psychological treatments such as cognitive therapy. Such therapy can be effective in most types of anxiety. If unsuccessful, short-term treatment with a benzodiazepine may be considered. Benzodiazepines can exert an effect very rapidly, possibly even after the first dose, and this makes them suitable for treating an acute reaction.[1] However, their use in chronic disorders such as generalised anxiety disorders is limited by serious problems of dependence (see under Diazepam, p.690). Tolerance may develop to the anxiolytic effects of benzodiazepines although this appears to be less likely than tolerance to the psychomotor effects. There do not appear to be clear advantages in terms of efficacy for any one benzodiazepine in the treatment of anxiety disorders.[2] However, adverse effects and pharmacokinetic parameters may influence choice.

Buspirone, an azaspirodecanedione, appears to have broadly similar efficacy to the benzodiazepines but a slower onset of action. It is reported to lack euphoriant effect, and may cause less sedation and dependence than the benzodiazepines. Its efficacy is reduced in patients who have had previous extensive use of benzodiazepines.[3-5]

Increasingly, antidepressants are considered preferable to benzodiazepines for the treatment of generalised anxiety disorders;[1,3,5-8] they are particularly appropriate when medium or long-term therapy is necessary or when depression is also present. It may be several weeks before their effects are apparent, therefore combined therapy with benzodiazepines may be required initially. Tricyclic antidepressants such as imipramine have demonstrated efficacy in the treatment of generalised anxiety disorders.[1,2,5,7,8] SSRIs have been used as alternatives to the tricyclics although they have been less well studied in the treatment of generalised anxiety disorders.[2,9,10] The noradrenaline and serotonin reuptake inhibitor venlafaxine may also be used. These newer drugs are safer in overdose and are associated with less severe adverse effects than the tricyclics and consequently are becoming the antidepressants of choice in generalised anxiety disorders.[2]

Beta blockers may be useful for the control of the physical symptoms of anxiety.[10] There is little evidence to support the efficacy of antihistamines such as hydroxyzine in anxious patients,[1,3] and the use of antihistamines solely for their sedative effect in anxiety is not considered appropriate. Antipsychotics have been used by some in severe anxiety for their sedative effects; long-term use should be avoided because of the risk of tardive dyskinesia.

Anxiety may be present with other disorders such as depression in **mixed anxiety and depressive disorders**, the management of which is discussed under Depression on p.279.

1. Ballenger JC, *et al.* Consensus statement on generalized anxiety disorder from the International Consensus Group on Depression and Anxiety. *J Clin Psychiatry* 2001; **62** (suppl 11): 53–8.
2. Sramek JJ, *et al.* Generalised anxiety disorder: treatment options. *Drugs* 2000; **62:** 1635–48.
3. Lader M. Treatment of anxiety. *BMJ* 1994; **309:** 321–4.
4. Nutt DJ. The psychopharmacology of anxiety. *Br J Hosp Med* 1996; **55:** 187–91.
5. Rickels K, Rynn M. Pharmacotherapy of generalized anxiety disorder. *J Clin Psychiatry* 2002; **63** (suppl 14): 9–16.
6. Lader M, *et al.* Royal College of Psychiatrists. Guidelines for the management of patients with generalised anxiety. *Psychiatr Bull* 1992; **16:** 560–5.
7. Gorman JM. Treating generalized anxiety disorder. *J Clin Psychiatry* 2003; **64** (suppl 2): 24–9.
8. Kapczinski F, *et al.* Antidepressants for generalized anxiety disorder. Available in The Cochrane Library; Issue 1. Chichester: John Wiley; 2004.
9. Feighner JP. Overview of antidepressants currently used to treat anxiety disorders. *J Clin Psychiatry* 1999; **60** (suppl 22): 18–22.
10. House A, Stark D. Anxiety in medical patients. *BMJ* 2002; **325:** 207–9.

**Obsessive-compulsive disorder.** Obsessive-compulsive disorder is associated with intrusive, recurrent, obsessional thoughts and/or repetitive compulsive behaviour (e.g. hand washing) performed in a ritualistic manner. A combination of pharmacological, behavioural, and psychosocial methods appears to have the most successful long-term outcome in its treatment. **Drug therapy** is based on antidepressants that inhibit reuptake of serotonin.[1-5] These include clomipramine, the SSRIs, and the serotonin and noradrenaline reuptake inhibitor venlafaxine. There is some evidence that clomipramine is more effective than the SSRIs but its adverse effects are more problematic.[3,5,6] It may take 4 to 6 weeks before any response is obtained and up to about 12 weeks to achieve an optimal effect.[2,7] If one serotonin reuptake inhibitor fails then another can be tried.[2-5] About 40 to 60% of patients do not respond to these drugs and of those who do, many do not experience complete remission.[3] The optimum duration of treatment in responders remains to be determined. Some suggest therapy for at least a year or longer[4,7,8] but many patients relapse when drug therapy is withdrawn and prolonged therapy may be necessary. It has been suggested that patients may be maintained on reduced dosage.[9] Gradual withdrawal over several months may be more successful if patients are also receiving behavioural therapy.[5]

Drugs such as buspirone, lithium, pindolol, and some antipsychotics including the atypicals have been tried as **adjuncts** when patients are refractory to serotonin reuptake inhibitors and behavioural therapy but results of such augmentation therapy have been variable.[2-5,8] Benzodiazepines have been tried as alternatives to serotonin reuptake inhibitors but they are unsuitable because of the problems associated with prolonged therapy.[8]

1. Piccinelli M, *et al.* Efficacy of drug treatment in obsessive-compulsive disorder: a meta-analytic review. *Br J Psychiatry* 1995; **166:** 424–43.
2. Carpenter LL, *et al.* A risk-benefit assessment of drugs used in the management of obsessive-compulsive disorder. *Drug Safety* 1996; **15:** 116–34.
3. Goodman WK. Obsessive-compulsive disorder: diagnosis and treatment. *J Clin Psychiatry* 1999; **60** (suppl 18): 27–32.
4. Stein DJ, *et al.* Obsessive-compulsive disorder. *Lancet* 2002; **360:** 397–405.
5. McDonough M, Kennedy N. Pharmacological management of obsessive-compulsive disorder: a review for clinicians. *Harv Rev Psychiatry* 2002; **10:** 127–37.
6. Ackerman DL, Greenland S. Multivariate meta-analysis of controlled drug studies for obsessive-compulsive disorder. *J Clin Psychopharmacol* 2002; **22:** 309–17.
7. March JS, *et al.* Expert Consensus Guideline Series: treatment of obsessive-compulsive disorder. *J Clin Psychiatry* 1997; **58** (suppl 4): 1–73.
8. Zohar J, *et al.* Current concepts in the pharmacological treatment of obsessive-compulsive disorder. *Drugs* 1992; **43:** 210–18.
9. Mundo E, *et al.* Long-term pharmacotherapy of obsessive-compulsive disorder: a double-blind controlled study. *J Clin Psychopharmacol* 1997; **17:** 4–10.

**Panic attacks.** Panic attacks are severe, sudden, unexpected, recurrent exacerbations of anxiety. During an attack there is a feeling of fear, terror, and impending doom or even death accompanied by autonomic symptoms. If behavioural or cognitive therapy fails in the management of panic disorders drug therapy can then be tried, but it may need to be prolonged as there is a high rate of relapse on discontinuation.[1] Antidepressants are the drugs of choice in the treatment of panic disorder. Tricyclic antidepressants or SSRIs can reduce the frequency of attacks and can often prevent them completely.[2-4] Efficacy is broadly comparable, although SSRIs may be associated with a lower incidence of serious adverse effects.[5-8] MAOIs such as phenelzine are also effective but dietary restrictions and serious adverse effects limit their use to patients unresponsive to tricyclics and SSRIs.[4,5] Other antidepressants are being evaluated in panic attacks.

It may take several weeks before the effects of antidepressants are seen and initially there may be an increase in anxiety and the frequency of panic attacks. Benzodiazepines are sometimes used as adjuncts until antidepressants exert their full effect.[4-7] Short courses of benzodiazepines may also be of use in patients who cannot tolerate, or who are refractory to, antidepressants,[2] but any benefit may be outweighed by the risk of dependence.[3] There is little evidence to support the use of beta blockers, but they may control physical symptoms. Other drugs that might produce beneficial effects in some patients include valproate[2,4,6] and possibly clonidine.[9]

1. Michels R, Marzuk PM. Progress in psychiatry. *N Engl J Med* 1993; **329:** 628–38.
2. Johnson MR, *et al.* Panic disorder: pathophysiology and drug treatment. *Drugs* 1995; **49:** 328–44.
3. Anonymous. Stopping panic attacks. *Drug Ther Bull* 1997; **35:** 58–62.
4. Bennett JA, *et al.* A risk-benefit assessment of pharmacological treatments for panic disorder. *Drug Safety* 1998; **18:** 419–30.
5. American Psychiatric Association. Practice guideline for the treatment of patients with panic disorder. *Am J Psychiatry* 1998; **155** (suppl): 1–34. Also available at: http://www.psych.org/psych_pract/treatg/pg/pg_panic.cfm (accessed 27/04/04)
6. Ballenger JC, *et al.* Consensus statement on panic disorder from the International Consensus Group on Depression and Anxiety. *J Clin Psychiatry* 1998; **59** (suppl 8): 47–54.
7. Kasper S, Resinger E. Panic disorder: the place of benzodiazepines and selective serotonin reuptake inhibitors. *Eur Neuropsychopharmacol* 2001; **11:** 307–21.
8. Bakker A, *et al.* SSRIs vs TCAs in the treatment of panic disorder: a meta-analysis. *Acta Psychiatr Scand* 2002; **106:** 163–7.
9. Puzantian T, Hart LL. Clonidine in panic disorder. *Ann Pharmacother* 1993; **27:** 1351–3.

**Phobic disorders.** Phobic disorders consist of an irrational or exaggerated fear of, and a wish to avoid, specific objects, activities, or situations. As there is a strong link between **agoraphobia** and panic attacks (see above) it is treated similarly. Simple or specific phobias are usually unresponsive to pharmacotherapy and respond better to behaviour therapy.

SSRIs, and particularly paroxetine, are considered to be the first choice for the treatment of **social anxiety disorder** (social phobia).[1-4] MAOIs such as phenelzine are also effective in social anxiety disorder and can improve anticipatory anxiety and functional disability;[5,6] however, their use is limited by dietary restrictions and serious adverse effects. Results with the reversible inhibitor of monoamine oxidase moclobemide have been variable.[1-4] The benzodiazepines bromazepam and clonazepam have also been reported to be of some benefit,[1,3-5,7] although benzodiazepines should be used with caution because of the risk of dependence and abuse.

Beta blockers may help to reduce the physical symptoms in **performance-related anxiety**.[3,5,7]


1. Ballenger JC, *et al.* Consensus statement on social anxiety disorder from the International Consensus Group on Depression and Anxiety. *J Clin Psychiatry* 1998; **59** (suppl 17): 54–60.
2. Liebowitz MR. Update on the diagnosis and treatment of social anxiety disorder. *J Clin Psychiatry* 1999; **60** (suppl 18): 22–6.
3. Sareen J, Stein M. A review of the epidemiology and approaches to the treatment of social anxiety disorder. *Drugs* 2000; **59:** 497–509.
4. Blanco C, *et al.* Pharmacotherapy of social anxiety disorder. *Biol Psychiatry* 2002; **51:** 109–20.
5. den Boer JA. Social phobia: epidemiology, recognition, and treatment. *BMJ* 1997; **315:** 796–800.
6. Hale AS. Anxiety. *BMJ* 1997; **314:** 1886–9.
7. Healy D. Social phobia in primary care. *Prim Care Psychiatry* 1995; **1:** 31–8.


**Post-traumatic stress disorder.** In post-traumatic stress disorder, anxiety is precipitated by recall of a traumatic experience. Patients may also suffer from negative symptoms such as avoidance, alienation, emotional numbness, and social withdrawal. The main treatment is psychotherapy.[1-5] Drug therapy is largely aimed at accompanying symptoms of anxiety or depression.[6] SSRIs are the treatment of choice for most of the symptoms of post-traumatic stress disorder.[2-4,7] Tricyclic antidepressants or, in refractory patients, MAOIs, may be used as alternatives to SSRIs to help reduce traumatic recollections and nightmares and to repress flashbacks.[1-4,7] The newer antidepressants nefazodone and venlafaxine have also been tried,[2-4,7] generally in patients refractory to SSRIs. Negative symptoms are usually resistant to pharmacotherapy. Some 8 to 12 weeks of treatment is generally thought necessary to judge the efficacy of treatment.[1,3,4] Antiepileptics such as carbamazepine and valproate appear to improve symptoms of hyper-reactivity, violent behaviour, and angry outbursts but only a small number of patients have been studied.[7] Lamotrigine may also relieve avoidance and intrusive symptoms although, again, patient numbers are small.[7] Benzodiazepines may be helpful for short-term management of anxiety and sleep disturbances (although some studies have failed to show benefit[6]) but they must be used with caution because of the risk of dependence and abuse,[2] and some do not favour their use, even short-term.[4]


1. McIvor RJ, Turner SW. Drug treatment in post-traumatic stress disorder. *Br J Hosp Med* 1995; **53:** 501–6.
2. Foa EB, *et al.* Treatment of posttraumatic stress disorder. *J Clin Psychiatry* 1999; **60** (suppl 16): 1–75.
3. Yehuda R. Post-traumatic stress disorder. *N Engl J Med* 2002; **346:** 108–14.
4. Ballenger JC, *et al.* Consensus statement on posttraumatic stress disorder from the International Consensus Group on Depression and Anxiety. *J Clin Psychiatry* 2000; **61** (suppl 5): 60–6.
5. Adshead G. Psychological therapies for post-traumatic stress disorder. *Br J Psychiatry* 2000; **177:** 144–8.
6. Stein DJ, *et al.* Pharmacotherapy for post traumatic stress disorder (PTSD). Available in The Cochrane Library; Issue 1. Chichester: John Wiley; 2004.
7. Hageman I, *et al.* Post-traumatic stress disorder: a review of psychobiology and pharmacotherapy. *Acta Psychiatr Scand* 2001; **104:** 411–22.


## Extrapyramidal disorders

Extrapyramidal disorders are movement disorders involving the brain's motor systems outside the pyramidal tract. They are usually characterised by akinesia (a loss of movement) or bradykinesia (abnormal slowness of movement) accompanied by an increase in muscle tone (typified by parkinsonism, p.1196); or by dyskinesias (abnormal involuntary movements), often accompanied by a reduction in muscle tone (see below for some examples). Drug-induced extrapyramidal disorders are discussed under Chlorpromazine, p.677.

**Ballism.** Ballism, sometimes called hemiballism or hemiballismus because it is usually unilateral, consists of involuntary flinging movements of the extremities and most often results from acute vascular infarction or haemorrhage of the subthalamic nucleus. It often improves spontaneously but dopamine-blocking antipsychotics such as haloperidol or dopamine-depleting drugs such as tetrabenazine may be needed to control severe symptoms. Surgery may be necessary in severe cases.

**Chorea.** Chorea is characterised by brief involuntary muscle contractions and an inability to sustain voluntary contractions. It may be related to neurological abnormalities in the caudate nucleus and putamen of the striatum as well as other basal ganglia structures. Overactivity of dopaminergic nigrostriatal pathways and depletion of gamma-aminobutyric acid (GABA) and acetylcholine may also play a part. Chorea may be an adverse effect of some drugs, including antipsychotics, levodopa, and oral contraceptives; it may also be a symptom of an underlying disorder such as systemic lupus erythematosus.

**Huntington's chorea** (Huntington's disease, progressive hereditary chorea) is a hereditary autosomal dominant disease characterised by chorea, behavioural disturbances, and a progressive decline in cognitive function culminating in dementia and death. The identification of a gene marker for Huntington's chorea now makes it possible to identify carriers of the abnormal gene. Symptoms usually appear in mid-life, with death following after about 15 years, although there are also juvenile-onset forms. Westphal variant, a form commonest in children, tends to be characterised more by rigidity than by chorea.

**Sydenham's chorea** (St Vitus' dance; Chorea Minor) is an acute, usually self-limiting, disorder with an autoimmune basis, characterised by chorea and behavioural disturbances. It commonly occurs about 6 months after rheumatic fever but is now rare since the incidence of rheumatic fever has declined. It may also arise during pregnancy (chorea gravidarum).

**Treatment of chorea** is symptomatic only and does not alter the progressive decline of Huntington's chorea; Sydenham's chorea resolves spontaneously within weeks or months but antibacterial prophylaxis to prevent recurrence of rheumatic fever (p.144) has been recommended. Other forms of chorea may resolve with treatment of the underlying disorder or withdrawal of any causative drug.

Tetrabenazine has been used effectively in chorea, although not all patients respond, and it may produce depression. The mode of action is thought to involve depletion of striatal dopamine. Reserpine, which has a similar action and effects, has also been used.

Phenothiazines such as chlorpromazine and fluphenazine have dopamine-receptor blocking activity and have also been used to treat chorea. Other antipsychotics with a similar mode of action that have been used include haloperidol, pimozide, sulpiride, and tiapride. Some atypical antipsychotics such as olanzapine and zotepine have also been tried. Adverse effects such as tardive dyskinesias may limit the use of antipsychotics, and doses should be kept as low as possible; attempts to control choreiform movements completely are not recommended. In addition to improving chorea, antipsychotics may also be of value in controlling the behavioural symptoms associated with Huntington's chorea; anxiolytics and antidepressants may also be of use.

Carbamazepine and lamotrigine have been tried with some degree of success in a limited number of patients. The use of drugs to increase GABA activity has been of little value. Implantation of human and porcine fetal neural cells is being studied.

References.


1. Marsden CD. Basal ganglia disease. *Lancet* 1982; **ii:** 1141–6.
2. Kremer B, *et al.* A worldwide study of the Huntington's disease mutation: the sensitivity and specificity of measuring CAG repeats. *N Engl J Med* 1994; **330:** 1401–6.
3. Furtado S, Suchowersky O. Huntington's disease: recent advances in diagnosis and management. *Can J Neurol Sci* 1995; **22:** 5–12.
4. Quinn N, Schrag A. Huntington's disease and other choreas. *J Neurol* 1998; **245:** 709–16.


**Tics.** Tics may manifest as sudden, involuntary, brief, isolated, repetitive movements which may be simple (e.g. eye blinking, nose twitching, or head jerking) or complex (e.g. touching, jumping, or kicking); they may also be sensory in nature or may present in a vocal or phonic way and may range from simple clearing of the throat to more complex symptoms such as echolalia (involuntary repetition of others speech) or coprolalia (involuntary and inappropriate swearing). Symptoms can usually be suppressed voluntarily and may increase with stress and decrease with distraction. Some tics persist during sleep. The most common cause is **Tourette's syndrome** (Gilles de la Tourette's syndrome), in which behavioural disturbances accompany the tics. It is mainly a genetic disorder with an onset during childhood but may also be precipitated by various substances (e.g. antipsychotics), trauma, streptococcal infection, or viral encephalitis.

Most patients' symptoms wax and wane and behavioural therapy and reassurance may be sufficient to resolve mild tics. Drug treatment may be necessary when tics are severe enough to cause discomfort or embarrassment. Clonidine, or alternatively guanfacine, are increasingly favoured for first-line treatment in patients with mild to moderate symptoms, because of a relative lack of serious adverse effects. However the greatest experience is with the classical antipsychotics pimozide or haloperidol, which often decrease the frequency and severity of tics and may improve any accompanying behavioural disturbances. Superiority of either drug in terms of efficacy or adverse effects has not been clearly demonstrated. It is usually recommended that doses are titrated to as low as possible bearing in mind that optimum treatment does not necessarily lead to the complete control of symptoms. The risk of developing serious adverse effects such as tardive dyskinesia with these drugs should be balanced against the perceived benefits of treatment. Medication can often be discontinued after a few years.

Alternative drugs may be required for those unresponsive to or intolerant of haloperidol or pimozide. Other drugs that are also used in the management of tics and/or behavioural aspects of Tourette's syndrome include sulpiride, baclofen, botulinum toxin, clonazepam, fluphenazine, levodopa, olanzapine, pergolide, risperidone, tiapride, tetrabenazine, and ziprasidone. Nicotine has been reported to produce benefit when used alone or with haloperidol in patients whose symptoms were not satisfactorily controlled with haloperidol alone.

For drugs used in the treatment of comorbid disorders commonly associated with Tourette's syndrome, such as obsessive-compulsive disorder and attention deficit hyperactivity disorder, see above and p.1583, respectively.

References.


1. Sandor P. Clinical management of Tourette's syndrome and associated disorders. *Can J Psychiatry* 1995; **40:** 577–83.
2. Peterson BS. Considerations of natural history and pathophysiology in the psychopharmacology of Tourette's syndrome. *J Clin Psychiatry* 1996; **57** (suppl 9): 24–34.
3. Robertson MM, Stern JS. Gilles de la Tourette syndrome. *Br J Hosp Med* 1997; **58:** 253–6.
4. Kurlan R. Treatment of tics. *Neurol Clin North Am* 1997; **15:** 403–9.
5. Peterson BS, Cohen DJ. The treatment of Tourette's syndrome: multimodal, developmental intervention. *J Clin Psychiatry* 1998; **59** (suppl 1): 62–74.
6. Scahill L, *et al.* Pharmacologic treatment of tic disorders. *Child Adolesc Psychiatr Clin North Am* 2000; **9:** 99–117.
7. Robertson MM, Stern JS. Gilles de la Tourette syndrome: symptomatic treatment based on evidence. *Eur Child Adolesc Psychiatry* 2000; **9** (suppl 1): 60–75.
8. Jiménez-Jiménez FJ, García-Ruiz PJ. Pharmacological options for the treatment of Tourette's disorder. *Drugs* 2001; **61:** 2207–20.
9. Singer HS. The treatment of tics. *Curr Neurol Neurosci Rep* 2001; **1:** 195–202.
10. Kossoff EH, Singer HS. Tourette syndrome: clinical characteristics and current management strategies. *Paediatr Drugs* 2001; **3:** 355–63.
11. Jankovic J. Tourette's syndrome. *N Engl J Med* 2001; **345:** 1184–92.
12. Leckman JF. Tourette's syndrome. *Lancet* 2002; **360:** 1577–86.
13. Lavenstein BL. Treatment approaches for children with Tourette's syndrome. *Curr Neurol Neurosci Rep* 2003; **3:** 143–8.


## Hypochondriasis

Hypochondriasis (hypochondriacal neurosis) is a morbid preoccupation with one's health characterised by a fear or belief that normal bodily sensations are indicative of serious disease. It persists despite medical reassurance and management is difficult. If hypochondriasis is secondary to a psychiatric disorder, particularly depression and some anxiety disorders, treatment aimed at the primary condition may also lead to resolution of the hypochondrial symptoms.

Cognitive and behavioural therapies may be useful in the treatment of hypochondriasis; drug treatment of primary hypochondriasis has been less well studied although antidepressants such as the SSRIs may be effective. Pimozide is used in the management of hypochondriacal psychoses such as delusions of parasitic infestation or sexually transmitted disease.

References.


1. Hamann K, Avnstorp C. Delusions of infestation treated by pimozide: a double-blind crossover clinical study. *Acta Derm Venereol (Stockh)* 1982; **62:** 55–8.
2. Lyell A. Delusions of parasitosis. *Br J Dermatol* 1983; **108:** 485–99.
3. Fallon BA, *et al.* The pharmacotherapy of hypochondriasis. *Psychopharmacol Bull* 1996; **32:** 607–11.
4. Goldmeier D. Psychological and sexual problems. In: Adler MW, ed. *ABC of sexually transmitted diseases.* 4th ed. London: BMJ Publishing Group, 1999; 63–5.
5. Perkins RJ. SSRI antidepressants are effective for treating delusional hypochondriasis. *Med J Aust* 1999; **170:** 140–1.
6. Barsky AJ. The patient with hypochondriasis. *N Engl J Med* 2001; **345:** 1395–9.
7. Magariños M, *et al.* Epidemiology and treatment of hypochondriasis. *CNS Drugs* 2002; **16:** 9–22.

### Psychoses

Psychoses and psychotic disorders are terms that have been used to describe a collection of severe psychiatric disorders in which the patient has disordered thinking and loses contact with reality due to delusions and/or hallucinations. There may be accompanying mood or behavioural disturbances. *Organic psychoses* arise from organic brain disease produced by toxic insults, metabolic disturbances, infections, or structural abnormalities and may be acute (delirium) or chronic (dementia) in nature.

**Disturbed behaviour.** Drug therapy is sometimes indicated for the immediate control of severely disturbed, agitated, or violent behaviour associated with a variety of conditions such as toxic delirium, brain damage, mania (see Bipolar Disorder, p.278), or other psychotic disorders. Antipsychotics and benzodiazepines, either alone or in combination, are commonly used for disturbed behaviour. There is little agreement on the best antipsychotic for these indications, selection depending mainly on the condition of the patient and the adverse effect profile of the drug.[1-4] Oral therapy should be tried first and parenteral therapy only given if this is ineffective or refused. The high-potency butyrophenone haloperidol is commonly used for **acutely disturbed behaviour** although it lacks any sedative effects and may be associated with severe extrapyramidal symptoms. The atypical antipsychotics such as olanzapine and risperidone are increasingly used in acute situations. Benzodiazepines such as diazepam and lorazepam are valuable sedatives for the disturbed or delirious patient. A combination of an antipsychotic and a benzodiazepine allows the use of lower doses of each drug.

Other drugs that have had some success in the control of symptoms such as agitation, aggression, rage, or violent behaviour include beta blockers, lithium, carbamazepine, and valproate. Buspirone and antidepressants such as the SSRIs and trazodone may also be useful.

Antipsychotics appear to be modestly effective for the control of disturbed behaviour associated with the **dementia** of chronic conditions such as Alzheimer's disease (p.1484).[5-10] However, antipsychotics can themselves precipitate confusion or exacerbate dementia and may hasten cognitive decline, increase the risk of falls, incontinence, and drowsiness, and interfere with the performance of motor skills.[11] Elderly patients with dementia, especially Lewy-body dementia, are reported to be highly susceptible to the extrapyramidal adverse effects of antipsychotics and the reaction can be life-threatening. Antipsychotics are used only after careful consideration of the causes of disturbed behaviour and the benefits and risks of antipsychotic treatment. Very low doses are given at first and increased gradually according to clinical response and development of adverse effects; the necessity for continued use is reviewed periodically. Again, there is no agreement over the choice of antipsychotic. Atypical antipsychotics such as olanzapine, quetiapine, and risperidone have been used and may be less likely to produce extrapyramidal symptoms but whether they are more effective remains to be determined. However, the UK Committee on Safety of Medicines have recommended[12] that risperidone and olanzapine should not be used to treat behavioural problems in elderly patients with dementia after analysis of placebo-controlled clinical studies revealed an increased risk of stroke with these 2 atypical antipsychotics. Guidelines for the management of behavioural and psychiatric symptoms in patients with dementia and a history of stroke or transient ischaemic attacks have been issued in the UK.[13] The sedative drug, clomethiazole, may be a useful alternative to antipsychotics for the control of agitated behaviour in elderly patients, generally causing fewer adverse effects; respiratory depression, excessive sedation, and dependence may, however, be a problem. Benzodiazepines are not generally indicated for the management of elderly demented patients because of the risks of dependence with continued use, disinhibiting effects, and the particular problems of these drugs in old people (see the Elderly, under Diazepam, p.692). They are not as effective as antipsychotics in reducing behavioural problems, but may be useful in short courses for the management of severe anxiety disorders, or given as required for patients who only have rare episodes of agitation.

The use of antipsychotics in the control of **disturbed behaviour in children** is controversial and can probably be justified only in severe cases resistant to other therapy.[14] Autistic and mentally retarded children are among those who may require antipsychotics on a short-term basis. Some suggest the use of high-potency antipsychotics such as haloperidol on the grounds that they are less likely to cause sedation or impair arousal, cognitive function, and learning; others have favoured a drug such as thioridazine which carries a lower risk of dystonic reactions, but thioridazine is no longer recommended for use in children because of cardiotoxic risks. The tendency of antipsychotics to lower the seizure threshold is an important consideration in autistic children who are at an increased risk of seizure disorders.

Antipsychotics and benzodiazepines have been used to control the symptoms of **drug-induced delirium**.[15] Psychosis in patients with Parkinson's disease may be particularly difficult to treat, since the extrapyramidal effects of classical antipsychotics can exacerbate the movement disorder; benefit has been reported with the atypical antipsychotic clozapine (which must be used with caution because of the risk of agranulocytosis) but results with other atypical antipsychotics such as risperidone and olanzapine have been mixed; quetiapine appears to be reasonably well tolerated.

Benzodiazepines such as lorazepam or midazolam have been used for palliative treatment of agitation and restlessness in patients with **terminal restlessness**;[16] levomepromazine has been used similarly. Antipsychotics may exacerbate the existing tendency to myoclonus and convulsions in these patients and may not produce adequate sedation in the terminal phase, but haloperidol may be used where sedation is not required.

Paraphilias and other **deviant sexual behaviour** are rare in women so treatment is focussed largely towards men; it consists mainly of psychotherapy and the use of libido-suppressing drugs such as the anti-androgens.[17] The use of such pharmacotherapy is controversial and involves not only medical but legal issues. Drugs used for their anti-androgenic action include cyproterone and medroxyprogesterone. Gonadorelin analogues have also been tried for suppression of libido. Medroxyprogesterone has also been used for the control of intrusive disinhibited sexual behaviour in elderly men with dementia. There have been some case reports of fluoxetine being used with some success in the control of fantasies associated with various paraphilias. The antipsychotic benperidol is used in some countries for the management of sexual deviations but its value is not established. In general few well-controlled blinded studies have been conducted into the pharmacological treatment of sexual offenders and there is no evidence that drug treatment reduces the rate of re-offending.


1. Fava M. Psychopharmacologic treatment of pathologic aggression. *Psychiatr Clin North Am* 1997; **20:** 427–51.
2. American Psychiatric Association. Practice guideline for the treatment of patients with delirium. *Am J Psychiatry* 1999; **156** (suppl): 1–20. Also available at: http://www.psych.org/psych_pract/treatg/pg/pg_delirium.cfm (accessed 27/04/04)
3. Davies T. Management of the acutely disturbed patient. *Prescribers' J* 1999; **39:** 129–35.
4. Lambert M, *et al.* Pharmacotherapy of first-episode psychosis. *Expert Opin Pharmacother* 2003; **4:** 717–50.
5. American Psychiatric Association. Practice guideline for the treatment of patients with Alzheimer's disease and other dementias of late life. *Am J Psychiatry* 1997; **154** (suppl): 1–39. Also available at: http://www.psych.org/psych_pract/treatg/pg/pg_dementia_32701.cfm (accessed 27/04/04)
6. Alexopoulos GS, *et al.* Treatment of agitation in older persons with dementia. *Postgrad Med* 1998; Apr (suppl): 1–88.
7. Ballard C, O'Brien J. Treating behavioural and psychological signs in Alzheimer's disease. *BMJ* 1999; **319:** 138–9.
8. Daniel DG. Antipsychotic treatment of psychosis and agitation in the elderly. *J Clin Psychiatry* 2000; **61** (suppl 14): 49–52.
9. Scottish Intercollegiate Guidelines Network. Interventions in the management of behavioural and psychological aspects of dementia: a national clinical guideline, pilot edition (February 1998). Available at: http://www.sign.ac.uk/pdf/sign22.pdf (accessed 27/04/04)
10. Anonymous. Drugs for disruptive features in dementia. *Drug Ther Bull* 2003; **41:** 1–4.
11. McShane R, *et al.* Do neuroleptic drugs hasten cognitive decline in dementia: prospective study with necropsy follow up. *BMJ* 1997; **314:** 266–70.
12. Atypical antipsychotic drugs and stroke message from Professor G Duff, Chairman of Committee on Safety of Medicines (CSM). Available at: http://www.mca.gov.uk/ourwork/monitorsafequalmed/safetymessages/antipsystoke_9304.pdf (accessed 27/04/04)
13. Working group for the Faculty of Old Age Psychiatry RCPsych, RCGP, BGS, and Alzheimer's Society, following CSM restriction on risperidone and olanzapine. Guidance for the management of behavioural and psychiatric symptoms in dementia and the treatment of psychosis in people with history of stroke/TIA. Available at: http://www.rcpsych.ac.uk/college/faculty/oap/professional/guidance_summary.htm (accessed 27/04/04)
14. Connor DF, Steingard RJ. A clinical approach to the pharmacotherapy of aggression in children and adolescents. *Ann N Y Acad Sci* 1996; **794:** 290–307.
15. Friedman JH, Factor SA. Atypical antipsychotics in the treatment of drug-induced psychosis in Parkinson's disease. *Mov Disord* 2000; **15:** 201–11.
16. Burke AL. Palliative care: an update on "terminal restlessness". *Med J Aust* 1997; **166:** 39–42.
17. Bradford JMW. Treatment of men with paraphilia. *N Engl J Med* 1998; **338:** 464–5.


**Mania.** Mania usually occurs as part of bipolar disorder. The treatment of acute attacks of mania including mention of the role of antipsychotics is described under Bipolar Disorder, p.278.

**Schizophrenia.** Schizophrenia is a complex disorder associated with a high morbidity; it may be a group of related syndromes rather than a single disorder. Schizophrenia begins most commonly in late adolescence to the early twenties and many patients develop a chronic illness with repeated relapses. The estimated prevalence is between 0.2 to 1% in the general population. The predominant clinical features of acute schizophrenia syndrome can be divided into psychotic features such as delusions and hallucinations, and disorganised features involving speech, thought, and behaviour (together often known as 'positive' symptoms). The main features of the chronic syndrome are apathy, lack of drive, and social withdrawal (so-called 'negative' symptoms). Positive symptoms tend to respond better to drug therapy than negative symptoms. The pathophysiological mechanism of schizophrenia is unclear. Since classical antipsychotics used in the treatment of schizophrenia block dopamine $D_2$ receptors in the midbrain it has been suggested that dopaminergic system overactivity may be involved. However, the efficacy of atypical antipsychotics such as clozapine (see below), which is a relatively weak dopamine $D_2$ inhibitor, has raised the possibility that an imbalance of other neurotransmitters such as serotonin may also be involved (see also Action, under Chlorpromazine, p.681).

The **treatment** of schizophrenia consists mainly of a combination of social therapy and antipsychotics.[1-14] Drug treatment must be started as soon as possible for best outcome. There is little difference in the efficacy of classical antipsychotics such as chlorpromazine and haloperidol. The atypical antipsychotic clozapine appears to be more effective than classical antipsychotics in the management of both positive and negative symptoms, but its use is restricted because it can cause potentially fatal agranulocytosis. Comparative studies have shown that other atypical antipsychotics are at least as effective on positive symptoms as the classical antipsychotics, although claims of greater effects on negative symptoms remain to be proven.

Choice of therapy depends on the risk of adverse effects (which vary between the different groups of antipsychotics), any past treatment, and, unfortunately, cost. UK guidelines issued by the National Institute for Clinical Excellence (NICE)[15] recommend that the oral atypical antipsychotics amisulpride, olanzapine, quetiapine, risperidone, and zotepine are considered as first-line treatments for patients with newly diagnosed schizophrenia. These atypical antipsychotics should also be considered in patients responding to classical antipsychotics but experiencing unacceptable extrapyramidal or other adverse effects and in those who have relapsed and who experienced poorly-controlled symptoms or unacceptable adverse effects with their previous therapy. However, classical antipsychotics are still widely used, since the diversity of their preparations (tablets, oral liquids, injections, and depot injections) and lower cost offer advantages over the atypical antipsychotics. NICE therefore does not recommend changing to an atypical in patients who are already adequately controlled by classical antipsychotic treatment without unacceptable adverse effects. Because risperidone and olanzapine have been associated with an increased risk of stroke when used in elderly patients with dementia, UK guidelines[16] recommend that other antipsychotics should be considered for patients with a history of stroke, transient ischaemic attacks, or other cerebrovascular disease even in the absence of dementia.

There is great interindividual variation in response to antipsychotics, and choosing the most appropriate one may require a trial of antipsychotics from different chemical groups and careful adjustment of dosage. The Royal College of Psychiatrists in the UK has issued advice for those considering the use of higher than normally recommended doses of antipsychotics (see under Administration in the Uses and Administration of Chlorpromazine, p.681). However, in recent years there has been a trend in favour of lower doses of antipsychotics, often with adjunctive benzodiazepines (see below). The use of more than one antipsychotic at the same time is not usually recommended.

About 30% of patients may have little or no response to classical antipsychotics while many others have only a partial response. Such **resistant schizophrenia** may be due to poor patient compliance, which is a major problem in schizophrenic patients; lack of compliance may be a result of adverse effects (see below for possible treatments) or because the patient experiences a relapse while on medication and is unable to maintain treatment.[17] A patient should not be considered resistant to therapy until at least 2 different antipsychotics (NICE also recommends that at least one of these should have been an atypical[11]) have each been given for an adequate trial period (at least 6 to 8 weeks). If other drugs are still ineffective clozapine may be tried; it should be given for at least 3 months before resorting to measures such as ECT or the use of adjunctive drugs (see below).

Following the initial control of schizophrenia with antipsychotics relapse rates are high in those who stop treatment, therefore **maintenance** therapy is probably warranted. Some recommend the use of lower doses of antipsychotics during maintenance to reduce adverse effects, although this may increase the risk of relapse. The decision to withdraw an antipsychotic completely in a stabilised patient is complex and depends on the number of previous psychotic episodes. In some cases maintenance therapy may need to be indefinite. Regular injections of long-acting depot antipsychotics are sometimes used for maintenance therapy especially if compliance is a problem.[18] They are particularly useful for patients living in the community, and may also be advantageous for those who respond poorly to therapy because of increased first-pass metabolism or intestinal malabsorption. Concern over the possibility of increased extrapyramidal effects and other adverse effects with depot antipsychotics has not been substantiated.

**Adjunctive drugs** have been used in schizophrenia either to augment antipsychotic therapy or reduce their adverse effects.[19] The short-term addition of a benzodiazepine to the initial treatment of acute episodes of schizophrenia can provide a useful extra sedative and anxiolytic effect. It may also allow a smaller dose of antipsychotic to be used and thereby reduce the likelihood of extrapyramidal effects.

The use of antimuscarinics for the treatment or prophylaxis of antipsychotic-induced extrapyramidal side-effects is controversial (see Extrapyramidal Disorders on p.677). They are particularly effective in the management of acute dystonic reactions but efficacy in parkinsonism may be minimal and little benefit has been demonstrated in akathisia. Fears that the long-term use of antimuscarinics increases the risk of tardive dyskinesia appear to be unfounded, although they may worsen the condition and should be discontinued if it develops. However, the side-effects of antimuscarinics may be troublesome and may be additive with the antimuscarinic actions of the antipsychotic. Antimuscarinics also have euphoric effects. Routine use of prophylactic antimuscarinics is therefore not indicated with the possible exception of short-term use in patients at high risk of developing dystonias, or in patients with a previous history of drug-induced dystonias. Antimuscarinics may be given on a short-term basis to treat dystonias.

Addition of lithium to antipsychotic treatment may be worthwhile in some patients who fail to respond to an antipsychotic alone, although there is the danger of an interaction (see p.303).

The value of treatment of depressive symptoms of schizophrenia with antidepressants is not established but the addition of antidepressants such as the tricyclics is considered worth a trial for depression occurring during the recovery phase after an acute episode of psychosis.

Carbamazepine has produced modest benefit in some patients with refractory schizophrenia, the main effect being a reduction in accompanying symptoms such as excitement, impulsivity, and aggression, but concomitant administration of carbamazepine and haloperidol has also resulted in reduced haloperidol concentrations and clinical deterioration in a few patients. Valproate has also been tried.

Propranolol in high doses has been reported to be beneficial in refractory schizophrenia but several controlled studies of adjunctive use have found slight or no benefit. However, it may be of use as an adjunct in patients who develop akathisia unresponsive to antimuscarinics.


1. Fleischhacker WW, Hummer M. Drug treatment of schizophrenia in the 1990s: achievements and future possibilities in optimising outcomes. *Drugs* 1997; **53:** 915–29.
2. Buckley PF. New dimensions in the pharmacologic treatment of schizophrenia and related psychoses. *J Clin Pharmacol* 1997; **37:** 363–78. Correction. *ibid.* 1998; **38:** 27.
3. American Psychiatric Association. Practice guideline for the treatment of patients with schizophrenia, 2nd edition (issued February 2004). Available at: http://www.psych.org/psych_pract/treatg/pg/SchizPG-Complete-Feb04.pdf (accessed 27/04/04)
4. McGrath J, Emmerson WB. Treatment of schizophrenia. *BMJ* 1999; **319:** 1045–8.
5. Campbell M, *et al.* The use of atypical antipsychotics in the management of schizophrenia. *Br J Clin Pharmacol* 1999; **47:** 13–22.
6. Pearsall R, *et al.* A new algorithm for treating schizophrenia. *Psychopharmacol Bull* 1998; **34:** 349–53.
7. Frankenburg FR. Choices in antipsychotic therapy in schizophrenia. *Harv Rev Psychiatry* 1999; **6:** 241–9.
8. Kane JM. Management strategies for the treatment of schizophrenia. *J Clin Psychiatry* 1999; **60** (suppl. 12): 13–17.
9. Kane JM. Pharmacologic treatment of schizophrenia. *Biol Psychiatry* 1999; **46:** 1396–1408.
10. Maguire GA. Comprehensive understanding of schizophrenia and its treatment. *Am J Health-Syst Pharm* 2002; **59** (suppl 5): S4–S11.
11. National Institute for Clinical Excellence. Schizophrenia: core interventions in the treatment and management of schizophrenia in primary and secondary care (issued December 2002). Available at: http://www.nice.org.uk/pdf/CG1NICEguideline.pdf (accessed 27/04/04)
12. Lambert TJR, Castle DJ. Pharmacological approaches to the management of schizophrenia. *Med J Aust* 2003; **178** (suppl): S57–S61.
13. American Academy of Child and Adolescent Psychiatry. Practice parameter for the assessment and treatment of children and adolescents with schizophrenia. *J Am Acad Child Adolesc Psychiatry* 2001; **40** (suppl 7): 4S–23S.
14. Freedman R. Schizophrenia. *N Engl J Med* 2003; **349:** 1738–49.
15. National Institute for Clinical Excellence. Guidance on the use of newer (atypical) antipsychotic drugs for the treatment of schizophrenia (issued June 2002). Available at: http://www.nice.org.uk/pdf/ANTIPSYCHOTICfinalguidance.pdf (accessed 27/04/04)
16. Working group for the Faculty of Old Age Psychiatry RCPsych, RCGP, BGS, and Alzheimer's Society, following CSM restriction on risperidone and olanzapine. Guidance for the management of behavioural and psychiatric symptoms in dementia and the treatment of psychosis in people with history of stroke/TIA. Available at: http://www.rcpsych.ac.uk/college/faculty/oap/professional/guidance_summary.htm (accessed 27/04/04/)
17. Pantelis C, Lambert TJR. Managing patients with "treatment-resistant" schizophrenia. *Med J Aust* 2003; **178** (suppl): S62–S66.
18. Altamura AC, *et al.* Intramuscular preparations of antipsychotics: uses and relevance in clinical practice. *Drugs* 2003; **63:** 493–512.
19. Johns CA, Thompson JW. Adjunctive treatments in schizophrenia: pharmacotherapies and electroconvulsive therapy. *Schizophr Bull* 1995; **21:** 607–19.


## Sedation

Since sedatives reduce excitement and anxiety, they may be used before or during various medical procedures to alleviate fear and produce a state of calmness in the patient. A practical aim for situations requiring **conscious sedation**, for example in *dentistry* or during investigative procedures such as *endoscopy*, may be the reduction or abolition of physiological and psychological responses to the stress without loss of consciousness, cooperation, or protective reflexes. A greater degree of sedation may be required for patients in *intensive care* and some consider that patients should be maintained asleep but easily rousable. The difference between sedatives and hypnotics is mainly dose related. The same drug or group of drugs can have both effects, larger doses being necessary for a hypnotic effect, that is to produce a state of sleep.

Some specific situations where sedation may be required are discussed below. The use of sedatives in premedication for anaesthesia is discussed on p.1296.

**Dental sedation.** Intravenous midazolam has largely superseded diazepam for sedation in dental procedures. However, midazolam needs to be given slowly in small increments as its sedative end-point is reached much more abruptly than with diazepam. Midazolam has a rapid onset of action and produces good anterograde amnesia, but the response in children may be poor. Full recovery can take several hours. Although benzodiazepines have no analgesic activity, concomitant use of analgesics is rarely required. In addition, use of opioid analgesics to supplement sedation and provide postoperative analgesia is not recommended because of the possibility of respiratory depression.

Inhaled nitrous oxide is a powerful analgesic and sedative, well tolerated by children, and relatively safe and simple to use, although there is some concern over its long-term effect on dental staff. It also requires a certain amount of patient cooperation.

Oral sedatives may also be used to provide dental sedation and are particularly useful to ensure that the patient has a restful night prior to the procedure. Those drugs used include the benzodiazepines diazepam, nitrazepam, and temazepam, and the antihistamines promethazine and alimemazine. Temazepam is preferred when it is important to minimise any residual effects.

**Endoscopy.** The practice of giving sedation routinely before endoscopy varies widely between and within countries. It is unclear whether sedation improves patient comfort and the ease of performing the procedure; there may be a failure to distinguish between the need for sedation and the need for analgesia in such procedures. Ultimately the acceptability of unsedated endoscopy differs from patient to patient and procedure to procedure, and it may be appropriate to offer patients the choice.

Intravenous benzodiazepines are commonly used for sedation during endoscopy. Midazolam is generally preferred to diazepam because of its shorter duration of action. Since hypoventilation and oxygen desaturation may occur with benzodiazepines and the procedure itself can lower oxygen saturation, some recommend the administration of prophylactic nasal oxygen in conjunction with oxygen saturation monitoring.

Intravenous opioid analgesics such as morphine and pethidine have also been given but they have largely been replaced by the newer shorter-acting opioids, for example fentanyl, which have faster recovery times. Combination of a benzodiazepine with an opioid analgesic is not advocated in the UK because of the increased risk of cardiorespiratory effects and, possibly, fatalities. However, in the USA, benzodiazepines have often been given with opioids, including pethidine, since such combinations may reduce gagging and increase patient tolerance.

Low-dose intravenous propofol has also been used for sedation as an alternative to, or in combination with, midazolam. However the risk of adverse effects may limit its use and require the presence of an anaesthetist.

The use of topical anaesthetics such as lidocaine should probably be reserved for those who prefer to undergo endoscopy without sedation as topical anaesthesia appears to serve little useful function in patients premedicated with benzodiazepines or opioids. There appears to be no practical difference between individual topical anaesthetics. Sprays are safer and may be more effective than lozenges, but even when using a spray it is difficult to anaesthetise the oropharyngeal region effectively.

References.


1. Arrowsmith JB, *et al.* Results from the American Society for Gastrointestinal Endoscopy/US Food and Drug Administration collaborative study on complication rates and drug use during gastrointestinal endoscopy. *Gastrointest Endosc* 1991; **37:** 421–7.
2. The Royal College of Surgeons of England Commission on the Provision of Surgical Services. *Report of the working party on guidelines for sedation by non-anaesthetists.* London: Royal College of Surgeons, 1993.
3. Williams TJ. Sedation in fibreoptic bronchoscopy. *BMJ* 1995; **310:** 872.
4. Sutherland FWH. Sedation in fibreoptic bronchoscopy. *BMJ* 1995; **310:** 872.
5. Charlton JE. Monitoring and supplemental oxygen during endoscopy. *BMJ* 1995; **310:** 886–7.
6. Ristikankare M, *et al.*. Is routinely given conscious sedation of benefit during colonoscopy? *Gastrointest Endosc* 1999; **49:** 566–72.
7. Davis DE, *et al.* Topical pharyngeal anesthesia does not improve upper gastrointestinal endoscopy in conscious sedated patients. *Am J Gastroenterol* 1999; **94:** 1853–6.
8. Bell GD. Premedication, preparation, and surveillance. *Endoscopy* 2000; **32:** 92–100.
9. Zuccaro G. Sedation and sedationless endoscopy. *Gastrointest Endosc Clin N Am* 2000; **10:** 1–20.
10. American Society for Gastrointestinal Endoscopy. Guidelines for the use of deep sedation and anesthesia for GI endoscopy. *Gastrointest Endosc* 2002; **56:** 613–17. Also available at: http://www.asge.org/gui/resources/manual/pe_deepsedation.asp (accessed 28/04/04)
11. Waring JP, *et al.* Guidelines for conscious sedation and monitoring during gastrointestinal endoscopy. *Gastrointest Endosc* 2003; **58:** 317–22. Also available at: http://www.asge.org/gui/resources/manual/cons_sed.asp (accessed 28/04/04)
12. British Society of Gastroenterology. Guidelines: safety and sedation during endoscopic procedures (issued September 2003). Available at: http://www.bsg.org.uk/clinical_prac/guidelines/sedation.htm (accessed 28/04/04)


**Intensive care.** Most patients in an intensive care unit require analgesia, sedation, or both during at least part of their stay. The required level of sedation may vary but, in general, many consider patients should be maintained asleep but easily rousable. Most sedatives and analgesics are given parenterally. Continuous intravenous infusion avoids the peaks and troughs of analgesia and sedation associated with intermittent intramuscular or intravenous administration, but to what extent it improves patient outcomes is unclear: sedation produced in this way may prolong the need for mechanical ventilation.

Opioid analgesics have both sedative and analgesic properties and are appropriate for sedation when pain is anticipated, although special care is required in those not artificially ventilated. The antitussive action of the opioids may also help ventilated patients to tolerate a tracheal tube. Morphine is a suitable opioid in many situations in intensive care but has a slow onset of action. If prolonged sedation is required analgesia can be obtained by a loading dose followed by a continuous infusion. Fentanyl has a short duration of action after single doses as a result of redistribution in the body. However, following repeated doses it is not a short-acting drug and therefore offers little advantage over morphine. Alfentanil has a short duration of action and has proved satisfactory in patients requiring overnight sedation but does not appear to offer any advantage over other opioids. In some patients, elimination and duration of action have been prolonged. It may be suitable for use at the start and end of prolonged periods of sedation to produce a rapid effect and to decrease the risk of prolonged respiratory depression respectively.

Not all patients require sedatives if sufficient analgesia is achieved, particularly after the first 24 to 48 hours, but most will require a balanced combination of analgesics and sedatives to relieve pain and anxiety. It is inappropriate to use high doses of opioids to achieve deep sedation and it is also inappropriate to use sedatives alone for patients who are in pain.

Benzodiazepines induce sleep and reduce anxiety and muscle tone; however, they do not provide analgesia. Although they produce profound amnesia, they often fail to achieve satisfactory sedation; doses that do achieve sedation often interfere with verbal contact with the patient. All benzodiazepines tend to produce cardiovascular and respiratory depression and care is required if they are used with opioids. Midazolam has a rapid onset and short duration of action following single doses, and has largely replaced diazepam as the benzodiazepine of choice for sedation. However, the half-life of midazolam can be substantially increased when given as a continuous intravenous infusion for long-term sedation in patients in intensive care. Lorazepam has also been used although onset of action may be slower than midazolam.

Flumazenil is a specific benzodiazepine antagonist and some suggest that it may be of use to assist the return of spontaneous respiration and consciousness in patients receiving benzodiazepines. Multiple doses may be required as it has a short duration of action. However, its routine use after prolonged benzodiazepine treatment is not usually recommended because of the risk of inducing withdrawal symptoms.

Propofol is used successfully in low doses for sedation in adults in intensive care, and weaning times in propofol-sedated patients on mechanical ventilation have been demonstrated to be shorter than those seen with midazolam. However, propofol is not recommended for use in children because of adverse effects (see p.1305).

Dexmedetomidine has recently been approved for use in intensive care as a sedative; it is also stated to have analgesic-sparing properties.

Ketamine has also been investigated for sedation in the intensive care setting and appears to be effective; it may be used with a benzodiazepine.

Rapid discontinuation of sedatives such as benzodiazepines, opioids, and propofol may lead to withdrawal symptoms, especially following high doses or prolonged sedation (more than 1 week). Doses should be tapered to prevent such symptoms.

Sedation and analgesia for **children** in intensive care is a subject of debate. Many of the regimens used appear to be similar to those used in adults or modifications of existing regimens for paediatric sedation. Drugs commonly used include midazolam and opioids such as fentanyl or morphine. However, there has been some concern over a report of encephalopathy associated with the prolonged use of midazolam with fentanyl for sedation in infants under intensive care (see Encephalopathy, under Effects on the Nervous System, p.691). As mentioned above, propofol is not recommended for children in intensive care. Withdrawal symptoms may also be a problem.

References.

1. Wolf AR. Neonatal sedation: more art than science. *Lancet* 1994; **344:** 628–9.
2. Barker DP, Rutter N. Neonatal sedation. *Lancet* 1994; **344:** 1362.
3. Wagner BKJ, O'Hara DA. Pharmacokinetics and pharmacodynamics of sedatives and analgesics in the treatment of agitated critically ill patients. *Clin Pharmacokinet* 1997; **33:** 426–53.
4. Lerch C, Park GR. Sedation and analgesia. *Br Med Bull* 1999; **55:** 76–95.
5. Bennett NR. Paediatric intensive care. *Br J Anaesth* 1999; **83:** 139–56.
6. Ostermann ME, *et al.* Sedation in the intensive care unit: a systematic review. *JAMA* 2000; **283:** 1451–9.
7. Society of Critical Care Medicine and American Society of Health-System Pharmacists. Clinical practice guidelines for the sustained use of sedatives and analgesics in the critically ill adult. *Am J Health-Syst Pharm* 2002; **59:** 150–78.

## Sleep disorders

The exact function of sleep is uncertain but it is believed to be involved in energy conservation and total body restoration and recuperation. Initially there is a period of light sleep (stages 1 and 2) followed by deep sleep (stages 3 and 4); this latter period is also known as slow-wave sleep. After stage 4, which occurs about 90 minutes after first falling asleep, there is a period of rapid-eye-movement (REM) sleep during which most dreams occur and EEG traces show high frequency waves. During a period of sleep there are several cycles of stages 1 to 4 followed by REM sleep, with periods of non-REM sleep becoming shorter and periods of REM sleep longer. It is the slow-wave sleep that is considered to be the more restorative. Most healthy adults sleep for single periods of between 7 to 9 hours a day. In old age there is less slow-wave sleep and sleep becomes more fragmented.

Sleep disorders include insomnia (see below), hypersomnia such as narcolepsy, p.1583, in which the timing, length, and quality of sleep is altered, and the parasomnias (see below) in which abnormal events occur during sleep.

**Insomnia.** Insomnia is the inability to achieve or maintain sleep and is the most common of the sleep disorders.[1-11] It often leaves sufferers feeling unrefreshed by sleep and may lead to impaired daytime performance.

- Transient insomnia may occur in those who normally sleep well and may be due to an alteration in the conditions that surround sleep, for example noise, or to an unusual pattern of rest as in shift work or travelling between time zones. It may also be associated with acute disorders.
- Short-term insomnia is often related to an emotional problem or more serious medical illness such as acute pain and may recur.
- Chronic insomnia may be attributed to an underlying psychiatric disorder, especially depression or anxiety, to alcohol or drug abuse, to certain drug treatments, to excessive caffeine intake, to daytime cat napping, or to physical causes such as pain, pruritus, or dyspnoea.

Management of insomnia requires resolution of any stressful precipitant or identification and treatment of any underlying causes, with an emphasis on non-pharmacological measures such as counselling, behavioural therapy, development of relaxation techniques, and avoidance of stimulant substances. Hypnotic drugs should ideally be reserved for short courses in the acutely distressed patient; they should be avoided in the elderly, and their use is rarely justified in children. Generally, hypnotics should be given at the lowest effective dose for as short a period as possible. In transient insomnia one or two doses of a short-acting hypnotic may be indicated, whereas in short-term insomnia intermittent doses of a short-acting hypnotic given for no more than 3 weeks may be appropriate. Routine use of hypnotics is undesirable. Tolerance can develop rapidly with continuous use and withdrawal following long-term use can lead to rebound insomnia and a withdrawal syndrome.

Benzodiazepines are generally regarded as the hypnotics of choice. They hasten sleep onset, decrease nocturnal awakenings, increase total sleeping time, and often impart a sense of deep and refreshing sleep. Slow-wave sleep and REM sleep are, however, reduced and the extra sleeping time is largely made up of relatively light sleep. A short-acting benzodiazepine such as temazepam is generally used when residual sedation is undesirable, if falling asleep is a problem, or, when necessary, in elderly patients. Longer-acting benzodiazepines such as nitrazepam are indicated when early waking is a problem and possibly when an anxiolytic effect is needed during the day or when some impairment of psychomotor function is acceptable.

Because of the hazard of dependence with benzodiazepines (see p.690), the UK Committee on Safety of Medicines (CSM)[12] has issued certain recommendations:

- they should be used to treat insomnia only when it is severe, disabling, or subjecting the individual to extreme distress
- they should be given in the lowest dose which controls symptoms (if possible, intermittently)
- they should not be continued beyond 4 weeks
- they should be withdrawn by gradual tapering of the dose to zero

Subsequently, the EU Committee on Proprietary Medicinal Products (CPMP) has recommended that the treatment period should be limited to 2 weeks when brotizolam, midazolam, or triazolam are used.[13]

Tolerance to the hypnotic effects of benzodiazepines develops rapidly, with sleep latency and pattern returning to pretreatment levels within a few weeks of starting treatment.

A number of other drugs have been used as alternatives to the benzodiazepines. Zaleplon, zopiclone, and zolpidem act on the same receptors or receptor subtypes as the benzodiazepines although structurally they are unrelated. Their short duration of action makes them more suitable for patients who have trouble falling asleep. The CPMP has recommended that treatment with zolpidem should be limited to a maximum of 4 weeks.[13] It remains to be proven whether these drugs offer any advantages over the benzodiazepines. Indeed, the CSM considers that zopiclone has the same potential for adverse psychiatric reactions, including dependence, as benzodiazepines.[14]

The use of cloral hydrate and its derivatives as hypnotics is now very limited. They have been used as alternatives to benzodiazepines in the elderly, although there is no convincing evidence of any special value in these patients. They used to be considered useful hypnotics for children but such use is rarely justified.

Clomethiazole has also been used as an alternative to benzodiazepines in the elderly. Nasal and conjunctival irritation may be troublesome, and the danger of overdosage and risk of dependence should be considered.

Some antihistamines have hypnotic properties and a number, including diphenhydramine, doxylamine, promethazine, and alimemazine, are marketed for insomnia. They may cause troublesome antimuscarinic effects and those with longer half-lives may cause hangover effects. Promethazine is also popular for use in children, but such use is not usually justified.

Barbiturates are no longer recommended as hypnotics because of their adverse effects. The CSM[15] has advised that barbiturates should only be used for insomnia that is severe and intractable when there are compelling reasons to, and then only in patients already taking barbiturates. It was also advised that attempts should be made to wean patients off barbiturate hypnotics. Similarly, compounds such as ethchlorvynol, glutethimide, and methaqualone are not recommended.

Alcohol is not recommended because it has a short weak hypnotic action, and rebound excitation can result in early morning insomnia. Its diuretic effects can interrupt sleep and chronic use can lead to rapid development of tolerance and addiction.

Tryptophan, sometimes in the form of dietary supplements, has enjoyed some popularity in the treatment of insomnia. Its efficacy is difficult to substantiate and, since the publication of reports linking tryptophan with the eosinophilic-myalgia syndrome, preparations indicated for insomnia have been withdrawn from the market in many countries.

Melatonin, a hormone believed to be involved in the maintenance of circadian rhythms, may be useful in the treatment of insomnias such as those due to **jet lag**[16] or other disorders (where it might act by resetting the body clock), and in the elderly. However, evidence for a direct hypnotic effect is less conclusive; its sleep-inducing properties are usually only seen after very high, supraphysiological concentrations have been attained.[6,7]

1. National Medical Advisory Committee. The management of anxiety and insomnia. A report by the National Medical Advisory Committee. Edinburgh: HMSO 1994.
2. Mendelson WB, Jain B. An assessment of short-acting hypnotics. *Drug Safety* 1995; **13:** 257–70.
3. NIH Technology Assessment Panel. Integration of behavioral and relaxation approaches into the treatment of chronic pain and insomnia. *JAMA* 1996; **276:** 313–18.
4. Kupfer DJ, Reynolds CF. Management of insomnia. *N Engl J Med* 1997; **336:** 341–6.
5. Ashton CH. Management of insomnia. *Prescribers' J* 1997; **37:** 1–10.
6. Wagner J, *et al.* Beyond benzodiazepines: alternative pharmacologic agents for the treatment of insomnia. *Ann Pharmacother* 1998; **32:** 680–91.
7. Nishino S, Mignot E. Drug treatment of patients with insomnia and excessive daytime sleepiness: pharmacokinetic considerations. *Clin Pharmacokinet* 1999; **37:** 305–30.
8. Holbrook AM, *et al.* The diagnosis and management of insomnia in clinical practice: a practical evidence-based approach. *Can Med Assoc J* 2000; **162:** 216–20.
9. Lenhart SE, Buysse DJ. Treatment of insomnia in hospitalized patients. *Ann Pharmacother* 2001; **35:** 1449–57.
10. Lavie P. Sleep disturbances in the wake of traumatic events. *N Engl J Med* 2001; **345:** 1825–32.
11. Grunstein R. Insomnia: diagnosis and management. *Aust Fam Physician* 2002; **31:** 995–1000.
12. Committee on Safety of Medicines. Benzodiazepines, dependence and withdrawal symptoms. *Current Problems 21* 1988.
13. Anonymous. Short-acting hypnotics: a comparative assessment. *WHO Drug Inf* 1993; **7:** 125–6.
14. Committee on Safety of Medicines. Zopiclone (Zimovane) and neuro-psychiatric reactions. *Current Problems 30* 1990.
15. Committee on Safety of Medicines/Medicines Control Agency. Barbiturate hypnotics: avoid whenever possible. *Current Problems* 1996; **22:** 7.
16. Herxheimer A, Petrie KJ. Melatonin for the prevention and treatment of jet lag. Available in The Cochrane Library; Issue 2. Chichester: John Wiley; 2004.

**Parasomnias.** Parasomnias are motor or autonomic disturbances that occur during sleep or are exaggerated by sleep. Some of the main parasomnias include nightmares, night terrors, sleepwalking (somnambulism), restless legs syndrome, periodic movements in sleep, nocturnal enuresis (p.475), bruxism (teeth grinding), head banging, and aggression during sleep. Parasomnias are common but rarely require treatment with drugs other than the symptomatic treatment of sleep-related medical problems. The management of some parasomnias is discussed briefly below.

The **restless legs syndrome** is characterised by an unpleasant creeping sensation deep in the legs with an irresistible urge to move them. The disorder is intermittent and begins during relaxation in the evenings and in bed. The aetiology of this condition is obscure and treatment has been largely empirical.[1-8] Drug treatment may not always be necessary and non-pharmacological methods such as good sleep hygiene should be tried initially.[4,6] There have been reports of efficacy with a wide range of treatments, although few have been well studied. Dopaminergic therapy has emerged as a common first-line treatment, a long-acting agonist being preferred in order to avoid the complications associated with levodopa. Anticonvulsants, such as carbamazepine, clonazepam, and gabapentin may be of use in those intolerant of dopamine agonists or in those who require additional medication. Other drugs that have been reported to be of benefit include some opioids, baclofen, clonidine, and the benzodiazepines. Iron supplementation may be effective if the syndrome is associated with iron deficiency.[5-7] Many patients with restless legs syndrome exhibit **periodic limb movements in sleep**,[5,6] characterised by repetitive periodic leg and foot jerking during sleep. Treatments tried are similar to those for the restless legs syndrome; clonazepam and levodopa are amongst the drugs shown to be of benefit.

Some **other parasomnias** have responded to treatment with benzodiazepines.[9,10] These include bruxism, head banging, aggression during sleep, night terrors, and sleep walking.

References.


1. Collado-Seidel V, *et al.* Aetiology and treatment of restless legs syndrome. *CNS Drugs* 1999; **12:** 9–20.
2. Hening W, *et al.* The treatment of restless legs syndrome and periodic limb movement disorder. *Sleep* 1999; **22:** 970–99.
3. Weimerskirch PR, Ernst ME. Newer dopamine agonists in the treatment of restless legs syndrome. *Ann Pharmacother* 2001; **35:** 627–30.
4. Clark MM. Restless legs syndrome *J Am Board Fam Pract* 2001; **14:** 368–74.
5. Odin P, *et al.* Restless legs syndrome. *Eur J Neurol* 2002; **9** (suppl 3): 59–67.
6. Stiasny K, *et al.* Clinical symptomatology and treatment of restless legs syndrome and periodic limb movement disorder. *Sleep Med Rev* 2002; **6:** 253–65.
7. Earley CJ. Restless legs syndrome. *N Engl J Med* 2003; **348:** 2103–9.
8. Schapira AH. Restless legs syndrome : an update on treatment options. *Drugs* 2004; **64:** 149–58.
9. Stores G. Dramatic parasomnias. *J R Soc Med* 2001; **94:** 173–6.
10. Wills L, Garcia J. Parasomnias: epidemiology and management. *CNS Drugs* 2002; **16:** 803–10.


## Abecarnil *(rINN)*

Abecarnilo; ZK-112119. Isopropyl 6-(benzyloxy)-4-(methoxymethyl)-9*H*-pyrido(3,4-*b*)indole-3-carboxylate.

$C_{24}H_{24}N_2O_4$ = 404.5.

*CAS — 111841-85-1.*

### Profile

Abecarnil is a beta-carboline compound reported to be a partial agonist at benzodiazepine receptors. It has been studied for its anxiolytic and anticonvulsant actions in anxiety disorders and alcohol withdrawal syndrome.

◊ References.


1. Krause W, *et al.* Pharmacokinetics and acute toleration of the β-carboline derivative abecarnil in man. *Arzneimittelforschung* 1990; **40:** 529–32.
2. Karara AH, *et al.* Pharmacokinetics of abecarnil in patients with renal insufficiency. *Clin Pharmacol Ther* 1996; **59:** 520–8.
3. Lydiard RB, *et al.* Abecarnil Work Group. A double-blind evaluation of the safety and efficacy of abecarnil, alprazolam, and placebo in outpatients with generalized anxiety disorder. *J Clin Psychiatry* 1997; **58** (suppl 11): 11–18.
4. Pollack MH, *et al.* Abecarnil for the treatment of generalized anxiety disorder: a placebo-controlled comparison of two dosage ranges of abecarnil and buspirone. *J Clin Psychiatry* 1997; **58** (suppl 11): 19–23.
5. Anton RF, *et al.* A double-blind comparison of abecarnil and diazepam in the treatment of uncomplicated alcohol withdrawal. *Psychopharmacology (Berl)* 1997; **131:** 123–9.
6. Rickels K, *et al.* A double-blind, placebo-controlled trial of abecarnil and diazepam in the treatment of patients with generalized anxiety disorder. *J Clin Psychopharmacol* 2000; **20:** 12–8.


## Acamprosate Calcium *(BANM, USAN, rINNM)*

Acamprosato de calcio; Acamprosatum Calcicum. Calcium 3-acetamido-1-propanesulphate.

$C_{10}H_{20}CaN_2O_8S_2$ = 400.5.

*CAS — 77337-76-9 (acamprosate); 77337-73-6 (acamprosate calcium).*

*ATC — N07BB03.*

**Pharmacopoeias.** In *Eur.* (see p.vi).

**Ph. Eur. 5.0** (Acamprosate Calcium). A white powder. Freely soluble in water; practically insoluble in alcohol and in dichloromethane. A 5% solution in water has a pH of 5.5 to 7.0.

### Adverse Effects

The main adverse effect of acamprosate is a dosage-related diarrhoea; nausea, vomiting, and abdominal pain occur less frequently. Other adverse effects have included pruritus, and occasionally a maculopapular rash; bullous skin reactions have occurred rarely. Depression and fluctuations in libido have also been reported.

**Effects on the skin.** A case of erythema multiforme in a woman with cirrhosis of the liver has been attributed to use of acamprosate[1] although both the diagnosis and any association with acamprosate has been seriously challenged.[2]


1. Fortier-Beaulieu M, *et al.* Possible association of erythema multiforme with acamprosate. *Lancet* 1992; **339:** 991.
2. Potgieter AS, Opsomer L. Acamprosate as cause of erythema multiforme contested. *Lancet* 1992; **340:** 856–7.


### Precautions

Acamprosate is contra-indicated in patients with renal or severe hepatic impairment.

**Renal impairment.** It is considered[1] likely that accumulation of acamprosate would occur with prolonged use of therapeutic doses in patients with renal impairment. It has been reported that the mean maximum concentration of acamprosate after a single 666-mg dose was 813 nanograms/mL in 12 patients with moderate or severe renal impairment compared with 198 nanograms/mL in 6 healthy subjects; values for the plasma elimination half-life were 47 and 18 hours, respectively.


1. Wilde MI, Wagstaff AJ. Acamprosate: a review of its pharmacology and clinical potential in the management of alcohol dependence after detoxification. *Drugs* 1997; **53:** 1038–53.


### Pharmacokinetics

Absorption of acamprosate from the gastrointestinal tract is slow but sustained and is subject to considerable interindividual variation. Steady-state concentrations are achieved after 7 days' administration. Bioavailability is reduced by administration with food. Acamprosate is not protein bound and although it is hydrophilic it is reported to cross the blood-brain barrier. Acamprosate does not appear to be metabolised and is excreted unchanged in the urine. The elimination half-life after oral administration has been reported to be about 33 hours.

◊ References.


1. Saivin S, *et al.* Clinical pharmacokinetics of acamprosate. *Clin Pharmacokinet* 1998; **35:** 331–45.


### Uses and Administration

Acamprosate has a chemical structure similar to that of gamma-aminobutyric acid (GABA) (p.1690). It is given by mouth as the calcium salt to prevent relapse in alcoholics who have been weaned off alcohol. The usual dose for patients weighing 60 kg or more is 666 mg of acamprosate calcium given three times daily; for patients less than 60 kg a dose of 666 mg may be given at breakfast followed by 333 mg at midday and 333 mg at night. Treatment should be started as soon as possible after alcohol withdrawal and maintained, even if the patient relapses, for the recommended period of 1 year.

**Alcohol dependence.** Acamprosate is considered to be of use as an adjunct to psychotherapy in maintaining abstinence after alcohol withdrawal in patients with alcohol dependence (p.1166). Reviews[1-4] of placebo-controlled studies conclude that acamprosate helps to prevent relapse and increase the number of drink-free days during a 1-year course of treatment and possibly for up to one year thereafter. Efficacy appears to be dose related but its effects in promoting abstinence may wane during treatment. Use with disulfiram or naltrexone may improve results but published data on combined treatment is relatively limited. Several mechanisms have been proposed to account for acamprosate's action including inhibition of neuronal hyperexcitability by antagonising excitatory amino acids such as glutamate.


1. Wilde MI, Wagstaff AJ. Acamprosate: a review of its pharmacology and clinical potential in the management of alcohol dependence after detoxification. *Drugs* 1997; **53:** 1038–53.
2. Anonymous. Acamprosate for alcohol dependence? *Drug Ther Bull* 1997; **35:** 70–2.
3. Mason BJ. Treatment of alcohol-dependent outpatients with acamprosate: a clinical review. *J Clin Psychiatry* 2001; **62** (suppl 20): 42–8.
4. Overman GP, *et al.* Acamprosate for the adjunctive treatment of alcohol dependence. *Ann Pharmacother* 2003; **37:** 1090–9.


### Preparations

**Proprietary Preparations** (details are given in Part 3)
***Arg.:*** Campral; ***Austral.:*** Campral; ***Austria:*** Campral; ***Belg.:*** Campral; ***Braz.:*** Campral; ***Chile:*** Campral; ***Denm.:*** Campral; ***Fr.:*** Aotal; ***Ger.:*** Campral; ***Hong Kong:*** Campral; ***Irl.:*** Campral; ***Mex.:*** Campral; ***Neth.:*** Campral; ***Norw.:*** Campral; ***Port.:*** Campral; ***S.Afr.:*** Sobrial; ***Singapore:*** Campral; ***Spain:*** Campral; Zulex; ***Swed.:*** Campral; ***Switz.:*** Campral; ***UK:*** Campral.

## Acecarbromal *(rINN)*

Acetcarbromal; Acetylcarbromal. *N*-Acetyl-*N*′-(2-bromo-2-ethylbutyryl)urea.

$C_9H_{15}BrN_2O_3$ = 279.1.

*CAS — 77-66-7.*

### Profile

Acecarbromal has similar actions to those of carbromal (p.674). It was formerly used for its sedative properties but the use of bromides is generally deprecated.

### Preparations

**Proprietary Preparations** (details are given in Part 3)
***USA:*** Paxarel†.

## Acepromazine *(BAN, rINN)*

Acepromazina. 10-(3-Dimethylaminopropyl)phenothiazin-2-yl methyl ketone.

$C_{19}H_{22}N_2OS$ = 326.5.

*CAS — 61-00-7.*

*ATC — N05AA04.*

## Acepromazine Maleate *(BANM, USAN, rINNM)*

Acetylpromazine Maleate; Maleato de acepromazina. 10-(3-Dimethylaminopropyl)phenothiazin-2-yl methyl ketone hydrogen maleate.

$C_{19}H_{22}N_2OS,C_4H_4O_4$ = 442.5.

*CAS — 3598-37-6.*

*ATC — N05AA04.*

**Pharmacopoeias.** In *US* for veterinary use only. Also in *BP(Vet).*

**BP(Vet) 2003** (Acepromazine Maleate). A yellow odourless or almost odourless crystalline powder. Soluble in water and in alcohol; freely soluble in chloroform; slightly soluble in ether. A 1% solution in water has a pH of 4.0 to 4.5.

**USP 27** (Acepromazine Maleate). pH of a 1% solution is between 4.0 and 5.5. Protect from light.

### Profile

Acepromazine is a phenothiazine with general properties similar to those of chlorpromazine (p.675). It has been given by mouth as the maleate in the treatment of anxiety disorders, hiccups, and nausea and vomiting. Acepromazine, as the base, has also been given in preparations for the management of insomnia.

### Preparations

**Proprietary Preparations** (details are given in Part 3)
***Denm.:*** Plegicil.
**Multi-ingredient:** ***Fr.:*** Noctran.

## Aceprometazine *(rINN)*

16-64 CB; Aceprometazina. 10-(2-Dimethylaminopropyl)phenothiazin-2-yl methyl ketone.

$C_{19}H_{22}N_2OS$ = 326.5.

*CAS — 13461-01-3.*

### Profile

Aceprometazine is a phenothiazine with general properties similar to those of chlorpromazine (p.675). It is available usually as the maleate in preparations for the management of insomnia.

### Preparations

**Proprietary Preparations** (details are given in Part 3)
**Multi-ingredient:** ***Fr.:*** Mepronizine; Noctran.

## Allobarbital *(USAN, rINN)*

Allobarbitone; Alobarbital; Diallylbarbitone; Diallylbarbituric Acid; Diallylmalonylurea; Diallymalum; NSC-9324. 5,5-Diallylbarbituric acid.

$C_{10}H_{12}N_2O_3$ = 208.2.

*CAS — 52-43-7.*

*ATC — N05CA21.*

### Profile

Allobarbital is a barbiturate with general properties similar to those of amobarbital (p.670). It has been used in combination preparations for the treatment of sleep disorders and pain but barbiturates are no longer considered appropriate for such purposes.

## Alprazolam *(BAN, USAN, rINN)*

Alprazolamum; U-31889. 8-Chloro-1-methyl-6-phenyl-4*H*-1,2,4-triazolo[4,3-*a*][1,4]benzodiazepine.

$C_{17}H_{13}ClN_4$ = 308.8.

*CAS — 28981-97-7 (alprazolam).*

*ATC — N05BA12.*

**Pharmacopoeias.** In *Chin., Eur.* (see p.vi), *Jpn,* and *US.*

**Ph. Eur. 5.0** (Alprazolam). A white crystalline powder. It exhibits polymorphism. Practically insoluble in water; sparingly soluble in alcohol and in acetone; freely soluble in dichloromethane. Protect from light.

**USP 27** (Alprazolam). A white to off-white crystalline powder. Insoluble in water; soluble in alcohol; sparingly soluble in acetone; freely soluble in chloroform; slightly soluble in ethyl acetate.

### Dependence and Withdrawal

As for Diazepam, p.690. Dependence may be a particular problem at the high doses used in the treatment of panic attacks.

## Adverse Effects and Treatment

As for Diazepam, p.690.

**Effects on the liver.** Abnormal liver enzyme values occurred on 2 occasions when alprazolam was added to the treatment regimen of a patient receiving phenelzine for depression.[1] It was not possible to say if this was due to alprazolam alone or a synergistic effect with phenelzine.

1. Roy-Byrne P, *et al.* Alprazolam-related hepatotoxicity. *Lancet* 1983; **ii:** 786–7.

**Effects on the skin.** There have been some reports of alprazolam-induced photosensitivity.[1,2]

1. Kanwar AJ, *et al.* Photosensitivity due to alprazolam. *Dermatologica* 1990; **181:** 75.
2. Watanabe Y, *et al.* Photosensitivity due to alprazolam with positive oral photochallenge test after 17 days administration. *J Am Acad Dermatol* 1999; **40:** 832–3.

## Precautions

As for Diazepam, p.691.

**Abuse.** High doses of alprazolam taken after maintenance doses of methadone produced a 'high' without pronounced sedation; the drug was also misused by nonopioid-drug abusers.[1] The usual urine toxicology screens for benzodiazepines often give false-negative results for alprazolam because of the extremely low concentrations of metabolites excreted, making abuse difficult to detect. A subsequent review[2] considered that the literature did not support the widely held belief that alprazolam had a greater liability for abuse than other benzodiazepines, but the possibility could not be discounted.

1. Weddington WW, Carney AC. Alprazolam abuse during methadone maintenance therapy. *JAMA* 1987; **257:** 3363.
2. Rush CR, *et al.* Abuse liability of alprazolam relative to other commonly used benzodiazepines: a review. *Neurosci Biobehav Rev* 1993; **17:** 277–85.

**Breast feeding.** The American Academy of Pediatrics[1] considers that, although the effect of alprazolam on breast-feeding infants is unknown, its use by mothers during breast feeding may be of concern since anxiolytic drugs do appear in breast milk and thus could conceivably alter CNS function in the infant both in the short and long term.

From a study[2] of the distribution of alprazolam into breast milk in 8 lactating women it was estimated that the average daily dose of alprazolam ingested by a breast-fed infant would range from 0.3 to 5 micrograms/kg or about 3% of a maternal dose.

1. American Academy of Pediatrics. The transfer of drugs and other chemicals into human milk. *Pediatrics* 2001; **108:** 776–89. Correction. *ibid.*; 1029. Also available at: http://aappolicy.aappublications.org/cgi/content/full/pediatrics%3b108/3/776 (accessed 28/04/04)
2. Oo CY, *et al.* Pharmacokinetics in lactating women: prediction of alprazolam transfer into milk. *Br J Clin Pharmacol* 1995; **40:** 231–6.

**Handling.** Care should be taken to prevent inhaling particles of alprazolam and exposing the skin to it.

**Hepatic impairment.** Alprazolam 1 mg by mouth was absorbed more slowly in 17 patients with alcoholic cirrhosis with no ascites than in 17 healthy subjects.[1] Mean peak alprazolam concentrations were achieved after 3.34 hours in the cirrhosis patients and 1.47 hours in the healthy subjects. Mean elimination half-life for cirrhosis patients was 19.7 hours compared with 11.4 hours for subjects from the healthy group. However, there were no significant differences in the maximum plasma concentrations achieved. The results indicate that alprazolam, in common with other benzodiazepines that undergo oxidative metabolism, would accumulate to a greater extent in patients with alcoholic liver disease than in healthy subjects; the daily dose of alprazolam may need to be reduced by half in this population.

1. Juhl RP, *et al.* Alprazolam pharmacokinetics in alcoholic liver disease. *J Clin Pharmacol* 1984; **24:** 113–19.

**Porphyria.** Alprazolam is considered to be unsafe in patients with porphyria because it has been shown to be porphyrinogenic in *in-vitro* systems.

## Interactions

As for Diazepam, p.692.

## Pharmacokinetics

Alprazolam is well absorbed from the gastrointestinal tract after oral administration, with peak plasma concentrations being achieved within 1 to 2 hours of a dose. The mean plasma half-life is 11 to 15 hours. Alprazolam is 70 to 80% bound to plasma protein. It is metabolised in the liver primarily to α-hydroxyalprazolam, which is reported to be approximately half as active as the parent compound, and to an inactive benzophenone; plasma concentrations of metabolites are very low. It is excreted in urine as unchanged drug and metabolites.

◊ References.

1. Greenblatt DJ, Wright CE. Clinical pharmacokinetics of alprazolam: therapeutic implications. *Clin Pharmacokinet* 1993; **24:** 453–71.
2. Wright CE, *et al.* Pharmacokinetics and psychomotor performance of alprazolam: concentration-effect relationship. *J Clin Pharmacol* 1997; **37:** 321–9.
3. Kaplan GB, *et al.* Single-dose pharmacokinetics and pharmacodynamics of alprazolam in elderly and young subjects. *J Clin Pharmacol* 1998; **38:** 14–21.

## Uses and Administration

Alprazolam is a short-acting benzodiazepine with general properties similar to those of diazepam (p.695). It is used in the short-term treatment of anxiety disorders in doses of 250 to 500 micrograms three times daily by mouth, increased where necessary to a total daily dose of 3 or 4 mg. In elderly or debilitated patients, an initial dose of 250 micrograms two or three times daily has been suggested. For doses in patients with hepatic impairment, see below.

Doses of up to 10 mg of alprazolam daily have been used in the treatment of panic attacks. A modified-release preparation of alprazolam is also available for once daily dosing.

**Administration in hepatic impairment.** Caution has been advised when using alprazolam in patients with hepatic impairment. In those with advanced liver disease, an initial dose of 250 micrograms two or three times daily has been suggested.

**Anxiety disorders.** The management of anxiety disorders, including the use of benzodiazepines, is discussed on p.663.

References.

1. Cross-National Collaborative Panic Study, Second Phase Investigators. Drug treatment of panic disorder: comparative efficacy of alprazolam, imipramine, and placebo. *Br J Psychiatry* 1992; **160:** 191–202.
2. Lepola UM, *et al.* Three-year follow-up of patients with panic disorder after short-term treatment with alprazolam and imipramine. *Int Clin Psychopharmacol* 1993; **8:** 115–18.
3. Pollack MH, *et al.* Long-term outcome after acute treatment with alprazolam or clonazepam for panic disorder. *J Clin Psychopharmacol* 1993; **13:** 257–63.
4. Woodman CL, *et al.* Predictors of response to alprazolam and placebo in patients with panic disorder. *J Affect Disord* 1994; **30:** 5–13.

**Depression.** Although they may be useful for associated anxiety, benzodiazepines are not usually considered appropriate for treatment of depression (p.279); however, some drugs such as alprazolam have been tried for this indication.[1]

1. Kravitz HM, *et al.* Alprazolam and depression: a review of risks and benefits. *J Clin Psychiatry* 1993; **54:** (suppl.): 78–84.

**Premenstrual syndrome.** Alprazolam has been reported[1-3] to have produced a marginal to good response in the premenstrual syndrome (p.1551) but others have not found it to be of benefit,[4] and the role of benzodiazepines is limited by their adverse effects. If benzodiazepines are selected it is recommended that in order to reduce the risk of dependence and withdrawal symptoms they should be carefully restricted to the luteal phase in selected patients.[5] Withdrawal symptoms may be more severe after short-acting drugs such as alprazolam. Antidepressant drugs such as SSRIs may be preferred.

1. Smith S, *et al.* Treatment of premenstrual syndrome with alprazolam: results of a double-blind, placebo-controlled, randomized crossover clinical trial. *Obstet Gynecol* 1987; **70:** 37–43.
2. Harrison WM, *et al.* Treatment of premenstrual dysphoria with alprazolam: a controlled study. *Arch Gen Psychiatry* 1990; **47:** 270–5.
3. Freeman EW, *et al.* A double-blind trial of oral progesterone, alprazolam, and placebo in treatment of severe premenstrual syndrome. *JAMA* 1995; **274:** 51–7.
4. Evans SM, *et al.* Mood and performance changes in women with premenstrual dysphoric disorder: acute effects of alprazolam. *Neuropsychopharmacology* 1998; **19:** 499–516.
5. Mortola JF. A risk-benefit appraisal of drugs used in the management of premenstrual syndrome. *Drug Safety* 1994; **10:** 160–9.

## Preparations

*USP 27:* Alprazolam Tablets.

**Proprietary Preparations** (details are given in Part 3)

***Arg.:*** Alplax; Becede; Bestrol; Krama; Prenadona; Prinox; PTA; Retan; Tensium; Thiprasolan; Tranquinal; Xanax; ***Austral.:*** Alprax; Kalma; Ralozam†; Xanax; ***Austria:*** Alpratyrol; Xanor; ***Belg.:*** Alpraz; Xanax; ***Braz.:*** Apraz; Frontal; Tranquinal; ***Canad.:*** Apo-Alpraz; Novo-Alprazol; Nu-Alpraz; Xanax; ***Chile:*** Adax; Grifoalpram; Prazam; Sanerva; Tricalma Retard; Zotran; ***Denm.:*** Alprox; Tafil; ***Fin.:*** Alprox; Xanor; ***Fr.:*** Xanax; ***Ger.:*** Cassadan; Esparon†; Tafil; Xanax; ***Gr.:*** Saturnil; Xanax; ***Hong Kong:*** Xanax; ***India:*** Alprax; Alprocontin; Pacyl; Zolam; ***Irl.:*** Alprox; Calmax; Gerax; Xanax; ***Israel:*** Alpralid; Alprox; Apox†; Xanagis; Xanax; ***Ital.:*** Alprazig; Frontal; Mialin; Valeans; Xanax; ***Malaysia:*** Apo-Alpraz; Xanax; ***Mex.:*** Neupax; Tafil; ***Neth.:*** Xanax; ***Norw.:*** Xanor; ***NZ:*** Xanax; ***Port.:*** Alpronax; Pazolam; Prazam; Unilan; Xanax; ***S.Afr.:*** Alzam; Anxirid; Azor; Drimpam; Panix†; Xanolam†; Xanor; Zopax; ***Singapore:*** Alzolam†; Apo-Alpraz; Dizolam; Xanax; Zacetin; ***Spain:*** Trankimazin; ***Swed.:*** Xanor; ***Switz.:*** Xanax; ***Thai.:*** Alcelam; Alnax; Anpress; Anzion; Dizolam; Marzolam; Mitranax; Pharnax; Siampraxol; Xanacine; Xanax; Xiemed; ***UK:*** Xanax; ***USA:*** Xanax.

**Multi-ingredient:** ***Arg.:*** Alplax Digest; Alplax Net; Novo Vegestabil; Tranquinal Soma.

# Amisulpride *(BAN, rINN)*

Amisulprida; Amisulpridum; DAN-216. 4-Amino-*N*-[(1-ethyl-2-pyrrolidinyl)methyl]-5-(ethylsulphonyl)-2-methoxybenzamide; (*RS*)-4-Amino-*N*-[(1-ethylpyrrolidin-2-yl)methyl]-5-(ethylsulfonyl)-o-anisamide.

$C_{17}H_{27}N_3O_4S$ = 369.5.

*CAS — 71675-85-9.*

*ATC — N05AL05.*

**Pharmacopoeias.** In *Eur.* (see p.vi).

**Ph. Eur. 5.0** (Amisulpride). A white or almost white crystalline powder. Practically insoluble in water; sparingly soluble in dehydrated alcohol; freely soluble in dichloromethane.

## Adverse Effects, Treatment, and Precautions

Although amisulpride may share some of the adverse effects seen with the classical antipsychotics (see Chlorpromazine, p.675), the incidence and severity of such effects may vary. Insomnia, anxiety, and agitation are common side-effects with amisulpride. Other less common effects include drowsiness and gastrointestinal disorders such as constipation, nausea, vomiting, and dry mouth. Allergic reactions, abnormal liver function tests, and seizures have been reported rarely.

Hyperprolactinaemia, which may result in galactorrhoea, amenorrhoea, impaired fertility, gynaecomastia, breast pain, and sexual dysfunction, has occurred with amisulpride treatment. Weight gain has also been noted. Dose-related extrapyramidal dysfunction may occur, but symptoms such as acute dystonia, parkinsonism, and akathisia are generally mild at licensed doses. Tardive dyskinesia has been reported after long-term use and there have been rare cases of neuroleptic malignant syndrome. Hypotension and bradycardia have been reported occasionally; QT prolongation, in rare cases leading to torsade de pointes, has also been noted. The risk of QT prolongation is increased by pre-existing conditions such as bradycardia, hypokalaemia, and congenital or acquired QT prolongation; patients should be reviewed for these conditions before starting amisulpride treatment. Certain medications may also increase the risk (see Interactions, below).

Amisulpride should not be given to patients with phaeochromocytoma or prolactin-dependent tumours. It should be used with caution in patients with severe renal impairment, or a history of epilepsy or Parkinson's disease. The risk of hypotension and sedation is increased in elderly patients.

Amisulpride may affect the performance of skilled tasks including driving.

Withdrawal symptoms have occurred rarely when amisulpride has been stopped abruptly; a gradual dose reduction may be appropriate when stopping amisulpride.

**Overdosage.** The effects of overdosage of amisulpride in 2 patients have been reported.[1] The first patient had taken about 3 g of amisulpride and an unknown amount of dosulepin and was found to have had a blood-amisulpride concentration of 9.63 micrograms/mL. Generalised convulsions, which resolved spontaneously, were followed by coma, motor restlessness, tachycardia, and slight prolongation of the QT interval. The patient was treated with gastric lavage and had recovered within 48 hours. The second patient, who had been found dead, had a blood-amisulpride concentration of 41.7 micrograms/mL.

1. Tracqui A, *et al.* Amisulpride poisoning: a report on two cases. *Hum Exp Toxicol* 1995; **14:** 294–8.

## Interactions

Amisulpride should not be given with drugs that may induce arrhythmias including torsade de pointes; such drugs include some antiarrhythmics, cisapride, thioridazine, erythromycin, and halofantrine. The risk of arrhythmias is also increased with drugs that produce bradycardia or hypokalaemia, including beta blockers, some calcium-channel blockers, clonidine, digoxin, guanfacine, potassium-depleting diuretics, pimozide, haloperidol, tricyclic antidepressants, and lithium; use of these drugs with amisulpride requires caution.

The central effects of other CNS depressants including alcohol may be enhanced by amisulpride. Amisulpride may also enhance the effects of antihypertensive drugs. The dopamine-blocking activity of amisulpride may antagonise the actions of dopaminergics such as levodopa.

### Pharmacokinetics

Amisulpride is absorbed from the gastrointestinal tract but bioavailability is reported to be only about 43 to 48%. An initial peak in plasma concentration has been reported to occur one hour after oral administration and a second higher one after 3 to 4 hours. Plasma protein binding is reported to be only about 16%. Metabolism is limited, with most of a dose appearing in the urine and faeces as unchanged drug. The terminal elimination half-life is about 12 hours.

### Uses and Administration

Amisulpride is a substituted benzamide atypical antipsychotic. It is reported to have a high affinity for dopamine $D_2$ and $D_3$ receptors. Amisulpride is used mainly in the management of psychoses such as schizophrenia (p.665) but in some countries it has also been tried in depression (p.279).

For acute psychotic episodes daily doses of between 400 and 800 mg may be given by mouth in 2 divided doses, increased if necessary to 1200 mg daily. For patients with predominantly negative symptoms daily doses between 50 and 300 mg are recommended. Daily doses of up to 300 mg may be given as a single dose. Amisulpride has also been given by intramuscular injection in doses of 400 mg daily.

◊ References.

1. Boyer P, *et al.* Treatment of negative symptoms in schizophrenia with amisulpride. *Br J Psychiatry* 1995; **166:** 68–72.
2. Möller H-J, *et al.* Improvement of acute exacerbations of schizophrenia with amisulpride: a comparison with haloperidol. *Psychopharmacology (Berl)* 1997; **132:** 396–401.
3. Loo H, *et al.* Amisulpride versus placebo in the medium-term treatment of the negative symptoms of schizophrenia. *Br J Psychiatry* 1997; **170:** 18–22.
4. Lecrubier Y, *et al.* Amisulpride Study Group. Amisulpride versus imipramine and placebo in dysthymia and major depression. *J Affect Disord* 1997; **43:** 95–103.
5. Smeraldi E. Amisulpride versus fluoxetine in patients with dysthymia or major depression in partial remission: a double-blind, comparative study. *J Affect Disord* 1998; **48:** 47–56.
6. Boyer P, *et al.* Amisulpride versus amineptine and placebo for the treatment of dysthymia. *Neuropsychobiology* 1999; **39:** 25–32.
7. Curran MP, Perry CM. Amisulpride: a review of its use in the management of schizophrenia. *Drugs* 2001; **61:** 2123–50.

**Administration in renal impairment.** For patients with renal impairment the dose of amisulpride should be reduced to half the normal dose for patients with a creatinine clearance (CC) of between 30 and 60 mL/minute and to one-third in patients with a CC between 10 and 30 mL/minute.

### Preparations

**Proprietary Preparations** (details are given in Part 3)
***Arg.:*** Enorden; ***Austral.:*** Solian; ***Austria:*** Solian; ***Belg.:*** Solian; ***Braz.:*** Socian; ***Chile:*** Socian; ***Fr.:*** Solian; ***Ger.:*** Solian; ***Hong Kong:*** Solian; ***Irl.:*** Solian; ***Israel:*** Solian; ***Ital.:*** Deniban; Solian; Sulamid; ***Norw.:*** Solian; ***Port.:*** Amitrex; Socian; ***S.Afr.:*** Solian; ***Singapore:*** Solian; ***Spain:*** Amilande; Solian; ***Switz.:*** Solian; ***UK:*** Solian.

## Amobarbital *(BAN, rINN)*

Amobarbitalum; Amylobarbitone; Pentymalum. 5-Ethyl-5-isopentylbarbituric acid.

$C_{11}H_{18}N_2O_3$ = 226.3.
*CAS — 57-43-2.*
*ATC — N05CA02.*

**Pharmacopoeias.** In *Chin., Eur.* (see p.vi), and *Jpn.*

**Ph. Eur. 5.0** (Amobarbital). A white crystalline powder. Very slightly soluble in water; freely soluble in alcohol; soluble in dichloromethane. Forms water-soluble compounds with alkali hydroxides and carbonates and with ammonia.

## Amobarbital Sodium *(BANM, rINNM)*

Amobarbital sódico; Amobarbitalum Natricum; Amylobarbitone Sodium; Barbamylum; Pentymalnatrium; Sodium Amobarbital; Soluble Amylobarbitone. Sodium 5-ethyl-5-isopentylbarbiturate.

$C_{11}H_{17}N_2NaO_3$ = 248.3.
*CAS — 64-43-7.*
*ATC — N05CA02.*

**Pharmacopoeias.** In *Chin., Eur.* (see p.vi), and *US.*
*Jpn* includes Amobarbital Sodium for Injection.

**Ph. Eur. 5.0** (Amobarbital Sodium). A white, hygroscopic, granular powder. Very soluble in carbon dioxide-free water (a small fraction may be insoluble); freely soluble in alcohol. A 10% solution in water has a pH of not more than 11.0. Store in airtight containers.

**USP 27** (Amobarbital Sodium). A white, odourless, hygroscopic, friable, granular powder. Very soluble in water; soluble in alcohol; practically insoluble in chloroform and in ether. Solutions decompose on standing; decomposition is accelerated by heat. pH of a 10% solution in water is not more than 11.0. Store in airtight containers.

**Incompatibility.** Amobarbital may be precipitated from preparations containing amobarbital sodium, depending on the concentration and pH. Amobarbital sodium has, therefore, been reported to be incompatible with many other drugs, particularly acids and acidic salts.

### Dependence and Withdrawal

The development of dependence is a high risk with amobarbital and other barbiturates and may occur after regular use even in therapeutic doses for short periods. Barbiturates should not therefore be discontinued abruptly, but should be withdrawn by gradual reduction of the dose over a period of days or weeks. A long-acting barbiturate such as phenobarbital may be substituted for a short- or intermediate-acting one, followed by gradual reduction of the phenobarbital dose.

Withdrawal symptoms are similar to those of alcohol withdrawal and are characterised after several hours by apprehension and weakness, followed by anxiety, headache, dizziness, irritability, tremors, nausea and vomiting, abdominal cramps, insomnia, distortion in visual perception, muscle twitching, and tachycardia. Orthostatic hypotension and convulsions may develop after a day or two, sometimes leading to status epilepticus. Hallucinations and delirium tremens may develop after several days followed by coma before the symptoms disappear or death occurs.

### Adverse Effects

Drowsiness, sedation, and ataxia are the most frequent adverse effects of amobarbital and other barbiturates and are a consequence of dose-related CNS depression. Other adverse effects include respiratory depression, headache, gastrointestinal disturbances, skin reactions, confusion, and memory defects. Paradoxical excitement and irritability may occur, particularly in children, the elderly, and patients in acute pain. Hypersensitivity reactions occur rarely and include skin rashes (erythema multiforme and exfoliative dermatitis, sometimes fatal, have been reported), hepatitis and cholestasis, and photosensitivity. Blood disorders, including megaloblastic anaemia after chronic use of barbiturates, have also occurred occasionally.

Neonatal intoxication, drug dependence, and symptoms resembling vitamin-K deficiency have been reported in infants born to mothers who received barbiturates during pregnancy. Congenital malformations have been reported in children of women who took barbiturates during pregnancy, but the causal role is a matter of some debate.

Nystagmus, miosis, slurred speech, and ataxia may occur with excessive doses of barbiturates. The toxic effects of overdosage result from profound central depression and include coma, respiratory and cardiovascular depression, with hypotension and shock leading to renal failure and death. Hypothermia may occur with subsequent pyrexia on recovery. Erythematous or haemorrhagic blisters reportedly occur in about 6% of patients, but are not characteristic solely of barbiturate poisoning.

Solutions of the sodium salts of barbiturates are extremely alkaline, and necrosis has followed subcutaneous injection. Intravenous injection may be hazardous; hypotension, shock, laryngospasm, and apnoea have occurred particularly after rapid administration. Gangrene has resulted from intra-arterial injection into an extremity.

**Overdosage.** A detailed review of drug-induced stupor and coma, including that caused by barbiturates.[1]

1. Ashton CH, *et al.* Drug-induced stupor and coma: some physical signs and their pharmacological basis. *Adverse Drug React Acute Poisoning Rev* 1989; **8:** 1–59.

### Treatment of Adverse Effects

Following an overdose of a barbiturate, endotracheal intubation may be necessary if the patient is unconscious. Administration of activated charcoal by mouth or nasogastric tube is advocated in patients who have ingested more than 10 mg/kg and present within 1 hour of ingestion; repeat doses may be necessary. Patients should be managed with intensive supportive therapy, with particular attention being paid to the maintenance of cardiovascular, respiratory, and renal functions, and to the maintenance of the electrolyte balance. Charcoal haemoperfusion can be lifesaving in the most severe cases and should be considered if there is no improvement after 24 hours of supportive care. The value of other measures aimed at the active removal of barbiturates is questionable.

### Precautions

Amobarbital and other barbiturates are best avoided in elderly and debilitated patients, in young adults, in children, and in those with depression.

Amobarbital is contra-indicated in patients with pulmonary insufficiency, sleep apnoea, pre-existing CNS depression or coma, and severe hepatic impairment, and should be given with caution to those with renal impairment. Barbiturates given to patients in pain may provoke a paradoxical excitatory reaction, unless an analgesic is given concomitantly. With continued use, tolerance develops to the sedative or hypnotic effects of the barbiturates to a greater extent than to their lethal effects. Barbiturates may cause drowsiness which may persist the next day; affected patients should not drive or operate machinery.

See under Adverse Effects, above, for the hazards of administration of barbiturates during pregnancy and under Breast Feeding, below, for cautions on their use in nursing mothers.

**Dependence** readily develops after use of barbiturates with a **withdrawal syndrome** on abrupt discontinuation (see under Dependence and Withdrawal, above).

Barbiturates are abused for their euphoriant effects.

**Breast feeding.** Small amounts of barbiturates are distributed into breast milk, and most authorities, such as the *British National Formulary*, consider that they should not be taken while breast feeding. The American Academy of Pediatrics notes[1] that the long-acting antiepileptic barbiturate, phenobarbital, has been associated with significant effects on some nursing infants, although it suggests that some other barbiturates may be compatible with breast feeding.

1. American Academy of Pediatrics. The transfer of drugs and other chemicals into human milk. *Pediatrics* 2001; **108:** 776–89. Correction. *ibid.*; 1029. Also available at: http://aappolicy.aappublications.org/cgi/content/full/pediatrics%3b108/3/776 (accessed 28/04/04)

**Porphyria.** Barbiturates including amobarbital have been associated with acute attacks of porphyria and are considered unsafe in porphyric patients.

### Interactions

Sedation or respiratory depression may be enhanced by drugs with CNS-depressant properties; in particular alcohol should be avoided. Barbiturates generally induce liver enzymes, and thus increase the rate of metabolism (and decrease the activity) of many other drugs as well as endogenous substances. Continued use may result in induction of their own metabolism. MAOIs may prolong the CNS depressant effects of some barbiturates, probably by inhibition of their metabolism. However, MAOIs, like other antidepressants, also reduce the convulsive threshold and thereby antagonise the anticonvulsant action of barbiturates.

For some further interactions involving barbiturates, see under Phenobarbital, p.368.

### Pharmacokinetics

Amobarbital is readily absorbed from the gastrointestinal tract. It is about 60% bound to plasma proteins. It has a half-life of about 20 to 25 hours which is considerably extended in neonates. It crosses the placenta and small amounts are distributed into breast milk. Amobarbital is metabolised in the liver; up to about 50% is excreted in the urine as 3′-hydroxyamylobarbital and up to about 30% as *N*-hydroxyamylobarbital, less than 1% appearing unchanged; up to about 5% is excreted in the faeces.

### Uses and Administration

Amobarbital is a barbiturate that has been used as a hypnotic and sedative. Its use can no longer be recommended because of its adverse effects and risk of dependence, although continued use may occasionally be considered necessary for severe intractable insomnia (p.667) in patients already taking it. The usual dose by mouth at bedtime was 100 to 200 mg of the base or 60 to 200 mg of the sodium salt. A more rapid onset of effect was obtained with the sodium salt.

Barbiturates with a longer action such as phenobarbital (p.367) are still used in epilepsy and those with a shorter action such as methohexital (p.1303) or thiopental (p.1309) for anaesthesia.

**Cerebrovascular disorders.** For reference to the use of barbiturate-induced coma in the management of patients with cerebral ischaemia, see p.1310.

**Epilepsy.** Amobarbital is used for specialised procedures in expert epilepsy centres only. It is given by deep intramuscular or slow intravenous injection as the sodium salt.

### Preparations

**USP 27:** Amobarbital Sodium for Injection; Secobarbital Sodium and Amobarbital Sodium Capsules.

**Proprietary Preparations** (details are given in Part 3)
***Austral.:*** Amytal; Neur-Amyl; ***Canad.:*** Amytal; ***Irl.:*** Amytal†; ***UK:*** Amytal; ***USA:*** Amytal.

**Multi-ingredient:** ***Arg.:*** Cuait N; ***Belg.:*** Bellanox†; ***Canad.:*** Tuinal†; ***Irl.:*** Tuinal†; ***S.Afr.:*** Repasmat†; ***Thai.:*** Ama; ***UK:*** Tuinal; ***USA:*** Tuinal.

## Amperozide *(BAN, rINN)*

Amperozida; FG-5606. 4-[4,4-Bis(4-fluorophenyl)butyl]-*N*-ethylpiperazine-1-carboxamide.

$C_{23}H_{29}F_2N_3O$ = 401.5.
*CAS — 75558-90-6 (amperozide); 75529-73-6 (amperozide hydrochloride).*

### Profile

Amperozide is an antipsychotic that has been used in veterinary medicine.

## Aprobarbital *(rINN)*

Allylisopropylmalonylurea; Allypropymal; Aprobarbitone. 5-Allyl-5-isopropylbarbituric acid.

$C_{10}H_{14}N_2O_3$ = 210.2.
*CAS — 77-02-1.*
*ATC — N05CA05.*

### Profile

Aprobarbital is a barbiturate with general properties similar to those of amobarbital (p.670). It has been used for the treatment of insomnia and as a sedative, but barbiturates are no longer considered appropriate for such purposes. Aprobarbital sodium was also formerly used.

### Preparations

**Proprietary Preparations** (details are given in Part 3)
***USA:*** Alurate†.

## Aripiprazole *(BAN, USAN, rINN)*

OPC-31; OPC-14597. 7-{4-[4-(2,3-Dichlorophenyl)-piperazin-1-yl]butoxy}-3,4-dihydroquinolin-2(1*H*)-one.
$C_{23}H_{27}Cl_2N_3O_2$ = 448.4.
*CAS — 129722-12-9.*

### Adverse Effects, Treatment, and Precautions

Although aripiprazole may share some of the adverse effects seen with the classical antipsychotics (see Chlorpromazine, p.675), the incidence and severity of such effects may vary. Common adverse effects with aripiprazole include headache, gastrointestinal disorders such as constipation, nausea, and vomiting, anxiety, insomnia, lightheadedness, and drowsiness. Weight gain has been reported; however, this appears to be slight. The incidence of extrapyramidal symptoms with aripiprazole is low with akathisia being most commonly reported. Tardive dyskinesia has been reported infrequently and there have been a few cases of neuroleptic malignant syndrome. Orthostatic hypotension may occur with aripiprazole treatment and consequently it should be used with caution in patients with cardiovascular or cerebrovascular disease, or in those with conditions that would predispose to hypotension.

Seizures are rare with aripiprazole but it should be used with care in those with a history of seizures.

Aripiprazole may affect the performance of skilled tasks.

◊ References.

1. Marder SR, *et al.* Aripiprazole in the treatment of schizophrenia: safety and tolerability in short-term, placebo-controlled trials. *Schizophr Res* 2003; **61:** 123–36.

**Effects on carbohydrate metabolism.** The increased risk of glucose intolerance and diabetes mellitus with some atypical antipsychotics and recommendations on monitoring are discussed under Adverse Effects in Clozapine, p.686.

### Interactions

The central effects of other CNS depressants including alcohol may be enhanced by aripiprazole. Aripiprazole may also enhance the effects of antihypertensive drugs.

Aripiprazole is metabolised by the cytochrome P450 isoenzymes CYP3A4 and CYP2D6. Ketoconazole, a potent CYP3A4 inhibitor, can increase aripiprazole plasma concentrations by about 60%; the manufacturers recommend that the dose of aripiprazole is reduced by half when given with ketoconazole. Similarly, the dose of aripiprazole should be halved when given with quinidine, a potent inhibitor of CYP2D6. The manufacturers advise that similar effects may occur with other potent inhibitors of these isoenzymes and recommend a reduced dose of aripiprazole in such combinations. Conversely, plasma concentrations of aripiprazole may decrease by about 70% when given with carbamazepine, a potent CYP3A4 inducer; the dose of aripiprazole should be doubled if carbamazepine is added to aripiprazole treatment.

### Pharmacokinetics

Aripiprazole is well absorbed from the gastrointestinal tract with peak concentrations reached in about 3 to 5 hours. It is metabolised mainly in the liver and pathways involved include dehydrogenation and hydroxylation, via the cytochrome P450 isoenzymes CYP3A4 and CYP2D6, and *N*-dealkylation, via CYP3A4. The major metabolite, dehydro-aripiprazole, is also active and represents about 40% of the plasma levels of aripiprazole. The elimination half-lives of aripiprazole and dehydro-aripiprazole are about 75 and 95 hours, respectively; in a minority of poor metabolisers the half-life of aripiprazole may be extended to about 146 hours. Protein binding of aripiprazole and its metabolite is about 99%. Elimination is predominantly in the faeces (55%), with about 25% of a dose appearing in the urine, mainly in the form of metabolites.

### Uses and Administration

Aripiprazole is an atypical antipsychotic that has serotonin $5\text{-}HT_{1A}$-receptor partial agonist and $5\text{-}HT_{2A}$-receptor antagonist properties as well as being a partial agonist at dopamine $D_2$ receptors. It is used in the management of schizophrenia and is also under investigation for bipolar disorder.

Aripiprazole is given by mouth in an initial dose of 10 or 15 mg once daily. The dose may be adjusted at intervals of not less than 2 weeks up to a maximum of 30 mg daily.

Dose adjustments of aripiprazole may be necessary in patients also taking potent inhibitors or inducers of cytochrome P450 isoenzymes. See Interactions, above for further details.

◊ References.

1. McGavin JK, Goa KL. Aripiprazole. *CNS Drugs* 2002; **16:** 779–86.
2. Goodnick PJ, Jerry JM. Aripiprazole: profile on efficacy and safety. *Expert Opin Pharmacother* 2002; **3:** 1773–81.
3. Taylor DM. Aripiprazole: a review of its pharmacology and clinical use. *Int J Clin Pract* 2003; **57:** 49–54.
4. Keck PE, McElroy SL. Aripiprazole: a partial dopamine D2 receptor agonist antipsychotic. *Expert Opin Invest Drugs* 2003; **12:** 655–62.
5. Bowles TM, Levin GM. Aripiprazole: a new atypical antipsychotic drug. *Ann Pharmacother* 2003; **37:** 687–94.
6. Keck PE, *et al.* A placebo-controlled, double-blind study of the efficacy and safety of aripiprazole in patients with acute bipolar mania. *Am J Psychiatry* 2003; **160:** 1651–8.

### Preparations

**Proprietary Preparations** (details are given in Part 3)
***Austral.:*** Abilify; ***UK:*** Abilify; ***USA:*** Abilify.

## Azaperone *(BAN, USAN, rINN)*

Azaperona; Azaperonum; R-1929. 4′-Fluoro-4-[4-(2-pyridyl)piperazin-1-yl]butyrophenone.
$C_{19}H_{22}FN_3O$ = 327.4.
*CAS — 1649-18-9.*

**Pharmacopoeias.** In *Eur.* (see p.vi) and *US* for veterinary use only.

**Ph. Eur. 5.0** (Azaperone for Veterinary Use). A white or almost white powder. It exhibits polymorphism. Practically insoluble in water; soluble in alcohol; freely soluble in acetone and in dichloromethane. Protect from light.

**USP 27** (Azaperone). M.p. 92° to 95°. Protect from light.

### Profile

Azaperone is a butyrophenone antipsychotic used as a tranquilliser in veterinary medicine.

## Barbital *(BAN, rINN)*

Barbitalum; Barbitone; Diemalum; Diethylmalonylurea. 5,5-Diethylbarbituric acid.
$C_8H_{12}N_2O_3$ = 184.2.
*CAS — 57-44-3.*
*ATC — N05CA04.*

**Pharmacopoeias.** In *Eur.* (see p.vi), *Jpn*, and *Pol.*

**Ph. Eur. 5.0** (Barbital). A white, crystalline powder or colourless crystals. Slightly soluble in water; soluble in boiling water and in alcohol. It forms water-soluble compounds with alkali hydroxides and carbonates and with ammonia.

## Barbital Sodium *(BANM, rINN)*

Barbital sódico; Barbitalum Natricum; Barbitone Sodium; Diemalnatrium; Soluble Barbitone. Sodium 5,5-diethylbarbiturate.
$C_8H_{11}N_2NaO_3$ = 206.2.
*CAS — 144-02-5.*
*ATC — N05CA04.*

**Pharmacopoeias.** In *Swiss.*

### Profile

Barbital is a barbiturate with general properties similar to those of amobarbital (p.670). It was formerly used for its hypnotic and sedative properties but barbiturates are no longer considered appropriate for such purposes.

### Preparations

**Proprietary Preparations** (details are given in Part 3)
***Mex.:*** Neurinase†.

## Benperidol *(BAN, USAN, rINN)*

Benperidolum; Benzperidol; CB-8089; McN-JR-4584; R-4584. 1-{1-[3-(4-Fluorobenzoyl)propyl]-4-piperidyl}benzimidazolin-2-one.
$C_{22}H_{24}FN_3O_2$ = 381.4.
*CAS — 2062-84-2.*
*ATC — N05AD07.*

**Pharmacopoeias.** In *Eur.* (see p.vi).

**Ph. Eur. 5.0** (Benperidol). A white or almost white powder. It exhibits polymorphism. Practically insoluble in water; slightly soluble in alcohol; soluble in dichloromethane; freely soluble in dimethylformamide. Protect from light.

### Profile

Benperidol is a butyrophenone with general properties similar to those of haloperidol (p.701). Doses of 0.25 to 1.5 mg daily in divided doses are given by mouth in the management of deviant sexual behaviour. Elderly or debilitated patients may require reduced doses of benperidol.

In some countries benperidol is given by mouth or parenterally for the treatment of psychotic conditions (p.665).

**Deviant sexual behaviour.** Results of a double-blind placebo-controlled crossover study demonstrated no difference between the effect of benperidol 1.25 mg daily, chlorpromazine 125 mg daily, or placebo on sexual drive and arousal in 12 paedophilic sexual offenders, except for a lower frequency of sexual thoughts with benperidol.[1] The effects of benperidol are unlikely to be sufficient to control severe forms of antisocial sexually deviant behaviour. The management of deviant sexual behaviour is discussed under Disturbed Behaviour on p.665.

1. Tennent G, *et al.* The control of deviant sexual behaviour by drugs: a double-blind controlled study of benperidol, chlorpromazine, and placebo. *Arch Sex Behav* 1974; **3:** 261–71.

**Pharmacokinetics.** References.

1. Furlanut M, *et al.* Pharmacokinetics of benperidol in volunteers after oral administration. *Int J Clin Pharmacol Res* 1988; **8:** 13–16.

### Preparations

**Proprietary Preparations** (details are given in Part 3)
***Belg.:*** Frenactil; ***Ger.:*** Glianimon; ***Gr.:*** Glianimon; ***Irl.:*** Anquil; ***Neth.:*** Frenactil; ***UK:*** Anquil†; Benquil.

## Bentazepam *(USAN, rINN)*

CI-718; QM-6008. 1,3,6,7,8,9-Hexahydro-5-phenyl-2*H*-[1]benzothieno[2,3-e]-1,4-diazepin-2-one.
$C_{17}H_{16}N_2OS$ = 296.4.
*CAS — 29462-18-8.*

### Profile

Bentazepam is a benzodiazepine with general properties similar to those of diazepam (p.690). It has been given by mouth, in usual doses of 25 mg every 8 hours, in the short-term treatment of anxiety disorders; it has also been used in insomnia.

**Effects on the liver.** Severe chronic active hepatitis has been reported in a 65-year-old man who had received long-term treatment with bentazepam.[1]

1. Andrade RJ, *et al.* Bentazepam-associated chronic liver disease. *Lancet* 1994; **343:** 860.

### Preparations

**Proprietary Preparations** (details are given in Part 3)
***Spain:*** Tiadipona.

## Brallobarbital *(rINN)*

Bralobarbital; UCB-5033. 5-Allyl-5-(2-bromoallyl)barbituric acid.
$C_{10}H_{11}BrN_2O_3$ = 287.1.
*CAS — 561-86-4.*

### Profile

Brallobarbital is a barbiturate with general properties similar to those of amobarbital (p.670). It has been used in preparations for the management of insomnia but barbiturates are no longer considered appropriate for such a purpose. Brallobarbital calcium has been used similarly.

### Preparations

**Proprietary Preparations** (details are given in Part 3)
**Multi-ingredient:** ***Belg.:*** Bellanox†; Vesparax†; ***Neth.:*** Vesparax†; ***Port.:*** Vesparax; ***S.Afr.:*** Vesparax†; ***Spain:*** Somatarax†.

## Bromazepam *(BAN, USAN, rINN)*

Bromazepamum; Ro-5-3350. 7-Bromo-1,3-dihydro-5-(2-pyridyl)-1,4-benzodiazepin-2-one.
$C_{14}H_{10}BrN_3O$ = 316.2.
*CAS — 1812-30-2.*
*ATC — N05BA08.*

**Pharmacopoeias.** In *Eur.* (see p.vi) and *Jpn.*

**Ph. Eur. 5.0** (Bromazepam). A white or yellowish crystalline powder. Practically insoluble in water; sparingly soluble in alcohol and in dichloromethane. Protect from light.

### Profile

Bromazepam is a benzodiazepine with general properties similar to those of diazepam (p.695). It has been used in the short-term treatment of anxiety disorders (p.663) occurring alone or associated with insomnia. A usual initial dose for anxiety is 6 to 18 mg daily in divided doses by mouth. Higher doses up to 60 mg daily have occasionally been given. Initial doses for elderly and debilitated patients should not exceed 3 mg daily in divided doses.

◊ References.

1. Kaplan SA, *et al.* Biopharmaceutical and clinical pharmacokinetic profile of bromazepam. *J Pharmacokinet Biopharm* 1976; **4:** 1–16.
2. Ochs HR, *et al.* Bromazepam pharmacokinetics: influence of age, gender, oral contraceptives, cimetidine, and propranolol. *Clin Pharmacol Ther* 1987; **41:** 562–70.
3. Erb T, *et al.* Preoperative anxiolysis with minimal sedation in elderly patients: bromazepam or clorazepate-dipotassium? *Acta Anaesthesiol Scand* 1998; **42:** 97–101.

### Preparations

**Proprietary Preparations** (details are given in Part 3)
***Arg.:*** Angular; Atemperator; Benedorm; Bromatanil; Creosedin; Equisedin; Estomina; Finaten; Lexotanil; Molival; Neurozepam; Nulastres; Octanyl; Sedatus; Sipcar; Tritopan; ***Austral.:*** Lexotan; ***Austria:*** Lexotanil; ***Belg.:*** Bromidem; Lexotan; ***Braz.:*** Bromazepan; Bromoxon; Brozepax; Calmex†; Deptran; Lexotan; Lucitan†; Nervium; Neurilan; Novazepam; Relaxil; Somalium; Uni Bromazepax; ***Canad.:*** Lectopam; ***Chile:*** Lexotanil; Totasedan; ***Denm.:*** Bromam; Lexotan; ***Fr.:*** Anxyrex; Lexomil; Quietiline; ***Ger.:*** Bromaz; Bromazanil; Bromazep; durazanil; Gityl; Lexostad; Lexotanil; neo OPT; Normoc; ***Gr.:*** Anconevron; Evagelin; Lexotanil; Notorium; Pascalium; ***Hong Kong:*** Akamon; Lexilium; Lexotan; ***Irl.:*** Lexotan; ***Israel:*** Lenitin; ***Ital.:*** Compendium; Lexotan; ***Malaysia:*** Akamon; ***Mex.:*** Bropamil; Lexotan; ***Neth.:*** Lexotanil; ***Port.:*** Bromalex; Lexotan; Ultramidol; ***S.Afr.:*** Brazepam; Bromaze; Lexotan; ***Singapore:*** Lexotan; ***Spain:*** Lexatin; ***Switz.:*** Lexotanil; ***Thai.:*** Lexotan; ***UK:*** Lexotan†.

**Multi-ingredient:** ***Arg.:*** Debridat B; Eudon; Faradil Novo; Fenatrop-A; Miopropan-T; Vegestabil Digest; Veralipral T; ***Braz.:*** Bromopirin; Sulpan; ***Ital.:*** Lexil.

## Bromisoval (rINN)

Bromisovalerylurea; Bromisovalum; Bromvalerylurea; Bromvaletone; Bromylum. N-(2-Bromo-3-methylbutyryl)urea.
$C_6H_{11}BrN_2O_2$ = 223.1.
*CAS — 496-67-3.*
*ATC — N05CM03.*

**Pharmacopoeias.** In *Jpn.*

### Profile

Bromisoval has actions and uses similar to those of carbromal (p.674) but the use of bromides is generally deprecated.

## Bromperidol (BAN, USAN, rINN)

Bromperidolum; R-11333. 4-[4-(p-Bromophenyl)-4-hydroxypiperidino]-4′-fluorobutyrophenone.
$C_{21}H_{23}BrFNO_2$ = 420.3.
*CAS — 10457-90-6.*
*ATC — N05AD06.*

**Pharmacopoeias.** In *Eur.* (see p.vi).

**Ph. Eur. 5.0** (Bromperidol). A white or almost white powder. Practically insoluble in water; slightly soluble in alcohol; sparingly soluble in dichloromethane and in methyl alcohol. Protect from light.

## Bromperidol Decanoate (BANM, USAN, rINNM)

Bromperidoli Decanoas; Decanoato de bromperidol; R-46541.
$C_{31}H_{41}BrFNO_3$ = 574.6.
*CAS — 75067-66-2.*

**Pharmacopoeias.** In *Eur.* (see p.vi).

**Ph. Eur. 5.0** (Bromperidol Decanoate). A white or almost white powder. Practically insoluble in water; soluble in alcohol; very soluble in dichloromethane. It melts at about 60°. Store at a temperature below 25°. Protect from light.

### Profile

Bromperidol is a butyrophenone with general properties similar to those of haloperidol (p.701). It is given in the treatment of schizophrenia (p.665) and other psychoses. Some bromperidol preparations are prepared with the aid of lactic acid and may be stated to contain bromperidol lactate. However, doses are expressed in terms of the equivalent amount of bromperidol. A usual dose is 1 to 15 mg daily by mouth, although up to 50 mg daily has been given. Elderly patients may require reduced doses of bromperidol. Bromperidol may also be given by intramuscular or intravenous injection.

The long-acting decanoate ester may be used for patients requiring long-term therapy with bromperidol. Doses are expressed in terms of bromperidol base; bromperidol decanoate 68.4 mg is approximately equivalent to 50 mg bromperidol base. Doses equivalent to up to 300 mg of bromperidol every 4 weeks have been given by deep intramuscular injection.

◊ References.

1. Benfield P, *et al.* Bromperidol: a preliminary review of its pharmacodynamic and pharmacokinetic properties, and therapeutic efficacy in psychoses. *Drugs* 1988; **35:** 670–84.

**Schizophrenia.** A systematic review[1] suggested that depot bromperidol had some benefits in schizophrenia but was less effective than depot haloperidol or fluphenazine.

1. Quraishi S, *et al.* Depot bromperidol decanoate for schizophrenia. Available in The Cochrane Library; Issue 2. Chichester: John Wiley; 2004.

### Preparations

**Proprietary Preparations** (details are given in Part 3)
***Arg.:*** Bromodol; ***Belg.:*** Impromen; ***Denm.:*** Bromidol†; ***Ger.:*** Impromen; Tesoprel; ***Ital.:*** Impromen; ***Neth.:*** Impromen; ***Thai.:*** Impromen.

## Brotizolam (BAN, USAN, rINN)

We-941; We-941-BS. 2-Bromo-4-(2-chlorophenyl)-9-methyl-6H-thieno[3,2-f][1,2,4]triazolo[4,3-a][1,4]diazepine.
$C_{15}H_{10}BrClN_4S$ = 393.7.
*CAS — 57801-81-7.*
*ATC — N05CD09.*

### Profile

Brotizolam is a short-acting benzodiazepine with general properties similar to those of diazepam (p.690). It is given by mouth for the short-term (up to 2 weeks) management of insomnia (p.667) in usual doses of 250 micrograms at night. The suggested dose for elderly and debilitated patients is 125 micrograms.

**Abuse.** Reference to abuse of brotizolam in Germany and Hong Kong.[1]

1. WHO. WHO expert committee on drug dependence: twenty-ninth report. *WHO Tech Rep Ser 856* 1995.

**Pharmacokinetics.** References.

1. Bechtel WD. Pharmacokinetics and metabolism of brotizolam in humans. *Br J Clin Pharmacol* 1983; **16:** 279S–283S.
2. Jochemsen R, *et al.* Pharmacokinetics of brotizolam in healthy subjects following intravenous and oral administration. *Br J Clin Pharmacol* 1983; **16:** 285S–290S.

### Preparations

**Proprietary Preparations** (details are given in Part 3)
***Austria:*** Lendorm; ***Belg.:*** Lendormin; ***Chile:*** Dormex; Noctilan; ***Denm.:*** Lendorm; ***Ger.:*** Lendormin; ***Israel:*** Bondormin; ***Ital.:*** Lendormin; Nimbisan†; ***Jpn:*** Lendormin; ***Mex.:*** Lindormin; ***Neth.:*** Lendormin; ***Port.:*** Lendormin; ***S.Afr.:*** Lendormin; ***Spain:*** Sintonal; ***Switz.:*** Lendormine.

# Buspirone Hydrochloride

*(BANM, USAN, rINNM)*

Hidrocloruro de buspirona; MJ-9022-1. 8-[4-(4-Pyrimidin-2-ylpiperazin-1-yl)butyl]-8-azaspiro[4.5]decane-7,9-dione hydrochloride.
$C_{21}H_{31}N_5O_2,HCl$ = 422.0.
*CAS — 36505-84-7 (buspirone); 33386-08-2 (buspirone hydrochloride).*
*ATC — N05BE01.*

**Pharmacopoeias.** In *US.*

**USP 27** (Buspirone Hydrochloride). A white crystalline powder. Very soluble in water; sparingly soluble in alcohol and in acetonitrile; freely soluble in dichloromethane and in methyl alcohol; very slightly soluble in ethyl acetate; practically insoluble in hexanes. Store in airtight containers at a temperature between 15° and 30°. Protect from light.

## Dependence and Adverse Effects

Dizziness, nausea, headache, nervousness, light-headedness, excitement, paraesthesias, sleep disturbances, chest pain, tinnitus, sore throat, and nasal congestion are amongst the most frequent adverse effects reported following the use of buspirone hydrochloride. Other adverse effects have included tachycardia, palpitations, drowsiness, confusion, seizures, dry mouth, fatigue, and sweating. A syndrome of restlessness appearing shortly after the start of treatment has been reported in a small number of patients given buspirone. Buspirone is reported to produce less sedation, and to have a lower potential for dependence, than the benzodiazepines.

**Effects on the nervous system.** Mild acute hypertension and panic were reported on two occasions after the addition of single 10-mg doses of buspirone to therapy with tricyclic antidepressants in a 40-year-old man with panic disorder. Adrenergic or serotonin dysfunction were postulated as possible mechanisms for the reaction.[1,2] Psychotic reactions associated with buspirone treatment have also been reported in a few patients.[3] There have also been isolated reports of mania,[4] and seizures have been reported, primarily in overdosage.[5]

1. Chignon JM, Lepine JP. Panic and hypertension associated with single dose of buspirone. *Lancet* 1989; **ii:** 46–7.
2. Norman TR, Judd FK. Panic attacks, buspirone, and serotonin function. *Lancet* 1989; **ii:** 615.
3. Friedman R. Possible induction of psychosis by buspirone. *Am J Psychiatry* 1991; **148:** 1606.
4. Price WA, Bielefeld M. Buspirone-induced mania. *J Clin Psychopharmacol* 1989; **9:** 150–1.
5. Catalano G, *et al.* Seizures associated with buspirone overdose: case report and literature review. *Clin Neuropharmacol* 1998; **21:** 347–50.

EXTRAPYRAMIDAL DISORDERS. There have been isolated reports of exacerbation or precipitation of movement disorders[1-4] associated with the use of buspirone. However, buspirone has also been reported to have been of benefit in some patients with tardive dyskinesia (see under Uses and Administration, below).

1. Hammerstad JP, *et al.* Buspirone in Parkinson's disease. *Clin Neuropharmacol* 1986; **9:** 556–60.
2. Ritchie EC, *et al.* Acute generalized myoclonus following buspirone administration. *J Clin Psychiatry* 1988; **49:** 242–3.
3. Strauss A. Oral dyskinesia associated with buspirone use in an elderly woman. *J Clin Psychiatry* 1988; **49:** 322–3.
4. LeWitt PA, *et al.* Persistent movement disorders induced by buspirone. *Mov Disord* 1993; **8:** 331–4.

## Precautions

Buspirone hydrochloride should be used with caution in patients with renal or hepatic impairment and is contra-indicated if the impairment is severe. It should not be used in patients with epilepsy or a history of such disorders. It does not exhibit cross-tolerance with benzodiazepines or other common sedatives or hypnotics and will not block symptoms of their withdrawal; they should, therefore, be gradually withdrawn before commencing treatment with buspirone. Buspirone may impair the patient's ability to drive or operate machinery.

**Diagnosis and testing.** Buspirone may interfere with diagnostic assays of urinary catecholamines.[1]

1. Cook FJ, *et al.* Effect of buspirone on urinary catecholamine assays. *N Engl J Med* 1995; **332:** 401.

**Hepatic impairment.** Caution has been advised when using buspirone in patients with liver disease. The mean peak plasma-buspirone concentration after a dose by mouth was about 16 times higher in cirrhotic patients than in controls[1] and the elimination half-life was prolonged about twofold. A secondary peak concentration was seen in some subjects, occurring between 4 and 24 hours after a dose in the cirrhotics and after between 2 and 8 hours in controls. Data from a multiple-dose study[2] suggested that there was accumulation of buspirone and its metabolite 1-(2-pyrimidinyl)-piperazine in hepatic impairment, but that plasma concentrations appeared to reach steady state after 3 days regardless of the state of liver function. The area under the curve and mean peak concentration for buspirone were both higher in patients with hepatic impairment than in healthy subjects, but there were no significant differences for its metabolites. Specific dosing recommendations could not be made for patients with hepatic impairment because of the high intra- and inter-subject variations in plasma-buspirone concentrations.

1. Dalhoff K, *et al.* Buspirone pharmacokinetics in patients with cirrhosis. *Br J Clin Pharmacol* 1987; **24:** 547–50.
2. Barbhaiya RH, *et al.* Disposition kinetics of buspirone in patients with renal or hepatic impairment after administration of single and multiple doses. *Eur J Clin Pharmacol* 1994; **46:** 41–7.

**Pregnancy and breast feeding.** In some *animal* studies, administration of large doses of buspirone during pregnancy has had adverse effects on survival and on birth and weanling weight. Manufacturer recommendations for use during pregnancy or breast feeding vary from avoid, if possible, to contra-indicated.

**Renal impairment.** As for hepatic impairment (above) caution is advised when giving buspirone to patients with renal impairment.[1,2] There is evidence of accumulation of buspirone and its metabolite following repeated administration but plasma concentrations appeared to reach steady state after 3 days regardless of the degree of renal function. At steady state both the area under the curve and maximum concentrations for buspirone and its metabolite were greater in patients with renal failure than in healthy subjects. The metabolite, but not the parent drug, was removed by haemodialysis. Specific dosing recommendations could not be made for patients with renal impairment because of the high intra- and inter-subject variations in buspirone plasma concentrations following repeated administration.

1. Caccia S, *et al.* Clinical pharmacokinetics of oral buspirone in patients with impaired renal function. *Clin Pharmacokinet* 1988; **14:** 171–7.
2. Barbhaiya RH, *et al.* Disposition kinetics of buspirone in patients with renal or hepatic impairment after administration of single and multiple doses. *Eur J Clin Pharmacol* 1994; **46:** 41–7.

## Interactions

The sedative effects of buspirone may be enhanced if taken with alcohol or other CNS depressants. Because of reports of increased blood pressure in patients receiving buspirone hydrochloride with an MAOI, the manufacturers of buspirone recommend that it should not be given with an MAOI.

The metabolism of buspirone is mediated by the cytochrome P450 isoenzyme CYP3A4 and therefore there is the potential for interactions between buspirone and other drugs that inhibit or act as a substrate for this enzyme. The dose of buspirone may need to be reduced if given at the same time as potent inhibitors of CYP3A4. Plasma concentrations of buspirone may be reduced by enzyme-inducing drugs such as rifampicin.

**Antibacterials.** Pretreatment with *erythromycin* in healthy subjects given buspirone resulted in mild to moderate side-effects associated with increased plasma concentrations of buspirone.[1]

Pretreatment with *rifampicin* greatly reduced plasma concentrations of buspirone in healthy subjects.[2] A reduced anxiolytic effect could be expected if buspirone is used with rifampicin or other potent inducers of the cytochrome P450 isoenzyme CYP3A4.

1. Kivistö KT, *et al.* Plasma buspirone concentrations are greatly increased by erythromycin and itraconazole. *Clin Pharmacol Ther* 1997; **62:** 348–54.
2. Lamberg TS, *et al.* Concentrations and effects of buspirone are considerably reduced by rifampicin. *Br J Clin Pharmacol* 1998; **45:** 381–5.

**Antidepressants.** Concomitant use of buspirone and *nefazodone* can raise plasma concentrations of buspirone. The US manufacturer of nefazodone recommends that the initial dose of buspirone be lowered (e.g. 2.5 mg daily) and subsequent dose adjustments of either drug should be based on clinical assessment. A possible serotonin syndrome (p.313) has been reported[1] in one patient following concomitant use of buspirone and *fluoxetine*.

1. Manos GH. Possible serotonin syndrome associated with buspirone added to fluoxetine. *Ann Pharmacother* 2000; **34:** 871–4.

**Antifungals.** Pretreatment with *itraconazole* in healthy subjects given buspirone resulted in mild to moderate side-effects associated with increased plasma concentrations of buspirone.[1]

1. Kivistö KT, *et al.* Plasma buspirone concentrations are greatly increased by erythromycin and itraconazole. *Clin Pharmacol Ther* 1997; **62:** 348–54.

**Antipsychotics.** For the effect of buspirone on serum concentrations of *haloperidol*, see under Chlorpromazine, p.680. For a report of potentially fatal gastrointestinal bleeding and marked hyperglycaemia following concomitant use of buspirone and *clozapine*, see under Clozapine, p.688.

**Antivirals.** Parkinson-like symptoms developed in a 54-year-old man taking a drug regimen that included buspirone, *indina-*

*vir*, and *ritonavir*.[1] It was suspected that ritonavir inhibited the metabolism of buspirone, which is mediated by the cytochrome P450 isoenzyme CYP3A4, leading to increased plasma concentrations of the latter. The inhibitory effect of indinavir on CYP3A4 was considered to be less than that of ritonavir. Symptoms resolved following a change in antiviral regimen and reduction in the dose of buspirone.

1. Clay PG, Adams MM. Pseudo-Parkinson disease secondary to ritonavir-buspirone interaction. *Ann Pharmacother* 2003; **37:** 202–5.

**Calcium-channel blockers.** Increases in buspirone plasma concentrations have been seen in healthy subjects pretreated with *diltiazem* or *verapamil*.[1]

1. Lamberg TS, *et al.* Effects of verapamil and diltiazem on the pharmacokinetics and pharmacodynamics of buspirone. *Clin Pharmacol Ther* 1998; **63:** 640–5.

**Grapefruit.** Grapefruit juice increased the plasma concentrations of buspirone in healthy subjects.[1]

1. Lilja JJ, *et al.* Grapefruit juice substantially increases plasma concentrations of buspirone. *Clin Pharmacol Ther* 1998; **64:** 655–60.

## Pharmacokinetics

Buspirone hydrochloride is rapidly absorbed from the gastrointestinal tract reaching peak plasma concentrations within 40 to 90 minutes after administration by mouth. Systemic bioavailability is low because of extensive first-pass metabolism, but may be increased on administration with food as this delays absorption from the gastrointestinal tract and thereby reduces presystemic clearance. Buspirone is about 95% bound to plasma proteins. Metabolism in the liver is extensive via the cytochrome P450 isoenzyme CYP3A4; hydroxylation yields several inactive metabolites and oxidative dealkylation produces 1-(2-pyrimidinyl)-piperazine which is reported to be about 25% as potent as the parent drug in one model of anxiolytic activity. The elimination half-life of buspirone is usually about 2 to 4 hours but half-lives of up to 11 hours have been reported. Buspirone is excreted mainly as metabolites in the urine, and also in the faeces.

◊ References.

1. Mahmood I, Sahajwalla C. Clinical pharmacokinetics and pharmacodynamics of buspirone, an anxiolytic drug. *Clin Pharmacokinet* 1999; **36:** 277–87.

## Uses and Administration

Buspirone hydrochloride is an azaspirodecanedione anxiolytic. It is reported to be largely lacking in sedative, anticonvulsant, and muscle relaxant actions.

Buspirone hydrochloride is given, in initial doses of 5 mg two or three times daily, in the short-term management of anxiety disorders. The dose may be increased in increments of 5 mg at 2- to 3-day intervals if required. The recommended maximum daily dose, to be administered in divided doses, is 45 mg in the UK and 60 mg in the USA.

◊ General reviews.

1. Fulton B, Brogden RN. Buspirone: an updated review of its clinical pharmacology and therapeutic applications. *CNS Drugs* 1997; **7:** 68–88.
2. Apter JT, Allen LA. Buspirone: future directions. *J Clin Psychopharmacol* 1999; **19:** 86–93.

**Action.** Buspirone has dopaminergic, noradrenergic, and serotonin-modulating properties[1] and its anxiolytic effects appear to be related to its action on serotonin (5-hydroxytryptamine, 5-HT) neurotransmission. Buspirone, and the related drugs gepirone (p.701) and ipsapirone (p.703), are partial agonists at $5\text{-HT}_{1A}$ receptors.[1,2] While such drugs may inhibit serotonin neurotransmission (most likely via $5\text{-HT}_{1A}$ autoreceptor stimulation), they may also have postsynaptic $5\text{-HT}_{1A}$ agonist activity and thus facilitate serotonin neurotransmission.[1] To complicate matters further, $5\text{-HT}_{1A}$ partial agonists have demonstrated both anxiolytic and anxiogenic properties in *animal* models of anxiety. Clinical studies have, however, shown that buspirone is effective in the treatment of generalised anxiety.[1,2]

Clinical studies with buspirone and gepirone suggest that $5\text{-HT}_{1A}$ partial agonists may be useful in the treatment of depression, possibly by downregulation of either $5\text{-HT}_{1A}$ or $5\text{-HT}_2$ receptors or both.[1] There is some suggestion that buspirone has an anti-aggressive action in humans; it is unclear whether this is mediated via dopaminergic or serotonergic mechanisms.

Buspirone also has characteristics of both a dopamine agonist and antagonist; this may result in stimulation of both growth hormone and prolactin secretion.[3]

1. Glitz DA, Pohl R. $5\text{-HT}_{1A}$ partial agonists: what is their future? *Drugs* 1991; **41:** 11–18.
2. Marsden CA. The pharmacology of new anxiolytics acting on 5-HT neurones. *Postgrad Med J* 1990; **66** (suppl 2): S2–S6.
3. Meltzer HY, *et al.* The effect of buspirone on prolactin and growth hormone secretion in man. *Arch Gen Psychiatry* 1983; **40:** 1099–1102.

**Administration in hepatic or renal impairment.** For cautions on the use of buspirone in patients with impaired liver or kidney function see under Precautions, above.

**Anxiety disorders.** Buspirone has been shown to be as effective as the benzodiazepines in the short-term treatment of generalised anxiety disorder (p.663) and to be less likely to cause sedation or psychomotor and cognitive impairment. It also appears to have a lower propensity for interaction with alcohol and a lower risk of abuse and dependence. However, its usefulness may be limited by a relatively slow response to treatment, which some commentators consider may take up to 2 to 4 weeks to appear. Its efficacy may be reduced in patients who have recently taken benzodiazepines. It appears to be ineffective in panic disorders and convincing evidence of efficacy in other anxiety disorders is lacking.

References.

1. Caven P. Drugs in focus: 5. buspirone. *Prescribers' J* 1992; **32:** 200–204.
2. Deakin JFW. A review of clinical efficacy of $5\text{-HT}_{1A}$ agonists in anxiety and depression. *J Psychopharmacol* 1993; **7:** 283–9.
3. Pecknold JC. A risk-benefit assessment of buspirone in the treatment of anxiety disorders. *Drug Safety* 1997; **16:** 118–32.
4. Fulton B, Brogden RN. Buspirone: an updated review of its clinical pharmacology and therapeutic applications. *CNS Drugs* 1997; **7:** 68–88.

**Bruxism.** SSRI-induced bruxism has been successfully controlled by adjunctive therapy with buspirone.[1,2]

1. Romanelli F, *et al.* Possible paroxetine-induced bruxism. *Ann Pharmacother* 1996; **30:** 1246–7.
2. Bostwick JM, Jaffee MS. Buspirone as an antidote to SSRI-induced bruxism in 4 cases. *J Clin Psychiatry* 1999; **60:** 857–60.

**Cerebellar ataxias.** In general the management of cerebellar ataxias is mainly supportive; buspirone has improved some symptoms of ataxia in a small study of patients with cerebellar cortical activity.[1]

1. Trouillas P, *et al.* Buspirone, a 5-hydroxytryptamine$_{1A}$ agonist, is active in cerebellar ataxia: results of a double-blind drug placebo study in patients with cerebellar cortical atrophy. *Arch Neurol* 1997; **54:** 749–52.

**Depression.** Buspirone has been investigated for augmentation of therapy with antidepressants with serotonin reuptake inhibiting activity in patients with refractory depression (p.279), but results have been variable.

References.

1. Fischer P, *et al.* Weak antidepressant response after buspirone augmentation of serotonin reuptake inhibitors in refractory severe depression. *Int Clin Psychopharmacol* 1998; **13:** 83–6.
2. Dimitriou EC, Dimitriou CE. Buspirone augmentation of antidepressant therapy. *J Clin Psychopharmacol* 1998; **18:** 465–9.
3. Landen M, *et al.* A randomized, double-blind, placebo-controlled trial of buspirone in combination with an SSRI in patients with treatment-refractory depression. *J Clin Psychiatry* 1998; **59:** 664–8.

**Disturbed behaviour.** Buspirone has been tried in various disorders for the control of symptoms such as agitation, aggression, and disruptive behaviour (see Disturbed Behaviour, p.665) but evidence of efficacy is limited. Nonetheless, in the management of dementia, some[1] consider that it might be worth trying in nonpsychotic patients with disturbed behaviour, especially those with mild symptoms or those intolerant and unresponsive to antipsychotics.

1. American Psychiatric Association. Practice guideline for the treatment of patients with Alzheimer's disease and other dementias of late life. *Am J Psychiatry* 1997; **154** (suppl): 1–39. Also available at: http://www.psych.org/psych_pract/treatg/pg/pg_dementia_32701.cfm (accessed 28/04/04)

**Extrapyramidal disorders.** Although there have been reports[1,2] that buspirone may improve symptoms of drug-induced dyskinesia (p.677), drugs with dopaminergic actions have mostly exacerbated symptoms and there are a few reports of extrapyramidal disorders with buspirone (see under Adverse Effects, above).

1. Moss LE, *et al.* Buspirone in the treatment of tardive dyskinesia. *J Clin Psychopharmacol* 1993; **13:** 204–9.
2. Bonifati V, *et al.* Buspirone in levodopa-induced dyskinesias. *Clin Neuropharmacol* 1994; **17:** 73–82.

**Substance dependence.** ALCOHOL. Despite an early study[1] suggesting that buspirone could reduce alcohol craving in alcohol dependent patients, later studies[2-4] have overall failed to confirm that buspirone improves abstinence or reduces alcohol consumption. Although some studies[3,5] have found that buspirone may improve certain psychopathological symptoms in these patients, others[4] have found no such benefit; a meta-analysis[6] of 5 studies favoured the former interpretation.

The management of alcohol withdrawal and abstinence is discussed on p.1166.

1. Bruno F. Buspirone in the treatment of alcoholic patients. *Psychopathology* 1989; **22** (suppl 1): 49–59.
2. George DT, *et al.* Buspirone does not promote long term abstinence in alcoholics. *Clin Pharmacol Ther* 1995; **57:** 161.
3. Malec E, *et al.* Buspirone in the treatment of alcohol dependence: a placebo-controlled trial. *Alcohol Clin Exp Res* 1996; **20:** 307–12.
4. Malcolm R, *et al.* A placebo-controlled trial of buspirone in anxious inpatient alcoholics. *Alcohol Clin Exp Res* 1992; **16:** 1007–13.
5. Kranzler HR, *et al.* Buspirone treatment of anxious alcoholics: a placebo-controlled trial. *Arch Gen Psychiatry* 1994; **51:** 720–31.
6. Malec TS, *et al.*. Efficacy of buspirone in alcohol dependence: a review. *Alcohol Clin Exp Res* 1996; **20:** 853–8.

NICOTINE. Buspirone has produced conflicting results[1-5] in the management of smoking cessation (p.1721). Although some studies suggest that in the short-term buspirone can increase the numbers of patients who are able to cease smoking, it does not necessarily decrease withdrawal symptoms.

1. West R, *et al.* Effect of buspirone on cigarette withdrawal symptoms and short-term abstinence rates in a smokers clinic. *Psychopharmacology (Berl)* 1991; **104:** 91–6.
2. Hilleman DE, *et al.* Effect of buspirone on withdrawal symptoms associated with smoking cessation. *Arch Intern Med* 1992; **152:** 350–2.
3. Hilleman DE, *et al.* Comparison of fixed-dose transdermal nicotine, tapered-dose transdermal nicotine, and buspirone in smoking cessation. *J Clin Pharmacol* 1994; **34:** 222–4.
4. Schneider NG, *et al.* Efficacy of buspirone in smoking cessation: a placebo-controlled trial. *Clin Pharmacol Ther* 1996; **60:** 568–75.
5. Farid P, Abate MA. Buspirone use for smoking cessation. *Ann Pharmacother* 1998; **32:** 1362–4.

**Tourette's syndrome.** Report[1] of a 42-year-old patient with Tourette's syndrome (p.664) refractory to antipsychotics who had a 70% reduction in tic severity during treatment with buspirone 30 mg daily. Worsening of symptoms was noted during the period in which buspirone was discontinued.

1. Dursun SM, *et al.* Buspirone treatment of Tourette's syndrome. *Lancet* 1995; **345:** 1366–7.

## Preparations

*USP 27:* Buspirone Hydrochloride Tablets.

**Proprietary Preparations** (details are given in Part 3)

***Arg.:*** Ansial; ***Austral.:*** Buspar; ***Austria:*** Buspar; ***Belg.:*** Buspar; ***Braz.:*** Ansienon; Ansitec; Buspanil; Buspar; Busprilt†; Seduspar†; ***Canad.:*** Buspar; Buspirex; Bustab†; ***Chile:*** Paxon; ***Denm.:*** Buspar; Stesiron; ***Fin.:*** Buspar; Stesiron; ***Fr.:*** Buspar; ***Ger.:*** Anxut; Bespar; Busp; ***Gr.:*** Anchocalm; Antipsichos; Bergamol; Bespar; Boronex; Epsilat; Hiremon; Hobatstress; Komasin; Lanamont; Lebilon; Ledion; Loxapin; Nadrifor; Nervostal; Neurorestol; Norbal; Pendium; Stressigal; Svitalark; Tensispes; Trafuril; Umolit; ***Hong Kong:*** Buspar; Kalmiren; ***India:*** Buscalm; ***Irl.:*** Buspar; ***Israel:*** Buspirol; Sorbon; ***Ital.:*** Axoren; Buspar; Buspimen; ***Mex.:*** Buspar; Neurosine†; ***Neth.:*** Buspar; ***Norw.:*** Buspar; Stesiron; ***NZ:*** Biron; Buspar; ***Port.:*** Ansiten; Busansil; Buscalma; Buspar; Establix; Itagil†; ***S.Afr.:*** Buspar; Pasrin; ***Singapore:*** Buspar†; ***Spain:*** Buspar; Buspisal†; Effiplen; Narol†; ***Swed.:*** Buspar; ***Switz.:*** Buspar; ***Thai.:*** Anxiolan; Barpil†; ***UK:*** Buspar; ***USA:*** Buspar.

---

## Butalbital *(USAN, rINN)*

Alisobumalum; Allylbarbital; Allylbarbituric Acid; Itobarbital; Tetrallobarbital. 5-Allyl-5-isobutylbarbituric acid.

$C_{11}H_{16}N_2O_3$ = 224.3.
*CAS — 77-26-9.*

NOTE. The name Butalbital has also been applied to talbutal, the *S*-butyl analogue, which was formerly used as a hypnotic and sedative.

Compounded preparations of butalbital may be represented by the following names:

- Co-bucafAPAP (*PEN*)—butalbital, paracetamol, and caffeine.

**Pharmacopoeias.** In *US.*

**USP 27** (Butalbital). A white odourless crystalline powder. Slightly soluble in cold water; soluble in boiling water; freely soluble in alcohol, in chloroform, and in ether; soluble in solutions of fixed alkalis and alkali carbonates. A saturated solution is acid to litmus.

### Profile

Butalbital is a barbiturate with general properties similar to those of amobarbital (p.670). It has been used mainly with analgesics in the treatment of occasional tension-type headaches (p.465), but other treatments are generally preferred.

### Preparations

*USP 27:* Butalbital and Aspirin Tablets; Butalbital, Acetaminophen, and Caffeine Capsules; Butalbital, Acetaminophen, and Caffeine Tablets; Butalbital, Aspirin, and Caffeine Capsules; Butalbital, Aspirin, and Caffeine Tablets; Butalbital, Aspirin, Caffeine, and Codeine Phosphate Capsules.

**Proprietary Preparations** (details are given in Part 3)

***Multi-ingredient: Canad.:*** Fiorinal; Fiorinal C; Tecnal; Tecnal C; Trianal; Trianal C; ***Chile:*** Cafergot-PB; ***Denm.:*** Gynergen Comp; ***Ital.:*** Optalidon; ***S.Afr.:*** Cafergot-PB; ***Spain:*** Cafergot-PB; ***Switz.:*** Cafergot-PB; ***USA:*** Amaphen with Codeine; Amaphen†; Americet; Anolor; Anoquan†; Ascomp with Codeine; Axocet†; B-A-C†; Bupap; Butex; Dolgic; Dolgic LQ; Endolor; Esgic; Esgic-Plus; Femcet†; Fioricet; Fioricet with Codeine; Fiorinal; Fiorinal with Codeine; Fiorpap†; Fiortal with Codeine†; Fiortal†; Isocet†; Lanorinal†; Margesic; Marten-Tab; Medigesic; Pacaps; Phrenilin; Promacet; Prominol; Pyridium Plus; Repan; Repan CF; Sedapap; Tencet; Tencon; Triad.

---

## Butobarbital *(BAN)*

Butethal; Butobarbitalum; Butobarbitone. 5-Butyl-5-ethylbarbituric acid.

$C_{10}H_{16}N_2O_3$ = 212.2.
*CAS — 77-28-1.*
*ATC — N05CA03.*

NOTE. Butobarbital should be distinguished from Butabarbital, which is Secbutabarbital (p.721).

### Dependence and Withdrawal

As for Amobarbital, p.670.

### Adverse Effects, Treatment, and Precautions

As for Amobarbital, p.670.

### Interactions
As for Amobarbital, p.670.

**Antibacterials.** Results suggesting that *metronidazole* alters the metabolism of butobarbital.[1]

1. Al Sharifi MA, *et al.* The effect of anti-amoebic drug therapy on the metabolism of butobarbitone. *J Pharm Pharmacol* 1982; **34:** 126–7.

### Pharmacokinetics
Butobarbital is metabolised in the liver mainly by hydroxylation; small amounts are excreted in the urine as unchanged drug. It has been reported to have a half-life of about 40 to 55 hours and to be about 26% bound to plasma proteins.

### Uses and Administration
Butobarbital is a barbiturate with general properties similar to those of amobarbital (p.670). Its use can no longer be recommended because of the risk of its adverse effects and of dependence, although continued use may occasionally be considered necessary for severe intractable insomnia (p.667) in patients already taking it. It is given by mouth in usual doses of 100 to 200 mg at night.

### Preparations
**Proprietary Preparations** (details are given in Part 3)
**UK:** Soneryl.

**Multi-ingredient: Fr.:** Hypnasmine; **Thai.:** Belloid†.

## Calcium Bromolactobionate
Bromolactobionato de calcio; Calcium Galactogluconate Bromide. Calcium bromide lactobionate hexahydrate.

$Ca(C_{12}H_{21}O_{12})_2,CaBr_2,6H_2O$ = 1062.6.

*CAS — 33659-28-8 (anhydrous calcium bromolactobionate).*

### Profile
Calcium bromolactobionate has sedative properties and has been given by mouth in the treatment of insomnia and nervous disorders. The use of bromides is generally deprecated.

**Overdosage.** Bromide intoxication has been reported[1] in a patient following overdosage with calcium bromolactobionate tablets.

1. Danel VC, *et al.* Bromide intoxication and pseudohyperchloremia. *Ann Pharmacother* 2001; **35:** 386–7.

### Preparations
**Proprietary Preparations** (details are given in Part 3)
**Chile:** Bromocalcio; Nervolta; Sedofantil; **Fr.:** Calcibronat; **Ital.:** Calcibronat; **Mex.:** Calcibronat.

## Camazepam (rINN)
SB-5833. 7-Chloro-2,3-dihydro-1-methyl-2-oxo-5-phenyl-1H-1,4-benzodiazepin-3-yl dimethylcarbamate.

$C_{19}H_{18}ClN_3O_3$ = 371.8.

*CAS — 36104-80-0.*
*ATC — N05BA15.*

### Profile
Camazepam is a benzodiazepine with general properties similar to those of diazepam (p.690). It has been given by mouth for the short-term treatment of anxiety disorders and insomnia.

### Preparations
**Proprietary Preparations** (details are given in Part 3)
**Spain:** Albego†.

## Captodiame Hydrochloride (BANM, pINNM)
Captodiame Hydrochloride; Hidrocloruro de captodiamo. 2-(4-Butylthiobenzhydrylthio)ethyldimethylamine hydrochloride.

$C_{21}H_{29}NS_2,HCl$ = 396.1.

*CAS — 486-17-9 (captodiame); 904-04-1 (captodiame hydrochloride).*
*ATC — N05BB02.*

### Profile
Captodiame hydrochloride has been given in doses of 50 mg three times daily by mouth for the treatment of anxiety disorders (p.663).

### Preparations
**Proprietary Preparations** (details are given in Part 3)
**Fr.:** Covatine.

## Carbromal (BAN, rINN)
Bromodiethylacetylurea; Karbromal. N-(2-Bromo-2-ethylbutyryl)urea.

$C_7H_{13}BrN_2O_2$ = 237.1.

*CAS — 77-65-6.*
*ATC — N05CM04.*

### Profile
Carbromal is a bromureide with general properties similar to those of the barbiturates (see Amobarbital, p.670). It was formerly used for its hypnotic and sedative properties. Chronic use of carbromal could result in bromide accumulation and symptoms resembling bromism (see Bromides, p.1662). The use of bromides is generally deprecated.

**Porphyria.** Carbromal has been associated with acute attacks of porphyria and is considered unsafe in porphyric patients.

## Carpipramine Hydrochloride (rINNM)
Hidrocloruro de carpipramina; PZ-1511. 1-[3-(10,11-Dihydro-5H-dibenz[b,f]azepin-5-yl)propyl]-4-piperidinopiperidine-4-carboxamide dihydrochloride monohydrate.

$C_{28}H_{38}N_4O,2HCl,H_2O$ = 537.6.

*CAS — 5942-95-0 (carpipramine); 7075-03-8 (anhydrous carpipramine hydrochloride).*

### Profile
Carpipramine is structurally related both to imipramine (p.300) and to butyrophenones such as haloperidol (p.701). It has been used in the management of anxiety disorders (p.663) and psychoses such as schizophrenia (p.665). Carpipramine is given as the hydrochloride although doses are expressed in terms of the base; carpipramine hydrochloride 60.2 mg is approximately equivalent to 50 mg carpipramine base. A usual dose is equivalent to 50 mg of the base three times daily by mouth, with a range of 50 to 400 mg daily.

**Porphyria.** Carpipramine is considered to be unsafe in patients with porphyria although there is conflicting experimental evidence of porphyrinogenicity.

### Preparations
**Proprietary Preparations** (details are given in Part 3)
**Fr.:** Prazinil.

## Chlordiazepoxide (BAN, rINN)
Chlordiazepoxidum; Clordiazepóxido; Methaminodiazepoxide. 7-Chloro-2-methylamino-5-phenyl-3H-1,4-benzodiazepine 4-oxide.

$C_{16}H_{14}ClN_3O$ = 299.8.

*CAS — 58-25-3.*
*ATC — N05BA02.*

**Pharmacopoeias.** In *Chin., Eur.* (see p.vi), *Jpn, Pol.,* and *US.*

**Ph. Eur. 5.0** (Chlordiazepoxide). An almost white or light yellow, crystalline powder. Practically insoluble in water; sparingly soluble in alcohol. Protect from light.

**USP 27** (Chlordiazepoxide). A yellow, practically odourless, crystalline powder. Insoluble in water; soluble 1 in 50 of alcohol, 1 in 6250 of chloroform, and 1 in 130 of ether. Store in airtight containers. Protect from light.

## Chlordiazepoxide Hydrochloride
(BANM, USAN, rINNM)

Chlordiazepoxidi Hydrochloridum; Hidrocloruro de clordiazepóxido; Methaminodiazepoxide Hydrochloride; NSC-115748; Ro-5-0690.

$C_{16}H_{14}ClN_3O,HCl$ = 336.2.

*CAS — 438-41-5.*
*ATC — N05BA02.*

**Pharmacopoeias.** In *Eur.* (see p.vi), *Pol.,* and *US.*

**Ph. Eur. 5.0** (Chlordiazepoxide Hydrochloride). A white or slightly yellow, slightly hygroscopic, crystalline powder. Soluble in water; sparingly soluble in alcohol. Store in airtight containers. Protect from light.

**USP 27** (Chlordiazepoxide Hydrochloride). A white or practically white, odourless, crystalline powder. Soluble in water; sparingly soluble in alcohol; insoluble in petroleum spirit. Store in airtight containers. Protect from light.

### Dependence and Withdrawal
As for Diazepam, p.690.

◊ For the purpose of withdrawal regimens, 15 mg of chlordiazepoxide is considered approximately equivalent to 5 mg of diazepam.

### Adverse Effects, Treatment, and Precautions
As for Diazepam, p.690.

**Hepatic impairment.** Progressive drowsiness began after 20 days of treatment with chlordiazepoxide in a woman with cirrhosis and hepatitis.[1] One week after stopping the drug the patient could not be roused, and full consciousness was not regained for another week. Accumulation of active metabolites of chlordiazepoxide may have been responsible for the prolonged stupor.

1. Barton K, *et al.* Chlordiazepoxide metabolite accumulation in liver disease. *Med Toxicol* 1989; **4:** 73–6.

**Porphyria.** Chlordiazepoxide has been associated with acute attacks of porphyria and is considered unsafe in porphyric patients.

### Interactions
As for Diazepam, p.692.

### Pharmacokinetics
Absorption of chlordiazepoxide is almost complete after oral administration; peak plasma concentrations are achieved after 1 to 2 hours. Absorption after intramuscular injection may be slow and erratic depending on the site of injection. Chlordiazepoxide is about 96% bound to plasma proteins. Reported values for the elimination half-life of chlordiazepoxide have ranged from about 5 to 30 hours, but its main active metabolite desmethyldiazepam (nordazepam, p.710) has a half-life of several days. Other pharmacologically active metabolites of chlordiazepoxide include desmethylchlordiazepoxide, demoxepam, and oxazepam (p.712). Chlordiazepoxide passes into the CSF and breast milk, and crosses the placenta. Unchanged drug and metabolites are excreted in the urine, mainly as conjugated metabolites.

◊ References.

1. Greenblatt DJ, *et al.* Clinical pharmacokinetics of chlordiazepoxide. *Clin Pharmacokinet* 1978; **3:** 381–94.

### Uses and Administration
Chlordiazepoxide is a benzodiazepine with general properties similar to those of diazepam (p.695). It is used in the short-term treatment of anxiety disorders (p.663) and insomnia (p.667). Chlordiazepoxide is also used in muscle spasm (p.1386), in alcohol withdrawal syndrome (p.1166), and for premedication (p.1296).

Chlordiazepoxide is given by mouth as the hydrochloride or the base; the doses given refer equally to both. It may also be administered by deep intramuscular or slow intravenous injection as the hydrochloride. Preparations formulated for intramuscular use are stated to be unsuitable for intravenous administration due to the formation of air bubbles in the solvent.

Elderly and debilitated patients should be given one-half or less of the usual adult dose.

The usual dose by mouth for the treatment of **anxiety** is up to 30 mg daily in divided doses; in severe conditions up to 100 mg daily has been given. For acute or severe anxiety an initial dose of 50 to 100 mg of the hydrochloride has been given by injection, followed if necessary by 25 to 50 mg three or four times daily.

For relief of **muscle spasm** a dose of 10 to 30 mg daily by mouth in divided doses is recommended, and 10 to 30 mg by mouth may be given before retiring for insomnia associated with anxiety.

For the control of the acute symptoms of **alcohol withdrawal** chlordiazepoxide or chlordiazepoxide hydrochloride may be given by mouth in a dose of 25 to 100 mg repeated as needed up to a maximum of 300 mg daily. For severe symptoms treatment may be initiated by injection of 50 to 100 mg, repeated if necessary after 2 to 4 hours.

Chlordiazepoxide hydrochloride has also been given for anaesthetic **premedication** in a dose of 50 to 100 mg intramuscularly one hour before surgery.

### Preparations
**BP 2003:** Chlordiazepoxide Capsules; Chlordiazepoxide Hydrochloride Tablets;
**USP 27:** Chlordiazepoxide and Amitriptyline Hydrochloride Tablets; Chlordiazepoxide Hydrochloride and Clidinium Bromide Capsules; Chlordiazepoxide Hydrochloride Capsules; Chlordiazepoxide Hydrochloride for Injection; Chlordiazepoxide Tablets.

**Proprietary Preparations** (details are given in Part 3)
**Arg.:** OCM; **Braz.:** Psicosedin; Tensil†; **Canad.:** Novo-Poxide†; **Denm.:** Klopoxid; Risolid; **Fin.:** Risolid; **Ger.:** Librium; Multum; Radepur; **Gr.:** Oasil; **Hong Kong:** Librium; **India:** Equilibrium; Librium; **Irl.:** Librium; **Israel:** Servium†; **Ital.:** Librium; Psicofar†; Reliberan; **Malaysia:** Benpine; Klorpo; **Mex.:** Kalmocaps; **NZ:** Novapam†; **Port.:** Paxium; **S.Afr.:** Librium; **Singapore:** Benpine; Klorpo; **Spain:** Huberplex; Omnalio; **Thai.:** Benpine; Epoxide; **UK:** Librium; Tropium; **USA:** Libritabs†; Librium; Mitran†; Reposans†.

**Multi-ingredient: Arg.:** Librax; Plafonyl; **Austria:** Limbitrol; Pantrop; **Belg.:** Librax†; Limbitrol†; **Braz.:** Limbitrol; Menostress†; Menotensil; **Canad.:** Apo-Chlorax; Corium†; Librax; **Chile:** Aero Itan; Aerogastrol; Antalin; Garceptol; Gaseofin; Gastrolen; Lerogin; Libraxin; Lironex; Morelin; No-Ref; Profisin; Sedogastrol; Tensoliv; Tranvagal; **Fin.:** Librax; Limbitrol; **Fr.:** Librax; **Ger.:** Limbatril†; **Hong Kong:** Bralix; Librax; Medocalum; **India:** Equirex; Normaxin; **Israel:** Librax†; Nirvaxal; **Ital.:** Diapatol; Librax; Limbitryl; Sedans; **Malaysia:** Apo-Chlorax; Liblan; **Port.:** Gabil†; Librax; **S.Afr.:** Librax; Limbitrol; **Singapore:** Apo-Chlorax; Chlobax; Librax; Medocalum; **Spain:** Psico Blocan; Relaxedans†; **Switz.:** Librax; Limbitrol; **Thai.:** Kenspa; Liblan†; Librax; Pobrax; Tumax; Zepobrax; **USA:** Clindex; Librax; Limbitrol.

### Chlormezanone (BAN, rINN)

Chlormethazanone; Chlormezanonum; Clormezanona. 2-(4-Chlorophenyl)-3-methylperhydro-1,3-thiazin-4-one 1,1-dioxide.

$C_{11}H_{12}ClNO_3S$ = 273.7.

*CAS — 80-77-3.*

*ATC — M03BB02.*

**Profile**

Chlormezanone has been used in the treatment of anxiety disorders and insomnia. It was also used in conditions associated with painful muscle spasm, often in compound preparations with analgesics; its mechanism of action is not clear but is probably related to its sedative effect. Chlormezanone was withdrawn from use in many countries following reports of serious skin reactions (see below).

**Effects on the skin.** Chlormezanone was responsible for 5 of 86 cases of fixed drug eruption detected in a Finnish hospital from 1971 to 1980.[1] In the period from 1981 to 1985 chlormezanone was responsible for 1 out of 77 such eruptions.[2] In a case control study[3] comparing drug use in 245 patients hospitalised because of toxic epidermal necrolysis or Stevens-Johnson syndrome and 1147 controls, 13 patients and one control were found to have taken chlormezanone. From these figures a high crude relative risk of 62 was calculated; the excess risk was estimated to be 1.7 cases per million users per week.

1. Kauppinen K, Stubb S. Fixed eruptions: causative drugs and challenge tests. *Br J Dermatol* 1985; **112:** 575–8.
2. Stubb S, *et al.* Fixed drug eruptions: 77 cases from 1981 to 1985. *Br J Dermatol* 1989; **120:** 583.
3. Roujeau J-C, *et al.* Medication use and the risk of Stevens-Johnson syndrome or toxic epidermal necrolysis. *N Engl J Med* 1995; **333:** 1600–7.

**Porphyria.** Chlormezanone has been associated with acute attacks of porphyria and is considered unsafe in porphyric patients.

#### Preparations

**Proprietary Preparations** (details are given in Part 3)
***Chile:*** Restoril.

**Multi-ingredient: *Braz.:*** Besaprin†; ***Chile:*** Adalgen; Calmosedan; Cardiosedantol; Diapam; Dioran; Dolnix; Dolonase; Dolorelax; Fibrorelax; Mesolona; Multisedil; Neo Butartrol; Promidan; Sedantol; Sedilit; Silrelax; Sin-Algin; ***S.Afr.:*** Arcanaflex†; Besenol†; Betaflex†; Lobak†; Myoflex†; Rexachlor†; ***Singapore:*** Relexic†.

### Chlorproethazine Hydrochloride (rINNM)

Hidrocloruro de clorproetazina; RP-4909 (chlorproethazine). 3-(2-Chlorophenothiazin-10-yl)-NN-diethylpropylamine hydrochloride.

$C_{19}H_{23}ClN_2S,HCl$ = 383.4.

*CAS — 84-01-5 (chlorproethazine); 4611-02-3 (chlorproethazine hydrochloride).*

*ATC — N05AA07.*

**Profile**

Chlorproethazine is a phenothiazine derivative differing chemically from chlorpromazine by the substitution of a diethyl for a dimethyl group. It has general properties similar to those of chlorpromazine (below) but has been used mainly as a muscle relaxant in the management of muscle spasm (p.1386). Although exposure of the skin to phenothiazines has been associated with sensitivity reactions, chlorproethazine hydrochloride has been applied topically with the warning to avoid direct exposure to sunlight. It has also been given by mouth or by intramuscular or slow intravenous injection.

#### Preparations

**Proprietary Preparations** (details are given in Part 3)
***Fr.:*** Neuriplege.

**Multi-ingredient: *Fr.:*** Neuriplege†.

## Chlorpromazine (BAN, rINN)

Clorpromazina. 3-(2-Chlorophenothiazin-10-yl)propyldimethylamine.

$C_{17}H_{19}ClN_2S$ = 318.9.

*CAS — 50-53-3.*

*ATC — N05AA01.*

**Pharmacopoeias.** In *Br.* and *US.*

**BP 2003** (Chlorpromazine). A white or creamy-white powder or waxy solid; odourless or almost odourless. M.p. 56° to 58°. Practically insoluble in water; freely soluble in alcohol and in ether; very soluble in chloroform. Protect from light.

**USP 27** (Chlorpromazine). A white crystalline solid with an amine-like odour. It darkens on prolonged exposure to light. Practically insoluble in water; soluble 1 in 3 of alcohol, 1 in 2 of chloroform, 1 in 3 of ether, and 1 in 2 of benzene; freely soluble in dilute mineral acids; practically insoluble in dilute alkali hydroxides. Store in airtight containers. Protect from light.

### Chlorpromazine Embonate (BANM, rINNM)

Chlorpromazine Pamoate; Embonato de clorpromazina. Chlorpromazine 4,4′-methylenebis(3-hydroxy-2-naphthoate).

$(C_{17}H_{19}ClN_2S)_2,C_{23}H_{16}O_6$ = 1026.1.

*ATC — N05AA01.*

### Chlorpromazine Hydrochloride (BANM, rINNM)

Aminazine; Chlorpromazini Hydrochloridum; Hidrocloruro de clorpromazina.

$C_{17}H_{19}ClN_2S,HCl$ = 355.3.

*CAS — 69-09-0.*

*ATC — N05AA01.*

**Pharmacopoeias.** In *Chin., Eur.* (see p.vi), *Int., Jpn, Pol., US,* and *Viet.*

**Ph. Eur. 5.0** (Chlorpromazine Hydrochloride). A white or almost white crystalline powder. It decomposes on exposure to air and light. Very soluble in water; freely soluble in alcohol. A freshly prepared 10% solution in water has a pH of 3.5 to 4.5. Store in airtight containers. Protect from light.

**USP 27** (Chlorpromazine Hydrochloride). A white or slightly creamy-white odourless crystalline powder. It darkens on prolonged exposure to light. Soluble 1 in 1 of water, 1 in 1.5 of alcohol, and 1 in 1.5 of chloroform; insoluble in ether and in benzene. Store in airtight containers. Protect from light.

**Dilution.** Solutions containing 2.5% of chlorpromazine hydrochloride may be diluted to 100 mL with 0.9% sodium chloride solution provided the pH of the saline solution is such that the pH of the dilution does not exceed the critical range of pH 6.7 to 6.8.[1] With saline of pH 7.0 or 7.2, the final solution had a pH of 6.4.

1. D'Arcy PF, Thompson KM. Stability of chlorpromazine hydrochloride added to intravenous infusion fluids. *Pharm J* 1973; **210:** 28.

**Incompatibility.** Incompatibility has been reported between chlorpromazine hydrochloride injection and several other compounds; precipitation of chlorpromazine base from solution is particularly likely if the final pH is increased. Compounds reported to be incompatible with chlorpromazine hydrochloride include aminophylline, amphotericin B, aztreonam, some barbiturates, chloramphenicol sodium succinate, chlorothiazide sodium, dimenhydrinate, heparin sodium, morphine sulfate (when preserved with chlorocresol), some penicillins, and remifentanil.

For a warning about incompatibility between chlorpromazine solution (Thorazine) and carbamazepine suspension (Tegretol), see p.353.

**Sorption.** There was a 41% loss of chlorpromazine hydrochloride from solution when infused for 7 hours via a plastic infusion set (cellulose propionate burette with polyvinyl chloride tubing), and a 79% loss after infusion for 1 hour from a glass syringe through silastic tubing.[1] Loss was negligible after infusion for 1 hour from a system comprising a glass syringe with polyethylene tubing.

1. Kowaluk EA, *et al.* Interactions between drugs and intravenous delivery systems. *Am J Hosp Pharm* 1982; **39:** 460–7.

### Adverse Effects

Chlorpromazine generally produces less central depression than the barbiturates or benzodiazepines, and tolerance to its initial sedative effects develops fairly quickly in most patients. It has antimuscarinic properties and may cause adverse effects such as dry mouth, constipation, difficulty with micturition, blurred vision, and mydriasis. Tachycardia, ECG changes (particularly Q- and T-wave abnormalities), and, rarely, cardiac arrhythmias may occur; hypotension (usually orthostatic) is common. Other adverse effects include delirium, agitation and, rarely, catatonic-like states, insomnia or drowsiness, nightmares, depression, miosis, EEG changes and convulsions, nasal congestion, minor abnormalities in liver function tests, inhibition of ejaculation, impotence, and priapism.

Hypersensitivity reactions include urticaria, exfoliative dermatitis, erythema multiforme, and contact sensitivity. A syndrome resembling systemic lupus erythematosus has been reported. Jaundice has occurred, and probably has an immunological origin. Prolonged therapy may lead to deposition of pigment in the skin, or more frequently the eyes; corneal and lens opacities have been observed. Pigmentary retinopathy has occurred only rarely with chlorpromazine. Photosensitivity reactions are more common with chlorpromazine than with other antipsychotics.

Various haematological disorders, including haemolytic anaemia, aplastic anaemia, thrombocytopenic purpura, leucocytosis, and a potentially fatal agranulocytosis have occasionally been reported; they may be manifestations of a hypersensitivity reaction. Most cases of agranulocytosis have occurred within 4 to 10 weeks of starting treatment, and symptoms such as sore throat or fever should be watched for and white cell counts instituted should they appear. Mild leucopenia has been stated to occur in up to 30% of patients on prolonged high dosage.

Extrapyramidal dysfunction and resultant disorders include acute dystonia, a parkinsonism-like syndrome, and akathisia; late effects include tardive dyskinesia and perioral tremor. The neuroleptic malignant syndrome may also occur.

Chlorpromazine alters endocrine and metabolic functions. Patients have experienced amenorrhoea, galactorrhoea, gynaecomastia, weight gain, and hyperglycaemia and altered glucose tolerance. Body temperature regulation is impaired and may result in hypo- or hyperthermia depending on environment. There have also been reports of hypercholesterolaemia.

There have been isolated reports of sudden death with chlorpromazine; possible causes include cardiac arrhythmias or aspiration and asphyxia due to suppression of the cough and gag reflexes.

Pain and irritation at the injection site may occur on injection. Nodule formation may occur after intramuscular administration.

Phenothiazines do not cause dependence of the type encountered with barbiturates or benzodiazepines. However, withdrawal symptoms have been seen following abrupt withdrawal from patients receiving prolonged and/or high-dose maintenance therapy.

Although the adverse effects of **other phenothiazines** are broadly similar in nature to those of chlorpromazine, their frequency and pattern tend to fall into 3 groups:

- group 1 (e.g. chlorpromazine, levomepromazine, and promazine) are generally characterised by pronounced sedative effects and moderate antimuscarinic and extrapyramidal effects
- group 2 (e.g. pericyazine, pipotiazine, and thioridazine) are generally characterised by moderate sedative effects, marked antimuscarinic effects, and fewer extrapyramidal effects than groups 1 or 3
- group 3 (e.g. fluphenazine, perphenazine, prochlorperazine, and trifluoperazine) are generally characterised by fewer sedative and antimuscarinic effects but more pronounced extrapyramidal effects than groups 1 or 2

Classical antipsychotics of **other chemical groups** tend to resemble the phenothiazines of group 3. They include the butyrophenones (e.g. benperidol, and haloperidol); diphenylbutylpiperidines (e.g. pimozide); thioxanthenes (flupentixol and zuclopenthixol); substituted benzamides (e.g. sulpiride); oxypertine; and loxapine.

**Carcinogenicity.** See Effects on Endocrine Function, below.

**Convulsions.** Treatment with antipsychotics can result in EEG abnormalities and lowered seizure threshold.[1,2] Seizures can be induced particularly in patients with a history of epilepsy or drug-induced seizures, abnormal EEG, previous electroconvulsive therapy, or pre-existing CNS abnormalities. The risk appears to be greatest at the start of antipsychotic therapy, or with high doses, or abrupt increases of dose, or with the use of more than one antipsychotic. The incidence of antipsychotic-induced convulsions is, however, probably less than 1%.

Phenothiazines with an aliphatic side-chain such as chlorpromazine, promazine, and triflupromazine appear to present a higher risk than those with a piperazine or piperidine moiety. Despite conflicting evidence, haloperidol appears to carry a relatively low risk of seizures. In general, the epileptic potential has been correlated with the propensity of the antipsychotic to cause sedation. The following drugs have been suggested when antipsychotic therapy is considered necessary in patients at risk of seizures or being treated for epilepsy: fluphenazine, haloperidol, molindone, and pimozide. Antipsychotic dosage should be increased slowly and the possibility of interactions with antiepileptic therapy considered (see under Interactions, below).

The atypical antipsychotic clozapine appears to be associated with a particularly high risk of seizures (see Effects on the Nervous System, p.686).

1. Cold JA, *et al.* Seizure activity associated with antipsychotic therapy. *DICP Ann Pharmacother* 1990; **24:** 601–6. Correction. *ibid.*; 1012.
2. Zaccara G, *et al.* Clinical features, pathogenesis and management of drug-induced seizures. *Drug Safety* 1990; **5:** 109–51.

**Effects on the blood.** The UK Committee on Safety of Medicines provided data on the reports it had received between July 1963 and January 1993 on agranulocytosis and neutropenia.[1] Several groups of drugs were commonly implicated, among them phenothiazines for which there were 87 reports of agranulocytosis (42 fatal) and 33 of neutropenia (22 fatal). The most frequently implicated phenothiazines were chlorpromazine with

51 reports of agranulocytosis (26 fatal) and 12 of neutropenia (2 fatal) and thioridazine with 20 reports of agranulocytosis (9 fatal) and 10 of neutropenia (none fatal).

1. Committee on Safety of Medicines/Medicines Control Agency. Drug-induced neutropenia and agranulocytosis. *Current Problems* 1993; **19:** 10–11.

**Effects on body-weight.** Most antipsychotic drugs are associated with weight gain. A meta-analysis[1] found evidence of weight gain in patients receiving both classical (chlorpromazine, fluphenazine, haloperidol, loxapine, perphenazine, thioridazine, tiotixene, or trifluoperazine) and atypical (clozapine, olanzapine, quetiapine, risperidone, sertindole, and ziprasidone) antipsychotics. Two drugs, molindone and pimozide, appeared in contrast to be associated with weight loss, although in the case of pimozide this could not be confirmed statistically. Placebo treatment was also associated with weight loss.

A separate review[2] calculated the average monthly weight gain associated with atypical antipsychotics to be: olanzapine (2.28 kg), zotepine (2.28 kg), quetiapine (1.76 kg), clozapine (1.72 kg), risperidone (0.96 kg), ziprasidone (0.80 kg). Weight gain occurred most frequently during the first 6 to 12 months of treatment. It was recommended that if weight gain was more than 2 kg during the first 2 weeks, a strict dietary regimen should be started immediately. However, more recent opinion is that a change of antipsychotic may be necessary. For further details, see under Effects on Carbohydrate Metabolism, in Clozapine, p.686.

1. Allison DB, *et al.* Antipsychotic-induced weight gain: a comprehensive research synthesis. *Am J Psychiatry* 1999; **156:** 1686–96.
2. Wetterling T. Bodyweight gain with atypical antipsychotics: a comparative review. *Drug Safety* 2001; **24:** 59–73.

**Effects on the cardiovascular system. Orthostatic hypotension** is a common problem in patients taking psychotropic drugs and is particularly pronounced with low-potency antipsychotics.[1]

Various **EEG changes** or frank **arrhythmias** have occurred in patients receiving antipsychotics. T-wave changes have been reported with low-potency antipsychotics; they are usually benign and reversible, and subject to diurnal fluctuations. Low-potency antipsychotics, particularly *thioridazine* and *mesoridazine*, and the high-potency drug *pimozide*, prolong the QT interval in a similar manner to class I antiarrhythmics such as quinidine or procainamide; their use is therefore contra-indicated in patients taking such antiarrhythmics. Droperidol, another high-potency drug, has also been reported to prolong the QT interval.[2] Thioridazine is most frequently discussed in case reports of psychotropic drug-induced torsade de pointes,[2] which has led to restrictions on its use (see Precautions and Uses and Administration of Thioridazine, p.724); *chlorpromazine* and *pimozide* have also been implicated. Torsade de pointes has also been reported following overdosage[3-5] with, or high intravenous[6] doses of, the high-potency antipsychotic *haloperidol*. There are also isolated reports of cardiac arrhythmias following attempts at rapid control with high doses of haloperidol.[7,8] *Melperone*, a butyrophenone antipsychotic related to haloperidol, has been reported to have class III electrophysiologic and antiarrhythmic activity.[9,10]

Sudden unexpected deaths have long been reported in patients receiving antipsychotics.[11] Whether this is due to the disease being treated or to the treatment is still unclear. However, in a retrospective cohort study[12] involving about 482 000 patients, analysis of 1487 sudden cardiac deaths indicated that patients receiving antipsychotics in doses of more than 100 mg of thioridazine or its equivalent had a 2.4-fold increase in the rate of sudden cardiac death, rising to a 3.53-fold increase in those patients with pre-existing severe cardiovascular disease. A later case-control study[13] in 5 UK psychiatric hospitals found that sudden unexplained death in psychiatric patients was associated with hypertension, ischaemic heart disease, and current treatment with thioridazine. Although several mechanisms have been suggested for the effect, prolongation of the QT interval has been implicated in a proportion of the cases.[11]

Results from a case-control study[14] have suggested that use of classical antipsychotics may be associated with an increased risk of idiopathic **venous thromboembolism.** The risk was most pronounced during the first 3 months of treatment, and was higher for low potency than high potency antipsychotics. This study did not examine the risk of venous thromboembolism with atypical antipsychotics, but see under Clozapine, p.686.

1. DiGiacomo J. Cardiovascular effects of psychotropic drugs. *Cardiovasc Rev Rep* 1989; **10:** 31–2, 39–41, and 47.
2. Reilly JG, *et al.* QTc-interval abnormalities and psychotropic drug therapy in psychiatric patients. *Lancet* 2000; **355:** 1048–52.
3. Zee-Cheng C-S, *et al.* Haloperidol and torsades de pointes. *Ann Intern Med* 1985; **102:** 418.
4. Henderson RA, *et al.* Life-threatening ventricular arrhythmia (torsades de pointes) after haloperidol overdose. *Hum Exp Toxicol* 1991; **10:** 59–62.
5. Wilt JL, *et al.* Torsade de pointes associated with the use of intravenous haloperidol. *Ann Intern Med* 1993; **119:** 391–4.
6. O'Brien JM, *et al.* Haloperidol-induced torsade de pointes. *Ann Pharmacother* 1999; **33:** 1046–50.
7. Mehta D, *et al.* Cardiac arrhythmia and haloperidol. *Am J Psychiatry* 1979; **136:** 1468–9.
8. Bett JHN, Holt GW. Malignant ventricular tachyarrhythmia and haloperidol. *BMJ* 1983; **287:** 1264.
9. Møgelvang JC, *et al.* Antiarrhythmic properties of a neuroleptic butyrophenone, melperone, in acute myocardial infarction. *Acta Med Scand* 1980; **208:** 61–4.
10. Hui WKK, *et al.* Melperone: electrophysiologic and antiarrhythmic activity in humans. *J Cardiovasc Pharmacol* 1990; **15:** 144–9.
11. Haddad PM, Anderson IM. Antipsychotic-related QTc prolongation, torsade de pointes and sudden death. *Drugs* 2002; **62:** 1649–71.
12. Ray WA, *et al.* Antipsychotics and the risk of sudden cardiac death. *Arch Gen Psychiatry* 2001; **58:** 1161–7.
13. Reilly JG, *et al.* Thioridazine and sudden unexplained death in psychiatric in-patients. *Br J Psychiatry* 2002; **180:** 515–22.
14. Zornberg GL, Jick H. Antipsychotic drug use and risk of first-time idiopathic venous thromboembolism: a case-control study. *Lancet* 2000; **356:** 1219–23.

**Effects on endocrine function.** Antipsychotics can alter the secretion of prolactin, growth hormone, and thyrotrophin from the anterior pituitary[1] via their ability to block central dopamine-$D_2$ receptors. Therapeutic doses of antipsychotics increase serum-prolactin concentrations; this effect occurs at lower doses and after shorter latent periods than the antipsychotic effects. However, raised prolactin concentrations have not always been observed after long-term use, suggesting that tolerance may develop to the hyperprolactinaemic effect. Serum prolactin declines to normal values within 3 weeks of stopping oral antipsychotic therapy but may remain raised for 6 months after discontinuation of intramuscular depots.[2]

The long-term consequences of gonadal hormone deficiency, secondary to raised prolactin concentrations, are considered a cause for concern.[2] Preliminary results from one group[3] indicated that over 40% of patients taking prolactin raising antipsychotics show osteopenia associated with hypogonadism. Long-term antipsychotic treatment has been shown to increase the incidence of mammary tumours in the *rat*. Although early studies[4,5] found little or no evidence that chronic use in humans alters the risk of breast cancer among women with schizophrenia a more recent retrospective cohort study[6] found a modest dose-related increase in the risk of breast cancer in women using antipsychotic dopamine antagonists. A similar increase was seen in women receiving antiemetic dopamine antagonists. Fears that pituitary abnormalities, including pituitary tumours,[7] might develop in patients on long-term phenothiazine therapy have not been confirmed.[8,9]

Antipsychotics can in some circumstances reduce both basal and stimulated growth-hormone secretion but attempts to use them to treat dysfunctions in growth-hormone regulation have not been successful.[1] Although a number of clinical studies show that acute administration of antipsychotics increased both basal and stimulated thyrotrophin secretion, the majority of studies find either no change or only a small increase in thyrotrophin secretion following long-term use.

A small study has suggested that thioridazine may be more likely than other antipsychotics to decrease serum concentrations of testosterone or luteinising hormone in men.[10] However, concentrations were within the normal range in most patients taking antipsychotics.[10]

See also Effects on Fluid and Electrolyte Homoeostasis, below and Effects on Sexual Function, below.

1. Gunnet JW, Moore KE. Neuroleptics and neuroendocrine function. *Ann Rev Pharmacol Toxicol* 1988; **28:** 347–66.
2. Wieck A, Haddad P. Hyperprolactinaemia caused by antipsychotic drugs. *BMJ* 2002; **324:** 250–2.
3. Howes O, Smith S. Hyperprolactinaemia caused by antipsychotic drugs: endocrine antipsychotic side effects must be systematically assessed. *BMJ* 2002; **324:** 1278.
4. Mortensen PB. The incidence of cancer in schizophrenic patients. *J Epidemiol Community Health* 1989; **43:** 43–7.
5. Mortensen PB. The occurrence of cancer in first admitted schizophrenic patients. *Schizophr Res* 1994; **12:** 185–94.
6. Wang PS, *et al.* Dopamine antagonists and the development of breast cancer. *Arch Gen Psychiatry* 2002; **59:** 1147–54.
7. Asplund K, *et al.* Phenothiazine drugs and pituitary tumors. *Ann Intern Med* 1982; **96:** 533.
8. Rosenblatt S, *et al.* Chronic phenothiazine therapy does not increase sellar size. *Lancet* 1978; **ii:** 319–20.
9. Lilford VA, *et al.* Long-term phenothiazine treatment does not cause pituitary tumours. *Br J Psychiatry* 1984; **144:** 421–4.
10. Brown WA, *et al.* Differential effects of neuroleptic agents on the pituitary-gonadal axis in men. *Arch Gen Psychiatry* 1981; **38:** 1270–2.

**Effects on the eyes.** Phenothiazines may induce a pigmentary retinopathy which is dependent on both the dose and the duration of treatment.[1] Those phenothiazine derivatives with piperidine side-chains such as thioridazine have a higher risk of inducing retinal toxicity than other phenothiazine derivatives, with relatively few cases reported for those with aliphatic side-chains such as chlorpromazine; the piperazine group does not appear to exert direct ocular toxicity.[2] The retinopathy may present either acutely, (sudden loss of vision associated with retinal oedema and hyperaemia of the optic disc), or chronically, (a fine pigment scatter appearing in the central area of the fundus, extending peripherally but sparing the macula). Chronic paracentral and pericentral scotomas may be found. Although pigmentary disturbances may progress after withdrawal of thioridazine, they are not always paralleled by deterioration in visual function; nonetheless, some cases have led to progressive chorioretinopathy.[3] The critical ocular toxic dose of thioridazine is reported to be 800 mg daily and the UK manufacturers recommend that a daily dose of 600 mg should not usually be exceeded. However, there is a report[4] of pigmentary retinopathy in a patient who received long-term thioridazine in daily doses not exceeding 400 mg; the total dose was 752 g.

Pigmentation may also occur in the cornea, lens, and conjunctiva following use of phenothiazines. It may occur in association with pigmentary changes in the skin and is dose-related. In a study of 100 Malaysian patients, ocular pigmentation was observed in slightly more than half of those who had received a total dose of chlorpromazine of 100 to 299 g and in 13 of 15 who had received 300 to 599 g.[5] All those who had received more than 600 g of chlorpromazine or thioridazine had ocular pigmentation. Cataract formation, mainly of an anterior polar variety, has been observed rarely, mainly in patients on chlorpromazine. It does not appear to be dose-related.[2]

A patient who had received fortnightly injections of fluphenazine for 10 years to an estimated total dose of 3.25 g, developed bilateral maculopathy following unprotected exposure of less than 2-minute's duration to a welding arc.[6] It was postulated that accumulation of phenothiazine in the retinal epithelium sensitised the patient to photic damage.

1. Spiteri MA, James DG. Adverse ocular reactions to drugs. *Postgrad Med J* 1983; **59:** 343–9.
2. Crombie AL. Drugs causing eye problems. *Prescribers' J* 1981; **21:** 222–7.
3. Marmor MF. Is thioridazine retinopathy progressive? Relationship of pigmentary changes to visual function. *Br J Ophthalmol* 1990; **74:** 739–42.
4. Lam RW, Remick RA. Pigmentary retinopathy associated with low-dose thioridazine treatment. *Can Med Assoc J* 1985; **132:** 737.
5. Ngen CC, Singh P. Long-term phenothiazine administration and the eye in 100 Malaysians. *Br J Psychiatry* 1988; **152:** 278–81.
6. Power WJ, *et al.* Welding arc maculopathy and fluphenazine. *Br J Ophthalmol* 1991; **75:** 433–5.

**Effects on fluid and electrolyte homoeostasis.** There have been occasional reports of water intoxication in patients taking antipsychotics. A review[1] of hyponatraemia and the syndrome of inappropriate antidiuretic hormone secretion associated with psychotropics summarised 20 such reports for antipsychotics in the literature. The drugs implicated were thioridazine (8 patients), haloperidol (3 reports), chlorpromazine, trifluoperazine, and fluphenazine (2 reports each), and flupentixol, tiotixene, and clozapine (1 report each). The majority of reports did not permit clear conclusions and, particularly in the cases of prolonged treatment, the role of the medication was unclear. However, at least 3 of the cases were well documented and supported the view that antipsychotics could cause hyponatraemia.

A report not considered by the above review described water retention and peripheral oedema associated with chlorpromazine.[2] A small controlled study[3] found that 5 of 10 evaluated patients receiving haloperidol decanoate had impaired fluid homoeostasis.

1. Spigset O, Hedenmalm K. Hyponatraemia and the syndrome of inappropriate antidiuretic hormone secretion (SIADH) induced by psychotropic drugs. *Drug Safety* 1995; **12:** 209–25.
2. Witz L, *et al.* Chlorpromazine induced fluid retention masquerading as idiopathic oedema. *BMJ* 1987; **294:** 807–8.
3. Rider JM, *et al.* Water handling in patients receiving haloperidol decanoate. *Ann Pharmacother* 1995; **29:** 663–6.

**Effects on lipid metabolism.** There are scant data implicating phenothiazines as a cause of elevated cholesterol and decreased high-density lipoprotein concentrations.[1] The possibility of such effects should nevertheless be considered in dyslipidaemic patients treated with these drugs.

1. Henkin Y, *et al.* Secondary dyslipidemia: inadvertent effects of drugs in clinical practice. *JAMA* 1992; **267:** 961–8.

**Effects on the liver.** Chlorpromazine and other phenothiazines may cause hepatocanalicular cholestasis often with hepatocyte damage suggestive of immunological liver injury.[1] Only a small number of patients taking the drug are affected and the onset is usually in the first 4 weeks of therapy. The drug or one of its metabolites may induce alteration in the liver-cell membrane so that it becomes antigenic; there is also good evidence for direct hepatotoxicity related to the production of free drug radical. There may be an individual idiosyncrasy in the metabolism of chlorpromazine and in the production of these radicals. A study has suggested that patients who have poor sulfoxidation status combined with unimpaired hydroxylation capacity may be most likely to develop jaundice with chlorpromazine.[2]

A preliminary study[3] showing a high incidence of gallstones in psychiatric inpatients in Japan found a correlation between the presence of gallstones and the duration of illness and use of antipsychotics. It was speculated that gallstones could be a consequence of phenothiazine-induced cholestasis.

1. Sherlock S. The spectrum of hepatotoxicity due to drugs. *Lancet* 1986; **ii:** 440–4.
2. Watson RGP, *et al.* A proposed mechanism for chlorpromazine jaundice—defective hepatic sulphoxidation combined with rapid hydroxylation. *J Hepatol* 1988; **7:** 72–8.
3. Fukuzako H, *et al.* Ultrasonography detected a higher incidence of gallstones in psychiatric inpatients. *Acta Psychiatr Scand* 1991; **84:** 83–5.

**Effects on sexual function.** The phenothiazines can cause both impotence and ejaculatory dysfunction.[1] Thioridazine has been frequently implicated, and in an early report 60% of 57 male patients taking the drug reported sexual dysfunction compared with 25% of 64 men taking other antipsychotics.[2] There are also several reports of priapism with phenothiazines;[1,3-5] alpha-adrenoceptor blocking properties of these compounds may be partly responsible. Male sexual dysfunction, including priapism, has been reported only rarely with other antipsychotics such as the butyrophenones, diphenylbutylpiperidines, and thioxanthenes.[6] Priapism has also been reported with clozapine[7] and other atypical antipsychotics. The effects of antipsychotics on female sexual function are less well studied. Orgasmic dysfunction has been reported with thioridazine, trifluoperazine, and fluphenazine.[8]

The effects of hyperprolactinaemia (see Effects on Endocrine Function, above) on sexual function are described on p.1315.


1. Beeley L. Drug-induced sexual dysfunction and infertility. *Adverse Drug React Acute Poisoning Rev* 1984; **3:** 23–42.
2. Kotin J, *et al.* Thioridazine and sexual dysfunction. *Am J Psychiatry* 1976; **133:** 82–5.
3. Baños JE, *et al.* Drug-induced priapism: its aetiology, incidence and treatment. *Med Toxicol* 1989; **4:** 46–58.
4. Chan J, *et al.* Perphenazine-induced priapism. *DICP Ann Pharmacother* 1990; **24:** 246–9.
5. Salado J, *et al.* Priapism associated with zuclopenthixol. *Ann Pharmacother* 2002; **36:** 1016–18.
6. Fabian J-L. Psychotropic medications and priapism. *Am J Psychiatry* 1993, **150:** 349–50.
7. Patel AG, *et al.* Priapism associated with psychotropic drugs. *Br J Hosp Med* 1996; **55:** 315–19.
8. Segraves RT. Psychiatric drugs and inhibited female orgasm. *J Sex Marital Ther* 1988; **14:** 202–7.


**Effects on the skin.** DEPOT INJECTION. Of 217 patients who received a combined total of 2354 depot antipsychotic injections 42 (19.4%) had local problems at the site of injection; 18 (8.3%) experienced chronic complications and 30 (13.8%) acute reactions.[1] Acute problems reported included 31 episodes of unusual pain, 21 of bleeding or haematoma, 19 of clinically important leakage of drug from injection site, 11 of acute inflammatory indurations, and 2 of transient nodules. Complications were more common in patients receiving concentrated preparations, higher doses, weekly injections, haloperidol decanoate or zuclopenthixol decanoate, and injection volumes greater than 1 mL and in those treated for more than 5 years. Chronic reactions were more common in patients aged over 50 years.


1. Hay J. Complications at site of injection of depot neuroleptics. *BMJ* 1995; **311:** 421.


PHOTOSENSITIVITY. Testing in 7 subjects taking chlorpromazine revealed that photosensitivity reactions manifested primarily as immediate erythema and that sensitivity was primarily to light in the long ultraviolet (UVA) and visible wavebands. Sensitivity to UVB was normal.[1]

The incidence of photosensitivity reactions to chlorpromazine has been given as 3%. However, a higher incidence of 16-25% has also been reported.[2]

See also Effects on the Eyes, above.


1. Ferguson J, *et al.* Further clinical and investigative studies of chlorpromazine phototoxicity. *Br J Dermatol* 1986; **115** (suppl 30): 35.
2. Harth Y, Rapoport M. Photosensitivity associated with antipsychotics, antidepressants and anxiolytics. *Drug Safety* 1996; **14:** 252–9.


PIGMENTATION. The pigment found in the skin of patients treated with chlorpromazine was considered[1] to be a chlorpromazine-melanin polymer formed in a light-catalysed anaerobic reaction. Hydrogen chloride liberated during the reaction could account for the skin irritation. Intracutaneous injection of a preparation of the polymer into 2 volunteers produced a bluish-purple discoloration which faded in 3 days.


1. Huang CL, Sands FL. Effect of ultraviolet irradiation on chlorpromazine II: anaerobic condition. *J Pharm Sci* 1967; **56:** 259–64.


**Extrapyramidal disorders.** Antipsychotics and a number of other drugs, including antiemetics such as metoclopramide and some antidepressants, can produce a range of dyskinesias or involuntary movement disorders involving the extrapyramidal motor system, including parkinsonism, akathisia, acute dystonia, and chronic tardive dyskinesia.[1-4] Such reactions are a major problem in the clinical management of patients receiving antipsychotics. Reactions of this type can occur with any antipsychotic, but (excluding tardive dyskinesia) are particularly prominent during treatment with high-potency drugs such as the tricyclic piperazines and butyrophenones. Antipsychotics such as clozapine carry a low risk of extrapyramidal effects and are therefore described as atypical antipsychotics. The incidence of tardive dyskinesia does appear to be minimal with clozapine, although there is less evidence for other atypical antipsychotics (but see also below).

Of 2811 patients studied[5] in the first few months of therapy with prochlorperazine (a drug with a high propensity to cause extrapyramidal reactions), 57 reported adverse effects, 16 of which involved the extrapyramidal system. There were 4 dystonic-dyskinesic reactions (an incidence of 1 in 464 and 1 in 707 for patients aged under and over 30 years respectively), 9 reports of parkinsonism (under 60 years, 1 in 1555; over 60 years, 1 in 159), and 3 reports of akathisia (1 in 562).

One explanation of extrapyramidal disorders is an imbalance between dopaminergic and cholinergic systems in the brain. However, this simple model fails to explain the co-existence of a variety of extrapyramidal effects, and several alternative mechanisms have been proposed.[2,6] Hypotheses based on interactions between different dopamine receptor types may help to explain the decreased tendency of some antipsychotic drugs to induce these reactions (see Action under Uses and Administration, below).

**Akathisia** is a condition of mental and motor restlessness in which there is an urge to move about constantly and an inability to sit or stand still. It is the most common motor side-effect of treatment with antipsychotics.[7] Acute akathisia is dose-dependent, usually develops within a few days of beginning treatment or following a rapid increase in dose, and usually improves if the drug is stopped or the dose reduced. *Antimuscarinics* appear to provide only limited benefit, although success may be more likely in patients with concomitant parkinsonism. A low dose of a *beta blocker* such as *propranolol* or a *benzodiazepine* may be helpful. Improvement has also been reported with *clonidine* and *amantadine* but the usefulness of these drugs may be limited by side-effects or development of tolerance, respectively. The tardive form, like tardive dyskinesia (see below), which appears after several months of treatment, does not respond to antimuscarinics and is difficult to treat.

Acute **dystonic reactions**, which mainly affect the muscles of the face, neck, and trunk and include jaw clenching (trismus), torticollis, and oculogyric crisis are reported to occur in up to 10% of patients taking antipsychotics. Laryngeal dystonia is rare, but potentially fatal.[8] Dystonias usually occur within the first few days of treatment or after a dosage increase but may also develop on withdrawal. They are transitory, and are most common in children and young adults. Dystonic reactions may be controlled by *antimuscarinics* or *antihistamines* such as *diphenhydramine* or *promethazine*.[9] *Benzodiazepines* such as *diazepam* can also be used. Prophylactic administration of antimuscarinics can prevent the development of dystonias, but routine use is not recommended as not all patients require them and tardive dyskinesia may be unmasked or worsened (see below); such a strategy should probably be reserved for short-term use in those at high risk of developing dystonic reactions, such as young adults starting treatment with high-potency antipsychotics or in patients with a previous history of drug-induced dystonias.[10,11] Some patients may develop tardive dystonia. A range of drugs has been tried in this condition but without consistent benefit.[12]

**Parkinsonism**, often indistinguishable from idiopathic Parkinson's disease (p.1196), may develop during therapy with antipsychotics, usually after the first few weeks or months of treatment. It is generally stated to be more common in adults and the elderly, although a retrospective study with haloperidol found an inverse relationship between drug-induced parkinsonism and age.[13] This parkinsonism is generally reversible on drug withdrawal or dose reduction, and may sometimes disappear gradually despite continued drug therapy. *Antimuscarinic* drugs are used to suppress the symptoms of parkinsonism.[14] However, they are often minimally effective and commonly cause adverse effects. Routine use for prophylaxis is not recommended because of the risk of unmasking or exacerbating tardive dyskinesia (see below). *Amantadine* is an alternative to the antimuscarinics.[14]

The central feature of **tardive dyskinesia** is orofacial dyskinesia characterised by protrusion of the tongue ('fly catching'), lipsmacking, sucking, lateral chewing, and pouting of the lips and cheeks. The trunk and limbs also become involved with choreiform movements such as repetitive 'piano-playing' hand movements, shoulder shrugging, foot tapping, or rocking movements. The prevalence of tardive dyskinesia among those receiving antipsychotics varies widely but up to 60% of patients may develop symptoms. In most cases the condition is mild and not progressive and tends to wax and wane. Although tardive dyskinesia usually develops after many years of antipsychotic therapy no clear correlation has been shown between development of the condition and the length of drug treatment or the type and class of drug. However, administration of *clozapine* does not appear to be associated with development of the condition and in some cases has resulted in improvement of established tardive dyskinesia (see Schizophrenia under Clozapine, p.689). Whether other atypical antipsychotics also have a lower incidence of tardive dyskinesia remains to be established, although there are some data to suggest that this may be the case.[15,16] Symptoms of tardive dyskinesia often develop after discontinuation of the antipsychotic or after dose reduction. Risk factors include old age, female sex, affective disorder, schizophrenia characterised by negative symptoms, and organic brain damage.

Suggested causes of tardive dyskinesia include dopaminergic overactivity, imbalance between dopaminergic and cholinergic activity, supersensitivity of postsynaptic dopamine receptors, presynaptic catecholaminergic hyperfunction, and alterations of the gamma-aminobutyric acid (GABA) system. This has led to trials with antidopaminergics, noradrenergic antagonists, cholinergic drugs, and GABAergic drugs as well as attempts to reverse postsynaptic supersensitivity with dopamine. Although many drugs have been tried in the treatment of tardive dyskinesia there have been relatively few double-blind studies. Reviews of tardive dyskinesia[15,17-19] have concluded that there appeared to be no reliable or safe treatment. Overall, standard antipsychotics appeared to be the most effective in masking symptoms of tardive dyskinesia but tolerance may develop and a worsening of the underlying pathophysiology by antipsychotics had to be assumed on theoretical grounds. Other drugs with antidopaminergic actions which were probably of comparable efficacy included *reserpine, oxypertine, tetrabenazine,* and *metirosine.* The next most effective drugs were considered to be noradrenergic antagonists such as *clonidine*. Some encouraging results had also been obtained with GABAergic drugs such as the *benzodiazepines, baclofen, progabide, valproate,* and *vigabatrin,* although a systematic review[20] of studies of some GABAergic drugs found the evidence unconvincing. The efficacy of cholinergics could not be confirmed. Dopaminergics and antimuscarinics mostly exacerbated symptoms but others[11] had commented that there was no convincing evidence that long-term use of antimuscarinics increased the risk of developing the condition. Other drugs whose value is unclear include *vitamin E,* although a study[21] found favourable results, and some calcium-channel blockers.[22]

In view of the unsatisfactory management of tardive dyskinesia, emphasis is placed on its prevention. Antipsychotics should be prescribed only when clearly indicated, should be given in the minimum dose, and continued only when there is evidence of benefit. Although drug holidays have been suggested for reducing the risk of tardive dyskinesia, the limited evidence indicates that interruptions in drug treatment may increase the risk of both persistent dyskinesia and psychotic relapse. Increasing the dose of antipsychotic generally improves the condition, but only temporarily. Options in the management of tardive dyskinesia include withdrawal of antimuscarinic therapy, and either withdrawal of the antipsychotic or reduction of the dosage to the minimum required or transfer to an atypical antipsychotic. Success is most likely in younger patients. Stopping the drug usually worsens the condition although symptoms often diminish or disappear over a period of weeks or sometimes a year or so. During withdrawal drugs such as *diazepam* or *clonazepam* may be given to alleviate symptoms. Although standard antipsychotics are effective their routine use to suppress symptoms is not recommended but they may be required for acute distressing or life-threatening reactions or in chronic tardive dyskinesia unresponsive to other treatment. In extremely severe resistant cases some have used an antipsychotic with *valproate* or *carbamazepine* or *reserpine* with *metirosine.*


1. Committee on Safety of Medicines/Medicines Control Agency. Drug-induced extrapyramidal reactions. *Current Problems* 1994; **20:** 15–16.
2. Ebadi M, Srinivasan SK. Pathogenesis, prevention, and treatment of neuroleptic-induced movement disorders. *Pharmacol Rev* 1995; **47:** 575–604.
3. Holloman LC, Marder SR. Management of acute extrapyramidal effects induced by antipsychotic drugs. *Am J Health-Syst Pharm* 1997; **54:** 2461–77.
4. Jiménez-Jiménez FJ, *et al.* Drug-induced movement disorders. *Drug Safety* 1997; **16:** 180–204.
5. Bateman DN, *et al.* Extrapyramidal reactions to metoclopramide and prochlorperazine. *Q J Med* 1989; **71:** 307–11.
6. Ereshefsky L, *et al.* Pathophysiologic basis for schizophrenia and the efficacy of antipsychotics. *Clin Pharm* 1990; **9:** 682–707.
7. Miller CH, Fleischhacker WW. Managing antipsychotic-induced acute and chronic akathisia. *Drug Safety* 2000; **22:** 73–81.
8. Koek RJ, Pi EH. Acute laryngeal dystonic reactions to neuroleptics. *Psychosomatics* 1989; **30:** 359–64.
9. van Harten PN, *et al.* Acute dystonia induced by drug treatment. *BMJ* 1999; **319:** 623–6.
10. WHO. Prophylactic use of anticholinergics in patients on long-term neuroleptic treatment: a consensus statement. *Br J Psychiatry* 1990; **156:** 412.
11. Barnes TRE. Comment on the WHO consensus statement. *Br J Psychiatry* 1990; **156:** 413–14.
12. Raja M. Managing antipsychotic-induced acute and tardive dystonia. *Drug Safety* 1998; **19:** 57–72.
13. Moleman P, *et al.* Relationship between age and incidence of parkinsonism in psychiatric patients treated with haloperidol. *Am J Psychiatry* 1986; **143:** 232–4.
14. Mamo DC, *et al.* Managing antipsychotic-induced parkinsonism. *Drug Safety* 1999; **20:** 269–75.
15. Casey DE. Tardive dyskinesia and atypical antipsychotic drugs. *Schizophr Res* 1999; **35** (suppl): S61–S66.
16. Kane JM. Tardive dyskinesia in affective disorders. *J Clin Psychiatry* 1999; **60** (suppl 5): 43–7.
17. Haag H, *et al.*, eds. Tardive Dyskinesia. *WHO Expert Series on Biological Psychiatry Volume 1.* Seattle: Hogrefe & Huber, 1992.
18. Egan MF, *et al.* Treatment of tardive dyskinesia. *Schizophr Bull* 1997; **23:** 583–609.
19. Najib J. Tardive dyskinesia: a review and current treatment options. *Am J Ther* 1999; **6:** 51–60.
20. Soares KVS, *et al.* Gamma-aminobutyric acid agonists for neuroleptic-induced tardive dyskinesia. Available in The Cochrane Library; Issue 1. Chichester: John Wiley; 2004.
21. Adler LA, *et al.* Long-term treatment effects of vitamin E for tardive dyskinesia. *Biol Psychiatry* 1998; **43:** 868–72.
22. Soares KVS, McGrath JJ. Calcium channel blockers for neuroleptic-induced tardive dyskinesia. Available in The Cochrane Library; Issue 2. Chichester: John Wiley; 2004.


**Neuroleptic malignant syndrome.** The neuroleptic malignant syndrome (NMS) is a potentially fatal reaction to a number of drugs including antipsychotics and other dopamine antagonists such as metoclopramide. The clinical **features** of the classic syndrome are usually considered to include hyperthermia, severe extrapyramidal symptoms including muscular rigidity, autonomic dysfunction, and altered levels of consciousness. Skeletal muscle damage may occur and the resulting myoglobinuria may lead to renal failure. However, there appear to be no universal criteria for the diagnosis of the syndrome. Some believe the classic syndrome to be the extreme of a range of effects associated with antipsychotics and have introduced the concept of milder variants or incomplete forms. Others consider it to be a rare idiosyncratic reaction and suggest that the term neuroleptic malignant syndrome should be reserved for the full blown reaction. Consequently, estimates of the **incidence** vary greatly and recent estimates have ranged from 0.02 to 2.5%. The mortality rate has been substantial; although it has decreased over the years with improved diagnosis and management this may also be due to the detection and inclusion of the milder or incomplete variants. Possible risk factors include dehydration, pre-existing organic brain disease, and a history of a previous episode; young males have also been reported to be particularly susceptible.

The **pathogenesis** of NMS is still unclear. Blockade of dopaminergic receptors in the corpus striatum is thought to cause muscular contraction and rigidity generating heat while blockade of dopaminergic receptors in the hypothalamus leads to impaired heat dissipation. Peripheral mechanisms such as vasomotor paralysis may also play a role. Also a syndrome resembling NMS has been seen following withdrawal of treatment with dopamine agonists such as levodopa (see p.1207). Symptoms develop rapidly over 24 to 72 hours and may occur days to months after initiation of antipsychotic medication or increase in dosage, but no consistent correlation with dosage or duration of therapy has been found. Symptoms may last for up to 14 days after cessation of oral antipsychotics, or for up to 4 weeks after cessation of depot preparations. All antipsychotics are capable of inducing the condition; depot preparations may, however, be associated with prolonged recovery from the syndrome if it develops, and hence a higher mortality rate. Concomitant use of lithium carbonate or antimuscarinics may increase the likelihood of developing the syndrome.

Antipsychotic medication should be withdrawn immediately once the diagnosis of the classic syndrome is made; this should be followed by symptomatic and supportive **therapy** including cooling measures, correction of dehydration, and treatment of cardiovascular, respiratory, and renal complications. Whether antipsychotics should be withdrawn from patients with mild attacks and how they should be managed is a matter of debate. The efficacy of specific drug therapy remains to be proven and justification for use is based mainly on case reports. *Dantrolene* was first used because of its effectiveness in malignant hyperthermia. It has a direct action on skeletal muscle and may be particularly effective for the reversal of hyperthermia of muscle origin. In contrast, dopaminergic agonists may resolve hyperthermia of central origin, restoring dopaminergic transmission and hence alleviating extrapyramidal symptoms. There have been isolated reports of success with *amantadine* and *levodopa* but *bromocriptine* is generally preferred. Any underlying psychosis may, however, be aggravated by dopaminergic drugs. In view of the differing modes of action of dantrolene and dopaminergics a combination of the two might be useful but any advantage remains to be demonstrated. *Antimuscarinics* are generally considered to be of little use and may aggravate the associated hyperthermia. *Benzodiazepines* may be used for sedation in agitated patients and may be of use against concomitant catatonia. ECT may be an alternative in refractory cases of NMS or when catatonic symptoms are present.

Re-introduction of antipsychotic therapy may be possible but is not always successful and extreme caution is advised. It has been recommended that a gap of at least 5 to 14 days should be left after resolution of the symptoms before attempting re-introduction.

References.


1. Wells AJ, *et al.* Neuroleptic rechallenge after neuroleptic malignant syndrome: case report and literature review. *Drug Intell Clin Pharm* 1988; **22:** 475–80.
2. Bristow MF, Kohen D. How "malignant" is the neuroleptic malignant syndrome? *BMJ* 1993; **307:** 1223–4.
3. Kornhuber J, Weller M. Neuroleptic malignant syndrome. *Curr Opin Neurol* 1994; **7:** 353–7.
4. Velamoor VR, *et al.* Management of suspected neuroleptic malignant syndrome. *Can J Psychiatry* 1995; **40:** 545–50.
5. Ebadi M, Srinivasan SK. Pathogenesis, prevention, and treatment of neuroleptic-induced movement disorders. *Pharmacol Rev* 1995; **47:** 575–604.
6. Bristow MF, Kohen D. Neuroleptic malignant syndrome. *Br J Hosp Med* 1996; **55:** 517–20.
7. Velamoor VR. Neuroleptic malignant syndrome: recognition, prevention and management. *Drug Safety* 1998; **19:** 73–82.
8. Adnet P, *et al.* Neuroleptic malignant syndrome. *Br J Anaesth* 2000; **85:** 129–35.


**Withdrawal.** Abrupt discontinuation of an antipsychotic may be accompanied by withdrawal symptoms, the most common of which are nausea, vomiting, anorexia, diarrhoea, rhinorrhoea, sweating, myalgias, paraesthesias, insomnia, restlessness, anxiety, and agitation.[1] Patients may also experience vertigo, alternate feelings of warmth and coldness, and tremor. Symptoms generally begin within 1 to 4 days of withdrawal and abate within 7 to 14 days. They are more severe and frequent when antimuscarinics are discontinued simultaneously.


1. Dilsaver SC. Withdrawal phenomena associated with antidepressant and antipsychotic agents. *Drug Safety* 1994; **10:** 103–14.


## Treatment of Adverse Effects

Following an overdose of chlorpromazine patients should be managed with intensive symptomatic and supportive therapy. Activated charcoal should be given by mouth if a substantial amount of the phenothiazine has been taken within 1 hour of presentation, provided that the airway can be protected; emptying the stomach by gastric lavage has sometimes been recommended. Dialysis is of little or no value in poisoning by phenothiazines.

Hypotension should be corrected by raising the patient's legs, or in severe cases by intravascular volume expansion. An inotrope such as dopamine may be considered in refractory cases. If a vasoconstrictor is considered necessary in the management of phenothiazine-induced hypotension the use of adrenaline or other sympathomimetics with high beta-adrenergic agonist properties should be avoided since the alpha-blocking effects of phenothiazines may impair the usual alpha-mediated vasoconstriction of these drugs, resulting in unopposed beta-adrenergic stimulation and increased hypotension.

The treatment of neuroleptic malignant syndrome and the difficulties of treating extrapyramidal side-effects, especially tardive dyskinesia, are discussed above.

## Precautions

Chlorpromazine and other phenothiazines are contra-indicated in patients with pre-existing CNS depression or coma, bone-marrow suppression, phaeochromocytoma, or prolactin-dependent tumours. They should be used with caution or not at all in patients with impaired liver, kidney, cardiovascular, cerebrovascular, and respiratory function and in those with angle-closure glaucoma, a history of jaundice, parkinsonism, diabetes mellitus, hypothyroidism, myasthenia gravis, paralytic ileus, prostatic hyperplasia, or urinary retention. Care is required in patients with epilepsy or a history of seizures as phenothiazines may lower the seizure threshold. Debilitated patients may be more prone to the adverse effects of phenothiazines as may the elderly, especially those with dementia.

The sedative effects of phenothiazines are most marked in the first few days of treatment; affected patients should not drive or operate machinery.

Phenothiazine effects on the vomiting centre may mask the symptoms of overdosage of other drugs, or of disorders such as gastrointestinal obstruction. Use at extremes of temperature may be hazardous since body temperature regulation is impaired by phenothiazines.

Regular eye examinations are advisable for patients receiving long-term phenothiazine therapy and avoidance of undue exposure to direct sunlight is recommended. Phenothiazines should be used with caution in the presence of acute infection or leucopenia. Blood counts are advised if the patient develops an unexplained infection or fever.

Phenothiazines are generally not recommended late in pregnancy; such use may be associated with intoxication of the neonate. Chlorpromazine may prolong labour and should be withheld until the cervix is dilated 3 to 4 cm. For other possible risks of phenothiazines during pregnancy, see below.

Patients should remain supine for at least 30 minutes after parenteral administration of chlorpromazine; blood pressure should be monitored.

Abrupt withdrawal of phenothiazine therapy is best avoided.

**AIDS.** Isolated reports[1,2] have suggested that patients with AIDS may be particularly susceptible to antipsychotic-induced extrapyramidal effects.


1. Hollander H, *et al.* Extrapyramidal symptoms in AIDS patients given low-dose metoclopramide or chlorpromazine. *Lancet* 1985; **ii:** 1186.
2. Edelstein H, Knight RT. Severe parkinsonism in two AIDS patients taking prochlorperazine. *Lancet* 1987; **ii:** 341–2.


**Asthma.** Findings of a retrospective case-control study[1] appeared to indicate that asthmatic patients who receive antipsychotics were at an increased risk of death or near death from asthma.


1. Joseph KS, *et al.* Increased morbidity and mortality related to asthma among asthmatic patients who use major tranquillisers. *BMJ* 1996; **312:** 79–82.


**Breast feeding.** The American Academy of Pediatrics[1] considers that the use of chlorpromazine by mothers during breast feeding may be of concern, since there have been reports of galactorrhoea in the mother and of drowsiness, lethargy, and declines in developmental scores in the infant. The *British National Formulary* considers that the use of antipsychotics such as chlorpromazine should be avoided by breast-feeding mothers unless absolutely necessary.

Chlorpromazine was detected[2] in all milk samples obtained from 4 lactating women at concentrations ranging from 7 to 98 nanograms/mL. Two of the women breast-fed their infants, but one infant showed no effects while the other was noted to be drowsy and lethargic; milk-chlorpromazine concentrations were 7 and 92 nanograms/mL, respectively.


1. American Academy of Pediatrics. The transfer of drugs and other chemicals into human milk. *Pediatrics* 2001; **108:** 776–89. Correction. *ibid.*; 1029. Also available at: http://aappolicy.aappublications.org/cgi/content/full/pediatrics%3b108/3/776 (accessed 28/04/04)
2. Wiles DH, *et al.* Chlorpromazine levels in plasma and milk of nursing mothers. *Br J Clin Pharmacol* 1978; **5:** 272–3.


**Children.** Few phenothiazines are recommended for use in children; in particular there have been concerns about the use of phenothiazine derivatives in infants (see Sudden Infant Death Syndrome, p.439). For reference to the use of chlorpromazine in infants suffering neonatal abstinence syndrome see Substance Dependence, Opioids, under Uses and Administration, below.

References.


1. Dyer KS, Woolf AD. Use of phenothiazines as sedatives in children: what are the risks? *Drug Safety* 1999; **21:** 81–90.


**Contact sensitisation.** Owing to the risk of contact sensitisation health workers should avoid direct contact with chlorpromazine; tablets should not be crushed and solutions should be handled with care.

**The elderly.** The risk of *hip fracture* has been reported to be increased in elderly patients given antipsychotics. A large case-control study in patients over 65 found that current users of antipsychotics had a twofold increase in the risk of hip fractures.[1] The effect was dose-related and the increased risk was similar for chlorpromazine, haloperidol, and thioridazine. It was suggested that antipsychotic-induced sedation or orthostatic hypotension could increase the risk of falls in elderly persons. A study in 12 schizophrenic patients receiving antipsychotics plus other drugs such as antimuscarinics or benzodiazepines has suggested that long-term treatment with antipsychotics may decrease bone mineralisation.[2] A later study suggested that any increased risk of falls might be due to an effect of antipsychotics on balance as thioridazine was found to increase sway in elderly but not young subjects.[3] A meta-analysis of forty studies[4] concluded that there was a small, but consistent, association between the use of most classes of psychotropic drugs, including antipsychotics, and falls. However, the evidence from these studies was based solely on observational data, with minimal adjustment for confounders, dosage, or duration of therapy.

There is some evidence[5,6] to suggest that the use of antipsychotics to manage behavioural complications of *dementia* may increase the rate of cognitive decline. Elderly patients with dementia, especially Lewy-body dementia, are reported to be highly susceptible to the extrapyramidal adverse effects of antipsychotic drugs,[7,8] and the reaction can be extremely serious, even fatal. If these drugs are to be used in elderly patients with dementia, then very low doses should be used, and special care should be taken if the dementia is suspected to be of the Lewy-body type since sudden life-threatening deterioration may occur.[9] Depot preparations should not be used and since dopamine $D_2$ receptors may be involved, it has been suggested that consideration could be given to using an antipsychotic such as clozapine that does not principally antagonise those receptors,[8] although it too is not without its problems.

For further discussion of the problems associated with the use of antipsychotics in disturbed behaviour in the elderly, see p.665.


1. Ray WA, *et al.* Psychotropic drug use and the risk of hip fracture. *N Engl J Med* 1987; **316:** 363–9.
2. Higuchi T, *et al.* Certain neuroleptics reduce bone mineralization in schizophrenic patients. *Neuropsychobiology* 1987; **18:** 185–8.
3. Liu Y, *et al.* Comparative clinical effects of thioridazine (THD) on fall risk on young and elderly subjects. *Clin Pharmacol Ther* 1995; **57:** 200.
4. Leipzig RM, *et al.* Drugs and falls in older people: a systematic review and meta-analysis: I. Psychotropic drugs. *J Am Geriatr Soc* 1999; **47:** 30–9.
5. McShane R, *et al.* Do neuroleptic drugs hasten cognitive decline in dementia? Prospective study with necropsy follow up. *BMJ* 1997; **314:** 266–70.
6. Holmes C, *et al.* Do neuroleptic drugs hasten cognitive decline in dementia? Carriers of apolipoprotein E ε4 allele seem particularly susceptible to their effects. *BMJ* 1997; **314:** 1411.
7. McKeith I, *et al.* Neuroleptic sensitivity in patients with senile dementia of Lewy body type. *BMJ* 1992; **305:** 673–8.
8. Piggott MA, *et al.* DRD2 Ser311/Cys311 polymorphism in schizophrenia. *Lancet* 1994; **343:** 1044–5. Correction. *ibid.*; 1170. [Title: Dopamine D2 receptors in demented patients with severe neuroleptic sensitivity.]
9. Committee on Safety of Medicines/Medicines Control Agency. Neuroleptic sensitivity in patients with dementia. *Current Problems* 1994; **20:** 6.


**Epilepsy.** See Convulsions under Adverse Effects, above.

**Folic acid deficiency.** Concentrations of folate in serum and erythrocytes were reduced in 15 patients receiving long-term treatment with chlorpromazine or thioridazine.[1] All the patients showed significant induction of hepatic microsomal enzymes. It was suggested that folate deficiency due to the induction of microsomal enzymes might subsequently limit enzyme induction and hence reduce drug metabolism, which could lead to symptoms of toxicity in patients apparently stabilised for a number of years. The dietary intake of patients on long-term treatment with enzyme-inducing drugs might be inadequate.


1. Labadarios D, *et al.* The effects of chronic drug administration on hepatic enzyme induction and folate metabolism. *Br J Clin Pharmacol* 1978; **5:** 167–73.


**Hypoparathyroidism.** There have been rare reports[1,2] of acute dystonic reactions associated with the use of phenothiazines in patients with untreated hypoparathyroidism. Caution was recommended in giving phenothiazine derivatives to patients with hypoparathyroidism and it was suggested that any acute reaction to such a drug should prompt investigation for some form of latent tetany.


1. Schaaf M, Payne CA. Dystonic reactions to prochlorperazine in hypoparathyroidism. *N Engl J Med* 1966; **275:** 991–5.
2. Gur H, *et al.* Acute dystonic reaction to methotrimeprazine in hypoparathyroidism. *Ann Pharmacother* 1996; **30:** 957–9.


**Pregnancy.** A review[1] of the use of phenothiazines in pregnancy concluded that there was no clear evidence that these drugs caused a significant increase in fetal malformations. Nevertheless it was considered advisable that if pregnant patients required such treatment, then a single phenothiazine should be used and that it should be one of the established drugs. Use during labour could be effective in controlling nausea and vomiting, but the effects of interactions should be considered, as should the possibility of lethargy and extrapyramidal effects in the neonate due to slow elimination.

Others[2] considered that the criteria for the selection of an antipsychotic for use in pregnant women did not differ from that used in nonpregnant women. It was also concluded that the benefits of continuing antipsychotic treatment at the minimum effective dose would usually outweigh any risks to the fetus.

A subsequent review[3] of the literature reported that women with schizophrenia are generally at increased risk for poor obstetric outcomes including preterm delivery, low birth-weight, and neonates who are small for their gestational age. It was also considered that there was an increased risk of congenital malformation when the fetus was exposed to phenothiazines during weeks 4 to 10 of gestation but this conclusion and the methods used to select the data to review have been criticised.[4]

1. McElhatton PR. The use of phenothiazines during pregnancy and lactation. *Reprod Toxicol* 1992; **6:** 475–90.
2. Trixler M, Tényi T. Antipsychotic use in pregnancy: what are the best treatment options? *Drug Safety* 1997; **16:** 403–10.
3. Patton SW, *et al.* Antipsychotic medication during pregnancy and lactation in women with schizophrenia: evaluating the risk. *Can J Psychiatry* 2002; **47:** 959–65.
4. Levinson A. Review: women with schizophrenia have poorer pregnancy outcomes than other women, but it is unclear whether antipsychotic medications affect their infants. *Evid Based Ment Health* 2003; **6:** 89.

**Renal impairment.** Phenothiazine-induced toxic psychosis occurred in 4 patients with chronic renal failure who had been given chlorpromazine.[1]

1. McAllister CJ, *et al.* Toxic psychosis induced by phenothiazine administration in patients with chronic renal failure. *Clin Nephrol* 1978; **10:** 191–5.

## Interactions

The most common interactions encountered with phenothiazines such as chlorpromazine are those resulting from use with drugs with similar pharmacological actions. Symptoms of CNS depression may be enhanced by other drugs with CNS-depressant properties including alcohol, general anaesthetics, hypnotics, anxiolytics, and opioids. When given with other drugs that produce orthostatic hypotension dosage adjustments may be necessary. However, it should be noted that phenothiazines have been reported to reduce the antihypertensive action of guanethidine and other adrenergic neurone blockers. As many phenothiazines possess antimuscarinic actions they may potentiate the adverse effects of other drugs with antimuscarinic actions, including tricyclic antidepressants and the antimuscarinic antiparkinsonian drugs that may be given to treat phenothiazine-induced extrapyramidal effects. In theory, antipsychotics with dopamine-blocking activity and dopaminergic drugs such as those used to treat parkinsonism may be mutually antagonistic. Concomitant use of metoclopramide may increase the risk of antipsychotic-induced extrapyramidal effects.

There is an increased risk of arrhythmias when antipsychotics are used with drugs that prolong the QT interval, including certain antiarrhythmics, some non-sedating antihistamines, antimalarials, and cisapride; the co-administration of diuretics that cause electrolyte imbalance (particularly hypokalaemia) may also have the same effect. There is also an increased risk of arrhythmia when tricyclic antidepressants are used with antipsychotics that prolong the QT interval.

Because of an increased risk of seizures the US manufacturers of chlorpromazine recommend discontinuation before the use of metrizamide for radiographic procedures.

◊ Most interactions with antipsychotics are as a result of additive pharmacological effects.[1] Since tolerance develops to many of these side-effects, interactions are likely to be most important in the early stages of combination therapy.

1. Livingston MG. Interactions that matter: 11 antipsychotic drugs. *Prescribers' J* 1987; **27** (Dec): 26–9.

**Alcohol.** Akathisia and dystonia occurred after consumption of alcohol by patients taking antipsychotics.[1] Alcohol might lower the threshold of resistance to neurotoxic side-effects.

1. Lutz EG. Neuroleptic-induced akathisia and dystonia triggered by alcohol. *JAMA* 1976; **236:** 2422–3.

**Antacids.** Studies in 6 patients showed that chlorpromazine plasma concentrations were significantly lower after administration of chlorpromazine with an aluminium hydroxide and magnesium trisilicate antacid gel (Gelusil) than after chlorpromazine alone.[1] *In-vitro* studies indicated that chlorpromazine was highly bound to the gel.

1. Fann WE, *et al.* Chlorpromazine: effects of antacids on its gastrointestinal absorption. *J Clin Pharmacol* 1973; **13:** 388–90.

**Antiarrhythmics.** There is an increased risk of arrhythmias when antipsychotics are given with other drugs that prolong the QT interval. It has been recommended that the use of pimozide or thioridazine with antiarrhythmics (especially amiodarone, disopyramide, procainamide, and quinidine) should be avoided. Use of haloperidol with amiodarone is also not recommended. A study[1] in healthy subjects has suggested that quinidine might increase plasma concentrations of haloperidol.

1. Young D, *et al.* Effect of quinidine on the interconversion kinetics between haloperidol and reduced haloperidol in humans: implications for the involvement of cytochrome P450IID6. *Eur J Clin Pharmacol* 1993; **44:** 433–8.

**Antibacterials.** Seven schizophrenic patients whose antitubercular therapy included *rifampicin* (in addition to isoniazid, and in some cases also ethambutol) had lower serum concentrations of haloperidol compared with tuberculotic schizophrenic patients receiving no antimycobacterials and with non-tuberculotic schizophrenics.[1] Pharmacokinetic studies involving some of these patients indicated accelerated haloperidol clearance in the presence of rifampicin. Abnormally high serum-haloperidol concentrations were observed in 3 of 18 patients treated with *isoniazid* alone.

Black galactorrhoea occurred in a patient receiving *minocycline*, perphenazine, amitriptyline hydrochloride, and diphenhydramine hydrochloride.[2] Simultaneous occurrence of phenothiazine-induced galactorrhoea and tetracycline-induced pigmentation was considered responsible.

Sudden cardiac deaths have been reported[3] in patients given *clarithromycin* and pimozide. The manufacturer of pimozide has recommended that pimozide should not be used with macrolide antibacterials.

1. Takeda M, *et al.* Serum haloperidol levels of schizophrenics receiving treatment for tuberculosis. *Clin Neuropharmacol* 1986; **9:** 386–97.
2. Basler RSW, Lynch PJ. Black galactorrhea as a consequence of minocycline and phenothiazine therapy. *Arch Dermatol* 1985; **121:** 417–18.
3. Flockhart DA, *et al.* A metabolic interaction between clarithromycin and pimozide may result in cardiac toxicity. *Clin Pharmacol Ther* 1996; **59:** 189.

**Anticoagulants.** For reference to the effects of some antipsychotics on the activity of anticoagulants, see under Warfarin, p.1026.

**Antidepressants.** Interactions between antipsychotics and *tricyclic antidepressants* are generally of two forms: either additive pharmacological effects such as antimuscarinic effects or hypotension, or pharmacokinetic interactions. Although not commonly reported in the literature additive antimuscarinic activity may be a significant risk especially in the elderly. Careful drug selection might help to prevent the development of serious adverse effects. Mutual inhibition of liver enzymes concerned with the metabolism of both the antipsychotic and the tricyclic antidepressant might result in increased plasma concentrations of either drug. In one study[1] addition of nortriptyline to chlorpromazine therapy produced an increase in plasma concentrations of chlorpromazine but this resulted in a paradoxical increase in agitation and tension.

There is an increased risk of arrhythmias when tricyclic antidepressants are given with other drugs that prolong the QT interval. It has been recommended that the use of pimozide or thioridazine with tricyclic antidepressants should be avoided.

Increased serum concentrations of haloperidol have occurred in patients given haloperidol with *fluoxetine*,[2] *fluvoxamine*,[3] or *nefazodone*. Isolated reports[4-9] of extrapyramidal symptoms, psychoneuromotor syndrome, stupor, bradycardia, and urinary retention associated with use of fluoxetine with antipsychotics suggest that fluoxetine might exacerbate the adverse effects of antipsychotics or produce additive toxicity. Similar CNS effects have been noted in subjects given perphenazine and *paroxetine*.[10] There has also been an isolated report of a patient who complained of amenorrhoea and galactorrhoea after fluvoxamine was added to loxapine therapy.[11] Significant increases in the plasma concentrations of thioridazine have occurred after use with fluvoxamine.[12]

Combinations of antipsychotics and *lithium* should be used with care. Lithium can reduce plasma-chlorpromazine concentrations and there is a report of ventricular fibrillation on withdrawal of lithium from concomitant therapy with chlorpromazine. Chlorpromazine has also been reported to enhance the excretion of lithium. Neurotoxic or extrapyramidal symptoms have been reported rarely in patients taking antipsychotics and lithium; these may be atypical cases of lithium toxicity or neuroleptic malignant syndrome. The above issues are discussed in detail, and references given, on p.303.

A patient on long-term trifluoperazine treatment developed neuroleptic malignant syndrome after a single dose of *venlafaxine*.[13] The authors noted that the manufacturers of venlafaxine have received a small number of similar reports after introduction of venlafaxine in patients receiving antipsychotics including molindone.

There have been occasional reports of sexual disinhibition in patients taking *tryptophan* with phenothiazines.

1. Loga S, *et al.* Interaction of chlorpromazine and nortriptyline in patients with schizophrenia. *Clin Pharmacokinet* 1981; **6:** 454–62.
2. Goff DC, *et al.* Elevation of plasma concentrations of haloperidol after the addition of fluoxetine. *Am J Psychiatry* 1991; **148:** 790–2.
3. Daniel DG, *et al.* Coadministration of fluvoxamine increases serum concentrations of haloperidol. *J Clin Psychopharmacol* 1994; **14:** 340–3.
4. Tate JL. Extrapyramidal symptoms in a patient taking haloperidol and fluoxetine. *Am J Psychiatry* 1989; **146:** 399–400.
5. Ahmed I, *et al.* Possible interaction between fluoxetine and pimozide causing sinus bradycardia. *Can J Psychiatry* 1993; **38:** 62–3.
6. Ketai R. Interaction between fluoxetine and neuroleptics. *Am J Psychiatry* 1993; **150:** 836–7.
7. Hansen-Grant S, *et al.* Fluoxetine-pimozide interaction. *Am J Psychiatry* 1993; **150:** 1751–2.
8. D'Souza DC, *et al.* Precipitation of a psychoneuromotor syndrome by fluoxetine in a haloperidol-treated schizophrenic patient. *J Clin Psychopharmacol* 1994; **14:** 361–3.
9. Benazzi F. Urinary retention with fluoxetine-haloperidol combination in a young patient. *Can J Psychiatry* 1996; **41:** 606–7.
10. Özdemir V, *et al.* Paroxetine potentiates the central nervous system side effects of perphenazine: contribution of cytochrome P4502D6 inhibition in vivo. *Clin Pharmacol Ther* 1997; **62:** 334–47.
11. Jeffries J, *et al.* Amenorrhea and galactorrhea associated with fluvoxamine in a loxapine-treated patient. *J Clin Psychopharmacol* 1992; **12:** 296–7.
12. Carrillo JA, *et al.* Pharmacokinetic interaction of fluvoxamine and thioridazine in schizophrenic patients. *J Clin Psychopharmacol* 1999; **19:** 494–9.
13. Nimmagadda SR, *et al.* Neuroleptic malignant syndrome after venlafaxine. *Lancet* 2000; **354:** 289–90.

**Antidiabetic drugs.** Since chlorpromazine may cause hyperglycaemia or impair glucose tolerance the dose of oral hypoglycaemics or of insulin may need to be increased in diabetics.

**Antiepileptics.** *Carbamazepine*, *phenobarbital*, and *phenytoin* are potent enzyme inducers and use may decrease plasma concentrations of antipsychotics or their active metabolites.[1-5] The clinical effect of any interaction has not been consistent; worsening, improvement, or no change in psychotic symptoms have all been noted. Delirium has been reported in a patient given haloperidol and carbamazepine.[6] Phenytoin might also exacerbate antipsychotic-induced dyskinesia.[7] Care should be taken when withdrawing enzyme-inducing antiepileptics as this may result in a rise in antipsychotic serum concentrations.[8]

The effect of antipsychotics on antiepileptic concentrations is discussed on p.356 (carbamazepine) and p.373 (phenytoin). It should also be remembered that antipsychotics may lower the seizure threshold.

1. Loga S, *et al.* Interactions of orphenadrine and phenobarbitone with chlorpromazine: plasma concentrations and effects in man. *Br J Clin Pharmacol* 1975; **2:** 197–208.
2. Linnoila M, *et al.* Effect of anticonvulsants on plasma haloperidol and thioridazine levels. *Am J Psychiatry* 1980; **137:** 819–21.
3. Jann MW, *et al.* Effects of carbamazepine on plasma haloperidol levels. *J Clin Psychopharmacol* 1985; **5:** 106–9.
4. Arana GW, *et al.* Does carbamazepine-induced reduction of plasma haloperidol levels worsen psychotic symptoms? *Am J Psychiatry* 1986; **143:** 650–1.
5. Ereshefsky L, *et al.* Thiothixene pharmacokinetic interactions: a study of hepatic enzyme inducers, clearance inhibitors, and demographic variables. *J Clin Psychopharmacol* 1991; **11:** 296–301.
6. Kanter GL, *et al.* Case report of a possible interaction between neuroleptics and carbamazepine. *Am J Psychiatry* 1984; **141:** 1101–2.
7. DeVeaugh-Geiss J. Aggravation of tardive dyskinesia by phenytoin. *N Engl J Med* 1978; **298:** 457–8.
8. Jann MW, *et al.* Clinical implications of increased antipsychotic plasma concentrations upon anticonvulsant cessation. *Psychiatry Res* 1989; **28:** 153–9.

**Antihistamines.** For the effect of a preparation containing chlorphenamine maleate and phenylpropanolamine hydrochloride on thioridazine, see Sympathomimetics (below). There is an increased risk of arrhythmias when antipsychotics are given with other drugs that prolong the QT interval. It has been recommended that the use of pimozide or thioridazine with antihistamines such as astemizole or terfenadine should be avoided.

**Antihypertensives.** For discussion of the interaction between phenothiazines and drugs with hypotensive properties, see Interactions, above. For a report of chlorpromazine enhancing the hyperglycaemic effect of diazoxide, see p.893. For reports of hypertension or dementia in patients given methyldopa and antipsychotics, see p.954.

**Antimalarials.** Pretreatment with single doses of *chloroquine sulfate, amodiaquine hydrochloride*, or *sulfadoxine with pyrimethamine* increased the plasma concentrations of chlorpromazine and 7-hydroxychlorpromazine, but not of chlorpromazine sulfoxide, in schizophrenic patients maintained on chlorpromazine.[1] The raised plasma concentrations appeared to be associated with a greater level of sedation.

There is an increased risk of arrhythmias when antipsychotics are given with other drugs that prolong the QT interval. It has been recommended that the use of antipsychotics, and pimozide in particular, with antimalarials such as *halofantrine, mefloquine*, or *quinine* should be avoided. For the possible effects of the use of quinidine with antipsychotics see Antiarrhythmics, above.

1. Makanjuola ROA, *et al.* Effects of antimalarial agents on plasma levels of chlorpromazine and its metabolites in schizophrenic patients. *Trop Geogr Med* 1988; **40:** 31–3.

**Antimigraine drugs.** A report[1] of a patient receiving loxapine who had a dystonic reaction within 15 minutes of subcutaneous administration of *sumatriptan* suggests that these two drugs might interact or potentiate each other's adverse effects. However, the patient had a previous history of dystonic reactions associated with haloperidol and was receiving benzatropine prophylactically. Furthermore, the dose of loxapine had been increased 2 days before the event and this may have predisposed the patient to dystonia.

1. Garcia G, *et al.* Dystonic reaction associated with sumatriptan. *Ann Pharmacother* 1994; **28:** 1199.

**Antiparkinsonian drugs.** Antiparkinsonian drugs are sometimes given with antipsychotics for the management of antipsychotic-induced side-effects including extrapyramidal disorders (see under Adverse Effects, above). Theoretically, dopaminergics such as *levodopa* and *bromocriptine* might induce or exacerbate psychotic symptoms. A study in 18 subjects and review of the literature suggested that bromocriptine can be used safely in patients at risk of psychotic illness provided they are clinically stable and maintained on antipsychotics.[1] Conversely, antipsychotics might antagonise the effects of dopaminergics; diminished therapeutic effects of levodopa have been noted with several antipsychotics (see p.1208) and thioridazine has been reported to oppose the prolactin-lowering action of bromocriptine (see p.1202).

Additive antimuscarinic side-effects are obviously a risk when antimuscarinic antiparkinsonian drugs are given with antipsychotics. Although these are generally mild, serious reactions have occurred. *Trihexyphenidyl*[2] and *orphenadrine*[3] have both been reported to decrease plasma concentrations of chlorpromazine, possibly by interfering with absorption from the gastrointestinal tract. Reports suggesting that antimuscarinics may antagonise the antipsychotic effects of antipsychotics at the neurotransmitter level require substantiating.

1. Perovich RM, *et al.* The behavioral toxicity of bromocriptine in patients with psychiatric illness. *J Clin Psychopharmacol* 1989; **9:** 417–22.
2. Rivera-Calimlim L, *et al.* Effects of mode of management on plasma chlorpromazine in psychiatric patients. *Clin Pharmacol Ther* 1973; **14:** 978–86.
3. Loga S, *et al.* Interactions of orphenadrine and phenobarbitone with chlorpromazine: plasma concentrations and effects in man. *Br J Clin Pharmacol* 1975; **2:** 197–208.

**Antipsychotics.** Elevated plasma levels of haloperidol were reported[1] in a patient being treated for schizophrenia when *chlorpromazine* or *clozapine* were also given.

1. Allen SA. Effect of chlorpromazine and clozapine on plasma concentrations of haloperidol in a patient with schizophrenia. *J Clin Pharmacol* 2000; **40:** 1296–7.

**Antivirals.** *Ritonavir* may increase the plasma concentration of some antipsychotics. The increases expected for pimozide were considered by the manufacturer of ritonavir to be large enough to recommend that these drugs should not be used together. Other classical antipsychotics predicted to have increases include haloperidol, perphenazine, and thioridazine and it was recommended that monitoring of drug concentrations and/or adverse effects were required when used with ritonavir.

**Beta blockers.** Chlorpromazine and propranolol may mutually inhibit each other's hepatic metabolism. *Propranolol* has been reported to increase plasma concentrations of chlorpromazine[1] and thioridazine,[2,3] and *pindolol* to increase plasma-thioridazine concentrations.[4] Neither beta blocker tested had a significant effect on haloperidol concentrations,[3,4] although there is a report of severe hypotension or cardiopulmonary arrest occurring on 3 occasions in a schizophrenic patient given haloperidol and propranolol concomitantly.[5] The clinical significance of antipsychotic-beta blocker interactions is unclear.

For the effect of chlorpromazine on propranolol, see under Beta Blockers, p.871.

There is an increased risk of arrhythmias when antipsychotics are given with other drugs that prolong the QT interval. The concomitant use of antipsychotics, and pimozide in particular, with *sotalol* should be avoided.

1. Peet M, *et al.* Pharmacokinetic interaction between propranolol and chlorpromazine in schizophrenic patients. *Lancet* 1980; **ii:** 978.
2. Silver JM, *et al.* Elevation of thioridazine plasma levels by propranolol. *Am J Psychiatry* 1986; **143:** 1290–2.
3. Greendyke RM, Kanter DR. Plasma propranolol levels and their effect on plasma thioridazine and haloperidol concentrations. *J Clin Psychopharmacol* 1987; **7:** 178–82.
4. Greendyke RM, Gulya A. Effect of pindolol administration on serum levels of thioridazine, haloperidol, phenytoin, and phenobarbital. *J Clin Psychiatry* 1988; **49:** 105–7.
5. Alexander HE, *et al.* Hypotension and cardiopulmonary arrest associated with concurrent haloperidol and propranolol therapy. *JAMA* 1984; **252:** 87–8.

**Buspirone.** The use of haloperidol with buspirone has resulted in increased serum haloperidol concentrations. However, while some[1] found the mean rise in serum-haloperidol concentrations to be 26%, that observed by others[2] was not statistically significant.

1. Goff DC, *et al.* An open trial of buspirone added to neuroleptics in schizophrenic patients. *J Clin Psychopharmacol* 1991; **11:** 193–7.
2. Huang HF, *et al.* Lack of pharmacokinetic interaction between buspirone and haloperidol in patients with schizophrenia. *J Clin Pharmacol* 1996; **36:** 963–9.

**Cimetidine.** Despite expectations that cimetidine might reduce the metabolism of chlorpromazine, mean steady-state plasma concentrations of chlorpromazine fell rather than rose in 8 patients given cimetidine for 7 days in addition to regular chlorpromazine therapy.[1] The explanation was probably that cimetidine interfered with chlorpromazine absorption. Excessive sedation, necessitating a reduction in chlorpromazine dosage, has been reported[2] after addition of cimetidine to the drug therapy of 2 chronic schizophrenics.

1. Howes CA, *et al.* Reduced steady-state plasma concentrations of chlorpromazine and indomethacin in patients receiving cimetidine. *Eur J Clin Pharmacol* 1983; **24:** 99–102.
2. Byrne A, O'Shea B. Adverse interaction between cimetidine and chlorpromazine in two cases of chronic schizophrenia. *Br J Psychiatry* 1989; **155:** 413–15.

**Cocaine.** The risk of antipsychotic-induced dystonic reactions may be increased in cocaine abusers. Dystonia occurred in 6 of 7 cocaine abusers treated with haloperidol.[1]

1. Kumor K, *et al.* Haloperidol-induced dystonia in cocaine addicts. *Lancet* 1986; **ii:** 1341–2.

**Desferrioxamine.** Loss of consciousness lasting 48 to 72 hours occurred in 2 patients given prochlorperazine during desferrioxamine therapy.[1] Prochlorperazine may enhance the removal of transition metals from brain cells by desferrioxamine.

1. Blake DR, *et al.* Cerebral and ocular toxicity induced by desferrioxamine. *Q J Med* 1985; **56:** 345–55.

**Disulfiram.** A psychotic patient, previously maintained with plasma-perphenazine concentrations of 2 to 3 nanomoles/mL on a dose of 8 mg twice daily by mouth, was readmitted with subtherapeutic plasma-perphenazine concentrations of less than 1 nanomole/mL, despite unchanged dosage, following disulfiram therapy.[1] The concentration of the sulfoxide metabolite of perphenazine was much increased. Following a change from oral to intramuscular perphenazine therapy there was a substantial clinical improvement associated with a return to therapeutic plasma concentrations of perphenazine and a fall in concentration of the metabolite. Disulfiram appears to greatly enhance biotransformation of oral perphenazine to inactive metabolites, but parenteral administration avoids the 'first-pass' effect in the liver.

1. Hansen LB, Larsen N-E. Metabolic interaction between perphenazine and disulfiram. *Lancet* 1982; **ii:** 1472.

**General anaesthetics.** A schizophrenic patient without a history of epilepsy who was receiving oral chlorpromazine and flupentixol depot injection had a convulsive seizure when given *enflurane* anaesthesia.[1]

1. Vohra SB. Convulsions after enflurane in a schizophrenic patient receiving neuroleptics. *Can J Anaesth* 1994; **41:** 420–2.

**Naltrexone.** Two patients maintained on thioridazine experienced intense sleepiness and lethargy after receiving 2 doses of naltrexone.[1]

1. Maany I, *et al.* Interaction between thioridazine and naltrexone. *Am J Psychiatry* 1987; **144:** 966.

**NSAIDs.** A report of severe drowsiness and confusion in patients given haloperidol with *indometacin*.[1]

1. Bird HA, *et al.* Drowsiness due to haloperidol/indomethacin in combination. *Lancet* 1983; **i:** 830–1.

**Opioid analgesics.** For reference to the effects of phenothiazines on *pethidine*, see p.81.

**Piperazine.** There has been an isolated report[1] of convulsions associated with the use of chlorpromazine in a child who had received piperazine several days earlier. Subsequent *animal*[1-3] studies produced conflicting evidence for an interaction and it was suggested[3] that an interaction would only be clinically significant when high concentrations of piperazine were reached in the body.

1. Boulos BM, Davis LE. Hazard of simultaneous administration of phenothiazine and piperazine. *N Engl J Med* 1969; **280:** 1245–6.
2. Armbrecht BH. Reaction between piperazine and chlorpromazine. *N Engl J Med* 1970; **282:** 1490–1.
3. Sturman G. Interaction between piperazine and chlorpromazine. *Br J Pharmacol* 1974; **50:** 153–5.

**Sympathomimetics.** For reference to the possible interaction between phenothiazines and *adrenaline*, see Treatment of Adverse Effects, above.

A 27-year-old woman with schizophrenia and T-wave abnormality of the heart,[1] receiving thioridazine 100 mg daily with procyclidine 2.5 mg twice daily, died from ventricular fibrillation within 2 hours of also taking a single dose of a preparation reported to contain chlorphenamine maleate 4 mg with *phenylpropanolamine hydrochloride* 50 mg (Contac C).

1. Chouinard G, *et al.* Death attributed to ventricular arrhythmia induced by thioridazine in combination with a single Contac C capsule. *Can Med Assoc J* 1978; **119:** 729–31.

**Tobacco smoking.** Smoking has been shown to decrease the incidence of chlorpromazine-induced sedation[1,2] and orthostatic hypotension.[2] Studies indicate that the clearance of chlorpromazine,[3] fluphenazine,[4] tiotixene,[5] and haloperidol[6] may be increased in patients who smoke. It has been suggested that some of the components of smoke may act as liver-enzyme inducers. The clinical significance of this effect is unclear but the possible need to use increased doses in smokers should be borne in mind.

1. Swett C. Drowsiness due to chlorpromazine in relation to cigarette smoking: a report from the Boston Collaborative Drug Surveillance Program. *Arch Gen Psychiatry* 1974; **31:** 211–13.
2. Pantuck EJ, *et al.* Cigarette smoking and chlorpromazine disposition and actions. *Clin Pharmacol Ther* 1982; **31:** 533–8.
3. Chetty M, *et al.* Smoking and body weight influence the clearance of chlorpromazine. *Eur J Clin Pharmacol* 1994; **46:** 523–6.
4. Ereshefsky L, *et al.* Effects of smoking on fluphenazine clearance in psychiatric inpatients. *Biol Psychiatry* 1985; **20:** 329–32.
5. Ereshefsky L, *et al.* Thiothixene pharmacokinetic interactions: a study of hepatic enzyme inducers, clearance inhibitors, and demographic variables. *J Clin Psychopharmacol* 1991; **11:** 296–301.
6. Jann MW, *et al.* Effects of smoking on haloperidol and reduced haloperidol plasma concentrations and haloperidol clearance. *Psychopharmacology (Berl)* 1986; **90:** 468–70.

**Vitamins.** Administration of ascorbic acid, for vitamin C deficiency, to a patient receiving fluphenazine for bipolar disorder was associated with a fall in serum concentrations of fluphenazine and a deterioration of behaviour.[1]

1. Dysken MW, *et al.* Drug interaction between ascorbic acid and fluphenazine. *JAMA* 1979; **241:** 2008.

**Xanthine-containing beverages.** Studies *in vitro* have shown precipitation of some antipsychotics from solution by addition of coffee and tea.[1,2] However, in a study of 16 patients taking antipsychotics no correlation could be found between plasma-antipsychotic concentrations or behaviour and tea or coffee consumption.[3]

1. Kulhanek F, *et al.* Precipitation of antipsychotic drugs in interaction with coffee or tea. *Lancet* 1979; **ii:** 1130.
2. Lasswell WL, *et al.* In vitro interaction of neuroleptics and tricyclic antidepressants with coffee, tea, and gallotannic acid. *J Pharm Sci* 1984; **73:** 1056–8.
3. Bowen S, *et al.* Effect of coffee and tea on blood levels and efficacy of antipsychotic drugs. *Lancet* 1981; **i:** 1217–18.

## Pharmacokinetics

Chlorpromazine is readily, although sometimes erratically, absorbed from the gastrointestinal tract; peak plasma concentrations are attained 2 to 4 hours after ingestion. It is subject to considerable first-pass metabolism in the gut wall and is also extensively metabolised in the liver and is excreted in the urine and bile in the form of numerous active and inactive metabolites; there is some evidence of enterohepatic recycling. Owing to the first-pass effect, plasma concentrations following oral administration are much lower than those after intramuscular administration. Moreover, there is very wide intersubject variation in plasma concentrations of chlorpromazine; no simple correlation has been found between plasma concentrations of chlorpromazine and its metabolites, and their therapeutic effect (see Administration under Uses and Administration, below). Paths of metabolism of chlorpromazine include hydroxylation and conjugation with glucuronic acid, *N*-oxidation, oxidation of a sulfur atom, and dealkylation. Although the plasma half-life of chlorpromazine itself has been reported to be about 30 hours, elimination of the metabolites may be very prolonged. There is limited evidence that chlorpromazine induces its own metabolism.

Chlorpromazine is about 95 to 98% bound to plasma proteins. It is widely distributed in the body and crosses the blood-brain barrier to achieve higher concentrations in the brain than in the plasma. Chlorpromazine and its metabolites also cross the placenta and are distributed into breast milk.

◊ References.

1. Rivera-Calimlim L, *et al.* Plasma chlorpromazine concentrations in children with behavioral disorders and mental illness. *Clin Pharmacol Ther* 1979; **26:** 114–21.
2. Furlanut M, *et al.* Chlorpromazine disposition in relation to age in children. *Clin Pharmacokinet* 1990; **18:** 329–31.
3. Caccia S, Garattini S. Formation of active metabolites of psychotropic drugs: an updated review of their significance. *Clin Pharmacokinet* 1990; **18:** 434–59.
4. Yeung PK-F, *et al.* Pharmacokinetics of chlorpromazine and key metabolites. *Eur J Clin Pharmacol* 1993; **45:** 563–9.

## Uses and Administration

Chlorpromazine is a phenothiazine antipsychotic. It has a wide range of activity arising from its depressant actions on the CNS and its alpha-adrenergic blocking and antimuscarinic activities. Chlorpromazine is a dopamine inhibitor; the turnover of dopamine in the brain is also increased. There is some evidence that the antagonism of central dopaminergic function, especially at the $D_2$-dopaminergic receptor, is related to therapeutic effect in psychotic conditions. Chlorpromazine possesses sedative properties but patients usually develop tolerance rapidly to the sedation. It has antiemetic, serotonin-blocking, and weak antihistaminic properties and slight ganglion-blocking activity. It inhibits the heat-regulating centre so that the patient tends to acquire the temperature of the surroundings (poikilothermy). Chlorpromazine can relax skeletal muscle.

Chlorpromazine is widely used in the management of psychotic conditions as well as in some non-psychotic disorders, such as:

- acute and chronic schizophrenia (p.665) in adults and children
- to reduce acute mania, as in bipolar disorder (p.278)
- control of severely disturbed, agitated, or violent behaviour in adults and children (p.665) and sometimes other psychiatric conditions
- in autistic children
- as an adjunct for the short-term treatment of severe anxiety (but see also p.663), and to reduce pre-operative anxiety in adults and children
- as an antiemetic in some forms of nausea and vomiting (p.1245) in adults and children; it is ineffective in motion sickness
- in the alleviation of intractable hiccup (below)
- as an adjunct in the treatment of tetanus in adults and children (p.149 and p.1398) and to control symptoms in acute intermittent porphyria (p.1040)

Chlorpromazine is administered by mouth as the hydrochloride and the embonate. For both salts, the doses are expressed as the hydrochloride; chlorpromazine embonate 144 mg is approximately equivalent to 100 mg chlorpromazine hydrochloride. Chlorpromazine is also given by injection as the hydrochloride and doses are expressed in terms of this salt. The base is given rectally as suppositories; doses are in terms of the base.

Dosage varies both with the individual and with the purpose for which the drug is being used. In most patients with **psychiatric conditions** *oral treatment* may be used from the start, typically commencing with a dosage of 25 mg of the hydrochloride, or its equivalent as the embonate, three times daily and increasing as necessary; daily doses of 75 mg may be given as a single dose at night. In some patients doses of 10 mg three times daily may be adequate. Maintenance doses, when required, usually range from 25 to 100 mg three times daily, although psychotic patients may require daily doses of up to 1 g or more.

For *parenteral use*, deep intramuscular injection is preferable, but diluted solutions have sometimes been given by slow intravenous infusion for indications such as tetanus, severe intractable hiccup, or nausea and vomiting associated with surgery. Subcutaneous injection is contra-indicated. After injection of chlorpromazine, patients should remain in the supine position for at least 30 minutes; blood pressure should be monitored. The usual dose by intramuscular injection is 25 to 50 mg repeated every 6 to 8 hours if required although oral therapy should be substituted as soon as possible.

If the oral and parenteral routes are not suitable chlorpromazine may be administered *rectally* as suppositories containing 100 mg of chlorpromazine base; this is stated to have an effect comparable with 40 to 50 mg of the hydrochloride by mouth or 20 to 25 mg intramuscularly. Up to 4 suppositories may be given in 24 hours.

Initial oral doses of chlorpromazine of one-third to one-half the usual adult dose have been recommended for *elderly* or *debilitated patients*; doses should be increased more gradually. Intramuscular doses in the elderly may need to be reduced to up to one-quarter of the usual dose.

Chlorpromazine hydrochloride may be given to *children* aged 1 to 12 years in a dose of 500 micrograms/kg every 4 to 6 hours by mouth or every 6 to 8 hours by intramuscular injection, but for psychiatric indications the oral dose for children aged over 5 years is usually one-third to one-half the adult dose. Daily doses should not normally exceed 40 mg of chlorpromazine hydrochloride for children aged 1 to 5 years or 75 mg for children over 5 years of age. Chlorpromazine may be given to infants under 1 year of age if considered to be life-saving. Suppositories containing 25 mg of chlorpromazine base are available in some countries for use in children.

Doses of 10 to 25 mg every 4 to 6 hours by mouth are recommended for control of **nausea and vomiting**. If necessary, an initial dose of 25 mg may be given by intramuscular injection, followed by 25 to 50 mg every 3 to 4 hours until vomiting stops.

If **intractable hiccup** does not respond to 25 to 50 mg three or four times daily by mouth for 2 to 3 days then 25 to 50 mg may be given intramuscularly; if this fails 25 to 50 mg in 500 to 1000 mL of 0.9% sodium chloride intravenous infusion should be given by slow intravenous infusion, with the patient supine, and careful monitoring of the blood pressure.

**Action.** The therapeutic effects of antipsychotics appear to be mediated, at least in part, by interference with dopamine transmission in the brain. Chlorpromazine, thioridazine, and thioxanthene derivatives have relatively equal affinity for $D_1$ or $D_2$ receptors, although their metabolites tend to be more potent as $D_2$ blockers.[1] Butyrophenones (such as haloperidol) and diphenylbutylpiperidines (such as pimozide) are relatively selective for $D_2$ receptors, and the substituted benzamides such as sulpiride are highly $D_2$-specific. Clozapine has complex actions; it is a relatively weak inhibitor of $D_2$ receptors but has a high affinity for a number of other receptors including $D_1$, $D_4$, and serotonin$_2$ (5-$HT_2$) receptors.[2] Other atypicals mostly share this profile of greater 5-$HT_2$ than $D_2$ antagonism.[2]

The traditional hypothesis of the action of antipsychotics has been that blockade of $D_2$ receptors in the limbic and cortical regions is responsible for the antipsychotic effects, and that extrapyramidal motor side-effects result from blockade of $D_2$ receptors in the striatum (a typical motor region of the basal ganglia).[3] Modification of prolactin secretion results from blockade of $D_2$ receptors in the anterior pituitary. However, this hypothesis cannot satisfactorily account for the pharmacological profiles of atypical antipsychotics and the debate concerning their mechanism of action continues. It has been suggested that the balance between 5-$HT_2$ and $D_2$ antagonism is important in determining 'atypicality' (but the atypical antipsychotic amisulpride lacks marked 5-$HT_2$ antagonism), or that rapid dissociation from the $D_2$ receptor may be the determining factor (but it is not clear that some atypicals such as risperidone meet this criterion).[2] Other systems, such as glutamate, may play a role in modulating effectiveness against negative versus positive symptoms;[2] it has been suggested that the calcium antagonist actions of the diphenylbutylpiperidines may also be important in this respect.[4]

Division of antipsychotics into low- and high-potency drugs is discussed under Administration, below. For reference to the actions of antipsychotics on neuroendocrine function, see Effects on Endocrine Function under Adverse Effects, above.

1. Ereshefsky L, *et al*. Pathophysiologic basis for schizophrenia and the efficacy of antipsychotics. *Clin Pharm* 1990; **9:** 682–707.
2. Remington G. Understanding antipsychotic 'atypicality': a clinical and pharmacological moving target. *J Psychiatry Neurosci* 2003; **28:** 275–84.
3. Anonymous. Now we understand antipsychotics? *Lancet* 1990; **336:** 1222–3.
4. Snyder SH. Drug and neurotransmitter receptors: new perspectives with clinical relevance. *JAMA* 1989; **261:** 3126–9.

**Administration.** The classical antipsychotics are often divided into:

- **low-potency** drugs (phenothiazines with an aliphatic or piperidine side-chain or thioxanthenes with an aliphatic side-chain)
- **high-potency** drugs (butyrophenones, diphenylbutylpiperidines, and phenothiazines or thioxanthenes with a piperazine side-chain).

At doses with equipotent antipsychotic activity, the low-potency drugs are more prone to cause sedation and antimuscarinic or α-adrenergic-blocking effects than the high-potency drugs. However, they are associated with a lower incidence of extrapyramidal effects, with the exception of tardive dyskinesia which is likely to occur to the same extent with all conventional antipsychotics.

*Equivalent doses* of antipsychotics quoted in the literature have varied considerably. In the UK the following daily doses of oral antipsychotics have been suggested to have approximately equipotent antipsychotic activity for doses up to the maximum licensed doses:

- chlorpromazine hydrochloride 100 mg
- clozapine 50 mg
- haloperidol 2 to 3 mg
- pimozide 2 mg
- risperidone 0.5 to 1 mg
- sulpiride 200 mg
- thioridazine 100 mg
- trifluoperazine 5 mg.

In specialist psychiatric units where very high doses are required the equivalent dose of haloperidol might be up to 10 mg. It should be noted that all patients receiving pimozide require an annual ECG and all those receiving more than 16 mg of pimozide daily require periodic ECGs (see p.715).

Suggested equipotent doses of intramuscular depot antipsychotics are:

- flupentixol decanoate 40 mg every 2 weeks
- fluphenazine decanoate 25 mg every 2 weeks
- haloperidol (as the decanoate) 100 mg every 4 weeks
- pipotiazine palmitate 50 mg every 4 weeks
- zuclopenthixol decanoate 200 mg every 2 weeks.

It has been noted[1] that *high doses* of antipsychotics (greater than the equivalent of 600 mg of chlorpromazine daily) are generally not necessary for the treatment (both initial and maintenance) of psychotic disorders, and may be associated with an increased risk of side-effects as well as with a diminished clinical response. However, if high doses of antipsychotics have to be used, then doses should be increased gradually with caution and under the supervision of a specialist with facilities for emergency resuscitation available. The Royal College of Psychiatrists in the UK has issued advice for those considering the use of high doses of antipsychotics.[2]

- When patients have failed to respond to recommended doses of two different antipsychotics the diagnosis, patient compliance, and the duration of treatment already given should be reviewed before increasing the dose
- Alternative approaches to treatment including the use of adjuvant therapy or clozapine should also be considered
- Contra-indications to high-dose therapy such as cardiac disease and hepatic and renal impairment and other risk factors such as obesity and old age should be borne in mind
- An ECG should be carried out to exclude QT prolongation and repeated every 1 to 3 months while the dose remains high. The dose should be reduced if a prolonged QT interval develops
- Regular checks on pulse, blood pressure, temperature, and hydration are also advised
- If possible dosage should be increased gradually at intervals of at least one week
- The use of high-dose therapy should be considered as a limited course. The patient should be reviewed regularly and the dose reduced back to accepted levels after 3 months if there has been no improvement

The existence of a *therapeutic range* (or therapeutic window) has not been demonstrated for most antipsychotics (with the possible exception of haloperidol[3]), and plasma concentrations of these drugs must be interpreted with caution.[1,3] Many factors make it difficult to establish a meaningful correlation between dose, plasma concentrations, and clinical improvement. These include incomplete absorption, first-pass effect, enzyme induction, the presence of active and inactive metabolites, ethnic group, smoking, and factors occurring at the receptor level.[3]

1. Baldessarini RJ, *et al*. Significance of neuroleptic dose and plasma level in the pharmacological treatment of psychoses. *Arch Gen Psychiatry* 1988; **45:** 77–91.
2. The Royal College of Psychiatrists. Consensus statement on the use of high dose antipsychotic medication. *Council Report CR26* London: Royal College of Psychiatrists, October 1993. Also in: Thompson C. Royal College of Psychiatrists' Consensus Panel. The use of high-dose antipsychotic medication. *Br J Psychiatry* 1994; **164:** 448–58.
3. Sramek JJ, *et al*. Neuroleptic plasma concentrations and clinical response: in search of a therapeutic window. *Drug Intell Clin Pharm* 1988; **22:** 373–80.

**Administration in children.** For reference to the use of lytic cocktails containing chlorpromazine, promethazine, and pethidine and the view that alternatives should be considered in children, see Lytic Coctails under Sedation, p.82.

**Bipolar disorder.** Patients with bipolar disorder (p.278) suffering from acute mania with coexisting psychotic features, agitation, or disruptive behaviour are usually treated with antipsychotics as they produce rapid control of symptoms. Classical antipsychotics such as chlorpromazine or haloperidol have been widely used, although use of atypical antipsychotics, such as clozapine or olanzapine, is growing.

**Chorea.** For a discussion of the management of various choreas, including mention of the use of phenothiazines such as chlorpromazine, see p.664.

**Dyspnoea.** It has been shown that in healthy subjects an oral dose of 25 mg of chlorpromazine hydrochloride can reduce exercise-induced breathlessness without affecting ventilation or causing sedation.[1] Some workers[2] have reported that chlorpromazine relieves air hunger in patients with advanced cancer and dyspnoea (p.74) unresponsive to other measures and, if required, can be used to sedate dying patients who have unrelieved distress. It is recommended that initial doses should be small; 12.5 mg by slow intravenous injection or 25 mg by suppository may be given.

1. O'Neill PA, *et al*. Chlorpromazine—a specific effect on breathlessness? *Br J Clin Pharmacol* 1985; **19:** 793–7.
2. Walsh D. Dyspnoea in advanced cancer. *Lancet* 1993; **342:** 450–1.

**Dystonia.** Antipsychotics such as phenothiazines, haloperidol, or pimozide are sometimes useful in the treatment of idiopathic dystonia (p.1209) in patients who have failed to respond to other drugs.[1] However, they often act non-specifically, damping down excessive movements by causing a degree of drug-induced parkinsonism and there is the risk of adding drug-induced extrapyramidal disorders to the dystonia being treated (see Extrapyramidal Disorders under Adverse Effects, above).

1. Marsden CD, Quinn NP. The dystonias. *BMJ* 1990; **300:** 139–44.

**Eclampsia and pre-eclampsia.** Drug combinations known as lytic cocktails have been used in many countries for the management of pre-eclampsia and imminent eclampsia. The cocktail has usually consisted of a combination of chlorpromazine, pethidine, and/or promethazine. However, phenothiazines are not generally recommended late in pregnancy and other treatments are preferred for hypertension (see Hypertension in Pregnancy, under Hypertension, p.825); the management of eclampsia, which is the convulsive phase, is discussed on p.352.

**Headache.** The phenothiazines chlorpromazine and prochlorperazine have been used in migraine to control severe nausea and vomiting unresponsive to antiemetics such as metoclopramide and domperidone (see p.464). Parenteral phenothiazines may also relieve the pain of severe migraine attacks unresponsive to parenteral dihydroergotamine or sumatriptan.

References.

1. Stiell IG, *et al.* Methotrimeprazine versus meperidine and dimenhydrinate in the treatment of severe migraine: a randomized, controlled trial. *Ann Emerg Med* 1991; **20:** 1201–5.
2. Jones EB, *et al.* Safety and efficacy of rectal prochlorperazine for the treatment of migraine in the emergency department. *Ann Emerg Med* 1994; **24:** 237–41.
3. Coppola M, *et al.* Randomized, placebo-controlled evaluation of prochlorperazine versus metoclopramide for emergency department treatment of migraine headache. *Ann Emerg Med* 1995; **26:** 541–6.
4. Jones J, *et al.* Intramuscular prochlorperazine versus metoclopramide as single-agent therapy for the treatment of acute migraine headache. *Am J Emerg Med* 1996; **14:** 262–4.
5. Kelly AM, *et al.* Intravenous chlorpromazine versus intramuscular sumatriptan for acute migraine. *J Accid Emerg Med* 1997; **14:** 209–11.
6. Bigal ME, *et al.* Intravenous chlorpromazine in the emergency department treatment of migraines: a randomized controlled trial. *J Emerg Med* 2002; **23:** 141–8.

**Hiccup.** A hiccup is an involuntary spasmodic contraction of the diaphragm which causes a sudden inspiration of air which is then checked abruptly by closure of the glottis. Hiccups often have a simple cause such as gastric distension and usually resolve spontaneously or respond to simple measures. Intractable hiccups may stem from a serious underlying cause such as brain disorders, metabolic or endocrine disturbances, CNS infections, and oesophageal or other gastrointestinal disorders. Other precipitants include anaesthesia or drug therapy.

Treatment of intractable hiccups should initially be aimed at controlling or removing the underlying cause including the relief of gastric distension or oesophageal obstruction.[1-4] Measures that raise carbon dioxide pressure such as breath holding, rebreathing, or alteration of normal respiratory rhythm can be effective. Stimulation of the pharynx can also interrupt hiccups and may explain the action of a host of remedies such as sipping iced water, gargling, and swallowing granulated sugar. Many drugs have been tried in the treatment of hiccups but evidence of efficacy is largely from anecdotal reports or uncontrolled studies. However, the following treatment protocol[5] has been formulated for intractable hiccups from a review of the early literature and the authors' experience:

- correct any metabolic abnormality, then granulated sugar should be swallowed dry; if this is successful the sugar should be repeated if hiccups recur
- if not effective, pass nasogastric tube, decompress stomach, then irritate pharynx; if successful, repeat if hiccups recur
- if stimulation is unsuccessful, give chlorpromazine 25 to 50 mg intravenously; repeat up to 3 times if necessary; if parenteral therapy is effective maintain on chlorpromazine by mouth for 10 days (some manufacturers recommend the use of oral therapy first and if symptoms persist for 2 to 3 days they then recommend one dose by the intramuscular route followed if necessary by a slow intravenous infusion of a dilute solution—see under Uses and Administration, above)
- if hiccups are not controlled by chlorpromazine give metoclopramide 10 mg intravenously and if successful maintain on metoclopramide by mouth for 10 days
- if metoclopramide is not effective give quinidine 200 mg by mouth 4 times daily
- if this fails consider left phrenic nerve block and crush.

In later discussions[1,3] chlorpromazine still emerged as the most consistently effective drug treatment; metoclopramide appeared to be an acceptable second choice and nifedipine an appropriate third choice,[3] although haloperidol was also considered to be of value.[1,4] Other phenothiazines that have been used for intractable hiccup include perphenazine and promazine. It was also considered that clonazepam, carbamazepine, phenytoin, and valproic acid might be of value, especially in neuropathic hiccups.[1] Further reports had described some beneficial results with amitriptyline, amantadine, and baclofen.

Other methods which have been used in the treatment of hiccups include swallowing a solution of lidocaine.

1. Howard RS. Persistent hiccups: if excluding or treating any underlying pathology fails try chlorpromazine. *BMJ* 1992; **305:** 1237–8.
2. Rousseau P. Hiccups. *South Med J* 1995; **88:** 175–81.
3. Friedman NL. Hiccups: a treatment review. *Pharmacotherapy* 1996; **16:** 986–95.
4. WHO. Hiccup. In: *Symptom relief in terminal illness.* Geneva: WHO, 1998.
5. Williamson BWA, Macintyre IMC. Management of intractable hiccup. *BMJ* 1977; **2:** 501–3.

**Lesch-Nyhan syndrome.** The Lesch-Nyhan syndrome is an inherited disorder caused by a complete deficiency of hypoxanthine-guanine phosphoribosyl transferase, an enzyme involved in purine metabolism. It is characterised by hyperuricaemia, spasticity, choreoathetosis, self-mutilation, and mental retardation. The hyperuricaemia (see p.412) can be controlled by drugs such as allopurinol but there appears to be no effective treatment for the neurological deficits. It has been suggested that the behavioural problems might be associated with alterations in the brain's dopamine system. There have been rare reports of improvement in self-mutilation in patients given antipsychotics or antiepileptics such as carbamazepine and gabapentin.

References.

1. Nyhan WL, Wong DF. New approaches to understanding Lesch-Nyhan disease. *N Engl J Med* 1996; **334:** 1602–4.

**Migraine.** See under Headache, above.

**Nausea and vomiting.** Many antipsychotics, with the notable exception of thioridazine, have antiemetic properties and have been used in the prevention and treatment of nausea and vomiting (p.1245) arising from a variety of causes such as radiation sickness, malignancy, and emesis caused by drugs, including antineoplastics and opioid analgesics. Reference to the risk to the fetus of antiemetic therapy with phenothiazines during pregnancy can be found under Precautions, above.

**Schizophrenia.** Classical antipsychotics such as chlorpromazine, haloperidol, and thioridazine have been the traditional drug treatment of choice for patients with schizophrenia (p.665); however, atypical antipsychotics may now be preferred as first-line therapy. There is little difference in efficacy between the classical antipsychotics, but thioridazine is now restricted to second-line treatment of schizophrenia because of the risk of cardiotoxicity.

**Substance dependence.** ALCOHOL. For advice against the use of antipsychotics for alcohol withdrawal, see p.1166.

OPIOIDS. In a discussion of neonatal abstinence syndrome (p.72), it was observed in 1986 that, although opioids, diazepam, and phenobarbital were widely used in the USA for the management of this condition, chlorpromazine had tended to be the preferred treatment in the UK.[1] This was still true as late as 1996, although practice varied widely.[2] The following dosage schedule has been suggested: chlorpromazine is initiated with a loading dose of 3 mg/kg, followed by a total maintenance dose of 3 mg/kg by mouth daily, divided into 4 or 6 doses. This dose may be increased by 3 mg/kg daily if withdrawal symptoms are particularly severe. Once stabilised a reduction in the dose of chlorpromazine by 2 mg/kg every third day is attempted. Complications of phenothiazine usage have been notably absent, although rarely seizures may occur.

1. Rivers RPA. Neonatal opiate withdrawal. *Arch Dis Child* 1986; **61:** 1236–9.
2. Morrison CL, Siney C. A survey of the management of neonatal opiate withdrawal in England and Wales. *Eur J Pediatr* 1996; **155:** 323–6.

**Taste disorders.** Disturbances of the sense of taste may be broadly divided into either loss or distortion of taste. Loss of taste may be either complete (ageusia) or partial (hypogeusia). Distortion of taste (dysgeusia) may occur as aliageusia in which stimuli such as food or drink produce an inappropriate taste or as phantogeusia in which an unpleasant taste is not associated with an external stimuli and is sometimes referred to as a gustatory hallucination. Taste disturbances have many causes including infections, metabolic or nutritional disturbances, radiation, CNS disorders, neoplasms, drug therapy, or may occur as a consequence of normal aging.[1] Management primarily consists of treatment of any underlying disorder. Withdrawal of offending drug therapy is commonly associated with resolution but occasionally effects persist and may require treatment.[2] Zinc or vitamin therapy has been used but there is insufficient evidence to indicate efficacy[1,3] for taste disturbances secondary to drug therapy or medical conditions that do not involve low zinc or vitamin concentrations. Phantogeusia might be linked to excessive activity of dopaminergic receptors as it has been reported[4] to respond to short-term treatment with small doses of antipsychotic drugs such as haloperidol or pimozide.

1. Schiffman SS. Taste and smell losses in normal aging and disease. *JAMA* 1997; **278:** 1357–62.
2. Henkin RI. Drug-induced taste and smell disorders: incidence, mechanisms and management related primarily to treatment of sensory receptor dysfunction. *Drug Safety* 1994; **11:** 318–77.
3. Heyneman CA. Zinc deficiency and taste disorders. *Ann Pharmacother* 1996; **30:** 186–7.
4. Henkin RI. Salty and bitter taste. *JAMA* 1991; **265:** 2253.

## Preparations

***BP 2003:*** Chlorpromazine Injection; Chlorpromazine Oral Solution; Chlorpromazine Suppositories; Chlorpromazine Tablets;
***USP 27:*** Chlorpromazine Hydrochloride Injection; Chlorpromazine Hydrochloride Oral Concentrate; Chlorpromazine Hydrochloride Syrup; Chlorpromazine Hydrochloride Tablets; Chlorpromazine Suppositories.

**Proprietary Preparations** (details are given in Part 3)
***Arg.:*** Ampliactil; Conrax; ***Austral.:*** Largactil; ***Austria:*** Largactil†; ***Belg.:*** Largactil†; ***Braz.:*** Amplictil; Clorpromaz; Longactil; ***Canad.:*** Chlorpromanyl; Largactil; ***Chile:*** Largactil; ***Denm.:*** Largactil; ***Fin.:*** Klorproman; ***Fr.:*** Largactil; ***Ger.:*** Propaphenin; ***Gr.:*** Largactil; Solidon; Zuledine; ***Hong Kong:*** Largactil; ***Irl.:*** Clonazine; Largactil; ***Israel:*** Taroctyl; ***Ital.:*** Largactil; Prozin; ***Malaysia:*** Matcine; ***Mex.:*** Largactil; ***Neth.:*** Largactil; ***Norw.:*** Largactil; ***NZ:*** Largactil; ***Port.:*** Largactil; Largatrex; ***S.Afr.:*** Largactil; ***Singapore:*** Matcine; ***Spain:*** Largactil; ***Swed.:*** Hibernal; ***Switz.:*** Chlorazin; Largactil†; ***Thai.:*** Chlorpromasit; Chlorpromed; Duncan; Matcine; Prozine; ***UK:*** Chloractil†; Largactil; ***USA:*** Thorazine.

**Multi-ingredient:** ***Arg.:*** 6 Copin; ***India:*** Trinicalm Forte; ***Spain:*** Diminex Balsamico†; Largatrex; ***Thai.:*** Ama.

---

## Chlorprothixene *(BAN, USAN, rINN)*

Clorprotixeno; N-714; Ro-4-0403. (*Z*)-3-(2-Chlorothioxanthen-9-ylidene)-*NN*-dimethylpropylamine.

$C_{18}H_{18}ClNS = 315.9.$
*CAS — 113-59-7.*
*ATC — N05AF03.*

**Pharmacopoeias.** In *Chin.*

## Chlorprothixene Hydrochloride *(BANM, rINNM)*

Chlorprothixeni Hydrochloridum; Hidrocloruro de clorprotixeno.

$C_{18}H_{19}Cl_2NS = 352.3.$
*ATC — N05AF03.*

**Pharmacopoeias.** In *Eur.* (see p.vi) and *Pol.*
**Ph. Eur. 5.0** (Chlorprothixene Hydrochloride). A white or almost white, crystalline powder. Soluble in water and in alcohol; slightly soluble in dichloromethane. A 1% solution in water has a pH of 4.4 to 5.2. Protect from light.

## Chlorprothixene Mesilate *(BANM, rINNM)*

Chlorprothixene Mesylate; Chlorprothixenium Mesylicum; Mesilato de clorprotixeno.

$C_{19}H_{22}ClNO_3S_2,H_2O = 430.0.$
*ATC — N05AF03.*

### Profile

Chlorprothixene is a thioxanthene antipsychotic with general properties similar to those of the phenothiazine, chlorpromazine (p.675). It is used mainly in the treatment of psychoses (p.665). Chlorprothixene is given as the acetate, the citrate, and the hydrochloride. Some preparations of chlorprothixene were prepared with the aid of lactic acid and were stated to contain chlorprothixene lactate. The mesilate was also used.

Chlorprothixene is usually given by mouth as the hydrochloride and doses are expressed in terms of this salt; the citrate is also given by mouth although doses are expressed in terms of the base. The acetate is given by injection with doses expressed in terms of the base. A usual initial dose by mouth for the treatment of psychoses is 15 to 50 mg three or four times daily, increased according to response; doses of up to 600 mg or more daily have been given in severe or resistant conditions. It may also be given intramuscularly or intravenously in single doses of up to 100 mg. Chlorprothixene should be used in reduced dosage for elderly or debilitated patients.

**Adverse effects.** A 59-year-old man receiving chlorprothixene (for the second time) for acute mania developed severe obstructive jaundice within a few days; he was also taking chlorpropamide, digoxin, and diuretics.[1] Chlorprothixene was considered the most likely cause of the jaundice, though chlorpropamide could not be excluded.

1. Ruddock DGS, Hoenig J. Chlorprothixene and obstructive jaundice. *BMJ* 1973; **1:** 231.

**Breast feeding.** The American Academy of Pediatrics[1] considers that, although the effect of chlorprothixene on breast-feeding infants is unknown, its use by mothers during breast feeding may be of concern since antipsychotics do appear in breast milk and thus could conceivably alter CNS function in the infant both in the short and long term.

Chlorprothixene and its sulfoxide metabolite were concentrated in the breast milk of 2 mothers receiving chlorprothixene 200 mg daily but it was calculated that the amount supplied to the nursing infant was only 0.1% of the maternal dose per kg body-weight.[2]

1. American Academy of Pediatrics. The transfer of drugs and other chemicals into human milk. *Pediatrics* 2001; **108:** 776–89. Correction. *ibid.*; 1029. Also available at: http://aappolicy.aappublications.org/cgi/content/full/pediatrics%3b108/3/776 (accessed 28/04/04)
2. Matheson I, *et al.* Presence of chlorprothixene and its metabolites in breast milk. *Eur J Clin Pharmacol* 1984; **27:** 611–13.

**Metabolism.** Studies on the metabolism of chlorprothixene in *animals* and man.[1] In addition to the major metabolite chlorprothixene-sulfoxide, 2 further urinary metabolites were identified, namely *N*-desmethylchlorprothixene-sulfoxide and chlorprothixene-sulfoxide-*N*-oxide.

1. Raaflaub J. Zum Metabolismus des Chlorprothixen. *Arzneimittelforschung* 1967; **17:** 1393–5.

## Preparations

**Proprietary Preparations** (details are given in Part 3)
***Austria:*** Truxal; Truxaletten; ***Denm.:*** Truxal; ***Fin.:*** Cloxan; Truxal; ***Ger.:*** Truxal; ***Israel:*** Truquil†; ***Neth.:*** Truxal; ***Norw.:*** Truxal; ***Swed.:*** Truxal; ***Switz.:*** Truxal; Truxaletten.

### Cinolazepam (*rINN*)

OX-373. 7-Chloro-5-(2-fluorophenyl)-2,3-dihydro-3-hydroxy-2-oxo-1*H*-1,4-benzodiazepine-1-propionitrile.

$C_{18}H_{13}ClFN_3O_2$ = 357.8.
*CAS — 75696-02-5.*
*ATC — N05CD13.*

#### Profile

Cinolazepam is a benzodiazepine derivative with general properties similar to those of diazepam (p.690) that has been used in the short-term management of sleep disorders in usual doses of 40 mg at night.

#### Preparations

**Proprietary Preparations** (details are given in Part 3)
***Austria:*** Gerodorm.

### Clocapramine Hydrochloride (*rINNM*)

Chlorcarpipramine Hydrochloride; Hidrocloruro de clocapramina; Y-4153. 1′-[3-(3-Chloro-10,11-dihydro-5*H*-dibenz[*b,f*]azepin-5-yl)propyl][1,4′-bipiperidine]-4′-carboxamide dihydrochloride monohydrate.

$C_{28}H_{37}ClN_4O,2HCl,H_2O$ = 572.0.
*CAS — 47739-98-0 (clocapramine); 28058-62-0 (clocapramine hydrochloride).*

**Pharmacopoeias.** In *Jpn.*

#### Profile

Clocapramine is a chlorinated derivative of carpipramine (p.674). The hydrochloride has been given by mouth in the treatment of schizophrenia.

◊ References.


1. Yamagami S. A crossover study of clocapramine and haloperidol in chronic schizophrenia. *J Int Med Res* 1985; **13:** 301–10.
2. Yamagami S, *et al.* A single-blind study of clocapramine and sulpiride in hospitalized chronic schizophrenic patients. *Drugs Exp Clin Res* 1988; **14:** 707–13.


## Clomethiazole (*BAN, rINN*)

Chlormethiazole; Clometiazol. 5-(2-Chloroethyl)-4-methyl-1,3-thiazole.

$C_6H_8ClNS$ = 161.7.
*CAS — 533-45-9.*
*ATC — N05CM02.*

**Pharmacopoeias.** In *Br.*

**BP 2003** (Clomethiazole). A colourless to slightly yellowish-brown liquid with a characteristic odour. Slightly soluble in water; miscible with alcohol, with chloroform, and with ether. A 0.5% solution in water has a pH of 5.5 to 7.0. Store at a temperature of 2° to 8°.

### Clomethiazole Edisilate (*BANM, rINNM*)

Chlormethiazole Edisylate; Chlormethiazole Ethanedisulphonate; Clomethiazole Edisylate (*USAN*); Edisilato de clometiazol; NEX-002. 5-(2-Chloroethyl)-4-methylthiazole ethane-1,2-disulphonate.

$(C_6H_8ClNS)_2,C_2H_6O_6S_2$ = 513.5.
*CAS — 1867-58-9.*
*ATC — N05CM02.*

**Pharmacopoeias.** In *Br.* and *Pol.*

**BP 2003** (Clomethiazole Edisilate). A white crystalline powder with a characteristic odour. Freely soluble in water; soluble in alcohol; practically insoluble in ether.

**Incompatibility.** Several studies have demonstrated that clomethiazole edisilate may permeate through or be sorbed onto plastics used in intravenous infusion bags or giving sets.[1-4] The drug may also react with and soften the plastic.[1] The manufacturers of clomethiazole edisilate have suggested that thrombophlebitis, fever, and headache reported in young children during prolonged infusions may have been due to reaction with plastic giving sets and silastic cannulae. Recommendations for intravenous use have therefore included the use of a motor-driven glass syringe in preference to a plastic drip set in small children, changing plastic drip sets at least every 24 hours when used in older patients, and use of teflon intravenous cannulas.


1. Lingam S, *et al.* Problems with intravenous chlormethiazole (Heminevrin) in status epilepticus. *BMJ* 1980; **280:** 155–6.
2. Tsuei SE, *et al.* Sorption of chlormethiazole by intravenous infusion giving sets. *Eur J Clin Pharmacol* 1980; **18:** 333–8.
3. Kowaluk EA, *et al.* Dynamics of clomethiazole edisylate interaction with plastic infusion systems. *J Pharm Sci* 1984; **73:** 43–7.
4. Lee MG. Sorption of four drugs to polyvinyl chloride and polybutadiene intravenous administration sets. *Am J Hosp Pharm* 1986; **43:** 1945–50.


#### Dependence and Withdrawal

Dependence may develop, particularly with prolonged use of higher than recommended doses of clomethiazole. Features of dependence and withdrawal are similar to those of barbiturates (see Amobarbital, p.670).

#### Adverse Effects, Treatment, and Precautions

Clomethiazole may produce nasal congestion and irritation, sneezing, and conjunctival irritation sometimes associated with a headache. Nasopharyngeal or bronchial secretions may be increased. Skin rashes and urticaria have also occurred and in rare cases bullous eruptions have been reported. Gastrointestinal disturbances including nausea and vomiting, have been reported following oral administration. Reversible increases in liver enzyme values and blood-bilirubin concentrations have also been noted. Clomethiazole may cause excessive drowsiness particularly in high doses; drowsiness may persist the next day, and patients affected should not drive or operate machinery. Paradoxical excitation or confusion may occur rarely. Anaphylaxis has been reported rarely with clomethiazole.

Excessive doses may produce coma, respiratory depression, hypotension, and hypothermia; pneumonia may follow increased respiratory secretion. Treatment is as for barbiturate overdose (see Amobarbital, p.670).

Clomethiazole is contra-indicated in patients with acute pulmonary insufficiency, and should be given with care to patients with chronic pulmonary insufficiency, or renal, liver, cerebral, or cardiac disease. Paradoxical worsening of epilepsy may occur in the Lennox Gastaut syndrome.

**Administration by intravenous infusion.** Severe adverse effects have followed the intravenous administration of clomethiazole, and intravenous preparations are no longer generally available. Facilities for intubation and resuscitation were required when clomethiazole was given intravenously and care taken to ensure that the patient's airway was maintained since there is a risk of mechanical obstruction during deep sedation. With too high a rate of infusion sleep induced with clomethiazole could lapse into deep unconsciousness and patients required close and constant observation. Rapid infusion has also caused transient apnoea and hypotension, and special care was needed in patients susceptible to cerebral or cardiac complications, including the elderly. With prolonged infusion there was also a risk of electrolyte imbalance due to the water load involved with the glucose vehicle. Recovery has been considerably delayed after prolonged infusion.

**Effects on the heart.** Cardiac arrest in 2 chronic alcoholics might have been associated with clomethiazole infusion.[1]


1. McInnes GT, *et al.* Cardiac arrest following chlormethiazole infusion in chronic alcoholics. *Postgrad Med J* 1980; **56:** 742–3.


**Overdosage.** A report of clomethiazole poisoning on 16 occasions in 13 patients, some of whom had also taken other drugs and alcohol.[1] There was increased salivation on 7 occasions; otherwise the clinical features were those of barbiturate poisoning. The highest plasma-clomethiazole concentration was 36 micrograms/mL, with the highest value in a conscious patient 11.5 micrograms/mL. All the patients survived following intensive supportive treatment as for barbiturate poisoning.


1. Illingworth RN, *et al.* Severe poisoning with chlormethiazole. *BMJ* 1979; **2:** 902–3.


**Parotitis.** Acute bilateral parotitis has been reported in a patient given clomethiazole.[1] The swelling disappeared after withdrawal of clomethiazole and recurred on rechallenge.


1. Bosch X, *et al.* Parotitis induced by chlormethiazole. *BMJ* 1994; **309:** 1620.


**Pregnancy.** There have been reports of neonates being adversely affected by clomethiazole given to their mothers for toxaemia of pregnancy.[1,2] Effects included sedation, hypotonia, and apnoea. In a report[1] it was suggested that the effects might have been due to a synergistic interaction between clomethiazole and diazoxide as these drugs were given to most of the mothers with affected infants.


1. Johnson RA. Adverse neonatal reaction to maternal administration of intravenous chlormethiazole and diazoxide. *BMJ* 1976; **1:** 943.
2. Wood C, Renou P. Sleepy and hypotonic neonates. *Med J Aust* 1978; **2:** 73.


#### Interactions

The sedative effects of clomethiazole are enhanced by CNS depressants such as alcohol, barbiturates, other hypnotics and sedatives, and antipsychotics.

**Alcohol.** Although clomethiazole is a popular choice for the treatment of alcohol withdrawal symptoms (p.1166), if it is given long-term, patients readily transfer dependency to it; if they also continue to abuse alcohol this may lead to severe self-poisoning with deep coma and potentially fatal respiratory depression.[1]


1. McInnes GT. Chlormethiazole and alcohol: a lethal cocktail. *BMJ* 1987; **294:** 592.


**Beta blockers.** Sinus bradycardia developed in an 84-year-old woman taking *propranolol* for hypertension 3 hours after she took a second dose of clomethiazole 192 mg.[1] Her pulse rate increased on discontinuation of propranolol and clomethiazole and later stabilised when she took propranolol with haloperidol.


1. Adverse Drug Reactions Advisory Committee (Australia). *Med J Aust* 1979; **2:** 553.


**Diazoxide.** For a report of severe adverse reactions in neonates born to mothers given clomethiazole and diazoxide, see Pregnancy under Adverse Effects, Treatment, and Precautions, above.

**Histamine $H_2$-antagonists.** A study of the pharmacokinetics of clomethiazole edisilate 1 g by mouth in 8 healthy subjects, before and after administration of *cimetidine* 1 g daily for 1 week, demonstrated that mean clearance of clomethiazole was reduced by 31% by cimetidine.[1] This was associated with an increase in the mean peak plasma concentration of the hypnotic from 2.664 to 4.507 micrograms/mL and an increase in the mean elimination half-life from 2.33 to 3.63 hours. After the original dose of clomethiazole subjects slept for 30 to 60 minutes, whereas after cimetidine, most slept for at least 2 hours.

Ranitidine did not significantly affect the pharmacokinetics of clomethiazole in a study in 7 healthy subjects.[2]


1. Shaw G, *et al.* Cimetidine impairs the elimination of chlormethiazole. *Eur J Clin Pharmacol* 1981; **21:** 83–5.
2. Mashford ML, *et al.* Ranitidine does not affect chlormethiazole or indocyanine green disposition. *Clin Pharmacol Ther* 1983; **34:** 231–3.


#### Pharmacokinetics

Clomethiazole is rapidly absorbed from the gastrointestinal tract, peak plasma concentrations occurring about 15 to 90 minutes after oral administration depending on the formulation used. It is widely distributed in the body and is reported to be 65% bound to plasma proteins. Clomethiazole is extensively metabolised, probably by first-pass metabolism in the liver with only small amounts appearing unchanged in the urine. The elimination half-life has been reported to be about 4 hours but this may be increased to 8 hours or longer in the elderly or in patients with hepatic impairment. Clomethiazole crosses the placenta and is distributed into breast milk.

**Hepatic impairment.** Studies in 8 patients with advanced cirrhosis of the liver and in 6 healthy men showed that the amount of unmetabolised clomethiazole reaching the circulation after an oral dose was about 10 times higher in the patients than in the controls.[1] Low concentrations in the controls were related to extensive first-pass metabolism in the liver.


1. Pentikäinen PJ, *et al.* Pharmacokinetics of chlormethiazole in healthy volunteers and patients with cirrhosis of the liver. *Eur J Clin Pharmacol* 1980; **17:** 275–84.


#### Uses and Administration

Clomethiazole is a hypnotic and sedative with anticonvulsant effects. It is used in the treatment of agitation and restlessness (see Disturbed Behaviour, p.665) in elderly patients, in the short-term management of severe insomnia (p.667) in the elderly, and in the treatment of acute alcohol withdrawal symptoms (p.1166). It was also given as an intravenous infusion in the management of status epilepticus (p.352) and impending or actual eclampsia (p.352); however, a parenteral formulation of clomethiazole no longer appears to be available.

In the UK, clomethiazole as Heminevrin (*AstraZeneca*) is available as capsules containing 192 mg of clomethiazole base and as syrup containing 250 mg of the edisilate in 5 mL. As a result of differences in the bioavailability of these preparations, 192 mg of the base in the capsules is considered therapeutically equivalent to 250 mg (5 mL) of the edisilate in the syrup, i.e. one capsule or 5 mL of syrup are equivalent in their effects.

The usual hypnotic dose of clomethiazole for **insomnia** is 1 or 2 capsules (192 or 384 mg of the base) or the equivalent. For **restlessness and agitation** in the elderly 1 capsule (192 mg of the base), or the equivalent dose as one of the other dosage forms, may be given 3 times daily.

Various clomethiazole regimens have been suggested for the treatment of **alcohol withdrawal**, usually starting with 9 to 12 capsules, or the equivalent, divided into 3 or 4 doses, on the first day, and gradually reducing the dosage over the following 5 days. Treatment should be carried out in hospital or in specialist centres, and administration for longer than 9 days is not recommended because of the risk of dependence (see above).

**Porphyria.** Clomethiazole is one of the drugs that has been used for seizure prophylaxis in patients with porphyria (p.353) who continue to experience convulsions while in remission.

**Stroke.** Clomethiazole has been studied[1] as a neuroprotective drug in the acute management of patients with stroke, but no beneficial effect on long-term outcome was demonstrated.

1. Wahlgren NG, *et al.* CLASS Study Group. Clomethiazole Acute Stroke Study (CLASS): results of a randomized, controlled trial of clomethiazole versus placebo in 1360 acute stroke patients. *Stroke* 1999; **30:** 21–8.

**Substance dependence.** For a discussion of the management of *opioid* withdrawal symptoms, including mention of the use of clomethiazole, see p.71.

## Preparations

***BP 2003:*** Clomethiazole Capsules; Clomethiazole Intravenous Infusion; Clomethiazole Oral Solution.

**Proprietary Preparations** (details are given in Part 3)

***Austral.:*** Hemineurin†; ***Austria:*** Distraneurin†; ***Belg.:*** Distraneurine; ***Denm.:*** Heminevrin; ***Fin.:*** Heminevrin; ***Ger.:*** Distraneurin; ***Gr.:*** Distraneurine; Heminevrin; ***Hong Kong:*** Heminevrin; ***Irl.:*** Heminevrin; ***Neth.:*** Distraneurine†; ***Norw.:*** Heminevrin; ***NZ:*** Hemineurin†; ***S.Afr.:*** Heminevrin†; ***Spain:*** Distraneurine; ***Swed.:*** Heminevrin; ***Switz.:*** Distraneurin; ***UK:*** Heminevrin.

# Cloral Betaine *(BAN, rINN)*

Chloral Betaine *(USAN)*; Cloral betaína; Compound 5107. An adduct of cloral hydrate and betaine.

$C_7H_{12}Cl_3NO_3,H_2O = 282.5.$

*CAS — 2218-68-0.*

## Profile

Cloral betaine rapidly dissociates in the stomach to release cloral hydrate and has actions and uses similar to those of cloral hydrate (below). It is given by mouth in the short-term management of insomnia (p.667), as tablets containing 707 mg (approximately equivalent to 414 mg of cloral hydrate). The usual hypnotic dose is one or two tablets taken at night with water or milk. The maximum daily dose is five tablets (equivalent to about 2 g of cloral hydrate). A reduction in dosage may be appropriate in frail elderly patients or in those with hepatic impairment.

## Preparations

**Proprietary Preparations** (details are given in Part 3)

***UK:*** Welldorm.

# Cloral Hydrate

Chloral Hydrate *(BAN)*; Chlorali Hydras; Cloral, hidrato de. 2,2,2-Trichloroethane-1,1-diol.

$C_2H_3Cl_3O_2 = 165.4.$

*CAS — 302-17-0.*

*ATC — N05CC01.*

**Pharmacopoeias.** In *Chin., Eur.* (see p.vi), *Int., Jpn, Pol., US,* and *Viet.*

**Ph. Eur. 5.0** (Chloral Hydrate). Colourless, transparent crystals. Very soluble in water; freely soluble in alcohol. A 10% solution in water has a pH of 3.5 to 5.5. Store in airtight containers.

**USP 27** (Chloral Hydrate). Colourless, transparent, or white crystals having an aromatic, penetrating, and slightly acrid odour. It volatilises slowly on exposure to air and melts at about 55°. Soluble 1 in 0.25 of water, 1 in 1.3 of alcohol, 1 in 2 of chloroform, and 1 in 1.5 of ether; very soluble in olive oil. Store in airtight containers.

**Incompatibility.** Cloral hydrate is reported to be incompatible with alkalis, alkaline earths, alkali carbonates, soluble barbiturates, borax, tannin, iodides, oxidising agents, permanganates, and alcohol (cloral alcoholate may crystallise out). It forms a liquid mixture when triturated with many organic compounds, such as camphor, menthol, phenazone, phenol, thymol, and quinine salts.

## Dependence and Withdrawal, Adverse Effects, and Treatment

Cloral hydrate has an unpleasant taste and is corrosive to skin and mucous membranes unless well diluted. The most frequent adverse effect is gastric irritation; abdominal distension and flatulence may also occur. CNS effects such as drowsiness, lightheadedness, ataxia, headache, and paradoxical excitement, hallucinations, nightmares, delirium, and confusion (sometimes with paranoia) occur occasionally. Hypersensitivity reactions include skin rashes (erythema multiforme and Stevens-Johnson syndrome have been reported with the related compound triclofos). Ketonuria may occur.

The effects of acute overdosage resemble acute barbiturate intoxication (see Amobarbital, p.670 and below), and are managed similarly. In addition the irritant effect may cause initial vomiting, and gastric necrosis leading to strictures. Cardiac arrhythmias have been reported. Jaundice may follow liver damage, and albuminuria may follow kidney damage.

Tolerance may develop and dependence may occur. Features of dependence and withdrawal are similar to those of barbiturates (see Amobarbital, p.670).

**Incidence of adverse effects.** In a drug surveillance programme,[1] side-effects of cloral hydrate, which were reversible, occurred in 2.3% of 1130 patients evaluated and included gastrointestinal symptoms (10 patients), CNS depression (20), and skin rash (5). In 1 patient the prothrombin time was increased; in 1 patient hepatic encephalopathy seemed to worsen; and bradycardia developed in 1 patient. In another such programme, side-effects occurred in about 2% of 5435 patients who received cloral hydrate.[2] Three reactions were described as life-threatening.

1. Shapiro S, *et al.* Clinical effects of hypnotics II: an epidemiologic study. *JAMA* 1969; **209:** 2016–20.
2. Miller RR, Greenblatt DJ. Clinical effects of chloral hydrate in hospitalized medical patients. *J Clin Pharmacol* 1979; **19:** 669–74.

**Carcinogenicity.** Cloral hydrate has been widely used as a sedative, especially in children. Concern over warnings that cloral hydrate was carcinogenic in *rodents*[1] has prompted some experts, including the American Academy of Pediatrics, to review the relative risks of the medical use of this drug.[2,3] The original warnings appear to have been based, in part, on the assumption that cloral hydrate was a reactive metabolite of trichloroethylene and was responsible for its carcinogenicity, but there is evidence to suggest that the carcinogenicity of trichloroethylene is due to a reactive intermediate epoxide metabolite. Studies *in vitro* indicate that choral hydrate can damage chromosomes in some mammalian test systems but there have been no studies of the carcinogenicity of cloral hydrate in humans. Some long-term studies in *mice* have linked cloral hydrate with the development of hepatic adenomas or carcinomas. However, it was noted that cloral hydrate was not the only sedative that had been shown to be a carcinogen in experimental *animals*. The American Academy of Pediatrics considered cloral hydrate to be an effective sedative with a low incidence of acute toxicity when given short-term as recommended and, although the information on carcinogenicity was of concern, it was not sufficient to justify the risk associated with the use of less familiar sedatives. There was no evidence in infants or children demonstrating that any of the available alternatives were safer or more effective. However, the use of repetitive dosing with cloral hydrate to maintain prolonged sedation in neonates and other children was of concern because of the potential for accumulation of drug metabolites and resultant toxicity.

1. Smith MT. Chloral hydrate warning. *Science* 1990; **250:** 359.
2. Steinberg AD. Should chloral hydrate be banned? *Pediatrics* 1993; **92:** 442–6.
3. American Academy of Pediatrics Committee on Drugs and Committee on Environmental Health. Use of chloral hydrate for sedation in children. *Pediatrics* 1993; **92:** 471–3.

**Effects on the CNS.** A 2-year-old child[1] experienced the first of 2 seizures 60 minutes after receiving cloral hydrate 70 mg/kg for sedation.

1. Muñoz M, *et al.* Seizures caused by chloral hydrate sedative doses. *J Pediatr* 1997; **131:** 787–8.

**Hyperbilirubinaemia.** Small retrospective studies[1] have suggested that prolonged administration of cloral hydrate in neonates may be associated with the development of hyperbilirubinaemia. This may possibly be related to the prolonged half-life of the metabolite trichloroethanol in neonates.

1. Lambert GH, *et al.* Direct hyperbilirubinemia associated with chloral hydrate administration in the newborn. *Pediatrics* 1990; **86:** 277–81.

**Overdosage.** The general management of poisoning with cloral hydrate resembles that for barbiturates (see, p.670). Activated charcoal has been recommended if more than 2 g has been taken by an adult within 1 hour of treatment, or 30 mg/kg in a child, provided the airway can be protected. Gastric lavage may be considered before giving charcoal in serious cases. Of 76 cases of cloral hydrate poisoning reported to the UK National Poisons Information Service, 47 were severe.[1] Of 39 adults, 12 had cardiac arrhythmias including 5 with cardiac arrest. Antiarrhythmic drugs were recommended unless obviously contra-indicated. Haemoperfusion through charcoal or haemodialysis was recommended for patients in prolonged coma. Cardiac arrhythmias and CNS depression were also major features of 12 cases of cloral hydrate overdosage reported from Australia.[2] Lidocaine was not always successful in controlling arrhythmias, but propranolol was successful in all 7 patients in whom it was used. It was noted that resistant arrhythmias, particularly ventricular fibrillation, ventricular tachycardia, and supraventricular tachycardia, were the usual cause of death in patients who had taken an overdosage of cloral hydrate. Although there had been no controlled studies of antiarrhythmic therapy in overdosage with cloral hydrate, the successful use of beta blockers appeared to be a recurring feature in reports in the literature.

Administration of flumazenil produced an increased level of consciousness, pupillary dilatation, and return of respiratory rate and blood pressure towards normal in a patient who had taken an overdosage of cloral hydrate.[3]

1. Wiseman HM, Hampel G. Cardiac arrhythmias due to chloral hydrate poisoning. *BMJ* 1978; **2:** 960.
2. Graham SR, *et al.* Overdose with chloral hydrate: a pharmacological and therapeutic review. *Med J Aust* 1988; **149:** 686–8.
3. Donovan KL, Fisher DJ. Reversal of chloral hydrate overdose with flumazenil. *BMJ* 1989; **298:** 1253.

## Precautions

Cloral hydrate should not be used in patients with marked hepatic or renal impairment or severe cardiac disease, and oral administration is best avoided in the presence of gastritis. As with all sedatives, it should be used with caution in those with respiratory insufficiency.

Cloral hydrate can cause drowsiness that may persist the next day; affected patients should not drive or operate machinery. Prolonged use and abrupt withdrawal of cloral hydrate should be avoided to prevent precipitation of withdrawal symptoms. Repeated administration in infants and children may lead to accumulation of metabolites and thereby increase the risk of adverse effects. Use is best avoided during pregnancy.

Cloral hydrate may interfere with some tests for urinary glucose or 17-hydroxycorticosteroids.

**Breast feeding.** The American Academy of Pediatrics[1] states that, although usually compatible with breast feeding, use of cloral hydrate by breast-feeding mothers has been reported to cause sleepiness in the infant.

1. American Academy of Pediatrics. The transfer of drugs and other chemicals into human milk. *Pediatrics* 2001; **108:** 776–89. Correction. *ibid.*; 1029. Also available at: http://aappolicy.aappublications.org/cgi/content/full/pediatrics%3b108/3/776 (accessed 28/04/04)

**Neonates.** The half-life of trichloroethanol, an active metabolite of cloral hydrate, is prolonged in neonates;[1] values of up to 66 hours have been reported in some studies. Short-term sedation in the neonate with single oral doses of 25 to 50 mg/kg of cloral hydrate is considered[1] to be probably relatively safe, but repeated administration carries the risk of accumulation of metabolites which may result in serious toxicity. Toxic reactions may occur even after the drug has been discontinued since the metabolites may accumulate for several days.

1. Jacqz-Aigrain E, Burtin P. Clinical pharmacokinetics of sedatives in neonates. *Clin Pharmacokinet* 1996; **31:** 423–43.

**Obstructive sleep apnoea.** Children with obstructive sleep apnoea could be at risk from life-threatening respiratory obstruction if cloral hydrate is used for sedation. Details of 2 such children who suffered respiratory failure following sedation with cloral hydrate for lung function studies have been reported.[1]

1. Biban P, *et al.* Adverse effect of chloral hydrate in two young children with obstructive sleep apnea. *Pediatrics* 1993; **92:** 461–3.

**Porphyria.** The UK manufacturer recommends that cloral hydrate should not be used in patients with porphyria, although some authorities consider it safe; caution would seem appropriate.

## Interactions

The sedative effects of cloral hydrate are enhanced by other CNS depressants such as alcohol (the 'Mickey Finn' of detective fiction), barbiturates, and other sedatives.

Cloral hydrate may alter the effects of coumarin anticoagulants (see Warfarin, p.1026). A hypermetabolic state, apparently due to displacement of thyroid hormones from their binding proteins, has been reported in patients given an intravenous dose of furosemide subsequent to cloral hydrate.

## Pharmacokinetics

Cloral hydrate is rapidly absorbed from the gastrointestinal tract and starts to act within 30 minutes of oral administration. It is widely distributed throughout the body. It is rapidly metabolised to trichloroethanol and trichloroacetic acid (p.1162) in the erythrocytes, liver, and other tissues. It is excreted partly in the urine as trichloroethanol and its glucuronide (urochloralic acid) and as trichloroacetic acid. Some is also excreted in the bile.

Trichloroethanol is the active metabolite, and passes into the CSF, into breast milk, and across the placenta. The half-life of trichloroethanol in plasma is reported to range from about 7 to 11 hours but is considerably prolonged in the neonate. Trichloroacetic acid has a plasma half-life of several days.

## Uses and Administration

Cloral hydrate is a hypnotic and sedative with properties similar to those of the barbiturates. It is used in the short-term management of insomnia (p.667) and has been used as a sedative for premedication (p.1296). In the USA it has been widely used for sedation of children before diagnostic, dental, or medical procedures (but see under Carcinogenicity above).

Externally, cloral hydrate has a rubefacient action and has been used as a counter-irritant.

Cloral hydrate is given by mouth as an oral liquid or as gelatin capsules with cloral hydrate dissolved in a suitable vehicle. It has also been dissolved in a bland fixed oil and given by enema or as suppositories.

It should not be given as tablets because of the risk of damage to the mucous membrane of the alimentary tract.

The usual hypnotic dose by mouth is 0.5 to 2 g given as a single dose at night; as a sedative 250 mg can be given three times daily to a maximum daily dose of 2 g. Oral dosage forms should be taken well diluted or with plenty of water or milk. Children may be given 30 to 50 mg/kg to a maximum single dose of 1 g as a hypnotic. A suggested sedative dose for premedication in children is 25 to 50 mg/kg to a maximum single dose of 1 g.

A reduction in dosage may be appropriate in frail elderly patients or in those with hepatic impairment.

Derivatives of cloral hydrate, such as cloral betaine (above), chloralose (p.1501), and dichloralphenazone (p.697), which break down in the body to yield cloral hydrate, have been used similarly.

◊ References.

1. McCarver-May DG, *et al.* Comparison of chloral hydrate and midazolam for sedation of neonates for neuroimaging studies. *J Pediatr* 1996; **128:** 573–6.
2. Napoli KL, *et al.* Safety and efficacy of chloral hydrate sedation in children undergoing echocardiography. *J Pediatr* 1996; **129:** 287–91.

### Preparations

*USP 27:* Chloral Hydrate Capsules; Chloral Hydrate Syrup.

**Proprietary Preparations** (details are given in Part 3)
***Austria:*** Chloraldurat†; ***Ger.:*** Chloraldurat; ***Switz.:*** Chloraldurat; Medianox; Nervifene; ***UK:*** Welldorm; ***USA:*** Aquachloral.

**Multi-ingredient:** ***Belg.:*** Babygencal†; Dentophar; Synthol†; ***Canad.:*** Analgesic Balm; ***Fr.:*** Bain de Bouche Lipha; Pipiol†; Sirop Teyssedre†; ***Ger.:*** Leukona-Sedativ-Bad†; ***Spain:*** Dentol Topico.

## Clorazepic Acid *(BAN)*

Clorazépico, ácido. 7-Chloro-2,3-dihydro-2,2-dihydroxy-5-phenyl-1*H*-1,4-benzodiazepine-3-carboxylic acid.

$C_{16}H_{11}ClN_2O_3$ = 314.7.

*CAS — 23887-31-2; 20432-69-3.*

## Clorazepate Monopotassium *(USAN)*

Abbott-39083; 4311-CB; Clorazepato monopotásico. Potassium 7-chloro-2,3-dihydro-2-oxo-5-phenyl-1*H*-1,4-benzodiazepine-3-carboxylate.

$C_{16}H_{10}ClKN_2O_3$ = 352.8.

*CAS — 5991-71-9.*

## Dipotassium Clorazepate *(BANM, rINN)*

Abbott-35616; AH-3232; 4306-CB; Clorazepate Dipotassium *(USAN)*; Clorazepato de dipotasio; Dikalii Clorazepas; Potassium Clorazepate. Compound of Potassium 7-chloro-2,3-dihydro-2-oxo-5-phenyl-1*H*-1,4-benzodiazepine-3-carboxylate with potassium hydroxide.

$C_{16}H_{11}ClK_2N_2O_4$ = 408.9.

*CAS — 57109-90-7.*

*ATC — N05BA05.*

**Pharmacopoeias.** In *Eur.* (see p.vi) and *US.*

**Ph. Eur. 5.0** (Dipotassium Clorazepate). A white or light yellow, crystalline powder. Solutions in water and in alcohol are unstable and should be used immediately. Freely soluble or very soluble in water; very slightly soluble in alcohol; practically insoluble in dichloromethane. Store in airtight containers. Protect from light.

**USP 27** (Clorazepate Dipotassium). A light yellow, crystalline powder which darkens on exposure to light. Soluble in water but, upon standing, may precipitate from the solution; slightly soluble in alcohol and in isopropyl alcohol; practically insoluble in acetone, in chloroform, in dichloromethane, in ether, and in benzene. Store under nitrogen in airtight containers. Protect from light.

### Dependence and Withdrawal

As for Diazepam, p.690.

### Adverse Effects, Treatment, and Precautions

As for Diazepam, p.690.

**Effects on the liver.** A report of jaundice and hepatic necrosis associated with clorazepate administration.[1]

1. Parker JLW. Potassium clorazepate (Tranxene)-induced jaundice. *Postgrad Med J* 1979; **55:** 908–910.

**Effects on the nervous system.** For reference to extrapyramidal disorders associated with administration of clorazepate, see Diazepam, p.691.

**Porphyria.** Clorazepate has been associated with acute attacks of porphyria and is considered unsafe in porphyric patients.

### Interactions

As for Diazepam, p.692.

### Pharmacokinetics

Clorazepate is decarboxylated rapidly at the low pH in the stomach to form desmethyldiazepam (nordazepam, see p.710), which is quickly absorbed.

◊ References.

1. Ochs HR, *et al.* Comparative single-dose kinetics of oxazolam, prazepam, and clorazepate: three precursors of desmethyldiazepam. *J Clin Pharmacol* 1984; **24:** 446–51.
2. Bertler Å, *et al.* Intramuscular bioavailability of chlorazepate as compared to diazepam. *Eur J Clin Pharmacol* 1985; **28:** 229–30.

### Uses and Administration

Clorazepate is a long-acting benzodiazepine with general properties similar to those of diazepam (p.695). It is mainly used in the short-term treatment of anxiety disorders (p.663), as an adjunct in the management of epilepsy, and in the alcohol withdrawal syndrome (p.1166).

Dipotassium clorazepate is usually given by mouth but preparations for intravenous or intramuscular administration are also available in some countries. Modified-release preparations are available in some countries for maintenance therapy.

In the UK, a usual dose of 15 mg of dipotassium clorazepate by mouth is given as a single dose at night for the treatment of **anxiety**; alternatively a dose of 7.5 mg may be given up to three times daily. In the USA rather higher doses have been recommended; 15 to 60 mg of dipotassium clorazepate may be given daily, in divided doses or as a single dose at night.

Up to 90 mg has been given daily in divided doses in the management of **epilepsy** or the **alcohol withdrawal syndrome**. Children aged between 9 and 12 years may be given a maximum of 60 mg daily in the management of epilepsy.

Reduced doses should be given in elderly or debilitated patients.

### Preparations

*USP 27:* Clorazepate Dipotassium Tablets.

**Proprietary Preparations** (details are given in Part 3)
***Arg.:*** Justum; Tencilan; ***Austral.:*** Tranxene†; ***Austria:*** Tranxilium; ***Belg.:*** Tranxene; Uni-Tranxene; ***Braz.:*** Tranxilene; ***Canad.:*** Novo-Clopate; Tranxene; ***Chile:*** Calner; Modival; Tranxilium; ***Denm.:*** Tranxen†; ***Fr.:*** Tranxene; ***Ger.:*** Tranxilium; ***Gr.:*** Tranxene; ***Hong Kong:*** Tranxene; ***Irl.:*** Tranxene; ***Israel:*** Tranxal; ***Ital.:*** Transene; ***Malaysia:*** Sanor; ***Mex.:*** Tranxene; ***Neth.:*** Tranxene; ***Port.:*** Medipax; Tranxene; ***S.Afr.:*** Tranxene; ***Singapore:*** Tranxene†; ***Spain:*** Nansius†; Tranxilium; ***Switz.:*** Tranxilium; ***Thai.:*** Anxielax; Cloramed; Cloraxene; Diposef; Dipot; Flulium; Manotran; Polizep; Pomadom; Posene; Sanor; Serene; Trancap; Tranclor; Trancon; Tranxene; Zetran; ***UK:*** Tranxene; ***USA:*** Gen-Xene†; Tranxene.

**Multi-ingredient:** ***Arg.:*** Euciton Complex; Maxitratobes; Vegestabil; ***Fr.:*** Noctran; ***Spain:*** Dorken.

## Clotiapine *(BAN, rINN)*

Clothiapine *(USAN)*; Clotiapina; HF-2159. 2-Chloro-11-(4-methylpiperazin-1-yl)dibenzo[*b,f*][1,4]thiazepine.

$C_{18}H_{18}ClN_3S$ = 343.9.

*CAS — 2058-52-8.*

*ATC — N05AX09.*

### Profile

Clotiapine is a dibenzothiazepine antipsychotic with general properties similar to those of the phenothiazines (see Chlorpromazine, p.675). It is used in a variety of psychiatric disorders including schizophrenia (p.665), mania (see Bipolar Disorder, p.278), and anxiety (p.663). It is given by mouth in doses of 10 to 200 mg daily in divided doses; doses of up to 360 mg daily have been given in severe or resistant psychoses. It may also be given by slow intravenous or deep intramuscular injection.

**Psychoses.** A systematic review[1] found that good evidence to support the use of clotiapine over other treatments in acute psychotic illness was lacking.

1. Carpenter S, Berk M. Clotiapine for acute psychotic illnesses. Available in The Cochrane Library; Issue 2. Chichester: John Wiley; 2004.

### Preparations

**Proprietary Preparations** (details are given in Part 3)
***Arg.:*** Etumina; ***Belg.:*** Etumine; ***Israel:*** Etumin/Entumin; ***Ital.:*** Entumin; ***S.Afr.:*** Etomine; ***Spain:*** Etumina; ***Switz.:*** Entumine.

## Clotiazepam *(rINN)*

Y-6047. 5-(2-Chlorophenyl)-7-ethyl-1,3-dihydro-1-methyl-2*H*-thieno[2,3-e]-1,4-diazepin-2-one.

$C_{16}H_{15}ClN_2OS$ = 318.8.

*CAS — 33671-46-4.*

*ATC — N05BA21.*

**Pharmacopoeias.** In *Jpn.*

### Profile

Clotiazepam is a short-acting thienodiazepine with general properties similar to those of diazepam (p.690). A usual daily dose for the short-term management of anxiety disorders (p.663) is 5 to 15 mg by mouth given in divided doses but up to 60 mg daily has been used. For insomnia (p.667) up to 20 mg has been given as a single dose at night.

◊ References.

1. Jibiki I, *et al.* Beneficial effect of high-dose clotiazepam on intractable auditory hallucinations in chronic schizophrenic patients. *Eur J Clin Pharmacol* 1994; **46:** 367–9.

**Effects on the liver.** Development of hepatitis in a 65-year-old woman was attributed to clotiazepam begun 7 months earlier.[1] The patient took triazolam and lorazepam without any apparent effect on the liver, and it was speculated that the hepatotoxic effect of clotiazepam was related to the thiophene ring present in the chemical structure.

1. Habersetzer F, *et al.* Clotiazepam-induced acute hepatitis. *J Hepatol* 1989; **9:** 256–9.

**Porphyria.** Clotiazepam is considered to be unsafe in patients with porphyria because it has been shown to be porphyrinogenic in *in-vitro* systems.

### Preparations

**Proprietary Preparations** (details are given in Part 3)
***Belg.:*** Clozan; ***Fr.:*** Veratran; ***Ger.:*** Trecalmo†; ***Ital.:*** Rizen; Tienor; ***Jpn:*** Rize; ***Spain:*** Distensan.

## Cloxazolam *(rINN)*

CS-370. 10-Chloro-11b-(2-chlorophenyl)-2,3,7,11b-tetrahydro-oxazolo[3,2-*d*][1,4]benzodiazepin-6(5*H*)-one.

$C_{17}H_{14}Cl_2N_2O_2$ = 349.2.

*CAS — 24166-13-0.*

*ATC — N05BA22.*

**Pharmacopoeias.** In *Jpn.*

### Profile

Cloxazolam is a long-acting benzodiazepine with general properties similar to those of diazepam (p.690). It has been given by mouth in doses of up to 12 mg daily in divided doses for the short-term treatment of anxiety disorders (p.663). A dose of 100 micrograms/kg may be used for premedication (p.1296).

### Preparations

**Proprietary Preparations** (details are given in Part 3)
***Arg.:*** Tolestan; ***Belg.:*** Akton; ***Braz.:*** Clozal; Elum; Olcadil; ***Hong Kong:*** Sepazon†; ***Port.:*** Cloxam; Olcadil; ***Switz.:*** Lubalix.

## Clozapine *(BAN, USAN, rINN)*

Clozapina; Clozapinum; HF-1854. 8-Chloro-11-(4-methylpiperazin-1-yl)-5*H*-dibenzo[*b,e*][1,4]diazepine.

$C_{18}H_{19}ClN_4$ = 326.8.

*CAS — 5786-21-0.*

*ATC — N05AH02.*

**Pharmacopoeias.** In *Chin., Eur.* (see p.vi), *Pol.*, and *US.*

**Ph. Eur. 5.0** (Clozapine). A yellow crystalline powder. Practically insoluble in water; soluble in alcohol; freely soluble in dichloromethane. It dissolves in dilute acetic acid.

**USP 27** (Clozapine). A yellow crystalline powder. Insoluble in water; soluble in alcohol, in acetone, and in chloroform; sparingly soluble in acetonitrile.

**Stability.** A suspension of clozapine 100 mg in 5 mL, made by crushing clozapine tablets and suspending the powder in a syrup-based mixture containing carboxymethylcellulose preserved with methyl hydroxybenzoate and propyl hydroxybenzoate (Guy's Hospital paediatric base formula), was considered to be stable for at least 18 days after preparation.[1]

1. Ramuth S, *et al.* A liquid clozapine preparation for oral administration in hospital. *Pharm J* 1996; **257:** 190–1.

### Adverse Effects and Treatment

Although clozapine may share some of the adverse effects seen with the classical antipsychotics (see Chlorpromazine, p.675), the incidence and severity of such effects may vary; antimuscarinic effects with clozapine may be more pronounced. Sedation and weight gain may also be more prominent. Clozapine can cause reversible neutropenia which may progress to a potentially fatal agranulocytosis; strict monitoring of white blood cell counts is essential (see Precautions, below). Eosinophilia may also occur.

Extrapyramidal disorders, including tardive dyskinesia appear to be rare with clozapine. Clozapine has little effect on prolactin secretion. Clozapine appears to have a greater epileptic potential than chlorpromazine but a comparable risk of cardiovascular effects such as tachycardia and orthostatic hypotension. In rare cases circulatory collapse with cardiac and respiratory arrest has occurred, and hypertension has also been reported. Clozapine is also associated with an increased risk of developing myocarditis that may, in rare cases, be fatal; cardiomyopathy and pericarditis have also been reported.

Additional side-effects of clozapine include dizziness, hypersalivation (particularly at night), headache, nausea, vomiting, constipation (which, in a few cases, has led to gastrointestinal obstruction and paralytic ileus), urinary incontinence and retention, anxiety, confusion, fatigue, and transient fever which must be distinguished from the signs of impending agranulocytosis. There have also been rare reports of dysphagia, parotid gland enlargement, delirium, thromboembolism, acute pancreatitis, hepatitis and cholestatic jaundice, and very rarely fulminant hepatic necrosis. Isolated cases of acute interstitial nephritis have been reported. Abnormalities of glucose homoeostasis and the onset of diabetes mellitus occur uncommonly; severe hyperglycaemia, sometimes leading to ketoacidosis, has been reported very rarely. Many of the adverse effects of clozapine are most common at the beginning of therapy and may be minimised by gradual increase in dosage.

**Effects on the blood.** Clozapine can cause reversible neutropenia which, if the drug is not withdrawn immediately, may progress to a potentially fatal **agranulocytosis**. Particular concern over this side-effect dates from 1975 when 17 cases of neutropenia or agranulocytosis, 8 of them fatal, were reported in Finland;[1] the calculated incidence[2] of agranulocytosis or severe granulocytopenia during this Finnish epidemic was 7.1 per 1000. These reports led to the withdrawal of clozapine in some countries or to restrictions in its use and intense haematological monitoring in others. Following studies demonstrating the efficacy of clozapine in severely ill schizophrenic patients unresponsive to adequate therapy with standard antipsychotics, the drug became available in the UK and USA in 1990 with strict procedures for monitoring of white blood cell counts. The UK Committee on Safety of Medicines provided data on the reports it had received between July 1963 and January 1993 on agranulocytosis and neutropenia.[3] Clozapine was one of the individual drugs most frequently implicated, with 14 reports of agranulocytosis (one fatal) and 119 of neutropenia (none fatal). Various estimates of the **incidence** of clozapine-associated agranulocytosis have been made; analysis of data from 11 555 patients who had received clozapine in the USA[4] showed a cumulative incidence of agranulocytosis of 8.0 per 1000 at 1 year and 9.1 per 1000 at 1½ years with the risk being increased in elderly patients. The majority of cases of agranulocytosis occurred within 3 months of the start of treatment with the risk peaking in the third month. The manufacturers report a lower incidence of agranulocytosis of 4.8 per 1000 patients for the first 6 months[5] and an annual rate of 0.8 per 1000 patients during the next 2.5 years. These figures were based on data on 56 000 patients in the USA who had received clozapine up to the end of March 1993. Analysis of data[6] on 6316 patients registered in the UK and Ireland between January 1990 and July 1994 to receive (although not necessarily given) clozapine produced a cumulative incidence of agranulocytosis of 0.7% during the first year and 0.8% over the whole study period. Most cases of agranulocytosis and neutropenia occurred during the first 6 to 18 weeks of treatment. The incidence of agranulocytosis (0.07%) and neutropenia (0.7%) seen during the second year of therapy was of the same order of magnitude noted for some phenothiazine antipsychotics.

These data[6] and comparable data from the USA[7] were considered to indicate that mandatory haematological monitoring (see Precautions, below) helped to reduce the risks of clozapine-induced neutropenia and agranulocytosis and associated deaths.

The mechanism for clozapine-induced agranulocytosis is unclear and may be the result of direct toxicity or an immune response.[8,9] **Predisposing factors** for development of agranulocytosis have not been identified, apart from a possible excess of cases in female patients and an increased risk with increasing age. Furthermore, both agranulocytosis and neutropenia do not appear to be dose-related effects with clozapine. A postulated higher incidence of agranulocytosis in patients of Jewish background may be related to genetic factors.[10] Africans and Afro-Caribbeans appear to be at increased risk of developing neutropenia[6] and it has been noted[11] that many patients from these ethnic groups are currently already excluded from treatment with clozapine because their normal white blood cell and neutrophil counts are below the recommended range for treatment (see Precautions, below).

Evidence would suggest that development of clozapine-induced leucopenia or granulocytopenia precludes **retreatment** with clozapine at any future date; in one series of 9 patients re-treated all again developed leucopenia or agranulocytosis.[12] In the USA patients who have had clozapine withdrawn because of moderate leucopenia (judged to be when counts fall to 2000 to 3000 cells/mm³) are considered eligible for a return to clozapine treatment when this count returns to normal; such patients are considered to have a five- or sixfold greater risk of agranulocytosis.[5]


1. Idänpään-Heikkilä J, *et al.* Agranulocytosis during treatment with clozapine. *Eur J Clin Pharmacol* 1977; **11:** 193–8.
2. Anderman B, Griffith RW. Clozapine-induced agranulocytosis: a situation report up to August 1976. *Eur J Clin Pharmacol* 1977; **11:** 199–201.
3. Committee on Safety of Medicines/Medicines Control Agency. Drug-induced neutropenia and agranulocytosis. *Current Problems* 1993; **19:** 10–11.
4. Alvir JMJ, *et al.* Clozapine-induced agranulocytosis: incidence and risk factors in the United States. *N Engl J Med* 1993; **329:** 162–7.
5. Finkel MJ, Arellano F. White-blood-cell monitoring and clozapine. *Lancet* 1995; **346:** 849.
6. Atkin K, *et al.* Neutropenia and agranulocytosis in patients receiving clozapine in the UK and Ireland. *Br J Psychiatry* 1996; **169:** 483–8.
7. Honigfeld G, *et al.* Reducing clozapine-related morbidity and mortality: 5 years experience with the Clozaril National Registry. *J Clin Psychiatry* 1998; **59** (suppl 3): 3–7.
8. Gerson SL, *et al.* Polypharmacy in fatal clozapine-associated agranulocytosis. *Lancet* 1991; **338:** 262–3.
9. Hoffbrand AV, *et al.* Mechanisms of clozapine-induced agranulocytosis. *Drug Safety* 1992; **7** (suppl 1): 1–60.
10. Leiberman JA, *et al.* HLA-B38, DR4, DQw3 and clozapine-induced agranulocytosis in Jewish patients with schizophrenia. *Arch Gen Psychiatry* 1990; **47:** 945–8.
11. Fisher N, Baigent B. Treatment with clozapine: black patients' low white cell counts currently mean that they cannot be treated. *BMJ* 1996; **313:** 1262.
12. Safferman AZ, *et al.* Rechallenge in clozapine-induced agranulocytosis. *Lancet* 1992; **339:** 1296–7.


**Effects on carbohydrate metabolism.** Treatment with clozapine may be associated with an increased risk of glucose intolerance and diabetes mellitus; a similar association has also been noted for some other atypical antipsychotics.

Data received by WHO indicated that up to December 2000, there had been 480 reports of glucose intolerance with clozapine, 253 with olanzapine, and 138 with risperidone.[1] In some cases weight gain was also reported, which may predispose to development of glucose intolerance. Other risk factors identified included an underlying diabetic condition, male gender, and the concomitant use of some medications including valproate, SSRIs, and buspirone. The authors recommended regular monitoring of weight, blood glucose, and blood lipids in patients receiving clozapine, olanzapine, and risperidone.

Glucose intolerance has also been reported for the atypical antipsychotic quetiapine.[2]

Other reviewers have also found similar evidence of an increased risk of diabetes with atypical antipsychotics.[3] In September 2003 the FDA therefore requested labelling changes for all atypical antipsychotics to include the following recommendations and warnings:

- patients with diabetes mellitus receiving atypical antipsychotics should be monitored regularly for worsening glucose control
- patients with risk factors for diabetes mellitus should undergo fasting blood glucose testing at the start of and during treatment with atypical antipsychotics
- all patients treated with atypical antipsychotics should be monitored during treatment and those who develop hyperglycaemia should undergo fasting blood glucose testing
- in some cases hyperglycaemia resolved on discontinuation but some patients required continuation of antidiabetic therapy despite withdrawal

However, the American Diabetes Association and several other American medical associations[4] consider that the risks vary between atypical antipsychotics and have recommended that this should be taken into account when prescribing. The risk of weight gain, diabetes, and dyslipidaemia was considered to be greatest for clozapine and olanzapine, with risperidone and quetiapine having intermediate effects, and aripiprazole and ziprasidone having little effect. They recommended that ***baseline monitoring*** should include:

- personal and family history of obesity, diabetes, dyslipidaemia, hypertension, or cardiovascular disease
- weight, height, and waist circumference
- blood pressure
- fasting blood glucose
- fasting lipid profile

Patients at risk for diabetes should receive an atypical drug with a lower propensity for weight gain and glucose intolerance. *Follow-up monitoring* should consist of reassessment of weight at 4, 8, and 12 weeks and it was recommended that a change of antipsychotic should be considered for any patient who gained more than 5% of their original weight during treatment. Fasting plasma glucose and blood pressure should be assessed at 3 months and annually or more frequently thereafter according to risk. Lipid levels should also be assessed after 3 months and, if normal, at 5-year intervals thereafter. Any patient with worsening glycaemia or dyslipidaemia should be changed to an antipsychotic that has not been associated with significant weight gain or diabetes.


1. Hedenmalm K, *et al.* Glucose intolerance with atypical antipsychotics. *Drug Safety* 2002; **25:** 1107–16.
2. Griffiths J, Springuel P. Atypical antipsychotics: impaired glucose metabolism. *Can Adverse Drug React News* 2001; **11:** 3–6.
3. Citrome LL, Jaffe AB. Relationship of atypical antipsychotics with development of diabetes mellitus. *Ann Pharmacother* 2003; **37:** 1849–57.
4. American Diabetes Association; American Psychiatric Association; American Association of Clinical Endocrinologists; North American Association for the Study of Obesity. Consensus development conference on antipsychotic drugs and obesity and diabetes. *Diabetes Care* 2004; **27:** 596–601.


**Effects on the cardiovascular system.** The Committee on Safety of Medicines (CSM)[1] in the UK issued a warning in November 1993 of the risk of **myocarditis** with clozapine. Three patients who died while taking clozapine had evidence of myocarditis. The CSM had also received one other report of myocarditis and one of cardiomyopathy associated with clozapine. The Australian Adverse Drug Reactions Advisory Committee (ADRAC) subsequently reported[2] another 5 cases of clozapine-associated myocarditis in November 1994. A later report[3] from Australia identified 15 cases of myocarditis, including 5 fatalities, between January 1993 and March 1999 (these figures were established using both data from ADRAC and the Australian manufacturers). Between September 1989 and December 1999 the FDA had received reports of 28 cases of myocarditis (18 fatal) and 41 of cardiomyopathy (10 fatal) temporally associated with clozapine use.[4] A review[5] by the pharmacovigilance authorities in New Zealand stated that by November 1999 the manufacturers Novartis had analysed 125 reports of myocarditis received worldwide including 35 fatalities; 53% had occurred during the first month of treatment but about 5% occurred more than 2 years after starting treatment. In a more recent reminder article,[6] the CSM has also commented that myocarditis occurs most commonly in the first 2 months whereas cardiomyopathy generally develops later in therapy. Pericarditis and pericardial effusions have also been reported. As myocarditis can be difficult to diagnose and confirmation is not always possible, the CSM recommended that if there was a high clinical suspicion of myocarditis, antipsychotic medication should be stopped. Presenting features might include persistent tachycardia at rest, heart failure, arrhythmia, or symptoms mimicking myocardial infarction or pericarditis. Patients who have developed clozapine-induced myocarditis or cardiomyopathy should not be re-exposed to clozapine.

There is also evidence that clozapine may be associated with fatal **thromboembolism**. The Swedish Adverse Reactions Advisory Committee had received reports[7] on 6 cases (5 fatal) of pulmonary embolism and 6 of venous thrombosis associated with clozapine treatment as of March 2000. The effect seemed to occur mainly in the first 3 months of treatment, and the majority of the cases involved men. However, analysis of data[8] from Germany and Switzerland suggests that the incidence of clozapine-associated thromboembolism is no different from that in psychiatric patients treated with classical antipsychotics or no antipsychotics at all (see also under Chlorpromazine, p.676).

There have been isolated reports[9,10] of **paradoxical hypertension** in patients receiving clozapine. Concomitant administration of atenolol has controlled the hypertension and allowed therapy with clozapine to be continued.

A small preliminary study[11] has suggested that **serum triglyceride concentrations** may be higher in patients taking clozapine than in those treated with conventional antipsychotics.

Some studies[12] have suggested that serious cardiovascular effects might occur more frequently and might be more severe in healthy subjects than in patients with schizophrenia. The manufacturers had requested that for the purpose of pharmacokinetic studies, clozapine should not be given to healthy subjects.

For further details of effects of clozapine on the cardiovascular system, see Benzodiazepines under Interactions, below.


1. Committee on Safety of Medicines/Medicines Control Agency. Myocarditis with antipsychotics: recent cases with clozapine (Clozaril). *Current Problems* 1993; **19:** 9–10.
2. Adverse Drug Reactions Advisory Committee. Clozapine and myocarditis. *Aust Adverse Drug React Bull* 1994; **13** (Nov): 14–15.
3. Kilian JG, *et al.* Myocarditis and cardiomyopathy associated with clozapine. *Lancet* 1999; **354:** 1841–5.
4. La Grenada L, *et al.* Myocarditis and cardiomyopathy associated with clozapine use in the United States. *N Engl J Med* 2001; **345:** 224–5.
5. New Zealand Medicines and Medical Devices Safety Authority. Potentially fatal complications of clozapine therapy: myocarditis, venous thromboembolism and constipation. Available at: http://www.medsafe.govt.nz/profs/puarticles/cloz1.htm (accessed 28/04/04)
6. Committee on Safety of Medicines/Medicines Control Agency. Clozapine and cardiac safety: updated advice for prescribers. *Current Problems* 2002; **28:** 8. Also available at: http://www.mca.gov.uk/ourwork/monitorsafequalmed/currentproblems/cpoct2002.pdf (accessed 28/04/04)
7. Hägg S, *et al.* Association of venous thromboembolism and clozapine. *Lancet* 2000; **355:** 1155–6.
8. Wolstein J, *et al.* Antipsychotic drugs and venous thromboembolism. *Lancet* 2000; **356:** 252.
9. Gupta S. Paradoxical hypertension associated with clozapine. *Am J Psychiatry* 1994; **151:** 148.
10. Ennis LM, Parker RM. Paradoxical hypertension associated with clozapine. *Med J Aust* 1997; **166:** 278.
11. Ghaeli P, Dufresne RL. Serum triglyceride levels in patients treated with clozapine. *Am J Health-Syst Pharm* 1996; **53:** 2079–81.
12. Pokorny R, *et al.* Normal volunteers should not be used for bioavailability or bioequivalence studies of clozapine. *Pharm Res* 1994; **11:** 1221.


**Effects on fluid and electrolyte homoeostasis.** Hyponatraemia has been reported to be associated with clozapine,[1] as with other antipsychotics (p.676). It was emphasised that hyponatraemia should be excluded as a possible trigger when considering the epileptogenic potential of clozapine.


1. Ogilvie AD, Croy MF. Clozapine and hyponatraemia. *Lancet* 1992; **340:** 672.


**Effects on the gastrointestinal tract.** The UK Committee on Safety of Medicines had received 20 reports of serious gastrointestinal reactions resembling obstruction associated with clozapine treatment as of March 1999, of which 3 were fatal.[1] These reactions were thought to be due to the antimuscarinic actions of clozapine and, therefore, more likely to occur when clozapine was taken together with other drugs with antimuscarinic actions such as tricyclic antidepressants, some antiparkinsonian drugs, and other antipsychotics; care was also warranted in those patients with a history of colonic disease or previous bowel surgery. It was also important to recognise and treat constipation in patients receiving clozapine to prevent the development of more serious complications such as obstruction and paralytic ileus.


1. Committee on Safety of Medicines/Medicines Control Agency. Clozapine (Clozaril) and gastrointestinal obstruction. *Current Problems* 1999; **25:** 5. Also available at: http://www.mca.gov.uk/ourwork/monitorsafequalmed/currentproblems/volume25mar.htm (accessed 28/04/04)


**Effects on the kidneys.** Acute interstitial nephritis developed in a 38-year-old woman after 11 days of treatment with clozapine 250 mg daily;[1] she recovered after stopping clozapine.


1. Elias TJ, *et al.* Clozapine-induced acute interstitial nephritis. *Lancet* 1999; **354:** 1180–1.


**Effects on the nervous system.** As with other antipsychotics (see Convulsions, p.675), clozapine can lower the seizure threshold and cause EEG abnormalities, although treatment with clozapine appears to be associated with a higher frequency of seizures. A review[1] of 1418 patients treated with clozapine in the USA between 1972 and 1988 found that 41 had experienced generalized tonic-clonic seizures. It was considered that the risk of clozapine-induced seizures was dose-related. The seizure frequency was calculated to be 1% at a dosage less than 300 mg daily, 2.7% at 300 to 599 mg daily, and 4.4% with a dosage of 600 mg or more daily. Six of the patients had been taking other drugs reported to lower the seizure threshold. Therapy with clozapine was continued in 31 of the 41 patients by reducing the total daily dose of clozapine; antiepileptic drug therapy was initiated in about half of the patients. The UK Committee on Safety of Medicines[2] considered that although the epileptogenic effect of clozapine was claimed to be dose-related, the metabolism and plasma concentrations of clozapine were highly variable and data from 8 cases reported to the Committee suggested that convulsions might possibly be related to high plasma concentrations in susceptible individuals. A low initial dosage followed by careful increases according to response and downward titration thereafter to a maintenance dose was recommended to avoid convulsions in susceptible individuals.

1. Devinsky O, *et al.* Clozapine-related seizures. *Neurology* 1991; **41:** 369–71.
2. Committee on Safety of Medicines. Convulsions may occur in patients receiving clozapine (Clozaril®, Sandoz). *Current Problems 31* 1991.

**Effects on the pancreas.** There have been isolated reports of pancreatitis associated with clozapine.[1,2] Pancreatitis has also been reported[3] following overdosage with clozapine.

1. Martin A. Acute pancreatitis associated with clozapine use. *Am J Psychiatry* 1992; **149:** 714.
2. Frankenburg FR, Kando J. Eosinophilia, clozapine, and pancreatitis. *Lancet* 1992; **340:** 251.
3. Jubert P, *et al.* Clozapine-related pancreatitis. *Ann Intern Med* 1994; **121:** 722–3.

**Hypersalivation.** Hypersalivation has been reported[1] to occur in up to 54% of patients receiving clozapine. The pathophysiology for this effect is unclear, but proposed mechanisms include action at muscarinic ($M_3$ and $M_4$) receptors, blockade of $\alpha_2$-adrenoceptors, or distortion of the swallowing reflex. Management strategies have included chewing gum to increase frequency of swallowing or reduction of clozapine dosage in stabilised patients; antimuscarinics or $\alpha_2$-agonists have been tried when other methods have failed. However, antimuscarinics could potentially exacerbate the antimuscarinic adverse effects of clozapine, and intranasal administration of ipratropium bromide has been tried as an alternative with beneficial results in one small uncontrolled study.[2]

1. Davydov L, Botts SR. Clozapine-induced hypersalivation. *Ann Pharmacother* 2000; **34:** 662–5.
2. Calderon J, *et al.* Potential use of ipatropium [sic] bromide for the treatment of clozapine-induced hypersalivation: a preliminary report. *Int Clin Psychopharmacol* 2000; **15:** 49–52.

**Neuroleptic malignant syndrome.** A review of the literature[1] suggested that clozapine may produce fewer extrapyramidal effects and a lower rise in creatine kinase concentrations than classical antipsychotics. The incidence of neuroleptic malignant syndrome with clozapine appeared to be similar to that with classical antipsychotics;[1] however, its presentation may differ, with fever and rigidity less frequent, and possibly less severe, but diaphoresis more common.[2]

1. Sachdev P, *et al.* Clozapine-induced neuroleptic malignant syndrome: a review and report of new cases. *J Clin Psychopharmacol* 1995; **15:** 365–71.
2. Karagianis JL, *et al.* Clozapine-associated neuroleptic malignant syndrome: two new cases and a review of the literature. *Ann Pharmacother* 1999; **33:** 623–30. Correction. *ibid.*; 1011.

**Withdrawal.** A report[1] of 3 patients who experienced delirium with psychotic symptoms shortly after discontinuation of clozapine. One of the patients had developed symptoms within 24 hours despite gradual withdrawal of clozapine over a 2-week period. All the patients responded rapidly to resumption of low doses of clozapine.

1. Stanilla JK, *et al.* Clozapine withdrawal resulting in delirium with psychosis: a report of three cases. *J Clin Psychiatry* 1997; **58:** 252–5.

## Precautions

Clozapine should not be given to patients with uncontrolled epilepsy, alcoholic or toxic psychoses, drug intoxication, or a history of circulatory collapse. It is contra-indicated in patients with bone-marrow suppression, myeloproliferative disorders, or any abnormalities of white blood cell count or differential blood count. It is also contra-indicated in patients with a history of drug-induced neutropenia or agranulocytosis with the exception of that due to chemotherapy. It should not be used with drugs that carry a high risk of bone-marrow suppression (see Interactions, below). Clozapine is contra-indicated in patients with severe renal impairment; caution is required in mild to moderate renal impairment. It should be used with caution in hepatic impairment and avoided in symptomatic or progressive liver disease or hepatic failure. Patients with a history of cardiac impairment or abnormal cardiac findings on examination should be referred to a specialist for further evaluation, which may include an ECG; treatment with clozapine should only then be started if the potential benefits clearly outweigh any risk. Clozapine should not be used in severe heart failure. Clozapine possesses antimuscarinic effects and consequently it is contra-indicated in patients with paralytic ileus; it should also be used with caution in benign prostatic hyperplasia and angle-closure glaucoma.

Clinical monitoring for hyperglycaemia has been recommended, especially in patients with or at risk of developing diabetes (see Effects on Carbohydrate Metabolism, above)

Monitoring the white blood cell and absolute neutrophil counts is mandatory during clozapine treatment and should be carried out in accordance with official recommendations; these may vary between countries (see Monitoring, below for further details). Patients or their carers should report the development of any infection or signs such as fever, sore throat, or flu-like symptoms which suggest infection.

Patients who develop tachycardia at rest, dyspnoea, or signs or symptoms of heart failure should be investigated immediately and clozapine treatment discontinued if a diagnosis of myocarditis is suspected.

Because of an increased risk of collapse due to orthostatic hypotension associated with initial titration of dosage of clozapine it is recommended that treatment should be initiated under close medical supervision. In addition, patients with Parkinson's disease should have their blood pressure monitored for the first weeks of treatment.

On planned withdrawal the dose of clozapine should be reduced gradually over at least a 1- to 2-week period in order to avoid the risk of rebound psychosis. If abrupt withdrawal is necessary then patients should be observed carefully.

Clozapine may affect the performance of skilled tasks such as driving.

**Breast feeding.** The American Academy of Pediatrics[1] considers that, although the effect of clozapine on breast-feeding infants is unknown, its use by mothers during breast feeding may be of concern since antipsychotic drugs do appear in breast milk and thus could conceivably alter CNS function in the infant both in the short and long term.

Clozapine appears to be distributed into breast milk in relatively high concentrations.[2] Concentrations in one mother were 63.5 nanograms/mL in breast milk and 14.7 nanograms/mL in plasma when receiving clozapine 50 mg daily and 115.6 nanograms/mL and 41.4 nanograms/mL, respectively when receiving 100 mg daily.

The manufacturers have also stated that studies in *animals* suggest that clozapine is excreted into breast milk and has an effect on nursing infants; they recommend that mothers receiving clozapine should not breast feed.

1. American Academy of Pediatrics. The transfer of drugs and other chemicals into human milk. *Pediatrics* 2001; **108:** 776–89. Correction. *ibid.*; 1029. Also available at: http://aappolicy.aappublications.org/cgi/content/full/pediatrics%3b108/3/776 (accessed 28/04/04)
2. Barnas C, *et al.* Clozapine concentrations in maternal and fetal plasma, amniotic fluid, and breast milk. *Am J Psychiatry* 1994; **151:** 945.

**Monitoring.** WHITE CELL COUNTS. A white blood cell count and a differential blood count must be performed before starting clozapine therapy and regularly throughout treatment. Treatment should not be started if the white blood cell count is less than 3500 cells/mm³ and the absolute neutrophil count (ANC) is less than 2000 cells/mm³, or if there is an abnormal differential count. Monitoring should continue throughout therapy and for 4 weeks after discontinuation.

In the EU, including the UK, monitoring is performed at weekly intervals for the first 18 weeks and then at least every 4 weeks thereafter.

- If during therapy the white blood cell count falls to between 3000 and 3500 cells/mm³ or the ANC falls to between 1500 and 2000 cells/mm³ then monitoring should be performed **twice weekly** until values stabilise or increase.
- Clozapine should be **withdrawn** immediately if the white blood cell count falls below 3000 cells/mm³ or the ANC drops below 1500 cells/mm³; counts should be monitored daily until they return to normal. Clozapine should not be restarted in these patients.

In the USA, white blood cell and ANC are monitored weekly for the first 6 months and then every 2 weeks thereafter.

- If during therapy the white blood cell count falls to between 3000 and 3500 cells/mm³ and the ANC is above 1500 cells/mm³ then monitoring should be performed **twice weekly**.
- If the white blood cell count falls below 3000 cells/mm³ or the ANC is below 1500 cells/mm³ then clozapine treatment should be **interrupted** and counts performed daily. Clozapine may be restarted if the white blood cell count recovers to above 3000 cells/mm³ and the ANC to above 1500 cells/mm³; in such cases monitoring should be increased to twice weekly until the white blood cell count is above 3500 cells/mm³. After recovery, weekly monitoring is recommended for the next 6 months.
- Clozapine should be **withdrawn** if the white blood cell count falls below 2000 cells/mm³ or the ANC drops below 1000 cells/mm³. Clozapine should not be restarted.

In patients with decreased white blood cell or ANC it is especially important that they or their carers report the development of any infection or signs such as fever, sore throat, or flu-like symptoms which suggest infection.

EOSINOPHIL COUNT. In the EU, clozapine should be withdrawn if the eosinophil count is greater than 3000 cells/mm³; it should only be restarted once the count has fallen to below 1000 cells/mm³.

Similar advice is given in the USA although the values differ: clozapine should be withdrawn if the eosinophil count is above 4000 cells/mm³ and restarted once the count has fallen to below 3000 cells/mm³.

PLATELET COUNT. European licensing information states that clozapine should be stopped if the platelet count falls below 50 000 cells/mm³.

TREATMENT BREAK. If treatment with clozapine is interrupted for reasons other than abnormal haematological values then more frequent monitoring may be required.

In the EU, patients who have taken clozapine for at least 18 weeks and stop therapy for more than 3 days but less than 4 weeks should resume weekly monitoring for the next 6 weeks before reducing to at least every 4 weeks if the counts are stable; a break of 4 weeks or more would require weekly monitoring for the next 18 weeks.

The manufacturers in the USA recommend that patients on clozapine for less than 6 months should be monitored weekly for an additional 6 months if therapy is interrupted for more than 1 month; those on longer term treatment would only need to resume weekly monitoring for 6 months if the break was greater than 1 year.

## Interactions

Clozapine may enhance the central effects of CNS depressants including alcohol, benzodiazepines, and MAOIs.

Clozapine should not be used concurrently with drugs which carry a high risk of bone-marrow suppression including carbamazepine, co-trimoxazole, chloramphenicol, penicillamine, sulfonamides, antineoplastics, or pyrazolone analgesics such as azapropazone. Long-acting depot antipsychotics should not be used with clozapine as they cannot be withdrawn rapidly should neutropenia occur. Additive effects may occur when clozapine is given with drugs that possess antimuscarinic, hypotensive, or respiratory depressant effects. Clozapine may reduce the effects of alpha-adrenoceptor agonists such as noradrenaline. The metabolism of clozapine is mediated mainly by the cytochrome P450 isoenzyme CYP1A2. Concomitant use of drugs that inhibit or act as a substrate to this isoenzyme may affect plasma concentrations of clozapine and the dose of clozapine may need to be altered. Increased plasma-clozapine concentrations, with an increased risk of adverse effects, may be seen in patients who suddenly stop smoking. Use with phenytoin or other enzyme-inducing drugs may accelerate the metabolism of clozapine and reduce its plasma concentrations.

◊ References.

1. Taylor D. Pharmacokinetic interactions involving clozapine. *Br J Psychiatry* 1997; **171:** 109–12.

**Antibacterials.** A patient with schizophrenia controlled with clozapine therapy had a tonic-clonic seizure 7 days after starting treatment with *erythromycin*.[1] It appeared that erythromycin had inhibited the metabolism of clozapine and raised its serum concentrations. Increased drowsiness and hypersalivation have been seen in a patient receiving clozapine and *ampicillin*; he recovered when ampicillin was replaced with doxycycline.[2]

Giving clozapine with *rifampicin* has resulted in decreased clozapine concentrations with consequent return of paranoid thoughts in a patient with a complicated history of schizophrenia.[3] An improvement was seen after rifampicin was replaced with ciprofloxacin. The interaction was thought to be due to the induction of cytochrome P450 isoenzymes, particularly CYP1A2, by rifampicin, resulting in the accelerated metabolism of clozapine.

1. Funderburg LG, *et al.* Seizure following addition of erythromycin to clozapine treatment. *Am J Psychiatry* 1994; **151:** 1840–1.
2. Csík V, Molnár J. Possible adverse interaction between clozapine and ampicillin in an adolescent with schizophrenia. *J Child Adolesc Psychopharmacol* 1994; **4:** 123–8.
3. Joos AAB, *et al.* Pharmacokinetic interaction of clozapine and rifampicin in a forensic patient with atypical mycobacterial infection. *J Clin Psychopharmacol* 1998; **18:** 83–5.

**Antidepressants.** Rises in serum concentrations of clozapine have been found in patients receiving clozapine after addition of *fluoxetine*[1] or *fluvoxamine*[2] to therapy. Increased serum concentrations of clozapine have also been reported when *paroxetine* or *sertraline* was added to therapy.[3] A possible serotonin syndrome (p.313) has been reported[4] in a patient receiving clomipramine after clozapine was gradually withdrawn from the treatment regimen, although the symptoms were also similar to those of clozapine withdrawal. There has been an isolated report[5] of a patient who developed myoclonic jerks 79 days after fluoxetine was added to treatment with clozapine and lorazepam, although some[6] doubt whether the effects were entirely due to an interaction. Giving clozapine with *lithium* may increase the risk of neuroleptic malignant syndrome. For reference to neurological reactions in patients receiving lithium with clozapine, see p.303.

1. Centorrino F, *et al.* Serum concentrations of clozapine and its major metabolites: effects of cotreatment with fluoxetine or valproate. *Am J Psychiatry* 1994; **151:** 123–5.
2. Jerling M, *et al.* Fluvoxamine inhibition and carbamazepine induction of the metabolism of clozapine: evidence from a therapeutic drug monitoring service. *Ther Drug Monit* 1994; **16:** 368–74.
3. Centorrino F, *et al.* Serum levels of clozapine and norclozapine in patients treated with selective serotonin reuptake inhibitors. *Am J Psychiatry* 1996; **153:** 820–2.
4. Zerjav-Lacombe S, Dewan V. Possible serotonin syndrome associated with clomipramine after withdrawal of clozapine. *Ann Pharmacother* 2001; **35:** 180–2.
5. Kingsbury SJ, Puckett KM. Effects of fluoxetine on serum clozapine levels. *Am J Psychiatry* 1995; **152:** 473.
6. Baldessarini RJ, *et al.* Effects of fluoxetine on serum clozapine levels. *Am J Psychiatry* 1995; **152:** 473–4.

**Antiepileptics.** Concomitant use of *phenytoin* or other *enzyme-inducing antiepileptics* may accelerate the metabolism of clozapine and reduce its plasma concentrations. Studies have found that addition of *sodium valproate* to clozapine therapy may increase[1] or decrease[2] plasma concentrations of clozapine. Although no increase in clozapine-related adverse effects or loss of control of psychotic symptoms were reported in these studies there has been a report[3] of a patient who experienced sedation, confusion, slurring of speech and other functional impairment after valproate was given with clozapine.

See also under Benzodiazepines, below.

1. Centorrino F, *et al.* Serum concentrations of clozapine and its major metabolites: effects of cotreatment with fluoxetine or valproate. *Am J Psychiatry* 1994; **151:** 123–5.
2. Finley P, Warner D. Potential impact of valproic acid therapy on clozapine disposition. *Biol Psychiatry* 1994; **36:** 487–8.
3. Costello LE, Suppes T. A clinically significant interaction between clozapine and valproate. *J Clin Psychopharmacol* 1995; **15:** 139–41.

**Antipsychotics.** Adding *risperidone* in a patient with schizoaffective disorder partially controlled by clozapine produced clinical improvement but was associated with a 74% rise in serum-clozapine concentrations over a 2-week period.[1] Although no adverse effects occurred in this patient, the potential for serious adverse effects requires caution if these drugs are used together. Neuroleptic malignant syndrome associated with concomitant use of clozapine and *haloperidol* has been reported.[2] See also under Chlorpromazine, p.680.

1. Tyson SC, *et al.* Pharmacokinetic interaction between risperidone and clozapine. *Am J Psychiatry* 1995; **152:** 1401–2.
2. Garcia G, *et al.* Neuroleptic malignant syndrome with antidepressant/antipsychotic drug combination. *Ann Pharmacother* 2001; **35:** 784–5.

**Antivirals.** Although the UK manufacturers of *ritonavir* state that it may increase plasma concentrations of clozapine with a resultant increase in the risk of toxicity, there is evidence to suggest that, in fact, ritonavir may decrease the plasma concentrations of clozapine.[1] Ritonavir has been noted to induce the cytochrome P450 isoenzyme CYP1A2 and hence, as clozapine is primarily metabolised via this isoenzyme, an acceleration of the metabolism of clozapine would be expected. US prescribing information has been amended accordingly.

1. Penzak SR, *et al.* Comment: significant interactions with new antiretrovirals and psychotropic drugs. *Ann Pharmacother* 1999; **33:** 1372–3.

**Benzodiazepines.** Concern has been expressed over reports of cardiorespiratory collapse in patients taking both clozapine and benzodiazepines.[1,2] In response, the manufacturers of clozapine outlined[3] similar cases reported to them in the USA. Of 7 cases of respiratory arrest or depression only 2 involved recent use of a benzodiazepine; among 26 cases of orthostatic hypotension with syncope reported during the first year the drug was marketed, only 8 included recent benzodiazepine use. The manufacturers concluded that an increased risk of such reactions in patients taking both drugs simultaneously was possible but not established, and advised caution when initiating clozapine therapy in patients taking benzodiazepines.

Hypersalivation associated with clozapine and benzodiazepines may be exacerbated when these drugs are used together. A patient[4] experienced increased hypersalivation, salivary thickening, and distension of the parotid glands when clonazepam was added to treatment with clozapine. Adverse effects reported in 5 other patients given clozapine and benzodiazepines together included hypersalivation, sedation, ataxia, and symptoms of delirium.[5,6]

1. Sassim N, Grohmann R. Adverse drug reactions with clozapine and simultaneous application of benzodiazepines. *Pharmacopsychiatry* 1988; **21:** 306–7.
2. Friedman LJ, *et al.* Clozapine—a novel antipsychotic agent. *N Engl J Med* 1991; **325:** 518.
3. Finkel MJ, Schwimmer JL. Clozapine—a novel antipsychotic agent. *N Engl J Med* 1991; **325:** 518–19.
4. Martin SD. Drug-induced parotid swelling. *Br J Hosp Med* 1993; **50:** 426.
5. Cobb CD, *et al.* Possible interaction between clozapine and lorazepam. *Am J Psychiatry* 1991; **148:** 1606–7.
6. Jackson CW, *et al.* Delirium associated with clozapine and benzodiazepine combinations. *Ann Clin Psychiatry* 1995; **7:** 139–41.

**Buspirone.** Potentially fatal gastrointestinal bleeding, accompanied by severe acidosis and hyperglycaemia, developed in a patient given buspirone with clozapine.[1] The patient had previously been receiving clozapine for over a year without adverse effect, and was subsequently maintained on clozapine alone without a recurrence of symptoms.

1. Good MI. Lethal interaction of clozapine and buspirone? *Am J Psychiatry* 1997; **154:** 1472–3.

**Histamine $H_2$-antagonists.** A patient stabilised on clozapine developed increased serum clozapine concentrations and signs of clozapine toxicity after starting treatment with *cimetidine.*[1] Cimetidine was withdrawn and ranitidine substituted without recurrence of toxicity.

1. Szymanski S, *et al.* A case report of cimetidine-induced clozapine toxicity. *J Clin Psychiatry* 1991; **52:** 21–2.

**Xanthines.** *Caffeine* may inhibit the metabolism of clozapine.[1,2] Care should be taken before stopping or starting caffeine-containing beverages in patients stabilised on clozapine treatment.

1. Carrillo JA, *et al.* Effects of caffeine withdrawal from the diet on the metabolism of clozapine in schizophrenic patients. *J Clin Psychopharmacol* 1998; **18:** 311–16.
2. Hägg S, *et al.* Effect of caffeine on clozapine pharmacokinetics in healthy volunteers. *Br J Clin Pharmacol* 2000; **49:** 59–63.

## Pharmacokinetics

Although clozapine is well absorbed from the gastrointestinal tract, its bioavailability is limited to about 50% by first-pass metabolism. Peak plasma concentrations are achieved an average of about 2.5 hours after oral administration. Clozapine is about 95% bound to plasma proteins and has a mean terminal elimination half-life of about 12 hours at steady state. It is almost completely metabolised and routes of metabolism include *N*-demethylation, hydroxylation, and *N*-oxidation; the desmethyl metabolite (norclozapine) has limited activity. The metabolism of clozapine is mediated mainly by the cytochrome P450 isoenzyme CYP1A2. Metabolites and trace amounts of unchanged drug are excreted mainly in the urine and also in the faeces. There is wide interindividual variation in plasma concentrations of clozapine and no simple correlation has been found between plasma concentrations and therapeutic effect.

◊ References.

1. Jann MW, *et al.* Pharmacokinetics and pharmacodynamics of clozapine. *Clin Pharmacokinet* 1993; **24:** 161–76.
2. Lin S-K, *et al.* Disposition of clozapine and desmethylclozapine in schizophrenic patients. *J Clin Pharmacol* 1994; **34:** 318–24.
3. Freeman DJ, Oyewumi LK. Will routine therapeutic drug monitoring have a place in clozapine therapy? *Clin Pharmacokinet* 1997; **32:** 93–100.
4. Olesen OV. Therapeutic drug monitoring of clozapine treatment: therapeutic threshold value for serum clozapine concentrations. *Clin Pharmacokinet* 1998; **34:** 497–502.
5. Guitton C, *et al.* Clozapine and metabolite concentrations during treatment of patients with chronic schizophrenia. *J Clin Pharmacol* 1999; **39:** 721–8.

**Bioavailability.** An increase in the plasma concentration of clozapine was noted in 10 patients when switched from an extemporaneous liquid formulation to conventional tablets.[1] Mean plasma concentrations increased from 329 to 629 nanograms/mL.

1. Coker-Adeyemi F, Taylor D. Clozapine plasma levels in patients switched from clozapine liquid to tablets. *Pharm J* 2002; **269:** 650–2.

## Uses and Administration

Clozapine is a dibenzodiazepine derivative described as an atypical antipsychotic. It has relatively weak dopamine receptor-blocking activity at $D_1$, $D_2$, $D_3$, and $D_5$ receptors but has a high affinity for the $D_4$ receptor. Clozapine possesses alpha-adrenergic blocking, antimuscarinic, antihistamine, antiserotonergic, and sedative properties.

Clozapine is used for the management of schizophrenia; however, because of the risk of agranulocytosis, it is reserved for patients who fail to respond to other antipsychotics, including other atypicals, or who experience severe neurological effects with such drugs. In the USA it may also be used for reducing the risk of recurrent suicidal behaviour in those with schizophrenia or schizoaffective disorder who are at chronic risk for suicidal behaviour. It is also used in the management of treatment-resistant psychoses associated with Parkinson's disease.

Clozapine use must be accompanied by strict procedures for the monitoring of white blood cell counts (see Precautions, above). To minimise the incidence of adverse effects, clozapine therapy should be introduced gradually, beginning with low doses and increasing according to response.

In the treatment of **schizophrenia**, including reducing the risk of suicidal behaviour, the usual dose by mouth is 12.5 mg once or twice on the first day followed by 25 mg once or twice on the second day. Thereafter the daily dosage may be increased gradually in increments of 25 to 50 mg to achieve a daily dose of up to 300 mg within 14 to 21 days (in the USA, up to 450 mg daily is permitted by the end of 2 weeks). Subsequent increments of 50 to 100 mg may be made once or twice weekly. Most patients respond to 200 to 450 mg daily; a daily dosage of 900 mg should not be exceeded. The total daily dose is given in divided doses; a larger proportion may be given at night. Once a therapeutic response has been obtained, a gradual reduction of dosage to a suitable maintenance dose may be possible. Daily maintenance doses of 200 mg or less may be given as a single dose in the evening. If clozapine is to be withdrawn this should be done gradually over a 1- to 2-week period. However, immediate discontinuation with careful observation is essential if neutropenia develops or if myocarditis is suspected (see Precautions, above).

Elderly patients may require lower doses of clozapine and it is recommended that treatment should be initiated with a dose of 12.5 mg on the first day and that subsequent dose increments should be restricted to 25 mg.

For patients who are restarting treatment after an interval of more than 2 days, 12.5 mg may be given once or twice on the first day. If that dose is well tolerated it may be possible to increase the dosage more quickly than on initiation. However, patients who previously experienced respiratory or cardiac arrest with initial dosing should be re-titrated with extreme caution after even 24 hours discontinuation. Additional monitoring of blood cell counts may also be required if treatment is interrupted, see Treatment Break, under Monitoring, above.

In the management of **psychoses in Parkinson's disease**, the initial dose of clozapine is no more than 12.5 mg once daily in the evening. Subsequent increases may be made in increments of 12.5 mg, with up to 2 increases each week; a dose of 50 mg daily should not be reached before the end of the second week. The usual dose ranges from 25 to 37.5 mg daily although some patients may require higher doses, up to a maximum of 100 mg daily. Increases above 50 mg should be made at weekly intervals.

The dose of clozapine may need to be adjusted if psychotic symptoms recur following increases in antiparkinsonian therapy: the dose may be increased in weekly increments of 12.5 mg to a maximum of 100 mg daily, as a single dose or in two divided doses.

As in patients with schizophrenia, planned withdrawal of clozapine should also be gradual, in decrements of 12.5 mg over 1 to 2 weeks, in patients with Parkinson's disease.

It is recommended that therapy with classical antipsychotics should be withdrawn gradually before treatment with clozapine is started.

Clozapine has also been given by intramuscular injection.

◊ References.

1. Fitton A, Heel RC. Clozapine: a review of its pharmacological properties, and therapeutic use in schizophrenia. *Drugs* 1990; **40:** 722–47.
2. Anonymous. Clozapine and loxapine for schizophrenia. *Drug Ther Bull* 1991; **29:** 41–2. Correction. *ibid.*; 52.
3. Baldessarini RJ, Frankenburg FR. Clozapine: a novel antipsychotic agent. *N Engl J Med* 1991; **324:** 746–54.
4. Hirsch SR, Puri BK. Clozapine: progress in treating refractory schizophrenia. *BMJ* 1993; **306:** 1427–8.
5. Taylor D. Clozapine—five years on. *Pharm J* 1995; **254:** 260–3.
6. Kerwin RW. Clozapine: back to the future for schizophrenia research. *Lancet* 1995; **345:** 1063–4.

**Action.** Antipsychotics are thought to work through inhibition of dopamine $D_2$-receptors (see p.681), but this hypothesis fails to explain the activity of the atypical antipsychotics such as clozapine. How clozapine produces its antipsychotic activity is not clear; it has a high affinity for a number of different receptors.[1]

1. Kerwin RW. The new atypical antipsychotics: a lack of extrapyramidal side-effects and new routes in schizophrenia research. *Br J Psychiatry* 1994; **164:** 141–8.

**Bipolar disorder.** Clozapine is of benefit for the treatment of mania in patients with bipolar disorder (p.278), and the use of atypical antipsychotics in the management of such patients is increasing. However, the adverse effects of clozapine may restrict its use.

**Dementia.** For mention that atypical antipsychotics such as clozapine might be more appropriate than classical antipsychotics for elderly patients with dementia, see the Elderly in Precautions for Chlorpromazine, p.678. For further discussion of the management of disturbed behaviour, see p.665.

**Parkinsonism.** Clozapine is used as an alternative to classical antipsychotics in the management of treatment-resistant psychosis in patients with Parkinson's disease (p.1196). Some neurologists even consider clozapine to be the antipsychotic of choice in these patients[1] although this remains to be determined. A review[2] in 1994 considered that there was little evidence to support clozapine as first choice given the quality of the available studies and the need for extensive monitoring. However a more recent double-blind, placebo-controlled study[3] demonstrated that low-dose clozapine treatment (up to 50 mg daily) significantly improved drug-induced psychosis without worsening parkinsonism. Adverse effects noted in this study were generally mild although in the clozapine group of 30 patients, there was one report of leucopenia. A similar study also reported benefit,[4] although 7 of 32 patients noted some aggravation of parkinsonism, usually mild and transient, while receiving clozapine. Adverse effects reported from other individuals have also included a patient with parkinsonism who experienced worsening of psychotic symptoms when her dose of clozapine was increased,[5] and the sudden return of psychosis in another patient with parkinsonism whose psychosis was successfully treated with clozapine for 5 years.[6]

1. Klein C, *et al.* Clozapine in Parkinson's disease psychosis: 5-year follow-up review. *Clin Neuropharmacol* 2003; **26:** 8–11.
2. Pfeiffer C, Wagner ML. Clozapine therapy for Parkinson's disease and other movement disorders. *Am J Hosp Pharm* 1994; **51:** 3047–53.
3. The Parkinson Study Group. Low-dose clozapine for the treatment of drug-induced psychosis in Parkinson's disease. *N Engl J Med* 1999; **340:** 757–63.
4. The French Clozapine Parkinson Study Group. Clozapine in drug-induced psychosis in Parkinson's disease. *Lancet* 1999; **353:** 2041–2.
5. Auzou P, *et al.* Worsening of psychotic symptoms by clozapine in Parkinson's disease. *Lancet* 1994; **344:** 955.
6. Greene P. Clozapine therapeutic plunge in patient with Parkinson's disease. *Lancet* 1995; **345:** 1172–3.

**Schizophrenia.** Clozapine is an effective antipsychotic for the management of schizophrenia (p.665) but its use is limited by its blood toxicity. Its effectiveness and superiority over classical antipsychotics was demonstrated by Kane *et al.* in a multicentre study.[1] Patients refractory to at least 3 different antipsychotics and who failed to improve after a single-blind trial of haloperidol, were randomised, double-blind, to treatment for 6 weeks with either clozapine, up to 900 mg daily, or chlorpromazine hydrochloride up to 1800 mg daily with benzatropine mesilate up to 6 mg daily. Of the 267 patients included in the evaluation, 5 of 141 (4%) improved with chlorpromazine and benzatropine, and 38 of 126 (30%) improved with clozapine. Clozapine was superior to chlorpromazine in the treatment of negative as well as positive symptoms. Reviews[2,3] of clozapine indicate that these findings have been well replicated both in subsequent studies and in clinical practice. It is, however, unclear for how long clozapine should initially be tried: although one study[4] identified new responses up to 12 months after initiation of therapy others have indicated that if improvement was not seen within the first 6 to 24 weeks, it was unlikely to occur.[2,5]

Clozapine has shown consistent clinical benefit in schizophrenic patients with persistent aggressive or violent behaviour.[2] Whether this is due to a sedative effect, a specific antiaggressive action, or just reflects an overall improvement in psychosis remains to be determined.

Clozapine also appears to reduce suicide risk in patients with refractory chronic schizophrenia.[6] The reported suicide rate of 0.05% per year in 6300 patients in the UK given clozapine since 1990 was considered to be tenfold less than expected.[7] A recent study[8] found it to be more effective than olanzapine in preventing suicide attempts in patients with schizophrenia or schizoaffective disorder at high risk.

Clozapine has been advocated for use in schizophrenic patients with moderate to severe tardive dyskinesia. It is still unclear whether clozapine can itself cause tardive dyskinesia but some patients with established tardive dyskinesia have experienced improvement in their symptoms when using clozapine.[9,10]

1. Kane J, *et al.* Clozapine for the treatment-resistant schizophrenic: a double-blind comparison with chlorpromazine. *Arch Gen Psychiatry* 1988; **45:** 789–96.
2. Buckley PF. New dimensions in the pharmacologic treatment of schizophrenia and related psychoses. *J Clin Pharmacol* 1997; **37:** 363–78. Correction. *ibid.* 1998; **38:** 27.
3. Wahlbeck K, *et al.* Clozapine versus typical neuroleptic medication for schizophrenia. Available in The Cochrane Library; Issue 2. Chichester: John Wiley; 2004.
4. Meltzer HY, *et al.* A prospective study of clozapine in treatment-resistant schizophrenic patients I: preliminary report. *Psychopharmacology (Berl)* 1989; **99:** S68–S72.
5. Conley RR, *et al.* Time to clozapine response in a standardized trial. *Am J Psychiatry* 1997; **154:** 1243–7.
6. Meltzer HY, Okayli G. Reduction of suicidality during clozapine treatment of neuroleptic-resistant schizophrenia: impact on risk-benefit assessment. *Am J Psychiatry* 1995; **152:** 183–90.
7. Kerwin RW. Clozapine: back to the future for schizophrenia research. *Lancet* 1995; **345:** 1063–4.
8. Meltzer HY, *et al.* Clozapine treatment for suicidality in schizophrenia: International Suicide Prevention Trial (InterSePT). *Arch Gen Psychiatry* 2003; **60:** 82–91. Correction. *ibid.* 735.
9. Tamminga CA, *et al.* Clozapine in tardive dyskinesia: observations from human and animal model studies. *J Clin Psychiatry* 1994; **55** (suppl B): 102–106.
10. Nair C, *et al.* Dose-related effects of clozapine on tardive dyskinesia among "treatment-refractory" patients with schizophrenia. *Biol Psychiatry* 1996; **39:** 529–30.

## Preparations

***USP 27:*** Clozapine Tablets.

**Proprietary Preparations** (details are given in Part 3)
***Arg.:*** Lapenax; Sequax; ***Austral.:*** Clopine; Clozaril; ***Austria:*** Lanolept; Leponex; ***Belg.:*** Leponex; ***Braz.:*** Leponex; Zolapin; ***Canad.:*** Clozaril; ***Chile:*** Leponex; ***Denm.:*** Leponex; ***Fin.:*** Froidir; Leponex; ***Fr.:*** Leponex; ***Ger.:*** Elcrit; Leponex; ***Gr.:*** Leponex; ***Hong Kong:*** Clozaril; ***India:*** Lozapin; Sizopin; ***Irl.:*** Clozaril; ***Israel:*** Leponex; Lozapine; ***Ital.:*** Leponex; ***Malaysia:*** Clozaril; ***Mex.:*** Clopsine; Leponex; ***Neth.:*** Leponex; ***Norw.:*** Leponex; ***NZ:*** Clopine; Clozaril; ***Port.:*** Leponex; ***S.Afr.:*** Leponex; ***Singapore:*** Clozaril; ***Spain:*** Leponex; ***Swed.:*** Leponex; ***Switz.:*** Leponex; ***Thai.:*** Clozaril; ***UK:*** Clozaril; ***USA:*** Clozaril.

---

# Cyamemazine *(rINN)*

Ciamemazina; Cyamepromazine; RP-7204. 10-(3-Dimethylamino-2-methylpropyl)phenothiazine-2-carbonitrile.

$C_{19}H_{21}N_3S$ = 323.5.
*CAS — 3546-03-0 (cyamemazine); 93841-82-8 (cyamemazine tartrate).*
*ATC — N05AA06.*

## Profile

Cyamemazine is a phenothiazine with general properties similar to those of chlorpromazine (p.675). It is available as a preparation for the management of a variety of psychiatric disorders including anxiety disorders (p.663) and aggressive behaviour (p.665).

Cyamemazine has been given by mouth as the base or the tartrate and by injection as the base. Doses are expressed in terms of the equivalent amount of cyamemazine base; cyamemazine tartrate 36.6 mg is approximately equivalent to cyamemazine base 25 mg. Doses have ranged from 25 to 600 mg daily by mouth, depending on the individual and the condition being treated; the daily dosage is given in 2 or 3 divided doses with the larger amount at night. Doses given by intramuscular injection have ranged from 25 to 200 mg daily.

Cyamemazine should be given in reduced dosage to elderly patients; the parenteral route is not recommended for the elderly.

## Preparations

**Proprietary Preparations** (details are given in Part 3)
***Fr.:*** Tercian; ***Port.:*** Tercian.

---

# Cyclobarbital *(BAN, rINN)*

Ciclobarbital; Cyclobarbitalum; Cyclobarbitone; Ethylhexabital; Hexemalum. 5-(Cyclohex-1-enyl)-5-ethylbarbituric acid.

$C_{12}H_{16}N_2O_3$ = 236.3.
*CAS — 52-31-3.*
*ATC — N05CA10.*

NOTE. The name ciclobarbital has sometimes been applied to hexobarbital.

# Cyclobarbital Calcium *(BANM, rINNM)*

Ciclobarbital cálcico; Ciclobarbital Calcium; Cyclobarbitalum Calcicum; Cyclobarbitone Calcium; Hexemalcalcium. Calcium 5-(cyclohex-1-enyl)-5-ethylbarbiturate.

$(C_{12}H_{15}N_2O_3)_2Ca$ = 510.6.
*CAS — 5897-20-1.*
*ATC — N05CA10.*

**Pharmacopoeias.** In *Pol.*

## Profile

Cyclobarbital is a barbiturate with general properties similar to those of amobarbital (p.670). The calcium salt has been used as a hypnotic but barbiturates are no longer considered appropriate for such purposes.

---

# Delorazepam *(pINN)*

Chlordesmethyldiazepam; Clordesmethyldiazepam. 7-Chloro-5-(2-chlorophenyl)-1,3-dihydro-2H-1,4-benzodiazepin-2-one.

$C_{15}H_{10}Cl_2N_2O$ = 305.2.
*CAS — 2894-67-9.*

## Profile

Delorazepam is a long-acting benzodiazepine with general properties similar to those of diazepam (p.690). It has been used in the short-term treatment of anxiety disorders, insomnia, and epilepsy, and for premedication.

**Administration in hepatic or renal impairment.** The pharmacokinetics of total delorazepam were unchanged in patients with renal failure undergoing haemodialysis compared with controls.[1] However, the apparent volume of distribution of unbound drug was smaller and the clearance slower. The volume of distribution and clearance of unchanged drug was also reduced in patients with liver disease.[2]

1. Sennesael J, *et al.* Pharmacokinetics of intravenous and oral chlordesmethyldiazepam in patients on regular haemodialysis. *Eur J Clin Pharmacol* 1991; **41:** 65–8.
2. Bareggi SR, *et al.* Effects of liver disease on the pharmacokinetics of intravenous and oral chlordesmethyldiazepam. *Eur J Clin Pharmacol* 1995; **48:** 265–8.

## Preparations

**Proprietary Preparations** (details are given in Part 3)
***Ital.:*** En†.

---

# Detomidine Hydrochloride *(BAN, USAN, rINNM)*

Demotidini Hydrochloridum; Hidrocloruro de detomidina; MPV-253-AII. 4-(2,3-Dimethylbenzyl)imidazole monohydrochloride.

$C_{12}H_{14}N_2,HCl$ = 222.7.
*CAS — 90038-01-0 (detomidine hydrochloride); 76631-46-4 (detomidine).*

**Pharmacopoeias.** In *Eur.* (see p.vi) for veterinary use only.

**Ph. Eur. 5.0** (Detomidine Hydrochloride for Veterinary Use). A white or almost white, hygroscopic, crystalline powder. Soluble in water; freely soluble in alcohol; practically insoluble in acetone; very slightly soluble in dichloromethane. Protect from moisture.

## Profile

Detomidine is an $\alpha_2$-adrenoceptor agonist with sedative, muscle relaxant, and analgesic properties. It is used as the hydrochloride in veterinary medicine.

---

# Dexmedetomidine Hydrochloride

*(BANM, USAN, rINNM)*

Hidrocloruro de dexmedetomidina; MPV-1440 (dexmedetomidine). (S)-4-[1-(2,3-Xylyl)ethyl]imidazole hydrochloride.

$C_{13}H_{16}N_2,HCl$ = 236.7.
*CAS — 113775-47-6 (dexmedetomidine); 145108-58-3 (dexmedetomidine hydrochloride).*

## Adverse Effects and Precautions

The most frequently observed adverse effect with dexmedetomidine is hypotension. Other common adverse effects include hypertension, nausea and vomiting, bradycardia, tachycardia, fever, hypoxia, and anaemia. Patients should be continuously monitored during administration. Dexmedetomidine should be used with caution in patients with advanced heart block, or hepatic or renal impairment, or in the elderly.

## Interactions

The effects of other CNS depressants may be enhanced by dexmedetomidine. Dexmedetomidine may also increase the effects of other vasodilators or negative chronotropic drugs.

## Pharmacokinetics

Dexmedetomidine is about 94% protein bound, but this has been reported to be significantly decreased in patients with hepatic impairment. Dexmedetomidine is almost completely metabolised by direct glucuronidation or by cytochrome P450 isoenzymes. It is excreted mainly as metabolites in the urine and faeces. The terminal elimination half-life is approximately 2 hours.

◊ References.

1. De Wolf AM, *et al.* The pharmacokinetics of dexmedetomidine in volunteers with severe renal impairment. *Anesth Analg* 2001; **93:** 1205–9.

## Uses and Administration

Dexmedetomidine is a selective alpha$_2$-adrenergic receptor agonist with anxiolytic, analgesic, and sedative properties. It is used as the hydrochloride for the sedation of mechanically ventilated patients in intensive care.

Dexmedetomidine hydrochloride is administered in sodium chloride 0.9% by intravenous infusion in a loading dose of 1 microgram/kg over 10 minutes, followed by a maintenance infusion of 0.2 to 0.7 micrograms/kg per hour for up to 24 hours. Reduced doses may be necessary in patients with hepatic or renal impairment, or in the elderly.

The racemate, medetomidine (p.706), is used as the hydrochloride in veterinary medicine.

◊ References.


1. Peden CJ, Prys-Roberts C. Dexmedetomidine—a powerful new adjunct to anaesthesia? *Br J Anaesth* 1992; **68:** 123–5.
2. Scheinin H, *et al.* Pharmacodynamics and pharmacokinetics of intramuscular dexmedetomidine. *Clin Pharmacol Ther* 1992; **52:** 537–46.
3. Aho M, *et al.* Comparison of dexmedetomidine and midazolam sedation and antagonism of dexmedetomidine with atipamezole. *J Clin Anesth* 1993; **5:** 194–203.
4. Kivistö KT, *et al.* Pharmacokinetics and pharmacodynamics of transdermal dexmedetomidine. *Eur J Clin Pharmacol* 1994; **46:** 345–9.
5. Venn RM, *et al.* Preliminary UK experience of dexmedetomidine, a novel agent for postoperative sedation in the intensive care unit. *Anaesthesia* 1999; **54:** 1136–42.
6. Bhana N, *et al.* Dexmedetomidine. *Drugs* 2000; **59:** 263–8.


### Preparations

**Proprietary Preparations** (details are given in Part 3)
***Arg.:*** Precedex; ***Austral.:*** Precedex; ***Braz.:*** Precedex; ***Israel:*** Precedex; ***Malaysia:*** Precedex; ***NZ:*** Precedex; ***Singapore:*** Precedex; ***USA:*** Precedex.

## Diazepam *(BAN, USAN, rINN)*

Diazepamum; LA-III; NSC-77518; Ro-5-2807; Wy-3467.
7-Chloro-1,3-dihydro-1-methyl-5-phenyl-2*H*-1,4-benzodiazepin-2-one.
$C_{16}H_{13}ClN_2O$ = 284.7.
*CAS — 439-14-5.*
*ATC — N05BA01.*

**Pharmacopoeias.** In *Chin., Eur.* (see p.vi), *Int., Jpn, Pol., US,* and *Viet.*

**Ph. Eur. 5.0** (Diazepam). A white or almost white, crystalline powder. Very slightly soluble in water; soluble in alcohol. Protect from light.

**USP 27** (Diazepam). An off-white to yellow, practically odourless, crystalline powder. Soluble 1 in 333 of water, 1 in 16 of alcohol, 1 in 2 of chloroform, and 1 in 39 of ether. Store in airtight containers. Protect from light.

**Incompatibility.** Incompatibility has been reported between diazepam and several other drugs. Manufacturers of diazepam injection (*Roche* and others) have advised against its admixture with other drugs.

**Sorption.** Substantial adsorption of diazepam onto some plastics may cause problems when administering the drug by continuous intravenous infusion. More than 50% of diazepam in solution may be adsorbed onto the walls of PVC infusion bags and their use should, therefore, be avoided. Administration sets should contain the minimum amount of PVC tubing and should not contain a cellulose propionate volume-control chamber. Suitable materials for infusion containers, syringes, and administration sets when administering diazepam include glass, polyolefin, polypropylene, and polyethylene.

References.


1. Cloyd JC, *et al.* Availability of diazepam from plastic containers. *Am J Hosp Pharm* 1980; **37:** 492–6.
2. Parker WA, MacCara ME. Compatibility of diazepam with intravenous fluid containers and administration sets. *Am J Hosp Pharm* 1980; **37:** 496–500.
3. Kowaluk EA, *et al.* Interactions between drugs and intravenous delivery systems. *Am J Hosp Pharm* 1982; **39:** 460–7.
4. Kowaluk EA, *et al.* Factors affecting the availability of diazepam stored in plastic bags and administered through intravenous sets. *Am J Hosp Pharm* 1983; **40:** 417–23.
5. Martens HJ, *et al.* Sorption of various drugs in polyvinyl chloride, glass, and polyethylene-lined infusion containers. *Am J Hosp Pharm* 1990; **47:** 369–73.


**Stability.** Care should be observed when diluting diazepam injections for infusion because of problems of precipitation. The manufacturer's directions should be followed regarding diluent and concentration of diazepam and all solutions should be freshly prepared.

### Dependence and Withdrawal

The development of dependence is common after regular use of benzodiazepines, even in therapeutic doses for short periods. Dependence is particularly likely in patients with a history of alcohol or drug abuse and in patients with marked personality disorders. Benzodiazepines should therefore be withdrawn by gradual reduction of the dose after regular use for even a few weeks; the time needed for withdrawal can vary from about 4 weeks to a year or more. The extent to which tolerance occurs has been debated but appears to involve psychomotor performance more often than anxiolytic effects. Drug-seeking behaviour is uncommon with therapeutic doses of benzodiazepines. High doses of diazepam and other benzodiazepines, injected intravenously, have been abused for their euphoriant effects.

**Benzodiazepine withdrawal syndrome.** Development of dependence to benzodiazepines cannot be predicted but risk factors include high dosage, regular continuous use, the use of benzodiazepines with a short half-life, use in patients with dependent personality characteristics or a history of drug or alcohol dependence, and the development of tolerance. The mechanism of dependence is unclear but may involve reduced gamma-aminobutyric acid (GABA) activity resulting from down-regulation of GABA receptors.

**Symptoms** of benzodiazepine withdrawal include anxiety, depression, impaired concentration, insomnia, headache, dizziness, tinnitus, loss of appetite, tremor, perspiration, irritability, perceptual disturbances such as hypersensitivity to physical, visual, and auditory stimuli and abnormal taste, nausea, vomiting, abdominal cramps, palpitations, mild systolic hypertension, tachycardia, and orthostatic hypotension. Rare and more serious symptoms include muscle twitching, confusional or paranoid psychosis, convulsions, hallucinations, and a state resembling delirium tremens. Broken sleep with vivid dreams and increased REM sleep may persist for some weeks after withdrawal of benzodiazepines.

Symptoms typical of withdrawal have been observed despite continued use of benzodiazepines and have been attributed either to the development of tolerance or, as in the case of very short-acting drugs such as triazolam, to rapid benzodiazepine elimination. Pseudowithdrawal has been reported in patients who believed incorrectly that their dose of benzodiazepine was being reduced. Benzodiazepine withdrawal syndrome can theoretically be distinguished from these reactions and from rebound phenomena (return of original symptoms at greater than pretreatment severity) by the differing **time course**. A withdrawal syndrome is characterised by its onset, by the development of new symptoms, and by a peak in intensity followed by resolution. Onset of withdrawal symptoms depends on the half-life of the drug and its active metabolites. Symptoms can begin within a few hours after withdrawal of a short-acting benzodiazepine, but may not develop for up to 3 weeks after stopping a longer-acting benzodiazepine. Resolution of symptoms may take several days or months. The dependence induced by short- and long-acting benzodiazepines appears to be qualitatively similar although withdrawal symptoms may be more severe with short-acting benzodiazepines. Rebound effects are also more likely with short-acting benzodiazepines. Rebound and withdrawal symptoms develop particularly rapidly with the very short-acting drug triazolam.

With increased awareness of the problems of benzodiazepine dependence, emphasis has been placed on **prevention** by proper use and careful patient selection. For example, the UK Committee on Safety of Medicines has recommended that benzodiazepines should be reserved for the short-term relief (2 to 4 weeks only) of anxiety that is severe, disabling, or subjecting the individual to unacceptable distress and is occurring alone or in association with insomnia or short-term psychosomatic, organic, or psychotic illness. These recommendations are similar to those of the UK Royal College of Psychiatrists.

**Withdrawal** from long-term benzodiazepine use should generally be encouraged. Established dependence can be difficult to treat; the patient should have professional and family support and behavioural therapy may be helpful. Withdrawal in a specialist centre may be required for some patients. Since abrupt withdrawal of benzodiazepines may result in severe withdrawal symptoms dosage should be tapered. The *British National Formulary* considers that benzodiazepines can be withdrawn in steps of about one-eighth of the daily dose every fortnight (range one-tenth to one-quarter). There are no comparative studies of the efficacy of various withdrawal schedules and in practice the protocol should be titrated against the response of the patient. Clinicians often favour transferring the patient to an equivalent dose of diazepam given at night and the following approximate dosage equivalents to *diazepam 5 mg* have been recommended in the UK:

- chlordiazepoxide 15 mg
- loprazolam 0.5 to 1 mg
- lorazepam 500 micrograms
- lormetazepam 0.5 to 1 mg
- nitrazepam 5 mg
- oxazepam 15 mg
- temazepam 10 mg

The daily dosage of diazepam can then be reduced in steps of 0.5 to 2.5 mg at fortnightly intervals. If troublesome abstinence effects occur the dose should be held level for a longer period before further reduction; increased dosage should be avoided if possible. It is better to reduce too slowly than too quickly. Time required for withdrawal can vary from about 4 weeks to a year or longer. In many cases the rate of withdrawal is best decided by the patient.

Adjuvant therapy should generally be avoided. Although a beta blocker may be given for prominent sympathetic overactivity the *British National Formulary* recommends that this be tried only if other measures fail; antidepressants should be used only for clinical depression or panic attacks. Antipsychotic drugs should be avoided as they may aggravate symptoms.

Symptoms gradually improve after withdrawal but postwithdrawal syndromes lasting for several weeks or months have been described. Continued support may be required for the first year after withdrawal to prevent relapse.

References.


1. Committee on Safety of Medicines. Benzodiazepines, dependence and withdrawal symptoms. *Current Problems 21* 1988.
2. Marriott S, Tyrer P. Benzodiazepine dependence: avoidance and withdrawal. *Drug Safety* 1993; **9:** 93–103.
3. Pétursson H. The benzodiazepine withdrawal syndrome. *Addiction* 1994; **89:** 1455–59.
4. Ashton H. The treatment of benzodiazepine dependence. *Addiction* 1994; **89:** 1535–41.
5. Royal College of Psychiatrists. *Benzodiazepines: risks, benefits or dependence—a re-evaluation.* Council Report CR59; London: January, 1997. Available at: http://www.rcpsych.ac.uk/publications/cr/council/cr59.pdf (accessed 28/04/04)
6. DoH. *Drug misuse and dependence: guidelines on clinical management.* London: The Stationery Office, 1999. Available at: http://www.dh.gov.uk/assetRoot/04/07/81/98/04078198.pdf (accessed 28/04/04)


### Adverse Effects

Drowsiness, sedation, muscle weakness, and ataxia are the most frequent adverse effects of diazepam use. They generally decrease on continued administration and are a consequence of CNS depression. Less frequent effects include vertigo, headache, confusion, depression (but see Effects on Mental Function, below), slurred speech or dysarthria, changes in libido, tremor, visual disturbances, urinary retention or incontinence, gastrointestinal disturbances, changes in salivation, and amnesia. Some patients may experience a paradoxical excitation which may lead to hostility, aggression, and disinhibition. Jaundice, blood disorders, and hypersensitivity reactions have been reported rarely. Respiratory depression and hypotension occasionally occur with high dosage and parenteral administration.

Pain and thrombophlebitis may occur with some intravenous formulations of diazepam; raised liver enzyme values have occurred.

Overdosage can produce CNS depression and coma or paradoxical excitation. However, fatalities are rare when taken alone.

Use of diazepam in the first trimester of pregnancy has occasionally been associated with congenital malformations in the infant but no clear relationship has been established. This topic is reviewed under Pregnancy below. Use of diazepam in late pregnancy has been associated with intoxication of the neonate.

**Carcinogenicity.** The International Agency for Research on Cancer concluded[1] that there was sufficient evidence from human studies that diazepam did not produce breast cancer, and that there was inadequate data to support its potential carcinogenicity at other sites. For most other benzodiazepines the lack of human studies meant that the carcinogenic risk to humans was not classifiable. However, there appeared to be sufficient evidence of carcinogenicity in *animal* studies for oxazepam to be classified as possibly carcinogenic in humans.


1. IARC/WHO. Some pharmaceutical drugs. *IARC monographs on the evaluation of carcinogenic risks to humans volume 66* 1996.


**Effects on body temperature.** Studies in healthy subjects[1,2] indicate that benzodiazepines can reduce body temperature. After a single dose of diazepam 10 mg by mouth in 11 subjects, body temperature on exposure to cold fell to a mean of 36.93° compared with 37.08° on exposure without the drug.[1] An 86-year-old woman developed hypothermia[3] after administration of nitrazepam 5 mg. After recovery she was mistakenly given another 5-mg dose of nitrazepam and again developed hypothermia. Midazolam (given as anaesthetic premedication) also produces modest decreases in core body temperature, which can be abolished by atropine,[4] but its effects are negligible compared with other elements of the anaesthetic regimen.[5]

Hypothermia has been reported in the neonates of mothers given benzodiazepines during the late stages of pregnancy.


1. Martin SM. The effect of diazepam on body temperature change in humans during cold exposure. *J Clin Pharmacol* 1985; **25:** 611–13.
2. Matsukawa T, *et al.* I.M. midazolam as premedication produces a concentration-dependent decrease in core temperature in male volunteers. *Br J Anaesth* 1997; **78:** 396–9.
3. Impallomeni M, Ezzat R. Hypothermia associated with nitrazepam administration. *BMJ* 1976; **1:** 223–4.
4. Matsukawa T, *et al.* Atropine prevents midazolam-induced core hypothermia in elderly patients. *J Clin Anesth* 2001; **13:** 504–8.
5. Kurz A, *et al.* Midazolam minimally impairs thermoregulatory control. *Anesth Analg* 1995; **81:** 393–8.


**Effects on endocrine function.** Galactorrhoea with normal serum-prolactin concentrations has been noted in 4 women taking benzodiazepines.[1] Gynaecomastia has been reported in a man taking up to 140 mg diazepam daily[2] and in 5 men taking diazepam in doses of up to 30 mg daily.[3] Serum-oestradiol concentrations were raised in the latter group. However, raised plasma-testosterone concentrations have also been observed in men taking diazepam 10 to 20 mg daily for 2 weeks.[4]


1. Kleinberg DL, *et al.* Galactorrhea: a study of 235 cases, including 48 with pituitary tumors. *N Engl J Med* 1977; **296:** 589–600.
2. Moerck HJ, Magelund G. Gynaecomastia and diazepam abuse. *Lancet* 1979; **i:** 1344–5.

3. Bergman D, *et al.* Increased oestradiol in diazepam related gynaecomastia. *Lancet* 1981; **ii:** 1225–6.
4. Argüelles AE, Rosner J. Diazepam and plasma-testosterone levels. *Lancet* 1975; **ii:** 607.

**Effects on the eyes.** Brown opacification of the lens occurred in 2 patients who took diazepam 5 mg or more daily by mouth over several years.[1] Severe visual field loss associated with very high doses (100 mg) of diazepam has also been described.[2]

1. Pau H. Braune scheibenförmige Einlagerungen in die Linse nach Langzeitgabe von Diazepam (Valium). *Klin Monatsbl Augenheilkd* 1985; **187:** 219–20.
2. Elder MJ. Diazepam and its effects on visual fields. *Aust N Z J Ophthalmol* 1992; **20:** 267–70.

**Effects on the liver.** Reports of cholestatic jaundice[1] in a patient and focal hepatic necrosis with intracellular cholestasis[2] in another associated with the use of diazepam.

1. Jick H, *et al.* Drug-induced liver disease. *J Clin Pharmacol* 1981; **21:** 359–64.
2. Tedesco FJ, Mills LR. Diazepam (Valium) hepatitis. *Dig Dis Sci* 1982; **27:** 470–2.

**Effects on mental function.** The effects of benzodiazepines on psychomotor performance in laboratory tests[1] are not easily extrapolated to the clinical situation. For example postoperative cognitive dysfunction in the elderly does not seem to be related to benzodiazepine concentration in the blood.[2]

Concern has been expressed over the possible effects of long-term benzodiazepine use on the brain. A detailed study[3] found that performance of tasks involving visual-spatial ability and sustained attention was poor in patients taking high doses of benzodiazepines for long periods of time. There was no evidence of impairment in global measures of intellectual functioning such as memory, flexibility, and simple reaction time. The authors could draw no conclusions about the effect of benzodiazepine withdrawal on these changes. A study of 17 long-term users of benzodiazepines has indicated a dose-dependent increase in cerebral ventricle size.[4]

Sexual fantasies have been reported in women sedated with intravenous diazepam or midazolam.[5] These appear to be dose-related.[6]

The view that benzodiazepines can cause depression, albeit infrequently, has been queried.[7]

Adverse effects of alprazolam on behaviour have also been reviewed.[8]

1. Woods JH, *et al.* Abuse liability of benzodiazepines. *Pharmacol Rev* 1987; **39:** 251–413.
2. Rasmussen LS, *et al.* Benzodiazepines and postoperative cognitive dysfunction in the elderly. *Br J Anaesth* 1999; **83:** 585–9.
3. Golombok S, *et al.* Cognitive impairment in long-term benzodiazepine users. *Psychol Med* 1988; **18:** 365–74.
4. Schmauss C, Krieg J-C. Enlargement of cerebrospinal fluid spaces in long-term benzodiazepine abusers. *Psychol Med* 1987; **17:** 869–73.
5. Dundee JW. Fantasies during sedation with intravenous midazolam or diazepam. *Med Leg J* 1990; **58:** 29–34.
6. Brahams D. Benzodiazepine sedation and allegations of sexual assault. *Lancet* 1989; **i:** 1339–40.
7. Patten SB, Love EJ. Drug-induced depression: incidence, avoidance and management. *Drug Safety* 1994; **10:** 203–19.
8. Cole JO, Kando JC. Adverse behavioral events reported in patients taking alprazolam and other benzodiazepines. *J Clin Psychiatry* 1993; **54** (suppl): 49–61.

**Effects on the nervous system.** There are a few isolated reports of extrapyramidal symptoms in patients taking benzodiazepines.[1-4] Benzodiazepines have been used to treat such symptoms induced by antipsychotics (see Chlorpromazine, p.677).

1. Rosenbaum AH, De La Fuente JR. Benzodiazepines and tardive dyskinesia. *Lancet* 1979; **ii:** 900.
2. Sandyk R. Orofacial dyskinesias associated with lorazepam therapy. *Clin Pharm* 1986; **5:** 419–21.
3. Stolarek IH, Ford MJ. Acute dystonia induced by midazolam and abolished by flumazenil. *BMJ* 1990; **300:** 614.
4. Joseph AB, Wroblewski BA. Paradoxical akathisia caused by clonazepam, clorazepate and lorazepam in patients with traumatic encephalopathy and seizure disorders: a subtype of benzodiazepine-induced disinhibition? *Behav Neurol* 1993; **6:** 221–3.

ENCEPHALOPATHY. Prolonged use of midazolam with fentanyl has been associated with encephalopathy in infants sedated under intensive care.[1]

1. Bergman I, *et al.* Reversible neurologic abnormalities associated with prolonged intravenous midazolam and fentanyl administration. *J Pediatr* 1991; **119:** 644–9.

**Effects on sexual function.** The sedative effects of benzodiazepines may reduce sexual arousal and lead to impotence in some patients. Conversely sexual performance may be improved by therapy if it was previously impaired by anxiety.

Increased libido and orgasmic function has been reported in 2 women after withdrawal of long-term benzodiazepine use.[1]

1. Nutt D, *et al.* Increased sexual function in benzodiazepine withdrawal. *Lancet* 1986; **ii:** 1101–2.

**Effects on skeletal muscle.** In a report[1] of 2 patients who developed rhabdomyolysis secondary to hyponatraemia it was suggested that the use of benzodiazepines might have contributed to the rhabdomyolysis. Of 8 reported cases of rhabdomyolysis associated with hyponatraemia, 5 had received benzodiazepines. Rhabdomyolysis associated with intravenous drug abuse of oral temazepam formulations has also been reported.[2]

1. Fernández-Real JM, *et al.* Hyponatremia and benzodiazepines result in rhabdomyolysis. *Ann Pharmacother* 1994; **28:** 1200–1.
2. Deighan CJ, *et al.* Rhabdomyolysis and acute renal failure resulting from alcohol and drug abuse. *Q J Med* 2000; **93:** 29–33.

**Effects on the skin.** There have been rare reports of cutaneous reactions to benzodiazepines, including contact dermatitis, fixed drug eruptions, toxic epidermal necrolysis, and Stevens-Johnson syndrome. Analysis by the Boston Collaborative Drug Surveillance Program of data on 15 438 patients hospitalised between 1975 and 1982 detected 2 allergic skin reactions attributed to diazepam among 4707 recipients of the drug.[1] A reaction rate of 0.4 per 1000 recipients was calculated from these figures.

1. Bigby M, *et al.* Drug-induced cutaneous reactions. *JAMA* 1986; **256:** 3358–63.

**Hypersensitivity.** Hypersensitivity reactions including anaphylaxis are very rare following use of diazepam. Reactions have been attributed to the polyethoxylated castor oil (p.1414) vehicle used for some parenteral formulations.[1] There is also a report of a type I hypersensitivity reaction to a lipid emulsion formulation of diazepam.[2]

See also under Effects on the Skin, above.

1. Hüttel MS, *et al.* Complement-mediated reactions to diazepam with Cremophor as solvent (Stesolid MR). *Br J Anaesth* 1980; **52:** 77–9.
2. Deardon DJ, Bird GLA. Acute (type 1) hypersensitivity to iv Diazemuls. *Br J Anaesth* 1987; **59:** 391.

**Local reactions.** Ischaemia and gangrene have been reported after accidental intra-arterial injection of diazepam.[1,2] Clinical signs may not occur until several days after the event. Pain and thrombophlebitis after intravenous administration may be similarly delayed. Local reactions after intravenous injection have been attributed to the vehicle, and have been observed more often when diazepam is given as a solution in propylene glycol than in polyethoxylated castor oil.[3] An emulsion of diazepam in soya oil and water has been associated with a lower incidence of local reactions.[3] Pain and phlebitis may also be caused by precipitation of diazepam at the site of infusion.[4] Arterial spasm experienced by a patient given diazepam intravenously was probably due to pressure from a cuff on the arm being inflated causing extravasation of diazepam out of the vein and into the radial artery.[5]

Local irritation has also been observed after rectal administration of diazepam.[6]

For a report of the exacerbation of diazepam-induced thrombophlebitis by penicillamine, see below.

1. Gould JDM, Lingam S. Hazards of intra-arterial diazepam. *BMJ* 1977; **2:** 298–9.
2. Rees M, Dormandy J. Accidental intra-arterial injection of diazepam. *BMJ* 1980; **281:** 289–90.
3. Olesen AS, Hüttel MS. Local reactions to iv diazepam in three different formulations. *Br J Anaesth* 1980; **52:** 609–11.
4. Hussey EK, *et al.* Correlation of delayed peak concentration with infusion-site irritation following diazepam administration. *DICP Ann Pharmacother* 1990; **24:** 678–80.
5. Ng Wing Tin L, *et al.* Arterial spasm after administration of diazepam. *Br J Anaesth* 1994; **72:** 139.
6. Hansen HC, *et al.* Local irritation after administration of diazepam in a rectal solution. *Br J Anaesth* 1989; **63:** 287–9.

**Overdosage.** Impairment of consciousness is fairly rapid in poisoning by benzodiazepines.[1] Deep coma or other manifestations of severe depression of brainstem vital functions are rare; more common is a sleep-like state from which the patient can be temporarily roused by appropriate stimuli. There is usually little or no respiratory depression, and cardiac rate and rhythm remain normal in the absence of anoxia or severe hypotension. Since tolerance to benzodiazepines develops rapidly, consciousness is often regained while concentrations of drug in the blood are higher than those which induced coma. Anxiety and insomnia can occur during recovery from acute overdosage, while a full-blown withdrawal syndrome, possibly with major convulsions, can occur in patients who have previously been chronic users.

During the years 1980 to 1989, 1576 fatal poisonings in Britain were attributed to benzodiazepines.[2] Of these, 891 were linked to overdosage with benzodiazepines alone and another 591 to overdosage combined with alcohol. A comparison of these mortality statistics with prescribing data for the same period, to calculate a toxicity index of deaths per million prescriptions, suggested that there were differences between the relative toxicities of individual benzodiazepines in overdosage. A later study of another 303 cases of benzodiazepine poisoning[3] supported these findings of differences in toxicity as well as pointing to the relative safety of the benzodiazepines in overdosage.

1. Ashton CH, *et al.* Drug-induced stupor and coma: some physical signs and their pharmacological basis. *Adverse Drug React Acute Poisoning Rev* 1989; **8:** 1–59.
2. Serfaty M, Masterton G. Fatal poisonings attributed to benzodiazepines in Britain during the 1980s. *Br J Psychiatry* 1993; **163:** 386–93.
3. Buckley NA, *et al.* Relative toxicity of benzodiazepines in overdose. *BMJ* 1995; **310:** 219–21.

## Treatment of Adverse Effects

The treatment of benzodiazepine overdosage is generally symptomatic and supportive. Activated charcoal may be given to those patients who have taken more than 1 mg/kg of diazepam (or its equivalent) and who present within 1 hour. Gastric lavage is generally not advocated in overdoses of benzodiazepines alone. The specific benzodiazepine antagonist, flumazenil, is rarely required and can be hazardous, particularly in mixed overdoses involving tricyclic antidepressants or in benzodiazepine-dependent patients (see p.1039). The *British National Formulary* recommends that flumazenil should be used on expert advice only although other authorities contra-indicate its use.

## Precautions

Diazepam should be avoided in patients with pre-existing CNS depression or coma, respiratory depression, acute pulmonary insufficiency, myasthenia gravis, or sleep apnoea, and used with care in those with chronic pulmonary insufficiency. Diazepam should be given with care to elderly or debilitated patients who may be more prone to adverse effects. Caution is required in patients with muscle weakness, or those with impaired liver or kidney function, who may require reduced doses; its use should be avoided in severe hepatic impairment. The sedative effects of diazepam are most marked during the first few days of use; affected patients should not drive or operate machinery (see also Driving, below). Monitoring of cardiorespiratory function is generally recommended when benzodiazepines are used for deep sedation.

Diazepam is not appropriate for the treatment of chronic psychosis or for phobic or obsessional states. Diazepam-induced disinhibition may precipitate suicide or aggressive behaviour and it should not, therefore, be used alone to treat depression or anxiety associated with depression; it should also be used with care in patients with personality disorders. Caution is required in patients with organic brain changes particularly arteriosclerosis. In cases of bereavement, psychological adjustment may be inhibited by diazepam.

Many manufacturers of diazepam and other benzodiazepines advise against their use in patients with glaucoma, but the rationale for this contra-indication is unclear.

For warnings on benzodiazepines during pregnancy and breast feeding, see below.

Dependence characterised by a withdrawal syndrome may develop after regular use of diazepam, even in therapeutic doses for short periods (see above); because of the risk of dependence, diazepam should be used with caution in patients with a history of alcohol or drug addiction.

Since hypotension and apnoea may occur when benzodiazepines are given intravenously it has been recommended that this route should only be used when facilities for reversing respiratory depression with mechanical ventilation are available. Patients should remain supine and under medical supervision for at least one hour after intravenous injection. Intravenous infusion is best undertaken in specialist centres with intensive care facilities where close and constant supervision can be undertaken.

**Administration.** INTRAVENOUS. A warning[1] that prolonged use of high-dose intravenous infusions of diazepam preparations containing benzyl alcohol can result in benzyl alcohol poisoning. (Such preparations should never be used in neonates—see p.1170.)

1. López-Herce J, *et al.* Benzyl alcohol poisoning following diazepam intravenous infusion. *Ann Pharmacother* 1995; **29:** 632.

**Breast feeding.** The American Academy of Pediatrics considers that benzodiazepine use by nursing mothers for long periods was a cause for concern; anxiolytic drugs appear in breast milk and could conceivably alter CNS function in the infant both in the short and long term.[1] Similarly, in the UK the Committee on Safety of Medicines has recommended[2] that benzodiazepines should not be given to lactating mothers. In one reviewer's opinion[3] the limited distribution into breast milk did not constitute a hazard to the breast-fed infant but the infant should be monitored for sedation and the inability to suckle. Another group has also reported a low incidence of toxicity and adverse effects in the breast-fed infants of mothers taking psychotropic drugs including benzodiazepines.[4] It has been suggested[5] that if a benzodiazepine must be used during breast feeding it would be preferable to use a short-acting drug with minimal distribution into breast milk and inactive metabolites; oxazepam, lorazepam, alprazolam, or midazolam might be suitable.

1. American Academy of Pediatrics. The transfer of drugs and other chemicals into human milk. *Pediatrics* 2001; **108:** 776–89. Correction. *ibid*; 1029. Also available at: http://aappolicy.aappublications.org/cgi/content/full/pediatrics%3b108/3/776 (accessed 28/04/04)

2. Committee on Safety of Medicines/Medicines Control Agency. Reminder: avoid benzodiazepines in pregnancy and lactation. *Current Problems* 1997; **23:** 10. Also available at: http://www.mca.gov.uk/ourwork/monitorsafequalmed/currentproblems/page2.htm (accessed 28/04/04)
3. McElhatton PR. The effects of benzodiazepine use during pregnancy and lactation. *Reprod Toxicol* 1994; **8:** 461–75.
4. Birnbaum CS, *et al.* Serum concentrations of antidepressants and benzodiazepines in nursing infants: a case series. Abstract: *Pediatrics* 1999; **104:** 104. Full version: http://pediatrics.aappublications.org/cgi/content/full/104/1/e11 (accessed 28/04/04)
5. Chisholm CA, Kuller JA. A guide to the safety of CNS-active agents during breastfeeding. *Drug Safety* 1997; **17:** 127–42.

**Cardiovascular disorders.** See under Respiratory System Disorders, below.

**Driving.** Most benzodiazepines can adversely affect parameters of driving performance in healthy subjects.[1] It is not entirely clear to what extent benzodiazepines contribute to the risk of driving accidents. A large case-control cohort study[2] in elderly drivers suggested that the risk of accidents was increased in those who took longer-acting benzodiazepines. However, younger drivers are more susceptible to the effects of benzodiazepines or zopiclone as a group;[3,4] the risk is increased by alcohol consumption.[3] Patients affected by drowsiness while taking benzodiazepines should not drive or operate machinery. In the UK, it is an offence to drive while unfit due to the influence of any drug, and benzodiazepines are considered to be the most likely psychotropic medication to impair driving performance, particularly the long-acting compounds.[5] However, it is also noted that drivers with psychiatric illnesses may be safer when well controlled with regular medication than when ill. Drowsiness often becomes less troublesome with continued use of these drugs.

1. Woods JH, *et al.* Abuse liability of benzodiazepines. *Pharmacol Rev* 1987; **39:** 251–413.
2. Hemmelgarn B, *et al.* Benzodiazepine use and the risk of motor vehicle crash in the elderly. *JAMA* 1997; **278:** 27–31.
3. Barbone F, *et al.* Association of road-traffic accidents with benzodiazepine use. *Lancet* 1998; **352:** 1331–6.
4. Vanakoski J, *et al.* Driving under light and dark conditions: effects of alcohol and diazepam in young and older subjects. *Eur J Clin Pharmacol* 2000; **56:** 453–8.
5. Driver and Vehicle Licensing Agency. For medical practitioners: at a glance guide to the current medical standards of fitness to drive. Available at: http://www.dvla.gov.uk/at_a_glance/ch4_psychiatric.htm (accessed 28/04/04)

**The elderly.** Old age may alter the distribution, elimination, and clearance of benzodiazepines.[1,2] Metabolic clearance of benzodiazepines metabolised principally by oxidation appears to be reduced but not clearance of those biotransformed by glucuronide conjugation or nitroreduction. Prolonged half-life in the elderly may be a result of such a decrease in clearance or of an increase in the volume of distribution. The clinical consequence of these changes depends on factors such as dosage schedule and extent of first-pass extraction by the liver.

Irrespective of pharmacokinetic changes, the elderly may exhibit increased sensitivity to acute doses of benzodiazepines.[1-3] Impairment of memory, cognitive function, and psychomotor performance and behaviour disinhibition may be more common than with younger patients.[4] Long-term use commonly exacerbates underlying dementia in elderly patients.[4]

The upshot of the pharmacokinetic and pharmacodynamic changes of benzodiazepines in the elderly is that adverse effects may be more frequent in these patients and lower doses are commonly required. An epidemiological study of persons 65 years and older found an increased rate of hip fracture among current users of long-acting benzodiazepines (*chlordiazepoxide, clorazepate, diazepam,* and *flurazepam*), but not among users of short-acting drugs (*alprazolam, bromazepam, lorazepam, oxazepam,* and *triazolam*).[5] A case-control study[6] of patients with falls leading to femur fractures suggested that the most important factor in increasing risk was the dose of benzodiazepine. However, another case-control study[7] found no correlation between hip fracture and benzodiazepines either as a group or according to half-life or to characterisation as an anxiolytic or a hypnotic; there might, though, be an increase in risk with lorazepam. There was also an increased risk associated with use of two or more benzodiazepines. Nonetheless, if use of a benzodiazepine is considered necessary in elderly patients, a short-acting drug is to be preferred. It should also be remembered that the elderly are at increased risk of sleep-related breathing disorders, such as sleep apnoea and the use of hypnotics such as benzodiazepines should be avoided in these patients (see Respiratory System Disorders, below).

1. Greenblatt DJ, *et al.* Implications of altered drug disposition in elderly: studies of benzodiazepines. *J Clin Pharmacol* 1989; **29:** 866–72.
2. Greenblatt DJ, *et al.* Clinical pharmacokinetics of anxiolytics and hypnotics in the elderly: therapeutic considerations. *Clin Pharmacokinet* 1991; **21:** 165–77 and 262–73.
3. Swift CG. Pharmacodynamics: changes in homeostatic mechanisms, receptor and target organ sensitivity in the elderly. *Br Med Bull* 1990; **46:** 36–52.
4. Juergens SM. Problems with benzodiazepines in elderly patients. *Mayo Clin Proc* 1993; **68:** 818–20.
5. Ray WA, *et al.* Benzodiazepines of long and short elimination half-life and the risk of hip fracture. *JAMA* 1989; **262:** 3303–7.
6. Herings RMC, *et al.* Benzodiazepines and the risk of falling leading to femur fractures: dosage more important than elimination half-life. *Arch Intern Med* 1995; **155:** 1801–7.
7. Pierfitte C, *et al.* Benzodiazepines and hip fractures in elderly people: case-control study. *BMJ* 2001; **322:** 704–8.

**Hangover effects.** Long-acting benzodiazepines accumulate in the body to a greater extent than ones with a shorter half-life. Although this might be expected to increase the frequency of daytime sedation and impairment of performance (so-called hangover effects) after a hypnotic dose, such a straightforward relationship has not always been observed in practice.[1]

Anterograde amnesia is more common with short-acting drugs such as triazolam; 'traveller's amnesia' has been used to describe amnesia in persons taking benzodiazepines for sleep disturbances resulting from jet lag.[2]

1. Greenblatt DJ, *et al.* Neurochemical and pharmacokinetic correlates of the clinical action of benzodiazepine hypnotic drugs. *Am J Med* 1990; **88** (suppl 3A): 18S–24S.
2. Meyboom RHB. Benzodiazepines and pilot error. *BMJ* 1991; **302:** 1274–5.

**High-altitude disorders.** Sleep may be impaired at high altitude due to frequent arousals associated with pronounced oxygen desaturation and periodic breathing. Traditional advice has been that sedatives should not be given at high altitude.[1] Caution may also be warranted at moderate altitudes especially in non-acclimatised climbers.[2] It has been argued that since diazepam, and possibly other sedatives, blunt the hypoxic ventilatory response, sleep hypoxaemia might be exacerbated. A small study[3] has suggested that small doses of a short-acting benzodiazepine, such as temazepam, might actually improve the subjective quality of sleep and reduce episodes of arterial desaturation without changing mean oxygen saturation. However the possibility of an interaction between acetazolamide taken for prophylaxis or treatment of acute mountain sickness and the benzodiazepine should be borne in mind; ventilatory depression in a mountain climber with acute mountain sickness was considered to be due to the potentiation of triazolam by acetazolamide.[4]

1. Sutton JR, *et al.* Insomnia, sedation, and high altitude cerebral oedema. *Lancet* 1979; **i:** 165.
2. Röggla G, *et al.* Effect of temazepam on ventilatory response at moderate altitude. *BMJ* 2000; **320:** 56.
3. Dubowitz G. Effect of temazepam on oxygen saturation and sleep quality at high altitude: randomised placebo controlled crossover trial. *BMJ* 1998; **316:** 587–9.
4. Masuyama S, *et al.* 'Ondine's curse': side effect of acetazolamide? *Am J Med* 1989; **86:** 637.

**Neonates.** A retrospective review of records from 63 infants given lorazepam or midazolam in a neonatal intensive-care unit indicated that there were 14 cases of adverse effects associated with benzodiazepine use (seizures in 6 cases, hypotension in 5, and respiratory depression in 3).[1] Seven of these were associated with intravenous bolus doses of lorazepam and the remainder with continuous midazolam infusions. Despite the limitations of the study, the incidence of adverse effects in this group seemed high, and the authors recommended that benzodiazepine use in neonates be accompanied by close monitoring.

1. Ng E, *et al.* Safety of benzodiazepines in newborns. *Ann Pharmacother* 2002; **36:** 1150–5.

**Nervous system disorders.** Benzodiazepines can reduce cerebral perfusion pressure and blood oxygenation to an extent that results in irreversible neurological damage in patients with head injuries. Consequently, they should be given with great care to such patients.[1,2] Their use should be avoided for the control of seizures in patients with head injuries or other acute neurological lesions as these patients can be managed effectively with phenytoin.

1. Eldridge PR, Punt JAG. Risks associated with giving benzodiazepines to patients with acute neurological injuries. *BMJ* 1990; **300:** 1189–90.
2. Papazian L, *et al.* Effect of bolus doses of midazolam on intracranial pressure and cerebral perfusion pressure in patients with severe head injury. *Br J Anaesth* 1993; **71:** 267–71.

EPILEPSY. As with other antiepileptic drugs,[1] there have been rare reports of benzodiazepines producing paradoxical exacerbation of seizures in patients with epilepsy.[2-5]

1. Guerrini R, *et al.* Antiepileptic drug-induced worsening of seizures in children. *Epilepsia* 1998; **39** (suppl 3): S2–S10.
2. Prior PF, *et al.* Intravenous diazepam. *Lancet* 1971; **2:** 434–5.
3. Tassinari CA, *et al.* A paradoxical effect: status epilepticus induced by benzodiazepines (Valium and Mogadon). *Electroencephalogr Clin Neurophysiol* 1971; **31:** 182.
4. Di Mario FJ, Clancy RR. Paradoxical precipitation of tonic seizures by lorazepam in a child with atypical absence seizures. *Pediatr Neurol* 1988; **4:** 249–51.
5. Borusiak P, *et al.* Seizure-inducing paradoxical reaction to antiepileptic drugs. *Brain Dev* 2000; **22:** 243–5.

**Porphyria.** Diazepam has been associated with acute attacks of porphyria and is considered unsafe in porphyric patients.

Intravenous diazepam has been used successfully, however, to control status epilepticus occurring after the acute porphyric attack. For a discussion of the management of seizures associated with acute porphyric attacks, see p.353.

**Pregnancy.** Benzodiazepines have been widely used in pregnant patients.[1] Use of benzodiazepines in the *third trimester* and during *labour* seems to be associated in some infants with neonatal withdrawal symptoms or the floppy infant syndrome. Also a small number exposed *in utero* to benzodiazepines have shown slow development in the early years but by 4 years of age most had developed normally, and for those that had not it was not possible to prove a cause-effect relationship with benzodiazepine exposure. In a meta-analysis[2] of live births following benzodiazepine use during the *first trimester* of pregnancy, pooled data from cohort studies showed no apparent association between benzodiazepine use and the risk of major malformations or oral cleft alone. There was, however, a small but significantly increased risk of oral cleft according to data from case-control studies. Although benzodiazepines did not appear to be a major human teratogen, use of ultrasonography was advised to rule out visible forms of cleft lip. The UK Committee on Safety of Medicines has recommended[3] that women of child-bearing potential prescribed benzodiazepines should be advised to contact the physician regarding discontinuation of the drug if they intend to become, or suspect that they are, pregnant.

1. McElhatton PR. The effects of benzodiazepine use during pregnancy and lactation. *Reprod Toxicol* 1994; **8:** 461–75.
2. Dolovich LR, *et al.* Benzodiazepine use in pregnancy and major malformations or oral cleft: meta-analysis of cohort and case-control studies. *BMJ* 1998; **317:** 839–43.
3. Committee on Safety of Medicines/Medicines Control Agency. Reminder: avoid benzodiazepines in pregnancy and lactation. *Current Problems* 1997; **23:** 10. Also available at: http://www.mca.gov.uk/ourwork/monitorsafequalmed/currentproblems/page2.htm (accessed 28/04/04)

**Respiratory system disorders.** Benzodiazepines may affect the control of ventilation during sleep and may worsen sleep apnoea or other sleep-related breathing disorders especially in patients with chronic obstructive pulmonary disease or cardiac failure.[1] Risk factors for sleep apnoea, which often goes undiagnosed, include old age, obesity, male sex, postmenopausal status in women, and a history of heavy snoring. Although benzodiazepines may reduce sleep fragmentation, their long-term use may result in conversion from partial to complete obstructive sleep apnoea in heavy snorers or in short repetitive central sleep apnoea in patients with recent myocardial infarction.

1. Guilleminault C. Benzodiazepines, breathing, and sleep. *Am J Med* 1990; **88** (suppl 3A): 25S–28S.

## Interactions

Enhanced sedation or respiratory and cardiovascular depression may occur if diazepam or other benzodiazepines are given with other drugs that have CNS-depressant properties; these include alcohol, antidepressants, sedative antihistamines, antipsychotics, general anaesthetics, other hypnotics or sedatives, and opioid analgesics. The sedative effect of benzodiazepines may also be enhanced by cisapride. Adverse effects may also be produced by use with drugs that interfere with the metabolism of benzodiazepines. Drugs that have been reported to alter the pharmacokinetics of benzodiazepines are discussed in detail below but few of these interactions are likely to be of clinical significance. Benzodiazepines such as diazepam which are metabolised primarily by hepatic microsomal oxidation may be more susceptible to pharmacokinetic changes than those eliminated primarily by glucuronide conjugation.

**Analgesics.** The peak plasma concentration of oxazepam was significantly decreased during administration of *diflunisal* in 6 healthy subjects, while the renal clearance of the glucuronide metabolite was reduced and its mean elimination half-life increased from 10 to 13 hours.[1] Diflunisal also displaced oxazepam from plasma protein binding sites *in vitro*. *Aspirin* shortened the time to induce anaesthesia with midazolam in 78 patients also possibly due to competition for plasma protein binding sites.[2] *Paracetamol* produced no significant change in plasma concentrations of diazepam or its major metabolite and only marginal changes in urine concentrations in 4 healthy subjects.[3]

Benzodiazepines such as diazepam, lorazepam, and midazolam may be used with opioid analgesics in anaesthetic or analgesic regimens. An additive sedative effect is to be expected[4] but there are also reports of severe respiratory depression with midazolam and *fentanyl*[5] or sudden hypotension with midazolam and fentanyl[6] or *sufentanil*.[7] The clearance of midazolam appears to be reduced by fentanyl,[8] possibly as a result of competitive inhibition of metabolism by the cytochrome P450 isoenzyme CYP3A. Careful monitoring is therefore required during use of midazolam with these opioids and the dose of both drugs may need to be reduced. Synergistic potentiation of the induction of anaesthesia has been reported between midazolam and fentanyl,[9] but one study has suggested that midazolam can reduce the analgesic effects of sufentanil.[10] Pretreatment with *morphine* or *pethidine* has decreased the rate of oral absorption of diazepam. This has been attributed to the effect of opioid analgesics on gastrointestinal motility.[11]

*Dextropropoxyphene* prolonged the half-life and reduced the clearance of alprazolam but not diazepam or lorazepam in healthy subjects.[12]

1. Van Hecken AM, *et al.* The influence of diflunisal on the pharmacokinetics of oxazepam. *Br J Clin Pharmacol* 1985; **20:** 225–34.
2. Dundee JW, *et al.* Aspirin and probenecid pretreatment influences the potency of thiopentone and the onset of action of midazolam. *Eur J Anaesthesiol* 1986; **3:** 247–51.
3. Mulley BA, *et al.* Interactions between diazepam and paracetamol. *J Clin Pharm* 1978; **3:** 25–35.
4. Tverskoy M, *et al.* Midazolam-morphine sedative interaction in patients. *Anesth Analg* 1989; **68:** 282–5.
5. Yaster M, *et al.* Midazolam-fentanyl intravenous sedation in children: case report of respiratory arrest. *Pediatrics* 1990; **86:** 463–7.

6. Burtin P, *et al.* Hypotension with midazolam and fentanyl in the newborn. *Lancet* 1991; **337:** 1545–6.
7. West JM, *et al.* Sudden hypotension associated with midazolam and sufentanil. *Anesth Analg* 1987; **66:** 693–4.
8. Hase I, *et al.* I.V. fentanyl decreases the clearance of midazolam. *Br J Anaesth* 1997; **79:** 740–3.
9. Ben-Shlomo I, *et al.* Midazolam acts synergistically with fentanyl for induction of anaesthesia. *Br J Anaesth* 1990; **64:** 45–7.
10. Luger TJ, Morawetz RF. Clinical evidence for a midazolam-sufentanil interaction in patients with major trauma. *Clin Pharmacol Ther* 1991; **49:** 133.
11. Gamble JAS, *et al.* Some pharmacological factors influencing the absorption of diazepam following oral administration. *Br J Anaesth* 1976; **48:** 1181–5.
12. Abernethy DR, *et al.* Interaction of propoxyphene with diazepam, alprazolam and lorazepam. *Br J Clin Pharmacol* 1985; **19:** 51–7.

**Antiarrhythmics.** An interaction between clonazepam and existing therapy with amiodarone was suspected in a 78-year-old man who experienced symptoms of benzodiazepine toxicity 2 months after starting with clonazepam 500 micrograms given at bedtime for restless leg syndrome;[1] symptoms resolved on withdrawal of clonazepam.

1. Witt DM, *et al.* Amiodarone-clonazepam interaction. *Ann Pharmacother* 1993; **27:** 1463–4.

**Antibacterials.** Both *erythromycin*[1] and *troleandomycin*[2] have been reported to inhibit the hepatic metabolism of triazolam in healthy subjects. Peak plasma-triazolam concentrations were increased, half-life prolonged, and clearance reduced. Troleandomycin prolonged the psychomotor impairment and amnesia produced by triazolam.[2] Loss of consciousness following erythromycin infusion in a child premedicated with midazolam was attributed to a similar interaction,[3] and increases in peak plasma concentrations of midazolam with profound and prolonged sedation have been reported following administration of erythromycin.[4] Use of midazolam with erythromycin should be avoided or the dose of midazolam reduced by 50 to 75%. The clearance of midazolam is also reduced by *clarithromycin*, with an approximate doubling of the benzodiazepine's oral bioavailability.[5] The manufacturers of *quinupristin/dalfopristin* state that it too may increase plasma concentrations of midazolam. *Roxithromycin* has been reported[6] to have some effects on the pharmacokinetics and pharmacodynamics of midazolam but these changes were not thought clinically relevant. However, it was recommended that as a precaution the lowest possible effective dose of midazolam should be used when given with roxithromycin. In another study[7] *azithromycin* did not appear to have any effect on the metabolism or psychomotor effects of midazolam.

There is an isolated report of significant rises in steady-state blood-midazolam concentration coinciding with administration of *ciprofloxacin*.[8] Also ciprofloxacin has been reported to reduce diazepam clearance and prolong its terminal half-life,[9] although psychometric tests did not show any changes in diazepam's pharmacodynamics. However, ciprofloxacin appears to have no effect on the pharmacokinetics or pharmacodynamics of temazepam.[10]

*Isoniazid* has been reported to increase the half-life of a single dose of diazepam[11] and triazolam[12] but not of oxazepam[12] in healthy subjects. In contrast, *rifampicin* has decreased the half-life of diazepam,[13] midazolam,[14] and nitrazepam[15] and more or less abolishes the effects of triazolam,[16] while *ethambutol* has no effect on diazepam pharmacokinetics.[11] In patients receiving therapy for tuberculosis with a combination of isoniazid, rifampicin, and ethambutol the half-life of a single diazepam dose was shortened and its clearance increased.[11] Thus the enzyme-inducing effect of rifampicin appears to predominate over the enzyme-inhibiting effect of isoniazid.

1. Phillips JP, *et al.* A pharmacokinetic drug interaction between erythromycin and triazolam. *J Clin Psychopharmacol* 1986; **6:** 297–9.
2. Warot D, *et al.* Troleandomycin-triazolam interaction in healthy volunteers: pharmacokinetic and psychometric evaluation. *Eur J Clin Pharmacol* 1987; **32:** 389–93.
3. Hiller A, *et al.* Unconsciousness associated with midazolam and erythromycin. *Br J Anaesth* 1990; **65:** 826–8.
4. Olkkola KT, *et al.* A potentially hazardous interaction between erythromycin and midazolam. *Clin Pharmacol Ther* 1993; **53:** 298–305.
5. Gorski JC, *et al.* The contribution of intestinal and hepatic CYP3A to the interaction between midazolam and clarithromycin. *Clin Pharmacol Ther* 1998; **64:** 133–43.
6. Backman JT, *et al.* A pharmacokinetic interaction between roxithromycin and midazolam. *Eur J Clin Pharmacol* 1994; **46:** 551–5.
7. Mattila MJ, *et al.* Azithromycin does not alter the effects of oral midazolam on human performance. *Eur J Clin Pharmacol* 1994; **47:** 49–52.
8. Orko R, *et al.* Intravenous infusion of midazolam, propofol and vecuronium in a patient with severe tetanus. *Acta Anaesthesiol Scand* 1988; **32:** 590–2.
9. Kamali F, *et al.* The influence of steady-state ciprofloxacin on the pharmacokinetics and pharmacodynamics of a single dose of diazepam in healthy volunteers. *Eur J Clin Pharmacol* 1993; **44:** 365–7.
10. Kamali F, *et al.* The influence of ciprofloxacin on the pharmacokinetics and pharmacodynamics of a single dose of temazepam in the young and elderly. *J Clin Pharm Ther* 1994; **19:** 105–9.
11. Ochs HR, *et al.* Diazepam interaction with antituberculous drugs. *Clin Pharmacol Ther* 1981; **29:** 671–8.
12. Ochs HR, *et al.* Differential effect of isoniazid on triazolam oxidation and oxazepam conjugation. *Br J Clin Pharmacol* 1983; **16:** 743–6.
13. Ohnhaus EE, *et al.* The effect of antipyrine and rifampin on the metabolism of diazepam. *Clin Pharmacol Ther* 1987; **42:** 148–56.
14. Backman JT, *et al.* Rifampin drastically reduces plasma concentrations and effects of oral midazolam. *Clin Pharmacol Ther* 1996; **59:** 7–13.
15. Brockmeyer NH, *et al.* Comparative effects of rifampin and/or probenecid on the pharmacokinetics of temazepam and nitrazepam. *Int J Clin Pharmacol Ther Toxicol* 1990; **28:** 387–93.
16. Villikka K, *et al.* Triazolam is ineffective in patients taking rifampicin. *Clin Pharmacol Ther* 1997; **61:** 8–14.

**Anticoagulants.** Plasma binding of diazepam and desmethyldiazepam was reduced, and free concentrations increased, immediately following *heparin* intravenously.[1]

Benzodiazepines do not usually interact with oral anticoagulants although there have been rare reports of altered anticoagulant activity.

1. Routledge PA, *et al.* Diazepam and N-desmethyldiazepam redistribution after heparin. *Clin Pharmacol Ther* 1980; **27:** 528–32.

**Antidepressants.** It has been recommended that the dosage of alprazolam should be reduced when given with *fluvoxamine*, as concomitant use has resulted in doubling of plasma-alprazolam concentrations.[1] Since plasma concentrations of bromazepam[2] and of diazepam[3] also appear to be affected by fluvoxamine, it has been suggested that patients taking fluvoxamine who require a benzodiazepine should preferentially receive one such as lorazepam, which has a different metabolic pathway.[3] Small studies suggest that *fluoxetine* can also increase plasma concentrations of alprazolam.[4,5] Fluoxetine appears to have a similar effect on diazepam but plasma concentrations of diazepam's active metabolite desmethyldiazepam are reduced and it is considered that the overall effect is likely to be minor.[6] The potential for a clinically significant interaction with *sertraline, paroxetine,* or *citalopram* is considered to be less.[7]

The manufacturers in the USA have reported that alprazolam may increase the steady-state plasma concentrations of *imipramine* and *desipramine*, although the clinical significance of such changes is unknown. For a suggestion that benzodiazepines may increase the oxidation of *amineptine* to a toxic metabolite, see under Effects on the Liver in Adverse Effects of Amitriptyline, p.282.

*Nefazodone* has been reported to raise concentrations of alprazolam and triazolam, resulting in increased sedation, and impairment of psychomotor performance.[8,9] Nefazodone may inhibit the oxidative metabolism of alprazolam and triazolam. Raised concentrations of midazolam have similarly been seen when given by mouth with nefazodone.[10] No interaction was reported with lorazepam, which is primarily eliminated by conjugation.

For reference to an isolated report of hypothermia after administration of diazepam and *lithium*, see p.303.

There have been occasional reports of sexual disinhibition in patients taking *tryptophan* with benzodiazepines.

1. Fleishaker JC, Hulst LK. A pharmacokinetic and pharmacodynamic evaluation of the combined administration of alprazolam and fluvoxamine. *Eur J Clin Pharmacol* 1994; **46:** 35–9.
2. Van Harten J, *et al.* Influence of multiple-dose administration of fluvoxamine on the pharmacokinetics of the benzodiazepines bromazepam and lorazepam: a randomized crossover study. *Eur Neuropsychopharmacol* 1992; **2:** 381.
3. Perucca E, *et al.* Inhibition of diazepam metabolism by fluvoxamine: a pharmacokinetic study in normal volunteers. *Clin Pharmacol Ther* 1994; **56:** 471–6.
4. Lasher TA, *et al.* Pharmacokinetic pharmacodynamic evaluation of the combined administration of alprazolam and fluoxetine. *Psychopharmacology (Berl)* 1991; **104:** 323–7.
5. Greenblatt DJ, *et al.* Fluoxetine impairs clearance of alprazolam but not of clonazepam. *Clin Pharmacol Ther* 1992; **52:** 479–86.
6. Lemberger L, *et al.* The effect of fluoxetine on the pharmacokinetics and psychomotor responses of diazepam. *Clin Pharmacol Ther* 1988; **43:** 412–19.
7. Sproule BA, *et al.* Selective serotonin reuptake inhibitors and CNS drug interactions: a critical review of the evidence. *Clin Pharmacokinet* 1997; **33:** 454–71.
8. Greene DS, *et al.* Coadministration of nefazodone (NEF) and benzodiazepines I: pharmacokinetic assessment. *Clin Pharmacol Ther* 1994; **55:** 141.
9. Kroboth P, *et al.* Coadministration of nefazodone and benzodiazepines II: pharmacodynamic assessment. *Clin Pharmacol Ther* 1994; **55:** 142.
10. Lam YWF, *et al.* Effect of antidepressants and ketoconazole on oral midazolam pharmacokinetics. *Clin Pharmacol Ther* 1998; **63:** 229.

**Antiepileptics.** *Carbamazepine*, *phenobarbital*, and *phenytoin* are all inducers of hepatic drug-metabolising enzymes. Therefore, in patients receiving long-term therapy with these drugs the metabolism of benzodiazepines may be enhanced. For oral midazolam the effects of carbamazepine or phenytoin may be sufficient to virtually abolish the effects of a standard dose, with a more than 90% reduction in peak serum concentrations of the benzodiazepine.[1] Interactions between benzodiazepines and these antiepileptics are further discussed on p.356 (carbamazepine) and p.374 (phenytoin). Results from a study[2] involving 66 children and adults receiving clobazam as adjunctive therapy for epilepsy showed a significant increase in clobazam clearance, leading to accumulation of its principle active metabolite *N*-desmethyl-clobazam, in the 16 patients also taking *felbamate*.

*Sodium valproate* has been reported to displace diazepam from plasma-protein binding sites.[3] Sporadic reports exist of adverse effects when valproate is given with clonazepam[4,5] with the development of drowsiness and, more seriously, absence status epilepticus, but the existence of an interaction is considered to be unproven.[6] Drowsiness has also been reported when valproate was given with nitrazepam.[7] Use of valproate semisodium with lorazepam has resulted in raised concentrations of lorazepam due to inhibition of glucuronidation of lorazepam.[8]

1. Backman JT, *et al.* Concentrations and effects of oral midazolam are greatly reduced in patients treated with carbamazepine or phenytoin. *Epilepsia* 1996; **37:** 253–7.
2. Contin M, *et al.* Effect of felbamate on clobazam and its metabolite kinetics in patients with epilepsy. *Ther Drug Monit* 1999; **21:** 604–8.
3. Dhillon S, Richens A. Valproic acid and diazepam interaction in vivo. *Br J Clin Pharmacol* 1982; **13:** 553–60.
4. Watson WA. Interaction between clonazepam and sodium valproate. *N Engl J Med* 1979; **300:** 678.
5. Browne TR. Interaction between clonazepam and sodium valproate. *N Engl J Med* 1979; **300:** 679.
6. Levy RH, Koch KM. Drug interactions with valproic acid. *Drugs* 1982; **24:** 543–56.
7. Jeavons PM, *et al.* Treatment of generalized epilepsies of childhood and adolescence with sodium valproate (Epilim). *Dev Med Child Neurol* 1977; **19:** 9–25.
8. Samara EE, *et al.* Effect of valproate on the pharmacokinetics and pharmacodynamics of lorazepam. *J Clin Pharmacol* 1997; **37:** 442–50.

**Antifungals.** Both a single dose and multiple doses of *ketoconazole* decreased the clearance of a single intravenous injection of chlordiazepoxide.[1] Studies[2-4] have shown that ketoconazole and *itraconazole* can produce marked pharmacokinetic interactions with midazolam or triazolam and greatly increase the intensity and duration of action of these benzodiazepines. The area under the plasma concentration-time curve for midazolam was increased by 15 times by ketoconazole and by 10 times by itraconazole while peak plasma concentrations of midazolam were increased fourfold and threefold respectively.[2] The area under the curve for triazolam was increased by 22 times by ketoconazole and by 27 times by itraconazole;[3] peak plasma concentrations of triazolam were increased about threefold by both antifungals. One study[5] indicated that the risk of interaction persists for several days after cessation of itraconazole therapy. It is recommended that the use of these antifungals with benzodiazepines should be avoided or that the dose of the benzodiazepine should be greatly reduced. A similar but less pronounced interaction occurs between *fluconazole* and midazolam[6] or triazolam;[7] nonetheless the dosage of the benzodiazepine should be reduced during concomitant use.

1. Brown MW, *et al.* Effect of ketoconazole on hepatic oxidative drug metabolism. *Clin Pharmacol Ther* 1985; **37:** 290–7.
2. Olkkola KT, *et al.* Midazolam should be avoided in patients receiving the systemic antimycotics ketoconazole or itraconazole. *Clin Pharmacol Ther* 1994; **55:** 481–5.
3. Varhe A, *et al.* Oral triazolam is potentially hazardous to patients receiving systemic antimycotics ketoconazole or itraconazole. *Clin Pharmacol Ther* 1994; **56:** 601–7.
4. Greenblatt DJ, *et al.* Interaction of triazolam and ketoconazole. *Lancet* 1995; **345:** 191.
5. Neuvonen PJ, *et al.* The effect of ingestion time interval on the interaction between itraconazole and triazolam. *Clin Pharmacol Ther* 1996; **60:** 326–31.
6. Ahonen J, *et al.* Effect of route of administration of fluconazole on the interaction between fluconazole and midazolam. *Eur J Clin Pharmacol* 1997; **51:** 415–19.
7. Varhe A, *et al.* Effect of fluconazole dose on the extent of fluconazole-triazolam interaction. *Br J Clin Pharmacol* 1996; **42:** 465–70.

**Antihistamines.** A suggestion[1] that a reduction in temazepam metabolism caused by *diphenhydramine* may have contributed to perinatal death after ingestion of these drugs by the mother.

1. Kargas GA, *et al.* Perinatal mortality due to interaction of diphenhydramine and temazepam. *N Engl J Med* 1985; **313:** 1417–18.

**Antivirals.** The non-nucleoside reverse transcriptase inhibitors *delavirdine* and *efavirenz*,[1] and HIV-protease inhibitors such as *indinavir, nelfinavir, ritonavir*,[1-3] and *saquinavir*[1,4] may inhibit the hepatic microsomal systems involved in the metabolism of some benzodiazepines. Prolonged administration of protease inhibitors may also *induce* these metabolic systems; interactions may therefore be complex and difficult to predict. Monitoring and dosage adjustments for the benzodiazepine may be needed, or the combination should be avoided. Benzodiazepines which should **not** be used with HIV-protease inhibitors include alprazolam, clorazepate, diazepam, estazolam, flurazepam, midazolam, and triazolam.

1. Antoniou T, Tseng AL. Interactions between recreational drugs and antiretroviral agents. *Ann Pharmacother* 2002; **36:** 1598–1613.
2. Greenblatt DJ, *et al.* Extensive impairment of triazolam and alprazolam clearance by short-term low-dose ritonavir: the clinical dilemma of concurrent inhibition and induction *J Clin Psychopharmacol* 1999; **19:** 293–6.
3. Greenblatt DJ, *et al.* Alprazolam-ritonavir interaction: implications for product labeling. *Clin Pharmacol Ther* 2000; **67:** 335–41.
4. Palkama VJ, *et al.* Effect of saquinavir on the pharmacokinetics and pharmacodynamics of oral and intravenous midazolam. *Clin Pharmacol Ther* 1999; **66:** 33–9.

**Beta blockers.** A clear pattern of interactions between benzodiazepines and beta blockers has not emerged. *Propranolol* may inhibit the metabolism of diazepam[1,2] and bromazepam,[3] and *metoprolol* may inhibit the metabolism of diazepam[1,4] or bromazepam[5] to some extent, although in many cases the effect on pharmacokinetics and pharmacodynamics is unlikely to be of clinical significance. No significant pharmacokinetic interaction has been seen between propranolol and alprazolam,[2] lorazepam,[2] or oxazepam,[6] although the rate of alprazolam absorption may be decreased.[2] Similarly no pharmacokinetic interaction has been seen between *atenolol* and diazepam,[1] *labetalol* and oxazepam,[6] or metoprolol and lorazepam.[5]

1. Hawksworth G, *et al.* Diazepam/β-adrenoceptor antagonist interactions. *Br J Clin Pharmacol* 1984; **17:** 69S–76S.
2. Ochs HR, *et al.* Propranolol interactions with diazepam, lorazepam, and alprazolam. *Clin Pharmacol Ther* 1984; **36:** 451–5.
3. Ochs HR, *et al.* Bromazepam pharmacokinetics: influence of age, gender, oral contraceptives, cimetidine, and propranolol. *Clin Pharmacol Ther* 1987; **41:** 562–70.
4. Klotz U, Reimann IW. Pharmacokinetic and pharmacodynamic interaction study of diazepam and metoprolol. *Eur J Clin Pharmacol* 1984; **26:** 223–6.
5. Scott AK, *et al.* Interaction of metoprolol with lorazepam and bromazepam. *Eur J Clin Pharmacol* 1991; **40:** 405–9.
6. Sonne J, *et al.* Single dose pharmacokinetics and pharmacodynamics of oral oxazepam during concomitant administration of propranolol and labetalol. *Br J Clin Pharmacol* 1990; **29:** 33–7.

**Calcium-channel blockers.** Peak plasma concentrations of midazolam were doubled and the elimination half-life of midazolam prolonged when midazolam was given to healthy subjects receiving *diltiazem* or *verapamil*.[1] A similar interaction has been demonstrated between diltiazem and triazolam.[2,3] Concomitant use should be avoided or the dose of these benzodiazepines reduced.

1. Backman JT, *et al.* Dose of midazolam should be reduced during diltiazem and verapamil treatments. *Br J Clin Pharmacol* 1994; **37:** 221–5.
2. Varhe A, *et al.* Diltiazem enhances the effects of triazolam by inhibiting its metabolism. *Clin Pharmacol Ther* 1996; **59:** 369–75.
3. Kosuge K, *et al.* Enhanced effect of triazolam with diltiazem. *Br J Clin Pharmacol* 1997; **43:** 367–72.

**Ciclosporin.** *In-vitro* studies suggested that ciclosporin could inhibit the metabolism of midazolam.[1] However, blood-ciclosporin concentrations in patients given ciclosporin to prevent graft rejection were considered too low to result in such an interaction.

1. Li G, *et al.* Is cyclosporin A an inhibitor of drug metabolism? *Br J Clin Pharmacol* 1990; **30:** 71–7.

**Clonidine.** Anxiety was reduced and sedation was enhanced when *clonidine* was given with flunitrazepam for premedication.[1]

1. Kulka PJ, *et al.* Sedative and anxiolytic interactions of clonidine and benzodiazepines. *Br J Anaesth* 1994; **72** (suppl 1): 81.

**Clozapine.** For reports of cardiorespiratory collapse and other adverse effects in patients taking benzodiazepines and clozapine, see p.688.

**Corticosteroids.** The metabolism of midazolam was increased in chronic users of *glucocorticoids*,[1] perhaps due to the induction of cytochrome P450 isoenzyme CYP3A4, or of enzymes responsible for glucuronidation. The changes were not considered clinically relevant if midazolam was given intravenously, but might be so if it were given by mouth.

1. Nakajima M, *et al.* Effects of chronic administration of glucocorticoid on midazolam pharmacokinetics in humans. *Ther Drug Monit* 1999; **21:** 507–13.

**Digoxin.** For the effects of alprazolam and diazepam on digoxin pharmacokinetics, see p.897.

**Disulfiram.** Evidence from healthy and alcoholic subjects suggests that chronic use of disulfiram can inhibit the metabolism of chlordiazepoxide and diazepam leading to a prolonged half-life and reduced clearance; there was little effect on the disposition of oxazepam.[1] No significant pharmacokinetic interaction was observed between disulfiram and alprazolam in alcoholic patients.[2] Temazepam toxicity, attributed to concomitant use of disulfiram and temazepam, has been reported.[3]

See also under Disulfiram, p.1682.

1. MacLeod SM, *et al.* Interaction of disulfiram with benzodiazepines. *Clin Pharmacol Ther* 1978; **24:** 583–9.
2. Diquet B, *et al.* Lack of interaction between disulfiram and alprazolam in alcoholic patients. *Eur J Clin Pharmacol* 1990; **38:** 157–60.
3. Hardman M, *et al.* Temazepam toxicity precipitated by disulfiram. *Lancet* 1994; **344:** 1231–2.

**Gastrointestinal drugs.** *Antacids* have variable effects on the absorption of benzodiazepines[1-6] but any resulting interaction is unlikely to be of major clinical significance.

Several studies, usually involving single doses of diazepam given to healthy subjects, have demonstrated that *cimetidine* can inhibit the hepatic metabolism of diazepam.[7-10] The clearance of diazepam has generally been decreased and the half-life prolonged. Some studies have also shown impaired metabolic clearance of the major metabolite, desmethyldiazepam (nordazepam). Cimetidine has also been reported to inhibit the metabolism of other benzodiazepines (generally those metabolised by oxidation) including alprazolam,[11,12] bromazepam,[13] chlordiazepoxide,[14] clobazam,[15,16] flurazepam,[17] midazolam,[18] nitrazepam,[19] and triazolam.[11,12] Cimetidine does not appear to inhibit the hepatic metabolism of lorazepam,[17] oxazepam,[17] or temazepam.[20] The clinical significance of these interactions between cimetidine and benzodiazepines remains dubious, and little effect on cognitive function or degree of sedation has been shown.

Most studies have failed to demonstrate an effect of *ranitidine* on the hepatic metabolism of diazepam,[21-24] although one study[25] reported an increase in the bioavailability of a single dose of midazolam given by mouth, and considered that an effect on hepatic clearance was more likely than an effect on absorption. These results were consistent with those of another study which demonstrated an enhanced sedative effect of midazolam in patients pretreated with ranitidine.[26] Ranitidine has been reported to have no effect on the pharmacokinetics of lorazepam[22] or on the sedative effect of temazepam[26] but has increased the bioavailability of triazolam.[27]

*Famotidine*[10] or *nizatidine*[24] do not appear to inhibit the hepatic metabolism of diazepam.

Oral diazepam was absorbed more rapidly after the intravenous administration of *metoclopramide*.[28] Enhanced motility of the gastrointestinal tract was implicated. *Cisapride* may also accelerate the absorption of diazepam.[29]

Studies of continuous *omeprazole* administration on the pharmacokinetics of a single intravenous dose of diazepam in healthy subjects indicate inhibition of diazepam metabolism in a similar manner to cimetidine.[30,31] Omeprazole decreases the clearance and prolongs the elimination half-life of diazepam; in addition both the formation and elimination of desmethyldiazepam appear to be decreased. The effects may be greater in rapid than in slow metabolisers of omeprazole[32] and vary between ethnic groups.[33] The clinical significance of the interaction remains to be established. *Lansoprazole*[34] and *pantoprazole*[35] have been reported not to affect the pharmacokinetics of diazepam.

1. Nair SG, *et al.* The influence of three antacids on the absorption and clinical action of oral diazepam. *Br J Anaesth* 1976; **48:** 1175–80.
2. Greenblatt DJ, *et al.* Influence of magnesium and aluminum hydroxide mixture on chlordiazepoxide absorption. *Clin Pharmacol Ther* 1976; **19:** 234–9.
3. Chun AHC, *et al.* Effect of antacids on absorption of clorazepate. *Clin Pharmacol Ther* 1977; **22:** 329–35.
4. Shader RI, *et al.* Impaired absorption of desmethyldiazepam from clorazepate by magnesium aluminum hydroxide. *Clin Pharmacol Ther* 1978; **24:** 308–15.
5. Greenblatt DJ, *et al.* Diazepam absorption: effect of antacids and food. *Clin Pharmacol Ther* 1978; **24:** 600–9.
6. Shader RI, *et al.* Steady-state plasma desmethyldiazepam during long-term clorazepate use: effect of antacids. *Clin Pharmacol Ther* 1982; **31:** 180–3.
7. Klotz U, Reimann I. Delayed clearance of diazepam due to cimetidine. *N Engl J Med* 1980; **302:** 1012–14.
8. Gough PA, *et al.* Influence of cimetidine on oral diazepam elimination with measurement of subsequent cognitive change. *Br J Clin Pharmacol* 1982; **14:** 739–42.
9. Greenblatt DJ, *et al.* Clinical importance of the interaction of diazepam and cimetidine. *N Engl J Med* 1984; **310:** 1639–43.
10. Locniskar A, *et al.* Interaction of diazepam with famotidine and cimetidine, two $H_2$-receptor antagonists. *J Clin Pharmacol* 1986; **26:** 299–303.
11. Abernethy DR, *et al.* Interaction of cimetidine with the triazolobenzodiazepines alprazolam and triazolam. *Psychopharmacology (Berl)* 1983; **80:** 275–8.
12. Pourbaix S, *et al.* Pharmacokinetic consequences of long term coadministration of cimetidine and triazolobenzodiazepines, alprazolam and triazolam, in healthy subjects. *Int J Clin Pharmacol Ther Toxicol* 1985; **23:** 447–51.
13. Ochs HR, *et al.* Bromazepam pharmacokinetics: influence of age, gender, oral contraceptives, cimetidine, and propranolol. *Clin Pharmacol Ther* 1987; **41:** 562–70.
14. Desmond PV, *et al.* Cimetidine impairs elimination of chlordiazepoxide (Librium) in man. *Ann Intern Med* 1980; **93:** 266–8.
15. Grigoleit H-G, *et al.* Pharmacokinetic aspects of the interaction between clobazam and cimetidine. *Eur J Clin Pharmacol* 1983; **25:** 139–42.
16. Pullar T, *et al.* The effect of cimetidine on the single dose pharmacokinetics of oral clobazam and N-desmethylclobazam. *Br J Clin Pharmacol* 1987; **23:** 317–21.
17. Greenblatt DJ, *et al.* Interaction of cimetidine with oxazepam, lorazepam, and flurazepam. *J Clin Pharmacol* 1984; **24:** 187–93.
18. Sanders LD, *et al.* Interaction of H2-receptor antagonists and benzodiazepine sedation: a double-blind placebo-controlled investigation of the effects of cimetidine and ranitidine on recovery after intravenous midazolam. *Anaesthesia* 1993; **48:** 286–92.
19. Ochs HR, *et al.* Cimetidine impairs nitrazepam clearance. *Clin Pharmacol Ther* 1983; **34:** 227–30.
20. Greenblatt DJ, *et al.* Noninteraction of temazepam and cimetidine. *J Pharm Sci* 1984; **73:** 399–401.
21. Klotz U, *et al.* Effect of ranitidine on the steady state pharmacokinetics of diazepam. *Eur J Clin Pharmacol* 1983; **24:** 357–60.
22. Abernethy DR, *et al.* Ranitidine does not impair oxidative or conjugative metabolism: noninteraction with antipyrine, diazepam, and lorazepam. *Clin Pharmacol Ther* 1984; **35:** 188–92.
23. Fee JPH, *et al.* Diazepam disposition following cimetidine or ranitidine. *Br J Clin Pharmacol* 1984; **17:** 617P–18P.
24. Klotz U, *et al.* Nocturnal doses of ranitidine and nizatidine do not affect the disposition of diazepam. *J Clin Pharmacol* 1987; **27:** 210–12.
25. Fee JPH, *et al.* Cimetidine and ranitidine increase midazolam bioavailability. *Clin Pharmacol Ther* 1987; **41:** 80–4.
26. Wilson CM, *et al.* Effect of pretreatment with ranitidine on the hypnotic action of single doses of midazolam, temazepam and zopiclone. *Br J Anaesth* 1986; **58:** 483–6.
27. Vanderveen RP, *et al.* Effect of ranitidine on the disposition of orally and intravenously administered triazolam. *Clin Pharm* 1991; **10:** 539–43.
28. Gamble JAS, *et al.* Some pharmacological factors influencing the absorption of diazepam following oral administration. *Br J Anaesth* 1976; **48:** 1181–5.
29. Bateman DN. The action of cisapride on gastric emptying and the pharmacokinetics of oral diazepam. *Eur J Clin Pharmacol* 1986; **30:** 205–8.
30. Gugler R, Jensen JC. Omeprazole inhibits elimination of diazepam. *Lancet* 1984; **i:** 969.
31. Andersson T, *et al.* Effect of omeprazole and cimetidine on plasma diazepam levels. *Eur J Clin Pharmacol* 1990; **39:** 51–4.
32. Andersson T, *et al.* Effect of omeprazole treatment on diazepam plasma levels in slow versus normal rapid metabolizers of omeprazole. *Clin Pharmacol Ther* 1990; **47:** 79–85.
33. Caraco Y, *et al.* Interethnic difference in omeprazole's inhibition of diazepam metabolism. *Clin Pharmacol Ther* 1995; **58:** 62–72.
34. Lefebvre RA, *et al.* Influence of lansoprazole treatment on diazepam plasma concentrations. *Clin Pharmacol Ther* 1992; **52:** 458–63.
35. Gugler R, *et al.* Lack of pharmacokinetic interaction of pantoprazole with diazepam in man. *Br J Clin Pharmacol* 1996; **42:** 249–52.

**General anaesthetics.** A synergistic interaction has been demonstrated for the hypnotic effects of midazolam and *thiopental*.[1] Although midazolam failed to produce anaesthesia at the doses used, the drug caused a twofold increase in the anaesthetic potency of thiopental. Similar synergistic interactions have been observed between midazolam and both *methohexital*[2] and *propofol*.[3,4] The interaction between midazolam and propofol could not be explained solely by alteration in free-plasma concentration of either drug,[5] although a later study[6] does suggest that propofol reduces the clearance of midazolam via its inhibitory effects on the metabolism of midazolam by the cytochrome P450 isoenzyme CYP3A4. It has been reported that midazolam can produce a marked reduction in the concentration of halothane required for anaesthesia.[7]

1. Short TG, *et al.* Hypnotic and anaesthetic action of thiopentone and midazolam alone and in combination. *Br J Anaesth* 1991; **66:** 13–19.
2. Tverskoy M, *et al.* Midazolam acts synergistically with methohexitone for induction of anaesthesia. *Br J Anaesth* 1989; **63:** 109–12.
3. McClune S, *et al.* Synergistic interaction between midazolam and propofol. *Br J Anaesth* 1992; **69:** 240–5.
4. Short TG, Chui PT. Propofol and midazolam act synergistically in combination. *Br J Anaesth* 1991; **67:** 539–45.
5. Teh J, *et al.* Pharmacokinetic interactions between midazolam and propofol: an infusion study. *Br J Anaesth* 1994; **72:** 62–5.
6. Hamaoka N, *et al.* Propofol decreases the clearance of midazolam by inhibiting CYP3A4: an in vivo and in vitro study. *Clin Pharmacol Ther* 1999; **66:** 110–7.
7. Inagaki Y, *et al.* Anesthetic interaction between midazolam and halothane in humans. *Anesth Analg* 1993; **76:** 613–7.

**Grapefruit juice.** Grapefruit juice has been reported to be able to increase the bioavailability of oral midazolam[1] or triazolam[2] and to raise peak plasma concentrations. However, these results have been contradicted by another study,[3] which found no evidence for an interaction.

1. Kupferschmidt HHT, *et al.* Interaction between grapefruit juice and midazolam in humans. *Clin Pharmacol Ther* 1995; **58:** 20–8.
2. Hukkinen SK, *et al.* Plasma concentrations of triazolam are increased by concomitant ingestion of grapefruit juice. *Clin Pharmacol Ther* 1995; **58:** 127–31.
3. Vanakoski J, *et al.* Grapefruit juice does not enhance the effects of midazolam and triazolam in man. *Eur J Clin Pharmacol* 1996; **50:** 501–8.

**Kava.** A patient whose medication included alprazolam, cimetidine, and terazosin became lethargic and disoriented after starting to take kava.[1] An interaction between kava and the benzodiazepine was suspected.

1. Almeida JC, Grimsley EW. Coma from the health food store: interaction between kava and alprazolam. *Ann Intern Med* 1996; **125:** 940–1.

**Levodopa.** For reference to the effects of benzodiazepines on levodopa, see p.1208.

**Neuromuscular blockers.** For reference to the effect of diazepam on neuromuscular blockade, see p.1401.

**Oral contraceptives.** Some studies with alprazolam,[1] chlordiazepoxide,[2] and diazepam[3] have supported suggestions that oral contraceptives may inhibit the biotransformation of benzodiazepines metabolised by oxidation, although no significant pharmacokinetic alterations have been observed with clotiazepam,[4] or triazolam.[1] The biotransformation of benzodiazepines metabolised by conjugation, such as lorazepam, oxazepam, or temazepam, may be enhanced[1,2] or unchanged.[5] No consistent correlation has been observed between the above pharmacokinetic changes and clinical effects. It has been observed[6] that psychomotor impairment due to oral diazepam was greater during the menstrual pause than during the 21-daily oral contraceptive cycle. This may have been due to an effect of oral contraceptives on diazepam absorption. Another study[7] noted that women taking oral contraceptives appeared to be more sensitive to psychomotor impairment following single oral doses of alprazolam, lorazepam, or triazolam, than controls. The effects of temazepam were minimal in both groups. Alterations in sedative or amnesic effect could not be established with any certainty.

1. Stoehr GP, *et al.* Effect of oral contraceptives on triazolam, temazepam, alprazolam, and lorazepam kinetics. *Clin Pharmacol Ther* 1984; **36:** 683–90.
2. Patwardhan RV, *et al.* Differential effects of oral contraceptive steroids on the metabolism of benzodiazepines. *Hepatology* 1983; **3:** 248–53.
3. Abernethy DR, *et al.* Impairment of diazepam metabolism by low-dose estrogen-containing oral-contraceptive steroids. *N Engl J Med* 1982; **306:** 791–2.
4. Ochs HR, *et al.* Disposition of clotiazepam: influence of age, sex, oral contraceptives, cimetidine, isoniazid and ethanol. *Eur J Clin Pharmacol* 1984; **26:** 55–9.
5. Abernethy DR, *et al.* Lorazepam and oxazepam kinetics in women on low-dose oral contraceptives. *Clin Pharmacol Ther* 1983; **33:** 628–32.
6. Ellinwood EH, *et al.* Effects of oral contraceptives on diazepam-induced psychomotor impairment. *Clin Pharmacol Ther* 1984; **35:** 360–6.
7. Kroboth PD, *et al.* Pharmacodynamic evaluation of the benzodiazepine-oral contraceptive interaction. *Clin Pharmacol Ther* 1985; **38:** 525–32.

**Penicillamine.** Phlebitis associated with intravenous diazepam resolved with local heat but recurred on two separate occasions after oral penicillamine.[1]

1. Brandstetter RD, *et al.* Exacerbation of intravenous diazepam-induced phlebitis by oral penicillamine. *BMJ* 1981; **283:** 525.

**Probenecid.** Probenecid increased the half-life of intravenous lorazepam in 9 healthy subjects.[1] Probenecid was considered to impair glucuronide formation selectively and thus the clearance of drugs like lorazepam. Probenecid has also shortened the time to induce anaesthesia with midazolam in 46 patients.[2] The effect was considered to be due to competition for plasma protein binding sites. Probenecid has also been reported[3] to reduce the clearance of nitrazepam but not of temazepam.

1. Abernethy DR, *et al.* Probenecid inhibition of acetaminophen and lorazepam glucuronidation. *Clin Pharmacol Ther* 1984; **35:** 224.
2. Dundee JW, *et al.* Aspirin and probenecid pretreatment influences the potency of thiopentone and the onset of action of midazolam. *Eur J Anaesthesiol* 1986; **3:** 247–51.
3. Brockmeyer NH, *et al.* Comparative effects of rifampin and/or probenecid on the pharmacokinetics of temazepam and nitrazepam. *Int J Clin Pharmacol Ther Toxicol* 1990; **28:** 387–93.

**Smooth muscle relaxants.** Intracavernosal *papaverine* produced prolonged erection in 2 patients who had been given intravenous diazepam as an anxiolytic before the papaverine.[1]

1. Vale JA, *et al.* Papaverine, benzodiazepines, and prolonged erections. *Lancet* 1991; **337:** 1552.

**Tobacco smoking.** The Boston Collaborative Drug Surveillance Program reported drowsiness as a side-effect of diazepam or chlordiazepoxide less frequently in smokers than non smokers.[1] Pharmacokinetic studies have, however, been divided between those indicating that smoking induces the hepatic metabolism of benzodiazepines and those showing no effect on benzodiazepine pharmacokinetics.[2] Hence, diminished end-organ responsiveness may in part account for the observed clinical effects. Concomitant consumption of large amounts of xanthine-containing beverages may decrease any enzyme-inducing effects of smoking.[3]

1. Boston Collaborative Drug Surveillance Program, Boston University Medical Center. Clinical depression of the central nervous system due to diazepam and chlordiazepoxide in relation to cigarette smoking and age. *N Engl J Med* 1973; **288:** 277–80.
2. Miller LG. Cigarettes and drug therapy: pharmacokinetic and pharmacodynamic considerations. *Clin Pharm* 1990; **9:** 125–35.
3. Downing RW, Rickels K. Coffee consumption, cigarette smoking and reporting of drowsiness in anxious patients treated with benzodiazepines or placebo. *Acta Psychiatr Scand* 1981; **64:** 398–408.

**Xanthines.** There are reports of *aminophylline* given intravenously reversing the sedation from intravenous diazepam,[1-3] although not always completely[2] nor as effectively as flumazenil.[4] Blockade of adenosine receptors by aminophylline has been postulated as the mechanism of this interaction.[3,5]

*Xanthine-containing beverages* may be expected to decrease the incidence of benzodiazepine-induced drowsiness because of their CNS-stimulating effects and their ability to induce hepatic drug-metabolising enzymes. However, decreased drowsiness has only sometimes been observed and the actions of xanthines may themselves be decreased by concomitant heavy tobacco smoking.[6,7]

1. Arvidsson SB, *et al.* Aminophylline antagonises diazepam sedation. *Lancet* 1982; **ii:** 1467.
2. Kleindienst G, Usinger P. Diazepam sedation is not antagonised completely by aminophylline. *Lancet* 1984; **i:** 113.
3. Niemand D, *et al.* Aminophylline inhibition of diazepam sedation: is adenosine blockade of GABA-receptors the mechanism? *Lancet* 1984; **i:** 463–4.
4. Sibai AN, *et al.* Comparison of flumazenil with aminophylline to antagonise midazolam in elderly patients. *Br J Anaesth* 1991; **66:** 591–5.
5. Henauer SA, *et al.* Theophylline antagonises diazepam-induced psychomotor impairment. *Eur J Clin Pharmacol* 1983; **25:** 743–7.
6. Downing RW, Rickels K. Coffee consumption, cigarette smoking and reporting of drowsiness in anxious patients treated with benzodiazepines or placebo. *Acta Psychiatr Scand* 1981; **64:** 398–408.
7. Ghoneim MM, *et al.* Pharmacokinetic and pharmacodynamic interactions between caffeine and diazepam. *J Clin Psychopharmacol* 1986; **6:** 75–80.

## Pharmacokinetics

Diazepam is readily and completely absorbed from the gastrointestinal tract, peak plasma concentrations occurring within about 30 to 90 minutes of oral administration. Diazepam is rapidly absorbed after administration as a rectal solution; peak plasma concentrations are achieved after about 10 to 30 minutes. Absorption may be erratic following intramuscular administration and lower peak plasma concentrations may be obtained compared with those following oral administration. Diazepam is highly lipid soluble and crosses the blood-brain barrier; it acts promptly on the brain, and its initial effects decrease rapidly as it is redistributed into fat depots and tissues.

Diazepam has a biphasic half-life with an initial rapid distribution phase followed by a prolonged terminal elimination phase of 1 or 2 days; its action is further prolonged by the even longer half-life of 2 to 5 days of its principal active metabolite, desmethyldiazepam (nordazepam). Diazepam and desmethyldiazepam accumulate on repeated administration and the relative proportion of desmethyldiazepam in the body increases with long-term use. No simple correlation has been found between plasma concentrations of diazepam or its metabolites and their therapeutic effect.

Diazepam is extensively metabolised in the liver, notably via the cytochrome P450 isoenzyme CYP2C19; in addition to desmethyldiazepam, its active metabolites include oxazepam, and temazepam. It is excreted in the urine, mainly in the form of free or conjugated metabolites. Diazepam is 98 to 99% bound to plasma proteins.

The plasma elimination half-life of diazepam and/or its metabolites is prolonged in neonates, in the elderly, and in patients with liver disease. In addition to crossing the blood-brain barrier, diazepam and its metabolites also cross the placental barrier and are distributed into breast milk.

◊ Reviews.

1. Bailey L, *et al.* Clinical pharmacokinetics of benzodiazepines. *J Clin Pharmacol* 1994; **34:** 804–11.

**The elderly.** For mention of pharmacokinetics in the elderly, see under Precautions, above.

**Hepatic impairment.** For reference to the altered pharmacokinetics of diazepam in patients with hepatic impairment see Administration in Hepatic Impairment, below.

**Absorption and plasma concentrations.** CHRONIC ORAL ADMINISTRATION. In 36 patients who had received diazepam 2 to 30 mg daily for periods from one month to 10 years, plasma-diazepam concentrations were directly related to dose and inversely related to age.[1] There was a close association between the plasma concentrations of diazepam and its metabolite desmethyldiazepam and both concentrations were independent of the duration of therapy. Plasma-diazepam concentration ranges were 0.02 to 1.01 micrograms/mL, and plasma-desmethyldiazepam concentration ranges were 0.055 to 1.765 micrograms/mL. A similar study[2] reached the same general conclusions.

1. Rutherford DM, *et al.* Plasma concentrations of diazepam and desmethyldiazepam during chronic diazepam therapy. *Br J Clin Pharmacol* 1978; **6:** 69–73.
2. Greenblatt DJ, *et al.* Plasma diazepam and desmethyldiazepam concentrations during long-term diazepam therapy. *Br J Clin Pharmacol* 1981; **1:** 35–40.

RECTAL. In 6 *adults* given diazepam 10 mg by mouth or as a solution (Valium injection) by rectum, mean bioavailability was 76 and 81%, respectively compared with the same dose by intravenous injection.[1] Bioavailability was lower with suppositories than with the solution given rectally. Studies support the use of rectal solution rather than suppositories in children.[2,3]

1. Dhillon S, *et al.* Bioavailability of diazepam after intravenous, oral and rectal administration in adult epileptic patients. *Br J Clin Pharmacol* 1982; **13:** 427–32.
2. Dhillon S, *et al.* Rectal absorption of diazepam in epileptic children. *Arch Dis Child* 1982; **57:** 264–7.
3. Sonander H, *et al.* Effects of the rectal administration of diazepam. *Br J Anaesth* 1985; **57:** 578–80.

**Distribution into breast milk.** Studies measuring concentrations of diazepam and desmethyldiazepam transferred from mother to infant via breast milk.[1,2]

See also under Precautions, above.

1. Erkkola R, Kanto J. Diazepam and breast-feeding. *Lancet* 1972; **i:** 1235–6.
2. Brandt R. Passage of diazepam and desmethyldiazepam into breast milk. *Arzneimittelforschung* 1976; **26:** 454–7.

**Metabolism.** Most benzodiazepines are highly lipophilic compounds requiring biotransformation before excretion from the body, and many form active metabolites that affect the duration of action. The benzodiazepines may be classified as long-, intermediate-, or short-acting compounds.[1]

- **Long-acting** benzodiazepines are either $N_1$-desalkyl derivatives (*delorazepam* and *nordazepam*) or are oxidised in the liver to $N_1$-desalkyl derivatives (benzodiazepines so oxidised include *chlordiazepoxide, clobazam, clorazepate, cloxazolam, diazepam, flurazepam, halazepam, ketazolam, medazepam, oxazolam, pinazepam, prazepam,* and *quazepam*). Clorazepate and prazepam may be considered as prodrugs since the metabolite is the expected active principle. Both parent drug and metabolites contribute to the activity of the other long-acting drugs. Further biotransformation of $N_1$-desalkylated metabolites proceeds much more slowly than for the parent drug, and they therefore accumulate in the body after a few days of treatment. The rate-limiting step of their metabolism (with the exception of the 1,5-derivatives) is C3-hydroxylation to the pharmacologically active oxazepam or its 2′-halogenated analogues.
- **Intermediate-acting** benzodiazepines are 7-nitrobenzodiazepines such as *clonazepam, flunitrazepam,* and *nitrazepam* which are metabolised by nitroreduction with no important known active metabolites. The metabolites of long- and intermediate-acting benzodiazepines require conjugation before excretion in the urine.
- **Short-acting** benzodiazepines include the C3-hydroxylated benzodiazepines such as *lorazepam, lormetazepam, oxazepam,* and *temazepam* which undergo rapid conjugation with glucuronic acid to water-soluble inactive metabolites that are excreted in the urine, and drugs such as *alprazolam, brotizolam, estazolam, etizolam, midazolam, tofisopam,* and *triazolam* which require oxidation involving aliphatic hydroxylation before subsequent conjugation. Although these hydroxylated metabolites may retain pharmacological activity, they are unlikely to contribute significantly to clinical activity because of their negligible plasma concentrations and rapid inactivation by glucuronidation.

Drug-metabolising capacity is influenced by many factors including genetics, age, sex, endocrine and nutritional status, smoking, disease, and concurrent drug therapy. This results in wide interindividual variation in both parent drug concentrations and metabolite-to-parent drug ratios.

1. Caccia S, Garattini S. Formation of active metabolites of psychotropic drugs: an updated review of their significance. *Clin Pharmacokinet* 1990; **18:** 434–59.

**Pregnancy.** The passage of diazepam across the placenta depends in part on the relative degrees of protein binding in mother and fetus. This in turn is influenced by factors such as stage of pregnancy and plasma concentrations of free fatty acids in mother and fetus.[1-6] Adverse effects may persist in the neonate for several days after birth because of immature drug-metabolising enzymes. Competition between diazepam and bilirubin for protein binding sites could result in hyperbilirubinaemia in the neonate.[7]

See also under Precautions, above.

1. Lee JN, *et al.* Serum protein binding of diazepam in maternal and foetal serum during pregnancy. *Br J Clin Pharmacol* 1982; **14:** 551–4.
2. Kuhnz W, Nau H. Differences in in vitro binding of diazepam and N-desmethyldiazepam to maternal and fetal plasma proteins at birth: relation to free fatty acid concentration and other parameters. *Clin Pharmacol Ther* 1983; **34:** 220–6.
3. Kanto J, *et al.* Accumulation of diazepam and N-demethyldiazepam in the fetal blood during the labour. *Ann Clin Res* 1973; **5:** 375–9.
4. Nau H, *et al.* Decreased serum protein binding of diazepam and its major metabolite in the neonate during the first postnatal week related to increased free fatty acid levels. *Br J Clin Pharmacol* 1984; **17:** 92–8.
5. Ridd MJ, *et al.* The disposition and placental transfer of diazepam in cesarean section. *Clin Pharmacol Ther* 1989; **45:** 506–12.
6. Idänpään-Heikkilä J, *et al.* Placental transfer and fetal metabolism of diazepam-$C^{14}$ in early human pregnancy. *Clin Pharmacol Ther* 1971; **12:** 293.
7. Notarianni LJ. Plasma protein binding of drugs in pregnancy and in neonates. *Clin Pharmacokinet* 1990; **18:** 20–36.

## Uses and Administration

Diazepam is a long-acting benzodiazepine with anticonvulsant, anxiolytic, sedative, muscle relaxant, and amnestic properties. Its actions are mediated by enhancement of the activity of gamma-aminobutyric acid (GABA), a major inhibitory neurotransmitter in the brain. Diazepam is used in the short-term treatment of severe anxiety disorders (p.663), as a hypnotic in the short-term management of insomnia (p.667), as a sedative (p.666) and premedicant (p.1296), as an anticonvulsant (particularly in the management of status epilepticus and febrile convulsions), in the control of muscle spasm, and in the management of withdrawal symptoms (see the references below).

Diazepam is **administered** orally, rectally, and parenterally with the risk of dependence very much influencing the dose and duration of treatment. Doses should be the lowest that can control symptoms and courses of treatment should be short, not normally exceeding 4 weeks, with diazepam being withdrawn gradually (see above). Elderly and debilitated patients should be given not more than one-half the usual adult dose. Dosage reduction may also be required in patients with hepatic or renal impairment.

*Oral* administration is appropriate for many indications and modified-release formulations are available in some countries. *Rectal* administration may be by suppository or rectal solution or gel. Diazepam is also given by deep intramuscular or slow intravenous injection, although absorption following *intramuscular injection* may be erratic and provides lower blood concentrations than those following oral administration. *Intravenous injection* should be carried out slowly into a large vein of the antecubital fossa at a recommended rate of no more than 1 mL of a 0.5% solution (5 mg) per minute. It is advisable to keep the patient in the supine position and under medical supervision for at least an hour after administration. Diazepam may be given by continuous *intravenous infusion*; because of the risk of precipitation of diazepam, solutions should be freshly prepared following the manufacturer's directions regarding diluent and concentration of diazepam. Diazepam is substantially adsorbed onto some plastics (see under Sorption, above). Facilities for resuscitation should always be available when diazepam is given intravenously.

Diazepam may be given for **severe anxiety** in *oral* doses of 2 mg three times daily to a maximum of 30 mg daily. A wider dose range of 4 to 40 mg daily in divided doses is used in the USA with children over 6 months of age receiving up to 10 mg daily. Diazepam may be given as a *rectal solution* in a dose of 500 micrograms/kg repeated after 12 hours if necessary or as *suppositories* in a dose of 10 to 30 mg. Diazepam may sometimes have to be given by intramuscular or intravenous *injection* when a dose of up to 10 mg may be used, repeated if necessary after 4 hours.

The benzodiazepines have a limited role in **insomnia** and diazepam is used for the short-term management of insomnia associated with anxiety. The *British National Formulary* recommends a dose of 5 to 15 mg by mouth at bedtime, although doses up to 30 mg are licensed. Doses of 1 to 5 mg at bedtime have been used in children to control **night terrors** and **sleepwalking**.

Diazepam may be given for **premedication** before general anaesthesia or to provide sedative cover for minor surgical or investigative procedures. Doses *by mouth* are in the range of 5 to 15 mg; a dose of 10 mg as a *rectal solution* may also be suitable. When given by intravenous *injection* the dose is usually 100 to 200 micrograms/kg. Some regard the perioperative use of diazepam in children undesirable since its effect and onset of action are unreliable and paradoxical effects may occur. Diazepam may also be given for **sedation** during minor surgical and medical procedures; doses of 10 to 20 mg, given by intravenous injection over 2 to 4 minutes are recommended.

Diazepam is used in a variety of **seizures**. It is given *by mouth* as an adjunct in some types of epilepsy; for this purpose, 2 to 60 mg may be given daily in divided doses. A *rectal gel* formulation is also available for adjunctive use in the management of episodes of increased seizure activity in patients with refractory epilepsy; doses range from 200 to 500 micrograms/kg, depending on age, repeated after 4 to 12 hours if necessary. For febrile convulsions, status epilepticus, and convulsions due to poisoning, administration of a *rectal solution* may be appropriate; suppositories are not suitable because absorption is too slow. Recommended doses for the rectal solution differ but a typical dose is 500 micrograms/kg for adults and children over 10 kg, repeated every 12 hours if necessary; if convulsions are not controlled by the first dose the use of other anticonvulsive measures is recommended. Alternatively, diazepam may be given *intravenously* to adults in a dose of 10 to 20 mg given at a rate of 5 mg/minute and repeated if necessary after 30 to 60 minutes. Other schedules involve administering smaller amounts more frequently or giving diazepam *intramuscularly*, though again absorption may be too slow. Once the seizures have been controlled, a slow intravenous infusion providing up to 3 mg/kg over 24 hours has been administered to protect against recurrence. Doses by intravenous or intramuscular injection in children are within the range of 200 to 300 micrograms/kg; alternatively 1 mg may be given for each year of age.

Diazepam may be given *by mouth* in daily divided doses of 2 to 15 mg to alleviate **muscle spasm**. The dose may be increased in severe spastic disorders, such as cerebral palsy, to up to 60 mg daily in adults or up to 40 mg daily in children. If given by intramuscular or slow intravenous *injection* the dose is 10 mg repeated if necessary after 4 hours. Larger doses are used in tetanus in adults and children with 100 to 300 micrograms/kg being given every 1 to 4 hours by intravenous injection. Alternatively 3 to 10 mg/kg may be given over 24 hours by continuous intravenous infusion or by nasoduodenal tube using a suitable liquid oral dose form. Diazepam may also be given by the rectal route as a *rectal solution* in a dose of 500 micrograms/kg for adults and children over 10 kg in weight, repeated every 12 hours if necessary.

Symptoms of the **alcohol withdrawal syndrome** may be controlled by diazepam given *by mouth* in a dose of 5 to 20 mg, repeated if required after 2 to 4 hours; another approach is to give 10 mg three or four times on the first day reducing to 5 mg three or four times daily as required. Diazepam may need to be given by *injection* if the symptoms are severe and if delirium tremens has developed; 10 to 20 mg by intramuscular or intravenous injection may be adequate, although some patients may require higher doses.

◊ Reviews.

1. Ashton H. Guidelines for the rational use of benzodiazepines: when and what to use. *Drugs* 1994; **48:** 25–40.

**Administration in hepatic impairment.** Oxidative metabolism of diazepam is apparently reduced in patients with hepatic impairment, resulting in a prolonged half-life and reduced clearance.[1-3] A reduction in dosage was generally required in these studies, but no specific advice is given in licensed information for the UK or USA.

1. Branch RA, *et al.* Intravenous administration of diazepam in patients with chronic liver disease. *Gut* 1976; **17:** 975–83.
2. Klotz U, *et al.* Disposition of diazepam and its major metabolite desmethyldiazepam in patients with liver disease. *Clin Pharmacol Ther* 1977; **21:** 430–6.
3. Ochs HR, *et al.* Repeated diazepam dosing in cirrhotic patients: cumulation and sedation. *Clin Pharmacol Ther* 1983; **33:** 471–6.

**Administration in renal impairment.** Diazepam and its metabolites are excreted in urine, and licensed drug information suggests that dosage reduction may be required in patients with renal impairment, but gives no specific advice on how to do this.

**Cardiac arrhythmias.** Although not considered to be an antiarrhythmic, diazepam has been tried with good effect in treating the cardiotoxicity of chloroquine poisoning (see p.449). However, diazepam has been reported to possess both antiarrhythmic and pro-arrhythmic properties, possibly depending on the dose.[1]

1. Kumagai K, *et al.* Antiarrhythmic and proarrhythmic properties of diazepam demonstrated by electrophysiological study in humans. *Clin Cardiol* 1991; **14:** 397–401.

**Chloroquine poisoning.** For reference to the possible use of diazepam to decrease the cardiotoxic effects of chloroquine, see p.449.

**Conversion and dissociative disorders.** Conversion and dissociative disorders (formerly known as hysteria) are characterised by physical symptoms that occur in the absence of organic disease. Medication has no part to play in the treatment of these disorders unless they are secondary to conditions such as depression or anxiety disorders requiring treatment in their own right.

There have been suggestions that sedatives such as diazepam or midazolam may be used to confirm the diagnosis of hysterical paralysis.[1,2] The test tends to exacerbate organic disease while psychiatric dysfunction may improve.

1. Ellis SJ. Diazepam as a truth drug. *Lancet* 1990; **336:** 752–3.
2. Keating JJ, *et al.* Hysterical paralysis. *Lancet* 1990; **336:** 1506–7.

**Disturbed behaviour.** For a discussion of the management of behaviour disturbances associated with various psychotic disorders, and the value of benzodiazepines, see p.665. Benzodiazepines may sometimes be useful in palliative care for the relief of terminal restlessness. Midazolam is often used although other benzodiazepines such as diazepam have also been tried.[1] A suggested dose for diazepam is 5 to 10 mg given slowly as a rectal solution and repeated every 8 to 12 hours. In practice, however, haloperidol may be preferred; a review suggested that benzodiazepines used alone might exacerbate the problem. If agitation was severe haloperidol or risperidone could be combined with lorazepam, reserving subcutaneous midazolam for refractory cases.[2]

1. Burke AL. Palliative care: an update on "terminal restlessness." *Med J Aust* 1997; **166:** 39–42.
2. Jakobsson M, Strang P. Midazolam (Dormicum) vid terminal oro och agitation: sistahandsalternativ i palliativ vård. *Lakartidningen* 1999; **96:** 2079–81.

**Dyspnoea.** Despite the hazards of use in patients with any form of respiratory depression or pulmonary insufficiency (see under Precautions, above) benzodiazepines such as diazepam have been tried in the treatment of dyspnoea (p.74), in the belief that reduction of an elevated respiratory drive may alleviate respiratory distress. However, benefits have not been confirmed. Benzodiazepines may be of use in patients with advanced cancer who have rapid shallow respiration. A daily dose of 5 to 10 mg has been suggested for diazepam.

**Eclampsia and pre-eclampsia.** Diazepam has been used for the initial control of impending or actual eclampsia (p.352), but magnesium sulfate is now generally the preferred treatment.

**Epilepsy and other convulsive disorders.** Some benzodiazepines such as diazepam are used for the control of status epilepticus (p.352), including status epilepticus in patients with porphyria (p.353—but see also under Porphyria in Precautions, above), and for febrile convulsions (p.353); diazepam has also been used in eclampsia (see above) and for neonatal seizures (p.353). Benzodiazepines such as clobazam and clonazepam may be employed in the management of epilepsy (p.349), but their long-term use is limited by problems of sedation, dependence, and tolerance to the antiepileptic effects. Diazepam has been used as an adjunct in the management of some types of epilepsy including myoclonus.

References.

1. Rosman NP, *et al.* A controlled trial of diazepam administered during febrile illnesses to prevent recurrence of febrile seizures. *N Engl J Med* 1993; **329:** 79–84.
2. Somerville ER, Antony JH. Position statement on the use of rectal diazepam in epilepsy. *Med J Aust* 1995; **163:** 268–9.
3. Uhari M, *et al.* Effect of acetaminophen and low intermittent doses of diazepam on prevention of recurrences of febrile seizures. *J Pediatr* 1995; **126:** 991–5.
4. Akinbi MS, Welty TE. Benzodiazepines in the home treatment of acute seizures. *Ann Pharmacother* 1999; **33:** 99–102.
5. Rey E, *et al.* Pharmacokinetic optimisation of benzodiazepine therapy for acute seizures: focus on delivery routes. *Clin Pharmacokinet* 1999; **36:** 409–24.
6. Ogutu BR, *et al.* Pharmacokinetics and anticonvulsant effects of diazepam in children with severe falciparum malaria and convulsions. *Br J Clin Pharmacol* 2002; **53:** 49–57.

**Extrapyramidal disorders.** For reference to the use of benzodiazepines in the treatment of antipsychotic-induced extrapyramidal disorders, see Chlorpromazine, p.677.

**Irritable bowel syndrome.** Although some benzodiazepines have been used in the management of irritable bowel syndrome (p.1244) there is no evidence to support their use in this condition.

**Mania.** Benzodiazepines have been used as short-term adjuncts in the initial control of manic episodes in patients with bipolar disorder (p.278) until lithium has achieved its full effect.

**Muscle spasm.** Diazepam and other benzodiazepines may be used for the relief of muscle spasm (p.1386) of various aetiologies including that secondary to muscle or joint inflammation or trauma, such as in acute **low back pain** (p.7), or resulting from **spasticity** (p.1386), **dystonias** (p.1209), **stiff-man syndrome** (see below), **cerebral palsy**, **poisoning**, or **tetanus** (p.1398). High doses are often required and treatment may be limited by adverse effects or by risk of dependence.

STIFF-MAN SYNDROME. Stiff-man syndrome is a rare condition characterised by painful intermittent spasms and rigidity of the axial and limb muscles. Its exact cause is unknown but there is some evidence to implicate autoantibodies against one of the enzymes involved in the synthesis of the neurotransmitter gamma-aminobutyric acid. It is frequently associated with auto-immune diseases and type 1 diabetes mellitus. Patients typically respond to benzodiazepines and this may be of use in the differential diagnosis of the syndrome. Diazepam has been the mainstay of treatment but clonazepam may also be of use, especially in familial startle disease, a rare congenital form of stiff-man syndrome. Although rigidity and spasms in stiff-man syndrome are not completely resolved by diazepam the degree of improvement can be sufficient to restore the functional level to near normal. However, large doses are often required and sedation might be a limiting factor in some patients. Other drugs which have been used when diazepam is ineffective or poorly tolerated include baclofen or sodium valproate but benefit may be less evident. There have been isolated anecdotal reports of improvement with vigabatrin, tiagabine, and gabapentin. Antiepileptics or baclofen may sometimes be combined with benzodiazepines. Corticosteroids may be of benefit, although any response may take several weeks, and the chronic nature of the disorder and the high incidence of type 1 diabetes mellitus may make their use problematic. Other attempts at immunomodulation such as plasmapheresis have yielded variable results; there is some evidence of the efficacy of immunoglobulins.

References.

1. Toro C, *et al.* Stiff-man syndrome. *Semin Neurol* 1994; **14:** 154–8.
2. Gerhardt CL. Stiff-man syndrome revisited. *South Med J* 1995; **88:** 805–808.
3. Stayer C, Meinck H-M. Stiff-man syndrome: an overview. *Neurologia* 1998; **13:** 83–8.
4. Levy LM, *et al.* The stiff-person syndrome - an autoimmune disorder affecting neurotransmission of γ-aminobutyric acid. *Ann Intern Med* 1999; **131:** 522–30.
5. Meinck H-M. Stiff man syndrome. *CNS Drugs* 2001; **15:** 515–26.
6. Dalakas MC, *et al.* High-dose intravenous immune globulin for stiff-person syndrome. *N Engl J Med* 2001; **345:** 1870–6.
7. Vasconcelos OM, Dalakas MC. Stiff-person syndrome. *Curr Treat Options Neurol* 2003; **5:** 79–90.

**Nausea and vomiting.** Benzodiazepines, particularly lorazepam, are used as adjuncts in the management of nausea and vomiting induced by cancer chemotherapy (p.1245), particularly anticipatory emesis.

**Parasomnias.** Parasomnias (p.667) rarely require treatment other than the symptomatic treatment of sleep-related medical problems. A number of parasomnias such as restless leg syndrome, sleepwalking, and night terrors have been reported to respond to benzodiazepines. Although the muscle relaxant and anxiolytic action of a benzodiazepine can be helpful in bruxism (teeth grinding) it has been recommended that they should only be prescribed on a short-term basis during the acute phase.

References.

1. Schenck CH, Mahowald MW. Long-term, nightly benzodiazepine treatment of injurious parasomnias and other disorders of disrupted nocturnal sleep in 170 adults. *Am J Med* 1996; **100:** 333–7.

**Premenstrual syndrome.** For mention of the limited role of benzodiazepines in the management of premenstrual syndrome, see p.1551.

**Schizophrenia.** Benzodiazepines may be useful adjuncts to antipsychotics in the initial management of schizophrenia (p.665).

**Substance dependence.** The benzodiazepines are used in the management of symptoms of *alcohol* withdrawal (p.1166), of *opioid* withdrawal (p.71), and of *cocaine* withdrawal (p.1375).

**Vertigo.** Although intravenous diazepam has been used to abort acute attacks of vertigo of peripheral origin (p.423), it can prolong compensation and recovery from vestibular lesions.[1]

1. Rascol O, *et al.* Antivertigo medications and drug-induced vertigo: a pharmacological review. *Drugs* 1995; **50:** 777–91.

## Preparations

***BP 2003:*** Diazepam Injection; Diazepam Oral Solution; Diazepam Rectal Solution; Diazepam Tablets;
***USP 27:*** Diazepam Capsules; Diazepam Extended-release Capsules; Diazepam Injection; Diazepam Tablets.

**Proprietary Preparations** (details are given in Part 3)
***Arg.:*** Cuadel; Daiv; Dezepan; Diactal; Dipezona; Glutasedan; Lembrol; Plidan; Rupediz; Saromet; Valium; ***Austral.:*** Antenex; Diazemuls†; Ducene; Valium; Valpam; ***Austria:*** Gewacalm; Psychopax; Stesolid; Umbrium; Valium; ***Belg.:*** Valium; ***Braz.:*** Ansilive; Calmociteno; Compaz; Diazelong†; Diazepan; Dienpax; Kiatrium; Letansil†; Noan; Pazolini; Somaplus; Uni Diazepax; Valium; Valix; ***Canad.:*** Diastat; Diazemuls; Novo-Dipam†; Valium; Vivol†; ***Chile:*** Elongal; Pacinax; ***Denm.:*** Apozepam; Hexalid; Stesolid; Valaxona; Valium; ***Fin.:*** Diapam; Medipam; Stesolid; ***Fr.:*** Novazam; Valium; ***Ger.:*** Diazep; Faustan; Lamra; Stesolid; Tranquase; Valiquid; Valium; Valocordin-Diazepam; ***Gr.:*** Apollonset; Atarviton; Stedon; Stesolid; ***Hong Kong:*** Diazemuls; Kratium; Stesolid; ***India:*** Calmpose; Elcion; Paxum; Placidox; Valium; ***Irl.:*** Anxicalm; Diazemuls; Stesolid; Valium; ***Israel:*** Assival; Diaz; Disopam†; Stesolid; Valium†; ***Ital.:*** Aliseum; Ansiolin; Diazemuls; Eridan†; Micronoan; Noan; Tranquirit; Valium; Vatran; ***Malaysia:*** Diapine; Diapo; ***Mex.:*** Alboral; Arzepam; AT-V; Benzyme†; Diapanil; Diatex; Farmin†; Freudal; Imepas†; Laxyl; Nerolid†; Onapan; Ortopsique; Paxate†; Prizem; Rayne†; Relasan†; Relazepam; Sedirer†; Seredyn†; Tandial; Valium; Vanzor†; Zepan†; Zeprat; ***Neth.:*** Valium; ***Norw.:*** Stesolid; Valium; Vival; ***NZ:*** D-Pam†; Diazemuls; Propam; Stesolid; ***Port.:*** Bialzepam; Metamidol; Stesolid; Unisedil; Valium; ***S.Afr.:*** Benzopin†; Betapam; Calmpose; Doval; Pax; Valium; ***Singapore:*** Diapine; Stesolid; Valium†; ***Spain:*** Aneurol; Aspaserine B6 Tranq; Calmaven†; Complutine; Diaceplex Simple†; Diaceplex†; Dicepin B6†; Drenian†; Gobanal; Pacium; Podium†; Sico Relax; Stesolid; Valium; Vincosedan; ***Swed.:*** Apozepam; Stesolid; Valium†; ***Switz.:*** Paceum; Psychopax; Stesolid; Valium; ***Thai.:*** Azepam; Diano; Diapam; Diapine; Dizan; Dizepam; Sipam; Stesolid; V Day Zepam; Valenium; Valium; Zopam; ***UK:*** Dialar; Diazemuls; Rimapam; Stesolid; Tensium; Valclair; Valium†; ***USA:*** Diastat; Valium.

**Multi-ingredient:** ***Arg.:*** Dafne; Dislembral; Faradil; Pasminox Somatico; Plidex; Tratobes; ***Austria:*** Betamed; Harmomed; ***Braz.:*** Dialudon; Dobesix†; Fastium†; Moderine; Nofagus†; ***Chile:*** Calmosedan; Cardiosedantol; Diapam; Mesolona; Multisedil; Promidan; Sedantol; Sedilit; ***Fin.:*** Gastrodyn comp; Nitrapamil†; Relapamil; Vertipam; ***India:*** Depsonil-DZ; ***Ital.:*** Gamibetal Plus; Spasen Somatico; Spasmeridan; Spasmomen Somatico; Valpinax; Valtrax; ***Mex.:*** Adepsique; Esbelcaps; Numencial; Qual; ***Port.:*** Gamibetal Compositum; ***Spain:*** Ansium; Edym Sedante†; Pertranquil†; Tepazepan; Tropargal; ***USA:*** Emergent-Ez.

---

## Dichloralphenazone *(BAN)*

Dicloralfenazona.

$C_{15}H_{18}Cl_6N_2O_5$ = 519.0.
*CAS — 480-30-8.*
*ATC — N05CC04.*

**Pharmacopoeias.** In *US.*

**USP 27** (Dichloralphenazone). A white microcrystalline powder with a slight odour characteristic of cloral hydrate. Freely soluble in water, in alcohol, and in chloroform; soluble in dilute acids. It is decomposed by dilute alkalis liberating chloroform.

### Profile

Dichloralphenazone dissociates on administration to form cloral hydrate and phenazone. It has the general properties of cloral hydrate (p.684), although it is less likely to cause gastric irritation after administration by mouth. Phenazone-induced skin eruptions may, however, occur (see p.82). Dichloralphenazone is used in some countries in combination preparations mainly for the treatment of tension and vascular headaches.

**Porphyria.** Dichloralphenazone has been associated with acute attacks of porphyria and is considered unsafe in porphyric patients.

### Preparations

***USP 27:*** Isometheptene Mucate, Dichloralphenazone, and Acetaminophen Capsules.

**Proprietary Preparations** (details are given in Part 3)

**Multi-ingredient:** ***USA:*** Duradrin; Isocom†; Isopap†; Midchlor†; Midrin; Migratine.

---

## Difebarbamate *(rINN)*

Difebarbamato. 1,3-Bis(3-butoxy-2-hydroxypropyl)-5-ethyl-5-phenylbarbituric acid dicarbamate ester.

$C_{28}H_{42}N_4O_9$ = 578.7.
*CAS — 15687-09-9.*

### Profile

Difebarbamate is a barbiturate with general properties similar to those of amobarbital (p.670). Tetrabamate, a complex of difebarbamate, febarbamate, and phenobarbital, has been used in the management of anxiety disorders but was also associated with the development of hepatitis. Furthermore barbiturates are not considered appropriate in the management of these conditions.

### Preparations

**Proprietary Preparations** (details are given in Part 3)
***Spain:*** Sevrium†.
**Multi-ingredient:** ***Fr.:*** Atrium†; ***Switz.:*** Atrium†.

---

## Dixyrazine

Dixirazina; UCB-3412. 2-(2-{4-[2-Methyl-3-(phenothiazin-10-yl)propyl]piperazin-1-yl}ethoxy)ethanol.

$C_{24}H_{33}N_3O_2S$ = 427.6.
*CAS — 2470-73-7.*
*ATC — N05AB01.*

### Profile

Dixyrazine is a phenothiazine with general properties similar to those of chlorpromazine (p.675). It has a piperazine side-chain. It is given by mouth for its antipsychotic, antiemetic, and sedative properties in doses ranging from 20 to 75 mg daily. Dixyrazine has also been given by injection.

◊ References.

1. Larsson S, *et al.* Premedication with intramuscular dixyrazine (Esucos®): a controlled double-blind comparison with morphine-scopolamine and placebo. *Acta Anaesthesiol Scand* 1988; **32:** 131–4.
2. Karlsson E, *et al.* The effects of prophylactic dixyrazine on postoperative vomiting after two different anaesthetic methods for squint surgery in children. *Acta Anaesthesiol Scand* 1993; **37:** 45–8.
3. Oikkonen M, *et al.* Dixyrazine premedication for cataract surgery: a comparison with diazepam. *Acta Anaesthesiol Scand* 1994; **38:** 214–17.
4. Feet PO, Götestam KG. Increased antipanic efficacy in combined treatment with clomipramine and dixyrazine. *Acta Psychiatr Scand* 1994; **89:** 230–4.
5. Oikkonen M, *et al.* CSF concentrations and clinical effects following intravenous dixyrazine premedication. *Eur J Clin Pharmacol* 1995; **47:** 445–7.

**Porphyria.** Dixyrazine is considered to be unsafe in patients with porphyria because it has been shown to be porphyrinogenic in *animals*.

### Preparations

**Proprietary Preparations** (details are given in Part 3)
***Austria:*** Esucos; ***Belg.:*** Esucos†; ***Denm.:*** Esucos†; ***Fin.:*** Esucos; ***Ital.:*** Esucos; ***Norw.:*** Esucos; ***Swed.:*** Esucos.

---

## Droperidol *(BAN, USAN, rINN)*

Droperidolum; McN-JR-4749; R-4749. 1-{1-[3-(4-Fluorobenzoyl)propyl]-1,2,3,6-tetrahydro-4-pyridyl}-benzimidazolin-2-one.

$C_{22}H_{22}FN_3O_2$ = 379.4.
*CAS — 548-73-2.*
*ATC — N01AX01; N05AD08.*

**Pharmacopoeias.** In *Eur.* (see p.vi), *Jpn*, and *US.*

**Ph. Eur. 5.0** (Droperidol). A white or almost white powder. It exhibits polymorphism. Practically insoluble in water; sparingly soluble in alcohol; freely soluble in dichloromethane and in dimethylformamide. Protect from light.

**USP 27** (Droperidol). A white to light tan amorphous or microcrystalline powder. Practically insoluble in water; soluble 1 in 140 of alcohol, 1 in 4 of chloroform, and 1 in 500 of ether. Store under nitrogen in airtight containers at a temperature of 8° to 15°. Protect from light.

### Adverse Effects, Treatment, and Precautions

As for Chlorpromazine, p.675. There is an increased risk of cardiotoxicity and prolongation of the QT interval (see p.676) with droperidol. Droperidol should not be used in patients with known or suspected QT prolongation; it should also be used with extreme caution in patients at risk of arrhythmias, including those with impairment of cardiac function, hypokalaemia or other electrolyte imbalance.

### Uses and Administration

Droperidol is a butyrophenone with general properties similar to those of haloperidol (p.702). The duration of action of droperidol has been reported to last about 2 to 4 hours although alteration of alertness may last 12 hours or longer.

One of the manufacturers of droperidol (*Janssen-Cilag*) voluntarily withdrew it from the market worldwide in March 2001 following reports of QT prolongation, serious ventricular arrhythmias, or sudden death in association with its use. However, in the USA, droperidol remains available from other manufacturers although its use is restricted to the management of nausea and vomiting following surgical or diagnostic procedures. It may also still be available, in some other countries, for use as a premedicant, as an adjunct in anaesthesia, and for the control of agitated patients in acute psychoses and in mania. It has also been used with an opioid analgesic such as fentanyl citrate to maintain patients in a state of neuroleptanalgesia in which they are calm and indifferent to the surroundings and able to cooperate with the surgeon. The longer duration of action of droperidol must be kept in mind when using it with such opioid analgesics.

For the prevention of postoperative **nausea and vomiting** a maximum initial dose of 2.5 mg intramuscularly or intravenously has been given; additional doses of 1.25 mg may be given if necessary. Children have been given a maximum initial dose of 100 micrograms/kg intramuscularly or intravenously.

### Preparations

***BP 2003:*** Droperidol Injection; Droperidol Tablets;
***USP 27:*** Droperidol Injection.

**Proprietary Preparations** (details are given in Part 3)
***Austral.:*** Droleptan; ***Austria:*** Dehydrobenzperidol†; ***Belg.:*** Dehydrobenzperidol†; ***Braz.:*** Droperdal; ***Canad.:*** Inapsine†; ***Denm.:*** Dehydrobenzperidol†; ***Fin.:*** Dehydrobenzperidol; ***Fr.:*** Droleptan; ***Ger.:*** Dehydrobenzperidol†; ***Gr.:*** Dehydrobenzperidol; ***Hong Kong:*** Dehydrobenzperidol†; ***India:*** Droperol; ***Irl.:*** Droleptan†; ***Ital.:*** Sintodian; ***Mex.:*** Dehydrobenzperidol†; ***Neth.:*** Dehydrobenzperidol†; ***Norw.:*** Dridol†; ***NZ:*** Droleptan; ***S.Afr.:*** Inapsin†; Paxical†; ***Spain:*** Dehidrobenzperidol; ***Swed.:*** Dridol†; ***Switz.:*** Dehydrobenzperidol†; ***Thai.:*** Dehydrobenzperidol†; ***UK:*** Droleptan†; ***USA:*** Inapsine.

**Multi-ingredient:** ***Arg.:*** Disifelit; ***Austria:*** Thalamonal†; ***Belg.:*** Thalamonal†; ***Braz.:*** Inoval†; Nilperidol; ***Ger.:*** Thalamonal†; ***Ital.:*** Leptofen; ***Neth.:*** Thalamonal†; ***USA:*** Innovar†.

---

## Estazolam *(USAN, rINN)*

Abbott-47631; D-40TA. 8-Chloro-6-phenyl-4*H*-1,2,4-triazolo[4,3-*a*]-1,4-benzodiazepine.

$C_{16}H_{11}ClN_4$ = 294.7.
*CAS — 29975-16-4.*
*ATC — N05CD04.*

**Pharmacopoeias.** In *Chin.* and *Jpn.*

### Dependence and Withdrawal

As for Diazepam, p.690.

### Adverse Effects, Treatment, and Precautions

As for Diazepam, p.690.

### Interactions

As for Diazepam, p.692.

### Pharmacokinetics

Peak plasma concentrations of estazolam are reached on average within 2 hours of oral administration. Estazolam is about 93% protein bound. Reported mean elimination half-lives have generally been in the range of 10 to 24 hours. Estazolam is extensively metabolised, mainly to 4-hydroxyestazolam and 1-oxoestazolam, which are considered inactive. These metabolites are excreted, either free or conjugated, in the urine with small amounts detected in the faeces. Only a small proportion of a dose is excreted as unchanged drug.

### Uses and Administration

Estazolam is a short-acting benzodiazepine with general properties similar to those of diazepam (p.695). It is given by mouth as a hypnotic in the short-term management of insomnia (p.667) in usual doses of 1 to 2 mg at night. Small or debilitated elderly patients may be given an initial dose of 0.5 mg.

### Preparations

**Proprietary Preparations** (details are given in Part 3)
***Arg.:*** Somnatrol; ***Braz.:*** Noctal; ***Denm.:*** Domnamid; ***Fr.:*** Nuctalon; ***Ital.:*** Esilgan; ***Jpn:*** Eurodin; ***Mex.:*** Tasedan; ***Port.:*** Kainever; ***USA:*** Prosom.

---

## Ethchlorvynol *(BAN, rINN)*

β-Chlorovinyl Ethyl Ethynyl Carbinol; Etclorvinol; *E*-Ethchlorvynol. 1-Chloro-3-ethylpent-1-en-4-yn-3-ol.

$C_7H_9ClO$ = 144.6.
*CAS — 113-18-8.*
*ATC — N05CM08.*

**Pharmacopoeias.** In *US.*

**USP 27** (Ethchlorvynol). A colourless to yellow, slightly viscous liquid having a characteristic pungent odour. It darkens on exposure to air and light. Immiscible with water; miscible with most organic solvents. Store in airtight containers of glass or polyethylene, using polyethylene-lined closures. Protect from light.

### Dependence and Withdrawal

Prolonged use of ethchlorvynol may lead to dependence similar to that with barbiturates (see Amobarbital, p.670).

### Adverse Effects

Side-effects of ethchlorvynol include gastrointestinal disturbances, dizziness, headache, unwanted sedation and other symptoms of CNS depression such as ataxia, facial numbness, blurred vision, and hypotension. Hypersensitivity reactions include skin rashes, urticaria, and occasionally, thrombocytopenia and cholestatic jaundice. Idiosyncratic reactions include excitement, severe muscular weakness, and syncope without marked hypotension.

Acute overdosage is characterised by prolonged deep coma, respiratory depression, hypothermia, hypotension, and relative bradycardia. Pancytopenia and nystagmus have occurred.

Pulmonary oedema has followed abuse by intravenous injection.

### Treatment of Adverse Effects

Treatment is as for barbiturate overdose (see Amobarbital, p.670). Haemoperfusion may be of value in the treatment of severe poisoning with ethchlorvynol.

### Precautions

Ethchlorvynol should be used with caution in patients with hepatic or renal impairment or with depression, in patients with severe uncontrolled pain, and, as with all sedatives, in those with impaired respiratory function. It may cause drowsiness; affected patients should not drive or operate machinery.

Excessively rapid absorption of ethchlorvynol in some patients has been reported to produce giddiness and ataxia; this may be reduced by administration with food.

**Porphyria.** Ethchlorvynol has been associated with acute attacks of porphyria and is considered unsafe in porphyric patients.

### Interactions

The effect of ethchlorvynol may be enhanced by alcohol, barbiturates, and other CNS depressants. Ethchlorvynol has been reported to decrease the effects of coumarin anticoagulants.

**Tricyclic antidepressants.** Transient delirium has been reported with the concomitant use of ethchlorvynol and amitriptyline but details of such an interaction do not appear to have been published in the literature.

### Pharmacokinetics

Ethchlorvynol is readily absorbed from the gastrointestinal tract, peak plasma concentrations usually occurring within 2 hours of ingestion. It is widely distributed in body tissues and is extensively metabolised in the liver, and possibly to some extent in the kidneys. It has a biphasic plasma half-life with a rapid initial phase and a terminal phase reported to last from 10 to 20 hours. Ethchlorvynol is excreted mainly in the urine as metabolites and their conjugates. Ethchlorvynol crosses the placenta.

### Uses and Administration

Ethchlorvynol is a hypnotic and sedative with some anticonvulsant and muscle relaxant properties. It is given by mouth for the short-term management of insomnia (p.667) but has been largely superseded by other drugs. Use for periods greater than one week is not recommended. The usual hypnotic dose is 500 mg at night but doses ranging from 200 mg to 1 g have been given. Administration with food has been recommended—see Precautions, above.

### Preparations

***USP 27:*** Ethchlorvynol Capsules.

**Proprietary Preparations** (details are given in Part 3)
***USA:*** Placidyl†.

## Ethyl Loflazepate *(rINN)*

CM-6912; Loflazepato de etilo. Ethyl 7-chloro-5-(2-fluorophenyl)-2,3-dihydro-2-oxo-1*H*-1,4-benzodiazepine-3-carboxylate.
$C_{18}H_{14}ClFN_2O_3$ = 360.8.
*CAS — 29177-84-2.*
*ATC — N05BA18.*

### Profile

Ethyl loflazepate is a long-acting benzodiazepine derivative with general properties similar to those of diazepam (p.690). It is used in the short-term treatment of anxiety disorders (p.663) in usual doses of 1 to 3 mg daily by mouth in a single dose or in divided doses.

### Preparations

**Proprietary Preparations** (details are given in Part 3)
***Arg.:*** Victan; ***Belg.:*** Victan; ***Fr.:*** Victan; ***Jpn:*** Meilax; ***Mex.:*** Victan; ***Port.:*** Victan; ***Thai.:*** Victan.

## Etifoxine Hydrochloride *(BANM, rINNM)*

Etifoxin Hydrochloride; Hidrocloruro de etifoxina; Hoe-36801. 6-Chloro-4-methyl-4-phenyl-3,1-benzoxazin-2-yl(ethyl)amine hydrochloride.
$C_{17}H_{17}ClN_2O,HCl$ = 337.2.
*CAS — 21715-46-8 (etifoxine); 56776-32-0 (etifoxine hydrochloride).*
*ATC — N05BX03.*

### Profile

Etifoxine hydrochloride is an anxiolytic used for the short-term treatment of anxiety (p.663). It is given by mouth in usual doses of 150 or 200 mg daily in 2 or 3 divided doses.

### Preparations

**Proprietary Preparations** (details are given in Part 3)
***Fr.:*** Stresam.

## Etizolam *(rINN)*

AHR-3219; Y-7131. 4-(2-Chlorophenyl)-2-ethyl-9-methyl-6*H*-thieno[3,2-*f*]-s-triazolo[4,3-*a*][1,4]diazepine.
$C_{17}H_{15}ClN_4S$ = 342.8.
*CAS — 40054-69-1.*
*ATC — N05BA19.*

**Pharmacopoeias.** In *Jpn.*

### Profile

Etizolam is a short-acting benzodiazepine derivative with general properties similar to those of diazepam (p.690). It is given by mouth for the short-term treatment of insomnia (p.667) and anxiety disorders (p.663) in doses of up to 3 mg daily in divided doses or as a single dose at night.

### Preparations

**Proprietary Preparations** (details are given in Part 3)
***Ital.:*** Depas; Pasaden; ***Jpn:*** Depas.

## Febarbamate *(rINN)*

Febarbamato; Go-560. 1-(3-Butoxy-2-carbamoyloxypropyl)-5-ethyl-5-phenylbarbituric acid.
$C_{20}H_{27}N_3O_6$ = 405.4.
*CAS — 13246-02-1.*
*ATC — M03BA05.*

### Profile

Febarbamate is a barbiturate with general properties similar to those of amobarbital (p.670). It has been used in the management of anxiety, insomnia, and alcohol withdrawal symptoms. However, barbiturates are no longer considered appropriate in the management of these conditions.

Tetrabamate, a complex of febarbamate, difebarbamate, and phenobarbital, has been used similarly but was associated with the development of hepatitis.

### Preparations

**Proprietary Preparations** (details are given in Part 3)
***Spain:*** G Tril†; Sevrium†.
**Multi-ingredient:** ***Fr.:*** Atrium†; ***Switz.:*** Atrium†.

## Fluanisone *(BAN, rINN)*

Fluanisona; Haloanisone; MD-2028; R-2028; R-2167. 4′-Fluoro-4-[4-(2-methoxyphenyl)piperazin-1-yl]butyrophenone.
$C_{21}H_{25}FN_2O_2$ = 356.4.
*CAS — 1480-19-9.*
*ATC — N05AD09.*

**Pharmacopoeias.** In *BP(Vet).*

**BP(Vet) 2003** (Fluanisone). White or almost white to buff-coloured, odourless or almost odourless crystals or powder. It exhibits polymorphism. M.p. 72° to 76°. Practically insoluble in water; freely soluble in alcohol, in chloroform, in ether, and in dilute solutions of organic acids. Protect from light.

### Profile

Fluanisone is a butyrophenone with general properties similar to those of haloperidol (p.701). It has been used in the management of agitated states in psychiatric patients and as anaesthetic premedication.

Fluanisone is used in veterinary medicine for neuroleptanalgesia.

## Fludiazepam *(rINN)*

ID-540. 7-Chloro-5-(2-fluorophenyl)-1,3-dihydro-1-methyl-2*H*-1,4-benzodiazepin-2-one.
$C_{16}H_{12}ClFN_2O$ = 302.7.
*CAS — 3900-31-0.*
*ATC — N05BA17.*

**Pharmacopoeias.** In *Jpn.*

### Profile

Fludiazepam is a short-acting benzodiazepine with general properties similar to those of diazepam (p.690). It has been used in the short-term treatment of anxiety disorders.

# Flunitrazepam *(BAN, USAN, rINN)*

Flunitrazepamum; Ro-5-4200. 5-(2-Fluorophenyl)-1,3-dihydro-1-methyl-7-nitro-1,4-benzodiazepin-2-one.
$C_{16}H_{12}FN_3O_3$ = 313.3.
*CAS — 1622-62-4.*
*ATC — N05CD03.*

**Pharmacopoeias.** In *Eur.* (see p.vi) and *Jpn.*

**Ph. Eur. 5.0** (Flunitrazepam). A white or yellowish crystalline powder. Practically insoluble in water; slightly soluble in alcohol; soluble in acetone. Protect from light.

### Dependence and Withdrawal

As for Diazepam, p.690.

### Adverse Effects, Treatment, and Precautions

As for Diazepam, p.690.

**Abuse.** A WHO review[1] concluded that flunitrazepam had a moderate abuse potential that might be higher than that of other benzodiazepines. It was reported that there was current evidence of widespread abuse of flunitrazepam among drug abusers, particularly among those who used opioids or cocaine.

Street names for flunitrazepam include: Circles, Forget me drug, Forget me pill, Getting roached, La Rocha, Lunch money drug, Mexican valium, Pingus, R-2, Reynolds, Rib, Roach-2, Roapies, Robutal, Roofies, Rope, Rophies, Row-shay, Ruffles, and Wolfies.[2]

Flunitrazepam is tasteless and odourless and has been misused to incapacitate the victim and produce amnesia in sexual assaults[3] and drug-facilitated rape ('date rape').[2] A 1-mg dose may produce impairment for 8 to 12 hours.[4] Some manufacturers have incorporated a blue dye into flunitrazepam tablets to increase visibility when placed into drinks but caution is still necessary as it has been reported that blue tropical drinks and punches are being used to overcome this.[2]


1. WHO expert committee on drug dependence: twenty-ninth report. *WHO Tech Rep Ser 856* 1995.
2. Office of National Drug Control Policy. Fact sheet: Rohypnol (01/03). Available at: http://www.whitehousedrugpolicy.gov/publications/factsht/rohypnol/rohypnol.pdf (accessed 28/04/04)
3. Simmons MM, Cupp MJ. Use and abuse of flunitrazepam. *Ann Pharmacother* 1998; **32:** 117–19.
4. Smith KM, *et al.* Club drugs: methylenedioxymethamphetamine, flunitrazepam, ketamine hydrochloride, and γ-hydroxybutyrate. *Am J Health-Syst Pharm* 2002; **59:** 1067–76.


**Breast feeding.** Concentrations in breast milk the morning after a single evening 2-mg dose of flunitrazepam were considered to be too low to produce clinical effects in breast-fed infants, although accumulation in the milk might occur after repeated administration.[1]


1. Kanto J, *et al.* Placental transfer and breast milk levels of flunitrazepam. *Curr Ther Res* 1979; **26:** 539–46.


**Local reactions.** Of 43 patients given a single intravenous dose of flunitrazepam 1 to 2 mg, two had local thrombosis 7 to 10 days later.[1] The incidence was lower than in those given diazepam [in solution]. However, there was little difference in the incidence of local reactions after intravenous administration of flunitrazepam and diazepam in another study.[2]


1. Hegarty JE, Dundee JW. Sequelae after the intravenous injection of three benzodiazepines—diazepam, lorazepam, and flunitrazepam. *BMJ* 1977; **2:** 1384–5.
2. Mikkelsen H, *et al.* Local reactions after iv injections of diazepam, flunitrazepam and isotonic saline. *Br J Anaesth* 1980; **52:** 817–19.


**Porphyria.** Flunitrazepam has been associated with acute attacks of porphyria and is considered unsafe in porphyric patients.

### Interactions

As for Diazepam, p.692.

### Pharmacokinetics

Flunitrazepam is readily absorbed from the gastrointestinal tract. About 77 to 80% is bound to plasma proteins. It is extensively metabolised in the liver and excreted mainly in the urine as metabolites (free or conjugated). Its principal metabolites are 7-aminoflunitrazepam and *N*-desmethylflunitrazepam; *N*-desmethylflunitrazepam is reported to be pharmacologically active. The elimination half-life of flunitrazepam is reported to be between 16 and 35 hours. Flunitrazepam crosses the placental barrier and is distributed into breast milk.

◊ References.


1. Davis PJ, Cook DR. Clinical pharmacokinetics of the newer intravenous anaesthetic agents. *Clin Pharmacokinet* 1986; **11:** 18–35.
2. Pariente-Khayat A, *et al.* Pharmacokinetics and tolerance of flunitrazepam in neonates and in infants. *Clin Pharmacol Ther* 1999; **66:** 136–9.


**Pregnancy.** Concentrations of flunitrazepam in umbilical-vein and umbilical-artery plasma were lower than those in maternal venous plasma about 11 to 15 hours after administration of flunitrazepam 1 mg to 14 pregnant women; concentrations in amniotic fluid were lower still.[1]


1. Kanto J, *et al.* Placental transfer and breast milk levels of flunitrazepam. *Curr Ther Res* 1979; **26:** 539–46.


### Uses and Administration

Flunitrazepam is a short-acting benzodiazepine with general properties similar to those of diazepam (p.695). It is used in the short-term management of insomnia (p.667), as a premedicant in surgical procedures, and for induction of anaesthesia (p.1296).

A usual dose for **insomnia** is 0.5 to 1 mg by mouth at night; up to 2 mg may be given if necessary. In elderly or debilitated patients the initial dose should not exceed 0.5 mg at night; up to 1 mg may be given if necessary.

A dose of 1 to 2 mg (15 to 30 micrograms/kg) has been given intramuscularly or by mouth for **premedication** or by slow intravenous injection for **induction** of general anaesthesia.

### Preparations

**Proprietary Preparations** (details are given in Part 3)
***Arg.:*** Parsimonil; Primum; Rohypnol; ***Austral.:*** Hypnodorm; Rohypnol†; ***Austria:*** Guttanotte; Rohypnol; Somnubene; ***Belg.:*** Rohypnol; ***Braz.:*** Fluserin†; Rohypnol; ***Chile:*** Ipnopen; Rohypnol; ***Denm.:*** Flunipam; Rohypnol; Ronal; ***Fr.:*** Narcozep; Rohypnol; ***Ger.:*** Fluni; Flunibeta; Flunimerck; Fluninoc; Rohypnol; ***Gr.:*** Hipnosedon; Ilman; Neo Nifalium; Vulbegal; ***Hong Kong:*** Absint; Rohypnol; ***Irl.:*** Rohypnol; ***Israel:*** Hypnodorm; Rohypnol†; ***Ital.:*** Darkene; Roipnol; Valsera; ***Mex.:*** Rohypnol; ***Neth.:*** Rohypnol; ***Norw.:*** Flunipam; Flutraz†; Rohypnol; ***Port.:*** Rohypnol; Sedex; ***S.Afr.:*** Hypnor; Insom†; Rohypnol; ***Spain:*** Rohipnol; ***Swed.:*** Fluscand; Rohypnol; ***Switz.:*** Rohypnol; ***Thai.:*** Rohypnol; ***UK:*** Rohypnol†.

## Flupentixol Decanoate *(BANM, rINNM)*

Decanoato de flupentixol; Flupenthixol Decanoate; (Z)-Flupenthixol Decanoate; *cis*-Flupenthixol Decanoate. (Z)-2-{4-[3-(2-Trifluoromethylthioxanthen-9-ylidene)propyl]piperazin-1-yl}ethyl decanoate.
$C_{33}H_{43}F_3N_2O_2S$ = 588.8.
*CAS — 2709-56-0 (flupentixol); 30909-51-4 (flupentixol decanoate).*
*ATC — N05AF01.*

**Pharmacopoeias.** In *Br.*
**BP 2003** (Flupentixol Decanoate). A yellow viscous oil. Very slightly soluble in water; soluble in alcohol; freely soluble in chloroform and in ether. Store at a temperature below −15° and protect from light.

### Flupentixol Hydrochloride *(BANM, rINNM)*

Flupenthixol Dihydrochloride; Flupenthixol Hydrochloride; Flupentixoli Dihydrochloridum; Hidrocloruro de flupentixol; LC-44 (flupentixol); N-7009 (flupentixol). 2-{4-[3-(2-Trifluoromethylthioxanthen-9-ylidene)propyl]piperazin-1-yl}ethanol dihydrochloride.
$C_{23}H_{25}F_3N_2OS,2HCl$ = 507.4.
*CAS — 2413-38-9.*
*ATC — N05AF01.*

**Pharmacopoeias.** In *Eur.* (see p.vi).
**Ph. Eur. 5.0** (Flupentixol Dihydrochloride; Flupentixol Hydrochloride BP 2003). A white or almost white powder. Very soluble in water; soluble in alcohol; practically insoluble in dichloromethane. A 1% solution in water has a pH of 2.0 to 3.0. Protect from light.

**Stability.** References.

1. Enever RP, *et al.* Flupenthixol dihydrochloride decomposition in aqueous solution. *J Pharm Sci* 1979; **68:** 169–71.
2. Li Wan Po A, Irwin WJ. The photochemical stability of cis- and trans-isomers of tricyclic neuroleptic drugs. *J Pharm Pharmacol* 1980; **32:** 25–9.

### Adverse Effects and Treatment

As for Chlorpromazine, p.675. Flupentixol is less likely to cause sedation, but extrapyramidal disorders are more frequent.

**Sudden death.** A report of sudden death in 3 patients who had received depot injections of flupentixol decanoate.[1]

1. Turbott J, Smeeton WMI. Sudden death and flupenthixol decanoate. *Aust N Z J Psychiatry* 1984; **18:** 91–4.

### Precautions

As for Chlorpromazine, p.678. Flupentixol is not recommended in states of excitement or overactivity, including mania.

**Porphyria.** Flupentixol is considered to be unsafe in patients with porphyria because it has been shown to be porphyrinogenic in *animals*.

### Interactions

As for Chlorpromazine, p.679.

### Pharmacokinetics

Flupentixol is readily absorbed from the gastrointestinal tract and is probably subject to first-pass metabolism in the gut wall. It is also extensively metabolised in the liver and is excreted in the urine and faeces in the form of numerous metabolites; there is evidence of enterohepatic recycling. Owing to the first-pass effect, plasma concentrations following oral administration are much lower than those following estimated equivalent doses of the intramuscular depot preparation. Moreover, there is very wide intersubject variation in plasma concentrations of flupentixol, but, in practice, no simple correlation has been found between plasma concentrations of flupentixol and its metabolites, and the therapeutic effect. Paths of metabolism of flupentixol include sulfoxidation, side-chain *N*-dealkylation, and glucuronic acid conjugation. It is widely distributed in the body, and crosses the blood-brain barrier. Flupentixol crosses the placental barrier and small amounts have been detected in breast milk.

The decanoate ester of flupentixol is very slowly absorbed from the site of intramuscular injection and is therefore suitable for depot injection. It is gradually released into the bloodstream where it is rapidly hydrolysed to flupentixol.

### Uses and Administration

Flupentixol is a thioxanthene antipsychotic with general properties similar to those of the phenothiazine, chlorpromazine (p.680). It has a piperazine side-chain. Flupentixol is used mainly in the treatment of schizophrenia (p.665) and other psychoses. Unlike chlorpromazine, an activating effect has been ascribed to flupentixol, and it is not indicated in overactive or manic patients. Flupentixol has also been used for its antidepressant properties.

Flupentixol is administered by mouth as the hydrochloride although doses are expressed in terms of the base; flupentixol hydrochloride 3.5 mg is approximately equivalent to flupentixol base 3 mg. Flupentixol is also given as the longer-acting decanoate ester by deep intramuscular injection. The long-acting preparation available in the UK contains flupentixol decanoate as the *cis(Z)*-isomer (see Action, below) and doses are expressed in terms of the amount of *cis(Z)*-flupentixol decanoate.

The usual initial dose by mouth for the treatment of **psychoses** is the equivalent of 3 to 9 mg of flupentixol twice daily adjusted according to the response; the maximum recommended dose is a total of 18 mg daily. The initial dose in elderly and debilitated patients may need to be reduced to a quarter or a half of the normal starting dose. If given by deep intramuscular injection, an initial test dose of 20 mg of the decanoate, as 1 mL of a 2% oily solution, is used. Then after at least 7 days and according to the patient's response, this may be followed by doses of 20 to 40 mg at intervals of 2 to 4 weeks. Shorter dosage intervals or greater amounts may be required according to the patient's response. The initial dose in elderly and debilitated patients may need to be reduced to a quarter or a half of the normal starting dose. If doses greater than 40 mg are considered necessary they should be divided between 2 separate injection sites. Another means of reducing the volume of fluid to be injected in patients requiring high-dose therapy with flupentixol decanoate is to give an injection containing 100 or 200 mg/mL of the decanoate (10 or 20%). The usual maintenance dose is between 50 mg every 4 weeks and 300 mg every 2 weeks but doses of up to 400 mg weekly have been given in severe or resistant conditions.

Flupentixol has also been given as the hydrochloride, by mouth, for the treatment of mild to moderate **depression**, with or without anxiety (p.279). The usual initial dose, expressed in terms of the equivalent amount of flupentixol, is 1 mg (0.5 mg in the elderly) daily, increased after 1 week to 2 mg (1 mg in the elderly) and then to a maximum of 3 mg (2 mg in the elderly) daily. Doses above 2 mg (1 mg in the elderly) should be given in 2 divided doses. The last dose of the day should be given no later than 4 p.m. and if no effect has been noted within 1 week of administration of the maximum dose, the treatment should be withdrawn.

**Action.** Patients with acute schizophrenic illnesses taking α-flupentixol [(Z)-flupentixol or *cis*-flupentixol] improved more after 3 weeks than patients who were taking equal doses of β-flupentixol [(E)-flupentixol or *trans*-flupentixol] or a placebo.[1] The α-isomer had more effect on the positive symptoms of the disease; this difference was less apparent for the negative symptoms. The difference in activity between the isomers was attributed to the greater dopamine-receptor blocking activity of the α-isomer rather than to differences in distribution.[2]

1. Johnstone EC, *et al.* Mechanism of the antipsychotic effect in the treatment of acute schizophrenia. *Lancet* 1978; **i:** 848–51.
2. Crow TJ, Johnstone EC. Mechanism of action of neuroleptic drugs. *Lancet* 1978; **i:** 1050.

**Substance dependence.** Depot flupentixol decanoate had been reported[1] to produce promising results as an aid in reducing *cocaine* usage (see Withdrawal, p.1375) but this was not confirmed in a double-blind controlled study.[2]

1. Gawin FH, *et al.* Flupentixol-induced aversion to crack cocaine. *N Engl J Med* 1996; **334:** 1340–1.
2. Evans SM, *et al.* Effect of flupenthixol on subjective and cardiovascular responses to intravenous cocaine in humans. *Drug Alcohol Depend* 2001; **64:** 271–83.

### Preparations

***BP 2003:*** Flupentixol Injection.

**Proprietary Preparations** (details are given in Part 3)
***Austral.:*** Fluanxol; ***Austria:*** Fluanxol; ***Belg.:*** Fluanxol; ***Canad.:*** Fluanxol; ***Chile:*** Fluanxol; ***Denm.:*** Fluanxol; ***Fin.:*** Fluanxol; ***Fr.:*** Fluanxol; ***Ger.:*** Fluanxol; ***Hong Kong:*** Fluanxol; ***India:*** Fluanxol; ***Irl.:*** Depixol; Fluanxol; ***Israel:*** Fluanxol; ***Malaysia:*** Fluanxol; ***Mex.:*** Fluanxol; ***Neth.:*** Fluanxol; ***Norw.:*** Fluanxol; ***NZ:*** Depixol†; Fluanxol; ***Port.:*** Fluanxol; ***S.Afr.:*** Fluanxol; ***Singapore:*** Fluanxol; ***Swed.:*** Fluanxol; ***Switz.:*** Fluanxol; ***Thai.:*** Fluanxol; ***UK:*** Depixol; Fluanxol.

**Multi-ingredient:** ***Austria:*** Deanxit; ***Belg.:*** Deanxit; ***Hong Kong:*** Deanxit; ***Ital.:*** Deanxit; ***Singapore:*** Deanxit; ***Spain:*** Deanxit; ***Switz.:*** Deanxit; ***Thai.:*** Deanxit.

## Fluphenazine *(BAN, rINN)*

Flufenazina. 2-{4-[3-(2-Trifluoromethylphenothiazin-10-yl)propyl]piperazin-1-yl}ethanol.
$C_{22}H_{26}F_3N_3OS$ = 437.5.
*CAS — 69-23-8.*
*ATC — N05AB02.*

### Fluphenazine Decanoate *(BANM, rINNM)*

Decanoato de flufenazina; Fluphenazini Decanoas.
$C_{32}H_{44}F_3N_3O_2S$ = 591.8.
*CAS — 5002-47-1.*
*ATC — N05AB02.*

**Pharmacopoeias.** In *Chin., Eur.* (see p.vi), *Int.*, and *US.*
**Ph. Eur. 5.0** (Fluphenazine Decanoate). A pale yellow viscous liquid or a yellow solid. Practically insoluble in water; very soluble in dehydrated alcohol and in dichloromethane; freely soluble in methyl alcohol. Protect from light.
**USP 27** (Fluphenazine Decanoate). Store in airtight containers. Protect from light.

### Fluphenazine Enantate *(BANM, rINNM)*

Enantato de flufenazina; Fluphenazine Enanthate; Fluphenazine Heptanoate; Fluphenazini Enantas.
$C_{29}H_{38}F_3N_3O_2S$ = 549.7.
*CAS — 2746-81-8.*
*ATC — N05AB02.*

**Pharmacopoeias.** In *Eur.* (see p.vi), *Int., Jpn*, and *US.*
**Ph. Eur. 5.0** (Fluphenazine Enantate). A pale yellow viscous liquid or a yellow solid. Practically insoluble in water; very soluble in dehydrated alcohol and in dichloromethane; freely soluble in methyl alcohol. Protect from light.
**USP 27** (Fluphenazine Enanthate). A pale yellow to yellow-orange, clear to slightly turbid, viscous liquid having a characteristic odour. Insoluble in water; soluble 1 in less than 1 of alcohol and of chloroform and 1 in 2 of ether. Stable in air at room temperature but unstable in strong light. Store in airtight containers. Protect from light.

### Fluphenazine Hydrochloride *(BANM, rINNM)*

Fluphenazini Hydrochloridum; Hidrocloruro de flufenazina.
$C_{22}H_{26}F_3N_3OS,2HCl$ = 510.4.
*CAS — 146-56-5.*
*ATC — N05AB02.*

**Pharmacopoeias.** In *Chin., Eur.* (see p.vi), *Int., Pol.*, and *US.*
**Ph. Eur. 5.0** (Fluphenazine Hydrochloride). A white or almost white, crystalline powder. Freely soluble in water; slightly soluble in alcohol and in dichloromethane. Protect from light.
**USP 27** (Fluphenazine Hydrochloride). A white or nearly white, odourless crystalline powder. Soluble 1 in 1.4 of water and 1 in 6.7 of alcohol; slightly soluble in acetone and in chloroform; practically insoluble in ether and in benzene. Store in airtight containers. Protect from light.

### Adverse Effects and Treatment

As for Chlorpromazine, p.675. Fluphenazine is less likely to cause sedation, hypotension, or antimuscarinic effects but is associated with a higher incidence of extrapyramidal effects.

**Effects on the liver.** A patient given 3 injections of a depot antipsychotic containing fluphenazine decanoate over a 2-week period developed jaundice 17 days after the first dose.[1] The patient developed indicators of severe liver toxicity, with extreme hyperbilirubinaemia and raised liver enzyme values, and remained very ill for the next 4 months. The patient showed cross-sensitivity to haloperidol but not to flupentixol.

See also under Chlorpromazine, p.676.

1. Kennedy P. Liver cross-sensitivity to antipsychotic drugs. *Br J Psychiatry* 1983; **143:** 312.

**Effects on the nervous system.** A significant incidence of akinesia, involuntary movement, autonomic disturbances, and drowsiness may occur in the first few hours following injection of fluphenazine decanoate and in the first 2 days following injection of fluphenazine enantate.[1]

1. Curry SH, *et al.* Unwanted effects of fluphenazine enanthate and decanoate. *Lancet* 1979; **i:** 331–2.

CONVULSIONS. For mention of fluphenazine as one of the antipsychotics suitable for patients at risk of seizures, see p.675.

**Overdosage.** A patient who took about 30 fluphenazine hydrochloride 2.5-mg tablets was treated with gastric lavage.[1] Twenty hours after hospital admission he experienced difficulty in breathing due to spasm of the respiratory muscles; other very severe extrapyramidal side-effects were also present. Muscle spasm was controlled by diazepam.

There were few ill-effects in a patient given intramuscular fluphenazine decanoate 50 mg every 4 hours, instead of the intended 4 weeks, to a total of 1050 mg.[2] About three weeks after the period of overdosage the patient had some degree of hypothermia and tachycardia, and after a further week parkinsonian signs appeared. No specific treatment was given.

1. Ladhani FM. Severe extrapyramidal manifestations following fluphenazine overdose. *Med J Aust* 1974; **2:** 26.
2. Cheung HK, Yu ECS. Effect of 1050 mg fluphenazine decanoate given intramuscularly over six days. *BMJ* 1983; **286:** 1016–17.

## Precautions

As for Chlorpromazine, p.678. Fluphenazine may exacerbate depression and therefore it is contra-indicated in severely depressed patients.

**Pregnancy.** Nasal congestion with severe rhinorrhoea, respiratory distress, vomiting, and extrapyramidal symptoms occurred in a neonate delivered to a mother who had received fluphenazine hydrochloride 10 to 20 mg daily throughout pregnancy.[1] Respiratory symptoms appeared to respond to pseudoephedrine.

1. Nath SP, *et al.* Severe rhinorrhea and respiratory distress in a neonate exposed to fluphenazine hydrochloride prenatally. *Ann Pharmacother* 1996; **30:** 35–7.

## Interactions

As for Chlorpromazine, p.679.

## Pharmacokinetics

Fluphenazine hydrochloride is absorbed following oral administration, and has a reported plasma half-life of 14.7 hours after doses by mouth. Fluphenazine decanoate and fluphenazine enantate are very slowly absorbed from the site of subcutaneous or intramuscular injection. They both gradually release fluphenazine into the body and are therefore suitable for use as depot injections.

◊ References[1-4] to the pharmacokinetics of fluphenazine.

The plasma half-life of fluphenazine after a single dose was 14.7 hours in 1 patient given the hydrochloride by mouth and 14.9 and 15.3 hours in 2 patients given the hydrochloride by intramuscular injection.[1] The half-life was 3.6 and 3.7 days in 2 patients given the enantate intramuscularly and 9.6 and 6.8 days in 2 patients given the decanoate intramuscularly. Peak plasma-fluphenazine concentrations occurred earlier in patients given fluphenazine decanoate compared with those who received the enantate. Fluphenazine sulfoxide and 7-hydroxyfluphenazine were identified in the urine and faeces.

1. Curry SH, *et al.* Kinetics of fluphenazine after fluphenazine dihydrochloride, enanthate and decanoate administration to man. *Br J Clin Pharmacol* 1979; **7:** 325–31.
2. Wistedt B, *et al.* Slow decline of plasma drug and prolactin levels after discontinuation of chronic treatment with depot neuroleptics. *Lancet* 1981; **i:** 1163.
3. Midha KK, *et al.* Kinetics of oral fluphenazine disposition in humans by GC-MS. *Eur J Clin Pharmacol* 1983; **25:** 709–11.
4. Marder SR, *et al.* Plasma levels of parent drug and metabolites in patients receiving oral and depot fluphenazine. *Psychopharmacol Bull* 1989; **25:** 479–82.

## Uses and Administration

Fluphenazine is a phenothiazine with general properties similar to those of chlorpromazine (p.680). It has a piperazine side-chain. Fluphenazine is used in the treatment of a variety of psychiatric disorders including schizophrenia (p.665), mania (see Bipolar Disorder, p.278), severe anxiety (p.663), and behavioural disturbances (p.665). Fluphenazine is given as the hydrochloride by mouth or sometimes by intramuscular injection; for both routes, doses are expressed in terms of fluphenazine hydrochloride. The longer-acting decanoate or enantate esters of fluphenazine are given by intramuscular or sometimes subcutaneous injection; for both esters, doses are expressed in terms of the ester.

The usual initial dose of the hydrochloride for the treatment of schizophrenia, mania, and other **psychoses** is 2.5 to 10 mg daily in two or three divided doses *by mouth*; the dose is then increased according to response up to a usual maximum of 20 mg daily (10 mg daily in the elderly), although higher doses have occasionally been given. Dosage may subsequently be reduced to a usual maintenance dose of 1 to 5 mg daily. Treatment is sometimes started with an initial *intramuscular* injection of 1.25 mg of the hydrochloride adjusted thereafter according to response. The usual initial intramuscular daily dose is 2.5 to 10 mg given in divided doses every 6 to 8 hours. In general the required parenteral doses of fluphenazine hydrochloride have been found to be approximately one-third to one-half of those given by mouth.

The long-acting decanoate or enantate esters of fluphenazine are usually given by deep intramuscular injection and are used mainly for the *maintenance* treatment of patients with schizophrenia or other chronic psychoses. The onset of action is usually within 1 to 3 days of injection and significant effects on psychosis are usually evident within 2 to 4 days. An initial dose of fluphenazine decanoate 12.5 mg (6.25 mg in the elderly) is given intramuscularly to assess the extrapyramidal effects. Subsequent adjustments in the amounts and the dosage interval should be made according to the patient's response; the amounts required may range from 12.5 to 100 mg and the intervals required may range from 2 weeks to 5 or 6 weeks. Lower doses may be possible in some patients (see Schizophrenia, below). If doses greater than 50 mg are considered necessary cautious increments should be made in steps of 12.5 mg. The enantate ester of fluphenazine has been given in a similar dose range.

Fluphenazine hydrochloride has also been given *by mouth* in doses of 1 mg twice daily, increased if necessary to 2 mg twice daily, for the short-term adjunctive management of severe **anxiety** or **behavioural disturbances**.

**Chorea.** For a discussion of the management of various choreas, including mention of the use of phenothiazines such as fluphenazine, see p.664.

References.

1. Terrence CF. Fluphenazine decanoate is the treatment of chorea: a double-blind study. *Curr Ther Res* 1976; **20:** 177–83.

**Schizophrenia.** References[1-3] to fluphenazine decanoate in schizophrenia (p.665) indicating that low doses (10 mg or less every 2 weeks) may be effective in some patients. Use of standard doses at greater intervals (6 weeks) has also been tried.[4] A systematic review of the use of depot fluphenazine in schizophrenia considered the evidence with regard to any advantage over oral use to be very limited.[5]

1. Kane JM, *et al.* Low-dose neuroleptic treatment of outpatient schizophrenics: I preliminary results for relapse rates. *Arch Gen Psychiatry* 1983; **40:** 893–6.
2. Marder SR, *et al.* Low- and conventional-dose maintenance therapy with fluphenazine decanoate: two-year outcome. *Arch Gen Psychiatry* 1987; **44:** 581–21.
3. Hogarty GE, *et al.* Dose of fluphenazine, familial expressed emotion, and outcome in schizophrenia: results of a two-year controlled study. *Arch Gen Psychiatry* 1988; **45:** 797–805.
4. Carpenter WT, *et al.* Comparative effectiveness of fluphenazine decanoate injections every 2 weeks versus every 6 weeks. *Am J Psychiatry* 1999; **156:** 412–18.
5. Adams CE, Eisenbruch M. Depot fluphenazine for schizophrenia. Available in The Cochrane Library; Issue 2. Chichester: John Wiley; 2004.

**Tourette's syndrome.** Fluphenazine has been tried[1] as an alternative to standard dopamine antagonists such as haloperidol or pimozide in the symptomatic management of Tourette's syndrome (p.664).

1. Singer HS, *et al.* Haloperidol, fluphenazine and clonidine in tourette syndrome: controversies in treatment. *Pediatr Neurosci* 1985–86; **12:** 71–4.

## Preparations

***BP 2003:*** Fluphenazine Decanoate Injection; Fluphenazine Tablets;
***USP 27:*** Fluphenazine Decanoate Injection; Fluphenazine Enanthate Injection; Fluphenazine Hydrochloride Elixir; Fluphenazine Hydrochloride Injection; Fluphenazine Hydrochloride Oral Solution; Fluphenazine Hydrochloride Tablets.

**Proprietary Preparations** (details are given in Part 3)

***Austral.:*** Anatensol; Modecate; ***Austria:*** Dapotum; ***Belg.:*** Sevinol; ***Braz.:*** Anatensol†; Flufenan; ***Canad.:*** Modecate; Moditen; ***Chile:*** Modecate; ***Denm.:*** Pacinol; Siqualone; ***Fin.:*** Pacinol; Siqualone; ***Fr.:*** Modecate; Moditen; ***Ger.:*** Dapotum; Lyogen; Lyorodin; Omca; ***Hong Kong:*** Modecate; ***India:*** Anatensol; ***Irl.:*** Modecate; ***Israel:*** Fludecate; Modecate†; Sediten†; Selecten†; ***Ital.:*** Anatensol; Moditen Depot; ***Malaysia:*** Deca; ***Mex.:*** Siqualine†; ***Neth.:*** Anatensol; ***Norw.:*** Siqualone; ***NZ:*** Modecate; ***Port.:*** Anatensol; Cenilene; Phenazin; ***S.Afr.:*** Fludecate†; Modecate; Modecate Acutum†; ***Singapore:*** Modecate; ***Spain:*** Modecate; ***Swed.:*** Pacinol; Siqualone; ***Switz.:*** Dapotum; ***Thai.:*** Deca; Fluzine; Modecate†; Phenazine; Potensone; ***UK:*** Modecate; Moditen; ***USA:*** Permitil†; Prolixin.

**Multi-ingredient:** ***Braz.:*** Diserim; ***Chile:*** Motitrel; ***Hong Kong:*** Motival†; ***Irl.:*** Motival; ***Ital.:*** Dominans; ***S.Afr.:*** Motival; ***Thai.:*** Motival†; ***UK:*** Motipress†; Motival.

# Flurazepam *(BAN, rINN)*

7-Chloro-1-(2-diethylaminoethyl)-5-(2-fluorophenyl)-1,3-dihydro-1,4-benzodiazepin-2-one.

$C_{21}H_{23}ClFN_3O$ = 387.9.
*CAS — 17617-23-1.*
*ATC — N05CD01.*

**Pharmacopoeias.** In *Jpn.*

# Flurazepam Monohydrochloride *(BANM, rINNM)*

Flurazepami Monohydrochloridum; Monohidrocloruro de flurazepam.

$C_{21}H_{23}ClFN_3O,HCl$ = 424.3.
*CAS — 36105-20-1.*
*ATC — N05CD01.*

**Pharmacopoeias.** In *Eur.* (see p.vi) and *Jpn.*

**Ph. Eur. 5.0** (Flurazepam Monohydrochloride). A white or almost white crystalline powder. Very soluble in water; freely soluble in alcohol. A 5% solution in water has a pH of 5.0 to 6.0. Protect from light.

# Flurazepam Dihydrochloride *(BANM, rINNM)*

Dihidrocloruro de flurazepam; Flurazepam Hydrochloride *(USAN)*; NSC-78559; Ro-5-6901.

$C_{21}H_{23}ClFN_3O,2HCl$ = 460.8.
*CAS — 1172-18-5.*
*ATC — N05CD01.*

**Pharmacopoeias.** In *Chin.* and *US.*

**USP 27** (Flurazepam Hydrochloride). An off-white to yellow crystalline powder. Is odourless or has a slight odour. Soluble 1 in 2 of water, 1 in 4 of alcohol, 1 in 90 of chloroform, 1 in 3 of methyl alcohol, 1 in 69 of isopropyl alcohol, 1 in 5000 of ether and of petroleum spirit, and 1 in 2500 of benzene. A solution in water is acid to litmus. Store in airtight containers. Protect from light.

## Dependence and Withdrawal

As for Diazepam, p.690.

## Adverse Effects, Treatment, and Precautions

As for Diazepam, p.690.

**Effects on the liver.** Reports of cholestatic jaundice following the use of flurazepam.[1,2]

1. Fang MH, *et al.* Cholestatic jaundice associated with flurazepam hydrochloride. *Ann Intern Med* 1978; **89:** 363–4.
2. Reynolds R, *et al.* Cholestatic jaundice induced by flurazepam hydrochloride. *Can Med Assoc J* 1981; **124:** 893–4.

**Effects on taste.** Flurazepam had been reported to cause dysgeusia.[1]

1. Willoughby JMT. Drug-induced abnormalities of taste sensation. *Adverse Drug React Bull* 1983 (June): 368–71.

**Porphyria.** Flurazepam has been associated with acute attacks of porphyria and is considered unsafe in porphyric patients.

**Renal impairment.** Five patients on maintenance haemodialysis developed encephalopathy attributed to flurazepam and diazepam.[1]

1. Taclob L, Needle M. Drug-induced encephalopathy in patients on maintenance haemodialysis. *Lancet* 1976; **ii:** 704–5.

## Interactions

As for Diazepam, p.692.

## Pharmacokinetics

Flurazepam is readily absorbed from the gastrointestinal tract. It undergoes extensive first-pass metabolism and is excreted in the urine, chiefly as conjugated metabolites. The major active metabolite is *N*-desalkylflurazepam, which is reported to have a half-life ranging from 47 to 100 hours or more.

**Metabolism.** The metabolism of flurazepam was studied in 4 healthy male subjects given 30 mg daily for 2 weeks.[1] A hydroxyethyl metabolite was present in the blood shortly after administration. The *N*-desalkyl metabolite, the major metabolite in the blood, had a half-life ranging from 47 to 100 hours. Steady-state concentrations were reached after 7 to 10 days and were about 5 to 6 times greater than those observed on day 1. Results from a study in 3 patients indicated that some metabolism of flurazepam may occur in the small bowel mucosa.[2]

1. Kaplan SA, *et al.* Blood level profile in man following chronic oral administration of flurazepam hydrochloride. *J Pharm Sci* 1973; **62:** 1932–5.
2. Mahon WA, *et al.* Metabolism of flurazepam by the small intestine. *Clin Pharmacol Ther* 1977; **22:** 228–33.

## Uses and Administration

Flurazepam is a long-acting benzodiazepine with general properties similar to those of diazepam (p.695). It is used as a hypnotic in the short-term management of insomnia (p.667). In the USA flurazepam is given as the dihydrochloride and doses are expressed in terms of this salt. Flurazepam dihydrochloride 30 mg is approximately equivalent to 25.3 mg of flurazepam. Doses of 15 to 30 mg by mouth at night are given. In the UK flurazepam is given as the monohydrochloride although doses are expressed in terms of the base; flurazepam monohydrochloride 32.8 mg is approximately equivalent to 30 mg of flurazepam. Doses equivalent to 15 to 30 mg of flurazepam at night are given. A maximum initial dose of 15 mg has been suggested in the UK and the USA for elderly or debilitated patients.

### Preparations

**BP 2003:** Flurazepam Capsules;
**USP 27:** Flurazepam Hydrochloride Capsules.

**Proprietary Preparations** (details are given in Part 3)
**Arg.:** Fordrim; **Austria:** Staurodorm; **Belg.:** Staurodorm; **Braz.:** Dalmadorm; **Canad.:** Dalmane; Novo-Flupam†; Somnol†; **Ger.:** Dalmadorm; Staurodorm Neu; **Hong Kong:** Dalmadorm; **India:** Fluraz; **Irl.:** Dalmane; **Ital.:** Dalmadorm; Felison; Flunox; Remdue; Valdorm; **Neth.:** Dalmadorm; **Port.:** Dalmadorm; Morfex; **S.Afr.:** Dalmadorm; **Singapore:** Dalmadorm; **Spain:** Dormodor; **Switz.:** Dalmadorm; **Thai.:** Dalmadorm; **UK:** Dalmane; **USA:** Dalmane.

## Fluspirilene *(BAN, USAN, rINN)*

Fluspirileno; Fluspirilenum; McN-JR-6218; R-6218. 8-[4,4-Bis(4-fluorophenyl)butyl]-1-phenyl-1,3,8-triazaspiro[4.5]decan-4-one.
$C_{29}H_{31}F_2N_3O$ = 475.6.
*CAS — 1841-19-6.*
*ATC — N05AG01.*

**Pharmacopoeias.** In *Eur.* (see p.vi).
**Ph. Eur. 5.0** (Fluspirilene). A white or almost white powder. It exhibits polymorphism. Practically insoluble in water; slightly soluble in alcohol; soluble in dichloromethane. Protect from light.

### Profile

Fluspirilene is a diphenylbutylpiperidine antipsychotic and has general properties similar to those of the phenothiazine, chlorpromazine (p.675). It is less likely to cause sedation. Fluspirilene has been given by deep intramuscular injection for the treatment of psychoses including schizophrenia (p.665). A usual initial dose is up to 2 mg weekly by deep intramuscular injection, increased according to the patient's response. Usual maintenance doses have ranged from 1 to 10 mg weekly although higher doses have been used in exceptional cases.

**Adverse effects.** References.

1. McCreadie RG, *et al.* Probable toxic necrosis after prolonged fluspirilene administration. *BMJ* 1979; **1:** 523–4.

**Schizophrenia.** A systematic review[1] found that evidence to support the use of depot fluspirilene over oral chlorpromazine or other deport antipsychotics in the treatment of schizophrenia was lacking.

1. Quraishi S, *et al.* Depot fluspirilene for schizophrenia. Available in The Cochrane Library; Issue 2. Chichester: John Wiley; 2004.

### Preparations

**Proprietary Preparations** (details are given in Part 3)
**Arg.:** Imap; **Belg.:** Imap; **Canad.:** Imap†; **Ger.:** Fluspi; Imap; kivat; **Irl.:** Redeptin; **Israel:** Imap†; **Neth.:** Imap.

## Gepirone Hydrochloride *(USAN, rINNM)*

BMY-13805-1; Hidrocloruro de gepirona; MJ-13805-1. 3,3-Dimethyl-N-{4-[4-(2-pyrimidinyl)-1-piperazinyl]butyl}glutarimide hydrochloride.
$C_{19}H_{29}N_5O_2,HCl$ = 395.9.
*CAS — 83928-76-1 (gepirone); 83928-66-9 (gepirone hydrochloride).*
*ATC — N06AX19.*

### Profile

Gepirone is structurally related to buspirone (p.672). It is being investigated as the hydrochloride for the treatment of depression. It has also been tried in anxiety disorders.

**Action.** Gepirone is a partial agonist at serotonin (hydroxytryptamine, 5-HT) receptors of the $5\text{-HT}_{1A}$ subtype. For reference to the actions and potential uses of such drugs, see Buspirone, p.673.

References.

1. Feiger AD. A double-blind comparison of gepirone extended release, imipramine, and placebo in the treatment of outpatient major depression. *Psychopharmacol Bull* 1996; **32:** 659–65.
2. Rickels K, *et al.* Gepirone and diazepam in generalized anxiety disorder: a placebo-controlled trial. *J Clin Psychopharmacol* 1997; **17:** 272–7.
3. Dogterom PP, *et al.* Pharmacokinetics of gepirone (Org 33062) in subjects with normal renal function and in patients with chronic renal dysfunction. *Clin Pharmacol Ther* 2002; **71:** P95.
4. Feiger AD, *et al.* Gepirone extended-release: new evidence for efficacy in the treatment of major depressive disorder. *J Clin Psychiatry* 2003; **64:** 243–9.
5. Robinson DS, *et al.* A review of the efficacy and tolerability of immediate-release and extended-release formulations of gepirone. *Clin Ther* 2003; **25:** 1618–33.
6. Timmer CJ, Sitsen JM. Pharmacokinetic evaluation of gepirone immediate-release capsules and gepirone extended-release tablets in healthy volunteers. *J Pharm Sci* 2003; **92:** 1773–8.

## Glutethimide *(BAN, rINN)*

Glutethimidum; Glutetimida; Glutetimide. 2-Ethyl-2-phenylglutarimide; 3-Ethyl-3-phenylpiperidine-2,6-dione.
$C_{13}H_{15}NO_2$ = 217.3.
*CAS — 77-21-4.*
*ATC — N05CE01.*

### Profile

Glutethimide is a piperidinedione hypnotic and sedative with effects broadly similar to those of the barbiturates (see Amobarbital, p.670). It also has antimuscarinic properties. It has been given for the short-term management of insomnia but it has been superseded by other drugs.

**Abuse.** A warning of the hazards associated with the abuse of glutethimide in a combination with codeine termed 'loads'.[1]

1. Sramek JJ, Khajawall A. "Loads". *N Engl J Med* 1981; **305:** 231.

**Porphyria.** Glutethimide has been associated with acute attacks of porphyria and is considered unsafe in porphyric patients.

## Halazepam *(BAN, USAN, rINN)*

Sch-12041. 7-Chloro-1,3-dihydro-5-phenyl-1-(2,2,2-trifluoroethyl)-1,4-benzodiazepin-2-one.
$C_{17}H_{12}ClF_3N_2O$ = 352.7.
*CAS — 23092-17-3.*
*ATC — N05BA13.*

### Profile

Halazepam is a benzodiazepine with general properties similar to those of diazepam (p.690). It has been given by mouth for the short-term treatment of anxiety disorders (p.663).

### Preparations

**Proprietary Preparations** (details are given in Part 3)
**Ital.:** Paxipam†; **Port.:** Pacinone; **Spain:** Alapryl.

# Haloperidol *(BAN, USAN, rINN)*

Aloperidolo; Haloperidolum; McN-JR-1625; R-1625. 4-[4-(4-Chlorophenyl)-4-hydroxypiperidino]-4′-fluorobutyrophenone.
$C_{21}H_{23}ClFNO_2$ = 375.9.
*CAS — 52-86-8.*
*ATC — N05AD01.*

**Pharmacopoeias.** In *Chin., Eur.* (see p.vi), *Int., Jpn, Pol., US,* and *Viet.*
**Ph. Eur. 5.0** (Haloperidol). A white or almost white powder. Practically insoluble in water; slightly soluble in alcohol, in dichloromethane, and in methyl alcohol. Protect from light.
**USP 27** (Haloperidol). A white to faintly yellowish amorphous or microcrystalline powder. Practically insoluble in water; soluble 1 in 60 of alcohol, 1 in 15 of chloroform, and 1 in 200 of ether. A saturated solution is neutral to litmus. Store in airtight containers. Protect from light.

**Dilution.** See Incompatibility, below.

**Incompatibility.** Formation of a precipitate was observed after dilution of haloperidol (as the lactate) in sodium chloride 0.9% injection when the final haloperidol concentration was 1 mg/mL or higher.[1]

Undiluted haloperidol (5 mg/mL) injection has been reported to be incompatible with heparin sodium (diluted in sodium chloride 0.9% or glucose 5% injection),[2] sodium nitroprusside (diluted in glucose 5%),[1] cefmetazole sodium,[3] and diphenhydramine.[4] A mixture of equal volumes of sargramostim 10 micrograms/mL and haloperidol (as the lactate) 200 micrograms/mL resulted in a precipitate at 4 hours.[5]

1. Outman WR, Monolakis J. Visual compatibility of haloperidol lactate with 0.9% sodium chloride injection or injectable critical-care drugs during simulated Y-site injection. *Am J Hosp Pharm* 1991; **48:** 1539–41.
2. Solomon DA, Nasinnyk KK. Compatibility of haloperidol lactate and heparin sodium. *Am J Hosp Pharm* 1982; **39:** 843–4.
3. Hutchings SR, *et al.* Compatibility of cefmetazole sodium with commonly used drugs during Y-site delivery. *Am J Health-Syst Pharm* 1996; **53:** 2185–8.
4. Ukhun IA. Compatibility of haloperidol and diphenhydramine in a hypodermic syringe. *Ann Pharmacother* 1995; **29:** 1168–9.
5. Trissel LA, *et al.* Visual compatibility of sargramostim with selected antineoplastic agents, anti-infectives, or other drugs during simulated Y-site injection. *Am J Hosp Pharm* 1992; **49:** 402–6.

**Stability.** Mention that a combination of the stabilisers benzyl alcohol and vanillin could protect haloperidol from photodegradation.[1]

1. Thoma K, Klimek R. Photostabilisation of drugs in dosage forms without protection from packaging materials. *Int J Pharmaceutics* 1991; **67:** 169–75.

## Haloperidol Decanoate *(BANM, USAN, rINNM)*

Decanoato de haloperidol; Haloperidoli Decanoas; R-13672.
$C_{31}H_{41}ClFNO_3$ = 530.1.
*CAS — 74050-97-8.*
*ATC — N05AD01.*

**Pharmacopoeias.** In *Eur.* (see p.vi).
**Ph. Eur. 5.0** (Haloperidol Decanoate). A white or almost white powder. It melts at about 42°. Practically insoluble in water; very soluble in alcohol, in dichloromethane, and in methyl alcohol. Store at a temperature below 25°. Protect from light.

### Adverse Effects, Treatment, and Precautions

As for Chlorpromazine, p.675. Haloperidol is less likely to cause sedation, hypotension, or antimuscarinic effects, but is associated with a higher incidence of extrapyramidal effects. Haloperidol should be used with great care in children and adolescents as they may be at increased risk of severe dystonic reactions. Patients with hyperthyroidism may also be at increased risk.

**Breast feeding.** The American Academy of Pediatrics[1] considers that the use of haloperidol by mothers during breast feeding may be of concern, since there have been reports of decline in developmental scores in breast-fed infants. The manufacturers also report that there have been isolated cases of extrapyramidal effects in breast-fed infants.

The concentration of haloperidol in breast milk of one mother who had received a mean daily dose of about 30 mg for 6 days was reported to be 5 nanograms/mL; on day 12 the concentration measured 9 hours after a 12-mg dose was 2 nanograms/mL.[2]

1. American Academy of Pediatrics. The transfer of drugs and other chemicals into human milk. *Pediatrics* 2001; **108:** 776–89. Correction. *ibid.*; 1029. Also available at: http://aappolicy.aappublications.org/cgi/content/full/pediatrics%3b108/3/776 (accessed 28/04/04)
2. Stewart RB, *et al.* Haloperidol excretion in human milk. *Am J Psychiatry* 1980; **137:** 849–50.

**Convulsions.** For mention of haloperidol as one of the antipsychotics suitable for patients at risk of seizures, see p.675.

**Effects on the liver.** Liver dysfunction with jaundice and eosinophilia developed in a 15-year-old male 4 weeks after administration of haloperidol and benzatropine mesilate.[1] This treatment was discontinued 2 weeks later but some symptoms lasted for 28 months. The reaction was suggestive of a drug-induced hypersensitivity reaction and haloperidol was the most likely cause. Haloperidol-induced liver injury was considered to be rare.

1. Dincsoy HP, Saelinger DA. Haloperidol-induced chronic cholestatic liver disease. *Gastroenterology* 1982; **83:** 694–700.

**Overdosage.** Symptoms of haloperidol overdosage in children have ranged from the expected, such as drowsiness, restlessness, confusion, marked extrapyramidal symptoms, and hypothermia,[1,2] to unexpected reactions such as bradycardia (possibly secondary to hypothermia)[1] and an episode of severe, delayed hypertension.[3]

Torsade de pointes has followed overdosage in adults (for references, see Effects on the Cardiovascular System under Chlorpromazine, p.676).

1. Scialli JVK, Thornton WE. Toxic reactions from a haloperidol overdose in two children: thermal and cardiac manifestations. *JAMA* 1978; **239:** 48–9.
2. Sinaniotis CA, *et al.* Acute haloperidol poisoning in children. *J Pediatr* 1978; **93:** 1038–9.
3. Cummingham DG, Challapalli M. Hypertension in acute haloperidol poisoning. *J Pediatr* 1979; **95:** 489–90.

**Porphyria.** Haloperidol is considered to be unsafe in patients with porphyria although there is conflicting experimental evidence of porphyrinogenicity.

**Retroperitoneal fibrosis.** Obstructive uropathy was noted in a 45-year-old woman who had received haloperidol 5 to 15 mg daily for 8 years.[1] Benzatropine was also taken during that time, and in the previous 5 years she had taken chlorpromazine and fluphenazine. A diagnosis of retroperitoneal fibrosis was made and was tentatively associated with long-term antipsychotic therapy.

1. Jeffries JJ, *et al.* Retroperitoneal fibrosis and haloperidol. *Am J Psychiatry* 1982; **139:** 1524–5.

**Toxic encephalopathy.** A report[1] of possible toxic encephalopathy following the use of high intravenous doses of haloperidol. The patient, who had a history of bipolar disorder and cerebrovascular accident, had been given increasing intravenous doses of haloperidol (up to 270 mg daily) to control post-surgical agitation. The encephalopathy had resolved 8 days after discontinuation of haloperidol.

1. Maxa JL, *et al.* Possible toxic encephalopathy following high-dose intravenous haloperidol. *Ann Pharmacother* 1997; **31:** 736–7.

### Interactions

As for Chlorpromazine, p.679.

Haloperidol must be used with extreme caution in patients receiving lithium; an encephalopathic syndrome has been reported following their concomitant use (see p.303).

**Pharmacokinetics**

Haloperidol is readily absorbed from the gastrointestinal tract. It is metabolised in the liver and is excreted in the urine and, via the bile, in the faeces; there is evidence of enterohepatic recycling. Owing to first-pass metabolism in the liver, plasma concentrations following oral administration are lower than those after intramuscular administration. Moreover, there is wide intersubject variation in plasma concentrations of haloperidol, but, in practice, no strong correlation has been found between plasma concentrations of haloperidol and its therapeutic effect. Paths of metabolism of haloperidol include oxidative *N*-dealkylation and reduction of the ketone group to form an alcohol known as reduced haloperidol. Haloperidol has been reported to have a plasma elimination half-life ranging from about 12 to 38 hours after oral administration. Haloperidol is about 92% bound to plasma proteins. It is widely distributed in the body and crosses the blood-brain barrier. Haloperidol is distributed into breast milk.

The decanoate ester of haloperidol is very slowly absorbed from the site of injection and is therefore suitable for depot injection. It is gradually released into the bloodstream where it is rapidly hydrolysed to haloperidol.

◊ References.

1. Kudo S, Ishizaki T. Pharmacokinetics of haloperidol: an update. *Clin Pharmacokinet* 1999 **37:** 435–56.

**Metabolites.** The clinical significance of the reduced metabolite of haloperidol has been much debated.[1,2] Its activity appears to be substantially less than that of the parent drug but there is some evidence for re-oxidation of reduced haloperidol to haloperidol.[1-3] Some studies suggest that nonresponders to haloperidol have elevated ratios of reduced haloperidol to haloperidol in the plasma, although other workers have reported contrary findings.[2] Pyridinium metabolites resulting from oxidation of haloperidol have been detected in the urine and there is concern that they may be neurotoxic in a manner similar to MPTP (p.1196), a compound which can induce irreversible parkinsonism.[4]

1. Sramek JJ, *et al.* Neuroleptic plasma concentrations and clinical response: in search of a therapeutic window. *Drug Intell Clin Pharm* 1988; **22:** 373–80.
2. Froemming JS, *et al.* Pharmacokinetics of haloperidol. *Clin Pharmacokinet* 1989; **17:** 396–423.
3. Chakraborty BS, *et al.* Interconversion between haloperidol and reduced haloperidol in healthy volunteers. *Eur J Clin Pharmacol* 1989; **37:** 45–8.
4. Eyles DW, *et al.* Quantitative analysis of two pyridinium metabolites of haloperidol in patients with schizophrenia. *Clin Pharmacol Ther* 1994; **56:** 512–20.

**Therapeutic drug monitoring.** Measurement of concentrations of haloperidol or reduced haloperidol in scalp hair has been suggested as a useful means of monitoring compliance.[1,2] Evidence for the existence of any relationship between plasma concentrations of haloperidol and therapeutic effect in schizophrenia has been discussed.[3]

1. Uematsu T, *et al.* Human scalp hair as evidence of individual dosage history of haloperidol: method and retrospective study. *Eur J Clin Pharmacol* 1989; **37:** 239–44.
2. Matsuno H, *et al.* The measurement of haloperidol and reduced haloperidol in hair as an index of dosage history. *Br J Clin Pharmacol* 1990; **29:** 187–94.
3. Ulrich S, *et al.* The relationship between serum concentration and therapeutic effect of haloperidol in patients with acute schizophrenia. *Clin Pharmacokinet* 1998; **34:** 227–63.

## Uses and Administration

Haloperidol is a butyrophenone with general properties similar to those of the phenothiazine, chlorpromazine (p.680). It is an antipsychotic with actions most closely resembling those of phenothiazines with a piperazine side-chain.

Haloperidol is used in the treatment of various psychoses including schizophrenia (p.665) and mania (see Bipolar Disorder, p.278), and in behaviour disturbances (p.665), in Tourette's syndrome and severe tics (p.664), in intractable hiccups (p.682), and in severe anxiety (p.663). Haloperidol has also been used for its antiemetic effect in the management of nausea and vomiting of various causes (p.1245).

Haloperidol is usually given by mouth or injection as the base or intramuscularly as the long-acting decanoate ester. Some haloperidol preparations are prepared with the aid of lactic acid and may be stated to contain haloperidol lactate. Doses are expressed in terms of the equivalent amount of haloperidol. Haloperidol decanoate 141 mg is approximately equivalent to 100 mg of haloperidol. Dosages should be reduced in elderly or debilitated patients; a usual starting dose is half the normal adult dose. Doses at the lower end of the scale are also advised for adolescents.

The usual initial dose *by mouth* for the treatment of **psychoses** and associated behaviour disorders is 0.5 to 5 mg two or three times daily. In severe or resistant psychoses doses of up to 100 mg daily may be required; doses above 100 mg daily have rarely been used. The dose should be reduced gradually according to response. Maintenance doses as low as 3 to 10 mg daily may be sufficient. A suitable initial dose for children by mouth is 25 to 50 micrograms/kg daily in two divided doses, increased cautiously, if necessary; a maximum daily dose of 10 mg has been recommended in the UK but in the USA the suggested maximum daily dose is 150 micrograms/kg as the manufacturer has stated that there is little evidence of behaviour improvement with daily doses of more than 6 mg.

For the control of acute psychotic conditions, haloperidol may be given *intramuscularly* in doses of 2 to 10 mg; subsequent doses may be given hourly until symptoms are controlled although dosage intervals of 4 to 8 hours may be adequate. For the emergency control of very severely disturbed patients, an initial intramuscular dose of no more than 18 mg is recommended. The *intravenous* route may also be used.

In patients already stabilised on an oral dose of haloperidol and requiring long-term therapy the long-acting decanoate ester may be given by *deep intramuscular* injection. The usual initial dose is the equivalent of 10 to 20 times the total daily dose of haloperidol by mouth, up to a maximum of 100 mg; if more than 100 mg is required for an initial dose the excess should be given after 3 to 7 days. Subsequent doses, usually given every 4 weeks, may be increased to up to 300 mg or more, according to the patient's requirements, both dose and dose interval being adjusted as required.

In the management of **nausea and vomiting** haloperidol has been given in usual doses of 0.5 to 2 mg daily by *intramuscular* injection. In palliative care haloperidol 1.5 mg may be given *by mouth* once or twice daily or by *subcutaneous* infusion (via a syringe driver) in doses of 2.5 to 10 mg over 24 hours.

A starting dose of 0.5 to 1.5 mg three times daily *by mouth* has been suggested for the management of **Tourette's syndrome** and severe **tics**. Up to about 10 mg daily may be needed in Tourette's syndrome, although requirements vary considerably and the dose must be very carefully adjusted to obtain the optimum response.

For intractable **hiccups** a suggested dose is 1.5 mg given three times daily *by mouth* adjusted according to response; alternatively 3 to 15 mg may be given daily by intramuscular or intravenous *injection* in divided doses.

A dose of 0.5 mg twice daily *by mouth* has been used as adjunctive treatment in the short-term management of severe **anxiety disorders**.

In palliative care, haloperidol has been given in a dose of 1 to 3 mg every 8 hours *by mouth* for the treatment of **restlessness and confusion**. It may also be given as a *subcutaneous* infusion in a dose of 5 to 15 mg over 24 hours.

**Ballism.** Dopamine-blocking antipsychotics such as haloperidol may sometimes be needed for the management of patients with ballism (p.664) when symptoms are severe.

**Chorea.** For a discussion of the management of various choreas, including mention of the use of haloperidol, see p.664.

**Dystonia.** Antipsychotics such as phenothiazines, haloperidol, or pimozide are sometimes useful in the treatment of idiopathic dystonia (p.1209) in patients who have failed to respond to other drugs. However, they often act non-specifically and there is the risk of adding drug-induced extrapyramidal disorders to the dystonia being treated (see Extrapyramidal Disorders under Adverse Effects of Chlorpromazine, p.677).

**Sneezing.** Report[1] of a patient whose intractable sneezing was controlled by haloperidol given in doses of up to 5 mg twice daily. Symptoms recurred when treatment was stopped after 5 weeks but responded again to 5 mg three times daily. On gradual reduction of dosage over 6 months the patient experienced no recurrence and had remained symptom-free after 6 months without medication.

1. Davison K. Pharmacological treatment for intractable sneezing. *BMJ* 1982; **284:** 1163–4.

**Stuttering.** Stuttering (stammering) is a disorder that affects the fluency of speech. Developmental stuttering usually occurs in early childhood and is more common in boys than girls. While stuttering may cease in some children after only a few months, it may become a chronic condition in others. Stuttering which starts during adulthood is rarer and may be the result of a neurological insult. It should also be remembered that stuttering may be drug induced. While stuttering may be greatly improved with intensive speech training the effectiveness of other forms of management such as hypnosis, psychotherapy, counselling, and drug therapy has been largely unconvincing.[1] Although many drugs have been used to treat stuttering a review of the literature[2] indicated that there were few adequate studies of their efficacy. Haloperidol was considered to be the most well studied drug and its efficacy had been demonstrated by several double-blind placebo-controlled studies. However, most patients needed to continue taking haloperidol to maintain improvement but few did so because of its adverse effects. Double-blind studies have on the whole failed to confirm reports of benefit for drugs such as bethanechol, beta blockers, and calcium-channel blockers although isolated patients may have marked improvement. Other drugs that have been studied and which might be of benefit include clomipramine,[3] SSRIs,[4] and atypical antipsychotics[4] such as olanzapine and risperidone; local anaesthetics and injections of botulinum toxin have also been tried.

1. Andrews G, *et al.* Stuttering. *JAMA* 1988; **260:** 1445.
2. Brady JP, *et al.* The pharmacology of stuttering: a critical review. *Am J Psychiatry* 1991; **148:** 1309–16.
3. Gordon CT, *et al.* A double-blind comparison of clomipramine and desipramine in the treatment of developmental stuttering. *J Clin Psychiatry* 1995; **56:** 238–42.
4. Costa D, Kroll R. Stuttering: an update for physicians. *Can Med Assoc J* 2000; **162:** 1849–55.

**Taste disorders.** For reference to the use of haloperidol in the treatment of taste disorders, see Chlorpromazine, p.682.

**Tourette's syndrome.** Many patients with Tourette's syndrome (p.664) do not require medication but when treatment is needed dopamine antagonists such as the antipsychotics haloperidol or pimozide are most commonly used. They often decrease the frequency and severity of tics and may improve any accompanying behavioural disturbances. However, superiority of either drug in terms of efficacy or adverse effects has not been clearly demonstrated.[1,2] Because of the potential for acute and long-term adverse effects it is usually recommended that doses are titrated to be as low as possible; the aim of treatment is not necessarily to control symptoms completely. Medication can often be discontinued after a few years.

1. Shapiro E, *et al.* Controlled study of haloperidol, pimozide, and placebo for the treatment of Gilles de la Tourette's syndrome. *Arch Gen Psychiatry* 1989; **46:** 722–30.
2. Sallee FR, *et al.* Relative efficacy of haloperidol and pimozide in children and adolescents with Tourette's disorder. *Am J Psychiatry* 1997; **154:** 1057–62.

### Preparations

***BP 2003:*** Haloperidol Capsules; Haloperidol Injection; Haloperidol Oral Solution; Haloperidol Tablets; Strong Haloperidol Oral Solution;
***USP 27:*** Haloperidol Injection; Haloperidol Oral Solution; Haloperidol Tablets.

**Proprietary Preparations** (details are given in Part 3)
***Arg.:*** Halopidol; Halozen; Neupram; Zetoridal; ***Austral.:*** Haldol; Serenace; ***Austria:*** Haldol; ***Belg.:*** Haldol; ***Braz.:*** Haldol; Halo; Haloper; Loperidol; Uni Haloper; ***Canad.:*** Haldol; Novo-Peridol; Peridol; ***Chile:*** Alternus; Haldol; ***Denm.:*** Serenase; ***Fin.:*** Serenase; ***Fr.:*** Haldol; ***Ger.:*** Buteridol†; Haldol; Haloneural; Haloper; Sigaperidol; ***Gr.:*** Aloperidin; Sevium; ***Hong Kong:*** Haldol; Serenace; ***India:*** Cizoren; Serenace; ***Irl.:*** Haldol; Serenace; ***Israel:*** Haldol; Haloper; Pericate; Peridor; ***Ital.:*** Bioperidolo†; Haldol; Serenase; ***Malaysia:*** Avant; Serenace; ***Mex.:*** Haldol; Haloperil; Kepsidol†; Pulsit†; ***Neth.:*** Haldol; ***Norw.:*** Haldol; ***NZ:*** Haldol; Serenace; ***Port.:*** Serenelfi; ***S.Afr.:*** Serenace; ***Singapore:*** Serenace; ***Swed.:*** Haldol; ***Switz.:*** Haldol; Sigaperidol; ***Thai.:*** H-Tab; Haldol; Halo-P; Halomed; Halopol; Haricon; Haridol; Perida; Polyhadol; Schizopol; Senorm†; Serenace†; Tensidol; ***UK:*** Dozic; Haldol; Serenace; ***USA:*** Haldol.

**Multi-ingredient:** ***Austria:*** Vesalium†; ***Belg.:*** Vesalium†; ***Fr.:*** Vesadol.

---

## Haloxazolam *(rINN)*

10-Bromo-11b-(2-fluorophenyl)-2,3,7,11b-tetrahydrooxazolo-[3,2-*d*][1,4]benzodiazepin-6(5*H*)-one.

$C_{17}H_{14}BrFN_2O_2$ = 377.2.

*CAS — 59128-97-1.*

**Pharmacopoeias.** In *Jpn.*

### Profile

Haloxazolam is a benzodiazepine with general properties similar to those of diazepam (p.690). It has been given by mouth as a hypnotic in the short-term management of insomnia.

## Hexobarbital (BAN, rINN)

Enhexymalum; Enimal; Hexobarbitalum; Hexobarbitone; Methexenyl; Methyl-cyclohexenylmethyl-barbitursäure; Methylhexabarbital. 5-(Cyclohex-1-enyl)-1,5-dimethylbarbituric acid.

$C_{12}H_{16}N_2O_3$ = 236.3.

*CAS — 56-29-1.*

*ATC — N01AF02; N05CA16.*

NOTE. The name ciclobarbital (see Cyclobarbital, p.689) has sometimes been applied to hexobarbital.

**Pharmacopoeias.** In *Eur.* (see p.vi).

**Ph. Eur. 5.0** (Hexobarbital). A white crystalline powder. Very slightly soluble in water; sparingly soluble in alcohol. Forms water-soluble compounds with alkali hydroxides and carbonates and with ammonia.

## Hexobarbital Sodium (BANM, rINNM)

Enhexymalnatrium; Hexenalum; Hexobarbital sódico; Hexobarbitalum Natricum; Hexobarbitone Sodium; Sodium Hexobarbital; Soluble Hexobarbitone. Sodium 5-(cyclohex-1-enyl)-1,5-dimethylbarbiturate.

$C_{12}H_{15}N_2NaO_3$ = 258.2.

*CAS — 50-09-9.*

*ATC — N01AF02; N05CA16.*

### Profile

Hexobarbital is a barbiturate with the general properties of amobarbital (p.670). It has been used as a hypnotic and sedative but barbiturates are no longer considered appropriate for such purposes.

## Homofenazine Hydrochloride (rINNM)

D-775 (homofenazine); HFZ (homofenazine); Hidrocloruro de homofenazina. 2-{Hexahydro-4-[3-(2-trifluoromethylphenothiazin-10-yl)propyl]-1,4-diazepin-1-yl}ethanol dihydrochloride.

$C_{23}H_{28}F_3N_3OS,2HCl$ = 524.5.

*CAS — 3833-99-6 (homofenazine); 1256-01-5 (homofenazine hydrochloride).*

### Profile

Homofenazine hydrochloride is a phenothiazine with general properties similar to those of chlorpromazine (p.675). It has been used in the management of neuropsychiatric disorders.

### Preparations

**Proprietary Preparations** (details are given in Part 3)

**Multi-ingredient:** ***Austria:*** Pelvichthol†.

## Ipsapirone Hydrochloride (BANM, USAN, rINNM)

Bay-q-7821; Hidrocloruro de ipsapirona; TVX-Q-7821. 2-[4-(4-Pyrimidin-2-ylpiperazin-1-yl)butyl]-1,2-benzothiazol-3(2*H*)-one 1,1-dioxide hydrochloride.

$C_{19}H_{23}N_5O_3S,HCl$ = 437.9.

*CAS — 95847-70-4 (ipsapirone); 92589-98-5 (ipsapirone hydrochloride).*

### Profile

Ipsapirone is structurally related to buspirone (p.672). It has been investigated as the hydrochloride for the treatment of anxiety disorders and depression.

**Action.** Ipsapirone is a partial agonist at serotonin (hydroxytryptamine, 5-HT) receptors of the $5\text{-HT}_{1A}$ subtype. For reference to the actions and potential uses of such drugs, see Buspirone, p.673.

References.

1. Cutler NR, *et al.* A double-blind, placebo-controlled study comparing the efficacy and safety of ipsapirone versus lorazepam in patients with generalized anxiety disorder: a prospective multicenter trial. *J Clin Psychopharmacol* 1993; **13:** 429–37.
2. Fuhr U, *et al.* Absorption of ipsapirone along the human gastrointestinal tract. *Br J Clin Pharmacol* 1994; **38:** 83–6.
3. Mandos LA, *et al.* Placebo-controlled comparison of the clinical effects of rapid discontinuation of ipsapirone and lorazepam after 8 weeks of treatment for generalized anxiety disorder. *Int Clin Psychopharmacol* 1995; **10:** 251–6.
4. Lapierre YD, *et al.* A Canadian multicenter study of three fixed doses of controlled-release ipsapirone in outpatients with moderate to severe major depression. *J Clin Psychopharmacol* 1998; **18:** 268–73.

## Ketazolam (BAN, USAN, rINN)

U-28774. 11-Chloro-8,12b-dihydro-2,8-dimethyl-12b-phenyl-4*H*-[1,3]oxazino[3,2-*d*][1,4]benzodiazepine-4,7(6*H*)-dione.

$C_{20}H_{17}ClN_2O_3$ = 368.8.

*CAS — 27223-35-4.*

*ATC — N05BA10.*

### Profile

Ketazolam is a long-acting benzodiazepine with general properties similar to those of diazepam (p.690). It is given by mouth in the short-term treatment of anxiety (p.663) in usual doses of 15 to 60 mg daily, either in divided doses or as a single dose at night. Reduced doses may be required in elderly or debilitated patients.

◊ References.

1. Angelini G, *et al.* Ketazolam, a new long-acting benzodiazepine, in the treatment of anxious patients: a multicenter study of 2,056 patients. *Curr Ther Res* 1989; **45:** 294–304.

### Preparations

**Proprietary Preparations** (details are given in Part 3)

***Arg.:*** Ansieten; ***Belg.:*** Solatran; Unakalm†; ***Chile:*** Ansietil; Sedatival; ***Ital.:*** Anseren; ***Neth.:*** Unakalm; ***Port.:*** Unakalm; ***S.Afr.:*** Solatran; ***Spain:*** Marcen; Sedotime; ***Switz.:*** Solatran.

# Levomepromazine (BAN, USAN, rINN)

CL-36467; CL-39743; Levomepromazina; Methotrimeprazine; RP-7044; SKF-5116; XP-03. (−)-*NN*-Dimethyl-3-(2-methoxyphenothiazin-10-yl)-2-methylpropylamine; 3-(2-Methoxyphenothiazin-10-yl)-2-methylpropyldimethylamine.

$C_{19}H_{24}N_2OS$ = 328.5.

*CAS — 60-99-1.*

*ATC — N05AA02.*

**Pharmacopoeias.** In *US.* Also in *BP(Vet).*

**BP(Vet) 2003** (Levomepromazine). A white or slightly cream-coloured odourless or almost odourless crystalline powder. Practically insoluble in water; slightly soluble in alcohol; freely soluble in chloroform and in ether. Protect from light.

**USP 27** (Methotrimeprazine). A fine white, practically odourless, crystalline powder. Soluble 1 in 10 of water, of alcohol, and of methyl alcohol, and 1 in 2 of chloroform; freely soluble in ether; sparingly soluble in alcohol at 25° but freely soluble in boiling alcohol. Store at a temperature of 25°, excursions permitted between 15° and 30°. Protect from light.

## Levomepromazine Hydrochloride

(BANM, USAN, rINNM)

Hidrocloruro de levomepromazina; Levomepromazini Hydrochloridum; Methotrimeprazine Hydrochloride.

$C_{19}H_{24}N_2OS,HCl$ = 364.9.

*CAS — 4185-80-2; 1236-99-3.*

*ATC — N05AA02.*

**Pharmacopoeias.** In *Eur.* (see p.vi) and *Pol.*

**Ph. Eur. 5.0** (Levomepromazine Hydrochloride). A white or very slightly yellow, slightly hygroscopic crystalline powder. It deteriorates on exposure to air and light. Freely soluble in water and in alcohol. Store in airtight containers. Protect from light.

**Incompatibility.** Levomepromazine hydrochloride is reported to be incompatible with alkaline solutions.

## Levomepromazine Maleate (BANM, USAN, rINNM)

Levomepromazini Maleas; Maleato de levomepromazina; Methotrimeprazine Hydrogen Maleate; Methotrimeprazine Maleate.

$C_{19}H_{24}N_2OS,C_4H_4O_4$ = 444.5.

*CAS — 7104-38-3.*

*ATC — N05AA02.*

**Pharmacopoeias.** In *Eur.* (see p.vi), *Jpn*, and *Pol.*

**Ph. Eur. 5.0** (Levomepromazine Maleate). A white or slightly yellowish crystalline powder. It deteriorates when exposed to air and light. Slightly soluble in water and in alcohol; sparingly soluble in dichloromethane. The supernatant of a 2% dispersion in water has a pH of 3.5 to 5.5. Protect from light.

## Adverse Effects, Treatment, and Precautions

As for Chlorpromazine, p.675, although it may be more sedating. See also the sedating antihistamines, p.419.

Levomepromazine may cause severe orthostatic hypotension, and patients receiving large initial doses, patients over 50 years of age, or those receiving injections, should be recumbent. Children are very susceptible to the hypotensive and sedative effects of levomepromazine.

## Interactions

As for Chlorpromazine, p.679.

**Antidepressants.** Although MAOIs have been used with phenothiazines without untoward effects the use of levomepromazine with MAOIs should probably be avoided as this combination has been implicated in 2 fatalities.[1,2]

1. Barsa JA, Saunders JC. A comparative study of tranylcypromine and pargyline. *Psychopharmacologia* 1964; **6:** 295–8.
2. McQueen EG. New Zealand committee on adverse drug reactions: fourteenth annual report 1979. *N Z Med J* 1980; **91:** 226–9.

## Pharmacokinetics

◊ In a study involving a total of 5 psychiatric patients peak plasma concentrations of levomepromazine were noted 1 to 4 hours after administration by mouth and 30 to 90 minutes after injection into the gluteal muscle.[1] About 50% of orally administered drug reached the systemic circulation. Although the metabolite levomepromazine sulfoxide could not be detected after a single intramuscular injection it was found in concentrations higher than unmetabolised levomepromazine after single and multiple oral dosage, both substances reaching a steady state in the plasma within 7 days of starting multiple dose oral therapy. Fluctuations in plasma concentration during multiple dose oral therapy indicated that until the correlation between acute side-effects and peak plasma concentration of levomepromazine had been further studied the total daily dose should be divided into 2 or 3 portions when larger doses of levomepromazine were given by mouth.

1. Dahl SG. Pharmacokinetics of methotrimeprazine after single and multiple doses. *Clin Pharmacol Ther* 1976; **19:** 435–42.

**Half-life.** In 8 psychiatric patients given levomepromazine 50 to 350 mg daily the plasma half-life showed wide variation, from 16.5 to 77.8 hours, and did not correlate with the dose given.[1]

1. Dahl SG, *et al.* Pharmacokinetics and relative bioavailability of levomepromazine after repeated administration of tablets and syrup. *Eur J Clin Pharmacol* 1977; **11:** 305–310.

## Uses and Administration

Levomepromazine is a phenothiazine with pharmacological activity similar to that of both chlorpromazine (p.680) and promethazine (p.440). It has antihistaminic actions (p.419) as well as CNS effects resembling those of chlorpromazine. It is also reported to have analgesic activity. It is used in the treatment of various psychoses including schizophrenia (p.665), as an analgesic for moderate to severe pain usually in non-ambulatory patients, and for premedication (p.1296). It is also used for the control of symptoms such as restlessness, agitation, and vomiting and as an adjunct to opioid analgesia in terminally ill patients.

Levomepromazine is also used in veterinary medicine.

Levomepromazine is given by mouth as the maleate or the hydrochloride or by injection as the hydrochloride. In the UK, doses such as those given below are expressed in terms of the appropriate salt. However, in some countries, the dose of levomepromazine may be expressed in terms of the base. The embonate has also been used. Care is required in elderly patients because of the risk of severe hypotension; if levomepromazine is given to such patients reduced doses may be necessary.

The usual initial dose of levomepromazine maleate for the treatment of **schizophrenia** is 25 to 50 mg daily by mouth; the daily dosage is usually divided into 3 portions with a larger portion taken at night. Doses of 100 to 200 mg have been given to non-ambulant patients increased gradually up to 1 g daily if necessary. Children are very susceptible to the hypotensive and sedative effects of levomepromazine: a suggested dose for a 10-year-old is 12.5 to 25 mg of the maleate daily in divided doses by mouth; a dose of 37.5 mg daily should not be exceeded.

When used in **palliative care** as an adjunct to analgesics in the management of severe terminal **pain** and for the control of **nausea and vomiting**, levomepromazine maleate may be given by mouth in a dose of 12.5 to 50 mg every 4 to 8 hours. The *British National Formulary* also includes a dose of levomepromazine maleate 6 to 25 mg given by mouth for the management of nausea and vomiting where first-line antiemetics have proved inadequate. Alternatively 12.5 to 25 mg of levomepromazine hydrochloride may be given intramuscularly every 6 to 8 hours but patients should remain in bed for at least the first few doses; doses of up to 50 mg have been given for severe agitation. Levomepromazine hydrochloride may also be given intravenously in similar doses following dilution with an equal volume of sodium chloride 0.9% injection. Alternatively it may be given, suitably diluted with sodium chloride 0.9% injection, by continuous subcutaneous infusion via a syringe driver; doses range from a total of 25 to 200 mg daily although lower doses of 5 to 25 mg daily may also be effective against nausea and vomiting and produce less sedation. Experience with parenteral administration of levomepromazine hydrochloride in children is limited but a dose of 0.35 to 3 mg/kg daily has been suggested.

Levomepromazine hydrochloride given intramuscularly has also been used in some countries for the control of acute pain and for postoperative analgesia.

Levomepromazine hydrochloride has also been given intramuscularly as a **premedicant**. In some countries levomepromazine is also licensed for use as an **anxiolytic** and **sedative**, and the management of other types of pain, including **labour pain**.

**Pain.** As levomepromazine appears to possess intrinsic analgesic activity in addition to its antiemetic and antipsychotic actions it has been used for the symptomatic control of restlessness and vomiting and as an adjunct to opioid analgesics in pain control (see Choice of Analgesic, p.2) in terminally ill patients.

References.

1. Oliver DJ. The use of methotrimeprazine in terminal care. *Br J Clin Pract* 1985; **39:** 339–40.
2. Patt RB, *et al.* The neuroleptics as adjuvant analgesics. *J Pain Symptom Manage* 1994; **9:** 446–53.
3. O'Neill J, Fountain A. Levomepromazine (methotrimeprazine) and the last 48 hours. *Hosp Med* 1999; **60:** 564–7.
4. Skinner J, Skinner A. Levomepromazine for nausea and vomiting in advanced cancer. *Hosp Med* 1999; **60:** 568–70.

HEADACHE. Similarly to chlorpromazine (p.682) and prochlorperazine (p.717), levomepromazine[1] has been effective in relieving the pain of severe migraine attacks.

1. Stiell IG, *et al.* Methotrimeprazine versus meperidine and dimenhydrinate in the treatment of severe migraine: a randomized, controlled trial. *Ann Emerg Med* 1991; **20:** 1201–5.

## Preparations

***BP 2003:*** Levomepromazine Injection; Levomepromazine Tablets;
***USP 27:*** Methotrimeprazine Injection.

**Proprietary Preparations** (details are given in Part 3)
***Arg.:*** Nozinan; Togrel; ***Austria:*** Nozinan; ***Belg.:*** Nozinan; ***Braz.:*** Levozine; Neozine; ***Canad.:*** Apo-Methoprazine; Novo-Meprazine; Nozinan; ***Chile:*** Sinogan; ***Denm.:*** Nozinan; ***Fin.:*** Levozin; Nozinan; ***Fr.:*** Nozinan; ***Ger.:*** Levium; Neurocil; Tisercin†; ***Gr.:*** Nozinan; Prazine; ***Irl.:*** Nozinan; ***Israel:*** Methozane; Nozinan; Ronexine; ***Ital.:*** Nozinan; ***Mex.:*** Levocina; Sinogan; ***Neth.:*** Nozinan; ***Norw.:*** Nozinan; ***NZ:*** Nozinan; ***Port.:*** Nozinan; ***Spain:*** Sinogan; ***Swed.:*** Nozinan; ***Switz.:*** Minozinan†; Nozinan; ***UK:*** Nozinan; ***USA:*** Levoprome†.

# Loprazolam Mesilate *(BANM, rINNM)*

HR-158; Loprazolam Mesylate; Loprazolam Methanesulphonate; Mesilato de loprazolam; RU-31158. 6-(2-Chlorophenyl)-2,4-dihydro-2-(4-methylpiperazin-1-ylmethylene)-8-nitroimidazo[1,2-*a*][1,4]benzodiazepin-1-one methanesulphonate monohydrate.

$C_{23}H_{21}ClN_6O_3,CH_4O_3S,H_2O = 579.0.$

*CAS — 61197-73-7 (loprazolam); 70111-54-5 (anhydrous loprazolam mesilate).*

*ATC — N05CD11.*

**Pharmacopoeias.** In *Br.*

**BP 2003** (Loprazolam Mesilate). A yellow crystalline powder. Slightly soluble in water, in alcohol, and in chloroform; very slightly soluble in ether.

## Dependence and Withdrawal

As for Diazepam, p.690.

◊ For the purpose of withdrawal regimens, 0.5 to 1 mg of loprazolam is considered roughly equivalent to 5 mg of diazepam.

## Adverse Effects, Treatment, and Precautions

As for Diazepam, p.690.

**Porphyria.** Loprazolam is considered to be unsafe in patients with porphyria because it has been shown to be porphyrinogenic in *in-vitro* systems.

## Interactions

As for Diazepam, p.692.

## Pharmacokinetics

◊ References.

1. Garzone PD, Kroboth PD. Pharmacokinetics of the newer benzodiazepines. *Clin Pharmacokinet* 1989; **16:** 337–64.
2. Dorling MC, Hindmarch I. Pharmacokinetic profile of loprazolam in 12 young and 12 elderly healthy volunteers. *Drugs Exp Clin Res* 2001; **27:** 151–9.

## Uses and Administration

Loprazolam is an intermediate-acting benzodiazepine with general properties similar to those of diazepam (p.695).

Loprazolam mesilate is usually used for its hypnotic properties in the short-term management of insomnia (p.667), in usual doses equivalent to 1 mg of loprazolam at night. Dosage may be increased to up to 2 mg if necessary. A starting dose of 0.5 mg increased to a maximum of 1 mg may be appropriate for elderly or debilitated patients.

## Preparations

***BP 2003:*** Loprazolam Tablets.

**Proprietary Preparations** (details are given in Part 3)
***Arg.:*** Dormonoct; ***Belg.:*** Dormonoct; ***Fr.:*** Havlane; ***Ger.:*** Sonin; ***Neth.:*** Dormonoct; ***Port.:*** Dormonoct; ***S.Afr.:*** Dormonoct; ***Spain:*** Somnovit.

# Lorazepam *(BAN, USAN, rINN)*

Lorazepamum; Wy-4036. 7-Chloro-5-(2-chlorophenyl)-1,3-dihydro-3-hydroxy-1,4-benzodiazepin-2-one.

$C_{15}H_{10}Cl_2N_2O_2 = 321.2.$

*CAS — 846-49-1.*

*ATC — N05BA06.*

**Pharmacopoeias.** In *Eur.* (see p.vi), *Jpn,* and *US.*

**Ph. Eur. 5.0** (Lorazepam). A white or almost white, crystalline powder. It exhibits polymorphism. Practically insoluble in water; sparingly soluble in alcohol; sparingly or slightly soluble in dichloromethane. Store in airtight containers. Protect from light.

**USP 27** (Lorazepam). A white or practically white, practically odourless powder. Insoluble in water; sparingly soluble in alcohol; slightly soluble in chloroform. Store in airtight containers. Protect from light.

**Incompatibility.** Visual incompatibility has been noted with lorazepam and sargramostim[1] or aztreonam.[2]

1. Trissel LA, *et al.* Visual compatibility of sargramostim with selected antineoplastic agents, anti-infectives, or other drugs during simulated Y-site injection. *Am J Hosp Pharm* 1992; **49:** 402–6.
2. Trissel LA, Martinez JF. Compatibility of aztreonam with selected drugs during simulated Y-site administration. *Am J Health-Syst Pharm* 1995; **52:** 1086–90.

**Solubility.** The solubility of lorazepam in fluids for intravenous administration (water, glucose injection, lactated Ringer's injection, and sodium chloride injection) was greatest in glucose injection (5%) at 62 micrograms/mL and lowest in sodium chloride injection (0.9%) at 27 micrograms/mL;[1] these differences in solubility appeared to be pH related. Commercial injections are reported to contain polyethylene glycol in propylene glycol to overcome this poor solubility. However, precipitation has been noted[2] in solutions prepared by dilution of lorazepam injection with sodium chloride injection (0.9%) to a concentration of 500 micrograms/mL. One group of workers[3] have reported that they had overcome such problems with precipitation by using glucose injection (5%) as a diluent and by avoiding final concentrations of lorazepam between 0.08 mg/mL and 1 mg/mL. It was suggested that the propylene glycol in the mixture might account for the unusual concentration effect. Such recommendations have been adopted by another group[4] although they observed that precipitation occurred if a formulation of lorazepam containing 4 mg/mL was used to prepare the injection; no precipitation was noted when a formulation containing 2 mg/mL was used. The group also commented that, in the USA, the manufacturers of lorazepam injection advise that admixtures should be prepared with the 2 mg/mL formulation only.

1. Newton DW, *et al.* Lorazepam solubility in and sorption from intravenous admixture solutions. *Am J Hosp Pharm* 1983; **40:** 424–7.
2. Boullata JI, *et al.* Precipitation of lorazepam infusion. *Ann Pharmacother* 1996; **30:** 1037–8.
3. Volles DF, *et al.* More on usability of lorazepam admixtures for continuous infusion. *Am J Health-Syst Pharm* 1996; **53:** 2753–4.
4. Levanda M. Noticeable difference in admixtures prepared from lorazepam 2 and 4 mg/ml. *Am J Health-Syst Pharm* 1998; **55:** 2305.

**Sorption.** Significant loss of lorazepam has been reported from solutions stored in PVC[1] or polypropylene[2] giving equipment; polyolefin[3] or glass[4] equipment appears to be more suitable.

1. Hoey LL, *et al.* Lorazepam stability in parenteral solutions for continuous intravenous administration. *Ann Pharmacother* 1996; **30:** 343–6.
2. Stiles ML, *et al.* Stability of deferoxamine mesylate, floxuridine, fluorouracil, hydromorphone hydrochloride, lorazepam, and midazolam hydrochloride in polypropylene infusion-pump syringes. *Am J Health-Syst Pharm* 1996; **53:** 1583–8.
3. Trissel LA, Pearson SD. Storage of lorazepam in three injectable solutions in polyvinyl chloride and polyolefin bags. *Am J Hosp Pharm* 1994; **51:** 368–72.
4. Martens HJ, *et al.* Sorption of various drugs in polyvinyl chloride, glass, and polyethylene-lined infusion containers. *Am J Hosp Pharm* 1990; **47:** 369–73.

## Dependence and Withdrawal

As for Diazepam, p.690.

◊ For the purpose of withdrawal regimens, 500 micrograms of lorazepam may be considered approximately equivalent to 5 mg of diazepam.

## Adverse Effects, Treatment, and Precautions

As for Diazepam, p.690. Pain and a sensation of burning have occurred following injection of lorazepam.

**Breast feeding.** The American Academy of Pediatrics[1] considers that, although the effect of lorazepam on breast-feeding infants is unknown, its use by mothers during breast feeding may be of concern since anxiolytic drugs do appear in breast milk and thus could conceivably alter CNS function in the infant both in the short and long term.

Free lorazepam concentrations in the breast milk of 4 lactating mothers ranged from 8 to 9 nanograms/mL four hours after receiving a 3.5-mg oral dose.[2] This represented about 15 to 26% of the concentration in plasma, and was probably sufficiently low to cause no adverse effects in breast-fed infants.

1. American Academy of Pediatrics. The transfer of drugs and other chemicals into human milk. *Pediatrics* 2001; **108:** 776–89. Correction. *ibid.*; 1029. Also available at: http://aappolicy.aappublications.org/cgi/content/full/pediatrics%3b108/3/776 (accessed 28/04/04)
2. Summerfield RJ, Nielsen MS. Excretion of lorazepam into breast milk. *Br J Anaesth* 1985; **57:** 1042–3.

**Effects on the blood.** A case of pancytopenia associated with oral lorazepam was reported[1] in 1988; only 5 instances of thrombocytopenia and none of leucopenia had been reported to the UK Committee on Safety of Medicines or the UK manufacturers over the previous 13 years.

1. El-Sayed S, Symonds RP. Lorazepam induced pancytopenia. *BMJ* 1988; **296:** 1332.

**Effects on fluid and electrolyte homoeostasis.** Inappropriate secretion of antidiuretic hormone related to ingestion of lorazepam was considered to be the cause of hyponatraemia in an 81-year-old woman.[1]

1. Engel WR, Grau A. Inappropriate secretion of antidiuretic hormone associated with lorazepam. *BMJ* 1988; **297:** 858.

**Effects on the nervous system.** For reference to extrapyramidal disorders associated with administration of lorazepam, see Diazepam, p.691.

**The elderly.** For discussion of the need for reduced dosage of benzodiazepines in elderly patients, including mention of lorazepam, see Diazepam, p.692.

**Formulation.** There have been reports of toxicity, presumed to be due to polyethylene glycol[1,2] or propylene glycol,[3] following prolonged parenteral administration of lorazepam; polyethylene glycol in propylene glycol is included as a solubiliser in lorazepam solutions. Diarrhoea in an infant given large enteral doses of lorazepam or diazepam solutions may have been due to the combined osmotic effect of polyethylene glycol and propylene glycol in these preparations.[4]

1. Laine GA, *et al.* Polyethylene glycol nephrotoxicity secondary to prolonged high-dose intravenous lorazepam. *Ann Pharmacother* 1995; **29:** 1110–4.
2. Tayar J *et al.* Severe hyperosmolar metabolic acidosis due to a large dose of intravenous lorazepam. *N Engl J Med* 2002; **346:** 1253–4.
3. Seay RE, *et al.* Possible toxicity from propylene glycol in lorazepam infusion. *Ann Pharmacother* 1997; **31:** 647–8. Woycik CL, Walker PC. Correction and comment: possible toxicity from propylene glycol in injectable drug preparations. *ibid.*: 1413.
4. Marshall JD, *et al.* Diarrhea associated with enteral benzodiazepine solutions. *J Pediatr* 1995; **126:** 657–9.

**Hepatic impairment.** Lorazepam is contra-indicated in severe hepatic impairment; patients with mild to moderate impairment may require reduced doses. Although the elimination half-life of lorazepam was increased in 13 patients with alcoholic cirrhosis compared with 11 control subjects, this was not associated with an impairment in systemic plasma clearance.[1] With the exception of a modest decrease in the extent of plasma protein binding, acute viral hepatitis had no effect on the disposition kinetics of lorazepam.

1. Kraus JW, *et al.* Effects of aging and liver disease on disposition of lorazepam. *Clin Pharmacol Ther* 1978; **24:** 411–19.

**Local reactions.** Of 40 patients given a single intravenous dose of lorazepam 4 mg three had local thrombosis 2 to 3 days later and 6 had local thrombosis 7 to 10 days later.[1] The incidence was lower than in those given diazepam [in solution].

1. Hegarty JE, Dundee JW. Sequelae after the intravenous injection of three benzodiazepines—diazepam, lorazepam, and flunitrazepam. *BMJ* 1977; **2:** 1384–5.

## Interactions

As for Diazepam, p.692.

## Pharmacokinetics

Lorazepam is readily absorbed from the gastrointestinal tract following oral administration, with a bioavailability of about 90%; peak plasma concentrations are reported to occur about 2 hours after an oral dose. The absorption profile after intramuscular injection is similar to that after administration by mouth.

Lorazepam is about 85% bound to plasma protein. It crosses the blood-brain barrier and the placenta; it is also distributed into breast milk. Lorazepam is metabolised in the liver to the inactive glucuronide, and excreted in urine. The elimination half-life has been reported to range from about 10 to 20 hours.

◊ References.

1. Greenblatt DJ. Clinical pharmacokinetics of oxazepam and lorazepam. *Clin Pharmacokinet* 1981; **6:** 89–105.

**Children.** References to the pharmacokinetics of lorazepam in children.

1. Relling MV, *et al.* Lorazepam pharmacodynamics and pharmacokinetics in children. *J Pediatr* 1989; **114:** 641–6.

NEONATES. References to slow elimination of lorazepam by neonates.

1. Cummings AJ, Whitelaw AGL. A study of conjugation and drug elimination in the human neonate. *Br J Clin Pharmacol* 1981; **12:** 511–15.
2. McDermott CA, *et al.* Pharmacokinetics of lorazepam in critically ill neonates with seizures. *J Pediatr* 1992; **120:** 479–83.
3. Reiter PD, Stiles AD. Lorazepam toxicity in a premature infant. *Ann Pharmacother* 1993; **27:** 727–9.

**Distribution.** Evidence that lorazepam undergoes enterohepatic recirculation with possible first-pass metabolism.[1]

1. Herman RJ, *et al.* Disposition of lorazepam in human beings: enterohepatic recirculation and first-pass effect. *Clin Pharmacol Ther* 1989; **46:** 18–25.

CNS. In a study involving 6 healthy subjects, peak plasma-lorazepam concentrations were reached 5 minutes after the end of a one-minute intravenous injection.[1] CNS effects, as measured by EEG activity, were not maximal until 30 minutes after injection; they declined to baseline values slowly over 5 to 8 hours in a similar manner to plasma concentrations. In contrast, CNS effects of diazepam were maximal immediately after the injection. They also declined more rapidly than lorazepam, but again in a similar way to plasma concentrations. Studies in *mice* suggested that the slow onset of action of lorazepam that has been reported by some is at least partly explained by a delay in passage from systemic blood into brain tissue.

1. Greenblatt DJ, *et al.* Kinetic and dynamic study of intravenous lorazepam; comparison with intravenous diazepam. *J Pharmacol Exp Ther* 1989; **250:** 134–40.

## Uses and Administration

Lorazepam is a short-acting benzodiazepine with general properties similar to those of diazepam (p.695). It is used in the short-term treatment of anxiety disorders (p.663), as a hypnotic in the short-term management of insomnia (p.667), and as an anticonvulsant in the management of status epilepticus (p.352). When used in the treatment of status epilepticus lorazepam has a prolonged antiepileptic action. It is also used for its sedative and amnestic properties in premedication and as an adjunct in regimens for the control of nausea and vomiting associated with cancer chemotherapy (p.1245).

Lorazepam is usually given by mouth or by injection as the base although the pivalate is available for oral administration in some countries. Sublingual tablets are used in some countries in doses similar to those for standard tablets. The intramuscular route is usually only used when oral or intravenous administration is not possible. Injections should usually be diluted before administration; intravenous injections should be given at a rate of not more than 2 mg/minute into a large vein. Lorazepam should be given in reduced dosage to elderly or debilitated patients; half the usual adult dose, or less, may be sufficient.

The usual dose of lorazepam by mouth for the treatment of **anxiety disorders** is 1 to 6 mg daily in 2 or 3 divided doses with the largest dose taken at night; up to 10 mg daily has been given. A dose of 25 to 30 micrograms/kg may be given by injection every 6 hours for acute anxiety. Lorazepam has also been used for **panic attacks**. A suggested dose in the *British National Formulary* is 3 to 5 mg daily. A single oral dose of 1 to 4 mg at bedtime may be given for **insomnia** associated with anxiety.

For **premedication** adults may be given a dose of 2 to 3 mg by mouth the night before the operation followed if necessary the next morning by a smaller dose. Alternatively, 2 to 4 mg may be given 1 to 2 hours before an operation. A dose of 50 micrograms/kg may be administered 30 to 45 minutes before the operation if given intravenously or 1 to 1½ hours before if given intramuscularly.

In the management of **status epilepticus** 4 mg may be given as a single intravenous dose; a dose of 2 mg has been suggested for children.

In patients receiving modestly emetogenic chemotherapy, lorazepam 1 to 2 mg by mouth may be added to antiemetic therapy with domperidone or metoclopramide, for the prophylaxis of **nausea and vomiting**. The addition of lorazepam may be helpful in the prevention of anticipatory symptoms because of its sedative and amnestic effects.

**Disturbed behaviour.** For a discussion of the management of behaviour disturbances associated with various psychotic disorders and the value of benzodiazepines, see p.665.

References.

1. Bieniek SA, *et al.* A double-blind study of lorazepam versus the combination of haloperidol and lorazepam in managing agitation. *Pharmacotherapy* 1998; **18:** 57–62.

**Nausea and vomiting.** References.

1. Malik IA, *et al.* Clinical efficacy of lorazepam in prophylaxis of anticipatory, acute, and delayed nausea and vomiting induced by high doses of cisplatin: a prospective randomized trial. *Am J Clin Oncol* 1995; **18:** 170–5.

**Premedication and sedation.** Lorazepam is used as a premedicant (p.1296) and as a sedative for therapeutic and investigative procedures such as dental treatment (p.666) and endoscopy (p.666), and also in intensive care (p.666).

References.

1. Maltais F, *et al.* A randomized, double-blind, placebo-controlled study of lorazepam as premedication for bronchoscopy. *Chest* 1996; **109:** 1195–8.

**Substance dependence.** Lorazepam has been used in the management of symptoms of alcohol withdrawal (p.1166).

References.

1. D'Onofrio G, *et al.* Lorazepam for the prevention of recurrent seizures related to alcohol. *N Engl J Med* 1999; **340:** 915–9.

## Preparations

***BP 2003:*** Lorazepam Injection; Lorazepam Tablets;
***USP 27:*** Lorazepam Injection; Lorazepam Oral Concentrate; Lorazepam Tablets.

**Proprietary Preparations** (details are given in Part 3)
***Arg.:*** Aplacasse; Emotival; Kalmalin; Microzepam; Nervistop L; Sedatival; Sidenar; Trapax; Tratenamin; ***Austral.:*** Ativan; ***Austria:*** Ergocalm†; Merlit; Temesta; ***Belg.:*** Loridem; Optisedine; Serenase; Temesta; Vigiten; ***Braz.:*** Anosedil†; Calmogenol†; Lorax; Lorazepan; Lorium†; Max-Pax; Mesmerin; ***Canad.:*** Ativan; Novo-Lorazem; Nu-Loraz; ***Chile:*** Abinol; Amparax; ***Denm.:*** Lorabenz; Temesta; ***Fin.:*** Temesta; ***Fr.:*** Equitam; Temesta; ***Ger.:*** duralozam; Laubeel; Pro Dorm†; Punktyl†; Somagerol; Tavor; Tolid; ***Gr.:*** Aripax; Dorm; Modium; Nifalin; Novhepar; Proneurit; Tavor; Titus; Trankilium; ***Hong Kong:*** Ativan; Lorans; Lorivan; ***India:*** Ativan; Calmese; Larpose; ***Irl.:*** Ativan; ***Israel:*** Lorivan; ***Ital.:*** Control; Lorans; Quait†; Tavor; ***Malaysia:*** Ativan; Lorans; ***Mex.:*** Ativan; Sinestron; ***Neth.:*** Temesta; ***NZ:*** Ativan†; Lorapam; Lorzem†; ***Port.:*** Ansilor; Lorenin; Lorsedal; ***S.Afr.:*** Ativan; Tranqipam; ***Singapore:*** Ativan; Lorans†; ***Spain:*** Divial†; Donix; Idalprem; Orfidal; Piralone†; Placinoral; Sedicepan; Sedizepan†; ***Swed.:*** Temesta; ***Switz.:*** Lorasifar; Sedazin; Temesta; ***Thai.:*** Anta; Anxira; Ativan; Lonza; Lora; Loramed; Lorapam; Lorazene; Lorazep; Ora; Tranavan; ***UK:*** Ativan; ***USA:*** Ativan.

**Multi-ingredient:** ***Austria:*** Somnium; ***Switz.:*** Somnium.

---

## Lormetazepam *(BAN, USAN, rINN)*

Wy-4082. *(RS)*-7-Chloro-5-(2-chlorophenyl)-1,3-dihydro-3-hydroxy-1-methyl-1,4-benzodiazepin-2-one.

$C_{16}H_{12}Cl_2N_2O_2$ = 335.2.
*CAS — 848-75-9.*
*ATC — N05CD06.*

**Pharmacopoeias.** In *Br.*

**BP 2003** (Lormetazepam). A white crystalline powder. Practically insoluble in water; soluble in alcohol and in methyl alcohol. Protect from light.

### Dependence and Withdrawal

As for Diazepam, p.690.

◊ For the purpose of withdrawal regimens, 0.5 to 1 mg of lormetazepam is considered approximately equivalent to 5 mg of diazepam.

### Adverse Effects, Treatment, and Precautions

As for Diazepam, p.690.

### Interactions

As for Diazepam, p.692.

### Pharmacokinetics

Lormetazepam is rapidly absorbed from the gastrointestinal tract and metabolised to the inactive glucuronide. The terminal half-life is reported to be about 11 hours.

◊ A brief review of the pharmacokinetics of lormetazepam.[1]

1. Greenblatt DJ, *et al.* Clinical pharmacokinetics of the newer benzodiazepines. *Clin Pharmacokinet* 1983; **8:** 233–52.

### Uses and Administration

Lormetazepam is a short-acting benzodiazepine with general properties similar to those of diazepam (p.695). It is mainly used as a hypnotic in the short-term management of insomnia (p.667) in usual doses of 0.5 to 1.5 mg by mouth at night. A dose of 500 micrograms is recommended for elderly or debilitated patients. Lormetazepam is also used in some countries for premedication (p.1296).

### Preparations

***BP 2003:*** Lormetazepam Tablets.

**Proprietary Preparations** (details are given in Part 3)
***Arg.:*** Dilamet; ***Austria:*** Noctamid; ***Belg.:*** Loramet; Noctamid; Octonox; Sedaben; Stilaze; ***Chile:*** Nocton; ***Denm.:*** Pronoctan; ***Fr.:*** Noctamide; ***Ger.:*** Ergocalm; Loretam; Noctamid; ***Gr.:*** Loramet; ***Hong Kong:*** Loramet; ***Irl.:*** Loramet†; Noctamid; ***Ital.:*** Minias; ***Neth.:*** Loramet; Noctamid; ***NZ:*** Noctamid; ***Port.:*** Noctamid; ***S.Afr.:*** Loramet; Noctamid; ***Singapore:*** Loramet; ***Spain:*** Aldosomnil; Loramet; Noctamid; Sedobrina†; ***Switz.:*** Loramet; Noctamid; ***Thai.:*** Loramet.

---

## Loxapine *(BAN, USAN, rINN)*

CL-62362; Loxapina; Oxilapine; SUM-3170. 2-Chloro-11-(4-methylpiperazin-1-yl)dibenz[*b,f*][1,4]oxazepine.

$C_{18}H_{18}ClN_3O$ = 327.8.
*CAS — 1977-10-2.*
*ATC — N05AH01.*

## Loxapine Hydrochloride *(BANM, rINNM)*

Hidrocloruro de loxapina.

$C_{18}H_{18}ClN_3O,HCl$ = 364.3.
*ATC — N05AH01.*

## Loxapine Succinate *(BANM, USAN, rINNM)*

CL-71563; Succinato de loxapina.

$C_{18}H_{18}ClN_3O,C_4H_6O_4$ = 445.9.
*CAS — 27833-64-3.*
*ATC — N05AH01.*

**Pharmacopoeias.** In *US.*

**USP 27** (Loxapine Succinate). A white to yellowish, odourless, crystalline powder. Store in airtight containers.

### Adverse Effects, Treatment, and Precautions

As for Chlorpromazine, p.675.

Other side-effects reported include nausea and vomiting, seborrhoea, dyspnoea, ptosis, headache, paraesthesia, flush, weight gain or loss, and polydipsia.

**Abuse.** A report of 3 cases of loxapine succinate abuse.[1]

1. Sperry L, *et al.* Loxapine abuse. *N Engl J Med* 1984; **310:** 598.

**Effects on carbohydrate metabolism.** Reversible nonketotic hyperglycaemia, coma, and delirium, developed in a patient receiving loxapine 150 mg daily in addition to lithium therapy.[1] Symptoms improved following discontinuation of loxapine, but subsequently recurred when the patient was given amoxapine. The causative agent may have been 7-hydroxyamoxapine, a common metabolite of both amoxapine and loxapine.

1. Tollefson G, Lesar T. Nonketotic hyperglycemia associated with loxapine and amoxapine: case report. *J Clin Psychiatry* 1983; **44:** 347–8.

**Mania.** A patient, initially diagnosed as suffering from schizophrenia, developed manic symptoms after receiving loxapine.[1] The diagnosis was revised to schizoaffective disorder but it was suspected that loxapine had a role in the emergence of the affective symptoms. As loxapine shares common metabolites with the antidepressant amoxapine it was suggested that an antidepressant effect might have been instrumental in the production of manic symptoms.

1. Gojer JAC. Possible manic side-effects of loxapine. *Can J Psychiatry* 1992; **37:** 669–70.

**Overdosage.** An 8-year-old child was treated with activated charcoal within 30 minutes of being given 375 mg of loxapine by accident.[1] The child became drowsy and was asleep but arousable one hour after ingestion. The degree of sedation appeared to peak after 3.75 hours and the child was discharged about 20 hours postingestion.

1. Tarricone NW. Loxitane overdose. *Pediatrics* 1998; **101:** 496.

**Porphyria.** Loxapine is considered to be unsafe in patients with porphyria because it has been shown to be porphyrinogenic in *in-vitro* systems.

### Interactions

As for Chlorpromazine, p.679.

### Pharmacokinetics

Loxapine is readily absorbed from the gastrointestinal tract. It is very rapidly and extensively metabolised and there is evidence for a first-pass effect. It is mainly excreted in the urine, in the form of its conjugated metabolites, with smaller amounts appearing in the faeces as unconjugated metabolites; a substantial proportion of a dose is excreted in the first 24 hours. The major metabolites of loxapine are the active 7- and 8-hydroxyloxapine, which are conjugated to the glucuronide or sulfate; other metabolites include hydroxyloxapine-*N*-oxide, loxapine-*N*-oxide, and hydroxydesmethylloxapine (hydroxyamoxapine). Loxapine is widely distributed and *animal* studies have indicated that it crosses the placenta and is distributed into breast milk.

### Uses and Administration

Loxapine is a dibenzoxazepine with general properties similar to those of the phenothiazine, chlorpromazine (p.680). It is given by mouth as the succinate and by intramuscular injection as the base in the treatment of psychoses; doses are expressed in terms of the base. Loxapine succinate 34 mg is approximately equivalent to 25 mg of loxapine.

The usual dose by mouth is 20 to 50 mg daily initially, in 2 divided doses, increased according to requirements over the next 7 to 10 days to 60 to 100 mg daily or more in 2 to 4 divided doses; the maximum recommended dose is 250 mg daily. Maintenance doses are usually in the range of 20 to 100 mg daily. For the control of acute conditions it is given by intramuscular injection in daily doses up to 300 mg in 2 or 3 divided doses. Reduced dosage may be required in elderly patients.

Loxapine has also been given by mouth as the hydrochloride.

**Disturbed behaviour.** For a discussion of the use and limitations of antipsychotics such as loxapine in patients with disturbed behaviour, see p.665.

References.

1. Carlyle W, *et al.* Aggression in the demented patient: a double-blind study of loxapine versus haloperidol. *Int J Clin Psychopharmacol* 1993; **8:** 103–8.

**Schizophrenia.** A brief review of loxapine[1] concluded that suggestions that loxapine was particularly effective in patients with paranoid schizophrenia (p.665) had not been confirmed. A subsequent systematic review considered that the limited evidence did not indicate a clear difference in its effects from other antipsychotics.[2]

1. Anonymous. Clozapine and loxapine for schizophrenia. *Drug Ther Bull* 1991; **29:** 41–2.
2. Fenton M, *et al.* Loxapine for schizophrenia. Available in The Cochrane Library; Issue 1. Chichester: John Wiley; 2004.

### Preparations

***USP 27:*** Loxapine Capsules.

**Proprietary Preparations** (details are given in Part 3)
***Belg.:*** Loxapac†; ***Canad.:*** Loxapac†; ***Denm.:*** Loxapac†; ***Fr.:*** Loxapac; ***Gr.:*** Loxapac; ***India:*** Loxapac; ***Irl.:*** Loxapac†; ***NZ:*** Loxapac†; ***Spain:*** Desconex; ***UK:*** Loxapac; ***USA:*** Loxitane.

## Magnesium Aspartate Hydrobromide

Hidrobromuro de aspartato magnésico. Magnesium L-aspartate hydrobromide trihydrate.

### Profile

Magnesium aspartate hydrobromide has been used as a sedative but the use of bromides is generally deprecated.

### Preparations

**Proprietary Preparations** (details are given in Part 3)
***Ger.:*** Vernelan†.

## Medazepam *(BAN, rINN)*

7-Chloro-2,3-dihydro-1-methyl-5-phenyl-1*H*-1,4-benzodiazepine.

$C_{16}H_{15}ClN_2$ = 270.8.
*CAS — 2898-12-6.*
*ATC — N05BA03.*

**Pharmacopoeias.** In *Jpn.*

## Medazepam Hydrochloride *(USAN)*

Ro-5-4556.

$C_{16}H_{15}ClN_2,HCl$ = 307.2.
*CAS — 2898-11-5.*
*ATC — N05BA03.*

### Profile

Medazepam is a long-acting benzodiazepine with properties similar to those of diazepam (p.690). It has been given by mouth for the short-term treatment of anxiety disorders (p.663). A usual dose is 10 to 30 mg daily in divided doses; in severe conditions up to 60 mg daily has been given. Reduced doses should be given in elderly or debilitated patients.

### Preparations

**Proprietary Preparations** (details are given in Part 3)
***Ger.:*** Rudotel; Rusedal.

**Multi-ingredient:** ***Ital.:*** Debrum; ***Spain:*** Nobritol.

## Medetomidine Hydrochloride *(BANM, USAN, rINNM)*

Hidrocloruro de medetomidina; MPV-785. (±)-4-[1-(2,3-Xylyl)ethyl]imidazole monohydrochloride.

$C_{13}H_{16}N_2,HCl$ = 236.7.
*CAS — 86347-15-1 (medetomidine hydrochloride); 86347-14-0 (medetomidine).*

### Profile

Medetomidine is an $\alpha_2$-adrenoceptor agonist with sedative, muscle relaxant, and analgesic properties. It is used as the hydrochloride in veterinary medicine.

Dexmedetomidine (p.689) is used as the hydrochloride in intensive care.

## Melperone Hydrochloride *(BANM, rINNM)*

FG-5111; Flubuperone Hydrochloride; Hidrocloruro de melperona; Methylperone Hydrochloride. 4′-Fluoro-4-(4-methylpiperidino)butyrophenone hydrochloride.

$C_{16}H_{22}FNO,HCl$ = 299.8.
*CAS — 3575-80-2 (melperone); 1622-79-3 (melperone hydrochloride).*
*ATC — N05AD03.*

### Profile

Melperone is a butyrophenone with general properties similar to those of haloperidol (p.701). It is given as the hydrochloride by mouth or by intramuscular injection for the management of psychoses such as schizophrenia (p.665) and in disturbed behaviour (p.665); doses are expressed as the hydrochloride. A usual dose by mouth is up to 400 mg daily in divided doses. In acute conditions it may be given intramuscularly in doses of 25 to 100 mg repeated to a usual maximum of 200 mg daily.

**Cardiac arrhythmias.** Melperone has been reported to have class III electrophysiologic and antiarrhythmic activity[1,2] but its clinical use as an antiarrhythmic would be limited by a high incidence of adverse effects.[2] For a discussion of the cardiovascular effects of antipsychotics in general, see under Chlorpromazine, p.676.

1. Møgelvang JC, *et al.* Antiarrhythmic properties of a neuroleptic butyrophenone, melperone, in acute myocardial infarction. *Acta Med Scand* 1980; **208:** 61–4.
2. Hui WKK, *et al.* Melperone: electrophysiologic and antiarrhythmic activity in humans. *J Cardiovasc Pharmacol* 1990; **15:** 144–9.

**Pharmacokinetics.** References.

1. Köppel C, *et al.* Gas chromatographic-mass spectrometric study of urinary metabolism of melperone. *J Chromatogr Biomed Appl* 1988; **427:** 144–50.

### Preparations

**Proprietary Preparations** (details are given in Part 3)
***Austria:*** Buronil; Neuril; ***Belg.:*** Buronil; ***Denm.:*** Buronil; ***Fin.:*** Buronil; Melpax; ***Ger.:*** Eunerpan; Harmosin; Mel-Puren; Melneurin; Melperomerck; ***Norw.:*** Buronil†; ***Port.:*** Bunil; ***Swed.:*** Buronil.

## Meprobamate *(BAN, rINN)*

Meprobamato; Meprobamatum; Meprotanum. 2-Methyl-2-propyltrimethylene dicarbamate.

$C_9H_{18}N_2O_4$ = 218.3.
*CAS — 57-53-4.*
*ATC — N05BC01.*

**Pharmacopoeias.** In *Eur.* (see p.vi), *US,* and *Viet.*

**Ph. Eur. 5.0** (Meprobamate). A white or almost white, crystalline or amorphous powder. Slightly soluble in water; freely soluble in alcohol.

**USP 27** (Meprobamate). A white powder having a characteristic odour. Slightly soluble in water; freely soluble in alcohol and in acetone; practically insoluble or insoluble in ether. Store in airtight containers.

### Dependence and Withdrawal

As for the barbiturates (see Amobarbital, p.670).

### Adverse Effects and Treatment

Drowsiness is the most frequent side-effect of meprobamate. Other effects include nausea, vomiting, diarrhoea, paraesthesia, weakness, and CNS effects such as headache, paradoxical excitement, dizziness, ataxia, and disturbances of vision. There may be hypotension, tachycardia, and cardiac arrhythmias. Hypersensitivity reactions occur occasionally. These may be limited to skin rashes, urticaria, and purpura or may be more severe with angioedema, bronchospasm, or anuria. Erythema multiforme or Stevens-Johnson syndrome, and exfoliative or bullous dermatitis have been reported.

Blood disorders including agranulocytosis, eosinophilia, leucopenia, thrombocytopenia, and aplastic anaemia have occasionally been reported.

Overdosage with meprobamate produces symptoms similar to those of barbiturate overdosage (see Amobarbital, p.670), and is managed similarly.

**Overdosage.** Two children aged 2 and 2.5 years recovered with conservative management alone following overdosage of meprobamate with bendroflumethiazide despite measured plasma-meprobamate concentrations of 170 and 158 micrograms/mL, respectively.[1] Although it had been recommended that haemoperfusion should be considered at plasma-meprobamate concentrations above 100 micrograms/mL, the authors considered that experience with adults suggested haemoperfusion should normally only be considered at plasma concentrations above 200 micrograms/mL.

1. Dennison J, *et al.* Meprobamate overdosage. *Hum Toxicol* 1985; **4:** 215–17.

### Precautions

Meprobamate should be used with caution in patients with hepatic or renal impairment, depression, muscle weakness, and, as with all sedatives, in patients with impaired respiratory function. Meprobamate should be given with care to elderly or debilitated patients. Meprobamate may induce seizures in patients with a history of epilepsy.

Meprobamate may cause drowsiness; affected patients should not drive or operate machinery.

**Breast feeding.** The *British National Formulary* considers that the use of meprobamate should be avoided in breast feeding mothers as concentrations in milk may exceed maternal plasma concentrations fourfold and may cause drowsiness in the infant.

**Porphyria.** Meprobamate has been associated with acute attacks of porphyria and is considered unsafe in porphyric patients.

**Pregnancy.** Studies on the use of meprobamate during pregnancy.

1. Milkovich L, van den Berg BJ. Effects of prenatal meprobamate and chlordiazepoxide hydrochloride on human embryonic and fetal development. *N Engl J Med* 1974; **291:** 1268–71.
2. Crombie DL, *et al.* Fetal effects of tranquilizers in pregnancy. *N Engl J Med* 1975; **293:** 198–9.
3. Hartz SC, *et al.* Antenatal exposure to meprobamate and chlordiazepoxide in relation to malformations, mental development, and childhood mortality. *N Engl J Med* 1975; **292:** 726–8.

### Interactions

The sedative effects of meprobamate are enhanced by CNS depressants including alcohol. Meprobamate is capable of inducing hepatic microsomal enzyme systems involved in drug metabolism: the metabolism of other drugs may be enhanced if given concurrently.

### Pharmacokinetics

Meprobamate is readily absorbed from the gastrointestinal tract and peak plasma concentrations occur 1 to 3 hours after ingestion. Meprobamate is widely distributed. It is extensively metabolised in the liver and is excreted in the urine mainly as an inactive hydroxylated metabolite and its glucuronide conjugate. About 10% of a dose is excreted unchanged. Meprobamate has a half-life reported to range from about 6 to 17 hours, although this may be prolonged after chronic administration.

It diffuses across the placenta and appears in breast milk at concentrations of up to 4 times those in the maternal plasma.

### Uses and Administration

Meprobamate is a carbamate with hypnotic, sedative, and some muscle relaxant properties, although in therapeutic doses its sedative effect rather than a direct action may be responsible for muscle relaxation. It has been used in the short-term treatment of anxiety disorders (p.663) and also for the short-term management of insomnia (p.667) but has largely been superseded by other drugs. Meprobamate has sometimes been used, alone or in combination with an analgesic, in the management of muscle spasm (p.1386) and painful musculoskeletal disorders but such use is no longer considered appropriate.

The usual anxiolytic dose is 400 mg by mouth three or four times daily to a maximum of 2.4 g daily. In elderly patients, no more than half the usual adult dose has been suggested.

### Preparations

***USP 27:*** Meprobamate Oral Suspension; Meprobamate Tablets.

**Proprietary Preparations** (details are given in Part 3)
***Austral.:*** Equanil†; ***Austria:*** Cyrpon; Epikur; Microbamat; Miltaun; Pertranquil†; ***Belg.:*** Pertranquil; Reposo-Mono; Sanobamat†; ***Canad.:*** Equanil†; Novo-Mepro†; ***Fr.:*** Equanil; Norgagil†; Novalm†; ***Ger.:*** Visano N; Visano-mini N; ***Israel:*** Mepro; ***Ital.:*** Quanil; ***S.Afr.:*** Equanil; ***Spain:*** Dapaz†; Oasil Simes†; ***Swed.:*** Restenil†; ***Switz.:*** Meprodil; ***UK:*** Meprate†; ***USA:*** Equanil†; Miltown; Neuramate.

**Multi-ingredient:** ***Arg.:*** Hidromens; ***Belg.:*** Spasmosedine†; ***Canad.:*** 282 Mep; Equagesic†; ***Chile:*** Butartrol; ***Fin.:*** Anervan; Crampiton; Potentol; ***Fr.:*** Kaologeais; Mepronizine; Palpipax; Precyclan; ***Mex.:*** Artrilan; ***Norw.:*** Anervan; ***Port.:*** Vitasma; ***S.Afr.:*** Acugesil†; Adco-Payne; Antipyn Forte; Ban Pain; Briscopyn†; Dynapayne†; Equagesic†; Go-Pain; Maxadol Forte†; Megapyn; Meprogesic; Mepromol; Nopyn; Noralget; Painagon; Painrite†; Pynmed; Salterpyn; Spectrapain Forte; Stilpane; Stopayne; Supragesic; Synaleve; Tenston; Trinagesic; Vacudol Forte; Xeramax; Xerogesic; ***Swed.:*** Anervan; ***UK:*** Equagesic†; Paxidal; ***USA:*** Equagesic†; Micrainin.

## Mesoridazine *(BAN, USAN, rINN)*

Mesuridazine; NC-123; TPS-23. 10-[2-(1-Methyl-2-piperidyl)ethyl]-2-(methylsulphinyl)phenothiazine.

$C_{21}H_{26}N_2OS_2$ = 386.6.
*CAS — 5588-33-0.*
*ATC — N05AC03.*

## Mesoridazine Besilate *(BANM, rINNM)*

Bencenosulfonato de mesoridazina; Mesoridazine Benzenesulphonate; Mesoridazine Besylate; Mesoridazine Benzenesulphonate.

$C_{21}H_{26}N_2OS_2,C_6H_6O_3S$ = 544.7.
*CAS — 32672-69-8 (mesoridazine besilate).*
*ATC — N05AC03.*

**Pharmacopoeias.** In *US.*

**USP 27** (Mesoridazine Besylate). A white to pale yellowish powder having not more than a faint odour. Soluble 1 in 1 of water, 1 in 11 of alcohol, 1 in 3 of chloroform, and 1 in 6300 of ether; freely soluble in methyl alcohol. pH of a freshly prepared 1 in 100 solution is between 4.2 and 5.7. Store in airtight containers. Protect from light.

### Adverse Effects, Treatment, and Precautions

As for Chlorpromazine, p.675. Mesoridazine has been shown to prolong the QT interval in a dose-related manner which increases the risk of life-threatening arrhythmias such as torsade de pointes and sudden death; consequently its use has been restricted. Details of these restrictions are given under Precautions of Thioridazine, the parent drug of mesoridazine (see p.724).

For all patients starting mesoridazine it is recommended that a baseline ECG and potassium screening are performed. These tests should also be repeated periodically, especially during periods of dosage adjustment.

**Breast feeding.** The American Academy of Pediatrics[1] considers that, although the effect of mesoridazine on breast-feeding infants is unknown, its use by mothers during breast feeding may be of concern since antipsychotic drugs do appear in breast milk and thus could conceivably alter CNS function in the infant both in the short and long term.

1. American Academy of Pediatrics. The transfer of drugs and other chemicals into human milk. *Pediatrics* 2001; **108:** 776–89. Correction. *ibid.*; 1029. Also available at: http://aappolicy.aappublications.org/cgi/content/full/pediatrics%3b108/3/776 (accessed 28/04/04)

### Interactions

As for Chlorpromazine, p.679. Use of mesoridazine with other drugs known to prolong the QT interval is contra-indicated.

### Pharmacokinetics

Mesoridazine is a metabolite of thioridazine (p.724).

### Uses and Administration

Mesoridazine is a phenothiazine with general properties similar to those of chlorpromazine (p.680). It has a piperidine side-chain and is a metabolite of thioridazine (p.724).

The use of mesoridazine is restricted to the treatment of schizophrenia (p.665) in patients who fail to show an adequate response to treatment with other antipsychotics. Its use in other psychiatric disorders was abandoned after it was felt that there was an unacceptable balance of risks and benefits as a result of its cardiotoxic potential.

For all patients starting mesoridazine it is recommended that a baseline ECG and potassium screening are performed. These tests should also be repeated periodically, especially during periods of dosage adjustment.

Mesoridazine is usually given as the besilate but the doses are expressed in terms of the base mesoridazine besilate 35.2 mg is approximately equivalent to 25 mg mesoridazine. The usual initial dose for the treatment of schizophrenia is 50 mg three times daily by mouth; doses may be adjusted to 100 to 400 mg daily according to response. Mesoridazine may also be given intramuscularly in an initial dose of 25 mg repeated after 30 to 60 minutes if necessary; up to 200 mg daily has been given.

### Preparations

***USP 27:*** Mesoridazine Besylate Injection; Mesoridazine Besylate Oral Solution; Mesoridazine Besylate Tablets.

**Proprietary Preparations** (details are given in Part 3)
***Canad.:*** Serentil†; ***USA:*** Serentil.

## Methaqualone *(BAN, USAN, rINN)*

Cl-705; CN-38703; Metacualona; Methachalonum; Methaqualonum; QZ-2; R-148; TR-495. 2-Methyl-3-o-tolylquinazolin-4-(3*H*)-one.

$C_{16}H_{14}N_2O$ = 250.3.
*CAS — 72-44-6 (methaqualone); 340-56-7 (methaqualone hydrochloride).*
*ATC — N05CM01.*

**Pharmacopoeias.** In *Eur.* (see p.vi).

**Ph. Eur. 5.0** (Methaqualone). A white or almost white, crystalline powder. Very slightly soluble in water; soluble in alcohol; dissolves in dilute sulfuric acid. Protect from light.

### Profile

Methaqualone is a quinazoline derivative with hypnotic and sedative properties. It has been given by mouth in the short-term management of insomnia but the use of methaqualone for this purpose is no longer considered appropriate. It has also been given with diphenhydramine for an enhanced effect.

Methaqualone has been withdrawn from the market in many countries because of problems with abuse.

Adverse effects and symptoms of overdosage are similar to those of barbiturates (see Amobarbital, p.670) although cardiac and respiratory depression reportedly occur less frequently.

### Preparations

**Proprietary Preparations** (details are given in Part 3)
**Multi-ingredient: *Switz.:*** Toquilone compositum.

## Methylpentynol *(BAN, rINN)*

Meparfynol; Methylparafynol; Metilpentinol. 3-Methylpent-1-yn-3-ol.

$C_6H_{10}O$ = 98.14.
*CAS — 77-75-8.*
*ATC — N05CM15.*

### Profile

Methylpentynol is a hypnotic and sedative. It has been given as a hypnotic in the short-term management of insomnia.

## Mexazolam *(rINN)*

CS-386; Methylcloxazolam. 10-Chloro-11b-(2-chlorophenyl)-2,3,7,11b-tetrahydro-3-methyloxazolo[3,2-*d*][1,4]benzodiazepin-6(5*H*)-one.

$C_{18}H_{16}Cl_2N_2O_2$ = 363.2.
*CAS — 31868-18-5.*

### Profile

Mexazolam is a benzodiazepine with general properties similar to those of diazepam (p.690). It has been given by mouth for its anxiolytic and sedative properties.

### Preparations

**Proprietary Preparations** (details are given in Part 3)
***Port.:*** Sedoxil.

# Midazolam *(BAN, rINN)*

Midazolamum; Ro-21-3971. 8-Chloro-6-(2-fluorophenyl)-1-methyl-4*H*-imidazo[1,5-*a*][1,4]benzodiazepine.

$C_{18}H_{13}ClFN_3$ = 325.8.
*CAS — 59467-70-8.*
*ATC — N05CD08.*

**Pharmacopoeias.** In *Eur.* (see p.vi).

**Ph. Eur. 5.0** (Midazolam). A white or yellowish crystalline powder. Practically insoluble in water; freely soluble in alcohol and in acetone; soluble in methyl alcohol. Protect from light.

## Midazolam Hydrochloride *(BANM, USAN, rINNM)*

Hidrocloruro de midazolam; Ro-21-3981/003.

$C_{18}H_{13}ClFN_3,HCl$ = 362.2.
*CAS — 59467-96-8.*
*ATC — N05CD08.*

**Incompatibility.** The visual compatibility of midazolam hydrochloride with a range of drugs was studied over a period of 4 hours.[1] A white precipitate was formed immediately with dimenhydrinate, pentobarbital sodium, perphenazine, prochlorperazine edisilate, and ranitidine hydrochloride. Similar incompatibility has been reported[2,3] with furosemide, thiopental, and parenteral nutrition solutions. Other workers[4] have reported that a precipitate is formed with midazolam hydrochloride if the resultant mixture has a pH of 5 or more.

1. Forman JK, Souney PF. Visual compatibility of midazolam hydrochloride with common preoperative injectable medications. *Am J Hosp Pharm* 1987; **44:** 2298–9.
2. Chiu MF, Schwartz ML. Visual compatibility of injectable drugs used in the intensive care unit. *Am J Health-Syst Pharm* 1997; **54:** 64–5.
3. Trissel LA, *et al.* Compatibility of parenteral nutrient solutions with selected drugs during simulated Y-site administration. *Am J Health-Syst Pharm* 1997; **54:** 1295–300.
4. Swart EL, *et al.* Compatibility of midazolam hydrochloride and lorazepam with selected drugs during simulated Y-site administration. *Am J Health-Syst Pharm* 1995; **52:** 2020–2.

**Stability.** The manufacturers have stated that solutions of midazolam hydrochloride in sodium chloride 0.9%, glucose 5%, or glucose 4% with sodium chloride 0.18% are stable at room temperature for up to 24 hours, and similar solutions containing the equivalent of 0.5 mg/mL of the base were stable for 36 days[1] when stored in glass bottles at temperatures of 4° to 6°, 24° to 26°, and 39° to 41°. Other workers[2] found that a solution containing midazolam hydrochloride equivalent to 1 mg/mL of the base in sodium chloride 0.9% was stable for at least 10 days when stored in PVC bags. The manufacturer advises against admixture with Compound Sodium Lactate Intravenous Infusion (Hartmann's solution) as the potency of midazolam is reduced.

1. Pramar YV, *et al.* Stability of midazolam hydrochloride in syringes and i.v. fluids. *Am J Health-Syst Pharm* 1997; **54:** 913–15.
2. McMullin ST, *et al.* Stability of midazolam hydrochloride in polyvinyl chloride bags under fluorescent light. *Am J Health-Syst Pharm* 1995; **52:** 2018–20.

## Midazolam Maleate *(BANM, USAN, rINNM)*

Maleato de midazolam; Ro-21-3981/001.

$C_{18}H_{13}ClFN_3,C_4H_4O_4$ = 441.8.
*CAS — 59467-94-6.*
*ATC — N05CD08.*

## Dependence and Withdrawal

As for Diazepam, p.690.

◊ Withdrawal symptoms occurred[1] in 2 children following discontinuation of midazolam, which had been used for sedation during mechanical ventilation.

1. van Engelen BGM, *et al.* Benzodiazepine withdrawal reaction in two children following discontinuation of sedation with midazolam. *Ann Pharmacother* 1993; **27:** 579–81.

## Adverse Effects, Treatment, and Precautions

As for Diazepam, p.690. There have been reports of life-threatening adverse respiratory and cardiovascular events occurring after administration of midazolam; when giving midazolam the precautions given below should be observed to lessen the risk of such reactions. Pain, tenderness, and thrombophlebitis have occurred following injection of midazolam. Hiccups have been reported.

◊ Death due to respiratory depression, hypotension, or cardiac arrest has been reported in patients given intravenous midazolam for conscious sedation.[1] Within about 6 months of its introduction in the USA in May 1986, 13 fatalities due to cardiorespiratory depression had been reported (higher doses were used initially in the USA than those in the UK). By January 1988, 66 deaths had been reported, although in November 1987 the adult dosage recommendation had been reduced to 70 micrograms/kg and to 50 micrograms/kg for elderly patients. Fatalities have also occurred in the UK [where the dose is 70 micrograms/kg, reduced in the elderly] with 4 deaths reported to the UK Committee on Safety of Medicines by November 1987.

While it appears that midazolam and diazepam produce very similar degrees of hypoventilation and oxygen desaturation when used in equivalent doses,[2] the sedative end-point does appear to be reached more abruptly with midazolam.[3] Appropriate precautions should therefore be taken:

- facilities for resuscitation should always be available when intravenous midazolam is used
- respiratory and cardiac function should be monitored continuously
- the dose of midazolam should be carefully titrated against the response of the patient and the manufacturer's recommendations concerning speed of administration be observed
- particular care, including a reduction in midazolam dosage, is required in patients also receiving opioid analgesics, in the elderly and children, and in patients with compromised cardiorespiratory function
- similar warnings apply to the use of oral midazolam where it is available.

The availability of the benzodiazepine antagonist, flumazenil, should not be an encouragement to use larger doses of midazolam.[1]

Since endoscopy of the upper gastrointestinal tract can itself reduce oxygen saturation, some workers have advocated the prophylactic administration of nasal oxygen during this procedure for those patients at particular risk as outlined above.

1. Anonymous. Midazolam—is antagonism justified? *Lancet* 1988; **ii:** 140–2.
2. Bell GD. Review article: premedication and intravenous sedation for upper gastrointestinal endoscopy. *Aliment Pharmacol Ther* 1990; **4:** 103–22.
3. Ryder W, Wright PA. Dental sedation: a review. *Br Dent J* 1988; **165:** 207–16.

**Breast feeding.** The American Academy of Pediatrics[1] considers that, although the effect of midazolam on breast-feeding infants is unknown its use by mothers during breast feeding may be of concern since psychotropic drugs do appear in breast milk and thus could conceivably alter CNS function in the infant both in the short and long term.

Midazolam could not be detected in breast milk from 11 mothers the morning after either the first or the fifth nightly 15-mg dose by mouth.[2] Additional study of 2 mothers found that midazolam and its hydroxy-metabolite disappeared rapidly from milk with undetectable concentrations at 4 hours. The mean milk to plasma ratio for midazolam was 0.15 in 6 paired samples.

1. American Academy of Pediatrics. The transfer of drugs and other chemicals into human milk. *Pediatrics* 2001; **108:** 776–89. Correction. *ibid.*; 1029. Also available at: http://aappolicy.aappublications.org/cgi/content/full/pediatrics%3b108/3/776 (accessed 28/04/04)
2. Matheson I, *et al.* Midazolam and nitrazepam in the maternity ward: milk concentrations and clinical effects. *Br J Clin Pharmacol* 1990; **30:** 787–93.

**Children.** An intravenous bolus injection of midazolam in children already receiving intravenous morphine after cardiac surgery produced an undesirable transient fall in cardiac output.[1] It was suggested that for patients already receiving other drugs which provide sedation the use of midazolam in the early postoperative period should be limited to a continuous infusion. Similarly, it has been recommended[2] that bolus intravenous administration of midazolam should be avoided in neonates due to the occurrence of hypotension.

The initial dosage of midazolam used for continuous intravenous sedation may need to be reduced in critically ill children under 3 years of age since the plasma clearance of midazolam appears to be reduced in these patients.[3]

1. Shekerdemian L, *et al.* Cardiovascular effects of intravenous midazolam after open heart surgery. *Arch Dis Child* 1997; **76:** 57–61.
2. Jacqz-Aigrain E, Burtin P. Clinical pharmacokinetics of sedatives in neonates. *Clin Pharmacokinet* 1996; **31:** 423–43.
3. Hughes J, *et al.* Steady-state plasma concentrations of midazolam in critically ill infants and children. *Ann Pharmacother* 1996; **30:** 27–30.

**Effects on mental function.** For discussion of the adverse effects of benzodiazepines on mental function, including reports of sexual fantasies in women sedated with intravenous midazolam, see Diazepam, p.691.

**Effects on the nervous system.** For reference to acute dystonia associated with administration of midazolam, see Diazepam, p.691.

ENCEPHALOPATHY. For a report of prolonged use of midazolam with fentanyl being associated with encephalopathy in infants sedated under intensive care, see Diazepam, p.691.

MYOCLONUS. Myoclonic twitching of all four limbs was noted[1] in 6 of 102 neonates who received a continuous intravenous infusion of midazolam at a rate of 30 to 60 micrograms/kg per hour. Myoclonus ceased a few hours after discontinuing the infusion and never recurred. No ictal activity was detected in EEGs recorded during the myoclonus.

1. Magny JF, *et al.* Midazolam and myoclonus in neonate. *Eur J Pediatr* 1994; **153:** 389–90.

**The elderly.** Sedation with midazolam in elderly subjects needed only about half the dose necessary to produce comparable effects in younger subjects.[1] Pharmacodynamic differences due to age suggested an increase in sensitivity of the CNS to midazolam in the elderly subjects.

1. Albrecht S, *et al.* The effect of age on the pharmacokinetics and pharmacodynamics of midazolam. *Clin Pharmacol Ther* 1999; **65:** 630–9.

**Hepatic impairment.** For the precautions to be observed in patients with impaired liver function, see under Pharmacokinetics, below.

**Renal impairment.** Five patients with severe renal impairment experienced prolonged sedation when given midazolam; this was attributed to accumulation of conjugated metabolites.[1]

1. Bauer TM, *et al.* Prolonged sedation due to accumulation of conjugated metabolites of midazolam. *Lancet* 1995; **346:** 145–7.

### Interactions

As for Diazepam, p.692.

### Pharmacokinetics

Absorption of midazolam is rapid, peak plasma concentrations being achieved within 20 to 60 minutes of administration depending on the route. Extensive first-pass metabolism results in a low systemic bioavailability after oral administration. Bioavailability is higher, but variable, after intramuscular injection; figures of more than 90% are often cited.

Midazolam is lipophilic at physiological pH. It crosses the placenta and is distributed into breast milk (but see above). Midazolam is about 96% bound to plasma proteins.

Midazolam usually has a short elimination half-life of about 2 hours although half-lives longer than 7 hours have been reported in some patients. The half-life of midazolam is also prolonged in neonates, in the elderly, and in patients with liver disorders.

Midazolam is metabolised in the liver via the cytochrome P450 isoenzyme CYP3A4. The major metabolite, 1-hydroxymidazolam (alpha-hydroxymidazolam) has some activity; its half-life is less than 1 hour. Midazolam metabolites are excreted in the urine, mainly as glucuronide conjugates.

◊ Reviews.

1. Garzone PD, Kroboth PD. Pharmacokinetics of the newer benzodiazepines. *Clin Pharmacokinet* 1989; **16:** 337–64.

**Children.** In a study[1] of the pharmacokinetics of midazolam in children the bioavailability of a dose of 0.15 mg/kg was 100, 87, 27, and 18% after administration by the intravenous, intramuscular, oral, and rectal routes, respectively. The oral bioavailability was reduced to 16 and 15% after increasing the dose to 0.45 and 1 mg/kg, respectively. There was bioequivalence between the 0.15 mg/kg intramuscular dose and the 0.45 mg/kg oral dose from 45 to 120 minutes after administration. Absorption from the rectal route gave lower serum-midazolam concentrations than the oral route at the 0.15 mg/kg dose.

Midazolam appears to be absorbed rapidly when given by the intranasal route to children with mean maximum plasma concentrations being achieved within about 12 minutes;[2-4] values of 30% and 55% have been reported for the bioavailability[3,4] but methods to optimise nasal delivery have resulted in higher bioavailability in studies in adults (see below). A study comparing intranasal, intravenous, and rectal administration of midazolam to children found that plasma concentrations from 45 minutes after intranasal and intravenous administration were similar; those following rectal administration were consistently less than after these other 2 routes.[2] Possible reasons suggested by the authors for this included the effect that the wide interindividual variations in rectal pH may have had on the absorption of midazolam.

Another study has investigated the relationship between intravenous dose and plasma-midazolam concentrations in children.[5]

See also Children under Precautions, above.

1. Payne K, *et al.* The pharmacokinetics of midazolam in paediatric patients. *Eur J Clin Pharmacol* 1989; **37:** 267–72.
2. Malinovsky J-M, *et al.* Plasma concentrations of midazolam after iv, nasal or rectal administration in children. *Br J Anaesth* 1993; **70:** 617–20.
3. Rey E, *et al.* Pharmacokinetics of midazolam in children: comparative study of intranasal and intravenous administration. *Eur J Clin Pharmacol* 1991; **41:** 355–7.
4. Kauffman RE, *et al.* Intranasal absorption of midazolam. *Clin Pharmacol Ther* 1995; **57:** 209.
5. Tolia V, *et al.* Pharmacokinetic and pharmacodynamic study of midazolam in children during esophagogastroduodenoscopy. *J Pediatr* 1991; **119:** 467–71.

NEONATES. References to the pharmacokinetics of midazolam in neonates. See also Children under Precautions, above.

1. Jacqz-Aigrain E, *et al.* Pharmacokinetics of midazolam in critically ill neonates. *Eur J Clin Pharmacol* 1990; **39:** 191–2.
2. Jacqz-Aigrain E, *et al.* Pharmacokinetics of midazolam during continuous infusion in critically ill neonates. *Eur J Clin Pharmacol* 1992; **42:** 329–32.
3. Burtin P, *et al.* Population pharmacokinetics of midazolam in neonates. *Clin Pharmacol Ther* 1994; **56:** 615–25.
4. Jacqz-Aigrain E, Burtin P. Clinical pharmacokinetics of sedatives in neonates. *Clin Pharmacokinet* 1996; **31:** 423–43.
5. Harte GJ, *et al.* Haemodynamic responses and population pharmacokinetics of midazolam following administration to ventilated, preterm neonates. *J Paediatr Child Health* 1997 **33:** 335–8.
6. Lee TC, *et al.* Population pharmacokinetic modeling in very premature infants receiving midazolam during mechanical ventilation: midazolam neonatal pharmacokinetics. *Anesthesiology* 1999; **90:** 451–7.
7. de Wildt SN, *et al.* Pharmacokinetics and metabolism of intravenous midazolam in preterm infants. *Clin Pharmacol Ther* 2001; **70:** 525–31.

**Half-life.** Data collected from 7 studies involving 90 subjects has suggested that the prolonged midazolam half-lives reported in a small number of patients are secondary to increases in the volume of distribution and not a result of alterations in clearance and metabolism.[1] Prolongation of the half-life of midazolam has been reported[2] in 2 patients following sustained infusion for status epilepticus.

1. Wills RJ, *et al.* Increased volume of distribution prolongs midazolam half-life. *Br J Clin Pharmacol* 1990; **29:** 269–72.
2. Naritoku DK, Sinha S. Prolongation of midazolam half-life after sustained infusion for status epilepticus. *Neurology* 2000 **54:** 1366–8.

**Intranasal administration.** Plasma concentrations of midazolam sufficient to induce conscious sedation are rapidly attained following intranasal administration.[1] Although bioavailability of up to 55% had previously been obtained in children following intranasal administration (see above), slow administration and other methods to optimise nasal delivery had resulted in a bioavailability of 83% in adults.[2,3] Similar techniques should be developed for use in children.

1. Burstein AH, *et al.* Pharmacokinetics and pharmacodynamics of midazolam after intranasal administration. *J Clin Pharmacol* 1997; **37:** 711–18.
2. Björkman S, *et al.* Pharmacokinetics of midazolam given as an intranasal spray to adult surgical patients. *Br J Anaesth* 1997; **79:** 575–80.
3. Knoester PD, *et al.* Pharmacokinetics and pharmacodynamics of midazolam administered as a concentrated intranasal spray: a study in healthy volunteers. *Br J Clin Pharmacol* 2002; **53:** 501–7.

**Liver disorders.** The pharmacokinetics of midazolam in patients with advanced cirrhosis of the liver were characterised by an increase in oral systemic bioavailability[1] and by a decrease in clearance with consequent prolongation of elimination half-life.[1,2] Dosage may need to be reduced. Metabolism of midazolam has been demonstrated, however, in the anhepatic period of liver transplantation indicating extrahepatic metabolism (see below).

1. Pentikäinen PJ, *et al.* Pharmacokinetics of midazolam following intravenous and oral administration in patients with chronic liver disease and in healthy subjects. *J Clin Pharmacol* 1989; **29:** 272–7.
2. MacGilchrist AJ, *et al.* Pharmacokinetics and pharmacodynamics of intravenous midazolam in patients with severe alcoholic cirrhosis. *Gut* 1986; **27:** 190–5.

**Metabolism.** For a discussion of the metabolism of benzodiazepines, see Diazepam, p.695. Midazolam appears to be metabolised by at least 3 different cytochrome P450 isoenzymes which are found in the liver and in the kidney.[1] Variations in the activity of these enzymes might account for some of the interindividual differences in pharmacokinetics and pharmacodynamics seen with midazolam.[2] However, a study[3] in patients undergoing liver transplantation has indicated that the small intestine is a significant site for the first-pass metabolism of midazolam, metabolism presumably being catalysed by the cytochrome P450 isoenzyme CYP3A4 found in intestinal mucosa.

1. Wandel C, *et al.* Midazolam is metabolized by at least three different cytochrome P450 enzymes. *Br J Anaesth* 1994; **73:** 658–61.
2. Lown KS, *et al.* The erythromycin breath test predicts the clearance of midazolam. *Clin Pharmacol Ther* 1995; **57:** 16–24.
3. Paine MF, *et al.* First-pass metabolism of midazolam by the human intestine. *Clin Pharmacol Ther* 1996; **60:** 14–24.

**Sublingual administration.** High bioavailability (about 75%) and reliable plasma concentrations have been achieved following sublingual administration of midazolam.[1]

1. Schwagmeier R, *et al.* Midazolam pharmacokinetics following intravenous and buccal administration. *Br J Clin Pharmacol* 1998; **46:** 203–6.

### Uses and Administration

Midazolam is a short-acting benzodiazepine with general properties similar to those of diazepam (p.695), except that it has a more potent amnestic action. It is mainly used for sedation in minor surgical or investigative procedures, for premedication, and for induction of general anaesthesia. When midazolam is used as a premedicant or for conscious sedation, onset of sedation occurs at about 15 minutes after intramuscular injection reaching a peak at 30 to 60 minutes, and within about 3 to 5 minutes after intravenous injection. When given intravenously as an anaesthetic induction agent, anaesthesia is induced in about 2 to 2.5 minutes; onset of action is more rapid when premedication with an opioid analgesic has been given.

Since the sedative end-point is reached abruptly with midazolam, dosage must be titrated carefully against the response of the patient; lower doses of midazolam are required when it is used in conjunction with opioid analgesics. Respiratory and cardiac function should be monitored continuously, and facilities for resuscitation should always be available. It is advisable to keep the patient supine during intravenous administration and throughout the procedure. The doses given below are, except where specified, the usual adult doses: midazolam should be given in reduced doses to **elderly** or **debilitated patients**.

Midazolam is used as the hydrochloride for oral, parenteral, and rectal administration; the maleate may also be given orally. All doses are given in terms of the base; midazolam hydrochloride 8.3 mg or midazolam maleate 10.2 mg are both approximately equivalent to 7.5 mg midazolam base.

A usual total **sedative** dose for dental and minor surgical and other procedures ranges from 2.5 to 7.5 mg (about 70 micrograms/kg) *intravenously*; an initial dose of 2 mg over 30 seconds has been suggested, with further incremental doses of 0.5 to 1 mg at intervals of 2 minutes if required until the desired end-point is reached. In the USA a suggested initial dose of up to 2.5 mg is given intravenously over at least 2 minutes and repeated if necessary after an additional 2 minutes or more to a usual maximum total dose of 5 mg.

Sedation in children aged 6 months and over may be achieved by mouth. A single *oral* dose of 250 to 500 micrograms/kg, up to a maximum of 20 mg, is recommended although younger patients (6 months to less than 6 years) may require up to 1 mg/kg. If the *intravenous* route is more suitable, doses of 50 to 100 micrograms/kg up to a total dose of 600 micrograms/kg (but not exceeding 6 mg) are recommended in children aged 6 months to 5 years; children aged 6 to 12 years may be given 25 to 50 micrograms/kg up to a total dose of 400 micrograms/kg (or a maximum of 10 mg). Initial doses should be given over 2 to 3 minutes and an additional interval of at least 2 minutes is recommended before giving further doses. *Rectal* midazolam is also used in some countries for sedation in children over 6 months of age; doses range from 300 to 500 micrograms/kg as a single dose. The *intramuscular* route should only be used in children in exceptional cases as such injections are painful; usual doses ranging from 50 to 150 micrograms/kg have been suggested for intramuscular use in children aged 1 to 15 years.

Patients in **intensive care** who require continuous sedation (p.666) can be given midazolam by *intravenous infusion*. An initial loading dose of 30 to 300 micrograms/kg may be given by intravenous infusion over 5 minutes to induce sedation; in the USA a lower dose of 10 to 50 micrograms/kg is recommended. The maintenance dose required varies considerably but a dose of between 20 and 200 micrograms/kg per hour has been suggested. The loading dose should be reduced or omitted, and the maintenance dose reduced, for patients with hypovolaemia, vasoconstriction, or hypothermia. The need for continuous administration should be reassessed on a daily basis to reduce the risk of accumulation and prolonged recovery. Sedation can also be achieved by giving intermittent *intravenous bolus injections* of midazolam; doses of 1 to 2 mg may be given, and repeated, until the desired level of sedation has been reached. Midazolam is also used in children in intensive care who require sedation. In those over 6 months, an initial loading dose of 50 to 200 micrograms/kg is given by *slow intravenous injection*; maintenance doses are given as an intravenous infusion and range from 60 to 120 micrograms/kg per hour. Neonates with a gestational age of greater than 32 weeks and infants up to 6 months may be given midazolam by intravenous infusion in a dose of 60 micrograms/kg per hour; neonates with a gestational age of less than 32 weeks should be started on 30 micrograms/kg per hour. Loading doses are not recommended in infants under 6 months.

Abrupt withdrawal should be avoided after prolonged administration.

Midazolam is given *intramuscularly* as a **premedicant** about 20 to 60 minutes before surgery. The usual dose is about 5 mg; doses range from 70 to 100 micrograms/kg. Children aged 6 months and over may be premedicated with *oral* midazolam in similar doses to those used for sedation (see above). The *rectal* route is used for premedication in some countries; total doses recommended in the UK in children over 6 months range from 300 to 500 micrograms/kg. The *intramuscular* route is also authorised in children aged 1 to 15 years in doses of 80 to 200 micrograms/kg; however, as before, this route should only be used in exceptional circumstances.

The usual dose of midazolam for **induction of anaesthesia** (p.1296) is about 150 to 200 micrograms/kg by slow *intravenous injection* in premedicated patients and at least 300 micrograms/kg in those who have not received a premedicant. Additional doses may be needed to complete induction; up to 600 micrograms/kg has been used in resistant cases. Further incremental doses of midazolam of about 25% of the induction dose have also been given as a component of the regimens used for the maintenance of anaesthesia during short surgical procedures. A dose of 150 micrograms/kg has been recommended for the induction of anaesthesia in children over 7 years of age.

Midazolam is also given for sedation in **combined anaesthesia** by *intravenous injection* in a dose of 30 to 100 micrograms/kg repeated as required or by *intravenous infusion* in a dose of 30 to 100 micrograms/kg every hour.

Midazolam maleate is also given *by mouth* for the short-term management of **insomnia**; the usual dose is the equivalent of midazolam 7.5 to 15 mg at night.

◊ References.


1. Blumer JL. Clinical pharmacology of midazolam in infants and children. *Clin Pharmacokinet* 1998; **35:** 37–47.
2. Marshall J, *et al.* Pediatric pharmacodynamics of midazolam oral syrup. *J Clin Pharmacol* 2000; **40:** 578–89.


**Administration.** The rectal,[1] intranasal,[1-5] and sublingual[1,6] routes have all been proposed as alternatives to parenteral administration of midazolam.

Intranasal midazolam has caused intense burning, irritation, and lachrymation on instillation, and use of a lidocaine nasal spray has been advocated before administering midazolam to children.[7] The use of midazolam spray intranasally in adults would be impractical and uncomfortable because of the large volume required. It has therefore been tried as a nebulised solution.[8]


1. Wong L, McQueen KD. Midazolam routes of administration. *DICP Ann Pharmacother* 1991; **25:** 476–7.
2. Theroux MC, *et al.* Efficacy of intranasal midazolam in facilitating suturing of lacerations in preschool children in the emergency department. *Pediatrics* 1993; **91:** 624–7.
3. Louon A, *et al.* Sedation with nasal ketamine and midazolam for cryotherapy in retinopathy of prematurity. *Br J Ophthalmol* 1993; **77:** 529–30.
4. Bates BA, *et al.* A comparison of intranasal sufentanil and midazolam to intramuscular meperidine, promethazine, and chlorpromazine for conscious sedation in children. *Ann Emerg Med* 1994; **24:** 646–51.
5. Ljungman G, *et al.* Midazolam nasal spray reduces procedural anxiety in children. *Pediatrics* 2000; **105:** 73–8.
6. Karl HW, *et al.* Transmucosal administration of midazolam for premedication of pediatric patients: comparison of the nasal and sublingual routes. *Anesthesiology* 1993; **78:** 885–91.
7. Lugo RA, *et al.* Complication of intranasal midazolam. *Pediatrics* 1993; **92:** 638.
8. Hodgson PE, *et al.* Administration of nebulized intranasal midazolam to healthy adult volunteers: a pilot study. *Br J Anaesth* 1994; **73:** 719P.


INTRATHECAL. See Pain, below.

**Conversion and dissociative disorders.** For reference to the use of midazolam in the diagnosis of conversion disorders, such as hysterical paralysis, see p.696.

**Convulsions.** Benzodiazepines such as diazepam or lorazepam given parenterally are often tried first to control status epilepticus (p.352). Midazolam has been used as an alternative.[1] It may be of value when intravenous access is difficult as effective concentrations of midazolam can be obtained after intramuscular injection.[2,3] The *British National Formulary* considers it to be the benzodiazepine of choice when a continuous subcutaneous infusion is required for the control of convulsions, such as in palliative care, and states that it may be given in an initial dose of 20 to 40 mg every 24 hours. Intravenous midazolam has been used in some centres[4] for status epilepticus refractory to diazepam, lorazepam, or phenytoin but reviews of the literature[5] reveal that evidence of efficacy is limited mainly to uncontrolled studies and anecdotal reports. The intranasal[6,7] and buccal[8] routes have also been used for the management of seizures. The *British National Formulary* states that a single dose of midazolam may be given by theses routes and recommends a dose of 10 mg for the buccal route and a dose of 200 micrograms/kg when given intranasally.


1. Hanley DF, *et al.* Use of midazolam in the treatment of refractory status epilepticus. *Clin Ther* 1998; **20:** 1093–1105.
2. Bauer J, Elger CE. Management of status epilepticus in adults. *CNS Drugs* 1994; **1:** 26–44.
3. Towne AR, DeLorenzo RJ. Use of intramuscular midazolam for status epilepticus. *J Emerg Med* 1999; **17:** 323–8.
4. Bebin M, Bleck TP. New anticonvulsant drugs: focus on flunarizine, fosphenytoin, midazolam and stiripentol. *Drugs* 1994; **48:** 153–71.
5. Denzel D, Burstein AH. Midazolam in refractory status epilepticus. *Ann Pharmacother* 1996; **30:** 1481–3.
6. Wallace SJ. Nasal benzodiazepines for management of acute childhood seizures? *Lancet* 1997; **349:** 222.
7. Lahat E, *et al.* Intranasal midazolam for childhood seizures. *Lancet* 1998; **352:** 620.
8. Scott RC, *et al.* Buccal midazolam and rectal diazepam for treatment of prolonged seizures in childhood and adolescence: a randomised trial. *Lancet* 1999; **353:** 623–6.


**Disturbed behaviour.** For a discussion of the palliative treatment of terminal restlessness with benzodiazepines such as midazolam, see p.665.

**Dyspnoea.** Midazolam has been suggested[1] as an alternative to chlorpromazine in patients with advanced cancer and intractable dyspnoea (p.74) to relieve air hunger and to sedate dying patients who have unrelieved distress. Suggested[2] initial doses are 2.5 to 5 mg subcutaneously or 10 mg administered by infusion over a period of 24 hours, increased as necessary.


1. Walsh D. Dyspnoea in advanced cancer. *Lancet* 1993; **342:** 450–1.
2. Davis CL. ABC of palliative care: breathlessness, cough, and other respiratory problems. *BMJ* 1997; **315:** 931–4.


**Hiccup.** A protocol for the management of intractable hiccups may be found under Chlorpromazine, p.682. Midazolam given intravenously or subcutaneously has been reported[1] to have been effective in 2 patients with metastatic cancer who had hiccups unresponsive to conventional treatment. However, it has been noted[1,2] that benzodiazepines such as midazolam may exacerbate or precipitate hiccups.


1. Wilcock A, Twycross R. Midazolam for intractable hiccup. *J Pain Symptom Manage* 1996; **12:** 59–61.
2. Rousseau P. Hiccups. *South Med J* 1995; **88:** 175–81.


**Insomnia.** For discussion of the management of insomnia including limitations on the use of benzodiazepines and a recommendation that the period of treatment with midazolam should be limited to 2 weeks, see p.667.

References.


1. Monti JM, *et al.* The effect of midazolam on transient insomnia. *Eur J Clin Pharmacol* 1993; **44:** 525–7.


**Pain.** The conventional use of benzodiazepines in pain management is as muscle relaxants to relieve pain associated with skeletal muscle spasm (see under Choice of Analgesic, p.2). Midazolam has been studied[1-5] for use as an intrathecal analgesic but efficacy has been inconsistent.


1. Cripps TP, Goodchild CS. Intrathecal midazolam and the stress response to upper abdominal surgery. *Clin J Pain* 1988; **4:** 125–8.
2. Serrao JM, *et al.* Intrathecal midazolam for the treatment of chronic mechanical low back pain: a controlled comparison with epidural steroid in a pilot study. *Pain* 1992; **48:** 5–12.
3. Baaijens PFJ, *et al.* Intrathecal midazolam for the treatment of chronic mechanical low back pain: a randomized double-blind placebo-controlled study. *Br J Anaesth* 1995; **74** (suppl 1): 143.
4. Valentine JMJ, *et al.* The effect of intrathecal midazolam on post-operative pain. *Eur J Anaesthesiol* 1996; **13:** 589–93.
5. Batra YK, *et al.* Addition of intrathecal midazolam to bupivacaine produces better post-operative analgesia without prolonging recovery. *Int J Clin Pharmacol Ther* 1999; **37:** 519–23.


**Premedication and sedation.** Midazolam is used as a premedicant (p.1296) and as a sedative for therapeutic and investigative procedures such as dental treatment (p.666) and endoscopy (see below). It is also used to provide continuous sedation in patients in intensive care (p.666) although a systematic review has raised concerns about such use in neonates.

References.


1. Sandler ES, *et al.* Midazolam versus fentanyl as premedication for painful procedures in children with cancer. *Pediatrics* 1992; **89:** 631–4.
2. Stenhammar L, *et al.* Intravenous midazolam in small bowel biopsy. *Arch Dis Child* 1994; **71:** 558.
3. Jacqz-Aigrain E, *et al.* Placebo-controlled trial of midazolam sedation in mechanically ventilated newborn babies. *Lancet* 1994; **344:** 646–50.
4. Mitchell V, *et al.* Comparison of midazolam with trimeprazine as an oral premedicant for paediatric anaesthesia. *Br J Anaesth* 1995; **74** (suppl 1): 94–5.
5. McCarver-May DG, *et al.* Comparison of chloral hydrate and midazolam for sedation of neonates for neuroimaging studies. *J Pediatr* 1996; **128:** 573–6.
6. Zedie N, *et al.* Comparison of intranasal midazolam and sufentanil premedication in pediatric outpatients. *Clin Pharmacol Ther* 1996; **59:** 341–8.
7. McErlean M, *et al.* Midazolam syrup as a premedication to reduce the discomfort associated with pediatric intravenous catheter insertion. *J Pediatr* 2003; **142:** 429–30.
8. TREC Collaborative Group. Rapid tranquillisation for agitated patients in emergency psychiatric rooms: a randomised trial of midazolam versus haloperidol plus promethazine. *BMJ* 2003; **327:** 708–11.
9. Ng E, *et al.* Intravenous midazolam infusion for sedation of infants in the neonatal intensive care unit. Available in The Cochrane Library; Issue 2. Chichester: John Wiley; 2004.


ENDOSCOPY. Intravenous benzodiazepines such as diazepam or midazolam are often the preferred drugs for sedation in patients undergoing endoscopy (p.666). They are sometimes used with opioid analgesics for sedation.[1]

A reduced dose of midazolam was required for endoscopy when it was given as a bolus intravenous injection rather than as a slow intravenous titration. A study in 788 patients undergoing endoscopy found that a mean dose of 4.65 mg of midazolam given as a bolus intravenous injection was safe and effective in patients under 70 years of age whereas a mean dose of 1.89 mg was sufficient for patients over 70 years of age.[2] Furthermore, topical pharyngeal anaesthesia was not required with these doses of midazolam. Intravenous bolus administration is also easier to administer and associated with less oxygen desaturation than titrating the dose.[3] Another study found that even lower doses of midazolam (35 micrograms/kg) were effective as premedication before gastroscopy, and were associated with fewer complications than higher doses (70 micrograms/kg).[4]

Intranasal[5] and oral[6] midazolam have also been tried for sedation before endoscopy, particularly in children.


1. Bahal-O'Mara N, *et al.* Sedation with meperidine and midazolam in pediatric patients undergoing endoscopy. *Eur J Clin Pharmacol* 1994; **47:** 319–23.
2. Smith MR, *et al.* Small bolus injections of intravenous midazolam for upper gastrointestinal endoscopy: a study of 788 consecutive cases. *Br J Clin Pharmacol* 1993; **36:** 573–8.
3. Morrow JB, *et al.* Sedation for colonoscopy using a single bolus is safe, effective, and efficient: a prospective, randomized, double-blind trial. *Am J Gastroenterol* 2000; **95:** 2242–7.
4. Campo R, *et al.* Efficacy of low and standard midazolam doses for gastroscopy: a randomized, double-blind study. *Eur J Gastroenterol Hepatol* 2000; **12:** 187–90.
5. Fishbein M, *et al.* Evaluation of intranasal midazolam in children undergoing esophagogastroduodenoscopy. *J Pediatr Gastroenterol Nutr* 1997; **25:** 261–6.
6. Martinez JL, *et al.* A comparison of oral diazepam versus midazolam, administered with intravenous meperidine, as premedication to sedation for pediatric endoscopy. *J Pediatr Gastroenterol Nutr* 2002; **35:** 51–8.


## Preparations

**BP 2003:** Midazolam Injection.

**Proprietary Preparations** (details are given in Part 3)

***Arg.:*** Dalam; Dormicum; Dormid; Drimnorth; Gobbizolam; Ormir; Rem; ***Austral.:*** Hypnovel; ***Austria:*** Dormicum; ***Belg.:*** Dormicum; ***Braz.:*** Dormire; Dormium; Dormonid; Zolidan; ***Canad.:*** Versed; ***Chile:*** Dormonid; Noctura; ***Denm.:*** Dormicum; ***Fin.:*** Dormicum; ***Fr.:*** Hypnovel; Versed; ***Ger.:*** Dormicum; Midaselect; ***Gr.:*** Dormicum; ***Hong Kong:*** Dormicum; ***India:*** Fulsed; ***Irl.:*** Hypnovel; ***Israel:*** Dormicum; Midazol; Midolam; ***Ital.:*** Ipnovel; ***Malaysia:*** Fulsed; ***Mex.:*** Dormicum; ***Neth.:*** Dormicum; ***Norw.:*** Dormicum; ***NZ:*** Hypnovel; ***Port.:*** Dormicum; Zolamid; ***S.Afr.:*** Dormicum; ***Singapore:*** Dormicum; Fulsed; ***Spain:*** Dormicum; ***Swed.:*** Dormicum; ***Switz.:*** Dormicum; ***Thai.:*** Dormicum; Midazol; ***UK:*** Hypnovel; ***USA:*** Versed.

---

## Molindone Hydrochloride *(BANM, USAN, rINNM)*

EN-1733A; Hidrocloruro de molindona. 3-Ethyl-1,5,6,7-tetrahydro-2-methyl-5-(morpholinomethyl)indol-4-one hydrochloride.

$C_{16}H_{24}N_2O_2,HCl = 312.8.$

*CAS — 7416-34-4 (molindone); 15622-65-8 (molindone hydrochloride).*

*ATC — N05AE02.*

**Pharmacopoeias.** In *US.*

**USP 27** (Molindone Hydrochloride). pH of a 1% solution in water is between 4.0 and 5.0. Store in airtight containers. Protect from light.

### Adverse Effects, Treatment, and Precautions

As for Chlorpromazine, p.675. Molindone hydrochloride is less likely to cause hypotension than chlorpromazine and extrapyramidal effects may be frequent but less severe. The incidence of sedation is intermediate between that of chlorpromazine and of phenothiazines with a piperazine side-chain. Weight gain or loss may occur, but weight loss appears to be more prominent (see p.676).

**Convulsions.** For mention of molindone as one of the antipsychotics suitable for patients at risk of seizures, see p.675.

**Effects on the liver.** A report of hepatotoxicity, associated with a flu-like syndrome, in a patient given molindone.[1] Symptoms and liver-enzyme values returned to normal on discontinuation of the drug and recurred on rechallenge with low doses. The effect was probably due to a hypersensitivity reaction.


1. Bhatia SC, *et al.* Molindone and hepatotoxicity. *Drug Intell Clin Pharm* 1985; **19:** 744–6.


### Interactions

As for Chlorpromazine, p.679.

### Pharmacokinetics

Molindone is readily absorbed after oral administration, peak concentrations of unchanged molindone being obtained within about 1.5 hours. It is rapidly and extensively metabolised and a large number of metabolites have been identified. It is excreted in the urine and faeces almost entirely in the form of its metabolites. The pharmacological effect from a single oral dose is reported to last for 24 to 36 hours.

◊ References.


1. Zetin M, *et al.* Bioavailability of oral and intramuscular molindone hydrochloride in schizophrenic patients. *Clin Ther* 1985; **7:** 169–75.


### Uses and Administration

Molindone is an indole derivative with general properties similar to those of the phenothiazine, chlorpromazine (p.680). It is given as the hydrochloride for the treatment of psychoses including schizophrenia (p.665).

The usual dose of molindone hydrochloride by mouth is 50 to 75 mg daily initially, increased in 3 or 4 days to 100 mg daily; in severe or resistant conditions doses of up to 225 mg daily may be required. The maintenance dosage can range from 15 to 225 mg daily according to severity of symptoms. The daily dosage is usually divided into 3 or 4 portions.

Molindone should be given in reduced dosage to elderly or debilitated patients.

**Psychiatric disorders.** A systematic review[1] found that molindone appeared to be effective in mental illness but evidence of differences from other classical antipsychotics was lacking.

1. Bagnall A-M, *et al.* Molindone for schizophrenia and severe mental illness. Available in The Cochrane Library; Issue 2. Chichester: John Wiley; 2004.

### Preparations

***USP 27:*** Molindone Hydrochloride Tablets.

**Proprietary Preparations** (details are given in Part 3)
***Hong Kong:*** Moban†; ***USA:*** Moban.

## Moperone Hydrochloride *(rINNM)*

Hidrocloruro de moperona; Methylperidol Hydrochloride; R-1658 (moperone). 4′-Fluoro-4-(4-hydroxy-4-*p*-tolylpiperidino)butyrophenone hydrochloride.
$C_{22}H_{26}FNO_2,HCl$ = 391.9.
*CAS — 1050-79-9 (moperone); 3871-82-7 (moperone hydrochloride).*
*ATC — N05AD04.*

### Profile

Moperone is a butyrophenone with general properties similar to those of haloperidol (p.701). It has been given by mouth for the treatment of psychoses.

## Mosapramine *(rINN)*

Clospipramine; Mosapramina; Y-516. (±)-1′-[3-(3-Chloro-10,11-dihydro-5*H*-dibenz[*b,f*]azepin-5-yl)propyl]hexahydrospiro[imidazo[1,2-*a*]pyridine-3(2*H*),4′-piperidin]-2-one.
$C_{28}H_{35}ClN_4O$ = 479.1.
*CAS — 89419-40-9.*
*ATC — N05AX10.*

### Profile

Mosapramine is an antipsychotic that has been tried in the treatment of schizophrenia.

◊ References.

1. Ishigooka J, *et al.* Pilot study of plasma concentrations of mosapramine, a new iminodibenzyl antipsychotic agent, after multiple oral administration in schizophrenic patients. *Curr Ther Res* 1994; **55:** 331–42.
2. Takahashi N, *et al.* Comparison of risperidone and mosapramine addition to neuroleptic treatment in chronic schizophrenia. *Neuropsychobiology* 1999; **39:** 81–5.

## Nemonapride *(rINN)*

Emonapride; Nemonaprida; YM-09151-2. (±)-*cis*-*N*-(1-Benzyl-2-methyl-3-pyrrolidinyl)-5-chloro-4-(methylamino)-*o*-anisamide.
$C_{21}H_{26}ClN_3O_2$ = 387.9.
*CAS — 93664-94-9.*

### Profile

Nemonapride is a substituted benzamide antipsychotic with general properties similar to those of sulpiride (p.722). It is given by mouth in the treatment of schizophrenia in usual doses of 9 to 36 mg daily in divided doses; up to 60 mg daily may be given if necessary.

◊ References.

1. Satoh K, *et al.* Effects of nemonapride on positive and negative symptoms of schizophrenia. *Int Clin Psychopharmacol* 1996; **11:** 279–81.

### Preparations

**Proprietary Preparations** (details are given in Part 3)
***Jpn:*** Emilace.

## Nimetazepam *(rINN)*

Menifazepam; S-1530. 1,3-Dihydro-1-methyl-7-nitro-5-phenyl-1,4-benzodiazepin-2-one.
$C_{16}H_{13}N_3O_3$ = 295.3.
*CAS — 2011-67-8.*

### Profile

Nimetazepam is a benzodiazepine with the general properties of diazepam (p.690). It has been given by mouth for the short-term management of insomnia. It appears to have been subject to abuse, especially in South East Asia.

# Nitrazepam *(BAN, USAN, rINN)*

Nitrazepamum; NSC-58775; Ro-4-5360; Ro-5-3059. 1,3-Dihydro-7-nitro-5-phenyl-2*H*-1,4-benzodiazepin-2-one.
$C_{15}H_{11}N_3O_3$ = 281.3.
*CAS — 146-22-5.*
*ATC — N05CD02.*

**Pharmacopoeias.** In *Chin., Eur.* (see p.vi), *Int., Jpn,* and *Pol.*
**Ph. Eur. 5.0** (Nitrazepam). A yellow, crystalline powder. Practically insoluble in water; slightly soluble in alcohol. Protect from light.

### Dependence and Withdrawal

As for Diazepam, p.690.

◊ For the purpose of withdrawal regimens, 5 mg of nitrazepam may be considered approximately equivalent to 5 mg of diazepam.

### Adverse Effects, Treatment, and Precautions

As for Diazepam, p.690.

**Effects on the digestive system.** Two children given nitrazepam as part of their antiepileptic therapy developed drooling, eating difficulty, and aspiration pneumonia; symptoms improved in one patient when the dosage of nitrazepam was reduced.[1] Manometric studies indicated that the onset of normal cricopharyngeal relaxation in swallowing was delayed in these patients until after hypopharyngeal contraction, resulting in impaired swallowing and spillover of material into the trachea. Other workers[2] have found similar effects on swallowing and cricopharyngeal relaxation in children given nitrazepam. The deaths of 6 epileptic children under 5 years of age who were treated with nitrazepam have been reported.[3] Three of the deaths were unexpected, and in view of the previous reports of swallowing difficulties and aspiration, it was recommended that the use of nitrazepam in young children be restricted to those in whom seizure control fails to improve with other antiepileptics. Another study[4] also found an apparently increased risk of death, especially in young patients with intractable epilepsy, associated with nitrazepam therapy.

1. Wyllie E. *et al.* The mechanism of nitrazepam-induced drooling and aspiration. *N Engl J Med* 1986; **314:** 35–8.
2. Lim HCN, *et al.* Nitrazepam-induced cricopharyngeal dysphagia, abnormal esophageal peristalsis and associated bronchospasm: probable cause of nitrazepam-related sudden death. *Brain Dev* 1992; **14:** 309–14.
3. Murphy JV, *et al.* Deaths in young children receiving nitrazepam. *J Pediatr* 1987; **111:** 145–7.
4. Rintahaka PJ, *et al.* Incidence of death in patients with intractable epilepsy during nitrazepam treatment. *Epilepsia* 1999; **40:** 492–6.

**Porphyria.** Nitrazepam has been associated with acute attacks of porphyria and is considered unsafe in porphyric patients.

### Interactions

As for Diazepam, p.692.

### Pharmacokinetics

Nitrazepam is fairly readily absorbed from the gastrointestinal tract, although there is some individual variation. It is about 87% bound to plasma proteins. It crosses the blood-brain and the placental barriers and traces are found in breast milk. Nitrazepam is metabolised in the liver, mainly by nitroreduction followed by acetylation; none of the metabolites possess significant activity. It is excreted in the urine in the form of its metabolites (free or conjugated) with only small amounts of a dose appearing unchanged. Up to about 20% of an oral dose is found in the faeces. Mean elimination half-lives of 24 to 30 hours have been reported.

**Distribution into breast milk.** A mean milk-to-plasma ratio of 0.27 was obtained after administration of nitrazepam 5 mg for 5 nights to 9 puerperal women.[1] The degree of nitrazepam accumulation in milk over the study period was similar to that in plasma.

1. Matheson I, *et al.* Midazolam and nitrazepam in the maternity ward: milk concentrations and clinical effects. *Br J Clin Pharmacol* 1990; **30:** 787–93.

**Hepatic impairment.** A study of the pharmacokinetics of intravenous nitrazepam in 12 patients with cirrhosis of the liver compared with 9 healthy subjects aged 22 to 49 years and 8 healthy elderly subjects aged 67 to 76 years.[1] The mean elimination half-life of nitrazepam was 26 hours in young and 38 hours in elderly subjects, the difference, which was not significant, being chiefly due to the greater volume of distribution in elderly subjects. Although there was also no significant difference between young and elderly subjects in percentage of unbound nitrazepam (13.0 and 13.9% respectively) there was a substantially higher unbound fraction in the patients with cirrhosis, the mean value being 18.9%, and clearance of unbound nitrazepam was reduced relative to healthy subjects.

1. Jochemsen R, *et al.* Effect of age and liver cirrhosis on the pharmacokinetics of nitrazepam. *Br J Clin Pharmacol* 1983; **15:** 295–302.

**Metabolism.** Although the acetylation of the reduced metabolite of nitrazepam has been reported to be controlled by acetylator phenotype,[1] no significant differences between either half-life or residual effects of nitrazepam were observed in slow and fast acetylators.[2]

1. Karim AKMB, Price Evans DA. Polymorphic acetylation of nitrazepam. *J Med Genet* 1976; **13:** 17–19.
2. Swift CG, *et al.* Acetylator phenotype, nitrazepam plasma concentrations and residual effects. *Br J Clin Pharmacol* 1980; **9:** 312P–313P.

### Uses and Administration

Nitrazepam is an intermediate-acting benzodiazepine with general properties similar to those of diazepam (p.695). It is used as a hypnotic in the short-term management of insomnia (p.667) and is reported to act in 30 to 60 minutes to produce sleep lasting for 6 to 8 hours. Nitrazepam has also been used in epilepsy, notably for infantile spasms (see below).

The usual dose by mouth for insomnia is 5 mg at night, although 10 mg may be required in some patients. Elderly or debilitated patients should not be given more than half of the normal adult dose.

**Epilepsy.** Benzodiazepines are sometimes employed in the management of epilepsy (p.349), but their long-term use is limited by problems of sedation, dependence, and tolerance to the antiepileptic effects. Nitrazepam has perhaps been most useful in the treatment of infantile spasms (as for example in West's syndrome) and the so-called infantile myoclonic seizures. Doses of 125 micrograms/kg twice daily, increased gradually to 250 to 500 micrograms/kg twice daily (or the same total daily dose given as 3 divided doses) have been suggested. There has been concern, however, over swallowing difficulties with subsequent aspiration and reports of unexpected death associated with the use of nitrazepam in young children (see Effects on the Digestive System under Adverse Effects, above).

### Preparations

***BP 2003:*** Nitrazepam Oral Suspension; Nitrazepam Tablets.

**Proprietary Preparations** (details are given in Part 3)
***Austral.:*** Alodorm; Mogadon; ***Austria:*** Mogadon; ***Belg.:*** Mogadon†; ***Braz.:*** Nitrapan; Nitrazepan†; Nitrazepol; Sonebon; Sonotrat†; ***Canad.:*** Mogadon; Nitrazadon; ***Denm.:*** Apodorm; Dumolid†; Mogadon; Pacisyn; ***Fin.:*** Insomin; ***Fr.:*** Mogadon; ***Ger.:*** Dormalon; Dormo-Puren; Eatan N; Imeson; Mogadan; Nitrazep†; Novanox; Radedorm; ***Hong Kong:*** Mogadon; ***India:*** Hypnotex; Nitavan; Nitravet; ***Irl.:*** Mogadon; Somnite; ***Israel:*** Numbon; ***Ital.:*** Mogadon; ***Malaysia:*** Mogadon; ***Neth.:*** Mogadon; ***Norw.:*** Apodorm; Mogadon; ***NZ:*** Insoma; Nitrados; ***S.Afr.:*** Arem; Mogadon; Ormodon; Paxadorm; ***Singapore:*** Dima†; Nitrados; ***Spain:*** Nitrazepan†; Pelson†; Serenade†; ***Swed.:*** Apodorm; Mogadon; ***Switz.:*** Mogadon; ***Thai.:*** Nitrados; ***UK:*** Mogadon; Remnos; Somnite.

**Multi-ingredient:** ***Arg.:*** Cavodan.

## Nordazepam *(rINN)*

A-101; Demethyldiazepam; Desmethyldiazepam; *N*-Desmethyldiazepam; Nordiazepam; Ro-5-2180. 7-Chloro-1,3-dihydro-5-phenyl-2*H*-1,4-benzodiazepin-2-one.
$C_{15}H_{11}ClN_2O$ = 270.7.
*CAS — 1088-11-5.*
*ATC — N05BA16.*

### Profile

Nordazepam is a long-acting benzodiazepine with the general properties of diazepam (p.690). It is the principal active metabolite of a number of benzodiazepines and has a half-life of 2 to 5 days. It is given by mouth in doses of up to 15 mg daily for the short-term treatment of anxiety disorders (p.663) and insomnia (p.667).

**Porphyria.** Nordazepam is considered to be unsafe in patients with porphyria because it has been shown to be porphyrinogenic in *animals* or *in-vitro* systems.

### Preparations

**Proprietary Preparations** (details are given in Part 3)
***Belg.:*** Calmday; ***Fr.:*** Nordaz; ***Ger.:*** Tranxilium N; ***Ital.:*** Madar; ***Neth.:*** Calmday; ***Port.:*** Sopax; ***Singapore:*** Nordaz; ***Switz.:*** Vegesan†.

# Olanzapine *(BAN, USAN, rINN)*

LY-170053; Olanzapina. 2-Methyl-4-(4-methyl-1-piperazinyl)-10*H*-thieno[2,3-*b*][1,5]benzodiazepine.
$C_{17}H_{20}N_4S$ = 312.4.
*CAS — 132539-06-1.*
*ATC — N05AH03.*

**Stability.** A suspension of olanzapine 1 mg/mL, made by crushing olanzapine tablets and suspending the powder in a syrup-based mixture containing carboxymethylcellulose preserved with methyl hydroxybenzoate and propyl hydroxybenzoate (Guy's Hospital paediatric base formula) was considered to be stable for 2 weeks when stored in a refrigerator.[1]

1. Harvey EJ, *et al.* The preparation and stability of a liquid olanzapine preparation for oral administration in hospitals. *Pharm J* 2000; **265:** 275–6.

### Adverse Effects, Treatment, and Precautions

Although olanzapine may share some of the adverse effects seen with the classical antipsychotics (see Chlorpromazine, p.675), the incidence and severity of such effects may vary. The most frequent adverse effects with olanzapine are somnolence and weight gain; hyperprolactinaemia is also common, but usually asymptomatic. Increased appetite, dizziness, elevated plasma glucose, triglyceride, and liver enzyme valves, eosinophilia, oedema, orthostatic hypotension, and mild transient antimuscarinic effects such as constipation and dry mouth are also relatively common. Speech difficulty has also been reported. More severe abnormalities of glucose homoeostasis occur uncommonly; severe hyperglycaemia, or exacerbation of pre-existing diabetes, sometimes leading to ketoacidosis or coma, has been reported. Clinical monitoring for hyperglycaemia has been recommended, especially in patients with or at risk of developing diabetes. Olanzapine has been associated with a low incidence of extrapyramidal symptoms including tardive dyskinesia although extrapyramidal symptoms may be more likely at high doses. Neuroleptic malignant syndrome has been reported rarely.

Patients receiving olanzapine intramuscularly should be closely observed for 2 to 4 hours for hypotension, bradyarrhythmia, and hypoventilation.

The antimuscarinic effects of olanzapine contra-indicate its use in patients with angle-closure glaucoma; caution is also advised in those with conditions such as benign prostatic hyperplasia or paralytic ileus. Olanzapine is also not recommended in Parkinson's disease since its use has commonly been associated with an increase in parkinsonian symptoms and hallucinations. It should be used with caution in patients with hepatic impairment, or a history of blood dyscrasias, bone marrow depression, myeloproliferative disease, or convulsions. Those with diabetes mellitus, or risk factors for its development, should be carefully monitored. It is recommended that blood pressure is periodically assessed in elderly patients.

Olanzapine may affect the performance of skilled tasks such as driving.

Withdrawal symptoms have occurred rarely when olanzapine has been stopped abruptly; a gradual dose reduction may be appropriate when stopping olanzapine.

◊ References.

1. Beasley CM, *et al.* Safety of olanzapine. *J Clin Psychiatry* 1997; **58** (suppl 10): 13–17.
2. Biswasl PN, *et al.* The pharmacovigilance of olanzapine: results of a post-marketing surveillance study on 8858 patients in England. *J Psychopharmacol* 2001; **15:** 265–71.

**Breast feeding.** The UK manufacturer states that at steady state the estimated mean exposure of breast-fed infants of mothers taking olanzapine would be 1.8% of the maternal dose and have recommended that patients should not breast-feed if they are taking olanzapine.

**Cerebrovascular disorders.** The UK Committee on Safety of Medicines[1] have recommended that olanzapine should not be used to treat behavioural problems in elderly patients with dementia after analysis of placebo-controlled studies revealed an increased risk of stroke and a twofold increase in all-cause mortality. It was considered that the risk may not be confined to use in dementia and should be considered relevant to any patient with a history of stroke or transient ischaemic attack or other risk factors for cerebrovascular disease, including hypertension, diabetes, current smoking, or atrial fibrillation.

1. Atypical antipsychotic drugs and stroke message from Professor G Duff, Chairman of Committee on Safety of Medicines (CSM). Available at: http://www.mca.gov.uk/ourwork/monitorsafequalmed/safetymessages/antipsystoke_9304.pdf (accessed 28/04/04)

**Dementia.** For a recommendation that olanzapine should not be used to treat behavioural problems in elderly patients with dementia, see under Cerebrovascular Disorders, above.

**Effects on the blood.** A review[1] has described 11 reports of olanzapine-associated haematotoxicity that included 3 cases of agranulocytosis, 6 of neutropenia, and 2 of leucopenia. In most cases, the haematotoxicity developed within the first month of treatment and patients recovered after olanzapine withdrawal. There was a history of clozapine-associated haematotoxicity in 5 patients. It was suggested that white blood cell counts should be monitored periodically during olanzapine treatment.

Olanzapine has also apparently delayed recovery of granulocyte counts in patients with clozapine-induced granulocytopenia who were switched to olanzapine before blood counts had returned to the normal range.[2]

There has been a case report of thrombocytopenia associated with olanzapine treatment. The patient improved on discontinuation of olanzapine but subsequently had a similar episode associated with benzatropine therapy.[3]

1. Tolosa-Vilella C, *et al.* Olanzapine-induced agranulocytosis: a case report and review of the literature. *Prog Neuropsychopharmacol Biol Psychiatry* 2002; **26:** 411–4.
2. Flynn SW, *et al.* Prolongation of clozapine-induced granulocytopenia associated with olanzapine. *J Clin Psychopharmacol* 1997; **17:** 494–5.
3. Bogunovic O, Viswanathan R. Thrombocytopenia possibly associated with olanzapine and subsequently with benztropine mesylate. *Psychosomatics* 2000; **41:** 277–88.

**Effects on carbohydrate metabolism.** The increased risk of glucose intolerance and diabetes mellitus with some atypical antipsychotics and recommendations on monitoring are discussed under Adverse Effects in Clozapine, p.686.

Further references for such effects associated with olanzapine use are given below; in some cases the outcome was fatal.

1. Bettinger TL, *et al.* Olanzapine-induced glucose dysregulation. *Ann Pharmacother* 2000; **34:** 865–7.
2. Roefaro J, Mukherjee SM. Olanzapine-induced hyperglycemic nonketonic coma. *Ann Pharmacother* 2001: **35:** 300–302.
3. Bonanno DG, *et al.* Olanzapine-induced diabetes mellitus. *Ann Pharmacother* 2001; **35:** 563–5.
4. Ragucci KR, Wells BJ. Olanzapine-induced diabetic ketoacidosis. *Ann Pharmacother* 2001; **35:** 1556–8.
5. Koller E, *et al.* Atypical antipsychotic drugs and hyperglycemia in adolescents. *JAMA* 2001; **286:** 2547–8.
6. Anonymous. Olanzapine (Zyprexa) and diabetes. *Current Problems* 2002; **28:** 3. Also available at: http://www.mca.gov.uk/ourwork/monitorsafequalmed/currentproblems/cpapril2002.pdf (accessed 28/04/04)
7. Koro CE, *et al.* Assessment of independent effect of olanzapine and risperidone on risk of diabetes among patients with schizophrenia: population based nested case-control study. *BMJ* 2002; **325:** 243–5.

**Effects on the liver.** A report[1] of acute hepatocellular cholestatic jaundice that developed in a 78-year-old women 13 days after starting treatment with olanzapine.

1. Jadallah KA, *et al.* Acute hepatocellular-cholestatic liver injury after olanzapine therapy. *Ann Intern Med* 2003; **138:** 357–8.

**Effects on the nervous system.** A 31-year-old woman with a complicated medical history suffered three generalised tonic-clonic seizures after 13 days' therapy with olanzapine.[1] She recovered after treatment with phenytoin. Another patient with Huntington's disease also suffered a severe generalised tonic-clonic seizure following treatment with olanzapine 30 mg daily for 1 month.[2] Olanzapine was continued but carbamazepine was added; there was no recurrence of the seizure.

1. Lee JW, *et al.* Seizure associated with olanzapine. *Ann Pharmacother* 1999; **33:** 554–6.
2. Bonelli RM. Olanzapine-associated seizure. *Ann Pharmacother* 2003; **37:** 149–50.

**Effects on the pancreas.** There have been isolated reports of pancreatitis associated with olanzapine.[1,2]

1. Doucette DE, *et al.* Olanzapine-induced acute pancreatitis. *Ann Pharmacother* 2000; **34:** 1128–31.
2. Hagger R, *et al.* Olanzapine and pancreatitis. *Br J Psychiatry* 2000; **177:** 567.

**Effects on sexual function.** Priapism has been reported[1] in a patient receiving olanzapine.

1. Deirmenjian JM, *et al.* Olanzapine-induced reversible priapism: a case report. *J Clin Psychopharmacol* 1998; **18:** 351–3.

**Extrapyramidal disorders.** A report of 2 isolated cases of tardive dyskinesia associated with olanzapine treatment.[1]

1. Herrán A, Vázquez-Barquero JL. Tardive dyskinesia associated with olanzapine. *Ann Intern Med* 1999; **131:** 72.

**Mania.** Although it has been used in the treatment of bipolar disorder, olanzapine has been associated with reports of mania in both schizophrenic and bipolar patients.[1-4] A report sponsored by the manufacturers noted that no association was seen in pooled data from 2 placebo controlled studies involving 254 bipolar patients.[5]

1. Lindenmayer J-P, Klebanov R. Olanzapine-induced manic-like syndrome. *J Clin Psychiatry* 1998; **59:** 318–19.
2. Fitz-Gerald MJ, *et al.* Olanzapine-induced mania. *Am J Psychiatry* 1999; **156:** 1114.
3. Aubry J-M, *et al.* Possible induction of mania and hypomania by olanzapine or risperidone: a critical review of reported cases. *J Clin Psychiatry* 2000; **61:** 649–55.
4. Henry C, Demotes-Mainard J. Olanzapine-induced mania in bipolar disorders. *J Psychiatry Neurosci* 2002; **27:** 200–201.
5. Baker RW, *et al.* Placebo-controlled trials do not find association of olanzapine with exacerbation of bipolar mania. *J Affect Disord* 2003; **73:** 147–53.

**Neuroleptic malignant syndrome.** Cases of neuroleptic malignant syndrome associated with olanzapine therapy.[1-3]

1. Filice GA, *et al.* Neuroleptic malignant syndrome associated with olanzapine. *Ann Pharmacother* 1998; **32:** 1158–9.
2. Nyfort-Hansen K, Alderman CP. Possible neuroleptic malignant syndrome associated with olanzapine. *Ann Pharmacother* 2000; **34:** 667.
3. Kogoj A, Velikonja I. Olanzapine induced neuroleptic malignant syndrome–a case review. *Hum Psychopharmacol* 2003; **18:** 301–9.

**Overdosage.** A 2½-year-old boy was found sleeping and difficult to arouse after taking one or two 7.5-mg olanzapine tablets.[1] His reported symptoms included agitation, aggressive behaviour, miosis, hypersalivation, tachycardia, and ataxia; he recovered after 24 hours. A later review[2] identified 29 fatalities associated with olanzapine overdose, but evidence of a direct causative relationship was limited.

1. Yip L, *et al.* Olanzapine toxicity in a toddler. *Pediatrics* 1998; **102:** 1494.
2. Chue P, Singer P. A review of olanzapine-associated toxicity and fatality in overdose. *J Psychiatry Neurosci* 2003; **28:** 253–61.

**Parkinsonism.** Worsening of motor function has been reported[1-4] in patients with parkinsonism following olanzapine administration.

1. Graham JM, *et al.* Olanzapine in the treatment of hallucinosis in idiopathic Parkinson's disease: a cautionary note. *J Neurol Neurosurg Psychiatry* 1998 **65:** 774–7.
2. Molho ES, Factor SA. Worsening of motor features of parkinsonism with olanzapine. *Mov Disord* 1999; **14:** 1014–16.
3. Goetz CG, *et al.* Olanzapine and clozapine: comparative effects on motor function in hallucinating PD patients. *Neurology* 2000; **55:** 789–94.
4. Manson AJ, *et al.* Low-dose olanzapine for levodopa induced dyskinesias. *Neurology* 2000; **55:** 795–9.

**Pregnancy.** The manufacturer has reviewed both prospective and retrospective cases of pregnancies that have been exposed to olanzapine treatment.[1] Of the 37 prospective pregnancies, there were 14 therapeutic abortions (with no reported abnormality in the fetus), 3 spontaneous abortions (again with no reported abnormality in the fetus), and 1 still-birth. The remaining 19 pregnancies included 16 normal births without complications and 1 premature birth; the 2 other births were complicated by post-term deliveries. Eleven retrospective cases were also identified and included 2 cases of major malformation (dysplastic kidney and Down's syndrome), 1 case of fetal death following an overdose by the mother, and 1 case each of neonatal convulsion and sudden infant death.

1. Goldstein DJ, *et al.* Olanzapine-exposed pregnancies and lactation: early experience. *J Clin Psychopharmacol* 2000; **20:** 399–403.

## Interactions

The central effects of other CNS depressants including alcohol may be enhanced by olanzapine. Olanzapine may antagonise the actions of dopaminergics. Neutropenia may be more common when olanzapine is given with valproate. There is a theoretical risk of QT prolongation when olanzapine is given with other drugs that are known to cause this effect.

The metabolism of olanzapine is mediated to some extent by the cytochrome P450 isoenzyme CYP1A2. Use with drugs that inhibit, induce, or act as a substrate to this isoenzyme may affect plasma concentrations of olanzapine and a dose adjustment of olanzapine may be required. The CYP1A2 inhibitor fluvoxamine significantly inhibits the metabolism of olanzapine. The clearance of olanzapine is increased by tobacco smoking and carbamazepine.

## Pharmacokinetics

Olanzapine is well absorbed from the gastrointestinal tract after oral administration but undergoes considerable first-pass metabolism. Peak plasma concentrations are achieved about 5 to 8 hours after oral administration and about 15 to 45 minutes after intramuscular administration. Olanzapine is about 93% bound to plasma proteins. It is extensively metabolised in the liver primarily by direct glucuronidation and by oxidation mediated through the cytochrome P450 isoenzymes CYP1A2 and, to a lesser extent, CYP2D6. The two major metabolites 10-*N*-glucuronide and 4′-*N*-desmethyl olanzapine appear to be inactive. About 57% of a dose is excreted in the urine, mainly as metabolites and about 30% appears in the faeces. The plasma elimination half-life has been variously reported to be about 30 to 38 hours; half-lives tend to be longer in female than in male patients. Olanzapine is distributed into breast milk.

◊ References.

1. Callaghan JT, *et al.* Olanzapine: pharmacokinetic and pharmacodynamic profile. *Clin Pharmacokinet* 1999; **37:** 177–93.

## Uses and Administration

Olanzapine is a thienobenzodiazepine atypical antipsychotic. It has affinity for serotonin, muscarinic, histamine-$H_1$, and adrenergic ($\alpha_1$) receptors as well as various dopamine receptors.

Olanzapine is used for the management of schizophrenia and for the treatment of moderate to severe mania associated with bipolar disorder.

In the UK the usual initial dose for **schizophrenia** is 10 mg daily as a single dose *by mouth*; thereafter dosage adjustments of 5 mg daily may be made according to response at intervals of not less than 24 hours to within the range of 5 to 20 mg daily. In the USA the starting dose is 5 to 10 mg daily and it is recommended that dosage adjustments beyond 10 mg daily are made at intervals of not less than one week. However, it is recommended that doses above 10 mg daily should be given only after clinical reassessment.

For the treatment of **acute manic episodes** a recommended initial dose is 10 or 15 mg daily by mouth as monotherapy or 10 mg if given as part of combination therapy; dosage adjustments of 5 mg may subsequently be made at intervals of not less than 24 hours if necessary to within the range 5 to 20 mg daily. If a response is achieved, therapy may continue at the same dosage to prevent recurrence. For **prevention of recurrence** in patients whose manic episodes have responded previously to olanzapine the recommended starting dose is 10 mg daily.

For the **rapid control of agitation and disturbed behaviour** in patients with schizophrenia or mania olanzapine may be given *intramuscularly* in an initial dose of 5 to 10 mg, followed by 5 to 10 mg as required after 2 hours. Not more than three injections should be given in any 24-hour period and the maximum daily dose, including olanzapine given by mouth, should not exceed 20 mg. Parenteral administration may be used for up to a maximum of 3 days but transfer to oral therapy should be initiated as soon as possible.

The metabolism of olanzapine might be slower in female, elderly, or non-smoking patients; if more than one of these factors is present a lower initial dose (e.g. 5 mg daily if given by mouth) and a more gradual dose escalation should be considered. The intramuscular dose should be reduced by half in the elderly. See below for doses in patients with hepatic or renal impairment.

**Administration in hepatic or renal impairment.** A starting dose of 5 mg daily of olanzapine by mouth may be necessary for patients with renal impairment; for patients with moderate hepatic insufficiency the starting dose should be 5 mg daily, and only increased with caution. An initial intramuscular dose of 5 mg should be considered for patients with renal or hepatic impairment; for patients with moderate hepatic insufficiency the starting dose should only be increased with caution.

**Bipolar disorder.** Olanzapine is of benefit for the treatment of mania, with or without psychosis, in patients with bipolar disorder (p.278) and the use of atypical antipsychotics in the management of such patients is increasing. However, there have been individual case reports of olanzapine-induced mania (see above). There is also increasing interest in the use of olanzapine for the depressive phase of bipolar disorder, and for other forms of resistant depression. In some countries olanzapine is available as a fixed-dose combination with fluoxetine for use in the former condition.

References.

1. Shelton RC, *et al.* A novel augmentation strategy for treating resistant major depression. *Am J Psychiatry* 2001; **158:** 131–4.
2. Rendell JM, *et al.* Olanzapine alone or in combination for acute mania. Available in The Cochrane Library; Issue 2. Chichester: John Wiley; 2004.

**Parkinsonism.** Olanzapine is associated with a relatively low incidence of extrapyramidal disorders and is therefore being studied[1] for use in the treatment of psychosis in patients with Parkinson's disease (see Disturbed Behaviour, p.665). However, there have been a number of reports of adverse effects including exacerbation of the movement disorder (see above).

1. Wolters EC, *et al.* Olanzapine in the treatment of dopaminomimetic psychosis in patients with Parkinson's disease. *Neurology* 1996; **47:** 1085–7.

**Schizophrenia.** Studies suggest that olanzapine is as effective as haloperidol against positive symptoms of schizophrenia (p.665) and more effective against negative symptoms in the short-term and possibly in the long-term,[1-5] although a systematic review considered the evidence equivocal.[6] Quality of life has also been judged to be greater in patients treated with olanzapine.[7] In comparative studies, extrapyramidal symptoms have been less frequent with olanzapine than haloperidol and fewer patients have discontinued treatment with olanzapine. There are few published comparisons with other atypical antipsychotics, but one study[8] has suggested that response of negative symptoms might be greater than with risperidone; patients in this study were also more likely to maintain their initial response with olanzapine and less likely to experience extrapyramidal effects, although risperidone had been given in doses higher than usually used clinically. Olanzapine's efficacy in the treatment of patients with refractory schizophrenia remains to be determined.

1. Beasley CM, *et al.* Olanzapine HGAD Study Group. Olanzapine versus placebo and haloperidol: acute phase results of the North American double-blind olanzapine trial. *Neuropsychopharmacology* 1996; **14:** 111–23.
2. Beasley C, *et al.* Olanzapine versus haloperidol: long-term results of the multi-center international trial. *Eur Neuropsychopharmacol* 1996; **6** (suppl 3): 59.
3. Beasley CM, *et al.* Olanzapine versus haloperidol: acute phase results of the international double-blind olanzapine trial. *Eur Neuropsychopharmacol* 1997; **7:** 125–37.
4. Tollefson GD, *et al.* Olanzapine versus haloperidol in the treatment of schizophrenia and schizoaffective and schizophreniform disorders: results of an international collaborative trial. *Am J Psychiatry* 1997; **154:** 457–65.
5. Bhana N, *et al.* Olanzapine: an updated review of its use in the management of schizophrenia. *Drugs* 2001; **61:** 111–61.
6. Duggan L, *et al.* Olanzapine for schizophrenia. Available in The Cochrane Library; Issue 2. Chichester: John Wiley; 2004.
7. Hamilton SH, *et al.* Olanzapine versus placebo and haloperidol: quality of life and efficacy results of the North American double-blind trial. *Neuropsychopharmacology* 1998; **18:** 41–9.
8. Tran PV, *et al.* Double-blind comparison of olanzapine versus risperidone in the treatment of schizophrenia and other psychotic disorders. *J Clin Psychopharmacol* 1997; **17:** 407–18.

**Stuttering.** Olanzapine may be of benefit in the treatment of stuttering (p.702).[1]

1. Lavid N, *et al.* Management of child and adolescent stuttering with olanzapine: three case reports. *Ann Clin Psychiatry* 1999; **11:** 233–6.

**Tourette's syndrome.** When treatment is required for tics and behavioural disturbances in Tourette's syndrome (p.664) haloperidol or pimozide are commonly used but olanzapine has also been tried.[1-3]

1. Stamenkovic M, *et al.* Effective open-label treatment of tourette's disorder with olanzapine. *Int Clin Psychopharmacol* 2000; **15:** 23–8.
2. Onofrj M, *et al.* Olanzapine in severe Gilles de la Tourette syndrome: a 52-week double-blind cross-over study vs. low-dose pimozide. *J Neurol* 2000; **247:** 443–6.
3. Budman CL, *et al.* An open-label study of the treatment efficacy of olanzapine for Tourette's disorder. *J Clin Psychiatry* 2001; **62:** 290–4.

## Preparations

**Proprietary Preparations** (details are given in Part 3)
***Arg.:*** Midax; Zyprexa; ***Austral.:*** Zyprexa; ***Austria:*** Zyprexa; ***Belg.:*** Zyprexa; ***Braz.:*** Zyprexa; ***Canad.:*** Zyprexa; ***Chile:*** Zyprexa; ***Denm.:*** Zyprexa; ***Fin.:*** Zyprexa; ***Fr.:*** Zyprexa; ***Ger.:*** Zyprexa; ***Gr.:*** Zyprexa; ***Hong Kong:*** Zyprexa; ***India:*** Joyzol; Olexa; ***Irl.:*** Zyprexa; ***Israel:*** Zyprexa; ***Ital.:*** Zyprexa; ***Malaysia:*** Zyprexa; ***Mex.:*** Zyprexa; ***Neth.:*** Zyprexa; ***Norw.:*** Zyprexa; ***NZ:*** Zyprexa; ***Port.:*** Zyprexa; ***S.Afr.:*** Zyprexa; ***Singapore:*** Zyprexa; ***Spain:*** Zyprexa; ***Swed.:*** Zyprexa; ***Switz.:*** Zyprexa; ***Thai.:*** Zyprexa; ***UK:*** Zyprexa; ***USA:*** Zyprexa.

**Multi-ingredient:** ***USA:*** Symbyax.

# Oxazepam *(BAN, USAN, rINN)*

Oxazepamum; Wy-3498. 7-Chloro-1,3-dihydro-3-hydroxy-5-phenyl-1,4-benzodiazepin-2-one.

$C_{15}H_{11}ClN_2O_2$ = 286.7.

*CAS — 604-75-1.*

*ATC — N05BA04.*

**Pharmacopoeias.** In *Chin., Eur.* (see p.vi), *Pol.,* and *US.*

**Ph. Eur. 5.0** (Oxazepam). A white or almost white crystalline powder. Practically insoluble in water; slightly soluble in alcohol and in dichloromethane. Protect from light.

**USP 27** (Oxazepam). A creamy-white to pale yellow, practically odourless powder. Practically insoluble in water; soluble 1 in 220 of alcohol, 1 in 270 of chloroform, and 1 in 2200 of ether. pH of a 2% suspension in water is between 4.8 and 7.0.

## Dependence and Withdrawal

As for Diazepam, p.690.

◊ For the purpose of withdrawal regimens, 15 mg of oxazepam is considered approximately equivalent to 5 mg of diazepam.

## Adverse Effects, Treatment, and Precautions

As for Diazepam, p.690.

**Hepatic impairment.** All benzodiazepines should be used with caution in patients with hepatic impairment, but short acting ones such as oxazepam may be preferred.

Seven patients with acute viral hepatitis, 6 with cirrhosis of the liver, and 16 age-matched healthy control subjects received a single dose of oxazepam 15 or 45 mg by mouth.[1] Urinary excretion rates and plasma elimination patterns were unaltered in patients with acute and chronic parenchymal liver disease. Oxazepam 15 mg was also administered three times daily by mouth for 2 weeks to 2 healthy subjects and to 2 patients with cirrhosis and did not appear to accumulate in any of the four.

1. Shull HJ, *et al.* Normal disposition of oxazepam in acute viral hepatitis and cirrhosis. *Ann Intern Med* 1976; **84:** 420–5.

**Porphyria.** Oxazepam is considered to be unsafe in patients with porphyria although there is conflicting experimental evidence of porphyrinogenicity.

**Renal impairment.** Pharmacokinetic studies suggesting that, in general, the dosage of oxazepam does not need adjusting in patients with renal impairment.[1-3]

1. Murray TG, *et al.* Renal disease, age, and oxazepam kinetics. *Clin Pharmacol Ther* 1981; **30:** 805–9.
2. Busch U, *et al.* Pharmacokinetics of oxazepam following multiple administration in volunteers and patients with chronic renal disease. *Arzneimittelforschung* 1981; **31:** 1507–11.
3. Greenblatt DJ, *et al.* Multiple-dose kinetics and dialyzability of oxazepam in renal insufficiency. *Nephron* 1983; **34:** 234–8.

**Thyroid disorders.** There was a reduction in half-life and an increase in the apparent oral clearance of oxazepam in 7 hyperthyroid patients.[1] In 6 hypothyroid patients there was no overall change in oxazepam elimination, although 5 of the 6 complained of drowsiness despite a relatively low dose (15 mg).

1. Scott AK, *et al.* Oxazepam pharmacokinetics in thyroid disease. *Br J Clin Pharmacol* 1984; **17:** 49–53.

## Interactions

As for Diazepam, p.692.

## Pharmacokinetics

Oxazepam is well absorbed from the gastrointestinal tract and reaches peak plasma concentrations about 2 hours after ingestion. It crosses the placenta and has been detected in breast milk. Oxazepam is about 85 to 97% bound to plasma proteins and has been reported to have an elimination half-life ranging from about 3 to 21 hours. It is largely metabolised to the inactive glucuronide which is excreted in the urine.

**Pregnancy.** A study on the placental passage of oxazepam and its metabolism in 12 women given a single dose of oxazepam 25 mg during labour.[1] Oxazepam was readily absorbed and peak plasma concentrations were in the same range as those reported in healthy males and non-pregnant females given the same dose, although the plasma half-life (range 5.3 to 7.8 hours in 8 subjects studied) was shorter than that reported for non-pregnant subjects. Oxazepam was detected in the umbilical vein of all 12 patients with the ratio between umbilical to maternal vein concentration of oxazepam reaching a value of about 1.35 and remaining constant beyond a dose-delivery time of 3 hours. All of the babies had a normal Apgar score value. The oxazepam plasma half-life in the newborns was about 3 to 4 times that in the mothers, although in 3 the plasma concentration of oxazepam conjugate rose during the first 6 to 10 hours after delivery indicating the ability of the neonate to conjugate oxazepam.

1. Tomson G, *et al.* Placental passage of oxazepam and its metabolism in mother and newborn. *Clin Pharmacol Ther* 1979; **25:** 74–81.

## Uses and Administration

Oxazepam is a short-acting benzodiazepine with general properties similar to those of diazepam (p.695). It is used in the short-term management of anxiety disorders (p.663) and insomnia (p.667) associated with anxiety. Oxazepam is also used for the control of symptoms associated with alcohol withdrawal (p.1166). Oxazepam is usually given as the base but the hemisuccinate has been used in some multi-ingredient preparations.

The usual dose of oxazepam for the treatment of anxiety or for control of symptoms of alcohol withdrawal is 15 to 30 mg three or four times daily by mouth. A suggested initial dose for elderly or debilitated patients is 10 mg three times daily increased if necessary up to 10 to 20 mg three or four times daily. For the treatment of insomnia associated with anxiety oxazepam 15 to 25 mg may be given one hour before retiring; up to 50 mg may occasionally be necessary.

**Administration in renal impairment.** For a suggestion that dosage adjustment of oxazepam may not be necessary in patients with renal impairment, see Renal Impairment, above.

## Preparations

***BP 2003:*** Oxazepam Tablets;
***USP 27:*** Oxazepam Capsules; Oxazepam Tablets.

**Proprietary Preparations** (details are given in Part 3)
***Arg.:*** Pausafren T; ***Austral.:*** Alepam; Murelax; Serepax; ***Austria:*** Adumbran; Anxiolit; Oxahexal; Praxiten; ***Belg.:*** Seresta; Tranquo; ***Canad.:*** Novoxapam†; Serax†; ***Chile:*** Serepax; ***Denm.:*** Alopam; Oxabenz; Oxapax; Serepax; ***Fin.:*** Alopam; Opamox; Oxamin; Oxepam; ***Fr.:*** Seresta; ***Ger.:*** Adumbran; Azutranquil; durazepam; Mirfudorm; Noctazepam; oxa; Praxiten; Sigacalm; Uskan; ***India:*** Serepax; ***Israel:*** Vaben; ***Ital.:*** Limbial; Oxapam†; Serpax; ***Neth.:*** Seresta; ***Norw.:*** Alopam; Serepax†; Sobril; ***NZ:*** Benzotran†; Ox-Pam; Serepax†; ***Port.:*** Serenal; ***S.Afr.:*** Medopam†; Noripam; Purata; Serepax; ***Spain:*** Adumbran; ***Swed.:*** Oxascand; Sobril; ***Switz.:*** Anxiolit; Seresta; Uskan†; ***USA:*** Serax.

**Multi-ingredient:** ***Arg.:*** Cavodan; Pankreoflat Sedante; ***Austria:*** Anxiolit plus; ***Chile:*** Novalona; ***Fin.:*** Spasmo-Oxepam†; ***Ital.:*** Persumbrax†; ***Port.:*** Sedioton; ***Spain:*** Novo Aerofil Sedante; Suxidina.

# Oxazolam *(rINN)*

Oxazolazepam. 10-Chloro-2,3,7,11b-tetrahydro-2-methyl-11b-phenyloxazolo[3,2-*d*][1,4]benzodiazepin-6(5*H*)-one.

$C_{18}H_{17}ClN_2O_2$ = 328.8.

*CAS — 24143-17-7.*

**Pharmacopoeias.** In *Jpn.*

## Profile

Oxazolam is a long-acting benzodiazepine with general properties similar to those of diazepam (p.690). It has been given by mouth for the short-term treatment of anxiety disorders.

Oxazolam has also been used as a premedicant in general anaesthesia.

### Preparations

**Proprietary Preparations** (details are given in Part 3)
***Hong Kong:*** Serebon†.

## Oxypertine *(BAN, USAN, rINN)*

Oxipertina; Win-18501-2. 5,6-Dimethoxy-2-methyl-3-[2-(4-phenylpiperazin-1-yl)ethyl]indole.
$C_{23}H_{29}N_3O_2$ = 379.5.
*CAS — 153-87-7 (oxypertine); 40523-01-1 (oxypertine hydrochloride).*
*ATC — N05AE01.*

### Profile

Oxypertine is an indole derivative with general properties similar to those of the phenothiazine, chlorpromazine (p.675). It has been given by mouth in the treatment of various psychoses including schizophrenia, mania, and disturbed behaviour, and of severe anxiety.

## Paraldehyde

Paracetaldehyde; Paraldehído; Paraldehydum. The trimer of acetaldehyde; 2,4,6-Trimethyl-1,3,5-trioxane.
$(C_2H_4O)_3$ = 132.2.
*CAS — 123-63-7.*
*ATC — N05CC05.*

**Pharmacopoeias.** In *Eur.* (see p.vi) and *US.*

**Ph. Eur. 5.0** (Paraldehyde). A colourless or slightly yellow, transparent liquid. It solidifies on cooling to form a crystalline mass. It may contain a suitable amount of an antoxidant. Relative density 0.991 to 0.996. F.p. is 10° to 13°; not more than 10% distils below 123° and not less than 95% below 126°. Soluble in water but less soluble in boiling water; miscible with alcohol and with volatile oils. Store in small well-filled airtight containers. Protect from light.

**USP 27** (Paraldehyde). A colourless transparent liquid with a strong characteristic, but not unpleasant or pungent, odour. It is subject to oxidation to form acetic acid. It may contain a suitable stabiliser. Specific gravity is about 0.99. It has a congealing temperature of not lower than 11° and distils completely between 120° and 126°. Soluble 1 in 10 of water v/v, but only 1 in 17 of boiling water v/v; miscible with alcohol, with chloroform, with ether, and with volatile oils. Store in well-filled airtight containers of not more than 30 mL at a temperature not exceeding 25°. Protect from light. It must not be used more than 24 hours after opening the container.

**Incompatibility.** Paraldehyde exerts a solvent action upon rubber, polystyrene, and styrene-acrylonitrile copolymer and should not be administered in plastic syringes made with these materials.

An evaluation of the compatibility of paraldehyde with plastic syringes and needle hubs concluded that, if possible, all-glass syringes should be used with paraldehyde.[1] Needles with plastic hubs could be used. Polypropylene syringes with rubber-tipped plastic plungers (Plastipak), or glass syringes with natural rubber-tipped plastic plungers (Glaspak) were acceptable only for the immediate administration or measurement of paraldehyde doses.

1. Johnson CE, Vigoreaux JA. Compatibility of paraldehyde with plastic syringes and needle hubs. *Am J Hosp Pharm* 1984; **41:** 306–8.

**Stability.** Paraldehyde decomposes on storage, particularly after the container has been opened. The administration of partly decomposed paraldehyde is **dangerous**. It must not be used if it has a brownish colour or a sharp penetrating odour of acetic acid.

### Dependence and Withdrawal

Prolonged use of paraldehyde may lead to dependence, especially in alcoholics. Features of dependence and withdrawal are similar to those of barbiturates (see Amobarbital, p.670).

### Adverse Effects and Treatment

Paraldehyde decomposes on storage and deaths from corrosive poisoning have followed the use of such material. Paraldehyde has an unpleasant taste and imparts a smell to the breath; it may cause skin rashes.

Oral and rectal administration of paraldehyde may cause gastric or rectal irritation. Intramuscular injection is painful and associated with tissue necrosis, sterile abscesses, and nerve damage. Intravenous administration is extremely hazardous since it may cause pulmonary oedema and haemorrhage, hypotension and cardiac dilatation, and circulatory collapse; thrombophlebitis is also associated with intravenous use.

Overdosage results in rapid laboured breathing owing to damage to the lungs and to acidosis. Nausea and vomiting may follow an overdose by mouth. Respiratory depression and coma as well as hepatic and renal damage may occur. Treatment is as for barbiturate overdose (see Amobarbital, p.670).

### Precautions

Paraldehyde should not be given to patients with gastric disorders and it should be used with caution, if at all, in patients with bronchopulmonary disease or hepatic impairment. It should not be given rectally in the presence of colitis. Old paraldehyde must never be used.

Paraldehyde must be well diluted before oral or rectal administration; if it is deemed essential to give paraldehyde intravenously it must be well diluted and given very slowly with extreme caution (see also Adverse Effects, above and Uses, below). Intramuscular injections may be given undiluted but care should be taken to avoid nerve damage. Plastic syringes should be avoided (see Incompatibility, above).

### Interactions

The sedative effects of paraldehyde are enhanced by CNS depressants such as alcohol, barbiturates, and other sedatives. A few case reports suggest that disulfiram may enhance the toxicity of paraldehyde; concomitant use is not recommended.

### Pharmacokinetics

Paraldehyde is generally absorbed readily, although absorption is reported to be slower after rectal than after oral or intramuscular administration. It is widely distributed and has a reported half-life of 4 to 10 hours. About 80% of a dose is metabolised in the liver probably to acetaldehyde, which is oxidised by aldehyde dehydrogenase to acetic acid. Unmetabolised drug is largely excreted unchanged through the lungs; only small amounts appear in the urine. It crosses the placental barrier and is distributed into breast milk.

### Uses and Administration

Paraldehyde is a hypnotic and sedative with antiepileptic effects. However, because of the hazards associated with its administration, its tendency to react with plastic, and the risks associated with its deterioration, it has largely been superseded by other drugs. It is still occasionally used to control status epilepticus (p.352) resistant to conventional treatment. Given rectally or intramuscularly it causes little respiratory depression and is therefore useful where facilities for resuscitation are poor.

At low temperature it solidifies to form a crystalline mass. If it solidifies, the whole should be liquefied before use.

A usual dose for adults is 10 to 20 mL given rectally as a 10% solution in sodium chloride 0.9% solution or diluted with 1 or 2 parts of oil. Doses of 5 to 10 mL are also occasionally given intramuscularly up to a maximum of 20 mL daily with not more than 5 mL being given at any one site. Recommended doses rectally or intramuscularly in children are: up to 3 months, 0.5 mL; 3 to 6 months, 1 mL; 6 to 12 months, 1.5 mL; 1 to 2 years, 2 mL; 3 to 5 years, 3 to 4 mL; 6 to 12 years, 5 to 6 mL.

Paraldehyde has been given by slow intravenous infusion in specialist centres with intensive care facilities but this method of administration is not usually recommended; it must be diluted in sodium chloride 0.9% before use.

Paraldehyde has been given by mouth; it should always be well diluted to avoid gastric irritation.

### Preparations

***BP 2003:*** Paraldehyde Injection.

**Proprietary Preparations** (details are given in Part 3)
***USA:*** Paral.

## Penfluridol *(BAN, USAN, rINN)*

McN-JR-16341; R-16341. 4-(4-Chloro-3-trifluoromethylphenyl)-1-[3-(p,p′-difluorobenzhydryl)propyl]piperidin-4-ol.
$C_{28}H_{27}ClF_5NO$ = 524.0.
*CAS — 26864-56-2.*
*ATC — N05AG03.*

**Pharmacopoeias.** In *Chin.*

### Profile

Penfluridol is a diphenylbutylpiperidine antipsychotic and shares the general properties of the phenothiazine, chlorpromazine (p.675). Following oral administration it has a prolonged duration of action that lasts for about a week. It is used in the treatment of various psychoses including schizophrenia (p.665).

The usual dose of penfluridol for the treatment of chronic psychoses is 20 to 60 mg weekly by mouth. Doses of up to 250 mg once a week may be required in severe or resistant conditions.

### Preparations

**Proprietary Preparations** (details are given in Part 3)
***Austria:*** Semap; ***Belg.:*** Semap; ***Braz.:*** Semap; ***Denm.:*** Semap; ***Fr.:*** Semap; ***Gr.:*** Flupidol; ***Israel:*** Semap; ***Mex.:*** Semap; ***Neth.:*** Semap; ***Switz.:*** Semap.

## Pentobarbital *(BAN, rINN)*

Aethaminalum; Mebubarbital; Mebumal; Pentobarbitalum; Pentobarbitone. 5-Ethyl-5-(1-methylbutyl)barbituric acid.
$C_{11}H_{18}N_2O_3$ = 226.3.
*CAS — 76-74-4.*
*ATC — N05CA01.*

**Pharmacopoeias.** In *Eur.* (see p.vi) and *US.*

**Ph. Eur. 5.0** (Pentobarbital). Colourless crystals or a white crystalline powder. Very slightly soluble in water; freely soluble in dehydrated alcohol. It forms water-soluble compounds with alkali hydroxides and carbonates, and with ammonia.

**USP 27** (Pentobarbital). A white or practically white, practically odourless, fine powder. Very slightly soluble in water and in carbon tetrachloride; soluble 1 in 4.5 of alcohol, 1 in 4 of chloroform, and 1 in 10 of ether; very soluble in acetone and in methyl alcohol; soluble in benzene. Store in airtight containers.

## Pentobarbital Calcium *(BANM, rINNM)*

Pentobarbital cálcico; Pentobarbitone Calcium. Calcium 5-ethyl-5-(1-methylbutyl)barbiturate.
$(C_{11}H_{17}N_2O_3)_2Ca$ = 490.6.
*ATC — N05CA01.*

**Pharmacopoeias.** In *Jpn.*

## Pentobarbital Sodium *(BANM, rINNM)*

Aethaminalum-Natrium; Ethaminal Sodium; Mebumalnatrium; Pentobarbital sódico; Pentobarbitalum Natricum; Pentobarbitone Sodium; Sodium Pentobarbital; Soluble Pentobarbitone. Sodium 5-ethyl-5-(1-methylbutyl)barbiturate.
$C_{11}H_{17}N_2NaO_3$ = 248.3.
*CAS — 57-33-0.*
*ATC — N05CA01.*

**Pharmacopoeias.** In *Eur.* (see p.vi) and *US.*

**Ph. Eur. 5.0** (Pentobarbital Sodium). A white, hygroscopic, crystalline powder. Very soluble in water. A 10% solution in water has a pH of 9.6 to 11.0 when freshly prepared. Store in airtight containers.

**USP 27** (Pentobarbital Sodium). White, crystalline granules or white powder. Is odourless or has a slight characteristic odour. Very soluble in water; freely soluble in alcohol; practically insoluble in ether. pH of a 10% solution in water is between 9.8 and 11.0. Solutions decompose on standing, the decomposition being accelerated at higher temperatures. Store in airtight containers.

**Incompatibility.** Pentobarbital may be precipitated from preparations containing pentobarbital sodium, depending on the concentration and pH. Pentobarbital sodium has, therefore, been reported to be incompatible with many other drugs particularly acids and acidic salts.

### Dependence and Withdrawal

As for Amobarbital, p.670.

### Adverse Effects, Treatment, and Precautions

As for Amobarbital, p.670.

### Interactions

As for Amobarbital, p.670.

### Pharmacokinetics

Following oral or rectal administration pentobarbital is well absorbed from the gastrointestinal tract, and is reported to be about 60 to 70% bound to plasma protein. The elimination half-life appears to be dose dependent and reported values have ranged from 15 to 50 hours. Pentobarbital is metabolised in the liver, mainly by hydroxylation, and excreted in the urine mainly as metabolites.

### Uses and Administration

Pentobarbital is a barbiturate that has been used as a hypnotic and sedative. It has general properties and uses similar to those of amobarbital (p.670). It has been used as a sedative and in the short-term management of insomnia (p.667) but barbiturates are not considered appropriate for such purposes. Pentobarbital sodium, given orally or by deep intramuscular or slow intravenous injection, has been used for premedication in anaesthetic procedures (p.1296), but the use of barbiturates for pre-operative sedation has been replaced by other drugs. Pentobarbital is usually given as the sodium salt, although pentobarbital itself and its calcium salt have both been used.

A usual dose of pentobarbital sodium given at night for insomnia is 100 mg by mouth or up to 200 mg rectally. A dose of 20 mg of the sodium salt has been given by mouth 3 or 4 times daily as a sedative; alternatively, 30 mg has been given rectally 2 to 4 times daily.

**Cerebrovascular disorders.** For reference to the use of barbiturate-induced coma in the management of patients with cerebral ischaemia, see p.1310. See also p.833 for reference to the use of barbiturates in the management of raised intracranial pressure.

**Status epilepticus.** Anaesthesia in conjunction with assisted ventilation may be instituted to control refractory tonic-clonic status epilepticus (p.352). A short-acting barbiturate such as thiopental is usually used, but pentobarbital has been used similarly.

### Preparations

***BP 2003:*** Pentobarbital Tablets;
***USP 27:*** Pentobarbital Elixir; Pentobarbital Sodium Capsules; Pentobarbital Sodium Injection.

**Proprietary Preparations** (details are given in Part 3)
***Braz.:*** Hypnol†; ***Canad.:*** Nembutal; Nova Rectal†; ***Hong Kong:*** Nembutal; ***Thai.:*** Nembutal; ***USA:*** Nembutal.

**Multi-ingredient:** ***Arg.:*** Dimaval; ***Canad.:*** Cafergot-PB; ***USA:*** Cafatine-PB.

## Perazine Dimalonate

P-725 (perazine); Pemazine Dimalonate; Perazina, dimalonato de. 10-[3-(4-Methylpiperazin-1-yl)propyl]phenothiazine dimalonate.
$C_{20}H_{25}N_3S,2C_3H_4O_4$ = 547.6.
*CAS — 84-97-9 (perazine); 14777-25-4 (perazine dimalonate).*
*ATC — N05AB10.*

**Pharmacopoeias.** *Pol.* includes only an injection of the dimalonate. It also includes a monograph for Perazine Dimaleate.

### Profile

Perazine dimalonate is a phenothiazine with general properties similar to those of chlorpromazine (p.675) and is used for the treatment of psychotic conditions. It has a piperazine side-chain. It is given by mouth as the dimalonate although doses are expressed in terms of the base; perazine dimalonate 40.3 mg is approximately equivalent to perazine base 25 mg. Usual doses are the equivalent of 50 to 600 mg of the base daily; up to 1000 mg daily has been given in resistant cases. It may also be given intramuscularly.

**Adverse effects.** A report of 5 patients receiving perazine dimalonate who developed acute axonal neuropathies of superficial nerve fibres after exposure to sunlight.[1]

1. Roelcke U, *et al.* Acute neuropathy in perazine-treated patients after sun exposure. *Lancet* 1992; **340:** 729–30.

### Preparations

**Proprietary Preparations** (details are given in Part 3)
**Ger.:** Taxilan; **Neth.:** Taxilan†.

## Pericyazine *(BAN)*

Periciazine *(pINN)*; Periciazina; Propericiazine; RP-8909; SKF-20716. 10-[3-(4-Hydroxypiperidino)propyl]phenothiazine-2-carbonitrile; 1-[3-(2-Cyanophenothiazin-10-yl)propyl]piperidin-4-ol.

$C_{21}H_{23}N_3OS$ = 365.5.
*CAS — 2622-26-6.*
*ATC — N05AC01.*

### Adverse Effects, Treatment, and Precautions

As for Chlorpromazine, p.675. Sedation and orthostatic hypotension may be marked.

### Interactions

As for Chlorpromazine, p.679.

### Uses and Administration

Pericyazine is a phenothiazine with general properties similar to those of chlorpromazine (p.680). It has a piperidine side-chain. It is used in the treatment of various psychoses including schizophrenia (p.665) and disturbed behaviour (p.665), and in the short-term management of severe anxiety (p.663).

Pericyazine is usually given as the base but the mesilate and tartrate have also been used.

The usual dose by mouth for the treatment of severe anxiety, agitation, aggression, or impulsive behaviour is 15 to 30 mg daily given in 2 divided doses, the larger amount in the evening. In schizophrenia and severe psychoses initial doses of 75 mg daily may be given in divided doses, increased if necessary, at weekly intervals by steps of 25 mg, to a maximum of 300 mg daily.

A recommended initial daily dose by mouth in children over one year is 500 micrograms for a child of 10 kg; for heavier children this initial dose may be increased by 1 mg for each additional 5 kg, to a maximum total of 10 mg daily. Thereafter the dose may be gradually increased according to response but the daily maintenance dose should not exceed twice the initial dose.

Elderly subjects should be given reduced doses: a recommended initial dose is 5 to 10 mg daily for anxiety or behaviour disorders and 15 to 30 mg daily for schizophrenia or psychosis, both in divided doses.

### Preparations

**Proprietary Preparations** (details are given in Part 3)
**Arg.:** Neuleptil; **Austral.:** Neulactil; **Austria:** Neuleptil; **Belg.:** Neuleptil†; **Braz.:** Neuleptil; **Canad.:** Neuleptil; **Chile:** Neuleptil; **Denm.:** Neulactil; **Fin.:** Neulactil; **Fr.:** Neuleptil; **Hong Kong:** Neulactil; **Irl.:** Neulactil; **Israel:** Neuleptil; **Ital.:** Neuleptil; **Neth.:** Neuleptil; **Norw.:** Neulactil†; **NZ:** Neulactil; **S.Afr.:** Neulactil; **Spain:** Nemactil; **Switz.:** Neuleptil†; **UK:** Neulactil.

## Perospirone Hydrochloride *(rINNM)*

SM-9018. *cis*-N-{4-[4-(1,2-Benzisothiazol-3-yl)-1-piperazinyl]butyl}-1,2-cyclohexanedicarboximide hydrochloride.

$C_{23}H_{30}N_4O_2S,HCl$ = 463.0.
*CAS — 150915-41-6 (perospirone); 129273-38-7 (perospirone hydrochloride).*

### Profile

Perospirone is an atypical antipsychotic used in the treatment of schizophrenia. Perospirone hydrochloride is given by mouth. Usual doses range from 12 to 48 mg daily given in 3 divided doses.

◊ References.

1. Onrust SV, McClellan K. Perospirone. *CNS Drugs.* 2001; **15:** 329–37.

### Preparations

**Proprietary Preparations** (details are given in Part 3)
**Jpn:** Lullan.

## Perphenazine *(BAN, rINN)*

Perfenazina; Perphenazinum. 2-{4-[3-(2-Chlorophenothiazin-10-yl)propyl]piperazin-1-yl}ethanol.

$C_{21}H_{26}ClN_3OS$ = 404.0.
*CAS — 58-39-9.*
*ATC — N05AB03.*

**Pharmacopoeias.** In *Chin., Eur.* (see p.vi), *Jpn, Pol.,* and *US. Jpn* also includes the maleate.

**Ph. Eur. 5.0** (Perphenazine). A white or yellowish-white crystalline powder. Practically insoluble in water; soluble in alcohol; freely soluble in dichloromethane; dissolves in dilute solutions of hydrochloric acid. Protect from light.

**USP 27** (Perphenazine). A white to creamy-white odourless powder. M.p. 94° to 100°. Practically insoluble in water; soluble 1 in 7 of alcohol and 1 in 13 of acetone; freely soluble in chloroform. Store in airtight containers. Protect from light.

**Incompatibility.** Perphenazine has been reported to be incompatible with cefoperazone sodium[1] and with midazolam hydrochloride (see p.707).

1. Gasca M, *et al.* Visual compatibility of perphenazine with various antimicrobials during simulated Y-site injection. *Am J Hosp Pharm* 1987; **44:** 574–5.

## Perphenazine Decanoate *(BANM, rINNM)*

Decanoato de perfenazina. 2-{4-[3-(2-Chlorophenothiazin-10-yl)propyl]piperazin-1-yl}ethyl decanoate.

$C_{31}H_{44}ClN_3O_2S$ = 558.2.
*ATC — N05AB03.*

## Perphenazine Enantate *(BANM, rINNM)*

Enantato de perfenazina; Perphenazine Enanthate; Perphenazine Heptanoate. 2-{4-[3-(2-Chlorophenothiazin-10-yl)propyl]piperazin-1-yl}ethyl heptanoate.

$C_{28}H_{38}ClN_3O_2S$ = 516.1.
*CAS — 17528-28-8.*
*ATC — N05AB03.*

### Adverse Effects, Treatment, and Precautions

As for Chlorpromazine, p.675. Perphenazine has been associated with a lower frequency of sedation, but a higher incidence of extrapyramidal symptoms.

**Breast feeding.** The American Academy of Pediatrics[1] considers that, although the effect of perphenazine on breast-feeding infants is unknown, its use by mothers during breast feeding may be of concern since antipsychotics do appear in breast milk and thus could conceivably alter CNS function in the infant both in the short and long term.

The distribution of perphenazine into breast milk was studied[2] in a mother who was receiving perphenazine 24 mg daily, later reduced to 16 mg daily, by mouth. Breast feeding was started after it was estimated that a breast-fed infant would ingest about 0.1% of a maternal dose. Treatment with perphenazine lasted for 3.5 months and during this period the child thrived normally and no drug-induced symptoms were seen.

1. American Academy of Pediatrics. The transfer of drugs and other chemicals into human milk. *Pediatrics* 2001; **108:** 776–89. Correction. *ibid.*; 1029. Also available at: http://aappolicy.aappublications.org/cgi/content/full/pediatrics%3b108/3/776 (accessed 28/04/04)
2. Olesen OV, *et al.* Perphenazine in breast milk and serum. *Am J Psychiatry* 1990; **147:** 1378–9.

### Interactions

As for Chlorpromazine, p.679.

### Pharmacokinetics

Perphenazine is well absorbed following oral administration and undergoes some first-pass metabolism, resulting in a relative bioavailability of about 60 to 80%. It is widely distributed and crosses the placenta. Perphenazine is extensively metabolised; up to 70% is excreted in the urine mainly as metabolites, with about 5% being excreted in the faeces. Perphenazine decanoate and perphenazine enantate are slowly absorbed from the site of intramuscular injection. They gradually release perphenazine into the body and are therefore suitable for use as depot injections.

◊ Perphenazine 5 or 6 mg given intravenously had a plasma half-life from 8.4 to 12.3 hours in a study of 4 schizophrenic patients and 4 healthy subjects.[1] Considerable fluctuations in plasma-perphenazine concentrations were observed 3 to 5 hours after administration before the exponential elimination phase. Plasma concentrations were undetectable after a 6-mg oral dose in 4 healthy subjects and only low plasma concentrations of its sulfoxide metabolite could be detected; this was attributed to a marked first-pass effect. Systemic availability was variable and poor in 4 schizophrenic patients given perphenazine 12 mg three times daily. However, it was considered that oral therapy should be on an 8-hour dosage regimen. Intramuscular injection of perphenazine enantate 50 or 100 mg every 2 weeks gave plasma-perphenazine concentrations similar to those after continuous oral administration but with a high initial absorption within 2 to 3 days associated with the most serious CNS adverse effects.

1. Hansen CE, *et al.* Clinical pharmacokinetic studies of perphenazine. *Br J Clin Pharmacol* 1976; **3:** 915–23.

**Metabolism.** In a study in 12 healthy subjects there was a clear difference in the disposition of a single oral dose of perphenazine between poor and extensive hydroxylators of debrisoquine.[1]

1. Dahl-Puustinen M-L, *et al.* Disposition of perphenazine is related to polymorphic debrisoquin hydroxylation in human beings. *Clin Pharmacol Ther* 1989; **46:** 78–81.

### Uses and Administration

Perphenazine is a phenothiazine with general properties similar to those of chlorpromazine (p.680). It has a piperazine side-chain. It is used in the treatment of various psychoses including schizophrenia (p.665) and mania (see Bipolar Disorder, p.278) as well as disturbed behaviour (p.665) and in the short-term, adjunctive management of severe anxiety (p.663). Perphenazine is also used for the management of postoperative or chemotherapy-induced nausea and vomiting (p.1245) and for the treatment of intractable hiccup (p.682).

Perphenazine is usually given as the base by mouth and sometimes by intramuscular or intravenous injection. Long-acting decanoate or enantate esters of perphenazine, available in some countries, are given by intramuscular injection.

The usual initial dose for the treatment of **schizophrenia, mania, and other psychoses** is 4 mg three times daily by mouth. The dose is adjusted according to response up to a usual maximum of 24 mg daily although up to 64 mg daily has occasionally been used in hospitalised patients. Similar doses have been used for the management of **severe agitated or violent behaviour** or in **severe anxiety**. Perphenazine has sometimes been used in preparations with tricyclic antidepressants such as amitriptyline in the treatment of anxiety with depression.

For the **control of nausea and vomiting** the usual dose by mouth is 4 mg three times daily but up to 8 mg three times daily may be required.

Perphenazine may be given by *intramuscular injection* for control of acute psychotic symptoms or for severe nausea and vomiting. An initial dose of 5 or 10 mg is followed, if necessary, by 5 mg every 6 hours to a maximum of 15 to 30 mg daily.

Perphenazine, diluted to a concentration of 500 micrograms/mL in sodium chloride 0.9%, is occasionally given by *intravenous injection* in divided doses, not more than 1 mg being administered every 1 to 2 minutes; the maximum intravenous dose is 5 mg. The intravenous route of administration is usually reserved for the control of severe vomiting or intractable hiccup. Perphenazine has also been given by continuous infusion.

The long-acting decanoate or enantate esters of perphenazine are administered by deep intramuscular injection in doses ranging from about 50 to 300 mg of ester given at intervals of 2 to 4 weeks.

Elderly subjects should be given reduced doses of perphenazine or its esters but it should be noted that perphenazine is not indicated for the management of agitation and restlessness in the elderly.

### Preparations

**BP 2003:** Perphenazine Tablets;
**USP 27:** Perphenazine and Amitriptyline Hydrochloride Tablets; Perphenazine Injection; Perphenazine Oral Solution; Perphenazine Syrup; Perphenazine Tablets.

**Proprietary Preparations** (details are given in Part 3)
**Austria:** Decentan; **Belg.:** Trilafon; **Canad.:** Trilafon; **Denm.:** Trilafon; **Fin.:** Peratsin; **Fr.:** Trilifan; **Ger.:** Decentan; **Irl.:** Fentazin†; **Israel:** Perphenan; **Ital.:** Trilafon; **Mex.:** Leptopsique; Trilafon; Zerfenazin†; **Neth.:** Trilafon; **Norw.:** Trilafon; **S.Afr.:** Trilafon; **Spain:** Decentan; **Swed.:** Trilafon; **Switz.:** Trilafon; **Thai.:** Conazine; Pernamed; Pernazine; Perzine; Porazine; **UK:** Fentazin; **USA:** Trilafon.

**Multi-ingredient: Arg.:** Karile; Mutabon D; **Canad.:** Elavil Plus†; Etrafon†; PMS-Levazine†; Triavil; **Chile:** Mutabon D; **Fin.:** Pertriptyl; **Gr.:** Minitran; **Irl.:** Triptafen†; **Ital.:** Mutabon; **Mex.:** Adepsique; **Port.:** Mutabon; **S.Afr.:** Etrafon; **Spain:** Mutabase; **Thai.:** Anxipress-D; Neuragon; **UK:** Triptafen; **USA:** Etrafon; Triavil.

### Phenazepam

Fenazepam. 7-Bromo-5-(2-chlorophenyl)-1,3-dihydro-2*H*-1,4-benzodiazepin-2-one.

$C_{15}H_{10}BrClN_2O$ = 349.6.

*CAS — 51753-57-2.*

### Profile

Phenazepam is a benzodiazepine with general properties similar to those of diazepam (p.690). It is used in the short-term treatment of anxiety disorders and as an anticonvulsant.

---

### Phenprobamate *(BAN, rINN)*

Fenprobamato; MH-532; Proformiphen. 3-Phenylpropyl carbamate.

$C_{10}H_{13}NO_2$ = 179.2.

*CAS — 673-31-4.*

*ATC — M03BA01.*

### Profile

Phenprobamate is a carbamate with general properties similar to those of meprobamate (p.706). It has been used for its anxiolytic and muscle relaxant actions.

### Preparations

**Proprietary Preparations** (details are given in Part 3)

**Multi-ingredient:** ***Switz.:*** Dolo-Prolixan†.

---

## Pimozide *(BAN, USAN, rINN)*

McN-JR-6238; Pimozida; Pimozidum; R-6238. 1-{1-[4,4-Bis(4-fluorophenyl)butyl]-4-piperidyl}benzimidazolin-2-one; 1-{1-[3-(4,4′-Difluorobenzhydryl)propyl]-4-piperidyl}benzimidazolin-2-one.

$C_{28}H_{29}F_2N_3O$ = 461.5.

*CAS — 2062-78-4.*

*ATC — N05AG02.*

**Pharmacopoeias.** In *Eur.* (see p.vi), *Pol.,* and *US.*

**Ph. Eur. 5.0** (Pimozide). A white or almost white powder. Practically insoluble in water; slightly soluble in alcohol; soluble in dichloromethane; sparingly soluble in methyl alcohol. Protect from light.

**USP 27** (Pimozide). A white crystalline powder. Insoluble in water; soluble 1 in 1000 of alcohol, of ether, and of methyl alcohol, 1 in 100 of acetone, 1 in 10 of chloroform, and 1 in more than 1000 of 0.1N hydrochloric acid. Store in airtight containers. Protect from light.

### Adverse Effects, Treatment, and Precautions

As for Chlorpromazine, p.675.

Extrapyramidal symptoms may be more common than with chlorpromazine, whereas pimozide may be less likely to cause sedation, hypotension, or antimuscarinic effects.

Ventricular arrhythmias and other ECG abnormalities, such as prolongation of the QT interval and T-wave changes, have been associated with the use of pimozide; an ECG should therefore be performed before treatment and repeated annually or earlier if indicated. In the UK, periodic assessment of cardiac function is recommended for patients receiving more than 16 mg daily. If repolarisation changes appear or arrhythmias develop, the need for continuing treatment with pimozide should be reviewed; at the very least dose reduction and close supervision are advised. Pimozide is contra-indicated in patients with pre-existing prolongation of the QT interval, or a family history of congenital QT prolongation, and in patients with a history of cardiac arrhythmias. Electrolyte disturbances such as hypokalaemia or hypomagnesaemia in patients receiving pimozide may lead to cardiotoxicity.

**Effects on the cardiovascular system.** The UK Committee on Safety of Medicines (CSM) has received reports of ventricular arrhythmias and other ECG abnormalities such as prolongation of the QT interval and T-wave changes associated with the use of pimozide.[1,2] In August 1990 they had received 13 reports of sudden unexpected death since 1971; many of these patients had no evidence of pre-existing cardiac disease, and 7 were under 30 years of age. Five of the 13 were also taking other antipsychotics. Most cases were associated with doses greater than 20 mg daily and many had had the dose increased rapidly, possibly resulting in substantial tissue accumulation. By February 1995 the CSM had received a total of 40 reports (16 fatal) of serious cardiac reactions most of which involved arrhythmias.

See also under Chlorpromazine, p.676.

1. Committee on Safety of Medicines. Cardiotoxic effects of pimozide. *Current Problems 29* 1990.
2. Committee on Safety of Medicines/Medicines Control Agency. Cardiac arrhythmias with pimozide (Orap). *Current Problems* 1995; **21:** 2.

### Interactions

As for Chlorpromazine, p.679. The risk of arrhythmias with pimozide may be increased by other drugs that prolong the QT interval including some antiarrhythmics, other antipsychotics (including depot preparations), tricyclic antidepressants, the antihistamines terfenadine and astemizole, antimalarials, and cisapride; concomitant use should be avoided. Use with drugs that induce electrolyte disturbances, such as diuretics, should also be avoided.

The concomitant use of drugs that inhibit the cytochrome P450 isoenzyme CYP3A4 is contra-indicated; the resultant decrease in the metabolism of pimozide may lead to increased plasma concentrations and hence greater risk of cardiac arrhythmias. CYP3A4 inhibitors include the macrolide antibacterials such as clarithromycin, erythromycin, and troleandomycin; the azole antifungals including itraconazole and ketoconazole; the HIV-protease inhibitors ritonavir, saquinavir, indinavir, and nelfinavir; nefazodone, and zileuton. The metabolism of pimozide may also be inhibited by grapefruit juice and concomitant use should be avoided.

Pimozide is also metabolised by CYP2D6, albeit to a lesser extent, and *in vitro* data indicate that the CYP2D6 inhibitor quinidine may reduce the metabolism of pimozide; the UK manufacturers contra-indicate the use of such inhibitors with pimozide. The isoenzyme CYP1A2 may also be involved in the metabolism of pimozide and consequently there is a theoretical possibility of interactions with CYP1A2 inhibitors.

**Antibacterials.** Two sudden deaths have occurred in patients on high-dose pimozide treatment when *clarithromycin* was also given. In a study[1] in healthy volunteers elevated pimozide plasma concentrations were recorded after pretreatment with clarithromycin.

1. Desta Z, *et al.* Effect of clarithromycin on the pharmacokinetics and pharmacodynamics of pimozide in healthy poor and extensive metabolisers of cytochrome P450 2D6 (CYP2D6). *Clin Pharmacol Ther* 1999; **65:** 10–20.

### Pharmacokinetics

Following oral administration, more than half of a dose of pimozide is reported to be absorbed. It undergoes significant first-pass metabolism. Peak plasma concentrations have been reported after 4 to 12 hours and there is a considerable interindividual variation in the concentrations achieved. Pimozide is metabolised in the liver mainly by *N*-dealkylation and excreted in the urine and faeces, both unchanged and in the form of metabolites. Metabolism is mediated mainly by the cytochrome P450 isoenzyme CYP3A4 and to a lesser extent by CYP2D6; CYP1A2 may also be involved. Pimozide has a long terminal half-life generally considered to be about 55 hours, although half-lives of up to 150 hours have been noted in some patients.

### Uses and Administration

Pimozide is a diphenylbutylpiperidine antipsychotic and is structurally similar to the butyrophenones. It is a long-acting antipsychotic with general properties similar to those of the phenothiazine, chlorpromazine (p.680), although it also has some calcium-blocking activity. Pimozide is given by mouth in the management of psychoses including schizophrenia, paranoid states, and monosymptomatic hypochondria (p.664) and in Tourette's syndrome. An ECG should be performed in all patients before starting treatment with pimozide (see Adverse Effects, Treatment, and Precautions, above).

For **schizophrenia**, treatment is usually initiated with a dose of 2 mg daily adjusted thereafter according to response in increments of 2 to 4 mg at intervals of not less than one week. A maximum daily dose of 20 mg should not be exceeded. It is usually given as a single daily dose.

In **monosymptomatic hypochondria** and **paranoid psychoses** the initial dose is 4 mg daily adjusted as above to a maximum daily dose of 16 mg.

For the treatment of **Tourette's syndrome** an initial dose of 1 to 2 mg daily is recommended, increased to a maximum of 10 mg daily or 200 micrograms/kg daily.

Pimozide treatment should start at half the standard dosage in elderly patients.

**Chorea.** Antipsychotics such as pimozide have some action against choreiform movements (p.664) as well as being of use to control the behavioural disturbances of Huntington's chorea.

References.

1. Shannon KM, Fenichel GM. Pimozide treatment of Sydenham's chorea. *Neurology* 1990; **40:** 186.

**Dystonia.** Antipsychotics such as phenothiazines, haloperidol, or pimozide are sometimes useful in the treatment of idiopathic dystonia (p.1209) in patients who have failed to respond to other drugs.[1] In very severe dystonia combination therapy may be required. Pimozide in gradually increasing doses up to 12 mg daily with tetrabenazine and trihexyphenidyl is sometimes effective. However, antipsychotics often act non-specifically and there is the risk of adding drug-induced extrapyramidal disorders to the dystonia being treated (see Extrapyramidal Disorders under Adverse Effects of Chlorpromazine, p.677).

1. Marsden CD, Quinn NP. The dystonias. *BMJ* 1990; **300:** 139–44.

**Schizophrenia.** A systematic review[1] concluded that pimozide appears to be of similar efficacy to other classical antipsychotics in the treatment of schizophrenia (p.665). There was no evidence that it was particularly useful for those with delusional disorders or with predominantly negative symptoms.

1. Sultana A, McMonagle T. Pimozide for schizophrenia or related psychoses. Available in The Cochrane Library; Issue 2. Chichester: John Wiley; 2004.

**Taste disorders.** For reference to the use of pimozide in the treatment of taste disorders, see Chlorpromazine, p.682.

**Tourette's syndrome.** Tourette's syndrome (p.664) is a disorder characterised by motor and vocal tics and behavioural disturbances. Many patients with Tourette's syndrome do not require medication but when treatment is needed dopamine antagonists such as the antipsychotics haloperidol or pimozide[1,2] have been most commonly used. They often decrease the frequency and severity of tics and may improve any accompanying behavioural disturbances. However, superiority of either drug in terms of efficacy or adverse effects has not been clearly demonstrated. Because of the potential for acute and long-term adverse effects it is usually recommended that doses are titrated to as low as possible; the aim of treatment is not necessarily to control symptoms completely. Medication can often be discontinued after a few years.

1. Shapiro E, *et al.* Controlled study of haloperidol, pimozide, and placebo for the treatment of Gilles de la Tourette's syndrome. *Arch Gen Psychiatry* 1989; **46:** 722–30.
2. Sallee FR, *et al.* Relative efficacy of haloperidol and pimozide in children and adolescents with Tourette's disorder. *Am J Psychiatry* 1997; **154:** 1057–62.

### Preparations

***BP 2003:*** Pimozide Tablets;
***USP 27:*** Pimozide Tablets.

**Proprietary Preparations** (details are given in Part 3)

***Arg.:*** Orap; ***Austral.:*** Orap; ***Austria:*** Orap; ***Belg.:*** Orap; ***Braz.:*** Orap; ***Canad.:*** Orap; ***Chile:*** Orap; ***Denm.:*** Orap; ***Fr.:*** Orap; ***Ger.:*** Antalon†; Orap; ***Gr.:*** Pirium; ***Hong Kong:*** Orap; ***India:*** Orap; ***Irl.:*** Orap; ***Israel:*** Orap; ***Ital.:*** Orap; ***Jpn:*** Orap; ***Neth.:*** Orap; ***Norw.:*** Orap†; ***NZ:*** Orap; ***S.Afr.:*** Orap; ***Singapore:*** Orap†; ***Spain:*** Orap; ***Swed.:*** Orap†; ***Switz.:*** Orap†; ***Thai.:*** Orap; Pizide; ***UK:*** Orap; ***USA:*** Orap.

---

### Pinazepam *(rINN)*

7-Chloro-1,3-dihydro-5-phenyl-1-(prop-2-ynyl)-2*H*-1,4-benzodiazepin-2-one.

$C_{18}H_{13}ClN_2O$ = 308.8.

*CAS — 52463-83-9.*

*ATC — N05BA14.*

### Profile

Pinazepam is a long-acting benzodiazepine with general properties similar to those of diazepam (p.690). It is given by mouth in doses of 5 to 20 mg daily in divided doses for the short-term treatment of anxiety disorders (p.663). Doses of 2.5 to 5 mg at night have been used in the treatment of insomnia (p.667).

### Preparations

**Proprietary Preparations** (details are given in Part 3)

***Hong Kong:*** Domar; ***Ital.:*** Domar; ***Singapore:*** Domar; ***Spain:*** Duna; ***Thai.:*** Domar.

---

## Pipamperone (BAN, USAN, rINN)

Floropipamide; McN-JR-3345; R-3345. 1-[3-(4-Fluorobenzoyl)propyl]-4-piperidinopiperidine-4-carboxamide.
$C_{21}H_{30}FN_3O_2$ = 375.5.
*CAS — 1893-33-0.*
*ATC — N05AD05.*

## Pipamperone Hydrochloride (BANM, rINNM)

Hidrocloruro de pipamperona.
$C_{21}H_{30}FN_3O_2,2HCl$ = 448.4.
*CAS — 2448-68-2.*
*ATC — N05AD05.*

### Profile

Pipamperone is a butyrophenone with general properties similar to those of haloperidol (p.701). It is given by mouth as the hydrochloride for the treatment of psychoses. Doses are expressed in terms of the base; pipamperone hydrochloride 47.8 mg is approximately equivalent to 40 mg of pipamperone. Starting doses equivalent to 20 mg of the base have been given daily, increased gradually thereafter according to response; doses of 360 mg or more have been given daily in divided doses.

### Preparations

**Proprietary Preparations** (details are given in Part 3)
***Belg.:*** Dipiperon; ***Denm.:*** Dipiperon; ***Fr.:*** Dipiperon; ***Ger.:*** Dipiperon; ***Gr.:*** Dipiperon R-3345; ***Ital.:*** Piperonil; ***Neth.:*** Dipiperon; ***Switz.:*** Dipiperon.

## Piperacetazine (USAN, rINN)

PC-1421; Piperacetazina. 10-{3-[4-(2-Hydroxyethyl)piperidino]propyl}phenothiazin-2-yl methyl ketone.
$C_{24}H_{30}N_2O_2S$ = 410.6.
*CAS — 3819-00-9.*

### Profile

Piperacetazine is a phenothiazine antipsychotic that has been used as a sedative in veterinary medicine.

## Pipotiazine (BAN, rINN)

Pipothiazine; Pipotiazina; RP-19366. 10-{3-[4-(2-Hydroxyethyl)piperidino]propyl}-*NN*-dimethylphenothiazine-2-sulphonamide; 2-{4-[3-(2-Dimethylsulphamoylphenothiazin-10-yl)propyl]piperazin-1-yl}ethanol.
$C_{24}H_{33}N_3O_3S_2$ = 475.7.
*CAS — 39860-99-6.*
*ATC — N05AC04.*

## Pipotiazine Palmitate (BANM, USAN, rINNM)

IL-19552; Palmitato de pipotiazina; Pipothiazine Palmitate; RP-19552.
$C_{40}H_{63}N_3O_4S_2$ = 714.1.
*CAS — 37517-26-3.*
*ATC — N05AC04.*

### Adverse Effects, Treatment, and Precautions

As for Chlorpromazine, p.675.

**Effects on mental function.** Manic symptoms developed in a schizophrenic patient following administration of pipotiazine palmitate. Symptoms recurred on subsequent rechallenge.[1]

1. Singh AN, Maguire J. Pipothiazine palmitate induced mania. *BMJ* 1984; **289:** 734.

### Pharmacokinetics

Pipotiazine palmitate is very slowly absorbed from the site of intramuscular injection. It gradually releases pipotiazine into the body and is therefore suitable for use as a depot injection.

### Uses and Administration

Pipotiazine is a phenothiazine with general properties similar to those of chlorpromazine (p.680). It has a piperidine side-chain. It is used in the treatment of schizophrenia (p.665) and other psychoses. Pipotiazine is given by mouth as the base and by deep intramuscular injection as the palmitate ester; oral doses are expressed as the base and parenteral doses are expressed as the ester.

A usual oral dose of pipotiazine for the treatment of psychoses is 5 to 20 mg daily in a single dose; in severe psychoses higher doses have been given for brief periods.

The long-acting palmitate ester of pipotiazine is given by deep intramuscular injection. An initial test dose of 25 mg is followed by a further 25 to 50 mg after 4 to 7 days. The dosage is then adjusted in increments of 25 to 50 mg according to response at intervals of 4 weeks. Usual maintenance doses of 50 to 100 mg are given at average intervals of 4 weeks; the maximum recommended dose is 200 mg every 4 weeks.

Pipotiazine should be given in reduced dosage to elderly patients; a starting dose of 5 to 10 mg has been suggested for pipotiazine palmitate intramuscular injections.

**Schizophrenia.** A systematic review[1] concluded that depot pipotiazine palmitate appeared to be no different in terms of efficacy or adverse effects to other antipsychotics given orally or by depot injection.

1. Quraishi S, David A. Depot pipothiazine palmitate and undecylenate for schizophrenia. Available in The Cochrane Library; Issue 2. Chichester: John Wiley; 2004.

### Preparations

**Proprietary Preparations** (details are given in Part 3)
***Arg.:*** Piportyl L4; ***Belg.:*** Piportil†; ***Braz.:*** Piportil; ***Canad.:*** Piportil L4; ***Chile:*** Piportyl; ***Fr.:*** Piportil; ***Hong Kong:*** Piportil†; ***Irl.:*** Piportil; ***Mex.:*** Piportil L4; ***Neth.:*** Piportil; ***NZ:*** Piportil; ***Singapore:*** Piportil; ***Spain:*** Lonseren; ***Switz.:*** Piportil†; ***UK:*** Piportil.

## Prazepam (BAN, USAN, rINN)

Prazepamum; W-4020. 7-Chloro-1-(cyclopropylmethyl)-1,3-dihydro-5-phenyl-2*H*-1,4-benzodiazepin-2-one.
$C_{19}H_{17}ClN_2O$ = 324.8.
*CAS — 2955-38-6.*
*ATC — N05BA11.*

**Pharmacopoeias.** In *Eur.* (see p.vi) and *Jpn*.

**Ph. Eur. 5.0** (Prazepam). A white to almost white crystalline powder. Practically insoluble in water; sparingly soluble in dehydrated alcohol; freely soluble in dichloromethane. Protect from light.

### Profile

Prazepam is a long-acting benzodiazepine with general properties similar to those of diazepam (p.690). After oral administration, prazepam undergoes extensive first-pass metabolism in the liver to oxazepam (p.712) and desmethyldiazepam (nordazepam, p.710). Desmethyldiazepam is largely responsible for the pharmacological activity of prazepam. The usual dose by mouth for the short-term treatment of anxiety disorders (p.663) is 30 mg daily as a single nightly dose or in divided doses; in severe conditions up to 60 mg daily has been given. In elderly or debilitated patients, treatment should be initiated with a daily dose of no more than 15 mg.

**Breast feeding.** The American Academy of Pediatrics[1] considers that, although the effect of prazepam on breast-feeding infants is unknown, its use by mothers during breast feeding may be of concern since anxiolytic drugs do appear in breast milk and thus could conceivably alter CNS function in the infant both in the short and long term.

The ratio of desmethyldiazepam in plasma to that in breast milk of 5 lactating women given prazepam 20 mg three times daily for 3 days was 9.6 from measurements 12 hours after the last dose.[2] It was estimated that a breast-fed infant of a mother on continuous prazepam therapy would ingest the equivalent of about 4% of the daily maternal dose.

1. American Academy of Pediatrics. The transfer of drugs and other chemicals into human milk. *Pediatrics* 2001; **108:** 776–89. Correction. *ibid.*; 1029. Also available at: http://aappolicy.aappublications.org/cgi/content/full/pediatrics%3b108/3/776 (accessed 28/04/04)
2. Brodie RR, *et al.* Concentrations of N-descyclopropylmethylprazepam in whole-blood, plasma, and milk after administration of prazepam to humans. *Biopharm Drug Dispos* 1981; **2:** 59–68.

**Pharmacokinetics.** References.

1. Ochs HR, *et al.* Comparative single-dose kinetics of oxazolam, prazepam, and clorazepate: three precursors of desmethyldiazepam. *J Clin Pharmacol* 1984; **24:** 446–51.

**Porphyria.** Prazepam is considered to be unsafe in patients with porphyria because it has been shown to be porphyrinogenic in *in-vitro* systems.

### Preparations

**Proprietary Preparations** (details are given in Part 3)
***Austria:*** Demetrin; ***Belg.:*** Lysanxia; ***Fr.:*** Lysanxia; ***Ger.:*** Demetrin; Mono Demetrin; ***Gr.:*** Centrac; ***Irl.:*** Centrax; ***Ital.:*** Prazene; Trepidan; ***Neth.:*** Reapam; ***Port.:*** Demetrin; ***S.Afr.:*** Demetrin; ***Switz.:*** Demetrin; ***Thai.:*** Pozapam; Prasepine.

# Prochlorperazine (BAN, rINN)

Chlormeprazine; Prochlorpemazine; Proclorperazina. 2-Chloro-10-[3-(4-methylpiperazin-1-yl)propyl]phenothiazine.
$C_{20}H_{24}ClN_3S$ = 373.9.
*CAS — 58-38-8.*
*ATC — N05AB04.*

**Pharmacopoeias.** In *US.*

**USP 27** (Prochlorperazine). A clear, pale yellow, viscous liquid, sensitive to light. Very slightly soluble in water; freely soluble in alcohol, in chloroform, and in ether. Store in airtight containers. Protect from light.

## Prochlorperazine Edisilate (BANM, rINNM)

Chlormeprazine Edisylate; Edisilato de proclorperazina; Prochlorpemazine Edisylate; Prochlorperazine Edisylate; Prochlorperazine Ethanedisulphonate. Prochlorperazine ethane-1,2-disulphonate.
$C_{20}H_{24}ClN_3S,C_2H_6O_6S_2$ = 564.1.
*CAS — 1257-78-9.*
*ATC — N05AB04.*

**Pharmacopoeias.** In *US.*

**USP 27** (Prochlorperazine Edisylate). A white to very light yellow odourless crystalline powder. Soluble 1 in 2 of water and 1 in 1500 of alcohol; insoluble in chloroform and in ether. Solutions in water are acid to litmus. Store in airtight containers. Protect from light.

**Incompatibility.** See under Prochlorperazine Mesilate, below.

## Prochlorperazine Maleate (BANM, rINNM)

Chlormeprazine Maleate; Maleato de proclorperazina; Prochlorpemazine Maleate; Prochlorperazine Dihydrogen Maleate; Prochlorperazine Dimaleate; Prochlorperazini Maleas.
$C_{20}H_{24}ClN_3S,2C_4H_4O_4$ = 606.1.
*CAS — 84-02-6.*
*ATC — N05AB04.*

**Pharmacopoeias.** In *Eur.* (see p.vi), *Jpn, Pol.*, and *US.*

**Ph. Eur. 5.0** (Prochlorperazine Maleate). A white or pale yellow, crystalline powder. Very slightly soluble in water and in alcohol. A freshly prepared saturated solution in water has a pH of 3.0 to 4.0. Protect from light.

**USP 27** (Prochlorperazine Maleate). A white or pale yellow, practically odourless, crystalline powder. Practically insoluble in water; soluble 1 in 1200 of alcohol; slightly soluble in warm chloroform. Its saturated solution is acid to litmus. Store in airtight containers. Protect from light.

## Prochlorperazine Mesilate (BANM, rINNM)

Chlormeprazine Mesylate; Mesilato de proclorperazina; Prochlorpemazine Mesylate; Prochlorperazine Dimethanesulphonate; Prochlorperazine Mesylate; Prochlorperazine Methanesulphonate; Prochlorperazini Mesylas.
$C_{20}H_{24}ClN_3S,2CH_3SO_3H$ = 566.2.
*CAS — 5132-55-8.*
*ATC — N05AB04.*

**Pharmacopoeias.** In *Br.*

**BP 2003** (Prochlorperazine Mesilate). A white or almost white, odourless or almost odourless powder. Very soluble in water; sparingly soluble in alcohol; slightly soluble in chloroform; practically insoluble in ether. A 2% solution in water has a pH of 2.0 to 3.0. Protect from light.

**Incompatibility.** Incompatibility has been reported between the edisilate or mesilate salts of prochlorperazine and several other compounds: these include aminophylline, amphotericin B, ampicillin sodium, aztreonam, some barbiturates, benzylpenicillin salts, calcium gluconate, cefalotin sodium, cefmetazole sodium, chloramphenicol sodium succinate, chlorothiazide sodium, dimenhydrinate, heparin sodium, hydrocortisone sodium succinate, midazolam hydrochloride, and some sulfonamides. Incompatibility between prochlorperazine edisilate and morphine sulfate has been attributed to phenol present in some formulations of the opioid.[1,2] Incompatibility has been reported on dilution of prochlorperazine edisilate injection with sodium chloride injection containing methyl hydroxybenzoate and propyl hydroxybenzoate as preservatives.[3] The problem did not occur with unpreserved sodium chloride or when benzyl alcohol was used as preservative. Prochlorperazine mesilate syrup has been reported to be incompatible with magnesium trisilicate mixture.[4]

1. Stevenson JG, Patriarca C. Incompatibility of morphine sulfate and prochlorperazine edisylate in syringes. *Am J Hosp Pharm* 1985; **42:** 2651.
2. Zuber DEL. Compatibility of morphine sulfate injection and prochlorperazine edisylate injection. *Am J Hosp Pharm* 1987; **44:** 67.
3. Jett S, *et al.* Prochlorperazine edisylate incompatibility. *Am J Hosp Pharm* 1983; **40:** 210.
4. Greig JR. Stemetil syrup and magnesium trisilicate. *Pharm J* 1986; **237:** 504.

### Adverse Effects, Treatment, and Precautions

As for Chlorpromazine, p.675. Prochlorperazine may cause less sedation and fewer antimuscarinic effects but extrapyramidal effects may be more frequent. Severe dystonic reactions have followed the use of prochlorperazine, particularly in children and adolescents. It should therefore be used with extreme care in children.

In addition, in the UK, parenteral use in children is not recommended. Local irritation has occurred after the use of buccal tablets of prochlorperazine maleate.

**Effects on the cardiovascular system.** Hypertension has been reported[1] in some patients given prochlorperazine intravenously for prophylaxis of cisplatin-induced nausea and vomiting.

1. Roche H, *et al.* Hypertension and intravenous antidopaminergic drugs. *N Engl J Med* 1985; **312:** 1125–6.

**Effects on the mouth.** Reports of ulceration and soreness of the lip and tongue associated with use of prochlorperazine maleate oral tablets.[1,2] The erosive cheilitis resolved after withdrawal of prochlorperazine and recurred on rechallenge.

1. Duxbury AJ, *et al.* Erosive cheilitis related to prochlorperazine maleate. *Br Dent J* 1982; **153:** 271–2.
2. Reilly GD, Wood ML. Prochlorperazine—an unusual cause of lip ulceration. *Acta Derm Venereol (Stockh)* 1984; **64:** 270–1.

### Interactions

As for Chlorpromazine, p.679.

### Pharmacokinetics

◊ The pharmacokinetics of prochlorperazine was studied in 8 healthy subjects following doses of 6.25 and 12.5 mg intravenously, and 25 mg by mouth.[1] There was a marked interindividual variation in pharmacokinetics following intravenous administration but no evidence of dose-dependent pharmacokinetics; mean terminal half-lives were 6.8 hours for the higher and 6.9 hours for the lower dose. The apparent volume of distribution was very high and plasma clearance values were apparently greater than liver plasma flow, suggesting that the liver may not be the only site of metabolism. After oral administration prochlorperazine concentrations were detectable in only 4 of the 8 subjects due in part to a low bioavailability but also to the lack of sensitivity of the high-pressure liquid chromatographic assay used. The time to peak plasma concentration varied from 1.5 to 5 hours, and the peak concentrations varied from 1.6 to 7.6 nanograms/mL. Bioavailability was estimated to range from 0 to 16%. A low bioavailability due to high first-pass metabolism would be expected because of the high plasma clearance of prochlorperazine.

1. Taylor WB, Bateman DN. Preliminary studies of the pharmacokinetics and pharmacodynamics of prochlorperazine in healthy volunteers. *Br J Clin Pharmacol* 1987; **23:** 137–42.

**Buccal administration.** Both single- and multiple-dose studies indicated that bioavailability of prochlorperazine maleate was greater after buccal administration than after oral administration.[1] Doses of 3 mg twice daily by the buccal route and 5 mg three times daily by mouth produced similar steady-state plasma-prochlorperazine concentrations.

1. Hessell PG, *et al.* A comparison of the availability of prochlorperazine following im buccal and oral administration. *Int J Pharmaceutics* 1989; **52:** 159–64.

## Uses and Administration

Prochlorperazine is a phenothiazine antipsychotic with general properties similar to those of chlorpromazine (p.680). It has a piperazine side-chain. Prochlorperazine and its salts are widely used in the prevention and treatment of nausea and vomiting (p.1245) including that associated with migraine or drug-induced emesis. They are also used for the short-term symptomatic relief of vertigo (p.423) as occurs in Ménière's disease (p.422) or labyrinthitis, and in the management of schizophrenia (p.665), mania (see Bipolar Disorder, p.278), and other psychoses. Prochlorperazine has been used as an adjunct in the short-term management of severe anxiety (p.663).

Prochlorperazine base is generally administered by the rectal route and prochlorperazine maleate by the oral or buccal routes, while prochlorperazine edisilate and mesilate are given orally or parenterally.

Depending on the country or the manufacturer, doses of prochlorperazine are expressed either as the base or the salt. Prochlorperazine edisilate 7.5 mg, prochlorperazine maleate 8 mg, or prochlorperazine mesilate 7.6 mg are approximately equivalent to 5 mg of prochlorperazine. Most doses in the UK, including the rectal doses, are expressed in terms of the maleate or mesilate, while most doses in the USA are expressed in terms of the base. As a result there is a disparity in the dosage recommendations for these countries, with the doses in the USA tending to be higher.

Reduced dosage may be required in elderly patients.

For **nausea and vomiting** doses are as follows:

- in the UK, the usual dose *by mouth* for prevention is 5 to 10 mg of the maleate or mesilate (roughly equivalent to about 3 to 6.5 mg of the base) two or three times daily. Similar doses may be given by the *rectal* route
- for the treatment of nausea and vomiting, recommended UK doses are 20 mg of the maleate or mesilate *by mouth*, 12.5 mg of the mesilate by deep *intramuscular* injection, or the equivalent of prochlorperazine maleate 25 mg *rectally* as suppositories; further doses, preferably by mouth, are given if necessary. The recommended *buccal* dose of prochlorperazine maleate for the management of nausea and vomiting is 3 to 6 mg twice daily
- in the USA the dose *by mouth* for the control of nausea and vomiting is the equivalent of 5 to 10 mg of the base (as edisilate or maleate) given 3 or 4 times daily; alternatively the equivalent of 10 mg of the base twice daily or 15 mg once daily of the base (both as the maleate) may be taken as modified-release capsules. The recommended *intramuscular* dosage is the equivalent of 5 to 10 mg of the base (as edisilate) given every 3 to 4 hours if necessary, up to a total of 40 mg of the base daily. The *rectal* dose is 25 mg of the base given twice daily. In the management of severe nausea and vomiting the equivalent of 2.5 to 10 mg of prochlorperazine (as the edisilate) may be given by slow *intravenous* injection or infusion at a rate not exceeding 5 mg/minute; doses should not exceed 40 mg daily.

For treatment of **psychoses** the following doses have been given:

- in the UK, prochlorperazine maleate or mesilate may be given *by mouth* in a dose of 12.5 mg twice daily for 7 days adjusted gradually to 75 to 100 mg daily according to response; some patients may be maintained on doses of 25 to 50 mg daily. The equivalent of prochlorperazine maleate 25 mg two or three times daily may be given by the *rectal* route or 12.5 to 25 mg of the mesilate two or three times daily by deep *intramuscular* injection
- in the USA prochlorperazine is given as the maleate or edisilate in usual initial doses equivalent to 5 to 10 mg of the base 3 or 4 times daily *by mouth* adjusted according to response up to a maximum of 150 mg of base daily. In acute disturbances it may be given by deep *intramuscular* injection as the edisilate in doses equivalent to 10 to 20 mg of the base and repeated every 2 to 6 hours if necessary.

There are similar discrepancies with **children's doses**. Owing to the risk of severe extrapyramidal reactions, prochlorperazine should be used with extreme caution in children: in particular it is not recommended for those weighing less than 10 kg or below 1 year of age. Where use in children is unavoidable, UK sources have suggested that 250 micrograms/kg of the maleate or mesilate may be given two or three times daily by mouth for the prevention and treatment of nausea and vomiting; the intramuscular and rectal routes are considered unsuitable. In contrast, in the USA oral, rectal, and intramuscular routes have all been advocated. The usual oral or rectal antiemetic dose ranges up to 7.5 mg of the base or its equivalent daily in children weighing 10 to 13 kg; in children 14 to 17 kg, up to 10 mg daily; from 18 to 39 kg, up to 15 mg daily. Higher doses have been given for psychoses. The suggested intramuscular dose for children in the USA is the equivalent of about 130 micrograms/kg of base given as a single deep intramuscular injection of the edisilate.

Doses of 5 to 10 mg of the maleate or mesilate (or, in the USA, the equivalent of 5 mg of the base) up to 3 or 4 times daily by mouth have been used for short-term adjunctive management of **severe anxiety disorders**. A modified-release preparation may be given in doses similar to those used in nausea and vomiting.

Prochlorperazine is also used in the UK in the treatment of **vertigo** including that due to Ménière's disease. It is given *by mouth* in doses of 15 to 30 mg of the maleate or mesilate daily in divided doses; after several weeks the dose may be gradually reduced to 5 to 10 mg daily. The recommended *buccal* dose of prochlorperazine maleate for the treatment of vertigo due to Ménière's disease is 3 to 6 mg twice daily.

**Headache.** The phenothiazines chlorpromazine and prochlorperazine have been used in migraine to control severe nausea and vomiting unresponsive to antiemetics such as metoclopramide and domperidone (see p.464). Parenteral phenothiazines may also relieve the pain of severe migraine attacks unresponsive to parenteral dihydroergotamine or sumatriptan. In comparative studies[1,2] prochlorperazine appears to have been more effective in relieving migraine headache and nausea and vomiting than metoclopramide when these drugs were given parenterally. Prochlorperazine was shown to be effective in aborting intractable migraine in children in a small uncontrolled study.[3]

For further references to the use of phenothiazines in the management of migraine, see under Chlorpromazine, p.682.

1. Coppola M, *et al.* Randomized, placebo-controlled evaluation of prochlorperazine versus metoclopramide for emergency department treatment of migraine headache. *Ann Emerg Med* 1995; **26:** 541–6.
2. Jones J, *et al.* Intramuscular prochlorperazine versus metoclopramide as single-agent therapy for the treatment of acute migraine headache. *Am J Emerg Med* 1996; **14:** 262–4.
3. Kabbouche MA, *et al.* Tolerability and effectiveness of prochlorperazine for intractable migraine in children. *Pediatrics* 2001; **107:** 767. Full version: http://pediatrics.aappublications.org/cgi/content/full/107/4/e62 (accessed 28/04/04)

## Preparations

***BP 2003:*** Prochlorperazine Buccal Tablets; Prochlorperazine Injection; Prochlorperazine Oral Solution; Prochlorperazine Tablets;
***USP 27:*** Prochlorperazine Edisylate Injection; Prochlorperazine Maleate Tablets; Prochlorperazine Oral Solution; Prochlorperazine Suppositories.

**Proprietary Preparations** (details are given in Part 3)
***Austral.:*** Stemetil; Stemzine; ***Canad.:*** Nu-Prochlor; Stemetil; ***Denm.:*** Stemetil; ***Fin.:*** Stemetil; ***Hong Kong:*** Dhaperazine; Stella†; Stemetil; ***India:*** Emidoxyn; Stemetil; ***Irl.:*** Buccastem; Stemetil; ***Ital.:*** Stemetil; ***Malaysia:*** Dhaperazine; Nautisol; Prochlor; Stemetil; ***Neth.:*** Stemetil; ***Norw.:*** Stemetil; ***NZ:*** Antinaus; Buccastem; Stemetil; ***S.Afr.:*** Mitil; Scripto-Metic; Stemetil; ***Singapore:*** Dhaperazine; Prochlor; Stemetil; ***Swed.:*** Stemetil; ***Thai.:*** Proclozine; Stemetil; ***UK:*** Buccastem; Proziere; Stemetil; ***USA:*** Compazine; Compro.

**Multi-ingredient:** ***Ital.:*** Difmetre.

# Promazine Embonate *(BANM, rINNM)*

Embonato de promazina; Promazine Pamoate; Propazinum (promazine).
$(C_{17}H_{20}N_2S)_2,C_{23}H_{16}O_6$ = 957.2.
*CAS — 58-40-2 (promazine).*
*ATC — N05AA03.*

## Promazine Hydrochloride *(BANM, rINNM)*

Hidrocloruro de promazina; Promazini Hydrochloridum. NN-Dimethyl-3-phenothiazin-10-ylpropylammonium chloride.
$C_{17}H_{20}N_2S,HCl$ = 320.9.
*CAS — 53-60-1.*
*ATC — N05AA03.*

**Pharmacopoeias.** In *Eur.* (see p.vi), *Pol.*, and *US.*

**Ph. Eur. 5.0** (Promazine Hydrochloride). A white or almost white, slightly hygroscopic, crystalline powder. Very soluble in water, in alcohol, and in dichloromethane. A freshly prepared 5% solution in water has a pH of 4.2 to 5.2. Protect from light.

**USP 27** (Promazine Hydrochloride). A white or slightly yellow, practically odourless, crystalline powder. It oxidises upon prolonged exposure to air and acquires a pink or blue colour. Soluble 1 in 3 of water; freely soluble in chloroform. pH of a 1 in 20 solution is between 4.2 and 5.2. Store in airtight containers. Protect from light.

**Incompatibility.** Incompatibility has been reported between promazine hydrochloride and several other compounds: these include aminophylline, some barbiturates, benzylpenicillin potassium, chlortetracycline, chlorothiazide sodium, dimenhydrinate, heparin sodium, hydrocortisone sodium succinate, phenytoin sodium, prednisolone sodium phosphate, and sodium bicarbonate.

**Sorption.** A study[1] of drug loss from intravenous delivery systems reported an 11% loss of promazine hydrochloride from solution when infused for 7 hours via a plastic infusion set, and a 59% loss after infusion for one hour from a glass syringe through silastic tubing. Loss was negligible after infusion for one hour from a system comprising a glass syringe with polyethylene tubing.

1. Kowaluk EA, *et al.* Interactions between drugs and intravenous delivery systems. *Am J Hosp Pharm* 1982; **39:** 460–7.

**Stability.** A study of the stability of promazine diluted to a 0.1% infusion in sodium chloride 0.9% or glucose 5% found that solutions in glucose 5% remained stable for up to 6 days at 4°, and at room temperature, provided they were stored in the dark.[1] However, with sodium chloride 0.9% as the diluent deterioration of the promazine was observed 24 hours after preparation, even when stored in the dark, and after 8 hours when exposed to light. Temperature had no effect on degradation rate.

1. Tebbett IR, *et al.* Stability of promazine as an intravenous infusion. *Pharm J* 1986; **237:** 172–4.

## Adverse Effects, Treatment, and Precautions

As for Chlorpromazine, p.675.

**Pregnancy.** An increased incidence of neonatal jaundice coincided with the increased use of promazine.[1] A decrease in the incidence of jaundice was noted 3 months after the total withdrawal of the drug from the hospital although restriction of its use during labour had no impact.

1. John E. Promazine and neonatal hyperbilirubinaemia. *Med J Aust* 1975; **2:** 342–4.

## Interactions

As for Chlorpromazine, p.679.

## Pharmacokinetics

The pharmacokinetics of promazine appear to be generally similar to those of chlorpromazine (p.680).

## Uses and Administration

Promazine is a phenothiazine with general properties similar to those of chlorpromazine (p.680). It has relatively weak antipsychotic activity and is not generally used for the management of psychoses. It is mainly used for the short-term management of agitated or disturbed behaviour (p.665). It has also been given for the alleviation of nausea and vomiting (p.1245). Promazine is given as the hydrochloride by mouth, intramuscularly, or by slow intravenous injection (the latter in concentrations not exceeding 25 mg/mL). Promazine has also been given by mouth as the embonate.

For the treatment of **agitated behaviour**, promazine is given in doses equivalent to 100 to 200 mg of the hydrochloride four times daily by mouth or 50 mg by intramuscular injection repeated if necessary after 6 to 8 hours. It has also been given by slow intravenous injection for severely agitated hospitalised patients.

A dose of 25 to 50 mg every 4 to 6 hours by mouth has been given for the control of **nausea and vomiting**; it has also been given by intramuscular injection for this indication.

Promazine should be given in reduced dosage to elderly or debilitated subjects; 25 mg by mouth of the hydrochloride initially, increasing, if necessary, to 50 mg four times daily has been suggested for the control of agitation and restlessness in the elderly; for intramuscular injection a dose of 25 mg may be sufficient.

### Preparations

***BP 2003:*** Promazine Injection; Promazine Oral Suspension; Promazine Tablets;
***USP 27:*** Promazine Hydrochloride Injection; Promazine Hydrochloride Oral Solution; Promazine Hydrochloride Syrup; Promazine Hydrochloride Tablets.

**Proprietary Preparations** (details are given in Part 3)
***Austral.:*** Sparine†; ***Belg.:*** Prazine; ***Denm.:*** Sparine; ***Fin.:*** Sparine; ***Ger.:*** Protactyl; Sinophenin; ***Gr.:*** Sparine; ***Irl.:*** Sparine†; ***Ital.:*** Talofen; ***S.Afr.:*** Sparine†; ***Switz.:*** Prazine; ***UK:*** Sparine†; ***USA:*** Prozine; Sparine†.

## Propionylpromazine

Dipropimazine; Propionilpromazina; Propiopromazine.
*CAS — 3568-24-9.*

### Profile

Propionylpromazine is a phenothiazine antipsychotic used for sedation and premedication in veterinary medicine.

## Prothipendyl Hydrochloride *(BANM, rINNM)*

D-206; Hidrocloruro de protipendilo; Phrenotropin. *NN*-Dimethyl-3-(pyrido[3,2-*b*][1,4]benzothiazin-10-yl)propylamine hydrochloride monohydrate.
$C_{16}H_{19}N_3S,HCl,H_2O = 339.9$.
*CAS — 303-69-5 (prothipendyl); 1225-65-6 (anhydrous prothipendyl hydrochloride).*
*ATC — N05AX07.*

### Profile

Prothipendyl is an azaphenothiazine with general properties similar to those of chlorpromazine (p.675). It is given by mouth as the hydrochloride in doses of 40 to 80 mg two to four times daily for the treatment of psychoses and agitation, and as an adjunct to analgesics in the treatment of severe pain. Prothipendyl hydrochloride may also be given by injection.

### Preparations

**Proprietary Preparations** (details are given in Part 3)
***Austria:*** Dominal; ***Belg.:*** Dominal; ***Ger.:*** Dominal.

## Proxibarbal *(rINN)*

HH-184; Proxibarbital. 5-Allyl-5-(2-hydroxypropyl)barbituric acid.
$C_{10}H_{14}N_2O_4 = 226.2$.
*CAS — 2537-29-3.*
*ATC — N05CA22.*

**Pharmacopoeias.** In *Pol.*

### Profile

Proxibarbal is a barbiturate with general properties similar to those of amobarbital (p.670). It has been used as a sedative in the management of anxiety disorders. It has also been used in the treatment of headache. However, barbiturates are not considered appropriate in the management of these conditions. Proxibarbal has been associated with severe hypersensitivity-induced thrombocytopenia.

### Preparations

**Proprietary Preparations** (details are given in Part 3)
***Fr.:*** Centralgol†.

## Pyrithyldione *(rINN)*

Didropyridinum; NU-903; Piritildiona. 3,3-Diethylpyridine-2,4(1*H*,3*H*)-dione.
$C_9H_{13}NO_2 = 167.2$.
*CAS — 77-04-3.*
*ATC — N05CE03.*

### Profile

Pyrithyldione has been given in preparations with diphenhydramine in the short-term management of insomnia but there have been reports of agranulocytosis associated with the use of this combination.

### Preparations

**Proprietary Preparations** (details are given in Part 3)
**Multi-ingredient: *Belg.:*** Dorment†.

## Quazepam *(BAN, USAN, rINN)*

Sch-16134. 7-Chloro-5-(2-fluorophenyl)-1,3-dihydro-1-(2,2,2-trifluoroethyl)-1,4-benzodiazepine-2-thione.
$C_{17}H_{11}ClF_4N_2S = 386.8$.
*CAS — 36735-22-5.*
*ATC — N05CD10.*

**Pharmacopoeias.** In *US.*

**USP 27** (Quazepam). Off-white to yellowish powder.

### Dependence and Withdrawal

As for Diazepam, p.690.

### Adverse Effects, Treatment, and Precautions

As for Diazepam, p.690.

**Breast feeding.** The American Academy of Pediatrics[1] considers that, although the effect of quazepam on breast-feeding infants is unknown, its use by mothers during breast feeding may be of concern since psychotropic drugs do appear in breast milk and thus could conceivably alter CNS function in the infant both in the short and long term.

However, a study in 4 women given a single 15-mg dose of quazepam found that only about 0.1% of the dose was excreted over 48 hours in breast milk, as quazepam and its 2 major metabolites.[2]

1. American Academy of Pediatrics. The transfer of drugs and other chemicals into human milk. *Pediatrics* 2001; **108:** 776–89. Correction. *ibid.*; 1029. Also available at: http://aappolicy.aappublications.org/cgi/content/full/pediatrics%3b108/3/776 (accessed 28/04/04)
2. Hilbert JM, *et al.* Excretion of quazepam into human breast milk. *J Clin Pharmacol* 1984; **24:** 457–62.

### Interactions

As for Diazepam, p.692.

### Pharmacokinetics

Quazepam is readily absorbed from the gastrointestinal tract after administration by mouth, peak plasma concentrations being reached in about 2 hours. It is metabolised extensively in the liver. The principal active metabolites are 2-oxoquazepam and *N*-desalkyl-2-oxoquazepam (*N*-desalkylflurazepam) which have elimination half-lives of about 39 and 73 hours respectively, compared with a half-life of 39 hours for quazepam. Further hydroxylation occurs and quazepam is excreted in urine and faeces mainly as conjugated metabolites.

Quazepam and its two active metabolites are more than 95% bound to plasma proteins. Quazepam and its metabolites are distributed into breast milk.

### Uses and Administration

Quazepam is a long-acting benzodiazepine with general properties similar to those of diazepam (p.695). It is given by mouth as a hypnotic in the short-term management of insomnia (p.667), in an initial dose of 15 mg at night; in elderly or debilitated patients and some other patients this can be reduced to 7.5 mg.

### Preparations

***USP 27:*** Quazepam Tablets.

**Proprietary Preparations** (details are given in Part 3)
***Ital.:*** Quazium; ***Jpn:*** Doral; ***Port.:*** Prosedar; ***S.Afr.:*** Dormet†; ***Spain:*** Quiedorm; ***USA:*** Doral.

## Quetiapine Fumarate *(BANM, USAN, pINNM)*

Fumarato de quetiapina; ICI-204636; ZD-5077; ZM-204636. 2-[2-(4-Dibenzo[*b,f*][1,4]thiazepin-11-yl-1-piperazinyl)ethoxy]ethanol fumarate (2:1) salt.
$(C_{21}H_{25}N_3O_2S)_2,C_4H_4O_4 = 883.1$.
*CAS — 111974-69-7 (quetiapine); 111974-72-2 (quetiapine fumarate).*

### Adverse Effects, Treatment, and Precautions

Although quetiapine may share some of the adverse effects seen with the classical antipsychotics (see Chlorpromazine, p.675), the incidence and severity of such effects may vary. The most frequent adverse effects with quetiapine are somnolence, dizziness, constipation, orthostatic hypotension, dry mouth, and raised liver enzyme values. Quetiapine has been associated with a low incidence of extrapyramidal symptoms. Rises in prolactin concentrations may be less than with chlorpromazine. Weight gain particularly during early treatment has also been noted. Clinical monitoring for hyperglycaemia has been recommended, especially in patients with or at risk of developing diabetes. Neuroleptic malignant syndrome is rare with quetiapine but tardive dyskinesia may occur after long-term treatment. Tachycardia, and, occasionally, syncope have been reported; prolongation of the QT interval is rarely significant. Leucopenia, neutropenia, and eosinophilia have also been reported with quetiapine.

Other adverse effects have included mild asthenia, anxiety, fever, hypertension, myalgia, rhinitis, dyspepsia, rises in plasma-triglyceride and cholesterol concentrations, and reduced plasma-thyroid hormone concentrations. There have been rare reports of seizures, hypersensitivity reactions including angioedema, priapism, and peripheral oedema.

Asymptomatic changes in the lens of the eye have occurred in patients during long-term treatment with quetiapine; cataracts have developed in *dogs* during chronic dosing studies. In the USA it is recommended that patients should have an eye examination to detect cataract formation when starting therapy with quetiapine and every 6 months during treatment.

Quetiapine should be used with caution in patients with hepatic or renal impairment, with cardiovascular disease or other conditions predisposing to hypotension, or with a history of seizures.

Quetiapine may affect the performance of skilled tasks including driving.

**Effects on carbohydrate metabolism.** The increased risk of glucose intolerance and diabetes mellitus with some atypical antipsychotics including quetiapine and recommendations for monitoring are discussed under Adverse Effects in Clozapine, p.686.

**Hyperventilation.** A report of hyperventilation and respiratory alkalosis associated with quetiapine administration.[1]

1. Shelton PS, *et al.* Hyperventilation associated with quetiapine. *Ann Pharmacother* 2000; **34:** 335–7.

**Mania.** A 26-year-old man with schizophrenia developed manic symptoms after starting treatment with quetiapine; the symptoms resolved when quetiapine was withdrawn.[1]

1. Lykouras L, *et al.* Manic symptoms associated with quetiapine treatment. *Eur Neuropsychopharmacol* 2003; **13:** 135–6.

**Overdosage.** Hypotension, tachycardia, and somnolence were the main clinical events observed in a patient who had ingested an overdose of 3 g of quetiapine.[1] Tachycardia of an unexpectedly long duration was also noted. Management was symptomatic, including maintenance of fluids. Asymptomatic prolongation of the QT interval was observed in another patient who had ingested a 2 g overdose of quetiapine.[2] Her treatment regimen also included risperidone, and the authors warned that considerable QT interval prolongation may occur when patients overdose on quetiapine while taking therapeutic doses of risperidone.

A subsequent report[3] has described a case series of 18 patients who ingested from 500 mg to 24 g of quetiapine either alone (6 patients) or with other drugs (12). Quetiapine overdosage was primarily associated with CNS and respiratory depression and sinus tachycardia. Four of the 18 patients required mechanical ventilation but no deaths occurred. The corrected QT interval, but not the QT interval, was prolonged, but apart from sinus tachycardia no patient had a dysrhythmia. Seizures occurred in 2 patients and delirium in 3. The patient who took 24 g of quetiapine was found to have had a peak blood concentration of 20.48 micrograms/mL. She had presented 1.5 hours after ingestion and was intubated and treated with gastric lavage followed by activated charcoal. About 2.5 hours later she had a generalised tonic-clonic seizure. The patient was discharged after 40 hours without sequelae.

1. Beelen AP, *et al.* Asymptomatic QTc prolongation associated with quetiapine fumarate overdose in a patient being treated with risperidone. *Hum Exp Toxicol* 2001; **20:** 215–19.
2. Pollak PT, Zbuk K. Quetiapine fumarate overdose: clinical and pharmacokinetic lessons from extreme conditions. *Clin Pharmacol Ther* 2000; **68:** 92–7.
3. Balit CR, *et al.* Quetiapine poisoning: a case series. *Ann Emerg Med* 2003; **42:** 751–8.

### Interactions

The central effects of other CNS depressants, including alcohol, may be enhanced by quetiapine. Quetiapine should be used with caution in patients also receiving antihypertensives or drugs that prolong the QT interval. Quetiapine may antagonise the actions of dopaminergics such as levodopa.

CYP3A4 is the main isoenzyme responsible for cytochrome P450 mediated metabolism of quetiapine and caution is advised when quetiapine is used with potent inhibitors of CYP3A4 such as erythromycin, fluconazole, itraconazole, and ketoconazole; lower doses of quetiapine should be used when given with such inhibitors. Conversely, enzyme inducers such as carbamazepine and phenytoin may decrease the plasma concentrations of quetiapine, and higher doses of quetiapine may be necessary. Thioridazine has also been reported to increase the clearance of quetiapine.

**Antipsychotics.** For a report of asymptomatic QT prolongation associated with quetiapine in a patient also receiving *risperidone*, see under Overdosage, above.

## Pharmacokinetics

Quetiapine is well absorbed following oral administration and widely distributed throughout the body. Peak plasma concentrations are reached in about 1.5 hours. It is about 83% bound to plasma proteins. Quetiapine is extensively metabolised in the liver by sulfoxidation mediated mainly by the cytochrome P450 isoenzyme CYP3A4 and by oxidation. It is excreted mainly as inactive metabolites, about 73% of a dose appearing in the urine and about 20% in the faeces. The elimination half-life has been reported to be about 6 to 7 hours.

◊ References.

1. DeVane CL, Nemeroff CB. Clinical pharmacokinetics of quetiapine: an atypical antipsychotic. *Clin Pharmacokinet* 2001; **40:** 509–22.

## Uses and Administration

Quetiapine fumarate is a dibenzothiazepine atypical antipsychotic. It is reported to have affinity for serotonin ($5-HT_2$), histaminergic ($H_1$), and adrenergic ($\alpha_1$ and $\alpha_2$) receptors as well as dopamine $D_2$ receptors. Quetiapine is used in the treatment of schizophrenia and of mania associated with bipolar disorder.

Quetiapine is given by mouth as the fumarate although doses are expressed in terms of the base; 28.8 mg of quetiapine fumarate is approximately equivalent to 25 mg of quetiapine base. The usual initial dose in **schizophrenia** is the equivalent of 25 mg of the base twice daily on day one, 50 mg twice daily on day two, 100 mg twice daily on day three, and 150 mg twice daily on day four. The dosage is then adjusted according to response to a usual range of 300 to 450 mg daily given in 2 or 3 divided doses, although 150 mg daily may be adequate for some patients. The maximum recommended dose is 750 mg daily.

In the treatment of **mania**, the initial dose is 50 mg twice daily on day one, 100 mg twice daily on day two, 150 mg twice daily on day three, and 200 mg twice daily on day four. The dose may then be adjusted to a usual range of 400 to 800 mg daily, although, in some patients, 200 mg daily may be adequate. Increments in dosage should be no greater than 200 mg daily.

Quetiapine should be given in reduced doses to the elderly; a recommended starting dose is 25 mg daily increased in steps of 25 to 50 mg daily according to response. Reduced doses are also recommended in patients with hepatic or renal impairment, see below.

**Administration in hepatic or renal impairment.** Quetiapine should be given in reduced doses to patients with hepatic impairment; a recommended starting dose is 25 mg daily increased in steps of 25 to 50 mg daily according to response. The UK manufacturers recommend a similar reduction in patients with renal impairment.

**Bipolar disorder.** Quetiapine may be of benefit for the treatment of mania in patients with bipolar disorder (p.278) and the use of atypical antipsychotics in the management of such patients is increasing. However, there have been individual case reports of quetiapine-induced mania (see above).

References.

1. Sajatovic M, *et al.* Quetiapine alone and added to a mood stabilizer for serious mood disorders. *J Clin Psychiatry* 2001; **62:** 728–32.
2. Vieta E, *et al.* Quetiapine in the treatment of rapid cycling bipolar disorder. *Bipolar Disord* 2002; **4:** 335–40.
3. Delbello MP, *et al.* A double-blind, randomized, placebo-controlled study of quetiapine as adjunctive treatment for adolescent mania. *J Am Acad Child Adolesc Psychiatry* 2002; **41:** 1216–23.
4. Altamura AC, *et al.* Efficacy and tolerability of quetiapine in the treatment of bipolar disorder: preliminary evidence from a 12-month open-label study. *J Affect Disord* 2003; **76:** 267–71.

**Parkinsonism.** Quetiapine has been tried as an antipsychotic in patients with parkinsonism (see under Disturbed Behaviour, p.665).

**Schizophrenia.** A systematic review[1] noted that although the short-term benefits of quetiapine for positive and negative symptoms of schizophrenia appeared comparable with classical antipsychotics, and the incidence of extrapyramidal effects was low (equivalent to placebo), conclusions were necessarily limited by high drop-out rates in the studies considered.

1. Srisurapanont M, *et al.* Quetiapine for schizophrenia. Available in The Cochrane Library; Issue 2. Chichester: John Wiley; 2004.

## Preparations

**Proprietary Preparations** (details are given in Part 3)
***Arg.:*** Seroquel; ***Austral.:*** Seroquel; ***Austria:*** Seroquel; ***Belg.:*** Seroquel; ***Braz.:*** Seroquel; ***Canad.:*** Seroquel; ***Chile:*** Norsic; Quetidin; Seroquel; ***Denm.:*** Seroquel; ***Fin.:*** Seroquel; ***Ger.:*** Seroquel; ***Gr.:*** Seroquel; ***Hong Kong:*** Seroquel; ***Irl.:*** Seroquel; ***Israel:*** Seroquel; ***Ital.:*** Seroquel; ***Malaysia:*** Seroquel; ***Mex.:*** Seroquel; ***Neth.:*** Seroquel; ***Norw.:*** Seroquel; ***NZ:*** Seroquel; ***Port.:*** Alzen; Seroquel; ***S.Afr.:*** Seroquel; ***Singapore:*** Seroquel; ***Spain:*** Seroquel; ***Switz.:*** Seroquel; ***Thai.:*** Seroquel; ***UK:*** Seroquel; ***USA:*** Seroquel.

---

## Raclopride *(BAN, rINN)*

A-40664 (raclopride tartrate); FLA-870; Racloprida. (*S*)-3,5-Dichloro-*N*-(1-ethylpyrrolidin-2-ylmethyl)-2-hydroxy-6-methoxybenzamide.

$C_{15}H_{20}Cl_2N_2O_3$ = 347.2.

*CAS — 84225-95-6 (raclopride); 98185-20-7 (raclopride tartrate).*

### Profile

Raclopride is a substituted benzamide related to sulpiride (p.722). It has been investigated for the treatment of psychoses. Since it binds selectively and with high affinity to $D_2$ dopaminergic receptors raclopride labelled with carbon-11 has been tried as a tracer in computerised tomographic studies of neurological disorders associated with dysfunction of brain $D_2$ dopaminergic receptors.

---

# Risperidone *(BAN, USAN, rINN)*

R-64766; Risperidona; Risperidonum. 3-{2-[4-(6-Fluoro-1,2-benzisoxazol-3-yl)piperidino]ethyl}-6,7,8,9-tetrahydro-2-methylpyrido[1,2-*a*]pyrimidin-4-one.

$C_{23}H_{27}FN_4O_2$ = 410.5.

*CAS — 106266-06-2.*

*ATC — N05AX08.*

**Pharmacopoeias.** In *Eur.* (see p.vi).

**Ph. Eur. 5.0** (Risperidone). A white or almost white powder. It exhibits polymorphism. Practically insoluble in water; sparingly soluble in alcohol; freely soluble in dichloromethane; dissolves in dilute acid solutions. Protect from light.

## Adverse Effects, Treatment, and Precautions

Although risperidone may share some of the adverse effects seen with the classical antipsychotics (see Chlorpromazine, p.675), the incidence and severity of such effects may vary. Risperidone is reported to be less likely to cause sedation or extrapyramidal effects (see also Uses and Administration, below) but agitation may occur more frequently. Other common reactions include insomnia, anxiety, and headache. Dyspepsia, nausea, abdominal pain, constipation, blurred vision, sexual dysfunction including priapism, urinary incontinence, rash and other allergic reactions, drowsiness, concentration difficulties, dizziness, fatigue, and rhinitis have been reported less commonly. In addition to orthostatic hypotension, hypertension has been reported infrequently. Other adverse effects with risperidone include cerebrovascular accidents, tachycardia, weight gain, oedema, increased liver enzyme values, and mild decreases in neutrophil or thrombocyte counts. Risperidone may cause dose-dependent increases in prolactin levels. In rare cases, hyperglycaemia and a worsening of diabetes mellitus has also been reported. Clinical monitoring for hyperglycaemia has been recommended, especially in patients with or at risk of developing diabetes. Other rare effects include seizures, body temperature dysregulation, neuroleptic malignant syndrome, and tardive dyskinesia.

Risperidone should be used with caution in patients with cardiovascular disease including conditions associated with QT prolongation; caution is also recommended in patients with Parkinson's disease or epilepsy, and in patients with hepatic or renal impairment.

Risperidone may affect the performance of skilled tasks such as driving.

Gradual withdrawal of risperidone is recommended because of the risk of withdrawal symptoms with abrupt cessation.

**Breast feeding.** From the study of concentrations of risperidone in the breast milk of one mother it was estimated that a breast-fed infant would receive the daily equivalent of 4.3% of the weight-adjusted maternal dose.[1]

1. Hill RC, *et al.* Risperidone distribution and excretion into human milk: case report and estimated infant exposure during breast-feeding. *J Clin Psychopharmacol* 2000; **20:** 285–6.

**Cerebrovascular disorders.** Following analysis of data from controlled trials there was evidence that the use of risperidone in elderly patients with dementia appeared to be associated with an increased risk of cerebrovascular adverse effects such as stroke and transient ischaemic attacks. In 4 studies, involving 764 such patients treated with risperidone, there were 29 cases of cerebrovascular adverse events, 4 fatal, versus 7 cases (1 fatal) in 466 patients given placebo. Postmarketing data for elderly dementia patients, representing over 2.4 million patient-years of exposure, included 37 cases, of which 16 were fatal.[1]

The UK Committee on Safety of Medicines[2] have therefore recommended that risperidone should not be used to treat behavioural problems in elderly patients with dementia. It was considered that the risk may not be confined to use in dementia and should be considered relevant to any patient with a history of stroke or transient ischaemic attack or other risk factors for cerebrovascular disease, including hypertension, diabetes, current smoking, or atrial fibrillation.

1. Janssen-Ortho Inc./Health Canada. Important drug safety information: Risperdal (risperidone) and cerebrovascular adverse events in placebo-controlled dementia trials (issued 11/10/02). Available at: http://www.hc-sc.gc.ca/hpfb-dgpsa/tpd-dpt/risperdal1_e.html (accessed 28/04/04)
2. Atypical antipsychotic drugs and stroke message from Professor G Duff, Chairman of Committee on Safety of Medicines (CSM). Available at: http://www.mca.gov.uk/ourwork/monitorsafequalmed/safetymessages/antipsystoke_9304.pdf (accessed 28/04/04)

**Dementia.** For a recommendation that risperidone should not be used to treat behavioural problems in elderly patients with dementia, see under Cerebrovascular Disorders, above.

**Effects on carbohydrate metabolism.** The increased risk of glucose intolerance and diabetes mellitus with some atypical antipsychotics including risperidone and recommendations for monitoring are discussed under Adverse Effects in Clozapine, p.686.

**Effects on the liver.** A report of 2 cases of hepatotoxicity associated with risperidone.[1] An idiosyncratic reaction to risperidone was suspected in another patient who developed hepatotoxicity after receiving only 2 doses of risperidone.[2]

1. Fuller MA, *et al.* Risperidone-associated hepatotoxicity. *J Clin Psychopharmacol* 1996; **16:** 84–5.
2. Phillips EJ, *et al.* Rapid onset of risperidone-induced hepatotoxicity. *Ann Pharmacother* 1998; **32:** 843.

**Effects on the skin.** A patient developed facial and periorbital oedema 2 weeks after her dose of risperidone reached 6 mg daily.[1] The oedema subsided when the dose was halved but recurred shortly after it was again increased to 6 mg. She had previously had a similar reaction to lithium and there was also a family history of angioedema.

1. Cooney C, Nagy A. Angio-oedema associated with risperidone. *BMJ* 1995; **311:** 1204.

**Extrapyramidal disorders.** In reports of 3 cases of tardive dystonia associated with risperidone therapy,[1,2] onset ranged from 3 to 8 months after starting the drug. Dyskinesia has also been reported 5 days after the withdrawal of risperidone and citalopram.[3]

1. Vercueil L, Foucher J. Risperidone-induced tardive dystonia and psychosis. *Lancet* 1999; **353:** 981.
2. Krebs MO, Olie JP. Tardive dystonia induced by risperidone. *Can J Psychiatry* 1999; **44:** 507–508.
3. Miller LJ. Withdrawal-emergent dyskinesia in a patient taking risperidone/citalopram. *Ann Pharmacother* 2000; **34:** 269.

**Mania.** All of 6 patients with bipolar schizoaffective disorder experienced onset or worsening of manic symptoms shortly after beginning treatment with risperidone.[1] Symptoms resolved in some patients but others required the addition of valproate to treatment. Since this report, additional cases[2] of risperidone-induced mania have been published.

1. Dwight MM, *et al.* Antidepressant activity and mania associated with risperidone treatment of schizoaffective disorder. *Lancet* 1994; **344:** 554–5.
2. Zolezzi M, Badr MG. Risperidone-induced mania. *Ann Pharmacother* 1999; **33:** 380–1.

**Neuroleptic malignant syndrome.** Neuroleptic malignant syndrome (p.677) has occasionally been associated with risperidone.[1-3]

1. Sharma R, *et al.* Risperidone-induced neuroleptic malignant syndrome. *Ann Pharmacother* 1996; **30:** 775–8.
2. Tarsy D. Risperidone and neuroleptic malignant syndrome. *JAMA* 1996; **275:** 446.
3. Reeves RR, *et al.* Neuroleptic malignant syndrome during a change from haloperidol to risperidone. *Ann Pharmacother* 2001; **35:** 698–701.

**Overdosage.** A 3½-year-old child developed extrapyramidal symptoms after accidental ingestion of a single 4-mg tablet of risperidone.[1] The child was initially treated with gastric lavage, activated charcoal, and sorbitol; extrapyramidal symptoms responded to treatment with diphenhydramine and the child recovered completely. The need to monitor for and treat hypotension following overdosage with risperidone was highlighted in a report[2] of a 15-year-old girl who took 40 mg of risperidone.

1. Cheslik TA, Erramouspe J. Extrapyramidal symptoms following accidental ingestion of risperidone in a child. *Ann Pharmacother* 1996; **30:** 360–3.
2. Himstreet JE, Daya M. Hypotension and orthostasis following a risperidone overdose. *Ann Pharmacother* 1998; **32:** 267.

## Interactions

The central effects of other CNS depressants, including alcohol, may be enhanced by risperidone. Risperidone may also enhance the effects of antihypertensives. There may be an increased risk of QT prolongation when risperidone is given with other drugs that are known to cause this effect. Risperidone may antagonise the actions of levodopa and other dopaminergics.

Carbamazepine has been shown to decrease the antipsychotic fraction (risperidone plus 9-hydroxyrisperidone) of risperidone and a similar effect may be seen with other enzyme inducers. Fluoxetine may increase the plasma concentrations of the antipsychotic fraction by raising the concentration of risperidone. Dose adjustment of risperidone may be necessary in such situations.

**Antipsychotics.** For a report suggesting that risperidone might increase plasma concentrations of *clozapine*, see p.688. For a report of asymptomatic QT prolongation associated with *quetiapine* in a patient also receiving risperidone, see under Overdosage of Quetiapine, p.718.

**Antivirals.** Dystonia and worsening of tremors were reported one week after adding *indinavir* and *ritonavir* to treatment with risperidone in a patient with AIDS;[1] he recovered once all 3 drugs were withdrawn and following treatment with clonazepam. An early exposure to risperidone, indinavir, and ritonavir had not resulted in any extrapyramidal side-effects. The authors considered this to reflect the patient's relatively short exposure to risperidone at the time.

1. Kelly DV, *et al.* Extrapyramidal symptoms with ritonavir/indinavir plus risperidone. *Ann Pharmacother* 2002; **36:** 827–30.

## Pharmacokinetics

Risperidone is readily absorbed after oral doses, peak plasma concentrations being reached within 1 to 2 hours. It is extensively metabolised in the liver by hydroxylation to its main active metabolite, 9-hydroxyrisperidone; oxidative *N*-dealkylation is a minor metabolic pathway. Hydroxylation is mediated by the cytochrome P450 isoenzyme CYP2D6 and is the subject of genetic polymorphism. Excretion is mainly in the urine and, to a lesser extent, in the faeces. Risperidone and 9-hydroxyrisperidone are about 90% and 77% bound to plasma proteins, respectively. Both are distributed into breast milk.

**Metabolism.** Although the hydroxylation of risperidone is subject to genetic polymorphism, the pharmacokinetics and effects of the active antipsychotic fraction (risperidone plus 9-hydroxyrisperidone) have been reported to vary little between extensive and poor metabolisers.[1] A mean value of 19.5 hours has been reported for the terminal elimination half-life of the active fraction following oral administration of risperidone.[1]

1. Huang M-L, *et al.* Pharmacokinetics of the novel antipsychotic agent risperidone and the prolactin response in healthy subjects. *Clin Pharmacol Ther* 1993; **54:** 257–68.

## Uses and Administration

Risperidone is a benzisoxazole atypical antipsychotic, reported to be an antagonist at dopamine $D_2$ and serotonin (5-$HT_2$), adrenergic ($\alpha_1$ and $\alpha_2$), and histamine ($H_1$) receptors. It is given by mouth for the treatment of schizophrenia and other psychoses and in the short-term treatment of mania associated with bipolar disorder. Risperidone may also be given by deep intramuscular injection for maintenance therapy in patients tolerant to oral antipsychotics.

For **schizophrenia** the usual initial daily dose of risperidone by mouth is 2 mg; this may be increased to 4 mg daily on the second day, and subsequently adjusted further as required in increments or decrements of 1 or 2 mg daily, generally at intervals of not less than one week, although other titration regimens have been employed. Most patients benefit from doses of 4 to 6 mg daily. Risperidone may be given once daily or in 2 divided doses. Extrapyramidal symptoms may be more likely with doses above 10 mg daily; the US manufacturer does not recommend daily doses above 6 mg if divided into 2 doses, although higher doses are permitted if given as a single dose. The maximum recommended dose is 16 mg daily.

An initial dose of 500 micrograms twice daily by mouth slowly increased in steps of 500 micrograms twice daily, if necessary, to a dose of 1 to 2 mg twice daily is recommended for the elderly or debilitated patients.

The long-acting formulation of risperidone should be given by deep intramuscular injection every 2 weeks. Patients with no history of risperidone use should be given risperidone by mouth for several days to assess tolerability. Treatment may then be started as follows:

- patients not stabilised on risperidone: 25 mg every 2 weeks
- patients stabilised on oral risperidone for at least 2 weeks in doses of 4 mg daily or less: 25 mg every 2 weeks
- patients stabilised on oral risperidone for at least 2 weeks in doses above 4 mg daily: 37.5 mg every 2 weeks
- elderly patients should be given a maximum of 25 mg every 2 weeks

Oral risperidone should be continued for the first 3 weeks after the first injection.

Dose increases of 12.5 mg, every 4 weeks, to a maximum of 50 mg every 2 weeks may be considered a minimum of 4 weeks after the previous adjustment; the clinical effects of a dose adjustment may not be seen for at least 3 weeks after the change.

For the treatment of **acute manic episodes** a recommended initial dose is 2 to 3 mg once daily by mouth. Dosage adjustments of 1 mg daily may be made at intervals of not less than 24 hours up to a total of 6 mg daily. The initial dosage regimen in elderly or debilitated patients should be reduced as for schizophrenia (see above).

Reduced doses are recommended in patients with hepatic or renal impairment, see below.

**Action.** Risperidone is described as an atypical antipsychotic but although it has a lower propensity to produce parkinsonism, dystonias and akathisias have been reported.[1] (See also Extrapyramidal Disorders, above.) The traditional hypothesis is that antipsychotics work through inhibition of dopamine $D_2$ receptors and that extrapyramidal motor side-effects result from blockade of $D_2$ receptors in the striatum (see p.681). Like clozapine, risperidone has a high affinity for 5-$HT_2$ receptors and, like haloperidol, it has a high affinity for dopamine $D_2$ receptors. Risperidone also binds to alpha-adrenergic and histamine $H_1$ sites. It is unclear whether risperidone's antipsychotic effect is due to activity at dopamine $D_2$ receptors or at another site. It has been suggested[1] that other potent effects of risperidone may be counterbalancing the $D_2$ activity to produce its atypicality.

1. Kerwin RW. The new atypical antipsychotics: a lack of extrapyramidal side-effects and new routes in schizophrenia research. *Br J Psychiatry* 1994; **164:** 141–8.

**Administration in hepatic or renal impairment.** The recommended initial oral dose of risperidone in patients with renal or hepatic impairment is 500 micrograms twice daily; this may be slowly increased in steps of 500 micrograms twice daily, if necessary, to a dose of 1 to 2 mg twice daily.

Patients with schizophrenia who tolerate an oral dose of risperidone of at least 2 mg daily may be switched to the long-acting formulation of risperidone. A dose of 25 mg by deep intramuscular injection every 2 weeks is recommended.

**AIDS.** Risperidone was used successfully to control HIV- or AIDS-related psychosis in 21 patients some of whom also had manic symptoms.[1] No extrapyramidal symptoms were reported during treatment. For reports suggesting that risperidone can induce or exacerbate manic symptoms in patients with schizoaffective disorders, see under Mania in Adverse Effects, above. For an interaction between risperidone and antiretroviral therapy in a patient with AIDS see under Interactions, above.

1. Singh AN, *et al.* Treatment of HIV-related psychotic disorders with risperidone: a series of 21 cases. *J Psychosom Res* 1997; **42:** 489–93.

**Anxiety disorders.** Although there have been anecdotal reports[1,2] of improvement following the addition of risperidone to treatment in patients with obsessive-compulsive disorder refractory to conventional treatment, there has also been a report[3] of a patient whose obsessive-compulsive behaviour recurred when he was treated with risperidone for tardive dyskinesia.

1. Jacobsen FM. Risperidone in the treatment of affective illness and obsessive-compulsive disorder. *J Clin Psychiatry* 1995; **56:** 423–9.
2. McDougle CJ, *et al.* Risperidone addition in fluvoxamine-refractory obsessive-compulsive disorder: three cases. *J Clin Psychiatry* 1995; **56:** 526–8.
3. Remington G, Adams M. Risperidone and obsessive-compulsive symptoms. *J Clin Psychopharmacol* 1994; **14:** 358–9.

**Bipolar disorder.** Risperidone may be of benefit for the treatment of mania in patients with bipolar disorder (p.278) and the use of atypical antipsychotics in the management of such patients is increasing. However, there have been individual case reports of risperidone-induced mania (see above).

References.

1. Segal J, *et al.* Risperidone compared with both lithium and haloperidol in mania: a double-blind randomized controlled trial. *Clin Neuropharmacol* 1998; **21:** 176–80.
2. Sachs GS, *et al.* Combination of a mood stabilizer with risperidone or haloperidol for treatment of acute mania: a double-blind, placebo-controlled comparison of efficacy and safety. *Am J Psychiatry* 2002; **159:** 1146–54.
3. Yatham LN, *et al.* Mood stabilisers plus risperidone or placebo in the treatment of acute mania: international, double-blind, randomised controlled trial. *Br J Psychiatry* 2003; **182:** 141–7. Correction. *ibid.*; 369.

**Disturbed behaviour.** Risperidone has been used for the management of behavioural disturbances[1,2] in patients with dementia (p.665), but such use in elderly patients is no longer recommended in the UK because of reports of an increased risk of cerebrovascular accident (see under Adverse Effects, above). Further, although there have been anecdotal reports[3] of efficacy in patients with Lewy-body dementia, other reports[4] suggest that these patients are likely to be just as sensitive to risperidone as to standard antipsychotics (see the Elderly in Precautions for Chlorpromazine, p.678).

Results from a short-term study[5] have also suggested that risperidone is effective in reducing behavioural disturbances in children with autism, but it has been pointed out that the marked hyperprolactinaemia induced by risperidone could lead to hypogonadism, and deleterious effects on adolescent bones.[6]

1. DeDeyn PP, *et al.* A randomized trial of risperidone, placebo, and haloperidol for behavioral symptoms of dementia. *Neurology* 1999; **53:** 946–55.
2. Falsetti AE. Risperidone for control of agitation in dementia patients. *Am J Health-Syst Pharm* 2000; **57:** 862–70.
3. Allen RL, *et al.* Risperidone for psychotic and behavioural symptoms in Lewy body dementia. *Lancet* 1995; **346:** 185.
4. McKeith IG, *et al.* Neuroleptic sensitivity to risperidone in Lewy body dementia. *Lancet* 1995; **346:** 699.
5. Research Units on Pediatric Psychopharmacology Autism Network. Risperidone in children with autism and serious behavioral problems. *N Engl J Med* 2002; **347:** 314–21.
6. Valiquette G. Risperidone in children with autism and serious behavioral problems. *N Engl J Med* 2002; **347:** 1890–1.

**Dystonias.** Antipsychotics are sometimes useful in the treatment of idiopathic dystonia (p.1209) in patients who have failed to respond to treatment with levodopa or antimuscarinics, but as with classical antipsychotics there is the risk of adding drug-induced extrapyramidal effects to the dystonia. Risperidone has been reported to be of benefit in a few patients with idiopathic segmental dystonia partly insensitive to haloperidol.[1]

1. Zuddas A, Cianchetti C. Efficacy of risperidone in idiopathic segmental dystonia. *Lancet* 1996; **347:** 127–8.

**Parkinsonism.** There have been conflicting reports of the use of risperidone as an antipsychotic in a small number of patients with Parkinson's disease (see also Disturbed Behaviour, p.665). While some patients found that risperidone ameliorated levodopa-induced hallucinations without worsening extrapyramidal symptoms,[1,2] others reported that risperidone produced a substantial worsening of symptoms.[2,3]

1. Meco G, *et al.* Risperidone for hallucinations in levodopa-treated Parkinson's disease patients. *Lancet* 1994; **343:** 1370–1.
2. Leopold NA. Risperidone treatment of drug-related psychosis in patients with parkinsonism. *Mov Disord* 2000; **15:** 301–4.
3. Ford B, *et al.* Risperidone in Parkinson's disease. *Lancet* 1994; **344:** 681.

**Schizophrenia.** Risperidone is claimed to produce a relatively low incidence of extrapyramidal effects and to have efficacy against both positive and negative symptoms of schizophrenia. Most of the earlier studies compared risperidone with haloperidol but, of these, some of the major studies[1-3] were criticised for potential methodological flaws[4,5] and it was difficult to determine any difference in efficacy including effect on negative symptoms. A more recent systematic review[6] suggested that risperidone's benefits over haloperidol or other classical antipsychotics were marginal; although it did appear to reduce the risk of extrapyramidal effects compared with haloperidol, the latter produces a relatively high incidence of such effects. Furthermore, the risk of extrapyramidal effects with risperidone appears to be dose dependent:[7] although similar to that for placebo overall, at doses of more than 10 mg the risk appears to approach that associated with haloperidol. In the few comparative studies with other atypical antipsychotics risperidone has appeared to be of similar efficacy to clozapine.[8] However, another systematic review[9] concluded that such equivalence with clozapine cannot be assumed. For a comparative study with olanzapine, see p.712. There is insufficient evidence to indicate whether risperidone is effective for treatment-resistant or poorly responsive patients but there is some evidence that patients stabilised on risperidone may be less likely to relapse.[10]

1. Chouinard G, *et al.* A Canadian multicenter placebo-controlled study of fixed doses of risperidone and haloperidol in the treatment of chronic schizophrenic patients. *J Clin Psychopharmacol* 1993; **13:** 25–40.

2. Marder SR, Meibach RC. Risperidone in the treatment of schizophrenia. *Am J Psychiatry* 1994; **151:** 825–35.
3. Peuskens J, *et al.* Risperidone Study Group. Risperidone in the treatment of patients with chronic schizophrenia: a multi-national, multi-centre, double-blind, parallel-group study versus haloperidol. *Br J Psychiatry* 1995; **166:** 712–26.
4. Livingston MG. Risperidone. *Lancet* 1994; **343:** 457–60.
5. Musser WS, Kirisci L. Critique of the Canadian multicenter placebo-controlled study of risperidone and haloperidol. *J Clin Psychopharmacol* 1995; **15:** 226–8.
6. Hunter RH, *et al.* Risperidone versus typical antipsychotic medication for schizophrenia. Available in The Cochrane Library; Issue 2. Chichester: John Wiley; 2004.
7. Owens DGC. Extrapyramidal side effects and tolerability of risperidone: a review. *J Clin Psychiatry* 1994; **55** (suppl 5): 29–35.
8. Klieser E, *et al.* Randomized, double-blind, controlled trial of risperidone versus clozapine in patients with chronic schizophrenia. *J Clin Psychopharmacol* 1995; **15** (suppl 1): 45S–51S.
9. Gilbody SM, *et al.* Risperidone versus other atypical antipsychotic medication for schizophrenia. Available in The Cochrane Library; Issue 2. Chichester: John Wiley; 2004.
10. Csernansky JG, *et al.* A comparison of risperidone and haloperidol for the prevention of relapse in patients with schizophrenia. *N Engl J Med* 2002; **346:** 16–22.

**Stuttering.** Risperidone 0.5 to 2 mg daily was found to be of benefit in the management of stuttering in a placebo controlled study[1] involving 16 patients but there has also been a case report[2] of a patient whose stuttering returned during treatment with risperidone.

1. Maguire GA, *et al.* Risperidone for the treatment of stuttering. *J Clin Psychopharmacol* 2000; **20:** 479–82.
2. Lee H-J, *et al.* A case of risperidone-induced stuttering. *J Clin Psychopharmacol* 2001; **21:** 115–16.

**Tourette's syndrome.** When treatment is required for tics and behavioural disturbances in Tourette's syndrome (p.664) haloperidol or pimozide are commonly used but risperidone has also been tried.[1-3]

1. Bruun RD, Budman CL. Risperidone as a treatment for Tourette's syndrome. *J Clin Psychiatry* 1996; **57:** 29–31.
2. Bruggeman R, *et al.* Risperidone versus pimozide in Tourette's disorder: a comparative double-blind parallel-group study. *J Clin Psychiatry* 2001; **62:** 50–6.
3. Scahill L, *et al.* A placebo-controlled trial of risperidone in Tourette syndrome. *Neurology* 2003; **60:** 1130–5.

## Preparations

**Proprietary Preparations** (details are given in Part 3)

***Arg.:*** Dropicine; Risperdal; Risperin; Sequinan; ***Austral.:*** Risperdal; ***Austria:*** Belivon; Risperdal; ***Belg.:*** Risperdal; ***Braz.:*** Risperdal; Viverdal; Zargus; ***Canad.:*** Risperdal; ***Chile:*** Dagotil; Goval; Radigen; Risperdal; Spiron; ***Denm.:*** Risperdal; ***Fin.:*** Risperdal; ***Fr.:*** Risperdal; ***Ger.:*** Risperdal; ***Gr.:*** Risperdal; ***Hong Kong:*** Risperdal; ***India:*** Rispid; ***Irl.:*** Risperdal; ***Israel:*** Risperdal; ***Ital.:*** Belivon; Risperdal; ***Jpn:*** Risperdal; ***Malaysia:*** Risperdal; ***Mex.:*** Risperdal; ***Neth.:*** Risperdal; ***Norw.:*** Risperdal; ***NZ:*** Risperdal; ***Port.:*** Risperdal; ***S.Afr.:*** Risperdal; ***Singapore:*** Risperdal; ***Spain:*** Risperdal; ***Swed.:*** Risperdal; ***Switz.:*** Risperdal; ***Thai.:*** Risperdal; ***UK:*** Risperdal; ***USA:*** Risperdal.

---

## Ritanserin *(BAN, USAN, rINN)*

R-55667; Ritanserina. 6-{2-[4-(4,4′-Difluorobenzhydrylidene)piperidino]ethyl}-7-methyl[1,3]thiazolo[3,2-*a*]pyrimidin-5-one.

$C_{27}H_{25}F_2N_3OS$ = 477.6.

*CAS — 87051-43-2.*

### Profile

Ritanserin is a serotonin antagonist that has been studied in a variety of disorders including anxiety disorders, depression, and schizophrenia. It is reported to have little sedative action.

**Action.** Ritanserin is a relatively selective antagonist at serotonin (5-hydroxytryptamine, 5-HT) receptors of the 5-$HT_2$ subtype, although it also has appreciable affinity for 5-$HT_{1C}$ receptors.[1] Unlike ketanserin (p.943), it does not block $\alpha_1$-adrenergic receptors. Ritanserin has anxiolytic activity; it also hastens the onset of slow-wave sleep although sleep may be impaired on withdrawal.

Ritanserin may interfere with platelet function[2,3] but has been reported to have no significant effect on blood pressure, blood flow, or heart rate in patients with hypertension.[2,4] Features characteristic of class III antiarrhythmic activity have also been noted.[2]

1. Marsden CA. The pharmacology of new anxiolytics acting on 5-HT neurones. *Postgrad Med J* 1990; **66** (suppl 2): S2–S6.
2. Stott DJ, *et al.* The effects of the 5$HT_2$ antagonist ritanserin on blood pressure and serotonin-induced platelet aggregation in patients with untreated essential hypertension. *Eur J Clin Pharmacol* 1988; **35:** 123–9.
3. Wagner B, *et al.* Effect of ritanserin, a 5-hydroxytryptamine$_2$-receptor antagonist, on platelet function and thrombin generation at the site of plug formation in vivo. *Clin Pharmacol Ther* 1990; **48:** 419–23.
4. Chau NP, *et al.* Comparative haemodynamic effects of ketanserin and ritanserin in the proximal and distal upper limb circulations of hypertensive patients. *Eur J Clin Pharmacol* 1989; **37:** 215–20.

**Schizophrenia.** Ritanserin has produced some beneficial effects[1,2] when tried in small numbers of patients with schizophrenia (p.665).

1. Duinkerke SJ, *et al.* Ritanserin, a selective 5-$HT_{2/1C}$ antagonist, and negative symptoms in schizophrenia: a placebo-controlled double-blind trial. *Br J Psychiatry* 1993; **163:** 451–5.
2. Wiesel F-A, *et al.* An open clinical and biochemical study of ritanserin in acute patients with schizophrenia. *Psychopharmacology (Berl)* 1994; **114:** 31–8.

**Substance dependence.** Despite some encouraging preliminary data[1] suggesting that ritanserin might influence the desire to drink alcohol, subsequent studies[2,3] have failed to support a role for ritanserin in patients with *alcohol* dependence (p.1166).

1. Meert TF. Ritanserin and alcohol abuse and dependence. *Alcohol Alcohol* 1994; **2** (suppl): 523–30.
2. Johnson BA, *et al.* Ritanserin Study Group. Ritanserin in the treatment of alcohol dependence—a multi-center clinical trial. *Psychopharmacology (Berl)* 1996; **128:** 206–15.
3. Wiesbeck GA, *et al.* The effects of ritanserin on mood, sleep, vigilance, clinical impression, and social functioning in alcohol-dependent individuals. *Alcohol Alcohol* 2000; **35:** 384–9.

---

## Romifidine *(BAN, rINN)*

Romifidina; STH-2130. 2-Bromo-6-fluoro-*N*-(1-imidazolin-2-yl)aniline.

$C_9H_9BrFN_3$ = 258.1.

*CAS — 65896-16-4.*

### Profile

Romifidine is an $\alpha_2$-adrenoceptor agonist with sedative, muscle relaxant, and analgesic properties and is used in veterinary medicine.

---

## Secbutabarbital *(rINN)*

Butabarbital; Butabarbitone; Secbutobarbital *(BAN)*; Secbutobarbitone. 5-sec-Butyl-5-ethylbarbituric acid.

$C_{10}H_{16}N_2O_3$ = 212.2.

*CAS — 125-40-6.*

NOTE. Butabarbital should be distinguished from Butobarbital (p.673).

**Pharmacopoeias.** In *US.*

**USP 27** (Butabarbital). A white, odourless, crystalline powder. Very slightly soluble in water; soluble in alcohol, in chloroform, in ether, and in aqueous solutions of alkali hydroxides and carbonates. Store in airtight containers.

## Secbutabarbital Sodium *(rINNM)*

Butabarbital Sodium; Secbutabarbital sódico; Secbutobarbital Sodium *(BANM)*; Secbutobarbitone Sodium; Secumalnatrium; Sodium Butabarbital. Sodium 5-sec-butyl-5-ethylbarbiturate.

$C_{10}H_{15}N_2NaO_3$ = 234.2.

*CAS — 143-81-7.*

**Pharmacopoeias.** In *US.*

**USP 27** (Butabarbital Sodium). A white powder. Soluble 1 in 2 of water, 1 in 7 of alcohol, and 1 in 7000 of chloroform; practically insoluble in absolute ether. pH of a 10% solution in water is between 10.0 and 11.2. Store in airtight containers.

### Profile

Secbutabarbital is a barbiturate with general properties similar to those of amobarbital (p.670). It was used as a hypnotic and sedative although barbiturates are no longer considered appropriate for such purposes. For the short-term management of insomnia (p.667) it was usually given as the sodium salt in doses of 50 to 100 mg by mouth at night; as a sedative 15 to 30 mg has been given 3 or 4 times daily. Secbutabarbital base has also been given.

### Preparations

***USP 27:*** Butabarbital Sodium Elixir; Butabarbital Sodium Tablets.

**Proprietary Preparations** (details are given in Part 3)
***Canad.:*** Butisol†; ***USA:*** Butisol.

**Multi-ingredient:** ***USA:*** Butibel; Urelief Plus.

---

## Secobarbital *(rINN)*

Meballymal; Quinalbarbitone; Secobarbitalum; Secobarbitone. 5-Allyl-5-(1-methylbutyl)barbituric acid.

$C_{12}H_{18}N_2O_3$ = 238.3.

*CAS — 76-73-3.*

*ATC — N05CA06.*

**Pharmacopoeias.** In *US.*

**USP 27** (Secobarbital). A white amorphous or crystalline odourless powder. Very slightly soluble in water; freely soluble in alcohol, in ether, and in solutions of fixed alkali hydroxides and carbonates; soluble in chloroform; soluble 1 in 8.5 of 0.5N sodium hydroxide. A saturated solution in water has a pH of about 5.6. Store in airtight containers.

## Secobarbital Sodium *(BAN, rINNM)*

Meballymalnatrium; Quinalbarbitone Sodium; Secobarbital sódico; Secobarbitalum Natricum; Secobarbitone Sodium. Sodium 5-allyl-5-(1-methylbutyl)barbiturate.

$C_{12}H_{17}N_2NaO_3$ = 260.3.

*CAS — 309-43-3.*

*ATC — N05CA06.*

**Pharmacopoeias.** In *Chin.* and *US.*

**USP 27** (Secobarbital Sodium). A white odourless hygroscopic powder. Very soluble in water; soluble in alcohol; practically insoluble in ether. pH of a 10% solution in water is between 9.7 and 10.5. Solutions decompose on standing, heat accelerating the decomposition. Store in airtight containers.

**Incompatibility.** Secobarbital may be precipitated from preparations containing secobarbital sodium depending on the concentration and pH. Secobarbital sodium has, therefore, been reported to be incompatible with many other drugs, particularly acids and acidic salts.

### Dependence and Withdrawal

As for Amobarbital, p.670.

### Adverse Effects, Treatment, and Precautions

As for Amobarbital, p.670.

**Breast feeding.** No adverse effects have been observed in breast-feeding infants whose mothers were receiving secobarbital, and the American Academy of Pediatrics considers[1] that it is therefore usually compatible with breast feeding. However, for the view that barbiturates should not be used in women who are breast feeding, see under Amobarbital, p.670.

1. American Academy of Pediatrics. The transfer of drugs and other chemicals into human milk. *Pediatrics* 2001; **108:** 776–89. Correction. *ibid.*; 1029. Also available at: http://aappolicy.aappublications.org/cgi/content/full/pediatrics%3b108/3/776 (accessed 28/04/04)

**Industrial exposure.** Exposure to secobarbital sodium among 6 workers in the pharmaceutical industry resulted in absorption of substantial amounts of the drug, with blood concentrations approaching those expected after a therapeutic dose.[1] There continued to be evidence of absorption, despite protective masks to reduce inhalation, and it appeared that substantial absorption was taking place through the skin.

1. Baxter PJ, *et al.* Exposure to quinalbarbitone sodium in pharmaceutical workers. *BMJ* 1986; **292:** 660–1.

**Porphyria.** Secobarbital has been associated with acute attacks of porphyria and is considered unsafe in porphyric patients.

### Interactions

As for Amobarbital, p.670.

### Pharmacokinetics

Secobarbital is well absorbed from the gastrointestinal tract following oral doses and is reported to be about 46 to 70% bound to plasma proteins. The mean elimination half-life is reported to be 28 hours. It is metabolised in the liver, mainly by hydroxylation, and excreted in urine as metabolites and a small amount of unchanged drug.

### Uses and Administration

Secobarbital is a barbiturate that has been used as a hypnotic and sedative. It has general properties similar to those of amobarbital (p.670). As a hypnotic in the short-term management of insomnia (p.667) it was usually given by mouth in a dose of 100 mg of the sodium salt at night, but barbiturates are no longer considered appropriate for such use.

Secobarbital sodium has also been given by mouth or by intramuscular or intravenous injection for premedication in anaesthetic procedures (p.1296) but the use of barbiturates for preoperative sedation has been replaced by other drugs.

### Preparations

***USP 27:*** Secobarbital Elixir; Secobarbital Sodium and Amobarbital Sodium Capsules; Secobarbital Sodium Capsules; Secobarbital Sodium for Injection; Secobarbital Sodium Injection.

**Proprietary Preparations** (details are given in Part 3)
***Canad.:*** Seconal†; ***Irl.:*** Seconal†; ***S.Afr.:*** Seconal†; ***UK:*** Seconal; ***USA:*** Seconal.

**Multi-ingredient:** ***Belg.:*** Bellanox†; Vesparax†; ***Canad.:*** Tuinal†; ***Irl.:*** Tuinal†; ***Neth.:*** Vesparax†; ***Port.:*** Vesparax; ***S.Afr.:*** Vesparax†; ***Spain:*** Somatarax†; ***UK:*** Tuinal; ***USA:*** Tuinal.

---

## Sertindole *(BAN, USAN, rINN)*

Lu-23-174; Sertindol. 1-(2-{4-[5-Chloro-1-(*p*-fluorophenyl)indol-3-yl]piperidino}ethyl)-2-imidazolidinone.

$C_{24}H_{26}ClFN_4O$ = 440.9.

*CAS — 106516-24-9.*

*ATC — N05AE03.*

### Adverse Effects, Treatment, and Precautions

Although sertindole may share some of the adverse effects seen with the classical antipsychotics (see Chlorpromazine, p.675), the incidence and severity of such effects may vary. Sertindole is associated with a low incidence of extrapyramidal symptoms and does not appear to cause sedation. Prolactin elevation may be less frequent. Other adverse effects have included peripheral oedema, rhinitis, dyspnoea, sexual dysfunction, dizziness, dry mouth, orthostatic hypotension, weight gain, and paraesthesia. Hyperglycaemia, convulsions, and tardive dyskinesia are uncommon.

Marketing of sertindole has been restricted because of cardiac arrhythmias and sudden cardiac deaths associated with its use (see below). Since sertindole has been associated with prolongation of the QT interval, usually during the first 3 to 6 weeks of treatment, it is recommended that patients should have an ECG before the start of therapy and periodically during treatment. Patients with pre-existing prolongation of the QT interval or a family history of congenital QT prolongation should not be given sertindole and sertindole should be discontinued if such prolongation occurs during treatment. In addition, sertindole is contraindicated in patients with a history of cardiovascular disease, heart failure, cardiac hypertrophy, arrhythmias, or bradycardia. Sertindole should not be given to patients with uncorrected hypokalaemia or hypomagnesaemia. It is also recommended that blood pressure should be monitored during dose titration and in early maintenance therapy.

Sertindole is contra-indicated in patients with severe hepatic impairment. It should be used with caution in the elderly and in patients with Parkinson's disease, mild to moderate hepatic impairment, or a history of seizures.

Sertindole may affect the performance of skilled tasks including driving.

The manufacturers recommend that sertindole is gradually stopped because of the risk of withdrawal symptoms with abrupt cessation.

**Effects on the cardiovascular system.** The manufacturer has stated that in clinical studies prolongation of the QT interval is common in patients given sertindole with the effect being greater at the upper end of the dose range. In addition, the QT interval is prolonged to a greater extent than that seen with some other antipsychotics. QT interval prolongation is a known risk factor for the development of serious arrhythmias such as torsade de pointes although such arrhythmias are uncommon with sertindole.

In evidence presented to the FDA it was reported that as of 1st June 1996 there had been 27 deaths, 16 due to adverse cardiac events, among the 2194 patients given sertindole in clinical studies.[1] By the end of November 1998, the UK Committee on Safety of Medicines (CSM) was aware of 36 suspected adverse drug reactions with a fatal outcome, 9 of which originated in the UK.[2] There had also been 13 reports of serious but non-fatal cardiac arrhythmias in the UK. Although not all the fatalities were related to sudden cardiac events, at the time the CSM considered that, given the number of serious arrhythmias and sudden cardiac deaths, the risk-benefit ratio of sertindole was no longer favourable. The drug was withdrawn from the market in the UK and subsequently in a number of other countries, although it remained available on a named-patient basis. However, in 2001, the issue was re-evaluated by the CSM and the European advisory body, the Committee on Proprietary Medicinal Products, and it was recommended that sertindole could be reintroduced in Europe under certain restrictions.[3] Initially sertindole should only be prescribed to patients enrolled in clinical studies to ensure that they are carefully selected and monitored. In the UK, sertindole was remarketed in September 2002.

1. Barnett AA. Safety concerns over antipsychotic drug, sertindole. *Lancet* 1996; **348:** 256.
2. Committee on Safety of Medicines/Medicines Control Agency. Suspension of availability of sertindole (Serdolect). *Current Problems* 1999; **25:** 1. Also available at: http://www.mca.gov.uk/ourwork/monitorsafequalmed/currentproblems/volume25feb.htm (accessed 28/04/04)
3. Committee on Safety of Medicines/Medicines Control Agency. Restricted re-introduction of the atypical antipsychotic sertindole (Serdolect). Available at: http://www.mca.gov.uk/ourwork/monitorsafequalmed/safetymessages/serdolect3.htm (accessed 28/04/04)

### Interactions

The risk of arrhythmias with sertindole may be increased by other drugs which prolong the QT interval and concomitant use should be avoided. Sertindole should be given with caution with drugs that produce electrolyte disturbances; monitoring of serum potassium is recommended if giving with potassium-depleting diuretics.

Sertindole may antagonise the effects of dopaminergics.

Sertindole is extensively metabolised by the cytochrome P450 isoenzymes of the group CYP3A and by CYP2D6. The use of potent inhibitors of CYP3A such as indinavir, itraconazole, and ketoconazole with sertindole is contra-indicated. Minor increases in sertindole plasma concentrations have been noted in patients also given macrolide antibacterials or calcium-channel blockers which also inhibit CYP3A; however, despite the small increase, the use of these CYP3A4 inhibitors with sertindole is also not recommended. Fluoxetine and paroxetine, potent inhibitors of CYP2D6, have increased plasma concentrations of sertindole by a factor of 2 to 3 and lower maintenance doses of sertindole may be required. In contrast, enzyme inducers such as rifampicin, carbamazepine, phenytoin, and phenobarbital may decrease sertindole levels by a factor of 2 to 3; in such cases, higher doses of sertindole may be required.

### Pharmacokinetics

Sertindole is slowly absorbed with peak concentrations occurring about 10 hours after oral administration. It is about 99.5% bound to plasma proteins and readily crosses the placenta. Sertindole is extensively metabolised in the liver by the cytochrome P450 isoenzymes CYP2D6 and CYP3A. There is moderate intersubject variation in the pharmacokinetics of sertindole due to polymorphism in the isoenzyme CYP2D6. Poor metabolisers, deficient in this isoenzyme, may have plasma concentrations of sertindole 2 to 3 times higher than other patients. The two major metabolites identified, dehydrosertindole and norsertindole, appear to be inactive. Sertindole and its metabolites are excreted slowly, mainly in the faeces with a minor amount appearing in the urine. The mean terminal half-life is about 3 days.

### Uses and Administration

Sertindole is an atypical antipsychotic that is an antagonist at central dopamine ($D_2$), serotonin ($5\text{-}HT_2$), and adrenergic ($\alpha_1$) receptors. It is used in the treatment of schizophrenia (p.665) in patients who are unable to tolerate at least one other antipsychotic. In addition, sertindole should only be prescribed to patients enrolled in clinical studies to ensure adequate monitoring especially regular ECG measurements (see Adverse Effects, above).

Sertindole is given by mouth in an initial dose of 4 mg once daily, increased gradually by 4 mg every 4 or 5 days to a usual maintenance dose of 12 to 20 mg given once daily. The maximum dose is 24 mg daily. Slower dose titration and lower maintenance doses are advisable for the elderly and patients with mild to moderate hepatic impairment.

If therapy is interrupted for 1 week or more, the dose of sertindole should be re-titrated. An ECG should also be taken before re-starting sertindole.

### Preparations

**Proprietary Preparations** (details are given in Part 3)
***Austria:*** Serdolect†; ***Denm.:*** Serdolect†; ***Ger.:*** Serdolect†; ***Norw.:*** Serdolect†; ***Switz.:*** Serdolect; ***UK:*** Serdolect.

---

## Sulpiride *(BAN, USAN, rINN)*

Sulpiridum. *N*-(1-Ethylpyrrolidin-2-ylmethyl)-2-methoxy-5-sulphamoylbenzamide.
$C_{15}H_{23}N_3O_4S = 341.4$.
*CAS — 15676-16-1 (sulpiride).*
*ATC — N05AL01.*

**Pharmacopoeias.** In *Chin., Eur.* (see p.vi), and *Jpn.*

**Ph. Eur. 5.0** (Sulpiride). A white or almost white crystalline powder. Practically insoluble in water; slightly soluble in alcohol and in dichloromethane; sparingly soluble in methyl alcohol. It dissolves in dilute solutions of mineral acids and in alkali hydroxides.

## Levosulpiride *(rINN)*

Levosulpride; L-Sulpiride.
$C_{15}H_{23}N_3O_4S = 341.4$.
*CAS — 23672-07-3.*
*ATC — N05AL07.*

### Adverse Effects, Treatment, and Precautions

As for Chlorpromazine, p.675.

Sleep disturbances, overstimulation, and agitation may occur. Extrapyramidal effects appear to be as frequent as with chlorpromazine but have usually been mild. Whether sulpiride is less likely to cause tardive dyskinesia remains to be established. Sulpiride is less likely to cause sedation than chlorpromazine and antimuscarinic effects are minimal. Cardiovascular effects such as hypotension are generally rare although they may occur with overdosage.

Sulpiride should be given with care to manic or hypomanic patients in whom it may exacerbate symptoms.

**Breast feeding.** Sulpiride may be distributed into breast milk in relatively large amounts and the *British National Formulary* recommends that its use should be avoided in mothers wishing to breast feed.

On the fifth day after starting D-sulpiride, DL-sulpiride, or L-sulpiride in a dose of 50 mg twice daily, mean concentrations of sulpiride in breast milk from 45 lactating women were 840 nanograms/mL, 850 nanograms/mL, and 810 nanograms/mL respectively.[1]

1. Polatti F. Sulpiride isomers and milk secretion in puerperium. *Clin Exp Obstet Gynecol* 1982; **9:** 144–7.

**Effects on the cardiovascular system.** Sulpiride 100 mg by mouth caused an attack of hypertension in 6 of 26 hypertensive patients; in 4 it induced a rise in urinary excretion of vanillylmandelic acid and catecholamines.[1] A transient rise in blood pressure and catecholamines after administration of sulpiride occurred in 3 patients who were found to have a phaeochromocytoma; another patient probably had a phaeochromocytoma. The means by which sulpiride provoked hypertension were not known but appeared to be due to a noradrenergic effect. Sulpiride should be avoided during the treatment of phaeochromocytoma, and prescribed with great care in hypertensive patients.

1. Corvol P, *et al.* Poussées hypertensives déclenchées par le sulpiride. *Sem Hop Paris* 1974; **50:** 1265–9.

**Porphyria.** Sulpiride is considered to be unsafe in patients with porphyria because it has been shown to be porphyrinogenic in *animals*.

**Renal impairment.** For the precautions to be observed in patients with impaired renal function, see under Uses and Administration, below.

### Interactions

As for Chlorpromazine, p.679

**Gastrointestinal drugs.** Giving sulpiride with therapeutic doses of *sucralfate* or an *antacid* containing aluminium and magnesium hydroxides to 6 healthy subjects reduced the mean oral bioavailability of sulpiride by 40 and 32%, respectively.[1] When sulpiride was given 2 hours after the antacid or sucralfate (each in 2 subjects), the reduction in bioavailability was about 25%. This interaction was expected to be clinically significant, and it was recommended that sulpiride should be given before, rather than with or after, sucralfate or antacids.

1. Gouda MW, *et al.* Effect of sucralfate and antacids on the bioavailability of sulpiride in humans. *Int J Pharmaceutics* 1984; **22:** 257–63.

### Pharmacokinetics

Sulpiride is slowly absorbed from the gastrointestinal tract; bioavailability is low and subject to interindividual variation. It is rapidly distributed to the tissues but passage across the blood-brain barrier is poor. Sulpiride is less than 40% bound to plasma proteins and is reported to have a plasma half-life of about 8 to 9 hours. It is excreted in the urine and faeces, chiefly as unchanged drug. Sulpiride is distributed into breast milk.

◊ References.

1. Wiesel F-A, *et al.* The pharmacokinetics of intravenous and oral sulpiride in healthy human subjects. *Eur J Clin Pharmacol* 1980; **17:** 385–91.
2. Bressolle F, *et al.* Sulpiride pharmacokinetics in humans after intramuscular administration at three dose levels. *J Pharm Sci* 1984; **73:** 1128–36.
3. Bressolle F, *et al.* Absolute bioavailability, rate of absorption, and dose proportionality of sulpiride in humans. *J Pharm Sci* 1992; **81:** 26–32.

### Uses and Administration

Sulpiride is a substituted benzamide antipsychotic that is reported to be a selective antagonist of central dopamine ($D_2$, $D_3$, and $D_4$) receptors. It is also claimed to have mood elevating properties.

Sulpiride is mainly used in the treatment of psychoses such as schizophrenia. It has also been given in the management of Tourette's syndrome, anxiety disorders (p.663), vertigo (p.423), and benign peptic ulceration. Levosulpiride, the L-isomer of sulpiride, has been used similarly to sulpiride.

In the treatment of schizophrenia initial doses of 200 to 400 mg of sulpiride are given twice daily by mouth, increased if necessary up to a maximum of 1.2 g twice daily in patients with mainly positive symptoms or up to a total of 800 mg daily in patients with mainly negative symptoms. Sulpiride is also given in some countries by intramuscular injection, in usual doses ranging from 200 to 800 mg daily. A daily dose of 3 to 5 mg/kg may be given by mouth to children over 14 years of age. Lower initial doses have been recommended in elderly patients, subsequently adjusted as required. Dosage adjustment is also advised in patients with renal impairment (see below).

◊ Reviews.

1. Caley CF, Weber SS. Sulpiride: an antipsychotic with selective dopaminergic antagonist properties. *Ann Pharmacother* 1995; **29:** 152–60.
2. Mauri MC, *et al.* A risk-benefit assessment of sulpiride in the treatment of schizophrenia. *Drug Safety* 1996; **14:** 288–98.

**Administration in renal impairment.** A single intravenous dose of sulpiride 100 mg was administered to 6 healthy subjects with normal renal function (creatinine clearance greater than 90 mL/minute) and to three groups of 6 patients each with creatinine clearances (CC) in the ranges 30 to 60, 10 to 30, and less than 10 mL/minute.[1] There was a progressive diminution in the rate of elimination and an increase in half-life with decreasing renal function. The mean plasma elimination half-lives were 5.90, 11.02, 19.27, and 25.96 hours in the four groups, respectively.

In the UK it has been recommended that the dose be reduced to two-thirds of the normal amount in patients with CC of 30 to 60 mL/minute, to half the normal dose where CC is 10 to 30 mL/minute, and to one-third where CC is less than 10 mL/minute; alternatively, the dosage interval can be prolonged by a factor of 1.5, 2, and 3, respectively. However, the *British National Formulary* suggests that sulpiride should be avoided if possible in moderate renal impairment.

1. Bressolle F, *et al.* Pharmacokinetics of sulpiride after intravenous administration in patients with impaired renal function. *Clin Pharmacokinet* 1989; **17:** 367–73.

**Chorea.** Antipsychotics have some action against choreiform movements (p.664) as well as being of use to control the behavioural disturbances of Huntington's chorea. Although sulpiride was found to have produced an overall reduction in abnormal movements in 11 patients with Huntington's chorea when compared with placebo in a double-blind study[1] there was generally no accompanying functional improvement and patients with mild disease tended to worsen when taking sulpiride.

1. Quinn N, Marsden CD. A double blind trial of sulpiride in Huntington's disease and tardive dyskinesia. *J Neurol Neurosurg Psychiatry* 1984; **47:** 844–7.

**Gastrointestinal disorders.** Although sulpiride is used in some countries as an adjunct in the treatment of peptic ulcer disease (p.1246) it is not among the more usual drugs used for this indication. Efficacy has also been claimed for sulpiride or levosulpiride in a variety of other gastrointestinal disorders, including irritable bowel disease (p.1244), gastrointestinal motility disorders (p.1241), and nausea and vomiting (p.1245), but again they are not among the drugs usually considered for use in these conditions.

**Lactation.** Drug therapy has been used occasionally to stimulate lactation in breast-feeding mothers, although mechanical stimulation of the nipple remains the primary method. Dopamine antagonists such as sulpiride can produce modest increases in breast milk production[1-3] although metoclopramide has been more widely used (see p.1317). However, there is concern about the adverse effects of these drugs. As sulpiride appears in breast milk in relatively large amounts and may be associated with adverse effects in the infant it has been recommended that it should not be used to enhance milk production.[4]

1. Aono T, *et al.* Effect of sulpiride on poor puerperal lactation. *Am J Obstet Gynecol* 1982; **143:** 927–32.
2. Ylikorkala O, *et al.* Sulpiride improves inadequate lactation. *BMJ* 1982; **285:** 249–51.
3. Ylikorkala O, *et al.* Treatment of inadequate lactation with oral sulpiride and buccal oxytocin. *Obstet Gynecol* 1984; **63:** 57–60.
4. Pons G, *et al.* Excretion of psychoactive drugs into breast milk: pharmacokinetic principles and recommendations. *Clin Pharmacokinet* 1994; **27:** 270–89.

**Schizophrenia.** A systematic review[1] of the use of sulpiride for schizophrenia (p.665) or serious mental illness concluded that while sulpiride might be as effective as the classical antipsychotics for schizophrenia and appeared to produce few adverse effects, evidence of its value for treating negative symptoms was lacking. Comparisons with the atypical antipsychotic drugs were also lacking.

1. Soares BGO, *et al.* Sulpiride for schizophrenia. Available in The Cochrane Library; Issue 2. Chichester: John Wiley; 2004.

**Tourette's syndrome.** When treatment is needed for tics and behavioural disturbances in Tourette's syndrome (p.664) dopamine antagonists such as the antipsychotics haloperidol or pimozide are most commonly used but sulpiride has also been tried.[1]

1. Robertson MM, *et al.* Management of Gilles de la Tourette syndrome using sulpiride. *Clin Neuropharmacol* 1990; **13:** 229–35.

### Preparations

***BP 2003:*** Sulpiride Tablets.

**Proprietary Preparations** (details are given in Part 3)

***Arg.:*** Nivelan; Vipral; ***Austria:*** Dogmatil; Meresa; ***Belg.:*** Dogmatil; Levopraid; ***Braz.:*** Dogmatil; Equilid; ***Chile:*** Aplacid; Dislep; Sanblex; Sulpilan; ***Denm.:*** Dogmatil; Sulpril†; ***Fin.:*** Suprium; ***Fr.:*** Aiglonyl; Dogmatil; Synedil; ***Ger.:*** Arminol; Desisulpid†; Dogmatil; Intrasil†; Meresa; neogama; neogama D novo; Sulp; Sulpivert; Vertigo-Meresa; vertigo-neogama; ***Gr.:*** Calmoflorine; Darleton; Dogmatyl; Eclorion; Nufarol; Nylipark; Restful; Stamoneyrol; Valirem; ***Hong Kong:*** Dogmatil; Sulpiren†; ***Irl.:*** Dolmatil; ***Israel:*** Modal; ***Ital.:*** Championyl; Dobren; Equilid; Levobren; Levopraid; Normum†; ***Jpn:*** Dogmatyl; ***Mex.:*** Dogmatil†; Ekilid; Pontiride; Rimastine; ***Neth.:*** Dogmatil; ***Port.:*** Dogmatil; Lisopride; ***S.Afr.:*** Eglonyl; Espiride; ***Singapore:*** Dogmatil†; ***Spain:*** Digton; Dogmatil; Guastil; Lebopride; Pausedal; Psicocen; Sulkine; Tepavil; ***Switz.:*** Dogmatil; ***UK:*** Dolmatil; Sulparex†; Sulpitil; Sulpor.

**Multi-ingredient:** ***Arg.:*** Alplax Digest; Novo Vegestabil; Tranquinal Soma; Vegestabil; ***Braz.:*** Bromopirin; Sulpan; ***Mex.:*** Numencial; ***Spain:*** Ansium; Roter Complex†; Sirodina; Tepazepan.

## Sultopride Hydrochloride *(rINNM)*

Hidrocloruro de sultoprida; LIN-1418. *N*-(1-Ethylpyrrolidin-2-ylmethyl)-5-ethylsulphonyl-2-methoxybenzamide hydrochloride.

$C_{17}H_{26}N_2O_4S,HCl = 390.9.$

*CAS — 53583-79-2 (sultopride); 23694-17-9 (sultopride hydrochloride).*

*ATC — N05AL02.*

### Profile

Sultopride is a substituted benzamide with general properties similar to those of sulpiride (above). It is used in the emergency management of agitation in psychotic or aggressive patients (see Disturbed Behaviour, p.665) and in psychoses such as schizophrenia (p.665). It is given as the hydrochloride but doses are expressed in terms of the base; sultopride hydrochloride 441 mg is approximately equivalent to 400 mg sultopride. For acute agitation it may be given in doses of 400 to 800 mg daily by mouth or intramuscularly. In psychoses daily doses of 400 to 1200 mg have been given by mouth; up to 800 mg daily has been given intramuscularly. For chronically aggressive patients, maintenance doses of sultopride 400 to 600 mg daily may be given.

Ventricular arrhythmias, including torsade de pointes, have been reported. It has been recommended that sultopride should not be used in patients with bradycardia.

**Porphyria.** Sultopride is considered to be unsafe in patients with porphyria because it has been shown to be porphyrinogenic in *in-vitro* systems.

### Preparations

**Proprietary Preparations** (details are given in Part 3)

***Belg.:*** Barnetil; ***Fr.:*** Barnetil; ***Ital.:*** Barnotil; ***Port.:*** Barnetil.

## Tandospirone Citrate *(BANM, USAN, rINNM)*

Citrato de tandospirona; Metanopirone Citrate; SM-3997 (tandospirone or tandospirone citrate). (1R*,2S*,3R*,4S*)-*N*-{4-[4-(2-Pyrimidinyl)-1-piperazinyl]butyl}-2,3-norbornanedicarboximide citrate.

$C_{21}H_{29}N_5O_2,C_6H_8O_7 = 575.6.$

*CAS — 87760-53-0 (tandospirone); 112457-95-1 (tandospirone citrate).*

### Profile

Tandospirone, a partial agonist at serotonin (5-HT) receptors of the $5\text{-}HT_{1A}$ subtype, is an anxiolytic structurally related to buspirone (p.672). It also has antidepressant actions. Tandospirone citrate is given by mouth in usual doses of 30 mg daily in divided doses.

◊ References.

1. Sumiyoshi T, *et al.* The effect of tandospirone, a serotonin(1A) agonist, on memory function in schizophrenia. *Biol Psychiatry* 2001; **49:** 861–8.
2. Yamada K, *et al.* Clinical efficacy of tandospirone augmentation in patients with major depressive disorder: a randomized controlled trial. *Psychiatry Clin Neurosci* 2003; **57:** 183–7.

### Preparations

**Proprietary Preparations** (details are given in Part 3)

***Jpn:*** Sediel.

# Temazepam *(BAN, USAN, rINN)*

ER-115; 3-Hydroxydiazepam; K-3917; Ro-5-5345; Temazepamum; Wy-3917. 7-Chloro-1,3-dihydro-3-hydroxy-1-methyl-5-phenyl-1,4-benzodiazepin-2-one.

$C_{16}H_{13}ClN_2O_2 = 300.7.$

*CAS — 846-50-4.*

*ATC — N05CD07.*

**Pharmacopoeias.** In *Eur.* (see p.vi), *Pol.*, and *US.*

**Ph. Eur. 5.0** (Temazepam). A white or almost white crystalline powder. Practically insoluble in water; sparingly soluble in alcohol; freely soluble in dichloromethane. Protect from light.

**USP 27** (Temazepam). A white or nearly white crystalline powder. Very slightly soluble in water; sparingly soluble in alcohol. Protect from light.

## Dependence and Withdrawal

As for Diazepam, p.690.

◊ For the purpose of withdrawal regimens, 10 mg of temazepam may be considered approximately equivalent to 5 mg of diazepam.

## Adverse Effects, Treatment, and Precautions

As for Diazepam, p.690.

**Abuse.** Liquid-filled temazepam *capsules* (known on the street as 'eggs') were widely abused on the illicit drugs market, the liquid gel lending itself to intravenous administration.[1] This formulation was, therefore, replaced in a number of countries by tablets or semi-solid gel-filled capsules, which were intended to be difficult to inject even after heating or diluting the gel in various solvents.[2] In spite of this there is evidence of intravenous or intra-arterial abuse of these capsules,[3-5] and there are reports of ischaemia, in some cases necessitating amputation.[6-8] The *tablets* may also be liable to abuse; there has been a report of death following intravenous injection of a solution containing crushed temazepam tablets.[9] The manufacturers of a temazepam *elixir* considered that, because of its viscosity and its low strength relative to the liquid in the capsules, it had a low potential for intravenous abuse.[10] Nonetheless, there have been reports[3] of some drug abusers injecting large quantities of diluted elixir.

For mention of rhabdomyolysis associated with abuse of temazepam, see Effects on Skeletal Muscle, under Diazepam, p.691.

1. Farrell M, Strang J. Misuse of temazepam. *BMJ* 1988; **297:** 1402.
2. Launchbury AP. Temazepam abuse. *Pharm J* 1990; **244:** 749.
3. Ruben SM, Morrison CL. Temazepam misuse in a group of injecting drug users. *Br J Addict* 1992; **87:** 1387–92.
4. Scott RN, *et al.* Intra-arterial temazepam. *BMJ* 1992; **304:** 1630.
5. Adiseshiah M, *et al.* Intra-arterial temazepam. *BMJ* 1992; **304:** 1630.
6. Blair SD, *et al.* Leg ischaemia secondary to non-medical injection of temazepam. *Lancet* 1991; **338:** 1393–4.
7. Fox R, *et al.* Misuse of temazepam. *BMJ* 1992; **305:** 253.
8. Feeney GFX, Gibbs HH. Digit loss following misuse of temazepam. *Med J Aust* 2002; **176:** 380.
9. Vella EJ, Edwards CW. Death from pulmonary microembolization after intravenous injection of temazepam. *BMJ* 1993; **307:** 26.
10. Drake J, Ballard R. Misuse of temazepam. *BMJ* 1988; **297:** 1402.

**Breast feeding.** The American Academy of Pediatrics[1] considers that, although the effect of temazepam on breast-feeding infants is unknown, its use by mothers during breast feeding may be of concern since psychotropic drugs do appear in breast milk and thus could conceivably alter CNS function in the infant both in the short and long term.

Temazepam was detected in breast milk in only one of 10 lactating mothers given temazepam as a bedtime sedative;[2] temazepam was given in a dose of 10 to 20 mg and milk concentrations were measured about 15 hours after a dose. The authors considered that breast-fed neonates would receive negligible amounts of temazepam.

1. American Academy of Pediatrics. The transfer of drugs and other chemicals into human milk. *Pediatrics* 2001; **108:** 776–89. Correction. *ibid.*; 1029. Also available at: http://aappolicy.aappublications.org/cgi/content/full/pediatrics%3b108/3/776 (accessed 28/04/04)
2. Lebedevs TH, *et al.* Excretion of temazepam in breast milk. *Br J Clin Pharmacol* 1992; **33:** 204–6.

**Effects on the skin.** Generalised lichenoid drug eruption that had persisted for 5 months in an elderly patient receiving therapy including temazepam resolved within 10 days of discontinuing the benzodiazepine.[1] Bullous eruptions associated with temazepam overdose have also been reported.[2]

1. Norris P, Sounex TS. Generalised lichenoid drug eruption associated with temazepam. *BMJ* 1986; **293:** 510.
2. Verghese J, Merino J. Temazepam overdose associated with bullous eruptions. *Acad Emerg Med* 1999; **6:** 1071.

**Hepatic impairment.** All benzodiazepines should be used with caution in patients with hepatic impairment, and the manufacturers in the UK advise that temazepam should be avoided in severe cases. However, short-acting benzodiazepines such as temazepam may pose less risk in patients with hepatic impairment; in a study of 15 patients with cirrhosis and 16 healthy subjects, liver disease had no significant effect on the pharmacokinetic parameters or pattern of elimination of temazepam.[1]

1. Ghabrial H, *et al.* The effects of age and chronic liver disease on the elimination of temazepam. *Eur J Clin Pharmacol* 1986; **30:** 93–7.

## Interactions

As for Diazepam, p.692.

## Pharmacokinetics

Temazepam is fairly readily absorbed from the gastrointestinal tract, although the exact rate of absorption depends on the formulation. It is about 96% bound to plasma protein. Mean elimination half-lives of about 8 to 15 hours or longer have been reported. It is excreted mainly in the urine in the form of its inactive glucuronide conjugate together with small amounts of the demethylated derivative, oxazepam, also in conjugated form.

◊ The elimination half-life was significantly longer at 16.8 hours among 17 women given temazepam 30 mg compared with 12.3 hours among 15 men.[1] The total clearance was also lower among women. After correction for differences in protein binding, unbound clearance was still lower in women than men but there was no significant effect of age on this parameter. Time to peak plasma concentration and volume of distribution were not affected by the age or sex of the subjects.

1. Divoll M, *et al.* Effect of age and gender on disposition of temazepam. *J Pharm Sci* 1981; **70:** 1104–7.

**Absorption and plasma concentration.** Various oral temazepam formulations have been available worldwide. These included powder-filled hard gelatin capsules, liquid-filled soft gelatin capsules, semi-solid gel-filled soft gelatin capsules, and an elixir. There has been considerable debate over the comparative absorption profiles of temazepam from these formulations which have, in some cases, been modified over the years. It should be noted that pharmacokinetic studies of temazepam do not always clearly state the formulation used.

Temazepam 30 mg was given as a premedicant to 80 patients undergoing surgery in the form of capsules [type not stated] or elixir.[1] Mean peak plasma concentrations of about 800 nanograms/mL occurred 30 minutes after administration of either formulation although there was wide interindividual variation in plasma concentrations. The evidence corresponded with previous suggestions that a plasma concentration of about 250 nanograms/mL or more was required to ensure sedation. The presence or absence of anxiety did not influence the absorption of the preparations.

1. Hosie HE, Nimmo WS. Temazepam absorption in patients before surgery. *Br J Anaesth* 1991; **66:** 20–4.

**Distribution into CSF.** A study in 13 male patients demonstrating a correlation between the unbound concentration of temazepam in plasma and the amount of temazepam detected in CSF.[1] The mean CSF to total plasma temazepam concentration ratio was 5.2.

1. Badcock NR. Plasma and cerebrospinal fluid concentrations of temazepam following oral drug administration. *Eur J Clin Pharmacol* 1990; **38:** 153–5.

**Metabolism.** References.

1. Locniskar A, Greenblatt DJ. Oxidative versus conjugative biotransformation of temazepam. *Biopharm Drug Dispos* 1990; **11:** 499–506.

## Uses and Administration

Temazepam is a short-acting benzodiazepine with general properties similar to those of diazepam (p.695). It is used as a hypnotic in the short-term management of insomnia (p.667) and for premedication before surgical or investigative procedures (p.1296).

A usual dose for insomnia is 10 to 20 mg by mouth at night; exceptionally, doses up to 40 mg may be required. For premedication the usual dose is 20 to 40 mg by mouth given half to one hour beforehand. The *British National Formulary* states that children may be given 1 mg/kg for premedication, to a maximum total dose of 30 mg.

Temazepam should be given in reduced dosage to elderly or debilitated patients; one-half the usual adult dose, or less, may be sufficient.

**Administration.** For reference to the various formulations of oral temazepam that have been used, see Abuse under Adverse Effects, Treatment, and Precautions, above.

**Administration in the elderly.** In a small study[1] a dose of temazepam of 7.5 mg was found to be adequate for the short-term management of insomnia in elderly patients.

1. Vgontzas AN, *et al.* Temazepam 7.5 mg: effects on sleep in elderly insomniacs. *Eur J Clin Pharmacol* 1994; **46:** 209–13.

## Preparations

***BP 2003:*** Temazepam Oral Solution; Temazepam Tablets;
***USP 27:*** Temazepam Capsules.

**Proprietary Preparations** (details are given in Part 3)
***Austral.:*** Euhypnos; Nocturne; Nomapam†; Normison; Temaze; Temtabs; ***Austria:*** Levanxol; Remestan; ***Belg.:*** Euhypnos; Levanxol†; Normison; Temador†; ***Canad.:*** Restoril; ***Denm.:*** Normison†; ***Fin.:*** Normison; Tenox; ***Fr.:*** Normison; ***Ger.:*** Norkotral Tema; Planum; Pronervon T; Remestan; temazep; ***Gr.:*** Normison; ***Irl.:*** Euhypnos; Normison; Nortem; Temazine†; Tenox; ***Ital.:*** Euipnos; Normison; ***Neth.:*** Normison; ***NZ:*** Euhypnos; Normison†; Somapam; ***Port.:*** Normison; ***S.Afr.:*** Normison; Z-Pam†; ***Switz.:*** Normison; ***Thai.:*** Euhypnos; ***UK:*** Euhypnos†; Normison†; ***USA:*** Restoril.

## Tetrazepam *(BAN, pINN)*

CB-4261; Tetrazepamum. 7-Chloro-5-(cyclohex-1-enyl)-1,3-dihydro-1-methyl-2*H*-1,4-benzodiazepin-2-one.

$C_{16}H_{17}ClN_2O$ = 288.8.
*CAS — 10379-14-3.*
*ATC — M03BX07.*

**Pharmacopoeias.** In *Eur.* (see p.vi) and *Pol.*

**Ph. Eur. 5.0** (Tetrazepam). A light yellow or yellow crystalline powder. Practically insoluble in water; soluble in acetonitrile; freely soluble in dichloromethane. Protect from light.

### Profile

Tetrazepam is a benzodiazepine with general properties similar to those of diazepam (p.690). It is used for its muscle relaxant properties in the treatment of muscle spasm (p.1386). The usual initial dose is 25 to 50 mg by mouth increased, if necessary, to 150 mg or more daily.

**Pharmacokinetics.** References.

1. Bun H, *et al.* Plasma levels and pharmacokinetics of single and multiple dose of tetrazepam in healthy volunteers. *Arzneimittelforschung* 1987; **37:** 199–202.

**Porphyria.** Tetrazepam is considered to be unsafe in patients with porphyria because it has been shown to be porphyrinogenic in *in-vitro* systems.

### Preparations

**Proprietary Preparations** (details are given in Part 3)
***Austria:*** Myolastan; ***Belg.:*** Myolastan; ***Fr.:*** Megavix; Myolastan; Panos; ***Ger.:*** Mobiforton; Musapam; Musaril; Muskelat; Myospasmal; Rilex; Tepam†; Tethexal; Tetra-saar; Tetramdura; Tetrazep; ***Mex.:*** Miolastan; ***Spain:*** Myolastan.

## Thioproperazine Mesilate *(BANM, rINNM)*

Mesilato de tioproperazina; RP-7843; SKF-5883; Thioproperazine Dimethanesulphonate; Thioproperazine Mesylate; Thioproperazine Methanesulphonate. *NN*-Dimethyl-10-[3-(4-methylpiperazin-1-yl)propyl]phenothiazine-2-sulphonamide dimethanesulphonate.

$C_{22}H_{30}N_4O_2S_2,2CH_4O_3S$ = 638.8.
*CAS — 316-81-4 (thioproperazine); 2347-80-0 (thioproperazine mesilate).*
*ATC — N05AB08.*

**Pharmacopoeias.** In *Fr.*

### Profile

Thioproperazine is a phenothiazine with general properties similar to those of chlorpromazine (p.675). It has a piperazine side-chain. It is used in the treatment of schizophrenia (p.665), mania (see Bipolar Disorder, p.278), and other psychoses. Thioproperazine is given as the mesilate although doses are expressed in terms of the base; thioproperazine mesilate 7.2 mg is approximately equivalent to 5 mg of thioproperazine. Initial daily doses of 5 mg are given by mouth, increased as necessary; the usual effective dosage is 30 to 40 mg daily. In severe or resistant cases daily doses of 90 mg or more have been given.

### Preparations

**Proprietary Preparations** (details are given in Part 3)
***Belg.:*** Majeptil†; ***Canad.:*** Majeptil; ***Fr.:*** Majeptil†; ***Gr.:*** Majeptil; ***Mex.:*** Majeptil; ***Spain:*** Majeptil.

## Thioridazine *(BAN, USAN, rINN)*

Thioridazinum; Tioridazina; TP-21. 10-[2-(1-Methyl-2-piperidyl)ethyl]-2-methylthiophenothiazine.

$C_{21}H_{26}N_2S_2$ = 370.6.
*CAS — 50-52-2.*
*ATC — N05AC02.*

**Pharmacopoeias.** In *Eur.* (see p.vi) and *US.*

**Ph. Eur. 5.0** (Thioridazine). A white or almost white powder. Practically insoluble in water; soluble in alcohol; very soluble in dichloromethane; freely soluble in methyl alcohol. Protect from light.

**USP 27** (Thioridazine). A white to slightly yellow crystalline or micronised powder; odourless or having a faint odour. Practically insoluble in water; freely soluble in dehydrated alcohol and in ether; very soluble in chloroform. Protect from light.

## Thioridazine Hydrochloride *(BANM, rINNM)*

Hidrocloruro de tioridazina; Thioridazini Hydrochloridum.

$C_{21}H_{26}N_2S_2,HCl$ = 407.0.
*CAS — 130-61-0.*
*ATC — N05AC02.*

**Pharmacopoeias.** In *Chin., Eur.* (see p.vi), *Jpn, Pol.,* and *US.*

**Ph. Eur. 5.0** (Thioridazine Hydrochloride). A white or almost white, crystalline powder. Freely soluble in water and in methyl alcohol; soluble in alcohol. A 1% solution in water has a pH of 4.2 to 5.2. Protect from light.

**USP 27** (Thioridazine Hydrochloride). A white to slightly yellow granular powder having a slight odour. Freely soluble in water, in chloroform, and in methyl alcohol; insoluble in ether. pH of a 1% solution in water is between 4.2 and 5.2. Store in airtight containers. Protect from light.

**Incompatibility.** For a warning about incompatibility between thioridazine hydrochloride solution (Mellaril) and carbamazepine suspension (Tegretol), see p.353.

### Adverse Effects and Treatment

As for Chlorpromazine, p.675.

Thioridazine has been associated with a higher incidence of antimuscarinic effects, but lower incidence of extrapyramidal symptoms than chlorpromazine. It may also be less sedating. However, it is more likely to induce hypotension and there is an increased risk of cardiotoxicity and dose-related prolongation of the QT interval. Because of this and the consequent danger of life-threatening arrhythmias such as torsade de pointes and sudden death, its use is restricted (see Precautions and Uses and Administration, below). Sexual dysfunction also appears to be more frequent with thioridazine.

Pigmentary retinopathy characterised by diminution of visual acuity, brownish colouring of vision, and impairment of night vision has been seen particularly in patients taking large doses.

**Effects on the cardiovascular system.** Between 1964 and 2001, the UK Committee on Safety of Medicines received 42 reports of suspected heart rate and rhythm disorders associated with thioridazine.[1] There were 21 fatalities reported out of 39 cases where the outcome was known.

See also under Chlorpromazine, p.676.

1. Committee on Safety of Medicines/Medicines Control Agency. QT interval prolongation with antipsychotics. *Current Problems* 2001; **27:** 4. Also available at: http://www.mca.gov.uk/ourwork/monitorsafequalmed/currentproblems/cpfeb2001.pdf (accessed 28/04/04)

**Hypersensitivity.** Pruritus and erythematous rash on the genitals of a woman following sexual intercourse were found to be due to thioridazine present in the seminal fluid of her husband, who was receiving 100 mg daily at night.[1]

1. Sell MB. Sensitization to thioridazine through sexual intercourse. *Am J Psychiatry* 1985; **142:** 271–2.

**Overdosage.** Rhabdomyolysis has been reported in a patient after overdosage with thioridazine.[1] Twenty-four hours after taking 9.4 g of thioridazine the patient presented with difficulty in moving and speaking. On examination he had swelling and tenderness over his upper arms, thighs, and calves. Ataxia and transient dysarthria were attributed to generalised muscle weakness. Other effects were consistent with antimuscarinic effects of thioridazine. He had no signs of neuroleptic malignant syndrome but his urine contained myoglobin. The patient was treated with gastric lavage, activated charcoal, and rehydration. Serum biochemistry returned to normal over one week and the muscle tenderness and weakness disappeared.

1. Nankivell BJ, *et al.* Rhabdomyolysis induced by thioridazine. *BMJ* 1994; **309:** 378.

### Precautions

As for Chlorpromazine, p.678. Thioridazine should not be used in patients with clinically significant cardiac disorders, uncorrected hypokalaemia or other electrolyte imbalance, with known or suspected QT prolongation or a family history of QT prolongation, or with a history of ventricular arrhythmias including torsade de pointes. Use is also contra-indicated in patients known to have reduced activity of the cytochrome P450 isoenzyme CYP2D6, which is responsible for thioridazine metabolism. Use with drugs liable to interfere with the metabolism of thioridazine, of other drugs known to prolong the QT interval, and of drugs likely to cause electrolyte imbalance should also be avoided (see under Interactions, below).

For all patients starting thioridazine it is recommended that a baseline ECG and electrolyte screening are performed. An ECG should also be repeated before each dose increase, one week after the maximum therapeutic dose has been reached, and at 6-monthly intervals in those who continue treatment. Serum electrolyte concentrations should also be monitored periodically during treatment and any imbalance corrected.

**Porphyria.** Thioridazine has been associated with acute attacks of porphyria and is considered unsafe in porphyric patients.

### Interactions

As for Chlorpromazine, p.679. The metabolism of thioridazine is mediated by the cytochrome P450 isoenzyme CYP2D6; thioridazine itself is also an inhibitor of CYP2D6. Therefore, there is the potential for interactions between thioridazine and other drugs that inhibit or act as a substrate for this enzyme; such drugs should not be given with thioridazine. Some examples include antiarrhythmics, certain antidepressants including the SSRIs and tricyclics, certain antipsychotics, beta blockers, HIV-protease inhibitors, and opiates.

Use with other drugs known to prolong the QT interval such as class IA and class III antiarrhythmics, tricyclic antidepressants, and some other antipsychotics should also be avoided, as should the co-administration of those drugs known to cause electrolyte imbalance.

### Pharmacokinetics

The pharmacokinetics of thioridazine appear to be generally similar to those of chlorpromazine (p.680). Thioridazine is metabolised by the cytochrome P450 isoenzyme CYP2D6. Its main active metabolite is mesoridazine (p.706); the metabolite, sulforidazine, also has some activity. Thioridazine and its active metabolites are reported to be highly bound to plasma proteins. The plasma half-life of thioridazine has been estimated to be about 4 to 10 hours.

◊ References.

1. Mårtensson E, Roos B-E. Serum levels of thioridazine in psychiatric patients and healthy volunteers. *Eur J Clin Pharmacol* 1973; **6:** 181–6.
2. Axelsson R, Mårtensson E. Serum concentration and elimination from serum of thioridazine in psychiatric patients. *Curr Ther Res* 1976; **19:** 242–65.

**Metabolism.** In 10 psychiatric patients stabilised on thioridazine, therapy was replaced by equipotent doses of the side-chain sulfoxide (mesoridazine) and side-chain sulfone (sulforidazine) metabolites of thioridazine.[1] Both metabolites were shown to have an antipsychotic effect, the dose of each required being about two-thirds that of thioridazine. The serum half-lives were thioridazine 21 hours, mesoridazine 16 hours, and sulforidazine 13 hours. Apathy, depression, and restlessness gradually developed during treatment with the 2 metabolites and they could not be used for any length of time. Extrapyramidal symptoms, hypersalivation, and drowsiness were more common with the metabolites; 2 patients had epileptic seizures, and one receiving sulforidazine developed probable cholestatic jaundice.

There is some evidence that the metabolism of thioridazine is influenced by debrisoquine hydroxylation phenotype.[2] A single-dose study in 19 healthy male subjects demonstrated slower formation of mesoridazine, and hence higher serum-thioridazine concentrations in poor debrisoquine hydroxylators compared with extensive hydroxylators. Formation of thioridazine ring-sulfoxide appeared to be compensatorily increased in slow hydroxylators.

1. Axelsson R. On the serum concentrations and antipsychotic effects of thioridazine, thioridazine side-chain sulfoxide and thioridazine side-chain sulfone, in chronic psychotic patients. *Curr Ther Res* 1977; **21:** 587–605.
2. von Bahr C, *et al.* Plasma levels of thioridazine and metabolites are influenced by the debrisoquin hydroxylation phenotype. *Clin Pharmacol Ther* 1991; **49:** 234–40.

### Uses and Administration

Thioridazine is a phenothiazine with general properties similar to those of chlorpromazine (p.680). It has a piperidine side-chain and, unlike chlorpromazine, has little antiemetic activity.

The use of thioridazine is restricted to the treatment of schizophrenia (p.665) in patients who fail to show an adequate response to treatment with other antipsychotics. Its use in other psychiatric disorders was abandoned after it was felt that there was an unacceptable balance of risks and benefits as a result of its cardiotoxic potential.

For all patients starting thioridazine it is recommended that a baseline ECG and electrolyte screening are performed. An ECG should also be repeated before each dose increase, one week after the maximum therapeutic dose has been reached, and at 6-monthly intervals in those who continue treatment. Serum electrolyte concentrations should also be monitored periodically during treatment and any imbalance corrected.

Thioridazine is administered by mouth as the hydrochloride or the base, and given in terms of either. In the UK, for example, doses of oral liquid preparations are given in terms of the base, whereas those of the tablets are given as the hydrochloride. In the USA all doses are given in terms of the hydrochloride. Thioridazine base 22.8 mg is approximately equivalent to 25 mg of thioridazine hydrochloride.

In the treatment of schizophrenia thioridazine should be started at the lowest recommended dose and slowly titrated upwards. A usual daily dosage range for outpatients is 50 to 300 mg, which may be given in divided doses. In the UK the maximum licensed dose is 600 mg daily in hospitalised patients but up to 800 mg daily is permitted in the USA; such doses should be reduced once effective control is achieved. It is recommended that increases in doses should be no more than 100 mg weekly.

Thioridazine should be given in lower initial doses to patients with a low body-mass or those with hepatic or renal impairment; dosage increases should also be more gradual.

In those patients who require withdrawal of thioridazine, the dose should be gradually reduced over 1 to 2 weeks to avoid symptoms such as gastrointestinal disorders, dizziness, anxiety, and insomnia that are sometimes seen after abrupt discontinuation of high-dose or long-term treatment.

### Preparations

***BP 2003:*** Thioridazine Oral Solution; Thioridazine Oral Suspension; Thioridazine Tablets;
***USP 27:*** Thioridazine Hydrochloride Oral Solution; Thioridazine Hydrochloride Tablets; Thioridazine Oral Suspension.

**Proprietary Preparations** (details are given in Part 3)
***Arg.:*** Meleril; ***Austral.:*** Aldazine; Melleril; ***Austria:*** Melleretten†; Melleril; ***Belg.:*** Melleril; ***Braz.:*** Melleril; ***Canad.:*** Mellaril†; Novo-Ridazine†; ***Chile:*** Meleril; Simultan; Tinsenol; ***Denm.:*** Melleril; ***Fin.:*** Melleril; Orsanil; ***Fr.:*** Melleril; ***Ger.:*** Melleretten; Melleril; ***Gr.:*** Melleril; ***Hong Kong:*** Melleril; ***India:*** Thioril; ***Irl.:*** Melleril; Melzine; Thiozine; ***Israel:*** Melleril†; Ridazin; ***Ital.:*** Mellerette†; Melleril; ***Malaysia:*** Aldazine; Melleril; ***Mex.:*** Melleril; ***Neth.:*** Melleretten; Melleril; ***Norw.:*** Melleril; ***NZ:*** Aldazine; Melleril; ***Port.:*** Melleril; ***S.Afr.:*** Melleril; ***Spain:*** Meleril; ***Swed.:*** Mallorol; ***Switz.:*** Mellerettes; Melleril; ***Thai.:*** Calmaril; Dazine; Ridazine; Thiomed; Thiosia; ***UK:*** Melleril; Rideril; ***USA:*** Mellaril.

**Multi-ingredient:** ***Ital.:*** Visergil†; ***Spain:*** Visergil†.

## Tiapride Hydrochloride *(BAN, rINNM)*

FLO-1347; Hidrocloruro de tiaprida; Tiapridi Hydrochloridum.
*N*-(2-Diethylaminoethyl)-2-methoxy-5-methylsulphonylbenzamide hydrochloride.
$C_{15}H_{24}N_2O_4S,HCl = 364.9$.
*CAS — 51012-32-9 (tiapride); 51012-33-0 (tiapride hydrochloride).*
*ATC — N05AL03.*

**Pharmacopoeias.** In *Eur.* (see p.vi).

**Ph. Eur. 5.0** (Tiapride Hydrochloride). A white or almost white crystalline powder. Very soluble in water; slightly soluble in dehydrated alcohol; soluble in methyl alcohol. A 5% solution in water has a pH of 4.0 to 6.0.

### Adverse Effects, Treatment, and Precautions

As for Chlorpromazine, p.675.

**Effects on the cardiovascular system.** Torsade de pointes developed following a single dose of tiapride in an elderly patient with cardiac disease, a known risk factor for such arrhythmias.[1]

1. Iglesias E, *et al.* Tiapride-induced torsade de pointes. *Am J Med* 2000; **109:** 509.

### Interactions

As for Chlorpromazine, p.679.

### Pharmacokinetics

Tiapride is rapidly absorbed following oral administration and excreted largely unchanged in the urine. The plasma half-life is reported to range from 3 to 4 hours.

◊ The steady-state pharmacokinetics of tiapride have been studied in 5 elderly patients with tardive dyskinesia, and in 2 patients with Huntington's chorea.[1] All patients received tiapride 100 mg three times daily by mouth for 7 days. The mean peak plasma concentration of tiapride was 1.47 micrograms/mL, achieved a mean of 1.4 hours after dosing, and the mean elimination half-life was 3.8 hours. These values did not differ significantly from those previously reported in younger healthy subjects, although renal clearance was slightly lower in these patients. About half of the dose of tiapride was excreted unchanged by the kidney; a metabolite, probably *N*-monodesethyltiapride was detected in the urine but its identity was not confirmed.

1. Roos RAC, *et al.* Pharmacokinetics of tiapride in patients with tardive dyskinesia and Huntington's disease. *Eur J Clin Pharmacol* 1986; **31:** 191–4.

### Uses and Administration

Tiapride is a substituted benzamide with general properties similar to those of sulpiride (p.722).

It is usually given as the hydrochloride in the management of behaviour disorders and to treat dyskinesias. Doses are expressed in terms of the equivalent amount of tiapride; tiapride hydrochloride 222.2 mg is approximately equivalent to 200 mg of tiapride base. Doses of 200 to 400 mg daily by mouth are usually given, although higher daily doses have been used, in particular in the management of dyskinesias. Tiapride hydrochloride has also been given by intramuscular or intravenous injection.

**Disturbed behaviour.** For a discussion of the management of disturbed behaviour including limitations on the use of antipsychotics, see p.665.

References.

1. Gutzmann H, *et al.* Measuring the efficacy of psychopharmacological treatment of psychomotoric restlessness in dementia: clinical evaluation of tiapride. *Pharmacopsychiatry* 1997; **30:** 6–11.

**Extrapyramidal disorders.** Tiapride has been tried in the treatment of antipsychotic-induced tardive dyskinesia (p.677), but as with all antipsychotics improvement may only be short-term.

Tiapride has also been tried in the treatment of Tourette's syndrome (p.664).

For reference to the use of tiapride in suppressing the adverse effects of levodopa on respiration, see p.1206.

CHOREA. Antipsychotics have some action against choreiform movements as well as being of use to control the behavioural disturbances of Huntington's chorea. For a discussion of the management of various choreas, see p.664.

References to the use of tiapride.

1. Roos RAC, *et al.* Tiapride in the treatment of Huntington's chorea. *Acta Neurol Scand* 1982; **65:** 45–50.
2. Deroover J, *et al.* Tiapride versus placebo: a double-blind comparative study in the management of Huntington's chorea. *Curr Med Res Opin* 1984; **9:** 329–38.

**Substance dependence.** An early review[1] concluded that the role of tiapride in acute *alcohol* withdrawal (p.1166) was likely to be limited as patients at risk of severe reactions would still require adjunct therapy for the control of hallucinations and seizures. Following detoxification tiapride appeared to help to some degree to alleviate distress, improve abstinence and drinking behaviour, and facilitate reintegration within society.[2] Interest in its use with carbamazepine continues.[3]

1. Peters DH, Faulds D. Tiapride: a review of its pharmacology and therapeutic potential in the management of alcohol dependence syndrome. *Drugs* 1994; **47:** 1010–32.
2. Shaw GK, *et al.* Tiapride in the prevention of relapse in recently detoxified alcoholics. *Br J Psychiatry* 1994; **165:** 515–23.
3. Franz M, *et al.* Treatment of alcohol withdrawal: tiapride and carbamazepine versus clomethiazole: a pilot study. *Eur Arch Psychiatry Clin Neurosci* 2001; **251:** 185–92.

### Preparations

**Proprietary Preparations** (details are given in Part 3)
***Arg.:*** Etiles; ***Austria:*** Delpral; ***Belg.:*** Tiapridal; ***Braz.:*** Tiapridal; ***Chile:*** Sereprid; ***Fr.:*** Clemental; Equilium; Tiapridal; ***Ger.:*** Tiapridex; ***Hong Kong:*** Tiapridal; ***Israel:*** Doparid; ***Ital.:*** Italprid; Luxoben†; Sereprile; ***Jpn:*** Gramalil; ***Neth.:*** Tiapridal; ***Port.:*** Normagit; Tiapridal; ***Singapore:*** Tiapridal†; ***Spain:*** Tiaprizal; ***Switz.:*** Tiapridal.

## Timiperone *(rINN)*

DD-3480; Timiperona. 4′-Fluoro-4-[4-(2-thioxo-1-benzimidazolinyl)piperidino]butyrophenone.
$C_{22}H_{24}FN_3OS = 397.5$.
*CAS — 57648-21-2.*

### Profile

Timiperone is a butyrophenone with general properties similar to those of haloperidol (p.701). It has been used by mouth in the treatment of schizophrenia. Timiperone has also been given by injection.

## Tiotixene *(BAN, rINN)*

NSC-108165; P-4657B; Thiothixene *(USAN)*; Tiotixeno. (*Z*)-*NN*-Dimethyl-9-[3-(4-methylpiperazin-1-yl)propylidene]thioxanthene-2-sulphonamide.
$C_{23}H_{29}N_3O_2S_2 = 443.6$.
*CAS — 5591-45-7; 3313-26-6 (tiotixene Z-isomer).*
*ATC — N05AF04.*

**Pharmacopoeias.** In *US.*

**USP 27** (Thiothixene). White to tan, practically odourless, crystals. Practically insoluble in water; soluble 1 in 110 of dehydrated alcohol, 1 in 2 of chloroform, and 1 in 120 of ether; slightly soluble in acetone and in methyl alcohol. Store in airtight containers. Protect from light.

## Tiotixene Hydrochloride *(BANM, rINNM)*

CP-12252-1; Hidrocloruro de tiotixeno; Thiothixene Hydrochloride *(USAN)*.
$C_{23}H_{29}N_3O_2S_2,2HCl,2H_2O = 552.6$.
*CAS — 58513-59-0 (anhydrous tiotixene hydrochloride); 49746-04-5 (anhydrous tiotixene hydrochloride, Z-isomer); 22189-31-7 (tiotixene hydrochloride dihydrate); 49746-09-0 (tiotixene hydrochloride dihydrate, Z-isomer).*
*ATC — N05AF04.*

**Pharmacopoeias.** In *US,* which permits both the dihydrate and the anhydrous form.

**USP 27** (Thiothixene Hydrochloride). It contains two molecules of water of hydration or is anhydrous ($C_{23}H_{29}N_3O_2S_2,2HCl = 516.5$). A white or practically white crystalline powder having a slight odour. Soluble 1 in 8 of water, 1 in 270 of dehydrated alcohol, and 1 in 280 of chloroform; practically insoluble in acetone, in ether, and in benzene. Store in airtight containers. Protect from light.

**Stability.** A combination of the stabilisers hydroxyquinoline sulfate and vanillin could protect tiotixene from photodegradation.[1]

1. Thoma K, Klimek R. Photostabilization of drugs in dosage forms without protection from packaging materials. *Int J Pharmaceutics* 1991; **67:** 169–75.

### Adverse Effects, Treatment, and Precautions

As for Chlorpromazine, p.675. Tiotixene is less likely to cause sedation but extrapyramidal disorders are more frequent.

### Interactions

As for Chlorpromazine, p.679.

### Pharmacokinetics

◊ In 15 adequately controlled schizophrenic patients receiving tiotixene 15 to 60 mg daily in 2, 3, or 4 divided doses by mouth, plasma concentrations were found to be in the relatively narrow range of 10 to 22.5 nanograms/mL 126 to 150 minutes after the last daily dose despite the fourfold difference in dosage.[1] Investigations in a further 5 patients indicated that peak plasma concentrations were obtained about 1 to 3 hours after a dose, indicating rapid absorption with an absorption half-time of about 30 minutes. There was an early plasma half-life of about 210 minutes and a late half-life of about 34 hours; resurgence of drug concentrations in some subjects might have been due to enterohepatic recycling.

1. Hobbs DC, *et al.* Pharmacokinetics of thiothixene in man. *Clin Pharmacol Ther* 1974; **16:** 473–8.

**Metabolism.** A study[1] indicating that tiotixene may induce its own metabolism.

1. Bergling R, *et al.* Plasma levels and clinical effects of thioridazine and thiothixene. *J Clin Pharmacol* 1975; **15:** 178–86.

### Uses and Administration

Tiotixene is a thioxanthene antipsychotic with general properties similar to those of the phenothiazine, chlorpromazine (p.680). It has a piperazine side-chain. It is used in the treatment of various psychoses including schizophrenia (p.665). Tiotixene is given by mouth as the base or hydrochloride and by intramuscular injection as the hydrochloride. Doses are expressed in terms of the base. Tiotixene 1 mg is approximately equivalent to 1.2 mg of tiotixene hydrochloride.

The usual initial dose is 2 mg three times daily by mouth (or 5 mg twice daily in more severe conditions) gradually increasing to 20 to 30 mg daily if necessary; once-daily dosage may be adequate. In severe or resistant psychoses doses of up to 60 mg daily may be given. The usual initial intramuscular dose is 4 mg two to four times daily increased if necessary to a maximum of 30 mg daily.

Tiotixene should be given in reduced dosage to elderly or debilitated patients.

### Preparations

***USP 27:*** Thiothixene Capsules; Thiothixene Hydrochloride for Injection; Thiothixene Hydrochloride Injection; Thiothixene Hydrochloride Oral Solution.

**Proprietary Preparations** (details are given in Part 3)
***Austral.:*** Navane; ***Braz.:*** Navane†; ***Canad.:*** Navane; ***Hong Kong:*** Navane; ***Neth.:*** Navane; ***NZ:*** Thixit; ***Thai.:*** Navane†; ***USA:*** Navane.

## Tofisopam *(rINN)*

EGYT-341; Tofizopam. 1-(3,4-Dimethoxyphenyl)-5-ethyl-7,8-dimethoxy-4-methyl-5*H*-2,3-benzodiazepine.
$C_{22}H_{26}N_2O_4 = 382.5$.
*CAS — 22345-47-7.*
*ATC — N05BA23.*

**Pharmacopoeias.** In *Jpn.*

### Profile

Tofisopam is a 2,3-benzodiazepine related structurally to the 1,4-benzodiazepines such as diazepam (p.690) and sharing some of the same actions. It is reported, however, to be largely lacking in the sedative, anticonvulsant, and muscle relaxant properties of the conventional benzodiazepines. Tofisopam has been given by mouth in the short-term treatment of anxiety disorders.

### Preparations

**Proprietary Preparations** (details are given in Part 3)
***Hung.:*** Grandaxin; ***Thai.:*** Grandaxin.

## Triazolam *(BAN, USAN, rINN)*

Clorazolam; U-33030. 8-Chloro-6-(2-chlorophenyl)-1-methyl-4*H*-[1,2,4]triazolo[4,3-*a*][1,4]benzodiazepine.
$C_{17}H_{12}Cl_2N_4 = 343.2$.
*CAS — 28911-01-5.*
*ATC — N05CD05.*

**Pharmacopoeias.** In *Chin.* and *US.*

**USP 27** (Triazolam). A white to off-white, practically odourless, crystalline powder. Practically insoluble in water and in ether; soluble 1 in 1000 of alcohol, 1 in 25 of chloroform, and 1 in 600 of 0.1N hydrochloric acid.

### Dependence and Withdrawal

As for Diazepam, p.690.

## Adverse Effects and Treatment

As for Diazepam, p.690.

**Effects on the liver.** A 44-year-old man developed severe pruritus with jaundice which subsequently proved fatal. Liver histology showed intense cholestasis. Triazolam was considered to be the most likely precipitant.[1]

1. Cobden I, *et al.* Fatal intrahepatic cholestasis associated with triazolam. *Postgrad Med J* 1981; **57:** 730–1.

**Effects on mental function.** The effects of triazolam on mental function have been controversial since van der Kroef first described in 1979 a range of symptoms including anxiety, amnesia, depersonalisation and derealisation, depression, paranoia, and severe suicidal tendencies that he had observed in 25 patients and attributed to the administration of triazolam.[1] This led to suspension of triazolam in the Netherlands (re-approved in 1990) and removal of the 1-mg tablet from other markets. Continued reporting of similar symptoms of cognitive impairment with triazolam resulted in discontinuation of the 500-microgram dosage form in several countries in 1987 and 1988 and in a gradual reduction of recommended dosage from 1 mg at night down to 125 to 250 micrograms at night. Triazolam was withdrawn from the UK[2] and some other markets in 1991. Opinion still remains divided over the adverse effects of triazolam, the main issues being its propensity to cause side-effects relative to other benzodiazepines and whether its risk-benefit ratio is acceptable to justify its continued use.[3,4]

Others[5] have reviewed spontaneous adverse effects reported to the FDA in the USA for triazolam, temazepam, and flurazepam. Daytime sedation was noted with all three, but triazolam caused more agitation, confusion, hallucinations, and amnesia. Such effects occurred frequently with the 250-microgram dose as well as with the 500-microgram dose. Similar results were obtained after analysis of reports for triazolam and temazepam in the first 7 years of marketing, although the possibility that selection factors were producing higher reporting rates for triazolam could not be entirely excluded.[6] A study[7] gave triazolam 500 micrograms, lormetazepam 2 mg, or placebo, to groups of 40 patients for 25 nights and observed the greatest frequency of daytime anxiety, panic, derealisation, and paranoia with triazolam. Another[8] found a greater total number of reports of memory impairment or amnesia after nightly administration of triazolam 500 micrograms compared with temazepam 30 mg. Triazolam also impaired delayed, but not immediate, memory recall. Similar cases of memory impairment occurring with triazolam at doses of 125 and 250 micrograms have reportedly been submitted to the UK Committee on Safety of Medicines.[2] The emergence of daytime symptoms after more than a few days' treatment with triazolam could be attributed to rebound or withdrawal phenomena occurring as a result of rapid elimination of the drug.

As regards the risk-benefit ratio of triazolam some workers have questioned the hypnotic efficacy of the drug at a dose of 250 micrograms and consider that reduction of the dose has decreased efficacy more than side-effects.[3]

In defence of triazolam, the FDA and the manufacturers (Upjohn) have considered epidemiological studies which, unlike the FDA spontaneous reporting scheme, have been unable to demonstrate a substantial difference in its adverse effects compared with other benzodiazepines except, perhaps, in the incidence of amnesia.[9] Retrospective studies[10,11] claiming similar findings have been the subject of criticism.[12-14] Other workers have cited studies indicating benefit of triazolam 250 micrograms for the treatment of insomnia.[15] A review by the US Institute of Medicine found that triazolam was safe when given in a dose of 250 micrograms daily for 7 to 10 days but called for studies of lower doses and of long-term use.[16]

1. Van der Kroef C. Reactions to triazolam. *Lancet* 1979; **ii:** 526.
2. Anonymous. The sudden withdrawal of triazolam—reasons and consequences. *Drug Ther Bull* 1991; **29:** 89–90.
3. O'Donovan MC, McGuffin P. Short acting benzodiazepines. *BMJ* 1993; **306:** 945–6.
4. Ghaeli P, *et al.* Triazolam treatment controversy. *Ann Pharmacother* 1994; **28:** 1038–40.
5. Bixler EO, *et al.* Adverse reactions to benzodiazepine hypnotics: spontaneous reporting system. *Pharmacology* 1987; **35:** 286–300.
6. Wysowski DK, Barash D. Adverse behavioral reactions attributed to triazolam in the Food and Drug Administration's spontaneous reporting system. *Arch Intern Med* 1991; **151:** 2003–8.
7. Adam K, Oswald I. Can a rapidly-eliminated hypnotic cause daytime anxiety? *Pharmacopsychiatry* 1989; **22:** 115–19.
8. Bixler EO, *et al.* Next-day memory impairment with triazolam use. *Lancet* 1991; **337:** 827–31.
9. Drucker RF, MacLeod N. Benzodiazepines. *Pharm J* 1989; **243:** 508.
10. Hindmarch I, *et al.* Adverse events after triazolam substitution. *Lancet* 1993; **341:** 55.
11. Rothschild AJ, *et al.* Triazolam and disinhibition. *Lancet* 1993; **341:** 186.
12. Hawley CJ, *et al.* Adverse events after triazolam substitution. *Lancet* 1993; **341:** 567.
13. Vela-Bueno A. Adverse events after triazolam substitution. *Lancet* 1993; **341:** 567.
14. Kales A, *et al.* Adverse events after triazolam substitution. *Lancet* 1993; **341:** 567–8.
15. Gillin JC, Byerley WF. Diagnosis and management of insomnia. *N Engl J Med* 1990; **323:** 487.
16. Ault A. FDA advisers find no major Halcion dangers. *Lancet* 1997; **350:** 1760.

## Precautions

As for Diazepam, p.691.

**Hepatic impairment.** Cirrhosis decreased the apparent oral clearance of triazolam to an extent depending on the severity of the liver disease.[1] An initial dose of 125 micrograms was suggested for patients with severe liver dysfunction. It was suggested that the relative lack of effect that mild to moderate cirrhosis had on the metabolism of oral triazolam might be due to some first-pass metabolism occurring in the intestinal wall.[2]

1. Kroboth PD, *et al.* Nighttime dosing of triazolam in patients with liver disease and normal subjects: kinetics and daytime effects. *J Clin Pharmacol* 1987; **27:** 555–60.
2. Robin DW, *et al.* Triazolam in cirrhosis: pharmacokinetics and pharmacodynamics. *Clin Pharmacol Ther* 1993; **54:** 630–7.

**Renal impairment.** Peak plasma-triazolam concentrations were lower in 11 dialysis patients compared with 11 controls.[1] It was postulated that a relatively high basal gastric acid secretion in dialysis patients could result in hydrolysis and opening of the ring structure of triazolam effectively reducing its systemic availability. Administration of an antacid could reverse this effect. Renal failure had no other effect on the pharmacokinetics of triazolam which could probably be given in usual doses.

1. Kroboth PD, *et al.* Effects of end stage renal disease and aluminium hydroxide on triazolam pharmacokinetics. *Br J Clin Pharmacol* 1985; **19:** 839–42.

## Interactions

As for Diazepam, p.692.

## Pharmacokinetics

Triazolam is rapidly and nearly completely absorbed from the gastrointestinal tract, peak plasma concentrations being achieved within 2 hours of administration by mouth. Triazolam has a plasma elimination half-life ranging from 1.5 to 5.5 hours. It is reported to be about 89% bound to plasma proteins. Hydroxylation of triazolam in the liver is mediated by the cytochrome P450 isoenzyme CYP3A4. Triazolam is excreted in the urine mainly in the form of its conjugated metabolites with only small amounts appearing unchanged.

◊ Reviews of the pharmacokinetics of triazolam.

1. Garzone PD, Kroboth PD. Pharmacokinetics of the newer benzodiazepines. *Clin Pharmacokinet* 1989; **16:** 337–64.

## Uses and Administration

Triazolam is a short-acting benzodiazepine with general properties similar to those of diazepam (p.695). It is used as a hypnotic in the short-term management of insomnia (p.667) in doses of 125 to 250 micrograms at night for no more than 2 weeks; doses of up to 500 micrograms at night have been used for resistant cases but these may be associated with an increased risk of severe adverse effects (see Effects on Mental Function, above). Initial doses of 125 micrograms at night have been suggested for elderly or debilitated subjects, increased up to a maximum of 250 micrograms only if necessary.

**Administration in hepatic or renal impairment.** See under Precautions, above.

## Preparations

***USP 27:*** Triazolam Tablets.

**Proprietary Preparations** (details are given in Part 3)
***Austral.:*** Halcion; ***Austria:*** Halcion; ***Belg.:*** Halcion; ***Braz.:*** Halcion; ***Canad.:*** Apo-Triazo; Halcion; Novo-Triolam†; ***Chile:*** Balidon; Somese; ***Denm.:*** Halcion; Rilamir; ***Fin.:*** Halcion; ***Fr.:*** Halcion; ***Ger.:*** Halcion; ***Gr.:*** Halcion; ***Hong Kong:*** Halcion; ***Irl.:*** Halcion; Trilam; ***Israel:*** Halcion; ***Ital.:*** Halcion; Songar; ***Malaysia:*** Somese; ***Mex.:*** Halcion; ***Neth.:*** Halcion; ***NZ:*** Halcion; Hypam†; Trycam†; ***Port.:*** Halcion; ***S.Afr.:*** Halcion; ***Singapore:*** Somese†; ***Spain:*** Halcion; ***Swed.:*** Halcion; ***Switz.:*** Halcion; ***Thai.:*** Halcion; Trycam; ***USA:*** Halcion.

# Triclofos Sodium *(BANM, USAN, rINNM)*

Sch-10159; Sodium Triclofos; Triclofós sódico. Sodium 2,2,2-trichloroethyl hydrogen orthophosphate.
$C_2H_3Cl_3NaO_4P$ = 251.4.
*CAS — 306-52-5 (triclofos); 7246-20-0 (triclofos sodium).*
*ATC — N05CM07.*

**Pharmacopoeias.** In *Br.* and *Jpn.*

**BP 2003** (Triclofos Sodium). A white or almost white, odourless or almost odourless, hygroscopic powder. Freely soluble in water; slightly soluble in alcohol; practically insoluble in ether. A 2% solution in water has a pH of 3.0 to 4.5.

## Dependence and Withdrawal, Adverse Effects, Treatment, and Precautions

As for Cloral Hydrate, p.684 but causes fewer gastrointestinal disturbances. Also, triclofos sodium is not corrosive to skin and mucous membranes.

## Interactions

As for Cloral Hydrate, p.684.

## Pharmacokinetics

Triclofos sodium is rapidly hydrolysed to trichloroethanol, peak serum concentrations being achieved within about one hour after oral administration. For the pharmacokinetics of trichloroethanol, see Cloral Hydrate, p.684.

## Uses and Administration

Triclofos sodium has hypnotic and sedative actions similar to those of cloral hydrate (p.684) but it is more palatable and causes less gastric irritation. It is given by mouth in the short-term management of insomnia (p.667).

The usual adult dose as a hypnotic is 1 to 2 g at night. A suggested hypnotic dose for children up to 1 year of age is 25 to 30 mg/kg; children aged 1 to 5 years may be given single doses of 250 to 500 mg, and children aged 6 to 12 years may be given single doses of 0.5 to 1 g.

## Preparations

***BP 2003:*** Triclofos Oral Solution.

**Proprietary Preparations** (details are given in Part 3)
***India:*** Tricloryl; ***Irl.:*** Tricloryl; ***Israel:*** Triclonam.

# Trifluoperazine Hydrochloride

*(BANM, rINNM)*

Hidrocloruro de trifluoperazina; Trifluoperazini Hydrochloridum; Triphthazinum. 10-[3-(4-Methylpiperazin-1-yl)propyl]-2-trifluoromethylphenothiazine dihydrochloride.
$C_{21}H_{24}F_3N_3S,2HCl$ = 480.4.
*CAS — 117-89-5 (trifluoperazine); 440-17-5 (trifluoperazine hydrochloride).*
*ATC — N05AB06.*

**Pharmacopoeias.** In *Chin., Eur.* (see p.vi), *Pol.,* and *US.*

**Ph. Eur. 5.0** (Trifluoperazine Hydrochloride). A white to pale yellow, hygroscopic, crystalline powder. Freely soluble in water; soluble in alcohol; practically insoluble in ether. A 10% solution in water has a pH of 1.6 to 2.5. Protect from light.

**USP 27** (Trifluoperazine Hydrochloride). A white to pale yellow, practically odourless, crystalline powder. Soluble 1 in 3.5 of water, 1 in 11 of alcohol, and 1 in 100 of chloroform; insoluble in ether and in benzene. pH of a 1 in 20 solution is between 1.7 and 2.6. Store in airtight containers. Protect from light.

## Adverse Effects, Treatment, and Precautions

As for Chlorpromazine, p.675. Trifluoperazine is less likely to cause sedation, hypotension, hypothermia, or antimuscarinic effects but is associated with a higher incidence of extrapyramidal effects particularly when the daily dose exceeds 6 mg.

**Breast feeding.** The American Academy of Pediatrics[1] considers that, although the effect of trifluoperazine on breast-feeding infants is unknown, its use by mothers during breast feeding may be of concern since antipsychotic drugs do appear in breast milk and thus could conceivably alter CNS function in the infant both in the short and long term.

1. American Academy of Pediatrics. The transfer of drugs and other chemicals into human milk. *Pediatrics* 2001; **108:** 776–89. Correction. *ibid.*; 1029. Also available at: http://aappolicy.aappublications.org/cgi/content/full/pediatrics%3b108/3/776 (accessed 29/04/04)

## Interactions

As for Chlorpromazine, p.679.

## Pharmacokinetics

◊ The pharmacokinetics of trifluoperazine as a single 5-mg dose by mouth in 5 healthy subjects have been studied.[1] Peak plasma concentrations of trifluoperazine were reached from 1.5 to 4.5 hours after ingestion and varied widely between subjects, ranging from 0.53 to 3.09 nanograms/mL. Elimination of trifluoperazine was multiphasic; the mean elimination half-life was estimated to be 5.1 hours over the period from 4.5 to 12 hours after ingestion, while the mean apparent terminal elimination half-life was estimated to be 12.5 hours.

1. Midha KK, *et al.* Kinetics of oral trifluoperazine disposition in man. *Br J Clin Pharmacol* 1983; **15:** 380–2.

## Uses and Administration

Trifluoperazine is a phenothiazine antipsychotic with general properties similar to those of chlorpromazine (p.680). It has a piperazine side-chain.

Trifluoperazine is used in the treatment of a variety of psychiatric disorders including schizophrenia (p.665), severe anxiety (p.663), and disturbed behaviour (p.665). It is also used for the control of nausea and vomiting (p.1245).

Trifluoperazine is given as the hydrochloride but its doses are expressed in terms of the base. Trifluoperazine 1 mg is approximately equivalent to 1.2 mg of trifluoperazine hydrochloride. A modified-release preparation is also available in some countries; the total daily dosage, as given below, may be administered in a single dose by mouth. Trifluoperazine should be given in reduced dosage to elderly or debilitated patients.

The usual initial dose for the treatment of schizophrenia and other **psychoses** is 2 to 5 mg twice daily *by mouth*, gradually increased to a usual range of 15 to 20 mg daily; in severe or resistant psychoses daily doses of 40 mg or more have been given. For the control of acute psychotic symptoms it may be given by deep *intramuscular* injection in a dose of 1 to 2 mg, repeated if necessary at intervals of not less than every 4 hours; more than 6 mg daily is rarely required. The initial dose for use in *children* is up to 5 mg daily by mouth in divided doses adjusted according to age, body-weight, and response, or 1 mg given once or twice daily by intramuscular injection.

For the control of **nausea and vomiting** the usual adult dose *by mouth* is 1 or 2 mg twice daily; up to 6 mg daily may be given in divided doses. *Children* aged 3 to 5 years may be given up to 1 mg daily in divided doses; this may be increased to a maximum of 4 mg daily in children aged 6 to 12 years.

When used as an adjunct in the short-term management of **severe anxiety disorders** doses are similar to those used for the control of nausea and vomiting.

### Preparations

***BP 2003:*** Trifluoperazine Tablets;
***USP 27:*** Trifluoperazine Hydrochloride Injection; Trifluoperazine Hydrochloride Syrup; Trifluoperazine Hydrochloride Tablets.

**Proprietary Preparations** (details are given in Part 3)
***Arg.:*** Stelazine; ***Austral.:*** Stelazine; ***Austria:*** Jatroneural†; ***Braz.:*** Stelazine; ***Canad.:*** Novo-Flurazine†; Stelazine†; Terfluzine†; ***Fr.:*** Terfluzine†; ***Ger.:*** Jatroneural†; ***Gr.:*** Stelazine; Stelium; ***India:*** Trinicalm; ***Irl.:*** Stelazine; ***Israel:*** Terfluzine†; ***Ital.:*** Modalina; ***Mex.:*** Flupazine; Sedisan†; Stelazine; ***Neth.:*** Terfluzine†; ***NZ:*** Stelazine; ***S.Afr.:*** Stelazine; ***Spain:*** Eskazine; ***Thai.:*** Psyrazine; Trifumed; Triplex; ***UK:*** Stelazine; ***USA:*** Stelazine†.

**Multi-ingredient:** ***Arg.:*** Cuait D; Cuait N; Stelapar; ***Braz.:*** Stelapar; ***Canad.:*** Stelabid; ***India:*** Sycot; Trinicalm Forte; Trinicalm Plus; ***Irl.:*** Parstelin†; Stelabid†; ***Ital.:*** Parmodalin; ***Mex.:*** Stelabid.

## Trifluperidol *(BAN, USAN, rINN)*

McN-JR-2498; R-2498. 4′-Fluoro-4-[4-hydroxy-4-(3-trifluoromethylphenyl)piperidino]butyrophenone.

$C_{22}H_{23}F_4NO_2$ = 409.4.
*CAS — 749-13-3.*
*ATC — N05AD02.*

## Trifluperidol Hydrochloride *(BANM, rINNM)*

Hidrocloruro de trifluperidol.

$C_{22}H_{23}F_4NO_2$,HCl = 445.9.
*CAS — 2062-77-3.*
*ATC — N05AD02.*

### Profile

Trifluperidol is a butyrophenone with general properties similar to those of haloperidol (p.701), and has been used as the hydrochloride in the treatment of psychoses including schizophrenia.

### Preparations

**Proprietary Preparations** (details are given in Part 3)
***Ger.:*** Triperidol†; ***India:*** Triperidol.

## Triflupromazine *(BAN, rINN)*

Fluopromazine; Triflupromazina. *NN*-Dimethyl-3-(2-trifluoromethylphenothiazin-10-yl)propylamine.

$C_{18}H_{19}F_3N_2S$ = 352.4.
*CAS — 146-54-3.*
*ATC — N05AA05.*

**Pharmacopoeias.** In *US.*

**USP 27** (Triflupromazine). A light amber viscous oily liquid that crystallises into large irregular crystals during prolonged storage. Practically insoluble in water. Store in airtight containers. Protect from light.

## Triflupromazine Hydrochloride *(BANM, rINNM)*

Fluopromazine Hydrochloride; Hidrocloruro de triflupromazina.

$C_{18}H_{19}F_3N_2S$,HCl = 388.9.
*CAS — 1098-60-8.*
*ATC — N05AA05.*

**Pharmacopoeias.** In *US.*

**USP 27** (Triflupromazine Hydrochloride). A white to pale tan crystalline powder having a slight characteristic odour. Soluble 1 in less than 1 of water and of alcohol and 1 in 1.7 of chloroform; soluble in acetone; insoluble in ether. Store in glass containers. Protect from light.

### Profile

Triflupromazine hydrochloride is a phenothiazine with general properties similar to those of chlorpromazine (p.675). It is used mainly in the management of psychoses (p.665) and the control of nausea and vomiting (p.1245). Triflupromazine hydrochloride is usually given by injection but in some countries preparations are available for administration by mouth.

In the management of psychosis, the usual dose is 60 to 150 mg daily by intramuscular injection. For the control of nausea and vomiting 5 to 15 mg is given intramuscularly and repeated after 4 hours if necessary up to a maximum of 60 mg daily; a dose of 1 mg to a maximum total daily dose of 3 mg may be given intravenously.

A suggested intramuscular dose for children over 2½ years of age is 200 to 250 micrograms/kg daily up to a maximum of 10 mg daily.

Reduced doses should be used in elderly or debilitated patients.

### Preparations

***USP 27:*** Triflupromazine Hydrochloride Injection; Triflupromazine Hydrochloride Tablets; Triflupromazine Oral Solution.

**Proprietary Preparations** (details are given in Part 3)
***Austria:*** Psyquil; ***Ger.:*** Psyquil; ***India:*** Siquil; ***Neth.:*** Siquil†; ***USA:*** Vesprin†.

## Valnoctamide *(USAN, rINN)*

McN-X-181; NSC-32363; Valnoctamida. 2-Ethyl-3-methylvaleramide.

$C_8H_{17}NO$ = 143.2.
*CAS — 4171-13-5.*
*ATC — N05CM13.*

### Profile

Valnoctamide, an isomer of valpromide (p.380), has been given by mouth in the treatment of anxiety disorders.

◊ References.

1. Bialer M, *et al.* Pharmacokinetics of a valpromide isomer, valnoctamide, in healthy subjects. *Eur J Clin Pharmacol* 1990; **38:** 289–91.
2. Barel S, *et al.* Stereoselective pharmacokinetic analysis of valnoctamide in healthy subjects and in patients with epilepsy. *Clin Pharmacol Ther* 1997; **61:** 442–9.

**Interactions.** For a discussion of the potential interaction between carbamazepine and valnoctamide, see Antiepileptics, p.356.

## Veralipride *(rINN)*

Veraliprida. *N*-[(1-Allyl-2-pyrrolidinyl)methyl]-5-sulphamoyl-2-veratramide.

$C_{17}H_{25}N_3O_5S$ = 383.5.
*CAS — 66644-81-3.*
*ATC — N05AL06.*

### Profile

Veralipride is a substituted benzamide antipsychotic. It has been used in the treatment of cardiovascular and psychological symptoms associated with the menopause; the usual dose by mouth is 100 mg daily for 20 days repeated at intervals of 7 to 10 days.

**Menopausal disorders.** HRT with oestrogens is the mainstay of treatment for acute symptoms associated with the menopause (see p.1540) but when it is considered to be unsuitable a variety of other drugs including veralipride have been tried.[1]

1. Young RL, *et al.* Management of menopause when estrogen cannot be used. *Drugs* 1990; **40:** 220–30.

**Porphyria.** Veralipride is considered to be unsafe in patients with porphyria because it has been shown to be porphyrinogenic in *in-vitro* systems.

### Preparations

**Proprietary Preparations** (details are given in Part 3)
***Arg.:*** Veralipral; ***Belg.:*** Agreal; ***Braz.:*** Agreal; ***Chile:*** Agreal; ***Fr.:*** Agreal; ***Hong Kong:*** Agreal†; ***Ital.:*** Agradil; Veralipril; ***Mex.:*** Aclimafel; Veraligral; ***Port.:*** Agreal; ***Spain:*** Agreal; Faltium†.

**Multi-ingredient:** ***Arg.:*** Veralipral T.

## Vinylbital *(BAN, rINN)*

Butyvinal; JD-96; Vinilbital; Vinylbitone; Vinymalum. 5-(1-Methylbutyl)-5-vinylbarbituric acid.

$C_{11}H_{16}N_2O_3$ = 224.3.
*CAS — 2430-49-1.*
*ATC — N05CA08.*

### Profile

Vinylbital is a barbiturate with general properties similar to those of amobarbital (p.670). It was used as a hypnotic but barbiturates are no longer considered appropriate for such use.

## Zaleplon *(BAN, USAN, rINN)*

CL-284846; L-846; LJC-10846; ZAL-846; Zaleplón. 3′-(3-Cyanopyrazolo[1,5-*a*]pyrimidin-7-yl)-*N*-ethylacetanilide.

$C_{17}H_{15}N_5O$ = 305.3.
*CAS — 151319-34-5.*
*ATC — N05CF03.*

### Dependence and Withdrawal

As for Diazepam, p.690.

### Adverse Effects, Treatment, and Precautions

As for Diazepam, p.690. Zaleplon should be used with caution and in reduced doses in patients with hepatic impairment, and should be avoided where this is severe.

Treatment of overdose is largely supportive. Activated charcoal may be given orally within one hour of ingestion of more than 50 mg zaleplon by adults, or 1 mg/kg by children. Flumazenil may be considered in cases of severe CNS depression.

◊ References.

1. Israel AG, Kramer JA. Safety of zaleplon in the treatment of insomnia. *Ann Pharmacother* 2002; **36:** 852–9.

**Abuse.** In a controlled study in healthy patients with a history of drug abuse, zaleplon was shown to have a comparable abuse potential to that of the benzodiazepine, triazolam.[1]

1. Rush CR, *et al.* Zaleplon and triazolam in humans: acute behavioral effects and abuse potential. *Psychopharmacology (Berl)* 1999; **145:** 39–51.

**Breast feeding.** The manufacturers of zaleplon advise that it should not be given to breast-feeding mothers since, although only a small amount is excreted into breast milk, the effect on the nursing infant is not known.

Zaleplon was detected in the breast milk of 5 lactating women who had been given a 10-mg dose.[1] The milk-to-plasma concentration ratio for zaleplon was about 0.5.

1. Darwish M, *et al.* Rapid disappearance of zaleplon from breast milk after oral administration to lactating women. *J Clin Pharmacol* 1999; **39:** 670–4.

### Interactions

As for Diazepam, p.692. Zaleplon is primarily metabolised by aldehyde oxidase and use with inhibitors of this enzyme, such as cimetidine, may result in increased plasma concentrations of zaleplon (see Uses and Administration, below). Zaleplon is also partly metabolised by the cytochrome P450 isoenzyme CYP3A4 and, consequently, caution is advised when zaleplon is given with drugs that are substrates for, or potent inhibitors of, this isoenzyme. Cimetidine is also an inhibitor of CYP3A4 and thus inhibits both the primary and secondary metabolic pathways of zaleplon.

Use with rifampicin or other potent enzyme-inducing drugs may accelerate the metabolism of zaleplon and reduce its plasma concentrations.

### Pharmacokinetics

Zaleplon is rapidly absorbed from the gastrointestinal tract with peak plasma concentrations reached in about one hour after oral administration. A heavy meal or one with a high-fat content delays absorption and reduces peak concentrations. Bioavailability is about 30% due to significant first-pass hepatic metabolism. Zaleplon is metabolised primarily by aldehyde oxidase to form 5-oxo-zaleplon and, to a lesser extent, by the cytochrome P450 isoenzyme CYP3A4 to desethylzaleplon, which is further metabolised by aldehyde oxidase to 5-oxo-desethylzaleplon. The plasma-elimination half-life of zaleplon is approximately 1 hour. About 70% of a dose is excreted in the urine as these inactive metabolites or their glucuronides; less than 1% is excreted unchanged. About 17% of a dose is eliminated in the faeces, mainly as 5-oxo-zaleplon. Zaleplon is distributed into breast milk.

◊ References.

1. Greenblatt DJ, *et al.* Comparative kinetics and dynamics of zaleplon, zolpidem, and placebo. *Clin Pharmacol Ther* 1998; **64:** 553–61.
2. Drover D, *et al.* Pharmacokinetics, pharmacodynamics, and relative pharmacokinetic/pharmacodynamic profiles of zaleplon and zolpidem. *Clin Ther* 2000; **22:** 1443–61.

## Uses and Administration

Zaleplon is a pyrazolopyrimidine that is reported to have similar sedative properties to the benzodiazepines (see Diazepam, p.695). It is used as a hypnotic in the short-term management of insomnia. Zaleplon has a rapid onset and short duration of action. The usual dose is 10 mg at bedtime although the US manufacturer notes that occasional patients may require 20 mg. Elderly or debilitated patients or those also taking cimetidine should be given 5 mg. For dosages in patients with hepatic impairment, see below.

**Administration in hepatic impairment.** The dose of zaleplon should be reduced to 5 mg at bedtime in patients with mild to moderate hepatic impairment; it should not be given to those with severe impairment.

**Insomnia.** Zaleplon is a pyrazolopyrimidine hypnotic. Although not related structurally to the benzodiazepines it appears to act by binding selectively to the benzodiazepine type I receptor (BZ1- or $\omega_1$-receptors) on the GABA subtype A complex. Zaleplon reduces sleep latency but has little effect on sleep duration; it is rapidly absorbed and eliminated and consequently residual effects the next day are said to be minimal. These characteristics make it best suited for the treatment of patients with insomnia (p.667) who have difficulty falling asleep; zaleplon can either be taken at bedtime or during the night if a patient has trouble falling back to sleep, provided they are assured of at least 4 hours uninterrupted sleep.

References.


1. Anonymous. Zaleplon for insomnia. *Med Lett Drugs Ther* 1999; **41:** 93–4.
2. Danjou P, *et al.* A comparison of the residual effects of zaleplon and zolpidem following administration 5 to 2 h before awakening. *Br J Clin Pharmacol* 1999; **48:** 367–74.
3. Elie R, *et al.* Sleep latency is shortened during 4 weeks of treatment with zaleplon, a novel nonbenzodiazepine hypnotic. *J Clin Psychiatry* 1999; **60:** 536–44.
4. Dooley M, Plosker GL. Zaleplon: a review of its use in the treatment of insomnia. *Drugs* 2000; **60:** 413–45.
5. George CFP. Pyrazolopyrimidines. *Lancet* 2001; **358:** 1623–6.
6. Terzano MG, *et al.* New drugs for insomnia: comparative tolerability of zopiclone, zolpidem and zaleplon. *Drug Safety* 2003; **26:** 261–82.


## Preparations

**Proprietary Preparations** (details are given in Part 3)
***Arg.:*** Hegon; Hipnodem; ***Belg.:*** Sonata; ***Braz.:*** Sonata; ***Canad.:*** Starnoc; ***Chile:*** Noctiplon; Plenidon; Rhem; Somnipax; ***Denm.:*** Sonata; ***Fin.:*** Sonata; ***Ger.:*** Sonata; ***Gr.:*** Sonata; ***India:*** Zaplon; ***Irl.:*** Sonata; ***Ital.:*** Sonata; Zerene; ***Mex.:*** Sonata; ***Spain:*** Sonata; ***Swed.:*** Sonata; ***Switz.:*** Sonata; ***UK:*** Sonata; ***USA:*** Sonata.

---

# Ziprasidone *(BAN, rINN)*

Ziprasidona. 5-{2-[4-(1,2-Benzisothiazol-3-yl)-1-piperazinyl]ethyl}-6-chloro-2-indolinone.
$C_{21}H_{21}ClN_4OS = 412.9.$
*CAS — 146939-27-7 (ziprasidone).*
*ATC — N05AE04.*

# Ziprasidone Hydrochloride *(BANM, USAN, rINNM)*

CP-88059; CP-88059-1.
$C_{21}H_{21}ClN_4OS,HCl,H_2O = 467.4.$
*CAS — 138982-67-9.*
*ATC — N05AE04.*

# Ziprasidone Mesilate *(BANM, rINNM)*

CP-88059/27; Ziprasidone Mesylate *(USAN)*.
$C_{21}H_{21}ClN_4OS,CH_4O_3S,3H_2O = 563.1.$
*CAS — 199191-69-0.*
*ATC — N05AE04.*

## Adverse Effects, Treatment, and Precautions

Although ziprasidone may share some of the adverse effects seen with the classical antipsychotics (see Chlorpromazine, p.675), the incidence and severity of such effects may vary. Frequent adverse effects with ziprasidone include somnolence, rash or urticaria, gastrointestinal disturbances, dizziness, flu-like symptoms, hypertension, headache, agitation, confusion, and dyspnoea. Orthostatic hypotension may be a problem, particularly when starting treatment. Ziprasidone may increase prolactin levels and weight gain has also been noted. Sexual dysfunction has been reported infrequently. Extrapyramidal symptoms may occur, and tardive dyskinesia may develop with prolonged use. There have also been infrequent or rare cases of cholestatic jaundice, hepatitis, seizures, blood dyscrasias including leucopenia and thrombocytopenia, hyperlipidaemia, and hyperglycaemia or altered glucose tolerance.

Ziprasidone has been associated with dose-related prolongation of the QT interval. Because of this and the consequent danger of life-threatening arrhythmias such as torsade de pointes and sudden death, its use is contra-indicated in patients with a history of QT prolongation or cardiac arrhythmias, with recent acute myocardial infarction, or with decompensated heart failure. Use with drugs liable to interfere with the metabolism of ziprasidone, of other drugs known to prolong the QT interval, and of drugs likely to cause electrolyte imbalance should also be avoided.

For all patients starting ziprasidone, it is recommended that baseline serum potassium and magnesium screening should be performed. Serum electrolytes should be monitored in patients who commence diuretic therapy during ziprasidone treatment. Patients who present during ziprasidone treatment with symptoms that might indicate torsade de pointes (e.g. dizziness, palpitations, or syncope) should be further evaluated.

Ziprasidone should be used with caution in patients with a history of seizures, cerebrovascular disease, or conditions which predispose to hypotension.

Ziprasidone may affect the performance of skilled tasks including driving.

**Effects on carbohydrate metabolism.** The increased risk of glucose intolerance and diabetes mellitus with some atypical antipsychotics and recommendations on monitoring are discussed under Adverse Effects in Clozapine, p.686.

## Interactions

Use of ziprasidone with other drugs known to prolong the QT interval is contra-indicated.

The metabolism of ziprasidone is mediated by the cytochrome P450 isoenzyme CYP3A4. Therefore, there is the potential for interactions between ziprasidone and other drugs that induce, inhibit, or act as a substrate for this enzyme, and such drugs should not be given concomitantly.

Ziprasidone may enhance the effects of other CNS depressants and certain antihypertensives; it may antagonise the effects of levodopa and dopamine agonists.

## Pharmacokinetics

Ziprasidone is well absorbed following oral administration with peak plasma concentrations being reached after 6 to 8 hours. Following intramuscular administration, peak plasma levels are reached within 1 hour. The presence of food may double the absorption. Plasma protein binding is about 99%. Ziprasidone is extensively metabolised by aldehyde oxidase (about 66% of the original dose ) and by the cytochrome P450 isoenzyme CYP3A4. The terminal elimination half-life has been reported to be about 7 hours. Ziprasidone is excreted predominantly as metabolites in the faeces (66%) and urine (20%); less than 5% appears as unchanged drug.

◊ References.


1. Various. The pharmacokinetics of ziprasidone. *Br J Clin Pharmacol* 2000; **49** (suppl 1): 1S–76S.


## Uses and Administration

Ziprasidone is an atypical antipsychotic used for the treatment of schizophrenia. It is reported to have affinity for adrenergic ($\alpha_1$), histamine ($H_1$), and serotonin ($5\text{-}HT_2$) receptors as well as dopamine ($D_2$) receptors. Ziprasidone hydrochloride is given by mouth in an initial dose of 20 mg twice daily with food. Doses may be increased if necessary at intervals of not less than 2 days up to 80 mg twice daily. For maintenance, doses as low as 20 mg twice daily may be effective.

For acute agitation in patients with schizophrenia, ziprasidone may be given as the mesilate by intramuscular injection. Doses are expressed as the base: ziprasidone mesilate 13.6 mg is approximately equivalent to 10 mg of ziprasidone base. The recommended dose is 10 to 20 mg as required up to a maximum of 40 mg daily. Patients should be switched to oral therapy as soon as possible.

**Bipolar disorder.** Ziprasidone has been shown to be effective in the management of acute mania in patients with bipolar disorder[1] but it may also be associated with the induction of mania or hypomania in such patients.[2]


1. Keck PE, *et al.* Ziprasidone in the treatment of acute bipolar mania: a three-week, placebo-controlled, double-blind, randomized trial. *Am J Psychiatry* 2003; **160:** 741–8.
2. Baldassano CF, *et al.* Ziprasidone-associated mania: a case series and review of the mechanism. *Bipolar Disord* 2003; **5:** 72–5.


**Schizophrenia.** A systematic review[1] of the effectiveness and safety of ziprasidone in patients with schizophrenia (p.665) found that from the limited data available ziprasidone was as effective as haloperidol; it was less likely to provoke extrapyramidal disorders but appeared to cause more nausea and vomiting, and pain at the site of injection. Comparisons with other atypical antipsychotics were lacking. A comparative study[2] of intramuscular ziprasidone compared with intramuscular haloperidol also demonstrated a favourable outcome in patients with acute psychoses.


1. Bagnall A-M, *et al.* Ziprasidone for schizophrenia and severe mental illness. Available in The Cochrane Library; Issue 2. Chichester: John Wiley; 2004.
2. Brook S, *et al.* Intramuscular ziprasidone compared with intramuscular haloperidol in the treatment of acute psychosis. *J Clin Psychiatry* 2000; **61:** 933–41.


**Tourette's syndrome.** When treatment is required for tics and behavioural disturbances in Tourette's syndrome (p.664) haloperidol or pimozide are commonly used but ziprasidone has also been tried.[1]


1. Sallee FR, *et al.* Ziprasidone treatment of children and adolescents with Tourette's syndrome: a pilot study. *J Am Acad Child Adolesc Psychiatry* 2000; **39:** 292–9.


## Preparations

**Proprietary Preparations** (details are given in Part 3)
***Arg.:*** Zeldox; ***Braz.:*** Zeldox†; ***Chile:*** Zeldox; ***Denm.:*** Zeldox; ***Irl.:*** Geodon; ***Israel:*** Geodon; ***Norw.:*** Zeldox; ***Swed.:*** Zeldox; ***USA:*** Geodon.

---

# Zolazepam Hydrochloride *(BANM, USAN, rINNM)*

CI-716; Hidrocloruro de zolazepam. 4-(o-Fluorophenyl)-6,8-dihydro-1,3,8-trimethylpirazole[3,4-e][1,4]diazepin-7(1H)-one monohydrochloride.
$C_{15}H_{15}FN_4O,HCl = 322.8.$
*CAS — 31352-82-6 (zolazepam); 33754-49-3 (zolazepam hydrochloride).*

**Pharmacopoeias.** In *US* for veterinary use only.

**USP 27** (Zolazepam Hydrochloride). A white to off-white crystalline powder. Freely soluble in water and in 0.1N hydrochloric acid; slightly soluble in chloroform; practically insoluble in ether; soluble in methyl alcohol. pH of a 10% solution in water is between 1.5 and 3.5. Store in airtight containers.

## Profile

Zolazepam hydrochloride is a benzodiazepine with general properties similar to those of diazepam (p.695). It is used with tiletamine (p.1310) for general anaesthesia in veterinary medicine.

---

# Zolpidem Tartrate *(BANM, USAN, rINNM)*

SL-80.0750 (zolpidem); SL-80.0750-23N; Tartrato de zolpidem; Zolpidem Hemitartrate; Zolpidemi Tartras. *N,N*-Dimethyl-2-(6-methyl-2-*p*-tolylimidazo[1,2-*a*]pyridin-3-yl)acetamide hemitartrate.
$(C_{19}H_{21}N_3O)_2,C_4H_6O_6 = 764.9.$
*CAS — 82626-48-0 (zolpidem); 99294-93-6 (zolpidem tartrate).*
*ATC — N05CF02.*

**Pharmacopoeias.** In *Eur.* (see p.vi) and *Pol.*

**Ph. Eur. 5.0** (Zolpidem Tartrate). A white or almost white hygroscopic crystalline powder. Slightly soluble in water; practically insoluble in dichloromethane; sparingly soluble in methyl alcohol. Store in airtight containers. Protect from light.

## Dependence and Withdrawal

As for Diazepam, p.690.

**Withdrawal symptoms.** A 37-year-old male suffered a generalised tonic-clonic seizure after zolpidem was abruptly stopped.[1] He had himself escalated the dose from 10 mg to 130 mg daily over 2 months. The patient recovered after being started on a benzodiazepine dosage tapering programme. Symptoms attributed to daytime abstinence following excessive night-time doses have been reported[2] in 2 patients and included anxiety, tremor, sweating, nausea, gastric and abdominal pain, swallowing difficulties, tachycardia, and tachypnoea. The patients had increased their doses because of the development of tolerance to the hypnotic effect but had begun to experience muscle twitches and myoclonic jerks.


1. Gilbert DL, Staats PS. Seizure after withdrawal from supratherapeutic doses of zolpidem tartrate, a selective omega I benzodiazepine receptor agonist. *J Pain Symptom Manage* 1997; **14:** 118–20.
2. Cavallaro R, *et al.* Tolerance and withdrawal with zolpidem. *Lancet* 1993; **342:** 374–5.


## Adverse Effects, Treatment, and Precautions

As for Diazepam, p.690.

Treatment of overdose is largely supportive. Activated charcoal may be given orally within one hour of ingestion of 100 mg zolpidem or more by adults, or more than 5 mg by children. Alternatively, gastric lavage may be considered in adults if they present within 1 hour of a potentially life-threatening overdose. Flumazenil may be considered in cases of severe CNS depression.

◊ Reviews.


1. Darcourt G, *et al.* The safety and tolerability of zolpidem—an update. *J Psychopharmacol* 1999; **13:** 81–93.


**Abuse.** Chronic abuse has been reported in a patient with depression who obtained a stimulant effect when taking large doses of zolpidem.[1] Tolerance also developed. See also under Dependence and Withdrawal, above.


1. Gericke CA, Ludolph AC. Chronic abuse of zolpidem. *JAMA* 1994; **272:** 1721–2.


**Breast feeding.** No adverse effects have been observed in breast-feeding infants whose mothers were receiving zolpidem, and the American Academy of Pediatrics considers[1] that it is therefore usually compatible with breast feeding.

In 5 lactating women given a 20-mg dose of zolpidem, the amount of drug excreted in breast milk after 3 hours ranged between 0.76 and 3.88 micrograms, which represented 0.004 to 0.019% of the dose.[2] No detectable (below 0.5 nanograms/mL) zolpidem was found in subsequent milk samples.


1. American Academy of Pediatrics. The transfer of drugs and other chemicals into human milk. *Pediatrics* 2001; **108:** 776–89. Correction. *ibid.*; 1029. Also available at: http://aappolicy.aappublications.org/cgi/content/full/pediatrics%3b108/3/776 (accessed 29/04/04)
2. Pons G, *et al.* Zolpidem excretion in breast milk. *Eur J Clin Pharmacol* 1989; **37:** 245–8.

**Effects on the liver.** Hepatitis developed on two separate occasions in a 53-year-old woman following the use of zolpidem for insomnia.[1]

1. Karsenti D, *et al.* Hepatotoxicity associated with zolpidem treatment. *BMJ* 1999; **318:** 1179.

**Effects on mental function.** Psychotic reactions, which may not subsequently be recalled, have been reported in patients taking therapeutic doses of zolpidem.[1-4]

1. Ansseau M, *et al.* Psychotic reactions to zolpidem. *Lancet* 1992; **339:** 809.
2. Iruela LM, *et al.* Zolpidem-induced macropsia in anorexic woman. *Lancet* 1993; **342:** 443–4.
3. Brodeur MR, Stirling AL. Delirium associated with zolpidem. *Ann Pharmacother* 2001; **35:** 1562–4.
4. Anonymous. Seeing things with zolpidem. *Aust Adverse Drug React Bull* 2002; **21:** 3. Also available at: http://www.tga.health.gov.au/docs/pdf/aadrbltn/aadr0202.pdf (accessed 06/05/04)

**Overdosage.** A retrospective analysis of 344 cases of acute overdosage with zolpidem reported to the Paris Poison Center and the manufacturers Synthelabo has been published.[1] The ingested dose, where known, ranged from 10 to 1400 mg, and the most common adverse effect was drowsiness (in 89 patients). Other adverse effects probably associated with the overdosage included coma in 4 patients and vomiting in 7. Recovery was usually rapid when overdosage involved only zolpidem. It was recommended that patients who had ingested more than 100 mg of zolpidem should undergo gastric lavage and should be monitored for at least 12 hours (see also above). Although it has been shown that flumazenil[2] can effectively antagonise the CNS effects of zolpidem the authors of this analysis[1] found that in general it was not required.

1. Garnier R, *et al.* Acute zolpidem poisoning—analysis of 344 cases. *J Toxicol Clin Toxicol* 1994; **32:** 391–404.
2. Patat A, *et al.* Flumazenil antagonizes the central effects of zolpidem, an imidazopyridine hypnotic. *Clin Pharmacol Ther* 1994; **56:** 430–6.

## Interactions

As for Diazepam, p.692.

**Antidepressants.** A 16-year-old girl who had been taking *paroxetine* 20 mg daily for 3 days began to hallucinate and became disorientated one hour after taking zolpidem 10 mg at night. The delirium cleared spontaneously 4 hours later without treatment.[1] When questioned, at least one other of the author's patients receiving this combination reported transient visual hallucinations. Other isolated cases of visual hallucinations have been reported in patients taking zolpidem with antidepressants including *bupropion, desipramine, fluoxetine, sertraline*, and *venlafaxine*.[2]

1. Katz SE. Possible paroxetine-zolpidem interaction. *Am J Psychiatry* 1995; **152:** 1689.
2. Elko CJ, *et al.* Zolpidem-associated hallucinations and serotonin reuptake inhibition: a possible interaction. *J Toxicol Clin Toxicol* 1998; **36:** 195–203.

**Antifungals.** Use of *ketoconazole* with zolpidem has resulted in increased plasma concentrations, and an enhanced sedative effect, of zolpidem, albeit only modest.[1] The use of zolpidem with *fluconazole*[1] or *itraconazole*[1,2] has resulted in small, non-significant changes in the pharmacokinetics and sedative effects of zolpidem.

1. Greenblatt DJ, *et al.* Kinetic and dynamic interaction study of zolpidem with ketoconazole, itraconazole, and fluconazole. *Clin Pharmacol Ther* 1998; **64:** 661–71.
2. Luurila H, *et al.* Effect of itraconazole on the pharmacokinetics and pharmacodynamics of zolpidem. *Eur J Clin Pharmacol* 1998; **54:** 163–6.

**Antivirals.** HIV-protease inhibitors such as *ritonavir* may increase plasma concentrations of zolpidem with a risk of extreme sedation and respiratory depression; use together is not recommended.

**Rifampicin.** Rifampicin reduced the hypnotic effect of zolpidem in a study in 8 healthy female subjects.[1] The area under the curve for zolpidem was reduced by 73% after administration of rifampicin and the peak plasma concentration by 58%. The elimination half-life of zolpidem was reduced from 2.5 to 1.6 hours. Similar effects could be expected with other potent inducers of the cytochrome P450 isoenzyme CYP3A4 such as carbamazepine and phenytoin.

1. Villikka K, *et al.* Rifampin reduces plasma concentrations and effects of zolpidem. *Clin Pharmacol Ther* 1997; **62:** 629–34.

**Valproic acid.** A 47-year-old man with a history of bipolar disorder, who was receiving citalopram and zolpidem, had episodes of somnambulism after he was additionally given valproic acid for treatment of manic symptoms.[1] The episodes stopped on withdrawal of valproic acid and returned on rechallenge. An interaction between zolpidem and valproic acid was suspected.

1. Sattar SP, *et al.* Somnambulism due to probable interaction of valproic acid and zolpidem. *Ann Pharmacother* 2003; **37:** 1429–33.

## Pharmacokinetics

Zolpidem is rapidly absorbed from the gastrointestinal tract after oral administration, peak plasma concentrations being reached within 3 hours. Zolpidem undergoes first-pass metabolism and an absolute bioavailability of about 70% has been reported. Zolpidem has an elimination half-life of about 2.5 hours and is approximately 92% bound to plasma proteins. It is metabolised primarily by the cytochrome P450 isoenzyme CYP3A4; the inactive metabolites of zolpidem are excreted in the urine and faeces. Zolpidem is distributed into breast milk.

◊ References.

1. Salvà P, Costa J. Clinical pharmacokinetics and pharmacodynamics of zolpidem: therapeutic implications. *Clin Pharmacokinet* 1995; **29:** 142–53.
2. von Moltke LL, *et al.* Zolpidem metabolism in vitro: responsible cytochromes, chemical inhibitors, and vivo correlations. *Br J Clin Pharmacol* 1999; **48:** 89–97.
3. Drover D, *et al.* Pharmacokinetics, pharmacodynamics, and relative pharmacokinetic/pharmacodynamic profiles of zaleplon and zolpidem. *Clin Ther* 2000; **22:** 1443–61.

## Uses and Administration

Zolpidem tartrate is an imidazopyridine that is reported to have similar sedative properties to the benzodiazepines (see Diazepam, p.695), but minimal anxiolytic, muscle relaxant, and anticonvulsant properties. It has a rapid onset and short duration of action, and is used as a hypnotic in the short-term management of insomnia. The usual dose by mouth is 10 mg taken immediately before retiring. In elderly or debilitated patients, treatment should be limited to a dose of 5 mg at night. Doses should also be reduced in patients with hepatic impairment, see below.

**Administration in hepatic impairment.** In patients with hepatic impairment, treatment with zolpidem tartrate should be initiated with a dose of 5 mg at night; the dose may be increased to 10 mg, if necessary, in those under 65 years. The UK manufacturer contra-indicates the use of zolpidem in patients with severe impairment.

**Catatonia.** Anecdotal reports[1,2] suggesting that zolpidem may be a useful test in the diagnosis of catatonia.

1. Thomas P, *et al.* Test for catatonia with zolpidem. *Lancet* 1997; **349:** 702.
2. Zaw ZF, Bates GDL. Replication of zolpidem test for catatonia in an adolescent. *Lancet* 1997; **349:** 1914.

**Insomnia.** Zolpidem is an imidazopyridine with strong sedative actions, but only minor anxiolytic, muscle relaxant, or anticonvulsant properties. Some degree of amnesia has been reported. Zolpidem appears to act by binding to the benzodiazepine receptor component of the GABA receptor complex. It has, however, a selective affinity for the subtype of benzodiazepine receptors prevalent in the cerebellum (BZ1- or $\omega_1$-receptors) as opposed to those more commonly found in the spinal cord (BZ2- or $\omega_2$-receptors) or in the peripheral tissues (BZ3- or $\omega_3$-receptors). Zolpidem has a rapid onset and short duration of hypnotic action and at usual doses decreases time to sleep onset and increases duration of sleep with little apparent effect on sleep stages (see Insomnia, p.667). Reviews agree that clinical studies have shown zolpidem to have hypnotic activity superior to placebo and generally similar to comparative benzodiazepines. Although it does not appear to produce rebound insomnia to any great extent, there appears to be little evidence that zolpidem offers any advantage over short-acting benzodiazepines in terms of residual effects the next day, or its potential to induce tolerance or withdrawal symptoms or dependence (see also under Dependence and Withdrawal, above).

References.

1. Langtry HD, Benfield P. Zolpidem: a review of its pharmacodynamic and pharmacokinetic properties and therapeutic potential. *Drugs* 1990; **40:** 291–313.
2. Lobo BL, Greene WL. Zolpidem: distinct from triazolam? *Ann Pharmacother* 1997; **31:** 625–32.
3. Nowell PD, *et al.* Benzodiazepines and zolpidem for chronic insomnia: a meta-analysis of treatment efficacy. *JAMA* 1997; **278:** 2170–7.
4. Holm KJ, Goa KL. Zolpidem: an update of its pharmacology, therapeutic efficacy and tolerability in the treatment of insomnia. *Drugs* 2000; **59:** 865–89.
5. Terzano MG, *et al.* New drugs for insomnia: comparative tolerability of zopiclone, zolpidem and zaleplon. *Drug Safety* 2003; **26:** 261–82.

**Parkinsonism.** Although preliminary findings[1] in 10 patients suggested that zolpidem might improve symptoms of Parkinson's disease concern has been expressed[2] over the risk of falls associated with zolpidem-induced drowsiness and the serious consequences for these patients. Benefit has also been reported[3] in the treatment of antipsychotic-induced parkinsonism in one patient with symptoms of repetitive persistent gross tremors of the hands.

1. Daniele A, *et al.* Zolpidem in Parkinson's disease. *Lancet* 1997; **349:** 1222–3.
2. Lavoisy J, Marsac J. Zolpidem in Parkinson's disease. *Lancet* 1997; **350:** 74.
3. Farver DK, Khan MH. Zolpidem for antipsychotic-induced parkinsonism. *Ann Pharmacother* 2001; **35:** 435–7.

## Preparations

**Proprietary Preparations** (details are given in Part 3)

***Arg.:*** Somit; Sumenan; ***Austral.:*** Stilnox; ***Austria:*** Ivadal; ***Belg.:*** Stilnoct; ***Braz.:*** Lioram; Stilnox; ***Chile:*** Adormix; Dormilam; Dormosol; Somnil; Somnipron; Somno; Sucedal; ***Denm.:*** Eanox; Nimadorm; Stilnoct; ***Fin.:*** Stella; Stilnoct; ***Fr.:*** Ivadal†; Stilnox; ***Ger.:*** Bikalm; Stilnox; Zodormdura; Zolpi-Lich; Zolpinox; ***Gr.:*** Stilnox; ***Hong Kong:*** Stilnox; ***India:*** Ambiz; Zleep; ***Irl.:*** Nytamel; Stilnoct; Zolnod; ***Israel:*** Stilnox; Zodorm; ***Ital.:*** Ivadal†; Niotal; Nottem; Stilnox; ***Jpn:*** Myslee; ***Malaysia:*** Stilnox; ***Mex.:*** Stilnox; ***Neth.:*** Stilnoct; ***Norw.:*** Stilnoct; ***Port.:*** Cymerion; Stilnox; ***S.Afr.:*** Stilnox; ***Singapore:*** Stilnox; ***Spain:*** Cedrol†; Dalparan; Stilnox; ***Swed.:*** Stilnoct; ***Switz.:*** Stilnox; ***Thai.:*** Stilnox; ***UK:*** Stilnoct; ***USA:*** Ambien.

# Zopiclone *(BAN, rINN)*

27267-RP; Zopiclona; Zopiclonum. 6-(5-Chloro-2-pyridyl)-6,7-dihydro-7-oxo-5*H*-pyrrolo[3,4-*b*]pyrazin-5-yl 4-methylpiperazine-1-carboxylate.

$C_{17}H_{17}ClN_6O_3$ = 388.8.

*CAS — 43200-80-2.*

*ATC — N05CF01.*

**Pharmacopoeias.** In *Eur.* (see p.vi) and *Pol.*

**Ph. Eur. 5.0** (Zopiclone). A white or slightly yellowish powder. Practically insoluble in water and in alcohol; sparingly soluble in acetone; freely soluble in dichloromethane. It dissolves in dilute mineral acids. Protect from light.

## Dependence and Withdrawal

As for Diazepam, p.690.

◊ Reports[1,2] of zopiclone dependence and associated withdrawal symptoms on dosage reduction or cessation of use.

1. Jones IR, Sullivan G. Physical dependence on zopiclone: case reports. *BMJ* 1998; **316:** 117.
2. Sikdar S. Physical dependence on zopiclone. *BMJ* 1998; **317:** 146.

## Adverse Effects, Treatment, and Precautions

As for Diazepam, p.690. A bitter or metallic taste in the mouth has been the most frequently reported side-effect with zopiclone.

Treatment of overdose is largely supportive. Activated charcoal may be given orally within one hour of ingestion of more than 150 mg zopiclone by adults, or 1.5 mg/kg by children. Alternatively gastric lavage may be considered in adults if they present within 1 hour of a potentially life-threatening overdose. Flumazenil has been used in cases of severe CNS depression.

**Incidence of adverse effects.** In a French postmarketing survey[1] of 20 513 patients treated with zopiclone the most commonly reported adverse events were bitter taste (3.6%), dry mouth (1.6%), difficulty arising in the morning (1.3%), sleepiness (0.5%), nausea (0.5%) and nightmares (0.5%). The UK Committee on Safety of Medicines (CSM)[2] had received 122 reports of adverse reactions to zopiclone over a period of about one year since the product's introduction in November 1989. A fifth of these were neuropsychiatric reactions, a proportion similar to that found with other hypnotics. Many of these reactions were potentially serious and involved hallucinations (3 auditory and 2 visual), amnesia (4 cases) and behavioural disturbances (10, including 3 cases of aggression). Most reactions started immediately or shortly after the first dose and improved rapidly on stopping the drug. Three patients had difficulty in stopping treatment, 2 because of withdrawal symptoms and one due to repeated rebound insomnia. The CSM considered that, although differing structurally from the benzodiazepines, zopiclone has the same potential for adverse psychiatric reactions, including dependence. As with the benzodiazepines it should be reserved for patients with severe sleep disturbance and its duration of use limited to 28 days; care should also be taken in the elderly, those who have a history of previous psychiatric illness, or who are prone to drug abuse.

1. Allain H, *et al.* Postmarketing surveillance of zopiclone in insomnia: analysis of 20,513 cases. *Sleep* 1991; **14:** 408–13.
2. Committee on Safety of Medicines. Zopiclone (Zimovane) and neuro-psychiatric reactions. *Current Problems 30* 1990.

**Administration.** Results in 9 healthy subjects given zopiclone indicated a significant delay in onset of action when the drug was taken in the supine, as opposed to the standing, position; this was associated with a prolongation of more than 20 minutes in the lag time before absorption began.[1] In order to obtain a rapid and complete hypnotic effect from zopiclone the tablet should be swallowed in the standing position.

1. Channer KS, *et al.* The effect of posture at the time of administration on the central depressant effects of the new hypnotic zopiclone. *Br J Clin Pharmacol* 1984; **18:** 879–86.

**Driving.** For reference to the increased risk of road-traffic accidents for drivers taking zopiclone, see p.692.

**Hepatic impairment.** Zopiclone was given in a dose of 7.5 mg to 7 cirrhotic patients and 8 healthy subjects; a further 2 cirrhotic patients received 3.75 mg.[1] Mean peak plasma concentrations were similar in healthy subjects and those with hepatic impairment following equivalent doses but time to peak plasma concentration was 4 hours in the latter as compared with 2 hours in the healthy subjects. Elimination was greatly prolonged in cirrhotic patients, in whom the mean plasma half-life was 8.53 hours compared with 3.5 hours. The CNS-depressant effects of zopiclone were delayed in the cirrhotic patients in a way consistent with the pharmacokinetic changes. There was also some evidence of an increased response in these patients. The authors recommended caution when administering zopiclone to patients with severe hepatic disease; the manufacturers contra-indicate the use of zopiclone in such patients.

1. Parker G, Roberts CJC. Plasma concentrations and central nervous system effects of the new hypnotic agent zopiclone in patients with chronic liver disease. *Br J Clin Pharmacol* 1983; **16:** 259–65.

**Overdosage.** Consciousness was rapidly regained after intravenous flumazenil administration in a patient who had taken an overdosage of zopiclone.[1] However, fatalities following zopiclone overdose have also been reported.[2,3]

1. Ahmad Z, *et al.* Diagnostic utility of flumazenil in coma with suspected poisoning. *BMJ* 1991; **302:** 292.
2. Boniface PJ, Russell SGG. Two cases of fatal zopiclone overdose. *J Anal Toxicol* 1996; **20:** 131–3.
3. Meatherall RC. Zopiclone fatality in a hospitalized patient. *J Forensic Sci* 1997; **42:** 340–3.

## Interactions

As for Diazepam, p.692. Concomitant use of rifampicin or other potent inducers of the cytochrome P450 isoenzyme CYP3A4, such as carbamazepine or phenytoin, is likely to reduce the effects of zopiclone.

**Antibacterials.** In a study in healthy subjects *erythromycin* increased the rate of absorption of zopiclone and prolonged its elimination.[1] In another study[2] in 8 healthy subjects *rifampicin* was associated with an 82% reduction in the area under the curve for zopiclone. The peak plasma concentration of zopiclone was reduced from 76.9 to 22.5 nanograms/mL and the elimination half-life from 3.8 to 2.3 hours.

1. Aranko K, *et al.* The effect of erythromycin on the pharmacokinetics and pharmacodynamics of zopiclone. *Br J Clin Pharmacol* 1994; **38:** 363–7.
2. Villikka K, *et al.* Concentrations and effects of zopiclone are greatly reduced by rifampicin. *Br J Clin Pharmacol* 1997; **43:** 471–4.

## Pharmacokinetics

Zopiclone is rapidly absorbed and widely distributed following administration by mouth. It has an elimination half-life of 3.5 to 6.5 hours and is reported to be about 45 to 80% bound to plasma proteins. Zopiclone is extensively metabolised in the liver; the 2 major metabolites, the less active zopiclone *N*-oxide and the inactive *N*-desmethylzopiclone, are excreted mainly in the urine. About 50% of a dose is converted by decarboxylation to inactive metabolites, which are partly eliminated via the lungs as carbon dioxide. Only about 5% of a dose appears unchanged in the urine and about 16% appears in the faeces. Excretion of zopiclone in the saliva may explain reports of a bitter taste. It is also distributed into breast milk.

◊ Reviews.

1. Fernandez C, *et al.* Clinical pharmacokinetics of zopiclone. *Clin Pharmacokinet* 1995; **29:** 431–41.

**Distribution into breast milk.** Zopiclone was distributed into breast milk in 12 lactating women in concentrations about half those in plasma.[1] The calculated dose that would be received by a neonate was 1.5 micrograms/kg, corresponding to 1.2% of the maternal dose.

1. Matheson I, *et al.* The excretion of zopiclone into breast milk. *Br J Clin Pharmacol* 1990; **30:** 267–71.

## Uses and Administration

Zopiclone is a cyclopyrrolone that is reported to have similar sedative, anxiolytic, muscle relaxant, amnestic, and anticonvulsant properties to those of the benzodiazepines (see Diazepam, p.695). Like diazepam, its actions are mediated by enhancement of the activity of gamma-aminobutyric acid (GABA) in the brain. Zopiclone is reported to bind to the benzodiazepine receptor component of the GABA receptor complex but at a different site to the benzodiazepines. It has a short duration of action.

Zopiclone is used as a hypnotic in the short-term management of insomnia. The usual dose is 7.5 mg by mouth before retiring. In elderly patients, treatment should be initiated with a dose of 3.75 mg before retiring. Reduced doses are also recommended in patients with hepatic or renal impairment, see below.

Eszopiclone, the (+)-isomer of zopiclone, is being studied for the management of insomnia.

**Administration in hepatic or renal impairment.** In those with renal impairment or mild to moderate hepatic impairment, treatment with zopiclone should be initiated with a dose of 3.75 mg before retiring. It should not be given to patients with severe hepatic impairment.

**Insomnia.** Zopiclone has a similar pharmacological and pharmacokinetic profile to the short-acting benzodiazepines. It is claimed to initiate sleep rapidly, without reduction of total rapid-eye-movement (REM) sleep, and then sustain it with preservation of normal slow-wave sleep (see Insomnia, p.667). It is generally considered to be as effective as a hypnotic as the benzodiazepines. Rebound insomnia has occurred but does not appear to be common. Residual effects the next day may be less pronounced after zopiclone than after short-acting benzodiazepines but there appears to be little evidence that zopiclone offers any clinical advantage in terms of its potential to induce tolerance, withdrawal symptoms, or dependence. For recommendations of the UK Committee on Safety of Medicines concerning its use as a hypnotic, see under Adverse Effects, Treatment, and Precautions, above.

References.

1. Noble S, *et al.* Zopiclone: an update of its pharmacology, clinical efficacy and tolerability in the treatment of insomnia. *Drugs* 1998; **55:** 277–302.
2. Hajak G. A comparative assessment of the risks and benefits of zopiclone: a review of 15 years' clinical experience. *Drug Safety* 1999; **21:** 457–69.
3. Terzano MG, *et al.* New drugs for insomnia: comparative tolerability of zopiclone, zolpidem and zaleplon. *Drug Safety* 2003; **26:** 261–82.

## Preparations

**Proprietary Preparations** (details are given in Part 3)
***Arg.:*** Foltran; Imovane; Insomnium; ***Austral.:*** Imovane; ***Austria:*** Imovane†; Somnal; ***Belg.:*** Imovane; ***Braz.:*** Imovane; Neurolil; Serenex†; ***Canad.:*** Imovane; Rhovane; ***Chile:*** Alpaz; Imovane; Losopil; Nuctane; Zedax; Zetix; Zometic; ***Denm.:*** Imoclone; Imovane; Imozop; ***Fin.:*** Imovane; Zopinox; ***Fr.:*** Imovane; Noctirex†; ***Ger.:*** espa-dorm; Optidorm; Somnosan; Ximovan; Zodurat; Zop; Zopi-Puren; Zopicalm; Zopiclodura; ***Gr.:*** Imovane; ***Hong Kong:*** Amvey; Eurovan; Imovane; Zolief; Zomni; ***India:*** Zonap; ***Irl.:*** Zileze; Zimoclone; Zimovane; Zopitan; Zorclone; ***Israel:*** Imovane; Nocturno; ***Ital.:*** Imovane; ***Malaysia:*** Imovane; ***Mex.:*** Imovane; ***Neth.:*** Imovane; ***Norw.:*** Imovane; ***NZ:*** Imovane; Zo-Tab†; ***S.Afr.:*** Alchera; Imovane; Z-Dorm; Zopimed; ***Singapore:*** Imovane; ***Spain:*** Datolan; Limovan; Siaten; Zopicalma; ***Swed.:*** Imovane; ***Switz.:*** Imovane; ***UK:*** Zileze; Zimovane.

---

# Zotepine *(BAN, rINN)*

Zotepina. 2-[(8-Chlorodibenzo[*b,f*]-thiepin-10-yl)oxy]-*N,N*-dimethylethylamine.

$C_{18}H_{18}ClNOS$ = 331.9.

*CAS — 26615-21-4.*

*ATC — N05AX11.*

## Adverse Effects, Treatment, and Precautions

Although zotepine may share some of the adverse effects seen with the classical antipsychotics (see Chlorpromazine, p.675), the incidence and severity of such effects may vary. Common adverse effects include asthenia, headache, hypotension and, less commonly, orthostatic hypotension, tachycardia, gastrointestinal disturbances, elevated liver-enzyme values, leucopenia, agitation, anxiety, dizziness, insomnia, somnolence, rhinitis, sweating, and blurred vision. Other less common reactions include thrombocytopenia, hyperglycaemia, convulsions, sexual dysfunction, and urinary incontinence. Extrapyramidal symptoms have been reported and tardive dyskinesia may occur with prolonged therapy. Neuroleptic malignant syndrome has been reported rarely. Prolactin levels may be increased and weight gain has been noted.

Zotepine can prolong the QT interval and patients with pre-existing prolongation of the QT interval should not be given the drug. It should be used with caution in patients at risk of developing arrhythmias; in such patients an ECG should be performed before starting treatment. Electrolytes should also be measured and any imbalance corrected. Monitoring of ECG and electrolytes should be continued during treatment especially at each dose increase. Zotepine may also increase the heart rate and, consequently, it should be used with care in patients with angina pectoris due to coronary artery disease. Caution is also recommended in patients with other cardiovascular disorders such as severe hypertension.

Zotepine has uricosuric properties and should not be given to patients with acute gout or a history of nephrolithiasis. It should not be used in patients with a personal or family history of epilepsy unless the potential benefit outweighs the risk of convulsions. Zotepine has antimuscarinic actions and should be used with caution in patients with disorders such as benign prostatic hyperplasia, urinary retention, and paralytic ileus. It should also be used with caution in patients with hepatic impairment. Weekly monitoring of liver function is recommended for at least the first 3 months of therapy in patients with hepatic impairment. Zotepine may exacerbate the symptoms of Parkinson's disease.

Zotepine may affect the performance of skilled tasks including driving.

The manufacturers recommend that zotepine is gradually stopped because of the risk of withdrawal symptoms with abrupt cessation.

## Interactions

Zotepine may enhance the effects of other CNS depressants; the risk of seizures is particularly increased when zotepine is given with high doses of other antipsychotics and the combination is not recommended. Zotepine may also enhance the effects of antihypertensives.

The risk of arrhythmias with zotepine may be increased by use with other drugs that prolong the QT interval or cause hypokalaemia. Use of zotepine with fluoxetine or diazepam may lead to increased plasma concentrations of zotepine.

## Pharmacokinetics

Zotepine is absorbed from the gastrointestinal tract and peak plasma concentrations have been achieved 2 to 3 hours after oral administration. It undergoes extensive first-pass metabolism to the equipotent metabolite norzotepine and inactive metabolites. CYP1A2 and CYP3A4 are the major cytochrome P450 isoenzymes involved in the metabolism of zotepine. Protein binding of zotepine and norzotepine is 97%. Zotepine is excreted mainly in the urine and faeces as metabolites and has an elimination half-life of about 14 hours.

## Uses and Administration

Zotepine is an atypical antipsychotic that, in addition to its antagonist action at central dopamine ($D_1$ and $D_2$) receptors, binds to serotonin ($5\text{-}HT_2$), adrenergic ($\alpha_1$), and histamine ($H_1$) receptors and inhibits noradrenaline reuptake. It is given by mouth in the treatment of schizophrenia in an initial dose of 25 mg three times daily increased at intervals of 4 days according to response to a maximum dose of 100 mg three times daily. There is an appreciable increase in the incidence of seizures at total daily doses above the recommended maximum of 300 mg. For elderly patients the recommended starting dose is 25 mg given twice daily increased gradually up to a maximum of 75 mg twice daily. Doses should also be reduced in patients with hepatic or renal impairment, see below.

**Administration in hepatic or renal impairment.** For patients with renal or hepatic impairment the recommended starting dose of zotepine is 25 mg given twice daily increased gradually up to a maximum of 75 mg twice daily.

**Schizophrenia.** A systematic review[1] of short-term studies of zotepine for schizophrenia (p.665) concluded tentatively that it was as effective as classical antipsychotics and might be of benefit in patients with negative symptoms; in addition it seemed less likely to provoke extrapyramidal disorders. Comparisons with atypical antipsychotics were too scanty for a meaningful comparison to be drawn.

1. Fenton M, *et al.* Zotepine for schizophrenia. Available in The Cochrane Library; Issue 2. Chichester: John Wiley; 2004.

## Preparations

**Proprietary Preparations** (details are given in Part 3)
***Austria:*** Nipolept; ***Ger.:*** Nipolept; ***Jpn:*** Lodopin; ***UK:*** Zoleptil.

---

# Zuclopenthixol *(BAN, rINN)*

AY-62021 (clopenthixol or clopenthixol hydrochloride); Z-Clopenthixol; *cis*-Clopenthixol; α-Clopenthixol; N-746 (clopenthixol or clopenthixol hydrochloride); NSC-64087 (clopenthixol); Zuclopentixol. (*Z*)-2-{4-[3-(2-Chloro-10*H*-dibenzo[*b,e*]thiin-10-ylidene)propyl]piperazin-1-yl}ethanol.

$C_{22}H_{25}ClN_2OS$ = 401.0.

*CAS — 53772-83-1 (zuclopenthixol); 982-24-1 (clopenthixol).*

*ATC — N05AF05.*

NOTE. Clopenthixol (*BAN, INN, USAN*) is the racemic mixture.

## Zuclopenthixol Acetate *(BANM, rINNM)*

Acetato de zuclopentixol.

$C_{24}H_{27}ClN_2O_2S$ = 443.0.

*CAS — 85721-05-7.*

*ATC — N05AF05.*

**Pharmacopoeias.** In *Br.*

**BP 2003** (Zuclopenthixol Acetate). A yellowish, viscous oil. Very slightly soluble in water; very soluble in alcohol, in dichloromethane, and in ether. Store at a temperature not exceeding −20°. Protect from light.

## Zuclopenthixol Decanoate *(BANM, rINNM)*

Decanoato de zuclopentixol; Zuclopenthixoli Decanoas.

$C_{32}H_{43}ClN_2O_2S$ = 555.2.

*CAS — 64053-00-5.*

*ATC — N05AF05.*

**Pharmacopoeias.** In *Eur.* (see p.vi).

**Ph. Eur. 5.0** (Zuclopenthixol Decanoate). A yellow viscous oily liquid. Very slightly soluble in water; very soluble in alcohol and in dichloromethane. Store under an inert gas in airtight containers at a temperature not exceeding −20°. Protect from light.

## Zuclopenthixol Hydrochloride *(BANM, rINNM)*

Hidrocloruro de zuclopentixol. Zuclopenthixol dihydrochloride.

$C_{22}H_{25}ClN_2OS,2HCl$ = 473.9.

*CAS — 58045-23-1.*

*ATC — N05AF05.*

**Pharmacopoeias.** In *Br.*

**BP 2003** (Zuclopenthixol Hydrochloride). An off-white granular powder. Very soluble in water; sparingly soluble in alcohol; slightly soluble in chloroform; very slightly soluble in ether. A 1% solution in water has a pH of 2.0 to 3.0. Protect from light.

**Stability.** References.

1. Li Wan Po A, Irwin WJ. The photochemical stability of cis- and trans-isomers of tricyclic neuroleptic drugs. *J Pharm Pharmacol* 1980; **32:** 25–9.

## Adverse Effects, Treatment, and Precautions

As for Chlorpromazine, p.675. Zuclopenthixol is less likely to cause sedation. It should not be used in apathetic or withdrawn states.

**Porphyria.** Zuclopenthixol is considered to be unsafe in patients with porphyria because it has been shown to be porphyrinogenic in *animals*.

## Interactions

As for Chlorpromazine, p.679.

## Pharmacokinetics

Zuclopenthixol is absorbed following oral administration with peak plasma concentrations occurring 3 to 6 hours after a dose. The biological half-life is reported to be about 1 day. It is mainly excreted in the faeces as unchanged zuclopenthixol and its *N*-dealkylated metabolite. Small amounts of drug or metabolites cross the placenta and are distributed into breast milk. Following intramuscular injection the acetate and decanoate esters of zuclopenthixol are hydrolysed to release zuclopenthixol. Zuclopenthixol acetate has a relatively quick onset of action after injection, and has a duration of action of 2 to 3 days; it is, therefore, useful for the control of acute psychotic symptoms while avoiding repeated injections. The decanoate has a much longer duration of action and is a suitable depot preparation for maintenance treatment.

**Metabolism.** Determination of metaboliser phenotype with regard to cytochrome P450 isoenzyme CYP2D6 appeared to be of limited value in patients receiving zuclopenthixol as interindividual variation appeared to be the main factor affecting dose to serum concentration ratios.[1]

1. Linnet K, Wiborg O. Influence of Cyp2D6 genetic polymorphism on ratios of steady-state serum concentration to dose of the neuroleptic zuclopenthixol. *Ther Drug Monit* 1996; **18:** 629–34.

## Uses and Administration

Zuclopenthixol is a thioxanthene of high potency with general properties similar to the phenothiazine, chlorpromazine (p.680). It has a piperazine side-chain.

Zuclopenthixol is used for the treatment of schizophrenia, mania (see Bipolar Disorder, p.278), and other psychoses. It may be particularly suitable for agitated or aggressive patients who may become over-excited with flupentixol. Zuclopenthixol hydrochloride is usually administered by mouth with doses expressed in terms of the base; zuclopenthixol hydrochloride 11.8 mg is approximately equivalent to 10 mg of zuclopenthixol. Zuclopenthixol hydrochloride has also been given intramuscularly. Zuclopenthixol acetate and zuclopenthixol decanoate are given by deep intramuscular injection; doses are expressed in terms of the ester. The acetate ester has an onset of action shortly after injection and a duration of action of 2 to 3 days; it is used for the initial treatment of acute psychoses and for exacerbations of chronic psychoses. The longer-acting decanoate ester is used for the maintenance treatment of chronic psychoses.

The usual initial oral dose of the hydrochloride for the treatment of psychoses is the equivalent of 20 to 30 mg of the base daily in divided doses; in severe or resistant schizophrenia up to 150 mg daily has been given. The usual maintenance dose is 20 to 50 mg daily.

The usual dose of zuclopenthixol acetate is 50 to 150 mg by deep intramuscular injection repeated, if necessary, after 2 or 3 days. Some patients may need an additional injection between 1 and 2 days after the first dose. Zuclopenthixol acetate is not intended for maintenance treatment; not more than four injections should be given in a course of treatment and the total dose should not exceed 400 mg. When maintenance therapy is required, zuclopenthixol hydrochloride by mouth may be introduced 2 to 3 days after the last injection of zuclopenthixol acetate, or intramuscular injections of the decanoate (see below) commenced with the last injection of the acetate.

The long-acting decanoate should be given by deep intramuscular injection; treatment is usually started with a test dose of 100 mg. This may be followed after at least one week by a dose of 200 to 500 mg or more, repeated at intervals of 1 to 4 weeks, and adjusted according to response. Injection volumes greater than 2 mL should be divided between 2 separate injection sites. The maximum recommended dose of zuclopenthixol decanoate is 600 mg weekly.

Elderly or debilitated patients should be given reduced doses of zuclopenthixol. The manufacturers state that the dose of the hydrochloride or the decanoate may need to be reduced to one-quarter or one-half of the normal initial dose; in addition, the maximum single dose of the acetate should be limited to 100 mg.

**Administration in hepatic or renal impairment.** The manufacturers recommend that for zuclopenthixol acetate, half the normal recommended dose should be used for patients with hepatic impairment; a dosage reduction is considered to be unnecessary in patients with renal impairment but where there is renal failure half the normal dosage is recommended.

**Schizophrenia.** A systematic review[1] comparing zuclopenthixol decanoate with other depot antipsychotic preparations considered that although it may induce more adverse effects, limited data suggested it might offer advantages such as lower relapse rates and increased acceptability in the treatment of schizophrenia (p.665) and similar serious mental illnesses. A similar review[2] of the use of zuclopenthixol acetate in the management of acute psychiatric illness found, however, that evidence of additional benefit over other antipsychotics was lacking.

1. Coutinho E, *et al.* Zuclopenthixol decanoate for schizophrenia and other serious mental illnesses. Available in The Cochrane Library; Issue 2. Chichester: John Wiley; 2004.
2. Fenton M, *et al.* Zuclopenthixol acetate in the treatment of acute schizophrenia and similar serious mental illnesses. Available in The Cochrane Library; Issue 2. Chichester: John Wiley; 2004.

## Preparations

***BP 2003:*** Zuclopenthixol Acetate Injection; Zuclopenthixol Decanoate Injection; Zuclopenthixol Tablets.

**Proprietary Preparations** (details are given in Part 3)
***Austral.:*** Clopixol; ***Austria:*** Cisordinol; ***Belg.:*** Clopixol; ***Braz.:*** Clopixol; ***Canad.:*** Clopixol; ***Chile:*** Cisordinol; ***Denm.:*** Cisordinol; ***Fin.:*** Cisordinol; ***Fr.:*** Clopixol; ***Ger.:*** Ciatyl-Z; ***Gr.:*** Clopixol; ***Hong Kong:*** Clopixol; ***India:*** Clopixol; ***Irl.:*** Clopixol; ***Israel:*** Clopixol; ***Ital.:*** Clopixol; ***Malaysia:*** Clopixol; ***Mex.:*** Clopixol; ***Neth.:*** Cisordinol; ***Norw.:*** Cisordinol; ***NZ:*** Clopixol; ***Port.:*** Cisordinol; ***S.Afr.:*** Clopixol; ***Singapore:*** Clopixol; ***Spain:*** Cisordinol; Clopixol; ***Swed.:*** Cisordinol; ***Switz.:*** Clopixol; ***Thai.:*** Clopixol; ***UK:*** Clopixol.

# Blood Products Plasma Expanders and Haemostatics


Anaemias, p.732
Aplastic anaemia, p.732
Haemolytic anaemia, p.733
Iron-deficiency anaemia, p.733
Megaloblastic anaemia, p.734
Normocytic-normochromic anaemia, p.734
Sideroblastic anaemia, p.734
Haemoglobinopathies, p.734
Sickle-cell disease, p.734
β-Thalassaemia, p.735
Haemostasis and Fibrinolysis, p.735
Disseminated intravascular coagulation, p.737
Haemorrhagic disorders, p.737
Neonatal intraventricular haemorrhage, p.740
Neutropenia, p.740


This chapter describes the management of blood disorders including anaemias, haemorrhagic disorders, and neutropenia. It covers blood, blood products and substitutes, and colloid plasma expanders; crystalloid plasma expanders are generally solutions of sodium chloride (p.1233) or glucose (p.1432) or both. Also included in the chapter are haemostatic drugs and erythropoietin and other colony-stimulating factors.

## Anaemias

Anaemia is usually understood to mean a lowering of haemoglobin concentration, red cell count, or packed cell volume to below 'normal' values, but the criteria for normality are difficult to establish. WHO's suggested definition of anaemia in populations living at around sea level is a haemoglobin concentration below:

- 13 g per 100 mL in men
- 12 g per 100 mL in women
- 11 g per 100 mL in pregnant women
- 12 g per 100 mL in children aged 12 to 14 years
- 11.5 g per 100 mL in children aged 5 to 11 years
- 11 g per 100 mL in children aged 6 to 59 months

However, because of individual variation, some apparently normal individuals have blood haemoglobin concentrations below these values, while others may be above these values and still be effectively anaemic.

Reduction in overall haemoglobin concentrations may be due just to fewer red cells with the cells retaining normal amounts of haemoglobin (normochromic anaemia), or the amount of haemoglobin in the cells may be reduced (hypochromic anaemia). Red cells themselves may be reduced in size (microcytic), enlarged (macrocytic), or normal in size (normocytic).

The immediate cause of anaemia may be decreased red cell production (due to defective proliferation and/or maturation of red cells from their precursors in bone marrow), increased red cell destruction (i.e. haemolysis), or loss of red cells from the circulation due to haemorrhage, either occult or overt. These conditions may occur due to underlying disease, nutritional deficiency, congenital disorders, or toxicity due to drugs or other substances and the cause must always be sought before an appropriate treatment can be determined.

The symptoms of anaemia are as variable as its causes but may include fatigue, pallor, dyspnoea, palpitations, headache, faintness or lightheadedness, tinnitus, anorexia and gastrointestinal disturbances, and loss of libido; tachycardia, heart failure, and retinal haemorrhage may occur in severe anaemia.

The treatment of anaemia depends upon its type and cause. Some of the principal types are classified in Table 1, below, and their management is discussed in more detail under the relevant headings. Sickle-cell disease and β-thalassaemia are discussed under Haemoglobinopathies.

**Table 1.** Types of anaemias.

| Classification | Anaemia | Mean cell volume | Haemoglobin | Associated with |
|---|---|---|---|---|
| Microcytic | Iron-deficiency anaemia | Decreased (or normal in early stages) | Hypochromic | Blood loss, malabsorption, inadequate iron intake |
| | Hereditary sideroblastic anaemia | Decreased | Hypochromic | |
| | Thalassaemias | Decreased | Hypochromic | |
| Macrocytic | Megaloblastic anaemia | Increased | Normochromic | Vitamin $B_{12}$ deficiency, folate deficiency (including drug induced) |
| | Acquired sideroblastic anaemia | Increased | Hypochromic | Alcoholism, drug or other toxicity |
| Normocytic | Normocytic-normochromic anaemia | Normal | Normochromic | Anaemia of chronic disorders, bone-marrow disorders (including aplastic anaemia), malignancy, renal failure, endocrine disorders, prematurity |
| Haemolytic | Haemolytic anaemia | Increased | | Immune disorders, drug toxicity, hereditary disorders |
| | Sickle-cell anaemia | | | |

### Aplastic anaemia

Aplastic anaemia is characterised by pancytopenia and hypoplasia of the bone marrow, with less than 25% of the marrow occupied by haematopoietic cells but without evident fibrosis or malignant infiltration. It is relatively rare, although it may be somewhat more common in the Far East, and is predominantly seen in younger adults. Some forms, such as Fanconi's anaemia, are inherited but most are acquired from various causes, including the effects of cytotoxic drugs or radiation, idiosyncratic reactions to other drugs, seronegative fulminant hepatitis, or auto-immune reactions. All cell lines are affected and patients consequently develop thrombocytopenia and neutropenia as well as anaemia, and symptoms include bleeding syndromes and infections as well as typical symptoms of anaemia.

Although spontaneous recovery has occurred, untreated aplastic anaemia is usually fatal. Management may be divided into supportive care and attempts to restore bone-marrow function and has been the subject of guidelines and reviews.[1,2]

**Supportive care**. Supportive care involves the prevention and treatment of infection (see Infections in Immunocompromised Patients, p.131), the control of haemorrhage with platelet concentrates, and where necessary, infusions of red blood cells (with platelets to prevent haemorrhage) for anaemia. Transfusions should be minimised in candidates for bone marrow transplant (see below).

**Restoration of bone-marrow function.** In patients aged under 40 years with severe disease and with a suitable HLA-matched donor, bone marrow transplantation has been considered the treatment of choice. Ideally this should be performed early before the patient has received too many transfusions, which increase the risk of rejection, and before infection develops. Transfusion of cord blood from an HLA-identical sibling can also produce permanent engraftment, and may be associated with less acute graft-versus-host disease than bone marrow transplantation.[2]

In patients unsuitable for bone marrow transplantation, or where a suitable donor is not available, treatment with immunosuppressants may be tried. About 50% of patients are reported to respond to a course of antilymphocyte immunoglobulin, and the addition of ciclosporin further improves response rates to between 60 and 80% and 5-year survival to between 75 and 90%.[1,2] However, one long-term study[3] providing follow-up data for 11 years has found no significant difference in survival between regimens of antilymphocyte immunoglobulin with or without ciclosporin.[3] Response to antilymphocyte immunoglobulin may not occur until about 3 months after the course,[2] and despite these good rates of response with the addition of ciclosporin, relapse is not uncommon.[4] A second course of antilymphocyte immunoglobulin is recommended if there is no response, or there is relapse, after 3 months.[2] Ciclosporin is continued after a response has occurred and until the blood count has been stable for at least 6 months; it may then be slowly withdrawn, usually over many months and depending on blood counts.[2] Ciclosporin has been used alone but is less effective than antilymphocyte immunoglobulin.[1] Good response rates have been reported from combined regimens including a granulocyte colony-stimulating factor.[5] However, there are concerns about long-term use and the role of these factors is still under investigation.[2] Oxymetholone was used extensively before the availability of antilymphocyte immunoglobulin and ciclosporin. It can increase the response to antilymphocyte immunoglobulin alone, but it can be hepatotoxic and causes virilisation, and is generally used for patients who have failed several courses of antilymphocyte immunoglobulin with ciclosporin, or where this regimen cannot be used.[2] Mycophenolate mofetil is under investigation in patients who are ineligible for bone marrow transplantation and refractory to standard immunosuppressive therapy.[2] Cyclophosphamide is commonly used in preparation for bone marrow transplantation and complete remission has also been reported with high-dose cyclophosphamide alone.[6,7] However, a randomised trial[8] of high-dose cyclophosphamide plus ciclosporin compared with conventional immunosuppression was stopped early when a higher mortality was observed in those receiving cyclophosphamide. Further follow-up[9] also found that relapse rates were no different.

Overall, the results of immunosuppression seem to be comparable to those of bone marrow transplantation, except perhaps in children,[10] who generally respond less well to immunosuppressants. Responses are often partial, but this may be sufficient to free the patient from dependency on transfusions and intensive antibacterial cover, and is considered well worth achieving. Some groups have preferred immunosuppression for initial therapy even in patients suitable for transplantation, reserving the transplant for salvage in nonresponders or relapse.[11] Such an approach has been reported to result in a 5-year survival of some 80%, but there is concern that patients treated with immunosuppression retain some underlying defect in marrow function, as many patients subsequently develop leukaemias or myelodysplasias.[1,12,13]

In moderate disease, or where immunosuppression fails, other drugs that have been tried include normal immunoglobulins, although it has been suggested that responses are uncommon.[12] The availability of recombinant haematopoietic growth factors has led to trials of colony-stimulating factors in a few patients,[14-16] but although some responses have occurred during therapy there is no evidence of sustained remission. The use of colony-stimulating factors alone has been criticised[17] on the grounds that such treatment delays bone marrow transplantation or immunosuppressive therapy and thus reduces the chance of a successful outcome. They may, however, have a role with immunosuppressive therapy (see above).


1. Young NS. Acquired aplastic anemia. *Ann Intern Med* 2002; **136:** 534–46.
2. Marsh JCW, *et al.* Guidelines for the diagnosis and management of acquired aplastic anaemia. *Br J Haematol* 2003; **123:** 782–801.
3. Frickhofen N, *et al.* Antithymocyte globulin with or without cyclosporin A: 11-year follow-up of a randomized trial comparing treatments of aplastic anemia. *Blood* 2003; **101:** 1236–42.
4. Rosenfeld S, *et al.* Antithymocyte globulin and cyclosporine for severe aplastic anemia: association between hematologic response and long-term outcome. *JAMA* 2003; **289:** 1130–5.
5. Bacigalupo A, *et al.* Antilymphocyte globulin, cyclosporine, prednisolone, and granulocyte colony-stimulating factor for severe aplastic anemia: an update of the GITMO/EBMT study on 100 patients. *Blood* 2000; **95:** 1931–4.
6. Brodsky RA, *et al.* Complete remission in severe aplastic anemia after high-dose cyclophosphamide without bone marrow transplantation. *Blood* 1996; **87:** 491–4.
7. Brodsky RA, *et al.* Durable treatment-free remission after high-dose cyclophosphamide therapy for previously untreated severe aplastic anemia. *Ann Intern Med* 2001; **135:** 477–83.
8. Tisdale JF, *et al.* High-dose cyclophosphamide in severe aplastic anaemia: a randomised trial. *Lancet* 2000; **356:** 1554–9.
9. Tisdale JF, *et al.* Late complications following treatment for severe aplastic anemia (SAA) with high-dose cyclophosphamide (Cy): follow-up of a randomized trial. *Blood* 2002; **100:** 4668–70.
10. Webb DKH, *et al.* Acquired aplastic anaemia: still a serious disease. *Arch Dis Child* 1991; **66:** 858–61.
11. Crump M, *et al.* Treatment of adults with severe aplastic anemia: primary therapy with antithymocyte globulin (ATG) and rescue of ATG failures with bone marrow transplantation. *Am J Med* 1992; **92:** 596–602.
12. Moore MAS, Castro-Malaspina H. Immunosuppression in aplastic anemia—postponing the inevitable? *N Engl J Med* 1991; **324:** 1358–60.
13. Socié G, *et al.* Malignant tumors occurring after treatment of aplastic anemia. *N Engl J Med* 1993; **329:** 1152–7.
14. Vadhan-Raj S, *et al.* Stimulation of myelopoiesis in patients with aplastic anemia by recombinant human granulocyte-macrophage colony-stimulating factor. *N Engl J Med* 1988; **319:** 1628–34.
15. Kurzrock R, *et al.* Very low doses of GM-CSF administered alone or with erythropoietin in aplastic anemia. *Am J Med* 1992; **93:** 41–8.
16. Geissler K, *et al.* Effect of interleukin-3 on responsiveness to granulocyte-colony-stimulating factor in severe aplastic anemia. *Ann Intern Med* 1992; **117:** 223–5.
17. Marsh JCW, *et al.* Haemopoietic growth factors in aplastic anaemia: a cautionary note. *Lancet* 1994; **344:** 172–3.


### Haemolytic anaemia

The normal life span of an erythrocyte is about 120 days; a haemolytic state is defined as a reduction in this mean life span due to premature destruction of red cells, either intravascularly, or more commonly after sequestration by the spleen or liver. Healthy bone marrow can compensate for even quite severe haemolysis by increased erythropoiesis; however, if the red cell survival-time is less than 15 days, or if the bone marrow is abnormal, or there is a deficiency of folate, iron, or other necessary nutrients, then compensation will be inadequate and haemolytic anaemia will result. In addition to typical symptoms of anaemia (above) patients frequently exhibit jaundice and splenomegaly, while the increased erythropoiesis results in reticulocytosis (elevated counts of immature red cells).

Haemolytic anaemias may be either congenital or acquired. The congenital disorders include those due to membrane defects in the erythrocyte such as spherocytosis or elliptocytosis; those due to enzyme defects (including the various forms of glucose-6-phosphate dehydrogenase (G6PD) deficiency); and those due to haemoglobin defects (haemoglobinopathies) including sickle-cell disease and β-thalassaemia (below).

The acquired haemolytic anaemias arise from numerous causes but may be divided into immune and non-immune types. The immune types include some drug-induced haemolytic anaemias (including those produced by penicillins, rifampicin, and methyldopa); auto-immune haemolytic anaemia (further classified into warm or cold depending on the temperature at which the red cell antibodies are most active); and haemolytic disease of the newborn (see p.1608). The non-immune types include haemolysis due to infections such as malaria; chemically-induced haemolysis (due to a direct effect on the red cell rather than an immunologically-mediated one, and including the effects of toxins such as copper and arsenic as well as some snake venoms, and drugs such as amphotericin B, dapsone, and sulfasalazine); and the effects of mechanical trauma.

**Treatment** of haemolytic anaemia depends on the underlying cause, although general supportive measures (bed rest, transfusion if haemodynamic abnormalities make it necessary, and supplementation with folate) will be similar in all poorly-compensated patients. Well compensated haemolysis may require no treatment at all, although clearly elucidation and, where possible, removal of the cause is desirable.

Hereditary haemolytic disorders such as spherocytosis mostly respond well to splenectomy, although milder forms may not require treatment. In patients with G6PD deficiency, treatment consists essentially of avoidance of drugs or foodstuffs likely to provoke haemolysis.

Acquired haemolytic anaemia is best treated by identification and where possible elimination of any underlying cause. Most drug-induced haemolytic anaemias respond rapidly to discontinuation of the offending substance.

Auto-immune haemolytic anaemias require treatment aimed at maintaining the patient and controlling haemolysis. Although treatment may need to be prolonged, in many patients with idiopathic disease antibodies eventually disappear or decrease to insignificant titres after months or years. The auto-immune haemolytic anaemias may be secondary to other disorders including leukaemias, lymphomas, and systemic lupus erythematosus; correction of the underlying disease often results in marked improvement of accompanying haemolysis.

In patients with warm auto-immune haemolytic anaemia initial treatment is with corticosteroids.[1] A typical initial dose is prednisone or prednisolone 1 to 1.5 mg/kg by mouth daily. The onset of response is usually rapid and most patients demonstrate benefit within 10 to 14 days. The initial effective dose of corticosteroid should be continued until a satisfactory response has been obtained, and once there is haematologic stabilisation the dose may be gradually reduced. Many patients will require low-dose maintenance therapy. If symptoms do not respond to tolerable doses of corticosteroids splenectomy should be considered. Alternative approaches include the use of vinblastine- or vincristine-loaded platelets,[2] or intravenous infusions of high-dose normal immunoglobulin.[3,4] Immunosuppressants such as azathioprine may be considered in patients refractory to other therapy; responses are reportedly variable, but they sometimes permit reduction of corticosteroid maintenance doses. There are some reports of benefit from the use of danazol.[1] Transfusion is problematic in these patients because of the difficulty in establishing compatibility between patient and donor.[5,6] Nonetheless, transfusion may be life-saving in acute disease, and the least incompatible blood should be used.

In patients with cold auto-immune haemolytic anaemias such as cold haemagglutinin disease it is additionally important to keep the patient warm. Corticosteroids and splenectomy are generally of no benefit in these patients (although there may be a responsive subgroup[7]), but treatment with chlorambucil 2 to 4 mg daily by mouth may produce a response. Blood transfusion should be avoided if possible, and if given it should be preferably via a warming coil and infused slowly.


1. Petz LD. Treatment of autoimmune hemolytic anemias. *Curr Opin Hematol* 2001; **8:** 411–16.
2. Ahn YS, *et al.* Treatment of autoimmune hemolytic anemia with vinca-loaded platelets. *JAMA* 1983; **249:** 2189–94.
3. Mitchell CA, *et al.* High dose intravenous gammaglobulin in Coombs positive hemolytic anemia. *Aust N Z J Med* 1987; **17:** 290–4.
4. Blanchette VS, *et al.* Role of intravenous immunoglobulin G in autoimmune hematologic disorders. *Semin Hematol* 1992; **29:** 72–82.
5. Salama A, *et al.* Red blood cell transfusion in warm-type autoimmune haemolytic anaemia. *Lancet* 1992; **340:** 1515–17.
6. Garratty G, Petz LD. Transfusing patients with autoimmune haemolytic anaemia. *Lancet* 1993; **341:** 1220.
7. Silberstein LE, *et al.* Cold hemagglutinin disease associated with IgG cold-reactive antibody. *Ann Intern Med* 1987; **106:** 238–42.


### Iron-deficiency anaemia

The iron content of the body is normally kept constant by regulation of the amount absorbed to balance the amount lost. If loss is increased, and/or intake inadequate, a negative iron-balance may lead by degrees to depletion of body iron stores, iron deficiency, and eventually to anaemia. Iron requirements are increased during infancy, puberty, pregnancy, and during menstruation, and iron-deficiency anaemias are most common in women and children; the most common cause in adult males and postmenopausal women is blood loss, usually from the gastrointestinal tract.

Iron deficiency usually results in a microcytic, hypochromic anaemia, but the diagnosis of iron deficiency should be confirmed, if there is any doubt, by measurement of serum ferritin, erythrocyte protoporphyrin, or total iron binding capacity (transferrin). Iron therapy can begin once deficiency is confirmed, but the underlying cause of the deficiency should still be sought and treated.

**Treatment.** The prevention and control of iron-deficiency anaemias has been reviewed.[1,2] Almost all iron-deficiency anaemias respond readily to treatment with iron. The treatment of choice is oral administration of a ferrous salt (ferrous iron is better absorbed than ferric iron). Many iron compounds have been used for this purpose, but do not offer any real advantage over the simple ferrous fumarate, gluconate, or sulfate salts. The usual adult dose is sufficient of these salts to supply about 100 to 200 mg of elemental iron daily (for the elemental iron content of various iron salts, see p.1436). A rise in haemoglobin concentration of about 0.1 g or more per 100 mL daily is considered a positive response. Haemoglobin response is greatest in the first few weeks of therapy and is proportional to the severity of the original anaemia. Once haemoglobin concentrations have risen to the normal range, iron therapy should be continued for a further 3 months to aid replenishment of iron stores.

Oral iron has been given with agents, such as ascorbic acid, that enhance iron absorption significantly if given in large enough doses, but such combinations may increase the incidence of adverse effects. Modified-release preparations have been used in patients intolerant of ordinary formulations of iron but some consider them therapeutically ineffective.

Failure to respond to oral iron after about 3 weeks of therapy may be indicative of non-compliance, continued blood loss with inadequate replacement of iron, malabsorption, wrong diagnosis, or other complicating factors, and the treatment should be reassessed.

Parenteral iron therapy is rarely indicated, may produce severe adverse effects, and should be reserved for patients who are genuinely intolerant of oral iron, persistently non-compliant, who have gastrointestinal disorders exacerbated by oral iron therapy, continuing blood loss too severe for oral treatment to provide sufficient iron, or for those unable to absorb iron adequately from the gastrointestinal tract. The most common parenteral forms are iron sorbitol (given intramuscularly), iron sucrose (given intravenously), and iron dextran (given intravenously, in which case the complete iron requirement may be given as a single infusion, or intramuscularly).

Exceptionally, in patients with profound anaemia, blood transfusion may be necessary to restore dangerously low concentrations of haemoglobin. This may be the case, for example, in elderly patients with long-standing iron deficiency leading to heart failure. However, transfusion should always be avoided if possible.

**Prophylaxis.** Prophylaxis may be desirable in some groups at risk of iron deficiency and consequent anaemia, and may include therapy with oral iron supplements, measures to improve dietary iron intake, fortification of food staples, or control of infection.

WHO[2] recommends that universal supplementation of iron and folic acid should be implemented for pregnant women, starting as soon as possible after gestation starts and continuing for the rest of the pregnancy. WHO also recommends that where anaemia prevalence is above 40%, women of child-bearing age and lactating women should be given 3 months of iron and folic acid supplementation. However, the US Preventive Services Task Force has reviewed the subject of iron supplementation during pregnancy,[3] and concluded that there was insufficient evidence for or against routine supplementation.[4]

Iron supplementation is accepted in menorrhagia, after gastrectomy, and in the management of low birth-weight infants such as the premature. Iron deficiency in infants and children may result in developmental delay that is reversible with iron supplements.[5] WHO has suggested[2] that where the diet does not include foods fortified with iron or where anaemia prevalence is above 40%, iron supplementation should be given to all children between 6 and 23 months of age; for children aged 24 months and above, a 3-month course of iron supplementation should be given where the anaemia prevalence is above 40%.

The usual prophylactic dose in adults is sufficient of a ferrous salt to provide about 60 to 120 mg of elemental iron daily. Doses of around 1 to 2 mg/kg of elemental iron daily (up to 30 mg) have been suggested for prophylaxis in children.

Dietary measures, such as addition of vitamin-C-rich foods, or other enhancers of iron absorption including iron in the form of haem (found in meat or fish) to the diet, and control of parasitic infections such as hookworm (which are responsible for considerable occult blood loss), are particularly important for the general community in developing countries. Fortification of food staples poses technical problems as iron salts react with food components and may produce rancidity or other undesirable changes on storage. Nonetheless, wheat flour, bread, and milk products are often so fortified, and consideration has been given to fortification of salt, sugar, rice, and fish sauce.


1. Frewin R, *et al.* ABC of clinical haematology. Iron deficiency anaemia. *BMJ* 1997; **314:** 360–3.

2. World Health Organization. *Iron deficiency anaemia assessment, prevention, and control: a guide for programme managers.* Geneva: WHO, 2001. Available at: http://www.who.int/nut/documents/ida_assessment_prevention_control.pdf (accessed 23/06/04)
3. US Preventive Services Task Force. Routine iron supplementation during pregnancy: review article. *JAMA* 1993; **270:** 2848–54.
4. US Preventive Services Task Force. Routine iron supplementation during pregnancy: policy statement. *JAMA* 1993; **270:** 2846–8.
5. Idjradinata P, Pollitt E. Reversal of developmental delays in iron-deficient anaemic infants treated with iron. *Lancet* 1993; **341:** 1–4.

## Megaloblastic anaemia

The megaloblastic anaemias are characterised by macrocytosis (an increased mean cell volume) and the production of distinctive morphological changes and abnormal maturation in developing haematopoietic cells in the bone marrow: white cell and platelet lines are affected as well as erythroid precursors, and in severe cases anaemia may be associated with leucopenia and thrombocytopenia. Megaloblastic anaemia is a consequence of impaired DNA biosynthesis in the bone marrow, usually due to a deficiency of vitamin $B_{12}$ (cobalamins) or folate, both of which are essential for this process. Although the haematological symptoms of $B_{12}$ deficiency and folate deficiency are similar it is important to distinguish between them since the use of folate alone in $B_{12}$-deficient megaloblastic anaemia may improve haematological symptoms without preventing aggravation of accompanying neurological symptoms, and may lead to severe nervous system sequelae such as subacute combined degeneration of the spinal cord. Where it is desirable to commence therapy immediately, combined treatment for both deficiencies may be started once suitable samples have been taken to permit diagnosis of the deficiency, and the patient converted to the appropriate treatment once the cause of the anaemia is known.

**Vitamin $B_{12}$ deficiency anaemia.** Vitamin $B_{12}$ deficiency and its associated symptoms may be due to malabsorption (including following gastrectomy), dietary deficiency (mainly in strict vegetarians), competition with intestinal bacteria or parasites, or to the effect of drugs such as nitrous oxide. In populations of northern European origin pernicious anaemia, in which atrophy of the gastric mucosa results in a lack of the intrinsic factor essential for $B_{12}$ absorption, is the most frequent cause. Owing to large body stores of the vitamin it may take several years for signs of deficiency to manifest once the defect in absorption occurs.

In addition to megaloblastic anaemia, vitamin $B_{12}$ deficiency may result in neurological damage, including peripheral neuropathy and effects on mental function ranging from mild neurosis to dementia.

TREATMENT. The treatment is with vitamin $B_{12}$, almost always by the intramuscular or sometimes the deep subcutaneous route since in most patients absorption from the gastrointestinal tract is inadequate. Hydroxocobalamin is generally preferred to cyanocobalamin since it need be given less often. Regimens may vary, but hydroxocobalamin 1 mg every few days for 6 to 8 doses will restore normal body stores of the vitamin. The haematological response to therapy is rapid, with improvement in most parameters and symptoms beginning within 48 hours. Neurological abnormalities may take much longer to respond, and may not do so completely.

PROPHYLAXIS. Where the defect in $B_{12}$ handling is irreversible, as in pernicious anaemia, maintenance therapy must continue for life to prevent a recurrence of the deficiency. Therapy must also be given prophylactically after total gastrectomy or total ileal resection, or where gastrointestinal surgery is shown to have impaired absorption of the vitamin. Typically, injection of hydroxocobalamin 1 mg every 2 to 3 months is used. In patients in whom injection is not possible, 1 to 2 mg may be given daily by mouth, since a few micrograms may be absorbed by passive diffusion. In patients whose diet supplies inadequate $B_{12}$, deficiency may be prevented, in the absence of other causes, by much lower oral doses given as a supplement; up to 150 micrograms of cyanocobalamin daily has been recommended.

**Folate-deficiency anaemia.** Deficiency of folate may be due to inadequate diet, or malabsorption syndromes (such as coeliac disease or sprue), to increased utilisation (as in pregnancy, one of the most common causes of megaloblastic anaemia, or the increased haematopoiesis of haemolytic syndromes), to increased urinary loss or loss due to haemodialysis, or to an adverse effect of alcohol, antiepileptics, or other drugs. The clinical features of folate-deficient megaloblastic anaemia are similar to those of disease due to vitamin-$B_{12}$ deficiency except that the accompanying severe neuropathy does not occur, and deficiency may develop much more rapidly. Deficiency may also be associated with neural tube defects (p.1430) if it occurs in pregnancy.

TREATMENT. Once folate deficiency has been established the usual treatment in the UK is folic acid 5 mg by mouth daily. Lower doses of 0.25 to 1 mg are suggested in the USA. It is customary to continue therapy for at least 4 months, the time necessary for complete red cell replacement. In patients with malabsorption, therapy may require higher doses, up to 15 mg of folic acid daily. As in $B_{12}$-deficiency anaemia, the response to therapy is rapid.

PROPHYLAXIS. Long-term maintenance is rarely needed, except in a few patients in whom the underlying cause of folate deficiency cannot be treated (for example in some severe haemolytic syndromes). Doses of 5 mg daily or even weekly have been suggested for prophylaxis in patients undergoing dialysis or with chronic haemolytic states, depending on the diet and rate of haemolysis; a dose of 400 micrograms daily is recommended in the USA.

For primary prophylaxis of megaloblastic anaemia in pregnancy, folic acid is given in the UK in usual doses of 200 to 500 micrograms daily, often with a ferrous salt for prophylaxis of iron deficiency.

Drugs which act as inhibitors of dihydrofolate reductase, such as methotrexate, may produce severe megaloblastic anaemia which cannot be reversed by therapy with folic acid. The adverse effects of such drugs may be largely prevented or reversed by therapy with folinic acid, which can be incorporated into folate metabolism without the need for reduction by the inhibited enzyme. For details of such 'folinic acid rescue', see under Folinic Acid, p.1431.

General references.

1. Hoffbrand V, Provan D. ABC of clinical haematology: macrocytic anaemias. *BMJ* 1997; **314:** 430–33.
2. Wickramasinghe SN. Folate and vitamin $B_{12}$ deficiency and supplementation. *Prescribers' J* 1997; **37:** 88–95.

## Normocytic-normochromic anaemia

Anaemias in which red cell size and cellular haemoglobin are not significantly different from normal (normocytic-normochromic anaemias) form a substantial proportion of all cases. Such anaemias are usually secondary to another disease and include the anaemia of chronic disorders (associated with chronic infection such as tuberculosis, malignancy, inflammatory disorders such as inflammatory bowel disease, polymyalgia rheumatica, rheumatoid arthritis, and systemic lupus erythematosus), anaemia of renal failure, anaemia of prematurity, anaemia associated with endocrine disorders such as hypothyroidism or hypopituitarism, and anaemias associated with primary bone-marrow failure (including aplastic anaemia, above, pure red cell aplasia, marrow fibrosis or infiltration as in myelodysplasia or leukaemia, and marrow failure associated with AIDS). Iron-deficiency anaemia, which is usually classified as microcytic and hypochromic may in fact be neither, particularly in the early stages, and should be differentiated from anaemia of chronic disease. The latter is also accompanied by changes in iron metabolism, notably sequestration of iron in reticuloendothelial cells: plasma iron is low but in contrast to iron deficiency the total iron binding capacity is reduced and serum ferritin is often increased.

The **treatment** of most of these anaemias is essentially that of the underlying disease. Blood transfusion has been given when anaemia is severe. In patients with anaemia of renal failure, which is due at least in part to decreased erythropoietin production by the damaged kidney, regular subcutaneous or intravenous injection of recombinant human erythropoietins (epoetin alfa or epoetin beta) can completely reverse the anaemia. Epoetins may also have a role in anaemia of prematurity and some drug-induced anaemias, and have been investigated in patients with the anaemia of chronic disease and some other normocytic-normochromic anaemias.

## Sideroblastic anaemia

The sideroblastic anaemias are characterised by a population of hypochromic red cells in the presence of increased serum-iron concentrations, and abnormal erythroid precursors, known as ring sideroblasts, in the bone marrow. They are associated with abnormalities in porphyrin biosynthesis leading to diminished production of haem, and increased cellular iron uptake. Sideroblastic anaemias may be of various types, and are classified as acquired or hereditary.

**Acquired sideroblastic anaemia.** Acquired sideroblastic anaemia may either be idiopathic, or secondary to either a drug or toxin (such as alcohol, isoniazid, chloramphenicol, or lead) or to a disease (including hypothyroidism, rheumatoid arthritis, haemolytic or megaloblastic anaemias, leukaemias, and lymphomas). The treatment of the secondary forms is essentially the treatment of the underlying disease or removal of the precipitating cause. The anaemia is usually mild and often macrocytic.

Patients with idiopathic disease usually have only mild anaemia, and most require no treatment. Although rarely suffering from vitamin $B_6$ deficiency a few patients will respond at least partially to high doses of pyridoxine by mouth, up to 400 mg daily, and a trial is considered worthwhile in all patients. If patients become symptomatic, transfusion may be required, but should be kept to a minimum because of the problems of iron overload. All patients with sideroblastic anaemia must have their serum-iron and -ferritin concentrations regularly monitored, and be given desferrioxamine by regular bolus injection when there is evidence of iron overload.

**Hereditary sideroblastic anaemia.** The hereditary forms of the disease appear to be sex-linked, and almost always manifest themselves in males. The anaemia may be more severe than in acquired sideroblastic anaemia, and is usually microcytic.

A trial of pyridoxine is considered worthwhile as some forms are responsive, but in many cases there is no benefit. Some patients develop gradually increasing iron loads, and may eventually develop haemosiderosis; to prevent this, regular venesection or the use of desferrioxamine are indicated if there is evidence of iron accumulation.

## Haemoglobinopathies

Haemoglobinopathies are clinical abnormalities due to altered structure, function, or production of haemoglobin. Human haemoglobins are tetramers, constructed of 4 globin chains each enfolding an iron-containing haem moiety: two of these globins are of the 'α-like' types (globins α or ζ) and two are 'non-α' (types β, γ, δ, or ε). The normal major adult haemoglobin, haemoglobin A, comprises two α and two β chains, while the predominant fetal haemoglobin, haemoglobin F (also present in minute amounts in normal adults), is composed of two α and two γ globins. The erythroblast inherits two genes for the production of α globin and one for β globin production from each parent, and a mutation in a single α gene will therefore affect only 25% of the haemoglobin produced, whereas a single β mutation will affect 50%: the β-haemoglobinopathies, due to defective β globin production, are therefore more likely to produce symptoms, and the most widespread forms are the β-thalassaemias and sickle-cell disease, which are discussed below.

## Sickle-cell disease

Sickle-cell disease is a haemoglobinopathy (see above) in which a structural abnormality in the β globin chain results in the formation of an abnormal haemoglobin, haemoglobin S. In the deoxygenated state haemoglobin S is less soluble and polymerises into rod-like fibres, and cells containing high concentrations of haemoglobin S subsequently become deformed into a sickle shape. Normal haemoglobins may be incorporated into the polymer but some, such as fetal haemoglobin (haemoglobin F), are not included; increasing concentrations of these in the red cell reduce the rate of sickling.

The heterozygous form, sickle-cell trait, is generally asymptomatic except in conditions of extreme anoxia, although characteristic abnormalities of renal function (inadequate concentration of the urine) may be present. As with thalassaemia trait (see below) it is more common in populations of tropical origin, and has been postulated to offer a degree of protection against malaria. In the homozygous form a varying degree of haemolytic anaemia is present, accompanied by increased erythropoiesis. In addition to shortened survival, the decreased flexibility of the deformed erythrocytes can lead to occlusion of the microvasculature, and sickle-cell crisis. The latter may manifest as excruciating pain due to infarction of the blood supply to the bones, or infarction of other organs including lung, liver, kidney, penis (leading to priapism), and brain (stroke). An acute chest syndrome occurs in many patients, and may be fatal. It is a form of acute lung injury associated with infarction, fat embolism, and infection, and may progress to acute respiratory distress syndrome.

Occasionally a large proportion of red cell mass may become trapped in the spleen or liver (sequestration crisis) with death due to gross anaemia. Chronic complications include skin ulceration, renal failure, retinal detachment, and increased susceptibility to infection.

**Treatment** of sickle-cell disease is essentially symptomatic.[1-4] Young children should receive prophylactic penicillin and pneumococcal vaccine, to reduce the risk of infection (see Spleen Disorders, p.146). Infection should be treated early, and folate supplementation given if necessary since the increased erythropoiesis resulting from chronic haemolysis may increase folate requirements.

Sickle-cell crisis requires hospitalisation, with the use of large volumes of intravenous fluids for dehydration, analgesia including opioids for pain (see p.8), and treatment of any concurrent infection. Oxygen should be given if the patient is hypoxaemic. Where crisis affects a vital organ with life-threatening or potentially disabling consequences partial exchange transfusion should be carried out promptly, as no other therapy exists. Where rapid enlargement of spleen or liver indicates a sequestration crisis, transfusion is also important to avoid fatal anaemia.

Maintenance transfusion is rarely indicated, although it may be given to patients who have already had a stroke; measures to avoid iron overload such as phlebotomy or desferrioxamine chelation are necessary in patients receiving regular transfusions. Prophylactic transfusions in children at high risk has been reported[5] to reduce the incidence of first stroke but the risks and benefits of treatment must be carefully considered. Splenectomy may be recommended in the management of recurrent splenic sequestration.

Research into specific therapy for sickling has produced some promising results.[6] Because haemoglobin F is known to protect against sickling, considerable interest has centred on attempts to stimulate fetal haemoglobin production. Most studies have used hydroxycarbamide. Initial trials showed some elevation in mean fetal haemoglobin concentrations, but responses were very variable. However, a subsequent randomised controlled study in 299 patients[7] reported that therapy with hydroxycarbamide caused a 44% reduction in the median annual rate of painful crises. The beneficial effects did not become evident for several months. Observational follow-up of 233 patients in this group,[8] for up to 9 years, suggested that hydroxycarbamide also reduced mortality. Beneficial effects have also been reported in initial studies in children.[9-11] However, the potential toxicity of long-term therapy with hydroxycarbamide (especially in children) remains a concern. Use of hydroxycarbamide with erythropoietin has been reported to increase fetal haemoglobin concentrations further in one study,[12] although not in another using a different dosage regimen.[13] A short-chain fatty acid, butyric acid, which has a low order of toxicity, has been reported to stimulate fetal haemoglobin in patients with sickle-cell disease when given by infusion as arginine butyrate.[14] Other drugs under investigation include clotrimazole, decitabine, inhaled nitric oxide, and the nonionic surfactant poloxamer 188. There is also some investigation into gene therapy.

As in thalassaemia (see below), bone marrow transplantation is potentially curative in a small minority of patients, but the indications for transplantation are much less well established, and its use and benefits remain a matter for debate.[15-17]


1. Steinberg MH. Management of sickle cell disease. *N Engl J Med* 1999; **340:** 1021–30.
2. Ballas SK. Sickle cell anaemia: progress in pathogenesis and treatment. *Drugs* 2002; **62:** 1143–72.
3. American Academy of Pediatrics Section on Hematology/Oncology Committee on Genetics. Health supervision for children with sickle cell disease. *Pediatrics* 2002; **109:** 526–35. Also available at: http://aappolicy.aappublications.org/cgi/reprint/pediatrics;109/3/526.pdf (accessed 23/06/04)
4. Claster S, Vichinsky EP. Managing sickle cell disease. *BMJ* 2003; **327:** 1151–5.
5. Adams RJ, *et al.* Prevention of a first stroke by transfusions in children with sickle cell anemia and abnormal results on transcranial doppler ultrasonography. *N Engl J Med* 1998; **339:** 5–11.
6. Bunn HF. Pathogenesis and treatment of sickle cell disease. *N Engl J Med* 1997; **337:** 762–9.
7. Charache S, *et al.* Effect of hydroxyurea on the frequency of painful crises in sickle cell anemia. *N Engl J Med* 1995; **332:** 1317–22.
8. Steinberg MH, *et al.* Effect of hydroxyurea on mortality and morbidity in adult sickle cell anemia: risks and benefits up to 9 years of treatment. *JAMA* 2003; **289:** 1645–51. Correction. *ibid.*; **290:** 756.
9. Scott JP, *et al.* Hydroxyurea therapy in children severely affected with sickle cell disease. *J Pediatr* 1996; **128:** 820–8.
10. Ferster A, *et al.* Hydroxyurea for treatment of severe sickle cell anemia: a pediatric clinical trial. *Blood* 1996; **88:** 1960–4.
11. Wang WC, *et al.* A two-year pilot trial of hydroxyurea in very young children with sickle-cell anemia. *J Pediatr* 2001; **139:** 790–6.
12. Rodgers GP, *et al.* Augmentation by erythropoietin of the fetal-hemoglobin response to hydroxyurea in sickle cell disease. *N Engl J Med* 1993; **328:** 73–80.
13. Goldberg MA, *et al.* Treatment of sickle cell anemia with hydroxyurea and erythropoietin. *N Engl J Med* 1990; **323:** 366–72.
14. Perrine SP, *et al.* A short-term trial of butyrate to stimulate fetal-globin-gene expression in the β-globin disorders. *N Engl J Med* 1993; **328:** 81–6.
15. Davies SC, Roberts IAG. Bone marrow transplant for sickle cell disease—an update. *Arch Dis Child* 1996; **75:** 3–6.
16. Walters MC, *et al.* Bone marrow transplantation for sickle cell disease. *N Engl J Med* 1996; **335:** 369–76.
17. Platt OS, Guinan EC. Bone marrow transplantation in sickle cell anemia—the dilemma of choice. *N Engl J Med* 1996; **335:** 426–8.


## β-Thalassaemia

β-Thalassaemia is a haemoglobinopathy (above) that is due to a deficiency in β globin production accompanied by normal production of α globin chains that, in the absence of sufficient partner chains, are insoluble and precipitate out in erythrocytes and erythroid precursors as large cellular inclusions. These interfere with red cell maturation resulting in ineffective haematopoiesis, retard the passage of red cells from the bone marrow, and create a tendency for those red cells that do mature to be trapped and destroyed in the spleen. The condition is therefore characterised by a hypochromic, microcytic anaemia accompanied by haemolysis. In the heterozygous form, where only one of the β globin genes is affected (known as thalassaemia trait or thalassaemia minor) the anaemia is mild and clinically insignificant. There is some evidence that patients with this form of the disease experience a degree of protection from malaria, which may account for the more frequent distribution of the trait in the populations of areas such as the Mediterranean, parts of Africa, and Asia.

The more severe forms of the disease (known as thalassaemia intermedia if haemoglobin levels are high enough not to require regular transfusion, or thalassaemia major in transfusion-dependent patients) occur in homozygous patients who inherit a defective β globin gene from both parents. Severe anaemia develops in the first year of life as fetal haemoglobin production (which does not involve a β globin) is replaced by the production of adult haemoglobin. The anaemia stimulates erythropoietin production, and if not corrected massive proliferation of red cell precursors develops within, and eventually beyond, the bone marrow, resulting in recurrent bone fractures, deformity of the skull due to expansion of the marrow spaces, and compression of vital structures such as the spinal cord with consequent paresis. Other symptoms include splenomegaly and hypersplenism (resulting in neutropenia and thrombocytopenia), increased susceptibility to infection, and hypermetabolism which may lead to folate deficiency because of the increased folate requirement. If untreated, death in patients with thalassaemia major usually occurs by the 2nd or 3rd year.

**Treatment**. The mainstay of treatment for severe β-thalassaemia has been regular blood transfusion to correct the anaemia. Transfusions should be started as early as possible in life once it is clear that anaemia is severe enough to warrant them. Transfusion of washed or frozen red cells every 6 to 8 weeks is usually required, to maintain haemoglobin values of between 9 and 14 g per 100 mL; a sudden increase in transfusion requirements is a sign of hypersplenism, which may be an indication for splenectomy although this should be avoided if possible below the age of 5 because of the increased risk of infection. For a discussion of antibacterial prophylaxis in splenectomised patients, see Spleen Disorders, p.146.

If anaemia is corrected by transfusion, growth and development proceed fairly normally in thalassaemic children. However, because the body lacks a mechanism for the excretion of excess iron, repeated transfusion invariably results in iron overload (p.1035), leading eventually to haemochromatosis. The consequences of haemochromatosis include liver dysfunction, endocrine dysfunction (failure of the adolescent growth spurt, hypogonadism, sometimes diabetes and hypothyroidism), and particularly heart disease (pericarditis, heart failure, and arrhythmias). If unchecked, the iron build-up usually leads to death (mainly through heart failure or arrhythmia) by the time patients reach their mid-20s. The accumulation of iron can be retarded by the chelator desferrioxamine and regular systemic use has been shown to improve survival in thalassaemic children,[1] and to protect against the cardiac complications of iron overload. The greatest increase in iron excretion may be seen in patients given the drug by continuous subcutaneous infusion rather than intramuscular bolus. There is some suggestion that intensive desferrioxamine therapy can improve impaired organ function,[1] but it is considered preferable to begin chelation therapy as early as possible (in practice usually not before 3 years of age) to try to prevent organ damage developing in the first place. Better iron excretion is achieved if patients are given ascorbic acid 100 to 200 mg daily in addition to desferrioxamine (but see under Interactions for Desferrioxamine, p.1034). Patients with thalassaemia may have increased folate requirements and folate supplementation may also be necessary. Although it is not yet certain how much chelation therapy will prolong survival the fact that a nearly normal iron balance can be achieved long term seems hopeful. Deferiprone has been used as an oral alternative to desferrioxamine,[2,3] but may not be effective in the longer term;[4] it may have a role in patients for whom desferrioxamine therapy is unsuitable.

In addition to the essentially symptomatic treatment of thalassaemia a very few patients may be candidates for bone marrow transplantation where suitable facilities and compatible donors exist; if transplantation is carried out before organ damage is marked, successfully transplanted patients are apparently cured and can lead a normal life.[5,6] Gene therapy is also under investigation.

An alternative approach using hydroxycarbamide in an attempt to stimulate fetal haemoglobin production and 'mop up' some of the excess α globin chains has been tried experimentally but results have been mixed. Results of an initial study in patients given butyric acid (as an arginine butyrate infusion) for the same purpose appeared more promising[7] although a subsequent study failed to show any benefit.[8]


1. Olivieri NF, Brittenham GM. Iron-chelating therapy and the treatment of thalassemia. *Blood* 1997; **89:** 739–61. Correction. *ibid.*; 2621.
2. Olivieri NF, *et al.* Iron-chelation therapy with oral deferiprone in patients with thalassemia major. *N Engl J Med* 1995; **332:** 918–22.
3. Nathan DG. An orally active iron chelator. *N Engl J Med* 1995; **332:** 953–4.
4. Olivieri NF, *et al.* Long-term safety and effectiveness of iron-chelation therapy with deferiprone for thalassemia major. *N Engl J Med* 1998; **339:** 417–23.
5. Lucarelli G, *et al.* Marrow transplantation in patients with thalassemia responsive to iron chelation therapy. *N Engl J Med* 1993; **329:** 840–4.
6. Lawson SE, *et al.* Bone marrow transplantation for β-thalassaemia major: the UK experience in two paediatric centres. *Br J Haematol* 2003; **120:** 289–95.
7. Perrine SP, *et al.* A short-term trial of butyrate to stimulate fetal-globin-gene expression in the β-globin disorders. *N Engl J Med* 1993; **328:** 81–6.
8. Sher GD, *et al.* Extended therapy with intravenous arginine butyrate in patients with β-hemoglobinopathies. *N Engl J Med* 1995; **332:** 1606–10.


## Haemostasis and Fibrinolysis

Haemostasis is the physiological response that occurs when blood vessels are damaged. It results in coagulation (formation of a blood clot) and thus arrests bleeding. The initial response is the formation of a plug of platelets which adhere both to the injured tissue and to each other. The vessel injury, with factors released by the platelets, trigger a series of reactions (the coagulation 'cascade') mediated by proteins circulating in the plasma (blood clotting factors). This results in formation of an insoluble fibrin clot that reinforces the initial platelet plug. Regulatory mechanisms come into operation to prevent widespread coagulation. Lysis of the clot (fibrinolysis) then occurs when wound healing and tissue repair are underway.

**Platelet aggregation**. Platelets usually circulate in plasma in an inactive form. Contact with damaged endothelium causes them to become activated and to adhere to the site of injury. This adhesion is partly mediated by binding of von Willebrand factor, a plasma protein that also acts as a carrier for factor VIII, to a glycoprotein (termed GPIb) on the platelet membrane surface. Substances are secreted by the activated platelets which cause further platelet aggregation (adenosine diphosphate and thromboxane $A_2$) and vasoconstriction (serotonin and thromboxane $A_2$). Thromboxane $A_2$ secreted by platelets is derived from arachidonic acid. The enzyme cyclo-oxygenase is required for the synthesis of thromboxane $A_2$ and this enzyme is inhibited by the **antiplatelet drugs** aspirin and sulfinpyrazone. Aspirin binds irreversibly to the enzyme and therefore the antiplatelet effect lasts for the lifetime of the platelet. Sulfinpyrazone is a reversible inhibitor of the enzyme. Platelet aggregation involves interaction of fibrinogen with a receptor, glycoprotein IIb/IIIa, on the platelet surface. Antiplatelet drugs such as abciximab act by blocking this receptor. In addition to their action in forming the initial haemostatic plug, platelets are also involved in coagulation by providing a surface on which interactions between clotting factors take place, resulting in more efficient coagulation.

**Coagulation**. The series of reactions that results in formation of a fibrin clot may be conveniently considered as two pathways, the *intrinsic* pathway (initiated within the blood) and the *extrinsic* pathway (initiated by substances extraneous to the blood). While this distinction is useful for understanding *in-vitro* coagulation and is the basis for tests that are specific for each pathway (see below), the mechanism of *in-vivo* coagulation is not so segregated and factors appearing in one pathway are also necessary for reactions in the other pathway. The intrinsic and extrinsic pathways of coagulation and the *in-vivo* pathways are discussed further below and are represented in summary form in Figure 1, p.737 and Figure 2, p.738 respectively. Factors circulate in the blood in an inactive form and are activated by cleavage of peptide bonds. The numerals attached to the factors reflect the order in which they were discovered and not their importance or position in the chain of reaction. The letter 'a' after a factor name or number denotes the activated form. Factors involved in blood coagulation are listed in Table 2, below. Once the coagulation cascade is initiated, activated factors act in positive feedback mechanisms to amplify the activation steps thus producing rapid coagulation. Cofactors are necessary as they increase the speed of the reactions. Other components necessary for coagulation are calcium ions and a membrane surface. Calcium ions are required for nearly all the reactions. Many of the activation steps, notably those involving factors VII, IX, and X, take place on a membrane surface provided by tissue factor or platelets. Factors bind to phospholipids on the membrane surface.

The *extrinsic* pathway is initiated when *tissue factor* (factor III) is released from damaged tissue. This forms a complex with *factor VII* and factor VIIa and directly activates *factor X*. The *intrinsic* pathway is initiated when blood comes into contact with a negatively charged surface. *Factor XII* interacts with high molecular weight kininogen (Fitzgerald factor) and prekallikrein (Fletcher factor) to produce *kallikrein* which activates factor XII. The active factor XIIa then activates *factor XI* which in turn activates *factor IX*. Factor IXa, with activated *factor VIII* (VIIIa) as a cofactor, converts *factor X* to factor Xa. The extrinsic and intrinsic pathways therefore converge with the activation of factor X. Factor Xa, with activated *factor V* (Va) as a cofactor, converts prothrombin to thrombin with the subsequent formation of a *fibrin* gel which is stabilised by *factor XIIIa* to form a stable clot.

The dependence on calcium ions of many steps in the coagulation cascade allows coagulation *in vitro* to be blocked by the addition of calcium chelators, such as sodium citrate, to collected blood. When collected blood is tested for coagulation function, addition of calcium ions allows clotting to proceed. Tests of coagulation function include activated partial thromboplastin time (APTT), which is a measure of the activity of the intrinsic system, prothrombin time (PT), a measure of the activity of the extrinsic system, and thrombin clotting time, which measures the conversion of fibrinogen to fibrin.

The factors involved in initiating the *in-vitro intrinsic* pathway, that is prekallikrein, factor XII, and possibly factor XI, are probably not important in *in-vivo* blood coagulation as deficiency of any of these factors is not associated with a serious bleeding disorder. The important step in initiating the clotting cascade *in vivo* is release of *tissue factor* (factor III) from damaged tissue. As has already been mentioned, tissue factor forms a complex with *factor VII* and factor VIIa that activates *factor X*. Factor Xa activates *prothrombin* resulting in formation of a *fibrin clot* which occurs as described above under the *in-vitro* systems. To enhance coagulation, various positive feedback mechanisms and other clotting factors operate to increase production of activated factors VII and X. For example, formation of factor VIIa is amplified by factor VIIa itself and by factor Xa. Formation of factor Xa is amplified by factor IXa produced by the action of thrombin on factor XI.

**Table 2.** Proteins involved in blood coagulation and in fibrinolysis.

| | Proteins | Synonyms |
|---|---|---|
| Blood coagulation | Factor I | Fibrinogen |
| | Factor II* | Prothrombin |
| | Factor III | Tissue thromboplastin; tissue factor |
| | Factor IV | Calcium ion |
| | Factor V | Ac-globulin; labile factor; proaccelerin |
| | Factor VI (unassigned) | |
| | Factor VII* | Proconvertin; SPCA; stable factor |
| | Factor VIII | Antihaemophilic factor; AHF |
| | Factor IX* | Christmas factor; plasma thromboplastin component; PTC |
| | Factor X* | Stuart factor; Stuart-Prower factor |
| | Factor XI | Plasma thromboplastin antecedent; PTA |
| | Factor XII | Hageman factor |
| | Factor XIII | Fibrin stabilising factor; FSF |
| | von Willebrand factor | Factor VIII-related antigen; vWF |
| | High molecular weight kininogen | HMWK; Fitzgerald factor |
| | Prekallikrein | Fletcher factor |
| Fibrinolysis | Plasminogen | |
| | Prourokinase | |
| | Tissue plasminogen activator | tPA |
| | Antithrombin III | Major antithrombin; AT-III; Heparin cofactor |
| | Protein C* | Autoprothrombin |
| | Protein S* | |
| | $\alpha_2$-Antiplasmin | |

* denotes vitamin K-dependent factor

**Regulation of coagulation.** The process of blood coagulation is regulated to ensure that it remains localised at the site of injury and does not result in more widespread clotting. This is achieved by dilution of clotting factors in flowing blood, by rapid hepatic clearance of many activated factors or products, and by natural anticoagulant mechanisms, which include antithrombin III, protein C, and protein S (see Figure 2). *Antithrombin III* inhibits the serine protease clotting factors, that is, thrombin, IXa, Xa, XIa, and XIIa. Antithrombin III is activated by binding to glycosaminoglycans, such as heparan glycosaminoglycan and dermatan sulfate, present in vascular endothelium. Heparin and low-molecular-weight heparins act as **anticoagulants** by binding antithrombin III at a specific binding site and enhancing its inhibitory effect on the serine protease clotting factors. At therapeutic doses of heparin the factors inhibited are thrombin and factor Xa. Low-dose heparin, such as that given for the prophylaxis of thromboembolism, inhibits factor Xa. Very high doses of heparin have a direct inhibitory effect on antithrombin III. Heparinoids which lack the specific binding site for antithrombin III do not have the anticoagulant properties of heparin. Low-molecular-weight heparins have a higher ratio of anti-factor-Xa to antithrombin activity than heparin and therefore mainly inhibit factor Xa.

*Proteins C and S* are both vitamin K-dependent plasma proteins. Protein C circulates in plasma in an inactive form. It is activated by contact with thrombin that is bound to thrombomodulin, a receptor located on the surface of endothelial cells. Activated protein C inhibits factors Va and VIIIa and therefore slows blood clotting. Protein S acts as a cofactor in this inhibition.

Vitamin K is essential for the activities of factors II, VII, IX, and X. It is also essential for the activity of proteins C and S. These factors contain glutamic acid residues that undergo carboxylation in the liver, a reaction requiring reduced vitamin K as a cofactor. This carboxylation step allows the factors to bind calcium, a reaction necessary for their function in the clotting cascade. Deficiency of vitamin K or the use of **oral anticoagulants** (which are vitamin K antagonists) therefore impairs the function of these clotting factors. Oral anticoagulants have no effect on circulating clotting factors and thus the time required before the anticoagulant effect is seen depends on the individual clearance rate of the factor.

**Fibrinolysis** is the mechanism of clot dissolution. It is mediated by *plasminogen*, which circulates in plasma in an inactive form; conversion to its active form, *plasmin*, occurs when plasminogen binds to fibrin in the presence of a *plasminogen activator* (see Figure 2). Plasmin, a *proteolytic enzyme*, digests fibrin clots and hydrolyses other proteins, including factors II, V, VIII, and XII. As fibrin is lysed, plasmin is released which is inhibited by $\alpha_2$-antiplasmin to prevent a systemic lytic state developing. There are two types of plasminogen activator, *tissue plasminogen activator* (tPA), which originates from the endothelium, and *urokinase*, which is activated from prourokinase. Activators of prourokinase include plasmin. Tissue plasminogen activator binds to fibrin and thus activates plasminogen bound to fibrin much more rapidly than circulating plasminogen; therefore the fibrinolytic action of tissue plasminogen activator is fibrin specific. Urokinase does not bind to fibrin, and therefore its fibrinolytic action is not fibrin specific, although it is activated by plasmin that is bound to fibrin. *In vivo*, fibrinolysis is almost entirely due to the activity of tissue plasminogen activator. The two types of plasminogen activator with their different modes of action provide the basis for the specificity of **thrombolytics** (the so-called 'clot specific' effect), which act by promoting the conversion of plasminogen to plasmin. The tissue plasminogen activators alteplase and duteplase are fibrin-specific thrombolytics, and streptokinase and urokinase are fibrin-nonspecific. The **antifibrinolytic drugs** aminocaproic acid and tranexamic acid act primarily by blocking the binding of plasminogen and plasmin to fibrin thereby preventing

**Figure 1.** Simplified representation of *in-vitro* coagulation.

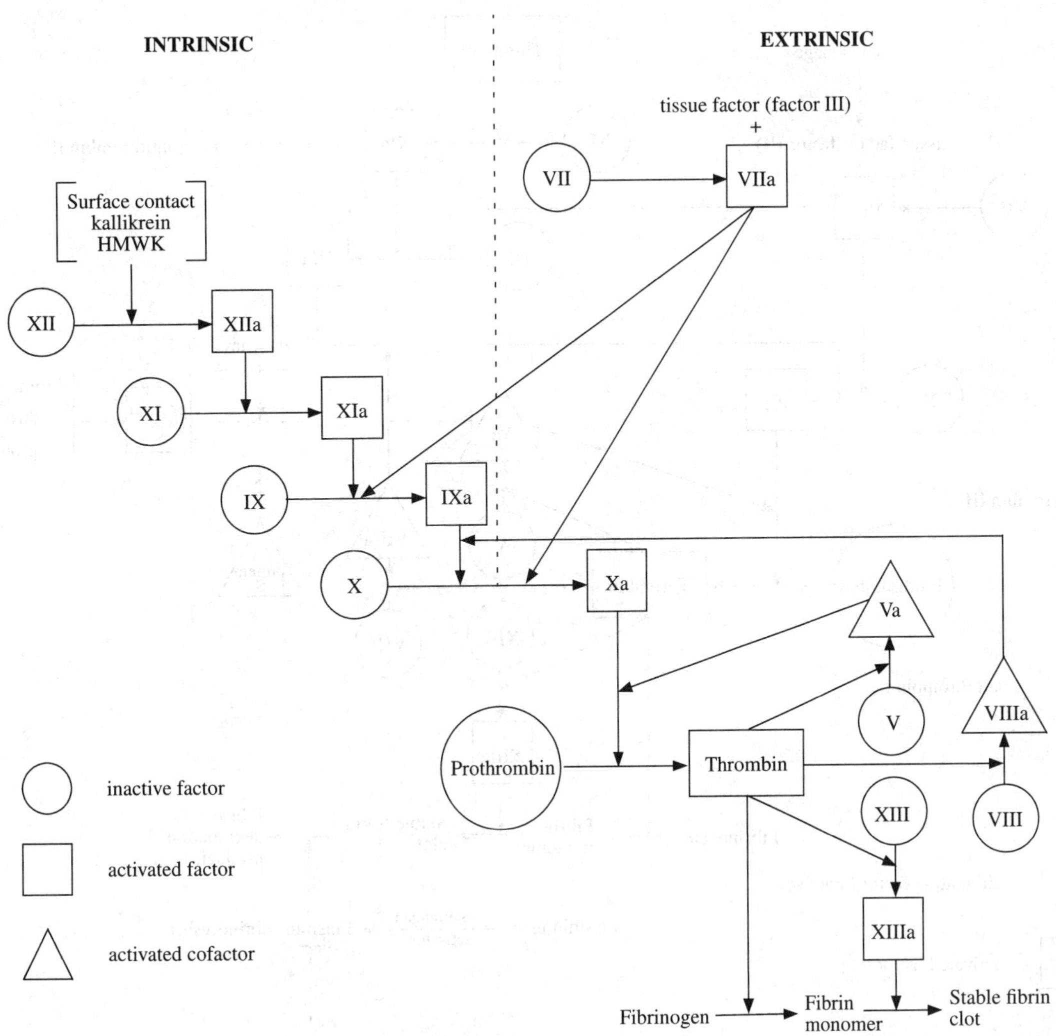


the breakdown of fibrin clots. Aprotinin, an inhibitor of proteolytic enzymes, acts as a **haemostatic** by inhibiting the action of plasmin and therefore preventing the breakdown of fibrin clots. Other drugs acting as haemostatics include batroxobin, which is reported to promote the production of fibrin from fibrinogen and etamsylate which has a stabilising effect on the capillary wall. Drugs such as oxidised cellulose, calcium alginate, collagen, and gelatin act by providing a physical meshwork within which clotting can occur. Adrenaline, adrenalone, and noradrenaline produce haemostasis by causing vasoconstriction. Drugs with astringent properties such as alum, ferric chloride, silver nitrate, and trichloroacetic acid are also used for haemostasis. The use of haemostatics may be considered when bleeding cannot be controlled by direct measures such as the application of pressure, suture or ligation, or electrocoagulation.

Dysfunction of the haemostatic mechanisms or the systems regulating haemostasis produces haemorrhagic (below) or thromboembolic (p.837) disorders.

◊ General references.

1. Furie B, Furie BC. Molecular and cellular biology of blood coagulation. *N Engl J Med* 1992; **326:** 800–806.
2. Dahlbäck B. Blood coagulation. *Lancet* 2000; **355:** 1627–32.

## Disseminated intravascular coagulation

Disseminated intravascular coagulation (DIC) is an acute or chronic syndrome resulting from an underlying condition that causes pathological stimulation of coagulation at some point in the coagulation pathway (above); thrombin generation triggered by uncontrolled tissue factor is probably the predominant factor in most cases. Causes include obstetric emergencies (placental abruption, eclampsia), infection (notably Gram-negative septicaemia), neoplasms, trauma (head injury, burns), venomous snake bites, transfusion of incompatible blood, liver disease, and various vascular causes.

Stimulation of coagulation leads to microvascular thrombosis that produces widespread tissue ischaemia and may lead to ischaemia of major organs. Simultaneously, secondary activation of the fibrinolytic system and consumption of coagulation factors produces bleeding, which is often the predominant manifestation. Symptoms are therefore very variable and include those of bleeding, such as spontaneous bruising, prolonged bleeding from intravenous puncture sites, and gastrointestinal and pulmonary haemorrhage, and those of thrombosis, such as acute renal failure, venous thromboembolism, skin necrosis, liver failure, cerebral infarction, acute respiratory distress, and coma. Some cases may be asymptomatic.

**Treatment** of DIC is aimed primarily at the underlying cause since the condition will not resolve until the underlying trigger is removed. Recovery is often fairly rapid once treatment is started. Supportive therapy to ensure adequate hydration and tissue oxygenation is also vital. These measures may be sufficient in patients with asymptomatic DIC. Most patients with symptomatic DIC also require plasma and other blood components including platelets and cryoprecipitate as necessary to replace coagulation factors and arrest bleeding. Heparin has been used in the management of DIC with the aim of switching off the coagulatory mechanisms. Although benefit has been shown with some underlying causes, heparin may worsen bleeding and its use in DIC is considered by some to be controversial. Where bleeding is the main clinical problem, heparin should only be given if replacement of coagulation factors fails to stop the bleeding. Where the risk of bleeding is relatively minor and thrombosis predominates, heparin may be appropriate. Other measures that have been tried in limited numbers of patients include use of a low-molecular-weight heparin, a thrombin inhibitor such as antithrombin III, and protein C.

General references.

1. Rubin RN, Colman RW. Disseminated intravascular coagulation: approach to treatment. *Drugs* 1992; **44:** 963–71.
2. Baglin T. Disseminated intravascular coagulation: diagnosis and treatment. *BMJ* 1996; **312:** 683–7.
3. Frewin R, *et al.* ABC of clinical haematology. Haematological emergencies. *BMJ* 1997; **314:** 1333–6.
4. de Jonge E, *et al.* Current drug treatment strategies for disseminated intravascular coagulation. *Drugs* 1998; **55:** 767–77.
5. Levi M, ten Cate H. Disseminated intravascular coagulation. *N Engl J Med* 1999; **341:** 586–92.
6. Toh CH, Dennis M. Disseminated intravascular coagulation: old disease, new hope. *BMJ* 2003; **327:** 974–7.

## Haemorrhagic disorders

Haemorrhage is bleeding from any part of the vascular system. The mechanisms responsible for haemostasis and its control, that is, platelet aggregation, blood coagulation, and fibrinolysis, are described under Haemostasis and Fibrinolysis, above. Dysfunction of any of these systems may produce a haemorrhagic disorder, as discussed below. The dysfunction may be an inherited disorder or it may be acquired as a result of disease or a medical or surgical procedure.

**Inherited haemorrhagic disorders.** Inherited disorders that lead to abnormal bleeding include platelet and vascular disorders, and disturbances in clotting factors.

Inherited *platelet disorders* are rare; they include

- Bernard-Soulier syndrome (a lack of platelet GPIb receptor)
- thrombasthenia (defective glycoproteins IIb and IIIa)
- storage pool disease (lack of platelet ADP)

Disorders of *vascular function* include

- hereditary telangiectasia

**Figure 2.** Simplified representation of *in-vivo* coagulation and fibrinolysis

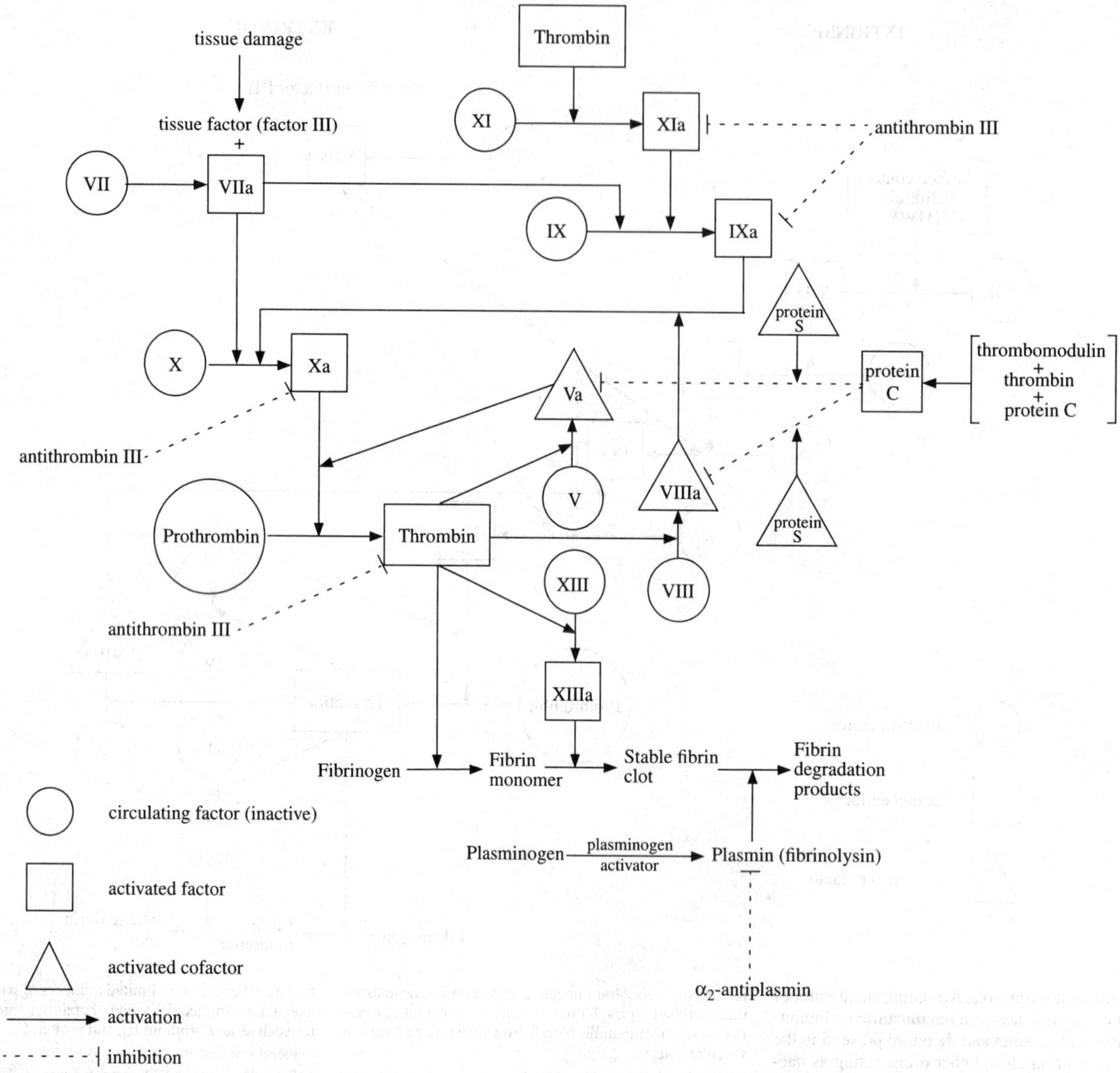

The most common inherited haemorrhagic disorders are due to absent, reduced, or malfunctioning *clotting factors*. The most important are

- **haemophilia A**
- **haemophilia B**
- **von Willebrand's disease**

Hereditary deficiency of all the clotting factors (other than calcium and thromboplastin) has been described although the incidence and clinical significance varies.

**Haemophilia A** (classical haemophilia, factor VIII deficiency) is the most common of the serious hereditary bleeding disorders. It is an X-linked recessive disorder and therefore with rare exceptions males are affected and females are carriers. The condition is due to deficiency of factor VIII; severity of bleeding is related to the residual factor level. The condition is severe when there is less than 1% of normal factor VIII activity, moderate when the factor VIII concentration is 1 to 5% of normal, and mild when the factor concentration is greater than 5%. Clots are slow to form and break up easily, and bleeding following trauma or surgery may continue for days or weeks. In moderate and severe haemophilia A bleeding may occur into major joints producing long-term joint destruction, a major cause of morbidity in haemophilia. Other frequent sites of bleeding are large muscles, and renal and intestinal tracts. CNS haemorrhage may also occur, especially after trauma.

Treatment of bleeding episodes depends on the severity of the haemophilia.[1-5] Patients with mild haemophilia may be satisfactorily treated with desmopressin, which produces an increase in factor VIII and von Willebrand factor. Desmopressin also stimulates release of plasminogen activator, and an antifibrinolytic, such as tranexamic acid, may be given at the same time to inhibit the enhanced fibrinolytic activity. Desmopressin is usually given intravenously; it can be given intranasally, but the factor VIII response is less predictable than with the injection.[6]

Desmopressin is ineffective in patients with more severe haemophilia A, and treatment of bleeding episodes in these patients requires replacement with a factor VIII preparation. The amount of factor given depends on the severity of bleeding.

In addition to use of factor VIII to treat bleeding episodes, it may also be given prophylactically in situations where haemorrhage may be anticipated, for example following trauma, and before surgery. Patients with haemophilia should also not be given intramuscular injections (because of potential muscle damage and bleeding into muscle) unless they are given during a period when the patient is covered by replacement factor. Dental extraction and other oral surgical procedures are examples of situations that may be followed by bleeding lasting days and weeks. Oral secretions, which can cause clot lysis, contribute to this bleeding. Patients undergoing dental or oral surgery should be given factor VIII and an antifibrinolytic, usually tranexamic acid, before the procedure. The antifibrinolytic should be continued for five days following the procedure. Fibrin glue[7] and topical aminocaproic acid[8] or tranexamic acid[9] are methods that have also been used.

An alternative method of management has been practised in Sweden since 1958 where continuous prophylaxis with factor VIII is given to patients with severe haemophilia with the aim of preventing arthropathy. Therapy is started at 1 to 2 years of age and the factor VIII concentration is maintained at a level of at least 1% of normal. Patients who began receiving prophylaxis before the age of 2 have had almost no bleeding episodes and joints have remained normal for up to 11 years of follow-up.[10,11] This approach has subsequently been adopted in a number of other countries.

There are various factor VIII preparations available that vary in activity and source.[12] Most products were previously derived from pooled donor plasma and were associated with transmission of viruses including HIV (leading to the subsequent development of AIDS), hepatitis B, and other hepatitis viruses. The introduction of products treated with heat or chemicals, and efforts to screen the donor material from which factor VIII is obtained, seem to have overcome problems with transmission of HIV and hepatitis B, although there is concern that non-lipid-enveloped viruses such as human parvovirus B19 and hepatitis A may still be transmitted. It is recommended that patients not already immune should be vaccinated against hepatitis A and B. Factor VIII produced by recombinant DNA technology may avoid the dangers of possible viral transmission (but see under Factor VIII, Transmission of Infections, p.751) and is therefore the factor VIII preparation of choice. There are some reports[13,14] that high-purity factor VIII preparations slow the decline in CD4 count in HIV-positive patients, although the evidence is conflicting.[15]

A complication of replacement therapy in haemophilia is the development of antibodies to factor VIII. Antibodies are more likely to develop in young patients with severe haemophilia, but on rare occasions can also arise in patients with mild haemophilia. An incidence of 10 to 15% is frequently cited, although prospective studies are lacking and it has been suggested that this is an underestimate.[16] A number of strategies have been developed to overcome the resulting immune tolerance to treatment.[1,2,4,17] Continued treatment with high-dose factor VIII may produce a clinical response and a decline in antibody formation in patients with a low antibody titre. Porcine factor VIII may be useful at least in the short term, although with longer use antibodies to the porcine material can develop in turn. When high titre, highly responding, antibodies are present, bleeding episodes are managed with the use of factor VIII inhibitor bypassing fraction or recombinant factor VIIa, which bypasses the factor VIII-dependent step in the coagulation cascade. Immune tolerance induction therapy may be used to try to eradicate these antibodies; various regimens have been used based on regular doses of factor VIII over prolonged periods, sometimes with immunosuppression by cyclophosphamide, immunomodulation by normal immunoglobulin, or extracorporeal immunoadsorption.

A future development that may provide a clinical cure for haemophilia is gene therapy.[18,19] Gene therapy for haemophilia A and B is being investigated and successful treatment has been carried out in an *animal* model with conversion to less severe haemophilia.

**Haemophilia B** (Christmas disease, factor IX deficiency) is less common than haemophilia A. The condition is due to deficiency of factor IX. The clinical features are identical to haemophilia A. Treatment follows the same principles as haemophilia A, bleeding episodes being treated with factor IX replacement.[1,4] Mild or moderate disease may be treated with fresh frozen plasma. Factor IX preparations derived from plasma, however, contain other clotting factors in addition to factor IX (such as the activated factors IX, X, and XII) and are therefore potentially associated with thromboembolic complications (mainly in patients with liver disease). Antifibrinolytic drugs, which may sometimes be used concurrently, increase the risk of thromboembolism further, and should be used with care. Highly purified factor IX preparations have been developed which do not contain other clotting factors and therefore may be expected to avoid this risk of thromboembolism. It has been suggested that these preparations should be used when very large amounts of replacement factor are required, or the risk of thrombotic complications is otherwise high.[1,3] Recently, a recombinant factor IX has been introduced.

Inhibitors to factor IX can be produced although the incidence is lower than the inhibition seen in haemophilia A. As in patients with haemophilia A, vaccination against hepatitis A and hepatitis B is recommended for all haemophiliacs not already immune.

As mentioned under haemophilia A, gene therapy is under investigation as a possible clinical cure.

**von Willebrand's disease** is due to deficiency of von Willebrand factor, a plasma protein that stimulates platelet aggregation and acts as a carrier for factor VIII, protecting it from premature destruction. Deficiency therefore slows clotting by reducing the platelet response to injury and reducing levels of factor VIII. There are many different types, and severity ranges from severe haemorrhagic disease to asymptomatic disease. Bleeding episodes in patients with mild to moderate forms of the disease may be managed with desmopressin, which increases levels of von Willebrand factor and factor VIII.[1,20-22] However, some forms of von Willebrand's disease do not respond to desmopressin therapy and in these patients, and in those with more severe disease, factor VIII concentrates are used; the very highly purified factor VIII preparations or recombinant forms should not be used as they do not contain appreciable amounts of von Willebrand factor and are thus ineffective. Cryoprecipitate (obtained from a very small donor pool to reduce the risk of transmission of infection) may also be used. Antifibrinolytic drugs may be used in open bleeding and in dental or oral surgery as for haemophilia A. A recombinant activated factor VII preparation has been developed that may also be used.

**OTHER INHERITED DISORDERS.** *Factor XI deficiency* is quite common in Jews of eastern European origin. Spontaneous bleeding is rare. Bleeding following trauma or surgery is generally mild and infusion of fresh frozen plasma is usually sufficient to maintain haemostasis. A factor XI concentrate is available.

*Inherited deficiencies of other clotting factors* are rare. Concentrates of factors II, VII, and X are available. Fresh frozen plasma or cryoprecipitate may be used in factor XIII deficiency.

**Acquired haemorrhagic disorders.** Bleeding disorders sometimes arise due to disturbances in either clotting factors or platelets or to vascular wall defects occurring as a result of a disease or a medical or surgical procedure. Disturbances and defects may also be drug induced. In some conditions, including renal and liver disease, cardiopulmonary bypass procedures, or following massive blood transfusion, disturbances in many of the homoeostatic mechanisms occur simultaneously producing complex haemorrhagic disorders, sometimes referred to as complex acquired coagulopathies.

One of the commoner causes of haemorrhagic disorder caused by **disturbance of clotting factors** is overdose with heparin, oral anticoagulants, or thrombolytics. Heparin overdose is rarely accompanied by serious haemorrhage. Stopping treatment is usually sufficient; protamine sulfate, which reverses the action of heparin, may be given. Bleeding in patients on oral anticoagulants is more difficult to control as the patient remains anticoagulated for several days after treatment is stopped. Local measures may be sufficient, although in life-threatening haemorrhage administration of phytomenadione (vitamin $K_1$), a concentrate of factors II, VII, IX, and X, or fresh frozen plasma may be necessary (see Treatment of Adverse Effects under Warfarin Sodium, p.1023). Overdose with a thrombolytic, such as streptokinase or urokinase, may be managed with an antifibrinolytic drug (for example aminocaproic acid or tranexamic acid), aprotinin, and packed red blood cells.

**Deficiencies in clotting factors** may occur in several diseases. Disorders producing a deficiency of vitamin K will lead to reduced levels of clotting factors (see also under Haemostasis and Fibrinolysis, above). Vitamin K deficiency due to impaired absorption, metabolism, or synthesis may occur in small bowel disease, biliary obstruction, or liver disease. Vitamin K deficiency in neonates produces vitamin K deficiency bleeding (p.1468). Vitamin K deficiency is treated by administration of vitamin K, although this is not always effective in patients with liver diseases. Rarely, deficiencies in clotting factors may be caused by the development of antibodies against a particular factor; factor VIII is the factor most frequently affected.

**Disturbances in platelet function** can give rise to a haemorrhagic disorder.[23] Sometimes the bleeding disorder is due to abnormally functioning platelets, such as occurs in renal failure or following the administration of some drugs (for example, aspirin and high doses of beta-lactam antibacterials). More often the bleeding disorder is due to a reduction is the number of platelets, that is, **thrombocytopenia.** Thrombocytopenia may occur in a wide range of disorders and can result from decreased production, increased destruction, or abnormal splenic sequestration of platelets. Decreased platelet production may occur in bone marrow diseases such as leukaemias and aplastic anaemia, chronic alcohol toxicity, and some viral illnesses. Decreased platelet production also occurs after bone marrow transplantation. Some drugs, for example thiazide diuretics and many antineoplastics, also reduce platelet production. Increased destruction of platelets occurs in many disorders including idiopathic thrombocytopenic purpura (p.1082), neonatal alloimmune thrombocytopenia, sepsis, disseminated intravascular coagulation (above), and thrombotic thrombocytopenic purpura and haemolytic-uraemic syndrome (see Thrombotic Microangiopathies, p.758). Many drugs also cause increased platelet destruction; they include aminosalicylic acid, cimetidine, digitalis, furosemide, heparin, methyldopa, paracetamol, and sulfonamides. Thrombocytopenia as a result of abnormal splenic sequestration may occur in hypersplenism from any cause. Thrombocytopenia also occurs in a few very rare congenital abnormalities such as Fanconi's anaemia and the Wiskott-Aldrich syndrome.

In thrombocytopenia, the severity of bleeding depends on the platelet count; clotting is impaired following surgery or trauma and spontaneous bleeding may occasionally occur when the platelet count is less than $50 \times 10^9$/litre. Treatment is management of the underlying disorder where appropriate or discontinuation of therapy with the offending drug. If surgery is contemplated or haemorrhage occurs and the platelet count is less than $50 \times 10^9$/litre or a platelet abnormality is manifested by a prolonged bleeding time, platelet transfusion may be given. Patients requiring long-term treatment may develop antibodies to HLA with repeated transfusions from random donors, which results in impaired responsiveness to subsequent transfusion; these patients should receive platelets obtained from a single donor for each transfusion. When thrombocytopenia is a result of increased platelet destruction, the condition is usually refractory to platelet transfusion. Oprelvekin (interleukin-11) has recently been introduced for the treatment of thrombocytopenia. Other haematopoietic growth factors under investigation include interleukin-3 and -6, and thrombopoietin.

**Complex acquired coagulopathies** can arise in many surgical settings, such as cardiopulmonary bypass procedures and liver transplantation, as well as with, or following, infection, massive blood transfusion, prolonged hypotension, and renal failure.

In renal failure the bleeding tendency is related to the degree and duration of uraemia. The bleeding defect is the result of platelet dysfunction and clotting factor deficiencies. There may also be mild thrombocytopenia. Correction of anaemia and dialysis seems to improve the bleeding disorder. If bleeding occurs, desmopressin and conjugated oestrogens may be used. Cryoprecipitate and platelet transfusions may be necessary in life-threatening haemorrhage.

In liver disease the haemorrhagic disorder is a result of impaired synthesis of clotting factors, thrombocytopenia, and impaired clearance of activated clotting factors. Desmopressin has been used to control bleeding episodes. Patients undergoing liver transplantation frequently develop a bleeding disorder as a result of the procedure itself as well as from the existing haemostatic defect. Small studies on the use of aprotinin in liver transplant patients have generally shown reductions in blood loss.

Various drugs including desmopressin, epoprostenol, tranexamic acid, aminocaproic acid, aprotinin, and nafamostat have been investigated for their effect on blood loss in patients undergoing surgery. Most of the investigations have been in surgery that involves cardiopulmonary bypass, a procedure that may be complicated by a postperfusion syndrome that includes impairment of haemostasis and pulmonary dysfunction. Aprotinin is the only agent that has shown a consistent effect in decreasing perioperative blood loss,[24] perhaps due to preservation of platelet function mediated by inhibition of plasmin. Desmopressin may be effective in those patients with excessive bleeding after cardiac surgery.[25]


1. Seremetis SV, Aledort LM. Congenital bleeding disorders: rational treatment options. *Drugs* 1993; **45:** 541–7.
2. Hoyer LW. Hemophilia A. *N Engl J Med* 1994; **330:** 38–47.
3. Berntorp E, *et al.* Modern treatment of haemophilia. *Bull WHO* 1995; **73:** 691–701.
4. Bolton-Maggs PH, Pasi KJ. Haemophilias A and B. *Lancet* 2003; **361:** 1801–9.
5. World Health Organization. *Delivery of treatment for haemophilia.* Geneva: WHO, 2002.
Available at: http://whqlibdoc.who.int/hq/2002/WHO_WFH_ISTH_WG_02.6.pdf (accessed 23/06/04)
6. Rose EH, Aledort LM. Nasal spray desmopressin (DDAVP) for mild hemophilia A and von Willebrand disease. *Ann Intern Med* 1991; **114:** 563–8.
7. Baudo F, *et al.* Management of oral bleeding in haemophilic patients. *Lancet* 1988; **ii:** 1082.
8. Casdorph DL. Topical aminocaproic acid in hemophiliac patients undergoing dental extraction. *DICP Ann Pharmacother* 1990; **24:** 160–1.
9. Sindet-Pedersen S, *et al.* Management of oral bleeding in haemophilic patients. *Lancet* 1988; **ii:** 566.
10. Nilsson IM, *et al.* Twenty-five years' experience of prophylactic treatment in severe haemophilia A and B. *J Intern Med* 1992; **232:** 25–32.
11. Aledort LM. Prophylaxis: the next haemophilia treatment. *J Intern Med* 1992; **232:** 1–2.
12. United Kingdom Haemophilia Centre Directors Organisation Executive Committee. Guidelines on therapeutic products to treat haemophilia and other hereditary coagulation disorders. *Haemophilia* 1997; **3:** 63–77.
13. Hilgartner MW, *et al.* Purity of factor VIII concentrates and serial CD4 counts. *Lancet* 1993; **341:** 1373–4.
14. Seremetis SV, *et al.* Three-year randomised study of high-purity or intermediate-purity factor VIII concentrates in symptom-free HIV-seropositive haemophiliacs: effects on immune status. *Lancet* 1993; **342:** 700–703.
15. Schwarz HP, *et al.* High-purity factor concentrates in prevention of AIDS. *Lancet* 1994; **343:** 478–9.
16. Ehrenforth S, *et al.* Incidence of development of factor VIII and factor IX inhibitors in haemophiliacs. *Lancet* 1992; **339:** 594–8.
17. Ho AYL, *et al.* Immune tolerance therapy for haemophilia. *Drugs* 2000; **60:** 547–54.
18. Lozier JN, Brinkhous KM. Gene therapy and the hemophilias. *JAMA* 1994; **271:** 47–51.
19. Brownlee GG. Prospects for gene therapy of haemophilia A and B. *Br Med Bull* 1995; **51:** 91–105.
20. Scott JP, Montgomery RR. Therapy of von Willebrand disease. *Semin Thromb Hemost* 1993; **19:** 37–47.
21. Castaman G, Rodeghiero F. Current management of von Willebrand's disease. *Drugs* 1995; **50:** 602–14.
22. Mannucci PM. How I treat patients with von Willebrand disease. *Blood* 2001; **97:** 1915–19.
23. Liesner RJ, Machin SJ. ABC of clinical haematology: platelet disorders. *BMJ* 1997; **314:** 809–12.
24. Royston D. Perioperative bleeding. *Lancet* 1993; **341:** 1629.
25. Cattaneo M, Mannucci PM. Desmopressin and blood loss after cardiac surgery. *Lancet* 1993; **342:** 812.

### Neonatal intraventricular haemorrhage

Intraventricular haemorrhage, also referred to as periventricular or periventricular-intraventricular haemorrhage, is bleeding from vessels in or around the ventricles of the brain. It is the major cause of death in very low birth-weight neonates and affects up to 60% of neonates weighing less than 1500 g. Intraventricular haemorrhage is rare in neonates over 32 weeks' gestation, since the vessels which bleed involute early in the third trimester. Intraventricular haemorrhage usually develops within the first 3 days of life. The haemorrhage may be graded from 1 to 4 according to severity, the higher numbered grades being the most severe and most likely to produce the long-term consequences of impaired motor and mental function. The aetiology is probably multifactorial and may include fluctuations in cerebral blood flow due to failure of autoregulatory mechanisms and tissue damage caused by oxygen free-radicals.

Once intraventricular haemorrhage has occurred **treatment** is supportive and includes correction of anaemia, hypotension, and acidaemia, and management of raised intracranial pressure. As intraventricular haemorrhage is a major risk factor for impaired motor and mental development **prevention** is very important. Numerous interventions aim to reduce its incidence and include prevention of premature births, avoidance of hypercapnia, correction of major haemodynamic disturbances, and correction of coagulation abnormalities. Various drugs have also been tried including corticosteroids, etamsylate, indometacin, pancuronium, phenobarbital, vitamin E, and vitamin K. Some of these drugs have been administered to the mother antenatally since the development of intraventricular haemorrhage may be related to perinatal events.

Administration of corticosteroids to pregnant women at risk of preterm delivery is recommended to prevent neonatal respiratory distress syndrome (p.1084) and may also reduce the incidence of intraventricular haemorrhage.[1] A review of data from 12 controlled studies involving antenatal corticosteroid administration (primarily to prevent respiratory distress syndrome)[2] suggested that the risk of intraventricular haemorrhage was also reduced but this was based on limited data. Further studies[3,4] have supported this finding, although none has involved randomised administration of corticosteroids. The mechanism for the beneficial effect of corticosteroids is not clear but avoidance of neonatal hypotension has been suggested.[3]

Etamsylate limits capillary bleeding through its action on hyaluronic acid and initial studies showed a reduction in intraventricular haemorrhage. A subsequent study[5] showed little evidence of benefit on short-term follow-up, although confidence intervals were wide. Follow-up[6] of these infants at 2 years of age found that etamsylate had not reduced the risk of death, impairment, or disability.

Indometacin may reduce cerebral blood flow as a result of vasoconstriction, reduce oxygen free-radical damage, and accelerate maturation of blood vessels around the ventricles. Early studies produced conflicting results but a later larger multicentre study[7] showed a reduction in both incidence and severity although there was an unusually large number of neonates with severe intraventricular haemorrhage in the control group.[8] A concern with the use of indometacin is the possibility that it may produce cerebral ischaemia due to its vasoconstrictor action and therefore increase the risk of developmental handicaps.[8] A review[9] of studies of prophylactic indometacin concluded that more studies of possible adverse effects and long-term outcome are needed before indometacin can be recommended for routine use. However, follow-up of the infants included in the multicentre study at the ages of 3 years,[10] 4.5 years,[11] and 8 years,[12] reported no adverse effects on cognitive or motor development.

Pancuronium abolishes non-synchronous respiration and therefore stabilises both cerebral and arterial blood flow velocity and some studies have shown a reduction in intraventricular haemorrhage in mechanically ventilated neonates (see Intensive Care, p.1398). However, other studies have produced conflicting results and routine use in all ventilated neonates is not recommended.

Phenobarbital was also suggested to act by stabilising fluctuations in cerebral blood flow, and studies of use in neonates show similarly inconsistent results with many showing no benefit. A meta-analysis[13] concluded that postnatal phenobarbital could not be recommended as prophylaxis, and was associated with an increased need for mechanical ventilation. Initial studies of antenatal phenobarbital were more promising with a decrease in severity of haemorrhage being reported.[14] However, a larger randomised study[15] in 610 women failed to show any effect of antenatal phenobarbital on incidence or severity of intraventricular haemorrhage. A concern with the use of phenobarbital in the perinatal period is that it may lower Apgar scores and produce respiratory depression. A meta-analysis[16] also did not support the maternal use of phenobarbital.

Vitamin E protects polyunsaturated fatty acids and thus membranes from oxidation. As oxygen free-radical damage may contribute to the development of intraventricular haemorrhage, vitamin E may have a role in its prevention. Results have been conflicting. Some studies have shown a reduction in incidence of intraventricular haemorrhage and a review of studies suggested vitamin E may be useful in the smallest, most susceptible neonates.[17] However, larger studies and studies to assess long-term outcome are needed.

The activity of vitamin K-dependent coagulation factors is reduced in neonates and thus antenatal administration of vitamin K to mothers has been tried as a means of preventing intraventricular haemorrhage. However, results of studies have not been promising. Most trials have been too small to produce conclusive results and a larger randomised controlled study[18] in 139 mothers failed to find any benefit from vitamin K prophylaxis.

Plasma volume expansion using fresh frozen plasma or a plasma substitute has also been thought to reduce intraventricular haemorrhage by stabilising the circulation, but a prospective multicentre study found no evidence of reduction in haemorrhage[19] or subsequent death and disability[20] after the use of plasma or gelatin as volume expanders.


1. NIH Consensus Development Panel. Effect of corticosteroids for fetal maturation on perinatal outcomes. *JAMA* 1995; **273:** 413–18.
2. Crowley P, *et al.* The effect of corticosteroid administration before preterm delivery: an overview of the evidence from controlled trials. *Br J Obstet Gynaecol* 1990; **97:** 11–25.
3. Garland JS, *et al.* Effect of maternal glucocorticoid exposure on risk of severe intraventricular hemorrhage in surfactant-treated preterm infants. *J Pediatr* 1995; **126:** 272–9.
4. Ment LR, *et al.* Antenatal steroids, delivery mode, and intraventricular hemorrhage in preterm infants. *Am J Obstet Gynecol* 1995; **172:** 795–800.
5. The EC Ethamsylate Trial Group. The EC randomised controlled trial of prophylactic ethamsylate for very preterm neonates: early mortality and morbidity. *Arch Dis Child* 1994; **70:** F201–F205.
6. Elbourne D, *et al.* Randomised controlled trial of prophylactic etamsylate: follow up at 2 years of age. *Arch Dis Child Fetal Neonatal Ed* 2001; **84:** F183–F187.
7. Ment LR, *et al.* Low-dose indomethacin and prevention of intraventricular haemorrhage: a multicenter randomized trial. *Pediatrics* 1994; **93:** 543–50.
8. Volpe JJ. Brain injury caused by intraventricular hemorrhage: is indomethacin the silver bullet for prevention? *Pediatrics* 1994; **93:** 673–6.
9. Fowlie PW. Prophylactic indomethacin: systematic review and meta-analysis. *Arch Dis Child* 1996; **74:** F81–F87.
10. Ment LR, *et al.* Neurodevelopment outcome at 36 months' corrected age of preterm infants in the multicenter indomethacin intraventricular hemorrhage prevention trial. *Pediatrics* 1996; **98:** 714–18.
11. Ment LR, *et al.* Outcome of children in the indomethacin intraventricular hemorrhage prevention trial. *Pediatrics* 2000; **105:** 485–91.
12. Vohr BR, *et al.* School-age outcomes of very low birth weight infants in the indomethacin intraventricular hemorrhage prevention trial. Abstract: *Pediatrics* 2003; **111:** 874. Full version: http://pediatrics.aappublications.org/cgi/content/full/111/4/e340 (accessed 23/06/04)
13. Whitelaw A. Postnatal phenobarbitone for the prevention of intraventricular hemorrhage in preterm infants. Available in The Cochrane Library; Issue 2. Chichester: John Wiley; 2004.
14. Barnes ER, Thompson DF. Antenatal phenobarbital to prevent or minimize intraventricular hemorrhage in the low-birthweight neonate. *Ann Pharmacother* 1993; **27:** 49–52.
15. Shankaran S, *et al.* The effect of antenatal phenobarbital therapy on neonatal intracranial hemorrhage in preterm infants. *N Engl J Med* 1997; **337:** 466–71.
16. Crowther CA, Henderson-Smart DJ. Phenobarbital prior to preterm birth for preventing neonatal periventricular haemorrhage. Available in The Cochrane Library; Issue 2. Chichester: John Wiley; 2004.
17. Poland RL. Vitamin E for prevention of perinatal intracranial hemorrhage. *Pediatrics* 1990; **85:** 865–7.
18. Thorp JA, *et al.* Antepartum vitamin K and phenobarbital for preventing intraventricular hemorrhage in the premature newborn: a randomized, double-blind, placebo-controlled trial. *Obstet Gynecol* 1994; **83:** 70–6.
19. The Northern Neonatal Nursing Initiative Trial Group. A randomized trial comparing the effect of prophylactic intravenous fresh frozen plasma, gelatin or glucose on early mortality and morbidity in preterm babies. *Eur J Pediatr* 1996; **155:** 580–8.
20. Northern Neonatal Nursing Initiative Trial Group. Randomized trial of prophylactic early fresh-frozen plasma or gelatin or glucose in preterm babies: outcome at 2 years. *Lancet* 1996; **348:** 229–32.


### Neutropenia

A circulating neutrophil count below $1.5 \times 10^9$/litre is usually regarded as abnormal and neutrophil counts below $0.5 \times 10^9$/litre are associated with increased risk of infections. Neutropenia may be a result of reduced production, increased peripheral destruction, or increased peripheral pooling of neutrophils, and can be inherited or acquired.

**Inherited** forms of neutropenia are rare and include congenital agranulocytosis (Kostmann's syndrome: severe persistent neutropenia with frequent and severe infections that start in infancy) and cyclic neutropenia (fluctuating periods of neutropenia accompanied by fever, mouth ulceration, and serious infection).

Granulocyte colony-stimulating factors have been shown to reduce the incidence of severe infections and have improved substantially the quality of life of patients with congenital neutropenias although there are some concerns over their safety. Before the development of colony-stimulating factors various treatments including plasma, glucocorticoids, androgens, and lithium were tried in patients with severe congenital neutropenias with the aim of stimulating neutrophil production. However, none was particularly effective.

There are many causes of **acquired** neutropenia. Drugs are a common cause, either by direct toxicity to the bone marrow, or by immune-mediated marrow suppression or peripheral destruction. Drugs that cause dose-related direct toxicity include cytotoxic and immunosuppressive drugs, flucytosine, ganciclovir, and zidovudine. Drugs that appear to cause neutropenia by immune-mediated mechanisms include sulfur-containing drugs (such as captopril, co-trimoxazole, and some antithyroid drugs), clozapine, penicillins, and cephalosporins. Patients with drug-induced neutropenia usually present with fever of sudden onset, sore throat, mouth ulcers, headache, and malaise. This condition is also known as **agranulocytosis**. Other causes of acquired neutropenia include serious bacterial and viral infections, radiotherapy, neoplasms that invade bone marrow, and some auto-immune disorders.

The management of acquired neutropenia includes the treatment of any contributory condition. Drug-induced neutropenia is usually managed by withdrawal of the offending drug. In idiosyncratic reactions readministration of the implicated drug should be avoided, since abrupt neutropenia will usually be precipitated. Colony-stimulating factors can be used to manage drug-induced neutropenia.

In all neutropenic patients onset of fever is indicative of serious infection and is treated immediately with empirical antibacterial therapy as described on p.131.

◊ General references.


1. Anonymous. Drug-induced agranulocytosis. *Drug Ther Bull* 1997; **35:** 49–52.
2. Provan D, O'Connell S. Management of the neutropenic patient. *Prescribers' J* 1999; **39:** 144–53.


## Albumin

Albúmina.

*ATC — B05AA01.*

**Pharmacopoeias.** Many pharmacopoeias have monographs including *Eur.* (see p.vi) and *US.*

**Ph. Eur. 5.0** (Human Albumin Solution; Albumini Humani Solutio). An aqueous solution of protein obtained from the plasma of healthy donors; the plasma is tested for the absence of hepatitis B surface antigen and antibodies against HIV-1 and HIV-2 and hepatitis C virus. It is prepared as a concentrated solution containing 15 to 25% of total protein or as an isotonic solution containing 3.5 to 5% of total protein; not less than 95% of the total protein is albumin. A suitable stabiliser, such as sodium octanoate or *N*-acetyltryptophan or a combination of the two, may be added but no antimicrobial preservative is added. It contains not more than 160 mmol of sodium per litre and not more than 200 micrograms of aluminium per litre. The solution is sterilised by filtration and distributed aseptically into containers which are sealed to prevent contamination and maintained at 59° to 61° for not less than 10 hours. Finally, the containers are incubated for not less than 14 days at 30° to 32° or for not less than 4 weeks at 20° to 25° and examined visually for signs of microbial contamination. It should be stored in a colourless glass container and protected from light.

A clear, almost colourless, yellow, amber, or green slightly viscous liquid. A solution in sodium chloride 0.9% containing 1% protein has a pH of 6.7 to 7.3.

The BP 2003 gives Albumin and Human Albumin as approved synonyms.

**USP 27** (Albumin Human). A sterile, nonpyrogenic, preparation of serum albumin obtained by fractionating material (blood, plasma, serum, or placentas) from healthy human donors, the source material being tested for the absence of hepatitis B surface antigen. It is made by a process that yields a product that is safe for intravenous use. It contains 4, 5, 20, or 25% of serum albumin and not less than 96% of the total protein is albumin. It may contain sodium acetyltryptophanate with or without sodium caprylate as a stabilising agent; it contains no added antimicrobial agent. It contains 130 to 160 mmol of sodium per litre. It is a practically odourless, moderately viscous, clear, brownish fluid. It should be stored in airtight containers.

## Adverse Effects and Precautions

Adverse reactions to albumin infusion occur rarely and include nausea and vomiting, increased salivation, and febrile reactions. Allergic reactions, including severe anaphylactic shock, are possible. Rapid increases in circulatory volume can cause vascular overload, haemodilution, and pulmonary oedema. Solutions containing albumin 20 or 25% are hyperosmotic and draw fluid from the extravascular compartment. Heating to about 60° in the presence of a stabiliser during preparation has reduced the risk of transmitting some viral infections.

Infusion of albumin solutions is contra-indicated in patients with severe anaemia or heart failure. They should be given with caution to patients with hypertension or low cardiac reserve. Dehydrated patients may require additional fluids. Injured or postoperative patients should be observed carefully following the administration of albumin as the rise in blood pressure may result in bleeding from previously undetected sites.

◊ Volume expansion with albumin (a colloid) has been widely used in critically ill patients, although its use has never been formally tested in large controlled studies. A systematic review based on available studies up to March 1998 (relatively small, old trials that recorded only a small number of deaths) suggested that albumin was of no benefit in critically ill patients with hypovolaemia, burns, or hypoalbuminaemia, and that it might be linked to increased mortality.[1] The authors of the review stressed that these results should be treated with caution but nevertheless called for an urgent reconsideration of the use of albumin in critically ill patients. The review was severely criticised[2] and while it was recognised that albumin has probably been overused in the past it was considered that more studies were required to define the effect of albumin on mortality.[3-5] An update[6] to the review, including some more recent studies, came to the same conclusions as the original review. Another review,[7] however, found that the use of albumin did not significantly affect mortality; this meta-analysis had broader criteria and included studies that were considered to be relevant but that had been excluded by the other review.

Pharmacovigilance data reported to albumin suppliers over 3 years (1998 to 2000) has also been analysed.[8] During this period of heightened awareness about possible adverse effects of albumin, due to the publication of the 1998 review, a total of $1.62 \times 10^7$ doses of 40 g had been distributed. Serious adverse effects possibly or probably related to albumin were found to be rare, and no death was classified as probably related to albumin use. Nevertheless, further well-designed trials are still considered to be needed, and a large study comparing albumin with sodium chloride 0.9% in approximately 7000 critically ill patients is underway.

On a broader level, debate continues about the relative merits and risks of such colloid solutions, compared with those of crystalloids such as glucose or sodium chloride solutions, in the management of hypovolaemia and shock (p.835).


1. Cochrane Injuries Group Albumin Reviewers. Human albumin administration in critically ill patients: systematic review of randomised controlled trials. *BMJ* 1998; **317:** 235–40.
2. Various. Human albumin administration in critically ill patients. *BMJ* 1998; **317:** 882–6. [Letters.]
3. Tomlin M. Albumin usage in the critically ill. *Pharm J* 1998; **261:** 193.
4. McClelland B. Albumin: don't confuse us with the facts. *BMJ* 1998; **317:** 829–30.
5. Committee on Safety of Medicines/Medicines Control Agency. The safety of human albumin. *Current Problems* 1999; **25:** 11. Available at: http://www.mca.gov.uk/ourwork/monitorsafequalmed/currentproblems/volume25jun.htm (accessed 23/06/04)
6. The Albumin Reviewers. Human albumin solution for resuscitation and volume expansion in critically ill patients. Available in The Cochrane Library; Issue 2. Chichester: John Wiley; 2004.
7. Wilkes MM, Navickis RJ. Patient survival after human albumin administration: a meta-analysis of randomized, controlled trials. *Ann Intern Med* 2001; **135:** 149–64.
8. Vincent J-L, *et al.* Safety of human albumin—serious adverse events reported worldwide in 1998–2000. *Br J Anaesth* 2003; **91:** 625–30.


**Aluminium toxicity.** Albumin solutions may contain appreciable amounts of aluminium. Marked increases in plasma-aluminium concentrations have been demonstrated in patients receiving large volumes by infusion and accumulation of aluminium may occur in patients with renal impairment.[1-3] In the UK albumin solutions with an aluminium content of less than 200 micrograms/litre are available for use in patients undergoing dialysis and premature infants.


1. Milliner DS, *et al.* Inadvertent aluminum administration during plasma exchange due to aluminum contamination of albumin-replacement solutions. *N Engl J Med* 1985; **312:** 165–7.
2. Maher ER, *et al.* Accumulation of aluminium in chronic renal failure due to administration of albumin replacement solutions. *BMJ* 1986; **292:** 306.
3. Maharaj D, *et al.* Aluminium bone disease in patients receiving plasma exchange with contaminated albumin. *BMJ* 1987; **295:** 693–6.


**Dilution.** If concentrated albumin solutions are to be diluted before administration, a suitable solution such as sodium chloride 0.9% or glucose 5% must be used. Albumin 25% that was erroneously diluted with water to produce a hypo-osmolar albumin 5% solution has produced severe haemolysis and renal failure in patients undergoing plasmapheresis,[1,2] including a fatality in one patient.[3]


1. Steinmuller DR. A dangerous error in the dilution of 25 percent albumin. *N Engl J Med* 1998; **338:** 1226.
2. Pierce LR, *et al.* Hemolysis and renal failure associated with use of sterile water for injection to dilute 25% human albumin solution. *Am J Health-Syst Pharm* 1998; **55:** 1057,1062, 1070.
3. Anonymous. Hemolysis associated with 25% human albumin diluted with sterile water—United States, 1994–1998. *MMWR* 1999; **48:** 157–9.


**Transmission of infections.** There has been concern that albumin preparations may carry a potential risk of transmission of viral and subviral particles, notably Creutzfeldt-Jakob disease. In 1993, *Pasteur-Mérieux* (one of the largest producers of blood products) withdrew all products containing albumin derived from placental blood[1] due to uncertainty regarding the adequacy of screening procedures for placentas as a source. It was considered that the agent responsible for Creutzfeldt-Jakob disease might be contained in placentas from women who have been treated with growth hormone derived from cadaver pituitaries. More recently, the production of blood products (including albumin) using plasma from UK donors has been phased out due to the possible risk of transmission of Creutzfeldt-Jakob disease.


1. Anonymous. Placental-derived albumin preparations withdrawn. *WHO Drug Inf* 1994; **8:** 29–30.


## Uses and Administration

Albumin is the major protein involved in maintaining colloid osmotic pressure in the blood. It also binds a number of endogenous and exogenous substances including bilirubin, steroid hormones, and many, mainly acidic, drugs.

Albumin solutions are used for plasma volume replacement and to restore colloid osmotic pressure. They have been used in conditions such as burns, severe acute albumin loss, and acute hypovolaemic shock (p.835). They are also used as an exchange fluid in therapeutic plasmapheresis. Concentrated albumin solutions are used in neonatal hyperbilirubinaemia associated with haemolytic disease of the newborn (p.1608). They have also been suggested for short-term management of hypoproteinaemia in hepatic disease and in diuretic-resistant patients with nephrotic syndrome but are of little value in chronic hypoproteinaemias. Albumin preparations labelled with technetium-99m are used as radiopharmaceuticals in scanning of the heart, lung, liver, spleen, bone marrow (p.1525) and gas-filled albumin microspheres are available for enhancing cardiac ultrasound imaging.

Albumin solutions are usually available as 4.5% or 5% solutions, which are iso-osmotic with plasma, and as 20% or 25% solutions which, being hyperosmotic with respect to plasma, cause a movement of fluid from the extravascular to the intravascular compartment. These concentrated solutions may be used undiluted or may be diluted with a suitable solution, commonly sodium chloride 0.9% or glucose 5%. Adequate hydration should be maintained in patients receiving hyperosmotic solutions of albumin.

The amount of albumin solution administered will depend upon the clinical condition of the patient and the response to treatment. The following doses have been suggested: in acute hypovolaemic shock an initial dose of 25 g of albumin for adults (for example, 500 mL of a 5% solution or 100 mL of a 25% solution) and up to about 1 g/kg for children; in hypoproteinaemia a maximum daily dose of 2 g/kg; and in neonatal hyperbilirubinaemia a dose of 1 g/kg before exchange transfusion.

A suggested rate of infusion is 1 to 2 mL/minute (5% solution) or 1 mL/minute (25% solution) although high rates may be needed in the treatment of shock.

Albumin solutions should not be used for parenteral nutrition.

◊ References.


1. Erstad BL, *et al.* The use of albumin in clinical practice. *Arch Intern Med* 1991; **151:** 901–11.
2. Tomlin M. Albumin usage on intensive care. *Pharm J* 1997; **259:** 856–9. Comment including corrections—Dash C, *et al. ibid.* 1998; **260:** 88–9.
3. McClelland DBL. Human albumin solutions. In Contreras M, ed. *ABC of transfusion*. 3rd ed. London: BMJ Books, 1998: 45–8.


## Preparations

**Ph. Eur.:** Human Albumin Solution;
**USP 27:** Albumin Human.

**Proprietary Preparations** (details are given in Part 3)
***Austral.:*** Albumex; ***Belg.:*** Albuman†; ***Braz.:*** Albumax; Albuminar; Albunex†; Beribumin; Blaubimax; Blaubumin; Blauinfuion†; Green-A KGCC†; OPV†; Pilmolite†; Pulmolite†; Zenalb; ***Canad.:*** Plasbumin; ***Chile:*** Plasbumin; ***Ger.:*** Humanalbin; ***Hong Kong:*** Albuminar; Albutein; Biseko; Buminate; Plasbumin; Zenalb†; ***Irl.:*** Albuminar†; ***Israel:*** Albuminar; Plasbumin; ***Ital.:*** Albital; Albuman; Albutein; Endalbumin†; Haimalbumin†; Seralbuman†; ***Malaysia:*** Albutein; Buminate; Plasbumin; Zenalb; ***Mex.:*** Albital; Albumar; Albumyn; Biomina†; Probi-Albumin; Seralbumin; Vanderbumin†; ***Norw.:*** Infosan†; ***NZ:*** Albumex; ***S.Afr.:*** Albusol; ***Singapore:*** Albutein; Buminate†; Plasbumin; Zenalb; ***Spain:*** Plasbumin; ***Switz.:*** Albuman; ***Thai.:*** Albuman†; Albutein; Buminate; Zenalb; ***UK:*** Alba; Albutein; Zenalb; ***USA:*** Albumarc; Albuminar; Albutein; Buminate; Plasbumin.

**Multi-ingredient:** ***Denm.:*** Tisseel Duo Quick; ***Swed.:*** Tisseel Duo Quick.

## Aminaphthone

Aminaftona; Aminaftone; Aminaphtone; Aminonaphthone. 2-Hydroxy-3-methylnaphtho-1,4-hydroquinone 2-(4-aminobenzoate); 3-Methylnaphthalene-1,2,4-triol 2-(4-aminobenzoate).

$C_{18}H_{15}NO_4$ = 309.3.
*CAS — 14748-94-8.*

### Profile

Aminaphthone is a haemostatic. Daily doses of 150 to 225 mg by mouth have been used.

### Preparations

**Proprietary Preparations** (details are given in Part 3)
***Braz.:*** Capilarema; ***Ital.:*** Capillarema; ***Port.:*** Capilarema; ***Spain:*** Capilarema.

## Aminocaproic Acid *(BAN, USAN, rINN)*

Ácido aminocaproico; Acidum Aminocaproicum; CL-10304; CY-116; EACA; Epsilon Aminocaproic Acid; JD-177; NSC-26154. 6-Aminohexanoic acid.

$C_6H_{13}NO_2$ = 131.2.
*CAS — 60-32-2.*
*ATC — B02AA01.*

**Pharmacopoeias.** In *Eur.* (see p.vi), *Pol.*, and *US.*

**Ph. Eur. 5.0** (Aminocaproic Acid). A white, crystalline powder or colourless crystals. Freely soluble in water; slightly soluble in alcohol. A 20% solution in water has a pH of 7.5 to 8.0.

**USP 27** (Aminocaproic Acid). A fine, white, odourless or practically odourless, crystalline powder. Soluble 1 in 3 of water and 1 in 450 of methyl alcohol; slightly soluble in alcohol; practically insoluble in chloroform and in ether; freely soluble in acids and in alkalis. Its solutions are neutral to litmus. Store in airtight containers.

### Adverse Effects

Adverse effects associated with aminocaproic acid include dose-related gastrointestinal disturbances, dizziness, tinnitus, headache, nasal and conjunctival congestion, and skin rashes. Aminocaproic acid may cause muscle damage. This has usually occurred with high doses given for prolonged periods; renal failure may develop. Thrombotic complications have been reported, although they are usually a consequence of inappropriate use. If aminocaproic acid is given by rapid intravenous administration it can produce hypotension, bradycardia, and arrhythmias. There have been reports of a few patients suffering from convulsions, dry ejaculation, or cardiac and hepatic damage.

**Effects on the blood.** Very high doses of aminocaproic acid (36 g or more daily) have been given intravenously in the management of subarachnoid haemorrhage. One study[1] reported rebleeding and excessive intra-operative bleeding and suggested that this was due to an antiplatelet effect of the aminocaproic acid. However, a comment on this report[2] pointed out that any antiplatelet effect was independent of its antifibrinolytic action and that this effect could only aggravate rebleeding, if it occurs, rather than initiating it.


1. Glick R, *et al.* High dose ε-aminocaproic acid prolongs the bleeding time and increases rebleeding and intraoperative hemorrhage in patients with subarachnoid hemorrhage. *Neurosurgery* 1981; **9:** 398–401.
2. Kassell NF. Comment. *Neurosurgery* 1981; **9:** 401.

**Effects on the muscles.** There have been a number of cases of reversible myopathy reported with aminocaproic acid,[1-4] associated with daily doses ranging from 10 to 49 g and treatment durations of about 1 to 3 months. In some patients myoglobinuria or acute tubular necrosis also occurred. Suggested mechanisms for the reaction have included a direct dose-related effect on the muscle fibre[2] or a defect in aerobic energy provision induced by aminocaproic acid.[3]

1. Brown JA, *et al.* Myopathy induced by epsilon-aminocaproic acid. *J Neurosurg* 1982; **57:** 130–4.
2. Vanneste JAL, van Wijngaarden GK. Epsilon-aminocaproic acid myopathy. *Eur Neurol* 1982; **21:** 242–8.
3. Van Renterghem D, *et al.* Epsilon amino caproic acid myopathy: additional features. *Clin Neurol Neurosurg* 1984; **86:** 153–7.
4. Seymour BD, Rubinger M. Rhabdomyolysis induced by epsilon-aminocaproic acid. *Ann Pharmacother* 1997; **31:** 56–8.

## Precautions

As for Tranexamic Acid, p.760.

The range of adverse effects that have been noted with aminocaproic acid indicates that caution is required in patients with renal or cardiac disorders. Should treatment be prolonged, it is advisable to monitor creatine phosphokinase values for signs of muscle damage.

**Renal impairment.** High anion gap metabolic acidosis developed in a 65-year-old woman with sepsis and acute renal failure who received aminocaproic acid for a haemorrhagic coagulopathy.[1] The acidosis improved temporarily following haemodialysis and resolved after withdrawal of aminocaproic acid and systemic alkalinisation. Although the dose of aminocaproic acid had been reduced because of renal impairment, it was suggested that more conservative dosing and close monitoring may be indicated in such patients.

1. Budris WA, *et al.* High anion gap metabolic acidosis associated with aminocaproic acid. *Ann Pharmacother* 1999; **33:** 308–11.

## Pharmacokinetics

Aminocaproic acid is readily absorbed when given by mouth and peak plasma concentrations are reached within 2 hours. It is widely distributed and is rapidly excreted in the urine, mainly unchanged, with a terminal elimination half-life of approximately 2 hours.

## Uses and Administration

Aminocaproic acid is an antifibrinolytic used similarly to tranexamic acid (p.761) in the treatment and prophylaxis of haemorrhage associated with excessive fibrinolysis. It has also been used in the prophylaxis of hereditary angioedema (p.761).

A plasma concentration of about 130 micrograms/mL is considered to be necessary for effective inhibition of fibrinolysis and the recommended dosage schedules are aimed at producing and maintaining this concentration for as long as is necessary. For the treatment and prophylaxis of haemorrhage, aminocaproic acid may be given by mouth in an initial dose of 4 to 5 g, followed by 1 to 1.25 g every hour. Alternatively, the same dose may be given intravenously as a 2% solution; the initial dose (4 to 5 g) should be given over one hour followed by a continuous infusion of 1 g/hour. Up to 8 hours of treatment is often sufficient. Should treatment need to be extended, then the maximum dose over 24 hours should not normally exceed 24 g. Care is required when aminocaproic acid is used in patients with renal impairment and dosage should be reduced.

## Preparations

**USP 27:** Aminocaproic Acid Injection; Aminocaproic Acid Syrup; Aminocaproic Acid Tablets.

**Proprietary Preparations** (details are given in Part 3)
***Arg.:*** Ipsilon; ***Austral.:*** Amicar; ***Braz.:*** Ipsilon; ***Canad.:*** Amicar; ***Fr.:*** Hexalense; ***India:*** Hemocid; ***Ital.:*** Caprolisin; ***Mex.:*** Amicar; ***NZ:*** Amicar; ***Port.:*** Epsicaprom; ***S.Afr.:*** Amicar†; ***Spain:*** Caproamin; ***USA:*** Amicar.

**Multi-ingredient:** ***Braz.:*** Eaca Balsamico; Expectovac; Ginurovac; ***Spain:*** Caprofides Hemostatico.

## Aminomethylbenzoic Acid

Aminometilbenzoico, ácido; PAMBA. 4-Aminomethylbenzoic acid.

$C_8H_9NO_2$ = 151.2.
*CAS — 56-91-7.*
*ATC — B02AA03.*

### Profile

Aminomethylbenzoic acid is an antifibrinolytic with actions and uses similar to those of tranexamic acid (p.760). It is given by mouth, by intramuscular injection, or intravenously by slow injection or infusion.

### Preparations

**Proprietary Preparations** (details are given in Part 3)
***Austria:*** Gumbix; ***Ger.:*** Gumbix; Pamba.

## Ancestim *(USAN, rINN)*

r-metHuSCF; SCF; Stem Cell Factor. N-L-Methionyl-1–165-haematopoietic cell growth factor KL (human clone V19.8:hSCF162), dimer.
*CAS — 163545-26-4.*
*ATC — L03AA12.*

### Adverse Effects and Precautions

Injection site reactions commonly occur with the use of ancestim. Other skin reactions, including pruritus, rash, and urticaria, are less frequent. Systemic hypersensitivity reactions also commonly occur and may be life-threatening. Premedication with antihistamines (both $H_1$- and $H_2$-antagonists) and an inhaled beta$_2$ agonist bronchodilator should be used, and the patient observed for at least one hour after administration of ancestim. Tachycardia and respiratory symptoms including pharyngitis, dyspnoea, and cough, have also been reported.

### Uses and Administration

Ancestim is a recombinant human stem cell factor. It is used with filgrastim (p.753) to mobilise peripheral blood progenitor cells. The dose of ancestim is 20 micrograms/kg daily by subcutaneous injection; the injections of ancestim and filgrastim must be given at separate sites.

◊ References.

1. Chin-Yee IH, *et al.* Optimising parameters for peripheral blood leukapheresis after r-metHuG-CSF (filgrastim) and r-metHuSCF (ancestim) in patients with multiple myeloma: a temporal analysis of CD34(+) absolute counts and subsets. *Bone Marrow Transplant* 2002; **30:** 851–60.
2. Prosper F, *et al.* Mobilization of peripheral blood progenitor cells with a combination of cyclophosphamide, r-metHuSCF and filgrastim in patients with breast cancer previously treated with chemotherapy. *Leukemia* 2003; **17:** 437–41.
3. To LB, *et al.* Successful mobilization of peripheral blood stem cells after addition of ancestim (stem cell factor) in patients who had failed a prior mobilization with filgrastim (granulocyte colony-stimulating factor) alone or with chemotherapy plus filgrastim. *Bone Marrow Transplant* 2003; **31:** 371–8.

### Preparations

**Proprietary Preparations** (details are given in Part 3)
***Austral.:*** Stemgen; ***Canad.:*** Stemgen.

## Antithrombin III *(BAN, rINN)*

Antithrombin III Human; Antitrombina III; AT-III; Heparin Cofactor; Heparin Cofactor I; Major Antithrombin.
*CAS — 52014-67-2.*
*ATC — B01AB02.*

**Pharmacopoeias.** Many pharmacopoeias have monographs including *Eur.* (see p.vi).

**Ph. Eur. 5.0** (Human Antithrombin III Concentrate; Antithrombinum III Humanum Densatum). A preparation of a glycoprotein fraction obtained from human plasma that inactivates thrombin in the presence of an excess of heparin. The plasma is obtained from healthy donors and is tested for the absence of hepatitis B surface antigen and antibodies against HIV-1 and HIV-2 and hepatitis C virus. The method of preparation includes a step or steps that have been shown to remove or to inactivate known agents of infection. The antithrombin III concentrate is passed through a bacteria-retentive filter, distributed into sterile containers, and immediately frozen. The preparation is freeze-dried and the containers sealed under vacuum or in an atmosphere of inert gas. No antimicrobial preservative is added but a suitable stabiliser (such as albumin) may be added. When reconstituted in the volume of solvent stated on the label, the resulting solution contains not less than 25 international units of antithrombin III per mL.

A white, hygroscopic, friable solid or powder. Store in airtight containers. Protect from light.

### Units

The potency of antithrombin III is expressed in international units and preparations may be assayed using the second International Standard for antithrombin concentrate (1997); each ampoule contains 4.7 international units of functional activity and 5.1 international units of antigenic activity.

### Uses and Administration

Antithrombin III is a protein in plasma; it is the major endogenous inhibitor of thrombin and other activated clotting factors including factors IX, X, XI, and XII (p.735), and is the cofactor through which heparin (p.929) exerts its effect. Genetic and acquired deficiency of antithrombin III occurs and is associated with susceptibility to thromboembolic disorders.

Antithrombin III is given intravenously in the management of acute thrombotic episodes and for prophylaxis during surgery and pregnancy in patients with antithrombin III deficiency. The aim of therapy is to restore plasma-antithrombin III concentrations to at least 80% of normal. The dose, frequency of administration, and duration of therapy are individualised for each patient taking into account the patient's pretreatment concentration and presence of active coagulation. A usual initial dose is about 30 to 50 international units/kg.

A recombinant human antithrombin III preparation is being developed.

◊ Reviews.

1. Rosenberg RD, ed. Role of antithrombin III in coagulation disorders: state-of-the-art review. *Am J Med* 1989; **87** (3B): 1S–67S.
2. Harper PL. The clinical use of antithrombin concentrate in septicaemia. *Br J Hosp Med* 1994; **52:** 571–4.

**Septicaemia.** Antithrombin III has been used in septicaemia (p.144) in an attempt to manage the pro-coagulant state that occurs. Initial small studies reported a reduction in mortality[1] but a large controlled study[2] found that treatment with antithrombin III had no effect on 28-day mortality. Although there was a trend towards benefit in patients who did not receive heparin, the use of antithrombin III and heparin was associated with an increased risk of haemorrhage. A further small observational study and meta-analysis found no benefit from the use of antithrombin III in septicaemia.[3]

1. Eisele B, *et al.* Antithrombin III in patients with severe sepsis: a randomized, placebo-controlled, double-blind multicenter trial plus a meta-analysis on all randomized, placebo-controlled, double-blind trials with antithrombin III in severe sepsis. *Intensive Care Med* 1998; **24:** 663–72.
2. Warren BL, *et al.* High-dose antithrombin III in severe sepsis: a randomized controlled trial. *JAMA* 2001; **286:** 1869–78. Correction. *ibid.* 2002; **287:** 192.
3. Messori A, *et al.* Antithrombin III in patients admitted to intensive care units: a multicenter observational study. *Crit Care* 2002; **6:** 447–51.

### Preparations

**Ph. Eur.:** Human Antithrombin III Concentrate.

**Proprietary Preparations** (details are given in Part 3)
***Austral.:*** Thrombotrol-VF; ***Austria:*** Atenativ; Athimbin P†; Kybernin P; Thrombhibin; ***Braz.:*** Kybernin; ***Canad.:*** Thrombate; ***Denm.:*** Atenativ; ***Fin.:*** Atenativ; ***Fr.:*** Aclotine; ***Ger.:*** AT III; Atenativ; Kybernin; ***Gr.:*** Kybernin P; ***Hong Kong:*** Thrombate†; ***Ital.:*** Anbin; Atenativ; Kybernin P; ***Jpn:*** Neuart; ***Neth.:*** Atenativ; ***Norw.:*** Atenativ; ***NZ:*** Thrombotrol; ***Spain:*** Anbin; Atenativ; Kybernin P; ***Swed.:*** Atenativ; ***Switz.:*** Atenativ; Kybernin; ***USA:*** Thrombate III.

## Aprotinin *(BAN, USAN, rINN)*

Aprotinina; Aprotininum; Bayer A-128; Riker 52G; RP-9921.
*CAS — 9087-70-1.*
*ATC — B02AB01.*

**Description.** Aprotinin is a single-chain polypeptide derived from bovine tissues consisting of 58 amino-acid residues and having a molecular weight of about 6500.

**Pharmacopoeias.** In *Chin.* and *Eur.* (see p.vi). *Eur.* also includes a concentrated solution.

**Ph. Eur. 5.0** (Aprotinin). A polypeptide consisting of 58 amino acids that inhibits the activity of several proteolytic enzymes such as chymotrypsin, kallikrein, plasmin, and trypsin. It contains not less than 3 Ph. Eur. units/mg calculated with reference to the dried substance. An almost white, hygroscopic powder. Soluble in water and in isotonic solutions; practically insoluble in organic solvents. Store in airtight containers. Protect from light.

**Ph. Eur. 5.0** (Aprotinin Concentrated Solution). A solution of aprotinin containing not less than 15 Ph. Eur. units/mL. A clear colourless solution. Store in airtight containers. Protect from light.

**Incompatibility.** Aprotinin is reported to be incompatible with corticosteroids, heparin, tetracyclines, and nutrient solutions containing amino acids or fat emulsions.

### Units

The potency of aprotinin is expressed in terms of kallikrein (kallidinogenase) inactivator units (KIU) or of trypsin inactivation (Ph. Eur. units). One KIU is contained in 140 nanograms of aprotinin. One Ph. Eur. unit is approximately equivalent to 1800 KIU.

Potency has also been expressed in terms of plasmin inactivation (antiplasmin units).

### Adverse Effects and Precautions

Aprotinin is usually well tolerated. Side-effects that have been observed include bronchospasm, gastrointestinal disturbances, skin rashes, and tachycardia; most of these effects are considered to be hypersensitivity reactions. Anaphylaxis has occasionally occurred as has local thrombophlebitis.

◊ Aprotinin has been used to reverse resistance to subcutaneous insulin. After one year's successful treatment of a diabetic patient with aprotinin and insulin given subcutaneously,[1] loss of effect from the aprotinin was accompanied by development of lipohypertrophy; this was not seen during prior or subsequent use of insulin alone. On continuing treatment glomerulonephritis was detected. It was suggested that development of antibodies against aprotinin might explain these effects.

1. Boag F, *et al.* Lipohypertrophy and glomerulonephritis after the use of aprotinin in an insulin-dependent diabetic. *N Engl J Med* 1985; **312:** 245–6.

**Disseminated intravascular coagulation.** Fatal disseminated intravascular coagulation has been reported in a patient after the use of intraoperative autotransfusion and aprotinin during surgery.[1] Activation of the clotting system occurs during autotransfusion although this usually causes no systemic adverse effects. While there were other possible causes, it was suggested that aprotinin could have contributed to deposition of fibrin microthrombi in the microvasculature and prevented subsequent fibrinolysis.

1. Milne AA, *et al.* Disseminated intravascular coagulation after aortic aneurysm repair, intraoperative salvage autotransfusion, and aprotinin. *Lancet* 1994; **344:** 470–1.

**Effects on coagulation tests.** In patients receiving heparin, aprotinin may prolong the activated clotting time when measured by some methods, but this may not represent increased anticoagulation. It has been recommended that an alternative to the activated clotting time should be used to monitor heparin therapy when aprotinin is used concurrently.

It should also be noted that aprotinin injection and heparin injection are pharmaceutically incompatible.

**Effects on the respiratory system.** Acute respiratory distress syndrome developed in a 24-year-old male 2 hours after the start of an intravenous infusion of aprotinin for bleeding after tonsillectomy.[1] Mechanical ventilation was required for 4 days.

1. Vucicevic Z, Suskovic T. Acute respiratory distress syndrome after aprotinin infusion. *Ann Pharmacother* 1997; **31:** 429–32.

**Hypersensitivity.** Acute allergic reactions were noted[1] in 2 of 136 courses of aprotinin; one patient experienced acute anaphylaxis, the other an acute urticarial reaction. Such patients might be detected by challenging their reactivity using aprotinin eye drops as an alternative to intradermal testing. However, a severe anaphylactic reaction occurred[2] in a patient after the intravenous administration of aprotinin despite negative ocular sensitivity tests. Repeat use of aprotinin (2 months after the initial dose) has produced anaphylactic shock in a 3-year-old boy.[3] In a study[4] of 248 re-exposures to aprotinin in 240 patients undergoing cardiac surgery, there were 7 cases of anaphylactic reactions ranging from mild to severe with a higher incidence of reactions occurring in those patients re-exposed within 6 months of the previous dose. It has been suggested that re-exposure should be avoided for at least 6 months,[4] that a test dose be used in all patients,[4] and that histamine $H_1$- and $H_2$-antagonists should be given before re-exposure to aprotinin to ameliorate severe anaphylactic reactions.[4,5]

1. Freeman JG, *et al.* Serial use of aprotinin and incidence of allergic reactions. *Curr Med Res Opin* 1983; **8:** 559–61.
2. LaFerla GA, Murray WR. Anaphylactic reaction to aprotinin despite negative ocular sensitivity tests. *BMJ* 1984; **289:** 1176–7.
3. Wüthrich B, *et al.* IgE-mediated anaphylactic reaction to aprotinin during anaesthesia. *Lancet* 1992; **340:** 173–4.
4. Dietrich W, *et al.* Prevalence of anaphylactic reactions to aprotinin: analysis of two hundred forty-eight reexposures to aprotinin in heart operations. *J Thorac Cardiovasc Surg* 1997: **113:** 194–201.
5. Lamparter-Schummert B, *et al.* Aprotinin re-exposure in patients undergoing repeat cardiac surgery: effect of prophylaxis with H1- and H2-receptor antagonists. *Br J Anaesth* 1995; **74** (suppl 2): 3.

## Interactions

**Heparin.** For comment on the use of aprotinin with heparin, see Effects on Coagulation Tests, above.

**Neuromuscular blockers.** For potentiation of the activity of neuromuscular blockers by aprotinin, see p.1401.

## Pharmacokinetics

Aprotinin, being a polypeptide, is inactivated in the gastrointestinal tract. After intravenous use, it is excreted in the urine as inactive degradation products. The terminal elimination half-life is about 7 to 10 hours.

**Renal impairment.** The terminal elimination half-life of aprotinin was reported as 13.3 and 14.9 hours, respectively, in two patients with chronic renal impairment given aprotinin by intravenous infusion over 30 minutes.[1]

1. Müller FO, *et al.* Pharmacokinetics of aprotinin in two patients with chronic renal impairment. *Br J Clin Pharmacol* 1996; **41:** 619–20.

## Uses and Administration

Aprotinin is a haemostatic. It is an inhibitor of proteolytic enzymes including chymotrypsin, kallikrein (kallidinogenase), plasmin, and trypsin.

Aprotinin is used in the treatment of haemorrhage associated with raised plasma concentrations of plasmin. It is also used to reduce blood loss and transfusion requirements in patients at high risk of major blood loss during and following open-heart surgery with extracorporeal circulation. Aprotinin has been tried in the management of pancreatitis (p.1726) because of the postulated role of proteolytic enzymes in this condition. Aprotinin is applied topically as a component of fibrin glues (p.753).

It is recommended that because of the risk of hypersensitivity reactions a test dose of 10 000 KIU should be given at least 10 minutes before the therapeutic dose. In the treatment of haemorrhage, 500 000 to 1 000 000 KIU of aprotinin is given by slow intravenous injection or infusion at a maximum rate of 100 000 KIU/minute with the patient in the supine position. This may be followed by 200 000 KIU every hour until the haemorrhage is controlled.

In open-heart surgery, the test dose is followed by a loading dose given after induction of anaesthesia but before incision; 2 000 000 KIU is given intravenously over 20 to 30 minutes. The loading dose is followed by a continuous infusion of 500 000 KIU/hour until the end of the operation. An additional dose of 2 000 000 KIU is added to the prime volume of the extracorporeal circuit. In patients with septic endocarditis, a dose of 3 000 000 KIU is added to the prime volume of the circuit and the continuous infusion may be continued into the early postoperative period. The total amount of aprotinin used is usually no more than 7 000 000 KIU. A regimen using half the dose for loading, maintenance, and to prime the circuit, may be used in low-risk patients.

**Haemorrhagic disorders.** Aprotinin is indicated in the treatment of life-threatening haemorrhage caused by raised plasma concentrations of plasmin. It is used alone, or with tranexamic acid or aminocaproic acid, in the treatment of severe bleeding arising from overdosage with thrombolytics.

It is also used to reduce blood loss in patients undergoing surgery, including that involving cardiopulmonary bypass.[1-3] (See also Complex Acquired Coagulopathies under Haemorrhagic Disorders, p.737.)

Cardiac surgery may be complicated by a postperfusion syndrome that includes impairment of haemostasis and pulmonary dysfunction. This syndrome has been interpreted as a 'whole-body inflammatory response'. The beneficial effect of aprotinin on haemostasis during cardiopulmonary bypass has been attributed, not to an antifibrinolytic action, but to a preservation of platelet function, possibly mediated by inhibition of plasmin.[2-7] Aprotinin has reduced blood loss and transfusion requirements in patients undergoing both primary and repeat cardiac surgery.[1,8,9] The usual dosage regimen is given under Uses and Administration, above. In addition, 500 000 KIU may be added to each litre of whole blood given during the operation.[4,5]

A slightly different dosage regimen has been used in a group of patients undergoing heart-valve replacement for infective endocarditis.[10] Other workers have investigated the use of reduced dosage regimens omitting the loading dose, including the administration of aprotinin in the priming volume alone.[11-15]

Encouraging reductions in blood loss have been obtained in some patients undergoing liver transplantation,[16,17] peripheral vascular surgery,[18] orthopaedic surgery,[19] and lung transplantation,[20] but it has been advised that until risks such as postoperative thromboembolic disease and loss of graft patency have been investigated aprotinin should be used with caution.[21]

Aprotinin is a component of fibrin glues (p.753), also known as fibrin sealants or tissue glues, that are applied topically in the control of bleeding or as a suture system. The other components of these glues include fibrinogen, factor XIII, and other plasma proteins, mixed with calcium and thrombin immediately prior to use.

1. Davis R, Whittington R. Aprotinin: a review of its pharmacology and therapeutic efficacy in reducing blood loss associated with cardiac surgery. *Drugs* 1995; **49:** 954–83.
2. Robert S, *et al.* Aprotinin. *Ann Pharmacother* 1996; **30:** 372–80.
3. Dobkowski WB, Murkin JM. A risk-benefit assessment of aprotinin in cardiac surgical procedures. *Drug Safety* 1998; **18:** 21–41.
4. van Oeveren W, *et al.* Effects of aprotinin on hemostatic mechanisms during cardiopulmonary bypass. *Ann Thorac Surg* 1987; **44:** 640–5.
5. Royston D, *et al.* Effect of aprotinin on need for blood transfusion after repeat open-heart surgery. *Lancet* 1987; **ii:** 1289–91.
6. Anonymous. Can drugs reduce surgical blood loss? *Lancet* 1988; **i:** 155–6.
7. van Oeveren W, *et al.* Platelet preservation by aprotinin during cardiopulmonary bypass. *Lancet* 1988; **i:** 644.
8. Bidstrup BP, *et al.* Aprotinin therapy in cardiac operations: a report on use in 41 cardiac centers in the United Kingdom. *Ann Thorac Surg* 1993; **55:** 971–6.
9. Laupacis A, Fergusson D. Drugs to minimize perioperative blood loss in cardiac surgery: meta-analyses using perioperative blood transfusion as the outcome. *Anesth Analg* 1997; **85:** 1258–67.
10. Bidstrup BP, *et al.* Effect of aprotinin on need for blood transfusion in patients with septic endocarditis having open-heart surgery. *Lancet* 1988; **i:** 366–7.
11. Locatelli A, *et al.* Aprotinin in cardiac surgery. *Lancet* 1991; **338:** 254.
12. Carrel T, *et al.* Low-dose aprotinin for reduction of blood loss after cardiopulmonary bypass. *Lancet* 1991; **337:** 673.
13. Vandenvelde C, *et al.* Low-dose aprotinin for reduction of blood loss after cardiopulmonary bypass. *Lancet* 1991; **337:** 1157–8.
14. Bailey CR, Wielogorski AK. Randomised placebo controlled double blind study of two low dose aprotinin regimens in cardiac surgery. *Br Heart J* 1994; **71:** 349–53.
15. Levy JH, *et al.* A multicenter, double-blind, placebo-controlled trial of aprotinin for reducing blood loss and the requirement for donor-blood transfusion in patients undergoing repeat coronary artery bypass graftings. *Circulation* 1995; **92:** 2236–44.
16. Neuhaus P, *et al.* Effect of aprotinin on intraoperative bleeding and fibrinolysis in liver transplantation. *Lancet* 1989; **ii:** 924–5.
17. Mallett SV, *et al.* Aprotinin and reduction of blood loss and transfusion requirements in orthotopic liver transplantation. *Lancet* 1990; **336:** 886–7.
18. Thompson JF, *et al.* Aprotinin in peripheral vascular surgery. *Lancet* 1990; **335:** 911.
19. Janssens M, *et al.* High-dose aprotinin reduces blood loss in patients undergoing total hip replacement surgery. *Anesthesiology* 1994; **80:** 23–9.
20. Jaquiss RDB, *et al.* Use of aprotinin in pediatric lung transplantation. *J Heart Lung Transplant* 1995; **14:** 302–7.
21. Hunt BJ, Yacoub M. Aprotinin and cardiac surgery. *BMJ* 1991; **303:** 660–1.

## Preparations

***BP 2003:*** Aprotinin Injection.

**Proprietary Preparations** (details are given in Part 3)

***Arg.:*** Quagu-Test; ***Austral.:*** Trasylol; ***Austria:*** Pantinol; Trasylol; ***Belg.:*** Iniprol†; Trasylol; ***Braz.:*** Trasylol; ***Canad.:*** Trasylol; ***Chile:*** Trasylol; ***Denm.:*** Trasylol; ***Fin.:*** Trasylol; ***Fr.:*** Antagosan†; Trasylol; ***Ger.:*** Antagosan†; Trasylol; ***Hong Kong:*** Trasylol; ***Israel:*** Protosol; ***Ital.:*** Antagosan†; Fase†; Kir Richter†; Trasylol†; ***Malaysia:*** Trasylol; ***Mex.:*** Protinin; Trasylol; ***Neth.:*** Trasylol; ***NZ:*** Trasylol; ***S.Afr.:*** Trasylol; ***Singapore:*** Trasylol; ***Spain:*** Trasylol; ***Swed.:*** Trasylol; ***Switz.:*** Trasylol; ***Thai.:*** Trasylol; ***UK:*** Trasylol; ***USA:*** Trasylol.

**Multi-ingredient:** ***Arg.:*** Dunason; Maxus; Optilac; Tissucol; Tissucol Duo Quick; ***Austral.:*** Tisseel Duo; ***Austria:*** Beriplast; TachoComb; Tissucol; Tissucol Duo Quick; ***Belg.:*** Tissucol†; ***Braz.:*** Beriplast P; Tissucol†; ***Canad.:*** Tisseel; ***Chile:*** Beriplast P; ***Denm.:*** Tisseel Duo Quick; ***Fin.:*** Beriplast†; Tisseel Duo Quick; ***Fr.:*** Beriplast; Biocol†; Tissucol; ***Ger.:*** Beriplast; TachoComb; Tissucol Duo S; Tissucol Fibrinkleber tiefgefroren†; Tissucol-Kit; ***Hong Kong:*** Beriplast P; TachoComb; Tisseel; ***Irl.:*** Tisseel†; ***Israel:*** Beriplast P; Tisseel; ***Ital.:*** Tissucol; ***Mex.:*** Beriplast P†; ***Spain:*** Tissucol Duo; ***Swed.:*** Tisseel Duo Quick; ***Switz.:*** Beriplast P; Tissucol; Tissucol Duo S; ***Thai.:*** TachoComb; ***UK:*** Tisseel.

## Batroxobin *(rINN)*

Batroxobina.

*CAS — 9039-61-6 (batroxobin); 9001-13-2 (haemocoagulase).*

*ATC — B02BX03.*

### Profile

Batroxobin is an enzyme obtained from the venom of the viper *Bothrops atrox*. It has also been obtained from *Bothrops moojeni* and a similar preparation is derived from *Bothrops jararaca*.

Batroxobin is reported to act on fibrinogen to produce a fibrin monomer that can be converted by thrombin to a fibrin clot. It is used both as a haemostatic and, in larger doses, to induce a hypofibrinogen state in the management of thromboembolic disorders. When used as a haemostatic it is usually given with a factor-X activator; such a combined preparation is known as haemocoagulase (hemocoagulase). Batroxobin may be administered parenterally or by local application.

### Preparations

**Proprietary Preparations** (details are given in Part 3)

***Austria:*** Defibrase; Reptilase; ***Fr.:*** Reptilase; ***India:*** Reptilase; ***Ital.:*** Botropase; Reptilase†; ***Port.:*** Reptilase; ***Spain:*** Reptilase†.

## Blood

Sangre.

**Pharmacopoeias.** Many pharmacopoeias have monographs including *US*.

**USP 27** (Whole Blood). It is obtained from suitable human donors and is collected under rigid aseptic precautions. It contains acid citrate dextrose, citrate phosphate dextrose, citrate phosphate dextrose with adenine, or heparin sodium as an anticoagulant. It may consist of blood from which the antihaemophilic factor has been removed, in which case it is termed 'Modified'. It should be stored in hermetically-sealed sterile containers at 1° to 6° (with a range of not more than 2°) except during transport when the temperature may be 1° to 10°. The expiration date is not later than 48 hours after withdrawal (heparin anticoagulant), not later than 21 days after withdrawal (acid citrate dextrose or citrate phosphate dextrose), or not later than 35 days after withdrawal (citrate phosphate dextrose with adenine).

It is a deep red, opaque liquid from which the corpuscles readily settle upon standing for 24 to 48 hours, leaving a clear, yellowish or pinkish supernatant layer of plasma.

The USP 27 gives the names ACD Whole Blood, CPD Whole Blood, CPDA-1 Whole Blood, and Heparin Whole Blood, which specify the anticoagulant used.

## Adverse Effects

The rapid transfusion of large volumes of whole blood may overload the circulation and cause pulmonary oedema. Repeated transfusions of blood, as in thalassaemia, may lead to iron overload. Transfusion of very large volumes of citrated blood can lead to hypocalcaemia which is not usually a problem unless there is hepatic impairment or hypothermia. Hyperkalaemia may occur but on its own is rarely clinically significant. Hypothermia may result from rapid transfusion of large volumes of cooled blood and may, in combination with hypocalcaemia, hyperkalaemia, and resultant acidosis, lead to cardiac toxicity. Disseminated intravascular coagulation may also occur in patients receiving large-volume transfusions.

The transfusion of incompatible blood causes haemolysis, possibly with renal failure. Pyrexia, rigors, and urticaria may be due to antibodies towards a number of blood components. Severe allergic reactions and anaphylaxis may occur.

**Transmission of infections**. The use of blood, blood components, or blood products has been associated with the transmission of viruses, most notably transmission of the hepatitis B virus and HIV; other reports of transmission include cytomegalovirus, hepatitis C and possibly other hepatitis viruses, HTLV-I and -II, and the agent causing Creutzfeldt-Jakob disease. Transmission of bacterial and parasitic diseases is also possible including syphilis, Chagas' disease, and malaria.

The main methods of minimising the risk of transmission of infection are by rigorous selection of blood donors and by microbiological screening tests. Contamination during collection and processing is minimised by using closed systems and by strict aseptic technique. Some organisms cannot survive storage under refrigeration, for example staphylococci, while others, like malaria parasites, can survive storage in blood at 4° for at least a week. Treatment of blood products with heat or chemicals can inactivate some organisms including some viruses, in particular HIV-I, but blood and blood components cannot be treated in either of these ways. Patients receiving multiple transfusions of pooled plasma products are at increased risk of contracting infections and can be offered immunological protection, for example hepatitis B vaccine.

◊ Reviews.


1. Donaldson MDJ, *et al.* Massive blood transfusion. *Br J Anaesth* 1992; **69:** 621–30.
2. Contreras M, Mollison PL. Immunological complications of transfusion. In: Contreras M, ed. *ABC of transfusion.* 3rd ed. London: BMJ Books, 1998: 53–7.
3. Barbara JAJ, Contreras M. Infectious complications of blood transfusion: bacteria and parasites. In: Contreras M. ed. *ABC of transfusion.* 3rd ed. London: BMJ Books, 1998: 58–61.
4. Barbara JAJ, Contreras M. Infectious complications of blood transfusion: viruses. In: Contreras M. ed. *ABC of transfusion.* 3rd ed. London: BMJ Books, 1998: 62–6.
5. McClelland DBL, ed. *Handbook of transfusion medicine: Blood Transfusion Services of the United Kingdom.* 3rd ed. London: The Stationery Office, 2001.
6. Regan F, Taylor C. Blood transfusion medicine. *BMJ* 2002; **325:** 143–7.


**Creutzfeldt-Jakob disease.** While there is no proof that transmission of Creutzfeldt-Jakob disease by blood or blood products has occurred,[1] it is recognised that there is a need for further assessment of the potential risk of transmission of new variant Creutzfeldt-Jakob disease by such products.[2] As precautionary measures, production of blood products using plasma from UK donors has been phased out and in some countries (including the UK) leucocytes are removed from donated blood (a procedure that early evidence suggests may remove infectivity).

Concern at the risk of transmitting Creutzfeldt-Jakob disease by albumin prepared from placental blood has led to restriction on this source of albumin (see p.741).


1. Wilson K, *et al.* Risk of acquiring Creutzfeldt-Jakob disease from blood transfusions: systematic review of case-control studies. *BMJ* 2000; **321:** 17–19.
2. Barbara J, Flanagan P. Blood transfusion risk: protecting against the unknown. *BMJ* 1998; **316:** 717–18.


**Effects on leucocytes.** A study of 50 patients in an intensive care unit found that 45 of them developed leucocytosis following transfusion of packed red blood cells.[1] The leucocytosis, which was accounted for by neutrophils, occurred immediately after transfusion and persisted for 12 hours.


1. Fenwick JC, *et al.* Blood transfusion as a cause of leucocytosis in critically ill patients. *Lancet* 1994; **344:** 855–6.


**Effects on the lungs.** A rare but life-threatening complication of transfusion of blood or other plasma-containing products is acute lung injury.[1] The symptoms, which usually develop 1 to 6 hours after the start of infusion, are those of acute respiratory distress syndrome but usually resolve within about 2 to 4 days with vigorous supportive therapy. The presence of HLA-specific antileucocyte antibodies in plasma from multiparous female donors appears to play a role in initiating the reaction.


1. Popovsky MA, *et al.* Transfusion-related acute lung injury: a neglected, serious complication of hemotherapy. *Transfusion* 1992: **32:** 589–92.


**Graft-versus-host disease.** Acute graft-versus-host disease (see Haematopoietic Stem Cell Transplantation, p.1344) has been reported in both immunocompromised and apparently immunocompetent patients following blood transfusion.[1-4] The reaction can be severe and fatal. Symptoms include fever, rash, hepatomegaly and abnormal liver function tests, diarrhoea, and pronounced pancytopenia. Infusion of products containing viable lymphocytes appears to be responsible and patients considered to be at risk may be given products depleted of viable lymphocytes by irradiation. Risk factors are incompletely defined. High-risk groups include bone marrow transplant recipients, patients with congenital immunodeficiencies, and possibly also premature infants undergoing exchange transfusions and patients receiving intensive chemotherapy for Hodgkin's disease. Immunocompetent patients who share an HLA haplotype with HLA-homozygous blood donors also appear to be at increased risk. A study in Japan[5] found that fresh and consanguineous blood transfusion was a major risk factor and that others were cardiovascular surgery, cancer, and being male.


1. Anonymous. Transfusions and graft-versus-host disease. *Lancet* 1989; **i:** 529–30.
2. Anderson KC, Weinstein HJ. Transfusion-associated graft-versus-host disease. *N Engl J Med* 1990; **323:** 315–21.
3. Webb DKH. Irradiation in the prevention of transfusion associated graft-versus-host disease. *Arch Dis Child* 1995; **73:** 388–9.
4. Williamson LM. Transfusion associated graft versus host disease and its prevention. *Heart* 1998; **80:** 211–12.
5. Takahashi K, *et al.* Analysis of risk factors for post-transfusion graft-versus-host disease in Japan. *Lancet* 1994; **343:** 700–2.


**Malignant neoplasms.** Blood transfusion is reported to have immunosuppressant effects, and several retrospective studies have suggested that perioperative blood transfusion in patients undergoing surgical resection of their tumours may be associated with an increased rate of tumour recurrence and decreased long-term survival.[1-5] This has been supported by experimental *animal* data.[6] However, the association has not been found in other studies[7,8] and at present there is insufficient data from prospective studies on which to base clinical recommendations.

Blood transfusions have also been associated with increased risk of non-Hodgkin's lymphoma in some studies, although it has been pointed out[9] that confounding factors could account for both the positive and negative associations that have been reported.


1. Burrows L, Tartter P. Effect of blood transfusions on colonic malignancy recurrence rate. *Lancet* 1982; **ii:** 662.
2. Blumberg N, *et al.* Relation between recurrence of cancer of the colon and blood transfusion. *BMJ* 1985; **290:** 1037–9.
3. Blumberg N, *et al.* Association between transfusion of whole blood and recurrence of cancer. *BMJ* 1986; **293;** 530–3.
4. Jackson RM, Rice DH. Blood transfusions and recurrence in head and neck cancer. *Ann Otol Rhinol Laryngol* 1989; **98:** 171–3.
5. Blumberg N, *et al.* The relationship of blood transfusion, tumor staging, and cancer recurrence. *Transfusion* 1990; **30:** 291–4.
6. Waymack JP, Chance WT. Effect of blood transfusions on immune function: IV effect on tumor growth. *J Surg Oncol* 1988; **39:** 159–64.
7. Blair SD, Janvrin SB. Relation between cancer of the colon and blood transfusion. *BMJ* 1985; **290:** 1516–17.
8. Frankish PD, *et al.* Relation between cancer of the colon and blood transfusion. *BMJ* 1985; **290:** 1827.
9. Alexander FE. Blood transfusion and risk of non-Hodgkin lymphoma. *Lancet* 1997; **350:** 1414–15.


## Precautions

Whole blood should generally not be transfused unless the ABO and Rh groups of the patient's and the donor's blood have been verified and a compatibility check made between the patient's serum and the donor's red cells (see under Blood Groups, below).

The Rh group of the recipient should always be determined and ideally all patients should be transfused with blood of homologous Rh groups.

To reduce the possibility of cardiac arrest from cardiac hypothermia when large volumes are used or the blood is transfused rapidly, and to minimise postoperative shivering, stored blood should be carefully warmed to about 37° before transfusion.

Whole blood should not be given to patients with chronic anaemia who have a normal or elevated plasma volume.

Drugs should *not* be added to blood.

Transfusion of blood from donors who have recently been receiving drug treatment may be hazardous to the recipient.

◊ Guidelines[1-3] for accepting blood from donors who have been receiving drugs have been published.


1. Ferner RE, *et al.* Drugs in donated blood. *Lancet* 1989; **ii:** 93–4.
2. Stichtenoth DO, *et al.* Blood donors on medication: are deferral periods necessary? *Eur J Clin Pharmacol* 2001; **57:** 433–40.
3. US Armed Services Blood Program Office. Drug and medication impact on blood donor eligibility (revised January 16, 2003). Available at: http://www.tricare.osd.mil/asbpo/library/policies/index.htm (accessed 23/06/04)


**Blood groups.** The chief blood group systems are the ABO system and the Rhesus system.

In simple terms red blood cells carry on their surface genetically determined antigens. A person with antigen A, B, A plus B, or neither is classified as group A, B, AB, or O respectively. Such persons will have, in their serum, antibodies to B, A, neither, or both respectively—anti-B (β), anti-A (α), or anti-B plus anti-A (α + β). Administration of blood containing red cells from a person of group A to a person with anti-A results in agglutination or possibly haemolysis. For the determination of the ABO group the agglutinogens of the red cells and the agglutinins of the serum are determined by testing against known standards.

In the Rhesus system many persons carry an antigen (Rh-positive) which stimulates antibody formation in Rh-negative persons; subsequent exposure to Rh-positive blood causes haemolysis.

Many variants of these systems, and other systems, are recognised.

## Uses and Administration

Blood is a complex fluid with many functions including the maintenance of hydration of the tissues, maintenance of body temperature, and the transport within the body of gases, ions, nutrients, hormones, enzymes, antibodies, waste products of metabolism, and drugs.

The main components of blood are plasma, red blood cells (erythrocytes), white blood cells (leucocytes), and platelets. The leucocytes are classified according to their morphological appearance into granulocytes, lymphocytes, and monocytes. The granulocytes are further classified as neutrophils, eosinophils, and basophils, according to the characteristics of their granules. The term polymorphonuclear leucocytes can be applied to granulocytes in general but applies in particular to neutrophils. Serum is the fluid which remains once blood or plasma has clotted; it is in effect plasma with fibrinogen removed.

Whole blood is used as a source of red cell concentrates, clotting factors, platelets, plasma and plasma fractions, and immunoglobulins, each of which has specific indications for use. Because of the risks involved in transfusing whole blood and the need for economy in its use, the appropriate blood component should be used whenever possible.

Whole blood may be used where replacement of plasma proteins as well as red blood cells is needed, for example following acute blood loss during surgery and severe haemorrhage. It may also be used to supplement the circulation during cardiac bypass surgery.

The amount of whole blood transfused and the rate at which it is given depend upon the patient's age and general condition, upon the state of their circulatory system, and upon the therapeutic indication for transfusion.

The expression 'unit of blood' generally represents a volume of about 510 mL, including anticoagulant. For blood preparations a unit generally refers to the quantity of a blood component obtained from 1 unit of whole blood. Specific units of activity are used for some blood components.

The haemoglobin concentration of the blood of the average adult is raised by about 1 g per 100 mL by the transfusion of 1 unit of whole blood.

◊ Reviews and guidelines for the use of blood and blood components.


1. Contreras M, ed. *ABC of transfusion*. 3rd ed. London: BMJ Books, 1998.
2. Goodnough LT, *et al.* Transfusion medicine: blood transfusion. *N Engl J Med* 1999; **340:** 438–47.
3. McClelland DBL, ed. *Handbook of transfusion medicine: Blood Transfusion Services of the United Kingdom.* 3rd ed. London: The Stationery Office, 2001.

4. World Health Organization. *The clinical use of blood in medicine, obstetrics, paediatrics, surgery and anaesthesia, trauma and burns.* Geneva: World Health Organization, 2001. Also available at: http://whqlibdoc.who.int/publications/2001/9241545399.pdf (accessed 23/06/04)
5. Australian Red Cross Blood Service. *Transfusion medicine manual 2003: blood transfusion practice and clinical use of blood in Australia.* Fitzroy: Australian Red Cross Blood Service, 2003. Also available at: http://svc127.bne077v.server-web.com/documents/uploaded//Transfusion_1-127.pdf (accessed 23/06/04)
6. Council of Europe. *Guide to the preparation, use and quality assurance of blood components.* 9th ed. Strasbourg: Council of Europe Publishing, 2003.
7. British Committee for Standards in Haematology Transfusion Task Force. Transfusion guidelines for neonates and older children. *Br J Haematol* 2004; **124:** 433–53. Also available at: http://www.bcshguidelines.com/pdf/Neonates_124_4_2004.pdf (accessed 23/06/04)

**Autologous blood transfusion.** Reviews and guidelines regarding autologous blood transfusion, the procedure of a patient acting as his own blood donor, the blood usually being collected shortly before elective surgery or salvaged during the surgical procedure.[1-7]

1. The National Blood Resource Education Program Expert Panel. The use of autologous blood. *JAMA* 1990; **263:** 414–17.
2. British Committee for Standards in Haematology Blood Transfusion Task Force. Guidelines for autologous transfusion I: preoperative autologous donation. *Transfus Med* 1993; **3:** 307–16. Also available at: http://www.bcshguidelines.com/pdf/TFM307.pdf (accessed 23/06/04)
3. British Committee for Standards in Haematology Blood Transfusion Task Force. Guidelines for autologous transfusion II: perioperative haemodilution and cell salvage. *Br J Anaesth* 1997; **78:** 768–71. Also available at: http://www.bcshguidelines.com/pdf/bja768.pdf (accessed 23/06/04)
4. Gillon J, Thomas DW. Autologous transfusion. In: Contreras M, ed. *ABC of transfusion.* 3rd ed. London: BMJ Books, 1998: 23–8.
5. Goodnough LT, *et al.* Transfusion medicine: blood conservation. *N Engl J Med* 1999; **340:** 525–33.
6. McClelland DBL, ed. *Handbook of transfusion medicine: Blood Transfusion Services of the United Kingdom.* 3rd ed. London: The Stationery Office, 2001.
7. Vanderlinde ES, *et al.* Autologous transfusion. *BMJ* 2002; **324:** 772–5.

### Preparations

**USP 27:** Whole Blood.

---

## Calcium Alginate

Alginato cálcico; E404.
*CAS — 9005-35-0.*
*ATC — B02BC08.*

### Profile

Calcium alginate is the calcium salt of alginic acid, a polyuronic acid composed of residues of D-mannuronic and L-guluronic acids. It may be obtained from seaweeds, mainly species of *Laminaria.* Calcium alginate is used as an absorbable haemostatic and for the promotion of wound healing (p.1139); it is also used in the form of a mixed calcium-sodium salt of alginic acid as a fibre made into a dressing or packing material. Calcium ions in the calcium alginate fibres are exchanged for sodium ions in the blood and exudate to form a hydrophilic gel.

Alginic acid and its calcium and sodium salts are widely used in the food industry.

◊ References.

1. Thomas S, Tucker CA. Sorbsan in the management of leg ulcers. *Pharm J* 1989; **243:** 706–9.
2. Anonymous. Scalpel and seaweed, nurse. *Lancet* 1990; **336:** 914.
3. Henderson NJ, *et al.* A randomised trial of calcium alginate swabs to control blood loss in 3–5-year-old children. *Br Dent J* 1998; **184:** 187–90. Correction. *ibid.*; 526.

### Preparations

**Proprietary Preparations** (details are given in Part 3)
***Arg.:*** Kaltostat; Tegagen; ***Austral.:*** Hydroheal Algin†; Kaltostat; Melgisorb; Sorbsan; ***Fr.:*** Algosteril; Coalgan; Sorbalgon; Sorbsan†; Stop Hemo; Trophiderm†; ***Ger.:*** Algosteril; Urgosorb; ***Irl.:*** Kaltostat; ***Ital.:*** Algosteril†; Cutinova Alginate; Kaltostat; Sorbsan; ***S.Afr.:*** Kaltostat; ***Switz.:*** Stop Hemo†; ***UK:*** Algosteril; Comfeel Seasorb; Kaltostat; Sorbsan.

**Multi-ingredient:** ***Arg.:*** Comfeel Purilon; Comfeel Seasorb; ***Fr.:*** Amivia; Askina Sorb; Comfeel Seasorb; Melgisorb; Purilon; Urgosorb; ***Israel:*** Kaltocarb; Kaltostat; ***Port.:*** Carboflex; Kaltostat; ***UK:*** Comfeel Plus; Seasorb Soft.

---

## Carbazochrome *(rINN)*

Adrenochrome Monosemicarbazone; Carbazocromo. 3-Hydroxy-1-methyl-5,6-indolinedione semicarbazone.
$C_{10}H_{12}N_4O_3$ = 236.2.
*CAS — 69-81-8 (carbazochrome); 13051-01-9 (carbazochrome salicylate); 51460-26-5 (carbazochrome sodium sulfonate).*
*ATC — B02BX02.*

**Pharmacopoeias.** *Jpn* includes Carbazochrome Sodium Sulfonate ($C_{10}H_{11}N_4NaO_5S,3H_2O$ = 376.3).

### Profile

Carbazochrome, an oxidation product of adrenaline, has been given as a haemostatic by mouth and by injection; it appears to be given as the dihydrate. It has also been used as the salicylate and the sodium sulfonate.

### Preparations

**Proprietary Preparations** (details are given in Part 3)
***Braz.:*** Adrenoplasma; Adrenoxil; ***Ger.:*** Adrenoxyl; ***Hong Kong:*** Adona; Adrezon†; ***India:*** Siochrome; Styptocid; ***Ital.:*** Adona; ***Jpn:*** Adona; ***Port.:*** Adrenoxil; ***Thai.:*** Neo-Hesna.

**Multi-ingredient:** ***India:*** Cadisper C; Siochrome; Styptocid; ***Ital.:*** Fleboside; ***Mex.:*** Hemosin-K; ***Spain:*** Cromoxin K; Flebeside; Perfus Multivitaminico; Quercetol Hemostatico†; Quercetol K†.

---

## Darbepoetin Alfa *(BAN, USAN, rINN)*

Darbepoetina alfa; NESP; Novel Erythropoiesis Stimulating Protein. 30-L-Asparagine-32-L-threonine-87-L-valine-88-L-asparagine-90-L-threonineerythropoietin (human).
*CAS — 209810-58-2.*
*ATC — B03XA02.*

### Adverse Effects and Precautions

As for Epoetins, p.747.

### Pharmacokinetics

Following subcutaneous injection the bioavailability of darbepoetin alfa is about 37% and absorption is slow. It undergoes extensive metabolism, with a terminal half-life of 21 hours after intravenous, and 49 hours after subcutaneous, use.

### Uses and Administration

Darbepoetin alfa is an analogue of the endogenous protein hormone erythropoietin with similar properties to the epoetins (p.748). It is used in the management of anaemia associated with chronic renal failure (see Normocytic-normochromic Anaemia, p.734) and for anaemia caused by chemotherapy in patients with non-myeloid malignancies.

For anaemia associated with chronic renal failure in adults and children aged 11 years and older, darbepoetin alfa is given by subcutaneous or intravenous injection in an initial dose of 450 nanograms/kg once weekly, as a single injection. The dose should be adjusted at intervals of not less than 4 weeks, according to response, until the target haemoglobin concentration is achieved. Maintenance doses may be given once every 1 or 2 weeks.

For anaemia in patients with non-myeloid malignancies, darbepoetin alfa is given subcutaneously in an initial dose of 2.25 micrograms/kg once weekly. If the response is inadequate after 4 to 6 weeks, the dose may be increased to 4.5 micrograms/kg once weekly, and continued until approximately 4 weeks after the end of chemotherapy. However, if the response is still inadequate 4 weeks after doubling the dose, further therapy with darbepoetin alfa may not be effective.

◊ Reviews.

1. Ibbotson T, Goa KL. Darbepoetin alfa. *Drugs* 2001; **61:** 2097–2104.
2. Joy MS. Darbepoetin alfa: a novel erythropoiesis-stimulating protein. *Ann Pharmacother* 2002; **36:** 1183–92.
3. Cvetkovic RS, Goa KL. Darbepoetin alfa in patients with chemotherapy-related anaemia. *Drugs* 2003; **63:** 1067–74.

### Preparations

**Proprietary Preparations** (details are given in Part 3)
***Austral.:*** Aranesp; ***Austria:*** Aranesp; ***Denm.:*** Aranesp; ***Fin.:*** Aranesp; ***Fr.:*** Aranesp; ***Ger.:*** Aranesp; ***Gr.:*** Aranesp; ***Irl.:*** Aranesp; ***Israel:*** Aranesp; ***Ital.:*** Nespo; ***Neth.:*** Aranesp; ***Norw.:*** Aranesp; ***Port.:*** Aranesp; ***Spain:*** Aranesp; ***Swed.:*** Aranesp; ***UK:*** Aranesp; ***USA:*** Aranesp.

---

## Dextran 1 *(BAN, rINN)*

Dextrán 1; Dextranum 1.
*CAS — 9004-54-0 (dextran).*
*ATC — B05AA05.*

**Pharmacopoeias.** In *Eur.* (see p.vi) and *US.*

**Ph. Eur. 5.0** (Dextran 1 for Injection). A low-molecular-weight fraction of dextran, consisting of a mixture of isomalto-oligosaccharides. It is obtained by hydrolysis and fractionation of dextrans produced by fermentation of sucrose using a certain strain or substrains of *Leuconostoc mesenteroides.* The average relative molecular mass is about 1000.

A white or almost white, hygroscopic powder. Very soluble in water; very slightly soluble in alcohol.

**USP 27** (Dextran 1). A low-molecular-weight fraction of dextran, consisting of a mixture of isomalto-oligosaccharides. It is obtained by controlled hydrolysis and fractionation of dextrans produced by fermentation of certain strains of *Leuconostoc mesenteroides,* in the presence of sucrose. It is a glucose polymer in which the linkages between glucose units are almost exclusively α-1,6. Its weight average molecular weight is about 1000.

A white to off-white, hygroscopic powder. Very soluble in water; sparingly soluble in alcohol. pH of a 15% solution in water is between 4.5 and 7.0. Store at a temperature between 4° and 30°.

### Uses and Administration

Dextran 1 is used to prevent severe anaphylactic reactions to infusions of dextran. It is reported to occupy the binding sites of dextran-reactive antibodies and so prevent the formation of large immune complexes with higher molecular weight dextrans.

Dextran 1 is given in usual doses of 20 mL of a solution containing 150 mg/mL by intravenous injection about 1 to 2 minutes before the infusion of the higher molecular weight dextran; the interval should not exceed 15 minutes. A suggested dose for children is 0.3 mL/kg. The dose of dextran 1 should be repeated if further infusions of dextran are required more than 48 hours after the initial dose.

◊ Two large multicentre studies (involving about 29 200 and 34 950 patients) have suggested that dextran 1 prevented anaphylactic reactions by hapten inhibition in a dose-dependent way.[1,2] It did not reduce the incidence of mild reactions, which are not generally mediated by antibodies. Another large study[3] comparing the effects of giving dextran 1 either 2 minutes before injection of dextran 40 or 70 or mixed with the injection, was discontinued after the occurrence of 2 severe reactions in the admixture group. A comparison[4] of severe anaphylactic reactions to dextran infusion during the period 1983 to 1992 (when prophylaxis with dextran 1 was used) with reactions reported during the period 1975 to 1979 (no prophylaxis) found that the use of dextran 1 was associated with a 35-fold reduction in severe anaphylactic reactions to dextran infusion.

There were 21, 20, and 2 adverse reactions to dextran 1 in the first 3 studies respectively, including nausea, skin reactions, bradycardia, and hypotension. Apart from one patient, reactions to dextran 1 were mild and were considered to be of minor clinical importance. In the fourth study, side-effects to dextran 1 were reported in approximately one case per 100 000 doses.

1. Ljungström K-G, *et al.* Prevention of dextran-induced anaphylactic reactions by hapten inhibition I: a Scandinavian multicenter study on the effects of 10 mL dextran 1, 15% administered before dextran 70 or dextran 40. *Acta Chir Scand* 1983; **149:** 341–8.
2. Renck H, *et al.* Prevention of dextran-induced anaphylactic reactions by hapten inhibition III: Scandinavian multicenter study on the effects of 20 mL dextran 1, 15% administered before dextran 70 or dextran 40. *Acta Chir Scand* 1983; **149:** 355–60.
3. Renck H, *et al.* Prevention of dextran-induced anaphylactic reactions by hapten inhibition II: a comparison of the effects of 20 mL dextran 1, 15% administered either admixed to or before dextran 70 or dextran 40. *Acta Chir Scand* 1983; **149:** 349–53.
4. Ljungström K-G. Hapten inhibition of dextran reactions. Ten years' experience with dextran 1. *Br J Anaesth* 1995; **74** (suppl 1): 127.

### Preparations

**Proprietary Preparations** (details are given in Part 3)
***Austral.:*** Promit; ***Austria:*** Praedex; Promit; ***Denm.:*** Promiten; ***Fr.:*** Promit†; ***Ger.:*** Promit; ***Norw.:*** Promiten; ***S.Afr.:*** Promit; ***Swed.:*** Promiten; ***Switz.:*** Promit; ***USA:*** Promit.

---

## Dextran 40 *(BAN, USAN, rINN)*

Dextrán 40; Dextranum 40; LMD; LMWD; Low-molecular-weight Dextran; LVD.
*CAS — 9004-54-0 (dextran).*
*ATC — B05AA05.*

**Pharmacopoeias.** In *Chin., Jpn, Pol.,* and *US.*
*Eur.* (see p.vi) and *Jpn* describe Dextran 40 for Injection.

**Ph. Eur. 5.0** (Dextran 40 for Injection). A mixture of polysaccharides, principally of the α-1,6-glucan type, obtained by hydrolysis and fractionation of dextrans produced by fermentation of sucrose using a certain strain or substrains of *Leuconostoc mesenteroides.* The average relative molecular mass is about 40 000.

A white or almost white powder. Very soluble in water; very slightly soluble in alcohol.

**USP 27** (Dextran 40). It is derived by controlled hydrolysis and fractionation of polysaccharides elaborated by the fermentative action of certain strains of *Leuconostoc mesenteroides* on a sucrose substrate. It is a glucose polymer in which the linkages between glucose units are almost entirely of the α-1:6 type. Its weight average molecular weight is in the 35 000 to 45 000 range. A 10% solution in water has a pH of 4.5 to 7.0. Store at a temperature of 25°, excursions permitted between 15° and 30°.

**Incompatibility.** Incompatibilities may arise from the slightly acid pH of dextran 40 preparations.

### Adverse Effects, Treatment, and Precautions

As for Dextran 70, p.746.

Rapid renal excretion of dextran 40 in patients with reduced urine flow can result in high urinary concentrations which increase urinary viscosity and may cause oliguria or acute renal failure. Therefore, infusions of dextran 40 are contra-indicated in renal disease with oliguria; should anuria or oliguria occur during treatment dextran 40 should be withdrawn. Dehydration should preferably be corrected before administration of dextran 40. Dextran 40 can cause capillary oozing of wound surfaces.

**Effects on the kidneys.** Acute renal failure has been associated with dextran 40[1-3] and less frequently with dextran 70.[1] The mechanism of the effect is still unclear[2-5] but low-molecular-weight dextran has been cited[1] as a common cause of drug-induced acute renal failure. Dextran should be withheld if the urine output falls during administration and diuresis induced with diuretics and a high fluid intake. Plasmapheresis has been used successfully to remove dextran from the circulation.[2]

1. Feest TG. Low molecular weight dextran: a continuing cause of acute renal failure. *BMJ* 1976; **2:** 1300.
2. Moran M, Kapsner C. Acute renal failure associated with elevated plasma oncotic pressure. *N Engl J Med* 1987; **317:** 150–3.
3. Druml W, *et al.* Dextran-40, acute renal failure, and elevated plasma oncotic pressure. *N Engl J Med* 1988; **318:** 252–3.
4. Stein HD. Dextran-40, acute renal failure, and elevated plasma oncotic pressure. *N Engl J Med* 1988; **318:** 253.
5. Moran M, Kapsner C. Dextran-40, acute renal failure, and elevated plasma oncotic pressure. *N Engl J Med* 1988; **318:** 253–4.

**Effects on the lungs.** In a study[1] of 45 women undergoing gynaecological surgery, 25 received 400 to 500 mL of a 10% solution of dextran 40 intraperitoneally for prevention of adhesions. After 5 to 7 days, 12 of the dextran group and none of the controls had a pleural effusion visible on chest X-ray. The effusions were small to moderate, asymptomatic, and resolved without treatment.

1. Adoni A, *et al.* Postoperative pleural effusion caused by dextran. *Int J Gynaecol Obstet* 1980; **18:** 243–74.

**Hypersensitivity.** For reports of anaphylactic reactions associated with administration of dextran 40, see Dextran 70, below, and Dextran 1, above.

### Pharmacokinetics

After intravenous infusion dextran 40 is slowly metabolised to glucose. About 70% of a dose is excreted unchanged in the urine within 24 hours. A small amount is excreted into the gastrointestinal tract and eliminated in the faeces.

### Uses and Administration

Dextran 40 is a plasma volume expander used in the management of hypovolaemic shock (p.835). As a 10% solution, dextran 40 exerts a slightly higher colloidal osmotic pressure than plasma proteins and thus produces a greater expansion of plasma volume than dextrans of a higher molecular weight, although the expansion may have a shorter duration because of more rapid renal excretion. Dextran 40 also reduces blood viscosity and inhibits sludging or aggregation of red blood cells. It is used in the prophylaxis and treatment of postoperative thromboembolic disorders, in conditions where improved circulatory flow is required, and as a priming solution during extracorporeal circulation.

Dextran 40 is given by intravenous infusion as a 10% solution in sodium chloride 0.9% or glucose 5%. Doses depend on the clinical condition of the patient.

In shock, a maximum of 20 mL/kg during the first 24 hours has been recommended; the first 10 mL/kg may be given by rapid intravenous infusion. Doses of up to 10 mL/kg may be given daily thereafter for up to 5 days. Dehydration should preferably be corrected before dextran 40 is administered.

In the treatment of thromboembolic disorders a suggested regimen is 500 to 1000 mL over 4 to 6 hours on the first day, then 500 mL over 4 to 6 hours on the next and subsequent alternate days for not more than 10 days.

For prophylaxis of postoperative thromboembolic disorders, 500 mL over 4 to 6 hours may be given during or at the end of surgery and the dose repeated on the next day; treatment may be continued in high risk patients on alternate days for up to 10 days.

Infants may be given up to 5 mL/kg and children up to 10 mL/kg.

A dose of 10 to 20 mL/kg has been added to extracorporeal perfusion fluids.

Dextran 40 is also an ingredient of artificial tears.

**Venous thromboembolism.** Dextran 40 is only one of a variety of drugs that have been used for the prophylaxis of venous thromboembolism (p.839) resulting from surgical operations. In hip replacement surgery[1] warfarin and dextran 40 gave similar protection whereas in general surgery[2] heparin was better than dextran 40 in preventing deep-vein thrombosis. Dextran 40 was considerably less effective than a combination of antithrombin III and heparin in total knee arthroplasty.[3]

1. Harris WH, *et al.* Prevention of venous thromboembolism following total hip replacement: warfarin vs dextran 40. *JAMA* 1972; **220:** 1319–22.
2. Gruber UF, *et al.* Prevention of postoperative thromboembolism by dextran 40, low doses of heparin, or xantinol nicotinate. *Lancet* 1977; **i:** 207–10.
3. Francis CW, *et al.* Prevention of venous thrombosis after total knee arthroplasty: comparison of antithrombin III and low-dose heparin with dextran. *J Bone Joint Surg Am* 1990; **72-A;** 976–82.

### Preparations

***BP 2003:*** Dextran 40 Intravenous Infusion;
***USP 27:*** Dextran 40 in Dextrose Injection; Dextran 40 in Sodium Chloride Injection.

**Proprietary Preparations** (details are given in Part 3)
***Austral.:*** Rheomacrodex†; ***Austria:*** Elorheo; Laevodex†; Onkovertin N†; Rheofusin; Rheomacrodex; ***Braz.:*** Isodex†; Rheomacrodex†; ***Canad.:*** Gentran 40; Rheomacrodex†; ***Denm.:*** Rheomacrodex; ***Fr.:*** Plasmacair†; Rheomacrodex†; ***Ger.:*** Infukoll M 40; Longasteril 40; Onkovertin N†; Rheomacrodex; Thomaedex 40†; ***Gr.:*** Rheomacrodex; ***Israel:*** Rheomacrodex; ***Ital.:*** Eudextran; Plander R; Solplex 40; ***Mex.:*** Rheomacrodex; ***Norw.:*** Rheomacrodex; ***Port.:*** Neodextril 40†; ***S.Afr.:*** Rheomacrodex; ***Spain:*** Rheomacrodex; ***Swed.:*** Perfadex; Rheomacrodex; ***Switz.:*** Rheomacrodex; ***Thai.:*** Onkovertin; ***UK:*** Gentran 40; Rheomacrodex†; ***USA:*** Gentran 40; Rheomacrodex.

**Multi-ingredient:** ***Braz.:*** Volumax D 40; ***Canad.:*** Ocutears†; ***Port.:*** Bas-Dextrano.

## Dextran 60

Dextrán 60.
*ATC — B05AA05.*

**Pharmacopoeias.** *Eur.* (see p.vi) describes Dextran 60 for Injection.

**Ph. Eur. 5.0** (Dextran 60 for Injection). A mixture of polysaccharides, principally of the α-1,6-glucan type, obtained by hydrolysis and fractionation of dextrans produced by fermentation of sucrose using a certain strain or substrains of *Leuconostoc mesenteroides*. The average relative molecular mass is about 60 000.

A white or almost white powder. Very soluble in water; very slightly soluble in alcohol.

**Incompatibility.** Incompatibilities may arise from the slightly acid pH of dextran 60 preparations.

### Profile

Dextran 60 is a plasma volume expander with actions and uses similar to those of dextran 70 (below). It is given by intravenous infusion as a 3 or 6% solution in sodium chloride 0.9% or a mixture of electrolytes.

Dextran 60 is also used topically for dry eyes.

### Preparations

**Proprietary Preparations** (details are given in Part 3)
***Austria:*** Laevodex†; Macrodex; Onkovertin†; ***Fr.:*** Dialens†; Hemodex†; ***Ger.:*** Macrodex; Onkovertin†; Thomaedex 60†; ***Mex.:*** Rescuesol; ***Norw.:*** Plasmodex; ***Swed.:*** Plasmodex; ***Switz.:*** Dialens.

## Dextran 70 *(BAN, USAN, rINN)*

Dextrán 70; Dextranum 70; Polyglucin (dextran).
*CAS — 9004-54-0 (dextran).*
*ATC — B05AA05.*

**Pharmacopoeias.** In *Chin., Jpn, Pol.,* and *US.*
*Eur.* (see p.vi) describes Dextran 70 for Injection.

**Ph. Eur. 5.0** (Dextran 70 for Injection). A mixture of polysaccharides, principally of the α-1,6-glucan type, obtained by hydrolysis and fractionation of dextrans produced by fermentation of sucrose using a certain strain or substrains of *Leuconostoc mesenteroides*. The average relative molecular mass is about 70 000.

A white or almost white powder. Very soluble in water; very slightly soluble in alcohol.

**USP 27** (Dextran 70). It is derived by controlled hydrolysis and fractionation of polysaccharides elaborated by the fermentative action of certain appropriate strains of *Leuconostoc mesenteroides* on a sucrose substrate. It is a glucose polymer in which the linkages between glucose units are almost entirely of the α-1:6 type. Its weight average molecular weight is in the 63 000 to 77 000 range. A 6% solution in water has a pH of 4.5 to 7.0. Store at a temperature of 25°, excursions permitted between 15° and 30°.

**Incompatibility.** Incompatibilities may arise from the slightly acid pH of dextran 70 preparations.

**Storage.** Crystals may form in solutions of dextran if they are stored at low temperatures. These may be redissolved by warming for a short time.

### Adverse Effects and Treatment

Infusions of dextrans may occasionally produce hypersensitivity reactions such as fever, nasal congestion, joint pains, urticaria, hypotension, and bronchospasm. Severe anaphylactic reactions occur rarely and may be fatal. Dextran-reactive antibodies may arise in response to dietary or bacterial polysaccharides in patients who have not previously received dextran. Nausea and vomiting have also been reported. These reactions are treated symptomatically after withdrawal of the dextran.

Dextran 1 (p.745) may be used to block the formation of dextran-reactive antibodies and hence the hypersensitivity reactions.

**Effects on the blood.** Disseminated intravascular coagulation and acute respiratory distress syndrome developed following hysteroscopy during which 1200 mL of dextran 70 was used to dilate the uterus.[1] The large volume used was considered to have contributed to the reaction by increasing the systemic absorption of the dextran solution.

1. Jedeikin R, *et al.* Disseminated intravascular coagulopathy and adult respiratory distress syndrome: life-threatening complications of hysteroscopy. *Am J Obstet Gynecol* 1990; **162:** 44–5.

**Effects on the kidneys.** For a report of acute renal failure associated with use of dextran 70, see Dextran 40, above.

**Hypersensitivity.** In a retrospective study of allergic reactions to dextran 40 and dextran 70 reported in Sweden from 1970 to 1979,[1] there were 478 reports of reactions, 458 of which were considered to be due to dextran, out of 1 365 266 infusions given. There was a male to female ratio of 1.5 to 1 for all reactions and a ratio of 3 to 1 for the most severe reactions. The mean age of the patients was higher in those with severe reactions. Of the 28 fatal reactions, 27 occurred within 5 minutes of the start of the infusion and 25 when less than 25 mL had been infused. Three of the fatal reactions occurred after a test dose of only 0.5 to 1 mL and it was strongly recommended that such test doses should not be used.

An anaphylactic reaction has also been reported[2] more than 75 minutes after intraperitoneal instillation. After successful symptomatic treatment symptoms recurred 20 minutes later, due to slow absorption of dextran from the peritoneal cavity. No further reaction occurred after removal of 200 mL of intraperitoneal fluid by culdocentesis.

Anaphylactoid reactions after BCG vaccination have been attributed to hypersensitivity to dextran in the formulation.[3,4]

The use of dextran 1 for the prevention of hypersensitivity reactions is discussed under that monograph (p.745).

1. Ljungström K-G, *et al.* Adverse reactions to dextran in Sweden 1970–1979. *Acta Chir Scand* 1983; **149:** 253–62.
2. Borten M, *et al.* Recurrent anaphylactic reaction to intraperitoneal dextran 75 used for prevention of postsurgical adhesions. *Obstet Gynecol* 1983; **61:** 755–7.
3. Rudin C, *et al.* Anaphylactoid reaction to BCG vaccination. *Lancet* 1991; **337:** 377.
4. Pönnighaus JM, *et al.* Hypersensitivity to dextran in BCG vaccine. *Lancet* 1991; **337:** 1039.

### Precautions

Dextran infusions produce a progressive dilution of oxygen-carrying capacity, coagulation factors, and plasma proteins and may overload the circulation. They are therefore contra-indicated in patients with severe heart failure, bleeding disorders such as hypofibrinogenaemia or thrombocytopenia, or renal failure and should be used with caution in patients with renal impairment, haemorrhage, chronic liver disease, or those at risk of developing pulmonary oedema or heart failure. Central venous pressure should be monitored during the initial period of infusion to detect fluid overload. Also patients should be watched closely during the early part of the infusion period, and the infusion stopped immediately if signs of anaphylactic reactions appear. Infusions should also be stopped if there are signs of oliguria or renal failure. The haematocrit should not be allowed to fall below 30% and all patients should be observed for early signs of bleeding complications. The bleeding time may be increased especially in patients receiving large volumes of dextrans. Deficiency of coagulation factors should be corrected and fluid and electrolyte balance maintained. Dehydration should be corrected before or at least during dextran infusions, in order to maintain an adequate urine flow.

The anticoagulant effect of heparin may be enhanced by dextran.

The higher molecular weight dextrans may interfere with blood grouping and cross-matching of blood, while the lower molecular weight dextrans may interfere with some methods. Therefore, whenever possible, a sample of blood should be collected before giving the dextran infusion and kept frozen in case such tests become necessary.

The presence of dextran may interfere with the determination of glucose, bilirubin, or protein in blood or urine.

### Pharmacokinetics

After intravenous infusion dextrans with a molecular weight of less than 50 000 are excreted unchanged by the kidney. Dextrans with a molecular weight greater than 50 000 are slowly metabolised to glucose. Small amounts of dextrans are excreted into the gastrointestinal tract and eliminated in the faeces.

About 50% of dextran 70 is excreted unchanged in the urine within 24 hours.

### Uses and Administration

Dextran 70 is a plasma volume expander used in the management of hypovolaemic shock (p.835). As a 6% solution dextran 70 exerts a colloidal osmotic pressure similar to that of plasma proteins and thus produces less expansion of plasma volume than dextrans of a lower molecular weight, although the expansion may have a longer duration because of less rapid renal excretion. Dextran 70 also reduces blood viscosity and inhibits sludging or aggregation of red blood cells. It is used in the prophylaxis of postoperative thromboembolic disorders (p.839).

Dextran 70 is given by intravenous infusion as a 6% solution in sodium chloride 0.9% or glucose 5%.

Doses depend on the severity of the plasma loss and on the degree of haemoconcentration.

In shock, the usual initial dose for rapid expansion of plasma volume is 500 to 1000 mL infused at a rate of 20 to 40 mL/minute. A suggested maximum dose is

20 mL/kg during the first 24-hour period and 10 mL/kg per day thereafter; treatment should not continue for longer than 3 days. Patients may also require administration of blood, coagulation factors, and electrolytes.

For the prophylaxis of pulmonary embolism or venous thrombosis in moderate- to high-risk patients undergoing surgery, a dose of 500 to 1000 mL may be given over 4 to 6 hours either during or immediately after surgery. A dose of 500 mL should be given on the next day and in high-risk patients on subsequent alternate days for up to 2 weeks after the operation.

A 32% solution of dextran 70 has been instilled into the uterus in a dose of 50 to 100 mL as a rinsing and dilatation fluid to aid hysteroscopy.

Dextran 70 is also an ingredient of artificial tears.

### Preparations

***BP 2003:*** Dextran 70 Intravenous Infusion;
***USP 27:*** Dextran 70 in Dextrose Injection; Dextran 70 in Sodium Chloride Injection.

**Proprietary Preparations** (details are given in Part 3)
***Austral.:*** Hyskon; Macrodex†; ***Canad.:*** Gentran 70; Hyskon†; Macrodex†; ***Denm.:*** Macrodex; RescueFlow; ***Ger.:*** Hyskon†; Longasteril 70; RescueFlow; ***Israel:*** Macrodex; ***Ital.:*** Plander; Solplex 70; ***Mex.:*** Macrodex; ***Norw.:*** Macrodex; RescueFlow; ***Port.:*** Neodextril 70; ***S.Afr.:*** Macrodex; ***Spain:*** Macrodex†; ***Swed.:*** Macrodex; RescueFlow; ***Switz.:*** Macrodex; ***UK:*** Gentran 70; Macrodex†; RescueFlow; ***USA:*** Gentran 70; Hyskon; Macrodex.

**Multi-ingredient:** ***Arg.:*** Alcon Lagrimas; ***Austral.:*** Bion Tears†; Poly-Tears; Tears Naturale; Visine Advanced Relief; ***Belg.:*** Alcon Adequad; Lacrystat; Tears Naturale; ***Braz.:*** Lacrima; Lacrima Plus; Volumax D 70; ***Canad.:*** Aquasite†; Bion Tears; Tears Naturale; ***Chile:*** Naphtears; Nicotears; Tears Naturale; ***Denm.:*** Dacriosol; ***Ger.:*** Isopto Naturale†; ***Gr.:*** Tears Natural; ***Hong Kong:*** Bion Tears; ***Irl.:*** Tears Naturale; ***Israel:*** Tears Naturale; ***Ital.:*** Dacriosol; ***Malaysia:*** Dacrolux; Tears Naturale; ***Norw.:*** Tears Naturale; ***NZ:*** Poly-Tears; Tears Naturale; Visine Advanced Relief; ***Port.:*** Tears Naturale; ***S.Afr.:*** Tears Naturale; ***Singapore:*** Bion Tears; Dacrolux; Tears Naturale; ***Spain:*** Dacrolux; Tears Humectante; ***Swed.:*** Bion Tears; Tears Naturale†; ***Switz.:*** Tears Naturale; ***Thai.:*** Bion Tears; Tears Naturale; ***UK:*** Tears Naturale; ***USA:*** Advanced Relief Visine; Aquasite; Bion Tears; Lacri-Tears; LubriTears; Moisture Drops; Nature's Tears; Ocucoat; Tears Naturale; Tears Renewed.

## Dextran 75 *(BAN, USAN, rINN)*

Dextrán 75; Dextranum 75.
*CAS — 9004-54-0 (dextran).*
*ATC — B05AA05.*

### Profile

Dextran 75 consists of dextrans (glucose polymers) of weight average molecular weight about 75 000 that are derived from the dextrans produced by the fermentation of sucrose by means of a certain strain of *Leuconostoc mesenteroides*.

Dextran 75 is a plasma volume expander with actions and uses similar to dextran 70 (p.746). It is given by intravenous infusion as a 6% solution in sodium chloride 0.9% or glucose 5%.

## Dextran 110 *(BAN, rINN)*

Dextrán 110; Dextranum 110.
*CAS — 9004-54-0 (dextran).*
*ATC — B05AA05.*

### Profile

Dextran 110 consists of dextrans (glucose polymers) of weight average molecular weight about 110 000 that are derived from dextrans produced by the fermentation of sucrose by means of a certain strain of *Leuconostoc mesenteroides*.

Dextran 110 is a plasma volume expander with actions and uses similar to dextran 70 (p.746). It has been given by intravenous infusion as a 6% solution.

# Epoetins

Epoetinas.
*ATC — B03XA01.*

**Description.** Erythropoietin is a glycosylated protein hormone and a haematopoietic growth factor produced primarily in the kidneys.

Erythropoietin for clinical use is produced by recombinant DNA technology and the name epoetin is often applied to such material. Epoetin alfa, epoetin beta, epoetin gamma, and epoetin omega are recombinant human erythropoietins derived from a cloned human erythropoietin gene. All have the same 165 amino acid sequence but differ in the glycosylation pattern. Epoetin delta is a recombinant human erythropoietin derived from a genetically engineered continuous human cell line. It has the same amino acid sequence and glycosylation pattern as human erythropoietin.

**Pharmacopoeias.** *Eur.* (see p.vi) includes Erythropoietin Concentrated Solution.

**Ph. Eur. 5.0** (Erythropoietin Concentrated Solution). A clear or slightly turbid colourless solution, containing 0.05 to 1% of glycoproteins indistinguishable from naturally occurring human erythropoietin in terms of amino acid sequence and glycosylation pattern. It has a potency of not less than 100 000 units per mg of active substance. Store in airtight containers below −20° and avoid repeated freezing and thawing.

## Epoetin Alfa *(BAN, USAN, rINN)*

EPO. 1–165-Erythropoietin (human clone λHEPOFL13 protein moiety), glycoform α.
*CAS — 113427-24-0.*
*ATC — B03XA01.*

## Epoetin Beta *(BAN, USAN, rINN)*

BM-06.019; EPOCH. 1–165-Erythropoietin (human clone λHEPOFL13 protein moiety), glycoform β.
*CAS — 122312-54-3.*
*ATC — B03XA01.*

## Epoetin Delta *(USAN, rINN)*

GA-EPO; HMR-4396. 1–165-Erythropoietin (human HMR4396), glycoform δ.
*CAS — 261356-80-3.*
*ATC — B03XA01.*

## Epoetin Gamma *(BAN, rINN)*

BI-71.052. 1–165-Erythropoietin (human clone λHEPOFL13 protein moiety), glycoform γ.
*CAS — 130455-76-4.*
*ATC — B03XA01.*

## Epoetin Omega *(rINN)*

1–165-Erythropoietin (human clone λHEPOFL13 protein moiety), glycoform ω.
*CAS — 148363-16-0.*
*ATC — B03XA01.*

**Stability.** Proprietary preparations of recombinant human erythropoietin may contain albumin or amino acids for stability. Administration to neonates may necessitate making very dilute solutions. A study of the stability of epoetin alfa in various intravenous fluids[1] found that a minimum of 0.05% protein was required to prevent loss of drug from solutions containing epoetin alfa 0.1 units/mL. In another study,[2] 0.0125% albumin was sufficient to prevent loss of drug from a solution containing epoetin alfa 100 units/mL.

1. Ohls RK, Christensen RD. Stability of human recombinant epoetin alfa in commonly used neonatal intravenous solutions. *Ann Pharmacother* 1996; **30:** 466–8.
2. Widness JA, Schmidt RL. Comment: epoetin alfa loss with NaCl 0.9% dilution. *Ann Pharmacother* 1996; **30:** 1501–2.

### Adverse Effects

Headache, hypertension, and seizures have been reported in patients treated with recombinant human erythropoietin particularly in those with poor renal function. These adverse effects are probably associated with haemodynamic changes produced by the increase in haematocrit. In patients with normal or low blood pressure there have been isolated reports of hypertensive crisis with encephalopathy-like symptoms, including headache and confusion, and generalised seizures. Other adverse effects include thrombosis at vascular access sites and clotting in the dialyser, transient increases in the platelet count, flu-like symptoms including chills and myalgia, hyperkalaemia, and skin rashes. There have been rare reports of anaphylactoid reactions. Pure red cell aplasia has been reported rarely in patients with chronic renal failure (see below).

◊ General references.

1. Macdougall IC. Adverse reactions profile: erythropoietin in chronic renal failure. *Prescribers' J* 1992; **32:** 40–4.

**Effects on the blood.** Changes in rheological properties of the blood following recombinant human erythropoietin therapy were attributed to high red cell aggregation, possibly due to hyperfibrinogenaemia.[1] The increased viscosity could have contributed to an early kidney graft thrombosis in 1 patient[2] and a delay in the onset of graft function in 7 others.[3] Pre-operative haemodilution was suggested as a possible solution.[3]

Pure red cell aplasia has been reported rarely in patients with chronic renal failure after months to years of treatment with epoetin alfa; most patients have been found to have antibodies to epoetins.[4] The effect appears to be brand specific[5-7] and associated particularly with the subcutaneous use of preparations containing polysorbate 80 as a stabiliser.[8]

1. Koppensteiner R, *et al.* Changes in determinants of blood rheology during treatment with haemodialysis and recombinant human erythropoietin. *BMJ* 1990; **300:** 1626–7.
2. Zaoui P, *et al.* Early thrombosis in kidney grafted into patient treated with erythropoietin. *Lancet* 1988; **ii:** 956.
3. Wahlberg J, *et al.* Haemodilution in renal transplantation in patients on erythropoietin. *Lancet* 1988; **ii:** 1418.
4. Casadevall N, *et al.* Pure red-cell aplasia and antierythropoietin antibodies in patients treated with recombinant erythropoietin. *N Engl J Med* 2002; **346:** 469–75.
5. Gershon SK, *et al.* Pure red-cell aplasia and recombinant erythropoietin. *N Engl J Med* 2002; **346:** 1584–5.
6. Casadevall N, Mayeux P. Pure red-cell aplasia and recombinant erythropoietin. *N Engl J Med* 2002; **346:** 1585. Correction. *ibid.*; **347:** 458.
7. Macdougall IC. Pure red cell aplasia with anti-erythropoietin antibodies occurs more commonly with one formulation of epoetin alfa than another. *Curr Med Res Opin* 2004; **20:** 83–6.
8. Janssen-Ortho. Important drug safety information: Eprex (epoetin alfa) sterile solution revised prescribing information for patients with chronic renal failure (January 13, 2004). Available at: http://www.hc-sc.gc.ca/hpfb-dgpsa/tpd-dpt/eprex3_hpc_e.html (accessed 23/06/04)

**Effects on electrolytes.** Hyperkalaemia and hyperphosphataemia may occur in patients receiving recombinant human erythropoietin. However, hypophosphataemia has also been reported in cirrhotic patients given erythropoietin before autologous blood donation.[1]

1. Kajikawa M, *et al.* Recombinant human erythropoietin and hypophosphatemia in patients with cirrhosis. *Lancet* 1993; **341:** 503–4.

**Effects on mental function.** Visual hallucinations occurred in 4 patients during treatment with recombinant human erythropoietin, stopped when treatment was withdrawn, and re-occurred in 2 patients when erythropoietin was reinstituted.[1] Commenting on these and a further 7 cases,[2] the manufacturers considered the reaction to be extremely rare and that the contribution of concurrent medication could not be discounted. In two groups of dialysis patients treated with recombinant human erythropoietin, 15 of 134 and 2 of 103 experienced visual hallucinations.[3] Increasing age appeared to be a risk factor.

1. Steinberg H. Erythropoietin and visual hallucinations. *N Engl J Med* 1991; **325:** 285.
2. Stead RB. Erythropoietin and visual hallucinations. *N Engl J Med* 1991; **325:** 285.
3. Steinberg H, *et al.* Erythropoietin and visual hallucinations in patients on dialysis. *Psychosomatics* 1996; **37:** 556–63.

**Effects on the skin.** Skin rashes may occur during treatment with recombinant human erythropoietin.

Pseudoporphyria cutanea tarda, a photosensitivity disorder, has been reported in 2 children undergoing peritoneal dialysis and receiving erythropoietin.[1] However, it was pointed out that this disorder has occurred in adults undergoing dialysis and the children were also receiving other potentially photosensitising drugs.

1. Harvey E, *et al.* Pseudoporphyria cutanea tarda: two case reports on children receiving peritoneal dialysis and erythropoietin therapy. *J Pediatr* 1992; **121:** 749–52.

**Effects on the spleen.** Aggravation of splenomegaly was reported in 2 patients with myeloproliferative disorders following use of recombinant human erythropoietin.[1] Splenic infarction has been reported in a patient with aplastic anaemia given erythropoietin.[2]

1. Iki S, *et al.* Adverse effect of erythropoietin in myeloproliferative disorders. *Lancet* 1991; **337:** 187–8.
2. Imashuku S, *et al.* Splenic infarction after erythropoietin therapy. *Lancet* 1993; **342:** 182–3.

**Effects of subcutaneous injection.** More pain at the injection site was experienced by patients given subcutaneous injections of epoetin alfa than in those given epoetin beta.[1,2] It was suggested that different excipients in the two formulations could be responsible.[1,2]

1. Frenken LAM, *et al.* Assessment of pain after subcutaneous injection of erythropoietin in patients receiving haemodialysis. *BMJ* 1991; **303:** 288.
2. Lui SF, *et al.* Pain after subcutaneous injection of erythropoietin. *BMJ* 1991; **303:** 856.

**Treatment of adverse effects.** Venesection successfully reduced the blood pressure in 4 patients with life-threatening hypertension unresponsive to antihypertensive therapy associated with recombinant human erythropoietin treatment.[1]

1. Fahal IH, *et al.* Phlebotomy for erythropoietin-associated malignant hypertension. *Lancet* 1991; **337:** 1227.

### Precautions

Recombinant human erythropoietin should be used with caution in patients with hypertension, a history of seizures, thrombocytosis, chronic hepatic impairment, ischaemic vascular disease, or in patients with malignant tumours. Hypertension should be well controlled before treatment is started and the blood pressure monitored during treatment.

Response to recombinant human erythropoietin may be diminished by iron deficiency, infection or inflammatory disorders, haemolysis, or aluminium intoxication. Anaemia due to folic acid and vitamin $B_{12}$ deficiencies should also be excluded, since these may also reduce the response. Patients developing sudden lack of efficacy should be investigated. If pure red cell aplasia is diagnosed treatment should be discontinued and testing for epoetin antibodies considered; patients should not be transferred to another epoetin.

Patients undergoing dialysis may require increased doses of heparin in view of the increase in packed cell volume.

Platelet counts and serum-potassium concentrations should be monitored regularly.

Dosage must be carefully controlled to avoid too fast an increase in haematocrit and recommended haematocrit levels should not be exceeded due to the increased risk of thrombotic events.

◊ A study[1] involving 1233 patients undergoing haemodialysis and suffering from heart failure or ischaemic heart disease found that erythropoietin in doses sufficient to increase haematocrit to 42% (within the normal range) was associated with lack of benefit and a trend towards increased mortality when compared with administration in doses sufficient to maintain a lower haematocrit of around 30%. However, these results are difficult to interpret, since within each group, increased haematocrit was associated with lower mortality, despite the between-group differences. The possibility that intravenous iron supplementation might have contributed to these adverse results was considered, but commentators suggested that until further data was available aiming for a haematocrit of 33 to 36%, and using intravenous iron supplementation where necessary, was still appropriate.[2]

1. Besarab A, *et al.* The effects of normal as compared with low hematocrit values in patients with cardiac disease who are receiving hemodialysis and epoetin. *N Engl J Med* 1998; **339:** 584–90.
2. Adamson JW, Eschbach JW. Erythropoietin for end-stage renal disease. *N Engl J Med* 1998; **339:** 625–7.

**Abuse.** Comments have been published on the dangers of the abuse of recombinant human erythropoietin by athletes as an alternative to 'blood doping'.[1-3] Haematocrit may continue to rise for several days after administration of recombinant human erythropoietin, possibly reaching dangerously high levels. Lack of medical supervision and fluid loss during endurance events increase the risk of serious adverse consequences of changes in blood viscosity produced by such misuse.

1. Scott WC. The abuse of erythropoietin to enhance athletic performance. *JAMA* 1990; **264:** 1660.
2. Adamson JW, Vapnek D. Recombinant erythropoietin to improve athletic performance. *N Engl J Med* 1991; **324:** 698–9.
3. Kennedy MC. Newer drugs used to enhance sporting performance. *Med J Aust* 2000; **173:** 314–17.

**Resistance.** Many factors may contribute to a poor response to recombinant human erythropoietin (see Precautions, above). A study in patients with anaemia of end-stage renal disease[1] found that inadequate dialysis was associated with a reduced response to erythropoietin treatment. Antibodies to recombinant human erythropoietin have also been reported.[2] Delayed clinical response to recombinant human erythropoietin in a patient[3] could have been due to an inherited subclinical pyruvate kinase deficiency.

1. Ifudu O, *et al.* The intensity of hemodialysis and the response to erythropoietin in patients with end-stage renal disease. *N Engl J Med* 1996; **334:** 420–5.
2. Peces R, *et al.* Antibodies against recombinant human erythropoietin in a patient with erythropoietin-resistant anemia. *N Engl J Med* 1996; **335:** 523–4.
3. Zachée P, *et al.* Pyruvate kinase deficiency and delayed clinical response to recombinant human erythropoietin treatment. *Lancet* 1989; **i:** 1327–8.

## Pharmacokinetics

Epoetin alfa and epoetin beta exhibit some differences in their pharmacokinetics, possibly due to differences in glycosylation and in the formulation of the commercial preparations.

Epoetin alfa is slowly and incompletely absorbed after subcutaneous injection, and a bioavailability of about 10 to 50% relative to intravenous administration has been reported. Peak concentrations after epoetin alfa intravenously are attained within 15 minutes, and within 4 to 24 hours following subcutaneous injection.

The elimination half-life of epoetin alfa after intravenous administration has been reported to be 4 to 16 hours in patients with chronic renal failure; the half-life is generally less in patients with normal renal function. An estimated elimination half-life of about 24 hours has been reported for epoetin alfa given subcutaneously.

Epoetin beta is similarly slowly and incompletely absorbed after subcutaneous injection, and its absolute bioavailability has been reported to be 23 to 42%. Peak serum concentrations are attained within 12 to 28 hours of subcutaneous administration. An elimination half-life of 4 to 12 hours has been reported following intravenous administration and a terminal half-life of 13 to 28 hours following subcutaneous administration.

◊ References.

1. Macdougall IC, *et al.* Clinical pharmacokinetics of epoetin (recombinant human erythropoietin). *Clin Pharmacokinet* 1991; **20:** 99–113.
2. Halstenson CE, *et al.* Comparative pharmacokinetics and pharmacodynamics of epoetin alfa and epoetin beta. *Clin Pharmacol Ther* 1991; **50:** 702–12.
3. Gladziwa U, *et al.* Pharmacokinetics of epoetin (recombinant human erythropoietin) after long term therapy in patients undergoing haemodialysis and haemofiltration. *Clin Pharmacokinet* 1993; **25:** 145–53.
4. Montini G, *et al.* Pharmacokinetics and hematologic response to subcutaneous administration of recombinant human erythropoietin in children undergoing long-term peritoneal dialysis: a multicenter study. *J Pediatr* 1993; **122:** 297–302.
5. Brown MS, *et al.* Single-dose pharmacokinetics of recombinant human erythropoietin in preterm infants after intravenous and subcutaneous administration. *J Pediatr* 1993; **122:** 655–7.

## Uses and Administration

Erythropoietin is a glycosylated protein hormone and a haematopoietic growth factor. It is secreted primarily by the kidneys, although a small amount is produced in extrarenal sites such as the liver. Erythropoietin regulates erythropoiesis by stimulating the differentiation and proliferation of erythroid precursors, stimulating the release of reticulocytes into the circulation, and stimulating the synthesis of cellular haemoglobin. The release of erythropoietin is promoted by hypoxia or anaemia, and up to 1000 times the normal serum-erythropoietin concentration may be reached under these conditions; this response may be impaired in some disease states such as chronic renal failure. The haematological response to erythropoietin is reduced if there is an inadequate supply of iron.

Epoetin alfa and epoetin beta are recombinant human erythropoietins available for clinical use that have the same pharmacological actions as endogenous erythropoietin. They are used in the management of anaemia associated with chronic renal failure in dialysis and predialysis patients; they may reduce or obviate the need for blood transfusions in these patients. They are also used in the management of chemotherapy-induced anaemia in patients with non-myeloid malignant disease. Epoetin alfa is used in zidovudine-related anaemia in HIV-positive patients. Epoetin beta is used in the management of anaemia of prematurity. Recombinant human erythropoietin is also being evaluated in the management of other types of normocytic-normochromic anaemias, including that associated with inflammatory disorders such as rheumatoid arthritis. In all patients, iron status should be monitored and supplementation provided if necessary.

Epoetin alfa and epoetin beta may also be used in patients with moderate anaemia (but no iron deficiency) before elective surgery to increase the yield of blood collected for autologous blood transfusion. Epoetin alfa may also be used in such patients to reduce the need for allogeneic blood transfusion.

In the management of **anaemia of chronic renal failure** epoetin alfa or epoetin beta may be given subcutaneously or intravenously, depending on the formulation. The aim of treatment is to increase the haemoglobin concentration to 10 to 12 g per 100 mL or to increase the haematocrit to 30 to 36%. The rate of rise in haemoglobin should be gradual to minimise side-effects such as hypertension; a rate not exceeding 2 g per 100 mL per month is suggested.

*Epoetin alfa* may be given by intravenous injection over at least 1 minute; slow intravenous injection over 5 minutes may be used in patients who experience flu-like symptoms as side-effects. Epoetin alfa may also be given subcutaneously, but preparations that contain polysorbate 80 should only be given intravenously in this group of patients (see Effects on the Blood, above). In predialysis and haemodialysis patients, a recommended initial dose of epoetin alfa is 50 international units/kg three times weekly; a higher initial dose of 50 to 100 units/kg three times weekly has been suggested in the USA. Doses may be increased at 4-week intervals in increments of 25 units/kg three times weekly until the target is reached. In patients on peritoneal dialysis an initial dose of 50 units/kg given intravenously twice weekly may be used. Once the target is reached doses may need to be adjusted, and even decreased, for maintenance therapy.

The usual total weekly maintenance dose of epoetin alfa in predialysis patients is 50 to 100 units/kg given in three divided doses, and in haemodialysis patients it is about 75 to 300 units/kg given in three divided doses. In predialysis patients a total weekly dose of 600 units/kg should not be exceeded. In patients on peritoneal dialysis, the usual total weekly maintenance dose is 50 to 100 units/kg given intravenously in two divided doses.

In children, epoetin alfa may be given intravenously to those on haemodialysis at an initial dose of 50 units/kg three times weekly. The dose may be increased at 4-week intervals in increments of 25 units/kg three times weekly until a target haemoglobin concentration of 9.5 to 11 g per 100 mL is reached; the usual total weekly maintenance dose given in three divided doses is: 225 to 450 units/kg for those weighing less than 10 kg; 180 to 450 units/kg for those weighing 10 to 30 kg; and 90 to 300 units/kg for those weighing over 30 kg.

*Epoetin beta* is used similarly in the management of anaemia of chronic renal failure in dialysis and predialysis patients. It may be given subcutaneously or by intravenous injection over 2 minutes. The following dosages may be used in adults and children. For subcutaneous injection the initial dose is 60 units/kg weekly for 4 weeks; the total weekly dose may be divided to be given in daily doses or three times a week. For intravenous injection the initial dose is 40 units/kg three times weekly for 4 weeks; the dose may then be increased to 80 units/kg three times weekly. Thereafter the dose of epoetin beta may be increased at 4-week intervals, for both subcutaneous and intravenous injection, in increments of 60 units/kg weekly in divided doses, until the target haemoglobin concentration or haematocrit is reached. A total weekly dose of 720 units/kg of epoetin beta should not be exceeded. For maintenance, the dose is halved initially and then adjusted every 1 to 2 weeks according to response. The weekly subcutaneous maintenance dose may be divided into 1, 3, or 7 doses; in patients stabilised on a once-weekly administration, it may be possible to adjust to a single dose every 2 weeks.

In patients with **non-myeloid malignant disease** receiving chemotherapy, epoetin alfa or epoetin beta may be given by subcutaneous injection in an initial dose of 150 units/kg three times weekly. The dose may be increased after 4 or 8 weeks, if necessary, to 300 units/kg three times weekly. If the response is still inadequate after 4 weeks at this higher dose, treatment should be discontinued. As alternative regimens, the total weekly dose of epoetin beta may be given as a single dose or divided into 3 to 7 doses. The rate of rise in haemoglobin should be gradual; a rate not exceeding 2 g per 100 mL per month is suggested. After the end of chemotherapy, epoetin alfa or epoetin beta may be continued for up to one month.

To increase the yield of **autologous blood**, epoetin alfa or epoetin beta may be used with iron supplementation. The dose depends on the volume of blood required for collection and on factors such as the patient's whole blood volume and haematocrit. Suggested regimens are: epoetin alfa 600 units/kg given intravenously twice weekly starting 3 weeks before surgery; or up to 800 units/kg of epoetin beta intravenously, or up to 600 units/kg subcutaneously, twice weekly for 4 weeks before surgery. To reduce the need for allogeneic blood transfusion epoetin alfa may be given in a dose of 600 units/kg subcutaneously once weekly starting 3 weeks before surgery, with a fourth dose given on the day of surgery; alternatively, when the time before surgery is short, 300 units/kg subcutaneously daily may be given for 10 days before surgery, on the day of surgery, and for 4 days after.

In **HIV-positive patients** on zidovudine therapy, epoetin alfa may be beneficial if the endogenous serum-erythropoietin concentration is 500 milliunits/mL or less. Epoetin alfa is given by subcutaneous or intravenous injection in an initial dose of 100 units/kg three times weekly for 8 weeks. The dose may then be increased every 4 to 8 weeks by 50 to 100 units/kg three times weekly according to response. However, patients are unlikely to benefit from doses above 300 units/kg three times weekly if this dose has failed to elicit a satisfactory response.

In the management of **anaemia of prematurity** epoetin beta is given subcutaneously in a dose of 250 units/kg three times weekly. Treatment should be started as early as possible and continued for 6 weeks.

◊ Reviews.


1. Markham A, Bryson HM. Epoetin alfa: a review of its pharmacodynamic and pharmacokinetic properties and therapeutic use in nonrenal applications. *Drugs* 1995; **49:** 232–54.
2. Dunn CJ, Markham A. Epoetin beta: a review of its pharmacological properties and clinical use in the management of anaemia associated with chronic renal failure. *Drugs* 1996; **51:** 299–318.
3. Beguin Y. A risk-benefit assessment of epoetin in the management of anaemia associated with cancer. *Drug Safety* 1998; **19:** 269–82.
4. Cheer SM, Wagstaff AJ. Epoetin beta: a review of its clinical use in the treatment of anaemia in patients with cancer. *Drugs* 2004; **64:** 323–46.


**Administration to neonates.** Recombinant human erythropoietin may be given to neonates for anaemia of prematurity (see Anaemias, below). It is usually administered by subcutaneous injection. Administration by intravenous infusion in total parenteral nutrition solutions produced satisfactory results in a group of 20 neonates.[1] Enteral administration was reported in one small study[2] to increase plasma-erythropoietin concentrations and peak reticulocyte counts, but in another larger study[3] it had no effect.

For a warning about diluting recombinant human erythropoietin solutions, see Stability, above.


1. Ohls RK, *et al.* Pharmacokinetics and effectiveness of recombinant erythropoietin administered to preterm infants by continuous infusion in total parenteral nutrition solution. *J Pediatr* 1996; **128:** 518–23.
2. Ballin A, *et al.* Erythropoietin, given enterally, stimulates erythropoiesis in premature infants. *Lancet* 1999; **353:** 1849.
3. Juul SE. Enterally dosed recombinant human erythropoietin does not stimulate erythropoiesis in neonates. *J Pediatr* 2003; **143:** 321–6.


**Anaemias.** Epoetins are used in normocytic-normochromic anaemias (p.734) associated with low endogenous erythropoietin concentrations.

Clinical studies have shown the effectiveness of epoetins in correcting the anaemia of end-stage renal disease in patients maintained by haemodialysis,[1,2] and they are also effective in anaemia in predialysis patients. Although several factors contribute to the aetiology of the anaemia, including blood loss associated with dialysis, the main cause is inadequate production of erythropoietin in the kidney. Consistently good results have been obtained with epoetins not only for correction of anaemia but also for quality of life and exercise capacity[3,4] and for improvements in haemostatic[5] and cardiorespiratory function.[6] Guidelines have been introduced for their use in chronic renal failure.[7]

Over 90% of patients with renal anaemia respond to treatment with epoetins.[8] Many factors may contribute to a poor response (see Precautions, above) and the patient should always be investigated and the cause corrected where possible.[8,9]

Epoetins may be administered intravenously or subcutaneously. Epoetin given subcutaneously produces lower but more sustained plasma concentrations and comparative studies have shown that total weekly maintenance doses are reduced by between 23 and 52% with subcutaneous rather than intravenous administration.[10,11] The subcutaneous route is thus preferred especially in patients not on haemodialysis. The frequency of administration may also be important in maximising the response to treatment;[12] daily subcutaneous administration has been reported to give a better response than the same total weekly dose given two or three times a week.[2] Intraperitoneal administration has also been investigated.[13]

Epoetins are also used to treat anaemias from other causes. Epoetins may be used for zidovudine-induced anaemia in AIDS patients, in chemotherapy-induced anaemia in patients with non-myeloid malignant disease (see Anaemia, p.496), and in anaemia of prematurity.[14-22] Epoetins have a potential application for other anaemias associated with impaired or insufficient erythropoietin production, such as anaemias in infants with bronchopulmonary dysplasia[23,24] and infants with haemolytic disease of the newborn,[25,26] postpartum anaemia,[27,28] and in arthritis[29-31] and inflammatory bowel disease.[32-34]


1. Winearls C. Treatment of anaemia in renal failure. *Prescribers' J* 1992; **32:** 238–44.
2. De Marchi S, *et al.* Erythropoietin and the anemia of chronic diseases. *Clin Exp Rheumatol* 1993; **11:** 429–44.
3. Canadian Erythropoietin Study Group. Association between recombinant human erythropoietin and quality of life and exercise capacity of patients receiving haemodialysis. *BMJ* 1990; **300:** 573–8.
4. Evans RW, *et al.* The quality of life of hemodialysis recipients treated with recombinant human erythropoietin. *JAMA* 1990; **263:** 825–30.
5. Moia M, *et al.* Improvement in the haemostatic defect of uraemia after treatment with recombinant human erythropoietin. *Lancet* 1987; **ii:** 1227–9.
6. Macdougall IC, *et al.* Long-term cardiorespiratory effects of amelioration of renal anaemia by erythropoietin. *Lancet* 1990; **335:** 489–93. Correction. *ibid.*; 614.
7. National Kidney Foundation. K/DOQI clinical practice guidelines for anemia of chronic kidney disease, 2000. *Am J Kidney Dis* 2001; **37** (suppl 1): S182–S238. Also available at: http://www.kidney.org/professionals/kdoqi/guidelines_updates/doqi_upex.html (accessed 23/06/04)
8. Macdougall IC. Poor response to erythropoietin. *BMJ* 1995; **310:** 1424–5.
9. Koury MJ. Investigating erythropoietin resistance. *N Engl J Med* 1993; **328:** 205–6.
10. Zachée P. Controversies in selection of epoetin dosages: issues and answers. *Drugs* 1995; **49:** 536–47.
11. Kaufman JS, *et al.* Subcutaneous compared with intravenous epoetin in patients receiving hemodialysis. *N Engl J Med* 1998; **339:** 578–83.
12. Abraham PA, *et al.* Controversies in determination of epoetin (recombinant human erythropoietin) dosages. *Clin Pharmacokinet* 1992; **22:** 409–15.
13. Taylor CA, *et al.* Clinical pharmacokinetics during continuous ambulatory peritoneal dialysis. *Clin Pharmacokinet* 1996; **31:** 293–308.
14. Bechensteen AG, *et al.* Erythropoietin, protein, and iron supplementation and the prevention of anaemia of prematurity. *Arch Dis Child* 1993; **69:** 19–23.
15. Maier RF, *et al.* The effect of epoetin beta (recombinant human erythropoietin) on the need for transfusion in very-low-birth-weight infants. *N Engl J Med* 1994; **330:** 1173–8.
16. Strauss RG. Erythropoietin and neonatal anemia. *N Engl J Med* 1994; **330:** 1227–8.
17. Shannon KM, *et al.* Recombinant human erythropoietin stimulates erythropoiesis and reduces erythrocyte transfusions in very low birth weight preterm infants. *Pediatrics* 1995; **95:** 1–8.
18. Wilimas JA, Crist WM. Erythropoietin—not yet a standard treatment for anemia of prematurity. *Pediatrics* 1995; **95:** 9–10.
19. Wandstrat TL, Kaplan B. Use of erythropoietin in premature neonates: controversies and the future. *Ann Pharmacother* 1995; **29:** 166–73.
20. Williamson P, *et al.* Blood transfusions and human recombinant erythropoietin in premature newborn infants. *Arch Dis Child* 1996; **75:** F65–F68.
21. Strauss RG. Recombinant erythropoietin for the anemia of prematurity: still a promise, not a panacea. *J Pediatr* 1997; **131:** 653–5.
22. Ohls RK, *et al.* The effect of erythropoietin on the transfusion requirements of preterm infants weighing 750 grams or less: a randomized, double-blind, placebo-controlled study. *J Pediatr* 1997; **131:** 661–5.
23. Ohls RK, *et al.* A randomized, double-blind, placebo-controlled trial of recombinant erythropoietin in treatment of the anemia of bronchopulmonary dysplasia. *J Pediatr* 1993; **123:** 996–1000.
24. Al-Kharfy T, *et al.* Erythropoietin therapy in neonates at risk of having bronchopulmonary dysplasia and requiring multiple transfusions. *J Pediatr* 1996; **129:** 89–96.
25. Ohls RK, *et al.* Recombinant erythropoietin as treatment for the late hyporegenerative anemia of Rh hemolytic disease. *Pediatrics* 1992; **90:** 678–80.
26. Scaradavou A, *et al.* Suppression of erythropoiesis by intrauterine transfusions in hemolytic disease of the newborn: use of erythropoietin to treat the late anemia. *J Pediatr* 1993; **123:** 279–84.
27. Huch A, *et al.* Recombinant human erythropoietin in the treatment of postpartum anemia. *Obstet Gynecol* 1992; **80:** 127–31.
28. Breymann C, *et al.* Use of recombinant human erythropoietin in combination with parenteral iron in the treatment of postpartum anaemia. *Eur J Clin Invest* 1996; **26:** 123–30.
29. Pincus T, *et al.* Multicenter study of recombinant human erythropoietin in correction of anemia in rheumatoid arthritis. *Am J Med* 1990; **89:** 161–8.
30. Murphy EA, *et al.* Study of erythropoietin in treatment of anaemia in patients with rheumatoid arthritis. *BMJ* 1994; **309:** 1337–8.
31. Peeters HRM, *et al.* Effect of recombinant human erythropoietin on anaemia and disease activity in patients with rheumatoid arthritis and anaemia of chronic disease: a randomised placebo controlled double blind 52 weeks clinical trial. *Ann Rheum Dis* 1996; **55:** 739–44.
32. Schreiber S, *et al.* Recombinant erythropoietin for the treatment of anemia in inflammatory bowel disease. *N Engl J Med* 1996; **334:** 619–23.
33. Gasché C, *et al.* Intravenous iron and erythropoietin for anemia associated with Crohn disease: a randomized, controlled trial. *Ann Intern Med* 1997; **126:** 782–7.
34. Dohil R, *et al.* Recombinant human erythropoietin for treatment of anemia for chronic disease in children with Crohn's disease. *J Pediatr* 1998; **132:** 155–9.


**Surgery.** Concern over the safety of blood transfusions and the need to conserve blood supplies has led to interest in methods of reducing blood use in surgery. Recombinant human erythropoietin has been used to increase the number of units harvested for autologous transfusion and to reduce transfusion requirements.[1] It has also been used as an alternative to blood transfusions.[2-4]


1. Goodnough LT, *et al.* Erythropoietin therapy. *N Engl J Med* 1997; **336:** 933–8.
2. Green D, Handley E. Erythropoietin for anemia in Jehovah's Witnesses. *Ann Intern Med* 1990; **113:** 720–1.
3. Busuttil D, Copplestone A. Management of blood loss in Jehovah's Witnesses. *BMJ* 1995; **311:** 1115–16.
4. Cothren C, *et al.* Blood substitute and erythropoietin therapy in a severely injured Jehovah's Witness. *N Engl J Med* 2002; **346:** 1097–8.


## Preparations

**Proprietary Preparations** (details are given in Part 3)

***Arg.:*** Eprex; Hemax; Pronivel; Recormon; ***Austral.:*** Eprex; ***Austria:*** Culat; Erypo; NeoRecormon; Recormon; ***Belg.:*** Eprex; NeoRecormon; Recormon†; ***Braz.:*** Eprex; Eritina; Eritromax; Hemax-Eritron; Mepotin; Recormon; Tinax; ***Canad.:*** Eprex; ***Chile:*** Eprex; Hypercrit; Recormon; ***Denm.:*** Eprex; NeoRecormon; Recormon†; ***Fin.:*** Eprex; NeoRecormon; ***Fr.:*** Eprex; NeoRecormon; Recormon†; ***Ger.:*** Eprex; Erypo; NeoRecormon; Recormon†; ***Gr.:*** Eprex; NeoRecormon; ***Hong Kong:*** Eprex; Recormon; ***India:*** Wepox; ***Irl.:*** Eprex; NeoRecormon; Recormon†; ***Israel:*** Eprex; Recormon; ***Ital.:*** Epoxitin; Eprex; Eritrogen†; Globuren; NeoRecormon; ***Jpn:*** Epogin; Espo; ***Malaysia:*** Eprex; ***Mex.:*** Bioyetin; Epomax; Eprex; Exetin-A; Hypercrit; Recormon; ***Neth.:*** Eprex; ***Norw.:*** Eprex; NeoRecormon; Recormon†; ***NZ:*** Eprex; Recormon; ***Port.:*** NeoRecormon; Recormon; ***S.Afr.:*** Eprex; Recormon; Repotin; ***Singapore:*** Eprex; Recormon; ***Spain:*** Epopen; Eprex; Erantin†; NeoRecormon; ***Swed.:*** Eprex; NeoRecormon; ***Switz.:*** Eprex; Recormon; ***Thai.:*** Eprex; Hemax; Recormon; ***UAE:*** Epotin; ***UK:*** Eprex; NeoRecormon; ***USA:*** Epogen; Procrit.

# Etamsylate *(BAN, rINN)*

Cyclonamine; E-141; Etamsilato; Etamsylatum; Ethamsylate *(USAN)*; MD-141. Diethylammonium 2,5-dihydroxybenzenesulphonate.

$C_{10}H_{17}NO_5S = 263.3.$

*CAS — 2624-44-4.*

*ATC — B02BX01.*

**Pharmacopoeias.** In *Eur.* (see p.vi) and *Pol.*

**Ph. Eur. 5.0** (Etamsylate). A white or almost white, crystalline powder. It shows polymorphism. Very soluble in water; soluble in dehydrated alcohol; practically insoluble in dichloromethane; freely soluble in methyl alcohol. A 10% solution in water has a pH of 4.5 to 5.6. Store in airtight containers. Protect from light.

## Adverse Effects and Precautions

Nausea, headache, and skin rash have occurred after administration of etamsylate. Transient hypotension has been reported following intravenous injection.

**Porphyria.** Etamsylate is considered to be unsafe in patients with porphyria because it has been shown to be porphyrinogenic in *animals*.

## Pharmacokinetics

Etamsylate is absorbed from the gastrointestinal tract. It is excreted unchanged, mainly in the urine. Etamsylate is distributed into breast milk.

## Uses and Administration

Etamsylate is a haemostatic that appears to maintain the stability of the capillary wall and correct abnormal platelet adhesion. It is given for the prophylaxis and control of haemorrhages from small blood vessels.

For short-term blood loss in menorrhagia a dose of 500 mg is given by mouth four times daily during menstruation. For the prophylaxis and treatment of periventricular haemorrhage in low birth-weight neonates 12.5 mg/kg is given by intramuscular or intravenous injection every 6 hours. For the control of haemorrhage following surgery etamsylate may be given to adults by mouth, or by intramuscular or intravenous injection in a dose of 250 to 500 mg; this dose may be repeated every 4 to 6 hours as necessary.

**Menorrhagia.** When administered during menstruation to women with idiopathic menorrhagia (p.1567), etamsylate was as effective as mefenamic acid in reducing uterine blood loss in 1 study,[1] but was ineffective in another.[2] A review, which included published and unpublished results from these and 2 earlier studies, reported that etamsylate produced about a 10 to 15% reduction in menstrual blood loss.[3]


1. Chamberlain G, *et al.* A comparative study of ethamsylate and mefenamic acid in dysfunctional uterine bleeding. *Br J Obstet Gynaecol* 1991; **98:** 707–11.
2. Bonnar J, Sheppard BL. Treatment of menorrhagia during menstruation: randomised controlled trial of ethamsylate, mefenamic acid, and tranexamic acid. *BMJ* 1996; **313:** 579–82.
3. Coulter A, *et al.* Treating menorrhagia in primary care: an overview of drug trials and a survey of prescribing practice. *Int J Technol Assess Health Care* 1995; **11:** 456–71.


**Neonatal intraventricular haemorrhage.** Etamsylate is one of several drugs that have been tried in the prevention of intraventricular haemorrhage in very low birth-weight infants (p.740). In a multicentre, placebo-controlled, double-blind study,[1] etamsylate was given in an initial dose of 12.5 mg/kg intravenously or intramuscularly within 1 hour of delivery, followed by the same dose intravenously every 6 hours for 4 days to a total dose of 200 mg/kg. Of 330 infants who had had no evidence of haemorrhage soon after delivery, the subsequent incidence of haemorrhage in the 162 who received etamsylate was reduced, particularly the more extensive grades when compared with the 168 who received placebo. Of a further 30 infants with evidence of periventricular haemorrhage before treatment, 21 were given etamsylate and 9 placebo; treatment with etamsylate limited the extension of bleeding. There was also a reduction in patent ductus arteriosus in the treated infants. However, a more recent study using the same dosage regimen,[2] showed little benefit on short-term follow-up. It was considered that the study size may have been too small and the drug administered too late; the initial dose was given within 4 hours of birth whereas, in the previous study, treatment was started within 1 hour of birth. Follow-up[3] of these infants at 2 years of age found that etamsylate had not reduced the risk of death, impairment, or disability.


1. Benson JWT, *et al.* Multicentre trial of ethamsylate for prevention of periventricular haemorrhage in very low birthweight infants. *Lancet* 1986; **ii:** 1297–1300.
2. The EC Ethamsylate Trial Group. The EC randomised controlled trial of prophylactic ethamsylate for very preterm neonates: early mortality and morbidity. *Arch Dis Child* 1994; **70:** F201–F205.
3. Elbourne D, *et al.* Randomised controlled trial of prophylactic etamsylate: follow up at 2 years of age. *Arch Dis Child Fetal Neonatal Ed* 2001; **84:** F183–F187.

## Preparations

**Proprietary Preparations** (details are given in Part 3)
**Arg.:** Impedil; **Belg.:** Dicynone; **Braz.:** Dicinone; **Chile:** Om-Dicynone; **Fr.:** Dicynone; **Ger.:** Altodor†; **India:** Alstat; Ethacid; Ethasyl; Hemsyl; **Irl.:** Dicynene; **Ital.:** Dicynone; Eselin; **Mex.:** Dicynone; **Singapore:** Dicynone†; **Spain:** Dicinone; Hemo 141; **Switz.:** Dicynone; **UK:** Dicynene.

# Etherified Starches

Almidón, éteres de; HES; Hydroxyethyl Starch. 2-Hydroxyethyl ether starch.

*CAS — 9005-27-0.*

*ATC — B05AA07.*

**Description.** Etherified starches are starches that are composed of more than 90% of amylopectin and that have been etherified to varying extents. In hetastarch (*BAN, USAN*) an average of 7 to 8 of the hydroxy groups in each 10 D-glucopyranose units of starch polymer have been converted into $OCH_2CH_2OH$ groups, whereas in pentastarch (*BAN, USAN*) an average of 4 to 5 of the hydroxy groups in each 10 D-glucopyranose units of the starch polymer have been converted to $OCH_2CH_2OH$ groups. Etherified starches also vary in terms of average molecular weight and the position of etherification within the glucopyranose unit.

**Incompatibility.** Hetastarch is incompatible with many compounds including a number of injectable antibacterials.

References.

1. Wohlford JG, Fowler MD. Visual compatibility of hetastarch with injectable critical-care drugs. *Am J Hosp Pharm* 1989; **46:** 995–6.
2. Wohlford JG, *et al.* More information on the visual compatibility of hetastarch with injectable critical-care drugs. *Am J Hosp Pharm* 1990; **47:** 297–8.

## Adverse Effects and Precautions

Hypersensitivity reactions including anaphylactic reactions have occurred after infusion of etherified starches.

Precautions that should be observed with plasma expanders are described under Dextran 70, p.746, and these should be considered when etherified starches are used. There does not appear to be any interference with blood grouping and cross-matching of blood.

**Effects on the blood.** Use of plasma expanders causes dilution of clotting factors and may also have direct effects on coagulation. Coagulopathy and haemorrhage has been reported in neurosurgical patients,[1,2] in a patient with coagulation defects,[3] and in a Jehovah's Witness[4] in whom large volumes of hetastarch solution were used during major orthopaedic surgery. It was suggested that hetastarch should probably be avoided in neurosurgical patients in whom the prevention of intracranial haemorrhage is critical, and in patients with a pre-existing bleeding disorder. Acquired type I von Willebrand's disease has been associated with the use of pentastarch.[5]

1. Symington BE. Hetastarch and bleeding complications. *Ann Intern Med* 1986; **105:** 627–8.
2. Damon L, *et al.* Intracranial bleeding during treatment with hydroxyethyl starch. *N Engl J Med* 1987; **317:** 964–5.
3. Abramson N. Plasma expanders and bleeding. *Ann Intern Med* 1988; **108:** 307.
4. Lockwood DNJ, *et al.* A severe coagulopathy following volume replacement with hydroxyethyl starch in a Jehovah's Witness. *Anaesthesia* 1988; **43:** 391–3.
5. Jonville-Béra A-P, *et al.* Acquired type I von Willebrand's disease associated with highly substituted hydroxyethyl starch. *N Engl J Med* 2001; **345:** 622–3.

**Effects on the kidneys.** Osmotic-nephrosis-like lesions found at biopsy in some transplanted kidneys have been attributed to use of solutions of etherified starches in the donor patient.[1] Such use has also been reported to impair immediate graft function.[2] However, another study[3] found no association between the use of these solutions in the donor patient and osmotic-nephrosis-like lesions or delayed graft function.

1. Legendre CH, *et al.* Hydroxyethylstarch and osmotic-nephrosis-like lesions in kidney transplantation. *Lancet* 1993; **342:** 248–9.
2. Cittanova ML, *et al.* Effect of hydroxethylstarch in brain-dead kidney donors on renal function in kidney-transplant recipients. *Lancet* 1996; **348:** 1620–22.
3. Coronel B, *et al.* Hydroxyethylstarch and renal function in kidney transplant recipients. *Lancet* 1997; **349:** 884.

**Effects on the skin.** Pruritus has been reported after infusion of etherified starches. A review[1] indicated that severe pruritus developed in 32% of patients and occurred, usually on the trunk, 3 days to 15 weeks after administration; the mean duration was nearly 9 weeks. Prolonged pruritus lasting more than 2 years has been reported.[2] Others[3] have reported a much lower incidence. The reaction is dose-dependent and usually refractory to treatment. There are individual reports of response to capsaicin.[4] Etherified starches have been shown to accumulate in the skin and other tissues but are eliminated over time.[5] Marked and persistent periocular swelling developed in a patient following 15 daily infusions of hetastarch.[6] Abnormal accumulation of hetastarch was found in the periocular tissues.

1. Gall H, *et al.* Persistierender Pruritus nach Hydroxyäthylstärke-Infusionen. *Hautarzt* 1993; **44:** 713–16.
2. Cox NH, Popple AW. Persistent erythema and pruritus, with a confluent histiocytic skin infiltrate, following the use of a hydroxyethylstarch plasma expander. *Br J Dermatol* 1996; **134:** 353–7.
3. Murphy M, *et al.* The incidence of hydroxyethyl starch-associated pruritus. *Br J Dermatol* 2001; **144:** 973–6.
4. Szeimies R-M, *et al.* Successful treatment of hydroxyethyl starch-induced pruritus with topical capsaicin. *Br J Dermatol* 1994; **131:** 380–2.
5. Sirtl C, *et al.* Tissue deposits of hydroxyethyl starch (HES): dose-dependent and time-related. *Br J Anaesth* 1999; **82:** 510–15.
6. Kiehl P, *et al.* Decreased activity of acid α-glucosidase in a patient with persistent periocular swelling after infusions of hydroxyethyl starch. *Br J Dermatol* 1998; **138:** 672–77.

## Pharmacokinetics

Etherified starches consist of mixtures of molecules with a range of molecular weights and with varying degrees of etherification. After intravenous infusion the molecules with a molecular weight of less than 50 000 are readily excreted unchanged by the kidney; larger molecules are metabolised and eliminated more slowly. The rate of metabolism depends upon the size of the molecule and the degree and position of etherification, with a high molecular weight, high degree of etherification, and etherification predominantly at the C2 position leading to a slower rate of metabolism and hence a longer duration of action. About 33% of a dose of high-molecular-weight hetastarch (weight average molecular weight 450 000) and about 70% of a dose of medium-molecular-weight pentastarch (weight average molecular weight 250 000) is excreted in the urine in 24 hours.

◊ References.

1. Mishler JM, *et al.* Changes in the molecular composition of circulating hydroxyethyl starch following consecutive daily infusions in man. *Br J Clin Pharmacol* 1979; **7:** 505–9.
2. Mishler JM, *et al.* Post-transfusion survival of hydroxyethyl starch 450/0.70 in man: a long-term study. *J Clin Pathol* 1980; **33:** 155–9.
3. Yacobi A, *et al.* Pharmacokinetics of hydroxyethyl starch in normal subjects. *J Clin Pharmacol* 1982; **22:** 206–12.

## Uses and Administration

Etherified starches are plasma volume expanders used in the management of hypovolaemic shock (p.835). Those most commonly used include high-molecular-weight hetastarch (weight average molecular weight 450 000 to 480 000) and medium-molecular-weight pentastarch (weight average molecular weight 200 000 to 250 000). Other etherified starches that are used include low-molecular-weight pentastarch and medium-molecular-weight hexastarch, which has a degree of etherification between that of pentastarch and hetastarch. A higher molecular weight hetastarch is also available. Iso-oncotic solutions of etherified starches, for example, 6% hetastarch or 6% medium-molecular-weight pentastarch, exert a similar colloidal osmotic pressure to human albumin, and when given by intravenous infusion produce an expansion of plasma volume slightly in excess of the infused volume. Hyperoncotic solutions, for example 10% medium-molecular-weight pentastarch, produce an expansion of plasma volume of about 1.5 times the infused volume. The duration of effect depends on the characteristics of the starch used; for 6% hetastarch the effect lasts for 24 to 36 hours.

Etherified starches are given intravenously as solutions in sodium chloride 0.9% or other electrolytes; concentrations used are usually 6 or 10%, although 3% solutions are also available for some. The dose and rate of infusion depend on the amount of fluid lost and degree of haemoconcentration; usual doses are in the range of 500 to 2500 mL daily, depending on the preparation used, and the infusion rate may be up to about 20 mL/kg per hour if necessary.

Hetastarch, hexastarch, and pentastarch increase the erythrocyte sedimentation rate when added to whole blood. They are therefore used in leucopheresis procedures to increase the yield of granulocytes. Doses of 250 to 700 mL may be added to venous blood in the ratio 1 part to at least 8 parts of whole blood in such procedures. Up to 2 such procedures per week and a total of 7 to 10 have been reported to be safe.

Hetastarch and hexastarch have also been used in extracorporeal perfusion fluids.

◊ References.

1. Treib J, *et al.* An international view of hydroxyethyl starches. *Intensive Care Med* 1999; **25:** 258–68.

**Administration in children.** A 6% solution of a low-molecular-weight etherified starch (average molecular weight 200 000) was considered effective and safe when compared with human albumin in the management of volume replacement in children under 3 years of age undergoing cardiac surgery.[1]

1. Boldt J, *et al.* Volume replacement with hydroxyethyl starch solutions in children. *Br J Anaesth* 1993; **70:** 661–5.

**Stroke.** Haemodilution with pentastarch has been tried in patients with acute ischaemic stroke (p.836) in an attempt to improve reperfusion of the brain by lowering blood viscosity. However, one study was terminated early when an excess mortality was noted in the haemodilution group.[1] The early fatalities occurred almost exclusively in patients with severe strokes; cerebral oedema was the main cause of death within one week of the onset of symptoms. Among the survivors neurological recovery was better among those who received haemodilution.

1. Hemodilution in Stroke Study Group. Hypervolemic hemodilution treatment of stroke: results of a randomized multicenter trial using pentastarch. *Stroke* 1989; **20:** 317–23.

## Preparations

**Proprietary Preparations** (details are given in Part 3)
**Arg.:** Hemohes; Infukoll HES; **Austria:** Elohast; Expafusin; Expahes; HAES-steril; Hyperhes; Isohes; Osmohes; Plasmasteril; Varihes; Voluven; **Belg.:** Elohaes†; HAES-steril†; Plasmasteril†; **Braz.:** Pentaspan; Plasmasteril†; **Canad.:** Pentaspan; **Chile:** Hemohes; **Denm.:** HAES-steril; Voluven; **Fin.:** HAES-steril; Hemohes; Plasmafusin; Voluven; **Fr.:** Elohes†; Heafusine; Hesteril; **Ger.:** Expafusin; Haemofusin; HAES-Rheopond; HAES-steril; Hemohes; HyperHAES; Infukoll HES; Plasmafusin; Plasmasteril; Rheohes; Serag-HAES; Voluven; **Gr.:** HAES-steril; **Israel:** HAES-sterile; **Ital.:** HAES-steril; Voluven; **Jpn:** Hespander; **Malaysia:** HAES-steril; **Mex.:** HAES-steril; Pentaspan; **Norw.:** HAES-steril; Voluven; **NZ:** Pentaspan; **Port.:** HAES-steril; Hemohes; HyperHAES; Voluven; **S.Afr.:** HAES-steril; **Singapore:** HAES-steril; Hemohes; **Spain:** Elohes; Expafusin†; HAES Esteril; Hesteril; Voluven; **Swed.:** HAES-steril; Hemohes; Voluven; **Switz.:** Elohast†; Expahes; HAES-steril; Hemohes; Isohes; Plasmasteril; Varihes; Voluven; **Thai.:** HAES-steril; Hespander; **UK:** Elohaes; HAES-steril; Hemohes; Hespan†; HyperHAES; Pentaspan†; Voluven; **USA:** Hespan; Pentaspan.

**Multi-ingredient: Norw.:** Hemohes; **Spain:** Hemohes.

# Factor VII

Proconvertin; SPCA; Stable Factor.

*ATC — B02BD05.*

**Description.** Factor VII is a plasma protein involved in blood coagulation. It may be obtained from human plasma or produced by recombinant DNA technology. The name Eptacog Alfa (Activated) is in use for a recombinant factor VIIa.

**Pharmacopoeias.** Many pharmacopoeias have monographs including *Eur.* (see p.vi).

**Ph. Eur. 5.0** (Human Coagulation Factor VII; Factor VII Coagulationis Humanus; Dried Factor VII Fraction BP 2003). A plasma protein fraction that contains the single-chain glycoprotein factor VII and may also contain small amounts of the activated form, the two-chain derivative factor VIIa, as well as coagulation factors II, IX, and X, and protein C and protein S. It is prepared from human plasma obtained from blood from healthy donors; the plasma is tested for the absence of hepatitis B surface antigen and antibodies against HIV-1 and HIV-2 and hepatitis C virus. The method of preparation is designed to minimise activation of any coagulation factor and includes a step or steps that have been shown to remove or inactivate known agents of infection. The factor VII fraction is dissolved in a suitable liquid, passed through a bacteria-retentive filter, distributed aseptically into the final containers, and immediately frozen. The preparation is freeze-dried and the containers sealed under vacuum or under an inert gas. Heparin, antithrombin, and other auxiliary substances such as a stabiliser may be added. No antimicrobial preservative is added. The specific activity is not less than 2 international units of factor VII per mg of protein before the addition of any protein stabiliser. When reconstituted as stated on the label the resulting solution contains not less than 15 international units/mL.

A white, pale yellow, green, or blue hygroscopic powder or friable solid. Store in airtight containers. Protect from light.

### Eptacog Alfa (Activated) (*BAN, rINN*)

Blood-coagulation factor VII (human clone λHVII2463 protein moiety).

*CAS — 102786-52-7; 102786-61-8;.*

*ATC — B02BD08.*

## Units

The potency of factor VII is expressed in international units and preparations may be assayed using the International Standard for blood coagulation factor VII concentrate, human (1998).

The potency of factor VIIa (activated factor VII) is expressed in international units and preparations may be assayed using the first International Standard for blood coagulation factor VIIa concentrate (1993).

### Adverse Effects and Precautions

Administration of factor VIIa (activated factor VII) may be associated with minor skin reactions, fever, headache, and changes in blood pressure. Factor VIIa should be used with caution in patients with conditions associated with circulating tissue factor, such as advanced atherosclerosis, crush injury, or septicaemia, since there is a risk of precipitating thrombosis or disseminated intravascular coagulation.

### Uses and Administration

Factor VII may be used as replacement therapy in patients with rare genetic deficiencies of factor VII.

Factor VIIa (activated factor VII) is used to treat bleeding episodes and to prevent bleeding associated with surgery in patients with haemophilia A or haemophilia B (p.737) who have developed antibodies to factor VIII or factor IX, respectively. It may also be used in acquired haemophilia, congenital factor VII deficiency, and Glanzmann's thrombasthenia. Factor VIIa may also be useful in patients with von Willebrand's disease. Factor VIIa is given as the recombinant form, eptacog alfa (activated). Eptacog alfa (activated) 100 micrograms is equivalent to 5000 international units.

In the treatment of bleeding episodes in patients with haemophilia, an initial dose of eptacog alfa (activated) 90 micrograms/kg is given by intravenous bolus injection. Further doses may be given as required to achieve and maintain haemostasis, initially every 2 to 3 hours. The dose may then be adjusted (effective doses have ranged from 35 to 120 micrograms/kg), or the dosing interval increased, according to response. Treatment may need to be continued for up to 3 weeks or more following serious bleeding episodes. A similar regimen may be used in patients with haemophilia when they undergo an invasive procedure or surgery, in which case the initial dose should be given immediately before the intervention.

In factor VII deficiency, the usual dose of eptacog alfa (activated) for treating bleeding episodes due to surgery or invasive procedures is 15 to 30 micrograms/kg every 4 to 6 hours until haemostasis is achieved.

In Glanzmann's thrombasthenia that is refractory to platelet transfusions, the usual dose of eptacog alfa (activated) for treating bleeding episodes or preventing bleeding due to surgery or invasive procedures is 90 micrograms/kg every 2 hours; at least 3 doses should be given.

◊ Reviews.

1. Poon MC. Use of recombinant factor VIIa in hereditary bleeding disorders. *Curr Opin Hematol* 2001; **8:** 312–18.
2. Midathada MV, *et al.* Recombinant factor VIIa in the treatment of bleeding. *Am J Clin Pathol* 2004; **121:** 124–37.

### Preparations

**Ph. Eur.:** Human Coagulation Factor VII.

**Proprietary Preparations** (details are given in Part 3)
***Arg.:*** NovoSeven; ***Austral.:*** NovoSeven; ***Austria:*** NovoSeven; ***Belg.:*** NovoSeven; ***Braz.:*** NovoSeven; ***Canad.:*** NiaStase; ***Denm.:*** NovoSeven; ***Fin.:*** NovoSeven; ***Fr.:*** Acset†; NovoSeven; ***Ger.:*** NovoSeven; ***Hong Kong:*** NovoSeven; ***Irl.:*** NovoSeven; ***Israel:*** NovoSeven; ***Ital.:*** NovoSeven; Provertin-UM TIM 3; ***Jpn:*** NovoSeven; ***Malaysia:*** NovoSeven; ***Neth.:*** NovoSeven; ***Norw.:*** NovoSeven; ***NZ:*** NovoSeven; ***S.Afr.:*** NovoSeven; ***Singapore:*** NovoSeven; ***Spain:*** NovoSeven; ***Swed.:*** NovoSeven; ***Switz.:*** NovoSeven; ***Thai.:*** NovoSeven; ***UK:*** NovoSeven; ***USA:*** NovoSeven.

**Multi-ingredient:** ***Spain:*** Hemofactor HT†.

## Factor VIII

AHF; Antihaemophilic Factor.

*ATC — B02BD02.*

**Description.** Factor VIII is a plasma protein involved in blood coagulation. It may be obtained from human plasma or produced by recombinant DNA technology. The names Moroctocog Alfa (see below) and Octocog Alfa (see below) are in use for recombinant factor VIII.

**Pharmacopoeias.** Many pharmacopoeias have monographs including *Eur.* (see p.vi) and *US.*

**Ph. Eur. 5.0** (Human Coagulation Factor VIII; Factor VIII Coagulationis Humanus; Dried Factor VIII Fraction BP 2003). A plasma protein fraction that contains the glycoprotein coagulation factor VIII with varying amounts of von Willebrand factor, depending on the method of preparation. It is prepared from human plasma obtained from blood from healthy donors; the plasma is tested for the absence of hepatitis B surface antigen and antibodies against HIV-1 and HIV-2 and hepatitis C virus. The method of preparation includes a step or steps that have been shown to remove or inactivate known agents of infection. The factor VIII fraction is dissolved in an appropriate liquid, passed through a bacteria-retentive filter, distributed aseptically into the final containers, and immediately frozen. The preparation is freeze-dried and the containers sealed under vacuum or under an inert gas. Auxiliary substances such as a stabiliser may be added. No antimicrobial preservative is added. The specific activity is not less than 1 international unit of factor VIII:C per mg of total protein before the addition of any protein stabiliser. When reconstituted as stated on the label the resulting solution contains not less than 20 international units of factor VIII:C per mL.

A white or pale yellow hygroscopic powder or friable solid. Store in airtight containers. Protect from light.

**Ph. Eur. 5.0** (Human Coagulation Factor VIII (rDNA); Factor VIII Coagulationis Humanus (ADNr)). A freeze-dried preparation of glycoproteins having the same activity as coagulation factor VIII in human plasma. It is prepared as full-length factor VIII (octocog alfa), or as a shortened two-chain structure (relative molecular mass 90 000 and 80 000), in which the B-domain has been deleted from the heavy chain (moroctocog alfa). Full-length human rDNA coagulation factor VIII contains 25 potential *N*-glycosylation sites, 19 in the B-domain of the heavy chain, 3 in the remaining part of the heavy chain (relative molecular mass 90 000) and 3 in the light chain (relative molecular mass 80 000).

Human coagulation factor VIII (rDNA) is produced by recombinant DNA technology in mammalian cell culture. Auxiliary substances such as a stabiliser may be added. A white or slightly yellow powder or friable mass. pH of the reconstituted preparation is 6.5 to 7.5. Protect from light.

**USP 27** (Antihemophilic Factor). A sterile freeze-dried powder containing the factor VIII fraction prepared from units of human venous plasma that have been tested for the absence of hepatitis B surface antigen, obtained from whole-blood donors and pooled; it may contain heparin sodium or sodium citrate. It contains not less than 100 units per g of protein. Unless otherwise specified it should be stored at 2° to 8° in hermetically-sealed containers. It should be used within 4 hours of reconstitution and should be administered with equipment that includes a filter.

A white or yellowish powder. On reconstitution it is opalescent with a slight blue tinge or is a yellowish liquid.

**USP 27** (Cryoprecipitated Antihemophilic Factor). A sterile frozen concentrate of human antihaemophilic factor prepared from the cryoprotein fraction, rich in factor VIII, of human venous plasma obtained from suitable whole-blood donors from a single unit of plasma derived from whole blood or by plasmapheresis, collected and processed in a closed system. It contains no preservative. It has an average potency of not less than 80 units per container. It should be stored at or below −18° in hermetically-sealed containers. It should be thawed to 20° to 37° before use; this liquid should be stored at room temperature and used within 6 hours of thawing; it should also be used within 4 hours of opening the container and administered with equipment that includes a filter.

A yellowish frozen solid. On thawing it becomes a very viscous, yellow, gummy liquid.

### Moroctocog Alfa *(BAN, rINN)*

(1—742)-(1637—1648)-Blood-coagulation factor VIII (human reduced) complex with 1649—2332-blood-coagulation factor VIII (human reduced).

**Pharmacopoeias.** *Eur.* (see p.vi) includes under the title Human Coagulation Factor VIII (rDNA) (see above).

### Octocog Alfa *(BAN, rINN)*

Bay-w-6240; Factor VIII (rDNA). Blood-coagulation factor VIII (human), glycoform α.

*CAS — 139076-62-3;.*

**Pharmacopoeias.** *Eur.* (see p.vi) includes under the title Human Coagulation Factor VIII (rDNA) (see above).

### Units

The potency of factor VIII is expressed in international units and preparations may be assayed using the sixth International Standard for blood coagulation factor VIII concentrate, human (1998).

### Adverse Effects and Precautions

Allergic reactions may sometimes follow the use of factor VIII preparations and chills, urticaria, and fever experienced by some patients may be allergic manifestations. Headache may occur. There is the possibility of intravascular haemolysis in patients with blood groups A, B, or AB receiving high doses or frequently repeated doses of factor VIII preparations due to the content of blood group isoagglutinins; also massive doses of some preparations may produce hyperfibrinogenaemia. Such risks should be reduced with more highly purified preparations.

Factor VIII preparations have been associated with the transmission of some viral infections, including hepatitis B and C, and more notably transmission of HIV. Strenuous efforts are now undertaken to screen the donor material from which factor VIII material is obtained and new methods of manufacture have also been introduced with the aim of inactivating any viruses present. Vaccination against hepatitis B is recommended for patients not already immune. Recombinant preparations are also available.

Some patients develop antibodies to factor VIII and, although large doses of preparations of both factor VIII and factor IX or porcine or highly purified factor VIII concentrates may be effective in the management of such patients, some patients remain resistant to treatment.

**Effects on blood platelets.** Thrombocytopenia was associated with administration of porcine factor VIII concentrate in 2 patients.[1] Platelet aggregation was noted in addition in 1 patient. Platelet counts improved when treatment with factor VIII was withdrawn.

1. Green D, Tuite GF. Declining platelet counts and platelet aggregation during porcine VIII:C infusions. *Am J Med* 1989; **86:** 222–4.

**Resistance.** Some patients with haemophilia A develop inhibitory antibodies to factor VIII. The risk is highest within the first 20 to 100 treatments. Low-titre antibodies are usually transient and overcome by increased or continuing treatment with factor VIII. With high-titre highly responding antibodies, however, bleeding episodes may need to be managed with factor VIII inhibitor bypassing fraction (activated prothrombin complex concentrate), or recombinant factor VIIa. Highly responding antibodies can be eradicated by immune tolerance regimens, using regular infusion of factor concentrates over long periods, with additional immunosuppression and immuno-adsorption in some cases.[1]

There have also been reports of lack of effect with the use of the recombinant factor VIII, moroctocog alfa, for prophylaxis, in patients who have no evidence of antibodies to factor VIII.[2]

1. Bolton-Maggs PHB, Pasi KJ. Haemophilias A and B. *Lancet* 2003; **361:** 1801–9.
2. Wyeth Canada. Important safety information about Refacto® (moroctocog alfa), antihemophilic factor (recombinant) [BDDr-FVIII] (September 15, 2003). Available at: http://www.hc-sc.gc.ca/hpfb-dgpsa/tpd-dpt/refacto_hpc_e.html (accessed 23/06/04)

**Transmission of infections.** Treatment with heat or chemicals and efforts to screen the donor material from which factor VIII and other clotting factors are obtained seem to have overcome problems with transmission of HIV and hepatitis B and C, although there is concern that non-lipid-enveloped viruses, such as human parvovirus B19 and hepatitis A, may still be transmitted. A solvent-detergent-treated factor VIII product[1-4] and a similar factor IX product[4] have been associated with reports of hepatitis A in patients with haemophilia and vaccination against hepatitis A has been recommended for patients treated with these factor preparations. Plasma-derived factor VIII preparations or recombinant preparations containing added albumin may carry a risk of transmission of Creutzfeldt-Jakob disease (see under Blood, p.744). It has been pointed out[5] that, since recombinant factor VIII is prepared from mammalian cell lines, there is a theoretical risk of transmission of infection with recombinant preparations.

1. Prowse C. Hepatitis A virus infection: no conclusive link to factor VIII. *BMJ* 1993; **307:** 561–2.
2. Thomas DP. Viral contamination of blood products. *Lancet* 1994; **343:** 1583–4.
3. Colvin BT. Viral contamination of blood products. *Lancet* 1994; **344:** 405.
4. Anonymous. Hepatitis A among persons with hemophilia who received clotting factor concentrate—United States, September-December 1995. *JAMA* 1996; **275:** 427–8.
5. Foster PR, *et al.* Hepatitis C and haemophilia. *BMJ* 1995; **311:** 754–5.

### Pharmacokinetics

◊ References.

1. Messori A, *et al.* Clinical pharmacokinetics of factor VIII in patients with classic haemophilia. *Clin Pharmacokinet* 1987; **13:** 365–80.
2. Björkman S, *et al.* Pharmacokinetics of factor VIII in humans: obtaining clinically relevant data from comparative studies. *Clin Pharmacokinet* 1992; **22:** 385–95.

### Uses and Administration

Factor VIII is used as replacement therapy in patients with haemophilia A (p.737), a genetic deficiency of factor VIII.

Preparations of factor VIII may be derived from human plasma or recombinant sources. They are used to control bleeding episodes in the treatment of patients with haemophilia A and to prevent bleeding episodes in such patients undergoing dental and surgical procedures. They may also be used for long-term prophylaxis in patients with severe haemophilia A.

Preparations of factor VIII are given by slow intravenous infusion. The dosage of factor VIII should be determined for each patient and will vary with the circumstances involving bleeding or type of surgery to be performed. In adults, a dose of 1 unit/kg has been reported to raise the plasma concentration of factor VIII by about 2% (of normal). A suggested formula to calculate, approximately, the dose required for a given effect is:

units = wt (kg) × 0.5 × % desired increase (of normal)

Recommended doses vary depending on the preparation used, but the following have been suggested: for mild to moderate haemorrhage the plasma concentration of factor VIII should be raised to 20 to 30% of normal, usually achieved with a single dose of 10 to 15 units/kg; for more serious haemorrhage or minor surgery it should be raised to 30 to 50% of normal, achieved with a usual initial dose of 15 to 25 units/kg followed by 10 to 15 units/kg every 8 to 12 hours if required; and for severe haemorrhage or major surgery an increase to 80 to 100% of normal may be necessary, achieved with a usual initial dose of 40 to 50 units/kg followed by 20 to 25 units/kg every 8 to 12 hours.

For prophylaxis in severe haemophilia A, doses of 10 to 50 units/kg every 2 or 3 days, as required, may be used.

In patients with inhibitory antibodies to human factor VIII, a porcine factor VIII preparation may be used in doses of 25 to 100 units/kg depending upon the severity of the haemorrhage.

Cryoprecipitate is an alternative source of clotting factors and contains factor VIII, factor XIII, von Willebrand's factor, fibrinogen, and fibronectin. Some factor VIII concentrates also contain von Willebrand's factor and these preparations or cryoprecipitate may be used in the management of von Willebrand's disease. Commercial very highly purified and recombinant factor VIII preparations do not contain appreciable amounts of von Willebrand's factor and are thus ineffective.

**Administration.** Surgical prophylaxis or significant haemorrhage in patients with haemophilia A is usually managed with injections of factor VIII given intravenously every 8 to 12 hours. Continuous intravenous infusion prevents wide fluctuations in factor VIII plasma concentrations and has been used successfully following major surgery in patients with haemophilia.[1-3]

1. Bona RD, *et al.* The use of continuous infusion of factor concentrates in the treatment of hemophilia. *Am J Hematol* 1989; **32:** 8–13.
2. Martinowitz U, *et al.* Adjusted dose continuous infusion of factor VIII in patients with haemophilia A. *Br J Haematol* 1992; **82:** 729–34.
3. Hawkins TE, *et al.* Treatment of haemophilia A by continuous factor VIII infusion. *Aust N Z J Med* 1995; **25:** 37–9.

## Preparations

***Ph. Eur.:*** Human Coagulation Factor VIII; Human Coagulation Factor VIII (rDNA);
***USP 27:*** Antihemophilic Factor; Cryoprecipitated Antihemophilic Factor.

**Proprietary Preparations** (details are given in Part 3)
***Arg.:*** Emoclot; Fanhdi; Haemoctin SDH; Hemofil M; Immunate; Koate-DVI; Monarc-M; Recombinate; ReFacto; ***Austral.:*** AHF; Kogenate; Recombinate; ReFacto; ***Austria:*** Beriate; Haemate P; Helixate; Immunate; Kogenate; Monoclate-P; Octanate; Recombinate; ReFacto; ***Belg.:*** Kogenate†; Recombinate†; ReFacto; ***Braz.:*** Beriate P; Emoclot†; Fatori 8Y; Haemate P; Immunate†; Koate; Kryobulin†; Monoclate-P; Vueffe; ***Canad.:*** Koate-HP†; Kogenate; Recombinate; ***Chile:*** Fanhdi; Koate-DVI; Octanate; ***Denm.:*** Bioclate†; Haemate; Helixate; Kogenate; Monoclate-P; Nordiate†; Recombinate; ReFacto; ***Fin.:*** Amofil; Helixate†; Recombinate; ReFacto; ***Fr.:*** Factane; Helixate; Hemofil M; Kogenate; Monoclate-P; Recombinate; ReFacto; ***Ger.:*** Beriate P; Bioclate†; Fanhdi; Haemate; Haemoctin SDH; Helixate; Hemofil; Immunate; Kogenate; Monoclate-P; Octanate; Profilate; Recombinate; ReFacto; ***Gr.:*** Hemofil M; Kogenate; Recombinate; Refacto; ***Hong Kong:*** Alphanate; Haemate P; Hemofil M; Koate-DVI; Recombinate; ***Irl.:*** Haemate P; Kogenate; Monoclate-P; ReFacto; ***Israel:*** Haemate P; Haemoctin SDM; Hemofil M; Hyate:C; Koate-HP; Monarc-M; Monoclate-P; Omrixate; Profilate; ***Ital.:*** Alphanate; Beriate P; Emoclot; Fanhdi; Haemate; Helixate; Hemofil M; Immunate; Koate-HS†; Kogenate; Kryobulin TIM 3-I†; Recombinate; ReFacto; Uman-Cry DI; Vueffe; ***Jpn:*** Recombinate; ***Malaysia:*** Alphanate; Hemofil; Koate-DVI; ***Mex.:*** Emoclot; Koate-DVI; Koate-HP†; Monoclate-P†; ***Neth.:*** Haemate; Helixate; Kogenate; ***Norw.:*** Kogenate; Octavi†; Octonativ-M†; ***NZ:*** AHF; Kogenate; Recombinate; ***Port.:*** Fanhdi; Haemoctin SDH; Hemofil M†; Kogenate†; Recombinate†; ReFacto; ***S.Afr.:*** Haemosolvate; ***Singapore:*** Alphanate; Fanhdi; Haemoctin SDH; Hemofil M†; Koate-DVI; ***Spain:*** Beriate P; Bioclate†; Criostat SD 2†; Fanhdi; Haemate; Helixate; Hemofil M; Kogenate; Kryobulin TIM 3†; Monoclate-P; Recombinate; ReFacto; ***Swed.:*** Beriate P; Haemate; Helixate; Hemofil M; Immunate; Kogenate; Monoclate-P; Octonativ-M; Recombinate; ReFacto; ***Switz.:*** Beriate P; Haemate HS; Helixate; Hyate:C†; Immunate; Kogenate; Kryobuline S-TIM 3†; Premofil M†; Recombinate; ReFacto; ***Thai.:*** Alphanate; Method M; ***UK:*** Advate; Alphanate; Beriate P; Bioclate†; Fanhdi; Haemate P; Helixate; Hemofil HT†; Hemofil M; Hyate:C; Kogenate; Liberate; Monoclate-P; Recombinate; ReFacto; Replenate; ***USA:*** Advate; Alphanate; Bioclate; Helixate; Hemofil M; Humate-P; Hyate:C; Koate-DVI; Koate-HP†; Kogenate; Monarc-M; Monoclate-P; Recombinate; ReFacto.

**Multi-ingredient:** ***Fr.:*** Innobrand.

## Factor VIII Inhibitor Bypassing Fraction

Activated Prothrombin Complex Concentrate; Anti-inhibitor Coagulant Complex; Complejo coagulante antiinhibidor del factor VIII.

*ATC — B02BD03.*

### Adverse Effects and Precautions

Allergic reactions may follow the administration of preparations having factor VIII inhibitor bypassing activity. Rapid infusion may cause headache, flushing, and changes in blood pressure and pulse rate.

It should not be given if disseminated intravascular coagulation is suspected or if there are signs of fibrinolysis. It should be used with caution in patients with liver disease.

As with other plasma-derived products, there is a risk of transmission of infection.

### Uses and Administration

Preparations with factor VIII inhibitor bypassing activity are prepared from human plasma. They are used in patients with haemophilia A (p.737) who have antibodies to factor VIII and in patients with acquired antibodies to factor VIII. The dose is administered intravenously and depends on the preparation used.

### Preparations

**Proprietary Preparations** (details are given in Part 3)
***Arg.:*** Feiba TIM 4; ***Austria:*** Feiba S-TIM 4; ***Belg.:*** Autoplex T†; Feiba†; ***Braz.:*** Feiba†; ***Canad.:*** Feiba; ***Denm.:*** Feiba; ***Fin.:*** Feiba; ***Fr.:*** Feiba; ***Ger.:*** Autoplex; Feiba S-TIM 4; ***Hong Kong:*** Feiba TIM 4; ***Israel:*** Anti-Inhibitor Coagulant Complex (Autoplex T)†; Feiba; ***Ital.:*** Feiba; ***Malaysia:*** Autoplex T; ***S.Afr.:*** Feiba TIM 4; ***Singapore:*** Autoplex T†; ***Spain:*** Autoplex T†; Feiba TIM 4; ***Swed.:*** Autoplex; Feiba; ***Switz.:*** Feiba; ***UK:*** Anti-inhibitor Coagulant Complex†; Autoplex†; Defix; Feiba; ***USA:*** Autoplex T; Feiba.

# Factor IX

Christmas Factor; Plasma Thromboplastin Component; PTC.

*ATC — B02BD04.*

**Description.** Factor IX is a plasma protein involved in blood coagulation. It may be obtained from human plasma or produced by recombinant DNA technology. The name Nonacog Alfa is in use for recombinant factor IX.

**Pharmacopoeias.** Many pharmacopoeias have monographs including *Eur.* (see p.vi) and *US.*

**Ph. Eur. 5.0** (Human Coagulation Factor IX; Factor IX Coagulationis Humanus; Dried Factor IX Fraction BP 2003). A plasma protein fraction containing coagulation factor IX, prepared by a method that effectively separates it from other prothrombin complex factors (factors II, VII, and X). It is prepared from human plasma obtained from healthy donors; the plasma is tested for the absence of hepatitis B surface antigen and antibodies against HIV-1 and HIV-2 and hepatitis C virus. The method of preparation is designed to maintain functional integrity of factor IX, to minimise activation of any coagulation factor, and includes a step or steps that have been shown to remove or inactivate known agents of infection. The factor IX fraction is dissolved in a suitable liquid, passed through a bacteria-retentive filter, distributed aseptically into the final containers, and immediately frozen. The preparation is freeze-dried and the containers are sealed under vacuum or under an inert gas. Heparin, antithrombin, or other auxiliary substances such as a stabiliser may be included. No antimicrobial preservative is added. The specific activity is not less than 50 international units of factor IX per mg of total protein before the addition of any protein stabiliser. The dried product is a white or pale yellow hygroscopic powder or friable solid. Store in airtight containers. Protect from light. When reconstituted as stated on the label the resulting solution contains not less than 20 international units/mL.

**Ph. Eur. 5.0** (Human Prothrombin Complex; Prothrombinum Multiplex Humanum; Dried Prothrombin Complex BP 2003). It contains factor IX with variable amounts of coagulation factors II, VII, and X. It is prepared by fractionation of human plasma obtained from blood from healthy donors; the plasma is tested for the absence of hepatitis B surface antigen and antibodies against HIV-1 and HIV-2 and hepatitis C virus. The method of preparation is designed in particular to minimise thrombogenicity and includes a step or steps that have been shown to remove or inactivate known agents of infection. The prothrombin complex fraction is dissolved in a suitable liquid, sterilised by filtration, distributed aseptically into final containers, and immediately frozen. The preparation is freeze-dried and the containers are sealed under vacuum or under an inert gas. No antimicrobial preservative is added. Heparin, antithrombin, and other auxiliary substances such as a stabiliser may be added. The potency of the preparation is not less than 0.6 international units of factor IX per mg of total protein before the addition of any protein stabiliser. The dried product is a white or slightly coloured, very hygroscopic, powder or friable solid. Store in airtight containers. Protect from light. When reconstituted as stated on the label the resulting solution contains not less than 20 international units/mL.

**USP 27** (Factor IX Complex). A sterile freeze-dried powder consisting of partially purified factor IX fraction, as well as concentrated factor II, VII, and X fractions of venous plasma obtained from healthy human donors. It contains no preservatives. It should be stored at 2° to 8° in hermetically-sealed containers. It should be used within 4 hours after reconstitution and administered with equipment that includes a filter.

## Nonacog Alfa *(BAN, USAN, rINN)*

Blood-coagulation factor IX (human), glycoform α; Blood-coagulation factor IX (synthetic human); .

*CAS — 113478-33-4; 181054-95-5;.*
*ATC — B02BD09.*

### Units

The activity of factor IX is expressed in terms of international units and preparations may be assayed using the third International Standard for blood coagulation factor IX concentrate, human (1996).

### Adverse Effects and Precautions

Allergic reactions may follow the use of factor IX preparations and there may be chills, fever, and urticaria. Other adverse effects include nausea and vomiting, headache, and flushing particularly after rapid administration. Intravascular coagulation and thrombosis have been reported, mainly in patients with liver disease, and factor IX should be used with care in patients at risk of thromboembolism or disseminated intravascular coagulation. The risk should be less with more highly purified preparations.

As with other plasma derivatives there is a possibility of transmitting viral infection, although selection of donors and heat or chemical treatments of products are used to minimise the risk. Vaccination against hepatitis B is recommended for patients not already immune.

Antibodies to factor IX may develop rarely.

**Effects on blood coagulation.** Some factor IX preparations derived from plasma contain other clotting factors in addition to factor IX (such as the activated factors IX, X, and XII) and administration of these preparations has the potential to produce thromboembolic complications. Reports of thrombosis[1] and intravascular coagulation[2,3] have generally been associated with the use of these factor IX preparations in patients with liver disease, although there has been a report[4] of deep-vein thrombosis in a patient with normal hepatic function who had been given factor IX postoperatively. Highly purified factor IX preparations which do not contain other clotting factors may be expected to avoid this risk of thromboembolism.

1. Blatt PM, *et al.* Thrombogenic materials in prothrombin complex concentrates. *Ann Intern Med* 1974; **81:** 766–70.
2. Gazzard BG, *et al.* Coagulation factor concentrate in the treatment of the haemorrhagic diathesis of fulminant hepatic failure. *Gut* 1974; **15:** 993–8.
3. Cederbaum AI, *et al.* Intravascular coagulation with use of human prothrombin complex concentrates. *Ann Intern Med* 1976; **84:** 683–7.
4. Machin SJ, Miller BR. Thrombosis and factor-IX concentrates. *Lancet* 1978; **i:** 1367.

**Effects on the heart.** Myocardial infarction has occurred in patients receiving factor IX concentrates[1-3] and may be associated with the large doses employed.[4]

1. Fuerth JH, Mahrer P. Myocardial infarction after factor IX therapy. *JAMA* 1981; **245:** 1455–6.
2. Schimpf K, *et al.* Myocardial infarction complicating activated prothrombin complex concentrate substitution in patient with haemophilia A. *Lancet* 1982; **ii:** 1043.
3. Gruppo RA, *et al.* Fatal myocardial necrosis associated with prothrombin-complex-concentrate therapy in hemophilia A. *N Engl J Med* 1983; **309:** 242–3.
4. Lusher JM. Myocardial necrosis after therapy with prothrombin-complex concentrate. *N Engl J Med* 1984; **310:** 464.

**Transmission of infections.** For a report of hepatitis A in a patient receiving a solvent-detergent-treated factor IX preparation, see under Adverse Effects and Precautions of Factor VIII, p.751.

### Uses and Administration

Factor IX is used as replacement therapy in patients with haemophilia B (Christmas disease), a genetic deficiency of factor IX (p.737).

There are two forms of factor IX preparation derived from plasma; one is of high purity, the other is rich in other clotting factors. A recombinant factor IX preparation, nonacog alfa, is also available. Preparations that contain other factors as well as factor IX may sometimes be useful for the treatment of bleeding due to deficiencies of factors II, VII, and X, as well as IX, and in the preparation of such patients for surgery; they may also be used for immediate reversal of coumarin anticoagulants and in the management of patients with haemophilia A who have antibodies to factor VIII.

Factor IX is given by slow intravenous infusion. In patients with factor IX deficiency the dosage should be determined for each patient and will vary with the preparation used and the circumstances of bleeding or type of surgery to be performed. Suggested target factor IX concentrations vary considerably.

### Preparations

***Ph. Eur.:*** Human Coagulation Factor IX; Human Prothrombin Complex; ***USP 27:*** Factor IX Complex.

**Proprietary Preparations** (details are given in Part 3)
***Arg.:*** Aimafix; Benefix; Immunine; Protromplex; ***Austral.:*** Benefix; Monofix-VF; ***Austria:*** Benefix; Beriplex; Immunine; Octanine; Prothromplex S-TIM 4; ***Belg.:*** Benefix†; ***Braz.:*** Bebulin†; Benefix; Berinin; Beriplex PN; Immunine†; Konyne†; Mononine; Prothromplex-T†; Replenine; ***Canad.:*** Immunine; ***Chile:*** Benefix; Octanyne; ***Denm.:*** Benefix; Immunine; Mononine; ***Fin.:*** Bemofil; ***Fr.:*** Benefix; Betafact; Kaskadil; Mononine; ***Ger.:*** Alphanine†; Benefix; Berinin; Beriplex PN; Immunine; Mononine; Octanine; PPSB Konzentrat S-TIM; Prothrombinkomplex BaWu; Prothromplex S-TIM 4†; ***Gr.:*** Benefix; Betafact; ***Hong Kong:*** Alphanine; Konyne 80†; Profilnine; Proplex T; ***Irl.:*** Mononine; ***Israel:*** Betafact; Konyne†; Profilnine; Proplex; Replenine; ***Ital.:*** Aimafix; Alphanine; Bebulin TIM 3†; Benefix; Immunine; Mononine; Protromplex TIM 3; Uman-Complex DI; ***Malaysia:*** Alphanine; Profilnine; Proplex T; Replenine VF; ***Mex.:*** Benefix; Berinin P†; Konyne 80; ***Neth.:*** Mononine; ***Norw.:*** Nanotiv†; Octanyne†; ***NZ:*** Monofix; Prothrombinex; ***S.Afr.:*** Haemosolvex; Prothromplex-T TIM 4; ***Singapore:*** Alphanine; Profilnine; Proplex T†; Replenine; ***Spain:*** Bebulin TIM 4†; Benefix; Immunine; Mononine; Proplex T†; Prothromplex; ***Swed.:*** Benefix; Immunine; Mononine; Nanotiv; ***Switz.:*** Benefix; Berinin HS; Immunine; Prothromplex Total S-TIM 4; ***Thai.:*** Alphanine; Profilnine; ***UK:*** Alphanine; Benefix; Beriplex PN†; Hipfix; Mononine; Proplex†; Prothromplex†; Replenine; ***USA:*** Alphanine; Bebulin VH; Benefix; Konyne 80†; Mononine; Profilnine; Proplex T.

**Multi-ingredient:** ***Spain:*** Hemofactor HT†.

## Factor XIII

Fibrin-stabilising Factor; FSF.

*ATC — B02BD07.*

### Profile

Factor XIII is used as replacement therapy in patients with a genetic deficiency of factor XIII. Dosage of factor XIII is based on the degree of deficiency and the condition of the patient. For prophylaxis of haemorrhage approximately 10 units/kg may be given intravenously every 4 weeks. For pre-operative use, a dose of up to 35 units/kg may be given immediately before the operation and followed by approximately 10 units/kg daily for 5 days or until the wound is healed. For the treatment of severe bleeding episodes 10 to 20 units/kg should be given daily.

Cryoprecipitate is also used as a source of factor XIII.

Factor XIII is also a component of fibrin glues (see Fibrin, p.753).

**Inflammatory bowel disease.** Some patients with inflammatory bowel disease may be deficient in factor XIII, possibly due to increased intestinal blood loss seen in severe ulcerative colitis or increased mucosal deposition of factor XIII in Crohn's disease. Factor XIII concentrate given intravenously has produced beneficial results in 12 patients with active ulcerative colitis resistant to conventional therapy with corticosteroids and mesalazine[1] and has also been associated with healing of intractable fistulae in 3 of 4 patients with Crohn's disease.[2]

1. Lorenz R, *et al.* Factor XIII substitution in ulcerative colitis. *Lancet* 1995; **345:** 449–50.
2. Oshitani N, *et al.* Treatment of Crohn's disease fistulas with coagulation factor XIII. *Lancet* 1996: **347:** 119–20.

### Preparations

***Ph. Eur.:*** Fibrin Sealant Kit.

**Proprietary Preparations** (details are given in Part 3)
***Austria:*** Fibrogammin; ***Braz.:*** Fibrogammin; ***Ger.:*** Fibrogammin; ***Hong Kong:*** Fibrogammin P; ***Israel:*** Fibrogammin P; ***UK:*** Fibrogammin P.

**Multi-ingredient:** ***Arg.:*** Tissucol; Tissucol Duo Quick; ***Austral.:*** Tisseel Duo; ***Austria:*** Beriplast; Tissucol; Tissucol Duo Quick; ***Braz.:*** Beriplast P; ***Canad.:*** Tisseel; ***Chile:*** Beriplast P; ***Denm.:*** Tisseel Duo Quick; ***Fin.:*** Beriplast†; Tisseel Duo Quick; ***Fr.:*** Beriplast; Biocol†; Tissucol; ***Ger.:*** Beriplast; Tissucol Duo S; Tissucol Fibrinkleber tiefgefroren†; Tissucol-Kit; ***Hong Kong:*** Beriplast P; Tisseel; ***Irl.:*** Tisseel†; ***Israel:*** Tisseel; ***Mex.:*** Beriplast P†; ***Spain:*** Tissucol Duo; ***Swed.:*** Tisseel Duo Quick; ***Switz.:*** Beriplast P; Tissucol; Tissucol Duo S; ***UK:*** Tisseel.

## Fibrin

Fibrina.

**Pharmacopoeias.** Many pharmacopoeias have monographs for fibrin preparations including *Eur.* (see p.vi).

**Ph. Eur. 5.0** (Fibrin Sealant Kit; Fibrini Glutinum). It is composed of two components, a fibrinogen concentrate containing human fibrinogen (component 1), and a human thrombin preparation (component 2). The kit may also contain other ingredients, such as human factor XIII, a fibrinolysis inhibitor, or calcium ions. Stabilisers such as human albumin may be added. The human constituents are obtained from plasma for fractionation and the method of preparation includes a step or steps that have been shown to remove or inactivate known agents of infection. The constituents are passed through a bacteria-retentive filter and distributed aseptically into sterile containers. Containers of freeze-dried constituents are sealed under vacuum or filled with oxygen-free nitrogen or other suitable inert gas before sealing. No antimicrobial preservative is added. When thawed or reconstituted as stated on the label, the fibrinogen concentrate contains not less than 40 g per litre of clottable protein; the activity of the thrombin preparation varies over a wide range (approximately 4 to 1000 international units/mL). Protect from light.

### Uses and Administration

Fibrin glue is prepared by mixing solutions containing fibrinogen, factor XIII, and often other clotting components with thrombin and calcium ions usually, with the addition of aprotinin to inhibit fibrinolysis. It is used as a haemostatic to control haemorrhage during surgical procedures or as a spray to bleeding surfaces.

A dry artificial sponge of human fibrin, prepared by clotting with human thrombin a foam of a solution of human fibrinogen and known as human fibrin foam, has been used similarly.

◊ Reviews.

1. Dunn CJ, Goa KL. Fibrin sealant: a review of its use in surgery and endoscopy. *Drugs* 1999; **58:** 863–86.

**Adverse effects.** Fatal neurotoxicity has been reported[1] following the use of a fibrin sealant during neurosurgical procedures. The toxicity may have been due to the presence of tranexamic acid as a stabiliser in the formulation, and such formulations should not be used in surgical operations where contact with the CSF or dura mater could occur.[2]

1. Committee on Safety of Medicines/Medicines Control Agency. Quixil human surgical sealant: reports of fatal reactions. *Current Problems* 1999; **25:** 19. Also available at: http://www.mca.gov.uk/ourwork/monitorsafequalmed/currentproblems/cpvol25dpg7.htm (accessed 23/06/04)
2. Committee on Safety of Medicines/Medicines Control Agency. Quixil human surgical sealant: update on fatal neurotoxic reactions. *Current Problems* 2000; **26:** 10. Also available at: http://www.mca.gov.uk/ourwork/monitorsafequalmed/currentproblems/cpsept2000.pdf (accessed 23/06/04)

### Preparations

***Ph. Eur.:*** Fibrin Sealant Kit.

**Proprietary Preparations** (details are given in Part 3)
***Braz.:*** Fibrinol†; ***Ital.:*** Hemofibrine Spugna†.

**Multi-ingredient:** ***Arg.:*** Tissucol; Tissucol Duo Quick; ***Austral.:*** Tisseel Duo; ***Austria:*** Tissucol; Tissucol Duo Quick; ***Belg.:*** Tissucol†; ***Braz.:*** Tissucol†; ***Canad.:*** Tisseel; ***Denm.:*** Tisseel Duo Quick; ***Fin.:*** Beriplast†; Tisseel Duo Quick; ***Fr.:*** Biocol†; Tissucol; ***Ger.:*** Beriplast; Tissucol Duo S; Tissucol Fibrinkleber tiefgefroren†; Tissucol-Kit; ***Hong Kong:*** Tisseel; ***Irl.:*** Tisseel†; ***Israel:*** Beriplast P; Tisseel; ***Ital.:*** Tissucol; ***Mex.:*** Beriplast P†; ***Spain:*** Tissucol Duo; ***Swed.:*** Tisseel Duo Quick; ***Switz.:*** Beriplast P; Tissucol; Tissucol Duo S; ***UK:*** Tisseel.

## Fibrinogen

Factor I; Fibrinógeno.

*ATC — B02BB01; B02BC10.*

**Pharmacopoeias.** Many pharmacopoeias have monographs including *Eur.* (see p.vi).

**Ph. Eur. 5.0** (Human Fibrinogen; Fibrinogenum Humanum). It contains the soluble constituent of human plasma that is transformed to fibrin on addition of thrombin. It is obtained from plasma for fractionation and the method of preparation includes a step or steps that have been shown to remove or inactivate known agents of infection. Stabilisers, including protein such as human albumin, salts, and buffers may be added. No antimicrobial preservative is added. When dissolved in the volume of solvent stated on the label, the solution contains not less than 10 g/litre of fibrinogen.

A white or pale yellow hygroscopic powder or friable solid. Store in airtight containers. Protect from light.

### Profile

Fibrinogen has been used to control haemorrhage associated with low blood-fibrinogen concentration in afibrinogenaemia or hypofibrinogenaemia but the use of plasma or cryoprecipitate is usually preferred. It has also been used in disseminated intravascular coagulation (p.737). Fibrinogen is a component of fibrin glue (see Fibrin, above).

Fibrinogen labelled with radionuclides has also been used in diagnostic procedures.

### Preparations

***Ph. Eur.:*** Fibrin Sealant Kit; Human Fibrinogen.

**Proprietary Preparations** (details are given in Part 3)
***Austria:*** Haemocomplettan; ***Ger.:*** Haemocomplettan; ***Gr.:*** Haemocomplettan-P; ***Ital.:*** Fibrinomer†; Uman-Fibrin†; ***Switz.:*** Haemocomplettan; ***UK:*** Haemocomplettan†.

**Multi-ingredient:** ***Arg.:*** Tissucol; Tissucol Duo Quick; ***Austral.:*** Tisseel Duo; ***Austria:*** Beriplast; TachoComb; Tissucol; Tissucol Duo Quick; ***Braz.:*** Beriplast P; Tissucol†; ***Canad.:*** Tisseel; ***Chile:*** Beriplast P; ***Denm.:*** Tisseel Duo Quick; ***Fin.:*** Beriplast†; Tisseel Duo Quick; ***Fr.:*** Beriplast; Biocol†; Tissucol; ***Ger.:*** Beriplast; TachoComb; Tissucol Duo S; Tissucol Fibrinkleber tiefgefroren†; Tissucol-Kit; ***Hong Kong:*** Beriplast P; TachoComb; Tisseel; ***Israel:*** Beriplast P; Tisseel; ***Mex.:*** Beriplast P†; ***Spain:*** Tissucol Duo; ***Swed.:*** Tisseel Duo Quick; ***Switz.:*** Beriplast P; Tissucol; Tissucol Duo S; ***Thai.:*** Fibrin Glue; TachoComb; ***UK:*** Tisseel.

## Filgrastim *(BAN, USAN, rINN)*

r-metHuG-CSF. A recombinant human granulocyte colony-stimulating factor.

*CAS — 121181-53-1.*
*ATC — L03AA02.*

### Pegfilgrastim *(BAN, rINN)*

Filgrastim conjugated with monomethoxy polyethylene glycol.

*CAS — 208265-92-3.*
*ATC — L03AA13.*

**Incompatibility.** References.

1. Trissel LA, Martinez JF. Compatibility of filgrastim with selected drugs during simulated Y-site administration. *Am J Hosp Pharm* 1994; **51:** 1907–13.

**Stability.** Solutions of filgrastim must not be diluted with sodium chloride solutions as precipitation will occur. Glucose 5% solution may be used if dilution is necessary. However, filgrastim in diluted solution may be adsorbed onto glass or plastic materials and so it should not be diluted below the recommended minimum concentration (2 micrograms/mL). Also, to protect from adsorption, solutions that are diluted to concentrations of filgrastim below 15 micrograms/mL must have albumin added to give a final concentration of 2 mg/mL.

### Adverse Effects

The main adverse effects of granulocyte colony-stimulating factors such as filgrastim during short-term treatment are musculoskeletal pain and dysuria. Hypersensitivity reactions have been reported rarely. In patients receiving long-term treatment the most frequent adverse effects are bone pain and musculoskeletal pain. Other side-effects include splenic enlargement, thrombocytopenia, anaemia, epistaxis, headache, diarrhoea, and cutaneous vasculitis. There have been reports of pulmonary infiltrates leading to respiratory failure or acute respiratory distress syndrome.

Preparations of filgrastim may contain sorbitol as an excipient; care is advisable in patients with hereditary fructose intolerance.

Colony-stimulating factors are fetotoxic in *animal* studies.

◊ General references.

1. Vial T, Descotes J. Clinical toxicity of cytokines used as haemopoietic growth factors. *Drug Safety* 1995; **13:** 371–406.

**Disseminated intravascular coagulation.** Long-term treatment with granulocyte colony-stimulating factor in a 7-year-old boy with HIV infection and zidovudine-induced neutropenia produced evidence of disseminated intravascular coagulation on 2 occasions.[1]

1. Mueller BU, *et al.* Disseminated intravascular coagulation associated with granulocyte colony-stimulating factor therapy in a child with human immunodeficiency virus infection. *J Pediatr* 1995; **126:** 749–52.

**Effects on the bones.** Bone mineral loss and osteoporosis have been reported in children with severe congenital neutropenia receiving granulocyte colony-stimulating factor for long periods.[1,2] However, the role of granulocyte colony-stimulating factor in producing this effect is uncertain since bone mineral loss may be a feature of the underlying disease.

1. Bishop NJ, *et al.* Osteoporosis in severe congenital neutropenia treated with granulocyte colony-stimulating factor. *Br J Haematol* 1995; **89:** 927–8.
2. Yakisan E, *et al.* High incidence of significant bone loss in patients with severe congenital neutropenia (Kostmann's syndrome). *J Pediatr* 1997; **131:** 592–7.

**Effects on the eyes.** Subretinal haemorrhage resulting in irreversible loss of vision in one eye occurred in a 4-year-old girl who received filgrastim and nartograstim for chemotherapy-induced neutropenia and for mobilising peripheral blood stem cells.[1] It was postulated that the colony-stimulating factor reactivated a primary ocular inflammation probably caused by an infection.

1. Matsumura T, *et al.* Subretinal haemorrhage after granulocyte colony-stimulating factor. *Lancet* 1997; **350:** 336. Correction. *ibid.*; 1406.

**Effects on the lungs.** There have been reports of exacerbation of chemotherapy-induced pulmonary toxicity in patients receiving granulocyte colony-stimulating factor with bleomycin[1,2] and cyclophosphamide.[3] The patients were also receiving other antineoplastics. However, analysis of 2 randomised controlled studies failed to show increased pulmonary toxicity when granulocyte colony-stimulating factor was added to bleomycin therapy[4,5] and it has been suggested[5] that confounding factors, including the use of other antineoplastics, may account for the increased pulmonary toxicity.

1. Matthews JH. Pulmonary toxicity of ABVD chemotherapy and G-CSF in Hodgkin's disease: possible synergy. *Lancet* 1993; **342:** 988.
2. Dirix LY, *et al.* Pulmonary toxicity and bleomycin. *Lancet* 1994; **344:** 56.
3. van Woensel JBM, *et al.* Acute respiratory insufficiency during doxorubicin, cyclophosphamide, and G-CSF therapy. *Lancet* 1994; **344:** 759–60.

4. Bastion Y, *et al.* Possible toxicity with the association of G-CSF and bleomycin. *Lancet* 1994; **343:** 1221–2.
5. Bastion Y, Coiffier B. Pulmonary toxicity of bleomycin: is G-CSF a risk factor? *Lancet* 1994; **344:** 474.

**Effects on the skin.** Skin reactions may occur in patients given colony-stimulating factors. In a study in women with inflammatory breast cancer, a pruritic skin reaction developed at the subcutaneous injection site in all 7 given granulocyte-macrophage colony-stimulating factor.[1] Exacerbation of psoriasis[2] and precipitation or exacerbation of neutrophilic dermatoses including Sweet's syndrome,[3,4] pyoderma gangrenosum,[5] and neutrophilic eccrine hidradenitis[6] have been reported following granulocyte colony-stimulating factor.

1. Steger GG, *et al.* Cutaneous reactions to GM-CSF in inflammatory breast cancer. *N Engl J Med* 1992; **327:** 286.
2. Kavanaugh A. Flare of psoriasis and psoriatic arthritis following treatment with granulocyte colony-stimulating factor. *Am J Med* 1996; **101:** 567.
3. Petit T, *et al.* Lymphoedema-area-restricted Sweet syndrome during G-CSF treatment. *Lancet* 1996; **347:** 690.
4. Garty BZ, *et al.* Sweet syndrome associated with G-CSF treatment in a child with glycogen storage disease type Ib. *Pediatrics* 1996; **97:** 401–3.
5. Johnson ML, Grimwood RE. Leukocyte colony-stimulating factors: a review of associated neutrophilic dermatoses and vasculitides. *Arch Dermatol* 1994; **130:** 77–81.
6. Bachmeyer C, *et al.* Neutrophilic eccrine hidradenitis induced by granulocyte colony-stimulating factor. *Br J Dermatol* 1998; **139:** 354–5.

**Effects on the thyroid.** Reversible thyroid dysfunction has been reported in patients with pre-existing thyroid antibodies during treatment with granulocyte-macrophage colony-stimulating factor,[1] but not with granulocyte colony-stimulating factor.[2] However, clinical hypothyroidism has been reported in a patient with no history of thyroid dysfunction or thyroid antibodies during treatment with granulocyte colony-stimulating factor.[3]

1. Hoekman K, *et al.* Reversible thyroid dysfunction during treatment with GM-CSF. *Lancet* 1991; **338:** 541–2.
2. van Hoef MEHM, Howell A. Risk of thyroid dysfunction during treatment with G-CSF. *Lancet* 1992; **340:** 1169–70.
3. de Luis DA, Romero E. Reversible thyroid dysfunction with filgrastim. *Lancet* 1996; **348:** 1595–6.

**Inflammatory disorders.** Reactivation of various inflammatory disorders including rheumatoid arthritis[1] and pseudogout[2,3] has been reported following granulocyte colony-stimulating factors. For further reports of reactivation of sites of inflammation, see under Effects on the Eyes and Effects on the Skin, above.

1. Vildarsson B, *et al.* Reactivation of rheumatoid arthritis and development of leukocytoclastic vasculitis in a patient receiving granulocyte colony-stimulating factor for Felty's syndrome. *Am J Med* 1995; **98:** 589–91.
2. Sandor V, *et al.* Exacerbation of pseudogout by granulocyte colony-stimulating factor. *Ann Intern Med* 1996; **125:** 781.
3. Teramoto S, *et al.* Increased synovial interleukin-8 and interleukin-6 levels in pseudogout associated with granulocyte colony-stimulating factor. *Ann Intern Med* 1998; **129:** 424–5.

## Precautions

Since granulocyte colony-stimulating factors such as filgrastim can promote growth of myeloid cells *in vitro* their use in myeloid malignancies has been contra-indicated, although recently colony-stimulating factors have been used in some patients with myeloid diseases without stimulation of malignant cells. However, caution is required when they are used in patients with any pre-malignant or malignant myeloid condition. They should not be used from 24 hours before until 24 hours after cytotoxic chemotherapy due to the sensitivity of rapidly dividing myeloid cells.

The complete blood count should be monitored regularly during therapy with granulocyte colony-stimulating factors. Treatment should be withdrawn in patients who develop signs of pulmonary infiltrates. Bone density should be monitored in patients with osteoporosis who are receiving long-term treatment with filgrastim.

## Uses and Administration

Filgrastim is a granulocyte colony-stimulating factor that acts as a haematopoietic growth factor stimulating the development of granulocytes. It is used to treat or prevent neutropenia in patients receiving myelosuppressive cancer chemotherapy and to reduce the period of neutropenia in patients undergoing bone marrow transplantation (p.496). It is also used to mobilise peripheral blood progenitor cells for use as an alternative to bone marrow transplantation, in the management of chronic neutropenia (congenital, cyclic, or idiopathic), and for persistent neutropenia in patients with advanced HIV infection.

Filgrastim may be given intravenously or subcutaneously. Doses may be expressed in micrograms or in units; 10 micrograms is equivalent to 1 million units.

As an adjunct to antineoplastic therapy, filgrastim is given in a dose of 5 micrograms/kg daily starting not less than 24 hours after the last dose of antineoplastic. It can be given as a single daily subcutaneous injection, as a continuous intravenous or subcutaneous infusion, or as a daily intravenous infusion over 15 to 30 minutes. Treatment is continued until the neutrophil count has stabilised within the normal range which may take up to 14 days or more. A formulation of filgrastim conjugated with monomethoxy polyethylene glycol (pegfilgrastim) may also be used to reduce the incidence of neutropenia associated with antineoplastic therapy; it is given by subcutaneous injection in a single dose of 6 mg, given not less than 24 hours after the last dose of antineoplastic.

The initial dose of filgrastim following bone marrow transplantation is 10 micrograms/kg daily, adjusted according to response. This may be given by intravenous infusion over 30 minutes, intravenous infusion over 4 hours, or by continuous intravenous or subcutaneous infusion over 24 hours.

For mobilisation of peripheral blood progenitor cells, a dose of 10 micrograms/kg daily of filgrastim may be given subcutaneously as a single daily injection or by continuous infusion; if given after myelosuppressive chemotherapy this dose is halved to 5 micrograms/kg daily by subcutaneous injection.

In patients with congenital neutropenia the initial dose is 12 micrograms/kg daily and in patients with idiopathic or cyclic neutropenia the initial dose is 5 micrograms/kg daily. In these forms of neutropenia the dose is given subcutaneously in single or divided doses and should be adjusted according to response.

In patients with HIV infection and persistent neutropenia the initial dose is 1 microgram/kg daily by subcutaneous injection. The dose may be titrated up to a maximum of 4 micrograms/kg daily until a normal neutrophil count is achieved and then adjusted for maintenance according to response. Maintenance doses of 300 micrograms daily on 1 to 7 days a week have been used.

The filgrastim doses described above for patients receiving antineoplastic therapy and for chronic neutropenias may also be given to children.

◊ Colony-stimulating factors or haematopoietic growth factors are naturally occurring glycoprotein growth factors (cytokines) that promote the proliferation and differentiation of haematopoietic precursors. Many colony-stimulating factors have been identified that stimulate development of different cell lines. These include: ancestim (p.742); erythropoietin (see Epoetins, p.747); granulocyte colony-stimulating factors; granulocyte-macrophage colony-stimulating factors such as molgramostim (p.756); thrombopoietin (p.760); interleukin-3 (p.755); and oprelvekin (interleukin-11) (p.757). Other factors under investigation include macrophage colony-stimulating factors.

◊ References.

1. Frampton JE, *et al.* Filgrastim: a review of its pharmacological properties and therapeutic efficacy in neutropenia. *Drugs* 1994; **48:** 731–60.
2. American Society of Clinical Oncology. Recommendations for the use of hematopoietic colony-stimulating factors: evidence-based, clinical practice guidelines. *J Clin Oncol* 1994; **12:** 2471–2508. Also available at: http://www.asco.org/asco/downloads/Use_of_hematopoietic_Colony_Stimulating_Factors_Evidence_Based.pdf (accessed 23/06/04)
3. American Society of Clinical Oncology. Update of recommendations for the use of hematopoietic colony-stimulating factors: evidence-based clinical practice guidelines. *J Clin Oncol* 1996; **14:** 1957–60.
4. Nemunaitis J. A comparative review of colony-stimulating factors. *Drugs* 1997; **54:** 709–29.
5. Ozer H, *et al.* 2000 Update of recommendations for the use of hematopoietic colony-stimulating factors: evidence-based, clinical practice guidelines. *J Clin Oncol* 2000; **18:** 3558–85. Also available at: http://www.jco.org/cgi/reprint/18/20/3558.pdf (accessed 23/06/04)
6. Dale DC, ed. Filgrastim anniversary supplement: reviewing 10 years of clinical experience, a seminar-in-print. *Drugs* 2002; **62** (suppl 1): 1–98.
7. Curran MP, Goa KL. Pegfilgrastim. *Drugs* 2002; **62:** 1207–13.

**Aplastic anaemia.** Colony-stimulating factors, including granulocyte colony-stimulating factors, have been tried in a few patients with aplastic anaemia (p.732).

**Infections.** It has been suggested[1] that colony-stimulating factors may be useful as adjuncts to antibacterials or antifungals in patients with severe infections and defects in phagocytic cell function. Such defects may occur in patients with diabetes mellitus or AIDS. Addition of granulocyte colony-stimulating factor to conventional therapy improved clinical outcome of foot infection in a small study in diabetic patients[2] and 3 of 4 patients with AIDS and resistant oral candidiasis responded to treatment with granulocyte-macrophage colony-stimulating factor.[3] A controlled study in 258 patients with advanced HIV infection found that prophylactic administration of granulocyte colony-stimulating factor reduced the incidence of severe neutropenia and also suggested that the incidence and duration of bacterial infections was reduced.[4]

Granulocyte colony-stimulating factors have also been tried as an adjunct to conventional therapy in chronic viral hepatitis.[5]

1. Khwaja A, Linch DC. Haemopoietic growth factors in the treatment of infection in non-neutropenic patients. *J Antimicrob Chemother* 1994; **33:** 679–83.
2. Gough A, *et al.* Randomised placebo-controlled trial of granulocyte-colony stimulating factor in diabetic foot infection. *Lancet* 1997; **350:** 855–9.
3. Capetti A, *et al.* Employment of recombinant human granulocyte-macrophage colony stimulating factor in oesophageal candidiasis in AIDS patients. *AIDS* 1995; **9:** 1378–9.
4. Kuritzkes DP, *et al.* Filgrastim prevents severe neutropenia and reduces infective morbidity in patients with advanced HIV infection: results of a randomized, multicenter, controlled trial. *AIDS* 1998; **12:** 65–74.
5. Pardo M, *et al.* Treatment of chronic hepatitis C with cirrhosis with recombinant human granulocyte colony-stimulating factor plus recombinant interferon-alpha. *J Med Virol* 1995; **45:** 439–44.

**Neutropenia.** Granulocyte colony-stimulating factors are used in the management of neutropenia (p.740). They are used to treat or prevent antineoplastic-induced neutropenia and have also been tried in patients with neutropenia induced by a wide range of other drugs.[1-6] They may be used for long-term treatment in patients with chronic neutropenias.[7] Short-term administration has been tried in a few preterm neonates with neutropenia and severe infections and increases in neutrophil counts have been reported in some,[8,9] though not in others.[10] There has also been a preliminary report that prophylaxis with filgrastim may reduce the incidence of sepsis in critically-ill neonates with neutropenia.[11] Granulocyte colony-stimulating factors have also been tried with mixed results in neonates with the rare condition of alloimmune neutropenia.[12-14]

1. Gerson SL, *et al.* Granulocyte colony-stimulating factor for clozapine-induced agranulocytosis. *Lancet* 1992; **340:** 1097.
2. Wyatt S, *et al.* Filgrastim for mesalazine-associated neutropenia. *Lancet* 1993; **341:** 1476.
3. Teitelbaum AH, *et al.* Filgrastim (r-met HuG-CSF) reversal of drug-induced agranulocytosis. *Am J Med* 1993; **95:** 245–6.
4. Geibig CB, Marks LW. Treatment of clozapine- and molindone-induced agranulocytosis with granulocyte colony-stimulating factor. *Ann Pharmacother* 1993; **27:** 1190–2.
5. Chia HM, *et al.* Filgrastim for low-dose, captopril-induced agranulocytosis. *Lancet* 1993; **342:** 304.
6. Gales BJ, Gales MA. Granulocyte-colony stimulating factor for sulfasalazine-induced agranulocytosis. *Ann Pharmacother* 1993; **27:** 1052–4.
7. Bonilla MA, *et al.* Long-term safety of treatment with recombinant human granulocyte colony-stimulating factor (r-metHuG-CSF) in patients with severe congenital neutropenias. *Br J Haematol* 1994; **88:** 723–30.
8. Bedford Russell AR, *et al.* Granulocyte colony stimulating factor treatment for neonatal neutropenia. *Arch Dis Child* 1995; **72:** F53–F54.
9. Carr R, Modi N. Haemopoietic colony stimulating factors for preterm neonates. *Arch Dis Child* 1997; **76:** F128–F133.
10. Schibler KR, *et al.* A randomized, placebo-controlled trial of granulocyte colony-stimulating factor administration to newborn infants with neutropenia and clinical signs of early-onset sepsis. *Pediatrics* 1998; **102:** 6–13.
11. Kocherlakota P, La Gamma EF. Preliminary report: rhG-CSF may reduce the incidence of neonatal sepsis in prolonged preeclampsia-associated neutropenia. *Pediatrics* 1998; **102:** 1107–11.
12. Gilmore MM, *et al.* Treatment of alloimmune neonatal neutropenia with granulocyte colony-stimulating factor. *J Pediatr* 1994; **125:** 948–51.
13. Bedu A, *et al.* Failure of granulocyte colony-stimulating factor in alloimmune neonatal neutropenia. *J Pediatr* 1995; **127:** 508.
14. Rodwell RL, *et al.* Granulocyte colony stimulating factor treatment for alloimmune neonatal neutropenia. *Arch Dis Child* 1996; **75:** F57–F58.

## Preparations

**Proprietary Preparations** (details are given in Part 3)
***Arg.:*** Filgen; Neupogen; Neutromax; ***Austral.:*** Neulasta; Neupogen; ***Austria:*** Neupogen; ***Belg.:*** Neupogen; ***Braz.:*** Granulen; Granulokine; ***Canad.:*** Neupogen; ***Chile:*** Neupogen; Neutromax; ***Denm.:*** Neupogen; ***Fin.:*** Neupogen; ***Fr.:*** Neulasta; Neupogen; ***Ger.:*** Neupogen; ***Gr.:*** Granulokine; ***Hong Kong:*** Neupogen; ***Irl.:*** Neupogen; ***Israel:*** Neupogen; ***Ital.:*** Granulokine; Neupogen; ***Jpn:*** Gran; ***Mex.:*** Neupogen; ***Neth.:*** Neupogen; ***Norw.:*** Neupogen; ***NZ:*** Neupogen; ***Port.:*** Neulasta; Neupogen; ***S.Afr.:*** Neupogen; ***Singapore:*** Neupogen; ***Spain:*** Granulokine†; Neupogen; ***Swed.:*** Neupogen; ***Switz.:*** Neupogen; ***Thai.:*** Neupogen; Neutromax; ***UK:*** Neulasta; Neupogen; ***USA:*** Neulasta; Neupogen.

# Gelatin

Gelatina.

*ATC — B05AA06.*

**Grades.** Gelling grades of gelatin are usually graded by gel strength, expressed as 'Bloom value', 'Bloom strength', or 'Bloom rating'.

**Pharmacopoeias.** In *Chin., Eur.* (see p.vi), *Int., Jpn, Pol.,* and *Viet.* Also in *USNF.*

The gelatin described in some pharmacopoeias is not necessarily suitable for preparations for parenteral use or for other special purposes.

**Ph. Eur. 5.0** (Gelatin). A purified protein obtained either by partial acid hydrolysis (type A), by partial alkaline hydrolysis (type

B), or by enzymatic hydrolysis of collagen from animals (including fish and poultry); it may also be a mixture of different types. The hydrolysis leads to gelling and non-gelling product grades. Gelling grades are characterised by the gel strength (Bloom value). It is not suitable for parenteral use or for other special purposes.

A faintly yellow or light yellowish-brown solid, usually occurring as translucent sheets, shreds, powder, or granules.

Gelling grades of gelatin swell in cold water and on heating give a colloidal solution which on subsequent cooling forms a more or less firm gel. Gelatin is practically insoluble in common organic solvents. Different gelatins form aqueous solutions that vary in clarity and colour. A 1% solution in water at about 55° has a pH of 3.8 to 7.6. Protect from heat and moisture.

**USNF 22** (Gelatin). It is obtained by the partial hydrolysis of collagen derived from the skin, white connective tissue, and bones of animals. Gelatin derived from an acid-treated precursor is known as Type A, and gelatin derived from an alkali-treated precursor is known as Type B.

Faintly yellow or amber sheets, flakes, or shreds, or a coarse to fine powder, the colour varying in depth according to the particle size. A solution has a slight, characteristic, bouillon-like odour. It is stable in air when dry, but is subject to microbial decomposition when moist or in solution. Gelatin swells and softens when immersed in cold water, gradually absorbing 5 to 10 times its weight of water. Soluble in hot water, in 6N acetic acid, and in a hot mixture of glycerol and water; insoluble in alcohol, in chloroform, in ether, and in fixed and volatile oils.

**Incompatibility.** A white precipitate was formed immediately when vancomycin injection was administered through a giving set containing modified fluid gelatin solution.[1]


1. Taylor A, Hornbrey P. Incompatibility of vancomycin and gelatin plasma expanders. *Pharm J* 1991; **246:** 466.


## Adverse Effects

Hypersensitivity reactions including anaphylactic reactions have occurred after the infusion of gelatin or its derivatives. Rapid infusion of gelatin derivatives may directly stimulate the release of histamine and other vasoactive substances.

For adverse reactions associated with the topical use of gelatin, see Haemostasis under Uses and Administration, below.

**Effects on the kidneys.** Acute renal failure developed in a patient undergoing aortobifemoral graft surgery who received modified fluid gelatin, blood transfusion, and diuretics following a fall in urine output.[1,2] The conclusion that gelatin was the most likely cause of the renal failure was contested[3-5] on the basis of previous experience and other major contributory factors such as diminished intravascular volume and reduced organ perfusion.


1. Hussain SF, Drew PJT. Acute renal failure after infusion of gelatins. *BMJ* 1989; **299:** 1137–8.
2. Drew PJT, Hussain SF. Acute renal failure after infusion of gelatin. *BMJ* 1989; **299:** 1400. Correction. *ibid.*; 1531.
3. Frazer RS, Macmillan RR. Acute renal failure after infusion of gelatin. *BMJ* 1989; **299:** 1399.
4. Fawcett WJ. Acute renal failure after infusion of gelatin. *BMJ* 1989; **299:** 1399.
5. Wilkins RG. Acute renal failure after infusion of gelatin. *BMJ* 1989; **299:** 1399–1400.


**Hypersensitivity.** Ten severe anaphylactoid reactions to an infusion of a modified fluid gelatin were reported over a period of 3 years.[1] Some hypersensitivity reactions associated with vaccine administration in children have also been attributed to the use of gelatin as an excipient.[2]

For reports of fatal reactions in asthmatic patients following administration of gelatin derivatives, see Polygeline, p.759.


1. Blanloeil Y, *et al.* Accidents anaphylactoïdes sévères après perfusion d'une gélatine fluide modifiée en solution équilibrée *Therapie* 1983; **38:** 539–46.
2. Kumagai T, *et al.* Gelatin-specific humoral and cellular immune responses in children with immediate- and nonimmediate-type reactions to live measles, mumps, rubella, and varicella vaccines. *J Allergy Clin Immunol* 1997; **100:** 130–4.


## Precautions

When gelatin or its derivatives are used as plasma expanders the precautions under Dextran 70 (p.746) should be considered. There does not appear to be any interference with blood grouping and cross-matching of blood.

When gelatin is used as an absorbable haemostatic the precautions under Oxidised Cellulose (p.757) should be considered.

## Pharmacokinetics

Following infusion of modified fluid gelatin (succinylated gelatin), 75% of the dose is excreted in the urine in 24 hours. The half-life is about 4 hours.

## Uses and Administration

Gelatin is a protein that has both clinical and pharmaceutical uses.

Gelatin is used as a haemostatic in surgical procedures as an absorbable film or sponge and can absorb many times its weight of blood. It is also employed as a plasma volume expander similarly to the dextrans in hypovolaemic shock (p.835). A 4% solution of a modified fluid gelatin (succinylated gelatin) has been infused in doses of 500 to 1000 mL. It may also be used in the form of a gelatin-derived polymer, see Polygeline, p.759.

Gelatin rods may be employed to temporarily block tear outflow in the diagnosis of dry eye (p.1576).

Gelatin is used in the preparation of pastes, pastilles, suppositories, tablets, and hard and soft capsule shells. It is also used for the microencapsulation of drugs and other industrial materials. It has been used as a vehicle for injections: Pitkin's Menstruum, which consists of gelatin, glucose, and acetic acid, has been used in a modified form for heparin while hydrolysed gelatin has been used for corticotropin. Gelatin is an ingredient of preparations used for the protection of stoma and lesions.

**Haemostasis.** Gelatin acts as a haemostatic (p.735) by providing a physical meshwork within which clotting can occur.

Gelatin powder may be applied dry to wound beds and may be most useful when mixed with saline or thrombin and applied to bone. Gelatin sponge can be applied dry or soaked in saline or thrombin solutions. When applied to skin wounds the gelatin liquefies within 2 to 5 days; when implanted into tissues it is absorbed within 4 to 6 weeks. Adverse reactions include an increased incidence of infection, compression of surrounding tissue due to fluid absorption, granuloma formation, and fibrosis. Generally, gelatin sponges cause little tissue reaction and can be applied to bone, dura, and pleural tissue.

References.


1. Larson PO. Topical hemostatic agents for dermatologic surgery. *J Dermatol Surg Oncol* 1988; **14:** 623–32.


**Neonatal intraventricular haemorrhage.** Plasma volume expansion in preterm neonates has been thought to help prevent neonatal intraventricular haemorrhage (p.740). However, a study using plasma or gelatin as plasma volume expanders,[1,2] found no evidence of a decreased risk of such haemorrhage or subsequent death or disability.


1. The Northern Neonatal Nursing Initiative Trial Group. A randomized trial comparing the effect of prophylactic intravenous fresh frozen plasma, gelatin or glucose on early mortality and morbidity in preterm babies. *Eur J Pediatr* 1996; **155:** 580–8.
2. Northern Neonatal Nursing Initiative Trial Group. Randomised trial of prophylactic early fresh-frozen plasma or gelatin or glucose in preterm babies: outcome at 2 years. *Lancet* 1996; **348:** 229–32.


## Preparations

**USP 27:** Absorbable Gelatin Film; Absorbable Gelatin Sponge.

**Proprietary Preparations** (details are given in Part 3)

***Arg.:*** Gelafundin; Infukoll; ***Austral.:*** Gelfilm; Gelfoam; Gelofusine; ***Austria:*** Gelofusin; ***Belg.:*** Gelfoam; Gelofusine; Geloplasma†; Willospon†; ***Braz.:*** Colagenan; Gelfoam; Hisocel†; ***Canad.:*** Gelfilm; Gelfoam; ***Chile:*** Gelfoam; Gelofusine; ***Fin.:*** Gelofusine; ***Fr.:*** Bloxang; Epiphane†; Gel-Phan; Gelofusine; Hydrocoll; Orangel†; ***Ger.:*** Gelafundin; Gelafusal-N in Ringer-acetat; Gelaspon; Gelastypt; stypro; Thomaegelin; ***Gr.:*** Gelofusine; ***Hong Kong:*** Gelafundin†; Gelfilm†; Gelfoam; Gelofusine; ***India:*** Seraccel; ***Israel:*** Gelfoam; ***Ital.:*** Cutanplast; Eufusin; Spongostan†; ***Malaysia:*** Gelfoam; ***Neth.:*** Gelfilm; Gelfoam; Willospon; ***NZ:*** Gelfilm; Gelfoam; Gelofusine; ***Port.:*** Epiphane 7†; Gelafundina†; Gelofusine; ***S.Afr.:*** Gelofusine; ***Singapore:*** Gelfoam; Gelofusine; ***Spain:*** Espongostan†; Geloplasma†; ***Switz.:*** Gelfoam†; Physiogel; ***Thai.:*** Gelafundin; Gelofusine; ***UK:*** Geloflex†; Gelofusine; Volplex; ***USA:*** Gelfilm; Gelfoam.

**Multi-ingredient:** ***Arg.:*** Megaplus; ***Austral.:*** Orabase; Orahesive; Stomahesive; ***Austria:*** Gelacet; ***Canad.:*** Orabase; Orahesive; ***Fr.:*** Gelodiet; Gelogastrine†; Plasmagel†; Plasmion; Rectopanbiline; ***Ger.:*** Gelacet N; Gerontamin†; ***Irl.:*** Orabase; ***Israel:*** Orabase; ***Ital.:*** Solecin; ***NZ:*** Orabase; Stomahesive; ***Port.:*** Combiderm†; Dagragel; Varihesive; ***S.Afr.:*** Granuflex; ***Switz.:*** Gelacet; Varihesive Hydroactive†; ***UK:*** Orabase; Orahesive; Stomahesive; ***USA:*** Dome-Paste.

## Haemoglobin

Hemoglobina.

## Hemoglobin Glutamer *(rINN)*

Haemoglobin Glutamer.

NOTE. The species of origin and average molecular mass should be indicated (e.g. hemoglobin glutamer-250 (bovine) indicates a polymerised haemoglobin of bovine origin with an average mass of 250 kD).

### Profile

Haemoglobin has the property of reversible oxygenation and is the respiratory pigment of blood. Solutions of haemoglobin or modified haemoglobin are being investigated as blood substitutes.

Hemoglobin glutamer-250 (bovine) (HBOC-201; haemoglobin-based oxygen carrier-201) is a polymerised bovine haemoglobin that is used for the treatment of anaemia in surgical patients.

Hemoglobin glutamer-200 (bovine) (HBOC-301) is used in veterinary medicine for the treatment of anaemia in dogs.

◊ The structure of haemoglobin gives a non-linear oxygen dissociation curve; almost maximum oxygen saturation occurs in normal arterial blood without the need for oxygen-enriched air. Thus the use of haemoglobin solutions for emergency use appears logical. Initial *animal* experiments with haemoglobin from haemolysed erythrocytes resulted in serious renal damage but haemoglobin is not itself nephrotoxic and the development of stroma-free haemoglobin solutions reduced this toxicity. However, once released from the erythrocytes, haemoglobin loses its ability to hold 2,3-diphosphoglycerate, which is essential for the delivery of oxygen, and haemoglobin, being a small molecule, is rapidly excreted by the kidneys. Various methods have been tried to overcome these problems; addition of pyridoxine 5-phosphate and formation of crosslinked haemoglobin restore the oxygen affinity to that of whole blood and polymerisation or microencapsulation in a lipid membrane extend the half-life. Polymerisation has the added advantages that this process is virucidal and also lowers the osmolality of the solution permitting higher concentrations to be used. There are, however, reservations concerning haemoglobin solutions as blood substitutes; blood itself must be available for their production, although expired blood may be employed and there is also concern about impairment of immune mechanisms. The development of recombinant human haemoglobin may overcome these problems and may allow further modification of the haemoglobin molecule.

References.


1. Anonymous. Blood substitutes: has the right solution been found? *Lancet* 1986; **i:** 717–18.
2. Urbaniak SJ. Artificial blood. *BMJ* 1991; **303:** 1348–50.
3. Jones JA. Red blood cell substitutes: current status. *Br J Anaesth* 1995; **74:** 697–703.
4. Mallick A, Bodenham AR. Modified haemoglobins as oxygen-transporting blood substitutes. *Br J Hosp Med* 1996; **55:** 443–8.
5. Lowe KC. Red cell substitutes. In: Contreras M, ed. *ABC of transfusion*. 3rd ed. London: BMJ Books, 1998: 71–5.
6. Remy B, *et al.* Red blood cell substitutes: fluorocarbon emulsions and haemoglobin solutions. *Br Med Bull* 1999; **55:** 277–98.


### Preparations

**Proprietary Preparations** (details are given in Part 3)

**Multi-ingredient:** ***Belg.:*** Aperop†; ***India:*** Blosyn; Globac-Z; Haem Up.

## Interleukin-3

Interleucina 3.

### Profile

Interleukin-3 (IL-3) is a cytokine that acts as a colony-stimulating factor. It is under investigation in the management of myelosuppression associated with cancer chemotherapy and following bone marrow transplantation. A fusion molecule with granulocyte-macrophage colony-stimulating factor, known as milodistim (PIXY-321), is also under investigation.

## Lenograstim *(BAN, USAN, rINN)*

rG-CSF. A recombinant human granulocyte colony-stimulating factor.

*CAS — 135968-09-1.*

*ATC — L03AA10.*

**Stability.** Solutions of colony-stimulating factors may be adsorbed onto glass or plastic materials. Solutions of lenograstim should not be diluted below the minimum recommended concentration for the formulation used.

## Adverse Effects and Precautions

As for Filgrastim, p.753.

## Uses and Administration

Lenograstim is a granulocyte colony-stimulating factor with actions and uses similar to those of filgrastim (p.754). It is used to treat or prevent neutropenia in patients receiving myelosuppressive cancer chemotherapy and to reduce the period of neutropenia in patients undergoing bone marrow transplantation (p.496). It is also used to mobilise peripheral blood progenitor cells for use as an alternative to bone marrow transplantation.

Lenograstim may be given in a dose of 150 micrograms/m$^2$ (19.2 million international units/m$^2$) daily to patients after bone marrow transplantation and also to patients established on antineoplastic therapy; in post-transplant patients it is given by intravenous infusion over 30 minutes or by subcutaneous injection, and in patients on antineoplastics it is given subcutaneously. Treatment is given until the neutrophil count has stabilised within the normal range, but a maximum treatment period of 28 consecutive days should not be exceeded.

For mobilisation of peripheral blood progenitor cells after cytotoxic chemotherapy a dose of 150 micrograms/m² (19.2 million international units/m²) daily may be administered by subcutaneous injection starting the day after completion of chemotherapy. When used alone, or in healthy donors, a dose of 10 micrograms/kg (1.28 million international units/kg) daily is given subcutaneously for 4 to 6 days.

◊ References.

1. Frampton JE, *et al.* Lenograstim: a review of its pharmacological properties and therapeutic efficacy in neutropenia and related clinical settings. *Drugs* 1995; **49:** 767–93.
2. Dunn CJ, Goa KL. Lenograstim: an update of its pharmacological properties and use in chemotherapy-induced neutropenia and related clinical settings. *Drugs* 2000; **59:** 681–717.

## Preparations

**Proprietary Preparations** (details are given in Part 3)
***Arg.:*** Granocyte; Leumostin; ***Austral.:*** Granocyte; ***Austria:*** Granocyte; ***Belg.:*** Granocyte; ***Braz.:*** Granocyte; ***Denm.:*** Granocyte; ***Fin.:*** Granocyte; ***Fr.:*** Granocyte; ***Ger.:*** Granocyte; ***Gr.:*** Granocyte; ***Irl.:*** Granocyte; ***Israel:*** Granocyte; ***Ital.:*** Granocyte; Myelostim; ***Jpn:*** Neutrogin; ***Malaysia:*** Granocyte; ***Neth.:*** Granocyte; ***Norw.:*** Granocyte; ***NZ:*** Granocyte; ***Port.:*** Granocyte; ***S.Afr.:*** Granocyte; ***Singapore:*** Granocyte; ***Spain:*** Euprotin; Granocyte; ***Swed.:*** Granocyte; ***Switz.:*** Granocyte; ***Thai.:*** Granocyte; ***UK:*** Granocyte.

## Leucocytes

Leucocitos.

**Description.** Preparations of leucocytes contain granulocytes with a variable content of red blood cells, lymphocytes, and platelets. Depending on the method of collection they may also contain dextran or hetastarch.

### Adverse Effects and Precautions

Leucocyte transfusions may cause severe transfusion reactions and fever. As with other blood products, there is a risk of transmission of infection. Severe lung reactions including fluid overload with pulmonary oedema are a particular problem in patients with active pulmonary infections.

Red blood cell compatibility testing is necessary because of the content of red blood cells. Graft-versus-host disease may occur in immunosuppressed recipients, and may be avoided by irradiating the product before administration.

### Uses and Administration

Transfusion of leucocytes has been used in patients with severe granulocytopenia and infection which has not been controlled by treatment with appropriate antimicrobials. Transfusion of $1 \times 10^{10}$ granulocytes once or twice daily has been suggested as an effective dose. Daily transfusions for at least 3 to 4 days are usually advised. Hydrocortisone and chlorphenamine may be given intravenously before transfusion to reduce the severity of adverse reactions.

◊ References.

1. Brozović B, *et al.* Platelet and granulocyte transfusions. In: Contreras M, ed. *ABC of transfusion.* 3rd ed. London: BMJ Books, 1998: 17–22.

## Preparations

**Proprietary Preparations** (details are given in Part 3)
***Ger.:*** LeukoNorm.

## Metacresolsulfonic Acid-Formaldehyde

*m*-Cresolsulphonic acid-formaldehyde condensation product; Dicresulene polymer; Metacresolsulphonic Acid-Formaldehyde; Policresolsulfonato; Polycresolsulfonate. Dihydroxydimethyldiphenylmethanedisulphonic acid polymer; Methylenebis(hydroxytoluenesulphonic acid) polymer.
$(C_{15}H_{16}O_8S_2)_n$.
*CAS — 9011-02-3.*

### Profile

Preparations of metacresolsulfonic acid-formaldehyde are highly acidic and are used as topical haemostatics and antiseptics. There are a number of vaginal preparations.

## Preparations

**Proprietary Preparations** (details are given in Part 3)
***Denm.:*** Nelex†; ***Fin.:*** Nelex†; ***Fr.:*** Negatol; ***Ger.:*** Albothyl; ***Hong Kong:*** Albothyl; ***Ital.:*** Negatol; ***Malaysia:*** Albothyl; ***Mex.:*** Albothyl; ***Port.:*** Nelex; ***S.Afr.:*** Nelex; ***Singapore:*** Albothyl; ***Spain:*** Negatol†; ***Swed.:*** Nelex†; ***Switz.:*** Negatol; Negatol Dental; ***Thai.:*** Albothyl†.

# Molgramostim *(BAN, USAN, rINN)*

Sch-39300. A recombinant human granulocyte-macrophage colony-stimulating factor; Colony-stimulating factor 2 (human clone $pHG_{25}$ protein moiety reduced).
*CAS — 99283-10-0.*
*ATC — L03AA03.*

**Pharmacopoeias.** *Eur.* (see p.vi) includes a concentrated solution.

**Ph. Eur. 5.0** (Molgramostim Concentrated Solution; Molgramostimi Solutio Concentrata). A solution of a protein having the structure of the granulocyte-macrophage colony-stimulating factor which is produced and secreted by various human blood cell types. It contains not less than 2.0 mg of protein per mL. A clear, colourless liquid. Store in airtight containers at a temperature below −65°. Protect from light.

**Stability.** Solutions of molgramostim may be adsorbed onto glass and plastic materials and therefore should not be diluted below the recommended minimum concentration of 7 micrograms/mL.

## Adverse Effects

Granulocyte-macrophage colony-stimulating factors such as molgramostim may cause transient hypotension and flushing, bone pain and musculoskeletal pain, fever and chills, dyspnoea, rash, fatigue, and gastrointestinal effects. Antibodies have been detected. Anaphylactic reactions, pleural and pericardial effusion, and cardiac arrhythmias have been reported rarely.

Colony-stimulating factors are fetotoxic in *animal* studies.

◊ General references.

1. Vial T, Descotes J. Clinical toxicity of cytokines used as haemopoietic growth factors. *Drug Safety* 1995; **13:** 371–406.

**Antibodies.** Antibodies have been reported in patients following administration of granulocyte-macrophage colony-stimulating factors produced in yeast[1] or in *Escherichia coli*.[2] Such factors are nonglycosylated or only partially glycosylated. A study[2] in 20 nonimmunocompromised patients given *E. coli*-derived granulocyte-macrophage colony-stimulating factors found that antibodies that were associated with reduced biological effectiveness developed in 95% of the patients. Only 1 of 8 immunocompromised patients given the colony-stimulating factor developed antibodies.

1. Gribben JG, *et al.* Development of antibodies to unprotected glycosylation sites on recombinant human GM-CSF. *Lancet* 1990; **335:** 434–7.
2. Ragnhammar P, *et al.* Induction of anti-recombinant human granulocyte-macrophage colony-stimulating factor (Escherichia coli-derived) antibodies and clinical effects in nonimmunocompromised patients. *Blood* 1994; **84:** 4078–87.

**Effects on the skin.** See under Filgrastim, p.754.

**Effects on the thyroid.** See under Filgrastim, p.754.

**Hypoalbuminaemia.** In a series of 9 patients given prolonged treatment with granulocyte-macrophage colony-stimulating factor for myelodysplasia or aplastic anaemia, 4 developed hypoalbuminaemia that was symptomatic in 2 of the patients.[1]

1. Kaczmarski RS, Mufti GJ. Hypoalbuminaemia after prolonged treatment with recombinant granulocyte macrophage colony stimulating factor. *BMJ* 1990; **301:** 1312–13.

## Precautions

Since granulocyte-macrophage colony-stimulating factors such as molgramostim can promote growth of myeloid cells *in vitro* their use in myeloid malignancies has been contra-indicated, although recently colony-stimulating factors have been used in some patients with myeloid diseases without stimulation of malignant cells. However, caution is required when they are used in patients with any pre-malignant or malignant myeloid condition. They should not be used from 24 hours before until 24 hours after cytotoxic chemotherapy or radiotherapy due to the sensitivity of rapidly dividing myeloid cells.

Granulocyte-macrophage colony-stimulating factors should be used with caution in patients with pulmonary disease as they may be predisposed to dyspnoea. Treatment should be withdrawn in patients who develop signs of pulmonary infiltrates. Caution is also necessary in patients with fluid retention or heart failure as fluid retention may be aggravated.

The complete blood count should be monitored regularly during therapy.

## Uses and Administration

Molgramostim is a granulocyte-macrophage colony-stimulating factor (GM-CSF) that acts as a haematopoietic growth factor stimulating the development of white blood cells, particularly granulocytes, macrophages, and monocytes. It is used to treat or prevent neutropenia in patients receiving myelosuppressive cancer chemotherapy and to reduce the period of neutropenia in patients undergoing bone marrow transplantation (p.496). It is also used to reduce ganciclovir-induced neutropenia (p.635).

As an adjunct to antineoplastic therapy, molgramostim is given by subcutaneous injection, starting 24 hours after the last dose of antineoplastic, in a dose of 5 to 10 micrograms/kg (60 000 to 110 000 international units/kg) daily. Treatment should be continued for 7 to 10 days.

Following bone marrow transplantation, molgramostim may be given by intravenous infusion over 4 to 6 hours in a dose of 10 micrograms/kg (110 000 international units/kg) daily. Treatment should be initiated the day after bone marrow transplantation and continued for up to 30 days depending on the neutrophil count.

For the management of ganciclovir-induced neutropenia, molgramostim may be given by subcutaneous injection in a dose of 5 micrograms/kg (60 000 international units/kg) daily. After 5 doses have been given the dose of molgramostim should be adjusted according to the neutrophil count.

The maximum dose for any indication should not exceed 10 micrograms/kg (110 000 international units/kg) daily.

Granulocyte colony-stimulating factors such as filgrastim (p.753) are also used. Macrophage colony-stimulating factors such as mirimostim are under investigation.

◊ General references.

1. American Society of Clinical Oncology. Recommendations for the use of hematopoietic colony-stimulating factors: evidence-based, clinical practice guidelines. *J Clin Oncol* 1994; **12:** 2471–2508. Also available at: http://www.asco.org/asco/downloads/Use_of_hematopoietic_Colony_Stimulating_Factors_Evidence_Based.pdf (accessed 23/06/04)
2. American Society of Clinical Oncology. Update of recommendations for the use of hematopoietic colony-stimulating factors: evidence-based clinical practice guidelines. *J Clin Oncol* 1996; **14:** 1957–60.
3. Nemunaitis J. A comparative review of colony-stimulating factors. *Drugs* 1997; **54:** 709–29.
4. Ozer H, *et al.* 2000 Update of recommendations for the use of hematopoietic colony-stimulating factors: evidence-based, clinical practice guidelines. *J Clin Oncol* 2000; **18:** 3558–85. Also available at: http://www.jco.org/cgi/reprint/18/20/3558.pdf (accessed 23/06/04)

**Aplastic anaemia.** Colony-stimulating factors, including granulocyte-macrophage colony-stimulating factors, have been tried in a few patients with aplastic anaemia (p.732).

**Infections.** See under Filgrastim, p.754.

**Respiratory disorders.** Pulmonary alveolar proteinosis is a rare diffuse lung disease that may result from impaired alveolar macrophage function caused by neutralising autoantibodies. It is characterised by excessive surfactant accumulation, and is usually managed with whole-lung lavage. Several months' therapy with granulocyte-macrophage colony-stimulating factor has been reported to induce remission in a number of these patients.[1-5]

1. Barraclough RM, Gillies AJ. Pulmonary alveolar proteinosis: a complete response to GM-CSF therapy. *Thorax* 2001; **56:** 664–5.
2. Seymour JF, *et al.* Therapeutic efficacy of granulocyte-macrophage colony-stimulating factor in patients with idiopathic acquired alveolar proteinosis. *Am J Respir Crit Care Med* 2001; **163:** 524–31.
3. Schoch OD, *et al.* BAL findings in a patient with pulmonary alveolar proteinosis successfully treated with GM-CSF. *Thorax* 2002; **57:** 277–80.
4. Romero A, *et al.* GM-CSF therapy in pulmonary alveolar proteinosis. *Thorax* 2002; **57:** 837.
5. Khanjari F, *et al.* GM-CSF and proteinosis. *Thorax* 2003; **58:** 645.

**Wounds and ulcers.** Molgramostim modifies several mechanisms involved in wound healing and is being investigated in non-healing wounds and ulcers (p.1139). It has been tried as an incubation solution for skin grafts,[1] and by perilesional injection[2,3] and topical application.[4] Molgramostim has been used as a mouthwash to relieve severe recurrent aphthous mouth ulcers in a small number of patients with AIDS.[5]

1. Pojda Z, Struzyna J. Treatment of non-healing ulcers with rhGM-CSF and skin grafts. *Lancet* 1994; **343:** 1100.
2. Marques da Costa R, *et al.* Quick healing of leg ulcers after molgramostim. *Lancet* 1994; **344:** 481–2.
3. Wheeler G, Brodie GN. GM-CSF and wound healing. *Med J Aust* 1998; **168:** 580.
4. Pieters RC, *et al.* Molgramostim to treat SS-sickle cell leg ulcers. *Lancet* 1995; **345:** 528.
5. Herranz P, *et al.* Successful treatment of aphthous ulcerations in AIDS patients using topical granulocyte-macrophage colony-stimulating factor. *Br J Dermatol* 2000; **142:** 171–6.

## Preparations

**Proprietary Preparations** (details are given in Part 3)
***Arg.:*** Growgen-GM; Leucomax; ***Austria:*** Leucomax; ***Belg.:*** Leucomax; ***Braz.:*** Gramostim; Leucocitim; ***Chile:*** Leucomax; ***Denm.:*** Leucomax; ***Fin.:*** Leucomax; ***Fr.:*** Leucomax†; ***Ger.:*** Leucomax; ***Gr.:*** Leucomax; Mielogen; ***Hong Kong:*** Leucomax; ***Irl.:*** Leucomax; ***Israel:*** Leucomax; ***Ital.:*** Leucomax; Mielogen; ***Malaysia:*** Leucomax; ***Mex.:*** Gramal; Leucomax; ***Neth.:*** Leucomax; ***Norw.:*** Leucomax; ***NZ:*** Leucomax; ***Port.:*** Leucomax†; ***S.Afr.:*** Leucomax; ***Singapore:*** Leucomax†; ***Spain:*** Leuco-

max; *Swed.:* Leucomax; *Switz.:* Leucomax; *Thai.:* Leucomax; *UK:* Leucomax.

## Naftazone *(BAN, rINN)*

Naftazona. 1,2-Naphthoquinone 2-semicarbazone.
$C_{11}H_9N_3O_2$ = 215.2.
*CAS — 15687-37-3.*

### Profile

Naftazone is a haemostatic used in venous insufficiency and in capillary haemorrhage. It is given by mouth in doses of up to 30 mg daily. It was formerly given by injection.

### Preparations

**Proprietary Preparations** (details are given in Part 3)
***Belg.:*** Mediaven; ***Fr.:*** Etioven; ***Spain:*** Metorene†; ***Switz.:*** Mediaven.

## Nartograstim *(rINN)*

A recombinant human granulocyte colony-stimulating factor; N-L-Methionyl-1-L-alanine-3-L-threonine-4-L-tyrosine-5-L-arginine-17-L-serine colony-stimulating factor (human clone 1034).
*CAS — 134088-74-7.*

### Profile

Nartograstim is a granulocyte colony-stimulating factor with properties similar to those of filgrastim (p.753). It has been given by intravenous or subcutaneous injection in the management of neutropenia.

## Oprelvekin *(USAN, rINN)*

Oprelvekina. 2-178-Interleukin 11 (human clone pXM/IL-11).
$C_{854}H_{1411}N_{253}O_{235}S_2$ = 19047.0.
*CAS — 145941-26-0.*
*ATC — L03AC02.*

### Adverse Effects and Precautions

Fluid retention may occur producing oedema and dyspnoea; caution is required when giving oprelvekin to patients with a history or signs of heart failure. Dilutional anaemia may occur. Fluid balance and electrolytes should be monitored in patients receiving long-term diuretic therapy. Transient atrial arrhythmias commonly occur. Other adverse effects include exfoliative dermatitis, mild blurred vision, and conjunctival injection. Hypersensitivity reactions, including anaphylaxis, have been reported with the use of oprelvekin. Papilloedema has been reported, and oprelvekin should be used with caution in patients with pre-existing papilloedema or tumours involving the CNS.

Fetotoxicity has been reported in *animals*.

**Effects on the eyes.** Papilloedema has been reported in patients treated with oprelvekin, and was found to be a dose-limiting adverse effect in a study of safety and pharmacokinetics in children.[1]

1. Wyeth-Ayerst. Neumega (oprelvekin), August 24, 2001. Available at: http://www.fda.gov/medwatch/SAFETY/2001/neumega.htm (accessed 23/06/04)

### Uses and Administration

Oprelvekin, a recombinant human interleukin-11, is a platelet growth factor that stimulates the proliferation and maturation of megakaryocytes and thus increases the production of platelets. Oprelvekin is given by subcutaneous injection in a dose of 50 micrograms/kg daily to prevent severe antineoplastic-induced thrombocytopenia in patients with non-myeloid malignancies. The initial dose should be given 6 to 24 hours after the last dose of antineoplastic, and continued up to a maximum of 21 days. Treatment with oprelvekin should be stopped at least 2 days before starting the next planned cycle of chemotherapy.

Oprelvekin is under investigation for the treatment of Crohn's disease.

◊ References.

1. Tepler I, *et al.* A randomized placebo-controlled trial of recombinant human interleukin-11 in cancer patients with severe thrombocytopenia due to chemotherapy. *Blood* 1996; **87:** 3607–14.
2. Isaacs C, *et al.* Randomized placebo-controlled study of recombinant human interleukin-11 to prevent chemotherapy-induced thrombocytopenia in patients with breast cancer receiving dose-intensive cyclophosphamide and doxorubicin. *J Clin Oncol* 1997; **15:** 3368–77.

### Preparations

**Proprietary Preparations** (details are given in Part 3)
***Arg.:*** Neumega; ***Braz.:*** Neumega; ***Chile:*** Neumega; ***Mex.:*** Neumega; ***USA:*** Neumega.

# Oxidised Cellulose

Cellulosic Acid; Celulosa oxidada; Oxidized Cellulose.
*CAS — 9032-53-5.*
*ATC — B02BC02.*

**Description.** Oxidised cellulose is a sterile polyanhydroglucuronic acid, prepared by the oxidation of a suitable form of cellulose.

**Pharmacopoeias.** In *US* which also includes Oxidized Regenerated Cellulose.

**USP 27** (Oxidized Cellulose). It contains not less than 16% and not more than 24% of carboxyl groups, calculated on the dried basis. It is a slightly off-white gauze or lint with a slight, charred odour. Insoluble in water and in acids; soluble in dilute alkalis. Store at a temperature not exceeding 8°. Protect from direct sunlight.

**USP 27** (Oxidized Regenerated Cellulose). It contains 18 to 24% of carboxyl groups calculated on the dried basis. It is a slightly off-white knit fabric, with a slight odour. Insoluble in water and in dilute acids; soluble in dilute alkalis. Store at a temperature between 15° and 30°. Protect from direct sunlight.

### Adverse Effects and Precautions

Foreign body reactions may occur after the use of oxidised cellulose or oxidised regenerated cellulose. Headache, burning, and stinging have been reported and sneezing has been noted after use in epistaxis. Oxidised cellulose swells on contact with a bleeding surface; this could result in tissue necrosis, nerve damage, obstruction, or vascular stenosis if packed closely, especially into bony cavities, or if wrapped tightly around blood vessels. To minimise such complications the removal of excess material should be considered after haemostasis is achieved, and oxidised cellulose should always be removed after use near the spinal cord or optic nerve. Oxidised cellulose should not be used in packing or implantation in fractures since it may interfere with bone regeneration or cause cyst formation. It should not be used as a surface dressing, except for immediate control of haemorrhage, as it inhibits epithelialisation.

Oxidised cellulose should be used as the dry material as moistening will reduce its ability to absorb blood. Silver nitrate or other escharotic chemicals should not be applied before use as cauterisation might inhibit absorption of oxidised cellulose. Thrombin is inactivated by the low pH of oxidised cellulose; it is recommended that oxidised cellulose should not be impregnated with other haemostatics or antibacterials.

### Uses and Administration

Oxidised cellulose and oxidised regenerated cellulose are absorbable haemostatics (p.735). When applied to a bleeding surface, they swell to form a gelatinous mass which aids in the formation of a clot. It is gradually absorbed by the tissues, usually within 2 to 7 days. Complete absorption of large amounts of such material may take 6 weeks or more. These materials also have a weak bactericidal action. They are used in surgery as adjuncts in the control of moderate bleeding where suturing or ligation is impracticable or ineffective; they should not be used to control haemorrhage from large arteries. The gauze, lint, or knitted material should be laid on the bleeding surface or held firmly against the tissues until haemostasis is achieved; removal should then be considered (see Adverse Effects and Precautions, above). Oxidised cellulose should be used as the dry material as moistening will reduce its ability to absorb blood.

### Preparations

**Proprietary Preparations** (details are given in Part 3)
***Fr.:*** Interceed†; Surgicel; ***Ger.:*** Interceed†; Tabotamp†; ***Hong Kong:*** Seal On; ***Irl.:*** Alltracel P; Premdoc; Seal-On; Traumacel P; ***Ital.:*** Tabotamp†; ***UK:*** Interceed†; Oxycel; Surgicel†; ***USA:*** Oxycel; Surgicel.

**Multi-ingredient:** ***Fr.:*** Promogran; ***Irl.:*** Alltracel S; ***UK:*** Seal-On.

## Oxypolygelatin

Oxipoligelatina.

### Profile

Oxypolygelatin is a polymer derived from gelatin (p.754). It is used as a 5.5% solution as a plasma volume expander. There have been reports of anaphylaxis.

### Preparations

**Proprietary Preparations** (details are given in Part 3)
***Arg.:*** Gelifundol; ***Austria:*** Gelifundol; ***Ger.:*** Gelifundol; ***Hong Kong:*** Gelifundol; ***S.Afr.:*** Gelifundol; ***Thai.:*** Gelifundol.

# Plasma

**Pharmacopoeias.** Many pharmacopoeias have monographs including *Eur.* (see p.vi).

**Ph. Eur. 5.0** (Human Plasma for Fractionation; Plasma Humanum ad Separationem). The liquid part of human blood remaining after separation of the cellular elements from whole blood or collected in an apheresis procedure; it is intended for the manufacture of plasma-derived products. It is obtained from healthy donors and is tested for the absence of hepatitis B surface antigen and antibodies against HIV-1 and HIV-2 and hepatitis C virus.

A light yellow to green, clear or slightly turbid liquid, without visible signs of haemolysis. Frozen plasma should be stored at or below −20°; it may still be used for fractionation if the temperature is between −20° and −15° for not more than a total of 72 hours without exceeding −15° on more than one occasion as long as the temperature is at all times −5° or lower.

**Ph. Eur. 5.0** (Human Plasma (Pooled and Treated for Virus Inactivation); Plasma Humanum Collectum Deinde Conditum ad Viros Exstinguendos). A frozen or freeze-dried, sterile, non-pyrogenic preparation obtained from human plasma derived from donors belonging to the same ABO blood group. The plasma used complies with the requirements for Human Plasma for Fractionation (above). The method of preparation is designed to minimise activation of any coagulation factor and includes a step or steps that have been shown to inactivate known agents of infection.

The frozen preparation, after thawing, is a clear or slightly opalescent liquid free from solid and gelatinous particles. The freeze-dried preparation is an almost white or slightly yellow powder or friable solid.

### Adverse Effects and Precautions

As for Blood, p.744, though with a low risk of transmitting cell-associated viruses. However, the production of blood products using plasma from UK donors has been phased out due to the possible risk of transmission of Creutzfeldt-Jakob disease.

### Uses and Administration

Fresh frozen plasma contains useful amounts of clotting factors. It should be reserved for patients with proven abnormalities in blood coagulation (see Haemorrhagic Disorders, p.737). Indications include congenital deficiencies in clotting factors for which specific concentrates are unavailable, severe multiple clotting factor deficiencies for example in patients with liver disease, rapid reversal of the action of coumarin anticoagulants, and disseminated intravascular coagulation. It may be used following massive blood transfusion when there is evidence of coagulation deficiency but its value for routine prophylaxis against abnormal bleeding tendencies in patients receiving massive blood transfusions is contentious except where clotting abnormalities have been confirmed. It has also been used in the treatment of thrombotic thrombocytopenic purpura and as a source of plasma proteins.

The amount of fresh frozen plasma transfused depends on the required level of clotting factors. A unit of fresh frozen plasma refers to the quantity of plasma obtained from 1 unit of whole blood; this generally represents a volume of about 250 mL, including anticoagulant.

Fresh frozen plasma should not be used as a volume expander or as a nutritional source.

Therapeutic plasma exchange or plasmapheresis (see below) are used in a wide variety of disorders.

Plasma is used for the production of various blood products including albumin, antithrombin III, blood clotting factors, immunoglobulins, and platelets. Other preparations include cryoprecipitate depleted plasma from which approximately half the fibrinogen, factor VIII, and fibronectin has been removed, and single donor plasma which is not frozen. A solvent-detergent-treated plasma preparation is available.

◊ References.

1. Fresh-frozen Plasma, Cryoprecipitate, and Platelets Administration Practice Guidelines Development Task Force of the College of American Pathologists. Practice parameter for the use of fresh-frozen plasma, cryoprecipitate, and platelets. *JAMA* 1994; **271:** 777–81.
2. Cohen H, *et al.* Plasma, plasma products, and indications for their use. In: Contreras M, ed. *ABC of transfusion.* 3rd ed. London; BMJ Books, 1998: 40–44.
3. British Committee for Standards in Haematology, Blood Transfusion Task Force. Guidelines for the use of fresh-frozen plasma, cryoprecipitate and cryosupernatant. *Br J Haematol* 2004; **126:** 11–28. Also available at: http://www.bcshguidelines.com/pdf/freshfrozen_280604.pdf (accessed 06/07/04)

**Hereditary angioedema.** For a mention of fresh frozen plasma being used in hereditary angioedema, see p.761.

**Neonatal intraventricular haemorrhage.** Plasma volume expansion in preterm neonates has been thought to help prevent neonatal intraventricular haemorrhage (p.740). However, a study using plasma or gelatin as plasma volume expanders,[1,2] found no evidence of a decreased risk of such haemorrhage or subsequent death or disability.


1. The Northern Neonatal Nursing Initiative Trial Group. A randomized trial comparing the effect of prophylactic intravenous fresh frozen plasma, gelatin or glucose on early mortality and morbidity in preterm babies. *Eur J Pediatr* 1996; **155:** 580–8.
2. Northern Neonatal Nursing Initiative Trial Group. Randomised trial of prophylactic early fresh-frozen plasma or gelatin or glucose in preterm babies: outcome at 2 years. *Lancet* 1996; **348:** 229–32.


**Plasma exchange.** Therapeutic plasma exchange or plasmapheresis are procedures in which plasma is selectively removed from the body while the cellular constituents of blood are retained. They have been tried in a number of disorders, including many with an immunological basis, when conventional treatment has not been successful. The aim is removal or reduction of those constituents of plasma causing or aggravating a disease or replacement of deficient plasma factors if the deficiency is the cause of the disorder. Although the two terms are commonly used synonymously, plasmapheresis generally involves the removal of small volumes of plasma, whereas plasma exchange removes larger volumes which must be replaced with a suitable fluid. Volume and frequency of plasma exchange is determined by the pathophysiology of the undesirable plasma constituent. For example, removal of antibody usually requires exchange of 1.5 times the estimated plasma volume (3 to 4 litres) repeated daily or on alternate days until the desired reduction is obtained. The replacement fluid used depends on the volume and the condition being treated; albumin solutions, plasma expanders, or sodium chloride 0.9% are frequently used, whereas in conditions where there is deficiency of a plasma factor replacement of blood components such as immunoglobulins may be required. Fresh frozen plasma has been used as a replacement fluid but is associated with a high incidence of adverse effects and is generally reserved for the management of thrombotic thrombocytopenic purpura. Technological developments, such as the use of specific adsorbents and the use of multiple filters with different pore sizes, may enable removal of only the desired constituent and avoid removal and subsequent replacement of total plasma.

References.


1. Urbaniak SJ, Robinson EA. Therapeutic apheresis. In: Contreras M, ed. *ABC of transfusion*. 3rd ed. London: BMJ Books, 1998: 67–70.


**Thrombotic microangiopathies.** Thrombotic thrombocytopenic purpura and haemolytic-uraemic syndrome are both syndromes characterised by intravascular platelet clumping.[1-3] Thrombocytopenia also occurs and fragmentation of erythrocytes, partly caused by the red cells passing through areas of the microvasculature occluded by the platelet aggregation, leads to microvascular haemolytic anaemia. In **thrombotic thrombocytopenic purpura** (TTP) the platelet aggregation is extensive and obstructs the vessels of various organs producing ischaemia or even infarction. The CNS, notably the brain, is often the area predominantly affected although some degree of renal involvement may occur. It is an uncommon disorder; adult women, in whom the condition presents as a chronic relapsing illness, are slightly more frequently affected.

In **haemolytic-uraemic syndrome** (HUS) the platelet aggregation is relatively less widespread and less severe and mainly affects the renal microvasculature although extra-renal manifestations may also occur. The primary consequences of HUS are hypertension and acute renal insufficiency or ultimately, if untreated, renal failure. Most cases of HUS occur in early childhood and follow a diarrhoeal illness caused by *Shigella dysenteriae* or *Escherichia coli*. However, the condition is becoming increasingly recognised in adults, particularly the elderly. Some cases may be drug induced. With appropriate symptomatic therapy HUS is typically a self-limiting disease with spontaneous recovery although fatalities have been known.

The supportive **management** of both syndromes follows similar lines.[1,3] In HUS, or TTP with renal symptoms, special attention needs to be directed towards the prevention of renal failure. Hypovolaemia should be corrected, with careful control of fluid and electrolyte balance and hypertension. Haemodialysis will be needed if renal failure develops. Severe anaemia requires blood transfusion, but platelet transfusion should be avoided.

Plasma exchange (plasmapheresis) is considered to be the mainstay of therapy for TTP.[1-3] The optimal regimen has not been determined, but it is usually performed daily. There is also some debate about the preferred fluid replacement; plasma exchange using cryosupernatant (the plasma remaining after cryoprecipitate is prepared, and which is depleted of von Willebrand factor) may be more efficacious than fresh frozen plasma.[3] When plasma exchange is not available, infusion of fresh frozen plasma may be used.[1,3] In HUS, there is some debate over the use of plasma exchange or infusion. Some consider that these have no proven benefit in HUS[2,3] but others[1] have challenged this belief.

Antiplatelet therapy and corticosteroids are often given, although neither has been adequately investigated and antiplatelets such as ticlopidine and clopidogrel have been reported to cause TTP (see p.1011). Aspirin and dipyridamole have been used, but are not recommended when profound thrombocytopenia is present because of the potential bleeding risk, without proven benefit. However, low-dose aspirin may be used when platelet counts have recovered following plasma exchange in TTP.[1,3] Some reports have described improved outcome in both syndromes with corticosteroids.[4] They are often used with plasma exchange in TTP.[1,3] However, a randomised, double-blind trial[5] in children with HUS failed to show any difference between oral corticosteroids and placebo in terms of haematological or neurological recovery, although renal function appeared to improve more rapidly in those receiving corticosteroids.

Other drugs may also be tried, particularly in refractory TTP. Some treatments that have been reported to be beneficial in case reports or small series include normal immunoglobulin,[1] azathioprine,[1] ciclosporin,[1,3] cyclophosphamide,[3] and vincristine.[1-3] The monoclonal antibody, rituximab, is under investigation.[2] The use of a protein-A immuno-adsorption column may be considered in the management of TTP associated with malignancy or bone marrow transplantation.[3] Administration of epoprostenol may be tried in order to inhibit platelet-endothelial interactions and to help promote diuresis but again has not been subject to controlled studies; anecdotal evidence presents both favourable[6,7] and negative[8,9] results. Alteplase has been used successfully in one patient with HUS.[10] Splenectomy may also be considered.[1,3]


1. Elliott MA, Nichols WL. Thrombotic thrombocytopenic purpura and hemolytic uremic syndrome. *Mayo Clin Proc* 2001; **76:** 1154–62.
2. Moake JL. Thrombotic microangiopathies. *N Engl J Med* 2002; **347:** 589–600.
3. British Society for Haematology. Guidelines on the diagnosis and management of the thrombotic microangiopathic haemolytic anaemias. *Br J Haematol* 2003; **120:** 556–73. Also available at: http://www.bcshguidelines.com/pdf/BJH556.pdf (accessed 23/06/04)
4. Bell WR, *et al.* Improved survival in thrombotic thrombocytopenic purpura-hemolytic uremic syndrome: clinical experience in 108 patients. *N Engl J Med* 1991; **325:** 398–403.
5. Perez N, *et al.* Steroids in the hemolytic uremic syndrome. *Pediatr Nephrol* 1998; **12:** 101–4.
6. Fitzgerald GA, *et al.* Intravenous prostacyclin in thrombotic thrombocytopenic purpura. *Ann Intern Med* 1981; **95:** 319–22.
7. Payton CD, *et al.* Successful treatment of thrombotic thrombocytopenic purpura by epoprostenol infusion. *Lancet* 1985; **i:** 927–8.
8. Budd GT, *et al.* Prostacyclin therapy of thrombotic thrombocytopenic purpura. *Lancet* 1980: **ii:** 915.
9. Johnson JE, *et al.* Ineffective epoprostenol therapy for thrombotic thrombocytopenic purpura. *JAMA* 1983; **250:** 3089–91.
10. Kruez W, *et al.* Successful treatment of haemolytic-uraemic syndrome with recombinant tissue-type plasminogen activator. *Lancet* 1993; **341:** 1665–6.


## Preparations

**Proprietary Preparations** (details are given in Part 3)
***Austria:*** Octaplas; ***Ger.:*** Octaplas; ***Ital.:*** Octaplas; ***Norw.:*** Octaplas; ***Switz.:*** Octaplas; ***UK:*** Octaplas.

# Plasma Protein Fraction

Fracción proteica del plasma.

**Pharmacopoeias.** Many pharmacopoeias have monographs including *US.*

**USP 27** (Plasma Protein Fraction). A sterile preparation of serum albumin and globulin obtained by fractionating material (blood, plasma, or serum) from healthy human donors, the source material being tested for the absence of hepatitis B surface antigen. It contains 5% of protein; not less than 83% of the total protein is albumin; not more than 17% is alpha and beta globulins; not more than 1% has the electrophoretic properties of gamma globulin. It contains sodium acetyltryptophanate with or without sodium caprylate as a stabilising agent but no antimicrobial preservative. It contains 130 to 160 mmol/litre of sodium, and not more than 2 mmol/litre of potassium. A solution in 0.15M sodium chloride containing 1% protein has a pH between 6.7 and 7.3. It should be used within 4 hours of opening the container.

## Profile

Plasma protein fraction consists mainly of albumin with a small proportion of globulins; it does not contain blood-clotting factors. It has properties and uses similar to those of other albumin solutions (p.741). It is given intravenously as a solution containing 5% of total protein. The amount of plasma protein fraction administered will depend upon the clinical condition of the patient. For most indications an initial infusion of up to 500 mL for adults has been suggested at a rate not normally exceeding 10 mL/minute. Patients with normal blood volume may require slower rates of administration to prevent excessive volume expansion. In hypoproteinaemia administration of 1 to 1.5 litres of a 5% solution will provide 50 to 75 g of protein. A suggested dose in infants and small children for shock with dehydration is up to 33 mL/kg given at a rate of up to 5 to 10 mL/minute.

As with other albumin solutions, plasma protein fraction should not be used for parenteral nutrition.

## Preparations

***USP 27:*** Plasma Protein Fraction.

**Proprietary Preparations** (details are given in Part 3)
***Austria:*** Biseko; ***Braz.:*** Plasmanate†; ***Canad.:*** Plasmanate†; ***Ger.:*** Biseko; ***Hong Kong:*** Plasmanate†; Protenate†; ***Israel:*** Plasmanate; ***Ital.:*** Haimaserum†; Plasmaviral†; PPS; Uman-Serum; ***Malaysia:*** Plasmanate; ***S.Afr.:*** Bioplasma FDP; ***Singapore:*** Plasmanate†; ***Thai.:*** Biseko; ***USA:*** Plasma-Plex; Plasmanate; Plasmatein†; Protenate.

**Multi-ingredient:** ***Belg.:*** Tissucol†; ***Fin.:*** Tisseel Duo Quick; ***Ger.:*** Tissucol Duo S; Tissucol Fibrinkleber tiefgefroren†; Tissucol-Kit; ***Ital.:*** Tissucol; ***Swed.:*** Tisseel Duo Quick; ***Switz.:*** Tissucol Duo S.

# Platelets

Plaquetas.

**Pharmacopoeias.** Many pharmacopoeias have monographs including *US.*

**USP 27** (Platelet Concentrate). It contains the platelets taken from plasma obtained, in a single procedure, by whole blood collection, plasmapheresis, or plateletpheresis from a single suitable human donor. The platelets are suspended in a specified volume (20 to 30 mL, or 30 to 50 mL) of the original plasma. The suspension contains not less than $5.5 \times 10^{10}$ platelets/unit in not less than 75% of the units tested. It should be stored in hermetically-sealed sterile containers at 20° to 24° (30 to 50 mL volume), or at 1° to 6° (20 to 30 mL volume) except during transport when the temperature may be 1° to 10°. The expiration time is not more than 72 hours from the time of collection of the source material. Continuous gentle agitation must be maintained if stored at 20° to 24°. The suspension must be used within 4 hours of opening the container and should be administered with equipment that contains a filter.

## Adverse Effects and Precautions

Transmission of infection has been associated with the transfusion of blood products including platelets (p.744). Since platelets are stored at room temperature there is increased risk of bacterial infection following transfusion. Transfusion reactions including fever and urticaria are not uncommon. Recipients of multiple transfusions of platelet concentrates from random donors may develop antibodies to HLA which result in impaired responsiveness to subsequent transfusions. Use of leucocyte-depleted platelet concentrates reduces the incidence of transfusion reactions and of HLA sensitisation. Platelet concentrates prepared from RhD-positive donors should generally not be given to RhD-negative women of child-bearing potential. Ideally platelet concentrates should also be ABO-compatible with the recipient.

**ABO compatibility.** A discussion[1] of ABO incompatibility and platelet transfusions concluded that, while ABO compatibility is desirable, it is better to transfuse incompatible platelets than none at all. However, acute haemolysis has occurred[2] after transfusion of platelet concentrate with high-titre anti-A. Increased use of single-donor, machine-harvested material from panels of regular platelet donors should make screening for high-titre isoagglutinins more practical.[1]


1. Anonymous. ABO incompatibility and platelet transfusion. *Lancet* 1990; **335:** 142–3.
2. Murphy MF, *et al.* Acute haemolysis after ABO-incompatible platelet transfusion. *Lancet* 1990; **335:** 974–5.


**HLA antibodies.** Platelets obtained from single donors have been used in patients receiving multiple transfusions of platelet concentrates to reduce the formation of antibodies to HLA. Leucocyte-depleted platelets and UVB-irradiated platelets have also been tried. A study[1] in 530 patients found that the incidence of platelet refractoriness was reduced from 13% of those patients receiving pooled platelet concentrates to 3% and 5% of those receiving leucocyte-depleted and UVB-irradiated platelets, respectively. Some guidelines[2] have recommended that although HLA alloimmunisation and platelet refractoriness may be reduced by the use of leucocyte-depleted platelets, there is no convincing evidence of clinical benefit from routine use.


1. The Trial to Reduce Alloimmunization to Platelets Study Group. Leukocyte reduction and ultraviolet B irradiation of platelets to prevent alloimmunization and refractoriness to platelet transfusions. *N Engl J Med* 1997; **337:** 1861–9.
2. British Committee for Standards in Haematology, Blood Transfusion Task Force. Guidelines on the clinical use of leucocyte-depleted blood components. *Transfus Med* 1998; **8:** 59–71. Also available at: http://www.bcshguidelines.com/pdf/trans129.pdf (accessed 23/06/04)


## Uses and Administration

Blood platelets assist in the haemostatic process (p.735) by aggregating to form a platelet thrombus, and by releasing factors involved in initiating coagulation.

Transfusions of platelet concentrates are given to patients with thrombocytopenic haemorrhage (see p.737). They are also given prophylactically to reduce the frequency of haemorrhage in thrombocytopenia associated with the chemotherapy of neoplastic disease (see p.496).

◊ References.

1. Fresh-frozen Plasma, Cryoprecipitate, and Platelets Administration Practice Guidelines Development Task Force of the College of American Pathologists. Practice parameter for the use of fresh-frozen plasma, cryoprecipitate, and platelets. *JAMA* 1994; **271:** 777–81.
2. Brozović B, *et al.* Platelet and granulocyte transfusions. In: Contreras M, ed. *ABC of transfusion.* 3rd ed. London: BMJ Books, 1998: 17–22.
3. Schiffer CA, *et al.* Platelet transfusion for patients with cancer: clinical practice guidelines of the American Society of Clinical Oncology. *J Clin Oncol* 2001; **19:** 1519–38. Also available at: http://www.jco.org/cgi/reprint/19/5/1519.pdf (accessed 23/06/04)
4. British Committee for Standards in Haematology, Blood Transfusion Task Force. Guidelines for the use of platelet transfusions. *Br J Haematol* 2003; **122:** 10–23. Also available at: http://www.bcshguidelines.com/pdf/platelettrans040703.pdf (accessed 23/06/04)

### Preparations

***USP 27:*** Platelet Concentrate.

## Polygeline *(BAN, pINN)*

Poligelina; Polygelinum.

*CAS — 9015-56-9.*

*ATC — B05AA10.*

**Description.** Polygeline is a polymer prepared by cross-linking polypeptides derived from denatured gelatin with a di-isocyanate to form urea bridges.

**Incompatibility.** Intravenous preparations of polygeline contain calcium ions and are incompatible with citrated blood.

### Adverse Effects

As for Gelatin, p.755.

**Hypersensitivity.** Fatal reactions following polygeline infusion have been reported in 2 patients with bronchial asthma.[1,2] In both cases, the patients were undergoing epidural analgesia with bupivacaine. Polygeline was administered to correct hypotension which had not responded to infusion of crystalloids. Both patients developed refractory bronchospasm and cardiac arrhythmias and died despite intensive resuscitation attempts. One patient also developed focal seizures.[2]

The manufacturer recommends that prophylaxis with histamine $H_1$- and $H_2$-antagonists should be given to patients with known allergic conditions such as asthma. Similar advice has been offered[3] for patients undergoing anaesthesia and receiving polygeline following findings of an increased incidence of severe histamine-related reactions in such patients.

1. Freeman MK. Fatal reaction to haemaccel. *Anaesthesia* 1979; **34:** 341–3.
2. Barratt S, Purcell GJ. Refractory bronchospasm following "Haemaccel" infusion and bupivacaine epidural anaesthesia. *Anaesth Intensive Care* 1988; **16:** 208–11.
3. Lorenz W, *et al.* Incidence and clinical importance of perioperative histamine release: randomised study of volume loading and antihistamines after induction of anaesthesia. *Lancet* 1994; **343:** 933–40.

### Precautions

Precautions that should be observed with plasma expanders are described under Dextran 70, p.746, and these should be considered when polygeline is used for this purpose.

Polygeline preparations contain calcium ions and therefore should be used with caution in patients being treated with cardiac glycosides.

**Renal impairment.** In a study[1] in 52 patients with normal or impaired renal function given 500 mL of polygeline 3.5% about 50% of the dose was excreted in the urine within 48 hours in those with normal renal function. Excretion of polygeline in those with renal impairment, based on the patient's glomerular filtration rate (GFR), was found to be:

- GFR 31 to 90 mL/minute: unimpaired
- GFR 11 to 30 mL/minute: slightly reduced
- GFR 2 to 10 mL/minute: reduced to 27% in 48 hours
- GFR 0.5 to 2 mL/minute: reduced to 9.3% in 48 hours.

The mean half-life of the elimination phase was 505 minutes in those with adequate renal function, increasing to 985 minutes in those with end-stage renal failure. Polygeline 500 mL of 3.5% solution could be given twice weekly for 1 to 2 months even in patients with total anuria.

1. Köhler H, *et al.* Elimination of hexamethylene diisocyanate cross-linked polypeptides in patients with normal or impaired renal function. *Eur J Clin Pharmacol* 1978; **14:** 405–12.

### Pharmacokinetics

Like gelatin, polygeline is excreted mainly in the urine. The half-life is about 5 hours.

### Uses and Administration

Polygeline is a plasma volume expander used as a 3.5% solution with electrolytes in the management of hypovolaemic shock (p.835). The rate of infusion depends on the condition of the patient and does not normally exceed 500 mL in 60 minutes although it may be greater in emergencies. Initial doses for hypovolaemic shock usually consist of 500 to 1000 mL; up to 1500 mL of blood loss can be replaced by polygeline alone. Patients losing greater volumes of blood will require blood transfusion as well as plasma expanders.

Polygeline is also used in extracorporeal perfusion fluids, as a perfusion fluid for isolated organs, as fluid replacement in plasma exchange, and as a carrier solution for insulin. For plasma exchange, up to 2 litres of polygeline may be given as sole replacement fluid.

### Preparations

**Proprietary Preparations** (details are given in Part 3)

***Arg.:*** Haemaccel; ***Austral.:*** Haemaccel; ***Austria:*** Haemaccel; ***Belg.:*** Haemaccel; ***Braz.:*** Haemaccel†; ***Chile:*** Haemaccel; ***Denm.:*** Haemaccel†; ***Fin.:*** Haemaccel†; ***Fr.:*** Haemaccel†; ***Ger.:*** Haemaccel; ***Gr.:*** Haemaccel; ***Hong Kong:*** Haemaccel; ***India:*** Haemaccel; ***Irl.:*** Haemaccel; ***Israel:*** Haemaccel; ***Ital.:*** Emagel; Gelplex; ***Malaysia:*** Haemaccel; ***Mex.:*** Haemaccel; ***Neth.:*** Haemaccel; ***Norw.:*** Haemaccel; ***NZ:*** Haemaccel; ***Port.:*** Haemaccel; ***S.Afr.:*** Haemaccel; ***Singapore:*** Haemaccel†; ***Spain:*** Hemoce†; ***Swed.:*** Haemaccel†; ***Switz.:*** Haemaccel; ***Thai.:*** Haemaccel; ***UK:*** Haemaccel†.

## Protein C

Proteína C.

*ATC — B01AD12.*

## Drotrecogin Alfa (Activated) *(BAN, rINN)*

LY-203638. Blood coagulation factor XIV (human).

*CAS — 98530-76-8.*

*ATC — B01AD10.*

### Adverse Effects and Precautions

As with other plasma-derived products, protein C preparations carry a risk of transmission of infection. Hypersensitivity reactions have been reported infrequently.

Drotrecogin alfa (activated), a recombinant activated protein C used in the management of severe sepsis, may increase the risk of severe bleeding episodes. It is contra-indicated in patients with active internal bleeding and should be used with caution when there is increased risk of bleeding.

### Uses and Administration

Protein C is an endogenous inhibitor of blood coagulation (see Haemostasis and Fibrinolysis, p.735). A preparation of protein C purified from human plasma is used in the management of thromboembolic disorders in patients with congenital deficiency of protein C. It is given by intravenous injection in an initial dose of 60 to 80 international units/kg, adjusted according to response.

Drotrecogin alfa (activated) is a recombinant activated protein C that is used in the management of severe sepsis. It is given by intravenous infusion in a dose of 24 micrograms/kg per hour for 96 hours.

**Severe sepsis.** Severe sepsis (sepsis associated with acute organ dysfunction; see Septicaemia, p.144) involves a systemic inflammatory response, inappropriate coagulation, and impaired fibrinolysis. These contribute to the development of disseminated intravascular coagulation (DIC) and microvascular thrombosis (p.737). Endogenous protein C becomes depleted as it is activated in an attempt to restore homoeostasis. In the small number of cases that have been reported,[1-3] protein C replacement appeared to improve rate of survival and clinical outcome in the management of purpura fulminans and DIC in severe meningococcaemia. Drotrecogin alfa (activated) has been studied in the management of severe sepsis and found to reduce mortality, but with an increased risk of serious bleeding events.[4,5] The efficacy of drotrecogin alfa (activated) does not appear to depend on the identity of the infective organism.[6]

1. Rintala E, *et al.* Protein C in the treatment of coagulopathy in meningococcal disease. *Lancet* 1996; **347:** 1767.
2. Smith OP, *et al.* Use of protein-C concentrate, heparin, and haemodiafiltration in meningococcus-induced purpura fulminans. *Lancet* 1997; **350:** 1590–3.
3. Alberio L, *et al.* Protein C replacement in severe meningococcemia: rationale and clinical experience. *Clin Infect Dis* 2001; **32:** 1338–46. Correction. *ibid.*; 1803.
4. Bernard GR, *et al.* Efficacy and safety of recombinant human activated protein C for severe sepsis. *N Engl J Med* 2001; **344:** 699–709.
5. Lyseng-Williamson KA, Perry CM. Drotrecogin alfa (activated). *Drugs* 2002; **62:** 617–30.
6. Opal SM, *et al.* Systemic host responses in severe sepsis analyzed by causative microorganism and treatment effects of drotrecogin alfa (activated). *Clin Infect Dis* 2003; **37:** 50–8.

### Preparations

**Proprietary Preparations** (details are given in Part 3)

***Austral.:*** Xigris; ***Denm.:*** Ceprotin; ***Fin.:*** Ceprotin; ***Fr.:*** Ceprotin; Protexel; Xigris; ***Ger.:*** Ceprotin; ***Irl.:*** Xigris; ***Ital.:*** Ceprotin; ***NZ:*** Xigris; ***Spain:*** Ceprotin; ***Swed.:*** Ceprotin; ***UK:*** Ceprotin; Xigris; ***USA:*** Xigris.

## Red Blood Cells

Eritrocitos.

**Pharmacopoeias.** Many pharmacopoeias have monographs including *US.*

**USP 27** (Red Blood Cells). The remaining red blood cells of whole human blood from suitable donors, from which plasma has been removed. It is prepared not later than 21 days after the blood has been withdrawn except that the period may be 35 days if the anticoagulant used was acid citrate dextrose adenine solution. If intended for extended manufacturer's storage at or below −65° it contains a portion of the plasma sufficient to ensure cell preservation, or a cryophylactic substance. It should be stored in hermetically-sealed sterile containers; store if unfrozen at 1° to 6° (with a range of not more than 2°) except during transport when the temperature may be 1° to 10°. The expiration date of unfrozen Red Blood Cells is not later than that of the whole human blood from which it is derived if plasma has not been removed, unless the hermetic seal is broken, in which case it should be used within 24 hours. The expiration date of frozen Red Blood Cells is not later than 3 years after the date of collection of the source blood when stored at or below −65° and not later than 24 hours after removal from −65° provided that it is then stored at the temperature for unfrozen Red Blood Cells. Red Blood Cells should be administered using equipment incorporating a filter.

Dark red in colour when packed and may show a slight creamy layer on the surface and a small supernatant layer of yellow or opalescent plasma.

### Adverse Effects and Precautions

As for Blood, p.744.

**Antibody formation.** Patients with sickle-cell anaemia frequently require repeated transfusions of red blood cells. Alloimmunisation is a common problem in these patients. Alloantibodies were detected in 32 of 107 black patients with sickle-cell anaemia who had received red cell transfusions compared with 1 of 19 non-black patients who had received transfusions for other chronic anaemias.[1] The incidence of antibody formation was related to the number of transfusions received. An analysis of the red cell phenotypes suggested that the high rate of alloimmunisation among patients with sickle-cell anaemia could be due to racial differences between donors and recipients.

1. Vichinsky EP, *et al.* Alloimmunization in sickle cell anemia and transfusion of racially unmatched blood. *N Engl J Med* 1990; **322:** 1617–21.

### Uses and Administration

Transfusions of red blood cells are given for the treatment of severe anaemia without hypovolaemia (p.732).

Red blood cells are also used for exchange transfusion in babies with haemolytic disease of the newborn (p.1608). Red cells may be used with volume expanders for acute blood loss of less than half of the blood volume; if more than half of the blood volume has been lost, whole blood should be used.

Other red blood cell products are available. Concentrated red cells in an optimal additive solution containing sodium chloride, adenine, glucose, and mannitol has reduced viscosity and an extended shelf-life. Leucocyte-depleted red cells may be used in patients who have developed antibodies to previous transfusions or in whom development of antibodies is undesirable. Frozen, thawed, and washed red cell concentrates in which plasma proteins are removed in addition to leucocytes and platelets may be used in patients with rare antibodies.

◊ References.

1. Davies SC, Williamson LM. Transfusion of red cells. In: Contreras M, ed. *ABC of transfusion.* 3rd ed. London: BMJ Books, 1998: 10–16.
2. British Committee for Standards in Haematology, Blood Transfusion Task Force. Guidelines on the clinical use of leucocyte-depleted blood components. *Transfus Med* 1998; **8:** 59–71. Also available at: http://www.bcshguidelines.com/pdf/trans129.pdf (accessed 23/06/04)
3. British Committee for Standards in Haematology, Blood Transfusion Task Force. Guidelines for the clinical use of red cell transfusions. *Br J Haematol* 2001; **113:** 24–31. Also available at: http://www.bcshguidelines.com/pdf/bjh2701.pdf (accessed 23/06/04)

### Preparations

***USP 27:*** Red Blood Cells.

**Proprietary Preparations** (details are given in Part 3)

**Multi-ingredient:** ***Arg.:*** Vulnofilin Compuesto.

## Sargramostim (BAN, USAN, rINN)

BI-61.012; rhu GM-CSF. A recombinant human granulocyte-macrophage colony-stimulating factor; 23-L-Leucinecolony-stimulating factor 2 (human clone $pHG_{25}$ protein moiety).

*CAS — 123774-72-1.*

*ATC — L03AA09.*

**Pharmacopoeias.** In *US.*

**USP 27** (Sargramostim). A highly purified glycosylated protein consisting of 127 amino acids, produced by recombinant DNA synthesis in yeast culture. Store in sealed containers at a temperature of −20° or below.

**Stability.** Solutions of sargramostim may be adsorbed onto glass or plastic materials and so albumin must be added to give a final concentration of 1 mg/mL to solutions that are diluted to concentrations of sargramostim below 10 micrograms/mL.

### Adverse Effects and Precautions

As for Molgramostim, p.756.

### Uses and Administration

Sargramostim is a granulocyte-macrophage colony-stimulating factor with actions and uses similar to those of molgramostim (p.756). It is used to treat or prevent neutropenia in patients receiving myelosuppressive cancer chemotherapy and to reduce the period of neutropenia in patients undergoing bone marrow transplantation (p.496). It is also used after bone marrow transplantation when engraftment is delayed or has failed, or to mobilise autologous peripheral blood progenitor cells for an alternative to bone marrow transplantation.

As an adjunct to antineoplastic therapy, sargramostim is given by intravenous infusion over 4 hours in a dose of 250 micrograms/m² daily for up to 42 days as required.

After bone marrow transplantation, sargramostim may be given in a dose of 250 micrograms/m² daily by intravenous infusion over 2 hours. When engraftment is delayed or has failed, a course of sargramostim 250 micrograms/m² daily for 14 days may be used. The dose can be repeated after a 7-day interval if engraftment has not occurred. A third course of 500 micrograms/m² daily for 14 days may be tried after another 7-day interval if needed, but further dose escalation is unlikely to be of benefit.

For mobilisation of peripheral blood progenitor cells a dose of 250 micrograms/m² daily is given by continuous intravenous infusion over 24 hours or by subcutaneous injection.

**HIV infection and AIDS.** Sargramostim is under investigation in the management of HIV infection (p.621). There is some evidence to suggest that it may help to decrease and suppress viral load, and increase CD4+ cell counts. It may do this by enhancing the activity of antiretroviral drugs and increasing the resistance of monocytes to HIV infection.[1-3]


1. Skowron G, *et al.* The safety and efficacy of granulocyte-macrophage colony-stimulating factor (sargramostim) added to indinavir- or ritonavir-based antiretroviral therapy: a randomized double-blind, placebo-controlled trial. *J Infect Dis* 1999; **180:** 1064–71.
2. Brites C, *et al.* A randomized, placebo-controlled trial of granulocyte-macrophage colony-stimulating factor and nucleoside analogue therapy in AIDS. *J Infect Dis* 2000; **182:** 1531–5.
3. Angel JB, *et al.* Phase III study of granulocyte-macrophage colony-stimulating factor in advanced HIV disease: effect on infections, CD4 cell counts and HIV suppression. *AIDS* 2000; **14:** 387–95.


### Preparations

***USP 27:*** Sargramostim for Injection.

**Proprietary Preparations** (details are given in Part 3)
***USA:*** Leukine.

## Thrombin

Factor IIa; Trombina.

*CAS — 9002-04-4.*

*ATC — B02BC06; B02BD30.*

**Pharmacopoeias.** Many pharmacopoeias have monographs including *US.*

**USP 27** (Thrombin). A sterile, freeze-dried powder derived from bovine plasma containing the protein substance prepared from prothrombin through interaction with added thromboplastin in the presence of calcium. It is capable, without the addition of other substances, of causing the clotting of whole blood, plasma, or a solution of fibrinogen. It should be stored at 2° to 8°. Once reconstituted, solutions should be used within a few hours of preparation. The label should state that the prepared solution should not be injected into or otherwise allowed to enter large blood vessels.

A white to greyish, amorphous substance dried from the frozen state.

### Adverse Effects and Precautions

Hypersensitivity reactions, including anaphylaxis, have occurred rarely. Thrombin solutions must not be injected into blood vessels.

**Effects on the blood.** Repeated exposure to thrombin preparations of bovine origin has led to the development of antibodies to bovine thrombin and factor V with cross-reactivity, in some cases, to human factors.[1-3] The presence of inhibitors to human factors may produce bleeding abnormalities and interfere with clotting measurements.


1. Rapaport SI, *et al.* Clinical significance of antibodies to bovine and human thrombin and factor V after surgical use of bovine thrombin. *Am J Clin Pathol* 1992; **97:** 84–91.
2. Bänninger H, *et al.* Fibrin glue in surgery: frequent development of inhibitors of bovine thrombin and human factor V. *Br J Haematol* 1993; **85:** 528–32.
3. Ortel TL, *et al.* Topical thrombin and acquired coagulation factor inhibitors: clinical spectrum and laboratory diagnosis. *Am J Hematol* 1994; **45:** 128–35.


### Uses and Administration

Thrombin is a protein substance produced *in vivo* from prothrombin that converts soluble fibrinogen into insoluble fibrin thus producing coagulation.

Thrombin of either human or bovine origin is applied topically to control bleeding from capillaries and small venules. It is applied directly to the bleeding surface either as a solution or dry powder. It may also be used with absorbable gelatin sponge during surgical procedures.

Thrombin is a component of fibrin glue (p.753).

### Preparations

***Ph. Eur.:*** Fibrin Sealant Kit;
***USP 27:*** Thrombin.

**Proprietary Preparations** (details are given in Part 3)
***Austral.:*** Thrombostat; ***Canad.:*** Thrombostat; ***Ger.:*** Thrombocoll†; ***NZ:*** Thrombostat; ***S.Afr.:*** Tisseel; ***Singapore:*** Thrombostat†; ***USA:*** Thrombinar; Thrombogen; Thrombostat.

**Multi-ingredient:** ***Arg.:*** Tissucol; Tissucol Duo Quick; ***Austral.:*** Tisseel Duo; ***Austria:*** Beriplast; TachoComb; Tissucol; Tissucol Duo Quick; ***Belg.:*** Tissucol†; ***Braz.:*** Beriplast P; Tissucol†; ***Canad.:*** Tisseel; ***Chile:*** Beriplast P; ***Denm.:*** Tisseel Duo Quick; ***Fin.:*** Beriplast†; Tisseel Duo Quick; ***Fr.:*** Beriplast; Biocol†; Tissucol; ***Ger.:*** Beriplast; TachoComb; Tissucol Duo S; Tissucol Fibrinkleber tiefgefroren†; Tissucol-Kit; ***Hong Kong:*** Beriplast P; TachoComb; Tisseel; ***Irl.:*** Tisseel†; ***Israel:*** Beriplast P; Quixil; Tisseel; ***Ital.:*** Tissucol; ***Mex.:*** Beriplast P†; ***Spain:*** Tissucol Duo; ***Swed.:*** Tisseel Duo Quick; ***Switz.:*** Beriplast P; Tissucol; Tissucol Duo S; ***Thai.:*** Fibrin Glue; TachoComb; ***UK:*** Tisseel.

## Thromboplastin

Cytozyme; Thrombokinase; Tromboplastina.

### Profile

Tissue thromboplastin (tissue factor; factor III) is a membrane glycoprotein that is released from damaged tissue and initiates coagulation. The term thromboplastin may also be applied to other related substances with similar activity. Commercial preparations may contain tissue extracts comprising a variety of such substances.

Preparations of thromboplastin have been used as haemostatics. A preparation of thromboplastin derived from rabbit brain is employed in the determination of the prothrombin time for the control of anticoagulant therapy (for further details see under Warfarin Sodium, p.1028).

### Preparations

**Proprietary Preparations** (details are given in Part 3)
**Multi-ingredient:** ***Braz.:*** Claudemor; ***Port.:*** Claudemor.

## Thrombopoietin

Trombopoyetina.

### Profile

Thrombopoietin is a naturally occurring colony-stimulating factor that regulates thrombopoiesis. Recombinant thrombopoietin is under investigation for the management of thrombocytopenia in patients receiving myelosuppressive chemotherapy. A form of recombinant thrombopoietin conjugated with polyethylene glycol (pegacaristim, PEG-megakaryocyte growth and development factor, PEG-MGDF) has also been investigated.

◊ References.


1. Basser RL, *et al.* Thrombopoietic effects of pegylated recombinant human megakaryocyte growth and development factor (PEG-rHuMGDF) in patients with advanced cancer. *Lancet* 1996; **348:** 1279–81.
2. Fanucchi M, *et al.* Effects of polyethylene glycol-conjugated recombinant human megakaryocyte growth and development factor on platelet counts after chemotherapy for lung cancer. *N Engl J Med* 1997; **336:** 404–9.
3. Vadhan-Raj S, *et al.* Stimulation of megakaryocyte and platelet production by a single dose of recombinant human thrombopoietin in patients with cancer. *Ann Intern Med* 1997; **126:** 673–81.
4. Kaushansky K. Thrombopoietin: platelets on demand? *Ann Intern Med* 1997; **126:** 731–3.
5. Kaushansky K. Thrombopoietin. *N Engl J Med* 1998; **339:** 746–54.
6. Archimbaud E, *et al.* A randomized, double-blind, placebo-controlled study with pegylated recombinant human megakaryocyte growth and development factor (PEG-rHuMGDF) as an adjunct to chemotherapy for adults with de novo acute myeloid leukemia. *Blood* 1999; **94:** 3694–3701.
7. Vadhan-Raj S, *et al.* Recombinant human thrombopoietin attenuates carboplatin-induced severe thrombocytopenia and the need for platelet transfusions in patients with gynecologic cancer. *Ann Intern Med* 2000; **132:** 364–8.
8. Vadhan-Raj S, *et al.* Safety and efficacy of transfusions of autologous cryopreserved platelets derived from recombinant human thrombopoietin to support chemotherapy-associated severe thrombocytopenia: a randomised cross-over study. *Lancet* 2002; **359:** 2145–52.


## Tranexamic Acid (BAN, USAN, rINN)

Ácido tranexámico; Acidum Tranexamicum; AMCA; *trans*-AMCHA; CL-65336. *trans*-4-(Aminomethyl)cyclohexanecarboxylic acid.

$C_8H_{15}NO_2$ = 157.2.

*CAS — 1197-18-8.*

*ATC — B02AA02.*

**Pharmacopoeias.** In *Chin., Eur.* (see p.vi), and *Jpn.*

**Ph. Eur. 5.0** (Tranexamic Acid). A white crystalline powder. Freely soluble in water and in glacial acetic acid; practically insoluble in alcohol and in acetone. A 5% solution in water has a pH of 7.0 to 8.0.

**Incompatibility.** Solutions of tranexamic acid are incompatible with benzylpenicillin.

### Adverse Effects

Tranexamic acid appears to be well tolerated. It can produce dose-related gastrointestinal disturbances. Hypotension has occurred, particularly after rapid intravenous administration. Thrombotic complications have been reported in patients receiving tranexamic acid, but these are usually a consequence of its inappropriate use (see Precautions, below).

Manufacturers of tranexamic acid report that there have been a few instances of transient disturbance of colour vision associated with its use.

◊ A patient undergoing regular peritoneal dialysis for Epstein's syndrome developed ligneous conjunctivitis, gingival hyperplasia, and peritoneal protein loss associated with the use of tranexamic acid.[1]


1. Diamond JP, *et al.* Tranexamic acid-associated ligneous conjunctivitis with gingival and peritoneal lesions. *Br J Ophthalmol* 1991; **75:** 753–4.


**Effects on the skin.** A widespread, patchy rash with associated blisters, considered on skin biopsy to be a fixed-drug eruption, occurred in a 33-year-old woman.[1] Tranexamic acid, which she had taken for 8 years and which had been well tolerated, was identified as the causative agent. Desensitisation was unsuccessful. Tranexamic acid was also suspected as being the cause of a fixed-drug eruption in a 36-year-old woman.[2] Pruritic, vesicle-bullous lesions appeared within a few hours of starting tranexamic acid and the lesions resolved completely 3 days after discontinuing therapy even though other drug treatment was continued.


1. Kavanagh GM, *et al.* Tranexamic acid (Cyklokapron®)-induced fixed-drug eruption. *Br J Dermatol* 1993; **128:** 229–30.
2. Carrión-Carrión C, *et al.* Bullous eruption induced by tranexamic acid. *Ann Pharmacother* 1994; **28:** 1305–6.


### Precautions

Tranexamic acid should not be used in patients with active intravascular clotting because of the risk of thrombosis. Patients with a predisposition to thrombosis are also at risk if given antifibrinolytic therapy. Haemorrhage due to disseminated intravascular coagulation should therefore not be treated with antifibrinolytic compounds unless the condition is predominantly due to disturbances in fibrinolytic mechanisms; tranexamic acid has been used when the latter conditions are met, but with careful monitoring and anticoagulant cover.

Lysis of existing extravascular clots may be inhibited in patients receiving tranexamic acid. Clots in the renal system can lead to intrarenal obstruction, so caution is required in patients with haematuria. Doses of tranexamic acid should be reduced in patients with renal impairment (see under Uses and Administration, below). The manufacturers recommend that regular eye examinations and liver function tests should be performed if tranexamic acid is used long term.

Some studies have suggested that tranexamic acid when given to patients after a subarachnoid haemorrhage increases the incidence of cerebral ischaemic complications (see Haemorrhagic Disorders under Uses, below).

Rapid intravenous administration may be associated with adverse effects (see above).

## Interactions

Drugs with actions on haemostasis should be given with caution to patients on antifibrinolytic therapy. The potential for thrombus formation may be increased by oestrogens, for example, or the action of the antifibrinolytic antagonised by compounds such as thrombolytics.

## Pharmacokinetics

Tranexamic acid is absorbed from the gastrointestinal tract with peak plasma concentrations occurring after about 3 hours. Bioavailability is about 30 to 50%. Tranexamic acid is widely distributed throughout the body and has very low protein binding. It diffuses across the placenta and is distributed into breast milk. Tranexamic acid has a plasma elimination half-life of about 2 hours. It is excreted in the urine mainly as unchanged drug.

◊ References.


1. Andersson L, *et al.* Role of urokinase and tissue activator in sustaining bleeding and the management thereof with EACA and AMCA. *Ann N Y Acad Sci* 1968; **146:** 642–56.
2. Kullander S, Nilsson IM. Human placental transfer of an antifibrinolytic agent (AMCA). *Acta Obstet Gynecol Scand* 1970; **49:** 241–2.
3. Pilbrant Å, *et al.* Pharmacokinetics and bioavailability of tranexamic acid. *Eur J Clin Pharmacol* 1981; **20:** 65–72.


## Uses and Administration

Tranexamic acid is an antifibrinolytic drug that inhibits breakdown of fibrin clots. It acts primarily by blocking the binding of plasminogen and plasmin to fibrin; direct inhibition of plasmin occurs only to a limited degree. Tranexamic acid is used in the treatment and prophylaxis of haemorrhage associated with excessive fibrinolysis. It is also used in the prophylaxis of hereditary angioedema.

Tranexamic acid is given by mouth and by slow intravenous injection or continuous infusion. Parenteral administration is usually changed to oral administration after a few days. Alternatively, an initial intravenous injection may be followed by continuous infusion. Oral doses are 1 to 1.5 g (or 15 to 25 mg/kg) 2 to 4 times daily. When given by slow intravenous injection doses are 0.5 to 1 g (or 10 mg/kg) 3 times daily. Tranexamic acid is administered by continuous infusion at a rate of 25 to 50 mg/kg daily. These doses are used in the short term for haemorrhage. Tranexamic acid is given for prolonged periods in hereditary angioedema in doses of 1 to 1.5 g by mouth 2 or 3 times daily.

Children may be given doses of 25 mg/kg by mouth or 10 mg/kg intravenously usually administered 2 or 3 times daily.

Reduced doses are recommended for patients with renal impairment (see below).

Solutions of tranexamic acid have been applied topically, for example as a bladder irrigation or mouthwash.

**Administration in renal impairment.** Reduced doses of tranexamic acid are recommended by the manufacturers for patients with renal impairment, based on the serum-creatinine concentration (SCC):

- SCC 120 to 250 micromoles/litre: 15 mg/kg twice daily orally, or 10 mg/kg twice daily intravenously
- SCC 250 to 500 micromoles/litre: 15 mg/kg once daily orally, or 10 mg/kg once daily intravenously
- SCC higher than 500 micromoles/litre: 7.5 mg/kg once daily or 15 mg/kg once every 48 hours orally, or 5 mg/kg once daily or 10 mg/kg once every 48 hours intravenously (some manufacturers contra-indicate use in severe renal impairment)

**Haemorrhagic disorders.** Tranexamic acid, aminocaproic acid, and aminomethylbenzoic acid are structurally related synthetic antifibrinolytic drugs that block the binding of plasminogen and plasmin to fibrin, thereby preventing dissolution of the haemostatic plug. Tranexamic acid is also a direct, but weak, inhibitor of plasmin.[1,2] A plasma concentration of tranexamic acid of 5 to 10 micrograms/mL has been considered necessary for effective inhibition of fibrinolysis.[1]

Antifibrinolytics are used to control haemorrhage that is considered to be caused by excessive fibrinolysis. Antifibrinolytic therapy may also be indicated in the prevention of rebleeding in some haemorrhagic conditions, the rationale being to retard dissolution of the haemostatic plug formed in response to vascular injury.[1,2]

In haemorrhage caused by a congenital or acquired deficiency of blood coagulation factors (p.737), haemostatic drugs have a secondary role and may be useful in reducing requirements of factor concentrates.[2] The most established use of antifibrinolytics in these conditions is in the prophylaxis of bleeding after dental procedures in haemophiliacs.[1,2] A standard regimen is the intravenous administration of tranexamic acid 10 mg/kg given preoperatively with factor VIII or factor IX. Tranexamic acid is continued postoperatively in a dose of 25 mg/kg 3 or 4 times daily by mouth for up to 8 days. Some workers have found that local treatment with a 4.8% solution of tranexamic acid as a mouthwash is a useful addition to systemic therapy.[3] A similar approach using tranexamic acid mouthwashes has been used to reduce the risk of bleeding after oral surgery in patients on anticoagulant therapy.[4] Tranexamic acid may prove beneficial in patients with other congenital bleeding disorders such as $\alpha_2$-antiplasmin deficiency.[5,6] Aminocaproic acid has been tried in a few patients with hereditary haemorrhagic telangiectasia with mixed results.[7,8] Benefit from treatment with aminocaproic acid or tranexamic acid has been reported in coagulopathies associated with thrombocytopenia[9,10] and acute promyelocytic leukaemia.[11]

Tranexamic acid and aminocaproic acid have each been used in an attempt to prevent rebleeding in patients with subarachnoid haemorrhage (see Stroke, p.836), particularly if surgery is to be delayed. However, while rebleeding may be reduced, there can be an increase in the incidence of cerebral ischaemic complications resulting in little overall improvement in outcome.[1] Paradoxically, rebleeding has been noted in patients given high doses of aminocaproic acid after subarachnoid haemorrhage (see Adverse Effects, Effects on the Blood, under Aminocaproic Acid, p.741). Possible methods of overcoming the ischaemic complications have included the administration of drugs such as nimodipine[12] or nicardipine[13] or the use of aprotinin with a low-dose regimen of tranexamic acid.[14]

Tranexamic acid has been used to control haemorrhage of gastrointestinal origin. In a meta-analysis[15] of 6 studies, involving a total of 1267 patients given tranexamic acid for acute upper gastrointestinal haemorrhage, treatment with tranexamic acid was associated with a 20 to 30% decrease in the rate of rebleeding, a 30 to 40% decrease in the need for surgery, and a 40% decrease in mortality. However, the validity of the results of one study included in the analysis has been disputed.[16,17] The management of bleeding associated with peptic ulcer disease and varices is discussed on p.1246 and p.1716, respectively.

Tranexamic acid or aminocaproic acid have been suggested to control bleeding in many other conditions. These include haemorrhage after surgical or other procedures including prostatectomy, bladder surgery, and cervical conisation, perioperative blood loss in cardiac surgery, and other conditions associated with excessive fibrinolysis such as menorrhagia (see below), epistaxis, and placental abruption.


1. Verstraete M. Clinical application of inhibitors of fibrinolysis. *Drugs* 1985; **29:** 236–61.
2. Verstraete M. Haemostatic drugs. In: Bloom AL, Thomas DP, eds. *Haemostasis and thrombosis.* 2nd ed. London: Churchill Livingstone, 1987: 607–17.
3. Sindet-Pedersen S, *et al.* Management of oral bleeding in haemophilic patients. *Lancet* 1988; **ii:** 566.
4. Sindet-Pedersen S, *et al.* Hemostatic effect of tranexamic acid mouthwash in anticoagulant-treated patients undergoing oral surgery. *N Engl J Med* 1989; **320:** 840–3.
5. Koie K, *et al.* $\alpha_2$-Plasmin-inhibitor deficiency (Miyasato disease). *Lancet* 1978; **ii:** 1334–6.
6. Kettle P, Mayne EE. A bleeding disorder due to deficiency of $\alpha_2$-antiplasmin. *J Clin Pathol* 1985; **38:** 428–9.
7. Saba HI, *et al.* Brief report: treatment of bleeding in hereditary hemorrhagic telangiectasia with aminocaproic acid. *N Engl J Med* 1994; **330:** 1789–90.
8. Korzenik JR, *et al.* Treatment of bleeding in hereditary hemorrhagic telangiectasia with aminocaproic acid. *N Engl J Med* 1994; **331:** 1236.
9. Warrell RP, Kempin SJ. Treatment of severe coagulopathy in the Kasabach-Merritt syndrome with aminocaproic acid and cryoprecipitate. *N Engl J Med* 1985; **313:** 309–12.
10. Poon M-C, *et al.* Epsilon-aminocaproic acid in the reversal of consumptive coagulopathy with platelet sequestration in a vascular malformation of Klippel-Trenaunay syndrome. *Am J Med* 1989; **87:** 211–13.
11. Avvisati G, *et al.* Tranexamic acid for control of haemorrhage in acute promyelocytic leukaemia. *Lancet* 1989; **ii:** 122–4.
12. van Gijn J. Subarachnoid haemorrhage. *Lancet* 1992; **339:** 653–5.
13. Beck DW, *et al.* Combination of aminocaproic acid and nicardipine in treatment of aneurysmal subarachnoid hemorrhage. *Stroke* 1988; **19:** 63–7.
14. Spallone A, *et al.* Low-dose tranexamic acid combined with aprotinin in the pre-operative management of ruptured intracranial aneurysms. *Neurochirurgia (Stuttg)* 1987; **30:** 172–6.
15. Henry DA, O'Connell DL. Effects of fibrinolytic inhibitors on mortality from upper gastrointestinal haemorrhage. *BMJ* 1989; **298:** 1142–6.
16. Brown C, Rees WDW. Drug treatment for acute upper gastrointestinal bleeding. *BMJ* 1992; **304:** 135–6.
17. Barer D. Drug treatment for acute upper gastrointestinal bleeding. *BMJ* 1992; **304:** 383.


**Hereditary angioedema.** Hereditary angioedema, formerly known as hereditary angioneurotic oedema, is a rare autosomal dominant disease caused by either a deficiency of complement C1 esterase inhibitor or, more rarely, a lack of functioning inhibitor.[1,2] The disease presents as episodic attacks of oedema, usually of the extremities and face, and often involving the gastrointestinal mucosa producing abdominal pain. A non-pruritic rash may also occur. A few patients develop life-threatening laryngeal oedema. Attacks generally last about 1 to 3 days and may occur as frequently as weekly or there may be years between attacks. The first attack may occur at any age although initial presentation in childhood is most common. Trauma, especially dental surgery, illness, and emotional stress may provoke an attack although often there is no precipitating factor.

Treatment of the acute attack is essentially supportive. If laryngeal oedema is present adrenaline, antihistamines, and corticosteroids may be given (as for Anaphylactic Shock, p.855) even though patients with hereditary angioedema often fail to respond adequately to them. The mainstay of treatment of an acute attack is replacement therapy with complement C1 esterase inhibitor. Fresh frozen plasma has been used although there is a risk of initially exacerbating the oedema due to the presence of other complements in the plasma. Tracheostomy or tracheal intubation may be necessary.

Once the acute attack has subsided most patients will not require further treatment, but those who experience life-threatening attacks, repeated episodes of swelling around the face or neck, or incapacitating attacks require long-term prophylactic therapy. A synthetic androgen (danazol or stanozolol) or an antifibrinolytic (aminocaproic acid or tranexamic acid) is effective for long-term prophylaxis. Danazol and stanozolol raise serum concentrations of C1 esterase inhibitor possibly by enhancing its synthesis in the liver. Aminocaproic acid and tranexamic acid may act by inhibiting plasmin activation. A synthetic androgen is often preferred because these seem to be more effective than antifibrinolytics. In children, however, androgens are generally avoided because of their adverse effects.

Short-term prophylaxis may be used in situations expected to provoke an attack, such as surgery or dental work. Complement C1 esterase inhibitor is given 6 to 12 hours before the procedure, or fresh frozen plasma may be used if this is not available. Alternatively, a synthetic androgen or antifibrinolytic may be used, but these must be started several days before the procedure and continued for 2 days after.

Therapies under investigation for the management of hereditary angioedema include a recombinant complement C1 esterase inhibitor, icatibant (a bradykinin receptor antagonist), and DX-88 (an inhibitor of human plasma kallikrein).


1. Nzeako UC, *et al.* Hereditary angioedema: a broad review for clinicians. *Arch Intern Med* 2001; **161:** 2417–29.
2. Fay A, Abinun M. Current management of hereditary angio-oedema (C'1 esterase inhibitor deficiency). *J Clin Pathol* 2002; **55:** 266–70.


**Menorrhagia.** Tranexamic acid is used in women with menorrhagia (p.1567) who do not require contraception or hormonal therapy. It reduces uterine blood loss in such women when used during menstruation.[1-3] A comparative trial[1] found tranexamic acid to be more effective than the NSAID mefenamic acid, a commonly used treatment for the condition. It is also more effective than cyclical norethisterone[2] (although less so than a progesterone-releasing intra-uterine device[3]). A review,[4] which included these and some other studies, reported that tranexamic acid reduces menstrual blood loss by about 34 to 59% over 2 to 3 cycles.


1. Bonnar J, Sheppard BL. Treatment of menorrhagia during menstruation: randomised controlled trial of ethamsylate, mefenamic acid, and tranexamic acid. *BMJ* 1996; **313:** 579–82.
2. Preston JT, *et al.* Comparative study of tranexamic acid and norethisterone in the treatment of ovulatory menorrhagia. *Br J Obstet Gynaecol* 1995; **102:** 401–406.
3. Milsom I, *et al.* A comparison of flurbiprofen, tranexamic acid, and a levonorgestrel-releasing intrauterine contraceptive device in the treatment of idiopathic menorrhagia. *Am J Obstet Gynecol* 1991; **164:** 879–83.
4. Wellington K, Wagstaff AJ. Tranexamic acid: a review of its use in the management of menorrhagia. *Drugs* 2003; **63:** 1417–33.


## Preparations

***BP 2003:*** Tranexamic Acid Injection; Tranexamic Acid Tablets.

**Proprietary Preparations** (details are given in Part 3)

***Austral.:*** Cyklokapron; ***Austria:*** Cyklo-F; Cyklokapron; ***Belg.:*** Exacyl; ***Braz.:*** Transamin; ***Canad.:*** Cyklokapron; ***Chile:*** Espercil; ***Denm.:*** Cyklokapron; ***Fin.:*** Caprilon; Cyklokapron; ***Fr.:*** Exacyl; Spotof; ***Ger.:*** Anvitoff; Cyklokapron; Ugurol†; ***Gr.:*** Transamin; ***Hong Kong:*** Cyklokapron; Transamin; ***India:*** Traxamic; ***Irl.:*** Cyklokapron; ***Israel:*** Hexakapron; ***Ital.:*** Tranex; Ugurol; ***Jpn:*** Transamin; ***Malaysia:*** Transamin; Tren; ***Neth.:*** Cyklo-F; Cyklokapron; ***Norw.:*** Cyklokapron; ***NZ:*** Cyklokapron; ***S.Afr.:*** Cyklokapron; ***Singapore:*** Cyklokapron; ***Spain:*** Amchafibrin; ***Swed.:*** Cyklo-F; Cyklokapron; ***Switz.:*** Anvitoff; Cyklokapron; ***Thai.:*** Tramic; Transamin; ***UK:*** Cyklokapron; ***USA:*** Cyklokapron.

# Bone Modulating Drugs

Bone and Bone Disease, p.762
Ectopic ossification, p.762
Malignant neoplasms of the bone, p.762
Osteogenesis imperfecta, p.762
Osteomalacia, p.762
Osteoporosis, p.763
Paget's disease of bone, p.764
Renal osteodystrophy, p.764
Rickets, p.765
Parathyroid Disorders, p.765
Hyperparathyroidism, p.765
Hypoparathyroidism, p.765

The processes of bone turnover, and the regulation of body calcium, are intimately connected. The concentration of calcium in plasma is normally kept within a narrow range (p.1217). It is regulated by the absorption and excretion of calcium, and also by modulation of the normal resorption and formation of bone and hence the movement of calcium to and from the skeletal reservoir. The endogenous substances, parathyroid hormone, calcitonin, and vitamin D, are involved in the regulation of calcium homoeostasis.

Calcitonins and the bisphosphonates inhibit bone resorption and thus have a hypocalcaemic effect. They are therefore used in the treatment of conditions associated with increased bone resorption, such as osteoporosis and Paget's disease of bone, and in the management of hypercalcaemia, especially that associated with malignancy (p.1218). Bisphosphonates have a high affinity for bone and radioactively labelled bisphosphonates are used as bone scanning agents. Gallium nitrate also inhibits bone resorption, and is used for Paget's disease of bone and hypercalcaemia of malignancy.

Parathyroid hormone, or synthetic analogues such as teriparatide, which have a hypercalcaemic effect, are under investigation to promote bone formation. Teriparatide has replaced the native hormone in the differential diagnosis of hypoparathyroidism and pseudohypoparathyroidism.

The inorganic fluoride salts, which can promote bone formation when given in appropriate doses, are discussed in the chapter on Nutritional Agents (see Sodium Fluoride, p.1444).

## Bone and Bone Disease

The skeleton acts as mechanical support and protection to softer tissues and organs. It is also important in electrolyte homoeostasis, acting as a reservoir of certain ions and minerals such as calcium, phosphorus, and magnesium.

Bone has two components: an organic matrix, called **osteoid**, consisting mainly of collagen, and a mineral phase deposited through that matrix; the latter, comprising about 70% of the skeletal mass, is composed chiefly of hydroxyapatite (a complex crystalline salt of calcium and phosphate). There are two structural forms known in mature bone, namely cortical (lamellar) bone, which has a dense, continuous structure, and trabecular (cancellous) bone, which has a 'spongy' structure of linked plates and is associated with high bone turnover and growth. The peripheral or appendicular parts of the skeleton are predominantly cortical bone, while the axial or central parts, such as the spine and pelvis, contain substantial amounts of trabecular bone.

Bone is a dynamic tissue: once new bone has been laid down it is subject to a continual process of formation and resorption called **remodelling**. Remodelling takes place along bone surfaces and is carried out by bone cells (osteoclasts and osteoblasts) that originate in the marrow and share common origins with blood cells. Stimulated by physical or chemical signals, **osteoclasts** dig a cavity into the bone (bone resorption); they are then replaced by **osteoblasts** that synthesise new osteoid to fill the cavity (bone formation) and may help to promote its subsequent mineralisation. The actions of these two types of bone cell are closely linked, and agents that suppress resorption ultimately decrease bone formation too. However, at any given time there is a deficit in potential bone mass, the **remodelling space**, which represents sites of bone resorption that have not yet been filled in. Any stimulus that affects bone turnover by altering the recruitment of osteoblasts and osteoclasts to remodelling will result in an increase or decrease in the remodelling space, until a new steady state is achieved, and this will be seen as a decrease or increase in bone mass.

Bone also contains **osteocytes**, which are cells derived from osteoblasts thought to be involved in the movement of minerals.

Bone cells are controlled by systemic hormones including parathyroid hormone, 1,25-dihydroxycholecalciferol (calcitriol), and calcitonin and local regulators such as bone morphogenetic proteins and interleukin-1; vitamin K is also thought to have a role, and bone cells are affected by other hormones including corticosteroids and sex hormones.

**Bone diseases** may be due to defects in the production of osteoid or its mineralisation, or to an imbalance in resorption and formation of bone.

### Ectopic ossification

Ectopic ossification (heterotopic ossification) is a condition in which mature bone develops in non-skeletal tissues, commonly the connective tissue of muscles. It occurs following local trauma, for example after joint dislocation or surgery such as total hip replacement, and also after neurological damage such as severe head or spinal cord injuries. Ectopic bone formation usually starts about 2 weeks after the injury, though symptoms, which include localised pain, swelling, and restriction of movement, may not appear for 8 to 10 weeks. A congenital form of ectopic ossification, myositis ossificans progressiva, also occurs but is rare.

Ectopic ossification should be distinguished from the calcification of soft tissue which may occur in connective tissue disorders or in parathyroid disorders due to high circulating concentrations of calcium and or phosphate; in these conditions calcification occurs without bone formation.

Treatment of established ectopic bone is limited to surgical resection. Patients at high risk of ectopic bone formation should therefore receive prophylaxis with radiotherapy, physiotherapy, or drug therapy. While prophylaxis does not always prevent the development of ectopic ossification, it can decrease its occurrence and severity. Prophylactic measures should be begun as early as possible and for orthopaedic surgery may be started before the operation. Prophylaxis is also required if mature ectopic bone is to be surgically excised in order to minimise the rate of recurrence. NSAIDs appear to significantly reduce the incidence of ectopic bone formation,[1-4] possibly by inhibiting the synthesis of osteoactive prostaglandins. Studies suggest that NSAID prophylaxis is of similar effectiveness to radiotherapy.[5-8] Bisphosphonates that inhibit the mineralisation of the deposited bone, such as etidronate, have also been used[9-11] but they do not prevent the formation of the osteoid matrix. Also when etidronate is discontinued, some mineralisation can occur, resulting in delayed ectopic ossification, though it is usually less severe.

1. Schmidt SA, *et al.* The use of indomethacin to prevent the formation of heterotopic bone after total hip replacement: a randomized, double-blind clinical trial. *J Bone Joint Surg Am* 1988; **70A:** 834–8.
2. Pagnani MJ, *et al.* Effect of aspirin on heterotopic ossification after total hip arthroplasty in men who have osteoarthrosis. *J Bone Joint Surg Am* 1991; **73A:** 924–9.
3. Knelles D, *et al.* Prevention of heterotopic ossification after total hip replacement: a prospective, randomised study using acetylsalicylic acid, indomethacin and fractional or single-dose irradiation. *J Bone Joint Surg Br* 1997; **79B:** 596–602.
4. Neal B, *et al.* Non-steroidal anti-inflammatory drugs for preventing heterotopic bone formation after hip arthroplasty. Available in The Cochrane Library; Issue 2. Chichester: John Wiley; 2004.
5. Moore KD, *et al.* Indomethacin versus radiation therapy for prophylaxis against heterotopic ossification in acetabular fractures: a randomised, prospective study. *J Bone Joint Surg Br* 1998; **80:** 259–63.
6. Kölbl O, *et al.* Preoperative irradiation versus the use of nonsteroidal anti-inflammatory drugs for prevention of heterotopic ossification following total hip replacement: the results of a randomized trial. *Int J Radiat Oncol Biol Phys* 1998; **42:** 397–401.
7. Sell S, *et al.* The suppression of heterotopic ossifications: radiation versus NSAID therapy-a prospective study. *J Arthroplasty* 1998; **13:** 854–9.
8. Kienapfel H, *et al.* Prevention of heterotopic bone formation after total hip arthroplasty: a prospective randomised study comparing postoperative radiation therapy with indomethacin medication. *Arch Orthop Trauma Surg* 1999; **119:** 296–302.
9. Finerman GAM, Stover SL. Heterotopic ossification following hip replacement or spinal cord injury: two clinical studies with EHDP. *Metab Bone Dis Relat Res* 1981; **4 & 5:** 337–42.
10. Banovac K, *et al.* Intravenous disodium etidronate therapy in spinal cord injury patients with heterotopic ossification. *Paraplegia* 1993; **31:** 660–6.
11. van Kuijk AA, *et al.* Neurogenic heterotopic ossification in spinal cord injury. *Spinal Cord* 2002; **40:** 313–26.

### Malignant neoplasms of the bone

The bisphosphonates and calcitonins are used to control the hypercalcaemia that often accompanies malignant disease (p.1218). Bisphosphonates are also used in metastatic bone disease (p.513) to control bone pain and to reduce skeletal complications such as fractures. Evidence of the ability of bisphosphonates to prevent the development of bone metastases is conflicting.

### Osteogenesis imperfecta

Osteogenesis imperfecta (brittle bone syndrome) is a heterogeneous inherited disorder of connective tissue characterised by bone fragility, osteopenia, short stature, joint laxity, teeth defects, and hearing abnormalities. It may be classified into 4 forms, I-IV, which vary in clinical severity, and radiological and genetic aspects.[1]

Orthopaedic treatment and physical activity programmes form the basis of therapy: at present there is no curative drug therapy. Calcitonins were commonly used, but their use has declined.[1] Beneficial effects have been reported with growth hormone,[2,3] especially in moderate forms of the disease.[1] Bisphosphonates have yielded substantial improvements in chronic pain, bone mineral density, fracture rate and mobility,[4-10] without significant adverse effects, and may be especially beneficial in severe osteogenesis imperfecta.[1] They may also be useful for associated immobilisation hypercalcaemia.[11] Bone marrow transplantation and the potential of antisense gene therapy are being investigated.[1,3]

1. Antoniazzi F, *et al.* Osteogenesis imperfecta: practical treatment guidelines. *Pediatr Drugs* 2000; **2:** 465–88.
2. Antoniazzi F, *et al.* Growth hormone treatment in osteogenesis imperfecta with quantitative defect of type I collagen synthesis. *J Pediatr* 1996; **129:** 432–9.
3. Marini JC, Gerber NL. Osteogenesis imperfecta: rehabilitation and prospects for gene therapy. *JAMA* 1997; **277:** 746–50.
4. Bembi B, *et al.* Intravenous pamidronate treatment in osteogenesis imperfecta. *J Pediatr* 1997; **131:** 622–5.
5. Shaw NJ. Bisphosphonates in osteogenesis imperfecta. *Arch Dis Child* 1997; **77:** 92–3.
6. Glorieux FH, *et al.* Cyclic administration of pamidronate in children with severe osteogenesis imperfecta. *N Engl J Med* 1998; **339:** 947–52.
7. Plotkin H, *et al.* Pamidronate treatment of severe osteogenesis imperfecta in children under 3 years of age. *J Clin Endocrinol Metab* 2000; **85:** 1846–50.
8. Åström E, Söderhäll S. Beneficial effect of long term intravenous bisphosphonate treatment of osteogenesis imperfecta. *Arch Dis Child* 2002; **86:** 356–64.
9. Falk MJ, *et al.* Intravenous bisphosphonate therapy in children with osteogenesis imperfecta. *Pediatrics* 2003; **111:** 573–8.
10. Devogelaer J-P. New uses of bisphosphonates: osteogenesis imperfecta. *Curr Opin Pharmacol* 2002; **2:** 748–53.
11. Williams CJC, *et al.* Hypercalcaemia in osteogenesis imperfecta treated with pamidronate. *Arch Dis Child* 1997; **76:** 169–70.

### Osteomalacia

Osteomalacia occurs when there is impaired mineralisation of the bone matrix resulting in 'soft' bones. Patients usually present with bone pain and muscle weakness and may have subclinical fractures. **Rickets** refers to defective mineralisation of growing bone and is therefore restricted to children;[1] it is associated with retarded growth, skeletal deformities, teeth defects, and muscle hypotonia.

Inadequate bone mineralisation is usually caused by vitamin D deficiency or its abnormal metabolism, but may also be due to phosphate depletion, calcium deficiency, or a primary disorder of bone matrix such as hypophosphatasia in which a deficiency of alkaline phosphatase results in an increase in pyrophosphate, an inhibitor of bone mineralisation. Some drugs including various antiepileptics (p.371), etidronate, and aluminium salts, can interfere with bone mineralisation and cause osteomalacia. Osteomalacia also occurs in renal osteodystrophy associated with chronic renal failure (see below).

Several hereditary disorders are associated with the development of rickets including vitamin D-pseudodeficiency rickets (vitamin D-dependent rickets), in which there is impaired synthesis of 1,25-dihydroxycholecalciferol (Type I) or receptor resistance to 1,25-dihydroxycholecalciferol (Type II), and X-linked hypophosphataemic rickets.[2]

Treatment of osteomalacia and rickets is primarily aimed at correcting any underlying deficiency. Vitamin D substances, calcium, or phosphate supplements can be given by mouth as appropriate but doses require careful individual adjustment to maintain calcium and phosphate concentrations within normal limits. A variety of forms or analogues of vitamin D are available. For the treatment of simple vitamin D deficiency colecalciferol or ergocalciferol are generally preferred. If malabsorption is suspected, larger doses or parenteral administration may be necessary, but where large doses are required it may be preferable to use one of the more potent forms of vitamin D such as calcitriol. Simple calcium deficiency may be a more important cause of rickets than vitamin D deficiency in some populations. A study in African children with rickets found that their calcium intake was low and that they responded better to calcium supplementation, with or without vitamin D, than to vitamin D alone.[3]

Type I vitamin D-pseudodeficiency rickets requires replacement therapy with calcitriol. In Type II disease, resistance to calcitriol treatment may be so extreme that only very large supplements of calcium may be effective.[2,4] X-linked hypophosphataemic rickets is considered to be best treated with combined phosphate supplementation and calcitriol.[2,5] There has also been some interest in the use of growth hormone in children with hypophosphataemic rickets.[6] A form of hypophosphataemic rickets, rickets of prematurity (p.1232), may occur in small, premature infants fed exclusively on breast milk, and phosphate supplementation with concomitant calcium and vitamin D has been suggested in such cases.


1. Wharton B, Bishop N. Rickets. *Lancet* 2003; **362:** 1389–1400.
2. Glorieux FH. Rickets, the continuing challenge. *N Engl J Med* 1991; **325:** 1875–7.
3. Thacher TD, *et al.* A comparison of calcium, vitamin D, or both for nutritional rickets in Nigerian children. *N Engl J Med* 1999; **341:** 563–8.
4. Hochberg Z, *et al.* Calcium therapy for calcitriol-resistant rickets. *J Pediatr* 1992; **121:** 803–8.
5. Verge CF, *et al.* Effects of therapy in X-linked hypophosphatemic rickets. *N Engl J Med* 1991; **325:** 1843–8.
6. Shaw NJ, *et al.* Growth hormone and hypophosphataemic rickets. *Arch Dis Child* 1995; **72:** 543–4.


## Osteoporosis

Osteoporosis is a disease characterised by low bone mass and microarchitectural deterioration of bone tissue, leading to enhanced bone fragility and risk of fracture,[1,2] particularly of the long bones (distal forearm and neck of the femur) and the vertebrae. Although bone formation outstrips resorption in youth, accumulated small deficits from remodelling (see Bone and Bone Disease, above) result in a gradual loss of bone mass after the third decade. Primary osteoporosis is therefore usually an age-related disease. It can affect both sexes, though women are at greater risk because bone loss is accelerated, to a variable degree, after the menopause. Osteoporosis can also be secondary to diseases such as thyrotoxicosis, hypogonadism, Cushing's syndrome, hypoparathyroidism, and rheumatoid arthritis, or to drugs such as corticosteroids (p.1069), gonadorelin analogues (p.1325), and heparin (p.928).[3] Also, immobility, especially in younger patients, can result in osteoblastic failure with an increase in osteoclastic resorption and the development of osteoporosis. Other risk factors for osteoporosis include smoking, high alcohol intake, physical inactivity, thin body type, early menopause, and a family history of osteoporosis.[4,5]

Patients are usually asymptomatic until fractures occur, and up to half of vertebral fractures may also be asymptomatic. Fractures may result in pain, deformity (kyphosis, loss of height), and disability. Currently, the most reliable method of assessing osteoporosis and fracture risk is measurement of bone mass density (BMD), usually by dual energy X-ray absorptiometry.[1] WHO have defined osteoporosis as a BMD 2.5 standard deviations or more below the young adult mean, and severe osteoporosis (established osteoporosis) as this BMD in the presence of one or more fragility fractures.[1,6] There is no universally agreed policy on screening for osteoporosis,[7] but measurement of BMD should be considered in those thought to be at risk of osteoporosis if the result is likely to affect treatment decisions.[5,6,8] Different approaches to the management of osteoporosis have been suggested, including changes in life-style, interventions to reduce falls, the use of drugs to either decrease bone resorption or stimulate bone formation.[5,9-16] Because bone remodelling is a coupled process decreases in resorption ultimately reduce the rate of bone formation, and antiresorptive drugs can therefore only produce modest increases in bone mass. Trials with such drugs must be sufficiently prolonged to determine whether an increase in bone mass represents more than just a constriction in the remodelling space.[17] Moreover, experience with fluoride indicates that increases in BMD do not always equate to decreases in fracture risk,[18,19] and so there is a need to show that drugs decrease fracture rate. In addition, the optimum timing and duration of drug therapy to optimise the benefits on bone and minimise the risks is not known, particularly for the prevention of primary osteoporosis.

**Prevention** is the most effective method of dealing with osteoporosis as once bone mass has decreased it is difficult to replace.

- Optimising peak bone mass is therefore important; regular moderate weight-bearing exercise and adequate dietary calcium during growth[20,21] have been advocated.
- After the third decade of life, interventions should be aimed at reducing the rate of bone loss. This includes life-style modifications such as avoiding smoking,[22] moderation of alcohol intake, improving diet to ensure an adequate calcium and vitamin D intake (see under Human Requirements, p.1226 and p.1462), and regular weight-bearing exercise.[3,23-25]
- Secondary causes of osteoporosis should be identified and treated as appropriate.[5]
- Antiresorptive drugs may be considered.

In postmenopausal women, HRT (p.1540) was initially considered first-line,[26] as its antiresorptive action has been shown to preserve BMD and decrease fracture risk.[27] However, results from the Women's Health Initiative and Million Women studies suggested that long-term use of HRT could increase the risk of breast and some other cancers (see p.1536), while not benefiting cardiovascular risk reduction or cognitive function. The UK Committee on Safety of Medicines (CSM) has thus recommended that HRT no longer be considered as a first-line therapy for the prevention of osteoporosis in women aged over 50 years and at increased risk of fractures;[28] it remains an option for those intolerant of or refractory to other therapies, and for prevention of osteoporosis in women with premature menopause until the age of 50.

Alternative antiresorptive drugs for the prevention of postmenopausal osteoporosis include tibolone,[26] raloxifene,[3,8,26,27,29,30] and bisphosphonates such as alendronate, etidronate, and risedronate.[3,8,26,27,29] There is good evidence that these drugs prevent loss of bone mineral density in postmenopausal osteoporotic women. However, as yet there is little experience of the use of these drugs for prevention of osteoporosis in women with normal BMD, or for women with osteopenia but no fracture, as most trials have been conducted in women with established osteoporosis.[31]

In postmenopausal women, the effects of calcium supplementation (about 1 g of calcium daily by mouth) have been conflicting; some studies have reported a reduction in bone loss[32-34] but others have found calcium supplements to be of little benefit.[35] However, a subsequent meta-analysis[36] found that increasing calcium intake by diet or supplements potentiated the effect of oestrogens and calcitonins on bone, confirming that an adequate intake of calcium is important when antiresorptive drugs are being used. Calcium and vitamin D supplements reduce fracture risk in elderly institutionalised persons, who should be offered such treatment.[25]

The use of calcitonins as prophylactic drugs has been limited by the necessity for parenteral administration. However, intranasal spray formulations of calcitonin (salmon) have been developed and oral formulations are under investigation.

Other drugs that have been reported to have favourable effects on bone mass in postmenopausal women include thiazide diuretics,[3] tamoxifen, intermittent teriparatide, diclofenac,[37] and potassium bicarbonate.

**Treatment.** In patients with osteoporosis with or without fragility fractures (established osteoporosis), treatment involves supportive therapy and interventions to prevent further bone loss and reduce the risk of fractures.[5,6,9-16]

- Supportive therapy in the acute phase of a fracture includes pain relief, physiotherapy, and appropriate orthopaedic management of fracture of long bones; surgery is required for the majority of hip fractures.[14]
- Life-style modifications and drugs to prevent further bone loss and fractures are similar to those outlined above, and the boundary between treatment and prevention (of further problems) is often blurred. In the elderly, interventions to reduce the risk of falls may be important,[38] and measures to protect the patient should falls occur may also be considered.[39]

In postmenopausal women with established osteoporosis, HRT increases bone mass and reduces the incidence of fractures[3,25] and has been an option in various guidelines.[26] However, as in prevention (above) the risks and benefits have been reassessed, and use to treat osteoporosis is now seen as inappropriate. The CSM and others recommend[2,3,28] that HRT should be reserved for the short-term treatment of menopausal symptoms, with a bone-sparing effect regarded as an added benefit.[2]

The major *antiresorptive* treatments are thus, as mentioned above for prevention, bisphosphonates or raloxifene. The bisphosphonates, such as alendronate, etidronate, and risedronate, have been shown to increase bone mass and decrease fracture rate in established osteoporosis.[2,3,27,29,31] Improvements in bone mass and fracture rate have also been shown with raloxifene.[40] Combination therapy of bisphosphonates with HRT or raloxifene has increased BMD but with no effect on fracture risk reduction.[29]

Calcitonins may also have an adjunctive role. It has been suggested that, in particular, the analgesic effects of calcitonins may be advantageous in patients with acute pain due to osteoporotic fractures.[8]

Studies using the vitamin D substance calcitriol for the treatment of osteoporosis have produced conflicting results; although some have reported an increase in spinal bone density[41] and a reduction in the rate of new vertebral fractures,[42] others have found no significant effects.[43]

Vitamin D supplements have shown beneficial effects in the elderly, and it is considered that they may have a particular role in frail or housebound individuals, who are at high risk of vitamin D deficiency and resulting hyperparathyroidism.[13,14,16,25]

Postmenopausal osteoporosis has also been treated with drugs that *promote bone formation*. Fluoride stimulates osteoblasts and increases the density of trabecular bone and has been given as sodium fluoride or sodium monofluorophosphate. However, increases in BMD with fluoride have not always resulted in decreased fracture rate, and may even be associated with increased bone fragility; thus, the role of fluoride remains unclear.[6,13,15,16,44] Anabolic steroids have been tried but have considerable adverse effects. Teriparatide has been found to increase BMD and decrease the risk of vertebral and non-vertebral fractures.[45] Strontium ranelate, given with calcium and vitamin D supplements, has been found to reduce the risk of vertebral fractures.[46] Other drugs that have been investigated for postmenopausal osteoporosis include mecasermin and ipriflavone. There is some suggestion that HMG-CoA reductase inhibitors have the potential to reduce fracture risk, but data are conflicting, and further trials are needed.[47,48]

There is less evidence to guide decisions on the management of osteoporosis in **men**[49-52] than in postmenopausal women. In hypogonadal men with osteoporosis, testosterone replacement therapy should be used.[51] In eugonadal men, there are concerns regarding the potential long-term adverse effects of exogenous testosterone. Therefore, in men with idiopathic osteoporosis, bisphosphonates may be the treatment of choice.[51] Calcium and vitamin D supplements do not affect the rate of bone mineral loss in healthy men with adequate diets.[53] However, there is some evidence that, as for women, elderly men may benefit from vitamin D supplements and calcium.[54] Other drugs that have been reported to have favourable effects on BMD in men include thiazides,[55] somatropin,[56] and teriparatide.[19,57]


1. WHO. Assessment of fracture risk and its application to screening for postmenopausal osteoporosis. *WHO Tech Rep Ser 843* 1994.
2. Åkesson K. New approaches to pharmacological treatment of osteoporosis. *Bull WHO* 2003; **81:** 657–64.
3. Follin SL, Hansen LB. Current approaches to the prevention and treatment of postmenopausal osteoporosis. *Am J Health-Syst Pharm* 2003; **60:** 883–904.
4. Dempster DW, Lindsay R. Pathogenesis of osteoporosis. *Lancet* 1993; **341:** 797–801.
5. Peel N, Eastell R. Osteoporosis. *BMJ* 1995; **310:** 989–92.
6. Kanis JA, *et al.* Guidelines for diagnosis and management of osteoporosis. *Osteoporosis Int* 1997; **7:** 390–406.
7. Fogelman I. Screening for osteoporosis. *BMJ* 1999; **319:** 1148–9.
8. Gourlay M, *et al.* Strategies for the prevention of hip fracture. *Am J Med* 2003; **115:** 309–17. Correction. *ibid.*; 509.
9. Riggs BL, Melton LJ. The prevention and treatment of osteoporosis. *N Engl J Med* 1992; **327:** 620–7.
10. Lindsay R. Prevention and treatment of osteoporosis. *Lancet* 1993; **341:** 801–5.
11. Conference Report. Consensus Development Conference: diagnosis, prophylaxis, and treatment of osteoporosis. *Am J Med* 1993; **94:** 646–50.
12. Khosla S, Riggs BL. Treatment options for osteoporosis. *Mayo Clin Proc* 1995; **70:** 978–82.
13. Anonymous. Managing osteoporosis. *Drug Ther Bull* 1996; **34:** 45–8.

14. Compston JE. Osteoporosis: management of established disease. *Prescribers' J* 1997; **37:** 119–24.
15. Gibaldi M. Prevention and treatment of osteoporosis: does the future belong to hormone replacement therapy? *J Clin Pharmacol* 1997; **37:** 1087–99.
16. Eastell R. Treatment of postmenopausal osteoporosis. *N Engl J Med* 1998; **338:** 736–46.
17. Heaney RP. Interpreting trials of bone-active agents. *Am J Med* 1995; **98:** 329–30.
18. Kleerekoper M, Schein JR. Comparative safety of bone remodeling agents with a focus on osteoporosis therapies. *J Clin Pharmacol* 2001; **41:** 239–50.
19. Rosen CJ, Bilezikian JP. Clinical review 123: Hot Topic: anabolic therapy for osteoporosis. *J Clin Endocrinol Metab* 2001; **86:** 957–64.
20. Johnston CC, *et al.* Calcium supplementation and increases in bone mineral density in children. *N Engl J Med* 1992; **327:** 82–7.
21. Lloyd T, *et al.* Calcium supplementation and bone mineral density in adolescent girls. *JAMA* 1993; **270:** 841–4.
22. Law MR, Hackshaw AK. A meta-analysis of cigarette smoking, bone mineral density and risk of hip fracture: recognition of a major effect. *BMJ* 1997; **315:** 841–6.
23. Nelson ME, *et al.* Effects of high intensity strength training on multiple risk factors for osteoporotic fractures: a randomized controlled trial. *JAMA* 1994; **272:** 1909–14.
24. Gregg EW, *et al.* Physical activity and osteoporotic fracture risk in older women. *Ann Intern Med* 1998; **129:** 81–8.
25. Anonymous. Lifestyle advice for fracture prevention. *Drug Ther Bull* 2002; **40:** 83–6.
26. Royal College of Physicians. *Osteoporosis: clinical guidelines for prevention and treatment.* London: Royal College of Physicians, 1999. Also available at: http://www.rcplondon.ac.uk/files/osteosummary.pdf (accessed 23/05/04) Update available at: http://www.rcplondon.ac.uk/pubs/wp_osteo_update.htm (accessed 23/05/04)
27. Eichner SF, *et al.* Comparing therapies for postmenopausal osteoporosis prevention and treatment. *Ann Pharmacother* 2003; **37:** 711–24.
28. Further advice on safety of HRT: risk:benefit unfavourable for first-line use in prevention of osteoporosis—message from Professor G Duff, Chairman of Committee on Safety of Medicines (CSM). Available at: http://medicines.mhra.gov.uk/ourwork/monitorsafequalmed/safetymessages/hrtepinet_31203.pdf (accessed 23/05/04)
29. Delmas PD. Treatment of postmenopausal osteoporosis. *Lancet* 2002; **359:** 2018–26.
30. Anonymous. Raloxifene to prevent postmenopausal osteoporosis. *Drug Ther Bull* 1999; **37:** 33–6.
31. Sambrook PN, *et al.* Preventing osteoporosis: outcomes of the Australian Fracture Prevention Summit. *Med J Aust* 2002; **176** (suppl): S1–S16.
32. Reid IR, *et al.* Effect of calcium supplementation on bone loss in postmenopausal women. *N Engl J Med* 1993; **328:** 460–4. Correction. *ibid.*; **329:** 1281.
33. Aloia JF, *et al.* Calcium supplementation with and without hormone replacement therapy to prevent postmenopausal bone loss. *Ann Intern Med* 1994; **120:** 97–103.
34. Reid IR, *et al.* Long-term effects of calcium supplementation on bone loss and fractures in postmenopausal women: a randomized controlled trial. *Am J Med* 1995; **98:** 331–5.
35. Riis B, *et al.* Does calcium supplementation prevent postmenopausal bone loss? *N Engl J Med* 1987; **316:** 173–7.
36. Nieves JW, *et al.* Calcium potentiates the effects of estrogen and calcitonin on bone mass: review and analysis. *Am J Clin Nutr* 1998; **67:** 18–24.
37. Bell NH, *et al.* Diclofenac sodium inhibits bone resorption in postmenopausal women. *Am J Med* 1994; **96:** 349–53.
38. Dargent-Molina P, *et al.* Fall-related factors and risk of hip fracture: the EPIDOS prospective study. *Lancet* 1996; **348:** 145–9.
39. Lauritzen JB, *et al.* Effect of external hip protectors on hip fractures. *Lancet* 1993; **341:** 11–13.
40. Clemett D, Spencer CM. Raloxifene: a review of its use in postmenopausal osteoporosis. *Drugs* 2000; **60:** 379–411.
41. Gallagher JC, Goldgar D. Treatment of postmenopausal osteoporosis with high doses of synthetic calcitriol: a randomized controlled study. *Ann Intern Med* 1990; **113:** 649–55.
42. Tilyard MW, *et al.* Treatment of postmenopausal osteoporosis with calcitriol or calcium. *N Engl J Med* 1992; **326:** 357–62.
43. Ott SM, Chesnut CH. Calcitriol treatment is not effective in postmenopausal osteoporosis. *Ann Intern Med* 1989; **110:** 267–74.
44. Haguenauer D, *et al.* Fluoride for treating postmenopausal osteoporosis. Available in The Cochrane Library; Issue 2. Chichester: John Wiley; 2004.
45. Neer RM, *et al.* Effect of parathyroid hormone (1-34) on fractures and bone mineral density in postmenopausal women with osteoporosis. *N Engl J Med* 2001; **344:** 1434–41.
46. Meunier PJ, *et al.* The effects of strontium ranelate on the risk of vertebral fracture in women with postmenopausal osteoporosis. *N Engl J Med* 2004; **350:** 459–68.
47. Hennessy S, Strom BL. Statins and fracture risk. *JAMA* 2001; **285:** 1888–9.
48. Cushenberry LM, de Bittner MR. Potential use of HMG-CoA reductase inhibitors for osteoporosis. *Ann Pharmacother* 2002; **36:** 671–8.
49. Anderson DC. Osteoporosis in men. *BMJ* 1992; **305:** 489–90.
50. Seeman E. The dilemma of osteoporosis in men. *Am J Med* 1995; **98** (suppl 2A): 76S–88S.
51. Eastell R, *et al.* Management of male osteoporosis: report of the UK Consensus Group. *Q J Med* 1998; **91:** 71–92.
52. Bilezikian JP. Osteoporosis in men. *J Clin Endocrinol Metab* 1999; **84:** 3431–4.
53. Orwoll ES, *et al.* The rate of bone mineral loss in normal men and the effects of calcium and cholecalciferol supplementation. *Ann Intern Med* 1990; **112:** 29–34.
54. Dawson-Hughes B, *et al.* Effect of calcium and vitamin D supplementation on bone density in men and women 65 years of age and older. *N Engl J Med* 1997; **337:** 670–6.
55. Wasnich R, *et al.* Effect of thiazide on rates of bone mineral loss: a longitudinal study. *BMJ* 1990; **301:** 1303–5. Correction. *ibid.* 1991; **302:** 218.
56. Gillberg P, *et al.* Two years of treatment with recombinant human growth hormone increases bone mineral density in men with idiopathic osteoporosis. *J Clin Endocrinol Metab* 2002; **87:** 4900–6.
57. Slovik DM, *et al.* Restoration of spinal bone in osteoporotic men by treatment with human parathyroid hormone (1–34) and 1,25-dihydroxyvitamin D. *J Bone Miner Res* 1986; **1:** 377–81.

### Paget's disease of bone

Paget's disease of bone (osteitis deformans) is characterised by excessive and disorganised bone resorption and formation. It may affect one or more bones, usually the cranium, spine, clavicles, pelvis, or long bones, but in most patients the majority of the skeleton is uninvolved. Paget's disease occurs in about 3 to 4% of the population over 40 years of age and its frequency increases with age. Patients are often asymptomatic, but some present with musculoskeletal and bone pain, or with bone weakness and deformity that can result in fractures. Other complications include hearing loss, nerve compression (especially of the spinal cord), and, in severe disease, heart failure due to increased skeletal vascularity.

Patients who are asymptomatic and in whom the sites of disease are associated with little or no risk of complications do not require any treatment. Bone or joint pain may be treated with NSAIDs or paracetamol. Therapy with drugs that reduce bone resorption,[1-3] such as the calcitonins and bisphosphonates, is indicated if bone pain is persistent or to prevent further progression of the disease, especially if complications such as spinal-cord compression are present or there is a risk of such complications. Such treatment is suppressive and while osteolytic lesions may be healed, the underlying disorder is not cured. Drug therapy is guided by monitoring biochemical improvement in disease activity.

Bisphosphonates give symptomatic relief and heal osteolytic lesions. In contrast to the short-lived effects of calcitonins, which generally need to be given continuously to suppress disease activity,[3] disease activity may be reduced for several months, or years, after bisphosphonate therapy has ceased; therefore, bisphosphonates have largely superseded the calcitonins.[2,4,5] Initial experience was with etidronate, but bisphosphonates that have less effect on bone mineralisation, such as alendronate, clodronate, pamidronate, risedronate, or tiludronate may be preferred.[3-6]

Use of a calcitonin with a bisphosphonate has been reported to induce a better response than either drug given alone,[7] but some consider that such combinations should be reserved for patients only partially responsive to a single drug.[1] Others suggest that a calcitonin may be useful in the first few weeks of bisphosphonate therapy for more rapid relief of bone pain.[3] When given consecutively, results have been conflicting.[8,9]

Plicamycin, a cytotoxic antibiotic with particular activity against osteoclasts, is highly effective in the treatment of Paget's disease of bone when given daily by intravenous infusion for 5 to 10 days. However, it is associated with severe toxicity and is therefore now avoided or reserved for patients refractory to other drugs.[3,10]

Studies with gallium nitrate,[5,11] another inhibitor of bone resorption, have indicated beneficial effects in the treatment of Paget's disease of bone. Ipriflavone has also been tried.[5]

In selected patients, orthopaedic surgery such as hip replacement or correction of a bone deformity may be appropriate. A calcitonin or bisphosphonate is usually given 1 to 3 months before surgery in order to reduce bone vascularity (thus minimising blood loss during the operation) and also to prevent development of postoperative hypercalcaemia of immobilisation.

1. Gennari C, *et al.* Management of osteoporosis and Paget's disease: an appraisal of the risks and benefits of drug treatment. *Drug Safety* 1994; **11:** 179–95.
2. Hosking D, *et al.* Paget's disease of bone: diagnosis and management. *BMJ* 1996; **312:** 491–4.
3. Delmas PD, Meunier PJ. The management of Paget's disease of bone. *N Engl J Med* 1997; **336:** 558–66.
4. Roux C, Dougados M. Treatment of patients with Paget's disease of bone. *Drugs* 1999; **58:** 823–30.
5. Hadjipavlou AG, *et al.* Paget's disease of the spine and its management. *Eur Spine J* 2001; **10:** 370–84.
6. Drake WM, *et al.* Consensus statement on the modern therapy of Paget's disease of bone from a Western Osteoporosis Alliance Symposium. *Clin Ther* 2001; **23:** 620–6.
7. O'Donoghue DJ, Hosking DJ. Biochemical response to combination of disodium etidronate with calcitonin in Paget's disease. *Bone* 1987; **8:** 219–25.
8. Perry HM, *et al.* Alternate calcitonin and etidronate disodium therapy for Paget's bone disease. *Arch Intern Med* 1984; **144:** 929–33.
9. Rico H, *et al.* Biochemical assessment of acute and chronic treatment of Paget's bone disease with calcitonin and calcium with and without biphosphonate. *Bone* 1988; **9:** 63–6.
10. Ryan WG, *et al.* Apparent cure of Paget's disease of bone. *Am J Med* 1990; **89:** 825–6.
11. Bockman RS, *et al.* A multicenter trial of low dose gallium nitrate in patients with advanced Paget's disease of bone. *J Clin Endocrinol Metab* 1995; **80:** 595–602.

### Renal osteodystrophy

Patients with chronic renal failure (p.1222) may develop complex changes to bone known as renal osteodystrophy.[1-3] Reduced vitamin D metabolism and consequent hypocalcaemia, plus lowered phosphate excretion, result in inadequate bone mineralisation with the development of *osteomalacia* (see above); excessive production of parathyroid hormone leads to secondary hyperparathyroidism (see below) and increased bone turnover. The latter leads in turn to *osteitis fibrosa*, a condition characterised by an abundance of osteoclasts, osteoblasts, and osteocytes, and the deposition of fibrous tissue in the bone marrow.

In patients with chronic renal failure on dialysis, the accumulation of aluminium from either the dialysis water supply or from the use of aluminium-containing phosphate binders may also have adverse effects on bone (see Aluminium Hydroxide, p.1249) and is associated with the development of osteomalacia and *adynamic bone disease* (suppression of remodelling). Osteosclerosis and osteoporosis may also occur.[3]

Most patients are asymptomatic at presentation and **treatment** is aimed at controlling the plasma concentrations of calcium, phosphate, and parathyroid hormone.[2,4] Severe hyperphosphataemia should be corrected first to reduce the risk of metastatic calcification which may be aggravated by the use of vitamin D compounds which increase calcium absorption.

*Hyperphosphataemia* is initially controlled with a low-phosphate diet but many patients, especially those on dialysis, also need an oral phosphate binder to complex with dietary phosphate in the gastrointestinal tract and reduce its absorption.[2,5]

Calcium salts such as the carbonate or acetate are effective phosphate binders[6,7] and have been found to suppress hyperparathyroidism. Calcium salts also raise plasma-calcium concentrations and reduce acidosis but hypercalcaemia can occur;[8,9] the use of dialysis fluids with a lower calcium content has been suggested for these patients.[2,10]

Alternatively, aluminium hydroxide may be given but relatively large doses are required and as mentioned above, aluminium accumulation can lead to osteomalacia and adynamic bone disease in patients with impaired renal function. Long-term use is not generally recommended,[2] and alternative drugs are probably preferable.

Sevelamer, a polymer capable of binding phosphate, may also be given.[4,11]

Vitamin D compounds that do not require renal hydroxylation such as calcitriol or its synthetic analogue, alfacalcidol, are the drugs of choice for correcting the *hypocalcaemia* and also contribute to the control of *secondary hyperparathyroidism*;[2] calcium supplements may also occasionally be required. Newer vitamin D analogues for secondary hyperparathyroidism related to chronic renal failure include doxercalciferol, paricalcitol, and falecalcitriol. Use of alfacalcidol in the early stages of renal failure, before dialysis is required, has been reported to improve subclinical bone disease.[12] Calcitriol or its analogues are given orally; the dose is adjusted according to response but must be carefully monitored as the dose required for adequate suppression of parathyroid hormone secretion may be close to that which causes hypercalcaemia. It has also been recommended that a close watch should be kept on renal function since deterioration may be accelerated by calcitriol, an effect that may be independent of any induced hypercalcaemia.[13]

Patients unresponsive to drug therapy or who develop hypercalcaemia (which may itself accelerate the decline in renal function) may require sub-total parathyroidectomy.[1,2] Alternatively, the administration of calcitriol as intermittent intravenous infusions (3 times a week during haemodialysis) has been reported to be effective in reducing plasma concentrations of parathyroid hormone and ameliorating osteitis fibrosa in some patients with moderate to severe secondary hyperparathyroidism due to chronic renal failure who had failed to respond adequately to oral calcitriol.[14] Bisphosphonates can be used in the acute management of hypercalcaemia,[11] but seem to be of little benefit in the long-term treatment of hyperparathyroidism.

Patients with *adynamic bone disease* related to aluminium retention require removal of aluminium from the body; desferrioxamine has been used to mobilise aluminium before haemodialysis.[15] Use of aluminium-containing phosphate binders is clearly undesirable in such patients, and it has also been suggested that vitamin D compounds should not be given because they decrease the proliferation of osteoblasts.[3]

1. Malluche HH, Faugere M-C. Renal osteodystrophy. *N Engl J Med* 1989; **321:** 317–19.

2. Gower P. Prevention of bone disease in chronic renal failure. *Prescribers' J* 1992; **32:** 245–51.
3. Hruska KA, Teitelbaum SL. Renal osteodystrophy. *N Engl J Med* 1995; **333:** 166–74.
4. Ho LT, Sprague SM. Renal osteodystrophy in chronic renal failure. *Semin Nephrol* 2002; **22:** 488–93.
5. Coburn JW, Salusky IB. Control of serum phosphorus in uremia. *N Engl J Med* 1989; **320:** 1140–42.
6. Mak RHK, *et al.* Suppression of secondary hyperparathyroidism in children with chronic renal failure by high dose phosphate binders: calcium carbonate versus aluminium hydroxide. *BMJ* 1985; **291:** 623–7.
7. Slatopolsky E, *et al.* Calcium carbonate as a phosphate binder in patients with chronic renal failure undergoing dialysis. *N Engl J Med* 1986; **315:** 157–61.
8. Stein HD, *et al.* Calcium carbonate as a phosphate binder. *N Engl J Med* 1987; **316:** 109–10.
9. Raine AEG, Oliver DO. Management of hyperphosphataemia in renal dialysis patients. *Lancet* 1987; **i:** 633–4.
10. Slatopolsky E, *et al.* Calcium carbonate as a phosphate binder. *N Engl J Med* 1987; **316:** 110.
11. Elder G. Pathophysiology and recent advances in the management of renal osteodystrophy. *J Bone Miner Res* 2002; **17:** 2094–2105.
12. Hamdy NAT, *et al.* Effect of alfacalcidol on natural course of renal bone disease in mild to moderate renal failure. *BMJ* 1995; **310:** 358–63.
13. Chan JCM, *et al.* A prospective, double-blind study of growth failure in children with chronic renal insufficiency and the effectiveness of treatment with calcitriol versus dihydrotachysterol. *J Pediatr* 1994; **124:** 520–8.
14. Andress DL, *et al.* Intravenous calcitriol in the treatment of refractory osteitis fibrosa of chronic renal failure. *N Engl J Med* 1989; **321:** 274–9.
15. McCarthy JT, *et al.* Clinical experience with desferrioxamine in dialysis patients with aluminium toxicity. *Q J Med* 1990; **74:** 257–76.

### Rickets

See Osteomalacia, above.

## Parathyroid Disorders

Parathyroid hormone, secreted by the parathyroid gland, maintains concentrations of ionised calcium in extracellular fluid within normal limits. It acts directly on the kidney to enhance renal reabsorption of calcium, to increase phosphate excretion, and to promote the conversion of vitamin D to its active metabolite, 1,25-dihydroxycholecalciferol, which in turn, enhances calcium absorption from the gastrointestinal tract. Parathyroid hormone also acts on bone, to accelerate bone resorption and the release of calcium and phosphate into the extracellular fluid. Secretion of parathyroid hormone is primarily regulated by the extracellular concentration of ionised calcium; hypocalcaemia stimulates secretion whereas hypercalcaemia has an inhibitory effect. 1,25-Dihydroxycholecalciferol can also suppress parathyroid hormone secretion.

Disorders of parathyroid hormone secretion cause a disruption of calcium homoeostasis and in the long-term, may result in bone disease.

### Hyperparathyroidism

Primary hyperparathyroidism is a disorder of parathyroid hormone hypersecretion usually caused by adenomas or hyperplasia of the parathyroid glands. Patients are commonly asymptomatic but may have signs of hypercalcaemia (p.1218); nephrolithiasis may also be present. Secondary hyperparathyroidism occurs in response to hypocalcaemia as in chronic renal failure (p.1222) and if prolonged may progress to autonomous hypersecretion by the parathyroid gland (tertiary hyperparathyroidism).

Severe hypercalcaemia requires immediate treatment, but is rare in primary hyperparathyroidism. In the long-term, the treatment of choice for primary and tertiary hyperparathyroidism is usually surgical parathyroidectomy;[1-3] in patients with asymptomatic primary hyperparathyroidism no therapy may be necessary,[1] but the precise indications for surgery have been subject to debate.[3,4] The treatment of secondary hyperparathyroidism is usually aimed at the underlying cause of the hypocalcaemia; for example, for the treatment of secondary hyperparathyroidism associated with chronic renal disease, see Renal Osteodystrophy, above.

Drug treatment plays only a modest role in primary hyperparathyroidism. Oral phosphate supplements have been given in the short-term to alleviate hypercalciuria and hypercalcaemia. Bisphosphonates can be used in the acute management of hypercalcaemia, but seem to be of little benefit in the long-term treatment of hyperparathyroidism.[5] Although calcitonins have a rapid hypocalcaemic effect it is usually short-lived; they are therefore generally given as an adjunct with other therapy such as a bisphosphonate.[4] Oestrogens have been reported to reduce the rate of bone turnover and perhaps plasma-concentrations of calcium in postmenopausal women with primary hyperparathyroidism.[3,6,7] Calcium receptor agonists (calcimimetics) are under development for hyperparathyroidism.[8] Use of parathyroid hormone peptides to induce autoantibodies against parathyroid hormone resulted in improvement in hypercalcaemia in a woman with parathyroid carcinoma.[9]

1. Consensus Development Conference Panel. Diagnosis and management of asymptomatic primary hyperparathyroidism: consensus development conference statement. *Ann Intern Med* 1991; **114:** 593–7.
2. Scott-Coombes DM, Lynn JA. Surgical treatment of parathyroid disease. *Br J Hosp Med* 1997; **57:** 488–91.
3. Marx SJ. Hyperparathyroid and hypoparathyroid disorders. *N Engl J Med* 2000; **343:** 1863–75. Correction. *ibid.*; **344:** 696.
4. Kearns AE, Thompson GB. Medical and surgical management of hyperparathyroidism. *Mayo Clin Proc* 2002; **77:** 87–91. Correction. *ibid.*; 298.
5. Al Zahrani A, Levine MA. Primary hyperparathyroidism. *Lancet* 1997; **349:** 1233–8.
6. Marcus R, *et al.* Conjugated estrogens in the treatment of postmenopausal women with hyperparathyroidism. *Ann Intern Med* 1984; **100:** 633–40.
7. Selby PL, Peacock M. Ethinyl estradiol and norethindrone in the treatment of primary hyperparathyroidism in postmenopausal women. *N Engl J Med* 1986; **314:** 1481–5.
8. Silverberg SJ, *et al.* Short-term inhibition of parathyroid hormone secretion by a calcium-receptor agonist in patients with primary hyperparathyroidism. *N Engl J Med* 1997; **337:** 1506–10.
9. Bradwell AR, *et al.* Control of hypercalcaemia of parathyroid carcinoma by immunisation. *Lancet* 1999; **353:** 370–3.

### Hypoparathyroidism

Hypoparathyroidism occurs when there is a deficiency of parathyroid hormone secretion due to lack of parathyroid gland development or destruction of the gland, for example by auto-immune disease or surgical removal.[1] Other factors that may lead to a deficiency in parathyroid hormone include hypomagnesaemia and parathyroid adenomas. Where the deficiency results from resistance to parathyroid hormone the condition is termed pseudohypoparathyroidism. Parathyroid hormone, as teriparatide, is used in the differential diagnosis of hypoparathyroidism and pseudohypoparathyroidism. Hypoparathyroidism leads to hypocalcaemia and hyperphosphataemia, though in some patients these may not become significant until there is an increased calcium demand as in pregnancy.

Treatment is aimed at correcting the hypocalcaemia (p.1218); in patients with hypocalcaemic tetany the parenteral administration of calcium salts may be necessary. In the long-term, treatment is usually with oral vitamin D compounds which increase the intestinal absorption of calcium; calcium supplements may be required if dietary calcium is inadequate. Calcium concentrations and renal function require careful monitoring, especially since the lack of parathyroid hormone results in an increase in the renal excretion of calcium and the risk of nephrolithiasis.

Beneficial effects on plasma-calcium concentrations have been reported following the use of thiazide diuretics to reduce the urinary excretion of calcium.[2,3] However, these effects tended to be modest and thiazide diuretics have not been found to be effective in all patients with hypoparathyroidism;[4] adverse effects such as metabolic alkalosis may also be a problem.[5]

Teriparatide also has potential in the treatment of hypoparathyroidism. In one study,[6] it maintained serum calcium in the normal range and decreased urine calcium excretion. Good results have been reported following transplantation of parathyroid cells depleted of antigen-bearing cells in a few patients with postsurgical hypoparathyroidism.[7,8] It was considered that this might prove a promising technique in the future.

1. Marx SJ. Hyperparathyroid and hypoparathyroid disorders. *N Engl J Med* 2000; **343:** 1863–75. Correction. *ibid.*; **344:** 696.
2. Porter RH, *et al.* Treatment of hypoparathyroid patients with chlorthalidone. *N Engl J Med* 1978; **298:** 577–81.
3. Newman GH, *et al.* Effect of bendrofluazide on calcium reabsorption in hypoparathyroidism. *Eur J Clin Pharmacol* 1984; **27:** 41–6.
4. Gertner JM, Genel M. Chlorthalidone for hypoparathyroidism. *N Engl J Med* 1978; **298:** 1478.
5. Barzel US. Chlorthalidone for hypoparathyroidism. *N Engl J Med* 1978; **298:** 1478.
6. Winer KK, *et al.* Synthetic human parathyroid hormone 1-34 vs calcitriol and calcium in the treatment of hypoparathyroidism: results of a short-term randomized crossover trial. *JAMA* 1996; **276:** 631–6.
7. Decker GAG, *et al.* Allotransplantation of parathyroid cells. *Lancet* 1995; **345:** 124. Correction. *ibid.*; 464.
8. Hasse C, *et al.* Parathyroid allotransplantation without immunosuppression. *Lancet* 1997; **350:** 1296–7.

## Alendronic Acid *(BAN, rINN)*

Ácido alendrónico; AHButBP; Aminohydroxybutylidene Diphosphonic Acid. 4-Amino-1-hydroxybutane-1,1-diylbis(phosphonic acid).

$C_4H_{13}NO_7P_2$ = 249.1.
*CAS — 66376-36-1.*
*ATC — M05BA04.*

## Alendronate Sodium *(USAN, rINNM)*

Alendronato sódico; G-704650; L-670452; MK-0217; MK-217; Monosodium alendronate; Natrii Alendronas; Sodium Alendronate *(BANM)*. Sodium trihydrogen (4-amino-1-hydroxybutylidene)diphosphonate trihydrate.

$C_4H_{12}NNaO_7P_2,3H_2O$ = 325.1.
*CAS — 121268-17-5.*
*ATC — M05BA04.*

**Pharmacopoeias.** In *Eur.* (see p.vi).

**Ph. Eur. 5.0** (Sodium Alendronate). A white or almost white crystalline powder. Soluble in water; practically insoluble in dichloromethane; very slightly soluble in methyl alcohol. A 1% solution in water has a pH of 4.0 to 5.0.

### Adverse Effects and Precautions

As for the bisphosphonates in general, p.766. Gastrointestinal symptoms such as abdominal pain, dyspepsia, diarrhoea or constipation are the most frequent adverse effects. Severe oesophageal reactions such as oesophagitis, erosions, and ulceration have occurred (see below); patients should be advised to stop taking the tablets and seek medical attention if they develop symptoms such as dysphagia, new or worsening heartburn, pain on swallowing, or retrosternal pain. Peptic ulceration has been reported.

Alendronate should not be given to patients with abnormalities of the oesophagus or other factors that might delay oesophageal emptying, or those unable to stand or sit upright for at least 30 minutes. It should be used with caution in patients with upper gastrointestinal abnormalities. To minimise the risk of oesophageal reactions:

- patients should be instructed to swallow alendronate tablets whole with plenty of water (not less than 200 mL), in an upright position (standing or sitting). Mineral water with a high concentration of calcium should be avoided
- tablets should be taken on rising for the day, on an empty stomach, at least 30 minutes before breakfast and any other oral medication
- patients should remain upright after taking the tablets, and should not lie down before eating the first meal of the day
- alendronate should not be taken at bedtime, or before getting up for the day

Hypocalcaemia should be corrected before starting alendronate therapy.

**Effects on the eyes.** For reports of ocular effects with the bisphosphonates, including alendronate, see under Bisphosphonates, p.767.

**Effects on the kidneys.** Renal failure has been associated with the aminobisphosphonates, including alendronate, see under Bisphosphonates, p.767.

**Effects on the liver.** Hepatitis[1,2] and hepatocellular damage with raised liver enzyme concentrations[3,4] have been reported following therapy with alendronate.

1. Lieverse RJ. Hepatitis after alendronate. *Neth J Med* 1998; **53:** 271–2.
2. Carrère C, *et al.* Hépatite aiguë sévère imputable á l'alendronate. *Gastroenterol Clin Biol* 2002; **26:** 179–80.
3. Halabe A, *et al.* Liver damage due to alendronate. *N Engl J Med* 2000; **343:** 365.
4. de la Serna Higuera C, *et al.* Lesión hepatocelular inducida por alendronato. *Gastroenterol Hepatol* 2001; **24:** 244–6.

**Effects on the oesophagus.** Between September 1995 and March 1996 the UK Committee on Safety of Medicines (CSM) had received 10 reports of adverse effects on the oesophagus in patients receiving alendronate sodium.[1] Of these, 4 were of oesophageal reflux, 4 of oesophagitis, and 2 of oesophageal ulceration. As of March 1996, worldwide an estimated 475 000 patients had received alendronate and 199 patients had oesophageal reactions reported to the manufacturer, of which 51 were serious or severe.[2] Endoscopic findings included erosions, ulcerations, exudative inflammation, and thickening of the oesophagus. Bleeding was rare, and oesophageal perforation was not reported. Most oesophageal reactions occurred within 1 week to 2 months of starting alendronate therapy. Recovery occurred when alendronate was stopped; however, it was considered important that patients be followed up for the possible development of strictures.[2] In about 60% of the cases where the information was available, alendronate had not been taken in accordance with the precautions for use (see above).

The CSM subsequently noted[3] that it had continued to receive reports of reactions; by July 1998 there had been 97 reports in the UK, in 1 case associated with a fatality. It was estimated that 1 to 2% of patients might experience oesophageal reactions even when following the precautions for use. Some have reported a much higher incidence of unacceptable upper gastrointestinal symptoms in clinical practice.[4] However, a large placebo-controlled trial of alendronate did not find any increase in upper gastrointestinal events in patients taking alendronate.[5]


1. Committee on Safety of Medicines/Medicines Control Agency. Oesophageal reactions with alendronate sodium (Fosamax). *Current Problems* 1996; **22:** 5.
2. de Groen PC, *et al.* Esophagitis associated with the use of alendronate. *N Engl J Med* 1996; **335:** 1016–21.
3. Committee on Safety of Medicines/Medicines Control Agency. Reminder: severe oesophageal reactions with alendronate sodium (Fosamax). *Current Problems* 1998; **24:** 13. Also available at: http://medicines.mhra.gov.uk/ourwork/monitorsafequalmed/currentproblems/volume24aug.htm (accessed 23/05/04)
4. Kelly R, Taggart H. Incidence of gastrointestinal side effects due to alendronate is high in clinical practice. *BMJ* 1997; **315:** 1235.
5. Bauer DC, *et al.* Upper gastrointestinal tract safety profile of alendronate: the fracture intervention trial. *Arch Intern Med* 2000; **160:** 517–25.


**Hypersensitivity.** Allergic reactions to bisphosphonates do occur but appear to be rare, see p.767

## Interactions

As for the bisphosphonates in general, p.767.

## Pharmacokinetics

Like other bisphosphonates, alendronate is poorly absorbed after oral administration. Absorption is decreased by food, especially by products containing calcium or other polyvalent cations. Bioavailability is about 0.4% when taken half an hour before food, reduced from 0.7% in the fasting state; absorption is negligible when taken up to 2 hours after a meal. About half of the absorbed portion is excreted in the urine; the remainder is sequestered to bone for a prolonged period. Bisphosphonates do not appear to be metabolised.

◊ References.


1. Gertz BJ, *et al.* Studies of the oral bioavailability of alendronate. *Clin Pharmacol Ther* 1995; **58:** 288–98.
2. Cocquyt V, *et al.* Pharmacokinetics of intravenous alendronate. *J Clin Pharmacol* 1999; **39:** 385–93.
3. Porras AG, *et al.* Pharmacokinetics of alendronate. *Clin Pharmacokinet* 1999; **36:** 315–28.


## Uses and Administration

Alendronate is an aminobisphosphonate with general properties similar to those of the other bisphosphonates (p.767). It is a potent inhibitor of bone resorption and is licensed as the sodium salt in osteoporosis and Paget's disease of bone. It has also been given in the treatment of bone metastases and hypercalcaemia of malignancy.

Alendronate sodium is given by mouth, and the specific instructions for its administration (see Adverse Effects and Precautions, above) should be followed to minimise adverse effects and permit adequate absorption. Doses are expressed in terms of alendronic acid; alendronate sodium 1.3 mg is approximately equivalent to 1 mg of alendronic acid. The usual dosage for the treatment of osteoporosis in men and women is 10 mg daily. Postmenopausal women may be given 5 mg daily for prophylaxis. Alendronic acid may also be given once weekly to postmenopausal women in a dose of 70 mg for treatment of osteoporosis, or 35 mg for prophylaxis. Alendronate is used for the treatment and prevention of corticosteroid-induced osteoporosis in a dose of 5 mg daily; postmenopausal women who do not receive HRT should be given 10 mg daily. In adults with Paget's disease of bone the usual dose is 40 mg daily for 6 months; treatment may be repeated if necessary after an interval of a further 6 months.

Alendronic acid has also been given by intravenous infusion.

**Administration.** Alendronate once-weekly was considered to be therapeutically equivalent to once-daily dosing in both the treatment[1,2] and prevention[3] of osteoporosis, although both the design and the conclusions of the treatment study[1] were considered to have weaknesses.[4] Tolerability of a once-weekly regimen was comparable to placebo in one study[5] and to once-daily dosing in another.[6]


1. Schnitzer T, *et al.* Therapeutic equivalence of alendronate 70 mg once-weekly and alendronate 10 mg daily in the treatment of osteoporosis. *Aging (Milano)* 2000; **12:** 1–12.
2. The Alendronate Once-Weekly Study Group. Two-year results of once-weekly administration of alendronate 70 mg for the treatment of postmenopausal osteoporosis. *J Bone Miner Res* 2002; **17:** 1988–96.
3. Luckey MM, *et al.* Therapeutic equivalence of alendronate 35 milligrams once weekly and 5 milligrams daily in the prevention of postmenopausal osteoporosis. *Obstet Gynecol* 2003; **101:** 711–21.
4. Tsun EC, Heck AM. Intermittent dosing of alendronate. *Ann Pharmacother* 2001; **35:** 1471–5.
5. Greenspan S, *et al.* Tolerability of once-weekly alendronate in patients with osteoporosis: a randomized, double-blind, placebo-controlled study. *Mayo Clin Proc* 2002; **77:** 1044–52.
6. Simon JA, *et al.* Patient preference for once-weekly alendronate 70 mg versus once-daily alendronate 10 mg: a multicenter, randomized, open-label, crossover study. *Clin Ther* 2002; **24:** 1871–86.


**Malignant neoplasms of the bone.** Bisphosphonates are of benefit in some patients with metastatic bone disease (p.513). An open study with alendronate given intravenously suggested that it might be useful in such circumstances,[1] while a randomised dose-response study[2] found that single intravenous doses of alendronate 5 mg or more effectively lowered serum-calcium concentrations in patients with hypercalcaemia of malignancy.


1. Attardo-Parrinello G, *et al.* Effects of a new aminodiphosphonate (aminohydroxybutylidene diphosphonate) in patients with osteolytic lesions from metastases and myelomatosis: comparison with dichloromethylene diphosphonate. *Arch Intern Med* 1987; **147:** 1629–33.
2. Nussbaum SR, *et al.* Dose-response study of alendronate sodium for the treatment of cancer-associated hypercalcemia. *J Clin Oncol* 1993; **11:** 1618–23.


**Hyperparathyroidism.** Bisphosphonates have been used to inhibit bone resorption in the treatment of hypercalcaemia associated with hyperparathyroidism (p.765), but seem to be of little benefit for long-term treatment.

References.


1. Rossini M, *et al.* Effects of oral alendronate in elderly patients with osteoporosis and mild primary hyperparathyroidism. *J Bone Miner Res* 2001; **16:** 113–19.
2. Parker CR, *et al.* Alendronate in the treatment of primary hyperparathyroid-related osteoporosis: a 2-year study. *J Clin Endocrinol Metab* 2002; **87:** 4482–9.
3. Chow CC, *et al.* Oral alendronate increases bone mineral density in postmenopausal women with primary hyperparathyroidism. *J Clin Endocrinol Metab* 2003; **88:** 581–7.


**Osteoporosis.** The use of alendronate for the prevention and treatment of osteoporosis (p.763) has been reviewed.[1] In randomised controlled trials of up to 3 years duration, alendronate increased bone mass density of the spine, hip, and total body in postmenopausal women with osteoporosis,[2-4] those with osteoporosis and existing vertebral fractures,[5,6] and those without osteoporosis.[7,8] In postmenopausal women without osteoporosis, alendronate increased bone mass density, but not quite to the same extent as HRT.[7,9] Continuous long-term therapy appears to be more effective than short-term treatment in terms of skeletal benefits,[9-11] but a residual effect on bone mineral density remains for several years after stopping treatment,[9-11] despite resumption of bone loss after withdrawal of alendronate.[11,12] Where incidence of vertebral fracture was the primary end-point, alendronate reduced the incidence of new vertebral and nonvertebral fractures in women with prior fractures.[5,6,13] In women without prior fractures, alendronate reduced the incidence of clinical fractures in those with osteoporosis,[13,14] but not in those with higher bone mass density.[14] Alendronate is also used in men with osteoporosis; in a 2-year randomised trial it was found to increase bone mineral density and help prevent vertebral fractures.[15]

Alendronate also increases bone mass density in men and women receiving oral corticosteroids at doses equivalent to at least 7.5 mg prednisone daily,[16] and may be of some benefit in reducing bone loss after heart transplantation.[17]


1. Sharpe M, *et al.* Alendronate: an update of its use in osteoporosis. *Drugs* 2001; **61:** 999–1039.
2. Chesnut CH, *et al.* Alendronate treatment of the postmenopausal osteoporotic woman: effect of multiple dosages on bone mass and bone remodeling. *Am J Med* 1995; **99:** 144–52.
3. Liberman UA, *et al.* Effect of oral alendronate on bone mineral density and the incidence of fractures in postmenopausal osteoporosis. *N Engl J Med* 1995; **333:** 1437–43.
4. Tucci JR, *et al.* Effect of three years of oral alendronate treatment in postmenopausal women with osteoporosis. *Am J Med* 1996; **101:** 488–501.
5. Black DM, *et al.* Randomised trial of effect of alendronate on risk of fracture in women with existing vertebral fractures. *Lancet* 1996; **348:** 1535–41.
6. Ensrud KE, *et al.* Treatment with alendronate prevents fractures in women at highest risk: results from the Fracture Intervention Trial. *Arch Intern Med* 1997; **157:** 2617–24.
7. Hosking D, *et al.* Prevention of bone loss with alendronate in postmenopausal women under 60 years of age. *N Engl J Med* 1998; **338:** 485–92.
8. McClung M, *et al.* Alendronate prevents postmenopausal bone loss in women without osteoporosis: a double-blind, randomized, controlled trial. *Ann Intern Med* 1998; **128:** 253–61.
9. Ravn P, *et al.* Alendronate and estrogen-progestin in the long-term prevention of bone loss: four-year results from the early postmenopausal intervention cohort study: a randomized, controlled trial. *Ann Intern Med* 1999; **131:** 935–42.
10. Tonino RP, *et al.* Skeletal benefits of alendronate: 7-year treatment of postmenopausal osteoporotic women. *J Clin Endocrinol Metab* 2000; **85:** 3109–15.
11. Bone HG, *et al.* Ten years' experience with alendronate for osteoporosis in postmenopausal women. *N Engl J Med* 2004; **350:** 1189–99.
12. Ravn P, *et al.* Alendronate in early postmenopausal women: effects on bone mass during long-term treatment and after withdrawal. *J Clin Endocrinol Metab* 2000; **85:** 1492–7.
13. Black DM, *et al.* Fracture risk reduction with alendronate in women with osteoporosis: the fracture intervention trial. *J Clin Endocrinol Metab* 2000; **85:** 4118–24.
14. Cummings SR, *et al.* Effect of alendronate on risk of fracture in women with low bone density but without vertebral fractures: results from the Fracture Intervention Trial. *JAMA* 1998; **280:** 2077–82.
15. Orwoll E, *et al.* Alendronate for the treatment of osteoporosis in men. *N Engl J Med* 2000; **343:** 604–10.
16. Saag KG, *et al.* Alendronate for the prevention and treatment of glucocorticoid-induced osteoporosis. *N Engl J Med* 1998; **339:** 292–9.
17. Shane E, *et al.* Alendronate versus calcitriol for the prevention of bone loss after cardiac transplantation. *N Engl J Med* 2004; **350:** 767–76.


**Paget's disease of bone.** Bisphosphonates may be indicated to control the excessive and disorganised resorption and formation of bone that occurs in Paget's disease of bone (p.764).

References.


1. Adami S, *et al.* Effects of two oral doses of alendronate in the treatment of Paget's disease of bone. *Bone* 1994; **15:** 415–17.
2. Reid LR, *et al.* Biochemical and radiologic improvement in Paget's disease of bone treated with alendronate: a randomized, placebo-controlled trial. *Am J Med* 1996; **101:** 341–8.
3. Siris E, *et al.* Comparative study of alendronate versus etidronate for the treatment of Paget's disease of bone. *J Clin Endocrinol Metab* 1996; **81:** 961–7.


**Polymyositis and dermatomyositis.** Alendronate has been reported to be effective in the treatment of calcinosis[1] associated with juvenile dermatomyositis (p.1086).


1. Mukamel M, *et al.* New insight into calcinosis of juvenile dermatomyositis: study of composition and treatment. *J Pediatr* 2001; **138:** 763–6.


## Preparations

**Proprietary Preparations** (details are given in Part 3)
***Arg.:*** Alenato; Arendal; Berlex; Brek; Elandur; Findeclin; Fosamax; Lafedam; Marvil; Maxtral; Phostarac; Regenesis; Silidral; ***Austral.:*** Fosamax; ***Austria:*** Fosamax; ***Belg.:*** Fosamax; ***Braz.:*** Alendil; Bonalen; Cleveron; Endronax; Fosamax; Minusorb; Norvic†; Osdron†; Ossomax†; Ostenan; Osteoform; Osteoral; Osteotrat; Recalfe; Terost; ***Canad.:*** Fosamax; ***Chile:*** Aldrox; Arendal; Fosamax; Fosval; Holadren; Leodrin; Oseotal; Osteofem; Osteosan; ***Denm.:*** Fosamax; ***Fin.:*** Fosamax; ***Fr.:*** Fosamax; ***Ger.:*** Fosamax; ***Gr.:*** Fosamax; ***Hong Kong:*** Fosamax; ***India:*** Bifosa; ***Irl.:*** Fosamax; ***Israel:*** Fosalan; Maxibone; ***Ital.:*** Adronat; Alendros; Dronal; Fosamax; Genalen; ***Jpn:*** Onclast; ***Malaysia:*** Fosamax; ***Mex.:*** Fosamax; ***Neth.:*** Fosamax; ***Norw.:*** Fosamax; ***NZ:*** Fosamax; ***Port.:*** Adronat; Fosamax; ***S.Afr.:*** Fosamax; ***Singapore:*** Fosamax; ***Spain:*** Fosamax; ***Swed.:*** Fosamax; ***Switz.:*** Fosamax; ***Thai.:*** Fosamax; ***UK:*** Fosamax; ***USA:*** Fosamax.

# Bisphosphonates

Bifosfonatos; Biphosphonates; Diphosphonates.

Bisphosphonates are analogues of pyrophosphate, in which the central oxygen atom is replaced by a carbon atom with two further substituents—see Figure 1, p.767. Like pyrophosphate they have a strong affinity for bone. The bisphosphonates are used chiefly for their antiresorptive and hypocalcaemic properties (see Uses and Administration, below).

## Adverse Effects, Treatment, and Precautions

Bisphosphonates may cause gastrointestinal disturbances including abdominal pain, nausea and vomiting, and diarrhoea or constipation. Existing gastrointestinal problems may be exacerbated, and oral bisphosphonates should generally be given with care or avoided if acute upper gastrointestinal inflammation is present. Abdominal pain may be more frequent with aminobisphosphonates such as alendronate and oesophagitis has occurred.

Disturbances in serum electrolytes may occur, most commonly hypocalcaemia and hypophosphataemia. Bisphosphonates may cause musculoskeletal pain and headache. Hypersensitivity reactions have occurred rarely; angioedema, rashes, and pruritus have been reported. Other rare adverse effects include blood disorders such as leucopenia and disturbances in liver enzyme values.

Transient fever and flu-like symptoms are common with infusions of ibandronate and pamidronate. There may be local reactions, including thrombophlebitis, following parenteral administration.

Impairment of renal function has been reported with bisphosphonates, particularly when given parenterally. As a result their use should generally be avoided in pa-

**Figure 1.** Comparative structures of the bisphosphonates.

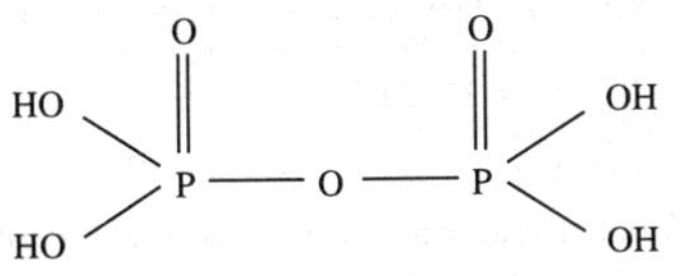

Pyrophosphate

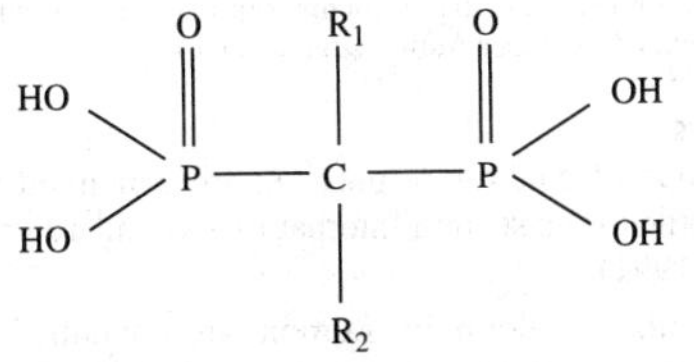

Generic structure of a bisphosphonate

| $R_1$ | $R_2$ | Name |
|---|---|---|
| $C_3H_6.NH_2$ | OH | Alendronic Acid |
| Cl | Cl | Clodronic Acid |
| $CH_3$ | OH | Etidronic Acid |
| $C_2H_4.NCH_3.C_5H_{11}$ | OH | Ibandronic Acid |
| $C_7H_{13}.NH$ | H | Incadronic Acid |
| H | H | Medronic Acid |
| $C_5H_{10}.NH_2$ | OH | Neridronic Acid |
| H | OH | Oxidronic Acid |
| $C_2H_4.NH_2$ | OH | Pamidronic Acid |
| $CH_2.C_5H_4N$ | OH | Risedronic Acid |
| $S.C_6H_4Cl$ | H | Tiludronic Acid |
| $CH_2.C_3H_3N_2$ | OH | Zoledronic Acid |

tients with moderate to severe renal impairment and they should be used with care in those with lesser degrees of renal impairment.

Etidronate interferes with bone mineralisation, especially at higher doses, which can result in osteomalacia and an increased incidence of fracture. Etidronate should be discontinued if a fracture occurs, until healing is complete. It has also been associated with a flare in bone pain in some patients with Paget's disease. Impaired mineralisation is much less marked at usual doses of other bisphosphonates.

Overdosage with bisphosphonates would be likely to result in symptoms of hypocalcaemia; if necessary, parenteral infusion of a calcium salt could be given. Administration of milk or antacids, to bind the bisphosphonate and minimise absorption, has been suggested for oral overdosage.

There is no clinical experience with bisphosphonates in pregnancy and they are generally contra-indicated; bisphosphonates have been associated with skeletal abnormalities in the fetus when given to pregnant *animals*.

◊ Reviews.

1. Adami S, Zamberlan N. Adverse effects of bisphosphonates: a comparative review. *Drug Safety* 1996; **14:** 158–70.
2. Kherani RB, *et al.* Long-term tolerability of the bisphosphonates in postmenopausal osteoporosis: a comparative review. *Drug Safety* 2002; **25:** 781–90.

**Effects on the eyes.** Ocular effects have been associated with bisphosphonates. Although adverse ocular reactions to pamidronate appeared to be rare, the manufacturers were aware of 23 cases up to September 1993 that were possibly associated with the drug.[1] The reactions included anterior uveitis in 7 patients and unilateral episcleritis or scleritis in 3. In one previously reported case,[2] bilateral iritis was associated with risedronate and subsequently pamidronate in a patient who had earlier received etidronate without ill-effect. There have been subsequent reports of unilateral and bilateral scleritis with pamidronate, requiring discontinuation of the drug.[3] Similarly, alendronate has been associated with scleritis[4] and anterior uveitis.[5,6] Scleritis and uveitis have also been reported with risedronate;[7,8] etidronate and clodronate have caused abnormal or blurred vision.[7] The Australian Adverse Drug Reactions Advisory Committee was aware of 38 reports of serious ocular reactions to bisphosphonates as of April 2004; these were associated with pamidronate or alendronate in 18 cases each, and risedronate or zoledronate in 1 case each.[8] Most reports were of inflammatory reactions such as uveitis, iritis, scleritis, episcleritis, or optic neuritis, and occurred a median of 3 weeks after starting therapy. The risk might be higher with intravenous bisphosphonates, but the frequency of reports was thought to relate mostly to usage.[8] Patients who have ocular pain or vision loss while taking bisphosphonates should have the drug discontinued and be referred to an ophthalmologist.[7]

1. Macarol V, Fraunfelder FT. Pamidronate disodium and possible ocular adverse drug reactions. *Am J Ophthalmol* 1994; **118:** 220–4.
2. Siris ES. Bisphosphonates and iritis. *Lancet* 1993; **341:** 436–7.
3. Fraunfelder FW, *et al.* Scleritis and other ocular side effects associated with pamidronate disodium. *Am J Ophthalmol* 2003; **135:** 219–22.
4. Mbekeani JN, *et al.* Ocular inflammation associated with alendronate therapy. *Arch Ophthalmol* 1999; **117:** 837–8.
5. Malik AR, *et al.* Bilateral acute anterior uveitis after alendronate. *Br J Ophthalmol* 2002; **86:** 1443.
6. Salmen S, *et al.* Nongranulomatous anterior uveitis associated with alendronate therapy. *Invest Clin* 2002; **43:** 49–52.
7. Fraunfelder FW, Fraunfelder FT. Bisphosphonates and ocular inflammation. *N Engl J Med* 2003; **348:** 1187–8.
8. Adverse Drug Reactions Advisory Committee (ADRAC). Bisphosphonates and ocular inflammation. *Aust Adverse Drug React Bull* 2004; **23:** 7–8. Also available at: http://www.tga.gov.au/adr/aadrb/aadr0404.htm (accessed 23/05/04)

**Effects on the kidneys.** Renal failure was associated with the intravenous administration of etidronate to 2 patients with hypercalcaemia of malignancy.[1] One had been given a high dose (1 g) by short intravenous infusion on two successive days and the other had an elevated serum-creatinine concentration before administration. A third patient given clodronate also developed renal failure but had a slightly raised serum-creatinine concentration before administration. Others[2] commented that with smaller doses of etidronate or clodronate (up to 300 mg daily) by intravenous infusion over 2 to 3 hours, renal impairment had not been seen in more than 40 patients treated. They noted a trend towards raised creatinine concentrations which was reversed when etidronate infusions were discontinued. Another group[3] found increased serum-creatinine concentrations after the first infusion of etidronate when compared with placebo, but not after subsequent infusions. An overdose of parenteral etidronate led to acute renal failure in one patient.[4] Pamidronate has been associated with nephrotoxicity,[5] proteinuria,[6] and acute tubular necrosis.[7] Over a period of 2 years, 72 cases of renal failure associated with intravenous zoledronic acid were reported to the FDA.[8] There has also been a report of acute renal failure with alendronate treatment in a patient with myeloma.[9]

1. Bounameaux HM, *et al.* Renal failure associated with intravenous diphosphonates. *Lancet* 1983; **i:** 471.
2. Kanis JA, *et al.* Effects of intravenous diphosphonates on renal function. *Lancet* 1983; **i:** 1328.
3. Hasling C, *et al.* Etidronate disodium for treating hypercalcaemia of malignancy: a double blind placebo-controlled study. *Eur J Clin Invest* 1986; **16:** 433–7.
4. O'Sullivan TL, *et al.* Acute renal failure associated with the administration of parenteral etidronate. *Ren Fail* 1994; **16:** 767–73.
5. Lockridge L, *et al.* Pamidronate-associated nephrotoxicity in a patient with Langerhans' histiocytosis. *Am J Kidney Dis* 2002; **40:** E2.
6. Desikan R, *et al.* Nephrotic proteinuria associated with high-dose pamidronate in multiple myeloma. *Br J Haematol* 2002; **119:** 496–9.
7. Banerjee D, *et al.* Short-term, high-dose pamidronate-induced acute tubular necrosis: the postulated mechanisms of bisphosphonate nephrotoxicity. *Am J Kidney Dis* 2003; **41:** E18.
8. Chang JT, *et al.* Renal failure with the use of zoledronic acid. *N Engl J Med* 2003; **349:** 1676–8.
9. Zazgornik J, *et al.* Acute renal failure and alendronate. *Nephrol Dial Transplant* 1997; **12:** 2797–8.

**Effects on the respiratory system.** Bronchospasm induced by bisphosphonates has been reported in 2 patients who were aspirin-sensitive asthmatics. The first patient complained of shortness of breath and wheezing 10 minutes after the start of an infusion of clodronate while the second developed similar symptoms 2 days after the start of cyclical therapy with etidronate by mouth. Oral rechallenge in both patients resulted in a fall in the forced expiratory values at 1 second.[1] The reaction in these 2 patients was not considered to be immune-mediated.

1. Rolla G, *et al.* Bisphosphonate-induced bronchoconstriction in aspirin-sensitive asthma. *Lancet* 1994; **343:** 426–7.

**Hypersensitivity.** Bisphosphonates may rarely cause hypersensitivity reactions such as angioedema, urticaria, and pruritus. Reports include a severe allergic reaction to sodium medronate in the form of a radiopharmaceutical,[1] and mild skin rashes in 2 patients given pamidronate by mouth.[2] There has also been a report of erythroderma with lesions of the mucous membranes being associated with clodronate administration in one patient,[3] and severe epidermal necrosis may have been associated with tiludronate in another.[4] A possibly drug-related rash has also been reported in a patient receiving alendronate.[5] Two patients experiencing cutaneous reactions to pamidronate or clodronate were able to continue oral clodronate after desensitisation.[6]

1. Elliott AT, *et al.* Severe reaction to diphosphonate: implications for treatment of Paget's disease. *BMJ* 1988; **297:** 592–3.
2. Mautalen CA, *et al.* Side effects of disodium aminohydroxypropylidenediphosphonate (APD) during treatment of bone diseases. *BMJ* 1984; **288:** 828–9.
3. Pajus I, *et al.* Erythroderma after clodronate treatment. *BMJ* 1993; **307:** 484.
4. Roux C, *et al.* Long-lasting dermatological lesions after tiludronate therapy. *Calcif Tissue Int* 1992; **50:** 378–80.
5. Chesnut CH, *et al.* Alendronate treatment of the postmenopausal osteoporotic woman: effect of multiple dosages on bone mass and bone remodeling. *Am J Med* 1995; **99:** 144–52.
6. Phillips EJ, *et al.* Allergic reactions to bisphosphonates: a report of three cases and an approach to management. *J Clin Pharmacol* 1998; **38:** 842–86.

## Interactions

The bisphosphonates are not well absorbed from the gastrointestinal tract, and administration with food further impairs their absorption.

Compounds containing aluminium, calcium, iron, or magnesium, including antacids and mineral supplements and some osmotic laxatives, can also impair the absorption of bisphosphonates given by mouth.

It has been suggested that the use of certain bisphosphonates with NSAIDs may result in an increased incidence of gastrointestinal or renal adverse effects.

There may be additive hypocalcaemic effects with aminoglycosides.

**Aminoglycosides.** A report of a patient who developed persisting severe hypocalcaemia after treatment with clodronate and *netilmicin*. Bisphosphonates and aminoglycosides can induce hypocalcaemia by different mechanisms and care should be taken when administering them simultaneously.[1]

1. Pedersen-Bjergaard U, Myhre J. Severe hypocalcaemia after treatment with diphosphonate and aminoglycoside. *BMJ* 1991; **302:** 295. Correction. *ibid.*; 791.

## Pharmacokinetics

The bisphosphonates are poorly absorbed following oral administration, with bioavailabilities in the fasting state ranging from about 0.7% (alendronate; risedronate) to up to 6% (etidronate; tiludronate). Absorption is reduced by food, especially by products containing calcium or other polyvalent cations. They have a high affinity for bone, with about 50% of an absorbed dose sequestered to ossified tissues and retained in the body for prolonged periods. Excretion is in the urine, as unchanged drug; they do not appear to be metabolised.

## Uses and Administration

The bisphosphonates inhibit bone resorption and thus have a hypocalcaemic effect. They are pyrophosphate analogues which have a high affinity for the hydroxyapatite of bone, and which inhibit bone resorption by osteoclasts; because of the coupling of resorption and formation this results in an overall reduction in remodelling and bone turnover (see Bone and Bone Disease, p.762). Their antiresorptive potency varies widely. The bisphosphonates also inhibit the formation and dissolution of hydroxyapatite crystals and thus have the potential to interfere with bone mineralisation. The degree to which the bisphosphonates inhibit mineralisation in clinical practice varies; disodium etidronate is the most potent inhibitor of those now in general clinical use.

Because bone resorption increases plasma-calcium concentrations, the bisphosphonates are used as adjuncts to the treatment of severe hypercalcaemia, especially when associated with malignancy. They are also used in disorders associated with excessive bone resorption and turnover, such as Paget's disease of bone and osteoporosis, as well as in the management of bone metastases. Etidronate has been used in the prevention and treatment of ectopic ossification.

Because of the affinity of bisphosphonates for bone, complexes labelled with radioactive technetium-99m (see p.1525) have been used diagnostically as bone scanning agents.

Bisphosphonates have been given by intravenous infusion or by mouth. In the latter case food should be avoided for a suitable period before and after administration, especially products with a high calcium content such as milk.

◊ References.

1. Compston JE. The therapeutic use of bisphosphonates. *BMJ* 1994; **309:** 711–15.

2. Rosen CJ, Kessenich CR. Comparative clinical pharmacology and therapeutic use of bisphosphonates in metabolic bone diseases. *Drugs* 1996; **51:** 537–51.
3. Brown DL, Robbins R. Developments in the therapeutic applications of bisphosphonates. *J Clin Pharmacol* 1999; **39:** 651–60.
4. Shoemaker LR. Expanding role of bisphosphonate therapy in children. *J Pediatr* 1999; **134:** 264–7.
5. Hillner BE, *et al.* American Society of Clinical Oncology 2003 update on the role of bisphosphonates and bone health issues in women with breast cancer. *J Clin Oncol* 2003; **21:** 4042–57. Correction. *ibid.* 2004; **22:** 1351.
6. Homik J, *et al.* Bisphosphonates for steroid induced osteoporosis. Available in The Cochrane Library; Issue 2. Chichester: John Wiley; 2004.


**Complex regional pain syndrome.** Osteoporosis is one of the features of complex regional pain syndrome (p.5). Bisphosphonates may be of benefit in controlling associated pain in some patients.[1,2]


1. Schott GD. Bisphosphonates for pain relief in reflex sympathetic dystrophy? *Lancet* 1997; **350:** 1117. Correction. *ibid.* 1998; **351:** 682.
2. Forouzanfar T, *et al.* Treatment of complex regional pain syndrome type I. *Eur J Pain* 2002; **6:** 105–22.


**Ectopic ossification.** The only treatment for established ectopic ossification (p.762) is surgery, but drugs have been used for prophylaxis or prevention of recurrence. Bisphosphonates that are potent inhibitors of mineralisation such as etidronate have been advocated for this purpose, but they do not prevent the formation of the osteoid matrix and delayed mineralisation may occur once they are withdrawn.

**Hypercalcaemia.** In patients with severe symptomatic hypercalcaemia restoration and maintenance of adequate hydration and urine flow is essential, and helps to reduce plasma-calcium concentrations by promoting calcium diuresis. In hypercalcaemia of malignancy (p.1218) therapy with inhibitors of bone resorption such as the bisphosphonates is used. Pamidronate has been widely used; zoledronic acid has shown promising results. Although sustained, the action of bisphosphonates is not particularly rapid; they may be used with a calcitonin where both rapid and prolonged diminution of plasma-calcium concentration is desired.

**Hyperparathyroidism.** Bisphosphonates have been used to inhibit bone resorption in the treatment of hypercalcaemia associated with hyperparathyroidism (p.765), but seem to be of little benefit for long-term treatment.

**Malignant neoplasms of the bone.** There is good evidence that some bisphosphonates are of benefit in patients with metastatic bone disease (p.513) not only to control bone pain and to manage the attendant hypercalcaemia, but also to reduce skeletal complications such as fractures. It has been suggested that given the strength of the evidence, treatment with bisphosphonates should be begun at first diagnosis of bone metastases, and continued until no longer clinically relevant.[1] There is also much interest in the use of bisphosphonates to prevent the development of bone metastases; however, preliminary evidence of their efficacy is conflicting. Specific references may be found under the individual drugs.


1. Ross JR, *et al.* Systematic review of role of bisphosphonates on skeletal morbidity in metastatic cancer. *BMJ* 2003; **327:** 469–72. Correction. *ibid.* 2004; **328:** 384.


**Osteogenesis imperfecta.** Bisphosphonates have been tried in osteogenesis imperfecta (p.762), but orthopaedic treatment and physical activity programmes form the basis of therapy.

**Osteoporosis.** Bisphosphonates are used in the prevention and treatment of postmenopausal and corticosteroid-induced osteoporosis (p.763). Both alendronate and etidronate have been shown to be effective in terms of effect on bone mass density. There is less evidence for a consequent reduction in fracture rates, although this has been shown for alendronate in postmenopausal osteoporosis (see p.766). Alendronate is given continuously, whereas etidronate is given intermittently, alternating with a calcium supplement; both drugs are administered orally. Although there is less evidence for their efficacy in men with idiopathic osteoporosis, some consider bisphosphonates are the preferred treatment for this condition.

**Paget's disease of bone.** Paget's disease of bone (p.764) is characterised by excessive and disorganised bone resorption and formation. Not all patients require treatment, and pain can be managed in some with NSAIDs or paracetamol. Bisphosphonates may be indicated if bone pain is persistent or to prevent further progression of the disease particularly if there is a risk of complications.

---

## Bone Morphogenetic Proteins

BMP; Proteínas morfogenéticamente óseas.

*ATC — M05BC01 (BMP-2); M05BC02 (BMP-7).*

### Dibotermin Alfa *(USAN, rINN)*

hrBMP-2; rhBMP-2. Human recombinant bone morphogenetic protein 2.

*CAS — 246539-15-1.*

### Eptotermin Alfa *(rINN)*

hrBMP-7; OP-1; Osteogenic Protein-1. Human recombinant bone morphogenetic protein 7.

*CAS — 129805-33-0.*

#### Profile

Bone morphogenetic proteins (BMPs) are growth factors that promote ectopic bone formation and can be extracted from demineralised bone matrix. Several have been identified and developed for use in orthopaedic and reconstructive surgery; some have been produced by recombinant technology.

Osteogenic protein 1 (OP-1, BMP-7, eptotermin alfa) is a recombinant form used in adults for the treatment of non-union of tibia of at least 9 months duration in cases where autograft has failed or is unfeasible. Dibotermin alfa, another recombinant form, is used as an adjunct to standard care for the treatment of acute tibia fractures in adults, as an implant containing 12 mg. Osteogenin (BMP-3) is under investigation.

◊ References.


1. Anonymous. New bone? *Lancet* 1992; **339:** 463–4.
2. Reddi AH. Bone morphogenetic proteins, bone marrow stromal cells, and mesenchymal cells: Maureen Owen revisited. *Clin Orthop* 1995; (313): 115–19.
3. Croteau S, *et al.* Bone morphogenetic proteins in orthopedics: from basic science to clinical practice. *Orthopedics* 1999; **22:** 686–95.
4. Groeneveld EH, Burger EH. Bone morphogenetic proteins in human bone regeneration. *Eur J Endocrinol* 2000; **142:** 9–21.
5. Valentin-Opran A, *et al.* Clinical evaluation of recombinant human bone morphogenetic protein-2. *Clin Orthop* 2002; **395:** 110–20.
6. Govender S, *et al.* Recombinant human bone morphogenetic protein-2 for treatment of open tibial fractures: a prospective, controlled, randomized study of four hundred and fifty patients. *J Bone Joint Surg Am* 2002; **84:** 2123–34.
7. Johnsson R, *et al.* Randomized radiostereometric study comparing osteogenic protein-1 (BMP-7) and autograft bone in human noninstrumented posterolateral lumbar fusion. *Spine* 2002; **27:** 2654–61.


#### Preparations

**Proprietary Preparations** (details are given in Part 3)
***Spain:*** Osigraft; ***UK:*** InductOs.

---

## Calcitonins

Calcitoninas.

*ATC — H05BA01; H05BA02; H05BA03.*

### Calcitonin (Human)

Calcitonina (humana); Calcitonin-human; Human Calcitonin.

$C_{151}H_{226}N_{40}O_{45}S_3$ = 3417.8.

*CAS — 21215-62-3.*

*ATC — H05BA03 (Human Synthetic).*

**Description.** Calcitonin (human) is a synthetic polypeptide comprising 32 amino acids in the same linear sequence as in naturally occurring human calcitonin.

**Pharmacopoeias.** In *Swiss.*

### Calcitonin (Pork) *(BANM)*

Calcitonina (cerdo).

*CAS — 12321-44-7.*

*ATC — H05BA02 (Pork Natural).*

NOTE. The synonym thyrocalcitonin and the CAS number 9007-12-9 have been used for calcitonin that is often of pork origin.

**Description.** Calcitonin (pork) is a polypeptide hormone obtained from pork thyroid.

### Calcitonin (Salmon) *(BAN)*

Calcitonina (salmón); Calcitonin-salmon; Calcitoninum Salmonis; Salcatonin; Salmon Calcitonin; SCT-1.

$C_{145}H_{240}N_{44}O_{48}S_2$ = 3431.9.

*CAS — 47931-85-1.*

*ATC — H05BA01 (Salmon Synthetic).*

NOTE. There may be some confusion between the terms Salcatonin and Calcitonin (Salmon) (Salmon Calcitonin; Calcitonin-salmon) although in practice these names appear to be used for the same substance.

- The Ph. Eur. 5.0 defines Calcitonin (Salmon) as a synthetic polypeptide having the structure of salmon calcitonin I.
- Calcitonin (Salmon)/Salcatonin (*BAN*) is defined as a *component* of natural salmon calcitonin. The BP 2003 defines Calcitonin (Salmon)/Salcatonin as a synthetic polypeptide having the structure determined for salmon calcitonin I.
- In the USA, Calcitonin (*USAN*) includes calcitonin (human) and calcitonin (salmon). Salcatonin is there understood to be a synthetic polypeptide structurally similar to natural salmon calcitonin (Calcitonin Salmon (Synthesis)). The US manufacturers use Calcitonin-salmon for a synthetic polypeptide with the same structure as calcitonin of salmon origin.

**Pharmacopoeias.** In *Eur.* (see p.vi).

**Ph. Eur. 5.0** (Calcitonin (Salmon)). A white or almost white powder. Freely soluble in water. Store at 2° to 8°. If the substance is sterile store in a sterile, airtight, tamper-proof container. Protect from light.

### Elcatonin *(rINN)*

[Aminosuberic Acid 1,7]-eel Calcitonin; [$Asu^{1,7}$]-E-CT; Carbocalcitonin; Elcatonina. 1-Butyric acid-7-(L-2-aminobutyric acid)-26-L-aspartic acid-27-L-valine-29-L-alaninecalcitonin (salmon).

$C_{148}H_{244}N_{42}O_{47}$ = 3363.8.

*CAS — 60731-46-6.*

*ATC — H05BA04.*

**Description.** Elcatonin is a synthetic analogue of eel calcitonin.

**Pharmacopoeias.** In *Jpn.*

**Incompatibility.** Like some other peptide drugs, calcitonin may be adsorbed onto the plastic of intravenous giving sets; it has been suggested that solutions for intravenous infusion should contain some protein to prevent the sorption and consequent loss of potency (see under Administration, below).

#### Units

0.8 units of calcitonin, porcine, are contained in one ampoule of the second International Standard Preparation (1991).

128 units of calcitonin, salmon, are contained in approximately 20 micrograms of freeze-dried purified synthetic salmon calcitonin, with mannitol 2 mg in one ampoule of the second International Standard Preparation (1989).

17.5 units of calcitonin, human, are contained in one ampoule of the second International Standard Preparation (1991).

There is also a first International Standard Preparation (1989) of elcatonin.

Potency of calcitonins is estimated by comparing the hypocalcaemic effect, in *rats*, with that of the standard preparation, and is expressed in international or MRC units which are considered to be equivalent. One manufacturer states that 100 international units by this assay is equivalent to 1 mg of porcine or human calcitonin, and to 25 micrograms of salmon calcitonin although other, slightly different, equivalencies have been cited for other preparations. However, although 1 unit of pork calcitonin, 1 unit of salmon calcitonin, and 1 unit of human calcitonin should give the same response in humans this is not necessarily the case. Clinically, doses of pork and salmon calcitonin are expressed in units whereas those of human calcitonin can be expressed by weight, probably a reflection of its purity.

Doses of calcitonin considered approximately equivalent in practice are:

- 80 units of pork calcitonin
- 50 units of salmon calcitonin
- 0.5 mg of human calcitonin

#### Adverse Effects, Treatment, and Precautions

Calcitonins may cause nausea, vomiting, diarrhoea, dizziness, flushing, and tingling of the hands. These reactions are dose dependent, usually transient, and occur more often with intravenous administration. Other adverse effects have included skin rash, an unpleasant taste, abdominal pain, urinary frequency, and tremor. A diabetogenic effect has been reported rarely. Inflammatory reactions at the injection site have been reported with some calcitonins, and rhinitis and other local reactions have been reported with nasal formulations. Transient hypocalcaemia may occur after injections of calcitonin.

Calcitonins should be given with care to patients with renal impairment (see below) or heart failure. If children receive calcitonin it should preferably be for short periods and bone growth should be monitored.

Circulating antibodies may develop after several months of use but resistance does not necessarily follow (see also below). In patients with a history of allergy, a skin test has been advised before use as hypersensitivity reactions, including anaphylaxis, have occurred.

Calcitonin has inhibited lactation in *animals*.

Nausea and vomiting may be reduced by administration at bedtime or by prior administration of an antiemetic.

Calcitonin (pork) may contain trace amounts of thyroid hormones, but clinical effects are unlikely in most patients.

**Antibody formation.** Long-term treatment with heterologous calcitonins may lead to the formation of neutralising antibodies. This appears to be common in patients given calcitonin (pork) or, to a lesser extent, calcitonin (salmon). Calcitonin (human) is less immunogenic than pork or salmon, but a study[1] has also detected antibodies to human calcitonin in 1 of 33 women with postmenopausal osteoporosis after 6 months of therapy.

The degree to which such antibodies affect therapeutic activity is uncertain. Some studies have suggested a significant loss of therapeutic activity in patients who developed neutralising antibodies to calcitonin (salmon),[2] or a restoration in activity following a switch from salmon to human calcitonin in such patients;[3] equally, others have presented evidence that the activity of calcitonin (salmon) was not reduced by the development of antibodies to the drug.[4]

1. Grauer A, *et al.* Formation of neutralizing antibodies after treatment with human calcitonin. *Am J Med* 1993; **95:** 439–42.
2. Grauer A, *et al.* In vitro detection of neutralizing antibodies after treatment of Paget's disease of bone with nasal salmon calcitonin. *J Bone Miner Res* 1990; **5:** 387–91.
3. Muff R, *et al.* Efficacy of intranasal human calcitonin in patients with Paget's disease refractory to salmon calcitonin. *Am J Med* 1990; **89:** 181–4.
4. Reginster JY, *et al.* Influence of specific anti-salmon calcitonin antibodies on biological effectiveness of nasal salmon calcitonin in Paget's disease of bone. *Scand J Rheumatol* 1990; **19:** 83–6.

**Effect on glucose metabolism.** A single subcutaneous injection of calcitonin (salmon) has been reported to increase blood-glucose concentrations,[1] but long-term treatment with calcitonins was considered unlikely to cause diabetes.[2] Nevertheless, deterioration in diabetic control has been noted in a patient given calcitonin (pork)[3] and postprandial release of insulin was abolished by intravenous salmon calcitonin in 8 patients with duodenal ulcers.[4]

1. Gattereau A, *et al.* Hyperglycaemic effect of synthetic salmon calcitonin. *Lancet* 1977; **ii:** 1076–7.
2. Evans IMA, *et al.* Hyperglycaemic effect of synthetic salmon calcitonin. *Lancet* 1978; **i:** 280.
3. Thomas DW, *et al.* Deterioration in diabetic control during calcitonin therapy. *Med J Aust* 1979; **2:** 699–70.
4. Jonderko K. Effect of calcitonin on gastric emptying in patients with an active duodenal ulcer. *Gut* 1989; **30:** 430–5.

**Gynaecomastia.** A 62-year-old man developed painful gynaecomastia on two occasions following treatment with calcitonin (salmon) administered by subcutaneous injection.[1]

1. Vankrunkelsven PJ, Thijs MM. Salcatonin and gynaecomastia. *Lancet* 1994; **344:** 482.

## Interactions

There is a theoretical possibility that dosage adjustments may be required in patients receiving cardiac glycosides who are given injections of calcitonin, because of the effects of the latter on serum calcium.

## Pharmacokinetics

Calcitonins are rapidly inactivated when given orally. After injection, calcitonins are quickly metabolised, primarily in the kidneys but also in blood and peripheral tissues. The inactive metabolites and a small proportion of unchanged drug are excreted in the urine. The half-life of calcitonin (human) is stated to be 60 minutes and that of calcitonin (salmon) about 70 to 90 minutes.

Calcitonins are also absorbed through the nasal and rectal mucosa. Although figures have varied widely, about 3% of an intranasal dose of calcitonin (salmon) is reported to be bioavailable compared with the same dose given by intramuscular injection, with peak plasma concentrations occurring after about 30 to 40 minutes compared with 15 to 25 minutes after the parenteral dose.

◊ After the subcutaneous injection of 19.9 micrograms of synthetic calcitonin (salmon) in 16 healthy subjects,[1] absorption was rapid with an absorption half-life of 23.4 minutes. The maximum mean plasma concentration was 384 picograms/mL at 60 minutes after which excretion was fairly rapid with an elimination half-life of 87 minutes. These results and those from previously reported investigations of salmon, human, and porcine calcitonin could not easily be compared, especially since different assay methods had been used. Nevertheless it was concluded that bioavailability from subcutaneous and intramuscular injection sites was good; that dosage may need to be adjusted in renal insufficiency because of low metabolic clearance rate; and that the higher potency of calcitonin (salmon) is due to higher intrinsic activity at the receptor site rather than to pharmacokinetic differences. The US manufacturers have cited a half-life of 1.02 hours after a single subcutaneous injection of calcitonin (human) 500 micrograms. The plasma elimination half-life of elcatonin was about 4.8 hours after intramuscular injection in healthy subjects.[2]

Calcitonins are absorbed following intranasal or rectal administration. Peak plasma concentrations of calcitonin (salmon) were achieved 20 to 60 minutes after administration by nasal spray in doses ranging from 200 to 400 units.[3] In another study[4] calcitonin (salmon) 200 units, repeated once after 3 hours, was given by nasal spray or suppository to healthy subjects. Absorption was prompt and the total amount absorbed was similar with either route. However, whereas intranasal administration produced low peaks with calcitonin (salmon) still detectable in the blood after 3 to 5 hours, rectal administration produced peak plasma concentrations about 6 to 8 times higher but the drug was undetectable within 2 hours; plasma concentrations were lower than those found after injection. Another group[5] found calcitonin (human) to be poorly absorbed when given intranasally to healthy subjects. Absorption from nasal powder or spray solutions was improved by the presence of the surfactants dihydrofusinate or glycocholate.

Investigations carried out in 4 osteoporotic patients[6] suggested that the rectal administration of calcitonin (salmon) could provide 65% of the bioavailability of intramuscular administration.

1. Nüesch E, Schmidt R. Comparative pharmacokinetics of calcitonins. In: Pecile A, ed. *Calcitonin international congress series no. 540.* Amsterdam: Excerpta Medica, 1980: 352–64.
2. Sergre G, *et al.* Pharmacokinetics of carbocalcitonin in humans. *Clin Trials J* 1986; **23** (suppl 1): 23–8.
3. Kurose H, *et al.* Intranasal absorption of salmon calcitonin. *Calcif Tissue Int* 1987; **41:** 249–51.
4. Buclin T, *et al.* The effect of rectal and nasal administration of salmon calcitonin in normal subjects. *Calcif Tissue Int* 1987; **41:** 252–8.
5. Pontiroli AE, *et al.* Nasal administration of glucagon and human calcitonin to healthy subjects: a comparison of powders and spray solutions and of different enhancing agents. *Eur J Clin Pharmacol* 1989; **37:** 427–30.
6. Gennari C, *et al.* Pharmacodynamic activity of synthetic salmon calcitonin in osteoporotic patients: comparison between rectal and intramuscular administration: pilot study. *Curr Ther Res* 1993; **53:** 301–8.

## Uses and Administration

Calcitonin is a hormone produced by mammalian thyroid parafollicular cells or the ultimobranchial gland in non-mammalian vertebrates. In man its secretion and biosynthesis are regulated by the plasma-calcium concentration. It has a hypocalcaemic action that is due primarily to inhibition of osteoclastic bone resorption; of less importance is a direct effect on the kidneys resulting in increased urinary excretion of calcium and phosphorus. Calcitonin contains 32 amino acids; the sequence varies according to the species. Naturally occurring calcitonin (pork), synthetic calcitonin (salmon), and synthetic calcitonin (human) are in clinical use; calcitonin (salmon) is the most potent. Elcatonin, a synthetic derivative of eel calcitonin, is available in some countries.

Calcitonins are used in the treatment of diseases characterised by high bone turnover such as Paget's disease of bone. They are also given as an adjunct in the treatment of severe hypercalcaemia, especially that associated with malignancy. Some calcitonins are used in the management of osteoporosis, and osteolysis and bone pain due to malignancies of bone.

Calcitonins are generally given by subcutaneous or intramuscular injection; some have been given intranasally, rectally, or by intravenous infusion.

In **Paget's disease of bone** the usual dose range for calcitonin (pork) by subcutaneous or intramuscular injection is 80 units three times weekly to 160 units daily in single or divided doses; patients with bone pain or nerve compression syndromes may be given 80 or 160 units daily for 3 to 6 months. For calcitonin (salmon) the range is 50 units three times weekly to 100 units daily in single or divided doses by subcutaneous or intramuscular injection. Calcitonin (human) is usually given by subcutaneous or intramuscular injection in a dose range of 0.5 mg two or three times weekly to 0.5 mg daily; severe cases may require up to 1 mg daily.

As an adjunct to the treatment of **hypercalcaemia**, calcitonins have a rapid effect which is greatest in patients with an increased bone turnover. Calcitonin (pork) may be given in a dose of 4 units/kg daily by intramuscular or subcutaneous injection according to the patient's needs. In severe hypercalcaemia larger doses of calcitonin may be more conveniently administered as the more potent calcitonin (salmon), given by subcutaneous or intramuscular injection in a dose of 5 to 10 units/kg daily in one or two divided doses or up to 400 units every 6 or 8 hours. Doses greater than 8 units/kg every 6 hours are considered to have no additional benefit. In the emergency treatment of hypercalcaemic crisis, calcitonin (salmon) has also been given intravenously: a suggested dose is 5 to 10 units/kg daily, diluted in 500 mL of sodium chloride 0.9% and given by slow intravenous infusion over at least 6 hours (see also under Administration below for the problems of intravenous administration). Calcitonin (human) has also been given intravenously for acute hypercalcaemia.

Calcitonin (salmon) is used in the treatment of **postmenopausal osteoporosis** in a dose of 100 units daily or every other day by subcutaneous or intramuscular injection, or 200 units daily intranasally by nasal spray, alternating nostrils each day. Supplementary calcium (equivalent to at least 600 mg of elemental calcium daily) and, if necessary, vitamin D (400 units daily) should also be given.

Calcitonin (salmon) has also been used for the control of **bone pain due to malignant neoplasms**. The usual dose by intramuscular or subcutaneous injection is 200 units every 6 hours or 400 units every 12 hours for up to 48 hours. The treatment course may be repeated as appropriate.

Oral formulations of calcitonin (salmon) are being studied.

**Administration.** Calcitonins have poor oral bioavailability and administration is usually by subcutaneous or intramuscular injection. To improve patient acceptability, especially in diseases requiring long-term drug therapy such as osteoporosis or Paget's disease of bone, alternative methods of administration have been investigated.

Calcitonin (salmon) has proved effective when given intranasally in usual doses of 50 to 200 units daily (for references, see Osteoporosis below), and intranasal products for osteoporosis are available. Suppositories containing 300 units of calcitonin (salmon) have been used in the management of hypercalcaemia; one suppository being administered three times daily (total daily dose of 900 units).[1,2] Daily doses of 100 units of calcitonin (salmon) by suppository have been tried in postmenopausal osteoporosis[3] and in patients with bone pain.[4]

Calcitonins have been given by intravenous infusion, but this is rarely necessary and may cause more side-effects. If intravenous administration is essential, it has been suggested[5] that some protein must be present in the solution to prevent adsorption onto the plastic of the giving set. However, in practice this does not seem to be the case; in the UK, manufacturer's recommendations are for dilution with normal saline, while acknowledging that such dilution results in a loss of potency, and dosage is adjusted accordingly. Presumably dilution with a protein-containing solution would allow lower doses to be used. The manufacturers do specify that solutions for infusion should be prepared immediately before use and that glass or hard plastic containers should not be used.

1. Thiébaud D, *et al.* Effectiveness of salmon calcitonin administered as suppositories in tumor-induced hypercalcemia. *Am J Med* 1987; **82:** 745–50.
2. Thiébaud D, *et al.* Fast and effective treatment of malignant hypercalcemia: combination of suppositories of calcitonin and a single infusion of 3-amino 1-hydroxypropylidene-1-bisphosphonate. *Arch Intern Med* 1990; **150:** 2125–8.
3. Gonnelli S, *et al.* Effect of rectal salmon calcitonin treatment on bone mass and bone turnover in patients with established postmenopausal osteoporosis: a 1-year crossover study. *Curr Ther Res* 1993; **54:** 458–65.
4. Mannarini M, *et al.* Analgesic effect of salmon calcitonin suppositories in patients with bone pain. *Curr Ther Res* 1994; **55:** 1079–83.
5. Stevenson JC. Current management of malignant hypercalcaemia. *Drugs* 1988; **36:** 229–38.

**Administration in renal impairment.** Calcitonins are metabolised mainly in the kidneys and pharmacokinetic studies (see above) have indicated that the dosage of calcitonins may need to be reduced in patients with renal insufficiency, but there have been no specific guidelines.

**Hypercalcaemia.** Calcitonins can be used in the management of moderate to severe symptomatic hypercalcaemia (p.1218) in addition to rehydration and diuresis. Because of their rapid effect, they may be particularly useful in life-threatening hypercalcaemia. However, although they have a rapid effect it is usually short-lived; calcitonins are therefore generally given as an adjunct with other therapy such as a bisphosphonate.

References.

1. Ralston SH, *et al.* Treatment of cancer associated hypercalcaemia with combined aminohydroxypropylidene diphosphonate and calcitonin. *BMJ* 1986; **292:** 1549–50.
2. Thiébaud D, *et al.* Effectiveness of salmon calcitonin administered as suppositories in tumor-induced hypercalcemia. *Am J Med* 1987; **82:** 745–50.

3. Thiébaud D, *et al.* Fast and effective treatment of malignant hypercalcemia: combination of suppositories of calcitonin and a single infusion as 3-amino 1-hydroxypropylidene-1-bisphosphonate. *Arch Intern Med* 1990; **150:** 2125–8.
4. Kaul S, Sockalosky JJ. Human synthetic calcitonin therapy for hypercalcemia of immobilization. *J Pediatr* 1995; **126:** 825–7.

**Malignant neoplasms of the bone.** Calcitonins may be useful adjuvants in the treatment of malignant disease involving the bone (p.513), not only to correct hypercalcaemia of malignancy, but also to relieve bone pain and osteolysis. The analgesic properties of calcitonins (see Pain, below) may play some part in this, although relief of bone pain has also been seen with bisphosphonates, suggesting that if such actions are of significance, they are not the sole reason for pain relief.

**Osteogenesis imperfecta.** There have been reports[1,2] of beneficial effects with calcitonins in the treatment of osteogenesis imperfecta (p.762).

1. Castells S, *et al.* Therapy of osteogenesis imperfecta with synthetic salmon calcitonin. *J Pediatr* 1979; **95:** 807–11.
2. Nishi Y, *et al.* Effect of long-term calcitonin therapy by injection and nasal spray on the incidence of fractures in osteogenesis imperfecta. *J Pediatr* 1992; **121:** 477–80.

**Osteoporosis.** Calcitonins may be used in the prevention and treatment of osteoporosis (p.763). In postmenopausal osteoporosis they are usually second-line agents. However, they may be particularly useful in women with high-turnover osteoporosis, and in those with bone pain due to vertebral crush fractures. References to the use of calcitonins for postmenopausal osteoporosis[1-10] and corticosteroid-induced osteoporosis[11] are given below.

1. Reginster JY, *et al.* 1-Year controlled randomised trial of prevention of early postmenopausal bone loss by intranasal calcitonin. *Lancet* 1987; **ii:** 1481–3.
2. MacIntyre I, *et al.* Calcitonin for prevention of postmenopausal bone loss. *Lancet* 1988; **i:** 900–2.
3. Pun KK, Chan LWL. Analgesic effect of intranasal salmon calcitonin in the treatment of osteoporotic vertebral fractures. *Clin Ther* 1989; **11:** 205–9.
4. Overgaard K, *et al.* Effect of salcatonin given intranasally on early postmenopausal bone loss. *BMJ* 1989; **299:** 477–9.
5. Overgaard K, *et al.* Discontinuous calcitonin treatment of established osteoporosis—effects of withdrawal of treatment. *Am J Med* 1990; **89:** 1–6.
6. Overgaard K, *et al.* Effect of salcatonin given intranasally on bone mass and fracture rates in established osteoporosis: a dose response study. *BMJ* 1992; **305:** 556–61.
7. Reginster JY, *et al.* A 5-year controlled randomized study of prevention of postmenopausal trabecular bone loss with nasal salmon calcitonin and calcium. *Eur J Clin Invest* 1994; **24:** 565–9.
8. Reginster JY, *et al.* A double-blind, placebo-controlled, dose-finding trial of intermittent nasal salmon calcitonin for prevention of postmenopausal lumbar spine bone loss. *Am J Med* 1995; **98:** 452–8.
9. Downs RW, *et al.* Comparison of alendronate and intranasal calcitonin for treatment of osteoporosis in postmenopausal women. *J Clin Endocrinol Metab* 2000; **85:** 1783–8.
10. Chesnut CH, *et al.* A randomized trial of nasal spray salmon calcitonin in postmenopausal women with established osteoporosis: the prevent recurrence of osteoporotic fractures study. *Am J Med* 2000; **109:** 267–76.
11. Cranney A, *et al.* Calcitonin for preventing and treating corticosteroid-induced osteoporosis. Available in The Cochrane Library; Issue 2. Chichester: John Wiley; 2004.

**Paget's disease of bone.** Patients with Paget's disease of bone (p.764) may require no treatment or just analgesics alone, but calcitonins may be indicated if bone pain is persistent or to prevent further progression of the disease. However, the bisphosphonates have largely superseded the calcitonins in this role. References.

1. Nagant de Deuxchaisnes C, *et al.* New modes of administration of salmon calcitonin in Paget's disease. *Clin Orthop* 1987; **217:** 56–71.
2. Muff R, *et al.* Efficacy of intranasal human calcitonin in patients with Paget's disease refractory to salmon calcitonin. *Am J Med* 1990; **89:** 181–4.

**Pain.** In addition to bone pain associated with malignancy and with bone disorders such as Paget's disease, calcitonins may also have other analgesic properties. Beneficial results have been seen in various painful conditions,[1-4] including complex regional pain syndrome and phantom limb pain.

1. Jaeger H, Maier C. Calcitonin in phantom limb pain: a double-blind study. *Pain* 1992; **48:** 21–7.
2. Mannerini M, *et al.* Analgesic effect of salmon calcitonin suppositories in patients with bone pain. *Curr Ther Res* 1994; **55:** 1079–83.
3. Wall GC, Heyneman CA. Calcitonin in phantom limb pain. *Ann Pharmacother* 1999; **33:** 499–501.
4. Appelboom T. Calcitonin in reflex sympathetic dystrophy syndrome and other painful conditions. *Bone* 2002; **30** (suppl): 84S–86S.

## Preparations

***BP 2003:*** Calcitonin (Salmon) Injection.

**Proprietary Preparations** (details are given in Part 3)
***Arg.:*** Anguilce; Calsynar; Citonina; Osmil; Salmocalcin; ***Austral.:*** Calcitare†; Calsynar†; Miacalcic; ***Austria:*** Calcitonin; Calco; Casalm; Cibacalcin; Elcimen; Miacalcic; Ucecal; ***Belg.:*** Calsynar; Cibacalcine†; Miacalcic; Steocalcin; ***Braz.:*** Acticalcin; Calsynar; Cibacalcina; Miacalcic; Serocalcin; Staporos†; Turbocalcin†; ***Canad.:*** Calcimar; Caltine; Miacalcin; ***Chile:*** Calfosina; Calnisan; Miacalcic; ***Denm.:*** Miacalcic; ***Fin.:*** Miacalcic; ***Fr.:*** Cadens; Calcitar†; Calsyn; Cibacalcine; Miacalcic; ***Ger.:*** Azucalcit; Calci; Calcimonta†; Calsynar; Calsynar Lyo†; Casalm; Cibacalcin; Karil; Osteos; Ostostabil; ***Gr.:*** Alciton; Calciplus; Calco; Calsynar; Genecalcin; Iricalcin; Latonina; Miacalcic; Miadenil; Neostesin; Norcalcin; Nylex; Osticalcin; Ostifix; Ostosalm; Rafacalcin; Salmoten; Tendolon; Tosicalcin; ***Hong Kong:*** Calsynar†; Miacalcic; Osteocalcin; Osteostabil†; ***India:*** Zycalcit; ***Irl.:*** Calsynar†; ***Israel:*** Calsynar†; Cibacalcin†; Miacalcic; Salco; ***Ital.:*** Aima-Calcin†; Biocalcin; Calciben; Calcinil†; Calciosint; Calcioton; Calcitar†; Calcitonina; Calco; Carbicalcin; Catonin; Cibacalcin†; Ipocalcin; Isi-Calcin†; Miacalcic; Miadenil; Osteocalcin; Osteotonina; Osteovis; Porostenina†; Quosten†; Rulicalcin; Salmocalcin†; Salmofar; Sical†; Sintocalcin†; Stalcin†; Steocin; Tonocalcin; Turbocalcin; ***Jpn:*** Calcitoran; ***Malaysia:*** Menocal; Miacalcic; Osteocalcin; ***Mex.:*** Endocal; Miacalcic; Oseum; Serocalcin†; Tonocalcin; ***Neth.:*** Cibacalcin†; ***Norw.:*** Miacalcic; ***NZ:*** Miacalcic; ***Port.:*** Bionocalcin†; Calcimon; Calogen; Calsyn; Cibacalcina; Miacalcic; Osseocalcina; Ostosalm; Salcat; Tonocaltin; ***S.Afr.:*** Miacalcic; ***Singapore:*** Calco; Menocal; Miacalcic; Osteocalcin†; ***Spain:*** Bionocalcin†; Calogen; Calsynar; Carbicalcin; Cibacalcina†; Diatin; Kalsimin†; Miacalcic; Oseototal; Ospor; Osteobion; Sical; Tonocaltin; Ucecal; ***Swed.:*** Cibacalcin†; Miacalcic; ***Switz.:*** Cibacalcine†; Miacalcic; ***Thai.:*** Calco; Miacalcic; Osteocalcin; Ostostabil†; Tonocalcin; ***UK:*** Calsynar†; Forcaltonin†; Miacalcic; ***USA:*** Calcimar; Miacalcin; Osteocalcin.

---

# Cinacalcet Hydrochloride *(USAN, rINNM)*

AMG-073 (cinacalcet). *N*-[(1*R*)-1-(Naphthalen-1-yl)ethyl]-3-[3-(trifluoromethyl)phenyl]propan-1-amine hydrochloride.

$C_{22}H_{22}F_3N,HCl = 393.9.$

*CAS — 364782-34-3.*

## Profile

Cinacalcet is a calcimimetic agent that increases the sensitivity to extracellular calcium of the calcium-sensing receptors of the parathyroid gland, which regulate parathyroid hormone secretion; this results in a reduction in parathyroid hormone secretion as well as a decrease in serum calcium. Cinacalcet hydrochloride is given by mouth in the treatment of **secondary hyperparathyroidism** in patients with chronic kidney disease on haemodialysis. Doses are expressed in terms of the base; cinacalcet hydrochloride 33 mg is approximately equivalent to 30 mg cinacalcet. The initial dose is 30 mg once daily, increased at intervals of 2 to 4 weeks by 30 mg to a maximum of 180 mg. It is also used for the treatment of **hypercalcaemia** in patients with parathyroid carcinoma in an initial dose of 30 mg twice daily, increased sequentially at intervals of 2 to 4 weeks to a maximum of 90 mg three or four times daily. Hypocalcaemia can occur; serum calcium and intact parathyroid hormone concentrations should be monitored regularly, especially in patients with a history of seizure disorders or hepatic impairment. Other adverse effects include gastrointestinal disturbances, myalgia, dizziness, hypertension, asthenia, anorexia, and non-cardiac chest pain.

◊ References.

1. Franceschini N, *et al.* Cinacalcet HCl: a calcimimetic agent for the management of primary and secondary hyperparathyroidism. *Expert Opin Invest Drugs* 2003; **12:** 1413–21.
2. Shoback DM, *et al.* The calcimimetic cinacalcet normalizes serum calcium in subjects with primary hyperparathyroidism. *J Clin Endocrinol Metab* 2003; **88:** 5644–9.
3. Block GA, *et al.* Cinacalcet for secondary hyperparathyroidism in patients receiving hemodialysis. *N Engl J Med* 2004; **350:** 1516–25.

## Preparations

**Proprietary Preparations** (details are given in Part 3)
***USA:*** Sensipar.

---

# Clodronic Acid *(BAN, USAN, rINN)*

Acide clodronique; Ácido clodrónico; Acidum clodronicum; $Cl_2MBP$; $Cl_2MDP$; DkhMDF. (Dichloromethylene)diphosphonic acid.

$CH_4Cl_2O_6P_2 = 244.9.$

*CAS — 10596-23-3.*

*ATC — M05BA02.*

## Disodium Clodronate

177501; BM-06.011; Clodronate Disodium *(USAN)*; Clodronate Sodium; Clodronato disódico; Dichloromethane Diphosphonate Disodium; Dichloromethylene Diphosphonate Disodium; Sodium Clodronate *(BANM)*; ZK-0091106. Disodium (dichloromethylene)diphosphonate tetrahydrate.

$CH_2Cl_2Na_2O_6P_2,4H_2O = 360.9.$

*CAS — 22560-50-5.*

*ATC — M05BA02.*

## Adverse Effects and Precautions

As for the bisphosphonates in general, p.766. Gastrointestinal symptoms following oral dosage may be reduced by giving the drug in divided doses rather than as a single daily dose. Reversible increases in liver enzyme values and moderate leucopenia have been seen in a few patients. Monitoring of hepatic and renal function and white cell counts is advised. Disodium clodronate has precipitated bronchospasm, even in patients with no history of asthma. Transient proteinuria has been reported immediately after intravenous infusion.

**Effects on the eyes.** For reports of ocular effects associated with the bisphosphonates, including clodronate, see under Bisphosphonates, p.767.

**Effects on the kidneys.** For mention of renal failure developing in a patient with slightly raised serum-creatinine concentrations who subsequently received an intravenous infusion of clodronate, see under Bisphosphonates, p.767.

**Effects on the respiratory system.** For a report of bronchospasm in an aspirin-sensitive asthmatic, induced by an infusion of clodronate, see p.767.

**Hypersensitivity.** Allergic reactions to bisphosphonates are rare. For published reports of cutaneous reactions associated with clodronate administration, see p.767.

## Interactions

As for the bisphosphonates in general, p.767.

**Aminoglycosides.** A patient developed persisting severe hypocalcaemia after treatment with clodronate and *netilmicin*. Bisphosphonates and aminoglycosides can induce hypocalcaemia by different mechanisms and care should be taken when giving them together.[1]

1. Pedersen-Bjergaard U, Myhre J. Severe hypocalcaemia after treatment with diphosphonate and aminoglycoside. *BMJ* 1991; **302:** 295. Correction. *ibid.*; 791.

## Pharmacokinetics

Disodium clodronate is poorly absorbed from the gastrointestinal tract and absorption is reduced by food, especially products containing calcium or other polyvalent cations; bioavailability is only 1 to 4%. Following absorption or intravenous administration it is cleared rapidly from the blood with a reported plasma half-life of only about 2 hours, but has a high affinity for bone. Over 70% of an intravenous dose is excreted unchanged in the urine within 24 hours, the remainder being sequestered to bone tissue. Disodium clodronate is not metabolised.

◊ References.

1. Conrad KA, Lee SM. Clodronate kinetics and dynamics. *Clin Pharmacol Ther* 1981; **30:** 114–20.
2. Yakatan GJ, *et al.* Clodronate kinetics and bioavailability. *Clin Pharmacol Ther* 1982; **31:** 402–10.
3. Ylitalo P, *et al.* Comparison of pharmacokinetics of clodronate after single and repeated doses. *Int J Clin Pharmacol Ther* 1999; **37:** 294–300.

**Bioavailability.** Enhanced bioavailability tablets of disodium clodronate are available in some countries, the licensed dose of which is 35% less than the dose of the standard formulation (see below). However, an open, randomised, crossover study in 88 subjects found that a 1040-mg dose of the new formulation provided only 52% of the bioavailable dose of 1600 mg of the standard capsule formulation.[1]

1. Lapham G, *et al.* Bioavailability of two clodronate formulations. *Br J Hosp Med* 1996; **56:** 231–3.

## Uses and Administration

Clodronate is a bisphosphonate with general properties similar to those of the other bisphosphonates (p.767). It inhibits bone resorption, but appears to have less effect on bone mineralisation than etidronate at comparable doses.

Disodium clodronate is used as an adjunct in the treatment of severe hypercalcaemia, especially when associated with malignancy. In addition, it is used in the treatment of osteolytic bone metastases.

It is administered by slow intravenous infusion or by mouth, as a single daily dose or in 2 divided doses; food should be avoided for at least 1 hour before or after an oral dose. Doses are expressed in terms of anhydrous disodium clodronate; 124.9 mg of disodium clodronate tetrahydrate is approximately equivalent to 100 mg of anhydrous substance. Disodium clodronate is available in capsules of 400 mg and standard tablets of 800 mg. Tablets of disodium clodronate 520 mg are also available in some countries, and have a greater bioavailability than the capsules or standard tablets; one such tablet of disodium clodronate 520 mg is approximately equivalent to two capsules each containing disodium clodronate 400 mg or one 800-mg standard tablet (but see Bioavailability, above).

In the management of osteolytic lesions, hypercalcaemia, and bone pain associated with **skeletal metastases** in patients with breast cancer or multiple myeloma, disodium clodronate 1.6 g daily has been given by mouth as capsules or standard tablets, and may be increased if necessary to a maximum of 3.2 g daily. Alternatively a dose of 1.04 g daily, increased if necessary up to 2.08 g daily, may be given as enhanced bioavailability tablets.

In **hypercalcaemia of malignancy** disodium clodronate is given by intravenous infusion over not less than 2 hours in a dose of 300 mg daily on successive days until normocalcaemia is achieved; duration of treatment should not exceed 10 days. Alternatively, it may be given as a single intravenous infusion of 1.5 g in 500 mL of infusion solution administered over a period of 4 hours. Once serum-calcium concentrations have been reduced to an acceptable level, maintenance therapy may be given by mouth in similar doses to those used for initial oral treatment of metastases.

◊ General references.


1. Plosker GL, Goa KL. Clodronate: a review of its pharmacological properties and therapeutic efficacy in resorptive bone disease. *Drugs* 1994; **47:** 945–82.


**Administration in renal impairment.** Some manufacturers recommend that *intravenous* infusion of clodronate should be avoided in patients with moderate to severe renal impairment (serum creatinine greater than 440 micromoles/litre). Others recommend, where multiple infusions are given, adjustment according to creatinine clearance (CC) as follows:

- mild renal impairment (CC 50 to 80 mL/minute): 25% reduction in dose
- moderate renal impairment (CC 10 to 50 mL/minute): 25 to 50% dose reduction
- severe impairment (CC below 10 mL/minute): contra-indicated

For the *oral* dosage form the following adjustments may be made:

- CC between 10 and 30 mL/minute: 50% dose reduction
- CC below 10 mL/minute (or serum creatinine greater than 440 micromoles/litre): contra-indicated

**Hypercalcaemia.** Treatment with bisphosphonates may be considered in patients with moderate to severe symptomatic hypercalcaemia of malignancy (p.1218) in addition to rehydration and diuresis.

References.


1. Urwin GH, *et al.* Treatment of the hypercalcaemia of malignancy with intravenous clodronate. *Bone* 1987; **8** (suppl 1): S43–S51.
2. Ralston SH, *et al.* Comparison of three intravenous bisphosphonates in cancer-associated hypercalcaemia. *Lancet* 1989; **ii:** 1180–2.
3. Rostom AY. Clodronate as outpatient treatment for hypercalcaemia. *Lancet* 1990; **336:** 1390.
4. O'Rourke NP, *et al.* Effective treatment of malignant hypercalcaemia with a single intravenous infusion of clodronate. *Br J Cancer* 1993; **67:** 560–3.
5. Elomaa I, Blomqvist C. Clodronate and other bisphosphonates as supportive therapy in osteolysis due to malignancy. *Acta Oncol* 1995; **34:** 629–36.
6. Shah S, *et al.* Is there a dose response relationship for clodronate in the treatment of tumour induced hypercalcaemia? *Br J Cancer* 2002; **86:** 1235–7.
7. Roemer-Bécuwe C, *et al.* Safety of subcutaneous clodronate and efficacy in hypercalcaemia of malignancy: a novel route of administration. *J Pain Symptom Manage* 2003; **26:** 843–8.


**Hyperparathyroidism.** Bisphosphonates have been used to inhibit bone resorption in the treatment of hypercalcaemia associated with hyperparathyroidism (p.765) but seem to be of little benefit for long-term treatment.

References.


1. Shane E, *et al.* Effects of dichloromethylene diphosphonate on serum and urinary calcium in primary hyperparathyroidism. *Ann Intern Med* 1981; **95:** 23–7.
2. Douglas DL, *et al.* Drug treatment of primary hyperparathyroidism: use of clodronate disodium. *BMJ* 1983; **286:** 587–90.
3. Hamdy NAT, *et al.* Clodronate in the medical management of hyperparathyroidism. *Bone* 1987; **8** (suppl 1): S69–77.


**Malignant neoplasms of the bone.** Bisphosphonates are of benefit in some patients with metastatic bone disease (p.513) not only to manage bone pain and hypercalcaemia, but to reduce skeletal complications such as fractures. Clodronate is licensed for such use in many countries. Whether bisphosphonates can prevent the development of new skeletal metastases is unclear.

References.


1. Kanis JA, *et al.* Clodronate decreases the frequency of skeletal metastases in women with breast cancer. *Bone* 1996; **19:** 663–7.
2. McCloskey EV, *et al.* A randomized trial of the effect of clodronate on skeletal morbidity in multiple myeloma. *Br J Haematol* 1998; **100:** 317–25.
3. Diel IJ, *et al.* Reduction in new metastases in breast cancer with adjuvant clodronate treatment. *N Engl J Med* 1998; **339:** 357–63.
4. Kristensen B, *et al.* Oral clodronate in breast cancer patients with bone metastases: a randomized study. *J Intern Med* 1999; **246:** 67–74.
5. Hurst M, Noble S. Clodronate: a review of its use in breast cancer. *Drugs Aging* 1999; **15:** 143–67.
6. Saarto T, *et al.* Adjuvant clodronate treatment does not reduce the frequency of skeletal metastases in node-positive breast cancer patients: 5-year results of a randomized controlled trial. *J Clin Oncol* 2001; **19:** 10–17.
7. Tubiana-Hulin M, *et al.* Essai comparatif randomisé en double aveugle clodronate oral 1600 mg/j versus placebo chez des patientes avec métastases osseuses de cancer du sein: double-blinded controlled study comparing clodronate versus placebo in patients with breast cancer bone metastases. *Bull Cancer* 2001; **88:** 701–7.
8. Powles T, *et al.* Randomized, placebo-controlled trial of clodronate in patients with primary operable breast cancer. *J Clin Oncol* 2002; **20:** 3219–24.


**Osteoporosis.** Bisphosphonates are used for the prevention and treatment of osteoporosis (p.763).

References.


1. Rossini M, *et al.* Intramuscular clodronate therapy in postmenopausal osteoporosis. *Bone* 1999; **24:** 125–9.
2. Filipponi P, *et al.* Intermittent versus continuous clodronate administration in postmenopausal women with low bone mass. *Bone* 2000; **26:** 269–74.
3. McCloskey E, *et al.* Effects of clodronate on vertebral fracture risk in osteoporosis: a 1-year interim analysis. *Bone* 2001; **28:** 310–15.
4. Välimäki MJ, *et al.* Prevention of bone loss by clodronate in early postmenopausal women with vertebral osteopenia: a dose-finding study. *Osteoporosis Int* 2002; **13:** 937–47.


**Paget's disease of bone.** Patients with Paget's disease of bone (p.764) may require no treatment or just analgesics, but bisphosphonates may be indicated if bone pain is persistent or to prevent further progression of the disease.

References.


1. Yates AJP, *et al.* Intravenous clodronate in the treatment and retreatment of Paget's disease of bone. *Lancet* 1985; **i:** 1474–7.
2. Gray RES, *et al.* Duration of effect of oral diphosphonate therapy in Paget's disease of bone. *Q J Med* 1987; **64:** 755–67.
3. Broggini M, *et al.* Short courses of intravenous clodronate in the treatment of Paget's disease of bone: a long-term follow-up trial. *Int J Clin Pharmacol Res* 1993; **13:** 301–4.
4. Khan SA, *et al.* Duration of response with oral clodronate in Paget's disease of bone. *Bone* 1996; **18:** 185–90.


## Preparations

**Proprietary Preparations** (details are given in Part 3)
***Austral.:*** Bonefos; ***Austria:*** Ascredar; Bonefos; Lodronat; ***Belg.:*** Bonefos; Ostac; ***Braz.:*** Bonefos; Ostac; ***Canad.:*** Bonefos; Ostac; ***Chile:*** Lodronat; ***Denm.:*** Bonefos; Loron†; ***Fin.:*** Bonefos; ***Fr.:*** Clastoban; Lytos; ***Ger.:*** Bonefos; Ostac; ***Gr.:*** Ostac; ***Hong Kong:*** Bonefos; Ostac; ***Irl.:*** Bonefos; Loron; ***Israel:*** Bonefos; Ostac; ***Ital.:*** Clasteon; Clodron; Clody; Difosfonal; Dolkin; Moticlod; Niklod; Ossiten; Osteostab; ***Malaysia:*** Bonefos; ***Neth.:*** Bonefos; Ostac; ***Norw.:*** Bonefos; Ostac†; ***NZ:*** Ostac†; ***Port.:*** Bonefos; Ostac; ***S.Afr.:*** Ostac; ***Singapore:*** Bonefos; Ostac†; ***Spain:*** Bonefos; Hemocalcin†; Mebonat; ***Swed.:*** Bonefos†; Ostac; ***Switz.:*** Bonefos†; Ostac; ***Thai.:*** Bonefos; ***UK:*** Bonefos; Loron.

# Etidronic Acid *(BAN, USAN, rINN)*

Ácido etidrónico. 1-Hydroxyethylidenedi(phosphonic acid).
$C_2H_8O_7P_2$ = 206.0.
*CAS — 2809-21-4.*
*ATC — M05BA01.*

## Disodium Etidronate *(BANM)*

EHDP; Etidronate Disodium *(USAN)*; Etidronato disódico. Disodium dihydrogen (1-hydroxyethylidene)diphosphonate.
$C_2H_6Na_2O_7P_2$ = 250.0.
*CAS — 7414-83-7.*
*ATC — M05BA01.*

NOTE. Other etidronic acid sodium salts are designated as etidronate monosodium, etidronate trisodium, and etidronate tetrasodium. The name sodium etidronate is used only where the salt cannot be identified more precisely.

**Pharmacopoeias.** In *US.*

**USP 27** (Etidronate Disodium). Store in airtight containers. pH of a 1% solution in water is between 4.2 and 5.2.

## Adverse Effects and Precautions

As for the bisphosphonates in general, p.766. Unlike the newer bisphosphonates etidronate produces marked impairment of bone mineralisation at high therapeutic doses. An increase in bone pain may occur in patients with Paget's disease. Impairment of bone mineralisation may result in osteomalacia and fractures have been reported. If a fracture occurs etidronate should be discontinued until healing is complete. Hyperphosphataemia may occur, usually at high doses, but generally resolves 2 to 4 weeks after therapy. There have been reports of paraesthesias and peripheral neuropathy. Transient loss or alteration of taste has been reported mainly during and after intravenous infusion.

**Effects on the eyes.** For reports of ocular effects associated with the bisphosphonates, including etidronate, see under Bisphosphonates, p.767.

**Effects on the gastrointestinal tract.** Oral etidronate was not associated with an increased incidence of upper gastrointestinal problems in a retrospective cohort study.[1] There was also no evidence of an increased incidence of gastrointestinal effects when given with NSAIDs or corticosteroids.


1. van Staa T, *et al.* Upper gastrointestinal adverse events and cyclical etidronate. *Am J Med* 1997; **103:** 462–7.


**Effects on the kidneys.** Bisphosphonates are excreted by the kidneys, thus caution is advised in patients with renal impairment. When given by intravenous infusion for the treatment of hypercalcaemia of malignancy they have been reported to affect renal function adversely; hypercalcaemia or malignancy may also have contributed. For reports of renal failure associated with etidronate administration see under Bisphosphonates, p.767.

**Effects on the respiratory system.** For a report of bronchospasm induced by etidronate in an aspirin-sensitive asthmatic, see p.767.

**Hypersensitivity.** Allergic reactions to bisphosphonates do occur but appear to be rare (see p.767).

## Interactions

As for the bisphosphonates in general, p.767.

◊ For a lack of apparent interaction between cyclical etidronate and corticosteroids or NSAIDs see under Effects on the Gastrointestinal Tract, above.

## Pharmacokinetics

Following doses by mouth, absorption is variable and appears to be dose dependent. At usual dosage ranges about 1 to 6% of a dose of disodium etidronate is absorbed. Absorption is reduced by food, especially by products containing calcium or other polyvalent cations. Disodium etidronate is rapidly cleared from the blood and has been reported to have a plasma half-life of 1 to 6 hours. It is not metabolised. About 50% is excreted in the urine within 24 hours, the remainder being sequestered to bone and slowly eliminated. The half-life of disodium etidronate in bone exceeds 90 days. Unabsorbed disodium etidronate appears in the faeces.

## Uses and Administration

Etidronate is a bisphosphonate with general properties similar to those of the other bisphosphonates (p.767). It inhibits the growth and dissolution of hydroxyapatite crystals in bone and may also directly impair osteoclast activity. It diminishes bone resorption and thus reduces bone turnover.

Disodium etidronate is used as an adjunct in the treatment of severe hypercalcaemia, especially when associated with malignancy. It is also given in bone disorders in which excessive bone resorption is a problem, such as Paget's disease of bone and osteoporosis. In addition, it may be used for the prevention and treatment of ectopic (heterotopic) ossification and the management of malignancies of bone. A chelate of etidronate with radioactive technetium-99m (p.1525) is used diagnostically as a bone scanning agent and a similar compound with rhenium-186 for the palliation of bone metastases in prostate cancer (see below).

Disodium etidronate is administered by intravenous infusion over at least 2 hours, or by mouth, usually as a single daily dose. Food should be avoided for 2 hours before and after oral administration.

In the treatment of **Paget's disease**, disodium etidronate is given by mouth in a usual initial dose of 5 mg/kg daily for not more than 6 months. Doses above 10 mg/kg daily should be reserved for severe disease and should not be given for more than 3 months at a time. The maximum dose is 20 mg/kg daily. The response to disodium etidronate may be slow in onset and may continue for several months after cessation of therapy. Therefore, further treatment should only be given after a drug-free interval of at least 3 months and after evidence of relapse; it should not be continued for more than the duration of the initial treatment.

In the treatment of **hypercalcaemia of malignancy** the recommended dose of disodium etidronate by slow intravenous infusion is 7.5 mg/kg daily for 3 successive days, although infusions may be continued for up to 7 days if necessary. This daily dose should be diluted in at least 250 mL of sodium chloride 0.9% and infused over at least 2 hours. There should be at least a 7-day interval between courses of treatment. Once serum-calcium concentrations have been reduced to an acceptable level, maintenance therapy with disodium etidronate 20 mg/kg daily by mouth for 30 days may be started on the day after the last intravenous dose; treatment may be extended to a maximum of 90 days.

For the prevention and treatment of **ectopic ossification** complicating hip replacement disodium etidronate has been given by mouth in a dose of 20 mg/kg daily for 1 month before and 3 months after the operation. For ectopic ossification due to spinal cord injury it has been given in a dose of 20 mg/kg daily for 2 weeks followed by 10 mg/kg daily for 10 weeks.

For the treatment of **osteoporosis**, the prevention of bone loss in postmenopausal women, and the prevention and treatment of corticosteroid-induced osteoporosis, etidronate is given in an intermittent or cyclical regimen with a calcium salt; disodium etidronate 400 mg is given by mouth daily for 14 days followed by the equivalent of 500 mg of elemental calcium by mouth for 76 days. Treatment has continued for 3 years in most patients; the optimum duration of treatment has not been established.

**Administration in renal impairment.** Some manufacturers have recommended that disodium etidronate should not be given *intravenously* to patients with serum-creatinine concentrations greater than 50 mg/litre, and that doses may need to be reduced in those with concentrations between 25 and 49 mg/litre. Reduced *oral* doses are similarly recommended in mild renal impairment, and avoidance in moderate to severe impairment.

**Ectopic ossification.** Bisphosphonates that inhibit bone mineralisation such as disodium etidronate have been used to prevent ectopic ossification (p.762).

References.

1. Finerman GAM, Stover SL. Heterotopic ossification following hip replacement or spinal cord injury: two clinical studies with EHDP. *Metab Bone Dis Relat Res* 1981; **4 & 5:** 337–42.
2. Banovac K, *et al.* Intravenous disodium etidronate therapy in spinal cord injury patients with heterotopic ossification. *Paraplegia* 1993; **31:** 660–6.
3. Banovac K. The effect of etidronate on late development of heterotopic ossification after spinal cord injury. *J Spinal Cord Med* 2000; **23:** 40–4.

**Hypercalcaemia.** Treatment with bisphosphonates (including etidronate although other bisphosphonates may be preferred) may be considered in patients with moderate to severe symptomatic hypercalcaemia of malignancy (p.1218) in addition to rehydration and diuresis.

References.

1. Hasling C, *et al.* Etidronate disodium for treating hypercalcaemia of malignancy: a double blind, placebo-controlled study. *Eur J Clin Invest* 1986; **16:** 433–7.
2. Ringenberg QS, Ritch PS. Efficacy of oral administration of etidronate disodium in maintaining normal serum calcium levels in previously hypercalcemic cancer patients. *Clin Ther* 1987; **9:** 318–25.
3. Ralston SH, *et al.* Comparison of three intravenous bisphosphonates in cancer-associated hypercalcaemia. *Lancet* 1989; **ii:** 1180–2.
4. Singer FR, *et al.* Treatment of hypercalcaemia of malignancy with intravenous etidronate: a controlled, multicenter study. *Arch Intern Med* 1991; **151:** 471–6. Correction. *ibid.*; 2008.

**Hyperparathyroidism.** Bisphosphonates have been used to inhibit bone resorption in the treatment of hypercalcaemia associated with hyperparathyroidism (p.765) but seem to be of little benefit in long-term treatment.

References.

1. Licata AA, O'Hanlon E. Treatment of hyperparathyroidism with etidronate disodium. *JAMA* 1983; **249:** 2063–4.

**Malignant neoplasms of the bone.** Bisphosphonates are of benefit in some patients with metastatic bone disease (p.513). Rhenium-186-labelled etidronate is used for the palliation of painful bone metastases of prostate cancer.

References.

1. Carey PO, Lippert MC. Treatment of painful prostatic bone metastases with oral etidronate disodium. *Urology* 1988; **32:** 403–7.
2. Smith JA. Palliation of painful bone metastases from prostate cancer using sodium etidronate: results of a randomized, prospective, double-blind, placebo-controlled study. *J Urol (Baltimore)* 1989; **141:** 85–7.
3. Han SH, *et al.* The Placorhen study: a double-blind, placebo-controlled, randomized radionuclide study with $^{186}$Re-etidronate in hormone-resistant prostate cancer patients with painful bone metastases. *J Nucl Med* 2002; **43:** 1150–6.

**Osteoporosis.** Bisphosphonates are used in the prevention and treatment of osteoporosis (p.763). For the treatment of postmenopausal osteoporosis, disodium etidronate is given in an intermittent or cyclical regimen;[1-4] additive effects with oestrogen have been described.[5,6] Similar cyclical regimens are used in the prevention of early postmenopausal bone loss.[7,8] Etidronate is also effective in both men and women for the prevention and treatment of corticosteroid-induced osteoporosis.[9-11] There is some interest in the use of etidronate to treat idiopathic vertebral osteoporosis in men.[12]

1. Storm T, *et al.* Effect of intermittent cyclical etidronate therapy on bone mass and fracture rate in women with postmenopausal osteoporosis. *N Engl J Med* 1990; **322:** 1265–71.
2. Watts NB, *et al.* Intermittent cyclical etidronate treatment of postmenopausal osteoporosis. *N Engl J Med* 1990; **323:** 73–9.
3. Harris ST, *et al.* Four-year study of intermittent cyclic etidronate treatment of postmenopausal osteoporosis: three years of blinded therapy followed by one year of open therapy. *Am J Med* 1993; **95:** 557–67.
4. Miller PD, *et al.* Cyclical etidronate in the treatment of postmenopausal osteoporosis: efficacy and safety after seven years of treatment. *Am J Med* 1997; **103:** 468–76.
5. Wimalawansa SJ. Combined therapy with estrogen and etidronate has an additive effect on bone mineral density in the hip and vertebrae: four-year randomized study. *Am J Med* 1995; **99:** 36–42.
6. Wimalawansa SJ. A four-year randomized controlled trial of hormone replacement and bisphosphonate, alone or in combination, in women with postmenopausal osteoporosis. *Am J Med* 1998; **104:** 219–26.
7. Herd RJM, *et al.* The prevention of early postmenopausal bone loss by cyclical etidronate therapy: a 2-year, double-blind, placebo-controlled study. *Am J Med* 1997; **103:** 92–9.
8. Meunier PJ, *et al.* Prevention of early postmenopausal bone loss with cyclical etidronate therapy. *J Clin Endocrinol Metab* 1997; **82:** 2784–91.
9. Struys A, *et al.* Cyclical etidronate reverses bone loss of the spine and proximal femur in patients with established corticosteroid-induced osteoporosis. *Am J Med* 1995; **99:** 235–42.
10. Adachi JD, *et al.* Intermittent etidronate therapy to prevent corticosteroid-induced osteoporosis. *N Engl J Med* 1997; **337:** 382–7.
11. Pitt P, *et al.* A double blind placebo controlled study to determine the effects of intermittent cyclical etidronate on bone mineral density in patients on long term oral corticosteroid treatment. *Thorax* 1998; **53:** 351–6.
12. Anderson FH, *et al.* Effect of intermittent cyclical disodium etidronate therapy on bone mineral density in men with vertebral fractures. *Age Ageing* 1997; **26:** 359–65.

**Paget's disease of bone.** Patients with Paget's disease of bone (p.764) may require no treatment or just analgesics, but bisphosphonates such as etidronate may be indicated if bone pain is persistent or to prevent further progression of the disease.

References.

1. Johnston CC, *et al.* Review of fracture experience during treatment of Paget's disease of bone with etidronate disodium (EHDP). *Clin Orthop* 1983; **172:** 186–94.
2. Preston CJ, *et al.* Effective short term treatment of Paget's disease with oral etidronate. *BMJ* 1986; **292:** 79–80.
3. Gibbs CJ, *et al.* Osteomalacia in Paget's disease treated with short term, high dose sodium etidronate. *BMJ* 1986; **292:** 1227–9.
4. Perry HM, *et al.* Alternate calcitonin and etidronate disodium therapy for Paget's bone disease. *Arch Intern Med* 1984; **144:** 929–33.

## Preparations

***USP 27:*** Etidronate Disodium Tablets.

**Proprietary Preparations** (details are given in Part 3)
***Arg.:*** Difosfen; ***Austral.:*** Didronel; ***Austria:*** Didronel; ***Belg.:*** Didronel; Osteodidronel; ***Braz.:*** Bonemass†; ***Canad.:*** Didronel; ***Chile:*** Osteotop; ***Denm.:*** Didronate; ***Fin.:*** Didronate; ***Fr.:*** Didronel; ***Ger.:*** Didronel; Diphos; ***Gr.:*** Anfozan; Dralen; Etiplus; Feminoflex; Ostedron; Ostogene; Ostopor; Somaflex; Sviroxit; ***Hong Kong:*** Didronel; ***India:*** Dronate-OS; ***Irl.:*** Didronel; ***Israel:*** Didronel; ***Ital.:*** Didronel; Etidron; ***Jpn:*** Didronel; ***Norw.:*** Didronate†; ***NZ:*** Didronel†; Etidrate; ***Port.:*** Didronel; ***S.Afr.:*** Didronel†; ***Singapore:*** Difosfen; ***Spain:*** Difosfen; Osteum; ***Swed.:*** Didronate; ***Switz.:*** Didronel; ***UK:*** Didronel; ***USA:*** Didronel.

**Multi-ingredient:** ***Arg.:*** Squam; ***Austral.:*** Didrocal; ***Canad.:*** Didrocal; ***Denm.:*** Didronate Calcium; ***Fin.:*** Didronate + Calcium; ***Ger.:*** Didronel Kit; ***Irl.:*** Didronel PMO; ***Ital.:*** Didro-Kit†; ***Neth.:*** Didrokit; ***Norw.:*** Didronate + Calsium; ***Swed.:*** Didronate + Calcium; ***UK:*** Didronel PMO.

# Gallium Nitrate *(USAN)*

Galio, nitrato de; NSC-15200; WR-135675.
$Ga(NO_3)_3,9H_2O = 417.9.$
*CAS — 13494-90-1 (anhydrous gallium nitrate); 135886-70-3 (gallium nitrate nonahydrate).*

## Adverse Effects, Treatment, and Precautions

Gallium nitrate may produce serious nephrotoxicity, especially when given as a brief intravenous infusion; administration by continuous infusion, with adequate hydration, may reduce the incidence of renal damage. Serum creatinine should be monitored during therapy and treatment discontinued if it exceeds 25 mg/litre. Gallium nitrate should be given with great care and in reduced doses, if at all, to patients with existing renal impairment.

Gastrointestinal disturbances, rashes, metallic taste, visual and auditory disturbances, anaemia, hypophosphataemia, and hypocalcaemia have also been reported.

**Effects on the nervous system.** Although it has been suggested, given the chemical similarity of gallium to aluminium, that repeated administration, particularly in the presence of renal impairment, might lead to severe neurotoxicity,[1] studies in *rats* do not provide any evidence of central neurological abnormalities.[2]

1. Altmann P, Cunningham J. Hazards of gallium for the treatment of Paget's disease of bone. *Lancet* 1990; **335:** 477.
2. Matkovic V, *et al.* Hazards of gallium for Paget's disease of bone. *Lancet* 1990; **335:** 1099.

## Uses and Administration

Gallium nitrate is an inorganic metallic salt with hypocalcaemic properties. It acts to decrease bone resorption by osteoclasts, with a lesser and probably indirect increase in bone formation, and a consequent decline in serum calcium.

Gallium nitrate is used in the treatment of hypercalcaemia associated with malignant neoplasms and has been investigated in other disorders associated with abnormally enhanced bone turnover, such as Paget's disease of bone. For the treatment of hypercalcaemia of malignancy doses of 100 to 200 mg/m$^2$ may be given daily for up to 5 days, diluted in 1 litre of sodium chloride 0.9% or glucose 5% injection and infused intravenously over 24 hours. Treatment may be repeated after 2 to 4 weeks, if necessary. Adequate hydration before and during treatment is essential: a urinary output of at least 2 litres daily should be maintained, and renal function should be regularly monitored.

Gallium nitrate has been tried, with limited benefit, as an antineoplastic in the management of lymphomas and some solid neoplasms.

**Hypercalcaemia.** Gallium nitrate is used in the treatment of hypercalcaemia of malignancy (p.1218).[1,2]

1. Chitambar CR. Gallium nitrate revisited. *Semin Oncol* 2003; **30** (suppl): 1–4.
2. Leyland-Jones B. Treatment of cancer-related hypercalcemia: the role of gallium nitrate. *Semin Oncol* 2003; **30** (suppl); 13–19.

**Paget's disease of bone.** Beneficial results[1] were reported when gallium nitrate was given subcutaneously in doses of 250 or 500 micrograms/kg daily for 14 days to patients with advanced Paget's disease of bone (p.764). In this pilot multicentre study 14 days of gallium nitrate injections were followed by 4 weeks off medication and the cycle repeated once.

1. Bockman RS, *et al.* A multicenter trial of low dose gallium nitrate in patients with advanced Paget's disease of bone. *J Clin Endocrinol Metab* 1995; **80:** 595–602.

## Preparations

**Proprietary Preparations** (details are given in Part 3)
***USA:*** Ganite.

# Ibandronic Acid *(BAN, rINN)*

Ácido ibandrónico; BM-21.0955. [1-Hydroxy-3-(methylpentylamino)propylidene]diphosphonic acid.
$C_9H_{23}NO_7P_2 = 319.2.$
*CAS — 114084-78-5.*
*ATC — M05BA06.*

# Sodium Ibandronate *(BANM, rINNM)*

Ibandronate Sodium *(USAN)*; Ibandronato sódico.
$C_9H_{22}NNaO_7P_2,H_2O = 359.2.$
*CAS — 138926-19-9.*
*ATC — M05BA06.*

## Adverse Effects and Precautions

As for the bisphosphonates in general, p.766. Gastrointestinal symptoms such as abdominal pain, dyspepsia, and nausea are the most frequent adverse effects. Severe oesophageal reactions such as oesophagitis, and ulceration have occurred; patients should be advised to stop taking the tablets and seek medical attention if they develop symptoms such as new or worsening dysphagia, pain on swallowing, retrosternal pain, or heartburn. Gastric and duodenal ulceration have been reported. To minimise the risk of oesophageal reactions, precautions similar to those for alendronate (see p.765) should be observed. Hypocalcaemia should be corrected before starting ibandronate therapy. Transient fever after parenteral administration is common, and flu-like symptoms have been reported.

## Interactions

As for the bisphosphonates in general, p.767.

## Pharmacokinetics

Like other bisphosphonates, ibandronate is poorly absorbed after oral administration; absolute bioavailability is less than 1%. Absorption is decreased by food, especially by products containing calcium or other polyvalent cations. Bioavailability is reduced by about 90% when given with food, by about 30% when given half an hour before food, and by about 75% when given 2 hours after food. About half of the absorbed portion is sequestered to bone; the remainder is excreted in urine. Plasma protein binding is about 87%. Bisphosphonates do not appear to be metabolised, and the unabsorbed fraction of ibandronate is excreted unchanged in the faeces.

## Uses and Administration

Ibandronate is an aminobisphosphonate (p.766) that is a potent inhibitor of bone resorption. It is used as the sodium salt in hypercalcaemia of malignancy, and for the prevention of fracture and bone complications in patients with breast cancer and bone metastases. Ibandronate is also under investigation for the treatment and prevention of osteoporosis.

Sodium ibandronate is administered by intravenous infusion, the dose being expressed in terms of ibandronic acid. Sodium ibandronate 1.13 mg is approximately equivalent to 1 mg of ibandronic acid. For **hypercalcaemia of malignancy**, a single dose of the equivalent of 2 to 4 mg ibandronic acid is given, up to a maximum of 6 mg; it is diluted in 500 mL of sodium chloride 0.9% or glucose 5%, and infused over 2 hours.

For the prevention of skeletal events in patients with breast cancer and **bone metastases**, a single dose of the equivalent of 6 mg ibandronic acid is given, diluted as above, but infused over 1 hour. The dose is repeated every 3 to 4 weeks. Alternatively, ibandronic acid 50 mg daily may be given by mouth; specific instructions for its administration (see Precautions in Alendronate, p.765) should be followed to minimise adverse effects and permit adequate absorption.

◊ General references.

1. Dooley M, Balfour JA. Ibandronate. *Drugs* 1999; **57:** 101–108.

**Administration in renal impairment.** One manufacturer has stated that the dose of ibandronate should be adjusted on the basis of creatinine clearance (CC) as follows:

- mild or moderate renal impairment (CC equal to or greater than 30 mL/minute): no adjustment necessary
- CC below 30 mL/minute: *intravenous* (for the prevention of skeletal events), reduce to 2 mg every 3 to 4 weeks, infused over 1 hour; *oral*, reduce to 50 mg weekly.

**Hypercalcaemia.** Treatment with bisphosphonates such as ibandronate may be considered in patients with moderate to severe symptomatic hypercalcaemia of malignancy (p.1218) in addition to rehydration and diuresis.

References.


1. Pecherstorfer M, *et al.* Randomized phase II trial comparing different doses of the bisphosphonate ibandronate in the treatment of hypercalcemia of malignancy. *J Clin Oncol* 1996; **14:** 268–76.
2. Ralston SH, *et al.* Dose-response study of ibandronate in the treatment of cancer-associated hypercalcaemia. *Br J Cancer* 1997; **75:** 295–300.


**Malignant neoplasms of the bone.** Bisphosphonates are of benefit in some patients with metastatic bone disease (p.513) not only to manage bone pain and hypercalcaemia, but to reduce skeletal complications such as fractures. Ibandronate is licensed for such use in many countries. Whether bisphosphonates can prevent the development of new skeletal metastases is unclear.

References.


1. Coleman RE, *et al.* Double-blind, randomised, placebo-controlled, dose-finding study of oral ibandronate in patients with metastatic bone disease. *Ann Oncol* 1999; **10:** 311–16.


**Osteoporosis.** Ibandronate is under investigation for the prevention and treatment of osteoporosis (p.763).

References.


1. Ravn P, *et al.* The effect on bone mass and bone markers of different doses of ibandronate: a new bisphosphonate for the prevention and treatment of postmenopausal osteoporosis: a 1-year randomized, double-blind, placebo-controlled dose-finding study. *Bone* 1996; **19:** 527–33.
2. Thiébaud D, *et al.* Three monthly intravenous injections of ibandronate in the treatment of postmenopausal osteoporosis. *Am J Med* 1997; **103:** 298–307.
3. Tankó LB, *et al.* Oral weekly ibandronate prevents bone loss in postmenopausal women. *J Intern Med* 2003; **254:** 159–67.
4. Cooper C, *et al.* Efficacy and safety of oral weekly ibandronate in the treatment of postmenopausal osteoporosis. *J Clin Endocrinol Metab* 2003; **88:** 4609–15.
5. Stakkestad JA, *et al.* Intravenous ibandronate injections given every three months: a new treatment option to prevent bone loss in postmenopausal women. *Ann Rheum Dis* 2003; **62:** 969–75.
6. Ringe JD, *et al.* Intermittent intravenous ibandronate injections reduce vertebral fracture risk in corticosteroid-induced osteoporosis: results from a long-term comparative study. *Osteoporosis Int* 2003; **14:** 801–7.


### Preparations

**Proprietary Preparations** (details are given in Part 3)
***Arg.:*** Bandrobon; ***Austria:*** Bondronat; ***Denm.:*** Bondronat; ***Fin.:*** Bondronat†; ***Fr.:*** Bondronat; ***Ger.:*** Bondronat; ***Gr.:*** Bondronat; ***S.Afr.:*** Bondronat; ***Singapore:*** Bondronat; ***Spain:*** Bondronat; ***Swed.:*** Bondronat; ***Switz.:*** Bondronat; ***Thai.:*** Bondronat; ***UK:*** Bondronat; ***USA:*** Boniva.

## Imidazole Oxoglurate

Imidazol, cetoglutarato de; Imidazole Cetoglutarate; Imidazole α-Ketoglutarate; Imidazole 2-Oxoglutarate.

### Profile

Imidazole oxoglurate was used in the treatment of bone disorders and disorders of calcium metabolism; it was also used for its reported effects on platelet aggregation in the treatment of thrombotic disorders.

## Incadronic Acid *(rINN)*

Ácido incadrónico; Cimadronic Acid; YM-175. [(Cycloheptylamino)methylene]diphosphonic acid.
$C_8H_{19}NO_6P_2$ = 287.2.
*CAS — 124351-85-5.*

## Disodium Incadronate *(rINNM)*

Incadronato disódico. Disodium [(cycloheptylamino)methylene]diphosphonate.
$C_8H_{17}NNa_2O_6P_2$ = 331.2.
*CAS — 138330-18-4.*

### Profile

Incadronic acid is an aminobisphosphonate (p.766) that is a potent inhibitor of bone resorption. It is given by intravenous infusion as disodium incadronate for hypercalcaemia of malignancy in a dose of 10 mg over 2 to 4 hours; if necessary this dose may be repeated at intervals of no less than 1 week. Hypocalcaemia and hypotension may occur. Incadronate is under investigation for the treatment of bone metastases in patients with breast cancer.

◊ References.


1. Usui T, *et al.* Pharmacokinetics of incadronate, a new bisphosphonate, in healthy volunteers and patients with malignancy-associated hypercalcemia. *Int J Clin Pharmacol Ther* 1997; **35:** 239–44.


### Preparations

**Proprietary Preparations** (details are given in Part 3)
***Jpn:*** Bisphonal.

## Ipriflavone *(rINN)*

FL-113; Ipriflavona. 7-Isopropoxyisoflavone.
$C_{18}H_{16}O_3$ = 280.3.
*CAS — 35212-22-7.*
*ATC — M05BX01.*

### Profile

Ipriflavone is a synthetic isoflavonoid that inhibits resorption of bone and is available in some countries for the treatment of osteoporosis (p.763). It is given by mouth in a dose of 200 mg three times daily.

◊ References.[1-4] Despite earlier favourable reports, a prospective randomised controlled study in postmenopausal women with low bone mass failed to show prevention of bone loss or improvements in markers of bone metabolism with ipriflavone.[4] There was also a significant incidence of lymphopenia with the drug.


1. Agnusdei D, *et al.* Metabolic and clinical effects of ipriflavone in established post-menopausal osteoporosis. *Drugs Exp Clin Res* 1989; **15:** 97–104.
2. Hyodo T, *et al.* A study of the effects of ipriflavone administration on hemodialysis patients with renal osteodystrophy: preliminary report. *Nephron* 1991; **58:** 114–15.
3. Agnusdei D, *et al.* Effects of ipriflavone on bone mass and bone remodeling in patients with established postmenopausal osteoporosis. *Curr Ther Res* 1992; **51:** 82–91.
4. Alexandersen P, *et al.* Ipriflavone in the treatment of postmenopausal osteoporosis: a randomized controlled trial. *JAMA* 2001; **285:** 1482–8.


### Preparations

**Proprietary Preparations** (details are given in Part 3)
***Arg.:*** Ipriosten; ***Braz.:*** Osteoplus; Rebone; ***Ital.:*** Iprosten; Osteofix; ***Jpn:*** Osten.
**Multi-ingredient:** ***UK:*** Osteopro.

## Medronic Acid *(BAN, USAN, pINN)*

Ácido medrónico. Methylenebis(phosphonic acid).
$CH_6O_6P_2$ = 176.0.
*CAS — 1984-15-2.*

## Disodium Medronate *(BANM)*

Disodium Methylene Diphosphonate; MDP; Medronate Disodium *(USAN)*; Medronato disódico. Disodium dihydrogen methylenediphosphonate.
$CH_4Na_2O_6P_2$ = 220.0.
*CAS — 25681-89-4.*

### Profile

Medronate is a bisphosphonate with general properties similar to those of the other bisphosphonates (p.766). Like other members of the class it has a strong affinity for bone. Complexes of disodium medronate and stannous chloride or fluoride, or medronic acid, stannous chloride dihydrate, and ascorbic acid, are labelled with radioactive technetium-99m (p.1525) and used diagnostically as bone scanning agents; they are given intravenously.

**Hypersensitivity.** For reference to a severe allergic reaction attributed to the sodium medronate component of a radiopharmaceutical, see under Adverse Effects and Precautions of Bisphosphonates, p.767.

### Preparations

**Proprietary Preparations** (details are given in Part 3)
***Braz.:*** Medronate†.

## Neridronic Acid *(rINN)*

Acide neridronique; Ácido neridrónico; Acido neridronico; Acidum neridronicum; AHDP; AHHexBP; Aminohexane Diphosphonate. (6-Amino-1-hydroxyhexylidene)diphosphonic acid.
$C_6H_{17}NO_7P_2$ = 277.1.
*CAS — 79778-41-9.*

## Neridronate Sodium *(rINNM)*

### Profile

Neridronic acid is an aminobisphosphonate with similar properties to those of the bisphosphonates in general (p.766). It inhibits bone resorption and is given intravenously as the sodium salt in the management of osteogenesis imperfecta; it has been used in the treatment of malignant hypercalcaemia and diseases associated with excessive bone turnover such as Paget's disease of bone.

◊ Bisphosphonates are widely used in the treatment of osteogenesis imperfecta (p.762), Paget's disease of bone (p.764), osteoporosis (p.763), and hypercalcaemia of malignancy (p.1218).

References.


1. O'Rourke NP, *et al.* Treatment of malignant hypercalcaemia with aminohexane bisphosphonate (neridronate). *Br J Cancer* 1994; **69:** 914–17.
2. Filipponi P, *et al.* Paget's disease of bone: benefits of neridronate as a first treatment and in cases of relapse after clodronate. *Bone* 1998; **23:** 543–8.
3. Adami S, *et al.* Short-term intravenous therapy with neridronate in Paget's disease. *Clin Exp Rheumatol* 2002; **20:** 55–8.
4. Adami S, *et al.* Intravenous neridronate in adults with osteogenesis imperfecta. *J Bone Miner Res* 2003; **18:** 126–30.
5. Braga V, *et al.* Intravenous intermittent neridronate in the treatment of postmenopausal osteoporosis. *Bone* 2003; **33:** 342–5.


### Preparations

**Proprietary Preparations** (details are given in Part 3)
***Ital.:*** Nerixia.

## Oxidronic Acid *(BAN, USAN, pINN)*

Ácido oxidrónico. (Hydroxymethylene)diphosphonic acid.
$CH_6O_7P_2$ = 192.0.
*CAS — 15468-10-7.*

## Disodium Oxidronate

HMDP; Oxidronate Disodium; Oxidronate Sodium; Oxidronato disódico; Sodium Oxidronate *(BANM)*. Disodium (hydroxymethylene)diphosphonate.
$CH_4Na_2O_7P_2$ = 236.0.
*CAS — 14255-61-9.*

### Profile

Oxidronate is a bisphosphonate with general properties similar to those of the other bisphosphonates (p.766). Like other members of the class it has a strong affinity for bone, and a chelate of oxidronate with radioactive technetium-99m (p.1525) is used diagnostically as a bone scanning agent; it is given intravenously.

# Pamidronic Acid *(BAN, rINN)*

Ácido pamidrónico; Aminohydroxypropylidenebisphosphonate; APD. 3-Amino-1-hydroxypropylidenebis(phosphonic acid).
$C_3H_{11}NO_7P_2$ = 235.1.
*CAS — 40391-99-9.*
*ATC — M05BA03.*

## Disodium Pamidronate *(BANM)*

Aminohydroxypropylidenebisphosphonate Disodium; CGP-23339A; CGP-23339AE; Disodium Aminohydroxypropylidenediphosphonate; Pamidronate Disodium *(USAN)*; Pamidronato disódico. Disodium 3-amino-1-hydroxypropylidenebisphosphonate pentahydrate.
$C_3H_9NNa_2O_7P_2,5H_2O$ = 369.1.
*CAS — 109552-15-0 (disodium pamidronate pentahydrate); 57248-88-1 (anhydrous disodium pamidronate).*
*ATC — M05BA03.*

**Pharmacopoeias.** In *Br.*

**BP 2003** (Disodium Pamidronate). A white crystalline powder. Soluble in water and in 2M sodium hydroxide; sparingly soluble in 0.1M hydrochloric acid; practically insoluble in organic solvents. A 1% solution in water has a pH of 7.8 to 8.8.

## Adverse Effects and Precautions

As for the bisphosphonates in general, p.766.

Fever and flu-like symptoms (sometimes accompanied by malaise, rigors, fatigue, and flushes) are common during treatment with disodium pamidronate but generally resolve spontaneously. Severe local reactions and thrombophlebitis have followed administration as a bolus injection. Rare CNS effects include agitation, confusion, dizziness, somnolence, and insomnia. Seizures have been precipitated in a few patients. In addition to hypocalcaemia and hypophosphataemia (which are common), hypomagnesaemia, and rarely hypernatraemia, and hyperkalaemia or hypokalaemia have occurred. Hypotension and hypertension have been reported.

Pamidronate should be used with caution in those with cardiac disease because of the potential for fluid overload and in those who have had thyroid surgery because of the increased risk of hypocalcaemia. Serum electrolytes, calcium and phosphate should be monitored during therapy. Patients should be warned against driving or operating machinery after treatment if somnolence or dizziness occur. Pamidronate should not be administered by bolus injection.

**Effects on the eyes.** For reports of ocular effects with the bisphosphonates, including pamidronate, see under Bisphosphonates, p.767.

**Effects on the gastrointestinal tract.** The tolerability of pamidronate administered *by mouth* may depend to some extent on the particular formulation. Gastrointestinal disturbances (in 21.8%) and haematological abnormalities (in 9.4%) were the predominant side-effects associated with oral pamidronate in an open study of elderly patients.[1] Oesophagitis, noted earlier[2] in 4 of 49 patients given a different formulation, was not reported in this study.[1]


1. Spivacow FR, *et al.* Tolerability of oral pamidronate in elderly patients with osteoporosis and other metabolic bone diseases. *Curr Ther Res* 1996; **57:** 123–30.
2. Lufkin EG, *et al.* Pamidronate: an unrecognised problem in gastrointestinal tolerability. *Osteoporosis Int* 1994; **4:** 320–2.

**Effects on the kidneys.** Like other bisphosphonates (see under Bisphosphonates, p.767), pamidronate may cause adverse renal effects. The UK manufacturers note that there have been isolated cases of haematuria, acute renal failure, and deterioration of pre-existing renal disease. Renal function should be monitored during long-term pamidronate therapy, especially in patients with pre-existing renal disease or a predisposition to renal impairment.

**Hypersensitivity.** Allergic reactions to bisphosphonates are rare. Rash and pruritus occasionally follow pamidronate infusion. Mild skin rashes have also been reported in some patients taking pamidronate by mouth (see also under Bisphosphonates, p.767).

**Musculoskeletal effects.** Although pamidronate appears to be a less potent inhibitor of bone mineralisation than etidronate, mineralisation defects have been reported in patients with Paget's disease of bone receiving pamidronate.[1] The resultant osteomalacia was not associated with any adverse clinical effects. Pamidronate-induced osteopetrosis has also been reported.[2] Acute pseudogout arthritis occurred in a woman treated with pamidronate for acute hypercalcaemia, possibly due to deposition of calcium in the joints.[3] Severe bone pain occurred in more patients than expected when pamidronate was used for low bone density in cystic fibrosis;[4] an increase in proinflammatory cytokines was postulated as a mechanism for this effect.[5]

1. Adamson BB, *et al.* Mineralisation defects with pamidronate therapy for Paget's disease. *Lancet* 1993; **342:** 1459–60.
2. Whyte MP, *et al.* Bisphosphonate-induced osteopetrosis. *N Engl J Med* 2003; **349:** 457–63.
3. Malnick SDH *et al.* Acute pseudogout as a complication of pamidronate. *Ann Pharmacother* 1997; **31:** 499–500.
4. Haworth CS, *et al.* Severe bone pain after intravenous pamidronate in adult patients with cystic fibrosis. *Lancet* 1998; **352:** 1753–4.
5. Teramoto S, *et al.* Increased cytokines and pamidronate-induced bone pain in adults with cystic fibrosis. *Lancet* 1999; **353:** 750.

## Interactions

As for the bisphosphonates in general, p.767.

## Pharmacokinetics

After intravenous administration of disodium pamidronate, about 20 to 55% of the dose is excreted in the urine unchanged within 72 hours, while the remainder is mainly sequestered to bone and only very slowly eliminated. Renal clearance is slower in patients with severe renal impairment and infusion rates may need to be reduced (see below).

Disodium pamidronate is poorly absorbed (about 1 to 3%) from the gastrointestinal tract.

## Uses and Administration

Pamidronate is an aminobisphosphonate with general properties similar to those of the other bisphosphonates (p.767). It inhibits bone resorption, but appears to have less effect on bone mineralisation than etidronate at comparable doses.

Disodium pamidronate is used as an adjunct in the treatment of severe hypercalcaemia, especially when associated with malignancy. It is also used in the treatment of osteolytic lesions and bone pain in multiple myeloma or bone metastases associated with breast cancer. It may also be of benefit in bone disorders associated with excessive bone resorption, including Paget's disease of bone.

Disodium pamidronate is administered by slow intravenous infusion. The UK manufacturers recommend infusion at a rate not exceeding 60 mg/hour (or not exceeding 20 mg/hour in patients with established or suspected renal impairment) and at a concentration not exceeding 60 mg per 250 mL of sodium chloride 0.9%. In the USA, the recommended concentration of infusion and its rate of administration vary depending on the indication.

In **hypercalcaemia of malignancy** disodium pamidronate is given by slow intravenous infusion in a total dose of 15 to 90 mg according to the initial plasma-calcium concentration. In the UK, the total dose is given as a single infusion or in divided doses over 2 to 4 days. In the USA, the total dose is given as a single infusion, doses of 60 mg to 90 mg being given over 2 to 24 hours. Plasma-calcium concentrations generally start declining 24 to 48 hours after administration of pamidronate with normalisation within 3 to 7 days. Treatment may be repeated if normocalcaemia is not achieved within this time or if hypercalcaemia recurs.

In patients with **osteolytic lesions and bone pain** of multiple myeloma or bone metastases associated with breast cancer, disodium pamidronate may be given in doses of 90 mg by intravenous infusion every 3 to 4 weeks.

In the treatment of **Paget's disease** the dosage regimen in the UK is 30 mg by slow infusion once a week for 6 weeks (total dose 180 mg), or 30 mg in the first week then 60 mg every other week for 6 weeks (total dose 210 mg). These courses may be repeated every 6 months, and the total dose increased if necessary up to a maximum of 360 mg. Alternatively, the dose used in the USA is 30 mg by infusion over 4 hours, repeated on consecutive days to a total dose of 90 mg. This course is repeated when clinically indicated.

Disodium pamidronate has also been given by mouth.

◊ General references.

1. Fitton A, McTavish D. Pamidronate: a review of its pharmacological properties and therapeutic efficacy in resorptive bone disease. *Drugs* 1991; **41:** 289–318. Correction. *ibid.* 1992; **43:** 145.
2. Anonymous. Pamidronate. *Med Lett Drugs Ther* 1992; **34:** 1–2.
3. Kellihan MJ, Mangino PD. Pamidronate. *Ann Pharmacother* 1992; **26:** 1262–9.
4. Coukell AJ, Markham A. Pamidronate: a review of its use in the management of osteolytic bone metastases, tumour-induced hypercalcaemia and Paget's disease of bone. *Drugs Aging* 1998; **12:** 149–68.

**Administration in renal impairment.** Pharmacokinetic studies suggest that no dosage reduction of disodium pamidronate is required in patients with any degree of renal impairment.[1] However, UK manufacturers currently recommend that the rate of infusion be reduced to a maximum of 20 mg/hour for patients with established or suspected renal impairment; use in those with severe renal impairment (creatinine clearance less than 30 mL/minute) is not advised as clinical experience is limited.

1. Berenson JR, *et al.* Pharmacokinetics of pamidronate disodium in patients with cancer with normal or impaired renal function. *J Clin Pharmacol* 1997; **37:** 285–90.

**Gaucher disease.** Treatment with oral disodium pamidronate in doses of 600 mg daily in adults,[1] and 150 to 300 mg daily in children,[2] or intravenous disodium pamidronate in doses of 45 mg every 3 weeks,[3] has been reported to improve bone lesions of Gaucher disease (p.1649) in a few patients.

1. Harinck HIJ, *et al.* Regression of bone lesions in Gaucher's disease during treatment with aminohydroxypropylidene bisphosphonate. *Lancet* 1984; **ii:** 513.
2. Samuel R, *et al.* Aminohydroxy propylidine bisphosphonate (APD) treatment improves the clinical skeletal manifestations of Gaucher's disease. *Pediatrics* 1994; **94:** 385–9.
3. Ciana G, *et al.* Short-term effects of pamidronate in patients with Gaucher's disease and severe skeletal involvement. *N Engl J Med* 1997; **337:** 712.

**Hypercalcaemia.** In patients with moderate to severe symptomatic hypercalcaemia of malignancy (p.1218) treatment with bisphosphonates, of which pamidronate is one of the most effective, may be considered in addition to rehydration and diuresis.

References.

1. Thiébaud D, *et al.* Oral versus intravenous AHP,BP (APD) in the treatment of hypercalcemia of malignancy. *Bone* 1986; **7:** 247–53.
2. Morton AR, *et al.* Single dose versus daily intravenous aminohydroxypropylidene biphosphonate (APD) for the hypercalcaemia of malignancy. *BMJ* 1988; **296:** 811–14.
3. Ralston SH, *et al.* Comparison of three intravenous bisphosphonates in cancer-associated hypercalcaemia. *Lancet* 1989; **ii:** 1180–2.
4. Nussbaum SR, *et al.* Single-dose intravenous therapy with pamidronate for the treatment of hypercalcaemia of malignancy: comparison of 30-, 60-, and 90-mg dosages. *Am J Med* 1993; **95:** 297–304.
5. Kutluk MT, *et al.* Childhood cancer and hypercalcemia: report of a case treated with pamidronate. *J Pediatr* 1997; **130:** 828–31.

**Malignant neoplasms of the bone.** Bisphosphonates are of benefit in some patients with metastatic bone disease (p.513) not only to manage bone pain and hypercalcaemia, but to reduce skeletal complications such as fractures. Pamidronate is licensed for such use in many countries. Whether bisphosphonates can prevent the development of new skeletal metastases is unclear.

References.

1. Ripamonti C, *et al.* Role of pamidronate disodium in the treatment of metastatic bone disease. *Tumori* 1998; **84:** 442–55.
2. Theriault RL, *et al.* Pamidronate reduces lesions: a randomized, placebo-controlled trial. *J Clin Oncol* 1999; **17:** 846–54.
3. Lipton A, *et al.* Pamidronate prevents skeletal complications and is effective palliative treatment in women with breast carcinoma and osteolytic bone metastases: long term follow-up of two randomized, placebo-controlled trials. *Cancer* 2000; **88:** 1082–90.

**Osteogenesis imperfecta.** Pamidronate has produced some benefit in children with osteogenesis imperfecta (p.762).

**Paget's disease of bone.** Patients with Paget's disease of bone (p.764) may require no treatment or just analgesics, but bisphosphonates such as pamidronate may be indicated if bone pain is persistent or to prevent further progression of the disease. References to the use of disodium pamidronate in Paget's disease are given below.[1-3] Bisphosphonates have also been given in other bone diseases with a similar pathology, particularly increased osteoclastic resorption. For example, pamidronate has had beneficial effects in patients with fibrous dysplasia of bone, a rare congenital disease leading to osteolytic lesions.[4-6]

1. Crisp AJ. Pamidronate for Paget's disease of the bone. *Br J Hosp Med* 1995; **53:** 66–8.
2. Selby PL. Pamidronate in the treatment of Paget's disease. *Bone* 1999; **24:** 57S–58S.
3. Tucci JR, Bontha S. Intravenously administered pamidronate in the treatment of Paget's disease of bone. *Endocr Pract* 2001; **7:** 423–9. Correction. *ibid.* 2002; **8:** 78.
4. Liens D, *et al.* Long-term effects of intravenous pamidronate in fibrous dysplasia of bone. *Lancet* 1994; **343:** 953–4.
5. Zacharin M, O'Sullivan M. Intravenous pamidronate treatment of polyostotic fibrous dysplasia associated with the McCune Albright syndrome. *J Pediatr* 2000; **137:** 403–9.
6. Plotkin H, *et al.* Effect of pamidronate treatment in children with polyostotic fibrous dysplasia of bone. *J Clin Endocrinol Metab* 2003; **88:** 4569–75.

**Rheumatoid arthritis.** Intravenous[1] and oral[2] administration of pamidronate has reportedly produced some modification of disease in a few patients with rheumatoid arthritis (p.9). Continuous oral pamidronate therapy was shown to be effective in preserving and increasing bone mass in a 3-year randomised controlled trial involving 105 patients with rheumatoid arthritis.[3]

1. Eggelmeijer F, *et al.* Clinical and biochemical response to single infusion of pamidronate in patients with active rheumatoid arthritis: a double blind placebo controlled study. *J Rheumatol* 1994; **21:** 2016–20.
2. Maccagno A, *et al.* Double blind radiological assessment of continuous oral pamidronic acid in patients with rheumatoid arthritis. *Scand J Rheumatol* 1994; **23:** 211–14.
3. Eggelmeijer F, *et al.* Increased bone mass with pamidronate treatment in rheumatoid arthritis: results of a three-year randomized, double-blind trial. *Arthritis Rheum* 1996; **39:** 396–402.

## Preparations

***BP 2003:*** Disodium Pamidronate Intravenous Infusion.

**Proprietary Preparations** (details are given in Part 3)
***Arg.:*** Aminomux; ***Austral.:*** Aredia; Pamisol; ***Austria:*** Aredia; ***Belg.:*** Aredia; ***Braz.:*** Aredia; ***Canad.:*** Aredia; ***Chile:*** Aredia; ***Denm.:*** Aredia; ***Fin.:*** Aredia; ***Fr.:*** Aredia; Ostepam; ***Ger.:*** Aredia; ***Gr.:*** Aredia; ***Hong Kong:*** Aredia; ***India:*** Aredronet; ***Irl.:*** Aredia; ***Israel:*** Aredia; ***Ital.:*** Aredia; ***Malaysia:*** Aredia; ***Mex.:*** Aredia; ***Neth.:*** Aredia; ***Norw.:*** Aredia; ***NZ:*** Aredia; ***Port.:*** Aredia; Pamidran; ***S.Afr.:*** Aredia; ***Singapore:*** Aredia†; ***Spain:*** Aredia; ***Swed.:*** Aredia; ***Switz.:*** Aredia; ***Thai.:*** Aredia; ***UK:*** Aredia; ***USA:*** Aredia.

## Parathyroid Hormone *(USAN, pINN)*

ALX1-11 (human recombinant parathyroid hormone); Parathormone; Parathyrin; Paratirina; PTH.

*CAS — 9002-64-6; 68893-82-3 (human parathyroid hormone); 345663-45-8 (human recombinant parathyroid hormone).*

### Profile

Parathyroid hormone is a single-chain polypeptide isolated from the parathyroid glands. It contains 84 amino acids and in man the first (N-terminal) 34 appear to be responsible for the hormonal activity. The amino-acid sequence varies according to the source.

Endogenous parathyroid hormone is involved in the maintenance of plasma-calcium concentrations having a hypercalcaemic effect through its actions on bone, kidney, and indirectly on the gastrointestinal tract (see also under Parathyroid Disorders, p.765).

Exogenous parathyroid hormone was formerly used in acute hypoparathyroidism with tetany. It has also been used in the differential diagnosis of hypoparathyroidism and pseudohypoparathyroidism.

Synthetic preparations of the first 34 amino acids of human and bovine parathyroid hormones (PTH 1-34; teriparatide) are now used for diagnostic purposes, and for the treatment of osteoporosis (see Teriparatide, p.775).

# Risedronic Acid *(BAN, rINN)*

Ácido risedrónico. [1-Hydroxy-2-(3-pyridinyl)ethylidene]diphosphonic acid.

$C_7H_{11}NO_7P_2$ = 283.1.
*CAS — 105462-24-6.*
*ATC — M05BA07.*

## Risedronate Sodium *(BANM, USAN, rINNM)*

Monosodium Risedronate; NE-58095; Risedronato sódico; Sodium Risedronate. Sodium trihydrogen [1-hydroxy-2-(3-pyridyl)ethylidene]diphosphonate.

$C_7H_{10}NNaO_7P_2$ = 305.1.
*CAS — 115436-72-1.*
*ATC — M05BA07.*

## Adverse Effects and Precautions

As for the bisphosphonates in general, p.766. The most frequent adverse effects during risedronate therapy are arthralgia and gastrointestinal disturbances. To minimise the risk of gastrointestinal effects precautions similar to those for alendronate (see p.765) should be observed, although UK licensed information allows for the tablets to be taken other than on rising (but not at bedtime or within 2 hours of food or drink). Hypocalcaemia should be corrected before beginning risedronate therapy.

**Effects on the eyes.** For reports of ocular effects with the bisphosphonates, including risedronate, see under Bisphosphonates, p.767.

**Effects on the gastrointestinal tract.** Although, like other oral bisphosphonates, it is recommended that risedronate be taken with care (above) to avoid gastrointestinal effects, pooled analysis of 9 studies involving 10 068 patients receiving risedronate 5 mg daily indicated that the drug was not associated with an increased frequency of upper gastrointestinal effects, even among patients at increased risk due to active gastrointestinal disease or concomitant treatment with aspirin or NSAIDs.[1] However, it was noted that comprehensive postmarketing data will be required to see how these results are reflected in clinical practice.

1. Taggart H, *et al.* Upper gastrointestinal tract safety of risedronate: a pooled analysis of 9 clinical trials. *Mayo Clin Proc* 2002; **77:** 262–70. Correction. *ibid.*; 601.

## Interactions

As for the bisphosphonates in general, p.767.

## Pharmacokinetics

Like other bisphosphonates, risedronate is poorly absorbed after oral administration. Absorption is reduced by food, especially by products containing calcium or other polyvalent cations. The mean bioavailability is 0.63% in the fasting state, and is reduced by 30% when administered 1 hour before breakfast, and by 55% when administered half an hour before breakfast. Unabsorbed drug is eliminated unchanged in the faeces. Risedronate is not metabolised, and 50% of the absorbed dose is excreted unchanged in the urine within 24 hours. The remainder of the absorbed dose is apparently sequestered to bone for a prolonged period.

**Absorption.** Absorption of a single dose of risedronate was comparable when given 0.5 to 1 hour before breakfast or 2 hours after an evening meal in a study in healthy subjects.[1]

1. Mitchell DY, *et al.* The effect of dosing regimen on the pharmacokinetics of risedronate. *Br J Clin Pharmacol* 1999; **48:** 536–42.

## Uses and Administration

Risedronate is an aminobisphosphonate with similar properties to those of the bisphosphonates in general (p.767). It inhibits bone resorption and is used as the sodium salt in Paget's disease of bone and for prevention and treatment of postmenopausal or corticosteroid-induced osteoporosis.

Risedronate sodium is given by mouth, and the specific instructions for its administration (see Adverse Effects and Precautions, above) should be followed to minimise gastrointestinal adverse effects and permit adequate absorption. The recommended dosage for **Paget's disease** of bone is 30 mg once daily for 2 months. Treatment may be repeated if necessary after an interval of a further 2 months. The recommended dosage for the treatment or prevention of postmenopausal or corticosteroid-induced **osteoporosis** is 5 mg daily. Alternatively, for postmenopausal osteoporosis, 35 mg once weekly may be given.

◊ General references.

1. Crandall C. Risedronate: a clinical review. *Arch Intern Med* 2001; **161:** 353–60.
2. Dunn CJ, Goa KL. Risedronate: a review of its pharmacological properties and clinical use in resorptive bone disease. *Drugs* 2001; **61:** 685–712.

**Administration in renal impairment.** Renal clearance of risedronate significantly correlated to renal function in a pharmacokinetic study,[1] although the authors concluded that generally no dosage adjustment appears necessary for patients with mild to moderate renal impairment (creatinine clearance (CC) greater than 20 mL/minute). The manufacturer states that no dosage adjustment is necessary when CC is greater than 30 mL/minute; however, use of risedronate is contra-indicated in patients with severe renal impairment (CC less than 30 mL/minute).

1. Mitchell DY, *et al.* Effect of renal function on risedronate pharmacokinetics after a single oral dose. *Br J Clin Pharmacol* 2000; **49:** 215–22.

**Hyperparathyroidism.** Bisphosphonates have been used to inhibit bone resorption in the treatment of hypercalcaemia associated with hyperparathyroidism (p.765) but seem to be of little benefit in long-term treatment.

References.

1. Reasner CA, *et al.* Acute changes in calcium homeostasis during treatment of primary hyperparathyroidism with risedronate. *J Clin Endocrinol Metab* 1993; **77:** 1067–71.

**Malignant neoplasms of the bone.** Bisphosphonates are of benefit in some patients with metastatic bone disease (p.513).

References.

1. Roux C, *et al.* Biologic, histologic and densitometric effects of oral risedronate on bone in patients with multiple myeloma. *Bone* 1994; **15:** 41–9.

**Osteoporosis.** Bisphosphonates such as risedronate may be used for the prevention and treatment of osteoporosis (p.763).

References.

1. Delmas PD, *et al.* Bisphosphonate risedronate prevents bone loss in women with artificial menopause due to chemotherapy of breast cancer: a double-blind, placebo-controlled study. *J Clin Oncol* 1997; **15:** 955–62.
2. Mortensen L, *et al.* Risedronate increases bone mass in early postmenopausal population: two years of treatment plus one year of follow-up. *J Clin Endocrinol Metab* 1998; **83:** 396–402.
3. Fogelman I, *et al.* Risedronate reverses bone loss in postmenopausal women with low bone mass: results from a multinational, double-blind, placebo-controlled trial. *J Clin Endocrinol Metab* 2000; **85:** 1895–1900.
4. McClung MR, *et al.* Effect of risedronate on the risk of hip fracture in elderly women. *N Engl J Med* 2001; **344:** 333–40.
5. Harris ST, *et al.* Effect of combined risedronate and hormone replacement therapies on bone mineral density in postmenopausal women. *J Clin Endocrinol Metab* 2001; **86:** 1890–7.
6. Dougherty JA. Risedronate for the prevention and treatment of corticosteroid-induced osteoporosis. *Ann Pharmacother* 2002; **36:** 512–16.
7. Sickels JM, Nip C-S. Risedronate for the prevention of fractures in postmenopausal osteoporosis. *Ann Pharmacother* 2002; **36:** 664–70.
8. Watts NB, *et al.* Risedronate prevents new vertebral fractures in postmenopausal women at high risk. *J Clin Endocrinol Metab* 2003; **88:** 542–9.
9. Sorensen OH, *et al.* Long-term efficacy of risedronate: a 5-year placebo-controlled clinical experience. *Bone* 2003; **32:** 120–6.
10. Watts NB, *et al.* Use of matched historical controls to evaluate the anti-fracture efficacy of once-a-week risedronate. *Osteoporosis Int* 2003; **14:** 437–41.

**Paget's disease of bone.** Patients with Paget's disease of bone (p.764) may require no treatment or just analgesics, but bisphosphonates such as risedronate may be indicated if bone pain is persistent or to prevent further progression of the disease.

References.

1. Brown JP, *et al.* Risedronate in Paget's disease: preliminary results of a multicenter study. *Semin Arthritis Rheum* 1994; **23:** 272.
2. Miller PD, *et al.* A randomized, double-blind comparison of risedronate and etidronate in the treatment of Paget's disease of bone. *Am J Med* 1999; **106:** 513–20.
3. Brown JP, *et al.* Improvement of pagetic bone lesions with risedronate treatment: a radiologic study. *Bone* 2000; **26:** 263–7.

## Preparations

**Proprietary Preparations** (details are given in Part 3)
***Arg.:*** Actonel; Ribastamin; ***Austral.:*** Actonel; ***Austria:*** Actonel; ***Belg.:*** Actonel; ***Braz.:*** Actonel; ***Canad.:*** Actonel; ***Chile:*** Actonel; ***Fin.:*** Optinate; ***Fr.:*** Actonel; ***Ger.:*** Actonel; ***Hong Kong:*** Actonel; ***Irl.:*** Actonel; ***Israel:*** Actonel; ***Ital.:*** Actonel; Optinate; ***Neth.:*** Actonel; ***Norw.:*** Optinate; ***Port.:*** Actonel; ***S.Afr.:*** Actonel; ***Singapore:*** Actonel; ***Spain:*** Actonel; ***Swed.:*** Optinate; ***Switz.:*** Actonel; ***Thai.:*** Actonel; ***UK:*** Actonel; ***USA:*** Actonel.

---

## Strontium Ranelate

S-12911. 2-(2-Carboxy-4-cyano-5-[*N*,*N*-di(carboxymethyl)amino]thiophen-3-yl) acetic acid distrontium salt.

$C_{12}H_6N_2O_8SSr_2$ = 513.5.
*CAS — 135459-87-9.*

### Profile

Strontium ranelate stimulates bone formation as well as reducing bone resorption. It is under investigation for the treatment of osteoporosis.

**Osteoporosis.** Strontium ranelate, given orally in a dose of 2 g daily, with calcium and vitamin D supplements, has been found to reduce the risk of vertebral fractures in postmenopausal women with osteoporosis.[1]

1. Meunier PJ, *et al.* The effects of strontium ranelate on the risk of vertebral fracture in women with postmenopausal osteoporosis. *N Engl J Med* 2004; **350:** 459–68.

---

## Teriparatide *(USAN, rINN)*

(1-34) Human parathormone; (1-34) Human parathyroid hormone; 1-34 Parathormone (human); hPTH 1-34; Human parathormone (1-34); Human parathyroid hormone (1-34); Human PTH (1-34); LY-333334; Parathyroid hormone peptide (1-34); Teriparatida; Teriparatidum.

$C_{181}H_{291}N_{55}O_{51}S_2$.
*CAS — 52232-67-4.*
*ATC — H05AA02.*

## Teriparatide Acetate *(USAN, rINNM)*

Acetato de teriparatida.

$C_{181}H_{291}N_{55}O_{51}S_2,xH_2O,yC_2H_4O_2$.
*CAS — 99294-94-7 (teriparatide acetate).*
*ATC — H05AA02.*

### Adverse Effects and Precautions

Gastrointestinal disturbances, pain in the limb of injection, headache, and dizziness are the most common adverse effects in patients treated with subcutaneous teriparatide. Dizziness, vertigo, and syncope may be associated with transient orthostatic hypotension in some patients, particularly when beginning treatment. Those so affected should not drive or operate potentially hazardous machinery. Asthenia, arthralgia, and rhinitis may occur. Angina pectoris, depression, dyspnoea, leg cramps, pneumonia, urinary disorders, and sciatica have also been reported. A metallic taste, tingling of the extremities, and pain at the site of injection have occasionally been associated with the intravenous infusion of teriparatide acetate. It is a peptide and the possibility of systemic hypersensitivity reactions should be borne in mind. Hypercalcaemia may develop with teriparatide or the acetate and it is therefore contra-indicated in patients with pre-existing hypercalcaemia. It is also contra-indicated in those with metabolic bone disease including Paget's disease, hyperparathyroidism, and unexplained elevations of serum alkaline phosphatase.

Teriparatide is contra-indicated in patients with severe renal impairment and should be used with caution with those with moderate impairment.

There have been reports of osteosarcoma in *rats* given teriparatide. Patients who may be at increased risk, including those with a history of skeletal metastases or previous radiotherapy to the skeleton, should not receive it. In the UK treatment is also limited to a maximum of 18 months.

### Uses and Administration

Teriparatide is a synthetic polypeptide that consists of the 1-34 amino-acid biologically active N-terminal region of human parathyroid hormone (p.774). It is used in the treatment of established postmenopausal osteoporosis; 20 micrograms is given subcutaneously daily into the thigh or abdominal wall. Treatment is limited to a maximum of 18 months in the UK, although it has been used for up to 2 years in the USA. Teriparatide acetate has been given by intravenous infusion in the differential diagnosis of hypoparathyroidism and pseudohypoparathyroidism.

**Hypoparathyroidism.** Hypoparathyroidism is characterised by a deficiency in endogenous parathyroid hormone, whereas pseudohypoparathyroidism is characterised by resistance to the effects of parathyroid hormone (see p.765). Teriparatide acetate is used *diagnostically* to distinguish between these 2 conditions.[1] A synthetic 1-38 fragment of human parathyroid hormone (1-38 hPTH) has been used similarly.[2] Teriparatide has also been used to *treat* hypoparathyroidism.[3,4]

1. Mallette LE. Synthetic human parathyroid hormone 1-34 fragment for diagnostic testing. *Ann Intern Med* 1988; **109:** 800–4.
2. Kruse K, Kracht U. A simplified diagnostic test in hypoparathyroidism and pseudohypoparathyroidism type I with synthetic 1-38 fragment of human parathyroid hormone. *Eur J Pediatr* 1987; **146:** 373–7.
3. Winer KK, *et al.* Synthetic human parathyroid hormone 1-34 vs calcitriol and calcium in the treatment of hypoparathyroidism. *JAMA* 1996; **276:** 631–6.
4. Winer KK, *et al.* A randomized, cross-over trial of once-daily versus twice-daily parathyroid hormone 1-34 in treatment of hypoparathyroidism. *J Clin Endocrinol Metab* 1998; **83:** 3480–6.

**Osteoporosis.** Parathyroid hormone is capable of stimulating both formation and resorption of bone; at low doses the former effect predominates and may avoid the development of hypercalcaemia. These different actions appear to be modulated by different signalling pathways in the osteoblast, and there is much interest in developing a hormone fragment or analogue which would stimulate bone formation but not resorption.[1] Parathyroid hormone appears to have less effect on cortical than trabecular bone, suggesting that, although it may be helpful in preventing vertebral fractures, its impact on fractures of the proximal femur may be more limited. However, combination with an antiresorptive agent such as oestrogen or a bisphosphonate, the currently preferred treatments for osteoporosis (p.763), might protect other parts of the skeleton. References[2-9] to the use of teriparatide and other synthetic parathyroid hormone fragments in osteoporosis are given below.

1. Bonn D. Parathyroid hormone for osteoporosis. *Lancet* 1996; **347:** 50.
2. Finkelstein JS, *et al.* Parathyroid hormone for the prevention of bone loss induced by estrogen deficiency. *N Engl J Med* 1994; **331:** 1618–23.
3. Hodsman AB, *et al.* A randomized controlled trial to compare the efficacy of cyclical parathyroid hormone versus cyclical parathyroid hormone and sequential calcitonin to improve bone mass in postmenopausal women with osteoporosis. *J Clin Endocrinol Metab* 1997; **82:** 620–8.
4. Lindsay R, *et al.* Randomised controlled study of effect of parathyroid hormone on vertebral-bone mass and fracture incidence among postmenopausal women on oestrogen with osteoporosis. *Lancet* 1997; **350:** 550–5.
5. Finkelstein JS, *et al.* Prevention of estrogen deficiency-related bone loss with human parathyroid hormone-(1-34): a randomized controlled trial. *JAMA* 1998; **280:** 1067–73.
6. Lane NE, *et al.* Parathyroid hormone treatment can reverse corticosteroid-induced osteoporosis. *J Clin Invest* 1998; **102:** 1627–33.
7. Neer RM, *et al.* Effect of parathyroid hormone (1-34) on fractures and bone mineral density in postmenopausal women with osteoporosis. *N Engl J Med* 2001; **344:** 1434–41.
8. Anonymous. Teriparatide (Forteo) for osteoporosis. *Med Lett Drugs Ther* 2003; **45:** 9–10.
9. Cappuzzo KA, Delafuente JC. Teriparatide for severe osteoporosis. *Ann Pharmacother* 2004; **38:** 294–302.

### Preparations

**Proprietary Preparations** (details are given in Part 3)
***UK:*** Forsteo; ***USA:*** Forteo.

## Tiludronic Acid *(BAN, rINN)*

Ácido tiludrónico; ME-3737; SR-41319. {[(p-Chlorophenyl)thio]methylene}diphosphonic acid.

$C_7H_9ClO_6P_2S$ = 318.6.

*CAS — 89987-06-4.*

*ATC — M05BA05.*

### Tiludronate Sodium *(BANM, rINNM)*

Disodium Tiludronate; SR-41319B; Tiludronate Disodium *(USAN)*; Tiludronato sódico. Disodium dihydrogen {[(p-chlorophenyl)thio]methylene}diphosphonate hemihydrate.

$C_7H_7ClNa_2O_6P_2S,\frac{1}{2}H_2O$ = 371.6.

*CAS — 149845-07-8 (anhydrous tiludronate sodium); 155453-10-4 (tiludronate sodium hemihydrate).*

*ATC — M05BA05.*

### Adverse Effects and Precautions

As for the bisphosphonates in general, p.766.

**Effects on the skin.** As with other bisphosphonates, tiludronate has been associated with rash and pruritus. For reference to a case of massive epidermal necrosis possibly associated with tiludronate, see Hypersensitivity, under Bisphosphonates, p.767.

### Interactions

As for the bisphosphonates in general, p.767. Indometacin may increase the bioavailability of tiludronate two to fourfold; diclofenac does not appear to have this effect. Aspirin may decrease the bioavailability of tiludronate by 50%.

### Pharmacokinetics

Like other bisphosphonates tiludronate is poorly absorbed after oral doses. Absorption is reduced by food, especially by products containing calcium or other polyvalent cations. The oral bioavailability of tiludronate is about 6% in the fasting state, and is reduced by about 90% when administered within 2 hours of food. About half of the absorbed portion of tiludronate is sequestered to bone, and only very slowly excreted; the remainder is excreted unchanged in the urine.

### Uses and Administration

Tiludronate is a bisphosphonate with similar properties to those of the bisphosphonates in general (p.767). It inhibits bone resorption and is used for Paget's disease of bone.

It is given by mouth as tiludronate sodium, but doses are expressed in terms of the equivalent amount of tiludronic acid; 117 mg of tiludronate sodium is approximately equivalent to 100 mg of tiludronic acid. To ensure adequate absorption doses should be taken with plenty of water (at least 200 mL), at least 2 hours before or after meals. In Paget's disease of bone the usual dose is 400 mg once daily for 3 months, and this may be repeated if necessary after an interval of at least 3 months.

Tiludronate has been tried in postmenopausal osteoporosis, but results were disappointing.

**Paget's disease of bone.** Some references to the use of tiludronate in Paget's disease of bone (p.764).


1. McClung MR, *et al.* Tiludronate therapy for Paget's disease of bone. *Bone* 1995; **17** (suppl 5): 493S–6S.
2. Roux C, *et al.* Comparative prospective, double-blind, multicenter study of the efficacy of tiludronate and etidronate in the treatment of Paget's disease of bone. *Arthritis Rheum* 1995; **38:** 851–8.
3. Anonymous. Tiludronate for Paget's disease of bone. *Med Lett Drugs Ther* 1997; **39:** 65–6.
4. Fraser WD, *et al.* A double-blind, multicentre, placebo-controlled study of tiludronate in Paget's disease of bone. *Postgrad Med J* 1997; **73:** 496–502.


### Preparations

**Proprietary Preparations** (details are given in Part 3)
***Austral.:*** Skelid; ***Austria:*** Skelid; ***Belg.:*** Skelid; ***Braz.:*** Skelid†; ***Fin.:*** Skelid; ***Fr.:*** Skelid; ***Ger.:*** Skelid; ***Neth.:*** Skelid; ***Spain:*** Skelid; ***Swed.:*** Skelid; ***Switz.:*** Skelid; ***UK:*** Skelid; ***USA:*** Skelid.

## Zoledronic Acid *(BAN, USAN, rINN)*

Ácido zoledrónico; CGP-42446. (1-Hydroxy-2-imidazol-1-ylethylidene)diphosphonic acid.

$C_5H_{10}N_2O_7P_2$ = 272.1.

*CAS — 118072-93-8 (anhydrous zoledronic acid); 165800-06-6 (zoledronic acid monohydrate).*

*ATC — M05BA08.*

### Zoledronate Disodium *(BANM, USAN, rINNM)*

CGP-42446A; Zoledronato disódico. Disodium dihydrogen (1-hydroxy-2-imidazol-1-ylethylidene)diphosphonate tetrahydrate.

$C_5H_8N_2Na_2O_7P_2,4H_2O$ = 388.1.

*CAS — 165800-07-7.*

*ATC — M05BA08.*

### Zoledronate Trisodium *(BANM, USAN, rINNM)*

CGP-42446B; Zoledronato trisódico. Trisodium hydrogen (1-hydroxy-2-imidazol-1-ylethylidene)diphosphonate hydrate (5:2).

$C_5H_7N_2Na_3O_7P_2,2\frac{1}{2}H_2O$ = 383.1.

*CAS — 165800-08-8.*

*ATC — M05BA08.*

### Adverse Effects and Precautions

As for Pamidronate, p.773. It is important to ensure adequate hydration before and after administration of zoledronic acid.

**Effects on the eyes.** For reports of ocular effects with bisphosphonates, including zoledronate, see p.767.

**Effects on the kidneys.** Renal failure has been associated with the aminobisphosphonates, see under Bisphosphonates, p.767.

### Interactions

As for the bisphosphonates in general, p.767.

### Pharmacokinetics

After intravenous doses of zoledronic acid, about 23 to 55% of the dose is excreted in the urine unchanged, while the remainder is mainly adsorbed onto bone and only very slowly eliminated. Renal clearance is slower in patients with severe renal impairment (see Administration in renal impairment, below).

◊ References.


1. Chen T, *et al.* Pharmacokinetics and pharmacodynamics of zoledronic acid in cancer patients with bone metastases. *J Clin Pharmacol* 2002; **42:** 1228–36.


### Uses and Administration

Zoledronic acid is an aminobisphosphonate (p.766) that is a potent inhibitor of bone resorption. It is used for **hypercalcaemia of malignancy**, in a single dose of 4 mg administered by intravenous infusion over 15 minutes. The treatment may be repeated if necessary after at least 7 days at a dose of 8 mg. In the USA, however, it is stated that individual doses should not exceed 4 mg, because of the increased risk of adverse renal effects, including renal failure, reported in patients who have received doses of 8 mg.

Zoledronic acid is given for the prevention of skeletal events in patients with advanced **bone malignancies** (p.513) at a dose of 4 mg every 3 to 4 weeks. It is also under investigation for various other disorders of increased bone turnover such as Paget's disease of bone and osteoporosis.

◊ References.


1. Arden-Cordone M, *et al.* Antiresorptive effect of a single infusion of microgram quantities of zoledronate in Paget's disease of bone. *Calcif Tissue Int* 1997; **60:** 415–18.
2. Body JJ, *et al.* A dose-finding study of zoledronate in hypercalcemic cancer patients. *J Bone Miner Res* 1999; **14:** 1557–61.
3. Buckler H, *et al.* Single infusion of zoledronate in Paget's disease of bone: a placebo-controlled, dose-ranging study. *Bone* 1999; **24** (suppl): 81S–85S.
4. Major P, *et al.* Zoledronic acid is superior to pamidronate in the treatment of hypercalcemia of malignancy: a pooled analysis of two randomised, controlled clinical trials. *J Clin Oncol* 2001; **19:** 558–67.
5. Reid IR, *et al.* Intravenous zoledronic acid in postmenopausal women with low bone mineral density. *N Engl J Med* 2002; **346:** 653–61.
6. Wellington K, Goa KL. Zoledronic acid: a review of its use in the management of bone metastases and hypercalcaemia of malignancy. *Drugs* 2003; **63:** 417–37.


**Administration in renal impairment.** Despite the fact that renal clearance of zoledronic acid correlates to renal function, a pharmacokinetic study[1] concluded that no dosage adjustment appeared necessary in patients with mild to moderate renal impairment (creatinine clearance 50 to 80 mL/minute, and 10 to 50 mL/minute, respectively). The manufacturer states no adjustment is necessary, but defines the mild to moderate renal impairment in terms of serum creatinine less than 400 micromoles/litre or less than 4.5 mg per 100 mL for patients with hypercalcaemia of malignancy, and as less than 265 micromoles/litre or less than 3 mg per 100 mL in patients with advanced bone malignancies.


1. Skerjanec A, *et al.* The pharmacokinetics and pharmacodynamics of zoledronic acid in cancer patients with varying degrees of renal function. *J Clin Pharmacol* 2003; **43:** 154–62.


### Preparations

**Proprietary Preparations** (details are given in Part 3)
***Arg.:*** Zometa; ***Austral.:*** Zometa; ***Braz.:*** Zometa; ***Canad.:*** Zometa; ***Chile:*** Zometa; ***Denm.:*** Zometa; ***Fin.:*** Zometa; ***Fr.:*** Zometa; ***Ger.:*** Zometa; ***Gr.:*** Zometa; ***Hong Kong:*** Zometa; ***Irl.:*** Zometa; ***Israel:*** Zomera; ***Ital.:*** Zometa; ***Malaysia:*** Zometa; ***Norw.:*** Zometa; ***NZ:*** Zometa; ***Port.:*** Zometa; ***Singapore:*** Zometa; ***Spain:*** Zometa; ***Swed.:*** Zometa; ***Switz.:*** Zometa; ***Thai.:*** Zometa; ***UK:*** Zometa; ***USA:*** Zometa.

# Bronchodilators and Anti-asthma Drugs

This chapter includes many of those drugs used for their bronchodilator or anti-inflammatory properties in the management of reversible airways obstruction, as in asthma and some patients with chronic obstructive pulmonary disease.

The main bronchodilators discussed in this chapter are the sympathomimetic beta agonists (stimulants of beta-adrenoceptors), and the xanthines, primarily theophylline. The antimuscarinic bronchodilators ipratropium and oxitropium are also included. The major class of anti-inflammatory drugs, the corticosteroids, are discussed separately, on p.1068; other drugs considered to act on the processes of airway inflammation and which are included in this section include sodium cromoglicate and its analogues, and the various drugs that act on leukotriene synthesis and receptor binding, on platelet-activating factor (PAF), or on other aspects of the inflammatory cascade.

## Anti-asthma Drug Groups

**Antimuscarinics.** The parasympathetic nervous system plays a role in the regulation of bronchomotor tone, and antimuscarinic drugs have bronchodilator properties. The quaternary ammonium compounds ipratropium bromide and oxitropium bromide are the main antimuscarinic (anticholinergic) bronchodilators in current use; as well as reduced CNS effects they have less effect on mucociliary clearance than drugs such as atropine, which can produce accumulation of viscid lower airway secretions and a risk of mucus plugging in these patients. An antimuscarinic may be the bronchodilator of choice in the management of chronic obstructive pulmonary disease. In patients with asthma they are usually reserved for use in life-threatening acute asthma exacerbations.

Described in this chapter are


Ipratropium, p.787
Oxitropium, p.790
Tiotropium, p.806


**Beta agonists.** The sympathetic nervous system plays a role in the regulation of bronchomotor tone and beta$_2$-adrenoceptors in bronchial smooth muscle produce bronchodilatation when stimulated. This makes short-acting selective agonists of beta$_2$-adrenoceptors (beta$_2$ agonists; beta$_2$ stimulants), of which salbutamol is the paradigmatic example, first-line drugs for the relief of asthma symptoms. They are also widely used in the management of chronic obstructive pulmonary disease, although antimuscarinic bronchodilators may be preferred or used in addition. Long-acting beta$_2$ agonists are used in asthma in patients also requiring anti-inflammatory therapy.

Described in this chapter are


Bambuterol, p.781
Bitolterol, p.781
Clenbuterol, p.784
Fenoterol, p.785
Formoterol, p.786
Hexoprenaline, p.786
Isoetarine, p.787
Levosalbutamol, p.788
Orciprenaline, p.790
Pirbuterol, p.790
Procaterol, p.791
Reproterol, p.791
Rimiterol, p.791
Salbutamol, p.791
Salmeterol, p.795
Terbutaline, p.797
Tretoquinol, p.806
Tulobuterol, p.806


**Corticosteroids.** Corticosteroids are widely used for their anti-inflammatory (glucocorticoid) properties in the management of asthma, and may be beneficial in some patients with chronic obstructive pulmonary disease. Because of the potential adverse effects associated with prolonged systemic corticosteroid therapy, inhalation of corticosteroids with reduced systemic activity is widely employed; oral corticosteroids are preferably only used in short courses, and at relatively low doses, to gain control of the disease. The actions and uses of the corticosteroids are discussed in much greater detail in the section beginning on p.1068.

**Leukotriene inhibitors and antagonists.** Leukotrienes appear to play an important role in the inflammatory process of asthma, and a number of drugs may modify or inhibit this action. Leukotriene synthesis may be prevented by blockade of the enzyme 5-lipoxygenase with inhibitors such as zileuton. Alternatively, leukotriene antagonists such as zafirlukast may be used to block specific receptors (usually those of leukotriene $D_4$) and prevent their activation. These anti-leukotriene drugs have a role in the prophylactic management of asthma as an alternative when inhaled corticosteroids cannot be used in mild asthma, and as add-on therapy in more severe asthma.

Described in this chapter are


Amlexanox, p.781
Ibudilast, p.786
Montelukast, p.788
Pemirolast, p.790
Pranlukast, p.791
Zafirlukast, p.807
Zileuton, p.807


**Mast cell stabilisers.** The role of the mast cell in initiating an inflammatory cascade has long been recognised as important, and the best established of the mast cell stabilisers are sodium cromoglicate and nedocromil sodium. These compounds inhibit mast cell degranulation in response to antigens or other stimuli, and hence prevent the release of histamine, leukotrienes, and other inflammatory mediators. They are generally well tolerated and guidelines for the treatment of asthma mention their use for prophylactic therapy as an alternative, or a supplement, to corticosteroids, particularly in children. However, it is generally considered that the corticosteroids are more effective.

Described in this chapter are


Amlexanox, p.781
Ketotifen, p.788
Nedocromil, p.789
Pemirolast, p.790
Repirinast, p.791
Sodium Cromoglicate, p.795
Tranilast, p.806


**Xanthines.** Xanthines are drugs with complex actions that include, in varying degrees, relaxation of bronchial smooth muscle and relief of bronchospasm, as well as stimulant effects on respiration. Theophylline and its derivatives have long been used for their bronchodilator properties in the management of asthma and chronic obstructive pulmonary disease, but the narrow therapeutic range and the propensity for interactions with other drugs make theophylline a difficult drug to use, and it tends to be reserved for combination therapy in patients who cannot be managed with other bronchodilators (such as the beta$_2$ agonists) plus inhaled corticosteroids.

Described in this chapter are


Aminophylline, p.780
Bamifylline, p.781
Bufylline, p.781
Caffeine, p.782
Choline Theophyllinate, p.784
Diprophylline, p.784
Doxofylline, p.785
Etamiphylline Camsilate, p.785
Etofylline, p.785
Heptaminol Acefyllinate, p.786
Proxyphylline, p.791
Pyridofylline, p.791
Theobromine, p.798
Theophylline, p.798


## Management of Reversible Airways Obstruction

### Asthma

Asthma is a chronic inflammatory disease in which the patient suffers episodes of reversible airways obstruction due to bronchial hyperresponsiveness; in a few patients, inflammation may lead to irreversible obstruction. It is a common disorder occurring in about 5% of the adult population and more than 10% of children in developed countries. Fatalities can occur.[1]

The aetiology of asthma is poorly understood, but both genetic and environmental factors are believed to contribute to initiation and progression of the disease.[1,2] Resistance to airflow in asthma is increased by a number of abnormalities, including contraction of the airway smooth muscle, the presence of excessive secretions within the airway lumen, and inflammatory cell infiltration. The inflammation in chronic asthma causes remodelling, found as shedding and thickening of the airway epithelium, and hypertrophy and hyperplasia of smooth muscle.[1,2] Asthma may be described as extrinsic when it is associated with exposure to a specific allergen such as pollen or house-dust mite, or to a non-specific stimulus such as a chemical irritant or exercise. It may be described as intrinsic when no external precipitating factor is identifiable.

The principal symptoms of asthma are wheezing, dyspnoea (breathlessness), chest tightness, and cough, and these symptoms tend to be variable, intermittent, worse at night, and provoked by particular triggers. In an acute attack, the respiratory rate is rapid and tachycardia is common.[3,4] The peak expiratory flow (PEF) and forced expiratory volume in the first second ($FEV_1$) are decreased in asthma, and in a severe asthmatic attack the PEF is generally less than 50% of predicted values. Life-threatening features include exhaustion, cyanosis, bradycardia, hypotension, confusion, and coma.[3,4]

**Management of asthma**. As asthma is a chronic disease, management involves prophylactic measures to reduce inflammation and airway resistance and to maintain airflow, as well as specific regimens for the treatment of acute attacks. Measurements of lung function play an important part in determining treatment and patients are encouraged to monitor their own disease by using a simple peak flow meter to measure PEF and adjust their therapy accordingly.[3-5]

The standard drugs used in the management of asthma are the beta$_2$ agonists and corticosteroids.[3,4,6] Therapy is preferably given by inhalation to deliver the drugs to the desired site of action. This permits smaller dosages than would be required with oral administration, with a consequent reduction in side-effects. Systematic reviews[7,8] have found that hand-held inhaler devices including pressurised metered-dose inhalers, dry powder inhalers, and breath actuated pressurised metered-dose inhalers, are generally equally effective for the delivery of short-acting beta$_2$ agonists and corticosteroids in stable asthma. Spacer devices can be fitted to some metered-dose inhalers to act as reservoirs for the drug to make it easier for the patient to inhale each dose correctly. There is increasing use of metered-dose inhalers with spacer devices, and nebulisers tend to be reserved for patients who are unable or unwilling to use these devices, although the choice of spacer and method of use may substantially affect drug delivery.[9] A large volume spacer device is recommended for the inhalation of high doses of corticosteroids to reduce oropharyngeal deposition and systemic absorption.[3] Specially adapted or modified inhalation devices, as well as spacer devices, are also available to enable children to achieve a correct technique when using inhaled drug therapy, but alternative routes of delivery such as oral administration or nebulisation may be necessary for some infants and small children.[9]

*Beta$_2$ agonists* relax the bronchial smooth muscle to produce bronchodilatation by selectively stimulating beta$_2$-adrenergic receptors. Short-acting beta$_2$ agonists such as salbutamol or terbutaline are the initial drugs of choice for acute bronchospasm; if inhaled, they can have an almost immediate bronchodilating effect. The epidemics of increased asthma mortality associated with inhaled beta agonists (see under Fenoterol, p.785) receded some time ago and since then the way in which these compounds are used has changed. Doses have fallen and selective agonists are preferred (nonselective beta agonists such as isoprenaline no longer have a role), and there has been a change from regular use to use as required. Regular use of beta$_2$ agonists is mainly restricted to 'long-acting' beta$_2$ agonists such as salmeterol xinafoate in patients also requiring anti-inflammatory prophylactic treatment; a 'short-acting' beta$_2$ agonist should still be used as required.[3-5]

*Corticosteroids* are the most effective preventer therapy available for the management of asthma. They are used for their anti-inflammatory properties and to reduce bronchial hyperresponsiveness; they must be taken regularly to achieve maximum benefit. Corticosteroid therapy is recommended both for acute attacks and chronic asthma prophylaxis. Although the use of corticosteroids for the treatment of acute asthma attacks has been questioned,[10] meta-analysis suggests that they do speed the resolution of exacerbations and reduce the rate of relapse.[11,12]

In addition, *xanthines* such as aminophylline or theophylline, and *antimuscarinics* such as ipratropium bromide or oxitropium bromide may be given for their bronchodilating properties; there is disagreement concerning xanthine use in addition to bronchodilating therapy with beta$_2$ agonists for the management of acute severe asthma (see below). *Cromoglicate or nedocromil* may be used as an alternative to corticosteroids for the prophylaxis of less severe asthma or combined with other therapy. *Anti-leukotrienes* such as zafirlukast and zileuton are another alternative or adjunct to inhaled corticosteroids.

**Chronic asthma**. Advice for patients with chronic asthma includes avoidance of smoking, of allergens such as pollen, and of bronchoconstricting drugs such as beta blockers. Patients who have had asthma induced by aspirin and NSAIDs should also avoid these drugs. Skin testing to determine allergen sensitivity may be advisable. US guidelines[3] suggest consideration of immunotherapy to desensitise patients with poorly controlled disease unavoidably exposed to a precipitating allergen, but evidence of benefit from this approach is ambiguous, particularly for multiple allergen immunotherapy, and the potential adverse effects make it controversial (see under Allergen Immunotherapy, p.1650). UK guidelines[4] consider that although there is evidence of benefit from immunotherapy when compared with placebo, comparative studies with other asthma treatments are needed. Gastro-oesophageal reflux has been suggested as another exacerbating factor, but this has been disputed[13] and a review of acid suppressive therapy concluded this did not benefit asthma in most patients.[14]

Guidelines for drug therapy of chronic asthma have been issued in the UK[4] and in the USA[3,5] and are broadly similar. They provide for a stepwise approach, obtaining initial control with the early use of anti-inflammatory drugs at doses most appropriate for the severity of disease, and subsequently 'stepping-down' therapy as far as possible. Treatment strategies for the management of asthma in infants and young children are similar to those outlined for adults and older children though some modifications are usually made.

The recommendations for **adults and children over 5 years of age** with chronic asthma are as follows.

- Patients requiring only occasional relief from symptoms may be adequately managed with an inhaled short-acting beta$_2$ agonist such as salbutamol or terbutaline taken when needed, provided this is not more than once daily (Step 1; mild intermittent asthma).
- If the beta$_2$ agonist is required more than two or three times a week then regular inhalation of a corticosteroid such as beclometasone dipropionate or budesonide (100 to 400 micrograms twice daily) or fluticasone (50 to 200 micrograms twice daily) should be added. *Alternatives* are cromoglicate or nedocromil, anti-leukotrienes, or sustained-release oral theophylline, but these are less effective (Step 2; mild persistent asthma).
- If adequate control is not achieved, the preferred treatment is to supplement low-dose inhaled corticosteroids with a long-acting inhaled beta$_2$ agonist such as salmeterol xinafoate (Step 3; moderate persistent asthma). At this stage there are slight differences of emphasis between US and UK guidelines, but essentially, if a long-acting inhaled beta$_2$ agonist cannot be used, or there is only suboptimal or no response, there are a number of options either in addition to the long-acting inhaled beta$_2$ agonist or as an alternative: the inhaled corticosteroid can be increased to moderate doses such as 800 micrograms of beclometasone or budesonide, or 400 micrograms of fluticasone, daily (or 400 and 200 micrograms daily for children, respectively); another preventer therapy such as an anti-leukotriene, modified-release oral theophylline, or a modified-release oral beta$_2$ agonist for adults can be added; or both can be combined.
- For patients with persistent poor control of asthma despite use of inhaled moderate-dose corticosteroids and an additional drug (usually a long-acting inhaled beta$_2$ agonist), the next treatment option is to use high-dose inhaled corticosteroids (2000 micrograms of beclometasone or budesonide, or 1000 micrograms of fluticasone, daily for adults; 800 and 400 micrograms daily for children, respectively) (Step 4; severe persistent asthma). The UK guidelines also suggest trials of anti-leukotrienes, modified-release oral theophylline, or oral modified-release beta$_2$ agonists, as alternatives.
- If further control is needed, then a corticosteroid such as prednisolone may also be given by mouth in single daily doses (UK Step 5; US guidelines consider this part of Step 4).

A short 'rescue' course of oral prednisolone 30 to 60 mg may also be needed at any time and at any step for an acute exacerbation.

Treatment should be reviewed every 3 to 6 months and if the asthma is adequately controlled a stepwise reduction in treatment may be possible.

Recommendations for the management of chronic asthma in **children under 5 years of age** have also been issued in the UK[4] and USA.[3,5] There is limited information available for this age group, however, and some recommendations are based on extrapolations from studies in older children and adults. These guidelines also provide a stepwise approach to management.

- Step 1 involves the use of an inhaled short-acting beta$_2$ agonist as required, but not more than once daily.
- Should that not provide control, an inhaled corticosteroid is added (beclometasone or budesonide in doses of 200 to 400 micrograms daily, or fluticasone 100 to 200 micrograms daily). If a corticosteroid cannot be used, alternatives to be considered are anti-leukotrienes or, in the USA, cromoglicate (Step 2).
- If further control is necessary, UK guidelines recommend the addition of an anti-leukotriene to inhaled corticosteroids, for patients aged 2 to 5 years (those under 2 may be referred to a respiratory paediatrician). In the USA, the preferred treatment is to add an inhaled long-acting beta$_2$ agonist to a low-dose inhaled corticosteroid, or to raise the dose of the corticosteroid to moderate doses. *Alternatively*, an anti-leukotriene or theophylline could be added to low-dose inhaled corticosteroids, and for patients with recurring severe exacerbations, moderate doses of corticosteroids may be combined with one of these other drugs (Step 3).
- Further increasing the inhaled corticosteroid dose is then recommended, with an inhaled long-acting beta$_2$ agonist (US Step 4).

Similarly to adults and older children, a short course of oral prednisolone (1 to 2 mg/kg daily) may be needed for acute exacerbations of asthma. There is some evidence[15] to suggest that lower doses of prednisolone (500 micrograms/kg daily) may be as effective.

Treatment should be regularly reviewed and reduced in a stepwise manner if asthma is well controlled.

**Acute severe asthma** (status asthmaticus). An acute attack of severe asthma is potentially life-threatening and treatment should be instituted as soon as possible. UK guidelines provide guidance on the assessment and initial treatment of exacerbations of asthma in general practice and in the accident and emergency department. Acute severe attacks require admission to hospital, and the guidelines suggest the following regimen for the hospital management of **adults**.[4]

- Initially, oxygen should be given at the highest concentration available (40 to 60%) with a high flow rate.
- High doses of inhaled beta$_2$ agonists, such as salbutamol 5 mg or terbutaline 10 mg, should be administered via a nebuliser with oxygen or compressed air if oxygen is not available, or if neither of these is available, by multiple actuations of a metered-dose inhaler into a large spacer device.
- High doses of systemic corticosteroids are also required: for example, prednisolone 40 to 50 mg by mouth or hydrocortisone 100 mg intravenously, or both.
- If life-threatening features are present, or the initial response to beta$_2$ agonists is poor, ipratropium bromide (500 micrograms) can be added to the nebuliser. A single intravenous dose of magnesium sulfate (1.2 to 2 g infused over 20 minutes) may also be considered at this stage. The role of magnesium sulfate has not been fully established, however, and results of clinical studies have been conflicting. A meta-analysis concluded that its routine use was not justified, but that it might benefit some patients with severe exacerbations.[16]
- Subsequently, oxygen therapy should be continued as should corticosteroid treatment (prednisolone 40 to 50 mg daily by mouth or hydrocortisone 100 mg every 6 hours intravenously).
- Nebulised beta$_2$ agonists may be given every 4 to 6 hours. If the patient's condition has not improved after 15 to 30 minutes, the nebulised beta$_2$ agonist should be given more frequently (up to every 15 minutes, or in a continuous regimen such as salbutamol 10 mg continuously hourly) and ipratropium bromide (500 micrograms every 4 to 6 hours) added.
- If progress is still unsatisfactory, then an infusion of aminophylline (5 mg/kg over 20 minutes then 500 to 700 micrograms/kg per hour, monitoring blood concentrations if continued for more than 24 hours; the loading dose should not be given to patients already on maintenance oral therapy), or a parenteral beta$_2$ agonist may be considered, although there is limited evidence to support the routine use of either of these drugs.
- Patients who deteriorate further with drowsiness, unconsciousness, or respiratory arrest need intermittent positive-pressure ventilation.

Once lung function is stabilised the patient can be discharged taking oral prednisolone, inhaled corticosteroids, and bronchodilators.

UK guidelines suggest the following regimen for **children**.

- Immediate treatment involves the administration of oxygen, nebulised beta$_2$ agonists, and oral prednisolone (20 mg daily in children aged 2 to 5 years, and 30 to 40 mg daily in those more than 5 years of age, usually for up to 3 days; children already receiving maintenance oral corticosteroids should receive 2 mg/kg up to a maximum of 60 mg daily).
- If life-threatening features are present, or response to beta$_2$ agonists is poor, nebulised ipratropium bromide (250 micrograms) and intravenous hydrocortisone (4 mg/kg every 4 hours) may be added. Further treatment options to consider are intravenous salbutamol (15 micrograms/kg over 10 minutes followed by an infusion of 1 to 5 micrograms/kg per minute); intravenous aminophylline (5 mg/kg over 20 minutes then 1 mg/kg per hour; aminophylline should not be used before hospital admission, and the loading dose should not be given in children already receiving oral theophylline); and, for children more than 5 years of age, a single intravenous dose of magnesium sulfate (40 mg/kg to a maximum of 2 g over 20 minutes).

Subsequent management follows a similar routine to that in adults.

In the USA guidelines for acute severe asthma in adults and children are slightly different.[3] Although subcutaneous adrenaline or terbutaline has been used in the management of acute severe asthma, the guidelines suggest that the parenteral use of beta$_2$ agonists is of unproven value. Moreover, in contrast to the UK the intravenous administration of xanthines is not recommended. In compiling the UK guidelines the British Thoracic Society has taken the view that although most patients on maximal doses of nebulised beta$_2$ agonists and corticosteroids derive no additional benefit from intravenous aminophylline, some could obtain additional bronchodilatation; intravenous aminophylline was therefore recommended for patients with life-threatening unresponsive acute asthma attacks;[4] some trials in children support this.[17,18] In contrast, the most recent US guidelines issued by the National Asthma Education and Prevention Program do not recommend the use of xanthines as they are considered to offer no benefit over the optimal use of inhaled beta$_2$ agonists.[3] In consequence, in the US guidelines patients whose asthma cannot be managed with oxygen, inhaled beta$_2$ agonists and antimuscarinics, and systemic corticosteroids are suggested as candidates for intubation and mechanical ventilation. There have been mixed results from studies of the addition of antimuscarinics to beta$_2$ agonist therapy in acute asthma, and systematic reviews of trials in adults[19] and children[20] have been published. A review,[21] which included these and further controlled studies, concluded that the addition of multiple doses of inhaled ipratropium bromide provided additional improvement in lung function for patients with severe acute asthma, but that single-dose treatment was less effective in severe asthma and of no benefit in mild to moderate asthma.

**Investigational therapy**. A number of other therapeutic approaches for the management of asthma are currently under investigation.[22] Immunomodulators such as methotrexate, ciclosporin, and gold have been used for their anti-inflammatory, immunosuppressant, and corticosteroid-sparing properties: their use must be balanced against their potentially serious adverse effects and they are therefore reserved for individual patients with chronic severe asthma dependent on systemic corticosteroid therapy.[23]

Interestingly, furosemide administered by inhalation has been found to protect against bronchoconstriction induced by exercise[24] and external stimuli,[25,26] but was not effective in improving bronchial hyperresponsiveness in a 4-week study,[27] and provided no additional benefit when added to salbutamol for the treatment of acute asthma in a small study in children.[28] Any clinical application has yet to be determined.[22] There has been some interest in heparin given by inhalation,[22,29,30] and nebulised lidocaine may be of some benefit;[22,31,32] intravenous lidocaine or oral mexiletine have been shown to block reflex bronchoconstriction.[33]

There is increasing study of the cellular mechanisms of inflammation in asthma and ways of controlling them. Phosphodiesterase type-4 is an enzyme that hydrolyses cyclic adenosine monophosphate (cyclic AMP), stimulating the release of acute inflammatory mediators and immune responses; it is found in airways smooth muscle, pulmonary nerves, and inflammatory and immune cells relevant to the pathogenesis of asthma. Phosphodiesterase type-4 inhibitors are under investigation for their anti-inflammatory and bronchodilator activity.[34] The thromboxane $A_2$ antagonist, seratrodast, is being tried for its effects on pulmonary function and mucus secretion. Interleukin-4 is a cytokine that stimulates a range of inflammatory processes in asthma, and soluble recombinant interleukin-4 receptor (IL-4R; rhuIL-4R) is being investigated[35] as an antagonist to bind and neutralise interleukin-4. Anti-IgE therapies are being studied in allergen-induced asthma; the monoclonal antibody omalizumab[36] is available for use in selected patients.

There have been some studies of the use of helium-oxygen mixtures in acute asthma. These mixtures have a lower density than air and so could reduce airway resistance and respiratory work, and improve deposition of nebulised bronchodilators. However, a systematic review[37] of 7 trials concluded that evidence to support the use of helium-oxygen mixtures in moderate to severe exacerbations of asthma was lacking.

**Pregnancy**. It is particularly important that asthma should be well controlled during pregnancy; where this is achieved asthma has no important effects on pregnancy, labour, or the fetus.[4,38]

Inhalation has particular advantages as a means of drug administration during pregnancy because the therapeutic action can be achieved without the need for plasma drug concentrations liable to have a pharmacological effect on the fetus. Systemic treatment should not be withheld if indicated, however, although there is insufficient information to support the use of anti-leukotrienes, except as continued treatment in women who were taking these before pregnancy for asthma not controlled by other medications.[4]

Severe exacerbations can have an adverse effect on pregnancy and should be treated promptly with conventional therapy, including oral or parenteral administration of corticosteroids, oxygen, and nebulisation of a $beta_2$ agonist.[4] Prednisolone is a suitable corticosteroid for oral use since very little of the drug reaches the fetus.[38]

1. Tattersfield AE, *et al.* Asthma. *Lancet* 2002; **360:** 1313–22.
2. Busse WW, Lemanske RF. Asthma. *N Engl J Med* 2001; **344:** 350–62.
3. National Asthma Education and Prevention Program. *Expert Panel Report 2: guidelines for the diagnosis and management of asthma.* Bethesda: National Heart, Lung, and Blood Institute, 1997. Available at: http://www.nhlbi.nih.gov/guidelines/asthma/asthgdln.pdf (accessed 20/04/04)
4. Scottish Intercollegiate Guidelines Network/The British Thoracic Society. British guideline on the management of asthma. *Thorax* 2003; **58** (suppl 1): i1–i94. Revised edition April 2004 available at: http://www.sign.ac.uk/pdf/sign63.pdf (accessed 21/04/04)
5. National Asthma Education and Prevention Program. Expert Panel Report: guidelines for the diagnosis and management of asthma update on selected topics—2002. *J Allergy Clin Immunol* 2002; **110** (suppl): S141–S219. Also available at: http://www2.us.elsevierhealth.com/scripts/om.dll/serve?action=searchDB&searchDBfor=iss&id=jai021105b (accessed 20/04/04)
6. Lipworth BJ. Modern drug treatment of chronic asthma. *BMJ* 1999; **318:** 380–4.
7. Brocklebank D, *et al.* Systematic review of clinical effectiveness of pressurised metered dose inhalers versus other hand held inhaler devices for delivering corticosteroids in asthma. *BMJ* 2001; **323:** 896–900.
8. Ram FSF, *et al.* Pressurised metered dose inhalers versus all other hand-held inhaler devices to deliver beta-2 agonist bronchodilators for non-acute asthma. Available in The Cochrane Library; Issue 1. Chichester: John Wiley; 2004.
9. O'Callaghan C, Barry PW. How to choose delivery devices for asthma. *Arch Dis Child* 2000; **82:** 185–7.
10. McFadden ER, Hejal R. Asthma. *Lancet* 1995; **345:** 1215–20.
11. Rowe BH, *et al.* Early emergency department treatment of acute asthma with systemic corticosteroids. Available in The Cochrane Library; Issue 1. Chichester: John Wiley; 2004.
12. Rowe BH, *et al.* Corticosteroids for preventing relapse following acute exacerbations of asthma. Available in The Cochrane Library; Issue 1. Chichester: John Wiley; 2004.
13. Field SK. A critical review of the studies of the effects of simulated or real gastroesophageal reflux on pulmonary function in asthmatic adults. *Chest* 1999; **115:** 848–56.
14. Coughlan JL, *et al.* Medical treatment for reflux oesophagitis does not consistently improve asthma control: a systematic review. *Thorax* 2001; **56:** 198–204.
15. Langton Hewer S, *et al.* Prednisolone in acute childhood asthma: clinical responses to three dosages. *Respir Med* 1998; **92:** 541–6.
16. Rowe BH, *et al.* Magnesium sulfate for treating exacerbations of acute asthma in the emergency department. Available in The Cochrane Library; Issue 1. Chichester: John Wiley; 2004.
17. Yung M, South M. Randomised controlled trial of aminophylline for severe acute asthma. *Arch Dis Child* 1998; **79:** 405–10.
18. Ream RS, *et al.* Efficacy of IV theophylline in children with severe status asthmaticus. *Chest* 2001; **119:** 1480–8.
19. Stoodley RG, *et al.* The role of ipratropium bromide in the emergency management of acute asthma exacerbation: a metaanalysis of randomized clinical trials. *Ann Emerg Med* 1999; **34:** 8–18.
20. Plotnick LH, Ducharme FM. Combined inhaled anticholinergics and beta2-agonists for initial treatment of acute asthma in children. Available in The Cochrane Library; Issue 1. Chichester: John Wiley; 2004.
21. Rodrigo GJ, Rodrigo C. The role of anticholinergics in acute asthma treatment: an evidence-based evaluation. *Chest* 2002; **121:** 1977–87.
22. Floreani AA, Rennard SI. Experimental treatments for asthma. *Curr Opin Pulm Med* 1997; **3:** 30–41.
23. Kon OM, Barnes N. Immunosuppressive treatment in asthma. *Br J Hosp Med* 1997; **57:** 383–6.
24. Munyard P, *et al.* Inhaled frusemide and exercise-induced bronchoconstriction in children with asthma. *Thorax* 1995; **50:** 677–9.
25. Bianco S, *et al.* Protective effect of inhaled furosemide on allergen-induced early and late asthmatic reactions. *N Engl J Med* 1989; **321:** 1069–73.
26. Seidenberg J, *et al.* Inhaled frusemide against cold air induced bronchoconstriction in asthmatic children. *Arch Dis Child* 1992; **67:** 214–17.
27. Yates DH, *et al.* Effect of acute and chronic inhaled furosemide on bronchial hyperresponsiveness in mild asthma. *Am J Respir Crit Care Med* 1995; **152:** 2173–5.
28. González-Sánchez R, *et al.* Furosemide plus albuterol compared with albuterol alone in children with acute asthma. *Allergy Asthma Proc* 2002; **23:** 181–4.
29. Diamant Z, *et al.* Effect of inhaled heparin on allergen-induced early and late asthmatic responses in patients with atopic asthma. *Am J Respir Crit Care Med* 1996; **153:** 1790–5.
30. Tutluoğlu B, *et al.* Effects of heparin on hypertonic potassium chloride—induced bronchoconstriction. *Ann Pharmacother* 2001; **35:** 1161–5.
31. Hunt LW, *et al.* Effect of nebulized lidocaine on severe glucocorticoid-dependent asthma. *Mayo Clin Proc* 1996; **71:** 361–8.
32. Decco ML, *et al.* Nebulized lidocaine in the treatment of severe asthma in children: a pilot study. *Ann Allergy Asthma Immunol* 1999; **82:** 29–32.
33. Groeben H, *et al.* Intravenous lidocaine and oral mexiletine block reflex bronchoconstriction in asthmatic subjects. *Am J Respir Crit Care Med* 1996; **154:** 885–8.
34. Giembycz MA. Phosphodiesterase 4 inhibitors and the treatment of asthma: where are we now and where do we go from here? *Drugs* 2000; **59:** 193–212.
35. Steinke JW, Borish L. Th2 cytokines and asthma: interleukin-4: its role in the pathogenesis of asthma, and targeting it for asthma treatment with interleukin-4 receptor antagonists. *Respir Res* 2001; **2:** 66–70.
36. Easthope S, Jarvis B. Omalizumab. *Drugs* 2001; **61:** 253–60.
37. Rodrigo GJ, *et al.* Use of helium-oxygen mixtures in the treatment of acute asthma: a systematic review. *Chest* 2003; **123:** 891–6.
38. Nelson-Piercy C. Asthma in pregnancy. *Thorax* 2001; **56:** 325–8.

### Chronic obstructive pulmonary disease

Chronic obstructive pulmonary disease (COPD, chronic obstructive lung disease, chronic obstructive airways disease) covers a range of disorders of progressive airflow limitation including chronic bronchitis and emphysema. Unlike asthma, the obstruction of airflow, indicated by an abnormal decline in the forced expiratory volume in one second ($FEV_1$), is more or less continuous and largely irreversible. Chronic obstructive pulmonary disease is a common disorder, frequently associated with cigarette smoking; infections, environmental pollution, and occupational dust exposure may also have an aetiological role.

- In *chronic bronchitis* there is enlargement of the mucous glands and an increase in the number of goblet cells within the bronchial mucosa, which leads to an increase in mucus production and thickening of the bronchial wall. Patients suffer from a chronic productive cough with excessive sputum production. They may also experience dyspnoea, bronchospasm, and frequent respiratory-tract infections. In severe cases (chronic obstructive bronchitis, small airways disease), irreversible narrowing of the airways leads to a disabling condition in which there is cyanosis, hypoxia, hypercapnia, and right-sided heart failure (cor pulmonale, see below); such patients have been described as 'blue bloaters'.
- *Emphysema* is an abnormal permanent enlargement of air spaces distal to the terminal bronchioles accompanied by destruction of the alveolar wall and without obvious fibrosis. There is excessive airway collapse upon expiration and irreversible airways obstruction. Dyspnoea is a prominent symptom; a productive cough, wheezing, recurrent respiratory infection, and a marked loss of weight may also be noted. Patients may hyperventilate to maintain oxygen levels in the blood and have been called 'pink puffers' in contrast to the 'blue bloaters' of the classic bronchitic presentation. Rarely, emphysema can be caused by a hereditary deficiency of $alpha_1$ antitrypsin ($alpha_1$-proteinase inhibitor), see p.1651.
- Patients with severe COPD can develop *cor pulmonale* (heart disease secondary to disease of the lungs and respiratory system) with pulmonary hypertension, right ventricular hypertrophy, and right heart failure.[1] Cor pulmonale is more often associated with chronic bronchitis than with emphysema.

**Management of COPD**. Although there is less consensus than for asthma, guidelines for the treatment of COPD have been issued in a number of countries.[2-4] The most important therapeutic intervention is encouraging those patients who smoke to stop; psychological support and adjunctive drug therapy may be required (see Smoking Cessation, p.1721). Prevention of respiratory infection should be considered, and influenza vaccination is recommended.[2-4] Pneumococcal vaccination has also been recommended,[3,4] although its value in these patients has not been unequivocally established.[2]

Drug treatment is primarily symptomatic and palliative using bronchodilators, corticosteroids, and oxygen therapy. Purulent sputum indicates a respiratory infection (see under Exacerbations, below).

First-line drug therapy for the treatment of COPD consists of bronchodilators to alleviate bronchospasm and any reversible component of the airways obstruction. Either an inhaled *antimuscarinic*, such as ipratropium bromide, or a short-acting *$beta_2$ agonist*, is suggested as the initial bronchodilator.[2-4] $Beta_2$ agonists, have a more rapid action, but there is some suggestion that antimuscarinics have a more prolonged effect.[2] Nevertheless, patients vary in their responsiveness and a $beta_2$ agonist should be tried in those who do not respond well to an antimuscarinic, and vice versa.[2] In mild disease inhaled bronchodilators can be used on an as-needed basis.[2-4] In moderate and more severe disease, therapeutic options include the regular use of these bronchodilators either alone[2,3] or in combination,[2-4] or the addition of long-acting bronchodilators such as the $beta_2$ agonist salmeterol or the antimuscarinic tiotropium.[2,4] A *xanthine* such as theophylline by mouth may also be considered and has been given in addition to inhaled agents.[2,4,5] Theophylline has been reported to improve respiratory muscle function in patients with COPD and may have positive cardiac inotropic effects which could be of value in cor pulmonale.

Meta-analysis has suggested that only about 10% of COPD patients receiving optimal bronchodilator therapy exhibit a substantial further response to oral *corticosteroids*.[6] Some guidelines[3] recommend that patients requiring frequent bronchodilator therapy should receive a trial of prednisolone 20 to 50 mg daily by mouth for 2 weeks; an increase in $FEV_1$ of more than 15% from baseline is considered evidence of responsiveness. In patients showing an objective response, these guidelines suggest the continued use of corticosteroids, preferably by the inhaled route as this is associated with fewer adverse effects. However, a large study[7] found that the response to such a trial of oral prednisolone was unrelated to the change in $FEV_1$ and health status over the following 3 years of treatment with either inhaled fluticasone or placebo. Other guidelines[2,4] have therefore concluded that a short course of oral corticosteroid is a poor predictor of long-term response to inhaled therapy, and do not recommend this assessment. Whether corticosteroids improve the long-term outcome of COPD remains to be confirmed. Inhaled corticosteroids have been reported to reduce the rate of exacerbation.[8] However, meta-analyses using essentially the same studies have come to different conclusions regarding the effect, if any, on the rate of decline in $FEV_1$. One analysis[9] found no association, while another[10] reported that inhaled corticosteroids slowed the rate of decline, and that high-dose regimens had a greater effect. Guidelines[2-4] recommend regular treatment with inhaled corticosteroids for symptomatic patients with severe disease and repeated exacerbations of COPD.

In patients with severe COPD and persistent hypoxaemia, supplemental *oxygen* provided on an almost continuous long-term basis at home has been found to improve survival and alleviate complications such as cor pulmonale, polycythaemia and neuropsychological impairment.[11,12] Guidelines recommend the institution of oxygen therapy in patients whose resting $PaO_2$ is less than 55 mmHg (about 7.3 kPa), or whose arterial-oxygen saturation is less than about 90%.[2-4] Non-invasive nocturnal ventilation (via a mask) may be of benefit in some patients.[13]

The use of *mucolytics* or *expectorants* is controversial. Although meta-analysis has suggested a modest benefit in reducing exacerbations,[14] and some guidelines[4] allow for the use of mucolytics, other guidelines[2,3] do not consider there to be sufficient evidence to recommend them. Improved pulmonary function has been reported in patients given aerosolised surfactant.[15]

*Surgery* may be used in selected patients with end-stage disease who remain symptomatic despite optimal medical treatment. Bullectomy may be used in emphysema to remove a large bulla that does not contribute to gas exchange.[2,4,16] Lung transplantation (p.1347) may be used in very advanced COPD,[2,4] particularly in patients with idiopathic emphysema or $alpha_1$ antitrypsin deficiency.[16] In severe emphysema with hyperinflation and obvious target areas, lung volume reduction surgery is being investigated;[2,16] it may be a better option than medical therapy to reduce mortality in patients with predominantly upper-lobe disease and low exercise capacity.[4,17]

*Investigational* approaches to COPD include blocking various mediators of the inflammatory processes with, for example, inhibitors of phosphodiesterase, neutrophil elastase, and matrix metalloproteinases.[18]

**Exacerbations**. Patients with COPD frequently suffer acute exacerbations of their symptoms, and may require hospitalisation. Treatment options include maximal bronchodilators, antibacterials, systemic corticosteroids, and oxygen as necessary, with appropriate management of any associated cardiovascular disorder.[2-4,19,20] Systemic corticosteroids are widely used, despite limited evidence of clinical benefit. Studies[21,22] of severe acute exacerbation requiring hospitalisation have found systemic corticosteroids to improve lung function and reduce the length of hospital stay. However, the most effective dose and duration of treatment is yet to be established,[23] although one study[21] found that a 2-week course was as effective as a longer course of 8 weeks. There is also no evidence of long-term benefit.[21,22] The use of *antibacterials* for acute exacerbations has long been controversial, but meta-analysis suggests that a modest benefit exists,[24] mainly in patients with more severe disease (see also Bronchitis, p.122). Guidelines recommend their use on an empirical basis where signs of infection are present[2-4,19] but do not support prophylactic antibacterial cover for those with recurrent acute exacerbations.[2-4] *Oxygen* therapy is required in patients with hypoxia; the goal is to maintain oxygen saturation above 90% but prevent increasing $CO_2$ retention.[2,4] Relatively low oxygen concentrations (beginning at about 25%) are advised in these generally hypercapnic patients, as high concentrations may impair ventilation and respiratory drive.[3] *Respiratory stimulants* such as doxapram[25] are of limited use but may be considered when non-invasive ventilation is unavailable or inappropriate.[4] Despite intensive therapy, some patients progress to respiratory muscle fatigue and require ventilatory support.


1. Weitzenblum E. Chronic cor pulmonale. *Heart* 2003; **89:** 225–30.
2. NHLBI/WHO global initiative for chronic obstructive lung disease (GOLD) workshop panel. Global strategy for the diagnosis, management, and prevention of chronic obstructive pulmonary disease, updated 2003. Available at: http://www.goldcopd.com/revised.pdf (accessed 20/04/04)
3. Australian Lung Foundation, Thoracic Society of Australia and New Zealand. The COPDX plan: Australian and New Zealand Guidelines for the management of chronic obstructive pulmonary disease 2003. *Med J Aust* 2003; **178** (suppl): S1–S39.
4. The National Collaborating Centre for Chronic Conditions. Chronic obstructive pulmonary disease: national clinical guideline on management of chronic obstructive pulmonary disease in adults in primary and secondary care. *Thorax* 2004; **59** (suppl 1): i1–i232. Also available at: http://www.nice.org.uk/cat.asp?c=104441 (accessed 20/04/04)
5. Ram FSF, *et al.* Oral theophylline for chronic obstructive pulmonary disease. Available in The Cochrane Library; Issue 1. Chichester: John Wiley; 2004.
6. Callahan CM, *et al.* Oral corticosteroid therapy for patients with stable chronic obstructive pulmonary disease. *Ann Intern Med* 1991; **114:** 216–23.
7. Burge PS, *et al.* Prednisolone response in patients with chronic obstructive pulmonary disease: results from the ISOLDE study. *Thorax* 2003; **58:** 654–8.
8. Alsaeedi A, *et al.* The effects of inhaled corticosteroids in chronic obstructive pulmonary disease: a systematic review of randomized placebo-controlled trials. *Am J Med* 2002; **113:** 59–65.
9. Highland KB, *et al.* Long-term effects of inhaled corticosteroids on $FEV_1$ in patients with chronic obstructive pulmonary disease: a meta-analysis. *Ann Intern Med* 2003; **138:** 969–73. Correction. *ibid.*; **139:** 873.
10. Sutherland ER, *et al.* Inhaled corticosteroids reduce the progression of airflow limitation in chronic obstructive pulmonary disease: a meta-analysis. *Thorax* 2003; **58:** 937–41.
11. Medical Research Council Working Party. Long-term domiciliary oxygen therapy in chronic hypoxic cor pulmonale complicating chronic bronchitis and emphysema. *Lancet* 1981; **i:** 681–6.
12. Nocturnal Oxygen Therapy Trial Group. Continuous or nocturnal oxygen therapy in hypoxemic chronic obstructive lung disease: a clinical trial. *Ann Intern Med* 1980; **93:** 391–8.
13. Elliott MW. Non-invasive ventilation in chronic obstructive pulmonary disease. *Br J Hosp Med* 1997; **57:** 83–6.
14. Poole PJ, Black PN. Mucolytic agents for chronic bronchitis or chronic obstructive pulmonary disease. Available in The Cochrane Library; Issue 1. Chichester: John Wiley; 2004.
15. Anzueto A, *et al.* Effects of aerosolized surfactant in patients with stable chronic bronchitis: a prospective randomized controlled trial. *JAMA* 1997; **278:** 1426–31.
16. Meyers BF, Patterson GA. Chronic obstructive pulmonary disease 10: bullectomy, lung volume reduction surgery, and transplantation for patients with chronic obstructive pulmonary disease. *Thorax* 2003; **58:** 634–8.
17. National Emphysema Treatment Trial Research Group. A randomized trial comparing lung-volume–reduction surgery with medical therapy for severe emphysema. *N Engl J Med* 2003; **348:** 2059–73.
18. Barnes PJ. New therapies for chronic obstructive pulmonary disease. *Thorax* 1998; **53:** 137–47.
19. Snow V, *et al.* Evidence base for management of acute exacerbations of chronic obstructive pulmonary disease. *Ann Intern Med* 2001; **134:** 595–9.
20. Hall CS, *et al.* Acute exacerbations in chronic obstructive pulmonary disease: current strategies with pharmacological therapy. *Drugs* 2003; **63:** 1481–8.
21. Niewoehner DE, *et al.*. Effect of systemic glucocorticoids on exacerbations of chronic obstructive pulmonary disease. *N Engl J Med* 1999; **340:** 1941–7.
22. Davies L, *et al.* Oral corticosteroids in patients admitted to hospital with exacerbations of chronic obstructive pulmonary disease: a prospective randomised controlled trial. *Lancet* 1999; **354:** 456–60.
23. Singh JM, *et al.* Corticosteroid therapy for patients with acute exacerbations of chronic obstructive pulmonary disease: a systematic review. *Arch Intern Med* 2002; **162:** 2527–36.
24. Saint S, *et al.* Antibiotics in chronic obstructive pulmonary disease exacerbations: a meta-analysis. *JAMA* 1995; **273:** 957–60.
25. Greenstone M, Lasserson TJ. Doxapram for ventilatory failure due to exacerbations of chronic obstructive pulmonary disease. Available in The Cochrane Library; Issue 1. Chichester: John Wiley; 2004.


## Acefylline Piperazine *(BAN, rINN)*

Acepifylline; Piperazine Theophylline Ethanoate. Piperazine bis(theophyllin-7-ylacetate) (1:1).

$(C_9H_{10}N_4O_4)_2,C_4H_{10}N_2 = 562.5.$

*CAS — 18833-13-1; 18428-63-2.*

*ATC — R03DA09.*

### Profile

Acefylline piperazine is a derivative of theophylline (p.798) that has been used for its bronchodilator effects.

### Preparations

**Proprietary Preparations** (details are given in Part 3)
***India:*** Etophylate.

**Multi-ingredient:** ***India:*** Cadiphylate.

## Aminophylline *(BAN, pINN)*

Aminofilina; Aminophyllinum; Euphyllinum; Metaphyllin; Theophyllaminum; Theophylline and Ethylenediamine; Theophylline Ethylenediamine Compound; Theophyllinum et Ethylenediaminum. A mixture of theophylline and ethylenediamine (2:1), its composition approximately corresponding to the formula below.

$(C_7H_8N_4O_2)_2,C_2H_4(NH_2)_2 = 420.4.$

*CAS — 317-34-0 (anhydrous aminophylline).*

*ATC — R03DA05.*

**Pharmacopoeias.** In *Eur.* (see p.vi), *Int., US,* and *Viet.* Some pharmacopoeias include anhydrous and hydrated aminophylline in one monograph. Some pharmacopoeias do not specify the hydration state.

**Ph. Eur. 5.0** (Theophylline-ethylenediamine; Aminophylline BP 2003). It contains 84.0 to 87.4% of anhydrous theophylline and 13.5 to 15.0% of anhydrous ethylenediamine. A white or slightly yellowish powder, sometimes granular. Freely soluble in water (the solution becomes cloudy through absorption of carbon dioxide); practically insoluble in dehydrated alcohol. Store in airtight containers. Protect from light.

**USP 27** (Aminophylline). It is anhydrous or contains not more than two molecules of water of hydration. It contains not less than 84.0 and not more than 87.4% of anhydrous theophylline. It consists of white or slightly yellowish granules or powder, having a slight ammoniacal odour. Upon exposure to air it gradually loses ethylenediamine and absorbs carbon dioxide with the liberation of theophylline. One g dissolves in 25 mL of water to give a clear solution; 1 g dissolved in 5 mL of water crystallises upon standing, but redissolves when a small amount of ethylenediamine is added; insoluble in alcohol and in ether. Its solutions are alkaline to litmus. Store in airtight containers.

## Aminophylline Hydrate *(BANM, pINNM)*

Aminofilina hidratada.

$(C_7H_8N_4O_2)_2,C_2H_4(NH_2)_2,2H_2O = 456.5.$

*CAS — 49746-06-7 (aminophylline dihydrate).*

*ATC — R03DA05.*

**Pharmacopoeias.** In *Chin., Eur.* (see p.vi), *Jpn, Pol., US,* and *Viet.* Some pharmacopoeias include anhydrous and hydrated aminophylline in one monograph. Some pharmacopoeias do not specify the hydration state.

**Ph. Eur. 5.0** (Theophylline-ethylenediamine Hydrate; Aminophylline Hydrate BP 2003). It contains 84.0 to 87.4% of anhydrous theophylline and 13.5 to 15.0% of anhydrous ethylenediamine. A white or slightly yellowish powder, sometimes granular. Freely soluble in water (the solution becomes cloudy through absorption of carbon dioxide); practically insoluble in dehydrated alcohol. Store in well-filled airtight containers. Protect from light.

**USP 27** (Aminophylline). It is anhydrous or contains not more than two molecules of water of hydration. It contains not less than 84.0 and not more than 87.4% of anhydrous theophylline. It consists of white or slightly yellowish granules or powder, having a slight ammoniacal odour. Upon exposure to air it gradually loses ethylenediamine and absorbs carbon dioxide with the liberation of theophylline. One g dissolves in 25 mL of water to give a clear solution; 1 g dissolved in 5 mL of water crystallises upon standing, but redissolves when a small amount of ethylenediamine is added; insoluble in alcohol and in ether. Its solutions are alkaline to litmus. Store in airtight containers.

**Incompatibility.** Aminophylline solutions should not be allowed to come into contact with metals.

Solutions of aminophylline are alkaline and if the pH falls below 8, crystals of theophylline will deposit.[1] Drugs known to be unstable in alkaline solutions, or that would lower the pH below the critical value, should not be mixed with aminophylline.


1. Edward M. pH—an important factor in the compatibility of additives in intravenous therapy. *Am J Hosp Pharm* 1967; **24:** 440–9.


### Adverse Effects, Treatment, and Precautions

As for Theophylline, p.798. Hypersensitivity has been associated with the ethylenediamine content.

**Porphyria.** Aminophylline is considered to be unsafe in patients with porphyria because it has been shown to be porphyrinogenic in *animals* or *in-vitro* systems.

### Interactions

As for Theophylline, p.800.

### Pharmacokinetics

Aminophylline, a complex of theophylline with ethylenediamine, readily liberates theophylline in the body. The pharmacokinetics of theophylline are discussed on p.803.

◊ Studies in healthy subjects suggested that ethylenediamine does not affect the pharmacokinetics of theophylline after oral or intravenous administration.[1,2]


1. Aslaksen A, *et al.* Comparative pharmacokinetics of theophylline and aminophylline in man. *Br J Clin Pharmacol* 1981; **11:** 269–73.
2. Caldwell J, *et al.* Theophylline pharmacokinetics after intravenous infusion with ethylenediamine or sodium glycinate. *Br J Clin Pharmacol* 1986; **22:** 351–5.


### Uses and Administration

Aminophylline has the actions and uses of theophylline (see p.804) and is used similarly as a bronchodilator in the management of asthma (p.777) and chronic obstructive pulmonary disease (p.779). Aminophylline is also used to relieve apnoea in neonates. It was formerly used in heart failure, and may occasionally have a role in patients with this condition who are also suffering from obstructive airways disease. Aminophylline is usually preferred to theophylline when greater solubility in water is required, particularly in intravenous formulations.

Aminophylline may be given in the anhydrous form or as the hydrate, and doses may be expressed as either; aminophylline hydrate 1.09 mg is approximately equivalent to 1 mg of aminophylline. The USP 27 specifies that aminophylline preparations should be labelled with respect to their anhydrous *theophylline* content. As the pharmacokinetics of theophylline are affected by a number of factors including age, smoking, disease, diet, and drug interactions, the dose of aminophylline must be carefully individualised and serum-theophylline concentrations monitored (see under Uses and Administration of Theophylline, p.804).

In the management of **acute severe bronchospasm**, aminophylline may be given intravenously by slow injection or infusion. To reduce adverse effects, the rate of intravenous administration of aminophylline should not exceed 25 mg/minute. In patients who have not been taking aminophylline, theophylline, or other xanthine-containing medication, a loading dose of 5 mg/kg ideal (lean) body-weight or 250 to 500 mg of aminophylline (25 mg/mL) may be given intravenously over 20 to 30 minutes by slow injection or infusion, followed by a maintenance infusion dose of 500 micrograms/kg per hour. Older patients and those with cor pulmonale, heart failure, or liver disease may require lower maintenance doses; smokers often need higher maintenance doses. A loading dose may not be considered necessary unless the patient's condition is deteriorating. Children (also not currently on xanthine medication) may be given the same loading dose per kg as adults; suggested maintenance doses are 1 mg/kg per hour for children aged 6 months to 9 years and 800 micrograms/kg per hour for children aged 10 to 16 years. The *American Hospital Formulary Service* suggests that the maintenance doses should be slightly higher for the first 12 hours of the infusion in both adults and children.

Intravenous aminophylline is best avoided in patients already taking theophylline, aminophylline, or other xanthine-containing medication but, if considered necessary, the serum-theophylline concentration should first be assessed and the initial loading dose should be calculated on the basis that each 600 micrograms/kg of aminophylline (equivalent to 500 micrograms/kg theophylline) will increase serum-theophylline concentration by 1 microgram/mL.

In the treatment of **acute bronchospasm** that does not require intravenous therapy, aminophylline has been given by mouth in conventional dosage forms; modified-release preparations are not suitable. Doses used have generally ranged from 100 to 300 mg three or four times daily after food.

In the management of **chronic bronchospasm** aminophylline may be given by mouth as conventional or as modified-release preparations. The modified-release products are generally preferred and a usual dose is aminophylline hydrate 225 to 450 mg twice daily by mouth. Therapy should be initiated with the lower dose and increased as appropriate. Retitration of the dosage is required if the patient is changed from one modified-release preparation to another as the bioavailability of modified-release aminophylline preparations may vary. Children (over 3 years) have been given modified-release aminophylline hydrate in doses of 12 mg/kg daily, increased after 1 week to 24 mg/kg daily, in 2 divided doses.

Intramuscular administration of aminophylline causes intense local pain and is not recommended.

Aminophylline has also been used as the hydrochloride.

**Administration.** RECTAL ADMINISTRATION. Absorption from aminophylline suppositories is erratic and this dose form has been associated with toxicity, hence the warnings that suppositories should not be used, especially in children. In the UK suppositories are no longer readily available and one hospital wishing to use the rectal route for apnoea in premature infants (see Neonatal Apnoea, p.806) achieved therapeutic plasma-theophylline concentrations with a specially formulated rectal gel.[1]

1. Cooney S, *et al.* Rectal aminophylline gel in treatment of apnoea in premature newborn babies. *Lancet* 1991; **337:** 1351.

**Erectile dysfunction.** For reference to the use of a cream containing aminophylline, isosorbide dinitrate, and co-dergocrine mesilate in the treatment of erectile dysfunction, see under Glyceryl Trinitrate, p.925.

**Methotrexate neurotoxicity.** For reference to the use of aminophylline or theophylline to relieve the acute neurotoxicity of methotrexate, see p.570.

**Reduction of body fat.** Cosmetic aminophylline cream has been promoted for its supposed ability to remove fat ('cellulite') from the thighs.[1] Concern has been raised about the potential for topical sensitisation.[2]

1. Dickinson BI, Gora-Harper ML. Aminophylline for cellulite removal. *Ann Pharmacother* 1996; **30:** 292–3.
2. Simon PA. Comment: aminophylline-containing cream. *Ann Pharmacother* 1996; **30:** 1341.

### Preparations

***BP 2003:*** Aminophylline Injection; Aminophylline Tablets;
***USP 27:*** Aminophylline Delayed-release Tablets; Aminophylline Injection; Aminophylline Oral Solution; Aminophylline Rectal Solution; Aminophylline Suppositories; Aminophylline Tablets.

**Proprietary Preparations** (details are given in Part 3)
***Arg.:*** Cardirenal; Fadafilina; Larjanfilina; ***Austria:*** Euphyllin; Mundiphyllin; ***Braz.:*** Aminoima; Aminoliv; Asmafin; Asmapen; Asmodrin; Asmoquinol; Eufilin†; Minoton; Unifilin; ***Canad.:*** Phyllocontin; ***Chile:*** Cardiomin; ***Denm.:*** Teofylamin; ***Fin.:*** Aminocont; Theophyllaminum†; ***Fr.:*** Planphylline†; ***Ger.:*** Phyllotemp; ***Hong Kong:*** Phyllocontin†; ***Irl.:*** Clonofilin†; Phyllocontin; ***Israel:*** Elixophyllin†; ***Ital.:*** Aminomal; Euphyllina; Tefamin; ***Jpn:*** Neophyllin; ***Mex.:*** Drafilyn-Z; ***Neth.:*** Euphyllin; ***Port.:*** Filotempo; ***S.Afr.:*** Peterphyllin†; Phyllocontin; ***Switz.:*** Aminomal†; Escophylline; Euphyllin; Phyllotemp; ***Thai.:*** Fileen; ***UK:*** Amnivent; Norphyllin†; Phyllocontin; ***USA:*** Phyllocontin†; Truphylline.

**Multi-ingredient:** ***Austria:*** Asthma-Hilfe; Limptar; Myocardon; ***Braz.:*** Alergo Filinal; Alergotox Expectorante†; Alergotox†; Dispneitrat; Teodrin†; ***Ger.:*** Limptar; ***Hong Kong:*** Asmeton; ***Mex.:*** Paliatil; ***Port.:*** Anti-Asmatico; Fluidin Antiasmatico†; ***S.Afr.:*** Diphenamill; Lotussin Expectorant; Repasma†; ***Spain:*** Angiosedante†; Lasa Antiasmatico†; ***Thai.:*** Asmeton; ***USA:*** Emergent-Ez; Mudrane GG-2†; Mudrane GG†; Mudrane†.

## Amlexanox *(BAN, USAN, rINN)*

AA-673; Amoxanox; CHX-3673. 2-Amino-7-isopropyl-5-oxo-5*H*-[1]benzopyrano[2,3-*b*]pyridine-3-carboxylic acid.

$C_{16}H_{14}N_2O_4$ = 298.3.
*CAS — 68302-57-8.*
*ATC — A01AD07; R03DX01.*

### Profile

Amlexanox has a stabilising action on mast cells resembling that of sodium cromoglicate (p.795) and is also a leukotriene inhibitor. It is administered by mouth in the management of asthma (p.777) and for allergic rhinitis (p.422); a dose of 25 or 50 mg three times daily has been suggested. Amlexanox is also given as a metered-dose nasal spray for allergic rhinitis.

Amlexanox is also applied as a 5% oral paste four times daily in the management of aphthous ulcers (see Mouth Ulceration, p.1245). A biodegradable oral disc designed to deliver amlexanox locally is also in development.

### Preparations

**Proprietary Preparations** (details are given in Part 3)
***Jpn:*** Solfa; ***USA:*** Aphthasol.

## Apafant *(USAN, rINN)*

WEB-2086; WEB-2086-BS. 4-{3-[4-(*o*-Chlorophenyl)-9-methyl-6*H*-thieno[3,2-*f*]-*s*-triazolo[4,3-*a*][1,4]diazepin-2-yl]propionyl}morpholine.

$C_{22}H_{22}ClN_5O_2S$ = 456.0.
*CAS — 105219-56-5.*

### Profile

Apafant is a platelet-activating factor antagonist that has been investigated for the prophylactic management of asthma. It has been tried in other conditions, including acute pancreatitis.

◊ References.

1. Brecht HM, *et al.* Pharmacodynamics, pharmacokinetics and safety profile of the new platelet-activating factor antagonist apafant in man. *Arzneimittelforschung* 1991; **41:** 51–9.

**Asthma.** In a study involving 106 patients with stable atopic asthma, apafant 40 mg by mouth three times daily was no more effective than placebo in reducing the requirement for inhaled corticosteroids.[1] It was concluded that these negative results, at a dose known to produce active concentrations in the airways, cast doubt on any role of platelet-activating factor in the pathogenesis of asthma (p.777).

1. Spence DPS, *et al.* The effect of the orally active platelet-activating factor antagonist WEB 2086 in the treatment of asthma. *Am J Respir Crit Care Med* 1994; **149:** 1142–8.

## Bambuterol Hydrochloride *(BANM, rINNM)*

Bambuteroli Hydrochloridum; Hidrocloruro de bambuterol; KWD-2183. (*RS*)-5-(2-*tert*-Butylamino-1-hydroxyethyl)-*m*-phenylene bis(dimethylcarbamate) hydrochloride.

$C_{18}H_{29}N_3O_5,HCl$ = 403.9.
*CAS — 81732-65-2 (bambuterol); 81732-46-9 (bambuterol monohydrochloride).*

**Pharmacopoeias.** In *Eur.* (see p.vi).

**Ph. Eur. 5.0** (Bambuterol Hydrochloride). A white or almost white crystalline powder. It exhibits polymorphism. Freely soluble in water; soluble in alcohol.

### Adverse Effects and Precautions

As for Salbutamol, p.791. Bambuterol is not recommended for patients with severe hepatic impairment as its metabolism would be unpredictable. The dose of bambuterol should be reduced in renal impairment (see below). It is unsuitable for the relief of acute bronchospasm or in patients with unstable respiratory disease.

**Effects on the heart.** A prescription event monitoring study found an excess risk of non-fatal heart failure in elderly patients receiving bambuterol, particularly in the first month of treatment.[1] See also under Salbutamol, p.792.

1. Martin RM, *et al.* Risk of non-fatal cardiac failure and ischaemic heart disease with long acting $\beta_2$ agonists. *Thorax* 1998; **53:** 558–62.

### Interactions

As for Salbutamol, p.792. Bambuterol inhibits plasma cholinesterases and can prolong the action of drugs such as suxamethonium (see Sympathomimetics, under Suxamethonium, p.1408) that are inactivated by these enzymes.

### Pharmacokinetics

Nearly 20% of a dose of bambuterol is absorbed from the gastrointestinal tract following oral administration. It is slowly metabolised in the body to its active metabolite, terbutaline; peak terbutaline concentrations are reported to occur about 4 to 7 hours after a dose of bambuterol as tablets. The slow rate at which metabolism occurs determines the prolonged duration of action of bambuterol of at least 24 hours. Hydrolysis of bambuterol to terbutaline and carbamic acid leads to inhibition of plasma-cholinesterase activity that can be correlated with plasma concentrations of terbutaline. For the metabolism and excretion of terbutaline, see p.797.

◊ References.

1. Sitar DS. Clinical pharmacokinetics of bambuterol. *Clin Pharmacokinet* 1996; **31:** 246–56.
2. Nyberg L, *et al.* Pharmacokinetics of bambuterol in healthy subjects. *Br J Clin Pharmacol* 1998; **45:** 471–8.
3. Bang U, *et al.* Pharmacokinetics of bambuterol in subjects homozygous for the atypical gene for plasma cholinesterase. *Br J Clin Pharmacol* 1998; **45:** 479–84.
4. Ahlström H, *et al.* Pharmacokinetics of bambuterol during oral administration to asthmatic children. *Br J Clin Pharmacol* 1999; **48:** 299–308.
5. Rosenborg J, *et al.* Pharmacokinetics of bambuterol during oral administration of plain tablets and solution to healthy adults. *Br J Clin Pharmacol* 2000; **49:** 199–206.

### Uses and Administration

Bambuterol is an inactive prodrug of terbutaline (p.797), a direct-acting sympathomimetic with predominantly beta-adrenergic activity and a selective action on beta$_2$ receptors (a beta$_2$ agonist). It has similar actions to those of salbutamol (p.793) except that it has a more prolonged duration of action (at least 24 hours). Bambuterol hydrochloride is used as a long-acting bronchodilator for persistent reversible airways obstruction in conditions such as asthma (p.777). The usual dose is 10 to 20 mg by mouth once daily at bedtime. Doses may need to be reduced in renal impairment (see below).

**Administration in renal impairment.** The manufacturer recommends that the initial dose of bambuterol hydrochloride should be halved in patients with renal impairment (glomerular filtration rate less than 50 mL/minute). Further doses should be adjusted according to response.

**Asthma.** References.

1. Fugleholm AM, *et al.* Therapeutic equivalence between bambuterol, 10 mg once daily, and terbutaline controlled release, 5 mg twice daily, in mild to moderate asthma. *Eur Respir J* 1993; **6:** 1474–8.
2. Gunn SD, *et al.* Comparison of the efficacy, tolerability and patient acceptability of once-daily bambuterol tablets against twice-daily controlled release salbutamol in nocturnal asthma. *Eur J Clin Pharmacol* 1995; **48:** 23–8.

### Preparations

**Proprietary Preparations** (details are given in Part 3)
***Austria:*** Bambec; ***Braz.:*** Bambec†; ***Denm.:*** Bambec; ***Fr.:*** Oxeol; ***Ger.:*** Bambec; ***Hong Kong:*** Bambec; ***India:*** Bambudil; ***Ital.:*** Bambec; ***Malaysia:*** Bambec; ***Norw.:*** Bambec; ***NZ:*** Bambec; ***Singapore:*** Bambec; ***Spain:*** Bambec; ***Swed.:*** Bambec; ***Switz.:*** Bambec†; ***Thai.:*** Bambec; ***UK:*** Bambec.

## Bamifylline Hydrochloride *(BANM, USAN, rINNM)*

AC-3810; BAX-2739Z; 8102-CB; CB-8102; Hidrocloruro de bamifilina. 8-Benzyl-7-[2-(*N*-ethyl-*N*-2-hydroxyethylamino)ethyl]theophylline hydrochloride.

$C_{20}H_{27}N_5O_3,HCl$ = 421.9.
*CAS — 2016-63-9 (bamifylline); 20684-06-4 (bamifylline hydrochloride).*
*ATC — R03DA08.*

### Profile

Bamifylline hydrochloride is a theophylline derivative (p.798) that is used for its bronchodilator properties in reversible airways obstruction. It is given by mouth in usual doses of 600 or 900 mg daily. It is also given rectally as suppositories, and by slow intravenous infusion.

### Preparations

**Proprietary Preparations** (details are given in Part 3)
***Belg.:*** Trentadil; ***Braz.:*** Bamifix; ***Fr.:*** Trentadil; ***Ital.:*** Airest; Bamifix; Bamixol; Briofil.

## Bitolterol Mesilate *(BANM, rINNM)*

Bitolterol Mesylate *(USAN)*; Mesilato de bitolterol; Win-32784. 4-[2-(*tert*-Butylamino)-1-hydroxyethyl]-*o*-phenylene di-*p*-toluate methanesulphonate.

$C_{28}H_{31}NO_5,CH_4O_3S$ = 557.7.
*CAS — 30392-40-6 (bitolterol); 30392-41-7 (bitolterol mesilate).*
*ATC — R03AC17.*

### Profile

Bitolterol is an inactive prodrug that is hydrolysed in the body to colterol, a direct-acting sympathomimetic with predominantly beta-adrenergic activity and a selective action on beta$_2$ receptors (a beta$_2$ agonist). It has similar properties to those of salbutamol (p.791).

It has been used as a bronchodilator in the management of diseases with reversible airways obstruction such as asthma (p.777) or in some patients with chronic obstructive pulmonary disease (p.779); administration by inhalation results in the rapid onset of bronchodilatation (2 to 4 minutes) with a duration of action of 5 or more hours.

Bitolterol has been given by inhalation via a metered-dose aerosol supplying 370 micrograms of bitolterol mesilate per inhalation. For the relief of bronchospasm the usual adult dose is 2 inhalations (740 micrograms) followed by a third inhalation (370 micrograms) if required. For the prevention of bronchospasm the usual adult dose is 2 inhalations (740 micrograms) every 8 hours. Maximum doses have been stated to be 3 inhalations (1110 micrograms) every 6 hours or 2 inhalations (740 micrograms) every 4 hours. In patients with asthma, as-required beta agonist therapy is preferable to regular use. An increased need for, or decreased duration of effect of, bitolterol indicates deterioration of asthma control and the need for review of therapy.

Alternatively, a 0.2% inhalation solution of bitolterol mesilate has been given by nebulisation.

### Preparations

**Proprietary Preparations** (details are given in Part 3)
***Ital.:*** Asmalene†; ***USA:*** Tornalate.

## Bufylline *(BAN)*

Ambuphylline *(USAN)*; Bufilina; Theophylline-aminoisobutanol. 2-Amino-2-methylpropan-1-ol theophyllinate.

$C_{11}H_{19}N_5O_3$ = 269.3.
*CAS — 5634-34-4.*
*ATC — R03DA10.*

### Profile

Bufylline is a theophylline derivative (p.798), which has been used for its bronchodilator effects as an ingredient of preparations promoted for coughs and other respiratory-tract disorders. The ethiodide has also been used.

### Preparations

**Proprietary Preparations** (details are given in Part 3)
**Multi-ingredient:** ***Braz.:*** Bronco-Ped†; Broncolex; EMS Expectorante; Revenil; Revenil Dospan; Revenil Expectorante†; ***Mex.:*** Isobutil; ***S.Afr.:*** Nethaprin Dospan; Nethaprin Expectorant.

## Caffeine (BAN)

Anhydrous Caffeine; Cafeína; Caféine; Coffeinum; Guaranine; Methyltheobromine; Théine. 1,3,7-Trimethylpurine-2,6(3H,1H)-dione; 1,3,7-Trimethylxanthine; 7-Methyltheophylline.

$C_8H_{10}N_4O_2$ = 194.2.

*CAS — 58-08-2.*

*ATC — N06BC01.*

NOTE. Compounded preparations of caffeine may be represented by the following names:

- Co-bucafAPAP (*PEN*)—butalbital, paracetamol, and caffeine.

**Pharmacopoeias.** In *Eur.* (see p.vi), *Int., Jpn, Pol., US,* and *Viet.* Some pharmacopoeias include caffeine and caffeine hydrate under one monograph.

**Ph. Eur. 5.0** (Caffeine). A white crystalline powder or silky white crystals. It sublimes readily. Sparingly soluble in water; freely soluble in boiling water; slightly soluble in dehydrated alcohol. It dissolves in concentrated solutions of alkali benzoates or salicylates.

**USP 27** (Caffeine). It is anhydrous or contains one molecule of water of hydration. An odourless white powder or white, glistening needles, usually matted together. The hydrate is efflorescent in air. The hydrate is soluble 1 in 50 of water, 1 in 75 of alcohol, 1 in 6 of chloroform, and 1 in 600 of ether. The hydrate should be stored in airtight containers.

## Caffeine Citrate (BANM)

Cafeína, citrato de; Citrated Caffeine; Coffeinum Citricum.

$C_8H_{10}N_4O_2,C_6H_8O_7$ = 386.3.

*CAS — 69-22-7.*

*ATC — N06BC01.*

## Caffeine Hydrate (BANM)

Cafeína hidrato; Caffeine Monohydrate; Coffeinum Monohydricum.

$C_8H_{10}N_4O_2,H_2O$ = 212.2.

*CAS — 5743-12-4.*

*ATC — N06BC01.*

**Pharmacopoeias.** In *Chin., Eur.* (see p.vi), *Int., Jpn, Pol., US,* and *Viet.* Some pharmacopoeias include caffeine and caffeine hydrate under one monograph.

**Ph. Eur. 5.0** (Caffeine Monohydrate; Caffeine Hydrate BP 2003). A white crystalline powder or silky white crystals. It sublimes readily. Sparingly soluble in water; freely soluble in boiling water; slightly soluble in dehydrated alcohol. It dissolves in concentrated solutions of alkali benzoates or salicylates.

**USP 27** (Caffeine). It is anhydrous or contains one molecule of water of hydration. An odourless white powder or white, glistening needles, usually matted together. The hydrate is efflorescent in air. The hydrate is soluble 1 in 50 of water, 1 in 75 of alcohol, 1 in 6 of chloroform, and 1 in 600 of ether. The hydrate should be stored in airtight containers.

**Stability.** References to the stability of caffeine and caffeine citrate.

1. Eisenberg MG, Kang N. Stability of citrated caffeine solutions for injectable and enteral use. *Am J Hosp Pharm* 1984; **41:** 2405–6.
2. Nahata MC, *et al.* Stability of caffeine injection in intravenous admixtures and parenteral nutrition solutions. *DICP Ann Pharmacother* 1989; **23:** 466–7.
3. Hopkin C, *et al.* Stability study of caffeine citrate. *Br J Pharm Pract* 1990; **12:** 133.
4. Donnelly RF, Tirona RG. Stability of citrated caffeine injectable solution in glass vials. *Am J Hosp Pharm* 1994; **51:** 512–14.

## Adverse Effects, Treatment, and Precautions

As for Theophylline, p.798.

Prolonged high intake of caffeine may lead to tolerance of some of the pharmacological actions and physical signs of withdrawal including irritability, lethargy, and headache may occur if intake is discontinued abruptly.

◊ General references.

1. Wills S. Drugs and substance misuse: caffeine. *Pharm J* 1994; **252:** 822–4.
2. Fredholm BB, *et al.* Actions of caffeine in the brain with special reference to factors that contribute to its widespread use. *Pharmacol Rev* 1999; **51:** 83–133.

**Breast feeding.** Studies examining the transfer of caffeine into breast milk after doses of 35 to 336 mg of caffeine by mouth have recorded peak maternal plasma concentrations of 2.4 to 4.7 micrograms/mL, peak maternal saliva concentrations of 1.2 to 9.2 micrograms/mL, and peak breast-milk concentrations of 1.4 to 7.2 micrograms/mL. At these concentrations in breast milk, the calculated daily caffeine ingestion by breast-fed infants ranged from 1.3 to 3.1 mg, which was not thought to present a hazard, although irritability and a poor sleeping pattern have been reported.[1-4]

The American Academy of Pediatrics[5] states that caffeine is excreted slowly by the infant and may be associated with irritability and poor sleeping pattern when ingested by breast-feeding mothers. However, no effects occur with moderate intake of caffeinated beverages (2 to 3 cups daily) and caffeine is usually compatible with breast feeding.

1. Tyrala EE, Dodson WE. Caffeine secretion into breast milk. *Arch Dis Child* 1979; **54:** 787–800.
2. Hildebrandt R, *et al.* Transfer of caffeine to breast milk. *Br J Clin Pharmacol* 1983; **15:** 612P.
3. Sagraves R, *et al.* Pharmacokinetics of caffeine in human breast milk after a single oral dose of caffeine. *Drug Intell Clin Pharm* 1984; **18:** 507.
4. Berlin CM, *et al.* Disposition of dietary caffeine in milk, saliva, and plasma of lactating women. *Pediatrics* 1984; **73:** 59–63.
5. American Academy of Pediatrics. The transfer of drugs and other chemicals into human milk. *Pediatrics* 2001; **108:** 776–89. Correction. *ibid.*; 1029. Also available at: http://aappolicy.aappublications.org/cgi/content/full/pediatrics%3b108/3/776 (accessed 20/04/04)

**Effects on the heart.** For a discussion of the effects of caffeine-containing beverages on cardiovascular risk factors, see p.1765.

**Effects on mental function.** A report of 6 cases of excessive daytime sleepiness associated with high caffeine intake.[1]

1. Regestein QR. Pathologic sleepiness induced by caffeine. *Am J Med* 1989; **87:** 586–8.

**Overdosage.** Reports and reviews of caffeine toxicity.

1. Kulkarni PB, Dorand RD. Caffeine toxicity in a neonate. *Pediatrics* 1979; **64:** 254–5.
2. Banner W, Czajka PA. Acute caffeine overdose in the neonate. *Am J Dis Child* 1980; **134:** 495–8.
3. Zimmerman PM, *et al.* Caffeine intoxication: a near fatality. *Ann Emerg Med* 1985; **14:** 1227–9.
4. Dalvi RR. Acute and chronic toxicity of caffeine: a review. *Vet Hum Toxicol* 1986; **28:** 144–50.
5. Rivenes SM, *et al.* Intentional caffeine poisoning in an infant. *Pediatrics* 1997; **99:** 736–8.

**Pregnancy.** In the USA, the FDA has advised pregnant women to limit their intake of caffeine and caffeine-containing beverages to a minimum, but this recommendation was based largely on *animal* studies and the effect of caffeine on the human fetus and fetal loss during pregnancy is controversial.[1] Although some studies found no evidence that moderate caffeine use increased the risk of spontaneous abortion,[2,3] others have reported conflicting results.[4,5] There is some evidence for an effect on fetal growth, but again it is not clear that this applies generally: a prospective population-based study in the UK found that a decreased birth-weight with increased caffeine intake was only significant in smokers.[6] The authors of this study concurred that a reduction in caffeine intake during pregnancy would be prudent, together with stopping smoking. An association between high maternal caffeine intake during pregnancy and an increased risk of the sudden infant death syndrome has also been reported,[7] although another study found no such association.[8]

1. Eskenazi B. Caffeine during pregnancy: grounds for concern? *JAMA* 1993; **270:** 2973–4.
2. Mills JL, *et al.* Moderate caffeine use and the risk of spontaneous abortion and intrauterine growth retardation. *JAMA* 1993; **269:** 593–7.
3. Klebanoff MA, *et al.* Maternal serum paraxanthine, a caffeine metabolite, and the risk of spontaneous abortion. *N Engl J Med* 1999; **341:** 1639–44.
4. Infante-Rivard C, *et al.* Fetal loss associated with caffeine intake before and during pregnancy. *JAMA* 1993; **270:** 2940–3.
5. Cnattingius S, *et al.* Caffeine intake and the risk of first-trimester spontaneous abortion. *N Engl J Med* 2000; **343:** 1839–45.
6. Cook DG, *et al.* Relation of caffeine intake and blood caffeine concentrations during pregnancy to fetal growth: prospective population based study. *BMJ* 1996; **313:** 1358–62.
7. Ford RPK, *et al.* Heavy caffeine intake in pregnancy and sudden infant death syndrome. *Arch Dis Child* 1998; **78:** 9–13.
8. Alm B, *et al.* Caffeine and alcohol as risk factors for sudden infant death syndrome. *Arch Dis Child* 1999; **81:** 107–11.

**Withdrawal.** Headache is a recognised symptom of caffeine withdrawal and even subjects who drink moderate amounts of coffee can develop headaches lasting 1 to 6 days when switched to a decaffeinated brand.[1] It has also been suggested that postoperative headache could be attributed to caffeine withdrawal as fasting patients are required to abstain from drinking tea or coffee before surgical procedures. Several studies[2-4] have found a positive association between postoperative headache and daily caffeine consumption, although there have also been negative findings.[5] A prospective study suggested that prophylactic intravenous administration of caffeine on the day of surgery reduced the likelihood of postoperative headache in patients at risk of caffeine withdrawal.[6]

1. van Dusseldorp M, Katan MB. Headache caused by caffeine withdrawal among moderate coffee drinkers switched from ordinary to decaffeinated coffee: a 12 week double blind trial. *BMJ* 1990; **300:** 1558–9.
2. Galletly DC, *et al.* Does caffeine withdrawal contribute to postanaesthetic morbidity? *Lancet* 1989; **i:** 1335.
3. Weber JG, *et al.* Perioperative ingestion of caffeine and postoperative headache. *Mayo Clin Proc* 1993; **68:** 842–5.
4. Nikolajsen L, *et al.* Effect of previous frequency of headache, duration of fasting and caffeine abstinence on perioperative headache. *Br J Anaesth* 1994; **72:** 295–7.
5. Verhoeff FH, Millar JM. Does caffeine contribute to postoperative morbidity? *Lancet* 1990; **336:** 632.
6. Weber JG, *et al.* Prophylactic intravenous administration of caffeine and recovery after ambulatory surgical procedures. *Mayo Clin Proc* 1997; **72:** 621–6.

## Interactions

Like theophylline (see p.800) caffeine undergoes extensive metabolism by hepatic microsomal cytochrome P450 isoenzyme CYP1A2, and is subject to numerous interactions with other drugs and substances which enhance or reduce its metabolic clearance.

◊ Reviews.

1. Carrillo JA, Benitez J. Clinically significant pharmacokinetic interactions between dietary caffeine and medications. *Clin Pharmacokinet* 2000; **39:** 127–53.

**Alcohol.** In a study of 8 healthy subjects given alcohol by mouth in a dose of 2.2 mL/kg, caffeine 150 mg by mouth did not antagonise the central effects of alcohol and, instead, a synergistic interaction occurred which further increased reaction time. The common practice of drinking coffee after drinking alcohol in order to sober up is not supported by these results.[1] Another study[2] found that some antagonism of the central effects of alcohol was produced by caffeine, although there was no reversal of subjective sensations of drunkenness; however the dose of caffeine in this study (400 mg) was considerably higher.

1. Oborne DJ, Rogers Y. Interactions of alcohol and caffeine on human reaction time. *Aviat Space Environ Med* 1983; **54:** 528–34.
2. Azcona O, *et al.* Evaluation of the central effects of alcohol and caffeine interaction. *Br J Clin Pharmacol* 1995; **40:** 393–400.

**Antiarrhythmics.** In 7 healthy subjects and 5 patients with cardiac arrhythmias, *mexiletine* in a single dose of 200 mg and a dose of 600 mg daily respectively, reduced the elimination of caffeine by 30 to 50%.[1] *Lidocaine, flecainide,* and *tocainide* had no effect on caffeine elimination in healthy subjects.[1]

1. Joeres R, Richter E. Mexiletine and caffeine elimination. *N Engl J Med* 1987; **317:** 117.

**Antibacterials.** Caffeine elimination half-life has been reported to be increased and clearance decreased by the concomitant administration of *ciprofloxacin,*[1-3] *enoxacin,*[2,3] and *pipemidic acid,*[2,3] whereas *lomefloxacin,*[4] *norfloxacin,*[2,3] and *ofloxacin*[2,3] had little or no effect on these parameters. Enoxacin had the greatest inhibitory effect on caffeine clearance.[2,3]

1. Healy DP, *et al.* Interaction between oral ciprofloxacin and caffeine in normal volunteers. *Antimicrob Agents Chemother* 1989; **33:** 474–8.
2. Harder S, *et al.* Ciprofloxacin-caffeine: a drug interaction established using in vivo and in vitro investigations. *Am J Med* 1989; **87** (suppl 5A): 89–91S.
3. Barnett G, *et al.* Pharmacokinetic determination of relative potency of quinolone inhibition of caffeine disposition. *Eur J Clin Pharmacol* 1990; **39:** 63–9.
4. Healy DP, *et al.* Lack of interaction between lomefloxacin and caffeine in normal volunteers. *Antimicrob Agents Chemother* 1991; **35:** 660–4.

**Antiepileptics.** The mean clearance of caffeine was increased and its half-life decreased in epileptic patients taking *phenytoin* compared with healthy controls, resulting in lower plasma-caffeine concentrations. Treatment with *carbamazepine* or *valproic acid* had no effect on the pharmacokinetics of caffeine.[1]

1. Wietholtz H, *et al.* Effects of phenytoin, carbamazepine, and valproic acid on caffeine metabolism. *Eur J Clin Pharmacol* 1989; **36:** 401–6.

**Antifungals.** In a single-dose study in healthy subjects, *terbinafine* 500 mg by mouth decreased the clearance and increased the elimination half-life of caffeine 3 mg/kg given intravenously. *Ketoconazole* 400 mg by mouth did not prolong the elimination of caffeine to a significant extent.[1]

1. Wahlländer A, Paumgartner G. Effect of ketoconazole and terbinafine on the pharmacokinetics of caffeine in healthy volunteers. *Eur J Clin Pharmacol* 1989; **37:** 279–83.

**Antigout drugs.** In a study in 2 healthy subjects, the plasma half-life of caffeine was essentially unchanged by 7 days' treatment with *allopurinol* 300 mg or 600 mg daily by mouth. However, allopurinol caused a specific, dose-dependent inhibition of the conversion of 1-methylxanthine to 1-methyluric acid.[1]

1. Grant DM, *et al.* Effect of allopurinol on caffeine disposition in man. *Br J Clin Pharmacol* 1986; **21:** 454–8.

**Gastrointestinal drugs.** *Cimetidine* 1 g daily by mouth reduced the systemic clearance of caffeine and prolonged its elimination half-life in 5 healthy subjects. Although the steady-state plasma-caffeine concentration would increase by approximately 70%, it was thought unlikely that this would produce adverse clinical effects.[1] However, in contrast a study in 11 children given cimetidine in doses of 11 to 36 mg/kg daily for gastritis found no evidence that it altered the metabolism of a dose of $^{13}$C-labelled caffeine.[2]

1. Broughton LJ, Rogers HJ. Decreased systemic clearance of caffeine due to cimetidine. *Br J Clin Pharmacol* 1981; **12:** 155–9.
2. Parker AC, *et al.* Lack of inhibitory effect of cimetidine on caffeine metabolism in children using the caffeine breath test. *Br J Clin Pharmacol* 1997; **43:** 467–70.

**Lithium.** For mention of the effect of caffeine on serum-lithium concentrations, see Xanthines, p.304.

**Sex hormones.** The clearance of caffeine has been reported to be reduced and its elimination half-life increased in women taking *oral contraceptives.*[1-3] This interaction was thought to be due to impairment of hepatic metabolism of caffeine by sex hormones and could result in increased accumulation of caffeine. Similar results have been reported[4] in a study of postmenopausal women given oestrogens for *hormone replacement therapy* and caffeine.

1. Patwardhan RV, *et al.* Impaired elimination of caffeine by oral contraceptive steroids. *J Lab Clin Med* 1980; **95:** 603–8.
2. Abernethy DR, Todd EL. Impairment of caffeine clearance by chronic use of low-dose oestrogen-containing oral contraceptives. *Eur J Clin Pharmacol* 1985; **28:** 425–8.

3. Balogh A, *et al.* Influence of ethinylestradiol-containing combination oral contraceptives with gestodene or levonorgestrel on caffeine elimination. *Eur J Clin Pharmacol* 1995; **48:** 161–6.
4. Pollock BG, *et al.* Inhibition of caffeine metabolism by estrogen replacement therapy in postmenopausal women. *J Clin Pharmacol* 1999; **39:** 936–40.


**Sympathomimetics.** Use of caffeine 400 mg with *phenylpropanolamine* 75 mg, both given orally as modified-release preparations, produced greater plasma-caffeine concentrations in healthy subjects than caffeine alone. Greater increases in blood pressure and more reports of physical side-effects occurred after the combination than after either drug alone.[1]


1. Lake CR, *et al.* Phenylpropanolamine increases plasma caffeine levels. *Clin Pharmacol Ther* 1990; **47:** 675–85.


**Theophylline.** For the effect of caffeine on the metabolism and elimination of theophylline, see p.802.

## Pharmacokinetics

Caffeine is absorbed readily after oral administration and is widely distributed throughout the body. It is also absorbed through the skin. Absorption after rectal administration by suppository may be slow and erratic. Absorption following intramuscular injection may be slower than after oral administration. Caffeine passes readily into the CNS and into saliva; low concentrations are also present in breast milk. Caffeine crosses the placenta.

In adults, caffeine is metabolised almost completely in the liver via oxidation, demethylation, and acetylation, and is excreted in the urine as 1-methyluric acid, 1-methylxanthine, 7-methylxanthine, 1,7-dimethylxanthine (paraxanthine), 5-acetylamino-6-formylamino-3-methyluracil (AFMU), and other metabolites with only about 1% unchanged. Neonates have a greatly reduced capacity to metabolise caffeine and it is largely excreted unchanged in the urine until hepatic metabolism becomes significantly developed, usually by about 6 months of age. Elimination half-lives are about 3 to 7 hours in adults but may be in excess of 100 hours in neonates.

**Metabolism and excretion.** The metabolism of caffeine has been shown to be dose dependent[1,2] with clearance decreasing as the dose is increased suggesting saturable metabolism. Four- to fivefold differences in plasma half-lives of caffeine are common among healthy people. The plasma half-life of caffeine is decreased by smoking[3] and by exercise,[4] and is increased by liver disease such as cirrhosis and viral hepatitis,[3,5] and in pregnancy.[3] The plasma half-life of caffeine is not affected by old age[6] or obesity.[7] Drug interactions also affect the pharmacokinetics of caffeine (see above).


1. Cheng WSC, *et al.* Dose-dependent pharmacokinetics of caffeine in humans: relevance as a test of quantitative liver function. *Clin Pharmacol Ther* 1990; **47:** 516–24.
2. Denaro CP, *et al.* Dose-dependency of caffeine metabolism with repeated dosing. *Clin Pharmacol Ther* 1990; **48:** 277–85.
3. Kalow W. Variability of caffeine metabolism in humans. *Arzneimittelforschung* 1985; **35:** 319–24.
4. Collomp K, *et al.* Effects of moderate exercise on the pharmacokinetics of caffeine. *Eur J Clin Pharmacol* 1991; **40:** 279–82.
5. Scott NR, *et al.* The pharmacokinetics of caffeine and its dimethylxanthine metabolites in patients with chronic liver disease. *Br J Clin Pharmacol* 1989; **27:** 205–13.
6. Blanchard J, Sawers SJA. Comparative pharmacokinetics of caffeine in young and elderly men. *J Pharmacokinet Biopharm* 1983; **11:** 109–26.
7. Abernethy DR, *et al.* Caffeine disposition in obesity. *Br J Clin Pharmacol* 1985; **20:** 61–6.


## Uses and Administration

Caffeine is a methylxanthine that, like theophylline (p.804), inhibits the enzyme phosphodiesterase and has an antagonistic effect at central adenosine receptors. It is a stimulant of the CNS, particularly the higher centres, and it can produce a condition of wakefulness and increased mental activity. It may also stimulate the respiratory centre, increasing the rate and depth of respiration. Its bronchodilating properties are weaker than those of theophylline. Caffeine facilitates the performance of muscular work and increases the total work which can be performed by a muscle. The diuretic action of caffeine is weaker than that of theophylline.

Caffeine is used as a mild CNS stimulant in usual doses of 50 to 100 mg by mouth, although doses of up to 200 mg may be used. A total dose of 1 g daily should not be exceeded. It is also frequently included in oral analgesic preparations with aspirin, paracetamol, or codeine in unit doses of about 15 to 65 mg but its clinical benefit is debated (see Pain, below). It is sometimes given with ergotamine in preparations for the treatment of migraine, usually in unit doses of 100 mg. Caffeine citrate has been used similarly.

Caffeine is also used in the short-term treatment of neonatal apnoea of prematurity (p.806). An initial dose for caffeine citrate is 20 mg/kg (equivalent to 10 mg/kg caffeine), followed by a maintenance dose of caffeine citrate 5 mg/kg daily. These doses are given either orally or by intravenous infusion. Serum concentrations of caffeine should be measured before starting treatment in infants who have already been treated with theophylline (which is metabolised to caffeine in infants) or whose mothers consumed caffeine before delivery; serious toxicity has been associated with serum concentrations greater than 50 micrograms/mL.

Caffeine and sodium benzoate and caffeine and sodium salicylate are readily soluble in water and have been used for the administration of caffeine by injection. Caffeine and sodium iodide (iodocaffeine) was formerly used in a similar manner.

Beverages of coffee, tea, and cola provide active doses of caffeine (see p.1765).

◊ General references.


1. Sawynok J. Pharmacological rationale for the clinical use of caffeine. *Drugs* 1995; **49:** 37–50.


**Asthma.** Caffeine's bronchodilating activity is about 40% that of theophylline[1] and doses of 5 or 10 mg/kg by mouth have been shown to produce an effect.[2,3] Because of its weak action other xanthines are generally recommended in asthma (p.777), but it may need to be avoided before tests of lung function.[4]


1. Gong H, *et al.* Bronchodilator effects of caffeine in coffee: a dose-response study of asthmatic subjects. *Chest* 1986; **89:** 335–42.
2. Becker AB, *et al.* The bronchodilator effects and pharmacokinetics of caffeine in asthma. *N Engl J Med* 1984; **310:** 743–6.
3. Bukowskyj M, Nakatsu K. The bronchodilator effect of caffeine in adult asthmatics. *Am Rev Respir Dis* 1987; **135:** 173–5.
4. Bara AI, Barley EA. Caffeine for asthma. Available in The Cochrane Library; Issue 1. Chichester: John Wiley; 2004.


**Diagnosis and testing.** Caffeine excretion assessed by measuring its urinary metabolites or by the exhalation of labelled $CO_2$ in breath following administration of $^{13}C$- or $^{14}C$-labelled caffeine has been used to develop liver function tests and to determine the activity of specific enzymes such as xanthine oxidase, P450 cytochromes, and polymorphic *N*-acetyltransferase.[1]

Caffeine administered orally has been used to assess acetylator status by determining the metabolic ratio of the metabolites 5-acetylamino-6-formylamino-1-methyluracil (AFMU) to 1-methylxanthine in urine,[2] but some have questioned its value.[3]


1. Kalow W, Tang B-K. The use of caffeine for enzyme assays: a critical appraisal. *Clin Pharmacol Ther* 1993; **53:** 503–14.
2. Hildebrand M, Seifert W. Determination of acetylator phenotype in caucasians with caffeine. *Eur J Clin Pharmacol* 1989; **37:** 525–6.
3. Notarianni LJ, *et al.* Caffeine as a metabolic probe: NAT2 phenotyping. *Br J Clin Pharmacol* 1996; **41:** 169–73.


**ECT.** In patients whose seizure duration is declining despite maximal ECT stimulation, pretreatment with high-dose intravenous caffeine increases seizure duration without affecting seizure threshold. Theophylline has been used similarly, see p.800. References.


1. Hinkle PE, *et al.* Use of caffeine to lengthen seizures in ECT. *Am J Psychiatry* 1987; **144:** 1143–8.
2. Coffey CE, *et al.* Caffeine augmentation of ECT. *Am J Psychiatry* 1990; **147:** 579–85.
3. Kelsey MC, Grossberg GT. Safety and efficacy of caffeine-augmented ECT in elderly depressives: a retrospective study. *J Geriatr Psychiatry Neurol* 1995; **8:** 168–72.


**Hypoglycaemia.** A single dose of caffeine 250 mg proved beneficial in augmenting warning symptoms and physiological responses to experimentally-induced hypoglycaemia in diabetic patients,[1] and was suggested as a potentially useful adjunct for diabetics who have difficulty in recognising the onset of hypoglycaemia (see Diabetic Emergencies, p.328). In a subsequent placebo-controlled crossover study caffeine 200 mg twice daily by mouth appeared to enhance the intensity of hypoglycaemic warning symptoms in patients with type 1 diabetes on a low-caffeine diet.[2]


1. Debrah K, *et al.* Effect of caffeine on recognition of and physiological responses to hypoglycaemia in insulin-dependent diabetes. *Lancet* 1996; **347:** 19–24.
2. Watson JM, *et al.* Influence of caffeine on the frequency and perception of hypoglycemia in free-living patients with type 1 diabetes. *Diabetes Care* 2000; **23:** 455–9.


**Orthostatic hypotension.** Caffeine has been of benefit in the treatment of orthostatic hypotension (p.1100) due to autonomic failure in some patients, especially for postprandial hypotension.[1-3] However, efficacy has only been demonstrated in mild cases and it is usually ineffective in severe cases.[4]


1. Onrot J, *et al.* Hemodynamic and humoral effects of caffeine in autonomic failure. *N Engl J Med* 1985; **313:** 549–54.
2. Hoeldtke RD, *et al.* Treatment of orthostatic hypotension with dihydroergotamine and caffeine. *Ann Intern Med* 1986; **105:** 168–73.
3. Tonkin AL. Postural hypotension. *Med J Aust* 1995; **162:** 436–8.
4. Mathias CJ. Orthostatic hypotension. *Prescribers' J* 1995; **35:** 124–32.


**Pain.** Caffeine has been widely used in analgesic preparations to enhance the effects of both non-opioid and opioid analgesics but is of debatable benefit (see under Choice of Analgesic, p.2). Some investigators have failed to show that caffeine offers any benefit[1,2] but others have shown that the adjuvant use of caffeine can increase analgesic activity.[3-7] A meta-analysis of 10 studies comparing paracetamol plus caffeine with paracetamol alone in women with postpartum uterine cramp found any benefit of the combination to be minimal.[8] A literature review[9] concluded that there was some evidence that caffeine may be useful as an analgesic adjuvant in relieving headache, but that the dose may need to be at least 65 mg and that these higher doses increase the risk of nervousness and dizziness. Evidence for the effects of caffeine in other types of pain, such as postpartum, postoperative, dental, rheumatic, and cancer pain, was inconclusive.

In the UK it is generally recommended that caffeine-containing analgesic preparations should not be used not only because of doubts about caffeine enhancing the analgesic effect but because it can add to gastrointestinal adverse effects and in large doses can itself cause headache.

Whether caffeine enhances the gastrointestinal absorption of ergotamine in preparations for the relief of migraine is not clear.


1. Winter L, *et al.* A double-blind, comparative evaluation of acetaminophen, caffeine, and the combination of acetaminophen and caffeine in outpatients with post-operative oral surgery pain. *Curr Ther Res* 1983; **33:** 115–22.
2. Sawynok J. Pharmacological rationale for the clinical use of caffeine. *Drugs* 1995; **49:** 37–50.
3. Laska EM, *et al.* Caffeine as an analgesic adjuvant. *JAMA* 1984; **251:** 1711–18.
4. Rubin A, Winter L. A double-blind randomized study of an aspirin/caffeine combination versus acetaminophen/aspirin combination versus acetaminophen versus placebo in patients with moderate to severe post-partum pain. *J Int Med Res* 1984; **12:** 338–45.
5. Schachtel BP, *et al.* Caffeine as an analgesic adjuvant: a double-blind study comparing aspirin with caffeine to aspirin and placebo in patients with sore throat. *Arch Intern Med* 1991; **151:** 733–7.
6. Migliardi JR, *et al.* Caffeine as an analgesic adjuvant in tension headache. *Clin Pharmacol Ther* 1994; **56:** 576–86.
7. Kraetsch HG, *et al.* Analgesic effects of propyphenazone in comparison to its combination with caffeine. *Eur J Clin Pharmacol* 1996; **49:** 377–82.
8. Zhang WY, Li Wan Po A. Analgesic efficacy of paracetamol and its combination with codeine and caffeine in surgical pain—a meta-analysis. *J Clin Pharm Ther* 1996; **21:** 261–82.
9. Zhang W-Y. A benefit-risk assessment of caffeine as an analgesic adjuvant. *Drug Safety* 2001; **24:** 1127–42.


POST-DURAL PUNCTURE HEADACHE. Intravenous caffeine sodium benzoate may relieve post-dural puncture headache (p.1368) which persists despite conservative therapy.

## Preparations

***BP 2003:*** Aspirin and Caffeine Tablets;
***USP 27:*** Acetaminophen and Caffeine Tablets; Acetaminophen, Aspirin, and Caffeine Tablets; Butalbital, Acetaminophen, and Caffeine Capsules; Butalbital, Acetaminophen, and Caffeine Tablets; Butalbital, Aspirin, and Caffeine Capsules; Butalbital, Aspirin, and Caffeine Tablets; Butalbital, Aspirin, Caffeine, and Codeine Phosphate Capsules; Caffeine and Sodium Benzoate Injection; Ergotamine Tartrate and Caffeine Suppositories; Ergotamine Tartrate and Caffeine Tablets; Propoxyphene Hydrochloride, Aspirin, and Caffeine Capsules.

**Proprietary Preparations** (details are given in Part 3)
***Arg.:*** Guarana; Percutafeine; ***Austral.:*** No Doz†; ***Austria:*** Coffekapton; ***Braz.:*** Percutafeine; ***Canad.:*** Wake-Up Tablets; ***Chile:*** Asafen Nueva Formula; Jaquedryl; ***Fin.:*** Cofi-Tabs; ***Fr.:*** Percutafeine; ***Ger.:*** Autonic†; Percoffedrinol N; ***Gr.:*** Cafcit; ***Port.:*** Bioregime SlimKit; ***S.Afr.:*** Doxypol†; Universal Concentration Tablets†; ***Spain:*** Durvitan; Prolert†; ***UK:*** Pro-Plus; ***USA:*** Cafcit; Caffedrine; Enerjets; Keep Alert; Lucidex; NoDoz; Quick Pep†; Stay Alert; Vivarin.

**Multi-ingredient:** ***Arg.:*** Alikal; Alzaten; Cafergot; Cafiaspirina; Cefalex; Dentolina Plus; Desenfriol; Dolanet; Dristan Analgesico; Dristan Compuesto; Enlinea; Falgos; Ferona; Geniol; Gripanil C; Ibu-Tetralgin; Ibumar Migra; Ibupirac Migra; Inmunogrip; Jaquedryl; Kiper; Mejoral Cafeina; Migra Dioxadol; Migral; Migral Compositum; Migral II; Mudagrip; Nulagrip C; Parsel; Polipectol; Reanima; Saridon; Sertinal; Tabcin Antigripal; Tetralgin; Tetralgin Novo; Trinitron; Uvasal; Yasta; Zilactin-E; ***Austral.:*** Cafergot; Dynamo†; Ergodryl; Migral†; No Doz Plus†; Travacalm; ***Austria:*** Adolorin; Asticol†; Avamigran; Cafergot; Capramin†; Coffo Selt; Coldadolin; Coldagrippin; Contraforte; Contralorin; Dihydergot; Dolmix; Dolomo; Duan; Eu-Med; Gastrotest†; Gerontin; Gewadal; Influvidon; Irocophan; Leaton fur Erwachsene; Lecikur; Lecivital; Melabon; Migradon; Migril; Montamed; Neo-Emedyl; Neokratin; Nervan; Nisicur; Panax†; Pasuma-Dragees; Rapidol; Ratiopyrin; Rilfit; Saridon; Secokapton; Sigmalin $B_6$; Sigmalin $B_6$ forte; Solukapton; Spalt; Synkapton; Systral C†; Thomapyrin; Tonopan; Vivimed; ***Belg.:*** Algostase; Antigriphine; Antigrippine Midy†; Asodal; Aspirine Duo; Cafergot; Croix Blanche; Dolviran; Eugrippine†; Finimal†; Guronsan; Kranit Nova; Lonarid N; Mann; Migraine-Kranit Nova†; Neomeritine†; Nevrine Codeine†; Optalidon; Panadeine†; Parmentier†; Perdolan Compositum; Saridon; ***Braz.:*** Adegrip†; Algi-Butazolon; Algi-Tanderil; Algiflex†; Alicura; Analgex C†; Anapirol†; Antigripine†; Asafen†; Aspirina Forte; Aspirisan†; Atagripe†; Banidor†; Benegrip†; Beserol; Cafergot†; Cafiaspirina; Carnabol; Cefaldina; Cefalium; Cefaliv; Cefunk†; Cheracap S; Cheracap†; Cibalena A; Coristina D; Coristina R; Coristina Reforcada†; Dalgex; Diclofetamol; Doralem†; Doralgina; Dorex†; Dorflex; Doribel; Doricin; Doridina; Doril†; Dorilax; Dorpinol†; Dorsedin; Dorserol†; Dorzone; Engov†; Excedrin; Flexdor; Fontol; Gerosenil†; Gripin C†; Gripionex†; Gripol C†; Gripol Composto†; Griptol†; Ioimbina Composta†; Itaiflex†; Melhoral; Migral†; Migraliv; Migrane; Mio-Citalgan; Miorrelax; Nasogrip; Neomigran; Neosaldina; Optalidon†; Ormigrein; Paceflex; Parcel; Posdrink; Redentil†; Relaflex†; Resfry; Resfry Infantil†; Resprax; Rielex; Sanacol†; Saridon; Sedagripe†; Sedalex; Sedalgina; Sedalmerck; Sedilax; Sedol; Sexormom†; Sulindor†; Superhist; Tacidina†; Tandene; Tanderalgin; Tandriflan; Tandrilax; Tensaldin; Termogripe C; Theopirina; Tonopan; Torsilax; Trilax; Veramon†; Vita Grip†; Vitalen C; ***Canad.:*** 217 Strong†; 217†; 222; 282; 282 Mep; 292; 692†; AC & C; Acet-2, Acet-3†; Acetaminophen with Codeine; Anacin; Anacin with Codeine†; Antidol; Arco Pain†; Astone†; Atasol-8, -15, -30; C2 with Codeine; Cafergot; Cafergot-PB; Dolomine†; Dristan†; Ergodryl; Excedrin; Exdol; Extra

Strength Acetaminophen with Codeine†; Fiorinal; Fiorinal C; Gravergol; Herbopyrine; Instantine; Lenoltec No 1, No 2, or No 3; Megral†; Midol Extra Strength; Midol Multi-Symptom†; Midol Original†; Midol Regular; Midol Traditional; Nervine†; Norgesic; Novo AC and C; Novo-Gesic C; Pain Aid; Sinugex†; Tecnal; Tecnal C; Triaminicin†; Trianal; Trianal C; Triatec-8; Tylenol No 1; Tylenol with Codeine No 2 or No 3; Wigraine†; ***Chile:*** Anacin; Cafergot-PB; Cafiaspirina; Cefalmin; Cheracol; Cinabel; Coldstat; Cotibin Flu; Dolorsin; Facitor; Feminosan; Fentos; Fredol; Gripasan Compuesto; Gripasan Nueva Formula; Gripexin Limonada Caliente; Gripexin Nueva Formula Compuesto; Kitadol Flu; Kitadol Flu Noche; Kitadol Max; Migragesic; Migranol; Migratam; Migratapsin; Migrax; Obleas Chinas; Panadol Plus; Panagesic Con Cafeina; Parsel; Piretanyl; Prefem; Saridon; Sedalmerck; Tapal-2; Tapsin 2 Analgesico; Tapsin Analgesico; Tapsin Compuesto; Tapsin Compuesto con Clorfenamina; Tapsin Compuesto Dia/Noche Plus; Trigesico; Ultrimin; Veradin; ***Denm.:*** Ergokoffin; Gynergen Comp; Kodamid; Koffisal; Letigen; Treo; ***Fin.:*** Anervan; Coldrex; Finrexin; Malvitona; Panadol Comp; Posivil; Somadril Comp; Treo; ***Fr.:*** Actron; Alepsal; Antigrippine a l'Aspirine†; Asproaccel; Asthmalgine†; Cefaline Hauth; Cefaline-Pyrazole; Cephyl; Cetafeine†; Claradol Cafeine; Diergospray; Dolidon†; Exidol; Finidol; Gelumaline; Guronsan; Gynergene Cafeine; Hordenol†; Kola Astier†; Lamaline; Mercalm; Metaspirine; Migralgine; Migwell†; Optalidon a la Noramidopyrine†; Polypirine; Prontalgine; Propofan; Rumicine†; Sedaspir; Suppomaline; Theinol; Vasobral; Veganine; ***Ger.:*** Alacetan; Aspirin forte; Azur; Azur compositum; Biovital Aktiv; Cafergot N; Chephapyrin N; Coffalon N; Coffeemed N; Coffetylin†; Copyrkal N; Ditonal N; Dolomo TN; Doppel-Spalt Compact; Dorocoff-ASS plus†; Entrodyn; Ergoffin; Eudorlin; Euvitan†; Fineural N†; Fohnetten N; Gewodin†; Grippostad C; HA-Tabletten N; Halloo-Wach N; Hermes ASS plus†; Hewedolor plus Coffein; Ilvico N†; Impletol†; Kola-Dallmann mit Lecithin†; Kola-Dallmann†; Melabon K†; Migranin; Neopyrin; Neuralgin; Neuramag P†; Neuranidal; Neuranidal Duo†; Novo Petrin; Octadon P; Optalidon N; Paracetamol plus; Procaneural; Prontopyrin plus; Quadronal ASS comp; Quadronal comp; Ratiopyrin; Reisegold; Ring N; Rio-Josipyrin N†; Rodavan†; Saridon; Systral C; Thomapyrin; Titralgan; Togal Kopfschmerzbrause + Vit C; Toximer C; ***Gr.:*** Cafergot; ***Hong Kong:*** Anacin; Antiflu Forte; Antiflu-N-Forte; Arfen Plus; Cafergot; Codoplex; Coldrex; Coltalin with Vit $B_1$; Cortal for Adults; Coryaid†; DF Multi-Symptom; Doloxene Compound†; Flu-Off; Gravergol; Metoplex; Midol†; Migril; Neosed†; Panadol Cold and Flu; Panadol Extra; Paramol Forte; Rhinocap; Saridon; Tonterin; Vasobral; ***Hung.:*** Quarelin; ***India:*** Alex; Carisoma Compound; Coldoff; Dristan Expectorant; Duoflam Plus; Micropyrin; Migranil; Pregnidoxin; Ralcidin; Sinarest; Zimalgin; ***Irl.:*** Anadin; Anadin Extra; Beechams Cold Relief†; Beechams Flu Plus; Cafergot†; Doloxene Compound†; Distan†; Feminax; Ilvico†; Maxilief; Migranat; Migril; Panadol Extra; Parahypon†; Solpadeine; Syndol; Tramil; Uniflu & Gregovite C†; Vivimed†; ***Israel:*** Anacin; Aspex; Cafergot; Coldex; Dexamol Plus; Novocalm; Rogaan; Rokacet; Rokacet Plus; Rokal; Rokal Plus; Temigran; ***Ital.:*** Alfazina†; Alsogil; Anticorizza; Antiflu; Antinevralgico Dr Knapp; Antireumina; Azerodol†; Cafergot; Caffalgina†; Cafiaspirina†; Difmetre; Drin; Fluvaleas†; Geyfritz; Influrem; Micranet; Mindol-Merck; Murri Antidolorifico; Neo Coricidin; Neo Nisidina-Fher; Neo-Cibalgina; Neo-Nevral; Neo-Optalidon; Neodone†; Odontalgico Dr. Knapp con Vit. B1; Omniadol†; Optalidon; Raffreddoremed; Saridon; Sedol; Triaminic; Vasobral; Verdal; Via Mal; Virdex; ***Malaysia:*** Cafergot; ***Mex.:*** Amgrip; Asafen; Bioflusin; Cafergot; Cantipal; Cheracol; Coricidin F; Corilin F; Darvon-N Compuesto; Dolocibal†; Ergocaf; LM6; Numonyl C; Parsel; Pirafrin; Piralgina; Saridon†; Sedalmerck; Sin-A Crud; Sydolil; Tempra MF; Togrisol; Tonopan; Trinergot; ***Neth.:*** Antigrippine; Cafergot; Daro Hoofdpijnpoeders†; Dolviran N; Femerital†; Finimal; Panadol Plus; Sanalgin; Saridon; Witte Kruis; ***Norw.:*** Anervan; Antineuralgica; B-Tonin†; Fanalgin; ***NZ:*** Cafergot; De Witts Pills; Ergodryl†; Migril†; ***Port.:*** Algik; Almigripe; Anadin Extra; Anti-Gripe; Asfeina; Bisolgrip T; Cafiaspirina; Casfen; Cephyl; Cofena†; Dolviran; Fluidin Adulto†; Gripetral; Guronsan; Higigripe†; Ilvico N†; Melhoral; Migretil; Optalidon; Salicylcafeina; Saridon N; Ugrilon†; Zimaina; ***S.Afr.:*** Abflex; Acugesil†; Acurate; Adco-Dol; Adco-Payne; Algist†; Analgen; Analgen-SA; Antiflu; Antipyn; Antipyn Forte; Arcanaflu†; Asalen; B-Dol; Ban Pain; Betapyn; Briscopyn†; Cafergot; Cafergot-PB; Cetamine†; Colcaps; Colcleer; Colphen; Colstat; Degoran C; Degoran Plus; Dequa-Flu; Docdol; Doloxene Co; Dynapayne†; Emprazil-A†; Endcol Cold & Flu; Famucaps; Flu-Stat; Flucol†; Flusin; Flutex; Forpyn; Go-Pain; Grippon; Histacon; Histamed Compound; Histodor; Ilvico; KPP; Lenadol; Lenapain; Maxadol Forte†; Megapyn; Mepromol; Merck-Flu; Migril; Nervade†; Nitroflu; Nomopain; Nopyn; Noralget; Painagon; Painrite†; Paxidal; Propain; Propain Forte; Pynclear; Pynmed; Pynstop; Redupon; Salterpyn; Sedapain; Sedinol; Sinucon; Spectrapain Forte; Stilpane; Stopayne; Suncodin; Supragesic; Synaleve†; Synap; Syndol; Tensolve; Tensopyn†; Tenston; Ultraviro C†; Vacudol Forte; Xeramax; Xerogesic; Xerotens; ***Singapore:*** Anacin; Beacons; Cafergot; Dhacold; Dhaflu†; Febs; Migril†; Pacofen; Panadol Extra; Picapan; ***Spain:*** AB FE; Abdominol; Actron Compuesto; Analgilasa; Antidoloroso Rudol†; Aspirina Plus; Beecham Lemon Miel†; Biodramina Cafeina; Cafergot; Cafergot-PB; Cafiaspirina; Cafinitrina; Calmante Vitaminado P G; Calmante Vitaminado PG Efervescente; Cerebrino; Cinfamar Cafeina; Coricidin; Desenfriol; Desenfriol C; Desenfriol D; Dolofarma; Dolviran; Doscafis; Farmacola†; Fenalgin†; Fiorinal Codeina; Fiorinal†; Frenadol Complex; Frialgina†; Hemicraneal; Hubergrip; Igril†; Ilvico; Mastia†; Mejoral Cafeina; Melabon; Meloka; Neocibalena; Okal; Optalidon; Pridio; Propyre T†; Quimpedor; Rinomicine; Rinomicine Activada; Saldeva; Salvarina; Saridon; Sedalmerck; Sinefricol†; Tonopan; Unidor; Vincidol; Yendol; ***Swed.:*** Anervan; Bamyl koffein; Bamyl S koffein; Cafergot; Koffazon; Lergigan comp; Magnecyl-koffein; Malvitona; Somadril Comp; Treo; Treo comp; Vitatonin; ***Switz.:*** Agorhino; Anaestalgin; Antemin compositum; Biovital Ginseng; Cafergot; Cafergot-PB; Caposan; Cerebrol; Cerebrol sans codeine; Comprimes analgesiques "S"; Contre-Douleurs; Contre-Douleurs C; Contre-Douleurs plus; Demodenal compositum†; Demoderhin†; Dialgine forte; Dihydergot; Dolostop; Dragees contre les maux de voyage no 537; Dramamine-compositum; Duremesan; Ergosanol a la cafeine†; Ergosanol special a la cafeine†; Ergosanol special†; Escalgin sans codeine; Escogripp sans codeine; Ganavit†; Gewodine; Grippalgine N; Gubamine†; Histacylettes; Itinerol $B_6$; Kafa; Medramine-$B_6$ Rectocaps†; Melabon N; Migraine-Kranit; Migrexa†; Migril†; Neo-Cibalgin†; Novidol†; Rhinocap; Sanalgin N; Saridon; Seranex sans codeine; Sinedal; Siniphen†; Sonotryl†; Spedralgin sans codeine; Thomapyrine; Tonopan; Vadol†; Viaggio†; ***Thai.:*** Avamigran; Cafergot; Degran; Poligot-CF; Polygot; ***UAE:*** Adol Compound; Adol Extra; ***UK:*** Alka XS Go; Alka-Seltzer XS; Anadin; Anadin Cold Control†; Anadin Extra; Andrews Answer†; Aqua Ban; Askit; Beechams Decongestant Plus with Paracetamol; Beechams Flu-Plus; Beechams Powders; Beechams Powders Capsules; Boost; Boots Cold & Flu Relief; Boots Tension Headache Relief†; Cafadol†; Cafergot; Calpol Extra†; Catarrh-Ex; Charabs†; Coda-Med†; Cold Relief; Cullens Headache Powders; De Witt's Analgesic; Do-Do ChestEze; Dolvan; Dristan†; E.P.†; Extra Power Pain Reliever; Feminax; Glykola; Hedex Extra; Koladex†; Labiton; Lem-Plus†; Lemsip Cold & Flu Combined Relief†; Lemsip Cold & Flu Max Strength Capsules; Lemsip Max Strength Sinus Relief; Migril; Mrs Cullen's Powders; Non-Drowsy Sudafed Dual Relief; Nurse Sykes Powders; Painex; Panadol Extra; Paracets Plus; Paxidal; PEP; Phensic; Phensic Dual Action†; Propain; Propain Plus; Resolve Extra; Ronpirin APCQ†; Solpadeine Plus; SP†; Syndol; Toptabs†; Ultramol; Uniflu with Gregovite C; Veganin; Yeast Vite; ***USA:*** Amaphen with Codeine; Amaphen†; Americet; Anacin; Anolor; Anoquan†; Aqua Ban; Aqua Ban Plus; Ascomp with Codeine; Aspirin Free Excedrin; B-A-C†; Bayer Extra Strength Back & Body Pain; Bayer Select Maximum Strength Headache†; BC; Buffets II†; Cafatine; Cafatine-PB; Cafergot; Cafetrate†; Cope; Darvon Compound; DHC Plus; Dolgic LQ; Endolor; Ercaf; Esgic; Esgic-Plus; Excedrin; Excedrin Migraine; Excedrin QuickTabs; Excedrin Tension Headache; Femcet†; Fioricet; Fioricet with Codeine; Fiorinal; Fiorinal with Codeine; Fiorpap†; Fiortal with Codeine†; Fiortal†; Gelpirin†; Gensan†; Goody's Headache Powders; Headrin Extra Strength; Histosal†; Hycomine Compound; Isocet†; Lanorinal†; Margesic; Maximum Strength Arthritien†; Medigesic; Norgesic; Orphengesic; P-A-C; Pacaps; Pain Reliever†; Painaid; Painaid ESF Extra-Strength Formula; Panlor DC; PC-Cap; Repan; Saleto; Saleto-D†; Scot-Tussin Original 5-Action; Sinapils†; Supac†; Synalgos-DC; Tencet; Triad; Trim-Elim; Tussirex; Vanquish; Wigraine.

## Choline Theophyllinate *(BAN, rINN)*

Oxtriphylline; Teofilinato de colina; Theophylline Cholinate.

$C_{12}H_{21}N_5O_3$ = 283.3.

*CAS — 4499-40-5.*

*ATC — R03DA02.*

**Pharmacopoeias.** In *Br., Chin.,* and *US.*

**BP 2003** (Choline Theophyllinate). A white crystalline powder, odourless or with a faint amine-like odour. It contains between 41.9% and 43.6% of choline and between 61.7% and 65.5% of theophylline, each calculated with reference to the dried substance. Very soluble in water; soluble in alcohol; very slightly soluble in chloroform and in ether. Store at a temperature not exceeding 25°. Protect from light.

**USP 27** (Oxtriphylline). A white crystalline powder, having an amine-like odour. It contains not less than 61.7% and not more than 65.5% of anhydrous theophylline. Soluble 1 in 1 of water; freely soluble in alcohol; very slightly soluble in chloroform. A 1% solution in water has a pH of about 10.3. Store in airtight containers.

### Profile

Choline theophyllinate is a theophylline salt that liberates theophylline (p.798) in the body; choline theophyllinate 1.57 mg is approximately equivalent in theophylline content to 1 mg of anhydrous theophylline. It is used as a bronchodilator for reversible airways obstruction. The usual maintenance dosage for adults is 800 to 1200 mg daily by mouth, in 3 or 4 divided doses, preferably after food to reduce gastrointestinal side-effects. Low doses (200 to 400 mg daily) should be given initially and gradually increased according to clinical response and serum-theophylline concentrations (see Uses and Administration of Theophylline, p.804). A suggested maintenance dosage for children aged 5 to 9 years is 200 to 400 mg in 4 divided doses, and for children aged 10 to 14 years, 400 to 800 mg daily in 4 divided doses. Children under 5 years of age may receive 24 to 36 mg/kg daily in 3 divided doses.

### Preparations

***BP 2003:*** Choline Theophyllinate Tablets;
***USP 27:*** Oxtriphylline Delayed-release Tablets; Oxtriphylline Extended-release Tablets; Oxtriphylline Oral Solution; Oxtriphylline Tablets.

**Proprietary Preparations** (details are given in Part 3)
***Austral.:*** Brondecon Elixir; ***Canad.:*** Choledyl; Novo-Triphyl†; Rouphylline†; ***Ger.:*** Euspirax; ***Gr.:*** Choledyl; ***Hong Kong:*** Rouphylline†; ***Irl.:*** Choledyl†; ***Norw.:*** Teovent†; ***S.Afr.:*** Choledyl†; ***Swed.:*** Teovent; ***USA:*** Choledyl.

**Multi-ingredient:** ***Austral.:*** Brondecon Expectorant; ***Canad.:*** Choledyl Expectorant; ***NZ:*** Broncelix; Brondecon†; Pharmacycare Cough Expectorant; ***Port.:*** Vitasma; ***Spain:*** Dimayon†; Tilfilin†.

## Clenbuterol Hydrochloride *(BANM, rINNM)*

Hidrocloruro de clenbuterol; NAB-365 (clenbuterol). 1-(4-Amino-3,5-dichlorophenyl)-2-*tert*-butylaminoethanol hydrochloride.

$C_{12}H_{18}Cl_2N_2O,HCl$ = 313.7.

*CAS — 37148-27-9 (clenbuterol); 21898-19-1 (clenbuterol hydrochloride).*

*ATC — R03AC14; R03CC13.*

NOTE. Clenbuterol has been referred to as angel dust; this name has also been used to describe illicit phencyclidine.

**Pharmacopoeias.** In *Chin.*

### Profile

Clenbuterol hydrochloride is a direct-acting sympathomimetic with predominantly beta-adrenergic activity and a selective action on $beta_2$ receptors (a $beta_2$ agonist). It has properties similar to those of salbutamol (p.791). It is used as a bronchodilator in the management of reversible airways obstruction, as in asthma (p.777) and in certain patients with chronic obstructive pulmonary disease (p.779). A usual dose is 20 micrograms twice daily by mouth; doses of up to 40 micrograms twice daily have occasionally been employed. Clenbuterol hydrochloride is also given by inhalation in usual doses of 20 micrograms three times daily. In patients with asthma, as-required beta agonist therapy is preferable to regular use. An increased need for, or decreased duration of effect of, clenbuterol indicates deterioration of asthma control and the need for review of therapy.

**Abuse.** Clenbuterol has been used illicitly in animal feeds in an attempt to promote weight gain and to increase muscle to lipid mass. Adverse effects typical of sympathomimetic activity have been attributed to such misuse both in farmers perpetrating such acts[1] and in innocent persons consuming meat products from affected animals.[2-4] Clenbuterol has been abused by sportsmen for its anabolic effects,[5] although it is doubtful as to whether it enhances performance.[6]


1. Dawson J. β Agonists put meat in the limelight again. *BMJ* 1990; **301:** 1238–9.
2. Martínez-Navarro JF. Food poisoning related to consumption of illicit β-agonist in liver. *Lancet* 1990; **336:** 1311.
3. Maistro S, *et al.* Beta blockers to prevent clenbuterol poisoning. *Lancet* 1995; **346:** 180.
4. Brambilla G, *et al.* Food poisoning following consumption of clenbuterol-treated veal in Italy. *JAMA* 1997; **278:** 635.
5. Anonymous. Muscling in on clenbuterol. *Lancet* 1992; **340:** 403.
6. Spann C, Winter ME. Effect of clenbuterol on athletic performance. *Ann Pharmacother* 1995; **29:** 75–7.


### Preparations

**Proprietary Preparations** (details are given in Part 3)
***Arg.:*** Bronq-C; Clembumar; Oxibron; ***Austria:*** Spiropent; ***Braz.:*** Ventilan†; ***Chile:*** Airum; Asmeren; Broncotosil; ***Ger.:*** Contraspasmin; Spiropent; ***Gr.:*** Spiropent; ***Hong Kong:*** Clenasma; ***Ital.:*** Broncodil†; Clenasma; Contrasmina†; Monores; Prontovent; Spiropent; ***Jpn:*** Spiropent; ***Mex.:*** Novegam; Oxyflux; Spiropent; ***Port.:*** Broncoterol; Cesbron; ***Spain:*** Spiropent; Ventolase.

**Multi-ingredient:** ***Arg.:*** Mucosolvon Compositum; Oxibron NF; ***Austria:*** Mucospas; ***Ger.:*** Spasmo-Mucosolvan; ***Mex.:*** Balsibron-C; Brogal Compositum; Brosolan-C; Broxofar Compuesto; Broxol Plus; Ebromin-P; Mucosolvan Compositum; Mucovibrol C; Sekretovit Ex; Septacin Ex; ***Port.:*** Clembroxol†; Mucospas; Ventoliber.

## Diprophylline *(BAN, rINN)*

Dihydroxypropyltheophyllinum; Diprofilina; Diprophyllinum; Dyphylline; Glyphyllinum; Hyphylline. 7-(2,3-Dihydroxypropyl)-1,3-dimethylxanthine; 7-(2,3-Dihydroxypropyl)theophylline.

$C_{10}H_{14}N_4O_4$ = 254.2.

*CAS — 479-18-5.*

*ATC — R03DA01.*

**Pharmacopoeias.** In *Chin., Eur.* (see p.vi), *Pol.,* and *US.*

**Ph. Eur. 5.0** (Diprophylline). A white crystalline powder. Freely soluble in water; slightly soluble in alcohol. Protect from light.

**USP 27** (Dyphylline). A white, odourless, amorphous or crystalline solid. Freely soluble in water; sparingly soluble in alcohol and in chloroform; practically insoluble in ether. A 1% solution in water has a pH of 5.0 to 7.5. Store in airtight containers.

### Adverse Effects, Treatment, and Precautions

As for Theophylline, p.798. Diprophylline is primarily excreted unchanged in the urine and should therefore be used with caution in patients with renal impairment. However, unlike theophylline, plasma concentrations of diprophylline are not greatly affected by changes in liver function or hepatic enzyme activity such as those produced by smoking, age, and heart failure.

**Breast feeding.** In a study of 20 lactating women given diprophylline by intramuscular injection,[1] diprophylline was found to concentrate in breast milk, with a milk to serum concentration ratio of about 2. However, it was felt that the quantity of diprophylline a breast-fed infant would ingest was unlikely to produce any pharmacological action unless the child was very sensitive. The American Academy of Pediatrics[2] also considers that the use of diprophylline is usually compatible with breast feeding.


1. Jarboe CH, *et al.* Dyphylline elimination kinetics in lactating women: blood to milk transfer. *J Clin Pharmacol* 1981; **21:** 405–10.
2. American Academy of Pediatrics. The transfer of drugs and other chemicals into human milk. *Pediatrics* 2001; **108:** 776–89. Correction. *ibid.*; 1029. Also available at: http://aappolicy.aappublications.org/cgi/content/full/pediatrics%3b108/3/776 (accessed 20/04/04)


### Interactions

Since diprophylline does not undergo metabolism by hepatic microsomal cytochrome P450 it does not exhibit the numerous interactions seen with theophylline (p.800). However, the possibility of synergistic effects should be borne in mind if it is prescribed with other xanthines.

**Probenecid.** Probenecid has been reported to decrease the clearance of diprophylline thus prolonging its half-life.[1-3]


1. May DC, Jarboe CH. Inhibition of clearance of dyphylline by probenecid. *N Engl J Med* 1981; **304:** 791.
2. May DC, Jarboe CH. Effect of probenecid on dyphylline elimination. *Clin Pharmacol Ther* 1983; **33:** 822–5.
3. Acara M, *et al.* Probenecid inhibition of the renal excretion of dyphylline in chicken, rat and man. *J Pharm Pharmacol* 1987; **39:** 526–30.


### Pharmacokinetics

Diprophylline is rapidly absorbed from the gastrointestinal tract and from the site of intramuscular injections. Diprophylline does not liberate theophylline in the body and is largely excreted unchanged in the urine with an elimination half-life of about 2 hours. Diprophylline is distributed into breast milk.

### Uses and Administration

Diprophylline is a theophylline derivative which is used similarly to theophylline (p.804) as a bronchodilator in reversible airways obstruction.

The usual dose of diprophylline by mouth is up to 15 mg/kg every 6 hours. It has also been given intramuscularly. Diprophylline is also an ingredient of preparations that have been promoted for coughs.

**Action.** Improvements in measurements of lung function after diprophylline in doses of 15 and 20 mg/kg by mouth were only one-third to one-half those obtained after theophylline 6 mg/kg by mouth.[1]

1. Furukawa CT, *et al.* Diphylline versus theophylline: a double-blind comparative evaluation. *J Clin Pharmacol* 1983; **23:** 414–18.

### Preparations

***USP 27:*** Dyphylline and Guaifenesin Elixir; Dyphylline and Guaifenesin Tablets; Dyphylline Elixir; Dyphylline Injection; Dyphylline Tablets.

**Proprietary Preparations** (details are given in Part 3)
***Austria:*** Austrophyllin; Isophyllen†; ***Ger.:*** Asthmolysin†; ***Gr.:*** Silbephylline; ***Ital.:*** Katasma; ***Port.:*** Neufil; ***USA:*** Dilor; Dylix; Lufyllin.

**Multi-ingredient:** ***Austria:*** Laevostrophan compositum†; ***Fr.:*** Ozothine a la Diprophylline; ***Ger.:*** Ozothin†; ***Israel:*** Philinal; Philinet; ***Ital.:*** Cort-Inal; ***Spain:*** Alergical Expect; Bronsal; Difilina Asmorax†; Novofilin; ***Switz.:*** Brosol†; Neo-Biphyllin†; ***UK:*** Noradran; ***USA:*** Dilor-G†; Dy-G; Dyflex-G; Dyline GG; Dyphylline-GG; Lufyllin-EPG; Lufyllin-GG; Panfil G.

## Doxofylline *(USAN, rINN)*

ABC 12/3; Doxofilina. 7-(1,3-Dioxolan-2-ylmethyl)theophylline.

$C_{11}H_{14}N_4O_4$ = 266.3.
*CAS — 69975-86-6.*
*ATC — R03DA11.*

### Profile

Doxofylline is a theophylline derivative (p.798) which is used as a bronchodilator in reversible airways obstruction. It is given by mouth in doses of up to 1200 mg daily. It may also be given by slow intravenous injection.

### Preparations

**Proprietary Preparations** (details are given in Part 3)
***Ital.:*** Ansimar.

## Etamiphylline Camsilate *(BANM, rINNM)*

Camsilato de etamifilina; Diétamiphylline Camphosulfonate; Etamiphylline Camsylate; Etamphyllin Camsylate. 7-(2-Diethylaminoethyl)-1,3-dimethylxanthine camphor-10-sulphonate; 7-(2-Diethylaminoethyl)theophylline camphor-10-sulphonate.

$C_{23}H_{37}N_5O_6S$ = 511.6.
*CAS — 314-35-2 (etamiphylline); 19326-29-5 (etamiphylline camsilate).*
*ATC — R03DA06.*

**Pharmacopoeias.** In *BP(Vet).*

**BP(Vet) 2003** (Etamiphylline Camsilate). A white or almost white powder with a faint camphoraceous odour. Very soluble in water; soluble in alcohol and in chloroform; very slightly soluble in ether. A 10% solution in water has a pH of 3.9 to 5.4.

### Profile

Etamiphylline camsilate is a derivative of theophylline (p.798) and has been used as a bronchodilator in reversible airways obstruction. Etamiphylline does not liberate theophylline in the body.

Etamiphylline and its dehydrocholate, hydrochloride, and methiodide salts have also been used.

### Preparations

**Proprietary Preparations** (details are given in Part 3)
***Spain:*** Solufilina; Solufilina Simple†.

**Multi-ingredient:** ***Spain:*** Solufilina Sedante†.

## Etofylline *(BAN, rINN)*

Aethophyllinum; Etofilina; Etofyllinum; Hydroxyaethyltheophyllinum; Hydroxyéthylthéophylline; Oxyetophylline. 7-(2-Hydroxyethyl)-1,3-dimethylxanthine; 3,7-Dihydro-7-(2-hydroxyethyl)-1,3-dimethyl-1*H*-purine-2,6-dione; 7-(2-Hydroxyethyl)theophylline.

$C_9H_{12}N_4O_3$ = 224.2.
*CAS — 519-37-9.*
*ATC — C04AD04.*

**Pharmacopoeias.** In *Eur.* (see p.vi).

**Ph. Eur. 5.0** (Etofylline). A white crystalline powder. Soluble in water; slightly soluble in alcohol. Protect from light.

### Profile

Etofylline is a derivative of theophylline (p.798) that is an ingredient of preparations promoted for various respiratory and cardiovascular disorders. It does not liberate theophylline in the body.

Etofylline nicotinate has also been used.

### Preparations

**Proprietary Preparations** (details are given in Part 3)
***S.Afr.:*** Theostat†.

**Multi-ingredient:** ***Austria:*** Apoplectal†; Instenon; Perphyllon†; ***Braz.:*** Geri-Kan H3†; ***Ger.:*** Coroverlan†; ***Hong Kong:*** Instenon; ***India:*** Albutamol; Bronchilet; Deriphyllin; Etyofil; Terphylin; ***S.Afr.:*** Actophlem; Alcophyllex; D-Tussin†; Dilinct; Solphyllex; Solphyllin; Theophen; Theophen Comp; ***Spain:*** Flebo Stop†; Vasperdil†; ***Switz.:*** Theo-Talusin†; ***Thai.:*** Instenon.

## Fenoterol *(BAN, USAN, rINN)*

1-(3,5-Dihydroxyphenyl)-2-(4-hydroxy-α-methylphenethylamino)ethanol.

$C_{17}H_{21}NO_4$ = 303.4.
*CAS — 13392-18-2.*
*ATC — G02CA03; R03AC04; R03CC04.*

## Fenoterol Hydrobromide *(BANM, rINNM)*

Fenoteroli Hydrobromidum; Hidrobromuro de fenoterol; TH-1165a. 1-(3,5-Dihydroxyphenyl)-2-(4-hydroxy-α-methylphenethylamino)ethanol hydrobromide.

$C_{17}H_{21}NO_4,HBr$ = 384.3.
*CAS — 1944-12-3.*
*ATC — G02CA03; R03AC04; R03CC04.*

**Pharmacopoeias.** In *Eur.* (see p.vi) and *Pol.*

**Ph. Eur. 5.0** (Fenoterol Hydrobromide). A white crystalline powder. Soluble in water and in alcohol. A 4% solution in water has a pH of 4.2 to 5.2. Protect from light.

### Adverse Effects and Precautions

As for Salbutamol, p.791.

**Increased mortality.** Since the introduction of metered-dose aerosols of beta agonists there have been two reported epidemics of increased morbidity and mortality in asthmatic patients associated with their use. The first occurred in the 1960s and was linked with the use of high-dose isoprenaline inhalers.[1] The use of isoprenaline was subsequently largely discontinued in favour of more selective beta$_2$ agonists.

The second epidemic occurred in New Zealand in the late 1970s and 1980s and was associated with the use of fenoterol.[1-5] When use of fenoterol fell in New Zealand, so too did the asthma mortality rate.[5] Heavy or regular use of fenoterol was implicated.[6,7] Fenoterol was also implicated in increased asthma morbidity and mortality in a study in Canada,[7] as was salbutamol, and results from Japan also suggested a relation between asthma deaths and excessive use of beta agonists, particularly fenoterol.[8] However, an analysis of the New Zealand deaths could not identify such a risk with beta agonists other than fenoterol.[5]

There is still debate about this second epidemic. The individual case control studies, including the one from Canada,[7] showed an increased morbidity and mortality in patients taking fenoterol, but a meta-analysis of the accumulated data to 1992 suggested that the increase in mortality in the patients taking beta$_2$ agonists was slight and only significant when administration was by nebulisation.[9] Also a working party of the UK Committee on Safety of Medicines considered[10] that a causal link between asthma mortality and beta-agonist use could neither be confirmed nor refuted.

Not surprisingly there are different views on the cause of the increased asthma mortality. The cardiotoxicity of the beta agonist might have to be considered, although evidence for such an effect is felt by some to be slight.[11] The severity of the asthma might have been a factor in two different ways. One hypothesis is that patients used more fenoterol because they had severe asthma and were already at increased risk of dying.[12] Another proposes that heavy beta-agonist use led to an increase in asthma severity[13] which could be explained by a down regulation of beta receptors.[14]

This may appear to be only of historical interest since mortality rates have fallen and current recommendations for the use of short-acting beta$_2$ agonists, which are generally more selective than fenoterol, are for them to be taken as required rather than on a regular basis; indeed increasing use of such drugs is seen as an indication to amend the treatment schedule. Moreover, the dose of fenoterol has been reduced in recent years. However, controversy over regular use of beta$_2$ agonists continues to be fed by conflicting studies of their benefit.[15,16] It is possible that some benefit exists in more severe disease, and current recommendations for asthma treatment do permit the regular use of long-acting beta$_2$ agonists in severe chronic asthma. It is not clear to what extent the same concerns, particularly of downregulation of beta receptors, apply to such therapy (see Tolerance, under Salmeterol, p.795).

1. Pearce N, *et al.* Beta agonists and asthma mortality: déjà vu. *Clin Exp Allergy* 1991; **21:** 401–10.
2. Crane J, *et al.* Prescribed fenoterol and death from asthma in New Zealand, 1981-83: case-control study. *Lancet* 1989; **i:** 917–22.
3. Pearce N, *et al.* Case-control study of prescribed fenoterol and death from asthma in New Zealand, 1977–81. *Thorax* 1990; **45:** 170–5.
4. Grainger J, *et al.* Prescribed fenoterol and death from asthma in New Zealand, 1981–7: a further case-control study. *Thorax* 1991; **46:** 105–111.
5. Pearce N, *et al.* End of the New Zealand asthma mortality epidemic. *Lancet* 1995; **345:** 41–4.
6. Sears MR, *et al.* Regular inhaled beta-agonist treatment in bronchial asthma. *Lancet* 1990; **336:** 1391–6.
7. Spitzer WO, *et al.* The use of β-agonists and the risk of death and near death from asthma. *N Engl J Med* 1992; **326:** 501–6.
8. Beasley R, *et al.* β-agonist therapy and asthma mortality in Japan. *Lancet* 1998; **351:** 1406–7.
9. Mullen M, *et al.* The association between β-agonist use and death from asthma: a meta-analytic integration of case control studies. *JAMA* 1993; **270:** 1842–5.
10. Committee on Safety of Medicines. Beta-agonist use in asthma: report from the CSM Working Party. *Current Problems 33* 1992.
11. Sears MR, Taylor DR. The β$_2$-agonist controversy: observations, explanations and relationship to asthma epidemiology. *Drug Safety* 1994; **11:** 259–83.
12. Fuller RW. Use of β$_2$ agonists in asthma: much ado about nothing? *BMJ* 1994; **309:** 795–6.
13. Sears MR. Asthma deaths in New Zealand. *Lancet* 1995; **345:** 655–6.
14. Tattersfield AE. Use of β$_2$ agonists in asthma: much ado about nothing? *BMJ* 1994; **309:** 794–5.
15. Chapman KR, *et al.* Regular vs as-needed inhaled salbutamol in asthma control. *Lancet* 1994; **343:** 1379–82.
16. Drazen JM, *et al.* Comparison of regularly scheduled with as-needed use of albuterol in mild asthma. *N Engl J Med* 1996; **335:** 841–7.

**Pulmonary oedema.** Pulmonary oedema has occurred in women given beta agonists, including fenoterol,[1] for premature labour. The risk factors, the most important of which is fluid overload, are discussed under Precautions for Salbutamol, on p.792.

1. Hawker F. Pulmonary oedema associated with β$_2$-sympathomimetic treatment of premature labour. *Anaesth Intensive Care* 1984; **12:** 143–51.

### Interactions

As for Salbutamol, p.792.

### Pharmacokinetics

Fenoterol is incompletely absorbed from the gastrointestinal tract and is also subject to extensive first-pass metabolism by sulfate conjugation. It is excreted in the urine and bile almost entirely as the inactive sulfate conjugate.

◊ References.

1. Rominger KL, Pollmann W. Vergleichende Pharmakokinetik von Fenoterol-Hydrobromid bei Ratte, Hund und Mensch. *Arzneimittelforschung* 1972; **22:** 1190–6.
2. Hildebrandt R, *et al.* Pharmacokinetics of fenoterol in pregnant and nonpregnant women. *Eur J Clin Pharmacol* 1993; **45:** 275–7.

### Uses and Administration

Fenoterol is a direct-acting sympathomimetic with beta-adrenoceptor stimulant activity largely selective for beta$_2$ receptors (a beta$_2$ agonist). It has actions and uses similar to those of salbutamol (p.793) and is used as a bronchodilator in the management of reversible airways obstruction, as occurs in asthma (p.777) and in some patients with chronic obstructive pulmonary disease (p.779). Following inhalation, fenoterol acts rapidly (2 to 3 minutes) and has a duration of action of about 6 to 8 hours.

In the management of **reversible airways obstruction,** fenoterol hydrobromide may be administered by inhalation in a dose of 1 or 2 inhalations of 100 micrograms up to 3 or 4 times daily; children over the age of 6 years will only normally require one inhalation (100 micrograms) up to 3 times daily. If symptoms are not adequately controlled with this low-dose inhaler then a high-dose inhaler administering 200 micrograms per inhalation has been employed in adults; 2 inhalations of 200 micrograms may be given up to 3 times daily. The dose should not exceed 400 micrograms every six hours or 1.6 mg in a 24-hour period; this high-dose inhaler is not recommended for children under 16 years of age. Current asthma guidelines recommend that inhaled short-acting beta$_2$ agonists such as fenoterol be used on an 'as-required', not regular, basis. In those patients requiring more than occasional use of fenoterol, anti-inflammatory therapy is also needed. An increased requirement for, or decreased duration of effect of, fenoterol indicates deterioration of asthma control and the need for increased anti-inflammatory therapy.

Fenoterol hydrobromide may be given as a nebulised solution; the usual dose for inhalation by this route is 200 to 400 micrograms, up to a maximum of 1.6 mg daily.

Fenoterol hydrobromide has also been used similarly to salbutamol in the management of **premature labour** (see p.794). A suggested dose, by intravenous infusion, has been 0.5 to 3 micrograms/minute, continued until contractions are suppressed, and followed by oral administration of 5 mg every 3 to 6 hours.

### Preparations

**BP 2003:** Fenoterol Pressurised Inhalation.

**Proprietary Preparations** (details are given in Part 3)
**Arg.:** Alveofen; Berotec; **Austral.:** Berotec; **Austria:** Berotec; Fenostad; **Belg.:** Berotec; **Braz.:** Berotec; Bromifen; Bromotec†; Fenozan; **Canad.:** Berotec; **Chile:** Berotec; Parsistene; **Denm.:** Berotec; **Fin.:** Berotec; **Fr.:** Berotec†; **Ger.:** Berotec; Partusisten; **Hong Kong:** Berotec; **Irl.:** Berotec†; **Ital.:** Dosberotec; **Malaysia:** Berotec; Feno; **Mex.:** Berotec; Partusisten; **Neth.:** Berotec; Partusisten; **Norw.:** Berotec; **NZ:** Berotec†; **Port.:** Berotec; **S.Afr.:** Berotec; **Singapore:** Berotec; **Spain:** Berotec; **Swed.:** Berotec; **Switz.:** Berotec; Partusisten†; **Thai.:** Berotec; **UK:** Berotec†.

**Multi-ingredient: Arg.:** Berodual; Duotec; **Austria:** Arelcant; Berodual; Berodualin; Ditec; **Belg.:** Duovent; **Braz.:** Duovent; Fymnal; **Canad.:** Duovent; **Chile:** Berodual; **Denm.:** Berodual; **Fin.:** Atrovent Comp; **Fr.:** Bronchodual; **Ger.:** Berodual; Berotec solvens†; Ditec; **Gr.:** Berodual; **Hong Kong:** Berodual; **Irl.:** Duovent; **Ital.:** Duovent; Iprafen; **Malaysia:** Berodual; Duovent; **Mex.:** Berodual; **Neth.:** Berodual; **NZ:** Duovent†; **Port.:** Berodual; **S.Afr.:** Atrovent Beta; Duovent; **Singapore:** Berodual; Duovent; **Spain:** Berodual; Crismol†; **Switz.:** Berodual; **Thai.:** Berodual; **UK:** Duovent.

## Fenspiride Hydrochloride *(USAN, rINNM)*

Decaspiride; Hidrocloruro de fenspirida; JP-428; NAT-333; NDR-5998A. 8-Phenethyl-1-oxa-3,8-diazaspiro[4.5]decan-2-one hydrochloride.

$C_{15}H_{20}N_2O_2,HCl = 296.8.$

*CAS — 5053-06-5 (fenspiride); 5053-08-7 (fenspiride hydrochloride).*

*ATC — R03BX01; R03DX03.*

### Profile

Fenspiride is reported to have bronchodilator and anti-inflammatory properties. It is given as the hydrochloride in asthma (p.777) and other respiratory disorders in usual doses of 160 to 240 mg daily by mouth in divided doses before meals. It has also been given rectally and by intramuscular or intravenous injection.

### Preparations

**Proprietary Preparations** (details are given in Part 3)
**Belg.:** Pneumorel†; **Fr.:** Pneumorel; **Hong Kong:** Pneumorel; **Ital.:** Espiran†; Fenspir†; Fluident†; Pneumorel; **Port.:** Fenspin; Pneumorel.

## Formoterol Fumarate *(BANM, USAN, rINNM)*

BD-40A; CGP-25827A; Eformoterol Fumarate; Fumarato de formoterol; YM-08316. (±)-2′-Hydroxy-5′-[(RS)-1-hydroxy-2-{[(RS)-p-methoxy-α-methylphenethyl]amino}ethyl]formanilide fumarate.

$(C_{19}H_{24}N_2O_4)_2,C_4H_4O_4 = 804.9.$

*CAS — 73573-87-2 (formoterol); 43229-80-7 (formoterol fumarate).*

*ATC — R03AC13.*

**Pharmacopoeias.** In *Jpn. Eur.* (see p.vi) includes the dihydrate.

**Ph. Eur. 5.0** (Formoterol Fumarate Dihydrate; Formoteroli Fumaras Dihydricus). A white or almost white or slightly yellow powder. Slightly soluble in water and in isopropyl alcohol; practically insoluble in acetonitrile; soluble in methyl alcohol. A 0.1% solution in water has a pH of 5.5 to 6.5. Protect from light.

### Adverse Effects and Precautions

As for Salbutamol, p.791. Inhalation of formoterol may be associated with paradoxical bronchospasm, and high doses have been associated with an increase in severe exacerbations of asthma.

Long-acting $beta_2$ agonists such as formoterol are not appropriate for the treatment of acute bronchospasm.

Conjunctival irritation and eyelid oedema have been reported in isolated cases.

◊ References.

1. Wilton LV, Shakir SA. A post-marketing surveillance study of formoterol (Foradil®): its use in general practice in England. *Drug Safety* 2002; **25:** 213–23.
2. Mann M, *et al.* Serious asthma exacerbations in asthmatics treated with high-dose formoterol. *Chest* 2003; **124:** 70–4.

**Tolerance.** Regular use of formoterol produced bronchodilator desensitisation,[1] and tachyphylaxis to bronchoprotection against methacholine,[2] effects that have been noted with other long-acting $beta_2$ agonists (see Salmeterol, p.795) and short-acting $beta_2$ agonists (see Salbutamol, p.792).

1. Newnham DM, *et al.* Bronchodilator subsensitivity after chronic dosing with eformoterol in patients with asthma. *Am J Med* 1994; **97:** 29–37.
2. Lipworth B, *et al.* Effects of treatment with formoterol on bronchoprotection against methacholine. *Am J Med* 1998; **104:** 431–8.

### Interactions

As for Salbutamol, p.792.

### Pharmacokinetics

Inhaled formoterol is rapidly absorbed. It is largely metabolised by glucuronidation and *O*-demethylation, with about 10% being excreted as unchanged drug. The terminal elimination half-life after inhalation is estimated to be 8 hours.

### Uses and Administration

Formoterol is a direct-acting sympathomimetic with predominantly beta-adrenoceptor stimulant activity specific to $beta_2$ receptors (a $beta_2$ agonist). It has properties similar to those of salbutamol (p.793), but like salmeterol (p.795) it has a prolonged duration of action of up to 12 hours; it is therefore not considered suitable for the symptomatic relief of acute attacks of bronchospasm. It is used when the regular administration of a long-acting $beta_2$ agonist is required for management of reversible airways obstruction, as in chronic asthma (p.777) or in some patients with chronic obstructive pulmonary disease (p.779).

Formoterol is given as the fumarate. A usual dose for adults and children aged 5 years or older is 12 micrograms of formoterol fumarate twice daily by inhalation from inhalational capsules, increased to 24 micrograms twice daily if necessary in severe disease. Usual doses from a metered-dose dry powder inhaler are 6 or 12 micrograms once or twice daily, increased if necessary in severe disease to 24 micrograms twice daily for adults or 12 micrograms twice daily for children aged 6 years and older. Similar doses have been given using a metered-dose aerosol. Treatment should be reassessed if this proves inadequate; in the UK, some preparations are licensed for additional short-term symptom relief, but such use is contrary to current asthma guidelines (see p.777). Doses of 80 micrograms have been given twice daily by mouth.

◊ Reviews.

1. Faulds D, *et al.* Formoterol: a review of its pharmacological properties and therapeutic potential in reversible obstructive airways disease. *Drugs* 1991; **42:** 115–37.
2. Bartow RA, Brogden RN. Formoterol: an update of its pharmacological properties and therapeutic efficacy in the management of asthma. *Drugs* 1998; **55:** 303–22.

**Asthma.** Formoterol is a long-acting $beta_2$ agonist (duration of action about 12 hours). Guidelines on the management of asthma, see p.777, generally recommend that the use of long-acting $beta_2$ agonists be reserved for patients with chronic asthma who have already progressed to inhaled corticosteroids; it is not a substitute for corticosteroids. Increasing data suggest that, apart from in severe exacerbations, adding a long-acting $beta_2$ agonist to standard dose inhaled corticosteroid therapy may be more effective than increasing the dose of corticosteroid. Formoterol may also be useful in controlling persistent nocturnal asthma or preventing exercise-induced attacks. There is some evidence that after prolonged use, protection against bronchoconstriction is reduced (see Tolerance, above), and high-dose therapy may be associated with an increased rate of severe exacerbations.

References.

1. van Noord JA, *et al.* Salmeterol versus formoterol in patients with moderately severe asthma: onset and duration of action. *Eur Respir J* 1996; **9:** 1684–8.
2. van der Molen T, *et al.* Effects of the long acting β agonist formoterol on asthma control in asthmatic patients using inhaled corticosteroids. *Thorax* 1996; **52:** 535–9.
3. Pauwels RA, *et al.* Effect of inhaled formoterol and budesonide on exacerbations of asthma. *N Engl J Med* 1997; **337:** 1405–11. Correction. *ibid.*; 1998; **338:** 139.
4. O'Byrne PM, *et al.* Low dose inhaled budesonide and formoterol in mild persistent asthma: the OPTIMA randomized trial. *Am J Respir Crit Care Med* 2001; **164:** 1392–7.

### Preparations

**Proprietary Preparations** (details are given in Part 3)
**Arg.:** Fordilen; Oxis; Xanol; **Austral.:** Foradile; Oxis; **Austria:** Foradil; Oxis; **Belg.:** Foradil; Oxis; **Braz.:** Fluir; Foradil; Oxis; **Canad.:** Foradil; Oxeze; **Denm.:** Foradil; Oxis; **Fin.:** Foradil; Oxis; **Fr.:** Foradil; **Ger.:** Foradil; Oxis; **Gr.:** Foradil; Oxeze; **Hong Kong:** Foradil; Oxis; **Irl.:** Foradil; Oxis; **Israel:** Foradil; Oxis; **Ital.:** Eolus; Foradil; Oxis; **Jpn:** Atock; **Malaysia:** Foradil; Oxis; **Mex.:** Foradil; Oxis; **Neth.:** Foradil; Oxis; **Norw.:** Foradil; Oxis; **NZ:** Foradil; Oxis; **Port.:** Asmatec; Foradil; Oxis; **S.Afr.:** Foradil; Oxis; **Singapore:** Foradil; Oxis; **Spain:** Broncoral; Foradil; Neblik; Oxis; **Swed.:** Foradil; Oxis; **Switz.:** Foradil; Oxis; **Thai.:** Oxis; **UK:** Foradil; Oxis; **USA:** Foradil.

**Multi-ingredient: Arg.:** Neumoterol; Symbicort; **Austral.:** Symbicort; **Austria:** Symbicort; **Belg.:** Symbicort; **Braz.:** Foraseq; Symbicort; **Chile:** Symbicort; **Denm.:** Symbicort; **Fin.:** Symbicort; **Fr.:** Symbicort; **Ger.:** Symbicort; **Hong Kong:** Symbicort; **India:** Foracort; **Irl.:** Symbicort; **Israel:** Symbicort; **Ital.:** Assieme; Sinestic; Symbiocort; **Neth.:** Symbicort; **Norw.:** Symbicort; **NZ:** Symbicort; **Port.:** Assieme; Symbicort; **Singapore:** Symbicort; **Spain:** Symbicort; **Swed.:** Symbicort; **Switz.:** Symbicort; **Thai.:** Symbicort; **UK:** Symbicort.

## Heptaminol Acefyllinate *(rINNM)*

Acéfyllinate d'Heptaminol; Acefyllinum Heptaminolum; Heptaminol, acefilinato de; Heptaminol Acephyllinate; Heptaminol Theophylline Ethanoate; Heptaminol Theophylline-7-acetate. The 6-amino-2-methylheptan-2-ol salt of theophyllin-7-ylacetic acid.

$C_8H_{19}NO,C_9H_{10}N_4O_4 = 383.4.$

*CAS — 5152-72-7; 10075-18-0.*

*ATC — C01DX08.*

### Profile

Heptaminol acefyllinate is a derivative of theophylline (p.798) that has been used for its bronchodilator and cardiovascular effects.

### Preparations

**Proprietary Preparations** (details are given in Part 3)

**Multi-ingredient: Braz.:** Sureptil; **Fr.:** Sureptil†; **Spain:** Clinadil Compositum; Diclamina.

## Hexoprenaline Hydrochloride *(BANM, rINNM)*

Hidrocloruro de hexoprenalina; ST-1512. *N,N′*-Hexamethylenebis[4-(2-amino-1-hydroxyethyl)pyrocatechol] dihydrochloride; *N,N′*-Hexamethylenebis[2-amino-1-(3,4-dihydroxyphenyl)ethanol] dihydrochloride.

$C_{22}H_{32}N_2O_6,2HCl = 493.4.$

*CAS — 3215-70-1 (hexoprenaline); 4323-43-7 (hexoprenaline dihydrochloride).*

*ATC — R03AC06; R03CC05.*

## Hexoprenaline Sulfate *(USAN, rINNM)*

Hexoprenaline Sulphate *(BANM)*; Sulfato de hexoprenalina. (±)-α,α′-[Hexamethylenebis(iminomethylene)]-bis[3,4-dihydroxybenzyl alcohol] sulfate (1:1).

$C_{22}H_{32}N_2O_6,H_2SO_4 = 518.6.$

*CAS — 32266-10-7.*

*ATC — R03AC06; R03CC05.*

### Profile

Hexoprenaline is a direct-acting sympathomimetic with predominantly beta-adrenergic activity selective to $beta_2$ receptors (a $beta_2$ agonist). It has properties similar to those of salbutamol (p.791) and is used as a bronchodilator in the treatment of reversible airways obstruction as occurs with asthma (p.777) and in some patients with chronic obstructive pulmonary disease (p.779). It has sometimes been used similarly to salbutamol in the management of premature labour (p.794).

Hexoprenaline is usually given as the hydrochloride or sulfate.

For bronchodilatation, usual doses of the salts are 0.5 to 1 mg three times daily by mouth or 200 to 400 micrograms by inhalation three to four times daily. In patients with asthma, as-required beta agonist therapy is preferable to regular use. An increased need for, or decreased duration of effect of, hexoprenaline indicates deterioration of asthma control and the need for review of therapy. Hexoprenaline salts have also been given parenterally.

In the management of premature labour an intravenous infusion of hexoprenaline sulfate can be given at an initial rate of about 300 nanograms/minute. Infusion may be preceded by slow intravenous injection of 10 micrograms as a loading dose over 5 to 10 minutes. A prolonged infusion of 75 nanograms/minute has been used when there is no cervical change.

### Preparations

**Proprietary Preparations** (details are given in Part 3)
**Arg.:** Argocian; **Austria:** Gynipral; Ipradol; **Chile:** Gynipral; **Hong Kong:** Ipradol; **S.Afr.:** Ipradol; **Spain:** Ipradol†; **Switz.:** Gynipral; **Thai.:** Ipradol.

## Ibudilast *(rINN)*

KC-404. 1-(2-Isopropylpyrazolo[1,5-*a*]pyridin-3-yl)-2-methyl-1-propanone.

$C_{14}H_{18}N_2O = 230.3.$

*CAS — 50847-11-5.*

*ATC — R03DC04.*

### Profile

Ibudilast is an orally active leukotriene antagonist and platelet-activating factor antagonist. It is given by mouth in the management of asthma (p.777) in a dose of 10 mg twice daily.

Ibudilast is also promoted for the management of dizziness secondary to impaired cerebral circulation following cerebral infarction, in doses of 10 mg three times daily.

### Preparations

**Proprietary Preparations** (details are given in Part 3)
**Jpn:** Ketas.

## Ipratropium Bromide *(BAN, USAN, rINN)*

Bromuro de ipratropio; Ipratropii Bromidum; Sch-1000; Sch-1000-Br-monohydrate. (1R,3r,5S,8r)-8-Isopropyl-3-[(±)-tropoyloxy]tropanium bromide monohydrate.

$C_{20}H_{30}BrNO_3,H_2O$ = 430.4.

*CAS — 22254-24-6 (anhydrous ipratropium bromide); 66985-17-9 (ipratropium bromide monohydrate).*

*ATC — R01AX03; R03BB01.*

**Pharmacopoeias.** In *Eur.* (see p.vi) and *Jpn.*

**Ph. Eur. 5.0** (Ipratropium Bromide). White or almost white crystalline powder. Soluble in water; slightly soluble in alcohol; freely soluble in methyl alcohol. The pH of a 1% solution in water is 5.0 to 7.5.

**Stability.** In a study[1] of the stability of admixtures of ipratropium and salbutamol nebuliser solutions equal ratio mixtures were found to retain more than 90% of their initial concentrations after storage for 5 days at 4° or 22° in the dark or at 22° under continuous fluorescent lighting.

1. Jacobson GA, Peterson GM. Stability of ipratropium bromide and salbutamol nebuliser admixtures. *Int J Pharm Pract* 1995; **3:** 169–73.

### Adverse Effects and Precautions

Ipratropium and other inhaled antimuscarinic bronchodilators may occasionally cause dry mouth, and rarely constipation and urinary retention. They should be used with care in prostatic hyperplasia. Acute angle-closure glaucoma has been reported with *nebulised* ipratropium; the mist or solution should not be allowed to enter the eyes, particularly in patients susceptible to glaucoma. As with other bronchodilators, paradoxical bronchospasm has occurred. Tachycardia, palpitations, and arrhythmias have been reported with ipratropium. Hypersensitivity reactions, including urticaria, angioedema, and anaphylaxis have occurred rarely.

Intranasal ipratropium has been associated with nasal dryness and epistaxis.

For details of the adverse effects of, and precautions for, antimuscarinics in general, see Atropine, p.477.

**Buccal ulceration.** A report[1] of inflammation and ulceration of the buccal mucosa associated with the use of an ipratropium bromide inhaler.

1. Spencer PA. Buccal ulceration with ipratropium bromide. *BMJ* 1986; **292:** 380.

**Effects on the eyes.** Although short-term studies in patients with angle-closure glaucoma and normal subjects indicate that inhalation of ipratropium alone has no effect on intra-ocular pressure, accommodation, or pupil diameter[1,2] there has been a report[3] of a patient with a history of glaucoma who developed angle-closure glaucoma after receiving ipratropium using a metered dose inhaler and nebulised salbutamol together. Angle-closure glaucoma,[4-6] pupillary dilatation,[6-8] and anisocoria (unequal dilatation of the pupils)[9] have been reported in patients receiving *nebulised* ipratropium, usually with salbutamol, through a poorly fitting face mask. The antimuscarinic effects of ipratropium can lead to impaired drainage of aqueous humour in the eyes of patients predisposed to angle-closure glaucoma; co-administration of salbutamol may intensify this problem by increasing the production of aqueous humour.[5] Studies[10,11] suggest that patients with a history of angle-closure glaucoma might be at an increased risk of developing glaucoma when nebulised ipratropium and salbutamol are used together.

1. Scheufler G. Ophthalmotonometry, pupil diameter and visual accommodation following repeated administration of Sch 1000 MDI in patients with glaucoma. *Postgrad Med J* 1975; **51** (suppl 7): 132.
2. Thumm HW. Ophthalmic effects of high doses of Sch 1000 MDI in healthy volunteers and patients with glaucoma. *Postgrad Med J* 1975; **51** (suppl 7): 132–3.
3. Hall SK. Acute angle-closure glaucoma as a complication of combined β-agonist and ipratropium bromide therapy in the emergency department. *Ann Emerg Med* 1994; **23:** 884–7.
4. Packe GE, *et al.* Nebulised ipratropium bromide and salbutamol causing closed-angle glaucoma. *Lancet* 1984; **ii:** 691.
5. Shah P, *et al.* Acute angle closure glaucoma associated with nebulised ipratropium bromide and salbutamol. *BMJ* 1992; **304:** 40–1.
6. Mulpeter KM, *et al.* Ocular hazards of nebulized bronchodilators. *Postgrad Med J* 1992; **68:** 132–3.
7. Roberts TE, Pearson DJ. Wide eyed and breathless. *BMJ* 1989; **299:** 1348.
8. Woelfle J, *et al.* Unilateral fixed dilated pupil in an infant after inhalation of nebulized ipratropium bromide. *J Pediatr* 2000; **136:** 423–4.
9. Lust K, Livingstone I. Nebulizer-induced anisocoria. *Ann Intern Med* 1998; **128:** 327.
10. Watson WTA, *et al.* Effect of nebulized ipratropium bromide on intraocular pressures in children. *Chest* 1994; **105:** 1439–41.
11. Kalra L, Bone MF. The effect of nebulized bronchodilator therapy on intraocular pressures in patients with glaucoma. *Chest* 1988; **93:** 739–41.

**Effects on the gastrointestinal tract.** Paralytic ileus developed shortly after initiation of ipratropium therapy in 2 patients, apparently due to the inadvertent swallowing of the drug during inhalation.[1,2] Both patients also had other predisposing factors for paralytic ileus (cystic fibrosis,[1] spastic diplegia[2]).

1. Mulherin D, FitzGerald MX. Meconium ileus equivalent in association with nebulised ipratropium bromide in cystic fibrosis. *Lancet* 1990; **355:** 552.
2. Markus HS. Paralytic ileus associated with ipratropium. *Lancet* 1990; **355:** 1224.

**Effects on the respiratory tract.** Antimuscarinics typically inhibit mucociliary clearance and inhibit secretions of the nose, mouth, pharynx, and bronchi. However, inhaled ipratropium bromide has virtually no effect on sputum viscosity or volume and, in contrast to atropine, it does not affect mucociliary function in the respiratory tract.[1,2]

1. Gross NJ. Ipratropium bromide. *N Engl J Med* 1988; **319:** 486–94.
2. Mann KV, *et al.* Use of ipratropium bromide in obstructive lung disease. *Clin Pharm* 1988; **7:** 670–80.

BRONCHOSPASM. Paradoxical bronchoconstriction occurring after the use of ipratropium was reported in 3 patients.[1] The authors of a further report[2] of paradoxical bronchoconstriction following nebulisation therapy with salbutamol and ipratropium suggested that this adverse effect may have been caused by benzalkonium chloride present in the nebuliser solutions. Nebuliser solutions of ipratropium in some countries contain benzalkonium chloride as a preservative. Solutions available in the UK are preservative-free but the manufacturers still recommend that the first doses of ipratropium nebuliser solution should be inhaled under medical supervision.

1. Connolly CK. Adverse reaction to ipratropium bromide. *BMJ* 1982; **285:** 934–5.
2. Boucher M, *et al.* Possible associations of benzalkonium chloride in nebulizer solutions with respiratory arrest. *Ann Pharmacother* 1992; **26:** 772–4.

**Effects on the urinary tract.** Treatment with nebulised ipratropium bromide has resulted in urinary retention in elderly men especially those with prostatic hyperplasia.[1,2]

1. Lozewicz S. Bladder outflow obstruction induced by ipratropium bromide. *Postgrad Med J* 1989; **65:** 260–1.
2. Pras E, *et al.* Urinary retention associated with ipratropium bromide. *DICP Ann Pharmacother* 1991; **25:** 939–40.

**Increased mortality.** A case-control study found an unexpected association between death from asthma and treatment with ipratropium, which was not explained by co-morbidity due to chronic obstructive airways disease.[1] A later retrospective cohort study[2] of elderly patients found no increase in all-cause mortality associated with the use of ipratropium for chronic obstructive pulmonary disease. In patients with asthma there was a slight increase in the risk of death, but this may have been due to the confounding effect of disease severity.

1. Guite HF, *et al.* Risk factors for death from asthma, chronic obstructive pulmonary disease, and cardiovascular disease after a hospital admission for asthma. *Thorax* 1999; **54:** 301–7.
2. Sin DD, Tu JV. Lack of association between ipratropium bromide and mortality in elderly patients with chronic obstructive airway disease. *Thorax* 2000; **55:** 194–7.

### Interactions

For interactions associated with antimuscarinics in general, see Atropine, p.477. However, these interactions are not usually seen with antimuscarinics, such as ipratropium, given by inhalation.

**Salbutamol.** For reference to nebulised salbutamol exacerbating the adverse effects of nebulised ipratropium in patients predisposed to angle-closure glaucoma, see under Effects on the Eyes, above.

### Pharmacokinetics

After inhalation, only a small amount of ipratropium reaches the systemic circulation. Some ipratropium is inadvertently swallowed but it is poorly absorbed from the gastrointestinal tract. Ipratropium and its metabolites are eliminated in the urine and faeces.

◊ References.

1. Ensing K, *et al.* Pharmacokinetics of ipratropium bromide after single dose inhalation and oral and intravenous administration. *Eur J Clin Pharmacol* 1989; **36:** 189–94.

### Uses and Administration

Ipratropium bromide is a quaternary ammonium antimuscarinic (p.777). It is used by inhalation as a bronchodilator in the treatment of reversible airways obstruction, as in asthma (p.777) and chronic obstructive pulmonary disease (p.779).

In the UK the dose of ipratropium bromide from the metered-dose aerosol is expressed in terms of the amount of drug released from the valve into the mouthpiece (20 micrograms) whereas in the USA it is expressed in terms of the dose emitted from the mouthpiece (18 micrograms); recommended doses therefore appear lower in the USA. For **reversible airways obstruction**, the usual UK dose by inhalation from a metered-dose aerosol is 20 or 40 micrograms three or four times daily; single doses of up to 80 micrograms may be required. Comparable doses are used in the USA, but it is recommended that the daily dose should not exceed 216 micrograms (12 inhalations). In children aged 6 to 12 years the usual dose is 20 or 40 micrograms three times daily, and below 6 years the usual dose is 20 micrograms three times daily. Dry powder inhalation capsules are also available for use in adults, the usual dose being 40 micrograms three or four times daily.

Ipratropium bromide may also be administered by inhalation as a nebulised solution in doses of 100 to 500 micrograms up to 4 times daily. In children aged 3 to 14 years the usual dose by nebuliser is 100 to 500 micrograms up to 3 times daily. Doses of 62.5 to 250 micrograms up to 3 times daily have been given to children 1 month to 3 years of age.

Ipratropium bromide, given intranasally, is also used in the management of rhinorrhoea associated with **rhinitis**. A dose of 42 micrograms is administered into each nostril by metered-dose nasal spray 2 or 3 times daily. In the UK this dose may be used in adults and children aged 12 years and older, but in the USA this dose may also be used for children aged 6 years and older. US licensing also permits doses of 84 micrograms into each nostril 3 or 4 times daily for adults, or 3 times daily for children aged 5 to 11 years, for up to 4 days when rhinorrhoea is associated with the common cold; doses of 84 micrograms may be given into each nostril 4 times daily for adults and children aged 5 years and older, for up to 3 weeks when rhinorrhoea is associated with seasonal allergic rhinitis.

**Rhinitis.** Ipratropium bromide is used intranasally for the treatment of rhinorrhoea in allergic and non-allergic rhinitis (p.422). It has also relieved rhinorrhoea and sneezing associated with the common cold.

References.

1. Georgitis JW, *et al.* Ipratropium bromide nasal spray in non-allergic rhinitis: efficacy, nasal cytological response and patient evaluation on quality of life. *Clin Exp Allergy* 1994; **24:** 1049–55.
2. Hayden FG, *et al.* Effectiveness and safety of intranasal ipratropium bromide in common colds: a randomized, double-blind, placebo-controlled trial. *Ann Intern Med* 1996; **125:** 89–97.
3. Dockhorn R, *et al.* Ipratropium bromide nasal spray 0.03% and beclomethasone nasal spray alone and in combination for the treatment of rhinorrhea in perennial rhinitis. *Ann Allergy Asthma Immunol* 1999; **82:** 349–59.

### Preparations

***BP 2003:*** Ipratropium Pressurised Inhalation.

**Proprietary Preparations** (details are given in Part 3)

***Arg.:*** Atrovent; Iprabron; ***Austral.:*** Apoven; Atrovent; Ipratrin; Ipravent; ***Austria:*** Atronase†; Atrovent; Itrop; ***Belg.:*** Atronase; Atrovent; ***Braz.:*** Alvent; Atrovent; Iprabon; Ipraneo; ***Canad.:*** Apo-Ipravent; Atrovent; Novo-Ipramide; ***Chile:*** Atrovent; Neorinol; ***Denm.:*** Atrovent; ***Fin.:*** Atrovent; ***Fr.:*** Atrovent; ***Ger.:*** Atrovent; Itrop; ***Gr.:*** Atrovent; ***Hong Kong:*** Atrovent; Ipravent; ***India:*** Ipravent; ***Irl.:*** Atrovent; Rinatec; ***Israel:*** Aerovent; Apovent; ***Ital.:*** Atem; Atrovent†; Rinovagos; ***Jpn:*** Atrovent; ***Malaysia:*** Atrovent; ***Mex.:*** Atrovent; ***Neth.:*** Atrovent; ***Norw.:*** Atrovent; Respontin; ***NZ:*** Atrovent; Ipra; ***Port.:*** Atrovent; ***S.Afr.:*** Atrovent; Ipvent; ***Singapore:*** Atrovent; ***Spain:*** Atrovent; Disne Asmol†; Narilet†; ***Swed.:*** Atrovent; ***Switz.:*** Atrovent; Rhinovent; ***Thai.:*** Atrovent; ***UK:*** Atrovent; Respontin; Rinatec; Tropiovent†; ***USA:*** Atrovent.

**Multi-ingredient:** ***Arg.:*** Berodual; Combivent; ***Austral.:*** Combivent; ***Austria:*** Arelcant; Berodual; Berodualin; Combivent; Di-Promal; ***Belg.:*** Combivent; Duovent; ***Braz.:*** Combivent; Duovent; ***Canad.:*** Combivent; Duovent; ***Chile:*** Berodual; Combivent; ***Denm.:*** Berodual; Combivent; ***Fin.:*** Atrodual; Atrovent Comp; ***Fr.:*** Bronchodual; Combivent; ***Ger.:*** Berodual; ***Gr.:*** Berodual; Berovent; ***Hong Kong:*** Berodual; Combivent; ***India:*** Duolin; ***Irl.:*** Combivent; Duovent; ***Ital.:*** Breva; Duovent; Iprafen; ***Malaysia:*** Berodual; Combivent; Duovent; ***Mex.:*** Berodual; Combivent; ***Neth.:*** Berodual; Combivent†; ***NZ:*** Combivent; Duolin; Duovent†; ***Port.:*** Berodual; Combivent; ***S.Afr.:*** Atrovent Beta; Combivent; Duovent; ***Singapore:*** Berodual; Combivent; Duovent; ***Spain:*** Berodual; Combivent; Crismol†; ***Swed.:*** Combivent; ***Switz.:*** Berodual; Dospir; ***Thai.:*** Berodual; Combivent; ***UK:*** Combivent; Duovent; ***USA:*** Combivent; DuoNeb.

---

## Isoetarine *(BAN, rINN)*

Isoetharine *(USAN)*; Win-3406. 1-(3,4-Dihydroxyphenyl)-2-isopropylaminobutan-1-ol.

$C_{13}H_{21}NO_3$ = 239.3.

*CAS — 530-08-5.*

*ATC — R03AC07; R03CC06.*

## Isoetarine Hydrochloride *(BANM, rINNM)*

Etyprenaline Hydrochloride; Hidrocloruro de isoetarina; Isoetharine Hydrochloride; *N*-Isopropylethylnoradrenaline Hydrochloride.

$C_{13}H_{21}NO_3,HCl$ = 275.8.

*CAS — 50-96-4; 2576-92-3.*

*ATC — R03AC07; R03CC06.*

**Pharmacopoeias.** In *US.*

**USP 27** (Isoetharine Hydrochloride). A white to off-white, odourless, crystalline solid. Soluble in water; sparingly soluble in alcohol; practically insoluble in ether. A 1% solution in water has a pH of 4.0 to 5.6. Store in airtight containers.

## Isoetarine Mesilate *(BANM, rINNM)*

Isoetharine Mesylate; Isoetharine Methanesulphonate; *N*-Isopropylethylnoradrenaline Mesylate; Mesilato de isoetarina.

$C_{13}H_{21}NO_3,CH_4O_3S = 335.4.$

*CAS — 7279-75-6.*

*ATC — R03AC07; R03CC06.*

**Pharmacopoeias.** In *US.*

**USP 27** (Isoetharine Mesylate). White or practically white, odourless, crystals. Freely soluble in water; soluble in alcohol; practically insoluble in acetone and in ether. A 1% solution in water has a pH of 4.5 to 5.5. Store in airtight containers.

### Profile

Isoetarine is a sympathomimetic with predominantly beta-adrenergic activity. It has actions similar to those of salbutamol (p.791) but is less selective for $beta_2$ adrenoceptors (for the actions of a non-selective beta agonist see Isoprenaline, p.940). Isoetarine has been used as a bronchodilator in the management of reversible airways obstruction.

Isoetarine is given by inhalation, as a nebulised solution of the hydrochloride in strengths up to 0.25%; a 1% solution can be administered by a hand nebuliser. It has also been given as an aerosol inhalation of the mesilate.

### Preparations

***USP 27:*** Isoetharine Inhalation Solution; Isoetharine Mesylate Inhalation Aerosol.

---

## Ketotifen Fumarate *(BANM, USAN, rINNM)*

Fumarato de ketotifeno; HC-20511 (ketotifen); Ketotifen Hydrogen Fumarate; Ketotifeni Hydrogenofumaras. 4-(1-Methylpiperidin-4-ylidene)-4*H*-benzo[4,5]cyclohepta-[1,2-*b*]thiophen-10(9*H*)-one hydrogen fumarate.

$C_{19}H_{19}NOS,C_4H_4O_4 = 425.5.$

*CAS — 34580-13-7 (ketotifen); 34580-14-8 (ketotifen fumarate).*

*ATC — R06AX17; S01GX08.*

**Pharmacopoeias.** In *Chin., Eur.* (see p.vi), and *Jpn.*

**Ph. Eur. 5.0** (Ketotifen Hydrogen Fumarate; Ketotifen Fumarate BP 2003). A white to brownish-yellow, fine crystalline powder. Sparingly soluble in water; very slightly soluble in acetonitrile; slightly soluble in methyl alcohol.

### Adverse Effects and Precautions

As for the antihistamines in general, p.419; drowsiness may be a problem, and dry mouth and dizziness may occur. Increased appetite and weight gain, and CNS stimulation, have been reported. Cystitis has occurred rarely, and isolated cases of severe skin reactions have been reported.

For precautions to be observed in asthmatic patients, see Sodium Cromoglicate, p.796. Exacerbation of asthma has been reported; existing anti-asthma treatment should be continued for at least 2 weeks after starting ketotifen therapy. It should not be used for the treatment of acute asthma attacks.

**Overdosage.** Overdoses of ketotifen ranging from 10 to 120 mg were reported in 8 patients.[1] Symptoms included drowsiness, confusion, dyspnoea, bradycardia or tachycardia, disorientation, and convulsions. Gastric lavage was performed in 6 patients, and all 8 recovered within 12 hours after supportive treatment.

In an overview of 21 cases of overdosage (including those reported above) the manufacturers stated that no serious signs or symptoms had been reported with doses below 20 mg, and there had been no fatalities.[2] The most serious effects reported had included unconsciousness, convulsions, bradycardia and tachycardia, and a severe hypotensive reaction. Management is essentially supportive and symptomatic.


1. Jefferys DB, Volans GN. Ketotifen overdose: surveillance of the toxicity of a new drug. *BMJ* 1981; **282:** 1755–6.
2. Le Blaye I, *et al.* Acute ketotifen overdosage: a review of present clinical experience. *Drug Safety* 1992; **7:** 387–92.


### Interactions

A reversible fall in the platelet count has been seen in a few patients receiving ketotifen with oral antidiabetics and it has been suggested that this combination should therefore be avoided. Since ketotifen has the properties of the antihistamines, it may potentiate the effects of other CNS depressant drugs such as alcohol, antihistamines, hypnotics, and sedatives. For the interactions of antihistamines in general, see p.421.

### Pharmacokinetics

Ketotifen fumarate is almost completely absorbed from the gastrointestinal tract following oral administration, but bioavailability is reported to be only about 50% due to hepatic first-pass metabolism. Peak plasma concentrations occur 2 to 4 hours after a dose by mouth. It is mainly excreted in the urine as inactive metabolites with a small amount of unchanged drug; the terminal elimination half-life is about 21 hours.

### Uses and Administration

Ketotifen has the properties of the antihistamines (p.421) in addition to a stabilising action on mast cells analogous to that of sodium cromoglicate (p.796). It is used in the prophylactic management of asthma, when it may take several weeks to exert its full effect; it should not be used to treat acute asthma attacks. Ketotifen is also used in the treatment of allergic conditions such as rhinitis (p.422) and conjunctivitis (p.421).

Ketotifen is given as the fumarate, but doses are expressed in terms of the base; ketotifen fumarate 1.38 mg is approximately equivalent to 1 mg of ketotifen.

Ketotifen fumarate is taken by mouth in doses equivalent to 1 mg of ketotifen twice daily with food, increased if necessary to 2 mg twice daily; 0.5 to 1 mg at night may be preferable for the first few days of treatment if drowsiness is likely to be a problem. Children over 2 or 3 years may be given the equivalent of 1 mg of ketotifen twice daily. A dose equivalent to 500 micrograms twice daily has been suggested for children between 6 months and 3 years of age.

Ketotifen fumarate has also been applied topically, as eye drops equivalent to 0.025% ketotifen; it has been used twice daily in adults, and in children aged 3 years and older.

**Action.** It has been suggested that the anti-allergic action of ketotifen was independent of its antihistaminic properties.[1] This might be due to its effect on responses to platelet-activating factor (PAF).[2] However, the significance of PAF in the pathogenesis of asthma has been questioned.


1. Greenwood C. The pharmacology of ketotifen. *Chest* 1982; **82** (suppl): 45S–8S.
2. Morley J, *et al.* Effects of ketotifen upon responses to platelet activating factor: a basis for asthma prophylaxis. *Ann Allergy* 1986; **56:** 335–40.


**Asthma.** Results of studies on the effectiveness of ketotifen in the treatment of asthma (p.777) have been conflicting; although some have found it effective in reducing symptoms[1-4] and in enabling a reduction in concomitant anti-asthmatic drug therapy,[2,4] others have reported no significant benefits,[5,6] and UK guidelines on the management of asthma consider ketotifen to be ineffective.[7] A study in children described as 'preasthmatic' (that is, being at high risk of developing asthma) suggested that long-term therapy with ketotifen decreased the risk of asthma onset.[8]


1. Paterson JW, *et al.* Evaluation of ketotifen (HC20-511) in bronchial asthma. *Eur J Clin Pharmacol* 1983; **25:** 187–93.
2. Tinkelman DG, *et al.* A multicenter trial of the prophylactic effect of ketotifen, theophylline, and placebo in atopic asthma. *J Allergy Clin Immunol* 1985; **76:** 487–97.
3. Miraglia Del Giudice M, *et al.* Study of the efficacy of ketotifen treatment in asthmatic children under 3 years of age. *Curr Ther Res* 1986; **40:** 685–93.
4. Rackham A, *et al.* A Canadian multicenter study with Zaditen (ketotifen) in the treatment of bronchial asthma in children aged 5 to 17 years. *J Allergy Clin Immunol* 1989; **84:** 286–96.
5. White MP, *et al.* Ketotifen in the young asthmatic—a double-blind placebo-controlled trial. *J Int Med Res* 1988; **16:** 107–13.
6. Volovitz B, *et al.* Efficacy and safety of ketotifen in young children with asthma. *J Allergy Clin Immunol* 1988; **81:** 526–30.
7. Scottish Intercollegiate Guidelines Network/The British Thoracic Society. British guideline on the management of asthma. *Thorax* 2003; **58** (suppl 1): i1–i94. Revised edition April 2004 available at: http://www.sign.ac.uk/pdf/sign63.pdf (accessed 21/04/04)
8. Bustos GJ, *et al.* Prevention of asthma with ketotifen in preasthmatic children: a three-year follow-up study. *Clin Exp Allergy* 1995; **25:** 568–73.


### Preparations

**Proprietary Preparations** (details are given in Part 3)

***Arg.:*** Antilerg; Ketocev; Ketokid; Respimex; Zaditen; ***Austria:*** Zaditen; ***Belg.:*** Zaditen; ***Braz.:*** Asdron; Asmalergin; Asmanon; Asmax; Asmen; Asmifen; Asmofen; Biatos; Broncoten; Nemesil†; Profilasmim-Ped; Uni Cetotifen; Zaditen; Zetitec; ***Canad.:*** Zaditen; Zaditor; ***Chile:*** Ketotisin; Oftaler; Zaditen; ***Denm.:*** Zaditen; ***Fin.:*** Zaditen; ***Fr.:*** Zaditen; ***Ger.:*** Airvitess†; Astifat; Ketof; Padiatifen; Zaditen; Zatofug; ***Gr.:*** Eucycline; Frenasma; Klevistamin; Labelphen; Nostimex; Orpidix; Pellexeme; Zaditen; ***Hong Kong:*** Amitone; Asmafen; Asmaten; Ketifen; Vidatifen; Zaditen; ***India:*** Ketasma; ***Irl.:*** Zaditen; ***Israel:*** Profiten; Zaditen; ***Ital.:*** Alleal; Chetofen; Ketoftil; Zaditen; ***Malaysia:*** Asmafen; Asumalife; Denerel; Dhatifen; Ketifen; Xidanef; Zaden; Zaditen; ***Mex.:*** Asmaral-K; Fin-A†; Hidroazer†; Kasmal; Nemodine†; Nomotec; Osaten; Saluket-H1; Ventisol; Waytifeno†; Zaditen; ***Neth.:*** Zaditen; ***Norw.:*** Zaditen; ***NZ:*** Asmafen; ***Port.:*** Cipanfeno; Quefeno; Zaditen; ***S.Afr.:*** Ketohexal; Zaditen; Zetofen; ***Singapore:*** Asmafen; Beatifen; Denerel†; Dhatifen; Erliten; Tofen; Zaditen; ***Spain:*** Ketasma; Zaditena; Zasten; ***Swed.:*** Zaditen; ***Switz.:*** Zaditen; ***Thai.:*** Asmanoc; Denerel; Ibis; Katifen; Kenefen; Keten; Ketifen; Keto; Ketofen; Ketotab†; Medkofen; Medotifen; Politifen; Servitifen†; Sykofen; Xidanef; Zadino; Zaditen; Zytofen; ***UAE:*** Asmafort; ***UK:*** Zaditen; ***USA:*** Zaditor.

**Multi-ingredient:** ***Arg.:*** Airbronal; Fatigan Bronquial; Inastmol.

---

## Levosalbutamol Hydrochloride *(rINNM)*

Hidrocloruro de levosalbutamol; Levalbuterol Hydrochloride (USAN). (*R*)-α[1]-[(*tert*-Butylamino)methyl]-4-hydroxy-*m*-xylene-α,α′-diol hydrochloride.

$C_{13}H_{21}NO_3,HCl = 275.8.$

*CAS — 34391-04-3 (levosalbutamol); 50293-90-8 (levosalbutamol hydrochloride).*

### Adverse Effects and Precautions

As for Salbutamol, p.791.

**Incidence of adverse effects.** Beta-adrenergic adverse effects (e.g. nervousness and increased heart rate) appeared less frequent with nebulised levosalbutamol 630 micrograms than with racemic salbutamol 2.5 mg.[1] There is preliminary evidence that the increased airway hyperresponsiveness occasionally seen with long-term racemic salbutamol (see Tolerance, p.792) may be due to the *S*(+)-enantiomer, and therefore might not occur with levosalbutamol.[2]


1. Nelson HS, *et al.* Improved bronchodilation with levalbuterol compared with racemic albuterol in patients with asthma. *J Allergy Clin Immunol* 1998; **102:** 943–52.
2. Perrin-Fayolle M. Salbutamol in the treatment of asthma. *Lancet* 1995; **346:** 1101.


### Interactions

As for Salbutamol, p.792.

### Pharmacokinetics

There is some systemic absorption of inhaled levosalbutamol. It appears to be stereochemically stable *in vivo* and not metabolised to *S*(+)-salbutamol. After a single dose levosalbutamol has a half-life of 3.3 hours.

**Metabolism.** There is evidence that levosalbutamol is metabolised faster than *S*(+)-salbutamol.

References.


1. Boulton DW, Fawcett JP. Enantioselective disposition of salbutamol in man following oral and intravenous administration. *Br J Clin Pharmacol* 1996; **41:** 35–40.
2. Lipworth BJ, *et al.* Pharmacokinetics and extrapulmonary $\beta_2$ adrenoceptor activity of nebulised racemic salbutamol and its R and S isomers in healthy volunteers. *Thorax* 1997; **52:** 849–52.
3. Gumbhir-Shah K, *et al.* Pharmacokinetic and pharmacodynamic characteristics and safety of inhaled albuterol enantiomers in healthy volunteers. *J Clin Pharmacol* 1998; **38:** 1096–1106.
4. Boulton DW, Fawcett JP. The pharmacokinetics of levosalbutamol: what are the clinical implications? *Clin Pharmacokinet* 2001; **40:** 23–40.


### Uses and Administration

Levosalbutamol, the *R*(−)-enantiomer of salbutamol (p.791), may be used as an alternative to racemic salbutamol for the management of asthma (p.777). It is given as the hydrochloride but doses are expressed in terms of the base; levosalbutamol hydrochloride 1.15 mg is approximately equivalent to levosalbutamol 1 mg. Usual doses equivalent to levosalbutamol 630 micrograms are inhaled three times daily as a nebulised solution, increased if necessary to 1.25 mg three times daily. Children aged 6 to 11 years may be given 310 micrograms three times daily. In patients with asthma, as-required beta agonist therapy is preferable to regular use. An increased need for, or decreased duration of effect of, levosalbutamol indicates deterioration of asthma control and the need for review of therapy.

◊ References.


1. Nelson HS, *et al.* Improved bronchodilation with levalbuterol compared with racemic albuterol in patients with asthma. *J Allergy Clin Immunol* 1998; **102:** 943–52.
2. Jenne JW. The debate on S-enantiomers of β-agonists: tempest in a teapot or gathering storm? *J Allergy Clin Immunol* 1998; **102:** 893–5.
3. Gawchick SM, *et al.* The safety and efficacy of nebulized levalbuterol compared with racemic albuterol and placebo in the treatment of asthma in pediatric patients. *J Allergy Clin Immunol* 1999; **103:** 615–21.
4. Anonymous. Levalbuterol for asthma. *Med Lett Drugs Ther* 1999; **41:** 51–3.
5. Truitt T, *et al.* Levalbuterol compared to racemic albuterol: efficacy and outcomes in patients hospitalized with COPD or asthma. *Chest* 2003; **123:** 128–35.
6. Carl JC, *et al.* Comparison of racemic albuterol and levalbuterol for treatment of acute asthma. *J Pediatr* 2003; **143:** 731–6.


**Action.** *In vitro,* levosalbutamol had slightly higher affinity than racemic salbutamol for $beta_1$ and $beta_2$ adrenoceptors.[1] The *S*(+)-enantiomer had low affinity for these receptors. All 3 were mildly selective for $beta_2$ adrenoceptors.


1. Penn RB, *et al.* Comparison of R-, S-, and RS-albuterol interaction with human $\beta_1$- and $\beta_2$-adrenergic receptors. *Clin Rev Allergy Immunol* 1996; **14:** 37–45.


### Preparations

**Proprietary Preparations** (details are given in Part 3)

***USA:*** Xopenex.

---

## Montelukast Sodium *(BANM, USAN, rINNM)*

L-706631; MK-476; Montelukast sódico. Sodium 1-[({(*R*)-*m*-[(*E*)-2-(7-chloro-2-quinolyl)-vinyl]-α-[*o*-(1-hydroxy-1-methylethyl)phenethyl]-benzyl}thio)methyl] cyclopropaneacetate.

$C_{35}H_{35}ClNNaO_3S = 608.2.$

*CAS — 158966-92-8 (montelukast); 151767-02-1 (montelukast sodium).*

*ATC — R03DC03.*

### Adverse Effects and Precautions

As for Zafirlukast, p.807.

◊ Suspected adverse effects reported to the UK Committee on Safety of Medicines following the launch of montelukast included oedema, agitation and restlessness, allergy including anaphylaxis, angioedema, and urticaria, chest pain, tremor, dry mouth, vertigo, and arthralgia.[1] Further suspected adverse effects included nightmares, sedation, palpitations, and increased sweating.[2]


1. Committee on Safety of Medicines/Medicines Control Agency. Leukotriene antagonists: a new class of asthma treatment. *Current Problems* 1998; **24:** 14. Also available at: http://www.mca.gov.uk/ourwork/monitorsafequalmed/currentproblems/volume24aug.htm (accessed 20/04/04)
2. Committee on Safety of Medicines/Medicines Control Agency. Leukotriene receptor antagonists: update on adverse reaction profiles. *Current Problems* 1999; **25:** 14. Also available at: http://www.mca.gov.uk/ourwork/monitorsafequalmed/currentproblems/volume25nov.htm (accessed 20/04/04)


**Churg-Strauss syndrome.** Churg-Strauss syndrome has been reported with the use of montelukast.[1-5] There has also been a report of relapse in a patient with Churg-Strauss syndrome who had been in complete remission when montelukast therapy was started.[5] For discussion of the unresolved role of leukotriene antagonists in this disorder and precautions to be observed, see under Zafirlukast, p.807.


1. Franco J, Artés MJ. Pulmonary eosinophilia associated with montelukast. *Thorax* 1999; **54:** 558–60.
2. Tuggey JM, Hosker HSR. Churg-Strauss syndrome associated with montelukast therapy. *Thorax* 2000; **55:** 805–6.
3. Meghjee SPL, White JS. Montelukast and Churg-Strauss syndrome. *Thorax* 2001; **56:** 244.
4. Gal AA, *et al.* Cutaneous lesions of Churg-Strauss syndrome associated with montelukast therapy. *Br J Dermatol* 2002; **147:** 618–19.
5. Solans R, *et al.* Montelukast and Churg-Strauss syndrome. *Thorax* 2002; **57:** 183–5.


**Hepatic and renal impairment.** Although there is some evidence of effects on the liver in patients receiving montelukast, and although it is largely eliminated by hepatic metabolism, montelukast (unlike zafirlukast) is not considered by its UK manufacturer to be contra-indicated in hepatic impairment, and no dose adjustment is considered necessary in mild to moderate hepatic impairment.

No dosage adjustment is anticipated to be necessary in patients with renal impairment.

## Interactions

The manufacturer recommends clinical monitoring when potent hepatic enzyme inducers such as phenytoin, phenobarbital, or rifampicin are given with montelukast.

**Corticosteroids.** For a report of peripheral oedema in a patient given montelukast and *prednisone*, see Leukotriene Antagonists, p.1073.

**Phenobarbital.** Peak serum concentrations after a single dose of montelukast 10 mg were reduced by 20% in 14 healthy subjects who took phenobarbital 100 mg daily for 14 days, and area under the serum concentration-time curve was reduced by 38%. However, it was not thought that montelukast doses would need adjustment if given with phenobarbital.[1]


1. Holland S, *et al.* Metabolism of montelukast (M) is increased by multiple doses of phenobarbital (P). *Clin Pharmacol Ther* 1998; **63:** 231.


## Pharmacokinetics

Peak plasma concentrations of montelukast are achieved in 2 to 4 hours after oral administration. The mean oral bioavailability is 64%. Montelukast is more than 99% bound to plasma proteins. It is extensively metabolised in the liver by cytochrome P450 isoenzymes CYP3A4, CYP2A6, and CYP2C9, and is excreted principally in the faeces via the bile. Metabolism was reduced and the elimination half-life prolonged in patients with mild to moderate hepatic impairment.

◊ References.


1. Knorr B, *et al.* Montelukast dose selection in 6- to 14-year-olds: comparison of single-dose pharmacokinetics in children and adults. *J Clin Pharmacol* 1999; **39:** 786–93.
2. Knorr B, *et al.* Montelukast dose selection in children ages 2 to 5 years: comparison of population pharmacokinetics between children and adults. *J Clin Pharmacol* 1999; **41:** 612–19.


## Uses and Administration

Montelukast is a selective leukotriene receptor antagonist with actions and uses similar to those of zafirlukast (p.807) although it is reported to have a longer duration of action. It is used as the sodium salt, but doses are expressed in terms of the base; montelukast sodium 10.37 mg is approximately equivalent to montelukast 10 mg.

In the management of chronic asthma (p.777), montelukast sodium is given in doses equivalent to 10 mg of montelukast once daily in the evening; children aged 6 to 14 years may be given the equivalent of 5 mg in the evening and children aged 6 months to 5 years may be given 4 mg. It should not be used to treat an acute asthma attack.

In the management of seasonal allergic rhinitis (p.422), the same doses of montelukast are given as for asthma, in adults and children from 2 years of age.

**Asthma.** Montelukast produced modest improvements compared with placebo in chronic asthma and exercise-induced asthma in both adults[1,2] and children.[3-5] In a systematic review[6] of trials comparing leukotriene receptor antagonists with inhaled corticosteroids for mild to moderate asthma, in which 9 of the 14 studies used montelukast, leukotriene antagonists were found to be less effective in maintaining asthma control. One study[7] has reported that the use of montelukast did permit reduction in the dose of concomitant inhaled corticosteroid. There is some evidence that montelukast may be more effective than inhaled salmeterol for the chronic treatment of exercise-induced asthma.[8,9] Montelukast has been reviewed,[10-12] and further general references for leukotriene antagonists can be found under Zafirlukast, p.807.

An intravenous form of montelukast is under investigation for the treatment of severe acute asthma.[13,14]


1. Leff JA, *et al.* Montelukast, a leukotriene-receptor antagonist, for the treatment of mild asthma and exercise-induced bronchoconstriction. *N Engl J Med* 1998; **339:** 147–52.
2. Reiss TF, *et al.* Montelukast, a once-daily leukotriene receptor antagonist, in the treatment of chronic asthma: a multicenter, randomized, double-blind trial. *Arch Intern Med* 1998; **158:** 1213–20.
3. Knorr B, *et al.* Montelukast for chronic asthma in 6- to 14-year-old children: a randomized, double-blind trial. *JAMA* 1998; **279:** 1181–6.
4. Kemp JP, *et al.* Montelukast once daily inhibits exercise-induced bronchoconstriction in 6- to 14-year-old children with asthma. *J Pediatr* 1998; **133:** 424–8.
5. Knorr B, *et al.* Montelukast, a leukotriene receptor antagonist, for the treatment of persistent asthma in children aged 2 to 5 years. Abstract: *Pediatrics* 2001; **108:** 754–5. Full version: http://pediatrics.aappublications.org/cgi/content/full/108/3/e48 (accessed 21/04/04)
6. Ducharme FM, Hicks GC. Anti-leukotriene agents compared to inhaled corticosteroids in the management of recurrent and/or chronic asthma in adults and children. Available in The Cochrane Library; Issue 1. Chichester: John Wiley; 2004.
7. Löfdahl C-G, *et al.* Randomised, placebo controlled trial of effect of a leukotriene receptor antagonist, montelukast, on tapering inhaled corticosteroids in asthma. *BMJ* 1999; **319:** 87–90.
8. Villaran C, *et al.* Montelukast versus salmeterol in patients with asthma and exercise-induced bronchoconstriction. *J Allergy Clin Immunol* 1999; **104:** 547–53.
9. Edelman JM, *et al.* Oral montelukast compared with inhaled salmeterol to prevent exercise-induced bronchoconstriction: a randomized, double-blind trial. *Ann Intern Med* 2000; **132:** 97–104.
10. Anonymous. Montelukast for persistent asthma. *Med Lett Drugs Ther* 1998; **40:** 71–3.
11. Anonymous. Montelukast and zafirlukast in asthma. *Drug Ther Bull* 1998; **36:** 65–8.
12. Jarvis B, Markham A. Montelukast: a review of its therapeutic potential in persistent asthma. *Drugs* 2000; **59:** 891–928.
13. Dockhorn RJ, *et al.* Comparison of the effects of intravenous and oral montelukast on airway function: a double blind, placebo controlled, three period, crossover study in asthmatic patients. *Thorax* 2000; **55:** 260–5.
14. Camargo CA, *et al.* A randomized controlled trial of intravenous montelukast in acute asthma. *Am J Respir Crit Care Med* 2003; **167:** 528–33.


**Gastrointestinal disorders.** Benefit has been reported[1] with the use of montelukast in patients with eosinophilic oesophagitis, a rare condition involving eosinophilic infiltration of the oesophagus with intermittent painful dysphagia.


1. Attwood SEA, *et al.* Eosinophilic oesophagitis: a novel treatment using montelukast. *Gut* 2003; **52:** 181–5.


**Rhinitis.** Montelukast relieved the symptoms of seasonal allergic rhinitis compared with placebo in 2 large studies.[1,2] However, a meta-analysis[3] of these and other studies of leukotriene antagonists (mainly montelukast) for management of allergic rhinitis concluded that while leukotriene antagonists were modestly more effective than placebo and of similar efficacy to antihistamines, in reducing nasal symptoms and improving rhinoconjunctivitis, they were less effective than corticosteroids even when used with antihistamines.


1. Philip G, *et al.* Montelukast for treating seasonal allergic rhinitis: a randomized, double-blind, placebo-controlled trial performed in the spring. *Clin Exp Allergy* 2002; **32:** 1020–8.
2. van Adelsberg J, *et al.* Randomized controlled trial evaluating the clinical benefit of montelukast for treating spring seasonal allergic rhinitis. *Ann Allergy Asthma Immunol* 2003; **90:** 214–22.
3. Wilson AM, *et al.* Leukotriene receptor antagonists for allergic rhinitis: a systematic review and meta-analysis. *Am J Med* 2004; **116:** 338–44.


## Preparations

**Proprietary Preparations** (details are given in Part 3)

***Arg.:*** Lukair; Singulair; ***Austral.:*** Singulair; ***Austria:*** Singulair; ***Belg.:*** Singulair; ***Braz.:*** Singulair; ***Canad.:*** Singulair; ***Chile:*** Singulair; ***Denm.:*** Singulair; ***Fin.:*** Singulair; ***Fr.:*** Singulair; ***Ger.:*** Singulair; ***Gr.:*** Singulair; ***Hong Kong:*** Singulair; ***India:*** Montair; ***Irl.:*** Singulair; ***Israel:*** Singulair; ***Ital.:*** Lukasm; Montegen; Singulair; ***Jpn:*** Kipress; ***Malaysia:*** Singulair; ***Mex.:*** Singulair; ***Neth.:*** Singulair; ***Norw.:*** Singulair; ***NZ:*** Singulair; ***Port.:*** Singulair; ***S.Afr.:*** Singulair; ***Singapore:*** Singulair; ***Spain:*** Singulair; ***Swed.:*** Singulair; ***Switz.:*** Singulair; ***Thai.:*** Singulair; ***UK:*** Singulair; ***USA:*** Singulair.

# Nedocromil Sodium *(BANM, USAN, rINNM)*

FPL-59002 (nedocromil); FPL-59002KC (nedocromil calcium); FPL-59002KP (nedocromil sodium); Nedocromilo sódico. Disodium 9-ethyl-6,9-dihydro-4,6-dioxo-10-propyl-4*H*-pyrano[3,2-g]quinoline-2,8-dicarboxylate.

$C_{19}H_{15}NNa_2O_7 = 415.3.$

*CAS — 69049-73-6 (nedocromil); 69049-74-7 (nedocromil sodium); 101626-68-0 (nedocromil calcium).*

NOTE. Nedocromil Calcium is also *USAN.*

## Adverse Effects and Precautions

Inhaled nedocromil sodium may cause headache, nausea, abdominal discomfort (mild and transient), and a bitter taste. Increased bronchospasm has occurred in a few patients. Eye drops may cause transient burning and stinging.

It should not be used for the treatment of acute asthma attacks. The general cautions described under sodium cromoglicate (see p.796) also apply.

**Incidence of adverse effects.** A review[1] of nedocromil sodium commented that adverse effects were infrequent, mild, and short-lived. The most common effect appeared to be an unpleasant or bitter taste which was experienced by 12 to 13% of patients, although less than 1% of patients discontinued treatment because of it. Other adverse effects included cough (in 7%), headache (6%), sore throat (5.7%), nausea (4%), and vomiting (1.7%).


1. Brogden RN, Sorkin EM. Nedocromil sodium: an updated review of its pharmacological properties and therapeutic efficacy in asthma. *Drugs* 1993; **45:** 693–715.


## Pharmacokinetics

Nedocromil sodium is poorly absorbed from the gastrointestinal tract. About 5% of the inhaled dose is absorbed from the lungs and is excreted unchanged in the urine and bile. The half-life is stated to range from about 1.5 to 3.3 hours.

◊ The extent of absorption or bioavailability of nedocromil sodium after inhalation in healthy subjects was 7 to 9% of the dose, including 2 to 3% oral absorption and 5 to 6% absorption from the respiratory tract.[1] Following inhalation of nedocromil sodium 4 mg the mean peak plasma concentration was 3.3 nanograms/mL in healthy subjects and 2.8 nanograms/mL in asthmatic patients, with peak values being reached at about 20 and 40 minutes respectively. The mean total urinary excretion after 24 hours following a single dose was 5.4% of the dose in healthy subjects and 2.3% in asthmatics.


1. Neale MG, *et al.* The pharmacokinetics of nedocromil sodium, a new drug for the treatment of reversible obstructive airways disease, in human volunteers and patients with reversible obstructive airways disease. *Br J Clin Pharmacol* 1987; **24:** 493–501.


## Uses and Administration

Nedocromil sodium has a stabilising action on mast cells resembling that of sodium cromoglicate (p.796) and is used similarly in the management of chronic asthma. It should not be used to treat an acute attack of asthma.

For **asthma**, nedocromil sodium is given by metered-dose aerosol inhalation. The usual dose is 4 mg inhaled four times daily which may be decreased to 4 mg twice daily once control of symptoms is achieved. Clinical improvement usually occurs within 2 to 4 weeks of beginning therapy.

Nedocromil sodium is also used topically in the treatment of **allergic conjunctivitis** and allergic **rhinitis**. For allergic conjunctivitis it is given as a 2% solution, instilled into each eye twice daily. This may be increased to 4 times daily if necessary, which is the usual dose in vernal keratoconjunctivitis. In allergic rhinitis nedocromil sodium is used as a 1% nasal spray: one spray is given into each nostril 4 times daily.

◊ General references.


1. Brogden RN, Sorkin EM. Nedocromil sodium: an updated review of its pharmacological properties and therapeutic efficacy in asthma. *Drugs* 1993; **45:** 693–715.
2. Parish RC, Miller LJ. Nedocromil sodium. *Ann Pharmacother* 1993; **27:** 599–606.


**Asthma.** Nedocromil sodium is generally considered to be an alternative to sodium cromoglicate in the management of asthma (p.777). Nedocromil has been shown to improve symptoms and reduce bronchodilator intake in adults[1] and children[2] with chronic asthma. It may be used before exercise to reduce exercise-induced bronchoconstriction,[3] and appears to be as effective as sodium cromoglicate for this indication.[4]


1. Edwards AM, Stevens MT. The clinical efficacy of inhaled nedocromil sodium (Tilade) in the treatment of asthma. *Eur Respir J* 1993; **6:** 35–41.

2. Armenio L, *et al.* Double blind, placebo controlled study of nedocromil sodium in asthma. *Arch Dis Child* 1993; **68:** 193–7.
3. Spooner CH, *et al.* Nedocromil sodium for preventing exercise-induced bronchoconstriction. Available in The Cochrane Library; Issue 1. Chichester: John Wiley; 2004.
4. Kelly K, *et al.* Nedocromil sodium versus sodium cromoglycate for preventing exercise-induced bronchoconstriction in asthmatics. Available in The Cochrane Library; Issue 1. Chichester: John Wiley; 2004.

**Cough.** For references indicating a positive response to sodium cromoglicate but not to nedocromil sodium in the management of cough induced by ACE inhibitor therapy, see Cough, p.796.

**Rhinitis and conjunctivitis.** Nedocromil has been used in the management of allergic rhinitis (p.422) and conjunctivitis (p.421). There is some evidence that nedocromil may be more effective than cromoglicate in the management of vernal keratoconjunctivitis (see p.797), but is less effective than fluorometholone.[1]

1. Tabbara KF, Al-Kharashi SA. Efficacy of nedocromil 2% versus fluorometholone 0.1%: a randomised, double masked trial comparing the effects on severe vernal keratoconjunctivitis. *Br J Ophthalmol* 1999; **83:** 180–4.

## Preparations

**Proprietary Preparations** (details are given in Part 3)
***Austral.:*** Tilade; ***Austria:*** Tilade; Tilarin; Tilavist; ***Braz.:*** Tilade; ***Canad.:*** Alocril; Mirezeᵻ; Tilade; ***Denm.:*** Tilade; Tilavist; ***Fin.:*** Tilade; Tilarin; Tilavist; ***Fr.:*** Tiladeᵻ; Tilavist; ***Ger.:*** Halamid; Irtan; Tilade; ***Gr.:*** Tilade; ***Hong Kong:*** Tilade; ***Irl.:*** Tilade; Tilavist; ***Israel:*** Tilade; Tilavist; ***Ital.:*** Kovilen; Kovinal; Tilade; Tilarin; Tilavist; ***Mex.:*** Irtanᵻ; Tilaireᵻ; ***Neth.:*** Tilade; Tilavist; ***Norw.:*** Tilavist; ***NZ:*** Tilade; Tilarinᵻ; Tilavistᵻ; ***Port.:*** Tilavist; ***S.Afr.:*** Tiladeᵻ; ***Singapore:*** Tilavistᵻ; ***Spain:*** Brionil; Cetimil; Tilad; Tilavist; ***Swed.:*** Tilavist; ***Switz.:*** Tilade; Tilarin; Tilavist; ***UK:*** Rapitil; Tilade; ***USA:*** Alocril; Tilade.

**Multi-ingredient:** ***Ital.:*** Zarent.

## Omalizumab *(BAN, USAN, rINN)*

rhuMab-E25.
*CAS — 242138-07-4.*
*ATC — R03DX05.*

### Adverse Effects and Precautions

Injection site reactions commonly occur with the use of omalizumab. Other adverse effects that have been reported include generalised pain, fatigue, arthralgia, dizziness, and earache. Hypersensitivity reactions such as urticaria, dermatitis, and pruritus can occur, and anaphylaxis has been reported rarely. The manufacturers have reported an increased incidence of malignancies in patients receiving omalizumab.

Omalizumab should not be used for the treatment of acute asthma attacks.

### Pharmacokinetics

Omalizumab is absorbed after subcutaneous injection with a bioavailability of about 62%, reaching peak serum concentrations after 7 to 8 days. It is removed by IgG and IgE clearance processes in the liver, with a serum elimination half-life of about 26 days. During treatment with omalizumab, the serum concentration of free IgE decreases but that of total IgE increases because the omalizumab-IgE complex has a slower elimination rate than free IgE.

### Uses and Administration

Omalizumab is a recombinant humanised monoclonal antibody that selectively binds to IgE. It inhibits the binding of IgE on the surface of mast cells and basophils, thus reducing the release of mediators of the allergic response. Omalizumab is used in the prophylactic management of allergic asthma (p.777). The dose depends on the patient's weight and pre-treatment serum-IgE concentrations, and ranges from 150 to 375 mg every 2 or 4 weeks subcutaneously. Not more than 150 mg should be given at one injection site. Total IgE concentrations rise during treatment (see Pharmacokinetics, above), remaining elevated for up to 1 year after discontinuation, and cannot be used to determine dosage.

Omalizumab is under investigation in the prophylactic management of seasonal allergic rhinitis.

◊ References.

1. Milgrom H, *et al.* Treatment of allergic asthma with monoclonal anti-IgE antibody. *N Engl J Med* 1999; **341:** 1966–73.
2. Ädelroth E, *et al.* Recombinant humanized mAb-E25, an anti-IgE mAb, in birch pollen-induced seasonal allergic rhinitis. *J Allergy Clin Immunol* 2000; **106:** 253–9.
3. Easthope S, Jarvis B. Omalizumab. *Drugs* 2001; **61:** 253–60.
4. Milgrom H, *et al.* Treatment of childhood asthma with anti-immunoglobulin E antibody (omalizumab). *Pediatrics* 2001; **108:** 462–3. Full version: http://pediatrics.aappublications.org/cgi/content/full/108/2/e36 (accessed 20/04/04)
5. Busse W, *et al.* Omalizumab, anti-IgE recombinant humanized monoclonal antibody, for the treatment of severe allergic asthma. *J Allergy Clin Immunol* 2001; **108:** 184–90.
6. Solèr M, *et al.* The anti-IgE antibody omalizumab reduces exacerbations and steroid requirement in allergic asthmatics. *Eur Respir J* 2001; **18:** 254–61. Correction *ibid.*; 739–40.
7. Casale TB, *et al.* Effect of omalizumab on symptoms of seasonal allergic rhinitis: a randomized controlled trial. *JAMA* 2001; **286:** 2956–67.
8. Lanier BQ, *et al.* Omalizumab is effective in the long-term control of severe allergic asthma. *Ann Allergy Asthma Immunol* 2003; **91:** 154–9.
9. Chervinsky P, *et al.* Omalizumab, an anti-IgE antibody, in treatment of adults and adolescents with perennial allergic rhinitis. *Ann Allergy Asthma Immunol* 2003; **91:** 160–7.

### Preparations

**Proprietary Preparations** (details are given in Part 3)
***USA:*** Xolair.

## Orciprenaline Sulfate *(rINNM)*

Metaproterenol Sulfate *(USAN)*; Metaproterenol Sulphate; Orciprenaline Sulphate *(BANM)*; Orciprenalini Sulfas; Sulfato de orciprenalina; Th-152. 1-(3,5-Dihydroxyphenyl)-2-isopropylaminoethanol sulphate; *N*-Isopropyl-*N*(β,3,5-trihydroxyphenethyl)ammonium sulphate.
$(C_{11}H_{17}NO_3)_2,H_2SO_4$ = 520.6.
*CAS — 586-06-1 (orciprenaline); 5874-97-5 (orciprenaline sulfate).*
*ATC — R03AB03; R03CB03.*

**Pharmacopoeias.** In *Eur.* (see p.vi), *Jpn, Pol.,* and *US.*

**Ph. Eur. 5.0** (Orciprenaline Sulphate). A white, slightly hygroscopic, crystalline powder. Freely soluble in water and in alcohol; practically insoluble in dichloromethane. A 10% solution in water has a pH of 4.0 to 5.5. Protect from light.

**USP 27** (Metaproterenol Sulfate). A white to off-white crystalline powder. Freely soluble in water. A 10% solution in water has a pH of 4.0 to 5.5. Store in airtight containers. Protect from light.

### Adverse Effects and Precautions

As for Salbutamol, p.791. Adverse effects are more common because of the non-selective beta agonist effect of orciprenaline. For the adverse effects and precautions pertaining to a non-selective beta agonist see Isoprenaline Sulfate, p.940.

### Interactions

As for Salbutamol, p.792.

### Pharmacokinetics

Following oral administration orciprenaline is absorbed from the gastrointestinal tract and undergoes extensive first-pass metabolism in the liver; about 40% of an oral dose is reported to reach the circulation unchanged. It is excreted in the urine primarily as metabolites.

### Uses and Administration

Orciprenaline sulfate is a direct-acting sympathomimetic with predominantly beta-adrenoceptor stimulant activity. It has actions and uses similar to those of salbutamol (p.793) but is less selective for beta$_2$ receptors.

Orciprenaline sulfate is used as a bronchodilator in the management of reversible airways obstruction, as in asthma (p.777) and in some patients with chronic obstructive pulmonary disease (p.779). However, more selective beta$_2$ agonists such as salbutamol or terbutaline are now preferred. Following inhalation, the onset of action is usually within 5 to 30 minutes and can last up to 6 hours, though there is wide variation.

A typical adult dose for the relief of acute **bronchospasm** has been 1 or 2 inhalations of orciprenaline sulfate 750 micrograms from a metered-dose aerosol, repeated if required after not less than 3 hours, up to a maximum of 12 inhalations (9 mg) in 24 hours. A suggested maximum dose within a 24-hour period for children is: under 6 years, up to 4 inhalations; 6 to 12 years, up to 8 inhalations. In patients with asthma, 'as-required' beta agonist therapy is preferable to regular use. An increased need for, or decreased duration of effect of, orciprenaline indicates deterioration of asthma control and the need for review of therapy.

Orciprenaline sulfate has also been inhaled in 5% solution from a hand nebuliser, the usual adult dose being 10 inhalations. If the solution is used with any other nebulising device such as an intermittent positive-pressure breathing (IPPB) apparatus the adult dose is 0.2 to 0.3 mL of a 5% solution diluted up to about 2.5 mL with physiological saline (i.e. dilution to a 0.4 to 0.6% solution) administered not more often than every 4 hours. Unit-dose vials containing a prediluted solution of orciprenaline sulfate 0.4 and 0.6% are also available for nebulisation by an IPPB device.

In the chronic management of reversible airways obstruction, orciprenaline sulfate has been given by mouth in a usual adult dose of 20 mg three or four times daily.

Orciprenaline sulfate has also been used similarly to isoprenaline (see p.940) for its cardiovascular effects in the treatment of **bradycardia** of various types, notably in AV heart block and sinus bradycardia. In such cases doses of up to 240 mg daily by mouth in divided doses, or 250 to 500 micrograms by slow intravenous injection have been given; orciprenaline sulfate may also be given by intravenous infusion, or intramuscular or subcutaneous injection.

### Preparations

***BP 2003:*** Orciprenaline Tablets;
***USP 27:*** Metaproterenol Sulfate Inhalation Aerosol; Metaproterenol Sulfate Inhalation Solution; Metaproterenol Sulfate Syrup; Metaproterenol Sulfate Tablets.

**Proprietary Preparations** (details are given in Part 3)
***Austral.:*** Alupent; ***Austria:*** Alupent; ***Belg.:*** Alupentᵻ; ***Canad.:*** Alupent; ***Fr.:*** Alupentᵻ; ***Ger.:*** Alupent; ***Gr.:*** Alupent; ***India:*** Alupent; ***Irl.:*** Alupent; ***Ital.:*** Alupent; ***Mex.:*** Alupentᵻ; ***NZ:*** Alupentᵻ; ***S.Afr.:*** Alupentᵻ; ***Spain:*** Alupentᵻ; ***Switz.:*** Alupentᵻ; ***Thai.:*** Alupent; ***UK:*** Alupent; ***USA:*** Alupent.

**Multi-ingredient:** ***Braz.:*** Bisolvon Complexᵻ; ***Chile:*** Broncodual Compuesto; Cloval Compuesto; Pulbronc; Solvanol; Tusabron; Vapoflu; ***Irl.:*** Alupent Expectorant; ***S.Afr.:*** Adco-Linctopent; Benylin Chesty; Bisolvon Linctus DA; Bronkese Compound; Flemeze; Silomat DA; ***Thai.:*** Silomat Compositumᵻ; ***UAE:*** Orcinol.

## Oxitropium Bromide *(BAN, rINN)*

Ba-253; Bromuro de oxitropio. 6,7-Epoxy-8-ethyl-3-[(*S*)-tropoyloxy]tropanium bromide; (3*s*,6*R*,7*S*,8*r*)-8-Ethyl-3-[(*S*)-tropoyloxy]-6,7-epoxytropanium bromide.
$C_{19}H_{26}BrNO_4$ = 412.3.
*CAS — 30286-75-0.*
*ATC — R03BB02.*

### Profile

Oxitropium bromide is a quaternary ammonium antimuscarinic with actions similar to those of ipratropium bromide (p.787), to which it is structurally related. It is used as a bronchodilator in the treatment of reversible airways obstruction, as in asthma (p.777) and chronic obstructive pulmonary disease (p.779). Doses of 200 micrograms by inhalation from a metered-dose aerosol have been given 2 or 3 times daily. Oxitropium bromide may also be given as a nebulised solution in doses of 1.5 mg inhaled 2 or 3 times daily; an effective single dose may range from 1 to 2 mg. *Animal* studies have shown reproductive toxicity with high doses of oxitropium, hence the manufacturer's recommendation that it should not be used during pregnancy.

### Preparations

**Proprietary Preparations** (details are given in Part 3)
***Belg.:*** Oxivent; ***Denm.:*** Oxiventᵻ; ***Fin.:*** Ventox; ***Fr.:*** Tersigat; ***Ger.:*** Ventilat; ***Irl.:*** Oxivent; ***Ital.:*** Oxivent; ***UK:*** Oxiventᵻ.

## Pemirolast Potassium *(USAN, rINNM)*

BL-5617; BMY-26517; Pemirolast potásico. Potassium 9-methyl-3-(1*H*-tetrazol-5-yl)-4*H*-pyrido[1,2-*a*]pyrimidin-4-one.
$C_{10}H_7KN_6O$ = 266.3.
*CAS — 69372-19-6 (pemirolast); 100299-08-9 (pemirolast potassium).*

### Profile

Pemirolast potassium has mast cell stabilising properties like sodium cromoglicate (p.795) and may also be a leukotriene inhibitor. It has been used in the treatment of chronic asthma (p.777) and in the prophylaxis of allergic rhinitis (p.422) and conjunctivitis (p.421). For asthma, the usual dose used for adults is 10 mg orally twice daily after food. Children aged 1 to 4 years are given 2.5 mg twice daily, and those aged 5 to 10 years are given 5 mg twice daily. For allergic rhinitis, these doses for adults and children are halved. Pemirolast potassium 0.1% ophthalmic solution is used 4 times daily in the prophylactic management of allergic conjunctivitis. Pemirolast potassium has no bronchodilator properties and should not be used for the treatment of acute asthma attacks.

◊ References.

1. Tinkelman DG, Berkowitz RB. A pilot study of pemirolast in patients with seasonal allergic rhinitis. *Ann Allergy* 1991; **66:** 162–5.
2. Hasegawa T, *et al.* Kinetic interaction between theophylline and a newly developed anti-allergic drug, pemirolast potassium. *Eur J Clin Pharmacol* 1994; **46:** 55–8.
3. Anonymous. New drugs for allergic conjunctivitis. *Med Lett Drugs Ther* 2000; **42:** 39–40.
4. Abelson MB, *et al.* Pemirolast potassium 0.1% ophthalmic solution is an effective treatment for allergic conjunctivitis: a pooled analysis of two prospective, randomized, double-masked, placebo-controlled, phase III studies. *J Ocul Pharmacol Ther* 2002; **18:** 475–88.
5. Shulman DG. Two mast cell stabilizers, pemirolast potassium 0.1% and nedocromil sodium 2%, in the treatment of seasonal allergic conjunctivitis: a comparative study. *Adv Therapy* 2003; **20:** 31–40.

### Preparations

**Proprietary Preparations** (details are given in Part 3)
***Jpn:*** Alegysal; ***USA:*** Alamast.

## Pirbuterol Acetate *(BANM, USAN, rINNM)*

Acetato de pirbuterol; CP-24314-14; Pyrbuterol Acetate. 2-*tert*-Butylamino-1-(5-hydroxy-6-hydroxymethyl-2-pyridyl)ethanol acetate.
$C_{12}H_{20}N_2O_3,C_2H_4O_2$ = 300.4.
*CAS — 38677-81-5 (pirbuterol); 65652-44-0 (pirbuterol acetate).*
*ATC — R03AC08; R03CC07.*

## Pirbuterol Hydrochloride *(BANM, USAN, rINNM)*

CP-24314-1; Hidrocloruro de pirbuterol; Pyrbuterol Hydrochloride. 2-*tert*-Butylamino-1-(5-hydroxy-6-hydroxymethyl-2-pyridyl)ethanol dihydrochloride.
$C_{12}H_{20}N_2O_3,2HCl$ = 313.2.
*CAS — 38029-10-6.*
*ATC — R03AC08; R03CC07.*

### Profile

Pirbuterol is a direct-acting sympathomimetic with predominantly beta-adrenoceptor stimulant activity and a selective action on beta$_2$ receptors (a beta$_2$ agonist). It has properties similar to those of salbutamol (p.791).

Pirbuterol is used for its bronchodilating properties. It is given as the acetate in the management of reversible airways obstruction, as in asthma (p.777) and in some patients with chronic obstructive pulmonary disease (p.779). Following inhalation, pirbuterol exerts an effect within 10 minutes which is reported to last at least 5 hours.

Pirbuterol is given by inhalation as the acetate but doses are expressed in terms of the base: pirbuterol acetate 250 micrograms is approximately equivalent to pirbuterol 200 micrograms. It is given via a metered-dose aerosol in a usual dose equivalent to pirbuterol 200 to 400 micrograms (1 to 2 inhalations) as required but not more often than every four hours. In patients with asthma, 'as-required' beta agonist therapy is preferable to regular use. An increased need for, or decreased duration of effect of, pirbuterol indicates deterioration of asthma control and the need for review of therapy.

Pirbuterol has also been given by mouth as the hydrochloride.

### Preparations

**Proprietary Preparations** (details are given in Part 3)
***Austria:*** Exirel; ***Belg.:*** Spirolair†; ***Canad.:*** Maxair†; ***Fr.:*** Maxair; ***Ger.:*** Zeisin†; ***Switz.:*** Maxair; ***USA:*** Maxair.

## Pranlukast *(BAN, rINN)*

ONO-1078. *N*-[4-Oxo-2-(1*H*-tetrazol-5-yl)-4*H*-1-benzopyran-8-yl]-*p*-(4-phenylbutoxy)benzamide.

$C_{27}H_{23}N_5O_4$ = 481.5.
*CAS — 103177-37-3.*
*ATC — R03DC02.*

### Profile

Pranlukast is a selective antagonist of the leukotriene $D_4$ receptor with similar properties to zafirlukast (p.807). It is used in the management of asthma (p.777) at a usual dose of pranlukast hydrate 225 mg twice daily in adults. In children with asthma, and weighing at least 12 kg, a dose of 3.5 mg/kg twice daily may be used, up to no more than the adult dose. In the management of allergic rhinitis (p.422) a usual dose of 225 mg twice daily is used in adults.

◊ References.


1. Tamaoki J, *et al.* Leukotriene antagonist prevents exacerbation of asthma during reduction of high-dose inhaled corticosteroid. *Am J Respir Crit Care Med* 1997; **155:** 1235–40.
2. Barnes NC, *et al.* Pranlukast, a novel leukotriene receptor antagonist: results of the first European, placebo-controlled, multicentre clinical study in asthma. *Thorax* 1997; **52:** 523–7.
3. Grossman J, *et al.* Results of the first US double-blind, placebo-controlled, multicenter clinical study in asthma with pranlukast, a novel leukotriene receptor antagonist. *J Asthma* 1997; **34:** 321–8.
4. Keam SJ, *et al.* Pranlukast: a review of its use in the management of asthma. *Drugs* 2003; **63:** 991–1019.


**Churg-Strauss syndrome.** Churg-Strauss syndrome has been reported with the use of pranlukast.[1,2] For discussion of the unresolved role of leukotriene antagonists in this disorder and precautions to be observed, see under Zafirlukast, p.807.


1. Kinoshita M, *et al.* Churg-Strauss syndrome after corticosteroid withdrawal in an asthmatic patient treated with pranlukast. *J Allergy Clin Immunol* 1999; **103:** 534–5.
2. Hayashi S, *et al.* Fulminant eosinophilic endomyocarditis in an asthmatic patient treated with pranlukast after corticosteroid withdrawal. Abstract: *Heart* 2001; **86:** 261. Full version: http://www.heartjnl.com/cgi/content/full/86/3/e7 (accessed 16/03/04)


### Preparations

**Proprietary Preparations** (details are given in Part 3)
***Jpn:*** Onon.

## Procaterol Hydrochloride *(BANM, USAN, rINNM)*

CI-888; Hidrocloruro de procaterol; OPC-2009. (±)-*erythro*-8-Hydroxy-5-(1-hydroxy-2-isopropylaminobutyl)quinolin-2(1*H*)-one hydrochloride; (±)-8-Hydroxy-5-[(1*R**,2*S**)-1-hydroxy-2-isopropylaminobutyl]-2-quinolone hydrochloride.

$C_{16}H_{22}N_2O_3$,HCl = 326.8.
*CAS — 72332-33-3 (procaterol); 59828-07-8 (procaterol hydrochloride).*
*ATC — R03AC16; R03CC08.*

NOTE. Commercial procaterol hydrochloride is the hemihydrate ($C_{16}H_{22}N_2O_3$,HCl,½$H_2O$ = 335.8).

**Pharmacopoeias.** In *Jpn. Chin.* includes the hemihydrate.

### Profile

Procaterol hydrochloride is a direct-acting sympathomimetic with predominantly beta-adrenoceptor stimulant activity selective to $beta_2$ receptors (a $beta_2$ agonist). It has properties similar to those of salbutamol (p.791) and it is used as a bronchodilator in the management of reversible airways obstruction, as in asthma (p.777) or in some patients with chronic obstructive pulmonary disease (p.779). Administration by oral inhalation produces an effect within 5 minutes and the effect can last up to 8 hours.

To relieve acute bronchospasm, 10 to 20 micrograms of procaterol hydrochloride is given by inhalation from a metered-dose aerosol up to 3 times daily. In patients with asthma, 'as-required' beta agonist therapy is preferable to regular use. An increased need for, or decreased duration of effect of, procaterol indicates deterioration of asthma control and the need for review of therapy. An inhalation solution containing 100 micrograms/mL has been given via a nebuliser in usual doses of 30 to 50 micrograms. Procaterol hydrochloride can also be given by mouth in doses of 50 micrograms once or twice daily.

### Preparations

**Proprietary Preparations** (details are given in Part 3)
***Hong Kong:*** Meptin; ***Ital.:*** Procadil; Propulm; ***Jpn:*** Meptin; ***Malaysia:*** Meptin; ***Port.:*** Onsudil; ***Singapore:*** Meptin; ***Spain:*** Onsukil; Promaxol†; ***Thai.:*** Caterol; Meptin.

## Proxyphylline *(BAN, rINN)*

Proxifilina; Proxyphyllinum. 7-(2-Hydroxypropyl)-1,3-dimethylxanthine; (*RS*)-1,3-Dimethyl-7-(2-hydroxypropyl)purine-2,6(3*H*,1*H*)-dione; 7-(2-Hydroxypropyl)theophylline.

$C_{10}H_{14}N_4O_3$ = 238.2.
*CAS — 603-00-9.*
*ATC — R03DA03.*

**Pharmacopoeias.** In *Eur.* (see p.vi).

**Ph. Eur. 5.0** (Proxyphylline). A white crystalline powder. Very soluble in water; soluble in alcohol. Protect from light.

### Profile

Proxyphylline is a derivative of theophylline (p.798) which is used as a bronchodilator and for its cardiovascular properties. Proxyphylline is readily absorbed from the gastrointestinal tract and it does not liberate theophylline in the body.

### Preparations

**Proprietary Preparations** (details are given in Part 3)
***Denm.:*** Neofyllin†; ***Mex.:*** Purofilina†.

**Multi-ingredient:** ***Austria:*** Asthma Efeum; Omega; ***Braz.:*** Santussal; ***Ger.:*** Antihypertonicum S; ***Spain:*** Novofilin; ***Switz.:*** Neo-Biphyllin†.

## Pyridofylline *(rINN)*

Piridofilina; Pyridophylline; Pyridoxine *O*-(Theophyllin-7-ylethyl)sulphate. 3-Hydroxy-4,5-bis(hydroxymethyl)-2-methylpyridine 2-(theophyllin-7-yl)ethyl sulphate.

$C_{17}H_{23}N_5O_9S$ = 473.5.
*CAS — 53403-97-7.*

### Profile

Pyridofylline is a derivative of theophylline (p.798) that has been used as an ingredient of preparations promoted for respiratory-tract disorders.

## Repirinast *(USAN, rINN)*

MY-5116. Isopentyl 5,6-dihydro-7,8-dimethyl-4,5-dioxo-4*H*-pyrano[3,2-*c*]quinoline-2-carboxylate.

$C_{20}H_{21}NO_5$ = 355.4.
*CAS — 73080-51-0.*

### Profile

Repirinast is an orally active anti-allergic with a stabilising action on mast cells resembling that of sodium cromoglicate (p.795). It has been given by mouth in the management of asthma (p.777).

◊ References.


1. Takagi K, *et al.* Lack of effect of repirinast on the pharmacokinetics of theophylline in asthmatic patients. *Eur J Clin Pharmacol* 1989; **37:** 301–3.
2. Patel PC, *et al.* The effect of repirinast on airway responsiveness to methacholine and allergen. *J Allergy Clin Immunol* 1992; **90:** 782–8.


### Preparations

**Proprietary Preparations** (details are given in Part 3)
***Jpn:*** Romet.

## Reproterol Hydrochloride *(BANM, USAN, rINNM)*

D-1959 (reproterol); Hidrocloruro de reproterol; W-2946M. 7-{3-[(3,5,β-Trihydroxyphenethyl)amino]propyl}theophylline hydrochloride.

$C_{18}H_{23}N_5O_5$,HCl = 425.9.
*CAS — 54063-54-6 (reproterol); 13055-82-8 (reproterol hydrochloride).*
*ATC — R03AC15; R03CC14.*

### Profile

Reproterol is a direct-acting sympathomimetic with predominantly beta-adrenergic activity and a selective action on $beta_2$ receptors (a $beta_2$ agonist). It has properties similar to those of salbutamol (p.791).

Reproterol hydrochloride is used as a bronchodilator in the management of reversible airways obstruction, as in asthma (p.777) and in some patients with chronic obstructive pulmonary disease (p.779).

For the relief of acute attacks of bronchospasm the usual dose of reproterol hydrochloride is 1 or 2 inhalations of 500 micrograms from a metered-dose aerosol repeated every 3 to 6 hours as required. For children of 6 to 12 years of age the suggested dose is one inhalation of 500 micrograms every 3 to 6 hours. In patients with asthma, 'as-required' beta agonist therapy is preferable to regular use. An increased need for, or decreased duration of effect of, reproterol indicates deterioration of asthma control and the need for review of therapy. It has also been given by mouth (adult doses are 10 to 20 mg three times daily), and by slow intravenous injection.

### Preparations

**Proprietary Preparations** (details are given in Part 3)
***Austria:*** Bronchospasmin; ***Ger.:*** Bronchospasmin; ***Ital.:*** Broncospasmine; ***Spain:*** Broncospasmin†; Epiferol†; ***Switz.:*** Bronchospasmine†; ***UK:*** Bronchodil†.

**Multi-ingredient:** ***Austria:*** Aarane†; Allergospasmin†; ***Ger.:*** Aarane N; Allergospasmin; ***Switz.:*** Aarane; Allergospasmine.

## Rimiterol Hydrobromide *(BANM, USAN, rINNM)*

Hidrobromuro de rimiterol; R-798; WG-253. *erythro*-3,4-Dihydroxy-α-(2-piperidyl)benzyl alcohol hydrobromide; *erythro*-(3,4-Dihydroxyphenyl) (2-piperidyl)methanol hydrobromide.

$C_{12}H_{17}NO_3$,HBr = 304.2.
*CAS — 32953-89-2 (rimiterol); 31842-61-2 (rimiterol hydrobromide).*
*ATC — R03AC05.*

### Profile

Rimiterol is a direct-acting sympathomimetic with predominantly beta-adrenergic activity and a selective action on $beta_2$ receptors (a $beta_2$ agonist). It has properties similar to those of salbutamol (p.791).

Rimiterol hydrobromide has been used as a bronchodilator for reversible airways obstruction, as in asthma (p.777) and in certain patients with chronic obstructive pulmonary disease (p.779). In patients with asthma, 'as-required' beta agonist therapy is preferable to regular use. An increased need for, or decreased duration of effect of, rimiterol indicates deterioration of asthma control and the need for review of therapy.

### Preparations

**Proprietary Preparations** (details are given in Part 3)
***Denm.:*** Pulmadil†; ***Neth.:*** Pulmadil†.

## Roflumilast *(USAN, rINN)*

B-9302-107; BY-217; BYK-20869. 3-(Cyclopropylmethoxy)-*N*-(3,5-dichloro-4-pyridyl)-4-(difluoromethoxy)benzamide.

$C_{17}H_{14}Cl_2F_2N_2O_3$ = 403.2.
*CAS — 162401-32-3.*

### Profile

Roflumilast is a phosphodiesterase type-4 inhibitor. It is under investigation in the treatment of asthma and chronic obstructive pulmonary disease.

◊ References.


1. Spina D. Phosphodiesterase-4 inhibitors in the treatment of inflammatory lung disease. *Drugs* 2003; **63:** 2575–94.


# Salbutamol *(BAN, rINN)*

AH-3365; Albuterol *(USAN)*; Salbutamolum; Sch-13949W. 2-*tert*-Butylamino-1-(4-hydroxy-3-hydroxymethylphenyl)ethanol.

$C_{13}H_{21}NO_3$ = 239.3.
*CAS — 18559-94-9.*
*ATC — R03AC02; R03CC02.*

**Pharmacopoeias.** In *Chin., Eur.* (see p.vi), *Int., US,* and *Viet.*

**Ph. Eur. 5.0** (Salbutamol). A white or almost white, crystalline powder. Sparingly soluble in water; soluble in alcohol. Protect from light.

**USP 27** (Albuterol). A white crystalline powder. Sparingly soluble in water; soluble in alcohol. Protect from light.

## Salbutamol Sulfate *(rINNM)*

Albuterol Sulfate *(USAN)*; Salbutamol Hemisulphate; Salbutamol Sulphate *(BANM)*; Salbutamoli Sulfas; Sulfato de salbutamol.

$(C_{13}H_{21}NO_3)_2,H_2SO_4$ = 576.7.
*CAS — 51022-70-9.*
*ATC — R03AC02; R03CC02.*

**Pharmacopoeias.** In *Chin., Eur.* (see p.vi), *Int., Jpn, Pol.,* and *US.*

**Ph. Eur. 5.0** (Salbutamol Sulphate). A white or almost white crystalline powder. Freely soluble in water; practically insoluble or very slightly soluble in alcohol and in dichloromethane. Protect from light.

**USP 27** (Albuterol Sulfate). A white or practically white powder. Freely soluble in water; slightly soluble in alcohol, in chloroform, and in ether. Protect from light.

**Stability.** For mention of the stability of a 1:1 mixture of salbutamol and ipratropium nebuliser solutions, see under Ipratropium, p.787.

## Adverse Effects

Salbutamol and other beta agonists may cause fine tremor of skeletal muscle (particularly the hands), palpitations, tachycardia, nervous tension, headaches, peripheral vasodilatation, and rarely muscle cramps. Inhalation causes fewer side-effects than systemic administration, and the more selective $beta_2$ agonists cause fewer side-effects than less selective beta agonists. Potentially serious hypokalaemia has been reported after large doses. Hypersensitivity reactions have occurred, including paradoxical bronchospasm, angioedema, urticaria, hypotension, and collapse.

The high doses of salbutamol used intravenously to delay premature labour have additionally been associated with nausea and vomiting, and with severe adverse cardiac and metabolic effects and pulmonary oedema.

For details of the adverse effects of sympathomimetics in general, including distinction between alpha, beta$_1$, and beta$_2$ agonist effects, see under Adrenaline, p.852.

**Effects on electrolytes and metabolism.** Salbutamol, in common with other beta$_2$-agonists, may cause *hypokalaemia* and *hyperglycaemia*. These effects are related to the dose and route of salbutamol employed; hypokalaemia is more common after parenteral and nebulised administration. Hypokalaemia may be potentiated by concomitant therapy with corticosteroids, diuretics, or xanthines, and by hypoxia; potassium concentrations should therefore be monitored in severe asthma.

**Effects on the eyes.** It has been suggested that salbutamol and to a greater extent ritodrine may contribute to retinopathy in the premature infant when used for premature labour.[1]

For reports of glaucoma precipitated by the combined administration of ipratropium bromide and salbutamol via a nebuliser, see Ipratropium Bromide, p.787.

1. Michie CA, *et al.* Do maternal β-sympathomimetics influence the development of retinopathy in the premature infant? *Arch Dis Child* 1994; **71:** F149.

**Effects on the heart.** The main adverse cardiac effect of salbutamol is tachycardia due to increased sympathetic effects on the cardiovascular system. Such tachycardia is dose dependent and is more common after systemic than inhaled therapy. It has been suggested that the increased metabolic demand produced by tachycardia, especially following oral beta$_2$ agonists, might predispose to heart failure or angina in some older patients.[1]

The decreased vagal (parasympathetic) stimulation, and consequently increased sympathetic dominance of cardiac function, plus a tendency to decreased baroreflex sensitivity, that may occur with beta$_2$ agonist inhalation are similar to the risk factors which predispose to ventricular tachyarrhythmias.[2] Hypokalaemia (see under Effects on Electrolytes and Metabolism above) induced by salbutamol may also lead to arrhythmias. The manufacturers note that cardiac arrhythmias, including atrial fibrillation, supraventricular tachycardia, and extrasystoles, have been reported with beta$_2$ agonists, usually in susceptible patients. See also Pregnancy, below.

1. Jenne JW. Can oral β$_2$ agonists cause heart failure? *Lancet* 1998; **352:** 1081–2.
2. Jartti T, *et al.* The acute effects of inhaled salbutamol on the beat-to-beat variability of heart rate and blood pressure assessed by spectral analysis. *Br J Clin Pharmacol* 1997; **43:** 421–8.

**Effects on mental function.** Visual hallucinations lasting for an hour have been reported[1] following administration of nebulised salbutamol to an elderly patient. At the time of the report the manufacturers were aware of 3 cases of hallucinations in children given oral salbutamol but no such reaction had been previously reported in adults given recommended doses.

1. Khanna PB, Davies R. Hallucinations associated with the administration of salbutamol via a nebuliser. *BMJ* 1986; **292:** 1430.

**Effects on the respiratory system.** Paradoxical bronchoconstriction has occasionally been reported following bronchodilating therapy. With nebuliser solutions, it has been suggested that the preservatives present could be responsible (see also under Ipratropium, p.787), or that the pH may contribute if non-neutral. In addition, regular use of beta$_2$ agonists such as salbutamol (as opposed to use on an as-needed basis) has been shown to increase airway hyperresponsiveness to various stimuli and to lead to the possible development of tolerance to the bronchoprotective effect (see below).

The increased risk of pulmonary oedema associated with salbutamol is mentioned under Pulmonary Oedema, below.

**Increased mortality.** The increased incidence of morbidity and mortality that occurred in asthmatic patients mainly involved fenoterol, but salbutamol has been implicated.[1] The debate on the relevance of beta agonist therapy to this increased morbidity and mortality is discussed under Fenoterol on p.785.

1. Spitzer WO, *et al.* The use of β-agonists and the risk of death or near death from asthma. *N Engl J Med* 1992; **326:** 501–6.

**Overdosage.** Reports of overdosage with salbutamol[1-4] have generally only described the features that may be expected such as tachycardia, CNS stimulation, tremor, hypokalaemia, and hyperglycaemia. Symptomatic treatment of the adverse effects has proved successful. The plasma-potassium concentration and pulse rate have been found to correlate with the plasma concentration of salbutamol.[5]

1. Morrison GW, Farebrother MJB. Overdose of salbutamol. *Lancet* 1973; **ii:** 681.
2. O'Brien IAD, *et al.* Hypokalaemia due to salbutamol overdosage. *BMJ* 1981; **282:** 1515–16.
3. Prior JG, *et al.* Self-poisoning with oral salbutamol. *BMJ* 1981; **282:** 1932.
4. Connell JMC, *et al.* Metabolic consequences of salbutamol poisoning reversed by propranolol. *BMJ* 1982; **285:** 779.
5. Lewis LD, *et al.* A study of self poisoning with oral salbutamol—laboratory and clinical features. *Hum Exp Toxicol* 1993; **12:** 397–401. Correction. *ibid.* 1994; **13:** 371.

**Pregnancy.** Most adverse effects associated with salbutamol in pregnancy relate to the cardiovascular and metabolic effects of the very high doses given by intravenous infusion in attempts to delay premature labour (see also under Pulmonary Oedema, below). Thus myocardial ischaemia on stopping an infusion[1] and unifocal ventricular ectopics associated with the hypokalaemic response to intravenous salbutamol[2] have been reported. A further report concerned congestive heart failure in a hypertensive woman.[3] Metabolic acidosis following salbutamol infusions in diabetic women has also been reported.[4,5]

1. Whitehead MI, *et al.* Myocardial ischaemia after withdrawal of salbutamol for pre-term labour. *Lancet* 1979; **ii:** 904.
2. Chew WC, Lew LC. Ventricular ectopics after salbutamol infusion for preterm labour. *Lancet* 1979; **ii:** 1383–4.
3. Whitehead MI, *et al.* Acute congestive cardiac failure in a hypertensive woman receiving salbutamol for premature labour. *BMJ* 1980; **280:** 1221–2.
4. Chapman MG. Salbutamol-induced acidosis in pregnant diabetics. *BMJ* 1977; **1:** 639–40.
5. Thomas DJB, *et al.* Salbutamol-induced diabetic ketoacidosis. *BMJ* 1977; **2:** 438.

**Pulmonary oedema.** Pulmonary oedema has occurred in women given beta$_2$ agonists, including salbutamol,[1,2] for premature labour. The risk factors, the most important of which is fluid overload, are discussed under Precautions, below.

1. Hawker F. Pulmonary oedema associated with β$_2$-sympathomimetic treatment of premature labour. *Anaesth Intensive Care* 1984; **12:** 143–51.
2. Pisani RJ, Rosenow EC. Pulmonary edema associated with tocolytic therapy. *Ann Intern Med* 1989; **110:** 714–18.

**Tolerance.** Some studies suggest that regular inhalation of a short-acting beta$_2$ agonist, although it continues to produce bronchodilatation, increases airway hyperresponsiveness and may reduce the protective effect against bronchoconstriction provoked by stimuli such as bradykinin, methacholine, or allergen.[1-5] Such tolerance is considered another argument against regular use of short-acting drugs.[1] Reduced bronchoprotective effects have also been demonstrated with long-acting beta$_2$ agonists (see Salmeterol, p.795). There is some evidence that for salbutamol the effect may be due to the *S*(+)-enantiomer,[6] which unlike the *R*(−)-enantiomer does not possess bronchodilating activity: stereoselective metabolism (see under Pharmacokinetics, below) means that regular use of the racemate could lead to accumulation of the *S*-enantiomer, which provides a possible mechanism for the effect.

1. Cockcroft DW, *et al.* Regular inhaled salbutamol and airway responsiveness to allergen. *Lancet* 1993; **342:** 833–7.
2. O'Connor BJ, *et al.* Tolerance to the nonbronchodilator effects of inhaled β$_2$-agonists in asthma. *N Engl J Med* 1992; **327:** 1204–8.
3. Cockcroft DW, *et al.* Regular use of inhaled albuterol and the allergen-induced late asthmatic response. *J Allergy Clin Immunol* 1995; **96:** 44–9.
4. Inman MD, O'Byrne PM. The effect of regular inhaled albuterol on exercise-induced bronchoconstriction. *Am J Respir Crit Care Med* 1996; **153:** 65–9.
5. Crowther SD, *et al.* Varied effects of regular salbutamol on airway responsiveness to inhaled spasmogens. *Lancet* 1997; **350:** 1450.
6. Perrin-Fayolle M. Salbutamol in the treatment of asthma. *Lancet* 1995; **346:** 1101.

## Precautions

Salbutamol and other beta agonists should be given with caution in hyperthyroidism, myocardial insufficiency, arrhythmias, susceptibility to QT-interval prolongation, hypertension, and diabetes mellitus (especially on intravenous administration—blood glucose should be monitored since ketoacidosis has been reported).

In *severe asthma* particular caution is also required to avoid inducing hypokalaemia as this effect may be potentiated by hypoxia or by concomitant use of other anti-asthma drugs (see Interactions, below); plasma-potassium concentrations should be monitored.

Beta$_2$ agonists such as salbutamol are not appropriate for use alone in the treatment of more than mild asthma (see under Asthma, p.777). Increasing need for, or decreased duration of effect of, inhaled salbutamol and other short-acting beta$_2$ agonists indicates deterioration of asthma control and the likely requirement for increased anti-inflammatory therapy.

In *women being treated for premature labour* the risk of pulmonary oedema means that the patient's state of hydration and cardiac and respiratory function should be monitored very carefully; the volume of infusion fluid should be kept to the minimum (normally using glucose 5% as the diluent), and beta$_2$-agonist therapy should be discontinued immediately and diuretic therapy instituted if signs of pulmonary oedema develop. Other risk factors for pulmonary oedema include multiple pregnancy and cardiac disease, which is a specific contra-indication; where cardiac disease is suspected assessment by a physician experienced in cardiology is needed. Eclampsia and severe pre-eclampsia are also contra-indications, with special care needed in mild to moderate pre-eclampsia. Other contra-indications include intra-uterine infection, intra-uterine fetal death, antepartum haemorrhage (which requires immediate delivery), placenta praevia, and cord compression; beta$_2$ agonists should not be used for threatened miscarriage. See also Uses and Administration, below.

For details of the precautions to be observed with sympathomimetics in general, see Adrenaline, p.853.

**Abuse.** Salbutamol inhalers have been subject to abuse, particularly by children and young adults.[1-5] This has occurred in both asthmatic and non-asthmatic individuals and has been thought to be for the effect of sympathetic stimulation and for the effect of the fluorocarbon propellants. The introduction of fluorocarbon-free inhalers should reduce the latter motivation, although not the former.

1. Brennan PO. Inhaled salbutamol: a new form of drug abuse? *Lancet* 1983; **ii:** 1030–1.
2. Thompson PJ, *et al.* Addiction to aerosol treatment: the asthmatic alternative to glue sniffing. *BMJ* 1983; **287:** 1515–16.
3. Brennan PO. Addiction to aerosol treatment. *BMJ* 1983; **287:** 1877.
4. Wickramasinghe H, Liebeschuetz HJ. Addiction to aerosol treatment. *BMJ* 1983; **287:** 1877.
5. O'Callaghan C, Milner AD. Aerosol treatment abuse. *Arch Dis Child* 1988; **63:** 70.

## Interactions

Use of salbutamol and other beta$_2$ agonists with corticosteroids, diuretics, or xanthines increases the risk of hypokalaemia, and monitoring of potassium concentrations is recommended in severe asthma, where such combination therapy is the rule (see also Effects on Electrolytes and Metabolism, above). For an outline of interactions associated with sympathomimetics in general, see Adrenaline, p.853.

**Antidepressants.** For an apparent interaction between terbutaline and *toloxatone*, a reversible inhibitor of monoamine oxidase type A (RIMA), see Sympathomimetics, p.309.

**Beta$_2$ agonists.** Patients receiving *salmeterol* may require salbutamol to control an acute attack of bronchospasm. One study indicated that the effects might be additive,[1] but another demonstrated that patients receiving salmeterol had reduced sensitivity to salbutamol and might need higher doses of the latter for acute relief.[2] However, a study in asthmatics admitted to a hospital emergency department with acute exacerbations of their illness, found that previous salmeterol therapy did not reduce the effectiveness of standard doses of salbutamol.[3] Others have also noted attenuation of the bronchoprotective effects of a beta$_2$ agonist (in this case, *fenoterol*) by salmeterol.[4]

1. Smyth ET, *et al.* Interaction and dose equivalence of salbutamol and salmeterol in patients with asthma. *BMJ* 1993; **306:** 543–5.
2. Grove A, Lipworth BJ. Bronchodilator subsensitivity to salbutamol after twice daily salmeterol in asthmatic patients. *Lancet* 1995; **346:** 201–6.
3. Korosec M, *et al.* Salmeterol does not compromise the bronchodilator response to albuterol during acute episodes of asthma. *Am J Med* 1999; **107:** 209–13.
4. van Veen A, *et al.* Regular use of long-acting β$_2$-adrenoceptor agonists attenuates the bronchoprotective efficacy of short-acting β$_2$-adrenoceptor agonists in asthma. *Br J Clin Pharmacol* 2000; **50:** 499P.

**Cardiac glycosides.** Hypokalaemia produced by beta$_2$ agonists may result in an increased susceptibility to digitalis-induced arrhythmias although salbutamol intravenously and by mouth can also decrease serum concentrations of *digoxin* (see Beta$_2$ Agonists, p.897).

**Corticosteroids.** Corticosteroids and beta$_2$ agonists may both produce falls in plasma potassium concentrations; there is evidence that such falls can be exacerbated by concomitant administration.[1] The possibility of enhanced hyperglycaemic effects from such a combination should also be borne in mind.

1. Taylor DR, *et al.* Interaction between corticosteroid and beta-agonist drugs: biochemical and cardiovascular effects in normal subjects. *Chest* 1992; **102:** 519–24.

**Diuretics.** Hypokalaemia is known to be a possible side-effect during treatment with beta$_2$ agonists such as salbutamol or terbutaline, and this may be enhanced during concomitant diuretic therapy;[1,2] in addition the arrhythmogenic potential of this interaction may be clinically important in patients with ischaemic heart disease.[1]

1. Lipworth BJ, *et al.* Prior treatment with diuretic augments the hypokalemic and electrocardiographic effects of inhaled albuterol. *Am J Med* 1989; **86:** 653–7.
2. Newnham DM, *et al.* The effects of frusemide and triamterene on the hypokalaemic and electrocardiographic responses to inhaled terbutaline. *Br J Clin Pharmacol* 1991; **32:** 630–2.

**Neuromuscular blockers.** Salbutamol given intravenously has been reported to enhance the neuromuscular blockade produced by *pancuronium* and by *vecuronium* (see Sympathomimetics, p.1402).

**Xanthines.** An enhanced hypokalaemic effect may occur during coadministration of salbutamol with *theophylline*.[1,2] See also under Terbutaline, p.797 and Sympathomimetics, under Theophylline, p.803 for the potentiation of other effects.

1. Whyte KF, *et al.* Salbutamol induced hypokalaemia: the effect of theophylline alone and in combination with adrenaline. *Br J Clin Pharmacol* 1988; **25:** 571–8.
2. Kolski GB, *et al.* Hypokalemia and respiratory arrest in an infant with status asthmaticus. *J Pediatr* 1988; **112:** 304–7.

## Pharmacokinetics

Salbutamol is readily absorbed from the gastrointestinal tract. It is subject to first-pass metabolism in the liver and possibly in the gut wall; the main metabolite is an inactive sulfate conjugate. Salbutamol is rapidly excreted in the urine as metabolites and unchanged drug; there is some excretion in the faeces. Salbutamol does not appear to be metabolised in the lung, therefore its ultimate metabolism and excretion following inhalation depends upon the delivery method used, which determines the proportion of inhaled salbutamol relative to the proportion inadvertently swallowed. It has been suggested that the majority of an inhaled dose is swallowed and absorbed from the gut.

The plasma half-life of salbutamol has been estimated to range from 4 to 6 hours.

◊ General references.

1. Walker SR, *et al.* The clinical pharmacology of oral and inhaled salbutamol. *Clin Pharmacol Ther* 1972; **13:** 861–7.
2. Hetzel MR, Clark TJH. Comparison of intravenous and aerosol salbutamol. *BMJ* 1976; **2:** 919.
3. Lin C, *et al.* Isolation and identification of the major metabolite of albuterol in human urine. *Drug Metab Dispos* 1977; **5:** 234–8.
4. Morgan DJ, *et al.* Pharmacokinetics of intravenous and oral salbutamol and its sulphate conjugate. *Br J Clin Pharmacol* 1986; **22:** 587–93.
5. Lipworth BJ, *et al.* Single dose and steady-state pharmacokinetics of 4 mg and 8 mg oral salbutamol controlled-release in patients with bronchial asthma. *Eur J Clin Pharmacol* 1989; **37:** 49–52.
6. Rey E, *et al.* Pharmacokinetics of intravenous salbutamol in renal insufficiency and its biological effects. *Eur J Clin Pharmacol* 1989; **37:** 387–9.
7. Hindle M, Chrystyn H. Determination of the relative bioavailability of salbutamol to the lung following inhalation. *Br J Clin Pharmacol* 1992; **34:** 311–15.
8. Milliez JM, *et al.* Pharmacokinetics of salbutamol in the pregnant woman after subcutaneous administration with a portable pump. *Obstet Gynecol* 1992; **80:** 182–5.

**Stereoselectivity.** The *R*(−)-enantiomer of salbutamol (levosalbutamol—p.788) is preferentially metabolised and is therefore cleared from the body more rapidly than the *S*(+)-enantiomer, which lacks bronchodilator activity but may be implicated in some of the adverse effects of salbutamol (see Tolerance, under Adverse Effects, above).

References.

1. Boulton DW, Fawcett JP. Enantioselective disposition of salbutamol in man following oral and intravenous administration. *Br J Clin Pharmacol* 1996; **41:** 35–40.
2. Boulton DW, *et al.* Transplacental distribution of salbutamol enantiomers at Caesarian section. *Br J Clin Pharmacol* 1997; **44:** 587–90.
3. Lipworth BJ, *et al.* Pharmacokinetics and extrapulmonary $\beta_2$ adrenoceptor activity of nebulised racemic salbutamol and its R and S isomers in healthy volunteers. *Thorax* 1997; **52:** 849–52.
4. Ward JK, *et al.* Enantiomeric disposition of inhaled, intravenous and oral racemic-salbutamol in man — no evidence of enantioselective lung metabolism. *Br J Clin Pharmacol* 2000; **49:** 15–22.

## Uses and Administration

Salbutamol is a direct-acting sympathomimetic with predominantly beta-adrenergic activity and a selective action on beta$_2$ receptors (a beta$_2$ agonist—p.777). This results in its bronchodilating action being more prominent than its effect on the heart.

Salbutamol and salbutamol sulfate are used as bronchodilators in the management of reversible airways obstruction, as in asthma and in some patients with chronic obstructive pulmonary disease. Salbutamol also decreases uterine contractility and may be given as the sulfate to arrest premature labour (below).

Administration by inhalation results in the rapid onset (within 5 to 15 minutes) of bronchodilatation, which lasts for about 3 to 6 hours. Following doses by mouth, the onset of action is within 30 minutes, with a peak effect between 2 to 3 hours after the dose, and a duration of action of up to 6 hours; modified-release preparations that have a longer duration of action are available.

Salbutamol is used as the base or sulfate in aerosol inhalers and as the sulfate in other preparations. The dosage is expressed in terms of salbutamol base; salbutamol sulfate 1.2 mg is approximately equivalent to 1 mg of salbutamol.

For the relief of **acute bronchospasm**, 1 or 2 inhalations of salbutamol 100 micrograms may be given from a conventional *metered-dose aerosol* as required, up to every 4 to 6 hours or 3 or 4 times daily. Two inhalations (1 or 2 in children) may also be given just prior to exertion for the prophylaxis of exercise-induced bronchospasm. (In the USA these inhalations may be expressed as supplying 100 micrograms, the amount delivered *into* the mouthpiece, or 90 micrograms, the amount delivered *from* the mouthpiece.) Current asthma guidelines (see p.777) recommend that inhaled short-acting beta$_2$ agonists such as salbutamol be used on an as-required, not regular, basis. In those patients requiring more than occasional use of salbutamol, anti-inflammatory therapy is also needed. An increased requirement for, or decreased duration of effect of, salbutamol indicates deterioration of asthma control and the need for increased anti-inflammatory therapy. Salbutamol sulfate is now available in chlorofluorocarbon (CFC)-free aerosols. Doses for these aerosols (expressed in terms of salbutamol) are the same as for conventional aerosols.

Salbutamol may also be inhaled as the sulfate from *inhalation capsules* or *discs* containing powder for inhalation, particularly by patients who experience difficulty in using aerosol formulations. Owing to differences in the relative bioavailability to the lungs between these dry powder systems and the inhalation aerosol a 200-microgram dose (expressed in terms of salbutamol) from an inhalation capsule or disc is approximately equivalent in activity to a 100-microgram dose from a conventional aerosol and the recommended doses are therefore usually twice those suggested for the aerosol.

When inhalation is ineffective, salbutamol may be given *by mouth* in a dose of 2 to 4 mg three or four times daily as the sulfate; some patients may require doses of up to 8 mg three or four times daily, but such increased doses are unlikely to be tolerated or to provide much extra benefit. Elderly patients should be given the lower doses initially. A dose of 1 to 2 mg three or four times daily is recommended for children aged 2 to 6 years or 2 mg three or four times daily for older children. Modified-release preparations are also available; a usual adult dose is 8 mg twice daily.

In more severe or unresponsive bronchospasm salbutamol sulfate may be given intermittently via a *nebuliser* in adults and children. Licensed doses are 2.5 to 5 mg of salbutamol repeated up to 4 times daily in adults and children older than 18 months of age; continuous administration is also possible, usually at a rate of 1 to 2 mg/hour. However, guidelines allow for more frequent administration or continuous administration at a higher rate in acute severe asthma (see under Asthma, p.777). Single-dose units of 0.1% or 0.2%, or a concentrated solution of salbutamol 0.5%, are available for this method of administration. Continuous administration is usually as a 0.005 to 0.01% solution in sodium chloride 0.9%. The efficacy of nebulised salbutamol in infants under 18 months of age is uncertain; the *British National Formulary* warns that transient hypoxaemia may occur but suggests a dose of 1.25 to 2.5 mg up to four times daily. Patients with asthma may require supplemental oxygen.

In acute severe asthma without life-threatening features where delivery via nebuliser is not available, 4 to 6 inhalations of salbutamol 100 micrograms from a metered-dose inhaler may be given at intervals of 10 to 20 minutes via a large volume spacer. In emergency life-threatening situations, 1 inhalation can be repeated 10 to 20 times by multiple actuations of a metered-dose inhaler into a spacer device.

In the management of a severe attack of bronchospasm a slow *intravenous injection* of salbutamol 250 micrograms as a solution containing 50 micrograms/mL as the sulfate may be required; alternatively salbutamol may be given by intravenous infusion of a solution containing 5 mg in 500 mL (10 micrograms/mL) at a usual rate of 3 to 20 micrograms/minute according to the patient's need; higher dosages have been used in patients with respiratory failure.

Salbutamol sulfate can also be given for bronchospasm by *subcutaneous* or *intramuscular* injection in doses of salbutamol 500 micrograms every 4 hours as required.

For the arrest of uncomplicated **premature labour** between 24 and 33 weeks of gestation salbutamol sulfate is given by *intravenous infusion* preferably with the aid of a syringe pump when the concentration should be 200 micrograms/mL of salbutamol, glucose 5% having been used for dilution. If no syringe pump is available then the infusion should be with a more dilute solution of 20 micrograms/mL in glucose 5%. The same dose is used as with the syringe pump. The recommended initial rate of infusion is 10 micrograms/minute increased at intervals of 10 minutes until there is a response; the rate is then increased slowly until contractions cease. The usual effective dose is 10 to 45 micrograms/minute. The infusion should be maintained at the rate at which contractions cease for 1 hour, then reduced by decrements of 50% at intervals of 6 hours. Prolonged therapy should be avoided as the risks to the mother (see Precautions, above) increase after 48 hours, and there is a lack of evidence of benefit from further treatment.

The maternal pulse should be monitored throughout the infusion and the rate adjusted to avoid a maternal heart rate of more than 140 beats/minute. A close watch should also be kept on the patient's state of hydration since fluid overload is considered to be a key risk factor for pulmonary oedema.

Salbutamol may subsequently be given *by mouth* in a dose of 4 mg three or four times daily but such usage is not recommended by the *British National Formulary*, given the problems with prolonged therapy already mentioned.

**Administration.** Beta$_2$ agonists are used extensively in the management of reversible airways obstruction. A common, effective, and convenient method of administration is by a pressurised aerosol inhaler. With this route of administration relief is provided rapidly and fewer systemic side-effects are likely to occur than with oral administration. It is important that patients using conventional inhalers employ the correct technique, which involves coordinating actuation of the aerosol with inhalation; if patients have difficulty with this, alternatives are available. Spacer devices may be used with inhalers. These are added on to the inhaler and reduce the velocity of the aerosol; also more propellant may evaporate before inhalation allowing a greater proportion of the drug to reach the lungs, and coordination of actuation of the aerosol and inhalation is less important. Breath-actuated aerosol inhalers and inhalers of dry powder are also available and are actuated by the patient's inspiration and thus avoid entirely the need for coordination of actuation and inhalation; however, inhalation of the dry powder has occasionally caused irritation of the throat or coughing.

The oral route can be used although generally a form of inhaled therapy as described above is preferable. Various formulations intended for oral administration are commercially available, including modified-release formulations. Nebulisation is an alternative method of delivery and this may be used in the management of severe acute attacks as may parenteral therapy.

Chlorofluorocarbon (CFC) propellants in pressurised aerosol inhalers are being replaced by hydrofluoroalkane (HFA) propellants. Conventional and breath-actuated HFA preparations are available. HFA aerosols may feel and taste different to CFC aerosols.

**Asthma.** Short-acting beta$_2$ agonists such as salbutamol form the initial therapy of chronic as well as acute asthma (p.777). High doses are used in acute asthma, but current recommendations for chronic asthma are for low doses to be inhaled as required rather than regularly. When patients with mild asthma find that symptomatic relief is needed more than 2 or 3 times a week, then that should be a sign for additional treatment with anti-inflammatory drugs. Increasing need for, or decreased effect of, short-acting beta$_2$ agonists indicates deteriorating asthma and the requirement for stepping up therapy. In one placebo-controlled study,[1] patients with stable asthma receiving regular high doses of a short-acting inhaled beta$_2$ agonist were able to reduce the dose considerably with no change in asthma control, lending further support to the recommendation for 'as-required' rather than regular use of these drugs. The discussion under Fenoterol on p.785 on the increased mortality that has been observed in asthma patients and the connection with asthma therapy includes a view that regular administration might have contributed to the increased mortality. However, a systematic review[2] of studies of short-acting beta$_2$ agonists, most of which used salbutamol, found no clear clinical advantage or detriment from regular use compared with taking them as required.


1. Harrison TW, *et al.* Randomised placebo controlled trial of $\beta$ agonist dose reduction in asthma. *Thorax* 1999; **54:** 98–102.
2. Walters EH, Walters J. Inhaled short acting beta2-agonist use in chronic asthma: regular versus as needed treatment. Available in The Cochrane Library; Issue 1. Chichester: John Wiley; 2004.


**Bronchiolitis.** Acute bronchiolitis (inflammation of the bronchioles associated with viral respiratory-tract infection, usually due to respiratory syncytial virus—see p.625) is a poorly defined respiratory condition seen in children. The diagnostic criteria, and the usual management, vary considerably from country to country. Beta$_2$ agonists such as salbutamol are widely prescribed in the USA, but not in the UK, and attempts to establish their benefits have produced conflicting results.[1] Modest benefit (but no difference in hospital admission rate) has been reported from a meta-analysis of bronchodilator therapy in general,[2] but a meta-analysis of beta$_2$ agonist therapy in bronchiolitis did not show it to be effective.[3] Some comparative studies have suggested that nebulised adrenaline is more effective than salbutamol.[4,5] However, one study in hospitalised children found no benefit from nebulised salbutamol in terms of improved oxygenation or length of hospital stay,[6] and another[7] found no difference in efficacy between nebulised adrenaline, salbutamol, and sodium chloride 0.9%.


1. Everard ML. Acute bronchiolitis—a perennial problem. *Lancet* 1996; **348:** 279–80.
2. Kellner JD, *et al.* Bronchodilators for bronchiolitis. Available in The Cochrane Library; Issue 1. Chichester: John Wiley; 2004.
3. Flores G, Horwitz RI. Efficacy of $\beta_2$-agonists in bronchiolitis: a reappraisal and meta-analysis. *Pediatrics* 1997; **100:** 233–9.
4. Reijonen T, *et al.* The clinical efficacy of nebulized racemic epinephrine and albuterol in acute bronchiolitis. *Arch Pediatr Adolesc Med* 1995; **149:** 686–92.
5. Menon K, *et al.* A randomized trial comparing the efficacy of epinephrine with salbutamol in the treatment of acute bronchiolitis. *J Pediatr* 1995; **126:** 1004–7.
6. Dobson JV, *et al.* The use of albuterol in hospitalized infants with bronchiolitis. *Pediatrics* 1998; **101:** 361–8.
7. Patel H, *et al.* A randomized, controlled trial of the effectiveness of nebulized therapy with epinephrine compared with albuterol and saline in infants hospitalized for acute viral bronchiolitis. *J Pediatr* 2002; **141:** 818–24.


**Chronic obstructive pulmonary disease.** Salbutamol and other beta$_2$ agonist bronchodilators form part of the first-line treatment of chronic obstructive pulmonary disease, although, as discussed on p.779, there is some evidence that an inhaled quaternary ammonium antimuscarinic, such as ipratropium bromide, may have slight advantages compared with a beta$_2$ agonist.

**Cough.** For a study indicating that inhaled salbutamol was ineffective in the treatment of children with recurrent cough, see under Beclometasone, p.1092.

**Hyperkalaemia.** Salbutamol can lower plasma-potassium concentrations by promoting intracellular uptake,[1,2] and this effect has been used in treating mild hyperkalaemia (p.1219) associated with chronic disorders such as renal failure[3,4] and hyperkalaemic periodic paralysis.[5] However, such use is controversial: the effects of salbutamol may be inconsistent[6] and some clinicians prefer to avoid the use of beta$_2$ agonists because of fears that large doses may induce cardiac arrhythmias.[7]


1. Bushe C. Salbutamol for hyperkalaemia. *Lancet* 1983; **ii:** 797.
2. Anonymous. Hyperkalaemia—silent and deadly. *Lancet* 1989; **i:** 1240.
3. Allon M, *et al.* Nebulized albuterol for acute hyperkalemia in patients on hemodialysis. *Ann Intern Med* 1989; **110:** 426–9.
4. McClure RJ, *et al.* Treatment of hyperkalaemia using intravenous and nebulised salbutamol. *Arch Dis Child* 1994; **70:** 126–8.
5. Wang P, Clausen T. Treatment of attacks in hyperkalaemic familial periodic paralysis by inhalation of salbutamol. *Lancet* 1976; **i:** 221–3.
6. Wong S-L, Maltz HC. Albuterol for the treatment of hyperkalemia. *Ann Pharmacother* 1999; **33:** 103–6.
7. Halperin ML, Kamel KS. Potassium. *Lancet* 1998; **352:** 135–40.


**Lymphangioleiomyomatosis.** Inhaled beta$_2$ agonists are often helpful in treating the reversible component of airway obstruction in women with pulmonary lymphangioleiomyomatosis, and a trial of treatment is warranted.[1,2] For mention of the use of medroxyprogesterone in this rare disease, see Respiratory Disorders, p.1558.


1. Johnson S. Lymphangioleiomyomatosis: clinical features, management and basic mechanisms. *Thorax* 1999; **54:** 254–64.
2. Johnson SR, Tattersfield AE. Clinical experience of lymphangioleiomyomatosis in the UK. *Thorax* 2000; **55:** 1052–7.


**Premature labour.** Premature labour (preterm labour) is the onset of labour before the expected date, resulting in delivery of an immature infant. Conventionally the definition includes women giving birth before 37 weeks' gestation but in practice most problems arise with births before 32 weeks or when the baby's birth-weight is less than 1.5 kg.[1] Risk factors for premature labour include infection, premature rupture of the membranes, cervical incompetence, and multiple pregnancy. There are few proven measures to prevent premature labour, but cervical cerclage may be used for cervical incompetence, and treatment of infections is being investigated.[1,2] In women with premature rupture of the membranes who have not gone into spontaneous labour there is some evidence that antibacterial therapy may be effective in delaying delivery and improving outcomes (see Premature Labour, p.143). In women who have a history of spontaneous premature delivery, there is some evidence to suggest that prophylactic hydroxyprogesterone caproate may reduce the risk for premature delivery in subsequent pregnancies.[3]

A diagnosis of premature labour is not always easy to make and evidence of cervical change should usually be present in addition to uterine activity.[2,4] Once a diagnosis has been established, a decision must be made as to whether to postpone delivery by the use of drugs that inhibit uterine contractions (tocolysis). It may not be considered appropriate to stop labour in some women. However, in patients of less than about 28 to 32 weeks' gestation without complications, attempts to postpone delivery are usually worth trying, if only in the short-term, to allow emergency treatment such as corticosteroids to be given to the mother to enhance the maturation of the fetal respiratory system (see Neonatal Respiratory Distress Syndrome, p.1084) and to enable the patient to be transferred to a specialised unit for preterm delivery.[1,2,4,5] Tocolysis is rarely considered necessary after 34 weeks' gestation, provided adequate neonatal support facilities are available.[2,4]

- The commonest tocolytics have historically been the beta-adrenoceptor agonists, which relax the smooth muscle of the uterus by stimulation of beta$_2$-adrenoceptors.[2,4] Nonselective agonists, for example orciprenaline and isoxsuprine, have been replaced by more selective beta$_2$ agonists such as ritodrine and salbutamol.[2] These can postpone labour for a few days and the preferred route for starting treatment is subcutaneous or intravenous infusion.[4] Oral or subcutaneous maintenance therapy with beta$_2$ agonists after successful treatment of an episode of acute premature labour produces no further benefit.[6] There is little evidence that beta$_2$ agonists significantly reduce perinatal mortality rates.[7] The patient may experience adverse cardiovascular and metabolic effects and, in particular, pulmonary oedema has been reported in some women given beta$_2$ agonists intravenously to suppress labour (see above). It is therefore essential that the patient's heart rate and state of hydration are carefully monitored throughout administration. In the event of caesarean section beta blockers may be needed to combat an increased tendency to uterine bleeding.
- In the USA, magnesium sulfate is the most widely used parenteral tocolytic, and is thought to act by calcium antagonism at the neuromuscular junction.[4] It is generally considered as effective as the beta$_2$ agonists.[4] However, a systematic review[8] has concluded that it is ineffective at delaying birth or preventing preterm birth, and it has been suggested that tocolytic use of magnesium may be associated with increased paediatric mortality—see p.1230. To decrease the risk of overdose, magnesium sulfate should only be administered from a controlled pump.[4] Oral magnesium has been tried but has not been shown to be effective.[4]
- Prostaglandins have a role in the induction of labour as mediators of uterine contractions and cervical softening and dilatation. Cyclo-oxygenase (prostaglandin-synthetase) inhibitors such as indometacin may therefore be given by mouth or rectally to inhibit premature labour.[2,4] Although this treatment is as effective as ritodrine,[9,10] a number of adverse effects on the fetus have been reported, such as constriction of the ductus arteriosus and consequent pulmonary hypertension, bronchopulmonary dysplasia, oligohydramnios (a deficiency in amniotic fluid volume), and fatal renal toxicity. A retrospective study suggested that antenatal indometacin therapy for premature labour increased the risk of prematurity-related complications,[11] but some consider the benefits to outweigh the potential risks.[12] Indometacin is therefore generally reserved as a second-line drug or given with other tocolytics for an additive effect.[4] Sulindac, a cyclo-oxygenase inhibitor which seems to have little placental transfer, may reduce the incidence of fetal side-effects.[13] More recently it has been suggested that the enzyme isoform cyclo-oxygenase-2 is associated with labour, while cyclo-oxygenase-1 is responsible for constant prostaglandin synthesis in body tissues. The selective cyclo-oxygenase-2 inhibitor nimesulide is under investigation for its potential in the prevention of premature labour.[14]
- More recently, calcium-channel blockers have been shown to be effective tocolytics, presumably by their action on myometrial calcium.[4] Most experience concerns nifedipine, which is at least as effective in delaying labour as beta$_2$ agonists or magnesium,[4,15,16] It has the advantage that it can be given by mouth,[4] and some favour its use as a first-line drug.[16,17] Nicardipine has also produced favourable results.[18]
- Atosiban is a peptide analogue of oxytocin with oxytocin antagonist properties. A pooled analysis[19] of three trials found atosiban to be as effective as beta agonists in the management of premature labour, with fewer maternal cardiovascular adverse effects, and some clinicians favour its use as a first-line tocolytic in preference to the traditional drugs.[17]
- Other drugs are under investigation. Application of patches of the nitric oxide donor glyceryl trinitrate to the abdomen to produce uterine relaxation is reported to be as effective as ritodrine treatment.[20]


1. Goldenberg RL, Rouse DJ. Prevention of premature birth. *N Engl J Med* 1998; **339:** 313–20.
2. Steer P, Flint C. Preterm labour and premature rupture of membranes. *BMJ* 1999; **318:** 1059–62.
3. Meis PJ, *et al.* Prevention of recurrent preterm delivery by 17 alpha-hydroxyprogesterone caproate. *N Engl J Med* 2003; **348:** 2379–85.
4. Katz VL, Farmer RM. Controversies in tocolytic therapy. *Clin Obstet Gynecol* 1999; **42:** 802–19.
5. Report of the second working group of the British Association of Perinatal Medicine. Guidelines for good practice in the management of neonatal respiratory distress syndrome. Guideline produced in November 1998, not valid beyond 2002. [awaiting update] Available at: http://www.bapm.org/documents/publications/rds.pdf (accessed 20/04/04)
6. Sanchez-Ramos L, *et al.* Efficacy of maintenance therapy after acute tocolysis: a meta-analysis. *Am J Obstet Gynecol* 1999; **181:** 484–90.
7. The Canadian Preterm Labor Investigators Group. Treatment of preterm labor with the beta-adrenergic agonist ritodrine. *N Engl J Med* 1992; **327:** 308–12.
8. Crowther CA, *et al.* Magnesium sulphate for preventing preterm birth in threatened preterm labour. Available in The Cochrane Library; Issue 1. Chichester: John Wiley; 2004.
9. Morales WJ, *et al.* Efficacy and safety of indomethacin versus ritodrine in the management of preterm labor: a randomized study. *Obstet Gynecol* 1989; **74:** 567–72.
10. Besinger RE, *et al.* Randomized comparative trial of indomethacin and ritodrine for the long-term treatment of preterm labor. *Am J Obstet Gynecol* 1991; **164:** 981–8.
11. Norton ME, *et al.* Neonatal complications after the administration of indomethacin for preterm labor. *N Engl J Med* 1993; **329:** 1602–7.
12. Macones GA, Robinson CA. Is there justification for using indomethacin in preterm labor? An analysis of neonatal risks and benefits. *Am J Obstet Gynecol* 1997; **177:** 819–24.
13. Carlan SJ, *et al.* Randomized comparative trial of indomethacin and sulindac for the treatment of refractory preterm labor. *Obstet Gynecol* 1992; **79:** 223–8.
14. Sawdy R, *et al.* Use of cyclo-oxygenase type-2-selective nonsteroidal anti-inflammatory agent to prevent preterm delivery. *Lancet* 1997; **350:** 265–6.
15. Ray JG. Meta-analysis of nifedipine versus beta-sympathomimetic agents for tocolysis during preterm labour. *J Soc Obstet Gynaecol Can* 1998; **20:** 259–69.
16. Tsatsaris V, *et al.* Tocolysis with nifedipine or beta-adrenergic agonists: a meta-analysis. *Obstet Gynecol* 2001; **97:** 840–7.
17. Slattery MM, Morrison JJ. Preterm delivery. *Lancet* 2002; **360:** 1489–97.
18. Jannet D, *et al.* Nicardipine versus salbutamol in the treatment of premature labor: a prospective randomized study. *Eur J Obstet Gynecol Reprod Biol* 1997; **73:** 11–16.
19. The Worldwide Atosiban versus Beta-agonists Study Group. Effectiveness and safety of the oxytocin antagonist atosiban versus beta-adrenergic agonists in the treatment of preterm labour. *Br J Obstet Gynaecol* 2001; **108:** 133–42.
20. Lees CC, *et al.* Glyceryl trinitrate and ritodrine in tocolysis: an international multicenter randomized study. *Obstet Gynecol* 1999; **94:** 403–8.


**Proctalgia fugax.** Inhalation of salbutamol from a metered-dose inhaler at the beginning of an attack has been shown to reduce the duration of pain in patients with proctalgia fugax.[1]


1. Eckardt VF, *et al.* Treatment of proctalgia fugax with salbutamol inhalation. *Am J Gastroenterol* 1996; **91:** 686–9.


## Preparations

***BP 2003:*** Salbutamol Injection; Salbutamol Nebuliser Solution; Salbutamol Oral Solution; Salbutamol Pressurised Inhalation; Salbutamol Tablets; ***USP 27:*** Albuterol Tablets.

**Proprietary Preparations** (details are given in Part 3)
***Arg.:*** Airomir; Airsalbu; Amocasin; Asmatol; Duopack; Medihaler; Microterol; Respiret; Salbutol; Ventolin; ***Austral.:*** Airomir; Asmol; Epaq; Respax; Respolin†; Ventolin; ***Austria:*** Buventol; Epaq†; Sultanol; Zaperin†; ***Belg.:*** Airomir; Ventolin; ***Braz.:*** Aero-Clenil†; Aero-Jet; Aero-Ped; Aerodine; Aerolin; Aerotamol; Aerotrat; Albulin†; Asmaliv; Broncodil†; Broncolin†; Broncosedol†; Dilamol; Mebutol†; Pneumolat†; Pulmoflux; Salburin; Salbutalin; Salbutam; Salbutamax; Salbutib†; Saltamol†; Sarolin†; Suxar†; Teoden; Tussiliv; ***Canad.:*** Airomir; Apo-Salvent; Asmavent†; Novo-Salmol; Ventodisk; Ventolin; ***Chile:*** Aero-Sal; Aerolin; Airomir; Asmavent; Broncoterol; Butotal; Fesema; Respolin; Sinasmal; ***Denm.:*** Airomir; Buventol; Salbudan; Salbulin†; Salbutard†; Salbuvent; Ventoline; Volmax; ***Fin.:*** Airomir; Buventol; Salbuvent; Ventoline; ***Fr.:*** Airomir; Asmasal; Buventol; Salbumol; Spreor; Ventexxair; Ventodisks; Ventoline; ***Ger.:*** Aerolind†; Apsomol; Arubendol†; Asthma-Spray†; Asthmalitan; Broncho Fertiginhalat; Broncho Inhalat; Bronchospray; Epaq; Loftan; Padiamol; Pentamol; Salbu; Salbuhexal; Salbulair; Salbulind; Salbupp; Salmundin; Salvent; Sultanol; Ventilastin; Volmac; ***Gr.:*** Aerolin; Asthmotrat; Salbunova; ***Hong Kong:*** Airomir; Apo-Salvent; Buto Asma; Respax†; Respolin; Respreve; Salamol; Salmol; Ventodisks; Ventolin; Ventomol; Volmax; Zenmolin; ***India:*** Asthalin; Salbetol; Salmaplon; Salsol; ***Irl.:*** Aerolin; Airomir; Asmasal; Gerivent; Salamol; Salomol†; Steri-Neb Salamol; Ventamol; Ventodisks; Ventolin; ***Israel:*** Aerolin; Ventolin; Volmax; ***Ital.:*** Aerotec; Broncovaleas; Salbufax; Salbutard; Ventmax; Ventolin; Volmax; ***Malaysia:*** Airomir; Asmovent; Beatolin; Buventol; Colin; Respolin; Salbuterol; Salmax; Salmol; Ventamol; Ventolin; Volmax; ***Mex.:*** Anebron†; Assal; Biorenyn; Brodil†; Butotal†; Cobamol; Exafil; Inspiryl†; Oladin; Salbulin†; Salbutalan; Ventolin; Volmax; Zibil; ***Neth.:*** Aerolin; Airomir; Ventolin; ***Norw.:*** Airomir; Buventol; Inspiryl†; Salbuvent†; Ventoline; ***NZ:*** Airomir; Asmol; Respax†; Respolin; Salbuvent†; Ventodisk†; Ventolin; Volmax; ***Port.:*** Ventilan; ***S.Afr.:*** Airomir; Asthavent; Breatheze; Bronchospray†; Cybutol; Salbulin; Venteze; Ventimax†; Ventodisk; Ventolin; Viavent†; Volmax†; ***Singapore:*** Airomir; Azmasol; Butahale; Buventol; Medolin†; Respolin; Sabutol; Salamol; Salmol; Venderol; Ventolin; Volmax; ***Spain:*** Aldobronquial; Asmasal; Buto Asma; Dipulmin†; Emican; Respiroma; Ventadur; Ventolin; ***Swed.:*** Airomir; Buventol; Inspiryl†; Ventoline; ***Switz.:*** Airomir; Butohaler†; Butovent†; Buventol; Ecovent; Servitamol†; Ventodisk; Ventolin; Volmax; ***Thai.:*** Airomir; Asmasal; Asthmolin; Butamol; Buto Asma; Butovent; Buventol; Medolin†; Respolin; Salbusian; Salbutac; Salmol; Saltamol†; Servitamol†; Venterol; Ventodisk†; Ventolin; Violin; Volmax; Zebu; ***UAE:*** Butalin; ***UK:*** Aerolin†; Airomir; Asmasal; Asmaven†; Kentamol; Maxivent†; Pulvinal Salbutamol; Rimasal†; Salamol; Salapin; Salbulin; Ventmax; Ventodisks; Ventolin; Volmax; ***USA:*** Accuneb; Proventil; Ventolin; Volmax†; VoSpire.

**Multi-ingredient: *Arg.:*** Beclasma; Combivent; Fatigan Bronquial; Salbutol Beclo; Ventide; Ventolin Compuesto; ***Austral.:*** Combivent; ***Austria:*** Combivent; Di-Promal; Ventide; ***Belg.:*** Combivent; ***Braz.:*** Aeroflux Edulito; Aerotide; Beclotamol†; Clenil Compositum; Combivent; Pneumolat Expectorante†; ***Canad.:*** Combivent; ***Chile:*** Aero-Plus; Aerosoma; Asmavent-B; Beclasma; Belomet; Broncoterol-B; Butotal B; Combivent; Herolan Aerosol; Ventide; ***Denm.:*** Combivent; ***Fin.:*** Atrodual; Redol Comp; ***Fr.:*** Combivent; ***Gr.:*** Berovent; ***Hong Kong:*** Combivent; Ventide; Ventolin Expectorant; ***India:*** Aerocort; Albutamol; Asthalin Expectorant; Bronchilet; Deletus A; Duolin; Kofarest; Mucolinc; Pulmo-Rest; Pulmo-Rest Expectorant; Theo-Asthalin; Ventorlin; ***Irl.:*** Combivent; ***Ital.:*** Breva; Clenil Compositum; Plenaer; Ventolin Espettorante; Ventolin Flogo; Zarent; ***Malaysia:*** Asmovent Expectorant; Beatolin Expectorant; Combivent; Ventamol Expectorant; Ventolin Expectorant; ***Mex.:*** Aerocrom†; Aeroflux; Combivent; Ventide; ***Neth.:*** Combivent†; ***NZ:*** Combivent; Duolin; ***Port.:*** Combivent; Propavente; ***S.Afr.:*** Combivent; ***Singapore:*** Clenil Compositum; Combivent; Ventide; ***Spain:*** Butosol; Combivent; ***Swed.:*** Combivent; ***Switz.:*** Dospir; ***Thai.:*** Almasal; Asmasal Expectorant; Biovent; Clenil Compositum; Combivent; Royalin; Salceryl†; Salmol Expectorant; Theosal†; Ventide; Ventolin Expectorant; ***UK:*** Aerocrom†; Combivent; Ventide†; ***USA:*** Combivent; DuoNeb.

## Salmeterol Xinafoate *(BANM, USAN, rINNM)*

GR-33343G; Salmaterol Xinafoate; Salmeterol 1-Hydroxy-2-naphthoate; Xinafoato de Salmeterol. (RS)-5-{1-Hydroxy-2-[6-(4-phenylbutoxy)hexylamino]ethyl}salicyl alcohol 1-hydroxy-2-naphthoate.

$C_{25}H_{37}NO_4,C_{11}H_8O_3$ = 603.7.

*CAS — 89365-50-4 (salmeterol); 94749-08-3 (salmeterol xinafoate).*

*ATC — R03AC12.*

### Adverse Effects and Precautions

As for Salbutamol, p.791. Inhalation of salmeterol may be associated with paradoxical bronchospasm, and it should not be used in patients who are not also receiving an inhaled corticosteroid.

Long-acting beta$_2$ agonists such as salmeterol are not appropriate for the treatment of acute bronchospasm or for patients whose asthma is deteriorating.

**Effects on the respiratory system.** Transient paradoxical bronchoconstriction with breathlessness, wheeze, or cough has been reported in 6 asthmatic patients following inhalation of salmeterol from a metered-dose aerosol but not after inhalation of the dry powder formulation by diskhaler.[1] The fluorocarbon propellants in the metered-dose aerosol were suspected as the irritants causing bronchoconstriction.

1. Wilkinson JRW, *et al.* Paradoxical bronchoconstriction in asthmatic patients after salmeterol by metered dose inhaler. *BMJ* 1992; **305:** 931–2.

**Effects on the skin.** A case has been reported in which an urticarial rash was demonstrated to be associated with inhaled salmeterol and in which the propellant as a cause was excluded. Although many urticarial reactions and a variety of rashes had been attributed to beta-agonist therapy their reproducibility had not always been documented.[1]

1. Hatton MQF, *et al.* Salmeterol rash. *Lancet* 1991; **337:** 1169–70.

**Tolerance.** As with short-acting beta$_2$ agonists (see Salbutamol, p.792), there is evidence that regular use of long-acting beta$_2$ agonists such as salmeterol produces tachyphylaxis to their protective effect against bronchoconstriction, as provoked by stimuli such as allergen, methacholine, or exercise.[1-4] The authors of a study of the long-term effect of salmeterol on exercise-induced asthma concluded that the decreased bronchoprotective effect over time was due to a decrease in duration of action (to less than 9 hours) rather than tachyphylaxis,[5] but this interpretation was criticised.[6,7] Whatever the mechanism, the reduced bronchoprotective effect is perhaps more of a concern with long-acting beta$_2$ agonists, since, unlike the short-acting beta$_2$ agonists, their use on a regular basis is recommended.[8] There is little evidence at present that symptomatic relief is significantly reduced by regular use of beta$_2$ agonists, or that patients using salmeterol are at increased risk of death[9,10] or severe (near fatal) attacks,[11] despite a suggestion that receptor downregulation induced by regular salmeterol might mean that patients required higher doses of inhaled beta$_2$ agonists to attain relief from an acute asthma attack[12] (see also Beta$_2$ Agonists, under Interactions of Salbutamol, p.792). Nevertheless, a study[13] of salmeterol that was stopped early, providing safety data on more than 26 000 patients, found that although it was not statistically significant there was a trend towards an increased risk of severe attacks or asthma-associated deaths, and that the risk might be higher in African-American patients and those patients not taking inhaled corticosteroids.

1. Cheung D, *et al.* Long-term effects of a long-acting $\beta_2$-adrenoceptor agonist, salmeterol, on airway hyperresponsiveness in patients with mild asthma. *N Engl J Med* 1992; **327:** 1198–1203.
2. Bhagat R, *et al.* Rapid onset of tolerance to the bronchoprotective effect of salmeterol. *Chest* 1995; **108:** 1235–9.
3. Booth H, *et al.* Salmeterol tachyphylaxis in steroid treated asthmatic subjects. *Thorax* 1996; **51:** 1100–4.
4. Simons FER, *et al.* Tolerance to the bronchoprotective effect of salmeterol in adolescents with exercise-induced asthma using concurrent inhaled glucocorticoid treatment. *Pediatrics* 1997; **99:** 655–9.
5. Nelson JA, *et al.* Effect of long-term salmeterol treatment on exercise-induced asthma. *N Engl J Med* 1998; **339:** 141–6.
6. Aziz I, Lipworth BJ. Exercise-induced asthma. *N Engl J Med* 1998; **339:** 1783.
7. Dickey BF, Adachi R. Exercise-induced asthma. *N Engl J Med* 1998; **339:** 1783–4.
8. Abisheganaden J, Bonshey HA. Long-acting inhaled $\beta_2$-agonists and the loss of "bronchoprotective" efficacy. *Am J Med* 1998; **104:** 494–7.
9. Castle W, *et al.* Serevent nationwide surveillance study: comparison of salmeterol with salbutamol in asthmatic patients who require regular bronchodilator treatment. *BMJ* 1993; **306:** 1034–7.
10. Mann RD, *et al.* Salmeterol: a study by prescription-event monitoring in a UK cohort of 15,407 patients. *J Clin Epidemiol* 1996; **49:** 247–50.
11. Williams C, *et al.* Case-control study of salmeterol and near-fatal attacks of asthma. *Thorax* 1998; **53:** 7–13.
12. Lipworth BJ. Airway subsensitivity with long-acting $\beta_2$-agonists: is there cause for concern? *Drug Safety* 1997; **16:** 295–308.
13. Anonymous. Salmeterol study halted. *WHO Drug Inf* 2003; **17:** 25.

### Interactions

As for Salbutamol, p.792.

◊ For a study suggesting a decreased effect of salbutamol in patients receiving salmeterol, as well as a report of additive effects, see Beta$_2$ Agonists under Interactions of Salbutamol, p.792.

### Pharmacokinetics

The manufacturers report that plasma concentrations of salmeterol are negligible after inhalation of therapeutic doses.

◊ Reviews.

1. Cazzola M, *et al.* Clinical pharmacokinetics of salmeterol. *Clin Pharmacokinet* 2002; **41:** 19–30.

### Uses and Administration

Salmeterol is a direct-acting sympathomimetic with beta-adrenoceptor stimulant activity and a selective action on beta$_2$ receptors (a beta$_2$ agonist). When given by oral inhalation, salmeterol acts as a bronchodilator. The onset of action is about 10 to 20 minutes but the full effect may not be apparent until after regular administration of several doses. Unlike short-acting beta$_2$ agonists (see Salbutamol, p.793), salmeterol is therefore not suitable for the symptomatic relief of an acute attack of bronchospasm. However, it is long-acting with a duration of action of about 12 hours and is indicated where the regular administration of a long-acting beta$_2$ agonist is required for persistent reversible airways obstruction, as in chronic asthma or in some patients with chronic obstructive pulmonary disease. It may be useful in protecting against nocturnal and exercise-induced asthma attacks. Short-acting beta$_2$ agonists (on an as-required basis) and regular anti-inflammatory therapy should continue to be used.

Salmeterol is used in the form of the xinafoate; doses are expressed in terms of the equivalent amount of salmeterol; salmeterol xinafoate 1.45 micrograms is approximately equivalent to salmeterol 1 microgram.

The usual dose is two inhalations of salmeterol 25 micrograms twice daily from a metered-dose aerosol; if necessary, up to 100 micrograms may be inhaled twice daily. Alternatively, a dry powder inhalation of 50 micrograms, or if necessary 100 micrograms, twice daily may be used. Children of 4 years and over may be given 50 micrograms of salmeterol twice daily by inhalation.

◊ Reviews.

1. Brogden RN, Faulds D. Salmeterol xinafoate: a review of its pharmacological properties and therapeutic potential in reversible obstructive airways disease. *Drugs* 1991; **42:** 895–912.
2. Meyer JM, *et al.* Salmeterol: a novel, long-acting beta$_2$-agonist. *Ann Pharmacother* 1993; **27:** 1478–87.
3. Bennett J, Tattersfield A. Drugs in focus: 15. Salmeterol. *Prescribers' J* 1995; **35:** 84–8.
4. Adkins JC, McTavish D. Salmeterol: a review of its pharmacological properties and clinical efficacy in the management of children with asthma. *Drugs* 1997; **54:** 331–54.

**Asthma.** Salmeterol is a long-acting beta$_2$ agonist (duration of action about 12 hours). Guidelines on the management of asthma, see p.777, generally recommend that salmeterol should be reserved for use in patients with chronic asthma who have already progressed to inhaled corticosteroids; it is not a substitute for corticosteroids. Evidence suggests that, apart from in severe exacerbations, adding a long-acting beta$_2$ agonist to standard dose inhaled corticosteroid therapy may be more effective than increasing the dose of corticosteroid. Salmeterol may also be useful in controlling persistent nocturnal asthma or preventing exercise-induced attacks. There is some evidence that after prolonged use, duration of protection against exercise-induced bronchoconstriction is reduced (see Tolerance, above).

References.

1. Fitzpatrick MF, *et al.* Salmeterol in nocturnal asthma: a double blind, placebo controlled trial of a long acting inhaled $\beta_2$ agonist. *BMJ* 1990; **301:** 1365–8.
2. Pearlman DS, *et al.* A comparison of salmeterol with albuterol in the treatment of mild-to-moderate asthma. *N Engl J Med* 1992; **327:** 1420–5.
3. Green CP, Price JF. Prevention of exercise induced asthma by inhaled salmeterol xinafoate. *Arch Dis Child* 1992; **67:** 1014–17.
4. Smyth ET, *et al.* Interaction and dose equivalence of salbutamol and salmeterol in patients with asthma. *BMJ* 1993; **306:** 543–5.
5. D'Alonzo GE, *et al.* Salmeterol xinafoate as maintenance therapy compared with albuterol in patients with asthma. *JAMA* 1994; **271:** 1412–16.
6. Greening AP, *et al.* Added salmeterol versus higher-dose corticosteroid in asthma patients with symptoms on existing inhaled corticosteroid. *Lancet* 1994; **344:** 219–24.
7. Woolcock A, *et al.* Comparison of addition of salmeterol to inhaled steroids with doubling of the dose of inhaled steroids. *Am J Respir Crit Care Med* 1996; **153:** 1481–8.
8. Wilding P, *et al.* Effect of long term treatment with salmeterol on asthma control: a double blind, randomised crossover study. *BMJ* 1997; **314:** 1441–6.
9. Simons FER, *et al.* A comparison of beclomethasone, salmeterol, and placebo in children with asthma. *N Engl J Med* 1997; **337:** 1659–65.
10. van Noord JA, *et al.* Addition of salmeterol versus doubling the dose of fluticasone propionate in patients with mild to moderate asthma. *Thorax* 1999; **54:** 207–12.
11. Shrewsbury S, *et al.* Meta-analysis of increased dose of inhaled steroid or addition of salmeterol in symptomatic asthma (MIASMA). *BMJ* 2000; **320:** 1368–73.
12. Johansson G, *et al.* Comparison of salmeterol/fluticasone propionate combination with budesonide in patients with mild-to-moderate asthma. *Clin Drug Invest* 2001; **21:** 633–42.
13. Heyneman CA, *et al.* Fluticasone versus salmeterol/low-dose fluticasone for long-term asthma control. *Ann Pharmacother* 2002; **36:** 1944–9.

**Chronic obstructive pulmonary disease.** Short-acting beta$_2$ agonists are used as bronchodilators in patients with chronic obstructive pulmonary disease (see p.779), although there is some evidence to suggest that an antimuscarinic might be preferable. Long-acting beta$_2$ agonists such as salmeterol may be used for maintenance therapy in moderate and more severe disease. Improvement in lung function and symptoms has been seen in such patients following regular treatment with inhaled salmeterol.[1,2] Additional benefit has been reported from the use of salmeterol with inhaled corticosteroids.[3]

1. Boyd G, *et al.* An evaluation of salmeterol in the treatment of chronic obstructive pulmonary disease (COPD). *Eur Respir J* 1997; **10:** 815–21.
2. Mahler DA, *et al.* Efficacy of salmeterol xinafoate in the treatment of COPD. *Chest* 1999; **115:** 957–65.
3. Calverley P, *et al.* Combined salmeterol and fluticasone in the treatment of chronic obstructive pulmonary disease: a randomised controlled trial. *Lancet* 2003; **361:** 449–56. Correction. *ibid.*; 1660.

### Preparations

**Proprietary Preparations** (details are given in Part 3)
***Arg.:*** Abrilar; Serevent; ***Austral.:*** Optrol†; Serevent; ***Austria:*** Serevent; ***Belg.:*** Serevent; ***Braz.:*** Serevent; ***Canad.:*** Serevent; ***Chile:*** Kolpovent; Serevent; Xemos; ***Denm.:*** Serevent; ***Fin.:*** Serevent; ***Fr.:*** Serevent; ***Ger.:*** Aeromax; Serevent; ***Gr.:*** Serevent; ***Hong Kong:*** Serevent; ***India:*** Salmeter; Serobid; ***Irl.:*** Serevent; ***Israel:*** Serevent; ***Ital.:*** Arial; Salmetedur; Seretide; Serevent; ***Malaysia:*** Serevent; ***Mex.:*** Serevent; ***Neth.:*** Serevent; ***Norw.:*** Serevent; ***NZ:*** Serevent; ***Port.:*** Dilamax; Serevent; Ultrabeta; Veraspir; ***S.Afr.:*** Serevent; ***Singapore:*** Serevent; ***Spain:*** Beglan; Betamican; Inaspir; Serevent; ***Swed.:*** Serevent; ***Switz.:*** Serevent; ***Thai.:*** Serevent; ***UK:*** Serevent; ***USA:*** Serevent.

**Multi-ingredient:** ***Arg.:*** Seretide; ***Austral.:*** Seretide; ***Austria:*** Seretide; Viani; ***Belg.:*** Seretide; ***Braz.:*** Seretide; ***Canad.:*** Advair; ***Chile:*** Brexotide; Seretide; ***Denm.:*** Seretide; ***Fin.:*** Seretide; ***Fr.:*** Seretide; ***Ger.:*** Atmadisc; Viani; ***Gr.:*** Seretide; Viani; ***Hong Kong:*** Seretide; ***India:*** Seroflo; ***Irl.:*** Seretide; ***Israel:*** Seretide; ***Ital.:*** Aliflus; ***Malaysia:*** Seretide; ***Mex.:*** Seretide; ***Neth.:*** Seretide; ***Norw.:*** Seretide; ***Port.:*** Brisomax; Maizar; Seretaide; ***S.Afr.:*** Seretide; ***Singapore:*** Seretide; ***Spain:*** Anasma; Inaladuo; Plusvent; Seretide; ***Swed.:*** Seretide; ***Switz.:*** Seretide; ***Thai.:*** Seretide; ***UK:*** Seretide; ***USA:*** Advair.

## Seratrodast *(USAN, rINN)*

A-73001; AA-2414; Abbott-73001; ABT-001. (±)-2,4,5-Trimethyl-3,6-dioxo-ζ-phenyl-1,4-cyclohexadiene-1-heptanoic acid.

$C_{22}H_{26}O_4$ = 354.4.

*CAS — 112665-43-7; 103186-19-2.*

*ATC — R03DX06.*

### Profile

Seratrodast is a thromboxane $A_2$ antagonist that is reported to reduce airway hyperresponsiveness. It is given by mouth in the prophylactic management of asthma (p.777), in single doses of 80 mg in the evening after food.

Adverse effects include gastrointestinal disturbances, drowsiness, headache, palpitations, and hepatitis. Hepatic function should be monitored and the drug should be withdrawn if hypersensitivity reactions such as rashes and pruritus occur, or if there is elevation of liver enzyme values. Seratrodast should be used with care in patients with pre-existing hepatic impairment. It is not suitable for the treatment of an acute asthmatic attack.

◊ References.

1. Tamaoki J, *et al.* Effect of a thromboxane $A_2$ antagonist on sputum production and its physicochemical properties in patients with mild to moderate asthma. *Chest* 2000; **118:** 73–9.

### Preparations

**Proprietary Preparations** (details are given in Part 3)
***Jpn:*** Bronica.

## Sodium Cromoglicate *(BANM, rINNM)*

Cromoglicato de sodio; Cromolyn Sodium *(USAN)*; Disodium Cromoglycate; FPL-670; Natrii Cromoglicas; Sodium Cromoglycate. Disodium 4,4′-dioxo-5,5′-(2-hydroxytrimethylenedioxy)di(4*H*-chromene-2-carboxylate).

$C_{23}H_{14}Na_2O_{11}$ = 512.3.

*CAS — 16110-51-3 (cromoglycic acid); 15826-37-6 (sodium cromoglicate).*

*ATC — A07EB01; R01AC01; R03BC01; S01GX01.*

**Pharmacopoeias.** In *Chin., Eur.* (see p.vi), *Int., Jpn,* and *US.*

**Ph. Eur. 5.0** (Sodium Cromoglicate). A white or almost white, hygroscopic, crystalline powder. Soluble in water; practically insoluble in alcohol. Store in airtight containers. Protect from light

**USP 27** (Cromolyn Sodium). A white, odourless, hygroscopic, crystalline powder. Soluble in water; insoluble in alcohol and in chloroform. Store in airtight containers.

## Adverse Effects

Inhalation of sodium cromoglicate may cause transient bronchospasm, wheezing, cough, nasal congestion, and irritation of the throat. Nausea, headache, dizziness, an unpleasant taste, and joint pain and swelling have been reported. Other reactions, which have sometimes occurred after treatment for several weeks or months, include aggravation of existing asthma, urticaria, rashes, pulmonary infiltrates with eosinophilia, dysuria, and urinary frequency. Severe reactions such as marked bronchospasm, laryngeal oedema, angioedema, and anaphylaxis have been reported rarely; these have sometimes been referred to as pseudo-allergic.

Intranasal use of sodium cromoglicate may cause transient irritation of the nasal mucosa, sneezing, and occasionally epistaxis. Nausea, skin rashes, and joint pains have occurred when it is taken by mouth. Transient burning and stinging have occasionally been reported following use of sodium cromoglicate eye drops.

**Formulation.** Some of the adverse effects reported with sodium cromoglicate may be due to its formulation: there is a view that some of the irritant effects reported on inhalation may be due to the use of dry powder inhalers. It has also been suggested that in some patients receiving sodium cromoglicate via a nebuliser, hypotonicity of the nebuliser solution may induce bronchospasm,[1] although others consider this debatable.[2] Nausea, bloating, abdominal cramps, and flatulence developed in a 24-year-old lactase-deficient woman 2 hours after the use of Intal (sodium cromoglicate) via a turbo-haler for exercise-induced asthma.[3] These symptoms recurred on rechallenge and were attributed to ingestion of lactose contained within the Intal capsules.

1. Chin TW, Nussbaum E. Detrimental effect of hypotonic cromolyn sodium. *J Pediatr* 1992; **120:** 641–3.
2. Rachelefsky GS, *et al.* Detrimental effects of hypotonic cromolyn sodium. *J Pediatr* 1992; **121:** 992.
3. Brandstetter RD, *et al.* Lactose intolerance associated with Intal capsules. *N Engl J Med* 1986; **315:** 1613–14.

## Precautions

Sodium cromoglicate has no role in the treatment of acute asthmatic attacks. Withdrawal of sodium cromoglicate may lead to recurrence of the symptoms of asthma. Should withdrawal be necessary it has been suggested that the dose be reduced gradually over a period of one week; patients in whom sodium cromoglicate therapy has permitted a reduction of corticosteroid dosage may require restoration of full corticosteroid cover.

Systemic corticosteroid therapy that has been reduced or discontinued in asthmatic patients may need to be reinstated if symptoms increase, during periods of stress such as infection, illness, trauma, or severe antigen challenge, or where airways obstruction impairs inhalation of sodium cromoglicate.

## Pharmacokinetics

Sodium cromoglicate is poorly absorbed from the gastrointestinal tract, with a reported bioavailability of only 1%. It has been reported that following inhalation as a fine powder only 8 to 10% of a dose is deposited in the lungs from where it is rapidly absorbed and excreted unchanged in the urine and bile. Less than 7% of an intranasal dose appears to be absorbed. The majority of an inhaled or an intranasal dose is swallowed and excreted unchanged in the faeces. About 0.03% of an ophthalmic dose is reported to be absorbed. The elimination half-life has been reported to be about 20 to 60 minutes after intravenous administration, but the elimination half-life following oral administration or inhalation is longer, being stated to be about 80 minutes.

◊ A study[1] in patients with exercise-induced asthma concluded that the plasma concentration of cromoglicate was almost certainly not related directly to its protective effect, although another study in asthmatic children given sodium cromoglicate by dry-powder inhalation, found both blood concentration and clinical response to be correlated with inhalation technique.[2]

1. Patel KR, *et al.* Plasma concentrations of sodium cromoglycate given by nebulisation and metered dose inhalers in patients with exercise-induced asthma: relationship to protective effect. *Br J Clin Pharmacol* 1986; **21:** 231–3.
2. Yahav Y, *et al.* Sodium cromoglycate in asthma: correlation between response and serum concentrations. *Arch Dis Child* 1988; **63:** 592–7.

## Uses and Administration

Sodium cromoglicate is used for the prevention of allergic reactions. Although its precise mode of action remains uncertain, it is believed to act primarily by preventing release of mediators of inflammation from sensitised mast cells through stabilisation of mast-cell membranes. It has no intrinsic antihistaminic action and has generally been considered to possess no bronchodilator activity.

Sodium cromoglicate can prevent the asthmatic response to a variety of allergic and non-allergic stimuli. It is used in the management of chronic asthma that cannot be managed with inhaled beta$_2$ agonists alone; it is not used for acute attacks of asthma.

Sodium cromoglicate is also used in the prophylaxis and treatment of seasonal and perennial allergic rhinitis and allergic conditions of the eye including acute and chronic allergic conjunctivitis and vernal keratoconjunctivitis. It has been given by mouth for the prevention of food allergies, in conjunction with dietary restriction, and is also used in the treatment of mastocytosis.

It is important that the regular administration of sodium cromoglicate is maintained both in the prophylactic control of asthma and in the management of other allergic conditions. Beneficial effects may take several weeks to become established.

In the prophylaxis of **asthma**, sodium cromoglicate is given by inhalation either as a dry powder, or as a nebulised solution, or from a metered-dose aerosol. The usual dose as dry powder or nebulised solution is 20 mg by inhalation 4 times daily increased, if necessary, to 6 or, for the powder, even to 8 times daily. Once the asthma has been stabilised it may be possible to reduce the dose. The usual dose by aerosol in the UK is 10 mg four times daily, increased to 6 to 8 times daily if necessary; it may be possible to reduce the dosage to 5 mg four times daily once the asthma has been stabilised. Additional doses as the aerosol or dry powder may be taken before exercise. Doses are administered from metered aerosols providing units of 5 mg. However, aerosols providing units of about 1 mg are also available in some countries and doses of about 2 mg four times daily have been used. The adequacy of this low dosage has been questioned (see under Administration, below) and in the UK the manufacturers have discontinued the 1-mg aerosol.

Inhalation of sodium cromoglicate may cause bronchospasm; separate inhalation of a beta$_2$ agonist such as salbutamol a few minutes beforehand should prevent this. Use of a combination product containing a beta$_2$ agonist is not recommended as this is liable to be used inappropriately for relief of bronchospasm rather than for its prophylactic effect.

For the prophylaxis of **allergic rhinitis**, approximately 2.5 or 5 mg as a 2 or 4% solution is administered as a spray into each nostril, usually up to 4 times daily. Prophylactic treatment for seasonal allergic rhinitis should begin 2 to 3 weeks before exposure to the offending allergen and should continue throughout the season. In **allergic conjunctivitis** sodium cromoglicate is used as drops of 2 or 4%, generally applied 4 to 6 times daily; a 4% eye ointment has been applied 2 to 3 times daily.

In **food allergy** and in **mastocytosis**, sodium cromoglicate may be given by mouth in doses of 200 mg four times daily before meals; children over 2 years may be given 100 mg four times daily. If satisfactory control is not achieved within 2 to 3 weeks the dosage may be increased, but should not exceed 40 mg/kg daily; a reduction in dosage may be possible once symptoms have been controlled.

**Action.** Sodium cromoglicate has a range of actions at cellular level that may be important for its protective effect in asthma. It is known as a mast cell stabiliser that inhibits the release of histamine and other inflammatory mediators from sensitised mast cells. Other reported actions include a direct effect on airway nerves[1,2] and antagonism[3] of substance P, which ties up with its inhibition of the effects of platelet activating factor (PAF).[4,5]

There have been a few reports[6-8] of sodium cromoglicate producing bronchodilatation. However, in practice other drugs with accepted bronchodilating activity are used for this effect in asthma treatment schedules, see p.777.

1. Barnes PJ. Asthma as an axon reflex. *Lancet* 1986; **i:** 242–5.
2. Dixon M, *et al.* The effects of sodium cromoglycate on lung irritant receptors and left ventricular cardiac receptors in the anaesthetized dog. *Br J Pharmacol* 1979; **67:** 569–74.
3. Page C. Sodium cromoglycate, a tachykinin antagonist? *Lancet* 1994; **343:** 70.
4. Morley J, *et al.* The platelet in asthma. *Lancet* 1984; **ii:** 1142–4.
5. Morley J. PAF and airway hyperreactivity: prospects for novel prophylactic anti-asthma drugs. In: *PAF, Platelets, and Asthma*, Basel, Birkhäuser Verlag, 1987: 87–95.
6. Horn CR, *et al.* Bronchodilator effect of disodium cromoglycate administered as a dry powder in exercise induced asthma. *Br J Clin Pharmacol* 1984; **18:** 798–801.
7. Weiner P, *et al.* Bronchodilating effect of cromolyn sodium in asthmatic patients at rest and following exercise. *Ann Allergy* 1984; **53:** 186–8.
8. Yuksel B, Greenough A. Bronchodilator effect of nebulized sodium cromoglycate in children born prematurely. *Eur Respir J* 1993; **6:** 387–90.

**Administration.** The effectiveness of sodium cromoglicate 2 mg four times daily by metered-dose aerosol inhaler has been reported by a number of controlled studies in adults and children with asthma.[1-5] However, although sodium cromoglicate 2 mg by inhalation from a metered-dose aerosol was reported[6] to be as effective as 20 mg inhaled as powder, the tenfold difference in dosage has been questioned,[7] and others have reported contrary results.[8,9] It has been suggested that an aerosol supplying 5 mg per metered dose (currently favoured in the UK, see above) would be preferable.[10] In a comparison of single-dose pretreatment from metered-dose inhalers, sodium cromoglicate 10 mg (2 × 5 mg puffs) was as effective as beclometasone dipropionate 200 micrograms in inhibiting bronchial responsiveness to histamine.[11]

Care is required if inhaled sodium cromoglicate is given via a spacer device; evidence suggests that these may greatly influence the amount of drug delivered, reducing it to one-third of the dose delivered by inhaler actuation in some cases.[12]

1. Geller-Bernstein C, Levin S. Sodium cromoglycate pressurised aerosol in childhood asthma. *Curr Ther Res* 1983; **34:** 345–9.
2. Wheatley D. Sodium cromoglycate in aerosol form in regular users of bronchodilator drugs. *Curr Med Res Opin* 1983; **8:** 333–7.
3. Rubin AE, *et al.* The treatment of asthma in adults using sodium cromoglycate pressurized aerosol: a double-blind controlled trial. *Curr Med Res Opin* 1983; **8:** 553–8.
4. Blumenthal MN, *et al.* A multicenter evaluation of the clinical benefits of cromolyn sodium aerosol by metered-dose inhaler in the treatment of asthma. *J Allergy Clin Immunol* 1988; **81:** 681–7.
5. Selcow JE, *et al.* Clinical benefits of cromolyn sodium aerosol (MDI) in the treatment of asthma in children. *Ann Allergy* 1989; **62:** 195–9.
6. Latimer KM, *et al.* Inhibition by sodium cromoglycate of bronchoconstriction stimulated by respiratory heat loss: comparison of pressurised aerosol and powder. *Thorax* 1984; **39:** 277–81.
7. Anonymous. Sodium cromoglycate aerosol. *Drug Ther Bull* 1982; **20:** 27.
8. Robson RA, *et al.* Sodium cromoglycate: spincaps or metered dose aerosol. *Br J Clin Pharmacol* 1981; **11:** 383–4.
9. Bar-Yishay E, *et al.* Duration of action of sodium cromoglycate on exercise induced asthma: comparison of 2 formulations. *Arch Dis Child* 1983; **58:** 624–7.
10. Tullett WM, *et al.* Dose-response effect of sodium cromoglycate pressurised aerosol in exercise induced asthma. *Thorax* 1985; **40:** 41–4.
11. Cockcroft DW, Murdock KY. Comparative effects of inhaled salbutamol, sodium cromoglycate, and beclomethasone dipropionate on allergen-induced early asthmatic responses, late asthmatic responses, and increased bronchial responsiveness to histamine. *J Allergy Clin Immunol* 1987; **79:** 734–40.
12. Barry PW, O'Callaghan C. Inhalational drug delivery from seven different spacer devices. *Thorax* 1996; **51:** 835–40.

**Asthma.** Sodium cromoglicate is used as a prophylactic agent in the management of chronic asthma (p.777), but in practice inhaled corticosteroids are preferred if regular prophylactic treatment is indicated, i.e. if the condition cannot be managed with occasional use of an inhaled beta$_2$ agonist alone. Even in children, in whom cromoglicate has tended to be more widely used, the trend is towards greater use of inhaled corticosteroids. However, guidelines still specify the use of cromoglicate or nedocromil as a valid alternative to inhaled corticosteroids in some circumstances.

Response to treatment with nebulised sodium cromoglicate was found to be age-related in a study of children under 2 years of age with recurrent or persistent wheezy bronchitis and a history of allergic symptoms.[1] It was effective in children of 12 to 24 months of age but not in those below 12 months. Similarly, nebulised sodium cromoglicate was no more effective than placebo in the treatment of a group of 31 infants with persistent wheezing aged under 1 year,[2] and long-term inhalation therapy was ineffective in children aged 1 to 4 years.[3]

1. Geller-Bernstein C, Levin S. Nebulised sodium cromoglycate in the treatment of wheezy bronchitis in infants and young children. *Respiration* 1982; **43:** 294–8.
2. Furfaro S, *et al.* Efficacy of cromoglycate in persistently wheezing infants. *Arch Dis Child* 1994; **71:** 331–4.
3. Tasche MJA, *et al.* Randomised placebo-controlled trial of inhaled sodium cromoglycate in 1-4-year-old children with moderate asthma. *Lancet* 1997; **350:** 1060–4. Correction. *ibid.* 1998; **351:** 376.

**Cogan's syndrome.** Sodium cromoglicate eye drops improved blurred vision in a patient with Cogan's syndrome (p.1078) of 18 years' duration.[1] Sodium cromoglicate capsules [by mouth] also reduced the frequency of fever attacks in this patient.

1. Carter F, Nabarro J. Cromoglycate for Cogan's syndrome. *Lancet* 1987; **i:** 858.

**Cough.** Sodium cromoglicate has been used with modest success by aerosol inhalation to suppress the cough associated with

ACE inhibitor therapy (p.843) in some patients.[1,2] However, inhalation of nedocromil sodium was not helpful in the treatment of ACE inhibitor induced cough in 6 diabetic patients.[3]


1. Keogh A. Sodium cromoglycate prophylaxis for angiotensin-converting enzyme inhibitor cough. *Lancet* 1993; **341:** 560.
2. Hargreaves MR, Benson MK. Inhaled sodium cromoglycate in angiotensin-converting enzyme inhibitor cough. *Lancet* 1995; **345:** 13–16.
3. Puolijoki H, Rekiaro M. Lack of effect of nedocromil sodium in ACE-inhibitor-induced cough. *Lancet* 1995; **345:** 394.


**Food allergy.** Oral sodium cromoglicate has been used in the prophylaxis of food allergy reactions (p.422). However, efficacy has not been unequivocally established.

**Mastocytosis.** Mastocytosis is a condition characterised by abnormal proliferation of mast cells and their accumulation in body tissues.[1-3] It occurs in cutaneous or systemic forms, the former most often manifesting as urticaria pigmentosa, the latter involving diverse organs and tissues including the bones, liver, spleen, lymph nodes, haematopoietic system, gastrointestinal tract, and also the skin.

Treatment is aimed at relieving symptoms and does not alter the course of the disease. A combination of $H_1$ and $H_2$-antagonist antihistamines is widely used to control cutaneous and gastrointestinal symptoms, while antimuscarinics may be useful for diarrhoea.[1] Patients should carry adrenaline for self-injection in the event of severe attacks.

Sodium cromoglicate has been tried in systemic mastocytosis in doses of 100 to 200 mg four times daily by mouth, generally with favourable results.[4-6] In a comparative study in 6 patients sodium cromoglicate 200 mg four times daily was indistinguishable from chlorphenamine 4 mg plus cimetidine 300 mg four times daily in relieving overall symptoms of systemic mastocytosis.[6] However, individual symptoms responded to varying degrees. A much higher dose of sodium cromoglicate of 100 mg/kg daily by mouth in divided doses was used with some success in a 5-year-old boy with systemic mastocytosis after lower doses had proved ineffective.[5] Responses to interferon alfa have been reported.[7,8]


1. Golkar L, Bernhard JD. Mastocytosis. *Lancet* 1997; **349:** 1379–85.
2. Hartmann K, Henz BM. Mastocytosis: recent advances in defining the disease. *Br J Dermatol* 2001; **144:** 682–95.
3. Carter MC, Metcalfe DD. Paediatric mastocytosis. *Arch Dis Child* 2002; **86:** 315–19.
4. Soter NA, *et al.* Oral disodium cromoglycate in the treatment of systemic mastocytosis. *N Engl J Med* 1979; **301:** 465–9.
5. Businco L, *et al.* Systemic mastocytosis in a 5-year-old child: successful treatment with disodium cromoglycate. *Clin Allergy* 1984; **14:** 147–52.
6. Frieri M, *et al.* Comparison of the therapeutic efficacy of cromolyn sodium with that of combined chlorpheniramine and cimetidine in systemic mastocytosis. *Am J Med* 1985; **78:** 9–14.
7. Kolde G, *et al.* Treatment of urticaria pigmentosa using interferon alpha. *Br J Dermatol* 1995; **133:** 91–4.
8. Lippert U, Henz BM. Long-term effect of interferon alpha treatment in mastocytosis. *Br J Dermatol* 1996; **134:** 1164–5.


**Rhinitis and conjunctivitis.** Many drugs, including sodium cromoglicate, are used in the management of allergic rhinitis (p.422) and conjunctivitis (p.421). There is some evidence that nedocromil[1] or lodoxamide[2] may be more effective than cromoglicate in the management of vernal keratoconjunctivitis.


1. El Hennawi M. A double-blind placebo controlled group comparative study of ophthalmic sodium cromoglycate and nedocromil sodium in the treatment of vernal keratoconjunctivitis. *Br J Ophthalmol* 1994; **78:** 365–9.
2. Leonardi A, *et al.* Effect of lodoxamide and disodium cromoglycate on tear eosinophil cationic protein in vernal keratoconjunctivitis. *Br J Ophthalmol* 1997; **81:** 23–6.


## Preparations

***BP 2003:*** Sodium Cromoglicate Eye Drops; Sodium Cromoglicate Powder for Inhalation;
***USP 27:*** Cromolyn Sodium Inhalation Powder; Cromolyn Sodium Inhalation Solution; Cromolyn Sodium Nasal Solution; Cromolyn Sodium Ophthalmic Solution.

**Proprietary Preparations** (details are given in Part 3)
***Arg.:*** Claroftal; Clo-5; Intal; Sificrom; ***Austral.:*** Cromese; Intal; Opticrom; Rynacrom; ***Austria:*** Acromax; Aeropaxyn; Allercrom†; Coldacron; Cromal; Cromoglin; Cromophtal; Dilospir; Intal; Lomusol; Opticrom†; Pulmosin†; Vividrin; ***Belg.:*** Lomudal; Lomusol; Opticrom; Vividrin†; ***Braz.:*** Cromabak†; Cromocato; Cromolerg; Intal; Maxicrom; Opticrom†; Rilan; ***Canad.:*** Apo-Cromolyn; Cromolyn; Gen-Cromolyn; Intal; Nalcrom; Novo-Cromolyn†; Opticrom; Rynacrom†; Solu-Crom; Vistacrom†; ***Chile:*** Oftacon; ***Denm.:*** Hexacroman; Lecrolyn; Lomudal; ***Fin.:*** Glinor; Lecrolyn; Lomudal; ***Fr.:*** Allergocomod; Cromabak; Cromadoses; Cromoptic; Cromosoft; Intercron; Lomudal; Lomusol; Multicrom; Nalcron; Ophtacalm; Opticron; ***Ger.:*** Acecromol; Alerg; Allergo-COMOD; Allergocrom; Allergoval; Colimune; Crom-Ophtal; Cromo; Cromoglicin; Cromohexal; Cromol†; Cromolind; Cromolyn†; Cromopp; Diffusyl; Dispacromil; DNCG; duracroman; Fenistil; Flenid; Flui-DNCG; Gelodrin†; Intal; Lomupren; Opticrom; Otriven H; Padiacrom; Pentacrom; Pentatop; Prothanon cromo†; Pulbil; Vividrin; ***Gr.:*** Allergojovis; Allergotin; Botastin; Crolidin; Cromolergin UD; Erystamine-K; Fluvet; Iopanchol; Kaosyl; Lomudal; Spaziron; Vividrin; Zineli; ***Hong Kong:*** Cromabak; Cusicrom†; Intal; Opticrom; Rynacrom M†; Stadaglicin; ***India:*** Cromal; Fintal; ***Irl.:*** Cromogen; Hay-Crom; Intal; Nalcrom; Opticrom; Rynacrom; Steri-Neb Cromogen†; Vividrin; ***Israel:*** Cromogen; Cromolyn; Cromoptic; Cromunal†; Cronase; Lomudal; Nalcrom†; Opticrom; Vicrom; ***Ital.:*** Acticrom; Cromantal; Cromosan; Cronacol†; Frenal; Frenal Rinologico†; Gaster†; Gastrofrenal; Glicacil†; Lomudal; Lomuspray; Nalcrom; Sificrom; ***Jpn:*** Intal; ***Malaysia:*** Allergocrom; Cusicrom; Intal; Opticrom; Stadaglicin; Vividrin; ***Mex.:*** Alercrom; Cusicrom†; Exaler; Intal; Maxicrom; Oftacon; Opticrom; Rynacrom; ***Mon.:*** Cromedil; ***Neth.:*** Allergocrom†; Lomudal; Lomusol; Nalcrom; Opticrom; Prevalin†; Vividrin; ***Norw.:*** Lecrolyn; Lomudal; ***NZ:*** Intal; Nalcrom; Opticrom; Optrex Hayfever Allergy; Rynacrom; Vicrom; ***Port.:*** Croglina; Cromex; Cusicrom; Fenolip; Intal; Opticrom; Rynacrom; ***S.Afr.:*** Cromal†; Cromogen†; Cromohexal; Hay-Crom†; Kiddicrom†; Lomudal†; Nalcrom†; Opticrom†; Rynacrom†; Stop-Allerg; Vividrin; ***Singapore:*** Cromabak; Cusicrom†; Intal; Opticrom; Rynacrom; Sificrom; Stadaglicin†; Vividrin; ***Spain:*** Alergocrom; Cromo Asma; Cusicrom; Farmacrom; Frenal; Gastrofrenal; Intal; Nalcrom†; Nebulasma; Nebulcrom; Oralcrom†; Poledin; Primover; Renocil; Rinilyn; Rinofrenal; Vividrin†; ***Swed.:*** Lecrolyn; Lomudal; Pollyferm; Rinil; ***Switz.:*** Cromodyn; Cromosol Ophta; Cromosol UD; Glicinal; Lomudal; Lomusol; Nalcrom; Opticrom; Vividrin; ***Thai.:*** Ifiral†; Intal; Lecrolyn; Opticrom; Rynacrom; Stadaglicin†; Vividrin; ***UK:*** Brol-eze†; Clariteyes; Clarityn; Cromogen; Hay-Crom; Hayfever Eye Drops; Intal; Nalcrom; Opticrom; Optrex Allergy; Pollenase Allergy; Rynacrom; Vivicrom; Vividrin; Viz-On†; ***USA:*** Crolom; Gastrocrom; Intal; Nasalcrom; Opticrom.

**Multi-ingredient:** ***Arg.:*** Duotec; Hyalcrom; Rinogel; ***Austria:*** Aarane†; Allergospasmin†; Ditec; ***Belg.:*** Lomusol plus Xylometazoline†; ***Denm.:*** Kombicrom†; ***Ger.:*** Aarane N; Allergospasmin; Ditec; Lomupren compositum; Vividrin comp†; ***Hong Kong:*** Rynacrom Compound†; ***Irl.:*** Rynacrom Compound†; ***Ital.:*** Cromozil; Rinofrenal; Visuglican; ***Malaysia:*** Rynacrom Compound; ***Mex.:*** Aerocrom†; ***Port.:*** Rinoglin; Rynacrom Composto†; ***Singapore:*** Rynacrom Compound†; ***Spain:*** Cromoftol†; Frenal Compositum; Rinofrenal Plus; ***Switz.:*** Aarane; Allergospasmine; Lomusol-X; ***Thai.:*** Rynacrom Compound; ***UK:*** Aerocrom†; Rynacrom Allergy†; Rynacrom Compound.

## Suplatast Tosilate *(rINN)*

IPD-1151T; Suplatast Tosylate; Suplatastum Tosilas; Tosilato de suplatast. (±)-(2-{[*p*-(3-Ethoxy-2-hydroxypropoxy)phenyl]carbamoyl}ethyl)dimethylsulphonium *p*-toluenesulphonate; (3-{[4-(3-Ethoxy-2-hydroxypropoxy)phenyl]amino}-3-oxopropyl)dimethylsulphonium *p*-toluenesulphonate.

$C_{23}H_{33}NO_7S_2$ = 499.6.
*CAS — 94055-76-2.*

### Profile

Suplatast tosilate is an anti-allergic given by mouth in the prophylactic management of asthma and other allergic conditions.

◊ References.


1. Sano Y, *et al.* Anti-inflammatory effect of suplatast tosilate on mild asthma. *Chest* 1997; **112:** 862–3.
2. Nihei Y, *et al.* Suplatast tosilate (IPD), a new immunoregulator, is effective in vitiligo treatment. *J Dermatol* 1998; **25:** 250–5.
3. Tamaoki J, *et al.* Effect of suplatast tosilate, a Th2 cytokine inhibitor, on steroid-dependent asthma: a double-blind randomised study. *Lancet* 2000; **356:** 273–8.


# Terbutaline Sulfate *(USAN, rINNM)*

KWD-2019; Sulfato de terbutalina; Terbutaline Sulphate *(BANM)*; Terbutalini Sulfas. 2-*tert*-Butylamino-1-(3,5-dihydroxyphenyl)ethanol sulphate.

$(C_{12}H_{19}NO_3)_2,H_2SO_4$ = 548.6.
*CAS — 23031-25-6 (terbutaline); 23031-32-5 (terbutaline sulfate).*
*ATC — R03AC03; R03CC03.*

**Pharmacopoeias.** In *Chin., Eur.* (see p.vi), *Jpn*, and *US.*

**Ph. Eur. 5.0** (Terbutaline Sulphate). A white or almost white crystalline powder. It exhibits polymorphism. Freely soluble in water; slightly soluble in alcohol.

**USP 27** (Terbutaline Sulfate). A white to grey-white crystalline powder; odourless or has a faint odour of acetic acid. Soluble in water and in 0.1N hydrochloric acid; insoluble in chloroform; slightly soluble in methyl alcohol. Store at 15° to 30°. Protect from light.

## Adverse Effects and Precautions

As for Salbutamol, p.791.

**Overdosage.** An overdose of terbutaline due to transcutaneous absorption has been reported following inappropriate topical application to skin infected with tinea.[1] Transcutaneous absorption should be considered especially when children with facial eczema or dermatitis are given terbutaline via a nebuliser and mask.


1. Ingrams GJ, Morgan FB. Transcutaneous overdose of terbutaline. *BMJ* 1993; **307:** 484.


**Pulmonary oedema.** Pulmonary oedema has occurred in women given $beta_2$ agonists, including terbutaline, for premature labour.[1] The risk factors, the most important of which is fluid overload, are discussed under Precautions for Salbutamol, p.792.


1. Hawker F. Pulmonary oedema associated with $\beta_2$-sympathomimetic treatment of premature labour. *Anaesth Intensive Care* 1984; **12:** 143–51.


**Tolerance.** As with other $beta_2$ agonists (see p.792) there is some evidence[1] that tolerance may develop to terbutaline when it is used regularly.


1. O'Connor BJ, *et al.* Tolerance to the nonbronchodilator effects of inhaled $\beta_2$-agonists in asthma. *N Engl J Med* 1992; **327:** 1204–8.


**Tooth erosion.** The pH of some inhaled powder formulations of anti-inflammatory and bronchodilator drugs (including terbutaline) was found to be below 5.5, and it was suggested that this might contribute to the dissolution of enamel surfaces of teeth.[1]


1. O'Sullivan EA, Curzon MEJ. Drug treatments for asthma may cause erosive tooth damage. *BMJ* 1998; **317:** 820.


## Interactions

As for Salbutamol, p.792.

**Xanthines.** The metabolic and cardiovascular responses to terbutaline infusion were significantly enhanced by *theophylline* in a study in 7 healthy subjects; in particular the fall in serum potassium was greater when both drugs were given.[1] Careful monitoring of serum potassium is recommended in severe asthma where theophylline and $beta_2$-agonists may be given together. Terbutaline conversely has an effect on theophylline. Terbutaline can reduce serum-theophylline concentrations by increasing its systemic clearance. This may, or may not, have clinical implications, as improved clinical scores have still occurred with combined therapy despite the theophylline concentration being lower than when used alone; if respiratory symptoms persist, an increase in dosage may be contemplated while monitoring theophylline side-effects and concentration.[2]


1. Smith SR, Kendall MJ. Potentiation of the adverse effects of intravenous terbutaline by oral theophylline. *Br J Clin Pharmacol* 1986; **21:** 451–3.
2. Garty M, *et al.* Increased theophylline clearance in asthmatic patients due to terbutaline. *Eur J Clin Pharmacol* 1989; **36:** 25–8.


## Pharmacokinetics

Terbutaline is variably absorbed from the gastrointestinal tract and about 60% of the absorbed dose undergoes first-pass metabolism by sulfate (and some glucuronide) conjugation in the liver and the gut wall. It is accordingly excreted in the urine partly as the inactive conjugates and partly as unchanged terbutaline, the ratio depending upon the route of administration. The half-life is reported to be about 3 to 4 hours. There is some placental transfer. Trace amounts are distributed into breast milk.

**Stereoselectivity.** Terbutaline, like many other sympathomimetics, exists in two stereoisometric forms but only the (−)-enantiomer of terbutaline is pharmacologically active. Pharmacokinetic studies have been conducted on the two enantiomers and on the racemate.

The oral bioavailability of (−)-terbutaline was 14.8%, which was similar to that of the racemate; the bioavailability of (+)-terbutaline was much lower at 7.5%. The difference in bioavailability between the two enantiomers was mainly due to a difference in absorption (about 75% and 50% respectively) although a small difference in subsequent first-pass metabolism also occurred, with the (+)-isomer undergoing slightly more metabolism. It appeared that the (+)-isomer governed the elimination behaviour, both first-pass metabolism and renal clearance, of the racemate whereas the (−)-isomer determined the absorption.[1]

Other studies have also demonstrated stereoselective sulfate conjugation of terbutaline with sulfation of the (+)-enantiomer being double that of the (−)-enantiomer.[2] The primary site of terbutaline sulfation for both enantiomers appears to be in the gut and is significantly correlated with the activity of catechol sulfotransferase.[3]


1. Borgström L, *et al.* Pharmacokinetic evaluation in man of terbutaline given as separate enantiomers and as the racemate. *Br J Clin Pharmacol* 1989; **27:** 49–56.
2. Walle T, Walle UK. Stereoselective sulphate conjugation of racemic terbutaline by human liver cytosol. *Br J Clin Pharmacol* 1990; **30:** 127–33.
3. Pacifici GM, *et al.* (+) and (−) terbutaline are sulphated at a higher rate in human intestine than in the liver. *Eur J Clin Pharmacol* 1993; **45:** 483–7.


## Uses and Administration

Terbutaline sulfate is a direct-acting sympathomimetic with predominantly beta-adrenergic activity and a selective action on $beta_2$ receptors (a $beta_2$ agonist). It has actions and uses similar to those of salbutamol (p.793).

Terbutaline is given as the sulfate for its bronchodilating properties in reversible airways obstruction, as occurs in asthma (p.777) and in some patients with chronic obstructive pulmonary disease (p.779). It also decreases uterine contractility and may be used to arrest premature labour (p.794).

After inhalation, the bronchodilating effect of terbutaline usually begins within 5 minutes and lasts for about 3 to 4 hours. The onset of action following oral administration is about 30 minutes and its duration is up to 8 hours; the maximum effect occurs 2 to 3 hours after the dose.

Current asthma guidelines (see p.777) recommend that inhaled short-acting $beta_2$ agonists such as terbutaline be used on an 'as-required', not regular, basis. In those patients requiring more than occasional use of terbutaline, anti-inflammatory therapy is also needed. An increased requirement for, or decreased duration of effect of, terbutaline indicates deterioration of asthma control and the need for increased anti-inflammatory therapy.

- To relieve **acute bronchospasm** in adults and children, 1 or 2 inhalations of terbutaline sulfate 250 micrograms can be taken as required from a *metered-dose aerosol* every 4 to 6 hours, to a maximum of 8 inhalations in 24 hours. (In the USA, these inhalations may be expressed as supplying 250 micrograms, the amount delivered into the mouthpiece, or 200 micrograms, the amount delivered from the mouthpiece.)

- A breath-actuated metered-dose *powder inhaler* delivering 500 micrograms of terbutaline sulfate per inhalation is also available. One inhalation of 500 micrograms is taken when required up to a maximum of 4 inhalations in 24 hours.
- When inhalation is ineffective, terbutaline sulfate may be given *by mouth*; for adults the usual initial dose is 2.5 or 3 mg three times daily increased to 5 mg three times daily as necessary. Children's doses may be calculated on the basis of body-weight; a dose of 75 micrograms/kg three times daily is suggested. A usual dose in children over 7 years of age is 2.5 mg two or three times daily. Modified-release tablets are also available; the usual adult dose is 7.5 mg twice daily.
- Severe or unresponsive bronchospasm may require the administration of terbutaline sulfate intermittently via a *nebuliser*. A usual dose is 2 to 5 mg for children and 5 to 10 mg for adults inhaled 2 to 4 times daily. Single-dose units or a suitable dilution of a concentrated solution containing terbutaline sulfate 1% are used for this purpose. For continuous administration, a suitable adult dose is 1 to 2 mg/hour of terbutaline sulfate given as a 0.01% nebuliser solution in sodium chloride 0.9%.

Guidelines also allow for beta$_2$ agonists to be given more frequently or by continuous administration at a higher rate in acute severe asthma (see under Asthma, p.777).

- In acute severe asthma without life-threatening features where delivery via nebuliser is not available, 4 to 6 inhalations of terbutaline sulfate 250 micrograms from a metered-dose inhaler may be given at intervals of 10 to 20 minutes via a large volume spacer. In emergency life-threatening situations, 1 inhalation can be repeated 10 to 20 times by multiple actuations of a metered-dose inhaler into a spacer device. In children over 5 years of age, inhalation from a metered-dose inhaler has been as effective as the same dose given by nebulisation.
- In the treatment of severe forms of bronchospasm, terbutaline sulfate may be given by subcutaneous, intramuscular, or slow intravenous *injection*; a dose of 250 to 500 micrograms may be given up to 4 times daily. A suggested dose by injection for children over 2 years of age is 10 micrograms/kg to a maximum total dose of 300 micrograms. Terbutaline sulfate may also be given by *intravenous infusion*, as a solution containing 3 to 5 micrograms/mL at a rate of 0.5 to 1 mL/minute for adults.

Terbutaline sulfate is also used to arrest uncomplicated **premature labour** between 24 and 33 weeks of gestation. It is given by *intravenous infusion* in glucose 5%, preferably by syringe pump when the concentration is 100 micrograms/mL. If no syringe pump is available then the concentration of the infusion should be 10 micrograms/mL. The recommended initial rate of infusion is 5 micrograms/minute increased by 2.5 micrograms/minute at intervals of 20 minutes until contractions stop. Usually, a rate of up to 10 micrograms/minute is sufficient; rates in excess of 20 micrograms/minute should not be used and if that maximum rate does not delay labour then the infusion should be stopped. The maternal pulse should be monitored throughout the infusion which should be adjusted to avoid a maternal heart rate of more than 135 to 140 beats/minute. A close watch should also be kept on the patient's state of hydration since fluid overload is considered to be a key risk factor for pulmonary oedema. Once contractions have ceased and the infusion has been given for 1 hour, the dose may be decreased by 2.5 micrograms/minute at 20-minute intervals to the lowest maintenance dose that produces continued suppression of contractions. After a further 12 hours, *oral* maintenance therapy with 5 mg three times daily may be started. However, such usage is not recommended by the *British National Formulary* as the risks to the mother (see Precautions under Salbutamol, p.792) increase after 48 hours, and furthermore there is a lack of evidence of benefit from further treatment. *Subcutaneous* doses of 250 micrograms four times daily have been given for a few days before oral treatment was commenced.

**Hypoglycaemia.** Administration of terbutaline 5 mg by mouth at night reduced the risk of nocturnal hypoglycaemia in a study in patients with type 1 diabetes.[1]

1. Saleh TY, Cryer PE. Alanine and terbutaline in the prevention of nocturnal hypoglycemia in IDDM. *Diabetes Care* 1997; **20:** 1231–6.

**Systemic capillary leak syndrome.** Systemic capillary leak syndrome is a rare disorder marked by shifts of plasma from the intravascular to the extracellular space, and is often fatal. Acute attacks are treated with intravenous fluid resuscitation, but there is some anecdotal evidence that treatment with terbutaline combined with aminophylline or theophylline, both by mouth, may be useful in preventing further attacks.[1-3] Infusion of epoprostenol has also been used in acute management.[4]

1. Droder RM, *et al.* Control of systemic capillary leak syndrome with aminophylline and terbutaline. *Am J Med* 1992; **92:** 523–6.
2. Amoura Z, *et al.* Systemic capillary leak syndrome: report on 13 patients with special focus on course and treatment. *Am J Med* 1997; **103:** 514–19.
3. Tahirkheli NK, Greipp PR. Treatment of the systemic capillary leak syndrome with terbutaline and theophylline: a case series. *Ann Intern Med* 1999; **130:** 905–9.
4. Fellows IW, *et al.* Epoprostenol in systemic capillary leak syndrome. *Lancet* 1988; **ii:** 1143.

**Urticaria.** Patients with various types of urticaria unresponsive to conventional therapy with antihistamines (see p.1138) have obtained benefit from treatment with a combination of terbutaline and ketotifen; the urticarias have included chronic idiopathic urticaria,[1] dermographism,[1] and cold urticaria.[1,2] Terbutaline on its own was relatively ineffective and the mechanism of the combination was believed to be due to a stabilising effect on mast cells.[1]

1. Saihan EM. Ketotifen and terbutaline in urticaria. *Br J Dermatol* 1981; **104:** 205–6.
2. Edge JA, Osborne JP. Terbutaline and ketotifen in cold urticaria in a child. *J R Soc Med* 1989; **82:** 439–40.

## Preparations

***BP 2003:*** Terbutaline Tablets;
***USP 27:*** Terbutaline Sulfate Inhalation Aerosol; Terbutaline Sulfate Injection; Terbutaline Sulfate Tablets.

**Proprietary Preparations** (details are given in Part 3)
***Arg.:*** Bricanyl; ***Austral.:*** Bricanyl; ***Austria:*** Bricanyl; Terbutastad; ***Belg.:*** Bricanyl; ***Braz.:*** Bricanyl; ***Canad.:*** Bricanyl; ***Chile:*** Bricanyl; ***Denm.:*** Bricanyl; ***Fin.:*** Bricanyl; ***Fr.:*** Bricanyl; ***Ger.:*** Aerodur; Arubendol; Asthmo-Kranit Mono†; Asthmoprotect; Bricanyl; Butaliret; Butalitab; Contimit; Terbul; Terbuturmant; ***Gr.:*** Dracanyl; ***Hong Kong:*** Ataline; Bricanyl; Dhatalin; Terbron; Tolbin; Vida-Butaline; ***India:*** Bricanyl; ***Irl.:*** Bricanyl; ***Israel:*** Bricalin; Terbulin; ***Ital.:*** Bricanyl; ***Malaysia:*** Ataline; Bricanyl; Bucanil; Butaline; Butanil; Terbron; Terbulin; ***Mex.:*** Bricanyl; Taziken; Terbuken†; ***Neth.:*** Bricanyl; ***Norw.:*** Bricanyl; ***NZ:*** Bricanyl; ***Port.:*** Bricanyl; ***S.Afr.:*** Bricanyl; ***Singapore:*** Ataline†; Bricanyl; Bucanil; Butylin†; Tolbin; ***Spain:*** Tedipulmo; Terbasmin; ***Swed.:*** Bricanyl; ***Switz.:*** Bricanyl; ***Thai.:*** Asmaline; Asthamsian; Ataline†; Bricanyl; Broncholine; Bronco Asmo; Bucaril; Med-Broncodil; Proasma-T; Sulterline; Terbron; Terbulin; Terbuno; Vacanyl; ***UK:*** Bricanyl; Monovent; ***USA:*** Brethaire†; Brethine; Bricanyl.

**Multi-ingredient:** ***Austria:*** Bricanyl comp; ***Braz.:*** Bricanyl Composto; Broncasmin Composto†; ***Ger.:*** Bricanyl comp; Eudur†; ***Hong Kong:*** Bricanyl Expectorant; ***India:*** Asmotone Plus; Bricarex; Bro-Zedex; Broncho-solvin; Grilinctus-BM; Mucosol; Tergil; Tergil-T; Terpect; Terphylin; Theobric; Tuspel Plus; ***Irl.:*** Bricanyl Expectorant; ***Mex.:*** Bricanyl EX; ***S.Afr.:*** Bronchoped; Bronchospect; ***Spain:*** Terbasmin Expectorante; ***Thai.:*** Bricanyl Expectorant; Cofbron; Med-Broncodil Expectorant; Terbosil; Terbron Expectorant; Terbulin Expectorant†.

## Theobromine *(BAN)*

Santheose; Teobromina; Theobrominum. 3,7-Dihydro-3,7-dimethylpurine-2,6(1*H*)-dione; 3,7-Dimethylxanthine.

$C_7H_8N_4O_2$ = 180.2.
*CAS — 83-67-0.*
*ATC — C03BD01; R03DA07.*

**Pharmacopoeias.** In *Eur.* (see p.vi) and *Pol.*

**Ph. Eur. 5.0** (Theobromine). A white powder. Very slightly soluble in water and in dehydrated alcohol; slightly soluble in ammonia. It dissolves in dilute solutions of alkali hydroxides and in mineral acids.

### Profile

Theobromine has the general properties of the other xanthines (see Theophylline, p.798). It has a weaker activity than theophylline or caffeine and has practically no stimulant effect on the CNS. Large doses can cause nausea and vomiting. Theobromine has been used for its bronchodilating properties and in the treatment of cardiovascular disorders. Theobromine and calcium salicylate (theosalicin), theobromine and sodium acetate, and theobromine and sodium salicylate (themisalum, theobromsal) have all been used similarly to theobromine.

Theobromine is the chief xanthine in the beverage cocoa (p.1765). It is also present in chocolate and in small amounts in tea. Theobroma oil may contain up to 2% theobromine.

### Preparations

**Proprietary Preparations** (details are given in Part 3)
**Multi-ingredient:** ***Austria:*** Asthma-Hilfe; ***Braz.:*** Urodonal†; ***Ger.:*** Angiocardyl N†; ***Spain:*** Propyre T†.

## Theophylline *(BAN)*

Anhydrous Theophylline; Teofilina; Teofillina; Theophyllinum. 3,7-Dihydro-1,3-dimethylpurine-2,6(1*H*)-dione; 1,3-Dimethylxanthine.

$C_7H_8N_4O_2$ = 180.2.
*CAS — 58-55-9.*
*ATC — R03DA04.*

**Pharmacopoeias.** In *Eur.* (see p.vi), *Jpn, Pol., US,* and *Viet.* Some pharmacopoeias include anhydrous and hydrated theophylline in one monograph.

**Ph. Eur. 5.0** (Theophylline). A white crystalline powder. Slightly soluble in water; sparingly soluble in dehydrated alcohol. It dissolves in solutions of alkali hydroxides, in ammonia, and in mineral acids.

**USP 27** (Theophylline). It contains one molecule of water of hydration or is anhydrous. It is a white, odourless, crystalline powder. Slightly soluble in water, more soluble in hot water; sparingly soluble in alcohol, in chloroform, and in ether; freely soluble in solutions of alkali hydroxides and in ammonia.

## Theophylline Hydrate *(BANM)*

Teofilina hidrato; Theophylline Monohydrate; Theophyllinum Monohydricum.

$C_7H_8N_4O_2,H_2O$ = 198.2.
*CAS — 5967-84-0.*
*ATC — R03DA04.*

**Pharmacopoeias.** In *Chin., Eur.* (see p.vi), *Pol., US,* and *Viet.* Some pharmacopoeias include anhydrous and hydrated theophylline in one monograph.

**Ph. Eur. 5.0** (Theophylline Monohydrate; Theophylline Hydrate BP 2003). A white crystalline powder. Slightly soluble in water; sparingly soluble in dehydrated alcohol. It dissolves in solutions of alkali hydroxides, in ammonia, and in mineral acids.

**USP 27** (Theophylline). It contains one molecule of water of hydration or is anhydrous. It is a white, odourless, crystalline powder. Slightly soluble in water, more soluble in hot water; sparingly soluble in alcohol, in chloroform, and in ether; freely soluble in solutions of alkali hydroxides and in ammonia.

**Stability.** Alcohol-free theophylline liquid repackaged in clear or amber polypropylene oral syringes could be stored at room temperature under continuous fluorescent lighting for at least 180 days without significant change in the concentration of theophylline.[1] However, it was recommended that solutions be protected from light because of the potential for discoloration.

1. Johnson CE, Drabik BT. Stability of alcohol-free theophylline liquid repackaged in plastic oral syringes. *Am J Hosp Pharm* 1989; **46:** 980–1.

### Adverse Effects

The side-effects commonly encountered with theophylline and xanthine derivatives irrespective of the route of administration, are gastrointestinal irritation and stimulation of the CNS. Serum concentrations of theophylline greater than 20 micrograms/mL (110 micromol/litre) are associated with an increased risk of adverse effects (but see below).

Theophylline may cause nausea, vomiting, abdominal pain, diarrhoea, gastro-oesophageal reflux, and other gastrointestinal disturbances, insomnia, headache, anxiety, restlessness, dizziness, tremor, and palpitations. Overdosage may also lead to agitation, diuresis and repeated vomiting (sometimes haematemesis) and consequent dehydration, cardiac arrhythmias including tachycardia, hypotension, electrolyte disturbances including profound hypokalaemia, hyperglycaemia, metabolic acidosis, convulsions, and death. Severe toxicity may not be preceded by milder symptoms. Convulsions, cardiac arrhythmias, and hypotension may follow intravenous injection, particularly if the injection is too rapid, and sudden deaths have been reported; the drug is too irritant for intramuscular use. Proctitis may follow repeated administration of suppositories.

◊ Adverse effects are uncommon at serum-theophylline concentrations of 5 to 10 micrograms/mL but begin to become more frequent at 15 micrograms/mL or above, and are greatly increased in frequency and severity at concentrations greater than 20 micrograms/mL.[1-3] The severity of toxicity is generally correlated with age, underlying disease, and serum-theophylline concentration, but a distinction has been made between acute and chronic theophylline intoxication; symptoms appear to occur at a lower theophylline concentration in chronic toxicity than following acute ingestion of large amounts.[1,2,4] Young infants and the elderly (over 60 years) appear to be at particular risk from chronic intoxication with theophylline.[5,6] Common clinical manifestations of theophylline toxicity following overdosage of aminophylline or theophylline include nausea, vomiting, diarrhoea, agitation, tremor, hypertonicity, hyperventilation, supraventricular and ventricular arrhythmias, hypotension, and seizures. Metabolic disturbances such as hypokalaemia, hyperglycaemia, hypophosphataemia, hypercalcaemia, metabolic acidosis, and respiratory alkalosis often occur.[1-3] Other toxic effects reported include dementia,[7] toxic psychosis,[8] symptoms of acute pancreatitis,[9] rhabdomyolysis[10-12] with associated renal failure,[10] and acute compartment syndrome.[13]

Serious toxic symptoms may not be preceded by minor symptoms. In acute intoxication with sustained-release preparations the onset of major toxic symptoms may be delayed for up to 24 hours[1] and prolonged monitoring of such patients is required. Patients have recovered despite serum-theophylline concentrations in excess of 200 micrograms/mL[11,13] but fatalities have occurred with much lower serum concentrations.[9,14,15] Mortality in severe poisoning may be as high as 10%.


1. Dawson AH, Whyte IM. The assessment and treatment of theophylline poisoning. *Med J Aust* 1989; **151:** 689–93.
2. Minton NA, Henry JA. Acute and chronic human toxicity of theophylline. *Hum Exp Toxicol* 1996; **15:** 471–81.
3. Hardy CC, Smith J. Adverse reactions profile: theophylline and aminophylline. *Prescribers' J* 1997; **37:** 96–101.
4. Olson KR, *et al.* Theophylline overdose: acute single ingestion versus chronic repeated overmedication. *Am J Emerg Med* 1985; **3:** 386–94.
5. Shannon M, Lovejoy FH. Effect of acute versus chronic intoxication on clinical features of theophylline poisoning in children. *J Pediatr* 1992; **121:** 125–30.
6. Shannon M. Predictors of major toxicity after theophylline overdose. *Ann Intern Med* 1993; **119:** 1161–7.
7. Drummond I. Aminophylline toxicity in the elderly. *BMJ* 1982; **285:** 779–80.
8. Wasser WG, *et al.* Theophylline madness. *Ann Intern Med* 1981; **95:** 191.
9. Burgan THS, *et al.* Fatal overdose of theophylline simulating acute pancreatitis. *BMJ* 1982; **284:** 939–40.
10. Macdonald JB, *et al.* Rhabdomyolysis and acute renal failure after theophylline overdose. *Lancet* 1985; **i:** 932–3.
11. Rumpf KW, *et al.* Rhabdomyolysis after theophylline overdose. *Lancet* 1985; **i:** 1451–2.
12. Modi KB, *et al.* Theophylline poisoning and rhabdomyolysis. *Lancet* 1985; **ii:** 160–1.
13. Lloyd DM, *et al.* Acute compartment syndrome secondary to theophylline overdose. *Lancet* 1990; **ii:** 312.
14. Whyte KF, Addis GJ. Toxicity of salbutamol and theophylline together. *Lancet* 1983; **ii:** 618–19.
15. Davies RJ, Hawkey CJ. Fatal theophylline toxicity precipitated by in situ pulmonary artery thrombosis. *Postgrad Med J* 1989; **65:** 49–50.


**Effects on carbohydrate metabolism.** Hyperglycaemia is a frequent feature of theophylline intoxication, and is thought to be secondary to theophylline-induced adrenal catecholamine release.[1,2] Whether the effects on blood glucose are significant at more modest serum concentrations of theophylline is unclear, although in 29 preterm infants, mean plasma-glucose concentrations were significantly higher after treatment with intravenous aminophylline and oral theophylline than in those not treated. Two of 15 treated infants developed clinically significant hyperglycaemia and glycosuria. It was recommended that plasma-glucose concentrations be monitored in preterm infants receiving theophylline.[3]


1. Kearney TE, *et al.* Theophylline toxicity and the beta-adrenergic system. *Ann Intern Med* 1985; **102:** 766–9.
2. Shannon M. Hypokalemia, hyperglycemia and plasma catecholamine activity after severe theophylline intoxication. *J Toxicol Clin Toxicol* 1994; **32:** 41–7.
3. Srinivasan G, *et al.* Plasma glucose changes in preterm infants during oral theophylline therapy. *J Pediatr* 1983; **103:** 473–6.


**Effects on electrolytes.** Hypokalaemia is a common metabolic disturbance in theophylline intoxication, but it has also been reported[1] in patients with plasma-theophylline concentrations within the therapeutic range. It is considered to be secondary to theophylline-induced adrenal catecholamine release, with cellular influx of potassium ions.[2] It is recommended[1] that plasma-potassium is monitored during intravenous theophylline therapy particularly if other drugs predisposing to hypokalaemia are also administered (see also Interactions, below). Hypophosphataemia[1,3] and hyponatraemia[1] can also occur at therapeutic plasma-theophylline concentrations. Hypomagnesaemia[4] and hypercalcaemia[5] have occurred in theophylline overdose.


1. Zantvoort FA, *et al.* Theophylline and serum electrolytes. *Ann Intern Med* 1986; **104:** 134–5.
2. Minton NA, Henry JA. Acute and chronic human toxicity of theophylline. *Hum Exp Toxicol* 1996; **15:** 471–81.
3. Laaban J-P, *et al.* Hypophosphatemia complicating management of acute severe asthma. *Ann Intern Med* 1990; **112:** 68–9.
4. Hall KW, *et al.* Metabolic abnormalities associated with intentional theophylline overdose. *Ann Intern Med* 1984; **101:** 457–62.
5. McPherson ML, *et al.* Theophylline-induced hypercalcemia. *Ann Intern Med* 1986; **105:** 52–4.


**Effects on the heart.** ARRHYTHMIAS. Theophylline or aminophylline can precipitate sinus tachycardia and supraventricular and ventricular premature contractions at therapeutic serum-theophylline concentrations[1] and in overdose.[2,3] Multifocal atrial tachycardia has also been associated with both theophylline overdose[2] and serum-theophylline concentrations within the generally accepted therapeutic range of 10 to 20 micrograms/mL.[4] Use of theophylline with beta-adrenoceptor stimulants by mouth is associated with a significant increase in the mean heart rate.[5,6]


1. Josephson GW, *et al.* Cardiac dysrhythmias during the treatment of acute asthma: a comparison of two treatment regimens by a double blind protocol. *Chest* 1980; **78:** 429–35.
2. Greenberg A, *et al.* Severe theophylline toxicity: role of conservative measures, antiarrhythmic agents, and charcoal hemoperfusion. *Am J Med* 1984; **76:** 854–60.
3. Minton NA, Henry JA. Acute and chronic human toxicity of theophylline. *Hum Exp Toxicol* 1996; **15:** 471–81.
4. Levine JH, *et al.* Multifocal atrial tachycardia: a toxic effect of theophylline. *Lancet* 1985; **i:** 12–14.
5. Coleman JJ, *et al.* Cardiac arrhythmias during the combined use of β-adrenergic agonist drugs and theophylline. *Chest* 1986; **90:** 45–51.
6. Conradson T-B, *et al.* Arrhythmogenicity from combined bronchodilator therapy in patients with obstructive lung disease and concomitant ischemic heart disease. *Chest* 1987; **91:** 5–9.


**Effects on the kidneys.** For a report of rhabdomyolysis-induced acute renal failure occurring after aminophylline overdose, see the general discussion on toxicity, above.

**Effects on mental function.** As mentioned in the general discussion on toxicity above, theophylline toxicity has been associated with reports of dementia and toxic psychosis, as well as the more common adverse effects of anxiety and restlessness.

LEARNING AND BEHAVIOUR PROBLEMS. Several small studies[1-3] have suggested that theophylline may be associated with learning and behaviour problems in children, especially those with a low IQ. However, the FDA has concluded[4] that such studies provide insufficient evidence to support an adverse effect of theophylline on learning behaviour or school performance. Other studies have found no marked behavioural side-effects that could be attributed to theophylline.[5,6] Additionally, academic achievement generally appeared to be unaffected by either asthma or by treatment with appropriate doses of theophylline.[7]


1. Furukawa CT, *et al.* Learning and behaviour problems associated with theophylline therapy. *Lancet* 1984; **i:** 621.
2. Springer C, *et al.* Clinical, physiologic, and psychologic comparison of treatment by cromolyn or theophylline in childhood asthma. *J Allergy Clin Immunol* 1985; **76:** 64–9.
3. Schlieper A, *et al.* Effect of therapeutic plasma concentrations of theophylline on behavior, cognitive processing, and affect in children with asthma. *J Pediatr* 1991; **118:** 449–55.
4. Anonymous. Theophylline and school performance. *FDA Drug Bull* 1988; **18:** 32–3.
5. Bender B, Milgrom H. Theophylline-induced behavior change in children: an objective evaluation of parents' perceptions. *JAMA* 1992; **267:** 2621–4.
6. Bender BG, *et al.* Neuropsychological behavioral changes in asthmatic children treated with beclomethasone dipropionate versus theophylline. *Pediatrics* 1998; **101:** 355–60.
7. Lindgren S, *et al.* Does asthma or treatment with theophylline limit children's academic performance? *N Engl J Med* 1992; **327:** 926–30.


**Effects on the nervous system.** CONVULSIONS. The risk of convulsions with acute theophylline toxicity is low at serum theophylline concentrations less than 60 micrograms/mL;[1] seizures are most likely in patients with peak concentrations above 100 micrograms/mL.[2] However, the risk of seizures is much greater after chronic overdosage;[1,2] seizure activity has been reported at serum concentrations just above or even within the therapeutic range.[3] Elderly patients or those with previous brain injury or neurological disease may be at increased risk,[2-4] although some have questioned the association.[1] The outcome of seizures appears to be variable: death and severe neurological deficit have occurred,[2,3] but other series have recorded recovery without serious morbidity.[4]


1. Paloucek FP, Rodvold KA. Evaluation of theophylline overdoses and toxicities. *Ann Emerg Med* 1988; **17:** 135–44.
2. Olson KR, *et al.* Theophylline overdose: acute single ingestion versus chronic repeated overmedication. *Am J Emerg Med* 1985; **3:** 386–94.
3. Bahls FH, *et al.* Theophylline-associated seizures with "therapeutic" or low toxic serum concentrations: risk factors for serious outcome in adults. *Neurology* 1991; **41:** 1309–12.
4. Covelli HD, *et al.* Predisposing factors to apparent theophylline-induced seizures. *Ann Allergy* 1985; **54:** 411–15.


**Effects on the skin.** For reports of cutaneous reactions to theophylline and aminophylline, see under Hypersensitivity, below.

**Effects on the urinary tract.** Although diuresis is more commonly seen, urinary retention has been reported in male patients during therapy with aminophylline[1] or theophylline.[2]


1. Owens GR, Tannenbaum R. Theophylline-induced urinary retention. *Ann Intern Med* 1981; **94:** 212–13.
2. Prakash M, Washburne JD. Theophylline and urinary retention. *Ann Intern Med* 1981; **94:** 823.


**Hypersensitivity.** Hypersensitivity reactions have been reported following oral or intravenous administration of aminophylline. Reactions include erythematous rash with pruritus,[1,2] erythroderma,[2] and exfoliative dermatitis.[3] Aminophylline can produce both type I (immediate) and type IV (delayed) hypersensitivity reactions, the latter being due to the ethylenediamine component and can be confirmed by skin patch tests.[1-3] If hypersensitivity to ethylenediamine is confirmed it is recommended that aminophylline is avoided and treatment continued with theophylline or another theophylline salt.[1,3,4] Hypersensitivity reactions to theophylline have been reported rarely but type I reactions have occurred.[4] An erythematous, maculopapular rash has been reported[5] during treatment with a modified-release theophylline preparation which did not occur when another modified-release theophylline product was given.


1. Hardy C, *et al.* Allergy to aminophylline. *BMJ* 1983; **286:** 2051–2.
2. Mohsenifar Z, *et al.* Two cases of allergy to aminophylline. *Ann Allergy* 1982; **49:** 281–2.
3. Nierenberg DW, Glazener FS. Aminophylline-induced exfoliative dermatitis: cause and implications. *West J Med* 1982; **137:** 328–31.
4. Gibb WRG. Delayed-type hypersensitivity to theophylline/aminophylline. *Lancet* 1985; **i:** 49.
5. Mendel S, *et al.* Dermatologic reaction to a sustained-release theophylline product. *Clin Pharm* 1985; **4:** 334–5.


**Hyperuricaemia.** In a study of 112 asthmatic patients receiving modified-release theophylline 200 to 400 mg 12-hourly, there was a significant correlation of serum-uric acid concentrations and serum-theophylline concentrations.[1] Gout has been reported in a woman receiving theophylline and aminophylline;[2] her serum-uric acid concentration was increased while receiving the xanthines, but subsequently fell when they were discontinued, and rose again when treatment was resumed.


1. Morita Y, *et al.* Theophylline increases serum uric acid levels. *J Allergy Clin Immunol* 1984; **74:** 707–12.
2. Toda K, *et al.* Gout due to xanthine derivatives. *Br J Rheumatol* 1997; **36:** 1131–2.


**Necrotising enterocolitis.** Although there have been reports of neonatal necrotising enterocolitis associated with oral theophylline and aminophylline administration,[1,2] a study of 275 infants concluded that theophylline did not significantly contribute to its development.[3] It has been suggested that the high osmolality of liquid feeds and drugs including oral theophylline preparations may be involved in the aetiology of necrotising enterocolitis.[4]


1. Robinson MJ, *et al.* Xanthines and necrotising enterocolitis. *Arch Dis Child* 1980; **55:** 494–5.
2. Williams AJ. Xanthines and necrotising enterocolitis. *Arch Dis Child* 1980; **55:** 973–4.
3. Davis JM, *et al.* Role of theophylline in pathogenesis of necrotizing enterocolitis. *J Pediatr* 1986; **109:** 344–7.
4. Watkinson M, *et al.* Hyperosmolar preparations for neonates. *Pharm J* 1987; **241:** 488.


**Withdrawal syndromes.** Episodes of apnoea beginning 28 hours after birth and increasing in frequency and severity over the next 4 days occurred in a neonate whose mother had taken aminophylline and theophylline throughout pregnancy. Measurement of serum-theophylline concentration showed the increasing apnoea was coincident with falling theophylline concentration and administration of theophylline to the infant resulted in resolution of apnoea; treatment was discontinued after 4 months.[1]

Worsening asthma control may occur when theophylline is withdrawn; there is some evidence of a rebound deterioration in lung function due to the development of tolerance.[2]


1. Horowitz DA, *et al.* Apnea associated with theophylline withdrawal in a term neonate. *Am J Dis Child* 1982; **136:** 73–4.
2. Bennett JA, *et al.* The airway effects of stopping regular oral theophylline in patients with asthma. *Br J Clin Pharmacol* 1998; **45:** 402–4.


## Treatment of Adverse Effects

After theophylline or aminophylline overdosage by mouth the stomach may be emptied by lavage if within 2 hours of the overdose. Elimination may be enhanced by repeated oral doses of activated charcoal regardless of the route of theophylline overdose (see below). An osmotic laxative may also be considered, especially if modified-release preparations have been taken. Treatment is symptomatic and supportive. Serum-theophylline concentrations should be monitored and if modified-release preparations have been taken monitoring should be prolonged. Metabolic abnormalities, particularly hypokalaemia, should be corrected; hypokalaemia may be so severe as to require intravenous infusion of potassium under ECG monitoring. In the non-asthmatic patient extreme tachycardia, hypokalaemia, and hyperglycaemia may be reversed by a non-selective beta blocker (see also below). Isolated convulsions may be controlled by the intravenous administration of diazepam or a barbiturate; phenytoin may not be effective. In the most refractory cases general anaesthesia, and neuromuscular blockade, with ventilation, may be required. Ventricular arrhythmias in a patient who is having convulsions may be best treated with disopyramide rather than lidocaine or mexiletine since the latter may exacerbate convulsions.

Charcoal haemoperfusion or haemodialysis may be required.

◊ Reviews.


1. Dawson AH, Whyte IM. The assessment and treatment of theophylline poisoning. *Med J Aust* 1989; **151:** 689–93.
2. Skinner MH. Adverse reactions and interactions with theophylline. *Drug Safety* 1990; **5:** 275–85.
3. Minton NA, Henry JA. Treatment of theophylline overdose. *Am J Emerg Med* 1996; **14:** 606–12.


**Activated charcoal.** Multiple-dose oral activated charcoal (p.1030) is considered the cornerstone of treatment for theophylline and xanthine poisoning. It reduces the absorption of orally administered theophylline, and also enhances the elimination of theophylline from the body even after absorption or intravenous xanthine administration. Aggressive antiemetic therapy may be required to allow administration and retention of activated charcoal, since theophylline toxicity causes protracted vomiting. A cathartic such as sorbitol may be given with the activated charcoal to aid elimination of theophylline, but can cause fluid and electrolyte disturbances. For oral theophylline overdose the use of gastric lavage before oral activated charcoal administration may not be better than activated charcoal alone.

References.


1. Neuvonen PJ, *et al.* Comparison of activated charcoal and ipecac syrup in prevention of drug absorption. *Eur J Clin Pharmacol* 1983; **24:** 557–62.
2. Berlinger WG, *et al.* Enhancement of theophylline clearance by oral activated charcoal. *Clin Pharmacol Ther* 1983; **33:** 351–4.
3. Mahutte CK, *et al.* Increased serum theophylline clearance with orally administered activated charcoal. *Am Rev Respir Dis* 1983; **128:** 820–2.
4. Park GD, *et al.* Effects of size and frequency of oral doses of charcoal on theophylline clearance. *Clin Pharmacol Ther* 1983; **34:** 663–6.
5. Goldberg MJ, *et al.* The effect of sorbitol and activated charcoal on serum theophylline concentrations after slow-release theophylline. *Clin Pharmacol Ther* 1987; **41:** 108–11.
6. Al-Shareef AH, *et al.* The effects of charcoal and sorbitol (alone and in combination) on plasma theophylline concentrations after a sustained-release formulation. *Hum Exp Toxicol* 1990; **9:** 179–82.
7. Minton NA, *et al.* Prevention of drug absorption in simulated theophylline overdose. *Hum Exp Toxicol* 1995; **14:** 170–4.


**Beta blockers.** Infusion of propranolol following theophylline overdose in 2 patients was associated with improvement in hyperglycaemia, hypokalaemia, tachycardia, and hypotension. Beta-adrenergic blockade may therefore be of benefit in the management of the metabolic changes of theophylline poisoning, especially in the non-asthmatic patient.[1,2] However, in asthmatic patients, beta blockers should be reserved for those with severe hypokalaemia or cardiac arrhythmias when mechanical ventilation is available as beta blockers can cause bronchoconstriction.[1,2] Propranolol reduces the clearance of theophylline (see under Interactions, below) and it has been suggested that a non-interacting beta blocker may be more appropriate.[3] Esmolol has been used successfully to manage cardiovascular symptoms of overdosage.[4]


1. Kearney TE, *et al.* Theophylline toxicity and the beta-adrenergic system. *Ann Intern Med* 1985; **102:** 766–9.
2. Amin DN, Henry JA. Propranolol administration in theophylline overdose. *Lancet* 1985; **i:** 520–1.
3. Farrar KT, Dunn AM. Beta-blockers in treatment of theophylline overdose. *Lancet* 1985; **i:** 983.
4. Seneff M, *et al.* Acute theophylline toxicity and the use of esmolol to reverse cardiovascular instability. *Ann Emerg Med* 1990; **19:** 671–3.


**Endoscopy.** Absorption is delayed following overdosage with modified-release oral preparations of aminophylline or theophylline and may be further prolonged by the formation of tablet aggregates, or bezoars, in the stomach.[1-3] Of 11 patients admitted with overdosage, one vomited a bezoar, 2 had bezoars removed at gastroscopy, and in one a bezoar was found at necropsy.[3] If bezoar formation occurs gastric lavage and activated charcoal will have little if any effect and the patient may appear to stabilise before experiencing increasing serum-theophylline concentration and clinical deterioration;[1,2] fatalities have been reported.[1] Endoscopy should be considered in cases of modified-release theophylline overdosage in which clinical signs and serial concentration measurements suggest continuing drug absorption.[2]


1. Coupe M. Self-poisoning with sustained-release aminophylline: a mechanism for observed secondary rise in serum theophylline. *Hum Toxicol* 1986; **5:** 341–2.
2. Cereda J-M, *et al.* Endoscopic removal of pharmacobezoar of slow release theophylline. *BMJ* 1986; **293:** 1143.
3. Smith WDF. Endoscopic removal of a pharmacobezoar of slow release theophylline. *BMJ* 1987; **294:** 125.


**Haemodialysis and haemoperfusion.** Extracorporeal theophylline removal techniques following overdosage of aminophylline or theophylline have been reviewed.[1] Neither peritoneal dialysis nor exchange transfusion produced a significant increase in the total body clearance of theophylline, whereas haemodialysis could be expected to double clearance, and haemoperfusion results in four- to sixfold increases in clearance. Charcoal haemoperfusion should be considered if the plasma-theophylline concentration exceeds 100 micrograms/mL in an acute intoxication, or 60 micrograms/mL in chronic overdose (40 micrograms/mL if there is significant respiratory or heart failure, or liver disease) though plasma concentrations alone should not determine its use (see under Adverse Effects, above). If there is intractable vomiting, arrhythmias, or seizures charcoal haemoperfusion should be commenced without delay. In most patients a 4-hour haemoperfusion allows significant clinical improvement, but treatment should continue until plasma concentrations are below 15 micrograms/mL. Plasma concentrations should be followed at least every 4 hours for the first 12 hours post-perfusion, as rebound increases have been noted on terminating perfusion. Haemodialysis may rarely be an alternative if haemoperfusion is not available, or in series with haemoperfusion if significant rhabdomyolysis is present. There has been a case report[2] of continuous venovenous haemofiltration used to treat severe theophylline toxicity.


1. Heath A, Knudsen K. Role of extracorporeal drug removal in acute theophylline poisoning: a review. *Med Toxicol* 1987; **2:** 294–308.
2. Henderson JH, *et al.* Continuous venovenous haemofiltration for the treatment of theophylline toxicity. *Thorax* 2001; **56:** 242–3.


## Precautions

Theophylline or aminophylline should be given with caution to patients with peptic ulceration, hyperthyroidism, hypertension, cardiac arrhythmias or other cardiovascular disease, or epilepsy, as these conditions may be exacerbated. They should also be given with caution to patients with heart failure, hepatic dysfunction or chronic alcoholism, acute febrile illness, and to neonates and the elderly, since in all of these circumstances theophylline clearance may be decreased, resulting in increases in serum-theophylline concentrations and serum half-life. Conversely, smoking increases theophylline clearance. Many drugs interact with theophylline; for details see Interactions, below.

Intravenous injections of theophylline or aminophylline must be administered very slowly to prevent dangerous CNS and cardiovascular side-effects resulting from the direct stimulant effect.

Dosage requirements of theophylline vary widely between subjects; in view of the many factors affecting theophylline pharmacokinetics, serum concentration monitoring is necessary to ensure concentrations are within the therapeutic range.

Patients should not be transferred from one modified-release theophylline or aminophylline preparation to another without clinical assessment and the measurement of serum-theophylline concentrations because of bioavailability differences.

**Acute febrile illness.** A reduction in theophylline clearance has been noted in patients presenting with acute respiratory illness[1] and appears to be associated with the severity of the underlying pulmonary disease and the rate of change in the patient's condition.[2] Caution has been advised in administering theophylline to patients with chronic obstructive pulmonary disease with acute exacerbations of a concomitant respiratory illness such as pneumonia since these patients appear most likely to exhibit altered theophylline metabolism.[2]

Similarly, a decrease in theophylline clearance and an increase in the incidence of adverse effects has been reported during acute viral infections such as influenza in children receiving theophylline therapy for chronic asthma.[3,4] Influenza vaccination has also been reported to reduce theophylline clearance (see Interactions, below). The mechanism by which theophylline metabolism is reduced in these patients may be related to increased interferon production during the acute febrile response. A dosage reduction of one half has been recommended[5] in children receiving chronic theophylline therapy who are febrile for more than 24 hours. Further dose adjustments should be based on serum-theophylline concentrations until the patients have recovered from their acute illness and are restabilised on their usual dosage. However, conflicting results have been reported and in one controlled study respiratory syncytial virus infection was found to have no significant effect on theophylline disposition in children.[6]


1. Vozeh S, *et al.* Changes in theophylline clearance during acute illness. *JAMA* 1978; **240:** 1882–4.
2. Richer M, Lam YWF. Hypoxia, arterial pH and theophylline disposition. *Clin Pharmacokinet* 1993; **25:** 283–99.
3. Chang KC, *et al.* Altered theophylline pharmacokinetics during acute respiratory viral illness. *Lancet* 1978; **i:** 1132–3.
4. Kraemer MJ, *et al.* Altered theophylline clearance during an influenza B outbreak. *Pediatrics* 1982; **69:** 476–80.
5. American Academy of Pediatrics Committee on Drugs. Precautions concerning the use of theophylline. *Pediatrics* 1992; **89:** 781–3.
6. Muslow HA, *et al.* Lack of effect of respiratory syncytial virus infection on theophylline disposition in children. *J Pediatr* 1992; **121:** 466–71.


**Age.** For the effects of age on the metabolism and excretion of theophylline see under Pharmacokinetics, below. Dosage regimens for infants are discussed under Administration in Infants, in Uses and Administration, below.

**Breast feeding.** From one study of 3 lactating women it was estimated that less than 1% of the total theophylline eliminated was found in breast milk.[1] Another study of 5 women estimated that a breast-fed infant would receive less than 10% of the maternal dose of theophylline.[2] These amounts were considered unlikely to cause toxicity, but it has been reported that irritability in one infant seemed to occur on the intermittent days when the mother took aminophylline. The American Academy of Pediatrics[3] states that theophylline is usually compatible with breast feeding, although it has noted that irritability has been reported in infants whose mothers were receiving theophylline.


1. Stec GP, *et al.* Kinetics of theophylline transfer to breast milk. *Clin Pharmacol Ther* 1980; **28:** 404–8.
2. Yurchak AM, Jusko WJ. Theophylline secretion into breast milk. *Pediatrics* 1976; **57:** 518–20.
3. American Academy of Pediatrics. The transfer of drugs and other chemicals into human milk. *Pediatrics* 2001; **108:** 776–89. Correction. *ibid.*; 1029. Also available at: http://aappolicy.aappublications.org/cgi/content/full/pediatrics%3b108/3/776 (accessed 21/04/04)


**ECT.** Patients receiving theophylline are at risk of prolonged seizures during ECT, and status epilepticus has been reported.[1,2] The ability of theophylline to prolong seizures has led to it being used as an adjunct in ECT.[3] Caffeine has been used similarly, see p.783.


1. Peters SG, *et al.* Status epilepticus as a complication of concurrent electroconvulsive and theophylline therapy. *Mayo Clin Proc* 1984; **59:** 568–70.
2. Rasmussen KG, Zorumski CF. Electroconvulsive therapy in patients taking theophylline. *J Clin Psychiatry* 1993; **54:** 427–31.
3. Leentjens AFG, *et al.* Facilitation of ECT by intravenous administration of theophylline. *Convuls Ther* 1996; **12:** 232–7.


**Porphyria.** Theophylline has been associated with acute attacks of porphyria and is considered unsafe in porphyric patients.

**Pregnancy.** It has been recommended[1] that serum-theophylline concentrations are measured at monthly intervals throughout pregnancy and 1 and 4 weeks after delivery since the pharmacokinetics of theophylline may be altered. An increase in the volume of distribution of theophylline, a decrease in plasma-protein binding, and a continuing decrease in clearance throughout pregnancy have been noted in some patients, especially during the later part of pregnancy,[2-4] but other studies have noted an increase in theophylline clearance during pregnancy.[1,5] Some studies have found that after delivery there is a return of clearance values to those existing before pregnancy,[2] while others have not.[4]

In a study of 12 neonates whose mothers received various theophylline preparations throughout their pregnancies[6] maternal, cord, and neonatal heelstick theophylline concentrations were not notably different, and ranged from 2.3 to 19.6 micrograms/mL. Transient jitteriness was seen in 2 neonates and tachycardia in one, at cord theophylline concentrations of 11.7 to 17 micrograms/mL. There were no instances of vomiting, seizure, arrhythmias, diarrhoea, or feeding disturbances, which had been reported previously.


1. Rubin PC. Prescribing in pregnancy: general principles. *BMJ* 1986; **293:** 1415–17.
2. Carter BL, *et al.* Theophylline clearance during pregnancy. *Obstet Gynecol* 1986; **68:** 555–9.
3. Frederiksen MC, *et al.* Theophylline pharmacokinetics in pregnancy. *Clin Pharmacol Ther* 1986; **40:** 321–8.
4. Gardner MJ, *et al.* Longitudinal effects of pregnancy on the pharmacokinetics of theophylline. *Eur J Clin Pharmacol* 1987; **31:** 289–95.
5. Romero R, *et al.* Pharmacokinetics of intravenous theophylline in pregnant patients at term. *Am J Perinatol* 1983; **1:** 31–5.
6. Labovitz E, Spector S. Placental theophylline transfer in pregnant asthmatics. *JAMA* 1982; **247:** 786–8.


**Renal impairment.** Theophylline is eliminated mainly by hepatic metabolism and usual doses of aminophylline or theophylline can be given to patients with renal impairment. In patients undergoing haemodialysis the clearance of theophylline is increased and its elimination half-life reduced; mean values of 84.8 and 83 mL/minute and 2.5 and 2.3 hours respectively have been reported.[1,2] Haemodialysis removes up to 40% of a dose of theophylline.[1] Peritoneal dialysis has little effect on the pharmacokinetics of theophylline removing about 3.2% of a dose.[1]


1. Lee C-SC, *et al.* Comparative pharmacokinetics of theophylline in peritoneal dialysis and hemodialysis. *J Clin Pharmacol* 1983; **23:** 274–80.
2. Anderson JR, *et al.* Effects of hemodialysis on theophylline kinetics. *J Clin Pharmacol* 1983; **23:** 428–32.


**Smoking.** Certain components of tobacco smoke, notably aromatic hydrocarbons, induce hepatic drug-metabolising enzymes and cigarette smoking has been reported[1-3] to increase theophylline clearance and shorten its elimination half-life. The effect of smoking may override factors that tend to decrease theophylline clearance, such as old age.[4] The duration of enzyme induction after stopping smoking is uncertain; theophylline clearance decreased by 38% after one week of abstinence from smoking in one study,[5] while others have found changes in clearance persisting for at least 3 months.[1] Tobacco chewing has also been reported to increase theophylline clearance,[6] but nicotine chewing gum appears to have no effect.[5]


1. Hunt SN, *et al.* Effect of smoking on theophylline disposition. *Clin Pharmacol Ther* 1976; **19:** 546–51.
2. Jusko WJ, *et al.* Enhanced biotransformation of theophylline in marihuana and tobacco smokers. *Clin Pharmacol Ther* 1978; **24:** 406–10.
3. Grygiel JJ, Birkett DJ. Cigarette smoking and theophylline clearance and metabolism. *Clin Pharmacol Ther* 1981; **30:** 491–6.
4. Cusack B, *et al.* Theophylline kinetics in relation to age: the importance of smoking. *Br J Clin Pharmacol* 1980; **10:** 109–14.
5. Lee BL, *et al.* Cigarette abstinence, nicotine gum, and theophylline disposition. *Ann Intern Med* 1987; **106:** 553–5.
6. Rockwood R, Henann N. Smokeless tobacco and theophylline clearance. *Drug Intell Clin Pharm* 1986; **20:** 624–5.


## Interactions

The toxic effects of theophylline, aminophylline, and other xanthines are additive. Use with other xanthine medications should therefore be avoided; if intravenous aminophylline is to be given for acute bronchospasm in patients who have been taking maintenance theophylline therapy, serum-theophylline concentrations should be measured first and the initial dose reduced as appropriate (see Uses and Administration, below).

Theophylline clearance may be reduced by interaction with other drugs including allopurinol, some antiarrhythmics, cimetidine, disulfiram, fluvoxamine, interferon alfa, macrolide antibacterials and quinolones, oral contraceptives, tiabendazole, and viloxazine, necessitating dosage reduction. Phenytoin and some other antiepileptics, ritonavir, rifampicin, and sulfinpyrazone may increase theophylline clearance, necessitating an increase in dose or dosing frequency. Xanthines can potentiate hypokalaemia caused by hypoxia or associated with the administration of beta$_2$-adrenoceptor stimulants (beta$_2$ agonists), corticosteroids, and diuretics. There is a risk of synergistic toxicity if theophylline is given with halothane or ketamine, and it may antagonise the effects of adenosine and of competitive neuromuscular blockers; lithium elimination may be enhanced with a consequent loss of effect. The interaction between theophylline and beta blockers is complex (see below) but concomitant use tends to be avoided on pharmacological grounds since beta blockers produce bronchospasm.

◊ Theophylline is metabolised by several hepatic cytochrome P450 isoenzymes, of which the most important seems to be CYP1A2.[1] Numerous drugs affect the metabolic clearance of theophylline and aminophylline,[2] but the variability in theophylline pharmacokinetics makes the clinical significance of these interactions difficult to predict. Giving theophylline with drugs that inhibit its metabolism should be avoided but, if unavoidable, the dose of theophylline should be halved and subsequently adjusted based on serum-theophylline monitoring.[3] Even when introducing medication for which no interaction is suspected, a check on the serum-theophylline concentration within 24 hours of beginning the new drug has been advised.[3]

Theophylline reduces liver plasma flow[4] and may therefore prolong the half-life and increase steady-state levels of hepatically eliminated drugs but it is claimed to have no effect on antipyrine clearance.[5]

1. Ha HR, *et al.* Metabolism of theophylline by cDNA-expressed human cytochromes P-450. *Br J Clin Pharmacol* 1995; **39:** 321–6.
2. Upton RA. Pharmacokinetic interactions between theophylline and other medication. *Clin Pharmacokinet* 1991; **20:** 66–80 (part I) and 135–50 (part II).
3. American Academy of Pediatrics Committee on Drugs. Precautions concerning the use of theophylline. *Pediatrics* 1992; **89:** 781–3.
4. Onrot J, *et al.* Reduction of liver plasma flow by caffeine and theophylline. *Clin Pharmacol Ther* 1986; **40:** 506–10.
5. Døssing M, *et al.* Effect of theophylline and salbutamol on hepatic drug metabolism. *Hum Toxicol* 1989; **8:** 225–8.

**Antiarrhythmics.** An increase in serum-theophylline concentration from 93.2 to 194.2 micromol/litre with symptoms of tachycardia, nervousness, and tremors occurred in a patient 9 days after starting *amiodarone* therapy.[1] Elevated theophylline concentrations and/or decreased clearance have also been reported following addition of *mexiletine* to theophylline therapy.[2-6] Amiodarone and mexiletine probably interact with theophylline through inhibition of its hepatic metabolism. *Tocainide* has also been found to impair theophylline metabolism resulting in a reduction in theophylline clearance but the effect was substantially smaller than that of mexiletine.[7] In one patient stabilised on theophylline therapy, an increase in the plasma-theophylline concentration with subsequent toxicity was noted following the initiation of treatment with *propafenone.*[8] See also under Calcium-channel Blockers, below.

1. Soto J, *et al.* Possible theophylline-amiodarone interaction. *DICP Ann Pharmacother* 1990; **24:** 1115.
2. Stanley R, *et al.* Mexiletine-theophylline interaction. *Am J Med* 1989; **86:** 733–4.
3. Ueno K, *et al.* Interaction between theophylline and mexiletine. *DICP Ann Pharmacother* 1990; **24:** 471–2.
4. Hurwitz A, *et al.* Mexiletine effects on theophylline disposition. *Clin Pharmacol Ther* 1991; **50:** 299–307.
5. Loi C-M, *et al.* Inhibition of theophylline metabolism by mexiletine in young male and female nonsmokers. *Clin Pharmacol Ther* 1991; **49:** 571–80.
6. Ueno K, *et al.* Mechanism of interaction between theophylline and mexiletine. *DICP Ann Pharmacother* 1991; **25:** 727–30.
7. Loi C-M, *et al.* The effect of tocainide on theophylline metabolism. *Br J Clin Pharmacol* 1993; **35:** 437–40.
8. Lee BL, Dohrmann ML. Theophylline toxicity after propafenone treatment: evidence for drug interaction. *Clin Pharmacol Ther* 1992; **51:** 353–5.

**Antibacterials.** IMIPENEM. Seizures have been reported in 3 patients receiving theophylline who were given imipenem,[1] although serum concentrations of theophylline were not affected.

1. Semel JD, Allen N. Seizures in patients simultaneously receiving theophylline and imipenem or ciprofloxacin or metronidazole. *South Med J* 1991; **84:** 465–8.

ISONIAZID. Isoniazid inhibits oxidative enzymes in the liver and has been found to impair the elimination of theophylline. Both clearance and volume of distribution of theophylline were reduced with an increase in serum-theophylline concentrations in healthy subjects after 14 days' pretreatment with isoniazid[1] and theophylline toxicity has been reported[2] in a patient one month after adding theophylline to isoniazid therapy.

1. Samigun, *et al.* Lowering of theophylline clearance by isoniazid in slow and rapid acetylators. *Br J Clin Pharmacol* 1990; **29:** 570–3.
2. Torrent J, *et al.* Theophylline-isoniazid interaction. *DICP Ann Pharmacother* 1989; **23:** 143–5.

MACROLIDES. There are conflicting reports of the effect of *erythromycin* on the pharmacokinetics of theophylline. Significant decreases in the clearance of theophylline and prolonged elimination half-life have been reported[1-3] but other studies have found no interaction.[4,5] It has also been noted that the serum concentrations and bioavailability of erythromycin may be reduced by theophylline.[6,7] The clearance of theophylline is also markedly decreased by *troleandomycin*,[8-10] but there have been reports that for clinical purposes the pharmacokinetics of theophylline do not seem to be significantly altered by *dirithromycin*,[11-13] *josamycin*,[9,14] *midecamycin*,[10,15,16] *rokitamycin*,[17] *roxithromycin*,[18] or *spiramycin*.[19] *Clarithromycin* also seems unlikely to have a significant effect in most patients, but in a few theophylline dosage may need to be adjusted.[20,21] In one case report, serum-theophylline concentrations fell over a few days following the withdrawal of *azithromycin*.[22]

1. Zarowitz BJM, *et al.* Effect of erythromycin base on theophylline kinetics. *Clin Pharmacol Ther* 1981; **29:** 601–5.
2. Renton KW, *et al.* Depression of theophylline elimination by erythromycin. *Clin Pharmacol Ther* 1981; **30:** 422–6.
3. May DC, *et al.* The effects of erythromycin on theophylline elimination in normal males. *J Clin Pharmacol* 1982; **22:** 125–30.
4. Maddux MS, *et al.* The effect of erythromycin on theophylline pharmacokinetics at steady state. *Chest* 1982; **81:** 563–5.
5. Hildebrandt R, *et al.* Lack of clinically important interaction between erythromycin and theophylline. *Eur J Clin Pharmacol* 1984; **26:** 485–9.
6. Iliopoulou A, *et al.* Pharmacokinetic interaction between theophylline and erythromycin. *Br J Clin Pharmacol* 1982; **14:** 495–9.
7. Paulsen O, *et al.* The interaction of erythromycin with theophylline. *Eur J Clin Pharmacol* 1987; **32:** 493–8.
8. Weinberger M, *et al.* Inhibition of theophylline clearance by troleandomycin. *J Allergy Clin Immunol* 1977; **59:** 228–31.
9. Brazier JL, *et al.* Retard d'élimination de la théophylline dû à la troléandomycine: absence d'effet de la josamycine. *Therapie* 1980; **35:** 545–9.
10. Lavarenne J, *et al.* Influence d'un nouveau macrolide, la midécamycine, sur les taux sanguins de théophylline. *Therapie* 1981; **36:** 451–6.
11. Bachmann K, *et al.* Changes in the steady-state pharmacokinetics of theophylline during treatment with dirithromycin. *J Clin Pharmacol* 1990; **30:** 1001–5.
12. Bachmann K, *et al.* Steady-state pharmacokinetics of theophylline in COPD patients treated with dirithromycin. *J Clin Pharmacol* 1993; **33:** 861–5.
13. McConnell SA, *et al.* Lack of effect of dirithromycin on theophylline pharmacokinetics in healthy volunteers. *J Antimicrob Chemother* 1999; **43:** 733–6.
14. Ruff F, *et al.* Macrolide et théophylline: absence d'interaction josamycine-théophylline. *Nouv Presse Med* 1981; **10:** 175.
15. Principi N, *et al.* Effect of miocamycin on theophylline kinetics in children. *Eur J Clin Pharmacol* 1987; **31:** 701–4.
16. Couet W, *et al.* Lack of effect of ponsinomycin on the plasma pharmacokinetics of theophylline. *Eur J Clin Pharmacol* 1989; **37:** 101–4.
17. Ishioka T. Effect of a new macrolide antibiotic, 3″-O-propionylleucomycin $A_5$ (rokitamycin) on serum concentrations of theophylline and digoxin in the elderly. *Acta Ther* 1987; **13:** 17–24.
18. Saint-Salvi B, *et al.* A study of the interaction of roxithromycin with theophylline and carbamazepine. *J Antimicrob Chemother* 1987; **20** (suppl B): 121–9.
19. Debruyne D, *et al.* Spiramycin has no effect on serum theophylline in asthmatic patients. *Eur J Clin Pharmacol* 1986; **30:** 505–7.
20. Bachand RT. Comparative study of clarithromycin and ampicillin in the treatment of patients with acute bacterial exacerbations of chronic bronchitis. *J Antimicrob Chemother* 1991; **27** (suppl A): 91–100.
21. Gillum JG, *et al.* Effect of combination therapy with ciprofloxacin and clarithromycin on theophylline pharmacokinetics in healthy volunteers. *Antimicrob Agents Chemother* 1996; **40:** 1715–16.
22. Pollak PT, Slayter KL. Reduced serum theophylline concentrations after discontinuation of azithromycin: evidence for an unusual interaction. *Pharmacotherapy* 1997; **17:** 827–9.

QUINOLONES. The fluoroquinolone antibacterials vary in their propensity to interact with theophylline. *Enoxacin* shows the strongest interaction and has been reported[1] to cause serious nausea and vomiting, tachycardia, and headaches, associated with unexpectedly high plasma-theophylline concentrations in patients with respiratory-tract infections. Studies,[2-5] mainly in healthy subjects, have found that enoxacin decreases theophylline clearance by up to 74%[3] with an increase in the elimination half-life and serum-theophylline concentration. A 50% decrease in theophylline clearance has been reported with *grepafloxacin*.[6]

*Ciprofloxacin*[2,7-9] and *pefloxacin*[2] interact with theophylline to a lesser extent than enoxacin, decreasing theophylline clearance by about 30%. Eight clinically important interactions between ciprofloxacin and theophylline had been reported to the UK Committee on Safety of Medicines[10] including 1 death. A ciprofloxacin-induced seizure has been reported[11] which may have been due to the combined inhibitory effects of the 2 drugs on GABA binding. It has been recommended that ciprofloxacin should not be used in patients treated with theophylline.[10]

*Norfloxacin*[4,12-14] and *ofloxacin*[4,12,15] have been reported to have minor effects on the pharmacokinetics of theophylline. Although their effects were usually considered not to be clinically significant, the US FDA had received 9 reports of theophylline toxicity associated with concomitant norfloxacin administration, including 1 death.[16] *Fleroxacin*,[17] *flumequine*,[18] *lomefloxacin*,[9,19,20] *moxifloxacin*,[21] and *rufloxacin*[22] have been reported to have no significant effect on the pharmacokinetics of theophylline in small studies in healthy subjects.

The mechanism of interaction involves a reduction in the metabolic clearance of theophylline due to inhibition of hepatic microsomal enzymes. However, the exact mechanism is unknown and it is difficult to predict which patients will be at risk. Extreme caution should be used when giving quinolones with theophylline, particularly in the elderly[16] and it may be advisable to use a non-interacting fluoroquinolone, although theophylline concentrations should still be monitored.

Of the non-fluorinated quinolones, *nalidixic acid*[2] has been reported not to affect theophylline clearance whereas *pipemidic acid* has markedly inhibited theophylline clearance.[20]

1. Wijnands WJA, *et al.* Enoxacin raises plasma theophylline concentrations. *Lancet* 1984; **ii:** 108–9.
2. Wijnands WJA, *et al.* The influence of quinolone derivatives on theophylline clearance. *Br J Clin Pharmacol* 1986; **22:** 677–83.
3. Beckmann J, *et al.* Enoxacin—a potent inhibitor of theophylline metabolism. *Eur J Clin Pharmacol* 1987; **33:** 227–30.
4. Sano M, *et al.* Inhibitory effect of enoxacin, ofloxacin and norfloxacin on renal excretion of theophylline in humans. *Eur J Clin Pharmacol* 1989; **36:** 323–4.
5. Koup JR, *et al.* Theophylline dosage adjustment during enoxacin coadministration. *Antimicrob Agents Chemother* 1990; **34:** 803–7.
6. Efthymiopoulos C, *et al.* Theophylline and warfarin interaction studies with grepafloxacin. *Clin Pharmacokinet* 1997; **33** (suppl 1): 39–46.
7. Nix DE, *et al.* Effect of multiple dose oral ciprofloxacin on the pharmacokinetics of theophylline and indocyanine green. *J Antimicrob Chemother* 1987; **19:** 263–9.
8. Schwartz J, *et al.* Impact of ciprofloxacin on theophylline clearance and steady-state concentrations in serum. *Antimicrob Agents Chemother* 1988; **32:** 75–7.
9. Robson RA, *et al.* Comparative effects of ciprofloxacin and lomefloxacin on the oxidative metabolism of theophylline. *Br J Clin Pharmacol* 1990; **29:** 491–3.
10. Bem JL, Mann RD. Danger of interaction between ciprofloxacin and theophylline. *BMJ* 1988; **296:** 1131.
11. Karki SD, *et al.* Seizure with ciprofloxacin and theophylline combined therapy. *DICP Ann Pharmacother* 1990; **24:** 595–6.
12. Sano M, *et al.* Comparative pharmacokinetics of theophylline following two fluoroquinolones co-administration. *Eur J Clin Pharmacol* 1987; **32:** 431–2.
13. Ho G, *et al.* Evaluation of the effect of norfloxacin on the pharmacokinetics of theophylline. *Clin Pharmacol Ther* 1988; **44:** 35–8.
14. Davis RL, *et al.* Effect of norfloxacin on theophylline metabolism. *Antimicrob Agents Chemother* 1989; **33:** 212–14.
15. Gregoire SL, *et al.* Inhibition of theophylline clearance by coadministered ofloxacin without alteration of theophylline effects. *Antimicrob Agents Chemother* 1987; **31:** 375–8.
16. Grasela TH, Dreis MW. An evaluation of the quinolone-theophylline interaction using the Food and Drug Administration spontaneous reporting system. *Arch Intern Med* 1992; **152:** 617–21.
17. Parent M, *et al.* Safety of fleroxacin coadministered with theophylline to young and elderly volunteers. *Antimicrob Agents Chemother* 1990; **34:** 1249–53.
18. Lacarelle B, *et al.* The quinolone, flumequine, has no effect on theophylline pharmacokinetics. *Eur J Clin Pharmacol* 1994; **46:** 477–8.
19. LeBel M, *et al.* Influence of lomefloxacin on the pharmacokinetics of theophylline. *Antimicrob Agents Chemother* 1990: **34:** 1254–6.
20. Staib AH, *et al.* Interaction of quinolones with the theophylline metabolism in man: investigations with lomefloxacin and pipemidic acid. *Int J Clin Pharmacol Ther Toxicol* 1989; **27:** 289–93.
21. Stass H, Kubitza D. Lack of pharmacokinetic interaction between moxifloxacin, a novel 8-methoxyfluoroquinolone, and theophylline. *Clin Pharmacokinet* 2001; **40** (suppl 1): 63–70.
22. Kinzig-Schippers M, *et al.* Absence of effect of rufloxacin on theophylline pharmacokinetics in steady state. *Antimicrob Agents Chemother* 1998; **42:** 2359–64.

RIFAMPICIN. Rifampicin induces hepatic oxidative enzymes and a dose of 600 mg daily by mouth for 6 to 14 days has been shown to increase mean plasma-theophylline clearance by 25 to 82% due to enhancement of hepatic theophylline metabolism. This increase in clearance is sufficient to require dosage adjustment in some patients,[1-4] including children.[5]

1. Straughn AB, *et al.* Effect of rifampin on theophylline disposition. *Ther Drug Monit* 1984; **6:** 153–6.
2. Robson RA, *et al.* Theophylline-rifampicin interaction: non-selective induction of theophylline metabolic pathways. *Br J Clin Pharmacol* 1984; **18:** 445–8.
3. Boyce EG, *et al.* The effect of rifampin on theophylline kinetics. *J Clin Pharmacol* 1986; **26:** 696–9.
4. Adebayo GE, *et al.* Attenuation of rifampicin-induced theophylline metabolism by diltiazem/rifampicin coadministration in healthy volunteers. *Eur J Clin Pharmacol* 1989; **37:** 127–31.
5. Brocks DR, *et al.* Theophylline-rifampin interaction in a pediatric patient. *Clin Pharm* 1986; **5:** 602–4.

TETRACYCLINES. *Tetracycline* weakly inhibited theophylline clearance after 5 days of therapy in 5 non-smoking adults with chronic obstructive airways disease[1] and theophylline toxicity has been reported[2] in a patient given a 10-day course of tetracycline during theophylline therapy. *Doxycycline* has been reported not to have any significant effect on theophylline pharmacokinetics in healthy subjects.[3]

1. Gotz VP, Ryerson GG. Evaluation of tetracycline on theophylline disposition in patients with chronic obstructive airways disease. *Drug Intell Clin Pharm* 1986; **20:** 694–7.

2. McCormack JP, *et al.* Theophylline toxicity induced by tetracycline. *Clin Pharm* 1990; **9:** 546–9.
3. Jonkman JHG, *et al.* No influence of doxycycline on theophylline pharmacokinetics. *Ther Drug Monit* 1985; **7:** 92–4.

**Antidepressants.** Significantly reduced clearance and increased plasma concentrations of theophylline have been reported when given with *viloxazine*.[1,2] The dosage of theophylline should be decreased and its plasma concentrations monitored when viloxazine is also prescribed.[2] The interaction probably involves competition between the two drugs for hepatic microsomal enzymes.

*Fluvoxamine* has also been associated with a significant reduction in theophylline clearance[3] and theophylline toxicity has been described in patients when fluvoxamine was added to their therapy.[4,5] This interaction which is due to potent liver enzyme inhibition[6] has been the subject of a warning by the UK Committee on Safety of Medicines[7] in which they issued the standard advice of avoiding the two drugs if at all possible and, where they could not be avoided, of giving half the dose of theophylline and monitoring plasma concentrations.

*Hypericum* may have decreased theophylline concentrations and increased the theophylline dosage requirement in one case report.[8] However, a study[9] in 12 healthy volunteers found that 15 days of treatment with hypericum did not significantly change theophylline pharmacokinetics.

For a mention of the effect of theophylline on the renal clearance of *lithium*, see Xanthines, under Interactions of Lithium, p.304.

1. Thomson AH, *et al.* Theophylline toxicity following coadministration of viloxazine. *Ther Drug Monit* 1988; **10:** 359–60.
2. Perault MC, *et al.* A study of the interaction of viloxazine with theophylline. *Ther Drug Monit* 1989; **11:** 520–2.
3. Donaldson KM, *et al.* The effect [of] fluvoxamine at steady state on the pharmacokinetics of theophylline after a single dose in healthy male volunteers. *Br J Clin Pharmacol* 1994; **37:** 492P.
4. Sperber AD. Toxic interaction between fluvoxamine and sustained release theophylline in an 11-year-old boy. *Drug Safety* 1991; **6:** 460–2.
5. Thomson AH, *et al.* Interaction between fluvoxamine and theophylline. *Pharm J* 1992; **249:** 137.
6. Rasmussen BB, *et al.* Selective serotonin reuptake inhibitors and theophylline metabolism in human liver microsomes: potent inhibition by fluvoxamine. *Br J Clin Pharmacol* 1995; **39:** 151–9.
7. Committee on Safety of Medicines/Medicines Control Agency. Fluvoxamine increases plasma theophylline levels. *Current Problems* 1994; **20:** 12.
8. Nebel A, *et al.* Potential metabolic interaction between St John's wort and theophylline. *Ann Pharmacother* 1999; **33:** 502.
9. Morimoto T, *et al.* Effect of St. John's wort on the pharmacokinetics of theophylline in healthy volunteers. *J Clin Pharmacol* 2004; **44:** 95–101.

**Antiepileptics.** *Phenytoin* markedly decreases the elimination half-life and increases the clearance of theophylline, probably due to hepatic enzyme induction, at therapeutic serum-phenytoin concentrations,[1-3] at subtherapeutic phenytoin concentrations,[2,4] and even in heavy smokers.[2] A preliminary report suggested that the serum concentration of phenytoin may be decreased simultaneously,[5] perhaps due to enzyme induction by theophylline[5] or reduced phenytoin absorption.[6] The interaction has been reported to occur within 5 to 14 days of taking phenytoin and theophylline, and theophylline clearance has increased by up to 350%, and reductions in serum half-life have ranged from 25 to 70% of initial values.[3,4]

*Carbamazepine* has also been observed to increase theophylline elimination. In one patient, theophylline serum half-life was decreased by approximately 24 to 60%, and clearance was increased by about 35 to 100% when carbamazepine was given.[2] In an 11-year-old girl theophylline-serum half-life was almost halved with loss of asthma control after 3 weeks of concurrent carbamazepine therapy.[7] In turn, theophylline has been reported to reduce the half-life of carbamazepine—see p.357.

Although *phenobarbital* was not found to have a significant effect on the pharmacokinetics of a single dose of theophylline given intravenously,[8] enhanced theophylline clearance has been seen in patients after longer periods of treatment with phenobarbital.[9,10] The magnitude of the changes in theophylline elimination appears to be smaller with phenobarbital than phenytoin. *Pentobarbital* in high doses has also been reported to increase theophylline metabolism.[11] A more recent study[12] has also shown that therapeutic doses of pentobarbital (100 mg daily) increase plasma clearance of theophylline by a mean of 40%, although this was subject to marked interindividual variations. Renal clearance was not affected, suggesting hepatic enzyme induction as the probable mechanism.

1. Marquis J-F, *et al.* Phenytoin-theophylline interaction. *N Engl J Med* 1982; **307:** 1189–90.
2. Reed RC, Schwartz HJ. Phenytoin-theophylline-quinidine interaction. *N Engl J Med* 1983; **308:** 724–5.
3. Sklar SJ, Wagner JC. Enhanced theophylline clearance secondary to phenytoin therapy. *Drug Intell Clin Pharm* 1985; **19:** 34–6.
4. Miller M, *et al.* Influence of phenytoin on theophylline clearance. *Clin Pharmacol Ther* 1984; **35:** 666–9.
5. Taylor JW, *et al.* The interaction of phenytoin and theophylline. *Drug Intell Clin Pharm* 1980; **14:** 638.
6. Hendeles L, *et al.* Decreased oral phenytoin absorption following concurrent theophylline administration. *J Allergy Clin Immunol* 1979; **63:** 156.
7. Rosenberry KR, *et al.* Reduced theophylline half-life induced by carbamazepine therapy. *J Pediatr* 1983; **102:** 472–4.
8. Piafsky KM, *et al.* Effect of phenobarbital on the disposition of intravenous theophylline. *Clin Pharmacol Ther* 1977; **22:** 336–9.
9. Jusko WJ, *et al.* Factors affecting theophylline clearances: age, tobacco, marijuana, cirrhosis, congestive heart failure, obesity, oral contraceptives, benzodiazepines, barbiturates, and ethanol. *J Pharm Sci* 1979; **68:** 1358–66.
10. Saccar CL, *et al.* The effect of phenobarbital on theophylline disposition in children with asthma. *J Allergy Clin Immunol* 1985; **75:** 716–19.
11. Gibson GA, *et al.* Influence of high-dose phenobarbital on theophylline pharmacokinetics: a case report. *Ther Drug Monit* 1985; **7:** 181–4.
12. Dahlqvist R, *et al.* Induction of theophylline metabolism by pentobarbital. *Ther Drug Monit* 1989; **11:** 408–10.

**Antifungals.** There have been reports that *ketoconazole* does not appear significantly to alter the pharmacokinetics of theophylline.[1,2] The manufacturer of *fluconazole* has, however, stated that plasma clearance of theophylline may be decreased by fluconazole. A 16% reduction in theophylline clearance has been reported[3] following oral fluconazole but fluconazole was considered to have only a minor inhibitory effect on theophylline metabolism and theophylline disposition was not significantly affected. Theophylline metabolism has been inhibited to a similar degree by *terbinafine*.[4]

1. Brown MW, *et al.* Effect of ketoconazole on hepatic oxidative drug metabolism. *Clin Pharmacol Ther* 1985; **37:** 290–7.
2. Heusner JJ, *et al.* Effect of chronically administered ketoconazole on the elimination of theophylline in man. *Drug Intell Clin Pharm* 1987; **21:** 514–17.
3. Konishi H, *et al.* Effect of fluconazole on theophylline disposition in humans. *Eur J Clin Pharmacol* 1994; **46:** 309–12.
4. Trépanier EF, *et al.* Effect of terbinafine on theophylline pharmacokinetics in healthy volunteers. *Antimicrob Agents Chemother* 1998; **42:** 695–7.

**Antigout drugs.** *Allopurinol* 300 mg by mouth daily for 7 days was found to have no effect on the pharmacokinetics of theophylline following a single intravenous dose of aminophylline[1,2] or following theophylline given by mouth to steady state.[1] However, allopurinol 600 mg by mouth daily for 28 days has been found to inhibit the metabolism of theophylline,[3] increasing the mean half-life by 25% after 14 days and 29% after 28 days and there has been a report of allopurinol increasing peak plasma-theophylline concentrations by 38% in one patient within 2 days of concomitant administration.[4]

*Probenecid* has been reported[5] to have no effect on the hepatic metabolism or total body clearance of theophylline in a single-dose study in healthy subjects.

*Sulfinpyrazone* 800 mg daily for 7 days increased the total plasma clearance of theophylline by 22% in healthy subjects due to selective induction of certain cytochrome P450 isoenzymes.[6]

1. Grygiel JJ, *et al.* Effects of allopurinol on theophylline metabolism and clearance. *Clin Pharmacol Ther* 1979; **26:** 660–7.
2. Vozeh S, *et al.* Influence of allopurinol on theophylline disposition in adults. *Clin Pharmacol Ther* 1980; **27:** 194–7.
3. Manfredi RL, Vesell ES. Inhibition of theophylline metabolism by long-term allopurinol administration. *Clin Pharmacol Ther* 1981; **29:** 224–9.
4. Barry M, Feely J. Allopurinol influences aminophenazone elimination. *Clin Pharmacokinet* 1990; **19:** 167–9.
5. Chen TWD, Patton TF. Effect of probenecid on the pharmacokinetics of aminophylline. *Drug Intell Clin Pharm* 1983; **17:** 465–6.
6. Birkett DJ, *et al.* Evidence for a dual action of sulphinpyrazone on drug metabolism in man: theophylline-sulphinpyrazone interaction. *Br J Clin Pharmacol* 1983; **15:** 567–9.

**Antineoplastics.** There has been a report of increased clearance of theophylline in 3 patients receiving *aminoglutethimide*.[1]

For reference to a possible interaction between theophylline and *lomustine*, see Lomustine, p.565.

1. Lønning PE, *et al.* Effect of aminoglutethimide on antipyrine, theophylline, and digitoxin disposition in breast cancer. *Clin Pharmacol Ther* 1984; **36:** 796–802.

**Antivirals.** A single injection of recombinant human *interferon alfa* reduced theophylline clearance by 33 to 81% in 8 of 9 subjects, resulting in a 1.5 to sixfold increase in the theophylline elimination half-life.[1] Injection of interferon alfa once daily for 3 days in 11 healthy subjects also reduced theophylline clearance and increased elimination half-life,[2] but the magnitude of the changes were of a similar order to normal intra-individual variation and the interaction was considered of minor clinical significance.

The manufacturers of *ritonavir* state that it substantially increases the clearance of theophylline; theophylline dosage may need to be increased to maintain efficacy.

There is evidence[3] that *aciclovir* inhibits theophylline metabolism, resulting in accumulation.

1. Williams SJ, *et al.* Inhibition of theophylline metabolism by interferon. *Lancet* 1987; **ii:** 939–41.
2. Jonkman JHG, *et al.* Effects of α-interferon on theophylline pharmacokinetics and metabolism. *Br J Clin Pharmacol* 1989; **27:** 795–802.
3. Maeda Y, *et al.* Inhibition of theophylline metabolism by aciclovir. *Biol Pharm Bull* 1996; **19:** 1591–5.

**Benzodiazepines.** For reference to the antagonism of benzodiazepine sedation by aminophylline, see Xanthines, under Interactions of Diazepam, p.695.

**Beta blockers.** *Propranolol* reduced theophylline clearance by 36% in healthy subjects given aminophylline intravenously. *Metoprolol* did not reduce clearance in the group as a whole, but a reduction was noted in some smokers whose theophylline clearance was initially high.[1] Propranolol is thought to exert a dose-dependent selective inhibitory effect on the separate cytochrome P450 isoenzymes involved in theophylline demethylation and 8-hydroxylation.[2] The less lipophilic beta blockers *atenolol*[3,4] and *nadolol*[4] had no significant effect on the pharmacokinetics of theophylline.

In general, however, beta blockers should be avoided in patients taking theophylline as they can dangerously exacerbate bronchospasm in patients with a history of asthma or chronic obstructive pulmonary disease.

1. Conrad KA, Nyman DW. Effects of metoprolol and propranolol on theophylline elimination. *Clin Pharmacol Ther* 1980; **28:** 463–7.
2. Miners JO, *et al.* Selectivity and dose-dependency of the inhibitory effect of propranolol on theophylline metabolism in man. *Br J Clin Pharmacol* 1985; **20:** 219–23.
3. Cerasa LA, *et al.* Lack of effect of atenolol on the pharmacokinetics of theophylline. *Br J Clin Pharmacol* 1988; **26:** 800–2.
4. Corsi CM, *et al.* Lack of effect of atenolol and nadolol on the metabolism of theophylline. *Br J Clin Pharmacol* 1990; **29:** 265–8.

**Caffeine.** Abstention from dietary methylxanthines by healthy subjects has resulted in faster elimination of theophylline.[1] While the addition of extra caffeine to the diet has been reported not to alter theophylline disposition,[2] some studies in healthy subjects have indicated that the ingestion of moderate amounts of caffeine (120 to 900 mg daily), which could be consumed by drinking several cups of coffee daily, can have a pronounced influence on the pharmacokinetics of theophylline.[3,4] In these latter studies the mean theophylline clearance was reduced by 23 and 29% with a corresponding increase in the elimination half-lives.

1. Monks TJ, *et al.* Influence of methylxanthine-containing foods on theophylline metabolism and kinetics. *Clin Pharmacol Ther* 1979; **26:** 513–24.
2. Monks TJ, *et al.* The effect of increased caffeine intake on the metabolism and pharmacokinetics of theophylline in man. *Biopharm Drug Dispos* 1981; **2:** 31–7.
3. Jonkman JHG, *et al.* The influence of caffeine on the steady-state pharmacokinetics of theophylline. *Clin Pharmacol Ther* 1991; **49:** 248–55.
4. Sato J, *et al.* Influence of usual intake of dietary caffeine on single-dose kinetics of theophylline in healthy human subjects. *Eur J Clin Pharmacol* 1993; **44:** 295–8.

**Calcium-channel blockers.** *Verapamil* has been reported[1] to decrease the clearance of theophylline by a mean of 14% in healthy subjects and although this was not considered to be clinically significant, symptoms of theophylline toxicity, associated with near doubling of the serum-theophylline concentration have occurred in a 76-year-old woman taking theophylline after 6 days of therapy with verapamil.[2] Studies in healthy subjects and asthmatic patients have produced conflicting results of the effect of *nifedipine* on the pharmacokinetics of theophylline. Reduced clearance[1] and an increase in the volume of distribution[3,4] of theophylline have been reported and both decreased[4] and increased[5] serum-theophylline concentrations; theophylline toxicity has been reported.[6,7] However, most studies have concluded that the effects of nifedipine are unlikely to be of clinical importance.[1,4,5,8]

Serum concentrations of theophylline have been reported to be increased by *diltiazem*[5] and reduced by *felodipine*;[9] neither of these effects were considered to be clinically significant.

1. Robson RA, *et al.* Selective inhibitory effects of nifedipine and verapamil on oxidative metabolism: effects on theophylline. *Br J Clin Pharmacol* 1988; **25:** 397–400.
2. Burnakis TG, *et al.* Increased serum theophylline concentrations secondary to oral verapamil. *Clin Pharm* 1983; **2:** 458–61.
3. Jackson SHD, *et al.* The interaction between iv theophylline and chronic oral dosing with slow release nifedipine in volunteers. *Br J Clin Pharmacol* 1986; **21:** 389–92.
4. Adebayo GI, Mabadeje AFB. Effect of nifedipine on antipyrine and theophylline disposition. *Biopharm Drug Dispos* 1990; **11:** 157–64.
5. Smith SR, *et al.* The influence of nifedipine and diltiazem on serum theophylline concentration-time profiles. *J Clin Pharm Ther* 1989; **14:** 403–8.
6. Parrillo SJ, Venditto M. Elevated theophylline blood levels from institution of nifedipine therapy. *Ann Emerg Med* 1984; **13:** 216–17.
7. Harrod CS. Theophylline toxicity and nifedipine. *Ann Intern Med* 1987; **106:** 480.
8. Spedini C, Lombardi C. Long-term treatment with oral nifedipine plus theophylline in the management of chronic bronchial asthma. *Eur J Clin Pharmacol* 1986; **31:** 105–6.
9. Bratel T, *et al.* Felodipine reduces the absorption of theophylline in man. *Eur J Clin Pharmacol* 1989; **36:** 481–5.

**Cannabis.** A search of the literature[1] revealed 2 studies, both published in the 1970s, that showed that marijuana smoking increased the clearance of theophylline.

1. Brown D. Influence on theophylline clearance. *Pharm J* 1994; **253:** 595.

**Corticosteroids.** In 3 patients with acute severe asthma given aminophylline intravenously, serum-theophylline concentrations rose rapidly from the therapeutic range to between 40 and 50 micrograms/mL when *hydrocortisone* was given intravenously.[1] In studies in healthy subjects, no significant changes in serum-theophylline concentrations were noted after the concomitant administration of hydrocortisone, *methylprednisolone*,[2] or *prednisone*[3] although there was a trend towards increased theophylline clearance during corticosteroid therapy.[2,3] In preterm neonates, exposure to *betamethasone in utero* stimulated the hepatic metabolism of theophylline,[4,5] but did not affect dosage requirements.

The possibility that adverse effects such as hypokalaemia may be potentiated by concomitant administration of theophylline and corticosteroids should be borne in mind.

1. Buchanan N, *et al.* Asthma—a possible interaction between hydrocortisone and theophylline. *S Afr Med J* 1979; 56: 1147–8.

2. Leavengood DC, *et al.* The effect of corticosteroids on theophylline metabolism. *Ann Allergy* 1983; **50:** 249–51.
3. Anderson JL, *et al.* Potential pharmacokinetic interaction between theophylline and prednisone. *Clin Pharm* 1984; **3:** 187–9.
4. Jager-Roman E, *et al.* Increased theophylline metabolism in premature infants after prenatal betamethasone administration. *Dev Pharmacol Ther* 1982; **5:** 127–35.
5. Baird-Lambert J, *et al.* Theophylline metabolism in preterm neonates during the first weeks of life. *Dev Pharmacol Ther* 1984; **7:** 239–44.

**Disulfiram.** In a study involving 20 recovering alcoholic patients, disulfiram decreased the plasma clearance and prolonged the elimination half-life of theophylline in a dose-dependent manner.[1] It was concluded that disulfiram exerts a dose-dependent inhibitory effect on the hepatic metabolism of theophylline and that, in order to minimise the risk of toxicity, the dosage of theophylline may need to be reduced by up to 50% during co-administration.

1. Loi C-M, *et al.* Dose-dependent inhibition of theophylline metabolism by disulfiram in recovering alcoholics. *Clin Pharmacol Ther* 1989; **45:** 476–86.

**Diuretics.** Although increased mean serum-theophylline concentrations were noted in 10 patients receiving continuous intravenous aminophylline infusions after intravenous injection of *furosemide*,[1] in 8 patients with chronic stable asthma, mean peak serum-theophylline concentrations were reduced from 12.14 micrograms/mL with placebo to 7.16 micrograms/mL when furosemide was given. Reduced concentrations were noted for up to 6 hours after furosemide administration.[2] Decreased theophylline concentrations were also noted in 4 neonates receiving oral or intravenous theophylline when given furosemide.[3] Serum-theophylline concentrations returned to normal when furosemide and theophylline were given more than 2 hours apart.

The possibility that adverse effects such as hypokalaemia may be potentiated if theophylline is given with diuretics should be borne in mind.

1. Conlon PF, *et al.* Effect of intravenous furosemide on serum theophylline concentration. *Am J Hosp Pharm* 1981; **38:** 1345–7.
2. Carpentiere G, *et al.* Furosemide and theophylline. *Ann Intern Med* 1985; **103:** 957.
3. Toback JW, Gilman ME. Theophylline-furosemide inactivation. *Pediatrics* 1983; **71:** 140–1.

**Gastrointestinal drugs.** Oral *antacids* do not appear to affect the total absorption of theophylline from the gut.[1-5] However, some studies have shown a reduction in the rate of absorption from both immediate-[1] and modified-release theophylline preparations[2] after antacids. Also an increase in peak serum-theophylline concentrations has been noted with certain modified-release formulations.[3]

*Cimetidine* inhibits the oxidative metabolism of theophylline reducing its clearance by 20 to 35% and prolonging its serum half-life;[6-8] toxic effects have been reported.[6] It has been recommended that the dose of aminophylline should be reduced by about one-third if given with cimetidine.[6] This inhibition of theophylline metabolism may be enhanced by liver disease,[9] but there is wide interindividual variation. The reduction in clearance may be greater in smokers.[10] Studies have suggested that *ranitidine* does not significantly inhibit theophylline metabolism,[11-14] even at very high doses.[15] However, there have been occasional reports of theophylline toxicity after concomitant ranitidine therapy.[16-18] *Famotidine*[19] has also been reported to not alter theophylline disposition but one small study found a significant decrease in theophylline clearance in some patients with chronic obstructive pulmonary disease.[20]

*Omeprazole, lansoprazole,* and *pantoprazole* generally have insignificant or no effect on theophylline clearance.[21,22] A modest increase in theophylline clearance in CYP2C19 poor metabolisers receiving omeprazole was not considered clinically relevant.[23]

1. Arnold LA, *et al.* Effect of an antacid on gastrointestinal absorption of theophylline. *Am J Hosp Pharm* 1979; **36:** 1059–62.
2. Shargel L, *et al.* Effect of antacid on bioavailability of theophylline from rapid and timed-release drug products. *J Pharm Sci* 1981; **70:** 599–602.
3. Darzentas LJ, *et al.* Effect of antacid on bioavailability of a sustained-release theophylline preparation. *Drug Intell Clin Pharm* 1983; **17:** 555–7.
4. Myhre KI, Walstad RA. The influence of antacid on the absorption of two different sustained-release formulations of theophylline. *Br J Clin Pharmacol* 1983; **15:** 683–7.
5. Muir JF, *et al.* Lack of effect of magnesium-aluminium hydroxide on the absorption of theophylline given as a pH-dependent sustained-release preparation. *Eur J Clin Pharmacol* 1993; **44:** 85–8.
6. Bauman JH, *et al.* Cimetidine-theophylline interaction: report of four patients. *Ann Allergy* 1982; **48:** 100–102.
7. Vestal RE, *et al.* Cimetidine inhibits theophylline clearance in patients with chronic obstructive pulmonary disease: a study using stable isotope methodology during multiple oral dose administration. *Br J Clin Pharmacol* 1983; **15:** 411–18.
8. Roberts RK, *et al.* Cimetidine-theophylline interaction in patients with chronic obstructive airways disease. *Med J Aust* 1984; **140:** 279–80.
9. Gugler R, *et al.* The inhibition of drug metabolism by cimetidine in patients with liver cirrhosis. *Klin Wochenschr* 1984; **62:** 1126–31.
10. Grygiel JJ, *et al.* Differential effects of cimetidine on theophylline metabolic pathways. *Eur J Clin Pharmacol* 1984; **26:** 335–40.
11. Breen KJ, *et al.* Effects of cimetidine and ranitidine on hepatic drug metabolism. *Clin Pharmacol Ther* 1982; **31:** 297–300.
12. Segger JS, *et al.* No evidence for interaction between ranitidine and theophylline. *Arch Intern Med* 1987; **147:** 179–80.
13. Adebayo GI. Effects of equimolar doses of cimetidine and ranitidine on theophylline elimination. *Biopharm Drug Dispos* 1989; **10:** 77–85.
14. Boehning W. Effect of cimetidine and ranitidine on plasma theophylline in patients with chronic obstructive airways disease treated with theophylline and corticosteroids. *Eur J Clin Pharmacol* 1990; **38:** 43–5.
15. Kelly HW, *et al.* Ranitidine at very large doses does not inhibit theophylline elimination. *Clin Pharmacol Ther* 1986; **39:** 577–81.
16. Fernandes E, Melewicz FM. Ranitidine and theophylline. *Ann Intern Med* 1984; **100:** 459.
17. Gardner ME, Sikorski GW. Ranitidine and theophylline. *Ann Intern Med* 1985; **102:** 559.
18. Hegman GW, Gilbert RP. Ranitidine-theophylline interaction—fact or fiction? *DICP Ann Pharmacother* 1991; **25:** 21–5.
19. Chremos AN, *et al.* Famotidine does not interfere with the disposition of theophylline in man: comparison to cimetidine. *Clin Pharmacol Ther* 1986; **39:** 187.
20. Dal Negro R, *et al.* Famotidine and theophylline pharmacokinetics: an unexpected cimetidine-like interaction in patients with chronic obstructive pulmonary disease. *Clin Pharmacokinet* 1993; **24:** 255–8.
21. Kokufu T, *et al.* Effects of lansoprazole on pharmacokinetics and metabolism of theophylline. *Eur J Clin Pharmacol* 1995; **48:** 391–5.
22. Dilger K, *et al.* Lack of drug interaction between omeprazole, lansoprazole, pantoprazole and theophylline. *Br J Clin Pharmacol* 1999; **48:** 438–44.
23. Cavuto NJ, *et al.* Effect of omeprazole on theophylline clearance in poor metabolizers of omeprazole. *Clin Pharmacol Ther* 1995; **57:** 215.

**General anaesthetics.** There have been several reports[1,2] of increased cardiotoxicity when patients taking theophylline were anaesthetised with *halothane.* There was also an early report of seizures and tachycardia attributed to an interaction between theophylline and *ketamine.*[3]

1. Barton MD. Anesthetic problems with aspirin-intolerant patients. *Anesth Analg* 1975; **54:** 376–80.
2. Richards W, *et al.* Cardiac arrest associated with halothane anesthesia in a patient receiving theophylline. *Ann Allergy* 1988; **61:** 83–4.
3. Hirschman CA, *et al.* Ketamine-aminophylline-induced decrease in seizure threshold. *Anesthesiology* 1982; **56:** 464–7.

**Leukotriene inhibitors and antagonists.** *Zileuton* prolongs the half-life and reduces the clearance of theophylline;[1] dosage of theophylline should be reduced to avoid toxicity when both drugs are given together, and plasma-theophylline concentrations should be monitored. Use of *zafirlukast* with theophylline decreased zafirlukast plasma concentrations but had no effect on theophylline plasma concentrations in clinical trials. However, toxic serum-theophylline concentrations occurred in one patient when zafirlukast was added to therapy, and recurred on rechallenge.[2] A dose of *montelukast* 10 mg daily did not affect the pharmacokinetics of theophylline, but doses of 200 mg and 600 mg daily reduced the maximum plasma concentration, area under the concentration-time curve, and elimination half-life of theophylline.[3]

1. Granneman GR, *et al.* Effect of zileuton on theophylline pharmacokinetics. *Clin Pharmacokinet* 1995; **29** (suppl 2): 77–83.
2. Katial RK, *et al.* A drug interaction between zafirlukast and theophylline. *Arch Intern Med* 1998; **158:** 1713–15.
3. Malmstrom K, *et al.* Effect of montelukast on single-dose theophylline pharmacokinetics. *Am J Ther* 1998; **5:** 189–95.

**Neuromuscular blockers.** For reference to resistance to neuromuscular block with pancuronium in patients receiving aminophylline, see Xanthines, p.1402.

**Oral contraceptives.** Oral contraceptives have been reported to decrease the clearance of theophylline by about 30%, and serum concentrations may be increased,[1-3] due to the inhibitory effects of oral contraceptives on hepatic P450 isoenzymes.

1. Tornatore KM, *et al.* Effect of chronic oral contraceptive steroids on theophylline disposition. *Eur J Clin Pharmacol* 1982; **23:** 129–34.
2. Gardner MJ, *et al.* Effects of tobacco smoking and oral contraceptive use on theophylline disposition. *Br J Clin Pharmacol* 1983; **16:** 271–80.
3. Roberts RK, *et al.* Oral contraceptive steroids impair the elimination of theophylline. *J Lab Clin Med* 1983; **101:** 821–5.

**Sympathomimetics.** The effect of beta-adrenoceptor agonists on the pharmacokinetics of theophylline is unclear. Whereas some studies have found that *orciprenaline*[1] or *terbutaline*[2] had no effect on theophylline disposition, others have shown an increase in theophylline clearance following *isoprenaline*[3,4] or *terbutaline.*[5,6]

Use of theophylline with beta-adrenoceptor agonists can potentiate adverse effects including hypokalaemia,[7,8] hyperglycaemia,[7] tachycardia,[7,8] hypertension,[7] and tremor.[9] Of 9 patients reported to the UK Committee on Safety of Medicines with hypokalaemia during such combined therapy, 4 had clinical sequelae of cardiorespiratory arrest, intestinal pseudo-obstruction, or confusion. Monitoring of serum-potassium concentrations was recommended in patients with severe asthma receiving concomitant treatment with beta-adrenoceptor agonists and xanthine derivatives.[10]

The possibility of an interaction with *phenylpropanolamine* should also be borne in mind, as it has been shown to reduce the clearance of theophylline significantly.[11]

1. Conrad KA, Woodworth JR. Orciprenaline does not alter theophylline elimination. *Br J Clin Pharmacol* 1981; **12:** 756–7.
2. Snidow J, *et al.* Acute effects of short-term subcutaneous terbutaline on theophylline disposition. *Eur J Clin Pharmacol* 1987; **32:** 191–3.
3. Hemstreet MP, *et al.* Effect of intravenous isoproterenol on theophylline kinetics. *J Allergy Clin Immunol* 1982; **69:** 360–4.
4. Griffith JA, Kozloski GD. Isoproterenol-theophylline interaction: possible potentiation by other drugs. *Clin Pharm* 1990; **9:** 54–7.
5. Danziger Y, *et al.* Reduction of serum theophylline levels by terbutaline in children with asthma. *Clin Pharmacol Ther* 1985; **37:** 469–71.
6. Garty M, *et al.* Increased theophylline clearance in asthmatic patients due to terbutaline. *Eur J Clin Pharmacol* 1989; **36:** 25–8.
7. Smith SR, Kendall MJ. Potentiation of the adverse effects of intravenous terbutaline by oral theophylline. *Br J Clin Pharmacol* 1986; **21:** 451–3.
8. Whyte KF, *et al.* Salbutamol induced hypokalaemia: the effect of theophylline alone and in combination with adrenaline. *Br J Clin Pharmacol* 1988; **25:** 571–8.
9. van der Vet APH, *et al.* Pharmacodynamics (lungfunction tests, tremor measurements and cAMP determinations) of a single dose of 0.5 mg terbutaline subcutaneously during sustained-release theophylline medication in patients with asthmatic bronchitis. *Int J Clin Pharmacol Ther Toxicol* 1986; **24:** 569–73.
10. Committee on Safety of Medicines. $\beta_2$ agonists, xanthines and hypokalaemia. *Current Problems 28* 1990.
11. Wilson HA, *et al.* Phenylpropanolamine significantly reduces the clearance of theophylline. *Am Rev Respir Dis* 1991; **143:** A629.

**Tacrine.** Results of a study in healthy subjects indicated that tacrine reduced theophylline clearance by about 50% and increased plasma-theophylline concentrations. Competitive inhibition by tacrine of theophylline metabolism was proposed.[1]

1. deVries TM, *et al.* Effect of multiple-dose tacrine administration on single-dose pharmacokinetics of digoxin, diazepam, and theophylline. *Pharm Res* 1993; **10** (suppl): S333.

**Tiabendazole.** Tiabendazole has been reported[1,2] to increase serum-theophylline concentrations and to decrease theophylline clearance. It has been recommended[2] that theophylline dosage should be reduced by 50% when tiabendazole therapy is initiated.

1. Sugar AM, *et al.* Possible thiabendazole-induced theophylline toxicity. *Am Rev Respir Dis* 1980; **122:** 501–3.
2. Lew G, *et al.* Theophylline-thiabendazole drug interaction. *Clin Pharm* 1989; **8:** 225–7.

**Ticlopidine.** Theophylline elimination half-life was increased and plasma clearance was decreased in 10 healthy subjects after the use of ticlopidine 500 mg daily by mouth for 10 days.[1]

1. Colli A, *et al.* Ticlopidine-theophylline interaction. *Clin Pharmacol Ther* 1987; **41:** 358–62.

**Vaccines.** Transient inhibition of the hepatic metabolism of theophylline, possibly secondary to interferon production, resulting in increased theophylline serum half-life and concentration has been reported after BCG vaccination[1] and influenza vaccination.[2,3] Other studies have not been able to confirm the interaction with influenza vaccine.[4-7] The differing findings are probably due to differences in vaccine; modern purified subvirion vaccines which do not induce interferon production do not appear to alter theophylline metabolism.[8,9]

1. Gray JD, *et al.* Depression of theophylline elimination following BCG vaccination. *Br J Clin Pharmacol* 1983; **16:** 735–7.
2. Renton KW, *et al.* Decreased elimination of theophylline after influenza vaccination. *Can Med Assoc J* 1980; **123:** 288–90.
3. Walker S, *et al.* Serum theophylline levels after influenza vaccination. *Can Med Assoc J* 1981; **125:** 243–4.
4. Goldstein RS, *et al.* Decreased elimination of theophylline after influenza vaccination. *Can Med Assoc J* 1982; **126:** 470.
5. Fischer RG, *et al.* Influence of trivalent influenza vaccine on serum theophylline levels. *Can Med Assoc J* 1982; **126:** 1312–13.
6. Britton L, Ruben FL. Serum theophylline levels after influenza vaccination. *Can Med Assoc J* 1982; **126:** 1375.
7. Patriarca PA, *et al.* Influenza vaccination and warfarin or theophylline toxicity in nursing-home residents. *N Engl J Med* 1983; **308:** 1601–2.
8. Stults BM, Hashisaki PA. Influenza vaccination and theophylline pharmacokinetics in patients with chronic obstructive lung disease. *West J Med* 1983; **139:** 651–4.
9. Winstanley PA, *et al.* Lack of effect of highly purified subunit influenza vaccination on theophylline metabolism. *Br J Clin Pharmacol* 1985; **20:** 47–53.

## Pharmacokinetics

Theophylline is rapidly and completely absorbed from liquid preparations, capsules, and uncoated tablets; the rate, but not the extent, of absorption is decreased by food, and food may also affect theophylline clearance. Modified-release preparations of theophylline can usually provide adequate plasma concentrations when given every 12 hours. However, there is a considerable variability in their absorption characteristics and in the effect of food. It is generally recommended that if a patient is transferred from one such preparation to another then the dose should be retitrated. Peak serum-theophylline concentrations occur 1 to 2 hours after ingestion of liquid preparations, capsules, and uncoated tablets, and generally about 4 hours after ingestion of modified-release preparations. Rectal absorption is rapid from enemas, but may be slow and erratic from suppositories. Absorption following intramuscular injection is slow and incomplete.

Theophylline is approximately 40% bound to plasma proteins, but in neonates, or adults with liver disease, binding is reduced. Optimum therapeutic serum concentrations are generally considered to range from 10 to 20 micrograms/mL (55 to 110 micromol/litre) although some consider a lower range appropriate (see Therapeutic Drug Monitoring, below).

Theophylline is metabolised in the liver to 1,3-dimethyluric acid, 1-methyluric acid (via the intermediate 1-methylxanthine), and 3-methylxanthine. Demethylation to 3-methylxanthine (and possibly to 1-methylxanthine) is catalysed by the cytochrome P450 isoenzyme CYP1A2; hydroxylation to 1-methyluric acid is catalysed by CYP2E1 and CYP3A3. The metabolites are excreted in the urine. In adults, about 10% of a dose of theophylline is excreted unchanged in the urine, but in neonates around 50% is excreted unchanged, and a large proportion is excreted as caffeine. Considerable interindividual differences in the rate of hepatic metabolism of theophylline result in large variations in clearance, serum concentrations, and half-lives. Hepatic metabolism is further affected by factors such as age, smoking, disease, diet, and drug interactions. The serum half-life of theophylline in an otherwise healthy, non-smoking asthmatic adult is 6 to 12 hours, in children 1 to 5 hours, in cigarette smokers 4 to 5 hours, and in neonates and premature infants 10 to 45 hours. The serum half-life of theophylline may be increased in the elderly and in patients with heart failure or liver disease.

Theophylline crosses the placenta; it is also distributed into breast milk.

**Absorption.** FOOD. Food has substantial but variable effects on the absorption of theophylline from modified-release formulations but it is difficult to predict whether a particular formulation will be affected.[1] Some formulations are not affected by the presence of food but for others increases or decreases in the rate and/or extent of absorption have been reported. The composition and fluid content of the food appears to be important and a rapid release of theophylline ('dose-dumping') has occurred with some formulations following a meal, especially one with a high fat content.

A diet high in protein and low in carbohydrate has been reported to increase theophylline clearance, and a low-protein, high-carbohydrate diet to decrease theophylline clearance.[2-6] The consumption of methylxanthines, particularly caffeine, in the diet may decrease theophylline clearance (see under Interactions, above).


1. Jonkman JHG. Food interactions with sustained-release theophylline preparations: a review. *Clin Pharmacokinet* 1989; **16:** 162–79.
2. Kappas A, *et al.* Influence of dietary protein and carbohydrate on antipyrine and theophylline metabolism in man. *Clin Pharmacol Ther* 1976; **20:** 643–53.
3. Feldman CH, *et al.* Effect of dietary protein and carbohydrate on theophylline metabolism in children. *Pediatrics* 1980; **66:** 956–62.
4. Feldman CH, *et al.* Interaction between nutrition and theophylline metabolism in children. *Ther Drug Monit* 1982; **4:** 69–76.
5. Juan D, *et al.* Effects of dietary protein on theophylline pharmacokinetics and caffeine and aminopyrine breath tests. *Clin Pharmacol Ther* 1986; **40:** 187–94.
6. Juan D, *et al.* Impairment of theophylline clearance by a hypocaloric low-protein diet in chronic obstructive pulmonary disease. *Ther Drug Monit* 1990; **12:** 111–14.


**Metabolism and excretion.** AGE. From about 1 year of age until adolescence, children have a rapid theophylline clearance.[1] Premature infants and those under 1 year of age have a slower clearance[2,3] due to immature metabolic pathways.[3-5] In neonates the capacity of hepatic cytochrome P450 enzymes is much reduced compared with older children and adults, and *N*-demethylation and oxidation reactions play a minor role in the metabolism of theophylline.[4-6] Neonates are, however, capable of methylating theophylline at the N7 position to form caffeine, which is present at about one-third the concentration of theophylline at steady state.[5,6] The proportion of theophylline excreted unchanged is also increased in premature neonates and decreases with age as hepatic enzyme systems develop.[6] More rapid clearance on the first day of life in premature neonates has been reported.[7]

Some studies have found a progressive decline in clearance throughout adult years[8] whereas others have not.[9] Similarly, some studies have noted a decreased clearance in the elderly[10,11] but others have found no significant change.[12,13]


1. Zaske DE, *et al.* Oral aminophylline therapy: increased dosage requirements in children. *JAMA* 1977; **237:** 1453–5.
2. Aranda JV, *et al.* Pharmacokinetic aspects of theophylline in premature newborns. *N Engl J Med* 1976; **295:** 413–16.
3. Kraus DM, *et al.* Alterations in theophylline metabolism during the first year of life. *Clin Pharmacol Ther* 1993; **54:** 351–9.
4. Grygiel JJ, Birkett DJ. Effect of age on patterns of theophylline metabolism. *Clin Pharmacol Ther* 1980; **28:** 456–62.
5. Tserng K-Y, *et al.* Theophylline metabolism in premature infants. *Clin Pharmacol Ther* 1981; **29:** 594–600.
6. Tserng K-Y, *et al.* Developmental aspects of theophylline metabolism in premature infants. *Clin Pharmacol Ther* 1983; **33:** 522–8.
7. Stile IL, *et al.* Pharmacokinetics of theophylline in premature infants on the first day of life. *Clin Ther* 1986; **8:** 336–41.
8. Randolph WC, *et al.* The effect of age on theophylline clearance in normal subjects. *Br J Clin Pharmacol* 1986; **22:** 603–5.
9. Wiffen JK, *et al.* Does theophylline clearance alter within the adult age range? *Br J Clin Pharmacol* 1984; **17:** 219P.
10. Antal EJ, *et al.* Theophylline pharmacokinetics in advanced age. *Br J Clin Pharmacol* 1981; **12:** 637–45.
11. Jackson SHD, *et al.* The relationship between theophylline clearance and age in adult life. *Eur J Clin Pharmacol* 1989; **36:** 29–34.
12. Bauer LA, Blouin RA. Influence of age on theophylline clearance in patients with chronic obstructive pulmonary disease. *Clin Pharmacokinet* 1981; **6:** 469–74.
13. Fox RW, *et al.* Theophylline kinetics in a geriatric group. *Clin Pharmacol Ther* 1983; **34:** 60–7.


ELIMINATION KINETICS. There is evidence that the elimination of theophylline is dose-dependent and that at high serum concentrations, a small change in dose of a theophylline preparation could cause a disproportionate increase in serum-theophylline concentration, due to a reduction in clearance.[1-3] However, it is not clear that this effect is clinically significant when serum-theophylline concentrations are within the therapeutic range.[4-8] It has also been suggested that repeated oral dosing of theophylline might result in a decrease of clearance compared with pre-treatment values.[9]


1. Weinberger M, Ginchansky E. Dose-dependent kinetics of theophylline disposition in asthmatic children. *J Pediatr* 1977; **91:** 820–4.
2. Tang-Liu DD-S, *et al.* Nonlinear theophylline elimination. *Clin Pharmacol Ther* 1982; **31:** 358–69.
3. Butcher MA, *et al.* Dose-dependent pharmacokinetics with single daily dose slow release theophylline in patients with chronic lung disease. *Br J Clin Pharmacol* 1982; **13:** 241–3.
4. Koëter GH, *et al.* Pharmacokinetics of sustained release theophylline in low and high multidose regimens. *Br J Clin Pharmacol* 1981; **12:** 647–51.
5. Rovei V, *et al.* Pharmacokinetics of theophylline: a dose-range study. *Br J Clin Pharmacol* 1982; **14:** 769–78.
6. Gundert-Remy U, *et al.* Non-linear elimination processes of theophylline. *Eur J Clin Pharmacol* 1983; **24:** 71–8.
7. Brown PJ, *et al.* Lack of dose dependent kinetics of theophylline. *Eur J Clin Pharmacol* 1983; **24:** 525–7.
8. Milavetz G, *et al.* Dose dependency for absorption and elimination rates of theophylline: implications for studies of bioavailability. *Pharmacotherapy* 1984; **4:** 216–20.
9. Efthimiou H, *et al.* Influence of chronic dosing on theophylline clearance. *Br J Clin Pharmacol* 1984; **17:** 525–30.


GENDER. A higher theophylline clearance and shorter elimination half-life has been reported in healthy premenopausal women than in healthy men, probably due to sex-related differences in hepatic metabolism.[1] Changes in the pharmacokinetics of theophylline in women have also been reported according to the stage of the menstrual cycle;[2,3] another study[4] found no changes.


1. Nafziger AN, Bertino JS. Sex-related differences in theophylline pharmacokinetics. *Eur J Clin Pharmacol* 1989; **37:** 97–100.
2. Bruguerolle B, *et al.* Influence of the menstrual cycle on theophylline pharmacokinetics in asthmatics. *Eur J Clin Pharmacol* 1990; **39:** 59–61.
3. Nagata K, *et al.* Increased theophylline metabolism in the menstrual phase of healthy women. *J Allergy Clin Immunol* 1997; **100:** 39–43.
4. Matsuki S, *et al.* Pharmacokinetic changes of theophylline and amikacin through the menstrual cycle in healthy women. *J Clin Pharmacol* 1999; **39:** 1256–62.


**Pregnancy and breast feeding.** For mention of the pharmacokinetics of theophylline during pregnancy and breast feeding, see under Precautions, above.

**Protein binding.** Albumin is the major plasma binding protein for theophylline, binding is pH-dependent, and the percentage of theophylline bound at physiological pH is reported to range from about 35 to 45%.[1,2] Some studies have found the plasma protein binding of theophylline to be concentration dependent,[3] but others have not confirmed this.[1,4] Protein binding has been reported to be slightly but significantly higher in patients with bronchial asthma than in healthy controls.[5] Reduced protein binding occurs in patients with hypoalbuminaemia;[6,7] it has also been found in obese subjects[8] possibly due to elevated concentrations of free fatty acids which can displace theophylline from binding sites.


1. Buss D, *et al.* Determinants of the plasma protein binding of theophylline in health. *Br J Clin Pharmacol* 1983; **15:** 399–405.
2. Brørs O, *et al.* Binding of theophylline in human serum determined by ultrafiltration and equilibrium dialysis. *Br J Clin Pharmacol* 1983; **15:** 393–7.
3. Gundert-Remy U, Hildebrandt R. Binding of theophylline and its metabolites to human plasma proteins. *Br J Clin Pharmacol* 1983; **16:** 573–4.
4. Buss DC, *et al.* Protein binding of theophylline. *Br J Clin Pharmacol* 1985; **19:** 529–31.
5. Trnavská Z. Theophylline protein binding. *Arzneimittelforschung* 1990; **40:** 166–9.
6. Leopold D, *et al.* The ex vivo plasma protein binding of theophylline in renal disease. *Br J Clin Pharmacol* 1985; **19:** 823–5.
7. Connelly TJ, *et al.* Characterization of theophylline binding to serum proteins in pregnant and nonpregnant women. *Clin Pharmacol Ther* 1990; **47:** 68–72.
8. Shum L, Jusko WJ. Effects of obesity and ancillary variables (dialysis time, drug, albumin, and fatty acid concentrations) on theophylline serum protein binding. *Biopharm Drug Dispos* 1989; **10:** 549–62.


**Therapeutic drug monitoring.** Dosage requirements of theophylline preparations vary widely between subjects and even vary with time in individuals, since serum-theophylline concentrations are influenced by various factors including disease states, concurrent medication, diet, smoking, and age. Serious toxicity is related to serum concentration and may not be preceded by minor symptoms. For these reasons it is recommended that serum-theophylline concentrations should be monitored. The generally accepted optimal serum concentration is between 10 and 20 micrograms/mL,[1-4] but this should be regarded as a guide and not a rigid barrier and clinical decisions should never be based solely on the serum concentration.[1] The therapeutic range in the treatment of neonatal apnoea is usually considered to be 5 to 15 micrograms/mL although some babies may respond at lower concentrations.[5] Some now consider that this is a more appropriate range in asthma (except perhaps acute severe asthma).[6] It has been suggested that pulmonary function tests provide a better guide in long-term therapy with theophylline.[7]

Serum-theophylline concentrations were originally measured by spectrophotometry but this is subject to considerable interference from other drugs. High performance liquid chromatography is now the method of choice when extreme accuracy is important and the enzyme multiplied immunoassay technique (EMIT) has become popular because of its rapidity and adaptability to processing large batches.[2] Devices are also available that provide serum-theophylline measurements within several minutes using monoclonal antibody technology.[2,8]

The use of salivary concentrations for monitoring theophylline dosage requirements has been tried, because it is noninvasive, but poor correlations between salivary- and serum-theophylline concentrations mean it has not gained general usage.


1. Hampson JP. The theophylline "therapeutic window"—fact or fallacy? *Pharm J* 1988; **241:** 722–4.
2. Bierman CW, Williams PV. Therapeutic monitoring of theophylline: rationale and current status. *Clin Pharmacokinet* 1989; **17:** 377–84.
3. Holford N, *et al.* Theophylline target concentration in severe airways obstruction—10 or 20 mg/L. A randomised concentration-controlled trial. *Clin Pharmacokinet* 1993; **25:** 495–505.
4. Pesce AJ, *et al.* Standards of laboratory practice: theophylline and caffeine monitoring. *Clin Chem* 1998; **44:** 1124–8.
5. Edwards C. Theophylline and caffeine. *Pharm J* 1986; **237:** 128–9.
6. Hardy CC, Smith J. Adverse reactions profile: theophylline and aminophylline. *Prescribers' J* 1997; **37:** 96–101.
7. Ashutosh K, *et al.* Use of serum theophylline level as a guide to optimum therapy in patients with chronic obstructive lung disease. *J Clin Pharmacol* 1990; **30:** 324–9.
8. Clifton GD, *et al.* Accuracy and time requirements for use of three rapid theophylline assay methods. *Clin Pharm* 1988; **7:** 462–6.


## Uses and Administration

Theophylline is a xanthine (p.777) and relaxes bronchial smooth muscle, relieves bronchospasm, and has a stimulant effect on respiration. It stimulates the myocardium and CNS, decreases peripheral resistance and venous pressure, and causes diuresis. It is still not clear how theophylline exerts these effects. Inhibition of phosphodiesterase with a resulting increase in intracellular cyclic adenosine monophosphate (cyclic AMP) occurs, and may play a role. Other proposed mechanisms of action include adenosine receptor antagonism, prostaglandin antagonism, and effects on intracellular calcium.

Theophylline is used as a bronchodilator in the management of reversible airways obstruction, such as in asthma. Although selective $beta_2$ adrenoceptor stimulants ($beta_2$ agonists) such as salbutamol are generally the preferred bronchodilators for initial treatment, theophylline is commonly used as an adjunct to $beta_2$ agonist and corticosteroid therapy in patients requiring an additional bronchodilating effect. Some patients with chronic obstructive pulmonary disease also exhibit a beneficial response to theophylline therapy. Theophylline is also used to relieve apnoea in neonates. It was formerly used in the treatment of heart failure, and may occasionally have a role in patients with this condition who are also suffering from asthma and bronchitis.

Theophylline may be given in the anhydrous form or as the hydrate. Doses of theophylline are usually expressed as anhydrous theophylline; theophylline hydrate 1.1 mg is approximately equivalent to 1 mg of theophylline.

The pharmacokinetics of theophylline may be altered by a number of factors including age, smoking, disease, diet, and drug interactions (see above under Precautions, Interactions, and Pharmacokinetics). Theophylline doses should therefore be adjusted for each individual patient according to clinical response, adverse effects, and serum-theophylline concentrations.

- Optimum **therapeutic serum concentrations** of theophylline are traditionally considered to range from 10 to 20 micrograms/mL (55 to 110 micromoles/litre) and toxic effects are more common above 20 micrograms/mL. A range of 5 to 15 micrograms/mL may be effective, and associated with fewer adverse effects.

For long-term administration, once a maintenance dose has been established, monitoring of serum-theophylline concentrations at 6- to 12-monthly intervals has been recommended.

In the management of **acute severe bronchospasm**, theophylline may be given by *intravenous infusion*, though usually aminophylline is preferred (see p.780). (Anhydrous theophylline 1 mg is approximately equivalent to 1.17 mg anhydrous aminophylline or 1.27 mg aminophylline hydrate.)

- In patients not currently receiving theophylline, aminophylline, or other xanthine-containing medications, a suggested loading dose of 4 to 5 mg/kg may be given by intravenous infusion over 20 to 30 minutes followed by a suggested maintenance dose of 400 micrograms/kg per hour. Lower doses should be used in the elderly and those with cor pulmonale, heart failure, or liver disease; smokers may require a higher maintenance dose. Dosage should be calculated in terms of lean or ideal body-weight. Some authorities do not consider a loading dose is necessary unless the patient's condition is deteriorating.
- Suggested doses for children (not taking theophylline or other xanthine medication) are theophylline 4 to 5 mg/kg by intravenous infusion over 20 to 30 minutes, followed by maintenance doses of: in children 1 to 9 years, 800 micrograms/kg per hour; in children over 9 years, 600 to 700 micrograms/kg per hour.
- Intravenous theophylline therapy is best avoided in patients already taking theophylline, aminophylline, or other xanthine-containing medication but, if considered necessary, serum-theophylline concentrations should be monitored and the initial dose should be calculated on the basis that each 500 micrograms of theophylline/kg of lean body-weight will result in an increase of serum-theophylline concentration of 1 microgram/mL.

In the treatment of **acute bronchospasm** that has not required intravenous therapy, theophylline has been given *by mouth* in conventional dosage forms; modified-release preparations are not suitable.

- In the USA, one suggested oral regimen for adults and children not currently taking theophylline or xanthine-containing products is 5 mg/kg, to produce an average peak serum concentration of 10 micrograms/mL, and followed by appropriate oral maintenance doses. These are given every 6 to 8 hours in adults, and every 4 to 6 hours in children. Doses should again be reduced in the elderly and those with cor pulmonale, heart failure, or liver disease; smokers may require a higher maintenance dose.

In the long-term management of **chronic bronchospasm**, theophylline may be given *by mouth* in doses ranging from 300 to 1000 mg daily in divided doses as conventional tablets, capsules, liquid preparations, or modified-release preparations. For conventional dosage forms the divided doses are generally given every 6 to 8 hours. However, modified-release preparations are more commonly used as they reduce adverse effects and the need for frequent dosing, especially in patients with a rapid theophylline clearance.

- A usual dose of modified-release theophylline is 175 to 500 mg every 12 hours, though the bioavailability of different modified-release theophylline preparations may not be comparable and retitration of dosage is required if the patient is changed from one modified-release preparation to another. The total dose of some modified-release preparations may be given as a single daily dose, for example, in the evening if nocturnal symptoms and early morning wheezing are a problem.
- Initially, low doses of theophylline should be given and they should be gradually adjusted according to clinical response and serum-theophylline measurements. In the USA a preferred approach to initial dosage titration, in adults and children weighing over 45 kg, may be to begin with 300 mg daily, in divided doses, for 3 days; if well tolerated to increase the total daily dose to 400 mg for 3 days, and then 600 mg for a further 3 days, before titrating to a final dose based on serum-theophylline concentrations.
- In the UK, suggested oral doses for children weighing 20 to 35 kg (about 6 to 12 years old) are approximately half the adult dose; dosage recommendations for children aged 2 to 6 years are scarce and inconsistent, but one manufacturer recommends approximately quarter the adult dose; use for chronic bronchospasm in children under 2 years is not recommended. In the USA, suggested daily doses in children weighing less than 45 kg and 1 year of age or older are 12 to 14 mg/kg (maximum 300 mg) for 3 days initially, increased, if well tolerated, to 16 mg/kg (maximum 400 mg) for 3 days, and then up to 20 mg/kg (maximum 600 mg), before titrating to a final dose based on serum-theophylline concentrations.

Intramuscular injection and administration by suppository are not recommended due to severe local irritation and slow unreliable absorption.

Theophylline is an ingredient of some preparations promoted for coughs.

There are topical cosmetic preparations containing theophylline derivatives, particularly aminophylline, that have been promoted for the local reduction of body fat (p.781).

Theophylline monoethanolamine (theophylline olamine), theophylline calcium salicylate, theophylline and sodium acetate (theophylline sodium acetate), theophylline sodium glycinate (theophylline sodium aminoacetate), theophylline calcium glycinate, and theophylline glycinate have all been used similarly to theophylline.

◊ General references.


1. Vasallo R, Lipsky JJ. Theophylline: recent advances in the understanding of its mode of action and uses in clinical practice. *Mayo Clin Proc* 1998; **73:** 346–54.


**Administration.** Various methods have been proposed for estimating theophylline pharmacokinetic parameters to enable optimisation of initial dosage but none should be substituted for the subsequent determination of serum-theophylline concentrations and clearance at steady state.[1-3]

It was noted in 1997 that dosage requirements for theophylline had declined relative to those of historical controls, apparently due to a downward shift in theophylline clearance in the US population (perhaps due to environmental changes, such as a decrease in exposure to tobacco smoke).[4] It was suggested that earlier dosage guidelines for theophylline needed to be revised in the light of these data, so that the initial dose did not exceed 300 mg daily by mouth—for an approach to initial dosage titration consonant with this view, see Uses and Administration, above.


1. Erdman SM, *et al.* An updated comparison of drug dosing methods part II: theophylline. *Clin Pharmacokinet* 1991; **20:** 280–92.
2. Hogue SL, Phelps SJ. Evaluation of three theophylline dosing equations for use in infants up to one year of age. *J Pediatr* 1993; **123:** 651–6.
3. Lee TC, *et al.* Theophylline population pharmacokinetics from routine monitoring data in very premature infants with apnoea. *Br J Clin Pharmacol* 1996; **41:** 191–200.
4. Asmus MJ, *et al.* Apparent decrease in population clearance of theophylline: implications for dosage. *Clin Pharmacol Ther* 1997; **62:** 483–9.


ADMINISTRATION IN INFANTS. Theophylline clearance is reduced in premature neonates and infants under 1 year of age due to an immature hepatic microsomal enzyme system (see under Metabolism and Excretion in Pharmacokinetics, above). Postconceptional age may have a slight influence on theophylline clearance but postnatal age is thought to be more significant.[1]

Theophylline dosage guidelines for infants under 1 year of age were suggested by the FDA[2] in 1985, but a number of clinicians considered that higher doses might be necessary.[1,3,4] Subsequent guidelines for oral theophylline,[5] issued in 1995, suggested a modified regimen: premature infants should receive initial doses of 1 mg/kg every 12 hours if less than 24 days postnatal age, or 1.5 mg/kg every 12 hours if more than 24 days; in full-term infants initial daily dosage (to be given in 3 or 4 divided doses) could be calculated on the basis of the equation:

$$\text{Daily dose (mg/kg)} = (0.2 \times \text{age in weeks}) + 5.0$$

Subsequent dosage should be adjusted based on steady-state serum-theophylline concentrations, which might take as long as 5 days to be achieved in premature neonates if a loading dose is not used.[5] The recommended serum concentrations were 5 to 10 micrograms/mL in neonates and 10 to 15 micrograms/mL in older infants. If a loading dose is considered necessary, 5 mg/kg (or 1 mg/kg for each 2 micrograms/mL increase in serum-theophylline concentration in those already receiving theophylline) has been suggested.

Other equations and models of population pharmacokinetics have been proposed for the calculation of appropriate theophylline doses in neonates.[6-8]


1. Gilman JT, Gal P. Inadequacy of FDA dosing guidelines for theophylline use in neonates. *Drug Intell Clin Pharm* 1986; **20:** 481–4.
2. Anonymous. Use of theophylline in infants. *FDA Drug Bull* 1985; **15:** 16–17.
3. Murphy JE, *et al.* New FDA guidelines for theophylline dosing in infants. *Clin Pharm* 1986; **5:** 16.
4. Kriter KE, Blanchard J. Management of apnea in infants. *Clin Pharm* 1989; **8:** 577–87.
5. Hendeles L, *et al.* Revised FDA labeling guideline for theophylline oral dosage forms. *Pharmacotherapy* 1995; **15:** 409–27.
6. Hogue SL, Phelps SJ. Evaluation of three theophylline dosing equations for use in infants up to one year of age. *J Pediatr* 1993; **123:** 651–6.
7. Lee TC, *et al.* Theophylline population pharmacokinetics from routine monitoring data in very premature infants with apnoea. *Br J Clin Pharmacol* 1996; **41:** 191–200.
8. Gagnon AJ. Aminophylline dosing in the treatment of apnea of prematurity—a commentary. *Pharmacotherapy* 1996; **16:** 317–18.


**Asthma.** Theophylline and its derivatives may be used in the treatment of chronic asthma (p.777) as an adjunct to beta$_2$ agonists and corticosteroid therapy when an additional bronchodilator is indicated. Modified-release preparations can be useful in the control of nocturnal asthma.

Evidence suggests[1,2] that adding low-dose oral theophylline to inhaled corticosteroids is as effective as increasing the dose of corticosteroid in patients with moderate asthma and persistent symptoms. A systematic review[3] of trials that compared theophylline with long-acting beta$_2$ agonists found that they were both effective for control of nocturnal asthma, but that long-acting beta$_2$ agonists may be more effective in reducing asthma symptoms, including night waking and the need for rescue medication, and are associated with fewer adverse effects.

The use of xanthines in acute asthma attacks is more controversial. UK guidelines permit the use of intravenous aminophylline in patients with severe or unresponsive acute asthma, whereas US guidelines do not consider xanthines have any benefit over the optimal use of beta agonists and consequently do not recommend their use (see p.777).


1. Evans DJ, *et al.* A comparison of low-dose inhaled budesonide plus theophylline and high-dose inhaled budesonide for moderate asthma. *N Engl J Med* 1997; **337:** 1412–18.
2. Ukena D, *et al.* Comparison of addition of theophylline to inhaled steroid with doubling of the dose of inhaled steroid in asthma. *Eur Respir J* 1997; **10:** 2754–60.
3. Shah L, *et al.* Long acting beta-agonists versus theophylline for maintenance treatment of asthma. Available in The Cochrane Library; Issue 1. Chichester: John Wiley; 2004.


**Cardiac arrhythmias.** Theophylline has been tried in various bradyarrhythmias, usually when other treatment has failed or is contra-indicated.[1-6]


1. Viskin S, *et al.* Aminophylline for bradyasystolic cardiac arrest refractory to atropine and epinephrine. *Ann Intern Med* 1993; **118:** 279–81.
2. Sra JS, *et al.* Comparison of cardiac pacing with drug therapy in the treatment of neurocardiogenic (vasovagal) syncope with bradycardia or asystole. *N Engl J Med* 1993; **328:** 1085–90.
3. Bertolet BD, *et al.* Theophylline for the treatment of atrioventricular block after myocardial infarction. *Ann Intern Med* 1995; **123:** 509–11.
4. Alboni P, *et al.* Effects of permanent pacemaker and oral theophylline in sick sinus syndrome: the THEOPACE study: a randomized controlled trial. *Circulation* 1997; **96:** 260–6.
5. Ling CA, Crouch MA. Theophylline for chronic symptomatic bradycardia in the elderly. *Ann Pharmacother* 1998; **32:** 837–9.
6. Cawley MJ, *et al.* Intravenous theophylline — an alternative to temporary pacing in the management of bradycardia secondary to AV nodal block. *Ann Pharmacother* 2001; **35:** 303–7.


**Cheyne-Stokes respiration.** Oral theophylline considerably reduced Cheyne-Stokes respiration (periodic breathing) and episodes of central apnoea in a study in 15 patients with stable heart failure and left ventricular systolic dysfunction.[1] This was associated with an improvement in arterial-oxygen saturation during sleep. There was no significant change in cardiac function, although pulmonary function did improve. Theophylline was also effective in a patient with Cheyne-Stokes respiration possibly related to diabetic autonomic neuropathy[2] (the use of the term Cheyne-Stokes respiration to describe this patient's respiratory disorder has been questioned[3,4]).


1. Javaheri S, *et al.* Effect of theophylline on sleep-disordered breathing in heart failure. *N Engl J Med* 1996; **335:** 562–7.
2. Pesek CA, *et al.* Theophylline therapy for near-fatal Cheyne-Stokes respiration: a case report. *Ann Intern Med* 1999; **130:** 427–30.
3. Sin DD, Bradley TD. Theophylline therapy for near-fatal Cheyne-Stokes respiration. *Ann Intern Med* 1999; **131:** 713.
4. Geigel EJ, Chediak AD. Theophylline therapy for near-fatal Cheyne-Stokes respiration. *Ann Intern Med* 1999; **131:** 713–14.


**Chronic obstructive pulmonary disease.** In the treatment of chronic obstructive pulmonary disease (p.779), the bronchodilators of first choice are usually either an antimuscarinic such as ipratropium bromide, or a beta$_2$ agonist such as salbutamol, given by inhalation. However the addition of a xanthine such as theophylline, administered by mouth, may be of value in some patients to maximise respiratory function and for its positive cardiac inotropic effects.

**ECT.** For mention of the use of theophylline as an adjunct to electroconvulsive therapy, see under Precautions, above.

**Erythrocytosis.** Erythrocytosis (secondary polycythaemia) is an absolute increase in red cell mass that may occur as a result of tissue hypoxia (as in chronic obstructive airways disease), or excessive erythropoietin production (as in some renal tumours or after renal transplant). Post-transplantation erythrocytosis is usually self-limiting but weekly phlebotomy may be required to avoid thromboembolic complications. Theophylline 8 mg/kg daily by mouth has been shown to reduce haematocrit, red cell mass, and serum-erythropoietin concentrations in post-transplantation erythrocytosis,[1,2] and was beneficial in up to 60% of patients.[2] However, there is evidence that an ACE inhibitor may be more effective than theophylline for this purpose.[3] Theophylline treatment may also reduce erythrocytosis associated with chronic obstructive pulmonary disease.[4] Beneficial effects have also been reported for losartan in both forms of erythrocytosis.


1. Bakris GL, *et al.* Effects of theophylline on erythropoietin production in normal subjects and in patients with erythrocytosis after renal transplantation. *N Engl J Med* 1990; **323:** 86–90.
2. Ilan Y, *et al.* Erythrocytosis after renal transplantation: the response to theophylline treatment. *Transplantation* 1994; **57:** 661–4.
3. Ok E, *et al.* Comparison of the effects of enalapril and theophylline on polycythemia after renal transplantation. *Transplantation* 1995; **59:** 1623–45.
4. Oren R, *et al.* Effect of theophylline on erythrocytosis in chronic obstructive pulmonary disease. *Arch Intern Med* 1997; **157:** 1474–8.


**Methotrexate neurotoxicity.** For reference to the use of aminophylline or theophylline to relieve the acute neurotoxicity of methotrexate, see p.570.

**Neonatal apnoea.** Apnoea of infancy has been defined as cessation of breathing either lasting 20 seconds or more or associated with bradycardia, cyanosis, pallor, and marked hypotonia, for which no specific cause can be identified.[1] Premature infants (less than 37 weeks' gestation) can exhibit periodic breathing with pathological apnoea (apnoea of prematurity); this usually resolves as the infant approaches term and the neurological systems controlling ventilation mature.[1,2]

The management of neonatal apnoea for which no underlying disorder can be found may involve supportive measures such as water beds and cardiorespiratory monitoring, or in some cases, drug therapy.

Administration of either caffeine (as the citrate) or theophylline has been found to reduce the number and severity of apnoeic episodes within 24 to 48 hours in premature infants;[3-7] it is important to rule out any underlying seizure disorder before beginning such therapy. Caffeine has a wider therapeutic index and fewer peripheral adverse effects than theophylline, and a longer half-life enabling once-daily administration, and is therefore preferred.[1,6] It may be effective in some children unresponsive to theophylline.[2] The oral route is generally preferred.[1] Appropriate serum concentrations have been considered to be 5 to 15 micrograms/mL for theophylline (see also under Administration in Infants, above) and 8 to 20 micrograms/mL for caffeine.[1] High doses of caffeine (to produce a desired serum concentration of 26 to 40 micrograms/mL) have been used to obtain a faster response (within 8 hours) without apparent side-effects.[5] During the first year of life, the elimination half-life of both caffeine and theophylline decreases significantly as the infant matures; regular monitoring of serum concentrations and constant dosage adjustments are therefore required.[1]

As the patient gets older or becomes asymptomatic (for at least 4 to 8 weeks), xanthine therapy can be withdrawn on a trial basis to see if apnoea will recur.

Use of doxapram may be considered for apnoea that does not respond to xanthine therapy.[1,2,7] It is as effective as theophylline, and may also be of benefit as an addition to xanthine therapy[8,9] but must be given by continuous intravenous infusion and blood pressure must be monitored for signs of hypertension.[2] Adverse effects such as irritability and convulsions may also be a problem.[2]


1. Kriter KE, Blanchard J. Management of apnea in infants. *Clin Pharm* 1989; **8:** 577–87.
2. Ruggins NR. Pathophysiology of apnoea in preterm infants. *Arch Dis Child* 1991; **66:** 70–73.
3. Murat I, *et al.* The efficacy of caffeine in the treatment of recurrent idiopathic apnea in premature infants. *J Pediatr* 1981; **99:** 984–9.
4. Autret E, *et al.* Comparaison de deux doses d'entretien différentes de caféine dans le traitment des apnées du prématuré. *Therapie* 1985; **40:** 235–9.
5. Scanlon JEM, *et al.* Caffeine or theophylline for neonatal apnoea? *Arch Dis Child* 1992; **67:** 425–8.
6. Henderson-Smart DJ, Steer P. Methylxanthine treatment for apnea in preterm infants. Available in The Cochrane Library; Issue 1. Chichester: John Wiley; 2004.
7. Hascoet J-M, *et al.* Risks and benefits of therapies for apnoea in premature infants. *Drug Safety* 2000; **23:** 363–79.
8. Eyal F, *et al.* Aminophylline versus doxapram in idiopathic apnea of prematurity: a double-blind controlled study. *Pediatrics* 1985; **75:** 709–13.
9. Peliowski A, Finer NN. A blinded, randomized, placebo-controlled trial to compare theophylline and doxapram for the treatment of apnea of prematurity. *J Pediatr* 1990; **116:** 648–53.


## Preparations

***USP 27:*** Theophylline and Guaifenesin Capsules; Theophylline and Guaifenesin Oral Solution; Theophylline Capsules; Theophylline Extended-release Capsules; Theophylline in Dextrose Injection; Theophylline Oral Solution; Theophylline Sodium Glycinate Elixir; Theophylline Sodium Glycinate Tablets; Theophylline Tablets; Theophylline, Ephedrine Hydrochloride, and Phenobarbital Tablets.

**Proprietary Preparations** (details are given in Part 3)

***Arg.:*** Aminofilin; Asmabiol; Crisasma; Drilyna; Nefoben; Teodosis; Teosona; Teosona Sol; Theo-Dur; ***Austral.:*** Austyn†; Nuelin; Theo-Dur†; ***Austria:*** Aerodyne; Afonilum; Euphyllin; Pulmidur; Respicur; Theohexal†; Theoplus; Theospirex; Unifyl; ***Belg.:*** Euphyllin; Theo-Dur†; Theolair; Theophyllard†; Xanthium; ***Braz.:*** Bermacia; Bronquiasma†; Codrinan; Talofilina; Teolong; Teophyl; Teoston; ***Canad.:*** Apo-Theo; Novo-Theophyl; Pulmophylline†; Quibron-T; Slo-Bid†; Theo-Dur; Theo-SR†; Theochron†; Theolair; Uniphyl; ***Chile:*** Elixine; ***Denm.:*** Nuelin; Pulmo-Timelets; Theo-Dur; UniXan; Uno-Lin; ***Fin.:*** Euphyllin; Nuelin; Retafyllin; Theo-Dur; Theofol; ***Fr.:*** Euphylline; Theolair†; Theostat; Xanthium; ***Ger.:*** Aerobin; Afonilum; Afonilum novo; afpred-THEO; Bronchoparat; Bronchoretard; Contiphyllin; Cronasma; Ditenate N†; duraphyllin; Etheophyl†; Euphyllin†; Euphylong; Myocardon N†; Perasthman N†; Pulmidur; Pulmo-Timelets; Solosin; theo; Theolair; Theophyllard†; Tromphyllin; Unilair; Uniphyllin; ***Gr.:*** Aberten; Novaphylline; Theo-Bros; Theo-Dur; Theoplus; Uniphyllin; ***Hong Kong:*** Apo-Theo†; Euphylong; Novo-Theophyl; Nuelin; Phenedrine†; Slo-Bid†; Slo-Theo; Theo-Dur; Theovent†; Uniphyl†; ***India:*** Phylobid; Phyloday; Theo PA; Unicontin; ***Irl.:*** Lasma†; Nuelin; Pro-Vent†; Slo-Phyllin; Theo-Dur†; Theolan†; Uniphyllin Continus; Zepholin; ***Israel:*** Asthma T†; Glyphyllin; Theotard; Theotrim; ***Ital.:*** Aminomal; Diffumal; Euphyllina; Frivent; Paidomal; Respicur; Tefamin; Teobid†; Teonova†; Theo-24; Theo-Dur; Theolair; Uni-Dur†; ***Jpn:*** Theolong; ***Malaysia:*** Apo-Theo; Nuelin; Numalin; Retafyllin; Theolin; ***Mex.:*** Elixofilina†; Slo-Bid; Teolong; Uni-Dur; ***Mon.:*** Dilatrane; Pneumogeine; Tedralan; ***Neth.:*** Euphylong†; Theolair; Theolin†; Unilair†; ***Norw.:*** Euphyllin†; Nuelin; Theo-Dur; ***NZ:*** Nuelin; Theo-Dur†; ***Port.:*** Eufilina; Lepobron; Teonibsa; Teovent; Unicontin; ***S.Afr.:*** Alcophyllin; Chronophyllin; Euphyllin; Microphyllin; Nuelin; Pulmophyllin; Theo-Dur†; Theoplus; Uni-Dur†; Uniphyl; ***Singapore:*** Apo-Theo; Austyn†; Nuelin; Retafyllin; Theo-Dur†; Theolin; Theoplus; ***Spain:*** Chantaline; Elixifilin; Eufilina; Histafilin; Neo Elixifilin†; Piridasmin†; Pulmeno; Teolixir; Teromol; Theo Max; Theo-Dur; Theolair; Theoplus; Unilong; Vent Retard; ***Swed.:*** Euphylong; Theo-Dur; ***Switz.:*** Euphyllin; Sodip-phylline; Theolair; Unifyl; Xantivent†; ***Thai.:*** Aerobin; Almarion; Asmasolon; Franol; Med-Phylline; Nuelin; Quibron†; Retafyllin; Temaco; Theo-Dur†; Theotrim; Xanthium; ***UAE:*** Theophar; ***UK:*** Lasma†; Nuelin; Slo-Phyllin; Theo-Dur†; Uniphyllin Continus; ***USA:*** Accurbron; Aerolate; Aquaphyllin; Asmalix; Elixomin; Elixophyllin; Quibron-T; Respbid; Slo-Bid; Slo-Phyllin; Sustaire; T-Phyl; Theo-24; Theo-Dur†; Theo-X; Theobid Duracaps; Theochron; Theolair; Theospan-SR†; Theovent; Uni-Dur†; Uniphyl.

**Multi-ingredient:** ***Arg.:*** Airbronal; Bronkasma; Bronquisedan; Dexa Aminofilin; Dexa Teosona; Fatigan Bronquial; Inastmol; Sedacris; ***Austria:*** Ambredin; Asthma 23 D; Bronchisan†; Perphyllon†; Thilocombin†; ***Braz.:*** Abacateirol†; Alergotox†; Asmatiron†; Bronquitos; CAM†; Endotussin; Filinasma†; Franol; Marax; ***Canad.:*** Tedral†; Theo-Bronc; ***Fin.:*** Theofol Comp; ***Fr.:*** Hypnasmine; ***Ger.:*** Broncho-Euphyllin; Eudur†; ***Hong Kong:*** Lipostabil†; ***India:*** Alergin; Asmapax; Asthmino; Deriphyllin; Etyofil; Marax; Tergil-T; Theo-Asthalin; Theobric; ***Irl.:*** Franol Expectorant; Franol†; ***Israel:*** Bronchophylline†; ***Malaysia:*** Asthma; Brondal; Grenin; ***Mex.:*** Aminoefedrison NF; ***Port.:*** Cosmaxil; Prelus; ***S.Afr.:*** Actophlem; Alcophyllex; Diatussin; Lipostabil†; Metaxol; Solphyllex; Solphyllin; Theophen; Theophen Comp; ***Spain:*** Novofilin; Teolixir Compositum; Winasma†; ***Switz.:*** Neo-Biphyllin†; ***Thai.:*** Almasal; Asianbron; Bronchil; Brondil; Mila-Asma; Polyphed; Qualiton; Theosal†; ***UK:*** Do-Do ChestEze; Franol; Franol Plus; Franolyn Expectorant†; ***USA:*** Elixophyllin-GG; Elixophyllin-KI; Glyceryl-T; Hydrophed; Marax; Primatene Dual Action†; Quadrinal; Quibron; Slo-Phyllin GG; Tedrigen; Theodrine; Theomax DF.

---

# Tiotropium Bromide *(BAN, rINN)*

BA-679; Ba-679BR; Bromuro de tiotropio. 6β,7β-Epoxy-3β-hydroxy-8-methyl-1αH,5αH-tropanium bromide di-2-thienylglycolate.

$C_{19}H_{22}BrNO_4S_2$ = 472.4.

*CAS — 139404-48-1 (anhydrous tiotropium bromide or tiotropium bromide hydrate); 136310-93-5 (anhydrous tiotropium bromide); 411207-31-3 (tiotropium bromide monohydrate).*

*ATC — R03BB04.*

## Profile

Tiotropium bromide is a quaternary ammonium antimuscarinic, structurally related to ipratropium (p.787), that has a prolonged bronchodilator action. It is used in the maintenance treatment of reversible airways obstruction, as in chronic obstructive pulmonary disease (p.779). Tiotropium bromide is given as inhalation powder in capsules containing 22.5 micrograms of tiotropium bromide monohydrate, equivalent to 18 micrograms of tiotropium, and supplying 10 micrograms of tiotropium from the mouthpiece of the inhaler device. The contents of one capsule are inhaled daily, at the same time each day.

◊ References.


1. O'Connor BJ, *et al.* Prolonged effect of tiotropium bromide on methacholine-induced bronchoconstriction in asthma. *Am J Respir Crit Care Med* 1996; **154:** 876–80.
2. Casaburi R, *et al.* The spirometric efficacy of once-daily dosing with tiotropium in stable COPD: a 13-week multicenter trial. *Chest* 2000; **118:** 1294–1302.
3. van Noord JA, *et al.* A randomised controlled comparison of tiotropium and ipratropium in the treatment of chronic obstructive pulmonary disease. *Thorax* 2000; **55:** 289–94.
4. Vincken W, *et al.* Improved health outcomes in patients with COPD during 1 yr's treatment with tiotropium. *Eur Respir J* 2002; **19:** 209–16.
5. Casaburi R, *et al.* A long-term evaluation of once-daily inhaled tiotropium in chronic obstructive pulmonary disease. *Eur Respir J* 2002; **19:** 217–24.
6. Donohue JF, *et al.* A 6-month, placebo-controlled study comparing lung function and health status changes in COPD patients treated with tiotropium or salmeterol. *Chest* 2002; **122:** 47–55.
7. Hvizdos KM, Goa KL. Tiotropium bromide. *Drugs* 2002; **62:** 1195–1203.


## Preparations

**Proprietary Preparations** (details are given in Part 3)
***Austral.:*** Spiriva; ***Chile:*** Spiriva; ***Irl.:*** Spiriva; ***Port.:*** Spiriva; ***UK:*** Spiriva; ***USA:*** Spiriva.

---

# Tranilast *(USAN, rINN)*

MK-341; N-5'. N-(3,4-Dimethoxycinnamoyl)anthranilic acid.

$C_{18}H_{17}NO_5$ = 327.3.

*CAS — 53902-12-8.*

## Adverse Effects and Precautions

Adverse effects reported with tranilast have included gastrointestinal disturbances, headache, drowsiness or insomnia, dizziness, malaise, and skin rashes and generalised pruritus. Rarely, liver function disturbance or jaundice, cystitis-like symptoms, anaemia, palpitations, oedema, facial flushing, and stomatitis may occur. Tranilast should be used with caution in patients with impaired hepatic function. Haematological monitoring is recommended.

The manufacturers advise against the use of tranilast in pregnancy because of teratogenicity in *animal* studies.

It should not be used for the treatment of acute asthma attacks. The general cautions described under sodium cromoglicate (p.796) also apply.

## Uses and Administration

Tranilast has a stabilising action on mast cells resembling that of sodium cromoglicate (p.796). It is also stated to inhibit collagen synthesis in fibroblasts. It is used in the prophylactic management of asthma (p.777) and in allergic rhinitis (p.422), conjunctivitis (p.421), and eczema (p.1135). It is also used in the management of keloids and hypertrophic scarring. Adults have been given 100 mg three times daily by mouth; 5 mg/kg daily in divided doses has been suggested for children. Eye drops containing tranilast 0.5% are administered four times daily for allergic conjunctivitis.

Tranilast has been investigated for the prevention of restenosis following coronary artery revascularisation procedures but was found to be ineffective.

**Sarcoidosis.** For a mention of possible benefit from tranilast in cutaneous sarcoidosis, see p.1087.

## Preparations

**Proprietary Preparations** (details are given in Part 3)
***Jpn:*** Rizaben.

---

# Tretoquinol Hydrochloride *(pINNM)*

AQ-110 (tretoquinol); Hidrocloruro de tretoquinol; Ro-07-5965; Trimethoquinol Hydrochloride; Trimetoquinol Hydrochloride. (−)-1,2,3,4-Tetrahydro-1-(3,4,5-trimethoxybenzyl)isoquinoline-6,7-diol hydrochloride monohydrate.

$C_{19}H_{23}NO_5,HCl,H_2O$ = 399.9.

*CAS — 30418-38-3 (tretoquinol); 18559-59-6 (anhydrous tretoquinol hydrochloride).*

*ATC — R03AC09; R03CC09.*

**Pharmacopoeias.** In *Jpn.*

## Profile

Tretoquinol is a direct-acting sympathomimetic reported to have a selective action on beta$_2$ receptors (a beta$_2$ agonist). It has properties similar to those of salbutamol (p.791). It is given as the hydrochloride for its bronchodilating properties in the management of reversible airways obstruction, as in asthma (p.777) or in some patients with chronic obstructive pulmonary disease (p.779). A usual dose by mouth is 2 to 4 mg of tretoquinol hydrochloride two to three times daily.

## Preparations

**Proprietary Preparations** (details are given in Part 3)
***Jpn:*** Inolin.

---

# Tulobuterol Hydrochloride *(BANM, rINNM)*

C-78; Hidrocloruro de tulobuterol; HN-078 (tulobuterol). 2-*tert*-Butylamino-1-*o*-chlorophenylethanol hydrochloride.

$C_{12}H_{18}ClNO,HCl$ = 264.2.

*CAS — 41570-61-0 (tulobuterol); 56776-01-3 (tulobuterol hydrochloride).*

*ATC — R03AC11; R03CC11.*

**Pharmacopoeias.** In *Jpn.*

## Profile

Tulobuterol is a direct-acting sympathomimetic with mainly beta-adrenergic activity and a selective action on beta$_2$ receptors (a beta$_2$ agonist). It has properties similar to those of salbutamol (p.791).

Tulobuterol is used as a bronchodilator in the management of reversible airways obstruction, as in asthma (p.777) and in some patients with chronic obstructive pulmonary disease (p.779). It is given by mouth as the hydrochloride. The initial oral dose in adults is 1 or 2 mg of tulobuterol hydrochloride twice daily, increased to 2 mg three times daily if necessary. A suggested dose for children is: 1 to 6 years, 0.25 to 0.5 mg twice daily; 6 to 10 years, 0.5 to 1 mg twice daily; 10 to 14 years, 1 to 1.5 mg twice daily. Tulobuterol has also been given as the base by inhalation from a metered-dose inhaler. A transdermal formulation of tulobuterol base is also available.

◊ References to the transdermal formulation of tulobuterol.


1. Uematsu T, *et al.* The pharmacokinetics of the $\beta_2$-adrenoceptor agonist, tulobuterol, given transdermally and by inhalation. *Eur J Clin Pharmacol.* 1993; **44:** 361–4.
2. Iikura Y, *et al.* Pharmacokinetics and pharmacodynamics of the tulobuterol patch, HN-078, in childhood asthma. *Ann Allergy* 1995; **74:** 147–51.


### Preparations

**Proprietary Preparations** (details are given in Part 3)
***Austria:*** Bremax; ***Belg.:*** Respacal; ***Ger.:*** Atenos; Brelomax; ***Jpn:*** Hokunalin; ***Mex.:*** Bremax†; ***Port.:*** Atenos; ***UK:*** Respacal†.

## Zafirlukast *(BAN, USAN, rINN)*

ICI-204219. Cyclopentyl 3-{2-methoxy-4-[(o-tolylsulfonyl)carbamoyl]benzyl}-1-methylindole-5-carbamate.
$C_{31}H_{33}N_3O_6S$ = 575.7.
*CAS — 107753-78-6.*
*ATC — R03DC01.*

### Adverse Effects and Precautions

Headache, an increased incidence of respiratory-tract infection (in the elderly), and gastrointestinal disturbances have been reported with zafirlukast and other leukotriene antagonists. Other adverse effects have included generalised pain, arthralgia, myalgia, fever, and dizziness. Elevations in liver enzyme values have occurred, and rarely, symptomatic hepatitis or hyperbilirubinaemia (see also below); fatalities have occurred. Hypersensitivity reactions, including rashes, urticaria, and angioedema, have been reported. There have also been rare reports of agranulocytosis, bleeding, bruising and oedema. There have been a few reports of systemic eosinophilia consistent with Churg-Strauss syndrome in patients receiving zafirlukast (see below); treatment should be withdrawn in these patients.

Zafirlukast and other leukotriene antagonists should not be used for the treatment of acute asthma attacks. Zafirlukast is contra-indicated in patients with hepatic impairment or cirrhosis.

**Churg-Strauss syndrome.** Pulmonary infiltrates and eosinophilia, resembling the Churg-Strauss syndrome, with dilated cardiomyopathy, were reported following the withdrawal of corticosteroid therapy in 8 patients receiving zafirlukast.[1] Symptoms responded to withdrawal of zafirlukast and treatment with corticosteroids, with or without cyclophosphamide. It has been suggested that the patients' original asthmatic symptoms had been part of an unrecognised vasculitic syndrome that was unmasked by the corticosteroid withdrawal.[2] However, others have reported Churg-Strauss syndrome associated with zafirlukast in patients who had not been receiving corticosteroids,[3,4] although these cases were not inconsistent with the view that treatment with leukotriene antagonists was coincidental.[5] Eosinophilic syndromes have also been reported for other anti-asthma drugs including inhaled fluticasone and sodium cromoglicate, evidence supporting a non-drug-related aetiology.[5] However, the increasing number of reports with zafirlukast and the other leukotriene antagonists, montelukast (see p.789) and pranlukast,[6] means that a particular class-effect cannot be ruled out.[7] It has been suggested that patients should be monitored carefully (e.g. by measuring erythrocyte sedimentation rate, C reactive protein, and eosinophil counts) if the introduction of an anti-asthma drug such as a leukotriene antagonist permits the reduction of oral corticosteroid dosage.[8] In addition, in patients with asthma and features of multisystem disease, the possibility of underlying Churg-Strauss syndrome (p.1078) may be worth considering.


1. Wechsler ME, *et al.* Pulmonary infiltrates, eosinophilia, and cardiomyopathy following corticosteroid withdrawal in patients with asthma receiving zafirlukast. *JAMA* 1998; **279:** 455–7.
2. Churg A, Churg J. Steroids and Churg-Strauss syndrome. *Lancet* 1998; **352:** 32–3.
3. Katz RS, Papernik M. Zafirlukast and Churg-Strauss syndrome. *JAMA* 1998; **279:** 1949.
4. Green RL, Vayonis AG. Churg-Strauss syndrome after zafirlukast in two patients not receiving systemic steroid treatment. *Lancet* 1999; **353:** 725–6.
5. Wechsler M, Drazen JM. Churg-Strauss syndrome. *Lancet* 1999; **353:** 1970.
6. Kinoshita M, *et al.* Churg-Strauss syndrome after corticosteroid withdrawal in an asthmatic patient treated with pranlukast. *J Allergy Clin Immunol* 1999; **103:** 534–5.
7. Green RL, Vayonis AG. Churg-Strauss syndrome. *Lancet* 1999; **353:** 1971.
8. D'Cruz DP, *et al.* Difficult asthma or Churg-Strauss syndrome? *BMJ* 1999; **318:** 475–6.


**Effects on the liver.** Severe hepatotoxicity has been associated with zafirlukast.[1-4] The Canadian manufacturer reported[4] in April 2004 that from worldwide postmarketing surveillance of zafirlukast there had been 46 reports of hepatitis, 14 of hepatic failure, 3 of which progressed to fulminant hepatitis, and 59 reports of other clinically significant hepatic dysfunction; 7 fatalities had occurred. In most, but not all, cases symptoms had abated and liver enzymes had returned to normal after stopping zafirlukast. It was important that prescribers, patients and/or their carers were alert to the signs and symptoms of hepatotoxicity. In Canada and in the USA, the manufacturers of zafirlukast advise stopping treatment if hepatotoxicity is suspected, and performing liver function tests; UK product information suggests that the decision to cease therapy should be based on an assessment of the individual benefits and potential risks.


1. Grieco AJ, Burstein-Stein J. Oral montelukast versus inhaled salmeterol to prevent exercise-induced bronchoconstriction. *Ann Intern Med* 2000; **133:** 392.
2. Reinus JF, *et al.* Severe liver injury after treatment with the leukotriene receptor antagonist zafirlukast. *Ann Intern Med* 2000; **133:** 964–8.
3. Danese S, *et al.* Severe liver injury associated with zafirlukast. *Ann Intern Med* 2001; **135:** 930.
4. AstraZeneca Canada. Important safety information regarding reports of serious hepatic events in patients receiving Accolate® (zafirlukast). Available at: http://www.hc-sc.gc.ca/hpfb-dgpsa/tpd-dpt/accolate_2_hpc_e.pdf (accessed 21/04/04)


**Lupus.** Zafirlukast was thought to be responsible for the development of lupus in a 9-year-old girl.[1]


1. Finkel TH, *et al.* Drug-induced lupus in a child after treatment with zafirlukast (Accolate). *J Allergy Clin Immunol* 1999; **103:** 533–4.


**Renal impairment.** The UK manufacturer states that zafirlukast should be used with caution in patients with moderate or severe renal impairment because of limited experience in this group. However, the US manufacturer mentions no such caution, and states that the pharmacokinetics of zafirlukast in patients with renal impairment do not appear to differ from those in patients with normal renal function. Only about 10% of a dose is reported to be excreted in the urine.

### Interactions

Zafirlukast is metabolised by hepatic cytochrome P450, specifically the CYP2C9 isoenzyme, and has been shown to inhibit the activity of isoenzymes CYP2C9 and CYP3A4. Therefore, concomitant use of other drugs that are metabolised by these hepatic enzymes may result in increases in plasma concentrations, and possibly, adverse effects. Patients receiving warfarin may develop prolongation of the prothrombin time and anticoagulant dosage should be adjusted accordingly. Erythromycin, terfenadine and theophylline may reduce plasma concentrations of zafirlukast; zafirlukast has rarely been reported to increase plasma-theophylline concentrations. Increased plasma concentrations of zafirlukast have been seen when given with high doses of aspirin.

### Pharmacokinetics

Peak plasma concentrations of zafirlukast occur about 3 hours after oral administration. The absolute bioavailability is uncertain, but administration with food reduces both the rate and extent of absorption, decreasing bioavailability by about 40%. Zafirlukast is about 99% bound to plasma proteins. It is extensively metabolised in the liver, predominantly by the cytochrome P450 isoenzyme CYP2C9, and excreted principally in faeces, as unchanged drug and metabolites. About 10% of a dose is excreted in urine as metabolites. The terminal elimination half-life of zafirlukast is about 10 hours. Studies in *animals* suggest that small amounts cross the placenta; it is also distributed in low concentrations into breast milk.

◊ Reviews.


1. Dekhuijzen PNR, Koopmans PP. Pharmacokinetic profile of zafirlukast. *Clin Pharmacokinet* 2002; **41:** 105–14.


### Uses and Administration

Zafirlukast is a selective antagonist of the leukotriene $D_4$ receptor (p.777), stimulation of which by circulating leukotrienes is thought to play a role in the pathogenesis of asthma. It suppresses both early and late bronchoconstrictor responses to inhaled antigens or irritants, but is not suitable for the management of acute attacks of asthma.

Zafirlukast is used in the management of chronic asthma. It is given by mouth in doses of 20 mg twice daily, taken at least 1 hour before or 2 hours after meals. Children aged 5 to 11 years may be given 10 mg twice daily.

◊ General references.


1. Lipworth BJ. Leukotriene-receptor antagonists. *Lancet* 1999; **353:** 57–62.
2. Dunn CJ, Goa KL. Zafirlukast: an update of its pharmacology and therapeutic efficacy in asthma. *Drugs* 2001; **61:** 285–315.
3. García-Marcos L, *et al.* Benefit-risk assessment of antileukotrienes in the management of asthma. *Drug Safety* 2003; **26:** 483–518.


**Asthma.** Zafirlukast produces modest improvement in mild-to-moderate asthma,[1,2] which was of a similar order to that seen with inhaled sodium cromoglicate in one study,[3] but less than that of inhaled salmeterol in another.[4] It has also been found to be less effective than inhaled fluticasone in persistent asthma.[5-7] Guidelines for the management of asthma (p.777) permit the use of zafirlukast as an alternative to inhaled corticosteroids in patients with mild persistent asthma, who cannot be managed with inhaled beta$_2$ agonists on an as-needed basis alone. It can also be considered for use in moderate or severe persistent asthma, usually added to standard therapy of inhaled corticosteroids and long-acting inhaled beta$_2$ agonists.


1. Suissa S, *et al.* Effectiveness of the leukotriene receptor antagonist zafirlukast for mild-to-moderate asthma: a randomized, double-blind, placebo-controlled trial. *Ann Intern Med* 1997; **126:** 177–83.
2. Fish JE, *et al.* Zafirlukast for symptomatic mild-to-moderate asthma: a 13-week multicenter study. *Clin Ther* 1997; **19:** 675–90.
3. Nathan RA, *et al.* Two first-line therapies in the treatment of mild asthma: use of peak flow variability as a predictor of effectiveness. *Ann Allergy Asthma Immunol* 1999; **82:** 497–503.
4. Busse W, *et al.* Comparison of inhaled salmeterol and oral zafirlukast in patients with asthma. *J Allergy Clin Immunol* 1999; **103:** 1075–80.
5. Busse W, *et al.* Fluticasone propionate compared with zafirlukast in controlling persistent asthma: a randomized double-blind, placebo-controlled trial. *J Fam Pract* 2001; **50:** 595–602.
6. Nathan RA, *et al.* A comparison of short-term treatment with inhaled fluticasone propionate and zafirlukast for patients with persistent asthma. *Am J Med* 2001; **111:** 195–202.
7. Brabson JH, *et al.* Efficacy and safety of low-dose fluticasone propionate compared with zafirlukast in patients with persistent asthma. *Am J Med* 2002; **113:** 15–21.


**Rhinitis.** Although it was reported to improve symptoms of seasonal allergic rhinitis (p.422) in one study,[1] zafirlukast 20 mg twice daily was not effective when compared with placebo and intranasal beclometasone in another.[2]


1. Donnelly AL, *et al.* The leukotriene $D_4$-receptor antagonist, ICI 204,219, relieves symptoms of acute seasonal allergic rhinitis. *Am J Respir Crit Care Med* 1995; **151:** 1734–9.
2. Pullerits T, *et al.* Randomized placebo-controlled study comparing a leukotriene receptor antagonist and a nasal glucocorticoid in seasonal allergic rhinitis. *Am J Respir Crit Care Med* 1999; **159:** 1814–18.


**Urticaria.** Leukotriene antagonists, such as zafirlukast, are reported to have some benefit in the management of chronic urticaria (p.1138).

### Preparations

**Proprietary Preparations** (details are given in Part 3)
***Arg.:*** Accolate; Vanticon; Zafarismal; ***Austral.:*** Accolate; ***Belg.:*** Accolate; Resma; ***Braz.:*** Accolate; ***Canad.:*** Accolate; ***Chile:*** Accolate; ***Fin.:*** Accolate; ***Hong Kong:*** Accolate; ***India:*** Zuvair; ***Irl.:*** Accolate; ***Israel:*** Accolate; ***Ital.:*** Accoleit; Zafirst; ***Mex.:*** Accolate; ***Port.:*** Accolate; ***S.Afr.:*** Accolate; ***Singapore:*** Accolate; ***Spain:*** Accolate; Aeronix; Azimax†; Olmoran; ***Switz.:*** Accolate; ***Thai.:*** Accolate; ***UK:*** Accolate; ***USA:*** Accolate.

## Zileuton *(BAN, USAN, rINN)*

A-64077; Abbott-64077; Zileutón. (±)-1-(1-Benzo[*b*]thien-2-ylethyl)-*N*-hydroxyurea.
$C_{11}H_{12}N_2O_2S$ = 236.3.
*CAS — 111406-87-2.*

**Pharmacopoeias.** In *US.*

**USP 27** (Zileuton). A white to off-white powder. Store in airtight containers. Protect from light.

### Adverse Effects and Precautions

Zileuton has been associated with raised liver enzyme values, gastrointestinal disturbances, urticaria, headache, and leucopenia in a few patients. It should not be used in patients with hepatic impairment or active liver disease. Hepatic transaminases should be monitored before, and periodically during, therapy.

Zileuton is not suitable for the treatment of acute asthma attacks.

### Interactions

Zileuton has been reported to impair the metabolism of some drugs metabolised via hepatic cytochrome P450, including propranolol, terfenadine, theophylline, and warfarin.

### Pharmacokinetics

Zileuton is reported to be well absorbed from the gastrointestinal tract following oral administration, with peak plasma concentrations occurring about 2 hours after a dose. It is apparently widely distributed and is about 93% bound to plasma proteins. It is extensively metabolised in the liver by the cytochrome P450 isoenzymes CYP1A2, CYP2C9, and CYP3A4, and excreted in the urine, largely as glucuronide metabolites. The elimination half-life is reported to be about 2 hours.

◊ References.


1. Wong SL, *et al.* The pharmacokinetics of single oral doses of zileuton 200 to 800 mg, its enantiomers, and its metabolites, in normal healthy volunteers. *Clin Pharmacokinet* 1995; **29** (suppl 2): 9–21.
2. Awni WM, *et al.* Pharmacokinetics and pharmacodynamics of zileuton after oral administration of single and multiple dose regimens of zileuton 600 mg in healthy volunteers. *Clin Pharmacokinet* 1995; **29** (suppl 2): 22–33.

3. Braeckman RA, *et al.* The pharmacokinetics of zileuton in healthy young and elderly volunteers. *Clin Pharmacokinet* 1995; **29** (suppl 2): 42–8.
4. Awni WM, *et al.* Population pharmacokinetics of zileuton, a selective 5-lipoxygenase inhibitor, in patients with rheumatoid arthritis. *Eur J Clin Pharmacol* 1995; **48:** 155–60.

## Uses and Administration

Zileuton is an orally active 5-lipoxygenase inhibitor that acts as a leukotriene inhibitor (p.777). It is used in the management of chronic asthma but has no bronchodilator properties and is not suitable for the management of acute attacks. Zileuton is given by mouth, in doses of 600 mg 4 times daily.

It has also been tried in some other disorders including arthritis, allergic rhinitis, and inflammatory bowel disease.

**Asthma.** Zileuton has been found to be of some benefit in asthma, including that provoked by cold air, exercise, and NSAIDs. US guidelines for the management of asthma (p.777) permit its use as an alternative to inhaled corticosteroids in patients with mild persistent asthma who cannot be managed with inhaled $beta_2$ agonists on an as-needed basis alone; it may also be added to inhaled corticosteroid therapy in moderate persistent asthma.

References.

1. Israel E, *et al.* The effects of a 5-lipoxygenase inhibitor on asthma induced by cold, dry air. *N Engl J Med* 1990; **323:** 1740–4.
2. Israel E, *et al.* The effect of inhibition of 5-lipoxygenase by zileuton in mild-to-moderate asthma. *Ann Intern Med* 1993; **119:** 1059–66.
3. McGill KA, Busse WW. Zileuton. *Lancet* 1996; **348:** 519–24.
4. Israel E, *et al.* Effect of treatment with zileuton, a 5-lipoxygenase inhibitor, in patients with asthma: a randomized controlled trial. *JAMA* 1996; **275:** 931–6.

**Inflammatory bowel disease.** Despite initial hopes that inhibition of lipoxygenase might prove of benefit in patients with ulcerative colitis,[1] a study in patients with mild or moderately active relapsing ulcerative colitis found that the symptomatic benefits of zileuton were confined to those not already receiving sulfasalazine.[2] A subsequent study showed zileuton was not significantly better than placebo in maintaining remission.[3] For a discussion of inflammatory bowel disease and its management, see p.1243.

1. Laursen LS, *et al.* Selective 5-lipoxygenase inhibition in ulcerative colitis. *Lancet* 1990; **335:** 683–5.
2. Laursen LS, *et al.* Selective 5-lipoxygenase inhibition by zileuton in the treatment of relapsing ulcerative colitis: a randomized double-blind placebo-controlled multicentre trial. *Eur J Gastroenterol Hepatol* 1994; **6:** 209–15.
3. Hawkey CJ, *et al.* A trial of zileuton versus mesalazine or placebo in the maintenance of remission of ulcerative colitis. *Gastroenterology* 1997; **112:** 718–24.

**Rhinitis.** A study in 8 patients with allergic rhinitis (p.422) found that a single dose of zileuton 800 mg reduced the response to a nasal antigen challenge 3 hours later,[1] including reduced sneezing and nasal congestion.

1. Knapp HR. Reduced allergen-induced nasal congestion and leukotriene synthesis with an orally active 5-lipoxygenase inhibitor. *N Engl J Med* 1990; **323:** 1745–8.

## Preparations

**Proprietary Preparations** (details are given in Part 3)
***USA:*** Zyflo.

# Cardiovascular Drugs

Cardiovascular Drug Groups, p.809
ACE inhibitors, p.809
Adrenergic neurone blockers, p.809
Alpha blockers, p.809
Angiotensin II receptor antagonists, p.809
Antiarrhythmics, p.809
Anticoagulants, p.810
Antiplatelet drugs, p.810
Beta blockers, p.810
Calcium-channel blockers, p.810
Cardiac inotropes, p.811
Centrally acting antihypertensives, p.811
Diuretics, p.811
Ganglion blockers, p.811
Lipid regulating drugs, p.811
Nitrates, p.811
Potassium-channel openers, p.812
Sympathomimetics, p.812
Thrombolytics, p.812
Vasodilators, p.812
Management of Cardiovascular Disorders, p.812
Advanced cardiac life support, p.812
Angina pectoris, p.813
Ascites, p.815
Atherosclerosis, p.815
Cardiac arrhythmias, p.816
Cardiomyopathies, p.818
Cardiovascular risk reduction, p.819
Cerebrovascular disease, p.820
Heart failure, p.820
High-altitude disorders, p.822
Hyperlipidaemias, p.823
Hypertension, p.825
Hypotension, p.828
Kawasaki disease, p.828
Myocardial infarction, p.828
Patent ductus arteriosus, p.830
Peripheral arterial thromboembolism, p.830
Peripheral vascular disease, p.831
Phaeochromocytoma, p.831
Pulmonary hypertension, p.832
Raised intracranial pressure, p.833
Raynaud's syndrome, p.833
Reperfusion and revascularisation procedures, p.834
Shock, p.835
Stroke, p.836
Thromboembolic disorders, p.837
Valvular heart disease, p.838
Venous thromboembolism, p.839

This chapter describes drugs used principally in the management of cardiovascular disorders, as well as the choice of treatment for a particular disorder. Blood products, plasma expanders, and haemostatics, which also have a role in cardiovascular disease, are described elsewhere (p.732).

## Cardiovascular Drug Groups

Although very diverse, cardiovascular drugs can be broadly classified according to their pharmacological action. Basic details of the major groups follow, together with lists of the drugs described in this chapter.

### ACE inhibitors

The main uses of ACE (angiotensin-converting enzyme) inhibitors are in the management of heart failure, hypertension, and myocardial infarction. Their actions and uses are discussed in more detail on p.842.

Described in this chapter are

Alacepril, p.856
Benazepril, p.867
Captopril, p.879
Cilazapril, p.883
Delapril, p.892
Enalapril, p.909
Enalaprilat, p.909
Fosinopril, p.919
Imidapril, p.938
Lisinopril, p.946
Moexipril, p.961
Perindopril, p.980
Quinapril, p.991
Ramipril, p.994
Spirapril, p.1003
Temocapril, p.1010
Teprotide, p.1010
Trandolapril, p.1016
Zofenopril, p.1029

### Adrenergic neurone blockers

Adrenergic neurone blockers are used in hypertension although they have largely been superseded by other drugs less likely to cause orthostatic hypotension. They have also been used in open-angle glaucoma.

Adrenergic neurone blockers act by selectively inhibiting transmission in postganglionic adrenergic nerves. They are believed to act mainly by preventing the release of noradrenaline at nerve endings; they cause the depletion of noradrenaline stores in peripheral sympathetic nerve terminals. They do not prevent the secretion of catecholamines by the adrenal medulla.

Described in this chapter are

Betanidine, p.872
Debrisoquine, p.891
Guabenxan, p.926
Guanadrel, p.926
Guanethidine, p.926
Guanoxan, p.927

### Alpha blockers

Alpha blockers are used mainly in the management of hypertension and to relieve urinary obstruction in benign prostatic hyperplasia.

Alpha blockers are also known as alpha-adrenergic antagonists or alpha-adrenergic receptor antagonists. Some have particular affinities for one of the subtypes of the alpha adrenoceptor. Drugs such as indoramin or prazosin are much more potent in blocking $alpha_1$ than $alpha_2$ adrenoceptors and are often termed selective $alpha_1$ blockers. Blockade of $alpha_1$ adrenoceptors inhibits the vasoconstriction induced by endogenous catecholamines. Both arteriolar and venous vasodilatation may occur resulting in a fall in blood pressure because of decreased peripheral resistance. Blockade of $alpha_2$ adrenoceptors with a selective drug such as yohimbine (p.1766) can conversely lead to a rise in blood pressure. With phenoxybenzamine and phentolamine, which broadly have similar affinities for both the $alpha_1$ and $alpha_2$ subtypes of receptor, any increase in blood pressure due to $alpha_2$ blockade is prevented by the inhibition of vasoconstriction caused by $alpha_1$ blockade. Alpha blockers also act at alpha adrenoceptors in nonvascular smooth muscle, for example in the bladder where alpha blockade produces decreased resistance to urinary outflow. Most alpha blockers are reversible or 'competitive' inhibitors of alpha adrenoceptors; phenoxybenzamine is an irreversible or 'non-competitive' alpha blocker and is particularly useful in phaeochromocytoma.

Described in this chapter are

Alfuzosin, p.856
Bunazosin, p.878
Doxazosin, p.908
Indoramin, p.939
Moxisylyte, p.962
Naftopidil, p.964
Phenoxybenzamine, p.981
Phentolamine, p.982
Prazosin, p.985
Tamsulosin, p.1009
Terazosin, p.1010
Tolazoline, p.1015
Urapidil, p.1018

References.

1. Frishman WH, Kotob F. Alpha-adrenergic blocking drugs in clinical medicine. *J Clin Pharmacol* 1999; **39:** 7–16.

### Angiotensin II receptor antagonists

Angiotensin II receptor antagonists are used in the management of hypertension; they may have a particular role in patients who develop cough with ACE inhibitors. Some are also used in diabetic nephropathy and some are under investigation in the management of heart failure. They act mainly by selective blockade of $AT_1$ receptors thus reducing the pressor effects of angiotensin II.

Described in this chapter are

Candesartan, p.878
Eprosartan, p.912
Irbesartan, p.940
Losartan, p.947
Olmesartan, p.975
Tasosartan, p.1009
Telmisartan, p.1010
Valsartan, p.1018

### Antiarrhythmics

Drugs used in the management of cardiac arrhythmias form a diverse group. Many of them, such as beta blockers (p.868), digoxin (p.895), lidocaine (p.1377), magnesium (p.1227), and phenytoin (p.370) have important actions in addition to their antiarrhythmic properties and thus, as well as being used in the treatment of cardiac arrhythmias, have a wide range of other clinical applications.

Various methods of classifying antiarrhythmics (formerly described as cardiac depressants) may be employed.

The most widely used **classification** of antiarrhythmics is that proposed by Vaughan Williams and later modified by Harrison. This classification is based largely on *in-vitro* electrophysiological effects of the drugs on myocardial cells. The action potential involved in the contraction of cardiac muscle consists of several phases (Figure 1, below) controlled by ionic movements across the myocardial cell membrane. When the cell is excited it becomes depolarised due to an increase in sodium conductance and a consequent fast influx of sodium ions (phase 0) lasting a few milliseconds, followed by a transient outward current probably carried by potassium ions (phase 1). A slow influx of ions, mainly calcium ions, forms phase 2 of the cardiac action potential which is known as the 'plateau' phase. The cell finally repolarises (phase 3) due to an increase in potassium conductance and an efflux of potassium ions which returns it to its initial resting membrane potential (phase 4).

**Figure 1.** The action potential.

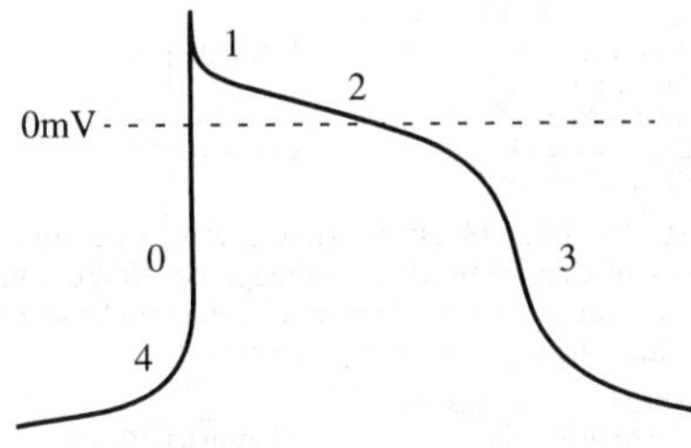


In specialised cardiac tissue such as the sino-atrial node and atrioventricular node the resting cell membrane spontaneously depolarises and initiates action potentials, due mainly to decreased potassium conductance. The tissues of the nodes are dependent predominantly on calcium transport for the depolarisation phase of the action potential, whereas the atria and ventricles are mainly sodium-dependent.

A typical normal ECG trace is shown in Figure 2, below.

**Figure 2.** A normal ECG trace.

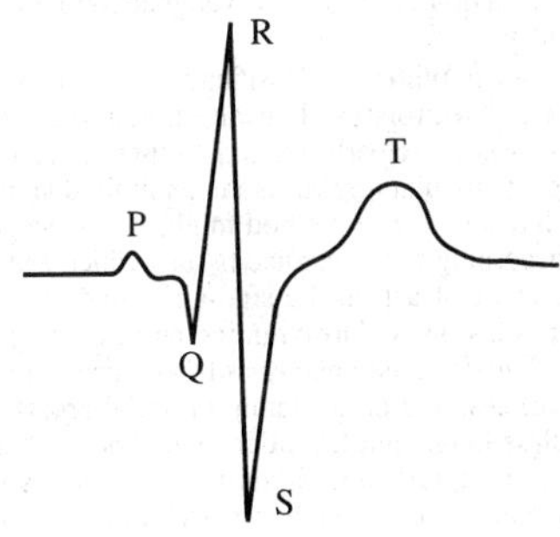


**Class I** includes drugs which directly interfere with depolarisation of the cell membrane (membrane-stabilising drugs) by blocking the fast inward current of sodium into cardiac cells; they also have local anaesthetic properties. They are subdivided into 3 further groups according to their effects on factors such as the duration of the cardiac action potential, the rate of change of the depolarisation phase of the cardiac action potential, the fibrillation threshold, conduction properties, and atrial and ventricular refractoriness.

*Class Ia* drugs slow the rate of change of the depolarisation phase of the action potential, moderately prolong the repolarisation phase, and prolong the PR, QRS, and QT intervals on ECG recording.

Described in this chapter are

Ajmaline, p.856
Cibenzoline, p.883
Disopyramide, p.903
Hydroquinidine, p.937
Pirmenol, p.984
Procainamide, p.987
Quinidine, p.991

*Class Ib* drugs have a limited effect on the rate of change of the depolarisation phase of the action potential, shorten the repolarisation phase, shorten the QT interval, and elevate the fibrillation threshold.

Described in this chapter are

Aprindine, p.864
Mexiletine, p.958
Tocainide, p.1014

*Class Ic* drugs markedly slow the rate of change of the depolarisation phase of the action potential, have little effect on the repolarisation phase, and markedly prolong the PR and QRS intervals.

Described in this chapter are

Encainide, p.910
Flecainide, p.916
Lorcainide, p.947
Pilsicainide, p.983
Propafenone, p.988

**Class II** drugs are characterised by beta-blocking activity, leading to a reduction in heart rate, myocardial contractility, and the rate of conduction of impulses through the conducting system.

Described in this chapter are

Beta blockers (but sotalol has predominantly class III activity), p.868
Bretylium, p.876

**Class III** drugs prolong the repolarisation phase of the action potential.

Described in this chapter are

Acecainide, p.848
Amiodarone, p.859
Azimilide, p.866
Bretylium, p.876
Cibenzoline, p.883
Dofetilide, p.906
Ibutilide, p.938
Nifekalant, p.972
Sotalol, p.1001

**Class IV** drugs block the slow inward calcium current (calcium-channel blockers) although not all drugs that fall into the broad general category of calcium-channel blockers share the same specific properties.

Described in this chapter are

Cibenzoline, p.883
Verapamil, p.1019

Many antiarrhythmics have actions typical of more than one class of compound making allocation to one specific class difficult. In some cases this results in multiple classification; an example is bretylium which has class II and III actions. However, in other cases a compound has been allocated to only one class even though it does display additional properties typical of another class; thus propafenone is usually recognised as a class Ic drug although it does possess some beta-blocking activity; beta blockers such as propranolol are traditionally described as class II drugs despite possessing some class I actions; sotalol has some class II actions typical of the beta blockers generally, but has predominantly class III activity and is usually described as a class III drug. Some drugs such as adenosine and digoxin do not fit into the Vaughan Williams classification at all.

The Vaughan Williams classification has been criticised because the electrophysiological action of the antiarrhythmic drugs is not clearly related to their effectiveness in treating a particular arrhythmia in an individual patient. A more clinically useful method might be to categorise the drugs according to the cardiac tissues which each affects. Thus drugs that act on the sino-atrial node include beta blockers, class IV antiarrhythmics, and cardiac glycosides such as digoxin; class I and class III antiarrhythmics act on the ventricles; and drugs acting on atrial arrhythmias include class Ia, Ic, and III antiarrhythmics and beta blockers. Class Ia and III antiarrhythmics act on accessory pathways and drugs acting on the atrioventricular node include class Ic and IV antiarrhythmics, beta blockers, and cardiac glycosides. A simplification of this scheme is to classify drugs into those that act on both ventricular and supraventricular arrhythmias such as amiodarone, beta blockers, disopyramide, procainamide, and quinidine, those that act mainly on ventricular arrhythmias such as lidocaine, mexiletine, and phenytoin, and those that act mainly on supraventricular arrhythmias such as verapamil.

References.


1. Vaughan Williams EM. Classification of antidysrhythmic drugs. *Pharmacol Ther* 1975; **1:** 115–38.
2. Harrison DC. Current classification of antiarrhythmic drugs as a guide to their rational clinical use. *Drugs* 1986; **31:** 93–5.
3. Frumin H, *et al.* Classification of antiarrhythmic drugs. *J Clin Pharmacol* 1989; **29:** 387–94.
4. Nattel S. Antiarrhythmic drug classifications: a critical appraisal of their history, present status, and clinical relevance. *Drugs* 1991; **41:** 672–701.
5. Vaughan Williams EM. Classifying antiarrhythmic actions: by facts or speculation. *J Clin Pharmacol* 1992; **32:** 964–77.


## Anticoagulants

Anticoagulants are used in the treatment and prophylaxis of thromboembolic disorders. They may be divided into direct anticoagulants such as the heparins, low-molecular-weight heparins, heparinoids, and direct thrombin inhibitors, and indirect anticoagulants such as the coumarin and indanedione derivatives.

### Direct anticoagulants

*Heparin* inhibits clotting of blood *in vitro* and *in vivo* by enhancing the action of antithrombin III. Antithrombin III, which is present in plasma, inhibits the activity of activated clotting factors including thrombin (factor IIa) and activated factor X (factor Xa). With normal therapeutic doses heparin has an inhibitory effect on both thrombin and factor Xa. The low doses that are given subcutaneously for the prophylaxis of thromboembolism have a selective effect on antithrombin III's inhibition of factor Xa. Very high doses are reported to reduce the activity of antithrombin III. Heparin also has some effect on platelet function, inhibits the formation of a stable fibrin clot, and has an antilipidaemic effect.

*Low-molecular-weight heparins* are salts of fragments of heparin produced by chemical or enzymatic depolymerisation of the heparin molecule. Commercially available low-molecular-weight heparins differ in their method of production, molecular-weight range, and degree of sulfation. Like heparin, these compounds enhance the action of antithrombin III but they are characterised by a higher ratio of anti-factor Xa to anti-factor IIa (antithrombin activity) than heparin. Although the possibility that such selective factor-Xa inhibition would result in antithrombotic activity without anticoagulant, and hence haemorrhagic, effects has not been confirmed by clinical experience, they have more predictable effects and require less monitoring than heparin. Low-molecular-weight heparins also have less effect on platelet aggregation than heparin.

*Direct thrombin inhibitors* such as bivalirudin, desirudin, and lepirudin are also used.

Described in this chapter are

Ardeparin, p.864
Argatroban, p.864
Bemiparin, p.867
Bivalirudin, p.875
Certoparin, p.882
Dalteparin, p.891
Desirudin, p.892
Enoxaparin, p.910
Heparin, p.927
Hirudin, p.931
Lepirudin, p.945
Low-molecular-weight Heparins, p.949
Melagatran, p.952
Nadroparin, p.963
Parnaparin, p.978
Reviparin, p.995
Tinzaparin, p.1013
Ximelagatran, p.952

The term *heparinoid* includes heparin derivatives and has also been used more loosely to include naturally occurring and synthetic highly sulfated polysaccharides of similar structure, such as danaparoid and dermatan sulfate. Some compounds have been described in many ways; some of the terms used include sulfated glucosaminoglycans, glycosaminoglycan polysulfate compounds, or sulfated mucopolysaccharides.

Described in this chapter are

Danaparoid, p.891
Dermatan Sulfate, p.892
Pentosan Polysulfate Sodium, p.979
Sodium Apolate, p.1000
Suleparoid, p.1009
Sulodexide, p.1009

### Indirect anticoagulants

Indirect anticoagulants act by depressing the hepatic vitamin K-dependent synthesis of coagulation factors II (prothrombin), VII, IX, and X, and of the anticoagulant protein C and its cofactor protein S. Warfarin, a coumarin, is the main drug used, but indanediones such as phenindione are also available. Since they act indirectly, they have no effect on existing clots. Also as the coagulation factors involved have half-lives ranging from 6 to 60 hours, several hours are required before an effect is observed. A therapeutic effect is usually apparent by 24 hours, but the peak effect may not be achieved until 2 or 3 days after a dose; the overall effect may last for 5 days.

Described in this chapter are

Acenocoumarol, p.848
Anisindione, p.863
Dicoumarol, p.894
Ethyl Biscoumacetate, p.914
Fluindione, p.918
Phenindione, p.981
Phenprocoumon, p.981
Tioclomarol, p.1013
Warfarin, p.1022

## Antiplatelet drugs

Platelet aggregation is important in haemostasis (p.735) and is also involved in thrombus formation, particularly in the arterial circulation. Antiplatelet drugs reduce platelet aggregation and are used to prevent further thromboembolic events in patients who have suffered myocardial infarction, ischaemic stroke or transient ischaemic attacks, or unstable angina, and for primary prevention of a thromboembolic event in patients at risk. Some are also used for the prevention of reocclusion or restenosis following angioplasty and bypass procedures.

Antiplatelet drugs act through a wide range of mechanisms. Aspirin (p.15) is the most widely used and studied; it acts by irreversibly inhibiting platelet cyclo-oxygenase and thus preventing synthesis of thromboxane $A_2$. Reversible cyclo-oxygenase inhibitors such as indobufen are also available, and thromboxane synthase inhibitors and thromboxane receptor antagonists have also been used.

Drugs that interfere with adenosine metabolism have an antiplatelet effect and those used include some prostaglandins, which act by increasing platelet cyclic adenosine monophosphate levels; the thienopyridines clopidogrel and ticlopidine, which interfere with adenosine diphosphate mediated platelet activation; and the adenosine reuptake inhibitor dipyridamole.

Thrombin inhibitors such as heparin and the hirudins have antiplatelet and anticoagulant effects. Glycoprotein IIb/IIIa-receptor antagonists, such as abciximab, eptifibatide, and tirofiban, interfere with the final step in platelet aggregation and are used in unstable angina and as adjuncts in reperfusion and revascularisation procedures.

Described in this chapter are

Abciximab, p.841
Cilostazol, p.884
Clopidogrel, p.888
Cloricromen, p.889
Dipyridamole, p.903
Ditazole, p.905
Eptifibatide, p.912
Indobufen, p.939
Lamifiban, p.944
Orbofiban, p.977
Picotamide, p.982
Sarpogrelate, p.996
Sibrafiban, p.996
Ticlopidine, p.1011
Tirofiban, p.1013
Trapidil, p.1016
Triflusal, p.1017
Xemilofiban, p.1029

References.


1. Schrör K. Antiplatelet drugs: a comparative review. *Drugs* 1995; **50:** 7–28.
2. Chong PH. Glycoprotein IIb/IIIa receptor antagonists in the management of cardiovascular diseases. *Am J Health-Syst Pharm* 1998; **55:** 2363–86.
3. Gershlick AH. Antiplatelet therapy. *Hosp Med* 2000; **61:** 15–23.
4. Sabatine MS, Jang I-K. The use of glycoprotein IIb/IIIa inhibitors in patients with coronary artery disease. *Am J Med* 2000; **109:** 224–37.


## Beta blockers

Beta blockers are competitive antagonists at beta-adrenergic receptor sites and are used in the management of cardiovascular disorders such as hypertension, angina pectoris, cardiac arrhythmias, myocardial infarction, and heart failure. They are also given to control symptoms of sympathetic overactivity in alcohol withdrawal, anxiety states, hyperthyroidism, and tremor and in the prophylaxis of migraine and of bleeding associated with portal hypertension. Some beta blockers are used as eye drops to reduce raised intra-ocular pressure in glaucoma and ocular hypertension. Their actions and uses are discussed in more detail on p.868.

Described in this chapter are

Acebutolol, p.848
Alprenolol, p.856
Amosulalol, p.862
Arotinolol, p.865
Atenolol, p.865
Befunolol, p.867
Betaxolol, p.873
Bevantolol, p.873
Bisoprolol, p.875
Bopindolol, p.875
Bucindolol, p.877
Bunitrolol, p.878
Bupranolol, p.878
Carazolol, p.880
Carteolol, p.880
Carvedilol, p.881
Celiprolol, p.881
Esmolol, p.913
Indenolol, p.939
Labetalol, p.943
Landiolol, p.945
Levobetaxolol, p.946
Levobunolol, p.946
Mepindolol, p.952
Metipranolol, p.955
Metoprolol, p.956
Nadolol, p.963
Nebivolol, p.964
Nipradilol, p.973
Oxprenolol, p.978
Penbutolol, p.979
Pindolol, p.983
Propranolol, p.989
Sotalol, p.1001
Talinolol, p.1009
Tertatolol, p.1011
Timolol, p.1012

## Calcium-channel blockers

The main use of calcium-channel blockers is in the management of angina pectoris and hypertension; some are also employed in cardiac arrhythmias.

Calcium-channel blockers, (calcium antagonists, calcium-entry blockers, or slow-channel blockers) inhibit the cellular influx of calcium that is responsible for maintenance of the plateau phase of the action potential. Thus calcium-channel blockers primarily affect tissues in which depolarisation is dependent upon calcium rather than sodium influx, such as vascular smooth muscle, myocardial cells, and cells within the sino-atrial (SA) and atrioventricular (AV) nodes. The main actions of the calcium-channel blockers include dilatation of coronary and peripheral arteries and arterioles with little or no effect on venous tone, a negative inotropic action, reduction of heart rate, and slowing of AV conduction. However, the effects of individual drugs, and therefore their uses, are modified by their selectivity of action at different tissue sites and by baroreceptor reflexes.

Traditionally, calcium-channel blockers have been classified according to their chemical structure; other methods of classification relate to the subtypes of calcium channels which they block, and their effects on heart rate. There are three major groups that are highly specific blockers of calcium channels.

**Dihydropyridine** calcium-channel blockers (such as nifedipine) act on slow, L-type channels. They have a greater selectivity for vascular smooth muscle than for myocardium and therefore their main effect is vasodilatation. They are non-rate-limiting, with little or no action at the SA or AV nodes, and negative inotropic activity is rarely seen at therapeutic doses. They are used for their antihypertensive and anti-anginal properties. Some dihydropyridine derivatives, for example nimodipine, cross the blood-brain barrier and are used in cerebral ischaemia.

**Benzothiazepine** calcium-channel blockers (such as diltiazem) and **phenylalkylamine** calcium-channel blockers (such as verapamil) also act on L-type channels but they have less selective vasodilator activity than dihydropyridine derivatives. They are classed as rate-limiting and have a direct effect on myocardium, causing depression of SA and AV nodal conduction. They are used for their antiarrhythmic, anti-anginal, and antihypertensive properties.

Drugs acting principally on the fast T-type calcium channels have also been investigated. Mibefradil, a benzimidazolyl-substituted tetraline derivative, is an example of this class. It is rate-limiting, and causes coronary and peripheral vasodilatation. However, it is no longer used clinically due to serious interactions with a wide range of drugs.

For further discussion of the actions and uses of the three main groups of calcium-channel blockers, see Nifedipine, p.966, Diltiazem, p.900, and Verapamil, p.1019, respectively.

Described in this chapter are


| | |
|---|---|
| Amlodipine, p.862 | Lacidipine, p.944 |
| Aranidipine, p.864 | Lercanidipine, p.946 |
| Azelnidipine, p.866 | Lidoflazine, p.946 |
| Barnidipine, p.866 | Manidipine, p.950 |
| Benidipine, p.868 | Mibefradil, p.959 |
| Bepridil, p.868 | Nicardipine, p.965 |
| Cilnidipine, p.884 | Nifedipine, p.966 |
| Diltiazem, p.900 | Nilvadipine, p.972 |
| Efonidipine, p.909 | Nimodipine, p.972 |
| Felodipine, p.914 | Nisoldipine, p.973 |
| Gallopamil, p.922 | Nitrendipine, p.973 |
| Isradipine, p.942 | Verapamil, p.1019 |


References.


1. Abernethy DR, Schwartz JB. Calcium-antagonist drugs. *N Engl J Med* 1999; **341:** 1447–57.
2. Eisenberg MJ, *et al.* Calcium channel blockers: an update. *Am J Med* 2004; **116:** 35–43.


## Cardiac inotropes

Positive cardiac inotropes increase the force of contraction of the myocardium and are therefore used in the management of acute and chronic heart failure. Some inotropes also increase or decrease the heart rate (positive or negative chronotropes), provide vasodilatation (inodilators), or improve myocardial relaxation (positive lusitropes), and these additional properties influence the choice of drug in specific situations. Drugs that are used predominantly for their inotropic effects include the cardiac glycosides and phosphodiesterase inhibitors; sympathomimetics are employed as inotropes but also have other important uses.

References.


1. Feldman AM. Classification of positive inotropic agents. *J Am Coll Cardiol* 1993; **22:** 1223–7.
2. Cuthbertson BH, *et al.* Inotropic agents in the critically ill. *Br J Hosp Med* 1996; **56:** 386–91.


**Cardiac glycosides**, such as digoxin, possess positive inotropic activity, which is mediated by inhibition of sodium-potassium adenosine triphosphatase (Na/K-ATPase). They also reduce conductivity in the heart, particularly through the atrioventricular node, and therefore have a negative chronotropic effect. The cardiac glycosides have very similar pharmacological effects but differ considerably in their speed of onset and duration of action. They are used to slow the heart rate in supraventricular arrhythmias, especially atrial fibrillation, and are also given in chronic heart failure.

Described in this chapter are


| | |
|---|---|
| Acetyldigoxin, p.851 | Digoxin, p.895 |
| Deslanoside, p.893 | Lanatoside C, p.945 |
| Digitalis Lanata Leaf, p.894 | Metildigoxin, p.955 |
| | Ouabain, p.977 |
| Digitalis Leaf, p.894 | Proscillaridin, p.990 |
| Digitoxin, p.894 | Strophanthin-K, p.1009 |


**Phosphodiesterase inhibitors** are potent inotropes; they also have vasodilator effects. They are used in the short-term treatment of severe heart failure; long-term oral therapy with some phosphodiesterase inhibitors has been associated with increased mortality.

Described in this chapter are


| | |
|---|---|
| Amrinone, p.862 | Olprinone, p.976 |
| Enoximone, p.911 | Pimobendan, p.983 |
| Milrinone, p.959 | Vesnarinone, p.1022 |


## Centrally acting antihypertensives

Centrally acting antihypertensives include $alpha_2$-adrenoceptor agonists such as clonidine and methyldopa. Stimulation of $alpha_2$ adrenoceptors in the CNS results in a reduction in sympathetic tone and a fall in blood pressure. Heart rate is also reduced. They are used in the management of hypertension, although other drugs with fewer adverse effects are generally preferred. Some have a role in the management of glaucoma.

Described in this chapter are


| | |
|---|---|
| Apraclonidine, p.864 | Guanfacine, p.927 |
| Brimonidine, p.876 | Methyldopa, p.953 |
| Clonidine, p.885 | Moxonidine, p.962 |
| Guanabenz, p.926 | Rilmenidine, p.996 |


## Diuretics

Diuretics promote the excretion of water and electrolytes by the kidneys. They are used in the treatment of heart failure or in hepatic, renal, or pulmonary disease when salt and water retention has resulted in oedema or ascites. Diuretics are also used, either alone, or in association with other drugs, in the treatment of hypertension, although the mechanism for their antihypertensive effect is poorly understood.

The principal groups of diuretics are as follows.

**Carbonic anhydrase inhibitors** are weak diuretics and are used mainly to reduce raised intra-ocular pressure.

Described in this chapter are


| | |
|---|---|
| Acetazolamide, p.849 | Dorzolamide, p.908 |
| Brinzolamide, p.877 | Methazolamide, p.953 |
| Diclofenamide, p.894 | |


**'Loop'** or **'high-ceiling' diuretics** produce an intense, dose-dependent diuresis of relatively short duration.

Described in this chapter are


| | |
|---|---|
| Azosemide, p.866 | Furosemide, p.919 |
| Bumetanide, p.877 | Piretanide, p.983 |
| Etacrynic Acid, p.913 | Torasemide, p.1015 |
| Etozolin, p.914 | |


**Osmotic diuretics** raise the osmolality of plasma and renal tubular fluid. They are used to reduce or prevent cerebral oedema, to reduce raised intra-ocular pressure, and in acute renal failure.

Described in this chapter are


| | |
|---|---|
| Isosorbide, p.941 | Mannitol, p.950 |


**Potassium-sparing diuretics** have a relatively weak diuretic effect and are normally used in conjunction with thiazide or loop diuretics. Canrenone, eplerenone, potassium canrenoate, and spironolactone are aldosterone antagonists and are particularly used in conditions where aldosterone contributes to the pathophysiology.

Described in this chapter are


| | |
|---|---|
| Amiloride, p.858 | Potassium Canrenoate, p.984 |
| Canrenone, p.879 | Spironolactone, p.1003 |
| Eplerenone, p.911 | Triamterene, p.1016 |


**Thiazides** (benzothiadiazines), such as bendroflumethiazide and hydrochlorothiazide, and certain other compounds, such as metolazone, with structural similarities to the thiazides, inhibit sodium and chloride reabsorption in the kidney tubules and produce a corresponding increase in potassium excretion.

Described in this chapter are


| | |
|---|---|
| Altizide, p.858 | Hydroflumethiazide, p.937 |
| Bemetizide, p.867 | Indapamide, p.938 |
| Bendroflumethiazide, p.867 | Mebutizide, p.951 |
| | Mefruside, p.951 |
| Benzthiazide, p.868 | Methyclothiazide, p.953 |
| Butizide, p.878 | Meticrane, p.955 |
| Chlorothiazide, p.882 | Metolazone, p.956 |
| Chlortalidone, p.882 | Polythiazide, p.984 |
| Clopamide, p.888 | Quinethazone, p.991 |
| Cyclopenthiazide, p.890 | Teclothiazide, p.1010 |
| Cyclothiazide, p.891 | Trichlormethiazide, p.1017 |
| Epitizide, p.911 | Tripamide, p.1018 |
| Hydrochlorothiazide, p.933 | Xipamide, p.1029 |


## Ganglion blockers

Ganglion blockers are nicotinic antagonists that inhibit the transmission of nerve impulses in both sympathetic and parasympathetic ganglia. Their antihypertensive action is due to sympathetic blockade, which produces peripheral vasodilatation; there is also a direct vasodilator effect on peripheral blood vessels.

Described in this chapter are


| | |
|---|---|
| Azamethonium, p.866 | Trimetaphan, p.1017 |
| Mecamylamine, p.951 | |


## Lipid regulating drugs

Lipid regulating drugs are used to modify blood lipid concentrations in the management of hyperlipidaemias and for the reduction of cardiovascular risk. The principal groups of lipid regulating drugs are the statins, fibrates, bile-acid binding resins, nicotinates, and omega-3 triglycerides.

The **statins** are inhibitors of 3-hydroxy-3-methylglutaryl-coenzyme A (HMG-CoA) reductase, the rate-determining enzyme for cholesterol synthesis. They reduce cholesterol by stimulating an increase in low-density-lipoprotein (LDL)-receptors on hepatocyte membranes, thereby increasing the clearance of LDL from the circulation. Their main effect is to reduce LDL-cholesterol, but they may also reduce triglycerides to a modest extent and increase high-density-lipoprotein (HDL)-cholesterol. They are generally considered to be the most effective lipid lowering drugs.

Described in this chapter are


| | |
|---|---|
| Atorvastatin, p.866 | Pitavastatin, p.984 |
| Cerivastatin, p.881 | Pravastatin, p.984 |
| Fluvastatin, p.918 | Rosuvastatin, p.996 |
| Lovastatin, p.949 | Simvastatin, p.997 |
| Mevastatin, p.958 | |


The **fibrates** include derivatives of fibric acid and related compounds. They inhibit the synthesis of cholesterol and bile acids, and enhance the secretion of cholesterol in bile. Their main effect is to reduce triglycerides by reducing the concentration of very-low-density lipoproteins (VLDL); they also increase HDL-cholesterol and have variable effects on LDL-cholesterol. They are used mainly in patients with hypertriglyceridaemia.

Described in this chapter are


| | |
|---|---|
| Bezafibrate, p.873 | Fenofibrate, p.915 |
| Ciprofibrate, p.884 | Gemfibrozil, p.923 |
| Clinofibrate, p.884 | Pirifibrate, p.984 |
| Clofibrate, p.884 | Simfibrate, p.997 |
| Etofylline Clofibrate, p.914 | Tocofibrate, p.1015 |


**Bile-acid binding resins** (bile-acid sequestrants) lower cholesterol by combining with bile acids in the gastrointestinal tract and preventing their reabsorption. This leads to an increased oxidation of cholesterol to replace the lost bile acids, and an increase in LDL-receptor synthesis on hepatocytes, resulting primarily in a reduction of LDL-cholesterol.

Described in this chapter are


| | |
|---|---|
| Colesevelam, p.889 | Colestyramine, p.889 |
| Colestilan, p.889 | Colextran, p.890 |
| Colestipol, p.889 | Divistyramine, p.905 |


**Nicotinates** include nicotinic acid (p.1441) and its derivatives. Nicotinic acid is a member of the vitamin B group and, in high doses, has beneficial effects on blood lipids; it reduces triglycerides and increases HDL-cholesterol, and may also modestly reduce LDL-cholesterol. Nicotinates are mainly used in hypertriglyceridaemia. Compounds derived from both nicotinic acid and clofibrate (nicotinate-fibrate derivatives) are also used.

Described in this chapter are


| | |
|---|---|
| Acipimox, p.851 | Nicofibrate, p.965 |
| Binifibrate, p.875 | Pirozadil, p.984 |
| Etofibrate, p.914 | Ronifibrate, p.996 |
| Niceritrol, p.965 | Tocoferil Nicotinate, p.1015 |


**Omega-3 triglycerides** are long-chain polyunsaturated fatty acids that primarily reduce triglycerides.

Described in this chapter are


Omega-3 Triglycerides, p.976


## Nitrates

Nitrates are peripheral and coronary vasodilators used in the management of angina pectoris, heart failure, and myocardial infarction. Some of them may also be used to control blood pressure during surgery. Nitrates are believed to exert their vasodilator effect through release of nitric oxide (p.973), which causes stimulation of guanylate cyclase in the vascular smooth muscle cells; this results in an increase in cyclic guanosine monophosphate. This nucleotide induces relaxation, probably by lowering the free calcium concentration in the cytosol. Nitrates are thus termed nitrovasodilators. In their action on vascular muscle, venous dilatation predominates over dilatation of the arterioles. Venous dilatation decreases venous return as a result of venous pooling, and lowers left ventricular diastolic volume and pressure (termed a reduction in preload). The smaller or less important dilatation of arterioles reduces both peripheral vascular resistance and left ventricular pressure at systole (termed a reduction in afterload). The consequent effect is a reduction in the primary determinants of myocardial oxygen demand. The effect on preload is not shared by beta blockers or calcium-channel blockers. Nitrates also have a coronary vasodilator effect which improves regional coronary blood flow to ischaemic areas resulting in improved oxygen supply to the myocardium.

Described in this chapter are

| | |
|---|---|
| Eritrityl Tetranitrate, p.913 | Pentaerithrityl Tetranitrate, p.979 |
| Glyceryl Trinitrate, p.923 | Propatylnitrate, p.989 |
| Isosorbide Dinitrate, p.941 | Sodium Nitroprusside, p.1000 |
| Isosorbide Mononitrate, p.942 | Tenitramine, p.1010 |
| Linsidomine, p.946 | |
| Molsidomine, p.961 | |

### Potassium-channel openers

Potassium-channel openers (potassium-channel activators) have been used in the management of hypertension; nicorandil is used in angina pectoris. They have a direct relaxant effect on smooth muscle. They act at potassium channels to allow cellular efflux of potassium which hyperpolarises the cell membrane and leads to a reduction in intracellular calcium. The reduction in intracellular calcium produces relaxation of smooth muscle. Activation of potassium channels in blood vessels produces vasodilatation. Potassium-channel openers may also have potential use in other conditions caused by smooth muscle contraction, for example asthma and urinary incontinence.

Described in this chapter are

| | |
|---|---|
| Cromakalim, p.890 | Pinacidil, p.983 |
| Nicorandil, p.965 | |

### Sympathomimetics

Sympathomimetics produce either direct or indirect stimulation of adrenergic receptors and have various actions depending on the specific receptors involved. Stimulation of alpha$_1$ receptors produces smooth muscle contraction. In the cardiovascular system this leads to vasoconstriction and increased blood pressure and in the eye to mydriasis. Other affected organs include the urinary sphincter and uterus. Stimulation of beta$_1$ receptors has an inotropic effect and also increases heart rate. Stimulation of beta$_2$ receptors leads to smooth muscle relaxation and produces vasodilatation.

Sympathomimetics have a wide range of uses. In cardiovascular disorders, they are mainly used for their alpha$_1$ and beta$_1$ properties to provide haemodynamic support in the management of acute heart failure and shock. Some sympathomimetics with alpha-agonist activity, such as phenylephrine (p.1126), pseudoephedrine (p.1129), and naphazoline (p.1124), are used to produce vasoconstriction of the nasal mucosa, for the symptomatic relief of nasal congestion. Apraclonidine (p.864) and brimonidine (p.876) are examples of drugs with alpha$_2$ agonist-properties that are used to lower intra-ocular pressure and treat glaucoma.

For further discussion of the actions of sympathomimetics in general, see Adrenaline, p.852.

Described in this chapter are

| | |
|---|---|
| Adrenaline, p.852 | Mephentermine, p.952 |
| Amezinium, p.858 | Metaraminol, p.952 |
| Arbutamine, p.864 | Methoxamine, p.953 |
| Denopamine, p.892 | Midodrine, p.959 |
| Dimetofrine, p.902 | Noradrenaline, p.974 |
| Dobutamine, p.905 | Norfenefrine, p.975 |
| Docarpamine, p.906 | Octodrine, p.975 |
| Dopamine, p.907 | Oxedrine, p.977 |
| Dopexamine, p.908 | Oxilofrine, p.977 |
| Etilefrine, p.914 | Pholedrine, p.982 |
| Gepefrine, p.923 | Prenalterol, p.986 |
| Ibopamine, p.937 | Xamoterol, p.1029 |
| Isoprenaline, p.940 | |

### Thrombolytics

Thrombolytics are used in the treatment of thromboembolic disorders such as myocardial infarction, peripheral arterial thromboembolism, and venous thromboembolism (deep-vein thrombosis and pulmonary embolism), and some may be used in ischaemic stroke. They are also used to clear blocked cannulas and shunts.

Thrombolytics activate plasminogen to form plasmin, a proteolytic enzyme that degrades fibrin and thus produces dissolution of clots. Some thrombolytics, such as alteplase, act only on fibrin-bound plasminogen and have little effect on circulating, unbound plasminogen; these thrombolytics are termed fibrin-specific agents. Thrombolytics, such as streptokinase, that affect circulating, unbound as well as fibrin-bound plasminogen are termed fibrin-nonspecific agents. Although it has been suggested that the degree of fibrin specificity should influence the risk of haemorrhage, the clinical significance of this has not been established (see Haemorrhage under Adverse Effects of Streptokinase, p.1006).

Described in this chapter are

| | |
|---|---|
| Alteplase, p.857 | Pamiteplase, p.978 |
| Anistreplase, p.863 | Plasminogen, p.984 |
| Defibrotide, p.892 | Reteplase, p.995 |
| Duteplase, p.909 | Saruplase, p.996 |
| Fibrinolysin, p.916 | Staphylokinase, p.1005 |
| Lanoteplase, p.945 | Streptokinase, p.1005 |
| Monteplase, p.961 | Tenecteplase, p.1010 |
| Nasaruplase, p.964 | Urokinase, p.1018 |
| Nateplase, p.964 | |

References.

1. Ross AM. New plasminogen activators: a clinical review. *Clin Cardiol* 1999; **22:** 165–71.
2. Verstraete M. Third-generation thrombolytic drugs. *Am J Med* 2000; **109:** 52–8.

### Vasodilators

Vasodilator is a broad term applied to a wide range of drugs that produce dilatation of blood vessels. The main groups of drugs producing vasodilatation are ACE inhibitors (p.842), nitrates (above), and direct-acting vasodilators.

**Direct-acting vasodilators** act predominantly on the arterioles reducing peripheral resistance and producing a fall in blood pressure. Their main use is in hypertension, although other drugs are generally preferred. Some of them are used in hypertensive crises.

Described in this chapter are

| | |
|---|---|
| Cadralazine, p.878 | Hydralazine, p.931 |
| Diazoxide, p.893 | Minoxidil, p.960 |
| Dihydralazine, p.899 | Todralazine, p.1015 |
| Endralazine, p.910 | Tolazoline, p.1015 |

**Other vasodilators** may be divided into those used for ischaemic heart disease and those used mainly for cerebral and peripheral vascular disorders. Some drugs originally regarded as vasodilators and used for cerebral and peripheral vascular disorders are now thought to improve microcirculatory flow disturbances by altering the rheological properties of blood or tissue metabolism.

Vasodilators used in Ischaemic Heart Disease

Described in this chapter are

| | |
|---|---|
| Carbocromen, p.880 | Fendiline, p.915 |
| Cinepazet, p.884 | Hexobendine, p.931 |
| Cloridarol, p.889 | Oxyfedrine, p.978 |
| Dilazep, p.900 | Trapidil, p.1016 |
| Etafenone, p.914 | Trimetazidine, p.1018 |

Vasodilators used in Cerebral and Peripheral Vascular Disorders

Described in this chapter are

| | |
|---|---|
| Azapetine, p.866 | Ifenprodil, p.938 |
| Bamethan, p.866 | Inositol Nicotinate, p.939 |
| Bencyclane, p.867 | Naftidrofuryl, p.964 |
| Buflomedil, p.877 | Nicotinyl Alcohol, p.966 |
| Butalamine, p.878 | Pentifylline, p.979 |
| Calcitonin Gene-related Peptide, p.878 | Pentoxifylline, p.979 |
| Cetiedil, p.882 | Pipratecol, p.983 |
| Cinepazide, p.884 | Propentofylline, p.989 |
| Cyclandelate, p.890 | Raubasine, p.994 |
| Di-isopropylammonium Dichloroacetate, p.900 | Xantinol Nicotinate, p.1029 |
| Fasudil, p.914 | |

## Management of Cardiovascular Disorders

Management of the main cardiovascular disorders is discussed below. These overviews focus on pharmacological therapy, but other options are also mentioned where they form an important part of treatment.

### Advanced cardiac life support

**Cardiac arrest** is the cessation of effective cardiac mechanical activity and is usually a result of ischaemic heart disease in adults and respiratory or circulatory failure in children. It may be associated with four arrhythmias, namely **ventricular fibrillation, pulseless ventricular tachycardia, asystole**, and **electromechanical dissociation (pulseless electrical activity)**. Ventricular fibrillation is the commonest in adults and asystole in children. In ventricular fibrillation and pulseless ventricular tachycardia there is chaotic electrical and mechanical activity; in asystole a total absence of both activities; and in electromechanical dissociation an absence of mechanical activity, or undetectable activity, in the presence of some electrical activity.

Cardiac arrest is an emergency situation[1,2] and should be treated with full life support measures.

International guidelines[3] for advanced life support and the immediate period of cardiac arrest have been published, developed by the American Heart Association in collaboration with various resuscitation councils, including the International Liaison Committee on Resuscitation. European[4] and UK[5] guidelines have also been published; these are based on the international guidelines and, apart from some differences in detail, are broadly similar.

In order to maintain cardiorespiratory function, basic life support (cardiopulmonary resuscitation) consisting of chest compression and ventilation (mouth-to-mouth/mask) should be started immediately and continued during the resuscitation attempt. Subsequent procedures will depend to some extent on the type of arrhythmia present. For the commonest, ventricular fibrillation, rapid defibrillation is of paramount importance and should not be delayed by other necessary measures such as the administration of oxygen, intubation, and the provision of intravenous access. Defibrillation is intended to produce momentary asystole and allow the natural pacemakers to resume normal activity. Adrenaline is given principally to increase the efficacy of basic life support rather than as an adjunct to defibrillation although evidence that it improves survival is limited; through its alpha agonist effects it increases myocardial and cerebral blood flow. A dose of 1 mg of adrenaline is regarded as the 'standard' dose. A higher dose of 5 mg has been used in some clinical trials, but there is no evidence that this dose is associated with an improvement in overall survival rate and it is not generally recommended. Vasopressin has been tried as an alternative although it has not been shown to be superior to adrenaline.[6,7] In the case of asystole, atropine may be given to block excess vagal tone. Amiodarone may be considered for ventricular tachycardia or fibrillation; lidocaine or procainamide are alternatives if amiodarone is not available. A study[8] comparing lidocaine with amiodarone for shock-resistant ventricular fibrillation found that survival to hospital admission was higher in those given amiodarone. Survival to discharge was not increased, however, but the study was not powered to assess this outcome. Other drugs that may be given during resuscitation attempts include buffering agents such as intravenous sodium bicarbonate for acidosis, and calcium, magnesium, or potassium salts for known deficiencies. Therapeutic hypothermia may be beneficial in patients who remain unconscious following resuscitation, and cooling to 32° to 34° has been recommended[9] in unconscious adults whose initial rhythm was ventricular fibrillation. Specific guidelines for the different types of arrhythmia are as follows.

**Ventricular fibrillation** and **pulseless ventricular tachycardia** are treated in the same way. The guidelines for **adults** emphasise that the first defibrillating shock must be administered as quickly as possible. In cases of witnessed cardiac arrest a precordial thump, which sometimes aborts the arrhythmia if given within 30 seconds of the loss of cardiac output, may be given before attaching the monitor/defibrillator, but the attachment of the defibrillator must not be delayed. The initial monophasic direct current shock (200J) is followed as necessary by a second (200J) and a third (360J) shock if the preceding shock is not successful; lower energies may be used for biphasic shocks. If the initial group of three shocks is unsuccessful, chest compression and ventilation should be continued and further shocks given. Adrenaline 1 mg intravenously should be administered before the next set of three shocks (each of 360J) but should not delay further defibrillation. Endotracheal administration of adrenaline may be used if intravenous access cannot be obtained. Doses 2 to 3 times greater than those given intravenously are suggested, although studies investigating this route have had mixed results.[10,11] A single dose of vasopressin (as argipressin) 40 units intravenously has been suggested[3] as an alternative to adrenaline, followed by further doses of adrenaline if required, but this is not universally recommended.[4,5] The cycle of adrenaline and up to three shocks (360J or equivalent) should be repeated as necessary. Amiodarone or other antiarrhythmics may be considered after the first cycle, provided that administration does not delay further shocks. Other drugs (such as those described above) may be used as appropriate. Meanwhile, the adrenaline and 3-shock cycles continue for as long as defibrillation is indicated. The total number of cycles is a matter of judgement but a resuscitation attempt may reasonably last for anything from 10 minutes to 1 hour.

Ventricular fibrillation in **children** is unusual; the basic management is the same as in adults, but the energies used for defibrillation and the doses of drugs used are different and a precordial thump is not generally given. The initial dose of adrenaline is 10 micrograms/kg by intravenous or intraosseous injection; for the second and subsequent doses, a higher dose of 100 micrograms/kg may be considered, although there is no evidence that this improves outcome. Endotracheal administration is an alternative route if an intravenous or intraosseous access cannot be obtained; the suggested endotracheal dose is 100 micrograms/kg for both initial and subsequent doses.

In survivors of ventricular fibrillation and pulseless ventricular tachycardia in whom it is considered there is a high risk of **recurrence**, implantable cardioverter defibrillators may be used. Drug therapy may also be used prophylactically (see Ventricular Tachycardia under Cardiac Arrhythmias, p.816).

**Asystole** and **electromechanical dissociation** have a much less favourable prognosis than ventricular fibrillation or pulseless ventricular tachycardia, although there are certain causes such as hypovolaemia, hypoxia, pneumothorax, pulmonary embolism, drug overdose, hypothermia, and electrolyte imbalances that may respond to treatment and these should be considered and the appropriate therapy given promptly once resuscitation has been instituted. As described above, a precordial thump may be appropriate if the cardiac arrest is witnessed. Once ventricular fibrillation or tachycardia is positively excluded, cardiopulmonary resuscitation should be instituted immediately and adrenaline 1 mg should be given intravenously every 3 to 5 minutes. In asystole a single dose of atropine 3 mg intravenously is also administered to block vagal activity.[4,5] In the international guidelines[3] atropine is recommended in repeated doses of 1 mg to a total of 0.04 mg/kg rather than as a single dose of 3 mg. Other drugs (such as buffering agents) may be considered. Cardiac pacing may be instituted once there is evidence of electrical activity. Resuscitation should generally continue for at least 20 to 30 minutes from the time of collapse; prolonged resuscitation is not usually undertaken as recovery rarely occurs after 15 minutes of asystole if there has been no response.

For **children** with asystole or electromechanical dissociation, the initial dose of adrenaline recommended is 10 micrograms/kg given by intravenous or intraosseous injection; as for ventricular fibrillation, higher doses have been used subsequently but are not generally recommended. Adrenaline may be given by the endotracheal route in doses of 100 micrograms/kg. Atropine is not generally used and a precordial thump is not recommended.


1. Eisenberg MS, Mengert TJ. Cardiac resuscitation. *N Engl J Med* 2001; **344:** 1304–13.
2. Vincent R. Resuscitation. *Heart* 2003; **89:** 673–80.
3. The American Heart Association in collaboration with the International Committee on Resuscitation (ILCOR). International guidelines 2000 for cardiopulmonary resuscitation and emergency cardiovascular care: a consensus on science. *Circulation* 2000; **102** (suppl I): I1–I384. Also published in *Resuscitation* 2000; **46:** 3–447.
4. European Resuscitation Council. European Resuscitation Council Guidelines 2000. *Resuscitation* 2001; **48:** 199–239. Also available at: http://www.erc.edu/index.php/doclibrary/en/12/1 (accessed 13/05/04)
5. Resuscitation Council (UK). Resuscitation Guidelines 2000. Available at: http://www.resus.org.uk/pages/guide.htm (accessed 13/05/04)
6. Stiell IG, *et al.* Vasopressin versus epinephrine for inhospital cardiac arrest: a randomised controlled trial. *Lancet* 2001; **358:** 105–9.
7. Wenzel V, *et al.* A comparison of vasopressin and epinephrine for out-of-hospital cardiopulmonary resuscitation. *N Engl J Med* 2004; **350:** 105–13.
8. Dorian P, *et al.* Amiodarone as compared with lidocaine for shock-resistant ventricular fibrillation. *N Engl J Med* 2002; **346:** 884–90. Correction. *ibid.*; **347:** 955.
9. Nolan JP, *et al.* Therapeutic hypothermia after cardiac arrest: an advisory statement by the advanced life support task force of the International Liaison Committee on Resuscitation. *Circulation* 2003; **108:** 118–21.
10. McCrirrick A, Monk CR. Comparison of i.v. and intra-tracheal administration of adrenaline. *Br J Anaesth* 1994; **72:** 529–32.
11. Raymondos K, *et al.* Absorption and hemodynamic effects of airway administration of adrenaline in patients with severe cardiac disease. *Ann Intern Med* 2000; **132:** 800–803.


## Angina pectoris

Angina pectoris is a syndrome that arises from an inadequate myocardial oxygen supply (myocardial ischaemia) and is part of the spectrum of coronary or ischaemic heart disease. The prominent symptom is transient precordial discomfort ranging from a mild ache to severe pain. Some patients may also experience dyspnoea, nausea, sweating, and left arm discomfort. Myocardial oxygen supply depends upon coronary blood flow, which normally increases to meet increased oxygen demands. Ischaemia occurs when blood flow either cannot be increased, or is reduced; this may be due to a fixed obstruction in the coronary arteries, vasoconstriction, thrombus formation, or platelet aggregation.

Three main types of angina have been described: stable angina; unstable angina; and Prinzmetal's angina. Although these are discrete groups, stable angina may become unstable, and Prinzmetal's angina may co-exist with stable or unstable angina.

**Stable angina** (effort angina) is angina which is usually precipitated by exertion and relieved by rest. It is often called chronic stable angina and as the name implies the frequency, intensity, and duration of the attacks are stable. The predominant underlying disorder is coronary atherosclerosis causing a fixed obstruction in one or more coronary arteries. While the restricted coronary blood flow is still adequate for oxygenation of the unstressed heart, it is not capable of being increased to meet the increase in myocardial oxygen demand that may occur during exercise, cold exposure, emotional stress, or after eating.

**Unstable angina** is an acute coronary syndrome intermediate between stable angina pectoris and myocardial infarction. Three subgroups are recognised: angina that presents from the beginning as severe and frequent attacks; an increase in the frequency, intensity, and/or duration of previously stable angina, often with diminishing responsiveness to sublingual nitrates (crescendo angina); and recurring or prolonged angina at rest. In unstable angina the decreased coronary artery blood flow is usually caused by disruption of an atherosclerotic plaque, which leads to platelet adhesion and aggregation, thrombus formation, and vasoconstriction, thus resulting in partial occlusion of one or more coronary arteries. The coronary blood flow can be so restricted that it does not meet the oxygenation demands of the unstressed heart, but the ischaemia is not sufficient to result in myocardial damage. Non-Q wave myocardial infarction is a closely related syndrome in which some myocardial injury occurs, but to a lesser extent than in acute myocardial infarction. Patients with the different acute coronary syndromes may present similarly and definitive diagnosis is only possible retrospectively once the results of biochemical measurements such as cardiac troponins or cardiac enzymes are available. However, patients without the characteristic ECG change of ST-segment elevation (non-ST elevation myocardial infarction) do not generally develop Q waves and management is as for unstable angina. Patients with unstable angina are at an increased risk of sudden death and myocardial infarction, and those with rest pain are at the greatest risk.

**Prinzmetal's angina** (variant angina) is a rare form of angina caused by coronary vasospasm and is often associated with atherosclerosis. It occurs spontaneously at rest and with greater frequency during the night or early hours of the morning. It is associated with transient ST-segment elevation and carries a risk of progression to myocardial infarction. Prolonged vasospasm may also lead to ventricular arrhythmias, heart block, or death.

In addition to the types of angina described above periods of **silent myocardial ischaemia** (asymptomatic transient myocardial ischaemia) in which there is no anginal pain have been identified during ECG monitoring. In some patients all ischaemic episodes are asymptomatic. However, asymptomatic ischaemic episodes also occur in patients with angina and seem to be more common than symptomatic episodes. It is not clear why some episodes of ischaemia are symptomatic while others are not.

**Treatment** depends on the type of angina and involves symptomatic management of acute anginal pain, antithrombotic therapy to prevent progression to myocardial infarction, and long-term management both to prevent angina attacks and to reduce the risk of other cardiovascular events. Anti-anginal treatment is used in both stable and unstable angina and is described in more detail below; it includes drug therapy (nitrates, beta blockers, calcium-channel blockers, and potassium-channel openers), percutaneous coronary interventions, and coronary artery bypass surgery. Antithrombotics are used in unstable angina and include anticoagulants and antiplatelets (see Treatment of Unstable Angina, below). Long-term measures to reduce cardiovascular risk are important in all patients, even when symptoms are controlled, and include antiplatelet therapy (which should be given to all patients unless contra-indicated), lipid lowering therapy, and lifestyle changes; these interventions are discussed in more detail under Cardiovascular Risk Reduction, p.819. Patients with ischaemic heart disease who undergo non-cardiac surgery are at risk of complications resulting from perioperative myocardial ischaemia.[1] Perioperative use of drugs such as beta blockers or mivazerol is under investigation.

Anti-anginal drugs act in a variety of ways. Glyceryl trinitrate and other organic *nitrates* have a vasodilator effect with venodilatation predominating over dilatation of the arterioles. Dilatation of veins decreases venous return as a result of venous pooling and lowers left ventricular diastolic volume and pressure (together termed a reduction in preload). The smaller or less important dilatation of arterioles reduces both peripheral vascular resistance and left ventricular pressure at systole (termed a reduction in afterload). The consequence of these effects is a reduction in myocardial oxygen demand. Also the vasodilator effect improves regional coronary blood flow to ischaemic areas, and alleviates coronary spasm. *Beta blockers* cause a slowing of the heart rate and reduction in contractility and therefore reduce myocardial oxygen demand. *Calcium-channel blockers* reduce the work of the heart by dilating peripheral arteries, and diltiazem and verapamil also slow the heart rate. Calcium-channel blockers also act on the coronary circulation preventing spasm. *Potassium-channel openers* act as coronary vasodilators, while nicorandil also has a nitrate component that may contribute to its effect.

Percutaneous transluminal coronary *angioplasty* is a means of mechanically dilating coronary arteries using a balloon that has been passed down a catheter and inflated at the appropriate sites, and is often used in conjunction with stenting. Nitrates and calcium-channel blockers may be given to alleviate coronary spasm due to the procedure. Coronary artery *bypass surgery* uses a vein or artery graft to bypass the occlusion. Both angioplasty and bypass surgery abolish or reduce episodes of angina in most patients but symptoms commonly recur over a period of time due to restenosis. Adjunctive therapy is therefore needed both to prevent short-term thromboembolic complications and long-term reocclusion (see Reperfusion and Revascularisation Procedures, p.834). Other interventions that have been tried in refractory angina include transmyocardial revascularisation and spinal cord stimulation.

**Treatment of stable angina.** Management of the patient with stable angina[2-6] primarily involves the use of anti-anginal drugs, antiplatelet therapy, and measures to reduce cardiovascular risk. Any contributory conditions, such as anaemia, should be identified and treated.

Treatment of infrequent angina episodes (less than about 2 attacks per week) usually consists of glyceryl trinitrate given when required, generally sublingually; alternatively, a buccal tablet or spray formulation may be used. Isosorbide dinitrate, in the form of sublingual tablets or spray, may be used, although it has a slower onset of action than glyceryl trinitrate. Glyceryl trinitrate in sublingual or buccal forms may also be used before an activity or circumstance that might precipitate an attack.

When episodes occur more frequently, sublingual glyceryl trinitrate, at least on its own, may no longer be appropriate, and regular symptomatic treatment has to be considered. Choice depends upon patient characteristics and any concurrent medical conditions.

Beta blockers are the mainstay of therapy. They are generally considered to be first-line treatment if sublingual glyceryl trinitrate is not adequate since they provide effective symptom control and have also been shown to reduce mortality in certain patients with high cardiovascular risk.[2,4,5] The different beta blockers appear to be equally effective in stable angina, although it has been suggested[7] that those with intrinsic sympathomimetic activity should be avoided.

A calcium-channel blocker may be used as an alternative, particularly in patients unable to tolerate beta blockers. Care is required in selecting an appropriate drug since the properties of dihydropyridine calcium-channel blockers (such as nifedipine) and rate-limiting calcium-channel blockers (diltiazem and verapamil) are not the same. Studies comparing long-acting calcium-channel blockers (verapamil[8] or modified-release nifedipine[9]) with beta blockers have shown similar outcomes in terms of symptom control and cardiovascular events. However, dihydropyridines may cause tachycardia and are less suitable than rate-limiting calcium-channel blockers for monotherapy; they should not be used without beta blockers in unstable angina.[3] Short-acting preparations of nifedipine have been associated with increased mortality and are not recommended (see under Adverse Effects of Nifedipine, p.966).

Regular nitrate therapy is a further alternative, and includes modified-release forms of glyceryl trinitrate, for example transdermal patches, and the long-acting nitrates such as isosorbide dinitrate or isosorbide mononitrate; it may be particularly suitable in patients with left ventricular dysfunction. Diminished effectiveness or tolerance occurs, particularly with nitrate preparations that produce sustained plasma concentrations, and dosage regimens including a nitrate-free period should be used (see Nitrate Tolerance, p.924).

Alternative drugs that may be used as monotherapy in the management of stable angina include potassium-channel openers such as nicorandil.

Where optimal therapy with a single drug fails to control symptoms, combination therapy may be used. There is additional benefit from concomitant nitrate and beta blocker therapy, since nitrates can moderate the excessive effects that beta blockers may have in increasing left ventricular diastolic volume and pressure and in inducing bradycardia. Calcium-channel blockers may also be used with nitrates; the combination of verapamil or diltiazem with a nitrate may be preferrable to a combination of nifedipine (or other dihydropyridine derivative) with nitrates as both nifedipine and nitrates cause reflex tachycardia, hypotension, and headaches.

Combination therapy with beta blockers and dihydropyridine calcium-channel blockers or diltiazem improves exercise tolerance[2] but adverse effects may be a problem. Verapamil should be avoided in such combinations as its use with a beta blocker increases the risk of impaired cardiac conduction (see p.1020). Caution with any combination of a calcium-channel blocker with a beta blocker is particularly necessary in patients with pre-existing conduction disorders or moderate to severe left ventricular dysfunction as the use of calcium-channel blockers may actually increase mortality.[10]

Triple therapy using a nitrate, a beta blocker, and a calcium-channel blocker may sometimes be used although it is likely to be associated with more adverse effects.

If medical treatment does not control the angina the patient should be investigated to determine suitability for coronary angioplasty or coronary artery bypass surgery.[11] Angioplasty is ideally suited to patients with single-vessel disease, good left ventricular function, and stable angina, although the technique is also used in patients with more complex disease, impaired left ventricular function, and unstable angina.[12] Coronary artery bypass surgery is generally the preferred technique in patients with disease of the left main coronary artery, three-vessel disease, or impaired left ventricular function.[13] Age and other clinical factors also influence the choice of technique; angioplasty may be favoured in the elderly and others with high operative risks.[12] The role of angioplasty in patients whose symptoms are controlled with medical treatment is less clear. A comparison of angioplasty and medical treatment in patients considered suitable for either strategy suggested that greater symptomatic improvement following angioplasty may not be maintained, and that the risk of death or non-fatal infarction may be greater than for patients receiving medical treatment alone;[14] however, quality of life may be better following angioplasty.[15]

**Treatment of unstable angina**. Unstable angina and non-ST segment elevation myocardial infarction are managed similarly.[16-24] Unstable angina is generally regarded as an emergency and those patients with a change in the pattern of previously stable angina or with recurring or prolonged angina at rest should be hospitalised. A resting ECG should be obtained to identify those patients with ST segment elevation who should be treated as for acute myocardial infarction (p.828). In patients without ST segment elevation, initial treatment is given to control the symptoms and reduce ischaemia and involves use of antiplatelets, heparin, nitrates, beta blockers, and possibly calcium-channel blockers. Subsequent therapy depends on the risk of progression and may involve glycoprotein IIb/IIIa inhibitors and urgent revascularisation. Once the patient has been stabilised, underlying risk factors should be identified and treated, and long-term anti-anginal therapy may be given.

Aspirin is routinely included in the initial treatment. It inhibits platelet aggregation and substantially reduces the incidence of myocardial infarction and death, although it has not been shown to reduce the number of ischaemic episodes or to relieve pain during the acute phase. Clopidogrel or ticlopidine may be alternatives if aspirin is not tolerated, although clopidogrel has fewer adverse effects and is generally preferred. Additional benefit has also been shown[25] with a combination of aspirin with clopidogrel, given for 3 to 12 months.

Heparin is generally given in addition to aspirin to reduce thrombin generation and fibrin formation. Both unfractionated heparin and low-molecular-weight heparin are of established benefit,[26-28] reducing the number of ischaemic episodes and major cardiovascular events during the acute phase, with sustained benefit in the longer term.[28] Unfractionated heparin is generally given by continuous infusion for at least 48 hours,[16,19,23] although it may also be effective subcutaneously.[29] Reactivation of unstable angina has been reported in patients discontinuing intravenous heparin;[30] combination with aspirin or gradual discontinuation may prevent this effect.[19] Low-molecular-weight heparins appear to be at least as safe and effective as unfractionated heparin and their advantages in terms of administration have led to their increasing use, although unfractionated heparin may be preferred in patients undergoing bypass surgery or percutaneous coronary intervention.[22] Prolonged use of low-molecular-weight heparins has been investigated,[31,32] but benefit has not been confirmed. Direct thrombin inhibitors such as lepirudin have also been tried;[33] compared with heparin, lepirudin led to fewer major cardiovascular events at 7 days but bleeding episodes were more common in the lepirudin group.

Nitrates are widely used although evidence from controlled trials is limited.[22,24] The initial treatment may be given intravenously to produce a fast response and to provide better dose control than can be achieved with other routes. Glyceryl trinitrate or isosorbide dinitrate are used. Generally, the intravenous route is only used during the acute phase, and once the patient is stabilised the infusion is withdrawn, usually within about 48 hours. Sublingual glyceryl trinitrate may be tried initially in patients with less severe symptoms.

Treatment with a beta blocker is started during the acute phase to reduce myocardial oxygen demand. Initially, the intravenous route may be used and then followed by oral administration. Beta blockers with intrinsic sympathomimetic activity do not reduce resting heart rate and are not recommended.[7,22,23]

Calcium-channel blockers may be added to therapy although they are generally reserved for patients with angina refractory to treatment with the above drugs. However, calcium-channel blockers are the drugs of choice if the angina has a vasospastic aetiology, for example in Prinzmetal's angina. The choice of calcium-channel blocker is described under the treatment of stable angina above.

Thrombolytics have been tried in unstable angina but do not improve outcome and are associated with an excess of bleeding complications; thrombolytic therapy is therefore not recommended in patients with unstable angina.[22,23]

Once the initial therapy has been started patients should be assessed for their risk of progressing to myocardial infarction and the need for additional treatment. Patients at high risk include those with recurrent ischaemia and those with raised cardiac troponins. Glycoprotein IIb/IIIa inhibitors such as abciximab, eptifibatide, and tirofiban are potent inhibitors of platelet aggregation and may have a role in patients at high risk. They are of established benefit in patients undergoing percutaneous coronary angioplasty (see Reperfusion and Revascularisation Procedures, p.834), but results in patients treated medically have been less consistent. A meta-analysis[34] of trials studying the efficacy of glycoprotein IIb/IIIa inhibitors in unstable angina or non-ST segment elevation myocardial infarction found that they reduced the risk of death or myocardial infarction in patients who were not scheduled for early revascularisation, particularly in those at high risk of progression, such as those with raised troponins. However, many of the patients included in the analysis did receive revascularisation and the use of glycoprotein IIb/IIIa inhibitors in patients not undergoing intervention remains questionable.[22] Whether all the glycoprotein IIb/IIIa inhibitors are effective is also unclear. Individual studies have reported beneficial results in patients receiving tirofiban and aspirin alone[35] or in combination with heparin therapy,[36] and with eptifibatide[37] in addition to standard therapy. However, a study with abciximab[38] in addition to aspirin and heparin failed to show any additional benefit.

Coronary angiography should be performed early in patients at high risk, including those in whom medical therapy fails to control symptoms, with urgent revascularisation where indicated.[39,40] In patients at lower risk, the benefits of early revascularisation are less well established; such patients should be assessed before discharge, usually with stress testing, and angiography should be performed as appropriate.

Following discharge, patients should continue to take aspirin and a beta blocker; continuation of clopidogrel for 9 months, in combination with aspirin, has also been recommended.[22,24] As in stable angina, measures to reduce cardiovascular risk should be adopted. Statins have been shown to reduce cardiovascular events when started early after admission for unstable angina,[41] or in patients with a history of unstable angina,[42] and should be considered. Some patients are given a long-acting nitrate for long-term prophylaxis, although nitrates have not been shown to protect against subsequent cardiovascular events. Long-term oral anticoagulation has been used but is not routine therapy, and studies of warfarin with aspirin have given mixed results.[43,44]

**Treatment of Prinzmetal's angina.** This should be treated like unstable angina with the addition of a calcium-channel blocker; the selection of an appropriate calcium-channel blocker is described above under the treatment of stable angina. Once stabilised, maintenance should include a nitrate, or calcium-channel blocker, or both to protect against further spasm. Surgery may be considered in some patients.

**Treatment of silent myocardial ischaemia.** Silent myocardial ischaemia has been recognised as a potential risk factor for future cardiovascular morbidity and mortality and research has been undertaken to assess whether suppressing such episodes can improve long-term outcome. Although many of the therapies used in angina reduce the incidence of silent ischaemia it is not yet clear whether complete suppression of ischaemia affects prognosis.[9,45-47] Other studies have suggested that periods of ischaemia may protect the heart during subsequent myocardial infarction[48] and further work is needed to reconcile these findings.

1. Eagle KA, *et al.* ACC/AHA guideline update for perioperative cardiovascular evaluation for noncardiac surgery: a report of the American College of Cardiology/American Heart Association Task Force on Practice Guidelines (Committee to Update the 1996 Guidelines on Perioperative Cardiovascular Evaluation for Noncardiac Surgery). Executive summary: *Circulation* 2002; **105:** 1257–67. Full version: http://www.acc.org/clinical/guidelines/perio/update/periupdate_index.htm (accessed 13/05/04)
2. North of England Stable Angina Guideline Development Group. North of England evidence based guidelines development project: summary version of evidence based guideline for the primary care management of stable angina. *BMJ* 1996; **312:** 827–32. Update available at: http://www.ncl.ac.uk/chsr/publications/guidelines/angina.pdf (accessed 13/05/04)
3. de Bono D. Investigation and management of stable angina: revised guidelines 1998. *Heart* 1999; **81:** 546–55.
4. Gibbons RJ, *et al.* ACC/AHA 2002 guideline update for the management of patients with chronic stable angina: a report of the American College of Cardiology/American Heart Association Task Force on Practice Guidelines (Committee on the Management of Patients With Chronic Stable Angina). Summary article: *Circulation* 2003; **107:** 149–58. Full version: http://www.americanheart.org/downloadable/heart/1044991838085StableAnginaNewFigs.pdf (accessed 13/05/04)
5. Scottish Intercollegiate Guidelines Network. Management of stable angina: a national clinical guideline (issued April 2001). Available at: http://www.show.scot.nhs.uk/sign/pdf/sign51.pdf (accessed 13/05/04)
6. Staniforth AD. Contemporary management of chronic stable angina. *Drugs Aging* 2001; **18:** 109–21.
7. Anonymous. Which beta-blocker? *Med Lett Drugs Ther* 2001; **43:** 9–11.
8. Rehnqvist N, *et al.* Effects of metoprolol vs verapamil in patients with stable angina pectoris: the Angina Prognosis Study in Stockholm (APSIS). *Eur Heart J* 1996; **17:** 76–81.
9. Dargie HJ, *et al.* Total Ischaemic Burden European Trial (TIBET): effects of ischaemia and treatment with atenolol, nifedipine SR and their combination on outcome in patients with chronic stable angina. *Eur Heart J* 1996; **17:** 104–12.
10. Packer M. Combined beta-adrenergic and calcium-entry blockade in angina pectoris. *N Engl J Med* 1989; **320:** 709–18.
11. Solomon AJ, Gersh BJ. Management of chronic stable angina: medical therapy, percutaneous transluminal coronary angioplasty, and coronary artery bypass graft surgery. *Ann Intern Med* 1998; **128:** 216–23.
12. Smith SC, *et al.* ACC/AHA guidelines for percutaneous coronary intervention: executive summary and recommendations: a report of the American College of Cardiology/American Heart Association Task Force on Practice Guidelines (Committee to Revise the 1993 Guidelines for Percutaneous Transluminal Coronary Angioplasty). *Circulation* 2001; **103:** 3019–41. Also available at: http://www.acc.org/clinical/guidelines/percutaneous%5Fexecsumm/perc_execsummPDF.pdf (accessed 13/05/04)
13. Eagle KA, *et al.* ACC/AHA guidelines for coronary artery bypass graft surgery: executive summary and recommendations: a report of the American College of Cardiology/American Heart Association Task Force on Practice Guidelines (Committee to Revise the 1991 Guidelines for Coronary Artery Bypass Graft Surgery). *Circulation* 1999; **100:** 1464–80. Available at: http://www.acc.org/clinical/guidelines/bypass/bypassexec.pdf (accessed 07/07/04)
14. RITA-2 trial participants. Coronary angioplasty versus medical therapy for angina: the second Randomised Intervention Treatment of Angina (RITA-2) trial. *Lancet* 1997; **350:** 461–8.
15. Pocock SJ, *et al.* Quality of life after coronary angioplasty or continued medical treatment for angina: three-year follow-up in the RITA-2 trial. *J Am Coll Cardiol* 2000; **35:** 907–14.
16. Waller D. Unstable angina and non-Q-wave myocardial infarction. *Prescribers' J* 1999; **39:** 193–201.
17. Yeghiazarians Y, *et al.* Unstable angina pectoris. *N Engl J Med* 2000; **342:** 101–14.
18. Fox KAA. Acute coronary syndromes: presentation—clinical spectrum and management. *Heart* 2000; **84:** 93–100.
19. Grubb NR, Fox KAA. Management of unstable angina. *Hosp Med* 2000; **61:** 489–94.
20. Ambrose JA, Dangas G. Unstable angina: current concepts of pathogenesis and treatment. *Arch Intern Med* 2000; **160:** 25–37.
21. Manhapra A, Borzak S. Treatment possibilities for unstable angina. *BMJ* 2000; **321:** 1269–75.
22. Braunwald E, *et al.* ACC/AHA guideline update for the management of patients with unstable angina and non-ST-segment elevation myocardial infarction: a report of the American College of Cardiology/American Heart Association Task Force on Practice Guidelines (Committee on the Management of Patients With Unstable Angina). Summary article [with minor clarifica-

tions]: *Circulation* 2002; **106:** 1893–1900. Full version: http://www.acc.org/clinical/guidelines/unstable/unstable.pdf (accessed 13/05/04)
23. British Cardiac Society Guidelines and Medical Practice Committee, and Royal College of Physicians Clinical Effectiveness and Evaluation Unit. Guideline for the management of patients with acute coronary syndromes without persistent ECG ST segment elevation. *Heart* 2001; **85:** 133–42.
24. Bertrand ME, *et al.* Management of acute coronary syndromes in patients presenting *without* persistent ST-segment elevation: the Task Force on the Management of Acute Coronary Syndromes of the European Society of Cardiology. *Eur Heart J* 2002; **23:** 1809–40. Corrections. *ibid.*; **24:** 485 and 1174–5. Also available at: http://www.escardio.org/NR/rdonlyres/19004FCF-9E1B-4563-8C76-0460CAAAE09C/0/acs_euhj02.pdf (accessed 13/05/04)
25. The Clopidogrel in Unstable Angina to Prevent Recurrent Events Trial Investigators. Effects of clopidogrel in addition to aspirin in patients with acute coronary syndromes without ST-segment elevation. *N Engl J Med* 2001; **345:** 494–502.
26. Oler A, *et al.* Adding heparin to aspirin reduces the incidence of myocardial infarction and death in patients with unstable angina: a meta-analysis. *JAMA* 1996; **276:** 811–15.
27. Eikelboom JW, *et al.* Unfractionated heparin and low-molecular-weight heparin in acute coronary syndrome without ST elevation: a meta-analysis. *Lancet* 2000; **355:** 1936–42.
28. Kaul S, Shah PK. Low molecular weight heparin in acute coronary syndrome: evidence for superior or equivalent efficacy compared with unfractionated heparin? *J Am Coll Cardiol* 2000; **35:** 1699–712.
29. Serneri GGN, *et al.* Randomised comparison of subcutaneous heparin, intravenous heparin, and aspirin in unstable angina. *Lancet* 1995; **345:** 1201–4. Correction. *ibid.*; **346:** 130.
30. Théroux P, *et al.* Reactivation of unstable angina after the discontinuation of heparin. *N Engl J Med* 1992; **327:** 141–5.
31. FRagmin and Fast Revascularisation during InStability in Coronary artery disease (FRISC II) Investigators. Long-term low-molecular-mass heparin in unstable coronary-artery disease: FRISC II prospective randomised multicentre study. *Lancet* 1999; **354:** 701–7. Correction. *ibid.*; 1478.
32. The Frax.I.S Study Group. Comparison of two treatment durations (6 days and 14 days) of a low molecular weight heparin with a 6-day treatment of unfractionated heparin in the initial management of unstable angina or non-Q wave myocardial infarction: FRAX.I.S (FRAxiparine in Ischaemic Syndrome). *Eur Heart J* 1999; **20:** 1553–62.
33. Organisation to Assess Strategies for Ischemic Syndromes (OASIS-2) Investigators. Effects of recombinant hirudin (lepirudin) compared with heparin on death, myocardial infarction, refractory angina, and revascularisation procedures in patients with acute myocardial ischaemia without ST elevation: a randomised trial. *Lancet* 1999; **353:** 429–38.
34. Boersma E, *et al.* Platelet glycoprotein IIb/IIIa inhibitors in acute coronary syndromes: a meta-analysis of all major randomised clinical trials. *Lancet* 2002; **359:** 189–98. Correction. *ibid.*; 2120.
35. The Platelet Receptor Inhibition in Ischemic Syndrome Management (PRISM) study Investigators. A comparison of aspirin plus tirofiban with aspirin plus heparin for unstable angina. *N Engl J Med* 1998; **338:** 1498–1505.
36. The Platelet Receptor Inhibition in Ischemic Syndrome Management in Patients Limited by Unstable Signs and Symptoms (PRISM-PLUS) Study Investigators. Inhibition of the platelet glycoprotein IIb/IIIa receptor with tirofiban in unstable angina and non-Q-wave myocardial infarction. *N Engl J Med* 1998; **338:** 1488–97.
37. The PURSUIT Trial Investigators. Inhibition of platelet glycoprotein IIb/IIIa with eptifibatide in patients with acute coronary syndromes. *N Engl J Med* 1998; **339:** 436–43.
38. The GUSTO IV-ACS Investigators. Effect of glycoprotein IIb/IIIa receptor blocker abciximab on outcome in patients with acute coronary syndromes without early coronary revascularisation: the GUSTO IV-ACS randomised trial. *Lancet* 2001; **357:** 1915–24.
39. FRagmin and Fast Revascularisation during InStability in Coronary artery disease (FRISC II) Investigators. Invasive compared with non-invasive treatment in unstable coronary-artery disease: FRISC II prospective randomised multicentre study. *Lancet* 1999; **354:** 708–15.
40. Cannon CP, *et al.* Comparison of early invasive and conservative strategies in patients with unstable coronary syndromes treated with the glycoprotein IIb/IIIa inhibitor tirofiban. *N Engl J Med* 2001; **344:** 1879–87.
41. Schwartz GG, *et al.* Effects of atorvastatin on early recurrent ischemic events in acute coronary syndromes: the MIRACL study: a randomized controlled trial. *JAMA* 2001; **285:** 1711–18.
42. Tonkin AM, *et al.* Effects of pravastatin in 3260 patients with unstable angina: results from the LIPID study. *Lancet* 2000; **356:** 1871–5.
43. The Organization to Assess Strategies for Ischemic Syndromes (OASIS) Investigators. Effects of long-term, moderate-intensity oral anticoagulation in addition to aspirin in unstable angina. *J Am Coll Cardiol* 2001; **37:** 475–84.
44. van Es RF, *et al.* Aspirin and coumadin after acute coronary syndromes (the ASPECT-2 study): a randomised controlled trial. *Lancet* 2002; **360:** 109–13.
45. Bertolet BD, Pepine CJ. Daily life cardiac ischaemia: should it be treated? *Drugs* 1995; **49:** 176–95.
46. Pepine CJ, *et al.* Effects of treatment on outcome in mildly symptomatic patients with ischaemia during daily life: the Atenolol Silent Ischaemia Study (ASIST). *Circulation* 1994; **90:** 762–8.
47. Davies RF, *et al.* Asymptomatic Cardiac Ischemia Pilot (ACIP) study two-year follow-up: outcomes of patients randomized to initial strategies of medical therapy versus revascularization. *Circulation* 1997; **95:** 2037–43.
48. Yellon DM, *et al.* Angina reassessed: pain or protector? *Lancet* 1996; **347:** 1159–62.

## Ascites

Ascites is the accumulation of fluid within the peritoneal cavity. Although it is not strictly a cardiovascular disorder, treatment depends mainly on cardiovascular drugs. Alcoholic hepatic cirrhosis is probably the commonest underlying cause in the western world; others include malignant neoplasms, heart failure, and tuberculosis. The following discussion is restricted mainly to **cirrhotic ascites**.

The mechanism of ascites formation in hepatic cirrhosis has been explained in terms of the underfill and overflow theories, and more recently, the vasodilatation hypothesis. Whatever the mechanism, ascites formation is linked to renal sodium and water retention partly as a result of increased circulating renin and aldosterone concentrations. Portal hypertension and hypoalbuminaemia may be contributory factors. More details may be found in reviews of the pathophysiology of ascites formation.[1-3]

Small amounts of ascitic fluid may go undetected but as it accumulates abdominal distension becomes apparent, and there is a feeling of discomfort. There may be respiratory distress and cardiac dysfunction in severe cases. Peripheral oedema may, or may not, be present. Renal dysfunction may progress to severe impairment (the hepatorenal syndrome). Patients are at risk of primary (spontaneous) bacterial peritonitis (p.140).

Management[1-8] depends on the severity of ascites but the mainstays are dietary sodium restriction and diuretic treatment. In mild to moderate ascites, sodium restriction alone may sometimes be effective but most patients also require diuretics. Bed rest has been advocated but not all workers consider its value proven. Response is monitored by measuring the daily reduction in body-weight. The diuretic of choice is the aldosterone antagonist spironolactone, with the addition of a loop diuretic such as furosemide if necessary. Amiloride or another potassium-sparing diuretic may be used as an alternative to spironolactone if adverse effects are a problem. Spironolactone together with furosemide from the outset has also been employed. In tense or refractory ascites, large-volume or total paracentesis (removal of ascitic fluid by drainage) is often used initially; patients may then be maintained on diuretics or repeated paracentesis may be used. Plasma volume replacement with albumin or dextrans after paracentesis is usual, particularly if large volumes are removed. Where ascites remains refractory or repeated paracentesis is not tolerated various shunting procedures have been tried, although their role is not established. In severe cases liver transplantation may be necessary.

In **malignant ascites**, that is ascites due to malignant neoplasms, paracentesis is often necessary but spironolactone may be of benefit in some patients.

1. Roberts LR, Kamath PS. Ascites and hepatorenal syndrome: pathophysiology and management. *Mayo Clin Proc* 1996; **71:** 874–81.
2. Stanley AJ, *et al.* Pathophysiology and management of portal hypertension 2: cirrhotic ascites. *Br J Hosp Med* 1997; **58:** 74–8.
3. Jalan R, Hayes PC. Hepatic encephalopathy and ascites. *Lancet* 1997; **350:** 1309–15.
4. Gerbes AL. Medical treatment of ascites in cirrhosis. *J Hepatol* 1993; **17** (suppl 2): S4–S9.
5. Runyon BA. Care of patients with ascites. *N Engl J Med* 1994; **330:** 337–42.
6. Bataller R, *et al.* Practical recommendations for the treatment of ascites and its complications. Drugs 1997; **54:** 571–80.
7. Krige JEJ, Beckingham IJ. ABC of diseases of liver, pancreas, and biliary system: portal hypertension–2. Ascites, encephalopathy, and other conditions. *BMJ* 2001; **322:** 416–18.
8. Ginès P, *et al.* Management of cirrhosis and ascites. *N Engl J Med* 2004; **350:** 1646–54.

## Atherosclerosis

Atherosclerosis is a pathological condition affecting medium and large arteries in which lipid-rich lesions (atheromas) develop in the intimal lining, leading to arterial dysfunction, obstruction of blood flow, and ischaemia. **Ischaemic heart disease** (coronary heart or coronary artery disease), which includes angina pectoris (p.813) and myocardial infarction (p.828), is the most common manifestation of atherosclerosis and in most industrialised countries ischaemic heart disease is a leading cause of death. Atherosclerosis of peripheral or cerebral arteries leads to peripheral vascular disease (p.831) or ischaemic stroke (p.836). Atherosclerotic diseases are thus a major cause of mortality and morbidity and the prevention and treatment of atherosclerosis has an important role in the management of these diseases.

Atherosclerosis is a progressive condition and various stages of atheroma development are recognised.[1,2] Early lesions include fatty streaks, which develop from infancy and are composed of lipid-filled macrophages (foam cells). These progress to fibrous plaques, which consist of a core of lipid and lipid-rich macrophages surrounded by a connective-tissue matrix. Plaques may undergo calcification and may become sufficiently large to obstruct the lumen of the artery. However, acute occlusion more commonly occurs as a result of thrombosis at the site of a plaque, due to endothelial denudation or disruption of the plaque (plaque rupture or fissuring) with exposure of the thrombogenic core. Endothelial dysfunction is an important underlying factor, promoting both the development of atheromas (atherogenesis) and subsequent thrombosis.[3,4] Although symptoms depend on the site of obstruction, atherosclerosis is essentially a generalised condition and patients with peripheral vascular disease, for example, are likely to develop or to have evidence of ischaemic heart disease also.

The management of atherosclerotic diseases involves treatment of the clinical manifestations (as discussed under the specific diseases) and measures to reduce the risk of cardiovascular events occurring (see Cardiovascular Risk Reduction, p.819). Some of the measures used to reduce risk, such as lipid regulating drugs or antihypertensives, may also reduce the progression of atherosclerosis. Other approaches have been targeted more directly at the atherosclerotic process, and some of these are discussed below.

*Oxidation* of low-density lipoprotein (LDL) is thought to be a crucial step in atherogenesis[5-7] and a number of studies have investigated the use of dietary antoxidants such as vitamins E and C and betacarotene (see Prophylaxis of Ischaemic Heart Disease, p.1420). Although some studies have found a reduction in the progression of atherosclerosis, others have not confirmed this finding, and several large studies have failed to find any effect on the risk of clinical events. Polyphenol compounds found in various foods, including red wine, have also received much attention for their possible role in the prevention of atherosclerosis.

*Hyperhomocysteinaemia* has been suggested as a risk factor for atherosclerosis, although its importance is not clear.[8] Interventions to reduce homocysteine, such as the use of folic acid or vitamin B supplements (see Ischaemic Heart Disease, p.1429), have been tried. Some effects on endothelial function have been noted, but there is as yet no evidence that clinical events are reduced, although a number of studies are ongoing.

*Inflammation* appears to have an important role in the development and progression of atherosclerosis, and in acute events due to plaque instability.[9] Various studies have shown an association between C-reactive protein, a marker of inflammation, and cardiovascular events, although its precise role is unclear.[8] Statins, which reduce lipids and have an established role in reducing clinical events, have also been shown to reduce the progression of atherosclerosis,[4] possibly through an effect on inflammation. Other non-lipid effects such as improvement of endothelial dysfunction, or an effect on thrombosis, have also been suggested.

Another possible cause of inflammation that has been investigated is infection,[10] and serological and pathological studies have found an association with a number of organisms. The evidence appears to be strongest for *Chlamydophila pneumoniae* (*Chlamydia pneumoniae*), although its precise role in the development or progression of atherosclerosis is unclear.[11] Treatment with antibacterials has been tried in patients with atherosclerotic disorders but any benefit has not yet been confirmed.[10,11] Some antibacterials may also have a direct anti-inflammatory action which may contribute to their effects.[11]

Chelation therapy with disodium edetate has been tried since calcium deposition has been proposed as another factor in the development of atherosclerosis; however, the benefits remain to be established (see p.1038).

Women have a lower risk of atherosclerotic disease than men of a comparable age, although the difference narrows with increasing age postmenopausally, and the use of HRT has therefore been investigated. HRT lowers lipid concentrations and some angiographic or ultrasound studies have shown beneficial effects on the progress of atherosclerosis, although others have failed to confirm these findings. However, controlled studies do not support a role for HRT in the prevention of cardiovascular disease in postmenopausal women (see Effects on the Cardiovascular System, p.1538).

Therapeutic angiogenesis (the development and growth of blood vessels) is also under investigation to improve myocardial perfusion. Preliminary studies of growth factor proteins, such as vascular endothelial growth factor (VEGF) and fibroblast growth factor (FGF), and gene therapy to stimulate VEGF production, have shown promise.[12,13]

1. Stary HC, *et al.* A definition of initial, fatty streak, and intermediate lesions of atherosclerosis: a report from the Committee on Vascular Lesions of the Council on Arteriosclerosis, American Heart Association. *Circulation* 1994; **89:** 2462–78.
2. Stary HC, *et al.* A definition of advanced types of atherosclerotic lesions and a histological classification of atherosclerosis: a report from the Committee on Vascular Lesions of the Council on Arteriosclerosis, American Heart Association. *Circulation* 1995; **92:** 1355–74.

3. Corti R, *et al.* The vulnerable plaque and acute coronary syndromes. *Am J Med* 2002; **113:** 668–80.
4. Grobbee DE, Bots ML. Statin treatment and progression of atherosclerotic plaque burden. *Drugs* 2003; **63:** 893–911.
5. Esterbauer H, *et al.* Lipid peroxidation and its role in atherosclerosis. *Br Med Bull* 1993; **49:** 566–76.
6. Witztum JL. The oxidation hypothesis of atherosclerosis. *Lancet* 1994; **344:** 793–5.
7. Diaz MN, *et al.* Antioxidants and atherosclerotic heart disease. *N Engl J Med* 1997; **337:** 408–16.
8. Hackam DG, Anand SS. Emerging risk factors for atherosclerotic vascular disease: a critical review of the evidence. *JAMA* 2003; **290:** 932–40.
9. Ross R. Atherosclerosis – an inflammatory disease. *N Engl J Med* 1999; **340:** 115–26.
10. Mehta JL, Romeo F. Inflammation, infection and atherosclerosis: do antibacterials have a role in the therapy of coronary artery disease? *Drugs* 2000; **59:** 159–70.
11. Higgins JP. Chlamydia pneumoniae and coronary artery disease: the antibiotic trials. *Mayo Clin Proc* 2003; **78:** 321–32.
12. Sellke FW, Simons M. Angiogenesis in cardiovascular disease: current status and therapeutic potential. *Drugs* 1999; **58:** 391–6.
13. Freedman SB, Isner JM. Therapeutic angiogenesis for coronary artery disease. *Ann Intern Med* 2002; **136:** 54–71.

## Cardiac arrhythmias

The heart acts as a pump and maintains circulation of the blood by alternate contraction and relaxation of cardiac muscle (the myocardium). It generally contracts at a rate of 70 to 75 beats/minute in a healthy 70-kg person at rest. The normal heart rhythm, known as *sinus rhythm*, originates in specialised cardiac cells, called *pacemaker cells*, in the *sino-atrial (SA)* or *sinus node* and has been defined as a sinus node rate of 60 to 100 beats/minute. Each heart beat or contraction is initiated by generation of an *action potential* (see Antiarrhythmics, p.809) in the SA node; the electrical impulse spreads over both atria, causing them to contract, and on to the *atrioventricular (AV) node*. From the AV node it spreads through the bundle of His and down the Purkinje fibres to the ventricles, causing them to contract. It is the movement of ions across the cardiac cell membrane that generates the action potential. The electrical changes involved can be recorded on an electrocardiogram (ECG). Other cardiac cells that are located outside the sinus node are also capable of initiating impulses. These cells, termed *ectopic pacemakers*, can be found in the atrioventricular junction and in the His-Purkinje system. The normal rate of impulse initiation by these ectopic pacemakers is less than that of the sinus node and therefore they do not normally initiate the heart beat. However, they may become dominant in certain circumstances such as: if the intrinsic rate of the ectopic pacemaker rises above that of the sinus node; if the sinus node rate falls below that of the ectopic pacemaker; or when a normal sinus node impulse is prevented from being conducted through the heart (heart block) leaving the ectopic pacemaker to fire at its own intrinsic rate.

A **cardiac arrhythmia** can be defined in simple terms as any abnormality of rate, regularity, or site of origin of the cardiac impulse or as a disturbance in conduction that causes an abnormal sequence of activation. Symptoms depend on the arrhythmia but may include fatigue, dyspnoea, dizziness, and syncope; sudden death may occur. **Palpitation** is a term used to describe an unacceptable awareness of the beating heart by the patient. This may occur normally in circumstances such as emotion, exercise, or stress or may occur in association with arrhythmias. Clinically, arrhythmias may be classified by presumed site of origin, namely as **supraventricular arrhythmias** (including **atrial arrhythmias** and **atrioventricular junctional arrhythmias**) or as **ventricular arrhythmias**. Classification can also be based on rate as either bradyarrhythmias (slow) or tachyarrhythmias (fast).

**Bradyarrhythmias** are caused by sinus node dysfunction, which either depresses impulse generation or disturbs the conduction of impulses from the sinus node to the atria.[1] **Atrioventricular block** indicates disturbance of conduction of the atrial impulse to the ventricles. In first-degree block the impulse is delayed. It is usually asymptomatic but may progress to second- or third-degree block. In second-degree block the impulse is blocked intermittently and in third-degree block there is a complete block. **Atrioventricular dissociation** indicates a condition in which ventricular activity is faster than, and independent of, the atrial activity. Bradyarrhythmias may be treated with either atropine or isoprenaline, although cardiac pacing is the treatment of choice.

For **tachyarrhythmias** a classification or diagnosis based on the precise mechanism of the arrhythmia would also be desirable but this is not always clear. In many of the clinically relevant arrhythmias, however, the mechanism is one of re-entry. Re-entry occurs when the initial impulse does not die out but continues to propagate and reactivate the heart.

**Diagnosis and management.** Cardiac arrhythmias can range from little more than asymptomatic ECG abnormalities through to severe or life-threatening events. Treatment can be with antiarrhythmics or with non-pharmacological methods.

The precise identification of an arrhythmia is not always easy, but is important for correct management. The inappropriate use of an antiarrhythmic for a specific arrhythmia can not only be ineffective but, in view of the proarrhythmic potential of most of them, may even be deleterious. Identification and diagnosis should be based on clinical symptoms and on characteristic ECG features as well as on other specialised tests and features relevant to individual arrhythmias. A typical normal ECG trace is shown in Figure 2, p.809. An arrhythmia with a narrow QRS complex is always supraventricular in origin whereas a broad QRS complex can indicate either a supraventricular or ventricular origin, hence the diagnostic difficulties.

**Ectopic beats, extrasystoles,** or **premature contractions** can arise in either the atria or the ventricles and, although their precise meaning and definition differs, for practical purposes they can be considered equivalent. Generally, they cause few or no symptoms and usually have no prognostic value although some patients suffer distressing symptoms or palpitations.

**Atrial fibrillation** is the commonest cardiac arrhythmia and has been the subject of reviews[2-9] and guidelines.[10] The mechanism of the arrhythmia in atrial fibrillation is one of re-entry. Atrial fibrillation is often associated with underlying cardiovascular disease, notably ischaemic or hypertensive heart disease and heart failure. Rheumatic heart disease is also an important cause, although this is now less common in developed countries. Other causes include hyperthyroidism and acute alcohol intoxication; atrial fibrillation is also relatively common following cardiothoracic surgery, but is usually self-limiting. In some patients there is no obvious cause, in which case the arrhythmia is described as 'lone' atrial fibrillation. Atrial fibrillation is characterised by an irregular and very rapid atrial rate (usually more than 300 beats/minute) and, as the atrioventricular node is incapable of conducting all the impulses adequately, the increased ventricular response results in a rapid and totally irregular ventricular rate. Atrial fibrillation has been classified in several ways, but in general patients with 2 or more episodes are considered to have recurrent atrial fibrillation; this may be classed as paroxysmal (intermittent) if the arrhythmia terminates spontaneously, or persistent (chronic) if it is sustained. Persistent atrial fibrillation that does not respond to cardioversion or where cardioversion is not attempted is classed as permanent. Although atrial fibrillation can cause distressing symptoms such as severe palpitations and exercise intolerance it is not usually immediately life-threatening; however, it does result in long-term morbidity and mortality. Left atrial dilatation and reduced cardiac output lead to stasis of blood in the left atrium, and this can result in thrombus formation and subsequent systemic embolisation, notably ischaemic stroke. Thromboembolic events are relatively rare in lone atrial fibrillation but the risk is very much increased in concomitant cardiovascular disease, especially so in rheumatic heart disease.

The two main options for the management of atrial fibrillation are cardioversion followed by the maintenance of sinus rhythm, or treatment to slow the increased ventricular response while allowing atrial fibrillation to continue. Anticoagulation may also be necessary to prevent thromboembolic episodes. Prophylactic treatment to prevent atrial fibrillation may be considered in patients undergoing cardiac surgery; beta blockers, sotalol, and amiodarone are effective.[11]

Rate control may have a role in the acute management of symptoms and in maintenance therapy.[12] Digoxin has traditionally been used to slow an increased ventricular rate and still has an important role in patients who also have heart failure. In general, however, beta blockers or rate-limiting calcium-channel blockers such as diltiazem or verapamil are preferred as they are usually considered more effective, especially for acute control and for controlling the increased rates that may occur during exercise. If necessary, a combination of digoxin with either a beta blocker or a calcium-channel blocker may be used. All these drugs act by slowing conduction through the atrioventricular node. They do not, however, have an antifibrillatory action and do not restore sinus rhythm. Amiodarone, which is used to restore rhythm, also provides some rate control, but adverse effects may limit its use; it may have a role in patients with heart failure. Catheter ablation of atrioventricular conduction pathways followed by permanent pacing may be necessary for rate control in patients intolerant or unresponsive to drug therapy.

Restoration of sinus rhythm may be achieved either by synchronised direct current cardioversion or by pharmacological cardioversion, but both methods must be preceded by anticoagulation unless fibrillation is of recent onset (less than 24 hours). Pharmacological cardioversion is most effective in atrial fibrillation of recent onset. Various classes of antiarrhythmic (see p.809 for an explanation of the classification of antiarrhythmics) have been used, although evidence for efficacy is limited in some cases.[10] Those that have been shown to be effective include the class Ic drugs flecainide and propafenone, and the class III drugs dofetilide, ibutilide, and azimilide; amiodarone, another class III drug, is also effective for cardioversion, but probably less so than some of the other drugs. The class Ia drugs disopyramide, procainamide, and quinidine, and sotalol, a beta blocker with additional class III effects, have been used, but there is less evidence to support their efficacy. Direct current cardioversion has the advantage of restoring sinus rhythm more rapidly and effectively than drugs but has the disadvantage that it needs to be performed under general anaesthesia. Adjunctive pharmacological therapy may be started before electrical cardioversion to increase the success of the procedure and to reduce the risk of early recurrence.[10]

Once sinus rhythm has been achieved, or in cases of paroxysmal atrial fibrillation, long-term maintenance drug therapy needs to be considered. The drugs used for this are broadly similar to those used for pharmacological cardioversion, namely the class I or class III antiarrhythmics. Again, there is limited evidence for many of the drugs used, and few comparative studies are available.[10] Choice of drug also needs to take into consideration any underlying heart disease, since this may be exacerbated by many of the drugs used. Amiodarone may be more effective than sotalol or class I drugs[13] but is generally considered a second-line choice due to its adverse effects; it may be particularly useful in patients with heart failure. Surgery or catheter ablation may have a role in some patients, and implantable defibrillators have also been used, but all of these methods have limitations.

The choice between rate and rhythm control depends on the characteristics of the patient. Rhythm control has been preferred since restoration of sinus rhythm both alleviates symptoms and was thought to reduce thromboembolic risk. However, in many patients relapse occurs, despite maintenance therapy, and the adverse effects of antiarrhythmic drugs are also a problem. Several studies comparing rate control with rhythm control in patients with atrial fibrillation that was either persistent or considered likely to recur have found no difference between the two strategies in terms of symptom control,[14] or clinical events, including mortality and morbidity,[15,16] and in such patients it appears that rate control is an acceptable option if initial rhythm control fails. However, in younger patients or those with specific underlying conditions, rhythm control is likely to still have an important role.

The problem of **thromboembolic** events, principally ischaemic stroke, resulting from atrial fibrillation has been the subject of several reviews[17-22] as well as being addressed in the general reviews quoted above. If atrial fibrillation has been present for 48 hours or more it is generally recognised that there is a potential risk of causing systemic embolisation once sinus rhythm is restored. It is therefore recommended that oral anticoagulation with warfarin should be given for 3 to 4 weeks before cardioversion is attempted. If immediate cardioversion is necessary, administration of intravenous heparin followed by transoesophageal echocardiography to exclude the presence of thrombi has been suggested.[10,23] Control of the ventricular rate as outlined above should also be undertaken during this period. Anticoagulation is usually continued for at least 3 to 4 weeks following successful cardioversion.[10,23]

Anticoagulation may also be undertaken for long-term **prophylaxis of stroke** in selected patients. The risk of stroke is increased about 17 times in atrial fibrillation associated with rheumatic heart disease and the benefits of long-term prophylaxis with warfarin are well-established. For non-rheumatic heart disease the risk is less, but is still increased by about fivefold and affects many more patients; however, the use of warfarin is more controversial. Meta-analyses of a number of studies have clearly demonstrated a beneficial effect of warfarin in the primary[24,25] and secondary[24] prevention of stroke in patients with non-rheumatic atrial fibrillation, and a cohort study[26] has reported similar findings. However, the benefit for primary prevention has been disputed.[27] The benefits of anticoagulation need to be balanced against the risk of increased bleeding episodes, notably stroke due to intracranial haemorrhage, induced by warfarin. The risk of thromboembolism is influenced by different factors and variables and should be assessed in all patients; oral anticoagulation is recommended for specific groups with high risk factors such as increasing age, ischaemic or hypertensive heart disease, heart failure, hyperthyroidism, or history or evidence of thromboembolism.[10,23,28] In lower risk patients, the risk of haemorrhage may outweigh any benefits of warfarin, and alternative strategies have been tried. Aspirin has been shown to reduce the risk of stroke, although most analyses[29-31] have concluded that it is less effective than warfarin. However, one review[32] has disputed this finding and suggested that the increased bleeding risk with warfarin outweighs any benefit. Aspirin is usually recommended[10,23] in low risk patients or in those at high risk for haemorrhage. Indobufen, another antiplatelet drug, has also been suggested[33] as a possible alternative. Several new anticoagulants are also being investigated, and results with the oral thrombin inhibitor ximelagatran[34] suggest it may be as effective as warfarin. A combination of low-dose warfarin with aspirin, however, has been shown[35,36] to be less effective than adjusted-dose warfarin and is not recommended.

**Atrial flutter** is an arrhythmia somewhat similar in nature to atrial fibrillation and has been discussed in reviews[37] and guidelines.[38] Like atrial fibrillation it is characterised by a rapid (about 300 beats/minute) atrial rate, although the atrial rhythm is more regular and organised, and by a corresponding increase in the ventricular rate. It is far less common than atrial fibrillation, to which it often degenerates if left untreated; it may revert to normal sinus rhythm in some cases. Unlike atrial fibrillation, atrial flutter has not been considered to carry an increased risk of thromboembolic episodes, but several studies have suggested this may not be the case.[39-41] Anticoagulation may therefore have a role in patients with recurrent or chronic atrial flutter,[37,38] and has been recommended prior to cardioversion.[23,38] Management strategies for atrial flutter are broadly similar to those outlined above for atrial fibrillation, namely controlling the increased ventricular response rate and cardioversion. However, in general terms drug therapy for either of these interventions is less successful in flutter than in fibrillation. Cardioversion with drug therapy has a relatively low success rate and cardiac pacing is usually used, which often results in a self-terminating atrial fibrillation. Synchronised direct current cardioversion may be used to restore sinus rhythm if pacing fails. Radiofrequency ablation may also be used,[38,42] and may be the treatment of choice if long-term therapy is required.[37]

Other atrial arrhythmias include **atrial premature beats** and various types of **atrial tachycardia**. Premature beats are usually asymptomatic but if symptoms are severe (the awareness of a pause between normal beats) beta blockers may be used. Atrial tachycardia may also be treated with beta blockers or rate-limiting calcium-channel blockers, but if it is due to digoxin toxicity, withdrawal of digoxin may be all that is required.[38]

**Paroxysmal supraventricular tachycardia** is a re-entry arrhythmia. The term paroxysmal atrial tachycardia was formerly used, but became obsolete when it was realised that many such arrhythmias arise in the atrioventricular junction rather than in atrial muscle.[43] The re-entry circuit can be either due to an accessory pathway between the atria and ventricles (atrioventricular reciprocating tachycardia) or re-entry can occur at the site of the node itself (atrioventricular nodal reciprocating tachycardia). It is a relatively common arrhythmia occurring in otherwise healthy individuals. It may resolve spontaneously, or reflex vagal stimulation by respiratory manoeuvres, prompt squatting, or pressure over one carotid sinus may restore normal sinus rhythm. If symptoms associated with the rapid heart rate are severe, treatment will be needed. For termination of paroxysmal supraventricular tachycardia adenosine given intravenously is often the drug of choice;[38,43,44] intravenous verapamil or diltiazem are alternatives.[38,45] Digoxin or beta blockers, also given intravenously, have been tried but appear to offer no advantage over adenosine or verapamil and are less effective.[43,44] Propafenone, flecainide, procainamide, and sotalol have also been used;[46] direct current cardioversion may be necessary in some cases. Long-term maintenance therapy to prevent recurrence is required in some patients. Oral drugs are used and may include beta blockers, digoxin, disopyramide, flecainide, propafenone, quinidine, or verapamil. Beta blockers, digoxin, and calcium-channel blockers such as verapamil act by delaying impulses along the atrioventricular conduction system and are usually first-line therapy.[38] Class I drugs act on atrial refractoriness; flecainide and propafenone, which are class Ic, are usually preferred.[38,45] Amiodarone may be used in patients with structural heart disease. Single-dose antiarrhythmic therapy may have a role in some patients with infrequent episodes.[38] However, for symptomatic patients in whom an accessory atrioventricular pathway is the cause or for atrioventricular nodal reentry tachycardia, radiofrequency ablation of the affected tissue is often the treatment of choice.[38,42,43,45,47,48]

Patients with the Wolff-Parkinson-White syndrome,[49] a congenital abnormality characterised by an accessory atrioventricular conduction pathway known as a Kent bundle, may be at special risk of developing atrial fibrillation or paroxysmal supraventricular tachycardia. Great care is necessary with the choice of antiarrhythmic in such patients and radiofrequency ablation may often be preferred.[38,42]

Supraventricular tachycardia can occur rarely *in utero* and is associated with hydrops fetalis and perinatal mortality and morbidity. Treatment is with antiarrhythmic drugs such as digoxin or flecainide given to the mother (transplacental therapy);[50,51] in resistant cases direct intraperitoneal or intravascular administration to the fetus may be necessary and amiodarone is often used.[50]

**Ventricular tachycardia** is a re-entry arrhythmia[52-56] often associated with underlying cardiovascular disease such as myocardial infarction or cardiomyopathies or with digoxin toxicity. The heart rate is about 120 to 250 beats/minute and the tachycardia, which arises in the ventricles below the atrioventricular node, can be paroxysmal, consisting of short self-terminating episodes, or can be sustained (lasting 30 seconds or longer). Although ventricular tachycardia can be asymptomatic (if the episodes are non-sustained) it is potentially a serious condition which may lead to reduced cardiac output, shock, and progression to **ventricular fibrillation**. It is one of the most common causes of sudden unexplained cardiac death.[57] The ECG trace of ventricular tachycardia has sometimes been confused with that of supraventricular tachycardia but since the treatments differ markedly, every effort should be made to obtain the correct diagnosis.

The initial treatment of ventricular tachycardia depends largely on the haemodynamic status of the patient. If the patient has sustained ventricular tachycardia or has pulseless non-sustained ventricular tachycardia, both of which tend to be associated with instability and a poorer prognosis, defibrillation, as outlined under Advanced Cardiac Life Support (p.812), should be initiated. In the more stable patient, intravenous drug therapy may be used for acute termination of the tachycardia. Lidocaine has been the drug of choice; other class I drugs such as disopyramide, flecainide, mexiletine, procainamide, propafenone, or quinidine are alternatives, as are bretylium, which has class II and class III activity, and the class III drug amiodarone. In some patients with non-sustained ventricular tachycardia, beta blockers may be effective and in one study[58] sotalol appeared to be superior to lidocaine for the acute termination of sustained tachycardia. Non-pharmacological methods of treatment include ablation either by radiofrequency or surgery, and electrical techniques such as pacing or cardioversion.

Following restoration of normal sinus rhythm maintenance therapy needs to be considered to prevent recurrences. Long-term prophylaxis is generally not warranted in low risk patients such as those who have experienced asymptomatic non-sustained ventricular tachycardia. Survivors of ventricular fibrillation and pulseless ventricular tachycardia have a high risk of recurrence of arrhythmia and either an implantable cardioverter defibrillator or drug therapy has been used in these patients prophylactically. However, studies comparing the two methods have found a greater reduction in mortality with implantable cardioverter defibrillators[59] and guidelines now recommend implantable defibrillators as preferred first-line therapy.[60,61] Drug therapy was formerly given empirically but if drugs are used choice is now generally guided by electrophysiological or electrocardiographic testing using programmed electrical stimulation or ambulatory monitoring. Drugs used have included class I drugs, beta blockers, sotalol, and amiodarone. The use of drug therapy in patients who have implantable cardioverter defibrillators to reduce activation of the device is also under investigation.

Ventricular arrhythmias may be associated with **heart disease** such as myocardial infarction or heart failure. Ventricular tachycardia and ventricular fibrillation are common early after **acute myocardial infarction**. Lidocaine has been given prophylactically after myocardial infarction to patients at high risk of ventricular fibrillation, but should probably be reserved for symptomatic patients.[56] Asymptomatic premature ventricular arrhythmias in subjects who have previously suffered a myocardial infarction are also common and are recognised as a risk factor for subsequent sudden cardiac death. However, a number of studies using class I antiarrhythmics have shown increased mortality with prophylactic use in such patients,[62,63] and increased mortality was also found in a study[64] using *d*-sotalol.

Meta-analyses[62,63] have concluded that the only class of drugs with proven benefit after myocardial infarction is the beta blockers. Some benefit has also been seen with amiodarone, and a meta-analysis[65] found a small reduction in total mortality suggesting that it might be of benefit after myocardial infarction in patients, such as those with heart failure, at high risk of arrhythmic death. Treatment with implantable cardioverter defibrillators may be more effective than drug therapy, particularly in patients with heart failure and symptomatic or non-symptomatic ventricular tachycardia,[59] and their use has been recommended[60,61] in such patients.

Implantable cardioverter defibrillators may also be considered in patients with hypertrophic cardiomyopathies and other structural heart disease who are at high risk for sudden cardiac death.[61] Attempts have been made to reduce deaths from ventricular arrhythmias in patients with severe **heart failure** (p.820); beneficial results have been reported with amiodarone but adverse effects may limit its use.

Drugs used to treat arrhythmias can have a **proarrhythmic** effect, that is they can exacerbate or induce arrhythmias of all types. **Torsade de pointes** is a potentially lethal ventricular tachycardia with a characteristic ECG pattern and is associated with prolongation of the QT interval; this may be congenital but is commonly drug-induced.[66-68] Drugs responsible include antiarrhythmics and several non-cardiac drugs[69-71] including phenothiazines, tricyclic antidepressants, antihistamines such as astemizole and terfenadine, antibacterials such as erythromycin, the antimalarial halofantrine, and the lipid lowering drug probucol. The ventricular tachycardia is often non-sustained, but may persist for long enough to cause syncope or it may even progress to ventricular fibrillation. If torsade de pointes is drug-induced, withdrawal and subsequent avoidance of the offending drug is mandatory. Electrolyte disturbances appear to contribute to torsade de pointes and initial therapy is with magnesium given intravenously together with temporary pacing of the atria or ventricles as appropriate. Isoprenaline may be given cautiously to increase the heart rate and shorten the QT interval, until pacing is instituted. Congenital long QT syndromes are usually treated with beta blockers and/or pacing.[67,68]


1. Mangrum JM, DiMarco JP. The evaluation and management of bradycardia. *N Engl J Med* 2000; **342:** 703–9.
2. Narayan SM, *et al.* Atrial fibrillation. *Lancet* 1997; **350:** 943–50.
3. Jung F, DiMarco JP. Treatment strategies for atrial fibrillation. *Am J Med* 1998; **104:** 272–86.
4. Falk RH. Atrial fibrillation. *N Engl J Med* 2001; **344:** 1067–78. Correction. *ibid.*; 1876.
5. Channer KS. Current management of symptomatic atrial fibrillation. *Drugs* 2001; **61:** 1425–37.
6. Peters NS, *et al.* Atrial fibrillation: strategies to control, combat, and cure. *Lancet* 2002; **359:** 593–603.
7. Nattel S, *et al.* New approaches to atrial fibrillation management: a critical review of a rapidly evolving field. *Drugs* 2002; **62:** 2377–97.
8. Blaauw Y, *et al.* Treatment of atrial fibrillation. *Heart* 2002; **88:** 432–7.
9. Markides V, Schilling RJ. Atrial fibrillation: classification, pathophysiology, mechanisms and drug treatment. *Heart* 2003; **89:** 939–43.
10. Fuster V, *et al.* ACC/AHA/ESC guidelines for the management of patients with atrial fibrillation: a report of the American College of Cardiology/American Heart Association Task Force on Practice Guidelines and the European Society of Cardiology Committee for Practice Guidelines and Policy Conferences (Committee to Develop Guidelines for the Management of Patients With Atrial Fibrillation). Executive summary: *J Am Coll Cardiol* 2001; **38:** 1231–66. Full text: http://www.americanheart.org/downloadable/heart/222_ja20017993p_1.pdf (accessed 13/05/04)
11. Crystal E, *et al.* Interventions on prevention of postoperative atrial fibrillation in patients undergoing heart surgery: a meta-analysis. *Circulation* 2002; **106:** 75–80.
12. Boriani G, *et al.* Rate control in atrial fibrillation: choice of treatment and assessment of efficacy. *Drugs* 2003; **63:** 1489–509.
13. The AFFIRM First Antiarrhythmic Drug Substudy Investigators. Maintenance of sinus rhythm in patients with atrial fibrillation: an AFFIRM substudy of the first antiarrhythmic drug. *J Am Coll Cardiol* 2003; **42:** 20–9.
14. Hohnloser SH, *et al.* Rhythm or rate control in atrial fibrillation—Pharmacological Intervention in Atrial Fibrillation (PIAF): a randomised trial. *Lancet* 2000; **356:** 1789–94.
15. The Atrial Fibrillation Follow-up Investigation of Rhythm Management (AFFIRM) Investigators. A comparison of rate control and rhythm control in patients with atrial fibrillation. *N Engl J Med* 2002; **347:** 1825–33.

16. Van Gelder IC, *et al.* A comparison of rate control and rhythm control in patients with recurrent persistent atrial fibrillation. *N Engl J Med* 2002; **347:** 1834–40.
17. Howard PA, Duncan PW. Primary stroke prevention in nonvalvular atrial fibrillation: implementing the clinical trial findings. *Ann Pharmacother* 1997; **31:** 1187–96.
18. Hardman SMC, Cowie MR. Anticoagulation in heart disease. *BMJ* 1999; **318:** 238–44.
19. Hart RG, Halperin JL. Atrial fibrillation and thromboembolism: a decade of progress in stroke prevention. *Ann Intern Med* 1999; **131:** 688–95.
20. Lip GYH. Thromboprophylaxis for atrial fibrillation. *Lancet* 1999; **353:** 4–6. Correction. *ibid.*; 1978.
21. Hankey GJ. Non-valvular atrial fibrillation and stroke prevention. *Med J Aust* 2001; **174:** 234–9.
22. Lip GYH, *et al.* ABC of antithrombotic therapy: antithrombotic therapy for atrial fibrillation. *BMJ* 2002; **325:** 1022–5.
23. Albers GW, *et al.* Antithrombotic therapy in atrial fibrillation. *Chest* 2001; **119** (suppl): 194S–206S.
24. Hart RG, *et al.* Antithrombotic therapy to prevent stroke in patients with atrial fibrillation: a meta-analysis. *Ann Intern Med* 1999; **131:** 492–501.
25. Benavente O, *et al.* Oral anticoagulants for preventing stroke in patients with non-valvular atrial fibrillation and no previous history of stroke or transient ischemic attacks. Available in The Cochrane Library; Issue 2. Chichester: John Wiley; 2004.
26. Go AS, *et al.* Anticoagulation therapy for stroke prevention in atrial fibrillation: how well do randomized trials translate into clinical practice? *JAMA* 2003; **290:** 2685–92.
27. Green CJ, *et al.* Anticoagulation in chronic nonvalvular atrial fibrillation: a critical appraisal and meta-analysis. *Can J Cardiol* 1997; **13:** 811–15.
28. Scottish Intercollegiate Guidelines Network. Antithrombotic therapy: a national clinical guideline (March 1999). Available at: http://www.show.scot.nhs.uk/sign/pdf/sign36.pdf (accessed 13/05/04)
29. The Atrial Fibrillation Investigators. The efficacy of aspirin in patients with atrial fibrillation: analysis of pooled data from 3 randomised trials. *Arch Intern Med* 1997; **157:** 1237–40.
30. Segal JB, *et al.* Anticoagulants or antiplatelet therapy for nonrheumatic atrial fibrillation and flutter. Available in The Cochrane Library; Issue 2. Chichester: John Wiley; 2004.
31. van Walraven C, *et al.* Oral anticoagulants vs aspirin in nonvalvular atrial fibrillation: an individual patient meta-analysis. *JAMA* 2002; **288:** 2441–8.
32. Taylor FC, *et al.* Systematic review of long term anticoagulation or antiplatelet treatment in patients with non-rheumatic atrial fibrillation. *BMJ* 2001; **322:** 321–6.
33. Morocutti C, *et al.* Indobufen versus warfarin in the secondary prevention of major vascular events in nonrheumatic atrial fibrillation. *Stroke* 1997; **28:** 1015–21.
34. Executive Steering Committee on behalf of the SPORTIF III Investigators. Stroke prevention with the oral direct thrombin inhibitor ximelagatran compared with warfarin in patients with non-valvular atrial fibrillation (SPORTIF III): randomised controlled trial. *Lancet* 2003; **362:** 1691–8.
35. Stroke Prevention in Atrial Fibrillation Investigators. Adjusted-dose warfarin versus low-intensity, fixed-dose warfarin plus aspirin for high-risk patients with atrial fibrillation: Stroke Prevention in Atrial Fibrillation III randomised clinical trial. *Lancet* 1996; **348:** 633–8.
36. Gulløv AL, *et al.* Fixed minidose warfarin and aspirin alone and in combination vs adjusted-dose warfarin for stroke prevention in atrial fibrillation: Second Copenhagen Atrial Fibrillation, Aspirin, and Anticoagulation Study. *Arch Intern Med* 1998; **158:** 1513–21.
37. Waldo AL. Treatment of atrial flutter. *Heart* 2000; **84:** 227–32.
38. Blomström-Lundqvist C, *et al.* ACC/AHA/ESC guidelines for the management of patients with supraventricular arrhythmias: a report of the American College of Cardiology/American Heart Association Task Force on Practice Guidelines and the European Society of Cardiology Committee for Practice Guidelines (Writing Committee to Develop Guidelines for the Management of Patients With Supraventricular Arrhythmias). Executive summary: *Circulation* 2003; **108:** 1871–909. Full text: http://www.americanheart.org/downloadable/heart/1062186010820SVAFullTextGLfinal.pdf (accessed 13/05/04)
39. Lanzarotti CJ, *et al.* Thromboembolism in chronic atrial flutter: is the risk underestimated? *J Am Coll Cardiol* 1997; **30:** 1506–11.
40. Wood KA, *et al.* Risk of thromboembolism in chronic atrial flutter. *Am J Cardiol* 1997; **79:** 1043–7.
41. Seidl K, *et al.* Risk of thromboembolic events in patients with atrial flutter. *Am J Cardiol* 1998; **82:** 580–3.
42. Morady F. Radio-frequency ablation as treatment for cardiac arrhythmias. *N Engl J Med* 1999; **340:** 534–44.
43. Ganz LI, Friedman PL. Supraventricular tachycardia. *N Engl J Med* 1995; **332:** 162–73.
44. Kugler JD, Danford DA. Management of infants, children, and adolescents with paroxysmal supraventricular tachycardia. *J Pediatr* 1996; **129:** 324–38.
45. Ferguson JD, DiMarco JP. Contemporary management of paroxysmal supraventricular tachycardia. *Circulation* 2003; **107:** 1096–9.
46. Pfammatter J-P, Bauersfeld U. Safety issues in the treatment of paediatric supraventricular tachycardias. *Drug Safety* 1998; **18:** 345–56.
47. Kuck K-H, Schlüter M. Junctional tachycardia and the role of catheter ablation. *Lancet* 1993; **341:** 1386–91.
48. Schilling RJ. Which patient should be referred to an electrophysiologist: supraventricular tachycardia. *Heart* 2002; **87:** 299–304.
49. Gaita F, *et al.* Wolff-Parkinson-White syndrome: identification and management. *Drugs* 1992; **43:** 185–200.
50. Owen P, Cameron A. Fetal tachyarrhythmias. *Br J Hosp Med* 1997; **58:** 142–4.
51. Simpson JM, Sharland GK. Fetal tachycardias: management and outcome of 127 consecutive cases. *Heart* 1998; **79:** 576–81.
52. Dancy M. Diagnosis and management of ventricular tachycardia. *Postgrad Med J* 1992; **68:** 406–14.
53. Campbell RWF. Ventricular ectopic beats and non-sustained ventricular tachycardia. *Lancet* 1993; **341:** 1454–8.
54. Shenasa M, *et al.* Ventricular tachycardia. *Lancet* 1993; **341:** 1512–19.
55. Welch PJ, *et al.* Management of ventricular arrhythmias: a trial-based approach. *J Am Coll Cardiol* 1999; **34:** 621–30.
56. Cannom DS, Prystowsky EN. Management of ventricular arrhythmias: detection, drugs, and devices. *JAMA* 1999; **281:** 172–9.
57. Huikuri HV, *et al.* Sudden death due to cardiac arrhythmias. *N Engl J Med* 2001; **345:** 1473–82.
58. Ho DSW, *et al.* Double-blind trial of lignocaine versus sotalol for acute termination of spontaneous sustained ventricular tachycardia. *Lancet* 1994; **344:** 18–23.
59. Ezekowitz JA, *et al.* Implantable cardioverter defibrillators in primary and secondary prevention: a systematic review of randomized, controlled trials. *Ann Intern Med* 2003; **138:** 445–52.
60. Gregoratos G, *et al.* ACC/AHA/NASPE 2002 guideline update for implantation of cardiac pacemakers and antiarrhythmia devices: a report of the American College of Cardiology/American Heart Association Task Force on Practice Guidelines (ACC/AHA/NASPE Committee to update the 1998 Pacemaker Guidelines). Summary article: *Circulation* 2002; **106:** 2145–61. Full text: http://www.americanheart.org/downloadable/heart/1032981283481CleanPacemakerFinalFT.pdf (accessed 13/05/04)
61. Priori SG, *et al.* Task Force on Sudden Cardiac Death of the European Society of Cardiology. *Eur Heart J* 2001; **22:** 1374–450. Correction. *ibid.* 2002; **23:** 257. Also available at: http://www.escardio.org/NR/rdonlyres/DFD1EBD3-1641-44AD-AFF2-3AA5898D59D4/0/suddendeath.pdf (accessed 12/05/04) Priori SG, *et al.* Update of the guidelines on sudden cardiac death of the European Society of Cardiology. *Eur Heart J* 2003; **24:** 13–15. http://www.escardio.org/NR/rdonlyres/59AB76B6-EC45-4115-904E-8C01C2B32FBE/0/02_update_scd.pdf (accessed 12/05/04)
62. Teo KK, *et al.* Effects of prophylactic antiarrhythmic drug therapy in acute myocardial infarction: an overview of results from randomized controlled trials. *JAMA* 1993; **270:** 1589–95.
63. McAlister FA, Teo KK. Antiarrhythmic therapies for the prevention of sudden cardiac death. *Drugs* 1997; **54:** 235–52.
64. Waldo AL, *et al.* Effect of d-sotalol on mortality in patients with left ventricular dysfunction after recent and remote myocardial infarction. *Lancet* 1996; **348:** 7–12. Correction. *ibid.*; 416.
65. Amiodarone Trials Meta-Analysis Investigators. Effect of prophylactic amiodarone on mortality after acute myocardial infarction and in congestive heart failure: meta-analysis of individual data from 6500 patients in randomised trials. *Lancet* 1997; **350:** 1417–24.
66. Ben-David J, Zipes DP. Torsades de pointes and proarrhythmia. *Lancet* 1993; **341:** 1578–82.
67. Viskin S. Long QT syndromes and torsade de pointes. *Lancet* 1999; **354:** 1625–33.
68. Khan IA. Clinical and therapeutic aspects of congenital and acquired long QT syndrome. *Am J Med* 2002; **112:** 58–66.
69. Thomas SHL. Drugs and the QT interval. *Adverse Drug React Bull* 1997; **182:** 691–4.
70. Doig JC. Drug-induced cardiac arrhythmias: incidence, prevention and management. *Drug Safety* 1997; **17:** 265–75.
71. Yap YG, Camm AJ. Drug induced QT prolongation and torsades de pointes. *Heart* 2003; **89:** 1363–72.


## Cardiomyopathies

Cardiomyopathy is a term used to describe diseases of the heart muscle associated with cardiac dysfunction. It has usually been used to describe conditions with an unknown cause (idiopathic) but specific heart muscle diseases where the cause is known are now often included in the definition.[1] Specific cardiomyopathies include those associated with systemic or pulmonary hypertension, ischaemic heart disease, valvular heart disease, congenital abnormalities, metabolic disorders, inflammatory or infectious diseases, and drug-induced conditions. Three distinct types of cardiomyopathy are generally recognised, namely dilated cardiomyopathy, hypertrophic cardiomyopathy, and restrictive cardiomyopathy; the dilated and hypertrophic forms are the two major types. A fourth type, arrhythmogenic right ventricular cardiomyopathy, may also occur. The management of the individual forms has been reviewed.[2-12]

In **dilated cardiomyopathy** (previously known as congestive cardiomyopathy) the main finding is systolic dysfunction with dilated and poorly contracting ventricles and a low cardiac output. The right, left, or both ventricles may be affected. Although there may be some ventricular hypertrophy, because of the dilatation there is no overall increase in the thickness of the ventricle walls. Dilated cardiomyopathy may be asymptomatic for some time but the initial manifestations are commonly those of heart failure; chest pain, systemic and pulmonary embolism, and arrhythmias may also occur. Management should generally follow the conventional strategies for heart failure (see p.820), including ACE inhibitors, diuretics, and beta blockers. Early studies[13-15] with beta blockers in patients with dilated cardiomyopathy demonstrated significant improvements in cardiac function and symptoms, together with prevention of clinical deterioration, but failed to demonstrate a significant effect on overall mortality. However, a further trial evaluating carvedilol therapy in patients with heart failure, including patients with dilated cardiomyopathy, was terminated early because mortality was significantly reduced in the carvedilol groups[16] and the CIBIS-II trial[17] using bisoprolol was also terminated early because of favourable results. A further long-term study[18] using metoprolol has also reported a significantly higher survival rate in those receiving metoprolol for up to 7 years. Although calcium-channel blockers are not usually used in heart failure, symptomatic improvement has also been reported with the calcium-channel blocker diltiazem.[19]

Patients with dilated cardiomyopathy may be at particular risk for systemic or pulmonary thromboembolism, due to blood stasis in the poorly contracting ventricle. Chronic oral anticoagulation has therefore been suggested, although current recommendations generally limit its use to those with atrial fibrillation, previous systemic embolism, or severe left ventricular dysfunction.[2,20] Arrhythmias should be treated as appropriate (see Cardiac Arrhythmias, p.816); amiodarone may be particularly suitable as it has no negative inotropic effect. Low-dose amiodarone has been tried in patients at high risk of sudden death, but its role has not yet been confirmed.[2,9]

A number of surgical treatments have been tried but cardiac transplantation remains the principal method of improving survival in these patients. Other therapies that have been tried include growth hormone, levothyroxine, pentoxifylline, levocarnitine, and immunosuppressants for presumed myocarditis.

In **hypertrophic cardiomyopathy** (previously known as obstructive cardiomyopathy) there is, as the name implies, ventricular hypertrophy but the ventricles are not dilated. This leads to diastolic dysfunction since diastolic filling is impaired by the stiff hypertrophied ventricular walls. It is an inherited condition occurring as an autosomal dominant trait and can occur at any age although presentation during the second decade of life is common. Patients may be asymptomatic or may experience chest pain, syncope, dyspnoea, or arrhythmias. Sudden death associated with emotional stress or exercise is not an uncommon finding and patients should avoid intense exercise. However, overall life expectancy is similar to that of the general population and many patients have little or no disability and do not require treatment.[6,12]

Patients should be investigated for the presence of any arrhythmias and treated appropriately (see Cardiac Arrhythmias, p.816) although this may not necessarily prevent sudden death. Atrial fibrillation is particularly important and is probably most effectively treated with amiodarone.[5,6,12] Anticoagulation should be considered in all patients with sustained atrial fibrillation.[4-6,12]

Beta blockers may be used for control of symptoms. They curtail emotion- or exercise-induced tachycardia. Anginal pain is also reduced and syncopal attacks may be prevented. Calcium-channel blockers (usually verapamil) also improve symptoms and exercise tolerance and may be considered in those who continue to have disabling symptoms or who are unable to tolerate beta blockers; however, verapamil may have adverse effects in patients with outflow obstruction and it should be used with caution in such patients.[10-12] In a crossover study,[21] exercise capacity was not improved by either verapamil or nadolol, although most patients preferred one or other of the drugs rather than placebo and quality of life did appear to be improved by verapamil. Other drugs that may provide symptomatic relief include disopyramide, which is used for its negative inotropic effect and is often given with beta blockers. Diuretics may be needed for congestive symptoms but may also reduce cardiac output. Surgery or septal ablation to reduce outflow obstruction may be of benefit in some patients whose symptoms are resistant to drug therapy.[4-6,10-12]

The risk of sudden death is difficult to assess, particularly in asymptomatic patients. Neither beta blockers nor verapamil, as used for possible symptomatic relief, prevent ventricular arrhythmias. However, there is some evidence[22] that high-dose therapy with beta blockers may improve survival in children with hypertrophic cardiomyopathy. Low-dose amiodarone may have a role in high risk patients, but adverse effects may limit its use;[10,12] implantable cardioverter-defibrillators are also used in some patients.[12,23]

In **restrictive cardiomyopathy** the filling of the ventricles is impaired, often due to endomyocardial fibrosis, resulting in predominantly diastolic dysfunction. Diuretics may improve congestive symptoms but should be used cautiously as they may decrease cardiac output. Arrhythmias should be treated if they are symptomatic and anticoagulation is advised, particularly in patients with atrial fibrillation, valvular disorders, or a low cardiac output.[7]


1. Richardson P, *et al.* Report of the 1995 World Health Organization/International Society and Federation of Cardiology Task Force on the definition and classification of cardiomyopathies. *Circulation* 1996; **93:** 841–2.
2. Dec GW, Fuster V. Idiopathic dilated cardiomyopathy. *N Engl J Med* 1994; **331:** 1564–75.
3. Burch M, Runciman M. Dilated cardiomyopathy. *Arch Dis Child* 1996; **74:** 479–81.
4. Elliott PM, McKenna WJ. Management of hypertrophic cardiomyopathy. *Br J Hosp Med* 1996; **55:** 419–23.
5. Spirito P, *et al.* The management of hypertrophic cardiomyopathy. *N Engl J Med* 1997; **336:** 775–85.
6. Maron BJ. Hypertrophic cardiomyopathy. *Lancet* 1997; **350:** 127–33.
7. Kushwaha SS, *et al.* Restrictive cardiomyopathy. *N Engl J Med* 1997; **336:** 267–76.
8. Oakley C. Aetiology, diagnosis, investigation, and management of cardiomyopathies. *BMJ* 1997; **315:** 1520–4.

9. Elliott P. Diagnosis and management of dilated cardiomyopathy. *Heart* 2000; **84:** 106–12.
10. McKenna WJ, Behr ER. Hypertrophic cardiomyopathy: management, risk stratification, and prevention of sudden death. *Heart* 2002; **87:** 169–76.
11. Maron BJ. Hypertrophic cardiomyopathy: a systematic review. *JAMA* 2002; **287:** 1308–20.
12. Maron BJ, *et al.* American College of Cardiology/European Society of Cardiology clinical expert consensus document on hypertrophic cardiomyopathy: a report of the American College of Cardiology Foundation Task Force on Clinical Expert Consensus Documents and the European Society of Cardiology Committee for Practice Guidelines. *J Am Coll Cardiol* 2003; **42:** 1687–713. Also published in *Eur Heart J* 2003; **24:** 1965–91. Also available at: http://www.escardio.org/NR/rdonlyres/D2085338-DDC0-4A7E-B4B5-F1F520DB5140/0/HCM_281003.pdf (accessed 12/05/04)
13. Waagstein F, *et al.* Beneficial effects of metoprolol in idiopathic dilated cardiomyopathy. *Lancet* 1993; **342:** 1441–6.
14. CIBIS Investigators and Committees. A randomized trial of β-blockade in heart failure: the cardiac insufficiency bisoprolol study (CIBIS). *Circulation* 1994; **90:** 1765–73.
15. The Metoprolol in Dilated Cardiomyopathy (MDC) Trial Study Group. 3-year follow-up of patients randomised in the metoprolol in dilated cardiomyopathy trial. *Lancet* 1998; **351:** 1180–1.
16. Packer M, *et al.* The effect of carvedilol on morbidity and mortality in patients with chronic heart failure. *N Engl J Med* 1996; **334:** 1349–55.
17. CIBIS-II Investigators and Committees. The Cardiac Insufficiency Bisoprolol Study II (CIBIS-II): a randomised trial. *Lancet* 1999; **353:** 9–13.
18. Di Lenarda A, *et al.* Long term survival effect of metoprolol in dilated cardiomyopathy. *Heart* 1998; **79:** 337–44.
19. Figulla HR, *et al.* Diltiazem improves cardiac function and exercise capacity in patients with idiopathic dilated cardiomyopathy: results of the Diltiazem in Dilated Cardiomyopathy Trial. *Circulation* 1996; **94:** 346–52.
20. Cheng JWM, Spinler SA. Should all patients with dilated cardiomyopathy receive chronic anticoagulation? *Ann Pharmacother* 1994; **28:** 604–9.
21. Gilligan DM, *et al.* A double-blind, placebo-controlled crossover trial of nadolol and verapamil in mild and moderately symptomatic hypertrophic cardiomyopathy. *J Am Coll Cardiol* 1993; **21:** 1672–9.
22. Östman-Smith I, *et al.* A cohort study of childhood hypertrophic cardiomyopathy: improved survival following high-dose beta-adrenoceptor antagonist treatment. *J Am Coll Cardiol* 1999; **34:** 1813–22.
23. Maron BJ, *et al.* Efficacy of implantable cardioverter-defibrillators for the prevention of sudden death in patients with hypertrophic cardiomyopathy. *N Engl J Med* 2000; **342:** 365–73.

## Cardiovascular risk reduction

Atherosclerotic cardiovascular disease includes ischaemic (coronary) heart disease (myocardial infarction and angina pectoris), ischaemic stroke, and peripheral vascular disease. Ischaemic heart disease, in particular, is a major cause of mortality in developed countries, and cardiovascular disease overall is associated with considerable morbidity. The benefits of a number of interventions are well established in patients at high risk of cardiovascular disease, and identification and treatment of such people is therefore an important healthcare strategy.[1-4]

Overall cardiovascular risk depends on a number of factors. Those who are at the highest risk are those with manifestations of atherosclerosis, particularly those who have already had a cardiovascular event such as a myocardial infarction or ischaemic stroke, but also those with symptoms of angina or peripheral vascular disease. The major modifiable risk factors identified through epidemiological studies are tobacco smoking, raised blood pressure, and raised blood-lipid concentrations;[5] other established risk factors include age, sex, left ventricular hypertrophy, and family history. Diabetics are also at considerable risk of ischaemic heart disease, even when treated, and aggressive therapy to reduce risk may be appropriate. Obesity, lack of exercise, abnormal blood clotting profile, and hyperhomocysteinaemia have also been associated with increased risk, although their relevance is less established.[6] Patients with abdominal obesity, hypertension, dyslipidaemia, and glucose intolerance are considered to have the **metabolic syndrome**, and are at increased risk of both cardiovascular disease and diabetes mellitus.[7]

The aim of cardiovascular risk reduction is to prevent clinical events occurring by abolishing or reducing any modifiable risk factors that are present. This requires both individual intervention, to identify and treat those at high risk, and also a population approach based on general health promotion and education to reduce the overall levels of risk factors in the general populace. Guidelines[1-3] have been published for identification and management at the individual level, including specific guidelines for women[8] and the elderly.[9] Since atheroma development may begin in childhood, approaches to risk reduction should also be considered from an early age.[10]

Lifestyle and dietary modifications are the mainstay of risk reduction, particularly at a population level, and include advice not to smoke, avoidance of obesity, increased exercise, moderation of alcohol intake, and a diet that is low in saturated fat and high in fruit, vegetables, and fish.[1-3,11-14] In unselected populations, these efforts probably produce only modest changes in risk factors,[15,16] and while the incidence of ischaemic heart disease is falling in many populations, the WHO MONICA project (Monitoring the Trends and Determinants in Cardiovascular Diseases) found only a weak association between changes in classic risk factors and changes in event rates.[17] In individuals with established modifiable risk factors, drug treatment may also be required. Smoking cessation should be encouraged in all smokers, and specific strategies are discussed on p.1721. Treatment of hypertension and hyperlipidaemias depends on their severity and the patient's overall risk and is discussed under the individual diseases (see p.825 and p.823, respectively). Assessment of risk is a complex procedure and risk and treatment tables are available to aid decisions about when to initiate therapy in patients without established cardiovascular disease.[1,18] Guidelines differ as to the level of risk at which treatment should be initiated; this is a matter of judgement and may depend on economic factors and the balance between benefit and risk of adverse effects in otherwise healthy people. Tight control of blood glucose is important in diabetic patients (see Diabetic Complications, p.326). Other interventions that may be of benefit in some individuals include antiplatelet therapy, reduction of lipids in those with normal lipid concentrations, and ACE inhibitors.

***Antiplatelet therapy*** has been investigated for primary and secondary prevention of various cardiovascular disorders. Numerous studies[19] have established that antiplatelet therapy reduces the risk of subsequent cardiovascular events but that the risk of bleeding is increased, and absolute benefit therefore depends on the individual level of risk. In patients with a previous vascular event, the use of antiplatelets for secondary prevention is well established.[1,2] Aspirin, given in the acute phase and continued long-term, reduces the risk of re-infarction and death following myocardial infarction and should be given indefinitely.[19] Long-term prophylaxis with aspirin also reduces the risk of future serious vascular events including stroke in patients who have suffered an ischaemic stroke or transient ischaemic attack,[19-22] regardless of age.[23] A number of studies also support the benefits of antiplatelets for primary prevention of cardiovascular events in individuals at high risk. Aspirin may reduce the risk of first myocardial infarction in patients with stable chronic angina.[24] The Thrombosis Prevention Trial[25] in males at high risk of developing occlusive vascular disease and the Hypertension Optimal Treatment (HOT) trial[26] in hypertensive patients have, more recently, confirmed that aspirin reduces the incidence of myocardial infarction in these at-risk groups, although both studies reported little or no effect on the overall incidence of stroke. The Primary Prevention Project,[27] a study in patients with at least one major risk factor, showed a reduction in cardiovascular mortality and in a composite of cardiovascular events including death, myocardial infarction, and stroke.

Primary prevention in healthy individuals is more controversial. Two large studies in the UK[28] and in the US[29] in healthy male physicians produced conflicting results. In the UK study there was no reduction in the incidence of fatal and non-fatal myocardial infarction in those who had taken aspirin, while the US study did show a reduction in subjects 50 years of age or older; both showed a slight non-significant increase in the number of disabling strokes which, in the US study, were attributed to cerebral haemorrhage. A large observational study in healthy US nurses[30] indicated that aspirin might reduce the risk of first myocardial infarction in women. However, meta-analyses[19,31,32] have concluded that for most healthy individuals, aspirin therapy is inappropriate.

Aspirin has been the most widely studied antiplatelet drug and appears to be effective over a range of doses (see p.18). Other antiplatelets may be used in those intolerant of aspirin; in the CAPRIE study,[33] clopidogrel was shown to be at least as effective as aspirin in reducing cardiovascular events, including myocardial infarction and stroke, in individuals at high risk. Dipyridamole given alone has been shown to be effective for secondary prevention of ischaemic stroke[34] and may be used in patients unable to tolerate aspirin. The combination of aspirin and dipyridamole has produced additive protective effects in stroke,[34,35] and there is also some evidence[36] for the use of other antiplatelet combinations in ischaemic heart disease. ***Oral anticoagulants*** may be more effective than antiplatelet therapy but the risk of bleeding is increased,[25,37] and they are generally only recommended in patients unable to take antiplatelets or where antiplatelets have been ineffective.

The benefits of ***lipid lowering therapy*** in individuals with hypercholesterolaemia is well established,[38-40] particularly in those at high risk of clinical events. However, a number of studies have also investigated the use of lipid lowering drugs in individuals with average rather than elevated cholesterol concentrations. In the Cholesterol and Recurrent Events (CARE) Trial[41,42] and the Long-term Intervention with Pravastatin in Ischaemic Disease (LIPID) study,[43] pravastatin was found to be of benefit for secondary prevention in patients with average cholesterol concentrations, while data from the WOSCOPS trials[44-46] indicate that pravastatin is also effective for primary prevention in moderate hypercholesterolaemia. Similar findings have been published for lovastatin in patients with average cholesterol levels.[47] Although most recent studies have used statins, beneficial effects for secondary prevention of ischaemic heart disease have also been reported for gemfibrozil[48] in men whose primary lipid abnormality was a low HDL-cholesterol level, and for omega-3 marine triglycerides[49] in a Mediterranean population.

There has been concern that there might be an association between low cholesterol concentrations and increased morbidity and mortality from non-cardiac causes including haemorrhagic stroke, cancer, accidents and suicide, and chronic respiratory, liver, and bowel disease.[50-55] However, meta-analyses have shown that statin therapy reduces all-cause mortality,[38] without significantly increasing non-illness mortality,[56] and such concerns appear to be unfounded.

The primary and secondary prevention studies have been predominantly in middle-aged men. Although some studies have suggested benefit in women[43,47,57,58] and in older individuals,[57,59] the numbers included have generally been too few to fully assess the effects of lipid lowering. The Heart Protection Study[60] confirmed the benefits of statins in both of these subgroups, and supports the recommendations for treatment in these patients.[8,9,61,62]

The use of ***ACE inhibitors*** has mainly been investigated in individuals with established cardiovascular disease. Studies[63,64] in patients with heart failure suggested that ACE inhibitors also reduced the risk of myocardial infarction, while in the HOPE study,[65] treatment with ramipril significantly reduced the rate of death, myocardial infarction, and stroke in patients at high risk for cardiovascular disease. A reduction in cardiovascular events was also found[66] in patients with stable ischaemic heart disease given perindopril. It is not clear whether the benefit seen is due to the reduction in blood pressure caused by ACE inhibitors, or whether they have additional effects. A study[67] using perindopril, alone or with a diuretic, found that the risk of recurrent stroke was reduced in patients with a history of stroke or transient ischaemic attack, irrespective of whether they had normal or raised blood pressure at study entry. ***Angiotensin II receptor antagonists*** may have similar benefits; a study[68] comparing losartan with a beta blocker in hypertensive patients with left ventricular hypertrophy found that there was a greater reduction in cardiovascular events with losartan despite a similar effect on blood pressure.

Women have a lower risk of atherosclerotic disease than men of a comparable age, although the difference narrows with increasing age postmenopausally, and the use of ***HRT*** has therefore been investigated. Some epidemiological studies have suggested that HRT lowers the risk of cardiovascular events, although other studies have produced conflicting results (see p.1540). However, randomised trials have failed to confirm a beneficial effect on clinical events[69] and HRT is no longer recommended[8] for either the primary or secondary prevention of cardiovascular disease in women.

Specific interventions to reduce the progression of atherosclerosis are discussed on p.815.

1. De Backer G, *et al.* European guidelines on cardiovascular disease prevention in clinical practice: third Joint Task Force of European and Other Societies on Cardiovascular Disease Prevention in Clinical Practice. Executive summary: *Eur Heart J* 2003; **24:** 1601–10. Full guidelines: *Eur J Cardiovasc Prev Rehabil* 2003; **10** (suppl 1): S1–S78. Also available at: http://www.escardio.org/NR/rdonlyres/A0EF5CA5-421B-45EF-A65C-19B9EC411261/0/CVD_Prevention_03_full.pdf (accessed 12/05/04)
2. Smith SC, *et al.* AHA/ACC guidelines for preventing heart attack and death in patients with atherosclerotic cardiovascular disease: 2001 update. A statement for healthcare professionals from the American Heart Association and the American College of Cardiology. *J Am Coll Cardiol* 2001; **38:** 1581–3. Also published in *Circulation* 2001; **104:** 1577–9. Also available at: http://www.acc.org/clinical/guidelines/atherosclerosis/atherosclerosis_pdf.pdf (accessed 13/05/04)
3. Pearson TA, *et al.* AHA guidelines for primary prevention of cardiovascular disease and stroke: 2002 update: consensus panel guide to comprehensive risk reduction for adult patients without coronary or other atherosclerotic vascular diseases. *Circulation* 2002; **106:** 388–91.

4. Wood D. Asymptomatic individuals—risk stratification in the prevention of coronary heart disease. *Br Med Bull* 2001; **59:** 3–16.
5. Khot UN, *et al.* Prevalence of conventional risk factors in patients with coronary heart disease. *JAMA* 2003; **290:** 898–904.
6. Kullo IJ, *et al.* Novel risk factors for atherosclerosis. *Mayo Clin Proc* 2000; **75:** 369–80.
7. Grundy SM, *et al.* Definition of metabolic syndrome: Report of the National Heart, Lung, and Blood Institute/American Heart Association conference on scientific issues related to definition. *Circulation* 2004; **109:** 433–8.
8. Mosca L, *et al.* Evidence-based guidelines for cardiovascular disease prevention in women. *Circulation* 2004; **109:** 672–93.
9. Williams MA, *et al.* Secondary prevention of coronary heart disease in the elderly (with emphasis on patients ≥75 years of age): an American Heart Association scientific statement from the Council on Clinical Cardiology Subcommittee on Exercise, Cardiac Rehabilitation, and Prevention. *Circulation* 2002; **105:** 1735–43.
10. Kavey R-EW, *et al.* American Heart Association guidelines for primary prevention of atherosclerotic cardiovascular disease beginning in childhood. *Circulation* 2003; **107:** 1562–6. Also published in *J Pediatr* 2003; **142:** 368–72.
11. Anonymous. Lifestyle measures to tackle atherosclerotic disease. *Drug Ther Bull* 2001; **39:** 21–4.
12. Mann JI. Diet and risk of coronary heart disease and type 2 diabetes. *Lancet* 2002; **360:** 783–9.
13. Hu FB, Willett WC. Optimal diets for prevention of coronary heart disease. *JAMA* 2002; **288:** 2569–78.
14. Hooper L, *et al.* Reduced or modified dietary fat for preventing cardiovascular disease. Available in The Cochrane Library; Issue 2. Chichester: John Wiley; 2004.
15. Ebrahim S, Davey Smith G. Systematic review of randomised controlled trials of multiple risk factor interventions for preventing coronary heart disease. *BMJ* 1997; **314:** 1666–74.
16. Ebrahim S, Davey Smith G. Multiple risk factor interventions for primary prevention of coronary heart disease. Available in The Cochrane Library; Issue 2. Chichester: John Wiley; 2004.
17. Kuulasmaa K, *et al.* Estimation of contribution of changes in classic risk factors to trends in coronary-event rates across the WHO MONICA Project populations. *Lancet* 2000; **355:** 675–87.
18. Wallis EJ, *et al.* Coronary and cardiovascular risk estimation for primary prevention: validation of a new Sheffield table in the 1995 Scottish health survey population. *BMJ* 2000; **320:** 671–6. Correction. *ibid.*; 1034.
19. Antithrombotic Trialists' Collaboration. Collaborative meta-analysis of randomised trials of antiplatelet therapy for prevention of death, myocardial infarction, and stroke in high risk patients. *BMJ* 2002; **324:** 71–86. Correction. *ibid.*; 141.
20. Albers GW, *et al.* Antithrombotic and thrombolytic therapy for ischemic stroke. *Chest* 2001; **119** (suppl): 300S–320S.
21. Wolf PA, *et al.* Preventing ischemic stroke in patients with prior stroke and transient ischemic attack: a statement for healthcare professionals from the Stroke Council of the American Heart Association. *Stroke* 1999; **30:** 1991–4.
22. Albers GW, *et al.* Supplement to the guidelines for the management of transient ischemic attacks: a statement from the Ad Hoc Committee on Guidelines for the Management of Transient Ischemic Attacks, Stroke Council, American Heart Association. *Stroke* 1999; **30:** 2502–11. Also available at: http://stroke.ahajournals.org/cgi/reprint/30/11/2502.pdf (accessed 21/05/04)
23. Sivenius J, *et al.* Antiplatelet treatment in elderly people with transient ischaemic attacks or ischaemic strokes. *BMJ* 1995; **310:** 25–6.
24. Juul-Möller S, *et al.* Double-blind trial of aspirin in primary prevention of myocardial infarction in patients with stable chronic angina pectoris. *Lancet* 1992; **340:** 1421–5.
25. The Medical Research Council's General Practice Research Framework. Thrombosis prevention trial: randomised trial of low-intensity oral anticoagulation with warfarin and low-dose aspirin in the primary prevention of ischaemic heart disease in men at increased risk. *Lancet* 1998; **351:** 233–41.
26. Hansson L, *et al.* Effects of intensive blood-pressure lowering and low-dose aspirin in patients with hypertension: principal results of the Hypertension Optimal Treatment (HOT) randomised trial. *Lancet* 1998; **351:** 1755–62.
27. Collaborative Group of the Primary Prevention Project. Low-dose aspirin and vitamin E in people at cardiovascular risk: a randomised trial in general practice. *Lancet* 2001; **357:** 89–95.
28. Peto R, *et al.* Randomised trial of prophylactic daily aspirin in British male doctors. *BMJ* 1988; **296:** 313–16.
29. Steering Committee of the Physicians Health Study Research Group. Final report on the aspirin component of the ongoing physicians' health study. *N Engl J Med* 1989; **321:** 129–35.
30. Manson JE, *et al.* A prospective study of aspirin use and primary prevention of cardiovascular disease in women. *JAMA* 1991; **266:** 521–7.
31. Sanmuganathan PS, *et al.* Aspirin for primary prevention of coronary heart disease: safety and absolute benefit related to coronary risk derived from meta-analysis of randomised trials. *Heart* 2001; **85:** 265–71.
32. Hayden M, *et al.* Aspirin for the primary prevention of cardiovascular events: a summary of the evidence for the U.S. Preventive Services Task Force. *Ann Intern Med* 2002; **136:** 161–72.
33. CAPRIE Steering Committee. A randomised, blinded, trial of clopidogrel versus aspirin in patients at risk of ischaemic events (CAPRIE). *Lancet* 1996; **348:** 1329–39.
34. Diener HC, *et al.* European Stroke Prevention Study 2: dipyridamole and acetylsalicylic acid in the secondary prevention of stroke. *J Neurol Sci* 1996; **143:** 1–13.
35. Wilterdink JL, Easton JD. Dipyridamole plus aspirin in cerebrovascular disease. *Arch Neurol* 1999; **56:** 1087–92.
36. Nappi J, Talbert R. Dual antiplatelet therapy for prevention of recurrent ischemic events. *Am J Health-Syst Pharm* 2002; **59:** 1723–35.
37. The Stroke Prevention in Reversible Ischemia Trial (SPIRIT) Study Group. A randomized trial of anticoagulants versus aspirin after cerebral ischemia of presumed arterial origin. *Ann Neurol* 1997; **42:** 857–65.
38. LaRosa JC, *et al.* Effect of statins on risk of coronary disease: a meta-analysis of randomized controlled trials. *JAMA* 1999; **282:** 2340–6.
39. Pignone M, *et al.* Use of lipid lowering drugs for primary prevention of coronary heart disease: meta-analysis of randomised trials. *BMJ* 2000; **321:** 983–6. Correction. *ibid.*; 1519.
40. Law MR, *et al.* Quantifying effect of statins on low density lipoprotein cholesterol, ischaemic heart disease, and stroke: systematic review and meta-analysis. *BMJ* 2003; **326:** 1423–7.
41. Sacks FM, *et al.* The effect of pravastatin on coronary events after myocardial infarction in patients with average cholesterol levels. *N Engl J Med* 1996; **335:** 1001–9.
42. Sacks FM, *et al.* Relationship between plasma LDL concentrations during treatment with pravastatin and recurrent coronary events in the Cholesterol and Recurrent Events Trial. *Circulation* 1998; **97:** 1446–52.
43. The Long-Term Intervention with Pravastatin in Ischaemic Disease (LIPID) Study Group. Prevention of cardiovascular events and death with pravastatin in patients with coronary heart disease and a broad range of initial cholesterol levels. *N Engl J Med* 1998; **339:** 1349–57.
44. Shepherd J, *et al.* Prevention of coronary heart disease with pravastatin in men with hypercholesterolemia. *N Engl J Med* 1995; **333:** 1301–7.
45. West of Scotland Coronary Prevention Group. West of Scotland Coronary Prevention Study: identification of high-risk groups and comparison with other cardiovascular intervention trials. *Lancet* 1996; **348:** 1339–42.
46. West of Scotland Coronary Prevention Study Group. Influence of pravastatin and plasma lipids on clinical events in the West of Scotland Coronary Prevention Study (WOSCOPS). *Circulation* 1998; **97:** 1440–5.
47. Downs JR, *et al.* Primary prevention of acute coronary events with lovastatin in men and women with average cholesterol levels: results of AFCAPS/TexCAPS. *JAMA* 1998; **279:** 1615–22.
48. Rubins HB, *et al.* Gemfibrozil for the secondary prevention of coronary heart disease in men with low levels of high-density lipoprotein cholesterol. *N Engl J Med* 1999; **341:** 410–18.
49. GISSI-Prevenzione Investigators. Dietary supplementation with n-3 polyunsaturated fatty acids and vitamin E after myocardial infarction: results of the GISSI-Prevenzione trial. *Lancet* 1999; **354:** 447–55.
50. Jacobs D, *et al.* Report of the conference on low blood cholesterol: mortality associations. *Circulation* 1992; **86:** 1046–60.
51. Davey Smith G, *et al.* Plasma cholesterol concentration and mortality: the Whitehall Study. *JAMA* 1992; **267:** 70–6.
52. Law MR, *et al.* Assessing possible hazards of reducing serum cholesterol. *BMJ* 1994; **308:** 373–9.
53. Newman TB, Hulley SB. Carcinogenicity of lipid-lowering drugs. *JAMA* 1996; **275:** 55–60.
54. Zureik M, *et al.* Serum cholesterol concentration and death from suicide in men: Paris prospective study I. *BMJ* 1996; **313:** 649–51.
55. Golomb BA. Cholesterol and violence: is there a connection? *Ann Intern Med* 1998; **128:** 478–87.
56. Muldoon MF, *et al.* Cholesterol reduction and non-illness mortality: meta-analysis of randomised clinical trials. *BMJ* 2001; **322:** 11–15.
57. Miettinen TA, *et al.* Cholesterol-lowering therapy in women and elderly patients with myocardial infarction or angina pectoris: findings from the Scandinavian Simvastatin Survival Study (4S). *Circulation* 1997; **96:** 4211–18.
58. Lewis SJ, *et al.* Effect of pravastatin on cardiovascular events in women after myocardial infarction: the Cholesterol and Recurrent Events (CARE) trial. *J Am Coll Cardiol* 1998; **32:** 140–6.
59. Lewis SJ, *et al.* Effect of pravastatin on cardiovascular events in older patients with myocardial infarction and cholesterol levels in the average range: results of the Cholesterol and Recurrent Events (CARE) trial. *Ann Intern Med* 1998; **129:** 681–9.
60. Heart Protection Study Collaborative Group. MRC/BHF Heart Protection Study of cholesterol lowering with simvastatin in 20 536 high-risk individuals: a randomised placebo-controlled trial. *Lancet* 2002; **360:** 7–22.
61. Mosca L, *et al.* Guide to preventive cardiology for women. *Circulation* 1999; **99:** 2480–4.
62. Grundy SM, *et al.* Cholesterol lowering in the elderly population. *Arch Intern Med* 1999; **159:** 1670–8.
63. Pfeffer MA, *et al.* Effect of captopril on mortality and morbidity in patients with left ventricular dysfunction after myocardial infarction: results of the Survival and Ventricular Enlargement Trial. *N Engl J Med* 1992; **327:** 669–77.
64. Yusuf S, *et al.* Effect of enalapril on myocardial infarction and unstable angina in patients with low ejection fractions. *Lancet* 1992; **340:** 1173–8.
65. The Heart Outcomes Prevention Evaluation Study Investigators. Effects of an angiotensin-converting-enzyme inhibitor, ramipril, on cardiovascular events in high-risk patients. *N Engl J Med* 2000; **342:** 145–53.
66. EURopean trial On reduction of cardiac events with Perindopril in stable coronary Artery disease Investigators. Efficacy of perindopril in reduction of cardiovascular events among patients with stable coronary artery disease: randomised, double-blind, placebo-controlled, multicentre trial (the EUROPA study). *Lancet* 2003; **362:** 782–8.
67. PROGRESS Collaborative Group. Randomised trial of a perindopril-based blood-pressure-lowering regimen among 6105 individuals with previous stroke or transient ischaemic attack. *Lancet* 2001; **358:** 1033–41. Corrections. *ibid.*; 1556 and 2002; **359:** 2120.
68. Dahlöf B, *et al.* Cardiovascular morbidity and mortality in the Losartan Intervention For Endpoint reduction in hypertension study (LIFE): a randomised trial against atenolol. *Lancet* 2002; **359:** 995–1003.
69. Humphrey LL, *et al.* Postmenopausal hormone replacement therapy and the primary prevention of cardiovascular disease. *Ann Intern Med* 2002; **137:** 273–84.

## Cerebrovascular disease

The term 'cerebrovascular disease' may cover disorders of the cerebral circulation such as ischaemic stroke and subarachnoid haemorrhage (see Stroke, below), but is often used to cover the rather vague concept of cerebrovascular insufficiency.

At one time it was believed that the dementia associated with Alzheimer's disease (p.1484) was due to cerebrovascular insufficiency and many drugs with vasodilator activity have been tried, but overall there is little convincing evidence of benefit.[1] Ergot derivatives such as co-dergocrine mesilate and nicergoline have been commonly used; however, any effectiveness is now attributed to their action as metabolic enhancers or nootropic drugs rather than to vasodilatation and their place in therapy has still to be established. The calcium-channel blocker nimodipine has shown benefit in some patients with dementia. Other vasodilators used have included buflomedil, cyclandelate, isoxsuprine, naftidrofuryl, pentoxifylline, and propentofylline.

1. Erkinjuntti T. Cerebrovascular dementia: pathophysiology, diagnosis and treatment. *CNS Drugs* 1999; **12:** 35–48.

## Heart failure

Heart failure is a clinical diagnosis made in a patient with a known or suspected cardiac disorder who presents with dyspnoea, fatigue, and oedema (peripheral and/or pulmonary). It may be graded as mild, moderate, or severe depending upon whether symptoms such as dyspnoea and fatigue appear on ordinary physical exertion, on little exertion, or at rest, respectively. Another grading system (that of the New York Heart Association) has four grades (grades I, II, III, IV), again partly classified on appearance of symptoms in relation to exertion (with grade IV representing the most severe form). The discussion that follows focuses on the chronic form of heart failure. The management of acute heart failure resulting in cardiogenic shock is covered under Shock, p.835.

Heart failure is a common condition[1] and is a consequence of cardiac abnormality, injury, or cardiovascular stress such as hypertension or valve disorders. Myocardial infarction is a leading cause of heart failure, and chronic myocardial ischaemia may also be a contributing factor. Other cardiovascular disorders that may lead to heart failure include cardiomyopathies and cor pulmonale. Infections causing myocardial damage, and cardiotoxicity arising from alcoholism or induced by drugs may also be precipitating factors. The increased demands put on the heart by chronic severe anaemia or hyperthyroidism can also be causes.

Traditionally, heart failure has been thought of in purely haemodynamic terms, as a condition in which the heart is unable to provide an adequate blood flow to meet the metabolic demands of the body. However, it is now appreciated that compensatory neurohormonal mechanisms play just as important a role in its development.[2-4] Echocardiography, the most useful investigative procedure in patients with heart failure, assesses haemodynamic factors; it allows assessment of ventricular function and ejection fraction, enables structural changes to be observed, and rapidly identifies patients with potentially correctable abnormalities such as valvular disease. Measurement of blood concentrations of brain natriuretic peptide has been suggested as another useful investigation;[5,6] this relates to the neurohormonal mechanisms involved.

Echocardiography can be used to divide patients into those with dysfunction of either the right or left ventricle (right- or left-sided heart failure), although dysfunction of both ventricles is likely to be present to some extent. In most patients, and especially in those with heart failure following myocardial infarction, the predominant finding is that of a dilated and poorly contracting left ventricle. This represents left ventricular systolic dysfunction, in which both the ejection fraction and the cardiac output are low. Isolated left ventricular diastolic dysfunction,[7] in which there is impaired ventricular filling but a normal ejection fraction, can also result in heart failure although this is less common; cardiac output may be normal but does not increase in response to exercise. Diastolic dysfunction is more common in the elderly and also occurs in some cardiomyopathies (see p.818); many patients have both diastolic and systolic dysfunction. Asymptomatic left ventricular dysfunction has been found in some patients, especially those in the early postmyocardial infarction period, and although these patients are not strictly defined as having heart failure, treatment may be given to prevent the development of full symptomatic disease.

Neurohormonal disturbances both result from, and contribute to, the deterioration in ventricular function.[3,4] Myocardial injury or impairment leads to an inability of the ventricles to empty adequately during systole. The resulting ventricular dilatation increases wall tension and initially leads to an increase in contraction while the decrease in cardiac output and blood pressure results in activation of the sympathetic nervous system, leading to an increase in the force and frequency of contraction. Reduced blood flow to the kidney also leads to activation of the renin-angiotensin-aldosterone system, resulting in vasoconstriction and fluid retention. At the same time, an increase in wall stress also occurs in the atria, leading to secretion of atrial natriuretic peptide; this inhibits the release of noradrenaline but also has direct vasodilator and natriuretic actions that lower the haemodynamic load on the heart. Thus, in the short term, compensation for myocardial injury can occur and cardiac output may be maintained. In the long term, these compensatory haemodynamic and neurohormonal mechanisms become ineffective. Ventricular dilatation progresses, the sympathetic nervous system and renin-angiotensin system are persistently activated, ventricular hypertrophy occurs, and ventricular function deteriorates progressively.

**Management**. Heart failure is a progressively disabling condition associated with considerable morbidity and mortality. Management is aimed therefore not only at providing symptomatic relief, but also at improving prognosis. Reviews[6,8-11] and guidelines[5,12-15] have been published concerning management; these are generally specific to heart failure due to left ventricular systolic dysfunction. The management of patients with diastolic dysfunction is less clear. In theory, this should differ from systolic dysfunction, but few trials have specifically studied such patients. While many of the early drug trials were based on a clinical diagnosis of heart failure and may have included patients with diastolic dysfunction, therapy for such patients is not established and the following discussion is specific for patients with systolic dysfunction unless stated otherwise.

Any underlying cause of heart failure should be corrected and certain non-pharmacological interventions may be beneficial. Weight reduction should be attempted in the overweight and moderate salt restriction may be undertaken. In acute heart failure bed rest may become necessary, but in controlled chronic heart failure exercise should be encouraged and specific exercise programmes may be of benefit.[5,16] Immunisation with influenza and pneumococcal vaccines is advised.[5,12-14] Drug therapy of heart failure is based on the use of diuretics, ACE inhibitors, cardiac glycosides, beta blockers, and vasodilators. Other drugs that may have a role include angiotensin II receptor antagonists and spironolactone.

***Diuretics*** have been the mainstay in the treatment of heart failure. They provide very effective symptomatic control in patients with peripheral or pulmonary oedema and rapidly relieve dyspnoea. If symptoms of fluid retention are only mild, a *thiazide diuretic*, such as *bendroflumethiazide* or *hydrochlorothiazide*, may be adequate. However, in most cases, especially in moderate or severe fluid retention, a *loop diuretic* such as *furosemide* will be necessary. Combination treatment with diuretics that behave synergistically by acting at different sites (the principle of sequential nephron blockade) may be needed in some patients, especially when there is diuretic resistance.[17,18] A loop diuretic with either a thiazide or metolazone is commonly used,[5] but severe fluid and electrolyte disturbances may occur, particularly with metolazone; loop diuretics with potassium-sparing diuretics have also been used. *Spironolactone* is an aldosterone antagonist and has diuretic and possibly additional effects, as discussed below.

However, diuretics are not a sufficient treatment on their own as clinical stability tends to deteriorate over time. In addition, although a meta-analysis[19] has suggested that diuretics have beneficial effects on symptoms and mortality, there have been no long-term trials assessing the effect of diuretics on prognosis, and drugs that have been shown to have a mortality benefit are also required.

***ACE inhibitors*** given orally produce clinical benefit in all stages of chronic heart failure additional to that seen with diuretics. They relieve symptoms such as dyspnoea and improve exercise tolerance. In addition, studies have demonstrated that ACE inhibitors improve survival and reduce the progression of mild or moderate heart failure to more severe stages.[20] ACE inhibitors may also be beneficial in asymptomatic left ventricular dysfunction.[21] The Studies of Left Ventricular Dysfunction (SOLVD)[22] trials indicated that ACE inhibitors, in this case enalapril, might protect against myocardial infarction, unstable angina, and cardiac death in patients with either symptomatic or asymptomatic heart failure. ACE inhibitors are now recommended,[12-15,23] therefore, in all patients with symptomatic heart failure due to left ventricular systolic dysfunction, including those whose symptoms are controlled with diuretic therapy. Some guidelines[14,15] recommend that ACE inhibitors should be given to all patients with significantly reduced left ventricular ejection fraction, whether or not they have symptoms.

ACE inhibitors have also been given to patients shortly after suffering myocardial infarction but before the development of symptomatic heart failure and appear to be beneficial. However, it is not yet clear which patients should receive such therapy or when it should be started (see Myocardial Infarction, p.828).

The precise mode of action of ACE inhibitors in heart failure is not completely understood but appears to be a result of both haemodynamic and neurohormonal mechanisms. They are vasodilators and cause both arteriolar and venous dilatation, mainly through reduction of angiotensin II formation. They also attenuate the ventricular dilatation and prevent the ventricular remodelling that develops after a myocardial injury. It has also been suggested that they may protect against the development of arrhythmias.[24]

***Cardiac glycosides*** such as *digoxin* or *digitoxin* have an extremely long history in the management of heart failure. They are positive inotropes and increase the contractility of the heart thereby increasing cardiac output. Additional effects in heart failure appear to be due to neuroendocrine suppression such as inhibition of the sympathetic nervous system and indirect arterial vasodilatation.

The benefit of cardiac glycosides in heart failure accompanied by atrial fibrillation is not disputed although their role in patients with sinus rhythm has been debated. There is evidence that withdrawal of digoxin from patients receiving diuretics (the PROVED trial)[25] or ACE inhibitors (the RADIANCE study)[26] carries a considerable risk of clinical deterioration if they are stable on such combination therapy. The large DIG study[27] found that digoxin, given in addition to diuretics and ACE inhibitors, improved symptoms but had no effect on mortality. Digoxin may therefore have a role in patients who remain symptomatic despite ACE inhibitor, diuretic, and beta-blocker therapy,[5,14,15,28,29] and in those unable to tolerate ACE inhibitors.[13]

***Beta blockers*** have negative inotropic properties and have generally been contra-indicated in patients with heart failure. However, persistent activation of the sympathetic nervous system is associated with disease progression and the benefit of beta blockers in the long-term management of heart failure is now established.[30-33] It is not clear whether all beta blockers are equally effective.[34] *Carvedilol*, *bisoprolol*, and *metoprolol* have shown positive effects on mortality and morbidity in patients with varying degrees of heart failure and are acceptable therapy, although a meta-analysis[35] in patients with mild to moderate heart failure has suggested that vasodilating beta blockers such as carvedilol have a greater effect on overall mortality than those that do not produce vasodilatation. A large study[36] comparing carvedilol with metoprolol also found a greater mortality reduction with carvedilol, although the equivalence of the doses used in the study has been questioned.[37] The role of beta blockers in severe heart failure is less established; a study with *bucindolol*[38] was stopped early because no mortality benefit was found, although carvedilol was found to reduce mortality in a similar study.[39] Beta blockers are now recommended[5,12-15] in all patients with clinically stable heart failure due to left ventricular systolic dysfunction and should be given in combination with ACE inhibitors and diuretics. However, they must be introduced cautiously since symptoms may initially worsen. Beta blockers also appear to be of value in heart failure due to idiopathic dilated cardiomyopathy (see Cardiomyopathies, p.818) and possibly in isolated diastolic dysfunction.

The effects of various ***vasodilators*** in heart failure have been studied in a series of Vasodilator-Heart Failure Trials (V-HeFT).[40] Oral nitrates, such as *isosorbide dinitrate*, produce a predominantly venous dilatation whereas *hydralazine* produces arterial vasodilatation, and they are thus used together. They alleviate peripheral vasoconstriction and produce symptomatic control, including a benefit on exercise tolerance, but are of somewhat limited efficacy in long-term control. A modest improvement in long-term survival has been noted but this effect is less than that seen with ACE inhibitors. Use of isosorbide dinitrate with hydralazine may be considered in patients with left ventricular dysfunction who are unable to tolerate ACE inhibitors; they may also be used as adjuncts in patients who remain symptomatic despite therapy with ACE inhibitors, diuretics, beta blockers, and digoxin.

***Angiotensin II receptor antagonists*** have been investigated both as alternatives to ACE inhibitors, and also in combination with ACE inhibitors to provide more complete blockade of the renin-angiotensin system. Although an early study[41] suggested that losartan improved mortality compared with enalapril, this was not confirmed in the larger ELITE II study,[42] although losartan was found to be better tolerated. Guidelines therefore continue to recommend ACE inhibitors as first-line therapy, although angiotensin II receptor antagonists may be used in those unable to tolerate ACE inhibitors; candesartan has been shown[43] to be of benefit in such patients. Studies using valsartan[44] or candesartan[45] with ACE inhibitors have suggested that there may be additional benefit, particularly in terms of hospitalisation for heart failure. The study with valsartan suggested that use with both ACE inhibitors and beta blockers might be detrimental, but this was not confirmed in the study with candesartan; however, the role of such therapy remains to be determined. In the ValHeFT study,[44] valsartan was added to standard therapy (including ACE inhibitors in most patients) and reduced the combined endpoint of death or hospitalisation for heart failure. However, the effect on mortality alone was not significant and in patients who were also receiving both ACE inhibitors and beta blockers mortality appeared to be increased.

Although the precise neurohormonal mechanisms leading to the development of heart failure are still not clear, there is evidence that raised levels of aldosterone may contribute to the pathophysiology.[46] ACE inhibitor therapy suppresses aldosterone production but this effect is not complete and the aldosterone antagonist ***spironolactone*** has been studied in combination with ACE inhibitors. In patients with severe heart failure, addition of low-dose spironolactone to therapy with ACE inhibitors and loop diuretics reduced the risk of death or hospitalisation,[47] and the use of spironolactone should therefore be considered in such patients.[5,12-15] However, the benefit in patients with less severe heart failure remains to be established, and all patients receiving spironolactone with ACE inhibitors must have their plasma-potassium concentrations closely monitored.

***Calcium-channel blockers***, like beta blockers, have generally been contra-indicated in heart failure because of their negative inotropic activity. Despite this, their use as adjuncts has been investigated but studies have failed to show any additional benefit in patients receiving standard therapy for heart failure. However, in both the PRAISE study[48] (using *amlodipine*) and the V-HeFT III study[49] (using *felodipine*), no adverse effect on morbidity or mortality was found. Amlodipine or felodipine might therefore be suitable as a treatment for angina or hypertension in patients with heart failure, although experience is limited with felodipine in severe heart failure.

***Phosphodiesterase inhibitors*** have a dual action being both positive inotropes and vasodilators. In theory, this is an attractive combination of mechanisms for use in heart failure but in general this group of drugs has not lived up to early expectations. Although short-term haemodynamic variables are improved, long-term oral use has been associated either with an unacceptable incidence of adverse effects (*amrinone*) or with an increased mortality rate (*enoximone*[50] and *milrinone*[51]). Thus, these phosphodiesterase inhibitors have been reserved for intravenous use in the short-term treatment of severe heart failure unresponsive to other treatment.[52-54] More recently introduced phosphodiesterase inhibitors include *vesnarinone*, and *pimobendan*, which also has calcium-sensitising properties. Initial studies with vesnarinone indicated a survival benefit but a larger trial[55] has shown an increased mortality in patients receiving vesnarinone. The place of these drugs in the management of heart failure remains unclear.

Although ***antiarrhythmics*** are not routinely recommended, those without a negative inotropic effect may have a role since sudden deaths have been attributed to ventricular arrhythmias in patients with severe heart failure. A meta-analysis[56] of 5 trials involving 1452 patients with symptomatic compensated heart failure indicated that *amiodarone* reduced the rate of arrhythmic or sudden death in high-risk patients and that this resulted in an overall reduction in mortality. However, amiodarone may have a number of adverse effects and it is not currently recommended in heart failure except in patients with symptomatic ventricular arrhythmias.

Several ***miscellaneous drugs***, such as *flosequinan* (an arterial and venous vasodilator), *epoprostenol* (a prostaglandin), and *xamoterol* (a partial $\beta_1$-adrenoceptor agonist) have been tried in heart failure but have proved either disappointing or have been associated with excessive toxicity or an increased mortality rate. The oral dopamine agonist *ibopamine* has also been used, but appears to increase mortality in patients with severe heart failure.[57] Other drugs that have been studied in heart failure include *candoxatril*, an endopeptidase inhibitor that acts by inhibiting the metabolism of atrial natriuretic peptide, and *endothelin antagonists* such as *bosentan*. *Omapatrilat*, a dual inhibitor of endopeptidase and angiotensin-converting enzyme, has shown some benefit,[58] but adverse effects may limit its use. *Tumour necrosis factor antagonists* such as *etanercept* and *infliximab* have been tried[59] since heart failure also appears to have an inflammatory component, but results have been disappointing and there have been reports[60] of exacerbation of heart failure in some patients. Although patients with heart failure are at increased risk of thromboembolism, the role of routine *antithrombotic* therapy remains unclear.[12,61]

Many patients with chronic heart failure experience exacerbations of their condition (decompensated heart failure) requiring hospitalisation.[62] Intravenous diuretics may be required for peripheral and pulmonary oedema. Intravenous nitrates and intravenous inotropes (such as dobutamine or milrinone) may be used to reduce filling pressures and increase cardiac output. Natriuretic peptides such as nesiritide, which has vasodilator properties, and levosimendan, a calcium-sensitiser with both vasodilator and inotropic actions, may also be used. Long-term intravenous inotropes may be required in some patients, but intermittent intravenous sympathomimetics may increase mortality and are not recommended.[14]

Some patients with refractory heart failure may be suitable for surgical management. Heart transplantation is the optimum surgical therapy but availability is limited and a number of methods for augmenting the heart muscle or reducing ventricular dilatation are being investigated.[63]


1. Krum H, Gilbert RE. Demographics and concomitant disorders in heart failure. *Lancet* 2003; **362:** 147–58.
2. Schrier RW, Abraham WT. Hormones and hemodynamics in heart failure. *N Engl J Med* 1999; **341:** 577–85.
3. Jackson G, *et al.* ABC of heart failure: pathophysiology. *BMJ* 2000; **320:** 167–70.
4. Terpening CM. Mediators of chronic heart failure: how drugs work. *Ann Pharmacother* 2001; **35:** 1066–74.
5. National Institute for Clinical Excellence. Chronic heart failure: management of chronic heart failure in adults in primary and secondary care (issued July 2003). Available at: http://www.nice.org.uk/pdf/CG5NICEguideline.pdf (accessed 13/05/04)
6. Cowie MR, Zaphiriou A. Management of chronic heart failure. *BMJ* 2002; **325:** 422–5.
7. Vasan RS. Diastolic heart failure. *BMJ* 2003; **327:** 1181–2.
8. Cleland JGF, *et al.* Successes and failures of current treatment of heart failure. *Lancet* 1998; **352** (suppl): 19–28.
9. Lonn E, McKelvie R. Drug treatment in heart failure. *BMJ* 2000; **320:** 1188–92. Correction. *ibid.*; **321:** 161.
10. Jessup M, Brozena S. Heart failure. *N Engl J Med* 2003; **348:** 2007–18.
11. DiBianco R. Update on therapy for heart failure. *Am J Med* 2003; **115:** 480–8.
12. Packer M, Cohn JN, eds. Consensus recommendations for the management of chronic heart failure. *Am J Cardiol* 1999; **83** (suppl 2A): 1A–38A.
13. Scottish Intercollegiate Guidelines Network. Diagnosis and treatment of heart failure due to left ventricular systolic dysfunction (February 1999). Available at: http://www.show.scot.nhs.uk/sign/pdf/sign35.pdf (accessed 13/05/04)
14. Hunt SA, *et al.* ACC/AHA guidelines for the evaluation and management of chronic heart failure in the adult: a report of the American College of Cardiology/American Heart Association Task Force on Practice Guidelines (Committee to Revise the 1995 Guidelines for the Evaluation and Management of Heart Failure). Executive Summary: *J Am Coll Cardiol* 2001; **38:** 2101–13. Full version: http://www.acc.org/clinical/guidelines/failure/hf_index.htm (accessed 13/05/04)
15. Task Force for the Diagnosis and Treatment of Chronic Heart Failure, European Society of Cardiology. Guidelines for the diagnosis and treatment of chronic heart failure. *Eur Heart J* 2001; **22:** 1527–60. Correction. *ibid.*; 2217–18. Also available at: http://www.escardio.org/NR/rdonlyres/83B0E854-D56A-47C1-988F-585F4EBFEAF8/0/CHF_diagnosis.pdf (accessed 12/05/04)
16. Piña IL, *et al.* Exercise and heart failure: a statement from the American Heart Association Committee on exercise, rehabilitation, and prevention. *Circulation* 2003; **107:** 1210–25. Also available at: http://www.circ.ahajournals.org/cgi/reprint/107/8/1210.pdf (accessed 21/05/04)
17. Ellison DH. The physiologic basis of diuretic synergism: its role in treating diuretic resistance. *Ann Intern Med* 1991; **114:** 886–94.
18. Krämer BK, *et al.* Diuretic treatment and diuretic resistance in heart failure. *Am J Med* 1999; **106:** 90–6.
19. Faris R, *et al.* Current evidence supporting the role of diuretics in heart failure: a meta analysis of randomised controlled trials. *Int J Cardiol* 2002; **82:** 149–58.
20. Garg R, Yusuf S. Overview of randomized trials of angiotensin-converting enzyme inhibitors on mortality and morbidity in patients with heart failure. *JAMA* 1995; **273:** 1450–6.
21. Nelson KM, Yeager BF. What is the role of angiotensin-converting enzyme inhibitors in congestive heart failure and after myocardial infarction? *Ann Pharmacother* 1996; **30:** 986–93.
22. The SOLVD Investigators. Effects of enalapril on mortality and the development of heart failure in asymptomatic patients with reduced left ventricular ejection fractions. *N Engl J Med* 1992; **327:** 685–91.
23. Eccles M, *et al.* North of England evidence based development project; guideline for angiotensin converting enzyme inhibitors in primary care management of adults with symptomatic heart failure. *BMJ* 1998; **316:** 1369–75.
24. Campbell RWF. ACE inhibitors and arrhythmias. *Heart* 1996; **76** (suppl 3): 79–82.
25. Uretsky NF, *et al.* Randomized study assessing the effect of digoxin withdrawal in patients with mild to moderate chronic congestive heart failure: results of the PROVED trial. *J Am Coll Cardiol* 1993; **22:** 955–62.
26. Packer M, *et al.* Withdrawal of digoxin from patients with chronic heart failure treated with angiotensin-converting-enzyme inhibitors. *N Engl J Med* 1993; **329:** 1–7.
27. The Digitalis Investigation Group. The effect of digoxin on mortality and morbidity in patients with heart failure. *N Engl J Med* 1997; **336:** 525–33.
28. Packer M. End of the oldest controversy in medicine: are we ready to conclude the debate on digitalis? *N Engl J Med* 1997; **336:** 575–6.
29. Riaz K, Forker AD. Digoxin use in congestive heart failure: current status. *Drugs* 1998; **55:** 747–58.
30. Abraham WT. β-Blockers: the new standard of therapy for mild heart failure. *Arch Intern Med* 2000; **160:** 1237–47.
31. Hart SM. Influence of β-blockers on mortality in chronic heart failure. *Ann Pharmacother* 2000; **34:** 1440–51.
32. Pritchett AM, Redfield MM. β-Blockers: new standard therapy for heart failure. *Mayo Clin Proc* 2002; **77:** 839–46.
33. Goldstein S. Benefits of β-blocker therapy for heart failure: weighing the evidence. *Arch Intern Med* 2002; **162:** 641–8.
34. Kukin ML. β-Blockers in chronic heart failure: considerations for selecting an agent. *Mayo Clin Proc* 2002; **77:** 1199–1206.
35. Bonet S, *et al.* β-Adrenergic blocking agents in heart failure: benefits of vasodilating and nonvasodilating agents according to patients' characteristics: a meta-analysis of clinical trials. *Arch Intern Med* 2000; **160:** 621–7.
36. Poole-Wilson PA, *et al.* Comparison of carvedilol and metoprolol on clinical outcomes in patients with chronic heart failure in the Carvedilol Or Metoprolol European Trial (COMET): randomised controlled trial. *Lancet* 2003; **362:** 7–13.
37. Dargie HJ. β-Blockers in heart failure. *Lancet* 2003; **362:** 2–3.
38. The Beta-Blocker Evaluation of Survival Trial Investigators. A trial of the beta-blocker bucindolol in patients with advanced chronic heart failure. *N Engl J Med* 2001; **344:** 1659–67.
39. Packer M, *et al.* Effect of carvedilol on survival in severe chronic heart failure. *N Engl J Med* 2001; **344:** 1651–8.
40. Cohn JN. Vasodilators in heart failure: conclusions from V-HeFT II and rationale for V-HeFT III. *Drugs* 1994; **47** (suppl 4): 47–58.
41. Pitt B, *et al.* Randomised trial of losartan versus captopril in patients over 65 with heart failure (Evaluation of Losartan in the Elderly Study, ELITE). *Lancet* 1997; **349:** 747–52.
42. Pitt B, *et al.* Effect of losartan compared with captopril on mortality in patients with symptomatic heart failure: randomised trial—the Losartan Heart Failure Survival Study ELITE II. *Lancet* 2000; **355:** 1582–7.
43. Granger CB, *et al.* Effects of candesartan in patients with chronic heart failure and reduced left-ventricular systolic function intolerant to angiotensin-converting-enzyme inhibitors: the CHARM-Alternative trial. *Lancet* 2003; **362:** 772–6.
44. Cohn JN, Tognoni G. A randomized trial of the angiotensin-receptor blocker valsartan in chronic heart failure. *N Engl J Med* 2001; **345:** 1667–75.
45. McMurray JJV, *et al.* Effects of candesartan in patients with chronic heart failure and reduced left-ventricular systolic function taking angiotensin-converting-enzyme inhibitors: the CHARM-Added trial. *Lancet* 2003; **362:** 767–71.
46. Struthers AD. Why does spironolactone improve mortality over and above an ACE inhibitor in chronic heart failure? *Br J Clin Pharmacol* 1999; **47:** 479–82.
47. Pitt B, *et al.* The effect of spironolactone on morbidity and mortality in patients with severe heart failure. *N Engl J Med* 1999; **341:** 709–17.
48. Packer M, *et al.* Effect of amlodipine on morbidity and mortality in severe chronic heart failure. *N Engl J Med* 1996; **335:** 1107–14.
49. Cohn JN, *et al.* Effect of the calcium antagonist felodipine as supplementary vasodilator therapy in patients with chronic heart failure treated with enalapril. V-HeFT III. *Circulation* 1997; **96:** 856–63.
50. Uretsky BF, *et al.* Multicenter trial of oral enoximone in patients with moderate to moderately severe congestive heart failure: lack of benefit compared with placebo. *Circulation* 1990; **82:** 774–80.
51. Packer M, *et al.* Effect of oral milrinone on mortality in severe chronic heart failure. *N Engl J Med* 1991; **325:** 1468–75.
52. Fischer TA, *et al.* Current status of phosphodiesterase inhibitors in the treatment of congestive heart failure. *Drugs* 1992; **44:** 928–45.
53. Packer M. The search for the ideal positive inotropic agent. *N Engl J Med* 1993; **329:** 210–2.
54. Nony P, *et al.* Evaluation of the effect of phosphodiesterase inhibitors on mortality in chronic heart failure patients: a meta-analysis. *Eur J Clin Pharmacol* 1994; **46:** 191–6.
55. Cohn JN, *et al.* A dose-dependent increase in mortality with vesnarinone among patients with severe heart failure. *N Engl J Med* 1998; **339:** 1810–16.
56. Amiodarone Trials Meta-Analysis Investigators. Effect of prophylactic amiodarone on mortality after acute myocardial infarction and in congestive heart failure: meta-analysis of individual data from 6500 patients in randomised trials. *Lancet* 1997; **350:** 1417–24.
57. Hampton JR, *et al.* Randomised study of effect of ibopamine on survival in patients with advanced severe heart failure. *Lancet* 1997; **349:** 971–7.
58. Packer M, *et al.* Comparison of omapatrilat and enalapril in patients with chronic heart failure: the Omapatrilat Versus Enalapril Randomized Trial of Utility in Reducing Events (OVERTURE). *Circulation* 2002; **106:** 920–6.
59. Henriksen PA, Newby DE. Therapeutic inhibition of tumour necrosis factor α in patients with heart failure: cooling an inflamed heart. *Heart* 2003; **89:** 14–8.
60. Kwon HJ, *et al.* Case reports of heart failure after therapy with a tumor necrosis factor antagonist. *Ann Intern Med* 2003; **138:** 807–11.
61. De Lorenzo F, *et al.* Blood coagulation in patients with chronic heart failure: evidence for hypercoagulable state and potential for pharmacological intervention. *Drugs* 2003; **63:** 565–76.
62. Nohria A, *et al.* Medical management of advanced heart failure. *JAMA* 2002; **287:** 628–40.
63. Taggart DP, Westaby S. Surgical management of heart failure. *BMJ* 1997; **314:** 453–4.


## High-altitude disorders

Rapid ascent (ascent without time to acclimatise) to high altitudes may produce a spectrum of illness (altitude illness) ranging from the usually benign acute mountain sickness to life-threatening pulmonary oedema and cerebral oedema. Factors influencing the development of altitude illness include rate of ascent, altitude attained, sleeping altitude, and length of stay at altitude. Individual susceptibility is also an important factor. Symptoms of altitude sickness commonly occur at altitudes above 2500 metres (8125 feet), although susceptible individuals may be affected at altitudes as low as 2000 metres (6500 feet).[1,2] Reported incidences at higher altitudes vary, but in general symptoms occur in about 50% of people ascending rapidly to altitudes of over 4000 metres (13 000 feet) and in about 75% of people at 4500 metres (14 625 feet); they are severe (pulmonary oedema or cerebral oedema) in about 4%.

**Symptoms** of **acute mountain sickness** include headache, which is worse in the supine position, nausea, vomiting, anorexia, lethargy, insomnia, and dizziness. These may develop during ascent, but characteristically occur 6 to 48 hours after arrival at altitude. They are usually short-lived and resolve after a few days at altitude. In a very few people symptoms persist for longer. Chronic mountain sickness, characterised by persistent severe hypoxia and polycythaemia, may develop during prolonged residence at high altitude. The discussion that follows is limited to management of the acute forms. A small proportion of people with acute mountain sickness suddenly deteriorate and develop pulmonary oedema or cerebral oedema, both of which may be life-threatening. Occasionally, pulmonary or cerebral oedema develops without symptoms of acute mountain sickness. Symptoms of **pulmonary oedema** include rapid onset of breathlessness and tachypnoea at rest, and a dry cough which may develop into haemoptysis. Symptoms of **cerebral oedema** include increasing headache, ataxia, mental disturbances, drowsiness and eventually coma. Pulmonary and cerebral oedema frequently occur together.

The **pathogenesis** of altitude illness is not fully understood, and it is not known whether the mechanisms of acute mountain sickness and pulmonary or cerebral oedema differ in nature or merely degree. Hypoxia, a result of the reduced partial pressure of oxygen at high altitudes, is considered the primary stimulus in the development of altitude illness.[1-3] When ascent to high altitudes occurs gradually, the bicarbonate concentration and the pH of extracellular fluid fall progressively. The falling pH increases the sensitivity of chemoreceptors to hypoxia and so permits greater ventilation, thus allowing acclimatisation. Rapid ascent to high altitudes does not allow time for these changes to occur and although the hypoxia stimulates hyperventilation, it produces a respiratory alkalosis which limits the ventilatory response to hypoxia. The hypoxaemia produced leads to neurohumoral and haemodynamic changes that ultimately result in the symptoms of altitude illness.[1] Symptoms are often worse at night when ventilation is reduced leading to a worsening of the hypoxaemia.

**Prophylaxis.** Altitude illness may be avoided by ascending to high altitudes slowly and thereby allowing time for acclimatisation. This may be achieved by spending several days at 1500 to 3000 metres and avoiding strenuous physical activity, thus allowing the body to adapt to the reduced oxygen pressure and to ascend above 3000 metres without sickness. Acclimatisation may also be achieved when going above 3000 metres by increasing the sleeping altitude by no more than 300 to 600 metres a day and by adding a rest day for every 1000 metres climbed;[1-3] slower rates of ascent than this have also been advised.

However, when time for acclimatisation is limited or when abrupt arrival at high altitude (for instance by air) cannot be avoided, drug prophylaxis may be considered. Prophylaxis should also be considered for those individuals who have developed symptoms on ascending to high altitudes on previous occasions.

*Acetazolamide* is the most frequently used drug[1-3] and has been shown[4] to effectively reduce the frequency of symptoms, although the optimum dose is not clear. It produces a mild metabolic acidosis which has the effect of stimulating chemoreceptors to produce an increase in the rate of respiration and tidal volume, and it therefore accelerates the process of acclimatisation. Although acetazolamide has diuretic actions it does not prevent fluid retention or prevent or protect against pulmonary or cerebral oedema. It improves sleep hypoxaemia and quality of sleep, reduces proteinuria, improves exercise performance, and reduces loss of muscle mass, probably by improving oxygen supply to the tissues.[5] Acetazolamide should be taken on the day of ascent or 1 or 2 days before ascent to altitudes above 3000 metres, and continued for several days at the higher altitudes.[1,3] However, there has been concern that the use of acetazolamide to prevent symptoms of acute mountain sickness may encourage too rapid an ascent and perhaps increase the risk of developing pulmonary or cerebral oedema.[5]

*Dexamethasone* has also been shown[4] to be effective in the prevention of acute mountain sickness. The rationale for its use is that mild cerebral oedema is thought to contribute to the symptoms of acute mountain sickness. However, as the side-effects associated with dexamethasone are more severe than those associated with acetazolamide, it is not considered suitable for routine prophylaxis; it may have a role if acetazolamide is unavailable or contra-indicated.[1-3] If it is used, dexamethasone should be started a few hours before ascent;[3] adverse effects may be fewer if the dose is tapered before stopping.[4]

*Nifedipine* has been shown to lower pulmonary artery pressure and to protect against pulmonary oedema in people susceptible to the development of pulmonary symptoms at altitude[6] but is not usually recommended for prophylaxis due to the risk of adverse effects.

Other drugs that have shown some benefit in small studies include *spironolactone*[4] and *ginkgo biloba*.[1,4] A study[7] with inhaled *salmeterol* suggested that it reduced the risk of pulmonary oedema in people considered to be at high risk. *Aspirin* was reported[8] to reduce the incidence of headache in a small study in people with a history of headache at high altitude.

**Treatment**. Once symptoms of altitude illness develop the course of action should be determined by the severity and nature of the symptoms.

When symptoms are *mild* and are not suggestive of pulmonary or cerebral oedema, rest and mild analgesics for headache are usually all that is required; symptoms resolve within a few days and further ascent is possible.[1-3] *Acetazolamide* may have some benefit in relieving symptoms[1,2,9] although studies have been small. If mild symptoms of pulmonary oedema are present, such as dyspnoea and cough, rest with supplementary oxygen and further oxygen at night may resolve the symptoms and allow further ascent; however signs and symptoms at altitude may be confusing and it is always safest to descend. The use of hypnotics at altitude is not generally advised since there is a risk that respiratory depression may further reduce oxygen saturation. However, a small study[10] using the short-acting benzodiazepine *temazepam* reported that sleep quality was improved without an alteration in mean oxygen saturation.

When symptoms are *moderate to severe*, and are progressing or suggestive of cerebral oedema, immediate descent is necessary.[1-3] Descending by as little as 400 to 500 metres is beneficial. Various drugs and therapies have been given to alleviate symptoms and to facilitate descent and should also be used when immediate descent is not possible. For example, *dexamethasone* can reduce the symptoms of acute mountain sickness and might be used in emergencies.[11,12] Portable hyperbaric chambers are available[13] and provide rapid but short-term improvement. They may be useful in combination with dexamethasone, which has a more sustained effect.[14]

If pulmonary oedema is present, oxygen, which relieves hypoxia and reduces pulmonary hypertension, should be given;[1-3] *nifedipine*, which suppresses the exaggerated hypoxic pulmonary vasoconstrictor response seen in people with pulmonary oedema, has provided benefit.[15] Positive-pressure expiration may also be useful;[2] it has the effect of increasing oxygen saturation and partial pressure of carbon dioxide at altitude. Inhalation of nitric oxide has also been reported to improve oxygenation but administration may not be feasible at altitude.[16]

People with cerebral oedema should be given *dexamethasone* and oxygen therapy.


1. Hackett PH, Roach RC. High-altitude illness. *N Engl J Med* 2001; **345:** 107–14.
2. Basnyat B, Murdoch DR. High-altitude illness. *Lancet* 2003; **361:** 1967–74.
3. Barry PW, Pollard AJ. Altitude illness. *BMJ* 2003; **326:** 915–9.
4. Dumont L, *et al.* Efficacy and harm of pharmacological prevention of acute mountain sickness: quantitative systematic review. *BMJ* 2000; **321:** 267–72.
5. Dickinson JG. Acetazolamide in acute mountain sickness. *BMJ* 1987; **295:** 1161–2.
6. Bärtsch P, *et al.* Prevention of high-altitude pulmonary edema by nifedipine. *N Engl J Med* 1991; **325:** 1284–9.
7. Sartori C, *et al.* Salmeterol for the prevention of high-altitude pulmonary edema. *N Engl J Med* 2002; **346:** 1631–6.
8. Burtscher M, *et al.* Aspirin for prophylaxis against headache at high altitudes: randomised, double blind, placebo controlled trial. *BMJ* 1998; **316:** 1057–8.
9. Grissom CK, *et al.* Acetazolamide in the treatment of acute mountain sickness: clinical efficacy and effect on gas exchange. *Ann Intern Med* 1992; **116:** 461–5.
10. Dubowitz G. Effect of temazepam on oxygen saturation and sleep quality at high altitude: randomised placebo controlled crossover trial. *BMJ* 1998; **316:** 587–9.
11. Ferrazzini G, *et al.* Successful treatment of acute mountain sickness with dexamethasone. *BMJ* 1987; **294:** 1380–2.
12. Levine BD, *et al.* Dexamethasone in the treatment of acute mountain sickness. *N Engl J Med* 1989; **321:** 1707–13.
13. Bärtsch P, *et al.* Treatment of acute mountain sickness by simulated descent: a randomised controlled trial. *BMJ* 1993; **306:** 1098–1101.
14. Keller H-R, *et al.* Simulated descent v dexamethasone in treatment of acute mountain sickness: a randomised trial. *BMJ* 1995; **310:** 1232–5.
15. Oelz O, *et al.* Nifedipine for high altitude pulmonary oedema. *Lancet* 1989; **2:** 1241–4. Correction. *ibid.* 1991; **337:** 556.
16. Scherrer U, *et al.* Inhaled nitric oxide for high-altitude pulmonary edema. *N Engl J Med* 1996; **334:** 624–9.


## Hyperlipidaemias

Hyperlipidaemia results from a disorder in the synthesis and degradation of plasma lipoproteins. Although the main concern has generally been the overall elevation of plasma lipids (hyperlipidaemia), it is now increasingly recognised that the balance of lipids in the plasma is also important, and the term dyslipidaemia is often used. Dyslipidaemias have genetic and other causes, and are often associated with a high-fat diet. Although patients with hyperlipidaemia may have symptoms that require treatment, the major concern is their increased risk of ischaemic heart disease.

The **lipids** that are of relevance in hyperlipidaemias are cholesterol, an essential component of cell membranes and a precursor of steroid hormone synthesis, and triglyceride, an important energy source. They are transported in the blood as lipoproteins.

**Lipoproteins** are complex particles[1,2] comprising a hydrophilic coat of phospholipids, free cholesterol, and specific polypeptides termed apolipoproteins (apoproteins) around a core of varying proportions of triglyceride and of cholesterol which is present as cholesteryl ester. The lipoproteins are characterised by their density, which in general increases as they are metabolised and the proportion of cholesteryl ester to triglyceride increases. Table 1, below, lists the principal lipoproteins and their associated lipids. The lowest density lipoproteins are the **chylomicrons** which transport triglyceride derived from dietary fat, and the **VLDL** (very low-density lipoproteins; pre-β lipoproteins) which transport endogenous triglyceride mainly synthesised in the liver, to peripheral tissues. The triglyceride is hydrolysed in the peripheral tissues by lipoprotein lipase, which is activated by apolipoprotein CII present in the lipoproteins. Both chylomicrons and VLDL are progressively depleted of triglyceride, yielding increasingly dense lipoprotein particles termed 'remnant' particles. Chylomicron remnants are cleared rapidly from plasma by the liver where they are metabolised, releasing free cholesterol. VLDL remnants, which include **IDL** (intermediate-density lipoproteins; broad β-lipoproteins), may also be cleared by the liver or converted to **LDL** (low-density lipoprotein; β-lipoprotein). **HDL** (high-density lipoproteins; α-lipoproteins) are synthesised in the liver and small intestine and have a role in the transport of cholesterol from the peripheral tissues back to the liver, where it is either utilised or excreted in the bile as bile acids and unesterified cholesterol. The majority is reabsorbed from the intestines and a small proportion is excreted in the faeces.

Defining hyperlipidaemia is difficult due to the marked variation in lipid concentrations between different populations. Apparently 'normal' lipid concentrations may still be associated with a significant risk of cardiovascular disease, and this may depend on which lipids are affected. Epidemiological data show a progressive and continuous relationship between plasma-cholesterol concentrations and mortality from ischaemic heart disease. The Framingham Study[3] found a 9% increase in death from cardiovascular disease for each 10 mg/dL (0.26 mmol/litre) rise in total plasma-cholesterol concentration. Plasma-cholesterol concentrations of 5.2 mmol/litre (200 mg/dL) or less are associated with a low risk of ischaemic heart disease. The increased risk is due mainly to raised LDL-cholesterol. In contrast, HDL-cholesterol is inversely associated with ischaemic heart disease. Low plasma concentrations of HDL-cholesterol (below 1 mmol/litre or 40 mg/dL) are generally associated with increased risk of ischaemic heart disease, whereas high concentrations are protective.[4] There also appears to be an association between plasma-triglyceride concentrations and risk of ischaemic heart disease. Some triglyceride-rich lipoproteins such as chylomicron remnant particles and IDL are atherogenic and the risk of heart disease increases as triglyceride concentrations increase in patients who also have high total cholesterol and low HDL-cholesterol concentrations. Hypertriglyceridaemia alone (greater than 2.3 mmol/litre or 200 mg/dL) may be an independent risk factor for ischaemic heart disease, but any clinical benefit from intervention to lower triglyceride levels is yet to be established.[5] Current US guidelines[2,6] suggest an LDL-cholesterol concentration of below 100 mg/dL as optimal, and a total cholesterol concentration of below 200 mg/dL as desirable, although evidence from more recent studies suggests that even lower concentrations may be beneficial.[16] However, the absolute risk for any individual also depends on other cardiovascular risk factors, including smoking and hypertension, and treatment decisions should in general be based on assessment of overall risk (see Cardiovascular Risk Reduction, p.819).

Hyperlipidaemias may result from a number of underlying defects and various methods have been used for classification.[7] A simple system is to divide them on the basis of whether raised serum cholesterol (hypercholesterolaemia), triglyceride (hypertriglyceridaemia), or both (mixed or combined hyperlipidaemia) is the predominant abnormality. Alternatively, the Frederickson/WHO method (see Table 2, below) describes them in terms of the lipoprotein abnormality (hyperlipoproteinaemia), although this is less useful clinically. Within these systems, primary hyperlipidaemias are those with an underlying genetic defect, whereas secondary hyperlipidaemias are caused by another disease state or by drug therapy. Primary and secondary causes of hyperlipidaemia may co-exist.

**Primary hyperlipidaemias** (see Table 3, p.824) may be monogenic, relating to a single genetic defect, but much more commonly they are due to the interaction of a number of genes with dietary and other factors (polygenic). Individuals with common, polygenic (multifactorial) hypercholesterolaemia tend to have only mild or moderate elevations of plasma-cholesterol, whereas those with monogenic hyperlipidaemias tend to have much higher plasma-lipid concentrations.

**Secondary hyperlipidaemias** may have various causes. Diseases producing hypertriglyceridaemia include diabetes mellitus, chronic renal failure, and bulimia. Hypercholesterolaemia can occur in hypothyroidism, nephrotic syndrome, biliary obstruction, and anorexia nervosa. Drugs that may produce hypertriglyceridaemia and/or hypercholesterolaemia include thiazide diuretics (in high doses), beta blockers, corticosteroids, and antivirals in patients with HIV infection. Excessive alcohol intake may produce elevated plasma-triglyceride concentrations.

The degree of hyperlipidaemia seen in patients with either primary or secondary hyperlipidaemia is influenced by various factors, including, importantly, diet. A diet rich in saturated fat and cholesterol and poor in fibre can produce hypercholesterolaemia. Obesity further predisposes to hyperlipidaemia. Other factors that may influence lipid concentrations include pregnancy, lack of exercise, and smok-

**Table 1.** Principal lipoproteins and associated lipids.

| Lipoprotein | Lipid |
|---|---|
| Chylomicron | Triglyceride |
| VLDL | Triglyceride |
| IDL | Cholesterol and triglyceride |
| LDL | Cholesterol |
| HDL | Cholesterol |

**Table 2.** Classification of hyperlipoproteinaemias.

| | | Plasma lipids affected | |
|---|---|---|---|
| WHO classification | Lipoproteins elevated | Cholesterol | Triglyceride |
| I | Chylomicrons | Normal or elevated | Elevated |
| IIa | LDL | Elevated | Normal |
| IIb | LDL and VLDL | Elevated | Elevated |
| III | VLDL with abnormally high cholesterol content | Elevated | Elevated |
| IV | VLDL | Normal or elevated | Elevated |
| V | Chylomicrons and VLDL | Elevated | Elevated |

**Table 3.** Primary hyperlipidaemias.

| | Lipoprotein Abnormality (WHO type) | Prevalence | Typical lipid concentrations (mmol/L) Cholesterol | Triglyceride | Risk of IHD | Pancreatitis |
|---|---|---|---|---|---|---|
| Common (polygenic) hypercholesterolaemia | IIa or IIb | Very common | 6.5 to 9.0 | < 2.3 | + | – |
| Familial hypercholesterolaemia | IIa or IIb | Moderately common | 7.5 to 16.0 | < 2.3 | +++ | – |
| Familial hypertriglyceridaemia | IV or V | Common | 6.5 to 12.0 | 10 to 30 | ? | ++ |
| Familial combined hyperlipidaemia | IIa, IIb, IV, or V | Common | 6.5 to 10.0 | 2.3 to 12.0 | ++ | – |
| Familial dysbetalipoproteinaemia or remnant hyperlipoproteinaemia | III | Uncommon | 9.0 to 14.0 | 9.0 to 14.0 | ++ | + |
| Abnormal lipoprotein lipase function | I | Rare | < 6.5 | 10.0 to 30.0 | – | +++ |

+ = elevated risk; – = no risk; ? = uncertain risk; IHD = ischaemic heart disease

ing. After myocardial infarction cholesterol levels may be temporarily reduced for several weeks; therefore, to measure the patient's usual level of cholesterol, blood samples should be taken within a few hours of the infarction.

The majority of people with hyperlipidaemia have plasma-lipid concentrations that are only mildly or moderately elevated, and they exhibit no **clinical symptoms**. At the other end of the spectrum, severe hypercholesterolaemia can cause tendon, tuberous, or planar xanthomas, xanthelasma, and arcus corneae; it is also associated with an increased risk of ischaemic stroke. Severe hypertriglyceridaemia can cause acute severe abdominal pain due to pancreatitis; hepatic and splenic enlargement, eruptive xanthomas, and lipaemia retinalis may also occur. However, the main concern in patients with hyperlipidaemias is the increased risk of ischaemic heart disease. In patients with very severe hypercholesterolaemia, such as familial hypercholesterolaemia, this may occur at a very young age; in those with the heterozygous form onset of heart disease during their 20s or 30s is not unusual, and in the rarer homozygous form ischaemic heart disease may develop by the age of 10.

**Treatment of hyperlipidaemias.** In patients with clinical symptoms, treatment is indicated to promote the regression or non-progression of disfiguring xanthomas, or to prevent attacks of acute pancreatitis in those with severe hypertriglyceridaemia. The main aim of treatment, however, particularly in patients with only mildly elevated lipids, is to reduce the risk of ischaemic heart disease.

Since the relationship between plasma-cholesterol concentrations and ischaemic heart disease is continuous, the level at which treatment with lipid regulating drugs should be started has been widely debated. Guidelines recommend that the decision to treat should be based on the overall risk profile of the patient and that other risk factors should also be treated (see Cardiovascular Risk Reduction, p.819). Specifically, British guidelines[8] advise that, in patients with cardiovascular disease or high cardiovascular risk, drug therapy should be added to dietary therapy if total plasma cholesterol remains above 5 mmol/litre and LDL-cholesterol above 3 mmol/litre despite dietary therapy. More recent European guidelines[9] suggest a target of total plasma cholesterol below 4.5 mmol/litre and LDL-cholesterol below 2.5 mmol/litre in patients with diabetes mellitus or established cardiovascular disease; patients with total cholesterol above 8 mmol/litre or LDL-cholesterol above 6 mmol/litre require treatment irrespective of their other risk factors. US guidelines[2,6] suggest that drug treatment should be considered if the LDL-cholesterol level is 190 mg/dL or higher. For patients with 2 or more risk factors, drug therapy should be considered if the LDL-cholesterol is 160 mg/dL or higher, and for those with existing cardiovascular disease, diabetes mellitus, or particularly high risk, drug therapy should be considered if LDL-cholesterol is 130 mg/dL or higher. The US guidelines also give target LDL-cholesterol levels of less than 160 mg/dL, less than 130 mg/dL, and less than 100 mg/dL, respectively, for the three risk groups. However, based on evidence from more recent studies, it has been suggested[16] that treatment may be appropriate in some very high risk patients at LDL-cholesterol concentrations below 100 mg/dL and that a goal of below 70 mg/dL may be reasonable. Although low HDL-cholesterol is an additional risk factor, the benefits of raising HDL-cholesterol are not established and no target is therefore specified in the current guidelines.

The main methods of treating hyperlipidaemias are dietary and lifestyle changes and the use of lipid regulating drugs.[2,6,8,9] Some surgical and other procedures may also be used in familial hypercholesterolaemia (see below).

**Dietary therapy** should be initiated in all patients with hyperlipidaemia and is based on weight reduction in the obese and a reduction in total fat intake. UK dietary recommendations[10] include a reduction in saturated fatty acids, restriction of *trans* fatty acids, and increased consumption of long-chain n-3 polyunsaturated fatty acids; the intake of cholesterol and n-6 polyunsaturated fatty acids should also be restricted. Similar recommendations have been made in the US.[6] Increased physical exercise is also recommended. Moderation of alcohol intake is advised, particularly in patients with hypertriglyceridaemia, in whom alcohol may precipitate pancreatitis. However, more rigorous diet than that often recommended may be necessary for diet alone to be of much value,[11] and most patients will require drug therapy to achieve target lipid concentrations. Patients at low cardiovascular risk should have a trial of dietary therapy before drugs are started, but in those with established cardiovascular disease or major risk factors drug therapy and dietary changes may be started at the same time.

The principal groups of **lipid regulating drugs** (hypolipidaemic drugs) are the statins, fibric acid derivatives and related compounds, bile-acid binding resins, nicotinic acid and its derivatives, and the omega-3 marine triglycerides.[1,12,13] *Statins* (HMG-CoA reductase inhibitors) reduce cholesterol by stimulating an increase in LDL-receptors on hepatocyte membranes, thereby increasing the clearance of LDL from the circulation. Their main effect is to reduce LDL-cholesterol, but they may also reduce triglycerides to a modest extent and increase HDL-cholesterol. They are generally considered to be the most effective lipid lowering drugs. *Fibrates* inhibit the synthesis of cholesterol and bile acids, and enhance the secretion of cholesterol in bile. Their main effect is to reduce triglycerides by reducing the concentration of VLDL; they also increase HDL-cholesterol and have variable effects on LDL-cholesterol. They are used mainly in patients with hypertriglyceridaemia. *Bile-acid binding resins* lower cholesterol by combining with bile acids in the gastrointestinal tract and preventing their reabsorption. This leads to an increased oxidation of cholesterol to replace the lost bile acids, and an increase in LDL-receptor synthesis on hepatocytes, resulting primarily in a reduction of LDL-cholesterol. *Nicotinic acid* inhibits production of VLDL in the liver; it lowers LDL-cholesterol and triglycerides and increases HDL-cholesterol, but adverse effects may limit its use. *Omega-3 triglycerides* primarily reduce triglycerides. *Other drugs* that may be used include cholesterol absorption inhibitors[14] such as ezetimibe; dietary supplements containing soluble fibre, such as guar gum or ispaghula, or plant stanols or sterols, may also be used to reduce cholesterol absorption. In postmenopausal women, oestrogen therapy reduces lipid concentrations, but the adverse effects may outweigh any benefit (see Effects on the Cardiovascular System, p.1538); soya protein may have a similar effect. Garlic supplements have also been promoted for hyperlipidaemia, although their effect appears to be modest.

Choice of therapy ideally depends upon the lipid profile of the individual patient since the drug groups differ in their effects on the different lipid components. In practice, most patients have common, polygenic hypercholesterolaemia, and can be treated effectively with statins as first-line therapy. Bile-acid binding resins or nicotinic acid may be alternatives, but are generally less well tolerated. Combination therapy may be required in some patients to reach target lipid concentrations, but the risk of adverse effects is increased in patients receiving statins and fibrates together (see Effects on Skeletal Muscle under Adverse Effects of Simvastatin, p.997). In patients with hypertriglyceridaemia, statins or fibrates may be used; resins should not be used alone since they may increase triglyceride concentrations.

Patients with the less common familial dyslipidaemias generally have higher lipid concentrations and require more intensive therapy. Specific treatment strategies are as follows:

- FAMILIAL HYPERCHOLESTEROLAEMIA. Patients with familial hypercholesterolaemia usually have very high plasma-cholesterol concentrations, which rarely respond adequately to diet alone and drug therapy is therefore often necessary in this high-risk group. Aggressive therapy may lead to regression of atherosclerotic lesions.[15] The first-line drugs are the statins. In severe cases combination therapy is usually required, such as a statin with a bile-acid binding resin. A low dose of the bile-acid binding resin may be sufficient. In the homozygous form of familial hypercholesterolaemia there may be a complete lack of functional LDL-receptors and drugs that act by increasing LDL-receptors, such as statins and bile-acid binding resins, may be ineffective. However, statins may be useful as adjunctive therapy in those patients who have some LDL-receptor function. In some forms of familial hypercholesterolaemia, and where plasma-cholesterol concentrations are very high, plasma-triglyceride concentrations may also be raised. In these cases a fibric acid derivative or nicotinic acid may be effective, and in more severe cases the combination of a bile-acid binding resin together with a fibric acid derivative or a statin may be used. In patients with the homozygous form liver transplantation is the most definitive treatment. Plasma exchange (weekly or fortnightly) or more selective procedures such as LDL apheresis, including the use of heparin to precipitate LDL (the HELP system—Heparin Extracorporeal LDL Precipitation) may also be used in combination with lipid regulating drugs. Gene therapy is under investigation as a treatment for familial hypercholesterolaemia.
- FAMILIAL HYPERTRIGLYCERIDAEMIA. In patients with familial hypertriglyceridaemia dietary therapy is generally adequate, but drugs may be required if there is a high risk of acute pancreatitis or if there is a family history of atherosclerosis. The risk of acute pancreatitis is high when plasma-triglyceride concentrations are above 20 mmol/litre. Nicotinic acid or the fibric acid derivatives, particularly gemfibrozil, are generally recommended and may be used in combination in severe cases. Omega-3 marine triglycerides may also be of value. In severe intractable hypertriglyceridaemia, particularly type V hyperlipoproteinaemia, norethisterone has been suggested for women or oxandrolone for men.
- FAMILIAL COMBINED HYPERLIPIDAEMIA. Drug therapy may be used in patients who do not respond to dietary therapy alone. The choice will depend on the predominant lipid abnormality. A statin is the first choice in cases where hypercholesterolaemia is predominant. A fibric acid derivative may be first choice when hypertriglyceridaemia predominates, and nicotinic acid is useful where plasma concentrations of triglyceride and cholesterol are elevated to a similar degree. Bile-acid binding

resins should not be used alone since they can aggravate hypertriglyceridaemia, but they may be useful with a triglyceride-lowering drug in some patients. Treatment with a combination of drugs that lowers both cholesterol and triglyceride concentrations may be required in some patients especially in those with markedly raised plasma concentrations of triglyceride or cholesterol, as treatment of these patients with drugs effective against only the predominant lipid may produce a rise in the plasma-concentrations of the other lipid. The choice of treatment in these cases is largely empirical as responses are not always predictable in individual patients.

- FAMILIAL DYSBETALIPOPROTEINAEMIA (remnant hyperlipoproteinaemia; remnant particle disease). In this lipid disorder the degree of hyperlipidaemia is usually severe and, although it may respond remarkably to dietary therapy, drug treatment is usually necessary. Fibric acid derivatives are the first-choice drugs. Statins or nicotinic acid may also be used.
- ABNORMAL LIPOPROTEIN LIPASE FUNCTION (chylomicronaemia). No drugs currently available are useful in this disorder. The condition is treated with severe restriction of dietary fat, and the diet may be supplemented by medium chain triglycerides to improve tolerability.


1. Chong PH, Bachenheimer BS. Current, new and future treatments in dyslipidaemia and atherosclerosis. *Drugs* 2000; **60:** 55–93.
2. The American Association of Clinical Endocrinologists Lipid Guidelines Committee. AACE medical guidelines for clinical practice for the diagnosis and treatment of dyslipidemia and prevention of atherogenesis. *Endocr Pract* 2000; **6:** 162–213. 2002 amended version available at: http://www.aace.com/clin/guidelines/lipids.pdf (accessed 13/05/04)
3. Anderson KM, *et al.* Cholesterol and mortality: 30 years of follow-up from the Framingham Study. *JAMA* 1987; **257:** 2176–80.
4. Hersberger M, von Eckardstein A. Low high-density lipoprotein cholesterol: physiological background, clinical importance and drug treatment. *Drugs* 2003; **63:** 1907–45.
5. Sattar N, *et al.* The end of triglycerides in cardiovascular risk assessment? *BMJ* 1998; **317:** 553–4.
6. Expert Panel on Detection, Evaluation, and Treatment of High Blood Cholesterol in Adults. Executive summary of the third report of the National Cholesterol Education Program (NCEP) expert panel on detection, evaluation, and treatment of high blood cholesterol in adults (Adult Treatment Panel III). *JAMA* 2001; **285:** 2486–97.
7. Beaumont JL, *et al.* Classification of hyperlipidaemias and hyperlipoproteinaemias. *Bull WHO* 1970; **43:** 891–915.
8. Wood D, *et al.* Joint British recommendations on prevention of coronary heart disease in clinical practice. *Heart* 1998; **80** (suppl 2): S1–S29.
9. De Backer G, *et al.* European guidelines on cardiovascular disease prevention in clinical practice: third Joint Task Force of European and Other Societies on Cardiovascular Disease Prevention in Clinical Practice. Executive summary: *Eur Heart J* 2003; **24:** 1601–10. Full guidelines: *Eur J Cardiovasc Prev Rehabil* 2003; **10** (suppl 1): S1–S78. Also available at: http://www.escardio.org/NR/rdonlyres/A0EF5CA5-421B-45EF-A65C-19B9EC411261/0/CVD_Prevention_03_full.pdf (accessed 12/05/04)
10. DoH. Nutritional aspects of cardiovascular disease. *Report on health and social subjects 46.* London: HMSO, 1994.
11. Ramsay LE, *et al.* Dietary reduction of serum cholesterol concentration: time to think again. *BMJ* 1991; **303:** 953–7.
12. Knopp RH. Drug treatment of lipid disorders. *N Engl J Med* 1999; **341:** 498–511.
13. Anonymous. Choice of lipid-regulating drugs. *Med Lett Drugs Ther* 2001; **43:** 43–8.
14. Sudhop T, von Bergmann K. Cholesterol absorption inhibitors for the treatment of hypercholesterolaemia. *Drugs* 2002; **62:** 2333–47.
15. Smilde TJ, *et al.* Effect of aggressive versus conventional lipid lowering on atherosclerosis progression in familial hypercholesterolaemia (ASAP): a prospective, randomised, double-blind trial. *Lancet* 2001; **357:** 577–81.
16. Grundy SM, *et al.* Implications of recent clinical trials for the National Cholesterol Education Program Adult Treatment Panel III Guidelines. *Circulation* 2004; **110:** 227–39.


## Hypertension

Hypertension, particularly essential or primary hypertension, is widespread and although usually asymptomatic, is a major risk factor for stroke and to some extent ischaemic heart disease. Control of hypertension is therefore a major aspect of cardiovascular risk reduction. National[1,2] and international[3,4] guidelines on management have been published.

**Definitions.** The term *blood pressure* generally means arterial blood pressure, that is the pressure of the blood on artery walls. It is usually measured indirectly in the brachial artery just above the elbow using an appropriately calibrated sphygmomanometer and is expressed in mmHg. Two measurements are made: *systolic* or maximum blood pressure (achieved during ventricular contraction of the heart) and *diastolic* or minimum blood pressure (achieved during ventricular dilatation). *Hypertension* means a higher than 'normal' blood pressure; it has been defined as the level of blood pressure above which intervention has been shown to reduce the associated cardiovascular risk. Many factors influence blood pressure, resulting in a bell-shaped distribution curve in the general population, and in consequence it is difficult to define an absolute norm. *Normal* adult blood pressure has been arbitrarily defined as a systolic pressure below 130 mmHg together with a diastolic pressure below 85 mmHg (i.e. below 130/85 mmHg), but more recent studies have suggested that optimal blood pressure, in terms of cardiovascular risk, may be lower than this. US guidelines[2] now define normal blood pressure as below 120/80 mmHg, while European[4] and British[1] guidelines classify this as optimal. Blood pressures of 130–139/85–89 mmHg are regarded as high normal[1,4] or are included in the classification of prehypertension.[2] Although hypertension was formerly defined in terms of diastolic blood pressure alone, it is now recognised that systolic pressure is also important in determining risk, and current guidelines give equal emphasis to both.

Blood pressure above 140 mmHg systolic, and/or 90 mmHg diastolic is generally considered to represent hypertension. Although classifications of mild, moderate, and severe hypertension have been widely used, these terms may be misleading since absolute cardiovascular risk is more important in determining the need for treatment and depends on other factors in addition to blood pressure. Most guidelines[1,3,4] therefore use a grading system to classify hypertension, as follows:

grade 1: 140–159/90–99 mmHg;
grade 2: 160–179/100–109 mmHg;
grade 3: ≥180/≥110 mmHg.

In the US guidelines,[2] stage 1 hypertension corresponds to grade 1, whereas stage 2 includes both grades 2 and 3.

When systolic and diastolic pressure fall into different categories the higher value is used for classification purposes. Classification and subsequent treatment decisions should be based on blood pressure measurements taken on several occasions over a period that varies according to the severity of hypertension. Ambulatory blood pressure monitoring may be used in some cases.[1,2,5] However, readings tend to be lower with ambulatory monitoring than with conventional measurement and normal and abnormal values are not yet clearly established, although recommendations have been made.[1,4,5]

In *malignant* or *accelerated hypertension* rapidly progressing severe hypertension is associated with retinopathy and often renal impairment.

*Isolated systolic hypertension* occurs mainly in the elderly and has been defined[1,4] as systolic pressure of 140 mmHg or more and diastolic pressure under 90 mmHg.

**Origins.** In the majority of cases of hypertension the cause is unknown, and such *primary* or *essential* hypertension is probably multifactorial in origin, with genotype, as well as external factors such as diet and body-weight, playing a role.[6] Hypertension may also be associated with surgery or pregnancy and is prevalent in diabetics. In a limited number of cases hypertension is *secondary* to some other condition, such as renal disease, Cushing's syndrome, phaeochromocytoma, or the adverse effects of drugs such as oestrogens, and such causes may be suspected particularly in resistant or malignant hypertension. Although treatment of the underlying condition will generally be desirable, the resultant hypertension will not necessarily be abolished by this.

**Management of hypertension.** Most of what follows relates to primary or essential hypertension in adults. Hypertensive crises and hypertension associated with surgery, diabetes, renal disease, or pregnancy are also discussed below under separate headings.

Hypertension may be discovered because of adverse vascular events, especially in the eyes, brain, kidneys, or heart, but is more often asymptomatic and only discovered on routine measurement of blood pressure. Once diagnosed, decisions have to be made about the need for treatment. It is well-established that hypertension is a risk factor for the development of stroke, heart failure, and renal damage, and to a lesser extent ischaemic heart disease, and a reduction in blood pressure is generally beneficial, although mortality remains higher than in non-hypertensives.[7] However, it is important to assess hypertension in the context of overall cardiovascular risk (see Cardiovascular Risk Reduction, p.819); additional considerations include the presence of target-organ disease, such as left ventricular hypertrophy or renal disease, and associated conditions such as other cardiovascular disease or diabetes. All patients with sustained hypertension of grade 2 or above can be considered at moderate to high risk and should be treated irrespective of other risk factors.[1,4] For patients with lower blood pressures, however, the decision to treat is more complex since the absolute cardiovascular risk may range from low to high depending on what other risk factors are present. Treatment of hypertension may involve both non-pharmacological and pharmacological interventions to reduce blood pressure, as well as assessment and treatment of any other cardiovascular risk factors; any co-existing diseases should also be treated. Guidelines on the management of hypertension may differ in detail, but reflect judgement on when intervention is justified.

**Non-pharmacological treatment**. Adopting a healthy lifestyle is beneficial for all individuals, and any patient with raised blood pressure should be encouraged to make lifestyle changes that will reduce their cardiovascular risk (see Cardiovascular Risk Reduction, p.819). Some of these changes may also reduce blood pressure,[6,8] and in those who are at low overall risk no other treatment may be needed; a trial of non-pharmacological treatment is recommended in most patients before initiating drug therapy.[1-4] Interventions that have been shown to reduce blood pressure include: reduction in excess weight; reduction in excess alcohol consumption; reduction in sodium intake; adequate exercise; reduced fat intake; and increased fruit and vegetable consumption. Other interventions that have been tried, but with less evidence of benefit, include: increased intake of potassium, magnesium, and calcium; increased polyunsaturated fat intake with reduced saturated fat intake; and relaxation therapies for stress reduction.

These lifestyle changes may also be promoted in the population as a whole, or in individuals most likely to develop hypertension, in strategies for the *primary prevention* of high blood pressure.

**Pharmacological treatment**. The main factors determining drug treatment relate to the blood pressure at which therapy should be initiated, the target blood pressure, and the most appropriate drug regimen to use.

*When to intervene* with antihypertensive drugs depend on a number of factors and guidelines take different approaches to this question. In patients with grade 1 or grade 2 hypertension, drug treatment is generally only initiated after an adequate period of observation, including blood pressure monitoring; the period depends on the level of risk but may be 3 months or longer. In the US guidelines,[2] all patients with sustained blood pressure above target levels (140/90 mmHg or 130/80 mmHg in diabetics or those with renal disease) despite lifestyle changes are recommended for drug treatment. In other guidelines,[1,4] the decision depends on both the measured blood pressure and the overall cardiovascular risk. Patients with sustained blood pressure of 180/110 mmHg or higher should receive prompt treatment. Those with values of 140/90 mmHg or above who are at high or very high overall risk should also receive prompt treatment.[4] If the overall risk is moderate, treatment should be initiated if the blood pressure remains at 140/90 mmHg or above after a period of monitoring; treatment may also be considered in those with lower risk.[4] The WHO/ISH guidelines[3] acknowledge that even low-risk individuals with blood pressures above 140/90 mmHg are likely to benefit from treatment, but suggests that those at higher risk should be given the highest priority. For *elderly patients* (over 60 years) the benefit of treating hypertension has been established in several trials.[9-12] Benefit is evident up to at least 80 years of age and a strict age limit to drug therapy is probably inappropriate. Guidelines therefore generally recommend that treatment decisions should not be based on age, although slower titration of drugs has been suggested[4] in older patients since they may be more susceptible to adverse effects. In the very old (those over 80 years) the benefit of initiating therapy is less clear,[13] although those already being treated should continue.[1]

*Target blood pressures* are controversial. There has been concern that over-aggressive reduction of diastolic pressure might increase the risk of ischaemic heart disease.[14] However, a more recent meta-analysis[15] suggested that any increased mortality at low blood pressures was not linked to antihypertensive therapy but may have been due to poor health as a cause of low blood pressure. The HOT study[16] found that effective control to maintain the diastolic pressure below 90 mmHg (at about 85 mmHg) reduced the rate of cardiovascular events, but lower pressures (of around 70 mmHg) did not provide any further benefit, while a more recent meta-analysis[17] found no evidence of a threshold for treatment benefit down to a blood pressure of at least 115/75 mmHg. Target blood pressures of below 140/90 mmHg[2,4] or below 140/85 mmHg[1] are now recommended. In diabetics the target is below 130/80 mmHg;[1-4] similar or lower targets should also be considered in non-diabetics with nephropathy.[1,2]

*The drug regimen* may include drugs from a number of groups that have antihypertensive effects. These groups have differing pharmacological actions although the precise mechanism is not understood in all cases. Thiazide diuretics and beta blockers have been the mainstay of drug therapy for hypertension, but the availability of other drug groups such as calcium-channel blockers, ACE inhibitors, alpha blockers, and angiotensin II receptor antagonists, as well as concern about the possible metabolic effects of thiazides and beta blockers, has led to increasing use of these newer drugs.

Choice of initial therapy has been controversial and depends on antihypertensive efficacy, safety, and long term effects on morbidity and mortality.[18,19] Studies such as the TOMHS[20] (comparing chlortalidone, acebutolol, amlodipine, enalapril, and doxazosin), and a similar study[21] (comparing hydrochlorothiazide, atenolol, diltiazem, captopril, prazosin, and clonidine), have shown that the main types of antihypertensive drug reduce blood pressure to a similar extent and in a similar proportion of patients, although the response may also depend on individual factors such as age[22] and race.[23] Angiotensin II receptor antagonists also effectively reduce blood pressure. However, it is now generally acknowledged that a single drug is unlikely to control blood pressure adequately and most patients will require more than one drug to reach their treatment target. Tolerance of the drug groups is also similar, although results from an interim analysis[24] of the ALLHAT study have suggested that the risk of developing heart failure may be greater with doxazosin than with chlortalidone. There has also been concern about the safety of short-acting dihydropyridine calcium-channel blockers, and they are no longer generally recommended for hypertension (see Effects on Mortality under Adverse Effects of Nifedipine, p.966); long-acting dihydropyridines, however, are of established benefit.

All of the main drug groups are therefore established as effective antihypertensives, but their effects on long-term mortality and morbidity have been less clear. Although the different drug groups have differing effects on several surrogate outcomes, such as left ventricular hypertrophy[25] and endothelial dysfunction,[26] the clinical significance of this has not been established. For a long time, only diuretics (particularly thiazides) and beta blockers had been adequately tested in long-term trials and were therefore preferred for initial therapy. However, further studies have suggested that other drug groups may be comparable. The very large ALLHAT study[27] found that there was no difference in all-cause mortality for those receiving a diuretic (chlortalidone), an ACE inhibitor (lisinopril), or a calcium-channel blocker (amlodipine), although some cause-specific outcomes varied. The LIFE study[28] confirmed that angiotensin II receptor antagonists also reduce both morbidity and mortality. A meta-analysis[29] including these and other large studies has supported the view that the major benefit is from the reduction in blood pressure and that there is little evidence that any of the drug classes provide additional benefit with regard to overall cardiovascular outcome.

Guidelines now therefore generally recommend that, in most patients, treatment should be initiated with the cheapest or most cost-effective drug;[1-3] this will often be a thiazide diuretic.[2,3] However, for many of the drug groups there are specific groups of patients who have been shown to derive additional benefit or in whom there are specific contra-indications. Compelling indications include the use of ACE inhibitors or angiotensin II receptor blockers in patients with nephropathy, diuretics or calcium-channel blockers in elderly patients, and beta blockers in patients who have had a myocardial infarction. Additional considerations include the lower efficacy of beta blockers and ACE inhibitors in Afro-Caribbean blacks.

Having decided what drug to use, treatment is started at the lowest recommended dose. If this is ineffective or only partially effective the dose may be increased (except in the case of thiazide diuretics where there is generally no additional benefit, but more adverse effects); alternatively another first-line drug may either be substituted (sequential therapy) or added. Two-drug combinations will control blood pressure in a higher proportion of patients and may be necessary in most patients to achieve optimal levels, although the effects of the two drugs may not be fully additive. Combination therapy also allows lower doses of the individual drugs to be used with a consequent reduction in adverse effects. Initial treatment with a low-dose combination may be considered in some patients.[2,4] The most effective combinations involve drugs that act on different physiological systems. Appropriate combinations therefore include: a diuretic plus either a beta blocker, an ACE inhibitor, or an angiotensin II receptor antagonist; and a calcium-channel blocker plus either an ACE inhibitor, an angiotensin II receptor antagonist, or (except with verapamil) a beta blocker. Alpha blockers may be used with any of the other classes but are usually reserved for third-line therapy unless specifically indicated for another reason. A 3-drug combination is often required, especially in severe hypertension. In patients who maintain an elevated diastolic blood pressure despite triple therapy the possibility of secondary hypertension should be considered, although factors such as non-compliance, NSAID use, or alcohol abuse may contribute to resistance.[30]

Other classes of antihypertensive drugs that are sometimes used include centrally acting drugs such as clonidine, methyldopa, and the less sedating moxonidine, and direct-acting vasodilators such as hydralazine and minoxidil. Older drugs like the adrenergic neurone blocker guanethidine and the rauwolfia alkaloid reserpine are rarely recommended now. Renin inhibitors, endopeptidase inhibitors, endothelin antagonists, and the aldosterone antagonist eplerenone are under investigation.

*Withdrawal of drug treatment.* It has been standard teaching that drug treatment for hypertension is continued indefinitely, but there have been some reports of successful withdrawal in selected patients.[31-33] If this is attempted, blood pressure must be closely monitored and lifestyle measures should be continued indefinitely.

**Hypertensive crises.** Patients with severe hypertension may be divided into those in whom there is evidence of rapid or progressive CNS, cardiovascular, or renal deterioration (hypertensive *emergencies*) and those with no evidence of target-organ damage (urgent hypertensive crises or hypertensive *urgencies*).[2,34,35] In the former case the goal is a reduction in mean arterial blood pressure by 25%, or a fall in diastolic blood pressure to 100 to 110 mmHg, over a period of several minutes to several hours depending on the clinical situation; intravenous therapy is often required although oral therapy may be adequate. In the latter case a drastic reduction in blood pressure is inappropriate and oral therapy is preferred, with the aim of a reduction in blood pressure over several hours to days. It should be remembered in both situations that a too rapid reduction of blood pressure may be detrimental and may lead to cerebral infarction and blindness, to deterioration in renal function, and to myocardial ischaemia.

If oral treatment can be given and there is no evidence of ongoing target-organ damage, standard initiation of antihypertensive therapy is appropriate, although the patient should be closely monitored. If there is no evidence of heart failure or asthma then a beta blocker has often been the treatment of choice.[36] Diuretics are less suitable since patients may initially be fluid depleted but they may be added after two to three days' treatment with other antihypertensive drugs to maintain blood pressure control.[36] Other drugs that have been used for a rapid effect include the centrally acting drug clonidine, the ACE inhibitor captopril, and the alpha blocker prazosin (especially when there are increased circulating catecholamines), but caution is needed since they may all lower blood pressure abruptly, and for this reason they are not generally recommended as initial therapy. Nifedipine and captopril have been administered sublingually for a faster onset,[37] but again care is needed since their rapid action may be detrimental. There appears to be no clearly defined clinical advantage for sublingual as opposed to oral administration and it is generally considered that nifedipine should not be used.[2,38]

In the emergency situation, when parenteral therapy is required, choice of therapy depends on concomitant clinical conditions.[39] Sodium nitroprusside has most often been the drug of choice, given by intravenous infusion.[40,41] Alternatives include intravenous labetalol, nicardipine, hydralazine (in eclampsia), glyceryl trinitrate (in patients with coronary ischaemia), phentolamine (in phaeochromocytoma and other states associated with catecholamine excess such as the MAOI-tyramine interaction), enalaprilat, esmolol, trimetaphan,[40,41] fenoldopam,[39] and urapidil.[42]

Hypertensive emergencies in children have been managed successfully with intravenous infusions of labetalol and/or sodium nitroprusside.[43]

**Hypertension during surgery.** Despite earlier concern over the risks of administering antihypertensive drugs to patients about to undergo surgery, substantial subsequent data have confirmed that it is not only safe but probably preferable to continue such medication up to and including the morning of surgery.[2,44,45]

Perioperative hypertension may occur as a result of surgery and frequently needs to be controlled with parenteral antihypertensives since oral administration in such patients may not be possible. The parenteral drug of choice is often sodium nitroprusside; others include glyceryl trinitrate (especially after coronary artery bypass), hydralazine, labetalol, enalaprilat, esmolol, fenoldopam, and nicardipine; diazoxide and methyldopa have also been used.[40,45]

**Hypertension in diabetic patients.** Hypertension occurs with twice the frequency in the diabetic compared with the nondiabetic population, and up to 50% of patients with type 2 diabetes mellitus become hypertensive.[46,47] The reasons proposed for this increased prevalence are controversial, but insulin resistance has been implicated.[48] In addition to being a major risk factor for atherosclerosis in large blood vessels, hypertension in diabetes appears to contribute to small vessel disease and is a risk factor for diabetic nephropathy and possibly for diabetic retinopathy. The UK Prospective Diabetes Study (UKPDS) Group has reported[49] that tight control of blood pressure (with a target of <150/85 mmHg) reduces the risk of diabetes-related death and diabetic complications, including diabetic retinopathy, in type 2 diabetics.

The threshold for intervention with drug treatment may be lower in diabetic than in non-diabetic hypertensive patients and treatment targets are also lower. An initial target of 140/80 mmHg has been suggested,[1] while a target below 130/80 mmHg may be optimal and is recommended in most guidelines;[1-4,50] the lower target is particularly advised in type 1 diabetics with nephropathy. All the main groups of antihypertensive drugs can be used in diabetics,[51] and most patients will require at least two drugs to achieve target blood pressure. ACE inhibitors have been particularly recommended, as there is evidence of benefit in preserving renal function in patients with nephropathy; they have been reported to decrease proteinuria and preserve glomerular filtration rate in diabetic patients independently of changes in systemic blood pressure.[52] Angiotensin II receptor antagonists are an alternative, particularly in type 2 diabetics. Diuretics and beta blockers have often been avoided because of their potential adverse effects on glucose and lipid metabolism, but are now generally considered a suitable choice. In the UKPDS treatment with an ACE inhibitor (captopril) or a beta blocker (atenolol) was equally effective in reducing the risk of diabetic complications, although the ACE inhibitor appeared to be better tolerated.[53] Although there has been concern regarding the safety of calcium-channel blockers, studies such as ALLHAT[27] have confirmed that long-acting calcium-channel blockers are also a suitable choice.

**Hypertension and renal disease.** Hypertension is closely linked with the kidney—the kidney may have a role in the pathogenesis of hypertension and it may also be a prime target of damage caused by hypertension. Both renal parenchymal disorders and renovascular disorders may be associated with hypertension. In the former, hypertension is often resistant to treatment and a combination of drugs, including vasodilators, may be required. Antihypertensive therapy is also important in these patients since it may slow the decline in renal function in patients with nephropathy.[54] There is some evidence that ACE inhibitors may have a greater protective effect than other antihypertensives,[55,56] and they have been recommended as the basis of therapy, usually in combination with a diuretic.[1,2,4] The effect of blood pressure reduction appears to be related to the degree of proteinuria, and studies have shown that patients with proteinuria higher than 1 g/day benefit from lower blood pressures.[56] Current guidelines[1,2,4] recommend a target blood pressure of below 130/80 mmHg in patients with nephropathy, with a lower target[1] of 125/75 mmHg in those with proteinuria of 1 g/day or over.

*Renovascular hypertension* has been defined as arterial hypertension resulting from obliteration or compression of one or both renal arteries, the commonest cause being stenosis due to atherosclerosis. Underperfusion of the kidney leads to increased release of renin and a consequent rise in blood pressure. However, the relationship between renovascular hypertension and renal artery stenosis is not clear cut; the two conditions may simply co-exist or hypertension may cause the stenosis rather than the other way round.[57,58]

Renovascular hypertension may be difficult to distinguish clinically, but carries a worse prognosis than essential hypertension, may be less amenable to treatment, carries a higher risk of progression to accelerated or malignant hypertension, and may result in irreversible ischaemic failure of the affected kidney.

Diagnostic methods used to detect renovascular hypertension include imaging studies such as ultrasonography and angiography, and functional tests such as the captopril-renin test (see under ACE inhibitors on p.846 for further details); renal scintigraphy with and without ACE inhibition is also used.

Blood pressure in renovascular hypertension can often be lowered by antihypertensive drugs.[59] However, medical treatment may not prevent progression of stenosis and there are concerns about possible harmful effects of blood pressure reduction on the function of the affected kidney.[57] Adverse effects on renal function are a particular concern with ACE inhibitors since, in patients with bilateral renal artery stenosis or stenosis to a solitary kidney, renal perfusion may be dependent on angiotensin II. Although some consider renovascular disease to be a contra-indication to the use of ACE inhibitors, they may be needed to control blood pressure in some patients. However, they should be used cautiously and in low doses[60] and renal function needs to be monitored with great care (see Precautions for ACE inhibitors, p.844). Renal angioplasty is an alternative to medical treatment and may be more effective;[61] surgery may also be used.

**Hypertension in pregnancy**. Hypertension in pregnancy may be life-threatening to both mother and fetus. It may be pre-existing or may develop for the first time during pregnancy when it may range from transient hypertension late in pregnancy through to pre-eclampsia and eclampsia. Definitions vary, but hypertension presenting before 20 weeks' gestation generally continues long-term and is considered chronic hypertension. Hypertension presenting after the twentieth week (gestational hypertension) may be transient hypertension (pregnancy-induced hypertension), chronic hypertension, or pre-eclampsia. Gestational hypertension is usually defined as a blood pressure of 140/90 mmHg or more on at least two occasions in a previously normotensive woman; it is considered transient hypertension if the blood pressure has returned to normal limits by the twelfth week postpartum.[62] In pre-eclampsia, increased blood pressure occurs together with proteinuria; abnormal coagulation, liver dysfunction, and oedema may also be present. Pre-eclampsia may progress to eclampsia, a convulsive phase.

Recommendations about the level of blood pressure that warrants treatment during pregnancy have been controversial. Most women with chronic hypertension will have grade 1 or grade 2 hypertension and a low risk of cardiovascular complications during the short period of pregnancy, and the benefits of treatment in such patients are not established. It is usually recommended that blood pressures of 170/110 mmHg or above should be treated; there is less agreement about lower limits but some suggest treatment of blood pressures of 140/90 mmHg or above.[63] However, in some cases of pre-existing hypertension it may be possible to withdraw treatment during pregnancy and only restart therapy if the blood pressure exceeds threshold values.[62,64] However, women with mild hypertension are at an increased risk of developing pre-eclampsia, regardless of whether they receive antihypertensives, and should be closely monitored.

Women with *pre-existing* hypertension usually continue their antihypertensive treatment although ACE inhibitors and angiotensin II receptor antagonists are contra-indicated in pregnancy. Methyldopa or beta blockers are effective first-line antihypertensives in mild to moderate hypertension and comparative studies have shown little difference between them in the outcome of pregnancy. However, methyldopa has the advantage of reassuring long-term safety results in the infant, whereas there have been concerns about fetal growth retardation with beta blockers, particularly with atenolol.[65-67] Nifedipine may also be used.[68] Diuretics are not generally recommended for controlling hypertension in pregnancy because of the theoretical risk of exacerbating the volume depletion of pre-eclampsia; however, they appear to be safe in practice and may be used if necessary.[1,62,64]

In patients with *pre-eclampsia* the aim of *treatment* is to prevent maternal complications while allowing fetal maturation; delivery is the definitive treatment.[69] Evidence to guide choice of therapy is limited.[70] Oral therapy may be appropriate although intravenous antihypertensives are used in acute pre-eclampsia or when delivery is imminent. For oral treatment methyldopa or a beta blocker is considered first-line. If this fails to reduce blood pressure adequately then it is usual to add a vasodilator such as hydralazine or prazosin;[71] a calcium-channel blocker such as nifedipine is also effective.[69,72] In the emergency control of hypertension in patients with severe pre-eclampsia or eclampsia intravenous hydralazine has been widely used, although it may be less effective than other drugs.[65] Intravenous labetalol and oral nifedipine are also used, and sodium nitroprusside may be required in some patients.[62,71] Other parenteral antihypertensives tried have included diazoxide, clonidine, and glyceryl trinitrate.[72]

The management of seizures associated with eclampsia is discussed on p.352.

*Prevention of pre-eclampsia*. It was hoped that prevention of pre-eclampsia might be possible by reducing the local platelet aggregation thought to be responsible for some of its manifestations. Several small studies suggested that low-dose aspirin reduced the risk of pregnancy-induced hypertension and intra-uterine growth retardation in high-risk patients.[73] However, larger studies in women at lower risk generally failed to confirm this benefit[74,75] and in one[75] the risk of placental abruption was higher in those taking aspirin. Findings of the CLASP (Collaborative Low-dose Aspirin Study in Pregnancy) multicentre study[76] involving over 9000 women considered to be at increased risk of pre-eclampsia or intra-uterine growth retardation did not support the routine prophylactic or therapeutic use of antiplatelet therapy in all such women. A further study[77] in high-risk women also failed to show any benefit, although aspirin appeared to be safe for mother and fetus. However, a systematic review[78] found that antiplatelet therapy provided a small to moderate benefit in patients at risk of developing pre-eclampsia, although further information was needed to establish which women were most likely to benefit. Calcium supplementation has also been shown[79] to reduce the risks of pregnancy-induced hypertension and pre-eclampsia, although its role is not yet established. Preliminary evidence suggests that supplementation with vitamins C and E may be beneficial in women at high risk, but confirmation is needed from larger studies.[80]


1. Williams B, *et al.* Guidelines for management of hypertension: report of the fourth working party of the British Hypertension Society, 2004—BHS IV. *J Hum Hypertens* 2004; **18:** 139–185. Also available at: http://www.hyp.ac.uk/bhs/pdfs/BHS_IV_Guidelines.pdf (accessed 13/05/04)
2. Chobanian AV, *et al.* Seventh report of the joint national committee on prevention, detection, evaluation, and treatment of high blood pressure (JNC 7). *Hypertension* 2003; **42:** 1206–52.
3. World Health Organization, International Society of Hypertension Writing Group. 2003 World Health Organization (WHO)/International Society of Hypertension (ISH) statement on management of hypertension. *J Hypertens* 2003; **21:** 1983–92.
4. European Society of Hypertension - European Society of Cardiology Guidelines Committee. 2003 European Society of Hypertension - European Society of Cardiology guidelines for the management of arterial hypertension. *J Hypertens* 2003; **21:** 1011–53. Also available at: http://www.eshonline.org/documents/2003_guidelines.pdf (accessed 13/05/04)
5. O'Brien E, *et al.* Use and interpretation of ambulatory blood pressure monitoring: recommendations of the British Hypertension Society. *BMJ* 2000; **320:** 1128–34.
6. Kornitzer M, *et al.* Epidemiology of risk factors for hypertension: implications for prevention and therapy. *Drugs* 1999; **57:** 695–712.
7. Andersson OK, *et al.* Survival in treated hypertension: follow up study after two decades. *BMJ* 1998; **317:** 167–71.
8. Writing Group of the PREMIER Collaborative Research Group. Effects of comprehensive lifestyle modification on blood pressure control: main results of the PREMIER clinical trial. *JAMA* 2003; **289:** 2083–93.
9. Staessen JA, *et al.* Randomised double-blind comparison of placebo and active treatment for older patients with isolated systolic hypertension. *Lancet* 1997; **350:** 757–64. Correction. *ibid.*; 1636.
10. Dahlöf B, *et al.* Morbidity and mortality in the Swedish Trial in Old Patients with Hypertension (STOP-Hypertension). *Lancet* 1991; **338:** 1281–5.
11. SHEP Cooperative Research Group. Prevention of stroke by antihypertensive drug treatment in older persons with isolated systolic hypertension: final results of the Systolic Hypertension in the Elderly Program (SHEP). *JAMA* 1991; **265:** 3255–64.
12. MRC Working Party. Medical Research Council trial of treatment of hypertension in older patients: principal results. *BMJ* 1992; **304:** 405–12.
13. Gueyffier F, *et al.* Antihypertensive drugs in very old people: a subgroup meta-analysis of randomised controlled trials. *Lancet* 1999; **353:** 793–6.
14. Staessen JA. Potential adverse effects of blood pressure lowering—J-curve revisited. *Lancet* 1996; **348:** 696–7.
15. Boutitie F, *et al.*J-shaped relationship between blood pressure and mortality in hypertensive patients: new insights from a meta-analysis of individual-patient data. *Ann Intern Med* 2002; **136:** 438–48.
16. Hansson L, *et al.* Effects of intensive blood-pressure lowering and low-dose aspirin in patients with hypertension: principal results of the Hypertension Optimal Treatment (HOT) randomised trial. *Lancet* 1998; **351:** 1755–62.
17. Prospective Studies Collaboration. Age-specific relevance of usual blood pressure to vascular mortality: a meta-analysis of individual data for one million adults in 61 prospective studies. *Lancet* 2002; **360:** 1903–13. Correction. *ibid.* 2003; **361:** 1060.
18. Brown MJ. Matching the right drug to the right patient in essential hypertension. *Heart* 2001; **86:** 113–20.
19. August P. Initial treatment of hypertension. *N Engl J Med* 2003; **348:** 610–17.
20. Neaton JD, *et al.* Treatment of mild hypertension study: final results. *JAMA* 1993; **270:** 713–24.
21. Materson BJ, *et al.* Single-drug therapy for hypertension in men: a comparison of six antihypertensive agents with placebo. *N Engl J Med* 1993; **328:** 914–21. Correction. *ibid.* 1994; **330:** 1689.
22. Bennet NE. Hypertension in the elderly. *Lancet* 1994; **344:** 447–9.
23. Kaplan NM. Ethnic aspects of hypertension. *Lancet* 1994; **344:** 450–2.
24. The ALLHAT Officers and Coordinators for the ALLHAT Collaborative Research Group. Major cardiovascular events in hypertensive patients randomized to doxazosin vs chlorthalidone: the Antihypertensive and Lipid-Lowering Treatment to Prevent Heart Attack Trial (ALLHAT). *JAMA* 2000; **283:** 1967–75.
25. Klingbeil AU, *et al.* A meta-analysis of the effects of treatment on left ventricular mass in essential hypertension. *Am J Med* 2003; **115:** 41–6.
26. Taddei S, *et al.* Effects of antihypertensive drugs on endothelial dysfunction: clinical implications. *Drugs* 2002; **62:** 265–84.
27. The ALLHAT Officers and Coordinators for the ALLHAT Collaborative Research Group. Major outcomes in high-risk hypertensive patients randomized to angiotensin-converting enzyme inhibitor or calcium channel blocker vs diuretic: The Antihypertensive and Lipid-Lowering Treatment to Prevent Heart Attack Trial (ALLHAT). *JAMA* 2002; **288:** 2981–97. Correction. *ibid.* 2003; **289:** 178.
28. Dahlöf B, *et al.* Cardiovascular morbidity and mortality in the Losartan Intervention For Endpoint reduction in hypertension study (LIFE): a randomised trial against atenolol. *Lancet* 2002; **359:** 995–1003.
29. Blood Pressure Lowering Treatment Trialists' Collaboration. Effects of different blood-pressure-lowering regimens on major cardiovascular events: results of prospectively-designed overviews of randomised trials. *Lancet* 2003; **362:** 1527–35.
30. Padfield PL. Resistant hypertension. *Prescribers' J* 1997; **37:** 69–76.
31. van den Bosch WJHM, *et al.* Withdrawal of antihypertensive drugs in selected patients. *Lancet* 1994; **343:** 1157.
32. Aylett MJ, *et al.* Withdrawing antihypertensive drugs. *Lancet* 1994; **343:** 1512.
33. Nelson MR, *et al.* Predictors of normotension on withdrawal of antihypertensive drugs in elderly patients: prospective study in second Australian national blood pressure study cohort. *BMJ* 2002; **325:** 815–17.
34. Calhoun DA, Oparil S. Treatment of hypertensive crisis. *N Engl J Med* 1990; **323:** 1177–83.
35. Vaughan CJ, Delanty N. Hypertensive emergencies. *Lancet* 2000; **356:** 411–17.
36. Semple PF. Emergency treatment of hypertension. *Prescribers' J* 1989; **29:** 62–9.
37. Anonymous. Hypertensive emergencies. *Lancet* 1991; **338:** 220–1.
38. Grossman E, *et al.* Should a moratorium be placed on sublingual nifedipine capsules for hypertensive emergencies and pseudoemergencies? *JAMA* 1996; **276:** 1328–31.
39. Grossman E, *et al.* Comparative tolerability profile of hypertensive crisis treatments. *Drug Safety* 1998; **19:** 99–122.
40. Gifford RW. Management of hypertensive crises. *JAMA* 1991; **266:** 829–35.
41. Kaplan NM. Management of hypertensive emergencies. *Lancet* 1994; **344:** 1335–8.
42. Hirschl MM. Guidelines for the drug treatment of hypertensive crises. *Drugs* 1995; **50:** 991–1000.
43. Deal JE, *et al.* Management of hypertensive emergencies. *Arch Dis Child* 1992; **67:** 1089–92.
44. Goldman L. Cardiac risks and complications of noncardiac surgery. *Ann Intern Med* 1983; **98:** 504–13.
45. Erstad BL, Barletta JF. Treatment of hypertension in the perioperative patient. *Ann Pharmacother* 2000; **34:** 66–79.
46. MacLeod MJ, McLay J. Drug treatment of hypertension complicating diabetes mellitus. *Drugs* 1998; **56:** 189–202.
47. Deedwania PC. Hypertension and diabetes: new therapeutic options. *Arch Intern Med* 2000; **160:** 1585–94.
48. Reaven GM, *et al.* Hypertension and associated metabolic abnormalities—the role of insulin resistance and the sympathoadrenal system. *N Engl J Med* 1996; **334:** 374–81.
49. UK Prospective Diabetes Study Group. Tight blood pressure control and risk of macrovascular and microvascular complications in type 2 diabetes: UKPDS 38. *BMJ* 1998; **317:** 703–13.
50. American Diabetes Association. Hypertension management in adults with diabetes. *Diabetes Care* 2004; **27** (suppl 1): S65–S67. Also available at: http://care.diabetesjournals.org/cgi/reprint/27/suppl_1/s65.pdf (accessed 13/05/04)
51. Kaplan NM. Management of hypertension in patients with type 2 diabetes mellitus: guidelines based on current evidence. *Ann Intern Med* 2001; **135:** 1079–83.
52. Kaisiske BL, *et al.* Effect of antihypertensive therapy on the kidney in patients with diabetes: a meta-regression analysis. *Ann Intern Med* 1993; **118:** 129–38.
53. UK Prospective Diabetes Study Group. Efficacy of atenolol and captopril in reducing risk of macrovascular and microvascular complications in type 2 diabetes: UKPDS 39. *BMJ* 1998; **317:** 713–20.
54. Salvetti A, *et al.* Renal protection and antihypertensive drugs: current status. *Drugs* 1999; **57:** 665–93.
55. Wright JT, *et al.* Effect of blood pressure lowering and antihypertensive drug class on progression of hypertensive kidney disease: results from the AASK trial. *JAMA* 2002; **288:** 2421–31.
56. Jafar TH, *et al.* Progression of chronic kidney disease: the role of blood pressure control, proteinuria, and angiotensin-converting enzyme inhibition: a patient-level meta-analysis. *Ann Intern Med* 2003; **139:** 244–52.
57. Derkx FHM, Schalekamp MADH. Renal artery stenosis and hypertension. *Lancet* 1994; **344:** 237–9.
58. Safian RD, Textor SC. Renal-artery stenosis. *N Engl J Med* 2001; **344:** 431–42.
59. Rosenthal T. Drug therapy of renovascular hypertension. *Drugs* 1993; **45:** 895–909.
60. Navis G, *et al.* ACE inhibitors and the kidney: a risk-benefit assessment. *Drug Safety* 1996; **15:** 200–211.
61. Nordmann AJ, *et al.* Balloon angioplasty or medical therapy for hypertensive patients with atherosclerotic renal artery stenosis? A meta-analysis of randomized controlled trials. *Am J Med* 2003; **114:** 44–50.
62. National High Blood Pressure Education Program Working Group on High Blood Pressure in Pregnancy. Report of the National High Blood Pressure Education Program Working Group on High Blood Pressure in Pregnancy. *Am J Obstet Gynecol* 2000; **183** (suppl): S1–S22. Also available from the National Institutes of Health at: http://www.nhlbi.nih.gov/health/prof/heart/hbp/hbp_preg.htm (accessed 13/05/04)
63. Rey É. Report of the Canadian Hypertension Society Consensus Conference: pharmacologic treatment of hypertensive disorders in pregnancy. *Can Med Assoc J* 1997; **157:** 1245–54.
64. Task Force on the Management of Cardiovascular Diseases During Pregnancy of the European Society of Cardiology. Expert consensus document on management of cardiovascular diseases during pregnancy. *Eur Heart J* 2003; **24:** 761–81. Also available at: http://www.escardio.org/NR/rdonlyres/

DFC7D44A-CC29-4971-8F43-20BCD2EE6754/0/ESC_ECD_ON_CVD_PREGNANCY.pdf (accessed 13/05/04)
65. Magee LA, *et al.* Management of hypertension in pregnancy. *BMJ* 1999; **318:** 1332–6.
66. Garovic VD. Hypertension in pregnancy: diagnosis and treatment. *Mayo Clin Proc* 2000; **75:** 1071–6.
67. Magee LA. Treating hypertension in women of child-bearing age and during pregnancy. *Drug Safety* 2001; **24:** 457–74.
68. Sibai BM. Treatment of hypertension in pregnant women. *N Engl J Med* 1996; **335:** 257–65.
69. Walker JJ. Pre-eclampsia. *Lancet* 2000; **356:** 1260–5.
70. Duley L. Pre-eclampsia and the hypertensive disorders of pregnancy. *Br Med Bull* 2003; **67:** 161–76.
71. Broughton Pipkin F, Rubin PC. Pre-eclampsia—the 'disease of theories'. *Br Med Bull* 1994; **50:** 381–96.
72. Mushambi MC, *et al.* Recent developments in the pathophysiology and management of pre-eclampsia. *Br J Anaesth* 1996; **76:** 133–48.
73. Imperiale TF, Petrulis AS. A meta-analysis of low-dose aspirin for the prevention of pregnancy-induced hypertensive disease. *JAMA* 1991; **266:** 260–4.
74. Italian Study of Aspirin in Pregnancy. Low-dose aspirin in prevention and treatment of intrauterine growth retardation and pregnancy-induced hypertension. *Lancet* 1993; **341:** 396–400.
75. Sibai BM, *et al.* Prevention of preeclampsia with low-dose aspirin in healthy, nulliparous pregnant women. *N Engl J Med* 1993; **329:** 1213–18.
76. CLASP (Collaborative Low-dose Aspirin Study in Pregnancy) Collaborative Group. CLASP: a randomised trial of low-dose aspirin for the prevention and treatment of pre-eclampsia among 9364 pregnant women. *Lancet* 1994; **343:** 619–29.
77. Caritis S, *et al.* Low-dose aspirin to prevent preeclampsia in women at high risk. *N Engl J Med* 1998; **338:** 701–5.
78. Duley L, *et al.* Antiplatelet agents for preventing pre-eclampsia and its complications. Available in The Cochrane Library; Issue 2. Chichester: John Wiley; 2004.
79. Atallah AN, *et al.* Calcium supplementation during pregnancy for preventing hypertensive disorders and related problems. Available in The Cochrane Library; Issue 2. Chichester: John Wiley; 2004.
80. Chappell LC, *et al.* Effect of antioxidants on the occurrence of pre-eclampsia in women at increased risk: a randomised trial. *Lancet* 1999; **354:** 810–16.

## Hypotension

As discussed under Hypertension (above) many factors influence blood pressure making it difficult to define an absolute norm. An arbitrary definition of *normal* adult blood pressure[1] is a systolic pressure below 130 mmHg together with a diastolic pressure below 85 mmHg (i.e. below 130/85 mmHg); a value of less than 120/80 mmHg has also been suggested.[2] Unlike hypertension, for which national and international guidelines have been developed, there does not appear to be an accepted definition of either low blood pressure or hypotension.

Despite such shortcomings over definition, the existence of several forms of hypotensive disease is recognised.

Hypotension can occur after haemorrhage or in other forms of shock and the management of this acute and potentially dangerous form of low blood pressure is usually with vasopressor sympathomimetics, notably noradrenaline or dopamine (see Shock, p.835). Another situation in which acute hypotension can develop is during anaesthesia and surgery; spinal or epidural block is associated with a greater risk than many other forms of anaesthesia. Again, sympathomimetics, and ephedrine particularly, are used as vasopressors[3] (see p.1120).

Chronic forms of hypotension also exist and include orthostatic (postural) hypotension and neurally mediated hypotension; both are important causes of syncope (fainting).[4] Drug therapy for orthostatic hypotension usually involves fludrocortisone (see p.1100). For neurally mediated hypotension, however, choice of therapy is less clear.[4-7]

Neurally mediated hypotension (neurocardiogenic syncope, neurally mediated reflex syncope, vasodepressor syncope, or vasovagal syncope) is a common cause of recurrent lightheadedness (presyncope) and syncope in persons with structurally normal hearts. It is characterised by a paradoxical neurocardiogenic reflex that ultimately results in vasodilatation, bradycardia, and hypotension. Avoidance of triggering events and an increase in dietary salt and electrolyte intake may be sufficient treatment in some patients,[4] but those with recurrent attacks may require drug therapy. Numerous drugs have been tried, but evidence of benefit is limited for most of them.[4,5] Fludrocortisone, a beta blocker (such as atenolol or metoprolol), and disopyramide are reported to be among the standard drugs used.[5-8] Selective serotonin reuptake inhibitors have been effective in some cases.[5-8] Benefit has also been reported with vasoconstrictors, including the alpha agonist midodrine.[5,9] Antimuscarinics, such as propantheline bromide, have also been tried.[6,8] In a few patients cardiac pacing may be required.

One contentious issue is whether general and non-specific symptoms of ill health such as mental and physical fatigue, depression, and anxiety can be attributed to a low blood pressure (for example, a systolic pressure below 110 mmHg or diastolic pressure below 60 mmHg).[10] In the UK and the USA such an association has never been accepted whereas in some European countries (e.g. Germany) a wide range of pharmaceutical preparations, usually containing a sympathomimetic, has been available for treatment. Some evidence has been presented to support the theory,[11,12] as well as to suggest a possible link between the chronic fatigue syndrome and neurally mediated hypotension,[13,14] although implications for treatment are far from clear.

1. Guidelines Subcommittee. 1999 World Health Organization–International Society of Hypertension guidelines for the management of hypertension. *J Hypertens* 1999; **17:** 151–83. Also available at: http://www.eshonline.org/documents/whoish99.pdf (accessed 13/05/04)
2. Chobanian AV, *et al.*. The seventh report of the joint national committee on prevention, detection, evaluation, and treatment of high blood pressure: the JNC 7 report. *JAMA* 2003; **289:** 2560–72. Correction. *ibid.*; **290:** 197.
3. McCrae AF, Wildsmith JAW. Prevention and treatment of hypotension during central neural block. *Br J Anaesth* 1993; **70:** 672–80.
4. Task Force on Syncope, European Society of Cardiology. Guidelines on management (diagnosis and treatment) of syncope. *Eur Heart J* 2001; **22:** 1256–306.
Also available at: http://www.escardio.org/NR/rdonlyres/4614BBA0-2AE9-414C-A44F-1369DD1A81CC/0/managementsyncope.pdf (accessed 14/05/04)
5. Benditt DG, *et al.* Pharmacotherapy of neurally mediated syncope. *Circulation* 1999; **100:** 1242–8.
6. Fenton AM, *et al.* Vasovagal syncope. *Ann Intern Med* 2000; **133:** 714–25.
7. Gatzoulis KA, Toutouzas PK. Neurocardiogenic syncope: aetiology and management. *Drugs* 2001; **61:** 1415–23.
8. Lazarus JC, Mauro VF. Syncope: pathophysiology, diagnosis, and pharmacotherapy. *Ann Pharmacother* 1996; **30:** 994–1005.
9. Ward CR, *et al.* Midodrine: a role in the management of neurocardiogenic syncope. *Heart* 1998; **79:** 45–9.
10. Mann A. Psychiatric symptoms and low blood pressure. *BMJ* 1992; **304:** 64–5.
11. Rosengren A, *et al.* Low systolic blood pressure and self perceived wellbeing in middle aged men. *BMJ* 1993; **306:** 243–6.
12. Barrett-Connor E, Palinkas LA. Low blood pressure and depression in older men: a population based study. *BMJ* 1994; **308:** 446–9.
13. Rowe PC, *et al.* Is neurally mediated hypotension an unrecognised cause of chronic fatigue? *Lancet* 1995; **345:** 623–4.
14. Bou-Holaigah I, *et al.* The relationship between neurally mediated hypotension and the chronic fatigue syndrome. *JAMA* 1995; **274:** 961–7.

## Kawasaki disease

Cardiac effects including coronary artery abnormalities are the major complications of Kawasaki disease, also known as mucocutaneous lymph node syndrome of childhood. Normal immunoglobulin and aspirin are used in its initial management, and antiplatelet therapy, usually with aspirin, may be continued long term to prevent coronary thrombosis. Further details concerning the overall management of Kawasaki disease are provided under Normal Immunoglobulins, p.1629.

## Myocardial infarction

Myocardial infarction is defined as necrosis of heart muscle caused by ischaemia.[1] It is part of the spectrum of acute coronary syndromes, which includes unstable angina, non-Q wave, and Q wave myocardial infarction. Although it has been suggested that any degree of myocardial necrosis should be defined as a myocardial infarction, since it indicates a worse prognosis, treatment differs depending on the degree of damage, and in practice the diagnosis of acute myocardial infarction is generally made on clinical grounds, determined by characteristic symptoms, ECG changes, and changes in biochemical markers. The following discussion relates to the management of acute myocardial infarction; the management of other acute coronary syndromes is discussed under Angina Pectoris (p.813).

Although the incidence may be declining, myocardial infarction remains a leading cause of mortality in western societies. The introduction of aspirin and thrombolytics has transformed the management of acute myocardial infarction, but a significant number of deaths are sudden deaths that occur within the first hour and therefore before treatment can be initiated. While new therapies for the management of acute myocardial infarction may further reduce in-hospital mortality, earlier recognition and presentation for treatment is important if survival is to be improved further, and primary prophylaxis in patients at risk or at a population level may also have a role (see Cardiovascular Risk Reduction, p.819). Patients who survive a myocardial infarction are at high risk for further cardiovascular events and also frequently develop complications such as arrhythmias, left ventricular failure, persistent angina, and venous thromboembolism. Management of acute myocardial infarction therefore involves both early treatment of the acute condition, and long-term therapy in survivors to reduce risk and to treat and prevent complications.

Myocardial ischaemia generally occurs as a result of coronary artery occlusion, usually due to thrombosis at the site of a recently ruptured atheromatous plaque; in a few patients coronary embolism or spasm, arteritis, spontaneous thrombosis, or a sudden severe rise in blood pressure, as in phaeochromocytoma, is responsible. The immediate consequence of coronary occlusion is myocardial ischaemia which leads to impaired contractility, arrhythmias, and eventually myocardial cell death. The lay term 'heart attack' describes both sudden cardiac death and myocardial infarction. Sudden death is usually due to ventricular fibrillation and most patients who are resuscitated from ventricular fibrillation develop features of myocardial infarction or have coronary artery disease. In many cases myocardial infarction is asymptomatic or 'silent' and is only diagnosed due to characteristic changes on the ECG.[2]

**Early management.** Guidelines[3-6] and reviews[7,8] emphasise the importance of rapid recognition and treatment of patients with acute myocardial infarction. The initial symptoms are usually chest pain, breathlessness, and sweating. The chest pain is typically severe and resembles that of angina pectoris, being precordial with radiation to the neck, lower jaw, and left arm; chest pain lasting more than 20 minutes is generally considered to indicate myocardial infarction, although this is absent in many patients. Other signs and symptoms include nausea and vomiting, bradycardia, hypotension, and apprehension. Characteristic ECG changes including ST segment elevation and left bundle branch block confirm the clinical diagnosis and guide initial treatment; elevation of biochemical markers such as troponins and cardiac enzymes develops later and is useful for confirming the diagnosis and determining prognosis.

Those patients with myocardial infarction who develop ventricular fibrillation very quickly have a high mortality and require rapid provision of life support measures. Ventricular fibrillation is treated by defibrillation followed by adrenaline and possibly antiarrhythmics if defibrillation alone is unsuccessful (see Advanced Cardiac Life Support, p.812, for further details). Paramedic ambulance teams experienced in defibrillation and programmes aimed at educating the public in the basic techniques of cardiopulmonary resuscitation have an important role. Patients with suspected myocardial infarction should be admitted to hospital and where possible managed in a coronary care unit.

The immediate priority in patients with myocardial infarction is administration of aspirin, followed by relief of pain and anxiety. Pain should be relieved with an opioid analgesic, usually diamorphine or morphine given intravenously (see Myocardial Infarction Pain, p.7); an antiemetic such as metoclopramide intravenously may also be necessary. Supplemental oxygen should also be given. An inhaled mixture of nitrous oxide and oxygen (Entonox) has sometimes been used to provide pain relief before arrival in hospital; sublingual glyceryl trinitrate or an alternative fast-acting nitrate may also be given. A benzodiazepine may be useful for anxiety.

In patients with confirmed myocardial infarction, rapid reperfusion is important since myocardial recovery depends on the duration of ischaemia. It is usually achieved with a thrombolytic such as streptokinase given intravenously and the antiplatelet drug aspirin by mouth. Aspirin should be given immediately since it is of benefit in both myocardial infarction and unstable angina. The thrombolytic should be given as soon as an ECG has been performed to confirm the diagnosis; alternatively, reperfusion may be achieved with angioplasty.

***Thrombolysis.*** Thrombolytics are given intravenously to break up the thrombus or clot and restore the patency of the coronary artery, thereby limiting infarct size and irreversible damage to the myocardium. Several large studies have established that thrombolytics can preserve left ventricular function and improve short-term and long-term mortality in patients with ECG evidence of ST elevation or new left bundle branch block (for more details see Ischaemic Heart Disease under Uses of Streptokinase, p.1008). The greatest benefit is seen in those given thrombolytics early;[9] mortality is significantly reduced in those receiving treatment within 6 hours of symptom onset, and there is also benefit up to 12 hours. In those presenting later than 12 hours, the benefits are less well established; there has been some evidence of early excess mortality due to cardiac rupture in some patients given late thrombolytics. Evidence of benefit in patients over the age of 75 years is also limited,[9] and a retrospective analysis[10] of thrombolytic therapy in older patients suggested that mortality may be increased in those over 75, although this has been challenged.[11] Guidelines therefore recommend that all patients presenting with an appropriate ECG within 12 hours of symptom onset should receive thrombolytic therapy, unless they have specific contra-indications (see Precautions under Streptokinase, p.1007); in those presenting later than 12 hours after symptom onset thrombolytics should generally only be given if there is evidence of ongoing ischaemia. The thrombolytic should be given as soon as possible; recommendations are for a delay of no more than 90 minutes between calling the medical services and administration ('call to needle' time),[3] and for no more than 30 minutes between admission to hospital and administration ('door to needle' time).[3,6] Prehospital thrombolysis is feasible and reduces the time to thrombolytic administration and short-term mortality.[12] Five-year follow-up of one study[13] has suggested that there is also a beneficial effect on long-term mortality.

Streptokinase has been the most widely used thrombolytic. Overall efficacy appears to be similar for all the drugs available and factors such as cost, method of administration, and contra-indications help to determine the choice. Different thrombolytic regimens and adjunctive therapies are being investigated in attempts to improve patency rates.[14] However, ensuring that a thrombolytic is given as soon as possible is probably more important than which is given.[15] If streptokinase or anistreplase, so-called antigenic thrombolytics, have been used recently, non-antigenic drugs such as alteplase or urokinase should be given.

The overall effectiveness of thrombolytics is limited by persistent coronary occlusion, re-occlusion, and infrequent but serious bleeding complications including intracranial haemorrhage. If reperfusion fails or re-occlusion occurs further thrombolytic therapy may be given or angioplasty may be performed.[3,16,17] Antiplatelet and antithrombin drugs are given as adjuncts to thrombolytics.

***Antiplatelet drugs.*** The value of giving aspirin by mouth as an antiplatelet drug was shown by the ISIS-2 study,[18] in which aspirin started during the first 24 hours after myocardial infarction reduced mortality and also reduced the incidence of re-infarction and stroke. Use with streptokinase proved to be more effective than either streptokinase or aspirin alone. Aspirin should therefore be taken as soon as possible when myocardial infarction is suspected and the tablet chewed so that some buccal absorption occurs. For patients with aspirin allergy, dipyridamole, clopidogrel, or ticlopidine are alternatives.[4,5] Additional antiplatelet therapy with glycoprotein IIb/IIIa inhibitors has also been investigated in an attempt to further improve outcomes. In patients receiving primary angioplasty, benefit has been shown with abciximab.[19,20] Studies have also shown improved rates of reperfusion when glycoprotein IIb/IIIa inhibitors are used with thrombolytics, but evidence of long-term benefit is limited. In patients with acute myocardial infarction, abciximab given as an adjunct to thrombolysis improved early patency rates,[21] but a further study[22] that assessed mortality found no benefit over thrombolysis alone at 30 days; similar results were found in a study[23] with eptifibatide. However, in the ASSENT-3 study,[24] combination of abciximab with half-dose tenecteplase and heparin resulted in a significant improvement in outcomes at 30 days, although bleeding rates were also significantly increased.

***Anticoagulants.*** Heparin was widely used in acute myocardial infarction before thrombolytics were available, but the necessity for adjuvant therapy with heparin in addition to aspirin is not certain. An overview of randomised studies[25] found that in patients receiving aspirin, addition of heparin (either intravenous or subcutaneous) produced a small reduction in mortality but was associated with an excess of major bleeds. The authors concluded that the routine addition of heparin to aspirin could not be justified. However, many centres administer parenteral heparin with or shortly after thrombolytic therapy to prevent the re-occlusion of the coronary artery often associated with thrombolysis. Alteplase appears to open occluded arteries more rapidly but to cause re-occlusion more often than streptokinase, and thus heparin is recommended[3,5] when alteplase is used; this may also apply for reteplase and tenecteplase. Low-molecular-weight heparins may be an alternative; in the ASSENT-3 study,[24] improved outcomes were reported in patients receiving a combination of tenecteplase with enoxaparin compared with those receiving tenecteplase with unfractionated heparin. Alternatives to heparin such as the thrombin inhibitors bivalirudin, desirudin, and lepirudin, have been investigated although results have been disappointing. Early studies reported increased bleeding and no additional benefit (see under Lepirudin, p.945). Later studies used lower doses and resulted in reduced bleeding, but no outcome benefit was found. The place of thrombin inhibitors is therefore not established, although they may be useful in patients who develop heparin-induced thrombocytopenia. Heparin is also given prophylactically to myocardial infarction patients at risk of developing left ventricular mural thrombosis with subsequent systemic embolisation. Patients with complications following myocardial infarction who are likely to be immobile for several days should also receive heparin prophylaxis.

***Angioplasty.*** Percutaneous transluminal coronary angioplasty is effective at re-opening occluded coronary arteries and immediate angioplasty (termed primary angioplasty) has been performed as an alternative method of reperfusion to thrombolysis. A review of randomised studies comparing primary angioplasty with thrombolysis concluded that primary angioplasty was associated with lower mortality and re-infarction rates both early (4 to 6 weeks) and late (6 to 18 months) after myocardial infarction.[26] Long-term follow-up in one study[27] has found that the benefit is maintained at 5 years. Observational studies[28,29] have suggested that thrombolysis and primary angioplasty offer similar efficacy. Where angioplasty is available it may be considered, particularly for patients in whom thrombolytics are contra-indicated or in patients at highest risk such as those with cardiogenic shock.[3-5] Since angioplasty is only available in specialised cardiac centres, thrombolysis will remain the method of reperfusion for the majority of patients. However, transfer to a specialised centre for angioplasty may be of benefit.[26] Angioplasty may also be considered when thrombolytic therapy has failed to unblock the artery (so-called 'rescue' angioplasty). The use of antithrombotic therapy and other treatments given with angioplasty to prevent re-occlusion and restenosis is discussed under Reperfusion and Revascularisation Procedures (p.834).

Thus, at present, standard early therapy for the majority of patients with myocardial infarction is streptokinase with aspirin, and possibly heparin. Other early treatments that have been tried include beta blockers, nitrates, ACE inhibitors, magnesium, and calcium-channel blockers.

***Beta blockers.*** In studies performed before the routine use of thrombolytics the intravenous administration of beta blockers, such as atenolol and metoprolol, in the early period following myocardial infarction was associated with a reduction in mortality. Contributory mechanisms were considered to be a reduction in size of infarction or number of re-infarctions and an antiarrhythmic effect, although the ISIS-1 study[30] suggested that beta blockers improved early survival by reducing the incidence of cardiac rupture. The role of beta blockers in the thrombolytic era is less certain, but an overview of randomised studies[31] indicated that early use of intravenous beta blockers definitely reduced mortality after myocardial infarction. They appear to be less widely used in the UK than in the US.[32]

***Nitrates.*** The use of intravenous nitrates (glyceryl trinitrate or sodium nitroprusside), started within 24 hours of the onset of pain, has been associated with a reduction in mortality in patients with acute myocardial infarction,[33] although this was before the routine use of thrombolytics. The empirical use of intravenous glyceryl trinitrate in the acute phase of myocardial infarction is widespread and appears to be safe, as was demonstrated in the GISSI-3 study;[34] these workers considered that glyceryl trinitrate could be given when clinically indicated in addition to thrombolysis, aspirin, and a beta blocker.

***ACE inhibitors.*** ACE inhibitors have an established role in the long-term management of patients following myocardial infarction, but their use in the early stages is more controversial (see p.847). A systematic review[35] of studies of ACE inhibitors started within the first 1 to 2 days after acute myocardial infarction found that 30-day mortality and the incidence of heart failure were reduced in those receiving ACE inhibitors, although the greatest absolute benefit was seen in high-risk patients such as those who had already developed heart failure. The American College of Cardiology and American Heart Association recommend that early treatment with an ACE inhibitor should be considered in all patients, except those with cardiogenic shock or persistent severe hypotension, and that treatment should be reviewed after a few weeks and continued in those with left ventricular dysfunction. Others[36,37] consider that routine early treatment with an ACE inhibitor in unselected patients is not warranted and such use should be reserved for patients with signs of heart failure. The European Society of Cardiology recognises that opinions differ and advocates the early use of an ACE inhibitor if symptoms of heart failure appear.[3]

***Magnesium.*** Magnesium has an important physiological role in maintaining the ion balance in muscle including the myocardium and it has been suggested that administration of magnesium in acute myocardial infarction might protect against both arrhythmias and reperfusion injury. Early studies[38,39] suggested some evidence of benefit, but the larger ISIS-4 study[40] and the MAGIC study[41] found no effect on mortality. Although differences in study design make conclusions difficult, the routine use of magnesium is not currently recommended.

***Calcium-channel blockers.*** Studies have not shown a reduction in mortality when calcium-channel blockers are given in the early phase of acute myocardial infarction. However, since myocardial stunning has been linked to intracellular calcium overload[42] there has been speculation that calcium-channel blockers might benefit patients about to undergo reperfusion. This is yet to be confirmed.

***Metabolic support.*** Infusions containing glucose, insulin, and potassium have been used in small numbers of patients with the aim of providing metabolic support in the acute phase of myocardial infarction. A meta-analysis of randomised controlled trials that were performed before the widespread use of thrombolytics found that mortality was reduced in recipients of glucose-insulin-potassium.[43] A pilot study[44] including patients treated with thrombolytics or primary angioplasty reported similar findings, but the results require confirmation in larger trials. Reduced mortality has also been reported in diabetic patients with myocardial infarction given insulin-glucose infusions (see Myocardial Infarction under Insulin, p.342).

**Long-term management.** Patients who survive the immediate post-myocardial infarction period remain at high risk for cardiovascular mortality. The main predictors of poor outcome are the extent of left ventricular dysfunction, residual myocardial ischaemia, and ventricular arrhythmias. Follow-up should include cardiac rehabilitation and the identification and modification of risk factors for ischaemic heart disease (see Cardiovascular Risk Reduction, p.819). Exercise testing, echocardiography, myocardial imaging techniques, and pharmacological stress testing (see Myocardial Imaging under Dipyridamole, p.903) can be used after myocardial infarction to help identify those at high risk for recurrent ischaemic events and to select patients needing coronary angiography.[3-5] In patients who develop angina soon after myocardial infarction, exercise testing may be unhelpful and potentially hazardous, although many will need angiography to determine whether angioplasty or bypass surgery is required.

Drug therapy is important in the long-term management of patients following myocardial infarction, both for symptom control and for secondary prevention.[45-47] *Aspirin*, given during the acute phase and then continued for one to two years, has been shown to reduce mortality and re-infarction rates. A meta-analysis[48] confirmed the benefit of prolonged antiplatelet treatment in the secondary prevention of myocardial infarction and patients should receive antiplatelet therapy indefinitely. Clopidogrel appears to be as effective as aspirin[49] and should be considered in patients intolerant of, or with contra-indications to, aspirin; ticlopidine or sulfinpyrazone may be alternatives. The routine long-term use of *oral anticoagulation* after acute myocardial infarction remains to be established. Although studies such as ASPECT[50] found some benefit with full dose anticoagulation, this was before the routine use of aspirin; later studies[51] suggested that cardiac events were similar in patients receiving anticoagulants or aspirin, but that anticoagulants caused more bleeding. Several studies have used a combination of anticoagulants and aspirin, with mixed results. Low-intensity anticoagulation and aspirin appears to have no benefit over aspirin alone;[52,53] however, medium-intensity anticoagulation (INR 2.0 to 2.5) and aspirin may be more effective than aspirin alone,[54,55] although, again, bleeding may be increased. Those at high risk of systemic embolism because of atrial fibrillation, heart failure, or mobile mural thrombus require prophylaxis with oral anticoagulants, but for other patients aspirin is preferred.[5,45] Long-term prophylactic treatment with oral *beta blockers* (most studies have used propranolol, metoprolol, or timolol) has reduced mortality and the rate of re-infarction.[56] In patients with no contra-indications to beta-blocker therapy (see Precautions, p.870) they are usually started before hospital discharge and continued for a minimum of one year; indefinite use has been recommended.[3-5] Although some only use them in patients with hypertension or angina pectoris following myocardial infarction, a survey of 201 752 patients who had suffered a myocardial infarction found that low-risk patients and those with conditions often considered to be contra-indications also benefited from administration of a beta blocker.[57] Beta blockers seem to be underused particularly in elderly patients even though there is clear evidence of benefit in this group.[58,59] *Calcium-channel blockers* are not routinely used in the long-term management of myocardial infarction, although in selected patients without heart failure verapamil or diltiazem may be of some benefit if beta blockers are contra-indicated. *ACE inhibitors* reduce left ventricular remodelling, a process which sometimes follows myocardial infarction and is a recognised precursor of symptomatic heart failure. Myocardial infarction patients with left ventricular dysfunction benefit from long-term oral administration of ACE inhibitors started early after infarction and continued for at least 4 to 6 weeks.[60,61] Long-term use of ACE inhibitors in patients without left ventricular dysfunction is less established, since less benefit has been found in this group. However, the HOPE study[62] found that treatment with ramipril significantly improved outcome in patients at high risk for cardiovascular disease, including patients with previous myocardial infarction but preserved left ventricular function, and some guidelines[45,46] therefore recommend that ACE inhibitors should be given long-term to all patients following myocardial infarction. Angiotensin II receptor antagonists may be an alternative; a study[63] comparing valsartan with captopril found that both were equally effective, although another study[64] comparing losartan with captopril suggested that ACE inhibitors should remain first-line. *Statins*, such as simvastatin and pravastatin, are effective in the primary and secondary prevention of myocardial infarction in patients with both high and average cholesterol concentrations and their use has been advocated in all patients who have suffered a myocardial infarction (see Cardiovascular Risk Reduction, p.819). Some patients, for example those with myocardial ischaemia or poor left ventricular function, may require the long-term administration of *nitrates*, but there is no evidence to support their routine use in all patients.[3,45] Patients with acute myocardial infarction may have magnesium deficiency and long-term treatment with *oral magnesium* has been tried, but in one study was associated with an increased risk of adverse cardiac events and could not be recommended for secondary prevention.[65]

Post-infarction problems such as heart failure (left ventricular dysfunction), angina pectoris, and arrhythmias are discussed on p.820, p.813, and p.816, respectively.


1. The Joint European Society of Cardiology/American College of Cardiology Committee. Myocardial infarction redefined—a consensus document of The Joint European Society of Cardiology/American College of Cardiology Committee for the redefinition of myocardial infarction. *Eur Heart J* 2000; **21:** 1502–13.
2. Sheifer SE, *et al.* Unrecognized myocardial infarction. *Ann Intern Med* 2001; **135:** 801–11.
3. The Task Force on the Management of Acute Myocardial Infarction of the European Society of Cardiology. Management of acute myocardial infarction in patients presenting with ST-segment elevation. *Eur Heart J* 2003; **24:** 28–66. Also available at: http://www.escardio.org/NR/rdonlyres/18AB1C95-7959-4D2D-A40E-BA51DE4052FA/0/AMI_02.pdf (accessed 12/05/04)
4. Ryan TJ, *et al.* ACC/AHA guidelines for the management of patients with acute myocardial infarction: a report of the American College of Cardiology/American Heart Association Task Force on Practice Guidelines (Committee on Management of Acute Myocardial Infarction). *J Am Coll Cardiol* 1996; **28:** 1328–1428.
5. Ryan TJ, *et al.* 1999 update: ACC/AHA guidelines for the management of patients with acute myocardial infarction: a report of the American College of Cardiology/American Heart Association Task Force on Practice Guidelines (Committee on Management of Acute Myocardial Infarction). *J Am Coll Cardiol* 1999; **34:** 890–911. Also available at: http://www.acc.org/clinical/guidelines/nov96/edits/amipdf99edits.pdf (accessed 07/07/04)
6. The American Heart Association in collaboration with the International Liaison Committee on Resuscitation (ILCOR). International guidelines 2000 for cardiopulmonary resuscitation and emergency cardiovascular care. Part 7: the era of reperfusion. Section 1: acute coronary syndromes (acute myocardial infarction). *Circulation* 2000; **102** (suppl I): I172–I203.
7. Gershlick AH. The acute management of myocardial infarction. *Br Med Bull* 2001; **59:** 89–112.
8. Maxwell S. Emergency management of acute myocardial infarction. *Br J Clin Pharmacol* 1999; **48:** 284–98.
9. Fibrinolytic Therapy Trialists' (FTT) Collaborative Group. Indications for fibrinolytic therapy in suspected acute myocardial infarction: collaborative overview of early mortality and major morbidity results from all randomised trials of more than 1000 patients. *Lancet* 1994; **343:** 311–22.
10. Thiemann DR, *et al.* Lack of benefit for intravenous thrombolysis in patients with myocardial infarction who are older than 75 years. *Circulation* 2000; **101:** 2239–46.
11. White HD. Thrombolytic therapy in the elderly. *Lancet* 2000; **356:** 2028–30.
12. Morrison LJ, *et al.* Mortality and prehospital thrombolysis for acute myocardial infarction: a meta-analysis. *JAMA* 2000; **283:** 2686–92.
13. Rawles JM. Quantification of the benefit of earlier thrombolytic therapy: five-year results of the Grampian Region Early Anistreplase Trial (GREAT). *J Am Coll Cardiol* 1997; **30:** 1181–6.
14. Wright RS, *et al.* Update on intravenous fibrinolytic therapy for acute myocardial infarction. *Mayo Clin Proc* 2000; **75:** 1185–91.
15. Collins R, *et al.* Aspirin, heparin, and fibrinolytic therapy in suspected acute myocardial infarction. *N Engl J Med* 1997; **336:** 847–60.
16. Goldman LE, Eisenberg MJ. Identification and management of patients with failed thrombolysis after acute myocardial infarction. *Ann Intern Med* 2000; **132:** 556–65.
17. de Belder MA. Acute myocardial infarction: failed thrombolysis. *Heart* 2001; **85:** 104–112.
18. Second International Study of Infarct Survival Collaborative Group. Randomised trial of intravenous streptokinase, oral aspirin, both, or neither among 17 187 cases of suspected acute myocardial infarction: ISIS-2. *Lancet* 1988; **ii:** 349–60.
19. Brener SJ, *et al.* Randomized, placebo-controlled trial of platelet glycoprotein IIb/IIIa blockade with primary angioplasty for acute myocardial infarction. *Circulation* 1998; **98:** 734–41.
20. Montalescot G, *et al.* Platelet glycoprotein IIb/IIIa inhibition with coronary stenting for acute myocardial infarction. *N Engl J Med* 2001; **344:** 1895–1903.
21. Antman EM, *et al.* Abciximab facilitates the rate and extent of thrombolysis: results of the Thrombolysis in Myocardial Infarction (TIMI) 14 trial. *Circulation* 1999; **99:** 2720–32.
22. The GUSTO V Investigators. Reperfusion therapy for acute myocardial infarction with fibrinolytic therapy or combination reduced fibrinolytic therapy and platelet glycoprotein IIb/IIIa inhibition: the GUSTO V randomised trial. *Lancet* 2001; **357:** 1905–14. Correction. *ibid.*; **358:** 512.
23. Brener SJ, *et al.* Eptifibatide and low-dose tissue plasminogen activator in acute myocardial infarction: the integrilin and low-dose thrombolysis in acute myocardial infarction (INTRO AMI) trial. *J Am Coll Cardiol* 2002; **39:** 377–86.
24. The Assessment of the Safety and Efficacy of a New Thrombolytic Regimen (ASSENT)-3 Investigators. Efficacy and safety of tenecteplase in combination with enoxaparin, abciximab, or unfractionated heparin: the ASSENT-3 randomised trial in acute myocardial infarction. *Lancet* 2001; **358:** 605–613.
25. Collins R, *et al.* Clinical effects of anticoagulant therapy in suspected acute myocardial infarction: systematic overview of randomised trials. *BMJ* 1996; **313:** 652–9.
26. Keeley EC, *et al.* Primary angioplasty versus intravenous thrombolytic therapy for acute myocardial infarction: a quantitative review of 23 randomised trials. *Lancet* 2003; **361:** 13–20.
27. Zijlstra F, *et al.* Long-term benefit of primary angioplasty as compared with thrombolytic therapy for acute myocardial infarction. *N Engl J Med* 1999; **341:** 1413–19.
28. Every NR, *et al.* A comparison of thrombolytic therapy with primary coronary angioplasty for acute myocardial infarction. *N Engl J Med* 1996; **335:** 1253–60.
29. Tiefenbrunn AJ, *et al.* Clinical experience with primary percutaneous transluminal coronary angioplasty compared with alteplase (recombinant tissue-type plasminogen activator) in patients with acute myocardial infarction: a report from the second National Registry of Myocardial Infarction (NRMI-2). *J Am Coll Cardiol* 1998; **31:** 1240–5.
30. First International Study of Infarct Survival Collaborative Group. Mechanisms for the early mortality reduction produced by beta-blockade started early in acute myocardial infarction: ISIS-1. *Lancet* 1988; **i:** 921–3.
31. Teo KK, *et al.* Effects of prophylactic antiarrhythmic drug therapy in acute myocardial infarction: an overview of results from randomized controlled trials. *JAMA* 1993; **270:** 1589–95.
32. Owen A. Intravenous β blockade in acute myocardial infarction. *BMJ* 1998; **317:** 226–7.
33. Yusuf S, *et al.* Effect of intravenous nitrates on mortality in acute myocardial infarction: an overview of the randomised trials. *Lancet* 1988; **i:** 1088–92.
34. Gruppo Italiano per lo Studio della Sopravvivenza nell'Infarto Miocardico. GISSI-3: effects of lisinopril and transdermal glyceryl trinitrate singly and together on 6-week mortality and ventricular function after acute myocardial infarction. *Lancet* 1994; **343:** 1115–22.
35. ACE Inhibitor Myocardial Infarction Collaborative Group. Indications for ACE inhibitors in the early treatment of acute myocardial infarction: systematic overview of individual data from 100 000 patients in randomized trials. *Circulation* 1998; **97:** 2202–12.
36. Ertl G, Jugdutt B. ACE inhibition after myocardial infarction: can megatrials provide answers? *Lancet* 1994; **344:** 1068–9.
37. Hall AS, *et al.* Inhibition of the renin-angiotensin system after acute myocardial infarction—treat first, select later? *Heart* 1996; **76** (suppl 3): 73–8.
38. Teo KK, *et al.* Effects of intravenous magnesium in suspected acute myocardial infarction: overview of randomised trials. *BMJ* 1991; **303:** 1499–1503.
39. Woods KL, *et al.* Intravenous magnesium sulphate in suspected acute myocardial infarction: results of the second Leicester Intravenous Magnesium Intervention Trial (LIMIT-2). *Lancet* 1992; **339:** 1553–8.
40. ISIS-4 (Fourth International Study of Infarct Survival) Collaborative Group. ISIS-4: a randomised factorial trial assessing early oral captopril, oral mononitrate, and intravenous magnesium sulphate in 58 050 patients with suspected acute myocardial infarction. *Lancet* 1995; **345:** 669–85.
41. The Magnesium in Coronaries (MAGIC) Trial Investigators. Early administration of intravenous magnesium to high-risk patients with acute myocardial infarction in the Magnesium in Coronaries (MAGIC) Trial: a randomised controlled trial. *Lancet* 2002; **360:** 1189–96.
42. Anonymous. Myocardial stunning. *Lancet* 1991; **337:** 585–6.
43. Fath-Ordoubadi F, Beatt KJ. Glucose-insulin-potassium therapy for treatment of acute myocardial infarction: an overview of randomized placebo-controlled trials. *Circulation* 1997; **96:** 1152–6.
44. Díaz R, *et al.* Metabolic modulation of acute myocardial infarction: the ECLA glucose-insulin-potassium pilot trial. *Circulation* 1998; **98:** 2227–34.
45. Scottish Intercollegiate Guidelines Network. Secondary prevention of coronary heart disease following myocardial infarction: a national clinical guideline (issued January 2000). Available at: http://www.show.scot.nhs.uk/sign/pdf/sign41.pdf (accessed 14/05/04)
46. North of England Evidence-based Guidelines Development Project. Prophylaxis for patients who have experienced a myocardial infarction: drug treatment, cardiac rehabilitation and dietary manipulation (issued April 2001). Available at: http://www.nice.org.uk/pdf/clinicalguidelinemiguidance yorknewcastle.pdf (accessed 14/05/04)
47. Maxwell S, Waring WS. Drugs used in secondary prevention after myocardial infarction: case presentation. *Br J Clin Pharmacol* 2000; **50:** 405–417.
48. Antithrombotic Trialists' Collaboration. Collaborative meta-analysis of randomised trials of antiplatelet therapy for prevention of death, myocardial infarction, and stroke in high risk patients. *BMJ* 2002; **324:** 71–86.
49. CAPRIE Steering Committee. A randomised, blinded, trial of clopidogrel versus aspirin in patients at risk of ischaemic events (CAPRIE). *Lancet* 1996; **348:** 1329–39.
50. Anticoagulants in the Secondary Prevention of Events in Coronary Thrombosis (ASPECT) Research Group. Effects of long-term oral anticoagulant treatment on mortality and cardiovascular morbidity after myocardial infarction. *Lancet* 1994; **343:** 499–503.
51. Julian DG, *et al.* A comparison of aspirin and anticoagulation following thrombolysis for myocardial infarction (the AFTER Study): a multicentre unblinded randomised clinical trial. *BMJ* 1996; **313:** 1429–31.
52. Coumadin Aspirin Reinfarction Study (CARS) Investigators. Randomised double-blind trial of fixed low-dose warfarin with aspirin after myocardial infarction. *Lancet* 1997; **350:** 389–96.
53. Fiore LD, *et al.* Department of Veterans Affairs Cooperative Studies Program Clinical Trial comparing combined warfarin and aspirin with aspirin alone in survivors of acute myocardial infarction: primary results of the CHAMP study. *Circulation* 2002; **105:** 557–63.
54. van Es RF, *et al.* Aspirin and coumadin after acute coronary syndromes (the ASPECT-2 study): a randomised controlled trial. *Lancet* 2002; **360:** 109–13.
55. Hurlen M, *et al.* Warfarin, aspirin, or both after myocardial infarction. *N Engl J Med* 2002; **347:** 969–74.
56. Freemantle N, *et al.* β Blockade after myocardial infarction: systematic review and meta regression analysis. *BMJ* 1999; **318:** 1730–7. Correction. *ibid.* 2000; **321:** 482.
57. Gottlieb SS, *et al.* Effect of beta-blockade on mortality among high-risk and low-risk patients after myocardial infarction. *N Engl J Med* 1998; **339:** 489–97.
58. Soumerai SB, *et al.* Adverse outcomes of underuse of β-blockers in elderly survivors of acute myocardial infarction. *JAMA* 1997; **277:** 115–21.
59. Krumholz HM, *et al.* National use and effectiveness of β-blockers for the treatment of elderly patients after acute myocardial infarction: National Cooperative Cardiovascular Project. *JAMA* 1998; **280:** 623–9. Correction. *ibid.* 1999; **281:** 37.
60. Latini R, *et al.* ACE inhibitor use in patients with myocardial infarction: summary of evidence from clinical trials. *Circulation* 1995; **92:** 3132–7.
61. Reynolds G, *et al.* What have the ACE-inhibitor trials in post-myocardial patients with left ventricular dysfunction taught us? *Eur J Clin Pharmacol* 1996; **49:** S35–S39.
62. The Heart Outcomes Prevention Evaluation Study Investigators. Effects of an angiotensin-converting-enzyme inhibitor, ramipril, on cardiovascular events in high-risk patients. *N Engl J Med* 2000; **342:** 145–53.
63. Pfeffer MA, *et al.* Valsartan, captopril, or both in myocardial infarction complicated by heart failure, left ventricular dysfunction, or both. *N Engl J Med* 2003; **349:** 1893–906. Correction. *ibid.* 2004; **350:** 203.
64. Dickstein K, *et al.* Effects of losartan and captopril on mortality and morbidity in high-risk patients after acute myocardial infarction: the OPTIMAAL randomised trial. *Lancet* 2002; **360:** 752–60.
65. Galløe AM, *et al.* Influence of oral magnesium supplementation on cardiac events among survivors of an acute myocardial infarction. *BMJ* 1993; **307:** 585–7.


### Patent ductus arteriosus

The ductus arteriosus is a vascular channel present in the fetal circulation that connects the pulmonary artery and the descending aorta. In some infants the ductus arteriosus fails to close, a condition known as persistent patent ductus arteriosus. Details of its management are given on p.49.

### Peripheral arterial thromboembolism

Occlusion of the peripheral arteries may occur due to embolism or thrombosis (see Thromboembolic Disorders, p.837). Sudden or acute occlusion causes reduction of blood flow to the distal portions of the limb and may lead to critical limb ischaemia. Emergency treatment with surgery or thrombolytic drugs is often required to restore blood flow and preserve the limb.

Acute peripheral arterial thromboembolism produces pain, pallor, and coldness in the affected limb. Numbness and paraesthesia may occur and if the clot is not removed, gangrene develops. Sudden onset is usually due to occlusion by an embolus. The heart is a frequent source of emboli; atrial fibrillation, cardiomyopathy, myocardial infarction, and valvular heart disease are all associated with peripheral arterial embolism. Peripheral arterial thrombosis often has a more gradual onset due to collateral vessels maintaining some perfusion of the limb. Thrombosis is usually the result of thrombus formation at a site of atheroma in an atherosclerotic artery; thus it may occur in patients with chronic occlusive arterial disease (see Peripheral Vascular Disease, p.831). Thrombosis is now more common than pure embolism although the two may co-exist.

Sudden arterial occlusion requires emergency treatment to restore circulation and to avoid gangrene and possible amputation of the limb. Where there is imminent danger to the limb surgery is necessary to rapidly restore blood flow. In patients with **embolism** in otherwise healthy arteries surgical removal of the embolus by catheter (embolectomy) is used and usually results in restoration of blood flow. Sudden arterial occlusion due to **thrombosis** where gangrene is imminent requires emergency bypass surgery to restore blood flow; surgical removal of a thrombus (thrombectomy) is not usually successful as most arterial thromboses are superimposed on atheromatous plaques, particularly in elderly patients, and thrombectomy adds to the intimal damage.

Where the risk from ischaemia is less acute, angiography may be performed to confirm the type of occlusion, and intra-arterial thrombolysis may be used as initial therapy, particularly if the cause is thrombotic.[1-4] This method is particularly useful for occlusion of smaller vessels, distal occlusions in surgically inaccessible small arteries, or in patients too ill to undergo surgery. However, it is a slower method of restoring blood flow and its use in limb-threatening ischaemia is controversial.[5] The TOPAS study[6] reported no significant difference in outcomes in patients with acute arterial occlusion treated initially with thrombolysis or surgery, although the rate of bleeding complications was higher with thrombolysis. It has therefore been suggested that thrombolysis may be appropriate for initial therapy in acute occlusion, providing this will not lead to an unacceptable delay in reperfusion.[7,8] However, others[9] consider that thrombolysis should not be used as first-line therapy due to the lack of significant benefit and the increased risk of bleeding.

Thrombolytics may be given intravenously, but intra-arterial administration of low doses of thrombolytics directly into the clot is often used. Despite the use of low doses the risk of major haemorrhage is still about 10%. Continuous intra-arterial infusion, pulse infusion, and different thrombolytics are used; the optimal technique and choice of thrombolytic are unclear. Alteplase, streptokinase, and urokinase are all used. Local treatment with low-dose streptokinase or urokinase infused into the clot is successful in about 50 to 80% of patients and recanalisation is sustained for a year in 50%. Thrombolytic therapy is more likely to be successful if it is begun soon after thrombosis occurs. If no lysis has occurred within the first 12 to 24 hours the procedure is unlikely to be successful, but where thrombolysis is occurring infusion has been continued for several days. There is rather less experience with alteplase; it is claimed to produce more rapid thrombolysis than streptokinase although studies have been too small to provide evidence of reduced limb loss or mortality.[1] On completion of thrombolytic therapy angiography should be repeated to identify the underlying abnormalities that caused the original occlusion. The lesions can then be treated by balloon angioplasty or surgical repair, and this should be done as soon as possible to avoid rethrombosis, which occurs in about 10 to 30% of patients.

Intra-arterial thrombolysis may also be used in conjunction with surgical techniques, particularly when surgery fails to restore blood flow due to distal occlusions.[10-13]

Adjunctive treatment with antithrombotics, such as heparin and aspirin, is often given to patients with peripheral arterial thromboembolism to prevent propagation of the clot and also to prevent postoperative thromboembolic complications. However, there is an increased risk of serious bleeding complications if heparin is used with thrombolytic therapy.[6] Glycoprotein IIb/IIIa-receptor antagonists, such as abciximab, have also been tried.[14] Where the occlusion has been due to embolism, the patient should be investigated for a possible source of emboli and long-term oral anticoagulation should be considered to prevent recurrent embolism.


1. Wolfe JH. Critical limb ischaemia. *Prescribers' J* 1994; **34:** 50–8.
2. Beattie DK, Davies AH. Management of the acutely ischaemic limb. *Br J Hosp Med* 1996; **55:** 204–8.
3. Ludlam CA, *et al.* Guidelines for the use of thrombolytic therapy. *Blood Coag Fibrinol* 1995; **6:** 273–85.
4. Callum K, Bradbury A. ABC of arterial and venous disease: acute limb ischaemia. *BMJ* 2000; **320:** 764–7. Correction. *ibid.*; 984.
5. Hawkins DW, Hirsh J. Antithrombotic drugs for thromboembolic disorders: a lesson in evidence-based medicine. *Am J Health-Syst Pharm* 1997; **54:** 1992–4.
6. Ouriel K, *et al.* A comparison of recombinant urokinase with vascular surgery as initial treatment for acute arterial occlusion of the legs. *N Engl J Med* 1998; **338:** 1105–15.
7. Working Party on Thrombolysis in the Management of Limb Ischemia. Thrombolysis in the management of lower limb peripheral arterial occlusion—a consensus document. *Am J Cardiol* 1998; **81:** 207–18.
8. Jackson MR, Clagett GP. Antithrombotic therapy in peripheral arterial occlusive disease. *Chest* 2001; **119** (suppl): 283S–299S.
9. Porter JM. Thrombolysis for acute arterial occlusion of the legs. *N Engl J Med* 1998; **338:** 1148–50.
10. Earnshaw JJ, Beard JD. Intraoperative use of thrombolytic agents. *BMJ* 1993; **307:** 638–9.
11. Chester JF, *et al.* Peroperative t-PA thrombolysis. *Lancet* 1991; **337:** 861–2.
12. Verstraete M. Use of thrombolytic drugs in non-coronary disorders. *Drugs* 1989; **38:** 801–21.
13. Anonymous. Non-coronary thrombolysis. *Lancet* 1990; **335:** 691–3.
14. Ansel GM, *et al.* Use of glycoprotein IIb/IIIa platelet inhibitors in peripheral vascular interventions. *Rev Cardiovasc Med* 2002; **3** (suppl 1): S35–S40.


## Peripheral vascular disease

The term peripheral vascular disease is often used for atherosclerotic or occlusive arterial disease but in its widest sense covers both arterial and venous disorders and may be due to atherosclerosis, vasospasm, or thromboembolism. Peripheral arterial occlusive disorders are the subject of the following discussion; for reviews of vasospastic arterial disorders see Raynaud's Syndrome (p.833), and for venous disorders see Venous Thromboembolism (p.839).

The commonest form of **occlusive arterial disease** is caused by atherosclerosis. It may well be only one manifestation of a generalised atherosclerotic process and sufferers also usually experience, or are at increased risk of, ischaemic heart disease. **Thromboangiitis obliterans** (Buerger's disease)[1] is also an occlusive arterial disease, but, rather than being caused by atherosclerosis, it is a result of inflammatory and proliferative lesions in medium and small arteries and veins of the limbs. The lesions are predominantly thrombotic in nature. It progresses more rapidly than atherosclerotic disease; severe ulceration and gangrene, necessitating amputation, may often occur. Sufferers are typically heavy smokers. **Intermittent claudication** is a major feature of occlusive arterial disease of the lower limbs and is characterised by pain that develops during exercise and which usually disappears at rest although it may persist in severe forms of disease. The pain is due to ischaemia (insufficient oxygen supply) resulting from the obstruction or vasoconstriction of peripheral arteries. Ischaemia may also result in trophic changes in the skin. In severe or advanced disease, ulceration of skin and tissues can occur and may even progress to gangrene. Although the cause of arterial obstruction is usually atherosclerosis, ischaemia is commonly precipitated by thrombosis. Smoking causes vasoconstriction and is frequently a contributory factor.

**Management**. Patients with occlusive arterial disease are at high risk of other cardiovascular events such as myocardial infarction and stroke, and treatment is important both to reduce this risk and to improve symptoms.[2-6] Measures to reduce cardiovascular risk (see p.819) include general lifestyle changes, antiplatelet therapy, treatment of hypertension and hyperlipidaemia, and smoking cessation. In the case of thromboangiitis obliterans, cessation of smoking is essential to halt progression of the disease. These measures do not generally improve symptoms in those with intermittent claudication, although supervised exercise programmes have been shown[7] to improve walking distance, and there is also some evidence[8] that lipid lowering therapy may do the same.

Many drugs have been employed for symptom control in occlusive arterial disease, but studies have often been unsatisfactory and their efficacy and/or overall place in management remains to be firmly established.[9]

*Vasodilators* have been the most commonly used drugs in intermittent claudication, although any purported benefit is probably due to mechanisms other than vasodilatation, such as actions on blood cells or changes in blood rheology. Vasodilators do not preferentially dilate the affected arteries, which may in any case be fully dilated already. Administration of vasodilators will result in dilatation of arteries supplying non-ischaemic tissues elsewhere in the body and thus blood may actually be diverted away from the affected ischaemic area—the so-called 'steal' phenomenon; this is a known risk with all vasodilators, but especially with powerful arterial vasodilators such as hydralazine and this type of drug is not suitable for use in peripheral arterial disease. Vasodilators that are used include *naftidrofuryl* and *pentoxifylline*; they may increase the time and distance walked before the onset of pain, but evidence of benefit is limited.[9,10] *Cilostazol*, which has antiplatelet and vasodilator effects, may also increase walking distance,[11] and it has been recommended in patients with disabling claudication.[12] Other vasodilators that have been promoted for the treatment of intermittent claudication include cinnarizine, cyclandelate, and inositol nicotinate; ketanserin, which inhibits vasoconstriction and also changes indices of blood rheology, has also been used.

Certain *prostaglandins* cause vasodilatation and prevent platelet aggregation and some may have a role in the presence of advanced disease or complications.[2,3] A beneficial effect on rest pain has been noted and some ulcers have either regressed or healed; in selected patients this form of therapy has avoided the need for amputation. Prostaglandins employed include *alprostadil* or *epoprostenol*, both intra-arterially or intravenously, *iloprost* intravenously, and *dinoprostone* topically. *Beraprost*, which is active orally, has also been used.

Other drugs that have shown positive results in small studies include ginkgo biloba,[9] levocarnitine[9,13] and sulodexide.[14] Local administration of growth factors[15] and gene therapy have also been tried.

If intermittent claudication is severe **non-pharmacological** techniques such as bypass surgery, endarterectomy, percutaneous transluminal angioplasty, or intravascular stenting should be considered. Following these procedures, treatment to prevent postoperative thrombosis and restenosis may be necessary (see Reperfusion and Revascularisation Procedures, p.834).

**Sudden** or **acute arterial occlusion** due to emboli or to thrombosis may occur in 10% of patients with atherosclerotic disease, but is rare in thromboangiitis obliterans. The initial approach has been surgical removal; dissolution of the thrombus using local or systemic thrombolytic therapy may be considered. For further details, see Peripheral Arterial Thromboembolism, p.830.


1. Olin JW. Thromboangiitis obliterans (Buerger's disease). *N Engl J Med* 2000; **343:** 864–9.
2. Hiatt WR. Medical treatment of peripheral arterial disease and claudication. *N Engl J Med* 2001; **344:** 1608–21.
3. Ouriel K. Peripheral arterial disease. *Lancet* 2001; **358:** 1257–64.
4. Regensteiner JG, Hiatt WR. Current medical therapies for patients with peripheral arterial disease: a critical review. *Am J Med* 2002; **112:** 49–57.
5. Burns P, *et al.* Management of peripheral arterial disease in primary care. *BMJ* 2003; **326:** 584–8.
6. Kim CK, *et al.* Pharmacological treatment of patients with peripheral arterial disease. *Drugs* 2003; **63:** 637–47.
7. Leng GC, *et al.* Exercise for intermittent claudication. Available in The Cochrane Library; Issue 2. Chichester: John Wiley; 2004.
8. Meade T, *et al.* Bezafibrate in men with lower extremity arterial disease: randomised controlled trial. *BMJ* 2002; **325:** 1139–43.
9. Moher D, *et al.* Pharmacological management of intermittent claudication: a meta-analysis of randomised trials. *Drugs* 2000; **59:** 1057–70.
10. Girolami B, *et al.* Treatment of intermittent claudication with physical training, smoking cessation, pentoxifylline, or nafronyl: a meta-analysis. *Arch Intern Med* 1999; **159:** 337–45.
11. Crouse JR, *et al.* Clinical manifestation of atherosclerotic peripheral arterial disease and the role of cilostazol in treatment of intermittent claudication. *J Clin Pharmacol* 2002; **42:** 1291–8.
12. Jackson MR, Clagett GP. Antithrombotic therapy in peripheral arterial occlusive disease. *Chest* 2001; **119** (suppl): 283S–299S.
13. Hiatt WR, *et al.* Propionyl-L-carnitine improves exercise performance and functional status in patients with claudication. *Am J Med* 2001; **110:** 616–22.
14. Coccheri S, *et al.* Sulodexide in the treatment of intermittent claudication: results of a randomized, double-blind, multicentre, placebo-controlled study. *Eur Heart J* 2002; **23:** 1057–65.
15. Lederman RJ, *et al.* Therapeutic angiogenesis with recombinant fibroblast growth factor-2 for intermittent claudication (the TRAFFIC study): a randomised trial. *Lancet* 2002; **359:** 2053–8.


## Phaeochromocytoma

Phaeochromocytoma is a rare catecholamine-secreting tumour of the adrenal medulla. Patients with phaeochromocytoma are usually hypertensive and suffer headache, palpitations, and excessive sweating; the hypertension may be either episodic or sustained. However, if the tumour is predominantly adrenaline-secreting, tachyarrhythmias may be associated with a normal or even decreased arterial pressure and if the tumour secretes mainly noradrenaline, vasoconstriction may lead to contraction of the venous pool and hypovolaemia. If the effects of the release of catecholamines are not controlled a life-threatening crisis ultimately ensues and may range from a shock-like syndrome with multiple organ failure to hypertensive crisis, depending on the predominance of the catecholamine secreted.

For a diagnosis of phaeochromocytoma, history and clinical symptoms are important, but a firm diagnosis requires further investigative techniques. Raised plasma or urinary concentrations of catecholamine metabolites indicate the presence of a tumour; measurement of urinary or plasma concentrations of adrenaline and noradrenaline may be necessary to confirm the diagnosis in some patients. The precise location of the tumour can be established by procedures such as computed tomography, magnetic resonance imaging, or scintigraphy with $^{131}$I-iobenguane ($^{131}$I-*m*-iodobenzylguanidine). Other tests that may be used include administration of drugs such as clonidine that suppress catecholamine release in normal patients but not in those with phaeochromocytoma. A glucagon stimulation test may also be used but other provocative tests are generally considered obsolete.

Although surgery to remove the tumour is the ultimate treatment goal, the initial step in management must be the prevention of the pressor and other effects of catecholamines. Alpha blockers, given by mouth, are the mainstay of therapy; they both reduce the blood pressure and allow the plasma volume to return to normal. Phenoxybenzamine is the alpha blocker of choice since the long-lasting, non-competitive blockade that it produces cannot be overridden by surges of catecholamine release, as may happen with competitive blockers. In patients who are unable to tolerate phenoxybenzamine, a selective alpha$_1$-adrenoceptor blocker such as prazosin may be used; it results in less tachycardia and may be preferable if the tumour is predominantly adrenaline-secreting, but hypotension may be a problem. Phentolamine may be given intravenously in patients with hypertensive crises. The initial dose of alpha blocker should be small and should be increased gradually until all signs of pressor activity are suppressed. Once, but not until, alpha blockade is successfully established, tachycardia can be controlled by the cautious use of a beta blocker. A beta$_1$-selective blocker is preferred so that peripheral beta$_2$-mediated vasodilatation is unaffected. α-Methyltyrosine, which suppresses catecholamine synthesis, may be tried in selected patients such as those resistant to alpha blockade or those in whom the effects of alpha or beta blockade may be undesirable.

Once the pressor effects of catecholamine secretion are controlled, surgery can be undertaken. Drugs used for premedication and anaesthesia should be chosen so as to avoid those which may cause pressor responses or tachycardia and ideally should suppress the adrenergic response to surgical stimuli. This will still not be adequate to prevent catecholamine release when the tumour is handled and potent vasodilators such as sodium nitroprusside or glyceryl trinitrate have been given intravenously to prevent dangerously high arterial pressures; the alpha blocker phentolamine has also been advocated although tachycardia is invariably a problem. Cardioselective beta blockers such as atenolol may be given, often in high dosage, to control tachycardia during surgery.

If it proves impossible to remove all the active tissue of a phaeochromocytoma during surgery, or in patients who are unsuitable for surgery or who have malignant phaeochromocytoma, maintenance therapy with alpha and beta blockade needs to be continued or α-methyltyrosine may be used. Alternatively, $^{131}$I-iobenguane has been given in high doses sufficient to cause radionecrosis; antineoplastic therapy has also been used.

References.


1. Klingler HC, *et al.* Pheochromocytoma. *Urology* 2001; **57:** 1025–32.
2. Pacak K, *et al.* Recent advances in genetics, diagnosis, localization, and treatment of pheochromocytoma. *Ann Intern Med* 2001; **134:** 315–29.


### Pulmonary hypertension

Pulmonary hypertension, unless otherwise specified, refers to pulmonary arterial pressure. Mean pulmonary artery pressure in a resting individual at sea level is normally about 15 mmHg and pulmonary hypertension is usually defined as a pressure above 25 mmHg; pressures will be correspondingly higher at higher altitudes.

Pulmonary hypertension has usually been classified as primary or secondary, although a wider classification system based on the underlying cause may now be used.[1-3] Primary pulmonary hypertension is uncommon and patients have no underlying disease known to cause an elevation of the pulmonary arterial pressure. Secondary pulmonary hypertension, in contrast, is far more prevalent and patients have some form of cardiopulmonary disorder that can lead to the development of pulmonary hypertension.

**Primary pulmonary hypertension** has been reviewed,[1,2,4-7] and guidelines for its management[3] have been published. It occurs in patients of all ages and in both sexes but women in the fourth decade of life are those typically seen. Initial complaints include dyspnoea on exertion, fatigue, and chest discomfort or pain. In advanced disease, cor pulmonale (an enlargement of the right ventricle due to either dilatation, hypertrophy, or both) occurs and may progress to right-sided heart failure. The pulmonary arteries may be affected by thromboembolic disease. Primary pulmonary hypertension is a progressive and incurable disease and patients appear to be prone to sudden death.

The aim of treatment is to decrease the pulmonary arterial pressure, preferably in conjunction with an increase in cardiac output. Many drugs with vasodilating effects have been investigated in pulmonary hypertension,[8,9] the rationale usually being based upon their application in systemic hypertension. Unfortunately, the vast majority have been unsatisfactory. Although most vasodilators do reduce pulmonary arterial pressure they are not selective for the pulmonary circulation and therefore also reduce systemic blood pressure producing undesirable, or sometimes intolerable, side-effects. Of the vasodilators studied, calcium-channel blockers and the prostaglandin epoprostenol have an established role.[3] Improved survival over a 5-year period has been noted in some patients treated with high-dose *calcium-channel blockers*.[10] However, not all patients respond and because of concerns about previously reported adverse effects in patients with primary pulmonary hypertension given these drugs it has been advised that an acute response test should be performed before embarking on long-term treatment.[3,9,10] Although oral calcium-channel blockers may be used for the test, shorter-acting vasodilators such as intravenous epoprostenol, intravenous adenosine, or inhaled nitric oxide, are generally employed.[3] *Epoprostenol* was originally introduced into the management of primary pulmonary hypertension to sustain patients long enough for them to have heart-lung transplantation but long-term therapy may also have a role as an alternative to transplantation,[11,12] and should be considered in patients who do not respond to standard therapy.[3] Sustained clinical improvement and improved survival have been reported in some patients given long-term intravenous therapy using portable infusion pumps.[13,14] Continuous intravenous infusion of the more stable analogue iloprost may be an alternative.[3,15] Another analogue, treprostinil, is given by continuous subcutaneous infusion[16] and may have a role in patients for whom intravenous treatment is not suitable. A small study[17] has reported the safe transfer of patients from epoprostenol to treprostinil therapy. Administration by inhalation is another alternative that has been tried; epoprostenol has been used, but iloprost has a longer action and may be preferred.[18-20] Another analogue, beraprost sodium, has been given orally,[21-23] but is not widely available. The oral endothelin receptor antagonist bosentan may also be used, and studies[24,25] have reported an improvement in haemodynamics and exercise capacity. Preliminary studies[26-28] with the phosphodiesterase inhibitor sildenafil have also reported beneficial responses, but further studies are needed to confirm these results.

Surgical intervention, and ultimately lung or heart-lung transplantation may be required in patients who do not respond to vasodilator therapy.[3] Oxygen therapy may be necessary in some patients.[3] Patients with primary pulmonary hypertension have an increased risk of thromboembolism and *oral anticoagulants* are recommended on a long term basis for most patients as they may improve survival.[3] *Diuretics*[3] and *digoxin*[3] are given as necessary for associated right-sided heart failure.

**Secondary pulmonary hypertension** occurs as a consequence of an established cardiopulmonary disorder and the clinical manifestations are dominated by those of the underlying condition. Chronic obstructive pulmonary disease is the commonest respiratory cause. Other lung disorders that may lead to pulmonary hypertension include: diseases of the lung parenchyma such as the respiratory distress syndromes, sarcoidosis, and cryptogenic fibrosing alveolitis; diseases affecting the pulmonary vessels such as thromboembolic disease and systemic lupus erythematosus; and connective tissue diseases such as scleroderma. Cardiac causes include disorders leading to impaired left ventricular function such as myocardial infarction or mitral valve disease.

Management of secondary pulmonary hypertension basically constitutes appropriate treatment of the underlying condition, although continuous intravenous epoprostenol may be of benefit in some patients.[29,30] Inhaled nitric oxide has been used in acutely ill patients,[31] and long-term use has also been reported.[32] Patients with underlying connective tissue disorders may require similar management to those with primary pulmonary hypertension.[33]

**Persistent pulmonary hypertension of the newborn**, sometimes also termed persistent fetal circulation, is, as the name implies, a form of pulmonary hypertension specifically affecting neonates. It can be primary in nature (that is, idiopathic, affecting infants with an anatomically normal heart and no pulmonary disease) or secondary, being associated with a number of cardiopulmonary conditions including congenital heart disease, diaphragmatic hernia, meconium aspiration, respiratory distress syndrome, or sepsis. The pulmonary hypertension and altered vasoreactivity lead to a right-to-left shunting of blood across the patent ductus arteriosus or foramen ovale and this often results in critical hypoxaemia.

Management generally involves high-frequency oscillatory ventilation (to achieve optimal lung inflation) and, if necessary, extracorporeal membrane oxygenation. Mechanical hyperventilation induces alkalosis and has decreased pulmonary arterial pressure and improved oxygenation in some patients.[34] Intravenous vasodilators have also been employed, but, as discussed above, their use is generally restricted because of their non-selectivity for the pulmonary circulation; inhaled *nitric oxide* which is a potent, selective pulmonary vasodilator, is now more widely used.[35] Studies[36-40] have shown that it can cause marked improvement in oxygenation and a reduction in the need for extracorporeal membrane oxygenation, but no effect on mortality has been demonstrated. Although there have been concerns that use of inhaled nitric oxide might adversely affect neurodevelopmental outcome more than conventional therapy, this has not been confirmed in infants followed up for up to 2 years.[41,42] Use of inhaled nitric oxide in combination with high-frequency oscillatory ventilation may have additional benefits.[43]

Of the vasodilators tried, *tolazoline* has been the most commonly employed. Inhaled *epoprostenol* has been used in a few neonates,[44,45] and this method of administration may overcome the problems of systemic vasodilatation. *Magnesium sulfate* intravenously has also been reported[46-48] to have potential use as a vasodilator, and intravenous *adenosine* has also been tried.[49]


1. Peacock AJ. Primary pulmonary hypertension. *Thorax* 1999; **54:** 1107–18.
2. Galiè N, Torbicki A. Pulmonary arterial hypertension: new ideas and perspectives. *Heart* 2001; **85:** 475–80.
3. British Cardiac Society Guidelines and Medical Practice Committee. Recommendations on the management of pulmonary hypertension in clinical practice. *Heart* 2001; **86** (suppl 1): I1-I13.
4. Gaine S. Pulmonary hypertension. *JAMA* 2000; **284:** 3160–8.
5. Klings ES, Farber HW. Current management of primary pulmonary hypertension. *Drugs* 2001; **61:** 1945–56.
6. Pass SE, Dusing ML. Current and emerging therapy for primary pulmonary hypertension. *Ann Pharmacother* 2002; **36:** 1414–23.
7. Runo JR, Loyd JE. Primary pulmonary hypertension. *Lancet* 2003; **361:** 1533–44.
8. Weir EK, *et al.* The acute administration of vasodilators in primary pulmonary hypertension: experience from the National Institutes of Health Registry on Primary Pulmonary Hypertension. *Am Rev Respir Dis* 1989; **140:** 1623–30.
9. Barnes PJ, Liu SF. Regulation of pulmonary vascular tone. *Pharmacol Rev* 1995; **47:** 87–131.
10. Rich S, *et al.* The effect of high doses of calcium-channel blockers on survival in primary pulmonary hypertension. *N Engl J Med* 1992; **327:** 76–81.
11. Herner SJ, Mauro LS. Epoprostenol in primary pulmonary hypertension. *Ann Pharmacother* 1999; **33:** 340–7.
12. Barst RJ. Treatment of primary pulmonary hypertension with continuous intravenous prostacyclin. *Heart* 1997; **77:** 299–301.
13. Higenbottam T, *et al.* Long term intravenous prostaglandin (epoprostenol or iloprost) for the treatment of severe pulmonary hypertension. *Heart* 1998; **80:** 151–5.
14. McLaughlin VV, *et al.* Survival in primary pulmonary hypertension: the impact of epoprostenol therapy. *Circulation* 2002; **106:** 1477–82.
15. Higenbottam TW, *et al.* Treatment of pulmonary hypertension with the continuous infusion of a prostacyclin analogue, iloprost. *Heart* 1998; **79:** 175–9.
16. Simonneau G, *et al.* Continuous subcutaneous infusion of treprostinil, a prostacyclin analogue, in patients with pulmonary arterial hypertension: a double-blind, randomized placebo-controlled trial. *Am J Respir Crit Care Med* 2002; **165:** 800–804.
17. Vachiéry J-L, *et al.* Transitioning from IV epoprostenol to subcutaneous treprostinil in pulmonary arterial hypertension. *Chest* 2002; **121:** 1561–5.
18. Olschewski H, *et al.* Inhaled iloprost to treat severe pulmonary hypertension: an uncontrolled trial. *Ann Intern Med* 2000; **132:** 435–43.
19. Hoeper MM, *et al.* Long-term treatment of primary pulmonary hypertension with aerosolized iloprost, a prostacyclin analogue. *N Engl J Med* 2000; **342:** 1866–70.
20. Olschewski H, *et al.* Inhaled iloprost for severe pulmonary hypertension. *N Engl J Med* 2002; **347:** 322–9.
21. Nagaya N, *et al.* Effect of orally active prostacyclin analogue on survival of outpatients with primary pulmonary hypertension. *J Am Coll Cardiol* 1999; **34:** 1188–92.
22. Vizza CD, *et al.* Long term treatment of pulmonary arterial hypertension with beraprost, an oral prostacyclin analogue. *Heart* 2001; **86:** 661–5.
23. Barst RJ, *et al.* Beraprost therapy for pulmonary arterial hypertension. *J Am Coll Cardiol* 2003; **41:** 2119–25.
24. Channick RN, *et al.* Effects of the dual endothelin-receptor antagonist bosentan in patients with pulmonary hypertension: a randomised placebo-controlled study. *Lancet* 2001; **358:** 1119–23.
25. Rubin LJ, *et al.* Bosentan therapy for pulmonary arterial hypertension. *N Engl J Med* 2002; **346:** 896–903. Correction. *ibid.*; 1258.
26. Watanabe H, *et al.* Sildenafil for primary and secondary pulmonary hypertension. *Clin Pharmacol Ther* 2002; **71:** 398–402.
27. Ghofrani HA, *et al.* Sildenafil for treatment of lung fibrosis and pulmonary hypertension: a randomised controlled trial. *Lancet* 2002; **360:** 895–900.
28. Ghofrani HA, *et al.* Combination therapy with oral sildenafil and inhaled iloprost for severe pulmonary hypertension. *Ann Intern Med* 2002; **136:** 515–22.
29. McLaughlin VV, *et al.* Compassionate use of continuous prostacyclin in the management of secondary pulmonary hypertension: a case series. *Ann Intern Med* 1999; **130:** 740–3.
30. Badesch DB, *et al.* Continuous intravenous epoprostenol for pulmonary hypertension due to the scleroderma spectrum of disease: a randomized, controlled trial. *Ann Intern Med* 2000; **132:** 425–34.
31. Cuthbertson BH, *et al.* Use of inhaled nitric oxide in British intensive therapy units. *Br J Anaesth* 1997; **78:** 696–700.
32. Vonbank K, *et al.* Controlled prospective randomised trial on the effects on pulmonary haemodynamics of the ambulatory long term use of nitric oxide and oxygen in patients with severe COPD. *Thorax* 2003; **58:** 289–93.

33. Sanchez O, *et al.* Treatment of pulmonary hypertension secondary to connective tissue diseases. *Thorax* 1999; **54:** 273–7.
34. Kinsella JP, Abman SH. Recent developments in the pathophysiology and treatment of persistent pulmonary hypertension of the newborn. *J Pediatr* 1995; **126:** 853–64.
35. Rennie JM, Bokhari SA. Recent advances in neonatology. *Arch Dis Child* 1999; **81:** F1–F4.
36. The Neonatal Inhaled Nitric Oxide Study Group. Inhaled nitric oxide in full-term and nearly full-term infants with hypoxic respiratory failure. *N Engl J Med* 1997; **336:** 597–604.
37. Roberts JD, *et al.* Inhaled nitric oxide and persistent pulmonary hypertension of the newborn. *N Engl J Med* 1997; **336:** 605–10.
38. Davidson D, *et al.* Inhaled nitric oxide for the early treatment of persistent pulmonary hypertension of the term newborn: a randomized, double-masked, placebo-controlled, dose-response, multicenter study. *Pediatrics* 1998; **101:** 325–34.
39. Wessel DL, *et al.* Improved oxygenation in a randomized trial of inhaled nitric oxide for persistent pulmonary hypertension of the newborn. Abstract: *Pediatrics* 1997; **100:** 888. Full version: http://pediatrics.aappublications.org/cgi/content/full/100/5/e7 (accessed 14/05/04)
40. Clark RH, *et al.* Low-dose nitric oxide therapy for persistent pulmonary hypertension of the newborn. *N Engl J Med* 2000; **342:** 469–74.
41. Rosenberg AA, *et al.* Longitudinal follow-up of a cohort of newborn infants treated with inhaled nitric oxide for persistent pulmonary hypertension. *J Pediatr* 1997; **131:** 70–5.
42. The Neonatal Inhaled Nitric Oxide Study Group. Inhaled nitric oxide in term and near-term infants: neurodevelopmental follow-up of the Neonatal Inhaled Nitric Oxide Study Group (NINOS). *J Pediatr* 2000; **136:** 611–17.
43. Kinsella JP, *et al.* Randomized, multicenter trial of inhaled nitric oxide and high-frequency oscillatory ventilation in severe, persistent pulmonary hypertension of the newborn. *J Pediatr* 1997; **131:** 55–62.
44. Bindl L, *et al.* Aerosolised prostacyclin for pulmonary hypertension in neonates. *Arch Dis Child Fetal Neonatal Ed* 1994; **71:** F214–F216.
45. Kelly LK, *et al.* Inhaled prostacyclin for term infants with persistent pulmonary hypertension refractory to inhaled nitric oxide. *J Pediatr* 2002; **141:** 830–2.
46. Abu-Osba YK, *et al.* Treatment of severe persistent pulmonary hypertension of the newborn with magnesium sulphate. *Arch Dis Child* 1992; **67:** 31–5.
47. Tolsa J-F, *et al.* Magnesium sulphate as an alternative and safe treatment for severe persistent pulmonary hypertension of the newborn. *Arch Dis Child Fetal Neonatal Ed* 1995; **72:** F184–F187.
48. Wu T-Z, *et al.* Persistent pulmonary hypertension of the newborn treated with magnesium sulfate in premature neonates. *Pediatrics* 1995; **96:** 472–4.
49. Konduri GG, *et al.* Adenosine infusion improves oxygenation in term infants with respiratory failure. *Pediatrics* 1996; **97:** 295–300.


## Raised intracranial pressure

The intracranial compartment consists of brain parenchyma, vascular tissue, and cerebrospinal fluid (CSF). Since the skull is a rigid structure a change in the volume of any one of these compartments will raise intracranial pressure. This may be due to the formation of cerebral oedema following head injury or around tumours, mass-lesions such as tumours or haemorrhage, CNS infections, or metabolic disorders. Other mechanisms that can raise intracranial pressure include increased dural sinus venous pressure, increased resistance to CSF outflow, and an increased rate of formation of CSF. In conditions such as benign intracranial hypertension there may be no obvious cause. Raised intracranial pressure (intracranial hypertension) can produce irreversible damage to the CNS and is potentially fatal; herniation of brain tissue can occur and reduced cerebral blood flow can lead to cerebral ischaemia. Symptoms of raised intracranial pressure include headache, which is frequently worse in the morning and may wake the patient from sleep, vomiting, drowsiness, and visual disturbances; most patients have papilloedema on examination.

There are several ways of reducing raised intracranial pressure, the choice of treatment being determined mainly by the underlying cause.[1-6] Whatever the cause, in acutely raised intracranial pressure the initial aim is to reduce the volume of the intracranial contents as quickly as possible to prevent brain damage. For patients with haematoma or tumours the treatment of choice is frequently surgery but other methods may be used to control intracranial pressure before surgery.

Intracranial pressure monitoring can be helpful in guiding therapy since reducing the intracranial pressure too far is also deleterious. Patients may be sedated to avoid elevations of intracranial pressure due to unnecessary movement but if this is ineffective the use of neuromuscular blockers such as pancuronium or atracurium with artificial ventilation should be considered. Hyperventilation reduces the intracranial pressure by constricting the cerebral blood vessels and controlled hyperventilation has been employed; however, it also reduces cerebral blood flow and routine use is not generally advised.[4,5] Raising the patient's head to promote venous drainage may be helpful. Although restriction of fluid intake has been advised, hypotension reduces cerebral blood flow and should be avoided, and intravenous fluids should therefore be given as required.[4,5] Removal of CSF through a ventricular catheter may also be effective. Controlled hypothermia has been used, but a review[7] of its use in head injury found no evidence that it improves outcome.

The mainstay of pharmacological treatment for acutely raised intracranial pressure is diuretic therapy, usually with an osmotic diuretic. Mannitol is most commonly used but urea, glycerol, sorbitol, and hypertonic glucose or sodium chloride solutions have also been employed.[3] Osmotic diuretics act by increasing the osmolality of plasma and drawing water out of the tissues, as well as by promoting an osmotic diuresis. They should not be given to patients with intracranial bleeding after head injury since they can exacerbate the bleeding,[6] and should also be avoided in patients who are already dehydrated. *Mannitol* decreases intracranial pressure and increases cerebral blood flow both by an osmotic effect and by decreasing blood viscosity.[4,8] It has been suggested for control of raised intracranial pressure of various origins including severe head injury,[4,5] and cerebral oedema in hepatic failure,[9] and is often used to control intracranial pressure prior to surgery. Mannitol has also produced beneficial responses in *children* with raised intracranial pressure from birth asphyxia,[10] diabetic ketoacidosis,[11] or Reye's syndrome.[12,13] Beneficial effects with osmotic diuretics such as mannitol or glycerol in patients following stroke have not been demonstrated (see Neuroprotection under Stroke, p.836). The use of osmotic diuretics to reduce intracranial pressure in patients with cerebral malaria is not routinely recommended and is controversial in other CNS infections.

In addition to its ability to lower intracranial pressure *glycerol* is reported to be able to increase blood flow to areas of brain ischaemia. It has been used by mouth or intravenously in an attempt to reduce cerebral oedema and raised intracranial pressure in a variety of conditions including Reye's syndrome[14] and meningitis;[15] it has been reported to be ineffective in hepatic coma.[16] Some patients have experienced severe adverse effects including haemolysis, haemoglobinuria, and renal failure. Strongly *hyperosmotic glucose* solutions (25 to 50%) have been used to reduce raised intracranial pressure and cerebral oedema caused by delirium or acute alcohol intoxication. *Hypertonic sodium chloride* has been shown to reduce intracranial pressure in several studies, although its place in therapy is not yet confirmed; it may have a role in resistant cases.[4,17]

If control is required for more than a few hours, repeated doses or continuous administration of osmotic diuretics may be necessary. Mannitol may accumulate with continuous infusion and repeated bolus doses are generally preferred.[5] Fluid and electrolyte balance and plasma osmolality should be closely monitored.

Loop diuretics such as *furosemide* are also effective and may be used as alternatives to osmotic diuretics, particularly where a sustained effect is required. They may increase the effect of osmotic diuretics and may be used as adjuncts, usually given after the osmotic diuretic. Furosemide decreases cerebral water content and possibly also reduces secretion of CSF. It may be preferred to mannitol in patients undergoing neurosurgery.[18]

*Corticosteroids* have an accepted and important role in the management of raised intracranial pressure associated with tumour-induced cerebral oedema. They may be used intravenously in high doses to control acutely raised intracranial pressure due to a rapidly expanding tumour. Lower doses are given orally for maintenance or where the onset of cerebral oedema is more insidious. Corticosteroids have also been tried in patients with head injury or stroke but their effectiveness is not proven and their adverse effects may outweigh any benefit. Further studies are needed to clarify their role in head injury.[19]

The use of barbiturate-induced coma with intravenous *thiopental* or *pentobarbital* for raised intracranial pressure has been controversial but it may be of benefit in patients refractory to conventional therapies.[4,5] In addition to their effect on intracranial pressure barbiturates may be able to protect the brain from ischaemia. *Trometamol* is reported to lower raised intracranial pressure in patients with head injury; it may do this by causing metabolic acidosis leading to vasoconstriction of cerebral vessels.[3]

**Benign intracranial hypertension** (pseudotumour cerebri) is a rare disorder of unknown cause in which there is a raised intracranial pressure in the absence of an intracranial mass or obstruction to CSF outflow. Patients are often obese and tend to be young and female. Although the condition is not life-threatening and is often self-limiting, it may be a chronic condition and treatment is required to prevent visual loss and to alleviate symptoms. Drug-induced intracranial hypertension may also occur. Management of mild symptoms usually involves diuretic treatment with furosemide, a thiazide, or acetazolamide. Corticosteroids may be used to control acute symptoms but long-term adverse effects limit their use. Repeated lumbar puncture to remove CSF may relieve symptoms and has been used every 2 to 5 days to induce remission. In patients who cannot be controlled medically, surgical methods such as lumboperitoneal shunting may be required. There has been an anecdotal report of beneficial effects with *octreotide* in a small number of patients.[20]

Acetazolamide has also been tried in the treatment of patients with chronically raised intracranial pressure due to cryptococcal meningitis.[21]


1. Lyons MK, Meyer FB. Cerebrospinal fluid physiology and the management of increased intracranial pressure. *Mayo Clin Proc* 1990; **65:** 684–707.
2. Woster PS, LeBlanc KL. Management of elevated intracranial pressure. *Clin Pharm* 1990; **9:** 762–72.
3. Nau R. Osmotherapy for elevated intracranial pressure: a critical reappraisal. *Clin Pharmacokinet* 2000; **38:** 23–40.
4. Marik PE, *et al.* Management of head trauma. *Chest* 2002; **122:** 699–711.
5. The Brain Trauma Foundation and the American Association of Neurological Surgeons, Joint Section on Neurotrauma and Critical Care. Guidelines for the management of severe traumatic brain injury. *J Neurotrauma* 2000; **17:** 449–554. Also available at: http://www2.braintrauma.org/guidelines/downloads/btf_guidelines_management.pdf (accessed 14/05/04)
6. Kirkham FJ. Non-traumatic coma in children. *Arch Dis Child* 2001; **85:** 303–12.
7. Gadkary CA, *et al.* Therapeutic hypothermia for head injury. Available in The Cochrane Library; Issue 2. Chichester: John Wiley; 2004.
8. Schrot RJ, Muizelaar JP. Mannitol in acute traumatic brain injury. *Lancet* 2002; **359:** 1633–4.
9. Canalese J, *et al.* Controlled trial of dexamethasone and mannitol for the cerebral oedema of fulminant hepatic failure. *Gut* 1982; **23:** 625–9.
10. Levene MI, Evans DH. Medical management of raised intracranial pressure after severe birth asphyxia. *Arch Dis Child* 1985; **60:** 12–16.
11. Bello FA, Sotos JF. Cerebral oedema in diabetic ketoacidosis in children. *Lancet* 1990; **336:** 64.
12. Shaywitz BA, *et al.* Prolonged continuous monitoring of intracranial pressure in severe Reye's syndrome. *Pediatrics* 1977; **59:** 595–605.
13. Newman SL, *et al.* Reye's syndrome: success of supportive care. *N Engl J Med* 1978; **299:** 1079.
14. Nahata MC, *et al.* Variations in glycerol kinetics in Reye's syndrome. *Clin Pharmacol Ther* 1981; **29:** 782–7.
15. Kilpi T, *et al.* Oral glycerol and intravenous dexamethasone in preventing neurologic and audiologic sequelae of childhood bacterial meningitis. *Pediatr Infect Dis J* 1995; **14:** 270–8.
16. Record CO, *et al.* Glycerol therapy for cerebral oedema complicating fulminant hepatic failure. *BMJ* 1975; **ii:** 540.
17. Qureshi AI, Suarez JI. Use of hypertonic saline solutions in treatment of cerebral edema and intracranial hypertension. *Crit Care Med* 2000; **28:** 3301–13.
18. Cottrell JE, *et al.* Furosemide- and mannitol-induced changes in intracranial pressure and serum osmolality and electrolytes. *Anesthesiology* 1977; **47:** 28–30.
19. Alderson P, Roberts I. Corticosteroids for acute traumatic brain injury. Available in The Cochrane Library; Issue 2. Chichester: John Wiley; 2004.
20. Antaraki A, *et al.* Octreotide in benign intracranial hypertension. *Lancet* 1993; **342:** 1170.
21. Johnston SRD, *et al.* Raised intracranial pressure and visual complications in AIDS patients with cryptococcal meningitis. *J Infect* 1992; **24:** 185–9.


## Raynaud's syndrome

Raynaud's syndrome is the most important form of vasospastic peripheral arterial disease and forms part of the spectrum of peripheral vascular disease (see p.831). Vasospastic arterial disorders occur due to an inappropriate response to temperature, resulting in vasoconstriction and/or vasospasm; Raynaud's syndrome, acrocyanosis, and chilblains are usually induced by cold, whereas erythromelalgia is caused by heat.

In **Raynaud's syndrome**, paroxysmal attacks of pallor and cyanosis, usually of the digits, occur in response to cold, or sometimes emotional stress. Erythema replaces the cyanosis as the attacks resolve. The cause of primary Raynaud's syndrome (Raynaud's disease) is unknown. Features identified include intense vasoconstriction or vasospasm, disturbance of sympathetic nerve supply, changes in circulating catecholamines, enhanced platelet aggregation, red cell deformability, and fibrinolysis. It is probable that not all cases are due to the same mechanism. It has been suggested that the underlying problem may not be an overreaction to the initial cold insult but a defect in the normal ensuing adaptive response. Secondary Raynaud's syndrome (Raynaud's phenomenon) frequently coexists with arterial occlusive disease such as thromboangiitis obliterans and connective tissue disorders, in particular scleroderma (systemic sclerosis). Trauma and certain drugs, notably beta blockers and ergotamine, may also be responsible for inducing secondary Raynaud's syndrome.

**Management**. In mild cases of Raynaud's syndrome, where attacks are infrequent and of limited severity, protective measures to keep warm are the mainstay of treatment; this involves wearing appropriate clothing and the use of appliances such as heated gloves. Smoking should be avoided because of the vasoconstriction caused. Any underlying or co-existing disease or cause in secondary Raynaud's syndrome should be treated. Drug therapy is indicated in more severe cases.[1-6] It is directed towards producing vascular smooth muscle relaxation and vasodilatation in order to improve resting blood flow, thereby reducing the extent of tissue ischaemia. Some drugs may also act by modifying platelet aggregation or blood rheology. Numerous drugs have been tried in Raynaud's syndrome, although only a few have an established role.

*Calcium-channel blockers* have been of benefit and are widely used in Raynaud's syndrome, but it is not entirely clear which of their pharmacological actions is responsible. Dihydropyridines are usually preferred; the most widely used and studied is *nifedipine*.

*Moxisylyte*, an alpha blocker with vasodilating activity, is also widely employed. Other alpha blockers, for example, phenoxybenzamine and prazosin as well as reserpine have been used although in some cases side-effects have limited their usefulness.

*Cinnarizine*, *naftidrofuryl*, *pentoxifylline*, and *nicotinic acid derivatives* such as inositol nicotinate have had widespread use in Raynaud's syndrome but evidence of efficacy is lacking. Topical vasodilators, including glyceryl trinitrate, have also been used.

In severe Raynaud's syndrome complicated by ulceration and gangrene, *prostaglandins* have been promising. *Alprostadil*, *epoprostenol*, and *iloprost* have been given by intravenous infusion. In some cases the beneficial effects have persisted for a few months after treatment and two or three infusions given at intervals over the winter months have prevented the severe complications of Raynaud's suffered in previous years. Iloprost orally has also been reported to reduce the severity of attacks. Prostaglandins applied topically in ulcerative cases include *dinoprostone*.

Small studies or anecdotal reports have noted variable effects with many *other drugs* including the ACE inhibitors captopril and enalapril, the serotonin reuptake inhibitors fluoxetine and venlafaxine, ketanserin, piracetam, sodium nitroprusside, calcitonin gene-related peptide, and losartan. None of these therapies appears, however, to have an established role.

**Acrocyanosis** is characterised by a persistent blue discoloration of the skin. There is an abnormal constriction of arterioles, even at normal environmental conditions and this is potentiated by cold. **Chilblains** are an inflammatory condition (perniosis) affecting the extremities and symptoms include erythema, pruritus, and ulceration; they may be acute or chronic. Chilblains occur more commonly in cold damp conditions. Acrocyanosis and chilblains do not generally require specific treatment; smoking cessation, protection from the cold, or symptomatic antipruritic treatment are often sufficient. However, if severe, the drugs described above under Raynaud's syndrome may be considered.

**Erythromelalgia** (sometimes also called erythermalgia) is a vasospastic condition usually provoked by heat although it may also be drug-induced or secondary to other conditions. It is characterised by painful, red extremities together with a burning sensation and increased skin temperature of the affected area. Thrombocythaemia is the most common underlying cause and, indeed, erythromelalgia may be the presenting feature of this disorder; in thrombocythaemia, arteriolar occlusion may occur as a result of platelet aggregation. Small doses of aspirin have produced considerable relief in some patients, presumably by preventing platelet aggregation. Beta blockers may also be of some help, and there are anecdotal reports of benefit with various other drugs.[7] Attacks should be prevented wherever possible by avoiding exposure to heat.


1. Belch JJF, Ho M. Pharmacotherapy of Raynaud's phenomenon. *Drugs* 1996; **52:** 682–95.
2. Black CM. Raynaud's phenomenon. *Prescribers' J* 1994; **34:** 125–33.
3. Isenberg DA, Black C. Raynaud's phenomenon, scleroderma, and overlap syndromes. *BMJ* 1995; **310:** 795–8.
4. Block JA, Sequeira W. Raynaud's phenomenon. *Lancet* 2001; **357:** 2042–8.
5. Wigley FM. Raynaud's Phenomenon. *N Engl J Med* 2002; **347:** 1001–8.
6. Bowling JCR, Dowd PM. Raynaud's disease. *Lancet* 2003; **361:** 2078–80.
7. Cohen JS. Erythromelalgia: new theories and new therapies. *J Am Acad Dermatol* 2000; **43:** 841–7.


### Reperfusion and revascularisation procedures

Atherosclerosis, leading to narrowing of arteries with a consequent reduction in blood flow, is the major underlying cause of a number of cardiovascular disorders, including angina pectoris (p.813), myocardial infarction (p.828), and peripheral vascular disease (p.831). Restoration of blood flow is the main aim of treatment for atherosclerosis, and various pharmacological and non-pharmacological methods are available for achieving reperfusion and revascularisation. Percutaneous coronary interventions,[1] such as balloon angioplasty (PTCA), stenting, and atherectomy, and surgical procedures such as coronary artery bypass grafting (CABG), are the main non-pharmacological methods used in the coronary circulation. Similar techniques are used for peripheral vascular and cerebrovascular disease.

The choice between pharmacological and interventional approaches, and which procedure to use, depends on various factors and is discussed under the individual diseases. Patients undergoing non-pharmacological procedures are at risk of further thromboembolic events, including myocardial infarction and ischaemic stroke, either shortly after the procedure due to perioperative thrombosis, or in the long term as a consequence of restenosis of the artery,[2] or progression of the underlying disease. Thus, adjunctive drug therapy is given with the aim of preventing both short- and long-term complications, and this is the focus of the following discussion. Patients who have undergone reperfusion or revascularisation procedures remain at high risk of further cardiovascular events, and require assessment and treatment to reduce their risk (see Cardiovascular Risk Reduction, p.819). Antithrombotic therapy is generally given to reduce the risk of perioperative thrombosis during percutaneous and surgical procedures.[3-6] Heparin is given during both coronary and peripheral bypass surgery, although its effects are often reversed at the end of the operation to reduce the risk of bleeding. It also has an established role during percutaneous procedures. Unfractionated heparin is given intravenously by continuous infusion, and the dose is adjusted according to clotting time. Relatively high doses are used, although lower doses have been investigated during percutaneous coronary intervention and are recommended when glycoprotein IIb/IIIa inhibitors are also used.[1,3] Low-molecular-weight heparins have also been tried but their role is not yet established.[1,3] Direct thrombin inhibitors such as bivalirudin may be used as an alternative to unfractionated heparin.[3] Bivalirudin appears to be as effective as unfractionated heparin in patients undergoing percutaneous coronary interventions,[7,8] while in another study there were fewer acute ischaemic events early after angioplasty when desirudin was given instead of heparin, but no longer term benefit was seen.[9]

Antiplatelet drugs also have an important role in preventing acute occlusion. Aspirin is most commonly used and is usually started around the time of angioplasty or bypass grafting and continued long-term as discussed further below; clopidogrel or ticlopidine may be alternatives in patients unable to tolerate aspirin.[3] Aspirin does not completely inhibit platelet function and more potent drugs have also been studied. Glycoprotein IIb/IIIa-receptor antagonists, given as adjuncts to heparin and aspirin, reduce the acute complications of percutaneous coronary interventions,[10] and long-term benefit has been shown with both abciximab and eptifibatide. They are of benefit following both elective and emergency procedures, although the evidence for tirofiban is limited to patients with acute coronary syndromes. Abciximab and eptifibatide also improve outcomes in patients receiving coronary stents.[11,12] Glycoprotein IIb/IIIa-receptor antagonists have therefore been recommended in all patients undergoing percutaneous procedures.[3,13]

Oral anticoagulants such as warfarin are not used routinely following percutaneous procedures or coronary bypass, although they may have a role in selected patients following peripheral artery bypass.[4] However, a study[14] comparing oral anticoagulants with aspirin following peripheral bypass surgery found no difference in reocclusion or mortality, but bleeding was higher in patients receiving anticoagulants.

Antithrombotic therapy is particularly important in patients who receive stents. Coronary stents (metallic mesh tubes that are inflated across a stenosis and thus permanently embedded in the vessel wall) are widely used as a routine adjunct to angioplasty to prevent both acute vessel closure and restenosis. Thrombotic occlusion occurring 2 to 14 days following stent implantation (subacute stent thrombosis) initially led to the use of intensive anticoagulation/antiplatelet regimens consisting of aspirin, dipyridamole, dextran, heparin, and warfarin.[15] However, studies have shown that antiplatelet therapy, in addition to optimal stent deployment and heparin during the procedure, effectively prevents thrombotic complications and is now preferred.[16] Although the initial studies used aspirin and ticlopidine, a regimen of aspirin with clopidogrel is better tolerated[17] and may be used as an alternative.[3] Glycoprotein IIb/IIIa-receptor antagonists have also been used with coronary stenting. Cilostazol has also been tried and may be effective,[18] although its place in therapy remains to be established. Heparin-coated stents are also used.[19]

Other acute complications during percutaneous coronary interventions include vasospasm, reperfusion injury, and arrhythmias. Nitrates[20] or calcium-channel blockers[20,21] may be used to reduce the risk of vasospasm, while various drugs are under investigation for cardioprotection.

Restenosis, including in-stent restenosis, is a specific long-term complication of percutaneous procedures, and the problem and its treatment have been reviewed.[20,22] Several pathological processes are believed to be responsible for the development of restenosis, and include platelet aggregation and thrombus formation, neointimal hyperplasia, elastic recoil, and vascular remodelling. This has led to the investigation of a wide variety of drugs in an attempt to prevent restenosis developing, although few have an established role.

The value of antiplatelet drugs in reducing major coronary events is well established following revascularisation procedures,[23,24] although whether they reduce the degree of restenosis following percutaneous interventions is less clear.[3] Conflicting results have been reported with aspirin, but it should be given to all patients unless contra-indicated to reduce the risk of further events.[3] Clopidogrel also reduces major coronary events,[25] but the effect on restenosis has not been assessed. Preliminary results with cilostazol suggest that it may have some effect,[18] but this remains to be confirmed. Heparin, low-molecular-weight heparins, and warfarin, have all been tried, but have not been shown to reduce restenosis.[22]

Lipid regulating drugs similarly have an established role in cardiovascular risk reduction, and their effects on restenosis have been investigated.[22] Fish oils appear to be ineffective, and studies with statins have also failed to show a reduction in restenosis following angioplasty, although they may be effective after stenting. Probucol has also shown some promise, although pretreatment appears to be necessary.

Various antiproliferative drugs have been tried, but again early positive results have not been confirmed in larger studies.[22] Drugs that have shown promise include lanreotide, trapidil, and tranilast, although larger trials with trapidil[26] or with tranilast[27] in patients receiving coronary stents found no benefit.

Although coronary stents improve outcome for percutaneous procedures, in-stent restenosis is a particular problem.[28,29] The pathological mechanism of restenosis appears to be primarily neointimal growth. The most promising treatments for in-stent restenosis are intracoronary radiotherapy, and drug-eluting stents. Intracoronary radiotherapy has reduced the rates of restenosis after angioplasty,[30] and after stenting.[31] Heparin-coated stents may reduce long-term stenosis,[19] and various other drugs are under investigation for delivery in a similar way. Both sirolimus-eluting stents[32,33] and paclitaxel-eluting stents[34] have been found to reduce neointimal proliferation and clinical events, including the need for repeat revascularisation procedures, although thrombosis may still occur. Local gene delivery is also under investigation as a possible treatment for restenosis.

Re-occlusion due to thrombosis or progression of atherosclerosis is a problem following bypass procedures; antithrombotic therapy[5] and statins[35] may reduce this risk. Intra-arterial administration of thrombolytics, directly into the clot, has been used in conjunction with surgery or angioplasty for acute occlusion of peripheral bypass grafts.[36]


1. Windecker S, Meier B. Intervention in coronary artery disease. *Heart* 2000; **83:** 481–90.
2. O'Meara JJ, Dehmer GJ. Care of the patient and management of complications after percutaneous coronary artery interventions. *Ann Intern Med* 1997; **127:** 458–71.
3. Popma JJ, *et al.* Antithrombotic therapy in patients undergoing percutaneous coronary intervention. *Chest* 2001; **119** (suppl): 321S–336S.
4. Jackson MR, Clagett GP. Antithrombotic therapy in peripheral arterial occlusive disease. *Chest* 2001; **119** (suppl): 283S-299S.
5. Stein PD, *et al.* Antithrombotic therapy in patients with saphenous vein and internal mammary artery bypass grafts. *Chest* 2001; **119** (suppl): 278S-282S.
6. Scottish Intercollegiate Guidelines Network. Antithrombotic therapy: a national clinical guideline (March 1999). Available at: http://www.show.scot.nhs.uk/sign/pdf/sign36.pdf (accessed 14/05/04)
7. Kong DF, *et al.* Clinical outcomes of bivalirudin for ischemic heart disease. *Circulation* 1999; **100:** 2049–53.
8. Lincoff AM, *et al.* Bivalirudin and provisional glycoprotein IIb/IIIa blockade compared with heparin and planned glycoprotein IIb/IIIa blockade during percutaneous coronary intervention: REPLACE-2 randomized trial. *JAMA* 2003; **289:** 853–63. Correction. *ibid.*; 1638.

9. Serruys PW, *et al.* A comparison of hirudin with heparin in the prevention of restenosis after coronary angioplasty. *N Engl J Med* 1995; **333:** 757–63.
10. Kong DF, Califf RM. Glycoprotein IIb/IIIa receptor antagonists in non-ST elevation acute coronary syndromes and percutaneous revascularisation: a review of trial reports. *Drugs* 1999; **58:** 609–20.
11. Topol EJ, *et al.* Outcomes at 1 year and economic implications of platelet glycoprotein IIb/IIIa blockade in patients undergoing coronary stenting: results from a multicentre randomised trial. *Lancet* 1999; **354:** 2019–24.
12. O'Shea JC, *et al.* Platelet glycoprotein IIb/IIIa integrin blockade with eptifibatide in coronary stent intervention. The ESPRIT Trial: a randomized controlled trial. *JAMA* 2001; **285:** 2468–73.
13. National Institute for Clinical Excellence. Guidance on the use of glycoprotein IIb/IIIa inhibitors in the treatment of acute coronary syndromes (issued September 2000). Available at: http://www.nice.org.uk/pdf/Nice+GLYCOPROTEIN+12+guidan.pdf (accessed 14/05/04)
14. Dutch Bypass Oral anticoagulants or Aspirin (BOA) Study Group. Efficacy of oral anticoagulants compared with aspirin after infrainguinal bypass surgery (The Dutch Bypass Oral anticoagulants or Aspirin study): a randomised trial. *Lancet* 2000; **355:** 346–51. Correction. *ibid.*; 1104.
15. Mauro LS, *et al.* Introduction to coronary artery stents and their pharmacotherapeutic management. *Ann Pharmacother* 1997; **31:** 1490–8.
16. Holmes DR, *et al.* ACC Expert Consensus document on coronary artery stents. *J Am Coll Cardiol* 1998; **32:** 1471–82.
17. Bertrand ME, *et al.* Double-blind study of the safety of clopidogrel with and without a loading dose in combination with aspirin compared with ticlopidine in combination with aspirin after coronary stenting: the Clopidogrel Aspirin Stent International Cooperative Study (CLASSICS). *Circulation* 2000; **102:** 624–9.
18. El-Beyrouty C, Spinler SA. Cilostazol for prevention of thrombosis and restenosis after intracoronary stenting. *Ann Pharmacother* 2001; **35:** 1108–13.
19. Serruys PW, *et al.* Randomised comparison of implantation of heparin-coated stents with balloon angioplasty in selected patients with coronary artery disease (Benestent II). *Lancet* 1998; **352:** 673–81. Correction. *ibid.*; 1478.
20. Landau C, *et al.* Percutaneous transluminal coronary angioplasty. *N Engl J Med* 1994; **330:** 981–93.
21. Vahanian A, Iung B. Role of calcium channel blockers in reducing acute ischaemia and preventing restenosis in PTCA. *Drugs* 1996; **52** (suppl 4): 9–16.
22. Garas SM, *et al.* Overview of therapies for prevention of restenosis after coronary interventions. *Pharmacol Ther* 2001; **92:** 165–78.
23. Antiplatelet Trialists' Collaboration. Collaborative overview of randomised trials of antiplatelet therapy—maintenance of vascular graft or arterial patency by antiplatelet therapy. *BMJ* 1994; **308:** 159–68.
24. Antithrombotic Trialists' Collaboration. Collaborative meta-analysis of randomised trials of antiplatelet therapy for prevention of death, myocardial infarction, and stroke in high risk patients. *BMJ* 2002; **324:** 71–86.
25. Mehta SR, *et al.* Effects of pretreatment with clopidogrel and aspirin followed by long-term therapy in patients undergoing percutaneous coronary intervention: the PCI-CURE study. *Lancet* 2001; **358:** 527–33.
26. Serruys PW, *et al.* The TRAPIST study: a multicentre randomized placebo controlled clinical trial of trapidil for prevention of restenosis after coronary stenting, measured by 3-D intravascular ultrasound. *Eur Heart J* 2001; **22:** 1938–47.
27. Holmes DR, *et al.* Results of Prevention of REStenosis with Tranilast and its Outcomes (PRESTO) trial. *Circulation* 2002; **106:** 1243–50.
28. Regar E, *et al.* Stent development and local drug delivery. *Br Med Bull* 2001; **59:** 227–48.
29. Fattori R, Piva T. Drug-eluting stents in vascular intervention. *Lancet* 2003; **361:** 247–9.
30. Verin V, *et al.* Endoluminal beta-radiation therapy for the prevention of coronary restenosis after balloon angioplasty. *N Engl J Med* 2001; **344:** 243–9.
31. Leon MB, *et al.* Localized intracoronary gamma-radiation therapy to inhibit the recurrence of restenosis after stenting. *N Engl J Med* 2001; **344:** 250–6.
32. Morice M-C, *et al.* A randomized comparison of a sirolimus-eluting stent with a standard stent for coronary revascularization. *N Engl J Med* 2002; **346:** 1773–80.
33. Moses JW, *et al.* Sirolimus-eluting stents versus standard stents in patients with stenosis in a native coronary artery. *N Engl J Med* 2003; **349:** 1315–23.
34. Stone GW, *et al.* A polymer-based, paclitaxel-eluting stent in patients with coronary artery disease. *N Engl J Med* 2004; **350:** 221–31.
35. The Post Coronary Artery Bypass Graft Trial Investigators. The effect of aggressive lowering of low-density lipoprotein cholesterol levels and low-dose anticoagulation on obstructive changes in saphenous-vein coronary-artery bypass grafts. *N Engl J Med* 1997; **336:** 153–62.
36. Greenberg RK, Ouriel K. A multi-modal approach to the management of bypass graft failure. *Vasc Med* 1998; **3:** 215–20.

## Shock

Shock is a complex clinical syndrome of multiple aetiologies but the common factor in all types of shock is a failure of the circulatory system to maintain cellular perfusion and function. A traditional approach has been to place the cause of shock into one of several basic groups. Commonly used groupings are hypovolaemic shock, cardiogenic shock, septic shock, and anaphylactic shock. These are the types discussed below.

*Hypovolaemic shock* results from fluid loss and can be due to a haemorrhagic or non-haemorrhagic cause. Haemorrhagic causes include severe gastrointestinal bleeding and traumatic injury, while non-haemorrhagic causes include severe vomiting and diarrhoea, polyuria, and burns. Hypovolaemia can also be present in other forms of shock; fluid loss from the vasculature may occur due to capillary leakage in septic or anaphylactic shock, while peripheral vasodilatation may lead to relative hypovolaemia.

*Cardiogenic shock* usually results from acute failure of the heart, leading to an inadequate stroke volume and reduced cardiac output. It has a number of causes, but is most commonly associated with acute myocardial infarction. Other cardiac causes include valvular heart disease, cardiomyopathies, and severe cardiac arrhythmias; episodes of acute heart failure may also occur in patients with chronic heart failure. Shock due to circulatory disorders such as massive pulmonary embolism is also sometimes classified as cardiogenic. Other forms of shock may also have a cardiac component.

*Septic shock* occurs as a complication of infectious disease and is described and defined in more detail under Septicaemia, p.144. Hypotension occurs primarily due to peripheral vasodilatation, but fluid loss and direct effects on the heart may also be involved.

*Anaphylactic shock* (p.855) is the result of a hypersensitivity reaction and is similar haemodynamically to septic shock.

The haemodynamic effects of shock thus result either from an absolute or relative reduction in plasma volume, or a reduction in cardiac output. Although compensatory mechanisms are initially able to restore the blood pressure, these become inadequate and patients in decompensated shock classically present with hypotension, tachycardia, and tachypnoea. Compensatory peripheral vasoconstriction leads to cold, clammy, cyanotic skin and impaired organ perfusion results in dulled mental alertness, which may progress to stupor or coma; oliguria or anuria, due to impaired renal perfusion, are also frequent. Pulmonary oedema may occur as a result of impaired cardiac output in cardiogenic shock. Complications of shock include disseminated intravascular coagulation due to platelet sludging and microvascular insufficiency, acute respiratory distress syndrome (previously termed 'shock lung') (p.1075), and acute renal failure. The terms multiple organ failure syndrome (MOFS) and multiple organ dysfunction syndrome (MODS) are applied to the consequences of shock where several organs or body systems have become hypoperfused and are unable to maintain their normal function.

**Management**. The management of shock can be divided into general supportive and symptomatic measures that may be applicable in all forms of shock, and primary specific therapies directed against any underlying cause.

General measures include correction of electrolyte disturbances, correction of hypovolaemia and hypotension, and improvement of cardiac output.[1] Pain and respiratory problems often accompany shock and may necessitate the administration of intravenous opioid analgesics and oxygen therapy.

Electrolyte disturbances (see Acid-base Balance, p.1217) should be managed conventionally; sodium bicarbonate may be required but should be reserved for severe acidosis.[1] An adequate diuresis should be maintained in order to prevent renal failure.

Correction of hypovolaemia is important in all forms of shock. Replacement fluids available include blood products and crystalloid or colloid plasma expanders,[2,3] and the choice is not always clear. In haemorrhage, although for initial therapy volume expansion is most important, where 40% or more of the total blood volume has been lost red cell replacement is necessary. This usually takes the form of packed red cells in conjunction with plasma expanders, with other plasma components as required for severe haemorrhage. In non-haemorrhagic hypovolaemia, the choice is between crystalloid and colloid plasma expanders, and there continues to be debate over their relative merits. Crystalloids (solutions containing solutes such as glucose or sodium chloride that can pass a semipermeable membrane) rapidly expand both the intravascular and extravascular compartments. Although it has been argued that this is necessary as the interstitial space becomes depleted in hypovolaemia, large volumes are required and the duration of effect is short as fluid is rapidly redistributed. Colloids (solutions containing large molecules such as albumin, dextrans, gelatins, and etherified starches, which do not pass semipermeable membranes) expand the intravascular space more effectively; they have a longer duration of effect and smaller volumes are required. This leads to less haemodilution, although the exact significance of this has been questioned. However, colloids may cause hypersensitivity reactions including anaphylaxis, and this has been raised as a potential concern.

Studies comparing the use of crystalloids and colloids in hypovolaemia have generally been of poor quality and the results are difficult to interpret. A systematic review[4] of trials in critically ill patients concluded that there was a small increase in mortality associated with the use of colloids. However, following considerable criticism,[5,6] an update of the review[7] modified these conclusions to state that there was no evidence of a mortality benefit with colloids and therefore no support for their continued use other than in clinical trials. A further review[8] looking specifically at the use of albumin solutions also suggested that there was an increased mortality in those receiving the colloid, but this review was also criticised.[9] In practice a mixture of colloids and crystalloids tends to be given. It is unclear whether there are any significant differences in outcome associated with the various colloid solutions available,[10] but use of albumin is now generally reserved for specific indications.

Successful correction of hypovolaemia may alleviate hypotension in some cases, but cardiac output may remain depressed and signs of impaired organ perfusion may persist, necessitating additional therapy. Further measures are also frequently needed if there is profound hypotension; blood pressure in shock can be extremely low (sometimes a systolic pressure of less than 70 mmHg) despite fluid replacement. In patients with profound **hypotension** or a **low cardiac output** sympathomimetics are usually employed.[11,12] Their precise effects on the vasculature vary and choice depends on individual patient characteristics and the type of shock.[13] In cardiogenic or hypovolaemic shock cardiac output is usually low but peripheral resistance is high and drugs that have predominantly inotropic effects are most suitable. Dopamine or dobutamine are often chosen. Dopamine has been widely used in all forms of shock, often in combination with other inotropes. At low doses it causes peripheral vasodilatation, which was thought to protect renal perfusion; however, any clinical benefit is unclear and at higher doses it causes vasoconstriction. Dobutamine causes peripheral vasodilatation and is useful where hypotension is not significant. Noradrenaline causes peripheral vasoconstriction and should be reserved for severe hypotension. It is particularly useful in septic shock where the cardiac output is usually high but peripheral resistance is low. It is often given in combination with more potent inotropes such as dobutamine or adrenaline. Adrenaline has also been used alone but renal artery vasoconstriction may limit its use, and it has also been reported to cause lactic acidosis.[14] Vasopressin may be useful[15] in patients with shock due to vasodilatation, such as septic shock or the late stages of other forms of shock, in whom resistance to sympathomimetics commonly occurs. Phosphodiesterase inhibitors such as amrinone and milrinone, which have positive inotropic activity, can also be considered in low cardiac output states;[11] like dopamine they also produce peripheral vasodilatation. Vasodilators such as intravenous glyceryl trinitrate or sodium nitroprusside can be beneficial for patients in shock with a low cardiac output but a high diastolic pressure (more than 110 mmHg),[12] and also in patients with pulmonary oedema.[1] They act by reducing cardiac afterload. Caution must however be observed because of the risk of precipitating hypotension.

In cardiogenic shock associated with **myocardial infarction**,[12,16,17] specific therapy to restore myocardial perfusion is also indicated (see p.828).

In **septic shock** appropriate antibacterial therapy should be given as outlined under Septicaemia on p.144. Methods of inhibiting endogenous mediators released in response to sepsis that are thought to be responsible for the haemodynamic effects are also under investigation but clinical benefits have not yet been demonstrated.[18,19]

Adrenaline is the cornerstone of management in **anaphylactic shock** (see p.855).

1. Hinds CJ, Watson D. ABC of intensive care: circulatory support. *BMJ* 1999; **318:** 1749–52.
2. Nolan JP, Parr MJA. Aspects of resuscitation in trauma. *Br J Anaesth* 1997; **79:** 226–40.
3. Nolan J. Fluid replacement. *Br Med Bull* 1999; **55:** 821–43.
4. Schierhout G, Roberts I. Fluid resuscitation with colloid or crystalloid solutions in critically ill patients: a systematic review of randomised trials. *BMJ* 1998; **316:** 961–4.
5. Watts J. Fluid resuscitation with colloid or crystalloid solutions. *BMJ* 1998; **317:** 277.
6. Wyncoll DLA, *et al.* Fluid resuscitation with colloid or crystalloid solutions. *BMJ* 1998; **317:** 278–9.
7. Alderson P, *et al.* Colloids versus crystalloids for fluid resuscitation in critically ill patients. Available in The Cochrane Library; Issue 2. Chichester: John Wiley; 2004.
8. Cochrane Injuries Group Albumin Reviewers. Human albumin administration in critically ill patients: systematic review of randomised controlled trials. *BMJ* 1998; **317:** 235–40.
9. Beale RJ, *et al.* Human albumin administration in critically ill patients. *BMJ* 1998; **317:** 884.
10. Bunn F, *et al.* Colloid solutions for fluid resuscitation. Available in The Cochrane Library; Issue 2. Chichester: John Wiley; 2004.
11. Barnard MJ, Linter SPK. Acute circulatory support. *BMJ* 1993; **307:** 35–41.

12. Califf RM, Bengtson JR. Cardiogenic shock. *N Engl J Med* 1994; **330:** 1724–30.
13. Cuthbertson BH, *et al.* Inotropic agents in the critically ill. *Br J Hosp Med* 1996; **56:** 386–91.
14. Day NPJ, *et al.* The effects of dopamine and adrenaline infusions on acid-base balance and systemic haemodynamics in severe infection. *Lancet* 1996; **348:** 219–23.
15. Dünser MW, *et al.* Management of vasodilatory shock: defining the role of arginine vasopressin. *Drugs* 2003; **63:** 237–56.
16. Hollenberg SM, *et al.* Cardiogenic shock. *Ann Intern Med* 1999; **131:** 47–59.
17. Hasdai D, *et al.* Cardiogenic shock complicating acute coronary syndromes. *Lancet* 2000; **356:** 749–56.
18. Glauser MP. The inflammatory cytokines: new developments in the pathophysiology and treatment of septic shock. *Drugs* 1996; **52** (suppl 2): 9–17.
19. Astiz ME, Rackow EC. Septic shock. *Lancet* 1998; **351:** 1501–5.


## Stroke

Stroke, sometimes called a cerebrovascular accident, is the major consequence of cerebrovascular disease and has been defined as an acute neurological dysfunction of vascular origin with sudden (within seconds) or at least rapid (within hours) occurrence of symptoms and signs corresponding to the involvement of focal areas of the brain.[1] If signs and symptoms persist for more than 24 hours the event is termed a completed stroke whereas if they disappear within a few minutes or hours, or at most within 24 hours, the event is termed a transient ischaemic attack.

Strokes may be ischaemic (infarction-related) or haemorrhagic.[2,3] **Ischaemic stroke** is by far the commonest type and may result from arterial occlusion caused by local thrombosis in the vessels of the brain at sites of atheroma or, more often, by thromboembolism arising from outside the brain and lodging in the cerebral vessels. An example of the latter is cardio-embolic infarction associated with atrial fibrillation or acute myocardial infarction. Such arterial occlusion results in inadequate cerebral perfusion, depriving the brain of glucose and oxygen, and leading to stroke. About 20% of patients with acute ischaemic stroke experience worsening of symptoms within a few days of onset. This is termed progressing stroke, stroke-in-evolution, or unstable stroke, and occurs when the thrombotic process is incomplete. **Transient ischaemic attacks** are acute episodes of focal neurological deficit or monocular visual loss (amaurosis fugax), mainly due to ischaemia associated with atherothrombosis, but unlike stroke they last less than 24 hours and often only minutes. They are usually of sudden onset with complete clinical recovery but a tendency to recur. Patients suffering these attacks are at an increased risk of stroke. **Haemorrhagic stroke** is secondary to subarachnoid or to intracerebral haemorrhage. *Subarachnoid haemorrhage* is bleeding into the fluid-filled subarachnoid space between the brain and the skull, and usually occurs after rupture of an aneurysm; other causes include arteriovenous malformations and hypertensive microaneurysms. *Intracerebral haemorrhage* is bleeding into the parenchyma of the brain, and may result from rupture of arteries damaged by chronic hypertension. Haemorrhage produces a focal haematoma causing a local increase in pressure which may lead to further bleeding and enlargement of the haematoma. The increase in pressure in the area of the haematoma may also produce local ischaemia.

Clinical presentation of stroke can vary enormously in severity and combination of signs and symptoms, and depends on the site of infarction or haemorrhage. Neurological deficits may include impairments to speech, balance, vision, touch sensation, and movement. Patients have been classed as major or minor stroke (reversible ischaemic neurological deficit) victims according to their degree of recovery at a given time after the stroke.

It is important to diagnose the type of stroke correctly because management is very different and what might be of benefit in patients with cerebral infarction might be dangerous in those with haemorrhage. Haemorrhagic stroke is typically of sudden onset with severe headaches, vomiting, and rapid deterioration of consciousness – all signs of raised intracranial pressure – but mild to moderate haemorrhage may be difficult to distinguish from infarction on the basis of clinical signs alone. Computed tomography (CT) is a surer way of distinguishing between haemorrhagic and ischaemic stroke. Magnetic resonance imaging may also be useful. Recent guidelines[4-7] have emphasised that, as in myocardial infarction, early recognition of symptoms and prompt evaluation and treatment of stroke are of vital importance. Where possible patients should be managed within a stroke unit.

Diagnosis of transient ischaemic attacks usually rests on the patient's history as these short attacks are seldom witnessed by a physician and there are no objective confirmatory tests.

Management of stroke can be divided into treatment of acute stroke, either ischaemic or haemorrhagic, and long-term treatment for secondary prevention. Symptomatic treatment of complications such as swallowing disorders or spasticity may also be required, but is not discussed here. Primary prevention may be considered in individuals at risk of ischaemic stroke. This includes those with atrial fibrillation, a major risk factor for stroke (see Cardiac Arrhythmias, p.816), and those with risk factors for atherosclerosis (see Cardiovascular Risk Reduction p.819); the role of endarterectomy in individuals with carotid artery stenosis is discussed under Secondary Prevention, below.

**Ischaemic stroke**. The treatment of acute ischaemic stroke has been reviewed[8-11] and guidelines[4-7] have been published. The aim is early reversal or limitation of the degree of brain dysfunction by treatment, given as soon as possible after the onset of symptoms, that will re-establish cerebral blood flow, limit ischaemic neuronal injury, and reduce cerebral oedema. General supportive measures include ensuring adequate oxygenation and fluid and electrolyte balances, avoiding hypercapnia and hyperglycaemia or hypoglycaemia, abolishing seizures, and treating fever. Control of hypertension is controversial since lowering the blood pressure may reduce cerebral perfusion and worsen ischaemia, and hypertension usually resolves spontaneously without treatment.[12] Antihypertensive therapy may be indicated in specific patients, such as those with severe hypertension or those being considered for thrombolytic therapy.

Specific therapy is limited but has mainly involved antithrombotic drugs and neuroprotectants. Antithrombotic therapy with antiplatelet drugs, heparin, and thrombolytics would be expected to be of benefit in the treatment of cerebral infarction and the re-establishment of cerebral blood flow. However, the evidence is limited and the presence of haemorrhage must be excluded and the risk of potentiating spontaneous secondary brain haemorrhage (haemorrhagic transformation) must be borne in mind. The use of neuroprotectants to limit the effects of ischaemia on brain tissue is also attractive, but results to date have been disappointing.

***Antiplatelet drugs.*** The rationale for using aspirin is based on its effectiveness in patients with myocardial infarction where the underlying vascular pathology is similar to that in ischaemic stroke. Aspirin has been evaluated in two large studies—the International Stroke Trial (IST)[13] and the Chinese Acute Stroke Trial (CAST).[14] The combined results of these studies[14] found that aspirin 160 mg[14] or 300 mg[13] daily started within 48 hours of symptom onset produced about 9 fewer deaths or non-fatal strokes per 1000 patients in the first few weeks following ischaemic stroke. Aspirin has therefore been recommended for patients with ischaemic stroke who are not receiving thrombolytic or anticoagulant therapy, and should be started within 48 hours of stroke onset.[4,5,7,15,16]

***Anticoagulants*** are not routinely recommended in the early management of acute ischaemic stroke, although they may have a role in selected patients.[4,5,16] Anticoagulation should prevent further thrombus formation and limit the size of the cerebral infarct; however, any benefit may be offset by an increase in intracranial haemorrhage, and a systematic review[17] has suggested there is no evidence to support routine use. The IST[13] which evaluated two dosages of heparin (5000 units or 12 500 units subcutaneously twice daily), found no benefit from either regimen and the higher dose particularly was associated with haemorrhagic stroke and bleeding. Another study,[18] comparing the low-molecular-weight heparin tinzaparin with aspirin, similarly found no benefit. It had been suggested that patients with cardio-embolic stroke were likely to benefit from heparin therapy,[19] even though there is a special risk of haemorrhagic transformation in these patients which means that early anticoagulation is often hazardous. However, the IST[13] failed to show any benefit in this group, and a study[20] of low-molecular-weight heparin in patients with acute ischaemic stroke and atrial fibrillation also showed no benefit. No improvement in outcome was reported after 3 months in a study of danaparoid given in acute ischaemic stroke.[21] A study[22] with ancrod found an improvement in outcome when given within 3 hours of stroke onset, but a further study was terminated due to lack of benefit. Although stroke-in-evolution has been considered as an indication for heparin therapy, the evidence for any benefit is poor.[15]

Low-dose subcutaneous heparin may be indicated to reduce the risk of venous thromboembolism (deep-vein thrombosis and pulmonary embolism) associated with stroke.

***Thrombolytics.*** Stroke is normally considered a contra-indication to the use of thrombolytics, and clearly they would be inappropriate in acute haemorrhagic stroke. However, when stroke is associated with thrombotic occlusion there is evidence, as with myocardial infarction, that a degree of neuronal recovery is possible if the occlusion is reversed sufficiently quickly[23,24] Studies using thrombolytics in acute stroke have had mixed results, and their role remains controversial. A study[25] with alteplase given within 3 hours of the onset of stroke (NINDS—National Institute of Neurological Disorders and Stroke rt-PA Stroke Trial) found that alteplase appeared to improve clinical outcome despite an increased incidence of symptomatic intracerebral haemorrhage. Patients treated with alteplase were more likely to have minimal or no disability 3 months following stroke,[25] and this benefit was maintained at 12 months.[26] However, there was no difference in mortality or rate of recurrence of stroke. On the basis of this study, most guidelines[4-7,15] now recommend alteplase for selected patients if it can be given within 3 hours of stroke onset. Studies of the use of alteplase outside the setting of a clinical trial have had mixed results.[27,28] Other thrombolytics, such as streptokinase, have generally produced less favourable results, and none of these are currently recommended. The intra-arterial administration of thrombolytics is under investigation and may be used in selected patients.[4,5,15]

Other attempts to improve cerebral blood flow have included haemodilution with *dextran* or *pentastarch,* but both of these approaches have been disappointing and they are not generally recommended.[4,5]

***Neuroprotection.*** Ischaemia leads to a complex series of biochemical changes, the 'ischaemic cascade', resulting eventually in cell necrosis. The process is incompletely understood, but steps include calcium influx and release of neurotransmitters. Drugs acting at different steps in this ischaemic cascade, sometimes termed neuroprotectants, have been tried in acute ischaemic stroke in the hope of limiting the damage caused by ischaemia. Results of studies so far have been largely disappointing, and no drug has yet been found to be effective. However, this is an area of active research and many trials of neuroprotectants are underway[29] with many focusing on starting treatment in the first few hours following ischaemic stroke.[30] Drugs that have been investigated include:

- *calcium-channel blockers* such as nimodipine. In addition to increasing cerebral blood flow they may prevent brain cell necrosis by limiting transcellular calcium influx, but results have been conflicting;
- *clomethiazole*, which may act through an agonist effect on GABA receptors;
- *citicoline*, a derivative of choline and cytidine, thought to prevent accumulation of toxic free fatty acids and to contribute to repair of damaged neuronal tissue;
- *edaravone*, a free-radical scavenger;
- *fibroblast growth factors* that stimulate blood vessel formation and tissue repair processes;
- *glycine antagonists*, such as gavestinel, which block neuronal influx of calcium;
- *lipid peroxidation inhibitors* such as tirilazad (also used in subarachnoid haemorrhage) and ebselen;
- *lubeluzole*, a glutamate antagonist;
- *magnesium sulfate*;
- *naftidrofuryl*, which has a direct effect on cerebral intracellular metabolism and protects cells against the results of ischaemia;
- *N-methyl-D-aspartate (NMDA)-receptor antagonists* such as aptiganel, dextrorphan, dextromethorphan, dizocilpine, and ketamine might reduce ischaemic neuronal injury by preventing fatal influx of calcium;
- *pentoxifylline* reduces viscosity of blood and this effect may be beneficial in ischaemic tissue.

Hypoxia and hypocapnia occur in some patients with ischaemic stroke and are likely to contribute to ischaemic injury both directly and via cerebral vasoconstriction. There are anecdotal reports and some small studies on the use of *hyperbaric oxygen therapy* but its clinical value remains unknown.

Cerebral oedema associated with ischaemic stroke may be a mixture of intracellular oedema associated with cell damage (part of the ischaemic cascade) and interstitial vasogenic oedema. Treatment with *corticosteroids* or hyperosmolar diuretics such as *glycerol* or *mannitol* in an attempt to reduce the cerebral oedema has been disappointing.[31]

***Long-term management.*** Patients who have had an ischaemic stroke or transient ischaemic attack are at risk of further stroke but are also at increased risk of other cardiovascular events, including myocardial infarction and sudden death. Long-term treatment for secondary prevention therefore has an important role.[32,33] All patients should be assessed for risk factors, including hypertension and atrial fibrillation, and these should be treated as appropriate. Blood screening should also be carried out for polycythaemia, thrombocytosis, and abnormal coagulation functions. Carotid endarterectomy is of established benefit for secondary prevention in patients with clinically significant carotid stenosis,[4,34] but its role in primary prevention is less clear.[35] Antithrombotic therapy may also have a specific role.

***Antiplatelet drugs.*** Long-term prophylaxis with aspirin reduces the risk of future serious vascular events including stroke in patients who have already suffered an ischaemic stroke or transient ischaemic attack,[15,36-38] regardless of age.[39] Medium doses of 75 to 325 mg of aspirin daily have been most widely studied[36] and an analysis of trials using aspirin over a dose range of 50 to 1500 mg daily found no relationship between dose and the reduction in risk of stroke.[40] In patients undergoing carotid endarterectomy the risk of stroke, myocardial infarction, and death over 3 months may be lower for those taking medium dose aspirin compared with higher doses.[41] Dipyridamole given alone has also been shown to be effective for secondary prevention of ischaemic stroke[42] and may be used in patients unable to tolerate aspirin; the combination of aspirin and dipyridamole has produced additive protective effects.[42] Earlier studies had produced conflicting results however, possibly due to differences in dose and formulation. A meta-analysis[43] concluded that the combination did reduce the risk of stroke more than aspirin alone, but that further study is needed. Clopidogrel[44] may also be used in patients unable to tolerate aspirin and appears to be at least as effective; ticlopidine is also effective[45-47] but adverse effects limit its use.

***Anticoagulants.*** Oral anticoagulants have an established role in patients with cardioembolic stroke, but their value in patients with non-cardioembolic stroke or with transient ischaemic attacks is unclear. One study[48] was terminated early because of a high rate of major bleeding complications in the patients receiving an oral anticoagulant, while another study[49] comparing warfarin with aspirin found no additional benefit with the anticoagulant, although bleeding was not significantly increased. Anticoagulants are therefore not generally recommended for secondary prevention in non-cardioembolic stroke[4,7,37] although they have been used in patients with recurrent symptoms despite antiplatelet therapy.[38]

**Subarachnoid haemorrhage.** Subarachnoid haemorrhage[50,51] is associated with high morbidity and mortality, early deaths being due to damage from initial bleeding, recurrence of bleeding, and infarction. Infarction is often a result of vasospasm which is one of the pathophysiological mechanisms that contributes to stopping the bleeding; clot formation and increasing intracranial pressure are other processes involved. Up to a quarter of patients with subarachnoid haemorrhage develop delayed cerebral ischaemia mainly between days 5 and 14 after the initial bleed, and again vasospasm may be a contributory factor. Early medical treatment aims to prevent delayed cerebral ischaemia, to prevent rebleeding, and to stabilise the patient. Surgical or endovascular interventions to clip or embolise the aneurysm or correct the arteriovenous malformation are then performed to prevent further haemorrhage. Plasma volume should be maintained to prevent delayed cerebral ischaemia; a fluid intake of 3 litres per day has been recommended. Nimodipine is of benefit and should be started as soon as possible after diagnosis of subarachnoid haemorrhage. There is some evidence[52] that papaverine may be useful in patients with refractory vasospasm. Antifibrinolytic drug therapy with tranexamic acid or aminocaproic acid has been used to prevent rebleeding, particularly if surgery is to be delayed, but a systematic review[53] found that any benefits were offset by an increase in poor outcomes due to cerebral ischaemia. Paradoxically, rebleeding has been noted in patients given high doses of aminocaproic acid after subarachnoid haemorrhage (see Effects on the Blood, under Adverse Effects of Aminocaproic Acid, p.741). Headache can be managed with analgesics such as paracetamol, dextropropoxyphene, or codeine; aspirin should be avoided. Localised haematomas may be amenable to surgical evacuation, and intraventricular thrombolytics have also been used.[54] Tirilazad, a lipid peroxidation inhibitor, may be given to male patients with subarachnoid haemorrhage, but is not suitable for females due to pharmacokinetic factors. It is thought to have a cytoprotective effect against radicals produced in response to tissue trauma.

**Intracerebral haemorrhage.** Outcome of intracerebral haemorrhage depends on the location and size of the haematoma (determined by computed tomography), on the level of consciousness, and on the progression of neurological signs, and development of increased intracranial pressure.[55,56] Any known cause of bleeding, such as warfarin anticoagulation, should be reversed. Blood pressure should be lowered when it is very high (>180 mmHg systolic[57]), but hypoperfusion should be avoided. Drugs such as labetalol, esmolol, or sodium nitroprusside have been used to reduce blood pressure. Surgical drainage of the haematoma may sometimes be possible. Instillation of a thrombolytic to improve aspiration of the haematoma has been reported.[58] Raised intracranial pressure must be controlled[57] (see p.833). Antiepileptic prophylaxis, usually with phenytoin, may be necessary in some patients.[57] Long-term management of risk factors, particularly hypertension, should be considered for secondary prevention.


1. WHO. Stroke—1989: recommendations on stroke prevention, diagnosis, and therapy: report of the WHO task force on stroke and other cerebrovascular disorders. *Stroke* 1989; **20:** 1407–31.
2. Bath PMW, Lees KR. ABC of arterial and venous disease: acute stroke. *BMJ* 2000; **320:** 920–3.
3. Warlow C, *et al.* Stroke. *Lancet* 2003; **362:** 1211–24. Correction. *ibid.* 2004; **363:** 402.
4. The European Stroke Initiative Executive Committee and the EUSI Writing Committee. European Stroke Initiative recommendations for stroke management – update 2003. *Cerebrovasc Dis* 2003; **16:** 311–37.
5. Adams HP, *et al.* Guidelines for the early management of patients with acute ischemic stroke: a scientific statement from the Stroke Council of the American Stroke Association. *Stroke* 2003; **34:** 1056–83. Also available at: http://stroke.ahajournals.org/cgi/reprint/34/4/1056.pdf (accessed 21/05/04)
6. The American Heart Association in collaboration with the International Committee on Resuscitation (ILCOR). International guidelines 2000 for cardiopulmonary resuscitation and emergency cardiovascular care: a consensus on science. Part 7: the era of reperfusion. Section 2: acute stroke. *Circulation* 2000; **102** (suppl I): I204–I216. Also published in *Resuscitation* 2000; **46:** 239–52.
7. The Intercollegiate Stroke Working Party. National clinical guidelines for stroke: second edition. London: Royal College of Physicians; 2004. Also available at: http://www.rcplondon.ac.uk/pubs/books/stroke/Stroke_guidelines_2ed.pdf (accessed 07/07/04)
8. Alberts MJ. Diagnosis and treatment of ischemic stroke. *Am J Med* 1999; **106:** 211–21.
9. Lindley RI. Drug therapy for acute ischaemic stroke: risks versus benefits. *Drug Safety* 1998; **19:** 373–82.
10. Hill MD, Hachinski V. Stroke treatment: time is brain. *Lancet* 1998; **352** (suppl 3): 10–14.
11. Brott T, Bogousslavsky J. Treatment of acute ischemic stroke. *N Engl J Med* 2000; **343:** 710–22.
12. Goldstein LB. Should antihypertensive therapies be given to patients with acute ischaemic stroke? *Drug Safety* 2000; **22:** 13–18.
13. International Stroke Trial Collaborative Group. The International Stroke Trial (IST): a randomised trial of aspirin, subcutaneous heparin, both, or neither among 19 435 patients with acute ischaemic stroke. *Lancet* 1997; **349:** 1569–81.
14. CAST (Chinese Acute Stroke Trial) Collaborative Group. CAST: randomised placebo-controlled trial of early aspirin use in 20 000 patients with acute ischaemic stroke. *Lancet* 1997; **349:** 1641–9.
15. Albers GW, *et al.* Antithrombotic and thrombolytic therapy for ischemic stroke. *Chest* 2001; **119** (suppl): 300S–320S.
16. Coull BM, *et al.* Anticoagulants and antiplatelet agents in acute ischemic stroke: report of the Joint Stroke Guideline Development Committee of the American Academy of Neurology and the American Stroke Association (a division of the American Heart Association). *Stroke* 2002; **33:** 1934–42. Also published in *Neurology* 2002; **59:** 13–22. Also available at: http://www.neurology.org/cgi/reprint/59/1/13.pdf (accessed 14/05/04)
17. Gubitz G, *et al.* Anticoagulants for acute ischaemic stroke. Available in The Cochrane Library; Issue 2. Chichester: John Wiley; 2004.
18. Bath PMW, *et al.* Tinzaparin in acute ischaemic stroke (TAIST): a randomised aspirin-controlled trial. *Lancet* 2001; **358:** 702–10. Correction. *ibid.*; 1276.
19. Sandercock PAG, *et al.* Antithrombotic therapy in acute ischaemic stroke: an overview of the completed randomised trials. *J Neurol Neurosurg Psychiatry* 1993; **56:** 17–25.
20. Berge E, *et al.* Low molecular-weight heparin versus aspirin in patients with acute ischaemic stroke and atrial fibrillation: a double-blind randomised study. *Lancet* 2000; **355:** 1205–10.
21. The Publications Committee for the Trial of ORG 10172 in Acute Stroke Treatment (TOAST) Investigators. Low molecular weight heparinoid, ORG 10172 (danaparoid), and outcome after acute ischemic stroke: a randomized controlled trial. *JAMA* 1998; **279:** 1265–72.
22. Sherman DG, *et al.* Intravenous ancrod for treatment of acute ischemic stroke: the STAT study: a randomized controlled trial. *JAMA* 2000; **283:** 2395–2403.
23. Tanne D, *et al.* Management of acute ischaemic stroke in the elderly: tolerability of thrombolytics. *Drugs* 2001; **61:** 1439–53.
24. Meschia JF, *et al.* Thrombolytic treatment of acute ischemic stroke. *Mayo Clin Proc* 2002; **77:** 542–51.
25. The National Institute of Neurological Disorders and Stroke rt-PA Stroke Study Group. Tissue plasminogen activator for acute ischemic stroke. *N Engl J Med* 1995; **333:** 1581–7.
26. Kwiatowski TG, *et al.* Effects of tissue plasminogen activator for acute ischemic stroke at one year. *N Engl J Med* 1999; **340:** 1781–7.
27. Albers GW, *et al.* Intravenous tissue-type plasminogen activator for treatment of acute stroke: the Standard Treatment with Alteplase to Reverse Stroke (STARS) Study. *JAMA* 2000; **283:** 1145–50.
28. Katzan IL, *et al.* Use of tissue-type plasminogen activator for acute ischemic stroke: the Cleveland area experience. *JAMA* 2000; **283:** 1151–8.
29. Lees KR. Neuroprotection. *Br Med Bull* 2000; **56:** 401–12.
30. Fisher M, Bogousslavsky J. Further evolution toward effective therapy for acute ischemic stroke. *JAMA* 1998; **279:** 1298–1303.
31. Anonymous. Treatment for stroke? *Lancet* 1991; **337:** 1129–31.
32. Straus SE, *et al.* New evidence for stroke prevention: scientific review. *JAMA* 2002; **288:** 1388–95.
33. MacWalter RS, Shirley CP. A benefit-risk assessment of agents used in the secondary prevention of stroke. *Drug Safety* 2002; **25:** 943–63.
34. Biller J, *et al.* Guidelines for carotid endarterectomy: a statement for healthcare professionals from a special writing group of the Stroke Council, American Heart Association. *Stroke* 1998; **29:** 554–62. Also available at: http://circ.ahajournals.org/cgi/reprint/97/5/501.pdf (accessed 21/05/04)
35. Benavente O, *et al.* Carotid endarterectomy for asymptomatic carotid stenosis: a meta-analysis. *BMJ* 1998; **317:** 1477–80.
36. Antithrombotic Trialists' Collaboration. Collaborative meta-analysis of randomised trials of antiplatelet therapy for prevention of death, myocardial infarction, and stroke in high risk patients. *BMJ* 2002; **324:** 71–86. Correction. *ibid.*; 141.
37. Wolf PA, *et al.* Preventing ischemic stroke in patients with prior stroke and transient ischemic attack: a statement for healthcare professionals from the Stroke Council of the American Heart Association. *Stroke* 1999; **30:** 1991–4.
38. Albers GW, *et al.* Supplement to the guidelines for the management of transient ischemic attacks: a statement from the Ad Hoc Committee on Guidelines for the Management of Transient Ischemic Attacks, Stroke Council, American Heart Association. *Stroke* 1999; **30:** 2502–11. Also available at: http://stroke.ahajournals.org/cgi/reprint/30/11/2502.pdf (accessed 21/05/04)
39. Sivenius J, *et al.* Antiplatelet treatment in elderly people with transient ischaemic attacks or ischaemic strokes. *BMJ* 1995; **310:** 25–6.
40. Johnson ES, *et al.* A metaregression analysis of the dose-response effect of aspirin on stroke. *Arch Intern Med* 1999; **159:** 1248–53.
41. Taylor DW, *et al.* Low-dose and high-dose acetylsalicylic acid for patients undergoing carotid endarterectomy: a randomised controlled trial. *Lancet* 1999; **353:** 2179–84.
42. Diener HC, *et al.* European Stroke Prevention Study 2: dipyridamole and acetylsalicylic acid in the secondary prevention of stroke. *J Neurol Sci* 1996; **143:** 1–13.
43. Wilterdink JL, Easton JD. Dipyridamole plus aspirin in cerebrovascular disease. *Arch Neurol* 1999; **56:** 1087–92.
44. CAPRIE Steering Committee. A randomised, blinded, trial of clopidogrel versus aspirin in patients at risk of ischaemic events (CAPRIE). *Lancet* 1996; **348:** 1329–39.
45. Hass WK, *et al.* A randomized trial comparing ticlopidine hydrochloride with aspirin for the prevention of stroke in high-risk patients. *N Engl J Med* 1989; **321:** 501–7.
46. Harbison JW. Ticlopidine versus aspirin for the prevention of recurrent stroke: analysis of patients with minor stroke from the ticlopidine aspirin stroke study. *Stroke* 1992; **23:** 1723–7.
47. Bellavance A. Efficacy of ticlopidine and aspirin for prevention of reversible cerebrovascular ischemic events: the ticlopidine aspirin stroke study. *Stroke* 1993; **24:** 1452–7.
48. The Stroke Prevention in Reversible Ischemia Trial (SPIRIT) Study Group. A randomized trial of anticoagulants versus aspirin after cerebral ischemia of presumed arterial origin. *Ann Neurol* 1997; **42:** 857–65.
49. Mohr JP, *et al.* A comparison of warfarin and aspirin for the prevention of recurrent ischemic stroke. *N Engl J Med* 2001; **345:** 1444–51.
50. van Gijn J. Subarachnoid haemorrhage. *Lancet* 1992; **339:** 653–5.
51. Bendok BR, *et al.* Treatment of aneurysmal subarachnoid hemorrhage. *Semin Neurol* 1998; **18:** 521–31.
52. Clouston JE, *et al.* Intraarterial papaverine infusion for cerebral vasospasm after subarachnoid hemorrhage. *Am J Neuroradiol* 1995; **16:** 27–38.
53. Roos YBWEM, *et al.* Antifibrinolytic therapy for aneurysmal subarachnoid haemorrhage. Available in The Cochrane Library; Issue 2. Chichester: John Wiley; 2004.
54. Rice TL, *et al.* Thrombolytic administration in the management of subarachnoid hemorrhage. *Am J Health-Syst Pharm* 2003; **60:** 1883–93.
55. Caplan LR. Intracerebral haemorrhage. *Lancet* 1992; **339:** 656–8.
56. Qureshi AI, *et al.* Spontaneous intracerebral hemorrhage. *N Engl J Med* 2001; **344:** 1450–60.
57. Broderick JP, *et al.* Guidelines for the management of spontaneous intracerebral hemorrhage: a statement for healthcare professionals from a special writing group of the Stroke Council, American Heart Association. *Stroke* 1999; **30:** 905–15. Also available at: http://stroke.ahajournals.org/cgi/reprint/30/4/905.pdf (accessed 21/05/04)
58. Andrews CO, Engelhard HH. Fibrinolytic therapy in intraventricular hemorrhage. *Ann Pharmacother* 2001; **35:** 1435–48.


### Thromboembolic disorders

The term thromboembolic disorder has been applied loosely to cardiovascular disorders associated with thrombus and embolus formation in blood vessels. A **thrombus** is a stationary blood clot composed of fibrin and platelets and other cellular elements. **Thrombosis** is occlusion of a vein or artery by a thrombus. An **embolus** is a fragment of blood clot, atheromatous material, or other foreign matter carried along in the bloodstream. Occlusion of a blood vessel by an embolus is termed **embolism** or **thromboembolism**.

Formation of blood clots in the body is the result of a coagulation cascade (see Haemostasis and Fibrinolysis, p.735). Under normal circumstances systemic coagulation is prevented by natural antithrombotic systems that limit blood clots to sites of vascular injury. Thromboembolic disorders occur when there is an imbalance between these systems. Three factors are involved, namely damage to the endothelial lining of blood vessels, reduced blood flow, or changes in the coagulation mechanisms of the blood. A further factor that increases the risk of clotting is the presence of an artificial surface in contact with the blood, for example mechanical heart valves, intravascular catheters, or during extracorporeal circulation procedures. Thromboembolism can occur in any part of the circulation, including the heart and the capillaries, but the characteristics of the thrombi, the consequences, and the management of thromboembolism depend to a large extent upon whether the arterial or venous system is involved.

The mainstay of management for thromboembolic disorders is antithrombotic drugs. These act at different points in the coagulation cascade and include anticoagulants and antiplatelet drugs, which are used to limit the extent of thrombosis or thromboembolism and to prevent further thromboembolic events occurring, and thrombolytics, which are used to lyse the clot.

**Arterial thromboembolism** is almost always a consequence of damage to the endothelium due to atherosclerosis (p.815); the atheroma may block the blood vessel or, more commonly, occlusion is a result of thrombus formation at a site of a recently ruptured atheromatous plaque. Arterial thrombi contain more platelets than venous thrombi and tend to remain fixed, but emboli may break off and occlude distal vessels. Arterial emboli may also result from thrombosis within the heart, for example due to arrhythmias or valvular heart disorders.

Thrombosis or thromboembolism in the arterial circulation produces ischaemia in the tissues perfused by the artery, which may lead to infarction. It may therefore result in myocardial infarction (p.828) or unstable angina (p.813) if it occurs in coronary arteries, stroke (p.836) if it occurs in cerebral arteries, or critical limb ischaemia if it occurs in peripheral arteries (p.830).

**Venous thromboembolism** (p.839) is usually a consequence of stasis of the blood, but other factors such as local trauma or coagulation activation are also required. Reduced venous blood flow occurs in many conditions, including obesity, heart failure, and during prolonged immobilisation. Abnormal clotting may occur in conditions such as malignancy, pregnancy, and the nephrotic syndrome, or during oestrogen therapy; it may also be due to inherited or acquired clotting disorders or thrombophilias (see below). Surgical operations are particularly associated with venous thromboembolism; trauma activates clotting factors and reduced blood flow may occur during the procedure and recovery period.

Venous thrombi have a 'red tail' of fibrin and red cells that may occlude the vein but which often separates to form an embolus; this is most likely during the early stages when the thrombus is only loosely attached. Thrombosis or thromboembolism in the venous circulation produces oedema or inflammation in the tissue drained by the affected vein. The commonest type of venous thrombosis is deep-vein thrombosis, which is associated especially with immobility and the postoperative period. Pulmonary embolism is the most serious complication of deep-vein thrombosis and occurs when part of the thrombus migrates in the circulation and becomes lodged in the pulmonary artery. Hypercoagulable states may result in deep-vein thrombosis or more generalised clotting in microvessels (microvessel thrombosis), such as thrombotic thrombocytopenic purpura or purpura fulminans (see Thrombotic Microangiopathies, p.758).

**Thrombophilias** are acquired or inherited disorders of the clotting system in which the antithrombotic mechanisms are impaired. Inherited deficiencies of antithrombin III, protein C and protein S all predispose to thromboembolism. Resistance to activated protein C has been identified as a major cause of inherited thrombophilia and appears to be due to a mutation in the factor V gene (factor V Leiden). A mutation in the prothrombin (factor II) gene is associated with increased concentrations of prothrombin and risk of thrombosis. Acquired thrombophilias may occur secondary to disorders such as malignancy, infection, or collagen-vascular disorders; in many cases antiphospholipid antibodies (such as lupus anticoagulant) are present. Hyperhomocysteinaemia is another risk factor and may have both inherited and acquired causes.

Inherited thrombophilias generally result in venous thromboembolism; this is often recurrent and may occur in unusual sites or at a young age. They often present when some further risk factor is present, such as pregnancy, use of combined oral contraceptives, or surgery, but the value of screening asymptomatic patients remains unclear. Acquired thrombophilias may lead to arterial or venous thromboembolism.

Patients with thrombophilias who develop thromboembolism should be treated conventionally, with anticoagulants or thrombolytics as appropriate. There continues to be debate regarding the duration of therapy, with some authorities recommending life-long anticoagulant therapy following a single episode and others recommending life-long therapy only in those with recurrent thrombosis. The optimum intensity of long-term anticoagulation in patients with thrombophilia is also debated. If anticoagulation is not continued, thromboprophylaxis should be given during high risk situations. Thromboprophylaxis is probably also necessary during pregnancy, particularly in women with antiphospholipid antibodies who are at risk for recurrent fetal loss (see Systemic Lupus Erythematosus, p.1088), but the risks to the fetus from anticoagulant therapy must also be considered (see Venous Thromboembolism, p.839).

References.


1. Haines ST, Bussey HI. Thrombosis and the pharmacology of antithrombotic agents. *Ann Pharmacother* 1995; **29:** 892–905.
2. Anonymous. Management of patients with thrombophilia. *Drug Ther Bull* 1995; **33:** 6–8.
3. WHO. Inherited thrombophilia: memorandum from a joint WHO/International Society on Thrombosis and Haemostasis meeting. *Bull WHO* 1997; **75:** 177–89.
4. Price DT, Ridker PM. Factor V Leiden mutation and the risks for thromboembolic disease: a clinical perspective. *Ann Intern Med* 1997; **127:** 895–903.
5. Rosendaal FR. Venous thrombosis: a multicausal disease. *Lancet* 1999; **353:** 1167–73.
6. Seligsohn U, Lubetsky A. Genetic susceptibility to venous thrombosis. *N Engl J Med* 2001; **344:** 1222–31.
7. Bauer KA. The thrombophilias: well-defined risk factors with uncertain therapeutic implications. *Ann Intern Med* 2001; **135:** 367–73.
8. Crowther MA, *et al.* A comparison of two intensities of warfarin for the prevention of recurrent thrombosis in patients with the antiphospholipid antibody syndrome. *N Engl J Med* 2003; **349:** 1133–8. Correction. *ibid.*; 2577.


## Valvular heart disease

Valvular heart disease affects the normal function of the heart and leads to disorders of blood circulation. The principal cause of valvular disease world-wide is rheumatic heart disease. Other causes include congenital abnormalities, cardiovascular disorders such as ischaemic heart disease and hypertension, and degenerative disorders. Any of the heart valves may be affected but disorders of the aortic and mitral valves are most significant; more than one valve may be involved in some patients.

The symptoms of valvular heart disease depend upon the valve that is affected, and whether the problem is stenosis or regurgitation. All valve disorders place a haemodynamic burden on the heart and ultimately lead to heart failure.[1] Other consequences include the development of pulmonary hypertension and arrhythmias. Infective endocarditis and thromboembolic disorders, in particular stroke or systemic embolism, are important complications.

The main aims of treatment in patients with valvular heart disease are to reduce symptoms, prevent complications, and reduce mortality. In symptomatic patients, standard treatment for heart failure (see p.820) may be of benefit, although improvement is not generally sustained. Choice of therapy depends upon the valve affected.[2] Vasodilators are generally contra-indicated in patients with aortic stenosis[3] since they may reduce blood pressure without increasing cardiac output; however, there has been a report[4] of the successful use of sodium nitroprusside to increase cardiac output in patients with aortic stenosis and decompensated heart failure. In severe aortic regurgitation, vasodilators have an established role; use of nifedipine has improved outcome in asymptomatic patients with severe aortic regurgitation.[5] Arrhythmias should be treated with standard antiarrhythmics (see p.816). Surgical treatment is necessary in most patients and generally involves valve replacement, although valve repair may be suitable in some cases, particularly for mitral regurgitation; balloon valvulotomy may have a role in some patients with stenosis.[6] Valve replacement alleviates symptoms but does not remove the risks of endocarditis or thromboembolism. Bioprosthetic (tissue) or mechanical valves may be used; the latter are longer lasting, but pose a greater risk for thromboembolism.

In asymptomatic patients and in those who have had valve replacement, the main aim of therapy is to prevent the complications of bacterial endocarditis and of systemic embolism from thrombus formation within the heart.[7] Antibacterial prophylaxis should be given to all patients with valvular heart disease as indicated (see Endocarditis, p.125). Long-term thromboembolism prophylaxis is only required in patients with another risk factor for embolisation, such as concurrent atrial fibrillation, a dilated left atrium, or previous systemic embolism,[6,8] and in those with mechanical replacement valves.

Long-term treatment with an oral anticoagulant such as warfarin is generally regarded as essential for patients with a mechanical prosthetic heart valve.[7,9] The risk of thromboembolism depends upon the type and position of the valve and the presence of other risk factors. In the UK, a target INR of 3.5 is recommended,[10] but there is evidence that lower intensities may be effective while reducing the risk of bleeding.[11,12] In the USA, the recommended target INR is 2.5 to 3.5, although a lower range of 2.0 to 3.0 may be adequate for most types of valves in the aortic position when there are no other risk factors.[6,13] The value of adding an antiplatelet drug to anticoagulant therapy in patients with artificial heart valves is less clear, although it has been suggested[14] that all patients with prosthetic valves should receive low-dose aspirin given its additional benefits in preventing cardiovascular disease. There is some evidence of reduced thromboembolism with aspirin, and with dipyridamole, in patients with prosthetic valves but the risk of bleeding is increased.[15] Adjunctive antiplatelet drugs may be considered for patients with additional risk factors such as embolism while on warfarin therapy, or ischaemic heart disease.[6,13] For some types of valve the use of aspirin with warfarin adjusted to maintain a lower INR may provide adequate anticoagulation without increasing the risk of bleeding.[13]

For patients with bioprosthetic heart valves anticoagulants are recommended for the first 3 months after replacement.[7,9] Thereafter, long-term oral anticoagulant therapy is generally considered necessary only for patients with risk factors such as atrial fibrillation, a dilated left atrium, left atrial thrombus, a history of systemic embolism, and possibly those with severe left ventricular dysfunction.[6,9,13] An INR of 2.0 to 3.0 appears adequate for patients with bioprosthetic heart valves. Low-dose aspirin should be considered in patients with bioprosthetic valves who do not require oral anticoagulants.[6,13]

For patients on long-term anticoagulation, interruption of therapy for surgical procedures or due to bleeding complications exposes patients to the risk of thromboembolism. A study[16] in patients with haemorrhage suggested that it is safe to withhold oral anticoagulants. For patients undergoing surgery, however, the evidence for either withholding anticoagulants or converting to heparin perioperatively is not conclusive.[8]

The use of anticoagulants is controversial in patients with infective endocarditis because of the substantial increase in risk of haemorrhage in these patients. Oral anticoagulants should generally be continued in patients who have prosthetic heart valves, unless complications occur.[8,9] Anticoagulation may also be considered for patients with endocarditis who have other risk factors for systemic embolism.

The haemodynamic changes that occur during **pregnancy** may complicate the management of women with valvular heart disease.[17] In addition, pregnancy is a known risk-factor for thromboembolism and patients with valvular heart disease who become pregnant are therefore at increased risk. However, long-term prophylaxis with an oral anticoagulant such as warfarin presents a problem since warfarin is generally contra-indicated in pregnancy (see Adverse Effects under Warfarin, p.1022). Women with mechanical prosthetic valves must continue anticoagulation but choice of therapy is unclear. A systematic review[18] found that continued use of oral anticoagulants increased the risk to the fetus, but that thromboembolic complications were higher with heparin. Guidelines therefore vary in their recommendations. It is usually recommended that subcutaneous heparin should be substituted for warfarin.[7,19] A dose of 17 500 to 20 000 units subcutaneously every 12 hours has been suggested;[19] intravenous administration is an alternative for women at high risk,[6] but low-dose subcutaneous heparin is not suitable since it provides inadequate protection against prosthetic valve thrombosis.[20] Ideally heparin should be started before conception, or as soon after as possible, and should be continued at least until the twelfth week to avoid the risk of warfarin embryopathy. If necessary, warfarin may then be reintroduced, although heparin is also recommended at term (to avoid an anticoagulated neonate). However, a retrospective study[21] suggested that outcomes were satisfactory following use of warfarin during the first trimester of pregnancy and some authorities[3] recommend continued use of oral anticoagulants throughout pregnancy in most patients, depending on the dose of warfarin. Low-molecular-weight heparins may also be an alternative to heparin in pregnant patients,[19] although there is less experience with their use. Low-dose aspirin may be used as an adjunct to subcutaneous heparin or warfarin in women at high risk of thromboembolism.[9,19]


1. Carabello BA, Crawford FA. Valvular heart disease. *N Engl J Med* 1997; **337:** 32–41.
2. Boon NA, Bloomfield P. The medical management of valvar heart disease. *Heart* 2002; **87:** 395–400.
3. Prendergast BD, *et al.* Valvular heart disease: recommendations for investigation and management. *J R Coll Physicians Lond* 1996; **30:** 309–15.

4. Khot UN, *et al.* Nitroprusside in critically ill patients with left ventricular dysfunction and aortic stenosis. *N Engl J Med* 2003; **348:** 1756–63.
5. Scognamiglio R, *et al.* Nifedipine in asymptomatic patients with severe aortic regurgitation and normal left ventricular function. *N Engl J Med* 1994; **331:** 689–94.
6. Bonow RO, *et al.* ACC/AHA guidelines for the management of patients with valvular heart disease. *Circulation* 1998; **98:** 1949–84. Also available at: http://www.americanheart.org/downloadable/heart/1018975856239 1998%20ACCAHA%20Valvular%20Heart%20Disease.pdf (accessed 21/05/04)
7. Coulshed DS, *et al.* Drug treatment associated with heart valve replacement. *Drugs* 1995; **49:** 897–911.
8. Salem DN, *et al.* Antithrombotic therapy in valvular heart disease. *Chest* 2001; **119** (suppl): 207S–219S.
9. Vongpatanasin W, *et al.* Prosthetic heart valves. *N Engl J Med* 1996; **335:** 407–16.
10. British Society for Haematology: British Committee for Standards in Haematology—Haemostasis and Thrombosis Task Force. Guidelines on oral anticoagulation: third edition. *Br J Haematol* 1998; **101:** 374–87. Also available at: http://www.bcshguidelines.com/pdf/bjh715.pdf (accessed 14/05/04)
11. Saour JN, *et al.* Trial of different intensities of anticoagulation in patients with prosthetic heart valves. *N Engl J Med* 1990; **322:** 428–32.
12. Cannegieter SC, *et al.* Optimal oral anticoagulant therapy in patients with mechanical heart valves. *N Engl J Med* 1995; **333:** 11–17.
13. Stein PD, *et al.* Antithrombotic therapy in patients with mechanical and biological prosthetic heart valves. *Chest* 2001; **119** (suppl): 220S–227S.
14. Tiede DJ, *et al.* Modern management of prosthetic valve anticoagulation. *Mayo Clin Proc* 1998; **73:** 665–80.
15. Massel D, Little SH. Risks and benefits of adding anti-platelet therapy to warfarin among patients with prosthetic heart valves: a meta-analysis. *J Am Coll Cardiol* 2001: **37:** 569–78.
16. Ananthasubramaniam K, *et al.* How safely and for how long can warfarin therapy be withheld in prosthetic heart valve patients hospitalized with a major hemorrhage? *Chest* 2001; **119:** 478–84.
17. Reimold SC, Rutherford JD. Valvular heart disease in pregnancy. *N Engl J Med* 2003; **349:** 52–9.
18. Chan WS, *et al.* Anticoagulation of pregnant women with mechanical heart valves: a systematic review of the literature. *Arch Intern Med* 2000; **160:** 191–6.
19. Ginsberg JS, *et al.* Use of antithrombotic agents during pregnancy. *Chest* 2001; **119** (suppl): 122S–131S.
20. Maternal and Neonatal Haemostasis Working Party of the Haemostasis and Thrombosis Task. Guidelines on the prevention, investigation and management of thrombosis associated with pregnancy. *J Clin Pathol* 1993; **46:** 489–96.
21. Sbarouni E, Oakley CM. Outcome of pregnancy in women with valve prostheses. *Br Heart J* 1994; **71:** 196–201.

## Venous thromboembolism

The term venous thromboembolism embraces both deep-vein thrombosis and pulmonary embolism; the two often co-exist and should be considered as a single clinical entity. In deep-vein thrombosis a thrombus forms, frequently in the pockets of valves, and blocks the veins of the lower limbs or main pelvic veins. Pulmonary embolism occurs when the thrombus or part of it migrates in the circulation and blocks the pulmonary artery. About 70% of patients with confirmed pulmonary embolism have thrombosis in their deep leg veins and about 40% of patients with confirmed deep-vein thrombosis have silent pulmonary embolism. Proximal deep-vein thrombosis is associated with a higher risk of pulmonary embolism than distal deep-vein thrombosis.

Venous thromboembolism is a common but underdiagnosed condition and the cause of considerable morbidity and mortality, especially among hospitalised patients. Various factors underlie the development of thrombosis and there are a number of conditions that predispose patients to venous thromboembolism (see Thromboembolic Disorders, p.837).

Symptoms of *deep-vein thrombosis* include a tender and swollen calf; increased temperature, cyanosis, and engorgement of the superficial veins of the affected limb; fever; and tachycardia. However, about half of all cases may be symptomless. In the longer term chronic venous insufficiency and venous ulceration often occur (post-phlebitic or post-thrombotic syndrome). As most clinical signs of deep-vein thrombosis are non-specific, the diagnosis should always be confirmed before committing a patient to long-term anticoagulation treatment. Noninvasive diagnostic techniques are usually adequate, although venography may be required in some patients.[1,2] Compression ultrasound is the preferred method, often combined with measurement of D-dimer concentrations; impedence plethysmography may also be used. *Pulmonary embolism* may present in a number of ways depending on its extent and duration. Acute massive embolism causes serious haemodynamic disturbance with a sudden reduction in cardiac output and circulatory collapse. The most common form of pulmonary embolism seen, however, is acute minor embolism where the patient may present with pleuritic pain, haemoptysis, dyspnoea, tachycardia, and fever. Diagnosis may involve perfusion/ventilation scans, angiography, or computed tomography (CT); echocardiography may also be used.[3,4]

**Prophylaxis of venous thromboembolism.** Prophylaxis with anticoagulants aims to prevent deep-vein thrombosis and hence pulmonary embolism in patients at risk. Ideally all medical and surgical hospital inpatients should be assessed for risk factors and should receive prophylaxis according to their degree of risk at least until discharge or, for those at higher risk, after discharge; however, considerable underuse has been reported.[5,6] A prophylactic regimen should be chosen for a particular patient after balancing the degree of risk against the potential complications of prophylaxis. Guidelines have been published in the UK[7,8] and the USA.[9]

Patients can be categorised as being at low, medium, or high risk of venous thromboembolism according to the duration and type of operation in those undergoing surgery, to age, and to the presence of other risk factors such as cancer, heart failure, and lung disease.[9,10] Low-risk patients include young patients undergoing short operative procedures. Older age, operations lasting longer than 30 minutes, and a history of thrombophilia or previous thromboembolism indicate medium risk. Orthopaedic surgery is associated with a high risk of venous thromboembolism in all patients. Other patients at high risk include those with multiple risk factors. Non-surgical patients are also at risk of thromboembolism, particularly if they are immobile, or have major trauma or spinal cord injury. Pregnancy is also a risk factor and is discussed in more detail below.

Methods of prophylaxis may be physical or pharmacological. Physical methods act by increasing venous blood flow and include elevation of the legs, early ambulation, graduated compression stockings, and intermittent pneumatic compression devices. Pharmacological methods generally involve anticoagulation with heparin, low-molecular-weight heparins, or an oral anticoagulant. Other therapies that have been used include antiplatelet drugs, dihydroergotamine, dextrans, antithrombin III, heparinoids such as danaparoid, and the direct thrombin inhibitor desirudin. Fondaparinux and the oral thrombin inhibitor ximelagatran are more recently introduced alternatives. Ancrod and argatroban have been used in patients who have developed heparin-induced thrombocytopenia or thrombosis.

For low-risk surgical patients measures such as early ambulation and the use of graduated compression stockings are generally considered adequate. Moderate- and high-risk patients require pharmacological methods, although physical methods (particularly intermittent compression devices) may be used in those who are at high risk from bleeding complications. Physical methods are not suitable in patients with significant peripheral vascular disease. In practice, a combination of mechanical methods (particularly graduated compression stockings) and pharmacological methods is often used, and may give better protection than either method alone.[8,9]

For moderate-risk patients, such as those undergoing general surgical procedures lasting more than 30 minutes, ***low-dose subcutaneous heparin*** ('standard heparin prophylaxis') is the most widely used pharmacological method, a typical regimen being 5000 units subcutaneously 2 hours pre-operatively, then every 8 or 12 hours post-operatively for 7 days or until the patient is mobile.[7] Subcutaneous low-molecular-weight heparins may be used as an alternative.[8] High-risk patients may require more aggressive prophylaxis with higher doses of low-molecular-weight heparin; higher doses of unfractionated heparin with laboratory monitoring (*adjusted-dose heparin*) or oral anticoagulants may also be used.

The use of low-dose subcutaneous heparin for surgical thromboembolism prophylaxis is well established. In an overview[11] of more than 70 randomised studies in 16 000 patients heparin reduced the risk of subclinical deep-vein thrombosis by 67% in general surgery, 68% in orthopaedic surgery, and 75% in urological surgery. There was also a 40% reduction in non-fatal cases of pulmonary embolism, a 64% reduction in fatal cases, and a 47% reduction of all cases. Surgical thromboembolism prophylaxis with heparin also decreased total mortality. Adjusted-dose heparin may be more effective in higher risk patients but the need for laboratory monitoring and the risk of bleeding complications limit its use.

***Low-molecular-weight heparins*** have a number of potential advantages over unfractionated heparin, including less frequent administration and no need for monitoring, and they are widely used. However, they have not been clearly shown to reduce the risk of bleeding and they may increase the risk of spinal haematoma in patients receiving spinal or epidural anaesthesia, which may limit their use. Generally, studies have shown low-molecular-weight heparins to be at least as effective as unfractionated or standard heparin, but a number of meta-analyses have come to differing conclusions regarding superiority. The evidence suggests that low-molecular-weight heparins are superior in orthopaedic surgery,[12-15] particularly with regard to proximal deep-vein thrombosis.[14] In general surgery both types of heparin appear to be of equivalent efficacy, although one analysis[13] reported that low-molecular-weight heparins were superior. A large study[16] showed low-molecular-weight heparins to be as effective as heparin for prophylaxis after major abdominal surgery and to be associated with fewer bleeding complications. Two meta-analyses of 45 studies[17] and 56 studies[18] respectively evaluated the efficacy of several prophylactic methods (such as aspirin, dextran, oral anticoagulants, heparin, heparin with dihydroergotamine, low-molecular-weight heparins, and intermittent pneumatic compression) against deep-vein thrombosis following major hip surgery and concluded that low-molecular-weight heparins should be the method of choice. Low-molecular-weight heparins may also be more effective than unfractionated heparin in patients with major trauma.[19]

The optimum duration of prophylaxis is unclear. Prophylaxis is usually only continued during hospitalisation but following orthopaedic surgery there is an increased risk for deep-vein thrombosis detected by venography up to a month after discharge, which may be reduced by low-molecular-weight heparin.[20,21] Although the clinical significance of this finding has been questioned,[22] extended prophylaxis may have a role, particularly in high-risk patients following orthopaedic surgery,[8,9] or in very high-risk general surgical patients.[8,9] A study[23] in patients undergoing surgery for cancer also found a reduction in thrombosis when enoxaparin was given for 4 weeks.

***Oral anticoagulants*** have not been so widely used as subcutaneous heparin although US guidelines[9] allow the use of adjusted-dose warfarin to give an international normalised ratio (INR — see Warfarin, p.1028 for further details) of 2.0 to 3.0 in patients having hip or knee replacement surgery and in selected high-risk general surgical patients. When compared[24] with low-molecular-weight heparin this 'less intense' regimen was slightly less effective in preventing deep-vein thrombosis after hip or knee replacements, but there were fewer bleeding complications with warfarin; warfarin was started on the evening of the day of surgery in an initial dose of 10 mg. A fixed 'minidose' warfarin regimen (1 mg daily) starting a mean of 20 days before surgery may be effective in gynaecological surgery[25] but not in patients having hip or knee joint replacements.[26,27] In another study[28] warfarin, in a two-stage regimen beginning 10 to 14 days before total hip replacement, was much more effective than external pneumatic compression in preventing proximal vein thrombi, but was less effective in preventing calf vein thrombosis. The dose of warfarin was adjusted to give an INR of 1.5 pre-operatively and 2.5 postoperatively.

***Antiplatelet drugs*** such as aspirin have been considered less effective antithrombotics than anticoagulants in the venous circulation and to be of limited value in preventing venous thromboembolism. An overview[29] of randomised trials of antiplatelet therapy (mainly aspirin) available up to March 1990 and a more recent placebo-controlled trial[30] of aspirin in patients having hip surgery have suggested that antiplatelets reduce the risk of venous thromboembolism and should thus be considered in high-risk patients. However, both reports have been criticised and, while some guidelines recommend the use of aspirin,[8] others suggest it should not be used alone since other methods are generally more effective.[9,31]

Of the ***other drugs*** tried for surgical thromboembolism prophylaxis, *dihydroergotamine* can reduce venous stasis by vasoconstriction of capacitance vessels and has enhanced postoperative prophylaxis when used in association with low-dose heparin, but there is a risk of peripheral ischaemia[7] and it is no longer widely used. *Dextrans* (dextran 70 or dextran 40) alone, or with dihydroergotamine, have also been used for prophylaxis, but their administration involves the infusion of 500 to 1000 mL of fluid, a procedure which is cumbersome and may interfere with fluid balance. *Antithrombin III* (an endogenous inhibitor of thrombin and the cofactor through which heparin acts) used together with heparin has reduced the risk of venous thromboembolism in patients undergoing total knee arthroplasty.[32] The direct thrombin inhibitor *desirudin* has also been shown to be effective and was reported to be superior to both low-dose subcutaneous heparin[33] and to a low-molecular-weight heparin[34] in patients undergoing hip replacement surgery. Bivalirudin has also been tried. The synthetic pentasaccharide *fondaparinux* has been reported[35] to be more effective than low-molecular-weight heparin for orthopaedic surgery, although bleeding may be increased and its role is not yet clear. *Ximelagatran*, an oral thrombin inhibitor, appears to be at least as effective as warfarin following knee replacement surgery.[36,37]

The role of prophylaxis of thromboembolism in the non-surgical setting is less established,[38] but a meta-analysis[39] suggested that low-dose subcutaneous heparin or low-molecular-weight heparin may be of benefit, and their use should be considered in patients at high risk.[8,9] One study[40] showed that very-low-dose warfarin (average daily dose of 2.6 mg) was safe and effective in patients receiving chemotherapy for metastatic breast cancer, a situation in which the high risk of thromboembolic disease is well recognised. Prophylaxis with low-molecular-weight heparin has been shown to be effective in patients with immobilisation of the leg,[41] and in acutely ill medical patients with risk factors for venous thromboembolism.[42] Standard unfractionated heparin prophylaxis, however, had no effect on mortality in patients admitted to hospital with infection.[43] Although some studies[44,45] have shown an increased risk of venous thromboembolism following prolonged travel, the role of prophylaxis is unclear; compression stockings and low-dose aspirin may be considered, while low-molecular-weight heparin may be required in those at high risk.[8]

**Treatment of venous thromboembolism.** Treatment of *deep-vein thrombosis*[2,46,47] aims to prevent the development of pulmonary embolism, to prevent extension of the thrombus, to reduce the risk of recurrence, and to reduce the long-term complications of chronic venous insufficiency and venous ulceration. Non-pharmacological therapy may include bed rest with the foot of the bed raised, limb exercise, and graduated compression stockings.[48] These measures may be adequate in patients with small thrombi confined to the calf veins, although this is controversial. Heparin and oral anticoagulants are the mainstay of treatment; they prevent further thrombosis while allowing natural thrombolytic mechanisms to act on the existing clot. Anticoagulants may be used in combination with non-pharmacological methods; graduated compression stockings may reduce the risk of post-phlebitic symptoms in patients receiving anticoagulants.[49] Thrombolytics, or very rarely surgical thrombectomy, may be used for very extensive thrombosis.[50]

Heparin has an immediate effect whereas oral anticoagulants such as warfarin take several days to achieve their full anticoagulant effect. Heparin is therefore used for initial therapy and oral anticoagulants are used for maintenance. Doses of unfractionated heparin and oral anticoagulants must be adjusted according to laboratory monitoring. In the initial treatment of deep-vein thrombosis, current UK recommendations[7] are for an intravenous loading dose of heparin 5000 units followed by 1000 to 2000 units/hour by continuous intravenous infusion or 15 000 units by subcutaneous injection every 12 hours. A meta-analysis suggested that heparin twice daily by subcutaneous injection is more effective and at least as safe as continuous intravenous heparin in the initial treatment of deep-vein thrombosis.[51] In the USA,[50] a similar 5000-unit loading dose has been suggested, followed by 1400 units/hour intravenously or 17 500 units every 12 hours subcutaneously. However, low-molecular-weight heparins have a number of advantages and are now generally preferred.[52] A number of meta-analyses[53-57] have shown them to be at least as effective and safe as unfractionated heparin in the treatment of deep-vein thrombosis and pulmonary embolism. They are also safe and effective for the outpatient treatment of deep-vein thrombosis[58] and have been recommended for outpatient treatment in patients with uncomplicated pulmonary embolism.[4]

Ancrod, argatroban, or the recombinant hirudin, lepirudin, may be used as an alternative to heparin in patients who have developed heparin-induced thrombocytopenia or thrombosis. A heparinoid such as danaparoid or a low-molecular-weight heparin may also be suitable, although there may be cross-reactivity.

Treatment with an oral anticoagulant (usually warfarin) may be started at the same time as heparin, or 3 to 4 days before it is discontinued. A standard loading dose is usually given, and dosage is then adjusted to maintain the INR within recommended limits.[50,52,59] Heparin should be continued until the INR has been in the therapeutic range for at least 2 days;[50,52,60] a period of about 5 days is usually adequate[61] if warfarin has been started on day 1. The optimum duration of oral anticoagulation is unclear. Thromboembolism is most likely to recur in patients with ongoing risk factors, but prevention of recurrence must be balanced against the risk of haemorrhagic complications. A meta-analysis[62] of studies comparing different lengths of treatment concluded that the risk of recurrence was reduced for as long as the oral anticoagulant was taken; however, the absolute risk of recurrence decreased over time, whereas the bleeding risk remained the same. For patients with transient risk factors, short-term treatment is generally preferred; a study[63] comparing treatment for 4 weeks with treatment for 3 months suggested that 4 weeks was adequate in patients with postoperative thromboembolism. For patients with ongoing risk factors or idiopathic venous thromboembolism, the situation is less clear. A study[64] in patients with idiopathic deep vein thrombosis found that the rate of recurrence following discontinuation of treatment was the same whether anticoagulation was given for 3 months or 1 year, suggesting that the longer duration of therapy only postponed recurrence. Guidelines for treatment reflect this uncertainty, with recommendations in the UK[59] and US,[50,52] showing considerable variation. For a first episode of venous thromboembolism in patients with reversible risk factors, such as surgery, trauma, or temporary immobilisation, suggestions range from 6 weeks to 3 to 6 months. For patients with idiopathic venous thromboembolism periods of 3 to 6 months or longer are recommended. Longer, possibly lifelong treatment may be considered in patients with repeated thromboembolic episodes or with a continuing risk factor.

The limitations of long-term oral anticoagulation, including bleeding complications and recurrent thromboembolism, have led to the investigation of other approaches. Low-molecular weight heparins may be more effective than continued warfarin in patients with recurrence during warfarin therapy;[65] they may also be more effective than warfarin as initial therapy in patients with cancer.[66] Use of lower-intensity warfarin regimens has been tried for extended prophylaxis, and may reduce the risk of recurrence compared with no therapy.[67] However, a study[68] comparing low- and high-intensity regimens found that the lower intensity regimen was less effective and did not reduce the risk of bleeding. Extended prophylaxis with ximelagatran has also been studied.[69] In patients who have contra-indications to anticoagulation or in whom thrombosis recurs despite anticoagulation, insertion of a vena caval filter may be appropriate.[50] The use of filters in conjunction with anticoagulation has also been investigated.[70] Although the incidence of pulmonary embolism was reduced during the first 12 days, no effect on mortality was shown at 2 years.

Therapy with thrombolytics such as streptokinase is controversial[71] but is generally reserved for very extensive thrombosis. Patients with more recent thrombi, incomplete occlusion, and proximal rather than distal thrombus location respond best.[72] Thrombolysis has not been shown to improve mortality in patients with deep-vein thrombosis and the main indication is to reduce the incidence of post-phlebitic syndrome. A study[73] using various thrombolytics found that systemic thrombolysis reduced the incidence of post-phlebitic syndrome but that the risk of bleeding was increased. Since thrombolytic activity fades when infusion stops, heparin followed by oral anticoagulation is given to prevent re-occlusion.

Minor *pulmonary embolism* is treated with heparin or low-molecular-weight heparin and oral anticoagulants as described for deep-vein thrombosis (above).[4,74] Fondaparinux may be an alternative to heparin,[75] but its use is not yet established. For more severe pulmonary embolism the initial bolus dose of heparin may be doubled[7] and heparin may be continued for 7 to 10 days.[50] An initial dose of unfractionated heparin may also be given before treatment with low-molecular-weight heparins.[4] Acute massive pulmonary embolism with major haemodynamic disturbance may be treated initially with thrombolytic therapy;[3,4] surgical methods such as embolectomy or percutaneous catheter fragmentation may be preferred in some patients.[76,77] Streptokinase, urokinase, and alteplase have all been shown to accelerate the lysis of pulmonary emboli and to decrease pulmonary vascular obstruction. However, their effects on mortality are uncertain and bleeding risk is increased,[78] and they are therefore not recommended in non-massive pulmonary embolism.[4] Comparisons between thrombolytics have been difficult because the doses used in different studies have not always been comparable. Probably more important than the choice of thrombolytic is ensuring that treatment starts quickly in patients where it is indicated.[74]

**Venous thromboembolism in children.** Venous thromboembolism is relatively rare in children and has differing epidemiology to that in adults.[79] Although guidelines[80] for its management have been published they generally rely on extrapolation from studies in adults.

**Venous thromboembolism in pregnancy.** Pregnancy is a known risk factor for venous thromboembolism and, although the absolute risk is low, pulmonary embolism is the commonest cause of maternal death during pregnancy in the UK. Anticoagulation during pregnancy may be necessary either to prevent or treat venous thromboembolism; continued anticoagulation may also be needed in pregnant patients at risk of systemic embolism because of valvular heart disease or prosthetic heart valves (see above).

Oral anticoagulants such as warfarin cross the placenta and may harm the fetus; they are generally contra-indicated during pregnancy. Heparin does not appear to cross the placenta and despite potential maternal complications such as osteoporosis and thrombocytopenia remains the anticoagulant of choice in pregnancy. Low-molecular-weight heparins appear to be as safe as unfractionated heparin during pregnancy[81] and may now be preferred.[82]

The management of venous thromboembolism in pregnancy has been reviewed[83-85] and guidelines have been published in the UK[86,87] and the US.[82] **Prophylactic anticoagulation** is not necessary in all pregnancies, but should be considered in women at special risk of venous thromboembolism either because of a history of thromboembolism and/or a thrombophilic abnormality such as inherited deficiency of antithrombin III, protein C, or protein S or acquired thrombophilia due to antiphospholipid antibodies in plasma. Patients must be managed individually and current strategies differ. In those women with a history of thromboembolism but without thrombophilic abnormalities some authors recommend prophylactic anticoagulation at delivery and for 6 weeks post partum provided there has been only one episode of thromboembolism and there are no additional risk factors; others advocate prophylaxis with subcutaneous heparin throughout pregnancy. However, a prospective study[88] has suggested that it is safe to withhold anticoagulation until after delivery in such patients, and this approach has been recommended.[82] Although standard low-dose heparin has been recommended, higher doses may be necessary during pregnancy.[82-84] Low-molecular-weight heparins may also be used.[82,84,87] Those with inherited or acquired thrombophilic abnormalities but no evidence of thrombosis do not necessarily require anticoagulation, but must be assessed carefully.

If acute venous thromboembolism occurs during pregnancy it should be **treated** with low-molecular-weight heparin or intravenous heparin as in non-pregnant patients (see above). Antenatal patients need to continue anticoagulation for the rest of their pregnancy, usually by substituting adjusted-dose subcutaneous heparin every 12 hours after 6 to 10 days of intravenous therapy; low-molecular-weight heparins may be an alternative.[50,84,86] Special care must be taken at delivery. Patients receiving full therapeutic doses of heparin should have their dose reduced or discontinued on the day of delivery; this may not be necessary in those on lower prophylactic doses of heparin. Low-molecular-weight heparins should be stopped 24 hours before planned delivery.[82] If possible patients receiving warfarin should be changed to heparin 2 or 3 weeks before labour or delivery and not later than 36 weeks' gestation. Anticoagulants should be continued after delivery, but can usually be stopped after 6 weeks; the total duration of treatment should be at least 3 months.[50,86]

During pregnancy, especially the third trimester, laboratory monitoring of anticoagulation may be less reliable because high procoagulant concentrations particularly of factor VIII and fibrinogen, may result in low activated partial thromboplastin time (APTT) values despite adequate heparin concentrations in plasma.


1. Kearon C, *et al*. Noninvasive diagnosis of deep venous thrombosis. *Ann Intern Med* 1998; **128:** 663–77.
2. Tovey C, Wyatt S. Diagnosis, investigation, and management of deep vein thrombosis. *BMJ* 2003; **326:** 1180–4.
3. European Society of Cardiology Task Force on Pulmonary Embolism. Guidelines on diagnosis and management of acute pulmonary embolism. *Eur Heart J* 2000; **21:** 1301–36. Also available at: http://www.escardio.org/NR/rdonlyres/1FB62735-A84B-43C0-B6DA-70F115E5090D/0/APE_euhj00.pdf (accessed 12/05/04)
4. British Thoracic Society Standards of Care Committee Pulmonary Embolism Guideline Development Group. British Thoracic Society guidelines for the management of suspected acute pulmonary embolism. *Thorax* 2003; **58:** 470–83. Also available at: http://www.brit-thoracic.org.uk/docs/PulmonaryembolismJUN03.pdf (accessed 14/05/04)
5. The Venous Thromboembolism Study Group of the Spanish Society of Clinical Pharmacology. Multicentre hospital drug utilization study on the prophylaxis of venous thromboembolism. *Br J Clin Pharmacol* 1994; **37:** 255–9.
6. Bratzler DW, *et al.* Underuse of venous thromboembolism prophylaxis for general surgery patients: physician practices in the community hospital setting. *Arch Intern Med* 1998; **158:** 1902–12.
7. Colvin BT, Barrowcliffe TW. The British Society for Haematology guidelines on the use and monitoring of heparin 1992: second revision. *J Clin Pathol* 1993; **46:** 97–103.

8. Scottish Intercollegiate Guidelines Network. Prophylaxis of venous thromboembolism: a national clinical guideline (October 2002). Available at: http://www.show.scot.nhs.uk/sign/pdf/sign62.pdf (accessed 14/05/04)
9. Geerts WH, *et al.* Prevention of venous thromboembolism. *Chest* 2001; **119** (suppl): 132S–175S.
10. Verstraete M. Prophylaxis of venous thromboembolism. *BMJ* 1997; **314:** 123–5.
11. Collins R, *et al.* Reduction in fatal pulmonary embolism and venous thrombosis by perioperative administration of subcutaneous heparin: overview of results of randomized trials in general, orthopedic, and urologic surgery. *N Engl J Med* 1988; **318:** 1162–73.
12. Nurmohamed MT, *et al.* Low-molecular-weight heparin versus standard heparin in general and orthopaedic surgery: a meta-analysis. *Lancet* 1992; **340:** 152–6.
13. Leizorovicz A, *et al.* Low molecular weight heparin in prevention of perioperative thrombosis. *BMJ* 1992; **305:** 913–20.
14. Anderson DR, *et al.* Efficacy and cost of low-molecular-weight heparin compared with standard heparin for the prevention of deep vein thrombosis after total hip arthroplasty. *Ann Intern Med* 1993; **119:** 1105–12.
15. Koch A, *et al.* Low molecular weight heparin and unfractionated heparin in thrombosis prophylaxis after major surgical intervention: update of previous meta-analyses. *Br J Surg* 1997; **84:** 750–9.
16. Kakkar VV, *et al.* Low molecular weight versus standard heparin for prevention of venous thromboembolism after major abdominal surgery. *Lancet* 1993; **341:** 259–65.
17. Simonneau G, Leizorovicz A. Prophylactic treatment of postoperative thrombosis: a meta-analysis of the results from trials assessing various methods used in patients undergoing major orthopaedic (hip and knee) surgery. *Clin Trials Meta-Analysis* 1993; **28:** 177–91.
18. Imperiale TF, Speroff T. A meta-analysis of methods to prevent venous thromboembolism following total hip replacement. *JAMA* 1994; **271:** 1780–5. Correction. *ibid.* 1995; **273:** 288.
19. Geerts WH, *et al.* A comparison of low-dose heparin with low-molecular-weight heparin as prophylaxis against venous thromboembolism after major trauma. *N Engl J Med* 1996; **335:** 701–7.
20. Eikelboom JW, *et al.* Extended-duration prophylaxis against venous thromboembolism after total hip or knee replacement: a meta-analysis of the randomised trials. *Lancet* 2001; **358:** 9–15.
21. Hull RD, *et al.* Extended out-of-hospital low-molecular-weight heparin prophylaxis against deep venous thrombosis in patients after elective hip arthroplasty: a systematic review. *Ann Intern Med* 2001; **135:** 858–69.
22. Anderson DR, *et al.* Enoxaparin as prophylaxis against thromboembolism after total hip replacement. *N Engl J Med* 1997; **336:** 585.
23. Bergqvist D, *et al.* Duration of prophylaxis against venous thromboembolism with enoxaparin after surgery for cancer. *N Engl J Med* 2002; **346:** 975–80.
24. Hull R, *et al.* A comparison of subcutaneous low-molecular-weight heparin with warfarin sodium for prophylaxis against deep-vein thrombosis after hip or knee implantation. *N Engl J Med* 1993; **329:** 1370–6.
25. Poller L, *et al.* Fixed minidose warfarin: a new approach to prophylaxis against venous thrombosis after major surgery. *BMJ* 1987; **295:** 1309–12.
26. Fordyce MJF, *et al.* Efficacy of fixed minidose warfarin prophylaxis in total hip replacement. *BMJ* 1991; **303:** 219–20.
27. Dale C, *et al.* Prevention of venous thrombosis with minidose warfarin after joint replacement. *BMJ* 1991; **303:** 224.
28. Francis CW, *et al.* Comparison of warfarin and external pneumatic compression in prevention of venous thrombosis after total hip replacement. *JAMA* 1992; **267:** 2911–15.
29. Antiplatelet Trialists' Collaboration. Collaborative overview of randomised trials of antiplatelet therapy—III: reduction in venous thrombosis and pulmonary embolism by antiplatelet prophylaxis among surgical and medical patients. *BMJ* 1994; **308:** 235–46.
30. Pulmonary Embolism Prevention (PEP) Trial Collaborative Group. Prevention of pulmonary embolism and deep vein thrombosis with low dose aspirin: Pulmonary Embolism Prevention (PEP) trial. *Lancet* 2000; **355:** 1295–1302.
31. Thomas DP. Thromboprophylaxis after replacement arthroplasty. *BMJ* 2001; **322:** 686–7.
32. Francis CW, *et al.* Prevention of venous thrombosis after total knee arthroplasty: comparison of antithrombin III and low-dose heparin with dextran. *J Bone Joint Surg (Am)* 1990; **72-A:** 976–82.
33. Eriksson BI, *et al.* Prevention of deep-vein thrombosis after total hip replacement: direct thrombin inhibition with recombinant hirudin, CGP 39393. *Lancet* 1996; **347:** 635–9.
34. Eriksson BI, *et al.* A comparison of recombinant hirudin with a low-molecular-weight heparin to prevent thromboembolic complications after total hip replacement. *N Engl J Med* 1997; **337:** 1329–35.
35. Bounameaux H, Perneger T. Fondaparinux: a new synthetic pentasaccharide for thrombosis prevention. *Lancet* 2002; **359:** 1710–11.
36. Francis CW, *et al.* Ximelagatran versus warfarin for the prevention of venous thromboembolism after total knee arthroplasty: a randomized, double-blind trial. *Ann Intern Med* 2002; **137:** 648–55.
37. Francis CW, *et al.* Comparison of ximelagatran with warfarin for the prevention of venous thromboembolism after total knee replacement. *N Engl J Med* 2003; **349:** 1703–12.
38. Lederle FA. Heparin prophylaxis for medical patients? *Ann Intern Med* 1998; **128:** 768–70.
39. Mismetti P, *et al.* Prevention of venous thromboembolism in internal medicine with unfractionated or low-molecular-weight heparins: a meta-analysis of randomised clinical trials. *Thromb Haemost* 2000; **83:** 14–19.
40. Levine M, *et al.* Double-blind randomised trial of very-low-dose warfarin for prevention of thromboembolism in stage IV breast cancer. *Lancet* 1994; **343:** 886–9.
41. Kock H-J, *et al.* Thromboprophylaxis with low-molecular-weight heparin in outpatients with plaster-cast immobilisation of the leg. *Lancet* 1995; **346:** 459–61.
42. Samama MM, *et al.* A comparison of enoxaparin with placebo for the prevention of venous thromboembolism in acutely ill medical patients. *N Engl J Med* 1999; **341:** 793–800.
43. Gårdlund B. Randomised, controlled trial of low-dose heparin for prevention of fatal pulmonary embolism in patients with infectious diseases. *Lancet* 1996; **347:** 1357–61.
44. Ferrari E, *et al.* Travel as a risk factor for venous thromboembolic disease: a case-control study. *Chest* 1999; **115:** 440–4.
45. Scurr JH, *et al.* Frequency and prevention of symptomless deep-vein thrombosis in long-haul flights: a randomised trial. *Lancet* 2001; **357:** 1485–9.
46. Shetty HG. Management of deep-vein thrombosis. *Prescribers' J* 1997; **37:** 166–72.
47. Lensing AWA, *et al.* Deep-vein thrombosis. *Lancet* 1999; **353:** 479–85.
48. McCollum C. Avoiding the consequences of deep vein thrombosis. *BMJ* 1998; **317:** 696.
49. Brandjes DPM, *et al.* Randomised trial of effect of compression stockings in patients with symptomatic proximal-vein thrombosis. *Lancet* 1997; **349:** 759–62.
50. Hirsh J, Hoak J. Management of deep vein thrombosis and pulmonary embolism: a statement for healthcare professionals. *Circulation* 1996; **93:** 2212–45.
51. Hommes DW, *et al.* Subcutaneous heparin compared with continuous intravenous heparin administration in the initial treatment of deep vein thrombosis. *Ann Intern Med* 1992; **116:** 279–84.
52. Hyers TM, *et al.* Antithrombotic therapy for venous thromboembolic disease. *Chest* 2001; **119** (suppl): 176S–193S.
53. Siragusa S, *et al.* Low-molecular-weight heparins and unfractionated heparin in the treatment of patients with acute venous thromboembolism: results of a meta-analysis. *Am J Med* 1996; **100:** 269–77.
54. Leizorovicz A. Comparison of the efficacy and safety of low molecular weight heparins and unfractionated heparin in the initial treatment of deep venous thrombosis: an updated meta-analysis. *Drugs* 1996; **52** (suppl 7): 30–7.
55. Gould MK, *et al.* Low-molecular-weight heparins compared with unfractionated heparin for treatment of acute deep venous thrombosis: a meta-analysis of randomized, controlled trials. *Ann Intern Med* 1999; **130:** 800–9.
56. van den Belt AGM, *et al.* Fixed dose subcutaneous low molecular weight heparins versus adjusted dose unfractionated heparin for venous thromboembolism. Available in The Cochrane Library; Issue 2. Chichester: John Wiley; 2004.
57. Dolovich LR, *et al.* A meta-analysis comparing low-molecular-weight heparins with unfractionated heparin in the treatment of venous thromboembolism: examining some unanswered questions regarding location of treatment, product type, and dosing frequency. *Arch Intern Med* 2000; **160:** 181–8.
58. Segal JB, *et al.* Outpatient therapy with low molecular weight heparin for the treatment of venous thromboembolism: a review of efficacy, safety, and costs. *Am J Med* 2003; **115:** 298–308.
59. British Society for Haematology: British Committee for Standards in Haematology—Haemostasis and Thrombosis Task Force. Guidelines on oral anticoagulation: third edition. *Br J Haematol* 1998; **101:** 374–87. Also available at: http://www.bcshguidelines.com/pdf/bjh715.pdf (accessed 14/05/04)
60. Ginsberg JS. Management of venous thromboembolism. *N Engl J Med* 1996; **335:** 1816–28.
61. Hull RD, *et al.* Heparin for 5 days as compared with 10 days in the initial treatment of proximal venous thrombosis. *N Engl J Med* 1990; **322:** 1260–4.
62. Hutten BA, Prins MH. Duration of treatment with vitamin K antagonists in symptomatic venous thromboembolism. Available in The Cochrane Library; Issue 2. Chichester: John Wiley; 2004.
63. Research Committee of the British Thoracic Society. Optimum duration of anticoagulation for deep-vein thrombosis and pulmonary embolism. *Lancet* 1992; **340:** 873–6.
64. Agnelli G, *et al.* Three months versus one year of oral anticoagulant therapy for idiopathic deep venous thrombosis. *N Engl J Med* 2001; **345:** 165–9.
65. Luk C, *et al.* Extended outpatient therapy with low molecular weight heparin for the treatment of recurrent venous thromboembolism despite warfarin therapy. *Am J Med* 2001; **111:** 270–3.
66. Lee AYY, *et al.* Low-molecular-weight heparin versus a coumarin for the prevention of recurrent venous thromboembolism in patients with cancer. *N Engl J Med* 2003; **349:** 146–53.
67. Ridker PM, *et al.* Long-term, low-intensity warfarin therapy for the prevention of recurrent venous thromboembolism. *N Engl J Med* 2003; **348:** 1425–34.
68. Kearon C, *et al.* Comparison of low-intensity warfarin therapy with conventional-intensity warfarin therapy for long-term prevention of recurrent venous thromboembolism. *N Engl J Med* 2003; **349:** 631–9.
69. Schulman S, *et al.* Secondary prevention of venous thromboembolism with the oral direct thrombin inhibitor ximelagatran. *N Engl J Med* 2003; **349:** 1713–21.
70. Decousus H, *et al.* A clinical trial of vena caval filters in the prevention of pulmonary embolism in patients with proximal deep-vein thrombosis. *N Engl J Med* 1998; **338:** 409–15.
71. Hawkins DW, Hirsh J. Antithrombotic drugs for thromboembolic disorders: a lesson in evidence-based medicine. *Am J Health-Syst Pharm* 1997; **54:** 1992–4.
72. Rogers LQ, Lutcher CL. Streptokinase therapy for deep vein thrombosis: a comprehensive review of the English literature. *Am J Med* 1990; **88:** 389–95.
73. Schweizer J, *et al.* Short- and long-term results after thrombolytic treatment of deep venous thrombosis. *J Am Coll Cardiol* 2000; **36:** 1336–43.
74. Riedel M. Acute pulmonary embolism 2: treatment. *Heart* 2001; **85:** 351–60.
75. The Matisse Investigators. Subcutaneous fondaparinux versus intravenous unfractionated heparin in the initial treatment of pulmonary embolism. *N Engl J Med* 2003; **349:** 1695–702.
76. Gulba DC, *et al.* Medical compared with surgical treatment for massive pulmonary embolism. *Lancet* 1994; **343:** 576–7.
77. Goldhaber SZ. Pulmonary embolism. *N Engl J Med* 1998; **339:** 93–104.
78. Dalen JE. The uncertain role of thrombolytic therapy in the treatment of pulmonary embolism. *Arch Intern Med* 2002; **162:** 2521–3.
79. David M, Andrew M. Venous thromboembolic complications in children. *J Pediatr* 1993; **123:** 337–46.
80. Monagle P, *et al.* Antithrombotic therapy in children. *Chest* 2001; **119** (suppl): 344S–370S.
81. Sanson B-J, *et al.* Safety of low-molecular-weight heparin in pregnancy: a systematic review. *Thromb Haemost* 1999; **81:** 668–72.
82. Ginsberg JS, *et al.* Use of antithrombotic agents during pregnancy. *Chest* 2001; **119** (suppl): 122S–131S.
83. Toglia MR, Weg JG. Venous thromboembolism during pregnancy. *N Engl J Med* 1996; **335:** 108–14.
84. Greer IA. Thrombosis in pregnancy: maternal and fetal issues. *Lancet* 1999; **353:** 1258–65.
85. Drife J. Thromboembolism. *Br Med Bull* 2003; **67:** 177–90.
86. Royal College of Obstetricians and Gynaecologists. Thromboembolic disease in pregnancy and the puerperium: acute management (April 2001 - [awaiting update]). Available at: http://www.rcog.org.uk/guidelines.asp?PageID=106&GuidelineID=20 (accessed 14/05/04)
87. Royal College of Obstetricians and Gynaecologists. Thromboprophylaxis during pregnancy, labour and after vaginal delivery (January 2004). Available at: http://www.rcog.org.uk/guidelines.asp?PageID=106&GuidelineID=62 (accessed 14/05/04)
88. Brill-Edwards P, *et al.* Safety of withholding heparin in pregnant women with a history of venous thromboembolism. *N Engl J Med* 2000; **343:** 1439–44.


---

# Abciximab *(BAN, USAN, rINN)*

c7E3; c7E3 Fab; 7E3. Immunoglobulin G (human-mouse monoclonal c7E3 clone p7E3$V_H$h$C_\gamma$4 Fab fragment anti-human platelet glycoprotein IIb/IIIa complex), disulphide with human-mouse monoclonal c7E3 clone p7E3$V_\kappa$h$C_\kappa$ light chain.

$C_{2101}H_{3229}N_{551}O_{673}S_{15}$ = 47455.4.

*CAS — 143653-53-6.*

*ATC — B01AC13.*

## Adverse Effects

Bleeding during the first 36 hours after administration is the most common adverse effect of abciximab. Other side-effects include hypotension, nausea and vomiting, back pain, chest pain, headache, haematoma, bradycardia, fever, cardiac tamponade, and thrombocytopenia. Hypersensitivity reactions (see Precautions, below) have occurred on repeated administration.

**Effects on the blood.** In clinical trials increased bleeding has been the most common adverse effect of abciximab, and this has also been reported[1] during clinical use. Thrombocytopenia is also a well documented adverse effect of abciximab therapy. In a review[2] of the major clinical trials of abciximab, mild thrombocytopenia was reported in 4.2% of patients and severe thrombocytopenia in 1.0%; patients also received treatment with heparin. There have also been a number of case reports of patients developing severe thrombocytopenia.[3] It is recommended that platelet counts should be monitored before and 2 hours after initiation of abciximab, and that the drug should be withdrawn if thrombocytopenia occurs.[3] However, pseudothrombocytopenia also occurs in some patients and should be excluded before withdrawing therapy.[4] Although there have been case reports, the incidence of thrombocytopenia does not appear to be increased with other glycoprotein IIb/IIIa receptor inhibitors,[2] and there have been reports of the successful use of eptifibatide[5] and tirofiban[6] in patients who developed thrombocytopenia with abciximab.


1. Cote AV, *et al.* Hemorrhagic and vascular complications after percutaneous coronary intervention with adjunctive abciximab. *Mayo Clin Proc* 2001; **76:** 890–6.
2. Dasgupta H, *et al.* Thrombocytopenia complicating treatment with intravenous glycoprotein IIb/IIIa receptor inhibitors: a pooled analysis. *Am Heart J* 2000; **140:** 206–11.
3. Bishara AI, Hagmeyer KO. Acute profound thrombocytopenia following abciximab therapy. *Ann Pharmacother* 2000; **34:** 924–30.
4. Sane DC, *et al.* Occurrence and clinical significance of pseudothrombocytopenia during abciximab therapy. *J Am Coll Cardiol* 2000; **36:** 75–83.
5. Rao J, Mascarenhas DAN. Successful use of eptifibatide as an adjunct to coronary stenting in a patient with abciximab-associated acute profound thrombocytopenia. *J Invasive Cardiol* 2001; **13:** 471–3.
6. Desai M, Lucore CL. Uneventful use of tirofiban as an adjunct to coronary stenting in a patient with a history of abciximab-associated thrombocytopenia 10 months earlier. *J Invasive Cardiol* 2000; **12:** 109–12.


## Precautions

Abciximab should not be given to patients who are actively bleeding or to patients at increased risk of haemorrhage. Such patients include: those with haemorrhagic disorders, including thrombocytopenia; those with cerebrovascular disorders, including intracerebral neoplasms, aneurysms, or arteriovenous malformation, and those with a history of stroke; those with uncontrolled hypertension; or those who have recently undergone major surgery or severe trauma. Other patients in whom caution is required include those with vasculitis, haemorrhagic retinopathy, acute pericarditis, or aortic dissection. Abciximab should be discontinued if serious uncontrolled bleeding occurs or emergency surgery is required. Abciximab should not be given to patients with severe renal impairment, or to those with severe hepatic impairment, in whom coagulation may be affected. Platelet counts should be monitored before and following administration of abciximab.

Antibodies may develop 2 to 4 weeks after administration of abciximab and hypersensitivity reactions could occur on administration of other monoclonal antibodies or following readministration of abciximab (see below). Hypersensitivity reactions have not been noted after a single administration but the possibility should be considered.

**Readministration.** Antibodies to abciximab develop in approximately 5.8% of patients following treatment and could lead to hypersensitivity reactions or to reduced efficacy if abciximab is readministered. In a retrospective study[1] in 164 patients who had received a second course of therapy with abciximab, efficacy was not affected and no allergic or anaphylactic reactions occurred. However, severe thrombocytopenia was noted in 4% of patients, and the incidence was highest in those receiving abciximab within 2 weeks of the first administration.

1. Madan M, *et al.* Efficacy of abciximab readministration in coronary intervention. *Am J Cardiol* 2000; **85:** 435–40.

## Interactions

There may be an increased risk of bleeding if abciximab is given with other drugs that affect bleeding, including anticoagulants, other antiplatelets, or thrombolytics.

## Pharmacokinetics

Following intravenous administration of abciximab free plasma concentrations fall rapidly due to binding to platelet receptors. Platelet function recovers over about 48 hours although abciximab may remain in the circulation for 15 days or more in a platelet-bound state.

## Uses and Administration

Abciximab is the Fab fragment of the chimeric monoclonal antibody 7E3. It binds to the glycoprotein IIb/IIIa receptor on the surface of platelets. This prevents binding of fibrinogen, von Willebrand factor, and other adhesive molecules to the receptor sites and inhibits platelet aggregation. It is used as an adjunct to heparin and aspirin therapy for the prevention of acute ischaemic complications in patients undergoing percutaneous transluminal coronary procedures including angioplasty, atherectomy, and stenting. It is also used in patients with unstable angina who are candidates for such procedures. It is under investigation in acute ischaemic stroke.

Abciximab is given intravenously as a bolus injection over 1 minute in a dose of 250 micrograms/kg followed immediately by an infusion of 0.125 micrograms/kg per minute (to a maximum dose of 10 micrograms/minute). For stabilisation in patients with unstable angina the bolus dose followed by the infusion should be started up to 24 hours before the possible intervention and continued for 12 hours after; for other patients the bolus should be given 10 to 60 minutes before the intervention followed by the infusion for 12 hours.

◊ General references.

1. Foster RH, Wiseman LR. Abciximab: an updated review of its use in ischaemic heart disease. *Drugs* 1998; **56:** 629–65.
2. Kleiman NS. A risk-benefit assessment of abciximab in angioplasty. *Drug Safety* 1999; **20:** 43–57.
3. Ibbotson T, *et al.* Abciximab: an updated review of its therapeutic use in patients with ischaemic heart disease undergoing percutaneous coronary revascularisation. *Drugs* 2003; **63:** 1121–63.

**Ischaemic heart disease.** Patients with ischaemic heart disease (stable angina, unstable angina, or myocardial infarction) may be treated medically or by various surgical or percutaneous interventions. **Percutaneous transluminal coronary angioplasty** is a non-pharmacological procedure employed in both the acute and long-term management of such patients to aid reperfusion and revascularisation (p.834). Heparin is usually given during the procedure to prevent perioperative thrombosis and aspirin is given as an antiplatelet drug to reduce long-term stenosis. Abciximab has a role as an *adjunct to heparin and aspirin* in various groups of patients undergoing angioplasty. In the EPIC study,[1] which included only patients at high risk for abrupt vessel closure, acute ischaemic events and complications of angioplasty were reduced but there was also a significant increase in bleeding complications. In those given abciximab as a bolus injection immediately before angioplasty followed by intravenous infusion for 12 hours there was also a reduction in restenosis at 6 months[2] and at 3 years.[3] Similar results were obtained in the EPILOG study,[4] which used a lower dose of heparin and included unselected patients. However, in the CAPTURE study,[5] in which abciximab was given for 18 to 24 hours before angioplasty and for 1 hour after, the initial benefit was not maintained at 6 months. Short-term benefit has also been reported[6] with abciximab in patients with acute myocardial infarction treated with primary angioplasty.

Coronary stenting is now widely used as an adjunct to angioplasty. In the EPISTENT study, the combination of *abciximab and stenting* reduced the rates of death and myocardial infarction compared with either treatment alone; this benefit was maintained at 30 days,[7] 6 months,[8] and at 1 year[9] follow-up. In patients with acute myocardial infarction treated with primary angioplasty and coronary stenting, abciximab improved outcomes both immediately following the procedure and at 6 months.[10]

Abciximab has also been tried as an **adjunct to medical treatment** alone in patients with acute coronary syndromes. Although other glycoprotein IIb/IIIa inhibitors have a role in patients with unstable angina who are not receiving angioplasty, a large study[11] with abciximab in such patients failed to show any benefit over placebo. In patients with acute myocardial infarction, abciximab given as an *adjunct to thrombolysis* (TIMI 14) improved early patency rates,[12] but a further study (GUSTO V)[13] found no benefit over thrombolysis alone at 30 days. However, in the ASSENT-3 study,[14] combination of abciximab with half-dose tenecteplase and heparin resulted in a significant improvement in outcomes at 30 days, although bleeding rates were also significantly increased.

1. The EPIC Investigators. Use of a monoclonal antibody directed against the platelet glycoprotein IIb/IIIa receptor in high-risk coronary angioplasty. *N Engl J Med* 1994; **330:** 956–61.
2. Topol EJ, *et al.* Randomised trial of coronary intervention with antibody against platelet IIb/IIIa integrin for reduction of clinical restenosis: results at six months. *Lancet* 1994; **343:** 881–6.
3. Topol EJ, *et al.* Long-term protection from myocardial ischemic events in a randomized trial of brief integrin $\beta_3$ blockade with percutaneous coronary intervention. *JAMA* 1997; **278:** 479–84.
4. The EPILOG Investigators. Platelet glycoprotein IIb/IIIa receptor blockade and low-dose heparin during percutaneous coronary revascularization. *N Engl J Med* 1997; **336:** 1689–96.
5. The CAPTURE Investigators. Randomised placebo-controlled trial of abciximab before and during coronary intervention in refractory unstable angina: the CAPTURE study. *Lancet* 1997; **349:** 1429–35. Correction. *ibid.*; **350:** 744.
6. Brener SJ, *et al.* Randomized, placebo-controlled trial of platelet glycoprotein IIb/IIIa blockade with primary angioplasty for acute myocardial infarction. *Circulation* 1998; **98:** 734–41.
7. The EPISTENT Investigators. Randomised placebo-controlled and balloon-angioplasty-controlled trial to assess safety of coronary stenting with use of platelet glycoprotein-IIb/IIIa blockade. *Lancet* 1998; **352:** 87–92.
8. Lincoff AM, *et al.* Complementary clinical benefits of coronary-artery stenting and blockade of platelet glycoprotein IIb/IIIa receptors. *N Engl J Med* 1999; **341:** 319–27.
9. Topol EJ, *et al.* Outcomes at 1 year and economic implications of platelet glycoprotein IIb/IIIa blockade in patients undergoing coronary stenting: results from a multicentre randomised trial. *Lancet* 1999; **354:** 2019–24. Correction. *ibid.* 2000; **355:** 1104.
10. Montalescot G, *et al.* Platelet glycoprotein IIb/IIIa inhibition with coronary stenting for acute myocardial infarction. *N Engl J Med* 2001; **344:** 1895–1903.
11. The GUSTO IV-ACS Investigators. Effect of glycoprotein IIb/IIIa receptor blocker abciximab on outcome in patients with acute coronary syndromes without early coronary revascularisation: the GUSTO IV-ACS randomised trial. *Lancet* 2001; **357:** 1915–24.
12. Antman EM, *et al.* Abciximab facilitates the rate and extent of thrombolysis: results of the Thrombolysis in Myocardial Infarction (TIMI) 14 trial. *Circulation* 1999; **99:** 2720–32.
13. The GUSTO V Investigators. Reperfusion therapy for acute myocardial infarction with fibrinolytic therapy or combination reduced fibrinolytic therapy and platelet glycoprotein IIb/IIIa inhibition: the GUSTO V randomised trial. *Lancet* 2001; **357:** 1905–14. Correction. *ibid.*; **358:** 512.
14. The Assessment of the Safety and Efficacy of a New Thrombolytic Regimen (ASSENT)-3 Investigators. Efficacy and safety of tenecteplase in combination with enoxaparin, abciximab, or unfractionated heparin: the ASSENT-3 randomised trial in acute myocardial infarction. *Lancet* 2001; **358:** 605–13.

## Preparations

**Proprietary Preparations** (details are given in Part 3)
***Arg.:*** ReoPro; ***Austral.:*** ReoPro; ***Austria:*** ReoPro; ***Belg.:*** ReoPro; ***Braz.:*** ReoPro; ***Canad.:*** ReoPro; ***Chile:*** ReoPro; ***Denm.:*** ReoPro; ***Fin.:*** ReoPro; ***Fr.:*** ReoPro; ***Ger.:*** ReoPro; ***Gr.:*** ReoPro; ***Hong Kong:*** ReoPro; ***India:*** ReoPro; ***Irl.:*** ReoPro; ***Israel:*** ReoPro; ***Ital.:*** ReoPro; ***Malaysia:*** ReoPro; ***Mex.:*** ReoPro; ***Neth.:*** ReoPro; ***Norw.:*** ReoPro; ***NZ:*** ReoPro; ***S.Afr.:*** ReoPro; ***Singapore:*** ReoPro; ***Spain:*** ReoPro; ***Swed.:*** ReoPro; ***Switz.:*** ReoPro; ***Thai.:*** ReoPro; ***UK:*** ReoPro; ***USA:*** ReoPro.

# Acadesine *(BAN, USAN, rINN)*

Acadesina; AICA Riboside; GP-1-110; GP-1-110-0. 5-Amino-1-(β-D-ribofuranosyl)imidazole-4-carboxamide.

$C_9H_{14}N_4O_5$ = 258.2.
*CAS — 2627-69-2.*
*ATC — C01EB13.*

## Profile

Acadesine is a purine nucleoside analogue reported to have cardioprotective effects. It has been investigated in the management of myocardial ischaemia, particularly in patients undergoing coronary artery bypass graft surgery. Acadesine may protect against further ischaemia by influencing metabolism in ischaemic cells, enhancing the release of adenosine in preference to inosine following the breakdown of adenosine monophosphate.

◊ References.

1. Europe/Canada Perioperative Ischemia Research Group. Multinational study of the effect of acadesine on major cardiovascular outcomes associated with CABG surgery. *J Am Coll Cardiol* 1993; **21** (suppl): 150A.
2. Leung JM, *et al.* An initial multicenter, randomized controlled trial on the safety and efficacy of acadesine in patients undergoing coronary artery bypass graft surgery. *Anesth Analg* 1994; **78:** 420–34.
3. Alkhulaifi AM, Pugsley WB. Role of acadesine in clinical myocardial protection. *Br Heart J* 1995; **73:** 304–5.
4. Mangano DT. Effects of acadesine on myocardial infarction, stroke, and death following surgery: a meta-analysis of the 5 international randomized trials. *JAMA* 1997; **277:** 325–32.

# ACE Inhibitors

Angiotensin-converting Enzyme Inhibitors; Inhibidores de la ECA.

There appear to be few significant differences between ACE inhibitors. They may be distinguished from each other by the presence or absence of a sulfhydryl group, whether they are prodrugs or not, their route of elimination, and their affinity for angiotensin-converting enzyme in vascular and other tissue, although whether these characteristics modify pharmacodynamics and therefore clinical efficacy is uncertain. Differences in these characteristics do however influence onset and duration of action of ACE inhibitors.

## Adverse Effects and Treatment

Many of the adverse effects of ACE inhibitors relate to their pharmacological action and all therefore have a similar spectrum of adverse effects. Some effects, such as taste disturbances and skin reactions, were at one time attributed to the presence of a sulfhydryl group (as in captopril) but have now also been reported with other ACE inhibitors; however, they may be more common with captopril.

The most common adverse effects are due to the vascular effects of ACE inhibitors and include hypotension, dizziness, fatigue, headache, and nausea and other gastrointestinal disturbances.

Pronounced hypotension may occur at the start of therapy with ACE inhibitors, particularly in patients with heart failure and in sodium- or volume-depleted patients (for example, those who have received previous diuretic therapy). Myocardial infarction and stroke have been reported and may relate to severe falls in blood pressure in patients with ischaemic heart disease or cerebrovascular disease. Other cardiovascular effects that have occurred include tachycardia, palpitations, and chest pain.

Deterioration in renal function, including increasing blood concentrations of urea and creatinine, may occur, and reversible acute renal failure has been reported. Renal effects are most common in patients with existing renal or renovascular dysfunction or heart failure, in whom vasodilatation reduces renal perfusion pressure; it may be aggravated by hypovolaemia. Proteinuria has also occurred and in some patients has progressed to nephrotic syndrome. Hyperkalaemia and hyponatraemia may develop due to decreased aldosterone secretion.

Other adverse effects include persistent dry cough and other upper respiratory tract symptoms, and angioedema; these may be related to effects on bradykinin or prostaglandin metabolism. Skin rashes (including erythema multiforme and toxic epidermal necrolysis) may occur; photosensitivity, alopecia, and other hypersensitivity reactions have also been reported.

Blood disorders have been reported with ACE inhibitors and include neutropenia and agranulocytosis (especially in patients with renal failure and in those with collagen vascular disorders such as systemic lupus erythematosus and scleroderma), thrombocytopenia, and anaemias.

Other less common adverse effects reported with ACE inhibitors include stomatitis, abdominal pain, pancreatitis, hepatocellular injury or cholestatic jaundice, muscle cramps, paraesthesias, mood and sleep disturbances, and impotence.

ACE inhibitors may be toxic to the fetus (see Pregnancy under Precautions, below).

Most of the adverse effects of ACE inhibitors are reversible on withdrawing therapy. Symptomatic hypotension, including that following overdosage, generally responds to volume expansion with an intravenous infusion of sodium chloride 0.9%.

◊ General reviews.


1. Parish RC, Miller LJ. Adverse effects of angiotensin converting enzyme (ACE) inhibitors: an update. *Drug Safety* 1992; **7:** 14–31.
2. Alderman CP. Adverse effects of the angiotensin-converting enzyme inhibitors. *Ann Pharmacother* 1996; **30:** 55–61.
3. Agusti A, *et al.* Adverse effects of ACE inhibitors in patients with chronic heart failure and/or ventricular dysfunction : meta-analysis of randomised clinical trials. *Drug Safety* 2003; **26:** 895–908.


**Angioedema.** See under Hypersensitivity, below.

**Cough.** Treatment with ACE inhibitors has been associated with the development of cough in up to 20% of hypertensive patients; cough may be less troublesome in those with heart failure,[1] although the incidence may be higher.[2] The cough is reported to be persistent, paroxysmal, and non-productive; it causes irritation of the throat, may be accompanied by voice changes (hoarseness or huskiness), and is often worse when lying down.[1,3,4] It is more common in women and non-smokers, and may be delayed in onset by weeks or even months.

The majority of reports of this adverse effect concern captopril and enalapril,[3,4] but it has also occurred in patients receiving many of the other ACE inhibitors,[5] suggesting that the effect is common to all drugs of this class.

The mechanism that produces the reaction is uncertain but appears to be related to the non-specific blockade of ACE since angiotensin II receptor antagonists are associated with a much lower incidence of cough.[6] The sensitivity of the cough reflex is increased.[7] Prostaglandins released in the respiratory tract have been proposed as mediators,[3] but other mediators such as bradykinin[8] or substance P,[9] both of which are substrates for ACE, have been suggested. However, attempts to demonstrate a link between the effects of ACE inhibitors on cough, and bronchial hyperreactivity of the type found in obstructive airways disease and asthma have produced conflicting evidence, with bronchial hyperreactivity being demonstrated in some studies[10] but not in others.[11]

Where the patient can tolerate the cough, it may be reasonable to continue treatment; in some cases reducing the dose may help. Spontaneous recovery or improvement in the cough has been reported.[12] Changing to an alternative ACE inhibitor is not advised since it is rarely effective.[7] Drugs that inhibit prostaglandin synthesis, including the NSAIDs sulindac[13] and indometacin,[14] have been reported to suppress the cough, but NSAIDs and ACE inhibitors may interact adversely (see under Interactions, below). The calcium-channel blocker nifedipine also reduced cough, although to a lesser extent than indometacin, possibly by a similar mechanism.[14] Inhaled bupivacaine,[15] inhaled sodium cromoglicate,[16,17] oral baclofen,[18] oral picotamide,[19] and oral ferrous sulfate,[20] have also been reported to be of help. However, in many patients there will be no alternative but to withdraw the ACE inhibitor.[4] Angiotensin II receptor antagonists may be a suitable alternative in patients with hypertension.


1. Anonymous. Cough caused by ACE inhibitors. *Drug Ther Bull.* 1994; **32:** 28 and 55–6.
2. Ravid D, *et al.* Angiotensin-converting enzyme inhibitors and cough: a prospective evaluation in hypertension and congestive heart failure. *J Clin Pharmacol* 1994; **34:** 1116–20.
3. Coulter DM, Edwards IR. Cough associated with captopril and enalapril. *BMJ* 1987; **294:** 1521–3.
4. Berkin KE, Ball SG. Cough and angiotensin converting enzyme inhibition. *BMJ* 1988; **296:** 1279–80.
5. Israili ZH, Hall WD. Cough and angioneurotic edema associated with angiotensin-converting enzyme inhibitor therapy. *Ann Intern Med* 1992; **117:** 234–42.
6. Pylypchuk GB. ACE inhibitor- versus angiotensin II blocker-induced cough and angioedema. *Ann Pharmacother* 1998; **32:** 1060–6.
7. Overlack A. ACE inhibitor-induced cough and bronchospasm. *Drug Safety* 1996; **15:** 72–8.
8. Ferner RE, *et al.* Effects of intradermal bradykinin after inhibition of angiotensin converting enzyme. *BMJ* 1987; **294:** 1119–20.
9. Morice AH, *et al.* Angiotensin-converting enzyme and the cough reflex. *Lancet* 1987; **ii:** 1116–18.
10. Bucknall CE, *et al.* Bronchial hyperreactivity in patients who cough after receiving angiotensin converting enzyme inhibitors. *BMJ* 1988; **296:** 86–8.
11. Boulet L-P, *et al.* Pulmonary function and airway responsiveness during long-term therapy with captopril. *JAMA* 1989; **261:** 413–16.
12. Reisin L, Schneeweiss A. Spontaneous disappearance of cough induced by angiotensin-converting enzyme inhibitors (captopril or enalapril). *Am J Cardiol* 1992; **70:** 398–9.
13. Nicholls MG, Gilchrist NL. Sulindac and cough induced by converting enzyme inhibitors. *Lancet* 1987; **i:** 872.
14. Fogari R, *et al.* Effects of nifedipine and indomethacin on cough induced by angiotensin-converting enzyme inhibitors: a double-blind, randomized, cross-over study. *J Cardiovasc Pharmacol* 1992; **19:** 670–3.
15. Brown RC, Turton CWG. Cough and angiotensin converting enzyme inhibition. *BMJ* 1988; **296:** 1741.
16. Keogh A. Sodium cromoglycate prophylaxis for angiotensin-converting enzyme inhibitor cough. *Lancet* 1993; **341:** 560.
17. Hargreaves MR, Benson MK. Inhaled sodium cromoglycate in angiotensin-converting enzyme inhibitor cough. *Lancet* 1995; **345:** 13–16.
18. Dicpinigaitis PV. Use of baclofen to suppress cough induced by angiotensin-converting enzyme inhibitors. *Ann Pharmacother* 1996; **30:** 1242–5.
19. Malini PL, *et al.* Thromboxane antagonism and cough induced by angiotensin-converting-enzyme inhibitor. *Lancet* 1997; **350:** 15–18.
20. Lee S-C, *et al.* Iron supplementation inhibits cough associated with ACE inhibitors. *Hypertension* 2001; **38:** 166–70.


**Effects on the blood.** A number of blood disorders have occurred in patients receiving ACE inhibitors, although there have been few reports in the literature. A reduction in haemoglobin concentration and haematocrit may occur but is not usually clinically significant (but see Erythrocytosis under Uses, below). Cases of neutropenia and agranulocytosis (particularly in patients with renal or collagen vascular disorders), and thrombocytopenia have been noted. Aplastic anaemia has also occurred[1,2] and may be fatal.[2]


1. Kim CR, *et al.* Captopril and aplastic anemia. *Ann Intern Med* 1989; **111:** 187–8.
2. Harrison BD, *et al.* Fatal aplastic anaemia associated with lisinopril. *Lancet* 1995; **346:** 247–8.


**Effects on the kidneys.** ACE inhibitors have complex effects on the kidney;[1,2] they have established renoprotective effects but also cause acute deterioration in renal function in some patients. These apparently contradictory effects are related to the action of ACE inhibitors on the renin-angiotensin-aldosterone system.

The renin-angiotensin-aldosterone system has an important role in maintaining normal renal blood flow and renal function. A reduction in renal perfusion, for example due to hypovolaemia, heart failure, or renal artery stenosis, leads to activation of this system and an increase in angiotensin II release. This results predominantly in post-glomerular renal vasoconstriction, which maintains renal glomerular pressure and thus glomerular filtration, despite the fall in renal blood flow.

In normal individuals with unrestricted sodium intake, the renin-angiotensin-aldosterone system is suppressed and ACE inhibitors have little effect on renal function. In patients with essential hypertension ACE inhibitors generally increase renal blood flow despite the reduction in arterial blood pressure, since this is exceeded by the effects of renal vasodilatation. However, filtration fraction falls since the pressure within the glomerulus is reduced, and there are only minor changes in glomerular filtration rate. The increase in renal blood flow is more pronounced during sodium restriction and in younger patients.

These effects are generally beneficial. However, in patients with reduced renal perfusion, glomerular filtration rate may be critically dependent on the renin-angiotensin-aldosterone system and the use of ACE inhibitors may provoke problems. Severe renal function loss or even anuria have been reported in patients with a single transplanted kidney with renal artery stenosis, or patients with bilateral renal artery disease. The stenotic kidney maintains its filtering capacity by preferential vasoconstriction of the efferent arterioles, a mechanism mainly mediated by the renin-angiotensin system; under ACE inhibition, vasodilatation of the efferent arterioles combined with the drop in arterial pressure can result in a critical decrease in filtration pressure. Hypovolaemia or sodium depletion, for example due to diuretics, also leads to activation of the renin-angiotensin-aldosterone system and predisposes patients to renal impairment. Most patients developing renal insufficiency have been using diuretics and sodium repletion can restore renal function despite continuation of ACE inhibition.

Patients with heart failure may also be at risk of a decline in renal function on long-term ACE inhibitor therapy. This is because in chronic heart failure, angiotensin-II mediated systemic and renal vasoconstriction is again important in the maintenance of renal perfusion pressure. The decline may be alleviated by reduction of the dosage of diuretics or liberalisation of dietary salt intake, despite continuation of the ACE inhibitor. An additional risk factor in elderly patients with heart failure is the high incidence of occult renovascular disease in these patients.[3]

Moderate impairment of renal function either before or during use of ACE inhibitors is not necessarily an indication to stop therapy. The effects of ACE inhibitors on renal function are generally reversible, and the reduction in filtration pressure may result in renoprotection. A review[4] of studies of the use of ACE inhibitors in patients with renal impairment found that those who initially lost renal function had the greatest long-term benefit.

In addition to pathophysiological effects ACE inhibitors may induce membranous glomerulopathy or interstitial nephritis. The former has been associated with captopril use, particularly at high doses, but is rare, and seems less likely to occur at the lower doses favoured today. The proteinuria usually clears without appreciable renal function loss irrespective of whether or not the drug is continued, although persistent proteinuria and renal function loss have been described. Proven interstitial nephritis has also been reported rarely, and may possibly be due to an allergic mechanism.


1. Navis G, *et al.* ACE inhibitors and the kidney: a risk-benefit assessment. *Drug Safety* 1996; **15:** 200–11.
2. Schoolwerth AC, *et al.* Renal considerations in angiotensin converting enzyme inhibitor therapy: a statement for healthcare professionals from the Council on the Kidney in Cardiovascular Disease and the Council for High Blood Pressure Research of the American Heart Association. *Circulation* 2001; **104:** 1985–91.
3. MacDowall P, *et al.* Risk of morbidity from renovascular disease in elderly patients with congestive cardiac failure. *Lancet* 1998; **352:** 13–16.
4. Bakris GL, Weir MR. Angiotensin-converting enzyme inhibitor-associated elevations in serum creatinine: is this a cause for concern? *Arch Intern Med* 2000; **160:** 685–93.


**Effects on the liver.** Hepatotoxicity has been reported with captopril,[1,2] and also with enalapril and lisinopril.[2] Most reports have been associated with captopril. In a report[1] of 3 cases of liver disease apparently caused or aggravated by captopril, it was noted that jaundice due to captopril is usually predominantly cholestatic in nature but acute hepatocellular injury has also been observed. Of 29 cases of liver dysfunction due to captopril and reported to the UK Committee on Safety of Medicines, 9 had hepatocellular jaundice, with 2 deaths; 8 were cholestatic jaundice, with 1 fatality; and 3 patients had hepatorenal syndrome, all of whom died. Worldwide, excluding the UK, 164 cases of hepatic adverse reactions had been notified to the WHO by January 1989. The incidence of such reactions is estimated at 0.09 per 1000 patients but this is likely to be an underestimate. Resolution may take a long time and captopril should be withdrawn immediately at the earliest hint of liver sensitivity.


1. Bellary SV, *et al.* Captopril and the liver. *Lancet* 1989; **ii:** 514.
2. Hagley MT, *et al.* Hepatotoxicity associated with angiotensin-converting enzyme inhibitors. *Ann Pharmacother* 1993; **27:** 228–31.


**Effects on the mouth.** Aphthous and tongue ulcers may occur during treatment with ACE inhibitors. There have been a few reports of a 'scalded mouth syndrome', described as similar to being scalded by hot liquids, associated with captopril,[1] enalapril,[1] and lisinopril[2] therapy.


1. Vlasses PH, *et al.* "Scalded mouth" caused by angiotensin-converting enzyme inhibitors. *BMJ* 1982; **284:** 1672–3.
2. Savino LB, Haushalter NM. Lisinopril-induced "scalded mouth syndrome." *Ann Pharmacother* 1992; **26:** 1381–2.


**Effects on the nervous system.** Encephalopathy and focal neurological signs,[1] and peripheral neuropathy,[2,3] including Guillain-Barré neuropathy,[3] have been reported in patients receiving captopril. Some CNS effects of captopril may be attributable to alterations in cerebral blood flow. In a study in patients with severe heart failure, cerebral blood flow in patients aged under 65 was improved by a single dose of captopril 12.5 mg, but in patients aged over 70 there was a 13% reduction.[4] Two patients in whom captopril 6.25 mg produced impaired consciousness and paraesthesias, and dizziness, blurred vision, and aphasia, were found to have stenosis of the carotid arteries.[5] Agitation, panic, extreme depression, and insomnia was reported in a patient 4 weeks after starting treatment with enalapril; depressive episodes recurred on rechallenge.[6] There have been reports of mania possibly precipitated by captopril,[7] and visual hallucinations have been reported in association with captopril and enalapril therapy.[8]


1. Rapoport S, Zyman P. Captopril and central nervous system effects. *Ann Intern Med* 1983; **98:** 1023.
2. Samanta A, Burden AC. Peripheral neuropathy due to captopril. *BMJ* 1985; **291:** 1172.
3. Chakraborty TK, Ruddell WSJ. Guillain-Barré neuropathy during treatment with captopril. *Postgrad Med J* 1987; **63:** 221–2.
4. Britton KE, *et al.* Angiotensin-converting-enzyme inhibitors and treatment of heart failure. *Lancet* 1985; **ii:** 1236.
5. Jensen H, *et al.* Carotid artery stenosis exposed by an adverse effect of captopril. *BMJ* 1986; **293:** 1073–4.
6. Ahmad S. Enalapril-induced acute psychosis. *DICP Ann Pharmacother* 1991; **25:** 558–9.
7. Peet M, Peters S. Drug-induced mania. *Drug Safety* 1995; **12:** 146–53.
8. Haffner CA, *et al.* Hallucinations as an adverse effect of angiotensin converting enzyme inhibition. *Postgrad Med J* 1993; **69:** 240.


**Effects on the pancreas.** The manufacturers of captopril, enalapril, and lisinopril have all been reported[1] to have data on file on drug-associated pancreatitis. In 1994 the UK Committee on Safety of Medicines[2] noted that there had been 23 reports of pancreatitis associated with ACE inhibitors (captopril 11, enalapril 10, fosinopril 1, and quinapril 1) although whether or not this was causal was not certain.


1. Dabaghi S. ACE inhibitors and pancreatitis. *Ann Intern Med* 1991; **115:** 330–1.
2. Committee on Safety of Medicines/Medicines Control Agency. Drug-induced pancreatitis. *Current Problems* 1994; **20:** 2–3.


**Effects on the respiratory system.** Cough is a recognised adverse effect of ACE inhibitors but evidence for a link with bronchial hyperreactivity or airways obstruction is controversial (see Cough, above). In reports of adverse respiratory reactions to ACE inhibitors submitted to the Swedish Adverse Drug Reactions Advisory Committee and to WHO, symptoms of airway obstruction such as dyspnoea, asthma, and bronchospasm occurred rarely, usually within the first few weeks of treatment.[1] However, the evidence for a causal link between ACE inhibitors and these symptoms was questioned.[2]

Severe nasal obstruction was associated with enalapril treatment in a 45-year-old woman with a history of mild rhinorrhoea and sneezing. Symptoms cleared within 2 days of stopping enalapril and recurred on rechallenge.[3]

There have been case reports of pneumonitis associated with treatment with captopril[4] and perindopril.[5]


1. Lunde H, *et al.* Dyspnoea, asthma, and bronchospasm in relation to treatment with angiotensin converting enzyme inhibitors. *BMJ* 1994; **308:** 18–21.
2. Inman WHW, *et al.* Angiotensin converting enzyme inhibitors and asthma. *BMJ* 1994; **308:** 593–4.
3. Fennerty A, *et al.* Enalapril-induced nasal blockage. *Lancet* 1986; **ii:** 1395–6.
4. Kidney JC, *et al.* Captopril and lymphocytic alveolitis. *BMJ* 1989; **299:** 981.
5. Benard A, *et al.* Perindopril-associated pneumonitis. *Eur Respir J* 1996; **9:** 1314–16.


**Effects on skeletal muscle.** Severe muscle pain and weakness, accompanied by morning stiffness, was reported[1] in a patient taking enalapril. Symptoms resolved within a few days of discontinuing the drug.


1. Leloët X, *et al.* Pseudopolymyalgia rheumatica during treatment with enalapril. *BMJ* 1989; **298:** 325.


**Effects on the skin.** Skin rashes may occur during treatment with ACE inhibitors; they have been reported in 1 to 6% of patients receiving captopril. Angioedema is also an adverse effect of ACE inhibitors (see Hypersensitivity, below). There have been reports of bullous pemphigoid,[1] hyperhidrosis,[2] Kaposi's sarcoma,[3] lichen planus,[4] onycholysis,[5,6] pemphigus,[7,8] and cutaneous hypersensitivity vasculitis[9] associated with administration of captopril. Onycholysis has also occurred with enalapril[10] and pemphigus with enalapril[11,12] and ramipril.[13] Lichen planus pemphigoides has been reported with ramipril.[14] A severe cutaneous reaction, resembling early mycosis fungoides, and possibly allergic in nature, has been reported following administration of captopril or enalapril.[15] Captopril has also been reported to exacerbate psoriasis.[16] Vulvovaginal pruritus with dysuria[17] has been noted in a patient receiving enalapril.


1. Mallet L, *et al.* Bullous pemphigoid associated with captopril. *DICP Ann Pharmacother* 1989; **23:** 63.
2. Morse MH. Hyperhidrosis: a possible side effect of captopril treatment. *BMJ* 1984; **289:** 1272.
3. Puppin D, *et al.* Kaposi's sarcoma associated with captopril. *Lancet* 1990; **336:** 1251–2.
4. Cox NH, *et al.* Lichen planus associated with captopril: a further disorder demonstrating the 'tin-tack' sign. *Br J Dermatol* 1989; **120:** 319–21.
5. Brueggemeyer CD, Ramirez G. Onycholysis associated with captopril. *Lancet* 1984; **i:** 1352–3.
6. Borders JV. Captopril and onycholysis. *Ann Intern Med* 1986; **105:** 305–6.
7. Parfrey PS, *et al.* Captopril-induced pemphigus. *BMJ* 1980; **281:** 194.
8. Butt A, Burge SM. Pemphigus vulgaris induced by captopril. *Br J Dermatol* 1995; **132:** 315–16.
9. Miralles R, *et al.* Captopril and vasculitis. *Ann Intern Med* 1988; **109:** 514.
10. Gupta S, *et al.* Nail changes with enalapril. *BMJ* 1986; **293:** 140.
11. Kuechle MK, *et al.* Angiotensin-converting enzyme inhibitor-induced pemphigus: three case reports and literature review. *Mayo Clin Proc* 1994; **69:** 1166–71.
12. Frangogiannis NG, *et al.* Pemphigus of the larynx and esophagus. *Ann Intern Med* 1995; **122:** 803–4.
13. Vignes S, *et al.* Ramipril-induced superficial pemphigus. *Br J Dermatol* 1996; **135:** 657–8.
14. Ogg GS, *et al.* Ramipril-associated lichen planus pemphigoides. *Br J Dermatol* 1997; **136:** 412–14.
15. Furness PN, *et al.* Severe cutaneous reactions to captopril and enalapril; histological study and comparison with early mycosis fungoides. *J Clin Pathol* 1986; **39:** 902–7.
16. Hamlet NW, *et al.* Does captopril exacerbate psoriasis? *BMJ* 1987; **295:** 1352.
17. Heckerling PS. Enalapril and vulvovaginal pruritus. *Ann Intern Med* 1990; **112:** 879–80.


**Gynaecomastia.** Painful unilateral gynaecomastia was reported in a patient with systemic lupus erythematosus and renal impairment who was given captopril for hypertension.[1] In view of reports of breast enlargement in women given penicillamine it was suggested that the sulfhydryl structure might be responsible; however, gynaecomastia has also been reported in two patients receiving enalapril,[2,3] which does not contain the sulfhydryl grouping.


1. Markusse HM, Meyboom RHB. Gynaecomastia associated with captopril. *BMJ* 1988; **296:** 1262–3.
2. Nakamura Y, *et al.* Gynaecomastia induced by angiotensin converting enzyme inhibitor. *BMJ* 1990; **300:** 541.
3. Llop R, *et al.* Gynecomastia associated with enalapril and diazepam. *Ann Pharmacother* 1994; **28:** 671–2.


**Hypersensitivity.** Some of the adverse effects of ACE inhibitors might be mediated by the immune system, but evidence of specific **hypersensitivity reactions** seems to be limited. The presence of an IgG antibody to captopril was demonstrated in the serum of 2 of 45 patients receiving the drug but the clinical significance was unclear.[1] A reaction resembling serum sickness was reported in a patient given captopril, with deposition of immune complexes in the glomerular basement membrane, and symptoms of rash, arthralgia, epidermolysis, fever, and lymphadenopathy.[2] Eosinophilia has also been reported in a number of patients.[3] The formation of antinuclear antibodies and lupus-like reactions have been described.[4,5]

Treatment with ACE inhibitors (enalapril, captopril, or lisinopril) has been associated with the development of **anaphylactoid reactions** in patients undergoing high-flux haemodialysis using polyacrylonitrile membrane (AN69).[6,7] The UK Committee on Safety of Medicines has advised that the combined use of ACE inhibitors and such membranes should be avoided.[8] Similar anaphylactoid reactions have occurred in patients taking ACE inhibitors while being treated for severe hypercholesterolaemia by extracorporeal removal of low-density lipoproteins (LDL-apheresis) with dextran sulfate columns.[9] These reactions are thought to be bradykinin-mediated. Prolonging the interval between the last dose of ACE inhibitor and dextran sulfate apheresis has averted the reaction;[10] successful prevention has also been reported with the bradykinin receptor antagonist icatibant.[11] Hypotensive reactions associated with blood transfusion through bedside leucoreduction filters in patients receiving ACE inhibitors have also been attributed to bradykinin.[12] There have also been rare reports of severe anaphylactoid reactions occurring during desensitisation with Hymenoptera venom (e.g. bee or wasp venom) in patients receiving ACE inhibitors.

**Angioedema**, a known adverse effect of ACE inhibitors,[13-16] is reported to occur in 0.1 to 0.2% of patients.[15,16] The incidence may be higher in black American[17] or Afro-Caribbean[18] patients. There is no evidence that it results from an immunological mechanism in these patients and it has been suggested that the effect is due to impaired kinin degradation. However, angioedema has been reported with lisinopril in a patient who had previously tolerated captopril.[19] The onset of angioedema has usually been within hours or at most a week of starting treatment with the ACE inhibitor,[15] but can occur after prolonged therapy for several months or years.[20-22] Visceral angioedema presenting as abdominal pain with diarrhoea, nausea, and vomiting, has also been reported.[23,24] If angioedema occurs the ACE inhibitor should be withdrawn and if there is swelling affecting the tongue, glottis, or larynx likely to cause airway obstruction, adrenaline should be given (see p.854). Angiotensin II receptor antagonists have been suggested as an alternative in patients unable to tolerate ACE inhibitors, but there have also been reports of angioedema associated with their use (see under Losartan Potassium, p.947).


1. Coleman JW, *et al.* Drug-specific antibodies in patients receiving captopril. *Br J Clin Pharmacol* 1986; **22:** 161–5.
2. Hoorntje SJ, *et al.* Serum-sickness-like syndrome with membranous glomerulopathy in patient on captopril. *Lancet* 1979; **ii:** 1297.
3. Kayanakis JG, *et al.* Eosinophilia during captopril treatment. *Lancet* 1980; **ii:** 923.
4. Schwartz D, *et al.* Enalapril-induced antinuclear antibodies. *Lancet* 1990; **336:** 187.
5. Pelayo M, *et al.* Drug-induced lupus-like reaction and captopril. *Ann Pharmacother* 1993; **27:** 1541–2.
6. Verresen L, *et al.* Angiotensin-converting-enzyme inhibitors and anaphylactoid reactions to high-flux membrane dialysis. *Lancet* 1990; **336:** 1360–2.
7. Tielmans C, *et al.* ACE inhibitors and anaphylactoid reactions to high-flux membrane dialysis. *Lancet* 1991; **337:** 370–1.
8. Committee on Safety of Medicines. Anaphylactoid reactions to high-flux polyacrylonitrile membranes in combination with ACE inhibitors. *Current Problems 33* 1992.
9. Olbricht CJ, *et al.* Anaphylactoid reactions, LDL apheresis with dextran sulphate, and ACE inhibitors. *Lancet* 1992; **340:** 908–9.
10. Keller C, *et al.* LDL-apheresis with dextran sulphate and anaphylactoid reactions to ACE inhibitors. *Lancet* 1993; **341:** 60–1.
11. Davidson DC, *et al.* Prevention with icatibant of anaphylactoid reactions to ACE inhibitor during LDL apheresis. *Lancet* 1994; **343:** 1575.
12. Quillen K. Hypotensive transfusion reactions in patients taking angiotensin-converting-enzyme inhibitors. *N Engl J Med* 2000; **343:** 1422–3.
13. Wood SM, *et al.* Angio-oedema and urticaria associated with angiotensin converting enzyme inhibitors. *BMJ* 1987; **294:** 91–2.
14. Hedner T, *et al.* Angio-oedema in relation to treatment with angiotensin converting enzyme inhibitors. *BMJ* 1992; **304:** 941–6.
15. Israili ZH, Hall WD. Cough and angioneurotic edema associated with angiotensin-converting enzyme inhibitor therapy: a review of the literature and pathophysiology. *Ann Intern Med* 1992; **117:** 234–42.
16. Vleeming W, *et al.* ACE inhibitor-induced angioedema. *Drug Safety* 1998; **18:** 171–88.
17. Brown NJ, *et al.* Black Americans have an increased rate of angiotensin converting enzyme inhibitor-associated angioedema. *Clin Pharmacol Ther* 1996; **60:** 8–13.
18. Gibbs CR, *et al.* Angioedema due to ACE inhibitors: increased risk in patients of African origin. *Br J Clin Pharmacol* 1999; **48:** 861–5.
19. McElligott S, *et al.* Angioedema after substituting lisinopril for captopril. *Ann Intern Med* 1992; **116:** 426–7.
20. Chin HL, Buchan DA. Severe angioedema after long-term use of an angiotensin-converting enzyme inhibitor. *Ann Intern Med* 1990; **112:** 312–13.
21. Edwards TB. Adverse effects of ACE inhibitors. *Ann Intern Med* 1993; **118:** 314.
22. Chu TJ, Chow N. Adverse effects of ACE inhibitors. *Ann Intern Med* 1993; **118:** 314.
23. Mullins RJ, *et al.* Visceral angioedema related to treatment with an ACE inhibitor. *Med J Aust* 1996; **165:** 319–21.
24. Byrne TJ, *et al.* Isolated visceral angioedema: an underdiagnosed complication of ACE inhibitors? *Mayo Clin Proc* 2000; **75:** 1201–4.


**Overdosage.** There have been reports of overdosage with captopril,[1,2] enalapril,[3-6] and lisinopril.[7,8] The main adverse effect is hypotension which usually responds to supportive treatment and volume expansion. Activated charcoal may be given in severe overdosage if the patient presents within 1 hour of ingestion. If hypotension persists, sympathomimetics may be given, although they are not usually required. Specific therapy with angiotensinamide (p.863) may be considered if conventional therapy is ineffective,[5,6,8] but it is not widely available. There has also been a report[9] of the successful use of naloxone following captopril overdosage.


1. Augenstein WL, *et al.* Captopril overdose resulting in hypotension. *JAMA* 1988; **259:** 3302–5.
2. Graham SR, *et al.* Captopril overdose. *Med J Aust* 1989; **151:** 111.
3. Waeber B, *et al.* Self poisoning with enalapril. *BMJ* 1984; **288:** 287–8.
4. Lau CP. Attempted suicide with enalapril. *N Engl J Med* 1986; **315:** 197.
5. Jackson T, *et al.* Enalapril overdose treated with angiotensin infusion. *Lancet* 1993; **341:** 703.
6. Newby DE, *et al.* Enalapril overdose and the corrective effect of intravenous angiotensin II. *Br J Clin Pharmacol* 1995; **40:** 103–4.
7. Dawson AH, *et al.* Lisinopril overdose. *Lancet* 1990; **335:** 487–8.
8. Trilli LE, Johnson KA. Lisinopril overdose and management with intravenous angiotensin II. *Ann Pharmacother* 1994; **28:** 1165–8.
9. Varon J, Duncan SR. Naloxone reversal of hypotension due to captopril overdose. *Ann Emerg Med* 1991; **20:** 1125–7.


## Precautions

ACE inhibitors should not be used in patients with aortic stenosis or outflow tract obstruction. They should not generally be used in patients with renovascular disease or suspected renovascular disease, but are occasionally necessary for severe resistant hypertension in such patients, when they should only be given with great caution and under close specialist supervision. It should be noted that the elderly, or patients with peripheral vascular diseases or generalised atherosclerosis, may be at high risk because they may have clinically silent renovascular disease. Renal function should be assessed in all patients before administration of ACE inhibitors and should be monitored during therapy. Patients with existing renal disease or taking high doses should be monitored regularly for proteinuria. Regular white blood cell counts may be necessary in patients with collagen vascular disorders, such as systemic lupus erythematosus and scleroderma, or in patients receiving immunosuppressive therapy, especially when they also have impaired renal function. ACE inhibitors should be used with caution in patients with a history of idiopathic or hereditary angioedema.

Patients with heart failure and patients who are likely to be sodium or water depleted (for example, those receiving treatment with diuretics or dialysis) may experience symptomatic hypotension during the initial stages of ACE inhibitor therapy. Treatment should therefore be started under close medical supervision, using a low dose and with the patient in a recumbent position to minimise this effect.

Anaphylactoid reactions have occurred in patients taking ACE inhibitors during haemodialysis using high-flux polyacrylonitrile membranes, during LDL-apheresis with dextran sulfate columns, and during desensitisation with wasp or bee venom (see Hypersensitivity under Adverse Effects, above).

ACE inhibitors have been reported to produce harmful effects in *animal* fetuses following large maternal doses and should not be used during pregnancy (see below).

**Diarrhoea.** Several reports have indicated that life-threatening hypotension and signs of renal failure may develop in patients receiving captopril[1-3] or enalapril[3] following volume depletion due to diarrhoea.


1. McMurray J, Matthews DM. Effect of diarrhoea on a patient taking captopril. *Lancet* 1985; **i:** 581.
2. Benett PR, Cairns SA. Captopril, diarrhoea, and hypotension. *Lancet* 1985; **i:** 1105.
3. McMurray J, Matthews DM. Consequences of fluid loss in patients treated with ACE inhibitors. *Postgrad Med J* 1987; **63:** 385–7.


**Ethnicity.** ACE inhibitors are less effective as antihypertensives in Afro-Caribbean black patients than in white patients. A similar difference appears to occur in heart failure; in a pooled analysis[1] of the Studies of Left Ventricular Dysfunction (SOLVD) treatment and prevention trials, treatment with enalapril significantly reduced the risk of hospitalisation for heart failure in white patients with left ventricular dysfunction, but not in similar black patients.


1. Exner DV, *et al.* Lesser response to angiotensin-converting-enzyme inhibitor therapy in black as compared with white patients with left ventricular dysfunction. *N Engl J Med* 2001; **344:** 1351–7.


**Hepatic cirrhosis.** It has been suggested that in patients with cirrhosis, captopril could cause a marked reduction in arterial pressure and severely compromise renal function, since maintenance of glomerular filtration rate might be mediated by angiotensin II in these patients.[1] This theory was supported by a report of a reduction in glomerular filtration rate in response to a fall in mean arterial pressure in 4 patients with resistant ascites secondary to hepatic cirrhosis.[2] The fall in mean arterial pressure was associated with postural hypotension and increasing encephalopathy. Severe confusion has also been reported in 2 patients with cirrhosis during treatment with captopril 6.25 to 12.5 mg three times daily.[3]


1. Ring T. Captopril and resistant ascites: a word of caution. *Lancet* 1983; **ii:** 165.
2. Wood LJ, *et al.* Adverse effects of captopril in treatment of resistant ascites, a state of functional bilateral renal artery stenosis. *Lancet* 1985; **ii:** 1008–9.
3. Jørgensen F, *et al.* Captopril and resistant ascites. *Lancet* 1983; **ii:** 405.


**Huntington's disease.** The condition of a woman with Huntington's disease deteriorated dramatically during treatment with captopril and improved on withdrawal of the drug.[1]


1. Goldblatt J, Bryer A. Huntington's disease: deterioration in clinical state during treatment with angiotensin converting enzyme inhibitor. *BMJ* 1987; **294:** 1659–60.


**Peripheral vascular disease.** Patients with peripheral vascular disease may have a high incidence of renal artery stenosis and are therefore at high risk of renal failure with ACE inhibitor therapy (see Effects on the Kidneys, above). Mild renal artery stenosis was found in 64 of 374 patients (17%) with peripheral vascular disease, and severe renal artery stenosis in 52 (14%); the stenosis was bilateral in 43 (12%).[1] Renal function should be carefully monitored in any patient with peripheral vascular disease who receives ACE inhibitors.


1. Salmon P, Brown MA. Renal artery stenosis and peripheral vascular disease: implications for ACE inhibitor therapy. *Lancet* 1990; **336:** 321.


**Pregnancy.** There is evidence from *animal* studies that administration of ACE inhibitors during pregnancy is associated with fetal toxicity and an increase in still-births.[1] In humans, the main effect of ACE inhibitors is on the kidneys. Several case reports have described the development of fetal renal failure, with oligohydramnios or neonatal anuria, in the offspring of mothers receiving captopril[2-4] or enalapril;[5,6] there have been fetal[4] and neonatal[3] deaths. A literature search up to the end of 1989 indicated that the use of ACE inhibitors during pregnancy can cause severe disturbances of fetal and neonatal renal function, long-lasting neonatal anuria, and pulmonary hypoplasia.[7] There are also 2 case reports in which maternal captopril[8] or enalapril[9] therapy, in association with other drugs, was associated with birth defects including defective ossification of the skull. A registry study[10] found that 2 of 19 infants exposed to ACE inhibitors during pregnancy had serious life-threatening conditions: one had prolonged anuria requiring dialysis; the other had microcephaly and a large occipital encephalocele.

The FDA has re-emphasised that ACE inhibitors can cause injury and even death to the developing fetus in the second and third trimester.[11] Use of ACE inhibitors in the first trimester appears to carry a lesser risk,[12-14] and there has been a report showing reversal of oligohydramnios following withdrawal of the ACE inhibitor.[6] However, a review of the available experimental and clinical data concluded that the use of ACE inhibitors should be avoided in all trimesters of pregnancy.[15]


1. Broughton Pipkin F, *et al.* Possible risk with captopril in pregnancy: some animal data. *Lancet* 1980; **i:** 1256.
2. Boutroy M-J, *et al.* Captopril administration in pregnancy impairs fetal angiotensin converting enzyme activity and neonatal adaptation. *Lancet* 1984; **ii:** 935–6.
3. Guignard JP, *et al.* Persistent anuria in a neonate: a side effect of captopril? *Int J Pediatr Nephrol* 1981; **2:** 133.
4. Knott PD, *et al.* Congenital renal dysgenesis possibly due to captopril. *Lancet* 1989; **i:** 451.
5. Schubiger G, *et al.* Enalapril for pregnancy-induced hypertension: acute renal failure in a neonate. *Ann Intern Med* 1988; **108:** 215–16. Correction. *ibid.:* 777.
6. Broughton Pipkin F, *et al.* ACE inhibitors in pregnancy. *Lancet* 1989; **ii:** 96–7.
7. Hanssens M, *et al.* Fetal and neonatal effects of treatment with angiotensin-converting enzyme inhibitors in pregnancy. *Obstet Gynecol* 1991; **78:** 128–35.
8. Duminy PC, Burger P du T. Fetal abnormality associated with use of captopril during pregnancy. *S Afr Med J* 1981; **60:** 805.
9. Mehta N, Modi N. ACE inhibitors in pregnancy. *Lancet* 1989; **ii:** 96.
10. Piper JM, *et al.* Pregnancy outcome following exposure to angiotensin-converting enzyme inhibitors. *Obstet Gynecol* 1992; **80:** 429–32.
11. Nightingale SL. Warnings on use of ACE inhibitors in second and third trimester of pregnancy. *JAMA* 1992; **267:** 2445.
12. Centers for Disease Control and Prevention. Postmarketing surveillance for angiotensin-converting enzyme inhibitor use during the first trimester of pregnancy—United States, Canada, and Israel, 1987-1995. *JAMA* 1997; **277:** 1193–4.
13. Lip GYH, *et al.* Angiotensin-converting-enzyme inhibitors in early pregnancy. *Lancet* 1997; **350:** 1446–7.
14. Steffensen FH, *et al.* Pregnancy outcome with ACE-inhibitor use in early pregnancy. *Lancet* 1998; **351:** 596.
15. Shotan A, *et al.* Risk of angiotensin-converting enzyme inhibition during pregnancy: experimental and clinical evidence, potential mechanisms, and recommendations for use. *Am J Med* 1994; **96:** 451–6.


## Interactions

Excessive hypotension may occur when ACE inhibitors are used concurrently with diuretics, other antihypertensives, or other agents, including alcohol, that lower blood pressure. An additive hyperkalaemic effect is possible in patients receiving ACE inhibitors with potassium-sparing diuretics, potassium supplements (including potassium-containing salt substitutes), or other drugs that can cause hyperkalaemia (such as ciclosporin or indometacin), and serum-potassium concentrations should be monitored. Potassium-sparing diuretics and potassium supplements should generally be stopped before initiating ACE inhibitors in patients with heart failure. However, ACE inhibitor therapy does not obviate the possible need for potassium supplementation in patients receiving potassium-wasting diuretics and potassium concentrations should also be monitored in these patients. The adverse effects of ACE inhibitors on the kidneys may be potentiated by other drugs, such as NSAIDs, that can affect renal function.

◊ General references.


1. Shionoiri H. Pharmacokinetic drug interactions with ACE inhibitors. *Clin Pharmacokinet* 1993; **25:** 20–58.
2. Mignat C, Unger T. ACE inhibitors: drug interactions of clinical significance. *Drug Safety* 1995; **12:** 334–7.


**Allopurinol.** For reports of reactions in patients taking captopril and allopurinol, see p.413.

**Antacids.** Administration of captopril with antacids reduced the bioavailability of captopril although this did not significantly alter the effects on blood pressure and heart rate.[1] The bioavailability of fosinopril, and possibly other ACE inhibitors, may also be reduced by concurrent antacid administration.


1. Mäntylä R, *et al.* Impairment of captopril bioavailability by concomitant food and antacid intake. *Int J Clin Pharmacol Ther Toxicol* 1984; **22:** 626–9.


**Antidiabetics.** Hypoglycaemia was noted in 3 type 1 diabetics when captopril was added to their therapeutic regimen; it was also seen in a type 2 diabetic, in whom withdrawal of hypoglycaemic drugs became necessary.[1] Subsequent study suggested that the effect was due to enhanced insulin sensitivity.[1] Similar instances of a reduction in blood sugar in both non-diabetic[2] and diabetic[3] patients given enalapril have occurred. Two case-control studies in diabetic patients receiving insulin or oral hypoglycaemics suggested that patients treated with ACE inhibitors were at increased risk of developing severe hypoglycaemia.[4,5] However, other studies in diabetic patients given captopril or enalapril have failed to find any significant alterations in blood-glucose control,[6,7] and ACE inhibitors are widely used in the treatment of hypertension in diabetic patients (see p.825) and also have a role in the management of diabetic complications such as nephropathy (see Kidney Disorders under Uses, below).


1. Ferriere M, *et al.* Captopril and insulin sensitivity. *Ann Intern Med* 1985; **102:** 134–5.
2. Helgeland A, *et al.* Enalapril, atenolol, and hydrochlorothiazide in mild to moderate hypertension: a comparative multicentre study in general practice in Norway. *Lancet* 1986; **i:** 872–5.
3. McMurray J, Fraser DM. Captopril, enalapril, and blood glucose. *Lancet* 1986; **i:** 1035.
4. Herings RMC, *et al.* Hypoglycaemia associated with use of inhibitors of angiotensin converting enzyme. *Lancet* 1995; **345:** 1195–8.
5. Morris AD, *et al.* ACE inhibitor use is associated with hospitalization for severe hypoglycemia in patients with diabetes. *Diabetes Care* 1997; **20:** 1363–7.
6. Passa P, *et al.* Enalapril, captopril, and blood glucose. *Lancet* 1986; **i:** 1447.
7. Winocour P, *et al.* Captopril and blood glucose. *Lancet* 1986; **ii:** 461.


**Azathioprine.** Leucopenia has been reported in a patient given captopril with azathioprine; the effect did not occur when either drug was given alone.[1] In a similar report, neutropenia in a patient receiving a regimen including azathioprine and captopril did not recur when captopril was reintroduced following withdrawal of azathioprine.[2]


1. Kirchertz EJ, *et al.* Successful low dose captopril rechallenge following drug-induced leucopenia. *Lancet* 1981; **i:** 1363.
2. Edwards CRW, *et al.* Successful reintroduction of captopril following neutropenia. *Lancet* 1981; **i:** 723.


**Ciclosporin.** An additive hyperkalaemic effect with ACE inhibitors and ciclosporin is possible. Also, acute renal failure has been reported in 2 patients receiving ciclosporin after renal transplantation following administration of enalapril.[1] Renal function recovered when the ACE inhibitor was withdrawn.


1. Murray BM, *et al.* Enalapril-associated acute renal failure in renal transplants: possible role of cyclosporine. *Am J Kidney Dis* 1990; **16:** 66–9.


**Digoxin.** For reports of an increase in serum-digoxin concentrations during therapy with ACE inhibitors, see p.896.

**Diuretics.** Excessive hypotension may occur when ACE inhibitors are used with diuretics. Deterioration in renal function has also been reported with *metolazone* (see p.956). Severe hyperkalaemia may occur if ACE inhibitors are used with *spironolactone* (see p.1004).

**Epoetins.** An additive hyperkalaemic effect may occur when ACE inhibitors are administered with epoetins. ACE inhibitors have also been reported to antagonise the haematopoietic effects of epoetins.

**General anaesthetics.** Marked hypotension may occur during general anaesthesia in patients receiving ACE inhibitors. In addition corrected cerebral blood flow was significantly lower in 11 patients who received captopril before general anaesthesia induced with thiopental and maintained with nitrous oxide and enflurane, than in 9 patients pretreated with metoprolol and 9 untreated controls.[1] Although there were no complications of anaesthesia associated with captopril pretreatment, discontinuation of ACE inhibitor therapy before anaesthesia should be considered. However, others have suggested[2] that since there is no clear evidence for stopping them, ACE inhibitors may be continued with care.


1. Jensen K, *et al.* Cerebral blood flow during anaesthesia: influence of pretreatment with metoprolol or captopril. *Br J Anaesth* 1989; **62:** 321–3.
2. Anonymous. Drugs in the peri-operative period: 4 – cardiovascular drugs. *Drug Ther Bull* 1999; **37:** 89–92.


**Gold salts.** The nitritoid reaction (flushing, nausea, dizziness, and hypotension associated with the first weeks of gold treatment) occurred soon after commencing treatment with an ACE inhibitor (captopril, lisinopril, or enalapril) in 4 patients who had been receiving sodium aurothiomalate for at least 2 years.[1]


1. Healey LA, Backes MB. Nitritoid reactions and angiotensin-converting-enzyme inhibitors. *N Engl J Med* 1989; **321:** 763.


**Interferons.** Severe granulocytopenia has been reported[1] in 3 patients with mixed cryoglobulinaemia treated with interferon alfa-2a who also received ACE inhibitors. The effect was considered to be due to synergistic haematological toxicity. However, in a further report,[2] 2 patients developed only mild granulocytopenia that was reversible despite continued therapy, while a third patient retained a normal granulocyte count.


1. Casato M, *et al.* Granulocytopenia after combined therapy with interferon and angiotensin-converting enzyme inhibitors: evidence for a synergistic hematologic toxicity. *Am J Med* 1995; **99:** 386–91.
2. Jacquot C, *et al.* Granulocytopenia after combined therapy with interferon and angiotensin-converting enzyme inhibitors: evidence for a synergistic hematologic toxicity. *Am J Med* 1996; **101:** 235–6.


**Interleukin-3.** Marked hypotension occurred in 3 patients[1] receiving ACE inhibitors who were given interleukin-3 following chemotherapy; blood pressure returned to normal when the ACE inhibitors were discontinued.


1. Dercksen MW, *et al.* Hypotension induced by interleukin-3 in patients on angiotensin-converting enzyme inhibitors. *Lancet* 1995; **345:** 448.


**Lithium.** For reports of lithium toxicity in patients taking ACE inhibitors, see p.303.

**NSAIDs.** *Indometacin* and possibly other NSAIDs, including aspirin, have been reported to reduce or abolish the hypotensive action of ACE inhibitors. A similar effect has been reported[1] with *rofecoxib*. NSAIDs cause sodium and water retention and thus may attenuate the effects of various antihypertensives. It has also been suggested that part of the hypotensive effect of ACE inhibitors is prostaglandin-dependent, which might explain this interaction with drugs such as NSAIDs that block prostaglandin synthesis. However, in a double-blind study designed to assess the role of prostaglandins,[2] indometacin did not influence the hypotensive effect of captopril or enalapril, suggesting that the effects on prostaglandins are not significant.

The possibility of an interaction between low-dose *aspirin* and ACE inhibitors has caused concern.[3-5] Retrospective analysis of some studies of ACE inhibitors in patients with heart failure following myocardial infarction suggested that outcome was poorer in those who were also receiving aspirin. A number of small studies have investigated the effects of concomitant aspirin and ACE inhibitors on haemodynamic parameters, but results have been conflicting and the clinical relevance of these findings is not clear. Given the well-established benefits of both ACE inhibitors and aspirin in patients with heart failure associated with ischaemic heart disease, it is generally recommended that patients should continue to receive treatment with both.[4,5] A systematic review[6] of long-term studies using ACE inhibitors came to a similar conclusion.

The combination of NSAIDs and ACE inhibitors may also have variable effects on renal function since they act at different parts of the glomerulus.[7] When given to patients whose kidneys are underperfused, for example because of heart failure, liver cirrhosis, or haemorrhage, renal function may deteriorate. However, specific patient groups without reduced renal perfusion may benefit from combining an NSAID with an ACE inhibitor.

*Indometacin*, and possibly other NSAIDs, may have an additive hyperkalaemic effect.


1. Brown CH. Effect of rofecoxib on the antihypertensive activity of lisinopril. *Ann Pharmacother* 2000; **34:** 1486.
2. Gerber JG, *et al.* The hypotensive action of captopril and enalapril is not prostacyclin dependent. *Clin Pharmacol Ther* 1993; **54:** 523–32.
3. Stys T, *et al.* Does aspirin attenuate the beneficial effects of angiotensin-converting enzyme inhibition in heart failure? *Arch Intern Med* 2000; **160:** 1409–13.
4. Mahé I, *et al.* Interaction between aspirin and ACE inhibitors in patients with heart failure. *Drug Safety* 2001; **24:** 167–82.
5. Olson KL. Combined aspirin/ACE inhibitor treatment for CHF. *Ann Pharmacother* 2001; **35:** 1653–8.
6. Teo KK, *et al.* Effects of long-term treatment with angiotensin-converting-enzyme inhibitors in the presence or absence of aspirin: a systematic review. *Lancet* 2002; **360:** 1037–43. Correction. *ibid.* 2003; **361:** 90.
7. Sturrock NDC, Struthers AD. Non-steroidal anti-inflammatory drugs and angiotensin converting enzyme inhibitors: a commonly prescribed combination with variable effects on renal function. *Br J Clin Pharmacol* 1993; **35:** 343–8.


**Probenecid.** Administration of probenecid to 4 healthy subjects during intravenous infusion of captopril caused increases in the steady-state plasma-captopril concentration. The interaction was considered to be due to a reduction of tubular secretion of captopril by probenecid.[1]


1. Singhvi SM, *et al.* Renal handling of captopril: effect of probenecid. *Clin Pharmacol Ther* 1982; **32:** 182–9.


## Pharmacokinetics

Most ACE inhibitors are given by mouth. Apart from captopril and lisinopril, they are generally prodrugs and following absorption undergo rapid metabolism by ester hydrolysis to the active diacid form; for example, enalapril is converted to enalaprilat. Metabolism occurs mainly in the liver. Excretion as active drug or active metabolite is principally in the urine; some, such as benazeprilat and fosinoprilat are also excreted via the biliary tract. Elimination of the diacid is polyphasic and there is a prolonged terminal elimination phase, which is considered to represent binding to the angiotensin-converting enzyme at a saturable binding site. This bound fraction does not contribute to accumulation of drug following multiple doses. The terminal elimination half-life does not therefore predict the kinetics observed with multiple dosing and the effective half-life for accumulation is the value usually quoted.

◊ Reviews.

1. Burnier M, Biollaz J. Pharmacokinetic optimisation of angiotensin converting enzyme (ACE) inhibitor therapy. *Clin Pharmacokinet* 1992; **22:** 375–84.
2. Hoyer J, *et al.* Clinical pharmacokinetics of angiotensin converting enzyme (ACE) inhibitors in renal failure. *Clin Pharmacokinet* 1993; **24:** 230–54.

## Uses and Administration

ACE inhibitors are antihypertensive drugs that act as vasodilators and reduce peripheral resistance. They inhibit angiotensin-converting enzyme (ACE), which is involved in the conversion of angiotensin I to angiotensin II. Angiotensin II stimulates the synthesis and secretion of aldosterone and raises blood pressure via a potent direct vasoconstrictor effect. ACE is identical to bradykininase (kininase II) and ACE inhibitors also reduce the degradation of bradykinin, which is a direct vasodilator and is also involved in the generation of prostaglandins. The pharmacological actions of ACE inhibitors are thought to be primarily due to the inhibition of the renin-angiotensin-aldosterone system, but since they also effectively reduce blood pressure in patients with low renin concentrations other mechanisms are probably also involved. ACE inhibitors produce a reduction in both preload and afterload in patients with heart failure. They also reduce left ventricular remodelling, a process that sometimes follows myocardial infarction. Normally, renal blood flow is increased without a change in glomerular filtration rate. ACE inhibitors also reduce proteinuria associated with glomerular kidney disease.

ACE inhibitors are used in the treatment of hypertension and heart failure and are given to improve survival following myocardial infarction and for the prophylaxis of cardiovascular events in patients with certain risk factors. They are also used in the treatment of diabetic nephropathy. Administration is generally by mouth.

In some hypertensive patients there may be a precipitous fall in blood pressure when starting therapy with an ACE inhibitor and the first dose should preferably be given at bedtime; if possible, any diuretic therapy should be stopped a few days beforehand and resumed later if necessary.

In patients with heart failure taking loop diuretics, severe first-dose hypotension is common on introduction of an ACE inhibitor, but temporary withdrawal of the diuretic may cause rebound pulmonary oedema. Thus treatment should be initiated with a low dose under close medical supervision.

**Action.** Although the main target for ACE inhibitors was initially thought to be the endocrine renin-angiotensin system in the circulation this mechanism alone cannot readily explain all the actions of ACE inhibitors.[1] Endogenous renin-angiotensin systems exist in many tissues and ACE inhibitors also have localised effects.[2] This may underlie some of the long-term effects of ACE inhibition, including improved endothelial function, increased arterial wall compliance, improved left ventricular function in heart failure, regression of vascular and left ventricular hypertrophy, and delayed progression of diabetic nephropathy. ACE inhibitors differ in their degree of binding to tissue ACE and in their tissue distribution, but the clinical significance of this is not clear. In one study[3] endothelial function improved with quinapril, which has high tissue specificity, but a similar effect was not seen with the less-specific enalapril, despite an earlier study[4] showing it to be effective.

ACE inhibitors also have effects on the kinin system and there is some evidence that the cardiovascular actions of ACE inhibitors also involve localised accumulation of kinins.[5-7] It has been suggested[8] that the free radical scavenging property of captopril may contribute to some of its actions, although not all studies have confirmed this effect.[9]

1. Tabibiazar R, *et al.* Formulating clinical strategies for angiotensin antagonism: a review of preclinical and clinical studies. *Am J Med* 2001; **110:** 471–80.
2. Zarnke KB, Feldman RD. Direct angiotensin converting enzyme inhibitor-mediated venodilation. *Clin Pharmacol Ther* 1996; **59:** 559–68.
3. Anderson TJ, *et al.* Comparative study of ACE-inhibition, angiotensin II antagonism, and calcium channel blockade on flow-mediated vasodilation in patients with coronary disease (BANFF study). *J Am Coll Cardiol* 2000; **35:** 60–6.
4. O'Driscoll G, *et al.* Improvement in endothelial function by angiotensin converting enzyme inhibition in insulin-dependent diabetes mellitus. *J Clin Invest* 1997; **100:** 678–84.
5. Linz W, *et al.* Contribution of kinins to the cardiovascular actions of angiotensin-converting enzyme inhibitors. *Pharmacol Rev* 1995; **47:** 25–49.
6. Bönner G. The role of kinins in the antihypertensive and cardioprotective effects of ACE inhibitors. *Drugs* 1997; **54** (suppl 5): 23–30.
7. Gainer JV, *et al.* Effect of bradykinin-receptor blockade on the response to angiotensin-converting-enzyme inhibitor in normotensive and hypertensive subjects. *N Engl J Med* 1998; **339:** 1285–92.
8. Chopra M, *et al.* Captopril: a free radical scavenger. *Br J Clin Pharmacol* 1989; **27:** 396–9.
9. Lapenna D, *et al.* Captopril has no significant scavenging antioxidant activity in human plasma in vitro or in vivo. *Br J Clin Pharmacol* 1996; **42:** 451–6.

**Bartter's syndrome.** Captopril has been reported to produce beneficial responses in patients with Bartter's syndrome[1-5] (p.1220), which is characterised by hyperaldosteronism, hypokalaemia, and hyperreninaemia, but with normal or reduced blood pressure.

1. Aurell M, Rudin A. Effects of captopril in Bartter's syndrome. *N Engl J Med* 1981; **304:** 1609.
2. Hené RJ, *et al.* Long-term treatment of Bartter's syndrome with captopril. *BMJ* 1982; **285:** 695.
3. James JM, Davies D. The use of captopril in Bartter's syndrome. *BMJ* 1984; **289:** 162.
4. Savastano A, *et al.* Treatment of Bartter's disease with captopril: a case report. *Curr Ther Res* 1986; **39:** 408–13.
5. Jest P, *et al.* Angiotensin-converting enzyme inhibition as a therapeutic principle in Bartter's syndrome. *Eur J Clin Pharmacol* 1991; **41:** 303–5.

**Diabetic complications.** Control of blood pressure plays a major role in the prevention of the sequelae of diabetes mellitus (p.326). ACE inhibitors have been reported[1] to reduce the risk of major cardiovascular events in patients, including a broad range of diabetics, with either a history of cardiovascular disease or at least one additional cardiovascular risk factor. Further analysis of the same study also suggested[2] that the ACE inhibitor could prevent the development of diabetes in non-diabetic patients, but these results require confirmation in a prospective study.

ACE inhibitors may also have benefits in a number of other diabetic complications. They have an established role in the management of nephropathy in patients with type 1 and type 2 diabetes (see Kidney Disorders, below).

It has been reported[3] that ACE inhibitors may reduce the progression of retinopathy in normotensive patients with type 1 diabetes mellitus. However, progression of retinopathy was a secondary end-point of the study and it was suggested that further studies were needed to confirm the beneficial results.

A preliminary report[4] has suggested that ACE inhibitors may improve peripheral neuropathy in diabetic patients, but again further studies are needed.

1. Heart Outcomes Prevention Evaluation (HOPE) Study Investigators. Effects of ramipril on cardiovascular and microvascular outcomes in people with diabetes mellitus: results of the HOPE study and MICRO-HOPE substudy. *Lancet* 2000; **355:** 253–9. Correction. *ibid.*; **356:** 860.
2. Yusuf S, *et al.* Ramipril and the development of diabetes. *JAMA* 2001; **286:** 1882–5.
3. Chaturvedi N, *et al.* Effect of lisinopril on progression of retinopathy in normotensive people with type 1 diabetes. *Lancet* 1998; **351:** 28–31.
4. Malik RA, *et al.* Effect of angiotensin-converting-enzyme (ACE) inhibitor trandolapril on human diabetic neuropathy: randomised double-blind controlled trial. *Lancet* 1998; **352:** 1978–81.

**Erythrocytosis.** Erythrocytosis (polycythaemia) may occur following renal transplantation and is usually treated by phlebotomy, although ACE inhibitors and theophylline (p.806) may be alternatives. Enalapril, in a dose of 10 mg daily by mouth, was reported to be more effective than theophylline in one study.[1] A second study[2] reported effective reductions in haematocrit with a dose of enalapril 2.5 mg daily. Beneficial responses have also been reported with captopril[3] and lisinopril.[4]

Beneficial reductions in packed cell volume and haemoglobin concentration have also been reported[5] in patients with altitude polycythaemia given enalapril in a dose of 5 mg daily.

1. Ok E, *et al.* Comparison of the effects of enalapril and theophylline on polycythemia after renal transplantation. *Transplantation* 1995; **59:** 1623–45.
2. Beckingham IJ, *et al.* A randomized placebo-controlled study of enalapril in the treatment of erythrocytosis after renal transplantation. *Nephrol Dial Transplant* 1995; **10:** 2316–20.
3. Hernández E, *et al.* Usefulness and safety of treatment with captopril in posttransplant erythrocytosis. *Transplant Proc* 1995; **27:** 2239–41.
4. MacGregor MS, *et al.* Treatment of postrenal transplant erythrocytosis. *Nephron* 1996; **74:** 517–21.
5. Plata R, *et al.* Angiotensin-converting-enzyme inhibition therapy in altitude polycythaemia: a prospective randomised trial. *Lancet* 2002; **359:** 663–6.

**Heart failure.** ACE inhibitors given orally produce clinical benefit in all stages of chronic heart failure (p.820) additional to that seen with diuretics. They relieve symptoms and improve survival and reduce the progression of mild or moderate heart failure to more severe stages. Thus, it is now recommended that all patients with heart failure due to left ventricular systolic dysfunction should receive ACE inhibitors, even if they are asymptomatic with diuretics alone. The studies that have shown a benefit with ACE inhibitors have tended to use higher doses than those used in practice. A study[1] with lisinopril found that higher doses reduced the combined end-point of death or hospitalisation more than low doses and were equally well tolerated, suggesting that higher doses should be used. However, studies with enalapril have failed to show a benefit of standard doses over lower doses,[2] or high doses over standard doses,[3] and the optimum dose in patients with heart failure remains to be established. Combination of ACE inhibitors with angiotensin II receptor antagonists to produce a more complete blockade of the renin-angiotensin system is also under investigation.[4] ACE inhibitors may also have a role in patients with asymptomatic left ventricular dysfunction, although this is less well established; their role in diastolic dysfunction is also not yet clear. ACE inhibitors may be beneficial in patients with heart failure associated with valve disorders.

The mechanism of action in heart failure is not established. ACE inhibitors have beneficial haemodynamic effects; they produce arterial and venous dilatation,[5] reducing both preload and afterload and thus improving cardiac output without increasing heart rate. Their neurohormonal effects also play a part,[6] as do their effects on cytokines. Further actions that may contribute include reduction of left ventricular hypertrophy, and an indirect action to prevent cardiac arrhythmias.[7,8]

Captopril and enalapril have both been used in infants with severe heart failure (see p.880, and p.910, respectively).

1. Packer M, *et al.* Comparative effects of low and high doses of the angiotensin-converting enzyme inhibitor, lisinopril, on morbidity and mortality in chronic heart failure. *Circulation* 1999; **100:** 2312–18.
2. The NETWORK investigators. Clinical outcome with enalapril in symptomatic chronic heart failure; a dose comparison. *Eur Heart J* 1998; **19:** 481–9.
3. Nanas JN, *et al.* Outcome of patients with congestive heart failure treated with standard versus high doses of enalapril: a multicenter study. *J Am Coll Cardiol* 2000; **36:** 2090–5.
4. Struckman DR, Rivey MP. Combined therapy with an angiotensin II receptor blocker and an angiotensin-converting enzyme inhibitor in heart failure. *Ann Pharmacother* 2001; **35:** 242–8.
5. Capewell S, *et al.* Acute and chronic arterial and venous effects of captopril in congestive cardiac failure. *BMJ* 1989; **299:** 942–5.
6. Deedwania PC. Angiotensin-converting enzyme inhibitors in congestive heart failure. *Arch Intern Med* 1990; **150:** 1798–1805.
7. Wesseling H, *et al.* Cardiac arrhythmias—a new indication for angiotensin-converting enzyme inhibitors? *J Hum Hypertens* 1989; **3** (suppl 1): 89–95.
8. Campbell RWF. ACE inhibitors and arrhythmias. *Heart* 1996; **76** (suppl 3): 79–82.

**Hypertension.** ACE inhibitors have an established role in the management of hypertension (p.825) and appear to have comparable effects to the other main groups of antihypertensives.[1] The Captopril Prevention Project (CAPPP) trial,[2] which compared captopril-based therapy with conventional beta blocker- or diuretic-based therapy, suggested that cardiovascular mortality was lower with captopril, although the risk of stroke was increased in those receiving captopril and overall mortality did not differ between the groups. In the large ALLHAT study,[3] which compared an ACE inhibitor with a calcium-channel blocker or a diuretic, overall mortality did not differ significantly between any of the groups, although there were slightly higher rates of stroke and heart failure in those given the ACE inhibitor compared with the diuretic group. ACE inhibitors are particularly recommended in diabetic patients with nephropathy as they have beneficial effects on the kidney, and also in patients with heart failure. Other advantages that have been suggested include their lack of adverse effects on serum lipids, a reduction in left ventricular hypertrophy,[4] and a reduction in plasma fibrinogen levels,[5] but the clinical significance of these effects is not established.

The antihypertensive actions of ACE inhibitors may be potentiated by drugs that activate the renin-angiotensin system. Hence, combination therapy with diuretics or with calcium-channel blockers may be particularly useful.

1. Blood Pressure Lowering Treatment Trialists' Collaboration. Effects of different blood-pressure-lowering regimens on major cardiovascular events: results of prospectively-designed overviews of randomised trials. *Lancet* 2003; **362:** 1527–35.
2. Hansson L, *et al.* Effect of angiotensin-converting-enzyme inhibition compared with conventional therapy on cardiovascular morbidity and mortality in hypertension: the Captopril Prevention Project (CAPPP) randomised trial. *Lancet* 1999; **353:** 611–16.
3. The ALLHAT Officers and Coordinators for the ALLHAT Collaborative Research Group. Major outcomes in high-risk hypertensive patients randomized to angiotensin-converting enzyme inhibitor or calcium channel blocker vs diuretic: The Antihypertensive and Lipid-Lowering Treatment to Prevent Heart Attack Trial (ALLHAT). *JAMA* 2002; **288:** 2981–97. Correction. *ibid.* 2003; **289:** 178.
4. Schmieder RE, *et al.* Reversal of left ventricular hypertrophy in essential hypertension: a meta-analysis of randomized double-blind studies. *JAMA* 1996; **275:** 1507–13.
5. Fogari R, *et al.* Effects of different antihypertensive drugs on plasma fibrinogen in hypertensive patients. *Br J Clin Pharmacol* 1995; **39:** 471–6.

DIAGNOSIS OF RENOVASCULAR HYPERTENSION. Captopril has been used to diagnose renovascular hypertension, the increase in plasma renin activity following blockade of the conversion of angiotensin I to angiotensin II being greater in renovascular hypertension than in primary hypertension.[1] However, a meta-analysis[2] of various tests used for the diagnosis of renovascular hypertension found that the accuracy of the captopril test is low when compared with imaging methods such as computed tomography or magnetic resonance angiography. Captopril is also used to enhance the sensitivity and specificity of renal scintigraphy.[3]

1. Muller FB, *et al.* The captopril test for identifying renovascular disease in hypertensive patients. *Am J Med* 1986; **80:** 633–44.

2. Vasbinder GBC, *et al.* Diagnostic tests for renal artery stenosis in patients suspected of having renovascular hypertension: a meta-analysis. *Ann Intern Med* 2001; **135:** 401–411.
3. Dowling RJ, *et al.* Imaging and stenting for renal artery stenosis. *Hosp Med* 1999; **60:** 329–34.

**Ischaemic heart disease.** ACE inhibitors have clinical benefits in patients with ischaemic heart disease and other atherosclerotic conditions. They have an established role in the treatment of patients after acute myocardial infarction (see below) and may also have a preventative effect; in the SAVE[1] and SOLVD[2] studies, administration of ACE inhibitors to patients with heart failure was noted to lead to a reduction in the incidence of myocardial infarction. In the HOPE study,[3] treatment with ramipril significantly reduced the rate of death, myocardial infarction, and stroke in patients at high risk for cardiovascular disease, and in the QUO VADIS study,[4] administration of quinapril for 1 year in patients following coronary artery bypass grafting reduced the incidence of clinical ischaemic events although there was no effect on ischaemia during exercise testing or Holter monitoring.

The mechanisms by which ACE inhibitors produce benefit in these patients is less clear. Although a direct action to reduce atherosclerosis (p.815) has been suggested, studies have failed to confirm this effect. In the TREND study,[5] administration of quinapril for 6 months was reported to improve endothelial dysfunction in patients with ischaemic heart disease, but apparently no effects on the progression of atherosclerosis or the incidence of cardiac events were found in the QUIET study[6] which used a lower dose of quinapril given for 3 years. In the PART-2 study,[7] ramipril had no effect on the progression of carotid atherosclerosis, while the PARIS study[8] found an increase in angiographic restenosis following administration of quinapril.

A lack of acute anti-ischaemic effect has been found with short-term administration of captopril and enalapril in patients with stable angina,[9] and with enalapril in Prinzmetal's angina;[10] however, a further study[11] in patients with stable angina reported an improvement in the results of maximal exercise testing following sublingual captopril administration.

1. Pfeffer MA, *et al.* Effect of captopril on mortality and morbidity in patients with left ventricular dysfunction after myocardial infarction: results of the Survival and Ventricular Enlargement Trial. *N Engl J Med* 1992; **327:** 669–77.
2. Yusuf S, *et al.* Effect of enalapril on myocardial infarction and unstable angina in patients with low ejection fractions. *Lancet* 1992; **340:** 1173–8.
3. The Heart Outcomes Prevention Evaluation Study Investigators. Effects of an angiotensin-converting-enzyme inhibitor, ramipril, on cardiovascular events in high-risk patients. *N Engl J Med* 2000; **342:** 145–53.
4. Oosterga M, *et al.* Effects of quinapril on clinical outcome after coronary artery bypass grafting (The QUO VADIS Study): QUinapril on Vascular Ace and Determinants of Ischemia. *Am J Cardiol* 2001; **87:** 542–6.
5. Mancini GBJ, *et al.* Angiotensin-converting enzyme inhibition with quinapril improves endothelial vasomotor dysfunction in patients with coronary artery disease: the TREND (Trial on Reversing Endothelial Dysfunction) study. *Circulation* 1996; **94:** 258–65.
6. Cashin-Hemphill L, *et al.* Angiotensin-converting enzyme inhibition as antiatherosclerotic therapy: no answer yet. *Am J Cardiol* 1999; **83:** 43–7.
7. MacMahon S, *et al.* Randomized, placebo-controlled trial of the angiotensin-converting enzyme inhibitor, ramipril, in patients with coronary or other occlusive arterial disease. *J Am Coll Cardiol* 2000; **36:** 438–43.
8. Meurice T, *et al.* Effect of ACE inhibitors on angiographic restenosis after coronary stenting (PARIS): a randomised, double-blind, placebo-controlled trial. *Lancet* 2001; **357:** 1321–4.
9. Longobardi G, *et al.* Failure of protective effect of captopril and enalapril on exercise and dipyridamole-induced myocardial ischemia. *Am J Cardiol* 1995; **76:** 255–8.
10. Guazzi M, *et al.* Ineffectiveness of angiotensin converting enzyme inhibition (enalapril) on overt and silent myocardial ischemia in vasospastic angina and comparison with verapamil. *Clin Pharmacol Ther* 1996; **59:** 476–81.
11. Gemici K, *et al.* The effects of sublingual administration of captopril on parameters of exercise test and neurohormonal activation in patients with stable angina pectoris. *Int J Angiol* 1998; **7:** 238–43.

**Kidney disorders.** The effects of ACE inhibitors on the kidney are complex. Although they may reduce renal function and should be used with caution in patients with renal impairment (see under Adverse Effects and Treatment, above), ACE inhibitors may also have beneficial effects in diabetic and nondiabetic renal disease. This is partly due to their antihypertensive action; the kidney is a prime target of damage caused by hypertension, and ACE inhibitors tend to improve renal haemodynamics in patients with hypertension and may slow the rate of loss of renal function. However, they may also have an antiproteinuric effect that is independent of their antihypertensive action.[1,2]

Most experience has been gained in patients with overt diabetic nephropathy (see Diabetic Complications, p.326), which is often associated with hypertension and may progress from microalbuminuria to the nephrotic syndrome and end-stage renal failure. The use of ACE inhibitors now appears to be of established benefit in these patients, whether they are hypertensive or normotensive or whether they have type 1 or type 2 diabetes mellitus. ACE inhibitors also slow progression of microalbuminuria in early diabetic nephropathy,[3,4] although it is not clear whether a specific antiproteinuric effect is involved; they have been recommended, in conjunction with tight glycaemic control, in all diabetic patients with microalbuminuria.[5] In normotensive type 2 diabetics with normal renal albumin excretion ACE inhibitor therapy has been reported[6] to reduce the progression to albuminuria, but further studies are needed to assess the clinical significance of this effect.

ACE inhibitors may also be of benefit in renal disease unrelated to diabetes, although their role is not yet established. Proteinuria is an important indicator of glomerular kidney disease (p.1080) of various causes and may range from asymptomatic to severe. A number of studies[7-13] have reported that ACE inhibitors reduce both proteinuria and the rate of decline of renal function in patients with various non-diabetic renal disorders, and a meta-analysis[14] concluded that ACE inhibitors are more effective than other antihypertensives in reducing the incidence of end-stage renal disease.

Patients with systemic sclerosis (see Scleroderma, p.1348) are considered to be at high risk of adverse effects from ACE inhibitors; however there is evidence that these drugs are of benefit in the management of scleroderma-associated hypertension and renal crisis.[15]

1. Kasiske BL, *et al.* Effect of antihypertensive therapy on the kidney in patients with diabetes: a meta-regression analysis. *Ann Intern Med* 1993; **118:** 129–38.
2. Lewis EJ, *et al.* The effect of angiotensin-converting-enzyme inhibition on diabetic nephropathy. *N Engl J Med* 1993; **329:** 1456–62.
3. Lovell HG. Angiotensin converting enzyme inhibitors in normotensive diabetic patients with microalbuminuria. Available in The Cochrane Library; Issue 2. Chichester: John Wiley; 2004.
4. The ACE Inhibitors in Diabetic Nephropathy Trialist Group. Should all patients with type 1 diabetes mellitus and microalbuminuria receive angiotensin-converting enzyme inhibitors? A meta-analysis of individual patient data. *Ann Intern Med* 2001; **134:** 370–9.
5. Mogensen CE, *et al.* Prevention of diabetic renal disease with special reference to microalbuminuria. *Lancet* 1995; **346:** 1080–4.
6. Ravid M, *et al.* Use of enalapril to attenuate decline in renal function in normotensive, normoalbuminuric patients with type 2 diabetes mellitus. *Ann Intern Med* 1998; **128:** 982–8.
7. Gansevoort RT, *et al.* Long-term benefits of the antiproteinuric effect of angiotensin-converting enzyme inhibition in nondiabetic renal disease. *Am J Kidney Dis* 1993; **22:** 202–6.
8. Hannedouche T, *et al.* Randomised controlled trial of enalapril and β blockers in non-diabetic chronic renal failure. *BMJ* 1994; **309:** 833–7.
9. Maschio G, *et al.* Effect of the angiotensin-converting-enzyme inhibitor benazepril on the progression of chronic renal insufficiency. *N Engl J Med* 1996; **334:** 939–45.
10. The GISEN Group (Gruppo Italiano di Studi Epidemiologici in Nefrologia). Randomised placebo-controlled trial of effect of ramipril on decline in glomerular filtration rate and risk of terminal renal failure in proteinuric, non-diabetic nephropathy. *Lancet* 1997; **349:** 1857–63.
11. Ruggenenti P, *et al.* Renal function and requirement for dialysis in chronic nephropathy patients on long-term ramipril: REIN follow-up trial. *Lancet* 1998; **352:** 1252–6.
12. Ruggenenti P, *et al.* Renoprotective properties of ACE-inhibition in non-diabetic nephropathies with non-nephrotic proteinuria. *Lancet* 1999; **354:** 359–64.
13. Agodoa LY, *et al.* Effect of ramipril vs amlodipine on renal outcomes in hypertensive nephrosclerosis: a randomized controlled trial. *JAMA* 2001; **285:** 2719–28.
14. Giatras I, *et al.* Effect of angiotensin-converting enzyme inhibitors on the progression of nondiabetic renal disease: a meta-analysis of randomized trials. *Ann Intern Med* 1997; **127:** 337–45.
15. Steen VD, *et al.* Outcome of renal crisis in systemic sclerosis: relation to availability of angiotensin converting enzyme (ACE) inhibitors. *Ann Intern Med* 1990; **113:** 352–7.

**Malignant neoplasms.** *Animal* and *in vitro* studies have suggested that ACE inhibitors may protect against the development of cancer, and there has been a case report[1] of regression of Kaposi's sarcoma in a patient treated with captopril. A retrospective cohort study[2] suggested that the incidence of cancer in hypertensive patients receiving ACE inhibitors was lower than expected. However, a subsequent case control study[3] in postmenopausal women found no evidence of a reduced risk of breast cancer associated with ACE inhibitor therapy.

1. Vogt B, Frey FJ. Inhibition of angiogenesis in Kaposi's sarcoma by captopril. *Lancet* 1997; **349:** 1148.
2. Lever AF, *et al.* Do inhibitors of angiotensin-I-converting enzyme protect against risk of cancer? *Lancet* 1998; **352:** 179–84.
3. Meier CR, *et al.* Angiotensin-converting enzyme inhibitors, calcium channel blockers, and breast cancer. *Arch Intern Med* 2000; **160:** 349–53.

**Migraine.** Observations that attacks of migraine occurred less frequently in hypertensive patients treated with lisinopril, were confirmed by a small placebo-controlled study[1] in 47 non-hypertensive patients with migraine (p.464).

1. Schrader H, *et al.* Prophylactic treatment of migraine with angiotensin converting enzyme inhibitor (lisinopril): randomised, placebo controlled, crossover study. *BMJ* 2001; **322:** 19–22.

**Myocardial infarction.** ACE inhibitors may be of benefit in both the prevention and treatment of myocardial infarction (p.828). They reduce left ventricular remodelling, a process which sometimes follows myocardial infarction and is a recognised precursor of symptomatic heart failure. Studies in patients with evidence of left ventricular dysfunction have shown benefit from long-term oral administration of ACE inhibitors such as captopril (the SAVE study),[1] ramipril (the AIRE and AIRE extension (AIREX) studies),[2-4] or trandolapril (the TRACE study)[5,6] started about 3 days, or more, after infarction, and long-term ACE inhibitors are now established therapy in such patients.[7,8]

Early treatment with ACE inhibitors as an adjunct to standard thrombolytic therapy is less well established. Favourable results have been reported in the GISSI-3[9] and the ISIS-4[10] studies where lisinopril and captopril, respectively, were given by mouth starting within 24 hours of the onset of chest pain and in the Chinese Cardiac Study[11] (CCS-1) where captopril was given by mouth within 36 hours of the onset of symptoms. In the GISSI-3 study the beneficial effects were maintained at 6 months.[12] However, the CONSENSUS II study was terminated early when it was found that enalapril, given intravenously as enalaprilat and begun within 24 hours of the onset of chest pain, did not improve survival during the 180 days after infarction.[13] A substudy on some of the patients did however suggest that they may have benefited from early treatment since left ventricular dilatation was attenuated.[14] An interaction between aspirin and enalapril was postulated as one of the reasons for the overall lack of benefit seen, and further analysis of the CONSENSUS II results found that the beneficial effect of enalapril was reduced in those patients already taking aspirin,[15] although a systematic overview[16] failed to support this finding. A systematic review of the CONSENSUS II, GISSI-3, ISIS-4, and CCS-1 studies found lower 30-day cumulative mortality and incidence of non-fatal heart failure among ACE inhibitor recipients.[17] However, the size of benefit in these studies of largely unselected patients is much smaller than in the studies of patients with left ventricular dysfunction, and there remains no clear consensus as to whether all patients should receive ACE inhibitors or only those who develop evidence of left ventricular dysfunction.

1. Pfeffer MA, *et al.* Effect of captopril on mortality and morbidity in patients with left ventricular dysfunction after myocardial infarction: results of the Survival and Ventricular Enlargement Trial. *N Engl J Med* 1992; **327:** 669–77.
2. The Acute Infarction Ramipril Efficacy (AIRE) Study Investigators. Effect of ramipril on mortality and morbidity of survivors of acute myocardial infarction with clinical evidence of heart failure. *Lancet* 1993; **342:** 821–8.
3. Hall AS, *et al.* Follow-up study of patients randomly allocated ramipril or placebo for heart failure after acute myocardial infarction: AIRE extension (AIREX) study. *Lancet* 1997; **349:** 1493–7.
4. Cleland JGF, *et al.* Effect of ramipril on morbidity and mode of death among survivors of acute myocardial infarction with clinical evidence of heart failure: a report from the AIRE study investigators. *Eur Heart J* 1997; **18:** 41–51.
5. Køber L, *et al.* A clinical trial of the angiotensin-converting-enzyme inhibitor trandolapril in patients with left ventricular dysfunction after myocardial infarction. *N Engl J Med* 1995; **333:** 1670–6.
6. Torp-Pedersen C, Køber L. Effect of ACE inhibitor trandolapril on life expectancy of patients with reduced left-ventricular function after acute myocardial infarction. *Lancet* 1999; **354:** 9–12.
7. Borghi C, Ambrosioni E. A risk-benefit assessment of ACE inhibitor therapy post-myocardial infarction. *Drug Safety* 1996; **14:** 277–87.
8. Murdoch DR, McMurray JJV. ACE inhibitors in acute myocardial infarction. *Hosp Med* 1998; **59:** 111–15.
9. Gruppo Italiano per lo Studio della Sopravvivenza nell'Infarto Miocardico. GISSI-3: effects of lisinopril and transdermal glyceryl trinitrate singly and together on 6-week mortality and ventricular function after acute myocardial infarction. *Lancet* 1994; **343:** 1115–22.
10. ISIS-4 (Fourth International Study of Infarct Survival) Collaborative Group. ISIS-4: a randomised factorial trial assessing early oral captopril, oral mononitrate, and intravenous magnesium sulphate in 58 050 patients with suspected acute myocardial infarction. *Lancet* 1995; **345:** 669–85.
11. Chinese Cardiac Study collaborative group. Oral captopril versus placebo among 13 634 patients with suspected acute myocardial infarction: interim report from the Chinese Cardiac Study (CCS-1). *Lancet* 1995; **345:** 686–7.
12. Gruppo Italiano per lo Studio della Sopravvivenza nell'Infarto Miocardico. Six-month effects of early treatment with lisinopril and transdermal glyceryl trinitrate singly and together withdrawn six weeks after acute myocardial infarction: the GISSI-3 trial. *J Am Coll Cardiol* 1996; **27:** 337–44.
13. Swedberg K, *et al.* Effects of the early administration of enalapril on mortality in patients with acute myocardial infarction: results of the Cooperative New Scandinavian Enalapril Survival Study II (CONSENSUS II). *N Engl J Med* 1992; **327:** 678–84.
14. Bonarjee VVS, *et al.* Attenuation of left ventricular dilatation after acute myocardial infarction by early initiation of enalapril therapy. *Am J Cardiol* 1993; **72:** 1004–9.
15. Nguyen KN, *et al.* Interaction between enalapril and aspirin on mortality after acute myocardial infarction: subgroup analysis of the Cooperative New Scandinavian Enalapril Survival Study II (CONSENSUS II). *Am J Cardiol* 1997; **79:** 115–19.
16. Latini R, *et al.* Clinical effects of early angiotensin-converting enzyme inhibitor treatment for acute myocardial infarction are similar in the presence and absence of aspirin: systematic overview of individual data from 96,712 randomized patients. *J Am Coll Cardiol* 2000; **35:** 1801–7.
17. ACE Inhibitor Myocardial Infarction Collaborative Group. Indications for ACE inhibitors in the early treatment of acute myocardial infarction: systematic overview of individual data from 100 000 patients in randomized trials. *Circulation* 1998; **97:** 2202–12.

**Raynaud's syndrome.** ACE inhibitors are among many drugs that have been tried in Raynaud's syndrome, a vasospastic peripheral vascular disease (p.831). Variable effects have been reported. In a patient with Raynaud's syndrome captopril improved blood circulation in the fingers both acutely and during long-term therapy with a dose of 37.5 mg daily; the effect was apparently related to its effects on kinins rather than inhibition of angiotensin II formation.[1] However, a double-blind crossover study in 15 patients with Raynaud's phenomenon given captopril 25 mg or placebo three times daily for 6 weeks found that the drug improved blood flow but not the frequency or severity of attacks,[2] and a similar study in patients given enalapril failed to find any subjective or objective benefits.[3]

There has also been a report[4] of a patient in whom peripheral ischaemia induced by ergotamine was rapidly reversed by captopril.

1. Miyazaki S, *et al.* Relief from digital vasospasm by treatment with captopril and its complete inhibition by serine proteinase inhibitors in Raynaud's phenomenon. *BMJ* 1982; **284:** 310–11.
2. Rustin MHA, *et al.* The effect of captopril on cutaneous blood flow in patients with primary Raynaud's phenomenon. *Br J Dermatol* 1987; **117:** 751–8.

3. Challenor VF, *et al.* Subjective and objective assessment of enalapril in primary Raynaud's phenomenon. *Br J Clin Pharmacol* 1991; **31:** 477–80.
4. Zimran A, *et al.* Treatment with captopril for peripheral ischaemia induced by ergotamine. *BMJ* 1984; **288:** 364.


**Stroke.** Antihypertensive therapy reduces the risk of stroke (p.836) in patients with hypertension. However, in patients who have had a stroke, antihypertensive therapy has often been avoided due to the perceived risk of reducing cerebral perfusion. A study[1] of blood-pressure lowering with the ACE inhibitor perindopril, alone or in combination with a diuretic, found that the risk of recurrent stroke was reduced in patients with a history of stroke or transient ischaemic attack, irrespective of whether they had a normal or raised blood pressure at study entry. The beneficial effects of ACE inhibitors in stroke may not be entirely due to their antihypertensive effects; in the HOPE study,[2] ramipril reduced the incidence of stroke in patients with high cardiovascular risk despite only a small reduction in blood pressure.

There have also been reports[3,4] that ACE inhibitors may reduce the risk of pneumonia in patients with a history of stroke, possibly by an effect on symptomless dysphagia.[5]


1. PROGRESS Collaborative Group. Randomised trial of a perindopril-based blood-pressure-lowering regimen among 6105 individuals with previous stroke or transient ischaemic attack. *Lancet* 2001; **358:** 1033–41. Corrections. *ibid.*; 1556 and 2002; **359:** 2120.
2. Bosch J, *et al.* Use of ramipril in preventing stroke: double blind randomised trial. *BMJ* 2002; **324:** 699–702.
3. Sekizawa K, *et al.* ACE inhibitors and pneumonia. *Lancet* 1998; **352:** 1069.
4. Arai T, *et al.* ACE inhibitors and pneumonia in elderly people. *Lancet* 1998; **352:** 1937–8.
5. Arai T, *et al.* ACE inhibitors and symptomless dysphagia. *Lancet* 1998; **352:** 115–6.


## Acebutolol *(BAN, USAN, rINN)*

(±)-3′-Acetyl-4′-(2-hydroxy-3-isopropylaminopropoxy)butyranilide.

$C_{18}H_{28}N_2O_4$ = 336.4.

*CAS — 37517-30-9.*

*ATC — C07AB04.*

### Acebutolol Hydrochloride *(BANM, rINNM)*

Acebutololi Hydrochloridum; Hidrocloruro de acebutolol; IL-17803A; M&B-17803A.

$C_{18}H_{28}N_2O_4$,HCl = 372.9.

*CAS — 34381-68-5.*

*ATC — C07AB04.*

**Pharmacopoeias.** In *Eur.* (see p.vi), *Jpn, Pol.,* and *US.*

**Ph. Eur. 5.0** (Acebutolol Hydrochloride). A white or almost white crystalline powder. Freely soluble in water and in alcohol; very slightly soluble in acetone and in dichloromethane. A 1% solution in water has a pH of 5.0 to 7.0. Protect from light.

**USP 27** (Acebutolol Hydrochloride). A white or almost white crystalline powder. Soluble in water and in alcohol; very slightly soluble in acetone and in dichloromethane; practically insoluble in ether. pH of a 1% solution in water is between 4.5 and 7.0. Store in airtight containers.

### Adverse Effects, Treatment, and Precautions

As for Beta Blockers, p.869.

**Breast feeding.** Acebutolol and its active metabolite diacetolol are distributed into breast milk and concentrations in milk are higher than those in maternal plasma.[1] Pharmacological effects in the neonate, including hypotension, bradycardia, and tachypnoea, have been reported,[1] and the American Academy of Pediatrics therefore considers[2] that acebutolol should be given with caution to breast-feeding mothers.


1. Boutroy MJ, *et al.* To nurse when receiving acebutolol: is it dangerous for the neonate? *Eur J Clin Pharmacol* 1986; **30:** 737–9.
2. American Academy of Pediatrics. The transfer of drugs and other chemicals into human milk. *Pediatrics* 2001; **108:** 776–89. Correction. *ibid.*; 1029. Also available at: http://aappolicy.aappublications.org/cgi/content/full/pediatrics%3b108/3/776 (accessed 06/07/04)


**Effects on the liver.** Six cases of hepatotoxicity associated with acebutolol were reported[1] in the USA to the FDA between 1985 and 1989. The syndrome consisted of markedly elevated transaminase concentrations, moderately elevated alkaline phosphatase concentrations, fever, and other constitutional symptoms. The duration of therapy before onset of symptoms ranged from 10 to 31 days; 5 patients received a daily dose of 400 mg; the dose was unspecified in the sixth patient. The syndrome resolved when acebutolol was discontinued but reappeared in 2 patients who were rechallenged.


1. Tanner LA, *et al.* Hepatic toxicity after acebutolol therapy. *Ann Intern Med* 1989; **111:** 533–4.


**Effects on respiratory function.** Bronchospasm is a recognised adverse effect of beta blockers, but other respiratory disorders have also been reported. Pleurisy and pulmonary granulomas developed in a patient receiving acebutolol and a diuretic; acebutolol was considered to be responsible.[1] Hypersensitivity pneumonitis has also been reported in a patient taking acebutolol.[2]


1. Wood GM, *et al.* Pleurisy and pulmonary granulomas after treatment with acebutolol. *BMJ* 1982; **285:** 936.
2. Akoun GM, *et al.* Acebutolol-induced hypersensitivity pneumonitis. *BMJ* 1983; **286:** 266–7.


**Hypersensitivity.** See Effects on Respiratory Function, above and Lupus, below.

**Lupus.** An increase in antinuclear antibodies has been observed with acebutolol.[1] A report of a lupus syndrome in an elderly patient receiving acebutolol and clonidine described remission of symptoms when acebutolol was withdrawn, but the high antinuclear antibody titre persisted for more than 9 months.[2]


1. Wilson JD. Antinuclear antibodies and cardiovascular drugs. *Drugs* 1980; **19:** 292–305.
2. Hourdebaigt-Larrusse P, *et al.* Une nouvelle observation de lupus induit par acébutolol. *Ann Cardiol Angeiol (Paris)* 1985; **34:** 421–3.


**Pregnancy.** Both acebutolol and its active metabolite diacetolol cross the placenta. In a study[1] in 29 pregnant women who had received acebutolol for at least one month before delivery, there was evidence of bradycardia in 12 of the 31 offspring and tachypnoea in 6.


1. Boutroy MJ, *et al.* Infants born to hypertensive mothers treated by acebutolol. *Dev Pharmacol Ther* 1982; **4** (suppl 1): 109–15.


### Interactions

The interactions associated with beta blockers are discussed on p.870.

### Pharmacokinetics

Acebutolol is well absorbed from the gastrointestinal tract, but undergoes extensive first-pass metabolism in the liver. Although the bioavailability of acebutolol is reported to be only about 40%, the major metabolite diacetolol is active. Following oral administration, peak plasma concentrations of acebutolol and diacetolol are reached in about 2 and 4 hours, respectively.

Acebutolol and diacetolol are widely distributed in the body, but they have low to moderate lipid solubility and penetration into the CSF is poor. They cross the placenta and higher concentrations are achieved in breast milk than in maternal plasma. Acebutolol is only about 26% bound to plasma proteins, but is about 50% bound to erythrocytes. The plasma elimination half-life for acebutolol and diacetolol is 3 to 4 hours and 8 to 13 hours respectively. Half-life values for acebutolol and diacetolol may be increased in the elderly and the half-life for diacetolol may be prolonged up to 32 hours in patients with severe renal impairment. Acebutolol and diacetolol are excreted in the urine and in the bile and may undergo enterohepatic recycling; acebutolol is also reported to be excreted directly from the intestinal wall. Acebutolol and diacetolol are removed by dialysis.

### Uses and Administration

Acebutolol is a cardioselective beta blocker (p.868). It is reported to have some intrinsic sympathomimetic activity and membrane stabilising properties.

Acebutolol is used in the management of hypertension (p.825), angina pectoris (p.813), and cardiac arrhythmias (p.816).

Acebutolol is used as the hydrochloride, but doses are usually expressed in terms of the base; 110.8 mg of acebutolol hydrochloride is equivalent to 100 mg of base. It is generally given by mouth although slow intravenous injection has been used for the emergency treatment of arrhythmias.

In **hypertension** the usual initial dose is 400 mg once daily or 200 mg twice daily by mouth, increased if necessary after 2 weeks according to response, to 400 mg twice daily. Doses up to 1.2 g daily in divided doses may be given.

The usual dose for **angina pectoris** is 400 mg once daily or 200 mg twice daily by mouth but up to 300 mg three times daily may be required and total daily doses of 1.2 g have been given.

The usual initial dose for **cardiac arrhythmias** is 200 mg twice daily by mouth, increased according to response; up to 1.2 g daily in divided doses has been required.

Reduced doses may be required in patients with impaired renal function (see below). Elderly patients may also require lower maintenance doses; doses greater than 800 mg daily should be avoided.

**Action.** Acebutolol is generally considered to be a cardioselective beta blocker but there has been considerable controversy as to the degree of its selectivity and the selectivity of its primary metabolite, diacetolol.[1-3] In a review of beta blockers,[4] acebutolol was stated to be less cardioselective than other drugs such as atenolol or metoprolol. It was proposed[5] that this may be because the metabolite accumulates during chronic dosage to reach concentrations which affect both $beta_1$ and $beta_2$ receptors since cardioselectivity is only a relative and dose-related phenomenon. This remains uncertain and there is some evidence[6] that at least after single doses, diacetolol is actually more cardioselective than acebutolol itself.


1. Whitsett TL, *et al.* Comparison of the $beta_1$ and $beta_2$ adrenoceptor blocking properties of acebutolol and propranolol. *Chest* 1982; **82:** 668–73.
2. Nair S, *et al.* The effect of acebutolol, a beta adrenergic blocking agent, and placebo on pulmonary functions in asthmatics. *Int J Clin Pharmacol Ther Toxicol* 1981; **19:** 519–26.
3. Leary WP, *et al.* Respiratory effects of acebutolol hydrochloride: a new selective beta-adrenergic blocking agent. *S Afr Med J* 1973; **47:** 1245–8.
4. Feely J, *et al.* Beta-blockers and sympathomimetics. *BMJ* 1983; **286:** 1043–7.
5. Feely J, Maclean D. New drugs: beta blockers and sympathomimetics. *BMJ* 1983; **286:** 1972.
6. Thomas MS, Tattersfield AE. Comparison of beta-adrenoceptor selectivity of acebutolol and its metabolite diacetolol with metoprolol and propranolol in normal man. *Eur J Clin Pharmacol* 1986; **29:** 679–83.


**Administration in renal impairment.** The dose of acebutolol should be reduced in patients with renal impairment. It is recommended that the dose should be reduced by 50% in patients with a creatinine clearance between 25 and 50 mL/minute and by 75% in those with a creatinine clearance of less than 25 mL/minute. The dose frequency should not exceed once daily.

### Preparations

***BP 2003:*** Acebutolol Capsules; Acebutolol Tablets;
***USP 27:*** Acebutolol Hydrochloride Capsules.

**Proprietary Preparations** (details are given in Part 3)

***Austria:*** Sectral†; ***Belg.:*** Sectral; ***Canad.:*** Monitan; Rhotral; Sectral; ***Chile:*** Beloc; Grifobutol; ***Denm.:*** Abutol†; Diasectral; ***Fin.:*** Diasectral; Espesil; ***Fr.:*** Sectral; ***Ger.:*** Neptal†; Prent; ***Hong Kong:*** Sectral; ***Irl.:*** Sectral; ***Israel:*** Sectral; ***Ital.:*** Acecor†; Prent; Sectral; ***Malaysia:*** Sectral; ***Neth.:*** Sectral; ***NZ:*** ACB; ***Port.:*** Prent; ***S.Afr.:*** Sectral; ***Singapore:*** ACB; Sectral; ***Spain:*** Sectral; ***Switz.:*** Sectral; ***UK:*** Sectral; ***USA:*** Sectral.

**Multi-ingredient:** ***Belg.:*** Sectrazide; ***Ger.:*** Sali-Prent; Tredalat; ***Hong Kong:*** Secadrex†; ***Neth.:*** Secadrex; ***S.Afr.:*** Secadrex†; ***Spain:*** Secadrex; ***UK:*** Secadrex.

## Acecainide Hydrochloride *(USAN, rINNM)*

*N*-Acetylprocainamide Hydrochloride; ASL-601; Hidrocloruro de acecainida; NAPA. 4′-[(2-Diethylaminoethyl)carbamoyl]-acetanilide hydrochloride.

$C_{15}H_{23}N_3O_2$,HCl = 313.8.

*CAS — 32795-44-1 (acecainide); 34118-92-8 (acecainide hydrochloride).*

### Profile

Acecainide is the acetylated form of procainamide (p.987) but has class III antiarrhythmic activity (p.809). It has been tried for the treatment of premature ventricular contractions and ventricular arrhythmias.

◊ References.


1. Harron DWG, Brogden RN. Acecainide (N-acetylprocainamide): a review of its pharmacodynamic and pharmacokinetic properties, and therapeutic potential in cardiac arrhythmias. *Drugs* 1990; **39:** 720–40.


## Acenocoumarol *(BAN, rINN)*

Acenocumarin; Acenocumarol; G-23350; Nicoumalone. (*RS*)-4-Hydroxy-3-[1-(4-nitrophenyl)-3-oxobutyl]coumarin.

$C_{19}H_{15}NO_6$ = 353.3.

*CAS — 152-72-7.*

*ATC — B01AA07.*

**Pharmacopoeias.** In *Br.* and *Pol.*

**BP 2003** (Acenocoumarol). An almost white to buff-coloured odourless or almost odourless powder. It exhibits polymorphism. Practically insoluble in water and in ether; slightly soluble in alcohol and in chloroform; dissolves in aqueous solutions of alkali hydroxides.

### Adverse Effects, Treatment, and Precautions

As for Warfarin Sodium, p.1022.

**Effects on the fetus.** Fetal outcome has been reported for a group of women who received acenocoumarol for anticoagulant prophylaxis of mechanical heart valves during pregnancy.[1] Fetal loss occurred in 13 of 61 pregnancies where oral anticoagulation was continued during the first trimester. No malformations were reported in the remaining neonates, although there was 1 case of hydrocephalus.

1. Meschengieser SS, *et al.* Anticoagulation in pregnant women with mechanical heart valve prostheses. *Heart* 1999; **82:** 23–6.

## Interactions

The interactions associated with oral anticoagulants are discussed in detail under warfarin (p.1023). Specific references to interactions involving acenocoumarol can be found there under the headings for the following drug groups: analgesics; antiarrhythmics; antibacterials; antidepressants; antifungals; antigout drugs; antihistamines; antineoplastics; antiplatelets; antivirals; diuretics; gastrointestinal drugs; immunosuppressants; lipid regulating drugs; prostaglandins; sex hormones; and vaccines.

## Pharmacokinetics

Acenocoumarol is readily absorbed from the gastrointestinal tract and is excreted chiefly in the urine mainly as metabolites. It is extensively bound to plasma proteins. Figures reported for elimination half-life vary; the UK manufacturer gives a range of 8 to 11 hours. Acenocoumarol crosses the placenta; only small quantities have been detected in breast milk. It is administered as a racemic mixture; the *R*-isomer is reported to be more potent. The stereo-isomers have different pharmacokinetics.

## Uses and Administration

Acenocoumarol is an orally administered coumarin anticoagulant with actions similar to those of warfarin (p.1028). It is used in the management of thromboembolic disorders (p.837). The usual dose is 8 to 12 mg on the first day and 4 to 8 mg on the second day; subsequent maintenance doses range from 1 to 8 mg depending on the response. Acenocoumarol is given in a single dose at the same time every day.

## Preparations

***BP 2003:*** Acenocoumarol Tablets.

**Proprietary Preparations** (details are given in Part 3)

***Arg.:*** Sintrom; ***Austria:*** Sintrom; ***Belg.:*** Sintrom; ***Canad.:*** Sintrom; ***Chile:*** Acenox; Coarol; Isquelium; Neo-Sintrom; ***Fr.:*** Mini-sintrom; Sintrom; ***Gr.:*** Sintrom; ***India:*** Acitrom; ***Israel:*** Sintrom; ***Ital.:*** Sintrom; ***Mex.:*** Sintrom; ***Neth.:*** Sintrom Mitis; ***Port.:*** Sintrom; ***Spain:*** Sintrom; ***Switz.:*** Sintrom; ***UK:*** Sinthrome.

---

# Acetazolamide *(BAN, rINN)*

Acetazolam; Acetazolamida; Acetazolamidum. 5-Acetamido-1,3,4-thiadiazole-2-sulphonamide; *N*-(5-Sulphamoyl-1,3,4-thiadiazol-2-yl)acetamide.

$C_4H_6N_4O_3S_2$ = 222.2.

*CAS — 59-66-5.*

*ATC — S01EC01.*

**Pharmacopoeias.** In *Chin., Eur.* (see p.vi), *Int., Jpn, Pol.,* and *US.*

**Ph. Eur. 5.0** (Acetazolamide). A white or almost white, crystalline powder. Very slightly soluble in water; slightly soluble in alcohol. It dissolves in dilute solutions of alkali hydroxides.

**USP 27** (Acetazolamide). A white to faintly yellowish-white, odourless, crystalline powder. Very slightly soluble in water; sparingly soluble in practically boiling water; slightly soluble in alcohol. Store in airtight containers.

## Acetazolamide Sodium *(BANM, rINNM)*

Acetazolamida sódica; Sodium Acetazolamide.

$C_4H_5N_4NaO_3S_2$ = 244.2.

*CAS — 1424-27-7.*

*ATC — S01EC01.*

**Stability.** Solutions of acetazolamide sodium in glucose 5% and sodium chloride 0.9% were stable for 5 days at 25° with a loss of potency of less than 7.2%.[1] At 5° the loss of potency in both solutions was less than 6% after 44 days of storage. Small reductions in pH were recorded, possibly due to the formation of acetic acid during the decomposition of acetazolamide. At −10° the loss in potency after 44 days of storage was less than 3% in both solutions. Results were similar in samples thawed in tap water and in a microwave oven.

An oral suspension of acetazolamide 25 mg/mL prepared from tablets with the aid of sorbitol solution 70% was stable for at least 79 days at 5°, 22°, and 30°. It was recommended that the formulation be maintained at pH 4 to 5 and stored in amber glass bottles.[2]

1. Parasrampuria J, *et al.* Stability of acetazolamide sodium in 5% dextrose or 0.9% sodium chloride injection. *Am J Hosp Pharm* 1987; **44:** 358–60.
2. Alexander KS, *et al.* Stability of acetazolamide in suspension compounded from tablets. *Am J Hosp Pharm* 1991; **48:** 1241–4.

## Adverse Effects

Acetazolamide can commonly cause malaise, fatigue, depression, excitement, headache, weight loss, and gastrointestinal disturbances. Drowsiness and paraesthesia involving numbness and tingling of the face and extremities are common particularly with high doses. Diuresis can be troublesome, but generally abates after a few days of continuous therapy. Acidosis may develop during treatment and is generally mild but severe metabolic acidosis has occasionally been reported, especially in elderly or diabetic patients or those with renal impairment.

Blood dyscrasias occur rarely and may include aplastic anaemia, agranulocytosis, leucopenia, thrombocytopenia, and thrombocytopenic purpura. Acetazolamide can give rise to crystalluria, renal calculi, and renal colic; renal lesions, possibly due to a hypersensitivity reaction, have also been reported. Other adverse reactions include allergic skin reactions, fever, thirst, dizziness, ataxia, alterations in taste, transient myopia, and tinnitus and hearing disturbances. Hypokalaemia may occur but is generally transient and rarely clinically significant.

Intramuscular injections are painful owing to the alkalinity of the solution.

◊ A retrospective review[1] of 222 patients with glaucoma indicated that those aged 40 years or less tolerated treatment with carbonic anhydrase inhibitors much better than older patients.

1. Shrader CE, *et al.* Relationship of patient age and tolerance to carbonic anhydrase inhibitors. *Am J Ophthalmol* 1983; **96:** 730–3.

**Effects on the blood.** Severe, often fatal, blood dyscrasias have been reported in patients taking acetazolamide. By 1989, the National Registry of Drug-Induced Ocular Side Effects in the USA[1] had received reports of haematological reactions possibly due to carbonic anhydrase inhibitors in 139 patients of which 50 (36%) were fatal. The majority of deaths were due to aplastic anaemia. Over half the reactions occurred during the first 6 months of therapy. There has been considerable debate over the value of periodic blood analysis in patients taking carbonic anhydrase inhibitors for prolonged periods;[2-7] the US National Registry has recommended[8] that initial and 6-monthly blood analysis should be undertaken.

1. Fraunfelder FT, Bagby GC. Possible hematologic reactions associated with carbonic anhydrase inhibitors. *JAMA* 1989; **261:** 2257.
2. Alm A, *et al.* Monitoring acetazolamide treatment. *Acta Ophthalmol (Copenh)* 1982; **60:** 24–34.
3. Johnson T, Kass MA. Hematologic reactions to carbonic anhydrase inhibitors. *Am J Ophthalmol* 1986; **101:** 128–9.
4. Zimran A, Beutler E. Can the risk of acetazolamide-induced aplastic anemia be decreased by periodic monitoring of blood cell counts? *Am J Ophthalmol* 1987; **104:** 654–8.
5. Lichter PR. Carbonic anhydrase inhibitors, blood dyscrasias, and standard-of-care. *Ophthalmology* 1988; **95:** 711–12.
6. Mogk LG, Cyrlin MN. Blood dyscrasias and carbonic anhydrase inhibitors. *Ophthalmology* 1988; **95:** 768–71.
7. Miller RD. Hematologic reactions to carbonic anhydrase inhibitors. *Am J Ophthalmol* 1985; **100:** 745–6.
8. Fraunfelder FT, *et al.* Hematologic reactions to carbonic anhydrase inhibitors. *Am J Ophthalmol* 1985; **100:** 79–81.

**Effects on electrolyte balance.** Acetazolamide has been reported to cause symptomatic metabolic acidosis in the elderly, in diabetic patients, and in those with renal impairment.[1-5] Raised plasma-acetazolamide concentrations have been reported in elderly patients, probably attributable to reduced renal function, and in 6 of 9 glaucoma patients this was associated with hyperchloraemic metabolic acidosis.[6] A single-dose study[7] in 4 elderly patients found that reduced acetazolamide clearance correlated with renal function. Urea and electrolyte concentrations should be measured before and during treatment with acetazolamide in the elderly and in other patients such as diabetics who may have renal impairment. The elderly may require reduced doses.

1. Maisey DN, Brown RD. Acetazolamide and symptomatic metabolic acidosis in mild renal failure. *BMJ* 1981; **283:** 1527–8.
2. Goodfield M, *et al.* Acetazolamide and symptomatic metabolic acidosis in mild renal failure. *BMJ* 1982; **284:** 422.
3. Reid W, Harrower ADB. Acetazolamide and symptomatic metabolic acidosis in mild renal failure. *BMJ* 1982; **284:** 1114.
4. Heller I, *et al.* Significant metabolic acidosis induced by acetazolamide: not a rare complication. *Arch Intern Med* 1985; **145:** 1815–17.
5. Parker WA, Atkinson B. Acetazolamide therapy and acid-base disturbance. *Can J Hosp Pharm* 1987; **40:** 31–4.
6. Chapron DJ, *et al.* Acetazolamide blood concentrations are excessive in the elderly: propensity for acidosis and relationship to renal function. *J Clin Pharmacol* 1989; **29:** 348–53.
7. Chapron DJ, *et al.* Influence of advanced age on the disposition of acetazolamide. *Br J Clin Pharmacol* 1985; **19:** 363–71.

**Effects on endocrine function.** Hirsutism occurred in a 2½-year-old girl after treatment for 16 months with acetazolamide for congenital glaucoma.[1] There was no evidence of virilisation.

1. Weiss IS. Hirsutism after chronic administration of acetazolamide. *Am J Ophthalmol* 1974; **78:** 327–8.

**Effects on the kidneys.** Large reductions in glomerular filtration rate were observed during treatment with carbonic anhydrase inhibitors in 3 type 1 diabetics with nephropathy and glaucoma.[1] Kidney function improved when the drug was withdrawn.

1. Skøtt P, *et al.* Effect of carbonic anhydrase inhibitors on glomerular filtration rate in diabetic nephropathy. *BMJ* 1987; **294:** 549.

**Effects on the liver.** For a report of liver damage associated with use of acetazolamide, see Hypersensitivity, below.

**Effects on the skin.** Rashes, including severe skin reactions such as erythema multiforme, Stevens-Johnson syndrome, and toxic epidermal necrolysis, have been reported during acetazolamide administration; the fact that acetazolamide is a sulfonamide-derivative has been suggested as a cause for these reactions. Photosensitivity has also been noted rarely.

Severe exacerbation of rosacea occurred in a patient taking acetazolamide for glaucoma; the rosacea improved on withdrawal of acetazolamide and relapsed again on its reintroduction.[1]

1. Shah P, *et al.* Severe exacerbation of rosacea by oral acetazolamide. *Br J Dermatol* 1993; **129:** 647–8.

**Extravasation.** Extravasation was reported in a patient following intravenous acetazolamide; this resulted in severe ulceration necessitating surgical procedures to repair the skin defect.[1] It was recommended that 1 to 2 mL of sodium citrate 3.8% should be injected subcutaneously near the site of extravasation in order to neutralise the alkaline effects of the acetazolamide injection.

1. Callear A, Kirkby G. Extravasation of acetazolamide. *Br J Ophthalmol* 1994; **78:** 731.

**Hypersensitivity.** A 54-year-old man with glaucoma who was treated with acetazolamide 500 mg daily for 26 days developed a generalised erythematous rash and became delirious, dehydrated, markedly jaundiced, with peripheral circulatory failure, and died from cholestatic jaundice with hepatic coma and anuria.[1] Drug-induced hypersensitivity and hepatitis due to acetazolamide was suspected.

Anaphylaxis has also been reported[2] following a single oral dose in a patient who had not previously received acetazolamide. However, the patient was hypersensitive to sulfonamides and the reaction may have been caused by cross sensitivity.

1. Kristinsson A. Fatal reaction to acetazolamide. *Br J Ophthalmol* 1967; **51:** 348–9.
2. Tzanakis N, *et al.* Anaphylactic shock after a single oral intake of acetazolamide. *Br J Ophthalmol* 1998; **82:** 588.

## Precautions

Acetazolamide is contra-indicated in the presence of sodium or potassium depletion, in hyperchloraemic acidosis, in conditions such as Addison's disease and adrenocortical insufficiency, and in marked hepatic or renal impairment. Encephalopathy may be precipitated in patients with hepatic dysfunction. It should not be used in chronic angle-closure glaucoma since it may mask deterioration of the condition. It should be given with care to patients likely to develop acidosis or with diabetes mellitus; severe metabolic acidosis may occur in the elderly and in patients with renal impairment. Acetazolamide may increase the risk of hyperglycaemia in diabetic patients. Periodic monitoring of plasma electrolytes and blood count is recommended during long-term therapy and patients should be cautioned to report any unusual skin rashes. Acetazolamide is teratogenic in *animals*.

**Breast feeding.** Acetazolamide has been detected in breast milk.[1] However, there have been no reports of adverse effects in breast-fed infants whose mothers were receiving acetazolamide and the American Academy of Pediatrics considers[2] that it is therefore usually compatible with breast feeding.

1. Söderman P, *et al.* Acetazolamide excretion into human breast milk. *Br J Clin Pharmacol* 1984; **17:** 599–600.
2. American Academy of Pediatrics. The transfer of drugs and other chemicals into human milk. *Pediatrics* 2001; **108:** 776–89. Correction. *ibid.*; 1029. Also available at: http://aappolicy.aappublications.org/cgi/content/full/pediatrics%3b108/3/776 (accessed 06/07/04)

**Diabetes mellitus.** For a brief discussion of metabolic acidosis in patients with diabetes, see Effects on Electrolyte Balance under Adverse Effects, above.

For a report of renal impairment in patients with diabetic nephropathy associated with carbonic anhydrase inhibitors, see Effects on the Kidneys under Adverse Effects, above.

**The elderly.** A single-dose study[1] of acetazolamide in 4 elderly subjects indicated that the elderly have a reduced capacity to clear acetazolamide from plasma correlating with creatinine clearance; that they have reduced plasma protein binding which offsets the reduced unbound clearance; and that these factors predispose the elderly to enhanced accumulation of acetazolamide in erythrocytes.

Plasma-acetazolamide concentrations exceeded the **therapeutic range** (5.0 to 10.0 micrograms/mL) in 9 of 12 elderly patients receiving acetazolamide for glaucoma or metabolic alkalosis.[2] Hyperchloraemic metabolic acidosis was detected in 6 of 9 glaucoma patients. The excessive plasma concentrations were attributed to age-related reductions in renal function. It was suggested that elderly patients may require reduced doses of acetazolamide.

For reports of symptomatic metabolic acidosis associated with use of acetazolamide in the elderly, see Effects on Electrolyte Balance under Adverse Effects, above.

1. Chapron DJ, *et al.* Influence of advanced age on the disposition of acetazolamide. *Br J Clin Pharmacol* 1985; **19:** 363–71.
2. Chapron DJ, *et al.* Acetazolamide blood concentrations are excessive in the elderly: propensity for acidosis and relationship to renal function. *J Clin Pharmacol* 1989; **29:** 348–53.

**Interference with laboratory estimations.** Acetazolamide interfered with an HPLC method of assay for theophylline[1] resulting in an unnecessary dose reduction and worsening apnoea in an infant. Other workers[2] pointed out that the interference depended on the solvent used in the extraction, and presented evidence to suggest that acetazolamide may not interfere with other assay methods for theophylline.

1. Mecrow IK, Goldie BP. Acetazolamide interferes with theophylline assay. *Lancet* 1987; **i:** 558.
2. Kelsey HC, *et al.* Interference by acetazolamide in theophylline assay depends on the method. *Lancet* 1987; **ii:** 403.

**Renal impairment.** For a brief discussion of metabolic acidosis in patients with renal impairment, see Effects on Electrolyte Balance under Adverse Effects, above.

## Interactions

By rendering the urine alkaline acetazolamide reduces the urinary excretion and so may enhance the effects of drugs such as amfetamines, ephedrine, and quinidine; urinary alkalinisation also reduces the effects of methenamine and its compounds. Acetazolamide may enhance antiepileptic-induced osteomalacia. Use of acetazolamide with aspirin may result in severe acidosis and increase CNS toxicity. Acetazolamide may affect fluid and electrolyte balance leading to interactions similar to those of the thiazide diuretics (see Hydrochlorothiazide, p.935). Unlike thiazides, acetazolamide may increase the excretion of lithium.

**Antacids.** *Sodium bicarbonate* therapy enhances the risk of renal calculus formation in patients taking acetazolamide.[1]

1. Rubenstein MA, Bucy JG. Acetazolamide-induced renal calculi. *J Urol (Baltimore)* 1975; **114:** 610–12.

**Antiepileptics.** For severe osteomalacia in patients taking acetazolamide with *phenytoin* and other antiepileptics, see p.374. Acetazolamide may increase serum concentrations of *carbamazepine*, see p.356.

**Benzodiazepines.** Ventilatory depression in a mountain climber with acute mountain sickness was considered to be due to the potentiation of *triazolam* by acetazolamide.[1]

1. Masuyama S, *et al.* 'Ondine's Curse': side effect of acetazolamide? *Am J Med* 1989; **86:** 637.

**Local anaesthetics.** For the effect of acetazolamide on *procaine*, see p.1383.

**Salicylates.** Salicylates have been shown to displace acetazolamide from plasma protein binding sites and reduce its renal clearance,[1] leading to elevated plasma-acetazolamide concentrations. In addition acidosis produced by acetazolamide may increase salicylate toxicity by enhancing salicylate tissue penetration.[2] Severe metabolic acidosis has been reported[3] in patients with normal renal function given acetazolamide with salicylates. Concurrent use of salicylates and acetazolamide should be avoided if possible, particularly if renal dysfunction is present. If the combination is used, patients should be carefully monitored for symptoms of CNS toxicity such as lethargy, confusion, somnolence, tinnitus, and anorexia.

1. Sweeney KR, *et al.* Toxic interaction between acetazolamide and salicylate: case report and a pharmacokinetic explanation. *Clin Pharmacol Ther* 1986; **40:** 518–24.
2. Anderson CJ, *et al.* Toxicity of combined therapy with carbonic anhydrase inhibitors and aspirin. *Am J Ophthalmol* 1978; **86:** 516–19.
3. Cowan RA, *et al.* Metabolic acidosis induced by carbonic anhydrase inhibitors and salicylates in patients with normal renal function. *BMJ* 1984; **289:** 347–8.

## Pharmacokinetics

Acetazolamide is fairly rapidly absorbed from the gastrointestinal tract with peak plasma concentrations occurring about 2 hours after administration by mouth. It has been estimated to have a plasma half-life of about 3 to 6 hours. It is tightly bound to carbonic anhydrase and high concentrations are present in tissues containing this enzyme, particularly red blood cells and the renal cortex; it is highly bound to plasma proteins. It is excreted unchanged in the urine and has been detected in breast milk.

◊ References.

1. Lehmann B, *et al.* The pharmacokinetics of acetazolamide in relation to its use in the treatment of glaucoma and to its effects as an inhibitor of carbonic anhydrases. *Adv Biosci* 1969; **5:** 197–217.

## Uses and Administration

Acetazolamide is an inhibitor of carbonic anhydrase with weak diuretic activity and is used mainly in the management of glaucoma. Other indications include epilepsy and high-altitude disorders.

By inhibiting the reaction catalysed by carbonic anhydrase in the renal tubules, acetazolamide increases the excretion of bicarbonate and of cations, chiefly sodium and potassium, and so promotes an alkaline diuresis. When given by mouth, its effect begins within 60 to 90 minutes and lasts for 8 to 12 hours.

Continuous administration of acetazolamide is associated with metabolic acidosis and an accompanying loss of diuretic activity. Therefore, although acetazolamide has been used as a diuretic, its effectiveness diminishes with continuous use and it has largely been superseded by drugs such as the thiazides or furosemide. For **diuresis** the usual dose is 250 to 375 mg by mouth and is given either daily or on alternate days; intermittent therapy is required for a continued effect.

By inhibiting carbonic anhydrase in the eye acetazolamide decreases the formation of aqueous humour and so decreases intra-ocular pressure. It is used in the preoperative management of angle-closure **glaucoma**, or as an adjunct in the treatment of open-angle glaucoma. In the treatment of glaucoma the usual dose is 250 to 1000 mg daily by mouth; divided doses should be used for amounts greater than 250 mg daily. Modified-release preparations are also available.

Acetazolamide is also used, either alone or in association with other antiepileptics, for the treatment of various forms of **epilepsy** in doses of 250 to 1000 mg daily by mouth. A dose for children with epilepsy is 8 to 30 mg/kg daily by mouth; the total daily dose should not exceed 750 mg.

When oral administration is impracticable, acetazolamide may be given parenterally as the sodium salt; acetazolamide sodium 275 mg is approximately equivalent to 250 mg of acetazolamide. It may be given by intramuscular injection but the intravenous route is preferred due to the alkalinity of the solution. Doses are similar to those given orally.

Acetazolamide is also used to prevent or ameliorate the symptoms of **high-altitude disorders**. Prompt descent will still be necessary if severe symptoms such as cerebral oedema or pulmonary oedema occur. The usual dose is 500 to 1000 mg daily by mouth.

**Epilepsy.** Acetazolamide may be used in the treatment of epilepsy (p.349) as an alternative or adjunct to first-line drugs for refractory partial seizures with or without secondary generalisation. It is also effective in a number of other refractory forms of epilepsy including atypical absence, tonic, atonic, myoclonic, and menstruation-related seizures (catamenial epilepsy).[1-3] Beneficial responses have also been reported with acetazolamide in combination with carbamazepine in refractory partial seizures.[4] It is believed to act by inhibition of carbonic anhydrase in glial cells in the CNS.[5] The major drawback to the chronic use of acetazolamide is the rapid development of tolerance,[5,6] but this may be delayed or prevented by using it as adjunctive therapy to other antiepileptics. Acetazolamide has been shown to have greater activity in children than in adults.[1]

1. Millichap JG. Acetazolamide in treatment of epilepsy. *Lancet* 1987; **ii:** 163.
2. Resor SR, Resor LD. Chronic acetazolamide monotherapy in the treatment of juvenile myoclonic epilepsy. *Neurology* 1990; **40:** 1677–81.
3. Reiss WG, Oles KS. Acetazolamide in the treatment of seizures. *Ann Pharmacother* 1996; **30:** 514–19.
4. Oles KS, *et al.* Use of acetazolamide as an adjunct to carbamazepine in refractory partial seizures. *Epilepsia* 1989; **30:** 74–8.
5. Rogawski MA, Porter RJ. Antiepileptic drugs: pharmacological mechanisms and clinical efficacy with consideration of promising developmental stage compounds. *Pharmacol Rev* 1990; **42:** 223–86.
6. Hankey GJ, Stewart-Wynne EG. Management of non-convulsive status epilepticus. *Lancet* 1987; **i:** 1427.

**Glaucoma.** Acetazolamide may be given orally or parenterally in the acute management of angle-closure glaucoma (p.1485) and to minimise rises in intra-ocular pressure associated with ocular surgery.[1,2] It may also be given orally in the long-term management of primary and secondary open-angle glaucoma but is usually used as a second-line drug and added to topical beta blockers. However, up to 50% of patients are unable to tolerate oral therapy because of adverse effects[3] although topical carbonic anhydrase inhibitors such as dorzolamide may be better tolerated. Attempts have been made to reduce the adverse effects of acetazolamide by modifying the dosage schedule. A single-dose study[4] showed that doses of acetazolamide greater than 63 mg produced no greater reductions in intra-ocular pressure in patients with ocular hypertension. Another study[5] reported that acetazolamide 250-mg tablets twice daily controlled intra-ocular pressure adequately while producing fewer adverse effects than 250 mg four times daily and it was suggested that there was no advantage in using the modified-release capsule formulation (500 mg twice daily). A study in patients with open-angle glaucoma[6] found that most patients were adequately controlled by a single night-time dose of acetazolamide 500 mg either as tablets or modified-release capsules. The night-time dose also reduced the severity of adverse effects compared with the same dose given in the morning, and could aid compliance.

1. Ladas ID, *et al.* Prophylactic use of acetazolamide to prevent intraocular pressure elevation following Nd-YAG laser posterior capsulotomy. *Br J Ophthalmol* 1993; **77:** 136–8.
2. Edmunds B, Canning CR. The effect of prophylactic acetazolamide in patients undergoing extensive retinal detachment repair. *Eye* 1996; **10:** 328–30.
3. Hurvitz LM, *et al.* New developments in the drug treatment of glaucoma. *Drugs* 1991; **41:** 514–32.
4. Friedland BR, *et al.* Short-term dose response characteristics of acetazolamide in man. *Arch Ophthalmol* 1977; **95:** 1809–12.
5. Ledger-Scott M, Hurst J. Comparison of the bioavailability of two acetazolamide formulations. *Pharm J* 1985; **235:** 451.
6. Joyce PW, Mills KB. Comparison of the effect of acetazolamide tablets and sustets on diurnal intraocular pressure in patients with chronic simple glaucoma. *Br J Ophthalmol* 1990; **74:** 413–16.

**High-altitude disorders.** Acetazolamide is the most frequently used drug for the prophylaxis of high-altitude disorders (p.822). It accelerates the process of acclimatisation, thus reducing the incidence of acute mountain sickness and associated symptoms such as headache, nausea, vomiting, and lethargy. The optimum dose is not clear. A systematic review[1] concluded that 750 mg daily effectively prevented acute mountain sickness, but that a dose of 500 mg daily was not effective. However, these conclusions have been criticised, and a subsequent controlled study[2] found that a dose of 125 mg twice daily reduced the incidence of acute mountain sickness by about 50%. Acetazolamide may also have some benefit in relieving symptoms once they have developed although experience is limited. It does not prevent or protect against pulmonary or cerebral oedema.

1. Dumont L, *et al.* Efficacy and harm of pharmacological prevention of acute mountain sickness: quantitative systematic review. *BMJ* 2000; **321:** 267–72.
2. Basnyat B, *et al.* Efficacy of low-dose acetazolamide (125 mg BID) for the prophylaxis of acute mountain sickness: a prospective, double-blind, randomized, placebo-controlled trial. *High Alt Med Biol* 2003; **4:** 45–52.

**Macular oedema.** For mention of the use of acetazolamide to treat macular oedema associated with uveitis, see Uveitis, p.1090.

**Ménière's disease.** In Ménière's disease (p.422) high concentrations of carbonic anhydrase are found in the labyrinth, and acetazolamide, a carbonic anhydrase inhibitor, has been tried for both diagnosis and treatment.[1] A dose of 500 mg by intravenous injection has been suggested for diagnosis of fluctuating Ménière's disease.[1] Treatment with the drug by mouth, however, has not been particularly effective and has been associated with a high incidence of adverse effects.[2]

1. Brookes GB. Ménière's disease: a practical approach to management. *Drugs* 1983; **25:** 77–89.
2. Brookes GB, Booth JB. Oral acetazolamide in Ménière's disease. *J Laryngol Otol* 1984; **98:** 1087–95.

**Neuromuscular disorders.** Acetazolamide may be of benefit in some neuromuscular disorders, including hypokalaemic periodic paralysis (p.1220). Doses of 375 to 500 mg daily were effective in 2 patients with severe paralysis and were well tolerated.[1] Preliminary observations in 5 other patients showed a striking improvement in 3. In a further 12 patients,[2] doses of 125 mg were given three times daily to children and 250 mg two to six times daily to adults. There was dramatic improvement in 10 of the 12 and this lasted for up to 43 months. Chronic weakness between attacks in 10 patients was improved in 8.

Acetazolamide may reduce the frequency of attacks in patients with hyperkalaemic periodic paralysis (p.1219). It has also been used in episodic ataxia.[3]

1. Resnick JS, *et al.* Acetazolamide prophylaxis in hypokalemic periodic paralysis. *N Engl J Med* 1968; **278:** 582–6.
2. Griggs RC, *et al.* Acetazolamide treatment of hypokalemic periodic paralysis: prevention of attacks and improvement of persistent weakness. *Ann Intern Med* 1970; **73:** 39–48.
3. Melberg A, *et al.* Loss of control after a cup of coffee. *Lancet* 1997; **350:** 1220.

**Raised intracranial pressure.** Acetazolamide has been used to reduce raised intracranial pressure (p.833). It has a role in the management of benign intracranial hypertension. It has also been tried in the treatment of immunocompromised patients with chronically raised intracranial pressure due to cryptococcal meningitis,[1] although a controlled trial[2] was terminated early due to serious adverse events possibly due to additive toxicity with amphotericin. However, acetazolamide was used successfully for long-term treatment in 2 immunocompetent patients[3] with raised intracranial pressure following fungal meningitis.

1. Johnston SRD, *et al.* Raised intracranial pressure and visual complications in AIDS patients with cryptococcal meningitis. *J Infect* 1992; **24:** 185–9.
2. Newton PN, *et al.* A randomized, double-blind, placebo-controlled trial of acetazolamide for the treatment of elevated intracranial pressure in cryptococcal meningitis. *Clin Infect Dis* 2002; **35:** 769–72.
3. Patel S, *et al.* Acetazolamide therapy and intracranial pressure. *Clin Infect Dis* 2002; **36:** 538.

### Preparations

***BP 2003:*** Acetazolamide Tablets;
***USP 27:*** Acetazolamide for Injection; Acetazolamide Tablets.

**Proprietary Preparations** (details are given in Part 3)
***Arg.:*** Diamox; ***Austral.:*** Diamox; ***Austria:*** Diamox; ***Belg.:*** Diamox; ***Braz.:*** Diamox; Zolamox; ***Canad.:*** Diamox; Novo-Zolamide†; ***Denm.:*** Diamox; Glaupax†; ***Fin.:*** Diamox; Odemin; ***Fr.:*** Defiltran; Diamox; ***Ger.:*** Diamox; Diuramid; Glaupax; ***Gr.:*** Diamox; ***Hong Kong:*** Diamox; ***India:*** Diamox; ***Irl.:*** Diamox; Glaupax†; ***Israel:*** Diamox; Uramox; ***Ital.:*** Diamox; ***Mex.:*** Acetadiazol; Akezol†; Diamox; ***Neth.:*** Diamox; Glaupax; ***Norw.:*** Diamox; Glaupax†; ***NZ:*** Diamox; ***Port.:*** Carbinib; ***S.Afr.:*** Azomid; Diamox†; ***Spain:*** Diamox†; Edemox; ***Swed.:*** Diamox; ***Switz.:*** Diamox; Glaupax; ***Thai.:*** Diamox; Glaupax†; ***UK:*** Diamox; ***USA:*** Dazamide; Diamox.

## Acetyldigoxin

Acetildigoxina; Desglucolanatoside C. 3β-[(*O*-3-*O*-Acetyl-2,6-dideoxy-β-D-*ribo*-hexopyranosyl-(1→4)-*O*-2,6-dideoxy-β-D-*ribo*-hexopyranosyl-(1→4)-2,6-dideoxy-β-D-*ribo*-hexopyranosyl)oxy]-12β,14-dihydroxy-5β,14β-card-20(22)-enolide (α-acetyldigoxin); 3β-[(*O*-4-*O*-Acetyl-2,6-dideoxy-β-D-*ribo*-hexopyranosyl-(1→4)-*O*-2,6-dideoxy-β-D-*ribo*-hexopyranosyl-(1→4)-2,6-dideoxy-β-D-*ribo*-hexopyranosyl)oxy]-12β,14-dihydroxy-5β,14β-card-20(22)-enolide (β-acetyldigoxin).

$C_{43}H_{66}O_{15}$ = 823.0.
*CAS — 5511-98-8 (α-acetyldigoxin); 5355-48-6 (β-acetyldigoxin).*
*ATC — C01AA02.*

### Profile

Acetyldigoxin is a cardiac glycoside with positive inotropic activity. It has the general properties of digoxin (p.895) and has been used similarly in the management of some cardiac arrhythmias (p.816) and in heart failure (p.820). Both the α- and β-isomers have been used in usual maintenance doses of 200 to 400 micrograms daily by mouth.

### Preparations

**Proprietary Preparations** (details are given in Part 3)
***Austria:*** Corotal; Lanatilin; Novodigal; Sandolanid†; ***Belg.:*** Novodigal†; ***Ger.:*** Digostada; Digotab; Digox; Digoxin "Didier"; Gladixol N†; Kardiamed†; Novodigal; Stillacor; ***Ital.:*** Cardioreg.

**Multi-ingredient: *Austria:*** Digi-Aldopur; Gladixol.

## Acipimox *(BAN, rINN)*

K-9321. 5-Methylpyrazine-2-carboxylic acid 4-oxide.

$C_6H_6N_2O_3$ = 154.1.
*CAS — 51037-30-0.*
*ATC — C10AD06.*

### Adverse Effects and Precautions

Acipimox may cause peripheral vasodilatation resulting in flushing, itching, and a sensation of heat. Rash and erythema may occur. Gastrointestinal disturbances including heartburn, epigastric pain, nausea, and diarrhoea have been reported, as well as headache, malaise, and dry eye. Urticaria, angioedema, and bronchospasm may occur rarely.

Acipimox is contra-indicated in patients with peptic ulcer disease. It should be used with caution in renal impairment (see under Uses and Administration, below).

◊ In a study involving 3009 hyperlipidaemic patients with type 2 diabetes,[1] adverse effects associated with acipimox occurred in 8.8%, resulting in withdrawal in 5.5% of patients. The most frequent adverse effects involved the skin (57.6%), gastrointestinal tract (25.8%), and CNS (9.7%). Labial oedema occurred in 3 cases and an urticarial eruption, collapse, and dyspnoea in another. The incidence of adverse effects was almost twice as high in females as in males, the difference being mainly due to a greater incidence of flushing, pruritus, and skin rashes. The incidence was not affected by age. There was a mean 15.3% reduction in fasting blood-glucose concentrations and an 8.5% reduction in glycosylated haemoglobin during treatment with acipimox.

1. Lavezzari M, *et al.* Results of a phase IV study carried out with acipimox in type II diabetic patients with concomitant hyperlipoproteinaemia. *J Int Med Res* 1989; **17:** 373–80.

### Pharmacokinetics

Acipimox is rapidly and completely absorbed from the gastrointestinal tract and peak plasma concentrations occur within 2 hours. It does not bind to plasma proteins and the plasma half-life is about 2 hours. It is not significantly metabolised and is excreted in the urine, largely unchanged.

### Uses and Administration

Acipimox is a lipid regulating drug related to nicotinic acid (p.1441). It is used to reduce cholesterol and triglycerides in the management of hyperlipidaemias (below), including type IIa, IIb, or IV hyperlipoproteinaemias.

Acipimox is given by mouth in a usual dose of 250 mg two or three times daily, taken with meals. Doses of up to 1200 mg daily have been used. The dose should be reduced in renal impairment (see below).

**Administration in renal impairment.** Acipimox is contra-indicated in patients with a creatinine clearance below 30 mL/minute. In patients with creatinine clearance between 30 and 60 mL/minute, the interval between doses should be increased.

**Hyperlipidaemias.** Acipimox is used in the management of hyperlipidaemias (p.823) and produces effects on plasma lipoproteins similar to those of nicotinic acid, although it may not be as potent in its lipid modifying effect. Acipimox was developed to overcome the problems of compliance resulting from nicotinic acid's adverse effects. Its primary action is thought to be the inhibition of lipolysis thus reducing the availability of free fatty acids for the hepatic production of very-low-density lipoprotein (VLDL), and this in turn leads to a decrease in low-density lipoprotein (LDL) production. Increases in high-density lipoprotein (HDL) may also occur. The overall effect is a reduction in VLDL-triglyceride and total triglyceride concentrations and an increase in HDL-cholesterol concentrations, but only a modest reduction in LDL-cholesterol or total-cholesterol concentrations.[1-6]

Acipimox has been shown to be effective in the treatment of hyperlipidaemias in diabetic patients, and has generally produced a reduction in blood-glucose concentrations.[5,6] A patient with type A insulin-resistance syndrome, who had diabetes and severe hypertriglyceridaemia with very high fasting insulin and non-esterified fatty acids, responded to treatment with acipimox 500 mg twice daily in a modified-release form.[7]

1. Sommariva D, *et al.* Changes in lipoprotein cholesterol and triglycerides induced by acipimox in type IV and type II hyperlipoproteinemic patients. *Curr Ther Res* 1985; **37:** 363–8.
2. Ball MJ, *et al.* Acipimox in the treatment of patients with hyperlipidaemia: a double blind trial. *Eur J Clin Pharmacol* 1986; **31:** 201–4.
3. Taskinen M-R, Nikkilä EA. Effects of acipimox on serum lipids, lipoproteins and lipolytic enzymes in hypertriglyceridemia. *Atherosclerosis* 1988; **69:** 249–55.
4. Crepaldi G, *et al.* Plasma lipid lowering activity of acipimox in patients with type II and type IV hyperlipoproteinaemia. *Atherosclerosis* 1988; **70:** 115–21.
5. Dulbecco A, *et al.* Effect of acipimox on plasma glucose levels in patients with non-insulin-dependent diabetes mellitus. *Curr Ther Res* 1989; **46:** 478–83.
6. Lavezzari M, *et al.* Results of a phase IV study carried out with acipimox in type II diabetic patients with concomitant hyperlipoproteinaemia. *J Int Med Res* 1989; **17:** 373–80.
7. Kumar S, *et al.* Suppression of non-esterified fatty acids to treat type A insulin resistance syndrome. *Lancet* 1994; **343:** 1073–4.

### Preparations

**Proprietary Preparations** (details are given in Part 3)
***Austria:*** Olbetam; ***Belg.:*** Olbetam; ***Braz.:*** Olbetam; ***Chile:*** Olbetam; ***Denm.:*** Olbetam; ***Ger.:*** Olbemox; ***Gr.:*** Olbetam; ***Hong Kong:*** Olbetam; ***Irl.:*** Olbetam; ***Israel:*** Olbetam; ***Ital.:*** Olbetam; ***Mex.:*** Olbetam†; ***Neth.:*** Nedios; Olbetam; ***NZ:*** Olbetam; ***S.Afr.:*** Olbetam; ***Singapore:*** Olbetam; ***Switz.:*** Olbetam; ***Thai.:*** Olbetam; ***UK:*** Olbetam.

## Adenosine *(BAN, USAN)*

Adenosina; Adenosinum; SR-96225. 6-Amino-9-β-D-ribofuranosyl-9*H*-purine.

$C_{10}H_{13}N_5O_4$ = 267.2.
*CAS — 58-61-7.*
*ATC — C01EB10.*

**Pharmacopoeias.** In *Eur.* (see p.vi) and *US.*

**Ph. Eur. 5.0** (Adenosine). A white crystalline powder. Slightly soluble in water; soluble in hot water; practically insoluble in alcohol and in dichloromethane; dissolves in dilute mineral acids.

**USP 27** (Adenosine). A white, odourless crystalline powder. Soluble in water; practically insoluble in alcohol. Store in airtight containers. Protect from light.

**Stability.** Adenosine was found to be stable[1] when it was mixed with glucose 5%, lactated Ringer's, sodium chloride 0.9%, or a mixture of glucose 5% and lactated Ringer's and stored in polypropylene syringes or PVC bags.

1. Ketkar VA, *et al.* Stability of undiluted and diluted adenosine at three temperatures in syringes and bags. *Am J Health-Syst Pharm* 1998; **55:** 466–70.

### Adverse Effects and Precautions

Adverse effects of adenosine are usually transient, lasting less than a minute, due to its very short plasma half-life. They include nausea, lightheadedness, flushing, headache, angina-like chest pain, and dyspnoea. Bronchospasm has been reported. Like other antiarrhythmics, adenosine may worsen arrhythmias. Bradycardia and heart block have been reported. The larger doses given by intravenous infusion may rarely produce hypotension and tachycardia.

Adenosine is contra-indicated in patients with second- or third-degree atrioventricular block or in those with sick sinus syndrome. It is also contra-indicated in asthmatic subjects and should be used with caution in patients with obstructive pulmonary disease. Intravenous infusion of adenosine should be used with caution in patients who may develop hypotensive complications such as those with autonomic dysfunction, pericarditis, or stenotic valvular heart disease. Patients with recent heart transplantation may have increased sensitivity to the cardiac effects of adenosine.

◊ Use of the University of Wisconsin solution [UW Solution; Belzer Solution] for the hypothermic storage of kidneys prior to transplantation has been associated with bradycardia, prolonged PR intervals, and heart block.[1,2] The solution contains hetastarch, allopurinol, glutathione, and adenosine. The adenosine was considered to be the arrhythmogenic factor. Some centres had used the solution to flush kidneys before implantation,[2] a use for which it was never intended.[3] When used properly the adenosine in solution is catabolised to hypoxanthine and inosine, which do not cause cardiac problems, but this takes some time in hypothermic conditions.[3]

1. Prien T, *et al.* Bradyarrhythmia with University of Wisconsin preservation solution. *Lancet* 1989; **i:** 1319–20.
2. Vanrenterghem Y, *et al.* University of Wisconsin preservation solute and bradyarrhythmia. *Lancet* 1989; **ii:** 745.
3. Belzer FO. Correct use of University of Wisconsin preservation solution. *Lancet* 1990; **335:** 362.

**Effects on the heart.** Adenosine may worsen arrhythmias. A prospective study[1] in 200 patients reported an incidence of atrial fibrillation of 12% following bolus injection of adenosine 12 mg used to terminate paroxysmal supraventricular tachycardia. Haemodynamically unstable proarrhythmia occurred in 2 patients with the Wolff-Parkinson-White syndrome and palpitations[2] after standard intravenous doses of adenosine were given.

Myocardial infarction was reported[3] in a patient with ischaemic heart disease who underwent stress imaging using adenosine.

1. Strickberger SA, *et al.* Adenosine-induced atrial arrhythmia: a prospective analysis. *Ann Intern Med* 1997; **127:** 417–22.
2. Exner DV, *et al.* Proarrhythmia in patients with the Wolff-Parkinson-White syndrome after standard doses of intravenous adenosine. *Ann Intern Med* 1995; **122:** 351–2.
3. Polad JE, Wilson LM. Myocardial infarction during adenosine stress test. Abstract: *Heart* 2002; **87:** 106. Full version: http://www.heartjnl.com/cgi/content/full/87/2/e2 (accessed 06/07/04)

**Effects on the respiratory system.** Acute exacerbation of asthma is well known following inhalation of adenosine. There have been reports of bronchospasm in patients with asthma[1,2] or a history of asthma[3] given adenosine intravenously and bronchospasm followed by respiratory failure in a patient with obstructive pulmonary disease.[4]

1. DeGroff CG, Silka MJ. Bronchospasm after intravenous administration of adenosine in a patient with asthma. *J Pediatr* 1994; **125:** 822–3.
2. Drake I, *et al.* Bronchospasm induced by intravenous adenosine. *Hum Exp Toxicol* 1994; **13:** 263–5.
3. Hintringer F, *et al.* Supraventricular tachycardia. *N Engl J Med* 1995; **333:** 323.
4. Burkhart KK. Respiratory failure following adenosine administration. *Am J Emerg Med* 1993; **11:** 249–50.

**Migraine.** A 35-year-old man with a history of migraine developed symptoms identical to those of his usual episodes of migraine immediately following two intravenous bolus doses of adenosine.[1]

1. Brown SGA, Waterer GW. Migraine precipitated by adenosine. *Med J Aust* 1995; **162:** 389–91.

### Interactions

Dipyridamole inhibits adenosine uptake and therefore may potentiate the action of adenosine; if use of the two drugs is essential the dosage of adenosine should be reduced. Theophylline and other xanthines are competitive antagonists of adenosine. The risk of atrioventricular block may be increased if adenosine is used with other drugs that slow atrioventricular conduction.

### Pharmacokinetics

Following intravenous administration adenosine is rapidly taken up by an active transport system into erythrocytes and vascular endothelial cells where it is metabolised to inosine and adenosine monophosphate. The plasma half-life is less than 10 seconds.

## Uses and Administration

Adenosine is an endogenous nucleoside involved in many biological processes. It acts as an antiarrhythmic by stimulating adenosine ($A_1$) receptors and slowing conduction through the atrioventricular node. It does not fit into the usual classification of antiarrhythmics (p.809). It also produces peripheral and coronary vasodilatation by stimulating adenosine ($A_2$) receptors.

Adenosine is used to restore sinus rhythm in the treatment of paroxysmal supraventricular tachycardia including that associated with the Wolff-Parkinson-White syndrome. It is also used for the differential diagnosis of broad or narrow complex supraventricular tachycardias and in myocardial imaging.

In the treatment of **paroxysmal supraventricular tachycardia**, the usual initial dose of adenosine is 3 mg by rapid intravenous injection. If this dose is ineffective within 1 to 2 minutes, 6 mg may be given and if necessary, 12 mg after a further 1 to 2 minutes. Higher initial doses of 6 mg have sometimes been used although these are not appropriate for heart transplant patients who have an increased sensitivity to adenosine. The above dosage regimen beginning with 3 mg is also used for differential **diagnosis of supraventricular tachycardias**. In children with paroxysmal supraventricular tachycardia, an initial dose of 50 to 100 micrograms/kg may be used; if this is not effective the dose may be increased by 50 to 100 micrograms/kg increments at 1 to 2 minute intervals until the arrhythmia is controlled or a dose of 300 micrograms/kg is reached.

In **myocardial imaging** adenosine is given by intravenous infusion in a dose of 140 micrograms/kg per minute for 6 minutes. The radionuclide is injected after 3 minutes of the infusion.

Adenosine triphosphate (p.1648), in the form of the disodium salt, has been used as an antiarrhythmic.

**Cardiac arrhythmias.** Adenosine is used for the termination of paroxysmal supraventricular tachycardia[1-4] (p.816), including that associated with the Wolff-Parkinson-White syndrome, and may often be the drug of choice. Following bolus intravenous injection of adenosine, there is a rapid response and the extremely short plasma half-life (less than 10 seconds) allows dosage titration every 1 to 2 minutes so that most episodes can be controlled within 5 minutes without the danger of drug accumulation.

Adenosine has been used successfully in pregnant women with paroxysmal supraventricular tachycardia[5-8] and cardioversion of fetal supraventricular tachycardia by direct fetal therapy with adenosine has been reported.[9,10]

Adenosine can be used for the differential **diagnosis** of broad complex tachycardia where the mechanism is not known.[1] If the cause is supraventricular, adenosine will terminate the arrhythmia or produce atrioventricular block to reveal the underlying atrial rhythm. If the cause is ventricular, adenosine will have no effect on the tachycardia, whereas if an alternative treatment such as verapamil is given to these patients severe hypotension and cardiac arrest can occur.


1. Faulds D, *et al.* Adenosine: an evaluation of its use in cardiac diagnostic procedures, and in the treatment of paroxysmal supraventricular tachycardia. *Drugs* 1991; **41:** 596–624.
2. Garratt CJ, *et al.* Adenosine and cardiac arrhythmias. *BMJ* 1992; **305:** 3–4.
3. Rankin AC, *et al.* Adenosine and the treatment of supraventricular tachycardia. *Am J Med* 1992; **92:** 655–64.
4. Anonymous. Adenosine for acute cardiac arrhythmias. *Drug Ther Bull* 1993; **31:** 49–50.
5. Mason BA, *et al.* Adenosine in the treatment of maternal paroxysmal supraventricular tachycardia. *Obstet Gynecol* 1992; **80:** 478–80.
6. Afridi I, *et al.* Termination of supraventricular tachycardia with intravenous adenosine in a pregnant woman with Wolff-Parkinson-White syndrome. *Obstet Gynecol* 1992; **80:** 481–3.
7. Hagley MT, Cole PL. Adenosine use in pregnant women with supraventricular tachycardia. *Ann Pharmacother* 1994; **28:** 1241–2.
8. Hagley MT, *et al.* Adenosine use in a pregnant patient with supraventricular tachycardia. *Ann Pharmacother* 1995; **29:** 938.
9. Blanch G, *et al.* Cardioversion of fetal tachyarrhythmia with adenosine. *Lancet* 1994; **344:** 1646.
10. Kohl T, *et al.* Direct fetal administration of adenosine for the termination of incessant supraventricular tachycardia. *Obstet Gynecol* 1995; **85:** 873–4.


**Ischaemic heart disease.** Adenosine produces coronary vasodilatation and may be used to provide a pharmacological stress in patients undergoing assessment of their ischaemic heart disease when exercise stress is inappropriate. It has been given to such patients being evaluated either by thallium-201 myocardial imaging[1] or by stress echocardiography.[2] Adenosine is also under investigation as an adjunct to prevent reperfusion injury in the management of acute myocardial infarction.[3]


1. Mohiuddin SM, *et al.* Thallium-201 myocardial imaging in patients with coronary artery disease: comparison of intravenous adenosine and oral dipyridamole. *Ann Pharmacother* 1992; **26:** 1352–7.
2. Martin TW, *et al.* Comparison of adenosine, dipyridamole, and dobutamine in stress echocardiography. *Ann Intern Med* 1992; **116:** 190–6.
3. Mahaffey KW, *et al.* Adenosine as an adjunct to thrombolytic therapy for acute myocardial infarction: results of a multicenter, randomized, placebo-controlled trial: the Acute Myocardial Infarction STudy of ADenosine (AMISTAD) trial. *J Am Coll Cardiol* 1999; **34:** 1711–20.


**Pulmonary hypertension.** A number of vasodilators have been tried in persistent pulmonary hypertension of the newborn (p.832), but their use is generally restricted by their non-selectivity for the pulmonary circulation. A randomised placebo-controlled study[1] in 18 term infants with persistent pulmonary hypertension indicated that intravenous infusion of adenosine improved oxygenation without causing hypotension or tachycardia; however, the study was too small to assess any effect on mortality and/or the need for extracorporeal membrane oxygenation.


1. Konduri GG, *et al.* Adenosine infusion improves oxygenation in term infants with respiratory failure. *Pediatrics* 1996; **97:** 295–300.


## Preparations

***USP 27:*** Adenosine Injection.

**Proprietary Preparations** (details are given in Part 3)
***Arg.:*** Euritsin; ***Austral.:*** Adenocor; Adenoscan; ***Austria:*** Adenoscan; Adrekar; ***Belg.:*** Adenocor; ***Braz.:*** Adenocard; ***Canad.:*** Adenocard; ***Denm.:*** Adenocor; ***Fin.:*** Adenocor; Adenoscan; ***Fr.:*** Adenoscan; Krenosin; ***Ger.:*** Adenoscan; Adrekar; ***Gr.:*** Adenocor; ***Hong Kong:*** Adenoscan; ***India:*** Adenoject; ***Irl.:*** Adenocor; ***Israel:*** Adenocor; ***Ital.:*** Adenoscan; Krenosin; ***Malaysia:*** Adenocor; ***Mex.:*** Krenosin; ***Neth.:*** Adenocor; Adenoscan; ***Norw.:*** Adenocor; ***NZ:*** Adenocor; ***Port.:*** Adenocor†; ***S.Afr.:*** Adenocor; ***Singapore:*** Adenocor; ***Spain:*** Adenocor; Adenoscan; ***Switz.:*** Krenosine; ***Thai.:*** Adenocor; ***UK:*** Adenocor; Adenoscan; ***USA:*** Adenocard; Adenoscan.

**Multi-ingredient:** ***Austria:*** Laevadosin†; Vitasic†; ***Braz.:*** Aminotox; Anekron; Betaliver; Biofigado†; Biohepax; Colinvintol†; Enterofigon†; Epacrosil†; Eparex†; Epativan B6; Epocler; Eviepar†; Figadobil†; Hepacitron†; Hepalin†; Hepatobe†; Hepofilina†; Hormo Hepatico; Jecohepat†; Necro B-6; ***Fr.:*** Vitacic; Vitaphakol†; ***Ger.:*** Hepatofalk†; Vitreolent plus†; ***Hong Kong:*** Hepatofalk†; ***Port.:*** Vitaphakol†; ***Spain:*** Vitaphakol; ***Switz.:*** Vitaphakol†.

# Adrenaline *(BAN)*

Epinephrine *(BAN, rINN)*; Epinefrina; Epinephrinum; Epirenamine; Levorenin; Suprarenin. *(R)*-1-(3,4-Dihydroxyphenyl)-2-methylaminoethanol.

$C_9H_{13}NO_3$ = 183.2.
*CAS — 51-43-4.*
*ATC — A01AD01; B02BC09; C01CA24; R01AA14; R03AA01; S01EA01.*

NOTE. Endogenous adrenaline and the monograph substance are the laevo isomer. ADN and EPN are codes approved by the BP 2003 for use on single unit doses of eye drops containing adrenaline where the individual container may be too small to bear all the appropriate labelling information.

**Pharmacopoeias.** In *Br., Chin., Fr., Int., It., Jpn, Pol., US,* and *Viet.*

*US* also includes the racemic substances Racepinephrine (Racepinefrine (*rINN*)) and Racepinephrine Hydrochloride (Racepinefrine Hydrochloride (*rINNM*)).

**BP 2003** (Adrenaline; Epinephrine). It may be prepared by synthesis or isolated from the medulla of the suprarenal glands of certain mammals and substantially freed from noradrenaline. A white or creamy-white, sphaero-crystalline powder. It darkens in colour on exposure to air and light. Sparingly soluble in water; practically insoluble in alcohol and in ether. It dissolves in solutions of mineral acids and in solutions of sodium or potassium hydroxide, but not in solutions of ammonia or of the alkali carbonates. It is unstable in neutral or alkaline solutions, which rapidly become red on exposure to air. Store in containers which are preferably filled with nitrogen. Protect from light.

**USP 27** (Epinephrine). A white to practically white, odourless, microcrystalline powder or granules, gradually darkening on exposure to light and air. With acids, it forms salts that are readily soluble in water, and the base may be recovered by the addition of ammonia water or alkali carbonates. Very slightly soluble in water and in alcohol; insoluble in chloroform, in ether, and in fixed and volatile oils. Solutions are alkaline to litmus. Store in airtight containers. Protect from light.

## Adrenaline Acid Tartrate *(BANM)*

Epinephrine Bitartrate *(rINNM)*; Adrenaline Bitartrate; Adrenaline Tartrate; Adrenalini Bitartras; Adrenalini Tartras; Adrenalinii Tartras; Adrenalinium Hydrogentartaricum; Bitartrato de epinefrina; Epinephrine Acid Tartrate *(BANM)*; Epinephrine Hydrogen Tartrate; Epirenamine Bitartrate.

$C_9H_{13}NO_3,C_4H_6O_6$ = 333.3.
*CAS — 51-42-3.*
*ATC — A01AD01; B02BC09; C01CA24; R01AA14; R03AA01; S01EA01.*

**Pharmacopoeias.** In *Eur.* (see p.vi), *Int., Pol., US,* and *Viet.*

**Ph. Eur. 5.0** (Adrenaline Tartrate; Adrenaline Acid Tartrate BP 2003; Epinephrine Acid Tartrate BP 2003). A white to greyish-white, crystalline powder. Freely soluble in water; slightly soluble in alcohol. Store in airtight containers, or preferably in a sealed tube under vacuum or under an inert gas. Protect from light.

**USP 27** (Epinephrine Bitartrate). A white, or greyish-white or light brownish-grey, odourless, crystalline powder. It slowly darkens on exposure to air and light. Soluble 1 in 3 of water; slightly soluble in alcohol; practically insoluble in chloroform and in ether. Its solutions in water are acid to litmus, having a pH of about 3.5. Store in airtight containers. Protect from light.

**Stability.** Studies on the stability of adrenaline injections.


1. Taylor JB, *et al.* Effect of sodium metabisulphite and anaerobic processing conditions on the oxidative degradation of adrenaline injection BP [1980]. *Pharm J* 1984; **232:** 646–8.


## Adrenaline Hydrochloride *(BANM)*

Epinephrine Hydrochloride *(BANM, rINNM)*; Hidrocloruro de epinefrina.

$C_9H_{13}NO_3,HCl$ = 219.7.
*CAS — 55-31-2.*
*ATC — A01AD01; B02BC09; C01CA24; R01AA14; R03AA01; S01EA01.*

## Adverse Effects

Adrenaline is a potent sympathomimetic and may exhibit the adverse effects typical of both alpha- and beta-adrenoceptor stimulation. It can thus produce a wide range of adverse effects, most of which mimic the results of excessive stimulation of the sympathetic nervous system. Side-effects such as anxiety, dyspnoea, hyperglycaemia, restlessness, palpitations, tachycardia (sometimes with anginal pain), tremors, sweating, hypersalivation, weakness, dizziness, headache, and coldness of extremities may occur even with low doses. Overdosage may cause cardiac arrhythmias and a sharp rise in blood pressure (sometimes leading to cerebral haemorrhage and pulmonary oedema); these effects may occur at normal dosage in susceptible subjects.

Since adrenaline does not readily cross the blood-brain barrier, its central effects, which encompass anxiety, fear, restlessness, insomnia, confusion, irritability, and psychotic states, may be largely a somatic response to its peripheral effects. Anorexia, nausea, and vomiting, may occur similarly.

The peripheral adverse effects of adrenaline are complex and mediated via its action on the various types of adrenergic receptor (see under Uses and Administration, below). Stimulation of alpha-adrenergic (mainly alpha$_1$) receptors produces vasoconstriction leading to hypertension, and this alpha-mediated hypertension may induce reflex bradycardia. On the other hand, stimulation of beta$_1$-adrenergic receptors in the heart produces tachycardia and cardiac arrhythmias. Finally, stimulation of beta$_2$ receptors produces vasodilatation with flushing and hypotension (apparent if the vasoconstricting alpha effects are blocked).

In relation to some of the other adverse effects of adrenaline, difficulty in micturition with urinary retention is a characteristic of alpha$_1$-receptor stimulation whereas muscle tremor and hypokalaemia are characteristics of beta$_2$-receptor stimulation.

The potent alpha-adrenergic effects of adrenaline may lead to gangrene following the vasoconstriction that is induced by infiltration of adrenaline-containing local anaesthetic solutions into digits. Extravasation of parenterally administered adrenaline similarly causes intense vasoconstriction, resulting in tissue necrosis and sloughing.

Topical application of adrenaline to mucosal surfaces also causes vasoconstriction, which may induce hypoxia leading to compensatory rebound congestion of the mucosa.

Inhalations of adrenaline have been associated with epigastric pain (caused by swallowing a portion of the inhalation and minimised by rinsing the mouth and throat with water after inhaling).

Adrenaline eye drops may produce severe smarting, blurred vision, and photophobia on instillation; they may also leave melanin-like deposits in the cornea and conjunctiva, and this has led to obstruction of the nasolachrymal ducts. Repeated ocular administration of adrenaline may cause oedema, hyperaemia, and inflammation of the eyes.

*Other sympathomimetics* have adverse effects that resemble those of adrenaline to a greater or lesser extent according to their relative agonist activities on the different receptors. For example, noradrenaline, whose alpha-adrenergic effects predominate, may produce severe hypertension, whereas isoprenaline, whose beta-adrenergic effects predominate, may produce severe tachycardia.

◊ Systemic side-effects may occasionally follow the local or topical administration of sympathomimetics, for example when used as eye drops for the treatment of glaucoma.[1] Psychiatric side-effects including hallucinations and paranoia have also occurred following both proper and improper use of sympathomimetics in decongestant preparations.[2]

1. Everitt DE, Avorn J. Systemic effects of medications used to treat glaucoma. *Ann Intern Med* 1990; **112:** 120–5.
2. Anonymous. Drugs that cause psychiatric symptoms. *Med Lett Drugs Ther* 1993; **35:** 65–70.

**Effects on the eyes.** In addition to the possibility of pigment deposition and local pain (see above) adrenaline eye drops have been associated with maculopathy. During 4 years, 15 patients showed reactions to adrenaline eye drops, usually 2% of the hydrochloride or acid tartrate, while some used 1% adrenaline borate complex (epinephryl borate).[1] Blurring and distortion of vision were followed by decreased visual acuity, and by the appearance of oedema and sometimes haemorrhage in the macular region. A few patients developed cysts near the fovea. These effects appeared within a few weeks of, or several months after, commencement of therapy and were usually reversible. All except 1 of the patients were aphakic (devoid of lens). In a study of 200 consecutive patients receiving adrenaline therapy, 23 were aphakic in one or both eyes, and 7 experienced these reactions to adrenaline.

1. Kolker AE, Becker B. Epinephrine maculopathy. *Arch Ophthalmol* 1968; **79:** 552–62.

**Effects on the heart.** A review of the arrhythmogenic effects of vasopressor sympathomimetics[1] concluded that dopamine and adrenaline were associated with the highest risk, mainly of dose-related sinus tachycardia and ventricular arrhythmias. However, the clinical significance of most arrhythmias occurring with dopamine was considered questionable; supraventricular or ventricular arrhythmias occurring with adrenaline were most likely in patients receiving general anaesthesia or with underlying disorders of cardiac conduction. The risk with noradrenaline was uncertain, though there are few clinical reports, while phenylephrine and methoxamine were thought unlikely to cause problems. Overall the frequency of serious problems with this class of drugs did not seem to be high, and benefits outweighed the risks in most patients.

Myocardial infarction has been reported in an 11-year-old boy treated with nebulised racepinefrine for symptoms of croup.[2]

1. Tisdale JE, *et al.* Proarrhythmic effects of intravenous vasopressors. *Ann Pharmacother* 1995; **29:** 269–81.
2. Butte MJ, *et al.* Pediatric myocardial infarction after racemic epinephrine administration. Abstract: *Pediatrics* 1999; **104:** 103–4. Full version: http://pediatrics.aappublications.org/cgi/content/full/104/1/e9 (accessed 06/07/04)

**Overdosage.** Inadvertent intravenous administration of a solution containing racepinefrine meant for nebulisation has been reported[1] in a 13-month-old infant. The infant received the equivalent of about 327 micrograms/kg of *l*-adrenaline. Marked pallor, pulselessness, and profound bradycardia ensued, but the child responded to cardiopulmonary resuscitation and was subsequently discharged with no evidence of long-term sequelae.

1. Kurachek SC, Rockoff MA. Inadvertent intravenous administration of racemic epinephrine. *JAMA* 1985; **253:** 1441–2.

## Treatment of Adverse Effects

Because of the short duration of the adverse effects of adrenaline, due to inactivation in the body, treatment of severe toxic reactions in hypersensitive patients or after overdose is primarily supportive. Prompt injection of a rapidly acting alpha blocker, such as phentolamine, followed by a beta blocker such as propranolol, has been tried to counteract the pressor and arrhythmogenic effects of adrenaline; rapidly-acting vasodilators such as glyceryl trinitrate have also been used.

**Digital injection.** Inadvertent digital injection of adrenaline from autoinjector devices may cause acute ischaemia. Phentolamine injection has been successfully used to reverse the vasoconstriction, and there has also been a report[1] of the use of iloprost infusion followed by a stellate ganglion block.

1. Barkhordarian AR, *et al.* Accidental digital injection of adrenaline from an autoinjector device. *Br J Dermatol* 2000; **143:** 1359.

## Precautions

Adrenaline should be used with great caution in patients who may be particularly susceptible to its cardiovascular actions, notably those with pre-existing arrhythmias or tachycardia, Prinzmetal's angina, thromboembolic disorders, or a history of ischaemic heart disease. Extreme care is also needed in conditions that predispose a patient to adverse effects on the heart, such as hyperthyroidism; elevated thyroid hormone concentrations may also enhance receptor sensitivity. The use of adrenaline is generally inappropriate where there is pre-existing hypertension and it increases the risk of ischaemia in the extremities of patients with occlusive vascular disease. Special care is also needed in the elderly who may have pre-existing coronary or cerebrovascular disease.

Particular care is needed if adrenaline is given to patients with diabetes mellitus (both because of its vasoconstrictor actions and because of its metabolic effects on blood glucose). It should be avoided in phaeochromocytoma. Adrenaline may delay the second stage of labour and some manufacturers recommend that it should not be used during this time.

Adrenaline eye drops are contra-indicated in angle-closure glaucoma unless an iridectomy has been carried out.

When adrenaline is used for circulatory support, correction of hypovolaemia, metabolic acidosis, and hypoxia or hypercapnia should be carried out beforehand or concomitantly.

Precautions that need to be observed for *other sympathomimetics* resemble those for adrenaline, but vary to a greater or lesser extent according to their relative agonist activities on the different receptors. For example, noradrenaline, whose alpha-adrenergic effects predominate, is a particular hazard in hypertension, whereas a beta-adrenergic agonist such as isoprenaline is a particular hazard in tachycardia. It also needs to be borne in mind that since non-catecholamine sympathomimetics have a longer duration of action than catecholamines, side-effects are more likely to be sustained and, in particular, that any rise in blood pressure is liable to be prolonged.

**Contact lenses.** Adrenochrome staining of soft-contact lenses of patients using adrenaline eye drops has been reported.[1] Melanin deposits may also become locked into the lens; such deposits may be broken down by hydrogen peroxide. The prodrug, dipivefrine hydrochloride (p.1681) has been used without staining soft lenses.

1. Ingram DV. Spoiled soft contact lenses. *BMJ* 1986; **292:** 1619.

**Infection.** An open study[1] in 23 patients critically ill with severe sepsis or malaria has suggested that the use of adrenaline as an inotrope and vasopressor in patients with severe infection causes the development of lactic acidosis. However, adrenaline is widely used in the treatment of septic shock, and others have pointed out that 20 of the patients had responded to fluids, a situation in which the use of inotropic or vasopressor support was considered questionable.[2]

1. Day NPJ, *et al.* The effects of dopamine and adrenaline infusions on acid-base balance and systemic haemodynamics in severe infection. *Lancet* 1996; **348:** 219–23. Correction. *ibid.*; 902.
2. Barry B, Bodenham A. Effects of dopamine and adrenaline infusions in severe infection. *Lancet* 1996; **348:** 1099–1100.

## Interactions

Interactions with adrenaline are complex and often hazardous; they stem primarily from its agonist actions on alpha and beta adrenoceptors.

Hazardous arrhythmias are a risk if adrenaline is used in patients anaesthetised with *cyclopropane, halothane,* or other *volatile anaesthetics* that sensitise the myocardium to its beta-adrenergic effects.

The vasoconstrictor and pressor effects of adrenaline, mediated by its alpha-adrenergic action, may be enhanced by drugs with similar effects, such as *ergot alkaloids* or *oxytocin*.

Because adrenaline increases blood pressure, special care is advisable in patients receiving *antihypertensive therapy*. Moreover, adrenaline specifically reverses the antihypertensive effects of *adrenergic neurone blockers* such as *guanethidine* with the risk of severe hypertension. Severe hypertension (followed by reflex bradycardia) may also develop if adrenaline is given with a *beta blocker (especially a non-selective beta blocker)* since the beta blocker opposes the beta-adrenergic action of adrenaline, leaving its alpha-adrenergic effect unopposed; for details see below. Conversely, the bronchoconstrictor effect of a *beta blocker (especially a non-selective beta blocker)* antagonises the $beta_2$ (bronchodilating) effect of adrenaline and constitutes a serious hazard. It should also be noted that in patients on non-cardioselective beta blockers, severe anaphylaxis may not respond to adrenaline (see below). Complex interactions also occur with *alpha blockers* such as *phenoxybenzamine* and *phentolamine* which oppose the alpha-adrenergic action of adrenaline leaving its beta-adrenergic effect unopposed, thus resulting in both antihypertensive and cardiac-accelerating effects; nevertheless, use is made of this blood pressure reduction to reverse hypertension in adrenaline overdosage (see also Treatment of Adverse Effects, above). For a warning concerning hypotension associated with adrenaline-induced reversal of alpha-blockade in phenothiazine overdosage, see Treatment of Adverse Effects of Chlorpromazine, p.678.

Although caution is still necessary, the action of adrenaline or noradrenaline may be only slightly enhanced by an *MAOI*, since they are direct acting and inactivation by uptake into nerves and tissues is not inhibited. Dangerous hypertensive interactions are, however, a risk if dopamine (which has indirect-acting properties) is given concomitantly with an *MAOI (including an RIMA)*. Hazardous hypertensive interactions are also a major risk if dexamfetamine, dopexamine, ephedrine, isometheptene, mephentermine, metaraminol, methylphenidate, phentermine, phenylephrine, phenylpropanolamine, pseudoephedrine, and many other sympathomimetics are used with an *MAOI (including an RIMA)*. For additional warnings see under Phenelzine (p.314) and Moclobemide (p.308).

Administration of adrenaline or noradrenaline with *tricyclic antidepressants* (which inhibit their reuptake) carries a risk of inducing hypertension and arrhythmias.

In the case of local anaesthetic preparations containing adrenaline there is no clinical evidence of dangerous interactions with either *tricyclic antidepressants* or *MAOIs*, but great care needs to be taken to avoid inadvertent intravenous administration of these local anaesthetic preparations.

The hypokalaemic effect of adrenaline may be potentiated by other drugs that cause potassium loss, including *corticosteroids, potassium-depleting diuretics*, and *aminophylline* or *theophylline*; patients receiving high doses of $beta_2$-adrenergic agonists with such drugs should have their plasma-potassium concentration monitored (see Interactions of Salbutamol, p.792). Hypokalaemia may also result in increased susceptibility to cardiac arrhythmias caused by *digoxin* and other *cardiac glycosides*.

In addition to their interactions with *MAOIs* (cited above) the interactions of *other sympathomimetics* resemble those of adrenaline to a greater or lesser extent, according to their relevant agonist activities on the different receptors. For some details of specific interactions see under individual monographs.

**Beta blockers.** Patients given adrenaline (including the low doses used with local anaesthetics) while receiving non-selective beta blockers such as *propranolol* can develop elevated blood pressure due to alpha-mediated vasoconstriction, followed by reflex bradycardia, and occasionally cardiac arrest;[1] the bronchodilator effects of adrenaline are also inhibited. In contrast, cardioselective beta blockers such as *metoprolol*, which act preferentially at $beta_1$-adrenergic receptors, do not prevent adrenaline-induced vasodilatation via $beta_2$ receptors, and in consequence blood pressure and heart rate change only minimally. *Carvedilol*, which also has alpha-blocking effects, has been reported to cause hypotension with dobutamine (see p.906). Low doses of cardioselective beta blockers do not appear to interfere with sympathomimetic (isoprenaline)-induced bronchodilatation,[2] although the effect of larger doses is uncertain.

Propranolol has also been shown to inhibit the favourable pressor and bronchodilator responses to adrenaline when given for anaphylaxis.[3] Thus, patients receiving long-term treatment with some non-cardioselective beta blockers who develop anaphylaxis may be relatively refractory to adrenaline.

1. Jay GT, Chow MSS. Interaction of epinephrine and β-blockers. *JAMA* 1995; **274:** 1830–2.

2. Decalmer PBS, *et al.* Beta blockers and asthma. *Br Heart J* 1978; **40:** 184–9.
3. Newman BR, Schultz LK. Epinephrine-resistant anaphylaxis in a patient taking propranolol hydrochloride. *Ann Allergy* 1981; **47:** 35–7.

**General anaesthetics.** Anaesthesia may sensitise the myocardium to the effects of sympathomimetics, and it has been suggested[1] that clinically important effects may occur if adrenaline is injected into the operation area to reduce bleeding. Use of a low dose of adrenaline appears to be safe in patients anaesthetised with *cyclopropane, halothane*, or similar volatile anaesthetics, although other factors likely to increase the irritability of the myocardium, such as carbon-dioxide retention, hypoxia, or the use of cocaine, should be avoided.[1,2] A maximum strength for the adrenaline solution of 1 in 100 000 given at a rate not exceeding 10 mL per 10 minutes or 30 mL per hour has been recommended[1,2] for *halothane* or *trichloroethylene* anaesthesia; it may also be safe with cyclopropane although the risk of arrhythmias is higher.[2]

Fatalities have, however, been reported[3] in patients undergoing surgery involving the use of halothane and adrenaline.

1. Anonymous. Anaesthetics and the heart. *Lancet* 1967; **i:** 484–5.
2. Katz RL, Epstein RA. The interaction of anesthetic agents and adrenergic drugs to produce cardiac arrhythmias. *Anesthesiology* 1968; **29:** 763.
3. Buzik SC. Fatal interaction? Halothane, epinephrine and tooth implant surgery. *Can Pharm J* 1990; **123:** 68–9 and 81.

**Local anaesthetics.** It is common practice to administer adrenaline with a local anaesthetic to produce vasoconstriction; the lowest effective concentration of adrenaline should be used. However, with *cocaine* there is a risk of cardiac arrhythmias and the use, for example, of cocaine and adrenaline paste in otolaryngology may be hazardous. See p.1375 for references to this interaction.

## Pharmacokinetics

As a result of enzymatic degradation in the gut and first-pass metabolism in the liver, adrenaline is almost totally inactive when given orally. Systemic absorption can occur after topical application for example of eye drops. Adrenaline acts rapidly following intramuscular and subcutaneous injection; this latter route is, however, sometimes considered to be slower and therefore less reliable and predictable for emergency use. Although absorption is slowed by local vasoconstriction it can be hastened by massaging the injection site.

Most adrenaline that is either injected into the body or released into the circulation from the adrenal medulla, is very rapidly inactivated by processes that include uptake into adrenergic neurones, diffusion, and enzymatic degradation in the liver and body tissues. The half-life of circulating adrenaline is only about 1 minute. One of the enzymes responsible for the chemical inactivation of adrenaline is catechol-*O*-methyltransferase (COMT), the other is monoamine oxidase (MAO). In general, adrenaline is methylated to metanephrine by COMT followed by oxidative deamination by MAO and eventual conversion to 4-hydroxy-3-methoxymandelic acid (formerly termed vanillylmandelic acid; VMA), or oxidatively deaminated by MAO and converted to 3,4-dihydroxymandelic acid which, in turn, is methylated by COMT, once again to 4-hydroxy-3-methoxymandelic acid; the metabolites are excreted in the urine mainly as their glucuronide and ethereal sulfate conjugates.

The ability of COMT to effect introduction of a methyl group is an important step in the chemical inactivation of adrenaline and similar catecholamines (in particular, noradrenaline). It means that the termination of the pharmacological response of catecholamines is not simply dependent upon MAO. In its role of neurotransmitter intraneuronal catecholamine (mainly noradrenaline) is, however, enzymatically regulated by MAO.

Adrenaline crosses the placenta to enter fetal circulation.

## Uses and Administration

Adrenaline is an endogenous substance that is produced in the adrenal medulla and has important physiological effects. It is also used pharmacologically as a direct-acting sympathomimetic; for an outline of the actions of sympathomimetics, see below. It has a somewhat more marked effect on beta adrenoceptors than on alpha adrenoceptors, and this property explains many aspects of its pharmacology; in addition, its actions vary considerably according to the dose given, and the consequent reflex compensating responses of the body.

In practice, major effects of adrenaline include increased speed and force of cardiac contraction (with lower doses this causes increased systolic pressure yet reduced diastolic pressure since overall peripheral resistance is lowered, but with higher doses both systolic and diastolic pressure are increased as stimulation of peripheral alpha receptors increases peripheral resistance); blood flow to skeletal muscle is increased (reduced with higher doses); there is relaxation of bronchial smooth muscle; metabolic effects result in hyperglycaemia as well as markedly increased oxygen consumption; blood flow in the kidneys, mucosa, and skin is reduced; there is little direct effect on cerebral blood flow.

Adrenaline has an important role in the management of acute allergic reactions and can be life-saving in patients with anaphylactic shock (below). It is also used in advanced cardiac life support (below). Adrenaline has been given subcutaneously in the treatment of acute asthma but more selective drugs are available, and it has no role in the chronic management of asthma (p.777). It has been given by nebulisation in severe croup (p.1079). Adrenaline is used for a number of other indications including the control of minor bleeding from the skin and mucous membranes, in ophthalmology chiefly for the management of open-angle (simple) glaucoma (p.1485), and also as an adjunct to local anaesthesia (p.1369). Adrenaline was formerly incorporated into creams used in the treatment of rheumatic and muscular disorders, and in rectal preparations used in the treatment of haemorrhoids. Racepinefrine (racemic adrenaline) and racepinefrine hydrochloride have been used for bronchodilatation.

Adrenaline is given by subcutaneous or intramuscular injection. In extreme emergencies, where a more rapid effect is required, adrenaline may be given as a dilute solution (1 in 10 000 or 1 in 100 000) by very slow intravenous injection or by slow intravenous infusion. Intraosseous administration, usually into the marrow of the tibia, is sometimes used as an alternative to the intravenous route. Adrenaline has sometimes been injected directly in the heart but current guidelines for the management of cardiac emergencies recommend administration via a central vein. Endotracheal administration is occasionally used when intravenous access cannot be obtained. Adrenaline may be applied topically and can be given by inhalation. Aqueous solutions of adrenaline are usually prepared using the acid tartrate or the hydrochloride but the dosage is generally stated in terms of the equivalent content of adrenaline. Adrenaline acid tartrate 1.8 mg or adrenaline hydrochloride 1.2 mg is approximately equivalent to 1 mg of adrenaline.

The usual dose of adrenaline in **anaphylactic shock** is 500 micrograms (0.5 mL of a 1 in 1000 solution) by intramuscular injection repeated as necessary every 5 minutes. A dose of 300 micrograms (0.3 mL of a 1 in 1000 solution) may be appropriate for emergency self-administration. Children's doses range from 120 to 250 micrograms depending on age; 50 micrograms may be used in infants under 6 months of age. If intravenous administration is required the dose is 500 micrograms for adults and 10 micrograms/kg for children, given as a more dilute 1 in 10 000 solution at a rate of 1 mL (100 micrograms) or less per minute.

In **advanced cardiac life support** the initial dose of adrenaline for adults is 1 mg intravenously (10 mL of a 1 in 10 000 solution), preferably into a central vein, and this may be repeated as often as every 2 to 3 minutes in some circumstances for up to an hour. Higher doses have been used but are no longer generally recommended. Children may be given intravenous doses of 10 micrograms/kg initially then 100 micrograms/kg. Intraosseous doses are the same as those used intravenously. Endotracheal doses for adults are 2 to 3 times the intravenous dose; children may be given 100 micrograms/kg.

Adrenaline relaxes the bronchial musculature and has sometimes been injected subcutaneously or intramuscularly in the management of **acute asthmatic attacks**. However, in general, the use of adrenaline in asthma has been superseded by beta$_2$ agonists, such as salbutamol, which can alleviate bronchospasm with fewer effects on the heart. If adrenaline is to be used, the adult dose is 0.3 to 0.5 mL of a 1 in 1000 aqueous solution (300 to 500 micrograms); children have received 0.01 mL/kg (10 micrograms/kg) to a maximum of 0.5 mL (500 micrograms). Aqueous solutions with an adrenaline content equivalent to 1 in 100 have occasionally been used by inhalation as a spray to alleviate asthmatic attacks; these solutions must never be confused with the weaker strength used for injection. Pressurised aerosols delivering metered doses equivalent to approximately 160 micrograms to 275 micrograms of adrenaline have also been used; adults have received 1 or 2 metered inhalations repeated, if necessary, after 3 hours.

Adrenaline is frequently added to **local anaesthetics** to retard diffusion and limit absorption, to prolong the duration of effect, and to lessen the danger of toxicity. A concentration of 1 in 200 000 (5 micrograms/mL) is usually used; adrenaline should not be added when procedures involve digits, ears, nose, penis, or scrotum owing to the risk of ischaemic tissue necrosis. A concentration of up to 1 in 80 000 (12.5 micrograms/mL) may be used in dental preparations where the total dose given is small.

Adrenaline constricts arterioles and capillaries and causes blanching when applied locally to mucous membranes and exposed tissues. It is used as an aqueous solution in strengths up to a 1 in 1000 dilution to check capillary **bleeding**, epistaxis, and bleeding from superficial wounds and abrasions, but it does not stop internal haemorrhage. It is usually applied as a spray or on pledgets of cotton wool or gauze.

In ophthalmology, adrenaline solutions of 0.5%, 1%, or 2% are used as eye drops instilled once or twice daily to reduce intra-ocular pressure in open-angle **glaucoma** and ocular hypertension. An adrenaline borate complex (epinephryl borate) is also used in ophthalmology.

### Actions of sympathomimetics

Sympathomimetics have actions similar to those that follow stimulation of postganglionic sympathetic (or adrenergic) nerves. The three naturally occurring sympathomimetics are adrenaline, noradrenaline, and dopamine. All three are catecholamines, i.e. their aromatic portion is catechol (which is characterised by hydroxy groups at adjacent positions of a benzene ring) and the aliphatic portion is an amine. Despite widespread use of the term 'adrenergic' for sympathetic nerves, the physiological functions of adrenaline itself are predominantly metabolic. It is noradrenaline that is the endogenous neurotransmitter at postganglionic sympathetic nerves. Dopamine acts peripherally on the renal, mesenteric, and coronary vascular beds. Both noradrenaline and dopamine also have key roles as neurotransmitters within the CNS, but (in common with adrenaline) are highly polar and cannot cross the blood-brain barrier.

These three catecholamines differ markedly in effect according to their specificity for different adrenergic receptors.

Adrenergic receptors are divided into alpha and beta adrenoceptors. These are then subdivided into alpha$_1$ (postsynaptic) and alpha$_2$ (mainly presynaptic) types, and into beta$_1$, beta$_2$, and beta$_3$ receptors. A third distinct group of receptors that occur primarily within the CNS are described as dopamine receptors and at least 5 subtypes are known (see p.1196); $D_1$ receptors also occur within renal, mesenteric, and coronary vascular beds.

Stimulation of these different receptors produces the following effects:

- stimulation of alpha$_1$ receptors produces vasoconstriction, particularly in the vessels of the skin and mucosa, abdominal viscera, and kidney; this results in an increase in blood pressure, sometimes with compensatory reflex bradycardia; alpha$_1$ stimulation also results in contraction of other smooth muscle, including the urinary sphincter and the uterus, and induces mydriasis in the eye
- stimulation of alpha$_2$ receptors appears to play a role in feedback inhibition of neurotransmitter release and may be involved in the inhibition of intestinal activity; it also plays a role in the inhibition of insulin secretion

- stimulation of beta$_1$ receptors produces an increase in the rate and force of contraction of the heart, increased conduction velocity, and greater automaticity
- stimulation of beta$_2$ receptors produces vasodilatation, bronchodilatation, uterine relaxation, and a decrease in gastrointestinal motility; it also results in release of insulin and enhances gluconeogenesis and glycogenolysis
- stimulation of beta$_3$ receptors is thought to have a role in lipolysis and thermogenesis
- stimulation of D$_1$ receptors produces vasodilatation of renal, mesenteric, and coronary vessels.

The pattern of activity of the three catecholamines is complex and influenced not only by receptor specificity, but also by feedback mechanisms and receptor distribution. In broad terms:

- adrenaline is a potent agonist at both alpha and beta receptors
- noradrenaline is a potent agonist at alpha and beta$_1$ receptors, but has little effect on beta$_2$ receptors
- dopamine in low doses activates D$_1$ receptors; in higher doses it activates beta$_1$ and then alpha receptors, and also provokes release of noradrenaline from nerve terminals.

Other sympathomimetic drugs are analogues of the catecholamines and according to their structure either act directly on adrenergic receptors (e.g. phenylephrine) or indirectly (e.g. ephedrine, which also has direct actions). Indirect actions are achieved by displacing noradrenaline from storage vesicles within the nerve terminals. In practice many sympathomimetics have both direct and indirect actions.

Catecholamines have a fleeting action and are inactive by mouth whereas their analogues have a prolonged action and are active by mouth; the analogues are also less polar than the catecholamines and can often cross the blood-brain barrier. This ability to cross the blood-brain barrier explains why some sympathomimetics (e.g. dexamfetamine) have marked central stimulant effects. It may also explain the seemingly paradoxical antihypertensive effect of alpha$_2$-adrenergic agonists (e.g. clonidine) since their central effects may outweigh their effects in vascular smooth muscle.

**Advanced cardiac life support.** Adrenaline has an important role in advanced cardiac life support (p.812) since, through its alpha agonist effects, it increases myocardial and cerebral blood flow and thereby the efficacy of cardiopulmonary resuscitation or basic life support procedures. This should increase, although there is no clinical trial evidence for benefit.[1] Depending on the arrhythmia that has led to cardiac arrest, treatment starts with cardiopulmonary resuscitation and defibrillation. If these measures fail to restore a conventional rhythm, the next step involves the use of adrenaline.

For **adults**, adrenaline is given in a dose of 1 mg ideally intravenously into a central vein. If such venous access is not practicable adrenaline may be given through a peripheral vein followed by a flush of 20 mL or more of sodium chloride injection; however, the response is slower than with central venous injection. This intravenous dose of 1 mg may be given approximately every 3 minutes[2,3] or 3 to 5 minutes[4] in further cycles of cardiopulmonary resuscitation and, if necessary, shocks. A higher dose of 5 mg or 100 micrograms/kg has been given but there is insufficient evidence of benefit for this to be recommended.[2-4] In ventricular fibrillation or pulseless ventricular tachycardia, a resuscitation attempt may reasonably last for anything from 10 minutes to 1 hour with adrenaline 1 mg intravenously being given every 3 minutes during this period. Where the arrest is associated with asystole it is unlikely that a response will be achieved after 15 minutes.

The initial dose of 1 mg is reported to be based on the dose that was given by intracardiac injection, so it would be expected that a higher dose would be required for intravenous administration. However, studies[5-8] have failed to show any survival benefit with the use of higher doses.

The intravenous dose for **children** is 10 micrograms/kg as the first dose; a higher dose of 100 micrograms/kg[2-4] or possibly 200 micrograms/kg,[4] may be used for the second and subsequent doses. However, as with adults the use of the higher dose is not routinely recommended and a retrospective study[9] found no improvement in outcome.

The intraosseous route is a practicable alternative to intravenous injection for adults as well as for children, although the guidelines only give doses for children, which are identical to those given intravenously. Alternatively, adrenaline can be given through the endotracheal tube that will have been inserted, but only if the intravenous or intraosseous administration is delayed. Endotracheal doses for adults should be 2 to 3 times those used intravenously; for children doses of 100 micrograms/kg have been suggested. The adrenaline solution should be diluted and administered deeply using a catheter; several rapid ventilations or inflations should follow. It is recognised that the endotracheal route is imperfect[2-4] and some workers consider it to be ineffective.[10]

Although covering a somewhat different clinical situation some guidelines also include resuscitation of newborn infants (during the first few hours after birth).[2-4] Adrenaline may be used when the heart rate remains below 60 beats/minute despite adequate ventilation and chest compression. The dose of adrenaline is 10 to 30 micrograms/kg, repeated every 3 to 5 minutes as required; it is administered intravenously (generally into the umbilical vein) or by the endotracheal route.


1. Morley P. Vasopressin or epinephrine: which initial vasopressor for cardiac arrests? *Lancet* 2001; **358:** 85–6.
2. European Resuscitation Council. European Resuscitation Council Guidelines 2000. *Resuscitation* 2001; **48:** 199–239. Also available at: http://www.erc.edu/index.php/doclibrary/en/12/1 (accessed 06/07/04)
3. Resuscitation Council (UK). Resuscitation Guidelines 2000. Available at: http://www.resus.org.uk/pages/guide.htm (accessed 06/07/04)
4. The American Heart Association in collaboration with the International Liaison Committee on Resuscitation (ILCOR). International guidelines 2000 for cardiopulmonary resuscitation and emergency cardiovascular care: a consensus on science. *Circulation* 2000; **102** (suppl I): I1–I384. Also published in *Resuscitation* 2000; **46:** 3–447.
5. Stiell IG, *et al.* High-dose epinephrine in adult cardiac arrest. *N Engl J Med* 1992; **327:** 1045–50.
6. Brown CG, *et al.* A comparison of standard-dose and high-dose epinephrine in cardiac arrest outside the hospital. *N Engl J Med* 1992; **327:** 1051–5.
7. Callaham M, *et al.* A randomized clinical trial of high-dose epinephrine and norepinephrine vs standard-dose epinephrine in prehospital cardiac arrest. *JAMA* 1992; **268:** 2667–72.
8. Gueugniaud P-Y, *et al.* A comparison of repeated high doses and repeated standard doses of epinephrine for cardiac arrest outside the hospital. *N Engl J Med* 1998; **339:** 1595–1601.
9. Carpenter TC, Stenmark KR. High-dose epinephrine is not superior to standard-dose epinephrine in pediatric in-hospital cardiopulmonary arrest. *Pediatrics* 1997; **99:** 403–8.
10. McCrirrick A, Monk CR. Comparison of i.v. and intra-tracheal administration of adrenaline. *Br J Anaesth* 1994; **72:** 529–32.


**Anaphylactic shock.** Anaphylactic shock is usually a type 1 hypersensitivity reaction (p.421) to various allergens such as drugs, foods, latex, and insect venoms. A clinically identical reaction can, however, be provoked by a type II mechanism, as in blood transfusion reactions, or a type III mechanism, as in drug-induced serum sickness reactions. It is a medical emergency and prompt treatment of laryngeal oedema, bronchospasm, and hypotension is necessary. Adrenaline causes bronchodilatation and peripheral vasoconstriction, reducing oedema and increasing blood pressure, and is the cornerstone of management.[1-9] However, it may not always be effective,[2] and its use is not without hazard.[10]

In early anaphylaxis, vasodilatation is the main pathological change and cardiac output and blood flow to skin and muscle may be increased enabling intramuscular absorption of adrenaline to be sufficiently rapid and effective. The subcutaneous route has been used, especially by patients treating themselves, but intramuscular absorption is more rapid and is generally preferred.[6,8,9] Prefilled syringes for intramuscular or subcutaneous administration of adrenaline are available for those known to be at high risk of developing anaphylactic shock. Such syringes mean that patients can self-administer their initial emergency treatment; they should still seek medical assistance as additional treatment may be required.[2] In the early stages adrenaline may be given by inhalation and is sometimes taken with an antihistamine.[11] However, this should not be a substitute for adrenaline injection in patients with a history of acute attacks, and the number of inhalations required may limit the use of this route in children.[12] As anaphylaxis progresses the intravascular volume becomes depleted, shock occurs, and at this stage the intravenous route is probably necessary to enable absorption.[1] However, this route is hazardous and should only be used in life-threatening situations.[6,8,10] The general principles used in the management of hypovolaemia and hypotension in shock are outlined on p.835.

The dose of adrenaline for intramuscular injection is usually 500 micrograms (0.5 mL of a 1 in 1000 solution), which may be repeated at 5-minute intervals, according to blood pressure and pulse, until improvement occurs. Some use lower doses of 200 to 500 micrograms (0.2 to 0.5 mL of a 1 in 1000 solution) for intramuscular or subcutaneous injection. A more dilute solution of 1 in 10 000 is used for slow intravenous administration when the dose is 500 micrograms (5 mL) given at a rate of 100 micrograms/minute (1 mL/minute), stopping when a response has been obtained.

Various adrenaline dosage regimens have been suggested for children.[2,3,5,8,9] In one widely used regimen, the intramuscular dose for children using the 1 in 1000 solution ranges from: 50 micrograms (0.05 mL) for those under 6 months; 120 micrograms (0.12 mL) for those aged 6 months to 6 years; and 250 micrograms (0.25 mL) for children aged 6 to 12 years. Doses of 150 or 300 micrograms may be given if an auto-injector is used, but may not be suitable for children weighing less than 15 kg. The intravenous dose for children, employing the 1 in 10 000 solution, is 10 micrograms/kg (0.1 mL/kg).

A slow intravenous injection of an antihistamine, such as chlorphenamine 10 to 20 mg, may be given immediately after the adrenaline and repeated over the subsequent 24 to 48 hours to prevent relapse. Although antihistamines are particularly effective in the management of angioedema, pruritus, and urticaria, they remain second-line treatment. Intravenous corticosteroids have little place in the immediate management of anaphylaxis, since their beneficial effects are delayed for several hours but in severely ill patients early administration of hydrocortisone 100 to 500 mg as the sodium succinate may help prevent deterioration after the primary treatment has been given. Also some consider that asthmatics who have relatively recently undergone regular corticosteroid treatment may benefit from hydrocortisone.[2] Patients should also receive oxygen as required.

Continuing deterioration with circulatory collapse, bronchospasm, or laryngeal oedema requires further treatment including intravenous fluids, a nebulised beta$_2$ agonist (such as salbutamol or terbutaline), intravenous aminophylline, assisted respiration (if necessary), and possibly, emergency tracheostomy.[6,7]

It should be remembered that patients receiving some non-cardioselective beta blockers may be relatively refractory to the effects of adrenaline used for anaphylactic shock (see under Interactions for Adrenaline, above); in such cases the use of a more selective beta$_2$ agonist such as salbutamol by intravenous injection should be considered. Glucagon is another alternative to adrenaline in such patients.[6,13]

Other measures to prevent anaphylaxis include desensitisation in patients who have reacted to bee or wasp venom.[14]


1. Fisher M. Treating anaphylaxis with sympathomimetic drugs. *BMJ* 1992; **305:** 1107–8.
2. Patel L, *et al.* Management of anaphylactic reactions to food. *Arch Dis Child* 1994; **71:** 370–5.
3. Fisher M. Treatment of acute anaphylaxis. *BMJ* 1995; **311:** 731–3. Correction. *ibid.*; 937.
4. Ewan PW. Treatment of anaphylactic reactions. *Prescribers' J* 1997; **37:** 125–32.
5. Ewan PW. Anaphylaxis. *BMJ* 1998; **316:** 1442–5. Correction. *ibid.*; 1587.
6. The American Heart Association in collaboration with the International Liaison Committee on Resuscitation. Guidelines 2000 for cardiopulmonary resuscitation and emergency cardiovascular care. Part 8: advanced challenges in resuscitation: section 3: special challenges in ECC. *Circulation* 2000; **102** (suppl I): I229–I252.
7. Drain KL, Volcheck GW. Preventing and managing drug-induced anaphylaxis. *Drug Safety* 2001; **24:** 843–53.
8. Project Team of the Resuscitation Council (UK). The emergency medical treatment of anaphylactic reactions for first medical responders and for community nurses (revised January 2002). Available at: http://www.resus.org.uk/pages/reaction.htm (accessed 06/07/04)
9. Anonymous. Injectable adrenaline for children. *Drug Ther Bull* 2003; **41:** 21–24.
10. Johnston SL, *et al.* Adrenaline given outside the context of life threatening allergic reactions. *BMJ* 2003; **326:** 589–90.
11. Hourihane JO'B, Warner JO. Management of anaphylactic reactions to food. *Arch Dis Child* 1995; **72:** 274.
12. Simons FER, *et al.* Can epinephrine inhalations be substituted for epinephrine injection in children at risk for systemic anaphylaxis? *Pediatrics* 2000; **106:** 1040–4.
13. Lang DM. Anaphylactoid and anaphylactic reactions: hazards of β-blockers. *Drug Safety* 1995; **12:** 299–304.
14. Frew AJ, *et al.* Injection immunotherapy. *BMJ* 1993; **307:** 919–23.


**Haemorrhage.** Adrenaline has a long history of being applied topically to check minor bleeding. It constricts arterioles and capillaries and causes blanching. Local injection of adrenaline under endoscopic control is highly effective in controlling bleeding peptic ulcers (p.1246), and has also been combined with other therapies such as a contact thermal probe.[1]


1. Chung SSC, *et al.* Randomised comparison between adrenaline injection alone and adrenaline injection plus heat probe treatment for actively bleeding ulcers. *BMJ* 1997; **314:** 1307–11.


**Priapism.** Aspiration of blood followed by intracavernosal irrigation with a dilute adrenaline solution was reported to be effective treatment for priapism in a group of young patients (age range, 3.9 to 18.3 years) with sickle-cell disease.[1]

For reference to adrenaline in low dosage and dilute solution being given by intracavernosal injection to reverse priapism caused by alprostadil, see p.1513.


1. Mantadakis E, *et al.* Outpatient penile aspiration and epinephrine irrigation for young patients with sickle cell anemia and prolonged priapism. *Blood* 2000; **95:** 78–82.


**Respiratory-tract disorders.** Nebulised adrenaline may be used to reverse airway obstruction in inflammatory disorders such as croup since it relieves inflammation and also causes bronchodilatation. Although some studies in acute viral bronchiolitis (see Respiratory Syncytial Virus Infection, p.625) have shown improvement in clinical scores,[1,2] randomised studies have failed to find any difference in outcome between infants treated with adrenaline and either salbutamol[3] or placebo,[4] and a systematic review[5] found insufficient evidence to support its use.

However, the *British National Formulary* states that for severe croup not effectively controlled with corticosteroids, nebulised adrenaline solution 1 in 1000 may be given with close clinical monitoring in a dose of 400 micrograms/kg (up to a maximum of 5 mg) repeated after 30 minutes if necessary. The effects of nebulised adrenaline are expected to last 2 to 3 hours.

There has also been a report[6] of the successful use of nebulised adrenaline in a 15-month-old child with airway inflammation secondary to the ingestion of sodium hypochlorite.


1. Reijonen T, *et al.* The clinical efficacy of nebulized racemic epinephrine and albuterol in acute bronchiolitis. *Arch Pediatr Adolesc Med* 1995; **149:** 686–92.
2. Menon K, *et al.* A randomized trial comparing the efficacy of epinephrine with salbutamol in the treatment of acute bronchiolitis. *J Pediatr* 1995; **126:** 1004–7.
3. Patel H, *et al.* A randomized, controlled trial of the effectiveness of nebulized therapy with epinephrine compared with albuterol and saline in infants hospitalized for acute viral bronchiolitis. *J Pediatr* 2002; **141:** 818–24.
4. Wainwright C, *et al.* A multicenter, randomized, double-blind, controlled trial of nebulized epinephrine in infants with acute bronchiolitis. *N Engl J Med* 2003; **349:** 27–35.

5. Hartling L, *et al.* Epinephrine for bronchiolitis. Available in The Cochrane Library; Issue 1. Chichester: John Wiley; 2004.
6. Ziegler D, Bent G. Caustic-induced upper airway obstruction responsiveness to nebulized adrenaline. *Pediatrics* 2001; **107:** 807–8.

## Preparations

**BP 2003:** Adrenaline Eye Drops; Adrenaline Injection; Adrenaline Solution; Bupivacaine and Adrenaline Injection; Dilute Adrenaline Injection 1 in 10,000; Lidocaine and Adrenaline Injection;
**USP 27:** Cocaine and Tetracaine Hydrochlorides and Epinephrine Topical Solution; Epinephrine Bitartrate for Ophthalmic Solution; Epinephrine Bitartrate Inhalation Aerosol; Epinephrine Bitartrate Ophthalmic Solution; Epinephrine Inhalation Aerosol; Epinephrine Inhalation Solution; Epinephrine Injection; Epinephrine Nasal Solution; Epinephrine Ophthalmic Solution; Epinephryl Borate Ophthalmic Solution; Lidocaine Hydrochloride and Epinephrine Injection; Prilocaine and Epinephrine Injection; Procaine Hydrochloride and Epinephrine Injection; Racepinephrine Inhalation Solution.

**Proprietary Preparations** (details are given in Part 3)
**Austral.:** Epipen; **Austria:** Epipen; Glycirenan†; Suprarenin; **Belg.:** Epipen†; **Braz.:** Drenalin; Nefrin; **Canad.:** Bronkaid†; Epi EZ†; Epifrin†; Epipen; Vaponefrin; **Denm.:** Epipen; **Fin.:** Epipen; **Fr.:** Anahelp; Anakit†; Anapen; Dyspne-Inhal†; Eppy†; **Ger.:** Anaphylaxie-Besteck†; Fastjekt; InfectoKrupp; Suprarenin; **Irl.:** Eppy; Simplene†; **Israel:** Epipen; **Ital.:** Eppy†; Fastjekt; **Mex.:** Pinadrina; **Norw.:** Epipen; **NZ:** Epipen; **Port.:** Anapen†; Epipen; **S.Afr.:** Ana-Guard†; Epipen; Eppy†; Simplene†; **Spain:** Adreject; **Swed.:** Epipen; Eppy; Glaufrin†; **Switz.:** Epipen; Gingi-Pak†; Medihaler-Epi†; Orostat†; Surgident†; **UK:** Anapen; Epipen; Eppy†; Simplene†; **USA:** AsthmaHaler Mist; AsthmaNefrin; Epifrin; Epinal; Epipen; Glaucon; microNefrin; Nephron; Primatene Mist; Primatene Mist Suspension; S-2; Sus-Phrine†.

**Multi-ingredient: Arg.:** Asmopul; Yanal; **Austral.:** Rectinol; **Belg.:** Glaucofrin†; **Braz.:** Novaboin†; **Canad.:** Ana-Kit†; E-Pilo†; **Denm.:** Suprexon†; **Fr.:** Glaucadrine†; Sirop Boin†; **Ger.:** Links-Glaukosan; Mydrial-Atropin; Suprexon†; **India:** Brovon; **Irl.:** Ganda; **Ital.:** Pilodren; Rinantipiol; **Neth.:** Glaucofrin†; Suprexon†; **NZ:** Ana-Kit†; **Port.:** Adrinex; **Spain:** Coliriocilina Adren Astr; Epistaxol; **Switz.:** Glaucadrine†; Haemocortin; Medi-Kord†; Suprexon†; **UK:** Brovon; Ganda†; **USA:** Ana-Kit; E-Pilo; Emergent-Ez.

*Used as an adjunct in:* **Arg.:** Caina G; Duracaine; Gobbicaina; Larjancaina; Xylocaina; **Austral.:** Citanest Dental; Lignospan; Marcain; Nurocain; Nurocain with Sympathin†; Scandonest; Xylocaine; **Austria:** Carbostesin; Neo-Xylestesin; Neo-Xylestesin forte and Neo-Xylestesin special; Scandonest; Septanest; Ubistesin; Ultracain Dental; Xylanaest; Xylocain; **Belg.:** Citanest; Marcaine; Xylocaine; **Braz.:** Bupiabbott Plus; Carbostesin†; Lidocabbott; Lidogeyer; Marcaina; Neocaina; Novabupi; Scandicaine†; Septanest†; Xylestesin; Xylocaina; **Canad.:** Astracaine; Citanest; Marcaine; Sensorcaine; Ultracaine D-S†; Xylocaine; **Denm.:** Carbocain; Marcain; Scandonest; Septanest; Septocaine; Xylocain; **Fin.:** Marcain; Ultracain D-Suprarenin; Xylocain; **Fr.:** Alphacaine; Duranest†; Marcaine; Predesic; Xylocaine; **Ger.:** Anaesthol†; Carbostesin; Lidocaton†; Meaverin "A" mit Adrenalin†; Ubistesin; Ultracain D-S; Ultracain Suprarenin; Xylestesin-A, Xylestesin centro; Xylestesin-S; Xylocain; Xylocitin; Xylonest; **Gr.:** Marcaine; Xylocaine; **Hong Kong:** Marcaine; Xylestin-A; Xylocaine; **India:** Gesicain; Xylocaine; **Irl.:** Marcain; Xylocaine; **Israel:** Kamacaine; Lidocadren; Marcaine; **Ital.:** Alfacaina; Bupicain; Bupiforan; Bupisen; Bupisolver; Bupixamol; Bupyl†; Carbocaina; Carbosen; Cartidont; Citocartin; Ecocain; Lident Adrenalina; Lident Andrenor; Lidomol; Marcaina; Mepi-Mynol†; Mepicain; Mepident; Mepiforan; Mepisolver; Mepivamol; Mepyl†; Molcain; Optocain; Primacaine; Scandonest; Septanest; Ubistesin; Ultracain D-S†; Xilo-Mynol†; Xylocaina; Xylonor; **Malaysia:** Marcain; **Mex.:** Buvacaina; Pisacaina; Xylocaina; **Neth.:** Citanest; Marcaine; Scandicaine; Ultracain D-S; Xylocaine; **Norw.:** Marcain; Septocaine; Xylocain; **NZ:** Marcain; Nurocain†; Xylocaine; **Port.:** Bupinostrum Adrenalina; Lidonostrum; Lincaina; Scandinibsa; Xilonibsa; **S.Afr.:** Lignospan Special; Macaine; Scandonest; Xylotox; **Singapore:** Xylocaine; **Spain:** Anestesia Loc Braun C/A†; Anestesia Topi Braun C/A; Articaina C/E; Meganest; Scandinibsa; Stoma Anestesia Dental†; Ultracain; Xilonibsa; Xylonor Especial; **Swed.:** Carbocain; Marcain; Xylocain; **Switz.:** Alphacaine; Carbostesin; Lidocaton†; Lignospan; Rapidocaine; Rudocaine; Scandonest; Septanest; Ubistesin; Ultracaine D-S; Xylestesin-S "special"; Xylocain; Xylonest; Xylonor†; **Thai.:** Lidocation; Lidocaton; Xylocaine; Xylotox; **UAE:** Ecocain; **UK:** Lignostab-A; Marcain; Septanest; Xylocaine; Xylotox; **USA:** Citanest; Duranest†; Marcaine; Octocaine; Sensorcaine; Septocaine; Xylocaine.

## Ajmaline

Ajmalina; Ajmalinum; Rauwolfine. (17*R*,21*R*)-Ajmalan-17,21-diol.
$C_{20}H_{26}N_2O_2$ = 326.4.
*CAS — 4360-12-7.*
*ATC — C01BA05.*

**Pharmacopoeias.** In *Jpn.*

### Adverse Effects

Ajmaline depresses the conductivity of the heart, and at high doses can cause heart block. At very high doses it may produce a negative inotropic effect. High doses may cause cardiac arrhythmias, coma, and death. Arrhythmias have also been reported after usual intravenous doses (see below). Adverse neurological effects have been reported including eye twitching, convulsions, and respiratory depression. Hepatotoxicity and agranulocytosis may occasionally occur.

**Effects on the heart.** Electrophysiologic study[1] in 1955 patients revealed that ajmaline 1 mg/kg given intravenously could induce arrhythmias; 63 developed a supraventricular arrhythmia and 7 an atrioventricular re-entrant tachycardia.

1. Brembilla-Perrot B, Terrier de la Chaise A. Provocation of supraventricular tachycardias by an intravenous class I antiarrhythmic drug. *Int J Cardiol* 1992; **34:** 189–98.

### Precautions

As for Quinidine, p.992.

### Interactions

**Antiarrhythmics.** Oral use of *quinidine* with ajmaline increased plasma concentrations of ajmaline considerably in 4 healthy subjects; the elimination half-life of ajmaline was increased about twofold.[1] The pharmacokinetics of quinidine did not seem to be affected by ajmaline.

1. Hori R, *et al.* Quinidine-induced rise in ajmaline plasma concentration. *J Pharm Pharmacol* 1984; **36:** 202–4.

### Uses and Administration

Ajmaline is an alkaloid obtained from the root of *Rauwolfia serpentina* (Apocynaceae). It is a class Ia antiarrhythmic (p.809) used in the treatment of supraventricular and ventricular arrhythmias (p.816) and for differential diagnosis of Wolff-Parkinson-White syndrome. Ajmaline is given by intravenous injection in a usual dose of 50 mg over at least 5 minutes. It may also be given by intravenous infusion, and has been given by mouth and by intramuscular injection.

Ajmaline has also been used as the hydrochloride, monoethanolate, and as the phenobarbital salt.

### Preparations

**Proprietary Preparations** (details are given in Part 3)
**Austria:** Gilurytmal; **Ger.:** Gilurytmal; Tachmalin†; **Ital.:** Aritmina†; **Spain:** Gilurytmal†.

**Multi-ingredient: Spain:** Diu Rauwiplus†.

## Alacepril *(rINN)*

DU-1219. *N*-{1-[(*S*)-3-Mercapto-2-methylpropionyl]-L-prolyl}-3-phenyl-L-alanine acetate.
$C_{20}H_{26}N_2O_5S$ = 406.5.
*CAS — 74258-86-9.*

### Profile

Alacepril is an ACE inhibitor (p.842) used in the treatment of hypertension (p.825). It is converted to captopril and desacetylalacepril (DU-1227) in the body following oral administration. It is given by mouth in a usual dose of 25 to 75 mg daily, as a single dose or in two divided doses.

### Preparations

**Proprietary Preparations** (details are given in Part 3)
**Jpn:** Cetapril.

## Alfuzosin Hydrochloride

*(BANM, USAN, rINNM)*

Alfuzosini Hydrochloridum; Hidrocloruro de alfuzosina; SL-77499-10; SL-77499 (alfuzosin). *N*-{3-[4-Amino-6,7-dimethoxyquinazolin-2-yl(methyl)amino]propyl}tetrahydro-2-furamide hydrochloride.
$C_{19}H_{27}N_5O_4$,HCl = 425.9.
*CAS — 81403-80-7 (alfuzosin); 81403-68-1 (alfuzosin hydrochloride).*
*ATC — G04CA01.*

**Pharmacopoeias.** In *Eur.* (see p.vi).

**Ph. Eur. 5.0** (Alfuzosin Hydrochloride). A white or almost white, slightly hygroscopic, crystalline powder. Freely soluble in water; sparingly soluble in alcohol; practically insoluble in dichloromethane. A 2% solution in water has a pH of 4.0 to 6.0. Store in airtight containers. Protect from light.

### Adverse Effects, Treatment, and Precautions

As for Prazosin Hydrochloride, p.985. Alfuzosin may be more selective for the urinary tract and vasodilator effects may be less frequent. It should be avoided in severe hepatic impairment.

◊ References.

1. Lukacs B, *et al.* Safety profile of 3 months' therapy with alfuzosin in 13,389 patients suffering from benign prostatic hypertrophy. *Eur Urol* 1996; **29:** 29–35.

### Interactions

As for Prazosin Hydrochloride, p.985.

### Pharmacokinetics

Alfuzosin is readily absorbed after oral administration and peak plasma concentrations generally occur 0.5 to 3 hours after a dose; bioavailability is about 64%. Absorption of the modified-release preparation is improved if given with food. It is extensively metabolised in the liver to inactive metabolites and excreted primarily in faeces via the bile. Only about 11% of a dose is excreted unchanged in the urine. Alfuzosin has a plasma elimination half-life of 3 to 5 hours. It is 90% bound to plasma proteins.

### Uses and Administration

Alfuzosin is an alpha$_1$-adrenoceptor blocker (p.809) with actions similar to those of prazosin (p.986). It is used in benign prostatic hyperplasia (p.1555) to relieve symptoms of urinary obstruction, including acute urinary retention, and has been tried in the treatment of hypertension.

Alfuzosin is given by mouth as the hydrochloride. Like other alpha$_1$-adrenoceptor blockers, it may cause collapse in some patients after the first dose, which should therefore be given just before bedtime to reduce the risk. Doses may need to be reduced in patients with hepatic or renal impairment (see below); the initial dose should also be reduced in the elderly.

In **benign prostatic hyperplasia,** the usual dose is 2.5 mg three times daily, increased to 10 mg daily if necessary. A modified-release preparation may also be used in a dose of 10 mg once daily.

In patients aged over 65 years catheterised for **acute urinary retention** associated with benign prostatic hyperplasia, a modified-release preparation may be given in a dose of 10 mg once daily for 3 to 4 days.

◊ References.

1. Jardin A, *et al.* Alfuzosin for treatment of benign prostatic hypertrophy. *Lancet* 1991; **337:** 1457–61.
2. Wilde MI, *et al.* Alfuzosin: a review of its pharmacodynamic and pharmacokinetic properties, and therapeutic potential in benign prostatic hyperplasia. *Drugs* 1993; **45:** 410–29.
3. McKeage K, Plosker GL. Alfuzosin: a review of the therapeutic use of the prolonged-release formulation given once daily in the management of benign prostatic hyperplasia. *Drugs* 2002; **62:** 633–53.
4. Lee M. Alfuzosin hydrochloride for the treatment of benign prostatic hyperplasia. *Am J Health-Syst Pharm* 2003; **60:** 1426–39. Correction. *ibid.* 2004; **61:** 437.

**Administration in hepatic or renal impairment.** In patients with mild to moderate hepatic impairment the initial dose of alfuzosin hydrochloride should be 2.5 mg daily, increased to 2.5 mg twice daily according to response; modified-release preparations are contra-indicated.

In patients with renal impairment, 2.5 mg twice daily should be given initially, adjusted according to response. Although the UK manufacturer advises caution with the use of modified-release preparations in severe renal impairment, a study[1] in patients with varying degrees of renal impairment (including severe) suggested that no dose reduction was necessary.

1. Marbury TC, *et al.* Pharmacokinetics and safety of a single oral dose of once-daily alfuzosin, 10 mg, in male subjects with mild to severe renal impairment. *J Clin Pharmacol* 2002; **42:** 1311–17.

### Preparations

**Proprietary Preparations** (details are given in Part 3)
**Arg.:** Dalfaz; UroXatral; **Austria:** Urion; Xatral; **Belg.:** Xatral; **Braz.:** Xatral†; **Chile:** UroXatral; **Denm.:** Xatral; **Fin.:** Xatral; **Fr.:** Urion; Xatral; **Ger.:** Urion; UroXatral; **Gr.:** Xatral; **Hong Kong:** Xatral; **Irl.:** Xatral; **Israel:** Xatral; **Ital.:** Benestan†; Mittoval; Xatral; **Malaysia:** Xatral; **Neth.:** Xatral; **Norw.:** Xatral; **Port.:** Benestan; **S.Afr.:** Xatral; **Singapore:** Xatral; **Spain:** Alfetim; Benestan; Dalfaz†; **Swed.:** Xatral; **Switz.:** Xatral; **Thai.:** Xatral; **UK:** Xatral; **USA:** UroXatral.

## Alprenolol *(BAN, rINN)*

1-(2-Allylphenoxy)-3-isopropylaminopropan-2-ol.
$C_{15}H_{23}NO_2$ = 249.3.
*CAS — 13655-52-2.*
*ATC — C07AA01.*

## Alprenolol Benzoate *(BANM, rINNM)*

Alprenololi Benzoas; Benzoato de alprenolol.
$C_{22}H_{29}NO_4$ = 371.5.
*ATC — C07AA01.*

## Alprenolol Hydrochloride *(BANM, USAN, rINNM)*

Alprenololi Hydrochloridum; H56/28; Hidrocloruro de alprenolol.
$C_{15}H_{23}NO_2$,HCl = 285.8.
*CAS — 13707-88-5.*
*ATC — C07AA01.*

**Pharmacopoeias.** In *Eur.* (see p.vi) and *Jpn.*

**Ph. Eur. 5.0** (Alprenolol Hydrochloride). A white crystalline powder or colourless crystals. Very soluble in water; freely soluble in alcohol and in dichloromethane. Protect from light.

### Profile

Alprenolol is a non-cardioselective beta blocker (p.868). It is reported to have intrinsic sympathomimetic activity and some membrane-stabilising properties.

Alprenolol has been given by mouth, as the benzoate or hydrochloride, in the management of hypertension, angina pectoris, and cardiac arrhythmias.

### Preparations

**Proprietary Preparations** (details are given in Part 3)
**Belg.:** Aptine†; **Denm.:** Aptin†; **Ger.:** Aptin†; **Norw.:** Aptin†; **Swed.:** Aptin N†.

## Alteplase (BAN, USAN, rINN)

Alteplasa; G-11035; G-11044; G-11021 (2-chain form); Recombinant Tissue-type Plasminogen Activator; rt-PA.

CAS — 105857-23-6.

ATC — B01AD02; S01XA13.

**Description.** Alteplase is a glycosylated protein of 527 residues having the amino acid sequence of human tissue plasminogen activator (t-PA) and produced by recombinant DNA technology.

**Pharmacopoeias.** In *US*. *Eur.* (see p.vi) includes Alteplase for Injection.

**Ph. Eur. 5.0** (Alteplase for Injection; Alteplasum ad Iniectabile). A sterile, freeze-dried preparation of alteplase, a tissue plasminogen activator produced by recombinant DNA technology. It has a potency of not less than 500 000 units/mg of protein. It is a white or slightly yellow powder or friable mass. The reconstituted preparation has a pH of 7.1 to 7.5. Store in colourless glass containers, under vacuum or an inert gas, at a temperature between 2° and 30°. Protect from light. Alteplase consists of 527 amino acids with carbohydrate moieties attached.

**USP 27** (Alteplase). A highly purified glycosylated serine protease with fibrin-binding properties and plasminogen-specific proteolytic activities. It is produced by recombinant DNA synthesis in mammalian cell culture. It has a potency of 522 000 to 667 000 USP units/mg of protein. Store in airtight containers in the frozen state at a temperature of −20° or below.

**Incompatibility and Stability.** Incompatibility has been reported[1] between alteplase and dobutamine, dopamine, glyceryl trinitrate, and heparin, although a subsequent study found no incompatibility between alteplase and glyceryl trinitrate.[2] Another study[3] found that dilution of a proprietary preparation of alteplase (Activase) to 0.09 and 0.16 mg/mL with glucose 5% resulted in precipitation of the drug. Alteplase is formulated with arginine as a solubilising agent, and dilution with glucose 5% to concentrations below 0.5 mg/mL of alteplase makes precipitation possible. Dilution with sodium chloride 0.9% is possible to concentrations down to 0.2 mg/mL before precipitation becomes a risk.

Studies[4,5] have suggested that a 1 mg/mL solution of alteplase retains its activity when frozen at −20° or below for up to 6 months.


1. Lee CY, *et al.* Visual and spectrophotometric determination of compatibility of alteplase and streptokinase with other injectable drugs. *Am J Hosp Pharm* 1990; **47:** 606–8.
2. Lam XM, *et al.* Stability and activity of alteplase with injectable drugs commonly used in cardiac therapy. *Am J Health-Syst Pharm* 1995; **52:** 1904–9.
3. Frazin BS. Maximal dilution of Activase. *Am J Hosp Pharm* 1990; **47:** 1016.
4. Calis KA, *et al.* Bioactivity of cryopreserved alteplase solutions. *Am J Health-Syst Pharm* 1999; **56:** 2056–7.
5. Wiernikowski JT, *et al.* Stability and sterility of recombinant tissue plasminogen activator at −30°C. *Lancet* 2000; **355:** 2221–2.


### Units

The activity of alteplase can be measured in terms of international units using the third International Standard for tissue plasminogen activator recombinant, human, established in 1999, although doses are generally expressed by weight.

### Adverse Effects, Treatment, and Precautions

As for Streptokinase, p.1005. Allergic reactions are less likely with alteplase than with streptokinase and repeated administration may be possible.

**Hypersensitivity.** An anaphylactoid reaction to alteplase occurred in a patient with a history of atopy.[1] For comment on this unexpected reaction, see Hypersensitivity under Adverse Effects of Streptokinase, p.1006.


1. Purvis JA, *et al.* Anaphylactoid reaction after injection of alteplase. *Lancet* 1993; **341:** 966–7.


**Thrombin generation.** Infusion of alteplase produces considerable thrombin generation which may result from direct activation of the coagulation system by plasmin or by positive feedback of the coagulation system by clot-bound thrombin. This excessive thrombin generation was considered a possible cause of myocardial infarction in a patient undergoing thrombolytic therapy with alteplase for venous thrombosis.[1] Infusion of streptokinase produced no evidence of excessive thrombin generation.


1. Baglin TP, *et al.* Thrombin generation and myocardial infarction during infusion of tissue-plasminogen activator. *Lancet* 1993; **341:** 504–5.


### Interactions

As for Streptokinase, p.1007.

**Glyceryl trinitrate.** Although thrombolytics and nitrates are both frequently used in acute myocardial infarction a report suggested that this combination may result in impaired thrombolysis. Concurrent intravenous administration of alteplase and glyceryl trinitrate to 36 patients with acute myocardial infarction produced lower plasma-antigen concentrations of tissue-plasminogen activator than alteplase given alone to 11 patients.[1] Reperfusion was sustained in only 44% of patients receiving both drugs compared with 91% of patients receiving alteplase alone. The authors of a subsequent study[2] suggested that these lower plasma concentrations may be due to increased hepatic metabolism of alteplase as a result of glyceryl trinitrate's effect of increasing hepatic blood flow.


1. Nicolini FA, *et al.* Concurrent nitroglycerin therapy impairs tissue-type plasminogen activator-induced thrombolysis in patients with acute myocardial infarction. *Am J Cardiol* 1994; **74:** 662–6.
2. Romeo F, *et al.* Concurrent nitroglycerin administration reduces the efficacy of recombinant tissue-type plasminogen activator in patients with acute anterior wall myocardial infarction. *Am Heart J* 1995; **130:** 692–7.


### Pharmacokinetics

Alteplase is cleared rapidly from the plasma, mainly by metabolism in the liver. It has an initial half-life of 4 to 5 minutes and a terminal half-life of about 40 minutes.

◊ References.


1. Krause J. Catabolism of tissue-type plasminogen activator (t-PA), its variants, mutants and hybrids. *Fibrinolysis* 1988; **2:** 133–42.


### Uses and Administration

Alteplase is a thrombolytic drug. It is a predominantly single-chain form of the endogenous enzyme tissue plasminogen activator and is produced by recombinant DNA technology. Like endogenous tissue plasminogen activator, alteplase converts fibrin-bound plasminogen to the active form plasmin, resulting in fibrinolysis and dissolution of clots. The mechanisms of fibrinolysis are discussed further under Haemostasis and Fibrinolysis on p.735. Alteplase has relatively little effect on circulating, unbound plasminogen and thus may be termed a fibrin-specific thrombolytic (see p.812).

Alteplase is used similarly to streptokinase (p.1007) in the treatment of thromboembolic disorders, particularly myocardial infarction (p.828) and venous thromboembolism (p.839), and to clear occluded catheters (see below). Alteplase may also be used in patients with acute ischaemic stroke (p.836).

In the treatment of acute **myocardial infarction**, alteplase is given intravenously as soon as possible after the onset of symptoms in a total dose of 100 mg; the total dose should not exceed 1.5 mg/kg in patients weighing less than 65 kg. The total dose may be given either over 1½ hours (accelerated or 'front-loaded' alteplase) or over 3 hours. The accelerated schedule has been recommended where administration is within 6 hours of myocardial infarction, while the 3-hour schedule has been recommended where administration is more than 6 hours after myocardial infarction. Administration over 1½ hours is as follows: 15 mg as an intravenous bolus, then 0.75 mg/kg, up to a maximum of 50 mg, by intravenous infusion over 30 minutes, followed by the remainder infused over the subsequent 60 minutes. Administration over 3 hours is as follows: 10 mg as an intravenous bolus, then 50 mg by intravenous infusion over 1 hour, followed by the remainder infused over the subsequent 2 hours.

In the treatment of **pulmonary embolism** a total dose of 100 mg is given; the total dose should not exceed 1.5 mg/kg in patients weighing less than 65 kg. The first 10 mg is given as an intravenous bolus and the remainder by intravenous infusion over 2 hours.

In acute **ischaemic stroke**, alteplase is given within 3 hours of the onset of symptoms in a dose of 0.9 mg/kg up to a maximum total dose of 90 mg. The dose is administered intravenously over 60 minutes with 10% being given as a bolus during the first minute.

To **restore function in central venous lines,** alteplase is instilled into the catheter at a concentration of 1 mg/mL. The usual dose is 2 mg, repeated after 2 hours if necessary. A total dose of 4 mg should not be exceeded. For children weighing between 10 and 30 kg, the dose is 110% of the internal lumen volume of the catheter, but should not exceed 2 mg, and may be repeated after 2 hours if necessary.

◊ General references.


1. Gillis JC, *et al.* Alteplase: a reappraisal of its pharmacological properties and therapeutic use in acute myocardial infarction. *Drugs* 1995; **50:** 102–36.
2. Wagstaff AJ, *et al.* Alteplase: a reappraisal of its pharmacology and therapeutic use in vascular disorders other than acute myocardial infarction. *Drugs* 1995; **50:** 289–316.


**Arterial and venous thromboembolism.** For the use of alteplase for arterial or venous thromboembolism in children, see Administration in children under Streptokinase, p.1007.

**Catheters and cannulas.** Alteplase has been used successfully to clear thrombi in central venous catheters.[1,2] Doses typically employed have been 2 mg injected as a bolus into the blocked catheter. Children have been treated similarly; in one study[3] where patients' weight started from 3 kg, doses ranged from 0.1 to 2.0 mg (as a 1 mg/mL solution), depending on the size of the catheter. A cohort study[4] used doses of 0.5 mg for children weighing 10 kg or under, and 1 to 2 mg above this weight, with a dwell time of 2 to 4 hours. In another report, two children[5] were successfully treated with intravenous alteplase in doses of 0.01 to 0.05 mg/kg per hour for venous thrombosis associated with indwelling intravascular catheters.

For reports covering the use of alteplase to treat intracardiac thrombosis resulting from the placement of central venous lines, see Intracardiac Thrombosis, below.


1. Paulsen D, *et al.* Use of tissue plasminogen activator for reopening of clotted dialysis catheters. *Nephron* 1993; **64:** 468–9.
2. Haire WD, *et al.* Urokinase versus recombinant tissue plasminogen activator in thrombosed central venous catheters: a double-blinded, randomized trial. *Thromb Haemost* 1994; **72:** 543–7.
3. Jacobs BR, *et al.* Recombinant tissue plasminogen activator in the treatment of central venous catheter occlusion in children. *J Pediatr* 2001; **139:** 593–6.
4. Choi M, *et al.* The use of alteplase to restore patency of central venous lines in pediatric patients: a cohort study. *J Pediatr* 2001; **139:** 152–6.
5. Doyle E, *et al.* Thrombolysis with low dose tissue plasminogen activator. *Arch Dis Child* 1992; **67:** 1483–4.


**Intracardiac thrombosis.** Alteplase has been used, in a dose of 100 mg given intravenously over two hours, for thrombosis of prosthetic heart valves.[1]

Alteplase has been used successfully in a neonate to treat intracardiac thrombosis associated with the use of a central venous line.[2] A dose of 500 micrograms/kg given over 10 minutes was followed by infusion of 200 micrograms/kg per hour for three days. In another report,[3] 4 preterm infants were treated successfully. All received 400 to 500 micrograms/kg of alteplase in a 20 to 30 minute bolus. This was followed in one case by a 3-hour infusion at 100 micrograms/kg per hour.


1. Astengo D, *et al.* Recombinant tissue plasminogen activator for prosthetic mitral-valve thrombosis. *N Engl J Med* 1995; **333:** 259.
2. Van Overmeire B, *et al.* Intracardiac thrombus formation with rapidly progressive heart failure in the neonate: treatment with tissue type plasminogen activator. *Arch Dis Child* 1992; **67:** 443–5.
3. Ferrari F, *et al.* Early intracardiac thrombosis in preterm infants and thrombolysis with recombinant tissue type plasminogen activator. *Arch Dis Child Fetal Neonatal Ed* 2001; **85:** F66–F69.


**Microvessel thrombosis.** Alteplase has been used in a number of conditions where the underlying pathology is occlusion of small blood vessels by microthrombi.

Purpura and loss of circulation in the hands of a patient recovering from **fulminant meningococcaemia**[1] responded to intra-arterial infusion of alteplase 20 to 40 micrograms/kg per hour for 22 hours in the right hand, and 20 micrograms/kg per hour for 11 hours in the left. Perfusion was successfully restored to both hands, and full function subsequently attained in them. Improvement was also achieved when alteplase was given to 2 infants with septic shock and purpura fulminans caused by meningococcal infection.[2]

Six patients[3] with ulcers caused by **livedoid vasculitis** and refractory to conventional treatment were treated with alteplase 10 mg infused intravenously over 4 hours daily for 14 days. Most ulcers healed rapidly; one patient required re-treatment with concomitant anticoagulation.

A 4-year-old girl[4] with **haemolytic-uraemic syndrome** (see under Thrombotic Microangiopathies, p.758) responded to treatment with an intravenous infusion of alteplase 200 micrograms/kg per hour for 5 hours, subsequently reduced to 50 micrograms/kg per hour for 14 days.

Alteplase use has been reviewed[5] and mixed results found, in patients with **veno-occlusive disease of the liver**, a serious complication of bone marrow transplantation that may be caused by diffuse thrombi in the hepatic venules. Although results in patients with established veno-occlusive disease have been disappointing,[6] one study[7] suggested that alteplase given early in the course of the disease improves response rate.


1. Keeley SR, *et al.* Tissue plasminogen activator for gangrene in fulminant meningococcaemia. *Lancet* 1991; **337:** 1359.
2. Zenz W, *et al.* Recombinant tissue plasminogen activator treatment in two infants with fulminant meningococcemia. *Pediatrics* 1995; **96:** 44–8.
3. Klein KL, Pittelkow MR. Tissue plasminogen activator for treatment of livedoid vasculitis. *Mayo Clin Proc* 1992; **67:** 923–33.
4. Kruez W, *et al.* Successful treatment of haemolytic uraemic syndrome with recombinant tissue-type plasminogen activator. *Lancet* 1993; **341:** 1665–6.
5. Terra SG, *et al.* A review of tissue plasminogen activator in the treatment of veno-occlusive liver disease after bone marrow transplantation. *Pharmacotherapy* 1997; **17:** 929–37.

6. Bearman SI, *et al.* Treatment of hepatic venocclusive disease with recombinant human tissue plasminogen activator and heparin in 42 marrow transplant patients. *Blood* 1997; **89:** 1501–6.
7. Schriber J, *et al.* Tissue plasminogen activator (tPA) as therapy for hepatotoxicity following bone marrow transplantation. *Bone Marrow Transplant* 1999; **24:** 1311–14.

**Ocular fibrinolysis.** Intra-ocular alteplase has been used to treat postoperative fibrinous deposits that can form after procedures such as surgery for cataracts[1] or glaucoma,[2] including cataracts in children.[3] Doses ranging from 6 to 25 micrograms have been used. Intra-ocular bleeding has occurred as a complication of such use.[2,4]

Intra-ocular alteplase has also been used for treatment of subhyaloid haemorrhage,[5,6] including that seen in shaken baby syndrome.[7]

1. Heiligenhaus A, *et al.* Recombinant tissue plasminogen activator in cases with fibrin formation after cataract surgery: a prospective randomised multicentre study. *Br J Ophthalmol* 1998; **82:** 810–15.
2. Lundy DC, *et al.* Intracameral tissue plasminogen activator after glaucoma surgery: indications, effectiveness, and complications. *Ophthalmology* 1996; **103:** 274–82.
3. Mehta JS, Adams GGW. Recombinant tissue plasminogen activator following paediatric cataract surgery. *Br J Ophthalmol* 2000; **84:** 983–6.
4. Azuara-Blanco A, Wilson RP. Intraocular and extraocular bleeding after intracameral injection of tissue plasminogen activator. *Br J Ophthalmol* 1998; **82:** 1345–6.
5. Schmitz K, *et al.* Therapy of subhyaloidal haemorrhage by intravitreal application of rtPA and $SF_6$ gas. *Br J Ophthalmol* 2000; **84:** 1324–5.
6. Koh HJ, *et al.* Treatment of subhyaloid haemorrhage with intravitreal tissue plasminogen activator and $C_3F_8$ gas injection. *Br J Ophthalmol* 2000; **84:** 1329–30.
7. Conway MD, *et al.* Intravitreal tPA and $SF_6$ promote clearing of premacular subhyaloid hemorrhages in shaken and battered baby syndrome. *Ophthalmic Surg Lasers* 1999; **30:** 435–41.

**Peripheral arterial thromboembolism.** Thrombolytics, including alteplase, may be used in the management of peripheral arterial thromboembolism (p.830). Alteplase has been injected intravenously or intra-arterially directly into the clot as an alternative to surgical treatment of the occlusion. It has also been infused intra-arterially to remove distal clots during a surgical procedure. Alteplase is claimed to produce more rapid thrombolysis than streptokinase although studies have been too small to provide evidence of reduced limb loss or mortality.[1] The most common dose range is 0.5 to 1 mg/hour given *intra-arterially*.[1-3]

An *intravenous* dose of 500 micrograms/kg per hour for the first hour followed by 250 micrograms/kg per hour until clot lysis occurred has been used in infants.[4] Treatment of arterial thrombosis in neonates has been reported, using doses of alteplase ranging from 100 to 500 micrograms/kg per hour *intravenously*.[5,6] However, a retrospective study[7] of 80 infants and children with arterial or venous thrombi found that although treatment with alteplase may be effective, it is associated with a low safety margin and an unknown risk-benefit ratio.

Where a thrombolytic is used to remove distal clots during a surgical procedure alteplase has been given *intra-arterially* as three doses of 5 mg at 10-minute intervals.[8]

1. Wolfe JH. Critical limb ischaemia. *Prescribers' J* 1994; **34:** 50–8.
2. Anonymous. Non-coronary thrombolysis. *Lancet* 1990; **335:** 691–3.
3. Ward AS, *et al.* Peripheral thrombolysis with tissue plasminogen activator: results of two treatment regimens. *Arch Surg* 1994; **129:** 861–5.
4. Zenz W, *et al.* Tissue plasminogen activator (alteplase) treatment for femoral artery thrombosis after cardiac catheterisation in infants and children. *Br Heart J* 1993; **70:** 382–5.
5. Weiner GM, *et al.* Successful treatment of neonatal arterial thromboses with recombinant tissue plasminogen activator. *J Pediatr* 1998; **133:** 133–6.
6. Farnoux C, *et al.* Recombinant tissue-type plasminogen activator therapy of thrombosis in 16 neonates. *J Pediatr* 1998; **133:** 137–40.
7. Gupta AA, *et al.* Safety and outcomes of thrombolysis with tissue plasminogen activator for treatment of intravascular thrombosis in children. *J Pediatr* 2001; **139:** 682–8.
8. Chester JF, *et al.* Peroperative t-PA thrombolysis. *Lancet* 1991; **337:** 861–2.

### Preparations

***USP 27:*** Alteplase for Injection.

**Proprietary Preparations** (details are given in Part 3)
***Arg.:*** Actilyse; ***Austral.:*** Actilyse; ***Austria:*** Actilyse; Besopartin; ***Belg.:*** Actilyse; ***Braz.:*** Actilyse; ***Canad.:*** Activase; ***Chile:*** Actilyse; ***Denm.:*** Actilyse; ***Fin.:*** Actilyse; ***Fr.:*** Actilyse; ***Ger.:*** Actilyse; ***Gr.:*** Actilyse; ***Hong Kong:*** Actilyse; ***India:*** Actilyse; ***Irl.:*** Actilyse; ***Israel:*** Actilyse; ***Ital.:*** Actilyse; Actiplas†; ***Malaysia:*** Actilyse; ***Mex.:*** Actilyse; ***Neth.:*** Actilyse; ***Norw.:*** Actilyse; ***NZ:*** Actilyse; ***Port.:*** Actilyse; ***S.Afr.:*** Actilyse; ***Singapore:*** Actilyse; ***Spain:*** Actilyse; ***Swed.:*** Actilyse; ***Switz.:*** Actilyse; ***Thai.:*** Actilyse; ***UK:*** Actilyse; ***USA:*** Activase.

## Altizide *(rINN)*

Althiazide *(USAN)*; Altizida; P-1779. 3-Allylthiomethyl-6-chloro-3,4-dihydro-2*H*-1,2,4-benzothiadiazine-7-sulphonamide 1,1-dioxide.
$C_{11}H_{14}ClN_3O_4S_3$ = 383.9.
*CAS — 5588-16-9.*

### Profile

Altizide is a thiazide diuretic (see Hydrochlorothiazide, p.933) that is used in the treatment of oedema and hypertension. It is frequently used with spironolactone.

### Preparations

**Proprietary Preparations** (details are given in Part 3)
***Multi-ingredient: Belg.:*** Aldactazine; ***Fr.:*** Aldactazine; Practazin; Prinactizide†; Spiroctazine; ***Port.:*** Aldactazine; ***Spain:*** Aldactacine.

## Amezinium Metilsulfate *(rINN)*

Amezinium Methylsulphate; Metilsulfato de amezinio. 4-Amino-6-methoxy-1-phenylpyridazinium methylsulphate.
$C_{12}H_{15}N_3O_5S$ = 313.3.
*CAS — 30578-37-1.*

### Profile

Amezinium metilsulfate is a sympathomimetic (see Adrenaline, p.852) used for its vasopressor effects in the treatment of hypotensive states (p.828). It is given by mouth in a usual dose of 10 mg up to three times daily. It has also been given by slow intravenous injection.

### Preparations

**Proprietary Preparations** (details are given in Part 3)
***Belg.:*** Regulton; ***Ger.:*** Regulton; Supratonin.

# Amiloride Hydrochloride

*(BANM, USAN, rINNM)*

Amiloridi Hydrochloridum; Amipramizide; Cloridrato de Amilorida; Hidrocloruro de amilorida; MK-870. *N*-Amidino-3,5-diamino-6-chloropyrazine-2-carboxamide hydrochloride dihydrate.
$C_6H_8ClN_7O,HCl,2H_2O$ = 302.1.
*CAS — 2609-46-3 (amiloride); 2016-88-8 (anhydrous amiloride hydrochloride); 17440-83-4 (amiloride hydrochloride dihydrate).*
*ATC — C03DB01.*

NOTE. Compounded preparations of amiloride hydrochloride may be represented by the following names:

- Co-amilofruse *(BAN)*—amiloride hydrochloride 1 part and furosemide 8 parts (w/w)
- Co-amilozide *(BAN)*—amiloride hydrochloride 1 part and hydrochlorothiazide 10 parts (w/w)
- Co-amilozide *(PEN)*—amiloride hydrochloride and hydrochlorothiazide.

**Pharmacopoeias.** In *Chin., Eur.* (see p.vi), *Int.*, and *US.*

**Ph. Eur. 5.0** (Amiloride Hydrochloride). A pale yellow to greenish-yellow powder. Slightly soluble in water and in dehydrated alcohol. Protect from light.

**USP 27** (Amiloride Hydrochloride). A yellow to greenish-yellow, odourless or practically odourless, powder. Slightly soluble in water; insoluble in acetone, in chloroform, in ether, and in ethyl acetate; freely soluble in dimethyl sulfoxide; sparingly soluble in methyl alcohol.

## Adverse Effects

Amiloride can cause hyperkalaemia, particularly in elderly patients, diabetics, and patients with renal impairment. Hyponatraemia has been reported in patients receiving amiloride with other diuretics. Amiloride may cause nausea, vomiting, abdominal pain, diarrhoea or constipation, paraesthesia, thirst, dizziness, skin rash, pruritus, weakness, muscle cramps, headache, and minor psychiatric or visual changes. Orthostatic hypotension and rises in blood-urea-nitrogen concentrations have been reported. Other adverse effects of amiloride may include alopecia, cough, dyspnoea, jaundice, encephalopathy, impotence, angina pectoris, arrhythmias, and palpitations.

**Effects on electrolyte balance.** There have been reports of metabolic acidosis associated with amiloride or triamterene[1] and with co-amilozide.[2]

1. Kushner RF, Sitrin MD. Metabolic acidosis: development in two patients receiving a potassium-sparing diuretic and total parenteral nutrition. *Arch Intern Med* 1986; **146:** 343–5.
2. Wan HH, Lye MDW. Moduretic-induced metabolic acidosis and hyperkalaemia. *Postgrad Med J* 1980; **56:** 348–50.

POTASSIUM. Hyperkalaemia is the main adverse effect when amiloride is given alone but may also occur when amiloride is given with a potassium-wasting diuretic. Severe hyperkalaemia has been reported during co-amilozide therapy, particularly in patients with renal impairment[1,2] and has been accompanied by metabolic acidosis in one such patient.[3]

1. Whiting GFM, *et al.* Severe hyperkalaemia with Moduretic. *Med J Aust* 1979; **1:** 409.
2. Jaffey L, Martin A. Malignant hyperkalaemia after amiloride/hydrochlorothiazide treatment. *Lancet* 1981; **i:** 1272.
3. Wan HH, Lye MDW. Moduretic-induced metabolic acidosis and hyperkalaemia. *Postgrad Med J* 1980; **56:** 348–50.

SODIUM. For reports of severe hyponatraemia in patients taking amiloride with potassium-wasting diuretics, see Hydrochlorothiazide, p.934.

**Effects on the skin.** For a report of photosensitivity reactions in patients taking co-amilozide, see Hydrochlorothiazide, p.934.

## Precautions

Amiloride has the same precautions as spironolactone with regard to hyperkalaemia (see p.1003). It should be discontinued at least 3 days before glucose-tolerance tests are performed in patients who may have diabetes mellitus because of the risks of provoking severe hyperkalaemia.

## Interactions

There is an increased risk of hyperkalaemia if amiloride is given with potassium supplements or with other potassium-sparing diuretics. Hyperkalaemia may also occur in patients receiving ACE inhibitors, angiotensin II receptor antagonists, NSAIDs, ciclosporin, or trilostane concomitantly. In patients receiving amiloride with NSAIDs or ciclosporin the risk of nephrotoxicity may also be increased. Diuretics may reduce the excretion of lithium and increase the risk of lithium toxicity, but this does not appear to occur with amiloride. Severe hyponatraemia may occur in patients receiving a potassium-sparing diuretic with a thiazide; this risk may be increased in patients receiving chlorpropamide. Amiloride may reduce the ulcer-healing properties of carbenoxolone. As with other diuretics, amiloride may enhance the effects of other antihypertensive drugs.

**Digoxin.** For the effects of amiloride on digoxin clearance, see p.897.

**Quinidine.** For a report of amiloride producing arrhythmias in patients receiving quinidine, see p.993.

## Pharmacokinetics

Amiloride is incompletely absorbed from the gastrointestinal tract; bioavailability is about 50% and is reduced by food. It is not significantly bound to plasma proteins and has a plasma half-life of 6 to 9 hours; the terminal half-life may be 20 hours or more. It is excreted unchanged by the kidneys.

◊ General references.

1. Weiss P, *et al.* The metabolism of amiloride hydrochloride in man. *Clin Pharmacol Ther* 1969; **10:** 401–6.

**Hepatic impairment.** In patients with acute hepatitis the terminal half-life of amiloride was 33 hours compared with 21 hours in healthy subjects.[1] The proportion of the dose excreted in the urine was increased from 49 to 80%.

1. Spahn H, *et al.* Pharmacokinetics of amiloride in renal and hepatic disease. *Eur J Clin Pharmacol* 1987; **33:** 493–8.

**Renal impairment.** Studies of the pharmacokinetics of amiloride[1,2] have reported an increase in terminal elimination half-life from 20 hours in healthy subjects to 100 hours in patients with end-stage renal disease. The natriuretic effect of amiloride was reduced[1] in patients with creatinine clearance below 50 mL/minute. In patients with renal impairment amiloride could aggravate potassium retention due to renal disease. Studies in elderly patients have demonstrated increased half-life[3] and steady-state concentrations[4] associated with reduced renal function.

1. Knauf H, *et al.* Limitation on the use of amiloride in early renal failure. *Eur J Clin Pharmacol* 1985; **28:** 61–6.
2. Spahn H, *et al.* Pharmacokinetics of amiloride in renal and hepatic disease. *Eur J Clin Pharmacol* 1987; **33:** 493–8.
3. Sabanathan K, *et al.* A comparative study of the pharmacokinetics and pharmacodynamics of atenolol, hydrochlorothiazide and amiloride in normal young and elderly subjects and elderly hypertensive patients. *Eur J Clin Pharmacol* 1987; **32:** 53–60.
4. Ismail Z, *et al.* The pharmacokinetics of amiloride-hydrochlorothiazide combination in the young and elderly. *Eur J Clin Pharmacol* 1989; **37:** 167–71.

## Uses and Administration

Amiloride is a weak diuretic that appears to act mainly on the distal renal tubules. It is described as potassium-sparing since, like spironolactone, it increases the excretion of sodium and reduces the excretion of potassium. Unlike spironolactone, however, it does not act by specifically antagonising aldosterone. Amiloride does not inhibit carbonic anhydrase. It takes effect about 2 hours after oral administration and its diuretic action reaches a peak in 6 to 10 hours and has been reported to persist for about 24 hours.

Amiloride diminishes the kaliuretic effects of other diuretics, and may produce an additional natriuretic effect. It is mainly used as an adjunct to thiazide diuretics such as hydrochlorothiazide and loop diuretics such as furosemide, to conserve potassium in those at risk from hypokalaemia during the long-term treatment of oedema associated with hepatic cirrhosis (including ascites, p.815) and heart failure (p.820). It is also used with other diuretics in the treatment of hypertension (p.825). Diuretic-induced hypokalaemia and its management, including the role of potassium-sparing diuretics such as amiloride, is discussed under Effects on Electrolyte Balance in the Adverse Effects of Hydrochlorothiazide, p.933. Amiloride is sometimes used to manage hypokalaemia in primary hyperaldosteronism (p.1005).

Amiloride by inhalation has also been investigated in the management of cystic fibrosis patients with lung disease (see below).

In the treatment of **oedema** amiloride is given by mouth as the hydrochloride and doses are expressed in terms of the anhydrous substance. 1 mg of anhydrous hydrochloride is approximately equivalent to 1.14 mg of the hydrated substance. Treatment may be started with a dose of 2.5 mg daily, increasing gradually to a usual dose of 5 to 10 mg daily. This may be increased, if necessary, to a maximum of 20 mg daily. Similar doses are used to reduce potassium loss in patients receiving thiazide or loop diuretics.

Potassium supplements should not be given.

**Cystic fibrosis.** Pulmonary disease is the major cause of mortality in cystic fibrosis (p.123). Experimental treatment aimed at modifying the pulmonary disease process has included the administration of amiloride by inhalation.[1,2] No evidence of pulmonary or systemic toxicity was seen in 14 patients treated for 25 weeks.[1] The mechanism of action is unclear but could be the sodium-channel blocking effect[1] or anti-inflammatory effects[3] of amiloride. Concern has been expressed[4] over possible consequences of the inhibition of endogenous urokinase by amiloride although others[5] considered this to be unlikely at the concentrations studied. However, the addition of amiloride to standard therapy has not produced significant clinical benefits.[6,7]


1. Knowles MR, *et al.* A pilot study of aerosolized amiloride for the treatment of lung disease in cystic fibrosis. *N Engl J Med* 1990; **322:** 1189–94.
2. App EM, *et al.* Acute and long-term amiloride inhalation in cystic fibrosis lung disease: a rational approach to cystic fibrosis therapy. *Am Rev Respir Dis* 1990; **141:** 605–12.
3. Gallo RL. Aerosolized amiloride for the treatment of lung disease in cystic fibrosis. *N Engl J Med* 1990; **323:** 996–7.
4. Henkin J. Aerosolized amiloride for the treatment of lung disease in cystic fibrosis. *N Engl J Med* 1990; **323:** 997.
5. Knowles MR, *et al.* Aerosolized amiloride for the treatment of lung disease in cystic fibrosis. *N Engl J Med* 1990; **323:** 997–8.
6. Graham A, *et al.* No added benefit from nebulized amiloride in patients with cystic fibrosis. *Eur Respir J* 1993; **6:** 1243–8.
7. Bowler IM, *et al.* Nebulised amiloride in respiratory exacerbations of cystic fibrosis: a randomised controlled trial. *Arch Dis Child* 1995; **73:** 427–30.


**Diabetes insipidus.** Thiazide diuretics are commonly used in nephrogenic diabetes insipidus (p.1314) and NSAIDs may also be employed; both result in an overall decrease in urine production. Addition of amiloride to hydrochlorothiazide has been reported to be at least as effective as hydrochlorothiazide plus indometacin in 5 patients.[1] In addition, amiloride obviated the need for potassium supplements. The combination of hydrochlorothiazide and amiloride was also effective and well tolerated in a group of 4 children with nephrogenic diabetes insipidus who were treated for up to 5 years.[2]


1. Knoers N, Monnens LAH. Amiloride-hydrochlorothiazide versus indomethacin-hydrochlorothiazide in the treatment of nephrogenic diabetes insipidus. *J Pediatr* 1990; **117:** 499–502.
2. Kirchlechner V, *et al.* Treatment of nephrogenic diabetes insipidus with hydrochlorothiazide and amiloride. *Arch Dis Child* 1999; **80:** 548–52.


**Renal calculi.** Patients with idiopathic hypercalciuria and a history of renal calculi are usually given a thiazide diuretic such as hydrochlorothiazide to reduce calcium excretion (p.936). In patients with calcium oxalate calculi an inherited cellular defect in oxalate transport may also be involved and this might be corrected by amiloride.[1]


1. Baggio B, *et al.* An inheritable anomaly of red-cell oxalate transport in "primary" calcium nephrolithiasis correctable with diuretics. *N Engl J Med* 1986; **314:** 599–604.


## Preparations

***BP 2003:*** Amiloride Tablets; Co-amilofruse Tablets; Co-amilozide Oral Solution; Co-amilozide Tablets;
***USP 27:*** Amiloride Hydrochloride and Hydrochlorothiazide Tablets; Amiloride Hydrochloride Tablets.

**Proprietary Preparations** (details are given in Part 3)

***Austral.:*** Amidal†; Kaluril; Midamor; Midoride†; ***Austria:*** Midamor; ***Canad.:*** Midamor; ***Denm.:*** Amikal; Nirulid; ***Fin.:*** Medamor; ***Fr.:*** Modamide; ***Hong Kong:*** Midamor†; ***Neth.:*** Midamor†; ***Norw.:*** Midamor†; ***NZ:*** Midamor; ***Swed.:*** Midamor; ***Switz.:*** Midamor; ***UK:*** Amilamont; Berkamil†; ***USA:*** Midamor.

**Multi-ingredient:** ***Arg.:*** Diflux; Errolon A; Furdiuren; Hidrenox A; Lasiride; Moducren; Moduretic; Nuriban A; Plenacor D; Prenomod; Ren-Ur; Vericordin Compuesto; ***Austral.:*** Amizide; Hydrozide†; Modizide†; Moduretic; ***Austria:*** Aldoretic; Amiloral/HCT; Amiloretik; Amilorid comp; Amilorid/HCT; Amilostad HCT; Lanuretic; Loradur; Moducrin; Moduretic; ***Belg.:*** Belidral; Frusamil; Kalten; Moduretic; ***Braz.:*** Amiretic; Diupress; Diurisa; Moduretic; ***Canad.:*** Apo-Amilzide; Moduret; Novamilor; Nu-Amilzide; ***Chile:*** Furdiuren; Hidrium; Hidropid; ***Denm.:*** Amilco; Amilohyd†; Buram; Frusamil; Hydronet†; Moduretic; Sparkal; ***Fin.:*** Amitrid; Diuramin; Diurex; Miloride; Moduretic; Sparkal; ***Fr.:*** Logirene; Moducren; Moduretic; ***Ger.:*** Amilocomp beta; Amiloretik; Amilorid comp; Amilorid/HCT; Amilozid; Aquaretic; Diaphal; Dignoretik†; Diursan; durarese; Esmalorid; Hydrocomp†; Modu-Puren†; Moducrin; Moduretik; Rhefluin†; Tensoflux; ***Gr.:*** Frumil; Ividol; Moduretic; Tiaden; ***Hong Kong:*** Amilco; Amithiazide; Apo-Amilzide; Frumil†; Hydrozide†; Moducren; Moduretic; Navispare; Sefaretic; ***India:*** Biduret; Frumil; ***Irl.:*** Amilco; Buram; Clonuretic†; Fru-Co; Frumil; Lasoride; Moducren; Moduret; Moduretic†; Navispare†; ***Israel:*** Kaluril; ***Ital.:*** Moduretic; ***Malaysia:*** Ami-Hydrotride; Amizide; Apo-Amilzide; Moduretic; ***Mex.:*** Moducren†; Moduretic; ***Neth.:*** Elkin†; Moducren†; Moduretic; ***Norw.:*** Moduretic Mite; Normorix; ***NZ:*** Amizide; Frumil; Hydrozide†; Moduretic†; ***Port.:*** Aldoretic; Amiloride Composto; Chibretico; Diurene; Moducren; Moduretic; ***S.Afr.:*** Acumod†; Adco-Retic; Aldoretic†; Amiloretic; Betaretic; Diutec†; Hexaretic; Moducren; Moduretic; Servatrin; ***Singapore:*** Apo-Amilzide; ***Spain:*** Ameride; Diuzine; Donicer†; Kalten; ***Swed.:*** Amiloferm; Moduretic; Normorix; Sparkal; ***Switz.:*** Agorex; Aldoretic†; Amilo-basan; Amilorid comp†; Betadiur; Co-Amilorid; Comilorid; Ecodurex; Escoretic; Frumil; Grodurex; Hydrolid†; Kalten; Moducren; Moduretic; Rhefluin; ***Thai.:*** Amilhydrozide†; Amilide†; Bilduretic; Hydrozide Plus; Hyperretic; Miduret; Milorex; Miretic; Modulan; Moduretic; Poli-Uretic; Renase; Sefaretic; ***UK:*** Amil-Co; Amilmaxco†; Aridil; Burinex A; Delvas†; Froop Co; Fru-Co; Frumil; Frusemek†; Kalten; Komil; Lasoride; Moducren; Moduret; Moduretic; Navispare; Synuretic†; ***USA:*** Moduretic.

---

# Amiodarone *(BAN, USAN, rINN)*

L-3428; SKF-33134-A. 2-Butylbenzofuran-3-yl 4-(2-diethylaminoethoxy)-3,5-di-iodophenyl ketone.

$C_{25}H_{29}I_2NO_3$ = 645.3.
*CAS — 1951-25-3.*
*ATC — C01BD01.*

## Amiodarone Hydrochloride *(BANM, rINNM)*

Amiodaroni Hydrochloridum; Hidrocloruro de amiodarona; 51087N.

$C_{25}H_{29}I_2NO_3,HCl$ = 681.8.
*CAS — 19774-82-4.*
*ATC — C01BD01.*

**Pharmacopoeias.** In *Chin.* and *Eur.* (see p.vi).

**Ph. Eur. 5.0** (Amiodarone Hydrochloride). A white or almost white, fine crystalline powder. Very slightly soluble in water; sparingly soluble in alcohol; freely soluble in dichloromethane; soluble in methyl alcohol. Store at a temperature not exceeding 30°. Protect from light.

**Adsorption.** There was a rapid fall in the concentration of solutions of amiodarone hydrochloride by 10% in 3 hours followed by a steady decrease to 60% of the initial concentration after 5 days' storage in flexible PVC bags at ambient temperature.[1] When amiodarone solutions were perfused through PVC giving sets the concentration had fallen to 82% after 15 minutes. Similar losses were not observed from solutions stored in glass or rigid PVC bottles, and the losses were attributed to the presence of the plasticiser, di-2-ethylhexylphthalate. Amiodarone may also leach out plasticisers such as di-2-ethylhexylphthalate, and it may be preferable to avoid use of final administration sets containing them in order to minimise patient exposure.


1. Weir SJ, *et al.* Sorption of amiodarone to polyvinyl chloride infusion bags and administration sets. *Am J Hosp Pharm* 1985; **42:** 2679–83.


**Incompatibility.** Amiodarone injection has been reported to be incompatible with aminophylline,[1] flucloxacillin,[2] heparin,[3] and sodium bicarbonate.[4] A further study[5] reported incompatibility with ampicillin/sulbactam sodium, ceftazidime sodium, digoxin, furosemide, imipenem/cilastatin sodium, magnesium sulfate, piperacillin sodium, piperacillin/tazobactam sodium, potassium phosphate, and sodium phosphate. The manufacturer states that it is incompatible with sodium chloride solutions.


1. Hasegawa GR, Eder JF. Visual compatibility of amiodarone hydrochloride injection with other injectable drugs. *Am J Hosp Pharm* 1984; **41:** 1379–80.
2. Taylor A, Lewis R. Amiodarone and injectable drug incompatibility. *Pharm J* 1992; **248:** 533.
3. Cairns CJ. Incompatibility of amiodarone. *Pharm J* 1986; **236:** 68.
4. Korth-Bradley JM. Incompatibility of amiodarone hydrochloride and sodium bicarbonate injections. *Am J Health-Syst Pharm* 1995; **52:** 2340.
5. Chalmers JR, *et al.* Visual compatibility of amiodarone hydrochloride injection with various intravenous drugs. *Am J Health-Syst Pharm* 2001; **58:** 504–6.


**Stability.** An oral suspension prepared from tablets[1] and containing amiodarone hydrochloride 5 mg/mL was stable for 3 months at 4° and 6 weeks at 25°.


1. Nahata MC. Stability of amiodarone in an oral suspension stored under refrigeration and at room temperature. *Ann Pharmacother* 1997; **31:** 851–2.


## Adverse Effects and Treatment

Adverse effects are common with amiodarone; many are dose-related and reversible with reduction in dose.

Adverse cardiovascular effects associated with amiodarone include severe bradycardia, sinus arrest, and conduction disturbances. Severe hypotension may follow intravenous administration particularly, though not exclusively, at rapid infusion rates. Amiodarone may also produce ventricular tachyarrhythmias; torsade de pointes appears to be less of a problem with amiodarone than other antiarrhythmics. Rarely, heart failure may be precipitated or aggravated.

Amiodarone is reported to reduce the peripheral transformation of levothyroxine ($T_4$) to tri-iodothyronine ($T_3$) and to increase the formation of reverse-$T_3$. It can affect thyroid function and may induce hypo- or hyperthyroidism.

There have been reports of severe pulmonary toxicity including pulmonary fibrosis and interstitial pneumonitis. These effects are usually reversible on withdrawal of amiodarone but are potentially fatal.

Amiodarone can adversely affect the liver. There may be abnormal liver function tests and cirrhosis or hepatitis; fatalities have been reported.

Prolonged treatment with amiodarone causes the development of benign yellowish-brown corneal microdeposits in the majority of patients, sometimes associated with coloured haloes of light; these are reversible on stopping therapy. Photosensitivity reactions are also common and more rarely blue-grey discoloration of the skin may occur.

Other adverse effects reported include benign intracranial hypertension, haemolytic or aplastic anaemia, peripheral neuropathy, paraesthesias, myopathy, ataxia, tremor, nausea, vomiting, a metallic taste, nightmares, headaches, sleeplessness, fatigue, and epididymitis.

Thrombophlebitis can occur if amiodarone is injected regularly or infused for prolonged periods into a peripheral vein. Rapid intravenous administration has been associated with anaphylactic shock, hot flushes, sweating, and nausea.

It has been suggested that amiodarone-induced phospholipidosis may explain some of its adverse effects. Amiodarone's iodine content contributes to its thyrotoxicity.

◊ Reviews of the adverse effects of amiodarone.


1. Naccarelli GV, *et al.* Adverse effects of amiodarone: pathogenesis, incidence and management. *Med Toxicol Adverse Drug Exp* 1989; **4:** 246–53.
2. Kerin NZ, *et al.* Long-term efficacy and toxicity of high- and low-dose amiodarone regimens. *J Clin Pharmacol* 1989; **29:** 418–23.
3. Perkins MW, *et al.* Intraoperative complications in patients receiving amiodarone: characteristics and risk factors. *DICP Ann Pharmacother* 1989; **23:** 757–63.
4. Vrobel TR, *et al.* A general overview of amiodarone toxicity: its prevention, detection, and management. *Prog Cardiovasc Dis* 1989; **31:** 393–426.
5. Morgan DJR. Adverse reactions profile: amiodarone. *Prescribers' J* 1991; **31:** 104–11.
6. Committee on Safety of Medicines/Medicines Control Agency. Amiodarone (Cordarone X). *Current Problems* 1996; **22:** 3–4.
7. Vorperian VR, *et al.* Adverse effects of low dose amiodarone: a meta-analysis. *J Am Coll Cardiol* 1997; **30:** 791–8.


**Effects on electrolytes.** Hyponatraemia associated with the syndrome of inappropriate secretion of antidiuretic hormone has been reported[1] in a patient following use of amiodarone for 6 months. The hyponatraemia resolved when amiodarone was discontinued.


1. Odeh M, *et al.* Hyponatremia during therapy with amiodarone. *Arch Intern Med* 1999; **159:** 2599–2600.


**Effects on the eyes.** Slit-lamp examination showed corneal abnormalities in 103 of 105 patients treated with amiodarone for 3 months to 7 years.[1] The most advanced abnormality comprised whorled patterns with uniform granular opacities. The corneal deposits became denser if amiodarone dosage was increased and regressed if dosage was reduced. Ocular symptoms were reported in only 12 patients. Photophobia was reported in 3 patients, while 2 had visual haloes, 1 had blurring of vision, and a further 6 had lid irritation. However, lid irritation was considered a photosensitive skin reaction and blurred vision was probably not due to amiodarone. No patient had any deterioration in visual acuity attributable to amiodarone. In 16 patients amiodarone was withdrawn with complete clearing of corneal abnormalities within 7 months and routine ophthalmological monitoring was considered unnecessary in patients without ocular symptoms. However, optic neuropathy[2] and neuritis with visual impairment have been reported in association with amiodarone and the manufacturers recommend that annual ophthalmological examinations should be performed.

A sicca syndrome with diminished tear and saliva production has been reported[3] during amiodarone treatment.

1. Ingram DV, *et al.* Ocular changes resulting from therapy with amiodarone. *Br J Ophthalmol* 1982; **66:** 676–9.
2. Feiner LA, *et al.* Optic neuropathy and amiodarone therapy. *Mayo Clin Proc* 1987; **62:** 702–17.
3. Dickinson EJ, Wolman RL. Sicca syndrome associated with amiodarone therapy. *BMJ* 1986; **293:** 510.

**Effects on the genitalia.** Epididymal swelling and scrotal pain have been reported with amiodarone.[1,2] Symptoms occurred 7 to 20 months after the start of treatment and resolved within 10 weeks despite continuation of amiodarone in some patients. In one patient[2] the concentration of desethylamiodarone in semen was five times the concentration in serum.

Brown discoloration of semen and sweat has also been associated with amiodarone therapy.[3]

1. Gasparich JP, *et al.* Non-infectious epididymitis associated with amiodarone therapy. *Lancet* 1984; **ii:** 1211–12.
2. Ward MJ, *et al.* Association of seminal desethylamiodarone concentration and epididymitis with amiodarone treatment. *BMJ* 1988; **296:** 19–20.
3. Adams PC, *et al.* Amiodarone in testis and semen. *Lancet* 1985; **i:** 341.

**Effects on the heart.** Amiodarone has the potential to provoke arrhythmias, but a review of the literature[1] indicated that the frequency of proarrhythmic events, including torsade de pointes, was low.

1. Hohnloser SH, *et al.* Amiodarone-associated proarrhythmic effects: a review with special reference to torsade de pointes tachycardia. *Ann Intern Med* 1994; **121:** 529–35.

**Effects on lipids.** Amiodarone increases phospholipid concentrations in tissues and this may be responsible for some of its adverse effects.[1] Although hyperlipidaemia may result from hypothyroidism, amiodarone can also increase serum-cholesterol concentrations independently of any effect on the thyroid.[2,3] The effect on triglyceride concentrations is not clear.[3]

1. Kodavanti UP, Mehendale HM. Cationic amphiphilic drugs and phospholipid storage disorder. *Pharmacol Rev* 1990; **42:** 327–54.
2. Wiersinga WM, *et al.* An increase in plasma cholesterol independent of thyroid function during long-term amiodarone therapy: a dose-dependent relationship. *Ann Intern Med* 1991; **114:** 128–32.
3. Lakhdar AA, *et al.* Long-term amiodarone therapy raises serum cholesterol. *Eur J Clin Pharmacol* 1991; **40:** 477–80.

**Effects on the liver.** Amiodarone-induced elevation of liver enzyme concentrations without clinical symptoms of hepatic dysfunction occurs in some patients.[1] However, hepatic injury which may be severe[2] and sometimes fatal[3-7] has been reported. Hepatitis and cirrhosis have occurred and histological changes resemble those in alcoholic liver disease. Severe reversible cholestasis with hyperbilirubinaemia has also been reported.[2] Hepatotoxicity may not occur for several years after starting amiodarone but rapidly progressive fatal hepatic failure has occurred[6] only one month after starting treatment. Liver enzymes may remain elevated and hepatic injury continue to develop for several months after discontinuing amiodarone. Acute hepatitis occurring within 24 hours of intravenous administration of amiodarone has been reported.[8] In a further patient,[9] acute hepatitis developed following intravenous amiodarone but did not recur with subsequent oral therapy, and it was suggested that the reaction may have been related to the vehicle used in the intravenous formulation.

1. Simon JB, *et al.* Amiodarone hepatotoxicity simulating alcoholic liver disease. *N Engl J Med* 1984; **311:** 167–72.
2. Morse RM, *et al.* Amiodarone-induced liver toxicity. *Ann Intern Med* 1988; **109:** 838–40.
3. Lim PK, *et al.* Neuropathy and fatal hepatitis in a patient receiving amiodarone. *BMJ* 1984; **288:** 1638–9.
4. Tordjman K, *et al.* Amiodarone and the liver. *Ann Intern Med* 1985; **102:** 411–12.
5. Rinder HM, *et al.* Amiodarone hepatotoxicity. *N Engl J Med* 1986; **314:** 318–19.
6. Lwakatare JM, *et al.* Fatal fulminating liver failure possibly related to amiodarone treatment. *Br J Hosp Med* 1990; **44:** 60–1.
7. Richer M, Robert S. Fatal hepatotoxicity following oral administration of amiodarone. *Ann Pharmacother* 1995; **29:** 582–6.
8. Pye M, *et al.* Acute hepatitis after parenteral amiodarone administration. *Br Heart J* 1988; **59:** 690–1.
9. James PR, Hardman SMC. Acute hepatitis complicating parenteral amiodarone does not preclude subsequent oral therapy. *Heart* 1997; **77:** 583–4.

**Effects on the lungs.** Pulmonary toxicity is one of the most severe adverse effects associated with amiodarone therapy and may occur in up to 10% of patients.[1] Interstitial and alveolar infiltration,[2] fibrosis,[3] and pneumonitis[4] have been reported. Patients often present with increasing dyspnoea, cough, and pleuritic chest pain. Most patients respond to withdrawal of amiodarone and, if necessary, treatment with corticosteroids[2] but fatalities have occurred.[3,5] Two patients with amiodarone pulmonary toxicity died less than 1 hour and 24 hours, respectively after pulmonary angiography.[6] Pulmonary toxicity appears to be dose-related[2] in some patients, but an immunological reaction occurring at low doses[4] appears to be the cause in others.

1. Martin WJ, Rosenow EC. Amiodarone pulmonary toxicity: recognition and pathogenesis. *Chest* 1988; **93:** 1067–75 (part 1) and 1242–8 (part 2).
2. Marchlinski FE, *et al.* Amiodarone pulmonary toxicity. *Ann Intern Med* 1982; **97:** 839–45.
3. Morera J, *et al.* Amiodarone and pulmonary fibrosis. *Eur J Clin Pharmacol* 1983; **24:** 591–3.
4. Venet A, *et al.* Five cases of immune-mediated amiodarone pneumonitis. *Lancet* 1984; **i:** 962–3.
5. Committee on Safety of Medicines. Recurrent ventricular tachycardia: adverse drug reactions. *BMJ* 1986; **292:** 50.
6. Wood DL, *et al.* Amiodarone pulmonary toxicity: report of two cases associated with rapidly progressive fatal adult respiratory distress syndrome after pulmonary angiography. *Mayo Clin Proc* 1985; **60:** 601–3.

**Effects on mental state.** Delirium occurred 17 days after starting amiodarone therapy in a 66-year-old man.[1] Mental status returned to normal on withdrawal of amiodarone.

1. Trohman RG, *et al.* Amiodarone-induced delirium. *Ann Intern Med* 1988; **108:** 68–9.

**Effects on the nervous system.** Of 10 patients treated with amiodarone for more than 2 years, 3 patients had evidence of peripheral neuropathy.[1] Initial results suggested that neuropathy correlated with high doses and high serum concentrations of amiodarone.

1. Fraser AG, McQueen INF. Adverse reactions during treatment with amiodarone hydrochloride. *BMJ* 1983; **287:** 612.

**Effects on the pancreas.** Pancreatitis has been reported[1] in a patient 4 days after the initiation of amiodarone therapy. Symptoms resolved following withdrawal of the drug but returned on re-exposure.

1. Bosch X, Bernadich O. Acute pancreatitis during treatment with amiodarone. *Lancet* 1997; **350:** 1300.

**Effects on the skin and hair.** The most common adverse skin reaction associated with amiodarone is photosensitivity. This is a phototoxic rather than a photoallergic reaction[1-3] and the wavelengths responsible extend from the long-wave ultraviolet (UVA) into the visible light range.[1] Affected patients should be advised to wear protective clothing and avoid exposure to sunlight. Topical sunblock preparations, such as those containing zinc or titanium oxides, may reduce the risk of reaction and a reduction in amiodarone dosage may also be useful.[1] Although pyridoxine has been reported[4] to protect against amiodarone-induced photosensitivity, results from a double-blind placebo-controlled study[5] indicated that it may enhance the photosensitivity. Photosensitivity may continue for several weeks after withdrawal of amiodarone due to its extensive distribution.

Blue-grey[2,3] and golden-brown[3] pigmentation of light-exposed skin have been reported during long-term amiodarone use. The pigmentation is usually slowly reversible on withdrawing amiodarone but may not completely disappear. The mean concentrations of amiodarone and its desethyl metabolite in light-exposed pigmented skin have been found to be 10 times the concentrations in non-exposed skin.[2] Discoloration of semen and sweat has also been noted (see Effects on the Genitalia, above).

Cutaneous vasculitis,[6,7] exfoliative dermatitis,[8] and fatal toxic epidermal necrolysis[9] have been reported. Alopecia[10,11] has been associated with amiodarone but increased hair growth,[3] possibly due to the vasodilator activity of amiodarone, has also been reported.

1. Ferguson J, *et al.* Prevention of amiodarone-induced photosensitivity. *Lancet* 1984; **ii:** 414.
2. Zachary CB, *et al.* The pathogenesis of amiodarone-induced pigmentation and photosensitivity. *Br J Dermatol* 1984; **110:** 451–6.
3. Ferguson J, *et al.* A study of cutaneous photosensitivity induced by amiodarone. *Br J Dermatol* 1985; **113:** 537–49.
4. Kaufmann G. Pyridoxine against amiodarone-induced photosensitivity. *Lancet* 1984; **i:** 51–2.
5. Mulrow JP, *et al.* Pyridoxine and amiodarone-induced photosensitivity. *Ann Intern Med* 1985; **103:** 68–9.
6. Starke ID, Barbatis C. Cutaneous vasculitis associated with amiodarone therapy. *BMJ* 1985; **291:** 940.
7. Gutierrez R, *et al.* Vasculitis associated with amiodarone treatment. *Ann Pharmacother* 1994; **28:** 537.
8. Moots RJ, Banerjee A. Exfoliative dermatitis after amiodarone treatment. *BMJ* 1988; **296:** 1332–3.
9. Bencini PL, *et al.* Toxic epidermal necrolysis and amiodarone treatment. *Arch Dermatol* 1985; **121:** 838.
10. Samanta A, *et al.* Adverse reactions during treatment with amiodarone hydrochloride. *BMJ* 1983; **287:** 503.
11. Samuel LM, *et al.* Amiodarone and hair loss. *Postgrad Med J* 1992; **68:** 771.

**Effects on thyroid function.** The majority of euthyroid patients receiving amiodarone remain clinically euthyroid. However, serum concentrations of thyroid hormones may be altered and can complicate the interpretation of thyroid function tests. Use of amiodarone results in a reduction of the peripheral conversion of thyroxine ($T_4$) to tri-iodothyronine ($T_3$) with a resulting increase in $T_4$, a modest fall in $T_3$, and an increase in reverse-$T_3$ concentrations; the basal serum-TSH (thyroid-stimulating hormone; thyrotrophin) concentration rises transiently during the first several months of treatment.[1-4]

Occasionally patients become clinically hypo- or hyperthyroid and the prevalence appears to correlate with dietary iodine intake. The incidence of hyperthyroidism in amiodarone-treated patients in West Tuscany, Italy, an area where iodine intake is low, was 9.6% compared with an incidence of 2% in similar patients in Worcester, USA, an area where iodine intake is normal. The incidence of hypothyroidism in these patients was 5% and 22% respectively.[1] Each 200-mg tablet of amiodarone contains about 75 mg of iodine.[1,5] This large iodine load probably contributes to the development of hypo- or hyperthyroidism in patients with an underlying subclinical thyroid defect. Auto-immune mechanisms may also contribute and antithyroid antibodies have developed during amiodarone therapy.

Assessment of thyroid function is recommended in patients before starting amiodarone treatment and periodically during treatment. Patients with amiodarone-induced hyperthyroidism may present with tachycardia, tremor, weight loss, nervousness, irritability, reappearance of angina, or a worsening of arrhythmia. An ultrasensitive TSH assay should be used to confirm the diagnosis of hypo- or hyperthyroidism.

Hypothyroidism is usually treated with levothyroxine starting with a low dose and gradually increasing until control is achieved; amiodarone may be continued.[1-4]

Hyperthyroidism may be treated with the thiourea drugs carbimazole, thiamazole, or propylthiouracil;[1-6] although withdrawal of amiodarone has been advocated it may be continued if necessary. Potassium perchlorate has also been used[5] with a thiourea to reduce the thyroid iodine load. Radio-iodine can be used[1] but may not be effective if the uptake of radio-iodine by the thyroid is low due to the iodine load from amiodarone. Corticosteroids may also be employed.[2-4] Thyroidectomy has been successfully used[7,8] in the treatment of resistant amiodarone-induced hyperthyroidism.

1. Figge HL, Figge J. The effects of amiodarone on thyroid hormone function: a review of the physiology and clinical manifestations. *J Clin Pharmacol* 1990; **30:** 588–95.
2. Kumar A, Borsey DQ. Amiodarone-related thyroid dysfunction. *Br J Hosp Med* 1994; **52:** 283–9.
3. Harjai KJ, Licata AA. Effects of amiodarone on thyroid function. *Ann Intern Med* 1997; **126:** 63–73.
4. Newman CM, *et al.* Amiodarone and the thyroid: a practical guide to the management of thyroid dysfunction induced by amiodarone therapy. *Heart* 1998; **79:** 121–7.
5. Reichert LJM, de Rooy HAM. Treatment of amiodarone induced hyperthyroidism with potassium perchlorate and methimazole during amiodarone treatment. *BMJ* 1989; **298:** 1547–8.
6. Davies PH, *et al.* Treatment of amiodarone induced thyrotoxicosis with carbimazole alone and continuation of amiodarone. *BMJ* 1992; **305:** 224–5.
7. Farwell AP, *et al.* Thyroidectomy for amiodarone-induced thyrotoxicosis. *JAMA* 1990; **263:** 1526–8.
8. Gough IR, Gough J. Surgical management of amiodarone-associated thyrotoxicosis. *Med J Aust* 2002; **176:** 128–9.

## Precautions

Amiodarone should not be given to patients with bradycardia, sino-atrial block, atrioventricular block or other severe conduction disorders (unless the patient has a pacemaker), severe hypotension, or severe respiratory failure. It may be used with caution in patients with heart failure. Electrolyte disorders should be corrected before starting treatment. The use of amiodarone should be avoided in patients with iodine sensitivity, or evidence or history of thyroid disorders. Patients taking amiodarone should avoid exposure to sunlight.

Thyroid function should be monitored regularly in order to detect amiodarone-induced hyper- or hypothyroidism. Thyroxine, tri-iodothyronine, and thyrotrophin (thyroid-stimulating hormone; TSH) concentrations should be measured; clinical assessment is important but is unreliable alone. See also Effects on Thyroid Function under Adverse Effects and Treatment, above.

Tests of liver and pulmonary function should also be carried out regularly in patients on long-term therapy. Ophthalmological examinations should be performed annually. Although urinary excretion is not a major route for the elimination of amiodarone or its metabolites, some have nevertheless advised caution in patients with moderate or severe renal impairment because of the possibility of iodine accumulation.

Intravenous injections of amiodarone should be given slowly: if prolonged or repeated infusions are envisaged, the use of a central venous catheter should be considered.

**Administration.** For the problems of controlling the delivery rate of amiodarone by intravenous infusion, see under Uses and Administration, below.

**Breast feeding.** Amiodarone is distributed into breast milk[1,2] and significant amounts may be ingested if infants are breast fed. The manufacturers therefore contra-indicate the use of amiodarone during breast feeding, and the American Academy of Pediatrics considers[3] that the use of amiodarone may be of concern due to the risk of hypothyroidism in the infant. In one study,[2] amiodarone was still detectable in breast milk several weeks after amiodarone was discontinued, suggesting that caution is still required. However, there has been a report[4] of an infant who was successfully breast fed with close monitoring of thyroid function; the mother discontinued amiodarone at delivery.

1. Pitcher D, *et al.* Amiodarone in pregnancy. *Lancet* 1983; **i:** 597–8.
2. Plomp TA, *et al.* Use of amiodarone during pregnancy. *Eur J Obstet Gynecol Reprod Biol* 1992; **43:** 201–7.

3. American Academy of Pediatrics. The transfer of drugs and other chemicals into human milk. *Pediatrics* 2001; **108:** 776–89. Correction. *ibid.*; 1029. Also available at: http://aappolicy.aappublications.org/cgi/content/full/pediatrics%3b108/3/776 (accessed 06/07/04)
4. Hall CM, McCormick KPB. Amiodarone and breast feeding. *Arch Dis Child Fetal Neonatal Ed* 2003; **88:** F255–F258.

**Porphyria.** Amiodarone is considered to be unsafe in patients with porphyria because it has been shown to be porphyrinogenic in *in-vitro* systems.

**Pregnancy.** Each 200-mg tablet of amiodarone contains about 75 mg of iodine. The uncertainty as to the effect of this iodine load on the fetus has largely limited the use of amiodarone in pregnancy since iodine freely crosses the placenta and may cause thyroid disorders in the fetus. There are reports[1-3] of the use of amiodarone during pregnancy without any adverse effects appearing in the neonate, although transient biochemical hyperthyroidism or hypothyroidism in 2 neonates has been reported.[4] Amiodarone and desethylamiodarone both cross the placenta and at delivery their respective concentrations in cord blood are about 10% and 25% of the maternal plasma concentrations.

1. Pitcher D, *et al.* Amiodarone in pregnancy. *Lancet* 1983; **i:** 597–8.
2. Robson DJ, *et al.* Use of amiodarone during pregnancy. *Postgrad Med J* 1985; **61:** 75–7.
3. Rey E, *et al.* Effects of amiodarone during pregnancy. *Can Med Assoc J* 1987; **136:** 959–60.
4. Plomp TA, *et al.* Use of amiodarone during pregnancy. *Eur J Obstet Gynecol Reprod Biol* 1992; **43:** 201–7.

## Interactions

Amiodarone should be used with caution with other drugs liable to induce bradycardia, such as beta blockers or calcium-channel blockers, and with other antiarrhythmic drugs. Use with arrhythmogenic drugs, for example phenothiazine antipsychotics, tricyclic antidepressants, halofantrine, and terfenadine, should be avoided. Amiodarone is metabolised by the cytochrome P450 isoenzyme CYP3A4 and interactions may occur with inhibitors of this enzyme, such as HIV-protease inhibitors, cimetidine and grapefruit juice. Enzyme inducers such as rifampicin and phenytoin may reduce amiodarone levels. In addition, amiodarone is an inhibitor of some cytochrome P450 isoenzymes, resulting in higher plasma concentrations of other drugs metabolised by these enzymes. Examples of these include ciclosporin, clonazepam, digoxin, flecainide, phenytoin, procainamide, quinidine, and warfarin.

◊ Reviews.

1. Marcus FI. Drug interactions with amiodarone. *Am Heart J* 1983; **106:** 924–30.
2. Lesko LJ. Pharmacokinetic drug interactions with amiodarone. *Clin Pharmacokinet* 1989; **17:** 130–40.

**Agalsidase.** For the effect of the use of amiodarone with *agalsidase alfa* or *beta*, see p.1651.

**Antibacterials.** Palpitations and activation of an implantable cardioverter defibrillator occurred[1] in a woman receiving amiodarone when *rifampicin* was added. Serum concentrations of amiodarone were reduced, probably due to induction of metabolising enzymes by rifampicin.

1. Zarembski DG, *et al.* Impact of rifampin on serum amiodarone concentrations in a patient with congenital heart disease. *Pharmacotherapy* 1999; **19:** 249–51.

**Antiepileptics.** The interaction between *phenytoin* and amiodarone resulting in increased plasma-phenytoin concentrations is widely recognised (see p.372). However, phenytoin is a hepatic enzyme inducer and has been reported[1] to decrease serum-amiodarone concentrations by 32 and 49% after 1 and 2 weeks of use.

1. Nolan PE, *et al.* Effect of phenytoin on the clinical pharmacokinetics of amiodarone. *J Clin Pharmacol* 1990; **30:** 1112–19.

**Antivirals.** A potential interaction has been suggested between amiodarone and HIV-protease inhibitors due to inhibition of amiodarone metabolism. Raised serum concentrations of amiodarone have been reported[1] in a patient who received *indinavir* for postexposure prophylaxis; no clinical signs of toxicity occurred.

1. Lohman JJHM, *et al.* Antiretroviral therapy increases serum concentrations of amiodarone. *Ann Pharmacother* 1999; **33:** 645–6.

**Grapefruit juice.** A study[1] in healthy subjects reported that grapefruit juice decreased the metabolism of amiodarone; the area under the plasma concentration-time curve (AUC) and the maximum plasma concentration of amiodarone were both increased.

1. Libersa CC, *et al.* Dramatic inhibition of amiodarone metabolism induced by grapefruit juice. *Br J Clin Pharmacol* 2000; **49:** 373–8.

**Histamine $H_2$-antagonists.** *Cimetidine* inhibits hepatic metabolism and an increase in the serum-amiodarone concentration has been reported[1] in 8 out of 12 patients given amiodarone and cimetidine.

1. Hogan C, *et al.* Cimetidine-amiodarone interaction. *J Clin Pharmacol* 1988; **28:** 909.

## Pharmacokinetics

Amiodarone is absorbed variably and erratically from the gastrointestinal tract. It is extensively distributed to body tissues and accumulates notably in muscle and fat; it has been reported to be approximately 96% bound to plasma proteins. The terminal elimination half-life is about 50 days with a range of about 20 to 100 days due to its extensive tissue distribution. On stopping prolonged amiodarone therapy a pharmacological effect is evident for a month or more. A major metabolite, desethylamiodarone, has antiarrhythmic properties. There is very little urinary excretion of amiodarone or its metabolites, the major route of excretion being in faeces via the bile; some enterohepatic recycling may occur. Amiodarone and desethylamiodarone are reported to cross the placenta and to be distributed into breast milk.

Following intravenous injection the maximum effect is achieved within 1 to 30 minutes and persists for 1 to 3 hours.

◊ Reviews.

1. Latini R, *et al.* Clinical pharmacokinetics of amiodarone. *Clin Pharmacokinet* 1984; **9:** 136–56.

## Uses and Administration

Amiodarone is predominantly a class III antiarrhythmic (p.809). It is used in the control of ventricular and supraventricular **arrhythmias**, including arrhythmias associated with Wolff-Parkinson-White syndrome. It has been tried for the prevention of arrhythmias in patients with myocardial infarction or heart failure.

Amiodarone is given by mouth as the hydrochloride in initial doses of 200 mg three times daily for a week, then 200 mg twice daily for a week, and then a usual maintenance dosage of 200 mg or less daily, according to response. Loading doses of up to 1.6 g daily for 1 to 3 weeks, followed by 600 to 800 mg daily for a month, and usual maintenance doses of up to 400 mg daily, are used in the USA. Consideration should be given to potential adverse effects, and patients should be given the minimum effective dose.

Amiodarone hydrochloride may be given intravenously where facilities for close monitoring of cardiac function and resuscitation are available. It is given by intravenous infusion usually in a dose of 5 mg/kg in 250 mL of glucose 5%, infused over 20 minutes to 2 hours; further doses may be given up to a maximum in 24 hours of 1.2 g in up to 500 mL of glucose 5%. Repeated infusions are preferably made through a central venous catheter. In emergencies it may also be given in doses of 150 to 300 mg in 10 to 20 mL of glucose 5% by slow intravenous injection over a period of not less than 3 minutes; a second injection should not be given until at least 15 minutes after the first.

◊ General references.

1. Gill J, *et al.* Amiodarone: an overview of its pharmacological properties, and review of its therapeutic use in cardiac arrhythmias. *Drugs* 1992; **43:** 69–110.
2. Podrid PJ. Amiodarone: reevaluation of an old drug. *Ann Intern Med* 1995; **122:** 689–70.
3. Swanton H. Amiodarone. *Br J Hosp Med* 1997; **58:** 329–32.
4. Goldschlager N, *et al.* Practical guidelines for clinicians who treat patients with amiodarone. *Arch Intern Med* 2000; **160:** 1741–8.
5. Anonymous. Using oral amiodarone safely. *Drug Ther Bull* 2003; **41:** 9–12. Correction. *ibid.*; 40.

**Administration.** Addition of amiodarone hydrochloride to an intravenous infusion solution reduces the drop size delivered[1,2] and the reduction in size is greater as the concentration of amiodarone is increased. This resulted[1] in a reduction of about 30% in the expected delivery rate when amiodarone hydrochloride 1.2 g was administered in 500 mL of glucose 5%. The reduction in drop size has been attributed to a reduction in surface tension caused by inclusion of Tween 80 (polysorbate 80) in the commercial injection.[1] Allowances should be made for the changes in drop size causing a reduction of the delivery rate of infusions of amiodarone hydrochloride.

1. Capps PA, Robertson AL. Influence of amiodarone injection on the delivery rate of intravenous fluids. *Pharm J* 1985; **234:** 14–15.
2. Chouhan UM, Lynch E. Amiodarone intravenous infusion. *Pharm J* 1985; **235:** 466.

**Advanced cardiac life support.** Cardiac arrest should be treated by the institution of full life support measures (see Advanced Cardiac Life Support, p.812). In cardiac arrest due to ventricular fibrillation or pulseless ventricular tachycardia that is refractory to rapid defibrillation, amiodarone may be considered after adrenaline. Doses used are higher than those recommended by the manufacturers. The UK guidelines[1] recommend an intravenous dose of 300 mg, with a further dose of 150 mg if necessary. This is followed by an infusion of 1 mg/minute for 6 hours and then 500 micrograms/minute, up to a total maximum daily dose of 2 g. In the US the maximum recommended dose[2] is 2.2 g in 24 hours. A study[3] in patients with cardiac arrest outside of hospital found that amiodarone improved survival to admission, while another study[4] found that it was more effective than lidocaine in this setting.

1. Resuscitation Council (UK). Resuscitation Guidelines 2000. Available at: http://www.resus.org.uk/pages/guide.htm (accessed 06/07/04)
2. The American Heart Association in collaboration with the International Committee on Resuscitation (ILCOR). International guidelines 2000 for cardiopulmonary resuscitation and emergency cardiovascular care: a consensus on science. *Circulation* 2000; **102** (suppl I): I1–I384. Also published in *Resuscitation* 2000; **46:** 3–447.
3. Kudenchuk PJ, *et al.* Amiodarone for resuscitation after out-of-hospital cardiac arrest due to ventricular fibrillation. *N Engl J Med* 1999; **341:** 871–8.
4. Dorian P, *et al.* Amiodarone as compared with lidocaine for shock-resistant ventricular fibrillation. *N Engl J Med* 2002; **346:** 884–90. Correction. *ibid.*; **347:** 955.

**Cardiac arrhythmias.** Amiodarone is an effective drug for the management of supraventricular and ventricular arrhythmias[1-4] (p.816). It is useful for the treatment of supraventricular arrhythmias associated with the Wolff-Parkinson-White syndrome[2,3] and for both the acute conversion and long-term management of atrial fibrillation.[3] It has been used orally and intravenously in infants and children[5,6] and has been given by various routes to terminate fetal arrhythmias.[7] However, the manufacturers warn that the injection contains benzyl alcohol as a preservative which, in other solutions, has been associated with fatalities in neonates due to the 'gasping syndrome' (hypotension, bradycardia, and cardiovascular collapse). It is also useful for controlling both atrial and ventricular arrhythmias associated with hypertrophic **cardiomyopathy**[2,3] and may reduce the incidence of sudden death in these patients. It is effective in the management of malignant ventricular arrhythmias, although there are few comparative studies with other antiarrhythmics,[1-3] and may also be used in the management of **cardiac arrest** (see Advanced Cardiac Life Support, above). Amiodarone has also been tried for its antiarrhythmic effect in the management of **heart failure** (see below).

Amiodarone has also been investigated in patients with asymptomatic ventricular arrhythmias following **myocardial infarction** (BASIS: the Basel Antiarrhythmic Study of Infarct Survival,[8,9] CAMIAT: the Canadian Amiodarone Myocardial Infarction Arrhythmia Trial,[10] and EMIAT: the European Myocardial Infarct Amiodarone Trial[11]). Improved mortality rates were reported in the BASIS study,[8,9] but neither CAMIAT[10] nor EMIAT[11] showed a reduction in total mortality, although both studies reported a reduction in risk of arrhythmic death. However, meta-analysis of studies using amiodarone found a small reduction in total mortality suggesting that it might be of benefit after myocardial infarction in patients, such as those with heart failure, at high risk of arrhythmic death.[12] In patients at lower risk the role of amiodarone is not as clear; early use of amiodarone in less-selected patients following myocardial infarction appeared to have no overall effect on mortality, although mortality was increased in the group of patients receiving a high dose.[13]

While amiodarone can cause torsade de pointes it appears to do so rarely[14,15] and patients who have experienced this form of ventricular tachycardia as a result of other antiarrhythmic therapy have been given amiodarone subsequently without a recurrence.[16] However, amiodarone has generally been withheld until other appropriate antiarrhythmics have been tried because of its toxicity and the difficulty of instituting and evaluating other therapies after discontinuation of amiodarone.[1,3] The lower doses of amiodarone employed in Europe may be more acceptable than the higher doses that have been used in the USA.

1. Mason JW. Amiodarone. *N Engl J Med* 1987; **316:** 455–66. Correction. *ibid.*; 760.
2. Counihan PJ, McKenna WJ. Risk-benefit assessment of amiodarone in the treatment of cardiac arrhythmias. *Drug Safety* 1990; **5:** 286–304.
3. Katritsis D, Camm AJ. Amiodarone in long term prophylaxis. *Drugs* 1991; **41** (suppl 2): 54–66.
4. Desai AD, *et al.* The role of intravenous amiodarone in the management of cardiac arrhythmias. *Ann Intern Med* 1997; **127:** 294–303. Correction. *ibid.* 1998; **128:** 505.
5. Shuler CO, *et al.* Efficacy and safety of amiodarone in infants. *Am Heart J* 1993; **125:** 1430–2.
6. Figa FH, *et al.* Clinical efficacy and safety of intravenous amiodarone in infants and children. *Am J Cardiol* 1994; **74:** 573–7.
7. Flack NJ, *et al.* Amiodarone given by three routes to terminate fetal atrial flutter associated with severe hydrops. *Obstet Gynecol* 1993; **82:** 714–16.
8. Burkart F, *et al.* Effect of antiarrhythmic therapy on mortality in survivors of myocardial infarction with asymptomatic complex ventricular arrhythmias: Basel Antiarrhythmic Study of Infarct Survival (BASIS). *J Am Coll Cardiol* 1990; **16:** 1711–18.
9. Pfisterer ME, *et al.* Long-term benefit of 1-year amiodarone treatment for persistent complex ventricular arrhythmias after myocardial infarction. *Circulation* 1993; **87:** 309–11.
10. Cairns JA, *et al.* Randomised trial of outcome after myocardial infarction in patients with frequent or repetitive ventricular premature depolarisations: CAMIAT. *Lancet* 1997; **349:** 675–82.
11. Julian DG, *et al.* Randomised trial of effect of amiodarone on mortality in patients with left-ventricular dysfunction after recent myocardial infarction: EMIAT. *Lancet* 1997; **349:** 667–74. Corrections. *ibid.*; 1180 and 1776.

12. Amiodarone Trials Meta-Analysis Investigators. Effect of prophylactic amiodarone on mortality after acute myocardial infarction and in congestive heart failure: meta-analysis of individual data from 6500 patients in randomised trials. *Lancet* 1997; **350:** 1417–24.
13. Elizari MV, *et al.* Morbidity and mortality following early administration of amiodarone in acute myocardial infarction. *Eur Heart J* 2000; **21:** 198–205.
14. Naccarelli GV, *et al.* Adverse effects of amiodarone: pathogenesis, incidence and management. *Med Toxicol Adverse Drug Exp* 1989; **4:** 246–53.
15. Hohnloser SH, *et al.* Amiodarone-associated proarrhythmic effects: a review with special reference to torsade de pointes tachycardia. *Ann Intern Med* 1994; **121:** 529–35.
16. Mattioni TA, *et al.* Amiodarone in patients with previous drug-mediated torsade de pointes: long-term safety and efficacy. *Ann Intern Med* 1989; **111:** 574–80.

**Heart failure.** Although antiarrhythmics are not routinely recommended in the management of heart failure (p.820), those such as amiodarone that have no significant negative inotropic effect may have a role in some patients since sudden deaths in patients with severe heart failure have been attributed to ventricular arrhythmias. In the GESICA study (Grupo de Estudio de la Sobrevida en la Insuficiencia Cardiaca en Argentina)[1] amiodarone appeared to reduce mortality in patients with severe chronic heart failure who were without symptomatic ventricular arrhythmias. An improvement in functional capacity was also noted. The decrease in mortality appeared to be greater than could be expected from antiarrhythmic activity alone. However, in the CHF-STAT study (Survival Trial of Antiarrhythmic Therapy in Congestive Heart Failure)[2] involving patients with heart failure and premature ventricular contractions, overall survival did not appear to be improved by amiodarone. A meta-analysis[3] including these and 3 further trials concluded that amiodarone reduced the rate of arrhythmic or sudden death in high-risk patients and that this resulted in an overall reduction in mortality. However, amiodarone may have a number of adverse effects and it is not currently recommended in heart failure except in patients with symptomatic ventricular arrhythmias.

1. Doval HC, *et al.* Randomised trial of low-dose amiodarone in severe congestive heart failure. *Lancet* 1994; **344:** 493–8.
2. Singh SN, *et al.* Amiodarone in patients with congestive heart failure and asymptomatic ventricular arrhythmia. *N Engl J Med* 1995; **333:** 77–82.
3. Amiodarone Trials Meta-Analysis Investigators. Effect of prophylactic amiodarone on mortality after acute myocardial infarction and in congestive heart failure: meta-analysis of individual data from 6500 patients in randomised trials. *Lancet* 1997; **350:** 1417–24.

### Preparations

***BP 2003:*** Amiodarone Intravenous Infusion; Amiodarone Tablets.

**Proprietary Preparations** (details are given in Part 3)
***Arg.:*** Amiocar; Angoten; Asulblan; Atlansil; Coronovo; Miotenk; Ritmocardyl; ***Austral.:*** Aratac; Cardinorm; Cordarone X; ***Austria:*** Sedacoron; ***Belg.:*** Cordarone; ***Braz.:*** Amiobal; Ancoron; Angiodarona; Angyton; Atlansil; Cor Mio; Diodarone; Miocoron; Miodarid; Miodarон; Taquicord†; ***Canad.:*** Cordarone; ***Chile:*** Atlansil; Cordarone; Ritmocardyl; ***Denm.:*** Cordarone; ***Fin.:*** Cordarone; ***Fr.:*** Corbionax; Cordarone; ***Ger.:*** Amiobeta; Amiod; Amiodarex; Amiodura; Amiogamma; Amiohexal; Cordarex; Cornaron; Tachydaron; ***Gr.:*** Angoron; ***Hong Kong:*** Cordarone; Sedacoron; ***India:*** Aldarone; Cordarone; Eurythmic; ***Irl.:*** Cordarone X; ***Israel:*** Amiodacore; Procor; ***Ital.:*** Amiodar; Cordarone; ***Malaysia:*** Aratac; Cordarone; ***Mex.:*** Braxan; Cardiorona†; Cordarone; Forken; Sinarona†; ***Neth.:*** Cordarone; ***Norw.:*** Cordarone; ***NZ:*** Aratac; Cordarone; ***Port.:*** Cordarone; Miodrone; ***S.Afr.:*** Cordarone X; Hexarone; ***Singapore:*** Aratac; Cordarone; ***Spain:*** Trangorex; ***Swed.:*** Cordarone; ***Switz.:*** Cordarone; Escodarone; Rivodarone; ***Thai.:*** Aratac; Cordarone; ***UAE:*** Amirone; ***UK:*** Amidox†; Amyben; Cordarone X; ***USA:*** Cordarone; Pacerone.

## Amlodipine Besilate *(BANM, rINNM)*

Amlodipine Besylate *(USAN)*; Amlodipini Besilas; Besilato de amlodipino; UK-48340-26; UK-48340-11 (amlodipine maleate). 3-Ethyl 5-methyl 2-(2-aminoethoxymethyl)-4-(2-chlorophenyl)-1,4-dihydro-6-methylpyridine-3,5-dicarboxylate monobenzenesulphonate.

$C_{20}H_{25}ClN_2O_5,C_6H_6O_3S = 567.1.$

*CAS — 88150-42-9 (amlodipine); 111470-99-6 (amlodipine besilate); 88150-47-4 (amlodipine maleate).*

*ATC — C08CA01.*

**Pharmacopoeias.** In *Eur.* (see p.vi).

**Ph. Eur. 5.0** (Amlodipine Besilate). A white or almost white powder. Slightly soluble in water and in isopropyl alcohol; sparingly soluble in dehydrated alcohol; freely soluble in methyl alcohol. Store in airtight containers. Protect from light.

### Adverse Effects, Treatment, and Precautions

As for dihydropyridine calcium-channel blockers (see Nifedipine, p.966).

**Incidence of adverse effects.** Of 1091 patients prescribed amlodipine for hypertension, 128 (11.7%) discontinued the drug because of adverse effects.[1] The commonest side-effects were ankle oedema, flushing, headache, skin rash, and fatigue.

1. Benson E, Webster J. The tolerability of amlodipine in hypertensive patients. *Br J Clin Pharmacol* 1995; **39:** 578P–579P.

**Heart failure.** Calcium-channel blockers are normally avoided in patients with heart failure but amlodipine has not been found to have any adverse effects on morbidity or mortality in patients with severe heart failure receiving the drug.[1] Therefore, it may be a suitable treatment for angina pectoris or hypertension in such patients. However, a study[2] in hypertensive patients (ALLHAT) found that amlodipine was less effective than the diuretic chlortalidone in preventing the development of heart failure.

1. Packer M, *et al.* Effect of amlodipine on morbidity and mortality in severe chronic heart failure. *N Engl J Med* 1996; **335:** 1107–14.
2. The ALLHAT Officers and Coordinators for the ALLHAT Collaborative Research Group. Major outcomes in high-risk hypertensive patients randomized to angiotensin-converting enzyme inhibitor or calcium channel blocker vs diuretic: The Antihypertensive and Lipid-Lowering Treatment to Prevent Heart Attack Trial (ALLHAT). *JAMA* 2002; **288:** 2981–97. Correction. *ibid.* 2003; **289:** 178.

### Interactions

As for dihydropyridine calcium-channel blockers (see Nifedipine, p.969).

### Pharmacokinetics

Amlodipine is well absorbed following oral administration with peak blood concentrations occurring after 6 to 12 hours. The bioavailability varies but is usually about 60 to 65%. Amlodipine is reported to be about 97.5% bound to plasma proteins. It has a prolonged terminal elimination half-life of 35 to 50 hours and steady-state plasma concentrations are not achieved until after 7 to 8 days of administration. Amlodipine is extensively metabolised in the liver; metabolites are mostly excreted in urine together with less than 10% of a dose as unchanged drug. Amlodipine is not removed by dialysis.

◊ General reviews.

1. Meredith PA, Elliott HL. Clinical pharmacokinetics of amlodipine. *Clin Pharmacokinet* 1992; **22:** 22–31.

**Absorption.** Results of studies involving 24 healthy subjects indicated that absorption of amlodipine from a capsule was equivalent to that from a solution, suggesting that the slow transfer of amlodipine into the blood is a property of the drug not of the dosage form; it was also shown that absorption was not affected by food.[1]

1. Faulkner JK, *et al.* Absorption of amlodipine unaffected by food: solid dose equivalent to solution dose. *Arzneimittelforschung* 1989; **39:** 799–801.

**Metabolism.** The metabolites of amlodipine have been characterised in *animals* and in human subjects.[1] Metabolism of amlodipine is complex and extensive, and in common with other dihydropyridines oxidation to the pyridine analogue represents a major step. About 5% of a dose was recovered from urine as unchanged amlodipine.

1. Beresford AP, *et al.* Biotransformation of amlodipine. *Arzneimittelforschung* 1989; **39:** 201–9.

### Uses and Administration

Amlodipine is a dihydropyridine calcium-channel blocker with actions similar to those of nifedipine (p.970). It is used in the management of hypertension (p.825) and angina pectoris (p.813).

Amlodipine is given by mouth as the besilate, but doses are usually expressed in terms of the base; amlodipine besilate 6.9 mg is approximately equivalent to 5 mg of amlodipine.

In hypertension the usual initial dose is 5 mg once daily, increased, if necessary, to 10 mg once daily. Similar doses are given in the treatment of stable angina and Prinzmetal's angina. Lower initial doses may be used in elderly patients and those with hepatic impairment (see below).

The (*S*)-isomer of amlodipine besilate has also been used.

◊ Reviews.

1. Murdoch D, Heel RC. Amlodipine: a review of its pharmacodynamic and pharmacokinetic properties, and therapeutic use in cardiovascular disease. *Drugs* 1991; **41:** 478–505.
2. Haria M, Wagstaff AJ. Amlodipine: a reappraisal of its pharmacological properties and therapeutic use in cardiovascular disease. *Drugs* 1995; **50:** 560–86.

**Administration in children.** Amlodipine has been used to reduce blood pressure in children and adolescents with hypertension. In a study[1] in 28 children aged 3 to 19 years, amlodipine 5 to 10 mg (approximately 0.2 to 0.3 mg/kg) once daily significantly reduced blood pressure; therapy was withdrawn in 5 patients due to oedema and flushing. Younger children may need higher doses than older children. In a study[2] in 21 patients aged 6 to 17 years, the mean dose required in children under 13 years was 0.29 mg/kg daily compared with 0.16 mg/kg daily for children 13 years and over. Another study[3] in 55 children aged 13 months to 20 years reported similar mean doses, but also found that many of the younger children needed twice daily dosing. Amlodipine was well tolerated in both studies.

1. Pfammatter JP, *et al.* Amlodipine once-daily in systemic hypertension. *Eur J Pediatr* 1998; **157:** 618–21.
2. Tallian KB, *et al.* Efficacy of amlodipine in pediatric patients with hypertension. *Pediatr Nephrol* 1999; **13:** 304–10.
3. Flynn JT, *et al.* Treatment of hypertensive children with amlodipine. *Am J Hypertens* 2000; **13:** 1061–6.

**Administration in hepatic impairment.** The clearance of amlodipine is reduced in patients with hepatic impairment and lower doses should be considered; an initial dose of 2.5 mg once daily has been recommended.

### Preparations

**Proprietary Preparations** (details are given in Part 3)
***Arg.:*** Amloc; Amlodine; Amlotens; Amze; Anexa; Angiofilina; Ateriosan; Calpres; Cardiorex; Coroval; Ilduc; Mitokor; Pelmec; Sinop; Terloc; Tervalon; Zundic; ***Austral.:*** Norvasc; ***Austria:*** Norvasc; ***Belg.:*** Amlor; ***Braz.:*** Amloprax; Amlovasc; Anlodibal; Cordarex; Cordipina; Inovec†; Lodipen; Lopiden†; Nemodine; Nicord; Norvasc; Pressat; Roxflan; Tensaliv; Tensodin; ***Canad.:*** Norvasc; ***Chile:*** Amdipin; Amloc; Avirin; Norvasc; Presilam; Terloc; ***Denm.:*** Norvasc; ***Fin.:*** Norvasc; ***Fr.:*** Amlor; ***Ger.:*** Norvasc; ***Gr.:*** Norvasc; ***Hong Kong:*** Norvasc; ***India:*** Amlodac; Amlopres; Calchek; Lama; Myodura; ***Irl.:*** Istin; ***Israel:*** Norvasc; ***Ital.:*** Antacal; Monopina; Norvasc; ***Jpn:*** Amlodin; Norvasc; ***Malaysia:*** Norvasc; ***Mex.:*** Norvas; ***Neth.:*** Norvasc; ***Norw.:*** Norvasc; ***NZ:*** Norvasc; ***Port.:*** Cardionox; Norvasc; ***S.Afr.:*** Norvasc; ***Singapore:*** Norvasc; ***Spain:*** Astudal; Norvas; ***Swed.:*** Norvasc; ***Switz.:*** Norvasc; ***Thai.:*** Amlopine; Norvasc; ***UK:*** Istin; ***USA:*** Norvasc.

**Multi-ingredient:** ***Arg.:*** Adrebloc; Amzepril; Coroval B; Pelmec Duo; Terloc Duo; ***Braz.:*** Sinergen; ***India:*** Amace-BP; ***USA:*** Caduet; Lotrel.

## Amosulalol Hydrochloride *(rINNM)*

Hidrocloruro de amosulalol; YM-09538. (±)-5-(1-Hydroxy-2-{[2-(o-methoxyphenoxy)ethyl]amino}ethyl)-o-toluenesulphonamide hydrochloride.

$C_{18}H_{24}N_2O_5S,HCl = 416.9.$

*CAS — 85320-68-9 (amosulalol); 70958-86-0 (amosulalol hydrochloride); 93633-92-2 (amosulalol hydrochloride).*

### Profile

Amosulalol is a beta blocker (p.868); it also has alpha-blocking activity. It has been given by mouth as the hydrochloride in the management of hypertension.

## Amrinone *(BAN, rINN)*

Amrinona; Inamrinone *(USAN)*; Win-40680. 5-Amino-3,4′-bipyridyl-6(1*H*)-one.

$C_{10}H_9N_3O = 187.2.$

*CAS — 60719-84-8.*

*ATC — C01CE01.*

**Pharmacopoeias.** In *US.*

**USP 27** (Inamrinone). A pale yellow to tan powder; odourless or with a faint odour. Practically insoluble in water and in chloroform; slightly soluble in methyl alcohol. Store at a temperature of 25°, excursions permitted between 15° and 30°. Protect from light.

## Amrinone Lactate *(BANM, rINNM)*

Lactato de amrinona.

$C_{10}H_9N_3O,C_3H_6O_3 = 277.3.$

*CAS — 75898-90-7.*

*ATC — C01CE01.*

**Incompatibility.** The manufacturer has reported that amrinone lactate injection is physically incompatible with glucose-containing solutions and with furosemide.

Precipitation occurred[1] when amrinone was mixed with sodium bicarbonate injection, probably because of the reduced solubility of amrinone in alkaline solutions.

1. Riley CM, Junkin P. Stability of amrinone and digoxin, procainamide hydrochloride, propranolol hydrochloride, sodium bicarbonate, potassium chloride, or verapamil hydrochloride in intravenous admixtures. *Am J Hosp Pharm* 1991; **48:** 1245–52.

### Adverse Effects

Amrinone produces gastrointestinal disturbances that may necessitate withdrawal of treatment. It produces dose-dependent thrombocytopenia. Hepatotoxicity may occur, particularly during long-term oral treatment. Hypotension and cardiac arrhythmias have been reported. Other adverse effects include headache, fever, chest pain, nail discoloration, and decreased tear production. Hypersensitivity reactions including myositis and vasculitis have been reported. Local pain and burning may occur at the site of intravenous injection.

The adverse effects associated with oral administration have made this route unacceptable and amrinone is now only employed intravenously for short-term use. Studies with other inotropic phosphodiesterase inhibitors have shown that their prolonged oral administration can increase the mortality rate.

◊ References.

1. Wynne J, *et al.* Oral amrinone in refractory congestive heart failure. *Am J Cardiol* 1980; **45:** 1245–9.

2. Wilmshurst PT, Webb-Peploe MM. Side effects of amrinone therapy. *Br Heart J* 1983; **49:** 447–51.
3. Wilmshurst PT, *et al.* The effects of amrinone on platelet count, survival and function in patients with congestive cardiac failure. *Br J Clin Pharmacol* 1984; **17:** 317–24.
4. Silverman BD, *et al.* Clinical effects and side effects of amrinone: a study of 24 patients with chronic congestive heart failure. *Arch Intern Med* 1985; **145:** 825–9.
5. Webster MWI, Sharpe DN. Adverse effects associated with the newer inotropic agents. *Med Toxicol* 1986; **1:** 335–42.
6. Mattingly PM, *et al.* Pancytopenia secondary to short-term, high-dose intravenous infusion of amrinone. *DICP Ann Pharmacother* 1990; **24:** 1172–4.
7. Ross MP, *et al.* Amrinone-associated thrombocytopenia: pharmacokinetic analysis. *Clin Pharmacol Ther* 1993; **53:** 661–7.

## Precautions

Amrinone should be used with caution in severe obstructive aortic or pulmonary valvular disease or in hypertrophic cardiomyopathy. Blood pressure and heart rate should be monitored during parenteral amrinone administration. The fluid and electrolyte balance should be maintained. Platelet counts and liver function should also be monitored.

## Pharmacokinetics

Amrinone is rapidly absorbed from the gastrointestinal tract although it is no longer given orally because of an unacceptable level of adverse effects when administered by this route. The half-life is variable and after intravenous administration has been reported to be about 4 hours in healthy subjects and about 6 hours in patients with heart failure. Binding to plasma proteins is generally low. Amrinone is partially metabolised in the liver and excreted in the urine as unchanged drug and metabolites; up to about 40% is excreted as unchanged drug after intravenous administration. About 18% of an orally administered dose has been detected in the faeces over 72 hours.

◊ General references.

1. Rocci ML, Wilson H. The pharmacokinetics and pharmacodynamics of newer inotropic agents. *Clin Pharmacokinet* 1987; **13:** 91–109. Correction. *ibid.* 1988; **14:** (contents page).

**Infants.** For reference to the pharmacokinetics of amrinone in neonates and infants, see under Uses and Administration, below.

**Renal impairment.** Studies in a child with multi-organ failure and anuria[1] and in 3 adults with anuria following cardiac surgery[2] have shown that amrinone is effectively removed by haemofiltration but clearance varies widely between patients. Non-renal clearance may also be altered in critically ill patients and monitoring of plasma-amrinone concentrations has been suggested.[2]

1. Lawless S, *et al.* Effect of continuous arteriovenous haemofiltration on pharmacokinetics of amrinone. *Clin Pharmacokinet* 1993; **25:** 80–2.
2. Hellinger A, *et al.* Elimination of amrinone during continuous veno-venous haemofiltration after cardiac surgery. *Eur J Clin Pharmacol* 1995; **48:** 57–9.

## Uses and Administration

Amrinone is a phosphodiesterase inhibitor which has vasodilator and positive inotropic properties. It is used in the management of heart failure (p.820). Although amrinone is effective when given orally this route has been associated with an unacceptable level of adverse effects, and the drug is now only given intravenously for the short-term management of heart failure unresponsive to other forms of therapy.

The mode of action has not been fully determined, but appears to involve an increase in cyclic adenosine monophosphate concentration secondary to inhibition of phosphodiesterase, leading to an increased contractile force in cardiac muscle.

Amrinone is administered intravenously as the lactate and doses are expressed in terms of the base. Amrinone lactate 1.48 mg is approximately equivalent to 1 mg of amrinone. The initial loading dose is 750 micrograms/kg by slow intravenous injection over 2 to 3 minutes. This is followed by a maintenance infusion, although the loading dose may be repeated after 30 minutes if necessary. Maintenance doses are 5 to 10 micrograms/kg per minute by infusion to a usual maximum total dose (including loading doses) of 10 mg/kg in 24 hours. Doses of up to 18 mg/kg daily have been used for short periods in a limited number of patients.

◊ General references.

1. Colucci WS, *et al.* New positive inotropic agents in the treatment of congestive heart failure: mechanisms of action and recent clinical developments. *N Engl J Med* 1986; **314:** 349–58.

**Administration in infants.** Pharmacokinetic and pharmacodynamic studies[1,2] in infants undergoing cardiac surgery indicated that the dose needed for infants to achieve a plasma-amrinone concentration of 2 to 7 micrograms/mL was an initial intravenous bolus of 3 to 4.5 mg/kg in divided doses followed by a continuous infusion of 10 micrograms/kg per minute. Neonates appear to eliminate amrinone more slowly than infants, possibly due to their immature renal function;[1,3] it was therefore suggested[1] that neonates should receive a similar bolus dose to infants, followed by a continuous infusion of 3 to 5 micrograms/kg per minute. In a further study[4] that included mainly infants and older children, amrinone clearance and volume of distribution varied widely between patients but did not appear to be related to age.

1. Lawless S, *et al.* Amrinone in neonates and infants after cardiac surgery. *Crit Care Med* 1989; **17:** 751–4.
2. Lawless ST, *et al.* The acute pharmacokinetics and pharmacodynamics of amrinone in pediatric patients. *J Clin Pharmacol* 1991; **31:** 800–3.
3. Laitinen P, *et al.* Pharmacokinetics of amrinone in neonates and infants. *J Cardiothorac Vasc Anesth* 2000; **14:** 378–82.
4. Allen-Webb EM, *et al.* Age-related amrinone pharmacokinetics in a pediatric population. *Crit Care Med* 1994; **22:** 1016–24.

## Preparations

**USP 27:** Inamrinone Injection.

**Proprietary Preparations** (details are given in Part 3)
***Belg.:*** Inocor†; ***Braz.:*** Inocor†; ***Canad.:*** Inocor†; ***Fr.:*** Inocor†; ***Ger.:*** Wincoram; ***India:*** Cardiotone; ***Israel:*** Inocor; ***Ital.:*** Inocor; ***Malaysia:*** Inocor; ***Port.:*** Inocor; ***Spain:*** Wincoram; ***Swed.:*** Inocor†; ***USA:*** Inocor.

---

# Ancrod *(BAN, USAN, rINN)*

*CAS — 9046-56-4.*
*ATC — B01AD09.*

**Description.** Ancrod is an enzyme obtained from the venom of the Malayan pit-viper (*Calloselasma rhodostoma = Agkistrodon rhodostoma*).

## Adverse Effects and Treatment

Haemorrhage may occur during treatment with ancrod and usually responds to its withdrawal. If haemorrhage is severe, cryoprecipitate can be used to raise plasma fibrinogen concentrations; plasma may be used if cryoprecipitate is not available. An antivenom has been used to neutralise ancrod.

Skin rash, transient chills, and fever have been reported with the use of ancrod.

## Precautions

As for Heparin, p.929.

Ancrod should not be given to patients with severe infections or disseminated intravascular coagulation. It should be used cautiously in patients with cardiovascular disorders that may be complicated by defibrination. It is very important that when ancrod is given by intravenous infusion it should be administered slowly to prevent the formation of large amounts of unstable fibrin.

Ancrod is not recommended during pregnancy; high doses in *animals* have caused placental haemorrhage and fetal death.

## Interactions

Ancrod should not be administered with antifibrinolytics such as aminocaproic acid or with plasma volume expanders such as dextrans.

## Uses and Administration

Ancrod is an anticoagulant. It reduces the blood concentration of fibrinogen by the cleavage of microparticles of fibrin which are rapidly removed from the circulation by fibrinolysis or phagocytosis. It reduces blood viscosity but has no effect on established thrombi. Haemostatic concentrations of fibrinogen are normally restored in about 12 hours and normal concentrations in 10 to 20 days.

Ancrod has been used in the treatment of thromboembolic disorders (p.837), particularly in deep-vein thrombosis and to prevent thrombosis after surgery in patients requiring anticoagulation but who have developed heparin-induced thrombocytopenia or thrombosis (see Venous Thromboembolism, p.839). It has been investigated in the treatment of ischaemic stroke and has also been given for priapism.

For treatment of thromboembolic disorders ancrod has been given by intravenous infusion. For the prevention of deep-vein thrombosis after surgery for fractured neck of a femur, it has been given by subcutaneous injection postoperatively. Resistance has developed to ancrod.

◊ References.

1. Cole CW, *et al.* Heparin-associated thrombocytopenia and thrombosis: optimal therapy with ancrod. *Can J Surg* 1990; **33:** 207–10.
2. Demers C, *et al.* Rapid anticoagulation using ancrod for heparin-induced thrombocytopenia. *Blood* 1991; **78:** 2194–7.
3. Wright JG, Geroulakos G. Ancrod: clinical indications and methods of use. *Semin Vasc Surg* 1996; **9:** 315–28.
4. Sherman DG, *et al.* Intravenous ancrod for treatment of acute ischemic stroke: the STAT study: a randomized controlled trial. *JAMA* 2000; **283:** 2395–2403.

## Preparations

**Proprietary Preparations** (details are given in Part 3)
***Austria:*** Arwin; ***Canad.:*** Arvin†; Viprinex†; ***Spain:*** Arvin†.

---

# Angiotensinamide *(BAN, rINN)*

Angiotensin Amide *(USAN)*; Angiotensinamida; NSC-107678. Asn-Arg-Val-Tyr-Val-His-Pro-Phe; [1-Asparagine,5-valine]angiotensin II.

$C_{49}H_{70}N_{14}O_{11}$ = 1031.2.
*CAS — 11128-99-7 (angiotensin II); 53-73-6 (angiotensinamide).*
*ATC — C01CX06.*

## Uses and Administration

Angiotensinamide is a vasopressor related to the naturally occurring peptide angiotensin II. It increases the peripheral resistance mainly in cutaneous, splanchnic, and renal blood vessels. The increased blood pressure is accompanied by a reflex reduction in heart rate, and cardiac output may also be reduced.

Angiotensinamide has been used in the treatment of hypotension associated with shock. It has also been given in the management of overdosage of ACE inhibitors, when conventional therapy has been ineffective.

Angiotensinamide should not be given to patients being treated with an MAOI or within 14 days of stopping such treatment as a hypertensive crisis may be precipitated.

◊ References.

1. Jackson T, *et al.* Enalapril overdose treated with angiotensin infusion. *Lancet* 1993; **341:** 703.
2. Newby DE, *et al.* Enalapril overdose and the corrective effect of intravenous angiotensin II. *Br J Clin Pharmacol* 1995; **40:** 103–4.
3. Yunge M, Petros A. Angiotensin for septic shock unresponsive to noradrenaline. *Arch Dis Child* 2000; **82:** 388–9.

---

# Anisindione *(BAN, rINN)*

Anisindiona. 2-(4-Methoxyphenyl)indan-1,3-dione.

$C_{16}H_{12}O_3$ = 252.3.
*CAS — 117-37-3.*

## Profile

Anisindione is an orally administered indanedione anticoagulant with actions similar to those of warfarin (p.1022). It has been used in the management of thromboembolic disorders (p.837) but, as the indanediones are generally more toxic than warfarin (see Phenindione, p.981), its use is limited.

During treatment with anisindione the urine may be coloured pink or orange.

## Preparations

**Proprietary Preparations** (details are given in Part 3)
***USA:*** Miradon†.

---

# Anistreplase *(BAN, USAN, rINN)*

Anisoylated Plasminogen Streptokinase Activator Complex; Anistreplasa; APSAC; BRL-26921. *p*-Anisoylated (human) lys-plasminogen streptokinase activator complex (1:1).

*CAS — 81669-57-0.*
*ATC — B01AD03.*

**Storage.** The manufacturer recommends that anistreplase should be stored at 2° to 8°.

## Adverse Effects, Treatment, and Precautions

As for Streptokinase, p.1005. Like streptokinase, anistreplase appears to be antigenic and may be neutralised by streptokinase antibodies.

**Back pain.** For references to back pain associated with anistreplase infusion, see under Streptokinase, p.1005.

## Interactions

As for Streptokinase, p.1007.

## Pharmacokinetics

Anistreplase is reported to be cleared from plasma at about half the rate of streptokinase and has a fibrinolytic half-life of about 90 minutes. It is metabolised to the plasminogen-streptokinase complex at a steady rate.

◊ References.

1. Gemmill JD, *et al.* A comparison of the pharmacokinetic properties of streptokinase and anistreplase in acute myocardial infarction. *Br J Clin Pharmacol* 1991; **31:** 143–7.

## Uses and Administration

Anistreplase is a thrombolytic drug. It consists of a complex of the lys-form of plasminogen and streptokinase with the addition of a *p*-anisoyl group. Following intravenous injection the anisoyl group undergoes deacylation at a steady rate to release the active complex which converts plasminogen to plasmin, a proteolytic enzyme that has fibrinolytic effects. The mechanisms of fibrinolysis are discussed further under Haemostasis and Fibrinolysis on p.735.

Anistreplase is used similarly to streptokinase (p.1007) in the treatment of acute myocardial infarction (p.828). It is given as a single intravenous injection in a dose of 30 units over 5 minutes, as soon as possible after the onset of symptoms.

### Preparations

**Proprietary Preparations** (details are given in Part 3)
***Austria:*** Eminase†; ***Belg.:*** Eminase; ***Canad.:*** Eminase†; ***Ger.:*** Eminase; ***Israel:*** Eminase; ***Ital.:*** Multilase†; ***Neth.:*** Eminase; ***Port.:*** Fibrit†; ***Spain:*** Iminase†; ***UK:*** Eminase†.

## Apraclonidine Hydrochloride

*(BANM, USAN, rINNM)*

AL-02145 (apraclonidine); *p*-Aminoclonidine Hydrochloride; Aplonidine Hydrochloride; Hidrocloruro de apraclonidina; NC-14. 2-[(4-Amino-2,6-dichlorophenyl)imino]imidazolidine hydrochloride; 2,6-Dichloro-*N*[1]-imidazolidin-2-ylidene-*p*-phenylenediamine hydrochloride.

$C_9H_{10}Cl_2N_4,HCl = 281.6.$

*CAS — 66711-21-5 (apraclonidine); 73218-79-8 (apraclonidine hydrochloride).*

*ATC — S01EA03.*

NOTE. APR is a code approved by the BP 2003 for use on single unit doses of eye drops containing apraclonidine hydrochloride where the individual container may be too small to bear all the appropriate labelling information.

**Pharmacopoeias.** In *US.*

**USP 27** (Apraclonidine Hydrochloride). A white to off-white, odourless to practically odourless powder. Soluble 1 in 34 of water, 1 in 74 of alcohol, and 1 in 13 of methyl alcohol; insoluble in chloroform, in ethyl acetate, and in hexanes. pH of a 1% solution in water is between 5.0 and 6.6. Store in airtight containers. Protect from light.

### Adverse Effects and Precautions

Adverse effects following perioperative instillation of apraclonidine into the eye include hyperaemia, lid retraction, conjunctival blanching, and mydriasis. Some patients may develop an exaggerated reduction in intra-ocular pressure. Following regular instillation an ocular intolerance reaction may occur, characterised by hyperaemia, ocular pruritus, increased lachrymation, ocular discomfort, and oedema of the lids and conjunctiva. Other adverse effects reported include dry mouth and nose, conjunctivitis, blurred vision, asthenia, headache, and taste disturbances. Systemic absorption may occur after application to the eye and may result in adverse effects similar to those of clonidine (p.885). Cardiovascular effects have been reported; therefore apraclonidine should be used with caution in patients with severe cardiovascular disease, including hypertension, and in patients with a history of vasovagal attacks. Drowsiness may also occur. Depression has rarely been associated with use of apraclonidine and it should be used with caution in depressed patients.

### Interactions

Systemic absorption may occur after topical administration of apraclonidine to the eye and there is a theoretical possibility of interactions similar to those reported with clonidine (p.886). Since the effects of apraclonidine on circulating catecholamines are unknown, the concomitant use of MAOIs is contra-indicated by the manufacturer; tricyclic and related antidepressants and systemic sympathomimetics should also be avoided or used with caution.

### Uses and Administration

Apraclonidine is an alpha$_2$-adrenoceptor agonist derived from clonidine (p.885). It reduces intra-ocular pressure when instilled into the eye and is used in patients undergoing eye surgery and as an adjunct in the management of glaucoma. The reduction in intra-ocular pressure begins within an hour of instillation and is maximal after about 3 to 5 hours.

Apraclonidine is used as the hydrochloride, but the strength of an ophthalmic solution is usually expressed in terms of the base. Apraclonidine hydrochloride 11.5 mg is approximately equivalent to 10 mg of apraclonidine.

To control or prevent a postoperative increase in intra-ocular pressure in patients undergoing anterior segment laser surgery, a 1% solution is instilled into the eye one hour before surgery and again immediately upon completion of surgery.

For short-term adjunctive therapy in patients with raised intra-ocular pressure not controlled by conventional therapy, a 0.5% solution may be instilled three times daily.

There is a loss of effect over time (tachyphylaxis) with apraclonidine and the benefit in most patients lasts for less than a month.

### Preparations

***USP 27:*** Apraclonidine Ophthalmic Solution.

**Proprietary Preparations** (details are given in Part 3)
***Arg.:*** Iopidine; ***Austral.:*** Iopidine; ***Austria:*** Iopidine; ***Belg.:*** Iopidine; ***Braz.:*** Iopidine; ***Canad.:*** Iopidine; ***Chile:*** Iopidine; ***Denm.:*** Iopidine; ***Fin.:*** Iopidine; ***Fr.:*** Iopidine; ***Ger.:*** Iopidine; ***Gr.:*** Iopidine; ***Hong Kong:*** Iopidine; ***Irl.:*** Iopidine; ***Israel:*** Iopidine; ***Ital.:*** Iopidine; ***Jpn:*** Iopidine; ***Malaysia:*** Iopidine; ***Mex.:*** Iopidine†; ***Norw.:*** Iopidine; ***NZ:*** Iopidine; ***Port.:*** Iopidine; ***S.Afr.:*** Iopidine; ***Singapore:*** Iopidine; ***Spain:*** Iopimax; ***Swed.:*** Iopidine; ***Switz.:*** Iopidine; ***UK:*** Iopidine; ***USA:*** Iopidine.

## Aprindine Hydrochloride *(BANM, USAN, rINNM)*

AC-1802; Compound 83846; Compound 99170 (aprindine); Hidrocloruro de aprindina. *N*-(3-Diethylaminopropyl)-*N*-indan-2-ylaniline hydrochloride; *NN*-Diethyl-*N'*-indan-2-yl-*N'*-phenyltrimethylenediamine hydrochloride.

$C_{22}H_{30}N_2,HCl = 358.9.$

*CAS — 37640-71-4 (aprindine); 33237-74-0 (aprindine hydrochloride).*

*ATC — C01BB04.*

### Adverse Effects and Precautions

Adverse effects of aprindine are usually dose-related and most commonly affect the CNS. They include tremor, vertigo, ataxia, diplopia, memory impairment, hallucinations, and convulsions. Gastrointestinal effects include nausea, vomiting, and bloating. There have been reports of agranulocytosis which may be fatal. Hepatitis and cholestatic jaundice have occasionally been reported; blood and liver function tests should be performed during treatment.

Aprindine is contra-indicated in patients with advanced heart failure or severe conduction disturbances. Some manufacturers have recommended that aprindine should not be used in patients with parkinsonism or convulsive disorders. It should be used with caution in patients with bradycardia, hypotension, and hepatic or renal impairment.

### Interactions

**Antiarrhythmics.** Steady-state plasma-aprindine concentrations increased in 2 patients after the initiation of *amiodarone* and coincided with the appearance of adverse effects.[1]

1. Southworth W, *et al.* Possible amiodarone-aprindine interaction. *Am Heart J* 1982; **104:** 323.

### Pharmacokinetics

Aprindine is readily absorbed from the gastrointestinal tract. It has a long plasma half-life, usually between 20 and 27 hours, and is about 85 to 95% bound to plasma proteins. It is excreted in the urine and the bile.

### Uses and Administration

Aprindine is a class Ib antiarrhythmic (p.809) used in the management of ventricular and supraventricular arrhythmias (p.816).

Aprindine is given as the hydrochloride in usual maintenance doses of 50 to 100 mg daily by mouth; up to 200 mg daily may be given. If necessary initial doses of up to 300 mg daily may be given under strict surveillance for the first 2 to 3 days. Therapy should be monitored by ECG during initial stabilisation of the dose and intermittently thereafter. It has also been given intravenously.

◊ References.

1. Danilo P. Aprindine. *Am Heart J* 1979; **97:** 119–24.

### Preparations

**Proprietary Preparations** (details are given in Part 3)
***Belg.:*** Fiboran; ***Fr.:*** Fiboran; ***Ger.:*** Amidonal†; ***Spain:*** Fiboran†.

## Aranidipine *(rINN)*

Aranidipino; MPC-1304. (±)-Acetonyl methyl 1,4-dihydro-2,6-dimethyl-4-(*o*-nitrophenyl)-3,5-pyridinedicarboxylate.

$C_{19}H_{20}N_2O_7 = 388.4.$

*CAS — 86780-90-7.*

### Profile

Aranidipine is a dihydropyridine calcium-channel blocker used in the management of hypertension.

### Preparations

**Proprietary Preparations** (details are given in Part 3)
***Jpn:*** Bec; Flaspas; Sapresta.

## Arbutamine Hydrochloride *(BANM, USAN, rINNM)*

GP-2-121-3 (arbutamine or arbutamine hydrochloride); Hidrocloruro de arbutamina. (*R*)-4-(1-Hydroxy-2-[4-(4-hydroxyphenyl)butylamino]ethyl)pyrocatechol hydrochloride.

$C_{18}H_{23}NO_4,HCl = 353.8.$

*CAS — 128470-16-6 (arbutamine); 125251-66-3 (arbutamine hydrochloride).*

*ATC — C01CA22.*

### Profile

Arbutamine hydrochloride is a sympathomimetic (see Adrenaline, p.852) with beta-agonist properties and like dobutamine (p.906) has been used for cardiac stress testing in patients unable to exercise. For such a purpose an initial dose of 100 nanograms/kg is given intravenously by a computer-controlled delivery system over 1 minute, and the heart rate response is measured. The device then calculates the difference between the desired and actual heart rate and adjusts the infusion rate accordingly up to a maximum rate of 800 nanograms/kg per minute and a maximum total dose of 10 micrograms/kg.

◊ References.

1. Anonymous. Arbutamine for stress testing. *Med Lett Drugs Ther* 1998; **40:** 19–20.

### Preparations

**Proprietary Preparations** (details are given in Part 3)
***Swed.:*** Genesa†; ***USA:*** Genesa.

## Ardeparin Sodium *(USAN, rINN)*

Ardeparina sódica; Wy-90493-RD.

*CAS — 9041-08-1.*

**Description.** Ardeparin sodium is prepared by peroxide degradation of heparin obtained from the intestinal mucosa of pigs. The end chain structure appears to be the same as the starting material with no unusual sugar residues present. The molecular weight of 98% of the components is between 2000 and 15 000 and the average molecular weight is about 5500 to 6500. The degree of sulfation is about 2.7 per disaccharide unit.

### Profile

Ardeparin sodium is a low-molecular-weight heparin (p.949) with anticoagulant activity that has been used for the prevention of postoperative venous thromboembolism.

### Preparations

**Proprietary Preparations** (details are given in Part 3)
***USA:*** Normiflo†.

## Argatroban *(BAN, USAN, rINN)*

Argipidine; DK-7419; GN-1600; MCI-9038; MD-805. (2*R*,4*R*)-4-Methyl-1-[(*S*)-*N*[2]-{[(*RS*)-1,2,3,4-tetrahydro-3-methyl-8-quinolyl]sulfonyl}arginyl]pipecolic acid.

$C_{23}H_{36}N_6O_5S = 508.6.$

*CAS — 74863-84-6 (anhydrous argatroban); 141396-28-3 (argatroban monohydrate).*

*ATC — B01AE03.*

### Adverse Effects and Precautions

The most common adverse effect of argatroban is bleeding. Hypersensitivity reactions have been reported.

Argatroban is contra-indicated in patients with active bleeding. It should be used with extreme caution in patients at increased risk of bleeding including those with haemorrhagic blood disorders or recent major bleeding, in those with severe hypertension or who have recently undergone major surgery.

If argatroban and warfarin are given together there is an effect on the measurement of the INR values. The manufacturer provides guidelines for interpreting the INR during the change from combined therapy to warfarin alone.

Argatroban should be used with caution in patients with hepatic impairment.

**Administration in the critically ill.** Four critically ill patients became excessively anticoagulated[1] when treatment with argatroban was initiated after cardiac surgery, despite use of only the recommended doses or lower. All four had relatively normal hepatic function. Clearance of the drug appeared to be prolonged after discontinuation. In a patient[2] who had no significant direct hepatic dysfunction but severe hepatic congestion secondary to acute renal failure, the effect of argatroban was prolonged and reduction in dose was necessary. Haemodialysis had little or no effect on clearance.

1. Reichert MG, *et al.* Excessive argatroban anticoagulation for heparin-induced thrombocytopenia. *Ann Pharmacother* 2003; **37:** 652–4.
2. de Denus S, Spinler SA. Decreased argatroban clearance unaffected by hemodialysis in anasarca. *Ann Pharmacother* 2003; **37:** 1237–40.

### Interactions

Use of argatroban with other anticoagulants, antiplatelets, or thrombolytics, may increase the risk of haemorrhage.

**Warfarin.** Although caution is necessary in interpreting the INR when argatroban and warfarin are given together (see Adverse Effects and Precautions, above), a study in healthy volunteers[1] showed no pharmacokinetic interaction.

1. Brown PM, Hursting MJ. Lack of pharmacokinetic interactions between argatroban and warfarin. *Am J Health-Syst Pharm* 2002; **59:** 2078–83.

## Pharmacokinetics

Argatroban is about 54% bound to plasma proteins. Metabolism, mainly hydroxylation and aromatisation, takes place in the liver, with the main metabolite having weak anticoagulant activity. Anticoagulant effects are seen immediately upon initiation of infusion; steady-state concentrations occur within 1 to 3 hours and are maintained until the infusion is stopped or the dose adjusted. The terminal elimination half-life of argatroban is between 39 and 51 minutes. It is excreted primarily in the faeces, via the bile as metabolites and as unchanged drug. About 16% of a dose is excreted unchanged in the urine, and at least 14% unchanged in faeces.

## Uses and Administration

Argatroban is a synthetic thrombin inhibitor with anticoagulant and antiplatelet activity. It is used for the treatment and prophylaxis of thromboembolism in patients with heparin-induced thrombocytopenia (see Effects on the Blood under Heparin, p.928), and as an adjunct in patients undergoing percutaneous coronary interventions (see Reperfusion and Revascularisation Procedures, p.834) who have or are at risk of heparin-induced thrombocytopenia. It has also been used in other thromboembolic disorders.

In the management of heparin-induced thrombocytopenia, argatroban is given by intravenous infusion in an initial dose of 2 micrograms/kg per minute, adjusted according to the activated partial thromboplastin time (APTT), to a maximum dose of 10 micrograms/kg per minute.

In percutaneous coronary interventions in patients at risk of or with heparin-induced thrombocytopenia, argatroban is given by intravenous infusion in an initial dose of 25 micrograms/kg per minute, and an intravenous injection of 350 micrograms/kg is given simultaneously over 3 to 5 minutes. Close monitoring by measurement of the activated clotting time (ACT) is required. If necessary, additional intravenous bolus doses of 150 micrograms/kg may be given, and the infusion rate adjusted to between 15 and 40 micrograms/kg per minute.

Doses should be reduced in patients with hepatic impairment (see below).

◊ References.

1. Kondo LM, *et al.* Argatroban for prevention and treatment of thromboembolism in heparin-induced thrombocytopenia. *Ann Pharmacother* 2001; **35:** 440–51.
2. McKeage K, Plosker GL. Argatroban. *Drugs* 2001; **61:** 515–22.
3. Verme-Gibboney CN, Hursting MJ. Argatroban dosing in patients with heparin-induced thrombocytopenia. *Ann Pharmacother* 2003; **37:** 970–5.

**Administration in hepatic impairment.** In patients with heparin-induced thrombocytopenia with hepatic impairment the initial dose of argatroban should be reduced. An initial dose of 500 nanograms/kg per minute is suggested in moderate hepatic impairment. Reversal of anticoagulant effects after stopping argatroban may take more than 4 hours, due to decreased clearance and increased elimination half-life. High doses of argatroban should not be used in patients with significant hepatic impairment undergoing percutaneous coronary interventions.

### Preparations

**Proprietary Preparations** (details are given in Part 3)
***Jpn:*** Novastan; ***USA:*** Argatroban.

---

## Arotinolol Hydrochloride *(rINNM)*

Hidrocloruro de arotinolol; S-596. (±)-5-[2-{[3-(*tert*-Butylamino)-2-hydroxypropyl]thio}-4-thiazolyl]-2-thiophenecarboxamide hydrochloride.
$C_{15}H_{21}N_3O_2S_3,HCl = 408.0.$
*CAS — 68377-92-4 (arotinolol); 68377-91-3 (arotinolol hydrochloride).*

**Pharmacopoeias.** In *Jpn.*

### Profile

Arotinolol is a non-cardioselective beta blocker (p.868); it also has alpha$_1$-blocking activity. It is used as the hydrochloride in the management of hypertension (p.825), angina pectoris (p.813), cardiac arrhythmias (p.816), and essential tremor (p.872). The usual dose is 20 mg daily by mouth in 2 divided doses although up to 30 mg daily may be given. The initial dose for essential tremor is 10 mg daily.

### Preparations

**Proprietary Preparations** (details are given in Part 3)
***Jpn:*** Almarl.

---

## Atenolol *(BAN, USAN, rINN)*

Atenololum; ICI-66082. 2-{*p*-[2-Hydroxy-3-(isopropylamino)propoxy]phenyl}acetamide.
$C_{14}H_{22}N_2O_3 = 266.3.$
*CAS — 29122-68-7; 60966-51-0.*
*ATC — C07AB03.*

NOTE. Compounded preparations of atenolol may be represented by the following names:

- Co-tenidone (*BAN*)—atenolol 4 parts and chlortalidone 1 part (w/w)
- Co-tenidone (*PEN*)—atenolol and chlortalidone.

**Pharmacopoeias.** In *Chin.*, *Eur.* (see p.vi), *Int.*, and *US.*

**Ph. Eur. 5.0** (Atenolol). A white or almost white powder. Sparingly soluble in water; soluble in dehydrated alcohol; slightly soluble in dichloromethane.

**USP 27** (Atenolol). White or practically white, odourless powder. Slightly soluble in water and in isopropyl alcohol; sparingly soluble in alcohol; freely soluble in methyl alcohol.

## Adverse Effects, Treatment, and Precautions

As for Beta Blockers, p.869.

**Breast feeding.** Atenolol is distributed into breast milk and there has been a report of cyanosis and bradycardia in a breast-fed neonate whose mother had been taking atenolol (see under Pharmacokinetics, below). The American Academy of Pediatrics therefore considers[1] that it should be given with caution to breast-feeding mothers.

1. American Academy of Pediatrics. The transfer of drugs and other chemicals into human milk. *Pediatrics* 2001; **108:** 776–89. Correction. *ibid.*; 1029. Also available at: http://aappolicy.aappublications.org/cgi/content/full/pediatrics%3b108/3/776 (accessed 06/07/04)

**Effects on the heart.** Beta blockers are used in the management of cardiac arrhythmias. However, atenolol 2.5 mg by intravenous injection induced atrial fibrillation in 6 of 12 predisposed patients.[1]

1. Rassmussen K, *et al.* Atrial fibrillation induced by atenolol. *Eur Heart J* 1982; **3:** 276–81.

**Effects on lipid metabolism.** For a report of acute pancreatitis due to hypertriglyceridaemia in a patient taking atenolol and metoprolol, see p.869.

**Effects on the liver.** Reversible cholestatic hepatitis occurred in a patient receiving atenolol[1] and hepatic dysfunction in another.[2]

1. Schwartz MS, *et al.* Atenolol-associated cholestasis. *Am J Gastroenterol* 1989; **84:** 1084–6.
2. Yusuf SW, Mishra RM. Hepatic dysfunction associated with atenolol. *Lancet* 1995; **346:** 192.

**Effects on vision.** Visual symptoms without headache were associated with atenolol for migraine prophylaxis in a patient who had experienced a similar reaction with nadolol.[1]

1. Kumar KL, Cooney TG. Visual symptoms after atenolol therapy for migraine. *Ann Intern Med* 1990; **112:** 712–13. Correction. *ibid.*; **113:** 257.

**Overdosage.** Ventricular asystole occurred in a man who had taken a massive overdose of atenolol.[1]

1. Stinson J, *et al.* Ventricular asystole and overdose with atenolol. *BMJ* 1992; **305:** 693.

## Interactions

The interactions associated with beta blockers are discussed on p.870.

## Pharmacokinetics

About 50% of a dose is absorbed following oral administration. Peak plasma concentrations are reached in 2 to 4 hours. Atenolol has low lipid solubility. It crosses the placenta and is distributed into breast milk where concentrations higher than those in maternal plasma have been achieved. Only small amounts are reported to cross the blood-brain barrier, and plasma-protein binding is minimal. The plasma half-life is about 6 to 7 hours. Atenolol undergoes little or no hepatic metabolism and is excreted mainly in the urine. It is removed by haemodialysis.

**Breast feeding.** Atenolol diffuses into breast milk in concentrations similar[1] to or higher[2] than those in maternal blood. Cyanosis and bradycardia associated with ingestion of atenolol in breast milk has been reported in a 5-day-old term infant. The baby improved when breast feeding was discontinued.[3]

1. Thorley KJ, McAinsh J. Levels of the beta-blockers atenolol and propranolol in the breast milk of women treated for hypertension in pregnancy. *Biopharm Drug Dispos* 1983; **4:** 299–301.
2. White WB, *et al.* Atenolol in human plasma and breast milk. *Obstet Gynecol* 1984; **63:** 42S–44S.
3. Schimmel MS, *et al.* Toxic effects of atenolol consumed during breast feeding. *J Pediatr* 1989; **114:** 476–8.

**Pregnancy.** In 6 women who had taken atenolol for at least 6 days up to the time of delivery concentrations of atenolol in maternal and umbilical serum were approximately equal. In a further woman who had discontinued treatment one day before delivery atenolol was not found in maternal or umbilical serum.[1] The half-life of atenolol in neonates born to mothers who had been receiving atenolol ranged from 10.5 to 34.6 hours (mean 16.1 hours) in a study of 35 term infants.[2] Atenolol concentrations were determined in cord blood and in neonatal blood 24 hours after delivery. The range of elimination rate was 4 times slower than in adults, a difference expected based on renal excretion of atenolol.

1. Melander A, *et al.* Transplacental passage of atenolol in man. *Eur J Clin Pharmacol* 1978; **14:** 93–4.
2. Rubin PC, *et al.* Atenolol elimination in the neonate. *Br J Clin Pharmacol* 1983; **16:** 659–62.

## Uses and Administration

Atenolol is a cardioselective beta blocker (p.868). It is reported to lack intrinsic sympathomimetic activity and membrane-stabilising properties.

Atenolol is used in the management of hypertension (p.825), angina pectoris (p.813), cardiac arrhythmias (p.816), and myocardial infarction (p.828). It may also be used in the prophylactic treatment of migraine (p.464).

In **hypertension** atenolol is given by mouth in a dose of 50 to 100 mg daily, as a single dose, although 50 mg daily is generally adequate. The full effect is usually evident within 1 to 2 weeks.

The usual dose for **angina pectoris** is 50 to 100 mg daily by mouth, given as a single dose or in divided doses. Although up to 200 mg daily has been given for angina pectoris additional benefit is not usually obtained from higher doses of atenolol.

For the emergency treatment of **cardiac arrhythmias** atenolol may be given by intravenous injection in a dose of 2.5 mg injected at a rate of 1 mg/minute, repeated if necessary every 5 minutes to a maximum total dosage of 10 mg. Alternatively atenolol may be given by intravenous infusion in a dose of 150 micrograms/kg given over 20 minutes. The injection or infusion procedure may be repeated every 12 hours if necessary. When control is achieved maintenance doses of 50 to 100 mg daily may be given by mouth.

Atenolol is also used in the early management of acute **myocardial infarction**. Treatment should be given within 12 hours of the onset of chest pain; atenolol 5 mg should be given by slow intravenous injection at a rate of 1 mg/minute and followed after 15 minutes with 50 mg by mouth, provided no adverse effects result; alternatively the intravenous dose may be repeated after 10 minutes followed by 50 mg by mouth after a further 10 minutes. A further 50 mg may be given by mouth after 12 hours, and subsequent dosage maintained, after a further 12 hours, with 100 mg daily.

In the prophylaxis of **migraine** a dose of 50 to 100 mg daily by mouth has been used.

Reduced doses may be required in patients with impaired renal function (see below).

**Administration in renal impairment.** The dose of atenolol should be reduced in patients with renal impairment, depending on the creatinine clearance (CC). Doses are as follows:

- CC 15 to 35 mL/minute: 50 mg daily by mouth or 10 mg once every two days intravenously
- CC less than 15 mL/minute: 25 mg daily or 50 mg on alternate days by mouth or 10 mg once every four days intravenously
- dialysis patients: 25 to 50 mg by mouth after each dialysis.

### Preparations

***BP 2003:*** Atenolol Injection; Atenolol Oral Solution; Atenolol Tablets; Co-tenidone Tablets;
***USP 27:*** Atenolol and Chlorthalidone Tablets; Atenolol Injection; Atenolol Oral Solution; Atenolol Tablets.

**Proprietary Preparations** (details are given in Part 3)
***Arg.:*** Atel; Atenoblock; Felobits; Myocord; Plenacor; Prenormine; Telvodin; Vericordin; ***Austral.:*** Anselol; Atehexal; Noten; Tenlol†; Tenormin; Tensig; ***Austria:*** Arcablock; Atehexal; Atenobene; Atenolan; Atenotyrol;

Betasyn; Tenormin; **Belg.:** Athenol; Blokium†; Tenormin; **Braz.:** Ablock; Angipress; Atecard; Ateneo; Atenol; Atenopress; Neotenol; Plenacor; **Canad.:** Apo-Atenol; Novo-Atenol; Nu-Atenol; Tenolin; Tenormin; **Chile:** Betacar; Grifotenol; Labotensil; Tenormin; **Denm.:** Atenet; Atenodan; Atenor; Myopax†; Tenormin; Uniloc; **Fin.:** Atenblock; Atenol; Tenoblock; Tenoprin; Uniloc†; **Fr.:** Betatop; Tenormine; Xaten†; **Ger.:** Ate; Ate Lich; Atebeta; Atehexal; Atendol; Ateno; Atenogamma; Atenomerck†; Atereal†; Blocotenol; Cuxanorm; Dignobeta†; duratenol; Evitocor; Falitonsin; Jenatenol; Juvental; Teno†; Tenormin; Tonoprotect†; **Gr.:** Azectol; Blocotenol; Fealin; Hemon; Mesonex; Neocardon; Synarome; Tenormin; Umoder; **Hong Kong:** Antipressan; Apo-Atenol; Ateno; Corotenol†; Hypernol; Lo-Ten; Normaten; Tenormin; Tredol; Vascoten; Velorin; **India:** Atecard; Beta; Lonol; Tenolol; Tenormin; Tensimin; **Irl.:** Amolin; Atecor; Ateni; Atenogen; Atenomel; Tenormin; Trantalol; **Israel:** Aponorm†; Normalol; Normiten; **Ital.:** Atenol; Atermin; Seles Beta; Tenomax; Tenormin; **Malaysia:** Apo-Atenol; Corotenol; Loten; Normaten; Noten; Oraday; Renotol; Tenormin; Ternolol; Uphanormin; Urosin; Vascoten; **Mex.:** Blotex; Tenormin; **Neth.:** Tenormin; **Norw.:** Alinor; Tenormin; Uniloc; **NZ:** Anselol; Lo-Ten; Tenormin†; **Port.:** Ancoren; Blokium; Tenormin; Tessifol; **S.Afr.:** Atenoblok; B-Vasc; Hexa-Blok; Ten-Bloka; Tenormin; **Singapore:** Alonet; Apo-Atenol; Hypernol; Normaten; Noten; Prenolol; Tenolol; Tenormin; Ternolol; Vascoten; Velorin; **Spain:** Blokium; Neatenol; Tanser; Tenormin; **Swed.:** Selinol; Tenormin; Uniloc; **Switz.:** Atenil; ateno-basan; Atesifar; Cardaxen; Primatenol; Selobloc†; Servitenol†; Tenat†; Tenormin; **Thai.:** Atenol; Coratol; Noten†; Oraday; Prenolol; Tenocor; Tenolol; Tenormin; Vascoten; Velorin; **UAE:** Tensotin; **UK:** Antipressan; Atenix; Tenormin; **USA:** Tenormin.

**Multi-ingredient: Arg.:** Atel C; Atel N; Plenacor D; Prenomod; Prenoretic; Vericordin Compuesto; **Austria:** Arcablock comp; Atenobene comp; Atenolan comp; Atenolol comp; Atenotyrol comp; Beta-Adalat; Nif-Ten; Polinorm; Tenoretic; **Belg.:** Beta-Adalat; Kalten; Tenif; Tenoretic; **Braz.:** Ablock Plus; Angipress CD; Atenoric; Nifelat; Tenoretic; **Canad.:** Tenoretic; **Chile:** Tenoretic; **Denm.:** Tenidon; Tenoretic; **Fin.:** Beta-Adalat†; Nif-Ten; **Fr.:** Beta-Adalate; Tenordate; Tenoretic; **Ger.:** Ate Lich comp; Atehexal comp; Atel; AteNif beta; Ateno comp; Atenogamma comp; Atenolol AL comp; Atenolol comp; Atenomerck comp†; Blocotenol comp; Bresben; Diu-Atenolol; duratenol comp; Evitocor plus†; Nif-Ten; Nifatenol; Sigabloc; Teneretic; TRI-Normin; **Hong Kong:** Nif-Ten; Target; Tenoret; Tenoretic; **India:** Atecard-D; Beta Nicardia; Cardif Beta; Cardules Plus; Depten; Nifetolol; Presolar; Tenoclor; Tenofed; Tenoric; **Irl.:** Ate-Nife†; Atenetic; Beta-Adalat; Cotenomel†; Nif-Ten; Tenoret; Tenoretic; **Ital.:** Ataclor†; Atenigron; Atinorm; Carmian; Clortanol; Diube; Eupres; Igroseles; Mixer; Nif-Ten; Nor-Pa; Normopress; Target; Tenolone; Tenoretic; **Malaysia:** Tenoret; Tenoretic; **Mex.:** Plenacor; Tenoretic; **Neth.:** Nif-Ten; Tenoretic; **NZ:** Tenoret†; Tenoretic†; **Port.:** Blokium Diu; Tenoretic; **S.Afr.:** Adco-Loten; Atenoblok Co; Tenchlor; Tenoretic; **Singapore:** Nif-Ten; Nifetex; Tenoret; Tenoretic; **Spain:** Betasit Plus†; Blokium Diu; Kalten; Neatenol Diu; Neatenol Diuvas; Normopresil; Tenoretic; **Switz.:** Atedurex; ateno-basan comp.; Beta-Adalat; Cardaxen plus; Co-Atenolol; Cotenolol; Cotesifar; Kalten; Nif-Atenil; Nif-Ten; Primatenol Plus; Tenoretic; **Thai.:** Tenoret; Tenoretic; **UK:** Atenix-Co; Beta-Adalat; Kalten; Tenben†; Tenchlor; Tenif; Tenoret; Tenoretic; Totaretic; **USA:** Tenoretic.

## Atorvastatin Calcium *(BANM, USAN, rINNM)*

Atorvastatina cálcica; CI-981. Calcium (βR,δR)-2-(p-fluorophenyl)-β,δ-dihydroxy-5-isopropyl-3-phenyl-4-(phenylcarbamoyl)pyrrole-1-heptanoic acid (1:2) trihydrate.

$C_{66}H_{68}CaF_2N_4O_{10},3H_2O$ = 1209.4.

*CAS — 134523-00-5 (atorvastatin); 134523-03-8 (atorvastatin calcium).*

### Adverse Effects and Precautions

As for Simvastatin, p.997.

◊ General references.

1. Black DM, *et al.* An overview of the clinical safety profile of atorvastatin (Lipitor), a new HMG-CoA reductase inhibitor. *Arch Intern Med* 1998; **158:** 577–84.

**Effects on the skin.** Toxic epidermal necrolysis apparently caused by atorvastatin has been reported.[1] The authors were not aware of this adverse effect previously having been associated with any of the statin lipid regulating drugs.

1. Pfeiffer CM, *et al.* Toxic epidermal necrolysis from atorvastatin. *JAMA* 1998; **279:** 1613–14.

### Interactions

As for Simvastatin, p.998.

### Pharmacokinetics

Atorvastatin is rapidly absorbed from the gastrointestinal tract. It has low absolute bioavailability of about 12% due to presystemic clearance in the gastrointestinal mucosa and/or first-pass metabolism in the liver, its primary site of action. Atorvastatin is metabolised by the cytochrome P450 isoenzyme CYP3A4 to a number of active metabolites. It is 98% bound to plasma proteins. The mean plasma elimination half-life of atorvastatin is about 14 hours although the half-life of inhibitory activity for HMG-CoA reductase is about 20 to 30 hours due to the contribution of the active metabolites. Atorvastatin is excreted as metabolites, primarily in the bile.

◊ Reviews.

1. Lennernäs H. Clinical pharmacokinetics of atorvastatin. *Clin Pharmacokinet* 2003; **42:** 1141–60.

### Uses and Administration

Atorvastatin, a 3-hydroxy-3-methylglutaryl coenzyme A (HMG-CoA) reductase inhibitor (a statin), is a lipid regulating drug with actions on plasma lipids similar to those of simvastatin (p.999). It is used to reduce LDL-cholesterol, apolipoprotein B, and triglycerides, and to increase HDL-cholesterol in the treatment of hyperlipidaemias (p.823), including hypercholesterolaemias and combined (mixed) hyperlipidaemia (type IIa or IIb hyperlipoproteinaemias), hypertriglyceridaemia (type IV), and dysbetalipoproteinaemia (type III). Atorvastatin can also be effective as adjunctive therapy in patients with homozygous familial hypercholesterolaemia who have some LDL-receptor function.

Atorvastatin is given by mouth as the calcium salt although doses are expressed in terms of the base; 10.82 mg of atorvastatin calcium trihydrate is equivalent to 10 mg of base. The usual initial dose is 10 to 20 mg of atorvastatin once daily; an initial dose of 40 mg daily may be used in patients who require a large reduction in LDL-cholesterol. The dose may be adjusted at intervals of 4 weeks up to a maximum of 80 mg daily.

Children and adolescents aged 10 to 17 years with heterozygous familial hypercholesterolaemia may be given atorvastatin in an initial dose of 10 mg once daily, adjusted according to response to a maximum of 20 mg once daily.

◊ General reviews.

1. Lea AP, McTavish D. Atorvastatin: a review of its pharmacology and therapeutic potential in the management of hyperlipidaemias. *Drugs* 1997; **53:** 828–47.
2. Malinowski JM. Atorvastatin: a hydroxymethylglutaryl-coenzyme A reductase inhibitor. *Am J Health-Syst Pharm* 1998; **55:** 2253–67.
3. Malhotra HS, Goa KL. Atorvastatin: an updated review of its pharmacological properties and use in dyslipidaemia. *Drugs* 2001; **61:** 1835–81.

### Preparations

**Proprietary Preparations** (details are given in Part 3)
**Arg.:** Ampliar; Ateroclar; Atorvastan; Lipibec; Lipifen; Lipitor; Lipocambi; Liponorm; Lipovastinklonal; Normalip; Vastina; Zarator; **Austral.:** Lipitor; **Austria:** Sortis; **Belg.:** Lipitor; **Braz.:** Citalor; Lipitor; **Canad.:** Lipitor; **Chile:** Atenfar; Dislipor; Hipolixan; Lipitor; Lipotropic; Lipox; Lowden; Zarator; Zurinel; **Denm.:** Zarator; **Fin.:** Lipitor; **Fr.:** Tahor; **Ger.:** Sortis; **Gr.:** Lipitor; Zarator; **Hong Kong:** Lipitor; **India:** Atorva; **Irl.:** Lipitor; **Israel:** Lipitor; **Ital.:** Lipitor; Torvast; Totalip; Xarator; **Malaysia:** Lipitor; **Mex.:** Lipitor; **Neth.:** Lipitor; **Norw.:** Lipitor; **NZ:** Lipitor; **Port.:** Zarator; **S.Afr.:** Lipitor; **Singapore:** Lipitor; **Spain:** Cardyl; Prevencor; Zarator; **Swed.:** Lipitor; **Switz.:** Sortis; **Thai.:** Lipitor; **UK:** Lipitor; **USA:** Lipitor.

**Multi-ingredient: USA:** Caduet.

## Azamethonium Bromide *(BAN, rINN)*

Pentamethazene Bromide; Pentaminum. 2,2′-Methyliminobis(diethyldimethylammonium) dibromide.

$C_{13}H_{33}Br_2N_3$ = 391.2.

*CAS — 60-30-0 (azamethonium); 306-53-6 (azamethonium bromide).*

### Profile

Azamethonium bromide is a ganglion blocker used in the treatment of hypertension.

## Azapetine Phosphate *(BANM)*

Azepine Phosphate; Ro-2-3248. 6-Allyl-6,7-dihydro-5H-dibenz[c,e]azepine dihydrogen phosphate.

$C_{17}H_{17}N,H_3PO_4$ = 333.3.

*CAS — 146-36-1 (azapetine); 130-83-6 (azapetine phosphate).*

*ATC — C04AX30.*

### Profile

Azapetine is a vasodilator that has been used, as the phosphate, in peripheral vascular disorders.

### Preparations

**Proprietary Preparations** (details are given in Part 3)
**Mex.:** Peridil.

## Azelnidipine *(rINN)*

CS-905. 3-[1-(Diphenylmethyl)-3-azetidinyl] 5-isopropyl (±)-2-amino-1,4-dihydro-6-methyl-4-(m-nitrophenyl)-3,5-pyridinedicarboxylate.

$C_{33}H_{34}N_4O_6$ = 582.6.

*CAS — 123524-52-7.*

### Profile

Azelnidipine is a long-acting dihydropyridine calcium-channel blocker used in the management of hypertension.

◊ Reviews.

1. Wellington K, Scott LJ. Azelnidipine. *Drugs* 2003; **63:** 2613–21.

## Azimilide Hydrochloride *(BANM, rINNM)*

Azimilide Dihydrochloride *(USAN)*; Hidrocloruro de azimilida; NE-10064. 1-{[5-(p-Chlorophenyl)furfurylidene]amino}-3-[4-(4-methyl-1-piperazinyl)butyl]hydantoin dihydrochloride.

$C_{23}H_{28}ClN_5O_3,2HCl$ = 530.9.

*CAS — 149908-53-2 (azimilide); 149888-94-8 (azimilide hydrochloride).*

### Profile

Azimilide hydrochloride is a class III antiarrhythmic (p.809) being studied in the management of supraventricular arrhythmias.

◊ References.

1. Clemett D, Markham A. Azimilide. *Drugs* 2000; **59:** 271–7.
2. Pritchett ELC, *et al.* Effects of azimilide on heart rate and ECG conduction intervals during sinus rhythm in patients with a history of atrial fibrillation. *J Clin Pharmacol* 2002; **42:** 388–94.
3. Connolly SJ, *et al.* Symptoms at the time of arrhythmia recurrence in patients receiving azimilide for control of atrial fibrillation or flutter: results from randomized trials. *Am Heart J* 2003; **146:** 489–93.
4. Singer I, *et al.* Azimilide decreases recurrent ventricular tachyarrhythmias in patients with implantable cardioverter defibrillators. *J Am Coll Cardiol* 2004; **43:** 39–43.
5. Camm AJ, *et al.* Mortality in patients after a recent myocardial infarction: a randomized, placebo-controlled trial of azimilide using heart rate variability for risk stratification. *Circulation* 2004; **109:** 990–6.

## Azosemide *(USAN, rINN)*

Azosemida; BM-02001; Ple-1053. 2-Chloro-5-(1H-tetrazol-5-yl)-4-(2-thenylamino)benzenesulphonamide.

$C_{12}H_{11}ClN_6O_2S_2$ = 370.8.

*CAS — 27589-33-9.*

### Profile

Azosemide is a diuretic with actions similar to those of furosemide (p.919) that has been used in the management of oedema.

### Preparations

**Proprietary Preparations** (details are given in Part 3)
**Ger.:** Luret†.

## Bamethan Sulfate *(USAN, rINNM)*

Bamethan Sulphate *(BANM)*; Sulfato de bametán. 2-Butylamino-1-(4-hydroxyphenyl)ethanol sulfate.

$(C_{12}H_{19}NO_2)_2,H_2SO_4$ = 516.6.

*CAS — 3703-79-5 (bamethan); 5716-20-1 (bamethan sulfate).*

*ATC — C04AA31.*

**Pharmacopoeias.** In *Jpn* and *Pol.*

### Profile

Bamethan sulfate is a vasodilator used in the management of peripheral vascular disorders.

Bamethan nicotinate and bamethan succinate have been used similarly.

### Preparations

**Proprietary Preparations** (details are given in Part 3)
**Arg.:** Dilartan; **Austria:** Provascul; **Braz.:** Vasculat; **Ger.:** Emasex A; **Spain:** Vasculat†.

**Multi-ingredient: Arg.:** Flaval; Nadem Forte; Vefluxan; **Fr.:** Escinogel; **Ger.:** Emasex-N; Medigel.

## Barnidipine Hydrochloride *(rINNM)*

Hidrocloruro de barnidipino; LY-198561; Mepirodipine Hydrochloride; YM-730; YM-09730-5. (+)-(3′S,4S)-1-Benzyl-3-pyrrolidinyl methyl 1,4-dihydro-2,6-dimethyl-4-(m-nitrophenyl)-3,5-pyridinedicarboxylate hydrochloride.

$C_{27}H_{29}N_3O_6,HCl$ = 528.0.

*CAS — 104713-75-9 (barnidipine); 104757-53-1 (barnidipine hydrochloride).*

*ATC — C08CA12.*

### Profile

Barnidipine is a dihydropyridine calcium-channel blocker with general properties similar to those of nifedipine (p.966). It is given by mouth as the hydrochloride in the management of hypertension (p.825). The initial dose is 5 to 10 mg once daily, increased, according to response, to a usual maintenance dose of 10 to 20 mg once daily.

◊ Reviews.

1. Malhotra HS, Plosker GL. Barnidipine. *Drugs* 2001; **61:** 989–96.

### Preparations

**Proprietary Preparations** (details are given in Part 3)
**Arg.:** Dilacor; **Jpn:** Hypoca; **Neth.:** Cyress; **Spain:** Libradin; **Thai.:** Hypoca.

### Befunolol Hydrochloride *(rINNM)*

BFE-60; Hidrocloruro de befunolol. 7-[2-Hydroxy-3-(isopropylamino)propoxy]-2-benzofuranyl methyl ketone hydrochloride.

$C_{16}H_{21}NO_4,HCl = 327.8.$
*CAS — 39552-01-7 (befunolol); 39543-79-8 (befunolol hydrochloride).*
*ATC — S01ED06.*

#### Profile

Befunolol is a beta blocker (p.868). It is used as the hydrochloride in the management of ocular hypertension and open-angle glaucoma (p.1485). Eye drops containing befunolol hydrochloride 0.25% or 0.5% are instilled twice daily.

#### Preparations

**Proprietary Preparations** (details are given in Part 3)
***Austria:*** Glauconex; ***Belg.:*** Glauconex†; ***Fr.:*** Bentos; ***Ger.:*** Glauconex†; ***Hong Kong:*** Bentos†; ***Ital.:*** Betaclar; ***Jpn:*** Bentos.

### Bemetizide *(BAN, rINN)*

Bemetizida; Diu-60. 6-Chloro-3,4-dihydro-3-(α-methylbenzyl)-2*H*-1,2,4-benzothiadiazine-7-sulphonamide 1,1-dioxide.

$C_{15}H_{16}ClN_3O_4S_2 = 401.9.$
*CAS — 1824-52-8.*

#### Profile

Bemetizide is a thiazide diuretic (see Hydrochlorothiazide, p.933) that is used, often with triamterene, in the treatment of oedema and hypertension.

#### Preparations

**Proprietary Preparations** (details are given in Part 3)
**Multi-ingredient:** ***Austria:*** Diucomb†; ***Belg.:*** Diucomb; ***Ger.:*** dehydro sanol tri; dehydro tri mite; Diucomb; ***Switz.:*** Diucomb†.

## Bemiparin Sodium *(BAN, rINN)*

*CAS — 9041-08-1.*
*ATC — B01AB12.*

**Description.** Bemiparin sodium is prepared by alkaline degradation of heparin obtained from the intestinal mucosa of pigs. The majority of the components have a 2-*O*-sulfo-4-enepyranosuronic acid structure at the non-reducing end and a 2-*N*,6-*O*-disulfo-D-glucosamine structure at the reducing end of their chain. The average relative molecular mass is about 3600 (3000 to 4200). The degree of sulfation is about 2 per disaccharide unit.

#### Units

As for Low-molecular-weight Heparins, p.949.

#### Adverse Effects, Treatment, and Precautions

As for Low-molecular-weight Heparins, p.949.

Severe bleeding with bemiparin sodium may be reduced by the intravenous administration of protamine sulfate; 1.4 mg of protamine sulfate is stated to inhibit the effects of 100 units of bemiparin.

#### Interactions

As for Low-molecular-weight Heparins, p.950.

#### Pharmacokinetics

Bemiparin sodium is rapidly absorbed following subcutaneous injection with a bioavailability of about 96%. Peak plasma activity is reached in about 2 to 4 hours, depending on the dose. The elimination half-life is about 5 to 6 hours.

#### Uses and Administration

Bemiparin sodium is a low-molecular-weight heparin (p.949) with anticoagulant activity. It is used for the prevention and treatment of venous thromboembolism (p.839), and to prevent clotting during extracorporeal circulation.

In the prophylaxis of **venous thromboembolism** during surgery, bemiparin sodium is given subcutaneously in a dose of 2500 units once daily, with the first dose given 2 hours before or 6 hours after surgery; the dose should be increased to 3500 units once daily in patients at high risk of thromboembolism. For treatment of thromboembolism, a dose of 115 units/kg is given subcutaneously once daily.

For the prevention of clotting in the extracorporeal circulation during haemodialysis, bemiparin sodium is administered into the arterial side of the dialyser in a single dose of 2500 units for patients weighing less than 60 kg and 3500 units for patients weighing more than 60 kg.

◊ References.


1. Kakkar VV, *et al.* A comparative double-blind, randomised trial of a new second generation LMWH (bemiparin) and UFH in the prevention of post-operative venous thromboembolism. *Thromb Haemost* 2000; **83:** 523–9.
2. Chapman TM, Goa KL. Bemiparin: a review of its use in the prevention of venous thromboembolism and treatment of deep vein thrombosis. *Drugs* 2003; **63:** 2357–77.


#### Preparations

**Proprietary Preparations** (details are given in Part 3)
***Spain:*** Hibor; ***UK:*** Zibor.

## Benazepril Hydrochloride

*(BANM, USAN, rINNM)*

CGS-14824A (benazepril or benazepril hydrochloride); Hidrocloruro de benazepril. {(3*S*)-3-[(1*S*)-1-Ethoxycarbonyl-3-phenylpropylamino]-2,3,4,5-tetrahydro-2-oxo-1*H*-1-benzazepin-1-yl}acetic acid hydrochloride; 1-Carboxymethyl-3-[1-ethoxycarbonyl-3-phenyl-(1*S*)-propylamino]-2,3,4,5-tetrahydro-1*H*-1(3*S*)-benzazepin-2-one hydrochloride.

$C_{24}H_{28}N_2O_5,HCl = 461.0.$
*CAS — 86541-75-5 (benazepril); 86541-74-4 (benazepril hydrochloride).*
*ATC — C09AA07.*

#### Adverse Effects, Treatment, and Precautions

As for ACE inhibitors, p.842.

#### Interactions

As for ACE inhibitors, p.845.

#### Pharmacokinetics

Benazepril acts as a prodrug of the diacid benazeprilat, its active metabolite. Following oral administration at least 37% of a dose of benazepril is absorbed. Benazepril is almost completely metabolised in the liver to benazeprilat. Peak plasma concentrations of benazeprilat following an oral dose of benazepril have been achieved after 1 to 2 hours in the fasting state or after 2 to 4 hours in the nonfasting state. Both benazepril and benazeprilat are about 95% bound to plasma proteins. Benazeprilat is excreted mainly in the urine; about 11 to 12% is excreted in the bile. The effective half-life for accumulation of benazeprilat is 10 to 11 hours following multiple doses of benazepril. The elimination of benazeprilat is slowed in renal impairment, although biliary excretion may compensate to some extent. Small amounts of benazepril and benazeprilat are distributed into breast milk.

◊ References.


1. Kaiser G, *et al.* Pharmacokinetics of the angiotensin converting enzyme inhibitor benazepril HCl (CGS 14 824A) in healthy volunteers after single and repeated administration. *Biopharm Drug Dispos* 1989; **10:** 365–76.
2. Kaiser G, *et al.* Pharmacokinetics of a new angiotensin-converting enzyme inhibitor, benazepril hydrochloride, in special populations. *Am Heart J* 1989; **117:** 746–51.
3. Kaiser G, *et al.* Pharmacokinetics and pharmacodynamics of the ace inhibitor benazepril hydrochloride in the elderly. *Eur J Clin Pharmacol* 1990; **38:** 379–85.
4. Macdonald N-J, *et al.* A comparison in young and elderly subjects of the pharmacokinetics and pharmacodynamics of single and multiple doses of benazepril. *Br J Clin Pharmacol* 1993; **36:** 201–4.


#### Uses and Administration

Benazepril is an ACE inhibitor (p.842). It is used in the treatment of hypertension (p.825) and heart failure (p.820).

Benazepril owes its activity to benazeprilat to which it is converted after oral administration. The haemodynamic effects are seen within 1 hour of a single oral dose and the maximum effect occurs after about 2 to 4 hours, although the full effect may not develop for 1 to 2 weeks during chronic dosing. The haemodynamic action lasts for about 24 hours, allowing once-daily dosing. Benazepril is given by mouth as the hydrochloride.

In the treatment of **hypertension**, the usual initial dose of benazepril hydrochloride is 10 mg once daily. An initial dose of 5 mg once daily is suggested for patients with renal impairment (see below) or who are receiving a *diuretic*; if possible the diuretic should be withdrawn 2 or 3 days before benazepril is started and resumed later if necessary.

The usual maintenance dose is 20 to 40 mg daily, which may be given in 2 divided doses if control is inadequate with a single dose; doses of up to 80 mg daily have been used.

In the treatment of **heart failure** the usual initial dose of benazepril hydrochloride is 2.5 mg once daily, adjusted according to response to a maximum dose of 20 mg daily.

**Administration in renal impairment.** In patients with a creatinine clearance of less than 30 mL/minute, the initial dose of benazepril hydrochloride for hypertension is 5 mg once daily and the maintenance dose should not exceed 40 mg daily.

#### Preparations

**Proprietary Preparations** (details are given in Part 3)
***Arg.:*** Boncordin; ***Austria:*** Cibacen†; ***Belg.:*** Cibacen; ***Braz.:*** Lotensin; ***Canad.:*** Lotensin; ***Denm.:*** Cibacen; ***Fr.:*** Briem; Cibacene; ***Ger.:*** Cibacen; ***Gr.:*** Cibacen; ***India:*** Benace; ***Irl.:*** Cibacen; ***Israel:*** Cibacen; ***Ital.:*** Cibacen; Tensanil; Zinadril; ***Mex.:*** Lotensin; ***Neth.:*** Cibacen; ***NZ:*** Cibacen†; ***S.Afr.:*** Cibace; ***Spain:*** Cibacen; Labopal; ***Switz.:*** Cibacen; ***USA:*** Lotensin.
**Multi-ingredient:** ***Arg.:*** Adrebloc; Amzepril; Coroval B; Pelmec Duo; Terloc Duo; ***Austria:*** Cibadrex†; ***Braz.:*** Lotensin H; ***Denm.:*** Cibadrex†; ***Fr.:*** Briazide; Cibadrex; ***Ger.:*** Cibadrex; ***India:*** Amace-BP; ***Ital.:*** Cibadrex; Tensadiur; Zinadiur; ***Neth.:*** Cibadrex; ***S.Afr.:*** Cibadrex; ***Switz.:*** Cibadrex; ***USA:*** Lotensin HCT; Lotrel.

### Bencyclane Fumarate *(rINNM)*

Bencyclane Hydrogen Fumarate; Fumarato de benciclano. 3-(1-Benzylcycloheptyloxy)-*NN*-dimethylpropylamine hydrogen fumarate.

$C_{19}H_{31}NO,C_4H_4O_4 = 405.5.$
*CAS — 2179-37-5 (bencyclane); 14286-84-1 (bencyclane fumarate).*
*ATC — C04AX11.*

#### Profile

Bencyclane fumarate is a vasodilator used in the management of peripheral (p.831) and cerebral vascular disorders (p.820) in usual doses of 100 to 200 mg three times daily by mouth. It has also been given intravenously.

Bencyclane acefyllinate has also been used.

#### Preparations

**Proprietary Preparations** (details are given in Part 3)
***Austria:*** Ludilat; ***Braz.:*** Fludilat; ***Ger.:*** Fludilat; ***Hong Kong:*** Fludilat†; ***Port.:*** Fludilat; Fluxema†; ***Thai.:*** Fludilat.
**Multi-ingredient:** ***Spain:*** Dilapres†.

## Bendroflumethiazide *(BAN, rINN)*

Bendrofluaz.; Bendrofluazide; Bendroflumethiazidum; Bendroflumetiazida; Benzydroflumethiazide; FT-81. 3-Benzyl-3,4-dihydro-6-trifluoromethyl-2*H*-1,2,4-benzothiadiazine-7-sulphonamide 1,1-dioxide.

$C_{15}H_{14}F_3N_3O_4S_2 = 421.4.$
*CAS — 73-48-3.*
*ATC — C03AA01.*

**Pharmacopoeias.** In *Chin., Eur.* (see p.vi), and *US.*

**Ph. Eur. 5.0** (Bendroflumethiazide). A white or almost white crystalline powder. Practically insoluble in water; soluble in alcohol; freely soluble in acetone.

**USP 27** (Bendroflumethiazide). A white to cream-coloured, finely divided, crystalline powder. Is odourless or has a slight odour. Practically insoluble in water; soluble 1 in 23 of alcohol and 1 in 200 of ether; freely soluble in acetone. Store in airtight containers.

#### Adverse Effects, Treatment, and Precautions

As for Hydrochlorothiazide, p.933.

**Breast feeding.** Bendroflumethiazide is used to suppress lactation (see Uses below). However, the American Academy of Pediatrics considers[1] that it is usually compatible with breast feeding.


1. American Academy of Pediatrics. The transfer of drugs and other chemicals into human milk. *Pediatrics* 2001; **108:** 776–89. Correction. *ibid.*; 1029. Also available at: http://aappolicy.aappublications.org/cgi/content/full/pediatrics%3b108/3/776 (accessed 06/07/04)


**Porphyria.** Bendroflumethiazide is considered to be unsafe in patients with porphyria because it has been shown to be porphyrinogenic in *animals* or *in-vitro* systems.

**Overdosage.** Tonic-clonic convulsions occurred in a previously healthy 14-year-old girl following ingestion of bendroflumethiazide 150 to 200 mg.[1] The convulsions were not associated with any measurable disturbance of serum electrolytes.


1. Hine KR, *et al.* Bendrofluazide convulsions. *Lancet* 1982; **i:** 564.

### Interactions

As for Hydrochlorothiazide, p.935.

### Pharmacokinetics

Bendroflumethiazide has been reported to be completely absorbed from the gastrointestinal tract and to have a plasma half-life of about 3 or 4 hours. It is highly bound to plasma proteins. There are indications that bendroflumethiazide is fairly extensively metabolised; about 30% is excreted unchanged in the urine.

◊ References.

1. Beermann B, *et al.* Pharmacokinetics of bendroflumethiazide. *Clin Pharmacol Ther* 1977; **22:** 385–8.
2. Beermann B, *et al.* Pharmacokinetics of bendroflumethiazide in hypertensive patients. *Eur J Clin Pharmacol* 1978; **13:** 119–24.

### Uses and Administration

Bendroflumethiazide is a thiazide diuretic with actions and uses similar to those of hydrochlorothiazide (p.935). It is used for hypertension (p.825), either alone or with other antihypertensives such as ACE inhibitors and beta blockers. It is also used for oedema, including that associated with heart failure (p.820), and with renal or hepatic disorders. Other indications have included the suppression of lactation.

Diuresis starts in about 2 hours after oral administration of bendroflumethiazide, peaks after about 3 to 6 hours, and lasts for 12 to 18 hours or longer.

In the treatment of **hypertension** bendroflumethiazide 2.5 mg daily, either alone or with other antihypertensives, is usually adequate although doses of up to 20 mg daily have sometimes been suggested.

In the treatment of **oedema** the usual initial dose is 5 to 10 mg by mouth daily or on alternate days; in some cases initial doses of up to 20 mg may be necessary. Maintenance dosage schedules have varied from 2.5 to 10 mg once to three times weekly in the UK to 2.5 to 5 mg daily or intermittently in the USA.

An initial dose for children is up to 400 micrograms/kg daily, reduced to 50 to 100 micrograms/kg for maintenance.

Doses of 5 mg twice daily for about 5 days have been used to **suppress lactation**.

In the management of **idiopathic hypercalciuria** (see Renal Calculi, p.936) the *British National Formulary* considers that, with increased fluid intake, a sufficient dose is 2.5 mg daily.

### Preparations

***BP 2003:*** Bendroflumethiazide Tablets;
***USP 27:*** Bendroflumethiazide Tablets; Nadolol and Bendroflumethiazide Tablets.

**Proprietary Preparations** (details are given in Part 3)
***Austral.:*** Aprinox; ***Canad.:*** Naturetin†; ***Denm.:*** Centyl; ***Fr.:*** Naturine†; ***Irl.:*** Centyl; ***Norw.:*** Centyl; ***NZ:*** Neo-NaClex; ***Swed.:*** Salures; ***Switz.:*** Sinesalin†; ***UK:*** Aprinox; Neo-NaClex; ***USA:*** Naturetin.

**Multi-ingredient:** ***Arg.:*** Hidromens; Pertenso; Sumal; ***Austria:*** Inderetic; Pressimedin†; Sali-Aldopur; Solgeretik†; ***Belg.:*** Inderetic; ***Braz.:*** Diserim; ***Canad.:*** Corzide†; ***Denm.:*** Centyl med Kaliumklorid; ***Fr.:*** Precyclan; Tensionorme; ***Ger.:*** Docidrazin; Dociretic; Pertenso N; Sali-Aldopur; Sotaziden N; Spirostada comp; Tensoflux; ***Irl.:*** Centyl K; Inderetic†; Low Centyl K; Prestim†; ***Neth.:*** Inderetic; ***Norw.:*** Centyl med Kaliumklorid; ***S.Afr.:*** Corgaretic; Inderetic; ***Spain:*** Betadipresan Diu; Neatenol Diu; Neatenol Diuvas; Spirometon; ***Swed.:*** Salures-K; ***Switz.:*** Corgaretic†; Inderetic; Pressimed†; Saluretin†; ***UK:*** Centyl K; Corgaretic†; Inderetic†; Inderex†; Neo-NaClex-K; Prestim; Tenben†; ***USA:*** Corzide; Rauzide.

## Benfluorex Hydrochloride *(BANM, pINNM)*

Benfluorexi Hydrochloridum; Hidrocloruro de benfluorex; JP-992; SE-780. 2-[α-Methyl-3-(trifluoromethyl)phenethylamino]ethyl benzoate hydrochloride.

$C_{19}H_{20}F_3NO_2,HCl$ = 387.8.
*CAS — 23602-78-0 (benfluorex); 35976-51-3 (± benfluorex); 23642-66-2 (benfluorex hydrochloride).*

**Pharmacopoeias.** In *Eur.* (see p.vi).

**Ph. Eur. 5.0** (Benfluorex Hydrochloride). A white or almost white powder. It exhibits polymorphism. Slightly soluble in water; sparingly soluble or soluble in alcohol; soluble in dichloromethane; freely soluble in methyl alcohol.

### Profile

Benfluorex hydrochloride is a lipid regulating drug used in the treatment of hyperlipidaemias (p.823). It has also been used as an adjunct in the management of type 2 diabetes mellitus (p.324).

Benfluorex hydrochloride is given in usual doses of 150 mg three times daily by mouth with meals.

### Preparations

**Proprietary Preparations** (details are given in Part 3)
***Fr.:*** Mediator; ***Hong Kong:*** Mediaxal; ***Ital.:*** Mediaxal; ***Malaysia:*** Mediaxal; ***Port.:*** Mediator; ***Singapore:*** Mediaxal; ***Spain:*** Modulator.

## Benidipine Hydrochloride *(rINNM)*

Hidrocloruro de benidipino; KW-3049; Nakadipine Hydrochloride. (±)-(R*)-3-[(R*)-1-Benzyl-3-piperidyl]methyl 1,4-dihydro-2,6-dimethyl-4-(m-nitrophenyl)-3,5-pyridinedicarboxylate hydrochloride.

$C_{28}H_{31}N_3O_6,HCl$ = 542.0.
*CAS — 105979-17-7 (benidipine); 91599-74-5 (benidipine hydrochloride).*
*ATC — C08CA15.*

### Profile

Benidipine is a dihydropyridine calcium-channel blocker with general properties similar to those of nifedipine (p.966). It is given by mouth as the hydrochloride in the management of hypertension (p.825) and angina pectoris (p.813). In hypertension, the usual dose is 2 to 4 mg once daily, increased to 8 mg once daily if necessary. In angina pectoris, the usual dose is 4 mg twice daily.

### Preparations

**Proprietary Preparations** (details are given in Part 3)
***India:*** Caritec; ***Jpn:*** Coniel.

## Benzthiazide *(BAN, rINN)*

Benztiazida; P-1393. 3-Benzylthiomethyl-6-chloro-2H-1,2,4-benzothiadiazine-7-sulphonamide 1,1-dioxide.

$C_{15}H_{14}ClN_3O_4S_3$ = 431.9.
*CAS — 91-33-8.*

### Profile

Benzthiazide is a thiazide diuretic with properties similar to those of hydrochlorothiazide (p.933). It is used for oedema, including that associated with heart failure (p.820), and has also been used for hypertension (p.825). It has been given alone but is often given with triamterene. The usual initial dose for oedema is 75 mg daily by mouth, although higher doses have been given. The dose is reduced for maintenance; intermittent dosing may be adequate.

### Preparations

**Proprietary Preparations** (details are given in Part 3)
***USA:*** Exna†.

**Multi-ingredient:** ***Switz.:*** Dyrenium compositum; ***UK:*** Dytide.

## Bepridil Hydrochloride *(BANM, USAN, rINNM)*

CERM-1978; Hidrocloruro de bepridil; Org-5730. N-Benzyl-N-(3-isobutoxy-2-pyrrolidin-1-ylpropyl)aniline hydrochloride monohydrate.

$C_{24}H_{34}N_2O,HCl,H_2O$ = 421.0.
*CAS — 64706-54-3 (bepridil); 49571-04-2 (bepridil); 64616-81-5 (anhydrous bepridil hydrochloride); 74764-40-2 (bepridil hydrochloride monohydrate).*
*ATC — C08EA02.*

### Profile

Bepridil is a calcium-channel blocker (p.810). It has similar properties to nifedipine (p.966) but reduces the heart rate and does not usually cause reflex tachycardia. It also has antiarrhythmic activity. It is not related chemically to other calcium-channel blockers such as diltiazem, nifedipine, or verapamil.

Bepridil is used as the hydrochloride in the management of angina pectoris (p.813). Ventricular arrhythmias, including torsade de pointes, and agranulocytosis have been associated with bepridil and, as a result, it is usually reserved for patients who have not responded adequately to other anti-anginal drugs. The usual initial dose is 200 mg of bepridil hydrochloride once daily by mouth, increased after 10 days to 300 mg once daily, if tolerated; the maximum dose is 400 mg once daily. Elderly patients and those with hepatic or renal impairment may require reduced doses and more frequent monitoring.

◊ References.

1. Hollingshead LM, *et al.* Bepridil: a review of its pharmacological properties and therapeutic use in stable angina pectoris. *Drugs* 1992; **44:** 835–57.
2. Awni WM, *et al.* Pharmacokinetics of bepridil and two of its metabolites in patients with end-stage renal disease. *J Clin Pharmacol* 1995; **35:** 379–83.

**Porphyria.** Bepridil is considered to be unsafe in patients with porphyria because it has been shown to be porphyrinogenic in *in-vitro* systems.

### Preparations

**Proprietary Preparations** (details are given in Part 3)
***Belg.:*** Cordium†; ***Fr.:*** Cordium†; Unicordium; ***USA:*** Vascor†.

# Beta Blockers

β-Bloqueantes.

Beta blockers (beta-adrenoceptor blocking drugs or antagonists) are competitive antagonists of catecholamines at beta-adrenergic receptors in a wide range of tissues. Although they have broadly similar properties they differ in their affinity for $beta_1$ or $beta_2$ receptor subtypes, intrinsic sympathomimetic activity, membrane-stabilising activity, blockade of alpha-adrenergic receptors, and pharmacokinetic properties including differences in lipid solubility (see Table 4, below, for some of these characteristics). These differences may affect the choice of drug in specific situations.

**Table 4.** Characteristics of beta blockers.

| Beta blocker | $Beta_1$ selectivity | Intrinsic sympathomimetic activity | Membrane-stabilising activity |
|---|---|---|---|
| Acebutolol | + | + | + |
| Alprenolol | 0 | + | 0 |
| Atenolol | + | 0 | 0 |
| Betaxolol | + | 0 | 0 |
| Bisoprolol | + | 0 | 0 |
| Carteolol | 0 | + | 0 |
| Carvedilol | 0 | 0 | 0 |
| Celiprolol | + | + | – |
| Esmolol | + | 0 | 0 |
| Labetalol | 0 | 0 | 0 |
| Levobunolol | 0 | 0 | 0 |
| Metipranolol | 0 | 0 | 0 |
| Metoprolol | + | 0 | 0 |
| Nadolol | 0 | 0 | 0 |
| Nebivolol | + | 0 | 0 |
| Oxprenolol | 0 | + | + |
| Penbutolol | 0 | 0 | 0 |
| Pindolol | 0 | ++ | 0 |
| Propranolol | 0 | 0 | ++ |
| Sotalol | 0 | 0 | 0 |
| Timolol | 0 | 0 | 0 |

0 = absent or low; + = moderate; ++ = high; – = no information

## Adverse Effects

Beta blockers are generally well tolerated and most adverse effects are mild. The most frequent and serious adverse effects are related to their beta-adrenergic blocking activity. Among the most serious adverse effects are heart failure, heart block, and bronchospasm. Troublesome subjective side-effects include fatigue and coldness of the extremities. Reactions may be more severe following intravenous than oral administration; ocular use has also been associated with systemic adverse effects. When beta blockers are used for long-term treatment of asymptomatic diseases such as hypertension, subjective side-effects may be an important determinant of patient compliance.

Cardiovascular effects include bradycardia and hypotension; heart failure or heart block may be precipitated in patients with underlying cardiac disorders. Abrupt withdrawal of beta blockers may exacerbate angina and may lead to sudden death. (For further details on withdrawal of beta blockers, see Precautions, below.) Reduced peripheral circulation can produce coldness of the extremities and may exacerbate peripheral vascular disease such as Raynaud's syndrome.

Bronchospasm, shortness of breath, and dyspnoea, may be precipitated in susceptible patients due to blockade of beta$_2$ receptors in bronchial smooth muscle. Drugs with selectivity for beta$_1$ receptors or with intrinsic sympathomimetic activity at beta$_2$ receptors may be less likely to induce bronchospasm (but see Precautions, below). Pneumonitis, pulmonary fibrosis, and pleurisy have also been reported.

CNS effects include headache, depression, dizziness, hallucinations, confusion, and sleep disturbances including nightmares. Coma and convulsions have been reported following beta-blocker overdosage. Beta blockers that are lipid soluble are more likely to enter the brain and would be expected to be associated with a higher incidence of CNS adverse effects, although this is not proven.

Fatigue is a common side-effect experienced with beta blockers. Paraesthesia, peripheral neuropathy, arthralgia, and myopathies, including muscle cramps, have been reported.

Adverse gastrointestinal effects include nausea and vomiting, diarrhoea, constipation, and abdominal cramping.

Beta blockers interfere with carbohydrate and lipid metabolism and can produce hypoglycaemia, hyperglycaemia, and changes in blood concentrations of triglycerides and cholesterol (see below for further details).

Skin rash, pruritus, exacerbation of psoriasis, and reversible alopecia have occurred with use of beta blockers.

Decreased tear production, blurred vision, and soreness are among the ocular symptoms that have been reported. Adverse effects specific to ocular use are also discussed below.

Haematological reactions include nonthrombocytopenic purpura, thrombocytopenia, and rarely agranulocytosis. Transient eosinophilia can occur.

Other adverse effects reported with some beta blockers include a lupus-like syndrome, male impotence, sclerosing peritonitis, and retroperitoneal fibrosis.

**Carcinogenicity.** An apparent excess of deaths from cancer was noted in elderly men, but not women, given atenolol during a trial of antihypertensive treatment.[1] However, two subsequent studies found no evidence of a link between atenolol and cancer.[2,3]


1. MRC Working Party. Medical Research Council trial of treatment of hypertension in older adults: principal results. *BMJ* 1992; **304:** 405–12.
2. Fletcher AE, *et al.* Cancer mortality and atenolol treatment. *BMJ* 1993; **306:** 622–3.
3. Hole DJ, *et al.* Incidence of and mortality from cancer in hypertensive patients. *BMJ* 1993; **306:** 609–11.


**Effects on bones and joints.** There have been a number of reports of arthralgia in patients receiving beta blockers. Five cases associated with the use of metoprolol had been reported to the FDA;[1] there had also been 6 reports of similar symptoms with propranolol, and 1 with atenolol. A case of polymyalgia rheumatic-like syndrome has also been reported.[2]


1. Sills JM, Bosco L. Arthralgia associated with β-adrenergic blockade. *JAMA* 1986; **255:** 198–9.
2. Snyder S. Metoprolol-induced polymyalgia-like syndrome. *Ann Intern Med* 1991; **114:** 96–7.


**Effects on carbohydrate metabolism.** The sympathetic nervous system is involved in the control of carbohydrate metabolism and beta blockers can interfere with carbohydrate and insulin regulation; both hypoglycaemia and hyperglycaemia have been reported.

Propranolol-induced hypoglycaemia was first noted in adult type 1 diabetic patients in the late 1960s. A review[1] of drug-induced hypoglycaemia found that most reports associated with beta blockers were in nondiabetic patients taking propranolol and undergoing regular haemodialysis, neonates of mothers who took propranolol until a few hours before delivery, infants who received propranolol, and both diabetic and nondiabetic patients on long-term propranolol who were nutritionally compromised or had liver disease. In addition, in type 1 diabetes mellitus beta blockers mask the adrenaline-mediated symptoms of hypoglycaemia such as tachycardia and tremor, and may delay recovery in patients given glucose for hypoglycaemia. In a long-term study[2] in type 2 diabetics, however, there was no difference in the incidence of hypoglycaemia in patients receiving captopril or atenolol and both significantly improved outcome. A case-control study[3] and a review[4] of the use of beta blockers in diabetic patients both concluded that the incidence of hypoglycaemia was not increased and that beta blockers were appropriate therapy for diabetics. Although there have been conflicting reports, most studies have suggested that cardioselective beta blockers with little or no lipophilicity are preferred in type 2 diabetics.[5]

A number of studies in hypertensive patients have reported that beta blockers may be associated with the development of hyperglycaemia,[6,7] and in some cases diabetes mellitus,[8-10] but again the established benefits of beta blockers generally outweigh this risk.[11]


1. Seltzer HS. Drug-induced hypoglycemia. *Endocrinol Metab Clin North Am* 1989; **18:** 163–83.
2. UK Prospective Diabetes Study Group. Efficacy of atenolol and captopril in reducing risk of macrovascular and microvascular complications in type 2 diabetes: UKPDS 39. *BMJ* 1998; **317:** 713–20.
3. Thamer M, *et al.* Association between antihypertensive drug use and hypoglycemia: a case-control study of diabetic users of insulin or sulfonylureas. *Clin Ther* 1999; **21:** 1387–1400.
4. Sawicki PT, Siebenhofer A. Betablocker treatment in diabetes mellitus. *J Intern Med* 2001; **250:** 11–17.
5. O'Byrne S, Feely J. Effects of drugs on glucose tolerance in non-insulin-dependent diabetics (part 1). *Drugs* 1990; **40:** 6–18.
6. Veterans Administration Cooperative Study Group on Antihypertensive Agents. Propranolol or hydrochlorothiazide alone for the initial treatment of hypertension IV: effect on plasma glucose and glucose tolerance. *Hypertension* 1985; **7:** 1008–16.
7. Pollare T, *et al.* Sensitivity to insulin during treatment with atenolol and metoprolol: a randomised, double blind study of effects on carbohydrate and lipoprotein metabolism in hypertensive patients. *BMJ* 1989; **298:** 1152–7.
8. Skarfors ET, *et al.* Do antihypertensive drugs precipitate diabetes in predisposed men? *BMJ* 1989; **298:** 1147–52.
9. Samuelsson O, *et al.* Diabetes mellitus in treated hypertension: incidence, predictive factors and the impact of non-selective beta-blockers and thiazide diuretics during 15 years treatment of middle-aged hypertensive men in the Primary Prevention Trial in Göteborg, Sweden. *J Hum Hypertens* 1994; **8:** 257–63.
10. Gress TW, *et al.* Hypertension and antihypertensive therapy as risk factors for type 2 diabetes mellitus. *N Engl J Med* 2000; **342:** 905–12.
11. Luna B, Feinglos MN. Drug-induced hyperglycemia. *JAMA* 2001; **286:** 1945–8.


**Effects on the circulation.** Hypotension is a recognised adverse effect of beta blockers, and severe reactions have been reported. Near-fatal shock occurred[1] within 40 minutes of acebutolol 400 mg being given to an elderly patient with chronic bronchitis and angina pectoris. Hypotension, leading to a rise in serum creatinine indicative of kidney ischaemia, occurred[2] in 2 women following a single oral dose of atenolol 100 mg or 2 oral doses of atenolol 50 mg; both had presented with severe hypertension, hyponatraemia, hypokalaemia, and high renin activity. Renal artery thrombosis believed to be due to the hypotensive effect of atenolol was reported[3] in a 70-year-old man with a history of circulatory and cardiac disorders. He had received atenolol 100 mg for treatment of moderate hypertension.


1. Tirlapur VG, *et al.* Shock syndrome after acebutolol. *Br J Clin Pract* 1986; **40:** 33–4.
2. Kholeif M, Isles C. Profound hypotension after atenolol in severe hypertension. *BMJ* 1989; **298:** 161–2.
3. Shaw AB, Gopalka SK. Renal artery thrombosis caused by antihypertensive treatment. *BMJ* 1982; **285:** 1617.


**Effects on the gastrointestinal tract.** Sclerosing peritonitis was noted as part of the 'oculomucocutaneous syndrome' that occurred with practolol. However, while both sclerosing peritonitis and retroperitoneal fibrosis have also been reported with a number of other beta blockers, including atenolol,[1,2] metoprolol,[3,4] oxprenolol,[5] propranolol,[6] sotalol,[7] and timolol,[8,9] a review[10] of 100 cases of retroperitoneal fibrosis concluded that beta blockers could not be considered as the cause.


1. Nielsen BV, Pedersen KG. Sclerosing peritonitis associated with atenolol. *BMJ* 1985; **290:** 518.
2. Johnson JN, McFarland J. Retroperitoneal fibrosis associated with atenolol. *BMJ* 1980; **280:** 864.
3. Thompson J, Julian DG. Retroperitoneal fibrosis associated with metoprolol. *BMJ* 1982; **284:** 83–4.
4. Clark CV, Terris R. Sclerosing peritonitis associated with metoprolol. *Lancet* 1983; **i:** 937.
5. McCluskey DR, *et al.* Oxprenolol and retroperitoneal fibrosis. *BMJ* 1980; **281:** 1459–60.
6. Pierce JR, *et al.* Propranolol and retroperitoneal fibrosis. *Ann Intern Med* 1981; **95:** 244.
7. Laakso M, *et al.* Retroperitoneal fibrosis associated with sotalol. *BMJ* 1982; **285:** 1085–6.
8. Baxter-Smith DC, *et al.* Sclerosing peritonitis in patient on timolol. *Lancet* 1978; **ii:** 149.
9. Rimmer E, *et al.* Retroperitoneal fibrosis associated with timolol. *Lancet* 1983; **i:** 300.
10. Pryor JP, *et al.* Do beta-adrenoceptor blocking drugs cause retroperitoneal fibrosis? *BMJ* 1983; **287:** 639–41.


**Effects on lipid metabolism.** The adrenergic system is involved in the control of lipid metabolism and beta blockers may therefore have effects on plasma-lipid concentrations. In general, beta blocker therapy results in increased concentrations of very-low-density lipoprotein and triglycerides, a reduction in high-density lipoprotein, and no change in low-density lipoprotein.[1] These effects may be less pronounced with beta$_1$ cardioselective drugs, beta blockers with intrinsic sympathomimetic activity, and beta blockers that also block alpha-adrenergic receptors. For example, pindolol,[2,3] a beta blocker with intrinsic sympathomimetic activity, and arotinolol[4] and carvedilol,[5] which possess alpha-adrenergic blocking properties, are reported to have no adverse effects on plasma-lipid concentrations, although acute pancreatitis due to severe hypertriglyceridaemia has been reported[6] in a patient treated with metoprolol followed by atenolol. However, the effects on lipid concentrations are generally fairly small, and a review of the subject[7] concluded that there was little or no evidence that such effects negated the beneficial effects of beta blockers on cardiovascular outcomes.


1. Krone W, Nägele H. Effects of antihypertensives on plasma lipids and lipoprotein metabolism. *Am Heart J* 1988; **116:** 1729–34.
2. Hunter Hypertension Research Group. Effects of pindolol, or a pindolol/clopamide combination preparation, on plasma lipid levels in essential hypertension. *Med J Aust* 1989; **150:** 646–52.
3. Terént A, *et al.* Long-term effect of pindolol on lipids and lipoproteins in men with newly diagnosed hypertension. *Eur J Clin Pharmacol* 1989; **36:** 347–50.
4. Sasaki J, *et al.* Effects of arotinolol on serum lipid and apolipoprotein levels in patients with mild essential hypertension. *Clin Ther* 1989; **11:** 580–3.
5. Hauf-Zachariou U, *et al.* A double-blind comparison of the effects of carvedilol and captopril on serum lipid concentrations in patients with mild to moderate essential hypertension and dyslipidaemia. *Eur J Clin Pharmacol* 1993; **45:** 95–100.
6. Durrington PN, Cairns SA. Acute pancreatitis: a complication of beta-blockade. *BMJ* 1982; **284:** 1016.
7. Weir MR, Moser M. Diuretics and β-blockers: is there a risk for dyslipidemia? *Am Heart J* 2000; **139:** 174–84.


**Effects following ophthalmic use.** Ophthalmic administration of beta blockers may produce the following localised effects: ocular irritation (including hypersensitivity), blepharitis, keratitis, decreased corneal sensitivity, visual disturbances, diplopia, photophobia, and ptosis. Uveitis has been reported with metipranolol eye drops.[1] A case of iris depigmentation has occurred[2] following the use of topical levobunolol. Older patients using topical beta blockers may be at greater risk of decreased corneal sensitivity or corneal anaesthesia with the consequent risk of keratitis.[3]

Systemic absorption may occur following the use of beta blockers in eye drops. Excess drug can drain into the lachrymal ducts to be absorbed through the nasal mucosa. Absorption also occurs via the ophthalmic and facial veins. Following such absorption the beta blocker reaches the systemic circulation without undergoing first-pass hepatic metabolism.

The main systemic effects associated with topical ocular administration of beta blockers are on the pulmonary, cardiovascular, and central nervous systems.[4,5]

Pulmonary effects that have been reported include acute pulmonary oedema associated with use of metipranolol eye drops,[6] and wheezing after a single dose of topical levobunolol, which developed into severe respiratory distress requiring hospitalisation after a second dose.[7] Myocardial infarction has been reported[8] shortly after a single dose of betaxolol eye drops; the patient was also taking atenolol and indapamide for hypertension. Systemic effects have also been reported in patients using timolol eye drops, including depression and bradycardia, with a rise in blood pressure and neurological signs of stroke following rapid withdrawal of the drops,[9] and severe nausea and vomiting, which resolved within a few days of withdrawal but recurred on rechallenge.[10] A number of cases of alopecia associated with ocular use of beta blockers have also been reported.[11]


1. Akingbehin T, Villada JR. Metipranolol-associated granulomatous anterior uveitis. *Br J Ophthalmol* 1991; **75:** 519–23.
2. Doyle E, Liu C. A case of acquired iris depigmentation as a possible complication of levobunolol eye drops. *Br J Ophthalmol* 1999; **83:** 1405–6.
3. Weissman SS, Asbell PA. Effects of topical timolol (0.5%) and betaxolol (0.5%) on corneal sensitivity. *Br J Ophthalmol* 1990; **74:** 409–12.
4. Everitt DE, Avorn J. Systemic effects of medications used to treat glaucoma. *Ann Intern Med* 1990; **112:** 120–5.
5. Vander Zanden JA, *et al.* Systemic adverse effects of ophthalmic β-blockers. *Ann Pharmacother* 2001; **35:** 1633–7.
6. Johns MD, Ponte CD. Acute pulmonary edema associated with ocular metipranolol use. *Ann Pharmacother* 1995; **29:** 370–3.
7. Stubbs GM. Betagan drops. *Med J Aust* 1994; **161:** 576.
8. Chamberlain TJ. Myocardial infarction after ophthalmic betaxolol. *N Engl J Med* 1989; **321:** 1342.
9. Rao MR, *et al.* Systemic hazards of ocular timolol. *Br J Hosp Med* 1993; **50:** 553.
10. Wolfhagen FHJ, *et al.* Severe nausea and vomiting with timolol eye drops. *Lancet* 1998; **352:** 373.
11. Fraunfelder FT, *et al.* Alopecia possibly secondary to topical ophthalmic β-blockers. *JAMA* 1990; **263:** 1493–4.

**Hypersensitivity.** For the suggestion that beta blockers may exacerbate anaphylactic reactions, see under Precautions, below.

**Overdosage.** Many cases of beta-blocker overdosage[1-3] are uneventful, but some patients develop severe and occasionally fatal cardiovascular depression. Effects can include bradycardia, cardiac conduction block, hypotension, heart failure, and cardiogenic shock. Convulsions, coma, respiratory depression, and bronchoconstriction can also occur, although infrequently. Most reports of serious toxic reactions following overdosage concern beta blockers with significant membrane-stabilising activity, such as propranolol or oxprenolol.[1] Overdosage of beta blockers with intrinsic sympathomimetic activity may present with tachycardia and hypertension.[2] Overdosage of sotalol, a beta blocker with class II and III antiarrhythmic properties, usually presents as ventricular tachyarrhythmia.[1,2]

1. Critchley JAJH, Ungar A. The management of acute poisoning due to β-adrenoceptor antagonists. *Med Toxicol* 1989; **4:** 32–45.
2. Pentel PR, Salerno DM. Cardiac drug toxicity: digitalis glycosides and calcium-channel and β-blocking agents. *Med J Aust* 1990; **152:** 88–94.
3. Taboulet P, *et al.* Pathophysiology and management of self-poisoning with beta-blockers. *Clin Toxicol* 1993; **31:** 531–51.

## Treatment of Adverse Effects

Beta blockers are generally well tolerated and adverse effects usually respond to a reduction in dose. In overdosage, administration of activated charcoal or gastric lavage should be considered if the patient presents within 1 hour of ingestion. Mild hypotension may respond to intravenous fluid administration. If hypotension continues, intravenous glucagon should be given; sympathomimetics may be used as an alternative or given with glucagon. Isoprenaline is the sympathomimetic of choice since it acts mainly at beta receptors, but other sympathomimetics may also be used. High doses may be required; infusion rates of up to 333 micrograms/minute of isoprenaline have been used. Atropine may be given intravenously for bradycardia; sympathomimetics or a cardiac pacemaker may also be required. $Beta_2$ agonists or xanthines may be given for bronchospasm; hypoglycaemia may respond to glucose or glucagon. Haemodialysis may be of benefit for severe overdosage with renally excreted beta blockers, but is usually unnecessary.

**Overdosage.** A patient who failed to respond to the usual management for beta-blocker overdosage (see above) responded to treatment with enoximone.[1] A dramatic response to calcium chloride has also been reported in a patient with electromechanical dissociation following propranolol overdosage.[2]

1. Hoeper MM, Boeker KHW. Overdose of metoprolol treated with enoximone. *N Engl J Med* 1996; **335:** 1538.
2. Brimacombe JR, *et al.* Propranolol overdose—a dramatic response to calcium chloride. *Med J Aust* 1991; **155:** 267–8.

## Precautions

Beta blockers should not be given to patients with bronchospasm or asthma or to those with a history of obstructive airways disease. This contra-indication generally applies even to those beta blockers considered to be cardioselective. However, cardioselective beta blockers may be used with extreme caution when there is no alternative treatment (see Obstructive Airways Disease, below). Other contra-indications include metabolic acidosis, cardiogenic shock, hypotension, severe peripheral arterial disease, sinus bradycardia, and second- or third-degree atrioventricular block; caution should be observed in first-degree block. Although beta blockers are used in the management of heart failure, they should not be given to patients with uncontrolled heart failure and treatment should be initiated with great care. Patients with phaeochromocytoma should not receive beta blockers without concomitant alpha-adrenoceptor blocking therapy.

Beta blockers may mask the symptoms of hyperthyroidism and of hypoglycaemia. They may unmask myasthenia gravis. Psoriasis may be aggravated. Chest pain has been reported in patients with Prinzmetal's angina. Patients with a history of anaphylaxis to an antigen may be more reactive to repeated challenge with the antigen while taking beta blockers (see Hypersensitivity, below).

Abrupt withdrawal of beta blockers has sometimes resulted in angina, myocardial infarction, ventricular arrhythmias, and death. Patients on long-term treatment with a beta blocker should have their medication discontinued gradually over a period of 1 to 2 weeks.

Cardiovascular drugs including beta blockers should generally be continued perioperatively although some authorities have advocated their gradual and temporary withdrawal in order to provide better control of the circulatory system. If beta blockers are not discontinued before anaesthesia, a drug such as atropine may be given to counter increases in vagal tone. Anaesthetics causing myocardial depression, such as ether, cyclopropane, and trichloroethylene, are best avoided. It is of the greatest importance that the anaesthetist is aware that beta blockers are being taken.

Use of beta blockers in pregnancy shortly before delivery has occasionally resulted in bradycardia and other adverse effects such as hypoglycaemia and hypotension in the neonate. Many beta blockers are distributed into breast milk.

Similar precautions should be observed when beta blockers are applied topically as eye drops since systemic absorption can occur.

**Contact lenses.** Beta blockers may reduce tear flow, leading to irritation of the eye in wearers of contact lenses and potentially to the dehydration of soft lenses.[1]

1. McGuire T. Drugs interfering with contact lenses. *Aust J Hosp Pharm* 1987; **17:** 55–6.

**Hypersensitivity.** There have been reports of several patients whose anaphylactic reactions to stings or other antigens were potentiated by beta blockers.[1-3] In addition, beta blockers may antagonise the effects of adrenaline in the management of anaphylaxis (see Interactions under Adrenaline, p.853).

1. Hannaway PJ, Hopper GDK. Severe anaphylaxis and drug-induced beta-blockade. *N Engl J Med* 1983; **308:** 1536.
2. Pedersen DL. Hymenoptera stings and beta-blockers. *Lancet* 1989; **ii:** 619.
3. Lang DM. Anaphylactoid and anaphylactic reactions: hazards of β-blockers. *Drug Safety* 1995; **12:** 299–304.

**Obstructive airways disease.** Beta blockers may precipitate bronchospasm and are generally contra-indicated in patients with obstructive airways disease.[1] However, systematic reviews have suggested that short-term use of cardioselective beta blockers does not produce adverse respiratory effects in patients with mild to moderate asthma[2] or chronic obstructive pulmonary disease.[3] The reviewers concluded that, given the established benefits of beta blockers in cardiovascular disorders, they should not be withheld in such patients, although patients should be carefully monitored since long-term effects were less clear.

1. Committee on Safety of Medicines/Medicines Control Agency. Reminder: beta-blockers contraindicated in asthma. *Current Problems* 1996; **22:** 2.
2. Salpeter S, *et al.* Cardioselective beta-blockers for reversible airway disease. Available in The Cochrane Library; Issue 2. Chichester: John Wiley; 2004.
3. Salpeter S, *et al.* Cardioselective beta-blockers for chronic obstructive pulmonary disease. Available in The Cochrane Library; Issue 2. Chichester: John Wiley; 2004.

**Pregnancy.** The use of a beta blocker from early in pregnancy has been associated with growth retardation of the fetus.[1] However, beta blockers are still considered one of the first-line drugs in mild to moderate hypertension in pregnancy. Many beta blockers cross the placenta and administration of beta blockers to pregnant women shortly before delivery has occasionally resulted in bradycardia and other adverse effects such as hypoglycaemia and hypotension in the neonate.

1. Butters L, *et al.* Atenolol in essential hypertension during pregnancy. *BMJ* 1990; **301:** 587–9.

**Withdrawal.** The abrupt withdrawal of beta blockers may lead to rebound hypertension or overshoot hypertension where the patient's blood pressure is higher than before treatment. Angina can be exacerbated, myocardial infarction induced, and fatalities have occurred.[1,2]

1. Houston MC, Hodge R. Beta-adrenergic blocker withdrawal syndromes in hypertension and other cardiovascular diseases. *Am Heart J* 1988; **116:** 515–23.
2. Psaty BM, *et al.* The relative risk of incident coronary heart disease associated with recently stopping the use of β-blockers. *JAMA* 1990; **263:** 1653–7.

## Interactions

Both pharmacodynamic and pharmacokinetic interactions have been reported with beta blockers. **Pharmacodynamic** interactions may occur with drugs whose actions enhance or antagonise the various effects of beta blockers at $beta_1$ and $beta_2$ receptors, including their antihypertensive effect, cardiodepressant effect, effect on carbohydrate metabolism, or effect on bronchial $beta_2$ receptors. The characteristics of the individual beta blocker must therefore be borne in mind when considering likely interactions. For more details on the characteristics of different beta blockers, see Uses and Administration, below. Drugs that enhance the antihypertensive effects of beta blockers, such as ACE inhibitors, calcium-channel blockers, and clonidine may be useful in controlling hypertension (but see below). Drugs that cause hypotension such as aldesleukin and general anaesthetics also enhance the antihypertensive effects of beta blockers while other drugs, for example NSAIDs, antagonise the antihypertensive effects. Use of beta blockers with other cardiac depressants such as antiarrhythmics and rate-limiting calcium-channel blockers can precipitate bradycardia and heart block. Sotalol is particularly prone to interactions with other drugs affecting cardiac conduction (see p.1002). Beta blockers may potentiate bradycardia due to digoxin. In diabetic patients beta blockers can reduce the response to insulin and oral hypoglycaemics through their effects on pancreatic beta receptors. Blockade of peripheral beta receptors interferes with the effects of sympathomimetics; patients on beta blockers, especially non-selective beta blockers, may develop elevated blood pressure if they are given adrenaline and the bronchodilator effects of adrenaline are also inhibited. The response to adrenaline given for anaphylaxis may be reduced in patients on long-term treatment with beta blockers (see Adrenaline, p.853).

**Pharmacokinetic** interactions occur with drugs that alter the absorption or metabolism of beta blockers. Although these interactions may alter the beta blocker plasma concentration, they are not usually clinically significant since there is no association between plasma concentrations and therapeutic effect or toxicity and there are wide interindividual differences in steady-state plasma concentrations of beta blockers. Drugs that reduce absorption include aluminium salts (but see also Antacids, below) and bile-acid binding resins such as colestyramine. Metabolism of some beta blockers can be increased by drugs such as barbiturates and rifampicin and decreased with drugs such as cimetidine, erythromycin, fluvoxamine, and hydralazine. Drugs that alter hepatic blood flow also affect metabolism of some beta blockers. For example, cimetidine and hydralazine decrease hepatic blood flow and this contributes to the decreased hepatic clearance seen with these drugs. Drugs that influence hepatic metabolism affect beta blockers that are extensively metabolised, such as labetalol, propranolol, and timolol, while beta blockers that are excreted largely unchanged, for example atenolol and nadolol, are unaffected.

Since systemic absorption can occur following ocular use of beta blockers the possibility of similar interactions should be considered.

◊ General references.

1. McDevitt DG. Interactions that matter: 12. β-adrenoceptor antagonists. *Prescribers' J* 1988; **28:** 25–30.
2. Blaufarb I, *et al.* β-Blockers: drug interactions of clinical significance. *Drug Safety* 1995; **13:** 359–70.

**Anaesthetics.** Beta blockers are usually continued perioperatively although the anaesthetist must be informed of their use (see Precautions, above). However, the hypotensive effects of beta blockers may be potentiated by general anaesthetics, and anaesthetics that cause myocardial depression, such as *ether, cyclopropane,* and *trichloroethylene* should preferably be avoided.

**Antacids.** Bioavailability of metoprolol was increased when given concurrently with an antacid containing aluminium and magnesium salts but the bioavailability of atenolol was reduced by concurrent administration of this antacid. Variable results on bioavailability of propranolol have been reported when aluminium hydroxide was given with propranolol.[1]

1. Gugler R, Allgayer H. Effects of antacids on the clinical pharmacokinetics of drugs: an update. *Clin Pharmacokinet* 1990; **18:** 210–19.

**Antiarrhythmics.** Use of beta blockers with antiarrhythmic drugs and other drugs affecting cardiac conduction can precipitate bradycardia and heart block.

Bradycardia, cardiac arrest, and ventricular fibrillation have been reported shortly after starting beta-blocker therapy in patients receiving *amiodarone.*[1] Concurrent administration of *flecainide* and propranolol produced additive negative inotropic effects on the heart and increased serum concentrations of both drugs.[2] In a pharmacokinetic study in 12 healthy males, giving *propafenone* with propranolol resulted in increases in serum-propranolol concentrations but only modest enhancement of beta-blocking activity.[3] An increase in serum-metoprolol concentration has been reported after concurrent administration of propafenone and metoprolol.[4] The metabolism of metoprolol may be decreased by *quinidine.*[5] Both quinidine and beta blockers have a negative inotropic action on the heart; bradycardia[6] and hypotension[7] have occurred in patients given quinidine with beta blockers.

For a report of reduced clearance of *disopyramide* by concomitant administration of atenolol, see p.905.

The interactions of sotalol are discussed on p.1002.


1. Lesko LJ. Pharmacokinetic drug interactions with amiodarone. *Clin Pharmacokinet* 1989; **17:** 130–40.
2. Holtzman JL, *et al.* The pharmacodynamic and pharmacokinetic interaction of flecainide acetate with propranolol: effects on cardiac function and drug clearance. *Eur J Clin Pharmacol* 1987; **33:** 97–9.
3. Kowey PR, *et al.* Interaction between propranolol and propafenone in healthy volunteers. *J Clin Pharmacol* 1989; **29:** 512–17.
4. Wagner F, *et al.* Drug interaction between propafenone and metoprolol. *Br J Clin Pharmacol* 1987; **24:** 213–20.
5. Leemann T, *et al.* Single-dose quinidine treatment inhibits metoprolol oxidation in extensive metabolizers. *Eur J Clin Pharmacol* 1986; **29:** 739–41.
6. Dinai Y, *et al.* Bradycardia induced by interaction between quinidine and ophthalmic timolol. *Ann Intern Med* 1985; **103:** 890–1.
7. Loon NR, *et al.* Orthostatic hypotension due to quinidine and propranolol. *Am J Med* 1986; **81:** 1101–4.


**Antibacterials.** Serum-atenolol concentrations in 6 healthy subjects were reduced by oral administration of a 1-g dose of *ampicillin*.[1] Plasma concentrations of propranolol,[2] metoprolol,[3] and bisoprolol[4] may be reduced by *rifampicin*.


1. Schäfer-Korting M, *et al.* Atenolol interaction with aspirin, allopurinol, and ampicillin. *Clin Pharmacol Ther* 1983; **33:** 283–8.
2. Shaheen O, *et al.* Influence of debrisoquin phenotype on the inducibility of propranolol metabolism. *Clin Pharmacol Ther* 1989; **45:** 439–43.
3. Bennett PN, *et al.* Effect of rifampicin on metoprolol and antipyrine kinetics. *Br J Clin Pharmacol* 1982; **13:** 387–91.
4. Kirch W, *et al.* Interaction of bisoprolol with cimetidine and rifampicin. *Eur J Clin Pharmacol* 1986; **31:** 59–62.


**Anticoagulants.** For the effect of beta blockers on the pharmacokinetics of some oral anticoagulants, see p.1026.

**Antidepressants.** Bradycardia and heart block, occurring shortly after starting *fluoxetine* therapy, have been reported in patients receiving metoprolol[1] and propranolol.[2] Possible mechanisms include impaired conduction through the atrioventricular node and inhibition by fluoxetine of the oxidative metabolism of beta blockers. Use of fluoxetine also increased the plasma concentration of carvedilol in patients with heart failure but no clinical effects were noted.[3]

*Fluvoxamine* inhibits oxidative metabolism, and increased plasma concentrations of propranolol have been noted in patients receiving fluvoxamine.


1. Walley T, *et al.* Interaction of metoprolol and fluoxetine. *Lancet* 1993; **341:** 967–8.
2. Drake WM, Gordon GD. Heart block in a patient on propranolol and fluoxetine. *Lancet* 1994; **343:** 425–6.
3. Graff DW, *et al.* Effect of fluoxetine on carvedilol pharmacokinetics, CYP2D6 activity, and autonomic balance in heart failure patients. *J Clin Pharmacol* 2001; **41:** 97–106.


**Antihypertensives.** An enhanced antihypertensive effect is seen when other antihypertensives are given with beta blockers. However, some combinations should be avoided (see Calcium-channel Blockers, below). Beta blockers can potentiate the severe orthostatic hypotension that may follow the initial dose of alpha blockers such as prazosin and can exacerbate rebound hypertension following withdrawal of clonidine treatment (see p.886).

**Antimalarials.** Antimalarials such as *halofantrine, mefloquine*, and *quinine* can cause cardiac conduction defects and caution is necessary if they are used with beta blockers. Cardiopulmonary arrest has occurred after a single dose of mefloquine in a patient taking propranolol.[1]


1. Anonymous. Mefloquine for malaria. *Med Lett Drugs Ther* 1990; **32:** 13–14.


**Antimigraine drugs.** For the effect of propranolol on *rizatriptan*, see p.471.

See also under Ergotamine Tartrate, p.468, for further interactions with drugs used in the treatment of migraine.

**Anxiolytics and antipsychotics.** Plasma concentrations of some beta blockers may be reduced by *barbiturates*.[1-3] Increased plasma-propranolol concentrations and bioavailability, and reduced metabolism, have been reported in healthy subjects also given *chlorpromazine*.[4]

See p.693 for the effect of beta blockers on the pharmacokinetics of some *benzodiazepines*.


1. Sotaniemi EA, *et al.* Plasma clearance of propranolol and sotalol and hepatic drug-metabolizing enzyme activity. *Clin Pharmacol Ther* 1979; **26:** 153–61.
2. Haglund K, *et al.* Influence of pentobarbital on metoprolol plasma levels. *Clin Pharmacol Ther* 1979; **26:** 326–9.
3. Seideman P, *et al.* Decreased plasma concentrations and clinical effects of alprenolol during combined treatment with pentobarbitone in hypertension. *Br J Clin Pharmacol* 1987; **23:** 267–71.
4. Vestal RE, *et al.* Inhibition of propranolol metabolism by chlorpromazine. *Clin Pharmacol Ther* 1979; **25:** 19–24.


**Calcium-channel blockers.** Use of calcium-channel blockers with beta blockers has resulted in hypotension, bradycardia, conduction defects, and heart failure.[1]

Beta blockers should be avoided in combination with rate-limiting calcium-channel blockers such as *verapamil* (see p.1020) and *diltiazem*. Although they are reportedly safe with dihydropyridines such as *nifedipine*,[2] heart failure and severe hypotension have been reported (see under Nifedipine, p.969). Reported pharmacokinetic interactions include increased plasma concentrations of propranolol and of metoprolol with concurrent use of diltiazem[3] or verapamil,[1] and increased plasma concentrations of propranolol with *nicardipine*.[4]


1. Lam YWF, Shepherd AMM. Drug interactions in hypertensive patients: pharmacokinetic, pharmacodynamic and genetic considerations. *Clin Pharmacokinet* 1990; **18:** 295–317.
2. Reid JL. First-line and combination treatment for hypertension. *Am J Med* 1989; **86** (suppl 4A): 2–5.
3. Tateishi T, *et al.* Effect of diltiazem on the pharmacokinetics of propranolol, metoprolol and atenolol. *Eur J Clin Pharmacol* 1989; **36:** 67–70.
4. Schoors DF, *et al.* Influence of nicardipine on the pharmacokinetics and pharmacodynamics of propranolol in healthy volunteers. *Br J Clin Pharmacol* 1990; **29:** 497–501.


**Cardiac glycosides.** For reference to an interaction between beta blockers and *digoxin*, see p.897.

**Ciclosporin.** For the effect of carvedilol on plasma-ciclosporin concentrations, see p.1355.

**Ergot derivatives.** *Nicergoline* enhanced the cardiac depressant action of propranolol in healthy subjects.[1]

For reports of enhanced vasoconstrictor action in patients taking *ergot alkaloids* and beta blockers, see p.468.


1. Boismare F, *et al.* Potentiation by an alpha-adrenolytic agent, nicergoline, of the cardiac effects of propranolol. *Methods Find Exp Clin Pharmacol* 1983; **5:** 83–8.


**Food.** A study[1] in healthy volunteers found that *grapefruit juice* greatly reduced the plasma concentration of celiprolol, although the mechanism of the interaction was unclear. A similar effect has also been reported[2] with *orange juice*.


1. Lilja JJ, *et al.* Itraconazole increases but grapefruit juice greatly decreases plasma concentrations of celiprolol. *Clin Pharmacol Ther* 2003; **73:** 192–8.
2. Lilja JJ, *et al.* Orange juice substantially reduces the bioavailability of the beta-adrenergic-blocking agent celiprolol. *Clin Pharmacol Ther* 2004; **75:** 184–90.


**Histamine $H_2$-antagonists.** Plasma concentrations of propranolol and metoprolol may be increased by *cimetidine*;[1] pharmacokinetic studies indicate that cimetidine exerts its effect by reducing hepatic blood flow and impairing beta blocker metabolism. Cimetidine has been reported to increase the bioavailability of labetalol,[1] and to increase the systemic effects of timolol eye drops.[2]


1. Smith SR, Kendall MJ. Ranitidine versus cimetidine: a comparison of their potential to cause clinically important drug interactions. *Clin Pharmacokinet* 1988; **15:** 44–56.
2. Ishii Y, *et al.* Drug interaction between cimetidine and timolol ophthalmic solution: effect on heart rate and intraocular pressure in healthy Japanese volunteers. *J Clin Pharmacol* 2000; **40:** 193–9.


**Local anaesthetics.** For details of the effect of beta blockers in reducing the clearance of *bupivacaine*, see p.1371, and of *lidocaine*, see p.1378. For the effects of propranolol with *cocaine*, see p.1375.

**Neuromuscular blockers.** For the effects of beta blockers on neuromuscular blockers, see under Atracurium, p.1401.

**NSAIDs.** The antihypertensive effect of beta blockers may be impaired by some NSAIDs, possibly due to their inhibition of renal synthesis of vasodilating prostaglandins. This interaction probably occurs with all beta blockers but may not occur with all NSAIDs. For example, *sulindac* appears to affect blood pressure control less than *indometacin*.[1]


1. Lam YWF, Shepherd AMM. Drug interactions in hypertensive patients: pharmacokinetic, pharmacodynamic and genetic considerations. *Clin Pharmacokinet* 1990; **18:** 295–317.


**Opioid analgesics.** Bioavailability of propranolol and metoprolol was increased in subjects given *dextropropoxyphene*.[1] Intravenous administration of *morphine* may increase serum concentrations of esmolol.[2]


1. Lundborg P, *et al.* The effect of propoxyphene pretreatment on the disposition of metoprolol and propranolol. *Clin Pharmacol Ther* 1981; **29:** 263–4.
2. Lowenthal DT, *et al.* Clinical pharmacology, pharmacodynamics and interactions with esmolol. *Am J Cardiol* 1985; **56:** 14F–17F.


**Oral contraceptives.** Plasma-metoprolol concentrations were increased in some women taking oral contraceptives.[1]


1. Kendall MJ, *et al.* Metoprolol pharmacokinetics and the oral contraceptive pill. *Br J Clin Pharmacol* 1982; **14:** 120–2.


**Parasympathomimetics.** For the effect of beta blockers on the response to *anticholinesterases*, see p.1493.

**Thyroid drugs.** For a discussion of thyroid status and its effect on plasma-propranolol concentrations and the effects of propranolol on *thyroid hormone* metabolism, see p.1601.

**Xanthines.** For details of reduced *theophylline* clearance in patients receiving beta blockers, see p.802.

## Pharmacokinetics

Beta blockers differ widely in their pharmacokinetic properties. Differences in lipid solubility contribute to these varying pharmacokinetic properties. Beta blockers with low lipid solubility (hydrophilic beta blockers) include atenolol and nadolol. Beta blockers with high lipid solubility (lipophilic beta blockers) include alprenolol and propranolol. Generally, those with low lipid solubility tend to be less readily absorbed from the gastrointestinal tract, to be less extensively metabolised, to have low plasma-protein binding, to have relatively long plasma half-lives, and to cross the blood-brain barrier less readily than beta blockers with high lipid solubility. Beta blockers cross the placenta and most are known to distribute into breast milk.

There is no clear correlation between plasma concentrations of beta blockers and therapeutic activity, especially when the beta blocker undergoes metabolism to active metabolites.

## Uses and Administration

Beta blockers are competitive antagonists of the effects of catecholamines at beta-adrenergic receptor sites and are used in a variety of disorders, especially those affecting the cardiovascular system.

Two main subtypes of beta-adrenergic receptors are recognised: $beta_1$ and $beta_2$. A $beta_3$ receptor has also been identified in adipose tissue, but its role remains unclear. $Beta_1$ receptors are found mainly in the heart while $beta_2$ receptors are found in noncardiac tissue, including bronchial tissue, peripheral blood vessels, uterus, and pancreas, although it is now recognised that in some organs, including the heart, both receptor subtypes are present. Blockade of $beta_1$ receptors reduces heart rate, myocardial contractility, and the rate of conduction of impulses through the conducting system. These effects are termed class II antiarrhythmic actions (p.809). Other effects of blockade of $beta_1$ receptors include suppression of adrenergic-induced renin release and lipolysis. Effects produced by blockade of $beta_2$ receptors include increased bronchial resistance and inhibition of catecholamine-induced glucose metabolism. $Beta_2$ receptors may also have a role in regulation of heart rate.

Beta blockers have different affinities for $beta_1$ or $beta_2$ receptors. While propranolol affects both $beta_1$ and $beta_2$ receptors, other drugs such as atenolol and metoprolol have greater affinity for $beta_1$ receptors and are described as cardioselective. However, selectivity is relative and, as doses are increased, activity at $beta_2$ receptors becomes clinically important.

Some beta blockers, such as acebutolol, celiprolol, oxprenolol, and pindolol, also possess intrinsic (partial) sympathomimetic activity in that they activate beta receptors in the absence of catecholamines and are therefore partial agonists. Beta blockers with intrinsic sympathomimetic activity produce less resting bradycardia than beta blockers without.

At high blood concentrations, propranolol and some other beta blockers also possess a membrane-stabilising effect. This effect may not be evident at therapeutic doses but may be important in overdose. Some beta blockers, such as carvedilol and labetalol, also block $alpha_1$ receptors and thus produce vasodilatation. Other beta blockers, such as bevantolol and celiprolol, also have vasodilator properties; various mechanisms, including $alpha_1$ blockade, $beta_2$ stimulation, and direct vasodilator activity may contribute to this effect. The non-cardioselective beta blocker sotalol also has class III antiarrhythmic activity.

Beta blockers are used in the treatment of hypertension (p.825), angina pectoris (p.813), cardiac arrhythmias (p.816), and myocardial infarction (p.828) and also have a role in heart failure (below). They are also used to control symptoms of sympathetic overactivity in the management of alcohol withdrawal (p.1166), in anxiety disorders (below), in hyperthyroidism (p.1594), and in tremor (below). Beta blockers are used in the prophylaxis of migraine (below) and of variceal bleeding associated with portal hypertension (p.1716). They are also used, with an alpha blocker, in the initial management of phaeochromocytoma (below). Some beta blockers are instilled as eye drops in the management of glaucoma and ocular hypertension (below).

◊ The selection of a specific beta blocker for an individual patient depends on the condition being treated and patient characteristics such as liver and kidney function or existing disease such as diabetes. Patient tolerability also varies for different beta blockers. The characteristics of the beta blocker, for example, $beta_1$ selectivity and intrinsic sympathomimetic activity may also influence selection, as may additional pharmacological properties such as vasodilator activity. However, the clinical significance of these properties is debated.

References.

1. Hampton JR. Choosing the right β-blocker: a guide to selection. *Drugs* 1994; **48:** 549–68.
2. Brown MJ. To β block or better block? *BMJ* 1995; **311:** 701–2.
3. Anonymous. Too many beta-blockers. *Drug Ther Bull* 1996; **34:** 49–52.
4. Anonymous. Which beta-blocker? *Med Lett Drugs Ther* 2001; **43:** 9–11.

**Anxiety disorders.** Beta blockers have been used in patients with various anxiety disorders,[1] including generalised anxiety disorders (p.663), panic attacks (p.663), and performance anxiety[1] (see under Phobic Disorders, p.663). However, their benefits do not appear to be particularly great and they are probably most useful in reducing symptoms such as tremor or palpitations that are mediated through beta stimulation. Improvement usually occurs within 1 to 2 hours with relatively low doses of beta blockers (propranolol 40 mg, oxprenolol 40 to 80 mg, nadolol 40 mg). Some patients require higher doses and longer periods of treatment for a beneficial effect.

1. Tyrer P. Current status of β-blocking drugs in the treatment of anxiety disorders. *Drugs* 1988; **36:** 773–83.

**Cardiomyopathy.** See Heart Failure, below.

**Cardiovascular risk reduction.** Although some authorities have recommended discontinuation of beta blockers pre-operatively (see Precautions, above), there is some evidence that peri-operative use may be protective in patients with evidence of cardiovascular disease. A systematic review[1] of trials with beta blockers, including studies with atenolol[2] and bisoprolol,[3] suggested a reduction in myocardial ischaemia, non-fatal myocardial infarction, and mortality from cardiovascular causes in patients at high cardiovascular risk undergoing major noncardiac surgery. Guidelines in the USA recommend[4] that beta blockers should be given perioperatively to patients undergoing vascular surgery who are currently taking beta blockers and to those who are shown to be at high risk of ischaemia. There is also some evidence[5,6] that pre-operative beta blockers may be of benefit in patients undergoing cardiac procedures.

Long-term therapy with beta blockers has an established role in reducing cardiovascular risk in patients who have had a myocardial infarction (p.828).

1. Auerbach AD, Goldman L. β-Blockers and reduction of cardiac events in noncardiac surgery: scientific review. *JAMA* 2002; **287:** 1435–44.
2. Mangano DT, *et al.* Effect of atenolol on mortality and cardiovascular morbidity after noncardiac surgery. *N Engl J Med* 1996; **335:** 1713–20. Correction. *ibid.* 1997; **336:** 1040.
3. Poldermans D, *et al.* The effect of bisoprolol on perioperative mortality and myocardial infarction in high-risk patients undergoing vascular surgery. *N Engl J Med* 1999; **341:** 1789–94.
4. Eagle KA, *et al.* ACC/AHA guideline update for perioperative cardiovascular evaluation for noncardiac surgery: a report of the American College of Cardiology/American Heart Association Task Force on Practice Guidelines (Committee to Update the 1996 Guidelines on Perioperative Cardiovascular Evaluation for Noncardiac Surgery). Executive Summary: *Circulation* 2002; **105:** 1257–67. Full version: http://www.americanheart.org/downloadable/heart/1013454973885perio_update.pdf (accessed 06/07/04)
5. Sharma SK, *et al.* Cardioprotective effect of prior β-blocker therapy in reducing creatine kinase-MB elevation after coronary intervention: benefit is extended to improvement in intermediate-term survival. *Circulation* 2000; **102:** 166–72.
6. Ferguson TB, *et al.* Preoperative β-blocker use and mortality and morbidity following CABG surgery in North America. *JAMA* 2002; **287:** 2221–7. Correction. *ibid.*; 3212.

**Extrapyramidal disorders.** Beta blockers (in low doses) have been suggested for the management of antipsychotic-induced akathisia (see under Chlorpromazine, p.677).

**Glaucoma and ocular hypertension.** Topical beta blockers are often the drugs of first choice[1] for the initial treatment and maintenance of open-angle glaucoma and other chronic glaucomas (p.1485). They are believed to inhibit beta receptors in the ciliary epithelium and reduce the secretion of aqueous humour. Clinical studies have established that betaxolol, carteolol, levobunolol, metipranolol, and timolol are effective, generally reducing intra-ocular pressure to a similar extent.[2-6] The possibility of systemic effects following topical use needs to be borne in mind (see above), especially in the elderly.[7]

Beta blockers have also been used for prophylaxis of postoperative ocular hypertension.[8,9]

1. Frishman WH, *et al.* Topical ophthalmic β-adrenergic blockade for the treatment of glaucoma and ocular hypertension. *J Clin Pharmacol* 1994; **34:** 795–803.
2. LeBlanc RP, *et al.* Timolol: long-term Canadian Multicentre Study. *Can J Ophthalmol* 1985; **20:** 128–30.
3. Stewart RH, *et al.* Betaxolol vs timolol: a six-month double-blind comparison. *Arch Ophthalmol* 1986; **104:** 46–8.
4. Geyer O, *et al.* Levobunolol compared with timolol: a four-year study. *Br J Ophthalmol* 1988; **72:** 892–6.
5. Krieglstein GK, *et al.* Levobunolol and metipranolol: comparative ocular hypotensive efficacy, safety, and comfort. *Br J Ophthalmol* 1987; **71:** 250–3.
6. Scoville B, *et al.* A double-masked comparison of carteolol and timolol in ocular hypertension. *Am J Ophthalmol* 1988; **105:** 150–4.
7. O'Donoghue E. β Blockers and the elderly with glaucoma: are we adding insult to injury? *Br J Ophthalmol* 1995; **79:** 794–6.
8. West DR, *et al.* Comparative efficacy of the β-blockers for the prevention of increased intraocular pressure after cataract extraction. *Am J Ophthalmol* 1988; **106:** 168–73.
9. Odberg T. Primary argon laser trabeculoplasty after pretreatment with timolol. *Acta Ophthalmol (Copenh)* 1990; **68:** 317–19.

**Heart failure.** Beta blockers have negative inotropic properties and have generally been contra-indicated in patients with heart failure (p.820). However, there is increasing evidence that they may in fact be of benefit since persistent activation of the sympathetic nervous system appears to be associated with disease progression. Reviews,[1-3] meta-analyses,[4,5] and long-term studies[6,7] have confirmed that the beta blockers bisoprolol, carvedilol, and metoprolol all improve mortality in patients with chronic heart failure, and beta blockers are now recommended in combination with ACE inhibitors and diuretics as part of standard therapy in patients with clinically stable, mild to moderate heart failure due to left ventricular systolic dysfunction. It is not clear whether all beta blockers are equally effective. A meta-analysis[8] has suggested that vasodilating beta blockers such as carvedilol have a greater effect on overall mortality than those that do not produce vasodilatation. A large study[9] comparing carvedilol with metoprolol also found a greater mortality reduction with carvedilol, although the equivalence of the doses used in the study has been questioned.[10] The optimum dose is also unclear; many patients are unable to tolerate the target doses used in clinical trials, but an analysis[11] of a study with metoprolol suggested that the mortality benefit was equal in those receiving low or high doses. The role of beta blockers in severe heart failure is less clear; a study with bucindolol[12] was stopped early because no mortality benefit was found, although carvedilol was found to reduce mortality in a similar study.[13] A retrospective analysis[14] of a study with metoprolol also suggested that patients with severe heart failure had a similar benefit to other patients.

Beta blockers may also be of value in some patients with heart failure due to cardiomyopathy (p.818). A number of beta blockers have provided symptomatic benefit in idiopathic dilated cardiomyopathy, and the heart failure trials that showed a mortality benefit included patients with dilated cardiomyopathy. In hypertrophic cardiomyopathy, beta blockers may be of value for symptomatic management to curtail tachycardia, reduce anginal pain, and prevent syncope.

1. Foody JM, *et al.* β-Blocker therapy in heart failure: scientific review. *JAMA* 2002; **287:** 883–9.
2. Pritchett AM, Redfield MM. β-Blockers: new standard therapy for heart failure. *Mayo Clin Proc* 2002; **77:** 839–46.
3. Goldstein S. Benefits of β-blocker therapy for heart failure: weighing the evidence. *Arch Intern Med* 2002; **162:** 641–8.
4. Lechat P, *et al.* Clinical effects of β-adrenergic blockade in chronic heart failure: a meta-analysis of double-blind, placebo-controlled, randomized trials. *Circulation* 1998; **98:** 1184–91.
5. Brophy JM, *et al.* β-Blockers in congestive heart failure: a Bayesian meta-analysis. *Ann Intern Med* 2001; **134:** 550–60.
6. CIBIS-II Investigators and Committees. The Cardiac Insufficiency Bisoprolol Study II (CIBIS-II): a randomised trial. *Lancet* 1999; **353:** 9–13.
7. MERIT-HF Study Group. Effect of metoprolol CR/XL in chronic heart failure: Metoprolol CR/XL Randomised Intervention Trial in Congestive Heart Failure (MERIT-HF). *Lancet* 1999; **353:** 2001–7.
8. Bonet S, *et al.* β-Adrenergic blocking agents in heart failure: benefits of vasodilating and nonvasodilating agents according to patients' characteristics: a meta-analysis of clinical trials. *Arch Intern Med* 2000; **160:** 621–7.
9. Poole-Wilson PA, *et al.* Comparison of carvedilol and metoprolol on clinical outcomes in patients with chronic heart failure in the Carvedilol Or Metoprolol European Trial (COMET): randomised controlled trial. *Lancet* 2003; **362:** 7–13.
10. Dargie HJ. β-Blockers in heart failure. *Lancet* 2003; **362:** 2–3.
11. Wikstrand J, *et al.* Dose of metoprolol CR/XL and clinical outcomes in patients with heart failure: analysis of the experience in metoprolol CR/XL randomized intervention trial in chronic heart failure (MERIT-HF). *J Am Coll Cardiol* 2002; **40:** 491–8.
12. The Beta-Blocker Evaluation of Survival Trial Investigators. A trial of the beta-blocker bucindolol in patients with advanced chronic heart failure. *N Engl J Med* 2001; **344:** 1659–67.
13. Packer M, *et al.* Effect of carvedilol on survival in severe chronic heart failure. *N Engl J Med* 2001; **344:** 1651–8.
14. Goldstein S, *et al.* Metoprolol controlled release/extended release in patients with severe heart failure: analysis of the experience in the MERIT-HF study. *J Am Coll Cardiol* 2001; **38:** 932–8.

**Hypotension.** A beta blocker (such as atenolol or metoprolol) is reported to be one of the standard drugs used in the management of neurally mediated hypotension (p.828). Beta blockers with partial agonist activity have been used in orthostatic hypotension due to autonomic failure (p.1100) but are potentially dangerous.

**Migraine.** Beta blockers (usually propranolol or metoprolol) are considered[1] by many to be the drugs of choice in patients requiring prophylactic treatment for migraine (p.464). Their mechanism of action in this disorder is not fully understood. Other beta blockers reported to be effective include atenolol, nadolol, and timolol; those with intrinsic sympathomimetic activity may not be effective.

Beta blockers may sometimes also be of benefit in patients with chronic tension-type headache (p.465).

Propranolol has been tried in the treatment of children with abdominal migraine (p.470).

1. Limmroth V, Michel MC. The prevention of migraine: a critical review with special emphasis on β-adrenoceptor blockers. *Br J Clin Pharmacol* 2001; **52:** 237–43.

**Peripheral vascular disease.** Beta blockers may cause coldness of the extremities and have been reported to induce secondary Raynaud's syndrome. However, they may be of some help in the management of erythromelalgia (see under Raynaud's Syndrome on p.833).

**Phaeochromocytoma.** Beta blockers are used, with an alpha blocker, in the initial management of phaeochromocytoma (p.831). Beta blockers reduce the responses to the beta-adrenoceptor stimulating effects of adrenaline. Treatment must be started with the alpha blocker and only when alpha blockade is successfully established can tachycardia be controlled by the cautious use of a beta blocker. A $beta_1$-selective blocker is preferred so that peripheral $beta_2$-mediated vasodilatation is unaffected. In most cases modest doses are sufficient although higher doses may be required for a tumour that is predominantly adrenaline-secreting.

**Tension-type headache.** See Migraine, above.

**Tetanus.** Autonomic overactivity, usually due to excessive catecholamine release, may occur as a complication of tetanus and is usually controlled with sedation (see p.1398). Beta blockers have also been used but may produce severe hypertension and are therefore not usually recommended. Labetalol has both alpha- and beta-blocking properties and intravenous labetalol has been used successfully to control the cardiovascular effects of tetanus,[1] although it has not been shown to offer any advantage over propranolol in this situation. Esmolol, a short-acting beta blocker has also been used.[2]

1. Domenighetti GM, *et al.* Hyperadrenergic syndrome in severe tetanus: extreme rise in catecholamines responsive to labetalol. *BMJ* 1984; **288:** 1483–4.
2. King WW, Cave DR. Use of esmolol to control autonomic instability of tetanus. *Am J Med* 1991; **91:** 425–8.

**Tremor.** Tremor is a rhythmical oscillation of part of the body caused by involuntary contraction of opposing muscles. It may occur during action, maintenance of posture, or at rest, and varies in frequency and amplitude. Resting tremor is associated mainly with parkinsonism (p.1196), whereas action tremor, which includes postural tremor and kinetic tremor, occurs in a wide variety of disorders. Treatment of the underlying disorder may remove the tremor. Drugs such as bronchodilators, tricyclic antidepressants, lithium, and caffeine may induce tremor; withdrawal of the causative drug usually alleviates the tremor. However, tremor often has no known underlying cause. Such tremor is referred to as essential tremor or benign essential tremor; it is usually postural and tends to affect the hands, head, voice, and sometimes the legs and trunk. It is exacerbated by emotional stress and anxiety. Essential tremor may appear at any age and is a lifelong condition that may progress with increasing age. In many cases there is a family history of the disorder (familial essential tremor).

Mild cases of essential tremor may not require regular drug treatment. Single doses of a beta blocker or a benzodiazepine may be useful in acute circumstances to control exacerbations provoked by stress. A single dose of propranolol usually produces a maximum effect after 1 to 2 hours and the effect may persist for several hours. Small amounts of alcohol may also provide effective temporary relief of essential tremor, although its regular use is obviously discouraged.

For more severe cases of essential tremor long-term drug treatment may be required (and may also be tried in other forms of tremor).[1-3] A beta blocker (usually a non-cardioselective beta blocker such as propranolol) is often the first drug used. Up to 70% of people have been reported to respond, although the average tremor reduction is only about 50 to 60%. The beneficial effect appears to be predominantly due to blockade of peripheral $beta_2$ receptors on extrafusal muscle fibres and muscle spindles, although there may also be a CNS effect. Adverse effects may be troublesome on long-term use. Primidone may also be tried[4] although there may be a high incidence of acute adverse reactions following initial doses. Concern has been expressed that patients may become tolerant to these drugs given long-term. However, 3 small studies found a reduced response on long-term therapy in only a few patients.[5-7] Local injection of botulinum A toxin has been tried in refractory essential tremor. Benzodiazepines, antimuscarinics, and dopaminergic antiparkinsonian drugs may be effective in some forms of tremor.[1] Other drugs that have shown some benefit include gabapentin, topiramate, theophylline, and ondansetron. In very severe disabling cases, surgery (thalamotomy or deep brain stimulation) may have to be considered.

1. Habib-ur-Rehman. Diagnosis and management of tremor. *Arch Intern Med* 2000; **160:** 2438–44.
2. Louis ED. Essential tremor. *N Engl J Med* 2001; **345:** 887–91.
3. Lyons K, *et al.* Benefits and risks of pharmacological treatments for essential tremor. *Drug Safety* 2003; **26:** 461–81.
4. Koller WC, Royse VL. Efficacy of primidone in essential tremor. *Neurology* 1986; **36:** 121–4.
5. Koller WC, Vetere-Overfield B. Acute and chronic effects of propranolol and primidone in essential tremor. *Neurology* 1989; **39:** 1587–8.
6. Calzetti S, *et al.* Clinical and computer-based assessment of long-term therapeutic efficacy of propranolol in essential tremor. *Acta Neurol Scand* 1990; **81:** 392–6.
7. Sasso E, *et al.* Primidone in the long-term treatment of essential tremor: a prospective study with computerized quantitative analysis. *Clin Neuropharmacol* 1990; **13:** 67–76.

## Betanidine Sulfate *(pINNM)*

Betanidine Sulphate *(BANM)*; Betanidini Sulfas; Bethanidine Sulfate *(USAN)*; Bethanidine Sulphate; BW-467-C-60; NSC-106563; Sulfato de betanidina. 2-Benzyl-1,3-dimethylguanidine sulphate.

$(C_{10}H_{15}N_3)_2,H_2SO_4$ = 452.6.

*CAS — 55-73-2 (betanidine); 114-85-2 (betanidine sulfate).*

*ATC — C02CC01.*

**Profile**
Betanidine is an antihypertensive with actions and uses similar to those of guanethidine (p.926), but it causes less depletion of noradrenaline stores. It has been given by mouth as the sulfate in the management of hypertension, and has also been tried in ventricular fibrillation.

## Betaxolol Hydrochloride

*(BANM, USAN, rINNM)*

ALO-1401-02; Betaxololi Hydrochloridum; Hidrocloruro de betaxolol; SL-75212-10. 1-{4-[2-(Cyclopropylmethoxy)ethyl]phenoxy}-3-isopropylaminopropan-2-ol hydrochloride.

$C_{18}H_{29}NO_3,HCl = 343.9.$

*CAS — 63659-18-7 (betaxolol); 63659-19-8 (betaxolol hydrochloride).*

*ATC — C07AB05; S01ED02.*

**Pharmacopoeias.** In *Eur.* (see p.vi) and *US.*

**Ph. Eur. 5.0** (Betaxolol Hydrochloride). A white or almost white crystalline powder. Very soluble in water; freely soluble in alcohol; soluble in dichloromethane. Protect from light.

**USP 27** (Betaxolol Hydrochloride). A white crystalline powder. Freely soluble in water, in alcohol, in chloroform, and in methyl alcohol. pH of a 2% solution in water is between 4.5 and 6.5. Store in airtight containers.

### Adverse Effects, Treatment, and Precautions

As for Beta Blockers, p.869.

### Interactions

The interactions associated with beta blockers are discussed on p.870.

### Pharmacokinetics

Betaxolol is completely absorbed from the gastrointestinal tract and undergoes only minimal first-pass metabolism, resulting in a high oral bioavailability of 80 to 90%. It has high lipid solubility. Betaxolol is about 50% bound to plasma proteins. It crosses the placenta and is distributed into breast milk where higher concentrations have been achieved than in maternal blood. The plasma elimination half-life of betaxolol ranges from 16 to 20 hours. The primary route of elimination is via hepatic metabolism and urinary excretion; only about 15% is excreted in the urine as unchanged drug.

**Pregnancy and breast feeding.** The pharmacokinetics of betaxolol were investigated in the perinatal period in 28 pregnant hypertensive patients receiving doses of 10 to 40 mg daily.[1] Pharmacokinetic values were similar to those observed in non-pregnant patients. Umbilical-cord concentrations were similar to maternal blood concentrations and showed a negative correlation between concentration in cord blood and timing of the last dose of betaxolol. Thus the betaxolol concentration in the newborn can be considerably reduced by discontinuing drug administration to the mother 16 to 18 hours before birth. The blood-betaxolol half-life in the neonates ranged from 14.8 to 38.5 hours. The mean apparent half-life in infants with gestational age less than 36 weeks was about 32% higher than in full-term neonates. Betaxolol concentrations in milk and/or colostrum were determined in 3 mothers. In all samples the milk-to-blood ratio was greater than 2.

1. Morselli PL, *et al.* Placental transfer and perinatal pharmacokinetics of betaxolol. *Eur J Clin Pharmacol* 1990; **38:** 477–83.

### Uses and Administration

Betaxolol is a cardioselective beta blocker (p.868). It is reported to lack intrinsic sympathomimetic activity and to have little membrane-stabilising activity.

Betaxolol is used as the hydrochloride in the management of hypertension (p.825), angina pectoris (p.813), and glaucoma (p.1485).

In **hypertension** betaxolol hydrochloride is given in initial doses of 10 to 20 mg as a single daily dose by mouth; doses may be increased if necessary after 1 to 2 weeks according to response, to 40 mg daily. Similar doses are used in **angina pectoris**.

Initial doses of 5 to 10 mg daily are suggested for elderly patients. Reduced dosages should also be used in patients with severe renal impairment (see below).

Eye drops containing the equivalent of 0.25 or 0.5% betaxolol as the hydrochloride are instilled twice daily to reduce raised intra-ocular pressure in ocular hypertension and open-angle **glaucoma**.

◊ General references.

1. Buckley MM-T, *et al.* Ocular betaxolol: a review of its pharmacological properties, and therapeutic efficacy in glaucoma and ocular hypertension. *Drugs* 1990; **40:** 75–90.

**Administration in renal impairment.** The clearance of betaxolol is reduced in patients with renal impairment and the dose may therefore need to be reduced. The UK manufacturer recommends that no dose adjustment is necessary in patients with a creatinine clearance of greater than 20 mL/minute, but that the initial dose in patients on dialysis should be 10 mg daily. The US manufacturer recommends an initial dose of 5 mg daily in patients with severe renal impairment or on dialysis; the dose may be increased by 5 mg every 2 weeks, to a maximum of 20 mg daily.

**Speech disorders.** A 50-year-old man who had stuttered since childhood obtained striking improvement in his stuttering when he was given betaxolol 20 mg daily for essential hypertension.[1]

1. Burris JF, *et al.* Betaxolol and stuttering. *Lancet* 1990; **335:** 223.

### Preparations

***BP 2003:*** Betaxolol Eye Drops, Solution; Betaxolol Eye Drops, Suspension;
***USP 27:*** Betaxolol Ophthalmic Solution; Betaxolol Tablets.

**Proprietary Preparations** (details are given in Part 3)
***Arg.:*** Betasel; Tonobexol; ***Austral.:*** Betoptic; Betoquin; ***Austria:*** Betoptic; Kerlone; ***Belg.:*** Betoptic; Kerlone; ***Braz.:*** Betoptic; ***Canad.:*** Betoptic; ***Chile:*** Bemaz; Beof; Betoptic; ***Denm.:*** Betoptic; Kerlon; ***Fin.:*** Betoptic; Kerlon; ***Fr.:*** Betoptic; Kerlone; ***Ger.:*** Betoptima; Kerlone; ***Gr.:*** Betoptic; Betoptic S; Eifel; Kerlone; Pertaxol; ***Hong Kong:*** Betoptic; Kerlone†; ***India:*** Optipres; ***Irl.:*** Betoptic; ***Israel:*** Betoptic; Kerlone; ***Ital.:*** Betoptic; Kerlon; ***Malaysia:*** Betoptic; Kerlone; ***Mex.:*** Beofta; Betoptic; Bex-Hepar†; ***Neth.:*** Kerlon; ***Norw.:*** Betoptic; ***NZ:*** Betoptic; ***Port.:*** Bertocil; Betoptic; Davixolol; ***S.Afr.:*** Betoptic; ***Singapore:*** Betoptic; Kerlone; ***Spain:*** Betoptic; Oxodal†; ***Swed.:*** Betoptic; Kerlon; ***Switz.:*** Betoptic S; Kerlon; ***Thai.:*** Betoptic; Kerlone†; ***UK:*** Betoptic; Kerlone†; ***USA:*** Betoptic; Kerlone.

### Bevantolol Hydrochloride *(BANM, USAN, rINNM)*

Cl-775; Hidrocloruro de bevantolol; NC-1400. 1-(3,4-Dimethoxyphenethylamino)-3-*m*-tolyloxypropan-2-ol hydrochloride.

$C_{20}H_{27}NO_4,HCl = 381.9.$

*CAS — 59170-23-9 (bevantolol); 42864-78-8 (bevantolol hydrochloride).*

*ATC — C07AB06.*

**Profile**
Bevantolol is a cardioselective beta blocker (p.868). It is reported to lack significant intrinsic sympathomimetic activity but has weak membrane-stabilising properties and also has vasodilator activity. It has been given by mouth as the hydrochloride in the management of hypertension and angina pectoris.

◊ References.

1. Frishman WH, *et al.* Bevantolol: a preliminary review of its pharmacodynamic and pharmacokinetic properties, and therapeutic efficacy in hypertension and angina pectoris. *Drugs* 1988; **35:** 1–21.

## Bezafibrate *(BAN, USAN, rINN)*

Bezafibrato; Bezafibratum; BM-15075; LO-44. 2-[4-(2-*p*-Chlorobenzamidoethyl)phenoxy]-2-methylpropionic acid.

$C_{19}H_{20}ClNO_4 = 361.8.$

*CAS — 41859-67-0.*

*ATC — C10AB02.*

**Pharmacopoeias.** In *Eur.* (see p.vi).

**Ph. Eur. 5.0** (Bezafibrate). A white or almost white, crystalline powder. It exhibits polymorphism. Practically insoluble in water; sparingly soluble in alcohol and in acetone; freely soluble in dimethylformamide; it dissolves in dilute solutions of alkali hydroxides.

### Adverse Effects and Precautions

The commonest adverse effects of bezafibrate therapy are gastrointestinal disturbances including anorexia, nausea, and gastric discomfort. Other adverse effects reported to occur less frequently include headache, dizziness, vertigo, fatigue, skin rashes, pruritus, photosensitivity, alopecia, impotence, anaemia, leucopenia, and thrombocytopenia. Raised serum-aminotransferase concentrations have occasionally been reported. Elevated creatine phosphokinase concentrations during bezafibrate therapy may be associated with a syndrome of myositis, myopathy, and rarely rhabdomyolysis; patients with hypoalbuminaemia resulting from nephrotic syndrome or with renal impairment may be at increased risk. Bezafibrate may increase the lithogenic index, and there have been isolated reports of gallstones. Although there is no direct evidence that the use of bezafibrate is associated with an increased frequency of this condition, fibrates as a class may be (see Gallstones, below).

Bezafibrate should not be given to patients with severe hepatic impairment, primary biliary cirrhosis, gallstones or gallbladder disorders, or hypoalbuminaemic states such as nephrotic syndrome. It should be used with caution in renal impairment (see under Uses and Administration, below).

**Effects on glucose metabolism.** There have been conflicting reports of the effects of fibrates on glucose metabolism in hyperlipidaemic diabetic patients.

Reductions in fasting blood-glucose concentrations and improved glucose tolerance have been reported during therapy with bezafibrate in type 2 diabetic patients with hyperlipidaemia,[1-3] and it has been suggested that bezafibrate may be a particularly suitable choice of lipid regulating drug in such patients.[4]

In a study of 14 diabetic patients[5] treated with gemfibrozil for 9 to 23 weeks control of diabetes was not generally impaired and appeared in some cases to be slightly improved. Another study in 20 patients[6] reported a slight increase in antidiabetic therapy requirements in 9 and a decrease in 1. A decrease in fasting and oral glucose tolerance test-stimulated glucose concentrations has been noted[7] in patients with impaired glucose tolerance but not in those with normal glucose tolerance. No reduction in insulin secretion was noted. Two other studies[8,9] found no clinically significant changes in glucose metabolism in stable diabetics taking gemfibrozil. In another,[10] gemfibrozil was associated with decreased hyperglycaemia in diabetics whose blood-glucose concentrations were not well controlled.

Use of gemfibrozil in patients receiving repaglinide is contra-indicated due to the risk of serious hypoglycaemia (see p.344).

1. Rüth E, Vollmar J. Verbesserung der diabeteseinstellung unter der therapie mit bezafibrat. *Dtsch Med Wochenschr* 1982; **107:** 1470–3.
2. Bruneder H, Klein HJ. Hyperlipoproteinämie und diabetes mellitus: langzeitbehandlung mit bezafibrat bei 115 patienten. *Med Welt* 1984; **35:** 357–60.
3. Ogawa S, *et al.* Bezafibrate reduces blood glucose in type 2 diabetes mellitus. *Metabolism* 2000; **49:** 331–4.
4. Jones IR, *et al.* Lowering of plasma glucose concentrations with bezafibrate in patients with moderately controlled NIDDM. *Diabetes Care* 1990; **13:** 855–63.
5. de Salcedo I, *et al.* Gemfibrozil in a group of diabetics. *Proc R Soc Med* 1976; **69** (suppl 2): 64–70.
6. Konttinen A, *et al.* The effect of gemfibrozil on serum lipids in diabetic patients. *Ann Clin Res* 1979; **11:** 240–5.
7. Testori GP, *et al.* Effect of gemfibrozil treatment on glucose tolerance in hypertriglyceridemic patients with normal or impaired glucose tolerance. *Curr Ther Res* 1990; **47:** 390–5.
8. Leaf DA, *et al.* The hypolipidemic effects of gemfibrozil in type V hyperlipidemia. *JAMA* 1989; **262:** 3154–60.
9. Pagani A, *et al.* Effect of short-term gemfibrozil administration on glucose metabolism and insulin secretion in non-insulin-dependent diabetics. *Curr Ther Res* 1989; **45:** 14–20.
10. Notarbartolo A, *et al.* Effects of gemfibrozil in hyperlipidemic patients with or without diabetes. *Curr Ther Res* 1993; **53:** 381–93.

**Effects on the kidneys.** Small increases in creatinine concentration are common during treatment with bezafibrate. However, there have also been reports of acute renal failure associated with treatment with bezafibrate,[1] and with clofibrate.[2,3] Renal failure may also occur due to rhabdomyolysis in patients receiving fibrates, see Effects on Skeletal Muscle, below.

1. Lipkin GW, Tomson CRV. Severe reversible renal failure with bezafibrate. *Lancet* 1993; **341:** 371.
2. Dosa S, *et al.* Acute-on-chronic renal failure precipitated by clofibrate. *Lancet* 1976; **i:** 250.
3. Cumming A. Acute renal failure and interstitial nephritis after clofibrate treatment. *BMJ* 1980; **281:** 1529–30.

**Effects on the nervous system.** Adverse effects on the peripheral nervous system have been reported with fibrates. Peripheral neuropathy has been reported[1] with bezafibrate, and was substantiated by nerve conduction studies. There has also been a report[2] of peripheral neuropathy with clofibrate, which resolved when therapy was withdrawn. In addition, the Adverse Drug Reactions Advisory Committee in Australia has received reports of paraesthesia occurring in 6 patients in association with gemfibrozil treatment.[3]

1. Ellis CJ, *et al.* Peripheral neuropathy with bezafibrate. *BMJ* 1994; **309:** 929.
2. Gabriel R, Pearce JMS. Clofibrate-induced myopathy and neuropathy. *Lancet* 1976; **ii:** 906.
3. Anonymous. Paraesthesia and neuropathy with hypolipidaemic agents. *Aust Adverse Drug React Bull* 1993; **12:** 6.

**Effects on the pancreas.** Acute pancreatitis has been reported[1] in a patient receiving bezafibrate, and recurred on 2 occasions when bezafibrate was restarted. There has also been a report[2] of acute pancreatitis in a patient receiving both fenofibrate and simvastatin, although simvastatin was considered more likely to be responsible.

1. Gang N, *et al.* Relapsing acute pancreatitis induced by re-exposure to the cholesterol lowering agent bezafibrate. *Am J Gastroenterol* 1999; **94:** 3626–8.
2. McDonald KB, *et al.* Pancreatitis associated with simvastatin plus fenofibrate. *Ann Pharmacother* 2002; **36:** 275–9.

**Effects on sexual function.** Sexual dysfunction has occurred with some fibrates. Impotence and loss of libido has been reported in 3 patients[1-3] during gemfibrozil treatment. In 2 of the men[1,2] bezafibrate did not produce this adverse effect. The UK Committee on Safety of Medicines was reported to be aware of a further 6 cases.[2] Of a further 3 cases of impotence associated with gemfibrozil reported from Spain, 1 patient had previously reacted similarly to clofibrate.[4] A systematic review,[5] including these and other reports, supported the conclusion that fibrates could cause erectile dysfunction.

1. Pizarro S, *et al.* Gemfibrozil-induced impotence. *Lancet* 1990; **336:** 1135.
2. Bain SC, *et al.* Gemfibrozil-induced impotence. *Lancet* 1990; **336:** 1389.
3. Bharani A. Sexual dysfunction after gemfibrozil *BMJ* 1992; **305:** 693.
4. Figueras A, *et al.* Gemfibrozil-induced impotence. *Ann Pharmacother* 1993; **27:** 982.
5. Rizvi K, *et al.* Do lipid-lowering drugs cause erectile dysfunction? A systematic review. *Fam Pract* 2002; **19:** 95–8.

**Effects on skeletal muscle.** Muscle disorders including myositis and myopathy are well known to occur with lipid regulating drugs such as fibrates.[1] Rhabdomyolysis, presenting as muscle pain with elevated creatine phosphokinase and myoglobinuria leading to renal failure, has also been reported but appears to be rare. Patients with renal impairment, and possibly with hypothyroidism, may be at increased risk of muscle toxicity. The UK Committee on Safety of Medicines has advised[1] that patients treated with fibrates should consult their doctor if they develop muscle pain, tenderness, or weakness, and treatment should be stopped if muscle toxicity is suspected clinically or if creatine phosphokinase is markedly raised or progressively rising.

Other lipid regulating drugs, particularly the statins, have also been associated with myopathy and the risk of muscle toxicity is increased if fibrates and statins are taken together; combination therapy may be necessary in some patients but careful monitoring is required.[2] There have been reports of rhabdomyolysis in patients taking gemfibrozil with statins (see Lipid Regulating Drugs under Interactions of Simvastatin, p.999).

1. Committee on Safety of Medicines/Medicines Control Agency. Rhabdomyolysis associated with lipid-lowering drugs. *Current Problems* 1995; **21:** 3.
2. Shek A, Ferrill MJ. Statin-fibrate combination therapy. *Ann Pharmacother* 2001; **35:** 908–917.

**Gallstones.** Fibrates, including fenofibrate[1-3] and gemfibrozil[4] have been reported to increase indices of bile lithogenicity, and some studies[5,6] have suggested an increased risk of gallstones in patients receiving fibrates, although this is not yet established. In the Helsinki Heart Study[7] no significant increase in gallstone operations was reported among 2051 patients taking gemfibrozil compared with 2030 taking placebo. However, a follow-up study[8] reported that cholecystectomies were consistently more common in those receiving gemfibrozil during the entire 8.5-year observation period.

1. Brown WV. Treatment of hypercholesterolaemia with fenofibrate: a review. *Curr Med Res Opin* 1989; **11:** 321–30.
2. Blane GF. Comparative toxicity and safety profile of fenofibrate and other fibric acid derivatives. *Am J Med* 1987; **83** (suppl 5B): 26–36.
3. Palmer RH. Effects of fibric acid derivatives on biliary lipid composition. *Am J Med* 1987; **83** (suppl 5B): 37–43.
4. Leiss O, *et al.* Effect of gemfibrozil on biliary lipid metabolism in normolipemic subjects. *Metabolism* 1985; **34:** 74–82.
5. Mamdani MM, *et al.* Is there an association between lipid-lowering drugs and cholecystectomy? *Am J Med* 2000; **108:** 418–21.
6. Caroli-Bosc F-X, *et al.* Role of fibrates and HMG-CoA reductase inhibitors in gallstone formation: epidemiological study in an unselected population. *Dig Dis Sci* 2001; **46:** 540–4.
7. Frick MH, *et al.* Helsinki Heart Study: primary-prevention trial with gemfibrozil in middle-aged men with dyslipidemia: safety of treatment, changes in risk factors, and incidence of coronary heart disease. *N Engl J Med* 1987; **317:** 1237–45.
8. Huttunen JK, *et al.* The Helsinki Heart Study: an 8.5-year safety and mortality follow-up. *J Intern Med* 1994; **235:** 31–9.

**Headache.** Severe recurrent headaches have been reported[1] in a patient receiving bezafibrate. The headaches started about 24 hours after therapy with bezafibrate began, and recurred about 1 hour after each dose. Headaches occurred 30 to 90 minutes after each dose of gemfibrozil in 2 patients.[2,3] In both patients, the headaches were accompanied by dry mouth, and in 1 also by blurred vision. The headaches stopped when gemfibrozil was withdrawn and recurred one week after re-exposure.

1. Hodgetts TJ, Tunnicliffe C. Bezafibrate-induced headache. *Lancet* 1989; **i:** 163.
2. Arellano F, *et al.* Gemfibrozil-induced headache. *Lancet* 1988; **i:** 705.
3. Alvarez-Sabin J, *et al.* Gemfibrozil-induced headache. *Lancet* 1988; **ii:** 1246.

**Photosensitivity.** For mention of cross-sensitivity between fibrates (bezafibrate, ciprofibrate, or fenofibrate) and ketoprofen, see p.51.

## Interactions

Bezafibrate and other fibrates may enhance the effects of oral anticoagulants; the dose of anticoagulant should be reduced when treatment with a fibrate is started, and then adjusted gradually if necessary. Recommendations concerning the amount that the anticoagulant dose should be reduced by vary between the manufacturers of the differing fibrates and are not always specified; the manufacturers of bezafibrate suggest a reduction of up to 50% in the dosage of anticoagulant. The mechanism of the interaction has not yet been determined. Fibrates have been reported to displace warfarin from protein binding sites but other mechanisms are probably also involved.

A number of other drugs may be displaced from plasma proteins by fibrates, including tolbutamide and other sulfonylurea antidiabetics, phenytoin, and, in patients with hypoalbuminaemia, furosemide. The interaction with antidiabetics is complex since bezafibrate has been shown to alter glucose tolerance in both diabetic and non-diabetic patients (see Effects on Glucose Metabolism, above). The dosage of antidiabetics may need adjusting during bezafibrate therapy.

There is an increased risk of myopathy if fibrates are used with statins (see Lipid Regulating Drugs under Interactions of Simvastatin, p.999).

Increased ciclosporin concentrations and associated nephrotoxicity have been reported when the drug was given with bezafibrate.

**Lipid regulating drugs.** The bioavailability of gemfibrozil was reduced by the concomitant administration of *colestipol*, but was unaffected when gemfibrozil was taken either 2 hours before or 2 hours after colestipol.[1]

For discussion of the interaction between fibrates and *statins*, see p.999.

1. Forland SC, *et al.* Apparent reduced absorption of gemfibrozil when given with colestipol. *J Clin Pharmacol* 1990; **30:** 29–32.

**NSAIDs.** Acute renal failure due to rhabdomyolysis in a patient has been attributed to an interaction between ciprofibrate and *ibuprofen.*[1] Ibuprofen was believed to have displaced ciprofibrate from protein binding sites. The use of radiological contrast media may also have been a contributory factor.

For mention of cross-sensitivity between fibrates (bezafibrate, ciprofibrate, or fenofibrate) and *ketoprofen*, see Photosensitivity under Adverse Effects of Ketoprofen, p.51.

1. Ramachandran S, *et al.* Acute renal failure due to rhabdomyolysis in presence of concurrent ciprofibrate and ibuprofen treatment. *BMJ* 1997; **314:** 1593.

## Pharmacokinetics

Bezafibrate is readily absorbed from the gastrointestinal tract. Plasma protein binding is about 95%. The plasma elimination half-life is about 2 hours. Most of a dose is excreted in the urine, about half as unchanged drug, the remainder as metabolites including the glucuronide conjugate. A small proportion of the dose appears in the faeces.

◊ References.

1. Abshagen U, *et al.* Disposition pharmacokinetics of bezafibrate in man. *Eur J Clin Pharmacol* 1979; **16:** 31–8.
2. Abshagen U, *et al.* Steady-state kinetics of bezafibrate and clofibrate in healthy female volunteers. *Eur J Clin Pharmacol* 1980; **17:** 305–8.

**The elderly.** In a study comparing the pharmacokinetics of bezafibrate in 19 elderly patients with younger healthy subjects,[1] maximum plasma concentrations were 1.6 times higher in the elderly group (median 12.1 mg/litre against 7.7 mg/litre) and half-life was increased by 3.8 times (median 6.6 hours against 1.7 hours). The differences could not be attributed solely to diminished renal function in elderly patients. Dosage adjustments in elderly patients should not therefore be based on renal function alone.

1. Neugebauer G, *et al.* Steady-state kinetics of bezafibrate retard in hyperlipidemic geriatric patients. *Klin Wochenschr* 1988; **66:** 250–6.

**Renal impairment.** The half-life of bezafibrate may be prolonged in patients with renal impairment (see under Uses and Administration, below).

## Uses and Administration

Bezafibrate, a fibric acid derivative, is a lipid regulating drug. It is used to reduce total cholesterol and triglycerides in the management of hyperlipidaemias (p.823), including type IIa, type IIb, type III, type IV, and type V hyperlipoproteinaemias. Bezafibrate and other fibrates reduce triglycerides by reducing the concentration of very-low-density lipoprotein (VLDL). They reduce low-density lipoprotein (LDL)-cholesterol to a lesser extent, although the effect is variable, and may also increase high-density lipoprotein (HDL)-cholesterol.

Bezafibrate is given in a usual dose of 200 mg three times daily by mouth taken with or after food; 200 mg twice daily may occasionally be adequate for maintenance particularly in the treatment of hypertriglyceridaemia. A modified-release tablet is also available and is given as a single daily dose of 400 mg.

The dose of bezafibrate should be reduced in patients with renal impairment (see below).

◊ General reviews.

1. Goa KL, *et al.* Bezafibrate: an update of its pharmacology and use in the management of dyslipidaemia. *Drugs* 1996; **52:** 725–53.

**Action.** Bezafibrate is a typical member of the fibric acid derivative group of drugs (the fibrates) used in the treatment of hyperlipidaemias (p.823). One of the primary actions of the fibrates is to promote the catabolism of triglyceride-rich lipoproteins, in particular very-low-density lipoproteins (VLDL), apparently mediated by an enhanced activity of lipoprotein lipase.[1] They may also interfere with the synthesis of VLDL, possibly by inhibiting hepatic acetyl coenzyme A carboxylase. The effect of fibrates on low-density lipoprotein (LDL)-cholesterol depends on the overall lipoprotein status of the patient but concentrations tend to decrease if high at baseline and increase if low at baseline. High-density lipoprotein (HDL)-cholesterol concentrations are increased, although there have been a few reports of unexpected falls in HDL-cholesterol with bezafibrate[2,3] and ciprofibrate.[4,5]

Fibrates have three actions on sterol metabolism:[1] they inhibit the synthesis of cholesterol, they inhibit the synthesis of bile acids, and they enhance the secretion of cholesterol in bile. It is these latter two effects which are responsible for the raised cholesterol saturation of bile, which may lead to the formation of gallstones in some patients (see Gallstones, under Adverse Effects, above).

1. Grundy SM, Vega GL. Fibric acids: effects on lipids and lipoprotein metabolism. *Am J Med* 1987; **83** (suppl 5B): 9–20.
2. Capps NE. Lipid profiles on fibric-acid derivatives. *Lancet* 1994; **344:** 684–5.
3. McLeod AJ, *et al.* Abnormal lipid profiles on fibrate derivatives. *Lancet* 1996; **347:** 261.
4. Chandler HA, Batchelor AJ. Ciprofibrate and lipid profile. *Lancet* 1994; **344:** 128–9.
5. McLeod AJ, *et al.* Ciprofibrate and lipid profile. *Lancet* 1994; **344:** 955.

**Administration in renal impairment.** The manufacturer has stated that conventional formulations of bezafibrate may be given to patients with renal impairment depending on creatinine clearance (CC). Doses are:

- CC 40 to 60 mL/minute, 400 mg daily
- CC 15 to 40 mL/minute, 200 mg daily or on alternate days
- CC less than 15 mL/minute, contra-indicated unless receiving dialysis
- dialysis patients, 200 mg on every third day.

In a study in patients with renal impairment[1] the half-life of bezafibrate was reported to be prolonged to 4.6 hours in 3 patients with CC greater than 40 mL/minute, 7.8 hours in 8 patients with CC of 20 to 40 mL/minute, and 20.1 hours in a patient with CC of 13 mL/minute. An accelerated decline in renal function was reported[2] in 2 patients with advanced chronic renal failure during bezafibrate therapy, and it was suggested that further dosage reductions would be necessary to avoid excessive plasma-bezafibrate concentrations in uraemic patients.

1. Anderson P, Norbeck H-E. Clinical pharmacokinetics of bezafibrate in patients with impaired renal function. *Eur J Clin Pharmacol* 1981; **21:** 209–14.
2. Williams AJ, *et al.* The short term effects of bezafibrate on the hypertriglyceridaemia of moderate to severe uraemia. *Br J Clin Pharmacol* 1984; **18:** 361–7.

**Cardiovascular risk reduction.** Lipid lowering therapy has an important role in patients at risk of cardiovascular disease (p.819). Although the evidence is less good than for statins, several studies have shown that fibrates may reduce both the progression of atherosclerosis and the incidence of cardiovascular events.

In the Bezafibrate Coronary Atherosclerosis Intervention Trial (BECAIT)[1,2] treatment with bezafibrate for 5 years in young men (less than 45 years of age) following myocardial infarction resulted in fewer coronary events and slowed the progression of focal coronary atherosclerosis when compared with placebo. However, in older men with peripheral vascular disease,[3] bezafibrate had no effect on the incidence of coronary events and stroke together, although the severity of intermittent claudication was reduced and, in men under 65 years, there were fewer non-fatal coronary events. In the Diabetes Atherosclerosis Intervention Study (DAIS),[4] fenofibrate reduced the angiographic progression of coronary atherosclerosis in type 2 diabetics, and there were also fewer clinical events in those receiving fenofibrate.

The best evidence for a reduction in cardiovascular events is for gemfibrozil. The Helsinki Heart Study[5] assessed gemfibrozil for the primary prevention of ischaemic heart disease in 4081 middle-aged men with hyperlipidaemia. There was an overall reduction of 34% in the incidence of fatal and non-fatal myocardial infarctions and cardiac deaths in the gemfibrozil group compared with the placebo group, with the greatest reduction seen during years 3 to 5. Follow-up for a further 3.5 years[6] suggested that long-term treatment with gemfibrozil seemed to postpone coronary events for about 5 years. The Veterans Affairs High-Density Lipoprotein Cholesterol Intervention Trial (VA-HIT)[7] assessed gemfibrozil for the secondary prevention of ischaemic heart disease in 2531 older men (mean age 64 years) whose primary lipid abnormality was a low HDL-cholesterol level. There was an overall reduction of 22% in the incidence of fatal and non-fatal myocardial infarctions and cardiac deaths in the gemfibrozil group compared with the placebo group, with the beneficial effects of gemfibrozil becoming apparent about 2 years after randomisation. There was also a reduction in the incidence of stroke.[8]

1. Ericsson C-G, *et al.* Angiographic assessment of effects of bezafibrate on progression of coronary artery disease in young male postinfarction patients. *Lancet* 1996; **347:** 849–53.
2. Ericsson C-G, *et al.* Effect of bezafibrate treatment over five years on coronary plaques causing 20% to 50% diameter narrowing (The Bezafibrate Coronary Atherosclerosis Intervention Trial (BECAIT)). *Am J Cardiol* 1997; **80:** 1125–9.
3. Meade T, *et al.* Bezafibrate in men with lower extremity arterial disease: randomised controlled trial. *BMJ* 2002; **325:** 1139–43.
4. Diabetes Atherosclerosis Intervention Study Investigators. Effect of fenofibrate on progression of coronary-artery disease in type 2 diabetes: the Diabetes Atherosclerosis Intervention Study, a randomised study. *Lancet* 2001; **357:** 905–910. Correction. *ibid.*; 1890.
5. Frick MH, *et al.* Helsinki Heart Study: primary-prevention trial with gemfibrozil in middle-aged men with dyslipidemia: safety of treatment, changes in risk factors, and incidence of coronary heart disease. *N Engl J Med* 1987; **317:** 1237–45.
6. Heinonen OP, *et al.* The Helsinki Heart Study: coronary heart disease incidence during an extended follow-up. *J Intern Med* 1994; **235:** 41–9.
7. Bloomfield Rubins H, *et al.* Gemfibrozil for the secondary prevention of coronary heart disease in men with low levels of high-density lipoprotein cholesterol. *N Engl J Med* 1999; **341:** 410–18.
8. Bloomfield Rubins H, *et al.* Reduction in stroke with gemfibrozil in men with coronary heart disease and low HDL cholesterol: The Veterans Affairs HDL Intervention Trial (VA-HIT). *Circulation* 2001; **103:** 2828–33.

### Preparations

**Proprietary Preparations** (details are given in Part 3)
***Arg.:*** Bezacur; Bezalip; Elpi Lip; Nebufur; ***Austria:*** Bezacur; Bezalip; Beza-stad; ***Belg.:*** Cedur; Eulitop; ***Braz.:*** Cedur; ***Canad.:*** Bezalip; ***Chile:*** Nimus; Oralipin; ***Denm.:*** Bezalip†; ***Fin.:*** Bezalip; ***Fr.:*** Befizal; ***Ger.:*** Azufibrat; Befibrat; Beza; Beza-Lande†; Beza-Puren; Bezabeta; Bezacur; Bezadoc; Bezagamma; Bezamerck; Bezapham; Cedur; Durabezur†; Lipox; Regadrin B; Sklerofibrat; ***Gr.:*** Bezalip; Getup; Verbital; ***Hong Kong:*** Azufibrat†; Bezalip; Zafibral; ***India:*** Bezalip; ***Israel:*** Bezalip; Norlip; ***Ital.:*** Bezalip; Hadiel; ***Jpn:*** Bezalip; ***Mex.:*** Bezafisal; Bezalex; Bezalip; Bionolip; Colser; Klestran; Lipocin; Redalip; Solibay; Wayfrato†; ***Neth.:*** Bezalip; ***NZ:*** Bezalip; Fibalip; ***Port.:*** Bezalip; ***S.Afr.:*** Bezalip; ***Singapore:*** Bezalip; Zafibral†; ***Spain:*** Difaterol; Eulitop; Reducterol; ***Swed.:*** Bezalip; ***Switz.:*** Cedur; ***Thai.:*** Bezalip; Bezamil; Polyzalip; Raset; ***UAE:*** Lipitrol; ***UK:*** Bezagen; Bezalip; Bezalip Mono; Liparol†; Zimbacol.

## Binifibrate *(rINN)*

Binifibrato. 2-(4-Chlorophenoxy)-2-methylpropionic acid ester with 1,3-dinicotinoyloxypropan-2-ol.

$C_{25}H_{23}ClN_2O_7$ = 498.9.

*CAS — 69047-39-8.*

### Profile

Binifibrate, a derivative of clofibrate (p.884) and nicotinic acid (p.1441), is a lipid regulating drug used in the treatment of hyperlipidaemias (p.823). The usual dose is 600 mg three times daily by mouth.

### Preparations

**Proprietary Preparations** (details are given in Part 3)
***Spain:*** Antopal; Biniwas; Clearon†.

## Bisoprolol Fumarate *(BANM, USAN, rINNM)*

Bisoprolol Hemifumarate; CL-297939; EMD-33512 (bisoprolol or bisoprolol fumarate); Fumarato de bisoprolol. 1-[4-(2-Isopropoxyethoxymethyl)phenoxy]-3-isopropylaminopropan-2-ol fumarate.

$(C_{18}H_{31}NO_4)_2,C_4H_4O_4$ = 767.0.

*CAS — 66722-44-9 (bisoprolol); 66722-45-0 (bisoprolol fumarate); 104344-23-2 (bisoprolol fumarate).*

*ATC — C07AB07.*

**Pharmacopoeias.** In *US.*

**USP 27** (Bisoprolol Fumarate). A white crystalline powder. Very soluble in water and in methyl alcohol; freely soluble in alcohol, in chloroform, and in glacial acetic acid; slightly soluble in acetone and in ethyl acetate. Store in airtight containers. Protect from light.

### Adverse Effects, Treatment, and Precautions

As for Beta Blockers, p.869.

### Interactions

The interactions associated with beta blockers are discussed on p.870.

### Pharmacokinetics

Bisoprolol is almost completely absorbed from the gastrointestinal tract and undergoes only minimal first-pass metabolism resulting in an oral bioavailability of about 90%. Peak plasma concentrations are reached 2 to 4 hours after oral administration. Bisoprolol is about 30% bound to plasma proteins. It has a plasma elimination half-life of 10 to 12 hours. Bisoprolol is moderately lipid-soluble. It is metabolised in the liver and excreted in urine, approximately 50% as unchanged drug and 50% as metabolites.

### Uses and Administration

Bisoprolol is a cardioselective beta blocker (p.868). It is reported to be devoid of intrinsic sympathomimetic and membrane-stabilising properties.

Bisoprolol is given as the fumarate in the management of hypertension (p.825) and angina pectoris (p.813). It is also used as an adjunct to standard therapy in patients with stable chronic heart failure (p.820).

In **hypertension** or **angina pectoris** the usual dose of bisoprolol fumarate is 5 to 10 mg by mouth as a single daily dose; the maximum recommended dose is 20 mg daily. A reduction in dose may be necessary in patients with hepatic or renal impairment (see below).

In **heart failure** the initial dose of bisoprolol fumarate is 1.25 mg once daily by mouth. If tolerated, the dose should be doubled after 1 week, and then increased gradually at 1 to 4 week intervals to the maximum dose tolerated; this should not exceed 10 mg once daily.

◊ References.

1. Johns TE, Lopez LM. Bisoprolol: is this just another beta-blocker for hypertension or angina? *Ann Pharmacother* 1995; **29:** 403–14.
2. CIBIS-II Investigators and Committees. The Cardiac Insufficiency Bisoprolol Study II (CIBIS-II): a randomised trial. *Lancet* 1999; **353:** 9–13.
3. McGavin JK, Keating GM. Bisoprolol: a review of its use in chronic heart failure. *Drugs* 2002; **62:** 2677–96.

**Administration in hepatic or renal impairment.** In patients with severe hepatic impairment or renal impairment (creatinine clearance less than 40 mL/minute) the US manufacturer recommends that the initial dose for hypertension should be 2.5 mg daily, and that the dose should be increased cautiously. The UK manufacturers recommend a maximum dose of 10 mg daily for both angina pectoris and hypertension in patients with severe hepatic impairment or with a creatinine clearance of less than 20 mL/minute.

### Preparations

***USP 27:*** Bisoprolol Fumarate and Hydrochlorothiazide Tablets; Bisoprolol Fumarate Tablets.

**Proprietary Preparations** (details are given in Part 3)
***Arg.:*** Concor; Corbis; ***Austral.:*** Bicor; ***Austria:*** Bisocor; Bisotyrol; Cardiocor; Concor; Darbalan; Nanalan; ***Belg.:*** Emconcor; Isoten; ***Braz.:*** Concor; ***Canad.:*** Monocor; ***Chile:*** Concor; ***Denm.:*** Bisocor; Cardicor; Emconcor; Monocor†; ***Fin.:*** Bisopral; Emconcor; Orloc; ***Fr.:*** Cardensiel; Cardiocor; Detensiel; Soprol; ***Ger.:*** Biso; Biso Lich; Biso-Puren; Bisobeta; Bisobloc; Bisogamma; Bisohexal; Bisomerck; Concor; Cordalin; Fondril; ***Gr.:*** Pactens; ***Hong Kong:*** Concor; ***India:*** Concor; ***Irl.:*** Bisocor; Bisopine; Cardicor; Emcor; Soprol; ***Israel:*** Bisolol; Cardiloc; Concor; ***Ital.:*** Concor; ***Malaysia:*** Concor; ***Neth.:*** Bisobloc†; Emcor; ***Port.:*** Concor; ***S.Afr.:*** Concor; ***Singapore:*** Concor; ***Spain:*** Emconcor; Euradal; Godal†; ***Swed.:*** Emconcor; ***Switz.:*** Bilol; Concor; ***Thai.:*** Concor; ***UK:*** Bipranix; Cardicor; Emcor; Monocor; Soloc; Vivacor; ***USA:*** Zebeta.

**Multi-ingredient:** ***Arg.:*** Ziac; ***Austria:*** Bisoprolol-HCT; Concor Plus; Darbalan Plus; Nanalan Plus; ***Belg.:*** Emcoretic; Maxsoten; ***Braz.:*** Biconcor; ***Chile:*** Ziac; ***Fin.:*** Emconcor Comp; ***Fr.:*** Lodoz; Wytens; ***Ger.:*** Bisomerck Plus; Concor Plus; Fondril HCT; ***Hong Kong:*** Lodoz; ***Mex.:*** Biconcor; ***Neth.:*** Emcoretic; ***Port.:*** Concor Plus; ***S.Afr.:*** Ziak; ***Spain:*** Emcoretic; ***Switz.:*** Concor Plus; ***UK:*** Monozide†; ***USA:*** Ziac.

## Bivalirudin *(BAN, USAN, rINN)*

BG-8967; Bivalirudina; Hirulog.

$C_{98}H_{138}N_{24}O_{33}$ = 2180.3.

*CAS — 128270-60-0.*

### Adverse Effects and Precautions

The most common adverse effect of bivalirudin is bleeding.

Bivalirudin is contra-indicated in patients with active major bleeding and should be used with caution in patients at increased risk of bleeding. It should not be given by intramuscular injection.

### Interactions

Use of bivalirudin with other anticoagulants or thrombolytics may increase the risk of bleeding.

### Pharmacokinetics

Bivalirudin is partly metabolised and partly excreted by the kidney. Following intravenous administration the plasma half-life is about 25 minutes in patients with normal renal function but is prolonged in renal impairment. Bivalirudin does not bind to plasma proteins and is removed by haemodialysis.

◊ References.

1. Robson R, *et al.* Bivalirudin pharmacokinetics and pharmacodynamics: effect of renal function, dose, and gender. *Clin Pharmacol Ther* 2002; **71:** 433–9.

### Uses and Administration

Bivalirudin, an analogue of the peptide hirudin (p.931), is a direct thrombin inhibitor. It is used as an anticoagulant in patients with unstable angina undergoing percutaneous transluminal coronary angioplasty (see Reperfusion and Revascularisation Procedures, p.834) and has also been investigated in unstable angina and myocardial infarction.

In the management of patients undergoing angioplasty, bivalirudin is started immediately before the procedure. The initial dose is 1 mg/kg by intravenous injection followed by an intravenous infusion of 2.5 mg/kg per hour for 4 hours. The infusion may be continued at a dose of 200 micrograms/kg per hour for up to 20 hours if required. Patients should also receive treatment with aspirin.

The dose of bivalirudin should be reduced in patients with renal impairment (see below).

◊ References.

1. Carswell CI, Plosker GL. Bivalirudin: a review of its potential place in the management of acute coronary syndromes. *Drugs* 2002; **62:** 841–70.
2. Sciulli TM, Mauro VF. Pharmacology and clinical use of bivalirudin. *Ann Pharmacother* 2002; **36:** 1028–41.

**Administration in renal impairment.** The infusion dose of bivalirudin should be reduced in patients with renal impairment and the activated clotting time should be monitored. Required adjustments according to glomerular filtration rate (GFR) are:

- GFR 30 to 59 mL/minute: reduce by 20%
- GFR 10 to 29 mL/minute: reduce by 60%
- dialysis-dependent patients: reduce by 90%

### Preparations

**Proprietary Preparations** (details are given in Part 3)
***NZ:*** Angiomax; ***USA:*** Angiomax.

## Bopindolol Malonate *(rINNM)*

Bopindolol Hydrogen Malonate; LT-31-200; Malonato de bopindolol. (±)-1-(*tert*-Butylamino)-3-[(2-methylindol-4-yl)oxy]propan-2-ol benzoate malonate.

$C_{23}H_{28}N_2O_3,C_3H_4O_4$ = 484.5.

*CAS — 62658-63-3 (bopindolol); 82857-38-3 (bopindolol malonate).*

*ATC — C07AA17.*

### Profile

Bopindolol is a non-cardioselective beta blocker (p.868). It is reported to possess some intrinsic sympathomimetic activity.

Bopindolol is given by mouth as the malonate but doses are expressed in terms of the base; 1.27 mg of bopindolol malonate is approximately equivalent to 1 mg of base. It is used in the management of hypertension (p.825) and angina pectoris (p.813) in daily doses equivalent to 0.5 to 2 mg of bopindolol by mouth.

◊ References.

1. Harron DWG, *et al.* Bopindolol: a review of its pharmacodynamic and pharmacokinetic properties and therapeutic efficacy. *Drugs* 1991; **41:** 130–49.

### Preparations

**Proprietary Preparations** (details are given in Part 3)
***Austria:*** Sandonorm; ***Ger.:*** Wandonorm; ***Switz.:*** Sandonorm.

**Multi-ingredient:** ***Switz.:*** Sandoretic.

## Bosentan *(BAN, USAN, rINN)*

Bosentano; Ro-47-0203/029. *p-tert*-Butyl-*N*-[6-(2-hydroxyethoxy)-5-(*o*-methoxyphenoxy)-2-(2-pyrimidinyl)-4-pyrimidinyl]benzenesulfonamide.

$C_{27}H_{29}N_5O_6S$ = 551.6.

*CAS — 147536-97-8 (anhydrous bosentan); 157212-55-0 (bosentan monohydrate).*

*ATC — C02KX01.*

### Adverse Effects

Adverse effects reported with bosentan include headache, nasopharyngitis, flushing, oedema, hypotension, palpitations, gastrointestinal disturbances, pruritus, fatigue, and anaemia. Dose-related increases in liver aminotransferases may also occur.

Bosentan is teratogenic in *animals.*

### Precautions

Bosentan is contra-indicated in patients with moderate to severe hepatic impairment. Liver-aminotransferase concentrations should be measured before starting therapy, at monthly intervals during therapy, and 2 weeks after any increase in dose; bosentan should not be given to patients with concentrations greater than 3 times the upper limit of normal, and the dose should be reduced or treatment withdrawn if abnormalities occur during treatment or if there are clinical signs of hepatotoxicity. Haemoglobin concentrations should be monitored every 3 months during therapy, more frequently at the start.

Bosentan should not be given to patients with hypotension. Although there is no evidence of rebound effects after discontinuation of bosentan, it is recommended that therapy should be withdrawn gradually.

Bosentan is teratogenic in *animals*.

### Interactions

Bosentan is metabolised by the cytochrome P450 isoenzymes CYP2C9 and CYP3A4 and is also an inducer of the same isoenzymes. Interactions may therefore occur with other drugs that are either metabolised by, or inhibit, these isoenzymes. Use with ciclosporin is contra-indicated since plasma concentrations of bosentan are significantly increased (see below). There is an increased risk of hepatotoxicity if bosentan is given with glibenclamide and the combination should be avoided; the hypoglycaemic effect of glibenclamide may also be reduced.

**Anticoagulants.** For reports of bosentan decreasing the anticoagulant effect of *warfarin*, see Endothelin Receptor Antagonists, p.1026.

**Ciclosporin.** For details of the complex interaction between bosentan and ciclosporin, see p.1355.

### Pharmacokinetics

Bosentan is absorbed from the gastrointestinal tract with an absolute bioavailability of about 50%. Peak plasma concentrations occur about 3 to 5 hours after an oral dose. It is more than 98% bound to plasma proteins, mainly to albumin. Bosentan is metabolised in the liver by the cytochrome P450 isoenzymes CYP2C9 and CYP3A4; one of the metabolites is active. Bosentan is excreted almost entirely as metabolites in the bile; less than 3% of an oral dose is excreted in the urine. The terminal elimination half-life is about 5 hours.

◊ References.

1. Weber C, *et al.* Multiple-dose pharmacokinetics, safety, and tolerability of bosentan, an endothelin receptor antagonist, in healthy male volunteers. *J Clin Pharmacol* 1999; **39:** 703–14.
2. van Giersbergen PLM, *et al.* Influence of mild liver impairment on the pharmacokinetics and metabolism of bosentan, a dual endothelin receptor antagonist. *J Clin Pharmacol* 2003; **43:** 15–22.

### Uses and Administration

Bosentan is an endothelin receptor antagonist used in the management of pulmonary hypertension (p.832). It has also been investigated in heart failure and in hypertension.

In pulmonary hypertension, bosentan is given by mouth in an initial dose of 62.5 mg twice daily, increased after 4 weeks to a maintenance dose of 125 mg twice daily.

◊ References.

1. Krum H, *et al.* The effect of an endothelin-receptor antagonist, bosentan, on blood pressure in patients with essential hypertension. *N Engl J Med* 1998; **338:** 784–90.
2. Sutsch G, *et al.* Short-term oral endothelin-receptor antagonist therapy in conventionally treated patients with symptomatic severe chronic heart failure. *Circulation* 1998; **98:** 2262–8.
3. Kenyon KW, Nappi JM. Bosentan for the treatment of pulmonary arterial hypertension. *Ann Pharmacother* 2003; **37:** 1055–62.

**Pulmonary hypertension.** Pulmonary hypertension (p.832) is a progressive and incurable disease associated with an increase in pulmonary arterial pressure. Treatment usually involves the use of vasodilators such as calcium-channel blockers or intravenous epoprostenol, but systemic effects limit their use. Patients with pulmonary hypertension have raised plasma concentrations of the potent vasoconstrictor endothelin I, and endothelin antagonists such as bosentan have therefore been tried. Studies[1,2] with oral bosentan have shown improvement in exercise tolerance and in time to clinical progression, although no effect on mortality has yet been demonstrated. Bosentan has also been studied[3] in children.

1. Channick RN, *et al.* Effects of the dual endothelin-receptor antagonist bosentan in patients with pulmonary hypertension: a randomised placebo-controlled study. *Lancet* 2001; **358:** 1119–23.
2. Rubin LJ, *et al.* Bosentan therapy for pulmonary arterial hypertension. *N Engl J Med* 2002; **346:** 896–903. Correction. *ibid.*; 1258.
3. Barst RJ, *et al.* Pharmacokinetics, safety, and efficacy of bosentan in pediatric patients with pulmonary arterial hypertension. *Clin Pharmacol Ther* 2003; **73:** 372–82.

### Preparations

**Proprietary Preparations** (details are given in Part 3)
***Austral.:*** Tracleer; ***Irl.:*** Tracleer; ***UK:*** Tracleer; ***USA:*** Tracleer.

## Bretylium Tosilate *(BAN, rINN)*

ASL-603; Bretylium Tosylate *(USAN)*; Tosilato de bretilio. (2-Bromobenzyl)ethyldimethylammonium toluene-4-sulphonate.

$C_{11}H_{17}BrN,C_7H_7O_3S = 414.4.$

*CAS — 59-41-6 (bretylium); 61-75-6 (bretylium tosilate).*

*ATC — C01BD02.*

**Pharmacopoeias.** In *Br.* and *US.*

**BP 2003** (Bretylium Tosilate). A white crystalline powder. M.p. about 98°. It exhibits polymorphism. Freely soluble in water, in alcohol, and in methyl alcohol. A 5% solution in water has a pH of 5.0 to 6.5. Store in airtight containers at a temperature not exceeding 25°. Protect from light.

**USP 27** (Bretylium Tosylate). A white, hygroscopic, crystalline powder. Freely soluble in water, in alcohol, and in methyl alcohol; practically insoluble in ether, in ethyl acetate, and in hexane. Store in airtight containers at a temperature of 25°, excursions permitted between 15° and 30°.

**Incompatibility.** Bretylium tosilate injection has been reported to be visually incompatible with propofol emulsion[1] and with warfarin sodium injection.[2]

1. Trissel LA, *et al.* Compatibility of propofol injectable emulsion with selected drugs during simulated Y-site administration. *Am J Health-Syst Pharm* 1997; **54:** 1287–92.
2. Bahal SM, *et al.* Visual compatibility of warfarin sodium injection with selected medications and solutions. *Am J Health-Syst Pharm* 1997; **54:** 2599–2600.

### Adverse Effects and Precautions

The most common adverse effect of bretylium is hypotension, which may be severe. Bretylium may also cause a transient initial increase in blood pressure and heart rate, and a worsening of cardiac arrhythmias due to a release of noradrenaline. Nausea and vomiting may occur particularly during rapid intravenous infusion. Intramuscular injection of bretylium can lead to local tissue necrosis and muscle atrophy, which can be avoided by limiting the volume and varying the site of the injection (see Uses and Administration, below). Bretylium should be given with care to patients with renal impairment and doses should be reduced. Caution is also required in patients with severe aortic stenosis or pulmonary hypertension in whom cardiac output may not increase in response to the fall in peripheral resistance produced by bretylium.

**Effects on body temperature.** Bretylium tosilate by intravenous infusion was considered to be the cause of hyperthermia in a 59-year-old-man.[1] Six similar cases had been reported to the manufacturer in the USA.

1. Thibault J. Hyperthermia associated with bretylium tosylate injection. *Clin Pharm* 1989; **8:** 145–6.

**Effects on the cardiovascular system.** Seven patients with recent myocardial infarction, 3 with and 4 without left ventricular failure, received bretylium tosilate 5 to 10 mg/kg intravenously.[1] Initial transient tachycardia and hypertension, and late sustained bradycardia, hypotension with decreased vascular resistance, and increased calf blood flow and venous capacitance occurred in all 7 patients. Bretylium should be used cautiously in patients with hypotension as it might cause a significant reduction in arterial pressure.

1. Chatterjee K, *et al.* Cardiovascular effects of bretylium tosylate in acute myocardial infarction. *JAMA* 1973; **223:** 757–60.

### Interactions

Bretylium may exacerbate arrhythmias caused by digitalis toxicity. If sympathomimetics are required to reverse bretylium-induced hypotension, great care should be exercised since their effects may be enhanced.

### Pharmacokinetics

Bretylium is incompletely absorbed from the gastrointestinal tract. It is well absorbed following intramuscular injection. It is not metabolised and is largely excreted unchanged in the urine. The half-life is reported to be between 4 and 17 hours in patients with normal renal function and is prolonged in patients with renal impairment. Bretylium is dialysable.

◊ Reviews.

1. Rapeport WG. Clinical pharmacokinetics of bretylium. *Clin Pharmacokinet* 1985; **10:** 248–56.

### Uses and Administration

Bretylium is a quaternary ammonium compound with class II and class III antiarrhythmic activity (p.809); it causes an initial release of noradrenaline and then blocks adrenergic transmission by preventing noradrenaline release from adrenergic nerve endings. It suppresses ventricular fibrillation and other ventricular arrhythmias, but its exact mode of action is unknown.

It may be given parenterally as the tosilate for the treatment of immediately life-threatening ventricular arrhythmias and for the short-term control of ventricular arrhythmias resistant to standard treatment (see p.816) although other drugs are generally preferred. If a positive response is to be seen in patients with ventricular fibrillation it usually occurs within minutes. However, a delay of up to several hours may occur before peak antiarrhythmic activity is achieved and therefore it should only be used in other ventricular arrhythmias if the arrhythmia is resistant to more rapidly acting drugs.

In immediately life-threatening ventricular arrhythmias such as **ventricular fibrillation** 5 to 10 mg/kg as an undiluted 5% (50 mg/mL) solution may be given by rapid intravenous injection, with other resuscitative measures and cardioversion, repeated as necessary at 15 to 30 minute intervals up to a total dose of 30 mg/kg.

For the control of **ventricular arrhythmias** that are not immediately life-threatening bretylium may be given under ECG monitoring by intramuscular or slow intravenous injection. The patient should be supine or closely observed for orthostatic hypotension. A dose of 5 to 10 mg/kg by either route may be repeated initially every 1 to 2 hours until the arrhythmia is controlled and subsequently every 6 to 8 hours for maintenance therapy. The patient should be changed to an oral antiarrhythmic as soon as possible. For intramuscular administration an undiluted 5% (50 mg/mL) solution is used; the site of intramuscular injections should be varied on repeated injection and not more than 5 mL should be given into any one site. Nausea and vomiting during intravenous administration can be avoided by giving the injection over not less than 8 minutes although a period of 15 to 30 minutes is preferred: the injection is diluted to 10 mg/mL with glucose 5% or sodium chloride 0.9%. Alternatively an intravenous infusion of 1 to 2 mg/minute may be used for maintenance therapy. The maximum daily dose by any route should not exceed 30 mg/kg.

Doses should be reduced in patients with renal impairment.

### Preparations

***BP 2003:*** Bretylium Injection;
***USP 27:*** Bretylium Tosylate in Dextrose Injection; Bretylium Tosylate Injection.

**Proprietary Preparations** (details are given in Part 3)
***Belg.:*** Bretylate†; ***Canad.:*** Bretylate†; ***Irl.:*** Bretylate†; ***Israel:*** Bretylate; ***S.Afr.:*** Bretylol; ***UK:*** Bretylate†.

## Brimonidine Tartrate *(BANM, USAN, rINNM)*

AGN-190342-LF; Tartrato de brimonidina; UK-14304-18. 5-Bromo-6-(2-imidazolin-2-ylamino)quinoxaline D-tartrate.

$C_{11}H_{10}BrN_5,C_4H_6O_6 = 442.2.$

*CAS — 59803-98-4 (brimonidine); 79570-19-7 (brimonidine tartrate).*

*ATC — S01EA05.*

### Adverse Effects and Precautions

As for Apraclonidine Hydrochloride, p.864.

### Interactions

As for Apraclonidine Hydrochloride, p.864.

### Uses and Administration

Brimonidine is an alpha$_2$-adrenoceptor agonist with actions and uses similar to those of apraclonidine (p.864). It is used to lower intra-ocular pressure in patients with open-angle glaucoma or ocular hypertension (p.1485), as an alternative to, or as an adjunct to, topical beta blocker therapy. The reduction in intra-ocular pressure is maximal about 2 hours after topical application.

Brimonidine is used as the tartrate. In the management of glaucoma or ocular hypertension a 0.15 or 0.2% solution is instilled two or three times daily.

◊ References.


1. Anonymous. Brimonidine—an alpha$_2$-agonist for glaucoma. *Med Lett Drugs Ther* 1997; **39:** 54–5.
2. Adkins JC, Balfour JA. Brimonidine: a review of its pharmacological properties and clinical potential in the management of open-angle glaucoma and ocular hypertension. *Drugs Aging* 1998; **12:** 225–41.


### Preparations

**Proprietary Preparations** (details are given in Part 3)

***Arg.:*** Alphagan; Brimopress; Oftalmotonil; ***Austral.:*** Alphagan; Enidin; ***Austria:*** Alphagan; ***Belg.:*** Alphagan; ***Braz.:*** Alphagan; ***Canad.:*** Alphagan; ***Chile:*** Agglad Ofteno; Alphagan; Brimopress; ***Denm.:*** Alphagan; ***Fin.:*** Alphagan; ***Fr.:*** Alphagan; ***Ger.:*** Alphagan; ***Gr.:*** Alphagan; ***Hong Kong:*** Alphagan; ***Irl.:*** Alphagan; ***Israel:*** Alphagan; ***Ital.:*** Alphagan; ***Malaysia:*** Alphagan; ***Mex.:*** Alphagan; ***NZ:*** Alphagan; ***Port.:*** Alphagan; ***S.Afr.:*** Alphagan; ***Singapore:*** Alphagan; ***Spain:*** Alphagan; ***Swed.:*** Alphagan; ***Switz.:*** Alphagan; ***Thai.:*** Alphagan; ***UK:*** Alphagan; ***USA:*** Alphagan.

## Brinzolamide *(BAN, USAN, rINN)*

AL-4862; Brinzolamida. (R)-4-(Ethylamino)-3,4-dihydro-2-(3-methoxypropyl)-2*H*-thieno[3,2-e]-1,2-thiazine-6-sulfonamide 1,1-dioxide.

$C_{12}H_{21}N_3O_5S_3$ = 383.5.

*CAS — 138890-62-7.*

*ATC — S01EC04.*

**Pharmacopoeias.** In *US.*

**USP 27** (Brinzolamide). A white or almost white powder. Insoluble in water; slightly soluble in alcohol and in methyl alcohol.

### Adverse Effects and Precautions

As for Dorzolamide, p.908.

### Uses and Administration

Brinzolamide is a carbonic anhydrase inhibitor with actions and uses similar to those of dorzolamide (p.908). It is used topically to reduce intra-ocular pressure in the management of open-angle glaucoma and ocular hypertension (p.1485), either alone or as adjunctive therapy with a topical beta blocker. A 1% suspension is instilled two or three times daily.

### Preparations

***USP 27:*** Brinzolamide Ophthalmic Suspension.

**Proprietary Preparations** (details are given in Part 3)

***Arg.:*** Azopt; ***Austral.:*** Azopt; ***Austria:*** Azopt; ***Belg.:*** Azopt; ***Braz.:*** Azopt; ***Canad.:*** Azopt; ***Chile:*** Azopt; ***Denm.:*** Azopt; ***Fin.:*** Azopt; ***Fr.:*** Azopt; ***Ger.:*** Azopt; ***Gr.:*** Azopt; ***Hong Kong:*** Azopt; ***Irl.:*** Azopt; ***Israel:*** Azopt; ***Ital.:*** Azopt; ***Mex.:*** Azopt; ***Norw.:*** Azopt; ***Port.:*** Azopt; ***Singapore:*** Azopt; ***Spain:*** Azopt; ***Swed.:*** Azopt; ***Switz.:*** Azopt; ***Thai.:*** Azopt; ***UK:*** Azopt; ***USA:*** Azopt.

## Bucindolol Hydrochloride *(BANM, USAN, rINNM)*

Hidrocloruro de bucindolol; MJ-13105-1. 2-[2-Hydroxy-3-(2-indol-3-yl-1,1-dimethylethylamino)propoxy]benzonitrile hydrochloride.

$C_{22}H_{25}N_3O_2$,HCl = 399.9.

*CAS — 71119-11-4 (bucindolol); 70369-47-0 (bucindolol hydrochloride).*

### Profile

Bucindolol is a non-cardioselective beta blocker (p.868). It is reported to possess weak alpha$_1$-blocking activity and direct vasodilating activity; the degree of intrinsic sympathomimetic activity is unclear. Bucindolol, as the hydrochloride, has been investigated in the management of hypertension, heart failure, and other cardiac disorders, but development has been discontinued.

◊ References.


1. The Beta-Blocker Evaluation of Survival Trial Investigators. A trial of the beta-blocker bucindolol in patients with advanced chronic heart failure. *N Engl J Med* 2001; **344:** 1659–67.


## Buflomedil Hydrochloride *(BANM, rINNM)*

Buflomedili Hydrochloridum; Hidrocloruro de buflomedil; LL-1656. 2′,4′,6′-Trimethoxy-4-(pyrrolidin-1-yl)butyrophenone hydrochloride.

$C_{17}H_{25}NO_4$,HCl = 343.8.

*CAS — 55837-25-7 (buflomedil); 35543-24-9 (buflomedil hydrochloride).*

*ATC — C04AX20.*

**Pharmacopoeias.** In *Eur.* (see p.vi).

**Ph. Eur. 5.0** (Buflomedil Hydrochloride). A white or almost white microcrystalline powder. Freely soluble in water; soluble in alcohol; very slightly soluble in acetone. A 5% solution in water has a pH of 5.0 to 6.5.

### Adverse Effects

Buflomedil has been reported to cause gastrointestinal disturbances, headache, vertigo, syncope, rash, pruritus, and paraesthesia. Overdosage may produce severe hypotension, tachycardia, and convulsions.

◊ References.


1. Bachand RT, Dubourg AY. A review of long-term safety data with buflomedil. *J Int Med Res* 1990; **18:** 245–52.


### Pharmacokinetics

Buflomedil hydrochloride is absorbed from the gastrointestinal tract and peak plasma concentrations are reached 1.5 to 4 hours following oral administration. Buflomedil is subject to first-pass metabolism; bioavailability is reported to be between 50 and 80%.

Buflomedil is widely distributed. Binding to plasma proteins is dose-dependent and varies between 60 and 80% at therapeutic concentrations. Buflomedil is metabolised in the liver and is mainly excreted in the urine both as unchanged drug and metabolites. The elimination half-life is about 2 to 3 hours. Elimination may be impaired in patients with renal or hepatic impairment.

### Uses and Administration

Buflomedil hydrochloride is a vasodilator used in the treatment of cerebrovascular (p.820) and peripheral vascular disease (p.831). Usual doses by mouth are 300 to 600 mg daily, by intramuscular injection up to 100 mg daily, by slow intravenous injection up to 200 mg daily, and by intravenous infusion up to 400 mg daily. In patients with hepatic or renal impairment, doses may need to be reduced (see below).

◊ References.


1. Clissold SP, *et al.* Buflomedil: a review of its pharmacodynamic and pharmacokinetic properties, and therapeutic efficacy in peripheral and cerebral vascular diseases. *Drugs* 1987; **33:** 430–60.
2. De Backer TLM, *et al.* Buflomedil for intermittent claudication. Available in The Cochrane Library; Issue 2. Chichester: John Wiley; 2004.


**Administration in hepatic and renal impairment.** In patients with hepatic impairment, or renal impairment with creatinine clearance below 40 mL/minute, the maximum recommended oral dose is 150 mg twice daily.

### Preparations

**Proprietary Preparations** (details are given in Part 3)

***Arg.:*** Arteriol; Buflomed; Lofton; ***Austria:*** Buflohexal; Buflomed; Buftyl; Loftyl; ***Belg.:*** Loftyl; ***Braz.:*** Bufedil; ***Chile:*** Loftyl; Vaselastic; ***Fr.:*** Fonzylane; Loftyl; ***Ger.:*** Bufedil; Buflo; Buflo-POS; Buflo-Puren; Buflo-Reu†; Buflohexal; Defluina; ***Hong Kong:*** Fonzylane; Irrodan; ***Ital.:*** Bufene†; Buflan; Buflocit; Buflofar; Bufoxin†; Emoflux†; Flomed; Flupress†; Irrodan; Loftyl; Medil†; Perfudan; Pirxane; ***Mex.:*** Loftyl; ***Neth.:*** Loftyl; ***Port.:*** Loftyl; ***S.Afr.:*** Loftyl; ***Spain:*** Lofton; Sinoxis; ***Switz.:*** Loftyl; ***Thai.:*** Irrodan.

**Multi-ingredient:** ***Arg.:*** Mimixin.

## Bumetanide *(BAN, USAN, rINN)*

Bumetanida; Bumetanidum; Ro-10-6338. 3-Butylamino-4-phenoxy-5-sulphamoylbenzoic acid.

$C_{17}H_{20}N_2O_5S$ = 364.4.

*CAS — 28395-03-1.*

*ATC — C03CA02.*

**Pharmacopoeias.** In *Chin., Eur.* (see p.vi), *Jpn,* and *US.*

**Ph. Eur. 5.0** (Bumetanide). A white crystalline powder. It exhibits polymorphism. Practically insoluble in water; soluble in alcohol and in acetone; slightly soluble in dichloromethane. It dissolves in dilute solutions of alkali hydroxides. Protect from light.

**USP 27** (Bumetanide). A practically white powder. Slightly soluble in water; soluble in alkaline solutions. Store in airtight containers at a temperature of 25°, excursions permitted between 15° and 30°. Protect from light.

### Adverse Effects

As for Furosemide, p.919. Bumetanide may cause muscle pain, particularly at high doses.

**Effects on the ears.** Early reports suggested that bumetanide might be less ototoxic than furosemide.[1] However, both drugs can cause deafness, especially when given in large doses to patients with renal impairment.


1. Ward A, Heel RC. Bumetanide: a review of its pharmacodynamic and pharmacokinetic properties and therapeutic use. *Drugs* 1984; **28:** 426–64.


**Effects on the muscles.** Bumetanide, particularly in high doses in patients with chronic renal impairment, may cause severe musculoskeletal pain. A curious muscle stiffness distinct from cramp, with tenderness to compression and pain on movement, was noted in 4 patients with end-stage renal failure.[1] The calf muscles were the first to be affected; shoulder girdle and thigh muscle tenderness also occurred in 2 patients, and 1 patient also had neck stiffness. The adverse effect appeared to be dose-related for the individual patients.


1. Barclay JE, Lee HA. Clinical and pharmacokinetic studies on bumetanide in chronic renal failure. *Postgrad Med J* 1975; **51** (suppl 6): 43–6.


**Effects on the skin.** Bullous pemphigoid developed in a patient approximately 6 weeks after starting bumetanide.[1] Healing occurred after withdrawal without the need for corticosteroid treatment.


1. Boulinguez S, *et al.* Bullous pemphigoid induced by bumetanide. *Br J Dermatol* 1998; **138:** 548–9.


### Precautions

Bumetanide's precautions and contra-indications are generally dependent on its effects on fluid and electrolyte balance and are similar to those of the thiazide diuretics (see Hydrochlorothiazide, p.935).

### Interactions

As for Furosemide, p.920.

### Pharmacokinetics

Bumetanide is almost completely and fairly rapidly absorbed from the gastrointestinal tract; the bioavailability is reported to be about 80 to 95%. It has a plasma elimination half-life of about 1 to 2 hours. It is about 95% bound to plasma proteins. About 80% of the dose is excreted in the urine, approximately 50% as unchanged drug, and 10 to 20% in the faeces.

◊ References to the pharmacokinetics of bumetanide in healthy subjects.


1. Halladay SC, *et al.* Diuretic effect and metabolism of bumetanide in man. *Clin Pharmacol Ther* 1977; **22:** 179–87.
2. Pentikäinen PJ, *et al.* Fate of [$^{14}$C]-bumetanide in man. *Br J Clin Pharmacol* 1977; **4:** 39–44.
3. Holazo AA, *et al.* Pharmacokinetics of bumetanide following intravenous, intramuscular, and oral administrations to normal subjects. *J Pharm Sci* 1984; **73:** 1108–13.
4. Ward A, Heel RC. Bumetanide: a review of its pharmacodynamic and pharmacokinetic properties and therapeutic use. *Drugs* 1984; **28:** 426–64.
5. McCrindle JL, *et al.* Effect of food on the absorption of frusemide and bumetanide in man. *Br J Clin Pharmacol* 1996; **42:** 743–6.


**Hepatic impairment.** In a study of 8 patients with chronic hepatic disease,[1] the diuretic response to bumetanide 1 mg was impaired but bumetanide excretion rates were normal.


1. Marcantonio LA, *et al.* The pharmacokinetics and pharmacodynamics of the diuretic bumetanide in hepatic and renal disease. *Br J Clin Pharmacol* 1983; **15:** 245–52.


**Renal impairment.** Renal excretion of bumetanide has been shown to be reduced in patients with chronic renal impairment with a subsequent attenuation of diuretic effect.[1-3] The cumulative pharmacodynamic effects of oral and intravenous doses were essentially similar in patients with renal impairment and transition from intravenous to oral maintenance regimens should pose no special problems.[2]


1. Marcantonio LA, *et al.* The pharmacokinetics and pharmacodynamics of the diuretic bumetanide in hepatic and renal disease. *Br J Clin Pharmacol* 1983; **15:** 245–52.
2. Lau HSH, *et al.* Kinetics, dynamics, and bioavailability of bumetanide in healthy subjects and patients with chronic renal failure. *Clin Pharmacol Ther* 1986; **39:** 635–45.
3. Howlett MR, *et al.* Metabolism of the diuretic bumetanide in healthy subjects and patients with renal impairment. *Eur J Clin Pharmacol* 1990; **38:** 583–6.


### Uses and Administration

Although chemically unrelated, bumetanide is a loop diuretic with actions and uses similar to those of furosemide (p.921). Bumetanide is used in the treatment of oedema associated with heart failure (p.820) and with renal and hepatic disorders. It is given in high doses in the management of oliguria due to renal failure or insufficiency. Bumetanide has also been used in hypertension (p.825).

Diuresis starts within about 30 minutes to an hour after a dose by mouth, reaches a maximum at 1 to 2 hours, and lasts for about 4 hours but may be prolonged to 6 hours after high doses; after intravenous injection its effects are evident within a few minutes and last for about 2 hours. As a general guide bumetanide 1 mg produces a diuretic effect similar to furosemide 40 mg although this should not be used for direct substitution at higher doses.

In the treatment of **oedema** the usual dose is 1 mg by mouth in the morning or early evening; a second dose may be given 6 to 8 hours later if necessary. A dose of 500 micrograms daily may be adequate in some elderly patients.

In refractory oedema higher doses may be necessary. An initial dose of 5 mg daily has been advocated, increased by 5 mg every 12 to 24 hours as required; however other sources have suggested a maximum total dose of 10 mg daily. Twice daily dosing may be preferred at higher doses. For maintenance therapy doses may be given daily or intermittently. In an emergency or when oral therapy cannot be given 0.5 to 1 mg may be administered by intramuscular or slow intravenous injection, subsequently adjusted according to response. A dose for pulmonary oedema is 1 to 2 mg by intravenous injection, repeated 20 minutes later if necessary. Alternatively, 2 to 5 mg may be given over 30 to 60 minutes in 500 mL of a suitable infusion fluid.

In the treatment of **hypertension** bumetanide has been given in doses of 0.5 to 1 mg daily by mouth, although higher doses have been used.

When very high doses of bumetanide are used careful laboratory control is essential as described under the uses for furosemide (p.921; high-dose therapy).

### Preparations

***BP 2003:*** Bumetanide and Slow Potassium Tablets; Bumetanide Injection; Bumetanide Oral Solution; Bumetanide Tablets;
***USP 27:*** Bumetanide Injection; Bumetanide Tablets.

**Proprietary Preparations** (details are given in Part 3)
***Arg.:*** Butinat; ***Austral.:*** Burinex; ***Austria:*** Burinex; ***Belg.:*** Burinex; ***Braz.:*** Burinax; ***Canad.:*** Burinex; ***Denm.:*** Burinex; ***Fin.:*** Burinex†; ***Fr.:*** Burinex; ***Ger.:*** Burinex; ***Gr.:*** Burinex; ***Hong Kong:*** Burinex†; ***Irl.:*** Burinex; ***Ital.:*** Fontego†; ***Malaysia:*** Burinex; ***Mex.:*** Bumedyl; Drenural; Durin†; Miccil; ***Neth.:*** Burinex; ***Norw.:*** Burinex; ***NZ:*** Burinex; ***S.Afr.:*** Burinex; ***Singapore:*** Burinex; ***Spain:*** Farmadiuril†; Fordiuran; ***Swed.:*** Burinex; ***Switz.:*** Burinex; ***Thai.:*** Burinex; ***UK:*** Betinex†; Burinex; ***USA:*** Bumex.

**Multi-ingredient:** ***Denm.:*** Buram; Burinex med kaliumklorid; ***Hong Kong:*** Burinex K†; ***Irl.:*** Buram; Burinex K; ***Malaysia:*** Burinex K; ***Norw.:*** Burinex K; ***S.Afr.:*** Burinex K; ***Singapore:*** Burinex K; ***UK:*** Burinex A; Burinex K.

## Bunazosin Hydrochloride *(rINNM)*

E-643; Hidrocloruro de bunazosina. 1-(4-Amino-6,7-dimethoxy-2-quinazolinyl)-4-butyrylhexahydro-1*H*-1,4-diazepine monohydrochloride.

$C_{19}H_{27}N_5O_3,HCl = 409.9.$

*CAS — 80755-51-7 (bunazosin); 52712-76-2 (bunazosin hydrochloride).*

**Pharmacopoeias.** In *Jpn.*

### Profile

Bunazosin is an alpha$_1$-adrenoceptor blocker (p.809) with general properties similar to those of prazosin (p.985). It is given by mouth as the hydrochloride in the management of hypertension in doses of up to 9 mg daily.

### Preparations

**Proprietary Preparations** (details are given in Part 3)
***Ger.:*** Andante; ***Jpn:*** Detantol; ***Thai.:*** Detantol.

## Bunitrolol Hydrochloride *(rINNM)*

Hidrocloruro de bunitrolol; Ko-1366 (bunitrolol). 2-(3-*tert*-Butylamino-2-hydroxypropoxy)benzonitrile hydrochloride.

$C_{14}H_{20}N_2O_2,HCl = 284.8.$

*CAS — 34915-68-9 (bunitrolol); 23093-74-5 (bunitrolol hydrochloride).*

### Profile

Bunitrolol is a beta blocker (p.868). It has been given as the hydrochloride by mouth in the management of cardiovascular disorders.

## Bupranolol Hydrochloride *(rINNM)*

B-1312; Hidrocloruro de bupranolol; KL-255. 1-*tert*-Butylamino-3-(6-chloro-*m*-tolyloxy)propan-2-ol hydrochloride.

$C_{14}H_{22}ClNO_2,HCl = 308.2.$

*CAS — 14556-46-8 (bupranolol); 15148-80-8 (bupranolol hydrochloride).*

*ATC — C07AA19.*

**Pharmacopoeias.** In *Jpn.*

### Profile

Bupranolol is a beta blocker (p.868). It is given as the hydrochloride in usual doses of 100 to 400 mg daily by mouth in the management of cardiovascular disorders.

Bupranolol eye drops have been used in the management of glaucoma.

### Preparations

**Proprietary Preparations** (details are given in Part 3)
***Ger.:*** Betadrenol.

**Multi-ingredient:** ***Austria:*** Beta-Isoket†; Betamed.

## Butalamine Hydrochloride *(BANM, rINNM)*

Hidrocloruro de butalamina; LA-1221. *NN*-Dibutyl-*N'*-(3-phenyl-1,2,4-oxadiazol-5-yl)ethylenediamine hydrochloride.

$C_{18}H_{28}N_4O,HCl = 352.9.$

*CAS — 22131-35-7 (butalamine); 56974-46-0 (butalamine hydrochloride).*

*ATC — C04AX23.*

### Profile

Butalamine hydrochloride is a vasodilator that has been used in the management of peripheral and cerebral vascular disorders.

### Preparations

**Proprietary Preparations** (details are given in Part 3)
***Ger.:*** Adrevil†; ***Spain:*** Suremt†.

## Butizide *(rINN)*

Buthiazide *(USAN)*; Butizida; Isobutylhydrochlorothiazide; Thiabutazide. 6-Chloro-3,4-dihydro-3-isobutyl-2*H*-1,2,4-benzothiadiazine-7-sulphonamide 1,1-dioxide.

$C_{11}H_{16}ClN_3O_4S_2 = 353.8.$

*CAS — 2043-38-1.*

### Profile

Butizide is a thiazide diuretic with properties similar to those of hydrochlorothiazide (p.933). It is used for oedema, including that associated with heart failure (p.820), and for hypertension (p.825).

Butizide has been given by mouth in maintenance doses of 5 to 10 mg daily, with other diuretics, for the treatment of oedema. It has also been given in doses of 2.5 to 7.5 mg daily for hypertension, with other antihypertensive drugs.

### Preparations

**Proprietary Preparations** (details are given in Part 3)
***Austria:*** Saltucin†; ***Ger.:*** Saltucin†.

**Multi-ingredient:** ***Austria:*** Aldactone Saltucin; Buti-Spirobene; Suprenoat†; Torrat†; ***Ger.:*** Aldactone Saltucin; Modenol; Torrat; Tri-Torrat; ***Hong Kong:*** Iso Triraupin†; Torrat; ***Ital.:*** Kadiur; Saludopin; ***Mex.:*** Aldazida; ***S.Afr.:*** Aldazide; ***Switz.:*** Aldozone; Sali-Spiroctan†; ***Thai.:*** Iso-Triraupin.

## Cadralazine *(BAN, rINN)*

Cadralazina; CGP-18684/E; ISF-2469. Ethyl 3-{6-[ethyl(2-hydroxypropyl)amino]pyridazin-3-yl}carbazate.

$C_{12}H_{21}N_5O_3 = 283.3.$

*CAS — 64241-34-5.*

*ATC — C02DB04.*

### Profile

Cadralazine is a vasodilator with actions and uses similar to those of hydralazine (p.931). It has been given in doses of 10 mg once daily by mouth in the management of hypertension (p.825).

◊ Reviews.

1. McTavish D, *et al.* Cadralazine: a review of its pharmacodynamic and pharmacokinetic properties, and therapeutic potential in the treatment of hypertension. *Drugs* 1990; **40:** 543–60.

◊ Unlike hydralazine, cadralazine is reported not to produce a lupus-like syndrome.[1,2]

1. Andersson OK. Cadralazine did not produce the SLE-syndrome when hydralazine did. *Eur J Clin Pharmacol* 1987; **31:** 741.
2. Mulder H. Conversion of drug-induced SLE-syndrome by the vasodilating agent cadralazine. *Eur J Clin Pharmacol* 1990; **38:** 303.

### Preparations

**Proprietary Preparations** (details are given in Part 3)
***Ital.:*** Cadraten; Cadrilan†.

## Cafedrine Hydrochloride *(BANM, pINNM)*

H-8351; Hidrocloruro de cafedrina; Kafedrin Hydrochloride. 7-[2-(β-Hydroxy-α-methylphenethylamino)ethyl]theophylline hydrochloride.

$C_{18}H_{23}N_5O_3,HCl = 393.9.$

*CAS — 58166-83-9 (cafedrine); 3039-97-2 (cafedrine hydrochloride).*

*ATC — C01CA21.*

### Profile

Cafedrine hydrochloride is a derivative of theophylline (p.798), used mainly in preparations with theodrenaline hydrochloride in the treatment of hypotensive states.

### Preparations

**Proprietary Preparations** (details are given in Part 3)

**Multi-ingredient:** ***Austria:*** Akrinor; ***Fr.:*** Praxinor; ***Ger.:*** Akrinor; ***S.Afr.:*** Akrinor; ***Spain:*** Bifort; ***Switz.:*** Akrinor†.

## Calcitonin Gene-related Peptide

CGRP; Péptido relacionado con el gen de la calcitonina.

### Profile

Calcitonin gene-related peptide is an endogenous peptide derived from the calcitonin gene. It has vasodilating activity and has been investigated in the management of peripheral vascular disease (Raynaud's syndrome), heart failure, and for ischaemia following neurosurgery for subarachnoid haemorrhage.

◊ References.

1. Johnston FG, *et al.* Effect of calcitonin-gene-related peptide on postoperative neurological deficits after subarachnoid haemorrhage. *Lancet* 1990; **335:** 869–72.
2. Shawkett S, *et al.* Prolonged effect of CGRP in Raynaud's patients: a double-blind randomised comparison with prostacyclin. *Br J Clin Pharmacol* 1991; **32:** 209–13.
3. Shekhar YC, *et al.* Effects of prolonged infusion of human alpha calcitonin gene-related peptide on haemodynamics, renal blood flow and hormone levels in congestive heart failure. *Am J Cardiol* 1991; **67:** 732–6.
4. European CGRP in Subarachnoid Haemorrhage Study Group. Effect of calcitonin-gene-related peptide in patients with delayed postoperative cerebral ischaemia after aneurysmal subarachnoid haemorrhage. *Lancet* 1992; **339:** 831–4.
5. Bunker CB, *et al.* Calcitonin gene-related peptide in treatment of severe peripheral vascular insufficiency in Raynaud's phenomenon. *Lancet* 1993; **342:** 80–2.
6. Feuerstein G, *et al.* Clinical perspectives of calcitonin gene related peptide pharmacology. *Can J Physiol Pharmacol* 1995; **73:** 1070–4.
7. Gherardini G, *et al.* Venous ulcers: improved healing by iontophoretic administration of calcitonin gene-related peptide and vasoactive intestinal peptide. *Plast Reconstr Surg* 1998; **101:** 90–3.

# Candesartan Cilexetil *(BANM, USAN, rINNM)*

Candesartán cilexetilo; CV-11974 (candesartan); H-212/91; TCV-116. Cyclohexyl carbonate ester of (±)-1-hydroxyethyl 2-ethoxy-1-[*p*-(*o*-1*H*-tetrazol-5-ylphenyl)benzyl]-7-benzimidazole-carboxylate.

$C_{33}H_{34}N_6O_6 = 610.7.$

*CAS — 139481-59-7 (candesartan); 145040-37-5 (candesartan cilexetil).*

*ATC — C09CA06.*

### Adverse Effects and Precautions

As for Losartan Potassium, p.947.

### Interactions

As for Losartan Potassium, p.948.

### Pharmacokinetics

Candesartan cilexetil is an ester prodrug that is hydrolysed during absorption from the gastrointestinal tract to the active form candesartan. The absolute bioavailability for candesartan is about 40% after administration of candesartan cilexetil as a solution and about 14% after administration as tablets. Peak plasma concentrations of candesartan occur about 3 to 4 hours after oral administration of tablets. Candesartan is more than 99% bound to plasma proteins. It is excreted in urine and bile mainly as unchanged drug and a small amount of inactive metabolites. The terminal elimination half-life is about 9 hours. Candesartan is not removed by haemodialysis.

◊ Reviews.

1. Gleiter CH, Mörike KE. Clinical pharmacokinetics of candesartan. *Clin Pharmacokinet* 2002; **41:** 7–17.

### Uses and Administration

Candesartan is an angiotensin II receptor antagonist with actions similar to those of losartan (p.948). It is used in the management of hypertension (p.825) and has also been investigated in heart failure.

Candesartan is administered by mouth as the ester prodrug candesartan cilexetil. Onset of its antihypertensive effect occurs about 2 hours after administration and the maximum effect is achieved within about 4 weeks after initiating therapy.

In the management of hypertension candesartan cilexetil is given in the UK in an initial dose of 8 mg once daily, adjusted according to response. The usual maintenance dose is 8 mg once daily with a maximum dose of 16 mg once daily. In the USA higher doses are used; the usual initial dose is 16 mg once daily with a maintenance dose of 8 to 32 mg daily as a single dose or in two divided doses. Lower initial doses should be considered in patients with intravascular volume depletion; in the UK an initial dose of 4 mg once daily is suggested. Patients with renal or hepatic impairment may also require lower initial doses (see below).

◊ Reviews.


1. Sever P, Ménard J, eds. Angiotensin II antagonism refined: candesartan cilexetil. *J Hum Hypertens* 1997; **11** (suppl 2): S1–S95.
2. McClellan KJ, Goa KL. Candesartan cilexetil: a review of its use in essential hypertension. *Drugs* 1998; **56:** 847–69.
3. Stoukides CA, *et al.* Candesartan cilexetil: an angiotensin II receptor blocker. *Ann Pharmacother* 1999; **33:** 1287–98.
4. See S, Stirling AL. Candesartan cilexetil: an angiotensin II-receptor blocker. *Am J Health-Syst Pharm* 2000; **57:** 739–46.
5. Easthope SE, Jarvis B. Candesartan cilexetil: an update of its use in essential hypertension. *Drugs* 2002; **62:** 1253–87.


**Administration in hepatic or renal impairment.** The dose of candesartan should be reduced in patients with hepatic impairment; in the UK candesartan is contra-indicated in severe hepatic impairment and an initial dose of 2 mg once daily is recommended in mild to moderate impairment.

Dosage reduction may also be considered in patients with renal impairment. In the UK an initial dose of 4 mg once daily is recommended, including for patients on haemodialysis; in the USA it is not considered necessary to reduce the initial dose in mild renal impairment.

## Preparations

**Proprietary Preparations** (details are given in Part 3)
***Arg.:*** Atacand; Dacten; Tiadyl; ***Austral.:*** Atacand; ***Austria:*** Atacand; Blopress; ***Belg.:*** Atacand; ***Braz.:*** Atacand; Blopress; ***Canad.:*** Atacand; ***Chile:*** Atacand; Bilaten; Blopress; Blox; ***Denm.:*** Atacand; ***Fin.:*** Atacand; ***Fr.:*** Atacand; Kenzen; ***Ger.:*** Atacand; Blopress; ***Gr.:*** Atacand; ***Hong Kong:*** Blopress; ***India:*** Candesar; ***Irl.:*** Atacand; ***Israel:*** Atacand; ***Ital.:*** Blopress; Ratacand; ***Jpn:*** Blopress; ***Malaysia:*** Atacand; Blopress; ***Mex.:*** Atacand; Blopress; ***Neth.:*** Atacand; ***Norw.:*** Atacand; ***NZ:*** Atacand; ***Port.:*** Atacand; Blopress; ***S.Afr.:*** Atacand; ***Singapore:*** Atacand; ***Spain:*** Atacand; Parapres; ***Swed.:*** Atacand; ***Switz.:*** Atacand; Blopress; ***Thai.:*** Blopress; ***UK:*** Amias; ***USA:*** Atacand.

**Multi-ingredient:** ***Arg.:*** Atacand-D; Tiadyl Plus; ***Austral.:*** Atacand Plus; ***Austria:*** Atacand Plus; Blopress Plus; ***Belg.:*** Atacand Plus; ***Braz.:*** Atacand HCT; ***Chile:*** Blopress D; Blox-D; ***Denm.:*** AtacandZid; Atazid; ***Fin.:*** Atacand Plus; ***Fr.:*** Cokenzen; Hytacand; ***Ger.:*** Atacand Plus; Blopress Plus; ***Irl.:*** Atacand Plus; ***Israel:*** Atacand Plus; ***Ital.:*** Blopresid; Ratacand Plus; ***Neth.:*** Atacand Plus; ***Norw.:*** Atacand Plus; ***Port.:*** Blopress 16 mg + 12,5 mg; Hytacand; ***S.Afr.:*** Atacand Plus; ***Singapore:*** Atacand Plus; ***Spain:*** Atacand Plus; Parapres Plus; ***Swed.:*** Atacand Plus; ***Switz.:*** Atacand Plus; Blopress Plus; ***Thai.:*** Blopress Plus; ***USA:*** Atacand HCT.

---

## Candoxatril *(BAN, USAN, rINN)*

Candoxatrilo; UK-79300. *cis*-4-{1-[(*S*)-2-(Indan-5-yloxycarbonyl)-3-(2-methoxyethoxy)propyl]cyclopentylcarbonylamino}cyclohexanecarboxylic acid.

$C_{29}H_{41}NO_7$ = 515.6.

*CAS — 118785-03-8; 123122-55-4.*

### Profile

Candoxatril is an ester prodrug that is hydrolysed in the body after oral administration to its active form candoxatrilat (UK-69578). Candoxatrilat is a neutral endopeptidase (neutral metalloendopeptidase) inhibitor. It is a potent inhibitor of the endopeptidase responsible for the metabolism of atrial natriuretic peptide (ANP) (p.964); inhibition of this enzyme results in raised ANP concentrations with consequent natriuresis and suppression of the renin-angiotensin-aldosterone system. Candoxatril has been studied in the management of hypertension and heart failure.

◊ References.


1. Newby DE, *et al.* Candoxatril improves exercise capacity in patients with chronic heart failure receiving angiotensin converting enzyme inhibition. *Eur Heart J* 1998; **19:** 1808–13.
2. Westheim AS, *et al.* Hemodynamic and neuroendocrine effects for candoxatril and frusemide in mild stable chronic heart failure. *J Am Coll Cardiol* 1999; **34:** 1794–1801.
3. Northridge DB, *et al.* Comparison of the short-term effects of candoxatril, an orally active neutral endopeptidase inhibitor, and frusemide in the treatment of patients with chronic heart failure. *Am Heart J* 1999; **138:** 1149–57.


---

## Canrenone *(USAN, pINN)*

Canrenona; SC-9376. 17-Hydroxy-3-oxo-17α-pregna-4,6-diene-21-carboxylic acid γ-lactone.

$C_{22}H_{28}O_3$ = 340.5.

*CAS — 976-71-6.*

*ATC — C03DA03.*

### Profile

Canrenone is a potassium-sparing diuretic with properties similar to those of spironolactone (p.1003) and is used in the treatment of refractory oedema associated with heart failure (p.820), renal, or hepatic disease, and in hypertension (p.825). It is a metabolite of both spironolactone and potassium canrenoate (p.984). It is given in usual doses of 50 to 200 mg daily by mouth. Doses of up to 300 mg daily may be required in some patients.

### Preparations

**Proprietary Preparations** (details are given in Part 3)
***Belg.:*** Contaren; ***Ital.:*** Luvion.

---

## Captopril *(BAN, USAN, rINN)*

Captoprilum; SQ-14225. 1-[(2*S*)-3-Mercapto-2-methylpropionyl]-L-proline.

$C_9H_{15}NO_3S$ = 217.3.

*CAS — 62571-86-2.*

*ATC — C09AA01.*

NOTE. Compounded preparations of captopril may be represented by the following names:

- Co-zidocapt (*BAN*)—captopril 2 parts and hydrochlorothiazide 1 part (w/w).

**Pharmacopoeias.** In *Chin., Eur.* (see p.vi), *Int., Jpn*, and *US.*

**Ph. Eur. 5.0** (Captopril). A white or almost white crystalline powder. Freely soluble in water, in dichloromethane, and in methyl alcohol. It dissolves in dilute solutions of alkali hydroxides. A 2% solution in water has a pH of 2.0 to 2.6. Store in airtight containers.

**USP 27** (Captopril). A white or off-white crystalline powder which may have a characteristic sulfide-like odour. Freely soluble in water, in alcohol, in chloroform, and in methyl alcohol. Store in airtight containers.

**Stability.** Although captopril itself is relatively stable[1] at temperatures up to 50°, and extemporaneously prepared powders (made by triturating the tablets with lactose) have been reported to be stable for at least 12 weeks at room temperature,[2] aqueous solutions are subject to oxidative degradation, mainly to captopril disulfide,[1] which increases[3] with increase in pH above 4. The manufacturers report that a liquid form of captopril prepared from pulverised tablets in distilled water containing 1 mg/mL retained 96.6% of the original concentration of drug after storage at room temperature for 5 days, but they advise that since it contains no preservative it should be used within 2 days of preparation.[4] Others have reported wide variations in stability depending upon the formulation. In one study[5] the shelf-life of a solution of captopril 1 mg/mL prepared from crushed tablets and tap water was estimated to be 27 days when stored at 5°. However, in another study[6] captopril was much less stable; in sterile water for irrigation captopril was stable for at least 3 days when stored at 5°, but in tap water it disappeared at a much faster rate. Increased stability has been reported following the addition of sodium ascorbate to the solution,[7] and with captopril powder rather than crushed tablets.[8] A 1 mg/mL preparation made with crushed tablets and undiluted syrup has also been reported to be stable for 30 days at 5° and may be more palatable than aqueous formulations.[9]


1. Lund W, Cowe HJ. Stability of dry powder formulations. *Pharm J* 1986; **237:** 179–80.
2. Taketomo CK, *et al.* Stability of captopril in powder papers under three storage conditions. *Am J Hosp Pharm* 1990; **47:** 1799–1801.
3. Timmins P, *et al.* Factors affecting captopril stability in aqueous solution. *Int J Pharmaceutics* 1982; **11:** 329–36.
4. Andrews CD, Essex A. Captopril suspension. *Pharm J* 1986; **237:** 734–5.
5. Pereira CM, Tam YK. Stability of captopril in tap water. *Am J Hosp Pharm* 1992; **49:** 612–15.
6. Anaizi NH, Swenson C. Instability of aqueous captopril solutions. *Am J Hosp Pharm* 1993; **50:** 486–8.
7. Nahata MC, *et al.* Stability of captopril in three liquid dosage forms. *Am J Hosp Pharm* 1994; **51:** 95–6.
8. Chan DS, *et al.* Degradation of captopril in solutions compounded from tablets and standard powder. *Am J Hosp Pharm* 1994; **51:** 1205–7.
9. Lye MYF, *et al.* Effects of ingredients on stability of captopril in extemporaneously prepared oral liquids. *Am J Health-Syst Pharm* 1997; **54:** 2483–7.


### Adverse Effects, Treatment, and Precautions

As for ACE inhibitors, p.842.

Captopril has been reported to cause false positive results in tests for acetone in urine.

**Incidence of adverse effects.** Results of postmarketing surveillance[1] in 30 515 hypertensive patients receiving captopril showed that 4.9% had their therapy discontinued because of adverse effects thought to be due to the drug. The mean initial daily dose was 46 mg; at final evaluation the mean daily dose was 58 mg. The adverse effect most commonly reported was headache (in 1.8%); others included dizziness (1.6%), rashes (1.1%), nausea (1.0%), taste disturbances (0.9%), and cough (0.8%). This study excluded patients with renal impairment but an earlier survey[2] in 6737 patients who received captopril alone or in combination found that rash and dysgeusia were more frequent in patients with renal impairment (occurring in 6.2% and 3.2% respectively of those receiving 150 mg daily or less of captopril) than in those with normal serum creatinine (4.3% and 2.2%). The frequency of both symptoms was somewhat higher in those given higher doses. Symptoms of hypotension occurred in about 5% of patients and were not influenced by dose or renal function. The cumulative frequency of withdrawal due to adverse effects was estimated at 5.8% in this study, which is similar to that in the larger survey. In another postmarketing surveillance study[3] involving more than 60 000 patients, captopril was withdrawn in 8.9% because of adverse effects.

For further reference to some of these adverse effects, see under ACE Inhibitors, p.842.


1. Schoenberger JA, *et al.* Efficacy, safety, and quality-of-life assessment of captopril antihypertensive therapy in clinical practice. *Arch Intern Med* 1990; **150:** 301–6.
2. Jenkins AC, *et al.* Captopril in hypertension: seven years later. *J Cardiovasc Pharmacol* 1985; **7** (suppl 1): S96–S101.
3. Chalmers D, *et al.* Postmarketing surveillance of captopril for hypertension. *Br J Clin Pharmacol* 1992; **34:** 215–23.


**Breast feeding.** Captopril is distributed into breast milk and the manufacturers advise that breast feeding should be avoided. However, a study[1] in 12 lactating women found that the concentration of captopril in breast milk was about 1% of maternal blood concentrations, suggesting that the amount ingested by the infant would be very low. No adverse effects were noted in the infants in this study, and the American Academy of Pediatrics considers[2] that captopril is therefore usually compatible with breast feeding.


1. Devlin RG, Fleiss PM. Captopril in human blood and breast milk. *J Clin Pharmacol* 1981; **21:** 110–113.
2. American Academy of Pediatrics. The transfer of drugs and other chemicals into human milk. *Pediatrics* 2001; **108:** 776–89. Correction. *ibid.*; 1029. Also available at: http://aappolicy.aappublications.org/cgi/content/full/pediatrics%3b108/3/776 (accessed 05/07/04)


**Porphyria.** Captopril is considered to be unsafe in patients with porphyria because it has been shown to be porphyrinogenic in *in-vitro* systems.

### Interactions

As for ACE inhibitors, p.845.

### Pharmacokinetics

About 60 to 75% of a dose of captopril is absorbed from the gastrointestinal tract and peak plasma concentrations are achieved within about an hour. Absorption has been reported to be reduced in the presence of food, but this may not be clinically relevant (see below). Captopril is about 30% bound to plasma proteins. It crosses the placenta and is found in breast milk at about 1% of maternal blood concentrations. It is largely excreted in the urine, 40 to 50% as unchanged drug, the rest as disulfide and other metabolites. The elimination half-life has been reported to be 2 to 3 hours but this is increased in renal impairment. Captopril is removed by haemodialysis.

◊ Reviews.


1. Duchin KL, *et al.* Pharmacokinetics of captopril in healthy subjects and in patients with cardiovascular diseases. *Clin Pharmacokinet* 1988; **14:** 241–59.


**Absorption.** The bioavailability and peak plasma concentrations of captopril have been shown to be reduced by 25 to 55% on administration with food in single dose studies[1-4] and with chronic dosing.[5] However, this may not be clinically significant since several studies[3,4,6] indicated that food intake had no effect on the antihypertensive activity of captopril.


1. Williams GM, Sugerman AA. The effect of a meal, at various times relative to drug administration, on the bioavailability of captopril. *J Clin Pharmacol* 1982; **22:** 18A.
2. Singhvi SM, *et al.* Effect of food on the bioavailability of captopril in healthy subjects. *J Clin Pharmacol* 1982; **22:** 135–40.
3. Mäntylä R, *et al.* Impairment of captopril bioavailability by concomitant food and antacid intake. *Int J Clin Pharmacol Ther Toxicol* 1984; **22:** 626–9.
4. Müller HM, *et al.* The influence of food intake on pharmacodynamics and plasma concentration of captopril. *J Hypertens* 1985; **3** (suppl 2): S135–6.
5. Öhman KP, *et al.* Pharmacokinetics of captopril and its effects on blood pressure during acute and chronic administration and in relation to food intake. *J Cardiovasc Pharmacol* 1985; **7** (suppl 1): S20–4.
6. Izumi Y, *et al.* Influence of food on the clinical effect of angiotensin I converting enzyme inhibitor (SQ 14225). *Tohoku J Exp Med* 1983; **139:** 279–86.


**Renal impairment.** A study of 9 patients with chronic renal failure undergoing dialysis found that peak plasma concentrations of captopril were 2.5 times higher and peak concentrations of the disulfide metabolites were 4 times higher than in patients with normal renal function following a single dose of captopril.[1] Peak concentrations occurred later in uraemic patients and the apparent half-life of total captopril was 46 hours in uraemic patients compared with 2.95 hours in patients with normal renal function.


1. Drummer OH, *et al.* The pharmacokinetics of captopril and captopril disulfide conjugates in uraemic patients on maintenance dialysis: comparison with patients with normal renal function. *Eur J Clin Pharmacol* 1987; **32:** 267–71.


### Uses and Administration

Captopril is a sulfhydryl-containing ACE inhibitor (p.842). It is used in the management of hypertension (p.825), in heart failure (p.820), following myocardial infarction (p.828), and in diabetic nephropathy (see Kidney Disorders, p.847).

Following oral administration captopril produces a maximum effect within 1 to 2 hours, although the full effect may not develop for several weeks during chronic dosing. The duration of action is dose-dependent and may persist for 6 to 12 hours.

In the treatment of **hypertension** the initial dose is 12.5 mg twice daily by mouth, increased gradually at intervals of 2 to 4 weeks according to the response. Since there may be a precipitous fall in blood pressure in some patients when starting therapy with an ACE inhibitor, the first dose should preferably be given at bedtime. An initial dose of 6.25 mg twice daily is recommended if captopril is given in addition to a *diuretic* or to elderly patients; if possible the diuretic should be stopped 2 or 3 days before introducing captopril. The usual maintenance dose is 25 to 50 mg twice daily and should not normally exceed 50 mg three times daily. If hypertension is not satisfactorily controlled at this dosage, addition of a second drug or substitution of an alternative drug should be considered. In the USA higher doses of up to 150 mg three times daily have been suggested for patients with hypertension uncontrolled by lower doses of captopril in conjunction with diuretic therapy.

In the treatment of **heart failure** severe first-dose hypotension on introduction of an ACE inhibitor is common in patients on loop diuretics, but their temporary withdrawal may cause rebound pulmonary oedema. Thus an initial dose of 6.25 to 12.5 mg of captopril is given by mouth under close medical supervision; the usual maintenance dose is 25 mg two or three times daily, and doses should not normally exceed 50 mg three times daily. Again, in the USA higher doses of up to 150 mg three times daily have been suggested.

Following **myocardial infarction**, captopril is used prophylactically in clinically stable patients with symptomatic or asymptomatic left ventricular dysfunction to improve survival, delay the onset of symptomatic heart failure, and reduce recurrent infarction. It may be started 3 days after myocardial infarction in an initial dose of 6.25 mg by mouth, increased over several weeks to 150 mg daily in divided doses if tolerated.

In **diabetic nephropathy** (microalbuminuria greater than 30 mg/day) in type 1 diabetics, 75 to 100 mg of captopril may be given daily, in divided doses, by mouth. Other antihypertensives may be used with captopril if a further reduction in blood pressure is required.

Doses may need to be reduced in patients with renal impairment (see below).

**Administration.** Captopril is generally given orally. Sublingual[1] and intravenous[2,3] administration has also been tried, but these routes are not established.

1. Angeli P, *et al.* Comparison of sublingual captopril and nifedipine in immediate treatment of hypertensive emergencies: a randomized, single-blind clinical trial. *Arch Intern Med* 1991; **151:** 678–82.
2. Savi L, *et al.* A new therapy for hypertensive emergencies: intravenous captopril. *Curr Ther Res* 1990; **47:** 1073–81.
3. Langes K, *et al.* Efficacy and safety of intravenous captopril in congestive heart failure. *Curr Ther Res* 1993; **53:** 167–76.

**Administration in children.** Experience with captopril in children is limited. The UK manufacturers have suggested an initial dose of 0.3 mg/kg increased as necessary to a maximum of 6 mg/kg daily given in two or three divided doses. They do not recommend captopril for the treatment of mild to moderate hypertension in children.

Captopril, given in an initial dose of 0.25 mg/kg daily, increased to up to 2.5 or 3.5 mg/kg daily in 3 divided doses has also been reported to produce benefit in infants with severe heart failure secondary to congenital defects (predominantly manifesting as left-to-right shunt).[1,2]

1. Scammell AM, *et al.* Captopril in treatment of infant heart failure: a preliminary report. *Int J Cardiol* 1987; **16:** 295–301.
2. Shaw NJ, *et al.* Captopril in heart failure secondary to a left to right shunt. *Arch Dis Child* 1988; **63:** 360–3.

**Administration in renal impairment.** The dose of captopril should be reduced or the dosage interval increased in patients with renal impairment, depending on their creatinine clearance (CC). The following doses have been suggested:

- CC 21 to 40 mL/minute: initial daily dose 25 mg and maximum daily dose 100 mg
- CC 10 to 20 mL/minute: initial daily dose 12.5 mg and maximum daily dose 75 mg
- CC below 10 mL/minute: initial daily dose 6.25 mg and maximum daily dose 37.5 mg

If a diuretic also needs to be given, a loop diuretic should be chosen rather than a thiazide.

**Nitrate tolerance.** For reference to the use of captopril as a sulfhydryl donor in the management of nitrate tolerance, see under Precautions for Glyceryl Trinitrate, p.924.

## Preparations

***BP 2003:*** Captopril Tablets;
***USP 27:*** Captopril and Hydrochlorothiazide Tablets; Captopril Tablets.

**Proprietary Preparations** (details are given in Part 3)
***Arg.:*** Antasten; ***Austral.:*** Acenorm; Capace†; Capoten; Captohexal; Enzace; Topace; ***Austria:*** Capace; Captomed; Captor; Captotyrol; Debax; Lopirin; ***Belg.:*** Capoten; ***Braz.:*** Aorten†; Capoten; Capotril; Capril; Captil; Captomed; Capton; Captopiril; Captotec; Captrizin; Catoprol; Ductopril; Hipocatril†; Hipoten; Normapril; Pressomax; Prilpressin; Venopril; ***Canad.:*** Apo-Capto; Capoten; Captril†; Novo-Captoril; Nu-Capto; ***Chile:*** Capoten; Properil; ***Denm.:*** Capoten; Captodan; Captol; Catonet; ***Fin.:*** Capoten; Captomin; Captostad; Lopril; ***Fr.:*** Captirex†; Captolane; Lopril; Oltens†; ***Ger.:*** ACE-Hemmer; Acenorm; Adocor; Capto; Capto-dura Cor†; Capto-dura M; Captobeta; Captodoc; Captoflux; Captogamma; Captohexal; Captomerck; Captoreal†; Cardiagen; cor tensobon; Coronorm; Epicordin; Esparil†; Lopirin; Mundil; Phamopril; Sansanal†; Sigacap Cor; Tensiomin; Tensiomin-Cor; Tensobon; Tensostad; ***Gr.:*** Capoten; Hypotensor; Neo-Ipertas; Normolose; Odupril; Pertacilon; Sancap; ***Hong Kong:*** Apo-Capto; Capocard; Capoten; Capril; Dexacap; Epsitron; Kimafan; Novo-Captoril; Rilcapton; Ropril; Tensiomin; ***India:*** Aceten; ***Irl.:*** Aceomel; Actopril; Capoten; Captor; Geroten; Tensopril; ***Israel:*** Aceril; Apocapen†; Capti; Inhibace; ***Ital.:*** Acepress; Aceprilex; Capoten; Merapril; Tenpril; ***Malaysia:*** Apo-Capto; Apuzin; Capoten; ***Mex.:*** Atrisol; Biodezil; Bugazon; Capotena; Captoser; Captral; Cardipril; Catona; Cryopril; Ecapresan; Ecapril†; Ecaten; Hipertex; Kenapril†; Kenolan; Keyerpril; Lenpryl; Lowpre†; Midrat; Novapres; Reductel; Romir; Toprilem; Tropisol†; ***Neth.:*** Capoten; ***Norw.:*** Capoten; ***NZ:*** Capoten; Captohexal; ***Port.:*** Calpix; Capoten; Carencil; Convertal; Hipertil; Hipotensil; Mereprine; Prilovase; Tensopril; Vidapril; ***S.Afr.:*** Aceten; Capace; Capoten; Captohexal; Captomax; Cardiace; Zapto; ***Singapore:*** Apo-Capto; Capoten; Catoplin; Katopril†; Ketanine; Pertacilon; Rilcapton†; Tensoprel; ***Spain:*** Alopresin; Capoten; Captosina; Cesplon; Dardex; Dilabar; Garanil; Tensoprel; ***Swed.:*** Capoten; ***Switz.:*** capto-basan; Captosol; Lopirin; Tensobon†; ***Thai.:*** Capoten; Epsitron; Gemzil; Tensiomin; ***UK:*** Acepril; Capoten; Ecopace; Hyteneze†; Kaplon; Tensopril; ***USA:*** Capoten.

**Multi-ingredient:** ***Austria:*** Capozide; Captocomp; Captoplus; Captopril Compositum; Co-Captopril; Veracapt; ***Braz.:*** Captotec + HCT; Hidropril; Lopril; ***Denm.:*** Capozid; ***Fr.:*** Captea; Ecazide; ***Ger.:*** ACE-Hemmer comp; Acenorm HCT; Adocomp; Capozide; Capto Comp; Capto Plus; Captobeta Comp; Captodoc Comp; Captogamma HCT; Captohexal Comp; Captopril Comp; Captopril HCT; Captopril Plus; Cardiagen HCT; Tensobon comp; ***Irl.:*** Capozide; Captor-HCT; Half Capozide; ***Ital.:*** Acediur; Aceplus; ***Mex.:*** Capozide; Co-Captral; ***Neth.:*** Aceplus†; Capozide; ***NZ:*** Capozide†; ***Port.:*** Lopiretic; Normotil; ***S.Afr.:*** Capozide; Captoretic; Zapto Co; ***Spain:*** Alopresin Diu; Cesplon Plus; Decresco; Dilabar Diu; Ecadiu; Ecazide; ***Swed.:*** Capozid†; ***Switz.:*** Capozide; Captosol comp; Tensobon comp; ***UK:*** Acezide; Capozide; Capto-Co; ***USA:*** Capozide.

---

## Carazolol *(BAN, rINN)*

BM-51052. 1-(Carbazol-4-yloxy)-3-isopropylaminopropan-2-ol.
$C_{18}H_{22}N_2O_2$ = 298.4.
*CAS — 57775-29-8.*

### Profile

Carazolol is a beta blocker (p.868). It is given in doses of 5 to 15 mg daily by mouth in the management of various cardiovascular disorders.

### Preparations

**Proprietary Preparations** (details are given in Part 3)
***Austria:*** Conducton; ***Ger.:*** Conducton.

---

## Carbocromen Hydrochloride *(rINNM)*

A-27053; AG-3; Cassella-4489; Chromonar Hydrochloride *(USAN)*; Hidrocloruro de carbocromeno; NSC-110430. Ethyl 3-(2-diethylaminoethyl)-4-methylcoumarin-7-yloxyacetate hydrochloride.
$C_{20}H_{27}NO_5,HCl$ = 397.9.
*CAS — 804-10-4 (carbocromen); 655-35-6 (carbocromen hydrochloride).*
*ATC — C01DX05.*

### Profile

Carbocromen hydrochloride is a vasodilator that has been used in ischaemic heart disease.

### Preparations

**Proprietary Preparations** (details are given in Part 3)
***Ger.:*** Intensain†; ***Ital.:*** Cardiocap†.

---

## Carperitide *(rINN)*

Carperitida.
*CAS — 89213-87-6.*

### Profile

Carperitide is a recombinant atrial natriuretic peptide (see p.964) used in the management of acute heart failure.

### Preparations

**Proprietary Preparations** (details are given in Part 3)
***Jpn:*** Hanp.

---

# Carteolol Hydrochloride

*(BANM, USAN, rINNM)*

Abbott-43326; Carteololi Hydrochloridum; Hidrocloruro de carteolol; OPC-1085. 5-(3-*tert*-Butylamino-2-hydroxypropoxy)-3,4-dihydroquinolin-2(1*H*)-one hydrochloride.
$C_{16}H_{24}N_2O_3,HCl$ = 328.8.
*CAS — 51781-06-7 (carteolol); 51781-21-6 (carteolol hydrochloride).*
*ATC — C07AA15; S01ED05.*

**Pharmacopoeias.** In *Chin., Eur.* (see p.vi), *Jpn,* and *US.*

**Ph. Eur. 5.0** (Carteolol Hydrochloride). White crystals or crystalline powder. Soluble in water; slightly soluble in alcohol; practically insoluble in dichloromethane; sparingly soluble in methyl alcohol. A 1% solution in water has a pH of 5.0 to 6.0. Store in airtight containers.

**USP 27** (Carteolol Hydrochloride). pH of a 1% solution in water is between 5.0 and 6.0.

## Adverse Effects, Treatment, and Precautions

As for Beta Blockers, p.869.

## Interactions

The interactions associated with beta blockers are discussed on p.870.

## Pharmacokinetics

Carteolol is well absorbed from the gastrointestinal tract with a peak plasma concentration being reached within 1 to 3 hours of oral administration. The bioavailability is about 85%. It has low lipid solubility. About 20 to 30% is protein bound. The plasma half-life is reported to be 5 to 6 hours. The major route of elimination is renal with 50 to 70% of a dose being excreted unchanged in the urine; carteolol therefore accumulates in patients with renal disease. Major metabolites are 8-hydroxycarteolol and glucuronic acid conjugates of carteolol and 8-hydroxycarteolol. The 8-hydroxycarteolol metabolite is active; its half-life is reported to be 8 to 12 hours.

## Uses and Administration

Carteolol is a non-cardioselective beta blocker (see p.868). It is reported to possess intrinsic sympathomimetic activity but lacks significant membrane-stabilising activity.

Carteolol is used as the hydrochloride in the management of glaucoma (p.1485), hypertension (p.825), and some cardiac disorders such as angina pectoris (p.813) and cardiac arrhythmias (p.816).

Eye drops containing carteolol hydrochloride 1% or 2% are instilled twice daily to reduce raised intra-ocular pressure in open-angle **glaucoma** and ocular hypertension.

In **hypertension** carteolol hydrochloride is given in initial doses of 2.5 mg once daily by mouth, increased, if necessary according to response, to 10 mg once daily; higher doses have also been used. In cardiac disorders such as **angina pectoris** and **arrhythmias** carteolol hydrochloride has been used in doses of up to 30 mg daily.

The oral dose of carteolol hydrochloride should be reduced in patients with renal impairment (see below).

◊ Reviews.

1. Chrisp P, Sorkin EM. Ocular carteolol: a review of its pharmacological properties, and therapeutic use in glaucoma and ocular hypertension. *Drugs Aging* 1992; **2:** 58–77. Correction. *ibid.* 1994; **4:** 62.

**Administration in renal impairment.** The oral dose of carteolol should be reduced in patients with renal impairment. A suggested regimen for patients with hypertension is to increase the dosage interval from 24 to 48 hours in patients with a creatinine clearance of 20 to 60 mL/minute and to 72 hours in patients with a creatinine clearance of less than 20 mL/minute.

## Preparations

***BP 2003:*** Carteolol Eye Drops;
***USP 27:*** Carteolol Hydrochloride Ophthalmic Solution; Carteolol Hydrochloride Tablets.

**Proprietary Preparations** (details are given in Part 3)
***Arg.:*** Elebloc; Glauteolol; Poenglaucol; Singlauc; ***Austria:*** Endak; ***Belg.:*** Carteol; ***Braz.:*** Elebloc†; ***Denm.:*** Arteoptic; ***Fin.:*** Arteoptic; ***Fr.:*** Cartea-bak; Carteol; Mikelan; ***Ger.:*** Arteoptic; Endak; ***Gr.:*** Fortinol; ***Hong Kong:*** Arteoptic; ***Irl.:*** Teoptic; ***Ital.:*** Carteol; ***Jpn:*** Mikelan; ***Neth.:*** Teoptic; ***Port.:*** Arteoptic; ***S.Afr.:*** Mikelan†; Teoptic; ***Spain:*** Arteolol; Elebloc;

Mikelan; **Swed.:** Arteoptic; **Switz.:** Arteoptic; **Thai.:** Arteoptic; **UK:** Teoptic; **USA:** Cartrol; Ocupress.

**Multi-ingredient: Belg.:** Carteopil; **Fr.:** Carpilo; **Switz.:** Arteopilo.

## Carvedilol *(BAN, USAN, rINN)*

BM-14190; Carvedilolum. 1-Carbazol-4-yloxy-3-[2-(2-methoxyphenoxy)ethylamino]propan-2-ol.

$C_{24}H_{26}N_2O_4$ = 406.5.

*CAS — 72956-09-3.*

*ATC — C07AG02.*

**Pharmacopoeias.** In *Eur.* (see p.vi).

**Ph. Eur. 5.0** (Carvedilol). A white or almost white crystalline powder. It exhibits polymorphism. Practically insoluble in water; slightly soluble in alcohol; practically insoluble in dilute acids.

### Adverse Effects, Treatment, and Precautions

As for Beta Blockers, p.869.

Liver function abnormalities, reversible on stopping treatment with carvedilol, have been reported rarely. Carvedilol is extensively metabolised in the liver and is not recommended in patients with hepatic impairment. Acute renal failure and renal abnormalities have been reported in patients with heart failure who also suffered from diffuse vascular disease and/or renal impairment. The risk of hypotension may be reduced by taking carvedilol with food to decrease the rate of absorption.

**Effects on the liver.** Pruritus and elevated serum transaminase concentrations occurred[1] in a man who had been taking carvedilol for 6 months. Carvedilol was discontinued and the liver function tests returned to normal within 3 weeks. However, pruritus recurred when the patient was started on metoprolol approximately 1 year later.

1. Hagmeyer KO, Stein J. Hepatotoxicity associated with carvedilol. *Ann Pharmacother* 2001; **35:** 1364–6.

### Interactions

The interactions associated with beta blockers are discussed on p.870.

### Pharmacokinetics

Carvedilol is well absorbed from the gastrointestinal tract but is subject to considerable first-pass metabolism in the liver; the absolute bioavailability is about 25%. Peak plasma concentrations occur 1 to 2 hours after an oral dose. It has high lipid solubility. Carvedilol is more than 98% bound to plasma proteins. It is extensively metabolised in the liver, primarily by the cytochrome P450 isoenzymes CYP2D6 and CYP2C9, and the metabolites are excreted mainly in the bile. The elimination half-life is about 6 to 10 hours. Carvedilol has been shown to accumulate in breast milk in *animals*.

◊ References.

1. McTavish D, *et al.* Carvedilol: a review of its pharmacodynamic and pharmacokinetic properties, and therapeutic efficacy. *Drugs* 1993; **45:** 232–58.
2. Morgan T. Clinical pharmacokinetics and pharmacodynamics of carvedilol. *Clin Pharmacokinet* 1994; **26:** 335–46.
3. Tenero D, *et al.* Steady-state pharmacokinetics of carvedilol and its enantiomers in patients with congestive heart failure. *J Clin Pharmacol* 2000; **40:** 844–53.

### Uses and Administration

Carvedilol is a non-cardioselective beta blocker (p.868). It has vasodilating properties, which are attributed mainly to its blocking activity at alpha$_1$ receptors; at higher doses calcium-channel blocking activity may contribute. It also has antoxidant properties. Carvedilol is reported to have no intrinsic sympathomimetic activity and only weak membrane-stabilising activity.

Carvedilol is used in the management of hypertension (p.825) and angina pectoris (p.813), and as an adjunct to standard therapy in symptomatic heart failure (p.820). It is also used to reduce mortality in patients with left ventricular dysfunction following myocardial infarction.

In **hypertension** carvedilol is given in an initial dose of 12.5 mg once daily by mouth, increased after two days to 25 mg once daily. Alternatively, an initial dose of 6.25 mg is given twice daily, increased after one to two weeks to 12.5 mg twice daily. The dose may be increased further, if necessary, at intervals of at least two weeks, to 50 mg once daily or in divided doses. A dose of 12.5 mg once daily may be adequate for elderly patients.

In **angina pectoris** an initial dose of 12.5 mg is given twice daily by mouth, increased after two days to 25 mg twice daily.

In **heart failure**, the initial dose is 3.125 mg twice daily by mouth. It should be taken with food to reduce the risk of hypotension. If tolerated, the dose should be doubled after two weeks to 6.25 mg twice daily and then increased gradually, at intervals of not less than two weeks, to the maximum dose tolerated; this should not exceed 25 mg twice daily in patients with severe heart failure or in those weighing less than 85 kg, or 50 mg twice daily in patients with mild to moderate heart failure weighing more than 85 kg.

In patients with **left ventricular dysfunction following myocardial infarction**, the initial dose is 6.25 mg twice daily, increased after 3 to 10 days, if tolerated, to 12.5 mg twice daily and then to a target dose of 25 mg twice daily. A lower initial dose may be used in symptomatic patients.

◊ References.

1. Ruffolo RR, *et al.* The pharmacology of carvedilol. *Eur J Clin Pharmacol* 1990; **38:** S82–S88.
2. McTavish D, *et al.* Carvedilol: a review of its pharmacodynamic and pharmacokinetic properties, and therapeutic efficacy. *Drugs* 1993: **45:** 232–58.
3. Morgan T. Clinical pharmacokinetics and pharmacodynamics of carvedilol. *Clin Pharmacokinet* 1994; **26:** 335–46.
4. Louis WJ, *et al.* A risk-benefit assessment of carvedilol in the treatment of cardiovascular disorders. *Drug Safety* 1994; **11:** 86–93.
5. Dunn CJ, *et al.* Carvedilol: a reappraisal of its pharmacological properties and therapeutic use in cardiovascular disorders. *Drugs* 1997; **54:** 161–85.
6. Frishman WH. Carvedilol. *N Engl J Med* 1998; **339:** 1759–65.
7. Keating GM, Jarvis B. Carvedilol: a review of its use in chronic heart failure. *Drugs* 2003; **63:** 1697–1741.

**Administration in children.** Several studies have reported the successful use of carvedilol in children with heart failure. A retrospective study[1] in 46 children aged 3 months to 19 years with heart failure due to dilated cardiomyopathy or congenital heart disease, found that carvedilol improved symptoms when given in addition to standard therapy. Carvedilol was initiated at a mean dose of 80 micrograms/kg daily, increased gradually to a mean maintenance dose of 460 micrograms/kg daily. In another study[2] in 15 children aged 6 weeks to 19 years, carvedilol was given in an initial dose of 90 micrograms/kg twice daily, increased to a target dose of 700 micrograms/kg daily. Symptoms and ejection fraction improved over 6 months, and 2 patients were removed from the transplant waiting list. A randomised, placebo-controlled, double-blind study[3] in 22 children with severe heart failure awaiting transplantation also reported that symptoms were improved with carvedilol, and 9 of 14 patients receiving carvedilol were removed from the transplant waiting list compared with none of those receiving placebo. The initial dose was 10 micrograms/kg daily, increased to a target dose of 200 micrograms/kg daily.

1. Bruns LA, *et al.* Carvedilol as therapy in pediatric heart failure: an initial multicenter experience. *J Pediatr* 2001; **138:** 505–11.
2. Läer S, *et al.* Carvedilol therapy in pediatric patients with congestive heart failure: a study investigating clinical and pharmacokinetic parameters. *Am Heart J* 2002; **143:** 916–22.
3. Azeka E, *et al.* Delisting of infants and children from the heart transplantation waiting list after carvedilol treatment. *J Am Coll Cardiol* 2002; **40:** 2034–8.

**Administration in the elderly.** The manufacturer of carvedilol recommends an initial dose of 12.5 mg daily in hypertension. A study in 16 elderly patients (mean age 70 years) given single doses of 12.5 mg and 25 mg found a high incidence of orthostatic hypotension[1] and the authors suggested that a starting dose lower than 12.5 mg may be necessary in elderly patients.

1. Krum H, *et al.* Postural hypotension in elderly patients given carvedilol. *BMJ* 1994; **309:** 775–6.

### Preparations

**Proprietary Preparations** (details are given in Part 3)

**Arg.:** Coritensil; Dilatrend; **Austral.:** Dilatrend; Kredex; **Austria:** Dilatrend; Hybridil; **Belg.:** Dimitone; Kredex; **Braz.:** Cardilol; Coreg; Dilatrend; Divelol; **Canad.:** Coreg; **Chile:** Betaplex; Blocar; Dilatrend; Dualten; Lodipres; **Denm.:** Dimitone; **Fin.:** Cardiol; **Fr.:** Kredex; **Ger.:** Dilatrend; Querto; **Gr.:** Dilatrend; **Hong Kong:** Dilatrend; **India:** Carloc; Carvil; **Irl.:** Eucardic; **Israel:** Dimitone; **Ital.:** Carvipress; Dilatrend; Kredex†; **Mex.:** Dilatrend; **Neth.:** Eucardic; **Norw.:** Dilatrend†; Kredex; **NZ:** Dilatrend; **Port.:** Dilbloc; Kredex†; **S.Afr.:** Carloc; Dilatrend; **Singapore:** Dilatrend; **Spain:** Coropres; Kredex†; **Swed.:** Eucardic†; Kredex; **Switz.:** Dilatrend; **Thai.:** Dilatrend; **UK:** Eucardic; **USA:** Coreg.

**Multi-ingredient: Austria:** Co-Dilatrend; Dilaplus.

## Celiprolol Hydrochloride

*(BANM, USAN, rINNM)*

Celiprololi Hydrochloridum; Hidrocloruro de celiprolol. 3-{3-Acetyl-4-[3-(*tert*-butylamino)-2-hydroxypropoxy]phenyl}-1,1-diethylurea hydrochloride.

$C_{20}H_{33}N_3O_4$,HCl = 416.0.

*CAS — 56980-93-9 (celiprolol); 57470-78-7 (celiprolol hydrochloride).*

*ATC — C07AB08.*

**Pharmacopoeias.** In *Eur.* (see p.vi).

**Ph. Eur. 5.0** (Celiprolol Hydrochloride). A white or very slightly yellow, crystalline powder. It exhibits polymorphism. Freely soluble in water and in methyl alcohol; soluble in alcohol; very slightly soluble in dichloromethane. Protect from light.

### Adverse Effects, Treatment, and Precautions

As for Beta Blockers, p.869.

Tremor and palpitations associated with intrinsic sympathomimetic activity at beta$_2$ receptors have been reported.

### Interactions

The interactions associated with beta blockers are discussed on p.870.

### Pharmacokinetics

Celiprolol is absorbed from the gastrointestinal tract in a non-linear fashion; the percentage of the dose absorbed increases with increasing dose. The plasma elimination half-life is about 5 to 6 hours. Celiprolol crosses the placenta. It has low lipid solubility and is about 25% bound to plasma proteins. Metabolism is minimal and celiprolol is mainly excreted unchanged in the urine and faeces.

### Uses and Administration

Celiprolol is a cardioselective beta blocker (p.868). It is reported to possess intrinsic sympathomimetic activity and direct vasodilator activity. Celiprolol is used as the hydrochloride in the management of hypertension (p.825) and angina pectoris (p.813). The usual dose of celiprolol hydrochloride is 200 to 400 mg once daily by mouth, before food. Reduced doses may be required in patients with renal impairment (see below).

◊ References.

1. Milne RJ, Buckley MM-T. Celiprolol: an updated review of its pharmacodynamic and pharmacokinetic properties, and therapeutic efficacy in cardiovascular disease. *Drugs* 1991; **41:** 941–69.
2. Anonymous. Celiprolol: theory and practice. *Lancet* 1991; **338:** 1426–7.
3. Anonymous. Celiprolol—a better beta blocker? *Drug Ther Bull* 1992; **30:** 35–6.
4. Kendall MJ, Rajman I. A risk-benefit assessment of celiprolol in the treatment of cardiovascular disease. *Drug Safety* 1994; **10:** 220–32.
5. Riddell J. Drugs in focus 18: celiprolol. *Prescribers' J* 1996; **36:** 165–8.

**Administration in renal impairment.** Celiprolol should not be given to patients with a creatinine clearance (CC) of less than 15 mL/minute. Patients with a CC between 15 and 40 mL/minute may be given 100 to 200 mg daily.

### Preparations

**Proprietary Preparations** (details are given in Part 3)

**Austria:** Selectol; **Belg.:** Selectol; **Chile:** Selectol; **Fin.:** Selectol; **Fr.:** Celectol; **Ger.:** Celipro; Selectol; **Gr.:** Selectol; **Hong Kong:** Selectol; **Irl.:** Selectol; **Ital.:** Cordiax; **Jpn:** Selectol; **Neth.:** Dilanorm; **NZ:** Celol; Selectol†; **Spain:** Cardem; **Switz.:** Selectol; **UK:** Celectol.

**Multi-ingredient: Austria:** Selecturon.

## Cerivastatin Sodium *(BANM, USAN, rINNM)*

Bay-W-6228; Cerivastatina sódica. Sodium {S-[R*,S*-(E)]}-7-[4-(4-fluorophenyl)-5-(methoxymethyl)-2,6-bis(1-methylethyl)-3-pyridinyl]-3,5-dihydroxy-6-heptenoate.

$C_{26}H_{33}FNNaO_5$ = 481.5.

*CAS — 143201-11-0.*

### Profile

Cerivastatin, a 3-hydroxy-3-methylglutaryl coenzyme A (HMG-CoA) reductase inhibitor (a statin), is a lipid regulating drug with actions on plasma lipids similar to those of simvastatin (p.999). It has been used in the treatment of hyperlipidaemias but was withdrawn from the market worldwide in 2001 following reports of severe muscle toxicity, particularly when given with gemfibrozil.

### Preparations

**Proprietary Preparations** (details are given in Part 3)
**Austral.:** Kazak†; Lipobay†; **Austria:** Lipobay†; Liposterol†; **Belg.:** Cholstat†; Lipobay†; **Braz.:** Lipobay†; **Canad.:** Baycol†; **Denm.:** Lipobay†; **Fin.:** Lipobay†; **Fr.:** Cholstat†; Staltor†; **Ger.:** Lipobay†; Zenas†; **Irl.:** Lipobay†; **Israel:** Lipogis†; **Ital.:** Cervasta†; Lipobay†; Stativa†; **Mex.:** Baycol; **Neth.:** Lipobay†; **Norw.:** Lipobay†; **Port.:** Colstat†; Lipobay†; **S.Afr.:** Baycol†; **Singapore:** Lipobay†; **Spain:** Lipobay†; Liposterol†; Vaslip†; Zenas†; **Swed.:** Lipobay†; **Switz.:** Lipobay†; **Thai.:** Lipobay†; **UK:** Lipobay†; **USA:** Baycol†.

## Certoparin Sodium *(BAN, rINN)*

Certoparin; Certoparina sódica.

**Description.** Certoparin sodium is prepared by amyl nitrite degradation of heparin obtained from the intestinal mucosa of pigs. The majority of the components have a 2-*O*-sulfo-α-L-idopyranosuronic acid structure at the non-reducing end and a 6-*O*-sulfo-2,5-anhydro-D-mannose structure at the reducing end of their chain. The molecular weight of 70% of the components is less than 10 000 and the average molecular weight is about 6000. The degree of sulfation is about 2 to 2.5 per disaccharide unit.

### Units

As for Low-molecular-weight Heparins, p.949.

### Adverse Effects, Treatment, and Precautions

As for Low-molecular-weight Heparins, p.949.

### Interactions

As for Low-molecular-weight Heparins, p.950.

### Pharmacokinetics

Certoparin sodium is rapidly and completely absorbed following subcutaneous injection. Peak plasma activity is reached within 2 to 4 hours. The half-life of anti-factor Xa activity is about 4 hours.

### Uses and Administration

Certoparin sodium is a low-molecular-weight heparin (p.949) with anticoagulant activity used for the prevention of postoperative venous thromboembolism (p.839). It is given by subcutaneous injection in a dose of 3000 units 1 to 2 hours before the procedure, followed by 3000 units daily for 7 to 10 days or until the patient is fully ambulant.

◊ References.


1. Kock H-J, *et al.* Thromboprophylaxis with low-molecular-weight heparin in outpatients with plaster-cast immobilisation of the leg. *Lancet* 1995; **346:** 459–61.
2. Adolf J, *et al.* Comparison of 3,000 IU aXa of the low molecular weight heparin certoparin with 5,000 IU aXa in prevention of deep vein thrombosis after total hip replacement. *Int Angiol* 1999; **18:** 122–6.
3. Harenberg J, *et al.* Fixed-dose, body weight-independent subcutaneous LMW heparin versus adjusted dose unfractionated intravenous heparin in the initial treatment of proximal venous thrombosis. *Thromb Haemost* 2000; **83:** 652–6.


### Preparations

**Proprietary Preparations** (details are given in Part 3)
**Austria:** Sandoparin; Troparin; **Ger.:** Mono-Embolex; **Switz.:** Sandoparine; **UK:** Alphaparin.

**Multi-ingredient: Austria:** Embolex; Troparin compositum; **Ger.:** Embolex NM.

## Cetiedil Citrate *(USAN, rINNM)*

Citrato de cetiedil. 2-(Perhydroazepin-1-yl)ethyl α-cyclohexyl-α-(3-thienyl)acetate dihydrogen citrate monohydrate.

$C_{20}H_{31}NO_2S,C_6H_8O_7,H_2O$ = 559.7.

*CAS — 14176-10-4 (cetiedil); 16286-69-4 (anhydrous cetiedil citrate).*

*ATC — C04AX26.*

### Profile

Cetiedil citrate is a vasodilator with antimuscarinic activity that has been used in the management of peripheral vascular disease.

### Preparations

**Proprietary Preparations** (details are given in Part 3)
**Fr.:** Stratene†; **Spain:** Huberdilat†.

## Chlorothiazide *(BAN, rINN)*

Chlorothiazidum; Clorotiazida. 6-Chloro-2*H*-1,2,4-benzothiadiazine-7-sulphonamide 1,1-dioxide.

$C_7H_6ClN_3O_4S_2$ = 295.7.

*CAS — 58-94-6.*

*ATC — C03AA04.*

**Pharmacopoeias.** In *Eur.* (see p.vi) and *US.*

**Ph. Eur. 5.0** (Chlorothiazide). A white or almost white crystalline powder. Very slightly soluble in water; slightly soluble in alcohol; sparingly soluble in acetone. It dissolves in dilute solutions of alkali hydroxides.

**USP 27** (Chlorothiazide). A white or practically white, odourless, crystalline powder. Very slightly soluble in water; practically insoluble in chloroform, in ether, and in benzene; freely soluble in dimethylformamide and dimethyl sulfoxide; slightly soluble in methyl alcohol and in pyridine. Store at a temperature of 25°, excursions permitted between 15° and 30°.

**Stability.** Alkaline solutions undergo decomposition due to hydrolysis upon standing or heating.

## Chlorothiazide Sodium *(BANM, USAN, rINNM)*

Clorotiazida sódica; Sodium Chlorothiazide.

$C_7H_5ClN_3NaO_4S_2$ = 317.7.

*CAS — 7085-44-1.*

*ATC — C03AA04.*

**Pharmacopoeias.** *US* includes Chlorothiazide Sodium for Injection.

**Incompatibility.** The alkaline nature of chlorothiazide in injectable form suggests that incompatibilities with acidic drugs could be expected; the US manufacturer states that the injection may be diluted with glucose or sodium chloride solutions.

### Adverse Effects, Treatment, and Precautions

As for Hydrochlorothiazide, p.933. Chlorothiazide sodium injection is alkaline: when administering chlorothiazide by intravenous infusion, care should be taken to ensure that extravasation does not occur.

**Breast feeding.** Chlorothiazide is distributed into breast milk in small amounts. A single 500 mg oral dose of chlorothiazide was given[1] to 11 lactating women and blood and milk samples taken after 1, 2, and 3 hours; all the samples had concentrations below 1 microgram/mL and it was calculated that an infant would receive no more than 1 mg of drug each day. The American Academy of Pediatrics states that no adverse effects have been observed in infants and therefore considers[2] that chlorothiazide is usually compatible with breast feeding.


1. Werthmann MW, Krees SV. Excretion of chlorothiazide in human breast milk. *J Pediatr* 1972; **81:** 781–3.
2. American Academy of Pediatrics. The transfer of drugs and other chemicals into human milk. *Pediatrics* 2001; **108:** 776–89. Correction. *ibid.*; 1029. Also available at: http://aappolicy.aappublications.org/cgi/content/full/pediatrics%3b108/3/776 (accessed 06/07/04)


### Interactions

As for Hydrochlorothiazide, p.935.

### Pharmacokinetics

Chlorothiazide is incompletely and variably absorbed from the gastrointestinal tract. It has been estimated to have a plasma half-life of 45 to 120 minutes although the clinical effects may last for up to about 12 hours. It is excreted unchanged in the urine. Chlorothiazide crosses the placental barrier and small amounts are reported to be distributed into breast milk.

### Uses and Administration

Chlorothiazide is a thiazide diuretic with actions and uses similar to those of hydrochlorothiazide (p.935). It is used for oedema, including that associated with heart failure (p.820), and for hypertension (p.825).

After oral administration of chlorothiazide diuresis usually occurs in about 2 hours, reaches a maximum at about 4 hours, and is maintained for 6 to 12 hours.

In the treatment of **oedema** the usual dose of chlorothiazide is 0.25 to 1 g by mouth once or twice daily; therapy on alternate days or on 3 to 5 days weekly may be adequate. The dose should not normally exceed 2 g daily.

In the treatment of **hypertension** the usual initial dose is 250 to 500 mg daily by mouth, given as a single or divided dose. A dose of 125 mg may be adequate in some patients. Patients may rarely require up to 1 g daily.

A dose of chlorothiazide in children is up to 25 mg/kg by mouth daily in two divided doses. Infants up to the age of 6 months may require up to 35 mg/kg daily in two divided doses.

Chlorothiazide has also been given intravenously as the sodium salt, in doses similar to those given by mouth. Chlorothiazide sodium 537 mg is approximately equivalent to 500 mg of chlorothiazide. It is not suitable for subcutaneous or intramuscular injection and extravasation should be avoided. The diuretic effect lasts for up to 2 hours following intravenous injection.

### Preparations

**USP 27:** Chlorothiazide Oral Suspension; Chlorothiazide Sodium for Injection; Chlorothiazide Tablets; Methyldopa and Chlorothiazide Tablets; Reserpine and Chlorothiazide Tablets.

**Proprietary Preparations** (details are given in Part 3)
**Austral.:** Chlotride†; **Denm.:** Chlotride†; **Irl.:** Saluric†; **Mex.:** Pahtlisan†; **Neth.:** Chlotride†; **Singapore:** Chlorzide; **USA:** Diurigen; Diuril.

**Multi-ingredient: Canad.:** Supres; **Ital.:** Ipogen†; **USA:** Aldoclor; Diupres.

## Chlortalidone *(BAN, rINN)*

Chlortalidonum; Chlorthalidone *(USAN)*; Clorotalidona; Clortalidona; G-33182; NSC-69200. 2-Chloro-5-(1-hydroxy-3-oxoisoindolin-1-yl)benzenesulphonamide.

$C_{14}H_{11}ClN_2O_4S$ = 338.8.

*CAS — 77-36-1.*

*ATC — C03BA04.*

NOTE. Compounded preparations of chlortalidone may be represented by the following names:

- Co-tenidone (*BAN*)—chlortalidone 1 part and atenolol 4 parts (w/w).

**Pharmacopoeias.** In *Chin., Eur.* (see p.vi), *Int.*, and *US.*

**Ph. Eur. 5.0** (Chlortalidone). A white or yellowish-white powder. Practically insoluble in water and in dichloromethane; slightly soluble in alcohol; soluble in acetone and in methyl alcohol. It dissolves in dilute solutions of alkali hydroxides.

**USP 27** (Chlorthalidone). A white or yellowish-white crystalline powder. Practically insoluble in water, in chloroform, and in ether; slightly soluble in alcohol; soluble in methyl alcohol.

### Adverse Effects, Treatment, and Precautions

As for Hydrochlorothiazide, p.933.

**Breast feeding.** Chlortalidone is distributed into breast milk, but a study[1] in 9 women given a dose of 50 mg daily found that the concentration in milk was only about 5% of that in the blood. However, caution was advised since chlortalidone elimination may be slower in neonates. The American Academy of Pediatrics considers[2] that chlortalidone is usually compatible with breast feeding.


1. Mulley BA, *et al.* Placental transfer of chlorthalidone and its elimination in maternal milk. *Eur J Clin Pharmacol* 1978; **13:** 129–31.
2. American Academy of Pediatrics. The transfer of drugs and other chemicals into human milk. *Pediatrics* 2001; **108:** 776–89. Correction. *ibid*; 1029. Also available at: http://aappolicy.aappublications.org/cgi/content/full/pediatrics%3b108/3/776 (accessed 06/07/04)


### Interactions

As for Hydrochlorothiazide, p.935.

**Anticoagulants.** For references to the interaction between *warfarin* and chlortalidone, see p.1026.

### Pharmacokinetics

Chlortalidone is erratically absorbed from the gastrointestinal tract and bioavailability varies according to the preparation used. It has a prolonged elimination half-life from plasma and blood of 40 to 60 hours and is highly bound to red blood cells; the receptor to which it is bound has been identified as carbonic anhydrase. Chlortalidone is much less strongly bound to plasma proteins. Chlortalidone is mainly excreted unchanged in the urine. It crosses the placental barrier and is distributed into breast milk.

◊ References.


1. Riess W, *et al.* Pharmacokinetic studies with chlorthalidone (Hygroton®) in man. *Eur J Clin Pharmacol* 1977; **12:** 375–82.
2. Fleuren HLJ, *et al.* Absolute bioavailability of chlorthalidone in man: a cross-over study after intravenous and oral administration. *Eur J Clin Pharmacol* 1979; **15:** 35–50.
3. Fleuren HLJ, *et al.* Dose-dependent urinary excretion of chlorthalidone. *Clin Pharmacol Ther* 1979; **25:** 806–12.
4. Mulley BA, *et al.* Pharmacokinetics of chlorthalidone: dependence of biological half life on blood carbonic anhydrase levels. *Eur J Clin Pharmacol* 1980; **17:** 203–7.


### Uses and Administration

Chlortalidone is a diuretic with actions and uses similar to those of the thiazide diuretics (see Hydrochlorothiazide, p.935) even though it does not contain a thiazide ring system. It is used for hypertension (p.825), and for oedema, including that associated with heart failure (p.820). Other indications include diabetes insipidus (p.1314).

Diuresis is initiated in about 2 hours and lasts for 48 to 72 hours.

The usual dose in the treatment of **hypertension** is 25 mg daily, given either alone or with other antihypertensives, increasing to 50 mg daily if necessary.

In the treatment of **oedema** the usual initial dose is 25 to 50 mg daily by mouth. In severe cases a daily dose of 100 to 200 mg may be given. If possible lower doses should be used for maintenance; 25 to 50 mg daily or on alternate days may be adequate.

A dose for children is up to 2 mg/kg daily on alternate days.

In **diabetes insipidus** an initial dose of 100 mg twice daily has been used, reduced to a maintenance dose of 50 mg daily.

In the US, a preparation is available with improved bioavailability; suggested doses range from 15 to 50 mg daily for hypertension and 30 to 120 mg daily for oedema.

## Preparations

***BP 2003:*** Chlortalidone Tablets; Co-tenidone Tablets;
***USP 27:*** Atenolol and Chlorthalidone Tablets; Chlorthalidone Tablets; Clonidine Hydrochloride and Chlorthalidone Tablets.

**Proprietary Preparations** (details are given in Part 3)
***Arg.:*** Euretico; Hygroton; ***Austral.:*** Hygroton; ***Austria:*** Hygroton; ***Belg.:*** Hygroton; ***Braz.:*** Clortalil; Clortil; Drenidra; Higroton; Neolidona; ***Canad.:*** Novo-Thalidone†; ***Denm.:*** Hygroton†; ***Fr.:*** Hygroton†; ***Ger.:*** Hydro-long; Hygroton; ***Gr.:*** Hygroton; ***Hong Kong:*** Hygroton; ***India:*** Hythalton; ***Israel:*** Aquadon; Hygroton†; ***Ital.:*** Igroton; Zambesil†; ***Malaysia:*** Hygroton; ***Mex.:*** Anilid†; Bioralin; Diuprol†; Hidrona; Higroton; ***Neth.:*** Hygroton; ***NZ:*** Hygroton; ***Port.:*** Hygroton; ***S.Afr.:*** Hygroton; ***Spain:*** Higrotona; ***Switz.:*** Hygroton; ***UK:*** Hygroton; ***USA:*** Hygroton; Thalitone.

**Multi-ingredient:** ***Arg.:*** Atel C; Bemplas; Hygroton-Reserpina; Prenoretic; ***Austria:*** Arcablock comp; Atenobene comp; Atenolan comp; Atenolol comp; Atenotyrol comp; Darebon; Polinorm; Selecturon; Tenoretic; Trasitensin; Trepress; ***Belg.:*** Logroton; Tenoretic; ***Braz.:*** Angipress CD; Atenoric; Diupress; Higroton Reserpina; Tenoretic; ***Canad.:*** Combipres†; Tenoretic; ***Chile:*** Tenoretic; ***Denm.:*** Tenidon; Tenoretic; ***Fr.:*** Logroton; Tenoretic; Trasitensine; ***Ger.:*** Ate Lich comp; Atehexal comp; Atel; Ateno comp; Atenogamma comp; Atenolol AL comp; Atenolol comp; Atenomerck comp†; Blocotenol comp; Combipresan; Darebon; Diu-Atenolol; duratenol comp; Evitocor plus†; Impresso; Prelis comp; Sigabloc; Teneretic; Trasitensin; Trepress; TRI-Normin; ***Hong Kong:*** Target; Tenoret; Tenoretic; ***India:*** Atecard-D; Catapres Diu; Tenoclor; Tenoric; ***Irl.:*** Atenetic; Cotenomel†; Tenoret; Tenoretic; ***Ital.:*** Ataclor†; Atenigron; Biotens†; Carmian; Clortanol; Diube; Eupres; Igroseles; Igroton-Lopresor; Igroton-Reserpina; Pressalolo Diuretico†; Target; Tenolone; Tenoretic; Trandiur; Trasitensin; ***Malaysia:*** Logroton; Tenoret; Tenoretic; ***Mex.:*** Higroton-Res; Tenoretic; ***Neth.:*** Logroton†; Tenoretic; ***NZ:*** Tenoret†; Tenoretic†; ***Port.:*** Blokium Diu; Tenoretic; ***S.Afr.:*** Adco-Loten; Atenoblok Co; Hygroton-Reserpine; Tenchlor; Tenoretic; ***Singapore:*** Tenoret; Tenoretic; ***Spain:*** Aldoleo; Betasit Plus†; Blokium Diu; Higrotona Reserpina; Normopresil; Resnedal†; Tenoretic; Trasitensin; ***Switz.:*** Atedurex; ateno-basan comp.; Cardaxen plus; Co-Atenolol; Cotenolol; Cotesifar; Hygroton-Reserpine; Logroton; Primatenol Plus; Sandoretic; Slow-Trasitensine; Tenoretic; Trasitensine†; Trepress†; ***Thai.:*** Tenoret; Tenoretic; ***UK:*** AtenixCo; Kalspare; Tenchlor; Tenoret; Tenoretic; Totaretic; ***USA:*** Clorpres; Combipres; Demi-Regroton; Regroton; Tenoretic.

---

## Cibenzoline *(BAN, rINN)*

Cibenzolina; Cifenline *(USAN)*; Ro-22-7796; Ro-22-7796/001 (cibenzoline succinate); UP-339-01. (±)-2-(2,2-Diphenylcyclopropyl)-2-imidazoline.

$C_{18}H_{18}N_2$ = 262.3.

*CAS — 53267-01-9 (cibenzoline); 100678-32-8 (cibenzoline succinate).*

*ATC — C01BG07.*

### Adverse Effects and Precautions

Cibenzoline may cause neurological and gastrointestinal side-effects including vertigo, tremor, nausea, vomiting, and diarrhoea. Other adverse effects include fatigue, visual disturbances, and hypoglycaemia. Like other antiarrhythmics it can cause arrhythmias and may reduce blood pressure.

Cibenzoline is contra-indicated in patients with heart block and severe heart failure. It should be used with caution in the elderly and in renal impairment, when doses should be reduced.

**Effects on the neuromuscular system.** A myasthenic syndrome with acute respiratory failure occurred after a cibenzoline overdose in a patient with renal impairment.[1]

1. Similowski T, *et al.* Neuromuscular blockade with acute respiratory failure in a patient receiving cibenzoline. *Thorax* 1997; **52:** 582–4.

**Hypoglycaemia.** Cibenzoline therapy was associated with severe hypoglycaemia in a 67-year-old patient.[1] The plasma-cibenzoline concentration was 1800 nanograms/mL which would probably be considered toxic since the accepted therapeutic trough range is 200 to 600 nanograms/mL.

1. Hilleman DE, *et al.* Cibenzoline-induced hypoglycemia. *Drug Intell Clin Pharm* 1987; **21:** 38–40.

### Interactions

**Histamine $H_2$-antagonists.** Increased blood concentrations and prolonged half-lives of cibenzoline occurred in healthy subjects given *cimetidine* but the clinical importance of this was unknown.[1] The interaction did not occur with *ranitidine*.

1. Massarella JW. The effects of cimetidine and ranitidine on the pharmacokinetics of cibenzoline. *Br J Clin Pharmacol* 1991; **31:** 481–3.

### Pharmacokinetics

Cibenzoline is well absorbed from the gastrointestinal tract following oral use, with a bioavailability of about 90%. It is about 50 to 60% bound to plasma proteins. About 60% of a dose is excreted unchanged in the urine and the elimination half-life is reported to be about 7 hours.

◊ References.

1. Brazzell RK, *et al.* Pharmacokinetics and pharmacodynamics of intravenous cibenzoline in normal volunteers. *J Clin Pharmacol* 1985; **25:** 418–23.
2. Massarella JW, *et al.* Pharmacokinetics of cibenzoline after single and repetitive dosing in healthy volunteers. *J Clin Pharmacol* 1986; **26:** 125–30.

### Uses and Administration

Cibenzoline is a class Ia antiarrhythmic that also has some class III and class IV properties (p.809). It is used in the management of ventricular and supraventricular arrhythmias (p.816). Cibenzoline is given by mouth as the succinate or intravenously as a mixture of the base and succinate, but doses for both routes are expressed in terms of the base; 145 mg of cibenzoline succinate is approximately equivalent to 100 mg of base. The usual dose of cibenzoline succinate by mouth is the equivalent of 260 to 390 mg cibenzoline daily. The usual initial intravenous dose is the equivalent of 1 mg/kg cibenzoline base over 2 minutes followed by 8 mg/kg over 24 hours by infusion, or by initiation of oral therapy. Dosage should be reduced in the elderly (below), and in renal impairment (below).

**Administration in the elderly.** The renal and non-renal clearance of cibenzoline was found to decrease with increasing age in healthy subjects.[1] The mean elimination half-life was 7 hours in the 20- to 30-year age group and 10.5 hours in the 70- to 80-year age group. The reduction in renal clearance was considered to be related to the decrease in creatinine clearance with increasing age. The results suggested that older patients may need lower doses than younger patients to maintain therapeutic plasma-cibenzoline concentrations. The manufacturers recommend a dosage of 130 mg daily in two divided doses in elderly patients.

1. Brazzell RK, *et al.* Age and cibenzoline disposition. *Clin Pharmacol Ther* 1984; **36:** 613–19.

**Administration in renal impairment.** A study[1] in patients with normal or impaired renal function has suggested that in renal impairment initial loading doses of cibenzoline may be equivalent to those used in normal renal function although maintenance doses should be reduced to about two-thirds of normal. Oral doses recommended by the manufacturers, based on creatinine clearance (CC), are as follows:

- CC 20 to 40 mL/min: the equivalent of 3 mg/kg daily
- CC 10 to 20 mL/min: the equivalent of 2.5 mg/kg daily

1. Aronoff G, *et al.* Bioavailability and kinetics of cibenzoline in patients with normal and impaired renal function. *J Clin Pharmacol* 1991; **31:** 38–44.

### Preparations

**Proprietary Preparations** (details are given in Part 3)
***Belg.:*** Cipralan; ***Fr.:*** Cipralan; Exacor; ***Jpn:*** Cibenol.

---

## Cicletanine *(BAN, USAN, rINN)*

(±)-BN-1270; (±)-Cycletanide; Win-90000. (±)-3-(*p*-Chlorophenyl)-1,3-dihydro-6-methylfuro[3,4-*c*]pyridin-7-ol.

$C_{14}H_{12}ClNO_2$ = 261.7.

*CAS — 89943-82-8;.*

*ATC — C03BX03.*

## Cicletanine Hydrochloride *(BANM, rINNM)*

Hidrocloruro de cicletanina.

$C_{14}H_{12}ClNO_2,HCl$ = 298.2.

*CAS — 89943-82-8;.*

*ATC — C03BX03.*

### Profile

Cicletanine hydrochloride is a diuretic with properties similar to those of the thiazide diuretics (see Hydrochlorothiazide, p.933). It is used in the treatment of hypertension (p.825) in a usual dose of 50 to 100 mg daily by mouth.

### Preparations

**Proprietary Preparations** (details are given in Part 3)
***Fr.:*** Tenstaten; ***Ger.:*** Justar.

---

## Cilazapril *(BAN, USAN, rINN)*

Cilazaprilum; Ro-31-2848 (anhydrous cilazapril); Ro-31-2848/006 (cilazapril monohydrate). (1*S*,9*S*)-9-[(*S*)-1-Ethoxycarbonyl-3-phenylpropylamino]-10-oxoperhydropyridazino[1,2-*a*][1,2]diazepine-1-carboxylic acid monohydrate.

$C_{22}H_{31}N_3O_5,H_2O$ = 435.5.

*CAS — 88768-40-5 (anhydrous cilazapril); 92077-78-6 (cilazapril monohydrate).*

*ATC — C09AA08.*

**Pharmacopoeias.** In *Eur.* (see p.vi).

**Ph. Eur. 5.0** (Cilazapril). A white or almost white crystalline powder. Slightly soluble in water; freely soluble in dichloromethane and in methyl alcohol. Protect from light.

### Adverse Effects, Treatment, and Precautions

As for ACE inhibitors, p.842.

### Interactions

As for ACE inhibitors, p.845.

### Pharmacokinetics

Cilazapril acts as a prodrug of the diacid cilazaprilat, its active metabolite. Following oral administration and absorption of cilazapril it is rapidly metabolised in the liver to cilazaprilat, the bioavailability of which is about 60%. Peak plasma concentrations of cilazaprilat occur within 2 hours of an oral dose of cilazapril. Cilazaprilat is eliminated unchanged in the urine. The effective half-life of cilazaprilat is reported to be 9 hours following once-daily dosing. The elimination of cilazaprilat is reduced in renal impairment. Both cilazapril and cilazaprilat are removed to a limited extent by haemodialysis.

◊ Reviews.

1. Kelly JG, O'Malley K. Clinical pharmacokinetics of the newer ACE inhibitors: a review. *Clin Pharmacokinet* 1990; **19:** 177–96.
2. Kloke HJ, *et al.* Pharmacokinetics and haemodynamic effects of the angiotensin converting enzyme inhibitor cilazapril in hypertensive patients with normal and impaired renal function. *Br J Clin Pharmacol* 1996; **42:** 615–20.

### Uses and Administration

Cilazapril is an ACE inhibitor (p.842). It is used in the treatment of hypertension (p.825) and heart failure (p.820).

Cilazapril owes its activity to cilazaprilat to which it is converted after oral administration. The haemodynamic effects are seen within 1 hour of a single oral dose and the maximum effect occurs after about 3 to 7 hours. The haemodynamic action persists for about 24 hours, allowing once-daily dosing. Cilazapril is given by mouth as the monohydrate, but doses are expressed in terms of the anhydrous substance. Cilazapril 1.04 mg as the monohydrate is approximately equivalent to 1 mg of anhydrous cilazapril.

In the treatment of **hypertension** the initial dose is 1 mg once daily. Since there may be a precipitous fall in blood pressure in some patients when starting therapy with an ACE inhibitor, the first dose should preferably be given at bedtime. Usual maintenance doses range from 2.5 to 5 mg daily. In the elderly, in patients with mild to moderate renal impairment, or those taking *diuretics*, a usual initial dose is 0.5 mg daily. If possible the diuretic should be withdrawn 2 to 3 days before cilazapril is started and resumed later if necessary.

In the treatment of **heart failure** severe first-dose hypotension on introduction of an ACE inhibitor is common in patients on loop diuretics, but their temporary withdrawal may cause rebound pulmonary oedema. Thus therapy should be initiated with a low dose under close medical supervision. Cilazapril is given in an initial dose of 0.5 mg once daily, increased if tolerated to a usual maintenance dose of 1 to 2.5 mg once daily. The usual maximum dose is 5 mg daily.

Reduced doses may be necessary in patients with renal impairment (see below).

◊ References.

1. Deget F, Brogden RN. Cilazapril: a review of its pharmacodynamic and pharmacokinetic properties, and therapeutic potential in cardiovascular disease. *Drugs* 1991; **41:** 799–820.

**Administration in renal impairment.** In patients with a creatinine clearance of 10 to 40 mL/minute, the initial dose of cilazapril is 0.5 mg once daily and the maintenance dose should not exceed 2.5 mg once daily. Cilazapril should be avoided in patients with a creatinine clearance below 10 mL/minute. In patients receiving haemodialysis, cilazapril should be given on the non-dialysis days and the dose should be adjusted according to response.

### Preparations

**Proprietary Preparations** (details are given in Part 3)
***Austral.:*** Inhibace†; ***Austria:*** Inhibace; ***Belg.:*** Inhibace; ***Braz.:*** Vascase; ***Canad.:*** Inhibace; ***Chile:*** Inhibace; ***Fr.:*** Justor; ***Ger.:*** Dynorm; ***Gr.:*** Vascace; ***Hong Kong:*** Inhibace; ***Irl.:*** Vascace; ***Israel:*** Vascace; ***Ital.:*** Inibace; Initiss; ***Jpn:*** Inhibace; ***Mex.:*** Inhibace; ***Neth.:*** Vascase; ***NZ:*** Inhibace; ***Port.:*** Inibace; Vascase; ***S.Afr.:*** Inhibace; ***Singapore:*** Inhibace; ***Spain:*** Inhibace; Inocar; ***Swed.:*** Inhibace; ***Switz.:*** Inhibace; ***Thai.:*** Inhibace; ***UK:*** Vascace.

**Multi-ingredient:** ***Austria:*** Inhibace Plus; ***Belg.:*** Co-Inhibace; ***Braz.:*** Vascase Plus; ***Canad.:*** Inhibace Plus; ***Chile:*** Inhibace Plus; ***Ger.:*** Dynorm Plus; ***Israel:*** Vascace Plus; ***Ital.:*** Inibace Plus; Initiss Plus; ***Neth.:*** Vascase Plus†; ***NZ:*** Inhibace Plus; ***Port.:*** Inibace Plus; Vascase Plus; ***S.Afr.:*** Inhibace Plus; ***Spain:*** Inhibace Plus; Inocar Plus; ***Swed.:*** Inhibace comp; ***Switz.:*** Inhibace Plus.

## Cilnidipine *(rINN)*

Cilnidipino; FRC-8653. (±)-(*E*)-Cinnamyl 2-methoxyethyl 1,4-dihydro-2,6-dimethyl-4-(*m*-nitrophenyl)-3,5-pyridinedicarboxylate.
$C_{27}H_{28}N_2O_7$ = 492.5.
*CAS — 132203-70-4.*
*ATC — C08CA14.*

### Profile

Cilnidipine is a dihydropyridine calcium-channel blocker (p.810) given by mouth in the management of hypertension (p.825). The usual dose is 5 to 10 mg once daily, increased to 20 mg once daily if necessary.

### Preparations

**Proprietary Preparations** (details are given in Part 3)
***Jpn:*** Atelec; Cinalong.

## Cilostazol *(BAN, USAN, pINN)*

OPC-21; OPC-13013. 6-[4-(1-Cyclohexyl-1*H*-tetrazol-5-yl)butoxy]-3,4-dihydrocarbostyril.
$C_{20}H_{27}N_5O_2$ = 369.5.
*CAS — 73963-72-1.*

### Adverse Effects and Precautions

Adverse effects of cilostazol include headache, dizziness, palpitations, and diarrhoea; oedema, nausea and vomiting, other cardiac arrhythmias, chest pain, rhinitis, ecchymosis, and skin rashes have also been reported.. Cardiovascular toxicity has been reported in *animal* studies of cilostazol, and prolonged oral use of other phosphodiesterase inhibitors (such as amrinone, p.862) for the treatment of heart failure has been associated with increased mortality. The use of cilostazol in patients with any degree of heart failure is therefore contra-indicated. In the UK, cilostazol is also contra-indicated in patients with a known predisposition to bleeding, a history of ventricular arrhythmias, QT interval prolongation, severe renal impairment, moderate to severe hepatic impairment, and in patients taking inhibitors of the cytochrome P450 isoenzymes CYP3A4 or CYP2C19 (see Interactions, below).

### Interactions

Cilostazol is extensively metabolised to active and inactive metabolites by cytochrome P450 isoenzymes, mainly CYP3A4 and to a lesser extent CYP2C19. Therefore use with other drugs that inhibit or are metabolised by these hepatic enzymes may result in changes in plasma concentrations of either drug and, possibly, adverse effects. Cilostazol should therefore be used with caution in patients taking drugs metabolised by these enzymes; in patients taking enzyme inhibitors it should be avoided or a reduced dose of 50 mg twice daily should be considered.

### Pharmacokinetics

Cilostazol is absorbed following oral administration and absorption is increased if taken with a high fat meal. Cilostazol is extensively metabolised in the liver by cytochrome P450 isoenzymes, mainly CYP3A4 and to a lesser extent CYP2C19, to both active and inactive metabolites; these are predominantly excreted in the urine (74%) with the remainder in the faeces (20%). The active metabolites have apparent elimination half-lives of 11 to 13 hours. Cilostazol is 95 to 98% protein bound.

### Uses and Administration

Cilostazol is a phosphodiesterase inhibitor with antiplatelet and vasodilating activity. It is used in the management of peripheral vascular disease (p.831).

The usual dose of cilostazol for the reduction of symptoms of intermittent claudication is 100 mg orally twice daily, at least 30 minutes before or 2 hours after food (but see also Interactions, above). Response to treatment may occur in 2 to 4 weeks, but up to 12 weeks may be required.

Cilostazol is under investigation for its antiplatelet effect following coronary stent implantation.

◊ Reviews.


1. Reilly MP, Mohler ER. Cilostazol: treatment of intermittent claudication. *Ann Pharmacother* 2001; **35:** 48–56.
2. El-Beyrouty C, Spinler SA. Cilostazol for prevention of thrombosis and restenosis after intracoronary stenting. *Ann Pharmacother* 2001; **35:** 1108–13.


**Peripheral vascular disease.** Intermittent claudication is a major feature of occlusive arterial disease of the lower limbs (a form of peripheral vascular disease, p.831) and is characterised by pain in the legs, which develops during exercise but usually disappears at rest. Many drugs have been used for symptom control, but none is of established benefit.

Several randomised, double-blind studies[1-3] have shown that cilostazol improves walking distances in patients with intermittent claudication, and one study[4] suggested that it was more effective than pentoxifylline. Cilostazol may therefore have a role for symptom control in patients with intermittent claudication.[5] However, long-term benefit has not been assessed and, since patients with intermittent claudication are at high risk of other cardiovascular events, appropriate therapy to reduce cardiovascular risk (p.819) is still required.


1. Money SR, *et al.* Effect of cilostazol on walking distances in patients with intermittent claudication caused by peripheral vascular disease. *J Vasc Surg* 1998; **27:** 267–75.
2. Beebe HG, *et al.* A new pharmacological treatment for intermittent claudication: results of a randomized, multicenter trial. *Arch Intern Med* 1999; **159:** 2041–50.
3. Strandness DE, *et al.* Effect of cilostazol in patients with intermittent claudication: a randomized, double-blind, placebo-controlled study. *Vasc Endovascular Surg* 2002; **36:** 83–91.
4. Dawson DL, *et al.* A comparison of cilostazol and pentoxifylline for treating intermittent claudication. *Am J Med* 2000; **109:** 523–30.
5. Crouse JR, *et al.* Clinical manifestation of atherosclerotic peripheral arterial disease and the role of cilostazol in treatment of intermittent claudication. *J Clin Pharmacol* 2002; **42:** 1291–8.


### Preparations

**Proprietary Preparations** (details are given in Part 3)
***Arg.:*** Pletaal; Trastocir; ***Braz.:*** Cebralat†; ***Chile:*** Artesol; ***Hong Kong:*** Pletaal; ***Jpn:*** Pletaal; ***Thai.:*** Pletaal; ***UK:*** Pletal; ***USA:*** Pletal.

## Cinepazet Maleate *(BANM, USAN, pINNM)*

Cinepazic Acid Ethyl Ester Maleate; Maleato de cinepazet. Ethyl 4-(3,4,5-trimethoxycinnamoyl)piperazin-1-ylacetate hydrogen maleate.
$C_{20}H_{28}N_2O_6,C_4H_4O_4$ = 508.5.
*CAS — 23887-41-4 (cinepazet); 50679-07-7 (cinepazet maleate).*
*ATC — C01DX14.*

### Profile

Cinepazet maleate is a vasodilator that has been used in angina pectoris.

## Cinepazide Maleate *(BANM, rINNM)*

Maleato de cinepazida; MD-67350. 1-(Pyrrolidin-1-ylcarbonylmethyl)-4-(3,4,5-trimethoxycinnamoyl)piperazine hydrogen maleate.
$C_{22}H_{31}N_3O_5,C_4H_4O_4$ = 533.6.
*CAS — 23887-46-9 (cinepazide); 26328-04-1 (cinepazide maleate).*
*ATC — C04AX27.*

### Profile

Cinepazide maleate is a vasodilator which has been used in peripheral vascular disorders, but has been withdrawn from the market in some countries following reports of agranulocytosis.

## Ciprofibrate *(BAN, USAN, rINN)*

Ciprofibrato; Ciprofibratum; Win-35833. 2-[4-(2,2-Dichlorocyclopropyl)phenoxy]-2-methylpropionic acid.
$C_{13}H_{14}Cl_2O_3$ = 289.2.
*CAS — 52214-84-3.*
*ATC — C10AB08.*

**Pharmacopoeias.** In *Eur.* (see p.vi).
**Ph. Eur. 5.0** (Ciprofibrate). A white or slightly yellow, crystalline powder. Practically insoluble in water; freely soluble in dehydrated alcohol; soluble in toluene. Store in airtight containers. Protect from light.

### Adverse Effects and Precautions

As for Bezafibrate, p.873.

### Interactions

As for Bezafibrate, p.874.

### Pharmacokinetics

Ciprofibrate is readily absorbed from the gastrointestinal tract; peak plasma concentrations occur within 1 to 4 hours. Ciprofibrate is highly protein bound. It is excreted in the urine as unchanged drug and as glucuronide conjugates. The elimination half-life varies from about 38 to 86 hours in patients on long-term therapy.

### Uses and Administration

Ciprofibrate, a fibric acid derivative, is a lipid regulating drug with actions on plasma lipids similar to those of bezafibrate (p.874).

It is used to reduce total cholesterol and triglycerides in the management of hyperlipidaemias (p.823), including type IIa, type IIb, type III, and type IV hyperlipoproteinaemias. The usual dose is 100 mg daily by mouth. The dose should be reduced in renal impairment (see below).

**Administration in renal impairment.** Ciprofibrate is contra-indicated in patients with severe renal impairment. The manufacturer has suggested reducing the dose to 100 mg every other day for patients with moderate renal impairment.

Renal clearance of ciprofibrate was reduced and elimination half-life approximately doubled in patients with severe renal impairment.[1] Mild renal impairment slowed the urinary excretion of ciprofibrate but not its extent. The clearance of ciprofibrate was unaffected by haemodialysis.


1. Ferry N, *et al.* The influence of renal insufficiency and haemodialysis on the kinetics of ciprofibrate. *Br J Clin Pharmacol* 1989; **28:** 675–81.


### Preparations

**Proprietary Preparations** (details are given in Part 3)
***Arg.:*** Estaprol; ***Belg.:*** Hyperlipen; ***Braz.:*** Oroxadin; ***Chile:*** Estaprol; ***Fr.:*** Lipanor; ***Gr.:*** Savilen; ***Israel:*** Lipanor; ***Malaysia:*** Modalim; ***Mex.:*** Oroxadin; ***Neth.:*** Modalim; ***Port.:*** Lipanor; ***Singapore:*** Modalim; ***Switz.:*** Hyperlipen; ***UK:*** Modalim.

## Clinofibrate *(rINN)*

Clinofibrato; S-8527. 2,2′-[Cyclohexylidenebis(4-phenyleneoxy)]bis[2-methylbutyric acid].
$C_{28}H_{36}O_6$ = 468.6.
*CAS — 30299-08-2.*

**Pharmacopoeias.** In *Jpn.*

### Profile

Clinofibrate, a fibric acid derivative (see Bezafibrate, p.873), is a lipid regulating drug used in the treatment of hyperlipidaemias (p.823). The usual dose is 200 mg three times daily by mouth.

### Preparations

**Proprietary Preparations** (details are given in Part 3)
***Jpn:*** Lipoclin.

## Clofibrate *(BAN, USAN, rINN)*

AY-61123; Clofibrato; Clofibratum; Ethyl *p*-Chlorophenoxyisobutyrate; Ethyl Clofibrate; ICI-28257; NSC-79389. Ethyl 2-(4-chlorophenoxy)-2-methylpropionate.
$C_{12}H_{15}ClO_3$ = 242.7.
*CAS — 637-07-0 (clofibrate); 882-09-7 (clofibric acid).*
*ATC — C10AB01.*

**Pharmacopoeias.** In *Chin., Eur.* (see p.vi), *Jpn*, and *US.*
**Ph. Eur. 5.0** (Clofibrate). A clear, almost colourless liquid. Very slightly soluble in water; miscible with alcohol.
**USP 27** (Clofibrate). A colourless to pale yellow liquid with a characteristic odour. Insoluble in water; soluble in alcohol, in acetone, in chloroform, and in benzene. Store in airtight containers. Protect from light.

## Aluminium Clofibrate *(BAN, rINN)*

Alufibrate; Aluminum Clofibrate; Clofibrato de aluminio. Bis[2-(4-chlorophenoxy)-2-methylpropionato]hydroxyaluminium.
$C_{20}H_{21}AlCl_2O_7$ = 471.3.
*CAS — 24818-79-9; 14613-01-5.*
*ATC — C10AB03.*

### Calcium Clofibrate *(rINN)*

Clofibrato de calcio.

$C_{20}H_{20}CaCl_2O_6$ = 467.4.

*CAS — 39087-48-4.*

### Magnesium Clofibrate *(rINN)*

Clofibrato de magnesio; Clomag; UR-112.

$C_{20}H_{20}Cl_2MgO_6$ = 451.6.

*CAS — 14613-30-0.*

#### Adverse Effects and Precautions

As for Bezafibrate, p.873.

Large-scale long-term studies have demonstrated an increased incidence of cholecystitis, gallstones, and sometimes pancreatitis in patients receiving clofibrate, and some studies, but not all, have indicated an increased incidence of certain cardiovascular disorders, including cardiac arrhythmias. The unexpected finding of an increased mortality rate in patients taking clofibrate in the WHO study (see below) produced serious concern over its long-term safety and the use of clofibrate is now generally restricted.

◊ Doubts over the safety of clofibrate for long-term prophylaxis were raised following 2 large-scale studies: the Coronary Drug Project[1] and the WHO Cooperative Trial.[2] The Coronary Drug Project showed that while clofibrate was generally well tolerated, there was an increased incidence of serious effects over the 5-year study period. These included cholelithiasis (3.0% against 1.3% with placebo), pulmonary embolism or thrombophlebitis (5.2% against 3.3%), arrhythmias other than atrial fibrillation, new cases of intermittent claudication, and new angina pectoris. Other findings included an increased incidence of palpable spleen, and enlarged, firm, or tender liver. Anticoagulant therapy was required in 37% more patients taking clofibrate than placebo. Further analysis of the results[3] showed that the incidence of cholelithiasis or cholecystitis over the first 6 years was 4.0% in the clofibrate group compared with 2.6% in the placebo group.

In the WHO study[2] there was a higher incidence of cholelithiasis and a slight excess of thromboembolism, but no evidence of an increased incidence of intermittent claudication. More importantly, the long-term safety of clofibrate was thrown into doubt by the finding that, although clofibrate reduced the incidence of non-fatal myocardial infarction, the overall death rate was higher in the clofibrate group than in the control groups. The excess deaths were related to a range of disorders with no single disorder predominating. Follow-up after 9.6 years[4] and 13.2 years[5] indicated that the excess of deaths from causes other than ischaemic heart disease was almost entirely confined to the period of exposure to clofibrate; the excess during the treatment period was 47% from all causes compared with 5% after treatment ended. The causes of death were spread over a range of malignant and non-malignant disorders.

1. The Coronary Drug Project Research Group. Clofibrate and niacin in coronary heart disease. *JAMA* 1975; **231:** 360–80.
2. Oliver MF, *et al.* A co-operative trial in the primary prevention of ischaemic heart disease using clofibrate. *Br Heart J* 1978; **40:** 1069–1118.
3. The Coronary Drug Project Research Group. Gall bladder disease as a side effect of drugs influencing lipid metabolism. *N Engl J Med* 1977; **296:** 1185–90.
4. Oliver MF, *et al.* WHO cooperative trial on primary prevention of ischaemic heart disease using clofibrate to lower serum cholesterol: mortality follow-up. *Lancet* 1980; **ii:** 379–85. Correction. *ibid.*; 490.
5. Oliver MF, *et al.* WHO cooperative trial on primary prevention of ischaemic heart disease using clofibrate to lower serum cholesterol: final mortality follow-up. *Lancet* 1984; **ii:** 600–604.

**Effects on the respiratory system.** Eosinophilic pneumonia has been reported[1] in a patient associated with the use of clofibrate.

1. Hendrickson RM, Simpson F. Clofibrate and eosinophilic pneumonia. *JAMA* 1982; **247:** 3082.

#### Interactions

As for Bezafibrate, p.874.

The manufacturers of clofibrate have suggested that, in patients taking oral anticoagulants, the dose of anticoagulant should be reduced by about 50% when treatment with clofibrate is started, and then adjusted gradually if necessary.

#### Pharmacokinetics

Clofibrate is readily absorbed from the gastrointestinal tract and is rapidly hydrolysed to its active metabolite, chlorophenoxyisobutyric acid (clofibric acid), which is at least 95% bound to plasma proteins. The plasma half-life of clofibric acid is about 18 to 22 hours. It is excreted in the urine, mainly in the form of a glucuronide conjugate.

◊ References.

1. Gugler R. Clinical pharmacokinetics of hypolipidaemic drugs. *Clin Pharmacokinet* 1978; **3:** 425–39.

#### Uses and Administration

Clofibrate, a fibric acid derivative, is a lipid regulating drug with actions on plasma lipids similar to those of bezafibrate (p.874). It is used to reduce triglycerides and possibly total cholesterol in the management of certain hyperlipidaemias (p.823), in particular type III hyperlipoproteinaemia. It may also be helpful in some patients with severe hypertriglyceridaemia due to type IV or type V hyperlipoproteinaemias. Because of the incidence of adverse effects during long-term treatment it should not be used for the prophylaxis of ischaemic heart disease (see under Adverse Effects, above).

The usual dose, by mouth, is 2 g daily in divided doses.

The aluminium, calcium, and magnesium salts of clofibrate have also been used in the treatment of hyperlipidaemias.

**Administration in renal impairment.** Clofibrate should generally be avoided in patients with renal impairment.

The plasma half-life of total clofibric acid has been reported[1] to be extended from about 17 hours in healthy subjects to a mean of about 130 hours in 5 patients with renal failure undergoing haemodialysis. A dose of 1 to 1.5 g of clofibrate per week effectively lowered plasma-triglyceride concentrations without causing toxicity in 11 hypertriglyceridaemic patients undergoing haemodialysis.[2]

1. Faed EM, McQueen EG. Plasma half-life of clofibric acid in renal failure. *Br J Clin Pharmacol* 1979; **7:** 407–10.
2. Goldberg AP, *et al.* Control of clofibrate toxicity in uraemic hypertriglyceridemia. *Clin Pharmacol Ther* 1977; **21:** 317–25.

**Neonatal jaundice.** Clofibrate has been found to be effective both in the treatment of jaundice in term infants and for prophylaxis in premature infants.[1] In a study involving 93 term infants with jaundice, clofibrate 50 mg/kg as a single oral dose reduced the intensity and duration of jaundice compared with placebo. As a prophylactic measure, clofibrate was shown to reduce the degree of jaundice in premature infants when the plasma concentration of clofibric acid reached 140 micrograms/mL within 24 hours of clofibrate administration. The dose required to achieve this was estimated to be 100 to 150 mg/kg.

1. Gabilan JC, *et al.* Clofibrate treatment of neonatal jaundice. *Pediatrics* 1990; **86:** 647–8.

#### Preparations

***BP 2003:*** Clofibrate Capsules;
***USP 27:*** Clofibrate Capsules.

**Proprietary Preparations** (details are given in Part 3)
***Arg.:*** Elpi; ***Austria:*** Arterioflexin; Regelan†; ***Belg.:*** Atromidin†; ***Braz.:*** Claripex AL†; ***Canad.:*** Atromid-S†; Novo-Fibrate†; ***Denm.:*** Atromidin†; ***Ger.:*** Regelan N†; ***Hong Kong:*** Atromid-S†; Lipilim; ***Irl.:*** Atromid-S†; ***Mex.:*** Atromid-S†; ***NZ:*** Atromid-S†; ***Port.:*** Atromid-S; ***S.Afr.:*** Atromid-S†; ***Spain:*** Neo Atromid†; ***Swed.:*** Atromidin†; ***Switz.:*** Regelan†; ***UK:*** Atromid-S†; ***USA:*** Atromid-S†.

**Multi-ingredient:** ***Braz.:*** Davistar†; Lipofacton; Sinteroid†; ***S.Afr.:*** Lipaten†; ***Spain:*** Arteriobrate†.

---

## Clonidine *(BAN, USAN, rINN)*

Clonidinum; ST-155-BS. 2-(2,6-Dichloroanilino)-2-imidazoline; 2,6-Dichloro-*N*-(imidazolidin-2-ylidene)aniline.

$C_9H_9Cl_2N_3$ = 230.1.

*CAS — 4205-90-7.*

*ATC — C02AC01; N02CX02; S01EA04.*

**Pharmacopoeias.** In *US.*

**USP 27** (Clonidine). A white to almost white, crystalline powder. Freely soluble in alcohol and in methyl alcohol. Store in airtight containers.

### Clonidine Hydrochloride *(BANM, USAN, rINNM)*

Clonidini Hydrochloridum; Hidrocloruro de clonidina; ST-155.

$C_9H_9Cl_2N_3$,HCl = 266.6.

*CAS — 4205-91-8.*

*ATC — C02AC01; N02CX02; S01EA04.*

**Pharmacopoeias.** In *Chin., Eur.* (see p.vi), *Jpn, Pol.,* and *US.*

**Ph. Eur. 5.0** (Clonidine Hydrochloride). A white or almost white crystalline powder. Soluble in water and in dehydrated alcohol. A 5% solution in water has a pH of 4.0 to 5.0.

**USP 27** (Clonidine Hydrochloride). pH of a 5% solution in water is between 3.5 and 5.5. Store in airtight containers at a temperature of 25°, excursions permitted between 15° and 30°.

#### Adverse Effects and Treatment

Drowsiness, dry mouth, dizziness, and headache commonly occur during the initial stages of therapy with clonidine. Constipation is also common, and other adverse effects which have been reported include depression, anxiety, fatigue, nausea, anorexia, parotid pain, sleep disturbances, vivid dreams, impotence and loss of libido, urinary retention or incontinence, slight orthostatic hypotension, and dry, itching, or burning sensations in the eye. Fluid retention may occur and is usually transient, but may be responsible for a reduction in the hypotensive effect during continued treatment. Clonidine may cause rashes and pruritus, and these are more common with the use of transdermal delivery systems. Less frequently, bradycardia, including sinus bradycardia with atrioventricular block, other ECG disturbances, heart failure, hallucinations, cramp, Raynaud's syndrome, gynaecomastia, and transient abnormalities in liver function tests have been reported. Large doses have been associated with initial increases in blood pressure and transient hyperglycaemia, although these do not persist during continued therapy.

Symptoms of overdosage include transient hypertension or profound hypotension, bradycardia, sedation, miosis, respiratory depression, convulsions, and coma. Treatment consists of general supportive measures. An alpha blocker may be given if necessary for hypertension, and atropine may be required for bradycardia and associated hypotension. Cardiac pacing may be needed rarely.

Sudden withdrawal of clonidine may produce rebound hypertension—see Precautions, below.

**Effects on the gastrointestinal tract.** Constipation is a relatively common adverse effect of clonidine, the US manufacturer reporting an incidence of about 10%. Several cases of ileus or pseudo-obstruction of the bowel in patients receiving clonidine have been reported;[1-3] withdrawal of clonidine was associated with a return of bowel function to normal. Abdominal pain mimicking acute appendicitis occurred in another patient prescribed clonidine; symptoms recurred on restarting the drug and subsided when it was withdrawn.[4]

1. Davidov M, *et al.* The antihypertensive effects of an imidazoline compound. *Clin Pharmacol Ther* 1967; **8:** 810–16.
2. Bear R, Steer K. Pseudo-obstruction due to clonidine. *BMJ* 1976; **1:** 197.
3. Bauer GE, Hellestrand KJ. Pseudo-obstruction due to clonidine. *BMJ* 1976; **1:** 769.
4. Mjörndal T, Mellbring G. Abdominal pain associated with clonidine. *BMJ* 1986; **292:** 174.

**Effects on the heart.** Clonidine has been associated with impaired atrioventricular conduction in a few patients,[1,2] although some of these may have had underlying conduction defects and had previously received digitalis, which may have contributed to their condition. Other ECG abnormalities may also occur. Sudden death has been reported in 3 children receiving clonidine and methylphenidate,[3,4] although the significance of these reports has been questioned.[5]

1. Kibler LE, Gazes PC. Effect of clonidine on atrioventricular conduction. *JAMA* 1977; **238:** 1930–2.
2. Abiuso P, Abelow G. Atrioventricular dissociation in a patient receiving clonidine. *JAMA* 1978; **240:** 108–9.
3. Maloney MJ, Schwam, JS. Clonidine and sudden death. *Pediatrics* 1995; **96:** 1176–7.
4. Fenichel RR. Combining methylphenidate and clonidine: the role of post-marketing surveillance. *J Child Adolesc Psychopharmacol* 1995; **5:** 155–6.
5. Blackman JA, *et al.* Clonidine and electrocardiograms. *Pediatrics* 1996; **98:** 1223–4.

**Effects on mental function.** There have been occasional reports of disturbed mental state in patients given clonidine.[1-3]

1. Lavin P, Alexander CP. Dementia associated with clonidine therapy. *BMJ* 1975; **1:** 628.
2. Enoch MD, Hammad GEM. Acute hallucinosis due to clonidine. *Curr Med Res Opin* 1977; **4:** 670–1.
3. Brown MJ, *et al.* Clonidine hallucinations. *Ann Intern Med* 1980; **93:** 456–7.

**Effects on the skin.** Skin reactions have been reported in up to 50% of patients receiving clonidine by a transdermal delivery system.[1] Localised erythema and irritation during early treatment are usually mild, but allergic contact dermatitis may develop.[2-4] Skin reactions may become commoner during prolonged treatment; although only mild skin reactions were observed in a trial of transdermal clonidine during 8 to 14 weeks of treatment in 15 patients, severe skin reactions occurred after an average of 20 weeks in 4 of 5 patients who continued treatment.[5] Despite a claim that skin reactions were due to a component in the delivery system and not to clonidine itself,[6] positive patch tests to clonidine have been obtained.[2,4] Subsequent reaction to oral clonidine in patients who develop skin reactions to the transdermal delivery system is reported to be rare.[7,8]

1. Carmichael AJ. Skin sensitivity and transdermal drug delivery: a review of the problem. *Drug Safety* 1994; **10:** 151–9.
2. Groth H, *et al.* Allergic skin reactions to transdermal clonidine. *Lancet* 1983; **ii:** 850–1.
3. McMahon FG, Weber MA. Allergic skin reactions to transdermal clonidine. *Lancet* 1983; **ii:** 851.
4. Boekhorst JC. Allergic contact dermatitis with transdermal clonidine. *Lancet* 1983; **ii:** 1031–2.
5. Dick JBC, *et al.* Skin reactions to long-term transdermal clonidine. *Lancet* 1987; **i:** 516.
6. Anonymous. Transdermal clonidine sensitiser identified? *Pharm J* 1984; **233:** 16.
7. Bigby M. Transdermal clonidine dermatitis. *JAMA* 1987; **258:** 1819.
8. Burris JF. Transdermal clonidine dermatitis. *JAMA* 1987; **258:** 1819–20.

PEMPHIGOID. Anogenital cicatricial pemphigoid has been reported[1] in a patient receiving long-term clonidine therapy.

1. van Joost T, *et al.* Drug-induced anogenital cicatricial pemphigoid. *Br J Dermatol* 1980; **102:** 715–18.

**Hypersensitivity.** See Effects on the Skin, above.

**Overdosage.** Analysis by the National Poisons Information Service[1] of poisoning by clonidine in 133 children and 37 adults revealed that there were no deaths but clinical features were often severe. Supportive measures were usually adequate but atropine was often needed for severe and persistent bradycardia. Forced diuresis was not advised because hypotension could be enhanced and there was no evidence that excretion of clonidine was increased.

Although naloxone has been suggested as an antidote for clonidine overdose, no reversal of the hypotensive effects of clonidine

300 micrograms was noted in 6 hypertensive subjects receiving naloxone by intravenous infusion.[2] In a retrospective analysis of 47 children with clonidine poisoning, only 3 of 19 given naloxone showed definite improvement;[3] it was concluded that naloxone is at best an inconsistent antidote for clonidine poisoning.

Severe symptoms of overdosage have also been reported following the ingestion of clonidine transdermal patches,[4] and following probable subcutaneous injection during filling of an epidural pump reservoir.[5]

1. Stein B, Volans GN. Dixarit overdose: the problem of attractive tablets. *BMJ* 1978; **2:** 667–8.
2. Rogers JF, Cubeddu LX. Naloxone does not antagonise the antihypertensive effect of clonidine in essential hypertension. *Clin Pharmacol Ther* 1983; **34:** 68–73.
3. Wiley JF, *et al.* Clonidine poisoning in young children. *J Pediatr* 1990; **116:** 654–8.
4. Raber JH, *et al.* Clonidine patch ingestion in an adult. *Ann Pharmacother* 1993; **27:** 719–22. Correction. *ibid.*; 1143.
5. Frye CB, Vance MA. Hypertensive crisis and myocardial infarction following massive clonidine overdose. *Ann Pharmacother* 2000; **34:** 611–15.

## Precautions

Clonidine should be used with caution in patients with cerebrovascular disease, ischaemic heart disease including myocardial infarction, renal impairment, occlusive peripheral vascular disorders such as Raynaud's disease, or those with a history of depression.

Clonidine causes drowsiness and patients should not drive or operate machinery where loss of attention could be dangerous.

Systemic effects also occur following epidural administration and patients should be closely monitored, particularly during the first few days of therapy.

Intravenous injections of clonidine should be given slowly to avoid a possible transient pressor effect especially in patients already receiving other antihypertensives such as guanethidine or reserpine.

**Withdrawal of clonidine therapy** should be gradual as sudden discontinuation may cause rebound hypertension, sometimes severe. Symptoms of increased catecholamine release such as agitation, sweating, tachycardia, headache, and nausea may also occur. Beta blockers can exacerbate the rebound hypertension and if clonidine is being used with a beta-blocking drug, it should not be discontinued until several days after the withdrawal of the beta blocker. Patients should be warned of the risk of missing a dose or stopping the drug without consulting their doctor and should carry a reserve supply.

Although hypotension may occur during anaesthesia in clonidine-treated patients clonidine should not be withdrawn; indeed, if necessary it should be given intravenously during the operation to avoid the risk of rebound hypertension.

**Abuse.** Despite its central effects and ability to cause a form of physical dependence, WHO rated the likelihood of abuse as very low.[1] However, clonidine may potentiate the psychoactive effects of morphine and abuse has been reported.[2]

1. WHO. WHO expert committee on drug dependence: twenty-fifth report. *WHO Tech Rep Ser 775* 1989.
2. Sullivan JT, *et al.* Does clonidine alter the abuse potential of morphine? *Clin Pharmacol Ther* 1995; **57:** 163.

**Diabetes mellitus.** The effects of clonidine on carbohydrate metabolism appear to be variable. Some studies suggest that clonidine does not affect carbohydrate metabolism in diabetic[1] or non-diabetic hypertensive patients,[2] although there has been a report of a diabetic patient in whom clonidine was associated with elevated fasting blood-glucose values,[3] and increased insulin requirements were noted in a diabetic child treated with clonidine for tics.[4] Conversely, clonidine was associated with severe hypoglycaemia in children when used as a provocative test for growth hormone deficiency (see Growth Retardation, below). However, a study in 10 diabetic hypertensive patients found that although clonidine impaired response to an acute glucose load, it did not significantly affect diabetic control over a 10-week period.[5] Problems may arise when clonidine is given to diabetics with autonomic neuropathy: both severe orthostatic hypotension[6] and paradoxical hypertension[7] have been reported.

For discussion of the use of clonidine in diabetic diarrhoea see below.

1. Nilsson-Ehle P, *et al.* Lipoproteins and metabolic control in hypertensive type II diabetics treated with clonidine. *Acta Med Scand* 1988; **224:** 131–4.
2. Molitch ME, *et al.* Effects of antihypertensive medications on carbohydrate metabolism. *Curr Ther Res* 1986; **39:** 398–407.
3. Okada S, *et al.* Effect of clonidine on insulin secretion: a case report. *J Int Med Res* 1986; **14:** 299–302.
4. Mimouni-Bloch A, Mimouni M. Clonidine-induced hyperglycemia in a young diabetic girl. *Ann Pharmacother* 1993; **27:** 980.
5. Guthrie GP, *et al.* Clonidine in patients with diabetes and mild hypertension. *Clin Pharmacol Ther* 1983; **34:** 713–17.
6. Moffat B. Postural hypotension induced by clonidine in insulin dependent diabetes. *BMJ* 1985; **290:** 822.
7. Young E, *et al.* Paradoxical hypertension from clonidine. *Ann Intern Med* 1984; **101:** 282–3.

**ECT.** Maximal ECT stimuli were unsuccessful in producing seizures in 4 of 7 treatment attempts in a 66-year-old patient receiving clonidine therapy.[1] It was suggested that clonidine may elevate the seizure threshold.

1. Elliott RL. Case report of a potential interaction between clonidine and electroconvulsive therapy. *Am J Psychiatry* 1983; **140:** 1237–8.

**Porphyria.** Clonidine hydrochloride has been associated with acute attacks of porphyria and is considered unsafe in porphyric patients.

## Interactions

The hypotensive effect of clonidine may be enhanced by diuretics, other antihypertensives, and drugs that cause hypotension. However, beta blockers may exacerbate rebound hypertension following clonidine withdrawal (see Precautions, above), and tricyclic antidepressants may antagonise the hypotensive effect. The sedative effect of clonidine may be enhanced by CNS depressants.

**Antidepressants.** Although tricyclic antidepressants commonly cause orthostatic hypotension, they may antagonise the hypotensive effects of clonidine. In a study[1] in 5 hypertensive patients receiving clonidine and a diuretic, *desipramine* 75 mg daily resulted in a loss of blood pressure control in 4. Increase in blood pressure generally occurred in the second week of treatment, but 1 patient had a dramatic rise in blood pressure within 24 hours of starting treatment. The mechanism is thought to be due to a central interaction between clonidine and the tricyclic antidepressant, although a peripheral effect cannot be completely excluded.[2] Loss of blood pressure control also occurred in a patient receiving guanfacine, another alpha$_2$-adrenoceptor agonist, when *amitriptyline* was given concomitantly.[3] The reaction recurred with *imipramine*. However, in another study clonidine was given to 11 patients receiving *amitriptyline* or *imipramine*, and 10 achieved good blood pressure control, although 4 developed an acute rise in blood pressure when methyldopa or guanethidine was added to the regimen.[4] *Maprotiline*[5] or *mianserin*[6] do not appear to interact with clonidine.

1. Briant RH, *et al.* Interaction between clonidine and desipramine in man. *BMJ* 1973; **1:** 522–3.
2. van Spanning HW, van Zwieten PA. The interference of tricyclic antidepressants with the central hypotensive effect of clonidine. *Eur J Pharmacol* 1973; **24:** 402–4.
3. Buckley M, Feely J. Antagonism of antihypertensive effect of guanfacine by tricyclic antidepressants. *Lancet* 1991; **337:** 1173–4.
4. Raftos J, *et al.* Clonidine in the treatment of severe hypertension. *Med J Aust* 1973; **1:** 786–93.
5. Gundert-Remy U, *et al.* Lack of interaction between the tetracyclic antidepressant maprotiline and the centrally acting antihypertensive drug clonidine. *Eur J Clin Pharmacol* 1983; **25:** 595–9.
6. Elliott HL, *et al.* Absence of an effect of mianserin on the actions of clonidine or methyldopa in hypertensive patients. *Eur J Clin Pharmacol* 1983; **24:** 15–19.

**Antipsychotics.** Acute, severe hypotension occurred in 2 agitated hypertensive patients following administration of clonidine and either *chlorpromazine* or *haloperidol*. Both patients had mitral insufficiency.[1]

1. Fruncillo RJ, *et al.* Severe hypotension associated with concurrent clonidine and antipsychotic medication. *Am J Psychiatry* 1985; **142:** 274.

**Dopaminergic antiparkinsonian drugs.** For a report of the inhibition of the therapeutic effect of *levodopa* by clonidine, see Antihypertensives, p.1208.

**Immunosuppressants.** For a report of clonidine increasing whole blood-*ciclosporin* concentrations, see p.1355.

## Pharmacokinetics

Following oral administration clonidine is well absorbed from the gastrointestinal tract, with peak plasma concentrations observed after about 3 to 5 hours. It is about 20 to 40% protein bound. About 50% of a dose is metabolised in the liver. It is excreted in the urine as unchanged drug and metabolites, 40 to 60% of an oral dose being excreted in 24 hours as unchanged drug; about 20% of a dose is excreted in the faeces, probably via enterohepatic circulation. The elimination half-life has been variously reported to range between 6 and 24 hours, extended to up to 41 hours in patients with renal impairment. Clonidine crosses the placenta and is distributed into breast milk.

It is absorbed through the skin; absorption is reported to be better when applied to the chest or arm than when applied to the thigh. Therapeutic plasma concentrations are achieved 2 or 3 days after application of a transdermal delivery system and are roughly equivalent to trough concentrations achieved after oral dosage. Therapeutic plasma concentrations are maintained for about 8 hours after removal of the delivery system and then decline slowly over several days.

◊ Reviews.

1. Lowenthal DT, *et al.* Clinical pharmacokinetics of clonidine. *Clin Pharmacokinet* 1988; **14:** 287–310.

**Pregnancy.** A study in 5 pregnant women treated with clonidine for pre-eclampsia[1] reported an average ratio of cord- to plasma-concentrations of 0.87, indicating placental transfer of clonidine.

1. Boutroy MJ, *et al.* Clonidine placental transfer and neonatal adaption. *Early Hum Dev* 1988; **17:** 275–86.

## Uses and Administration

Clonidine is an imidazoline antihypertensive that appears to act centrally to reduce sympathetic tone, resulting in a fall in diastolic and systolic blood pressure and a reduction in heart rate. The exact mechanism is unclear; clonidine stimulates alpha$_2$ adrenoceptors and central imidazoline receptors, but it is not known which receptors mediate which effects. It also acts peripherally, and this peripheral activity may be responsible for the transient increase in blood pressure seen during rapid intravenous administration as well as contributing to the hypotensive effect during chronic administration. Peripheral resistance is reduced during continuous treatment. Cardiovascular reflexes remain intact so orthostatic hypotension occurs infrequently.

Clonidine is used in the management of hypertension (p.825), including hypertensive crises, although other drugs with fewer adverse effects are now generally preferred. It may be given with a thiazide diuretic, but use with a beta blocker should be avoided where possible. Clonidine has also been used in the prophylactic treatment of migraine or recurrent vascular headaches (but see below) and in the treatment of menopausal flushing. It is used with opioids in the management of cancer pain (p.5) and has been tried for various other forms of pain (below). Other uses of clonidine have included the symptomatic treatment of opioid withdrawal (see under Substance Dependence, below), the diagnosis of phaeochromocytoma (below), and administration as eye drops in the management of glaucoma (p.1485). It has also been tried in Tourette's syndrome (below) and numerous other disorders.

Clonidine is used as the hydrochloride. When given by mouth, its haemodynamic effects appear in about 30 to 60 minutes, reaching a maximum after 2 to 4 hours and lasting up to 8 hours. Tolerance to clonidine has been reported. Withdrawal of clonidine should be gradual because of the risk of rebound hypertension.

In **hypertension**, the usual initial dose of clonidine hydrochloride is 50 to 100 micrograms three times daily by mouth (or in the US, 100 micrograms twice daily), increased every second or third day according to response; the usual maintenance dose is 300 to 1200 micrograms daily but doses of 1800 micrograms or more daily may sometimes be required. Modified-release preparations have been used. Clonidine may also be given by transdermal delivery systems that are applied once a week and deliver 100 to 300 micrograms of clonidine base daily at a constant rate.

Clonidine hydrochloride may be given by slow intravenous injection over 10 to 15 minutes in hypertensive crises, usually in doses of 150 to 300 micrograms. The effect usually appears within 10 minutes, but transient hypertension may precede hypotension if the injection is given too rapidly. The hypotensive effect reaches a maximum about 30 to 60 minutes after administration and the duration is about 3 to 7 hours; up to 750 micrograms may be given intravenously over 24 hours. Although oral administration does not produce a sufficiently rapid hypotensive effect for use in an emergency situation, a dose of 100 to 200 micrograms initially followed by 50 to 100 micrograms every hour until control of blood pressure is achieved or a maximum of 500 to 800 micrograms is reached, has been recommended for the control of severe hypertension.

In the prophylaxis of **migraine** or recurrent vascular headaches and in the treatment of **menopausal flush-**

**ing**, a dose of 50 micrograms twice daily by mouth has been used, increased, if there is no remission after 2 weeks, to 75 micrograms twice daily.

In the management of severe **cancer pain**, clonidine hydrochloride may be given by continuous epidural infusion with an opioid, in an initial dose of 30 micrograms/hour, adjusted according to response.

**Anxiety disorders.** Clonidine has been tried in various anxiety disorders but evidence of efficacy is limited. A review[1] of the use of clonidine in panic attacks (p.663) considered that it might be useful as a last-line anxiolytic in patients unresponsive to standard treatment as occasional success had been obtained in a few patients. There have also been isolated reports of small numbers of patients with post-traumatic stress disorder (p.664) who have benefited from treatment with clonidine.[2]


1. Puzantian T, Hart LL. Clonidine in panic disorder. *Ann Pharmacother* 1993; **27:** 1351–3.
2. Harmon RJ, Riggs PD. Clonidine for posttraumatic stress disorder in preschool children. *J Am Acad Child Adolesc Psychiatry* 1996; **35:** 1247–9.


**Cardiac arrhythmias.** Atrial fibrillation (p.816) is managed by treatment to slow the increased ventricular responses or by cardioversion. Control of ventricular rate is usually achieved with digoxin, beta blockers, or calcium-channel blockers but clonidine, which reduces sympathetic tone and thus reduces heart rate, has also been tried.[1-3]


1. Roth A, *et al.* Clonidine for patients with rapid atrial fibrillation. *Ann Intern Med* 1992; **116:** 388–90.
2. Scardi S, *et al.* Oral clonidine for heart rate control in chronic atrial fibrillation. *Lancet* 1993; **341:** 1211–12.
3. Simpson CS, *et al.* Clinical assessment of clonidine in the treatment of new-onset rapid atrial fibrillation; a prospective, randomized clinical trial. *Am Heart J* 2001; **142:** e3.


**Diarrhoea.** Some studies have shown that clonidine possesses antidiarrhoeal properties. Clonidine may stimulate $alpha_2$ adrenoceptors on enterocytes thus promoting fluid and electrolyte absorption and inhibiting anion secretion. It may also modify intestinal motility or rectal sphincter tone.

Most experience with clonidine is in diabetic diarrhoea (see Diabetic Complications, p.326). Clonidine 100 to 600 micrograms by mouth every 12 hours reduced diabetic diarrhoea in 3 patients with type 1 diabetes[1] and good results have also been reported in such patients when transdermal clonidine was used.[2,3] Benefit has also been reported in patients with symptoms of diabetic gastroparesis in addition to diarrhoea.[3,4] However, oral (but perhaps not transdermal) clonidine may worsen orthostatic hypotension in patients with diabetic diarrhoea and this may limit its usefulness.[5]


1. Fedorak RN, *et al.* Treatment of diabetic diarrhea with clonidine. *Ann Intern Med* 1985; **102:** 197–9.
2. Sacerdote A. Topical clonidine for diabetic diarrhea. *Ann Intern Med* 1986; **105:** 139.
3. Sacerdote AS. Topical clonidine and diabetic gastroparesis. *Ann Intern Med* 1990; **112:** 796.
4. Migliore A, *et al.* Diabetic diarrhea and clonidine. *Ann Intern Med* 1988; **109:** 170–1.
5. Ogbonnaya KI, Arem R. Diabetic diarrhea: pathophysiology, diagnosis, and management. *Arch Intern Med* 1990; **150:** 262–7.


**Extrapyramidal disorders.** There is limited evidence[1] from studies of small numbers of patients that clonidine might reduce symptoms of antipsychotic-induced akathisia and tardive dyskinesia (p.677). However, adverse effects such as sedation and hypotension may limit use.


1. Ahmed I, Takeshita J. Clonidine: a critical review of its role in the treatment of psychiatric disorders. *CNS Drugs* 1996; **6:** 53–70.


**Growth retardation.** Clonidine has been reported to be a stimulant of growth hormone release, presumably as a result of central alpha-adrenergic stimulation, and has been tried in the diagnosis and management of growth retardation (p.1314). It may be given orally as a provocative test for growth hormone deficiency,[1,2] particularly in children,[3] although some consider measurement of circulating somatomedins to be more useful than provocative tests. Caution is required when performing the test in children since severe hypoglycaemia has been reported.[4] Clonidine has also been tried in growth retardation, both in children with growth hormone deficiency and in short children without proven deficiency, but results have been contradictory and largely unsatisfactory.[5-7]


1. Gil-Ad I, *et al.* Oral clonidine as a growth hormone stimulation test. *Lancet* 1979; **ii:** 278–80.
2. Hoffman WH, *et al.* Relationship of plasma clonidine to growth hormone concentrations in children and adolescents. *J Clin Pharmacol* 1989; **29:** 538–42.
3. Hindmarsh PC, Swift PGF. An assessment of growth hormone provocation tests. *Arch Dis Child* 1995; **72:** 362–8.
4. Huang C, *et al.* Hypoglycemia associated with clonidine testing for growth hormone deficiency. *J Pediatr* 2001; **139:** 323–4.
5. Pintor C, *et al.* Clonidine treatment for short stature. *Lancet*; 1987; **i:** 1226–30.
6. Pescovitz OH, Tan E. Lack of benefit of clonidine treatment for short stature in a double-blind, placebo-controlled trial. *Lancet* 1988; **ii:** 874–7.
7. Allen DB. Effects of nightly clonidine administration on growth velocity in short children without growth hormone deficiency: a double-blind, placebo-controlled study. *J Pediatr* 1993; **122:** 32–6.


**Hyperactivity.** Drug treatment of attention deficit hyperactivity disorder (p.1583) is usually initiated with a central stimulant; clonidine has been tried mainly as an adjunct to stimulant therapy. A meta-analysis[1] of clonidine used to treat this disorder occurring alone or with other conditions, including tic disorders (see Tourette's Syndrome, below), concluded that clonidine may be a useful second-line treatment but is less effective than stimulants and is associated with many adverse effects. There have been reports[2] of sudden death when clonidine has been used with stimulants, but the role of the drugs in these events is unclear. A study[3] in children with both attention-deficit hyperactivity disorder and Tourette's syndrome found that clonidine used with methylphenidate was more effective than either drug alone, and only 1 child had evidence of adverse cardiac effects.


1. Connor DF, *et al.* A meta-analysis of clonidine for symptoms of attention-deficit hyperactivity disorder. *J Am Acad Child Adolesc Psychiatry* 1999; **38:** 1551–9.
2. Fenichel RR. Combining methylphenidate and clonidine: the role of post-marketing surveillance. *J Child Adolesc Psychopharmacol* 1995; **5:** 155–6.
3. The Tourette's Syndrome Study Group. Treatment of ADHD in children with tics: a randomized controlled trial. *Neurology* 2002; **58:** 527–36.


**Menopausal disorders.** Although HRT is the mainstay of treatment for menopausal disorders (p.1540) clonidine has been of some use in countering vasomotor symptoms in patients who cannot receive HRT;[1,2] however, some studies have failed to demonstrate a reduction in hot flushes. The adverse effects reported in normotensive women, including orthostatic hypotension, may mean that it is best reserved for women who are also hypertensive.

Clonidine has also been tried[3] for hot flushes in women receiving tamoxifen.


1. Young RL, *et al.* Management of menopause when estrogen cannot be used. *Drugs* 1990; **40:** 220–30.
2. Lucero MA, McCloskey WW. Alternatives to estrogen for the treatment of hot flashes. *Ann Pharmacother* 1997; **31:** 915–17.
3. Pandya KJ, *et al.* Oral clonidine in postmenopausal patients with breast cancer experiencing tamoxifen-induced hot flashes: a University of Rochester Cancer Center Community Clinical Oncology Program study. *Ann Intern Med* 2000; **132:** 788–93.


**Migraine.** Propranolol and pizotifen are probably the most well-established drugs for prophylaxis of migraine (p.464). Many other drugs have been used, including clonidine, but a review of clinical trials[1] indicated that it was a poor first choice and seemed unlikely to work even as a last resort. It has been used in patients whose attacks may be precipitated by tyramine-containing foods.


1. Anonymous. Clonidine in migraine prophylaxis—now obsolete. *Drug Ther Bull* 1990; **28:** 79–80.


**Orthostatic hypotension.** Clonidine has produced beneficial effects in a few patients with orthostatic hypotension (p.1100), including orthostatic hypotension due to autonomic neuropathy.[1] Its use in this condition is somewhat paradoxical as orthostatic hypotension may occur as an adverse effect of clonidine therapy.


1. Acott PD, *et al.* Effectiveness of clonidine in congenital orthostatic hypotension. *J Pediatr* 1990; **116:** 666–7.


**Pain.** Administration of opioids and local anaesthetics by the epidural or intrathecal routes can produce effective analgesia but adverse effects are common. Many other drugs, including clonidine, have been tried by these routes, alone or as adjuncts. Clonidine is thought to produce analgesia by a direct action on $alpha_2$ adrenoceptors in the spinal cord. Some studies[1,2] of clonidine given *epidurally* alone in a dose of 2 micrograms/kg or 150 micrograms have produced satisfactory pain relief, although duration of action was short. Higher doses have also been used.[3] Hypotension and sedation have been reported as frequent side-effects and an editorial on epidural clonidine[4] considered it unlikely that clonidine would be useful as a sole analgesic drug although it may have a role in combination with opioids and/or local anaesthetics. Clonidine has been given epidurally with various opioids and has produced satisfactory analgesia in postoperative pain,[5] neuropathic pain,[6] and labour pain;[7] the combination is also used in chronic pain due to cancer. Clonidine has also been given epidurally with local anaesthetics and enhanced analgesia has been reported in postoperative pain,[8] labour pain,[9] and in chronic pain.[10] Epidural clonidine combined with both an opioid and a local anaesthetic may increase the duration of analgesia during labour, but adverse effects on the fetal heartbeat may limit this use.[11] The combination of clonidine and bupivacaine has also produced enhanced analgesia in a study in children undergoing lower limb orthopaedic surgery;[12] clonidine was given epidurally in a dose of 2 micrograms/kg. Clonidine and bupivacaine have been given intrathecally[13] and may produce less urinary retention than the combination of morphine with bupivacaine.[14] Long-term intrathecal administration of clonidine with midazolam has also been used[15] and may be effective in refractory neuropathic or musculoskeletal pain.

Analgesia has also been reported following administration of clonidine by other routes. A study comparing *intravenous* and epidural clonidine 150 micrograms in 10 patients with back pain reported that intravenous clonidine produced better analgesia, although pain relief was poor following administration by either route.[16] However, a study[3] in postoperative patients using an initial dose of clonidine 8 micrograms/kg followed by bolus doses of 30 micrograms as required found that the epidural and intravenous routes were both effective but the epidural route produced less sedation. In another study,[17] *intramuscular* injection of clonidine 2 micrograms/kg was as effective as the same dose given epidurally for relief of postoperative pain. Clonidine has some effect when given *orally*[18-21] but the effect is much less marked than following parenteral administration. Premedication with oral clonidine has been reported to provide effective postoperative analgesia in children.[22] *Transdermal* clonidine has been tried for postoperative analgesia.[23] The *intra-articular* route has also been used.[24]

The role of clonidine in the management of pain remains to be established. For further discussion of pain and the management of its various types, see p.2.


1. Bonnet F, *et al.* Postoperative analgesia with extradural clonidine. *Br J Anaesth* 1989; **63:** 465–9.
2. Lund C, *et al.* Comparison of the effects of extradural clonidine with those of morphine on postoperative pain, stress responses, cardiopulmonary function and motor and sensory block. *Br J Anaesth* 1989; **63:** 516–19.
3. Bernard J-M, *et al.* Comparison of intravenous and epidural clonidine for postoperative patient-controlled analgesia. *Anesth Analg* 1995; **81:** 706–12.
4. Macdonald R. Extradural clonidine—the need for well designed controlled trials. *Br J Anaesth* 1994; **72:** 255–7.
5. Carabine UA, *et al.* Extradural clonidine infusions for analgesia after total hip replacement. *Br J Anaesth* 1992; **68:** 338–43.
6. Tamsen A, Gordh T. Epidural clonidine produces analgesia. *Lancet* 1984; **ii:** 231–2.
7. Buggy DJ, MacDowell C. Extradural analgesia with clonidine and fentanyl compared with 0.25% bupivacaine in the first stage of labour. *Br J Anaesth* 1996; **76:** 319–21.
8. Carabine UA, *et al.* Extradural clonidine and bupivacaine for postoperative analgesia. *Br J Anaesth* 1992; **68:** 132–5.
9. O'Meara ME, Gin T. Comparison of 0.125% bupivacaine with 0.125% bupivacaine and clonidine as extradural analgesia in the first stage of labour. *Br J Anaesth* 1993; **71:** 651–6.
10. Glynn C, O'Sullivan K. A double-blind randomised comparison of the effects of epidural clonidine, lignocaine and the combination of clonidine and lignocaine in patients with chronic pain. *Pain* 1995; **64:** 337–43.
11. Chassard D, *et al.* Extradural clonidine combined with sufentanil and 0.0625% bupivacaine for analgesia in labour. *Br J Anaesth* 1996; **77:** 458–62.
12. Lee JJ, Rubin AP. Comparison of a bupivacaine-clonidine mixture with plain bupivacaine for caudal analgesia in children. *Br J Anaesth* 1994; **72:** 258–62.
13. Bonnet F, *et al.* Prevention of tourniquet pain by spinal isobaric bupivacaine with clonidine. *Br J Anaesth* 1989; **63:** 93–6.
14. Gentili M, Bonnet F. Spinal clonidine produces less urinary retention than spinal morphine. *Br J Anaesth* 1996; **76:** 872–3.
15. Borg PAJ, Krijnen HJ. Long-term intrathecal administration of midazolam and clonidine. *Clin J Pain* 1996; **12:** 63–8.
16. Carroll D, *et al.* Single-dose, randomized, double-blind, double-dummy cross-over comparison of extradural and I.V. clonidine in chronic pain. *Br J Anaesth* 1993; **71:** 665–9.
17. Bonnet F, *et al.* Clonidine-induced analgesia in postoperative patients: epidural versus intramuscular administration. *Anesthesiology* 1990; **72:** 423–7.
18. Glynn CF, *et al.* Role of spinal noradrenergic system in transmission of pain in patients with spinal cord injury. *Lancet* 1986; **ii:** 1249–50.
19. Tan Y-M, Croese J. Clonidine and diabetic patients with leg pains. *Ann Intern Med* 1986; **105:** 633–4.
20. Petros AJ, Wright RMB. Epidural and oral clonidine in domiciliary control of deafferentation pain. *Lancet* 1987; **i:** 1034.
21. Benhamou D, *et al.* Addition of oral clonidine to postoperative patient-controlled analgesia with i.v. morphine. *Br J Anaesth* 1994; **72:** 537–40.
22. Mikawa K, *et al.* Oral clonidine premedication reduces postoperative pain in children. *Anesth Analg* 1996; **82:** 225–30.
23. Segal IS, *et al.* Clinical efficacy of oral transdermal clonidine combinations during the perioperative period. *Anesthesiology* 1991; **74:** 220–5.
24. Gentili M, *et al.* Intra-articular morphine and clonidine produce comparable analgesia but the combination is not more effective. *Br J Anaesth* 1997; **79:** 660–1.


**Phaeochromocytoma.** Clonidine acts centrally to suppress catecholamine release and may be used[1] in the diagnosis of phaeochromocytoma (p.831). Experience gained with the clonidine suppression test and a review of published studies indicated that it is of value in selected patients with moderately elevated plasma and/or urinary catecholamine concentrations.[2]


1. Bravo EL, *et al.* Clonidine-suppression test: a useful aid in the diagnosis of pheochromocytoma. *N Engl J Med* 1981; **305:** 623–6.
2. Lenz T, *et al.* Clonidine suppression test revisited. *Blood Press* 1998; **7:** 153–9.


**Premedication.** Clonidine has been given pre-operatively for its sedative, anxiolytic, and analgesic effects and to provide haemodynamic stability and reduce anaesthetic requirements; see Pain above for some further details. Pre-operative use has also been reported to reduce the incidence of postoperative vomiting in children[1] and in women.[2] Clonidine may attenuate the perioperative stress response and has been shown to reduce perioperative oxygen consumption, which is a marker of sympathetic activation.[3] It may also reduce the risk of perioperative myocardial ischaemia.[4]


1. Mikawa K, *et al.* Oral clonidine premedication reduces vomiting in children after strabismus surgery. *Can J Anaesth* 1995; **42:** 977–81.
2. Oddby-Muhrbeck E, *et al.* Effects of clonidine on postoperative nausea and vomiting in breast cancer surgery. *Anesthesiology* 2002; **96:** 1109–14.
3. Taittonen MT, *et al.* Effect of clonidine and dexmedetomidine premedication on perioperative oxygen consumption and haemodynamic state. *Br J Anaesth* 1997; **78:** 400–406.
4. Nishina K, *et al.* Efficacy of clonidine for prevention of perioperative myocardial ischemia: a critical appraisal and meta-analysis of the literature. *Anesthesiology* 2002; **96:** 323–9.


**Restless legs syndrome.** Numerous drugs have been tried for the treatment of restless legs syndrome (see Parasomnias, p.667). Symptomatic improvement has been reported with clonidine in a number of case studies[1,2] and small controlled trials,[3] but side-effects may limit its use.


1. Handwerker JV, Palmer RF. Clonidine in the treatment of "restless leg" syndrome. *N Engl J Med* 1985; **313:** 1228–9.

2. Zoe A, *et al.* High-dose clonidine in a case of restless legs syndrome. *Ann Pharmacother* 1994; **28:** 878–81.
3. Wagner ML, *et al.* Randomized, double-blind, placebo-controlled study of clonidine in restless legs syndrome. *Sleep* 1996; **19:** 52–8.

**Shivering.** Numerous drugs, including clonidine, have been tried for the treatment of postoperative shivering (p.1295). Clonidine's central and peripheral effects could both account for its antishivering activity, but some have suggested that it acts by resetting the central threshold for shivering. In preliminary studies a small intravenous dose of clonidine 75 micrograms or 30 micrograms stopped shivering after general anaesthesia[1] or epidural anaesthesia,[2] respectively. Clonidine given intra-operatively has also been reported to reduce the incidence of postoperative shivering.[3-5]

1. Joris J, *et al.* Clonidine and ketanserin both are effective treatment for postanesthetic shivering. *Anesthesiology* 1993; **79:** 532–9.
2. Capogna G, Celleno D. IV clonidine for post-extradural shivering in parturients: a preliminary study. *Br J Anaesth* 1993; **71:** 294–5.
3. Steinfath M, *et al.* Clonidine administered intraoperatively prevents postoperative shivering. *Br J Clin Pharmacol* 1995; **39:** 580P–581P.
4. Vanderstappen I, *et al.* The effect of prophylactic clonidine on postoperative shivering: a large prospective double-blind study. *Anaesthesia* 1996; **51:** 351–5.
5. Sia S. I.v. clonidine prevents post-extradural shivering. *Br J Anaesth* 1998; **81:** 145–6.

**Spasticity.** Clonidine, given alone or as an adjunct to baclofen, has been tried in patients with various forms of spasticity (p.1386) including those refractory to baclofen.[1-4]

1. Nance PW, *et al.* Clonidine in spinal cord injury. *Can Med Assoc J* 1985; **133:** 41–2.
2. Donovan WH, *et al.* Clonidine effect on spasticity: a clinical trial. *Arch Phys Med Rehabil* 1988; **69:** 193–4.
3. Sandford PR, *et al.* Clonidine in the treatment of brainstem spasticity: case report. *Am J Phys Med Rehabil* 1992; **71:** 301–3.
4. Middleton JW, *et al.* Intrathecal clonidine and baclofen in the management of spasticity and neuropathic pain following spinal cord injury: a case study. *Arch Phys Med Rehabil* 1996; **77:** 824–6.

**Substance dependence.** ALCOHOL. Although drug treatment of alcohol withdrawal (p.1166) is usually with a benzodiazepine, clonidine has sometimes been used to good effect,[1,2] although it does not have any effect on convulsions or delirium tremens[3] and should not be used as sole therapy.

1. Guthrie SK. The treatment of alcohol withdrawal. *Pharmacotherapy* 1989; **9:** 131–43.
2. Ip Yam PC, *et al.* Clonidine in the treatment of alcohol withdrawal in the intensive care unit. *Br J Anaesth* 1992; **68:** 106–8.
3. Anonymous. Alcohol problems in the general hospital. *Drug Ther Bull* 1991; **29:** 69–71.

OPIOID ANALGESICS. Clonidine has been reported to be useful in controlling withdrawal symptoms following abrupt discontinuation of opioids (p.71). However, a systematic review[1] of the use of alpha$_2$-adrenoceptor agonists, including clonidine, concluded that, for gradual withdrawal, they were no more effective than reducing doses of methadone over a period of around 10 days, and patients experienced more adverse effects and withdrew from treatment sooner with clonidine.

Clonidine has also been used with naltrexone to shorten the withdrawal syndrome, allowing withdrawal to be achieved within 6 days.[2] Subsequent modification to the regimen allowed 38 of 40 patients addicted to methadone to withdraw completely in 4 to 5 days.[3] Patients required a mean of 2.3 mg of clonidine on the first day which reduced, but did not abolish, symptoms. A further modification was reported allowing opioid withdrawal with minimal drop-out over 2 to 3 days.[4]

Clonidine has also been used in the management of neonatal abstinence syndrome (p.72) in infants born to opioid-addicted mothers maintained on methadone.[5,6] Benefit occurred in 6 of 7 such infants given an initial clonidine dose of 0.5 to 1 microgram/kg by mouth, increased over 1 to 2 days to 3 to 5 micrograms/kg daily in divided doses. Total length of treatment ranged from 6 to 17 days. The infant who failed to respond was born to a mother also receiving haloperidol, desipramine, and theophylline.[6]

1. Gowing L, *et al.* Alpha2 adrenergic agonists for the management of opioid withdrawal. Available in The Cochrane Library; Issue 1. Chichester: John Wiley; 2004
2. Charney DS, *et al.* Clonidine and naltrexone: a safe, effective, and rapid treatment of abrupt withdrawal from methadone therapy. *Arch Gen Psychiatry* 1982; **39:** 1327–32.
3. Charney DS, *et al.* The combined use of clonidine and naltrexone as a rapid, safe, and effective treatment of abrupt withdrawal from methadone. *Am J Psychiatry* 1986; **143:** 831–7.
4. Brewer C, *et al.* Opioid withdrawal and naltrexone induction in 48-72 hours with minimal drop-out, using a modification of the naltrexone-clonidine technique. *Br J Psychiatry* 1988; **153:** 340–3.
5. Hoder EL, *et al.* Clonidine in neonatal narcotic-abstinence syndrome. *N Engl J Med* 1981; **305:** 1284.
6. Hoder EL, *et al.* Clonidine treatment of neonatal narcotic abstinence syndrome. *Psychiatry Res* 1984; **13:** 243–51.

SMOKING. Nicotine dependence may be managed using behavioural or psychological counselling. In addition, nicotine replacement therapy (see Smoking Cessation, p.1721) can help alleviate withdrawal symptoms. A number of other drugs, including clonidine, have also been tried. A meta-analysis[1] found clonidine, given orally in doses of 150 to 450 micrograms daily, or transdermally in doses of 100 to 300 micrograms daily, to be effective; however adverse effects limit its usefulness and clonidine is usually reserved for second-line treatment in those who experience severe agitation and anxiety when stopping smoking.

Some individual studies have found clonidine to be more effective in women although the authors of the meta-analysis[1] recommended that these results be interpreted cautiously since some studies also found that women were less successful in giving up smoking unaided than men; treatment with clonidine, however, resulted in similar success rates in both men and women.

1. Gourlay SG, *et al.* Clonidine for smoking cessation. Available in The Cochrane Library; Issue 1. Chichester: John Wiley; 2004.

**Tourette's syndrome.** Clonidine is one of many drugs that have been tried in the management of Tourette's syndrome (see Tics under Extrapyramidal Disorders, p.664).

Disturbance of monoamine metabolism (including dopamine, noradrenaline, and serotonin) has been implicated in Tourette's syndrome. Clonidine is thought to reduce central noradrenergic activity and may also affect other neurochemical systems, and these properties may account for its beneficial effects in this disorder. Studies of clonidine in Tourette's syndrome have produced mixed results,[1-5] although this may reflect the difficulty in study design for a disease that can vary considerably in severity and presence of comorbid conditions and whose symptoms wax and wane. Nevertheless, clonidine is increasingly favoured for first-line treatment in patients with mild to moderate symptoms, because of a relative lack of serious adverse effects when compared to the commonly used antipsychotics pimozide and haloperidol. Clonidine has also been reported to successfully control symptoms in some children with Tourette's syndrome unresponsive to haloperidol.[1]

Clonidine has also been used with stimulants in children with Tourette's syndrome and attention-deficit hyperactivity disorder, although there have been concerns about the toxicity of such combinations (see Hyperactivity, above).

1. Cohen DJ, *et al.* Clonidine in Tourette's syndrome. *Lancet* 1979; **ii:** 551–3.
2. Shapiro AK, *et al.* Treatment of Gilles de la Tourette's syndrome with clonidine and neuroleptics. *Arch Gen Psychiatry* 1983; **40:** 1235–40.
3. Leckman JF, *et al.* Short- and long-term treatment of Tourette's syndrome with clonidine: a clinical perspective. *Neurology* 1985; **35:** 343–51.
4. Goetz CG, *et al.* Clonidine and Gilles de la Tourette's syndrome: double-blind study using objective rating methods. *Ann Neurol* 1987; **21:** 307–10.
5. Leckman JF, *et al.* Clonidine treatment of Gilles de la Tourette's syndrome. *Arch Gen Psychiatry* 1991; **48:** 324–8.

### Preparations

***BP 2003:*** Clonidine Injection; Clonidine Tablets;
***USP 27:*** Clonidine Hydrochloride and Chlorthalidone Tablets; Clonidine Hydrochloride Tablets.

**Proprietary Preparations** (details are given in Part 3)
***Arg.:*** Clonidural; ***Austral.:*** Catapres; ***Austria:*** Catapresan; Glausine; Isoglaucon; ***Belg.:*** Catapressan; Dixarit; ***Braz.:*** Atensina; Clonesina; Neo Clodil; ***Canad.:*** Catapres; Dixarit; ***Chile:*** Catapresan; ***Denm.:*** Catapresan; ***Fin.:*** Caprysin†; Catapresan; ***Fr.:*** Catapressan; ***Ger.:*** Aruclonin; Catapresan; Clonid-Ophtal; Clonistada; Dispaclonidin; Dixarit; Haemiton; Isoglaucon; Mirfat; Paracefan; ***Gr.:*** Catapresan; ***Hong Kong:*** Catapres; Dixarit; ***India:*** Arkamin; Catapres; ***Irl.:*** Catapres; Dixarit; ***Israel:*** Clonnirit; Normopresan; ***Ital.:*** Adesipress-TTS; Catapresan; Isoglaucon; ***Malaysia:*** Dixarit; ***Mex.:*** Catapresan; Epiclodina; ***Neth.:*** Catapresan; Dixarit; ***Norw.:*** Catapresan; ***NZ:*** Catapres; Dixarit; ***Port.:*** Catapresan; Edolglau; ***S.Afr.:*** Catapres†; Dixarit; Menograine; ***Singapore:*** Dixarit; ***Spain:*** Catapresan; Isoglaucon; ***Swed.:*** Catapresan; ***Switz.:*** Catapresan; ***Thai.:*** Catapres; ***UK:*** Catapres; Dixarit; ***USA:*** Catapres; Duraclon.

**Multi-ingredient:** ***Arg.:*** Bemplas; Pertenso; ***Canad.:*** Combipres†; ***Ger.:*** Combipresan; Haemiton compositum; ***India:*** Arkamin-H; Catapres Diu; ***Spain:*** Dilapres†; ***USA:*** Clorpres; Combipres.

## Clopamide *(BAN, USAN, rINN)*

Clopamida; DT-327. 4-Chloro-*N*-(2,6-dimethylpiperidino)-3-sulphamoylbenzamide; *cis*-3-(Aminosulphonyl)-4-chloro-*N*-(2,6-dimethyl-1-piperidinyl)benzamide.

$C_{14}H_{20}ClN_3O_3S$ = 345.8.
*CAS — 636-54-4.*
*ATC — C03BA03.*

### Profile

Clopamide is a diuretic with properties similar to those of the thiazide diuretics (see Hydrochlorothiazide, p.933) even though it does not contain a thiazide ring system. It is used for oedema, including that associated with heart failure (p.820), and for hypertension (p.825).

Diuresis starts in 1 to 2 hours, reaches a maximum in about 3 to 6 hours, and lasts for up to 24 hours.

In the treatment of oedema the usual dose is 10 to 40 mg daily by mouth; frequency may be reduced for maintenance. For hypertension doses of 5 to 10 mg daily, either alone, or with other antihypertensives have been used.

### Preparations

**Proprietary Preparations** (details are given in Part 3)
***Denm.:*** Adurix; ***Ger.:*** Brinaldix; ***India:*** Brinaldix.

**Multi-ingredient:** ***Austria:*** Brinerdin; Viskaldix; ***Belg.:*** Viskaldix; ***Braz.:*** Viskaldix; ***Chile:*** Viskaldix; ***Fr.:*** Viskaldix; ***Ger.:*** Briserin N; Viskaldix; ***Irl.:*** Viskaldix; ***Ital.:*** Brinerdina; ***Malaysia:*** Viskaldix; ***Neth.:*** Viskaldix; ***NZ:*** Viskaldix†; ***Port.:*** Brinerdine; ***S.Afr.:*** Brinerdin; ***Spain:*** Brinerdina; ***Switz.:*** Brinerdine; Viskaldix; ***Thai.:*** Bedin; Brinerdin; Hyperdine; Viskaldix; ***UK:*** Viskaldix.

## Clopidogrel Bisulfate *(USAN, rINNM)*

Bisulfato de clopidogrel; Clopidogrel Bisulphate *(BANM)*; Clopidogrel Hydrogen Sulphate; PCR-4099 (clopidogrel); SR-25990C. Methyl (*S*)-2-chlorophenyl(4,5,6,7-tetrahydrothieno[3,2-*c*]pyridin-5-yl)acetate bisulphate; Methyl (+)-(*S*)-α-(*o*-chlorophenyl)-6,7-dihydrothieno[3,2-*c*]pyridine-5(4*H*)-acetate sulphate.

$C_{16}H_{16}ClNO_2S,H_2SO_4$ = 419.9.
*CAS — 113665-84-2 (clopidogrel); 94188-84-8 (clopidogrel); 120202-66-6 (clopidogrel bisulfate).*
*ATC — B01AC04.*

**Pharmacopoeias.** In *US.*

**USP 27** (Clopidogrel Bisulfate). A white to off-white powder. Freely soluble in water and in methyl alcohol; practically insoluble in ether.

### Adverse Effects and Precautions

As for Ticlopidine, p.1011. The incidence of adverse effects, particularly blood dyscrasias, is lower with clopidogrel, although fatalities have been reported (see Effects on the Blood, p.1011).

**Effects on taste.** Loss of taste occurred in 2 patients 6 to 8 weeks after starting treatment with clopidogrel, but recovered fully when clopidogrel was withdrawn.[1] Rechallenge in 1 of the patients led to recurrence of the taste loss, which persisted when treatment was discontinued.

1. Golka K, *et al.* Reversible ageusia as an effect of clopidogrel treatment. *Lancet* 2000; **355:** 465–6.

### Interactions

Clopidogrel should be used with caution in patients receiving other drugs that increase the risk of bleeding, including anticoagulants, other antiplatelets, and NSAIDs.

### Pharmacokinetics

Clopidogrel is rapidly but incompletely absorbed after oral administration; absorption appears to be at least 50%. It is a prodrug and is extensively metabolised in the liver, mainly to the inactive carboxylic acid derivative. The active metabolite appears to be a thiol derivative but has not been identified in plasma. Clopidogrel and the carboxylic acid derivative are highly protein bound. Clopidogrel and its metabolites are excreted in urine and in faeces; after oral administration, about 50% of a dose is recovered from the urine and about 46% from the faeces.

### Uses and Administration

Clopidogrel is a thienopyridine antiplatelet drug used in thromboembolic disorders. It is an analogue of ticlopidine (p.1011) and acts by inhibiting adenosine diphosphate-mediated platelet aggregation. It is given prophylactically as an alternative to aspirin in patients at risk of thromboembolic disorders such as myocardial infarction (p.828), peripheral arterial disease (p.830), and stroke (p.836). Clopidogrel is also used with aspirin in the management of unstable angina (p.813), and has been tried as an alternative to ticlopidine in patients undergoing coronary stenting.

Clopidogrel is given by mouth as the bisulfate, but doses are expressed in terms of the base; 97.86 mg of clopidogrel bisulfate is equivalent to 75 mg of base.

For the **prophylaxis of thromboembolic events**, the usual dose of clopidogrel is 75 mg once daily.

In the management of **acute coronary syndromes**, including unstable angina and non-Q wave myocardial infarction, clopidogrel is given as a single 300-mg loading dose, followed by 75 mg once daily.

◊ Reviews.

1. Sharis PJ, *et al.* The antiplatelet effects of ticlopidine and clopidogrel. *Ann Intern Med* 1998; **129:** 394–405.
2. Jarvis B, Simpson K. Clopidogrel: a review of its use in the prevention of atherothrombosis. *Drugs* 2000; **60:** 347–77.
3. Solet DJ, *et al.* The role of adenosine 5′-diphosphate receptor blockade in patients with cardiovascular disease. *Am J Med* 2001; **111:** 45–53.

**Atherosclerotic disorders.** The use of aspirin to reduce the risk of cardiovascular events in patients with atherosclerotic vascular disorders is well established. Clopidogrel may have a role as an alternative. The CAPRIE trial[1] compared clopidogrel with aspirin in 19 185 patients at risk of ischaemic events, and found that clopidogrel reduced the risk of ischaemic stroke, myocardial infarction, or death from vascular causes to a greater extent than aspirin, although the absolute difference was small.

Clopidogrel has also been used with aspirin in patients with unstable angina. In the CURE trial,[2] the risk of cardiovascular death, myocardial infarction, or stroke was lower in patients treated with clopidogrel and aspirin, compared with those receiving aspirin alone. Clopidogrel was given in a loading dose of 300 mg, started within 24 hours of the onset of symptoms, followed by 75 mg daily for 3 to 12 months.


1. CAPRIE Steering Committee. A randomised, blinded, trial of clopidogrel versus aspirin in patients at risk of ischaemic events (CAPRIE). *Lancet* 1996; **348:** 1329–39.
2. The Clopidogrel in Unstable Angina to Prevent Recurrent Events Trial Investigators. Effects of clopidogrel in addition to aspirin in patients with acute coronary syndromes without ST-segment elevation. *N Engl J Med* 2001; **345:** 494–502. Correction. *ibid.*; 1716.


**Reperfusion and revascularisation procedures.** Coronary stents are being used increasingly to treat and prevent restenosis following angioplasty procedures (see p.834). Thrombotic occlusion commonly complicates their use and patients have been aggressively treated with a combination of antiplatelet drugs and anticoagulants. Recent studies, however, suggest that antiplatelet treatment alone may be adequate if the stent has been positioned correctly and the risk of thrombosis is considered to be low.

A regimen of long-term aspirin with ticlopidine for 4 weeks has been widely used. However, use of ticlopidine is associated with haematological toxicity and clopidogrel has been studied as an alternative. Observational studies[1,2] indicated that clopidogrel and ticlopidine produced similar benefits. In a subsequent randomised trial (CLASSICS),[3] in which clopidogrel was given in a dose of 75 mg daily for 28 days, with or without a 300-mg loading dose, the combination of clopidogrel with aspirin appeared to be as effective as ticlopidine with aspirin and was also better tolerated. Continuation of clopidogrel with aspirin for 12 months may provide additional benefit.[4]

Clopidogrel has also been given long-term in combination with aspirin following angioplasty (with or without stenting) in patients with unstable angina. In the PCI-CURE study,[5] the risk of major cardiovascular events was reduced in patients receiving clopidogrel and aspirin, compared with those receiving aspirin alone.


1. Mishkel GJ, *et al.*. Clopidogrel as adjunctive antiplatelet therapy during coronary stenting. *J Am Coll Cardiol* 1999; **34:** 1884–90.
2. Berger PB. Clopidogrel versus ticlopidine after intracoronary stent placement. *J Am Coll Cardiol* 1999; **34:** 1891–4.
3. Bertrand ME, *et al.* Double-blind study of the safety of clopidogrel with and without a loading dose in combination with aspirin compared with ticlopidine in combination with aspirin after coronary stenting: the Clopidogrel Aspirin Stent International Cooperative Study (CLASSICS). *Circulation* 2000; **102:** 624–9.
4. Steinhubl SR, *et al.* Early and sustained dual oral antiplatelet therapy following percutaneous coronary intervention: a randomized controlled trial. *JAMA* 2002; **288:** 2411–20. Correction. *ibid.* 2003; **289:** 987.
5. Mehta SR, *et al.* Effects of pretreatment with clopidogrel and aspirin followed by long-term therapy in patients undergoing percutaneous coronary intervention: the PCI-CURE study. *Lancet* 2001; **358:** 527–33.


### Preparations

**Proprietary Preparations** (details are given in Part 3)
***Arg.:*** Iscover; Nefazan; Plavix; ***Austral.:*** Iscover; Plavix; ***Austria:*** Plavix; ***Belg.:*** Plavix; ***Braz.:*** Iscover; Plavix; ***Canad.:*** Plavix; ***Chile:*** Artevil; Plavix; ***Denm.:*** Plavix; ***Fin.:*** Plavix; ***Fr.:*** Plavix; ***Ger.:*** Iscover; Plavix; ***Gr.:*** Iscover; Plavix; ***Hong Kong:*** Plavix; ***India:*** Noklot; ***Irl.:*** Plavix; ***Israel:*** Plavix; ***Ital.:*** Iscover; Plavix; ***Malaysia:*** Plavix; ***Mex.:*** Iscover; Plavix; ***Neth.:*** Plavix; ***Norw.:*** Plavix; ***NZ:*** Plavix; ***Port.:*** Iscover; Plavix; ***S.Afr.:*** Plavix; ***Singapore:*** Plavix; ***Spain:*** Iscover; Plavix; ***Swed.:*** Plavix; ***Switz.:*** Iscover†; Plavix; ***Thai.:*** Plavix; ***UK:*** Iscover; Plavix; ***USA:*** Plavix.

## Cloricromen *(rINN)*

Cloricromeno. Ethyl ({8-chloro-3-[2-(diethylamino)ethyl]-4-methyl-2-oxo-2*H*-1-benzopyran-7-yl}oxy)acetate.

$C_{20}H_{26}ClNO_5$ = 395.9.
*CAS — 68206-94-0.*
*ATC — B01AC02.*

### Profile

Cloricromen is an antiplatelet drug with vasodilating activity and is used in thromboembolic disorders (p.837). It is given as the hydrochloride in arterial vascular disorders where there is a risk of thrombosis. It may be given by mouth in a dose of 100 mg two or three times daily or intravenously in a dose of 30 mg daily.

### Preparations

**Proprietary Preparations** (details are given in Part 3)
***Ital.:*** Assogen†; Proendotel.

## Cloridarol *(rINN)*

Clobenfurol. α-(Benzofuran-2-yl)-α-(4-chlorophenyl)methanol.

$C_{15}H_{11}ClO_2$ = 258.7.
*CAS — 3611-72-1.*
*ATC — C01DX15.*

### Profile

Cloridarol is a vasodilator used in ischaemic heart disease in usual doses of 250 to 500 mg daily by mouth.

Ischaemic heart disease is discussed under Atherosclerosis (p.815) and the treatment of its clinical manifestations is described under Angina Pectoris (p.813) and Myocardial Infarction (p.828).

### Preparations

**Proprietary Preparations** (details are given in Part 3)
***Spain:*** Menoxicor†.

## Colesevelam Hydrochloride *(USAN, rINNM)*

GT31-104HB; Hidrocloruro de colesevelam. Allylamine polymer with epichlorohydrin (1-chloro-2,3-epoxypropane), [6-(allylamino)hexyl]trimethylammonium chloride and *N*-allyldecylamine, hydrochloride.
*CAS — 182815-44-7.*
*ATC — C10AC04.*

### Adverse Effects and Precautions

As for Colestyramine, p.889.

### Interactions

Colesevelam, like colestyramine (see p.890), has the potential to interfere with the absorption of other drugs. The plasma concentration of verapamil has been reported to be decreased when given with colesevelam.

◊ References.


1. Donovan JM, *et al.* Drug interactions with colesevelam hydrochloride, a novel, potent lipid-lowering agent. *Cardiovasc Drugs Ther* 2000; **14:** 681–90.


### Uses and Administration

Colesevelam hydrochloride is a nonabsorbable hydrogel. It binds bile acids in the intestine and has actions similar to those of colestyramine (p.890). It is used for the treatment of hypercholesterolaemia (p.823), particularly type IIa hyperlipoproteinaemia, either alone or with a statin. The usual dose is 3.75 g daily by mouth, as a single dose or in two divided doses, with meals. The dose may be increased to 4.375 g daily if required. When used with a statin, the dose is 2.5 to 3.75 g daily.

◊ References.


1. Davidson MH, *et al.* Colesevelam hydrochloride (Cholestagel): a new, potent bile acid sequestrant associated with a low incidence of gastrointestinal side effects. *Arch Intern Med* 1999; **159:** 1893–1900.
2. Aldridge MA, Ito MK. Colesevelam hydrochloride: a novel bile acid-binding resin. *Ann Pharmacother* 2001; **35:** 898–907.
3. Steinmetz KL. Colesevelam hydrochloride. *Am J Health-Syst Pharm* 2002; **59:** 932–9.


### Preparations

**Proprietary Preparations** (details are given in Part 3)
***USA:*** Welchol.

## Colestilan *(rINN)*

Colestimide. 2-Methylimidazole polymer with 1-chloro-2,3-epoxypropane.

$(C_4H_6N_2.C_3H_5ClO)_n$.
*CAS — 95522-45-5.*

### Profile

Colestilan, a bile-acid binding resin, is a lipid regulating drug with similar properties to colestyramine (p.889) used to reduce cholesterol in the management of hyperlipidaemias (p.823). It is given by mouth in a usual dose of 1.5 g twice daily.

### Preparations

**Proprietary Preparations** (details are given in Part 3)
***Jpn:*** Cholebine.

## Colestipol Hydrochloride

*(BANM, USAN, rINNM)*

Hidrocloruro de colestipol; U-26597A.
*CAS — 26658-42-4 (colestipol); 50925-79-6 (colestipol); 37296-80-3 (colestipol hydrochloride).*

**Pharmacopoeias.** In *Br.* and *US.*

**BP 2003** (Colestipol Hydrochloride). A copolymer of diethylenetriamine and epichlorohydrin (1-chloro-2,3-epoxypropane). Each g binds not less than 1.1 mEq and not more than 1.7 mEq of sodium cholate, calculated as the cholate binding capacity and with reference to the dried substance. Yellow to orange hygroscopic beads. Swells but does not dissolve in water and in dilute solutions of acids or alkalis. Practically insoluble in alcohol and in dichloromethane. The supernatant of a 10% w/w suspension in water has a pH of 6.0 to 7.5. Store in airtight containers.

**USP 27** (Colestipol Hydrochloride). A basic anion-exchange resin. It is the hydrochloride of a copolymer of diethylenetriamine and epichlorohydrin (1-chloro-2,3-epoxypropane). Each g binds not less than 1.1 mEq and not more than 1.6 mEq of sodium cholate, calculated as cholate binding capacity. Yellow to orange beads. Swells but does not dissolve in water or dilute aqueous solutions of acids or alkalis. Insoluble in common organic solvents. The supernatant of a 10% w/w suspension in water has a pH of 6.0 to 7.5. Store in airtight containers.

### Adverse Effects and Precautions

As for Colestyramine, p.889.

**Effects on thyroid function.** Reductions in total serum-thyroxine and thyroxine-binding globulin concentrations were found during routine monitoring of thyroid function in patients receiving colestipol and nicotinic acid, but were considered to be benign.[1]


1. Cashin-Hemphill L, *et al.* Alterations in serum thyroid hormonal indices with colestipol-niacin therapy. *Ann Intern Med* 1987; **107:** 324–9.


### Interactions

As for Colestyramine, p.890.

### Uses and Administration

Colestipol hydrochloride is a bile-acid binding resin. It is not absorbed from the gastrointestinal tract but binds bile acids in the intestines and has actions similar to those of colestyramine (p.890).

Colestipol hydrochloride is a lipid regulating drug and is used to reduce cholesterol in the treatment of hyperlipidaemias (p.823), particularly type IIa hyperlipoproteinaemia.

Colestipol hydrochloride is available as granules and is administered as a suspension in water or a flavoured vehicle. The initial dose is 5 g daily or twice daily, increasing gradually at intervals of 1 to 2 months to up to 30 g daily in a single dose or two divided doses as necessary.

In the USA, colestipol hydrochloride is also available as tablets; doses range from 2 to 16 g daily.

**Cardiovascular risk reduction.** Hyperlipidaemia is an established risk factor for atherosclerotic disease and lipid regulating drugs have an important role in cardiovascular risk reduction (p.819). Statins are the most widely used, but benefit has also been seen with other lipid regulating drugs. Colestipol on its own[1] or with nicotinic acid[2,3] has been reported to be effective in the prophylaxis of **ischaemic heart disease**. The Cholesterol-Lowering Atherosclerosis Study (CLAS)[2] in middle-aged men with progressive atherosclerosis who had undergone coronary bypass surgery showed that colestipol plus nicotinic acid reduced blood concentrations of total cholesterol, triglycerides, and low-density lipoprotein (LDL)-cholesterol, and increased those of high-density lipoprotein (HDL)-cholesterol. Drug treatment also reduced progression of atherosclerosis, development of new lesions in native coronary arteries, and changes in venous bypass grafts. Benefits were maintained after 4 years.[3]


1. Dorr AE, *et al.* Colestipol hydrochloride in hypercholesterolemic patients—effect on serum cholesterol and mortality. *J Chron Dis* 1978; **31:** 5–14.
2. Blankenhorn DH, *et al.* Beneficial effects of combined colestipol-niacin therapy on coronary atherosclerosis and coronary venous bypass grafts. *JAMA* 1987; **257:** 3233–40.
3. Cashin-Hemphill L, *et al.* Beneficial effects of colestipol-niacin on coronary atherosclerosis: a 4-year follow-up. *JAMA* 1990; **264:** 3013–17.


### Preparations

***BP 2003:*** Colestipol Granules;
***USP 27:*** Colestipol Hydrochloride for Oral Suspension.

**Proprietary Preparations** (details are given in Part 3)
***Austral.:*** Colestid; ***Belg.:*** Colestid; ***Canad.:*** Colestid; ***Denm.:*** Lestid; ***Fin.:*** Lestid; ***Ger.:*** Cholestabyl; Colestid; ***Irl.:*** Colestid; ***Israel:*** Colestid; ***Mex.:*** Colestid†; ***Neth.:*** Colestid; ***Norw.:*** Lestid; ***NZ:*** Colestid; ***Port.:*** Colestid; ***Spain:*** Colestid; ***Swed.:*** Lestid; ***Switz.:*** Colestid; ***UK:*** Colestid; ***USA:*** Colestid.

## Colestyramine *(BAN, rINN)*

Cholestyramine; Cholestyramine Resin; Colestiramina; Colestyraminum; MK-135.
*CAS — 11041-12-6.*
*ATC — C10AC01.*

**Pharmacopoeias.** In *Eur.* (see p.vi) and *US.*

**Ph. Eur. 5.0** (Colestyramine). A strongly basic anion-exchange resin in the chloride form, consisting of styrene-divinylbenzene copolymer with quaternary ammonium groups. Each g exchanges not less than 1.8 g and not more than 2.2 g of sodium glycocholate, calculated with reference to the dried material. A white or almost white, fine, hygroscopic powder. Insoluble in water, in alcohol, and in dichloromethane. A 1% suspension in water has a pH of 4.0 to 6.0 after standing for 10 minutes. Store in airtight containers.

**USP 27** (Cholestyramine Resin). A strongly basic anion-exchange resin containing quaternary ammonium functional groups which are attached to a styrene-divinylbenzene copolymer. Each g exchanges not less than 1.8 g and not more than 2.2 g of sodium glycocholate, calculated on the dried basis. It is used in the chloride form. A white to buff-coloured, hygroscopic, fine powder, odourless or has not more than a slight amine-like odour. It loses not more than 12% of its weight on drying. Insoluble in water, in alcohol, in chloroform, and in ether. A 1% slurry in water has a pH of 4.0 to 6.0. Store in airtight containers.

### Adverse Effects

The most common adverse effect of colestyramine is

constipation; faecal impaction may develop and haemorrhoids may be aggravated. Other gastrointestinal adverse effects include abdominal discomfort or pain, heartburn, flatulence, nausea, vomiting, and diarrhoea.

Colestyramine in high doses may cause steatorrhoea by interfering with the absorption of fats from the gastrointestinal tract and therefore decreased absorption of fat-soluble vitamins, such as vitamins A, D, E, and K, may occur. Chronic use of colestyramine may thus result in an increased bleeding tendency due to hypoprothrombinaemia associated with vitamin K deficiency; it also has a potential to cause osteoporosis due to impaired calcium and vitamin D absorption.

Colestyramine is the chloride form of an anion-exchange resin and prolonged use may produce hyperchloraemic acidosis, particularly in children.

Skin rashes and pruritus of the tongue, skin, and perianal region have occasionally occurred.

◊ Results of the Lipid Research Clinics Coronary Primary Prevention Trial[1] involving 3806 men given colestyramine or placebo for an average of 7.4 years showed that gastrointestinal adverse effects occurred frequently in both groups but especially in the colestyramine group. In the first year 68% of the colestyramine group experienced at least 1 gastrointestinal adverse effect compared with 43% of the placebo group; by the seventh year the incidence had diminished so that approximately equal percentages of patients were affected (29% and 26% respectively). Constipation and heartburn, especially, were more frequent in the colestyramine group which also reported more abdominal pain, belching or bloating, gas, and nausea. These adverse effects were usually not severe and could be dealt with by standard clinical means.

The incidence of malignant neoplasms was similar in the 2 groups although there were differences in incidence at some sites. In particular, there were 21 cases of malignancy in the gastrointestinal tract (8 fatal) in the colestyramine group compared with 11 cases (1 fatal) in the placebo group. The number of colon cancers was identical in both groups. However, the comment was made that 6 rare cancers of the buccal cavity or pharynx in the colestyramine group should not pass unnoticed.[2]

1. Lipid Research Clinics Program. The Lipid Research Clinics Coronary Primary Prevention Trial results. *JAMA* 1984; **251:** 351–64.
2. Oliver MF. Hypercholesterolaemia and coronary heart disease: an answer. *BMJ* 1984; **288:** 423–4.

## Precautions

Colestyramine powder should be given as a suspension in water or a flavoured vehicle to minimise the risk of oesophageal obstruction.

Colestyramine should not be used in patients with complete biliary obstruction as it is unlikely to be effective.

Because of the risk of vitamin deficiencies, supplements of vitamins A, D, E, and K should be considered during prolonged therapy with colestyramine; if given by mouth they need to be in a water-miscible form. Parenteral administration, particularly of vitamin K for hypoprothrombinaemia, may be necessary if a deficiency becomes established. Reduced serum-folate concentrations have also been reported in children with familial hypercholesterolaemia and supplementation with folic acid should be considered in such circumstances.

## Interactions

Colestyramine may delay or reduce the absorption of other drugs, particularly acidic drugs, administered concomitantly. Enterohepatic circulation may be reduced. Delayed or reduced absorption of thiazide diuretics, propranolol, digoxin and related glycosides, loperamide, phenylbutazone, barbiturates, oestrogens, progestogens, thyroid hormones, warfarin, and some antibacterials, has either been reported or may be expected. It is therefore recommended that other drugs should be taken at least 1 hour before, or 4 to 6 hours after, the administration of colestyramine.

## Uses and Administration

Colestyramine is a bile-acid binding resin and lipid regulating drug. It is used to reduce cholesterol in the treatment of hyperlipidaemias (p.823), particularly type IIa hyperlipoproteinaemia, and for the primary prevention of ischaemic heart disease (see Cardiovascular Risk Reduction, p.819) in middle-aged men with primary hypercholesterolaemia. Colestyramine is also used for the relief of diarrhoea associated with ileal resection, Crohn's disease, vagotomy, diabetic vagal neuropathy, and radiation, and to relieve the pruritus associated with the deposition in dermal tissue of excess bile acids in patients with partial biliary obstruction or primary biliary cirrhosis.

Colestyramine is not absorbed from the gastrointestinal tract but it adsorbs, and combines with, the bile acids in the intestine to form an insoluble complex that is excreted in the faeces. The normal reabsorption of bile acids is thus prevented and this leads to an increased oxidation of cholesterol to bile acids to replace those partially removed from the enterohepatic circulation, and an increased synthesis of low-density lipoprotein (LDL)-cholesterol receptors on hepatocytes. The overall effect is a reduction of total plasma-cholesterol concentration, mainly by lowering LDL-cholesterol; this may be accompanied by moderate increases in plasma triglyceride and high-density lipoprotein (HDL)-cholesterol concentrations. Since the uses of colestyramine are based upon the removal of intestinal bile acids it is unlikely that a response will be achieved in patients with complete biliary obstruction.

Colestyramine may be introduced gradually over 3 to 4 weeks to minimise gastrointestinal effects.

In hyperlipidaemias and diarrhoea the usual dose by mouth is 12 to 24 g daily, given either as a single dose or in up to 4 divided doses. Dosage should be adjusted according to the patient's response and may be increased to 36 g daily if necessary. Lower doses may be adequate in some forms of hyperlipidaemia.

In pruritus doses of 4 to 8 g daily are usually sufficient.

A dose of colestyramine for children over 6 years of age is 240 mg/kg daily in divided doses.

Colestyramine should be given as a suspension in water or a flavoured vehicle.

◊ General references.

1. LaRosa J. Review of clinical studies of bile acid sequestrants for lowering plasma lipid levels. *Cardiology* 1989; **76** (suppl 1): 55–64.
2. Shepherd J. Mechanism of action of bile acid sequestrants and other lipid-lowering drugs. *Cardiology* 1989; **76** (suppl 1): 65–74.
3. Ast M, Frishman WH. Bile acid sequestrants. *J Clin Pharmacol* 1990; **30:** 99–106.

**Administration in children.** Plasma-cholesterol concentrations were lowered in children given colestyramine alone[1] or with dietary restrictions[2,3] for periods ranging from 1 to 8 years. Long-term treatment with colestyramine had no adverse effects on physical growth[2,3] and development or sexual maturation.[2] However, compliance has been a problem with only 48% of patients complying with treatment after 8 years.[1]

1. West RJ, Lloyd JK. Long-term follow-up of children with familial hypercholesterolaemia treated with cholestyramine. *Lancet* 1980; **ii:** 873–5.
2. Glueck CJ, *et al.* Safety and efficacy of long-term diet and diet plus bile acid-binding resin cholesterol-lowering therapy in 73 children heterozygous for familial hypercholesterolemia. *Pediatrics* 1986; **78:** 338–48.
3. Tonstad S, *et al.* Efficacy and safety of cholestyramine therapy in peripubertal and prepubertal children with familial hypercholesterolemia. *J Pediatr* 1996; **129:** 42–9.

**Antibiotic-associated colitis.** Colestyramine binds *Clostridium difficile* toxins and has been tried as an alternative, or as an adjunct, to vancomycin or metronidazole in patients with diarrhoea associated with *C. difficile* toxins following antibiotic therapy (p.128). In general its use is not recommended.

**Biliary disorders.** Colestyramine is used to relieve diarrhoea associated with bile acid malabsorption (p.1241) and to manage pruritus and hypercholesterolaemia in patients with primary biliary cirrhosis (p.1761). Beneficial responses have also been reported with colestyramine in the management of congenital nonobstructive nonhaemolytic hyperbilirubinaemia (Crigler-Najjar disease) in 2 infants.[1,2] It has also produced a beneficial effect in a patient with sclerosing cholangitis.[3]

1. Arrowsmith WA, *et al.* Comparison of treatments for congenital nonobstructive nonhaemolytic hyperbilirubinaemia. *Arch Dis Child* 1975; **50:** 197–201.
2. Odièvre M, *et al.* Case of congenital nonobstructive, nonhaemolytic jaundice: successful long-term phototherapy at home. *Arch Dis Child* 1978; **53:** 81–2.
3. Polter DE, *et al.* Beneficial effect of cholestyramine in sclerosing cholangitis. *Gastroenterology* 1980; **79:** 326–33.

## Preparations

***BP 2003:*** Colestyramine Oral Powder;
***USP 27:*** Cholestyramine for Oral Suspension.

**Proprietary Preparations** (details are given in Part 3)
***Arg.:*** Questran; ***Austral.:*** Questran; ***Austria:*** Quantalan; ***Belg.:*** Questran; ***Braz.:*** Questran; ***Canad.:*** Novo-Cholamine; Questran; ***Denm.:*** Questran; ***Fin.:*** Questran; ***Fr.:*** Questran; ***Ger.:*** Colesthexal; Colestyr; Lipocol; Quantalan; Vasosan; ***Gr.:*** Questran; ***Hong Kong:*** Questran; ***Irl.:*** Questran; ***Israel:*** Chol-Less; Questran†; ***Ital.:*** Questran; ***Malaysia:*** Questran; ***Mex.:*** Questran†; ***Neth.:*** Questran; ***Norw.:*** Questran; ***NZ:*** Questran; ***Port.:*** Quantalan; ***S.Afr.:*** Questran; ***Singapore:*** Questran; Resincolestiramina; ***Spain:*** Lismol; Questran; Resincolestiramina; ***Swed.:*** Questran; ***Switz.:*** Quantalan; ***Thai.:*** Questran; Resincolestiramina; ***UK:*** Questran; ***USA:*** Locholest; Prevalite; Questran.

# Colextran Hydrochloride *(rINNM)*

DEAE-dextran Hydrochloride; Detaxtran Hydrochloride; Diethylaminoethyl-dextran Hydrochloride; Hidrocloruro de colextrán. Dextran 2-(diethylamino)ethyl ether hydrochloride.

*CAS — 9015-73-0 (colextran); 9064-91-9 (colextran hydrochloride).*

## Profile

Colextran hydrochloride, an anion-exchange resin that binds bile acids in the intestine, is a lipid regulating drug used in the treatment of hyperlipidaemias (p.823). It is given in a usual dose of 2 to 3 g daily by mouth in divided doses.

## Preparations

**Proprietary Preparations** (details are given in Part 3)
***Ital.:*** Dexide†; Nolipid†; Pulsar; Rationale; ***Spain:*** Dexide.

# Cromakalim *(BAN, rINN)*

BRL-34915. (±)-*trans*-3,4-Dihydro-3-hydroxy-2,2-dimethyl-4-(2-oxopyrrolidin-1-yl)-2*H*-chromene-6-carbonitrile.

$C_{16}H_{18}N_2O_3$ = 286.3.

*CAS — 94470-67-4 (cromakalim); 94535-50-9 (levcromakalim).*

## Profile

Cromakalim is a potassium-channel opening vasodilator (p.812). Cromakalim and its (−)-enantiomer, levcromakalim (lemakalim), have been investigated in the management of hypertension and have also been tried in patients with asthma.

◊ References.

1. Williams AJ, *et al.* Attenuation of nocturnal asthma by cromakalim. *Lancet* 1990; **336:** 334–6.
2. Suzuki S, *et al.* Antihypertensive effect of levcromakalim in patients with essential hypertension: study by 24-h ambulatory blood pressure monitoring. *Arzneimittelforschung* 1995; **45:** 859–64.

# Cyclandelate *(BAN, rINN)*

BS-572; Ciclandelato. 3,3,5-Trimethylcyclohexyl mandelate.

$C_{17}H_{24}O_3$ = 276.4.

*CAS — 456-59-7.*

*ATC — C04AX01.*

**Pharmacopoeias.** In *Chin.*

## Profile

Cyclandelate is a vasodilator used in the management of cerebrovascular (p.820) and peripheral vascular disorders (p.831). It is given by mouth in a dosage of up to 1.6 g daily in divided doses although a daily maintenance dose of 400 to 800 mg may be adequate.

## Preparations

**Proprietary Preparations** (details are given in Part 3)
***Belg.:*** Cyclospasmol; ***Canad.:*** Cyclospasmol†; ***Fin.:*** Cyclospasmol; ***Fr.:*** Cyclergine; Cyclospasmol†; Novodil†; Vascunormyl; ***Ger.:*** Natil; Spasmocyclon; ***India:*** Martispasmol; ***Ital.:*** Ciclospasmol; ***Port.:*** Cyclospasmol; ***Swed.:*** Cyclomandol.

# Cyclopenthiazide *(BAN, USAN, rINN)*

Ciclopentiazida; Cyclopenthiaz.; NSC-107679; Su-8341. 6-Chloro-3-cyclopentylmethyl-3,4-dihydro-2*H*-1,2,4-benzothiadiazine-7-sulphonamide 1,1-dioxide.

$C_{13}H_{18}ClN_3O_4S_2$ = 379.9.

*CAS — 742-20-1.*

*ATC — C03AA07.*

NOTE. Compounded preparations of cyclopenthiazide may be represented by the following names:

- Co-prenozide *(BAN)*—cyclopenthiazide 1 part and oxprenolol hydrochloride 640 parts (w/w).

**Pharmacopoeias.** In *Br.*

**BP 2003** (Cyclopenthiazide). A white, odourless or almost odourless powder. Practically insoluble in water; soluble in alcohol and in acetone; practically insoluble in chloroform; very slightly soluble in ether.

## Profile

Cyclopenthiazide is a thiazide diuretic with properties similar to those of hydrochlorothiazide (p.933). It is used for hypertension (p.825), and for oedema, including that associated with heart failure (p.820).

Diuresis is induced in 1 to 3 hours, reaches a maximum in 4 to 8 hours, and lasts up to about 12 hours.

In the treatment of hypertension the usual dose is 250 to 500 micrograms daily either alone, or with other antihypertensives. In the treatment of oedema the usual initial dose is 250 to 500 micrograms daily by mouth; up to 1 mg daily may be given in heart failure but higher doses rarely achieve any further benefit. The dose should be reduced to the lowest effective dose for maintenance.

**Porphyria.** Cyclopenthiazide is considered to be unsafe in patients with porphyria although there is conflicting experimental evidence of porphyrinogenicity.

### Preparations

***BP 2003:*** Cyclopenthiazide Tablets.

**Proprietary Preparations** (details are given in Part 3)
***NZ:*** Navidrex; Prothiazide†; ***UK:*** Navidrex.
**Multi-ingredient:** ***Hong Kong:*** Navispare; ***Irl.:*** Navispare†; Trasidrex†; ***S.Afr.:*** Trasidrex†; ***UK:*** Navispare; Trasidrex.

## Cyclothiazide (*BAN, USAN, rINN*)

Ciclotiazida; Compound 35483; MDi-193. 6-Chloro-3,4-dihydro-3-(norborn-5-en-2-yl)-2*H*-1,2,4-benzothiadiazine-7-sulphonamide 1,1-dioxide.

$C_{14}H_{16}ClN_3O_4S_2$ = 389.9.
*CAS — 2259-96-3.*
*ATC — C03AA09.*

### Profile

Cyclothiazide is a thiazide diuretic (see Hydrochlorothiazide, p.933) that has been used, usually in combination preparations, in the management of hypertension and oedema.

### Preparations

**Proprietary Preparations** (details are given in Part 3)
**Multi-ingredient:** ***Fr.:*** Cycloteriam†.

## Dalteparin Sodium (*BAN, USAN, rINN*)

Dalteparina sódica; Dalteparinum Natricum; Kabi-2165; Tedelparin Sodium.
*CAS — 9041-08-1.*
*ATC — B01AB04.*

**Pharmacopoeias.** In *Eur.* (see p.vi).

**Ph. Eur. 5.0** (Dalteparin Sodium). The sodium salt of a low-molecular-mass heparin that is obtained by nitrous acid depolymerisation of heparin from porcine intestinal mucosa. The majority of the components have a 2-*O*-sulfo-α-L-idopyranosuronic acid structure at the non-reducing end and a 6-*O*-sulfo-2,5-anhydro-D-mannitol structure at the reducing end of their chain. The mass-average molecular mass ranges between 5600 and 6400, with a characteristic value of about 6000. The mass percentage of chains lower than 3000 is not more than 13.0% and the mass percentage of chains higher than 8000 ranges between 15.0% and 25.0%. The degree of sulfation is 2.0 to 2.5 per disaccharide unit.

The potency is not less than 110 units and not more than 210 units of anti-factor Xa activity per mg with reference to the dried substance and the ratio of anti-factor Xa activity to anti-factor IIa activity is between 1.9 and 3.2.

### Units

As for Low-molecular-weight Heparins, p.949.

### Adverse Effects, Treatment, and Precautions

As for Low-molecular-weight Heparins, p.949.

Severe bleeding with dalteparin may be reduced by the slow intravenous injection of protamine sulfate; 1 mg of protamine sulfate is stated to inhibit the effects of 100 units of dalteparin sodium.

### Interactions

As for Low-molecular-weight Heparins, p.950.

### Pharmacokinetics

Dalteparin is almost completely absorbed after subcutaneous administration, with a bioavailability of about 87%. Peak plasma activity is reached in about 4 hours. The terminal half-life is about 2 hours following intravenous injection and 3 to 5 hours after subcutaneous injection. Dalteparin is excreted via the kidneys and the half-life is prolonged in patients with renal impairment.

### Uses and Administration

Dalteparin sodium is a low-molecular-weight heparin (p.949) with anticoagulant properties. It is used in the treatment and prophylaxis of venous thromboembolism (p.839) and to prevent clotting during extracorporeal circulation. It is also used in the management of unstable angina (p.813).

Dalteparin is administered by subcutaneous or intravenous injection. Doses are expressed in terms of units of anti-factor Xa activity.

For prophylaxis of **venous thromboembolism** during surgical procedures, dalteparin is usually started preoperatively. For patients at moderate risk of thrombosis 2500 units of dalteparin sodium are given by subcutaneous injection 1 to 2 hours before the procedure, followed by 2500 units once daily for 5 to 7 days or until the patient is fully ambulant. For patients at high risk, 2500 units are given 1 to 2 hours before and 8 to 12 hours after the procedure followed by 5000 units daily. Alternatively, 5000 units may be given the evening before surgery followed by 5000 units each subsequent evening. This dosage may be continued for up to 5 weeks following hip replacement surgery. A further option in patients undergoing hip replacement surgery is to omit the pre-operative dose; treatment is initiated with a dose of 2500 units given 4 to 8 hours postoperatively followed by 5000 units daily. For prophylaxis in medical patients, a dose of 5000 units once daily may be given for 14 days or longer.

In the treatment of established deep-vein thrombosis, pulmonary embolism, or both, dalteparin sodium is given subcutaneously in a dose of 200 units/kg daily. This may be given as a single dose or, in patients at higher risk of bleeding complications, in two divided doses. The maximum recommended dose is 18 000 units daily.

For prevention of clotting in the extracorporeal circulation during **haemodialysis** or **haemofiltration** in adults with chronic renal impairment an intravenous injection of dalteparin sodium 30 to 40 units/kg is followed by an intravenous infusion of 10 to 15 units/kg per hour. A single injection of 5000 units may be given for a haemodialysis or haemofiltration session lasting less than 4 hours. The dose of dalteparin sodium should be reduced in patients at high risk of bleeding complications or who are in acute renal failure; in such patients an intravenous injection of 5 to 10 units/kg is followed by an infusion of 4 to 5 units/kg per hour.

In the management of **unstable angina**, dalteparin sodium is given subcutaneously in a dose of 120 units/kg every 12 hours; the maximum recommended dose is 10 000 units every 12 hours. Treatment is continued for 5 to 8 days and low-dose aspirin should be given concomitantly. For patients who require treatment for longer than 8 days while awaiting a revascularisation procedure, a dose of 5000 units (7500 units in men weighing 70 kg or over and women weighing 80 kg or over) may be given every 12 hours for up to 45 days until the procedure is performed.

◊ References.


1. Dunn CJ, Sorkin EM. Dalteparin sodium: a review of its pharmacology and clinical use in the prevention and treatment of thromboembolic disorders. *Drugs* 1996; **52:** 276–305.
2. Howard PA. Dalteparin: a low-molecular-weight heparin. *Ann Pharmacother* 1997; **31:** 192–203.
3. Dunn CJ, Jarvis B. Dalteparin: an update of its pharmacological properties and clinical efficacy in the prophylaxis and treatment of thromboembolic disease. *Drugs* 2000; **60:** 203–37.


### Preparations

**Proprietary Preparations** (details are given in Part 3)
***Arg.:*** Ligofragmin; ***Austral.:*** Fragmin; ***Austria:*** Fragmin; ***Belg.:*** Fragmin; ***Braz.:*** Fragmin; ***Canad.:*** Fragmin; ***Chile:*** Fragmin; ***Denm.:*** Fragmin; ***Fin.:*** Fragmin; ***Fr.:*** Fragmine; ***Ger.:*** Fragmin; ***Gr.:*** Fragmin; ***Hong Kong:*** Fragmin; ***Israel:*** Fragmin; ***Ital.:*** Fragmin; ***Neth.:*** Fragmin; ***Norw.:*** Fragmin; ***NZ:*** Fragmin; ***Port.:*** Fragmin; ***S.Afr.:*** Fragmin; ***Singapore:*** Fragmin; ***Spain:*** Boxol; Fragmin; ***Swed.:*** Fragmin; ***Switz.:*** Fragmin; Low Liquemine†; ***UK:*** Fragmin; ***USA:*** Fragmin.

## Danaparoid Sodium (*BAN, USAN, rINN*)

Danaparoide sódico; Lomoparan; Org-10172.
*CAS — 83513-48-8.*
*ATC — B01AB09.*

**Description.** Danaparoid sodium is a low-molecular-weight heparinoid derived from porcine intestinal mucosa. It contains a mixture of the sodium salts of suleparoid (p.1009), dermatan sulfate (p.892), and chondroitin sulfate (p.1670) in an approximate ratio of 21:3:1. The average molecular weight is about 5500 to 6000.

### Adverse Effects and Treatment

Haemorrhage may occur after administration of danaparoid sodium, although there is a possible decreased risk of bleeding complications compared with heparin. Liver enzymes may be transiently elevated. Other adverse effects include hypersensitivity reactions, thrombocytopenia, and pain at the site of injection.

Protamine sulfate only partially neutralises the anticoagulant effect of danaparoid sodium and cannot be relied on to reverse bleeding associated with overdosage.

### Precautions

As for Heparin, p.929.

Danaparoid sodium should not be given to patients who have developed thrombocytopenia with heparin if they show cross-reactivity in an *in-vitro* test.

### Pharmacokinetics

After subcutaneous administration danaparoid sodium is well absorbed and peak anti-factor Xa activity is reached in approximately 4 to 5 hours. The elimination half-lives of anti-factor Xa and anti-factor IIa (antithrombin) activities are about 25 and 7 hours, respectively. Danaparoid sodium is excreted in the urine.

### Uses and Administration

Danaparoid sodium is a low-molecular-weight heparinoid. It is an anticoagulant and, like heparin (p.929), enhances the action of antithrombin III. Similarly to low-molecular-weight heparins (p.949) it is characterised by a higher ratio of anti-factor Xa to anti-factor IIa (antithrombin) activity than heparin, but is reported to be a much more selective inhibitor of factor Xa than the low-molecular-weight heparins. It was therefore hoped that danaparoid might be associated with a low incidence of bleeding complications, although this is yet to be established.

Danaparoid sodium is used in the prophylaxis of venous thromboembolism (p.839) in patients undergoing surgery. It may be used as an anticoagulant for prophylaxis or treatment in patients with heparin-induced thrombocytopenia providing there is no cross-reactivity. Danaparoid has been investigated in acute ischaemic stroke.

Doses of danaparoid sodium are expressed in terms of units of anti-factor Xa activity. In the prophylaxis of venous thromboembolism it is given by subcutaneous injection in a dose of 750 units twice daily for 7 to 10 days. The first dose should be given 1 to 4 hours before surgery.

For patients with heparin-induced thrombocytopenia requiring anticoagulation, danaparoid sodium is given intravenously. The initial bolus dose is 2500 units (or 1250 units for patients weighing less than 55 kg, or 3750 units for patients weighing more than 90 kg) followed by an infusion of 400 units/hour for 2 hours, then 300 units/hour for 2 hours, then 200 units/hour for 5 days. Monitoring of plasma anti-factor Xa activity is recommended for patients with renal impairment, or those weighing more than 90 kg.

◊ References.


1. Skoutakis VA. Danaparoid in the prevention of thromboembolic complications. *Ann Pharmacother* 1997; **31:** 876–87.
2. Wilde MI, Markham A. Danaparoid: a review of its pharmacology and clinical use in the management of heparin-induced thrombocytopenia. *Drugs* 1997; **54:** 903–24.
3. Ibbotson T, Perry CM. Danaparoid: a review of its use in thromboembolic and coagulation disorders. *Drugs* 2002; **62:** 2283–2314.


### Preparations

**Proprietary Preparations** (details are given in Part 3)
***Austral.:*** Orgaran; ***Austria:*** Orgaran; ***Belg.:*** Orgaran; ***Canad.:*** Orgaran; ***Fr.:*** Orgaran; ***Ger.:*** Orgaran; ***Neth.:*** Orgaran; ***NZ:*** Orgaran; ***Swed.:*** Orgaran; ***UK:*** Orgaran; ***USA:*** Orgaran.

## Debrisoquine Sulfate (*rINNM*)

Debrisoquin Sulfate (*USAN*); Debrisoquine Sulphate (*BANM*); Isocaramidine Sulphate; Ro-5-3307/1; Sulfato de debrisoquina. 1,2,3,4-Tetrahydroisoquinoline-2-carboxamidine sulphate.

$(C_{10}H_{13}N_3)_2,H_2SO_4$ = 448.5.
*CAS — 1131-64-2 (debrisoquine); 581-88-4 (debrisoquine sulfate).*
*ATC — C02CC04.*

**Pharmacopoeias.** In *Br.*

**BP 2003** (Debrisoquine Sulphate). A white, odourless or almost odourless, crystalline powder. Sparingly soluble in water; very slightly soluble in alcohol; practically insoluble in chloroform and in ether. A 3% solution in water has a pH of 5.3 to 6.8. Protect from light.

### Adverse Effects, Treatment, and Precautions

As for Guanethidine Monosulfate, p.927.

Diarrhoea is rare with debrisoquine sulfate. Abrupt cessation of treatment should be avoided as this may lead to rebound hypertension.

The metabolism of debrisoquine is subject to genetic polymorphism and non-metabolisers may show a marked response to doses that have little or no effect in metabolisers.

### Interactions

As for Guanethidine Monosulfate, p.927.

### Pharmacokinetics

Debrisoquine is rapidly absorbed from the gastrointestinal tract. The major metabolite is 4-hydroxydebrisoquine; metabolism is subject to genetic polymorphism.

◊ A study[1] in 15 hypertensive patients and 4 healthy subjects indicated that debrisoquine undergoes pre-systemic metabolism to 4-hydroxydebrisoquine, but the mechanism appears to be saturable and increases in the dose of debrisoquine could therefore produce disproportionate decreases in blood pressure. The estimated half-life of elimination for debrisoquine and 4-hydroxydebrisoquine ranged from 11.5 to 26 hours and from 5.8 to 14.5 hours respectively.

1. Silas JH, *et al.* The disposition of debrisoquine in hypertensive patients. *Br J Clin Pharmacol* 1978; **5:** 27–34.

**Genetic polymorphism.** Debrisoquine, along with sparteine and a number of other drugs, is a substrate for the cytochrome P450 isoenzyme CYP2D6, a polymorphic enzyme coded by a gene mapped to chromosome 22. Patients homozygous for the mutant allele are termed poor metabolisers and express little or no active enzyme. The prevalence of the poor-metaboliser phenotype is about 5% in most Caucasian populations, while studies in other genetic groups have indicated a range of about 2 to 10% although in some groups, such as the Japanese, poor metabolisers have yet to be identified. Poor metabolisers of debrisoquine are unable to 4-hydroxylate the drug adequately to its inactive metabolite and are thus prone to excessive hypotension. A number of other drugs are metabolised by the same enzyme, including: antidepressants such as amitriptyline, imipramine, and nortriptyline; other antihypertensives such as indoramin; antiarrhythmics such as encainide, flecainide, and propafenone; analgesics such as phenacetin; beta blockers such as metoprolol, propranolol, and timolol; hypoglycaemics such as phenformin; and opioids such as codeine and dextromethorphan. However, the clinical consequences of polymorphism in patients receiving these drugs depend on the relative activity and toxicity of parent drug and metabolite, and the availability and relative importance of other routes of metabolism. Determination of phenotype is generally performed by administration of a test drug such as debrisoquine and assay of parent drug and metabolite in urine collected over a defined period of time.

References.

1. Relling MV. Polymorphic drug metabolism. *Clin Pharm* 1989; **8:** 852–63.

### Uses and Administration

Debrisoquine is an antihypertensive with actions and uses similar to those of guanethidine (p.927), but it causes less depletion of noradrenaline stores. When given by mouth, debrisoquine is reported to act within about 4 to 10 hours and to have effects lasting for 9 to 24 hours. It is used in the management of hypertension (p.825), but has largely been superseded by other drugs.

Debrisoquine is given by mouth as the sulfate, but doses are usually expressed in terms of the base. Debrisoquine sulfate 12.8 mg is approximately equivalent to 10 mg of debrisoquine.

The usual initial dose is 10 to 20 mg once or twice daily. The daily dose is then increased by 10 to 20 mg, according to the severity of the condition, every 3 or 4 days. The usual maintenance dose is 20 to 120 mg daily, but 300 mg or more daily may be given.

For reference to the use of debrisoquine in identifying metabolic phenotypes, see Genetic Polymorphism, above.

## Defibrotide *(BAN, rINN)*

Defibrotida.

*ATC — B01AX01.*

### Profile

Defibrotide consists of polydeoxyribonucleotides from bovine lung; the molecular weights range between 45 000 and 55 000. Preparations derived from porcine tissues and with a lower molecular weight range are also used. Defibrotide has antithrombotic and fibrinolytic properties, although its mechanism of action is uncertain; it appears to increase levels of prostaglandin $E_2$ and prostacyclin, to alter platelet activity, and to increase tissue plasminogen activator function at the same time as decreasing activity of tissue plasminogen activator inhibitor. It is used in the management of thromboembolic disorders. Oral and parenteral formulations have been used in doses of up to 800 mg daily.

Defibrotide is being investigated for use in the treatment of hepatic veno-occlusive disease.

◊ References.

1. Palmer KJ, Goa KL. Defibrotide: a review of its pharmacodynamic and pharmacokinetic properties, and therapeutic use in vascular disorders. *Drugs* 1993; **45:** 259–94.

### Preparations

**Proprietary Preparations** (details are given in Part 3)
***Ital.:*** Noravid; Prociclide.

## Delapril Hydrochloride *(USAN, rINNM)*

Alindapril Hydrochloride; CV-3317; Hidrocloruro de delapril; Indalapril Hydrochloride; REV-6000A. Ethyl (*S*)-2-{[(*S*)-1-(carboxymethyl-2-indanylcarbamoyl)ethyl]amino}-4-phenylbutyrate hydrochloride.

$C_{26}H_{32}N_2O_5,HCl = 489.0$.

*CAS — 83435-66-9 (delapril); 83435-67-0 (delapril hydrochloride).*

*ATC — C09AA12.*

### Profile

Delapril is an ACE inhibitor (p.842). It is converted in the body to two metabolites to which it owes its activity. It is given by mouth as the hydrochloride in the treatment of hypertension (p.825), in usual maintenance doses of 30 to 60 mg daily in two divided doses.

### Preparations

**Proprietary Preparations** (details are given in Part 3)
***Braz.:*** Delakete; ***Ital.:*** Delaket; ***Jpn:*** Adecut; ***Malaysia:*** Cupressin; ***Singapore:*** Cupressin; ***Thai.:*** Cupressin.
**Multi-ingredient: *Ital.:*** Delapride; Dinapres.

## Denopamine *(rINN)*

Denopamina; TA-064. (−)-(*R*)-α-{[(3,4-Dimethoxyphenethyl)-amino]methyl}-*p*-hydroxybenzyl alcohol.

$C_{18}H_{23}NO_4 = 317.4$.

*CAS — 71771-90-9.*

### Profile

Denopamine is a sympathomimetic (see Adrenaline, p.852) with predominantly beta-adrenergic activity selective to beta$_1$ receptors. It acts as a partial agonist (see Xamoterol, p.1029) and is used for the treatment of heart failure (p.820). The usual dose is 15 to 30 mg daily by mouth in three divided doses.

### Preparations

**Proprietary Preparations** (details are given in Part 3)
***Jpn:*** Kalgut.

## Dermatan Sulfate

Chondroitin Sulfate B; Dermatán, sulfato de; Dermatan Sulphate; LMW-DS (depolymerised dermatan sulfate); MF-701; OP-370 (depolymerised dermatan sulfate).

*CAS — 24967-94-0 (dermatan sulfate).*

*ATC — B01AX04.*

## Dermatan Sulfate Sodium

Chondroitin Sulfate B Sodium; Dermatan Sulphate Sodium.

*CAS — 54328-33-5.*

*ATC — B01AX04.*

### Profile

Dermatan sulfate is a naturally occurring glycosaminoglycan used as an anticoagulant for prophylaxis of venous thromboembolism (p.839). It is given as the sodium salt in a dose of 100 to 300 mg daily by intramuscular injection. The dose may be increased to 300 mg twice daily in patients at high risk of thromboembolism, such as those undergoing major orthopaedic surgery.

Dermatan sulfate is a component of sulodexide (p.1009) and its sodium salt is a component of danaparoid sodium (p.891).

Dermatan sulfate is under investigation for the treatment of venous thromboembolism, heparin-induced thrombocytopenia, and to prevent clotting during haemodialysis. Low-molecular-weight (depolymerised) dermatan sulfate is also being studied.

◊ References.

1. Dawes J, *et al.* The pharmacokinetics of dermatan sulphate MF701 in healthy human volunteers. *Br J Clin Pharmacol* 1991; **32:** 361–6.
2. Lane DA, *et al.* Dermatan sulphate in haemodialysis. *Lancet* 1992; **339:** 334–5.
3. Cofrancesco E, *et al.* Dermatan sulphate in acute leukaemia. *Lancet* 1992; **339:** 1177–8.
4. Agnelli G, *et al.* Randomised, double-blind, placebo-controlled trial of dermatan sulphate for prevention of deep vein thrombosis in hip fracture. *Thromb Haemost* 1992; **67:** 203–8.
5. Gianese F, *et al.* The pharmacokinetics and pharmacodynamics of dermatan sulphate MF701 during haemodialysis for chronic renal failure. *Br J Clin Pharmacol* 1993; **35:** 335–9.
6. Legnani C, *et al.* Acute and chronic effects of a new low molecular weight dermatan sulphate (Desmin 370) on blood coagulation and fibrinolysis in healthy subjects. *Eur J Clin Pharmacol* 1994; **47:** 247–52.
7. Miglioli M, *et al.* Bioavailability of Desmin, a low molecular weight dermatan sulfate, after subcutaneous administration to healthy volunteers. *Int J Clin Lab Res* 1997; **27:** 195–8.
8. Taliani MR *et al.* Dermatan sulphate in patients with heparin-induced thrombocytopenia. *Br J Haematol* 1999; **104:** 87–9.
9. Di Carlo V, *et al.* Dermatan sulphate for the prevention of post-operative venous thromboembolism in patients with cancer. *Thromb Haemost* 1999; **82:** 30–4.

### Preparations

**Proprietary Preparations** (details are given in Part 3)
***Ital.:*** Aclotan; Mistral.

## Deserpidine *(BAN, rINN)*

Canescine; Deserpidina; 11-Desmethoxyreserpine; Raunormine; Recanescine. Methyl 11-demethoxy-*O*-(3,4,5-trimethoxybenzoyl)reserpate.

$C_{32}H_{38}N_2O_8 = 578.7$.

*CAS — 131-01-1.*

*ATC — C02AA05.*

### Profile

Deserpidine is an ester alkaloid isolated from the root of *Rauwolfia canescens*. It has properties similar to those described under reserpine (p.995) and has been used in the treatment of hypertension and psychoses.

### Preparations

**Proprietary Preparations** (details are given in Part 3)
**Multi-ingredient: *Hong Kong:*** Enduronyl; ***Ital.:*** Enduronil†; ***USA:*** Enduronyl†.

## Desirudin *(BAN, USAN, rINN)*

CGP-39393; Desirudina; Desulphatohirudin. 63-Desulfohirudin (*Hirudo medicinalis* isoform HV1).

$C_{287}H_{440}N_{80}O_{110}S_6 = 6963.4$.

*CAS — 120993-53-5.*

*ATC — B01AE01.*

### Adverse Effects and Precautions

The most common adverse effect of desirudin is bleeding. Hypersensitivity reactions have been reported. Local haematoma may occur if desirudin is administered by intramuscular injection and it should therefore not be given by this route.

Desirudin is contra-indicated in patients with active bleeding or irreversible coagulation disorders. It should be used with caution in patients with severe renal or hepatic impairment, severe hypertension, or bacterial endocarditis, and in those at increased risk of bleeding including those with haemorrhagic blood disorders, recent major bleeding, cerebrovascular disorders, or patients who have recently undergone major surgery, or biopsy or puncture of a noncompressible vessel. Teratogenicity has been observed in *animals*.

### Interactions

Use of desirudin with anticoagulants or drugs, such as aspirin and dipyridamole, that affect platelet function may increase the risk of bleeding. NSAIDs may also increase the risk of haemorrhage. Other drugs which affect the coagulation process and which may therefore increase the risk of haemorrhage include dextrans and thrombolytic enzymes such as streptokinase.

### Pharmacokinetics

Maximum plasma concentrations of desirudin are reached 1 to 3 hours after subcutaneous injection. Desirudin is metabolised and excreted by the kidney, and 40 to 50% of a dose is excreted unchanged in the urine. After subcutaneous or intravenous injection the terminal elimination half-life of desirudin is 2 to 3 hours.

◊ References.

1. Lefèvre G, *et al.* Effect of renal impairment on the pharmacokinetics and pharmacodynamics of desirudin. *Clin Pharmacol Ther* 1997; **62:** 50–9.

### Uses and Administration

Desirudin is a recombinant hirudin (p.931) that is a direct inhibitor of thrombin. It is used as an anticoagulant for the prevention of postoperative venous thromboembolism (p.839) in patients undergoing orthopaedic surgery. It has been investigated in arterial thromboembolic disorders such as myocardial infarction and unstable angina, and as an adjunct in angioplasty procedures (see under Uses and Administration of Lepirudin, p.945).

In the prevention of venous thromboembolism, desirudin is administered subcutaneously in a dose of 15 mg twice daily. The first dose is given 5 to 15 minutes before surgery, but after induction of regional block anaesthesia, if used, and then continued until the patient is fully ambulant, usually for 9 to a maximum of 12 days.

Response to desirudin should be monitored using activated partial thromboplastin time (APTT) in patients with renal or hepatic impairment, or increased risk of bleeding. Doses may need to be reduced in patients with renal impairment (see below).

◊ References.

1. Matheson AJ, Goa KL. Desirudin: a review of its use in the management of thrombotic disorders. *Drugs* 2000; **60:** 679–700.

**Administration in renal impairment.** Doses of desirudin may need to be reduced in patients with moderate to severe renal impairment. A suggested initial dose based on the patient's creatinine clearance (CC) is:

- CC 31 to 60 mL/minute: 5 mg twice daily
- CC less than 31 mL/minute: 1.7 mg twice daily

Further reductions in dose may be needed, depending on the APTT.

## Preparations

**Proprietary Preparations** (details are given in Part 3)
***Austral.:*** Revasc; ***Braz.:*** Revasc†; ***Fin.:*** Revasc†; ***Fr.:*** Revasc; ***Ger.:*** Revasc; ***Irl.:*** Revasc†; ***Norw.:*** Revasc; ***NZ:*** Revasc†; ***Spain:*** Revasc; ***Swed.:*** Revasc†; ***Switz.:*** Revasc; ***UK:*** Revasc†; ***USA:*** Iprivask.

## Deslanoside *(BAN, rINN)*

Deacetyl-lanatoside C; Desacetyl-lanatoside C; Deslanosídeo; Deslanósido; Deslanosidum. 3-[(O-β-D-Glucopyranosyl-(1→4)-O-2,6-dideoxy-β-D-*ribo*-hexopyranosyl-(1→4)-O-2,6-dideoxy-β-D-*ribo*-hexopyranosyl-(1→4)-O-2,6-dideoxy-β-D-*ribo*-hexopyranosyl)oxy]-12,14-dihydroxy-3β,5β,12β-card-20(22)-enolide.

$C_{47}H_{74}O_{19}$ = 943.1.
*CAS — 17598-65-1.*
*ATC — C01AA07.*

**Pharmacopoeias.** In *Chin., Eur.* (see p.vi), *Jpn,* and *US.*

**Ph. Eur. 5.0** (Deslanoside). A white, crystalline or finely crystalline hygroscopic powder. Practically insoluble in water; very slightly soluble in alcohol. In an atmosphere of low relative humidity, it loses water. Store in airtight, glass containers at a temperature below 10°. Protect from light.

**USP 27** (Deslanoside). Store in airtight containers at a temperature of 25°, excursions permitted between 15° and 30°. Protect from light.

### Profile

Deslanoside, a cardiac glycoside with positive inotropic activity, is a derivative of lanatoside C. It has the general properties of digoxin (p.895) and has been used similarly in the management of some cardiac arrhythmias (p.816) and in heart failure (p.820).

Deslanoside is usually reserved for emergency treatment although digoxin is generally preferred. Its effects occur about 5 to 10 minutes after intravenous administration and the full action on the heart is exerted after about 2 hours. It has a half-life of about 33 hours and its effects persist for 2 to 5 days.

A rapid digitalising dose of deslanoside is up to 1.6 mg given by intravenous injection as a single dose or in divided doses. Maintenance treatment with a cardiac glycoside given by mouth may be started within 12 hours of parenteral digitalisation with deslanoside.

## Preparations

***USP 27:*** Deslanoside Injection.

**Proprietary Preparations** (details are given in Part 3)
***Austria:*** Cedilanid†; ***Braz.:*** Cedilanide; Desacil†; ***Fr.:*** Cedilanide†.
**Multi-ingredient: *Braz.:*** Gratusminal†.

## Detajmium Bitartrate *(rINN)*

4-[3-(Diethylamino)-2-hydroxypropyl]ajmalinium hydrogen tartrate monohydrate.

$C_{31}H_{47}N_3O_9,H_2O$ = 623.7.
*CAS — 53862-81-0.*

### Profile

Detajmium is a class I antiarrhythmic (p.809). It is used, as the bitartrate, in the treatment of supraventricular and ventricular arrhythmias (p.816). The dose range is from 75 to 300 mg daily by mouth depending upon the arrhythmia.

## Preparations

**Proprietary Preparations** (details are given in Part 3)
***Ger.:*** Tachmalcor.

## Dextrothyroxine Sodium *(BANM, USAN, rINN)*

Dextrotiroxina sódica; Sodium Dextrothyroxine; 3,5,3′,5′-Tetraiodo-D-thyronine Sodium; D-Thyroxine Sodium. Sodium 4-O-(4-hydroxy-3,5-di-iodophenyl)-3,5-di-iodo-D-tyrosinate hydrate.

$C_{15}H_{10}I_4NNaO_4(+ xH_2O)$ = 798.9 (anhydrous).
*CAS — 51-49-0 (dextrothyroxine); 137-53-1 (anhydrous dextrothyroxine sodium); 7054-08-2 (dextrothyroxine sodium hydrate).*

### Profile

Dextrothyroxine is the D-isomer of levothyroxine (p.1600) and has similar actions, although it has only weak thyroid hormone activity. It also has lipid regulating properties and reduces elevated plasma-cholesterol concentrations, particularly the low-density lipoprotein (LDL) fraction.

Dextrothyroxine has been used as the sodium salt in the treatment of hypercholesterolaemia in type II hyperlipoproteinaemia, but its use is severely limited by cardiotoxicity.

Dextrothyroxine was formerly used to treat hypothyroidism.

## Preparations

**Proprietary Preparations** (details are given in Part 3)
***Canad.:*** Choloxin†; ***Ger.:*** Dynothel†; ***USA:*** Choloxin†.

# Diazoxide *(BAN, USAN, rINN)*

Diazóxido; Diazoxidum; NSC-64198; Sch-6783; SRG-95213. 7-Chloro-3-methyl-2H-1,2,4-benzothiadiazine 1,1-dioxide.

$C_8H_7ClN_2O_2S$ = 230.7.
*CAS — 364-98-7.*
*ATC — C02DA01; V03AH01.*

**Pharmacopoeias.** In *Eur.* (see p.vi), *Int.*, and *US.*

**Ph. Eur. 5.0** (Diazoxide). A white or almost white, fine or crystalline powder. Practically insoluble in water; slightly soluble in alcohol; freely soluble in dimethylformamide. It is very soluble in dilute solutions of alkali hydroxides.

**USP 27** (Diazoxide). White or cream-white crystals or crystalline powder. Practically insoluble to sparingly soluble in water and in most organic solvents; freely soluble in dimethylformamide; very soluble in strong alkaline solutions. Store at a temperature of 25°, excursions permitted between 15° and 30°.

## Adverse Effects

In addition to inappropriate hypotension and hyperglycaemia (which includes ketoacidosis and hyperosmolar nonketotic coma), adverse effects frequently include oedema due to salt and water retention, which may result in precipitation of heart failure. Other adverse effects include: dysgeusia, nausea, anorexia, and other gastrointestinal disturbances; mild hyperuricaemia; extrapyramidal symptoms; eosinophilia and thrombocytopenia; dyspnoea; hypertrichosis; and headache, dizziness, tinnitus, and blurred vision. Hypersensitivity has occurred, manifesting as rashes, leucopenia, and fever.

During intravenous therapy, particularly after large intravenous boluses, adverse effects may be associated with a too rapid reduction in blood pressure and include: coronary ischaemia leading to angina, cardiac arrhythmias, marked ECG changes, tachycardia, palpitations, and bradycardia; cerebral ischaemia leading to confusion, convulsions, loss of consciousness, and neurological deficit; renal impairment; and symptoms of vasodilatation.

Diazoxide may cause a burning sensation in the injected vein; extravasation of the alkaline solution is painful.

**Effects on the blood.** A 26-year-old man with hypertension developed reversible haemolytic anaemia when treated with diazoxide by mouth on 3 separate occasions.[1]

1. Best RA, Clink HM. Haemolysis associated with diazoxide, used for the control of hypertension. *Postgrad Med J* 1975; **51:** 402–4.

**Effects on the hair.** *Hirsutism* and *hypertrichosis* are different types of excessive hair growth, but the terms have often been used interchangeably. Hirsutism is androgen-related whereas hypertrichosis is thought to be independent of hormone stimulation. Hypertrichosis is acknowledged to be a frequent adverse effect of diazoxide in children receiving long-term treatment for idiopathic hypoglycaemia.[1] Two such children had unusually deep (low-pitched) voices as well as marked hypertrichosis.[2] A woman on continuous diazoxide therapy who developed so-called hirsutism without signs of virilisation had raised serum concentrations of androgens.[3]

*Alopecia* has been reported[4] in 4 infants born to mothers who had been on long-term treatment with diazoxide during pregnancy; the condition was still present to some extent when the infants were last observed at the ages of 5 months to 1 year.

1. Burton JL, *et al.* Hypertrichosis due to diazoxide. *Br J Dermatol* 1975; **93:** 707–11.
2. West RJ. Side effects of diazoxide. *BMJ* 1978; **2:** 506.
3. Hallengren B, Hökfelt B. Increase of serum androgens during diazoxide treatment. *Lancet* 1984; **ii:** 1044–5.
4. Milner RDG, Chouksey SK. Effects of fetal exposure to diazoxide in man. *Arch Dis Child* 1972; **47:** 537–43.

**Extrapyramidal effects.** In a study[1] of 100 hypertensive patients receiving diazoxide, the incidence of extrapyramidal symptoms was 15%.

1. Pohl JEF. Development and management of extrapyramidal symptoms in hypertensive patients treated with diazoxide. *Am Heart J* 1975; **89:** 401–2.

**Pancreatitis.** Ten patients with severe hypertension and renal failure were treated with diazoxide in a last attempt to avert nephrectomy; 1 patient developed acute pancreatitis and another diabetic ketoacidosis.[1] Both patients recovered from these effects when diazoxide was withdrawn.

1. De Broe M, *et al.* Oral diazoxide for malignant hypertension. *Lancet* 1972; **i:** 1397.

**Voice changes.** See Effects on the Hair, above.

## Treatment of Adverse Effects

Treatment is largely symptomatic. Severe hyperglycaemia may be corrected by giving insulin: less severe hyperglycaemia may respond to oral hypoglycaemics. Hypotension may be managed with intravenous fluids. Severe hypotension may require sympathomimetics. Antiparkinsonian drugs, such as procyclidine, have been given to control extrapyramidal effects while a diuretic may be required for salt and water retention. Diazoxide can be removed from the body by dialysis but recovery is relatively low owing to extensive protein binding.

## Precautions

Diazoxide should be used with care in patients with impaired cardiac or cerebral circulation and in patients with aortic coarctation, arteriovenous shunt, heart failure, or other cardiac disorders in which an increase in cardiac output could be detrimental. During prolonged therapy blood-glucose concentrations and blood pressure should be monitored and the blood should be examined regularly for signs of leucopenia and thrombocytopenia; in children, bone and psychological maturation, and growth, should be regularly assessed. Caution is necessary in patients with renal impairment.

If given during labour, diazoxide may cause cessation of uterine contractions and delay delivery unless oxytocin is given concomitantly.

**Pregnancy.** Transplacental transfer of diazoxide was considered[1] to be responsible for an inappropriately low plasma-insulin concentration in an infant whose mother had received diazoxide 150 mg daily for 47 days prior to delivery. For reference to alopecia in neonates whose mothers had received diazoxide during pregnancy, see Effects on the Hair under Adverse Effects, above.

For reports of sedation, hypotonia, hypoventilation, or apnoea among infants born to mothers given both diazoxide and clomethiazole edisilate for the treatment of toxaemia of pregnancy, see Precautions, Pregnancy, in Clomethiazole Edisilate, p.683.

1. Smith MJ, *et al.* Neonatal hyperglycaemia after prolonged maternal treatment with diazoxide. *BMJ* 1982; **284:** 1234.

## Interactions

The hyperglycaemic, hyperuricaemic, and hypotensive actions of diazoxide may be enhanced by diuretics. Use of diazoxide with other antihypertensives or vasodilators may lead to increased risk of hypotension.

**Chlorpromazine.** Chlorpromazine was reported[1] to enhance the hyperglycaemic effect of diazoxide in a 2-year-old child.

1. Aynsley-Green A, Illig R. Enhancement by chlorpromazine of hyperglycaemic action of diazoxide. *Lancet* 1975; **ii:** 658–9.

**Phenytoin.** For the effect of diazoxide on serum-phenytoin concentrations, see p.373.

## Pharmacokinetics

Diazoxide is readily absorbed from the gastrointestinal tract and more than 90% bound to plasma proteins, although protein binding is decreased in uraemic patients. Its plasma half-life has been estimated to range from about 20 to 45 hours but values of up to 60 hours have been reported. The half-life is reported to be prolonged in renal impairment and shorter for children. The plasma half-life greatly exceeds the duration of vascular activity. Diazoxide is partly metabolised in the liver and is excreted in the urine both unchanged and in the form of metabolites; only small amounts are recovered from the faeces. It crosses the placenta and the blood-brain barrier.

**Children.** A pharmacokinetic study[1] of diazoxide in 4 children with hypoglycaemia revealed a plasma half-life of 9.5 to 24 hours, which is considerably shorter than that in adults.

1. Pruitt AW, *et al.* Disposition of diazoxide in children. *Clin Pharmacol Ther* 1973; **14:** 73–82.

## Uses and Administration

Diazoxide increases the concentration of glucose in the plasma; it inhibits the secretion of insulin by the beta cells of the pancreas, and may increase the hepatic output of glucose. When given intravenously, it produces a fall in blood pressure by a vasodilator effect on the arterioles and a reduction in peripheral resistance. Diazoxide is closely related structurally to the thiazide diuretics, but has an antidiuretic action and thus produces fluid and electrolyte retention; a diuretic may be given concomitantly to reduce fluid retention.

Diazoxide is used by mouth in the management of intractable hypoglycaemia and intravenously in the management of hypertensive crises (p.825), particularly when first-line drugs such as sodium nitroprusside are ineffective or unsuitable. Diazoxide is not given by mouth in the chronic treatment of hypertension because of the severity of the adverse effects produced.

In **hypoglycaemia**, diazoxide is given in an initial dose of 3 to 5 mg/kg daily in 2 or 3 divided doses by mouth, then the dosage is adjusted according to response. Usual maintenance doses are from 3 to 8 mg/kg daily but total doses of up to 1 g daily have been given to adults with insulinomas (p.504). In neonates and infants, the initial dose is 5 to 10 mg/kg daily in 2 or 3 divided doses; usual maintenance doses have ranged from 8 to 15 mg/kg daily, although up to 20 mg/kg daily may be given to children with leucine-sensitive hypoglycaemia. The hyperglycaemic effect normally begins within 1 hour of administration and lasts for up to 8 hours.

In **hypertensive crises**, a bolus intravenous injection of 1 to 3 mg/kg is given within 30 seconds, up to a maximum dose of 150 mg, and repeated after 5 to 15 minutes if required.

Reduced doses may be necessary in patients with renal impairment.

### Preparations

***BP 2003:*** Diazoxide Injection; Diazoxide Tablets;
***USP 27:*** Diazoxide Capsules; Diazoxide Injection; Diazoxide Oral Suspension.

**Proprietary Preparations** (details are given in Part 3)
***Arg.:*** Proglicem; ***Belg.:*** Hyperstat†; ***Braz.:*** Glicemin†; Tensuril; ***Canad.:*** Hyperstat; Proglycem; ***Fr.:*** Hyperstat†; Proglicem; ***Ger.:*** Hypertonalum; Proglicem; ***Gr.:*** Hyperstat; Proglycem; ***Ital.:*** Hyperstat; Proglicem; ***Mex.:*** Hyperstat; Sefulken; ***Neth.:*** Hyperstat; Proglicem; ***S.Afr.:*** Hyperstat†; ***Spain:*** Hyperstat†; ***Swed.:*** Hyperstat; ***Switz.:*** Hyperstat†; Proglicem; ***UK:*** Eudemine; ***USA:*** Hyperstat; Proglycem.

## Diclofenamide *(BAN, rINN)*

Dichlorphenamide; Diclofenamida; Diclofenamidum. 4,5-Dichlorobenzene-1,3-disulphonamide.

$C_6H_6Cl_2N_2O_4S_2$ = 305.2.
*CAS — 120-97-8.*
*ATC — S01EC02.*

**Pharmacopoeias.** In *Chin., Jpn,* and *US.*

### Profile

Diclofenamide is an inhibitor of carbonic anhydrase with properties similar to those of acetazolamide (p.849). When given by mouth, its effect begins within 1 hour and lasts for 6 to 12 hours.

Diclofenamide is used to reduce intra-ocular pressure in glaucoma (p.1485). The usual initial dose is 100 to 200 mg by mouth, then 100 mg every 12 hours until the desired response is obtained, followed by a maintenance dose of 25 to 50 mg one to three times daily. Diclofenamide sodium has been given by injection.

### Preparations

***USP 27:*** Dichlorphenamide Tablets.

**Proprietary Preparations** (details are given in Part 3)
***Austral.:*** Daranide†; ***Austria:*** Glaucol†; ***Belg.:*** Oratrol; ***Denm.:*** Oralcon†; ***Gr.:*** Oratrol; ***Hong Kong:*** Oratrol†; ***Irl.:*** Daranide†; ***Ital.:*** Antidrasi; Fenamide; Glaumid; ***Spain:*** Glauconide; Oratrol†; ***Swed.:*** Oralcon†; ***Switz.:*** Oratrol†; ***USA:*** Daranide.

## Dicoumarol *(rINN)*

Bishydroxycoumarin; Dicoumarin; Dicumarol *(USAN)*; Melitoxin. 3,3′-Methylenebis(4-hydroxycoumarin).

$C_{19}H_{12}O_6$ = 336.3.
*CAS — 66-76-2.*
*ATC — B01AA01.*

**Pharmacopoeias.** In *Int.*

### Adverse Effects, Treatment, and Precautions

As for Warfarin Sodium, p.1022, although gastrointestinal side-effects are reported to occur more frequently. The absorption of dicoumarol is affected by food.

**Breast feeding.** No adverse effects have been observed in breast-feeding infants whose mothers were receiving dicoumarol, and the American Academy of Pediatrics considers[1] that it is therefore usually compatible with breast feeding.

1. American Academy of Pediatrics. The transfer of drugs and other chemicals into human milk. *Pediatrics* 2001; **108:** 776–89. Correction. *ibid.*; 1029. Also available at: http://aappolicy.aappublications.org/cgi/content/full/pediatrics%3b108/3/776 (accessed 06/07/04)

### Interactions

The interactions associated with oral anticoagulants are discussed in detail under warfarin (p.1023). Specific references to interactions involving dicoumarol can be found under the headings for the following drug groups: analgesics; antiarrhythmics; antibacterials; antidepressants; antidiabetics; antiepileptics; antigout drugs; anxiolytic sedatives; gastrointestinal drugs; lipid regulating drugs; sex hormones; and vitamins.

### Pharmacokinetics

Dicoumarol is slowly and erratically absorbed from the gastrointestinal tract and is extensively bound to plasma proteins. It is metabolised in the liver and is excreted in the urine, mainly as metabolites.

### Uses and Administration

Dicoumarol is an orally administered coumarin anticoagulant with actions similar to those of warfarin (p.1028). It is used in the management of thromboembolic disorders (p.837). The initial dose of dicoumarol is usually 200 to 300 mg with a daily maintenance dose according to coagulation tests of 25 to 200 mg.

Because of its unpredictability of response and high incidence of gastrointestinal effects, dicoumarol has been largely replaced by warfarin.

### Preparations

**Proprietary Preparations** (details are given in Part 3)
***Swed.:*** Apekumarol†.

## Digitalis Leaf

Digit. Fol.; Digit. Leaf; Digital, hoja de; Digitale Pourprée; Digitalis; Digitalis Folium; Digitalis Purpureae Folium; Feuille de Digitale; Fingerhutblatt; Folha de Dedaleira; Foxglove Leaf; Hoja de Digital.
*ATC — C01AA03.*

NOTE. The term 'digitalis' is often used to describe the entire class of cardiac glycosides.

**Pharmacopoeias.** In *Eur.* (see p.vi), *Jpn,* and *US.*

**Ph. Eur. 5.0** (Digitalis Leaf). The dried leaf of *Digitalis purpurea*. It contains not less than 0.3% of cardenolic glycosides, expressed as digitoxin, and calculated with reference to the drug dried at 100° to 105°. Protect from light and moisture.

**USP 27** (Digitalis). The dried leaf of *Digitalis purpurea* (Scrophulariaceae). The potency is such that, when assayed as directed, 100 mg is equivalent to not less than 1 USP unit. Store in containers that protect it from absorbing moisture.

### Profile

Digitalis leaf contains a number of cardiac glycosides with positive inotropic activity, including digitoxin, gitoxin, and gitaloxin. It has the general properties described under digoxin (p.895) and has been used similarly in the management of heart failure. However, when treatment with a cardiac glycoside is required a single glycoside is preferred to digitalis, and digoxin or digitoxin are most commonly used.

Digitalis is used in herbal and homoeopathic medicine.

### Preparations

***USP 27:*** Digitalis Capsules; Digitalis Tablets.

**Proprietary Preparations** (details are given in Part 3)
***Ger.:*** Digophton.

**Multi-ingredient:** ***Austria:*** Augentropfen Stulln; ***Ger.:*** Augentropfen Stulln Mono; Unguentum lymphaticum; ***Switz.:*** Augentonicum; Collypan.

## Digitalis Lanata Leaf

Austrian Digitalis; Austrian Foxglove; Digitalis lanata, hoja de; Digitalis Lanatae Folium; Woolly Foxglove Leaf.
*CAS — 17575-20-1 (lanatoside A).*

### Profile

Digitalis lanata leaf consists of the dried leaves of the woolly foxglove, *Digitalis lanata* (Scrophulariaceae), containing about 1 to 1.4% of a mixture of cardioactive glycosides, including digoxin, digitoxin, acetyldigoxin, acetyldigitoxin, lanatoside A, and deslanoside.

Digitalis lanata leaf is used as a source for the manufacture of digoxin and other glycosides.

◊ There have been reports[1] of toxicity following ingestion of dietary supplements contaminated with digitalis lanata.

1. Slifman NR, *et al.* Contamination of botanical dietary supplements by digitalis lanata. *N Engl J Med* 1998; **339:** 806–11.

## Digitoxin *(BAN, rINN)*

Digitaline Cristallisée; Digitoxina; Digitoxinum; Digitoxoside. 3β-[(O-2,6-Dideoxy-β-D-*ribo*-hexopyranosyl-(1→4)-O-2,6-dideoxy-β-D-*ribo*-hexopyranosyl-(1→4)-2,6-dideoxy-β-D-*ribo*-hexopyranosyl)oxy]-14β-hydroxy-5β-card-20(22)-enolide.

$C_{41}H_{64}O_{13}$ = 764.9.
*CAS — 71-63-6.*
*ATC — C01AA04.*

**Pharmacopoeias.** In *Chin., Eur.* (see p.vi), *Int., Jpn,* and *US.*

**Ph. Eur. 5.0** (Digitoxin). A white or almost white powder. Practically insoluble in water; slightly soluble in alcohol and in methyl alcohol; freely soluble in a mixture of equal volumes of chloroform and methyl alcohol. Protect from light.

**USP 27** (Digitoxin). A cardiotonic glycoside obtained from *Digitalis purpurea, Digitalis lanata* (Scrophulariaceae), or other suitable species of *Digitalis.* A white or pale buff-coloured, odourless, microcrystalline powder. Practically insoluble in water; soluble 1 in 150 of alcohol and 1 in 40 of chloroform; very slightly soluble in ether. Store in airtight containers.

**Adsorption.** Binding to an inline intravenous filter containing a cellulose ester membrane accounted for a reduction[1] in digitoxin concentration of up to 25% from solutions of digitoxin 200 micrograms in 50 mL of glucose 5% or sodium chloride 0.9%. Pretreatment of the filter with a polymer coating reduced adsorbance by about half.[2]

Digitoxin was found to be adsorbed onto glass and plastic in substantial amounts from simple aqueous solutions but not from solutions in 30% alcohol, or in plasma, or urine.[3]

1. Butler LD, *et al.* Effect of inline filtration on the potency of low-dose drugs. *Am J Hosp Pharm* 1980; **37:** 935–41.
2. Kanke M, *et al.* Binding of selected drugs to a "treated" inline filter. *Am J Hosp Pharm* 1983; **40:** 1323–8.
3. Molin L, *et al.* Solubility, partition, and adsorption of digitalis glycosides. *Acta Pharm Suec* 1983: **20:** 129–44.

### Adverse Effects, Treatment, and Precautions

As for Digoxin, below. Toxicity may be more prolonged after withdrawal of digitoxin because of the longer half-life.

◊ References.

1. Lely AH, van Enter CHJ. Large-scale digitoxin intoxication. *BMJ* 1970; **3:** 737–40.
2. Gilfrich H-J, *et al.* Treatment of massive digitoxin overdose by charcoal haemoperfusion and cholestyramine. *Lancet* 1978; **i:** 505.
3. Pond S, *et al.* Treatment of digitoxin overdose with oral activated charcoal. *Lancet* 1981; **ii:** 1177–8.
4. Kurowski V, *et al.* Treatment of a patient with severe digitoxin intoxication by Fab fragments of anti-digitalis antibodies. *Intensive Care Med* 1992; **18:** 439–42.
5. Schmitt K, *et al.* Massive digitoxin intoxication treated with digoxin-specific antibodies in a child. *Pediatr Cardiol* 1994; **15:** 48–9.

### Interactions

As for Digoxin, below. Since digitoxin is significantly metabolised in the liver it may be affected by drugs that induce microsomal enzymes, including rifampicin (see below) and antiepileptics such as phenobarbital.

**Antibacterials.** Acute heart failure has been reported in a patient taking digitoxin when treatment with *rifampicin* and isoniazid was started; plasma-digitoxin concentrations fell from a pretreatment steady-state value of 27 nanograms/mL to 10 nanograms/mL. The reduction in the digitoxin concentration was attributed to induction of digitoxin metabolism by rifampicin.[1]

Digitoxin toxicity has been described in 2 patients following addition of *azithromycin* to their therapy.[2]

1. Boman G, *et al.* Acute cardiac failure during treatment with digitoxin—an interaction with rifampicin. *Br J Clin Pharmacol* 1980; **10:** 89–90.
2. Thalhammer F, *et al.* Azithromycin-related toxic effects of digitoxin. *Br J Clin Pharmacol* 1998; **45:** 91–2.

**Antineoplastics.** A mean overall increase of 109% was seen in digitoxin clearance in 5 patients during concomitant treatment with *aminoglutethimide*. The interaction was attributed to the induction of hepatic enzymes by aminoglutethimide.[1]

1. Lønning PE, *et al.* Effect of aminoglutethimide on antipyrine, theophylline, and digitoxin disposition in breast cancer. *Clin Pharmacol Ther* 1984; **36:** 796–802.

**Calcium-channel blockers.** Steady-state plasma concentrations of digitoxin increased by an average of 35% over 2 to 3 weeks in 8 of 10 patients when *verapamil* 240 mg daily was added to their therapy. Total body clearance and extra-renal clearance of digitoxin were reduced by 27% and 29% respectively although renal excretion was unchanged. Plasma-digitoxin concentrations increased by a mean of 21% in 5 of 10 patients treated with *diltiazem* but were not increased by concomitant treatment with *nifedipine*.[1]

1. Kuhlman J. Effects of verapamil, diltiazem, and nifedipine on plasma levels and renal excretion of digitoxin. *Clin Pharmacol Ther* 1985; **38:** 667–73.

**Diuretics.** *Spironolactone* has been reported to decrease the half-life and the urinary elimination of unchanged digitoxin when given for at least 10 days to 8 patients on oral maintenance digitoxin therapy.[1] However, increased digitoxin half-life has been reported[2] in 3 healthy subjects when spironolactone was added to digitoxin therapy. The interaction was judged to be of minor clinical importance.


1. Wirth KE, *et al.* Metabolism of digitoxin in man and its modification by spironolactone. *Eur J Clin Pharmacol* 1976; **9:** 345–54.
2. Carruthers SG, Dujovne CA. Cholestyramine and spironolactone and their combination in digitoxin elimination. *Clin Pharmacol Ther* 1980; **27:** 184–7.


## Pharmacokinetics

Digitoxin is readily and completely absorbed from the gastrointestinal tract. Therapeutic plasma concentrations may range from 10 to 35 nanograms/mL but there is considerable interindividual variation. Digitoxin is more than 90% bound to plasma proteins. It is very slowly eliminated from the body and is metabolised in the liver. Most metabolites are inactive; the major active metabolite is digoxin. Enterohepatic recycling occurs and digitoxin is excreted in the urine, mainly as metabolites. It is also excreted in the faeces and this route becomes significant in renal impairment. Digitoxin has an elimination half-life of up to 7 days or more. The half-life is generally unchanged in renal impairment.

The pharmacokinetics of digitoxin may be affected by age and by concurrent diseases (see under Uses and Administration, below).

## Uses and Administration

Digitoxin is a cardiac glycoside with positive inotropic activity. It has actions similar to those of digoxin (below) and is used in the management of some cardiac arrhythmias (p.816) and in heart failure (p.820).

Digitoxin is the most potent of the digitalis glycosides and is the most cumulative in action. The onset of its action is slower than that of the other cardiac glycosides and it may therefore be less suitable than digoxin for rapid digitalisation; following oral administration its effects may be evident in about 2 hours and its full effects in about 12 hours. Its effects persist for about 3 weeks.

As described under digoxin, dosage should be carefully adjusted to the needs of the individual patient. Steady-state therapeutic plasma concentrations of digitoxin may range from 10 to 35 nanograms/mL; higher values may be associated with toxicity. In adults an initial dose of 600 micrograms of digitoxin by mouth may be given for rapid digitalisation, followed by 400 micrograms after 4 to 6 hours, then 200 micrograms every 4 to 6 hours as necessary; the maximum total dose is usually 1.6 mg. For slow digitalisation 200 micrograms may be given twice daily for 4 days. The maintenance dose varies from 50 to 300 micrograms once daily, the usual dose being 150 micrograms daily. (In the UK, the *British National Formulary* recommends 100 micrograms daily or on alternate days, increased to 200 micrograms daily if necessary.) Digitoxin may also be given in similar doses by slow intravenous injection when vomiting or other conditions prevent administration by mouth. It has also been given intramuscularly but injections may be irritant.

**Administration in children.** Children were found to have a greater volume of distribution of digitoxin than adults and a shorter mean half-life, although individual variation was considerable. The increase in total clearance in children compared with adults was attributed to greater metabolic clearance. Digitalisation doses of 20 micrograms/kg were well tolerated.[1]


1. Larsen A, Storstein L. Digitoxin kinetics and renal excretion in children. *Clin Pharmacol Ther* 1983; **33:** 717–26.


**Administration in the elderly.** Digitoxin half-life, apparent volume of distribution, and clearance were not found to differ in elderly subjects compared with young adults following intravenous injection in a single-dose study. The long half-life may make once weekly dosing possible in poorly compliant patients.[1]


1. Donovan MA, *et al.* The effect of age on digitoxin pharmacokinetics. *Br J Clin Pharmacol* 1981; **11:** 401–2.


**Administration in renal disease.** The pharmacokinetics of digitoxin were changed significantly in 5 patients with nephrotic syndrome. The apparent volume of distribution of digitoxin was increased and protein binding decreased. Such patients should be maintained at lower serum-digitoxin concentrations than other patients but will need larger doses because of the shortened serum half-life and the increased renal excretion of digitoxin and its cardioactive metabolites.[1]


1. Storstein L. Studies on digitalis VII: influence of nephrotic syndrome on protein binding, pharmacokinetics, and renal excretion of digitoxin and cardioactive metabolites. *Clin Pharmacol Ther* 1976; **20:** 158–66.


## Preparations

***BP 2003:*** Digitoxin Tablets;
***USP 27:*** Digitoxin Injection; Digitoxin Tablets.

**Proprietary Preparations** (details are given in Part 3)
***Austria:*** Digimerck; Ditaven; ***Belg.:*** Digitaline; ***Braz.:*** Digitaline; Variplastic†; ***Canad.:*** Digitaline†; ***Fr.:*** Digitaline†; ***Ger.:*** Coramedan; Digimed; Digimerck; Ditaven†; Tardigal; ***Hong Kong:*** Digitaline†; ***Norw.:*** Digitrin†; ***Swed.:*** Digitrin; ***USA:*** Crystodigin.

**Multi-ingredient:** ***Austria:*** Ditaven comp†; ***Switz.:*** Augentonicum; Optazine†.

The symbol † denotes a preparation no longer actively marketed

# Digoxin *(BAN, rINN)*

Digoxina; Digoxinum; Digoxosidum. 3β-[(O-2,6-Dideoxy-β-D-*ribo*-hexopyranosyl-(1→4)-O-2,6-dideoxy-β-D-*ribo*-hexopyranosyl-(1→4)-2,6-dideoxy-β-D-*ribo*-hexopyranosyl)oxy]-12β,14β-dihydroxy-5β-card-20(22)-enolide.

$C_{41}H_{64}O_{14}$ = 780.9.
*CAS — 20830-75-5.*
*ATC — C01AA05.*

**Pharmacopoeias.** In *Chin., Eur.* (see p.vi), *Int., Jpn, Pol.,* and *US.*

**Ph. Eur. 5.0** (Digoxin). A white or almost white powder or colourless crystals. Practically insoluble in water; slightly soluble in alcohol; freely soluble in a mixture of equal volumes of dichloromethane and methyl alcohol. Protect from light.

**USP 27** (Digoxin). A cardiotonic glycoside obtained from the leaves of *Digitalis lanata* (Scrophulariaceae). Clear to white, odourless, crystals, or a white, odourless, crystalline powder. Practically insoluble in water and in ether; slightly soluble in diluted alcohol and in chloroform; freely soluble in pyridine. Store in airtight containers.

## Adverse Effects

Digoxin and the other cardiac glycosides commonly produce adverse effects because the margin between the therapeutic and toxic doses is small; plasma concentrations of digoxin in excess of 2 nanograms/mL are considered to be an indication that the patient is at special risk although there is considerable interindividual variation. There have been many fatalities, particularly due to cardiac toxicity.

Nausea, vomiting, and anorexia may be among the earliest symptoms of digoxin toxicity or overdosage; diarrhoea and abdominal pain may occur. Certain neurological effects are also common symptoms of digoxin overdosage and include headache, facial pain, fatigue, weakness, dizziness, drowsiness, disorientation, mental confusion, bad dreams and more rarely delirium, acute psychoses, and hallucinations. Convulsions have been reported. Visual disturbances including blurred vision may occur; colour vision may be affected with objects appearing yellow or less frequently green, red, brown, blue, or white. Hypersensitivity reactions are rare; thrombocytopenia has been reported. The cardiac glycosides may have some oestrogenic activity and occasionally cause gynaecomastia at therapeutic doses.

Rapid intravenous injection of digoxin may cause vasoconstriction and transient hypertension. Intramuscular or subcutaneous injection can cause local irritation.

The most serious adverse effects are those on the heart. Toxic doses may cause or aggravate heart failure. Supraventricular or ventricular arrhythmias and defects of conduction are common and may be an early indication of excessive dosage, particularly in children. In general the incidence and severity of arrhythmias is related to the severity of the underlying heart disease. Almost any arrhythmia may ensue, but particular note should be made of supraventricular tachycardia, especially atrioventricular (AV) junctional tachycardia and atrial tachycardia with block. Ventricular arrhythmias including extrasystoles, sinoatrial block, sinus bradycardia, and AV block may also occur.

Hypokalaemia predisposes to digoxin toxicity; adverse reactions to digoxin may be precipitated if hypokalaemia occurs, for example following the prolonged administration of diuretics. Hyperkalaemia occurs in acute digoxin overdosage.

As digoxin has a shorter half-life than digitalis or digitoxin any toxic effects will tend to resolve more rapidly.

◊ General references to digitalis toxicity.


1. Beller GA, *et al.* Digitalis intoxication: a prospective clinical study with serum level concentrations. *N Engl J Med* 1971; **284:** 989–97.
2. Bullock RE, Hall RJC. Digitalis toxicity and poisoning. *Adverse Drug React Acute Poisoning Rev* 1982; **1:** 201–22.
3. Pentel PR, Salerno DM. Cardiac drug toxicity: digitalis glycosides and calcium-channel and β-blocking agents. *Med J Aust* 1990; **152:** 88–94.
4. Wells TG, *et al.* Age-related differences in digoxin toxicity and its treatment. *Drug Safety* 1992; **7:** 135–51.
5. Johnston GD. Adverse reaction profile: digoxin. *Prescribers' J* 1993; **33:** 29–35.
6. Kernan WN, *et al.* Incidence of hospitalization for digitalis toxicity among elderly Americans. *Am J Med* 1994; **96:** 426–31.
7. Li-Saw-Hee FL, Lip GYH. How safe is digoxin? *Adverse Drug React Bull* 1998; (Feb): 715–18.


**Effects on the blood.** Thrombocytopenia has been reported[1] in a small number of patients taking digoxin. An association between several cardiovascular drugs, including digitalis glycosides (digoxin and acetyldigoxin), and agranulocytosis was also found in an international study[2] although again the incidence was low.


1. George JN, *et al.* Drug-induced thrombocytopenia: a systematic review of published case reports. *Ann Intern Med* 1998; **129:** 886–90.
2. Kelly JP, *et al.* Risks of agranulocytosis and aplastic anemia in relation to the use of cardiovascular drugs: the international agranulocytosis and aplastic anemia study. *Clin Pharmacol Ther* 1991; **49:** 330–41.


**Effects in the elderly.** Elderly patients may be particularly susceptible to digoxin toxicity, even at therapeutic plasma concentrations.[1] Adverse effects reported in elderly patients with toxic plasma-digoxin concentrations have included chorea,[2] profuse watery diarrhoea,[3] and dysphagia with dysphonia.[4]


1. Miura T, *et al.* Effect of aging on the incidence of digoxin toxicity. *Ann Pharmacother* 2000; **34:** 427–32.
2. Mulder LJMM, *et al.* Generalised chorea due to digoxin toxicity. *BMJ* 1988; **296:** 1262.
3. Andrews PA, Wilkinson PR. Diarrhoea as a side effect of digoxin. *BMJ* 1990; **301:** 1398.
4. Cordeiro MF, Arnold KG. Digoxin toxicity presenting as dysphagia and dysphonia. *BMJ* 1991; **302:** 1025.


**Hypersensitivity.** Hypersensitivity reactions to cardiac glycosides are rare but skin reactions have been reported. An 86-year-old man developed a generalised, pruritic, erythematous rash following administration of digoxin intravenously.[1] The rash recurred following rechallenge with digoxin tablets.


1. Martin SJ, Shah D. Cutaneous hypersensitivity reaction to digoxin. *JAMA* 1994; **271:** 1905.


## Treatment of Adverse Effects

In *acute poisoning*, gastric lavage may be considered if the patient presents within one hour of ingestion. Repeated doses of activated charcoal may be given to reduce the absorption and enterohepatic recycling of cardiac glycosides; colestyramine and colestipol have also been tried. Attempts to remove cardiac glycosides by haemodialysis or peritoneal dialysis have generally been ineffective and the value of haemoperfusion is controversial. Forced diuresis with furosemide is generally ineffective and may be dangerous; serious electrolyte imbalance may result from the use of such potent diuretics.

Cardiac toxicity in acute or chronic poisoning should be treated under ECG control and serum electrolytes should be monitored. Antiarrhythmic treatment may be necessary and should be determined by the specific arrhythmia present (see p.816). Atropine is given intravenously to correct bradycardia and in patients with heart block. Pacing may be necessary if atropine is not effective. Potassium chloride may be given in hypokalaemic patients provided that renal function is normal and heart block is not present. Potassium has also been given to normokalaemic patients but caution is needed since hyperkalaemia can occur rapidly. Other electrolyte imbalances should be corrected.

In *massive overdosage* progressive hyperkalaemia occurs and is fatal unless reversed. Soluble insulin with glucose has been given and, if the hyperkalaemia is refractory, dialysis may be tried. Massive life-threatening overdosage has been treated successfully with digoxin-specific antibody fragments (p.1036).

For the treatment of *chronic poisoning* temporary withdrawal of digoxin or other cardiac glycosides may be all that is necessary, with subsequent doses adjusted according to the needs of the patient. Serum electrolytes should be measured and the ECG monitored. Potassium supplements should be given to correct hypokalaemia.

◊ References.


1. Allen NM, Dunham GD. Treatment of digitalis intoxication with emphasis on the clinical use of digoxin immune Fab. *DICP Ann Pharmacother* 1990; **24:** 991–8.
2. Dick M, *et al.* Digitalis intoxication recognition and management. *J Clin Pharmacol* 1991; **31:** 444–7.
3. Critchley JAJH, Critchley LAH. Digoxin toxicity in chronic renal failure: treatment by multiple dose activated charcoal intestinal dialysis. *Hum Exp Toxicol* 1997; **16:** 733–5.


## Precautions

Digoxin is generally contra-indicated in patients with hypertrophic obstructive cardiomyopathy unless there is severe cardiac failure, since the outflow obstruction may be worsened. It is also contra-indicated in patients with the Wolff-Parkinson-White syndrome or other evidence of an accessory pathway, especially if it is accompanied by atrial fibrillation, since ventricular tachycardia or fibrillation may be precipitated. Digoxin is not an appropriate form of therapy for any ventricular arrhythmia.

Digoxin toxicity is common and may result from raised plasma concentrations or an increase in sensitivity to digoxin. Almost any deterioration in the condition of the heart or circulation may increase the sensitivity to digoxin and it should be used with caution in all patients with cardiovascular disease. Early signs of digoxin toxicity should be watched for and the heart rate should generally be maintained above 60 beats per minute. Toxicity may result from administering loading doses too rapidly and from accumulation of maintenance doses as well as from acute poisoning. Even with intravenous administration a response may take a number of hours, and persistence of tachycardia is therefore not a reason to exceed the recommended intravenous dose.

Digoxin should be used with caution in partial heart block since complete heart block may be induced; it should also be used with care in sinus node disorders. Caution is also required in acute myocarditis (such as rheumatic carditis), in acute myocardial infarction, in advanced heart failure, and in severe pulmonary disease, due to the increased myocardial sensitivity. Digoxin may also enhance the occurrence of arrhythmias in patients undergoing cardioversion and should be withdrawn 1 to 2 days before such procedures if possible. If cardioversion is essential and digoxin has already been given, low energy shocks must be used.

Electrolyte imbalances may affect the sensitivity to digoxin, as may thyroid dysfunction. The effects of digoxin are enhanced by hypokalaemia, hypomagnesaemia, hypercalcaemia, hypoxia, and hypothyroidism and doses may need to be reduced until these conditions are corrected. Resistance to the effects of digoxin may occur in hyperthyroidism. Digoxin should be given with care, and possibly in reduced dosage, to patients who have received it or other cardiac glycosides within the previous 2 to 3 weeks.

Digoxin doses should generally be reduced and plasma-digoxin concentrations monitored in patients with renal impairment, in the elderly, and in premature infants (see Uses and Administration, below).

**Breast feeding.** Studies[1,2] have shown that digoxin is distributed into breast milk, although the amount was considered too small to have an effect on the child. No adverse effects have been observed in breast-feeding infants whose mothers were receiving digoxin, and the American Academy of Pediatrics considers[3] that it is therefore usually compatible with breast feeding.

1. Levy M, *et al.* Excretion of drugs in human milk. *N Engl J Med* 1997; **297:** 789.
2. Chan V, *et al.* Transfer of digoxin across the placenta and into breast milk. *Br J Obstet Gynaecol* 1978; **85:** 605–9.
3. American Academy of Pediatrics. The transfer of drugs and other chemicals into human milk. *Pediatrics* 2001; **108:** 776–89. Correction. *ibid.*; 1029. Also available at: http://aappolicy.aappublications.org/cgi/content/full/pediatrics%3b108/3/776 (accessed 06/07/04)

**Gastrointestinal disorders.** Absorption from tablet formulations of digoxin may be decreased due to inadequate dissolution in patients with malabsorption syndromes or small bowel resections and it has been recommended that liquid dosage forms of digoxin should be used in the latter case.[1] However, only 40 to 60% of a digoxin dose administered as elixir was absorbed in a patient with a small bowel resection[2] compared with about 80% in patients with normal gastrointestinal function, suggesting a need for slightly increased oral maintenance doses of digoxin in patients with resections. In a further patient with a similar resection[3] a therapeutic plasma-digoxin concentration was not achieved with any oral formulation.

1. Kumer KP, *et al.* Perspectives on digoxin absorption from small bowel resections. *Drug Intell Clin Pharm* 1983; **17:** 121–3.
2. Vetticaden SJ, *et al.* Digoxin absorption in a patient with short-bowel syndrome. *Clin Pharm* 1986; **5:** 62–4.
3. Ehrenpreis ED, *et al.* Malabsorption of digoxin tablets, gel caps, and elixir in a patient with an end jejunostomy. *Ann Pharmacother* 1994; **28:** 1239–40.

**Heart surgery.** Patients undergoing cardiac surgery appear to have increased sensitivity to digoxin toxicity and thus an increased risk of arrhythmias.[1] Digoxin has been found[2] to be no better than placebo in preventing postoperative arrhythmias after coronary artery bypass surgery, and actually induced supraventricular arrhythmias in 2 patients. Arrhythmias compatible with digoxin intoxication have occurred postoperatively[1] although serum-digoxin concentrations ranged from 0 to 2.8 nanograms/mL; therefore the arrhythmias may have been due to either the surgical procedures or to increased sensitivity to digoxin.

1. Rose MR, *et al.* Arrhythmias following cardiac surgery: relation to serum digoxin levels. *Am Heart J* 1975; **89:** 288–94.
2. Weiner B, *et al.* Digoxin prophylaxis following coronary artery bypass surgery. *Clin Pharm* 1986; **5:** 55–8.

**Interference with digoxin assays.** The presence of endogenous digoxin-like substances in neonates, and in patients with liver or kidney dysfunction may be responsible for elevated values or false-positive results in some plasma-digoxin assays.[1] Some patients may have antibodies that react with the assay system and produce falsely elevated values.[2]

A number of drugs may also interfere with plasma-digoxin assays; these include prednisolone[1] and the herbal medicine ginseng.[3] Raised serum-digoxin concentrations (but without signs of digoxin toxicity) were noted in an elderly man following the use of Siberian ginseng (*Eleutherococcus senticosus*). However, concentrations remained high even when digoxin was discontinued and returned to the therapeutic range only after the ginseng was stopped. Siberian ginseng contains eleutherosides, which are chemically related to cardiac glycosides such as digoxin, and the assay may have measured these compounds, or their derivatives, as well as digoxin. Although it has been suggested that this reaction may have been due to the substitution of the unrelated cardiotoxic herb *Periploca sepium*,[4] both ginseng and Siberian ginseng have been shown to interfere with some digoxin assays *in vitro* and *in vivo*.[5] Spironolactone may interfere with digoxin assays but may also produce changes in digoxin concentrations (see Diuretics under Interactions, below).

1. Yosselson-Superstine S. Drug interferences with plasma assays in therapeutic drug monitoring. *Clin Pharmacokinet* 1984; **9:** 67–89.
2. Liendo C, *et al.* A new interference in some digoxin assays: anti-murine heterophilic antibodies. *Clin Pharmacol Ther* 1996; **60:** 593–8.
3. McRae S. Elevated serum digoxin levels in a patient taking digoxin and Siberian ginseng. *Can Med Assoc J* 1996; **155:** 293–5.
4. Awang DVC. Siberian ginseng toxicity may be case of mistaken identity. *Can Med Assoc J* 1996; **155:** 1237.
5. Dasgupta A, *et al.* Effect of Asian and Siberian ginseng on serum digoxin measurement by five digoxin immunoassays. Significant variation in digoxin-like immunoreactivity among commercial ginsengs. *Am J Clin Pathol* 2003; **119:** 298–303.

**Pregnancy.** There is considerable evidence that digoxin crosses the placenta freely with serum-digoxin concentrations at term similar in the newborn and mother. No significant adverse effects attributed to digoxin have been noted in the fetus or neonate although adverse fetal effects, including fetal death, have been reported in mothers with digitalis toxicity. Some concern has been expressed that maternal digitalis therapy may occasionally cause low birth-weights in infants of mothers with heart disease, but the underlying disease might also be important.[1] The presence of endogenous digoxin-like immunoreactive substances in the serum of pregnant women and neonates could make the interpretation of digoxin assays difficult. In one study,[2] high concentrations of endogenous digoxin-like immunoreactivity in cord blood suggested that it might be synthesised during delivery, in which case the placental transfer of digoxin might be overestimated.

1. Rotmensch HH, *et al.* Management of cardiac arrhythmias during pregnancy: current concepts. *Drugs* 1987; **33:** 623–33.
2. Lupoglazoff JM, *et al.* Endogenous digoxin-like immunoreactivity during pregnancy and at birth. *Br J Clin Pharmacol* 1993; **35:** 251–4.

## Interactions

There may be interactions between digoxin and drugs which alter its absorption, interfere with its excretion, or have additive effects on the myocardium. Drugs which cause electrolyte disturbances increase the risk of toxicity from cardiac glycosides. Thiazides and loop *diuretics* cause hypokalaemia and also hypomagnesaemia which may lead to cardiac arrhythmias. Other causes of hypokalaemia include treatment with *corticosteroids, beta$_2$ agonists* (such as salbutamol), *amphotericin B, sodium polystyrene sulfonate, carbenoxolone*, and dialysis. Hypercalcaemia may also increase toxicity and intravenous administration of *calcium salts* is best avoided in patients taking cardiac glycosides. Serum-digoxin concentrations may be significantly increased by *quinidine*, *amiodarone*, and *propafenone* and reduction of digoxin dosage may be required. Other antiarrhythmic drugs may have additive effects on the myocardium increasing the likelihood of adverse effects; *beta blockers* may potentiate bradycardia due to digoxin. *Calcium-channel blockers* may increase digoxin concentrations.

◊ Reviews of drug interactions occurring with digoxin.

1. Rodin SM, Johnson BF. Pharmacokinetic interactions with digoxin. *Clin Pharmacokinet* 1988; **15:** 227–44.
2. Magnani B, Malini PL. Cardiac glycosides: drug interactions of clinical significance. *Drug Safety* 1995; **12:** 97–109.

**ACE inhibitors.** Although increased serum-digoxin concentrations have been reported in patients with severe chronic heart failure given *captopril*,[1] other studies have failed to confirm this effect.[2,3] Studies with various other ACE inhibitors have also failed to show any significant effect on serum-digoxin concentrations. However, ACE inhibitors may cause a deterioration in renal function and this could lead to an increase in serum-digoxin concentration due to impaired digoxin excretion.[4]

1. Cleland JGF, *et al.* Interaction of digoxin and captopril. *Br J Clin Pharmacol* 1984; **17:** 214P.
2. Magelli C, *et al.* Lack of effect of captopril on serum digoxin in congestive heart failure. *Eur J Clin Pharmacol* 1989; **36:** 99–100.
3. Rossi GP, *et al.* Effect of acute captopril administration on digoxin pharmacokinetics in normal subjects. *Curr Ther Res* 1989; **46:** 439–44.
4. Mignat C, Unger T. ACE inhibitors: drug interactions of clinical significance. *Drug Safety* 1995; **12:** 334–47.

**Alpha blockers.** *Prazosin*[1] has been reported to increase the mean plasma-digoxin concentration in patients receiving a maintenance dose of digoxin.

1. Çopur S, *et al.* Effects of oral prazosin on total plasma digoxin levels. *Fundam Clin Pharmacol* 1988; **2:** 13–17.

**Angiotensin II receptor antagonists.** In a study[1] in healthy volunteers, *telmisartan* increased peak serum-digoxin concentrations but trough concentrations were unaffected and it was suggested that the effect was unlikely to be clinically significant. No interaction was found when digoxin was administered concomitantly with *losartan*[2] or with *eprosartan*[3] in healthy volunteers.

1. Stangier J, *et al.* The effect of telmisartan on the steady-state pharmacokinetics of digoxin in healthy male volunteers. *J Clin Pharmacol* 2000; **40:** 1373–9.
2. de Smet M, *et al.* Effect of multiple doses of losartan on the pharmacokinetics of single doses of digoxin in healthy volunteers. *Br J Clin Pharmacol* 1995; **40:** 571–5.
3. Martin DE, *et al.* Lack of effect of eprosartan on the single dose pharmacokinetics of orally administered digoxin in healthy male volunteers. *Br J Clin Pharmacol* 1997; **43:** 661–4.

**Antiarrhythmics.** AMIODARONE. An interaction between digoxin and amiodarone resulting in increased plasma-digoxin concentrations has been reported[1-5] on several occasions; the concentration may be doubled.[5] An increase in serum-digoxin concentrations of 68 to 800% has been reported[2] during amiodarone therapy in children. The interaction does not appear to be due to a reduction in urinary excretion alone[3,4] and seems to be dose-related. It has been recommended[1,6] that the initial dose of digoxin should be halved when amiodarone is given concurrently.

1. Moysey JO, *et al.* Amiodarone increases plasma digoxin concentrations. *BMJ* 1981; **282:** 272.
2. Koren G, *et al.* Digoxin toxicity associated with amiodarone therapy in children. *J Pediatr* 1984; **104:** 467–70.
3. Douste-Blazy P, *et al.* Influence of amiodarone on plasma and urine digoxin concentrations. *Lancet* 1984; **i:** 905.
4. Mingardi G. Amiodarone and plasma digoxin levels. *Lancet* 1984; **i:** 1238.
5. Johnston A, *et al.* The digoxin-amiodarone interaction. *Br J Clin Pharmacol* 1987; **24:** 253P.
6. Naccarelli GV, *et al.* Adverse effects of amiodarone: pathogenesis, incidence and management. *Med Toxicol Adverse Drug Exp* 1989; **4:** 246–53.

DISOPYRAMIDE. Disopyramide appears to have no clinically significant effect on the pharmacokinetics of digoxin in healthy subjects[1,2] but has been reported to modify the cardiovascular effects of digoxin.[1]

1. Elliott HL, *et al.* Pharmacodynamic and pharmacokinetic evaluation of the interaction between digoxin and disopyramide. *Br J Clin Pharmacol* 1982; **14:** 141P.
2. Risler T, *et al.* On the interaction between digoxin and disopyramide. *Clin Pharmacol Ther* 1983; **34:** 176–80.

FLECAINIDE. Administration of flecainide 200 mg twice daily to 15 healthy subjects taking digoxin caused a mean increase of 24% in predose digoxin concentrations and of 13% in digoxin concentrations 6 hours after the digoxin dose.[1] It was considered that in most cases these increases in plasma-digoxin concentrations would not present a clinical problem, but that patients with higher plasma-digoxin concentrations or atrioventricular nodal dysfunction should be monitored.

1. Weeks CE, *et al.* The effect of flecainide acetate, a new antiarrhythmic, on plasma digoxin levels. *J Clin Pharmacol* 1986; **26:** 27–31.

PROPAFENONE. Increased serum-digoxin concentrations have been reported when propafenone is given concurrently.[1-4] There is considerable interindividual variation in the extent of the interaction; increases in serum-digoxin concentrations of up to 254% have been reported. If digoxin and propafenone are given concurrently, the dose of digoxin should be reduced and serum-digoxin concentration should be monitored.

1. Nolan PE, *et al.* Effects of coadministration of propafenone on the pharmacokinetics of digoxin in healthy volunteer subjects. *J Clin Pharmacol* 1989; **29:** 46–52.
2. Calvo MV, *et al.* Interaction between digoxin and propafenone. *Ther Drug Monit* 1989; **11:** 10–15.
3. Zalzstein E, *et al.* Interaction between digoxin and propafenone in children. *J Pediatr* 1990; **116:** 310–12.
4. Bigot M-C, *et al.* Serum digoxin levels related to plasma propafenone levels during concomitant treatment. *J Clin Pharmacol* 1991; **31:** 521–6.

QUINIDINE. Quinidine causes an increase in serum-digoxin concentration in almost all patients given the two drugs concurrently.[1-3] The serum-digoxin concentration may be increased by up to 500% but is usually approximately doubled.[1] Signs and symptoms of digoxin toxicity may occur although some workers[4] have suggested that these may be accounted for by an additive effect of the 2 drugs rather than by the effect on serum-digoxin concentration. The exact mechanism of interaction is not clear but a substantial decrease in the renal and nonrenal clearance of digoxin has been demonstrated.[5] The distribution volume of digoxin may also be reduced[2] reflecting impaired tissue binding, and there is increased systemic availability.[1] It is generally recommended that the dose of digoxin is halved in digitalised patients who are to be given quinidine.[2] Subsequently, serum-digoxin concentrations should be monitored, especially during the first 1 to 2 weeks after which the new steady-state digoxin concentration should be achieved.[2]

1. Bigger JT, Leahey EB. Quinidine and digoxin: an important interaction. *Drugs* 1982; **24:** 229–39.
2. Pedersen KE. Digoxin interactions: the influence of quinidine and verapamil on the pharmacokinetics and receptor binding of digitalis glycosides. *Acta Med Scand* 1985; **697** (suppl): 1–40.
3. Mordel A, *et al.* Quinidine enhances digitalis toxicity at therapeutic serum digoxin levels. *Clin Pharmacol Ther* 1993; **53:** 457–62.
4. Walker AM, *et al.* Drug toxicity in patients receiving digoxin and quinidine. *Am Heart J* 1983; **105:** 1025–8.
5. Hedman A, *et al.* Interactions in the renal and biliary elimination of digoxin: stereoselective difference between quinine and quinidine. *Clin Pharmacol Ther* 1990; **47:** 20–6.

VERAPAMIL. For a discussion on the interaction between digoxin and verapamil, see under Calcium-channel Blockers, below.

**Antibacterials.** Approximately 10% of patients receiving digoxin may metabolise 40% or more of the drug to cardio-inactive metabolites.[1] Gut flora contribute greatly to this process, and the administration of antibacterials such as *erythromycin* or *tetracycline* to these patients appears to reduce this metabolic process resulting in higher serum concentrations.[2] Digoxin toxicity has been reported in digitalised patients given erythromycin,[3,4] *azithromycin,*[5] *clarithromycin,*[6-8] and *roxithromycin.*[9] It has been postulated[5,10] that the macrolide antibacterials may also inhibit P-glycoprotein-mediated renal tubular secretion of digoxin. Oral *neomycin* may reduce serum-digoxin concentrations by reducing digoxin absorption.

*Rifampicin* may reduce serum-digitoxin concentrations by inducing its metabolism (see p.894) although a study[11] in healthy subjects suggested that the reduction in plasma-digoxin concentrations associated with rifampicin might rather be due to induction of intestinal P-glycoprotein. Digoxin is mainly excreted unchanged in the urine but rifampicin has been reported[12] to increase digoxin dose requirements substantially in 2 patients dependent on dialysis. When rifampicin was discontinued digoxin requirements fell by about 50%.

1. Doherty JE. A digoxin-antibiotic drug interaction. *N Engl J Med* 1981; **305:** 827–8.
2. Lindenbaum J, *et al.* Inactivation of digoxin by the gut flora: reversal by antibiotic therapy. *N Engl J Med* 1981; **305:** 789–94.
3. Maxwell DL, *et al.* Digoxin toxicity due to interaction of digoxin with erythromycin. *BMJ* 1989; **298:** 572.
4. Morton MR, Cooper JW. Erythromycin-induced digoxin toxicity. *DICP Ann Pharmacother* 1989; **23:** 668–70.
5. Ten Eick AP, *et al.* Possible drug interaction between digoxin and azithromycin in a young child. *Clin Drug Invest* 2000; **20:** 61–64.
6. Midoneck SR, Etingin OR. Clarithromycin-related toxic effects of digoxin. *N Engl J Med* 1995; **333:** 1505.
7. Nawarskas JJ, *et al.* Digoxin toxicity secondary to clarithromycin therapy. *Ann Pharmacother* 1997; **31:** 864–6.
8. Laberge P, Martineau P. Clarithromycin-induced digoxin intoxication. *Ann Pharmacother* 1997; **31:** 999–1002.
9. Corallo CE, Rogers IR. Roxithromycin-induced digoxin toxicity. *Med J Aust* 1996; **165:** 433–4.
10. Wakasugi H, *et al.* Effect of clarithromycin on renal excretion of digoxin: interaction with P-glycoprotein. *Clin Pharmacol Ther* 1998; **64:** 123–8.
11. Greiner B, *et al.* The role of intestinal P-glycoprotein in the interaction of digoxin and rifampin. *J Clin Invest* 1999; **104:** 147–53.
12. Gault H, *et al.* Digoxin-rifampin interaction. *Clin Pharmacol Ther* 1984; **35:** 750–4.

**Antidepressants.** In a study[1] in healthy volunteers, administration of digoxin concomitantly with an extract of *Hypericum* for 10 days resulted in a significant decrease in the plasma-digoxin concentration. It was suggested that the interaction might be due to induction of the P-glycoprotein transporter. In a study[2] in healthy male subjects, administration of *nefazodone* increased steady-state plasma-digoxin concentrations by approximately 30% but no adverse or clinical effects were associated with the increase. However, due to the narrow therapeutic range of digoxin, it was suggested that plasma-digoxin concentrations should be monitored in patients given nefazodone concomitantly. Similar recommendations have been made for *trazodone*.

1. Johne A, *et al.* Pharmacokinetic interaction of digoxin with an herbal extract from St John's wort (Hypericum perforatum). *Clin Pharmacol Ther* 1999; **66:** 338–45.
2. Dockens RC, *et al.* Assessment of pharmacokinetic and pharmacodynamic drug interactions between nefazodone and digoxin in healthy male volunteers. *J Clin Pharmacol* 1996; **36:** 160–7.

**Antidiabetics.** Subtherapeutic plasma-digoxin concentrations were noted in a diabetic woman receiving *acarbose* and digoxin concurrently.[1] The plasma concentration of digoxin increased to a therapeutic level when acarbose was discontinued. A study[2] in healthy volunteers suggested that the interaction was due to inhibition of the absorption of digoxin by acarbose.

1. Serrano JS, *et al.* A possible interaction of potential clinical interest between digoxin and acarbose. *Clin Pharmacol Ther* 1996; **60:** 589–92.
2. Miura T, *et al.* Impairment of absorption of digoxin by acarbose. *J Clin Pharmacol* 1998; **38:** 654–7.

**Antiepileptics.** *Phenytoin* caused a marked decrease in steady-state serum-digoxin concentrations when administered with digoxin and acetyldigoxin to 6 healthy subjects for 7 days.[1] Total digoxin clearance was increased by an average of 27% and elimination half-life was reduced by an average of 30%. This interaction may be more likely with digitoxin, since digitoxin is more dependent on the liver for elimination.

A brief report of an open study[2] in 12 subjects indicated a slight but significant decrease in digoxin bioavailability when *topiramate* was given concomitantly, although half-life and renal clearance of digoxin did not appear to be affected.

1. Rameis H. On the interaction between phenytoin and digoxin. *Eur J Clin Pharmacol* 1985; **29:** 49–53.
2. Liao S, Palmer M. Digoxin and topiramate drug interaction study in male volunteers. *Pharm Res* 1993; **10** (suppl): S405.

**Antifungals.** Two men given *itraconazole* while receiving digoxin developed signs and symptoms of digoxin toxicity and elevated serum-digoxin concentrations.[1,2] A further case report[3] suggested that the interaction was due to a reduction in the renal clearance of digoxin when itraconazole was given concomitantly.

Additive adverse effects due to hypokalaemia may occur when digoxin is given with *amphotericin B*.

1. Rex J. Itraconazole–digoxin interaction. *Ann Intern Med* 1992; **116:** 525.
2. Alderman CP, Jersmann HPA. Digoxin–itraconazole interaction. *Med J Aust* 1993; **159:** 838–9.
3. Alderman CP, Allcroft PD. Digoxin-itraconazole interaction: possible mechanisms. *Ann Pharmacother* 1997; **31:** 438–40.

**Antimalarials.** In 6 subjects given *quinine sulfate,* total body clearance of digoxin after an intravenous dose was decreased by 26%, primarily through a reduction in nonrenal clearance.[1] Increased urinary excretion of digoxin was consistent with alterations in the nonrenal clearance of digoxin and might be due to changes in the metabolism or biliary secretion of digoxin. Quinine increased the mean elimination half-life of digoxin from 34.2 to 51.8 hours but did not consistently change the volume of distribution.

An increase in the plasma-digoxin concentration, but without symptoms of toxicity, was noted in two women given *hydroxychloroquine* (for rheumatoid arthritis) in addition to long-term digoxin therapy.[2]

1. Wandell M, *et al.* Effect of quinine on digoxin kinetics. *Clin Pharmacol Ther* 1980; **28:** 425–30.
2. Leden I. Digoxin–hydroxychloroquine interaction? *Acta Med Scand* 1982; **211:** 411–12.

**Antineoplastics.** A study[1] in patients undergoing antineoplastic therapy found that the absorption of digoxin from tablets was reduced by an average of 46.5%, whereas that of digoxin from liquid-filled capsules was not significantly changed. Another study[2] in similar patients found that the steady-state concentration of digoxin following administration of acetyldigoxin was reduced, but that digitoxin concentrations were maintained. It was suggested that the interaction was due to reduced absorption of digitalis glycosides through the damaged gastrointestinal mucosa and that liquid-filled capsules or digitoxin might be preferred in these patients.

1. Bjornsson TD, *et al.* Effects of high-dose cancer chemotherapy on the absorption of digoxin in two different formulations. *Clin Pharmacol Ther* 1986; **39:** 25–8.
2. Kuhlmann J. Inhibition of digoxin absorption but not of digitoxin during cytostatic drug therapy. *Arzneimittelforschung* 1982; **32:** 698–704.

**Antithyroid drugs.** Reduced peak serum-digoxin concentrations were noted in 9 of 10 healthy subjects following administration of a single oral dose of *carbimazole* although conversely in the tenth subject digoxin concentrations rose.[1] Caution is also needed since changes in thyroid function may affect sensitivity to digoxin independently of serum concentrations (see Precautions, above).

1. Rao BR, *et al.* Influence of carbimazole on serum levels and haemodynamic effects of digoxin. *Clin Drug Invest* 1997; **13:** 350–4.

**Benzodiazepines.** Raised serum-digoxin concentrations have been reported in patients also taking *diazepam*[1] or *alprazolam.*[2,3] The clearance of digoxin was reduced by these benzodiazepines.

1. Castillo-Ferrando JR, *et al.* Digoxin levels and diazepam. *Lancet* 1980; **ii:** 368.
2. Tollefson G, *et al.* Alprazolam-related digoxin toxicity. *Am J Psychiatry* 1984; **141:** 1612–14.
3. Guven H, *et al.* Age-related digoxin-alprazolam interaction. *Clin Pharmacol Ther* 1993; **54:** 42–4.

**Beta$_2$ agonists.** A single intravenous[1,2] or oral[3] dose of *salbutamol* has been reported to decrease steady-state serum-digoxin concentrations by up to 16% and 22% respectively in healthy subjects. Although salbutamol had no significant effect on the concentration of digoxin in skeletal muscle, it was considered that increased binding to skeletal muscle could explain the interaction. Beta$_2$ agonists such as salbutamol can also cause hypokalaemia which may increase susceptibility to digoxin-induced arrhythmias.

1. Edner M, Jogestrand T. Effect of salbutamol on digoxin concentration in serum and skeletal muscle. *Eur J Clin Pharmacol* 1989; **36:** 235–8.
2. Edner M, *et al.* Effect of salbutamol on digoxin pharmacokinetics. *Eur J Clin Pharmacol* 1992; **42:** 197–201.
3. Edner M, Jogestrand T. Oral salbutamol decreases serum digoxin concentration. *Eur J Clin Pharmacol* 1990; **38:** 195–7.

**Beta blockers.** Beta blockers may increase the risk of heart block and bradycardia with digoxin. In addition, *carvedilol* has been reported[1-3] to increase plasma concentrations of digoxin, although the effect is generally small and probably not clinically significant. However, a study[4] in 8 children (aged 2 weeks to 7.8 years) found that the clearance of digoxin was approximately halved by carvedilol and 2 of the children developed digoxin toxicity.

1. Grunden JW, *et al.* Augmented digoxin concentrations with carvedilol dosing in mild-moderate heart failure. *Am J Ther* 1994; **1:** 157–161.
2. Wermeling DP, *et al.* Effects of long-term oral carvedilol on the steady-state pharmacokinetics of oral digoxin in patients with mild to moderate hypertension. *Pharmacotherapy* 1994; **14:** 600–6.
3. De Mey C, *et al.* Carvedilol increases the systemic bioavailability of oral digoxin. *Br J Clin Pharmacol* 1990; **29:** 486–90.
4. Ratnapalan S, *et al.* Digoxin-carvedilol interactions in children. *J Pediatr* 2003; **142:** 572–4.

**Calcium-channel blockers.** Studies on interactions between digoxin and calcium-channel blockers appear to show that *verapamil* increases plasma-digoxin concentrations[1-3] by up to 70%. The effect of *nifedipine* is not as clear. Although it has been reported[1] to produce a 45% increase in plasma-digoxin concentrations, other studies[4,5] have reported little or no increase and the interaction is unlikely to be of clinical significance for most patients. Studies on the interaction between digoxin and *diltiazem* have also produced conflicting results. Increases in plasma-digoxin concentrations of 20% and up to 59% have been reported[6,7] and an increase in metildigoxin concentrations[7] of up to 51%. However, other studies[8,9] have shown no diltiazem-induced change in digoxin pharmacokinetics or plasma concentration. *Bepridil,*[10] *gallopamil,*[1] *mibefradil,*[11] *nisoldipine,*[12] and *nitrendipine*[13] have all been reported to increase plasma-digoxin concentrations. Bepridil increased the concentration by 34% and it was recommended that patients given this combination be monitored carefully. *Felodipine*[14,15] and *isradipine*[3] have both been reported to increase peak serum-digoxin concentrations, but steady-state digoxin concentrations were not affected and the interactions were unlikely to be of clinical relevance.

The mechanism of interaction between calcium-channel blockers and digoxin is not completely understood but appears to be related to decreased renal and nonrenal clearance of digoxin. The pharmacodynamic effects of digoxin and calcium-channel blockers may also be additive.

1. Belz GG, *et al.* Interaction between digoxin and calcium antagonists and antiarrhythmic drugs. *Clin Pharmacol Ther* 1983; **33:** 410–17.
2. Pedersen KE, *et al.* Influence of verapamil on the inotropism and pharmacokinetics of digoxin. *Eur J Clin Pharmacol* 1983; **25:** 199–206.
3. Rodin SM, *et al.* Comparative effects of verapamil and isradipine on steady-state digoxin kinetics. *Clin Pharmacol Ther* 1988; **43:** 668–72.
4. Schwartz JB, Migliore PJ. Effect of nifedipine on serum digoxin concentration and renal digoxin clearance. *Clin Pharmacol Ther* 1984; **36:** 19–24.
5. Kleinbloesem CH, *et al.* Interactions between digoxin and nifedipine at steady state in patients with atrial fibrillation. *Ther Drug Monit* 1985; **7:** 372–6.
6. Rameis H, *et al.* The diltiazem-digoxin interaction. *Clin Pharmacol Ther* 1984; **36:** 183–9.
7. Oyama Y, *et al.* Digoxin-diltiazem interaction. *Am J Cardiol* 1984; **53:** 1480–1.
8. Beltrami TR, *et al.* Lack of effects of diltiazem on digoxin pharmacokinetics. *J Clin Pharmacol* 1985; **25:** 390–2.
9. Elkayam U, *et al.* Effect of diltiazem on renal clearance and serum concentration of digoxin in patients with cardiac disease. *Am J Cardiol* 1985; **55:** 1393–5.
10. Belz GG, *et al.* Digoxin and bepridil: pharmacokinetic and pharmacodynamic interactions. *Clin Pharmacol Ther* 1986; **39:** 65–71.
11. Siepmann M, *et al.* The interaction of the calcium antagonist RO 40-5967 with digoxin. *Br J Clin Pharmacol* 1995; **39:** 491–6.
12. Kirch W, *et al.* Influence of nisoldipine on haemodynamic effects and plasma levels of digoxin. *Br J Clin Pharmacol* 1986; **22:** 155–9.
13. Kirch W, *et al.* Nitrendipine increases digoxin plasma levels dose dependently. *J Clin Pharmacol* 1986; **26:** 553.
14. Rehnqvist N, *et al.* Pharmacokinetics of felodipine and effect on digoxin plasma levels in patients with heart failure. *Drugs* 1987; **34** (suppl 3): 33–42.
15. Dunselman PHJM, *et al.* Digoxin-felodipine interaction in patients with congestive heart failure. *Eur J Clin Pharmacol* 1988; **35:** 461–5.

**Diuretics.** *Amiloride* administration increased renal clearance of digoxin and reduced the extrarenal digoxin clearance in 6 healthy subjects after a single intravenous dose of digoxin.[1] Amiloride also inhibited the digoxin-induced positive inotropic effect, but the clinical implications in cardiac patients are unknown. A further study[2] failed to confirm this effect.

*Spironolactone* and its metabolites have been reported to interfere with serum-digoxin determinations by radio-immunoassay or fluorescence-polarisation immunoassay resulting in falsely elevated measurements.[3,4] The interference with digoxin assays is neither consistent nor predictable and falsely low readings have also been reported.[5] Serum-digoxin concentrations should be interpreted with caution when digoxin is given concomitantly with spironolactone or *canrenoate*, especially since spironolactone has also been reported to decrease digoxin clearance by a median of 26% resulting in a true increase in the serum-digoxin concentration.[6]

Diuretic therapy with *triamterene* in association with a thiazide or loop diuretic increased the mean serum-digoxin concentration; this interaction was considered unlikely to be of clinical importance, except perhaps in patients with renal impairment.[7]

1. Waldorff S, *et al.* Amiloride-induced changes in digoxin dynamics and kinetics: abolition of digoxin-induced inotropism with amiloride. *Clin Pharmacol Ther* 1981; **30:** 172–6.
2. Richter JP, *et al.* The acute effects of amiloride and potassium canrenoate on digoxin-induced positive inotropism in healthy volunteers. *Eur J Clin Pharmacol* 1993; **45:** 195–6.
3. Paladino JA, *et al.* Influence of spironolactone on serum digoxin concentration. *JAMA* 1984; **251:** 470–1.
4. Foukaridis GN. Influence of spironolactone and its metabolite canrenone on serum digoxin assays. *Ther Drug Monit* 1990; **12:** 82–4.
5. Steimer W, *et al.* Intoxication due to negative canrenone interference in digoxin drug monitoring. *Lancet* 1999; **354:** 1176–7.
6. Waldorff S, *et al.* Spironolactone-induced changes in digoxin kinetics. *Clin Pharmacol Ther* 1978; **24:** 162–7.
7. Impivaara O, Iisalo E. Serum digoxin concentrations in a representative digoxin-consuming adult population. *Eur J Clin Pharmacol* 1985; **27:** 627–32.

**Gastrointestinal drugs.** A number of gastrointestinal drugs can affect the absorption of digoxin by binding to it or by changing gastrointestinal motility. The problem has often been related to the bioavailability of the digoxin formulation and appears to be less important with currently used preparations. Some *antacids*,[1,2] particularly liquid formulations, and *adsorbents*[1] such as kaolin-pectin, can reduce the absorption of digoxin from the gastrointestinal tract and administration should probably be separated by at least 2 hours. *Activated charcoal*, and *ion-exchange resins* such as colestyramine and colestipol, also reduce digoxin absorption. *Sucralfate*[3] may also reduce the absorption of digoxin.

*Omeprazole* and possibly other gastric acid inhibitors may reduce the gastrointestinal metabolism and enhance the absorption of unchanged digoxin,[4] although the clinical relevance of this is uncertain.[5]

Drugs that increase gastrointestinal motility can reduce the absorption of digoxin, especially if digoxin is given as a slowly dissolving formulation. Reduced absorption of digoxin has occurred when digoxin and *metoclopramide* have been given concurrently,[6] and a similar effect has been reported with *cisapride*[7] and *tegaserod*.[8] Conversely, *anticholinergics* reduce motility, and propantheline has increased digoxin absorption.

*Sulfasalazine* has been found to impair the absorption of digoxin and to reduce the serum-digoxin concentration,[9] but the mechanism is unclear.

1. Rodin SM, Johnson BF. Pharmacokinetic interactions with digoxin. *Clin Pharmacokinet* 1988; **15:** 227–44.
2. Gugler R, Allgayer H. Effects of antacids on the clinical pharmacokinetics of drugs: an update. *Clin Pharmacokinet* 1990; **18:** 210–19.
3. Rey AM, Gums JG. Altered absorption of digoxin, sustained-release quinidine, and warfarin with sucralfate administration. *DICP Ann Pharmacother* 1991; **25:** 745–6.
4. Cohen AF, *et al.* Influence of gastric acidity on the bioavailability of digoxin. *Ann Intern Med* 1991; **115:** 540–5.
5. Oosterhuis B, *et al.* Minor effect of multiple dose omeprazole on the pharmacokinetics of digoxin after a single oral dose. *Br J Clin Pharmacol* 1991; **32:** 569–72.
6. Johnson BF, *et al.* Effect of metoclopramide on digoxin absorption from tablets and capsules. *Clin Pharmacol Ther* 1984; **36:** 724–30.
7. Kubler PA, *et al.* Possible interaction between cisapride and digoxin. *Ann Pharmacother* 2001; **35:** 127–8.
8. Zhou H, *et al.* The effects of tegaserod (HTF 919) on the pharmacokinetics and pharmacodynamics of digoxin in healthy subjects. *J Clin Pharmacol* 2001; **41:** 1131–9.
9. Juhl RP, *et al.* Effect of sulfasalazine on digoxin bioavailability. *Clin Pharmacol Ther* 1976; **20:** 387–94.

**Ginseng.** Siberian ginseng may interfere with plasma-digoxin assays (see under Precautions, above).

**Immunosuppressants.** Increased serum-digoxin concentrations with symptoms of toxicity have been reported in patients when *ciclosporin* was added to their digoxin therapy.[1,2]

1. Dorian P, *et al.* Digoxin-cyclosporine interaction: severe digitalis toxicity after cyclosporine treatment. *Clin Invest Med* 1988; **ii:** 108–12.
2. Robieux I, *et al.* The effects of cardiac transplantation and cyclosporine therapy on digoxin pharmacokinetics. *J Clin Pharmacol* 1992; **32:** 338–43.

**Lipid regulating drugs.** Small increases in plasma-digoxin concentrations have been reported with some *statins*, although the clinical significance is not clear. *Atorvastatin* at doses of 80 mg but not of 10 mg has been shown[1] to cause an increase in plasma-digoxin concentrations of approximately 20%. This may be due to the inhibition of P-glycoprotein-mediated secretion of digoxin in the intestine by atorvastatin.

1. Boyd RA, *et al.* Atorvastatin coadministration may increase digoxin concentrations by inhibition of intestinal P-glycoprotein-mediated secretion. *J Clin Pharmacol* 2000; **40:** 91–98.

**Neuromuscular blockers.** *Pancuronium* or *suxamethonium* may interact with digitalis glycosides resulting in an increased incidence of arrhythmias; the interaction is more likely with pancuronium.[1]

1. Bartolone RS, Rao TLK. Dysrhythmias following muscle relaxant administration in patients receiving digitalis. *Anesthesiology* 1983; **58:** 567–9.

**NSAIDs.** An increase in serum-digoxin concentration has been reported with *aspirin, ibuprofen, indometacin, fenbufen*, and *diclofenac*.[1] Potentially toxic serum-digoxin concentrations occurred in preterm infants[2] with patent ductus arteriosus on digoxin therapy when given indometacin by mouth in a mean total dose of 320 micrograms/kg; it was recommended that the dose of digoxin should be halved initially if indometacin is also given. Lack of increase in serum-digoxin concentrations has also been reported with concomitant aspirin or indometacin, as well as with *ketoprofen*, and *tiaprofenic acid*,[1] and also with *rofecoxib*,[3] but some of these studies were in healthy subjects and it is advised that digoxin therapy be monitored carefully whenever any NSAID is initiated or discontinued in digitalised patients.

1. Verbeeck RK. Pharmacokinetic drug interactions with nonsteroidal anti-inflammatory drugs. *Clin Pharmacokinet* 1990; **19:** 44–66.
2. Koren G, *et al.* Effects of indomethacin on digoxin pharmacokinetics in preterm infants. *Pediatr Pharmacol* 1984; **4:** 25–30.
3. Schwartz JI, *et al.* Effect of rofecoxib on the pharmacokinetics of digoxin in healthy volunteers. *J Clin Pharmacol* 2001; **41:** 107–112.

## Pharmacokinetics

The absorption of digoxin from the gastrointestinal tract is variable depending upon the formulation used. About 70% of the administered dose is absorbed from tablets which comply with BP or USP specifications, 80% is absorbed from an elixir, and over 90% is absorbed from liquid-filled soft gelatin capsules. The generally accepted therapeutic plasma concentration range is from 0.5 to 2.0 nanograms/mL but there is considerable interindividual variation. Digoxin has a large volume of distribution and is widely distributed in tissues, including the heart, brain, erythrocytes, and skeletal muscle. The concentration of digoxin in the myocardium is considerably higher than in plasma. From 20 to 30% is bound to plasma proteins. Digoxin has been detected in CSF and breast milk; it also crosses the placenta. It has an elimination half-life of 1.5 to 2 days.

Digoxin is mainly excreted unchanged in the urine by glomerular filtration and tubular secretion; reabsorption also occurs. Extensive metabolism has been reported in a minority of patients (see under Metabolism and Excretion, below). Excretion of digoxin is proportional to the glomerular filtration rate. After intravenous injection 50 to 70% of the dose is excreted unchanged. Digoxin is not removed from the body by dialysis, and only small amounts are removed by exchange transfusion and during cardiopulmonary bypass.

◊ Reviews of the clinical pharmacokinetics of digoxin.

1. Iisalo E. Clinical pharmacokinetics of digoxin. *Clin Pharmacokinet* 1977; **2:** 1–16.
2. Aronson JK. Clinical pharmacokinetics of digoxin 1980. *Clin Pharmacokinet* 1980; **5:** 137–49.
3. Mooradian AD. Digitalis: an update of clinical pharmacokinetics, therapeutic monitoring techniques and treatment recommendations. *Clin Pharmacokinet* 1988; **15:** 165–79.

**Absorption.** Studies in 6 healthy subjects demonstrated that ingestion of food decreased the rate but not the extent of absorption of concurrently administered digoxin.[1]

1. Johnson BF, *et al.* Effect of a standard breakfast on digoxin absorption in normal subjects. *Clin Pharmacol Ther* 1978; **23:** 315–19.

**Bioavailability.** Large variations in the content, disintegration, and dissolution of solid dosage forms of digoxin preparations have led to large variations in plasma concentrations from different proprietary preparations. Other factors involved in varying bioavailability include the pharmaceutical formulation and presentation (capsules, solution, or tablets), particle size, and biological factors. Serious problems occurred in the UK[1] in 1972 and in Israel[2] in 1975 following changes in the manufacturing procedure for Lanoxin leading to a twofold increase in bioavailability.

1. Anonymous. Therapeutic non-equivalence. *BMJ* 1972; **3:** 599–600.
2. Danon A, *et al.* An outbreak of digoxin intoxication. *Clin Pharmacol Ther* 1977; **21:** 643–6.

**Distribution and protein binding.** Digoxin has been reported to be 5 to 60% bound to plasma proteins,[1] depending partly on the method of measurement, but the figure is usually around 20%. Protein binding is reduced in patients undergoing haemodialysis; mean reductions of about 8 and 10% have been reported.[1,2] Injection of heparin has produced a similar reduction.[2]

Digoxin is widely distributed to tissues and serum-digoxin concentrations have been reported to be increased during immobilisation[3] and decreased during exercise[4,5] due to changes in binding to tissues such as skeletal muscle.

1. Storstein L. Studies on digitalis V: the influence of impaired renal function, hemodialysis, and drug interaction on serum protein binding of digitoxin and digoxin. *Clin Pharmacol Ther* 1976; **20:** 6–14.
2. Storstein L, Janssen H. Studies on digitalis VI: the effect of heparin on serum protein binding of digitoxin and digoxin. *Clin Pharmacol Ther* 1976; **20:** 15–23.
3. Pedersen KE, *et al.* Effects of physical activity and immobilization on plasma digoxin concentration and renal digoxin clearance. *Clin Pharmacol Ther* 1983; **34:** 303–8.
4. Joreteg T, Jogestrand T. Physical exercise and digoxin binding to skeletal muscle: relation to exercise intensity. *Eur J Clin Pharmacol* 1983; **25:** 585–8.
5. Joreteg T, Jogestrand T. Physical exercise and binding of digoxin to skeletal muscle—effect of muscle activation frequency. *Eur J Clin Pharmacol* 1984; **27:** 567–70.

**The elderly.** For references to alterations in the pharmacokinetics of digoxin in the elderly, see under Uses and Administration, below.

**Infants and neonates.** Digoxin has been widely used in the treatment of cardiac disorders in neonates and infants and its pharmacokinetics in this age group have been reviewed.[1,2] In full-term neonates or infants, 80 to 90% of a dose of digoxin given by mouth in liquid form is absorbed, with peak plasma concentrations occurring within 30 to 120 minutes. The rate of absorption may be slower in preterm and low birth-weight infants, with peak concentrations achieved at 90 to 180 minutes, and may be significantly reduced in severe heart failure and in malabsorption syndromes. After the intravenous administration of digoxin there is a rapid distribution phase with an apparent half-life of 20 to 40 minutes followed by a slower exponential decay of plasma concentrations. In full-term neonates, digoxin has an apparent volume of distribution of 6 to 10 litres/kg. Low birth-weight infants have a volume of distribution of 4.3 to 5.7 litres/kg while in older infants the volume may range from 10 to 22 litres/kg which is 1.5 to 2 times reported adult values. This large volume of distribution in full-term neonates and infants is thought to be due to increased tissue binding, a larger extracellular fluid volume, and slightly lower plasma protein binding.

The apparent plasma half-life in healthy and sick neonates is generally very long and may range from 20 to 70 hours in full-term neonates or from 40 to 180 hours in preterm neonates. Digoxin is eliminated at a considerably faster rate in infants than in neonates and, in parallel with maturation of kidney function, a marked increase in clearance rate is usually observed between the second and third month of life. The large apparent volume of distribution, higher clearance values, and greater concentrations of digoxin in the myocardial tissue and red cells of infants might justify the traditional assumption that infants tolerate digoxin better than adults and that higher doses are consequently needed in infants. However, studies have shown that in infants, as in adults, toxic signs become evident at plasma-digoxin concentrations above 3 nanograms/mL and that the therapeutic range may be 1.5 to 2 nanograms/mL.

1. Morselli PL, *et al.* Clinical pharmacokinetics in newborns and infants: age-related differences and therapeutic implications. *Clin Pharmacokinet* 1980; **5:** 485–527.
2. Besunder JB, *et al.* Principles of drug biodisposition in the neonate: a critical evaluation of the pharmacokinetic-pharmacodynamic interface. *Clin Pharmacokinet* 1988; **14:** 189–216 (part I) and 261–86 (part II).

**Metabolism and excretion.** Although digoxin is reported to be excreted mainly unchanged in the urine there is evidence to suggest that metabolism may sometimes be extensive. Metabolites that have been detected in the urine include digoxigenin, dihydrodigoxigenin, the mono- and bisdigitoxosides of digoxigenin, and dihydrodigoxin. Digoxigenin mono- and bisdigitoxosides are known to be cardioactive whereas dihydrodigoxin is probably much less active than digoxin.[1]

In about 10% of patients there is considerable reduction to cardio-inactive metabolites, chiefly dihydrodigoxin, and 40% or more of a dose may be excreted in the urine as dihydrodigoxin.[2-4] Bacterial flora in the gastrointestinal tract appear to be responsible for this metabolism and antibacterials can reduce the process. Oral digoxin formulations with a high bioavailability are mostly absorbed in the stomach and upper small intestine and little digoxin is available in the lower intestine for bacterial degradation to dihydrodigoxin.[4]

The excretion of digoxin is thought to be mediated by the efflux pump, P-glycoprotein,[5] which transports its substrates out of the cell. This may be the basis for some interactions hitherto poorly understood,[6] although the hypothesis has been questioned.[7]

1. Iisalo E. Clinical pharmacokinetics of digoxin. *Clin Pharmacokinet* 1977; **2:** 1–16.
2. Doherty JE. A digoxin-antibiotic drug interaction. *N Engl J Med* 1981; **305:** 827–8.
3. Rund DG, *et al.* Decreased digoxin cardioinactive-reduced metabolites after administration of an encapsulated liquid concentrate. *Clin Pharmacol Ther* 1983; **34:** 738–43.
4. Lofts F, *et al.* Digoxin metabolism to reduced products: clinical significance. *Br J Clin Pharmacol* 1986; **21:** 600P.
5. Tanigawara Y. Role of P-glycoprotein in drug disposition. *Ther Drug Monit* 2000; **22:** 137–40.
6. Fromm MF. P-glycoprotein: a defense mechanism limiting oral bioavailability and CNS accumulation of drugs. *Int J Clin Pharmacol Ther* 2000; **38:** 69–74.
7. Chiou WL, *et al.* A comprehensive account on the role of efflux transporters in the gastrointestinal absorption of 13 commonly used substrate drugs in humans. *Int J Clin Pharmacol Ther* 2001; **39:** 93–101.

**Renal impairment.** For references to alterations in the pharmacokinetics of digoxin in patients with renal impairment, see under Uses and Administration, below.

## Uses and Administration

Digoxin is a cardiac glycoside used in the management of supraventricular arrhythmias, particularly atrial fibrillation (p.816), and in heart failure (p.820).

The principal actions of digoxin are an increase in the force of myocardial contraction (positive inotropic activity) and a reduction in the conductivity of the heart, particularly in conduction through the atrioventricular (AV) node. Digoxin also has a direct action on vascular smooth muscle and indirect effects mediated primarily by the autonomic nervous system, and particularly by an increase in vagal activity. There are also reflex alterations in autonomic activity due to the effects on the circulation. Overall, these actions result in positive inotropic effects, negative chronotropic effects, and decreased AV nodal activity.

**Cardiac arrhythmias.** In atrial arrhythmias digoxin's actions cause a decrease in the conduction velocity through the AV node and an increase in the effective refractory period, thus reducing ventricular rate. In addition there is a decrease in the refractory period of the cardiac muscle and depression of the sinus node partly in response to the increase in vagal activity.

Digoxin is thus given to slow the increased ventricular rate that occurs in response to *atrial fibrillation*, although other drugs may be preferred; treatment is usually long term. In patients with the Wolff-Parkinson-White syndrome and atrial fibrillation, digoxin can cause rapid ventricular rates, and possibly ventricular fibrillation, and should be avoided. In *atrial flutter*, the ventricular rate is normally more difficult to control with digoxin. Direct current cardioversion is the preferred method of treatment, but treatment with digoxin may restore sinus rhythm, or it may convert the flutter to fibrillation and sinus rhythm may then be induced by subsequent withdrawal of digoxin. It may be given to relieve an attack of *paroxysmal supraventricular tachycardia* and has also been given to prevent further attacks.

**Heart failure.** Digoxin and other cardiac glycosides directly inhibit the activity of the enzyme sodium-potassium adenosine triphosphatase (Na/K-ATPase) which is required for the active transport of sodium from myocardial cells. The result is a gradual increase in the intracellular sodium concentration and a decrease in the intracellular potassium concentration. The increased concentration of sodium inside the cells leads, by stimulation of sodium-calcium exchange, to an increase in the intracellular calcium concentration with enhancement of mechanical contractile activity and an increased inotropic effect.

When used in heart failure the increased force of myocardial contraction results in increased cardiac output, decreased end-systolic volume, decreased heart size, and decreased end-diastolic pressure and volume. Increased blood flow through the kidneys results in diuresis with a reduction in oedema and blood volume. The decrease in pulmonary venous pressure relieves dyspnoea and orthopnoea. Digoxin may thus provide symptomatic improvement in patients with heart failure and is mainly used for adjunctive therapy.

**Dosage.** When given by mouth, digoxin may take effect within about 2 hours and the maximum effect may be reached in about 6 hours. Initially a loading dose may be given to digitalise the patient, although this may not be necessary in, for example, mild heart failure.

Dosage should be carefully adjusted to the needs of the individual patient. Factors which may be considered include the patient's age, lean body-mass, renal status, thyroid status, electrolyte balance, degree of tissue oxygenation, and the nature of the underlying cardiac or pulmonary disease. Bearing in mind the above factors, steady-state plasma-digoxin concentrations (in a sample taken at least 6 hours after a dose) of 0.5 to 2 nanograms/mL are generally considered acceptable. For reference to therapeutic drug monitoring, see below.

If rapid digitalisation is required then a loading dose is given to allow for the large volume of distribution. A total loading dose of 750 to 1500 micrograms of digoxin may be given by mouth during the initial 24-hour period, either as a single dose, or where there is less urgency or greater risk of toxicity, in divided doses at 6-hourly intervals. In some patients, for example those with mild heart failure, a loading dose may not be necessary, and digitalisation may be achieved more slowly with doses of 250 micrograms once or twice daily; steady-state plasma concentrations are achieved in about 7 days in patients with normal renal function. The usual maintenance dose of digoxin is 125 to 250 micrograms by mouth daily, but may range from 62.5 to 500 micrograms daily. In elderly patients therapy should generally be initiated gradually and with smaller doses (but see under Administration in the Elderly, below).

In urgent cases, provided that the patient has not received cardiac glycosides during the previous 2 weeks, digoxin may be given intravenously initially. The intravenous dose ranges from 500 to 1000 micrograms and generally produces a definite effect on the heart rate in about 10 minutes, reaching a maximum within about 2 hours. It is administered by intravenous infusion, either as a single dose given over 2 or more hours, or in divided doses each over 10 to 20 minutes. Maintenance treatment is then usually given by mouth. Digoxin has also been given intramuscularly but this route is not generally recommended since such injections may be painful and tissue damage has been reported. Digoxin should not be given subcutaneously as intense local irritation may occur.

Children's doses are complex. They are based on body-weight and the developmental stage of the child as well as on response. Premature infants are especially sensitive to digoxin but, along with all other neonates, infants, and children up to about 10 years of age, still require doses that are higher per kg body-weight than those used for adults. Preterm infants receive lower doses than full-term infants, while children aged 2 to 10 years require lower doses than children up to 2 years of age. As an indication of the doses employed, oral loading doses recommended by manufacturers in the UK range from 25 to 45 micrograms/kg over 24 hours and in the USA the range is 20 to 60 micrograms/kg; the range for intravenous loading doses given over 24 hours is 20 to 35 micrograms/kg in the UK and 15 to 50 micrograms/kg in the USA.

Doses should be reduced in patients with renal impairment (see below).

◊ General reviews on the actions and uses of digoxin and the other cardiac glycosides.


1. Opie LH. Digitalis and sympathomimetic stimulants. *Lancet* 1980; **i:** 912–18.
2. Taggart AJ, McDevitt DG. Digitalis: its place in modern therapy. *Drugs* 1980; **20:** 398–404.
3. Chamberlain DA. Digitalis: where are we now? *Br Heart J* 1985; **54:** 227–33.
4. Doherty JE. Clinical use of digitalis glycosides: an update. *Cardiology* 1985; **72:** 225–54.
5. Smith TW. Digitalis: mechanisms of action and clinical use. *N Engl J Med* 1988; **318:** 358–65.
6. Hampton JR. Digoxin. *Br J Hosp Med* 1997; **58:** 321–3.
7. Riaz K, Forker AD. Digoxin use in congestive heart failure: current status. *Drugs* 1998; **55:** 747–58.


**Administration in the elderly.** The volume of distribution of digoxin and the elimination half-life increase with age.[1] Therefore there are problems in giving digoxin to elderly patients since steady-state plasma concentrations may not be reached for up to 2 weeks. Fears of toxicity have led some practitioners to use a fixed 'geriatric' dose of 62.5 micrograms daily. However, such a dose can produce subtherapeutic concentrations.[2] The routine use of very low doses of digoxin in the elderly is inappropriate and dosage should be individualised.


1. McMurray J, McDevitt DG. Treatment of heart failure in the elderly. *Br Med Bull* 1990; **46:** 202–29.
2. Nolan L, *et al.* The need for reassessment of digoxin prescribing for the elderly. *Br J Clin Pharmacol* 1989; **27:** 367–70.


**Administration in renal impairment.** The pharmacokinetics of cardiac glycosides in patients with renal impairment have been reviewed.[1] The rate but not the extent of digoxin absorption is reduced in renal impairment but this is unlikely to be clinically important. Plasma-protein binding may also be reduced but since digoxin is poorly bound to these proteins and has a large apparent volume of distribution this also is unlikely to be important. The apparent volume of distribution is reduced by one-third to one-half and the loading dose of digoxin should therefore be reduced; an oral loading dose of 10 micrograms/kg is suggested. Non-renal clearance of digoxin is unaffected or only slightly reduced but renal clearance is reduced, the extent being closely related to creatinine clearance. The elimination half-life of digoxin is prolonged and it therefore takes longer to reach steady state and longer for toxicity to resolve. Because of the reduction in renal clearance of digoxin, maintenance doses must be reduced in line with renal function. Serum-digoxin concentration should be monitored although the presence of digoxin-like immunoreactive substances may make interpretation difficult. In addition, the presence of hyperkalaemia in patients with renal impairment may reduce sensitivity to the effects of digoxin.[2]

Since digoxin has such a large distribution volume, procedures such as peritoneal dialysis and haemodialysis remove only very small amounts of drug from the body and no dosage supplement is needed.


1. Aronson JK. Clinical pharmacokinetics of cardiac glycosides in patients with renal dysfunction. *Clin Pharmacokinet* 1983; **8:** 155–78.
2. Matzke GR, Frye RF. Drug administration in patients with renal insufficiency: minimising renal and extrarenal toxicity. *Drug Safety* 1997; **16:** 205–31.


**Therapeutic drug monitoring.** Digoxin has a narrow therapeutic index. It is generally considered that plasma-digoxin concentrations required for a therapeutic effect are usually between 0.5 and 2.0 nanograms/mL,[1-3] although some studies[4,5] have suggested that concentrations at the lower end of this range are adequate for heart failure. The factor for converting nanograms/mL to nanomoles/litre is 1.28.

Digoxin dosage can be calculated in uncomplicated cases by considering the patient's weight, renal function, and clinical status. Therapeutic drug monitoring is *not* considered to be necessary in patients with a satisfactory clinical response to conventional doses in the absence of signs or symptoms of toxicity.[1,2] Measurement of plasma-digoxin concentrations is useful if poor compliance is suspected, if response is poor or there is a deterioration in response without apparent reason, if renal function is fluctuating, when it is unknown if a cardiac glycoside has been previously taken, during drug interactions, and to confirm clinical toxicity.[1,3,6] A plasma concentration should never be considered in isolation and should be used with other patient data as an important component in clinical decision making. This is particularly important in the diagnosis of digoxin toxicity since signs and symptoms of toxicity may be difficult to distinguish from the underlying disease and can occur within the usual therapeutic range.

A number of factors may influence the response to digoxin and thus the interpretation of digoxin assays. These include renal impairment, extremes of age, thyroid disease, patient compliance, drug interactions, and electrolyte disturbances.[1-3,6] Variations in the bioavailability of different digoxin preparations have also caused problems. Renal impairment and hypokalaemia are two of the most important factors affecting dosage of digoxin and whenever plasma-digoxin concentrations are assayed renal function and plasma potassium should also be measured. The interpretation of digoxin assays is further confounded by the presence of digoxin-like immunoreactive substances in patients with renal or hepatic impairment, in pregnant women, and in neonates. Blood samples for digoxin assay should be taken at least 6 hours after a dose to allow for distribution.[1,3,6]

The usefulness of plasma-digoxin concentrations in the diagnosis of toxicity in children is unclear. For children older than 12 months the adult guidelines can probably be followed, and for younger children the trend for increased risk of toxicity at increased plasma-digoxin concentrations appears to hold but the threshold for toxicity may be higher, especially in children less than 3 months old.[1]


1. Aronson JK. Indications for the measurement of plasma digoxin concentrations. *Drugs* 1983; **26:** 230–42.
2. Lee TH, Smith TW. Serum digoxin concentration and diagnosis of digitalis toxicity: current concepts. *Clin Pharmacokinet* 1983; **8:** 279–85.
3. Aronson JK, Hardman M. Digoxin. *BMJ* 1992; **305:** 1149–52.
4. Adams KF, *et al.* Clinical benefits of low serum digoxin concentrations in heart failure. *J Am Coll Cardiol* 2002; **39:** 946–53.
5. Rathore SS, *et al.* Association of serum digoxin concentration and outcomes in patients with heart failure. *JAMA* 2003; **289:** 871–8.
6. Brodie MJ, Feely J. Practical clinical pharmacology: therapeutic drug monitoring and clinical trials. *BMJ* 1988; **296:** 1110–14.


## Preparations

***BP 2003:*** Digoxin Injection; Digoxin Tablets; Paediatric Digoxin Injection; Paediatric Digoxin Oral Solution;
***USP 27:*** Digoxin Elixir; Digoxin Injection; Digoxin Tablets.

**Proprietary Preparations** (details are given in Part 3)
***Arg.:*** Cardiogoxin; Digocard-G; Lanicor; Lanoxin; ***Austral.:*** Lanoxin; Sigmaxin; ***Austria:*** Lanicor; ***Belg.:*** Lanoxin; ***Braz.:*** Cardcor; Cimecard; Digoxil; Lanoxin; ***Canad.:*** Lanoxin; ***Fr.:*** Hemigoxine Nativelle; ***Ger.:*** Digacin; Dilanacin; Lanicor; Lenoxin; Novodigal; ***Hong Kong:*** Lanoxin; ***India:*** Cardioxin; Lanoxin; ***Irl.:*** Lanoxin; ***Israel:*** Lanoxin; ***Ital.:*** Digomal†; Eudigox; Lanoxin; ***Jpn:*** Digosin; ***Malaysia:*** Lanoxin; ***Mex.:*** Dogoxine†; Lanoxin; Mapluxin; ***Neth.:*** Lanoxin; ***Norw.:*** Lanoxin; ***NZ:*** Lanoxin; ***Port.:*** Lanoxin; ***S.Afr.:*** Lanoxin; Purgoxin; ***Singapore:*** Lanoxin; ***Spain:*** Lanacordin; ***Swed.:*** Lanacrist; Lanoxin; ***Switz.:*** Lanoxin†; ***Thai.:*** Grexin; Lanoxin; Toloxin; ***UK:*** Lanoxin; ***USA:*** Lanoxicaps; Lanoxin.

**Multi-ingredient: *Ger.:*** Crataelanat†.

---

## Dihydralazine Sulfate *(rINNM)*

Dihydralazine Sulphate *(BANM)*; Dihydralazini Sulfas Hydricus; Dihydralazinum Sulfuricum; Dihydrallazine Sulphate; Sulfato de dihidralazina. Phthalazine-1,4-diyldihydrazine sulphate hemipentahydrate.

$C_8H_{10}N_6,H_2SO_4,2\frac{1}{2}H_2O = 333.3.$
*CAS — 484-23-1 (dihydralazine); 7327-87-9 (dihydralazine sulfate).*
*ATC — C02DB01.*

**Pharmacopoeias.** In *Chin.* and *Eur.* (see p.vi). *Pol.* includes the anhydrous form.
*Swiss* includes dihydralazine mesilate.

**Ph. Eur. 5.0** (Dihydralazine Sulphate, Hydrated). A white or slightly yellow crystalline powder. Slightly soluble in water; practically insoluble in dehydrated alcohol. It dissolves in dilute mineral acids.

## Profile

Dihydralazine is a vasodilator with actions and uses similar to those of hydralazine (p.931). It is given by mouth as the sulfate. Dihydralazine sulfate hemipentahydrate 14.45 mg is approximately equivalent to 12.5 mg of anhydrous dihydralazine sulfate. In hypertension (p.825) the usual initial dose is the equivalent of 12.5 mg of anhydrous dihydralazine sulfate by mouth twice daily and the maximum recommended dose is 50 mg twice daily. Higher doses have been used in the management of heart failure.

Other salts of dihydralazine that have been used in oral preparations include the hydrochloride and the tartrate. The mesilate is given by injection.

**Porphyria.** Dihydralazine is considered to be unsafe in patients with porphyria because it has been shown to be porphyrinogenic in *animals* or *in-vitro* systems.

## Preparations

**Proprietary Preparations** (details are given in Part 3)
***Austria:*** Nepresol; ***Belg.:*** Nepresol; ***Denm.:*** Nepresol†; ***Fr.:*** Nepressol; ***Ger.:*** Depressan; Dihyzin†; Nepresol; ***Gr.:*** Nepresol; ***Hong Kong:*** Nepresol; ***India:*** Nepresol; ***Israel:*** Nepresol†; ***Malaysia:*** Nepresol; ***Neth.:*** Nepresol†; ***Norw.:*** Nepresol†; ***S.Afr.:*** Nepresol; ***Swed.:*** Nepresol; ***Switz.:*** Nepresol; ***Thai.:*** Nepresol.

**Multi-ingredient:** ***Austria:*** Adelphan-Esidrex; Elfanex†; ***Braz.:*** Adelfan-Esidrex; ***Ger.:*** Adelphan-Esidrix; Obsilazin N; Tri-Torrat; Triniton; ***Hong Kong:*** Adelphane-Esidrex; ***India:*** Adelphane; Adelphane-Esidrex; Beptazine; Beptazine-H; ***Israel:*** Pressunic Compositum†; ***Ital.:*** Ipogen†; ***Spain:*** Adelfan-Esidrex; ***Switz.:*** Adelphan-Esidrex.

---

## Di-isopropylammonium Dichloroacetate

Diisopropilamina, dicloroacetato de; Di-isopropylamine Dichloroacetate; Di-isopropylamine Dichloroethanoate; DIPA-DCA.

$C_8H_{17}Cl_2NO_2$ = 230.1.
*CAS — 660-27-5.*

## Profile

Di-isopropylammonium dichloroacetate is a vasodilator that has been given in peripheral and cerebral vascular disorders. Preparations containing it have sometimes been described as 'pangamic acid' (p.1727).

## Preparations

**Proprietary Preparations** (details are given in Part 3)
***Ger.:*** Disotat; Oxypangam; ***Mex.:*** Ditrei.

**Multi-ingredient:** ***Ger.:*** Neuro-Wied; ***Hong Kong:*** Liverall; ***Spain:*** Vitaber A E.

---

## Dilazep Hydrochloride *(rINNM)*

Asta C-4898; Hidrocloruro de dilazep. Perhydro-1,4-diazepin-1,4-diylbis(trimethylene 3,4,5-trimethoxybenzoate) dihydrochloride.

$C_{31}H_{44}N_2O_{10}$,2HCl = 677.6.
*CAS — 35898-87-4 (dilazep); 20153-98-4 (dilazep hydrochloride).*
*ATC — C01DX10.*

**Pharmacopoeias.** In *Jpn.*

## Profile

Dilazep hydrochloride is a vasodilator that has been used in ischaemic heart disease.

## Preparations

**Proprietary Preparations** (details are given in Part 3)
***India:*** Cormelian; ***Ital.:*** Cormelian†.

---

# Diltiazem Hydrochloride

*(BANM, USAN, rINNM)*

CRD-401; Diltiazemi Hydrochloridum; Hidrocloruro de diltiazem; Latiazem Hydrochloride; MK-793 (diltiazem malate). (+)-*cis*-3-Acetoxy-5-(2-dimethylaminoethyl)-2,3-dihydro-2-(4-methoxyphenyl)-1,5-benzothiazepin-4(5*H*)-one hydrochloride; (2*S*,3*S*)-5-(2-Dimethylaminoethyl)-2,3,4,5-tetrahydro-2-(4-methoxyphenyl)-4-oxo-1,5-benzothiazepin-3-yl acetate hydrochloride.

$C_{22}H_{26}N_2O_4S$,HCl = 451.0.
*CAS — 42399-41-7 (diltiazem); 33286-22-5 (diltiazem hydrochloride); 144604-00-2 (diltiazem malate).*
*ATC — C08DB01.*

**Pharmacopoeias.** In *Chin., Eur.* (see p.vi), *Jpn, Pol.,* and *US.*

**Ph. Eur. 5.0** (Diltiazem Hydrochloride). A white crystalline powder. Freely soluble in water, in dichloromethane, and in methyl alcohol; slightly soluble in dehydrated alcohol. The pH of a 1% solution in water is 4.3 to 5.3. Store in airtight containers. Protect from light.

**USP 27** (Diltiazem Hydrochloride). A white, odourless, crystalline powder, or small crystals. Freely soluble in water, in chloroform, in formic acid, and in methyl alcohol; sparingly soluble in dehydrated alcohol; insoluble in ether. Store in airtight containers. Protect from light.

## Adverse Effects

Treatment with diltiazem is generally well tolerated. Headache, ankle oedema, hypotension, dizziness, flushing, fatigue, and nausea and other gastrointestinal disturbances (including anorexia, vomiting, constipation or diarrhoea, taste disturbances, and weight gain) may occur. Gingival hyperplasia has been reported. Rashes, possibly due to hypersensitivity, are normally mild and transient, but in a few cases erythema multiforme or exfoliative dermatitis has developed; photosensitivity reactions may also occur. Transient elevations in liver enzyme values, and occasionally hepatitis, have been reported.

Diltiazem may depress cardiac conduction and has occasionally led to atrioventricular block, bradycardia, and rarely asystole or sinus arrest.

Overdosage with diltiazem may be associated with bradycardia, with or without atrioventricular conduction defects, and hypotension.

Diltiazem has been shown to cause teratogenicity in *animal* studies.

**Effects on mortality.** For discussion of the possibility that calcium-channel blockers might be associated with increased cardiovascular mortality, see under Adverse Effects of Nifedipine, p.966.

**Angioedema.** Periorbital angioedema, accompanied by pruritus or burning and erythema developed in 2 patients given diltiazem.[1]

1. Sadick NS, *et al.* Angioedema from calcium channel blockers. *J Am Acad Dermatol* 1989; **21:** 132–3.

**Effects on the blood.** Thrombocytopenia has been reported in association with diltiazem.[1,2]

1. Lehav M, Arav R. Diltiazem and thrombocytopenia. *Ann Intern Med* 1989; **110:** 327.
2. Michalets EL, Jackson DV. Diltiazem-associated thrombocytopenia. *Pharmacotherapy* 1997; **17:** 1345–8.

**Effects on carbohydrate metabolism.** Although raised blood-glucose concentrations and insulin requirements have been reported[1] in a patient with type 1 diabetes mellitus during diltiazem therapy, particularly at high doses, a study[2] in 11 obese black women, who were nondiabetic but had a family history of type 2 diabetes, failed to find any effect of diltiazem 240 mg daily on plasma-glucose and C-peptide concentrations, nor any clinical signs of glucose intolerance.

1. Pershadsingh HA, *et al.* Association of diltiazem therapy with increased insulin resistance in a patient with type I diabetes mellitus. *JAMA* 1987; **257:** 930–1.
2. Jones BJ, *et al.* Effects of diltiazem hydrochloride on glucose tolerance in persons at risk for diabetes mellitus. *Clin Pharm* 1988; **7:** 235–8.

**Effects on the ears.** There have been isolated reports[1] of tinnitus associated with several calcium-channel blockers including nifedipine, nicardipine, nitrendipine, diltiazem, verapamil, and cinnarizine.

1. Narváez M, *et al.* Tinnitus with calcium-channel blockers. *Lancet* 1994; **343:** 1229–30.

**Effects on the heart.** ATRIOVENTRICULAR BLOCK. Atrioventricular block appears to be uncommon in patients receiving diltiazem, but is potentially serious when it occurs. Prescription-event monitoring[1] of a cohort of 10 119 patients for 1 year revealed 22 reports of atrioventricular block during diltiazem treatment. At least 8 patients had third-degree heart block, and 12 required a pacemaker; 3 died within 72 hours of the onset of heart block. A high proportion of these patients were also receiving beta blockers, which is in line with other reports.[2,3] (See also Beta Blockers under Interactions, below.) There is some evidence that the incidence of this effect may depend on the serum concentration of diltiazem. In a study[4] in patients receiving diltiazem after myocardial infarction, patients with serum-diltiazem concentrations greater than 150 nanograms/mL were more likely to experience atrioventricular block than patients with concentrations of diltiazem below this value.

1. Waller PC, Inman WHW. Diltiazem and heart block. *Lancet* 1989; **i:** 617.
2. Hossack KF. Conduction abnormalities due to diltiazem. *N Engl J Med* 1982; **307:** 953–4.
3. Ishikawa T, *et al.* Atrioventricular dissociation and sinus arrest induced by oral diltiazem. *N Engl J Med* 1983; **309:** 1124–5.
4. Nattel S, *et al.* Determinants and significance of diltiazem plasma concentrations after acute myocardial infarction. *Am J Cardiol* 1990; **66:** 1422–8.

MYOCARDIAL INFARCTION. Results from at least one large multicentre study (the Multicenter Diltiazem Postinfarction Trial) suggest that diltiazem, although apparently of benefit after myocardial infarction in patients with normal left ventricular function (as indicated by absence of pulmonary congestion), was associated with an increased risk of cardiac death or non-fatal re-infarction in patients with impaired left ventricular function.[1] Long-term follow-up[2] indicated that diltiazem also increased the risk of late-onset heart failure in postinfarction patients with left ventricular dysfunction.

1. The Multicenter Diltiazem Postinfarction Trial Research Group. The effect of diltiazem on mortality and reinfarction after myocardial infarction. *N Engl J Med* 1988; **319:** 385–92.
2. Goldstein RE, *et al.* Diltiazem increases late-onset congestive heart failure in postinfarction patients with early reduction in ejection fraction. *Circulation* 1991; **83:** 52–60.

WITHDRAWAL. Life-threatening coronary vasospasm, which was fatal in one patient, occurred in 4 patients following coronary revascularisation for unstable angina.[1] Treatment with a calcium-channel blocker (diltiazem or nifedipine) had been discontinued between 8 and 18 hours before the procedure and this abrupt withdrawal was thought to be responsible for the rebound vasospasm. The coronary vasospasm was managed with glyceryl trinitrate and nifedipine.

Withdrawal of diltiazem over a 4-day period from a patient with stable angina pectoris was followed by recurrence of anginal attacks.[2] Ambulatory ECG monitoring confirmed worsening myocardial ischaemia that responded to re-introduction of diltiazem. Two further patients experienced a similar withdrawal effect.

1. Engelman RM, *et al.* Rebound vasospasm after coronary revascularization in association with calcium antagonist withdrawal. *Ann Thorac Surg* 1984; **37:** 469–72.
2. Subramanian VB, *et al.* Calcium antagonist withdrawal syndrome: objective demonstration with frequency-modulated ambulatory ST-segment monitoring. *BMJ* 1983; **286:** 520–1.

**Effects on the kidneys.** Diltiazem may be of benefit in various kidney disorders (see under Uses, below). However, there are a few reports of acute renal failure associated with diltiazem administration.[1,2] Acute interstitial nephritis has been proposed as a mechanism.[2,3]

1. ter Wee PM, *et al.* Acute renal failure due to diltiazem. *Lancet* 1984; **ii:** 1337–8.
2. Abadín JA, *et al.* Probable diltiazem-induced acute interstitial nephritis. *Ann Pharmacother* 1998; **32:** 656–8.
3. Achenbach V, *et al.* Acute renal failure due to diltiazem. *Lancet* 1985; **i:** 176.

**Effects on mental function.** By September 1989, the WHO collaborative programme for international drug monitoring had gathered 8 cases of mental depression (severe in 2) associated with diltiazem therapy.[1] Time of onset of symptoms varied from a few hours to a few months after starting treatment with diltiazem. There was some evidence that the problem might be dose-related as 5 of the 8 cases were receiving doses of 180 mg daily or more.

Psychoses have been reported rarely in association with diltiazem. A patient[2] who developed hallucinations (both auditory and visual) and paranoid delusions after 2 days of diltiazem therapy was subsequently treated with nifedipine without abnormal effects. Another patient[3] with bipolar affective disorder that had been well-controlled by lithium carbonate for some years developed acute psychosis with extrapyramidal symptoms of cogwheel rigidity and ataxia, which was thought to represent an interaction between diltiazem and lithium.

1. Biriell C, *et al.* Depression associated with diltiazem. *BMJ* 1989; **299:** 796.
2. Bushe CJ. Organic psychosis caused by diltiazem. *J R Soc Med* 1988; **81:** 296–7.
3. Binder EF. Diltiazem-induced psychosis and a possible diltiazem-lithium interaction. *Arch Intern Med* 1991; **151:** 373–4.

**Effects on the mouth.** A study involving 115 patients given nifedipine, diltiazem, or verapamil for at least 3 months indicated that gingival hyperplasia is an important side-effect that may occur with calcium-channel blockers.[1]

1. Steele RM, *et al.* Calcium antagonist-induced gingival hyperplasia. *Ann Intern Med* 1994; **120:** 663–4.

**Effects on the nervous system.** Akathisia has been reported in a patient the day after starting treatment with diltiazem. Symptoms disappeared when diltiazem was withdrawn and recurred on rechallenge after the third dose.[1] Similar symptoms in association with mania have also been reported in another patient given diltiazem.[2]

1. Jacobs MB. Diltiazem and akathisia. *Ann Intern Med* 1983; **99:** 794–5.
2. Brink DD. Diltiazem and hyperactivity. *Ann Intern Med* 1984; **100:** 459–60.

PARKINSONISM. Parkinsonism developed in an elderly patient with heart disease and hypertension when diltiazem was added to existing drug therapy.[1] Symptoms worsened over 3 months but improved significantly when diltiazem was slowly discontinued. On rechallenge severe tremor, impaired gait, and cogwheel rigidity recurred, but resolved when the drug was again discontinued except for slight residual cogwheel rigidity.

An acute parkinsonian syndrome also developed[2] in a patient taking lithium and tiotixene when diltiazem was added, and was thought to represent an interaction between lithium and diltiazem. See also Effects on Mental Function, above.

1. Dick RS, Barold SS. Diltiazem-induced parkinsonism. *Am J Med* 1989; **87:** 95–6.
2. Valdiserri EV. A possible interaction between lithium and diltiazem: case report. *J Clin Psychiatry* 1985; **46:** 540–1.

**Effects on the skin.** A variety of skin disorders have been associated with diltiazem therapy, including acute pustular dermatitis,[1-3] cutaneous vasculitis,[4,5] erythema multiforme,[6,7] pruritic macular rashes,[3,8] severe toxic erythema,[9] and subacute lupus erythematosus-like eruptions.[10] Analysis of cutaneous adverse reactions to diltiazem indicated that acne, rash, and urticaria were among the commonest.[11] There have also been a few reports of exfoliative dermatitis, erythema multiforme, Stevens Johnson syndrome, and toxic epidermal necrolysis.[3,11]

For a report of periorbital skin rash associated with diltiazem, see Angioedema, above.

Cross-sensitivity, manifest as a pruritic maculopapular rash, has been reported between diltiazem and amlodipine.[12]


1. Lambert DG, *et al.* Acute generalized exanthematous pustular dermatitis induced by diltiazem. *Br J Dermatol* 1988; **118:** 308–9.
2. Vicente-Calleja JM, *et al.* Acute generalized exanthematous pustulosis due to diltiazem: confirmation by patch testing. *Br J Dermatol* 1997; **137:** 837–9.
3. Knowles S, *et al.* The spectrum of cutaneous reactions associated with diltiazem: three cases and a review of the literature. *J Am Acad Dermatol* 1998; **38:** 201–6.
4. Carmichael AJ, Paul CJ. Vasculitic leg ulcers associated with diltiazem. *BMJ* 1988; **297:** 562.
5. Sheehan-Dare RA, Goodfield MJ. Severe cutaneous vasculitis induced by diltiazem. *Br J Dermatol* 1988; **119:** 134.
6. Berbis P, *et al.* Diltiazem associated erythema multiforme. *Dermatologica* 1989; **179:** 90.
7. Sanders CJG, Neumann HAM. Erythema multiforme, Stevens-Johnson syndrome, and diltiazem. *Lancet* 1993; **341:** 967.
8. Wirebaugh SR, Geraets DR. Reports of erythematous macular skin eruptions associated with diltiazem therapy. *DICP Ann Pharmacother* 1990; **24:** 1046–9.
9. Wakeel RA, *et al.* Severe toxic erythema caused by diltiazem. *BMJ* 1988; **296:** 1071.
10. Crowson AN, Magro CM. Diltiazem and subacute cutaneous lupus erythematosus-like lesions. *N Engl J Med* 1995; **333:** 1429.
11. Stern R, Khalsa JH. Cutaneous adverse reactions associated with calcium channel blockers. *Arch Intern Med* 1989; **149:** 829–32.
12. Baker BA, Cacchione JG. Dermatologic cross-sensitivity between diltiazem and amlodipine. *Ann Pharmacother* 1994; **28:** 118–19.


**Overdosage.** See under Treatment of Adverse Effects, below.

## Treatment of Adverse Effects

As for Nifedipine, p.968, but see also below.

Diltiazem and its metabolites are poorly dialysable.

**Overdosage.** The consequences and treatment of diltiazem overdosage are similar to nifedipine (p.968), although death and life-threatening complications might be more common with diltiazem.[1] Up to 1994, 6 cases of fatal overdose with diltiazem had been reported in the literature.[2] Measurement of diltiazem concentrations to assist in diagnosis and management of overdosage has been suggested,[2] but others[3] have disputed its value.

The following are individual reports of overdosage with diltiazem:

- A patient who took about 10.8 g of diltiazem developed hypotension and complete heart block. Dopamine, isoprenaline, and calcium chloride were required to maintain the blood pressure. The ECG reverted to sinus rhythm after 31 hours. The plasma-diltiazem concentration was 1670 nanograms/mL 43 hours after ingestion and fell to 12.1 nanograms/mL over a further 55.5 hours with an elimination half-life of 7.9 hours.[4]
- In a further case a patient took 5.88 g of diltiazem with alcohol, and developed severe junctional bradycardia, hypotension, and reduced cardiac function that did not respond to intravenous calcium gluconate. The maximum plasma-diltiazem concentration of 6090 nanograms/mL occurred 7 hours after presentation. About half of the dose was vomited after treatment with activated charcoal. The patient was treated with cardiac pacing and a dopamine infusion; he reverted to sinus rhythm within 24 hours, and a subsequent episode of atrial fibrillation was treated successfully with digoxin.[5]
- Charcoal haemoperfusion had a limited effect in improving the clearance of diltiazem in a patient who had taken 14.94 g of diltiazem.[6] The patient developed severe hypotension, complete heart block, and acute renal failure. Supportive care included cardiac pacing and numerous vasopressors including intravenous glucagon and infusions of dopamine, adrenaline, and noradrenaline.


1. Buckley NA, *et al.* Overdose with calcium channel blockers. *BMJ* 1994; **308:** 1639.
2. Roper TA. Overdose of diltiazem. *BMJ* 1994; **308:** 1571.
3. Lip GYH, Ferner RE. Overdose of diltiazem. *BMJ* 1994; **309:** 193.
4. Malcolm N, *et al.* Massive diltiazem overdosage: clinical and pharmacokinetic observations. *Drug Intell Clin Pharm* 1986; **20:** 888.
5. Ferner RE, *et al.* Pharmacokinetics and toxic effects of diltiazem in massive overdose. *Hum Toxicol* 1989; **8:** 497–9.
6. Williamson KM, Dunham GD. Plasma concentrations of diltiazem and desacetyldiltiazem in an overdose situation. *Ann Pharmacother* 1996; **30:** 608–11.


## Precautions

Diltiazem is contra-indicated in patients with the sick sinus syndrome, pre-existing second- or third-degree atrioventricular block, or marked bradycardia, and should be used with care in patients with lesser degrees of atrioventricular block or bradycardia. Diltiazem has been associated with the development of heart failure and great care is required in patients with impaired left ventricular function. Sudden withdrawal of diltiazem might be associated with an exacerbation of angina.

Treatment with diltiazem should commence with reduced doses in elderly patients and in patients with hepatic or renal impairment.

**Abuse.** Abuse of diltiazem by body builders and rugby players has been alleged. Such abuse is possibly because of evidence that diltiazem increases maximum oxygen consumption after training. A body builder who admitted to taking diltiazem in high doses suffered severe abdominal cramps.[1]


1. Richards H, *et al.* Use of diltiazem in sport. *BMJ* 1993; **307:** 940.


**Breast feeding.** Diltiazem is distributed into breast milk; in a woman receiving diltiazem 60 mg four times daily by mouth, concentrations in breast milk were similar to those in serum.[1] The manufacturers therefore recommend that diltiazem should generally be avoided during breast feeding. However, in another report,[2] a mother breast fed twins for at least 6 months while receiving diltiazem and no adverse effects were reported in the infants. Since there have been no reports of adverse effects, the American Academy of Pediatrics considers[3] that diltiazem is usually compatible with breast feeding.


1. Okada M, *et al.* Excretion of diltiazem in human milk. *N Engl J Med* 1985; **312:** 992–3.
2. Lubbe WF. Use of diltiazem during pregnancy. *N Z Med J* 1987; **100:** 121.
3. American Academy of Pediatrics. The transfer of drugs and other chemicals into human milk. *Pediatrics* 2001; **108:** 776–89. Correction. *ibid.*; 1029. Also available at: http://aappolicy.aappublications.org/cgi/content/full/pediatrics%3b108/3/776 (accessed 06/07/04)


**Porphyria.** Diltiazem is considered to be unsafe in patients with porphyria because it has been shown to be porphyrinogenic in *animals* or *in-vitro* systems.

**Renal impairment.** A patient with end-stage renal failure requiring haemodialysis developed hypotension, bradycardia, metabolic acidosis, hyperkalaemia, and acute congestive heart failure about 60 hours after his last haemodialysis.[1] The patient had been taking diltiazem 60 mg three times daily. The symptoms were attributed to diltiazem toxicity due to accumulation of diltiazem and its metabolites which are poorly dialysed and normally excreted partially in the urine.


1. Patel R, *et al.* Toxic effects of diltiazem in a patient with chronic renal failure. *J Clin Pharmacol* 1994; **34:** 273–4.


## Interactions

Increased depression of cardiac conduction with risk of bradycardia and atrioventricular block may occur when diltiazem is given with drugs such as amiodarone, beta blockers, digoxin, and mefloquine. Enhanced antihypertensive effect may occur with concomitant use of other antihypertensive drugs or drugs that cause hypotension such as aldesleukin and antipsychotics. Diltiazem is extensively metabolised in the liver by the cytochrome P450 isoenzyme CYP3A4 and may also inhibit the metabolism of drugs sharing the same pathway. Interactions may also be expected with enzyme inducers, such as carbamazepine, phenobarbital, phenytoin, and rifampicin, and with enzyme inhibitors, such as cimetidine.

**Antidepressants.** For a report of diltiazem increasing the bioavailability of *imipramine* and *nortriptyline*, see Calcium-channel Blockers under the Interactions of Amitriptyline, p.284.

**Antiepileptics.** For reports of diltiazem administration precipitating *carbamazepine* and *phenytoin* toxicity, see p.356 and p.374, respectively.

**Anxiolytics.** For the effect of diltiazem on plasma-*buspirone* concentrations, see p.673.

**Benzodiazepines.** For the effects of diltiazem on plasma concentrations of *midazolam* or *triazolam*, see Calcium-channel Blockers under Interactions of Diazepam, p.694.

**Beta blockers.** Profound bradycardia has been reported in a number of patients when diltiazem was prescribed with a beta blocker.[1,2] Diltiazem decreases the clearance of a single dose of *propranolol* or *metoprolol*, though not *atenolol*, and elevated concentrations of beta blocker may be responsible for the bradycardic effects.[3] This is unlikely to be the full story, however, since atenolol, which was unaffected in this study, has been implicated in producing bradycardia when diltiazem was added in a patient with myocardial ischaemia.[2]


1. Hassell AB, Creamer JE. Profound bradycardia after the addition of diltiazem to a β blocker. *BMJ* 1989; **298:** 675.
2. Nagle RE, *et al.* Diltiazem and heart block. *Lancet* 1989; **i:** 907.
3. Tateishi T, *et al.* Effect of diltiazem on the pharmacokinetics of propranolol, metoprolol and atenolol. *Eur J Clin Pharmacol* 1989; **36:** 67–70.


**Calcium-channel blockers.** For the effect of diltiazem and *nifedipine* on each others plasma concentrations, see p.969.

**Ciclosporin.** For reports of a potentially beneficial interaction between diltiazem and ciclosporin, see Transplantation under Uses and Administration, below.

**Corticosteroids.** Diltiazem has been reported to reduce the clearance of *methylprednisolone* (see Calcium-channel Blockers, p.1072).

**Digoxin.** For a discussion of interactions between digoxin and calcium-channel blockers including diltiazem, see p.897.

**General anaesthetics.** Two patients on diltiazem therapy developed impaired myocardial conduction during anaesthesia with *enflurane*;[1] one of the patients had severe sinus bradycardia that progressed to asystole. Additive cardiodepressant effects of diltiazem and enflurane were considered responsible.


1. Hantler CB, *et al.* Impaired myocardial conduction in patients receiving diltiazem therapy during enflurane anesthesia. *Anesthesiology* 1987; **67:** 94–6.


**Histamine $H_2$-antagonists.** *Cimetidine* caused increases in plasma-diltiazem concentrations and in plasma-deacetyldiltiazem concentrations in 6 subjects given a single dose of diltiazem 60 mg by mouth. *Ranitidine* produced a similar, though less marked effect.[1]


1. Winship LC, *et al.* The effect of ranitidine and cimetidine on single-dose diltiazem pharmacokinetics. *Pharmacotherapy* 1985; **5:** 16–19.


**Lithium.** Neurotoxicity has been reported in patients receiving lithium and diltiazem, see Effects on Mental Function and Parkinsonism under Effects on the Nervous System, above.

**Theophylline.** For the effect of diltiazem on plasma-theophylline concentrations, see p.802.

## Pharmacokinetics

Diltiazem is almost completely absorbed from the gastrointestinal tract following oral administration, but undergoes extensive first-pass hepatic metabolism. Peak plasma concentrations occur about 3 to 4 hours after a dose by mouth. The bioavailability has been reported to be about 40%, although there is considerable inter-individual variation in plasma concentrations. Diltiazem is about 80% bound to plasma proteins. It is distributed into breast milk. It is extensively metabolised in the liver, primarily by the cytochrome P450 isoenzyme CYP3A4; one of the metabolites, desacetyldiltiazem, has been reported to have 25 to 50% of the activity of the parent compound. The half-life of diltiazem is reported to be about 3 to 5 hours. About 2 to 4% of a dose is excreted in urine as unchanged diltiazem with the remainder excreted as metabolites in bile and urine. Diltiazem and its metabolites are poorly dialysable.

◊ General reviews.


1. Kelly JG, O'Malley K. Clinical pharmacokinetics of calcium antagonists: an update. *Clin Pharmacokinet* 1992; **22:** 416–33.


**Bioavailability.** Studies of the pharmacokinetics of diltiazem in healthy subjects after single and multiple doses,[1-3] indicated that bioavailability was increased after multiple doses, probably because of decreased presystemic elimination.[3]


1. Höglund P, Nilsson L-G. Pharmacokinetics of diltiazem and its metabolites after repeated multiple-dose treatments in healthy volunteers. *Ther Drug Monit* 1989; **11:** 543–50.
2. Höglund P, Nilsson L-G. Pharmacokinetics of diltiazem and its metabolites after repeated single dosing in healthy volunteers. *Ther Drug Monit* 1989; **11:** 551–7.
3. Höglund P, Nilsson L-G. Pharmacokinetics of diltiazem and its metabolites after single and multiple dosing in healthy volunteers. *Ther Drug Monit* 1989; **11:** 558–66.


**Renal impairment.** The pharmacokinetics of diltiazem and its major metabolite desacetyldiltiazem in patients with severe renal impairment were similar to those in patients with normal renal function.[1] Nevertheless, reduced doses may be necessary in patients with renal impairment (see under Uses and Administration below). See also under Precautions, above.


1. Pozet N, *et al.* Pharmacokinetics of diltiazem in severe renal failure. *Eur J Clin Pharmacol* 1983; **24:** 635–8.


## Uses and Administration

Diltiazem is a benzothiazepine calcium-channel blocker (p.810). It is a peripheral and coronary vasodilator with limited negative inotropic activity but its vasodilator properties are less marked than those of the dihydropyridine calcium-channel blocker nifedipine (p.966). Unlike nifedipine, diltiazem inhibits cardiac conduction, particularly at the sino-atrial and atrioventricular nodes.

Diltiazem hydrochloride is given by mouth in the management of angina pectoris (p.813) and hypertension (p.825) and is available in a number of formulations for administration once, twice, or three times daily. In some countries it is available for intravenous administration in the treatment of various cardiac arrhythmias (atrial fibrillation or flutter and paroxysmal supraventricular tachycardia) (p.816).

The variety of formulations means that dosage is dependent on the preparation used. Reduced doses may be required in the elderly or those with renal or hepatic impairment (see below).

In **angina pectoris** an initial dose is 60 mg by mouth three times daily (or 30 mg four times daily in the USA), increased if necessary to 360 mg daily; up to 480 mg daily has sometimes been given. Formulations suitable for once- or twice-daily administration may be used in doses of 120 to 480 mg daily; up to 540 mg daily has been given.

In **hypertension** diltiazem hydrochloride may be given as modified-release capsules or tablets. Depending on the formulation, an initial dose is 60 to 120 mg twice daily, increased as required to a maximum of 360 mg daily. Formulations suitable for once-daily administration may be given in similar daily doses, although up to 540 mg daily has been given.

In **cardiac arrhythmias** an initial dose of 250 micrograms/kg by bolus intravenous injection over 2 minutes has been suggested; a further dose of 350 micrograms/kg may be given after 15 minutes if the response is inadequate. Subsequent doses should be individualised for each patient. For those with atrial fibrillation or flutter, a continued reduction in heart rate may be achieved with an intravenous infusion of diltiazem hydrochloride after the bolus injection. An initial infusion rate of 5 to 10 mg/hour, may be increased as necessary in increments of 5 mg/hour up to a rate of 15 mg/hour. The infusion may be continued for up to 24 hours.

◊ General reviews.


1. Buckley MM-T, *et al.* Diltiazem: a reappraisal of its pharmacological properties and therapeutic use. *Drugs* 1990; **39:** 757–806.
2. Fisher M, Grotta J. New uses for calcium channel blockers: therapeutic implications. *Drugs* 1993; **46:** 961–75.
3. Weir MR. Diltiazem: ten years of clinical experience in the treatment of hypertension. *J Clin Pharmacol* 1995; **35:** 220–32.


**Action.** The haemodynamic and electrophysiological effects of diltiazem appear to resemble those of verapamil more than those of nifedipine.[1] It inhibits sino-atrial and atrioventricular nodal function in doses used clinically. The effects on sino-atrial function are more pronounced than those observed after verapamil. Diltiazem causes a decrease in the rate-pressure product indicating that decreased oxygen demand is a likely mechanism of action in relieving angina pectoris. Like verapamil, but unlike nifedipine, diltiazem does not appear to cause significant increases in coronary blood flow. The negative inotropic effect of diltiazem is presumably counteracted by afterload reduction.


1. Soward AL, *et al.* The haemodynamic effects of nifedipine, verapamil and diltiazem in patients with coronary artery disease: a review. *Drugs* 1986; **32:** 66–101.


**Administration in hepatic or renal impairment.** The dose of diltiazem hydrochloride may need to be reduced in patients with hepatic or renal impairment, and in the elderly. In the UK an initial dose of 120 mg daily is usually suggested, as a single dose or in 2 divided doses by mouth depending on the formulation. The dose should not be increased if the heart rate drops below 50 beats/minute.

**Anorectal disorders.** Beneficial responses to diltiazem reported[1,2] in 2 patients with *proctalgia fugax* may have been due to smooth muscle relaxation. The resting pressure of the internal anal sphincter was decreased by a mean of 20.6% in all but 1 of 13 subjects given a single 60-mg oral dose of diltiazem.[2] A small study[3] has compared oral with topical diltiazem in the management of *anal fissure* (p.1390). Despite a higher response rate with the topical drug, no significant difference in benefit was seen between the 2 routes. A subsequent study[4] suggested topical diltiazem (2%) might be of benefit in patients with anal fissure unresponsive to topical nitrates.


1. Boquet J, *et al.* Diltiazem for proctalgia fugax. *Lancet* 1986; **i:** 1493.
2. Jonard P, Essamri B. Diltiazem and internal anal sphincter. *Lancet* 1987; **i:** 754.
3. Jonas M, *et al.* A randomized trial of oral vs topical diltiazem for chronic anal fissures. *Dis Colon Rectum* 2001; **44:** 1074–8.
4. Jonas M, *et al.* Diltiazem heals glyceryl trinitrate-resistant chronic anal fissures: a prospective study. *Dis Colon Rectum* 2002; **45:** 1091–5.


**Cardiomyopathies.** Although calcium-channel blockers should be used with caution in patients with heart failure, symptomatic improvement has been reported in patients with dilated cardiomyopathy (p.818) given diltiazem.[1]


1. Figulla HR, *et al.* Diltiazem improves cardiac function and exercise capacity in patients with idiopathic dilated cardiomyopathy: results of the Diltiazem in Dilated Cardiomyopathy Trial. *Circulation* 1996; **94:** 346–52.


**Connective tissue and muscular disorders.** Subcutaneous deposition of calcium (calcinosis) can occur in a number of inflammatory conditions, particularly in juvenile dermatomyositis (see Polymyositis and Dermatomyositis, p.1086). Treatment of calcinosis is difficult, but there have been a number of reports of the successful use of diltiazem in children[1,2] and adults[3] with dermatomyositis, as well as in adults with CREST (calcinosis, Raynaud's phenomenon, esophageal dysmotility, sclerodactyly, telangiectasias) syndrome,[4] scleroderma,[5] and lupus panniculitis.[6] Another study,[7] however, found only a limited response in patients with systemic sclerosis.


1. Oliveri MB, *et al.* Regression of calcinosis during diltiazem treatment in juvenile dermatomyositis. *J Rheumatol* 1996; **23:** 2152–5.
2. Ichiki Y, *et al.* An extremely severe case of cutaneous calcinosis with juvenile dermatomyositis, and successful treatment with diltiazem. *Br J Dermatol* 2001; **144:** 894–7.
3. Vinen CS, *et al.* Regression of calcinosis associated with adult dermatomyositis following diltiazem therapy. *Rheumatology (Oxford)* 2000; **39:** 333–4.
4. Palmieri GMA, *et al.* Treatment of calcinosis with diltiazem. *Arthritis Rheum* 1995; **38:** 1646–54.
5. Dolan AL, *et al.* Diltiazem induces remission of calcinosis in scleroderma. *Br J Rheumatol* 1995; **34:** 576–8.
6. Morgan KW, *et al.* Calcifying lupus panniculitis in a patient with subacute cutaneous lupus erythematosus: response to diltiazem and chloroquine. *J Rheumatol* 2001; **28:** 2129–32.
7. Vayssairat M, *et al.* Clinical significance of subcutaneous calcinosis in patients with systemic sclerosis: does diltiazem induce its regression? *Ann Rheum Dis* 1998; **57:** 252–4.


**Kidney disorders.** Calcium-channel blockers may be of benefit in various forms of kidney disorder (see Nifedipine, p.971). Diltiazem has been reported to reduce urinary protein excretion without exacerbating pre-existing renal dysfunction in diabetic patients.[1,2] A small study[3] in 15 hypertensive patients with type 2 diabetes mellitus, albuminuria, and renal impairment found that diltiazem only reduced urinary albumin excretion when patients received a restricted dietary sodium intake of 50 mmol daily.

Diltiazem may also reduce the nephrotoxicity associated with certain drugs. Reduced nephrotoxicity has been reported when diltiazem is given to healthy subjects receiving netilmicin,[4] but diltiazem does not appear to modify the acute renal failure associated with tubular damage which may be caused by methotrexate.[5] Diltiazem may reduce ciclosporin-induced nephrotoxicity (see Transplantation, below).


1. Bakris GL. Effects of diltiazem or lisinopril on massive proteinuria associated with diabetes mellitus. *Ann Intern Med* 1990; **112:** 707–8.
2. Demarie BK, Bakris GL. Effects of different calcium antagonists on proteinuria associated with diabetes mellitus. *Ann Intern Med* 1990; **113:** 987–8.
3. Bakris GL, Smith A. Effects of sodium intake on albumin excretion in patients with diabetic nephropathy treated with long-acting calcium antagonists. *Ann Intern Med* 1996; **125:** 201–4.
4. Lortholary O, *et al.* Calcium antagonists and aminoglycoside nephrotoxicity. *Am J Med* 1990; **88:** 445.
5. Deray G, *et al.* The effects of diltiazem on methotrexate-induced nephrotoxicity. *Eur J Clin Pharmacol* 1989; **37:** 337–40.


**Migraine.** For reference to the use of calcium-channel blockers, including diltiazem, in the management of migraine, see under Nifedipine, p.971.

**Myocardial infarction.** Studies have not shown a reduction in mortality when calcium-channel blockers are given in the **early** phase of acute myocardial infarction (p.828). However, since myocardial stunning has been linked to intracellular calcium overload[1] there has been speculation that calcium-channel blockers might benefit patients about to undergo reperfusion. This is yet to be confirmed. Diltiazem started within 24 to 72 hours after the onset of infarction and continued for up to 14 days has been reported to protect against re-infarction and refractory angina in patients recovering from acute non-Q-wave infarction.[2] A pilot study[3] of intravenous diltiazem as an adjunct to thrombolysis in acute myocardial infarction also suggested a reduction in recurrent ischaemia; diltiazem was given intravenously for 48 hours, beginning at the same time as the thrombolytic, then continued orally for 4 weeks.

Calcium-channel blockers are not routinely used in the **long-term** management of myocardial infarction although in selected patients without heart failure verapamil or diltiazem may be of some benefit. In a study by the Multicenter Diltiazem Postinfarction Trial (MDPIT) research group,[4] diltiazem (target dose 240 mg daily) reduced 1-year mortality and re-infarction rates in patients without left ventricular dysfunction, but increased such adverse events in those with left ventricular dysfunction. Reanalysis of the Multicenter Diltiazem Postinfarction Trial provided further evidence that diltiazem should be avoided in postinfarction patients with left ventricular dysfunction.[5] Another study[6] in patients with acute myocardial infarction treated with thrombolysis found no reduction in mortality with diltiazem started 36 to 96 hours after infarction and continued for up to 6 months, although the incidence of non-fatal cardiac events was reduced. Patients with heart failure were excluded from the trial.


1. Anonymous. Myocardial stunning. *Lancet* 1991; **337:** 585–6.
2. Gibson RS, *et al.* Diltiazem and reinfarction in patients with non-Q-wave myocardial infarction: results of a double-blind, randomized, multicenter trial. *N Engl J Med* 1986; **315:** 423–9.
3. Théroux P, *et al.* Intravenous diltiazem in acute myocardial infarction: diltiazem as adjunctive therapy to activase (DATA) trial. *J Am Coll Cardiol* 1998; **32:** 620–8.
4. The Multicenter Diltiazem Postinfarction Trial Research Group. The effect of diltiazem on mortality and reinfarction after myocardial infarction. *N Engl J Med* 1988; **319:** 385–92.
5. Goldstein RE, *et al.* Diltiazem increases late-onset congestive heart failure in post-infarction patients with early reduction in ejection fraction. *Circulation* 1991; **83:** 52–60.
6. Boden WE, *et al.* Diltiazem in acute myocardial infarction treated with thrombolytic agents: a randomised placebo-controlled trial. *Lancet* 2000; **355:** 1751–6.


**Transplantation.** Diltiazem increases blood-ciclosporin concentrations when given by mouth in doses of 60 to 180 mg daily to transplant patients receiving ciclosporin therapy.[1-3] In consequence, ciclosporin doses can be reduced by about one-third, at a considerable saving in cost.[2,3] However, the effect may not occur in all patients,[4] and may vary with differing formulations,[5] and it has been suggested that blood-ciclosporin concentrations should be closely monitored if diltiazem is used for this purpose. In addition to this effect, which is apparently due to non-competitive inhibition of ciclosporin metabolism by diltiazem,[6] there is evidence of improved renal graft-function in patients given the combined therapy, suggesting that diltiazem may reduce ciclosporin-induced nephrotoxicity.[1,2]


1. Wagner K, Neumayer H-H. Prevention of delayed graft function in cadaver kidney transplants by diltiazem. *Lancet* 1985; **ii:** 1355–6.
2. Neumayer H-H, Wagner K. Diltiazem and economic use of cyclosporin. *Lancet* 1986; **ii:** 523.
3. Bourge RC, *et al.* Diltiazem-cyclosporine interaction in cardiac transplant recipients: impact on cyclosporine dose and medication costs. *Am J Med* 1991; **90:** 402–4.
4. Jones TE, Morris RG. Diltiazem does not always increase blood cyclosporin concentration. *Br J Clin Pharmacol* 1996; **42:** 642–4.
5. Jones TE, *et al.* Formulation of diltiazem affects cyclosporin-sparing activity. *Eur J Clin Pharmacol* 1997; **52:** 55–8.
6. Brockmöller J, *et al.* Pharmacokinetic interaction between cyclosporin and diltiazem. *Eur J Clin Pharmacol* 1990; **38:** 237–42.


## Preparations

***USP 27:*** Diltiazem Hydrochloride Extended-release Capsules; Diltiazem Hydrochloride Tablets.

**Proprietary Preparations** (details are given in Part 3)
***Arg.:*** Acalix; Diltenk; Diltiacor; Dilzen-G; Hart; Incoril; Kaltiazem; Ritmocit; Tilazem; ***Austral.:*** Auscard; Cardcal†; Cardizem; Coras; Diltahexal; Diltiamax†; Dilzem; Vasocardol; ***Austria:*** Cardiacton†; Corazem; Diltahexal; Diltiastad; Dilzatyrol; Dilzem; Gewazem; ***Belg.:*** Progor; Tildiem; ***Braz.:*** Angiolong; Balcor; Cardizem; Diltiacor; Diltipress; Diltizem†; Incoril; ***Canad.:*** Apo-Diltiaz; Cardizem; Novo-Diltazem; Nu-Diltiaz; Tiazac; ***Chile:*** Acasmul; Grifodilzem; Incoril; Tilazem; Tildiem; ***Denm.:*** Angiact†; Angicontin†; Cardil; Cardizem; Dilcor; Myonil; Tilker; UnoCardil†; Viazem; ***Fin.:*** Cardizem; Dilmin; Dilpral; Dilzem; ***Fr.:*** Bi-Tildiem; Deltazen; Diacor; Dilrene; Mono-Tildiem; Tildiem; ***Ger.:*** Corazet; Dil-Sanorania; Dilsal; Dilta; Diltabeta; Diltahexal; Diltapham; Diltaretard; Dilti; Diltiagamma; Diltiamerck†; Diltiuc; Dilzem; Dilzereal†; Dilzicardin; ***Gr.:*** Alfener; Cardil; Diltelan; Dilzanol; Dipen; Elvesil; Ergoclavin; Mavitalon; Rubiten; Ternel; Tildiem; Zilden; ***Hong Kong:*** Altiazem; Apo-Diltiaz; Cardium; Dilem†; Diltan; Dilzem†; Herbesser; Metazem†; Retalzem; Tildiem†; ***India:*** Dilcardia; Dilcontin; Dilzem; DTM; Iski; Kaizem; ***Irl.:*** Adizem; Diltam; Dilzem; Entrydil; Metazem†; Tildiem; ***Israel:*** Adizem; Dilatam; Levodex; ***Ital.:*** Altiazem; Angidil; Angipress; Angizem; Carzem†; Citizem; Diladel; Dilem; Diliter; Dilzene; Etyzem; Longazem; Tiakem†; Tiazen†; Tildiem; Zilden†; ***Jpn:*** Herbesser; ***Malaysia:*** Cardil; Cascor; Dilcard; Dilem; Herbesser; Mono-Tildiem; ***Mex.:*** Angiotrofin; Presoken†; Presoquim†; Tilazem; Waysen†; ***Neth.:*** Diloc; Surazem; Tiadil; Tildiem; ***Norw.:*** Cardizem; Diltikard†; Kardil†; Tilker; ***NZ:*** Cardizem; Dilcard; Dilzem; ***Port.:*** Alandiem; Balcor; Cal-Antagon; Dilfar; Dilongo; Diltiangina; Diltiem; Duplide†; Etizem; Herbesser; Pentilzeno†; Tiadil; ***S.Afr.:*** Diatil†; Dilatam; Tilazem; Zildem; ***Singapore:*** Altiazem†; Angizem†; Beatizem; Cardil; Cardium; Dilatam; Dilizem†; Herbesser; Metazem†; Mono-Tildiem; Tildiem†; ***Spain:*** Angiodrox; Cardiser; Carreldon; Clobendian; Convectal†; Corolater; Cronodine; Dilaclan; Diltiwas; Dinisor; Doclis; Lacerol; Masdil; Mdiltiwas†; Tilker; Trumsal; Uni Masdil; ***Swed.:*** Cardizem; Coramil; Viazem; ***Switz.:*** Coridil; Dilzem; Escozem; Tildiem; ***Thai.:*** Altiazem; Angizem; Cardil; Cascor; Denazox; Dilatam†; Dilem; Dilizem; Diltan†; Diltec; Dilzem; Ditizem; Herbesser; Medozem; Metazem†; Mono-Tildiem†; Tildiem†; ***UK:*** Adizem; Angiozem; Angitil; Calcicard; Dilcardia; Dilzem; Disogram; Horizem†; Metazem†; Optil; Slozem; Tildiem; Viazem; Zemtard; ***USA:*** Cardizem; Cartia; Dilacor; Diltia; Taztia; Tiamate†; Tiazac.

**Multi-ingredient:** ***Arg.:*** Lotrix; ***USA:*** Teczem.

---

## Dimetofrine Hydrochloride *(rINNM)*

Dimetophrine Hydrochloride; Hidrocloruro de dimetofrina. 4-Hydroxy-3,5-dimethoxy-α-[(methylamino)methyl]benzyl alcohol hydrochloride.

$C_{11}H_{17}NO_4,HCl = 263.7.$

*CAS — 22950-29-4 (dimetofrine); 22775-12-8 (dimetofrine hydrochloride).*

*ATC — C01CA12.*

### Profile

Dimetofrine hydrochloride is a sympathomimetic (see Adrenaline, p.852) which has been used for its vasopressor effects in the treatment of hypotensive states; it has been given by mouth or by intramuscular injection or intravenous infusion.

### Preparations

**Proprietary Preparations** (details are given in Part 3)
***Ital.:*** Pressamina.

**Multi-ingredient:** ***Ital.:*** Raffreddoremed.

## Dipyridamole (BAN, USAN, rINN)

Dipiridamol; Dipyridamolum; NSC-515776; RA-8. 2,2′,2″,2‴-[(4,8-Dipiperidinopyrimido[5,4-*d*]pyrimidine-2,6-diyl)dinitrilo]tetraethanol.

$C_{24}H_{40}N_8O_4$ = 504.6.

*CAS — 58-32-2.*

*ATC — B01AC07.*

**Pharmacopoeias.** In *Chin., Eur.* (see p.vi), *Jpn, Pol.,* and *US.*

**Ph. Eur. 5.0** (Dipyridamole). A bright yellow crystalline powder. Practically insoluble in water; soluble in dehydrated alcohol; freely soluble in acetone. It dissolves in dilute solutions of mineral acids. Protect from light.

**USP 27** (Dipyridamole). An intensely yellow, crystalline powder or needles. Slightly soluble in water; very soluble in chloroform, in alcohol, and in methyl alcohol; very slightly soluble in acetone and in ethyl acetate. Store in airtight containers. Protect from light.

### Adverse Effects, Treatment, and Precautions

Gastrointestinal disturbances, including nausea, vomiting, and diarrhoea, headache, dizziness, faintness, hypotension, facial flushing, and skin rash and other hypersensitivity reactions may occur after administration of dipyridamole. Dipyridamole can also induce chest pain or lead to a worsening of the symptoms of angina. Cardiac arrhythmias have been reported in patients given dipyridamole during thallium-201 imaging. Aminophylline may reverse some of the adverse effects.

Dipyridamole should be used with caution in patients with hypotension, unstable angina, aortic stenosis, recent myocardial infarction, heart failure, or coagulation disorders. Intravenous dipyridamole should not be given to patients with these conditions or to those with arrhythmias, conduction disorders, asthma, or a history of bronchospasm (but see Myocardial Imaging, below).

**Effects on the biliary tract.** Gallstones containing unconjugated dipyridamole were removed from 2 patients who had been taking dipyridamole for 15 and 10 years, respectively.[1] A gallstone containing unconjugated dipyridamole recurred in a patient who continued to take the drug after endoscopic removal of a similar stone 18 months earlier.[2]

1. Moesch C, *et al.* Biliary drug lithiasis: dipyridamole gallstones. *Lancet* 1992; **340:** 1352–3.
2. Sautereau D, *et al.* Recurrence of biliary drug lithiasis due to dipyridamole. *Endoscopy* 1997; **29:** 421–3.

**Effects on the heart.** Transient myocardial ischaemia occurred in 4 patients with unstable angina and multivessel coronary artery disease during oral treatment with dipyridamole.[1] See Myocardial Imaging, below, for additional reports.

1. Keltz TN, *et al.* Dipyridamole-induced myocardial ischemia. *JAMA* 1987; **257:** 1515–16.

**Effects on the muscles.** Symptoms resembling acute pseudopolymyalgia rheumatica developed in a patient taking dipyridamole.[1]

1. Chassagne P, *et al.* Pseudopolymyalgia rheumatica with dipyridamole. *BMJ* 1990; **301:** 875.

**Effects on taste.** A report of a disagreeable taste associated with other gastrointestinal symptoms occurring in a patient taking dipyridamole.[1] Two similar cases had been reported to the UK Committee on Safety of Medicines.

1. Willoughby JMT. Drug-induced abnormalities of taste sensation. *Adverse Drug React Bull* 1983; **100:** 368–71.

**Myocardial imaging.** Dipyridamole may be used in association with thallium-201 in myocardial stress imaging. Safety data from over 3900 patients has been summarised.[1] Adverse effects which occurred within 24 hours of dipyridamole intravenously (mean dose 0.56 mg/kg) were recorded. Ten patients had major adverse effects and 1820 patients experienced minor adverse effects. Myocardial infarction occurred in 4 patients, 3 of whom had unstable angina before thallium-201 myocardial scanning. Six patients developed acute bronchospasm, 4 of whom had a history of asthma or had wheezing before administration of dipyridamole. Adverse effects considered to be minor included chest pain in 19.7% of patients, ST-T-segment depression in 7.5%, ventricular extrasystoles in 5.2%, headache in 12.2%, dizziness in 11.8%, nausea in 4.6%, and hypotension in 4.6%. Aminophylline was effective in relieving symptoms of adverse effects in 97% of 454 patients.

Hypersensitivity reactions including anaphylaxis and angioedema have been reported.[2,3]

The UK manufacturers contra-indicate intravenous dipyridamole in patients with hypotension, unstable angina, aortic stenosis, recent myocardial infarction, heart failure, coagulation disorders, arrhythmias, conduction disorders, asthma, or a history of bronchospasm. However, a review[4] of pharmacological stress testing suggested that with appropriate patient selection and adequate monitoring, the incidence of life-threatening adverse reactions is negligible. It was also considered that dipyridamole-thallium-201 imaging could be safely performed in the early post-myocardial infarction period.

1. Ranhosky A, *et al.* The safety of intravenous dipyridamole thallium myocardial perfusion imaging. *Circulation* 1990; **81:** 1205–9.
2. Weinmann P, *et al.* Anaphylaxis-like reaction induced by dipyridamole during myocardial scintigraphy. *Am J Med* 1994; **97:** 488.
3. Angelides S, *et al.* Acute reaction to dipyridamole during myocardial scintigraphy. *N Engl J Med* 1999; **340:** 394.
4. Beller GA. Pharmacologic stress imaging. *JAMA* 1991; **265:** 633–8.

### Interactions

Dipyridamole may enhance the actions of oral anticoagulants due to its antiplatelet effect. It inhibits the reuptake of adenosine and may enhance its effects; the dose of adenosine must be reduced if the two drugs are given concomitantly. Dipyridamole may also inhibit the uptake of fludarabine and may reduce its efficacy.

The absorption of dipyridamole may be reduced by drugs such as antacids that increase gastric pH.

**Anticoagulants.** Dipyridamole may induce bleeding in patients receiving oral anticoagulants without altering prothrombin times (see Antiplatelets, under Warfarin, Interactions, p.1026).

**Xanthines.** Xanthines may antagonise some of the effects of dipyridamole due to their action as adenosine antagonists. *Aminophylline* may be used to reverse some of the adverse effects of dipyridamole. Administration of *caffeine* intravenously has been reported[1] to attenuate the haemodynamic response to dipyridamole and it has been suggested that caffeine should be avoided for at least 24 hours before the test in patients receiving dipyridamole for myocardial imaging.

1. Smits P, *et al.* Dose-dependent inhibition of the hemodynamic response to dipyridamole by caffeine. *Clin Pharmacol Ther* 1991; **50:** 529–37.

### Pharmacokinetics

Dipyridamole is incompletely absorbed from the gastrointestinal tract with peak plasma concentrations occurring about 75 minutes after oral administration. Dipyridamole is more than 90% bound to plasma proteins. A terminal half-life of 10 to 12 hours has been reported. Dipyridamole is metabolised in the liver and is mainly excreted as glucuronides in the bile. Excretion may be delayed by enterohepatic recirculation. A small amount is excreted in the urine. Dipyridamole is distributed into breast milk.

◊ References.

1. Mahony C, *et al.* Dipyridamole kinetics. *Clin Pharmacol Ther* 1982; **31:** 330–8.
2. Mahony C, *et al.* Plasma dipyridamole concentrations after two different dosage regimens in patients. *J Clin Pharmacol* 1983; **23:** 123–6.

### Uses and Administration

Dipyridamole is an adenosine reuptake inhibitor and phosphodiesterase inhibitor with antiplatelet and vasodilating activity and is used in thromboembolic disorders (p.837). Oral dipyridamole is used for the prophylaxis of thromboembolism following cardiac valve replacement (p.838) and in the management of stroke (below); it has also been used in the management of myocardial infarction (p.828). Dipyridamole administered intravenously results in marked coronary vasodilatation and is used in stress testing in patients with ischaemic heart disease (see below).

For the prophylaxis of **thromboembolism** following cardiac valve replacement, dipyridamole is given with an oral anticoagulant. The usual adult dose is 300 to 600 mg daily by mouth in divided doses before meals. Children have been given 5 mg/kg by mouth daily in divided doses.

For the secondary prevention of **stroke** or transient ischaemic attack dipyridamole is given as a modified-release preparation, alone or with aspirin, in a dose of 200 mg twice daily.

◊ General references.

1. FitzGerald GA. Dipyridamole. *N Engl J Med* 1987; **316:** 1247–57.
2. Gibbs CR, Lip GYH. Do we still need dipyridamole? *Br J Clin Pharmacol* 1998; **45:** 323–8.

**Myocardial imaging.** Perfusion abnormalities due to coronary artery disease are usually absent at rest but are present during stress, and stress imaging may therefore be used in the assessment of myocardial function. The stress is usually supplied by exercise, but when exercise is inappropriate pharmacological methods such as dipyridamole may be used.

Dipyridamole has been used with thallium-201 scintigraphy in adults and children and is usually given intravenously in a dose of 567 micrograms/kg over 4 minutes. Thallium-201 is given within 3 to 5 minutes following completion of the infusion of dipyridamole. Initial images are obtained 5 minutes after drug administration and delayed images are obtained 2.5 to 4 hours later. Dipyridamole (300 to 400 mg) has also been given as an oral suspension; thallium-201 is given about 45 minutes later to coincide with peak dipyridamole-serum concentrations.

Dipyridamole has also been used in echocardiography.[1,2] The intravenous dipyridamole dose used to obtain maximum sensitivity is often higher (750 to 840 micrograms/kg) than the dose used in scintigraphy.[1]

1. Beller GA. Pharmacologic stress imaging. *JAMA* 1991; **265:** 633–8.
2. Buchalter MB, *et al.* Dipyridamole echocardiography: the bedside stress test for coronary artery disease. *Postgrad Med J* 1990; **66:** 531–5.

**Stroke.** The value of long-term antiplatelet therapy with aspirin in patients who have suffered an ischaemic stroke or transient ischaemic attack is well-established, with a reduction in the risk of both stroke and other vascular events.[1] Early studies with dipyridamole, alone or in combination with aspirin, failed to show any benefit over aspirin alone. The European Stroke Prevention Study-2,[2] comparing aspirin and dipyridamole, alone or in combination, with placebo, found that both drugs reduced the risk of stroke and that the effects appeared to be additive. The study used a low dose of aspirin and a modified-release formulation of dipyridamole, which may explain the discrepancy with earlier studies.[3] However, subsequent meta-analyses,[3,4] while acknowledging that addition of dipyridamole does reduce the risk of stroke, have suggested that further studies are required to confirm an overall benefit.

1. Antiplatelet Trialists' Collaboration. Collaborative overview of randomised trials of antiplatelet therapy—I: prevention of death, myocardial infarction, and stroke by prolonged antiplatelet therapy in various categories of patients. *BMJ* 1994; **308:** 81–106. Correction. *ibid.*; 1540.
2. Diener HC, *et al.* European Stroke Prevention Study 2: dipyridamole and acetylsalicylic acid in the secondary prevention of stroke. *J Neurol Sci* 1996; **143:** 1–13.
3. Wilterdink JL, Easton JD. Dipyridamole plus aspirin in cerebrovascular disease. *Arch Neurol* 1999; **56:** 1087–92.
4. Antithrombotic Trialists' Collaboration. Collaborative meta-analysis of randomised trials of antiplatelet therapy for prevention of death, myocardial infarction, and stroke in high risk patients. *BMJ* 2002; **324:** 71–86. Correction. *ibid.*; 141.

### Preparations

***BP 2003:*** Dipyridamole Tablets;
***USP 27:*** Dipyridamole Injection; Dipyridamole Tablets.

**Proprietary Preparations** (details are given in Part 3)
***Arg.:*** Maxicardil; Persantin; ***Austral.:*** Persantin; ***Austria:*** Persantin; ***Belg.:*** Dipyridan; Persantine; ***Braz.:*** Fluxocor†; Persantin; Procor†; ***Canad.:*** Novo-Dipiradol; Persantine; ***Chile:*** Persantin; ***Denm.:*** Persantin; ***Fin.:*** Atrombin; Dipyrin; Persantin†; ***Fr.:*** Cleridium; Coronarine†; Perkod†; Persantine; Protangix†; ***Ger.:*** Curantyl N; Persantin†; ***Gr.:*** Adezan; Persantin; ***Hong Kong:*** Persantin; ***India:*** Persantin; ***Irl.:*** Persantin; ***Israel:*** Cardoxin; ***Ital.:*** Corosan; Novodil†; Persantin; ***Malaysia:*** Persantin; ***Mex.:*** Damosal†; Dipres†; Dirinol†; Lodimol†; Persantin; Pracem; Trepol; Trompersantin; Vadinar; ***Neth.:*** Persantin; ***Norw.:*** Persantin; ***NZ:*** Persantin; Pytazen; ***Port.:*** Persantin; ***S.Afr.:*** Persantin; Plato; ***Singapore:*** Persantin; Procardin†; ***Spain:*** Miosen†; Persantin; ***Swed.:*** Persantin; ***Switz.:*** Natyl†; Persantine†; ***Thai.:*** Agremol; Persantin; Posanin; ***UK:*** Persantin; ***USA:*** Persantine.

**Multi-ingredient:** ***Arg.:*** Agrenox; Licuamon; ***Austral.:*** Asasantin; ***Austria:*** Asasantin; Thrombohexal; Thrombosantin; ***Belg.:*** Aggrenox; ***Braz.:*** Persantin S†; Procor S†; Tromboxanil†; ***Canad.:*** Aggrenox; Asasantine†; ***Fin.:*** Asasantin; ***Fr.:*** Asasantine; ***Ger.:*** Asasantin; ***Gr.:*** Aggrenox; ***Hong Kong:*** Persantin Plus†; ***India:*** Dynasprin; ***Irl.:*** Asasantin; ***Ital.:*** Persumbrax†; ***Mex.:*** Asasantin; ***Neth.:*** Asasantin; ***Norw.:*** Asasantin; ***Port.:*** Aggrenox; ***S.Afr.:*** Asasantin; ***Spain:*** Asasantin†; ***Swed.:*** Asasantin; ***Switz.:*** Asasantine; ***UK:*** Asasantin; ***USA:*** Aggrenox.

## Disopyramide (BAN, USAN, rINN)

Disopiramida; Disopyramidum; SC-7031. 4-Di-isopropylamino-2-phenyl-2-(2-pyridyl)butyramide.

$C_{21}H_{29}N_3O$ = 339.5.

*CAS — 3737-09-5.*

*ATC — C01BA03.*

**Pharmacopoeias.** In *Eur.* (see p.vi) and *Jpn.*

**Ph. Eur. 5.0** (Disopyramide). A white or almost white powder. Slightly soluble in water; soluble in alcohol; freely soluble in dichloromethane. Protect from light.

### Disopyramide Phosphate (BANM, USAN, rINNM)

Disopyramidi Phosphas; Fosfato de disopiramida; SC-13957.

$C_{21}H_{29}N_3O,H_3PO_4$ = 437.5.

*CAS — 22059-60-5.*

**Pharmacopoeias.** In *Chin., Eur.* (see p.vi), *Pol.,* and *US.*

**Ph. Eur. 5.0** (Disopyramide Phosphate). A white or almost white powder. Soluble in water; sparingly soluble in alcohol; practically insoluble in dichloromethane. A 5% solution in water has a pH of 4.0 to 5.0. Protect from light.

**USP 27** (Disopyramide Phosphate). A white or practically white, odourless powder. Freely soluble in water; slightly soluble in alcohol; practically insoluble in chloroform and in ether. pH of a 5% solution in water is between 4.0 and 5.0. Store in airtight containers. Protect from light.

## Adverse Effects and Treatment

The adverse effects most commonly associated with disopyramide relate to its antimuscarinic properties and are dose-related. They include dry mouth, blurred vision, urinary hesitancy, impotence, and constipation; the most serious effect is urinary retention. Gastrointestinal effects which are less common include nausea, bloating, and abdominal pain. Other adverse effects reported include skin rashes, hypoglycaemia, dizziness, fatigue, muscle weakness, headache, and urinary frequency. Insomnia and depression have also been associated with disopyramide. There have been rare reports of psychosis, cholestatic jaundice, elevated liver enzymes, thrombocytopenia, and agranulocytosis. Disopyramide has cardiac depressant properties, and may induce cardiac arrhythmias particularly ventricular tachycardia and fibrillation, heart block and conduction disturbances, heart failure, and hypotension.

Over-rapid intravenous injection of disopyramide may cause profuse sweating and severe cardiovascular depression.

In overdose cardiovascular and antimuscarinic effects are pronounced, and there may be apnoea, loss of consciousness, loss of spontaneous respiration, and asystole. Treatment of overdosage is symptomatic and supportive. Activated charcoal may be considered if the patient presents within 1 hour of ingestion.

◊ A review of the adverse effects associated with the class Ia antiarrhythmic drugs disopyramide, procainamide, and quinidine, and their clinical management.[1]

1. Kim SY, Benowitz NL. Poisoning due to class IA antiarrhythmic drugs quinidine, procainamide and disopyramide. *Drug Safety* 1990; **5:** 393–420.

**Incidence of adverse effects.** During long-term therapy with disopyramide 400 to 1600 mg daily in 40 patients, 28 (70%) had one or more adverse effects.[1] Dry mouth occurred in 15 (38%), constipation in 12 (30%), blurred vision in 11 (28%), urinary hesitancy in 9 (23%), nausea in 9 (23%), impotence in 2 (5%), and dyspareunia in one patient (3%). In addition 3 of the 9 patients with pre-existing heart failure had worsening of their condition due to disopyramide. Adverse effects were sufficiently severe for disopyramide to be discontinued in 7 patients, and for dosage reductions in another 7.

1. Bauman JL, *et al.* Long-term therapy with disopyramide phosphate: side effects and effectiveness. *Am Heart J* 1986; **111:** 654–60.

**Effects on the blood.** Granulocytopenia was associated on 2 occasions with the use of disopyramide phosphate in a 61-year-old man.[1]

1. Conrad ME, *et al.* Agranulocytosis associated with disopyramide therapy. *JAMA* 1978; **240:** 1857–8.

**Effects on the eyes.** The antimuscarinic activity of disopyramide may cause adverse effects such as dilated pupils,[1] severe blurring of vision,[1] and acute glaucoma.[2,3] Disopyramide should be avoided in patients with glaucoma and used with caution if there is a family history of glaucoma.

1. Frucht J, *et al.* Ocular side effects of disopyramide. *Br J Ophthalmol* 1984; **68:** 890–1.
2. Trope GE, Hind VMD. Closed-angle glaucoma in patient on disopyramide. *Lancet* 1978, **i:** 329.
3. Ahmad S. Disopyramide: pulmonary complications and glaucoma. *Mayo Clin Proc* 1990; **65:** 1030–1.

**Effects on the heart.** Disopyramide has a strong negative inotropic effect and reversible heart failure has been reported[1] after its use. As many as 50% of patients with a previous history of heart failure may have a recurrence of the disease with an incidence of less than 5% in other patients.

As disopyramide can prolong the QT interval it can induce ventricular tachyarrhythmias. A case of fatal torsade de pointes has been reported.[2]

1. Podrid PJ, *et al.* Congestive heart failure caused by oral disopyramide. *N Engl J Med* 1980; **302:** 614–17.
2. Schattner A, *et al.* Fatal torsade de pointes following jaundice in a patient treated with disopyramide. *Postgrad Med J* 1989; **65:** 333–4.

**Effects on the liver.** Cholestatic jaundice with raised liver enzyme values has been associated with disopyramide.[1-3] Laboratory and clinical abnormalities disappear on withdrawal although liver enzyme values may remain elevated for several months.

Severe hepatocellular damage with disseminated intravascular coagulation[4] has also been reported.

1. Craxi A, *et al.* Disopyramide and cholestasis. *Ann Intern Med* 1980; **93:** 150–1.
2. Edmonds ME, Hayler AM. *Eur J Clin Pharmacol* 1980; **18:** 285–6.
3. Bakris GL, *et al.* Disopyramide-associated liver dysfunction. *Mayo Clin Proc* 1983; **58:** 265–7.
4. Doody PT. Disopyramide hepatotoxicity and disseminated intravascular coagulation. *South Med J* 1982; **75:** 496–8.

**Effects on mental state.** Agitation and distress leading to paranoia and auditory and visual hallucinations have been reported[1,2] in patients shortly after starting disopyramide therapy. Complete recovery occurred on withdrawal.

1. Falk RH, *et al.* Mental distress in patient on disopyramide. *Lancet* 1977; **i:** 858–9.
2. Padfield PL, *et al.* Disopyramide and acute psychosis. *Lancet* 1977; **i:** 1152.

**Effects on the nervous system.** Peripheral neuropathy affecting the feet and severe enough to prevent walking was associated with disopyramide in a 72-year-old patient.[1] There was gradual improvement on withdrawal of disopyramide with the patient being symptom-free after 4 months.

A 75-year-old woman with atrial fibrillation suffered a tonic-clonic seizure followed by respiratory arrest after receiving disopyramide 150 mg intravenously over a period of 10 minutes.[2] On recovery she complained of a dry mouth and blurred vision and it was considered that the seizure was caused by the antimuscarinic action of disopyramide, although it may have been due to a direct stimulant action.

1. Dawkins KD, Gibson J. Peripheral neuropathy with disopyramide. *Lancet* 1978; **i:** 329.
2. Johnson NM, *et al.* Epileptiform convulsion with intravenous disopyramide. *Lancet* 1978; **ii:** 848.

**Effects on sexual function.** Impotence associated with disopyramide was abolished when the patient's disopyramide plasma concentration was reduced from 14 to 3 micrograms/mL.[1] This effect was probably due to the antimuscarinic activity of disopyramide although the patient did not report any other antimuscarinic symptoms.

1. McHaffie DJ, *et al.* Impotence in patient on disopyramide. *Lancet* 1977; **i:** 859.

**Effects on the urinary tract.** In a report of 9 cases of urinary retention associated with disopyramide and a review of the literature,[1] it was noted that urinary retention secondary to disopyramide use was most likely to develop in male patients over the age of 65 in whom there was some pre-existing renal dysfunction; there was an increased risk in patients with evidence of prostatic hyperplasia.

1. Danziger LH, Horn JR. Disopyramide-induced urinary retention. *Arch Intern Med* 1983; **143:** 1683–6.

**Hypersensitivity.** Worsening of ventricular arrhythmia and an anaphylactoid reaction occurred in a 58-year-old man after a single dose of disopyramide 300 mg by mouth.[1] Two hours after the dose he complained of a swollen tongue and difficulty in breathing. He became cyanotic and was given diphenhydramine 25 mg intravenously, which resulted in improvement of his respiratory status.

1. Porterfield JG, *et al.* Respiratory difficulty after use of disopyramide. *N Engl J Med* 1980; **303:** 584.

**Hypoglycaemia.** Following reports to the manufacturer of hypoglycaemia associated with administration of disopyramide, 2 controlled studies were conducted in healthy subjects.[1] Disopyramide produced a small decrease in blood-glucose concentration but there were no symptoms of hypoglycaemia. It was considered that the glucose-lowering effect may be clinically significant in patients with hepatic or renal impairment.

1. Strathman I, *et al.* Hypoglycemia in patients receiving disopyramide phosphate. *Drug Intell Clin Pharm* 1983; **17:** 635–8.

**Overdosage.** A 2-year-old boy suffered hypotension, cardiac arrhythmias, and convulsions and died 28 hours after ingestion of 600 mg of disopyramide.[1] In a report[2] of 5 cases of fatal overdosage with disopyramide the most common clinical finding appeared to be an early loss of consciousness following an episode of respiratory arrest. Four of the patients initially responded to resuscitation but subsequently deteriorated rapidly, with cardiac arrhythmias and loss of spontaneous respiration; in 4 of the cases post-mortem examination demonstrated pulmonary congestion secondary to left ventricular failure.

1. Hutchison A, Kilham H. Fatal overdosage of disopyramide in a child. *Med J Aust* 1978; **2:** 335–6.
2. Hayler AM, *et al.* Fatal overdosage with disopyramide. *Lancet* 1978; **i:** 968–9.

## Precautions

Disopyramide is contra-indicated in patients with complete heart block or cardiogenic shock. It should be used with extreme caution in patients with other conduction disorders or uncompensated heart failure. If disopyramide is used to treat atrial tachycardia it may be necessary to pre-treat with digoxin (see Precautions for Quinidine, p.992). Hypokalaemia should be corrected before treatment with disopyramide is initiated. Care should be taken in patients susceptible to hypoglycaemia, including those with heart failure, hepatic or renal impairment, and patients taking drugs that affect glucose metabolism.

Intravenous injections of disopyramide should be given slowly to avoid hypotension and it is recommended that facilities for cardiac monitoring and defibrillation should be available when the injection is used.

Dosage reduction may be necessary in patients with hepatic or renal impairment and in patients with heart failure.

Owing to its antimuscarinic properties, disopyramide should be avoided in patients with glaucoma or a tendency to urinary retention, as in benign prostatic hyperplasia, and also in patients with myasthenia gravis due to the risk of precipitating a myasthenic crisis. It should be used with caution in patients with a family history of glaucoma.

◊ For dosage adjustments in the elderly and in patients with hepatic or renal impairment, see under Uses and Administration, below.

**Breast feeding.** Disopyramide is distributed into breast milk and milk to plasma ratios of 0.4, about 0.5, and 0.9 have been reported.[1-3] Disopyramide has been detected in the plasma of breast-fed infants, but was not associated with adverse effects. The American Academy of Pediatrics considers[4] that it is therefore usually compatible with breast feeding. However, the infant should be monitored for adverse effects, especially antimuscarinic effects.

1. MacKintosh D, Buchanan N. Excretion of disopyramide in human breast milk. *Br J Clin Pharmacol* 1985; **19:** 856–7.
2. Hoppu K, *et al.* Disopyramide and breast feeding. *Br J Clin Pharmacol* 1986; **21:** 553.
3. Barnett DB, *et al.* Disopyramide and its N-monodesalkyl metabolite in breast milk. *Br J Clin Pharmacol* 1982; **14:** 310–12.
4. American Academy of Pediatrics. The transfer of drugs and other chemicals into human milk. *Pediatrics* 2001; **108:** 776–89. Correction. *ibid.*; 1029. Also available at: http://aappolicy.aappublications.org/cgi/content/full/pediatrics%3b108/3/776 (accessed 06/07/04)

**Pregnancy.** No adverse effects were noted in a patient who received disopyramide 200 mg every 8 hours from 26 weeks' gestation until delivery,[1] although doses of 100 to 300 mg were associated with initiation of uterine contractions in another patient in week 32 of pregnancy.[2] A double-blind, placebo-controlled study[3] involving 20 women hospitalised for induction of labour confirmed that disopyramide induces uterine contractions. All 10 women given disopyramide 150 mg every 6 hours for 48 hours had initiation of contractions and in 8 delivery was induced. It was considered that disopyramide should not be used as an antiarrhythmic during pregnancy.

1. Shaxted EJ, Milton PJ. Disopyramide in pregnancy: a case report. *Curr Med Res Opin* 1979; **6:** 70–2.
2. Leonard RF, *et al.* Initiation of uterine contractions by disopyramide during pregnancy. *N Engl J Med* 1978; **299:** 84–5.
3. Tadmor OP, *et al.* The effect of disopyramide on uterine contractions during pregnancy. *Am J Obstet Gynecol* 1990; **162:** 482–6.

## Interactions

Disopyramide should be used cautiously with other cardiac depressants including beta blockers and other class I antiarrhythmics, and with other arrhythmogenic drugs. Disopyramide is metabolised by the cytochrome P450 isoenzyme CYP3A4 and interactions may occur with inhibitors or inducers of this enzyme and with other drugs metabolised by CYP3A4. Use of disopyramide with other antimuscarinic drugs produces enhanced antimuscarinic effects.

**Anti-anginals.** For reference to disopyramide reducing the effectiveness of sublingual *isosorbide dinitrate*, see p.941.

**Antiarrhythmics.** The cardiac depressant effects of disopyramide are additive to those of other class I antiarrhythmic drugs.[1] Disopyramide may prolong the QT interval, a factor associated with torsade de pointes, particularly when given with drugs that have a similar effect; this effect was noted in a few patients given *amiodarone* with disopyramide.[2] Also the serum concentration of disopyramide has been increased by *quinidine*;[3] there was a reciprocal decrease in the serum-quinidine concentration but this was less important clinically.

1. Ellrodt G, Singh BN. Adverse effects of disopyramide (Norpace): toxic interactions with other antiarrhythmic agents. *Heart Lung* 1980; **9:** 469–74.
2. Tartini R, *et al.* Dangerous interaction between amiodarone and quinidine. *Lancet* 1982; **i:** 1327–9.
3. Baker BJ, *et al.* Concurrent use of quinidine and disopyramide: evaluation of serum concentrations and electrocardiographic effects. *Am Heart J* 1983; **105:** 12–15.

**Antibacterials.** The metabolism of disopyramide may be increased by enzyme inducers such as *rifampicin*;[1,2] the increased clearance of disopyramide may lead to subtherapeutic plasma concentrations.

Conversely, elevation of serum-disopyramide concentrations may occur[3] when enzyme inhibitors are added to disopyramide therapy, and ventricular arrhythmias have been noted in patients given azithromycin,[4] clarithromycin,[5] and erythromycin.[3] Hypoglycaemia due to increased disopyramide concentrations has occurred in a patient given clarithromycin.[6]

1. Aitio M-L, *et al.* The effect of enzyme induction on the metabolism of disopyramide in man. *Br J Clin Pharmacol* 1981; **11:** 279–85.
2. Staum JM. Enzyme induction: rifampin-disopyramide interaction. *DICP Ann Pharmacother* 1990; **24:** 701–3.
3. Ragosta M, *et al.* Potentially fatal interaction between erythromycin and disopyramide. *Am J Med* 1989; **86:** 465–6.
4. Granowitz EV, *et al.* Potentially fatal interaction between azithromycin and disopyramide. *Pacing Clin Electrophysiol* 2000; **23:** 1433–5.

5. Paar D, *et al.* Life-threatening interaction between clarithromycin and disopyramide. *Lancet* 1997; **349:** 326–7.
6. Iida H, *et al.* Hypoglycemia induced by interaction between clarithromycin and disopyramide. *Jpn Heart J* 1999; **40:** 91–96.

**Antiepileptics.** The enzyme inducers *phenytoin*[1] and *phenobarbital* may increase the clearance of disopyramide.

1. Aitio M-L, *et al.* The effect of enzyme induction on the metabolism of disopyramide in man. *Br J Clin Pharmacol* 1981; **11:** 279–85.

**Beta blockers.** Beta blockers have negative inotropic effects that may be potentiated if they are given with disopyramide. A pharmacokinetic interaction may also occur with beta blockers since the clearance of disopyramide has been reported[1] to be reduced by about 16% during *atenolol* therapy.

1. Bonde J, *et al.* Atenolol inhibits the elimination of disopyramide. *Eur J Clin Pharmacol* 1985; **28:** 41–3.

## Pharmacokinetics

Disopyramide is readily and almost completely absorbed from the gastrointestinal tract, peak plasma concentrations being attained about 0.5 to 3 hours after oral administration.

Disopyramide is partially metabolised in the liver by the cytochrome P450 isoenzyme CYP3A4. The major metabolite is mono-*N*-dealkylated disopyramide which retains some antiarrhythmic and antimuscarinic activity. The major route of excretion is through the kidney, about 50% as the unchanged drug, 20% as the *N*-dealkylated metabolite, and 10% as other metabolites. About 10% is excreted in the faeces. The clearance of disopyramide does not appear to be influenced by urinary pH.

The therapeutic plasma concentration range is generally accepted as 2 to 6 micrograms/mL. Within this range, protein binding is reported to be 50 to 65%, but the degree of binding varies with the plasma concentration and this limits the usefulness of plasma concentration monitoring as a guide to therapy. Estimations of the plasma half-life of disopyramide range from about 4 to 10 hours. The half-life is increased in hepatic and renal impairment, and in heart failure.

Disopyramide crosses the placental barrier and is distributed into breast milk.

◊ Reviews.

1. Siddoway LA, Woosley RL. Clinical pharmacokinetics of disopyramide. *Clin Pharmacokinet* 1986; **11:** 214–22.

## Uses and Administration

Disopyramide is a class Ia antiarrhythmic (p.809) with a depressant action on the heart similar to that of quinidine (p.993). It also has antimuscarinic and negative inotropic properties.

Disopyramide is used in the management of supraventricular and ventricular **arrhythmias** (p.816).

It may be given by mouth as either the base or the phosphate or intravenously as the phosphate; doses are expressed in terms of the base. Disopyramide phosphate 1.3 g is approximately equivalent to 1 g of disopyramide. The usual oral dose is 300 to a maximum of 800 mg daily in divided doses adjusted according to response. A modified-release preparation can be used, enabling 12-hourly dosage intervals.

Disopyramide may be given by slow intravenous injection in a dose of 2 mg/kg to a maximum of 150 mg, at a rate not exceeding 30 mg/minute; this is followed by 200 mg by mouth immediately on completion of the injection and every 8 hours for 24 hours. If the arrhythmia recurs the intravenous injection may be repeated, but a total intravenous dose of 4 mg/kg (maximum, 300 mg) should not be exceeded in the first hour, nor should the total by both intravenous and oral routes exceed 800 mg in 24 hours. Alternatively, the initial intravenous injection may be followed by intravenous infusion of 400 micrograms/kg per hour (or 20 to 30 mg/hour) to a maximum of 800 mg daily. Patients receiving disopyramide intravenously or in high oral doses should be monitored by ECG.

Dosage reduction and/or increased dosage interval may be necessary in patients with hepatic or renal impairment (see below). Doses should also be adjusted in patients with heart failure to compensate for the prolonged half-life.

An optimum dosage regimen for children has not been fully established, but the following oral doses have been used: under 1 year, 10 to 30 mg/kg daily; age 1 to 4 years, 10 to 20 mg/kg daily; age 4 to 12 years, 10 to 15 mg/kg daily; age 12 to 18 years, 6 to 15 mg/kg daily.

◊ Reviews.

1. Brogden RN, Todd PA. Disopyramide: a reappraisal of its pharmacodynamic and pharmacokinetic properties, and therapeutic use in cardiac arrhythmias. *Drugs* 1987; **34:** 151–87.

**Action.** A study in 6 patients with atrial flutter suggested that the antiarrhythmic activity of racemic disopyramide resides in the S(+)-enantiomer.[1]

1. Lima JJ, *et al.* Antiarrhythmic activity and unbound concentrations of disopyramide enantiomers in patients. *Ther Drug Monit* 1990; **12:** 23–8.

**Administration in the elderly.** The clearance of disopyramide was reduced in elderly non-smoking patients compared with young subjects, but the reduction was less marked in elderly patients who smoked more than 20 cigarettes daily.[1] It was recommended that the dose of disopyramide should be reduced by about 30% in elderly non-smokers.

1. Bonde J, *et al.* The influence of age and smoking on the elimination of disopyramide. *Br J Clin Pharmacol* 1985; **20:** 453–8.

**Administration in hepatic impairment.** Dosage reduction should be considered for patients with hepatic impairment who have prolonged disopyramide plasma half-lives. Also the plasma concentration of $\alpha_1$-acid glycoprotein is significantly reduced in patients with liver cirrhosis[1,2] and its binding capacity for disopyramide is reduced.[1] This is associated with an increase in the free fraction of disopyramide such that measurement of total disopyramide in plasma may not be a safe indicator for dosing, and a therapeutic range 50% lower than in patients with normal hepatic function should be considered.[2]

1. Bonde J, *et al.* Kinetics of disopyramide in decreased hepatic function. *Eur J Clin Pharmacol* 1986; **31:** 73–7.
2. Echizen H, *et al.* Protein binding of disopyramide in liver cirrhosis and in nephrotic syndrome. *Clin Pharmacol Ther* 1986; **40:** 274–80.

**Administration in renal impairment.** Disopyramide is excreted mainly in the urine and alterations in its pharmacokinetics might be expected in renal impairment. A significant reduction in disopyramide clearance with an increase in elimination half-life has been observed[1] in patients with chronic renal failure and dosage reductions are generally recommended if creatinine clearance is less than 40 to 60 mL/minute. Patients with a creatinine clearance less than 40 mL/minute should not be given modified-release preparations of disopyramide.

At therapeutic concentrations disopyramide is not significantly removed by haemodialysis;[2] the half-life is similar both on and off dialysis (16.8 versus 16.1 hours). An increased free fraction of disopyramide has been observed[3] during haemodialysis associated with an elevation in free fatty acids in plasma and in such cases free plasma-disopyramide concentrations should be monitored.

1. Francois B, *et al.* Pharmacokinetics of disopyramide in patients with chronic renal failure. *Eur J Drug Metab Pharmacokinet* 1983; **8:** 85–92.
2. Sevka MJ, *et al.* Disopyramide hemodialysis and kinetics in patients requiring long-term hemodialysis. *Clin Pharmacol Ther* 1981; **29:** 322–6.
3. Horiuchi T, *et al.* Inhibitory effect of free fatty acids on plasma protein binding of disopyramide in haemodialysis patients. *Eur J Clin Pharmacol* 1989; **36:** 175–80.

**Hypotension.** Disopyramide is reported to be one of the standard drugs used in the management of neurally mediated hypotension (p.828).

References.

1. Milstein S, *et al.* Usefulness of disopyramide for prevention of upright tilt-induced hypotension-bradycardia. *Am J Cardiol* 1990; **65:** 1339–44.
2. Morillo CA, *et al.* A placebo-controlled trial of intravenous and oral disopyramide for prevention of neurally mediated syncope induced by head-up tilt. *J Am Coll Cardiol* 1993; **22:** 1843–8.
3. Bhaumick SK, *et al.* Oral disopyramide in the treatment of recurrent neurocardiogenic syncope. *Int J Clin Pract* 1997; **51:** 342.

## Preparations

***BP 2003:*** Disopyramide Capsules; Disopyramide Phosphate Capsules;
***USP 27:*** Disopyramide Phosphate Capsules; Disopyramide Phosphate Extended-release Capsules.

**Proprietary Preparations** (details are given in Part 3)
***Austral.:*** Norpace†; Rythmodan; ***Austria:*** Rythmodan; ***Belg.:*** Dirytmin†; Rythmodan; ***Braz.:*** Dicorantil; ***Canad.:*** Norpace†; Rythmodan; ***Denm.:*** Durbis; Norpace†; ***Fin.:*** Disomet; Durbis†; ***Fr.:*** Isorythm; Rythmodan; ***Ger.:*** Diso-Duriles; Disonorm†; Norpace; Rythmodul; ***Gr.:*** Rythmodan; ***Hong Kong:*** Norpace†; ***India:*** Norpace; ***Irl.:*** Rythmodan; ***Israel:*** Rythmical; ***Ital.:*** Ritmodan; ***Mex.:*** Dimodan; Disofarin†; ***Neth.:*** Dirytmin; Ritmoforine; Rythmodan; ***Norw.:*** Durbis; ***NZ:*** Rythmodan; ***Port.:*** Ritmodan; ***S.Afr.:*** Norpace; Rythmodan; ***Spain:*** Dicorynan; ***Swed.:*** Dirytmin; Durbis; ***Switz.:*** Norpace; ***Thai.:*** Norpace†; ***UK:*** Dirythmin†; Isomide†; Rythmodan; ***USA:*** Norpace.

## Ditazole (*rINN*)

Diethamphenazole; Ditazol; S-222. 2,2′-[(4,5-Diphenyloxazol-2-yl)imino]diethanol.

$C_{19}H_{20}N_2O_3$ = 324.4.
*CAS — 18471-20-0.*
*ATC — B01AC01.*

### Profile

Ditazole is an inhibitor of platelet aggregation used in the management of thromboembolic disorders (p.837) in doses of 400 mg two or three times daily by mouth.

### Preparations

**Proprietary Preparations** (details are given in Part 3)
***Port.:*** Fendazol; ***Spain:*** Ageroplas.

## Divistyramine

Divistiramina.

### Profile

Divistyramine, a bile-acid binding resin, is a lipid regulating drug that has been used similarly to colestyramine (p.889) in the treatment of hyperlipidaemias (p.823). It has also been used for the relief of pruritus in patients with partial biliary obstruction. It has been given by mouth in usual doses of 6 to 12 g daily as a suspension in a suitable vehicle.

### Preparations

**Proprietary Preparations** (details are given in Part 3)
***Switz.:*** Ipocol.

# Dobutamine Hydrochloride

*(BANM, USAN, rINNM)*

46236; Compound 81929 (dobutamine); Dobutamini Hydrochloridum; Hidrocloruro de dobutamina; LY-174008 (dobutamine tartrate). (±)-4-{2-[3-(4-Hydroxyphenyl)-1-methylpropylamino]ethyl}pyrocatechol hydrochloride.

$C_{18}H_{23}NO_3,HCl$ = 337.8.
*CAS — 34368-04-2 (dobutamine); 49745-95-1 (dobutamine hydrochloride); 101626-66-8 (dobutamine tartrate).*
*ATC — C01CA07.*

**Pharmacopoeias.** In *Chin.*, *Eur.* (see p.vi), *Jpn*, and *US*.

**Ph. Eur. 5.0** (Dobutamine Hydrochloride). A white or almost white crystalline powder. Sparingly soluble in water and in alcohol; soluble in methyl alcohol. Protect from light.

**USP 27** (Dobutamine Hydrochloride). A white to practically white crystalline powder. Sparingly soluble in water and in methyl alcohol; soluble in alcohol and in pyridine. Store in airtight containers at a temperature of 15° to 30°.

**Incompatibility.** Dobutamine is incompatible with alkaline solutions such as sodium bicarbonate 5% and alkaline drugs such as aminophylline, furosemide,[1] and thiopental sodium;[1] physical incompatibility with bumetanide, calcium gluconate, insulin, diazepam, and phenytoin has also been suggested. There have also been reports of incompatibility with alteplase,[2] heparin,[3] and warfarin sodium.[4]

1. Chiu MF, Schwartz ML. Visual compatibility of injectable drugs used in the intensive care unit. *Am J Health-Syst Pharm* 1997; **54:** 64–5.
2. Lee CY, *et al.* Visual and spectrophotometric determination of compatibility of alteplase and streptokinase with other injectable drugs. *Am J Hosp Pharm* 1990; **47:** 606–8.
3. Yamashita SK, *et al.* Compatibility of selected critical care drugs during simulated Y-site administration. *Am J Health-Syst Pharm* 1996; **53:** 1048–51.
4. Bahal SM, *et al.* Visual compatibility of warfarin sodium injection with selected medications and solutions. *Am J Health-Syst Pharm* 1997; **54:** 2599–2600.

## Adverse Effects

The principal adverse effects of dobutamine are dose-related increases in heart rate and blood pressure, ectopic beats, angina or chest pain, and palpitations; dosage should be reduced or temporarily stopped if they occur. Ventricular tachycardia may occur rarely. Other adverse effects that have occurred occasionally include hypotension, dyspnoea, paraesthesias, headache, nausea and vomiting, and leg cramps.

For the adverse effects of sympathomimetics in general, see Adrenaline, p.852.

**Effects on body temperature.** A 71-year-old woman with heart failure developed a fever on 2 separate occasions 8 to 12 hours after starting an infusion of dobutamine.[1]

1. Robison-Strane SR, Bubik JS. Dobutamine-induced fever. *Ann Pharmacother* 1992; **26:** 1523–4.

**Effects on the cardiovascular system.** For reference to severe cardiovascular complications of dobutamine stress echocardiography, see Diagnosis and Testing in Uses and Administration, below.

For reference to fatalities occurring in patients given dobutamine, see Heart Failure in Uses and Administration, below.

**Effects on the skin.** Troublesome pruritus of the scalp has been reported[1] to be associated with dobutamine infusion.

1. McCauley CS, Blumenthal MS. Dobutamine and pruritus of the scalp. *Ann Intern Med* 1986; **105:** 966.

**Hypersensitivity.** There has been a report[1] of redness, swelling, itching and a sensation of warmth around the site of infusion of dobutamine in a patient. These symptoms recurred when the infusion was given again one week later.

1. Cernek PK. Dermal cellulitis—a hypersensitivity reaction from dobutamine hydrochloride. *Ann Pharmacother* 1994; **28:** 964.

**Overdosage.** A patient received an accidental overdose[1] of dobutamine when given an intravenous infusion at a rate of more than 130 micrograms/kg per minute for 30 minutes, this being three times the recommended maximum. Characteristic side-effects of dobutamine such as emesis, palpitations, chest pain, dyspnoea, and paraesthesia developed together with urinary incontinence, an effect not previously associated with dobutamine.

1. Paulman PM, *et al.* Dobutamine overdose. *JAMA* 1990; **264:** 2386–7.

## Precautions

Dobutamine should be avoided or used only with great caution in patients with marked obstruction of cardiac ejection, such as idiopathic hypertrophic subaortic stenosis. It should also be used with caution in patients with acute myocardial infarction, and in cardiogenic shock complicated by severe hypotension. Hypovolaemia should be corrected before treatment.

For precautions to be observed with sympathomimetics in general, see Adrenaline, p.853.

**Interference with diagnostic tests.** Contamination of blood samples with dobutamine has been reported to produce falsely decreased creatinine values in an enzymatic test.[1] Colorimetric measurements of creatinine were not affected.

1. Daly TM, *et al.* "Bouncing" creatinine levels. *N Engl J Med* 1996; **334:** 1749–50.

## Interactions

Although it is less likely than adrenaline to produce ventricular arrhythmias, dobutamine should be used with extreme caution during anaesthesia with cyclopropane, halothane, and other volatile anaesthetics. The inotropic effects of dobutamine on the heart are reversed by beta blockade, and there may then be vasoconstriction and an increase in blood pressure due to dobutamine's alpha agonist effects.

For the interactions of sympathomimetics in general, see Adrenaline, p.853.

**Beta blockers.** Use of dobutamine with beta blockers may result in hypertension due to dobutamine's alpha-agonist action. However, marked hypotension occurred[1] in a patient taking *carvedilol* for heart failure when given dobutamine for worsening heart failure. It was suggested that the effect may have been due to blockade of $beta_1$ and alpha receptors by carvedilol, leaving the $beta_2$-mediated vasodilatation unopposed.

1. Lindenfeld J, *et al.* Hypotension with dobutamine: β-adrenergic antagonist selectivity at low doses of carvedilol. *Ann Pharmacother* 1999; **33:** 1266–9.

## Pharmacokinetics

Like adrenaline (p.854), dobutamine is inactive when given by mouth, and it is rapidly inactivated in the body by similar processes. It has a half-life of about 2 minutes. Conjugates of dobutamine and its major metabolite 3-*O*-methyldobutamine are excreted primarily in urine, with small amounts eliminated in the faeces.

◊ The primary mechanism of clearance of dobutamine appears to be distribution to other tissues, and not metabolism or elimination. It has a half-life of about 2 minutes and plasma concentrations of dobutamine reach steady state about 10 to 12 minutes after the start of an infusion. Dobutamine is used mainly for the short-term treatment of heart failure and any pharmacokinetic changes in this condition have no clinical implications in dosage titration.[1]

The pharmacokinetics of dobutamine and other cardiovascular drugs in children have been reviewed.[2]

1. Shammas FV, Dickstein K. Clinical pharmacokinetics in heart failure: an updated review. *Clin Pharmacokinet* 1988; **15:** 94–113.
2. Steinberg C, Notterman DA. Pharmacokinetics of cardiovascular drugs in children: inotropes and vasopressors. *Clin Pharmacokinet* 1994; **27:** 345–67.

## Uses and Administration

Dobutamine is a sympathomimetic (see Adrenaline, p.854) with direct effects on $beta_1$-adrenergic receptors, which confer upon it a prominent inotropic action on the heart. It also has some alpha- and $beta_2$-agonist properties. Dobutamine differs from dopamine in not having the specific dopaminergic properties of dopamine which induce renal mesenteric vasodilatation. However, like dopamine, the inotropic action of dobutamine on the heart is associated with less cardiac-accelerating effect than that of isoprenaline.

Dobutamine is used to increase the contractility of the heart in acute heart failure, as occurs in cardiogenic shock (p.835) and myocardial infarction (p.828); it is also used in septic shock. Other circumstances in which its inotropic activity may be useful are during cardiac surgery and positive end-expiratory pressure ventilation.

Dobutamine is given as the hydrochloride but doses are expressed in terms of the base; 1.12 micrograms of the hydrochloride is approximately equivalent to 1 microgram of base. It is administered by intravenous infusion as a dilute solution (0.25 to 5 mg/mL), in glucose 5% or sodium chloride 0.9%; other fluids may also be suitable and the manufacturers' guidelines should be consulted.

In the management of **acute heart failure**, dobutamine is given at a usual rate of 2.5 to 10 micrograms/kg per minute, according to the patient's heart rate, blood pressure, cardiac output, and urine output. A range of 0.5 up to 40 micrograms/kg per minute has occasionally been required. It has been recommended that treatment with dobutamine should be discontinued gradually.

Dobutamine is also used as an alternative to exercise in **cardiac stress testing**. A solution containing 1 mg/mL is employed for this purpose, given via an infusion pump. A dose of 5 micrograms/kg per minute is infused for 8 minutes; the dose is then increased by increments of 5 micrograms/kg per minute up to a usual maximum of 20 micrograms/kg per minute, with each dose being infused for 8 minutes before the next incremental increase; doses of up to 40 micrograms/kg per minute have sometimes been used. The ECG should be monitored continuously and the infusion terminated if arrhythmias, marked ST segment depression, or other adverse effects occur.

**Action.** *Animal* studies show that the ability of dobutamine to stimulate $alpha_1$- and $beta_2$-adrenergic receptors appears to be as great as its $beta_1$-stimulant properties, and it has been proposed that the inotropic action results from a combination of alpha-stimulant activity on myocardial $alpha_1$ receptors, a property residing mainly in the (−)-enantiomer, with $beta_1$ stimulation by the (+)-enantiomer; peripherally, alpha-mediated vasoconstriction would be opposed by the $beta_2$-agonist properties of the (+)-enantiomer, resulting in the net inotropic action with relatively little effect on blood pressure seen with the racemic mixture used clinically.[1]

Dobutamine has a thermogenic effect,[2] but using it to increase oxygen delivery and consumption and the cardiac index in critically ill patients did not improve patient outcome and in some cases might have been harmful.[3]

1. Ruffolo RR. The mechanism of action of dobutamine. *Ann Intern Med* 1984; **100:** 313–14.
2. Bhatt SB, *et al.* Effect of dobutamine on oxygen supply and uptake in healthy volunteers. *Br J Anaesth* 1992; **69:** 298–303.
3. Hayes MA, *et al.* Elevation of systemic oxygen delivery in the treatment of critically ill patients. *N Engl J Med* 1994; **330:** 1717–22.

**Administration in children.** Dobutamine and dopamine are both used for inotropic support in children. A study[1] in children undergoing cardiac surgery suggested that dobutamine may be preferred to dopamine since the latter could cause pulmonary vasoconstriction (see under Precautions for Dopamine, p.907). In preterm infants, one study[2] reported that dobutamine may have a greater effect on systemic blood flow than dopamine, but a systematic review[3] found that dopamine was more effective than dobutamine in the short-term treatment of hypotension although there was insufficient evidence of long-term benefit or safety with either drug for firm recommendations to be made.

1. Booker PD, *et al.* Comparison of the haemodynamic effects of dopamine and dobutamine in young children undergoing cardiac surgery. *Br J Anaesth* 1995; **74:** 419–23.
2. Osborn D, *et al.* Randomized trial of dobutamine versus dopamine in preterm infants with low systemic blood flow. *J Pediatr* 2002; **140:** 183–91.
3. Subhedar NV, Shaw NJ. Dopamine versus dobutamine for hypotensive preterm infants. Available in The Cochrane Library; Issue 2. Chichester: John Wiley; 2004.

**Diagnosis and testing.** Dynamic exercise is the established mode of stress for the assessment of cardiac function. In patients who are unable to exercise, a dobutamine infusion is one of the best alternative ways of producing a pharmacological stress.[1,2] Dobutamine stress echocardiography, which can often involve the additional administration of atropine, has been reported to be more sensitive than adenosine or dipyridamole stress echocardiography.[1,3] It also has a useful prognostic role.[4-7] However there have been instances of severe cardiovascular complications attributable to dobutamine.[8]

1. Cheitlin MD, *et al.* ACC/AHA/ASE 2003 guideline update for the clinical application of echocardiography: a report of the American College of Cardiology/American Heart Association Task Force on Practice Guidelines (ACC/AHA/ASE Committee to Update the 1997 Guidelines for the Clinical Application of Echocardiography). Summary article: *Circulation* 2003; **108:** 1146–62. Full text: http://www.americanheart.org/downloadable/heart/1060182581039Echocleanfulltext.pdf (accessed 06/07/04)
2. Marwick TH. Stress echocardiography. *Heart* 2003; **89:** 113–18.
3. Martin TW, *et al.* Comparison of adenosine, dipyridamole, and dobutamine in stress echocardiography. *Ann Intern Med* 1992; **116:** 190–6.
4. Poldermans D, *et al.* Dobutamine-atropine stress echocardiography and clinical data for predicting late cardiac events in patients with suspected coronary artery disease. *Am J Med* 1994; **97:** 119–25.
5. Cigarroa CG, *et al.* Dobutamine stress echocardiography identifies hibernating myocardium and predicts recovery of left ventricular function after coronary revascularization. *Circulation* 1993; **88:** 430–6.
6. Elhendy A, *et al.* Relation between ST segment elevation during dobutamine stress test and myocardial viability after a recent myocardial infarction. *Heart* 1997; **77:** 115–21.
7. Pingitore A, *et al.* Prognostic value of pharmacological stress echocardiography in patients with known or suspected coronary artery disease: a prospective, large-scale, multicenter, head-to-head comparison between dipyridamole and dobutamine test. *J Am Coll Cardiol* 1999; **34:** 1769–77.
8. Lattanzi F, *et al.* Dobutamine stress echocardiography: safety in diagnosing coronary artery disease. *Drug Safety* 2000; **22:** 251–62.

**Heart failure.** Dobutamine may be used in the management of acute heart failure, as discussed under Shock, p.835. It may also have a role as a bridge to transplantation in patients with severe chronic heart failure (p.820). In less severe cases, conflicting results have been reported. For example, one group reported[1] that pulsed therapy with dobutamine (30 minutes daily for 4 days each week for 3 weeks) could produce similar improvements to those achieved with exercise. However, sudden death occurred in patients receiving dobutamine as infusions for 48 hours per week, and another study[2] was halted for this reason.

1. Adamopoulos S, *et al.* Effects of pulsed β-stimulant therapy on β-adrenoceptors and chronotropic responsiveness in chronic heart failure. *Lancet* 1995; **345:** 344–9.
2. Dies F, *et al.* Intermittent dobutamine in ambulatory outpatients with chronic cardiac failure. *Circulation* 1986; **74:** (suppl II): 38.

## Preparations

***BP 2003:*** Dobutamine Intravenous Infusion;
***USP 27:*** Dobutamine for Injection; Dobutamine in Dextrose Injection; Dobutamine Injection.

**Proprietary Preparations** (details are given in Part 3)
***Arg.:*** Dobucard; Dobuject; Dobutrex; Duvig; ***Austral.:*** Dobutrex; ***Austria:*** Dobutrex†; Inotop; ***Belg.:*** Dobutrex; ***Braz.:*** Dobtan†; Dobutabbott; Dobutal; Dobutil; Dobuton; Dobutrex; Inotan†; ***Canad.:*** Dobutrex; ***Chile:*** Bagobutam; Dobutrex; ***Denm.:*** Dobuject†; Dobutrex; ***Fin.:*** Dobuject; Dobutrex; ***Fr.:*** Dobutrex; ***Ger.:*** Dobutrex†; ***Gr.:*** Inotrex; ***Hong Kong:*** Dobutrex; ***India:*** Dobutrex; ***Irl.:*** Dobutrex; Posiject; ***Israel:*** Butamine; Dobuject; Dobutam; Dobutrex†; ***Ital.:*** Dobutrex; Miozac; ***Malaysia:*** Dobucard; Dobutrex; ***Mex.:*** Cryobutol; Dobuject; Dobutrex; Kardion; Oxiken; ***Neth.:*** Dobutrex†; ***Norw.:*** Dobutrex; ***NZ:*** Dobutrex; ***Port.:*** Dobuject†; Dobutina; Inotrex; ***S.Afr.:*** Dobutrex; Posiject; ***Singapore:*** Dobuject; ***Spain:*** Dobucor; Dobutrex; ***Swed.:*** Dobuject†; Dobutrex; ***Switz.:*** Dobutrex; ***Thai.:*** Cardiject; Dobucard†; Dobuject; Dobutrex; ***UK:*** Dobutrex†; Posiject; ***USA:*** Dobutrex.

---

# Docarpamine *(rINN)*

Docarpamina; TA-870. (−)-(*S*)-2-Acetamido-*N*-(3,4-dihydroxyphenethyl)-4-(methylthio)butyramide bis(ethyl carbonate) ester.
$C_{21}H_{30}N_2O_8S$ = 470.5.
*CAS — 74639-40-0.*

## Profile

Docarpamine is an orally active prodrug of dopamine (p.907) that is used in the treatment of acute heart failure. The usual dose is 2.25 g of docarpamine daily by mouth, in 3 divided doses.

## Preparations

**Proprietary Preparations** (details are given in Part 3)
***Jpn:*** Tanadopa.

---

# Dofetilide *(BAN, USAN, rINN)*

Dofetilida; UK-68798. β-[(*p*-Methanesulfonamidophenethyl)methylamino]methanesulfono-*p*-phenetidide.
$C_{19}H_{27}N_3O_5S_2$ = 441.6.
*CAS — 115256-11-6.*
*ATC — C01BD04.*

## Adverse Effects and Precautions

Dofetilide may cause severe ventricular arrhythmias, including torsade de pointes, and should not be given to patients with congenital or acquired long QT syndromes. The dosage must be individualised according to QT interval and creatinine clearance; treatment should be initiated under ECG monitoring which must be continued for at least 3 days.

### Interactions

Dofetilide should not be given with other drugs that prolong the QT interval. Class I or class III antiarrhythmics should be stopped at least 3 half-lives before dofetilide is given. Dofetilide is metabolised to a small extent by the cytochrome P450 isoenzyme CYP3A4, and drugs or foods that inhibit this isoenzyme, such as macrolide antibacterials, protease inhibitors, diltiazem, and grapefruit juice, should be used with caution. Cimetidine, trimethoprim, ketoconazole, prochlorperazine, and megestrol, should not be given as they inhibit the renal excretion of dofetilide; verapamil is also contra-indicated as it too may substantially increase dofetilide concentrations.

◊ References.

1. Yamreudeewong W, *et al.* Potentially significant drug interactions of class III antiarrhythmic drugs. *Drug Safety* 2003; **26:** 421–38.

### Pharmacokinetics

The oral bioavailability of dofetilide is more than 90%. Peak plasma concentrations occur after 2 to 3 hours and steady state concentrations after 2 to 3 days. The terminal half-life is about 10 hours. Protein binding is 60 to 70%. Metabolism is mediated to a small extent by the cytochrome P450 isoenzyme CYP3A4. About 80% of a dose is excreted in the urine, mainly as unchanged drug, with about 20% as 5 minimally active or inactive metabolites. Renal elimination involves both glomerular filtration and active tubular secretion via the cation transport system. The clearance of dofetilide decreases with decreasing creatinine clearance.

### Uses and Administration

Dofetilide is a class III antiarrhythmic (p.809) used in the treatment of atrial fibrillation and flutter (p.816) in patients who are highly symptomatic. The initial dose in patients with a creatinine clearance greater than 60 mL/minute and corrected QT interval of 0.44 seconds or less is 500 micrograms twice daily; the maintenance dose must be reduced if the QT interval becomes prolonged after the first dose. Doses should be reduced in renal impairment (see below).

◊ References.

1. McClellan KJ, Markham A. Dofetilide: a review of its use in atrial fibrillation and atrial flutter. *Drugs* 1999; **58:** 1043–59.
2. Torp-Pedersen C, *et al.* Dofetilide in patients with congestive heart failure and left ventricular dysfunction. *N Engl J Med* 1999; **341:** 857–65.
3. Kalus JS, Mauro VF. Dofetilide: a class III-specific antiarrhythmic agent. *Ann Pharmacother* 2000; **34:** 44–56.

**Administration in renal impairment.** Doses of dofetilide should be reduced in patients with renal impairment based on creatinine clearance (CC). Initial doses are:

- CC 40 to 60 mL/minute: 250 micrograms twice daily.
- CC 20 to 39 mL/minute: 125 micrograms twice daily
- CC below 20 mL/minute: not recommended

### Preparations

**Proprietary Preparations** (details are given in Part 3)
***USA:*** Tikosyn.

## Dopamine Hydrochloride

*(BANM, USAN, pINNM)*

ASL-279; Dopamini Hydrochloridum; Hidrocloruro de dopamina; 3-Hydroxytyramine Hydrochloride. 4-(2-Aminoethyl)pyrocatechol hydrochloride.

$C_8H_{11}NO_2,HCl = 189.6.$

*CAS — 51-61-6 (dopamine); 62-31-7 (dopamine hydrochloride).*

*ATC — C01CA04.*

**Pharmacopoeias.** In *Chin., Eur.* (see p.vi), *Int., Jpn, Pol.,* and *US.*

**Ph. Eur. 5.0** (Dopamine Hydrochloride). A white or almost white crystalline powder. Freely soluble in water; soluble in alcohol; sparingly soluble in acetone and in dichloromethane. Store in airtight containers. Protect from light.

**USP 27** (Dopamine Hydrochloride). A white to off-white crystalline powder that may have a slight odour of hydrochloric acid. Freely soluble in water and in aqueous solutions of alkali hydroxides; insoluble in chloroform and in ether; soluble in methyl alcohol. pH of a 4% solution in water is between 3.0 and 5.5. Store in airtight containers.

**Incompatibility.** Dopamine is inactivated in alkaline solutions such as sodium bicarbonate 5% and is incompatible with alkaline drugs such as furosemide[1] and thiopental sodium;[1] incompatibility with insulin[2] and with alteplase[3] has also been reported, and the manufacturers state that it is incompatible with ampicillin and with amphotericin B, and that mixtures with gentamicin sulfate, cefalotin sodium, or oxacillin sodium should be avoided.

1. Chiu MF, Schwartz ML. Visual compatibility of injectable drugs used in the intensive care unit. *Am J Health-Syst Pharm* 1997; **54:** 64–5.
2. Yamashita SK, *et al.* Compatibility of selected critical care drugs during simulated Y-site administration. *Am J Health-Syst Pharm* 1996; **53:** 1048–51.
3. Lee CY, *et al.* Visual and spectrophotometric determination of compatibility of alteplase and streptokinase with other injectable drugs. *Am J Hosp Pharm* 1990; **47:** 606–8.

### Adverse Effects

The most common adverse effects of dopamine infusion are ectopic beats, tachycardia, anginal pain, palpitations, hypotension, vasoconstriction, nausea and vomiting, headache, and dyspnoea. More rarely, bradycardia and cardiac conduction abnormalities, piloerection, and azotaemia have been reported; hypertension has occurred, particularly in overdosage. Extravasation may lead to tissue necrosis and sloughing.

For the adverse effects of sympathomimetics in general, see Adrenaline, p.852.

**Effects on the endocrine system.** Dopamine infusion, even at low doses (2.5 micrograms/kg per minute) was found to decrease serum concentrations of prolactin in critically ill patients.[1] This was considered undesirable because of the immunomodulatory role of prolactin in the endocrine response to stress.

1. Bailey AR, Burchett KR. Effect of low-dose dopamine on serum concentrations of prolactin in critically ill patients. *Br J Anaesth* 1997; **78:** 97–9.

**Effects on the heart.** For mention of the arrhythmogenic effects of dopamine on the heart, see p.853.

**Ischaemia and gangrene.** Ischaemia and gangrene has been reported on several occasions following dopamine infusions.[1-4] Dopamine is converted to noradrenaline which is a known powerful vasoconstrictor and is also noted to be associated with vascular problems if extravasation occurs.

1. Alexander CS, *et al.* Pedal gangrene associated with the use of dopamine. *N Engl J Med* 1975; **293:** 591.
2. Julka NK, Nora JR. Gangrene aggravation after use of dopamine. *JAMA* 1976; **253:** 2812–13.
3. Boltax RS, *et al.* Gangrene resulting from infiltrated dopamine solution. *N Engl J Med* 1977; **296:** 823.
4. Maggi JC, *et al.* Gangrene in a neonate following dopamine therapy. *J Pediatr* 1982; **100:** 323–5.

### Treatment of Adverse Effects

Since the half-life of dopamine is only about 2 minutes most adverse effects can be corrected by discontinuing or reducing the rate of infusion. If these measures fail excessive vasoconstriction and hypertension may be treated with an alpha blocker such as phentolamine mesilate intravenously.

Relief from tissue necrosis and pain due to extravasation may be obtained by immediate infiltration with phentolamine (as for Noradrenaline, p.975).

**Ischaemia.** Topical glyceryl trinitrate ointment has been used successfully to improve capillary blood flow in patients with dopamine-induced ischaemia of the digits.[1,2]

1. Gibbs NM, Oh TE. Nitroglycerine ointment for dopamine induced peripheral digital ischaemia. *Lancet* 1983; **ii:** 290.
2. Coakley J. Nitroglycerin ointment for dopamine-induced peripheral ischaemia. *Lancet* 1983; **ii:** 633.

### Precautions

Dopamine should not be used in patients with phaeochromocytoma or hyperthyroidism, nor in the presence of uncorrected tachyarrhythmias or ventricular fibrillation. Care is required and low doses should be used in patients with shock secondary to myocardial infarction. Patients with a history of peripheral vascular disease are at increased risk of ischaemia of the extremities. Hypovolaemia should be corrected before beginning dopamine infusion.

For precautions to be observed with sympathomimetics in general, see Adrenaline, p.853.

**Children.** There have been reports of increased pulmonary artery pressure with the use of dopamine in children following cardiac surgery,[1] and in premature infants with hypotension.[2] It has therefore been suggested that dopamine should be used with caution in children at risk of developing pulmonary hypertension.

1. Booker PD, *et al.* Comparison of the haemodynamic effects of dopamine and dobutamine in young children undergoing cardiac surgery. *Br J Anaesth* 1995; **74:** 419–23.
2. Liet J-M, *et al.* Dopamine effects on pulmonary artery pressure in hypotensive preterm infants with patent ductus arteriosus. *J Pediatr* 2002; **140:** 373–5.

**Withdrawal.** There may be difficulty in weaning patients off dopamine. For example, there has been a report[1] of a patient in an intensive care unit with intra-abdominal sepsis who developed hypotension when withdrawal of dopamine was attempted. Withdrawal was made possible by substitution with ibopamine, a dopamine agonist.

1. Milner AR, *et al.* Ibopamine substitution in a dopamine-dependent patient. *Lancet* 1993; **342:** 1555.

### Interactions

Although it is less likely than adrenaline to produce ventricular arrhythmias, dopamine should be used with extreme caution during anaesthesia with cyclopropane, halothane, and other volatile anaesthetics. In patients treated with MAOIs, the dose of dopamine should be reduced substantially; a suggested starting dose is one-tenth of the usual dose.

For the interactions of sympathomimetics in general, see Adrenaline, p.853.

**Antiepileptics.** Following a report in 1976 to the FDA of hypotension in patients given *phenytoin* in addition to dopamine infusion, a study[1] of this potential interaction found that dopamine given by intravenous infusion with phenytoin infusion to *dogs,* did not alter the CNS effects of phenytoin nor result in hypotension and cardiovascular collapse. Large doses of phenytoin alone had a reproducible hypotensive effect that was reduced by dopamine, suggesting a possible supportive role in phenytoin-induced hypotension.

1. Smith RD, Lomas TE. Modification of cardiovascular responses to intravenous phenytoin by dopamine in dogs: evidence against an adverse interaction. *Toxicol Appl Pharmacol* 1978; **45:** 665–73.

**Dopaminergics.** Severe hypertension occurred[1] in a patient who had been receiving *selegiline* for Parkinson's disease when a dopamine infusion was started. Although selegiline is considered to be a selective monoamine oxidase type B inhibitor, at higher doses it also affects monoamine oxidase type A and could have reduced the metabolism of dopamine in this patient. Caution may be necessary if dopamine is given to patients who have been receiving selegiline within the previous 2 weeks.

1. Rose LM, *et al.* A hypertensive reaction induced by concurrent use of selegiline and dopamine. *Ann Pharmacother* 2000; **34:** 1020–4.

**Vasodilators.** Fatal hypotension occurred in a man given *tolazoline* in addition to dopamine.[1]

1. Carlon GC. Fatal association of tolazoline and dopamine. *Chest* 1979; **76:** 336.

### Pharmacokinetics

The vasoconstrictor properties of dopamine preclude its administration by the subcutaneous or intramuscular route. Like adrenaline (p.854) it is inactive when given by mouth, and it is rapidly inactivated in the body by similar processes, with a half-life of about 2 minutes. Dopamine is a metabolic precursor of noradrenaline and a proportion is excreted as the metabolites of noradrenaline. Nevertheless, the majority appears to be directly metabolised into dopamine-related metabolites.

◊ References.

1. Banner W, *et al.* Nonlinear dopamine pharmacokinetics in pediatric patients. *J Pharmacol Exp Ther* 1989; **249:** 131–3.
2. Padbury JF, *et al.* Pharmacokinetics of dopamine in critically ill newborn infants. *J Pediatr* 1990; **117:** 472–6.
3. Notterman DA, *et al.* Dopamine clearance in critically ill infants and children: effect of age and organ system dysfunction. *Clin Pharmacol Ther* 1990; **48:** 138–47.
4. Bhatt-Mehta V, *et al.* Dopamine pharmacokinetics in critically ill newborn infants. *Eur J Clin Pharmacol* 1991; **40:** 593–7.
5. Steinberg C, Notterman DA. Pharmacokinetics of cardiovascular drugs in children: inotropes and vasopressors. *Clin Pharmacokinet* 1994; **27:** 345–67.

### Uses and Administration

The catecholamine, dopamine, is a sympathomimetic (see Adrenaline, p.854) with both direct and indirect effects. It is formed in the body by the decarboxylation of levodopa, and is both a neurotransmitter in its own right (notably in the brain) and a precursor of noradrenaline. Dopamine differs from adrenaline and noradrenaline in dilating renal and mesenteric blood vessels and increasing urine output, apparently by a specific dopaminergic mechanism. This effect is predominant at low infusion rates (about 2 micrograms/kg per minute); at slightly higher infusion rates (around 2 to 10 micrograms/kg per minute) it also stimulates $beta_1$-adrenergic receptors in the myocardium, and at 10 to 20 micrograms/kg per minute the effects of alpha-adrenergic stimulation, such as vasoconstriction, predominate. The inotropic action of dopamine on the heart is associated with less cardiac-accelerating effect, and a lower incidence of arrhythmias, than that of isoprenaline.

Dopamine also inhibits release of prolactin from the anterior pituitary.

Dopamine is used in acute heart failure, as occurs in cardiogenic shock (p.835) and myocardial infarction (p.828); it is also used in renal failure (but see below, under Surgery and Intensive Care), in cardiac surgery, and in septic shock.

Dopamine is given as the hydrochloride by intravenous infusion as a dilute solution (usually 1.6 or 3.2 mg/mL, although more dilute solutions may be used where fluid expansion is not a problem), in glucose 5%, sodium chloride 0.9%, or other suitable diluents; many fluids are suitable and the manufacturers' data sheets or literature should be consulted. The initial rate is 1 to 5 micrograms/kg per minute, gradually increased by up to 5 to 10 micrograms/kg per minute according to the patient's blood pressure, cardiac output, and urine output. Up to 20 to 50 micrograms/kg per minute may be required in seriously ill patients; higher doses have been given. A reduction in urine flow, without hypotension, may indicate a need to reduce the dose. To avoid tissue necrosis dopamine is best administered into a large vein high up in a limb, preferably the arm. It has been recommended that on gradual discontinuation of dopamine care should be taken to avoid undue hypotension associated with very low dosage levels where vasodilatation could predominate.

**Surgery and intensive care.** As well as being used for its inotropic effect in cardiac surgery dopamine has been given in low doses for **renal protection** (sometimes termed 'renal-dose' dopamine) in patients at risk, such as those undergoing major surgery or in intensive care, and for the treatment of acute renal failure. However, the value of this use of dopamine as a renal protectant has been questioned and the evidence reviewed.[1,2] Studies in healthy *animals* and human subjects have shown that low-dose dopamine increases renal blood flow, natriuresis, diuresis, and possibly glomerular filtration rate. However, clinical studies have failed to convincingly demonstrate that low-dose dopamine is effective in either preventing acute renal failure in patients at high risk, or in improving renal function or outcome in patients with established acute renal failure. These studies were small, included uncontrolled case series, and often used surrogate markers rather than clinical outcome measures but a larger, placebo-controlled, randomised study[3] in critically-ill patients with early renal dysfunction also failed to show any benefit in those receiving dopamine. It was concluded[4] that dopamine has no role as a renal protectant in such patients, although further study is needed in patients with more severe renal failure.[5]


1. Denton MD, *et al.* "Renal-dose" dopamine for the treatment of acute renal failure: scientific rationale, experimental studies, and clinical trials. *Kidney Int* 1996; **49:** 4–14.
2. Kellum JA. The use of diuretics and dopamine in acute renal failure: a systematic review of the evidence. *Crit Care* 1997; **1:** 53–9.
3. Australian and New Zealand Intensive Care Society (ANZICS) Clinical Trials Group. Low-dose dopamine in patients with early renal dysfunction: a placebo-controlled randomised trial. *Lancet* 2000; **356:** 2139–43.
4. Galley HF. Renal-dose dopamine: will the message now get through? *Lancet* 2000; **356:** 2112–3. Correction. *ibid.* 2001; **357:** 890.
5. Romano G, Ferraccioli G. Usefulness of dopamine treatment in non-oliguric renal failure. *Lancet* 2001; **357:** 960.


## Preparations

***BP 2003:*** Dopamine Intravenous Infusion;
***USP 27:*** Dopamine Hydrochloride and Dextrose Injection; Dopamine Hydrochloride Injection.

**Proprietary Preparations** (details are given in Part 3)
***Arg.:*** Dopatropin; Hettytropin; Inotropin; Megadose; ***Belg.:*** Dynatra; ***Braz.:*** Dopabane; Dopacris; Revimine; Revivan; Vasomine; ***Canad.:*** Intropin; ***Denm.:*** Abbodop; Dopmin; Giludop; ***Fin.:*** Abbodop; Dopmin; ***Gr.:*** Giludop; ***Hong Kong:*** Dopaminex†; Intropin; ***India:*** Dopinga; ***Irl.:*** Intropin†; ***Israel:*** Docard; ***Ital.:*** Revivan; ***Jpn:*** Inovan; ***Malaysia:*** Dopmin; ***Mex.:*** Clorpamina; Drynalken; Drynalquin†; Heminat; Inotropisa; Zetarina; ***Neth.:*** Dynatra; ***Norw.:*** Abbodop; ***Port.:*** Cordodopa; Medopa; ***S.Afr.:*** Dynos†; Intropin; ***Singapore:*** Dopmin; Intropin†; ***Swed.:*** Abbodop; Giludop; Intropin; ***Thai.:*** Dopamex; Dopaminex; Dopmin; Inopin; ***USA:*** Intropin.

# Dopexamine Hydrochloride

*(BANM, USAN, rINNM)*

FPL-60278 (dopexamine); FPL-60278AR; Hidrocloruro de dopexamina. 4-{2-[6-(Phenethylamino)hexylamino]ethyl}pyrocatechol dihydrochloride.

$C_{22}H_{32}N_2O_2,2HCl = 429.4.$

*CAS — 86197-47-9 (dopexamine); 86484-91-5 (dopexamine dihydrochloride).*

*ATC — C01CA14.*

**Incompatibility.** Dopexamine is inactivated in alkaline solutions such as sodium bicarbonate 5%.

## Adverse Effects and Precautions

The most common adverse effect of dopexamine is tachycardia; transient hypotension may also occur. Other adverse effects include arrhythmias and ECG changes, exacerbation of heart failure, nausea and vomiting, tremor, headache, sweating, and dyspnoea.

Dopexamine should not be used in patients with left ventricular outlet obstruction such as aortic stenosis or in phaeochromocytoma or thrombocytopenic patients. It should be used with caution in patients with ischaemic heart disease or after myocardial infarction. Care is also required in the presence of hypokalaemia or hyperglycaemia. Pre-existing hypotension and reduced vascular resistance should be corrected before beginning dopexamine administration.

For the adverse effects of sympathomimetics in general, and precautions to be observed, see Adrenaline, p.852.

## Interactions

Dopexamine may potentiate the effects of noradrenaline and some other sympathomimetics by inhibiting neuronal uptake of noradrenaline.

For the interactions of sympathomimetics in general, see Adrenaline, p.853.

## Pharmacokinetics

Dopexamine has a short half-life in blood of about 6 to 7 minutes. It is excreted as metabolites in bile and in urine.

## Uses and Administration

Dopexamine is a sympathomimetic (see Adrenaline, p.854) with direct and indirect effects. It stimulates $beta_2$ adrenoceptors and peripheral dopamine receptors and also inhibits the neuronal reuptake of noradrenaline. These actions result in an increased cardiac output, peripheral vasodilatation, and an increase in renal and mesenteric blood flow.

Dopexamine hydrochloride is used to provide short-term haemodynamic support that may be required after cardiac surgery or in exacerbations of chronic heart failure. It is given as an intravenous infusion of either 400 or 800 micrograms/mL in glucose 5%, sodium chloride 0.9%, or other suitable diluents, through a central or large peripheral vein; more concentrated solutions may be given via a central vein but concentrations should not exceed 4 mg/mL. The initial dose is generally 0.5 micrograms/kg per minute and is then increased to 1 microgram/kg per minute; further increases, in increments of 0.5 to 1 microgram/kg per minute at intervals of not less than 15 minutes, may be made up to a total of 6 micrograms/kg per minute if necessary. Heart rate, blood pressure, urine output, and cardiac output should be monitored. On withdrawal, the dose of dopexamine hydrochloride should be reduced gradually.

◊ References.


1. Fitton A, Benfield P. Dopexamine hydrochloride. *Drugs* 1990; **39:** 308–30.
2. Anonymous. Dopexamine after cardiac surgery. *Drug Ther Bull* 1995; **33:** 30–2.


**Critical care.** Dopexamine has been reported to increase splanchnic blood flow and it has been used with the aim of preventing renal and gastrointestinal dysfunction in critically-ill patients.[1] Although there may be a reduction in ischaemic damage to the gut,[2] a study[3] in critically-ill patients failed to show any improvement in outcome with the use of dopexamine. Studies[4,5] using dopexamine to increase oxygen delivery in high-risk surgical patients have also failed to show any benefit in terms of postoperative mortality or organ function.


1. Lisbon A. Dopexamine, dobutamine, and dopamine increase splanchnic blood flow: what is the evidence? *Chest* 2003; **123** (suppl): 460S–463S.
2. Baguneid MS, *et al.* A randomized study to evaluate the effect of a perioperative infusion of dopexamine on colonic mucosal ischemia after aortic surgery. *J Vasc Surg* 2001; **33:** 758–63.
3. Ralph CJ, *et al.* A randomised controlled trial investigating the effects of dopexamine on gastrointestinal function and organ dysfunction in the critically ill. *Intensive Care Med* 2002; **28:** 884–90. Correction. *ibid*; 1001. [dose]
4. Takala J, *et al.* Effect of dopexamine on outcome after major abdominal surgery: a prospective, randomized, controlled multicenter study. *Crit Care Med* 2000; **28:** 3417–23.
5. Stone MD, *et al.* Effect of adding dopexamine to intraoperative volume expansion in patients undergoing major elective abdominal surgery. *Br J Anaesth* 2003; **91:** 619–24.


## Preparations

**Proprietary Preparations** (details are given in Part 3)
***Denm.:*** Dopacard; ***Fin.:*** Dopacard; ***Fr.:*** Dopacard; ***Ger.:*** Dopacard; ***Irl.:*** Dopacard; ***NZ:*** Dopacard†; ***Swed.:*** Dopacard; ***Switz.:*** Dopacard; ***UK:*** Dopacard.

# Dorzolamide Hydrochloride

*(BANM, USAN, rINNM)*

Hidrocloruro de dorzolamida; L-671152 (dorzolamide); MK-0507; MK-507. (4*S*,6*S*)-4-(Ethylamino)-5,6-dihydro-6-methyl-4*H*-thieno[2,3-*b*]thiopyran-2-sulphonamide 7,7-dioxide hydrochloride.

$C_{10}H_{16}N_2O_4S_3,HCl = 360.9.$

*CAS — 120279-96-1 (dorzolamide); 130693-82-2 (dorzolamide hydrochloride).*

*ATC — S01EC03.*

**Pharmacopoeias.** In *US.*

**USP 27** (Dorzolamide Hydrochloride). A white to off-white crystalline powder. Soluble in water. Store at 15° to 30°. Protect from light.

## Adverse Effects and Precautions

Local ocular adverse effects may occur with dorzolamide eye drops and include conjunctivitis, keratitis, burning or stinging, eyelid inflammation or irritation, and blurred vision. Dorzolamide may be absorbed systemically, resulting in adverse effects, precautions, and interactions similar to those of acetazolamide (see p.849). Other side-effects reported are headache, bitter taste, epistaxis, fatigue, and nausea.

## Uses and Administration

Dorzolamide is a carbonic anhydrase inhibitor with actions similar to those of acetazolamide (p.850). It is used topically in the management of open-angle **glaucoma** and ocular hypertension (p.1485), either alone or as adjunctive therapy with a topical beta blocker.

Dorzolamide is administered as eye drops containing dorzolamide hydrochloride equivalent to 2% of the base. When used as monotherapy the usual dose is one drop three times daily; a twice daily regimen is recommended when used with a beta blocker.

◊ References.


1. Martens-Lobenhoffer J, Banditt P. Clinical pharmacokinetics of dorzolamide. *Clin Pharmacokinet* 2002; **41:** 197–205.


## Preparations

**Proprietary Preparations** (details are given in Part 3)
***Arg.:*** Biodrop; Poenglausil; Trusopt; ***Austral.:*** Trusopt; ***Austria:*** Trusopt; ***Belg.:*** Trusopt; ***Braz.:*** Trusopt; ***Canad.:*** Trusopt; ***Chile:*** Glaucotensil; Trusopt; ***Denm.:*** Trusopt; ***Fin.:*** Trusopt; ***Fr.:*** Trusopt; ***Ger.:*** Trusopt; ***Gr.:*** Trusopt; ***Hong Kong:*** Trusopt; ***Irl.:*** Trusopt; ***Israel:*** Trusopt; ***Ital.:*** Trusopt; ***Malaysia:*** Trusopt; ***Mex.:*** Trusopt; ***Neth.:*** Trusopt; ***Norw.:*** Trusopt; ***NZ:*** Trusopt; ***Port.:*** Trusopt; ***S.Afr.:*** Trusopt; ***Singapore:*** Trusopt; ***Spain:*** Trusopt; ***Swed.:*** Trusopt; ***Switz.:*** Trusopt; ***Thai.:*** Trusopt; ***UK:*** Trusopt; ***USA:*** Trusopt.

**Multi-ingredient:** ***Arg.:*** Cosopt; Dorzoflax; Glaucotensil TD; Timed D; ***Austral.:*** Cosopt; ***Austria:*** Cosopt; Timsopt; ***Belg.:*** Cosopt; ***Braz.:*** Cosopt; ***Canad.:*** Cosopt; ***Chile:*** Cosopt; Dorsof T; Glaucotensil T; ***Denm.:*** Cosopt; ***Fin.:*** Cosopt; ***Fr.:*** Cosopt; ***Ger.:*** Cosopt; ***Gr.:*** Cosopt; ***Hong Kong:*** Cosopt; ***Irl.:*** Cosopt; ***Israel:*** Cosopt; ***Ital.:*** Cosopt; ***Mex.:*** Cosopt; ***Neth.:*** Cosopt; ***Norw.:*** Cosopt; ***NZ:*** Cosopt; ***S.Afr.:*** Cosopt; ***Singapore:*** Cosopt; ***Swed.:*** Cosopt; ***Switz.:*** Cosopt; ***Thai.:*** Cosopt; ***UK:*** Cosopt; ***USA:*** Cosopt.

# Doxazosin Mesilate *(BANM, rINNM)*

Doxazosin Mesylate *(USAN)*; Doxazosin Methanesulphonate; Mesilato de doxazosina; UK-33274-27. 1-(4-Amino-6,7-dimethoxyquinazolin-2-yl)-4-(1,4-benzodioxan-2-ylcarbonyl)piperazine methanesulphonate.

$C_{23}H_{25}N_5O_5,CH_3SO_3H = 547.6.$

*CAS — 74191-85-8 (doxazosin); 77883-43-3 (doxazosin mesilate).*

*ATC — C02CA04.*

### Adverse Effects, Treatment, and Precautions

As for Prazosin Hydrochloride, p.985.

**Effects on mental function.** For a report of acute psychosis associated with doxazosin administration, see under Adverse Effects of Prazosin Hydrochloride, p.985.

**Hypotension.** Six of 18 hypertensive patients had first-dose postural hypotension after receiving doxazosin 1 mg; three others had substantial but asymptomatic reductions in supine systolic blood pressure following the first dose.[1] The effect might have been exacerbated since all these patients were also receiving beta blockers or diuretics, or both. A further patient, who was also taking methyldopa, withdrew from the study with persistent postural hypotension.

1. Oliver RM, *et al.* The pharmacokinetics of doxazosin in patients with hypertension and renal impairment. *Br J Clin Pharmacol* 1990; **29:** 417–22.

**Urinary incontinence.** For reference to urinary incontinence associated with doxazosin, see under Adverse Effects of Prazosin Hydrochloride, p.985.

### Pharmacokinetics

Doxazosin is well absorbed after oral administration, peak plasma concentrations occurring 2 to 3 hours after a dose. Oral bioavailability is about 65%. It is extensively metabolised in the liver, and excreted in faeces as metabolites and a small amount of unchanged drug. Elimination from plasma is biphasic, with a mean terminal half-life of about 22 hours. The pharmacokinetics are not altered in patients with renal impairment. Doxazosin is about 98% bound to plasma proteins and is not removed by dialysis.

◊ Reviews.

1. Elliott HL, *et al.* Pharmacokinetic overview of doxazosin. *Am J Cardiol* 1987; **59:** 78G–81G.

### Uses and Administration

Doxazosin is an alpha$_1$-adrenoceptor blocker (p.809) with actions and uses similar to those of prazosin (p.986), but a longer duration of action. It is used in the management of hypertension (below), and in benign prostatic hyperplasia (p.1555) to relieve symptoms of urinary obstruction.

Doxazosin is given by mouth as the mesilate, but doses are usually expressed in terms of the base. Doxazosin mesilate 1.2 mg is approximately equivalent to 1 mg of doxazosin. Following an oral dose maximum reduction in blood pressure is reported to occur after 2 to 6 hours and the effects are maintained for 24 hours, permitting once daily dosage.

To avoid the risk of collapse which may occur in some patients after the first dose, the initial dose is 1 mg, preferably at bedtime. Dosage may be increased after 1 or 2 weeks according to response. Usual maintenance doses for hypertension are up to 4 mg once daily; doses of 16 mg daily should not be exceeded. For benign prostatic hyperplasia the usual maintenance dose is 2 to 4 mg daily; doses of 8 mg daily should not be exceeded.

◊ Reviews.

1. Fulton B, *et al.* Doxazosin: an update of its clinical pharmacology and therapeutic applications in hypertension and benign prostatic hyperplasia. *Drugs* 1995; **49:** 295–320.

**Hypertension.** Alpha blockers are among the drug groups that have been recommended as first-line therapy for hypertension (p.825). However, in the Antihypertensive and Lipid-Lowering Treatment to Prevent Heart Attack Trial (ALLHAT)[1] the doxazosin arm of the study was terminated early due to an increased incidence of heart failure in patients receiving doxazosin compared with those receiving chlortalidone.

1. The ALLHAT Officers and Coordinators for the ALLHAT Collaborative Research Group. Major cardiovascular events in hypertensive patients randomized to doxazosin vs chlorthalidone: the Antihypertensive and Lipid-Lowering Treatment to Prevent Heart Attack Trial (ALLHAT). *JAMA* 2000; **283:** 1967–75. Correction. *ibid.* 2002; **288:** 2976.

### Preparations

**Proprietary Preparations** (details are given in Part 3)

***Arg.:*** Cardura; Doxasin; Doxolbran; Prostazosina; Vazosin; ***Austral.:*** Cardura†; ***Austria:*** Doxazobene; Prostadilat; Supressin; ***Braz.:*** Carduran; Prodil; Unoprost; Zoflux; ***Canad.:*** Cardura; ***Chile:*** Alfadoxin; Angicon; Cardura; Dorbantil; ***Denm.:*** Carduran; ***Fr.:*** Zoxan; ***Ger.:*** Cardular; Diblocin; Doxa-Puren; Doxacor; Doxagamma; Doxazomerck; Uriduct; ***Gr.:*** Cardura; ***Hong Kong:*** Cardura; Doxasyn; ***India:*** Doxacard; ***Irl.:*** Cardura; ***Israel:*** Cadex; Cardoral; Doxaloc; ***Ital.:*** Benur; Cardura; Dedralen; Normothen; ***Jpn:*** Cardenalin; ***Malaysia:*** Cardura; ***Mex.:*** Cardura; ***Neth.:*** Cardura; ***Norw.:*** Carduran; ***NZ:*** Cardoxan; Dosan; ***S.Afr.:*** Cardura; ***Singapore:*** Cardura; ***Spain:*** Carduran; Doxatensa; Progandol; ***Swed.:*** Alfadil; ***Switz.:*** Cardura; ***Thai.:*** Cardura; Pencor; ***UK:*** Cardura; Doxadura; ***USA:*** Cardura.

## Duteplase *(rINN)*

Duteplasa; 245-L-Methionine Plasminogen Activator; SM-9527.

$C_{2736}H_{4174}N_{914}O_{824}S_{46}$ = 64529.0.

*CAS — 120608-46-0.*

### Profile

Duteplase is a thrombolytic drug. It is a biosynthetic derivative of endogenous tissue plasminogen activator and has been used similarly to alteplase (p.857) in the treatment of thromboembolic disorders, particularly acute myocardial infarction.

◊ References.

1. Hayashi H, *et al.* Effects of intravenous SM-9527 (double-chain tissue plasminogen activator) on left ventricular function in the chronic stage of acute myocardial infarction. *Clin Cardiol* 1993; **16:** 409–14.
2. Malcolm AD, *et al.* ESPRIT: a European study of the prevention of reocclusion after initial thrombolysis with duteplase in acute myocardial infarction. *Eur Heart J* 1996; **17:** 1522–31.

## Edaravone *(rINN)*

MCI-186; Norphenazone. 3-Methyl-1-phenyl-2-pyrazolin-5-one.

$C_{10}H_{10}N_2O$ = 174.2.

*CAS — 89-25-8.*

### Profile

Edaravone is a free-radical scavenger used in the management of acute ischaemic stroke (p.836). It is given by intravenous infusion in a dose of 30 mg twice daily, infused over 30 minutes, beginning within 24 hours of stroke onset and continued for up to 14 days.

◊ References.

1. Edaravone Acute Infarction Study Group. Effect of a novel free radical scavenger, edaravone (MCI-186), on acute brain infarction: randomized, placebo-controlled, double-blind study at multicenters. *Cerebrovasc Dis* 2003; **15:** 222–9.

### Preparations

**Proprietary Preparations** (details are given in Part 3)

***Jpn:*** Radicut.

## Efonidipine Hydrochloride *(rINNM)*

NZ-105; Serefodipine Hydrochloride. Cyclic 2,2-dimethyltrimethylene ester of 2-(*N*-benzylanilino)ethyl (±)-1,4-dihydro-2,6-dimethyl-4-(*m*-nitrophenyl)-5-phosphononicontinate hydrochloride .

$C_{34}H_{38}N_3O_7P,HCl$ = 668.1.

*CAS — 111011-63-3 (efonidipine); 111011-53-1 (efonidipine hydrochloride).*

### Profile

Efonidipine is a dihydropyridine calcium-channel blocker with general properties similar to those of nifedipine (p.966). It is used as the hydrochloride in the treatment of hypertension.

◊ References.

1. Tanaka H, Shigenobu K. Efonidipine hydrochloride: a dual blocker of L- and T-type $Ca^{2+}$ channels. *Cardiovasc Drug Rev* 2002; **20:** 81–92.

# Enalapril *(BAN, rINN)*

*N*-{*N*-[(*S*)-1-Ethoxycarbonyl-3-phenylpropyl]-L-alanyl}-L-proline.

$C_{20}H_{28}N_2O_5$ = 376.4.

*CAS — 75847-73-3.*

*ATC — C09AA02.*

## Enalapril Maleate *(BANM, USAN, rINNM)*

Enalaprili Maleas; Maleato de enalapril; MK-421. *N*-{*N*-[(*S*)-1-Ethoxycarbonyl-3-phenylpropyl]-L-alanyl}-L-proline hydrogen maleate.

$C_{20}H_{28}N_2O_5,C_4H_4O_4$ = 492.5.

*CAS — 76095-16-4.*

*ATC — C09AA02.*

**Pharmacopoeias.** In *Eur.* (see p.vi) and *US.*

**Ph. Eur. 5.0** (Enalapril Maleate). A white or almost white crystalline powder. Sparingly soluble in water; practically insoluble in dichloromethane; freely soluble in methyl alcohol. It dissolves in dilute solutions of alkali hydroxides. A 1% solution in water has a pH of 2.4 to 2.9. Protect from light.

**USP 27** (Enalapril Maleate). An off-white crystalline powder. Sparingly soluble in water; soluble in alcohol; freely soluble in dimethylformamide and in methyl alcohol; slightly soluble in semipolar organic solvents; practically insoluble in nonpolar organic solvents.

**Stability.** Enalapril has been reported[1,2] to be stable for at least 56 days in extemporaneously compounded oral liquids containing enalapril maleate 1 mg/mL in a number of vehicles.

1. Nahata MC, *et al.* Stability of enalapril maleate in three extemporaneously prepared oral liquids. *Am J Health-Syst Pharm* 1998; **55:** 1155–7.
2. Allen LV, Erickson MA. Stability of alprazolam, chloroquine phosphate, cisapride, enalapril maleate, and hydralazine hydrochloride in extemporaneously compounded oral liquids. *Am J Health-Syst Pharm* 1998; **55:** 1915–20.

## Enalaprilat *(BAN, USAN, rINN)*

Enalaprilic acid; MK-422. *N*-{*N*-[(*S*)-1-Carboxy-3-phenylpropyl]-L-alanyl}-L-proline dihydrate.

$C_{18}H_{24}N_2O_5,2H_2O$ = 384.4.

*CAS — 76420-72-9 (anhydrous enalaprilat); 84680-54-6 (enalaprilat dihydrate).*

**Pharmacopoeias.** In *US.*

**USP 27** (Enalaprilat). A white to nearly white, hygroscopic, crystalline powder. Soluble 1 in 200 of water, 1 in 40 of dimethylformamide, and 1 in 68 of methyl alcohol; very slightly soluble in alcohol, in acetone, and in hexane; practically insoluble in acetonitrile and in chloroform; slightly soluble in isopropyl alcohol.

**Incompatibility.** Enalaprilat was visually incompatible[1] with phenytoin sodium in sodium chloride 0.9%, producing a crystalline precipitate; there was also some visual evidence of incompatibility when mixed with amphotericin B in glucose 5%.

1. Thompson DF, *et al.* Visual compatibility of enalaprilat with selected intravenous medications during simulated Y-site injection. *Am J Hosp Pharm* 1990; **47:** 2530–1.

### Adverse Effects, Treatment, and Precautions

As for ACE inhibitors, p.842.

◊ Postmarketing surveillance for enalapril was carried out by prescription-event monitoring of 12 543 patients.[1] There were 374 skin events including facial oedema or angioedema in 29 (leading to withdrawal of treatment in 10), 15 cases of photosensitivity, and urticaria in 32 (leading to withdrawal in 5). Syncope and dizziness occurred in 155 and 483 patients respectively, sometimes in association with hypotension. Hypotension occurred in 218 patients, 71 in the first month. Treatment was stopped in 121 patients with hypotension, and dosage reduced in 36. Other adverse effects reported included headache in 310 patients, paraesthesias in 126, taste disturbances in 25, conjunctivitis in 67, tachycardia in 194, cough in 360, renal failure in 82, muscle cramp in 96, diarrhoea in 236, and nausea and vomiting in 326. Of 1098 deaths only 10, due to renal failure, were thought possibly related to enalapril therapy. Dysgeusia and skin reactions appeared to be less common than has been reported for captopril, but precise comparisons were difficult; the range of adverse effects was similar.[2]

Deafness was a possible side-effect of enalapril noted earlier;[2] it was reported in 19 of the 12 543 patients monitored, but only while they were taking enalapril, there being no record of deafness after treatment stopped.

For further reference to some of these adverse effects, see under ACE Inhibitors, p.842.

1. Inman WHW, *et al.* Postmarketing surveillance of enalapril I: results of prescription-event monitoring. *BMJ* 1988; **297:** 826–9.
2. Inman WHW, Rawson NSB. Deafness with enalapril and prescription event monitoring. *Lancet* 1987; **i:** 872.

**Breast feeding.** Following administration of a single dose of enalapril 20 mg to 5 lactating women enalaprilat was detected[1] in breast milk in concentrations of 1 to 2.3 nanograms/mL (mean peak 1.72 nanograms/mL); enalapril was also present (mean peak 1.74 nanograms/mL). This compared with peak serum values of 39 to 112 nanograms/mL for enalaprilat and 92 to 151 nanograms/mL for enalapril. Another study[2] found no detectable enalaprilat in the milk of 3 lactating women, while in a further woman[3] both enalapril and enalaprilat were detected, but the concentrations were low. Although enalapril and its metabolite are thus present in small amounts in breast milk it was calculated that the average total daily dose to the neonate would only be about 2 micrograms of enalaprilat.[1] The American Academy of Pediatrics[4] lists no reports of any clinical effect on the infant associated with the use of enalapril by breast-feeding mothers, and states that therefore it may be considered to be usually compatible with breast feeding.

1. Redman CWG, *et al.* The excretion of enalapril and enalaprilat in human breast milk. *Eur J Clin Pharmacol* 1990; **38:** 99.
2. Huttunen K, *et al.* Enalapril treatment of a nursing mother with slightly impaired renal function. *Clin Nephrol* 1989; **31:** 278.
3. Rush JE, *et al.* Comment. *Clin Nephrol* 1991; **35:** 234.
4. American Academy of Pediatrics. The transfer of drugs and other chemicals into human milk. *Pediatrics* 2001; **108:** 776–89. Correction. *ibid.*; 1029. Also available at: http://aappolicy.aappublications.org/cgi/content/full/pediatrics%3b108/3/776 (accessed 05/07/04)

**Porphyria.** Enalapril has been associated with acute attacks of porphyria and is considered unsafe in porphyric patients.

### Interactions

As for ACE inhibitors, p.845.

### Pharmacokinetics

Enalapril acts as a prodrug of the diacid enalaprilat, its active form, which is poorly absorbed by mouth. Following oral administration about 60% of a dose of enalapril is absorbed from the gastrointestinal tract and peak plasma concentrations are achieved within about 1 hour. Enalapril is extensively hydrolysed in the liver to enalaprilat; peak plasma concentrations of enalaprilat are achieved 3 to 4 hours after an oral dose of enalapril. Enalaprilat is 50 to 60% bound to plasma proteins. Following an oral dose, enalapril is excreted in the urine and in faeces, as enalaprilat and unchanged drug, with the urinary route predominating; more than 90% of an intravenous dose of enalaprilat is excreted in the urine. The elimination of enalaprilat is multiphasic but the effective half-life for accumulation following multiple doses of enalapril is reported to be about 11 hours in patients with normal renal function. Enalaprilat is removed by haemodialysis and by peritoneal dialysis.

◊ References.

1. MacFadyen RJ, *et al.* Enalapril clinical pharmacokinetics and pharmacokinetic-pharmacodynamic relationships: an overview. *Clin Pharmacokinet* 1993; **25:** 274–82.
2. Wells T, *et al.* The pharmacokinetics of enalapril in children and infants with hypertension. *J Clin Pharmacol* 2001; **41:** 1064–74.

**Renal impairment.** Comparison of the pharmacokinetics of enalapril in 6 diabetics with persistent proteinuria and glomerular filtration rates (GFR) of 44.1 to 58.4 mL/minute with those in 8 age-matched controls showed that in the diabetic group the peak serum concentration of enalaprilat was higher, the time to peak concentration longer, renal clearance lower, and the areas under the concentration/time curve greater than in controls.[1] Renal clearance of enalaprilat in the diabetics ranged from 56 to 66 mL/minute compared with 105 to 133 mL/minute in controls; clearance correlated with GFR.

1. Baba T, *et al.* Enalapril pharmacokinetics in diabetic patients. *Lancet* 1989; **i:** 226–7.

### Uses and Administration

Enalapril is an ACE inhibitor (p.842) used in the treatment of hypertension (p.825) and heart failure (p.820). It may also be given prophylactically to patients with asymptomatic left ventricular dysfunction to delay the onset of symptomatic heart failure, and has been used in patients with left ventricular dysfunction to reduce the incidence of coronary ischaemic events, including myocardial infarction (p.828).

Enalapril owes its activity to enalaprilat to which it is converted after oral administration. The haemodynamic effects are seen within 1 hour of a single oral dose and the maximum effect occurs after about 4 to 6 hours, although the full effect may not develop for several weeks during chronic dosing. The haemodynamic action lasts for about 24 hours, allowing once-daily dosing. Enalapril is given by mouth as the maleate.

Enalaprilat is not absorbed by mouth but is given by intravenous injection; its haemodynamic effects develop within 15 minutes of injection and reach a peak in 1 to 4 hours. The action lasts for about 6 hours at recommended doses. Enalaprilat is given as the dihydrate, but doses are expressed in terms of the anhydrous substance. Enalaprilat 1.38 mg as the dihydrate is approximately equivalent to 1.25 mg of anhydrous enalaprilat.

In the treatment of **hypertension**, an initial dose of 5 mg of enalapril maleate daily may be given by mouth. Since there may be a precipitous fall in blood pressure in some patients when starting therapy with an ACE inhibitor, the first dose should preferably be given at bedtime. An initial dose of 2.5 mg daily should be given to patients with renal impairment or to those who are receiving a *diuretic*; if possible, the diuretic should be withdrawn 2 or 3 days before enalapril is started and resumed later if necessary. The usual maintenance dose is 10 to 20 mg given once daily, although doses of up to 40 mg daily may be required in severe hypertension. It may be given in 2 divided doses if control is inadequate with a single dose.

When oral therapy of hypertension is impractical enalaprilat may be given in a dose of 1.25 mg by slow intravenous injection or infusion over at least 5 minutes, repeated every 6 hours if necessary; the initial dose should be halved in patients with renal impairment (creatinine clearance less than 30 mL/minute) or those who are receiving a diuretic.

In the management of **heart failure**, severe first-dose hypotension on introduction of an ACE inhibitor is common in patients on loop diuretics, but their temporary withdrawal may cause rebound pulmonary oedema. Thus treatment should be initiated with a low dose under close medical supervision. In patients with heart failure or asymptomatic left ventricular dysfunction enalapril maleate is given by mouth in an initial dose of 2.5 mg daily. The usual maintenance dose is 20 mg daily as a single dose or in 2 divided doses although up to 40 mg daily in 2 divided doses has been given.

**Administration in children.** Enalapril may be used in the management of hypertension in children.[1] The initial dose is 80 micrograms/kg once daily, with a maximum of 5 mg, adjusted according to response. Alternatively, children weighing 20 to below 50 kg may be given an initial dose of 2.5 mg once daily, increased to a maximum of 20 mg daily, while children weighing 50 kg or over may be given an initial dose of 5 mg once daily, increased to a maximum of 40 mg daily. Doses above 580 micrograms/kg or 40 mg daily have not been studied.

Enalapril has also been given to infants with severe heart failure in doses of 100 to 500 micrograms/kg daily as an oral suspension produced by suspending a crushed tablet in water.[2] In this study one infant, with severe myocarditis, developed hypotension and the drug had to be withdrawn; the remaining 7 showed clinical improvement on a mean enalapril dose of 260 micrograms/kg daily and were able markedly to reduce the dose of concomitant diuretic required. Another study in 10 infants found that enalapril was less bioavailable and probably had a shorter duration of action in infants than in adults, and that doses of 80 micrograms/kg daily were inadequate in the treatment of infant heart failure.[3] A larger study in 63 infants and children (median age 5.4 months) with heart failure found enalapril 360 micrograms/kg daily to be of benefit, whereas there was no improvement with a lower dose of 240 micrograms/kg daily.[4]

1. Wells T, *et al.* A double-blind, placebo-controlled, dose-response study of the effectiveness and safety of enalapril for children with hypertension. *J Clin Pharmacol* 2002; **42:** 870–80.
2. Frenneaux M, *et al.* Enalapril for severe heart failure in infancy. *Arch Dis Child* 1989; **64:** 219–23.
3. Lloyd TR, *et al.* Orally administered enalapril for infants with congestive heart failure: a dose-finding study. *J Pediatr* 1989; **114:** 650–4.
4. Leversha AM, *et al.* Efficacy and dosage of enalapril in congenital and acquired heart disease. *Arch Dis Child* 1994; **70:** 35–9.

### Preparations

***USP 27:*** Enalapril Maleate and Hydrochlorothiazide Tablets; Enalapril Maleate Tablets.

**Proprietary Preparations** (details are given in Part 3)
***Arg.:*** Defluin; Ecaprilat; Enalafel; Enaldun; Enatral; Enatrial; Gadopril; Glioten; Kinfil; Lotrial; Nalapril; Presi Regul; Priltenk; Renitec; Sulocten; Vapresan; ***Austral.:*** Alphapril; Amprace; Auspril; Enahexal; Renitec; ***Austria:*** Enac; Enalabene; Enaran; Enatyrol; Mepril; Regomed†; Renistad; Renitec; ***Belg.:*** Renitec; ***Braz.:*** Angiopril; Atens; Blootec†; Enalabal; Enalamed; Enalprin; Enapril†; Enaprotec; Enatec; Eupressin; Glioten; Hipertin; Lowpress; Maleapril†; Nalaprix; Neolapril; Pressel†; Pressotec; Renalapril; Renipress; Renitec; Sanvapress; Vasopril; ***Canad.:*** Vasotec; ***Chile:*** Bajaten; Enalten; Esalfon; Glioten; Grifopril; Hiperson; Hipoartel; Lotrial; Vasolat; ***Denm.:*** Aceren; Alacor; Alapren†; Corodil; Enadil; Renitec; ***Fin.:*** Enaloc; Enapress; Linatil; Renitec; ***Fr.:*** Renitec; ***Ger.:*** Benalapril; Corvo; Ena; Ena-Puren; Enabeta; enadura; Enahexal; Enal; Enalagamma; Enalind; Pres; Xanef; ***Gr.:*** Agioten; Analept; Antiprex; Erxetilan; Gnostocardin; Kaparlon-S; Kontic; Leovinezal; Megapress; Octorax; Ofnifenil; Rablas; Renitec; Stadelant; Supotron; Ulticadex; Virfen; Vitobel; ***Hong Kong:*** Anapril; Danssan; Renitec; ***India:*** BQL; EnAce; Envas; Nuril; ***Irl.:*** Ednyt; Enap; Innomel; Innovace; ***Israel:*** Convertin; Enaladex; ***Ital.:*** Converten; Enapren; Naprilene; ***Malaysia:*** Acetec; Invoril; Renitec; Zynace; ***Mex.:*** Bionafil; Blocatril; Enaladil; Enoval; Feliberal; Glioten; Imotoran; Kenopril; Lipraken; Norpril; Palane; Pulsol; Quimalan; Renitec; ***Neth.:*** Renitec; ***Norw.:*** Linatil; Renitec; ***NZ:*** Enahexal; Renitec; ***Port.:*** Balpril; Cetampril; Denapril; Hipten; Malen; Prilan; Renipril; Renitec; Tensazol; ***S.Afr.:*** Alapren; Ciplatec; Enap; Hypace; Pharmapress; Renitec; ***Singapore:*** Anapril; Corprilor; Daren; Enap; Enaril; Invoril; Korandil; Renaton; Renitec; ***Spain:*** Acetensil; Baripril; Bitensil; Clipto; Controlvas; Corprilor; Crinoren; Dabonal; Ditensor; Herten; Hipoartel; Iecatec; Insup; Nacor; Naprilene; Neotensin; Pressitan; Reca; Renitec; Ristalen†; ***Swed.:*** Linatil; Renitec; ***Switz.:*** Acepril; Enasifar; Enatec; Epril; Reniten; Vasocor; ***Thai.:*** Anapril; Enam; Enapril; Enaril; Invoril; Istopril; Korandil; Lapril; Nalopril; Naritec; Renitec; ***UAE:*** Narapril; ***UK:*** Ednyt†; Enacard†; Innovace; Pralenal; ***USA:*** Vasotec.

**Multi-ingredient:** ***Arg.:*** Co-Renitec; Defluin Plus; Gliotenzide; Lotrial D; Lotrix; Nikion; Presi Regul D; Vapresan Diur; ***Austral.:*** Renitec Plus; ***Austria:*** Co-Enaran; Co-Mepril; Co-Renitec; Enalapril/HCT; Renitec Plus; Synerpril; ***Belg.:*** Co-Renitec; ***Braz.:*** Atens H; Co-Pressotec; Co-Renitec; Enatec F; Eupressin H; Gliotenzide; Sinergen; Vasopril Plus; Yrelan†; ***Canad.:*** Vaseretic; ***Chile:*** Bajaten D; Enalten D; Enalten DN; Esalfon-D; Grifopril-D; Hiperson-D; Hipoartel H; Lotrial D; Normaten; Normaten Plus; ***Denm.:*** Co-Renitec; Corodil Comp; Synerpril; ***Fin.:*** Enaloc Comp; Linatil Comp; Renitec Comp; Renitec Plus; ***Fr.:*** Co-Renitec; ***Ger.:*** Pres plus; Renacor; ***Hong Kong:*** Co-Renitec; ***India:*** EnAce-D; Invozide; ***Irl.:*** Innozide; ***Israel:*** Naprizide; ***Ital.:*** Acesistem; Condiuren; Gentipress; Neoprex; Sinertec; Vasoretic; ***Mex.:*** Co-Renitec; ***Neth.:*** Co-Renitec; Renitec Plus; ***Norw.:*** Renitec Comp; ***NZ:*** Co-Renitec; ***Port.:*** Enatia; Laprilen; Renidur; Renipril Plus; ***S.Afr.:*** Co-Renitec; Enap-Co; Pharmapress Co; ***Singapore:*** Co-Renitec†; Enap HL; ***Spain:*** Acediur; Acetensil Plus; Baripril Diu; Bitensil Diu; Co-Renitec; Crinoretic; Dabonal Plus; Ditenside; Eneas; Enit; Hipoartel Plus; Neotensin Diu; Pressitan Plus; Renitecmax; Vipres; Zorail; ***Swed.:*** Enalapril Comp; Renitec Comp; Synerpril; ***Switz.:*** Co-Reniten; Reniten Plus; ***UK:*** Innozide; ***USA:*** Lexxel; Teczem; Vaseretic.

---

## Encainide Hydrochloride *(BANM, USAN, rINNM)*

Hidrocloruro de encainida; MJ-9067-1 (encainide). (±)-2′-[2-(1-Methyl-2-piperidyl)ethyl]-*p*-anisanilide hydrochloride.

$C_{22}H_{28}N_2O_2,HCl = 388.9.$

*CAS — 37612-13-8 (encainide); 66778-36-7 (encainide); 66794-74-9 (encainide hydrochloride).*

*ATC — C01BC08.*

### Profile

Encainide is a class Ic antiarrhythmic (p.809) and was used for the treatment of severe or life-threatening ventricular arrhythmias. It was withdrawn from the market as a result of an increase in mortality rates in post-infarction patients in the Cardiac Arrhythmia Suppression Trial (CAST) (p.918).

---

## Endralazine Mesilate *(BANM, rINNM)*

BQ-22-708; Compound 22-708; Endralazine Mesylate *(USAN)*; Mesilato de endralazina. 6-Benzoyl-5,6,7,8-tetrahydropyrido[4,3-c]pyridazin-3-ylhydrazone monomethanesulfonate.

$C_{14}H_{15}N_5O,CH_4O_3S = 365.4.$

*CAS — 39715-02-1 (endralazine); 65322-72-7 (endralazine mesilate).*

*ATC — C02DB03.*

### Profile

Endralazine is a vasodilator with properties similar to those of hydralazine (p.931). It has been used as the mesilate in the management of hypertension.

### Preparations

**Proprietary Preparations** (details are given in Part 3)
***Braz.:*** Arritlan†.

---

## Enoxaparin Sodium *(BAN, USAN, rINN)*

Enoxaparina sódica; Enoxaparinum Natricum; PK-10169; RP-54563.

*CAS — 9041-08-1; 679809-58-6.*

*ATC — B01AB05.*

**Pharmacopoeias.** In *Eur.* (see p.vi).

**Ph. Eur. 5.0** (Enoxaparin Sodium). The sodium salt of a low-molecular-mass heparin that is obtained by alkaline depolymerisation of the benzyl ester derivative of heparin from porcine intestinal mucosa. The majority of the components have a 4-enopyranose uronate structure at the non-reducing end of their chain. The mass-average molecular mass ranges between 3500 and 5500 with a characteristic value of about 4500. The degree of sulfation is about 2 per disaccharide unit.

The potency is not less than 90 units and not more than 125 units of anti-factor Xa activity per mg, with reference to the dried substance. The ratio of anti-factor Xa activity to anti-factor IIa activity is between 3.3 and 5.3.

### Units

As for Low-molecular-weight Heparins, p.949.

### Adverse Effects, Treatment, and Precautions

As for Low-molecular-weight Heparins, p.949.

Severe bleeding with enoxaparin may be reduced by the slow intravenous injection of protamine sulfate; 1 mg of protamine sulfate is stated to inhibit the effects of 1 mg (100 units) of enoxaparin sodium.

### Interactions

As for Low-molecular-weight Heparins, p.950.

### Pharmacokinetics

Enoxaparin is rapidly absorbed after subcutaneous injection with a bioavailability of about 92%. Peak plasma activity is reached within 1 to 5 hours. The elimination half-life is about 4 to 5 hours but anti-factor Xa activity persists for up to 24 hours following a 40-mg dose. Enoxaparin is metabolised in the liver and excreted in the urine, as unchanged drug and metabolites.

### Uses and Administration

Enoxaparin sodium is a low-molecular-weight heparin (p.949) with anticoagulant properties. It is used in the treatment and prophylaxis of venous thromboembolism (p.839) and to prevent clotting during extracorporeal circulation. It is also used in the management of unstable angina (p.813).

In the prophylaxis of **venous thromboembolism** during surgical procedures, enoxaparin sodium is given by subcutaneous injection; treatment is continued for 7 to 10 days or until the patient is ambulant. Patients at low to moderate risk are given 20 mg (2000 units) once daily with the first dose about 2 hours pre-operatively. In patients at high risk the dose should be increased to 40 mg (4000 units) once daily with the initial dose given about 12 hours before the procedure. Alternatively, a dose of 30 mg (3000 units) may be given subcutaneously twice daily, starting within 12 to 24 hours after operation. Following hip replacement surgery, enoxaparin may be continued in a dose of 40 mg once daily for a further 3 weeks. For the prophylaxis of thromboembolism in immobilised medical patients, the dose is 40 mg (4000 units) once daily for at least 6 days; treatment should be continued until the patient is fully ambulant, up to a maximum of 14 days.

For the treatment of deep-vein thrombosis enoxaparin sodium is given subcutaneously in a dose of 1 mg/kg (100 units/kg) every 12 hours, or 1.5 mg/kg (150 units/kg) once daily, for 5 days or until oral anticoagulation is established.

For prevention of clotting in the extracorporeal circulation during **haemodialysis**, enoxaparin sodium 1 mg (100 units) per kg is introduced into the arterial line of the circuit at the beginning of the dialysis session. A further dose of 0.5 to 1 mg (50 to 100 units) per kg may be given if required. The dose should be reduced in patients at high risk of haemorrhage.

In the management of **unstable angina**, enoxaparin sodium is given subcutaneously in a dose of 1 mg (100 units) per kg every 12 hours. Treatment is usually continued for 2 to 8 days and low-dose aspirin should be given concomitantly.

◊ References.

1. Noble S, *et al.* Enoxaparin: a reappraisal of its pharmacology and clinical applications in the prevention and treatment of thromboembolic disease. *Drugs* 1995; **49:** 388–410.
2. Noble S, Spencer CM. Enoxaparin: a review of its clinical potential in the management of coronary artery disease. *Drugs* 1998; **56:** 259–72.
3. Harvey DM, Offord RH. Management of venous and cardiovascular thrombosis: enoxaparin. *Hosp Med* 2000; **61:** 628–36.
4. Ibbotson T, Goa KL. Enoxaparin: an update of its clinical use in the management of acute coronary syndromes. *Drugs* 2002; **62:** 1407–31.
5. Fareed J, *et al.* Pharmacodynamic and pharmacokinetic properties of enoxaparin: implications for clinical practice. *Clin Pharmacokinet* 2003; **42:** 1043–57.

**Administration in infants and children.** Increasing numbers of infants and children are receiving anticoagulants for the management of thromboembolism. Few controlled studies have been carried out and recommendations for therapy have generally been adapted from adult guidelines. Low-molecular-weight heparins may have a number of advantages in children. Enoxaparin has been used for the treatment[1,2] and prophylaxis[2] of thromboembolism in children. Use in a preterm infant has also been reported.[3] Younger children may require a higher dose than older children. A regimen[4] for *treatment* of thromboembolism is:

- under 2 months of age: 1.5 mg/kg every 12 hours
- over 2 months of age: 1 mg/kg every 12 hours

Doses for *prophylaxis* are:

- under 2 months of age: 750 micrograms/kg every 12 hours
- over 2 months of age: 500 micrograms/kg every 12 hours

1. Massicotte P, *et al.* Low-molecular-weight heparin in pediatric patients with thrombotic disease: a dose finding study. *J Pediatr* 1996; **128:** 313–18.
2. Dix D, *et al.* The use of low molecular weight heparin in pediatric patients: a prospective cohort study. *J Pediatr* 2000; **136:** 439–45.
3. Dunaway KK, *et al.* Use of enoxaparin in a preterm infant. *Ann Pharmacother* 2000; **34:** 1410–13.
4. Monagle P, *et al.* Antithrombotic therapy in children. *Chest* 2001; **119** (suppl): 344S–370S.

### Preparations

**Proprietary Preparations** (details are given in Part 3)
***Arg.:*** Clexane; ***Austral.:*** Clexane; ***Austria:*** Lovenox; ***Belg.:*** Clexane; ***Braz.:*** Clexane; Flunox†; ***Canad.:*** Lovenox; ***Chile:*** Clexane; ***Denm.:*** Klexane; ***Fin.:*** Klexane; ***Fr.:*** Lovenox; ***Ger.:*** Clexane; ***Gr.:*** Clexane; ***Hong Kong:*** Clexane; ***India:*** Clexane; ***Irl.:*** Clexane; ***Israel:*** Clexane; ***Ital.:*** Clexane; Trombenox†; ***Malaysia:*** Clexane; ***Mex.:*** Clexane; ***Neth.:*** Clexane; ***Norw.:*** Klexane; ***NZ:*** Clexane; ***Port.:*** Lovenox; ***S.Afr.:*** Clexane; ***Singapore:*** Clexane; ***Spain:*** Clexane; Decipar; ***Swed.:*** Klexane; ***Switz.:*** Clexane; Lovenox†; ***Thai.:*** Clexane; ***UK:*** Clexane; ***USA:*** Lovenox.

## Enoximone *(BAN, USAN, rINN)*

Enoximona; Fenoximone; MDL-17043; MDL-19438; RMI-17043; YMDL-17043. 4-Methyl-5-[4-(methylthio)benzoyl]-4-imidazolin-2-one.

$C_{12}H_{12}N_2O_2S$ = 248.3.
*CAS — 77671-31-9.*
*ATC — C01CE03.*

**Incompatibility.** Crystal formation has been observed when enoximone injection was mixed in glass containers or syringes; the manufacturer recommends that only plastic containers or syringes are used for dilutions. The manufacturer also recommends that only sodium chloride 0.9% or water be used as diluents. Glucose solutions should not be used for dilution as crystal formation may occur.

### Adverse Effects

Long-term oral treatment with enoximone has been reported to increase the mortality rate and enoximone is now only employed intravenously for short-term use.

Enoximone may cause ventricular and supraventricular tachyarrhythmias, ectopic beats, and hypotension.

Adverse effects of enoximone affecting the gastrointestinal tract include diarrhoea, nausea, and vomiting. Other adverse effects include headache, insomnia, chills, oliguria, fever, urinary retention, and limb pain. There have been reports of thrombocytopenia and abnormal liver enzyme values.

**Effects on the nervous system.** Tonic-clonic convulsions have been reported[1] in a patient given enoximone 6 micrograms/kg per minute by intravenous infusion. The convulsions subsided when enoximone was discontinued.

1. Appadurai I, *et al.* Convulsions induced by enoximone administered as a continuous intravenous infusion. *BMJ* 1990; **300:** 613–14.

**Hyperosmolality.** Hyperosmolality occurred in an infant during intravenous infusion of enoximone 20 micrograms/kg per minute. The probable cause was propylene glycol in the enoximone injection providing a dose of 2.4 mg/kg per minute.[1]

1. Huggon I, *et al.* Hyperosmolality related to propylene glycol in an infant treated with enoximone infusion. *BMJ* 1990; **301:** 19–20.

### Precautions

Enoximone should be used with caution in patients with hypertrophic cardiomyopathy or severe obstructive aortic or pulmonary valvular disease.

Blood pressure, heart rate, ECG, fluid and electrolyte status, and renal function should be monitored during therapy. Platelet count and liver enzyme values should also be monitored.

The injection has a high pH (approximately 12) and must be diluted before use (but see Incompatibility, above). Extravasation should be avoided during administration.

Doses may need to be reduced in hepatic or renal impairment (see under Uses and Administration, below).

### Pharmacokinetics

Enoximone is absorbed from the gastrointestinal tract but it is no longer administered orally due to an increased mortality rate in some long-term studies. The plasma elimination half-life varies widely; it may be about 1 to 4 hours in healthy volunteers and about 3 to 8 hours in patients with heart failure, but longer times have been reported. Enoximone is about 85% bound to plasma proteins. It is metabolised in the liver and is excreted in the urine, mainly as metabolites. Following intravenous administration about 70% of a dose is excreted in the urine as metabolites and less than 1% as unchanged drug.

◊ General references.

1. Rocci ML, Wilson H. The pharmacokinetics and pharmacodynamics of newer inotropic agents. *Clin Pharmacokinet* 1987; **13:** 91–109. Correction. *ibid.* 1988; **14:** (contents page).
2. Booker PD, *et al.* Enoximone pharmacokinetics in infants. *Br J Anaesth* 2000; **85:** 205–10.

### Uses and Administration

Enoximone is a phosphodiesterase inhibitor similar to amrinone (p.863) with positive inotropic and vasodilator activity. It is given intravenously in the short-term management of heart failure. In some long-term studies it was given by mouth, but an increased mortality rate was reported.

The usual initial dose of enoximone by intravenous injection is 0.5 to 1.0 mg/kg given at a rate not greater than 12.5 mg/minute. This may be followed by doses of 0.5 mg/kg every 30 minutes until a satisfactory response is obtained or a total dose of 3 mg/kg has been given. Alternatively, the initial dose may be given as a continuous intravenous infusion in a dose of 90 micrograms/kg per minute over 10 to 30 minutes until the desired response is achieved.

For maintenance therapy the initial dose (up to a total of 3 mg/kg) may be repeated as required every 3 to 6 hours or a continuous or intermittent infusion may be given in a dose of 5 to 20 micrograms/kg per minute.

The total dose over 24 hours should not exceed 24 mg/kg.

Dosage may need to be reduced in patients with hepatic or renal impairment (see below).

◊ General references.

1. Vernon MW, *et al.* Enoximone: a review of its pharmacological properties and therapeutic potential. *Drugs* 1991; **42:** 997–1017.

**Administration in hepatic and renal impairment.** The elimination half-life of enoximone following intravenous administration was 2.16 hours in a patient with hepatic impairment and 1.33 hours in a patient with renal impairment. The mean elimination half-life in patients with normal hepatic and renal function was 1.26 hours. It was suggested that patients with renal impairment should be monitored and have plasma concentrations measured during continuous infusions and that in hepatic disease the dosage may need to be modified.[1] Similarly, in a study[2] in paediatric patients receiving intravenous enoximone clearance was reduced in those with renal or hepatic impairment and it was suggested that the infusion rate should be decreased in such patients.

1. Desager JP, *et al.* Plasma enoximone concentrations in cardiac patients. *Curr Ther Res* 1990; **47:** 743–52.
2. Booker PD, *et al.* Enoximone pharmacokinetics in infants. *Br J Anaesth* 2000; **85:** 205–10.

**Beta blocker overdosage.** Enoximone, given intravenously as a bolus dose of 0.5 mg/kg followed by an infusion of 15 micrograms/kg per minute, successfully increased the cardiac output and stroke volume in a woman who had ingested 10 g of metoprolol.[1] It was suggested that enoximone may be useful in such patients since its action does not involve the beta-adrenergic system.

1. Hoeper MM, Boeker KHW. Overdose of metoprolol treated with enoximone. *N Engl J Med* 1996; **335:** 1538.

**Heart failure.** Enoximone is one of several drugs that may be used in heart failure (p.820), but because of an increased mortality rate reported following long-term oral use it is only given intravenously for short-term management of heart failure unresponsive to other treatments. In a comparison of oral enoximone and placebo in patients with moderate to moderately severe heart failure,[1] enoximone was no better than placebo in improving exercise duration over the 16-week study period. Although the overall incidence of adverse effects was similar in the two groups, 5 patients receiving enoximone died compared with none in the placebo group.

1. Uretsky BF, *et al.* Multicenter trial of oral enoximone in patients with moderate to moderately severe congestive heart failure: lack of benefit compared with placebo. *Circulation* 1990; **82:** 774–80.

### Preparations

**Proprietary Preparations** (details are given in Part 3)
***Belg.:*** Perfan†; ***Fr.:*** Perfane; ***Ger.:*** Perfan; ***Irl.:*** Perfan†; ***Ital.:*** Perfan; ***Neth.:*** Perfan; ***UK:*** Perfan.

## Epitizide *(BAN, rINN)*

Epithiazide *(USAN)*; Epitizida; NSC-108164; P-2105. 6-Chloro-3,4-dihydro-3-(2,2,2-trifluoroethylthiomethyl)-2*H*-1,2,4-benzothiadiazine-7-sulphonamide 1,1-dioxide.

$C_{10}H_{11}ClF_3N_3O_4S_3$ = 425.9.
*CAS — 1764-85-8.*

### Profile

Epitizide is a thiazide diuretic (see Hydrochlorothiazide, p.933) used in the treatment of hypertension and oedema, often with triamterene.

### Preparations

**Proprietary Preparations** (details are given in Part 3)
**Multi-ingredient:** ***Belg.:*** Dyta-Urese†; ***Neth.:*** Dyta-Urese.

## Eplerenone *(USAN, rINN)*

SC-66110. 9,11α-Epoxy-17-hydroxy-3-oxo-17α-pregn-4-ene-7α,21-dicarboxylic acid γ-lactone methyl ester.

$C_{24}H_{30}O_6$ = 414.5.
*CAS — 107724-20-9.*

### Adverse Effects

As for Spironolactone, p.1003. Hypercholesterolaemia, hypertriglyceridaemia, and increases in liver enzymes have also occurred.

### Precautions

As for Spironolactone, p.1003.

### Interactions

Eplerenone is metabolised primarily by the cytochrome P450 isoenzyme CYP3A4, and increased plasma concentrations of eplerenone have occurred when inhibitors of this enzyme have been given. These include erythromycin, fluconazole, ketoconazole, saquinavir, and verapamil; grapefruit juice has a less marked effect. There is an increased risk of hyperkalaemia if eplerenone is given with potassium supplements or with other potassium-sparing diuretics. Hyperkalaemia may also occur in patients receiving ACE inhibitors, angiotensin II receptor antagonists, or NSAIDs. Diuretics may reduce the excretion of lithium and increase the risk of lithium toxicity.

### Pharmacokinetics

Peak plasma concentrations of eplerenone are reached approximatley 1.5 hours after an oral dose; they are dose proportional for doses of 25 to 100 mg, and less than proportional above 100 mg. Protein binding, primarily to $\alpha_1$-acid glycoprotein, is about 50%. Eplerenone metabolism is predominantly mediated by the cytochrome P450 isoenzyme CYP3A4; less than 5% of a dose is excreted unchanged. Approximately 32% of a dose is excreted in the faeces, and the remainder in the urine. The elimination half-life is about 4 to 6 hours. Eplerenone is not removed by dialysis.

### Uses and Administration

Eplerenone is an aldosterone antagonist with properties similar to those of spironolactone (p.1004) but with a higher selectivity for the aldosterone receptor. It is used in the management of hypertension (p.825) and heart failure (p.820).

In the management of **hypertension**, eplerenone may be given alone or with other antihypertensives. It is given by mouth in an initial dose of 50 mg daily, increasing if necessary to a maximum of 50 mg twice daily. In patients receiving CYP3A4 inhibitors (see Interactions, above), the initial dose should be reduced to 25 mg daily.

For the management of **heart failure** following myocardial infarction, eplerenone is given by mouth in an initial dose of 25 mg daily, increasing to 50 mg daily within 4 weeks if tolerated. Eplerenone should be withdrawn or the dose should be reduced to 25 mg daily, or on alternate days, if hyperkalaemia develops.

◊ References.


1. Zillich AJ, Carter BL. Eplerenone—a novel selective aldosterone blocker. *Ann Pharmacother* 2002; **36:** 1567–76.
2. Pitt B, *et al*, for the Eplerenone Post-Acute Myocardial Infarction Heart Failure Efficacy and Survival Study Investigators. Eplerenone, a selective aldosterone blocker, in patients with left ventricular dysfunction after myocardial infarction. *N Engl J Med* 2003; **348:** 1309–21. Correction. *ibid.*; 2271.


### Preparations

**Proprietary Preparations** (details are given in Part 3)
***USA:*** Inspra.

## Eprosartan Mesilate *(BANM, rINNM)*

Eprosartan Mesylate *(USAN)*; Mesilato de eprosartán; SKF-108566-J. (*E*)-2-Butyl-1-(*p*-carboxybenzyl)-α-2-thenylimidazole-5-acrylic acid methanesulfonate.

$C_{23}H_{24}N_2O_4S,CH_4O_3S$ = 520.6.

*CAS — 133040-01-4 (eprosartan); 144143-96-4 (eprosartan mesilate).*

*ATC — C09CA02.*

### Adverse Effects and Precautions

As for Losartan Potassium, p.947.

### Interactions

As for Losartan Potassium, p.948.

### Pharmacokinetics

Eprosartan is absorbed from the gastrointestinal tract with an absolute oral bioavailability of about 13%. Peak plasma concentrations occur about 1 to 2 hours after an oral dose in the fasted state; administration with food delays absorption but this is not clinically significant. Eprosartan is approximately 98% bound to plasma proteins. It is excreted in the bile and in the urine, primarily as the unchanged drug; following oral administration approximately 7% of the drug is excreted in the urine, with about 2% as the acyl glucuronide. The terminal elimination half-life is about 5 to 9 hours.

◊ References.


1. Martin DE, *et al.* Pharmacokinetics and protein binding of eprosartan in healthy volunteers and in patients with varying degrees of renal impairment. *J Clin Pharmacol* 1998; **38:** 129–37.
2. Tenero DM, *et al.* Effect of age and gender on the pharmacokinetics of eprosartan. *Br J Clin Pharmacol* 1998; **46:** 267–70.


### Uses and Administration

Eprosartan is an angiotensin II receptor antagonist with actions similar to those of losartan (p.948). It is used in the management of hypertension (p.825).

Eprosartan is given by mouth as the mesilate but doses are expressed in terms of the base; eprosartan mesilate 1.2 mg is approximately equivalent to 1 mg of eprosartan. The onset of antihypertensive effect occurs about 1 to 2 hours after administration and the maximum effect is achieved within 2 to 3 weeks after initiating therapy.

In the management of hypertension, eprosartan is given in an initial dose of 600 mg once daily. A lower initial dose of 300 mg once daily may be used in elderly patients over 75 years and has been recommended in renal or hepatic impairment (but see below). The dose should be adjusted according to response; the usual maintenance dose is 400 to 800 mg daily in a single dose or in two divided doses.

◊ Reviews.


1. McClellan KJ, Balfour JA. Eprosartan. *Drugs* 1998; **55:** 713–18.
2. Plosker GL, Foster RH. Eprosartan: a review of its use in the management of hypertension. *Drugs* 2000; **60:** 177–201.


**Administration in hepatic and renal impairment.** In the UK a lower initial dose of 300 mg daily of eprosartan is recommended in patients with renal impairment (creatinine clearance less than 60 mL/minute) or mild to moderate hepatic impairment; this seems to be due to lack of clinical experience in such patients. In the USA, however, no reduction in the initial dose is considered necessary in hepatic or renal impairment, but a maximum dose of 600 mg daily is recommended for patients with moderate or severe renal impairment.

### Preparations

**Proprietary Preparations** (details are given in Part 3)
***Austral.:*** Teveten; ***Austria:*** Teveten; ***Belg.:*** Teveten; ***Braz.:*** Teveten†; ***Canad.:*** Teveten; ***Denm.:*** Teveten; ***Fin.:*** Teveten; ***Fr.:*** Teveten; ***Ger.:*** Teveten; ***Gr.:*** Teveten; ***Irl.:*** Teveten; ***Ital.:*** Tevetenz; ***Neth.:*** Teveten; ***Norw.:*** Teveten; ***Port.:*** Teveten; ***Spain:*** Futuran; Navixen; Regulaten; Teveten; ***Swed.:*** Teveten; ***Switz.:*** Teveten; ***UK:*** Teveten; ***USA:*** Teveten.
**Multi-ingredient:** ***Austral.:*** Teveten Plus; ***USA:*** Teveten HCT.

## Eptifibatide *(BAN, rINN)*

C68-22; Eptifibatida; Integrelin; SB-1; Sch-60936. $N^6$-Amidino-$N^2$-(3-mercaptopropionyl)-L-lysylglycyl-L-α-aspartyl-L-tryptophyl-L-prolyl-L-cysteinamide, cyclic (1→6)-disulfide; $S^1,S^6$-Cyclo[$N^6$-carbamimidoyl-$N^2$-(3-sulfanylpropanoyl)-L-lysylglycyl-L-α-aspartyl-L-tryptophyl-L-prolyl-L-cysteinamide].

$C_{35}H_{49}N_{11}O_9S_2$ = 832.0.

*CAS — 148031-34-9; 157630-07-4.*

*ATC — B01AC16.*

### Adverse Effects

Bleeding is the most common adverse effect of eptifibatide. Hypotension has been reported. Antibodies to eptifibatide have not been detected.

**Effects on the blood.** Thrombocytopenia is an established adverse effect of the glycoprotein IIb/IIIa-receptor antagonist abciximab (see p.841) but appears to be less common with eptifibatide. However, there have been several reports[1-3] of severe thrombocytopenia associated with eptifibatide administration.


1. Paradiso-Hardy FL, *et al.* Severe thrombocytopenia possibly related to readministration of eptifibatide. *Catheter Cardiovasc Interv* 2001; **54:** 63–7.
2. Hongo RH, Brent BN. Association of eptifibatide and acute profound thrombocytopenia. *Am J Cardiol* 2001; **88:** 428–31.
3. Yoder M, Edwards RF. Reversible thrombocytopenia associated with eptifibatide. *Ann Pharmacother* 2002; **36:** 628–30.


### Precautions

As for Abciximab, p.841.

### Pharmacokinetics

Antiplatelet effects of eptifibatide persist for about 4 hours after stopping a continuous infusion. Plasma elimination half-life is about 2.5 hours. Eptifibatide is about 25% bound to plasma proteins. Renal clearance, as eptifibatide and metabolites excreted in the urine, accounts for about 50% of total body clearance.

### Uses and Administration

Eptifibatide is an antiplatelet drug that reversibly inhibits binding of fibrinogen, von Willebrand factor, and other adhesive molecules to the glycoprotein IIb/IIIa receptor of platelets. It is used, usually in combination with aspirin and heparin, in the management of unstable angina and in patients undergoing coronary angioplasty and stenting procedures.

In the management of **unstable angina**, eptifibatide is given in an initial dose of 180 micrograms/kg by intravenous injection, followed by 2 micrograms/kg per minute by intravenous infusion, for up to 72 hours. If percutaneous coronary intervention is performed during eptifibatide therapy, the infusion should be continued for 18 to 24 hours after the procedure, to a maximum total duration of 96 hours of therapy.

In patients undergoing **angioplasty**, though not presenting with unstable angina, eptifibatide is given in an initial dose of 180 micrograms/kg by intravenous injection immediately before the procedure, followed by 2 micrograms/kg per minute by intravenous infusion, with a second 180 micrograms/kg intravenous injection given 10 minutes after the first. The infusion should be continued until hospital discharge or for up to 18 to 24 hours; a minimum of 12 hours is recommended.

The dose of eptifibatide may need to be reduced in patients with renal impairment (see below).

◊ General references.


1. Goa KL, Noble S. Eptifibatide: a review of its use in patients with acute coronary syndromes and/or undergoing percutaneous coronary intervention. *Drugs* 1999; **57:** 439–62.
2. Gilchrist IC. Platelet glycoprotein IIb/IIIa inhibitors in percutaneous coronary intervention: focus on the pharmacokinetic-pharmacodynamic relationships of eptifibatide. *Clin Pharmacokinet* 2003; **42:** 703–20.


**Administration in renal impairment.** Eptifibatide should not be given to patients with severe renal impairment (creatinine clearance of less than 30 mL/minute) since there is limited experience with its use in such patients. The US manufacturer recommends that patients with a serum creatinine between 2.0 and 4.0 mg/dL should receive the same bolus doses as those with normal renal function but the infusion dose should be reduced to 1 microgram/kg per minute.

**Ischaemic heart disease.** Patients with acute coronary syndromes may be treated either medically or with percutaneous coronary interventions such as angioplasty or stenting. In patients with unstable angina (p.813), eptifibatide has been used as an adjunct to both medical and interventional therapy. In the PURSUIT study,[1] which compared eptifibatide with placebo in over 10 000 patients with ischaemic chest pain, the incidence of death and non-fatal myocardial infarction up to 30 days after treatment was reduced in those receiving eptifibatide; most patients also received aspirin and heparin and the number of percutaneous interventions was similar in each group.

Eptifibatide has also been of benefit in patients undergoing elective percutaneous interventions (see Reperfusion and Revascularisation Procedures, p.834). In the IMPACT-II study[2] of over 4000 patients undergoing elective or emergency percutaneous coronary revascularisation, the incidence of death, myocardial infarction, and further unplanned coronary intervention was reduced in those receiving eptifibatide compared with placebo. Similar results were also obtained in a further study (ESPRIT)[3] in patients who were undergoing percutaneous coronary revascularisation with stent implantation, and benefit was maintained at 6-month follow-up.[4]

Eptifibatide has also been tried as an adjunct to thrombolysis in patients with acute myocardial infarction. In a study (INTRO-AMI)[5] comparing eptifibatide and thrombolysis with thrombolysis alone, early patency rates were improved in those receiving eptifibatide but there was no significant difference in outcomes at 30 days.


1. The PURSUIT Trial Investigators. Inhibition of platelet glycoprotein IIb/IIIa with eptifibatide in patients with acute coronary syndromes. *N Engl J Med* 1998; **339:** 436–43.
2. The IMPACT-II Investigators. Randomised placebo-controlled trial of effect of eptifibatide on complications of percutaneous coronary intervention: IMPACT-II. *Lancet* 1997; **349:** 1422–8.
3. The ESPRIT Investigators. Novel dosing regimen of eptifibatide in planned coronary stent implantation (ESPRIT): a randomised, placebo-controlled trial. *Lancet* 2000; **356:** 2037–44. Correction. *ibid.* 2001; **357:** 1370.
4. O'Shea JC, *et al.* Platelet glycoprotein IIb/IIIa integrin blockade with eptifibatide in coronary stent intervention: the ESPRIT Trial: a randomized controlled trial. *JAMA* 2001; **285:** 2468–73.
5. Brener SJ, *et al.* Eptifibatide and low-dose tissue plasminogen activator in acute myocardial infarction: the integrilin and low-dose thrombolysis in acute myocardial infarction (INTRO AMI) trial. *J Am Coll Cardiol* 2002; **39:** 377–86.

### Preparations

**Proprietary Preparations** (details are given in Part 3)
***Belg.:*** Integrilin; ***Braz.:*** Integrilin†; ***Canad.:*** Integrilin; ***Chile:*** Integrilin; ***Denm.:*** Integrilin; ***Fin.:*** Integrilin; ***Fr.:*** Integrilin; ***Ger.:*** Integrilin; ***Gr.:*** Integrilin; ***Hong Kong:*** Integrilin; ***Irl.:*** Integrilin; ***Israel:*** Integrilin; ***Ital.:*** Integrilin; ***Malaysia:*** Integrilin; ***Neth.:*** Integrilin; ***Norw.:*** Integrilin; ***NZ:*** Integrilin; ***Port.:*** Integrilin†; ***S.Afr.:*** Integrilin; ***Singapore:*** Integrilin; ***Spain:*** Integrilin; ***Swed.:*** Integrilin; ***Switz.:*** Integrilin; ***Thai.:*** Integrilin; ***UK:*** Integrilin; ***USA:*** Integrilin.

## Eritrityl Tetranitrate *(rINN)*

Erythritol Tetranitrate; Erythrityl Tetranitrate *(USAN)*; Erythrol Nitrate; Erythrol Tetranitrate; Nitroerythrite; Nitroerythrol; NSC-106566; Tetranitrato de eritritilo; Tetranitrol. Butane-1,2,3,4-tetrol tetranitrate.

$C_4H_6(NO_3)_4$ = 302.1.
*CAS — 7297-25-8.*
*ATC — C01DA13.*

### Profile

Eritrityl tetranitrate is a vasodilator with general properties similar to those of glyceryl trinitrate (p.923). It has been used in angina pectoris.

Diluted eritrityl tetranitrate is a mixture of eritrityl tetranitrate and lactose or other suitable inert excipients, the excipients being added to minimise the risk of explosion.

**Handling.** Undiluted eritrityl tetranitrate can be exploded by percussion or excessive heat.

### Preparations

**Proprietary Preparations** (details are given in Part 3)
***Ital.:*** Cardilate†.

## Esmolol Hydrochloride

*(BANM, USAN, rINNM)*

ASL-8052; Hidrocloruro de esmolol. Methyl 3-[4-(2-hydroxy-3-isopropylaminopropoxy)phenyl]propionate hydrochloride.

$C_{16}H_{25}NO_4,HCl$ = 331.8.
*CAS — 81147-92-4 (esmolol); 84057-94-3 (esmolol); 103598-03-4 (esmolol); 81161-17-3 (esmolol hydrochloride).*
*ATC — C07AB09.*

**Incompatibility.** The manufacturers advise against admixture of esmolol hydrochloride with sodium bicarbonate because of incompatibility. There has also been a report[1] of immediate haze formation following admixture of esmolol hydrochloride with warfarin sodium.

1. Bahal SM, *et al.* Visual compatibility of warfarin sodium injection with selected medications and solutions. *Am J Health-Syst Pharm* 1997; **54:** 2599–2600.

### Adverse Effects, Treatment, and Precautions

As for Beta Blockers, p.869.

Hypotension is the most frequently reported adverse effect associated with the infusion of esmolol hydrochloride; it generally resolves within 30 minutes once the dosage is reduced or the infusion is discontinued. Local irritation at the site of infusion, inflammation, induration, and thrombophlebitis have occurred and necrosis is a hazard of extravasation. These local effects have occurred with concentrations of 20 mg/mL and it is recommended that concentrations should not exceed 10 mg/mL and that the infusion should not be made into a small vein.

**Effects on the CNS.** Generalised tonic-clonic seizures occurred in an elderly patient given esmolol hydrochloride.[1]

1. Das G, Ferris JC. Generalized convulsions in a patient receiving ultra short-acting beta-blocker infusion. *Drug Intell Clin Pharm* 1988; **22:** 484–5.

### Interactions

The interactions associated with beta blockers are discussed on p.870.

### Pharmacokinetics

Following intravenous administration esmolol is rapidly hydrolysed by esterases in the red blood cells. Steady-state blood concentrations are reached within 30 minutes with doses of 50 to 300 micrograms/kg per minute. The time to steady state may be reduced to 5 minutes by the administration of an appropriate loading dose. Blood concentrations are reported to decline in a biphasic manner with a distribution half-life of about 2 minutes and an elimination half-life of about 9 minutes. Esmolol has low lipid solubility and is about 55% bound to plasma proteins. It is excreted in urine, primarily as the de-esterified metabolite.

### Uses and Administration

Esmolol is a cardioselective short-acting beta blocker (p.868). It is reported to be lacking in intrinsic sympathomimetic and membrane-stabilising properties.

Esmolol is used as the hydrochloride in the management of supraventricular arrhythmias (p.816). It is also used for the control of hypertension (p.825) and tachycardia during the perioperative period.

Esmolol hydrochloride is given intravenously at a concentration not exceeding 10 mg/mL.

For the rapid temporary control of ventricular rate in patients with **supraventricular arrhythmias**, a loading dose of 500 micrograms/kg given over 1 minute is followed by an initial maintenance infusion of 50 micrograms/kg per minute for 4 minutes. If the response is satisfactory this maintenance infusion should be continued at 50 micrograms/kg per minute. If a suitable response is not obtained within the initial 5 minutes a further loading dose of 500 micrograms/kg over 1 minute may be given and the maintenance infusion may be increased to 100 micrograms/kg per minute for 4 minutes. This procedure may be repeated until a satisfactory response is obtained, increasing the maintenance infusion each time by 50 micrograms/kg per minute to a maximum of 200 micrograms/kg per minute. Little additional benefit is obtained from further increases in maintenance dosage. Once a satisfactory response is obtained infusion may be continued, if necessary, for up to 48 hours.

When transferring a patient to another antiarrhythmic drug, the infusion rate of esmolol hydrochloride is reduced by 50% thirty minutes after starting the alternative drug, and may be discontinued one hour after the second dose of that drug.

In the control of perioperative **hypertension** and/or **tachycardia**, esmolol hydrochloride may be given intravenously as follows: *during* anaesthesia, a loading dose of 80 mg over 15 to 30 seconds followed by an infusion of 150 micrograms/kg per minute, increased as necessary up to 300 micrograms/kg per minute; on *waking* from anaesthesia, an infusion of 500 micrograms/kg per minute for 4 minutes, followed by an infusion of 300 micrograms/kg per minute as required; *postoperatively*, a stepped dosage schedule, as described under control of supraventricular arrhythmias above, although maintenance infusions may be increased up to 300 micrograms/kg per minute as necessary.

◊ References.

1. Wiest D. Esmolol: a review of its therapeutic efficacy and pharmacokinetic characteristics. *Clin Pharmacokinet* 1995; **28:** 190–202.

### Preparations

**Proprietary Preparations** (details are given in Part 3)
***Arg.:*** Brevibloc; Dublon; ***Austral.:*** Brevibloc; ***Austria:*** Brevibloc; ***Belg.:*** Brevibloc†; ***Braz.:*** Brevibloc; ***Canad.:*** Brevibloc; ***Denm.:*** Brevibloc; ***Fin.:*** Brevibloc; ***Fr.:*** Brevibloc; ***Ger.:*** Brevibloc; ***Gr.:*** Brevibloc; ***Hong Kong:*** Brevibloc; ***India:*** Miniblock; ***Irl.:*** Brevibloc; ***Israel:*** Brevibloc; ***Ital.:*** Brevibloc; ***Malaysia:*** Brevibloc; ***Mex.:*** Brevibloc; ***NZ:*** Brevibloc; ***Port.:*** Brevibloc; ***S.Afr.:*** Brevibloc; ***Singapore:*** Brevibloc; ***Spain:*** Brevibloc; ***Swed.:*** Brevibloc; ***Switz.:*** Brevibloc; ***UK:*** Brevibloc; ***USA:*** Brevibloc.

## Etacrynic Acid *(BAN, rINN)*

Ácido etacrínico; Acidum Etacrynicum; Etacrynsäure; Ethacrynic Acid *(USAN)*; MK-595; NSC-85791. [2,3-Dichloro-4-(2-ethylacryloyl)phenoxy]acetic acid; [2,3-Dichloro-4-(2-methylene-1-oxobutyl)phenoxy]acetic acid.

$C_{13}H_{12}Cl_2O_4$ = 303.1.
*CAS — 58-54-8.*
*ATC — C03CC01.*

**Pharmacopoeias.** In *Chin., Eur.* (see p.vi), *Jpn, Pol.,* and *US.*

**Ph. Eur. 5.0** (Etacrynic Acid). A white or almost white, crystalline powder. Very slightly soluble in water; freely soluble in alcohol. It dissolves in ammonia and in dilute solutions of alkali hydroxides and carbonates.

**USP 27** (Ethacrynic Acid). A white or practically white, odourless or practically odourless, crystalline powder. Very slightly soluble in water; soluble 1 in 1.6 of alcohol, 1 in 6 of chloroform, and 1 in 3.5 of ether. Store at a temperature of 25°, excursions permitted between 15° and 30°.

## Sodium Etacrynate *(BANM, rINNM)*

Etacrinato sódico; Etacrynate Sodium; Ethacrynate Sodium *(USAN)*; Sodium Ethacrynate.

$C_{13}H_{11}Cl_2NaO_4$ = 325.1.
*CAS — 6500-81-8.*
*ATC — C03CC01.*

**Pharmacopoeias.** In *Chin.*
*Pol.* and *US* include sodium etacrynate for injection.

**Stability.** Solutions in water of sodium etacrynate containing the equivalent of etacrynic acid 0.1% have a pH of 6.3 to 7.7. Solutions are relatively stable at about pH 7 at room temperatures for short periods and less stable at higher pH values and temperatures. They are incompatible with solutions with a pH below 5. The injection should be protected from light.

### Adverse Effects

As for Furosemide, p.919. Gastrointestinal disturbances may be more common and severe with etacrynic acid; profuse watery diarrhoea is an indication for stopping therapy. Gastrointestinal bleeding has been associated with etacrynic acid. Tinnitus and deafness, particularly after high parenteral doses, may also be more common. Other adverse effects include confusion, fatigue, nervousness, and apprehension. Haematuria has been reported rarely.

Local irritation and pain may follow intravenous injection.

**Effects on carbohydrate metabolism.** Although etacrynic acid is generally considered to have less pronounced effects on carbohydrate metabolism than furosemide or the thiazide diuretics, adverse effects have been reported. Reductions in glucose tolerance[1] have been observed following etacrynic acid 200 mg daily for 6 weeks similar to those produced by hydrochlorothiazide 200 mg daily. The effect was most pronounced in diabetic patients. Hyperosmolar hyperglycaemic coma[2] and symptomatic hypoglycaemia with convulsions[3] have been reported in patients receiving high doses of etacrynic acid.

1. Russell RP, *et al.* Metabolic and hypotensive effects of ethacrynic acid: comparative study with hydrochlorothiazide. *JAMA* 1968; **205:** 11–16.
2. Cowley AJ, Elkeles RS. Diabetes and therapy with potent diuretics. *Lancet* 1978; **i:** 154.
3. Maher JF, Schreiner GE. Studies on ethacrynic acid in patients with refractory edema. *Ann Intern Med* 1965; **62:** 15–29.

**Effects on the ears.** Drug-induced deafness occurred in 2 of 184 patients given etacrynic acid intravenously.[1,2] Deafness accompanied by nystagmus was reported in a patient[3] following an intravenous infusion of etacrynic acid. Symptoms resolved within 1 hour. He had previously been taking furosemide and etacrynic acid orally.

1. Boston Collaborative Drug Surveillance Program. Drug-induced deafness: a cooperative study. *JAMA* 1973; **224:** 515–16.
2. Porter J, Jick H. Drug-induced anaphylaxis, convulsions, deafness, and extrapyramidal symptoms. *Lancet* 1977; **i:** 587–8.
3. Gomolin IH, Garshick E. Ethacrynic acid-induced deafness accompanied by nystagmus. *N Engl J Med* 1980; **303:** 702.

### Precautions

Etacrynic acid's precautions and contra-indications are generally dependent on its effects on fluid and electrolyte balance and are similar to those of the thiazide diuretics (see Hydrochlorothiazide, p.935). Etacrynic acid, especially in the form of dust, is irritating to the skin, eyes, and mucous membranes.

### Interactions

As for Furosemide, p.920. The risks of gastrointestinal bleeding may be enhanced by use of etacrynic acid with other gastric irritants or with anticoagulants.

**Anticoagulants.** For reference to the interaction between *warfarin* and etacrynic acid, see p.1026.

### Pharmacokinetics

Etacrynic acid is fairly rapidly absorbed from the gastrointestinal tract. The plasma half-life is 30 to 60 minutes. It is excreted both in the bile and the urine, partly unchanged and partly in the form of metabolites. It is extensively bound to plasma proteins.

### Uses and Administration

Although chemically unrelated, etacrynic acid is a loop diuretic with actions and uses similar to those of furosemide (p.921). Etacrynic acid is used in the treatment of oedema associated with heart failure (p.820) and with renal and hepatic disorders.

Diuresis is initiated within about 30 minutes after an oral dose, and lasts for about 6 to 8 hours; after intravenous injection of its sodium salt, the effects are evident within a few minutes and last for about 2 hours.

In the treatment of **oedema**, the usual initial dose is 50 mg by mouth in the morning. The dose may be increased, if necessary, by 25- to 50-mg increments daily to the minimum effective dose. Severe cases have required gradual titration of the dose up to a maximum of 400 mg daily, but the effective range is usually between 50 and 150 mg daily. Dosage of more than 50 mg daily should be given in divided doses. All doses should be taken with food. Maintenance doses may be taken daily or intermittently.

In emergencies, such as acute pulmonary oedema, or when oral therapy cannot be given, etacrynic acid may be given intravenously. It is administered as its salt, sodium etacrynate, but doses are expressed in terms of the acid. 10.7 mg of sodium etacrynate is approximately equivalent to 10 mg of etacrynic acid. The usual dose is 50 mg, or 0.5 to 1 mg/kg, as a 1 mg/mL solution in glucose 5% (provided the pH is above 5) or sodium chloride 0.9%, given by slow intravenous injection either directly or into the tubing of a running infusion. Should a subsequent injection be required the site should be changed to avoid thrombophlebitis. Single doses of 100 mg have been given intravenously in critical situations. It is not suitable for subcutaneous or intramuscular injection.

For children over 2 years of age an initial dose of etacrynic acid is 25 mg daily by mouth, cautiously increased as necessary by 25 mg daily.

If very high doses of etacrynic acid are used careful laboratory control is essential as described for furosemide (p.921; high-dose therapy).

### Preparations

**BP 2003:** Sodium Etacrynate Injection;
**USP 27:** Ethacrynate Sodium for Injection; Ethacrynic Acid Tablets.

**Proprietary Preparations** (details are given in Part 3)
***Austral.:*** Edecril; ***Austria:*** Edecrin; ***Canad.:*** Edecrin; ***Ger.:*** Hydromedin; Uregyt†; ***Irl.:*** Edecrin†; ***Ital.:*** Edecrin†; Reomax; ***Neth.:*** Edecrin†; ***NZ:*** Edecril†; ***Swed.:*** Edecrina; ***USA:*** Edecrin.

## Etafenone Hydrochloride *(rINNM)*

Hidrocloruro de etafenona; LG-11457. 2′-(2-Diethylaminoethoxy)-3-phenylpropiophenone hydrochloride.
$C_{21}H_{27}NO_2,HCl = 361.9.$
*CAS — 90-54-0 (etafenone); 2192-21-4 (etafenone hydrochloride).*
*ATC — C01DX07.*

### Profile

Etafenone hydrochloride is a vasodilator that has been used in ischaemic heart disease.

## Ethyl Biscoumacetate *(BAN, rINN)*

Aethylis Biscoumacetas; Biscumacetato de etilo; Ethyldicoumarol; Ethylis Biscoumacetas; Neodicumarinum. Ethyl bis(4-hydroxycoumarin-3-yl)acetate.
$C_{22}H_{16}O_8 = 408.4.$
*CAS — 548-00-5.*
*ATC — B01AA08.*

### Profile

Ethyl biscoumacetate is an orally administered coumarin anticoagulant with actions similar to those of warfarin (p.1028). It has been used in the management of thromboembolic disorders.

## Etilefrine Hydrochloride *(BANM, rINNM)*

Ethyladrianol Hydrochloride; Ethylnorphenylephrine Hydrochloride; Etilefrini Hydrochloridum; Hidrocloruro de etilefrina; M-I-36. 2-Ethylamino-1-(3-hydroxyphenyl)ethanol hydrochloride.
$C_{10}H_{15}NO_2,HCl = 217.7.$
*CAS — 709-55-7 (etilefrine); 943-17-9 (etilefrine hydrochloride).*
*ATC — C01CA01.*

**Pharmacopoeias.** In *Eur.* (see p.vi) and *Jpn.*

**Ph. Eur. 5.0** (Etilefrine Hydrochloride). A white or almost white, crystalline powder or colourless crystals. Freely soluble in water; soluble in alcohol; practically insoluble in dichloromethane. Store in airtight containers. Protect from light.

### Profile

Etilefrine is a direct-acting sympathomimetic (see Adrenaline, p.852) with $beta_1$-agonist properties, and some alpha- and $beta_2$-agonist actions. It is used for the treatment of hypotensive states. It is given as the hydrochloride by mouth in usual doses of 5 or 10 mg three times daily; modified-release dosage forms are also employed in doses of 25 mg once or twice daily. Etilefrine hydrochloride can also be given parenterally.

Etilefrine polistirex has been used in the management of rhinitis.

**Priapism.** Priapism is a common complication of sickle-cell disease (p.734) and is often treated with intracavernosal alpha agonists (see under Uses of Metaraminol, p.952). There have also been reports of the successful use of etilefrine, both by intracavernosal injection for acute treatment,[1,2] and orally for prophylaxis.[1-3]


1. Virag R, *et al.* Preventive treatment of priapism in sickle cell disease with oral and self-administered intracavernous injection of etilefrine. *Urology* 1996; **47:** 777–81.
2. Gbadoé AD, *et al.* Management of sickle cell priapism with etilefrine. *Arch Dis Child* 2001; **85:** 52–3.
3. Okpala I, *et al.* Etilefrine for the prevention of priapism in adult sickle cell disease. *Br J Haematol* 2002; **118:** 918–21.


### Preparations

**Proprietary Preparations** (details are given in Part 3)
***Arg.:*** Corcanfol; Effortil; Etil Adrianol; Menegradil; ***Austria:*** Agilo; Circupon; Effortil; ***Belg.:*** Effortil; ***Braz.:*** Efortil; ***Chile:*** Effortil; ***Fin.:*** Effortil; ***Fr.:*** Effortil†; ***Ger.:*** Adrenam; Bioflutin-N; Cardanat; Cardialgine; Circupon RR†; Circuvit E; Confidol†; Effortil; Eti-Puren; etil; Kreislauf Katovit†; Thomasin; Tonus-forte-Tablinen†; ***Gr.:*** Effortil; ***Ital.:*** Effortil; ***Mex.:*** Effortil; ***Norw.:*** Effortil; ***Port.:*** Effortil; ***S.Afr.:*** Effortil; ***Spain:*** Efortil; ***Swed.:*** Effortil; ***Switz.:*** Circupon†; Effortil; ***Thai.:*** Effortil; Efxine; Hyprosia.

**Multi-ingredient:** ***Austria:*** Agilan; Amphodyn; Effortil comp; Hypodyn; Influbene; ***Ger.:*** Agit plus; Amphodyn; Dihydergot plus; Effortil plus; Ergolefrin; Ergomimet plus; ***Switz.:*** Dihydergot plus; Effortil plus.

## Etofibrate *(rINN)*

Etofibrato. 2-Nicotinoyloxyethyl 2-(4-chlorophenoxy)-2-methylpropionate.
$C_{18}H_{18}ClNO_5 = 363.8.$
*CAS — 31637-97-5.*
*ATC — C10AB09.*

### Profile

Etofibrate, a derivative of clofibrate (p.884) and nicotinic acid (p.1441), is a lipid regulating drug used in the treatment of hyperlipidaemias (p.823). The usual dose is 500 mg daily by mouth.

### Preparations

**Proprietary Preparations** (details are given in Part 3)
***Austria:*** Lipo-Merz; ***Braz.:*** Tricerol; ***Chile:*** Lipo-Merz; ***Ger.:*** Lipo-Merz; ***Hong Kong:*** Lipo-Merz; ***Malaysia:*** Lipo-Merz; ***Mex.:*** Tricerol; ***Port.:*** Lipo-Merz; ***Singapore:*** Lipo-Merz; ***Spain:*** Afloyan†; ***Switz.:*** Lipo-Merz.

## Etofylline Clofibrate *(rINN)*

Clofibrato de etofilina; ML-1024; Theofibrate *(USAN)*. 2-(Theophyllin-7-yl)ethyl 2-(4-chlorophenoxy)-2-methylpropionate.
$C_{19}H_{21}ClN_4O_5 = 420.8.$
*CAS — 54504-70-0.*

### Profile

Etofylline clofibrate, a fibric acid derivative (see Bezafibrate, p.873), is a lipid regulating drug used in the treatment of hyperlipidaemias (p.823). The usual dose is 250 mg two or three times daily by mouth.

### Preparations

**Proprietary Preparations** (details are given in Part 3)
***Austria:*** Duolip; ***Ger.:*** Duolip; ***Hong Kong:*** Duolip; ***Malaysia:*** Duolip; ***Switz.:*** Duolip.

## Etozolin *(USAN, rINN)*

Etozolina; Gö-687; W-2900A. Ethyl (3-methyl-4-oxo-5-piperidinothiazolidin-2-ylidene)acetate.
$C_{13}H_{20}N_2O_3S = 284.4.$
*CAS — 73-09-6.*
*ATC — C03CX01.*

### Profile

Etozolin is a loop diuretic with properties similar to those of furosemide (p.919), but with a longer duration of action. It is used in the treatment of oedema and hypertension (p.825). Etozolin is reported to be rapidly metabolised to ozolinone which also has diuretic activity.

In the treatment of oedema an initial dose of 400 to 800 mg by mouth is followed by a maintenance dose of 400 mg daily or every 2 or 3 days. In the treatment of hypertension an initial dose of 400 mg daily for 2 days is followed by a maintenance dose of 200 mg daily or on alternate days.

◊ References.


1. Knauf H, *et al.* Pharmacodynamics and kinetics of etozolin/ozolinone in hypertensive patients with normal and impaired kidney function. *Eur J Clin Pharmacol* 1984; **26:** 687–93.
2. Beermann B, Grind M. Clinical pharmacokinetics of some newer diuretics. *Clin Pharmacokinet* 1987; **13:** 254–66.


### Preparations

**Proprietary Preparations** (details are given in Part 3)
***Ger.:*** Elkapin†; ***Ital.:*** Elkapin; ***Spain:*** Elkapin†.

## Ezetimibe *(BAN, USAN, rINN)*

Sch-58235. (3*R*,4*S*)-1-(*p*-Fluorophenyl)-3-[(3*S*)-3-(*p*-fluorophenyl)-3-hydroxypropyl]-4-(*p*-hydroxyphenyl)-2-azetidinone.
$C_{24}H_{21}F_2NO_3 = 409.4.$
*CAS — 163222-33-1.*
*ATC — C10AX09.*

### Adverse Effects and Precautions

Ezetimibe is generally well tolerated. The most common adverse effects include headache, abdominal pain, and diarrhoea; other gastro-intestinal disorders, hypersensitivity reactions including rash and angioedema, fatigue, chest pain, and arthralgia have also been reported. The risk of myalgia in patients receiving statins may be increased with ezetimibe.

Ezetimibe should be avoided in patients with moderate or severe hepatic impairment.

### Interactions

Colestyramine reduces the absorption of ezetimibe and should not be given at the same time of day. Ciclosporin has been reported to increase the plasma concentration of ezetimibe and patients receiving both drugs should be carefully monitored.

### Pharmacokinetics

Ezetimibe is rapidly absorbed when given orally and undergoes extensive conjugation in the small intestine and liver to an active glucuronide metabolite, which is the main circulating form. Both ezetimibe and the glucuronide are more than 90% bound to plasma proteins. Ezetimibe is excreted primarily in the faeces via bile and undergoes enterohepatic recycling; following an oral dose, about 78% is excreted in the faeces, mainly as ezetimibe, and about 11% is excreted in the urine, mainly as the glucuronide. The elimination half-life for both ezetimibe and the glucuronide is about 22 hours.

### Uses and Administration

Ezetimibe is an inhibitor of intestinal cholesterol absorption. It is used, alone or with statins, to reduce total cholesterol, low-density lipoprotein (LDL)-cholesterol, and apolipoprotein B in the management of hyperlipidaemias (p.823), and to reduce sitosterol and campesterol in patients with homozygous familial sitosterolaemia. It is given by mouth in a usual dose of 10 mg once daily.

◊ References.


1. Ezzet F, *et al.* The plasma concentration and LDL-C relationship in patients receiving ezetimibe. *J Clin Pharmacol* 2001; **41:** 943–9.
2. Kosoglou T, *et al.* Pharmacodynamic interaction between the new selective cholesterol absorption inhibitor ezetimibe and simvastatin. *Br J Clin Pharmacol* 2002; **54:** 309–319.
3. Sudhop T, von Bergmann K. Cholesterol absorption inhibitors for the treatment of hypercholesterolaemia. *Drugs* 2002; **62:** 2333–47.
4. Mauro VF, Tuckerman CE. Ezetimibe for management of hypercholesterolemia. *Ann Pharmacother* 2003; **37:** 839–48.


### Preparations

**Proprietary Preparations** (details are given in Part 3)
***Ger.:*** Ezetrol; ***UK:*** Ezetrol; ***USA:*** Zetia.

## Fasudil Hydrochloride *(rINNM)*

AT-877; HA-1077; Hidrocloruro de fasudil. Hexahydro-1-(5-isoquinolylsulfonyl)-1*H*-1,4-diazepine hydrochloride.
$C_{14}H_{17}N_3O_2S,HCl = 327.8.$
*CAS — 103745-39-7 (fasudil); 105628-07-7 (fasudil hydrochloride).*
*ATC — C04AX32.*

### Profile

Fasudil is a selective inhibitor of Rho-kinase, a protein kinase involved in contraction of vascular smooth muscle. Fasudil is used as the hydrochloride for its vasodilating properties in the management of cerebrovascular disorders including vasospasm following surgery for subarachnoid haemorrhage. It is under investigation for the treatment of angina pectoris and acute cerebral thrombosis.

◊ References.


1. Shibuya M, *et al.* Effect of AT877 on cerebral vasospasm after aneurysmal subarachnoid hemorrhage: results of a prospective placebo-controlled double-blind trial. *J Neurosurg* 1992; **76:** 571–7.
2. Masumoto A, *et al.* Suppression of coronary artery spasm by the Rho-kinase inhibitor fasudil in patients with vasospastic angina. *Circulation* 2002; **105:** 1545–7.
3. Shimokawa H, *et al.* Anti-anginal effect of fasudil, a Rho-kinase inhibitor, in patients with stable effort angina: a multicenter study. *J Cardiovasc Pharmacol* 2002; **40:** 751–61.


### Preparations

**Proprietary Preparations** (details are given in Part 3)
***Jpn:*** Eril.

## Felodipine *(BAN, USAN, rINN)*

Felodipino; Felodipinum; H-154/82. Ethyl methyl 4-(2,3-dichlorophenyl)-1,4-dihydro-2,6-dimethylpyridine-3,5-dicarboxylate.
$C_{18}H_{19}Cl_2NO_4 = 384.3.$
*CAS — 72509-76-3; 86189-69-7.*
*ATC — C08CA02.*

**Pharmacopoeias.** In *Eur.* (see p.vi) and *US.*

**Ph. Eur. 5.0** (Felodipine). A white or light yellow, crystalline powder. Practically insoluble in water; freely soluble in dehydrated alcohol, in acetone, in dichloromethane, and in methyl alcohol. Protect from light.

**USP 27** (Felodipine). A light yellow to yellow, crystalline powder. Insoluble in water; freely soluble in acetone and in methyl alcohol; very slightly soluble in heptane. Store in airtight containers. Protect from light.

### Adverse Effects, Treatment, and Precautions

As for dihydropyridine calcium-channel blockers (see Nifedipine, p.966).

### Interactions

As for dihydropyridine calcium-channel blockers (see Nifedipine, p.969).

### Pharmacokinetics

Felodipine is almost completely absorbed from the gastrointestinal tract after oral administration but undergoes extensive first-pass metabolism, with a bioavailability of about 15% (range 10 to 25%). It is extensively metabolised in the gut and the liver and is excreted almost entirely as metabolites, about 70% of a dose being excreted in urine and the remainder in faeces. The terminal elimination half-life is reported to be about 11 to 16 hours following oral administration of an immediate-release preparation, but longer with a modified-release formulation. Felodipine is about 99% bound to plasma proteins (mainly albumin).

◊ General reviews.

1. Dunselman PHJM, Edgar B. Felodipine clinical pharmacokinetics. *Clin Pharmacokinet* 1991; **21:** 418–30.

### Uses and Administration

Felodipine is a dihydropyridine calcium-channel blocker with actions similar to those of nifedipine (p.970). It is used in the management of hypertension (p.825) and angina pectoris (p.813).

Felodipine is given by mouth, generally in a modified-release formulation for administration once daily in the morning. In **hypertension** the usual initial dose is 5 mg daily by mouth, adjusted as required; the usual maintenance dose is 2.5 to 10 mg daily and doses above 20 mg daily are not usually needed. In **angina** the usual initial dose is 5 mg daily increased if necessary to 10 mg daily.

Lower doses may be required in the elderly and in patients with hepatic impairment (see below).

◊ Reviews.

1. Todd PA, Faulds D. Felodipine: a review of the pharmacology and therapeutic use of the extended release formulation in cardiovascular disorders. *Drugs* 1992; **44:** 251–77.
2. Walton T, Symes LR. Felodipine and isradipine: new calcium-channel-blocking agents for the treatment of hypertension. *Clin Pharm* 1993; **12:** 261–75.

**Administration in hepatic impairment.** In 9 patients with liver cirrhosis given felodipine 750 micrograms by intravenous infusion over 20 minutes and 10 mg by mouth as single doses on separate occasions the mean oral bioavailability was 17.1% which was not significantly different from published values in healthy subjects, but the maximum plasma concentrations were almost twice as high as normal, apparently due to reduced systemic clearance and volume of distribution.[1] The fact that bioavailability was not increased suggests that much pre-systemic metabolism takes place in the gut rather than the liver. Although increased adverse effects were not associated with the raised felodipine concentrations in this study it is recommended that therapy in cirrhotic patients be initiated at lower doses than in patients with normal liver function. The US manufacturer recommends that an initial dose of 2.5 mg once daily should be used in patients with hepatic impairment.

1. Regårdh CG, *et al.* Pharmacokinetics of felodipine in patients with liver disease. *Eur J Clin Pharmacol* 1989; **36:** 473–9.

### Preparations

***USP 27:*** Felodipine Extended-Release Tablets.

**Proprietary Preparations** (details are given in Part 3)
***Arg.:*** Munobal; Plendil; ***Austral.:*** Agon; Felodur; Plendil; ***Austria:*** Munobal; Plendil; ***Belg.:*** Plendil; Renedil; ***Braz.:*** Splendil; ***Canad.:*** Plendil; Renedil; ***Chile:*** Splendil; ***Denm.:*** Hydac; Plendil; Plendur; ***Fin.:*** Hydac; Plendil; ***Fr.:*** Flodil; ***Ger.:*** Felo-Puren; Felocor; Modip; Munobal; ***Gr.:*** Plendil; ***Hong Kong:*** Plendil; ***India:*** Felogard; ***Irl.:*** Plendil; ***Israel:*** Penedil; ***Ital.:*** Feloday; Plendil; Prevex; ***Jpn:*** Splendil; ***Malaysia:*** Plendil; ***Mex.:*** Munobal; Plendil; ***Neth.:*** Plendil; Renedil; ***Norw.:*** Plendil; ***NZ:*** Agon†; Felo; Plendil; ***Port.:*** Preslow; ***S.Afr.:*** Plendil; ***Singapore:*** Plendil; ***Spain:*** Fensel; Perfudal; Plendil; Preslow†; ***Swed.:*** Hydac†; Plendil; ***Switz.:*** Munobal; Plendil; ***Thai.:*** Plendil; ***UK:*** Felotens; Keloc; Plendil; Vascalpha; ***USA:*** Plendil.

**Multi-ingredient:** ***Arg.:*** Nikion; ***Austria:*** Logimax; Triapin; Unimax; ***Belg.:*** Logimat; ***Braz.:*** Yrelan†; ***Denm.:*** Logimax; ***Fin.:*** Logimax; Unimax; ***Fr.:*** Logimax; ***Ger.:*** Delmuno; Mobloc; Unimax; ***Hong Kong:*** Logimax; ***Israel:*** Logimax; ***Mex.:*** Logimax; ***Neth.:*** Logimax; Triapin; Unimax; ***Norw.:*** Logimax†; ***S.Afr.:*** Tri-Plen; ***Spain:*** Logimax; Unimest†; ***Swed.:*** Logimax; ***Switz.:*** Logimax; Unimax; ***UK:*** Triapin; ***USA:*** Lexxel.

## Fendiline Hydrochloride *(pINNM)*

Hidrocloruro de fendilina. *N*-(2-Benzhydrylethyl)-α-methylbenzylamine hydrochloride.

$C_{23}H_{25}N,HCl$ = 351.9.

*CAS — 13042-18-7 (fendiline); 13636-18-5 (fendiline hydrochloride).*

*ATC — C08EA01.*

### Profile

Fendiline hydrochloride is a calcium-channel blocker used as a vasodilator in ischaemic heart disease in usual doses of 150 mg daily, in divided doses, by mouth.

Ischaemic heart disease is discussed under Atherosclerosis (p.815) and the treatment of its clinical manifestations is described under Angina Pectoris (p.813) and Myocardial Infarction (p.828).

### Preparations

**Proprietary Preparations** (details are given in Part 3)
***Austria:*** Sensit; ***Ger.:*** Sensit; ***Gr.:*** Sensit; ***Ital.:*** Difmecor†; Olbiacor†; Sensit-F†.

## Fenofibrate *(BAN, rINN)*

Fenofibrato; Fenofibratum; LF-178; Procetofene. Isopropyl 2-[4-(4-chlorobenzoyl)phenoxy]-2-methylpropionate.

$C_{20}H_{21}ClO_4$ = 360.8.

*CAS — 49562-28-9.*

*ATC — C10AB05.*

**Pharmacopoeias.** In *Chin.* and *Eur.* (see p.vi).

**Ph. Eur. 5.0** (Fenofibrate). A white or almost white, crystalline powder. Practically insoluble in water; slightly soluble in alcohol; very soluble in dichloromethane. M.p. 79° to 82°. Protect from light.

### Adverse Effects and Precautions

As for Bezafibrate, p.873.

◊ The most common adverse effects in both long- and short-term studies of fenofibrate have been gastrointestinal disturbances, occurring in about 3 to 5% of patients.[1] Other adverse effects include dermatological, musculoskeletal, and neurological disorders. Fenofibrate has also been reported to increase indices of bile lithogenicity[1-3] and an increased risk of gallstones has been reported with fibrates (see Gallstones, under Adverse Effects of Bezafibrate, p.874).

For a report of the half-life being prolonged in patients with renal impairment, see Administration in Renal Impairment, under Uses and Administration, below.

1. Brown WV. Treatment of hypercholesterolaemia with fenofibrate: a review. *Curr Med Res Opin* 1989; **11:** 321–30.
2. Blane GF. Comparative toxicity and safety profile of fenofibrate and other fibric acid derivatives. *Am J Med* 1987; **83** (suppl 5B): 26–36.
3. Palmer RH. Effects of fibric acid derivatives on biliary lipid composition. *Am J Med* 1987; **83** (suppl 5B): 37–43.

### Interactions

As for Bezafibrate, p.874.

The manufacturers of fenofibrate suggest that in patients taking oral anticoagulants, the dose of anticoagulant should be reduced by about one-third when treatment with fenofibrate is started, and then adjusted gradually if necessary.

### Pharmacokinetics

Fenofibrate is readily absorbed from the gastrointestinal tract when taken with food; absorption is substantially reduced if fenofibrate is administered after an overnight fast. It is rapidly hydrolysed to its active metabolite fenofibric acid which is approximately 99% bound to plasma albumin. The plasma elimination half-life is about 20 hours. Fenofibric acid is excreted predominantly in the urine, mainly as the glucuronide conjugate, but also as a reduced form of fenofibric acid and its glucuronide. It is not removed by haemodialysis.

◊ References.

1. Chapman MJ. Pharmacology of fenofibrate. *Am J Med* 1987; **83** (suppl 5B): 21–5.

### Uses and Administration

Fenofibrate, a fibric acid derivative, is a lipid regulating drug with actions on plasma lipids similar to those of bezafibrate (p.874).

It is used to reduce low-density lipoprotein (LDL)-cholesterol, total cholesterol, triglycerides, and apolipoprotein B, and to increase high-density lipoprotein (HDL)-cholesterol, in the management of hyperlipidaemias (p.823), including type IIa, type IIb, type III, type IV, and type V hyperlipoproteinaemias.

Fenofibrate is given by mouth, usually in a micronised form that has improved bioavailability. The usual initial dose is 67 to 200 mg daily, as a single dose or in three divided doses, depending on the formulation. The dose should be adjusted according to response to a maximum dose of 267 mg daily. Children may be given a dose of 67 mg per 20 kg body-weight daily. A modified-release preparation is also available and is given in a dose of 54 to 160 mg daily (equivalent to 67 to 200 mg of micronised fenofibrate).

Fenofibrate may also be given in the non-micronised form; 67 mg of micronised fenofibrate is therapeutically equivalent to about 100 mg of non-micronised. The usual initial dose is 300 mg daily in divided doses with food. Doses may be adjusted according to response to between 200 and 400 mg daily. Children may be given 5 mg/kg daily.

◊ General references.

1. Balfour JA, *et al.* Fenofibrate: a review of its pharmacodynamic and pharmacokinetic properties and therapeutic use in dyslipidaemia. *Drugs* 1990; **40:** 260–90.
2. Adkins JC, Faulds D. Micronised fenofibrate: a review of its pharmacodynamic properties and clinical efficacy in the management of dyslipidaemia. *Drugs* 1997; **54:** 615–33.
3. Guay DRP. Micronized fenofibrate: a new fibric acid hypolipidemic agent. *Ann Pharmacother* 1999; **33:** 1083–1103.
4. Keating GM, Ormrod D. Micronised fenofibrate: an updated review of its clinical efficacy in the management of dyslipidaemia. *Drugs* 2002; **62:** 1909–44.

**Administration in renal impairment.** The plasma half-life of fenofibric acid has been shown to be prolonged to up to about 360 hours in patients with renal disease following a single dose of fenofibrate.[1] No correlation was found between the elimination half-life and serum creatinine concentrations or creatinine clearance. Fenofibrate metabolites were not removed by haemodialysis. Significant accumulation of fenofibric acid occurs on repeated daily dosing in renal impairment and fenofibrate is generally contra-indicated in patients with severe renal dysfunction. However, the UK manufacturers have stated that fenofibrate may be given in mild or moderate renal impairment in reduced doses. They have suggested doses of 134 mg of micronised fenofibrate daily for creatinine clearances of 20 to 60 mL/minute, and 67 mg daily for creatinine clearance less than 20 mL/minute. The US manufacturers advise an initial dose of 54 mg daily if the modified-release preparation is used.

1. Desager JP, *et al.* Effect of hemodialysis on plasma kinetics of fenofibrate in chronic renal failure. *Nephron* 1982; **31:** 51–4.

### Preparations

**Proprietary Preparations** (details are given in Part 3)
***Arg.:*** Fenobrate; Fenolip; Lipidil; Lipoplasmin; Minuslip; Procetoken; Qualecon; Sclerofin; ***Austria:*** Fenolip; Lipcor; Lipsin; ***Belg.:*** Fenogal; Lipanthyl; ***Braz.:*** Lipanon†; Lipidil†; ***Canad.:*** Apo-Feno; Lipidil; ***Chile:*** Lipidil; ***Fr.:*** Fegenor; Lipanthyl; Lipirex; Livesan†; Secalip; ***Ger.:*** CIL; durafenat; Fenobeta; Lipanthyl; Lipidil; Normalip pro; ***Gr.:*** Lipanthyl; Lipidil; Neo-Disterin; Planitrix; ***Hong Kong:*** Apo-Feno-Micro; Lexemin; Lipanthyl; Trolip; ***India:*** Lipicard; ***Irl.:*** Lipantil; ***Ital.:*** Fulcro; Lipanthyl; Lipidax†; Lipoclar†; Lipofene; Lipsin; Nolipax; Scleril; Tilene; Volutine; ***Malaysia:*** Lipanthyl; ***Mex.:*** Controlip; Lipidil; ***Port.:*** Catalip; Lipanthyl; Lipofen; ***S.Afr.:*** Lipsin; ***Singapore:*** Lexemin; Lipanthyl; ***Spain:*** Liparison; Secalip; ***Swed.:*** Lipanthyl; ***Switz.:*** Lipanthyl; ***Thai.:*** Lexemin; Lipanthyl; ***UK:*** Fenogal; Lipantil; Supralip; ***USA:*** Lofibra; Tricor.

## Fenoldopam Mesilate *(BANM, rINNM)*

Fenoldopam Mesylate *(USAN)*; Mesilato de fenoldopam; SKF-82526-j. 6-Chloro-2,3,4,5-tetrahydro-1-(*p*-hydroxyphenyl)-1*H*-3-benzazepine-7,8-diol methanesulfonate.

$C_{16}H_{16}ClNO_3,CH_4O_3S$ = 401.9.

*CAS — 67227-56-9 (fenoldopam); 67227-57-0 (fenoldopam mesilate).*

*ATC — C01CA19.*

**Pharmacopoeias.** In *US.*

**USP 27** (Fenoldopam Mesylate). A white to off-white powder. Soluble in water. Store in airtight containers at a temperature of 25°, excursions permitted between 15° and 30°. Protect from moisture.

**Incompatibility.** Physical incompatibility has been reported[1] with fenoldopam 80 micrograms/mL (as the mesilate) in 0.9% sodium chloride injection and the following drugs during simulated Y-site administration: aminophylline; ampicillin sodium; amphotericin B; bumetanide; cefoxitin sodium; dexamethasone sodium phosphate; diazepam; fosphenytoin sodium; furosemide; ketorolac trometamine; methohexital sodium; methylprednisolone sodium succinate; pentobarbital sodium; phenytoin sodium; prochlorperazine edisilate; sodium bicarbonate; and thiopental sodium.

1. Trissel LA, *et al.* Compatibility of fenoldopam mesylate with other drugs during simulated Y-site administration. *Am J Health-Syst Pharm* 2003; **60:** 80–5.

**Stability.** Fenoldopam mesilate, at concentrations ranging from 4 to 300 micrograms/mL in glucose 5% or sodium chloride 0.9%, has been reported[1] to be stable for 72 hours when stored at temperatures of 4° or 23°.

1. Trissel LA, *et al.* Stability of fenoldopam mesylate in two infusion solutions. *Am J Health-Syst Pharm* 2002; **59:** 846–8.

### Adverse Effects and Precautions

The adverse effects of fenoldopam are mainly due to vasodilatation and include hypotension, flushing, dizziness, headache, and reflex tachycardia. Nausea and vomiting, and ECG abnormalities have also been reported. Hypokalaemia has occurred and serum-electrolyte concentrations should be monitored during therapy. Fenoldopam may increase intra-ocular pressure and it should be used with caution in patients with glaucoma. Caution is also required in patients in whom hypotension could be deleterious, such as those with acute cerebral infarction or haemorrhage. Blood pressure and heart rate should be monitored.

**Effects on the heart.** Although fenoldopam is usually associated with reflex tachycardia, precipitous bradycardia occurred in 2 patients receiving fenoldopam infusion in a clinical study,[1] necessitating discontinuation of the drug.

1. Taylor AA, *et al.* Sustained hemodynamic effects of the selective dopamine-1 agonist, fenoldopam, during 48-hour infusions in hypertensive patients: a dose-tolerability study. *J Clin Pharmacol* 1999; **39:** 471–9.

## Interactions

The hypotensive effects of fenoldopam may be enhanced by other drugs with hypotensive actions. Beta blockers may block the reflex tachycardia that occurs with fenoldopam and concomitant use is not recommended.

## Pharmacokinetics

Steady-state plasma concentrations of fenoldopam are reached about 20 minutes after commencing continuous intravenous infusion. Fenoldopam is extensively metabolised with only about 4% of a dose being excreted unchanged. It is metabolised by conjugation (mainly glucuronidation, methylation, and sulfation). Fenoldopam and its metabolites are excreted predominantly in the urine, the remainder being excreted in the faeces. The elimination half-life of fenoldopam is about 5 minutes.

## Uses and Administration

Fenoldopam is a dopamine agonist that is reported to have a selective action at dopamine $D_1$-receptors, leading to vasodilatation. It is used in the short-term management of severe hypertension (below) and has also been tried in heart failure.

Fenoldopam is given intravenously as the mesilate, although doses are expressed in terms of the base; 1.31 micrograms of fenoldopam mesilate is equivalent to 1 microgram of base.

In the management of hypertensive crises, fenoldopam mesilate is given by continuous intravenous infusion as a solution containing 40 micrograms/mL of fenoldopam. The dose should be adjusted according to response, in usual increments of 50 to 100 nanograms/kg per minute at not less than 15-minute intervals. The usual dose range is from 100 to 1600 nanograms/kg per minute.

◊ Reviews.

1. Brogden RN, Markham A. Fenoldopam: a review of its pharmacodynamic and pharmacokinetic properties and intravenous clinical potential in the management of hypertensive urgencies and emergencies. *Drugs* 1997; **54:** 634–50.
2. Post JB, Frishman WH. Fenoldopam: a new dopamine agonist for the treatment of hypertensive urgencies and emergencies. *J Clin Pharmacol* 1998; **38:** 2–13.
3. Murphy MB, *et al.* Fenoldopam: a selective peripheral dopamine-receptor agonist for the treatment of severe hypertension. *N Engl J Med* 2001; **345:** 1548–57.

**Hypertension.** Fenoldopam has poor oral bioavailability and is usually given intravenously. It has a rapid onset of action and a short elimination half-life[1] and may thus be most suitable in patients requiring rapid blood pressure reduction. Comparative studies[2,3] with sodium nitroprusside in patients with severe hypertension requiring urgent therapy have shown fenoldopam to be effective in rapidly lowering blood pressure. Additionally, in contrast to nitroprusside, urine output, creatinine clearance, and sodium excretion were increased by fenoldopam in one of the studies.[2] Fenoldopam may therefore be particularly useful in the acute treatment of severe hypertension in patients with renal impairment.

For a discussion of the treatment of hypertension, including hypertensive crises, see p.825.

1. Weber RR, *et al.* Pharmacokinetic and pharmacodynamic properties of intravenous fenoldopam, a dopamine$_1$-receptor agonist, in hypertensive patients. *Br J Clin Pharmacol* 1988; **25:** 17–21.
2. Shusterman NH, *et al.* Fenoldopam, but not nitroprusside, improves renal function in severely hypertensive patients with impaired renal function. *Am J Med* 1993; **95:** 161–8.
3. Panacek EA, *et al.* Randomized, prospective trial of fenoldopam vs sodium nitroprusside in the treatment of acute severe hypertension. *Acad Emerg Med* 1995; **2:** 959–65.

**Radiocontrast nephrotoxicity.** Fenoldopam increases renal blood flow and has been tried to reduce the renal toxicity that may be associated with use of contrast media (see Effects on the Kidneys under Adverse Effects of Amidotrizoic Acid, p.1060). Small studies in patients at risk of renal toxicity have shown benefit with fenoldopam,[1,2] but larger randomised trials[3,4] have found no advantage with fenoldopam plus hydration compared with hydration using sodium chloride 0.45% alone.

1. Chu VL, Cheng JWM. Fenoldopam in the prevention of contrast media-induced acute renal failure. *Ann Pharmacother* 2001; **35:** 1278–82. Correction. *ibid.*; 1677.
2. Lepor NE. A review of contemporary prevention strategies for radiocontrast nephropathy: a focus on fenoldopam and N-acetylcysteine. *Rev Cardiovasc Med* 2003; **4** (suppl 1): S15–S20.
3. Allaqaband S, *et al.* Prospective randomized study of N-acetylcysteine, fenoldopam, and saline for prevention of radiocontrast-induced nephropathy. *Catheter Cardiovasc Interv* 2002; **57:** 279–83.
4. Stone GW, *et al.* Fenoldopam mesylate for the prevention of contrast-induced nephropathy: a randomized controlled trial. *JAMA* 2003; **290:** 2284–91.

### Preparations

***USP 27:*** Fenoldopam Mesylate Injection.

**Proprietary Preparations** (details are given in Part 3)
***Irl.:*** Corlopam; ***Ital.:*** Corlopam; ***USA:*** Corlopam.

---

## Fenquizone *(USAN, rINN)*

MG-13054. 7-Chloro-1,2,3,4-tetrahydro-4-oxo-2-phenylquinazoline-6-sulphonamide.
$C_{14}H_{12}ClN_3O_3S$ = 337.8.
*CAS — 20287-37-0.*
*ATC — C03BA13.*

## Fenquizone Potassium *(rINNM)*

Fenquizona potásica.
$C_{14}H_{12}ClN_3O_3S,K$ = 376.9.
*CAS — 52246-40-9.*
*ATC — C03BA13.*

### Profile

Fenquizone potassium is a diuretic that is used in the treatment of oedema and hypertension (p.825) in doses equivalent to 10 to 20 mg of fenquizone daily by mouth. 11.2 mg of the potassium salt is approximately equivalent to 10 mg of the base.

◊ References.

1. Beermann B, Grind M. Clinical pharmacokinetics of some newer diuretics. *Clin Pharmacokinet* 1987; **13:** 254–66.
2. Costa FV, *et al.* Hemodynamic and humoral effects of chronic antihypertensive treatment with fenquizone: importance of aldosterone response. *J Clin Pharmacol* 1990; **30:** 254–61.

### Preparations

**Proprietary Preparations** (details are given in Part 3)
***Ital.:*** Idrolone.

---

## Fibrinolysin

Fibrinolysin (Human) *(BAN, rINN)*; Fibrinase; Fibrinolisina (humana); Plasmin.
*CAS — 9001-90-5 (fibrinolysin); 9004-09-5 (human fibrinolysin).*
*ATC — B01AD05.*

NOTE. In *Martindale* the term fibrinolysin is used for the exogenous substance and plasmin for the endogenous substance.

### Profile

Fibrinolysin is a proteolytic enzyme derived from the activation of human plasminogen. Fibrinolysin derived from cattle (bovine fibrinolysin) and other animals is also available. Fibrinolysin converts fibrin into soluble products and also hydrolyses some other proteins. The role of plasmin (endogenous fibrinolysin) in the control of haemostasis is described further on p.735.

Fibrinolysin is used (generally as bovine fibrinolysin) in conjunction with deoxyribonuclease for the debridement of wounds. It was formerly given parenterally for the treatment of thrombotic disorders.

### Preparations

**Proprietary Preparations** (details are given in Part 3)
**Multi-ingredient:** ***Arg.:*** Clorfibrase; ***Austria:*** Fibrolan; ***Braz.:*** Cauterex; Dermofibrin C; Fibrabene; Fibrase; Gino-Cauterex; Gino-Fibrase; Procutan; ***Canad.:*** Elase-Chloromycetin†; Elase†; ***Chile:*** Elase; ***Fr.:*** Elase; ***Ger.:*** Fibrolan; ***Ital.:*** Elase; ***Malaysia:*** Elase; ***Mex.:*** Fibrase; Fibrase SA; ***Neth.:*** Elase; ***Spain:*** Parkelase Chloromycetin†; Parkelase†; ***Switz.:*** Fibrolan.

---

# Flecainide Acetate *(BANM, USAN, rINNM)*

Acetato de flecainida; Flecainidi Acetas; R-818. N-(2-Piperidylmethyl)-2,5-bis(2,2,2-trifluoroethoxy)benzamide acetate.
$C_{17}H_{20}F_6N_2O_3,C_2H_4O_2$ = 474.4.
*CAS — 54143-55-4 (flecainide); 54143-56-5 (flecainide acetate).*
*ATC — C01BC04.*

**Pharmacopoeias.** In *Eur.* (see p.vi) and *US.*

**Ph. Eur. 5.0** (Flecainide Acetate). A white or almost white, very hygroscopic crystalline powder. Soluble in water and in dehydrated alcohol; freely soluble in dilute acetic acid; practically insoluble in dilute hydrochloric acid. A 2.5% solution in water has a pH of 6.7 to 7.1. Protect from light.

**USP 27** (Flecainide Acetate). A white to slightly off-white crystalline powder; $pK_a$ is 9.3. Soluble in water; freely soluble in alcohol.

**Stability.** Storage of an extemporaneously prepared flecainide syrup in a refrigerator led to crystallisation of the drug and the administration of a toxic dose.[1] It was suggested that oral liquid formulations of flecainide should be freshly reconstituted from a powder before each dose.

1. Stuart AG, *et al.* Is there a genetic factor in flecainide toxicity? *BMJ* 1989; **298:** 117–18.

## Adverse Effects

The most common adverse effects caused by flecainide affect the CNS and include dizziness, visual disturbances, and lightheadedness. Nausea, vomiting, headache, tremor, peripheral neuropathy, ataxia, and paraesthesia may also occur. These effects are generally transient and respond to dosage reduction. Other adverse CNS effects that have been reported rarely include hallucinations, amnesia, confusion, depression, dyskinesias, and convulsions. Skin reactions, including rare cases of urticaria, have also occurred and there have been isolated cases of photosensitivity. Disturbances of liver function have been reported rarely. Corneal deposits, pulmonary fibrosis, and pneumonitis have occurred during long-term therapy. Cardiovascular effects are less common than those on the CNS, but can be serious and sometimes fatal. Ventricular tachyarrhythmias have been reported, particularly in patients with a history of ventricular tachyarrhythmias and taking high doses of flecainide. Chest pain and myocardial infarction have also occurred. Flecainide produced an increased mortality rate when it was assessed for the control of asymptomatic ventricular arrhythmias in patients who had previously suffered a myocardial infarction (see Cardiac Arrhythmias under Uses and Administration, below).

**Incidence of adverse effects.** In a report of the non-cardiac adverse effects of flecainide from 1 short-term and 3 longer term studies,[1] the most common adverse effects during both short- and long-term studies were dizziness and visual disturbances which occurred in about 30% of patients. Headache and nausea both occurred in about 10% of patients. Other adverse effects reported include dyspnoea, chest pain, asthenia, fatigue, and tremor. Therapy was discontinued due to non-cardiac adverse effects in 10% of patients in the short-term trial, and in 6% of those in the chronic studies. A review of 60 studies using flecainide[2] reported that non-cardiac side-effects (mainly gastrointestinal and CNS adverse effects) occurred in 12% of patients. The UK Committee on Safety of Medicines had received reports of neurological (4 patients with sensory neuropathy, 2 with ataxia), corneal (2 with corneal deposits), and pulmonary (3 with pulmonary fibrosis and pneumonitis) reactions associated with the long-term use of flecainide.[3]

1. Gentzkow GD, Sullivan JY. Extracardiac adverse effects of flecainide. *Am J Cardiol* 1984; **53:** 101B–105B.
2. Hohnloser SH, Zabel M. Short- and long-term efficacy and safety of flecainide acetate for supraventricular arrhythmias. *Am J Cardiol* 1992; **70:** 3A–10A.
3. Committee on Safety of Medicines. Multi-system adverse reactions following long-term flecainide therapy. *Current Problems* *31* 1991.

**Effects on the blood.** Severe granulocytopenia believed to be related to flecainide occurred in a 66-year-old man 3 months after starting therapy.[1] Haematological findings suggested an immune-mediated reaction in which flecainide binds to normal neutrophils with subsequent recognition by specific antibodies resulting in enhanced destruction of mature granulocytes in peripheral blood and bone marrow.

1. Samlowski WE, *et al.* Flecainide-induced immune neutropenia: documentation of a hapten-mediated mechanism of cell destruction. *Arch Intern Med* 1987; **147:** 383–4.

**Effects on the eyes.** In addition to visual disturbance, corneal deposits have been reported in association with flecainide.[1]

1. Ulrik H, *et al.* Corneal deposits associated with flecainide. *BMJ* 1991; **302:** 506–7.

**Effects on the heart.** Like many antiarrhythmics, flecainide can have proarrhythmic effects.[1,2] Further information is also given in Cardiac Arrhythmias under Uses and Administration, below.

1. Falk RH. Flecainide-induced ventricular tachycardia and fibrillation in patients treated for atrial fibrillation. *Ann Intern Med* 1989; **111:** 107–11.
2. Herre JM, *et al.* Inefficacy and proarrhythmic effects of flecainide and encainide for sustained ventricular tachycardia and ventricular fibrillation. *Ann Intern Med* 1990; **113:** 671–6.

**Effects on the liver.** Elevated liver enzymes and jaundice, reversible on stopping treatment, have been reported rarely in association with flecainide.

Conjugated hyperbilirubinaemia with jaundice developed in a newborn infant following maternal treatment with flecainide for fetal supraventricular tachycardia.[1]

1. Vanderhal AL, *et al.* Conjugated hyperbilirubinemia in a newborn infant after maternal (transplacental) treatment with flecainide acetate for fetal tachycardia and fetal hydrops. *J Pediatr* 1995; **126:** 988–90.

**Effects on the lungs.** There have been reports[1,2] of interstitial pneumonitis associated with flecainide.

1. Akoun GM, *et al.* Flecainide-associated pneumonitis. *Lancet* 1991; **337:** 49.
2. Hanston P, *et al.* Flecainide-associated interstitial pneumonitis. *Lancet* 1991; **337:** 371–2.

**Effects on mental state.** Dysarthria and visual hallucinations were associated with elevated plasma concentration of flecainide (2500 nanograms/mL) in a patient.[1] A serial rise and fall in plasma-bilirubin concentration during flecainide therapy also suggested possible direct hepatotoxicity.

1. Ramhamadany E, *et al.* Dysarthria and visual hallucinations due to flecainide toxicity. *Postgrad Med J* 1986; **62:** 61–2.

**Effects on the nervous system.** Peripheral neuropathy in a patient taking flecainide long term has been described;[1] symptoms regressed after drug withdrawal. The UK Committee on Safety of Medicines had received 4 other reports possibly associated with flecainide and 3 reports of aggravation of pre-existing neuropathy.[1]

1. Palace J, *et al.* Flecainide induced peripheral neuropathy. *BMJ* 1992; **305:** 810.

**Lupus erythematosus.** There has been a report[1] of a patient who developed painful eye movement during flecainide therapy. The pain resolved on withdrawal but recurred when flecainide was restarted, and was accompanied by lateral rectus spasm, a facial rash, and positive antinuclear factor, suggestive of lupus erythematosus.

1. Skander M, Isaacs PET. Flecainide, ocular myopathy, and antinuclear factor. *BMJ* 1985; **291:** 450.

## Treatment of Adverse Effects

In oral overdosage with flecainide activated charcoal may be considered if the patient presents within 1 hour of ingestion. Treatment is largely symptomatic and supportive and may need to be continued for extended periods of time because of the long half-life and the possibility of non-linear elimination at very high doses. Haemodialysis or haemoperfusion are unlikely to enhance elimination.

**Overdosage.** Life-threatening ventricular tachycardia occurred in a young woman after ingestion of flecainide acetate 3.8 g, diazepam 50 mg, loperamide 20 mg, and alcohol 100 g.[1] The serum-flecainide concentration on admission, 2 hours after the overdose, was 3700 nanograms/mL. Treatment included mechanical ventilation, intravenous dopamine and an intravenous sodium load for cardiogenic shock. The stomach was emptied by lavage followed by activated charcoal and diarrhoea was induced with mannitol. Forced diuresis was performed but probably had a negligible effect owing to the extensive distribution of flecainide into the tissues. The serum-flecainide concentration 9 hours after the overdose was 1680 nanograms/mL; it continued to decline thereafter at a slower rate.

Haemoperfusion failed to reduce flecainide intoxication in a patient with terminal renal failure managed by haemodialysis.[2]

1. Winkelmann BR, Leinberger H. Life-threatening flecainide toxicity: a pharmacodynamic approach. *Ann Intern Med* 1987; **106:** 807–14.
2. Braun J, *et al.* Failure of haemoperfusion to reduce flecainide intoxication: a case study. *Med Toxicol* 1987; **2:** 463–7.

## Precautions

Flecainide treatment should be instituted in hospitalised patients and pacing rescue should be available when it is used in patients with conduction defects. Its use is limited to serious or life-threatening arrhythmias and it should not be given to control asymptomatic arrhythmias especially in patients with a history of myocardial infarction (see Cardiac Arrhythmias under Uses and Administration, below). Flecainide has some negative inotropic activity and may precipitate or aggravate heart failure in patients with compromised left ventricular function; it should therefore be used with extreme caution, if at all, in patients with heart failure. Flecainide has been shown to increase the endocardial pacing threshold and should be used with caution in patients with pacemakers. Electrolyte imbalances should be corrected before initiating flecainide therapy. Reduction of dosage may be necessary in patients with renal impairment; extreme caution is needed in patients with pronounced hepatic impairment.

**Breast feeding.** Flecainide is distributed into breast milk but there have been no reports of infant exposure. Flecainide 100 mg every 12 hours by mouth was given to 11 healthy women, beginning 1 day after delivery and continuing for 5½ days.[1] The mean elimination half-life of flecainide from milk was 14.7 hours, very similar to the plasma elimination half-life. The mean milk to plasma ratios on study days 2 to 5 were 3.7, 3.2, 3.5, and 2.6 respectively but it was considered that the risk to breast-fed infants of ingesting toxic amounts of flecainide in breast milk would be very low. In another woman[2] who had been taking flecainide 100 mg twice daily since before pregnancy for ventricular arrhythmias, the ratio was 1.57 on day 5 postpartum and 2.18 on day 7. The American Academy of Pediatrics considers[3] flecainide to be usually compatible with breast feeding.

1. McQuinn RL, *et al.* Flecainide excretion in human breast milk. *Clin Pharmacol Ther* 1990; **48:** 262–7.
2. Wagner X, *et al.* Coadministration of flecainide acetate and sotalol during pregnancy: lack of teratogenic effects, passage across the placenta, and excretion in human breast milk. *Am Heart J* 1990; **119:** 700–2.
3. American Academy of Pediatrics. The transfer of drugs and other chemicals into human milk. *Pediatrics* 2001; **108:** 776–89. Correction. *ibid.*; 1029. Also available at: http://aappolicy.aappublications.org/cgi/content/full/pediatrics%3b108/3/776 (accessed 06/07/04)

**Pregnancy.** Flecainide crosses the placenta (see under Pharmacokinetics, below) and has been used for transplacental therapy of fetal cardiac arrhythmias (see under Uses and Administration, below). However, there has also been a report of hyperbilirubinaemia in an infant following maternal treatment with flecainide, (see Effects on the Liver, above).

## Interactions

Use of flecainide with other antiarrhythmics or arrhythmogenic drugs may increase the incidence of cardiac arrhythmias. Use with a beta blocker produces additive negative inotropic effects. Flecainide undergoes metabolism in the liver and its activity may be influenced by drugs that affect the enzymes, which include the cytochrome P450 isoenzyme CYP2D6, responsible for its metabolism.

**Antiarrhythmics.** *Amiodarone* increases the plasma-flecainide concentration when the two drugs are given together.[1] It has been recommended that the dose of flecainide should be reduced by about one-half, but because the effect of amiodarone differs widely between patients, plasma-flecainide concentrations should be monitored. The clearance of flecainide may be decreased by *quinidine* in patients who are extensive metabolisers, since quinidine inhibits the enzyme responsible for the metabolism of flecainide.[2] Cardiogenic shock and asystole occurred in 2 patients receiving flecainide when *verapamil* was added to their therapy.[3]

1. Shea P, *et al.* Flecainide and amiodarone interaction. *J Am Coll Cardiol* 1986; **7:** 1127–30.
2. Birgersdotter UM, *et al.* Stereoselective genetically-determined interaction between chronic flecainide and quinidine in patients with arrhythmias. *Br J Clin Pharmacol* 1992; **33:** 275–80.
3. Buss J, *et al.* Asystole and cardiogenic shock due to combined treatment with verapamil and flecainide. *Lancet* 1992; **340:** 546.

**Antimalarials.** *Quinine* has been reported[1] to inhibit metabolism of flecainide in healthy subjects without altering its renal elimination, resulting in a reduction of total clearance and prolongation of the elimination half-life.

1. Munafo A, *et al.* Altered flecainide disposition in healthy volunteers taking quinine. *Eur J Clin Pharmacol* 1990; **38:** 269–73.

**Beta blockers.** Use of flecainide and *propranolol* in healthy subjects increases the plasma concentration of both drugs. The negative inotropic effects of the two drugs on cardiac function are at most only additive, but treatment with this combination should be initiated with caution in patients with impaired left ventricular function.[1] Addition of *sotalol* to flecainide has produced profound bradycardia and atrioventricular block followed by cardiac arrest and death in a man with ventricular tachycardia.[2]

1. Holtzman JL, *et al.* The pharmacodynamic and pharmacokinetic interaction of flecainide acetate with propranolol: effects on cardiac function and drug clearance. *Eur J Clin Pharmacol* 1987; **33:** 97–9.
2. Warren R, *et al.* Serious interactions of sotalol with amiodarone and flecainide. *Med J Aust* 1990; **152:** 277.

**Digoxin.** For reference to an interaction between flecainide and digoxin leading to increased concentrations of digoxin, see Antiarrhythmics, under Interactions of Digoxin, p.896.

**Food.** Milk feeds reduced the absorption of flecainide in an infant who required a dose of 40 mg/kg daily to control supraventricular tachycardias. When milk feeds were replaced by glucose, the serum-flecainide concentration increased from 990 to 1824 nanograms/mL. Milk-fed infants on high doses of flecainide should have the dose reduced if milk is stopped or reduced.[1]

1. Russell GAB, Martin RP. Flecainide toxicity. *Arch Dis Child* 1989; **64:** 860–2.

**Histamine $H_2$-antagonists.** *Cimetidine* has been reported to increase the bioavailability of flecainide in healthy subjects, probably due to a decrease in the metabolism of flecainide. Elimination half-life and renal clearance were unchanged.[1]

1. Tjandra-Maga TB, *et al.* Altered pharmacokinetics of oral flecainide by cimetidine. *Br J Clin Pharmacol* 1986; **22:** 108–10.

## Pharmacokinetics

Flecainide is almost completely absorbed after oral administration and does not undergo extensive first-pass hepatic metabolism. Although absorption is not affected by food or antacids, milk may inhibit absorption in infants (see above). Flecainide is metabolised to 2 major metabolites, *m-O*-dealkylated flecainide and *m-O*-dealkylated lactam of flecainide, both of which may have some activity. Its metabolism appears to involve the cytochrome P450 isoenzyme CYP2D6 and is subject to genetic polymorphism (see Metabolism, below). Flecainide is excreted mainly in the urine, about 30% as unchanged drug and the remainder as metabolites. About 5% is excreted in the faeces. Excretion of flecainide is decreased in renal impairment, heart failure, and in alkaline urine. Haemodialysis removes only about 1% of an oral dose as unchanged flecainide.

The therapeutic plasma concentration range is generally accepted as 200 to 1000 nanograms/mL. The elimination half-life of flecainide is about 20 hours and it is about 40% bound to plasma proteins.

Flecainide crosses the placenta and is distributed into breast milk.

**Metabolism.** Oxidative metabolism is an important route of flecainide elimination.[1] It is mediated by the cytochrome P450 isoenzyme CYP2D6, which shows genetic polymorphism. The mean elimination half-life of flecainide in poor metabolisers (5 to 10% of the population) was found to be 11.8 hours compared with 6.8 hours in extensive metabolisers and the amounts of a dose excreted as unchanged drug in the urine were 51% and 31% respectively. These differences in pharmacokinetics will not usually be of clinical importance. However, in patients with renal impairment who are poor metabolisers, special care should be taken with dosage adjustments.

1. Mikus G, *et al.* The influence of the sparteine-debrisoquin phenotype on the disposition of flecainide. *Clin Pharmacol Ther* 1989; **45:** 562–7.

**Pregnancy.** A study of the pharmacokinetics of flecainide, given to a mother during the third trimester of pregnancy for the treatment of fetal supraventricular tachycardia,[1] indicated that close to term flecainide crosses the placenta easily without accumulating in fetal blood, but with a high concentration in the amniotic fluid.

See also Effects on the Liver, above.

1. Bourget P, *et al.* Flecainide distribution, transplacental passage and accumulation in the amniotic fluid during the third trimester of pregnancy. *Ann Pharmacother* 1994; **28:** 1031–4.

## Uses and Administration

Flecainide is a class Ic antiarrhythmic (p.809) used for the treatment of severe symptomatic ventricular arrhythmias such as sustained ventricular tachycardia; for premature ventricular contractions or non-sustained ventricular tachycardia resistant to other therapy; and for severe symptomatic supraventricular arrhythmias (atrioventricular nodal reciprocating tachycardia, arrhythmias associated with the Wolff-Parkinson-White syndrome, and paroxysmal atrial fibrillation in the absence of left ventricular dysfunction).

Flecainide is administered orally or intravenously as the acetate. Treatment should be started in hospital. A suggested therapeutic plasma concentration range is 200 to 1000 nanograms/mL.

In ventricular **arrhythmias** the usual initial dose of flecainide acetate by mouth is 100 mg twice daily; the maximum total dose is 400 mg daily although most patients will not need more than 300 mg daily. The dose should be adjusted after 3 to 5 days and reduced once control has been achieved. In supraventricular arrhythmias the usual initial dose is 50 mg twice daily by mouth with a maximum total dose of 300 mg daily.

For rapid control of arrhythmias flecainide acetate 2 mg/kg may be given intravenously over 10 to 30 minutes, to a maximum dose of 150 mg; the ECG should be monitored. If longer term parenteral therapy is necessary it is initiated by intravenous injection of 2 mg/kg over 30 minutes, as above, then continued by intravenous infusion of 1.5 mg/kg over the first hour, and 100 to 250 micrograms/kg per hour thereafter. The maximum cumulative dose in the first 24 hours should not exceed 600 mg. Infusion should not generally continue for more than 24 hours and oral therapy should be substituted as soon as possible.

The dose of flecainide should be reduced in renal impairment (see below).

Children may be given flecainide in initial oral doses of 50 mg/m² daily in divided doses for those aged under 6 months and 100 mg/m² daily for those aged over 6 months. A dose of 200 mg/m² daily should not be exceeded.

Flecainide has also been tried in the treatment of refractory neuropathic pain.

**Administration.** Flecainide is usually given by mouth or intravenously, but was reported to be rapidly and reliably absorbed after rectal administration as a solution in healthy subjects.[1] The mean time to achieve peak serum concentration was 0.67 hours and the mean bioavailability was 98%, compared with 1 hour and 78% for an oral solution and 4 hours and 81% for a tablet. The absorption of flecainide given rectally to 2 critically ill patients was good in one but poor in the other[2] and it was recommended that rectal administration be reserved for patients unresponsive to maximal parenteral therapy and in whom oral or nasogastric administration cannot be used.

1. Lie-A-Huen L, *et al.* Absorption kinetics of oral and rectal flecainide in healthy subjects. *Eur J Clin Pharmacol* 1990; **38:** 595–8.
2. Quattrocchi FP, Karim A. Flecainide acetate administration by enema. *DICP Ann Pharmacother* 1990; **24:** 1233–4.

**Administration in renal impairment.** In patients with renal impairment, doses of flecainide should be reduced. Patients with a creatinine clearance of 35 mL/minute or less should receive a maximum initial oral dose of 100 mg daily and plasma concentrations should be monitored; intravenous doses should be halved.

**Cardiac arrhythmias.** Flecainide is effective[1-4] in a number of cardiac arrhythmias (p.816). These include severe symptomatic ventricular and supraventricular arrhythmias including sustained ventricular tachycardia, premature ventricular contractions resistant to other therapy, atrioventricular nodal reciprocating tachycardias, arrhythmias associated with the Wolff-Parkinson-White syndrome, and paroxysmal atrial fibrillation. A role has been suggested[5] for flecainide given orally as a single loading dose in acute atrial fibrillation as an alternative to intravenous use.

Flecainide has also been used successfully to treat children, both alone[6-8] and also, in a small study,[9] with sotalol. Maternal administration of flecainide (transplacental therapy) has been successful in treating fetal arrhythmias.[10-13]

Although asymptomatic premature ventricular arrhythmias in subjects who have previously suffered a myocardial infarction are recognised as a risk factor for subsequent sudden cardiac death,[14] a large multicentre study in the USA, the Cardiac Arrhythmia Suppression Trial (CAST),[15,16] found that encainide, flecainide, and moracizine were all associated with increased mortality; it is now accepted that these drugs should not be used prophylactically in post-infarction patients with asymptomatic arrhythmias.

Flecainide has also been used in the diagnosis of Brugada syndrome.[17] This syndrome is characterised by syncope or aborted cardiac arrest due to ventricular tachycardia in the absence of organic heart disease, and is thought to be due to a deficiency in the inward sodium current in cardiac cells. Flecainide, because of its sodium-channel blocking action, exaggerates this deficiency and the resulting ST-segment elevation, and aids in diagnosis; it must not be used for treatment.

1. Hohnloser SH, Zabel M. Short- and long-term efficacy and safety of flecainide acetate for supraventricular arrhythmias. *Am J Cardiol* 1992; **70:** 3A–10A.
2. Anderson J, *et al.* Flecainide acetate for paroxysmal supraventricular tachyarrhythmias. *Am J Cardiol* 1994; **74:** 578–84.
3. Aliot E, *et al.* Comparison of the safety and efficacy of flecainide versus propafenone in hospital out-patients with symptomatic paroxysmal atrial fibrillation/flutter. *Am J Cardiol* 1996; **77:** 66A–71A.
4. Dorian P, *et al.* A randomized comparison of flecainide versus verapamil in paroxysmal supraventricular tachycardia. *Am J Cardiol* 1996; **77:** 89A–95A.
5. Alp NJ, *et al.* Randomised double blind trial of oral versus intravenous flecainide for the cardioversion of acute atrial fibrillation. *Heart* 2000; **84:** 37–40. Correction. *ibid.*; 331.
6. Till JA, *et al.* Treatment of refractory supraventricular arrhythmias with flecainide acetate. *Arch Dis Child* 1987; **62:** 247–52.
7. Till JA, *et al.* Use of flecainide in children. *Lancet* 1989; **ii:** 326.
8. O'Sullivan JJ, *et al.* Digoxin or flecainide for prophylaxis of supraventricular tachycardia in infants? *J Am Coll Cardiol* 1995; **26:** 991–4.
9. Price JF *et al.* Flecainide and sotalol: a new combination therapy for refractory supraventricular tachycardia in children <1 year of age. *J Am Coll Cardiol* 2002; **39:** 517–20.
10. Wren C, Hunter S. Maternal administration of flecainide to terminate and suppress fetal tachycardia. *BMJ* 1988; **296:** 249.
11. Perry JC, *et al.* Fetal supraventricular tachycardia treated with flecainide acetate. *J Pediatr* 1991; **118:** 303–5.
12. Smoleniec JS, *et al.* Intermittent fetal tachycardia and fetal hydrops. *Arch Dis Child* 1991; **66:** 1160–1.
13. Simpson JM, Sharland GK. Fetal tachycardias: management and outcome of 127 consecutive cases.*Heart* 1998; **79:** 576–81.
14. Task Force of the Working Group on Arrhythmias of the European Society of Cardiology. CAST and beyond: implications of the cardiac arrhythmias suppression trial. *Circulation* 1990; **81:** 1123–7. [Simultaneous publication occurred in *Eur Heart J* 1990; **11:** 194–9].
15. The Cardiac Arrhythmia Suppression Trial (CAST) Investigators. Preliminary report: effect of encainide and flecainide on mortality in a randomized trial of arrhythmia suppression after myocardial infarction. *N Engl J Med* 1989; **321:** 406–12.
16. Echt DS, *et al.* Mortality and morbidity in patients receiving encainide, flecainide, or placebo: The Cardiac Arrhythmia Suppression Trial. *N Engl J Med* 1991; **324:** 781–8.
17. Singleton CB, McGuire MA. The Brugada syndrome: a recently recognised genetic disease causing sudden cardiac death. *Med J Aust* 2000; **173:** 415–8.

**Pain.** Various drugs, including flecainide, have been tried for neuropathic pain (p.7) insensitive to opioid analgesics. Beneficial results were achieved with flecainide 100 mg twice daily by mouth in the control of severe pain associated with malignant infiltration of nerves.[1,2] A controlled trial of flecainide in neuropathic pain was abandoned[3] when an association between flecainide and increased mortality was found in a separate study in post-infarction patients. Nevertheless, flecainide may be of value in refractory neuropathic pain, usually as a second- or third-line drug in patients with advanced cancer, but with neither a history of, nor suspected, ischaemic heart disease.[4]

1. Dunlop R, *et al.* Analgesic effects of oral flecainide. *Lancet* 1988; **i:** 420–1.
2. Sinnott C, *et al.* Flecainide in cancer nerve pain. *Lancet* 1991; **337:** 1347.
3. Dunlop RJ, *et al.* Flecainide in cancer nerve pain. *Lancet* 1991; **337:** 1347.
4. Davis CL, Hardy JR. Palliative care. *BMJ* 1994; **308:** 1359–62.

### Preparations

***BP 2003:*** Flecainide Injection; Flecainide Tablets;
***USP 27:*** Flecainide Acetate Tablets.

**Proprietary Preparations** (details are given in Part 3)
***Arg.:*** Diondel; Tambocur; ***Austral.:*** Flecatab; Tambocor; ***Austria:*** Aristocor; ***Belg.:*** Tambocor; ***Canad.:*** Tambocor; ***Chile:*** Tambocor; ***Denm.:*** Tambocor; ***Fin.:*** Tambocor; ***Fr.:*** Flecaine; ***Ger.:*** Tambocor; ***Hong Kong:*** Tambocor; ***Irl.:*** Tambocor; ***Israel:*** Tambocor; ***Ital.:*** Almarytm; ***Malaysia:*** Tambocor; ***Mex.:*** Tambocor; ***Neth.:*** Tambocor; ***Norw.:*** Tambocor; ***NZ:*** Tambocor; ***Port.:*** Apocard†; ***S.Afr.:*** Tambocor; ***Singapore:*** Tambocor; ***Spain:*** Apocard; ***Swed.:*** Tambocor; ***Switz.:*** Tambocor; ***Thai.:*** Tambocor; ***UK:*** Tambocor; ***USA:*** Tambocor.

## Flosequinan *(BAN, USAN, rINN)*

BTS-49465; Flosequinán. 7-Fluoro-1-methyl-3-methylsulphinyl-4-quinolone.
$C_{11}H_{10}FNO_2S = 239.3.$
*CAS — 76568-02-0.*
*ATC — C01DB01.*

### Profile

Flosequinan is a direct-acting arteriovenous vasodilator that was used as an adjunct to the conventional treatment of heart failure, but was withdrawn from the market following findings of excess mortality.

◊ References.

1. Kamali F, Edwards C. Possible role of metabolite in flosequinan-related mortality. *Clin Pharmacokinet* 1995; **29:** 396–403.

## Fluindione *(rINN)*

Fluindiona; Fluorindione; LM-123. 2-(4-Fluorophenyl)indan-1,3-dione.
$C_{15}H_9FO_2 = 240.2.$
*CAS — 957-56-2.*

### Profile

Fluindione is an orally administered indanedione anticoagulant with actions similar to those of warfarin (p.1022). It is used in the management of thromboembolic disorders (p.837) but, as the indanediones are generally more toxic than warfarin (see phenindione, p.981), its use is limited.

The usual initial dose is 20 mg daily; the dose is then adjusted according to coagulation tests.

### Preparations

**Proprietary Preparations** (details are given in Part 3)
***Fr.:*** Previscan.

## Fluvastatin Sodium *(BANM, USAN, rINNM)*

Fluvastatina sódica; XU-62-320. Sodium (±)-(3R*,5S*,6E)-7-[3-(p-Fluorophenyl)-1-isopropylindol-2-yl]-3,5-dihydroxy-6-heptenoate.
$C_{24}H_{25}FNNaO_4 = 433.4.$
*CAS — 93957-54-1 (fluvastatin); 93957-55-2 (fluvastatin sodium).*

### Adverse Effects and Precautions

As for Simvastatin, p.997.

### Interactions

The interactions of statins with other drugs are described under simvastatin (p.998). Fluvastatin is metabolised mainly by the cytochrome P450 isoenzyme CYP2C9 and does not have the same interactions with enzyme inhibitors as simvastatin, although caution has been advised when such combinations are used. However, use with rifampicin, a CYP2C9 inducer, may reduce the bioavailability of fluvastatin by about 50%.

### Pharmacokinetics

Fluvastatin, unlike simvastatin or lovastatin, is active without the need for hydrolysis. It is rapidly and completely absorbed from the gastrointestinal tract and undergoes extensive first-pass metabolism in the liver, its primary site of action. Metabolism is mainly by the cytochrome P450 isoenzyme CYP2C9, with only a small amount metabolised by CYP3A4. An absolute bioavailability of about 24% has been reported. It is more than 98% bound to plasma proteins. About 90% is excreted in the faeces with only about 6% being excreted in the urine.

◊ General reviews.

1. Scripture CD, Pieper JA. Clinical pharmacokinetics of fluvastatin. *Clin Pharmacokinet* 2001; **40:** 263–81.

### Uses and Administration

Fluvastatin, a 3-hydroxy-3-methylglutaryl coenzyme A (HMG-CoA) reductase inhibitor (a statin), is a lipid regulating drug with actions on plasma lipids similar to those of simvastatin (p.999). It is used to reduce LDL-cholesterol, apolipoprotein B, and triglycerides, and to increase HDL-cholesterol, in the treatment of hyperlipidaemias (p.823), including hypercholesterolaemias and combined (mixed) hyperlipidaemia (type IIa or IIb hyperlipoproteinaemias). It is also given prophylactically to patients with ischaemic heart disease, including patients who have had a percutaneous coronary intervention.

Fluvastatin is given by mouth as the sodium salt, but doses are expressed in terms of the base; 21.06 mg of fluvastatin sodium is approximately equivalent to 20 mg of base. The usual initial dose is 20 to 40 mg of fluvastatin once daily in the evening. This may be increased, if necessary, at intervals of 4 weeks up to 80 mg daily, in two divided doses or as a once-daily modified-release preparation; patients requiring a large reduction in LDL-cholesterol may be started on the 80 mg daily dose. A dose of 80 mg daily may also be used in patients who have had a percutaneous coronary intervention.

◊ General reviews.

1. Deslypere JP. The role of HMG-CoA reductase inhibitors in the treatment of hyperlipidemia: a review of fluvastatin. *Curr Ther Res* 1995; **56:** 111–28.
2. Plosker GL, Wagstaff AJ. Fluvastatin: a review of its pharmacology and use in the management of hypercholesterolaemia. *Drugs* 1996; **51:** 433–59.
3. Schectman G, Hiatt J. Dose–response characteristics of cholesterol-lowering drug therapies: implications for treatment. *Ann Intern Med* 1996; **125:** 990–1000.
4. Langtry HD, Markham A. Fluvastatin: a review of its use in lipid disorders. *Drugs* 1999; **57:** 583–606.

### Preparations

**Proprietary Preparations** (details are given in Part 3)
***Arg.:*** Lescol; ***Austral.:*** Lescol; Vastin; ***Austria:*** Lescol; ***Belg.:*** Lescol; ***Braz.:*** Lescol; ***Canad.:*** Lescol; ***Denm.:*** Canef; Lescol; ***Fin.:*** Canef; Lescol; ***Fr.:*** Fractal; Lescol; ***Ger.:*** Cranoc; LOCOL; ***Gr.:*** Hovalin; Lescol; ***Hong Kong:*** Lescol; ***Irl.:*** Lescol; ***Israel:*** Lescol; ***Ital.:*** Lescol; Lipaxan; Primesin; ***Jpn:*** Lochol; ***Malaysia:*** Lescol; ***Mex.:*** Canef; Lescol; ***Neth.:*** Canef; Lescol; ***Norw.:*** Canef†; Lescol; ***NZ:*** Lescol; Vastin†; ***Port.:*** Canef; Cardiol; Lescol; ***S.Afr.:*** Lescol; ***Singapore:*** Lescol; ***Spain:*** Digaril; Lescol; Lymetel; Vaditon; ***Swed.:*** Canef; Lescol; ***Switz.:*** Lescol; ***Thai.:*** Lescol; ***UK:*** Lescol; ***USA:*** Lescol.

## Fondaparinux Sodium *(BAN, USAN, rINN)*

Fondaparin Sodium; Fondaparinux sódico; Org-31540; SR-90107A.
*CAS — 114870-03-0.*
*ATC — B01AX05.*

### Adverse Effects

As for Heparin, p.928.

### Treatment of Adverse Effects

If bleeding occurs fondaparinux should be stopped and appropriate therapy initiated. Unlike heparin, there is no specific antidote for fondaparinux (but see below).

**Overdosage.** Activated eptacog alfa (recombinant factor VIIa) given 2 hours after an injection of fondaparinux was found[1] in healthy subjects to normalise coagulation times and thrombin generation for up to 6 hours, suggesting that it may be useful to treat bleeding complications, or if acute surgery is needed.

1. Bijsterveld NR, *et al.* Ability of recombinant factor VIIa to reverse the anticoagulant effect of the pentasaccharide fondaparinux in healthy volunteers. *Circulation* 2002; **106:** 2550–54.

## Precautions

As for Heparin, p.929.

Fondaparinux should not be given to patients who have developed thrombocytopenia with heparin and who have a positive *in-vitro* platelet aggregation test (that is, cross-reactivity) in the presence of fondaparinux itself.

## Interactions

As for Heparin, p.929.

## Pharmacokinetics

Following subcutaneous injection fondaparinux sodium is rapidly and completely absorbed, with bioavailability of 100%. It is extensively bound in plasma, predominantly to antithrombin III. It is excreted in the urine, with 64 to 77% of a dose excreted unchanged. The elimination half-life is between 17 and 21 hours, but is prolonged in patients with renal impairment, in the elderly, and in those weighing less than 50 kg.

◊ References.

1. Donat F, *et al.* The pharmacokinetics of fondaparinux sodium in healthy volunteers. *Clin Pharmacokinet* 2002; **41** (suppl 2): 1–9.
2. Paolucci F, *et al.* Fondaparinux sodium mechanism of action: identification of specific binding to purified and human plasma-derived proteins. *Clin Pharmacokinet* 2002; **41** (suppl 2): 11–18.

**Pregnancy.** Although an *in vitro* study[1] reported that fondaparinux does not cross the placenta, a small study[2] in pregnant women who had received fondaparinux found that anti-factor Xa activity was elevated in umbilical cord blood, suggesting that a small amount of placental transfer had taken place.

1. Lagrange F, *et al.* Fondaparinux sodium does not cross the placental barrier: study using the in-vitro human dually perfused cotyledon model. *Clin Pharmacokinet* 2002; **41** (suppl 2): 47–9.
2. Dempfle C-EH. Minor transplacental passage of fondaparinux in vivo. *N Engl J Med* 2004; **350:** 1914–15.

## Uses and Administration

Fondaparinux is a synthetic pentasaccharide that acts as a selective inhibitor of activated factor X. It is used as the sodium salt as an anticoagulant in the prophylaxis of venous thromboembolism (p.839) in orthopaedic surgery, including extended prophylaxis in hip fracture.

Fondaparinux sodium is given by subcutaneous injection in a dose of 2.5 mg once daily, starting 6 to 8 hours after surgery and continued for 5 to 9 days, or up to 32 days in hip fracture.

Fondaparinux is under investigation in the initial treatment of venous thromboembolism, and for use in acute myocardial infarction, unstable angina, and coronary angioplasty.

◊ References.

1. Keam SJ, Goa KL. Fondaparinux sodium. *Drugs* 2002; **62:** 1673–85.
2. Tran AH, Lee G. Fondaparinux for prevention of venous thromboembolism in major orthopedic surgery. *Ann Pharmacother* 2003; **37:** 1632–43.
3. The Matisse Investigators. Subcutaneous fondaparinux versus intravenous unfractionated heparin in the initial treatment of pulmonary embolism. *N Engl J Med* 2003; **349:** 1695–1702.

## Preparations

**Proprietary Preparations** (details are given in Part 3)
***Austral.:*** Arixtra; ***Fr.:*** Arixtra; ***Hong Kong:*** Arixtra; ***NZ:*** Arixtra; ***Port.:*** Arixtra; ***Spain:*** Arixtra; ***Switz.:*** Arixtra; ***UK:*** Arixtra; ***USA:*** Arixtra.

# Fosinopril Sodium *(BANM, USAN, rINNM)*

Fosinopril sódico; SQ-28555. (4S)-4-Cyclohexyl-1-{[(RS)-2-methyl-1-(propionyloxy)propoxy]-(4-phenylbutyl)phosphinylacetyl}-L-proline sodium.

$C_{30}H_{45}NNaO_7P$ = 585.6.

*CAS — 97825-24-6 (fosinopril); 98048-97-6 (fosinopril); 88889-14-9 (fosinopril sodium).*

*ATC — C09AA09.*

## Adverse Effects, Treatment, and Precautions

As for ACE inhibitors, p.842.

## Interactions

As for ACE inhibitors, p.845.

## Pharmacokinetics

Fosinopril acts as a prodrug of the diacid fosinoprilat, its active metabolite. Following oral administration about 36% of a dose of fosinopril is absorbed. Fosinopril is rapidly and completely hydrolysed to fosinoprilat in both gastrointestinal mucosa and liver. Peak plasma concentrations of fosinoprilat are achieved about 3 hours after an oral dose of fosinopril. Fosinoprilat is more than 95% bound to plasma proteins. It is excreted both in urine and in the faeces via the bile; it has been detected in breast milk. The effective half-life for accumulation of fosinoprilat following multiple doses of fosinopril is about 11.5 hours in patients with hypertension and about 14 hours in patients with heart failure.

◊ References.

1. Singhvi SM, *et al.* Disposition of fosinopril sodium in healthy subjects. *Br J Clin Pharmacol* 1988; **25:** 9–15.
2. Kostis JB, *et al.* Fosinopril: pharmacokinetics and pharmacodynamics in congestive heart failure. *Clin Pharmacol Ther* 1995; **58:** 660–5.

**Renal impairment.** Total body clearance of fosinoprilat, the active metabolite of fosinopril, is slower in patients with renal impairment. However, pharmacokinetic studies in patients with varying degrees of impairment,[1-5] including those requiring dialysis, indicate that decreases in renal clearance may be compensated for, at least in part, by increases in hepatic clearance.

1. Hui KK, *et al.* Pharmacokinetics of fosinopril in patients with various degrees of renal function. *Clin Pharmacol Ther* 1991; **49:** 457–67.
2. Gehr TWB, *et al.* Fosinopril pharmacokinetics and pharmacodynamics in chronic ambulatory peritoneal dialysis patients. *Eur J Clin Pharmacol* 1991; **41:** 165–9.
3. Sica DA, *et al.* Comparison of the steady-state pharmacokinetics of fosinopril, lisinopril and enalapril in patients with chronic renal insufficiency. *Clin Pharmacokinet* 1991; **20:** 420–7.
4. Gehr TWB, *et al.* The pharmacokinetics and pharmacodynamics of fosinopril in haemodialysis patients. *Eur J Clin Pharmacol* 1993; **45:** 431–6.
5. Greenbaum R, *et al.* Comparison of the pharmacokinetics of fosinoprilat with enalaprilat and lisinopril in patients with congestive heart failure and chronic renal insufficiency. *Br J Clin Pharmacol* 2000; **49:** 23–31.

## Uses and Administration

Fosinopril is an ACE inhibitor (p.842). It is used in the treatment of hypertension (p.825) and heart failure (p.820).

Fosinopril owes its activity to fosinoprilat to which it is converted after oral administration. The haemodynamic effects are seen within 1 hour of a single oral dose and the maximum effect occurs after 2 to 6 hours, although the full effect may not develop for several weeks during chronic dosing. The haemodynamic action lasts for about 24 hours, allowing once-daily dosing. Fosinopril is given by mouth as the sodium salt.

In the treatment of **hypertension**, the initial dose of fosinopril sodium is 10 mg once daily. Since there may be a precipitous fall in blood pressure in some patients when starting therapy with an ACE inhibitor, the first dose should preferably be given at bedtime. Usual maintenance doses range from 10 to 40 mg once daily. In patients already receiving diuretic therapy the diuretic should be withdrawn if possible several days before commencing fosinopril, and resumed later if necessary.

In the management of **heart failure**, severe first-dose hypotension on introduction of an ACE inhibitor is common in patients on loop diuretics, but their temporary withdrawal may cause rebound pulmonary oedema. Thus treatment should be initiated with a low dose under close medical supervision. Fosinopril sodium is given in an initial dose of 10 mg once daily and, if well tolerated, increased to a maximum of 40 mg once daily. An initial dose of 5 mg may be given in patients at high risk of hypotension.

◊ Reviews.

1. Murdoch D, McTavish D. Fosinopril: a review of its pharmacodynamic and pharmacokinetic properties, and therapeutic potential in essential hypertension. *Drugs* 1992; **43:** 123–40.
2. Wagstaff AJ, *et al.* Fosinopril: a reappraisal of its pharmacology and therapeutic efficacy in essential hypertension. *Drugs* 1996; **51:** 777–91.
3. Davis R, *et al.* Fosinopril: a review of its pharmacology and clinical efficacy in the management of heart failure. *Drugs* 1997; **54:** 103–16.

## Preparations

**Proprietary Preparations** (details are given in Part 3)
***Austral.:*** Monopril; ***Austria:*** Fositens; ***Belg.:*** Fosinil; ***Braz.:*** Monopril; ***Canad.:*** Monopril; ***Chile:*** Monopril; ***Denm.:*** Monopril; ***Fr.:*** Fozitec; ***Ger.:*** Dynacil; Fosinorm; ***Gr.:*** Monopril; ***Hong Kong:*** Monopril; ***India:*** Fovas; ***Israel:*** Vasopril; ***Ital.:*** Eliten; Fosipres; Tensogard; ***Malaysia:*** Monopril; ***Mex.:*** Monopril; ***Neth.:*** NewAce; ***Norw.:*** Monopril†; ***Port.:*** Fositen; ***S.Afr.:*** Monopril; ***Singapore:*** Monopril; ***Spain:*** Fosinil; Fositens; Hicarlex†; Hiperlex; Tenso Stop; Tensocardil; ***Swed.:*** Monopril; ***Switz.:*** Fositen; ***Thai.:*** Monopril; ***UK:*** Staril; ***USA:*** Monopril.

**Multi-ingredient:** ***Austral.:*** Monoplus; ***Austria:*** Aceplus; Fosicomb; ***Belg.:*** Foside; ***Braz.:*** Monoplus; ***Fr.:*** Foziretic; ***Ger.:*** Dynacil comp; Fosinorm comp; ***Israel:*** Vasopril Plus; ***Ital.:*** Elidiur; Fosicombi; Tensozide; ***Neth.:*** Diurace; ***S.Afr.:*** Monozide; ***Spain:*** Fositens Plus; Hiperlex Plus; Tenso Stop Plus; ***Swed.:*** Monopril comp; ***Switz.:*** Fosicomp; ***USA:*** Monopril-HCT.

# Furosemide *(BAN, USAN, rINN)*

Frusemide; Furosemida; Furosemidum; LB-502. 4-Chloro-N-furfuryl-5-sulphamoylanthranilic acid.

$C_{12}H_{11}ClN_2O_5S$ = 330.7.

*CAS — 54-31-9.*

*ATC — C03CA01.*

NOTE. Compounded preparations of furosemide may be represented by the following names:

- Co-amilofruse (*BAN*)—furosemide 8 parts and amiloride hydrochloride 1 part (w/w).

**Pharmacopoeias.** In *Chin., Eur.* (see p.vi), *Int., Jpn, Pol., US,* and *Viet.*

**Ph. Eur. 5.0** (Furosemide). A white or almost white, crystalline powder. Practically insoluble in water and in dichloromethane; sparingly soluble in alcohol; soluble in acetone. It dissolves in dilute solutions of alkali hydroxides. Protect from light.

**USP 27** (Furosemide). A white to slightly yellow, odourless, crystalline powder. Practically insoluble in water; sparingly soluble in alcohol; freely soluble in acetone, in dimethylformamide, and in solutions of alkali hydroxides; very slightly soluble in chloroform; slightly soluble in ether; soluble in methyl alcohol. Store at a temperature of 25°, excursions permitted between 15° and 30°. Protect from light.

Solutions for injection are prepared with the aid of sodium hydroxide, giving solutions with a pH of 8.0 to 9.3.

**Incompatibility.** Solutions of furosemide for injection are alkaline and should not be mixed or diluted with glucose injection or other acidic solutions.

Furosemide injection has been reported[1] to be visually incompatible with injections of diltiazem hydrochloride, dobutamine hydrochloride, dopamine hydrochloride, labetalol hydrochloride, midazolam hydrochloride, milrinone lactate, nicardipine hydrochloride, and vecuronium bromide. Incompatibility has also been noted with parenteral nutrient solutions,[2] with cisatracurium besilate,[3] and with levofloxacin.[4]

1. Chiu MF, Schwartz ML. Visual compatibility of injectable drugs used in the intensive care unit. *Am J Health-Syst Pharm* 1997; **54:** 64–5.
2. Trissel LA, *et al.* Compatibility of parenteral nutrient solutions with selected drugs during simulated Y-site administration. *Am J Health-Syst Pharm* 1997; **54:** 1295–1300.
3. Trissel LA, *et al.* Compatibility of cisatracurium besylate with selected drugs during simulated Y-site administration. *Am J Health-Syst Pharm* 1997; **54:** 1735–41.
4. Saltsman CL, *et al.* Compatibility of levofloxacin with 34 medications during simulated Y-site administration. *Am J Health-Syst Pharm* 1999; **56:** 1458–9.

**Stability.** A study[1] showed that furosemide injection (10 mg/mL) in 25% human albumin solution was stable for 48 hours at room temperature when protected from light, and for 14 days under refrigeration. No bacterial or fungal growth was found.

1. Elwell RJ, *et al.* Stability of furosemide in human albumin solution. *Ann Pharmacother* 2002; **36:** 423–6.

## Adverse Effects

Most adverse effects of furosemide occur with high doses, and serious effects are uncommon. The most common adverse effect is fluid and electrolyte imbalance including hyponatraemia, hypokalaemia, and hypochloraemic alkalosis, particularly after large doses or prolonged use. Signs of electrolyte imbalance include headache, hypotension, muscle cramps, dry mouth, thirst, weakness, lethargy, drowsiness, restlessness, oliguria, cardiac arrhythmias, and gastrointestinal disturbances. Hypovolaemia and dehydration may occur, especially in the elderly. Because of their shorter duration of action, the risk of hypokalaemia may be less with loop diuretics such as furosemide than with thiazide diuretics. Unlike the thiazides, furosemide increases the urinary excretion of calcium and nephrocalcinosis has been reported in preterm infants.

Furosemide may cause hyperuricaemia and precipitate gout in some patients. It may provoke hyperglycaemia and glycosuria, but probably to a lesser extent than the thiazide diuretics.

Pancreatitis and cholestatic jaundice seem to occur more often than with the thiazides. Other adverse effects include blurred vision, yellow vision, dizziness, headache, and orthostatic hypotension. Other adverse effects occur rarely. Skin rashes and photosensitivity reactions may be severe; hypersensitivity reactions include interstitial nephritis and vasculitis; fever has also been reported. Bone marrow depression may occur: there have been reports of agranulocytosis, thrombocytopenia, and leucopenia. Tinnitus and deafness may occur, in particular during rapid high-dose parenteral furosemide. Deafness may be permanent, especially in patients taking other ototoxic drugs.

**Incidence of adverse effects.** In a survey of 553 hospital inpatients[1] receiving furosemide 220 patients (40%) experienced 480 adverse reactions. Electrolyte disturbances occurred in 130 (23.5%) patients and extracellular volume depletion in 50 (9%). Adverse reactions were more common in those with liver disease, and hepatic coma occurred in 20 patients with hepatic cirrhosis. A similar survey in 585 hospital inpatients[2] revealed 177 adverse effects in 123 (21%). These included volume depletion in 85 patients (14.5%), hypokalaemia in 21 (3.6%), and hyponatraemia in 6 (1%). Hypokalaemia was considered to be life-threatening in 2 patients. Hyperuricaemia occurred in 54 patients (9.2%), of whom 40 also had volume depletion, and clinical gout developed in 2.

1. Naranjo CA, *et al.* Frusemide-induced adverse reactions during hospitalization. *Am J Hosp Pharm* 1978; **35:** 794–8.
2. Lowe J, *et al.* Adverse reactions to frusemide in hospital inpatients. *BMJ* 1979; **2:** 360–2.

**Carcinogenicity.** See under Hydrochlorothiazide, p.933.

**Effects on the ears.** Ototoxicity and deafness during furosemide therapy is most frequently associated with elevated blood concentrations resulting from rapid intravenous infusion[1] or delayed excretion in patients with renal impairment.[2] Of 29 cases of furosemide-induced deafness reported to the FDA[3] in the USA, most patients had renal disease or had received the drug intravenously. Eight patients had also received another ototoxic drug. However, deafness occurred in 11 patients following oral use, and in 4 of these hearing loss occurred in the absence of renal disease or other ototoxic drugs. Hearing loss was generally transient, lasting from one-half to 24 hours, but permanent hearing loss occurred in 3 patients, one of whom had taken furosemide orally. Deafness was not always associated with high doses; six patients had received a total of 200 mg or less of furosemide.

See also Precautions, below.

1. Heidland A, Wigand ME. Einfluss hoher furosemiddosen auf die gehörfunktion bei urämie. *Klin Wochenschr* 1970; **48:** 1052–6.
2. Schwartz GH, *et al.* Ototoxicity induced by furosemide. *N Engl J Med* 1970; **282:** 1413–14.
3. Gallagher KL, Jones JK. Furosemide-induced ototoxicity. *Ann Intern Med* 1979; **91:** 744–5.

**Effects on electrolyte balance.** CALCIUM. Furosemide increases renal calcium excretion. There is a danger of hypocalcaemic tetany during furosemide use in hypoparathyroid patients[1] and it has also been reported[2] in a patient with latent hypoparathyroidism following thyroidectomy.

The decrease in serum-calcium concentrations could also induce hyperparathyroidism. In a study involving 36 patients with heart failure, furosemide was associated with elevations in both parathyroid hormone and alkaline phosphatase concentrations, possibly indicating accelerated bone remodelling such as that found in primary hyperparathyroidism.[3]

For reports of hypercalciuria, rickets, renal calculi, and hyperparathyroidism in neonates given furosemide, see Effects in Infants and Neonates, below.

1. Gabow PA, *et al.* Furosemide-induced reduction in ionized calcium in hypoparathyroid patients. *Ann Intern Med* 1977; **86:** 579–81.
2. Bashey A, MacNee W. Tetany induced by frusemide in latent hypoparathyroidism. *BMJ* 1987; **295:** 960–1.
3. Elmgreen J, *et al.* Elevated serum parathyroid hormone concentration during treatment with high ceiling diuretics. *Eur J Clin Pharmacol* 1980; **18:** 363–4.

MAGNESIUM, POTASSIUM, AND SODIUM. For discussions of the effects of diuretics on these electrolytes see under the Adverse Effects of Hydrochlorothiazide, p.933.

**Effects in infants and neonates.** Furosemide is commonly used in the treatment of cardiac and pulmonary disorders in premature infants and neonates. This age group appears to be particularly susceptible to adverse effects arising from the increase in urinary calcium excretion which occurs during long-term use. Increases in parathyroid hormone concentration[1,2] and evidence of bone resorption[1,3] support the suggestion that the increased calcium loss causes secondary hyperparathyroidism. There have been reports of decreased mineral content of bone,[1,3] rickets,[4] fractures,[3] and renal calcification.[1,5-7] An observation[5] that renal calcification could be reversed by the addition of a thiazide diuretic was supported by other workers.[6] There is evidence[8] that furosemide-related renal calcifications in very low birth-weight infants might be associated with long-term renal impairment. Renal calcification has also been reported following furosemide use in older infants.[9]

It has been suggested[10] that a sodium deficit in infants given furosemide for heart failure may contribute to a failure to thrive.

Concern has been expressed over the finding[11] that furosemide use in premature infants with respiratory distress syndrome increases the incidence of patent ductus arteriosus. The mechanism is thought to be connected with stimulation of renal prostaglandin $E_2$. However, the increased incidence of patent ductus arteriosus did not adversely affect the mortality in infants given furosemide, and a subsequent study[12] failed to find any increase in the incidence of patent ductus arteriosus in infants treated with furosemide compared with a control group. Paradoxically furosemide has been used in the management of delayed closure of ductus (see Patent Ductus Arteriosus under Uses and Administration, below). There is a possibility that furosemide may not be effective in infants receiving indometacin[13] but it can prevent the decline in urine output which occurs during indometacin use.[14,15]

1. Venkataraman PS, *et al.* Secondary hyperparathyroidism and bone disease in infants receiving long-term furosemide therapy. *Am J Dis Child* 1983; **187:** 1157–61.
2. Vileisis RA. Furosemide effect on mineral status of parenterally nourished premature neonates with chronic lung disease. *Pediatrics* 1990; **85:** 316–22.
3. Morgan MEI, Evans SE. Osteopenia in very low birthweight infants. *Lancet* 1986; **ii:** 1399–1400.
4. Chudley AE, *et al.* Nutritional rickets in 2 very low birthweight infants with chronic lung disease. *Arch Dis Child* 1980; **55:** 687–90.
5. Hufnagle KG, *et al.* Renal calcifications: a complication of long-term furosemide therapy in preterm infants. *Pediatrics* 1982; **70:** 360–3.
6. Noe HN, *et al.* Urolithiasis in pre-term neonates associated with furosemide therapy. *J Urol (Baltimore)* 1984; **132:** 93–4.
7. Pearse DM, *et al.* Sonographic diagnosis of furosemide-induced nephrocalcinosis in newborn infants. *J Ultrasound Med* 1984; **3:** 553–6.
8. Downing GJ, *et al.* Kidney function in very low birth weight infants with furosemide-related renal calcifications at ages 1 to 2 years. *J Pediatr* 1992; **120:** 599–604.
9. Alon US, *et al.* Nephrocalcinosis and nephrolithiasis in infants with congestive heart failure treated with furosemide. *J Pediatr* 1994; **125:** 149–51.
10. Salmon AP, *et al.* Sodium balance in infants with severe congestive heart failure. *Lancet* 1989; **ii:** 875.
11. Green TP, *et al.* Furosemide promotes patent ductus arteriosus in premature infants with respiratory-distress syndrome. *N Engl J Med* 1983; **308:** 743–8.
12. Yeh TF, *et al.* Early furosemide therapy in premature infants (≤ 2000 gm) with respiratory distress syndrome: a randomized controlled trial. *J Pediatr* 1984; **105:** 603–9.
13. Friedman Z, *et al.* Urinary excretion of prostaglandin E following the administration of furosemide and indomethacin to sick low-birth-weight infants. *J Pediatr* 1978; **93:** 512–15.
14. Yeh TF, *et al.* Furosemide prevents the renal side effects of indomethacin therapy in premature infants with patent ductus arteriosus. *J Pediatr* 1982; **101:** 433–7.
15. Nahata MC, *et al.* Furosemide can prevent decline in urine output in infants receiving indomethacin for patent ductus closure: a multidose study. *Infusion* 1988; **12:** 11–12 and 15.

**Effects on lipid metabolism.** Most studies into the effects of diuretics on blood-lipid concentrations have used thiazides (see Hydrochlorothiazide, p.934). The few studies into the effects of furosemide suggest that, like thiazides, it may adversely influence blood-lipid concentrations during short-term use.[1]

1. Ames RP. The effects of antihypertensive drugs on serum lipids and lipoproteins I: diuretics. *Drugs* 1986; **32:** 260–78.

## Precautions

Precautions and contra-indications for furosemide that are dependent on its effects on fluid and electrolyte balance are similar to those of the thiazide diuretics (see Hydrochlorothiazide, p.935). Although furosemide is used in high doses for oliguria due to chronic or acute renal impairment it should not be given in anuria or in renal failure caused by nephrotoxic or hepatotoxic drugs nor in renal failure associated with hepatic coma. Furosemide should not be given in pre-comatose states associated with hepatic cirrhosis. It should be used with care in patients with prostatic hyperplasia or impairment of micturition since it can precipitate acute urinary retention.

To reduce the risk of ototoxicity, the manufacturers recommend that furosemide should not be injected intravenously at a rate exceeding 4 mg/minute although the *British National Formulary* advises that a single dose of up to 80 mg may be given more rapidly.

Furosemide should be used with caution during pregnancy and breast feeding since it crosses the placenta and also appears in breast milk. Furosemide may compromise placental perfusion by reducing maternal blood volume; it may also inhibit lactation.

**Hepatic impairment.** In patients with chronic heart failure and moderate liver congestion, high-dose furosemide therapy could produce increases in liver enzymes suggestive of hepatitis.[1] Special care should be taken with the dosage and mode of administration of furosemide in such patients to avoid severe ischaemic liver damage caused by a drop in systemic blood pressure.

As with the thiazides, furosemide should be avoided in patients with severe hepatic impairment.

1. Lang I, *et al.* Furosemide and increases in liver enzymes. *Ann Intern Med* 1988; **109:** 845.

**Hypersensitivity.** Furosemide is a sulfur-containing diuretic and hypersensitivity reactions may occur, although they are rare; cross-reactivity with other sulfur-containing drugs is also possible. However, 2 patients who had in the distant past shown serious adverse reactions to sulfur-containing diuretics were successfully treated[1] with furosemide using a rechallenge protocol. They were given an initial dose of 50 micrograms which was increased gradually each day to 20 mg by day 10, and were discharged from hospital on a maintenance dose of 40 mg twice daily.

1. Earl G, *et al.* Furosemide challenge in patients with heart failure and adverse reactions to sulfa-containing diuretics. *Ann Intern Med* 2003; **138:** 358–9.

**Hypoparathyroidism.** For comments on the possibility of hypocalcaemic tetany in hypoparathyroid patients taking furosemide, see Effects on Electrolyte Balance, above.

**Infants and neonates.** Caution must be exercised in using furosemide in infants, particularly for extended periods. The immaturity of the renal system can result in unexpectedly high blood concentrations and extended half-lives. Fluid and electrolyte balances should therefore be monitored carefully. Neonates appear to be particularly susceptible to increases in urinary calcium concentrations following long-term furosemide use. There have also been reports[1] of an increased incidence of patent ductus arteriosus in infants given furosemide, although this did not adversely affect mortality.

Secondly, several studies[2-4] have shown furosemide to be a potent displacer of bilirubin from albumin binding sites and it should be used with caution in jaundiced infants. On a molar basis chlorothiazide, furosemide, and etacrynic acid were at least as potent as sulfafurazole in displacing bilirubin from albumin.[3] Doses of furosemide 1 mg/kg probably do not produce a significant increase in free bilirubin in most jaundiced infants,[3,4] although doses greater than 1.5 mg/kg or repeated dosing could potentially do so.[4] Chlorothiazide 15 to 20 mg/kg would not be an appropriate alternative to furosemide[3] since it could produce higher plasma bilirubin concentrations in jaundiced infants.

In addition, there is some evidence from an *in vitro* study[5] that bilirubin may displace furosemide from binding sites to a greater extent in neonates than in adults. The clearance of furosemide is much slower in neonates than in adults, with an eightfold prolongation in plasma half-life, and this should be taken into account during repeat dosing.[4]

1. Green TP, *et al.* Furosemide promotes patent ductus arteriosus in premature infants with the respiratory-distress syndrome. *N Engl J Med* 1983; **308:** 743–8.
2. Shankaran S, Poland RL. The displacement of bilirubin from albumin by furosemide. *J Pediatr* 1977; **90:** 642–6.
3. Wennberg RP, *et al.* Displacement of bilirubin from human albumin by three diuretics. *J Pediatr* 1977; **90:** 647–50.
4. Aranda JV, *et al.* Pharmacokinetic disposition and protein binding of furosemide in newborn infants. *J Pediatr* 1978; **93:** 507–11.
5. Viani A, Pacifici GM. Bilirubin displaces furosemide from serum protein: the effect is greater in newborn infants than adult subjects. *Dev Pharmacol Ther* 1990; **14:** 90–5.

**Porphyria.** Furosemide has been associated with acute attacks of porphyria and is considered unsafe in porphyric patients.

## Interactions

The interactions of furosemide that are due to its effects on fluid and electrolyte balance are similar to those of hydrochlorothiazide (see p.935).

Furosemide may enhance the nephrotoxicity of cephalosporin antibacterials such as cefalotin and can enhance the ototoxicity of aminoglycoside antibacterials and other ototoxic drugs.

**Antiepileptics.** The diuretic effect of furosemide has been shown to be substantially reduced by mixed antiepileptic therapy that included *phenytoin*.[1,2] The mean diuretic effect of furosemide 20 mg or 40 mg by mouth in patients on such therapy was 68% and 51% that of healthy controls respectively.[1]

For the effect of furosemide on *phenobarbital*, see p.369.

Symptomatic hyponatraemia has been associated with the use of furosemide or hydrochlorothiazide with *carbamazepine*.[3]

1. Ahmad S. Renal insensitivity to frusemide caused by chronic anticonvulsant therapy. *BMJ* 1974; **3:** 657–9.
2. Fine A, *et al.* Malabsorption of frusemide caused by phenytoin. *BMJ* 1977; **2:** 1061–2.
3. Yassa R, *et al.* Carbamazepine, diuretics, and hyponatremia: a possible interaction. *J Clin Psychiatry* 1987; **48:** 281–3.

**Diuretics.** Severe electrolyte disturbances may occur in patients given *metolazone* with furosemide.

**Hypnotics.** A syndrome of flushing, tachycardia, elevated blood pressure, and severe diaphoresis was reported following intravenous administration of furosemide to 6 patients who had received *cloral hydrate* orally during the preceding 24 hours.[1] The reaction recurred in 1 patient on a subsequent occasion when given both drugs but not when furosemide was used without cloral hydrate. A subsequent retrospective study[2] among 43 patients who had received both cloral hydrate and furosemide showed that 1 patient had suffered a similar reaction; of 2 further patients who had possibly been affected, 1 had subsequently taken both drugs without adverse effects. A similar interaction has been reported in an 8-year-old child.[3]

1. Malach M, Berman N. Furosemide and chloral hydrate: adverse drug interaction. *JAMA* 1975; **232:** 638–9.
2. Pevonka MP, *et al.* Interaction of chloral hydrate and furosemide: a controlled retrospective study. *Drug Intell Clin Pharm* 1977; **11:** 332–5.
3. Dean RP, *et al.* Interaction of chloral hydrate and intravenous furosemide in a child. *Clin Pharm* 1991; **10:** 385–7.

**Lithium.** For reports of a possible increase in plasma-lithium concentrations in patients receiving loop diuretics, see p.304.

**NSAIDs.** NSAIDs may antagonise the diuretic effect of furosemide and other diuretics.[1] Use of NSAIDs with diuretics may increase the risk of nephrotoxicity, although it has also been suggested that furosemide may protect against the renal effects of *indometacin* in infants (see Effects in Infants and Neonates, above).

1. Webster J. Interactions of NSAIDs with diuretics and β-blockers: mechanisms and clinical implications. *Drugs* 1985; **30:** 32–41.

**Probenecid.** Probenecid has been shown[1-4] to reduce the renal clearance of furosemide, and to reduce the diuretic effect.[2,3]

1. Honari J, *et al.* Effects of probenecid on furosemide kinetics and natriuresis in man. *Clin Pharmacol Ther* 1977; **22:** 395–401.
2. Odlind B, Beermann B. Renal tubular secretion and effects of furosemide. *Clin Pharmacol Ther* 1980; **27:** 784–90.
3. Smith DE, *et al.* Preliminary evaluation of furosemide-probenecid interaction in humans. *J Pharm Sci* 1980; **69:** 571–5.
4. Vree TB, *et al.* Probenecid inhibits the renal clearance of frusemide and its acyl glucuronide. *Br J Clin Pharmacol* 1995; **39:** 692–5.

**Tobacco.** The effects of tobacco smoking on the pharmacokinetics of furosemide have been reviewed.[1,2] Nicotine inhibits diuresis and diminishes the diuretic effect of furosemide. However, this effect is attenuated in habitual smokers.

1. Miller LG. Recent developments in the study of the effects of cigarette smoking on clinical pharmacokinetics and clinical pharmacodynamics. *Clin Pharmacokinet* 1989; **17:** 90–108.
2. Miller LG. Cigarettes and drug therapy: pharmacokinetic and pharmacodynamic considerations. *Clin Pharm* 1990; **9:** 125–35.

**Xanthines.** For the effect of furosemide on *theophylline*, see p.803.

## Pharmacokinetics

Furosemide is fairly rapidly absorbed from the gastro-intestinal tract; bioavailability has been reported to be about 60 to 70% but absorption is variable and erratic. The half-life of furosemide is up to about 2 hours although it is prolonged in neonates and in patients with renal and hepatic impairment. It is up to 99% bound to plasma albumin, and is mainly excreted in the urine, largely unchanged. There is also some excretion via the bile and non-renal elimination is considerably increased in renal impairment. Furosemide crosses the placental barrier and is distributed into breast milk. The clearance of furosemide is not increased by haemodialysis.

◊ The pharmacokinetics of furosemide have been extensively reviewed.[1-6] The development of an analytical method using HPLC with fluorescence has produced greater sensitivity and more consistent results. Absorption following oral use is erratic and is subject to large inter- and intra-individual variation. It is influenced by the dosage form, underlying disease processes, and by the presence of food. Furosemide absorption in patients with heart failure has been reported to be even more erratic than in healthy subjects. The bioavailability of furosemide from oral dosage forms is also highly variable with reported values ranging from 20 to 100%. It is influenced by factors affecting absorption but the poor solubility of furosemide does not appear to have a major influence on bioavailability and *in vitro* dissolution data may not reflect *in vivo* bioavailability. Bioavailability tends to be decreased by about 10% in patients with renal disease, and slightly increased in liver disease. Values are erratic in patients with heart disease.

Furosemide is highly bound to plasma proteins, almost exclusively to albumin. The proportion of free (unbound) furosemide is higher in patients with heart disease, renal impairment, and cirrhosis of the liver. Patients with liver disease also have an increased apparent volume of distribution which is proportionally greater than the observed decrease in protein binding. Patients with nephrotic syndrome have significant proteinuria and secondary hypoalbuminaemia. This results in reduced protein binding in the blood, particularly at higher blood concentrations, and binding to proteins present in the urine, which may account for the resistance to furosemide therapy reported in these patients.

A glucuronide metabolite of furosemide is produced in varying amounts. The site of metabolism is unknown at present. There is debate over another potential metabolite, 4-chloro-5-sulfamoyl anthranilic acid (CSA). It has been argued[3] that it is an artefact produced during the extraction procedures although there is some evidence to refute this.[4]

A half-life for furosemide in healthy subjects has generally been reported in the range of 30 to 120 minutes. In patients with end-stage renal disease the average half-life is 9.7 hours. The half-life may be slightly longer in patients with hepatic dysfunction and a range of 50 to 327 minutes has been reported in patients with heart failure. In severe multi-organ failure the half-life may range from 20 to 24 hours.

Furosemide clearance is influenced by age, underlying disease state, and drug interactions. Clearance reduces with increasing age, probably due to declining renal function. Renal impairment in renal or cardiac disease reduces renal clearance, although this may be compensated for by increases in non-renal clearance. Hepatic impairment has little impact on clearance. Renal and non-renal clearance may be reduced by probenecid and indometacin.

The effectiveness of furosemide as a diuretic depends upon it reaching its site of action, the renal tubules, unchanged. Approximately one-half to two-thirds of an intravenous dose or one-quarter to one-third of an oral dose are excreted unchanged, the difference being largely due to the poor bioavailability from the oral route. The effect of furosemide is more closely related to its urinary excretion than to the plasma concentration. Urinary excretion may be reduced in renal impairment due to reduced renal blood flow and reduced tubular secretion.

1. Cutler RE, Blair AD. Clinical pharmacokinetics of frusemide. *Clin Pharmacokinet* 1979; **4:** 279–96.
2. Benet LZ. Pharmacokinetics/pharmacodynamics of furosemide in man: a review. *J Pharmacokinet Biopharm* 1979; **7:** 1–27.
3. Hammarlund-Udenaes M, Benet LZ. Furosemide pharmacokinetics and pharmacodynamics in health and disease—an update. *J Pharmacokinet Biopharm* 1989; **17:** 1–46.
4. Ponto LLB, Schoenwald RD. Furosemide (frusemide): a pharmacokinetic/pharmacodynamic review (part I). *Clin Pharmacokinet* 1990; **18:** 381–408.
5. Ponto LLB, Schoenwald RD. Furosemide (frusemide): a pharmacokinetic/pharmacodynamic review (part II). *Clin Pharmacokinet* 1990; **18:** 460–71.
6. Vrhovac B, *et al.* Pharmacokinetic changes in patients with oedema. *Clin Pharmacokinet* 1995; **28:** 405–18.

**Infants and neonates.** The half-life of furosemide in term and preterm neonates is markedly prolonged compared with that in adults.[1,2] Half-lives of 4.5 to 46 hours have been reported and it has been suggested that the prolongation may be greater in preterm than in term neonates. This effect is due primarily to immature renal function and if repeated doses are necessary over a short period accumulation may occur.[1]

1. Besunder JB, *et al.* Principles of drug biodisposition in the neonate: a critical evaluation of the pharmacokinetic-pharmacodynamic interface (part II). *Clin Pharmacokinet* 1988; **14:** 261–86.
2. Aranda JV, *et al.* Pharmacokinetic disposition and protein binding of furosemide in newborn infants. *J Pediatr* 1978; **93:** 507–11.

## Uses and Administration

Furosemide is a potent diuretic with a rapid action. Like the other loop or high-ceiling diuretics it is used in the treatment of oedema associated with heart failure (below), including pulmonary oedema, and with renal and hepatic disorders (but see Precautions, above) and may be effective in patients unresponsive to thiazide diuretics. It is also used in high doses in the management of oliguria due to renal failure or insufficiency. Furosemide is also used in the treatment of hypertension (p.825), either alone or with other antihypertensives.

Furosemide inhibits the reabsorption of electrolytes primarily in the thick ascending limb of the loop of Henle and also in the distal renal tubules. It may also have a direct effect in the proximal tubules. Excretion of sodium, potassium, calcium, and chloride ions is increased and water excretion enhanced. It has no clinically significant effect on carbonic anhydrase. See Action, below, for further reference to its mechanism of action.

**Administration and dosage.** Furosemide's effects are evident within 30 minutes to 1 hour after a dose by mouth, peak at 1 to 2 hours, and last for about 4 to 6 hours; after intravenous injection its effects are evident in about 5 minutes and last for about 2 hours. It is given by mouth, usually in the morning. Alternatively it may be administered intramuscularly or intravenously as the sodium salt; doses are expressed in terms of furosemide base. 10.7 mg of furosemide sodium is approximately equivalent to 10 mg of furosemide base. The manufacturers recommend that whether by direct intravenous injection or by infusion the rate of intravenous administration should not exceed 4 mg/minute although the *British National Formulary* advises that a single dose of up to 80 mg may be given more rapidly.

Unlike the thiazide diuretics where, owing to their flat dose-response curve, very little is gained by increasing the dose, furosemide has a steep dose-response curve, which gives it a wide therapeutic range.

In the treatment of **oedema**, the usual initial dose is 40 mg once daily by mouth, adjusted as necessary according to response. Mild cases may respond to 20 mg daily or 40 mg on alternate days. Some patients may require doses of 80 mg or more daily given as one or two doses daily, or intermittently. Severe cases may require gradual titration of the furosemide dosage up to 600 mg daily. In an emergency or when oral therapy cannot be given, 20 to 50 mg of furosemide may be administered by slow intravenous injection; intramuscular injection may be given in exceptional cases but is not suitable for acute conditions. If necessary further doses may be given, increasing by 20-mg increments and not given more often than every 2 hours. If doses greater than 50 mg are required they should be given by slow intravenous infusion. For pulmonary oedema, if an initial slow intravenous injection of 40 mg does not produce a satisfactory response within one hour, a further 80 mg may be given slowly intravenously.

For children, the usual dose by mouth is 1 to 3 mg/kg daily up to a maximum of 40 mg daily; doses by injection are 0.5 to 1.5 mg/kg daily up to a maximum of 20 mg daily.

In the treatment of **hypertension**, furosemide is given in doses of 40 to 80 mg daily by mouth, either alone, or with other antihypertensives.

**High-dose therapy.** In the management of **oliguria** in acute or chronic renal failure where the glomerular filtration rate is less than 20 mL/minute but greater than 5 mL/minute, furosemide 250 mg diluted to 250 mL in a suitable diluent is infused over one hour. If urine output is insufficient within the next hour, this dose may be followed by 500 mg added to an appropriate infusion fluid, the total volume of which must be governed by the patient's state of hydration, and infused over about 2 hours. If a satisfactory urine output has still not been achieved within one hour of the end of the second infusion then a third dose of 1 g may be infused over about 4 hours. The rate of infusion should never exceed 4 mg/minute. In oliguric patients with significant fluid overload, the injection may be given without dilution directly into the vein, using a constant rate infusion pump with a micrometer screw-gauge adjustment; the rate of administration should still never exceed 4 mg/minute. Patients who do not respond to a dose of 1 g probably require dialysis. If the response to either method of administration is satisfactory, the effective dose (of up to 1 g) may then be repeated every 24 hours. Dosage adjustments should subsequently be made according to the patient's response. Alternatively, treatment may be maintained by mouth; 500 mg should be given by mouth for each 250 mg required by injection.

When used in chronic renal impairment, an initial dose of 250 mg may be given by mouth, increased, if necessary in steps of 250 mg every 4 to 6 hours to a maximum of 1.5 g in 24 hours; in exceptional cases up to 2 g in 24 hours may be given. Dosage adjustments should subsequently be made according to the patient's response.

During treatment with these high-dose forms of furosemide therapy, careful laboratory control is essential. Fluid balance and electrolytes should be carefully controlled and, in particular, in patients with shock, measures should be taken to correct the blood pressure and circulating blood volume, before commencing this type of treatment. High-dose furosemide therapy is contra-indicated in renal failure caused by nephrotoxic or hepatotoxic drugs, and in renal failure associated with hepatic coma.

**Action.** The mechanism of action of furosemide is not fully understood.[1] It appears to act primarily by inhibiting active reabsorption of chloride ions in the ascending limb of the loop of Henle. Urinary excretion of sodium, chloride, potassium, hydrogen, calcium, magnesium, ammonium, bicarbonate, and possibly phosphate is increased; the chloride excretion exceeds that of sodium and there is an enhanced exchange of sodium for potassium leading to greater excretion of potassium. The resulting low osmolality of the medulla inhibits the reabsorption of water by the kidney. There is a possibility that furosemide may also act at a more proximal site.

In addition to its diuretic actions, furosemide has been shown to increase peripheral venous capacitance and reduce forearm blood flow. It also reduces renal vascular resistance with a resultant increase in renal blood flow the degree of which is proportional to the initial resistance.

Furosemide has been shown to increase plasma-renin activity, plasma-noradrenaline concentrations, and plasma-arginine-vasopressin concentrations. Alterations in the renin-angiotensin-aldosterone system may play a part in the development of acute tolerance. Furosemide increases renal-prostaglandin concentrations but it is not known whether this is due to increased synthesis or inhibition of degradation or both. Prostaglandins appear to mediate the diuretic/natriuretic action. The primary effects appear to be alterations in renal haemodynamics with subsequent increases in electrolyte and fluid excretion.

The diuretic response to furosemide is related to the concentration in the urine, not to that in the plasma. Furosemide is delivered to the renal tubules by a non-specific organic acid pump in the proximal tubules.[1]

In some cases sodium intake may be sufficient to overcome the diuretic effect, and limiting sodium intake could restore responsiveness.[2]

1. Ponto LLB, Schaenwald RD. Furosemide (frusemide): a pharmacokinetic/pharmacodynamic review (part I). *Clin Pharmacokinet* 1990; **18:** 381–408.
2. Brater DC. Resistance to loop diuretics: why it happens and what to do about it. *Drugs* 1985; **30:** 427–43.

**Administration.** Continuous intravenous infusion of loop diuretics may be more effective than intermittent intravenous bolus injection and may provide a more consistent urine flow with fewer alterations in urine balance.[1] Bumetanide was more effective by continuous infusion than by bolus administration in 8 patients with severe chronic renal impairment.[2] In 20 patients with chronic heart failure requiring high-dose furosemide therapy, furosemide given by continuous infusion was more effective than the same dose by bolus injection.[3] The lower plasma concentrations associated with continuous infusion may also reduce the risk of toxicity.

1. Yelton SL, *et al.* The role of continuous infusion loop diuretics. *Ann Pharmacother* 1995; **29:** 1010–14.
2. Rudy DW, *et al.* Loop diuretics for chronic renal insufficiency: a continuous infusion is more efficacious than bolus therapy. *Ann Intern Med* 1991; **115:** 360–6.
3. Dormans TPJ, *et al.* Diuretic efficacy of high dose furosemide in severe heart failure: bolus injection versus continuous infusion. *J Am Coll Cardiol* 1996; **28:** 376–82.

**Ascites.** Dietary sodium restriction and diuretics are mainstays of the management of cirrhotic ascites (p.815). Spironolactone is usually the diuretic of first choice, but furosemide may be added to therapy as necessary.

**Asthma.** Furosemide administered by oral inhalation has been found to protect against bronchoconstriction induced by exercise[1] and external stimuli,[2,3] although it did not improve bronchial hyperresponsiveness in a 4-week study[4] and provided no additional benefit when added to salbutamol for the treatment of acute asthma in a small study in children.[5] A number of mechanisms have been suggested for the protective effect of furosemide, including inhibition of electrolyte transport across epithelium, inhibition of inflammatory mediators, or an effect on mast cell function.[6] The potential for clinical applications remains unclear[6] and furosemide is not a part of the accepted schedules for the treatment of asthma (p.777).

1. Munyard P, *et al.* Inhaled frusemide and exercise-induced bronchoconstriction in children with asthma. *Thorax* 1995; **50:** 677–9.
2. Bianco S, *et al.* Protective effect of inhaled furosemide on allergen-induced early and late asthmatic reactions. *N Engl J Med* 1989; **321:** 1069–73.
3. Seidenberg J, *et al.* Inhaled frusemide against cold air induced bronchoconstriction in asthmatic children. *Arch Dis Child* 1992; **67:** 214–17.
4. Yates DH, *et al.* Effect of acute and chronic inhaled furosemide on bronchial hyperresponsiveness in mild asthma. *Am J Respir Crit Care Med* 1995; **152:** 2173–5.
5. González-Sánchez R, *et al.* Furosemide plus albuterol compared with albuterol alone in children with acute asthma. *Allergy Asthma Proc* 2002; **23:** 181–4.
6. Floreani AA, Rennard SI. Experimental treatments for asthma. *Curr Opin Pulm Med* 1997; **3:** 30–41.

**Bronchopulmonary dysplasia.** Bronchopulmonary dysplasia is a major cause of chronic lung disease in infants. Treatment often involves the use of corticosteroids (see p.1077). Additional supportive therapy may include the use of diuretics such as furosemide.

Alternate-day therapy with furosemide 4 mg/kg by mouth has produced modest benefits in pulmonary status in the absence of a diuretic effect, and few adverse effects.[1] Improved pulmonary function has occurred in infants given furosemide 1 mg/kg parenterally following packed red blood cell transfusions, given to improve oxygen-carrying capacity.[2] The successful use of nebulised furosemide in a dose of 1 mg/kg has been reported;[3,4] again pulmonary status was improved without production of diuresis or renal side-effects. However, a single inhaled dose of 1 mg/kg failed to improve pulmonary mechanics in another study involving older infants with more severe disease.[5] Systematic reviews of the use of intravenous or oral,[6] or nebulised[7] diuretics in preterm infants with chronic lung disease concluded that, although there were improvements in pulmonary function, there was insufficient evidence to recommend routine use.

1. Rush MG, *et al.* Double-blind, placebo-controlled trial of alternate-day furosemide therapy in infants with chronic bronchopulmonary dysplasia. *J Pediatr* 1990; **117:** 112–18.
2. Stefano JL, Bhutani VK. Role of furosemide therapy after booster-packed erythrocyte transfusions in infants with bronchopulmonary dysplasia. *J Pediatr* 1990; **117:** 965–8.
3. Rastogi A, *et al.* Nebulized furosemide in infants with bronchopulmonary dysplasia. *J Pediatr* 1994; **125:** 976–9.
4. Prabhu VG, *et al.* Pulmonary function changes after nebulised and intravenous frusemide in ventilated premature infants. *Arch Dis Child* 1997; **77:** F32–F35.
5. Kugelman A, *et al.* Pulmonary effect of inhaled furosemide in ventilated infants with severe bronchopulmonary dysplasia. *Pediatrics* 1997; **99:** 71–5.
6. Brion LP, Primhak RA. Intravenous or enteral loop diuretics for preterm infants with (or developing) chronic lung disease. Available in The Cochrane Library; Issue 2. Chichester: John Wiley; 2004.
7. Brion LP, *et al.* Aerosolized diuretics for preterm infants with (or developing) chronic lung disease. Available in The Cochrane Library; Issue 2. Chichester: John Wiley; 2004.

**Haemolytic-uraemic syndrome.** Renal failure is a possible consequence of the haemolytic-uraemic syndrome (see Thrombotic Microangiopathies, p.758). Correction of any hypovolaemic state with adequate fluids and of oliguria by inducing diuresis with furosemide may be used to prevent this.

Of 54 children with haemolytic-uraemic syndrome given intravenous furosemide 2.5 to 4 mg/kg every 3 to 4 hours immediately after diagnosis 24% eventually required dialysis.[1] In contrast, a retrospective analysis of 39 patients treated conservatively showed that 82% had required dialysis. The results therefore suggested that high-dose furosemide could prevent the progression of oliguria to anuria in these patients by increasing urate clearance.

1. Rousseau E, *et al.* Decreased necessity for dialysis with loop diuretic therapy in hemolytic uremic syndrome. *Clin Nephrol* 1990; **34:** 22–5.

**Heart failure.** Diuretics have been the mainstay in the treatment of heart failure (p.820) but drugs such as ACE inhibitors that have been shown to improve mortality are now generally recommended for first-line therapy along with diuretics. Diuretics provide very effective symptomatic control in patients with peripheral or pulmonary oedema and rapidly relieve dyspnoea. If symptoms of fluid retention are only mild, a thiazide diuretic such as bendroflumethiazide or hydrochlorothiazide, may be adequate. However, in most cases, especially in moderate or severe fluid retention, a loop diuretic such as furosemide will be necessary. Combination treatment with diuretics that behave synergistically by acting at different sites (the principle of sequential nephron blockade), namely a loop diuretic with a thiazide or potassium-sparing diuretic, may be needed in some patients, especially when there is diuretic resistance.

Patients have been successfully treated using continuous intravenous infusions[1] or high doses (up to 8 g daily) of furosemide given by intravenous infusion[2,3] or by mouth.[3] A patient who was successfully maintained on intravenous furosemide at home has been described.[4] Combination of furosemide with thiazide diuretics[5] or metolazone[6,7] has been reported. There is a danger of overdiuresis with both of these strategies, and careful monitoring of electrolytes and renal function is essential.[8] Delivery of furosemide to the renal tubules may be enhanced by combined therapy with hydralazine[9] or captopril.[10] The use of captopril and furosemide may also correct hyponatraemia without fluid restriction.[11] In elderly patients not responding adequately to low-dose furosemide together with optimum doses of ACE inhibitors, increasing the dose of furosemide (to an average of 297 mg daily by mouth) has been reported[12] to be of benefit. However, caution is necessary when administering furosemide with antihypertensives and especially ACE inhibitors since these combinations can result in sudden and profound hypotension and renal toxicity. Low-dose dopamine infusion has been suggested as an alternative to high-dose furosemide infusion and may cause less toxicity. In a study[13] in patients with severe refractory heart failure receiving optimal therapy with ACE inhibitors, oral diuretics, nitrates, and digoxin, additional therapy with low-dose intravenous dopamine (4 micrograms/kg per minute) and low-dose oral furosemide (80 mg daily) was as effective as intravenous high-dose furosemide (10 mg/kg daily) but caused less hypokalaemia and renal impairment.

1. Lawson DH, *et al.* Continuous infusion of frusemide in refractory oedema. *BMJ* 1978; **2:** 476.
2. O'Rourke MF, *et al.* High-dose furosemide in cardiac failure. *Arch Intern Med* 1984; **144:** 2429.
3. Gerlag PGG, van Meijel JJM. High-dose furosemide in the treatment of refractory congestive heart failure. *Arch Intern Med* 1988; **148:** 286–91.
4. Hattersley AT, *et al.* Home intravenous diuretic therapy for patient with refractory heart failure. *Lancet* 1989; **i:** 446.
5. Channer KS, *et al.* Thiazides with loop diuretics for severe congestive heart failure. *Lancet* 1990; **335:** 922–3.
6. Aravot DJ, *et al.* Oral metolazone plus frusemide for home therapy in patients with refractory heart failure. *Lancet* 1989; **i:** 727.
7. Friedland JS, Ledingham JGG. Oral metolazone plus frusemide for home therapy in patients with refractory heart failure. *Lancet* 1989; **i:** 727–8.
8. Oster JR, *et al.* Combined therapy with thiazide-type and loop diuretic agents for resistant-sodium retention. *Ann Intern Med* 1983; **99:** 405–6.
9. Nomura A, *et al.* Effect of furosemide in congestive heart failure. *Clin Pharmacol Ther* 1981; **30:** 177–82.
10. Dzau VJ, Hollenberg NK. Renal response to captopril in severe heart failure: role of furosemide in natriuresis and reversal of hyponatremia. *Ann Intern Med* 1984; **100:** 777–82.
11. Hamilton RW, Buckalew VM. Sodium, water, and congestive heart failure. *Ann Intern Med* 1984; **100:** 902–4.
12. Waterer G, Donaldson M. High-dose frusemide for cardiac failure. *Lancet* 1995; **346:** 254.
13. Cotter G, *et al.* Increased toxicity of high-dose furosemide versus low-dose dopamine in the treatment of refractory congestive heart failure. *Clin Pharmacol Ther* 1997; **62:** 187–93.

**Hypercalcaemia.** Hypercalcaemia (p.1218) usually results from an underlying disease and long-term management involves treating the cause. However, if significant symptoms are present, treatment is necessary to reduce plasma-calcium concentrations. This primarily involves rehydration, but loop diuretics such as furosemide have been used following rehydration, to promote urinary calcium excretion.

**Patent ductus arteriosus.** The usual initial treatment for a haemodynamically significant ductus is reduction of fluid intake, correction of anaemia, support of respiration, and the administration of a diuretic. If that fails to control symptoms then indometacin is generally given to promote closure of the ductus (see p.49).

Furosemide is often the diuretic chosen. It is effective and widely used but there has been concern that it might delay closure (see Effects in Infants and Neonates under Adverse Effects, above). A systematic review[1] concluded that this did not seem to be the case, and that the diuretic might reduce adverse renal effects of indometacin; however, the evidence for this was limited and it was felt that there was not enough evidence to support the use of furosemide in infants treated with indometacin.

1. Brion LP, Campbell DE. Furosemide for prevention of morbidity in indomethacin-treated infants with patent ductus arteriosus. Available in The Cochrane Library; Issue 2. Chichester: John Wiley, 2004.

**Raised intracranial pressure.** Osmotic diuretics such as mannitol are first-line drugs for the management of raised intracranial pressure (p.833) but loop diuretics such as furosemide may be employed as adjuncts.

**Tinnitus.** Furosemide is one of many drugs that have been tried in tinnitus (p.1381), but although reported to be effective in some patients, it is rarely used because of problems with adverse effects.

## Preparations

***BP 2003:*** Co-amilofruse Tablets; Furosemide Injection; Furosemide Tablets;
***USP 27:*** Furosemide Injection; Furosemide Oral Solution; Furosemide Tablets.

**Proprietary Preparations** (details are given in Part 3)
***Arg.:*** Eliur; Errolon; Frecuental; Furagrand; Furital; Furix; Fursemida; Furtenk; Kolkin; Lasix; Nuriban; Viafurox; ***Austral.:*** Frusehexal; Frusid; Lasix; Uremide; Urex; ***Austria:*** Fural; Furohexal; Furon; Furostad; Furotyrol; Lasix; ***Belg.:*** Lasix; ***Braz.:*** Diuret†; Diurex†; Diurit†; Diurix; Fluxil; Furesin†; Furosan; Furosem; Furosetron; Furosix; Furozix; Fursemida; Lasix; Neosemid; Normotensor; ***Canad.:*** Lasix; Novo-Semide†; ***Chile:*** Asax; Lasix; ***Denm.:*** Diural; Furese; Furix; Furonet†; Impugan†; Lasix; ***Fin.:*** Furesis; Furomin; Lasix; Vesix; ***Fr.:*** Lasilix; ***Ger.:*** Diurapid; durafurid; Furanthril; Furo; Furo-BASF†; Furo-Puren; Furobeta; Furogamma; Furomed; Furorese; Furosal; Fusid; Hydro-rapid†; Lasix; Odemase; Sigasalur†; ***Gr.:*** Hydroflux; Lasix; ***Hong Kong:*** Dryptal†; Frusid†; Lasix; Urex; ***India:*** Diucontin-K; Frusenex; Lasix; ***Irl.:*** Lasix; ***Israel:*** Furovite†; Fusid; Lasix; Miphar; ***Ital.:*** Lasix; ***Malaysia:*** Dirine; Furmide; Lasix; Usix; ***Mex.:*** Biomisen; Butosali; Diurolan†; Edenol; Frudemisan†; Furmidal†; Furomil†; Furonex†; Furosan; Furoter†; Golan†; Henexal; Hidrasal†; Lasix; Osemin; Selectofur; Yuremid†; Zafimida; ***Neth.:*** Lasiletten; Lasix; ***Norw.:*** Diural; Furix; Lasix; ***NZ:*** Diurin; Frusid; Lasix; ***Port.:*** Aquedux; Lasix; Naqua; ***S.Afr.:*** Aquarid; Beurises; Lasix; Puresis; Uremide†; ***Singapore:*** Dirine; Frusid†; Lasix; ***Spain:*** Seguril; ***Swed.:*** Furix; Furoscand†; Impugan; Lasix; ***Switz.:*** Diuresal†; Diurix†; furo-basan; Furodrix; Furosifar; Fursol; Impugan; Lasix; Oedemex; ***Thai.:*** Aldic; Dirine; Frusid; Fudirine; Furetic; Furide; Furine; H-Mide; Hawkmide; Impugan; Lasix; Mediuresix; Urasin; ***UAE:*** Salurin; ***UK:*** Froop; Frumax†; Frusid; Frusol; Lasix; Rusyde; Tenkafruse†; ***USA:*** Lasix.

**Multi-ingredient:** ***Arg.:*** Diflux; Errolon A; Furdiuren; Lasilacton; Lasiride; Nuriban A; ***Austria:*** Furo-Aldopur; Furo-Spirobene; Furolacton; Hydrotrix; Lasilacton; Lasitace; Normotensin†; Spirono comp; ***Belg.:*** Frusamil; ***Braz.:*** Diurana; Diurisa; Furosemida Composta†; Hidrion; Lasilactona; Terbolan†; ***Chile:*** Furdiuren; Hidrium; Hidropid; ***Denm.:*** Frusamil; ***Fin.:*** Furesis comp; ***Fr.:*** Aldalix; Logirene; ***Ger.:*** Betasemid; Diaphal; duraspiron-comp; Furesis comp†; Furo-Aldopur; Furorese Comp; Hydrotrix; Osyrol Lasix; Spiro comp; Spiro-D; Spironolacton Plus; ***Gr.:*** Frumil; ***Hong Kong:*** Frumil†; ***India:*** Frumil; Lasilactone; Spiromide; ***Irl.:*** Diumide-K Continus; Fru-Co; Frumil; Lasoride; ***Ital.:*** Fluss 40; Lasitone; Spirofur; ***Mex.:*** Lasilacton; ***Neth.:*** Elkin†; ***NZ:*** Frumil; ***Spain:*** Salidur; ***Switz.:*** Frumil; Furocombin; Furosemid comp†; Furospir; Hydrotrix†; Lasilactone; ***UK:*** Aridil; Diumide-K Continus†; Froop Co; Fru-Co; Frumil; Frusemek†; Frusene; Komil; Lasikal; Lasilactone; Lasoride.

---

# Gallopamil Hydrochloride *(BANM, rINNM)*

D-600 (gallopamil); Hidrocloruro de galopamilo; Methoxyverapamil Hydrochloride. 5-[*N*-(3,4-Dimethoxyphenethyl)-*N*-methylamino]-2-(3,4,5-trimethoxyphenyl)-2-isopropylvaleronitrile hydrochloride.

$C_{28}H_{40}N_2O_5,HCl = 521.1.$

*CAS — 16662-47-8 (gallopamil); 16662-46-7 (gallopamil hydrochloride).*

*ATC — C08DA02.*

## Profile

Gallopamil is a calcium-channel blocker (see p.810) with antiarrhythmic activity and is chemically related to verapamil. It is used in the management of angina pectoris (p.813), cardiac arrhythmias (p.816), and hypertension (p.825). Gallopamil hydrochloride is given by mouth in doses of 25 to 50 mg every 6 to 12 hours up to a maximum total dose of 200 mg daily.

◊ General references.

1. Brogden RN, Benfield P. Gallopamil: a review of its pharmacodynamic and pharmacokinetic properties, and therapeutic potential in ischaemic heart disease. *Drugs* 1994; **47:** 93–115.

## Preparations

**Proprietary Preparations** (details are given in Part 3)
***Austria:*** Procorum; ***Ger.:*** Gallobeta; Procorum; ***Ital.:*** Algocor; Procorum; ***Mex.:*** Procorum; ***Thai.:*** Procorum.

## Gemfibrozil *(BAN, USAN, rINN)*

CI-719; Gemfibrozilo. 2,2-Dimethyl-5-(2,5-xylyloxy)valeric acid.

$C_{15}H_{22}O_3$ = 250.3.

*CAS — 25812-30-0.*

*ATC — C10AB04.*

**Pharmacopoeias.** In *Br., Chin.,* and *US.*

**BP 2003** (Gemfibrozil). A white or almost white, slightly waxy, crystalline solid. M.p. 58° to 61°. Practically insoluble in water; freely soluble in methyl alcohol. Protect from light.

**USP 27** (Gemfibrozil). A white waxy crystalline solid. M.p. 58° to 61°. Practically insoluble in water; soluble in alcohol, in methyl alcohol, and in chloroform. Store in airtight containers.

### Adverse Effects and Precautions

As for Bezafibrate, p.873.

**Incidence of adverse effects.** In the Helsinki Heart Study,[1] 11.3% of 2051 patients taking gemfibrozil reported various moderate to severe upper gastrointestinal tract symptoms during the first year of treatment compared with 7% of 2030 patients taking placebo. No differences were seen between gemfibrozil and placebo groups in haemoglobin concentrations, urinary-protein, or urinary-sugar concentrations.

There was no significant difference in the total number of cancers between the gemfibrozil and placebo groups nor in the number of operations for gallstones or for cataract surgery. A higher number of deaths in the gemfibrozil group was mainly due to accident or violence and intracranial haemorrhage.

A follow-up study[2] reported that gastrointestinal symptoms remained more common in patients taking gemfibrozil. Although there was no significant difference between the gemfibrozil and placebo groups cholecystectomies were consistently more common in those receiving gemfibrozil during the entire 8.5-year observation period. Cancer occurred equally in both groups, but there was increased mortality attributable to cancer in the gemfibrozil group, mainly during the last 1.5 years of follow-up.

1. Frick MH, *et al.* Helsinki Heart Study: primary-prevention trial with gemfibrozil in middle-aged men with dyslipidemia: safety of treatment, changes in risk factors, and incidence of coronary heart disease. *N Engl J Med* 1987; **317:** 1237–45.
2. Huttunen JK, *et al.* The Helsinki Heart Study: an 8.5-year safety and mortality follow-up. *J Intern Med* 1994; **235:** 31–9.

**Effects on the skin.** Psoriasis was exacerbated in a patient within 2 weeks of starting gemfibrozil therapy and recurred when gemfibrozil was subsequently reintroduced.[1]

1. Fisher DA, *et al.* Exacerbation of psoriasis by the hypolipidemic agent, gemfibrozil. *Arch Dermatol* 1988; **124:** 854–5.

### Interactions

As for Bezafibrate, p.874.

Use of gemfibrozil in patients receiving repaglinide is contra-indicated due to the risk of serious hypoglycaemia (see p.344).

### Pharmacokinetics

Gemfibrozil is readily absorbed from the gastrointestinal tract; peak concentrations in plasma occur within 1 to 2 hours; the half-life is about 1.5 hours. Plasma protein binding of gemfibrozil is about 98%. About 70% of a dose is excreted in the urine mainly as glucuronide conjugates of gemfibrozil and its metabolites; little is excreted in the faeces.

### Uses and Administration

Gemfibrozil, a fibric acid derivative, is a lipid regulating drug with actions on plasma lipids similar to those of bezafibrate (p.874).

Gemfibrozil is used to reduce total cholesterol and triglycerides in the management of hyperlipidaemias (p.823), including type IIa, type IIb, type III, type IV, and type V hyperlipoproteinaemias. It is also indicated for the primary prevention of ischaemic heart disease (see Cardiovascular Risk Reduction, p.819) in hyperlipidaemic middle-aged men who have not responded to dietary and other measures: in the USA this use is restricted to type IIb patients who also have low HDL-cholesterol concentrations. The usual dose, by mouth, is 1.2 g daily in 2 divided doses given 30 minutes before the morning and evening meals. The dosage range may vary between 0.9 and 1.5 g daily.

◊ Reviews.

1. Todd PA, Ward A. Gemfibrozil: a review of its pharmacodynamic and pharmacokinetic properties, and therapeutic use in dyslipidaemia. *Drugs* 1988; **36:** 314–39.
2. Spencer CM, Barradell LB. Gemfibrozil: a reappraisal of its pharmacological properties and place in the management of dyslipidaemia. *Drugs* 1996; **51:** 982–1018.

**Administration in renal impairment.** Although in the USA gemfibrozil is not recommended in patients with severe renal impairment, the UK manufacturer suggests that patients with renal impairment could be given a starting dose of 900 mg daily, adjusted according to response.

In a study[1] of the pharmacokinetics of gemfibrozil in 17 patients with stable chronic renal failure the mean plasma half-life was 1.8 and 1.9 hours after multiple and single doses respectively, which was comparable with that reported in patients with normal renal function. Gemfibrozil clearance was independent of renal function, but the kinetics of gemfibrozil metabolites were not evaluated.

Beneficial responses[2] were seen in lipid and lipoprotein concentrations in 5 of 6 uraemic patients treated with gemfibrozil 1200 mg daily for six months and in 6 nephrotic patients given gemfibrozil 800 mg daily for 4 months. No significant adverse effects or signs of organ toxicity were seen.

1. Evans JR, *et al.* The effect of renal function on the pharmacokinetics of gemfibrozil. *J Clin Pharmacol* 1987; **27:** 994–1000.
2. Manninen V, *et al.* Gemfibrozil treatment of dyslipidaemias in renal failure with uraemia or in the nephrotic syndrome. *Res Clin Forums* 1982; **4:** 113–18.

### Preparations

***BP 2003:*** Gemfibrozil Capsules; Gemfibrozil Tablets;
***USP 27:*** Gemfibrozil Capsules; Gemfibrozil Tablets.

**Proprietary Preparations** (details are given in Part 3)
***Arg.:*** Gedun; Hipolixan; Lopid; ***Austral.:*** Ausgem; Gemfibromax†; Gemhexal; Jezil; Lipazil; Lopid; ***Austria:*** Gevilon; ***Belg.:*** Lopid†; ***Braz.:*** Lopid; ***Canad.:*** Lopid; ***Chile:*** Grifogemzilo; Lipotril; Lopid; ***Denm.:*** Lopid; ***Fin.:*** Gevilon; Lopid; ***Fr.:*** Lipur; ***Ger.:*** Gemfi; Gevilon; ***Gr.:*** Amedran; Antilipid; Cholhepan; Dosamont; Drisofal; Entianthe; Fibrolip; Fibrospes; Gebrozil; Gemfolid; Gemlipid; Hobatolex; Lisolip; Lopid; Noxobran; Parnoxil; Prelisin; Renolip; Solulip; Terostrant; ***Hong Kong:*** Elmogan†; Gemnpid†; Gemzil; Ipolipid; Lipison; Lipistorol; Lipofor; Lopid; Lowin; Synbrozil; ***India:*** Lopid; Normolip; ***Irl.:*** Lopid; ***Ital.:*** Fibrocit; Fibros†; Gemlipid; Genlip; Genozil; Lipogen; Lipozid; Lopid; ***Malaysia:*** Brozil; Fibrol; Ipolipid; Lipistorol; Lipofor; Lopid; Mariston; ***Mex.:*** Lopid; ***Neth.:*** Lopid; ***NZ:*** Gemizol; Lopid†; ***Port.:*** Lipoite; Lopid; ***S.Afr.:*** Lopid; ***Singapore:*** Brozil; Gemd; Hidil; Ipolipid; Lipison; Lipofor; Lopid; Recozil; ***Spain:*** Bolutol; Decrelip; Litarek†; Lopid; Pilder; Taborcil†; Trialmin; ***Swed.:*** Lopid; ***Switz.:*** Gevilon; ***Thai.:*** Bisil; Chlorestrol; Deopid; Dropid; Gemfibril; Gozid; Hidil; Ipolipid†; Lipidys; Lipison; Lipolo; Lipozil; Locholes; Lopid; Manobrozil; Mariston; Norpid; Poli-Fibrozil; Polyxit; Tiba; ***UK:*** Lopid; ***USA:*** Lopid.

---

## Gepefrine Tartrate *(rINNM)*

Tartrato de gepefrina. (+)-(S)-*m*-(2-Aminopropyl)phenol tartrate.

$C_9H_{13}NO,C_4H_6O_6$ = 301.3.

*CAS — 18840-47-6 (gepefrine).*

*ATC — C01CA15.*

### Profile

Gepefrine is a sympathomimetic (see Adrenaline, p.852) that has been used as the tartrate in the treatment of hypotensive states.

### Preparations

**Proprietary Preparations** (details are given in Part 3)
***Ger.:*** Wintonin†.

---

## Glyceryl Trinitrate

Glonoin; Glyceroli Trinitratis; GTN; Nitroglicerina; Nitroglycerin; Nitroglycerol; NTG; Trinitrin; Trinitroglycerin. Propane-1,2,3-triol trinitrate.

$C_3H_5(NO_3)_3$ = 227.1.

*CAS — 55-63-0.*

*ATC — C01DA02; D03AX07.*

**Pharmacopoeias.** *Chin., Eur.* (see p.vi), *US,* and *Viet.* include glyceryl trinitrate as diluted solutions.

**Ph. Eur. 5.0** (Glyceryl Trinitrate Solution). An ethanolic solution containing 1 to 10% w/w of glyceryl trinitrate. It is a clear, colourless or slightly yellow solution. Miscible with dehydrated alcohol and with acetone.

Pure glyceryl trinitrate is practically insoluble in water; freely soluble in dehydrated alcohol; miscible with acetone.

Protect from light. Diluted solutions (1%) should be stored at 2° to 15°; more concentrated solutions may be stored at 15° to 20°.

**USP 27** (Diluted Nitroglycerin). A mixture of glyceryl trinitrate with lactose, glucose, alcohol, propylene glycol, or other suitable inert excipient, usually containing not more than 10% glyceryl trinitrate. When diluted in either alcohol or propylene glycol it is a clear, colourless, or pale yellow liquid. When diluted with lactose, it is a white odourless powder. Store in airtight containers at a temperature of 25°, excursions permitted between 15° and 30°. Prevent exposure to temperatures above 40°. Protect from light.

Undiluted glyceryl trinitrate is a white to pale yellow, thick, flammable, explosive liquid. Slightly soluble in water; soluble in alcohol, in acetone, in carbon disulfide, in chloroform, in dichloromethane, in ether, in ethyl acetate, in glacial acetic acid, in methyl alcohol, in benzene, in toluene, in nitrobenzene, and in phenol.

**Handling.** Undiluted glyceryl trinitrate can be exploded by percussion or excessive heat and only exceedingly small amounts should be isolated.

**Incompatibility.** Studies have found glyceryl trinitrate to be incompatible with phenytoin,[1] alteplase,[2] and levofloxacin.[3]

1. Klamerus KJ, *et al.* Stability of nitroglycerin in intravenous admixtures. *Am J Hosp Pharm* 1984; **41:** 303–5.
2. Lee CY, *et al.* Visual and spectrophotometric determination of compatibility of alteplase and streptokinase with other injectable drugs. *Am J Hosp Pharm* 1990; **47:** 606–8.
3. Saltsman CL, *et al.* Compatibility of levofloxacin with 34 medications during simulated Y-site administration. *Am J Health-Syst Pharm* 1999; **56:** 1458–9.

**Stability.** INTRAVENOUS SOLUTIONS. The loss of glyceryl trinitrate from solution by adsorption or absorption into some plastics of intravenous administration equipment has been recognised for some years,[1,2] although adsorption does not appear to occur to any great extent with polyolefin[3] or polyethylene.[4-6] It is not only infusion containers and plastic tubing that may be involved; some inline filters can adsorb glyceryl trinitrate.[7,8]

1. Grouthamel WG, *et al.* Loss of nitroglycerin from plastic intravenous bags. *N Engl J Med* 1978; **299:** 262.
2. Roberts MS, *et al.* The availability of nitroglycerin from parenteral solutions. *J Pharm Pharmacol* 1980; **32:** 237–44.
3. Wagenknecht DM, *et al.* Stability of nitroglycerin solutions in polyolefin and glass containers. *Am J Hosp Pharm* 1984; **41:** 1807–11.
4. Schaber DE, *et al.* Nitroglycerin adsorption to a combination polyvinyl chloride, polyethylene intravenous administration set. *Drug Intell Clin Pharm* 1985; **19:** 572–5.
5. Tracy TS, *et al.* Nitroglycerin delivery through a polyethylene-lined intravenous administration set. *Am J Hosp Pharm* 1989; **46:** 2031–5.
6. Martens HJ, *et al.* Sorption of various drugs in polyvinyl chloride, glass, and polyethylene-lined infusion containers. *Am J Hosp Pharm* 1990; **47:** 369–73.
7. Baaske DM, *et al.* Nitroglycerin compatibility with intravenous fluid filters, containers, and administration sets. *Am J Hosp Pharm* 1980; **37:** 201–5.
8. Kanke M, *et al.* Binding of selected drugs to a "treated" inline filter. *Am J Hosp Pharm* 1983; **40:** 1323–8.

TABLETS. Many studies have demonstrated that glyceryl trinitrate tablets are unstable and subject to considerable loss of potency in contact with packaging components such as adhesive labels, cotton and rayon fillers, and plastic bottles and caps. Both the Council of the Royal Pharmaceutical Society of Great Britain and the FDA in the USA have issued packaging and dispensing guidelines. Glyceryl trinitrate tablets should be dispensed only in glass containers sealed with a foil lined cap and containing no cotton wool wadding. In addition, the Council of the Royal Pharmaceutical Society of Great Britain recommends that no more than 100 tablets should be supplied and that the container should be labelled with an indication that any tablets should be discarded after 8 weeks in use.

### Adverse Effects

Glyceryl trinitrate may cause flushing of the face, dizziness, tachycardia, and throbbing headache. Large doses cause vomiting, restlessness, blurred vision, hypotension (which can be severe), syncope, and rarely cyanosis, and methaemoglobinaemia; impairment of respiration and bradycardia may ensue. Contact dermatitis has been reported in patients using topical glyceryl trinitrate preparations; local irritation and erythema may also occur. Preparations applied to the oral mucosa frequently produce a localised burning sensation.

Chronic poisoning may occur in industry but tolerance develops when glyceryl trinitrate is regularly handled and nitrate dependence can lead to severe withdrawal symptoms in subjects abruptly removed from chronic exposure. Loss of such tolerance is rapid and may cause poisoning on re-exposure. Tolerance may occur during clinical use and is usually associated with preparations that produce sustained plasma concentrations.

**Effects on the heart.** Tachycardia, hypotension, and bradycardia are recognised adverse cardiac effects of glyceryl trinitrate. Rarely reported adverse effects include asystole[1] and complete heart block.[2]

1. Ong EA, *et al.* Nitroglycerin-induced asystole. *Arch Intern Med* 1985; **145:** 954.
2. Lancaster L, Fenster PE. Complete heart block after sublingual nitroglycerin. *Chest* 1983; **84:** 111–12.

**Effects on taste.** A 61-year-old man experienced loss of bitter and salty taste sensations 2 weeks after addition of glyceryl trinitrate patches to his post-myocardial infarction drug regimen.[1] The patient experienced complete loss of taste after 6 weeks; his taste sensation returned to normal within 1 week of discontinuing glyceryl trinitrate patches. Taste sensation was again altered on rechallenge.

1. Ewing RC, *et al.* Ageusia associated with transdermal nitroglycerin. *Clin Pharm* 1989; **8:** 146–7.

**Hypersensitivity.** Contact dermatitis has been reported in patients using glyceryl trinitrate ointment and patches.[1] Both glyceryl trinitrate and formulation components may be involved in these reactions.

1. Carmichael AJ. Skin sensitivity and transdermal drug delivery: a review of the problem. *Drug Safety* 1994; **10:** 151–9.

**Intravenous administration.** Some formulations of glyceryl trinitrate for intravenous use may contain substantial quantities of alcohol in the solvent. There have been several reports of alcohol intoxication occurring in patients during high-dose intravenous glyceryl trinitrate infusion.[1-3] In a patient[3] who required glyceryl trinitrate 2 mg/minute, a blood-alcohol concentration of 2.67 mg/mL was reported. PVC tubing had been used for the infusion and it was suggested that adsorption of glyceryl trinitrate onto the tubing may have increased the dose requirement and thus the amount of alcohol given.

Propylene glycol is also used as a solvent in some formulations of glyceryl trinitrate. Infusion of solutions with propylene glycol can lead to hyperosmolarity: see under Propylene Glycol, p.1735, for details.


1. Shook TL, *et al.* Ethanol intoxication complicating intravenous nitroglycerin therapy. *Ann Intern Med* 1984; **101:** 498–9.
2. Daly TJ, *et al.* "Cocktail"-coronary care. *N Engl J Med* 1984; **310:** 1123.
3. Korn SH, Comer JB. Intravenous nitroglycerin and ethanol intoxication. *Ann Intern Med* 1985; **102:** 274.


## Treatment of Adverse Effects

Syncope and hypotension should be treated by keeping the patient in a recumbent position with the head lowered; pressor agents may be necessary in extreme hypotension. The administration of oxygen, with assisted respiration, may be necessary in severe poisoning and infusion of plasma expanders or suitable electrolyte solutions may be required to maintain the circulation. If methaemoglobinaemia occurs methylthioninium chloride may be given intravenously. In the case of severe poisoning with tablets the stomach should be emptied by lavage. If large amounts have been ingested within 1 hour, activated charcoal may be considered.

## Precautions

Glyceryl trinitrate should not be used in patients with severe hypotension, hypovolaemia, marked anaemia, heart failure due to obstruction (including constrictive pericarditis), or raised intracranial pressure due to head trauma or cerebral haemorrhage. Although it has been suggested that glyceryl trinitrate may increase intra-ocular pressure in patients with angle-closure glaucoma and should be avoided in such patients there appears to be no evidence for such a contra-indication.

Glyceryl trinitrate should be used with caution in patients with severe renal or severe hepatic impairment, hypothyroidism, malnutrition, or hypothermia. Metal-containing transdermal patches should be removed before cardioversion or diathermy.

**Nitrate tolerance.** Organic nitrates can lose their anti-anginal and anti-ischaemic effects in some patients.[1] Tolerance tends to develop in the majority of patients on continuous therapy and higher nitrate doses appear to induce attenuation to a greater degree than lower doses.[2]

The mechanisms of nitrate tolerance are incompletely understood. To exert their vasodilator effect organic nitrates must be converted to nitric oxide, a process which requires the presence of a sulfhydryl donor such as cysteine or another thiol. Repeated doses of a nitrate exhaust tissue stores of sulfhydryl groups and this is one mechanism that may account for the development of tolerance.[1,3] The activation of neurohormonal systems, which releases vasoconstrictor hormones that counteract the effects of organic nitrates, has also been proposed as a mechanism.[1,3] An increase in free-radical production during nitrate therapy has also been suggested,[1] as has the nitrate-induced expansion of plasma volume leading to reversal of the effects of nitrates on ventricular preload.[1]

One method used to avoid the development of tolerance is to provide a nitrate-free interval although rebound myocardial ischaemia may occur in some during the nitrate-free period.[1] With transdermal glyceryl trinitrate systems, the patch can be removed at night. For oral, buccal, and ointment preparations, the dose given at the end of the day can be omitted. Whether a nitrate-free interval is necessary for all patients has not been determined as many patients receiving continuous nitrates do not experience clinical tolerance. A transdermal patch with a higher release rate during the first than during the second part of a 24-hour period has been found not to prevent the development of tolerance.[4] Other methods investigated have included the administration of a sulfhydryl donor such as acetylcysteine, methionine, or captopril, and hydralazine, which may act by reducing neurohormonal activation, although none have found favour in clinical practice. Antioxidant effects of drugs, including carvedilol[5] and ascorbic acid,[6] are being studied.


1. Parker JD, Parker JO. Nitrate therapy for stable angina pectoris. *N Engl J Med* 1998; **338:** 520–31.
2. Flaherty JT. Nitrate tolerance: a review of the evidence. *Drugs* 1989; **37:** 523–50.
3. Maxwell SRJ, Kendall MJ. An update on nitrate tolerance: can it be avoided? *Postgrad Med J* 1992; **68:** 857–66.
4. Wiegand A, *et al.* Pharmacodynamic and pharmacokinetic evaluation of a new transdermal delivery system with a time-dependent release of glyceryl trinitrate. *J Clin Pharmacol* 1992; **32:** 77–84.
5. Watanabe H, *et al.* Randomized, double-blind, placebo-controlled study of carvedilol on the prevention of nitrate tolerance in patients with chronic heart failure. *J Am Coll Cardiol* 1998; **32:** 1194–1200.
6. Daniel TA, Nawarskas JJ. Vitamin C in the prevention of nitrate tolerance. *Ann Pharmacother* 2000; **34:** 1193–7.


**Transdermal patches.** An explosion occurred during defibrillation in a patient with a glyceryl trinitrate transdermal patch on the left side of the chest.[1] There was no visible injury to the patient. Subsequent studies suggested that this was caused by an electrical arc between the defibrillator paddle and the aluminium backing of the patch rather than explosion of the glyceryl trinitrate.

Although removal of transdermal patches prior to diathermy is usually recommended, a maximum rise in patch temperature of only 2.2° was reported when patches were exposed to a maximum power density of 800 watts/m². It was considered that exposure of transdermal patches to microwave diathermy, for example as part of physiotherapy treatment, was unlikely to cause direct thermal injury to the wearer.[2]


1. Babka JC. Does nitroglycerin explode? *N Engl J Med* 1983; **309:** 379.
2. Moseley H, *et al.* The influence of microwave radiation on transdermal delivery systems. *Br J Dermatol* 1990; **122:** 361–3.


## Interactions

The hypotensive effects of glyceryl trinitrate may be enhanced by alcohol, and by vasodilators and other drugs with hypotensive actions. The effectiveness of sublingual and buccal tablet preparations may be reduced by drugs that cause dry mouth since dissolution may be delayed.

**Anticoagulants.** For the effects of glyceryl trinitrate on *heparin*, see p.929.

**Antimuscarinics.** Delayed dissolution of glyceryl trinitrate tablets due to dry mouth has been reported in a patient taking *imipramine*[1] and in a patient treated with *atropine*;[2] this effect should be considered whenever glyceryl trinitrate sublingual tablets are given to patients taking other drugs that can cause dry mouth. Use of the lingual spray[2] rather than a sublingual tablet or addition of 1 mL of saline under the tongue[3] may be used to overcome the problem.


1. Robbins LJ. Dry mouth and delayed dissolution of sublingual nitro-glycerin. *N Engl J Med* 1983; **309:** 985.
2. Kimchi A. Dry mouth and delayed dissolution of nitroglycerin. *N Engl J Med* 1984; **310:** 1122.
3. Rasler FE. Ineffectiveness of sublingual nitroglycerin in patients with dry mucous membranes. *N Engl J Med* 1986; **314:** 181.


**Ergot alkaloids.** For the effects of glyceryl trinitrate on *dihydroergotamine*, see p.468.

**Sildenafil.** The concurrent use of nitrates and sildenafil is contra-indicated. Significant hypotension may occur because the vasodilator actions of nitrates are potentiated by sildenafil.[1] Deaths due to a possible interaction have been reported.[2]


1. Webb DJ, *et al.* Sildenafil citrate potentiates the hypotensive effects of nitric oxide donor drugs in male patients with stable angina. *J Am Coll Cardiol* 2000; **36:** 25–31.
2. Cheitlin MD, *et al.* Use of sildenafil (Viagra) in patients with cardiovascular disease. *J Am Coll Cardiol* 1999; **33:** 273–82. Correction. *ibid.*; **34:** 1850.


**Thrombolytics.** For the effects of glyceryl trinitrate on *alteplase*, see p.857.

## Pharmacokinetics

Glyceryl trinitrate is rapidly absorbed from the oral mucosa. It is also well absorbed from the gastrointestinal tract and through the skin. Bioavailability is less than 100% following administration by any of these routes due to pre-systemic clearance; bioavailability is further reduced after oral administration owing to extensive first-pass metabolism in the liver.

Therapeutic effect is apparent within 1 to 3 minutes of administration of sublingual tablets, sublingual spray, or buccal tablets; within 30 to 60 minutes of administration of an ointment or transdermal patch; and within 1 to 2 minutes after intravenous administration.

Duration of action is about 30 to 60 minutes with sublingual tablets or spray and 3 to 5 hours with modified-release buccal tablets. Transdermal patches are designed to release a stated amount of drug over 24 hours, while therapeutic effects following application of glyceryl trinitrate ointment 2% persist for up to 8 hours. Duration of action following intravenous administration is about 3 to 5 minutes.

Glyceryl trinitrate is widely distributed with a large apparent volume of distribution. It is taken up by smooth muscle cells of blood vessels and the nitrate group is cleaved to inorganic nitrite and then to nitric oxide. This reaction requires the presence of cysteine or another thiol. Glyceryl trinitrate also undergoes hydrolysis in plasma and is rapidly metabolised in the liver by glutathione-organic nitrate reductase to dinitrates and mononitrates. The dinitrates are less potent vasodilators than glyceryl trinitrate; the mononitrates may have some vasodilator activity.

◊ References.


1. Bogaert MG. Clinical pharmacokinetics of glyceryl trinitrate following the use of systemic and topical preparations. *Clin Pharmacokinet* 1987; **12:** 1–11.
2. Thadani U, Whitsett T. Relationship of pharmacokinetic and pharmacodynamic properties of the organic nitrates. *Clin Pharmacokinet* 1988; **15:** 32–43.
3. Ridout G, *et al.* Pharmacokinetic considerations in the use of newer transdermal formulations. *Clin Pharmacokinet* 1988; **15:** 114–31.
4. Hashimoto S, Kobayashi A. Clinical pharmacokinetics and pharmacodynamics of glyceryl trinitrate and its metabolites. *Clin Pharmacokinet* 2003; **42:** 205–21.


## Uses and Administration

Glyceryl trinitrate is a nitrovasodilator used in the management of angina pectoris (p.813), heart failure (p.820), and myocardial infarction (below). Other indications include inducing hypotension and controlling hypertension during surgery.

Glyceryl trinitrate is believed to exert its vasodilator effect through release of nitric oxide, which causes stimulation of guanylate cyclase in the vascular smooth muscle cells; this results in an increase in cyclic guanosine monophosphate. This nucleotide induces relaxation, probably by lowering the free calcium concentration in the cytosol. In its action on vascular muscle, venous dilatation predominates over dilatation of the arterioles. Venous dilatation decreases venous return as a result of venous pooling, and lowers left ventricular diastolic volume and pressure (termed a reduction in preload). The smaller or less important dilatation of arterioles reduces both peripheral vascular resistance and left ventricular pressure at systole (termed a reduction in afterload). The consequent effect is a reduction in the primary determinants of myocardial oxygen demand. The effect on preload is not shared by beta blockers or calcium-channel blockers. Glyceryl trinitrate also has a coronary vasodilator effect which improves regional coronary blood flow to ischaemic areas resulting in improved oxygen supply to the myocardium.

Glyceryl trinitrate may be administered by the sublingual, buccal, oral, transdermal, or intravenous route. The dose and choice of formulation depend upon the clinical situation.

In the management of **acute angina** glyceryl trinitrate is given as sublingual tablets, a sublingual aerosol spray, or buccal tablets, which all produce a rapid onset of therapeutic effect and provide rapid relief of anginal pain. These dosage forms may also be used before an activity or stress which might provoke an attack. One sublingual tablet (usual strength 300 to 600 micrograms) is placed under the tongue. The dose may be repeated as required but patients should be advised to seek medical care if pain persists after a total of 3 doses within 15 minutes. If an aerosol spray is used one or two sprays of 400 micrograms each are directed onto or under the tongue, then the mouth is closed; three sprays may be used if necessary. Buccal tablets of glyceryl trinitrate are placed between the upper lip and gum (see below for precautions to be observed during use). A dose of 1 or 2 mg is usually sufficient, although 3 mg may be needed in some cases.

In the long-term management of **stable angina** glyceryl trinitrate is given as modified-release tablets or capsules, transdermal formulations, or buccal tablets, which all provide a long duration of action. Dosage varies according to the specific formulation. In the UK, for example, modified-release oral tablets are available that allow doses of up to 12.8 mg to be given up to three times daily. The transdermal formulations available are ointments and patches. With the ointment a measured amount (½ to 2 inches of glyceryl trinitrate ointment 2%) is applied 3 or 4 times daily, or every 3 to 4 hours if necessary, to the chest, arm, thigh, or back. Transdermal patches applied to the chest, upper arm, or shoulder are more convenient. Patches are generally designed to release glyceryl trinitrate at a constant rate; they are available in a range of sizes, releasing an average of 2.5 to 20 mg of glyceryl trinitrate over 24 hours (0.1 to 0.8 mg/hour). A maximum daily dose of 20 mg has been suggested. Glyceryl trinitrate ointment and patches should be applied to a fresh area of skin and several days should elapse before re-application to formerly used sites. Buccal tablets are used in doses of 1 to 5 mg three times daily. The tablets are retained in the buccal cavity; the rate of dissolution of the tablet can be increased by touching the tablet with the tongue or drinking hot liquids. It is common practice to remove the tablets at bedtime because of the risk of aspiration. Also patients using buccal tablets should be advised to alternate placement sites and pay close attention to oral hygiene to reduce the risk of dental caries. The tablets are not intended to be chewed; if the buccal tablet is inadvertently swallowed, another may be placed in the buccal cavity.

Tolerance tends to develop in the majority of patients on continuous nitrate therapy and nitrate-free intervals are often employed to avoid this problem (see above under Precautions, Nitrate Tolerance for further details).

In the management of **unstable angina** glyceryl trinitrate may be given by intravenous infusion. Manufacturers' guidelines for dilution of glyceryl trinitrate injection specify glucose 5% or sodium chloride 0.9% as the diluent. During intravenous administration of glyceryl trinitrate there should be haemodynamic monitoring of the patient with the dose being adjusted gradually to produce the desired response. The plastic used in the infusion equipment may adsorb glyceryl trinitrate (see Stability, above) and allowance may have to be made for this. The usual initial dose for unstable angina is 5 to 10 micrograms/minute. Most patients respond to doses between 10 and 200 micrograms/minute. The sublingual and buccal routes may also be used; doses of up to 5 mg as buccal tablets may be required to relieve pain in patients with unstable angina.

In the management of acute **heart failure** glyceryl trinitrate is given intravenously in an initial dose of 5 to 25 micrograms/minute. Buccal tablets have been used in doses of 5 mg repeated as needed until symptoms are controlled. In chronic heart failure buccal tablets may be given in doses of 5 to 10 mg three times daily.

Glyceryl trinitrate is also used intravenously in acute **myocardial infarction**, and to induce hypotension or control hypertension during **surgery**. The initial dose is 5 to 25 micrograms/minute, adjusted according to response. The usual range is 10 to 200 micrograms/minute but some surgical patients may require up to 400 micrograms/minute.

Glyceryl trinitrate has also been used as transdermal patches in the prophylactic treatment of **phlebitis and extravasation** secondary to venous cannulation. One 5-mg patch is applied distal to the intravenous site; the patch should be replaced at a different skin site either daily or after 3 to 4 days, depending on the patch. This treatment should continue only as long as the intravenous infusion is maintained.

**Anal fissure.** Nitrates such as glyceryl trinitrate are being studied in the treatment of chronic anal fissure (p.1390) because of their ability to relax the anal sphincter. Topical application of glyceryl trinitrate ointment in concentrations of 0.2 to 0.8% has relieved pain and aided healing of anal fissures both in uncontrolled[1-3] and controlled studies,[4,5] although it may be less effective than injection with botulinum toxin.[6] One study[5] found that a concentration of 0.6% had no additional benefit over 0.2%. Follow-up[5,7] of some of the patients indicated that after 6 to 38 months most had not experienced further problems or had had occasional recurrences (relapses of about one-quarter to one-third) which in the majority of cases had responded to further topical treatment. A small placebo-controlled study specifically in children, however, did not find topical glyceryl trinitrate to be of benefit in this patient population.[8]

There is evidence that application of a glyceryl trinitrate patch may be as effective as topical application of a 0.2% ointment.[9]

Encouraging results have also been obtained in an uncontrolled study using a 1% ointment of isosorbide dinitrate.[10]

1. Gorfine SR. Topical nitroglycerin therapy for anal fissures and ulcers. *N Engl J Med* 1995; **333:** 1156–7.
2. Lund JN *et al.* Use of glyceryl trinitrate ointment in the treatment of anal fissure. *Br J Surg* 1996; **83:** 776–7.
3. Watson SJ, *et al.* Topical glyceryl trinitrate in the treatment of chronic anal fissure. *Br J Surg* 1996; **83:** 771–5.
4. Lund JN, Scholefield JH. A randomised, prospective, double-blind, placebo-controlled trial of glyceryl trinitrate ointment in treatment of anal fissure. *Lancet* 1997; **349:** 11–14. Correction. *ibid.*; 656.
5. Carapeti EA, *et al.* Randomised controlled trial shows that glyceryl trinitrate heals anal fissures, higher doses are not more effective, and there is a high recurrence rate. *Gut* 1999; **44:** 727–30.
6. Brisinda G, *et al.* A comparison of injections of botulinum toxin and topical nitroglycerin ointment for the treatment of chronic anal fissure. *N Engl J Med* 1999; **341:**65–9. Correction. *ibid.*; 624.
7. Lund JN, Scholefield JH. Follow-up of patients with chronic anal fissure treated with topical glyceryl trinitrate. *Lancet* 1998; **352:** 1681.
8. Kenny SE, *et al.* Double blind randomised controlled trial of topical glyceryl trinitrate in anal fissure. *Arch Dis Child* 2001; **85:** 404–7.
9. Zuberi BF, *et al.* A randomized trial of glyceryl trinitrate ointment and nitroglycerin patch in healing of anal fissures. *Int J Colorectal Dis* 2000; **15:** 243–5.
10. Schouten WR, *et al.* Pathophysiological aspects and clinical outcome of intra-anal application of isosorbide dinitrate in patients with chronic anal fissure. *Gut* 1996; **39:** 465–9.

**Erectile dysfunction.** Erectile dysfunction (p.1745) has been managed by the penile injection of drugs such as papaverine or alprostadil although oral treatment with drugs such as sildenafil is now available. Penile injections are not always acceptable to the patient and a number of studies have investigated topical therapies, mostly glyceryl trinitrate applied either as ointment or as a transdermal delivery system to the penis.[1-4] Such treatment can produce erections in some subjects, although response rates vary. However, patients must wear a condom to protect their partner against potential adverse effects resulting from the transfer of glyceryl trinitrate. The mechanism of action of glyceryl trinitrate is believed to be due to smooth muscle relaxation and vasodilatation which are necessary prerequisites for penile erection.

Topical application of a cream containing isosorbide dinitrate, co-dergocrine mesilate, and aminophylline produced satisfactory erections in 21 of 36 men with erectile dysfunction due to various causes.[5] Eight out of 9 men with erectile dysfunction of psychogenic origin reported a satisfactory response. However, another study[6] was abandoned after the cream produced no effect in 10 consecutive patients. A further study in 14 patients who received a total of 77 applications of the cream reported no benefit over placebo.[7] Topical treatment with a cream containing isosorbide dinitrate, co-dergocrine mesilate, and testosterone has also been tried for erectile dysfunction; in a study in 42 men with low sexual interest and low or slightly depressed testosterone levels, 28 reported beneficial results.[8]

It should be noted that topical nitrates must not be employed in patients already using sildenafil (see under Interactions, above).

1. Heaton JPW, *et al.* Topical glyceryl trinitrate causes measurable penile arterial dilation in impotent men. *J Urol (Baltimore)* 1990; **143:** 729–31.
2. Meyhoff HH, *et al.* Non-invasive management of impotence with transcutaneous nitroglycerin. *Br J Urol* 1992; **69:** 88–90.
3. Nunez BD, Anderson DC. Nitroglycerin ointment in the treatment of impotence. *J Urol (Baltimore)* 1993; **150:** 1241–3.
4. Anderson DC, Seifert CF. Topical nitrate treatment of impotence. *Ann Pharmacother* 1993; **27:** 1203–5.
5. Gomaa A, *et al.* Topical treatment of erectile dysfunction: randomised double blind placebo controlled trial of cream containing aminophylline, isosorbide dinitrate, and co-dergocrine mesylate. *BMJ* 1996; **312:** 1512–15.
6. Naude JH, Le Roux PJ. Topical treatment of erectile dysfunction did not show results. *BMJ* 1998; **316:** 1318.
7. Le Roux PJ, Naude JH. Topical vasoactive cream in the treatment of erectile failure: a prospective, randomized placebo-controlled trial. *BJU Int* 1999; **83:** 810–11.
8. Gomaa A, *et al.* The effect of topically applied vasoactive agents and testosterone versus testosterone in the treatment of erectile dysfunction in aged men with low sexual interest. *Int J Impot Res* 2001; **13:** 93–9.

**Gallstones.** Endoscopic removal of gallstones (p.1761) in a small series of 15 patients was facilitated by glyceryl trinitrate 1.2 to 3.6 mg applied as a spray to the tongue. Glyceryl trinitrate 1.2 mg was shown to relax the sphincter of Oddi to approximately 30% of its normal pressure.[1] The ability of glyceryl trinitrate to relax smooth muscle has also been employed to relieve biliary colic (p.4) in 3 patients with gallstones;[2] in one of these patients standard managements for the pain such as oral opioids had been only moderately effective.

1. Staritz M, *et al.* Nitroglycerine dilatation of sphincter of Oddi for endoscopic removal of bileduct stones. *Lancet* 1984; **i:** 956.
2. Hassel B. Treatment of biliary colic with nitroglycerin. *Lancet* 1993; **342:** 1305.

**Migraine.** Although use of glyceryl trinitrate may precipitate or exacerbate migraine (p.464) inhalation of glyceryl trinitrate at the onset of a migraine aura aborted attacks in a patient at risk of permanent neurological damage from migraine. Standard prophylactic therapy had previously been unsuccessful.[1]

1. Mitchell GK. Nitroglycerine by inhaler as treatment for migraine causing cerebral ischaemia. *Med J Aust* 1999; **171:** 336.

**Myocardial infarction.** The management of myocardial infarction (p.828) can involve numerous drug therapies including nitrates.

Nitrovasodilatation with intravenous glyceryl trinitrate or sodium nitroprusside, started within 24 hours of the onset of pain, has been associated with a reduction in mortality.[1] However, this was before the routine use of thrombolytics, and the role of nitrates in addition to standard treatment (with a thrombolytic, oral aspirin, and intravenous beta blocker) is less clear. The empirical use of intravenous glyceryl trinitrate in the acute phase of myocardial infarction is widespread and appears to be safe, as was demonstrated in the GISSI-3 study.[2] In this study glyceryl trinitrate was given by intravenous infusion during the first 24 hours, starting at 5 micrograms/minute and increasing by 5 to 20 micrograms/minute every 5 minutes for the first half hour until systolic blood pressure fell by at least 10% provided it remained above 90 mmHg; after 24 hours it was replaced by a transdermal patch providing 10 mg daily.

Some patients, for example those with myocardial ischaemia or poor left ventricular function, may require the long-term administration of nitrates, but recent studies have thrown doubt on their routine use. In the GISSI-3 study there was no significant benefit from the use of transdermal glyceryl trinitrate when assessed 6 weeks[2] and 6 months[3] post-infarction and in the ISIS-4 study[4] oral isosorbide mononitrate apparently had no effect on 35-day mortality.

1. Yusuf S, *et al.* Effect of intravenous nitrates on mortality in acute myocardial infarction: an overview of the randomised trials. *Lancet* 1988; **i:** 1088–92.
2. Gruppo Italiano per lo Studio della Sopravvivenza nell'Infarto Miocardico. GISSI-3: effects of lisinopril and transdermal glyceryl trinitrate singly and together on 6-week mortality and ventricular function after acute myocardial infarction. *Lancet* 1994; **343:** 1115–22.
3. Gruppo Italiano per lo Studio della Sopravvivenza nell'Infarto Miocardico. Six-month effects of early treatment with lisinopril and transdermal glyceryl trinitrate singly and together withdrawn six weeks after myocardial infarction: the GISSI-3 trial. *J Am Coll Cardiol* 1996; **27:** 337–44.
4. ISIS-4 (Fourth International Study of Infarct Survival) Collaborative Group. ISIS-4: a randomised factorial trial assessing early oral captopril, oral mononitrate, and intravenous magnesium sulphate in 58 050 patients with suspected acute myocardial infarction. *Lancet* 1995; **345:** 669–85.

**Obstetrics and gynaecology.** The smooth muscle relaxant properties of glyceryl trinitrate have been used in various obstetric or gynaecological situations although most reports are anecdotal or include small numbers of patients. The intravenous injection of glyceryl trinitrate 50 to 100 micrograms repeated to a total dose of 200 micrograms if necessary has produced sufficient uterine relaxation in postpartum women for the manual extraction of retained placentas.[1,2] Administration by sublingual spray has also been used successfully to facilitate breech extraction in a set of twins.[3]

Glyceryl trinitrate has been given as a sublingual spray to relax the cervix prior to IUD insertion. In a series of over 100 patients one or two doses of 400 micrograms sublingually were usually adequate.[4]

Beneficial results have been reported in women with possible premature labour (p.794) following application of glyceryl trinitrate patches to the abdomen,[5,6] and in one study[7] this was as effective as ritodrine infusion. However, another study[8] comparing glyceryl trinitrate and magnesium sulfate, both given intravenously, found that glyceryl trinitrate was associated with a higher failure rate and a greater reduction in maternal blood pressure.

Transdermal glyceryl trinitrate has been tried for controlling pain in severe and moderate-to-severe dysmenorrhoea[9,10] (p.6).

Glyceryl trinitrate has been given intravenously in the management of pre-eclampsia (see under Hypertension, p.825) and is reported to reduce blood pressure without compromising uterine blood flow.[11]

Isosorbide mononitrate administered vaginally has been found to produce cervical ripening[12] and may be an alternative to prostaglandins for this purpose before first trimester termination of pregnancy (p.1512).

1. DeSimone CA, *et al.* Intravenous nitro-glycerin aids manual extraction of a retained placenta. *Anesthesiology* 1990; **73:** 787.
2. Lowenwirt IP, *et al.* Safety of intravenous glyceryl trinitrate in management of retained placenta. *Aust N Z J Obstet Gynaecol* 1997; **37:** 20–4.
3. Greenspoon JS, Kovacic A. Breech extraction facilitated by glyceryl trinitrate sublingual spray. *Lancet* 1991; **338:** 124–5.
4. Yadava RP. Sublingual glyceryl trinitrate spray facilitates IUD insertion. *Br J Sex Med* 1990; **17:** 217.
5. Lees C, *et al.* Arrest of preterm labour and prolongation of gestation with glyceryl trinitrate, a nitric oxide donor. *Lancet* 1994; **343:** 1325–6.
6. Smith GN, *et al.* Randomised, double-blind, placebo controlled pilot study assessing nitroglycerin as a tocolytic. *Br J Obstet Gynaecol* 1999; **106:** 736–9.
7. Lees CC, *et al.* Glyceryl trinitrate and ritodrine in tocolysis: an international multicenter randomized study. *Obstet Gynecol* 1999; **94:** 403–8.
8. El-Sayed YY, *et al.* Randomized comparison of intravenous nitroglycerin and magnesium sulfate for treatment of preterm labor. *Obstet Gynecol* 1999; **93:** 79–83.
9. Pittrof R, *et al.* Crossover study of glyceryl trinitrate patches for controlling pain in women with severe dysmenorrhoea. *BMJ* 1996; **312:** 884.
10. The Transdermal Nitroglycerine/Dysmenorrhoea Study Group. Transdermal nitroglycerine in the management of pain associated with primary dysmenorrhoea: a multinational pilot study. *J Int Med Res* 1997; **25:** 41–4.
11. Grunewald C, *et al.* Effects of nitroglycerin on the uterine and umbilical circulation in severe preeclampsia. *Obstet Gynecol* 1995; **86:** 600–4.
12. Thomson AJ, *et al.* Randomised trial of nitric oxide donor versus prostaglandin for cervical ripening before first-trimester termination of pregnancy. *Lancet* 1998; **352:** 1093–6.

**Oesophageal motility disorders.** Achalasia is obstruction caused by failure of the lower oesophageal sphincter to relax and permit passage of food into the stomach. Nitrates such as isosorbide dinitrate have been reported to produce effective relaxation and to reduce symptoms when administered sublingually.

They have a role when mechanical dilatation of the sphincter or surgery are not feasible (see Oesophageal Motility Disorders, p.1246).

Nitrates may also be employed in oesophageal disorders such as variceal haemorrhage (see below).

**Peripheral vascular disease.** In peripheral vascular disease (p.831) nitrates have been tried as vasodilators and smooth muscle relaxants in order to improve resting blood flow. Glyceryl trinitrate has been applied topically in patients with Raynaud's syndrome[1-3] and in distal limb ischaemia[4] resulting in some benefit but this form of therapy is not widely used in these disorders.


1. Franks AG. Topical glyceryl trinitrate as adjunctive treatment in Raynaud's disease. *Lancet* 1982; **i:** 76–7.
2. Coppock JS, *et al.* Objective relief of vasospasm by glyceryl trinitrate in secondary Raynaud's phenomenon. *Postgrad Med J* 1986; **62:** 15–18.
3. Teh LS, *et al.* Sustained-release transdermal glyceryl trinitrate patches as a treatment for primary and secondary Raynaud's phenomenon. *Br J Rheumatol* 1995; **34:** 636–41.
4. Fletcher S, *et al.* Locally applied transdermal nitrate patches for the treatment of ischaemic rest pain. *Int J Clin Pract* 1997; **51:** 324–5.


**Pulmonary hypertension.** Glyceryl trinitrate reduces total pulmonary resistance in most patients with primary pulmonary hypertension (p.832).[1,2] However, other vasodilators such as calcium-channel blockers or epoprostenol are generally preferred for long-term treatment.


1. Pearl RG, *et al.* Acute hemodynamic effects of nitroglycerin in pulmonary hypertension. *Ann Intern Med* 1983; **99:** 9–13.
2. Weir EK, *et al.* The acute administration of vasodilators in primary pulmonary hypertension. *Am Rev Respir Dis* 1989; **140:** 1623–30.


**Quinine oculotoxicity.** Intravenous nitrate administration has been suggested for the management of quinine oculotoxicity (p.461) and its benefit may be due to an increase in retinal vascular bed flow.[1]


1. Moore D, *et al.* Research into quinine ocular toxicity. *Br J Ophthalmol* 1992; **76:** 703.


**Variceal haemorrhage.** The usual treatment in variceal haemorrhage (p.1716) is injection sclerotherapy or banding ligation which may be performed during the emergency endoscopy procedure. Where endoscopy is unavailable drug therapy may be used; it may also have a role when sclerotherapy fails and some have suggested that initial drug therapy may be preferable to sclerotherapy. Vasoconstrictors that are used include vasopressin and its analogue terlipressin, given together with glyceryl trinitrate which counteracts the adverse cardiac effects of vasopressin while potentiating its beneficial effects on portal pressure; somatostatin is also used.

Prophylaxis of a first bleed in patients with portal hypertension is controversial since about 70% of patients who have varices will never bleed. It is postulated that a reduction in portal pressure to below 12 mmHg is necessary to reduce the incidence of variceal bleeding and that treatment with beta blockers alone does not achieve this. More effective drugs are being sought and isosorbide mononitrate (as adjunctive therapy with a beta blocker) is under investigation, both for prophylaxis of a first bleed[1,2] and in the prevention of rebleeding.[3] Early emergency treatment (before endoscopy) with terlipressin given intravenously and glyceryl trinitrate transdermally controlled bleeding and lowered mortality rates in patients with gastrointestinal bleeding and a history or clinical signs of cirrhosis.[4] However, use of oral isosorbide mononitrate with somatostatin infusion for acute variceal bleeding was less effective than somatostatin alone and induced more adverse effects.[5]


1. Angelico M, *et al.* Isosorbide-5-mononitrate versus propranolol in the prevention of first bleeding in cirrhosis. *Gastroenterology* 1993; **104:** 1460–5.
2. Merkel C, *et al.* Randomised trial of nadolol alone or with isosorbide mononitrate for primary prophylaxis of variceal bleeding in cirrhosis. *Lancet* 1996; **348:** 1677–81.
3. Villanueva C, *et al.* Nadolol plus isosorbide mononitrate compared with sclerotherapy for the prevention of variceal rebleeding. *N Engl J Med* 1996; **334:** 1624–9.
4. Levacher S, *et al.* Early administration of terlipressin plus glyceryl trinitrate to control active upper gastrointestinal bleeding in cirrhotic patients. *Lancet* 1995; **346:** 865–8.
5. Junquera F, *et al.* Somatostatin plus isosorbide 5-mononitrate versus somatostatin in the control of acute gastro-oesophageal variceal bleeding: a double blind, randomised, placebo controlled clinical trial. *Gut* 2000; **46:** 127–32.


**Venepuncture.** Glyceryl trinitrate patches applied to skin adjacent to intravenous infusion sites are used in the prophylactic treatment of phlebitis and extravasation.[1]

Local application of glyceryl trinitrate 1 to 2 mg as ointment was found to be a useful aid to venepuncture in a study of 50 patients undergoing surgery,[2] but conflicting results have been reported in children and neonates.[3,4]


1. Tjon JA, Ansani NT. Transdermal nitroglycerin for the prevention of intravenous infusion failure due to phlebitis and extravasation. *Ann Pharmacother* 2000; **34:** 1189–92.
2. Hecker JF, *et al.* Nitroglycerine ointment as an aid to venepuncture. *Lancet* 1983; **i:** 332–3.
3. Vaksmann G, *et al.* Nitroglycerine ointment as aid to venous cannulation in children. *J Pediatr* 1987; **111:** 89–91.
4. Maynard EC, Oh W. Topical nitroglycerin ointment as an aid to insertion of peripheral venous catheters in neonates. *J Pediatr* 1989; **114:** 474–6.


## Preparations

***BP 2003:*** Glyceryl Trinitrate Sublingual Spray; Glyceryl Trinitrate Tablets; Glyceryl Trinitrate Transdermal Patches;
***USP 27:*** Nitroglycerin Injection; Nitroglycerin Ointment; Nitroglycerin Tablets.

**Proprietary Preparations** (details are given in Part 3)
***Arg.:*** Dauxona; Enetege; Minitran; Niglinar; Nitradisc; Nitroderm TTS; Nitrogray; ***Austral.:*** Anginine; Minitran; Nitradisc†; Nitro-Bid†; Nitro-Dur; Nitrolingual; Rectogesic; Transiderm-Nitro; ***Austria:*** Cordiplast; Deponit; Minitran; Nitro; Nitro Mack; Nitro Pohl; Nitro-Dur; Nitroderm; Nitrolingual; Nitronal†; Nitrong†; Perlinganit; ***Belg.:*** Deponit; Diafusor; Minitran; Nitroderm; Nitrodyl; Nitrolingual; Nitrong†; Nysconitrine; Trinipatch; Willlong; ***Braz.:*** Deponit†; Nitradisc†; Nitroderm TTS; Nitronal; Tridil; ***Canad.:*** Minitran; Nitro-Dur; Nitroject; Nitrol; Nitrolingual; Nitrong; Nitrostat; Transderm-Nitro; Tridil†; Trinipatch†; ***Chile:*** Angiolingual; Nitrocor; Nitroderm; Nitronal; ***Denm.:*** Buccard; Discotrine; Glytrin; Nitrolingual†; Nitromex; Nitrong†; Transiderm-Nitro†; ***Fin.:*** Deponit; Minitran; Nitro; Nitromex; Perlinganit; Transiderm-Nitro; ***Fr.:*** Cordipatch; Corditrine†; Diafusor; Discotrine; Epinitril; Lenitral; Natispray; Nitriderm TTS; Optizor†; Trinipatch; ***Ger.:*** Aquo-Trinitrosan; Corangin Nitrokapseln and Nitrospray; Coro-Nitro; Deponit; Gepan; Gilustenon†; MinitranS; neos nitro OPT; Nitradisc†; Nitrangin; Nitrangin forte†; Nitro Mack; Nitro Solvay; Nitro-Pflaster-ratiopharm TL; Nitroderm TTS; Nitrokapseln-ratiopharm†; Nitrokor; Nitrolingual; Nitronal†; Perlinganit; Trinitrosan; Turicard†; ***Gr.:*** Nitro Mack; Nitrodyl; Nitrolingual; Nitrong; Nitroretard-Faran; Pancoran; Sodemethin; Supranitrin; Trinipatch; Trinitrine Simple Laleuf; ***Hong Kong:*** Angised; Deponit; Glytrin†; Lenitral; Minitran†; Nitro Mack; Nitro Pohl; Nitro-Dur; Nitrocine; Nitroderm TTS; Nitroglyn†; Nitrolingual; Nitronal†; Nitropulse†; Nitrostat†; Tridil; ***India:*** Angised; Millisrol; Myonit; Myovin; Nitrocontin; Nitroderm TTS; Nitrogesic; ***Irl.:*** Angised†; Deponit; Epinitril; Glytrin; Nitro-Dur; Nitrocine; Nitrolingual; Nitromin; Nitronal; Suscard; Sustac; Transiderm-Nitro; Tridil†; ***Israel:*** Angised; Deponit; Nitrocine; Nitroderm TTS; Nitrolingual; Nitronal; Nitrovis†; Trinipatch; ***Ital.:*** Adesitrin; Deponit; Dermatrans; Epinitril; Minitran; Natispray; Nitro-Dur; Nitroderm TTS; Nitrosylon; Perganit; Top-Nitro; Triniplas; Trinitrina; Venitrin; ***Jpn:*** Millisrol; ***Malaysia:*** Deponit; Glytrin; Nitrocine; Nitroderm; ***Mex.:*** Anglix; Cardinit; Minitran; Nitradisc; Nitro-Dur; Nitroder†; Nitroderm TTS; ***Neth.:*** Deponit; Glytrin; Minitran; Nitro Pohl†; Nitro-Dur; Nitrolingual; Nitrostat; Transiderm-Nitro; Trinipatch; ***Norw.:*** Minitran; Nitro-Dur; Nitrolingual; Nitromex; Nitroven; Suscard†; Transiderm-Nitro; ***NZ:*** Anginine; Glytrin; Minitran; Nitroderm; Nitrolingual; Nitronal; ***Port.:*** Nitradisc; Nitro-Dur; Nitroderm TTS; Nitromint; Plastranit; Trinipatch; ***S.Afr.:*** Angised; Nitradisc†; Nitrocine; Nitroderm TTS†; Nitrolingual; Tridil; ***Singapore:*** Angised†; Deponit; Glytrin†; Lenitral†; Nitro Mack; Nitrocine; ***Spain:*** Cardiodisco†; Cordiplast; Dermatrans; Diafusor; Epinitril; Minitran; Nitradisc; Nitro-Dur; Nitroderm; Nitropacin†; Nitroplast; Nitrotard†; Solinitrina; Trinipatch; Trinispray; Vernies; ***Swed.:*** Glytrin; Minitran; Nitrolingual; Nitromex; Nitrong†; Perlinganit; Suscard; Transiderm-Nitro; ***Switz.:*** Deponit; Minitran; Natispray†; Niong retard†; Nitro Mack; Nitro-Dur; Nitroderm TTS; Nitrolingual; Nitromint†; Nitronal; Perlinganit; Trinitrine; ***Thai.:*** Amitacon; Angised; Deponit†; Glytrin; Minitran†; Nitradisc†; Nitro Mack; Nitrocine; Nitroderm; Nitroject; Willlong†; ***UK:*** Coro-Nitro; Deponit; Glytrin; Minitran; Nitro-Dur; Nitrocine; Nitrolingual; Nitromin; Nitronal; Percutol; Suscard; Sustac; Transiderm-Nitro; Trintek; ***USA:*** Deponit†; Minitran; Nitrek; Nitro-Bid; Nitro-Derm; Nitro-Dur; Nitro-Time; Nitrodisc; Nitrogard; Nitroglyn; Nitrol†; Nitrolingual; Nitrong; Nitro-Quick; Nitrostat; NitroTab; Transderm-Nitro; Transdermal-NTG; Tridil.

**Multi-ingredient:** ***Arg.:*** Trinitron; ***Austria:*** Myocardon; Spasmocor; ***Ger.:*** Angiocardyl N†; Nitrangin compositum; Nitro-cum†; Nitro-Praecordin N†; ***Spain:*** Cafinitrina; ***USA:*** Emergent-Ez.

---

## Guabenxan *(rINN)*

Guabenxán. (1,4-Benzodioxan-6-ylmethyl)guanidine.
$C_{10}H_{13}N_3O_2 = 207.2$.
*CAS — 19889-45-3.*

### Profile

Guabenxan is an antihypertensive with properties similar to guanethidine (below). It has been given by mouth as the sulfate.

---

## Guanabenz Acetate *(USAN, rINNM)*

Acetato de guanabenzo; NSC-68982 (guanabenz); Wy-8678 (guanabenz). (2,6-Dichlorobenzylideneamino)guanidine acetate.
$C_8H_8Cl_2N_4,C_2H_4O_2 = 291.1$.
*CAS — 5051-62-7 (guanabenz); 23256-50-0 (guanabenz acetate).*

**Pharmacopoeias.** In *Jpn* and *US*.

**USP 27** (Guanabenz Acetate). A white or almost white powder with not more than a slight odour. Sparingly soluble in water and in 0.1N hydrochloric acid; soluble in alcohol and in propylene glycol. A 0.7% solution in water has a pH of 5.5 to 7.0. Store in airtight containers. Protect from light.

### Adverse Effects and Precautions

As for Clonidine Hydrochloride, p.885.

**Overdosage.** Overdosage with guanabenz has been reported.[1] The main symptoms were lethargy, drowsiness, bradycardia, and hypotension. A 45-year-old woman who had taken 200 to 240 mg of guanabenz with alcohol recovered following gastric lavage and intravenous fluids; a 3-year-old child who had taken 12 mg of guanabenz responded to atropine and dopamine. Naloxone had little effect in either patient.


1. Hall AH, *et al.* Guanabenz overdose. *Ann Intern Med* 1985; **102:** 787–8.


### Interactions

As for Clonidine Hydrochloride, p.886.

### Pharmacokinetics

Following oral administration guanabenz is well absorbed and undergoes extensive first-pass metabolism. Peak plasma concentrations occur about 2 to 5 hours after a dose. It is about 90% bound to plasma proteins. Guanabenz is mainly excreted in urine, almost entirely as metabolites; about 10 to 30% is excreted in faeces. The average elimination half-life is reported to range from 4 to 14 hours.

### Uses and Administration

Guanabenz is an $alpha_2$-adrenoceptor agonist with actions and uses similar to those of clonidine (p.886). It is used in the management of hypertension (p.825), either alone or with other antihypertensives, particularly thiazide diuretics.

Guanabenz is given by mouth as the acetate, but doses are usually expressed in terms of the base. Guanabenz acetate 5 mg is approximately equivalent to 4 mg of guanabenz.

In hypertension, the usual dose is 4 mg twice daily initially; the daily dose may be increased by amounts of 4 to 8 mg every 1 to 2 weeks according to response. Doses of up to 32 mg twice daily have been used.

### Preparations

***USP 27:*** Guanabenz Acetate Tablets.

**Proprietary Preparations** (details are given in Part 3)
***Austria:*** Rexitene†; Wytensin†; ***Braz.:*** Lisapres; Tenelid†; ***USA:*** Wytensin.

---

## Guanadrel Sulfate *(USAN, rINNM)*

CL-1388R; Guanadrel Sulphate; Sulfato de guanadrel; U-28288D. 1-(Cyclohexanespiro-2′-[1′,3′]dioxolan-4′-ylmethyl)guanidine sulphate; 1-(1,4-Dioxaspiro[4.5]dec-2-ylmethyl)guanidine sulphate.
$(C_{10}H_{19}N_3O_2)_2,H_2SO_4 = 524.6$.
*CAS — 40580-59-4 (guanadrel); 22195-34-2 (guanadrel sulfate).*

**Pharmacopoeias.** In *US*.

**USP 27** (Guanadrel Sulfate). A white to off-white crystalline powder. Soluble in water; slightly soluble in alcohol and in acetone; sparingly soluble in methyl alcohol.

### Adverse Effects, Treatment, and Precautions

As for Guanethidine Monosulfate, below. Guanadrel has been reported to cause less diarrhoea, and less orthostatic hypotension on rising in the morning, than guanethidine, but orthostatic symptoms seem to occur with a similar frequency to guanethidine during the day.

### Interactions

As for Guanethidine Monosulfate, below.

### Pharmacokinetics

Guanadrel is rapidly and almost completely absorbed from the gastrointestinal tract, with a reported bioavailability of about 85%. It is widely distributed throughout the body and about 20% is bound to plasma proteins. It is reported not to cross the blood-brain barrier. Plasma concentrations decline in a biphasic manner: the half-life varies widely between individuals, in the initial phase from 1 to 4 hours, and in the terminal phase from 5 to 45 hours, with a mean of about 10 hours. Guanadrel is metabolised in the liver and about 85% is excreted in the urine over 24 hours as the unchanged drug and its metabolites. About 40 to 50% of the drug is excreted unchanged.

### Uses and Administration

Guanadrel is an antihypertensive with actions and uses similar to those of guanethidine (below). Following oral administration, guanadrel acts within 2 hours with the maximum effect after 4 to 6 hours. The hypotensive effect is reported to last for 4 to 14 hours following a single dose. It is used in the management of hypertension (p.825), although it has largely been superseded by other drugs less likely to cause orthostatic hypotension.

Guanadrel is given by mouth as the sulfate. The usual initial dose is 5 mg twice daily adjusted at weekly or monthly intervals according to the patient's response. The maintenance dose is normally in the range of 20 to 75 mg daily in two or more divided doses.

**Administration in renal impairment.** Renal and non-renal clearance of guanadrel was decreased in 16 patients with renal impairment compared with 6 healthy subjects, and this was reflected in a prolongation of the terminal elimination half-life from a mean of 3.69 hours to 6.8, 12.6, and 19.2 hours in patients with mild, moderate, and severe impairment. respectively.[1] It was suggested that the dose of guanadrel should be adjusted in patients with renal impairment, perhaps by giving the daily dose every 2 to 3 days in mild to moderate impairment and every 5 days in severe impairment.


1. Halstenson CE, *et al.* Disposition of guanadrel in subjects with normal and impaired renal function. *J Clin Pharmacol* 1989; **29:** 128–32.


### Preparations

***USP 27:*** Guanadrel Sulfate Tablets.

**Proprietary Preparations** (details are given in Part 3)
***USA:*** Hylorel†.

---

## Guanethidine Monosulfate *(USAN, rINNM)*

Guanethidine Monosulphate *(BANM)*; Guanethidini Monosulfas; Monosulfato de guanetidina; NSC-29863 (guanethidine hemisulfate); Su-5864 (guanethidine hemisulfate). 1-[2-(Perhydroazocin-1-yl)ethyl]guanidine monosulphate.
$C_{10}H_{22}N_4,H_2SO_4 = 296.4$.
*CAS — 55-65-2 (guanethidine); 60-02-6 (guanethidine hemisulfate); 645-43-2 (guanethidine monosulfate).*
*ATC — C02CC02; S01EX01.*

**Pharmacopoeias.** In *Eur.* (see p.vi), *Jpn*, and *US.*
*Chin.* includes the hemisulfate.

**Ph. Eur. 5.0** (Guanethidine Monosulphate). A colourless crystalline powder. Freely soluble in water; practically insoluble in alcohol. A 2% solution in water has a pH of 4.7 to 5.5. Protect from light.

**USP 27** (Guanethidine Monosulfate). A white to off-white crystalline powder. Very soluble in water; sparingly soluble in alcohol; practically insoluble in chloroform. A 2% solution in water has a pH of 4.7 to 5.7.

## Adverse Effects

The commonest side-effects with guanethidine are severe postural and exertional hypotension and diarrhoea which may be particularly troublesome during the initial stages of therapy and during dose adjustment. Dizziness, syncope, muscle weakness, and lassitude are liable to occur, especially on rising from sitting or lying. Orthostatic hypotension may be severe enough to provoke angina, renal impairment, and transient cerebral ischaemia. Other frequent side-effects are bradycardia, failure of ejaculation, fatigue, headache, and salt and water retention and oedema, which may be accompanied by breathlessness and may occasionally precipitate overt heart failure.

Nausea, vomiting, dry mouth, nasal congestion, parotid tenderness, blurring of vision, depression, myalgia, muscle tremor, paraesthesias, hair loss, dermatitis, disturbed micturition, priapism, aggravation or precipitation of asthma, and exacerbation of peptic ulcer disease have also been reported. Guanethidine may possibly cause anaemia, leucopenia, and thrombocytopenia.

When guanethidine is used as eye drops, common side-effects are conjunctival hyperaemia and miosis. Burning sensations and ptosis have also occurred. Superficial punctate keratitis has been reported particularly following prolonged use of high doses.

## Treatment of Adverse Effects

Withdrawal of guanethidine or reduction in dosage reverses many adverse effects. Diarrhoea may be controlled by reducing dosage or by giving codeine phosphate or antimuscarinics. If overdosage occurs the stomach should be emptied by lavage and activated charcoal may be given. Hypotension may respond to placing the patient in the supine position with the feet raised. If hypotension is severe it may be necessary to give intravenous fluid replacement and small doses of vasopressors may be given cautiously. The patient must be monitored for several days.

## Precautions

Guanethidine should not be given to patients with phaeochromocytoma, as it may cause a hypertensive crisis, or to patients with heart failure not caused by hypertension.

It should be used with caution in patients with renal impairment, cerebrovascular disorders, or ischaemic heart disease, or with a history of peptic ulcer disease or asthma. Exercise and heat may increase the hypotensive effect of guanethidine, and dosage requirements may be reduced in patients who develop fever.

There may be an increased risk of cardiovascular collapse or cardiac arrest in patients undergoing surgery while taking guanethidine, but authorities differ as to whether the drug should be discontinued before elective surgery. Some authorities have recommended discontinuation up to 2 or 3 weeks beforehand. In patients undergoing emergency procedures or where treatment has not been interrupted large doses of atropine should be given before induction of anaesthesia.

Patients undergoing treatment with eye drops containing guanethidine should be examined regularly for signs of conjunctival damage.

## Interactions

Patients taking guanethidine may show increased sensitivity to the action of adrenaline, amfetamine, and other sympathomimetics resulting in exaggerated pressor effects. The hypotensive effects may also be antagonised by tricyclic antidepressants, MAOIs, and phenothiazine derivatives and related antipsychotics (although phenothiazines may also exacerbate orthostatic hypotension, which may be more relevant clinically). In the UK the manufacturers suggest that MAOIs should be stopped at least 14 days before beginning guanethidine, although in the USA a minimum of a week has been recommended as adequate. It has been reported that oral contraceptives may reduce the hypotensive action of guanethidine. Concurrent use of digoxin or other digitalis derivatives with guanethidine may cause excessive bradycardia.

The hypotensive effects of guanethidine may be enhanced by thiazide diuretics, other antihypertensives, and levodopa. Alcohol may cause orthostatic hypotension in patients taking guanethidine.

## Pharmacokinetics

Guanethidine is variably and incompletely absorbed from the gastrointestinal tract with less than 50% of the dose reaching the systemic circulation. It is actively taken up into adrenergic neurones by the mechanism responsible for noradrenaline reuptake. A plasma concentration of 8 nanograms/mL is reported to be necessary for adrenergic blockade, but the dose required to achieve this varies between individuals due to differences in absorption and metabolism. Guanethidine is partially metabolised in the liver, and is excreted in the urine as metabolites and unchanged guanethidine. It has a terminal half-life of about 5 days. Guanethidine does not penetrate the blood-brain barrier significantly.

## Uses and Administration

Guanethidine is an antihypertensive that acts by selectively inhibiting transmission in postganglionic adrenergic nerves. It is believed to act mainly by preventing the release of noradrenaline at nerve endings. Guanethidine causes the depletion of noradrenaline stores in peripheral sympathetic nerve terminals but does not prevent the secretion of catecholamines by the adrenal medulla.

When given by mouth its maximal effects may take 1 to 3 weeks to appear on continued dosing and persist for 1 to 3 weeks after treatment has been stopped. It causes an initial reduction in cardiac output but its main hypotensive effect is to cause peripheral vasodilatation; it reduces the vasoconstriction which normally results from standing up and which is the result of reflex sympathetic nervous activity. In the majority of patients it reduces the standing blood pressure but has a less marked effect on the supine blood pressure. When applied topically to the eye guanethidine reduces the production of aqueous humour.

Guanethidine is used in the management of hypertension (p.825). Eye drops of guanethidine have been used for open-angle glaucoma (p.1485) and for lid retraction associated with hyperthyroidism. Guanethidine has also been used in the management of neuropathic pain syndromes (see below).

Guanethidine is used in the treatment of hypertension when other drugs have proved inadequate, although it has largely been superseded by other drugs less likely to cause orthostatic hypotension. Tolerance to guanethidine has occurred in some patients; this may be countered by concomitant diuretic therapy.

In **hypertension**, the usual initial dose of guanethidine monosulfate is 10 mg daily by mouth. This is increased by increments of 10 to 12.5 mg, not more often than every 5 to 7 days, according to response. The usual maintenance dose is 25 to 50 mg once daily.

Children have been given 200 micrograms/kg daily with increments of 200 micrograms/kg every 7 to 10 days until a satisfactory response is achieved.

Guanethidine monosulfate has been given intramuscularly in the treatment of hypertensive crises, including severe pre-eclampsia, but more suitable drugs are available. An intramuscular dose of 10 to 20 mg is reported to produce a fall in blood pressure within 30 minutes.

Eye drops containing guanethidine monosulfate have been used in the treatment of open-angle **glaucoma** (usually combined with adrenaline), and for the lid retraction that may accompany hyperthyroidism.

**Pain syndromes.** Sympathetic nerve blocks may be used in the management of acute or chronic pain associated with a well-defined anatomical site. Guanethidine is one of a number of drugs that have been used for intravenous regional sympathetic block in the management of neuropathic pain (see Complex Regional Pain Syndrome, p.5), to reduce pain and to maintain blood flow. However, a review of the literature and a double-blind trial[1] in patients with reflex sympathetic dystrophy failed to find any benefit from guanethidine. The trial had to be terminated early due to unacceptable adverse effects.

1. Jadad AR, *et al.* Intravenous regional sympathetic blockade for pain relief in reflex sympathetic dystrophy: a systematic review and a randomized, double-blind crossover study. *J Pain Symptom Manage* 1995; **10:** 13–20.

## Preparations

***BP 2003:*** Guanethidine Tablets;
***USP 27:*** Guanethidine Monosulfate Tablets.

**Proprietary Preparations** (details are given in Part 3)
***Austral.:*** Ismelin; ***Austria:*** Ismelin†; ***Fr.:*** Ismeline†; ***Ital.:*** Visutensil†; ***Mex.:*** Ismelin†; ***NZ:*** Ismelin†; ***S.Afr.:*** Ismelin†; ***Switz.:*** Ismelin†; ***UK:*** Ismelin; ***USA:*** Ismelin.

**Multi-ingredient:** ***Arg.:*** Normatensil; ***Austria:*** Thilodigon; ***Denm.:*** Suprexon†; ***Ger.:*** Esimil; Suprexon†; Thilodigon; ***Irl.:*** Ganda; ***Neth.:*** Suprexon†; ***Switz.:*** Suprexon†; ***UK:*** Ganda†; ***USA:*** Esimil.

---

# Guanfacine Hydrochloride *(BANM, USAN, rINNM)*

BS-100-141; Hidrocloruro de guanfacina; LON-798. N-Amidino-2-(2,6-dichlorophenyl)acetamide hydrochloride.
$C_9H_9Cl_2N_3O,HCl = 282.6.$
*CAS — 29110-47-2 (guanfacine); 29110-48-3 (guanfacine hydrochloride).*
*ATC — C02AC02.*

**Pharmacopoeias.** In *US.*

**USP 27** (Guanfacine Hydrochloride). Store in airtight containers. Protect from light.

## Adverse Effects and Precautions

As for Clonidine Hydrochloride, p.885. Rebound hypertension may occur but is delayed due to the longer half-life.

◊ Reviews.

1. Jerie P. Clinical experience with guanfacine in long-term treatment of hypertension, part II: adverse reactions to guanfacine. *Br J Clin Pharmacol* 1980; **10** (suppl 1): 157S–164S.
2. Board AW, *et al.* A postmarketing evaluation of guanfacine hydrochloride in mild to moderate hypertension. *Clin Ther* 1988; **10:** 761–75.

**Withdrawal.** Rapid reduction of the guanfacine dosage resulted in rebound hypertension leading to generalised seizures and coma in a 47-year-old patient with renal failure who was receiving haemodialysis.[1] Concomitant use of phenobarbital may have enhanced the metabolism of guanfacine and contributed to the development of the withdrawal effect.

1. Kiechel JR, *et al.* Pharmacokinetic aspects of guanfacine withdrawal syndrome in a hypertensive patient with chronic renal failure. *Eur J Clin Pharmacol* 1983; **25:** 463–6.

## Interactions

As for Clonidine Hydrochloride, p.886.

## Pharmacokinetics

Following oral administration guanfacine is rapidly absorbed, peak plasma concentrations occurring 1 to 4 hours after ingestion. The oral bioavailability is reported to be about 80%. It is about 70% bound to plasma proteins. It is excreted in urine as unchanged drug and metabolites; about 50% of a dose is reported to be eliminated unchanged. The normal elimination half-life ranges from 10 to 30 hours, tending to be longer in older patients.

**Renal impairment.** A study[1] in patients with normal or impaired renal function found that guanfacine clearance and serum concentrations were not significantly different in the 2 groups, suggesting that non-renal elimination plays an important role in patients with renal impairment.

1. Kirch W, *et al.* Elimination of guanfacine in patients with normal and impaired renal function. *Br J Clin Pharmacol* 1980; **10** (suppl 1): 33S–35S.

## Uses and Administration

Guanfacine is a centrally acting alpha$_2$-adrenoceptor agonist with actions and uses similar to those of clonidine (p.886). It is used in the management of hypertension (p.825), although other drugs are usually preferred. It may be used alone or with other antihypertensives, particularly thiazide diuretics. It has also been tried in the management of opioid withdrawal and in hyperactivity disorders.

Guanfacine is given by mouth as the hydrochloride, but doses are usually expressed in terms of the base. Guanfacine hydrochloride 1.15 mg is approximately equivalent to 1 mg of guanfacine. In hypertension the usual initial dose is 1 mg daily increasing after 3 to 4 weeks to 2 mg daily if necessary.

◊ Reviews.

1. Cornish LA. Guanfacine hydrochloride: a centrally acting antihypertensive agent. *Clin Pharm* 1988; **7:** 187–97.

**Tourette's syndrome.** Guanfacine may be used as an alternative to clonidine in the management of patients with mild to moderate symptoms of Tourette's syndrome (see Tics, p.664). First-line use of these drugs is increasingly favoured in such patients because of a relative lack of serious adverse effects when compared with the commonly used antipsychotics.

## Preparations

***USP 27:*** Guanfacine Tablets.

**Proprietary Preparations** (details are given in Part 3)
***Belg.:*** Estulic; ***Fr.:*** Estulic; ***Ger.:*** Estulic†; ***Irl.:*** Akfen†; ***Neth.:*** Estulic; ***USA:*** Tenex.

---

# Guanoxan Sulfate *(USAN, rINNM)*

3-01003; Guanoxan Sulphate *(BANM)*; Sulfato de guanoxano. 1-(1,4-Benzodioxan-2-ylmethyl)guanidine sulphate; 1-(2,3-Dihydro-1,4-benzodioxin-2-ylmethyl)guanidine sulphate.
$(C_{10}H_{13}N_3O_2)_2,H_2SO_4 = 512.5.$
*CAS — 2165-19-7 (guanoxan); 5714-04-5 (guanoxan sulfate).*
*ATC — C02CC03.*

## Profile

Guanoxan is an antihypertensive with properties similar to those of guanethidine (p.926). It has been used in the management of hypertension. Liver damage has followed treatment with guanoxan.

**Adverse effects.** Of 96 patients treated with guanoxan, 26 had some derangement of liver function tests, severe in 10; four of these developed jaundice and 1 of the 4 patients died from chronic hepatic necrosis.[1]

1. Cotton SG, Montuschi E. Guanoxan. *BMJ* 1967; **3:** 174.

---

# Heparin *(BAN)*

Heparina; Heparinum.
*CAS — 9005-49-6.*
*ATC — B01AB01; C05BA03; S01XA14.*

**Description.** Heparin is an anionic polysaccharide of mammalian origin with irregular sequence. It consists principally of alternating iduronate and glucosamine residues most of which are sulfated. It may be described as a sulfated glucosaminoglycan. Heparin has the characteristic property of delaying the clotting of freshly shed blood. It may be prepared from the lungs of oxen or the intestinal mucosa of oxen, pigs, or sheep.

Heparin is often described in the literature as standard heparin or unfractionated heparin to distinguish it from low-molecular-weight heparins.

## Heparin Calcium *(BANM)*

Calcium Heparin; Heparina cálcica; Heparinum Calcicum.
*CAS — 37270-89-6.*
*ATC — B01AB01; C05BA03; S01XA14.*

**Pharmacopoeias.** In *Eur.* (see p.vi), *Int.*, and *US.*

**Ph. Eur. 5.0** (Heparin Calcium). The potency of heparin calcium intended for parenteral administration is not less than 150 international units per mg and the potency of heparin calcium not intended for parenteral administration is not less than 120 international units per mg, both calculated with reference to the dried substance. A white or almost white, moderately hygroscopic powder. Freely soluble in water. A 1% solution in water has a pH of 5.5 to 8.0. Store in airtight containers.

**USP 27** (Heparin Calcium). The calcium salt of heparin with a potency, calculated on the dried basis, of not less than 140 USP units in each mg. USP heparin units are not equivalent to international units. The source of the material is usually the intestinal mucosa or other suitable tissues of domestic mammals used for food by man and should be stated on the label. A 1% solution in water has a pH of 5.0 to 7.5. Store in airtight containers at temperatures below 40°, preferably between 15 and 30°.

**Incompatibility.** See Heparin Sodium, below.

## Heparin Sodium *(BANM, rINN)*

Heparina sódica; Heparinum Natricum; Sodium Heparin; Soluble Heparin.

*CAS — 9041-08-1.*

*ATC — B01AB01; C05BA03; S01XA14.*

**Pharmacopoeias.** In *Chin., Eur.* (see p.vi), *Int., Jpn,* and *US.*

**Ph. Eur. 5.0** (Heparin Sodium). The potency of heparin sodium intended for parenteral administration is not less than 150 international units per mg and the potency of heparin sodium not intended for parenteral administration is not less than 120 international units per mg, both calculated with reference to the dried substance. A white or almost white, moderately hygroscopic powder. Freely soluble in water. A 1% solution in water has a pH of 5.5 to 8.0. Store in airtight containers.

**USP 27** (Heparin Sodium). The sodium salt of heparin with a potency, calculated on the dried basis, of not less than 140 USP units in each mg. USP heparin units are not equivalent to international units. The source of the material is usually the intestinal mucosa or other suitable tissues of domestic mammals used for food by man and should be stated on the label. A white or pale-coloured amorphous, odourless or almost odourless, hygroscopic powder. Soluble 1 in 20 of water. A 1% solution in water has a pH of 5.0 to 7.5. Store in airtight containers at temperatures below 40°, preferably between 15 and 30°.

**Incompatibility.** Incompatibility has been reported between heparin calcium or sodium and alteplase, amikacin sulfate, amiodarone hydrochloride, ampicillin sodium, aprotinin, benzylpenicillin potassium or sodium, cefalotin sodium, ciprofloxacin lactate, cytarabine, dacarbazine, daunorubicin hydrochloride, diazepam, dobutamine hydrochloride, doxorubicin hydrochloride, droperidol, erythromycin lactobionate, gentamicin sulfate, haloperidol lactate, hyaluronidase, hydrocortisone sodium succinate, kanamycin sulfate, meticillin sodium, netilmicin sulfate, some opioid analgesics, oxytetracycline hydrochloride, some phenothiazines, polymyxin B sulfate, streptomycin sulfate, tetracycline hydrochloride, tobramycin sulfate, vancomycin hydrochloride, and vinblastine sulfate. Heparin sodium has also been reported to be incompatible with cisatracurium besilate,[1] labetalol hydrochloride,[2] levofloxacin,[3] nicardipine hydrochloride,[4] reteplase,[5] and vinorelbine tartrate.[6] Although visually compatible,[7] cefmetazole sodium is reported to inactivate heparin sodium.

Glucose can have variable effects,[8,9] but glucose-containing solutions are generally considered suitable diluents for heparin. Incompatibility has also been reported between heparin and fat emulsion.

1. Trissel LA, *et al.* Compatibility of cisatracurium besylate with selected drugs during simulated Y-site administration. *Am J Health-Syst Pharm* 1997; **54:** 1735–41.
2. Yamashita SK, *et al.* Compatibility of selected critical care drugs during simulated Y-site administration. *Am J Health-Syst Pharm* 1996; **53:** 1048–51.
3. Saltsman CL, *et al.* Compatibility of levofloxacin with 34 medications during simulated Y-site administration. *Am J Health-Syst Pharm* 1999; **56:** 1458–9.
4. Chiu MF, Schwartz ML. Visual compatibility of injectable drugs used in the intensive care unit. *Am J Health-Syst Pharm* 1997; **54:** 64–5.
5. Committee on Safety of Medicines/Medicines Control Agency. Reteplase (Rapilysin): incompatibility with heparin. *Current Problems* 2000; **26:** 5. Also available at: http://medicines.mhra.gov.uk/ourwork/monitorsafequalmed/currentproblems/cpmay2000.pdf (accessed 06/07/04)
6. Balthasar JP. Concentration-dependent incompatibility of vinorelbine tartrate and heparin sodium. *Am J Health-Syst Pharm* 1999; **56:** 1891.
7. Hutching SR, *et al.* Compatibility of cefmetazole sodium with commonly used drugs during Y-site delivery. *Am J Health-Syst Pharm* 1996; **53:** 2185–8.
8. Anderson W, Harthill JE. The anticoagulant activity of heparins in dextrose solutions. *J Pharm Pharmacol* 1982; **34:** 90–6.
9. Wright A, Hecker J. Long term stability of heparin in dextrose-saline intravenous fluids. *Int J Pharm Pract* 1995; **3:** 253–5.

## Units

The fifth International Standard for unfractionated heparin was established in 1998. The USP 27 states that USP and international units are not equivalent, although doses expressed in either appear to be essentially the same.

## Adverse Effects

Heparin can give rise to haemorrhage as a consequence of its action. It can also cause thrombocytopenia, either through a direct effect or through an immune effect producing a platelet-aggregating antibody. Consequent platelet aggregation and thrombosis may therefore exacerbate the condition being treated. The incidence of thrombocytopenia is reported to be greater with bovine than porcine heparin.

Hypersensitivity reactions may occur, as may local irritant effects, and skin necrosis. Alopecia and osteoporosis resulting in spontaneous fractures have occurred after prolonged use of heparin.

**Effects on the adrenal glands.** Heparin inhibits the secretion of aldosterone which can cause hyperkalaemia.[1] Although all patients treated with heparin may develop reduced aldosterone concentrations, most are able to compensate through the renin-angiotensin system. Patients on prolonged heparin therapy or those unable to compensate, such as patients with diabetes mellitus or renal impairment or those on concomitant therapy with potassium-sparing drugs such as ACE inhibitors may present with symptoms. The UK Committee on Safety of Medicines suggests[2] that plasma-potassium concentration should be monitored in all patients with risk factors, particularly those receiving heparin for more than 7 days. The hyperkalaemia is usually transient or resolves when heparin is discontinued and treatment is not generally required; fludrocortisone was successfully used to treat resistant hyperkalaemia in a patient in whom continued heparin therapy was necessary.[3]

Adrenal insufficiency secondary to adrenal haemorrhage has also been associated with heparin; heparin-induced thrombocytopenia may be implicated.[4]

1. Oster JR, *et al.* Heparin-induced aldosterone suppression and hyperkalemia. *Am J Med* 1995; **98:** 575–86.
2. Committee on Safety of Medicines/Medicines Control Agency. Suppression of aldosterone secretion by heparin. *Current Problems* 1999; **25:** 6. Also available at: http://medicines.mhra.gov.uk/ourwork/monitorsafequalmed/currentproblems/cpvol25bsec2.htm (accessed 06/07/04)
3. Sherman DS, *et al.* Fludrocortisone for the treatment of heparin-induced hyperkalemia. *Ann Pharmacother* 2000; **34:** 606–10.
4. Dahlberg PJ, *et al.* Adrenal insufficiency secondary to adrenal hemorrhage: two case reports and a review of cases confirmed by computed tomography. *Arch Intern Med* 1990; **150:** 905–9.

**Effects on the blood.** *Haemorrhage* is a recognised risk with heparin.[1] The risk of major bleeding may be lower with continuous intravenous infusion than with intermittent intravenous injection; risk may increase with heparin dose and age.[2]

Heparin has been associated with the development of *thrombocytopenia.* The reported incidence has varied greatly; up to 6% appears to be a reasonable estimate[3,4] although up to 10% has also been quoted.[5] Thrombocytopenia induced by heparin may be of two types. The first is an acute, but usually mild, fall in platelet count occurring within 1 to 4 days of initiation of therapy and which often resolves without cessation of treatment. A direct effect of heparin on platelet aggregation appears to be responsible. The second type of thrombocytopenia, which has an immunological basis, is more serious. It usually occurs after 5 to 11 days of heparin although its onset may be more rapid in patients previously exposed to heparin;[6] delayed presentation up to 40 days after ceasing heparin has also been reported.[7-9] It is often associated with thromboembolic complications due to platelet-rich thrombi (the 'white clot syndrome') or, more rarely, bleeding. Of 34 cases of heparin-associated thrombocytopenia reported to the UK Committee on Safety of Medicines (CSM) from 1964 to 1989, bleeding or thromboembolic complications occurred in 11 patients, 7 of whom died.[3] This type of thrombocytopenia appears to occur more frequently with bovine heparin than with heparin from other species[10] and it has been proposed that in susceptible patients antibody reacts with heparin bound to platelets and endothelial cells.[11] Patients with lupus anticoagulant may also be more susceptible.[12] The reaction is independent of dose or route of administration; there are reports of thrombocytopenia after use of heparin flushes[13] or heparin-coated catheters.[14] The CSM recommend monitoring of platelet counts in patients given heparin for more than 5 days.[3] Patients previously exposed to heparin may be sensitised to it and after re-exposure should have a platelet count before the 5 days are up.[15]

The management of heparin-induced thrombocytopenia has been reviewed.[16,17] Heparin should be stopped immediately in those who develop thrombocytopenia. It should be noted, however, that thrombosis has occurred in patients whose reduction in platelet count was relatively mild and who may not be considered to be thrombocytopenic.[18-21] On withdrawal of heparin, a heparinoid such as danaparoid[22,23] may be tried, provided that an *in-vitro* platelet aggregation test is negative, i.e. there is no cross-reactivity with heparin. Alternatively, lepirudin,[23,24] a recombinant hirudin, or the thrombin inhibitor argatroban,[23,25] may be used. Low-molecular-weight heparins have been used; they are associated with a lower incidence of induced thrombocytopenia than unfractionated heparin[26] but the rate of cross-reactivity is high and they are not generally recommended.[23,25] Alternatively, oral anticoagulation may be started, although an increased risk of venous limb gangrene has been reported[27] with warfarin. Ancrod,[23,25] dermatan sulfate,[28] and fondaparinux[29] have also been used. Thrombocytopenia has been managed with aspirin and dipyridamole or with normal immunoglobulin.[30] A fibrinolytic such as urokinase has been used in a few cases of occlusive thrombosis.[31,32]

There may be a relationship between heparin-induced thrombocytopenia and skin necrosis (see below).

1. Walker AM, Jick H. Predictors of bleeding during heparin therapy. *JAMA* 1980; **244:** 1209–12.
2. Levine MN, *et al.* Hemorrhagic complications of anticoagulant treatment. *Chest* 2001; **119** (suppl): 108S–121S.
3. Committee on Safety of Medicines. Heparin-induced thrombocytopenia. *Current Problems 28* 1990.
4. Derlon A, *et al.* Thrombopénies induites par l'héparine: symptomatologie, détection, fréquence. *Therapie* 1988; **43:** 199–203.
5. Aster RH. Heparin-induced thrombocytopenia and thrombosis. *N Engl J Med* 1995; **332:** 1374–6.
6. Warkentin TE, Kelton JG. Temporal aspects of heparin-induced thrombocytopenia. *N Engl J Med* 2001; **344:** 1286–92.
7. Warkentin TE, Kelton JG. Delayed-onset heparin-induced thrombocytopenia and thrombosis. *Ann Intern Med* 2001; **135:** 502–6.
8. Rice L, *et al.* Delayed-onset heparin-induced thrombocytopenia. *Ann Intern Med* 2002; **136:** 210–5.
9. Warkentin TE, Bernstein RA. Delayed-onset heparin-induced thrombocytopenia and cerebral thrombosis after a single administration of unfractionated heparin. *N Engl J Med* 2003; **348:** 1067–9.
10. Bell WR, Royall RM. Heparin-associated thrombocytopenia: a comparison of three heparin preparations. *N Engl J Med* 1980; **303:** 902–7.
11. Cines DB, *et al.* Immune endothelial-cell injury in heparin-associated thrombocytopenia. *N Engl J Med* 1987; **316:** 581–9.
12. Auger WR, *et al.* Lupus anticoagulant, heparin use, and thrombocytopenia in patients with chronic thromboembolic pulmonary hypertension: a preliminary report. *Am J Med* 1995; **99:** 392–6.
13. Heeger PS, Backstrom JT. Heparin flushes and thrombocytopenia. *Ann Intern Med* 1986; **105:** 143.
14. Laster JL, *et al.* Thrombocytopenia associated with heparin-coated catheters in patients with heparin-associated antiplatelet antibodies. *Arch Intern Med* 1989; **149:** 2285–7.
15. Hunter JB, *et al.* Heparin induced thrombosis: an important complication of heparin prophylaxis for thromboembolic disease in surgery. *BMJ* 1993; **307:** 53–5.
16. Dager WE, White RH. Treatment of heparin-induced thrombocytopenia. *Ann Pharmacother* 2002; **36:** 489–503.
17. Messmore HL, *et al.* Benefit-risk assessment of treatments for heparin-induced thrombocytopenia. *Drug Safety* 2003; **26:** 625–41.
18. Phelan BK. Heparin-associated thrombosis without thrombocytopenia. *Ann Intern Med* 1983; **99:** 637–8.
19. Trono DP, *et al.* Thrombocytopenia and heparin-associated thrombosis. *Ann Intern Med* 1984; **100:** 464–5.
20. Ramirez-Lassepas M, Cipolle RJ. Heparin and thrombocytopenia. *Ann Intern Med* 1984; **100:** 613.
21. Hach-Wunderle V, *et al.* Heparin-associated thrombosis despite normal platelet counts. *Lancet* 1994; **344:** 469–70.
22. Wilde MI, Markham A. Danaparoid: a review of its pharmacology and clinical use in the management of heparin-induced thrombocytopenia. *Drugs* 1997; **54:** 903–24.
23. Januzzi JL, Jang I-K. Heparin induced thrombocytopenia: diagnosis and contemporary antithrombin management. *J Thromb Thrombolysis* 1999; **7:** 259–64.
24. Greinacher A, *et al.* Recombinant hirudin (lepirudin) provides safe and effective anticoagulation in patients with heparin-induced thrombocytopenia: a prospective study. *Circulation* 1999; **99:** 73–80.
25. Warkentin TE. Heparin-induced thrombocytopenia: pathogenesis, frequency, avoidance and management. *Drug Safety* 1997; **17:** 325–41.
26. Warkentin TE, *et al.* Heparin-induced thrombocytopenia in patients treated with low-molecular- weight heparin or unfractionated heparin. *N Engl J Med* 1995; **332:** 1330–5.
27. Warkentin TE, *et al.* The pathogenesis of venous limb gangrene associated with heparin-induced thrombocytopenia. *Ann Intern Med* 1997; **127:** 804–12.
28. Taliani MR, *et al.* Dermatan sulphate in patients with heparin-induced thrombocytopenia. *Br J Haematol* 1999; **104:** 87–9.
29. Parody R, *et al.* Fondaparinux (ARIXTRA®) as an alternative anti-thrombotic prophylaxis when there is hypersensitivity to low molecular weight and unfractionated heparins. *Haematologica* 2003; **88:** ECR32. Also available at: http://www.haematologica.org/e-cases/2003_11/ECR32.htm (accessed 06/07/04)
30. Frame JN, *et al.* Correction of severe heparin-associated thrombocytopenia with intravenous immunoglobulin. *Ann Intern Med* 1989; **111:** 946–7.
31. Krueger SK, *et al.* Thrombolysis in heparin-induced thrombocytopenia with thrombosis. *Ann Intern Med* 1985; **103:** 159.
32. Clifton GD, Smith MD. Thrombolytic therapy in heparin-associated thrombocytopenia with thrombosis. *Clin Pharm* 1986; **5:** 597–601.

**Effects on the bones.** Osteoporosis is a rare complication of long-term heparin therapy. Treatment and prophylaxis of thromboembolism in pregnancy is one of the few indications for long term use of heparin, so most reports and studies of heparin-induced osteoporosis have been in pregnant women.[1] The incidence of symptomatic osteoporosis in patients receiving heparin long term has been estimated to be about 2%.[1,2] Subclinical reduction in bone density occurs in up to one-third of patients,[2] but it is not possible to predict which of these patients will develop osteoporotic fractures. Pregnancy normally causes reversible bone demineralisation, so the combination of pregnancy and heparin therapy may therefore result in symptomatic osteoporosis in susceptible individuals.[1,3] Bone changes may be reversible.[1] Although some evidence suggests that bone demineralisation is dose- and duration-dependent, this has not been conclusively established.[1-3] Use of low-molecular-weight heparins may be associated with a lower risk of heparin-induced osteoporosis, but experience is limited.[1-3]

1. Nelson-Piercy C. Heparin-induced osteoporosis. *Scand J Rheumatol* 1998; **27** (suppl 107): 68–71.
2. Ginsberg JS, *et al.* Use of antithrombotic agents during pregnancy. *Chest* 2001; **119** (suppl): 122S–131S.
3. Farquharson RG. Heparin, osteoporosis and pregnancy. *Br J Hosp Med* 1997; **58:** 205–7.

**Effects on electrolytes.** See Effects on the Adrenal Glands, above.

**Effects on the liver.** Increases in transaminase values have been reported in patients given therapeutic[1-3] or prophylactic[3] doses of heparin. The abnormality usually resolved on discontinuation of heparin.

1. Sonnenblick M, *et al.* Hyper-transaminasemia with heparin therapy. *BMJ* 1975; **3:** 77.
2. Dukes GE, *et al.* Transaminase elevations in patients receiving bovine or porcine heparin. *Ann Intern Med* 1984; **100:** 646–50.
3. Monreal M, *et al.* Adverse effects of three different forms of heparin therapy: thrombocytopenia, increased transaminases, and hyperkalaemia. *Eur J Clin Pharmacol* 1989; **37:** 415–18.

**Effects on serum lipids.** Use of heparin leads to the release of lipoprotein lipase into the plasma. Postprandial lipidaemia is reduced due to increased hydrolysis of triglycerides into free fatty acids and glycerol. Raised concentrations of free fatty acids have been reported after heparin use but the magnitude of this effect may have been overestimated.[1] Rebound hyperlipidaemia may occur when heparin is withdrawn. With long-term use reserves of lipoprotein lipase may be depleted; severe hypertriglyceridaemia reported in a pregnant woman was attributed to long-term heparin prophylaxis that was thought to have resulted in lipoprotein lipase deficiency.[2]

1. Riemersma RA, *et al.* Heparin-induced lipolysis, an exaggerated risk. *Lancet* 1981; **ii:** 471.
2. Watts GF, *et al.* Lipoprotein lipase deficiency due to long-term heparinization presenting as severe hypertriglyceridaemia in pregnancy. *Postgrad Med J* 1991; **67:** 1062–4.

**Effects on sexual function.** There have been several reports of priapism associated with the use of heparin. The prognosis is poor, impotence following more often than in priapism of other aetiologies. The mechanism of heparin-induced priapism is unclear.[1]

1. Baños JE, *et al.* Drug-induced priapism: its aetiology, incidence and treatment. *Med Toxicol* 1989; **4:** 46–58.

**Effects on the skin.** Skin necrosis is a rare complication of heparin use.[1,2] It may be a localised reaction at the site of subcutaneous injection or possibly be related to heparin-induced thrombocytopenia (see Effects on the Blood, above). An immune mechanism may be responsible.

Eczematous plaque reactions have developed several days after initiation of subcutaneous heparin. A type IV hypersensitivity reaction has been implicated.[3] Low-molecular-weight heparins may be an alternative but cross-reactivity can occur.[4]

Recurrent fixed eczematous lesions have been attributed to heparin used intravenously during haemodialysis.[5]

1. Ulrick PJ, Manoharan A. Heparin-induced skin reaction. *Med J Aust* 1984; **140:** 287–9.
2. Fowlie J, *et al.* Heparin-associated skin necrosis. *Postgrad Med J* 1990; **66:** 573–5.
3. Bircher AJ, *et al.* Eczematous infiltrated plaques to subcutaneous heparin: a type IV allergic reaction. *Br J Dermatol* 1990; **123:** 507–14.
4. O'Donnell BF, Tan CY. Delayed hypersensitivity reactions to heparin. *Br J Dermatol* 1993; **129:** 634–6.
5. Mohammed KN. Symmetric fixed eruption to heparin. *Dermatology* 1995; **190:** 91.

## Treatment of Adverse Effects

Slight haemorrhage due to overdosage can usually be treated by withdrawing heparin. Severe bleeding may be reduced by the slow intravenous administration of protamine sulfate (p.1051). The dose is dependent on the amount of heparin to be neutralised and ideally should be titrated against assessments of the coagulability of the patient's blood. As heparin is being continuously excreted the dose should be reduced if more than 15 minutes have elapsed since heparin administration; for example, if protamine sulfate is given 30 minutes after heparin the dose may be reduced to about one-half. Not more than 50 mg of protamine sulfate should be injected for any one dose; patients should be carefully monitored as further doses may be required. The Ph. Eur. 5.0 specifies that 1 mg of protamine sulfate precipitates not less than 100 international units of heparin, but adds that this potency is based on a specific reference batch of heparin sodium. The UK manufacturer has stated that each mg of protamine sulfate will usually neutralise the anticoagulant effect of at least 80 international units of heparin (lung) or at least 100 international units of heparin (mucous). The US manufacturer has stated that each mg of protamine sulfate neutralises approximately 90 USP units of heparin (lung) or about 115 USP units of heparin (mucous).

**Thrombocytopenia.** For reference to the treatment of heparin-induced thrombocytopenia and associated thromboembolic complications, see Effects on the Blood under Adverse Effects, above.

## Precautions

Heparin should not be given to patients who are haemorrhaging. In general it should not be given to patients at serious risk of haemorrhage, although it has been used with very careful control; patients at risk include those with haemorrhagic blood disorders, thrombocytopenia, peptic ulcer disease, cerebrovascular disorders, bacterial endocarditis, severe hypertension, oesophageal varices, or patients who have recently undergone surgery at sites where haemorrhage would be an especial risk. Severe renal and hepatic impairment are considered by some to be contra-indications. Heparin should not be given by intramuscular injection. Since heparin has caused thrombocytopenia with severe thromboembolic complications, platelet counts should be monitored in patients receiving heparin for more than a few days. Heparin should be discontinued if thrombocytopenia develops. A test dose has been recommended for patients with a history of allergy.

Dosage of heparin may need to be reduced in the elderly; elderly women appear to be especially susceptible to haemorrhage after heparin administration.

**Catheters and cannulas.** Serum concentrations of sodium and potassium could be falsely elevated in samples obtained through heparin-bonded umbilical catheters due to release of benzalkonium chloride used in the manufacturing process of some catheters.[1] It was unknown if the amount released would be toxic to small premature neonates.

1. Gaylord MS, *et al.* Release of benzalkonium chloride from a heparin-bonded umbilical catheter with resultant factitious hypernatremia and hyperkalemia. *Pediatrics* 1991; **87:** 631–5.

**Hyperkalaemia.** For recommendations concerning the monitoring of patients susceptible to developing hyperkalaemia, such as those with diabetes mellitus or renal impairment, see Effects on the Adrenal Glands under Adverse Effects, above.

**Pregnancy.** Heparin does not cross the placenta, and therefore adverse effects on the fetus would not be expected.[1,2] A review[1] of the literature, however, indicated 2 spontaneous abortions and 17 still-births in 135 pregnancies exposed to heparin; 29 infants were premature, 10 of whom died. Another literature review[2] found adverse outcomes in 21.7% of heparin-treated patients, but this dropped to 10.4% when pregnancies with co-morbid conditions were excluded. A further drop to 3.6% was observed when cases of prematurity with normal outcome were also excluded. The death rate of 2.5% and prematurity rate of 6.8% in heparin-treated patients was similar to that found in the normal population. It was concluded that heparin appears safer for the fetus than warfarin when used during pregnancy. Similar results have also been reported with low-molecular-weight heparins; a systematic review[3] found an adverse outcome in 9.3% of 486 pregnancies in which low-molecular-weight heparin was used, but this dropped to 3.1% in women without comorbid conditions.

1. Hall JG, *et al.* Maternal and fetal sequelae of anticoagulation during pregnancy. *Am J Med* 1980; **68:** 122–40.
2. Ginsberg JS, Hirsh J. Optimum use of anticoagulants in pregnancy. *Drugs* 1988; **36:** 505–12.
3. Sanson B-J, *et al.* Safety of low-molecular-weight heparin in pregnancy: a systematic review. *Thromb Haemost* 1999; **81:** 668–72.

**Preservative.** The preservatives used in heparin preparations have been implicated in unwanted effects. Benzyl alcohol in heparinised flushing solutions has been suspected of causing toxicity in neonates (see p.1170). Chlorobutanol present in another heparin preparation caused a sharp fall in blood pressure (see Effects on the Cardiovascular System under Chlorobutanol, p.1176).

**Spinal anaesthesia.** Spinal and epidural haematomas, sometimes leading to paralysis, have occurred after spinal or epidural anaesthesia or analgesia in patients receiving heparin or low-molecular-weight heparins. The risk of haematoma appears to be higher in patients with indwelling epidural catheters or in those receiving concomitant therapy with drugs that affect haemostasis.[1] It is generally recommended that central nerve block should be avoided in patients receiving full-dose anticoagulation.[2] However, the use of prophylactic doses of anticoagulants with central nervous blockade is less clear.[2,3] The reported risk of haematoma with low-molecular-weight heparins has been higher in the USA where higher doses have been used for prophylaxis.[3] Recommendations to reduce the risk of spinal haematoma include waiting until after blockade has been completed to administer prophylactic heparin or low-molecular-weight heparin. Where anticoagulant prophylaxis has already been given, blockade should be delayed if possible until 4 to 6 hours after heparin, and the catheter should not be removed until 4 hours after heparin.[2] It is recommended that low-molecular-weight heparin should not be given within 8 to 10 hours before or after central nerve block or catheter removal.[2,3]

1. Wysowski DK, *et al.* Spinal and epidural hematoma and low-molecular-weight heparin. *N Engl J Med* 1998; **338:** 1774.
2. Armstrong RF, *et al.* Epidural and spinal anaesthesia and the use of anticoagulants. *Hosp Med* 1999; **60:** 491–6.
3. Dolenska S. Neuroaxial blocks and LMWH thromboprophylaxis. *Hosp Med* 1998; **59:** 940–3.

## Interactions

Heparin should be used with care with oral anticoagulants or drugs, such as aspirin and dipyridamole, that affect platelet function. NSAIDs may also increase the risk of haemorrhage. Other drugs that affect the coagulation process and which may therefore increase the risk of haemorrhage include dextrans, thrombolytic enzymes such as streptokinase, high doses of penicillins and some cephalosporins, some contrast media, asparaginase, and epoprostenol. Estimations of oral anticoagulant control may be modified by heparin's action on prothrombin.

**ACE inhibitors.** For reference to hyperkalaemia in patients on heparin and ACE inhibitors, see Effects on the Adrenal Glands under Adverse Effects, above.

**Alcohol.** Heavy drinkers were at greater risk of major heparin-associated bleeding than moderate drinkers or non-drinkers.[1]

1. Walker AM, Jick H. Predictors of bleeding during heparin therapy. *JAMA* 1980; **244:** 1209–12.

**Aprotinin.** For comment on the use of heparin with aprotinin, see Effects on Coagulation Tests under Aprotinin, p.743.

**Glyceryl trinitrate.** Glyceryl trinitrate has been reported to reduce the activity of heparin when both drugs are given simultaneously by the intravenous route.[1] This effect has been seen even at low doses of glyceryl trinitrate.[2] Propylene glycol present in the glyceryl trinitrate formulation may[3] or may not[1] contribute to the effect. No interaction was reported when glyceryl trinitrate was given immediately after heparin.[4]

1. Habbab MA, Haft JI. Heparin resistance induced by intravenous nitroglycerin. *Arch Intern Med* 1987; **147:** 857–60.
2. Brack MJ, *et al.* The effect of low dose nitroglycerine on plasma heparin concentrations and activated partial thromboplastin times. *Blood Coag Fibrinol* 1993; **4:** 183–6.
3. Col J, *et al.* Propylene glycol-induced heparin resistance during nitroglycerin infusion. *Am Heart J* 1985; **110:** 171–3.
4. Bode V, *et al.* Absence of drug interaction between heparin and nitroglycerin. *Arch Intern Med* 1990; **150:** 2117–19.

**Tobacco.** Reduced half-life and increased elimination of heparin have been reported in smokers compared with non-smokers.[1]

1. Cipolle RJ, *et al.* Heparin kinetics: variables related to disposition and dosage. *Clin Pharmacol Ther* 1981; **29:** 387–93.

## Pharmacokinetics

Heparin is not absorbed from the gastrointestinal tract. After intravenous or subcutaneous injection heparin is extensively bound to plasma proteins. It does not cross the placenta and it is not distributed into breast milk. The half-life of heparin depends on the dose and route of administration as well as the method of calculation and is subject to wide inter- and intra-individual variation; a range of 1 to 6 hours with an average of 1.5 hours has been cited. It may be slightly prolonged in renal impairment, decreased in patients with pulmonary embolism, and either increased or decreased in patients with liver disorders. Heparin is taken up by the reticuloendothelial system. It is excreted in the urine, mainly as metabolites, although, after administration of large doses, up to 50% may be excreted unchanged.

◊ References.

1. Estes JW. Clinical pharmacokinetics of heparin. *Clin Pharmacokinet* 1980; **5:** 204–20.
2. Kandrotas RJ. Heparin pharmacokinetics and pharmacodynamics. *Clin Pharmacokinet* 1992; **22:** 359–74.

## Uses and Administration

Heparin is an anticoagulant used principally in the treatment and prophylaxis of thromboembolic disorders (p.837). It is often described as standard heparin or unfractionated heparin to distinguish it from low-molecular-weight heparins (p.949).

It inhibits clotting of blood *in vitro* and *in vivo* through its action on antithrombin III. Antithrombin III, which is present in plasma, inhibits the activity of activated clotting factors including thrombin (factor IIa) and activated factor X (factor Xa); heparin increases the rate of this inhibition, but in a manner that is dependent on its dose. With normal therapeutic doses heparin has an inhibitory effect on both thrombin and factor Xa. Thus the conversion of fibrinogen to fibrin is blocked through the thrombin inhibition, while the conversion of prothrombin to thrombin is blocked by the inhibition of factor Xa. The low doses that are given subcutaneously for the prophylaxis of thromboembolism have a selective effect on antithrombin III's inhibition of factor Xa. Very high doses are reported to reduce the activity of antithrombin III. Heparin also has some effect on platelet function, inhibits the formation of a stable fibrin clot, and has an antilipidaemic effect. For an explanation of the coagulation cascade, see Haemostasis and Fibrinolysis, p.735.

Heparin is used in the treatment and prophylaxis of venous thromboembolism (deep-vein thrombosis and pulmonary embolism, p.839), especially prophylaxis in surgical patients and in those pregnant women at particular risk. It is also used in the management of arterial thromboembolism including that associated with unstable angina pectoris (p.813), myocardial infarction (p.828), acute peripheral arterial occlusion (p.830), and stroke (p.836). It is often used as a precursor to oral anticoagulation and is withdrawn once the oral anticoagulant is exerting its full effect.

Heparin has been tried in the treatment of disseminated intravascular coagulation. It is also used to prevent coagulation during haemodialysis and other extracorporeal circulatory procedures such as cardiopulmonary bypass. Other uses include the anticoagulation of blood for transfusion or blood samples and the flushing of catheters and cannulas to maintain patency.

Heparin and its salts are constituents of many topical preparations for the treatment of various inflammatory disorders.

**Administration and dosage**. Heparin is administered intravenously, preferably by continuous infusion, or by subcutaneous injection. It may be given as the calcium or sodium salt and it is generally accepted that there is little difference in their effects. Oral formulations of heparin are under investigation.

Doses of heparin for treatment (sometimes termed 'full-dose' heparin), and in some cases prophylaxis, of thromboembolism should be monitored and determined as discussed below under Control of Heparin Therapy. The subcutaneous doses of heparin commonly used for prophylaxis and often termed 'low-dose' subcutaneous heparin do not require routine monitoring. A test dose has been recommended for patients with a history of allergy. Although international and USP units are not strictly equivalent, doses expressed in either appear to be essentially the same. The following doses of heparin are broadly in line with British Society for Haematology guidelines.

For **treatment of venous thromboembolism**, an intravenous loading dose of 5000 to 10 000 units is followed by continuous intravenous infusion of 1000 to 2000 units/hour or subcutaneous injection of 15 000 units every 12 hours. Alternatively, intermittent intravenous injection of 5000 to 10 000 units every 4 to 6 hours is suggested in some product literature. Children and small adults are given a lower intravenous loading dose followed by maintenance with continuous intravenous infusion of 15 to 25 units/kg per hour or subcutaneous injection of 250 units/kg every 12 hours.

For **prophylaxis** of **postoperative venous thromboembolism**, subcutaneous doses used are 5000 units 2 hours before surgery then every 8 to 12 hours for 7 days or until the patient is ambulant. Similar doses are used to prevent thromboembolism during pregnancy in women with a history of deep-vein thrombosis or pulmonary embolism; the dosage may need to be increased to 10 000 units every 12 hours during the third trimester.

In the management of **unstable angina** or acute **peripheral arterial embolism,** heparin may be given by continuous intravenous infusion in the same doses as those recommended for the treatment of venous thromboembolism. Doses for the prevention of re-occlusion of the coronary arteries following thrombolytic therapy in **myocardial infarction** include 5000 units intravenously followed by 1000 units/hour intravenously with alteplase; a dose of 12 500 units subcutaneously every 12 hours for at least 10 days may be used to prevent mural thrombosis.

**Control of Heparin Therapy.** Treatment with full-dose heparin must be monitored to ensure that the dose is providing the required effect on antithrombin III. The most commonly used test to monitor the action of heparin is the activated partial thromboplastin time (APTT). The APTT of patients on full-dose heparin should generally be maintained at 1.5 to 2.5 times the control value although the optimum therapeutic range varies between individual laboratories depending on the APTT reagent in use. Regular monitoring is essential, preferably on a daily basis. Prophylaxis with low-dose subcutaneous heparin is not routinely monitored; the APTT is not significantly prolonged in these patients. A dose-adjusted regimen to maintain minimal prolongation of the APTT may be required in patients with malignancy or undergoing orthopaedic surgery to ensure adequate protection against thromboembolism. Other tests used include the activated clotting time (ACT). The value of measurements of heparin concentration in the blood remains to be established.

◊ General references to anticoagulation with heparin.


1. Hirsh J. Heparin. *N Engl J Med* 1991; **324:** 1565–74.
2. Freedman MD. Pharmacodynamics, clinical indications, and adverse effects of heparin. *J Clin Pharmacol* 1992; **32:** 584–96.
3. Hyers TM. Heparin therapy: regimens and treatment considerations. *Drugs* 1992; **44:** 738–49.
4. Colvin BT, Barrowcliffe TW. The British Society for Haematology guidelines on the use and monitoring of heparin 1992: second revision. *J Clin Pathol* 1993; **46:** 97–103.
5. Hirsh J, Fuster V. Guide to anticoagulant therapy part 1: heparin. *Circulation* 1994; **89:** 1449–68.
6. Hirsh J, *et al.* Heparin and low-molecular-weight heparin: mechanisms of action, pharmacokinetics, dosing, monitoring, efficacy, and safety. *Chest* 2001; **119** (suppl): 64S–94S.


**Action.** Heparin is well established as an anticoagulant and antithrombotic and acts primarily by binding to, and enhancing the activity of, antithrombin III. However, the physiological role of endogenous heparin has not been clearly defined, despite its presence in mast cells, its ability to interact with numerous proteins, and its close structural similarity to heparan sulfate (suleparoid) the ubiquitous cell-surface glycosaminoglycan.[1,2] Endogenous heparin activity may have a role in protecting against atherosclerosis.[3] Non-anticoagulant properties of heparin have been reported to include anti-inflammatory activity, with a possible application in, for example, asthma[4] or inflammatory bowel disease.[5] For mention of the use of aerosolised heparin with acetylcysteine to treat inhalation injury, see Burns, under Acetylcysteine, p.1113. A major obstacle to the use of heparin itself for non-anticoagulant purposes would be the risk of bleeding.


1. Lane DA, Adams L. Non-anticoagulant uses of heparin. *N Engl J Med* 1993; **329:** 129–30.
2. Page CP. Proteoglycans: the "Teflon" of the airways? *Thorax* 1997; **52:** 924–5.
3. Engelberg H. Actions of heparin in the atherosclerotic process. *Pharmacol Rev* 1996; **48:** 327–52.
4. Martineau P, Vaughan LM. Heparin inhalation for asthma. *Ann Pharmacother* 1995; **29:** 71–2.
5. Day R, Forbes A. Heparin, cell adhesion, and pathogenesis of inflammatory bowel disease. *Lancet* 1999; **354:** 62–5.


**Administration.** The activated partial thromboplastin time (APTT) is the test most commonly used to monitor intravenous full-dose heparin therapy. Heparin dosing algorithms have been developed[1,2] so that the time taken to achieve a therapeutic APTT and maintain the APTT in the therapeutic range (usually 1.5 to 2.5 times the control value) is shortened and thus the risk of recurrent thrombosis and major bleeding complications is reduced. Although use of ideal body-weight for dosage calculation in obese patients has been suggested, actual body-weight may be more appropriate,[3,4] but maximum bolus doses and infusion rates should be set, to avoid overdosage in morbidly obese patients.

However, the therapeutic ranges used in such algorithms are not applicable to all APTT reagents because different ones vary in their sensitivity to heparin.[5] The optimum therapeutic range therefore varies between individual laboratories depending on the APTT reagent used. Dosing algorithms may be adapted by calibrating the therapeutic APTT with heparin concentrations in patients receiving heparin.[5,6]

A weight-based algorithm for treatment doses of subcutaneous heparin in deep-vein thrombosis has also been proposed.[7]


1. Cruickshank MK, *et al.* A standard heparin nomogram for the management of heparin therapy. *Arch Intern Med* 1991; **151:** 333–7.
2. Raschke RA, *et al.* The weight-based heparin dosing nomogram compared with a "standard care" nomogram: a randomized controlled trial. *Ann Intern Med* 1993; **119:** 874–81.
3. Yee WP, Norton LL. Optimal weight base for a weight-based heparin dosing protocol. *Am J Health-Syst Pharm* 1998; **55:** 159–62.
4. Yee WP, Norton LL. Clarification of weight-based heparin protocol. *Am J Health-Syst Pharm* 2002; **59:** 1788.
5. Brill-Edwards P, *et al.* Establishing a therapeutic range for heparin therapy. *Ann Intern Med* 1993; **119:** 104–9.
6. Volles DF, *et al.* Establishing an institution-specific therapeutic range for heparin. *Am J Health-Syst Pharm* 1998; **55:** 2002–6.
7. Prandoni P, *et al.* Use of an algorithm for administering subcutaneous heparin in the treatment of deep venous thrombosis. *Ann Intern Med* 1998; **129:** 299–302.


**Catheters and cannulas.** Solutions of heparin sodium 10 or 100 units/mL in sodium chloride 0.9% are used for the flushing of intravenous catheters, cannulas, and other indwelling intravenous infusion devices used for intermittent administration (heparin locks). Several studies[1-6] and a meta-analysis[7] have, however, been unable to demonstrate any major advantage of either strength of heparin sodium solution over sodium chloride 0.9% alone in terms of maintenance of peripheral cannula patency or reduction in incidence of thrombophlebitis, and sodium chloride 0.9% is therefore recommended for cannulas intended to be in place for 48 hours or less. Reduced use of heparin flush solutions could minimise the risk of adverse effects to heparin such as thrombocytopenia and reduce the risk of incompatibilities with intravenously administered drugs.

Use of heparin-bonded catheters or the addition of heparin to intravenous fluids such as total parenteral nutrition solutions has also been tried in an attempt to maintain indwelling intravenous infusion devices (but see Catheters and Cannulas under Precautions, above). Continuous infusion of heparin-containing fluids may prolong the patency of peripheral arterial catheters.[7]

Central venous catheters are also subject to thrombus formation and their use may be complicated by vascular thrombosis and systemic infection. A meta-analysis[8] of prophylactic heparin used with central venous and pulmonary artery catheters suggested that heparin reduces catheter-related vascular thrombosis and may reduce catheter-related infection. This analysis included a range of heparin doses and methods of administration, as well as heparin-bonded catheters, and the authors suggest that further study is needed. Very low doses of warfarin (1 mg daily) may protect against thrombosis in patients with central venous catheters.[9]


1. Epperson EL. Efficacy of 0.9% sodium chloride injection with and without heparin for maintaining indwelling intermittent injection sites. *Clin Pharm* 1984; **3:** 626–9.
2. Hamilton RA, *et al.* Heparin sodium versus 0.9% sodium chloride injection for maintaining patency of indwelling intermittent infusion devices. *Clin Pharm* 1988; **7:** 439–43.
3. Lombardi TP, *et al.* Efficacy of 0.9% sodium chloride injection with or without heparin sodium for maintaining patency of intravenous catheters in children. *Clin Pharm* 1988; **7:** 832–6.
4. Shaw P, Baker D. Flushing solutions for indwelling intravenous catheters. *Pharm J* 1988; **241:** 122–3.
5. Garrelts JC, *et al.* Comparison of heparin and 0.9% sodium chloride injection in the maintenance of indwelling intermittent iv devices. *Clin Pharm* 1989; **8:** 34–9.
6. Nelson TJ, Graves SM. 0.9% Sodium chloride injection with and without heparin for maintaining peripheral indwelling intermittent-infusion devices in infants. *Am J Health-Syst Pharm* 1998; **55:** 570–3.
7. Randolph AG, *et al.* Benefit of heparin in peripheral venous and arterial catheters: systematic review and meta-analysis of randomised controlled trials. *BMJ* 1998; **316:** 969–75.
8. Randolph AG, *et al.* Benefit of heparin in central venous and pulmonary artery catheters: a meta-analysis of randomized controlled trials. *Chest* 1998; **113:** 165–71.
9. Bern MM, *et al.* Very low doses of warfarin can prevent thrombosis in central venous catheters: a randomized prospective trial. *Ann Intern Med* 1990; **112:** 423–8.


**Disseminated intravascular coagulation.** Heparin has been used with some success in disseminated intravascular coagulation (p.737) associated with a variety of conditions. However, this use is considered by some to be controversial and should be reserved for specific situations where the risk of bleeding is relatively minor in comparison with the possible beneficial effect on formation of microthromboses. The maximum dose given intravenously is usually 1000 units/hour because of the risk of bleeding.[1]


1. Colvin BT, Barrowcliffe TW. The British Society for Haematology guidelines on the use and monitoring of heparin 1992: second revision. *J Clin Pathol* 1993; **46:** 97–103.


**Extracorporeal circulation.** Anticoagulation with heparin is necessary during procedures such as cardiopulmonary bypass and haemodialysis and haemofiltration.[1] In the case of bypass, heparin is added to the crystalloid solution and any stored blood used for priming the bypass machine and is given intravenously before cannulation of the heart and major blood vessels. Activated clotting time (ACT) is monitored throughout. After bypass is discontinued, anticoagulation can be reversed with protamine but caution is advised because of potential toxicity on the cardiopulmonary circulation.

At the start of haemodialysis sessions patients generally receive a loading dose of heparin followed by continuous infusion into the exit line of the extracorporeal circuit until about one hour before the end of dialysis. The dose of heparin varies widely depending on body-weight, volume of the extracorporeal circulation, dialysis membrane biocompatibility, and pump speed.


1. Colvin BT, Barrowcliffe TW. The British Society for Haematology guidelines on the use and monitoring of heparin 1992: second revision. *J Clin Pathol* 1993; **46:** 97–103.


**Idiopathic thrombocytopenic purpura.** Subcutaneous administration of a low dose of heparin improved platelet counts in a small number of patients with idiopathic thrombocytopenic purpura (p.1082) that was resistant to standard corticosteroid therapy.[1] However, heparin may itself cause thrombocytopenia, even at very low doses (see Effects on the Blood under Adverse Effects, above).

1. Shen ZX, *et al.* Thrombocytopoietic effect of heparin given in chronic immune thrombocytopenic purpura. *Lancet* 1995; **346:** 220–1.

**Pregnancy.** Heparin is the anticoagulant of choice for use in pregnancy although it is not without risk for the fetus (see Pregnancy, under Precautions, above), and for the mother.

Guidelines on thrombosis associated with pregnancy have been published.[1,2] Pregnant women may require anticoagulation for the treatment or prophylaxis of venous thromboembolism (p.839), or for the prevention of systemic thromboembolism associated with prosthetic heart valves (p.838). Patients with a history of thromboembolism or a thrombophilic abnormality such as inherited deficiencies of antithrombin III, protein C, or protein S or acquired antiphospholipid antibodies may be at particular risk. Administration of heparin to women with antiphospholipid antibodies may also decrease the risk of fetal loss that has been associated with this disorder.[3-5]

1. Maternal and Neonatal Haemostasis Working Party of the Haemostasis and Thrombosis Task. Guidelines on the prevention, investigation and management of thrombosis associated with pregnancy. *J Clin Pathol* 1993; **46:** 489–96.
2. Ginsberg JS, *et al.* Use of antithrombotic agents during pregnancy. *Chest* 2001; **119** (suppl): 122S–131S.
3. Rosove MH, *et al.* Heparin therapy for pregnant women with lupus anticoagulant or anticardiolipin antibodies. *Obstet Gynecol* 1990; **75:** 630–4.
4. Rai R, *et al.* Randomised controlled trial of aspirin and aspirin plus heparin in pregnant women with recurrent miscarriage associated with phospholipid antibodies (or antiphospholipid antibodies). *BMJ* 1997; **314:** 253–7.
5. Empson M, *et al.* Recurrent pregnancy loss with antiphospholipid antibody: a systematic review of therapeutic trials. *Obstet Gynecol* 2002; **99:** 135–44.

**Reperfusion and revascularisation procedures.** Heparin is widely used in patients undergoing angioplasty or bypass surgery (p.834) to prevent perioperative thrombosis of the operated artery. It is frequently used in conjunction with aspirin or other antiplatelet drugs. However, it appears to have no role in the long-term prevention of restenosis, although heparin-coated stents may have potential benefits.

## Preparations

***BP 2003:*** Heparin Injection;
***USP 27:*** Anticoagulant Heparin Solution; Heparin Calcium Injection; Heparin Lock Flush Solution; Heparin Sodium Injection.

**Proprietary Preparations** (details are given in Part 3)
***Arg.:*** Calciparine; Cervep; Croneparina; Parinix; Riveparin; Serianon; Sobrius; Sodiparin; ***Austral.:*** Calcihep; Calciparine; Uniparin; ***Austria:*** Calciparin; Liquemin; Thrombophob; Thrombophob-S; Venoruton Heparin; ***Belg.:*** Calparine; Liquemine; ***Braz.:*** Disotron; Heptar; Liquemine; Trombofob; ***Canad.:*** Calcilean†; Hepalean; Hepalean-Lok; ***Fin.:*** Hepaflex; ***Fr.:*** Calciparine; ***Ger.:*** Calciparin; Depot-Thrombophob-N†; Essaven 60 000; Hemeran†; Hepa-Gel; Hepa-Salbe; Hepaplus; Hepathromb; Hepathrombin; Juwoment Sport†; Liquemin N; Perivar Venensalbe; Sportino; Thrombareduct; Thrombophob; Traumalitan; Trirutin†; Venalitan; Venelbin N†; Venoruton Emulgel; Vetren; ***Gr.:*** Hep Lok; Hepsal; Pump-Hep; ***Hong Kong:*** Lioton; ***India:*** Beparine; Thrombophob; ***Irl.:*** Calciparine; Hep-Rinse; Heplok; Hepsal; Minihep; Monoparin; Multiparin; Unihep; Uniparin†; ***Israel:*** Calciparin; ***Ital.:*** Ateroclar; Bioclaril; Calciparina; Calcipor†; Chemyparin†; Clarisco; Croneparina; Disebrin; Ecabil; Ecafast; Ecasolv; Emoklar; Epacalcica; Eparical; Eparinlider; Eparinovis; Eparven; Epsoclar; Epsodil; Eudipar; Flusolv; Hemofluss; Hepacal†; Isoclar; Lioton; Liquemin; Mica; Normoparin; Reoflus; Trombolisin; Zepac; ***Mex.:*** Helberina†; Heparth†; Inhepar; Proparin; ***Neth.:*** Calparine†; Minihep†; ***Norw.:*** Nycoheparin†; ***NZ:*** Minihep†; Monoparin; Multiparin; ***Port.:*** Calciparina; ***S.Afr.:*** Calciparine; Thrombophob; ***Spain:*** Calciparina; Menaven; ***Switz.:*** Calciparine; Demovarin; Gelparine; HepaGel; Lioton; Liquemine; Ruscovarin†; ***UK:*** Calciparine; Canusal; Hep-Flush†; Heplok†; Hepsal; Minihep†; Monoparin; Multiparin; Pump-Hep†; Unihep†; Uniparin†; ***USA:*** Hep-Lock; Hepflush.

**Multi-ingredient: *Arg.:*** Contractubex; Venostasin; ***Austria:*** Ambenat; Contractubex; Derivon; Ditaven comp†; Dolo-Menthoneurin; Dolobene; Etrat; Ichthalgan forte; Pasta Cool; Pertrombon; Thrombophob; Venobene; Venosin; Vetren; ***Braz.:*** Dolobene; Trombofob; Venalot H; Venostasin Composto†; ***Canad.:*** Lipactin; ***Fin.:*** Trombosol; ***Fr.:*** Cirkan a la Prednacinolone; Esberiven; ***Ger.:*** Arnica Kneipp Salbe†; Arnika plus†; Contractubex; Dolo-Menthoneurin; Dolobene; Enelbin-Salbe N; Essaven; Essaven Tri-Complex; Etrat Sportgel; Fibraflex†; Heparin Comp; Heparin Kombi-Gel; Heparin Plus; Ichthalgan; Kelofibrase; Lipactin; NeyGeront N (Revitorgan-Dilutionen N Nr 64); Ostochont; Pe-Ce Ven N†; Sensicutan; Trauma-Puren; Venengel; Venoplant AHS; Venostasin; ***Hong Kong:*** Contractubex; Dolobene; ***India:*** Beparine; Proctosedyl; Thrombophob; ***Ital.:*** Edeven; Essaven; Flebs; Idracemi Eparina†; Luxazone Eparina; Proctosoll; Reparil; Rubidiosin Composto†; Venotrauma; Via Mal Traumagel; Vit Eparin; Xantervit Eparina; ***Port.:*** DM Gel; Etrat†; ***S.Afr.:*** Essaven; Thrombophob†; ***Spain:*** Essavenon; Recto Menaderm†; Venacol; Venoplant†; ***Switz.:*** Assan; Assan-Thermo; Bonactin†; Butaparin; Contractubex; Dolo-Arthrosenex; Dolobene; Gorgonium; Hepabuzone; Heparinol; Hepathrombine; Keli-med; Keppur; Lipactin; Lyman; Phlebostasin compositum; Ralur; Roll-bene†; Sportium; Sportusal; Venalot†; Venoplant comp; Venoplant N; Venucreme; Venugel.

---

# Heparinoids

Heparinoides.

## Profile

The term heparinoid includes heparin derivatives and has also been used more loosely to include naturally occurring and synthetic highly-sulfated polysaccharides of similar structure. Such compounds have been described in many ways; some of the terms used include sulfated glucosaminoglycans; glycosaminoglycan polysulfate compounds; or sulfated mucopolysaccharides.

The following anticoagulants may be described as heparinoids: danaparoid sodium (p.891), dermatan sulfate (p.892), pentosan polysulfate sodium (p.979), sodium apolate (p.1000), suleparoid (p.1009), and sulodexide (p.1009).

Heparinoid preparations are available with uses ranging from anticoagulation to the alleviation of inflammation (applied topically); some are claimed to have hypolipidaemic properties.

The proprietary names listed in this monograph refer to preparations containing undefined or less readily defined heparinoids that are used in a range of conditions including musculoskeletal and joint disorders, haemorrhoids, lipid disorders, and thromboembolic disorders.

## Preparations

**Proprietary Preparations** (details are given in Part 3)
***Arg.:*** Fleboderma; Hemeran; Hirudoid; ***Austral.:*** Hirudoid; Lasonil; ***Austria:*** Hemeran; Hirudoid; Lasonil; ***Belg.:*** Hemeran; Hirudoid; Lasonil; ***Braz.:*** Ateroide†; Hirudoid; ***Chile:*** Hirudoid; ***Denm.:*** Hirudoid; ***Fin.:*** Hirudoid; ***Ger.:*** Etrat Sportsalbe MPS; Hirudoid; Lasonil N; ***Hong Kong:*** Bruise Cream; Hirudoid; ***India:*** Hirudoid; ***Ital.:*** Angioflux; Ateran; Ateroid; Ateroxide; Condral; Erevan; Glicamin; Gluparin†; Hirudoid; Lasonil; Lasoven; Lipostop†; Matrix; Provenal; Ravenol; Suloves†; Treparin; ***Neth.:*** Hirudoid; Lasonil; ***Norw.:*** Hirudoid; ***NZ:*** Hirudoid; ***Port.:*** Hemeran; Hirudoid; Lasonil; ***Singapore:*** Hirudoid; ***Spain:*** Dinoven; Hirudoid; ***Swed.:*** Hirudoid; ***Switz.:*** Hemeran; Hirudoid; ***Thai.:*** Hirudoid; Varidoid; ***UK:*** Bruiseze; Hirudoid; Lasonil.

**Multi-ingredient: *Arg.:*** Mantus; ***Austral.:*** Movelat; ***Austria:*** Bayolin; Lemuval; Mobilat; Mobilisin; Mobilisin plus; Moviflex; ***Belg.:*** Mobilat; Mobilisin; ***Braz.:*** Ateroide†; Etrat; Mobilat; Mobilisin Composto; Sinteroid†; ***Chile:*** Mobilat; Repariven; ***Fin.:*** Mobilat; Moviflex; ***Fr.:*** Lasonil†; ***Ger.:*** Dignowell†; Dolo Mobilat; Mobilat; Mobilat Aktiv; Mobilisin†; Sanaven; Thermo Mobilisin†; ***Hong Kong:*** Mobilat; Movilisin†; Prelloran; ***Israel:*** Lasonil†; ***Ital.:*** Artrocur†; Flebs; Flogogin†; Herbavit†; Lasonil H†; Lasoproct†; Lasoreuma†; Mobilat; Mobilisin; Traumal; ***Mex.:*** Mobilat; ***Neth.:*** Mobilat; ***NZ:*** Lasonil; Movelat; ***Port.:*** Anacal; Mobilat; Mobilisin; ***S.Afr.:*** Mobilat†; ***Singapore:*** Mobilat; ***Spain:*** Lasonil; Movilat; Movilisin; ***Switz.:*** Dolo-Veniten; Mobilat N; Mobilat†; Mobilisin; Prelloran; ***Thai.:*** Mobilat; Movelat; ***UK:*** Anacal; Movelat.

---

# Hexobendine Hydrochloride *(BANM, rINNM)*

Hidrocloruro de hexobendina; ST-7090. *NN'*-Ethylenebis(3-methylaminopropyl 3,4,5-trimethoxybenzoate) dihydrochloride.

$C_{30}H_{44}N_2O_{10},2HCl = 665.6.$

*CAS — 54-03-5 (hexobendine); 50-62-4 (hexobendine hydrochloride).*

*ATC — C01DX06.*

NOTE. Hexobendine is *USAN.*

## Profile

Hexobendine hydrochloride is a vasodilator used in ischaemic heart disease in usual doses of 180 to 270 mg daily, in divided doses, by mouth. It is also included in multi-ingredient preparations used in cerebrovascular disorders.

Ischaemic heart disease is discussed under Atherosclerosis (p.815) and the treatment of its clinical manifestations is described under Angina Pectoris (p.813) and Myocardial Infarction (p.828).

## Preparations

**Proprietary Preparations** (details are given in Part 3)
***Austria:*** Ustimon; ***Spain:*** Ustimon†.

**Multi-ingredient: *Austria:*** Instenon; ***Hong Kong:*** Instenon; ***Spain:*** Vasperdil†; ***Thai.:*** Instenon.

---

# Hirudin

Hirudina; Hirudine.

## Profile

Hirudin is a 65-amino-acid protein that is a direct inhibitor of thrombin. It has been extracted from leeches (p.945) and this form is used in various topical preparations for peripheral vascular disorders. Recombinant hirudins, such as desirudin (p.892) and lepirudin (p.945) and analogues of hirudin, such as bivalirudin (p.875), are used as anticoagulants.

## Preparations

**Proprietary Preparations** (details are given in Part 3)
***Austria:*** Exhirud; Irudil†; ***Fr.:*** Hirucreme; ***Ger.:*** Exhirud.

**Multi-ingredient: *Ger.:*** Haemo-Exhirud; ***Ital.:*** Hirudex.

---

# Hydralazine Hydrochloride

*(BANM, rINNM)*

Apressinum; Hidrocloruro de hidralazina; Hydralazini Hydrochloridum; Hydrallazine Hydrochloride; Idralazina. 1-Hydrazinophthalazine hydrochloride.

$C_8H_8N_4,HCl = 196.6.$

*CAS — 86-54-4 (hydralazine); 304-20-1 (hydralazine hydrochloride).*

*ATC — C02DB02.*

**Pharmacopoeias.** In *Chin., Eur.* (see p.vi), *Int., Jpn,* and *US.*

**Ph. Eur. 5.0** (Hydralazine Hydrochloride). A white or almost white, crystalline powder. Soluble in water; slightly soluble in alcohol; very slightly soluble in dichloromethane. A 2% solution in water has a pH of 3.5 to 4.2. Protect from light.

**USP 27** (Hydralazine Hydrochloride). A white to off-white, odourless, crystalline powder. Soluble 1 in 25 of water and 1 in 500 of alcohol; very slightly soluble in ether. A 2% solution in water has a pH of 3.5 to 4.2. Store in airtight containers at a temperature of 25°, excursions permitted between 15° and 30°.

**Stability.** Discoloration of hydralazine injection was observed on several occasions after storage in a syringe for up to 12 hours.[1] Hydralazine reacts with metals and therefore the injection should be prepared using a nonmetallic filter and should be used as quickly as possible after being drawn through a needle into a syringe.

A study of the rate of degradation of hydralazine hydrochloride, 1 mg/mL in sweetened, aqueous oral liquids showed that glucose, fructose, lactose, and maltose reduced the stability of the drug.[2] In solutions containing mannitol or sorbitol, there was less than 10% degradation of hydralazine after 3 weeks. The UK manufacturer states that contact with glucose causes hydralazine to be rapidly broken down and that hydralazine injection is therefore not compatible with glucose solutions.

1. Enderlin G. Discoloration of hydralazine injection. *Am J Hosp Pharm* 1984; **41:** 634.
2. Das Gupta V, *et al.* Stability of hydralazine hydrochloride in aqueous vehicles. *J Clin Hosp Pharm* 1986; **11:** 215–23.

## Adverse Effects

Adverse effects occur frequently with hydralazine, particularly tachycardia, palpitations, angina pectoris, severe headache, and gastrointestinal disturbances such as anorexia, nausea, vomiting, and diarrhoea. These adverse effects, together with flushing, dizziness, and nasal congestion, which occur less often, may be seen at the start of treatment, especially if the dose is increased quickly. They generally subside with continued treatment. Other less common adverse effects include orthostatic hypotension, fluid retention with oedema and weight gain, conjunctivitis, lachrymation, tremor, and muscle cramps.

Hydralazine may deplete pyridoxine in the body, and can produce peripheral neuropathy with numbness and tingling of the extremities. Occasionally, hepatotoxicity, blood dyscrasias, haemolytic anaemia, difficulty in urinating, glomerulonephritis, constipation, paralytic ileus, depression, and anxiety occur.

Hypersensitivity reactions including fever, chills, pruritus, and rashes have been reported, and eosinophilia may occur.

Following the prolonged use of large doses, antinuclear antibodies may develop and a condition resembling systemic lupus erythematosus may occur. The incidence is greater in slow acetylators, patients with renal impairment, women, and patients taking more than 100 mg of hydralazine daily. The symptoms usually disappear when the drug is withdrawn; some patients may require treatment with corticosteroids.

Following acute overdosage, hypotension, tachycardia, myocardial ischaemia, arrhythmias, shock, and coma may occur.

**Carcinogenicity.** Although earlier reports suggested that hydralazine might be carcinogenic, there was no evidence from a survey of 1978 patients with lung or colorectal cancer and 6807 controls that there was an increased risk of these neoplasms.[1]

1. Kaufman DW, *et al.* Hydralazine use in relation to cancers of the lung, colon, and rectum. *Eur J Clin Pharmacol* 1989; **36:** 259–64.

**Effects on the blood.** Three cases of thrombocytopenia were reported[1] in neonates whose mothers had been treated with hydralazine for some months before delivery. The thrombocytopenia and bleeding was transient with full recovery occurring within a few weeks. No adverse effects were noticed in the mothers.

1. Widerlöv E, *et al.* Hydralazine-induced neonatal thrombocytopenia. *N Engl J Med* 1980; **303:** 1235.

**Effects on the cardiovascular system.** Paradoxical severe hypertension developed after oral or intramuscular hydralazine on 3 occasions in a patient with renal artery stenosis.[1]

1. Webb DB, White JP. Hypertension after taking hydrallazine. *BMJ* 1980; **280:** 1582.

**Effects on the kidneys.** Rapidly progressive glomerulonephritis with focal and segmental lesions, usually accompanied by necrosis and crescent formation, has been reported in patients receiving hydralazine.[1-3] The condition is reported to be associated with the presence of antinuclear antibodies[3] and slow acetylator status,[2] factors associated with the development of hydralazine-induced lupus erythematosus.[4] However, renal involvement is much less common in drug-induced lupus,[4] and in a report of 15 such cases men and women and fast and slow acetylators were equally affected;[3] in addition the criteria for systemic lupus erythematosus were not usually fulfilled in these patients and it was suggested that the condition should be distinguished from lupus nephritis. Immediate withdrawal of hydralazine generally results in some improvement in renal function but complete recovery is uncommon; severe cases may require immunosuppressive therapy.[3]


1. Björck S, *et al.* Rapidly progressive glomerulonephritis after hydralazine. *Lancet* 1983; **ii:** 42.
2. Kincaid-Smith P, Whitworth JA. Hydralazine-associated glomerulonephritis. *Lancet* 1983; **ii:** 348.
3. Björck S, *et al.* Hydralazine-induced glomerulonephritis. *Lancet* 1985; **i:** 392.
4. Hughes GRV. Recent developments in drug-associated systemic lupus erythematosus. *Adverse Drug React Bull* 1987; (Apr.): 460–3.


**Effects on the skin.** Pruritus and skin rashes have been reported with hydralazine use.

A 59-year-old woman who had been taking hydralazine 25 mg three times daily for 6 months developed symptoms of Sweet's syndrome (erythematous plaques and nodules and haemorrhagic blisters).[1] Symptoms began to subside on withdrawal of hydralazine but recurred when hydralazine was reintroduced. The condition resolved on discontinuation of hydralazine and treatment with prednisolone.


1. Gilmour E, *et al.* Drug-induced Sweet's syndrome (acute febrile neutrophilic dermatosis) associated with hydralazine. *Br J Dermatol* 1995; **133:** 490–1.


**Lupus erythematosus.** Lupus erythematosus is a well-documented adverse effect of hydralazine therapy. Onset is typically delayed from 1 month to 5 years from the start of treatment, and the most common symptoms are arthralgia or arthritis, usually non-deforming, in up to 95% of patients, fever and myalgia in about 50%, and pleuropulmonary involvement, manifesting as pleurisy, pleural effusions, or pulmonary infiltrates in up to 30%.[1-3] Renal involvement is reported to be less common than in idiopathic systemic lupus erythematosus and there is some uncertainty as to whether the glomerulonephritis sometimes seen in patients receiving hydralazine should be considered lupus nephritis—see under Effects on the Kidneys, above. Nonetheless, a 20% incidence of renal involvement has been reported.[1] Other complications and symptoms that have been associated with lupus erythematosus in patients taking hydralazine include cutaneous vasculitis,[4-6] orogenital and cutaneous ulceration,[7] bilateral retinal vasculitis,[8] reactive hypoglycaemia (although the attribution is uncertain),[9] life-threatening cardiac tamponade,[10] and hoarseness and stridor secondary to vocal cord palsy, which progressed to respiratory arrest.[11] Skin rashes are reported to be less prominent than with the idiopathic form of the disease.[1] Fatalities have occurred,[12] but appear to be rare.

Estimates of the overall incidence of hydralazine-associated lupus erythematosus vary from about 1.2 to 5% or more.[13-16] The syndrome appears to occur only in patients who develop antinuclear antibodies while receiving hydralazine, but the incidence of positive antinuclear antibody tests is much higher than that of lupus, at up to 60%, so the presence of antinuclear antibodies alone is not diagnostic.[15] There is a strong relationship with drug dose,[14,16] acetylator status,[13,15,16] and patient gender,[16] the syndrome being more common in slow acetylators and women, and in patients receiving 100 mg daily or more.

Although it has been reported that hydralazine-associated lupus was more frequent in patients with the HLA-DR4 antigen[17] this was not confirmed by others[18] and subsequent work has suggested that the association is rather with the non-expressing or null forms of the adjacent complement C4 gene.[19] Hydralazine can inactivate complement C4 *in vitro*[20] and might exacerbate complement deficiency (which is known to be associated with idiopathic systemic lupus erythematosus) in patients with an already low level of C4 due to a null allele.[19]


1. Hughes GRV. Recent developments in drug-associated systemic lupus erythematosus. *Adverse Drug React Bull* 1987; (Apr.): 460–3.
2. Cohen MG, Prowse MV. Drug-induced rheumatic syndromes: diagnosis, clinical features and management. *Med Toxicol Adverse Drug Exp* 1989; **4:** 199–218.
3. Price EJ, Venables PJW. Drug-induced lupus. *Drug Safety* 1995; **12:** 283–90.
4. Bernstein RM, *et al.* Hydrallazine-induced cutaneous vasculitis. *BMJ* 1980; **280:** 156–7.
5. Peacock A, Weatherall D. Hydralazine-induced necrotising vasculitis. *BMJ* 1981; **282:** 1121–2.
6. Finlay AY, *et al.* Hydrallazine-induced necrotising vasculitis. *BMJ* 1981; **282:** 1703–4.
7. Neville E, *et al.* Orogenital ulcers, SLE and hydrallazine. *Postgrad Med J* 1981; **57:** 378–9.
8. Doherty M, *et al.* Hydralazine induced lupus syndrome with eye disease. *BMJ* 1985; **290:** 675.
9. Blackshear PJ, *et al.* Reactive hypoglycaemia and insulin autoantibodies in drug-induced lupus erythematosus. *Ann Intern Med* 1983; **99:** 182–4.
10. Anandadas JA, Simpson P. Cardiac tamponade, associated with hydralazine therapy, in a patient with rapid acetylator status. *Br J Clin Pract* 1986; **40:** 305–6.
11. Chong WK, *et al.* Acute laryngeal stridor with respiratory arrest in drug induced systemic lupus erythematosus. *BMJ* 1988; **297:** 660–1.
12. Sturman SG, *et al.* Fatal hydralazine-induced systemic lupus erythematosus. *Lancet* 1988; **ii:** 1304.
13. Bing RF, *et al.* Hydrallazine in hypertension: is there a safe dose? *BMJ* 1980; **281:** 353–4.
14. Freestone S, *et al.* Incidence of hydrallazine-associated autoimmune disease. *Br J Clin Pharmacol* 1982; **13:** 291P–292P.
15. Mansilla-Tinoco R, *et al.* Hydralazine, antinuclear antibodies, and the lupus syndrome. *BMJ* 1982; **284:** 936–9.
16. Cameron HA, Ramsay LE. The lupus syndrome induced by hydralazine: a common complication with low dose treatment. *BMJ* 1984; **289:** 410–12.
17. Batchelor JR, *et al.* Hydralazine-induced systemic lupus erythematosus: influence of HLA-DR and sex on susceptibility. *Lancet* 1980; **i:** 1107–9.
18. Brand C, *et al.* Hydralazine-induced lupus: no association with HLA-DR4. *Lancet* 1984; **i:** 462.
19. Speirs C, *et al.* Complement system protein C4 and susceptibility to hydralazine-induced systemic lupus erythematosus. *Lancet* 1989; **i:** 922–4.
20. Sim E, *et al.* Drugs that induce systemic lupus erythematosus inhibit complement component C4. *Lancet* 1984; **ii:** 422–4.


## Treatment of Adverse Effects

Withdrawal of hydralazine or dosage reduction reverses many of the adverse effects. Peripheral neuropathy has been reported to be alleviated by pyridoxine.

If overdosage occurs gastric lavage may be performed or activated charcoal may be given if the patient presents within 1 hour of ingestion. Symptomatic and supportive treatment, including plasma expanders for shock and a beta blocker for tachycardia, should be given as necessary. Hypotension may respond to placing the patient in the supine position with the feet raised. If possible, pressor drugs should be avoided. If a pressor is necessary, one should be chosen that will not cause tachycardia or exacerbate arrhythmias; adrenaline should not be used.

## Precautions

Hydralazine is contra-indicated in patients with severe tachycardia, dissecting aortic aneurysm, heart failure with high cardiac output, cor pulmonale, or myocardial insufficiency due to mechanical obstruction, for example aortic or mitral stenosis or constrictive pericarditis. Hydralazine is also contra-indicated in patients with idiopathic systemic lupus erythematosus and related disorders.

Hydralazine-induced vasodilatation produces myocardial stimulation. It should therefore be used with caution in patients with ischaemic heart disease since it can increase angina and it should not be given to patients following myocardial infarction until their condition has stabilised. Patients with suspected or confirmed ischaemic heart disease should be given hydralazine under cover of a beta blocker, which should be started a few days before hydralazine, in order to prevent myocardial stimulation. If given to patients with heart failure they should be monitored for orthostatic hypotension and tachycardia during the initial stages of therapy, preferably in hospital. If treatment with hydralazine is to be stopped in patients with heart failure it should generally be withdrawn gradually. Hydralazine should be used with caution in patients with cerebrovascular disorders.

The dose of hydralazine should be reduced or the dosage interval prolonged in patients with hepatic or renal impairment. Complete blood counts and antinuclear antibody determinations should be carried out about every 6 months during long-term therapy. Urine analysis (for microhaematuria and proteinuria) is also recommended.

Hydralazine is teratogenic in some species of *animals* and should therefore be avoided during the first two trimesters of pregnancy.

Patients may experience impaired reactions, especially at the start of therapy, and should not drive or operate machinery if affected.

**Breast feeding.** Hydralazine is distributed into breast milk in small amounts (see under Pregnancy, below) but no adverse effects have been seen in infants and the American Academy of Pediatrics therefore considers[1] hydralazine to be usually compatible with breast feeding.


1. American Academy of Pediatrics. The transfer of drugs and other chemicals into human milk. *Pediatrics* 2001; **108:** 776–89. Correction. *ibid.*; 1029. Also available at: http://aappolicy.aappublications.org/cgi/content/full/pediatrics%3b108/3/776 (accessed 06/07/04)


**Porphyria.** Hydralazine has been associated with acute attacks of porphyria and is considered unsafe in porphyric patients.

**Pregnancy.** Hydralazine should be avoided during the first two trimesters of pregnancy.

Hydralazine concentrations were found to be similar in maternal and umbilical-cord blood in a study of 6 women being treated with hydralazine for pronounced hypertension during pregnancy.[1] Hydralazine was determined in the breast milk of 1 mother, but amounts detected were unlikely to produce clinically relevant concentrations in the infant.

For a report of thrombocytopenia occurring in neonates following maternal treatment with hydralazine during pregnancy, see Effects on the Blood under Adverse Effects, above.


1. Liedholm H, *et al.* Transplacental passage and breast milk concentrations of hydralazine. *Eur J Clin Pharmacol* 1982; **21:** 417–19.


## Interactions

The hypotensive effect of hydralazine may be enhanced by other drugs with a hypotensive action. Severe hypotension may occur if hydralazine and diazoxide are given together. However, some interactions with antihypertensives may be beneficial: thiazide diuretics also counteract the fluid retention caused by hydralazine, and beta blockers diminish the cardiac-accelerating effects.

**Indometacin.** Indometacin 100 mg daily did not attenuate the hypotensive effect of hydralazine in a study[1] in 9 healthy subjects, but another study[2] showed that indometacin 200 mg daily did attenuate the hypotensive effect of hydralazine but not the effects on heart rate, renal or limb blood flow, or plasma-catecholamine concentration.


1. Jackson SHD, Pickles H. Indomethacin does not attenuate the effects of hydralazine in normal subjects. *Eur J Clin Pharmacol* 1983; **25:** 303–5.
2. Cinquegrani MP, Liang C. Indomethacin attenuates the hypotensive action of hydralazine. *Clin Pharmacol Ther* 1986; **39:** 564–70.


## Pharmacokinetics

Orally administered hydralazine is rapidly absorbed from the gastrointestinal tract but undergoes considerable first-pass metabolism by acetylation in the gastrointestinal mucosa and liver. The rate of metabolism is genetically determined and depends upon the acetylator status of the individual. The bioavailability of hydralazine has been reported to be about 35% in slow acetylators and less in fast acetylators; thus plasma concentrations after a given dose are higher in slow acetylators.

Peak plasma concentrations have been reported to occur after about one hour. Hydralazine is chiefly present in plasma as a hydrazone conjugate with pyruvic acid. Plasma protein binding is about 90%. The drug is widely distributed, notably into arterial walls.

Systemic metabolism in the liver is by hydroxylation of the ring system and conjugation with glucuronic acid; most sources suggest that *N*-acetylation is not of major importance in systemic clearance and that therefore acetylator status does not affect elimination. Hydralazine is excreted mainly in urine as metabolites.

The apparent average half-life for hydralazine has been reported to vary from about 45 minutes to about 8 hours, with a number of sources giving the average as about 2 to 4 hours. Some of the variation may be due to problems with the analytical procedures—see below. The half-life is prolonged in renal impairment and may be up to 16 hours in patients with a creatinine clearance of less than 20 mL/minute.

Hydralazine crosses the placenta and is distributed into breast milk.

◊ Attempts to describe the pharmacokinetics of hydralazine have been plagued by the instability of the drug itself in plasma and in alkaline solutions, and the instability of its circulating metabolites during analysis, and has meant that many techniques for the measurement of hydralazine have proved non-selective and yield overestimates of unchanged drug.[1] Studies using less selective methods have yielded an apparent bioavailability for oral hydralazine of 38 to 69% in slow acetylators and 22 to 32% in fast acetylators; in contrast, more selective assays have yielded values of 31 to 35% and 10 to 16% for slow and rapid acetylators respectively. Similarly, hydralazine plasma clearance is lower and the half-life longer when based upon the results of non-selective assay procedures; mean elimination half-life has ranged from 2.2 to 3.6 hours based upon these methods compared with 0.67 to 0.96 hours using a more selective assay. Improved pharmacokinetic data has indicated that while the first-pass effect is dependent upon acetylator phenotype, systemic clearance is only minimally dependent upon acetylation. The formation of the pyruvic acid hydrazone, which is without significant vasodilator activity, contributes to extrahepatic phenotype-independent clearance.

Although some workers have correlated the hypotensive effect of hydralazine with concentrations,[2] others have been unable to do so.[3] Moreover, the duration of hypotensive effect has been shown to exceed considerably that predicted from the rate of elimination.[4,5] Possible explanations are the accumulation of hydralazine at its sites of action in the arterial walls[6] or the existence of active metabolites.[7-9]

Concurrent intake of food has been found to enhance considerably the bioavailability of hydralazine[10] but food-related reductions in plasma-hydralazine concentrations with reduced vasodilator effect have also been reported.[11] The discrepancy was thought to be due to the greater specificity of the assay used in the latter study and to differences in the timing of food and hydralazine administration in the two studies.[12,13]


1. Ludden TM, *et al.* Clinical pharmacokinetics of hydralazine. *Clin Pharmacokinet* 1982; **7:** 185–205.
2. Zacest R, Koch-Weser J. Relation of hydralazine plasma concentration to dosage and hypotensive action. *Clin Pharmacol Ther* 1972; **13:** 420–5.
3. Talseth T, *et al.* Hydralazine slow-release: observations on serum profile and clinical efficacy in man. *Curr Ther Res* 1977; **21:** 157–68.
4. O'Malley K, *et al.* Duration of hydralazine action in hypertension. *Clin Pharmacol Ther* 1975; **18:** 581–6.
5. Shepherd AMM, *et al.* Hydralazine kinetics after single and repeated oral doses. *Clin Pharmacol Ther* 1980; **28:** 804–11.
6. Moore-Jones D, Perry HM. Radioautographic localization of hydralazine-1-$C_{14}$ in arterial walls. *Proc Soc Exp Biol Med* 1966; **122:** 576–9.
7. Barron K, *et al.* Comparative evaluation of the in vitro effects of hydralazine and hydralazine acetonide on arterial smooth muscle. *Br J Pharmacol* 1977; **61:** 345–9.
8. Haegele KD, *et al.* Identification of hydrallazine and hydrallazine hydrazone metabolites in human body fluids and quantitative in vitro comparisons of their smooth muscle relaxant activity. *Br J Clin Pharmacol* 1978; **5:** 489–94.
9. Reece PA, *et al.* Interference in assays for hydralazine in humans by a major plasma metabolite, hydralazine pyruvic acid hydrazone. *J Pharm Sci* 1978; **67:** 1150–3.
10. Melander A, *et al.* Enhancement of hydralazine bioavailability by food. *Clin Pharmacol Ther* 1977; **22:** 104–7.
11. Shepherd AMM, *et al.* Effect of food on blood hydralazine levels and response in hypertension. *Clin Pharmacol Ther* 1984; **36:** 14–18.
12. Melander A, *et al.* Concomitant food intake does enhance the bioavailability and effect of hydralazine. *Clin Pharmacol Ther* 1985; **38:** 475.
13. Shepherd AMM, *et al.* Concomitant food intake does enhance the bioavailability and effect of hydralazine. *Clin Pharmacol Ther* 1985; **38:** 475–6.


## Uses and Administration

Hydralazine is a direct-acting vasodilator that acts predominantly on the arterioles. It reduces blood pressure and peripheral resistance but produces fluid retention. Tachycardia and an increase in cardiac output occur mainly as a reflex response to the reduction in peripheral resistance. Hydralazine tends to improve renal and cerebral blood flow and its effect on diastolic pressure is more marked than on systolic pressure.

Hydralazine hydrochloride is given by mouth for the treatment of hypertension (p.825), usually with a beta blocker and a thiazide diuretic. In addition to an additive antihypertensive effect, this combination reduces the reflex tachycardia and fluid retention caused by hydralazine. It may be given intravenously in hypertensive crises. Hydralazine is also used with isosorbide dinitrate in the management of heart failure (but see Precautions, above). For further discussion of this use of hydralazine, see below.

The dose of hydralazine should be reduced or the dosage interval prolonged in patients with renal or hepatic impairment.

In **hypertension**, the usual initial dose of hydralazine hydrochloride is 40 to 50 mg daily by mouth in divided doses, increased according to response. In the UK it is recommended that the dose should not be increased above 100 mg daily without checking acetylator status, although the recommended maximum dose for hypertension is 200 mg daily; doses above 100 mg daily are associated with an increased incidence of lupus erythematosus, particularly in women and in slow acetylators.

In hypertensive crises, hydralazine hydrochloride is given in doses of 5 to 10 mg by slow intravenous injection, repeated if necessary after 20 to 30 minutes. Alternatively, it may be given by continuous intravenous infusion in an initial dose of 200 to 300 micrograms/minute; the usual maintenance dose range is 50 to 150 micrograms/minute. Hydralazine hydrochloride has also been given by intramuscular injection.

**Heart failure.** Hydralazine with isosorbide dinitrate may have a role in the management of patients with heart failure (p.820) in whom ACE inhibitors are contra-indicated or not tolerated. Although a meta-analysis of a number of studies[1] of vasodilator therapy for heart failure failed to show a benefit in terms of improved functional status or reduced mortality in patients given hydralazine alone, there is evidence from the Veterans Administration Cooperative Study[2] of reduced mortality from the use of hydralazine with nitrates. This has been confirmed in a second study (V-HeFTII),[3] although hydralazine with isosorbide dinitrate was less effective than enalapril.

If hydralazine is used in patients with heart failure it should be started under hospital supervision (see also Precautions, above). Doses used are generally higher than those given for hypertension; in the two studies,[2,3] the dose of hydralazine was increased gradually to 300 mg daily and that of isosorbide dinitrate to 160 mg daily, provided that they were tolerated. Both drugs were given by mouth in divided doses.

Hydralazine has also been tried in children with heart failure,[4,5] but experience is limited.


1. Mulrow CD, *et al.* Relative efficacy of vasodilator therapy in chronic congestive heart failure: implications of randomized trials. *JAMA* 1988; **259:** 3422–6.
2. Cohn JN, *et al.* Effect of vasodilator therapy on mortality in chronic congestive heart failure: results of a Veterans Administration cooperative study. *N Engl J Med* 1986; **314:** 1547–52.
3. Cohn JN, *et al.* A comparison of enalapril with hydralazine-isosorbide dinitrate in the treatment of chronic congestive heart failure. *N Engl J Med* 1991; **325:** 303–10.
4. Artman M, *et al.* Hemodynamic effects of hydralazine in infants with idiopathic dilated cardiomyopathy and congestive heart failure. *Am Heart J* 1987; **113:** 144–50.
5. Rao PS, Andaya WG. Chronic afterload reduction in infants and children with primary myocardial disease. *J Pediatr* 1986; **108:** 530–4.


## Preparations

***BP 2003:*** Hydralazine Injection; Hydralazine Tablets;
***USP 27:*** Hydralazine Hydrochloride Injection; Hydralazine Hydrochloride Oral Solution; Hydralazine Hydrochloride Tablets; Reserpine, Hydralazine Hydrochloride, and Hydrochlorothiazide Tablets.

**Proprietary Preparations** (details are given in Part 3)
***Arg.:*** Hidral; Hydrapres; ***Austral.:*** Alphapress; Apresoline; ***Braz.:*** Apresolina; Nepresol; ***Canad.:*** Apresoline; Novo-Hylazin; Nu-Hydral; ***Denm.:*** Apresolin†; ***Hong Kong:*** Apresoline; ***Irl.:*** Apresoline; ***Israel:*** Alphapress; ***Mex.:*** Apresolina; Bionobal; ***Neth.:*** Apresoline; ***Norw.:*** Apresolin; ***NZ:*** Apresoline; ***S.Afr.:*** Apresoline; Hyperphen; ***Spain:*** Hydrapres; ***Swed.:*** Apresolin; ***Thai.:*** Apresoline; Cesoline; ***UK:*** Apresoline; ***USA:*** Apresoline.

**Multi-ingredient:** ***Austria:*** Polinorm; Trepress; Triloc; ***Canad.:*** Ser-Ap-Es†; ***Ger.:*** Docidrazin; Impresso; Pertenso N; Treloc; Trepress; TRI-Normin; ***India:*** Corbetazine; ***Spain:*** Betadipresan; Betadipresan Diu; Neatenol Diuvas; Tensiocomplet; ***Switz.:*** Trepress†; ***Thai.:*** Hydrares; Hypery; Reser; Ser-Ap-Es; ***USA:*** Apresazide; Hydra-zide; Hydrap-ES; Marpres; Ser-Ap-Es; Tri-Hydroserpine.

# Hydrochlorothiazide *(BAN, rINN)*

Hidroclorotiazida; Hydrochlorothiazidum. 6-Chloro-3,4-dihydro-2*H*-1,2,4-benzothiadiazine-7-sulphonamide 1,1-dioxide.

$C_7H_8ClN_3O_4S_2$ = 297.7.

*CAS — 58-93-5.*

*ATC — C03AA03.*

NOTE. Compounded preparations of hydrochlorothiazide may be represented by the following names:

- Co-amilozide (*BAN*)—hydrochlorothiazide 10 parts and amiloride hydrochloride 1 part (w/w)
- Co-amilozide (*PEN*)—amiloride hydrochloride and hydrochlorothiazide
- Co-spironozide (*PEN*)—spironolactone and hydrochlorothiazide
- Co-triamterzide (*BAN*)—triamterene 2 parts and hydrochlorothiazide 1 part (w/w)
- Co-triamterzide (*PEN*)—triamterene and hydrochlorothiazide
- Co-zidocapt (*BAN*)—hydrochlorothiazide 1 part and captopril 2 parts (w/w).

**Pharmacopoeias.** In *Chin., Eur.* (see p.vi), *Int., Jpn, Pol., US,* and *Viet.*

**Ph. Eur. 5.0** (Hydrochlorothiazide). A white or almost white, crystalline powder. Very slightly soluble in water; sparingly soluble in alcohol; soluble in acetone. It dissolves in dilute solutions of alkali hydroxides.

**USP 27** (Hydrochlorothiazide). A white or practically white, practically odourless crystalline powder. Slightly soluble in water; insoluble in chloroform, in ether, and in dilute mineral acids; freely soluble in dimethylformamide, in *n*-butylamine, and in sodium hydroxide solution; sparingly soluble in methyl alcohol.

## Adverse Effects

Hydrochlorothiazide and other thiazide diuretics may cause a number of metabolic disturbances especially at high doses. They may provoke hyperglycaemia and glycosuria in diabetic and other susceptible patients. They may cause hyperuricaemia and precipitate attacks of gout in some patients. Administration of thiazide diuretics may be associated with electrolyte imbalances including hypochloraemic alkalosis, hyponatraemia, and hypokalaemia. Hypokalaemia intensifies the effect of digitalis on cardiac muscle and administration of digitalis or its glycosides may have to be temporarily suspended. Patients with cirrhosis of the liver are particularly at risk from hypokalaemia. Hyponatraemia may occur in patients with severe heart failure who are very oedematous, particularly with large doses in conjunction with restricted salt in the diet. The urinary excretion of calcium is reduced. Hypomagnesaemia has also occurred. Adverse changes in plasma lipids have also been noted but their clinical significance is unclear.

Signs of electrolyte imbalance include dry mouth, thirst, weakness, lethargy, drowsiness, restlessness, muscle pain and cramps, seizures, oliguria, hypotension, and gastrointestinal disturbances.

Other side-effects include anorexia, gastric irritation, nausea, vomiting, constipation, diarrhoea, sialadenitis, headache, dizziness, photosensitivity reactions, orthostatic hypotension, paraesthesia, impotence, and yellow vision. Hypersensitivity reactions include skin rashes, fever, pulmonary oedema, pneumonitis, anaphylaxis, and toxic epidermal necrolysis. Cholestatic jaundice, pancreatitis, and blood dyscrasias including thrombocytopenia and, more rarely, granulocytopenia, leucopenia, and aplastic and haemolytic anaemia have been reported.

Intestinal ulceration has occurred after the use of tablets containing thiazides with an enteric-coated core of potassium chloride (see also under Potassium, p.1232).

**Carcinogenicity.** Several studies have suggested that long-term diuretic therapy may be associated with the development of cancer. A meta-analysis[1] of 9 case control studies and 3 cohort studies found an increased risk of renal cell carcinoma in patients receiving diuretics, and a further retrospective study[2] found that the risk of colon cancer was also increased. While the risk is probably not significant in most patients, it was suggested[1,2] that it should be taken into consideration when choosing long-term therapy for younger patients.


1. Grossman E, *et al.* Does diuretic therapy increase the risk of renal cell carcinoma? *Am J Cardiol* 1999; **83:** 1090–3.
2. Tenenbaum A, *et al.* Is diuretic therapy associated with an increased risk of colon cancer? *Am J Med* 2001; **110:** 143–5.


**Effects on the blood.** There have been case reports of intravascular immune haemolysis in patients taking hydrochlorothiazide and methyldopa.[1-3] In each of these 3 cases the hydrochlorothiazide was identified as the probable cause of haemolysis on serological data, although methyldopa could have been a contributory factor. One of these patients died[3] during the haemolytic episode although post-mortem examination failed to reveal a cause of death.


1. Vila JM, *et al.* Thiazide-induced immune hemolytic anemia. *JAMA* 1976; **236:** 1723–4.
2. Garratty G, *et al.* Acute immune intravascular hemolysis due to hydrochlorothiazide. *Am J Clin Pathol* 1981; **76:** 73–8.
3. Beck ML, *et al.* Fatal intravascular immune hemolysis induced by hydrochlorothiazide. *Am J Clin Pathol* 1984; **81:** 791–4.


**Effects on electrolyte balance.** MAGNESIUM AND POTASSIUM. The clinical consequences of diuretic-induced hypokalaemia have been controversial.[1-3] Of major concern has been the possibility that diuretic-induced hypokalaemia could predispose to cardiac arrhythmias and sudden cardiac death in some patients, and it has been suggested that this could explain the lower than expected reduction in deaths due to ischaemic heart disease found in some hypertension trials. Indeed, some case-control studies[4,5] have suggested an association between an increased risk of sudden cardiac death and the use of thiazides or other non-potassium-sparing diuretics; the addition of a potassium supplement had little effect on this risk, whereas addition of a potassium-sparing diuretic to the thiazide lowered the risk.[4] However, no reduction in cardiac arrhythmias after the correction of hypokalaemia has been seen[6] nor any evidence of increased arrhythmias associated with diuretic-induced hypokalaemia.[7] Several reviews[8,9] have argued that there is no proof of a causal relationship between hypokalaemia and serious dysrhythmias and this was endorsed by a randomised study.[10]

It is generally agreed that routine potassium supplementation in patients taking diuretics is unnecessary; however, supplementation will be required if the serum-potassium concentration falls below 3.0 mmol/litre. Potassium replacement or conservation is also likely to be necessary in patients at risk from the cardiac effects of hypokalaemia[11] such as those with severe heart disease, those taking digitalis preparations or high doses of diuretics, and in patients with severe liver disease.

The amount of potassium in fixed combination diuretic and potassium preparations has long been considered insufficient to correct hypokalaemia and the effectiveness of oral potassium supplements in increasing body stores of potassium has been questioned.[12-14] Hypokalaemia may be overcome by adding a potassium-sparing diuretic such as amiloride or triamterene[15] to the regimen, but there is a danger of hyperkalaemia if they are used indiscriminately. The *routine* use of fixed-dose combination preparations of a thiazide or loop diuretic with a potassium-sparing diuretic is considered unnecessary.[16] Potassium-sparing diuretics will not correct the potassium deficit unrelated to diuretic therapy in patients with severe heart failure.[17] When thiazides are given with drugs that may induce hyperkalaemia, such as beta blockers, ACE inhibitors, or angiotensin II receptor antagonists, the diuretic-induced hypokalaemia may be ameliorated, but not necessarily corrected completely. Hypokalaemia has been reported[18-20] in patients taking fixed-dose combinations of thiazides and beta blockers.

Potassium supplementation alone may not be sufficient to correct hypokalaemia in patients who are also deficient in magnesium,[21] although it is unlikely to be of clinical significance.[22]

Magnesium depletion has also been implicated as a risk factor for arrhythmias.[9,23]

1. Materson BJ. Diuretic-associated hypokalemia. *Arch Intern Med* 1985; **145:** 1966–7.
2. Kaplan NM, *et al.* Potassium supplementation in hypertensive patients with diuretic-induced hypokalemia. *N Engl J Med* 1985; **312:** 746–9.
3. Kassirer JP, Harrington JT. Fending off the potassium pushers. *N Engl J Med* 1985; **312:** 785–7.
4. Siscovick DS, *et al.* Diuretic therapy for hypertension and the risk of primary cardiac arrest. *N Engl J Med* 1994; **330:** 1852–7.
5. Hoes AW, *et al.* Diuretics, β-blockers, and the risk for sudden cardiac death in hypertensive patients. *Ann Intern Med* 1995; **123:** 481–7.
6. Papademetriou V, *et al.* Diuretic-induced hypokalemia in uncomplicated systemic hypertension: effect of plasma potassium correction on cardiac arrhythmias. *Am J Cardiol* 1983; **52:** 1017–22.
7. Papademetriou V, *et al.* Thiazide therapy is not a cause of arrhythmia in patients with systemic hypertension. *Arch Intern Med* 1988; **148:** 1272–6.
8. Harrington JT, *et al.* Our national obsession with potassium. *Am J Med* 1982; **73:** 155–9.
9. Freis ED. Critique of the clinical importance of diuretic-induced hypokalemia and elevated cholesterol level. *Arch Intern Med* 1989; **149:** 2640–8.
10. Siegel D, *et al.* Diuretics, serum and intracellular electrolyte levels, and ventricular arrhythmias in hypertensive men. *JAMA* 1992; **267:** 1083–9.
11. Anonymous. Potassium-sparing diuretics—when are they really needed? *Drug Ther Bull* 1985; **23:** 17–20.
12. Jackson PR, *et al.* Relative potency of spironolactone, triamterene and potassium chloride in thiazide-induced hypokalaemia. *Br J Clin Pharmacol* 1982; **14:** 257–63.
13. Shenfield GM. Fixed combination drug therapy. *Drugs* 1982; **23:** 462–80.
14. Papademetriou V, *et al.* Effectiveness of potassium chloride or triamterene in thiazide hypokalemia. *Arch Intern Med* 1985; **145:** 1986–90.
15. Kohvakka A. Maintenance of potassium balance during long-term diuretic therapy in chronic heart failure patients with thiazide-induced hypokalemia: comparison of potassium supplementation with potassium chloride and potassium-sparing agents, amiloride and triamterene. *Int J Clin Pharmacol Ther Toxicol* 1988; **26:** 273–7.
16. Anonymous. Routine use of potassium-sparing diuretics. *Drug Ther Bull* 1991; **29:** 85–7.
17. Davidson C, *et al.* The effects of potassium supplements, spironolactone or amiloride on the potassium status of patients with heart failure. *Postgrad Med J* 1978; **54:** 405–9.
18. Skehan JD, *et al.* Hypokalaemia induced by a combination of a beta-blocker and a thiazide. *BMJ* 1982; **284:** 83.
19. Odugbesan O, *et al.* Hazards of combined beta-blocker/diuretic tablets. *Lancet* 1985; **i:** 1221–2.
20. Jacobs L. Hypokalaemia with beta-blocker/thiazide combinations. *J R Coll Gen Pract* 1986; **36:** 39.
21. Dyckner T. Relation of cardiovascular disease to potassium and magnesium deficiencies. *Am J Cardiol* 1990; **65:** 44–6.
22. Papademetriou V. Magnesium depletion and thiazide hypokalemia. *Arch Intern Med* 1986; **146:** 1026.
23. Ryan MP. Diuretics and potassium/magnesium depletion: directions for treatment. *Am J Med* 1987; **82** (suppl 3A): 38–47.

SODIUM. Diuretics are a common cause of hyponatraemia.[1-3] Dilutional hyponatraemia may occur in patients with heart failure, but hyponatraemia may also result from sodium depletion[1] or inappropriate antidiuretic hormone secretion.[4] Other suggested mechanisms include decreased renal clearance of free water, hypomagnesaemia, and intracellular potassium depletion.[3,5] There have been a number of reports suggesting that hyponatraemia may be a particular problem with combinations of hydrochlorothiazide and potassium-sparing diuretics,[6-8] especially in elderly patients. The effect may be exacerbated by the relatively high doses of thiazide present in some fixed-dose preparations.[9] The symptoms of hyponatraemia may be non-specific and include nausea, lethargy, weakness, mental confusion, and anorexia,[1,2] but it may be an important cause of morbidity.[2,5] Severe sequelae of hyponatraemia include tonic-clonic seizures[10] and clinical features resembling subarachnoid haemorrhage.[11,12] Some patients, especially the elderly, may be particularly susceptible to the hyponatraemic effects of thiazides, possibly as a result of inappropriate secretion of antidiuretic hormone.[4] Plasma electrolyte concentrations should be monitored in patients receiving long-term diuretic therapy.[3,10] Measurement of serum-sodium concentration and body-weight following a single dose of thiazide could be useful in identifying patients at increased risk of developing hyponatraemia.[5]

1. Roberts CJC, *et al.* Hyponatraemia: adverse effect of diuretic treatment. *BMJ* 1977; **1:** 210.
2. Kennedy PGE, *et al.* Severe hyponatraemia in hospital inpatients. *BMJ* 1978; **2:** 1251–3.
3. Walters EG, *et al.* Hyponatraemia associated with diuretics. *Br J Clin Pract* 1987; **41:** 841–4.
4. Sonnenblick M, *et al.* Thiazide-induced hyponatremia and vasopressin release. *Ann Intern Med* 1989; **110:** 751.
5. Friedman E, *et al.* Thiazide-induced hyponatremia: reproducibility by single dose rechallenge and an analysis of pathogenesis. *Ann Intern Med* 1989; **110:** 24–30.
6. Strykers PH, *et al.* Hyponatremia induced by a combination of amiloride and hydrochlorothiazide. *JAMA* 1984; **252:** 389.
7. Roberts CJC, *et al.* Hyponatraemia induced by a combination of hydrochlorothiazide and triamterene. *BMJ* 1984; **288:** 1962.
8. Millson D, *et al.* Hyponatraemia and Moduretic (amiloride plus hydrochlorothiazide). *BMJ* 1984; **289:** 1308–9.
9. Bayer AJ, *et al.* Plasma electrolytes in elderly patients taking fixed combination diuretics. *Postgrad Med J* 1986; **62:** 159–62.
10. Johnston C, *et al.* Hyponatraemia and Moduretic-grand mal seizures: a review. *J R Soc Med* 1989; **82:** 479–83.
11. Benfield GFA, *et al.* Dilutional hyponatraemia masquerading as subarachnoid haemorrhage in patient on hydrochlorothiazide/amiloride/timolol combined drug. *Lancet* 1986; **ii:** 341.
12. Bain PG, *et al.* Thiazide-induced dilutional hyponatraemia masquerading as subarachnoid haemorrhage. *Lancet* 1986; **ii:** 634.

**Effects on the gallbladder.** There is an increased risk of cholecystitis in patients taking thiazides, with some indication that risk increases with the duration of use;[1,2] some workers concluded that this increased risk was confined to patients with pre-existing gallstones.[2] In a study in 10 healthy subjects,[3] hydrochlorothiazide was found to induce modest changes in biliary lipid concentrations although it was not associated with supersaturation of the bile. These changes could not wholly explain any increase in gallbladder disease in patients taking thiazides. However, evidence is conflicting; other studies[4,5] have found no association between thiazides and cholecystitis, except possibly in women who are not overweight.[5]

1. Rosenberg L, *et al.* Thiazides and acute cholecystitis. *N Engl J Med* 1980; **303:** 546–8.
2. van der Linden W, *et al.* Acute cholecystitis and thiazides. *BMJ* 1984; **289:** 654–5.
3. Angelin B. Effect of thiazide treatment on biliary lipid composition in healthy volunteers. *Eur J Clin Pharmacol* 1989; **37:** 95–6.
4. Porter JB, *et al.* Acute cholecystitis and thiazides. *N Engl J Med* 1981; **304:** 954–5.
5. Kakar F, *et al.* Thiazide use and the risk of cholecystectomy in women. *Am J Epidemiol* 1986; **124:** 428–33.

**Effects on glucose metabolism.** The adverse effects of thiazides on glucose metabolism, such as insulin resistance, impaired glucose tolerance, precipitation of overt diabetes, and worsening of diabetic control, are well established but appear to be dose-related and may not be significant at lower doses (for example, hydrochlorothiazide 6.25 or 12.5 mg).[1] A study[2] in 16 non-diabetic hypertensive patients found that bendroflumethiazide, in a dose of 1.25 mg daily, had no effect on insulin sensitivity whereas a daily dose of 5 mg produced hepatic insulin resistance. Similarly, the high doses, for example bendroflumethiazide 5 mg twice daily, used in the Medical Research Council Study on Mild to Moderate Hypertension[3] resulted in an incidence of glucose intolerance that led to withdrawal from the study of 9.38 per 1000 patient-years in men and 6.01 per 1000 patient-years in women compared with 2.51 and 0.82 per 1000 patient-years respectively in patients taking placebo. A later prospective study[4] in non-diabetic hypertensive patients found that those taking thiazides [doses not specified] were at no greater risk for developing diabetes than those not receiving antihypertensive therapy. However, a prospective cohort study[5] in men aged between 50 and 60 found that those taking antihypertensive treatment (mainly thiazides, beta blockers, or both) showed an increase in blood glucose levels which was an independent risk factor for myocardial infarction, even when baseline insulin resistance was accounted for.

1. Neutel JM. Metabolic manifestations of low-dose diuretics. *Am J Med* 1996; **101** (suppl 3A): 71S–82S.
2. Harper R, *et al.* Effects of low dose versus conventional dose thiazide diuretic on insulin action in essential hypertension. *BMJ* 1994; **309:** 226–30.
3. Greenburg G. Adverse reactions to bendrofluazide and propranolol for the treatment of mild hypertension: report of Medical Research Council Working Party on Mild to Moderate Hypertension. *Lancet* 1981; **ii:** 539–43.
4. Gress TW, *et al.* Hypertension and antihypertensive therapy as risk factors for type 2 diabetes mellitus. *N Engl J Med* 2000; **342:** 905–12.
5. Dunder K, *et al.* Increase in blood glucose concentration during antihypertensive treatment as a predictor of myocardial infarction: population based cohort study. *BMJ* 2003; **326:** 681–4.

**Effects on the kidneys.** Thiazides can produce acute renal failure either from over-enthusiastic use producing sodium depletion and hypovolaemia or, occasionally, as a result of a hypersensitivity reaction.[1] Acute interstitial nephritis has been reported.[2,3] They can occasionally cause the formation of non-opaque urate calculi.[4]

1. Curtis JR. Diseases of the urinary system: drug-induced renal disorders: I. *BMJ* 1977; **2:** 242–4.
2. Linton AL, *et al.* Acute interstitial nephritis due to drugs: review of the literature with a report of nine cases. *Ann Intern Med* 1980; **93:** 735–41.
3. Anonymous. Case records of the Massachusetts General Hospital: case 42-1983. *N Engl J Med* 1983; **309:** 970–8.
4. Curtis JR. Diseases of the urinary system: drug-induced renal disorders: II. *BMJ* 1977; **2:** 375–7.

**Effects on lipids.** Thiazides have been reported to adversely affect the plasma-lipid profile in the short term by increasing concentrations of low-density and very-low-density lipoprotein cholesterol, as well as of triglycerides, but not of high-density lipoprotein cholesterol.[1] These effects are probably dose-related[2] and it has been argued that changes in plasma lipids are likely to be slight at the relatively low doses now used in hypertension. There is some evidence to suggest that these lipid changes may not persist long-term.[3] In the Treatment of Mild Hypertension Study (TOMHS),[4] plasma total cholesterol concentrations were increased after 12 months in patients receiving chlortalidone but this effect was no longer present after 24 months. Although there has been concern that any hyperlipidaemic effect might offset the benefits of treating hypertension in patients at risk of ischaemic heart disease, studies such as ALLHAT[5] have shown that thiazide-like diuretics (in this case chlortalidone) are as effective as other antihypertensives in reducing the incidence of cardiovascular events in patients with hypertension and at least one other risk factor for ischaemic heart disease.

1. Ames R. Effects of diuretic drugs on the lipid profile. *Drugs* 1988; **36** (suppl 2): 33–40.
2. Carlsen JE, *et al.* Relation between dose of bendrofluazide, antihypertensive effect, and adverse biochemical effects. *BMJ* 1990; **300:** 975–8.
3. Freis ED. Critique of the clinical importance of diuretic-induced hypokalemia and elevated cholesterol level. *Arch Intern Med* 1989; **149:** 2640–8.
4. Grimm RH, *et al.* Long-term effects on plasma lipids of diet and drugs to treat hypertension. *JAMA* 1996; **275:** 1549–56.
5. The ALLHAT Officers and Coordinators for the ALLHAT Collaborative Research Group. Major outcomes in high-risk hypertensive patients randomized to angiotensin-converting enzyme inhibitor or calcium channel blocker vs diuretic: The Antihypertensive and Lipid-Lowering Treatment to Prevent Heart Attack Trial (ALLHAT). *JAMA* 2002; **288:** 2981–97. Correction. *ibid.* 2003; **289:** 178.

**Effects on respiratory function.** Acute interstitial pneumonitis and acute pulmonary oedema are rare but potentially dangerous complications of thiazides and may be due to a hypersensitivity reaction. A number of cases have been reported,[1-7] frequently following a single dose of hydrochlorothiazide or chlorothiazide. The presenting symptoms could be mistakenly attributed to myocardial infarction.

1. Steinberg AD. Pulmonary edema following ingestion of hydrochlorothiazide. *JAMA* 1968; **204:** 167–9.
2. Beaudry C, Laplante L. Severe allergic pneumonitis from hydrochlorothiazide. *Ann Intern Med* 1973; **78:** 251–3.
3. Parfrey NA, Herlong HF. Pulmonary oedema after hydrochlorothiazide. *BMJ* 1984; **288:** 1880.
4. Watrigant Y, *et al.* Pneumopathie à l'hydrochlorothiazide d'évolution subaiguë: etude cytologique du lavage broncho-alvéolaire. *Rev Mal Respir* 1986; **4:** 227–9.
5. Klein MD. Noncardiogenic pulmonary edema following hydrochlorothiazide ingestion. *Ann Emerg Med* 1987; **16:** 901–3.
6. Bowden FJ. Non-cardiogenic pulmonary oedema after ingestion of chlorothiazide. *BMJ* 1989; **298:** 605.
7. Bernal C, Patarca R. Hydrochlorothiazide-induced pulmonary edema and associated immunologic changes. *Ann Pharmacother* 1999; **33:** 172–4.

**Effects on sexual function.** Adverse effects on sexual function have been reported in hypertensive patients receiving thiazides and other antihypertensives but it is not clear how much this is due to the underlying disease and how much is due to the drugs. In the Treatment of Mild Hypertension Study (TOMHS),[1] a double-blind randomised controlled trial that allocated patients to treatment with one of five groups of antihypertensives, the incidence of erectile dysfunction in men was relatively low but was highest in the diuretic group (chlortalidone treatment). The incidence was significantly higher in chlortalidone recipients than in placebo recipients at 24 months (17.1 and 8.1% respectively), but the difference was no longer significant at 48 months (18.3 and 16.7% respectively).

1. Grimm RH, *et al.* Long-term effects on sexual function of five antihypertensive drugs and nutritional hygienic treatment in hypertensive men and women: Treatment of Mild Hypertension Study (TOMHS). *Hypertension* 1997; **29:** 8–14.

**Effects on the skin.** A variety of rashes and skin reactions has been reported in patients taking thiazides. *Photosensitivity* reactions are among the most frequently reported skin reactions. In Australia[1] co-amilozide was the preparation most commonly implicated in photosensitivity reactions in reports to the Australian Drug Reactions Advisory Committee, although this may reflect the high usage of this preparation. The most likely mechanism is thought to be phototoxicity[1,2] involving mainly UVA radiation although UVB may be involved in some cases.[2] Chronic photosensitivity does not usually occur following withdrawal of the drug[2] although photosensitivity may persist for longer in some patients than in others.[2,3] Eruptions resembling *lichen planus*[4] and *subacute cutaneous lupus erythematosus*[5-7] may be due to photosensitivity reactions.

Other reported skin reactions include *vasculitis*,[8,9] *erythema multiforme*,[9] and *pseudoporphyria*.[10]

1. Stone K. Photosensitivity reactions to drugs. *Aust J Pharm* 1985; **66:** 415–18.
2. Addo HA, *et al.* Thiazide-induced photosensitivity: a study of 33 subjects. *Br J Dermatol* 1987; **116:** 749–60.
3. Robinson HN, *et al.* Thiazide diuretic therapy and chronic photosensitivity. *Arch Dermatol* 1985; **121:** 522–4.
4. Graham-Brown R. Lichen planus and lichen-planus-like reactions. *Br J Hosp Med* 1986; **36:** 281–4.
5. Jones SK, *et al.* Thiazide diuretic-induced subacute cutaneous lupus-like syndrome. *Br J Dermatol* 1985; **113** (suppl 29): 25.
6. Reed BR, *et al.* Subacute cutaneous lupus erythematosus associated with hydrochlorothiazide therapy. *Ann Intern Med* 1985; **103:** 49–51.
7. Darken M, McBurney EI. Subacute cutaneous lupus erythematosus-like drug eruption due to combination diuretic hydrochlorothiazide and triamterene. *J Am Acad Dermatol* 1988; **18:** 38–42.
8. Björnberg A, Gisslén H. Thiazides: a cause of necrotising vasculitis? *Lancet* 1965; **ii:** 982–3.
9. Hardwick N, Saxe N. Patterns of dermatology referrals in a general hospital. *Br J Dermatol* 1986; **115:** 167–76.
10. Motley RS. Pseudoporphyria due to Dyazide in a patient with vitiligo. *BMJ* 1990; **300:** 1468.

**Gout.** Thiazides have been associated with hyperuricaemia and gout in some patients. In the Medical Research Council Study on Mild to Moderate Hypertension,[1] a single-blinded trial, men receiving bendroflumethiazide had higher incidences of gout than those receiving placebo (12.23 and 1.03 per 1000 patient-years, respectively). The risk appears to be dose-related; in a retrospective study[2] in patients aged 65 or older receiving antihypertensive therapy, there was a significantly increased risk of starting antigout therapy in patients receiving the equivalent of 25 mg hydrochlorothiazide or more daily, but not in those receiving lower doses.

1. Greenburg G. Adverse reactions to bendrofluazide and propranolol for the treatment of mild hypertension: report of Medical Research Council Working Party on Mild to Moderate Hypertension. *Lancet* 1981; **ii:** 539–43.
2. Gurwitz JH, *et al.* Thiazide diuretics and the initiation of antigout therapy. *J Clin Epidemiol* 1997; **50:** 953–9.

**Withdrawal.** For a report of oedema following abrupt withdrawal of thiazides, see under Precautions, below.

## Treatment of Adverse Effects

Hypokalaemia in patients treated with thiazides may be avoided or treated by concurrent use of potassium or a potassium-sparing diuretic (but see the discussion on potassium supplements, under Effects on Electrolyte Balance in Adverse Effects, above). Hypokalaemia can also be reduced by moderate sodium restriction. With the exception of patients with conditions such as hepatic failure or renal disease, chloride deficiency is usually mild and does not require specific treatment. Apart from the rare occasions when it is life-threatening, dilutional hyponatraemia is best treated with water restriction rather than salt therapy; in true hyponatraemia, appropriate replacement is the treatment of choice (see p.1220).

In massive overdosage, treatment should be symptomatic and directed at fluid and electrolyte replacement. Use of activated charcoal should be considered if the patient presents within 1 hour of ingestion.

## Precautions

All diuretics produce changes in fluid and electrolyte balance (see Adverse Effects, above). They should be used with caution in patients with existing fluid and electrolyte disturbances or who are at risk from changes in fluid and electrolyte balance, such as the elderly. They should be avoided in patients with severe hepatic impairment, in whom encephalopathy may be precipitated. Patients with hepatic cirrhosis are also more likely to develop hypokalaemia. Hyponatraemia may occur in patients with severe heart failure who are very oedematous, particularly with large doses of thiazides and restricted salt intake. All patients should be carefully observed for signs of fluid and electrolyte imbalance, especially in the presence of vomiting or during parenteral fluid therapy. Thiazides should not be given to patients with Addison's disease.

Diuretics should also be given with caution in renal impairment since they can further reduce renal function. Most thiazides are not effective in patients with a creatinine clearance of less than 30 mL/minute. They should not be used in patients with severe renal impairment or anuria.

Thiazides may precipitate attacks of gout in susceptible patients. They may cause hyperglycaemia and aggravate or unmask diabetes mellitus. Blood-glucose concentrations should be monitored in patients taking antidiabetics, since requirements may change. Thiazides can reduce urinary excretion of calcium, sometimes resulting in mild hypercalcaemia; they should not be given to patients with pre-existing hypercalcaemia. There is a possibility that thiazides may exacerbate or activate systemic lupus erythematosus in susceptible patients. For a suggestion that thiazides may increase the risk of developing gallstones, see Effects on the Gallbladder, above.

Thiazides cross the placenta and there have been reports of neonatal jaundice, thrombocytopenia, and electrolyte imbalances following maternal use. Reductions in maternal blood volume could also adversely affect placental perfusion. Treatment with large doses can inhibit lactation.

**Breast feeding.** Hydrochlorothiazide has been shown to pass into breast milk. In a woman taking 50 mg hydrochlorothiazide daily, peak milk concentrations were found[1] 5 to 10 hours after a dose and were approximately 25% of peak blood concentrations. No drug could be detected in the infant's blood, and his serum electrolytes, blood glucose, and blood urea nitrogen were normal. The American Academy of Pediatrics considers[2] that hydrochlorothiazide is usually compatible with breast feeding.

1. Miller ME, *et al.* Hydrochlorothiazide disposition in a mother and her breast-fed infant. *J Pediatr* 1982; **101:** 789–91.
2. American Academy of Pediatrics. The transfer of drugs and other chemicals into human milk. *Pediatrics* 2001; **108:** 776–89. Correction. *ibid.*; 1029. Also available at: http://aappolicy.aappublications.org/cgi/content/full/pediatrics%3b108/3/776 (accessed 06/07/04)

**Hyperparathyroidism.** Hypertension is a complication of primary hyperparathyroidism but thiazides have often been withheld for fear of exacerbating hypercalcaemia. However, no differences in plasma-calcium concentrations were found in 13 patients who received thiazides intermittently for up to 18 months. It was therefore concluded that thiazides are not contra-indicated in such patients.[1] They should, however, be stopped before parathyroid function is tested.

1. Farquhar CW, *et al.* Failure of thiazide diuretics to increase plasma calcium in mild primary hyperparathyroidism. *Postgrad Med J* 1990; **66:** 714–16.

**Porphyria.** Hydrochlorothiazide has been associated with acute attacks of porphyria and is considered unsafe in porphyric patients.

**Withdrawal.** In patients with mild hypertension whose blood pressure is consistently controlled, reduction in dosage or withdrawal of antihypertensive drugs may be possible. Serious oedema occurred in 8 patients with controlled hypertension within 2 weeks of abrupt withdrawal of thiazide diuretics.[1] Thiazides were resumed and gradually tapered without recurrence of oedema.

1. Brandspigel K. Diuretic-withdrawal edema. *N Engl J Med* 1986; **314:** 515.

## Interactions

Many of the interactions of hydrochlorothiazide and other thiazides are due to their effects on fluid and electrolyte balance. Diuretic-induced hypokalaemia may enhance the toxicity of digitalis glycosides and may also increase the risk of arrhythmias with drugs that prolong the QT interval, such as astemizole, terfenadine, halofantrine, pimozide, and sotalol. Thiazides may enhance the neuromuscular blocking action of competitive neuromuscular blockers, such as atracurium, probably by their hypokalaemic effect. The potassium-depleting effect of diuretics may be enhanced by corticosteroids, corticotropin, beta$_2$ agonists such as salbutamol, carbenoxolone, amphotericin B, or reboxetine.

Diuretics may enhance the effect of other antihypertensives, particularly the first-dose hypotension that occurs with alpha blockers or ACE inhibitors. Orthostatic hypotension associated with diuretics may be enhanced by alcohol, barbiturates, or opioids. The antihypertensive effects of diuretics may be antagonised by drugs that cause fluid retention, such as corticosteroids, NSAIDs, or carbenoxolone; diuretics may enhance the nephrotoxicity of NSAIDs. Thiazides have been reported to diminish the response to pressor amines, such as noradrenaline, but the clinical significance of this effect is uncertain.

Thiazides should not usually be used with lithium since the association may lead to toxic blood concentrations of lithium. Other drugs for which increased toxicity has been reported when given with thiazides include allopurinol and tetracyclines. Thiazides may alter the requirements for hypoglycaemics in diabetic patients.

**Antibacterials.** Severe hyponatraemia has been reported in patients taking *trimethoprim* with co-amilozide[1] and hydrochlorothiazide.[2]

1. Eastell R, Edmonds CJ. Hyponatraemia associated with trimethoprim and a diuretic. *BMJ* 1984; **289:** 1658–9.
2. Hart TL, *et al.* Hyponatremia secondary to thiazide-trimethoprim interaction. *Can J Hosp Pharm* 1989; **42:** 243–6.

**Antiepileptics.** There has been a report of symptomatic hyponatraemia associated with the use of hydrochlorothiazide or furosemide and *carbamazepine*.[1]

1. Yassa R, *et al.* Carbamazepine, diuretics, and hyponatremia: a possible interaction. *J Clin Psychiatry* 1987; **48:** 281–3.

**Bile-acid binding resins.** Gastrointestinal absorption of both chlorothiazide and hydrochlorothiazide has been reported to be reduced by *colestipol* and *colestyramine*.[1-3] In a study in healthy subjects[2] colestyramine had the greatest effect on hydrochlorothiazide, decreasing absorption by 85% compared with a decrease of 43% with colestipol. Even when colestyramine was administered 4 hours after hydrochlorothiazide[3] reductions of absorption of at least 30 to 35% could be expected.

1. Kauffman RE, Azarnoff DL. Effect of colestipol on gastrointestinal absorption of chlorothiazide in man. *Clin Pharmacol Ther* 1973; **14:** 886–90.
2. Hunninghake DB, *et al.* The effect of cholestyramine and colestipol on the absorption of hydrochlorothiazide. *Int J Clin Pharmacol Ther Toxicol* 1982; **20:** 151–4.
3. Hunninghake DB, Hibbard DM. Influence of time intervals for cholestyramine dosing on the absorption of hydrochlorothiazide. *Clin Pharmacol Ther* 1986; **39:** 329–34.

**Calcium salts.** The milk-alkali syndrome, characterised by hypercalcaemia, metabolic alkalosis, and renal failure, developed in a patient taking chlorothiazide and moderately large doses of calcium carbonate.[1] Patients taking thiazides may be at increased risk of developing the syndrome because of their reduced ability to excrete excess calcium. Hypercalcaemia may also occur in patients taking thiazides with drugs that increase calcium levels, such as vitamin D.

1. Gora ML, *et al.* Milk-alkali syndrome associated with use of chlorothiazide and calcium carbonate. *Clin Pharm* 1989; **8:** 227–9.

**Dopaminergics.** For a report of increased *amantadine* toxicity associated with hydrochlorothiazide and triamterene, see p.1198.

**NSAIDs.** NSAIDs cause fluid retention and may antagonise the diuretic actions of thiazides.[1]

1. Webster J. Interactions of NSAIDs with diuretics and β-blockers: mechanisms and clinical implications. *Drugs* 1985; **30:** 32–41.

## Pharmacokinetics

Hydrochlorothiazide is fairly rapidly absorbed from the gastrointestinal tract. It is reported to have a bioavailability of about 65 to 70%. It has been estimated to have a plasma half-life of between about 5 and 15 hours and appears to be preferentially bound to red blood cells. It is excreted mainly unchanged in the urine. Hydrochlorothiazide crosses the placental barrier and is distributed into breast milk.

◊ References.

1. Beermann B, *et al.* Absorption, metabolism, and excretion of hydrochlorothiazide. *Clin Pharmacol Ther* 1976; **19:** 531–7.
2. Beermann B, Groschinsky-Grind M. Pharmacokinetics of hydrochlorothiazide in man. *Eur J Clin Pharmacol* 1977; **12:** 297–303.
3. Beermann B, Groschinsky-Grind M. Pharmacokinetics of hydrochlorothiazide in patients with congestive heart failure. *Br J Clin Pharmacol* 1979; **7:** 579–83.

## Uses and Administration

Hydrochlorothiazide and the other thiazide diuretics are used in the treatment of hypertension (p.825), either alone or with other antihypertensives such as ACE inhibitors and beta blockers. They are also used to treat oedema associated with heart failure (p.820) and with renal and hepatic disorders. Other indications have included the treatment of oedema accompanying the premenstrual syndrome (p.1551), the prevention of water retention associated with corticosteroids and oestrogens, the treatment of diabetes insipidus (below), and the prevention of renal calculus formation in patients with hypercalciuria (below).

Thiazides are moderately potent diuretics and exert their diuretic effect by reducing the reabsorption of electrolytes from the renal tubules, thereby increasing the excretion of sodium and chloride ions, and consequently of water. They act mainly at the beginning of the distal tubules. The excretion of other electrolytes, notably potassium and magnesium, is also increased. The excretion of calcium is reduced. They also reduce carbonic-anhydrase activity so that bicarbonate excretion is increased, but this effect is generally small compared with the effect on chloride excretion and does not appreciably alter the pH of the urine. They may also reduce the glomerular filtration rate.

Their hypotensive effect is probably partly due to a reduction in peripheral resistance; they also enhance the effects of other antihypertensives. Paradoxically, thiazides have an antidiuretic effect in patients with diabetes insipidus.

**Administration and dosage.** Thiazides are usually given in the morning so that sleep is not interrupted by diuresis. Diuresis starts in about 2 hours after the oral administration of hydrochlorothiazide, reaches a maximum in about 4 hours, and lasts for 6 to 12 hours.

The dosage of thiazides should be adjusted to the minimum effective dose. In general lower doses are required for the treatment of hypertension than for oedema, although the maximum therapeutic effect may not be seen for several weeks.

They may be given to patients with mild renal impairment, but thiazides are generally not effective at a creatinine clearance of less than 30 mL/minute.

Hydrochlorothiazide is given by mouth.

In the treatment of **hypertension** an initial dose of 12.5 mg may be sufficient, increasing to 25 to 50 mg daily if necessary, either alone or with other antihypertensives. Doses of up to 100 mg have been suggested but are rarely necessary.

In the treatment of **oedema** the usual dose is 25 to 100 mg daily, reduced to a dose of 25 to 50 mg daily or intermittently; in severe cases initial doses of up to 200 mg daily have been suggested, but the more powerful loop diuretics (see Furosemide, p.919) are preferred in such patients.

In the treatment of nephrogenic **diabetes insipidus** an initial dose of up to 100 mg daily may be used.

An initial dose for children has been 1 to 2 mg/kg daily in single or 2 divided doses. Infants under 6 months may need doses of up to 3 mg/kg daily.

For discussion of potassium supplementation in patients taking thiazide diuretics see Effects on Electrolyte Balance, under Adverse Effects, above.

**Bronchopulmonary dysplasia.** Bronchopulmonary dysplasia (p.1077) is a major cause of chronic lung disease in infants. Treatment often involves the use of corticosteroids. Additional supportive therapy has included the use of diuretics such as furosemide (p.922); results with hydrochlorothiazide or spironolactone have been more ambiguous. No beneficial effects on lung function or oxygenation were found in a study of 12 infants after 1 week of treatment with hydrochlorothiazide and spironolactone.[1] However, hydrochlorothiazide and spironolactone therapy was found to improve total respiratory system compliance with decreased lung damage and increased survival rate in 34 premature infants with bronchopulmonary dysplasia after 8 weeks of therapy.[2] In the latter study furosemide was also given if clinically indicated.


1. Engelhardt B, *et al.* Effect of spironolactone-hydrochlorothiazide on lung function in infants with chronic bronchopulmonary dysplasia. *J Pediatr* 1989; **114:** 619–24.
2. Albersheim SG, *et al.* Randomized, double-blind, controlled trial of long-term diuretic therapy for bronchopulmonary dysplasia. *J Pediatr* 1989; **115:** 615–20.


**Diabetes insipidus.** Thiazide diuretics are used in nephrogenic diabetes insipidus (p.1314), sometimes with potassium-sparing diuretics. For instance, hydrochlorothiazide with amiloride was effective in controlling nephrogenic diabetes insipidus in 5 boys and compared favourably with treatment with hydrochlorothiazide and indometacin.[1] Treatment was well tolerated in 4 patients. Abdominal pain and anorexia necessitated withdrawal of amiloride in the fifth patient after six months. The use of hydrochlorothiazide with amiloride also obviated the need for potassium supplements, which were required with hydrochlorothiazide and indometacin. The use of hydrochlorothiazide with amiloride was also effective and well tolerated in a group of 4 children with nephrogenic diabetes insipidus who were treated for up to 5 years.[2]


1. Knoers N, Monnens LAH. Amiloride-hydrochlorothiazide versus indomethacin-hydrochlorothiazide in the treatment of nephrogenic diabetes insipidus. *J Pediatr* 1990; **117:** 499–502.
2. Kirchlechner V, *et al.* Treatment of nephrogenic diabetes insipidus with hydrochlorothiazide and amiloride. *Arch Dis Child* 1999; **80:** 548–52.


**Hypoparathyroidism.** In hypoparathyroidism (p.765), treatment is usually with oral vitamin D compounds to correct the hypocalcaemia. Thiazides may be useful in some patients. Beneficial effects on serum-calcium concentrations in patients with hypoparathyroidism have been reported following chlortalidone plus dietary salt restriction,[1] and with bendroflumethiazide.[2] However, chlortalidone has not been found to be effective in all patients,[3] and the reduction in urinary calcium excretion by thiazides has been shown to be diminished in patients with hypoparathyroidism,[4] suggesting that this effect may be dependent on the presence of active parathyroid hormone. Care should be taken when giving diuretics to hypoparathyroid patients with coexisting adrenal insufficiency[3] or metabolic alkalosis.[5]


1. Porter RH, *et al.* Treatment of hypoparathyroid patients with chlorthalidone. *N Engl J Med* 1978; **298:** 577–81.
2. Newman GH, *et al.* Effect of bendrofluazide on calcium reabsorption in hypoparathyroidism. *Eur J Clin Pharmacol* 1984; **27:** 41–6.
3. Gertner JM, Genel M. Chlorthalidone for hypoparathyroidism. *N Engl J Med* 1978; **298:** 1478.
4. Middler S, *et al.* Thiazide diuretics and calcium metabolism. *Metabolism* 1973; **22:** 139–45.
5. Barzel US. Chlorthalidone for hypoparathyroidism. *N Engl J Med* 1978; **289:** 1478.


**Ménière's disease.** In Ménière's disease (p.422) there is an excess of endolymph fluid in the ear and diuretics such as hydrochlorothiazide have been used in attempts to relieve symptoms by reducing the amount of fluid.

**Osteoporosis.** Although some epidemiological studies have indicated beneficial effects of thiazides on bone (reduced rates of bone loss[1] and a reduced risk of hip fracture[2-5]) a comprehensive analysis involving 9704 women over the age of 65 years[6] showed only a small effect on bone mass, no effect on the risk for falls, and no overall protective effect against fractures. A further prospective study[7] reported a reduction in forearm fracture, but hip fracture was only reduced in postmenopausal women. Randomised, controlled studies[8,9] have confirmed that hydrochlorothiazide reduces bone loss, but again the effects were small. Thus, thiazides have no established role in the prevention or treatment of osteoporosis (p.763). They might, however, be useful to reduce hypercalciuria in patients taking glucocorticoids[10] but serum-potassium concentrations should be monitored closely.


1. Wasnich R, *et al.* Effect of thiazide on rates of bone mineral loss: a longitudinal study. *BMJ* 1990; **301:** 1303–5. Correction. *ibid.* 1991; **302:** 218.
2. Ray WA, *et al.* Long-term use of thiazide diuretics and risk of hip fracture. *Lancet* 1989; **i:** 687–90.
3. LaCroix AZ, *et al.* Thiazide diuretic agents and the incidence of hip fracture. *N Engl J Med* 1990; **322:** 286–90.
4. Felson DT, *et al.* Thiazide diuretics and the risk of hip fracture: results from the Framingham Study. *JAMA* 1991; **265:** 370–3.
5. Schoofs MWCJ, *et al.* Thiazide diuretics and the risk for hip fracture. *Ann Intern Med* 2003; **139:** 476–82.
6. Cauley JA, *et al.* Effects of thiazide diuretic therapy on bone mass, fractures, and falls. *Ann Intern Med* 1993; **118:** 666–73.
7. Feskanich D, *et al.* A prospective study of thiazide use and fractures in women. *Osteoporos Int* 1997; **7:** 79–84.
8. Reid IR, *et al.* Hydrochlorothiazide reduces loss of cortical bone in normal postmenopausal women: a randomized controlled trial. *Am J Med* 2000; **109:** 362–70.
9. LaCroix AZ, *et al.* Low-dose hydrochlorothiazide and preservation of bone mineral density in older adults: a randomized, double-blind, placebo-controlled trial. *Ann Intern Med* 2000; **133:** 516–26.
10. Lukert BP, Raisz LG. Glucocorticoid-induced osteoporosis: pathogenesis and management. *Ann Intern Med* 1990; **112:** 352–64.


**Renal calculi.** Normal urine contains calcium, oxalate, and phosphate in amounts greater than their normal aqueous solubility; this supersaturation is maintained by a variety of inhibitors of crystallisation, both organic and inorganic. However, increases in the concentrations of crystalline substances in the urine, or decreases in the relative proportions of crystallisation inhibitors, may render individuals susceptible to the formation of renal calculi (kidney stones).

Renal calculi consist of crystalline components arranged around an organic matrix. They are typically formed in the calices or renal pelvis, and may become lodged in the ureter. About 1 to 5% of the population are affected, and although some patients only ever develop a single stone, between 50 and 80% of patients experience recurrences. Calcium-containing stones (usually calcium oxalate and calcium phosphate in variable proportions) account for the vast majority of occurrences although stones of other compositions including cystine, uric acid, or magnesium ammonium phosphate, are occasionally seen.

Patients with renal calculi may be asymptomatic or may pass small stones with relatively little discomfort. However, passage of a larger stone down the ureter may be accompanied by excruciating pain (renal or ureteral colic), obstruction, and trauma; there may also be associated infection.

**Treatment.** Management of recurrent renal calculi has been reviewed.[1] Treatment of existing stones, if any, is essentially surgical, while medical treatment is aimed at prevention of recurrence.[1-3] In the acute episode analgesics may be required for the pain (see Biliary and Renal Colic, p.4) but if there is no obstruction, infection, or other complication, conservative treatment is favoured, with the patient being monitored radiographically over several weeks to see if the stone will pass of its own accord. Where intervention is considered necessary, it may be by endoscopic surgery, or shock wave lithotripsy,[1] in which focussed shock waves are used to shatter the stone. Antibacterials may be needed for infection (see p.153 for urinary-tract infections).

In the prevention of recurrence it is important to identify, and where possible correct, any underlying disease process or biochemical or anatomical abnormality. Certain general measures are also appropriate. Patients should drink a minimum of 3 litres of fluid daily in order to maintain an adequate volume of urine. In hot climates or working environments a higher volume of fluid should be taken.

Dietary restrictions may be appropriate in some cases.[2] Traditionally, dairy products and other foods rich in calcium, as well as calcium-containing antacids and vitamin D supplements, have been avoided in patients with calcium-containing stones. However, studies have found an inverse relationship between dietary calcium intake and the risk of stone formation in men[4] and in women,[5] and restriction of dietary calcium is probably not necessary.[6] Conversely, calcium supplements do appear to increase the risk of stone formation and should be avoided, although the reason for this difference is not clear.[5] Limitation of the intake of animal protein and oxalate-rich foods, is also probably appropriate in such patients,[7] and sodium restriction may also be beneficial.[1,2] Indeed, restriction of animal protein and sodium with normal calcium intake has been shown to provide greater long-term protection in men than a low-calcium diet.[8]

In patients with idiopathic hypercalciuria (i.e. when excessive calcium excretion cannot be linked to hyperparathyroidism, sarcoidosis, malignancy, or some other underlying condition) and a history of renal calculi a **thiazide diuretic** is usually given,[1] and a meta-analysis[9] has shown the effectiveness of such treatment. Hydrochlorothiazide or amiloride have also been reported to be of benefit in patients with a history of calcium oxalate stones due to a defect in oxalate transport,[10] while thiazides or oral phosphates have been found effective in decreasing urinary calcium excretion in patients with absorptive hypercalciuria.[11] Where thiazides are ineffective treatment with sodium cellulose phosphate may be considered, together with a magnesium supplement. Sodium cellulose phosphate is of value in patients with excessive intestinal calcium absorption.[12] Phosphate salts[12] or magnesium salts[13,14] which act as non-specific inhibitors of urinary crystallisation may also be used.

In patients with reduced citrate excretion, treatment with potassium citrate may be useful in preventing stone recurrence;[1,15] by increasing urinary pH, it may also be helpful in patients with uric acid stones. Allopurinol has also been suggested for prevention of both uric acid stones and, for calcium oxalate stones, particularly when there is hyperuricosuria.[16]

In patients with struvite (magnesium ammonium phosphate) stones, which are associated with bacterial infection and result from the action of bacterial urease, control may be difficult to achieve using antibacterials alone; acetohydroxamic acid, an inhibitor of bacterial urease, has been given as an adjunct.[17,18] Penicillamine may be of benefit in preventing cystine stones in patients with cystinuria (p.1049).


1. Bihl G, Meyers A. Recurrent renal stone disease—advances in pathogenesis and clinical management. *Lancet* 2001; **358:** 651–6.
2. Pearle MS. Prevention of nephrolithiasis. *Curr Opin Nephrol Hypertens* 2001; **10:** 203–9.
3. Pak CYC. Medical prevention of renal stone disease. *Nephron* 1999; **81** (suppl 1): S60–S65.
4. Curhan GC, *et al.* A prospective study of dietary calcium and other nutrients and the risk of symptomatic kidney stones. *N Engl J Med* 1993; **328:** 833–8.
5. Curhan GC, *et al.* Comparison of dietary calcium with supplemental calcium and other nutrients as factors affecting the risk for kidney stones in women. *Ann Intern Med* 1997; **126:** 497–504.
6. Coe FL, *et al.* Diet and calcium: the end of an era? *Ann Intern Med* 1997; **126:** 553–5.
7. Lemann J. Composition of the diet and calcium kidney stones. *N Engl J Med* 1993; **328:** 880–2.
8. Borghi L, *et al.* Comparison of two diets for the prevention of recurrent stones in idiopathic hypercalciuria. *N Engl J Med* 2002; **346:** 77–84.
9. Pearle MS, *et al.* Meta-analysis of randomized trials for medical prevention of calcium oxalate nephrolithiasis. *J Endourol* 1999; **13:** 679–85.
10. Baggio B, *et al.* An inheritable anomaly of red-cell oxalate transport in "primary" calcium nephrolithiasis correctable with diuretics. *N Engl J Med* 1986; **314:** 599–604.
11. Insogna KL, *et al.* Trichlormethiazide and oral phosphate therapy in patients with absorptive hypercalciuria. *J Urol (Baltimore)* 1989; **141:** 269–74.
12. Pak CYC. Formation of renal stones may be prevented by restoring normal urinary composition. *Proc Eur Dial Transplant Assoc* 1983; **20:** 371–85.
13. Melnick I, *et al.* Magnesium therapy for recurring calcium oxalate urinary calculi. *J Urol (Baltimore)* 1971; **105:** 119–22.
14. Johansson G, *et al.* Biochemical and clinical effects of the prophylactic treatment of renal calcium stones with magnesium hydroxide. *J Urol (Baltimore)* 1980; **124:** 770–4.
15. Pak CYC, Fuller C. Idiopathic hypocitraturic calcium-oxalate nephrolithiasis successfully treated with potassium citrate. *Ann Intern Med* 1986; **104:** 33–7.
16. Ettinger B, *et al.* Randomized trial of allopurinol in the prevention of calcium oxalate calculi. *N Engl J Med* 1986; **315:** 1386–9.
17. Martelli A, *et al.* Acetohydroxamic acid therapy in infected renal stones. *Urology* 1981; **17:** 320–2.
18. Williams JJ, *et al.* A randomized double-blind study of acetohydroxamic acid in struvite nephrolithiasis. *N Engl J Med* 1984; **311:** 760–4.


## Preparations

***BP 2003:*** Co-amilozide Oral Solution; Co-amilozide Tablets; Co-triamterzide Tablets; Hydrochlorothiazide Tablets;
***USP 27:*** Amiloride Hydrochloride and Hydrochlorothiazide Tablets; Bisoprolol Fumarate and Hydrochlorothiazide Tablets; Captopril and Hydrochlorothiazide Tablets; Enalapril Maleate and Hydrochlorothiazide Tablets; Hydrochlorothiazide Tablets; Methyldopa and Hydrochlorothiazide Tablets; Metoprolol Tartrate and Hydrochlorothiazide Tablets; Propranolol Hydrochloride and Hydrochlorothiazide Extended-release Capsules; Propranolol Hydrochloride and Hydrochlorothiazide Tablets; Reserpine and Hydrochlorothiazide Tablets; Reserpine, Hydralazine Hydrochloride, and Hydrochlorothiazide Tablets; Spironolactone and Hydrochlorothiazide Tablets; Timolol Maleate and Hydrochlorothiazide Tablets; Triamterene and Hydrochlorothiazide Capsules; Triamterene and Hydrochlorothiazide Tablets.

**Proprietary Preparations** (details are given in Part 3)
***Arg.:*** Diural; Diurex; Tandiur; ***Austral.:*** Dichlotride; Dithiazide; ***Austria:*** Dithiazid†; Esidrex; ***Belg.:*** Dichlotride†; Esidrex†; ***Braz.:*** Clorana; Diurepina; Diuretic; Diuretil; Diurezin; Drenol†; Hidroclorozil; Hidrofall; Neo Hidroclor; ***Canad.:*** Apo-Hydro; HydroDiuril; Novo-Hydrazide†; ***Chile:*** Hidroronol; ***Denm.:*** Dichlotride; ***Fin.:*** Hydrex; ***Fr.:*** Esidrex; ***Ger.:*** Disalunil; diu-melusin; Esidrix; HCT; HCT-Beta; HCT-ISIS; ***Hong Kong:*** Hydrozide; ***India:*** Esidrex; Selopres; ***Irl.:*** HydroSaluric†; ***Israel:*** Disothiazide; ***Ital.:*** Esidrex; ***Malaysia:*** Apo-Hydro; Dichlotride; Hydrozide; ***Mex.:*** Diclotride†; ***Neth.:*** Dichlotride†; Esidrex; ***Norw.:*** Dichlotride†; Esidrex; ***Port.:*** Dichlotride; ***S.Afr.:*** Dichlotride†; Hexazide; Ridaq; ***Singapore:*** Apo-Hydro; Di-Ertride; Didralin†; Hydrozide; ***Spain:*** Acuretic; Esidrex; Hidrosaluretil; ***Swed.:*** Dichlotride†; Esidrex; ***Switz.:*** Esidrex; ***Thai.:*** Dichlotride; Didralin†; Diuret-P; Hydrozide; Servithiazid†; ***UK:*** HydroSaluric†; ***USA:*** Esidrix; HydroDiuril; Microzide; Mictrin; Oretic.

**Multi-ingredient:** ***Arg.:*** Accuretic; Aldazida; Atacand-D; Avapro HCT; Co-Renitec; CoAprovel; Cozaarex D; Defluin Plus; Diovan D; Diubeloc; Gliotenzide; Hidrenox A; Losacor D; Lotrial D; Moducren; Moduretic; Niten D; Normatensil; Paxon-D; Plenacor D; Prenomod; Presi Regul D; Propayerst Plus; Ren-Ur; Tenopres D; Tensopril D; Tiadyl Plus; Tritace-HCT; Vapresan Diur; Vericordin Compuesto; Zestoretic; Ziac; ***Austral.:*** Accuretic; Amizide; Atacand Plus; Avapro HCT; Dyazide†; Hydrene; Hydrozide†; Karvezide; Micardis Plus; Modizide†; Moduretic; Monoplus; Renitec Plus; Teveten Plus; ***Austria:*** Accuzide; Acecomb; Aceplus; Adelphan-Esidrex; Aldoretic; Amiloral/HCT; Amiloretik; Amilorid comp; Amilorid/HCT; Amilostad HCT; Atacand Plus; Beloc comp; Bisoprolol-HCT; Blopress Plus; Capozide; Captoplus; Captopril Compositum; Cibadrex†; Co-Acetan; Co-Captopril; Co-Dilatrend; Co-Diovan; Co-Enaran; Co-Mepril; Co-Renitec; Concor Plus; Confit; Cosaar Plus; Darbalan Plus; Deverol mit Thiazid; Dilaplus; Diurid†; Dytide H; Elfanex†; Enalapril/HCT; Fosicomb; Hypren plus; Inderal comp†; Inhibace Plus; Lanuretic; Loradur; Metolol compositum†; Moducrin; Moduretic; Nanalan Plus; Renitec Plus; Resaltex†; Salodiur; Seloken retard Plus; Supergan†; Supracid; Synerpril; Triamteren comp; Triamteren/HCT; Triastad HCT; Triloc; Trioral/HCT; Tritazide; Valsartan/HCTZ; Zestoretic; ***Belg.:*** Accuretic; Atacand Plus; Belidral; Co-Diovane; Co-Inhibace; Co-Renitec; CoAprovel; Cozaar Plus; Dytenzide; Emcoretic; Foside; Kalten; Loortan Plus; Maxsoten; Maxzide†; Moduretic; Novazyd; Sectrazide; Selozide; Tritazide; Uractazide†; Zestoretic; Zok-Zid; ***Braz.:*** Ablock Plus; Accuretic†; Adelfan-Esidrex; Aldazida; Amiretic; Aprozide; Aradois H; Atacand HCT; Atens H; Biconcor; Captotec + HCT; Co-Pressotec; Co-Renitec; Corus H; Cotareg; Diovan HCT; Enatec F; Eupressin H; Gliotenzide; Hidropril; Hipress†; Hydromet; Hyzaar; Iguassina; Lisonotec; Lopril; Lotensin H; Moduretic; Monoplus; Naprix D; Neopress; Prinzide; Selopress; Tenadren; Triatec D; Vascase Plus; Vasopril Plus; Zestoretic; ***Canad.:*** Accuretic; Aldactazide; Aldoril†; Apo-Amilzide; Apo-Methazide; Apo-Triazide; Avalide; Diovan HCT; Dyazide†; Hydropres†; Hyzaar; Inderide†; Inhibace Plus; Micardis Plus; Moduret; Novamilor; Novo-Doparil†; Novo-Spirozine; Novo-Triamzide; Nu-Amilzide; Nu-Triazide; Prinzide; Ser-Ap-Es†; Timolide; Vaseretic; Viskazide; Zestoretic; ***Chile:*** Accuretic; Acerdil-D; Aratan D; Bajaten D; Blopress D; Blox-D; CoAprovel; Corodin D; Enalten D; Enalten DN; Esalfon-D; Grifopril-D; Hidroronol T; Hiperson-D; Hipoartel H; Hyzaar; Inhibace Plus; Losapres-D; Lotrial D; Micardis Plus; Normaten; Normaten Plus; Sanipresin-D; Simperten-D; Tareg-D; Tonotensil D; Uren; Vartalan D; Zestoretic; Ziac; ***Denm.:*** Amilco; Amilohyd†; AtacandZid; Atazid; Capozid; Cibadrex†; Co-Renitec; CoAprovel; Corodil Comp; Cozaar Comp; Diovan Comp; Fortzaar; Hydronet†; Moduretic; Sparkal; Synerpril; Triatec Comp; Vivazid; Zestoretic; Zok-Zid; ***Fin.:*** Accupro Comp; Acercomp; Amitrid; Atacand Plus; Cardace Comp; Cozaar Comp; Diovan Comp; Diuramin; Diurex; Emconcor Comp; Enaloc Comp; Linatil Comp; Lisipril Comp; Miloride; Moduretic; Renitec Comp; Renitec Plus; Selocomp ZOC; Sparkal; Vivatec Comp; ***Fr.:*** Acuilix; Briazide; Captea; Cibadrex; Co-Renitec; CoAprovel; Cokenzen; Cotareg; Ecazide; Fortzaar; Foziretic; Hytacand; Hyzaar; Koretic; Lodoz; MicardisPlus; Moducren; Moduretic; Nisisco; Prestole; Prinzide; PritorPlus; Wytens; Zestoretic; ***Ger.:*** Accuzide; ACE-Hemmer comp; Acenorm HCT; Acercomp; Adelphan-Esidrix; Adocomp; Amilocomp beta; Amiloretik; Amilorid comp; Amilorid/HCT; Amilozid; Aquaretic; Atacand Plus; Azumetop HCT; Barotonal; Beloc comp†; Beloc-Zok comp; Beta-Turfa; Betathiazid A†; Betathiazid†; Bisomerck Plus; Blopress Plus; Capozide; Capto Comp; Capto Plus; Captobeta Comp; Captodoc Comp; Captogamma HCT; Captohexal Comp; Captopril Comp; Captopril HCT; Captopril Plus; Cardiagen HCT; Cibadrex; Co-Diovan; CoAprovel; Concor Plus; Coric Plus; Corindocomb; Delix plus; Dignoretik†; Disalpin; Diu Venostasin; Diuretikum Verla; Diursan; Diutensat; Diutensat comp; Dociteren; duradiuret; durarese; Dynacil comp; Dynorm Plus; Dytide H; Esimil; Esiteren†; Fempress Plus; Fondril HCT; Fosinorm comp; Haemiton compositum; Hydrocomp†; Hypertorr†; Isoptin plus; Jenateren comp; Karvezide; Lorzaar plus; Manimon†; Meprolol Comp; Meto comp; Meto-comp†; meto-thiazid; Metobeta comp; Metodura comp; Metohexal comp; Metostad Comp; Modu-Puren†; Moducrin; Moduretik; Nephral; Pres plus; Propra comp; Provas comp; Renacor; Resaltex†; Rhefluin†; Risicordin; Sali-Puren; Spironothiazid; Tensobon comp; Thiazid-comp; Treloc; Tri-Thiazid; Tri-Thiazid Reserpin; Triampur compositum; Triamteren comp; Triamteren-H; Triamteren/HCT; Triarese; triazid; Triniton; Turfa; Veratide; Vesdil plus; ***Gr.:*** Ividol; Moduretic; Tiaden; ***Hong Kong:*** Adelphane-Esidrex; Amilco; Amithiazide; Apo-Amilzide; Apo-Triazide; Aprovel HCT; Betaloc Comp; Co-Diovan; Co-Renitec; Dyazide; Hydrozide†; Hyzaar; Lodoz; Moducren; Moduretic; Secadrex†; Sefaretic; Triam-Co; Trizid†; Zestoretic; ***India:*** Adelphane-Esidrex; Arkamin-H; Beptazine-H; Biduret; Ciplar-H; Cipril-H; EnAce-D; Invozide; Lisoril-5HT; Losacar-H; Zaart-H; ***Irl.:*** Accuretic; Amilco; Atacand Plus; Capozide; Captor-HCT; Carace Plus; Clonuretic†; Co-Betaloc; Co-Diovan; CoAprovel; Cozaar Comp; Dyazide; Half Capozide; Hydromet†; Innozide; MicardisPlus; Moducren; Moduret; Moduretic†; Zestoretic; ***Israel:*** Atacand Plus; Co-Diovan; Irban Plus; Kaluril; Naprizide; Ocsaar Plus; Tritace Comp; Vascace Plus; Vasopril Plus; ***Ital.:*** Accuretic; Acediur; Aceplus; Acequide; Acesistem; Aldactazide; Blopresid; Cibadrex; CoAprovel; Combisartan; Condiuren; Cotareg; Elidiur; Femipres Plus; Forzaar; Fosicombi; Gentipress; Hizaar; Idroquark; Inibace Plus; Initiss Plus; Karvezide; Losazid; Medozide; Moduretic; Nalapres; Neo-Lotan Plus; Neoprex; Prinzide; Quinazide; Ratacand Plus; Selozide; Sinertec; Spiridazide; Tensadiur; Tensozide; Triatec HCT; Uniprildiur; Vasoretic; Zestoretic; Zinadiur; ***Malaysia:*** Ami-Hydrotride; Amizide; Apo-Amilzide; Apo-Triazide; Co-Diovan; CoAprovel; Fortzaar; Hyzaar; Moduretic; ***Mex.:*** Biconcor; Capozide; Co-Captral; Co-Diovan; Co-Renitec; Diovan HCT†; Dyazide; Hyzaar; Moducren†; Moduretic; Prinzide; Selopres; Tritazide; Zestoretic; ***Neth.:*** Aceplus†; Acuzide; Atacand Plus; Capozide; Cibadrex; Co-Diovan; Co-Renitec; CoAprovel; Diurace; Dytenzide; Emcoretic; Hyzaar; Moducren†; Moduretic; Novazyd; Renitec Plus; Secadrex; Selokomb†; Tritazide; Vascase Plus†; Zestoretic; ***Norw.:*** Atacand Plus; CoAprovel; Cozaar Comp; Diovan Comp; Moduretic Mite; Normorix; Renitec Comp; Vivatec Comp; Zestoretic; ***NZ:*** Accuretic; Amizide; Capozide†; Co-Renitec; Dyazide†; Hydrozide†; Inhibace Plus; Moduretic†; Prinzide†; Triamizide; Trizid†; Zestoretic†; ***Port.:*** Acuretic; Aldoretic; Amiloride Composto; Blopress 16 mg + 12,5 mg; Chibretico; Co-Diovan; Co-Tareg; CoAprovel; Concor Plus; Cozaar Plus; Diurene; Dyazide; Enatia; Fortzaar; Hytacand; Inibace Plus; Laprilen; Lopiretic; Lortaan Plus; Micardis Plus; Moducren; Moduretic; Normotil; Ondolen; Prinzide; Renidur; Renipril Plus; Triam-Tiazida R; Triatec Composto; Vascase Plus; Zestoretic; ***S.Afr.:*** Accuretic; Acumod†; Adco-Retic; Aldoretic†; Amiloretic; Atacand Plus; Betaretic; Capozide; Captoretic; Cibadrex; Co-Diovan; Co-Micardis; Co-Renitec; CoAprovel; Cozaar Comp; Diutec†; Dyazide; Enap-Co; Fortzaar; Hexaretic; Inhibace Plus; Loretic†; Moducren; Moduretic; Monozide; Pharmapress Co; Renezide; Secadrex†; Servatrin; Urirex-K; Zapto Co; Zestoretic; Ziak; ***Singapore:*** Apo-Amilzide; Apo-Triazide; Atacand Plus; Co-Diovan; Co-Renitec†; CoAprovel; Dyazide†; Enap HL; Hyzaar; ***Spain:*** Acediur; Acetensil Plus; Adelfan-Esidrex; Alopresin Diu; Ameride; Atacand Plus; Baripril Diu; Bicetil; Bitensil Diu; Cesplon Plus; Co-Diovan; Co-Renitec; Co-Vals; CoAprovel; Cozaar Plus; Crinoretic; Dabonal Plus; Decresco; Dilabar Diu; Dilapres†; Ditenside; Diu Rauwiplus†; Diuzine; Doneka Plus; Donicer†; Ecadiu; Ecazide; Emcoretic; Flebo Stop†; Fortzaar; Fositens Plus; Hiperlex Plus; Hipoartel Plus; Inhibace Plus; Inocar Plus; Iricil Plus; Kalpress Plus; Kalten; Karvezide; Lidaltrin Diu; Micardis Plus; Miscidon; Miten Plus; Neotensin Diu; Parapres Plus; Pressitan Plus; Prinivil Plus; Pritor Plus; Renitecmax; Rulun; Secadrex; Secubar Diu; Selopresin; Tensikey Complex; Tensiocomplet; Tenso Stop Plus; Urocaudal Tiazida†; Zestoretic; ***Swed.:*** Accupro Comp; Amiloferm; Atacand Plus; Capozid†; CoAprovel; Cozaar Comp; Diovan Comp; Enalapril Comp; Hydromet†; Inhibace comp; Moduretic; Monopril comp; Normorix; Renitec Comp; Sparkal; Synerpril; Triatec Comp; Zestoretic; ***Switz.:*** Accuretic; Adelphan-Esidrex; Agorex; Aldoretic†; Amilo-basan; Amilorid comp†; Atacand Plus; Betadiur; Blopress Plus; Capozide; Captosol comp; Cibadrex; Co-Amilorid; Co-Diovan; Co-Reniten; CoAprovel; Comilorid; Concor Plus; Cosaar Plus; Dyazide; Ecodurex; Escoretic; Fosicomp; Grodurex; Hydrolid†; Inhibace Plus; Kalten; Moducren; Moduretic; Prinzide; Reniten Plus; Rhefluin; Spironothiazid†; Synureticum†; t/h-basan; Tensobon comp; Triatec Comp; Zestoretic; ***Thai.:*** Amilhydrozide†; Amilide†; Aprovel HCT; Bilduretic; Blopress Plus; Co-Diovan; Dazid; Dinazide; Dyazide†; Dyterene; Fortzaar; Hydrares; Hydrozide Plus; Hyperretic; Hypery; Hyzaar; Medeserpine Co; Miduret; Milorex; Miretic; Modulan; Moduretic; Poli-Uretic; Renase; Reser; Sefaretic; Ser-Ap-Es; Skezide†; ***UK:*** Accuretic; Acezide; Amil-Co; Amilmaxco†; Capozide; Capto-Co; Carace Plus; Co-Betaloc; CoAprovel; Cozaar Comp; Delvas†; Dyazide; Innozide; Kalten; MicardisPlus; Moducren; Moduret; Moduretic; Monozide†; Secadrex; Synuretic†; Triamaxco; Triamco; Zestoretic; ***USA:*** Accuretic; Aldactazide; Aldoril; Apresazide; Atacand HCT; Avalide; Benicar HCT; Capozide; Diovan HCT; Dyazide; Esimil; Hydra-zide; Hydrap-ES; Hydro-Serp; Hydropres; Hydroserpine; Hyzaar; Inderide; Lopressor HCT; Lotensin HCT; Marpres; Maxzide; Micardis HCT; Moduretic; Monopril-HCT; Prinzide; Ser-Ap-Es; Teveten HCT; Timolide; Tri-Hydroserpine; Uniretic; Vaseretic; Zestoretic; Ziac.

---

# Hydroflumethiazide *(BAN, rINN)*

Hidroflumetiazida; Hydroflumethiazidum; Trifluoromethylhydrothiazide. 3,4-Dihydro-6-trifluoromethyl-2*H*-1,2,4-benzothiadiazine-7-sulphonamide 1,1-dioxide.

$C_8H_8F_3N_3O_4S_2$ = 331.3.

*CAS — 135-09-1.*

*ATC — C03AA02.*

NOTE. Compounded preparations of hydroflumethiazide may be represented by the following names:

- Co-flumactone (*BAN*)—hydroflumethiazide and spironolactone in equal parts (w/w).

**Pharmacopoeias.** In *Br.* and *US.*

**BP 2003** (Hydroflumethiazide). White or almost white, odourless or almost odourless, glistening crystals or crystalline powder. Practically insoluble in water; soluble in alcohol; practically insoluble in chloroform and in ether.

**USP 27** (Hydroflumethiazide). A white to cream-coloured, odourless, finely divided crystalline powder. Very slightly soluble in water and in chloroform; soluble 1 in 39 of alcohol and 1 in 2500 of ether; freely soluble in acetone. A 1% dispersion in water has a pH of 4.5 to 7.5. Store in airtight containers.

## Adverse Effects, Treatment, and Precautions

As for Hydrochlorothiazide, p.933.

## Interactions

As for Hydrochlorothiazide, p.935.

## Pharmacokinetics

Hydroflumethiazide is incompletely but fairly rapidly absorbed from the gastrointestinal tract. It is reported to have a beta-phase biological half-life of about 17 hours and a metabolite with a longer half-life which is extensively bound to red blood cells. Hydroflumethiazide is excreted in the urine; its metabolite has also been detected in the urine.

◊ References.

1. Brørs O, *et al.* Pharmacokinetics of a single dose of hydroflumethiazide in health and in cardiac failure. *Eur J Clin Pharmacol* 1978; **14:** 29–37.

## Uses and Administration

Hydroflumethiazide is a thiazide diuretic with actions and uses similar to those of hydrochlorothiazide (p.935). It is used for oedema, including that associated with heart failure (p.820), and for hypertension (p.825).

Diuresis is initiated in about 2 hours and has been reported to last for up to 24 hours.

In the treatment of **oedema** the usual initial dose by mouth is 50 to 100 mg daily, in one or two divided doses, reduced to a dose of 25 to 50 mg on alternate days or intermittently. Doses of up to 200 mg daily may be required by some patients. In the treatment of **hypertension** the usual dose is 25 to 50 mg daily either alone, or with other antihypertensives. An initial dose of 12.5 mg may be used.

An initial dose for children is 1 mg/kg daily, reduced for maintenance.

## Preparations

***BP 2003:*** Hydroflumethiazide Tablets;
***USP 27:*** Hydroflumethiazide Tablets.

**Proprietary Preparations** (details are given in Part 3)
***USA:*** Diucardin†; Saluron.

**Multi-ingredient:** ***Irl.:*** Aldactide; ***S.Afr.:*** Protensin-M; ***UK:*** Aldactide; Spiro-Co†; ***USA:*** Salutensin.

---

## Hydroquinidine Hydrochloride

Dihydrochinidin Hydrochloride; Dihydroquinidine Hydrochloride; Hidroquinidina, hidrocloruro de; Hydroconchinine Hydrochloride. (8*R*,9*S*)-10,11-Dihydro-6′-methoxycinchonan-9-ol hydrochloride.

$C_{20}H_{26}N_2O_2$,HCl = 362.9.

*CAS — 1435-55-8 (hydroquinidine); 1476-98-8 (hydroquinidine hydrochloride).*

**Pharmacopoeias.** In *Fr.*

## Profile

Hydroquinidine is an antiarrhythmic with actions and uses similar to those of quinidine (p.991). It is given as the hydrochloride in a usual maintenance dose of 600 mg daily by mouth in divided doses.

Hydroquinidine alginate and quinalbital (the hydroquinidine salt of amobarbital) have also been used in the treatment of cardiac arrhythmias.

## Preparations

**Proprietary Preparations** (details are given in Part 3)
***Fr.:*** Serecor; ***Spain:*** Lentoquine.

---

# Ibopamine *(BAN, USAN, rINN)*

SB-7505; SKF-100168. 4-(2-Methylaminoethyl)-*o*-phenylene diisobutyrate.

$C_{17}H_{25}NO_4$ = 307.4.

*CAS — 66195-31-1.*

*ATC — C01CA16; S01FB03.*

## Ibopamine Hydrochloride *(BANM, rINNM)*

Hidrocloruro de ibopamina.

$C_{17}H_{25}NO_4$,HCl = 343.8.

*ATC — C01CA16; S01FB03.*

## Adverse Effects and Precautions

Ibopamine should not be used in patients with severe heart failure in whom, similarly to xamoterol (p.1029), it has been reported to increase the risk of death.

For the adverse effects of sympathomimetics in general, and precautions to be observed, see Adrenaline, p.852.

**Effects on the cardiovascular system.** A multicentre study (PRIME II) of the use of ibopamine in patients with severe (NYHA class III or IV) heart failure found that the drug was associated with an increased risk of death:[1] the study was stopped early. Subgroup analysis found that use of an antiarrhythmic drug was independently predictive of an adverse effect in ibopamine-treated patients. Excess mortality in heart failure has also been reported with dobutamine and xamoterol, and with flosequinan and the phosphodiesterase inhibitors amrinone, enoximone, milrinone, and vesnarinone, all of which produce positive inotropic effects through catecholamine-receptor stimulation or post-receptor pathway stimulation.[2] The association with antiarrhythmic therapy in the ibopamine study might reflect an interaction with amiodarone, the most commonly used antiarrhythmic in this study, or might simply be a marker for patients at risk of ibopamine-induced tachyarrhythmias.

1. Hampton JR, *et al.* Randomised study of effect of ibopamine on survival in patients with advanced severe heart failure. *Lancet* 1997; **349:** 971–7.

2. Niebauer J, Coats AJS. Treating chronic heart failure: time to take stock. *Lancet* 1997; **349:** 966–7.

## Interactions

It has been recommended that ibopamine should not be given to patients receiving amiodarone in the light of the increased mortality seen in the PRIME II study in patients receiving both drugs (see above), although it is not clear that this represents a genuine interaction.

For the interactions of sympathomimetics in general, see Adrenaline, p.853.

## Uses and Administration

Ibopamine is rapidly converted after oral administration to its active metabolite, epinine, which is a peripheral dopamine agonist with vasodilating properties and a weak positive inotropic effect; at high concentrations it has a stimulant action on alpha and beta adrenoceptors.

Ibopamine is used in the management of mild heart failure (p.820). It is given as the hydrochloride but doses are often expressed in terms of the base; 111.9 mg of hydrochloride is approximately equivalent to 100 mg of base. Doses of 100 to 200 mg by mouth two or three times daily have been used.

Ibopamine is also used topically as a mydriatic (p.476) in the form of eye drops containing ibopamine hydrochloride 2%.

## Preparations

**Proprietary Preparations** (details are given in Part 3)
***Austria:*** Escandine; ***Belg.:*** Idopamil†; Scandine; ***Braz.:*** Escandine; ***Ital.:*** Inopamil†; Scandine; Trazyl; ***Neth.:*** Inopamil; ***Port.:*** Scandine; ***Spain:*** Erfolgan†; Escandine.

## Ibutilide Fumarate *(BANM, USAN, rINNM)*

Fumarato de ibutilida; U-70226E. (±)-4′-[4-(Ethylheptylamino)-1-hydroxybutyl]methanesulfonanilide fumarate (2:1).

$(C_{20}H_{36}N_2O_3S)_2,C_4H_4O_4$ = 885.2.

*CAS — 122647-31-8 (ibutilide); 122647-32-9 (ibutilide fumarate).*

*ATC — C01BD05.*

### Adverse Effects

Adverse cardiovascular effects associated with ibutilide include heart block, hypotension, hypertension, and bradycardia. Like other antiarrhythmics it can cause arrhythmias, including torsade de pointes. Other adverse effects include nausea and vomiting.

**Effects on the kidneys.** Acute renal failure with biopsy evidence of acute tubular necrosis developed in a 52-year-old man shortly after he received 2 doses of ibutilide for an episode of atrial flutter.[1] Renal function returned to normal following 4 sessions of haemodialysis.

1. Franz M, *et al.* Acute renal failure after ibutilide. *Lancet* 1999; **353:** 467.

### Precautions

ECG monitoring should be carried out during, and for at least 4 hours after, administration of ibutilide. Electrolyte abnormalities should be corrected before treatment is started.

### Interactions

Use of ibutilide with other antiarrhythmics or drugs that prolong the QT interval should be avoided.

### Pharmacokinetics

Ibutilide is widely distributed in the body after intravenous administration. It has low plasma protein binding (about 40%) and undergoes extensive metabolism in the liver to form several metabolites. Ibutilide is excreted mainly in the urine as metabolites with about 19% being excreted in the faeces. The elimination half-life is reported to range from 2 to 12 hours.

### Uses and Administration

Ibutilide is a class III antiarrhythmic (p.809) used in the management of **atrial fibrillation** or **flutter** (p.816).

Ibutilide is given intravenously as the fumarate. The dose for patients weighing 60 kg or more is 1 mg given intravenously over 10 minutes. This dose may be repeated, if necessary, 10 minutes after completion of the first dose. The infusion should be stopped as soon as the arrhythmia is terminated. A dose of 10 micrograms/kg should be used in patients weighing less than 60 kg.

◊ References.

1. Foster RH, *et al.* Ibutilide: a review of its pharmacological properties and clinical potential in the acute management of atrial flutter and fibrillation. *Drugs* 1997; **54:** 312–30.
2. Granberry MC. Ibutilide: a new class III antiarrhythmic agent. *Am J Health-Syst Pharm* 1998; **55:** 255–60.
3. Howard PA. Ibutilide: an antiarrhythmic agent for the treatment of atrial fibrillation or flutter. *Ann Pharmacother* 1999; **33:** 38–47.

### Preparations

**Proprietary Preparations** (details are given in Part 3)
***Austria:*** Corvert; ***Braz.:*** Corvert†; ***Fin.:*** Corvert; ***Fr.:*** Corvert; ***Gr.:*** Corvert; ***Ital.:*** Corvert; ***Neth.:*** Corvert; ***Norw.:*** Corvert; ***Swed.:*** Corvert; ***Switz.:*** Corvert; ***USA:*** Corvert.

---

## Ifenprodil Tartrate *(rINNM)*

RC-61-91; Tartrato de ifenprodil. (±)-2-(4-Benzylpiperidino)-1-(4-hydroxyphenyl)propan-1-ol tartrate.

$(C_{21}H_{27}NO_2)_2,C_4H_6O_6$ = 801.0.

*CAS — 23210-56-2 (ifenprodil); 23210-58-4 (ifenprodil tartrate).*

*ATC — C04AX28.*

**Pharmacopoeias.** In *Jpn.*

### Profile

Ifenprodil tartrate is a vasodilator, with alpha-adrenoceptor blocking properties, used in peripheral vascular disease (p.831). It is given in usual doses of 40 to 60 mg daily by mouth or up to 15 mg daily by deep intramuscular injection, slow intravenous injection, or intravenous infusion.

### Preparations

**Proprietary Preparations** (details are given in Part 3)
***Fr.:*** Vadilex; ***Hong Kong:*** Vadilex†; ***Singapore:*** Vadilex†.

---

## Imidapril Hydrochloride *(BANM, rINNM)*

Hidrocloruro de imidapril; TA-6366. (*S*)-3-{*N*-[(*S*)-1-Ethoxycarbonyl-3-phenylpropyl]-L-alanyl}-1-methyl-2-oxoimidazoline-4-carboxylic acid hydrochloride.

$C_{20}H_{27}N_3O_6,HCl$ = 441.9.

*CAS — 89371-37-9 (imidapril); 89396-94-1 (imidapril hydrochloride).*

*ATC — C09AA16.*

### Adverse Effects, Treatment, and Precautions

As for ACE inhibitors, p.842.

### Interactions

As for ACE inhibitors, p.845.

### Pharmacokinetics

Imidapril acts as a prodrug of the diacid imidaprilat, its active metabolite. Following oral administration, imidapril is rapidly but incompletely absorbed; absorption is about 70% and is reduced in the presence of food. Imidapril is metabolised in the liver to imidaprilat. The bioavailability of imidaprilat is about 42% following oral imidapril administration, and peak plasma concentrations of imidaprilat are reached in about 7 hours. Both imidapril and imidaprilat are moderately bound to plasma proteins. About 40% of an oral dose is excreted in the urine, the rest in the faeces. The terminal half-life of imidaprilat is more than 24 hours. Imidapril and imidaprilat are removed by haemodialysis.

◊ References.

1. Hoogkamer JFW, *et al.* Pharmacokinetics of imidapril and its active metabolite imidaprilat following single dose and during steady state in patients with impaired liver function. *Eur J Clin Pharmacol* 1997; **51:** 489–91.
2. Hoogkamer JFW, *et al.* Pharmacokinetics of imidapril and its active metabolite imidaprilat following single dose and during steady state in patients with chronic renal failure. *Eur J Clin Pharmacol* 1998; **54:** 59–61.
3. Harder S, *et al.* Single dose and steady state pharmacokinetics and pharmacodynamics of the ACE-inhibitor imidapril in hypertensive patients. *Br J Clin Pharmacol* 1998; **45:** 377–80.

### Uses and Administration

Imidapril is an ACE inhibitor (p.842). It is used in the treatment of hypertension (p.825). Imidapril owes its activity to imidaprilat, to which it is converted after oral administration. The maximum haemodynamic effect occurs 6 to 8 hours after administration, although the full effect may not develop for several weeks during chronic dosing. Imidapril is given by mouth as the hydrochloride.

In the treatment of hypertension, the usual initial dose of imidapril hydrochloride is 5 mg once daily, before food. Since there may be a precipitous fall in blood pressure in some patients when starting therapy with an ACE inhibitor, the first dose should preferably be given at bedtime. An initial dose of 2.5 mg daily should be used in the elderly, in patients with renal or hepatic impairment, or in those receiving a *diuretic*; if possible, the diuretic should be withdrawn 2 or 3 days before imidapril is started and resumed later if necessary. The usual maintenance dose is 10 mg daily, although up to 20 mg daily may be given if required. The maximum dose for elderly patients is 10 mg daily.

### Preparations

**Proprietary Preparations** (details are given in Part 3)
***Arg.:*** Tanatril; ***Austria:*** Tanatril; ***Fin.:*** Tanatril; ***Fr.:*** Tanatril; ***Ger.:*** Tanatril; ***Gr.:*** Tanatril; ***Hong Kong:*** Tanatril; ***Ital.:*** Tanatril†; ***Jpn:*** Novarok; Tanatril; ***Port.:*** Cardipril; Tanatril; ***Singapore:*** Tanatril; ***Thai.:*** Tanatril; ***UK:*** Tanatril.

---

## Indapamide *(BAN, USAN, rINN)*

Indapamida; Indapamidum; SE-1520. 4-Chloro-*N*-(2-methylindolin-1-yl)-3-sulphamoylbenzamide.

$C_{16}H_{16}ClN_3O_3S$ = 365.8.

*CAS — 26807-65-8 (anhydrous indapamide).*

*ATC — C03BA11.*

**Pharmacopoeias.** In *Chin., Eur.* (see p.vi), and *US.*

**Ph. Eur. 5.0** (Indapamide). A white or almost white powder. Practically insoluble in water; soluble in alcohol. Protect from light.

**USP 27** (Indapamide). A white to off-white crystalline powder. Practically insoluble in water; soluble in alcohol, in glacial acetic acid, in acetonitrile, in ethyl acetate, and in methyl alcohol; very slightly soluble in chloroform and in ether.

### Adverse Effects, Treatment, and Precautions

As for Hydrochlorothiazide, p.933.

**Effects on carbohydrate and lipid metabolism.** Several studies have reported no changes in blood-glucose concentrations during indapamide treatment,[1-3] although elevated concentrations have been reported in individual patients.[4,5] There have been reports of increases in total cholesterol[2] and of no change.[3] No adverse biochemical changes were found in studies[6] of a modified-release preparation.

1. Velussi M, *et al.* Treatment of mild-to-moderate hypertension with indapamide in type II diabetics: midterm (six months) evaluation. *Curr Ther Res* 1988; **44:** 1076–86.
2. Prisant LM, *et al.* Biochemical, endocrine, and mineral effects of indapamide in black women. *J Clin Pharmacol* 1990; **30:** 121–6.
3. Leonetti G, *et al.* Long-term effects of indapamide: final results of a two-year Italian multicenter study in systemic hypertension. *Am J Cardiol* 1990; **65:** 674–714.
4. Slotkoff L. Clinical efficacy and safety of indapamide in the treatment of edema. *Am Heart J* 1983; **106:** 233–7.
5. Beling S, *et al.* Long term experience with indapamide. *Am Heart J* 1983; **106:** 258–62.
6. Weidmann P. Metabolic profile of indapamide sustained-release in patients with hypertension: data from three randomised double-blind studies. *Drug Safety* 2001; **24:** 1155–65.

**Effects on electrolyte balance.** It has been claimed that indapamide produces few adverse biochemical effects at the usual dose of 2.5 mg daily. However, by 2002, 164 cases of hyponatraemia had been reported to the Australian Adverse Drug Reactions Advisory Committee (ADRAC)[1], of which 68 also described hypokalaemia. Most patients were elderly women. A review[2] of some of these cases suggested that hyponatraemia was more commonly reported with indapamide than with chlorothiazide, although it was pointed out[3] that the true incidence cannot be determined from spontaneous reports. ADRAC recommends that indapamide should be used cautiously. It may be that indapamide has no clinical advantage over low-dose thiazide diuretics.

1. Australian Adverse Drug Reactions Advisory Committee. Indapamide and hyponatraemia. *Aust Adverse Drug React Bull* 2002; **21:** 11. Also available at: http://www.tga.health.gov.au/adr/aadrb/aadr0208.htm (accessed 06/07/04)
2. Chapman MD, *et al.* Hyponatraemia and hypokalaemia due to indapamide. *Med J Aust* 2002; **176:** 219–21.
3. Howes LG. Hyponatraemia and hypokalaemia caused by indapamide. *Med J Aust* 2002; **177:** 53–4.

**Effects on the kidneys.** Acute interstitial nephritis was associated with indapamide treatment in a 74-year-old patient.[1]

1. Newstead CG, *et al.* Interstitial nephritis associated with indapamide. *BMJ* 1990; **300:** 1344.

**Effects on the skin.** Sixteen cases of skin rash attributed to indapamide had been reported to the Netherlands Centre for Monitoring of Adverse Reactions to Drugs.[1] All patients had taken indapamide 2.5 mg daily for hypertension. The skin rash was accompanied by fever in 5 cases. In all cases the rash subsided within 14 days of withdrawal, and 11 patients subsequently took thiazides, furosemide, or clopamide without recurrence. Among 188 cases of skin rash attributed to indapamide reported to the WHO Collaborating Centre for International Drug Monitoring were 4 cases of erythema multiforme and 2 of epidermal necrolysis. A further case of toxic epidermal necrolysis was reported by independent authors.[2]

1. Stricker BHC, Biriell C. Skin reactions and fever with indapamide. *BMJ* 1987; **295:** 1313–14.
2. Black RJ, *et al.* Toxic epidermal necrolysis associated with indapamide. *BMJ* 1990; **301:** 1280–1.

### Interactions

As for Hydrochlorothiazide, p.935.

### Pharmacokinetics

Indapamide is rapidly and completely absorbed from the gastrointestinal tract. Elimination is biphasic with a half-life in whole blood of about 14 hours. Indapamide is strongly bound to red blood cells. It is extensively metabolised. About 60 to 70% of the dose has been reported to be excreted in the urine; only about 5 to 7% is excreted unchanged. About 16 to 23% of dose is excreted in the faeces. Indapamide is not removed by haemodialysis but does not accumulate in patients with renal impairment.

◊ References.

1. Beermann B, Grind M. Clinical pharmacokinetics of some newer diuretics. *Clin Pharmacokinet* 1987; **13:** 254–66.

### Uses and Administration

Indapamide is a diuretic with actions and uses similar to those of the thiazide diuretics (see Hydrochlorothiazide, p.935) even though it does not contain a thiazide ring system. It is used for hypertension (p.825), and also for oedema, including that associated with heart failure (p.820).

In some countries indapamide is described as the hemihydrate. In the treatment of **hypertension** the usual dose by mouth is 1.25 to 2.5 mg once daily, either alone, or with other antihypertensives; a modified-release preparation may be given in a dose of 1.5 mg daily. At higher doses the diuretic effect may become apparent without appreciable additional antihypertensive effect although the US manufacturers have suggested that the dose may be increased to 5 mg after 4 weeks. In the treatment of **oedema** the usual dose is 2.5 mg once daily increasing to 5 mg daily after 1 week if necessary.

◊ Reviews.

1. Chaffman M, *et al.* Indapamide: a review of its pharmacodynamic properties and therapeutic efficacy in hypertension. *Drugs* 1984; **28:** 189–235.

### Preparations

***BP 2003:*** Indapamide Tablets;
***USP 27:*** Indapamide Tablets.

**Proprietary Preparations** (details are given in Part 3)
***Arg.:*** Bajaten; Duremid; Natrilix; Noranat; ***Austral.:*** Dapa-Tabs; Indahexal; Insig; Napamide; Naride†; Natrilix; ***Austria:*** Fludex; ***Belg.:*** Fludex; ***Braz.:*** Natrilix; ***Canad.:*** Lozide; ***Chile:*** Indapress; ***Denm.:*** Fludex; Indacar; Natrilix; ***Fin.:*** Natrilix; ***Fr.:*** Fludex; ***Ger.:*** Inda-Puren; Natrilix; Sicco; ***Gr.:*** Fludex; Magniton-R; Transipen; ***Hong Kong:*** Agelan; Dapa-Tabs; Diflerix; Frumeron; Indalix; Millibar; Napamide†; Natrilix; ***India:*** Indocontin; Lorvas; Natrilix; ***Irl.:*** Agelan; Clonilix†; Inamide; Natrilix; ***Israel:*** Pamid; ***Ital.:*** Damide; Indaflex; Indamol; Indolin; Ipamix; Millibar; Natrilix; Pressural; Veroxil; ***Malaysia:*** Dapa; Diflerix; Natrilix; Rinalix; ***Neth.:*** Fludex; ***NZ:*** Napamide†; Naplin; Natrilix; ***Port.:*** Fludex; Fluidema; Tandix; ***S.Afr.:*** Dapamax; Daptril; Hydro-Less; Indalix; Lixamide; Natrilix; ***Singapore:*** Dapa-Tabs; Millibar; Napamide; Natrilix; Rinalix; ***Spain:*** Extur; Tertensif; ***Switz.:*** Fludapamide; Fludex; ***Thai.:*** Frumeron; Lorvas†; Napamide; Natrilix; ***UAE:*** Indanorm; ***UK:*** Natrilix; Nindaxa; ***USA:*** Lozol.

**Multi-ingredient:** ***Arg.:*** Preterax; ***Austral.:*** Coversyl Plus; ***Austria:*** Predonium; Preterax; ***Braz.:*** Preterax†; ***Fr.:*** Bipreterax; Preterax; ***Ger.:*** Coversum Combi; ***Hong Kong:*** Predonium; ***Irl.:*** Preterax; ***Ital.:*** Atinorm; Delapride; Dinapres; Nor-Pa; Normopress; Prelectal; Preterax; ***Neth.:*** Coversyl Plus; ***S.Afr.:*** Coversyl Plus; ***Singapore:*** Preterax; ***Switz.:*** Coversum Combi; ***UK:*** Coversyl Plus.

## Indenolol Hydrochloride *(BANM, rINNM)*

Hidrocloruro de indenolol; Sch-28316Z (indenolol); YB-2.

$C_{15}H_{21}NO_2,HCl = 283.8.$

*CAS — 60607-68-3 (indenolol); 68906-88-7 (indenolol hydrochloride).*

**Description.** Indenolol hydrochloride is a 2:1 tautomeric mixture of 1-(inden-7-yloxy)-3-isopropylaminopropan-2-ol hydrochloride and 1-(inden-4-yloxy)-3-isopropylaminopropan-2-ol hydrochloride.

**Pharmacopoeias.** In *Jpn.*

### Profile

Indenolol is a non-cardioselective beta blocker (p.868). It is reported to possess potent membrane-stabilising properties and intrinsic sympathomimetic activity.

Indenolol is used as the hydrochloride in the management of various cardiovascular disorders in doses of 30 to 180 mg daily by mouth.

### Preparations

**Proprietary Preparations** (details are given in Part 3)
***Ital.:*** Securpres.

## Indobufen *(rINN)*

Indobufén; K-3920. (±)-2-[4-(1-Oxo-isoindolin-2-yl)phenyl]butyric acid.

$C_{18}H_{17}NO_3 = 295.3.$

*CAS — 63610-08-2.*

*ATC — B01AC10.*

### Profile

Indobufen is an inhibitor of platelet aggregation used in various thromboembolic disorders (p.837) in doses of 200 to 400 mg daily by mouth given in 2 divided doses. It is also given parenterally as the sodium salt in similar doses. For patients over the age of 65, the dose should be reduced to 100 to 200 mg daily. Doses should also be reduced in renal impairment (see below).

◊ References.

1. Wiseman LR, *et al.* Indobufen: a review of its pharmacodynamic and pharmacokinetic properties, and therapeutic efficacy in cerebral, peripheral and coronary vascular disease. *Drugs* 1992; **44:** 445–64.
2. Bhana N, McClellan KJ. Indobufen: an updated review of its use in the management of atherothrombosis. *Drugs Aging* 2001; **18:** 369–88.

**Administration in renal impairment.** In patients with renal impairment the dose of indobufen should be reduced to 100 to 200 mg daily.

### Preparations

**Proprietary Preparations** (details are given in Part 3)
***Austria:*** Ibustrin; ***Ital.:*** Ibustrin; ***Mex.:*** Ibustrin; ***Port.:*** Ibustrin; ***Thai.:*** Ibustrin†.

## Indoramin Hydrochloride

*(BANM, USAN, rINNM)*

Hidrocloruro de indoramina; Wy-21901 (indoramin). *N*-[1-(2-Indol-3-ylethyl)-4-piperidyl]benzamide hydrochloride.

$C_{22}H_{25}N_3O,HCl = 383.9.$

*CAS — 26844-12-2 (indoramin); 33124-53-7 (indoramin hydrochloride); 38821-52-2 (indoramin hydrochloride).*

*ATC — C02CA02.*

**Pharmacopoeias.** In *Br.*

**BP 2003** (Indoramin Hydrochloride). A white or almost white powder. It exhibits polymorphism. Slightly soluble in water; sparingly soluble in alcohol; very slightly soluble in ether; soluble in methyl alcohol. A 2% suspension in water has a pH of 4.0 to 5.5. Protect from light.

### Adverse Effects, Treatment, and Precautions

The most common adverse effects in patients receiving indoramin are sedation and dizziness; dry mouth, nasal congestion, headache, fatigue, depression, weight gain (almost certainly due to fluid retention), and failure of ejaculation may also occur. Tachycardia does not seem to be a problem with therapeutic doses. Extrapyramidal disturbances have been reported.

Following overdosage, coma, convulsions, and hypotension may occur; hypothermia has been reported in *animals*. In acute poisoning appropriate symptomatic and supportive care should be given; if the patient presents within 1 hour, activated charcoal may be considered.

Indoramin should be avoided in patients with heart failure; it has been recommended that incipient heart failure should be controlled before giving indoramin. Caution should be observed in patients with hepatic or renal impairment, a history of depression, epilepsy, or Parkinson's disease. Elderly patients may respond to lower doses.

Because indoramin can cause drowsiness care should be taken in patients who drive or operate machinery.

**Effects on mental function.** Sleep disturbances and vivid dreams were reported during a study in hypertensive patients when indoramin was added to therapy with a thiazide diuretic and a beta blocker.[1]

1. Marshall AJ, *et al.* Evaluation of indoramin added to oxprenolol and bendrofluazide as a third agent in severe hypertension. *Br J Clin Pharmacol* 1980; **10:** 217–21.

**Overdosage.** A 43-year-old woman with a long history of heavy alcohol intake died after taking 100 tablets of indoramin 25 mg.[1] The main clinical features were deep sedation, respiratory depression, hypotension, and convulsions. Although the hypotension was satisfactorily controlled the CNS effects were resistant to treatment and proved fatal. Other clinical features included areflexia, metabolic acidosis, tachycardia, and later bradyarrhythmias.

1. Hunter R. Death due to overdose of indoramin. *BMJ* 1982; **285:** 1011.

### Interactions

The hypotensive effects of indoramin may be enhanced by diuretics and other antihypertensives. It has been reported that the ingestion of alcohol can increase the rate and extent of absorption and the sedative effects of indoramin (see below) and that indoramin should not be given to patients already receiving MAOIs.

**Alcohol.** In a study[1] in 9 healthy subjects alcohol 500 mg/kg significantly enhanced plasma-indoramin concentrations following an oral dose of 50 mg. The effect was most marked in the early period, corresponding to the absorptive phase. The mean maximum plasma-indoramin concentration was increased from 15.0 to 23.7 nanograms/mL by alcohol; the area under the concentration/time curve was increased by 25%. Alcohol did not affect the pharmacokinetics of intravenous indoramin. The results suggest that alcohol increases indoramin bioavailability either by enhancing absorption or reducing first-pass metabolism. The combination was more sedative than either drug alone.

1. Abrams SML, *et al.* Pharmacokinetic interaction between indoramin and ethanol. *Hum Toxicol* 1989; **8:** 237–41.

### Pharmacokinetics

Indoramin is readily absorbed from the gastrointestinal tract and undergoes extensive first-pass metabolism. It is reported to be about 90% bound to plasma proteins. It has a half-life of about 5 hours which is reported to be prolonged in elderly patients. It is extensively metabolised and is excreted mainly as metabolites in the urine and faeces. There is evidence to suggest that some metabolites may have some alpha-adrenoceptor blocking activity.

**The elderly.** The plasma half-life of indoramin in 5 healthy elderly subjects following a single oral dose ranged from 6.6 to 32.8 hours with a mean of 14.7 hours.[1] The increased half-life may have been caused by reduced clearance in elderly patients.

1. Norbury HM, *et al.* Pharmacokinetics of oral indoramin in elderly and middle-aged female volunteers. *Eur J Clin Pharmacol* 1984; **27:** 247–9.

### Uses and Administration

Indoramin is a selective and competitive $alpha_1$-adrenoceptor blocker (p.809) with actions similar to those of prazosin (p.986); it is also reported to have membrane-stabilising properties and to be a competitive antagonist at histamine $H_1$ and 5-hydroxytryptamine receptors. Indoramin is used in the management of hypertension (p.825), and in benign prostatic hyperplasia (p.1555) to relieve symptoms of urinary obstruction. It has also been used in the prophylactic treatment of migraine.

Indoramin is given by mouth as the hydrochloride, but doses are usually expressed in terms of the base. Indoramin hydrochloride 11.0 mg is approximately equivalent to 10 mg of indoramin.

In **hypertension**, the initial dose is 25 mg twice daily, increased in steps of 25 or 50 mg at intervals of 2 weeks to a maximum of 200 mg daily in 2 or 3 divided doses.

In **benign prostatic hyperplasia**, the initial dose is 20 mg twice daily, increased if necessary by 20 mg at 2-week intervals, to a maximum of 100 mg daily in divided doses.

Lower doses may be required in the elderly.

◊ Reviews.

1. Holmes B, Sorkin EM. Indoramin: a review of its pharmacodynamic and pharmacokinetic properties, and therapeutic efficacy in hypertension and related vascular, cardiovascular and airway diseases. *Drugs* 1986; **31:** 467–99.

**Migraine.** Propranolol and pizotifen are probably the most well-established drugs for prophylaxis of migraine (p.464). Many other drugs have been used including indoramin. In a double-blind study,[1] indoramin in a dose of 25 mg twice daily was reported to be as effective as dihydroergotamine mesilate in reducing the frequency of migraine attacks.

1. Pradalier A, *et al.* Etude comparative indoramine versus dihydroergotamine dans le traitement préventif de la migraine. *Therapie* 1988; **43:** 293–7.

### Preparations

***BP 2003:*** Indoramin Tablets.

**Proprietary Preparations** (details are given in Part 3)
***Austria:*** Wypresin; ***Fr.:*** Vidora; ***Ger.:*** Wydora; ***Irl.:*** Baratol; Doralese; ***S.Afr.:*** Baratol†; ***Spain:*** Orfidora†; ***UK:*** Baratol; Doralese.

## Inositol Nicotinate *(BAN, rINN)*

Inositol Niacinate *(USAN)*; Nicotinato de inositol; NSC-49506; Win-9154. *meso*-Inositol hexanicotinate; *myo*-Inositol hexanicotinate.

$C_{42}H_{30}N_6O_{12} = 810.7.$

*CAS — 6556-11-2.*

*ATC — C04AC03.*

**Pharmacopoeias.** In *Br.*

**BP 2003** (Inositol Nicotinate). A white or almost white, odourless or almost odourless powder. Practically insoluble in water, in alcohol, in acetone, and in ether; sparingly soluble in chloroform. It dissolves in dilute mineral acids.

### Profile

Inositol nicotinate is a vasodilator and is believed to be slowly hydrolysed to nicotinic acid (p.1441). It is given by mouth in the management of peripheral vascular disease (p.831). The usual dose is 3 g daily given in divided doses. The dose may be increased to 4 g daily if necessary.

Inositol nicotinate has been used in hyperlipidaemias.

### Preparations

***BP 2003:*** Inositol Nicotinate Tablets.

**Proprietary Preparations** (details are given in Part 3)
***Arg.:*** Evicyl; ***Ger.:*** Hamovannad; Hexanicit†; Nicolip; ***Irl.:*** Hexogen; Hexopal; ***Swed.:*** Hexanicit†; ***UK:*** Hexopal.

**Multi-ingredient:** ***Canad.:*** Formula Cl†; ***Ger.:*** Veno-Hexanicit†; Zellaforte N Plus; ***S.Afr.:*** Geratar†; ***Spain:*** Venosan†; ***Switz.:*** Hexafene†; Venosan†.

## Irbesartan *(BAN, USAN, rINN)*

BMS-186295; Irbesartán; SR-47436. 2-Butyl-3-[*p*-(*o*-1*H*-tetrazol-5-ylphenyl)benzyl]-1,3-diazaspiro[4.4]non-1-en-4-one.

$C_{25}H_{28}N_6O$ = 428.5.

*CAS — 138402-11-6.*

*ATC — C09CA04.*

**Pharmacopoeias.** In *US.*

**USP 27** (Irbesartan). A white to off-white, crystalline powder. Practically insoluble in water; slightly soluble in alcohol and in dichloromethane.

### Adverse Effects and Precautions

As for Losartan Potassium, p.947.

### Interactions

As for Losartan Potassium, p.948.

### Pharmacokinetics

Irbesartan is rapidly absorbed from the gastrointestinal tract with an oral bioavailability of 60 to 80%. Peak plasma concentrations of irbesartan occur 1.5 to 2 hours after an oral dose. Irbesartan is about 96% bound to plasma proteins. It undergoes some metabolism in the liver, primarily by the cytochrome P450 isoenzyme CYP2C9, to inactive metabolites. It is excreted as unchanged drug and metabolites in the bile and in urine; after oral or intravenous administration approximately 20% of the dose is excreted in the urine, with less than 2% as unchanged drug. The terminal elimination half-life is about 11 to 15 hours.

◊ References.


1. Sica DA, *et al.* The pharmacokinetics of irbesartan in renal failure and maintenance hemodialysis. *Clin Pharmacol Ther* 1997; **62:** 610–18.
2. Marino MR, *et al.* Pharmacokinetics and pharmacodynamics of irbesartan in healthy subjects. *J Clin Pharmacol* 1998; **38:** 246–55.
3. Marino MR, *et al.* Pharmacokinetics and pharmacodynamics of irbesartan in patients with hepatic cirrhosis. *J Clin Pharmacol* 1998; **38:** 347–56.
4. Vachharajani NN, *et al.* Oral bioavailability and disposition characteristics of irbesartan, an angiotensin antagonist, in healthy volunteers. *J Clin Pharmacol* 1998; **38:** 702–7.
5. Vachharajani NN, *et al.* The effects of age and gender on the pharmacokinetics of irbesartan. *Br J Clin Pharmacol* 1998; **46:** 611–13.
6. Sakarcan A, *et al.* The pharmacokinetics of irbesartan in hypertensive children and adolescents. *J Clin Pharmacol* 2001; **41:** 742–9.


### Uses and Administration

Irbesartan is an angiotensin II receptor antagonist with actions similar to those of losartan (p.948). It is used in the management of hypertension (p.825) including the treatment of renal disease in hypertensive type 2 diabetic patients (see Kidney Disorders, under Uses of Losartan, p.948). Irbesartan is also under investigation in heart failure.

Irbesartan is given by mouth. Following an oral dose the hypotensive effect peaks within 3 to 6 hours and persists for at least 24 hours. The maximum hypotensive effect is achieved within 4 to 6 weeks after initiating therapy.

In **hypertension**, irbesartan is given in a dose of 150 mg once daily increased, if necessary, to 300 mg once daily. A lower initial dose of 75 mg once daily may be considered in elderly patients over 75 years, for patients with intravascular volume depletion, and for those receiving haemodialysis. Children aged 6 to 12 years with hypertension may be given a dose of 75 mg once daily, increased to 150 mg once daily if necessary.

For the treatment of **renal disease** in hypertensive type 2 diabetics, irbesartan should be given in an initial dose of 150 mg once daily, increased to 300 mg once daily for maintenance.

◊ Reviews.


1. Gillis JC, Markham A. Irbesartan: a review of its pharmacodynamic and pharmacokinetic properties and therapeutic use in the management of hypertension. *Drugs* 1997; **54:** 885–902.
2. Brown MJ. Irbesartan treatment in hypertension. *Hosp Med* 1998; **59:** 808–11.
3. Markham A, *et al.* Irbesartan: an updated review of its use in cardiovascular disorders. *Drugs* 2000; **59:** 1187–1206.


### Preparations

**Proprietary Preparations** (details are given in Part 3)

***Arg.:*** Aprovel; Avapro; ***Austral.:*** Avapro; Karvea; ***Belg.:*** Aprovel; ***Braz.:*** Aprovel; Avapro; ***Canad.:*** Avapro; ***Chile:*** Aprovel; ***Denm.:*** Aprovel; ***Fin.:*** Aprovel; ***Fr.:*** Aprovel; ***Ger.:*** Aprovel; Karvea; ***Gr.:*** Aprovel; Karvea; ***Hong Kong:*** Aprovel; ***India:*** Irovel; ***Irl.:*** Aprovel; ***Israel:*** Irban; ***Ital.:*** Aprovel; Karvea; ***Malaysia:*** Aprovel; ***Mex.:*** Aprovel; Avapro; ***Neth.:*** Aprovel; ***Norw.:*** Aprovel; ***Port.:*** Aprovel; ***S.Afr.:*** Aprovel; ***Singapore:*** Aprovel; ***Spain:*** Aprovel; Karvea; ***Swed.:*** Aprovel; ***Switz.:*** Aprovel; ***Thai.:*** Aprovel; ***UK:*** Aprovel; ***USA:*** Avapro.

**Multi-ingredient:** ***Arg.:*** Avapro HCT; CoAprovel; ***Austral.:*** Avapro HCT; Karvezide; ***Belg.:*** CoAprovel; ***Braz.:*** Aprozide; ***Canad.:*** Avalide; ***Chile:*** CoAprovel; ***Denm.:*** CoAprovel; ***Fr.:*** CoAprovel; ***Ger.:*** CoAprovel; Karvezide; ***Hong Kong:*** Aprovel HCT; ***Irl.:*** CoAprovel; ***Israel:*** Irban Plus; ***Ital.:*** CoAprovel; Karvezide; ***Malaysia:*** CoAprovel; ***Neth.:*** CoAprovel; ***Norw.:*** CoAprovel; ***Port.:*** CoAprovel; ***S.Afr.:*** CoAprovel; ***Singapore:*** CoAprovel; ***Spain:*** CoAprovel; Karvezide; ***Swed.:*** CoAprovel; ***Switz.:*** CoAprovel; ***Thai.:*** Aprovel HCT; ***UK:*** CoAprovel; ***USA:*** Avalide.

## Isoprenaline *(BAN, rINN)*

Isoprenalina; Isopropylarterenol; Isopropylnoradrenaline; Isoproterenol. 1-(3,4-Dihydroxyphenyl)-2-isopropylaminoethanol.

$C_{11}H_{17}NO_3$ = 211.3.

*CAS — 7683-59-2.*

*ATC — C01CA02; R03AB02; R03CB01.*

### Isoprenaline Hydrochloride *(BANM, rINNM)*

Hidrocloruro de isoprenalina; Isoprenalini Hydrochloridum; Isopropylarterenol Hydrochloride; Isopropylnoradrenaline Hydrochloride; Isoproterenol Hydrochloride.

$C_{11}H_{17}NO_3,HCl$ = 247.7.

*CAS — 51-30-9.*

*ATC — C01CA02; R03AB02; R03CB01.*

**Pharmacopoeias.** In *Chin., Eur.* (see p.vi), *Int., Jpn,* and *US.*

**Ph. Eur. 5.0** (Isoprenaline Hydrochloride). A white or almost white crystalline powder. Freely soluble in water; sparingly soluble in alcohol; practically insoluble in dichloromethane. A 5% solution in water has a pH of 4.3 to 5.5. Store in airtight containers. Protect from light.

**USP 27** (Isoproterenol Hydrochloride). A white to practically white, odourless, crystalline powder. It gradually darkens on exposure to air and light. Soluble 1 in 3 of water and 1 in 50 of alcohol; less soluble in dehydrated alcohol; insoluble in chloroform and in ether. A 1% solution in water has a pH of about 5. Solutions become pink to brownish-pink on standing exposed to air and almost immediately so when made alkaline. Store in airtight containers. Protect from light.

### Isoprenaline Sulfate *(rINNM)*

Isoprenaline Sulphate *(BANM)*; Isoprenalini Sulfas; Isopropylarterenol Sulphate; Isopropylnoradrenaline Sulphate; Isoproterenol Sulfate; Sulfato de isoprenalina.

$(C_{11}H_{17}NO_3)_2,H_2SO_4,2H_2O$ = 556.6.

*CAS — 299-95-6 (anhydrous isoprenaline sulfate); 6700-39-6 (isoprenaline sulfate dihydrate).*

*ATC — C01CA02; R03AB02; R03CB01.*

**Pharmacopoeias.** In *Eur.* (see p.vi), *Int., Pol.,* and *US.*

**Ph. Eur. 5.0** (Isoprenaline Sulphate). A white or almost white crystalline powder. Freely soluble in water; very slightly soluble in alcohol. A 5% solution in water has a pH of 4.3 to 5.5. Store in airtight containers. Protect from light.

**USP 27** (Isoproterenol Sulfate). A white to practically white, odourless, crystalline powder. It gradually darkens on exposure to light and air. Soluble 1 in 4 of water; very slightly soluble in alcohol, in chloroform, in ether, and in benzene. A 1% solution in water has a pH of about 5. Solutions become pink to brownish-pink on standing exposed to air, and almost immediately so when made alkaline. Store in airtight containers. Protect from light.

### Adverse Effects and Precautions

The adverse effects of isoprenaline may include tachycardia and cardiac arrhythmias, palpitations, hypotension, tremor, headache, sweating, and facial flushing. Prolonged use of isoprenaline has been associated with swelling of the parotid glands. Special caution is needed in the presence of ischaemic heart disease, diabetes mellitus, and hyperthyroidism.

Prolonged use of isoprenaline tablets sublingually has been reported to cause severe damage to the teeth due to the acidic nature of the drug. Sublingual use or inhalation may colour the saliva or sputum red.

For the adverse effects of sympathomimetics in general, and precautions for their use, see Adrenaline, p.852.

**Increased mortality.** For a discussion of the increased mortality and morbidity that has sometimes been observed in asthmatic patients and reference to an early epidemic associated with isoprenaline inhalers, see Fenoterol, p.785.

### Interactions

Isoprenaline should not be used with other potent $beta_1$ agonists such as adrenaline.

For the interactions of sympathomimetics in general, see Adrenaline, p.853.

**Theophylline.** For reports of increased theophylline clearance following use of isoprenaline, see p.803.

### Pharmacokinetics

As a result of sulfate conjugation in the gut, isoprenaline is considerably less active after oral administration than after parenteral administration. It is absorbed through the oral mucosa and has accordingly been given sublingually, but absorption by this route remains very erratic. Isoprenaline in the body is resistant to metabolism by monoamine oxidase, but is metabolised by catechol-*O*-methyltransferase in the liver, lungs, and other tissues, this metabolite being subsequently conjugated before excretion in the urine. Whereas the sulfate conjugate of isoprenaline is inactive the methylated metabolite exhibits weak activity.

Following intravenous injection isoprenaline has a plasma half-life of about one to several minutes according to whether the rate of injection is rapid or slow; it is almost entirely excreted in the urine as unchanged drug and metabolites within 24 hours. A much slower onset of action and a more extended initial half-life has been demonstrated following oral administration. Isoprenaline is reported to have a duration of action of up to about 2 hours after inhalation; it has been shown that a large proportion of an inhaled dose is swallowed.

◊ References.


1. Blackwell EW, *et al.* The fate of isoprenaline administered by pressurized aerosols. *Br J Pharmacol* 1970; **39:** 194P–195P.
2. Conolly ME, *et al.* Metabolism of isoprenaline in dog and man. *Br J Pharmacol* 1972; **46:** 458–72.
3. Blackwell EW, *et al.* Metabolism of isoprenaline after aerosol and direct intrabronchial administration in man and dog. *Br J Pharmacol* 1974; **50:** 587–91.
4. Reyes G, *et al.* The pharmacokinetics of isoproterenol in critically ill pediatric patients. *J Clin Pharmacol* 1993; **33:** 29–34.


### Uses and Administration

Isoprenaline is a sympathomimetic (see Adrenaline, p.854) that acts almost exclusively on beta-adrenergic receptors. It stimulates the CNS. It has a powerful stimulating action on the heart and increases cardiac output, excitability, and rate; it also causes peripheral vasodilatation and produces a fall in diastolic blood pressure and usually maintains or slightly increases systolic blood pressure. In addition, isoprenaline has bronchodilating properties.

Isoprenaline has been used in a variety of cardiac disorders. It may be used for the temporary prevention or control of Stokes-Adams attacks although for long-term management the use of a pacemaker is preferable. Isoprenaline may be useful in severe bradycardia unresponsive to atropine, although again cardiac pacing is preferred. It has also been advocated as an adjunct for other cardiac disorders including shock (p.835) and torsade de pointes (see Cardiac Arrhythmias, p.816). It has been used in the diagnosis of congenital heart defects.

In the management of **cardiac disorders**, isoprenaline is usually given as the hydrochloride by slow intravenous infusion under ECG control. Infusion rates may range from 0.5 to 10 micrograms/minute depending on the clinical condition of the patient; 1 to 4 micrograms/minute may be adequate to correct bradycardia but rates of 4 to 8 micrograms/minute may be required for acute Stokes-Adams attacks. Isoprenaline hydrochloride can be given by intracardiac injection in extreme cases. It has also been given subcutaneously or intramuscularly in initial doses of 200 micrograms (as 1 mL of a 0.02% solution) and by slow intravenous injection in initial doses of 20 to 60 micrograms (as 1 to 3 mL of a 0.002% solution); doses are subsequently adjusted according to ventricular rate. Tablets of isoprenaline hydrochloride have been given orally or sublingually.

Isoprenaline has been used as a bronchodilator in the management of **reversible airways obstruction** but sympathomimetics with a selective action on $beta_2$ receptors, such as salbutamol, are now preferred (see Asthma, p.777). It has been given as the sulfate or hydrochloride usually by inhalation; sublingual tablets and intravenous injections have also been used.

### Preparations

***BP 2003:*** Isoprenaline Injection;

***USP 27:*** Acetylcysteine and Isoproterenol Hydrochloride Inhalation Solution; Isoproterenol Hydrochloride and Phenylephrine Bitartrate Inhalation

Aerosol; Isoproterenol Hydrochloride Inhalation Aerosol; Isoproterenol Hydrochloride Injection; Isoproterenol Hydrochloride Tablets; Isoproterenol Inhalation Solution; Isoproterenol Sulfate Inhalation Aerosol; Isoproterenol Sulfate Inhalation Solution.

**Proprietary Preparations** (details are given in Part 3)
***Arg.:*** Ciapar; Proterenal; ***Austral.:*** Isuprel; ***Austria:*** Ingelan; ***Belg.:*** Isuprel; Medihaler-Iso†; ***Canad.:*** Isuprel†; ***Fr.:*** Isuprel; ***Ger.:*** Ingelan; Kattwilon N†; ***Gr.:*** Isuprel; Saventrine; ***Hong Kong:*** Saventrine†; ***India:*** Autohaler; Isolin; ***Irl.:*** Saventrine; ***Israel:*** Isuprel; ***Neth.:*** Medihaler-Iso†; ***NZ:*** Isuprel; ***Port.:*** Medihaler-Iso†; ***S.Afr.:*** Imuprel; ***Singapore:*** Isuprel; Saventrine; ***Spain:*** Aleudrina; ***Thai.:*** Isuprel; ***UK:*** Saventrine†; ***USA:*** Isuprel; Medihaler-Iso.

**Multi-ingredient:** ***Arg.:*** Zantril; ***Austria:*** Ingelan; ***Ger.:*** Ingelan; ***Mex.:*** Isobutil; ***Port.:*** Prelus; ***Spain:*** Aldo Asma; Frenal Compositum; ***Switz.:*** Mucobronchyl†; ***USA:*** Norisodrine with Calcium Iodide.

---

## Isosorbide *(BAN, USAN, rINN)*

AT-101; Isosorbida; NSC-40725. 1,4:3,6-Dianhydro-D-glucitol.

$C_6H_{10}O_4$ = 146.1.

*CAS — 652-67-5.*

**Pharmacopoeias.** In *Jpn.*

*US* includes Isosorbide Concentrate.

**USP 27** (Isosorbide Concentrate). An aqueous solution containing 70.0 to 80.0% w/w of isosorbide. A colourless to slightly yellow liquid. Soluble in water and in alcohol. Store in airtight containers. Protect from light.

### Profile

Isosorbide is an osmotic diuretic with properties similar to those of mannitol (p.950). It is reported to cause less nausea and vomiting than other oral osmotic diuretics.

Isosorbide is used for short-term reduction of intra-ocular pressure in acute glaucoma or prior to surgery (p.1485). The usual dose is 1 to 3 g/kg by mouth 2 to 4 times daily. The onset of action is usually within 30 minutes and lasts for up to 5 or 6 hours.

### Preparations

***USP 27:*** Isosorbide Concentrate; Isosorbide Oral Solution.

**Proprietary Preparations** (details are given in Part 3)
***Braz.:*** Angil; ***Mex.:*** Biordin; Debisor; ***USA:*** Ismotic.

---

## Isosorbide Dinitrate *(BAN, USAN, rINN)*

Dinitrato de isosorbida; ISDN; Isosorbidi Dinitras; Sorbide Nitrate. 1,4:3,6-Dianhydro-D-glucitol 2,5-dinitrate.

$C_6H_8N_2O_8$ = 236.1.

*CAS — 87-33-2.*

*ATC — C01DA08; D03AX08.*

**Pharmacopoeias.** In *Chin., Jpn,* and *Pol.*

*Eur.* (see p.vi), *Int.,* and *US* include diluted isosorbide dinitrate.

**Ph. Eur. 5.0** (Isosorbide Dinitrate, Diluted). A dry mixture of isosorbide dinitrate and lactose monohydrate or mannitol. The solubility of the diluted product depends on the diluent and its concentration. Protect from light.

Undiluted isosorbide dinitrate is a fine, white, crystalline powder. Very slightly soluble in water; sparingly soluble in alcohol; very soluble in acetone.

**USP 27** (Diluted Isosorbide Dinitrate). A dry mixture of isosorbide dinitrate (usually about 25%) with lactose, mannitol, or other suitable inert excipients, the latter being added to minimise the risk of explosion. It may contain up to 1% of a suitable stabiliser such as ammonium phosphate. It is an ivory-white, odourless powder. Store in airtight containers.

Undiluted isosorbide dinitrate occurs as white crystalline rosettes. Very slightly soluble in water; sparingly soluble in alcohol; very soluble in acetone; freely soluble in chloroform.

**Handling.** Undiluted isosorbide dinitrate may explode if subjected to percussion or excessive heat.

**Stability.** The loss of isosorbide dinitrate from solution during infusion was found to be 30% with PVC plastic intravenous infusion sets but negligible when polyolefin or glass delivery systems were used.[1] Another study reported a 23% decrease in isosorbide dinitrate concentration after 24 hours of storage at 21° in PVC containers; most of the loss occurred in the first 6 hours. Loss of potency was not noted when isosorbide dinitrate was stored under similar conditions in glass bottles or polyethylene, nylon, and polypropylene laminated bags.[2]

1. Kowaluk EA, *et al.* Drug loss in polyolefin infusion systems. *Am J Hosp Pharm* 1983; **40:** 118–19.
2. Martens HJ, *et al.* Sorption of various drugs in polyvinyl chloride, glass, and polyethylene-lined infusion containers. *Am J Hosp Pharm* 1990; **47:** 369–73.

### Adverse Effects, Treatment, and Precautions

As for Glyceryl Trinitrate, p.923.

**Effects on the blood.** Haemolysis occurred in 2 patients with G6PD deficiency during treatment with isosorbide dinitrate.[1]

1. Aderka D, *et al.* Isosorbide dinitrate-induced hemolysis in G6PD-deficient subjects. *Acta Haematol (Basel)* 1983; **69:** 63–4.

**Headache.** The most common adverse effect of nitrate therapy is headache which usually decreases after a few days. There has been a report[1] of a severe continuous unilateral headache with an oculosympathetic paresis on the same side associated with isosorbide dinitrate therapy.

1. Mueller RA, Meienberg O. Hemicrania with oculosympathetic paresis from isosorbide dinitrate. *N Engl J Med* 1983; **308:** 458–9.

**Hypersensitivity.** Laryngeal oedema developed on two occasions in a woman following the use of isosorbide dinitrate spray;[1] nifedipine was also given sublingually which on the second occasion caused a noticeable increase in the laryngeal swelling induced by the nitrate.

1. Silfvast T, *et al.* Laryngeal oedema after isosorbide dinitrate spray and sublingual nifedipine. *BMJ* 1995; **311:** 232.

**Nitrate tolerance.** Continuous administration of organic nitrates is associated with tolerance to their haemodynamic effects; for an overview of nitrate tolerance, see under Precautions for Glyceryl Trinitrate, p.924.

A study in 12 patients with chronic stable angina[1] showed that following treatment for one week with isosorbide dinitrate 30 mg two or three times daily, treadmill-walking time was longer throughout a 5-hour testing period compared with placebo. In contrast, after treatment for one week with isosorbide dinitrate 30 mg four times daily, treadmill-walking time was prolonged at 1 hour but not at 3 or 5 hours. These results support the concept that clinical efficacy of isosorbide dinitrate is maintained if administered in a dose schedule which provides a nitrate-free or a low-nitrate period.

The effect of sublingual isosorbide dinitrate in patients receiving chronic therapy with isosorbide dinitrate was evaluated in 24 patients with angina.[2] Sublingual administration produced less reduction of aortic systolic pressure and left ventricular end-diastolic pressure and less dilatation of coronary artery diameter in patients who received chronic isosorbide dinitrate therapy compared with patients not receiving chronic therapy.

1. Parker JO, *et al.* Effect of intervals between doses on the development of tolerance to isosorbide dinitrate. *N Engl J Med* 1987; **316:** 1440–4.
2. Naito H, *et al.* Effects of sublingual nitrate in patients receiving sustained therapy of isosorbide dinitrate for coronary artery disease. *Am J Cardiol* 1989; **64:** 565–68.

**Oedema.** Reports of ankle oedema associated with isosorbide dinitrate therapy in 3 patients with heart failure.[1]

1. Rodger JC. Peripheral oedema in patients treated with isosorbide dinitrate. *BMJ* 1981; **283:** 1365–6.

### Interactions

As for Glyceryl Trinitrate, p.924.

**Disopyramide.** The effectiveness of sublingual isosorbide dinitrate was reduced in a patient taking disopyramide.[1] The interaction was considered to be due to diminished salivary secretions caused by the antimuscarinic action of disopyramide which inhibited the dissolution of the sublingual isosorbide dinitrate tablet.

1. Barletta MA, Eisen H. Isosorbide dinitrate-disopyramide phosphate interaction. *Drug Intell Clin Pharm* 1985; **19:** 764.

### Pharmacokinetics

Like glyceryl trinitrate, isosorbide dinitrate is readily absorbed from the oral mucosa. Isosorbide dinitrate is also readily absorbed when given by mouth but owing to extensive first-pass metabolism in the liver and presystemic clearance its bioavailability is reduced. Isosorbide dinitrate is also absorbed through the skin from an ointment basis.

Following sublingual administration, anti-anginal effect is apparent within 2 to 5 minutes and persists for about 1 to 2 hours. Following oral administration of conventional tablets, anti-anginal activity is present in less than 1 hour and lasts for 4 to 6 hours.

Isosorbide dinitrate is widely distributed with a large apparent volume of distribution. It is taken up by smooth muscle cells of blood vessels and the nitrate group is cleaved to inorganic nitrite and then to nitric oxide. It is also rapidly metabolised in the liver to the major active metabolites isosorbide 2-mononitrate and isosorbide 5-mononitrate (see Isosorbide Mononitrate, below).

After sublingual administration, isosorbide dinitrate has a plasma half-life of 45 to 60 minutes. Plasma half-lives of 20 minutes and 4 hours have been reported following intravenous and oral administration, respectively. During prolonged administration, the half-life is increased due to accumulation of the isosorbide 5-mononitrate metabolite which reduces hepatic isosorbide dinitrate extraction. Both primary metabolites have longer half-lives than the parent compound.

◊ References.

1. Abshagen U, *et al.* Pharmacokinetics and metabolism of isosorbide-dinitrate after intravenous and oral administration. *Eur J Clin Pharmacol* 1985; **27:** 637–44.
2. Straehl P, Galeazzi RL. Isosorbide dinitrate bioavailability, kinetics, and metabolism. *Clin Pharmacol Ther* 1985; **38:** 140–9.
3. Thadani U, Whitsett T. Relationship of pharmacokinetic and pharmacodynamic properties of the organic nitrates. *Clin Pharmacokinet* 1988; **15:** 32–43.
4. Schneider W, *et al.* Concentrations of isosorbide dinitrate, isosorbide-2-mononitrate and isosorbide-5-mononitrate in human vascular and muscle tissue under steady-state conditions. *Eur J Clin Pharmacol* 1990; **38:** 145–7.
5. Vogt D, *et al.* Pharmacokinetics and haemodynamic effects of ISDN following different dosage forms and routes of administration. *Eur J Clin Pharmacol* 1994; **46:** 319–24.
6. Bergami A, *et al.* Pharmacokinetics of isosorbide dinitrate in healthy volunteers after 24-hour intravenous infusion. *J Clin Pharmacol* 1997; **37:** 828–33.

### Uses and Administration

Isosorbide dinitrate is a vasodilator with general properties similar to those of glyceryl trinitrate (p.924). It is used in the management of angina pectoris (p.813) and of heart failure (p.820). It has also been investigated in myocardial infarction (p.828).

Isosorbide dinitrate may be administered by the sublingual, oral, transdermal, or intravenous route.

In **angina** isosorbide dinitrate may be given as sublingual tablets or spray for the relief of an acute attack, although glyceryl trinitrate may be preferred because it has a faster onset of action. Isosorbide dinitrate may also be used before an activity or stress which might provoke an attack. The usual dose in acute angina is 2.5 to 10 mg sublingually. As an alternative, one to three sprays (1.25 mg/spray) may be directed under the tongue.

Isosorbide dinitrate is also used in the long-term management of angina in oral doses of 20 to 120 mg daily in divided doses according to the patient's needs. Increases in dosage should be gradual to avoid side-effects. Up to 240 mg daily in divided doses may be necessary. Modified-release formulations may be used in equivalent doses. Transdermal preparations such as topical sprays or ointments may also be used.

Isosorbide dinitrate is given by intravenous infusion for unstable angina. The dose is titrated according to patient response; doses in the range of 2 to 12 mg/hour are usually suitable but up to 20 mg/hour may be necessary in some patients. The plastic used in the infusion equipment may adsorb isosorbide dinitrate (see Stability, above) and allowance may have to be made for this.

During percutaneous transluminal coronary angioplasty isosorbide dinitrate may be given by the intracoronary route to allow prolonged balloon inflation and to prevent or relieve coronary spasm. Only injections of isosorbide dinitrate which are approved for intracoronary administration should be given by this route as preparations intended for normal intravenous administration may contain additives that are harmful if injected into diseased coronary vessels. The usual dose is 1 mg as a bolus before balloon inflation. The maximum recommended dose is 5 mg within a 30-minute time period.

Isosorbide dinitrate is also used in the management of **heart failure**. It is given in doses of 5 to 15 mg sublingually every 2 to 3 hours, or in oral doses of 30 to 160 mg daily in divided doses. Oral doses of up to 240 mg daily may be required. The intravenous route may also be employed using the intravenous doses given above for angina.

◊ As well as being used in cardiovascular disorders, nitrates such as isosorbide dinitrate have been tried in a number of other conditions including anal fissure, erectile dysfunction, and oesophageal motility disorders such as achalasia and spasm. Further details of these uses are given under Glyceryl Trinitrate (p.925).

### Preparations

***BP 2003:*** Isosorbide Dinitrate Sublingual Tablets; Isosorbide Dinitrate Tablets;
***USP 27:*** Isosorbide Dinitrate Chewable Tablets; Isosorbide Dinitrate Extended-release Capsules; Isosorbide Dinitrate Extended-release Tablets; Isosorbide Dinitrate Sublingual Tablets; Isosorbide Dinitrate Tablets.

**Proprietary Preparations** (details are given in Part 3)
***Arg.:*** Isoket; Isordil; ***Austral.:*** Isordil; Sorbidin; ***Austria:*** Cedocard; Hexanitrat; Iso Mack; Isoket; Isostad; Sorbidilat†; Vasorbate; ***Belg.:*** Cedocard; Isordil; Sorbitrate†; ***Braz.:*** Dilatrat; Elantan†; Isocord; Isorbid; Isordil; ***Canad.:*** Apo-ISDN; Cedocard; Coradur†; Isordil†; Novo-Sorbide†; ***Denm.:*** Cardopax; Iso Mack; ***Fin.:*** Dinit; Nitrosid; ***Fr.:*** Isocard; Langoran; Risordan; ***Ger.:*** Corovliss†; Diconpin; Dignonitrat†; duranitrat; Iso Mack; Iso-Puren; Isodinit†; Isoket; Isostenase; Jenacard; Maycor; Nitro-Tablinen†; Nitrosorbon; TD Spray Iso Mack; ***Hong Kong:*** Apo-ISDN; Iso Mack; Isoket; Isordil; Isorem; Nitorol†; ***India:*** Isordil; Sorbitrate; ***Irl.:*** Cedocard†; Isoket; Isordil; Soni-Slo†; ***Israel:*** Cordil; Isocardide; Isoket; Isotard; ***Ital.:***

Carvasin; Diniket; Nitrosorbide; ***Jpn:*** Antup R; Nitorol; ***Malaysia:*** Apo-ISDN; Isoket; Isordil; Nitorol; Sorbidin; ***Mex.:*** Isoket; Isorbid; ***Neth.:*** Cedocard; Isordil; Prodicard†; ***Norw.:*** Sorbangil; ***NZ:*** Carvasin†; Coronex; ***Port.:*** Flindix; Isoket; Isopront; ***S.Afr.:*** Angi-Spray; Isoket; Isordil; ***Singapore:*** Apo-ISDN; Iso Mack; Isobin; Isoket; Isordil; Nitrosorbide†; ***Spain:*** Iso; Maycor†; ***Swed.:*** Sorbangil; ***Switz.:*** Acordin; Esconitro; Iso Mack; Isoday†; Isoket; Isosifar; Sorbidilat; ***Thai.:*** Angitrit; Cedocard†; Hartsorb; Iso Mack; Isobinate; Isoket; Isordil; Isorem; Isotrate; Izo; Sorbidin; Sorbitrate†; Sornil; ***UK:*** Angitak; Cedocard; Isocard†; Isoket; Isordil†; Sorbichew†; Sorbid†; Sorbitrate†; ***USA:*** Dilatrate; Isochron; Isordil; Sorbitrate.

**Multi-ingredient:** ***Austria:*** Beta-Isoket†; Viskenit; ***Ger.:*** Stenoptin.

## Isosorbide Mononitrate *(BAN, USAN, rINN)*

AHR-4698; BM-22145; IS-5-MN; Isosorbide-5-mononitrate; Isosorbidi Mononitras; Mononitrato de isosorbida. 1,4:3,6-Dianhydro-D-glucitol 5-nitrate.

$C_6H_9NO_6$ = 191.1.

*CAS — 16051-77-7.*

*ATC — C01DA14.*

**Pharmacopoeias.** *Eur.* (see p.vi) includes diluted isosorbide mononitrate.

**Ph. Eur. 5.0** (Isosorbide Mononitrate, Diluted). A dry mixture of isosorbide mononitrate and lactose monohydrate or mannitol. The solubility of the diluted product depends on the diluent and its concentration. Protect from light.

Undiluted isosorbide mononitrate is a white crystalline powder. Freely soluble in water, in alcohol, in acetone, and in dichloromethane.

### Adverse Effects, Treatment, and Precautions

As for Glyceryl Trinitrate, p.923.

Myalgia has been reported very rarely.

### Interactions

As for Glyceryl Trinitrate, p.924.

### Pharmacokinetics

Isosorbide mononitrate is readily absorbed from the gastrointestinal tract. Following oral administration of conventional tablets, peak plasma levels are reached in 30 minutes to 1 hour; onset of action occurs within 20 minutes and lasts for about 8 to 10 hours. Unlike isosorbide dinitrate, isosorbide mononitrate does not undergo first-pass hepatic metabolism and bioavailability is nearly 100%. Isosorbide mononitrate is widely distributed with a large apparent volume of distribution. It is taken up by smooth muscle cells of blood vessels and the nitrate group is cleaved to inorganic nitrite and then to nitric oxide. Isosorbide mononitrate is metabolised to inactive metabolites, including isosorbide and isosorbide glucuronide. Only about 2% of isosorbide mononitrate is excreted unchanged in the urine. An elimination half-life of about 4 to 5 hours has been reported.

◊ References.


1. Taylor T, *et al.* Isosorbide 5-mononitrate pharmacokinetics in humans. *Biopharm Drug Dispos* 1981; **2:** 255–63.
2. Thadani U, Whitsett T. Relationship of pharmacokinetic and pharmacodynamic properties of the organic nitrates. *Clin Pharmacokinet* 1988; **15:** 32–43.
3. McClennen W, *et al.* The plasma concentrations of isosorbide 5-mononitrate (5-ISMN) administered in an extended-release form to patients with acute myocardial infarction. *Br J Clin Pharmacol* 1995; **39:** 704–8.
4. Hutt V, *et al.* Evaluation of the pharmacokinetics and absolute bioavailability of three isosorbide-5-mononitrate preparations in healthy volunteers. *Arzneimittelforschung* 1995; **45:** 142–5.
5. Baxter T, Eadie CJ. Twenty-four hour plasma profile of sustained-release isosorbide mononitrate in healthy volunteers and in patients with chronic stable angina: two open label trials. *Br J Clin Pharmacol* 1997; **43:** 333–5.


### Uses and Administration

Isosorbide mononitrate is an active metabolite of the vasodilator isosorbide dinitrate and is used in the long-term management of angina pectoris (p.813) and heart failure (p.820). It has also been investigated in myocardial infarction (below).

The usual oral dose is 20 mg two or three times daily, although doses ranging from 20 to 120 mg daily have been given. Modified-release oral preparations have been developed for use in angina.

**Myocardial infarction.** Long-term management of myocardial infarction (p.828) can involve numerous drug therapies and some patients, for example those with myocardial ischaemia or poor left ventricular function, may require the long-term administration of nitrates, although recent studies have thrown doubt on their routine use. In the GISSI-3 study[1] there was no significant benefit from the use of transdermal glyceryl trinitrate when assessed 6 weeks post-infarction and in the ISIS-4 study[2] oral isosorbide mononitrate apparently had no effect on 35-day mortality.


1. Gruppo Italiano per lo Studio della Sopravvivenza nell'Infarto Miocardico. GISSI-3: effects of lisinopril and transdermal glyceryl trinitrate singly and together on 6-week mortality and ventricular function after acute myocardial infarction. *Lancet* 1994; **343:** 1115–22.
2. ISIS-4 (Fourth International Study of Infarct Survival) Collaborative Group. ISIS-4: a randomised factorial trial assessing early oral captopril, oral mononitrate, and intravenous magnesium sulphate in 58 050 patients with suspected acute myocardial infarction. *Lancet* 1995; **345:** 669–85.


**Termination of pregnancy.** For mention of the use of isosorbide mononitrate to ripen the cervix before termination of pregnancy, see Obstetrics and Gynaecology, under Glyceryl Trinitrate, p.925.

**Variceal haemorrhage.** For reference to the use of isosorbide mononitrate in the management of variceal haemorrhage, see under Glyceryl Trinitrate, p.926.

### Preparations

***BP 2003:*** Isosorbide Mononitrate Tablets; Prolonged-release Isosorbide Mononitrate Tablets.

**Proprietary Preparations** (details are given in Part 3)

***Arg.:*** Cilatron; Isolan; Medocor; Misordil; Monoket; Monotrin; ***Austral.:*** Duride; Imdur; Imtrate; Isomonit; Monodur; ***Austria:*** Corangin†; Elantan; Epicordin; Imdur†; Isomonat; Mono Mack; Monoket; Myocardon mono; Olicardin; Sorbimon†; ***Belg.:*** Pentacard†; Promocard; ***Braz.:*** Cardionil; Cincordil; Monocordil; Revange; ***Canad.:*** Imdur; Ismo†; ***Chile:*** Ismo; Mono Mack; ***Denm.:*** Fem-Mono; Imdur; Ismo†; Isodur; Isomonit†; ***Fin.:*** Imdur; Isangina; Ismexin; Ismox; Ormox; ***Fr.:*** Monicor; ***Ger.:*** Coleb; Conpin; Corangin; duramonitat; Elantan; IS 5 Mono; Ismo; Isomonit; Isomonoreal†; Moni; Monit-Puren; Mono Acis; mono corax; Mono Mack; Mono Maycor†; Mono Wolff; Monobeta; Monoclair; Monolong; Mononitrat; Monopur; Monostenase; Olicard; Orasorbil; Sigacora; Turimonit; ***Gr.:*** G-Dil; Imdur; Isomon; Monoginal; Monoket; Monorythm; Monosordil; Nitramin; Nitrilan; Procardol; ***Hong Kong:*** Corangin; Elantan; Imdur; Ismo; Isotrate†; Mono Mack; Monocinque; ***India:*** IHD; Ismo; Monicor; Monocontin; Monosorbitrate; Monotrate; ***Irl.:*** Elantan; Imdur; Isomel; Isomonit; Isotrate†; Sormon; ***Israel:*** Ismo†; Monocord; Monolong; Mononit; ***Ital.:*** Duronitrin; Elan; Ismo; Kiton; Leicester Retard; Monocinque; Monoket; Nitrex; Orasorbil†; Vasdilat; ***Malaysia:*** Elantan; Imdex; Imdur; ***Mex.:*** Elantan; Imdur; Mono Mack; ***Neth.:*** Ismo†; Mono Mack; Mono-Cedocard; Promocard; ***Norw.:*** Imdur; Ismo; Monoket; ***NZ:*** Corangin; Duride; Imdur†; Imtrate; Ismo; ***Port.:*** Amplexol; Imdur; Ismo; Monoket; Mononitril; Monopront; Orasorbil; ***S.Afr.:*** Angitrate; Elantan; Imdur; Ismo; ***Singapore:*** Elantan; Imdex; Imdur; Ismo†; Isotrate†; Mono Mack†; Monotrate†; ***Spain:*** Cardionil; Cardiovas; Coronur; Dolak; Isonitril; Olicard†; Pancardiol†; Percorina†; Pertil; Titrane†; Uniket; ***Swed.:*** Fem-Mono; Imdur; Ismo; Isodur; Monoket; ***Switz.:*** Corangine; Elantan†; Etimonis†; Imdur†; Ismo; ***Thai.:*** Elantan; Imdur; Ismo; Isopen; Mono Mack; Monolin; Monotrate; Pentacard†; ***UK:*** Angeze; Chemydur; Cibral; Dynamin; Elantan; Imdur; Isib; Ismo; Isodur; Isotard; Isotrate; MCR-50; Modisal; Monit; Mono-Cedocard†; Monomax; Trangina; Xismox; ***USA:*** Imdur; Ismo; Monoket.

**Multi-ingredient:** ***Braz.:*** Vasclin; ***India:*** Mono-A; Solosprin; ***UK:*** Imazin.

## Isradipine *(BAN, USAN, rINN)*

Isradipino; Isradipinum; PN-200-110. Isopropyl methyl 4-(2,1,3-benzoxadiazol-4-yl)-1,4-dihydro-2,6-dimethylpyridine-3,5-dicarboxylate.

$C_{19}H_{21}N_3O_5$ = 371.4.

*CAS — 75695-93-1.*

*ATC — C08CA03.*

**Pharmacopoeias.** In *Eur.* (see p.vi) and *US.*

**Ph. Eur. 5.0** (Isradipine). A yellow crystalline powder. Practically insoluble in water; freely soluble in acetone; soluble in methyl alcohol. Protect from light.

**USP 27** (Isradipine). A yellow fine crystalline powder. Protect from light.

**Stability.** An oral preparation of isradipine 1 mg/mL, prepared using the powder from capsules of isradipine suspended in syrup,[1] was stable when stored at 4° for up to 35 days after preparation.


1. MacDonald JL, *et al.* Stability of isradipine in an extemporaneously compounded oral liquid. *Am J Hosp Pharm* 1994; **51:** 2409–11.


### Adverse Effects, Treatment, and Precautions

As for dihydropyridine calcium-channel blockers (see Nifedipine, p.966).

◊ In a multicentre study[1] involving 74 patients allocated to antihypertensive therapy with isradipine 2.5 to 10 mg twice daily, and 72 allocated to treatment with hydrochlorothiazide, adverse effects were reported in 44 of the isradipine group but only 29 of the thiazide group. Flushing, palpitation, and oedema were more common in patients receiving isradipine, while headache, dizziness, and dyspnoea were reported in both groups with similar frequency. In another study,[2] spontaneously reported adverse effects occurred less frequently in patients taking isradipine (18.4% of 103 patients) than in those taking amlodipine (33.3% of 102 patients). In particular, ankle oedema was less frequent, severe, and prolonged with isradipine than with amlodipine. A multicentre study[3] comparing isradipine and enalapril antihypertensive therapy reported adverse effects in 51% of 71 patients taking isradipine and 45% of 64 patients taking enalapril. The commonest side-effects with isradipine were dizziness (14%), oedema (10%), fatigue (9%), headache (9%), and pruritus (7%).


1. Carlsen JE, Køber L. Blood pressure lowering effect and adverse events during treatment of arterial hypertension with isradipine and hydrochlorothiazide. *Drug Invest* 1990; **2:** 10–16.
2. Hermans L, *et al.* At equipotent doses, isradipine is better tolerated than amlodipine in patients with mild-to-moderate hypertension: a double-blind, randomized, parallel-group study. *Br J Clin Pharmacol* 1994; **38:** 335–40.
3. Johnson BF, *et al.* A multicenter comparison of adverse reaction profiles of isradipine and enalapril at equipotent doses in patients with essential hypertension. *J Clin Pharmacol* 1995; **35:** 484–92.


### Interactions

As for dihydropyridine calcium-channel blockers (see Nifedipine, p.969).

### Pharmacokinetics

Isradipine is almost completely absorbed from the gastrointestinal tract following a dose by mouth but undergoes extensive first-pass metabolism; the bioavailability is reported to be 15 to 24%. Peak plasma concentrations occur about 2 hours after oral administration. It is about 95% bound to plasma proteins. Isradipine is extensively metabolised in the liver, at least partly by the cytochrome P450 isoenzyme CYP3A4. About 70% of an oral dose is reported to be excreted as metabolites in urine, the remainder in faeces. The terminal elimination half-life is often stated to be about 8 hours although a value of less than 4 hours has also been reported.

◊ In single-dose and steady-state studies of the pharmacokinetics of isradipine in 9 hypertensive subjects using a specific high performance liquid chromatographic assay, isradipine was found to be rapidly absorbed with peak concentrations occurring 1.2 (steady state) to 1.5 (single dose) hours after administration.[1] The mean terminal elimination half-life at steady state was 3.8 hours, suggesting that duration of action is likely to be short and that isradipine would need to be administered at least twice daily. There was considerable interindividual variation in the pharmacokinetics. In an earlier study[2] in healthy subjects the effective half-life of isradipine was calculated to be 8.8 hours, but radiolabelled isradipine was used and the assay method might have been less specific for unchanged drug.


1. Shenfield GM, *et al.* The pharmacokinetics of isradipine in hypertensive subjects. *Eur J Clin Pharmacol* 1990; **38:** 209–11.
2. Tse FLS, Jaffe JM. Pharmacokinetics of PN 200-110 (isradipine), a new calcium antagonist, after oral administration in man. *Eur J Clin Pharmacol* 1987; **32:** 361–5.


**Hepatic impairment.** Systemic availability following a radiolabelled dose of isradipine 5 mg by mouth was no different at 15.6% in 7 patients with non-cirrhotic chronic liver disease from the value of 16.5% in 8 healthy subjects.[1] However, in 8 patients with cirrhosis of the liver availability was markedly increased to a mean of 36.9%; this was associated with decreased clearance (1.6 litres/minute, compared with 9.9 in controls). Terminal half-life, as measured after intravenous administration, was greater at 11.9 hours in cirrhotic patients than the 5.1 hours seen in controls.


1. Cotting J, *et al.* Pharmacokinetics of isradipine in patients with chronic liver disease. *Eur J Clin Pharmacol* 1990; **38:** 599–603.


### Uses and Administration

Isradipine is a dihydropyridine calcium-channel blocker with actions similar to those of nifedipine (p.970). It is used in the treatment of hypertension (p.825).

The usual initial dose of isradipine is 2.5 mg by mouth twice daily increased if necessary after 3 to 4 weeks to 5 mg twice daily. Some patients may require 10 mg twice daily. In elderly patients an initial dose of 1.25 mg twice daily may be preferable; a maintenance dose of 2.5 or 5 mg once daily may sometimes be sufficient. A reduced dose should also be considered in patients with hepatic or renal impairment (see below).

A modified-release preparation allowing once-daily dosing is available in some countries.

◊ Reviews.


1. Fitton A, Benfield P. Isradipine: a review of its pharmacodynamic and pharmacokinetic properties, and therapeutic use in cardiovascular disease. *Drugs* 1990; **40:** 31–74.
2. Walton T, Symes LR. Felodipine and isradipine: new calcium-channel blocking agents for the treatment of hypertension. *Clin Pharm* 1993; **12:** 261–75.
3. Brogden RN, Sorkin EM. Isradipine: an update of its pharmacodynamic and pharmacokinetic properties and therapeutic efficacy in the treatment of mild to moderate hypertension. *Drugs* 1995; **49:** 618–49.


**Administration in hepatic or renal impairment.** In patients with hepatic or renal impairment the UK manufacturer recommends an initial dose of isradipine of 1.25 mg twice daily. The dose may be increased as required, but a maintenance dose of 2.5 or 5 mg once daily may be sufficient in some patients.

## Preparations

**BP 2003:** Isradipine Tablets.

**Proprietary Preparations** (details are given in Part 3)

***Arg.:*** Dynacirc; ***Austria:*** Lomir; ***Belg.:*** Lomir; ***Braz.:*** Lomir; ***Chile:*** Dynacirc; ***Denm.:*** Lomir; ***Fin.:*** Lomir; ***Fr.:*** Icaz; ***Ger.:*** Lomir; Vascal; ***Gr.:*** Lomir; ***Hong Kong:*** Dynacirc; ***Ital.:*** Clivoten; Esradin; Lomir; ***Malaysia:*** Dynacirc; ***Mex.:*** Dynacirc; ***Neth.:*** Lomir; ***Norw.:*** Lomir; ***NZ:*** Dynacirc†; ***Port.:*** Dilatol; Lomir; ***S.Afr.:*** Dynacirc; ***Singapore:*** Dynacirc; ***Spain:*** Lomir; ***Swed.:*** Lomir; ***Switz.:*** Lomir; ***Thai.:*** Dynacirc; ***UK:*** Prescal; ***USA:*** Dynacirc.

## Ketanserin *(BAN, USAN, rINN)*

R-41468. 3-{2-[4-(4-Fluorobenzoyl)piperidino]ethyl}quinazoline-2,4(1*H*,3*H*)-dione.

$C_{22}H_{22}FN_3O_3$ = 395.4.

*CAS — 74050-98-9.*

*ATC — C02KD01.*

## Ketanserin Tartrate *(BANM, rINNM)*

R-49945; Tartrato de ketanserina.

$C_{22}H_{22}FN_3O_3,C_4H_6O_6$ = 545.5.

*CAS — 83846-83-7.*

*ATC — C02KD01.*

### Adverse Effects and Precautions

Ketanserin has been reported to cause sedation, fatigue, light-headedness, dizziness, headache, dry mouth, and gastrointestinal disturbances. Oedema has been reported rarely. In patients with predisposing factors such as QT prolongation, chronic use of ketanserin has been associated with the development of ventricular arrhythmias including torsade de pointes; ketanserin should be used with caution in patients taking antiarrhythmics and should not be used in second- or third-degree atrioventricular block. Care should be taken to avoid the development of hypokalaemia in patients taking ketanserin, for example if diuretics are given concomitantly.

Because ketanserin may cause drowsiness care should be taken in patients who drive or operate machinery.

Ketanserin is reported to be better tolerated in elderly than in younger patients.

### Interactions

The hypotensive effects of ketanserin may be enhanced by diuretics and other antihypertensives. Ketanserin should be used with caution in patients taking antiarrhythmics or drugs that cause hypokalaemia since the risk of arrhythmias is increased.

**Beta blockers.** Profound hypotension occurred in 2 patients one hour after taking ketanserin 40 mg by mouth.[1] Both patients were also taking a beta blocker which may have exacerbated the reaction.

1. Waller PC, *et al.* Profound hypotension after the first dose of ketanserin. *Postgrad Med J* 1987; **63:** 305–7.

### Pharmacokinetics

Ketanserin is rapidly absorbed from the gastrointestinal tract but has a bioavailability of about 50% due to first-pass hepatic metabolism. Peak plasma concentrations occur between 30 and 120 minutes after a dose by mouth. Ketanserin is about 95% bound to plasma proteins. The terminal half-life is stated to be between 13 and 18 hours but some studies report that following multiple doses the half-life is 19 to 29 hours. The metabolite ketanserinol has a terminal half-life of 31 to 35 hours following multiple doses, and it has been suggested that reconversion of ketanserinol to ketanserin may be responsible for the prolonged half-life of the parent compound during chronic administration.

Following oral administration about 68% of a dose is excreted in urine, and 24% in faeces, mainly as metabolites. Studies in *animals* suggest that ketanserin may cross the placenta and that some is present, together with metabolites, in breast milk.

◊ References.

1. Persson B, *et al.* Clinical pharmacokinetics of ketanserin. *Clin Pharmacokinet* 1991; **20:** 263–79.

### Uses and Administration

Ketanserin is a serotonin antagonist with a high affinity for peripheral serotonin-2 (5-$HT_2$) receptors and thus inhibits serotonin-induced vasoconstriction, bronchoconstriction, and platelet aggregation. It also has some alpha$_1$-antagonist and histamine $H_1$-antagonist properties, but the clinical significance of these is controversial.

Ketanserin is used in the management of hypertension (p.825) and has also been tried in a variety of other conditions (see below).

Ketanserin is given as the tartrate, but doses are usually expressed in terms of the base. Ketanserin tartrate 27.6 mg is approximately equivalent to 20 mg of ketanserin.

Ketanserin produces a gradual hypotensive effect when given orally, and 2 or 3 months of therapy may be required to produce the maximum reduction in blood pressure. Following intravenous injection a fall in blood pressure is generally produced in one or two minutes and lasts for 30 to 60 minutes.

In **hypertension** the usual initial dose is 20 mg twice daily by mouth, increasing, if necessary, after 1 month, to 40 mg twice daily. It has also been given by intravenous or intramuscular injection. The dose of ketanserin may need to be reduced or the dosage intervals increased in patients with hepatic impairment (see below).

◊ Reviews.

1. Brogden RN, Sorkin EM. Ketanserin: a review of its pharmacodynamic and pharmacokinetic properties, and therapeutic potential in hypertension and peripheral vascular disease. *Drugs* 1990; **40:** 903–49.

**Administration in hepatic impairment.** A study[1] in patients with cirrhosis found that the half-life and volume of distribution of ketanserin were decreased but the area under the concentration-time curve was markedly increased; the rate of metabolism was reduced. The results suggested that the dosage should be reduced or the dosage interval increased when ketanserin is given to patients with cirrhosis. A maximum dose of 20 mg twice daily by mouth has been suggested for patients with hepatic impairment.

1. Lebrec D, *et al.* Pharmacokinetics of ketanserin in patients with cirrhosis. *Clin Pharmacokinet* 1990; **19:** 160–6.

**Administration in renal impairment.** Results from a study in 12 patients with chronic renal impairment, of whom 6 required haemodialysis, suggested that no adjustment of the standard dose of ketanserin 20 mg twice daily was required in patients with renal impairment.[1]

1. Barendregt JNM, *et al.* Ketanserin pharmacokinetics in patients with renal failure. *Br J Clin Pharmacol* 1990; **29:** 715–23.

**Glaucoma and ocular hypertension.** Although ketanserin, as 0.5% eye drops, can reduce intra-ocular pressure in normal and glaucomatous eyes,[1,2] its value, if any, in the treatment of glaucoma and ocular hypertension remains to be determined.

1. Costagliola C, *et al.* Effect of topical ketanserin administration on intraocular pressure. *Br J Ophthalmol* 1993; **77:** 344–8.
2. Mastropasqua L, *et al.* Ocular hypotensive effect of topical ketanserin in timolol users. *Graefes Arch Clin Exp Ophthalmol* 1997; **235:** 130–5.

**Peripheral vascular disease.** Ketanserin is one of many drugs that have been tried in the management of peripheral vascular disease (p.831) but results have been contradictory. The multicentre Prevention of Atherosclerotic Complications with Ketanserin Trial (PACK),[1] involving 3899 patients with intermittent claudication, suggested that ketanserin might be of benefit in preventing limb amputation in some patients, although this was the result of subgroup analysis. Conflicting results have also been reported in patients with *Raynaud's syndrome*. A systematic review[2] found that ketanserin led to a small improvement in Raynaud's syndrome in patients with systemic sclerosis but that adverse effects increased; the authors concluded that ketanserin was not clinically beneficial in such patients.

Ketanserin has also been tried in other conditions associated with impaired peripheral blood flow: see Wounds and Ulcers, below.

1. Prevention of Atherosclerotic Complications with Ketanserin Trial Group. Prevention of atherosclerotic complications: controlled trial of ketanserin. *BMJ* 1989; **298:** 424–30. Correction. *ibid.*: 644.
2. Pope J, *et al.* Ketanserin for Raynaud's phenomenon in progressive systemic sclerosis. Available in The Cochrane Library; Issue 1. Chichester: John Wiley; 2004.

**Shivering.** Numerous drugs, including ketanserin, have been tried for the treatment of postoperative shivering (p.1295). Ketanserin 10 mg given intravenously has stopped shivering after general anaesthesia.[1,2]

1. Joris J, *et al.* Clonidine and ketanserin both are effective treatment for postanesthetic shivering. *Anesthesiology* 1993; **79:** 532–9.
2. Crisinel D, *et al.* Efficacité de la kétansérine sur le frisson postanesthésique. *Ann Fr Anesth Reanim* 1997; **16:** 120–5.

**Wounds and ulcers.** Systemic administration of ketanserin has been reported[1,2] to improve healing in various ulcers (p.1139) associated with impaired blood flow, although others have found little benefit.[3] Several placebo-controlled studies[4-6] have noted improved healing of decubitus, venous, and ischaemic ulcers following the application of ketanserin as a 2% ointment. However, when ketanserin was applied topically as a 2% gel to surgical wounds no improvement in healing rate was found and it was suggested that ketanserin is only of benefit where the blood supply is compromised.[7]

1. Roald OK, Seem E. Treatment of Raynaud's phenomenon with ketanserin in patients with connective tissue disorders. *BMJ* 1984; **289:** 577–8.
2. Rustin MHA, *et al.* Chronic leg ulceration with livedoid vasculitis, and response to oral ketanserin. *Br J Dermatol* 1989; **120:** 101–5.
3. Cox NH, Dufton PA. Treatment of Raynaud's phenomenon with ketanserin. *BMJ* 1984; **289:** 1078–9.
4. Tytgat H, van Asch H. Topical ketanserin in the treatment of decubitus ulcers: a double-blind study with 2% ketanserin ointment against placebo. *Adv Therapy* 1988; **5:** 143–52.
5. Roelens P. Double-blind placebo-controlled study with topical 2% ketanserin ointment in the treatment of venous ulcers. *Dermatologica* 1989; **178:** 98–102.
6. Janssen PAJ, *et al.* Use of topical ketanserin in the treatment of skin ulcers: a double-blind study. *J Am Acad Dermatol* 1989; **21:** 85–90.
7. Lawrence CM, *et al.* The effect of ketanserin on healing of fresh surgical wounds. *Br J Dermatol* 1995; **132:** 580–6.

### Preparations

**Proprietary Preparations** (details are given in Part 3)

***Arg.:*** Serefrex; ***Belg.:*** Sufrexal; ***Ital.:*** Perketan†; Serepress; Sufrexal†; ***Mex.:*** Sufrexal; ***Neth.:*** Ketensin; ***Port.:*** Sufrexal; ***Thai.:*** Sufrexal.

## Labetalol Hydrochloride

*(BANM, USAN, rINNM)*

AH-5158A; Hidrocloruro de labetalol; Ibidomide Hydrochloride; Labetaloli Hydrochloridum; Sch-15719W. 5-[1-Hydroxy-2-(1-methyl-3-phenylpropylamino)ethyl]salicylamide hydrochloride.

$C_{19}H_{24}N_2O_3,HCl$ = 364.9.

*CAS — 36894-69-6 (labetalol); 32780-64-6 (labetalol hydrochloride).*

*ATC — C07AG01.*

**Pharmacopoeias.** In *Eur.* (see p.vi) and *US.*

**Ph. Eur. 5.0** (Labetalol Hydrochloride). A white or almost white powder. Sparingly soluble in water and in alcohol; practically insoluble in dichloromethane. A 1% solution in water has a pH of 4.0 to 5.0.

**USP 27** (Labetalol Hydrochloride). A white to off-white powder. Soluble in water and in alcohol; insoluble in chloroform and in ether. A 1% solution in water has a pH of 4.0 to 5.0. Store in airtight containers at a temperature of 25°, excursions permitted between 15° and 30°. Protect from light.

**Incompatibility.** Labetalol hydrochloride is compatible with standard intravenous solutions such as glucose 5% and sodium chloride 0.9%. However, precipitation has been reported when labetalol hydrochloride is added to sodium bicarbonate injection 5%.[1] The precipitate is probably labetalol base.[2]

Incompatibilities have been reported with furosemide,[3] heparin,[4] insulin,[4] and thiopental.[3] In all cases a white precipitate formed immediately on mixing with labetalol hydrochloride 5 mg/mL (in glucose 5%). There has also been a report of immediate haze following admixture of labetalol hydrochloride (800 micrograms/mL) with warfarin sodium.[5]

1. Yuen P-HC, *et al.* Compatibility and stability of labetalol hydrochloride in commonly used intravenous solutions. *Am J Hosp Pharm* 1983; **40:** 1007–9.
2. Alam AS. Identification of labetalol precipitate. *Am J Hosp Pharm* 1984; **41:** 74.
3. Chiu MF, Schwartz ML. Visual compatibility of injectable drugs used in the intensive care unit. *Am J Health-Syst Pharm* 1997; **54:** 64–5.
4. Yamashita SK, *et al.* Compatibility of selected critical care drugs during simulated Y-site administration. *Am J Health-Syst Pharm* 1996; **53:** 1048–51.
5. Bahal SM, *et al.* Visual compatibility of warfarin sodium injection with selected medications and solutions. *Am J Health-Syst Pharm* 1997; **54:** 2599–2600.

### Adverse Effects

The adverse effects associated with beta blockers are described on p.869. Labetalol also has alpha-blocking activity which contributes to its adverse effects and these effects may predominate. Orthostatic hypotension may be a problem with high doses or at the start of treatment. Other effects associated with alpha blockade include dizziness, scalp tingling, and nasal congestion. Male sexual function may be impaired to a greater extent than with beta blockade alone. Muscle weakness, tremor, urinary retention, hepatitis, and jaundice have also been reported.

**Effects on the liver.** By 1990, the FDA had received 11 reports of hepatocellular damage associated with labetalol therapy.[1] Three patients died. Liver function should be monitored and labetalol discontinued in patients who develop liver function abnormalities. The *R,R*-isomer of labetalol, dilevalol, was withdrawn from the market because of hepatotoxicity.[2]

1. Clark JA, *et al.* Labetalol hepatotoxicity. *Ann Intern Med* 1990; **113:** 210–13.
2. Harvengt C. Labetalol hepatotoxicity. *Ann Intern Med* 1991; **114:** 341.

**Hypersensitivity.** Hypersensitivity reactions associated with labetalol may manifest as fever.[1,2] Anaphylactoid reaction to labetalol has also been reported.[3]

1. D'Arcy PF. Drug reactions and interactions: drug fever with labetalol. *Int Pharm J* 1987; **1:** 43–4.
2. Stricker BH, *et al.* Fever induced by labetalol. *JAMA* 1986; **256:** 619–20.
3. Ferree CE. Apparent anaphylaxis from labetalol. *Ann Intern Med* 1986; **104:** 729–30.

**Overdosage.** Acute oliguric renal failure developed after a short period of moderate hypotension in a patient who ingested labetalol 16 g. Renal function subsequently recovered.[1] Renal failure has also been reported[2] following ingestion of labetalol 6 g. The patient recovered following treatment with glucagon, isoprenaline, and dialysis.

1. Smit AJ, *et al.* Acute renal failure after overdose of labetalol. *BMJ* 1986; **293:** 1142–3.
2. Korzets A, *et al.* Acute renal failure associated with a labetalol overdose. *Postgrad Med J* 1990; **66:** 66–7.

### Precautions

As for Beta Blockers, p.870.

Because labetalol causes orthostatic hypotension it is recommended that injections are given to patients when they are lying down and that patients should remain lying down for the following 3 hours.

Labetalol should be withdrawn from patients who develop signs of hepatic impairment.

**Breast feeding.** Labetalol is distributed into breast milk, although it has been suggested[1] that the proportion of a maternal dose likely to be ingested by the infant is very low. In a study[2] in 25 patients, the mean concentration of labetalol in breast milk was less than in maternal plasma in patients receiving doses between 330 and 800 mg daily, although in 1 patient receiving 1200 mg daily a higher concentration was found in breast milk. In another study,[3] the concentration of drug in milk exceeded maternal plasma concentration in 2 of 3 mothers, and in 1 infant, the plasma-labetalol concentration was similar to that of the mother. However, no adverse effects have been reported in breast-feeding infants whose mothers were receiving labetalol, and the American Academy of Pediatrics considers[4] that it is therefore usually compatible with breast feeding.


1. Atkinson H, Begg EJ. Concentrations of beta-blocking drugs in human milk. *J Pediatr* 1990; **116:** 156.
2. Michael CA. Use of labetalol in the treatment of severe hypertension during pregnancy. *Br J Clin Pharmacol* 1979; **8** (suppl 2): 211S–215S.
3. Lunell NO, *et al.* Transfer of labetalol into amniotic fluid and breast milk in lactating women. *Eur J Clin Pharmacol* 1985; **28:** 597–9.
4. American Academy of Pediatrics. The transfer of drugs and other chemicals into human milk. *Pediatrics* 2001; **108:** 776–89. Correction. *ibid.*; 1029. Also available at: http://aappolicy.aappublications.org/cgi/content/full/pediatrics%3b108/3/776 (accessed 06/07/04)


## Interactions

The interactions associated with beta blockers are discussed on p.870.

## Pharmacokinetics

Labetalol is readily absorbed from the gastrointestinal tract, but is subject to considerable first-pass metabolism. Bioavailability varies widely between patients and may be increased in the presence of food. Peak plasma concentrations occur about 1 to 2 hours after an oral dose. Labetalol has low lipid solubility and only very small amounts appear to cross the blood-brain barrier in *animals*. It is about 50% protein bound. Labetalol crosses the placenta and is distributed into breast milk (see above). Labetalol is metabolised mainly in the liver, the metabolites being excreted in the urine together with only small amounts of unchanged labetalol; its major metabolite has not been found to have significant alpha- or beta-blocking effects. Excretion also occurs in the faeces via the bile. The elimination half-life at steady state is reported to be about 6 to 8 hours. Following intravenous infusion, the elimination half-life is about 5.5 hours. Labetalol is not removed by dialysis.

**The elderly.** Analysis[1] of data from 4 single-dose studies and 3 multidose studies indicated that age did not appear to be a significant factor in oral clearance in elderly patients receiving labetalol for long-term management of hypertension.


1. Rocci ML, *et al.* Effects of age on the elimination of labetalol. *Clin Pharmacokinet* 1989; **17:** 452–7.


**Pregnancy.** The concentration of labetalol has been found to be lower in amniotic fluid[1] and fetal plasma[2] than in maternal plasma. A ratio of infant to maternal drug concentration of 0.2 to 0.8 has been reported[2] based on concentration in infant cord blood at delivery [time since last maternal dose not stated]. In another study,[3] however, higher concentrations were found in cord plasma than in maternal plasma at delivery when infants were delivered 12 to 24 hours after the last maternal dose.

The half-life of labetalol was reported as 24 hours in a neonate of 37 weeks' gestation whose mother had received labetalol 600 mg daily for 11 weeks prior to delivery.[4]


1. Lunell NO, *et al.* Transfer of labetalol into amniotic fluid and breast milk in lactating women. *Eur J Clin Pharmacol* 1985; **28:** 597–9.
2. Michael CA. Use of labetalol in the treatment of severe hypertension during pregnancy. *Br J Clin Pharmacol* 1979; **8** (suppl 2): 211S–215S.
3. Boulton DW, *et al.* Transplacental distribution of labetalol stereoisomers at delivery. *Br J Clin Pharmacol* 1999; **47:** 573–4.
4. Haraldsson A, Geven W. Half-life of maternal labetalol in a premature infant. *Pharm Weekbl (Sci)* 1989; **11:** 229–31.


## Uses and Administration

Labetalol is a non-cardioselective beta blocker (p.868). It is reported to possess some intrinsic sympathomimetic and membrane-stabilising activity. In addition, it has selective $alpha_1$-blocking properties which decrease peripheral vascular resistance. The ratio of alpha- to beta-blocking activity has been estimated to be about 1:3 following oral administration and 1:7 following intravenous administration.

Labetalol is used as the hydrochloride in the management of hypertension (p.825). It is also used to induce hypotension during surgery. Labetalol decreases blood pressure more rapidly than other beta blockers; the full antihypertensive effect may be seen within 1 to 3 hours of an oral dose.

In **hypertension** labetalol hydrochloride is usually given in an initial dose of 100 mg twice daily by mouth with food, gradually increased if necessary according to response and standing blood pressure, to 200 to 400 mg twice daily; total daily doses of 2.4 g, in two to four divided doses, have occasionally been required. An initial dose of 50 mg twice daily has been recommended for elderly patients.

For the emergency treatment of hypertension labetalol hydrochloride may be given by slow intravenous injection. In the UK a dose of 50 mg is recommended, given over a period of at least 1 minute; if necessary this dose may be repeated at intervals of 5 minutes until a total of 200 mg has been given. In the USA an initial dose of 20 mg is recommended, given over 2 minutes; subsequent doses of 40 to 80 mg may be given every 10 minutes, if necessary, up to a maximum of 300 mg. Blood pressure should be monitored, and the patient should remain supine during intravenous administration and for 3 hours afterwards, to avoid excessive orthostatic hypotension. Following bolus intravenous injection a maximum effect is usually obtained within 5 minutes and usually lasts up to 6 hours, although it may extend as long as 18 hours.

Labetalol hydrochloride has also been given by intravenous infusion in usual doses of 2 mg/minute. Suggested concentrations for intravenous infusions are 1 mg/mL or 2 mg/3 mL of suitable diluent. In hypertension in pregnancy, labetalol infusion may be started at the rate of 20 mg/hour, then doubled every 30 minutes until a satisfactory response is obtained or a dose of 160 mg/hour is reached. In hypertension following myocardial infarction, labetalol infusion may be started at the rate of 15 mg/hour and gradually increased until a satisfactory response is obtained or a dose of 120 mg/hour is reached.

The initial dose in **hypotensive anaesthesia** is 10 to 20 mg intravenously, with increments of 5 to 10 mg if satisfactory hypotension is not achieved after 5 minutes. A higher initial dose may be required in patients who do not receive halothane anaesthesia.

**Action.** Labetalol has 2 optical centres; it is used as the racemic mixture of the 4 stereoisomers. The *R,R*- isomer is responsible for the beta-blocking activity and has limited alpha-blocking activity; it also has beta-adrenergic mediated peripheral vasodilating activity. The *S,R*-isomer has the most potent alpha-blocking activity. The *S,S*-isomer has some alpha-blocking activity and the *R,S*-isomer does not appear to have either alpha- or beta-adrenergic blocking effect.[1] The *R,R*-isomer, dilevalol, was withdrawn from the market because of hepatotoxicity.


1. Gold EH, *et al.* Synthesis and comparison of some cardiovascular properties of the stereoisomers of labetalol. *J Med Chem* 1982; **25:** 1363–70.


## Preparations

***BP 2003:*** Labetalol Injection; Labetalol Tablets;
***USP 27:*** Labetalol Hydrochloride Injection; Labetalol Hydrochloride Tablets.

**Proprietary Preparations** (details are given in Part 3)

***Austral.:*** Presolol; Trandate; ***Austria:*** Trandate; ***Belg.:*** Trandate; ***Canad.:*** Trandate; ***Chile:*** Trandate; ***Denm.:*** Trandate; ***Fin.:*** Albetol; ***Fr.:*** Trandate; ***Hong Kong:*** Trandate; ***Irl.:*** Trandate; ***Israel:*** Trandate; ***Ital.:*** Abetol†; Alfabetal†; Amipress†; Ipolab; Pressalolo†; Trandate; ***Malaysia:*** Tolbetol; Trandate; ***Neth.:*** Trandate; ***Norw.:*** Trandate; ***NZ:*** Hybloc; Trandate; ***Port.:*** Trandate; ***S.Afr.:*** Trandate; ***Singapore:*** Trandate†; ***Spain:*** Trandate; ***Swed.:*** Trandate; ***Switz.:*** Trandate; ***UK:*** Labrocol†; Trandate; ***USA:*** Normodyne; Trandate.

**Multi-ingredient:** ***Ital.:*** Biotens†; Pressalolo Diuretico†; Trandiur.

---

## Lacidipine *(BAN, USAN, rINN)*

GR-43659X; GX-1048; Lacidipino. Diethyl 4-{2-[(*tert*-butoxycarbonyl)vinyl]phenyl}-1,4-dihydro-2,6-dimethylpyridine-3,5-dicarboxylate.

$C_{26}H_{33}NO_6$ = 455.5.

*CAS — 103890-78-4.*

*ATC — C08CA09.*

**Pharmacopoeias.** In *Br.*

**BP 2003** (Lacidipine). A white to pale yellow crystalline powder. Practically insoluble in water; sparingly soluble in dehydrated alcohol; freely soluble in acetone and in dichloromethane.

## Adverse Effects, Treatment, and Precautions

As for dihydropyridine calcium-channel blockers (see Nifedipine, p.966).

## Interactions

As for dihydropyridine calcium-channel blockers (see Nifedipine, p.969).

## Pharmacokinetics

Lacidipine is rapidly but poorly absorbed from the gastrointestinal tract following oral administration and undergoes extensive first-pass metabolism; the bioavailability has been reported to be 2 to 9%, or 18.5% (range 4 to 52%) using a more sensitive assay method. It is more than 95% bound to plasma proteins. Lacidipine is eliminated by metabolism in the liver and metabolites are excreted mainly by the biliary route. About 70% of an oral dose is eliminated in the faeces, the remainder in the urine. The average steady-state terminal elimination half-life of lacidipine is 13 to 19 hours.

## Uses and Administration

Lacidipine is a dihydropyridine calcium-channel blocker with actions similar to those of nifedipine (p.970). It is used in the treatment of hypertension (p.825).

The usual initial dose of lacidipine is 2 mg once daily by mouth increased if necessary after 3 to 4 weeks or more to 4 mg daily; a further increase in dose to 6 mg daily may be necessary in some patients.

◊ Reviews.


1. Lee CR, Bryson HM. Lacidipine: a review of its pharmacodynamic and pharmacokinetic properties and therapeutic potential in the treatment of hypertension. *Drugs* 1994; **48:** 274–96.
2. Zanchetti A, ed. Cardiovascular advantages of a third generation calcium antagonist: symposium on lacidipine. *Drugs* 1999; **57** (suppl 1): 1–29.
3. McCormack PL, Wagstaff AJ. Lacidipine: a review of its use in the management of hypertension. *Drugs* 2003; **63:** 2327–56.


## Preparations

***BP 2003:*** Lacidipine Tablets.

**Proprietary Preparations** (details are given in Part 3)

***Arg.:*** Lacipil; Midotens; ***Belg.:*** Motens; ***Braz.:*** Lacipil; Midotens; ***Denm.:*** Midotens; ***Fr.:*** Caldine; ***Ger.:*** Motens; ***Gr.:*** Lacipil; Motens; ***Hong Kong:*** Lacipil; ***India:*** Sinopil; ***Ital.:*** Aponil; Lacipil; Lacirex; Ladip; Viapres; ***Malaysia:*** Lacipil; ***Mex.:*** Lacipil; Midotens; ***Neth.:*** Motens; ***Port.:*** Lacipil; Tens; ***Singapore:*** Lacipil; ***Spain:*** Lacimen; Lacipil; Motens; ***Swed.:*** Midotens†; ***Switz.:*** Motens; ***Thai.:*** Motens; ***UK:*** Motens.

---

## Lamifiban *(USAN, rINN)*

Lamifibán; Ro-44-9883; Ro-44-9883/000. ({1-[*N*-(*p*-Amidinobenzoyl)-L-tyrosyl]-4-piperidyl}oxy)acetic acid.

$C_{24}H_{28}N_4O_6$ = 468.5.

*CAS — 144412-49-7 (lamifiban); 243835-65-6 (lamifiban hydrochloride).*

## Profile

Lamifiban is a glycoprotein IIb/IIIa-receptor antagonist. It is under investigation as an antiplatelet drug given intravenously for the management of thromboembolic disorders, such as unstable angina and myocardial infarction.

◊ References.


1. Théroux P, *et al.* Platelet membrane receptor glycoprotein IIb/IIIa antagonism in unstable angina: the Canadian Lamifiban Study. *Circulation* 1996; **94:** 899–905.
2. The PARAGON Investigators. International, randomized, controlled trial of lamifiban (a platelet glycoprotein IIb/IIIa inhibitor), heparin, or both in unstable angina. *Circulation* 1998; **97:** 2386–95.
3. The PARADIGM Investigators. Combining thrombolysis with the platelet glycoprotein IIb/IIIa inhibitor lamifiban: results of the Platelet Aggregation Receptor Antagonist Dose Investigation and Reperfusion Gain in Myocardial Infarction (PARADIGM) trial. *J Am Coll Cardiol* 1998; **32:** 2003–10.
4. Global Organization Network (PARAGON)-B Investigators. Randomized, placebo-controlled trial of titrated intravenous lamifiban for acute coronary syndromes. *Circulation* 2002; **105:** 316–21.

### Lanatoside C (BAN, rINN)

Celanide; Celanidum; Lanatósido C; Lanatosidum C. 3-[(O-β-D-Glucopyranosyl-(1→4)-O-3-acetyl-2,6-dideoxy-β-D-ribo-hexopyranosyl-(1→4)-O-2,6-dideoxy-β-D-ribo-hexopyranosyl-(1→4)-O-2,6-dideoxy-β-D-ribo-hexopyranosyl)oxy]-12,14-dihydroxy-3β,5β,12β-card-20(22)-enolide.

$C_{49}H_{76}O_{20}$ = 985.1.

*CAS — 17575-22-3.*

*ATC — C01AA06.*

**Pharmacopoeias.** In *Jpn* and *Pol.*

#### Profile

Lanatoside C is a cardiac glycoside with positive inotropic activity. It is obtained from digitalis lanata leaf (p.894). It has general properties similar to those of digoxin (p.895) and has been used in the treatment of some cardiac arrhythmias and in heart failure.

Mixtures of lanatosides A, B, and C have also been used.

#### Preparations

**Proprietary Preparations** (details are given in Part 3)
***Arg.:*** Develanid; ***Austria:*** Cedilanid†.

### Landiolol Hydrochloride (rINNM)

ONO-1101. (−)-[(S)-2,2-Dimethyl-1,3-dioxolan-4-yl]methyl p-((S)-2-hydroxy-3-{[2-(4-morpholinecarboxamido)ethyl]amino}propoxy)hydrocinnamate hydrochloride.

$C_{25}H_{39}N_3O_8$,HCl = 546.1.

*CAS — 133242-30-5 (landiolol); 144481-98-1 (landiolol hydrochloride).*

#### Profile

Landiolol is a short-acting beta blocker given intravenously as the hydrochloride in the management of intra-operative cardiac arrhythmias.

◊ References.


1. Kitamura A, *et al.* Efficacy of an ultrashort-acting beta-adrenoceptor blocker (ONO-1101) in attenuating cardiovascular responses to endotracheal intubation. *Eur J Clin Pharmacol* 1997; **51:** 467–71.
2. Atarashi H, *et al.* Pharmacokinetics of landiolol hydrochloride, a new ultra-short-acting beta-blocker, in patients with cardiac arrhythmias. *Clin Pharmacol Ther* 2000; **68:** 143–50.


#### Preparations

**Proprietary Preparations** (details are given in Part 3)
***Jpn:*** Onoact.

### Lanoteplase (USAN, rINN)

BMS-200980; Lanoteplasa; Sun-9216. N-[$N^2$-(N-Glycyl-L-alanyl)-L-arginyl]-117-L-glutamine-245-L-methionine-(1-5)-(87-527)-plasminogen activator (human tissue-type protein moiety).

$C_{2184}H_{3323}N_{633}O_{666}S_{29}$ = 50032.5.

*CAS — 171870-23-8.*

#### Profile

Lanoteplase is a thrombolytic that has been investigated in acute myocardial infarction; development was stopped after an unacceptable rate of intracranial haemorrhage was found.

◊ References.


1. The InTIME-II Investigators. Intravenous NPA for the treatment of infarcting myocardium early: InTIME-II, a double-blind comparison of single-bolus lanoteplase vs accelerated alteplase for the treatment of patients with acute myocardial infarction. *Eur Heart J* 2000; **21:** 2005–13.


### Lappaconitine Hydrobromide

Allapinin. (1α,14α,16β)-20-Ethyl-1,14,16-trimethoxyaconitane-4,8,9-triol 4-[2-(acetylamino)benzoate] hydrobromide.

$C_{32}H_{44}N_2O_8$,HBr = 665.6.

*CAS — 97792-45-5.*

#### Profile

Lappaconitine hydrobromide is an antiarrhythmic drug.

### Leech

Blutegel; Hirudo; Sangsue; Sanguessugas; Sanguijuela; Sanguisuga.

**Description.** *Hirudo medicinalis* is the leech commonly used in medicine and is a fresh-water annelid.

NOTE. The substance described in the *Chin. P.* as Hirudo (Leech) is the dried body of *Whitmania pigra, Hirudo nipponica*, or *Whitmania acranulata.*

#### Profile

Leeches are used for withdrawing blood from congested areas and have been found to be of value in plastic surgery. The buccal secretion of the leech contains the anticoagulant hirudin (p.931). The part to be bitten may be moistened with sugar solution before applying the leech. Once used a leech should not be applied to another patient.

There have been reports of wound infection from *Aeromonas hydrophila* transmitted by leeches. Prolonged bleeding may occur from the site of attachment after removal of the leech.

◊ References.


1. Braidwood PS. The medicinal leech. *Pharm J* 1987; **239:** 766–7.
2. Abrutyn E. Hospital-associated infection from leeches. *Ann Intern Med* 1988; **109:** 356–8.
3. Adams SL. The medicinal leech; a page from the annelids of internal medicine. *Ann Intern Med* 1988; **109:** 399–405.
4. Menage MJ, Wright G. Use of leeches in a case of severe periorbital haematoma. *Br J Ophthalmol* 1991; **75:** 755–6.
5. Utley DS, *et al.* The failing flap in facial plastic and reconstructive surgery: role of the medicinal leech. *Laryngoscope* 1998; **108:** 1129–35.
6. Michalsen A, *et al.* Effect of leeches therapy (Hirudo medicinalis) in painful osteoarthritis of the knee: a pilot study. *Ann Rheum Dis* 2001; **60:** 986.


**Precautions.** Wound infection by *Aeromonas hydrophila*, an organism normally found in the gut of the leech, is a recognised complication of the use of leeches for decongestion after plastic surgery.[1] A 5-year retrospective study[2] in a French hospital found that *A. hydrophila* infections occurred more commonly in a unit where the leeches were kept in the tank which was filled with tap water and not disinfected regularly. Infections have caused minor wound drainage, cellulitis, abscess, tissue loss, and sepsis, and a case of meningitis secondary to *Aeromonas* infection has been reported.[3] Cephalosporins such as cefotaxime have been used for prophylaxis and treatment.

Other organisms have also caused cellulitis during treatment with leeches. *Aeromonas sobria* infection in a patient was treated with ceftazidime and ciprofloxacin.[4] *Serratia marcescens* infection in another patient was treated with ciprofloxacin.[5]


1. Lineaweaver WC, *et al.* Aeromonas hydrophila infections following use of medicinal leeches in replantation and flap surgery. *Ann Plast Surg* 1992; **29:** 238–44.
2. Sartor C, *et al.* Nosocomial infections with Aeromonas hydrophila from leeches. Abstract: *Clin Infect Dis* 2002; **35:** 111. Full version: http://www.journals.uchicago.edu/CID/journal/issues/v35n1/011371/011371.web.pdf (accessed 06/07/04)
3. Ouderkirk JP, *et al.* Aeromonas meningitis complicating medicinal leech therapy. Abstract: *Clin Infect Dis* 2004; **38:** 603. Full version: http://www.journals.uchicago.edu/CID/journal/issues/v38n4/32181/32181.web.pdf (accessed 06/07/04)
4. Fenollar F, *et al.* Unusual case of Aeromonas sobria cellulitis associated with the use of leeches. *Eur J Clin Microbiol Infect Dis* 1999; **18:** 72–3.
5. Pereira JA, *et al.* Leech-borne Serratia marcescens infection following complex hand injury. *Br J Plast Surg* 1998; **51:** 640–1.


## Lepirudin (BAN, rINN)

HBW-023; Lepirudina. 1-L-Leucine-2-L-threonine-63-desulfohirudin (*Hirudo medicinalis* isoform HV1).

$C_{287}H_{440}N_{80}O_{111}S_6$ = 6979.4.

*CAS — 138068-37-8.*

*ATC — B01AE02.*

### Adverse Effects and Precautions

The most frequent adverse effect of lepirudin is bleeding. Hypersensitivity reactions and fever have been reported. There have been reports of severe anaphylactic reactions, including death, with most occurring on re-exposure to lepirudin. There may be cross-reactivity with other hirudins or hirudin analogues.

Lepirudin should be used with caution in patients who are bleeding or at serious risk of bleeding including those with haemorrhagic blood disorders, recent major bleeding, cerebrovascular disorders, bacterial endocarditis, severe hypertension, or patients who have recently undergone major surgery or puncture of large vessels or organ biopsy.

### Interactions

Use of lepirudin with thrombolytics, oral anticoagulants, or drugs that affect platelet function may increase the risk of bleeding.

### Pharmacokinetics

Lepirudin is metabolised and excreted by the kidney. After intravenous administration about 45% of a dose is detected in the urine and about 35% is excreted unchanged. The terminal elimination half-life of lepirudin is about 1.3 hours. In patients with severe renal impairment the half-life may be prolonged to about 2 days.

**Breast feeding.** The concentration of hirudin was measured in the breast milk of a woman who was treated with lepirudin 50 mg subcutaneously twice daily for deep-vein thrombosis and heparin-induced thrombocytopenia.[1] Three hours after injection plasma concentrations of hirudin in the woman were 0.5 to 1 microgram/mL but no hirudin was detected in the breast milk.


1. Lindhoff-Last E, *et al.* Hirudin treatment in a breastfeeding woman. *Lancet* 2000; **355:** 467–8.


### Uses and Administration

Lepirudin is a recombinant hirudin (p.931) that is a direct inhibitor of thrombin. It is used as an anticoagulant in the management of thromboembolic disorders (p.837) in patients with heparin-induced thrombocytopenia. It is being investigated in arterial thromboembolic disorders such as myocardial infarction and unstable angina.

In the management of thromboembolism in patients with heparin-induced thrombocytopenia lepirudin is given in an initial dose of 400 micrograms/kg by slow intravenous injection. This is followed by a maintenance dose of 150 micrograms/kg per hour by continuous intravenous infusion, adjusted according to response, usually for 2 to 10 days. Doses must not exceed those based on a patient weight of 110 kg.

Doses of lepirudin should be reduced in patients with renal impairment and infusions should be avoided in those on haemodialysis (see below).

◊ Studies[1] have shown lepirudin to be effective for the management of venous thromboembolism in patients with heparin-induced thrombocytopenia. Recombinant hirudins are also under investigation as alternatives to heparin in the early management of myocardial infarction (p.828). Initial studies comparing heparin with the recombinant hirudins desirudin[2,3] (p.892) or lepirudin[4] had to be stopped because of higher than expected haemorrhagic stroke rates,[5,6] and subsequent studies using lower doses of desirudin[7,8] or lepirudin[9] failed to show a clear benefit over heparin. The role of hirudins therefore remains to be confirmed.

Desirudin has been investigated in unstable angina[10] (p.813) and studies in patients with acute ischaemic syndromes suggest that lepirudin is superior to heparin in preventing cardiovascular death, myocardial infarction, and refractory angina.[11,12] Desirudin has also been studied in patients undergoing percutaneous transluminal angioplasty[13] (p.834).


1. Greinacher A, *et al.* Recombinant hirudin (lepirudin) provides safe and effective anticoagulation in patients with heparin-induced thrombocytopenia: a prospective study. *Circulation* 1999; **99:** 73–80.
2. The Global Use of Strategies to Open Occluded Coronary Arteries (GUSTO) IIa Investigators. Randomized trial of intravenous heparin versus recombinant hirudin for acute coronary syndromes. *Circulation* 1994; **90:** 1631–7.
3. Antman EM, *et al.* Hirudin in acute myocardial infarction: safety report from the Thrombolysis and Thrombin Inhibition in Myocardial Infarction (TIMI) 9A trial. *Circulation* 1994; **90:** 1624–30.
4. Neuhaus K-L, *et al.* Safety observations from the pilot phase of the randomized r-Hirudin for Improvement of Thrombolysis (HIT-III) study: a study of the Arbeitsgemeinschaft Leitender Kardiologischer Krankenhausärzte (ALKK). *Circulation* 1994; **90:** 1638–42.
5. Zeymer U, Neuhaus K-L. Hirudin and excess bleeding: implications for future use. *Drug Safety* 1995; **12:** 234–9.
6. Conrad KA. Clinical pharmacology and drug safety: lessons from hirudin. *Clin Pharmacol Ther* 1995; **58:** 123–6.
7. The Global Use of Strategies to Open Occluded Coronary Arteries (GUSTO) IIb Investigators. A comparison of recombinant hirudin with heparin for the treatment of acute coronary syndromes. *N Engl J Med* 1996; **335:** 775–82.
8. Antman EM. Hirudin in acute myocardial infarction: thrombolysis and thrombin inhibition in myocardial infarction (TIMI) 9B trial. *Circulation* 1996; **94:** 911–21.
9. Neuhaus K-L, *et al.* Recombinant hirudin (lepirudin) for the improvement of thrombolysis with streptokinase in patients with acute myocardial infarction: results of the HIT-4 trial. *J Am Coll Cardiol* 1999; **34:** 966–73.
10. Topol EJ, *et al.* Recombinant hirudin for unstable angina pectoris: a multicenter, randomized angiographic trial. *Circulation* 1994; **89:** 1557–66.
11. Organization to Assess Strategies for Ischemic Syndromes (OASIS) Investigators. Comparison of the effects of two doses of recombinant hirudin compared with heparin in patients with acute myocardial ischemia without ST elevation: a pilot study. *Circulation* 1997; **96:** 769–77.
12. Organisation to Assess Strategies for Ischemic Syndromes (OASIS-2) Investigators. Effects of recombinant hirudin (lepirudin) compared with heparin on death, myocardial infarction, refractory angina, and revascularisation procedures in patients with acute myocardial ischaemia without ST elevation: a randomised trial. *Lancet* 1999; **353:** 429–38.
13. Serruys PW, *et al.* A comparison of hirudin with heparin in the prevention of restenosis after coronary angioplasty. *N Engl J Med* 1995; **333:** 757–63.


**Administration in renal impairment.** Doses of lepirudin should be reduced in patients with renal impairment. The initial dose is reduced to 200 micrograms/kg, and the maintenance infusion rate is reduced according to creatinine clearance (CC):

- CC 45 to 60 mL/minute: infusion rate 50% of normal rate
- CC 30 to 44 mL/minute: 30% of normal rate
- CC 15 to 29 mL/minute: 15% of normal rate
- CC below 15 mL/minute: infusion of lepirudin should be avoided, although further intravenous bolus doses of 100 micrograms/kg may be used on alternate days, according to response

### Preparations

**Proprietary Preparations** (details are given in Part 3)
***Austral.:*** Refludan†; ***Austria:*** Refludan; ***Belg.:*** Refludan†; ***Braz.:*** Refludan†; ***Canad.:*** Refludan; ***Denm.:*** Refludan; ***Fin.:*** Refludan; ***Fr.:*** Refludan; ***Ger.:*** Refludan; ***Gr.:*** Refludan; ***Irl.:*** Refludan; ***Ital.:*** Refludan; ***Neth.:*** Reflu-

dan; **Norw.:** Refludan; **Port.:** Refludan†; **S.Afr.:** Refludin†; **Spain:** Refludin; **Swed.:** Refludan; **Switz.:** Refludan; **UK:** Refludan; **USA:** Refludan.

## Lercanidipine Hydrochloride

*(BANM, USAN, rINNM)*

Hidrocloruro de lercanidipino; Masnidipine Hydrochloride; R-75; Rec-15-2375. (±)-2-[(3,3-Diphenylpropyl)methylamino]-1,1-dimethylethyl methyl 1,4-dihydro-2,6-dimethyl-4-(*m*-nitrophenyl)-3,5-pyridinedicarboxylate hydrochloride.

$C_{36}H_{41}N_3O_6,HCl = 648.2.$

*CAS — 100427-26-7 (lercanidipine); 132866-11-6 (lercanidipine hydrochloride).*

*ATC — C08CA13.*

### Adverse Effects, Treatment, and Precautions

As for dihydropyridine calcium-channel blockers (see Nifedipine, p.966).

### Interactions

As for dihydropyridine calcium-channel blockers (see Nifedipine, p.969).

### Pharmacokinetics

Lercanidipine is completely absorbed from the gastrointestinal tract following oral administration but undergoes extensive saturable first-pass metabolism. Bioavailability is low but is increased in the presence of food. Peak plasma concentrations occur about 1.5 to 3 hours after oral administration. Lercanidipine is rapidly and widely distributed. It is more than 98% bound to plasma proteins. Lercanidipine is extensively metabolised, primarily by the cytochrome P450 isoenzyme CYP3A4, mainly to inactive metabolites; about 50% of an oral dose is excreted in the urine. A terminal elimination half-life of about 2 to 5 hours has been reported, but studies using a more sensitive assay have suggested a value of 8 to 10 hours.

### Uses and Administration

Lercanidipine is a dihydropyridine calcium-channel blocker with actions similar to those of nifedipine (p.970). It is used in the treatment of hypertension (p.825).

Lercanidipine is given by mouth as the hydrochloride in a usual initial dose of 10 mg once daily before food, increased if necessary, after at least 2 weeks, to 20 mg daily.

◊ Reviews.


1. McClellan KJ, Jarvis B. Lercanidipine: a review of its use in hypertension. *Drugs* 2000; **60:** 1123–40.
2. Bang LM, *et al.* Lercanidipine : a review of its efficacy in the management of hypertension. *Drugs* 2003; **63:** 2449–72.


### Preparations

**Proprietary Preparations** (details are given in Part 3)
**Arg.:** Lercadip; **Austral.:** Zanidip; **Austria:** Zanidip; **Belg.:** Zanidip; **Braz.:** Zanidip; **Chile:** Zanidip; **Denm.:** Zanidip; **Fin.:** Zanidip; **Fr.:** Lercan; Zanidip; **Ger.:** Carmen; Corifeo; **Gr.:** Zanidip; **Hong Kong:** Zanidip; **Israel:** Vasodip; **Ital.:** Cardiovasc; Lercadip; Zanedip; **Neth.:** Lerdip; **Norw.:** Zanidip; **Port.:** Zanicor; **Singapore:** Zanidip; **Spain:** Lercadip; Lerzam; Zanidip; **Swed.:** Zanidip; **UK:** Zanidip.

## Levobetaxolol Hydrochloride

*(USAN, rINNM)*

AL-1577A (levobetaxolol or levobetaxolol hydrochloride); Hidrocloruro de levobetaxolol. (−)-(*S*)-1-{*p*-[2-(Cyclopropylmethoxy)ethyl]phenoxy}-3-isopropylaminopropan-2-ol hydrochloride.

$C_{18}H_{29}NO_3,HCl = 343.9.$

*CAS — 93221-48-8 (levobetaxolol); 116209-55-3 (levobetaxolol hydrochloride).*

### Adverse Effects, Treatment, and Precautions

As for Beta Blockers, p.869.

### Interactions

The interactions associated with beta blockers are discussed on p.870.

### Uses and Administration

Levobetaxolol, the *S*-isomer of betaxolol (p.873) is a cardioselective beta blocker (p.868). It is reported to lack intrinsic sympathomimetic activity and to have no significant membrane-stabilising properties.

Levobetaxolol is used as the hydrochloride to reduce raised intra-ocular pressure in open-angle glaucoma and ocular hypertension (p.1485). It is used topically as a suspension containing the equivalent of 0.5% levobetaxolol instilled twice daily.

### Preparations

**Proprietary Preparations** (details are given in Part 3)
**USA:** Betaxon.

## Levobunolol Hydrochloride

*(BANM, USAN, rINNM)*

(−)-Bunolol Hydrochloride; *l*-Bunolol Hydrochloride; Hidrocloruro de levobunolol; W-7000A. (−)-5-(3-*tert*-Butylamino-2-hydroxypropoxy)-1,2,3,4-tetrahydronaphthalen-1-one hydrochloride.

$C_{17}H_{25}NO_3,HCl = 327.8.$

*CAS — 47141-42-4 (levobunolol); 27912-14-7 (levobunolol hydrochloride).*

*ATC — S01ED03.*

**Pharmacopoeias.** In *Br.* and *US.*

**BP 2003** (Levobunolol Hydrochloride). A white or pinkish-white crystalline powder. Freely soluble in water; sparingly soluble in alcohol. A 5% solution in water has a pH of between 4.5 and 6.5. Protect from light.

**USP 27** (Levobunolol Hydrochloride). A white odourless crystalline powder. Soluble in water and in methyl alcohol; slightly soluble in alcohol and in chloroform. A 5% solution in water has a pH between 4.5 and 6.5.

### Adverse Effects, Treatment, and Precautions

As for Beta Blockers, p.869.

### Interactions

The interactions associated with beta blockers are discussed on p.870.

### Pharmacokinetics

Some systemic absorption is reported to occur following topical application to the eye. Following oral administration levobunolol is rapidly and almost completely absorbed from the gastrointestinal tract. It is extensively metabolised in the liver; the principal metabolite, dihydrolevobunolol, is reported to possess beta-blocking activity. The metabolites and some unchanged drug are excreted in the urine.

### Uses and Administration

Levobunolol is a non-cardioselective beta blocker (p.868). It is reported to lack intrinsic sympathomimetic activity and membrane-stabilising properties.

Levobunolol is used as the hydrochloride to reduce raised intra-ocular pressure in open-angle glaucoma and ocular hypertension (p.1485). It is usually used as a 0.5% ophthalmic solution instilled once or twice daily; alternatively a 0.25% solution may be instilled twice daily.

### Preparations

**BP 2003:** Levobunolol Eye Drops;
**USP 27:** Levobunolol Hydrochloride Ophthalmic Solution.

**Proprietary Preparations** (details are given in Part 3)
**Arg.:** Betagan; Levunolol; **Austral.:** Betagan; **Austria:** Vistagan; **Belg.:** Betagan; **Braz.:** Betagan; **Canad.:** Betagan; Ophtho-Bunolol; **Chile:** Betagen; **Denm.:** Betagan; **Fr.:** Betagan; **Ger.:** Vistagan; **Gr.:** Vistagan; **Hong Kong:** Betagan; **Irl.:** Betagan; **Israel:** Betagan; **Ital.:** Vistagan; **Malaysia:** Betagan; **Mex.:** Betagan; **NZ:** Betagan; **Port.:** Betagan; **S.Afr.:** Betagan; **Singapore:** Betagan; **Spain:** Betagan; **Swed.:** Betagan†; **Switz.:** Vistagan; **Thai.:** Betagan; **UK:** Betagan; **USA:** Ak-Beta; Betagan.

**Multi-ingredient: Canad.:** Probeta.

## Levosimendan *(USAN, rINN)*

Levosimendán; (−)-OR-1259. Mesoxalonitrile (−)-{*p*-[(*R*)-1,4,5,6-tetrahydro-4-methyl-6-oxo-3-pyridazinyl]phenyl}hydrazone.

$C_{14}H_{12}N_6O = 280.3.$

*CAS — 141505-33-1.*

*ATC — C01CX08.*

### Profile

Levosimendan is a cardiac inotrope and vasodilator with calcium-sensitising properties, used in the management of acute heart failure (p.820). It is given intravenously in a loading dose of 12 to 24 micrograms/kg over 10 minutes followed by a continuous infusion of 0.05 to 0.2 micrograms/kg per minute, adjusted according to response.

◊ References.


1. Figgitt DP, *et al.* Levosimendan. *Drugs* 2001; **61:** 613–27.
2. Follath F, *et al.* Efficacy and safety of intravenous levosimendan compared with dobutamine in severe low-output heart failure (the LIDO study): a randomised double-blind trial. *Lancet* 2002; **360:** 196–202.
3. McBride BF, White CM. Levosimendan: implications for clinicians. *J Clin Pharmacol* 2003; **43:** 1071–81.
4. Innes CA, Wagstaff AJ. Levosimendan: a review of its use in the management of acute decompensated heart failure. *Drugs* 2003; **63:** 2651–71.


### Preparations

**Proprietary Preparations** (details are given in Part 3)
**Fin.:** Simdax; **Norw.:** Simdax; **Spain:** Simdax; **Swed.:** Simdax.

## Lidoflazine *(BAN, USAN, rINN)*

Lidoflazina; McN-JR-7904; Ordiflazine; R-7904. 4-[3-(4,4′-Difluorobenzhydryl)propyl]piperazin-1-ylaceto-2′,6′-xylidide.

$C_{30}H_{35}F_2N_3O = 491.6.$

*CAS — 3416-26-0.*

### Profile

Lidoflazine is a calcium-channel blocker (p.810) that reduces atrioventricular conduction. It has been used in angina pectoris.

### Preparations

**Proprietary Preparations** (details are given in Part 3)
**India:** Clinium.

## Lifibrol *(USAN, rINN)*

K-12148. (±)-*p*-[4-(*p-tert*-Butylphenyl)-2-hydroxybutoxy]benzoic acid.

$C_{21}H_{26}O_4 = 342.4.$

*CAS — 96609-16-4.*

### Profile

Lifibrol is under investigation as a lipid regulating drug for the treatment of hypercholesterolaemia.

◊ References.


1. Schwandt P, *et al.* Safety and efficacy of lifibrol upon four-week administration to patients with primary hypercholesterolaemia. *Eur J Clin Pharmacol* 1994; **47:** 133–8.
2. Locker PK, *et al.* Lifibrol: a novel lipid-lowering drug for the therapy of hypercholesterolemia. *Clin Pharmacol Ther* 1995; **57:** 73–88.


## Linsidomine Hydrochloride *(rINNM)*

Hidrocloruro de linsidomina. 3-Morpholinosydnonimine hydrochloride.

$C_6H_{10}N_4O_2,HCl = 206.6.$

*CAS — 33876-97-0 (linsidomine); 16142-27-1 (linsidomine hydrochloride).*

*ATC — C01DX18.*

### Profile

Linsidomine is a nitrovasodilator and a metabolite of molsidomine (p.961). It is given as the hydrochloride via the intracoronary route in doses of 0.6 to 1 mg in the management of coronary artery spasm and to facilitate vasodilatation during coronary angiography. Additional doses may be required; the maximum total dose is 2 mg. It is also given by intravenous infusion in the management of unstable angina (p.813), in an initial dose of 1 mg/hour, adjusted according to response.

◊ References.


1. Delonca J, *et al.* Comparative efficacy of the intravenous administration of linsidomine, a direct nitric oxide donor, and isosorbide dinitrate in severe unstable angina: a French multicentre study. *Eur Heart J* 1997; **18:** 1300–6.


### Preparations

**Proprietary Preparations** (details are given in Part 3)
**Fr.:** Corvasal.

## Lisinopril *(BAN, USAN, rINN)*

L-154826; Lisinoprilum; MK-521. *N*-{*N*-[(*S*)-1-Carboxy-3-phenylpropyl]-L-lysyl}-L-proline dihydrate.

$C_{21}H_{31}N_3O_5,2H_2O = 441.5.$

*CAS — 76547-98-3 (anhydrous lisinopril); 83915-83-7 (lisinopril dihydrate).*

*ATC — C09AA03.*

**Pharmacopoeias.** In *Eur.* (see p.vi) and *US.*

**Ph. Eur. 5.0** (Lisinopril Dihydrate). A white or almost white crystalline powder. Soluble in water; practically insoluble in dehydrated alcohol and in acetone; sparingly soluble in methyl alcohol.

**USP 27** (Lisinopril). A white crystalline powder. Soluble 1 in 10 of water and 1 in 70 of methyl alcohol; practically insoluble in alcohol, in acetone, in acetonitrile, in chloroform, and in ether.

### Adverse Effects, Treatment, and Precautions

As for ACE inhibitors, p.842.

**Porphyria.** Lisinopril has been associated with acute attacks of porphyria and is considered unsafe in porphyric patients.

### Interactions

As for ACE inhibitors, p.845.

### Pharmacokinetics

Lisinopril is slowly and incompletely absorbed following oral administration. About 25% of a given dose is absorbed on average, but the absorption varies considerably between individuals, ranging from about 6 to 60%. It is already an active diacid and does not need to be metabolised *in vivo*. Peak concentrations in plasma are reported to occur after about 7 hours. Lisinopril is reported not to be significantly bound to plasma proteins. It is excreted unchanged in the urine. The effective half-life for accumulation following multiple doses is 12 hours in patients with normal renal function. Lisinopril is removed by haemodialysis.

◊ References.

1. Till AE, *et al.* The pharmacokinetics of lisinopril in hospitalized patients with congestive heart failure. *Br J Clin Pharmacol* 1989; **27:** 199–204.
2. Neubeck M, *et al.* Pharmacokinetics and pharmacodynamics of lisinopril in advanced renal failure: consequence of dose adjustment. *Eur J Clin Pharmacol* 1994; **46:** 537–43.

### Uses and Administration

Lisinopril is an ACE inhibitor (p.842). It is used in the treatment of hypertension (p.825) and heart failure (p.820), prophylactically after myocardial infarction (p.828), and in diabetic nephropathy (see Kidney Disorders, p.847).

The haemodynamic effects of lisinopril are seen within 1 to 2 hours of a single oral dose and the maximum effect occurs after about 6 hours, although the full effect may not develop for several weeks during chronic dosing. The haemodynamic action lasts for about 24 hours following once-daily dosing. Lisinopril is given by mouth as the dihydrate, but doses are expressed in terms of the anhydrous substance. Lisinopril 2.72 mg as the dihydrate is approximately equivalent to 2.5 mg of anhydrous lisinopril. The dose of lisinopril should be reduced in patients with renal impairment (see below).

In the treatment of **hypertension**, the usual initial dose is 10 mg daily. Since there may be a precipitous fall in blood pressure in some patients when starting therapy with an ACE inhibitor, the first dose should preferably be given at bedtime. Hypotension is particularly likely in patients with renovascular hypertension, volume depletion, heart failure, or severe hypertension and such patients should be given a lower initial dose of 2.5 to 5 mg once daily. Patients taking diuretics should have the diuretic withdrawn 2 or 3 days before lisinopril is started and resumed later if required; if this is not possible, an initial dose of 5 mg once daily should be given. The usual maintenance dose is 20 mg given once daily, though up to 80 mg daily may be given if necessary.

In the management of **heart failure**, severe first-dose hypotension on introduction of an ACE inhibitor is common in patients on loop diuretics, but their temporary withdrawal may cause rebound pulmonary oedema. Thus treatment should be initiated with a low dose under close medical supervision. Lisinopril is given in an initial dose of 2.5 mg daily. In the USA an initial dose of 5 mg daily is suggested. Usual maintenance doses range from 5 to 40 mg daily.

Following **myocardial infarction**, treatment with lisinopril may be started within 24 hours of the onset of symptoms in an initial dose of 5 mg once daily for two days, then increased to 10 mg once daily. An initial dose of 2.5 mg once daily is recommended for patients with a low systolic blood pressure.

In **diabetic nephropathy**, the initial dose is 2.5 mg once daily. In normotensive type 1 diabetics the maintenance dose is 10 mg daily, increased to 20 mg daily if necessary to achieve a sitting diastolic blood pressure below 75 mmHg. In hypertensive type 2 diabetics, the dose should be adjusted to achieve a sitting diastolic blood pressure below 90 mmHg.

◊ Reviews.

1. Lancaster SG, Todd PA. Lisinopril: a preliminary review of its pharmacodynamic and pharmacokinetic properties, and therapeutic use in hypertension and congestive heart failure. *Drugs* 1988; **35:** 646–69.
2. Goa KL, *et al.* Lisinopril: a review of its pharmacology and clinical efficacy in the early management of acute myocardial infarction. *Drugs* 1996; **52:** 564–88.
3. Goa KL, *et al.* Lisinopril: a review of its pharmacology and use in the management of the complications of diabetes mellitus. *Drugs* 1997; **53:** 1081–1105.
4. Simpson K, Jarvis B. Lisinopril: a review of its use in congestive heart failure. *Drugs* 2000; **59:** 1149–67.

**Administration in renal impairment.** In patients with renal impairment, the initial dose of lisinopril should be reduced depending on the creatinine clearance (CC) as follows:

- CC 31 to 80 mL/minute: 5 to 10 mg once daily
- CC 10 to 30 mL/minute: 2.5 to 5 mg once daily
- CC less than 10 mL/minute or on dialysis: 2.5 mg once daily

The dose should be adjusted according to response, to a maximum of 40 mg once daily.

### Preparations

***BP 2003:*** Lisinopril Tablets;
***USP 27:*** Lisinopril Tablets.

**Proprietary Preparations** (details are given in Part 3)
***Arg.:*** Doxapril; Lisinal; Sedotensil; Tensopril; Tersif; Zestril; ***Austral.:*** Fibsol; Liprace; Lisodur; Prinivil; Zestril; ***Austria:*** Acemin; Acetan; Hypomed; Lisinotyrol; Prinivil; ***Belg.:*** Novatec; Zestril; ***Braz.:*** Linopril†; Novral†; Prinivil; Vasojet; Zestril; Zinopril; ***Canad.:*** Prinivil; Zestril; ***Chile:*** Acerdil; Lipreren; Presokin; Tonotensil; Zestril; ***Denm.:*** Acepril; Lanatin; Vivatec; Zestril; ***Fin.:*** Lisipril; Vivatec; Zestril; ***Fr.:*** Prinivil; Zestril; ***Ger.:*** Acerbon; Coric; Lisi; Lisi Lich; Lisi-Puren; Lisibeta; Lisigamma; Lisihexal; Lisodura; ***Gr.:*** Adicanil; Axelvin; Gnostoval; Icoran; Leruze; Lisinospes; Nafordyl; Perenal; Press-12; Pressuril; Prinivil; Thriusedon; Vercol; Veroxil; Z-Bec; Zestril; ***Hong Kong:*** Acepril; Prinivil; Zestril; ***India:*** Cipril; Linoril; Linvas; Lipril; Lisoril; ***Irl.:*** Carace; Lisopress; Zesger; Zestan; Zestril; ***Israel:*** Tensopril; ***Ital.:*** Alapril; Prinivil; Zestril; ***Malaysia:*** Prinivil; Zestril; ***Mex.:*** Alfaken; Prinivil; Zestril; ***Neth.:*** Novatec; Zestril; ***Norw.:*** Vivatec; Zestril; ***NZ:*** Prinivil; Zestril; ***Port.:*** Ecapril; Farpresse; Lipril; Prinivil; Zestril; ***S.Afr.:*** Prinivil; Zestomax†; Zestril; Zetomax; ***Singapore:*** Lisoril; Prinivil; Zestril; ***Spain:*** Doneka; Iricil; Likenil; Prinivil; Secubar; Tensikey; Zestril; ***Swed.:*** Vivatec; Zestril; ***Switz.:*** Prinil; Zestril; ***Thai.:*** Lispril; Zestril; ***UK:*** Carace; Zestril; ***USA:*** Prinivil; Zestril.

**Multi-ingredient:** ***Arg.:*** Tensopril D; Zestoretic; ***Austria:*** Acecomb; Co-Acetan; Zestoretic; ***Belg.:*** Novazyd; Zestoretic; ***Braz.:*** Lisonotec; Prinzide; Zestoretic; ***Canad.:*** Prinzide; Zestoretic; ***Chile:*** Acerdil-D; Tonotensil D; Zestoretic; ***Denm.:*** Vivazid; Zestoretic; ***Fin.:*** Acercomp; Lisipril Comp; Vivatec Comp; ***Fr.:*** Prinzide; Zestoretic; ***Ger.:*** Acercomp; Coric Plus; ***Hong Kong:*** Zestoretic; ***India:*** Cipril-H; Lisoril-5HT; ***Irl.:*** Carace Plus; Zestoretic; ***Ital.:*** Nalapres; Prinzide; Zestoretic; ***Mex.:*** Prinzide; Zestoretic; ***Neth.:*** Novazyd; Zestoretic; ***Norw.:*** Vivatec Comp; Zestoretic; ***NZ:*** Prinzide†; Zestoretic†; ***Port.:*** Prinzide; Zestoretic; ***S.Afr.:*** Zestoretic; ***Spain:*** Doneka Plus; Iricil Plus; Prinivil Plus; Secubar Diu; Tensikey Complex; Zestoretic; ***Swed.:*** Zestoretic; ***Switz.:*** Prinzide; Zestoretic; ***UK:*** Carace Plus; Zestoretic; ***USA:*** Prinzide; Zestoretic.

---

## Lorcainide Hydrochloride *(BANM, USAN, rINNM)*

Hidrocloruro de lorcainida; Isocainide Hydrochloride; R-15889; Socainide Hydrochloride. 4′-Chloro-N-(1-isopropyl-4-piperidyl)-2-phenylacetanilide hydrochloride.

$C_{22}H_{27}ClN_2O,HCl = 407.4$.

*CAS — 59729-31-6 (lorcainide); 58934-46-6 (lorcainide hydrochloride).*

*ATC — C01BC07.*

### Profile

Lorcainide is a class Ic antiarrhythmic (p.809) that has been used for the management of ventricular and supraventricular arrhythmias. It has been given by mouth and by intravenous infusion as the hydrochloride.

---

## Losartan Potassium *(BANM, USAN, rINNM)*

DuP-753; E-3340; Losartán potásico; MK-0954. 2-Butyl-4-chloro-1-[p-(o-1H-tetrazol-5-ylphenyl)benzyl]imidazole-5-methanol potassium.

$C_{22}H_{22}ClKN_6O = 461.0$.

*CAS — 114798-26-4 (losartan); 124750-99-8 (losartan potassium).*

*ATC — C09CA01.*

### Adverse Effects

Adverse effects of losartan have been reported to be usually mild and transient, and include dizziness, headache, and dose-related orthostatic hypotension. Hypotension may occur particularly in patients with volume depletion (for example those who have received high-dose diuretics). Impaired renal function and, rarely, rash, urticaria, pruritus, angioedema, and raised liver enzyme values may occur. Hyperkalaemia, myalgia, and arthralgia have been reported. Losartan appears less likely than ACE inhibitors to cause cough. Other adverse effects that have been reported with angiotensin II receptor antagonists include respiratory-tract disorders, back pain, gastrointestinal disturbances, fatigue, and neutropenia.

◊ Reviews.

1. Mazzolai L, Burnier M. Comparative safety and tolerability of angiotensin II receptor antagonists. *Drug Safety* 1999; **21:** 23–33.

**Angioedema.** Angioedema is a recognised adverse effect of ACE inhibitors and is thought to be due to accumulation of bradykinins. However, several of the angiotensin II receptor antagonists (including losartan), which do not affect bradykinin levels, have been associated with reports[1-5] of angioedema. In some cases patients had previously experienced angioedema with ACE inhibitors and caution is advised when using angiotensin II receptor antagonists in such patients.[4,6]

1. Acker CG, Greenberg A. Angioedema induced by the angiotensin II blocker losartan. *N Engl J Med* 1995; **333:** 1572.
2. van Rijnsoever EW, *et al.* Angioneurotic edema attributed to the use of losartan. *Arch Intern Med* 1998; **158:** 2063–5.
3. Adverse Drug Reactions Advisory Committee. Angiotensin II receptor antagonists. *Aust Adverse Drug React Bull* 1999; **18:** 2.
4. Howes LG, Tran D. Can angiotensin receptor antagonists be used safely in patients with previous ACE inhibitor-induced angioedema? *Drug Safety* 2002; **25:** 73–6.
5. Irons BK, Kumar A. Valsartan-induced angioedema. *Ann Pharmacother* 2003; **37:** 1024–7.
6. Warner KK, *et al.* Angiotensin II receptor blockers in patients with ACE inhibitor-induced angioedema. *Ann Pharmacother* 2000; **34:** 526–8.

**Effects on the blood.** Symptomatic anaemia occurred[1] in a patient with a renal transplant 6 weeks after commencing therapy with losartan. Decreased haemoglobin concentrations have also been reported[2] in patients with severe renal impairment undergoing haemodialysis.

Immune thrombocytopenia has been reported[3] in a patient shortly after starting losartan.

1. Horn S, *et al.* Losartan and renal transplantation. *Lancet* 1998; **351:** 111.
2. Schwarzbeck A, *et al.* Anaemia in dialysis patients as a side-effect of sartanes. *Lancet* 1998; **352:** 286.
3. Ada S, *et al.* Immune thrombocytopenia after losartan therapy. *Ann Intern Med* 2002; **137:** 704.

**Effects on the liver.** Raised liver enzyme values have occurred rarely in patients receiving losartan. Severe, acute hepatotoxicity developed in a patient 1 month after losartan was substituted for enalapril because of ACE inhibitor-induced cough.[1] The patient recovered when losartan was withdrawn but symptoms and raised liver enzyme concentrations recurred following rechallenge. Acute, reversible hepatotoxicity also occurred in a patient who had been taking losartan 150 mg daily for 6 weeks.[2] A case of cholestatic jaundice associated with irbesartan therapy has also been reported;[3] the jaundice resolved slowly once irbesartan was withdrawn.

1. Bosch X. Losartan-induced hepatotoxicity. *JAMA* 1997; **278:** 1572.
2. Andrade RJ, *et al.* Hepatic injury associated with losartan. *Ann Pharmacother* 1998; **32:** 1371.
3. Hariraj R, *et al.* Prolonged cholestasis associated with irbesartan. *BMJ* 2000; **321:** 547.

**Effects on the skin.** Atypical cutaneous lymphoid infiltrates developed in 2 patients receiving losartan for hypertension.[1] In both cases the lesions disappeared within a few weeks of stopping the drug.

Henoch-Schönlein purpura has been reported[2,3] in patients taking losartan; in 1 case[2] the reaction recurred on rechallenge.

There has also been a report[4] of a number of patients in whom psoriasis either developed or was exacerbated following treatment with an angiotensin II receptor antagonist; the drugs involved included candesartan, irbesartan, losartan, and valsartan. In most cases the lesions regressed after the drug was withdrawn.

1. Viraben R, *et al.* Losartan-associated atypical cutaneous lymphoid hyperplasia. *Lancet* 1997; **350:** 1366.
2. Bosch X. Henoch-Schönlein purpura induced by losartan therapy. *Arch Intern Med* 1998; **158:** 191–2.
3. Brouard M, *et al.* Schönlein-Henoch purpura associated with losartan treatment and presence of antineutrophil cytoplasmic antibodies of x specificity. *Br J Dermatol* 2001; **145:** 362–3.
4. Marquart-Elbaz C, *et al.* Sartans, angiotensin II receptor antagonists, can induce psoriasis. *Br J Dermatol* 2002; **147:** 617–8.

**Effects on taste.** Taste disturbances, in some cases progressing to complete taste loss, have occurred[1,2] in patients receiving losartan for hypertension. In each case taste returned to normal after discontinuing losartan therapy.

1. Schlienger RG, *et al.* Reversible ageusia associated with losartan. *Lancet* 1996; **347:** 471–2.
2. Heeringa M, van Puijenbroek EP. Reversible dysgeusia attributed to losartan. *Ann Intern Med* 1998; **129:** 72.

**Hypersensitivity.** See Angioedema, and Effects on the Skin, above.

**Migraine.** Severe migraine has been reported[1] in a patient following administration of losartan. The patient had no history of migraine and symptoms recurred on rechallenge. However, angiotensin II receptor antagonists have also been reported to reduce the incidence of migraine (see under Uses and Administration, below).

1. Ahmad S. Losartan and severe migraine. *JAMA* 1995; **274:** 1266–7.

**Pancreatitis.** Acute pancreatitis has been reported[1,2] in 2 patients receiving losartan. However, 1 of the patients subsequently developed pancreatitis unrelated to losartan.[3] The other patient[2] had also developed acute pancreatitis during enalapril therapy. Acute pancreatitis has also been reported[4] with irbesartan; the patient was also taking hydrochlorothiazide but in a dose lower than that usually associated with thiazide-induced pancreatitis.


1. Bosch X. Losartan-induced acute pancreatitis. *Ann Intern Med* 1997; **127:** 1043–4.
2. Birck R, *et al.* Pancreatitis after losartan. *Lancet* 1998; **351:** 1178.
3. Bosch X. Correction: losartan, pancreatitis, and microlithiasis. *Ann Intern Med* 1998; **129:** 755.
4. Fisher AA, Bassett ML. Acute pancreatitis associated with angiotensin II receptor antagonists. *Ann Pharmacother* 2002; **36:** 1883–6.


**Vasculitis.** For mention of the development of Henoch-Schönlein purpura in patients receiving losartan see Effects on the Skin, above.

## Precautions

Losartan is contra-indicated in pregnancy (see below). It should be used with caution in patients with renal artery stenosis. Losartan is excreted in urine and in bile and reduced doses may therefore be required in patients with renal impairment and should be considered in patients with hepatic impairment. Patients with volume depletion (for example those who have received high-dose diuretic therapy) may experience hypotension; volume depletion should be corrected before starting therapy, or a low initial dose should be used. Since hyperkalaemia may occur, serum-potassium concentrations should be monitored, especially in the elderly and patients with renal impairment, and the concomitant use of potassium-sparing diuretics should generally be avoided.

**Diabetes mellitus.** Following reports of reduced awareness of hypoglycaemia in type 1 diabetic patients receiving losartan, a study[1] in healthy subjects found that losartan slightly attenuated the symptomatic and hormonal responses to hypoglycaemia. Although the clinical significance was not established, the authors recommended that losartan should be used with caution in diabetics with reduced awareness of hypoglycaemia. However, losartan and other angiotensin II receptor antagonists may have a role in type 2 diabetics with nephropathy (see Kidney Disorders under Uses, below).


1. Deininger E, *et al.* Losartan attenuates symptomatic and hormonal responses to hypoglycemia in humans. *Clin Pharmacol Ther* 2001; **70:** 362–9.


**Pregnancy.** Losartan is contra-indicated in pregnancy since it has been associated with fetal toxicity in *animal* studies and other drugs that act on the renin-angiotensin system, such as ACE inhibitors, have been associated with fetal toxicity in humans (see p.845). Oligohydramnios with subsequent fetal death occurred in a patient who received losartan during weeks 20 to 31 of pregnancy;[1] the effects on the fetus were similar to those reported with ACE inhibitors. A number of similar cases have subsequently been reported with losartan,[2,3] candesartan,[4] and valsartan.[3,5]


1. Saji H, *et al.* Losartan and fetal toxic effects. *Lancet* 2001; **357:** 363.
2. Lambot M-A, *et al.* Angiotensin-II-receptor inhibitors in pregnancy. *Lancet* 2001; **357:** 1619–20.
3. Martinovic J, *et al.* Fetal toxic effects and angiotensin-II-receptor antagonists. *Lancet* 2001; **358:** 241–2.
4. Hinsberger A, *et al.* Angiotensin-II-receptor inhibitors in pregnancy. *Lancet* 2001; **357:** 1620.
5. Briggs GG, Nageotte MP. Fatal fetal outcome with the combined use of valsartan and atenolol. *Ann Pharmacother* 2001; **35:** 859–61.


## Interactions

The antihypertensive effects of losartan may be potentiated by drugs or other agents that lower blood pressure. An additive hyperkalaemic effect is possible with potassium supplements, potassium-sparing diuretics, or other drugs that can cause hyperkalaemia; losartan and potassium-sparing diuretics should not generally be given together. Losartan and some other angiotensin II receptor antagonists are metabolised by cytochrome P450 isoenzymes and interactions may occur with drugs that affect these enzymes.

**Lithium.** For reference to a possible interaction between lithium and angiotensin II receptor antagonists, see p.303.

## Pharmacokinetics

Losartan is readily absorbed from the gastrointestinal tract following oral administration, but undergoes substantial first-pass metabolism resulting in a systemic bioavailability of about 33%. It is metabolised to an active carboxylic acid metabolite E-3174 (EXP-3174), which has greater pharmacological activity than losartan; some inactive metabolites are also formed. Metabolism is primarily by cytochrome P450 isoenzymes CYP2C9 and CYP3A4. Peak plasma concentrations of losartan and E-3174 occur about 1 hour and 3 to 4 hours, respectively, after an oral dose. Both losartan and E-3174 are more than 98% bound to plasma proteins. Losartan is excreted in the urine, and in the faeces via bile, as unchanged drug and metabolites. Following oral dosing about 4% of the dose is excreted unchanged in urine and about 6% is excreted in urine as the active metabolite. The terminal elimination half-lives of losartan and E-3174 are about 1.5 to 2.5 hours and 3 to 9 hours, respectively.

◊ References.


1. Ohtawa M, *et al.* Pharmacokinetics and biochemical efficacy after single and multiple oral administration of losartan, an orally active nonpeptide angiotensin II receptor antagonist, in humans. *Br J Clin Pharmacol* 1993; **35:** 290–7.
2. Lo M-W, *et al.* Pharmacokinetics of losartan, an angiotensin II receptor antagonist, and its active metabolite EXP3174 in humans. *Clin Pharmacol Ther* 1995; **58:** 641–9.
3. Csajka C, *et al.* Pharmacokinetic-pharmacodynamic profile of angiotensin II receptor antagonists. *Clin Pharmacokinet* 1997; **32:** 1–29.
4. Sica DA, *et al.* Pharmacokinetics and blood pressure response of losartan in end-stage renal disease. *Clin Pharmacokinet* 2000; **38:** 519–26.
5. Pedro AA, *et al.* The pharmacokinetics and pharmacodynamics of losartan in continuous ambulatory peritoneal dialysis. *J Clin Pharmacol* 2000; **40:** 389–95.


## Uses and Administration

Losartan is an angiotensin II receptor antagonist with antihypertensive activity due mainly to selective blockade of $AT_1$ receptors and the consequent reduced pressor effect of angiotensin II. It is used in the management of hypertension (p.825), particularly in patients who develop cough with ACE inhibitors and to reduce the risk of stroke in patients with left ventricular hypertrophy, and in the treatment of diabetic nephropathy (see Kidney Disorders, below). It has also been tried in heart failure (below) and in myocardial infarction (p.828).

Losartan is given by mouth as the potassium salt. The maximum hypotensive effect is achieved in about 3 to 6 weeks after initiating treatment.

In **hypertension** the usual dose is 50 mg once daily. The dose may be increased, if necessary, to 100 mg daily as a single dose or in two divided doses. An initial dose of 25 mg once daily should be given to patients with intravascular fluid depletion, and is recommended in the UK in the elderly over 75 years of age. Similar reductions may be appropriate in patients with hepatic or renal impairment (but see below).

Children aged 6 years or over with hypertension may be given an initial dose of 700 micrograms/kg once daily, with a maximum of 50 mg, adjusted according to response; doses higher than 1.4 mg/kg or 100 mg daily have not been studied.

In **diabetic nephropathy** losartan is given in an initial dose of 50 mg once daily, increased to 100 mg once daily depending on the blood pressure.

◊ Reviews.


1. Carr AA, Prisant LM. Losartan: first of a new class of angiotensin antagonists for the management of hypertension. *J Clin Pharmacol* 1996; **36:** 3–12.
2. Goa KL, Wagstaff AJ. Losartan potassium: a review of its pharmacology, clinical efficacy and tolerability in the management of hypertension. *Drugs* 1996; **51:** 820–45.
3. Schaefer KL, Porter JA. Angiotensin II receptor antagonists: the prototype losartan. *Ann Pharmacother* 1996; **30:** 625–36.
4. Burrell LM. A risk-benefit assessment of losartan potassium in the treatment of hypertension. *Drug Safety* 1997; **16:** 56–65.
5. McConnaughey MM, *et al.* Practical considerations of the pharmacology of angiotensin receptor blockers. *J Clin Pharmacol* 1999; **39:** 547–59.
6. Burnier M, Brunner HR. Angiotensin II receptor antagonists. *Lancet* 2000; **355:** 637–45.
7. Dina R, Jafari M. Angiotensin II-receptor antagonists: an overview. *Am J Health-Syst Pharm* 2000; **57:** 1231–41.
8. Rodgers JE, Patterson JH. Angiotensin II-receptor blockers: clinical relevance and therapeutic role. *Am J Health-Syst Pharm* 2001; **58:** 671–81. Correction. *ibid.*; 1658.


**Administration in hepatic and renal impairment.** The manufacturers of losartan in both the UK and the USA recommend a reduced initial dose of 25 mg daily in patients with hepatic impairment. However, in the UK a similar initial dose is also recommended in those with moderate to severe renal impairment (creatinine clearance less than 20 mL/minute), whereas in the USA dosage reduction is considered unnecessary.

**Erythrocytosis.** Like ACE inhibitors (p.846), losartan has been reported[1-5] to reduce the haematocrit in patients with erythrocytosis (p.806) following renal transplantation. Beneficial results have also been reported[6] in patients with erythrocytosis secondary to chronic obstructive pulmonary disease.


1. Klaassen RJL, *et al.* Losartan, an angiotensin-II receptor antagonist, reduces hematocrits in kidney transplant recipients with posttransplant erythrocytosis. *Transplantation* 1997; **64:** 780–2.
2. Navarro JF, *et al.* Effects of losartan on the treatment of posttransplant erythrocytosis. *Clin Nephrol* 1998; **49:** 370–2.
3. Julian BA, *et al.* Losartan, an angiotensin II type 1 receptor antagonist, lowers hematocrit in posttransplant erythrocytosis. *J Am Soc Nephrol* 1998; **9:** 1104–8.
4. Iñigo P, *et al.* Treatment with losartan in kidney transplant recipients with posttransplant erythrocytosis. *Transplant Proc* 1999; **31:** 2321.
5. Yildiz A, *et al.* Comparison of the effects of enalapril and losartan on posttransplantation erythrocytosis in renal transplant recipients: prospective randomized study. *Transplantation* 2001; **72:** 542–5.
6. Vlahakos DV, *et al.* Losartan reduces hematocrit in patients with chronic obstructive pulmonary disease and secondary erythrocytosis. *Ann Intern Med* 2001; **134:** 426–7.


**Heart failure.** Diuretics, ACE inhibitors, and beta blockers are the standard drugs used in the management of heart failure (p.820). Angiotensin II receptor antagonists have been studied as an alternative to ACE inhibitors since they may be better tolerated. In the ELITE study,[1] which compared losartan with captopril, both drugs had similar effects on renal function but other adverse effects were fewer with losartan and there was also a reduction in mortality in patients receiving losartan. However, the larger ELITE II study[2] failed to confirm any survival benefit with losartan. ACE inhibitors therefore remain first-line therapy, although angiotensin II receptor antagonists may have a role in patients unable to tolerate ACE inhibitors.[3,4] The combination of angiotensin II receptor antagonists with ACE inhibitors has also shown some benefit.[4] In the ValHeFT study,[5] valsartan was added to standard therapy (including ACE inhibitors in most patients) and reduced the combined end-point of death or hospitalisation for heart failure. However, the effect on mortality alone was not significant and in patients who were also receiving both ACE inhibitors and beta blockers mortality appeared to be increased. In the CHARM-Added trial,[6] however, addition of candesartan to therapy including an ACE inhibitor led to a reduction in cardiovascular events, and this was not affected by the use of beta blockers.


1. Pitt B, *et al.* Randomised trial of losartan versus captopril in patients over 65 with heart failure (Evaluation of Losartan in the Elderly Study, ELITE). *Lancet* 1997; **349:** 747–52.
2. Pitt B, *et al.* Effect of losartan compared with captopril on mortality in patients with symptomatic heart failure: randomised trial—the Losartan Heart Failure Survival Study ELITE II. *Lancet* 2000; **355:** 1582–7.
3. Granger CB, *et al.* Effects of candesartan in patients with chronic heart failure and reduced left-ventricular systolic function intolerant to angiotensin-converting-enzyme inhibitors: the CHARM-Alternative trial. *Lancet* 2003; **362:** 772–6.
4. Jong P, *et al.* Angiotensin receptor blockers in heart failure: meta-analysis of randomized controlled trials. *J Am Coll Cardiol* 2002; **39:** 463–70.
5. Cohn JN, Tognoni G. A randomized trial of the angiotensin-receptor blocker valsartan in chronic heart failure. *N Engl J Med* 2001; **345:** 1667–75.
6. McMurray JJV, *et al.* Effects of candesartan in patients with chronic heart failure and reduced left-ventricular systolic function taking angiotensin-converting-enzyme inhibitors: the CHARM-Added trial. *Lancet* 2003; **362:** 767–71.


**Kidney disorders.** ACE inhibitors have an established role in the management of type 1 and type 2 diabetics with nephropathy, whether or not they are hypertensive, and may also slow the progression of nephropathy in diabetics with microalbuminuria (see p.847). A number of studies have investigated the effects of angiotensin II receptor antagonists in type 2 diabetics with varying degrees of nephropathy. Both irbesartan[1,2] and losartan[3,4] have been reported to reduce the progression of nephropathy independently of their effect on blood pressure, and may have a role as an alternative to ACE inhibitors in such patients. A smaller study[5] using a combination of candesartan with lisinopril found that blood pressure and microalbuminuria were reduced more with combination therapy than with either drug alone. Benefit has also been reported[6] with a combination of losartan and trandolapril in patients with non-diabetic renal disease.


1. Lewis EJ, *et al.* Renoprotective effect of the angiotensin-receptor antagonist irbesartan in patients with nephropathy due to type 2 diabetes. *N Engl J Med* 2001; **345:** 851–60.
2. Parving H-H, *et al.* The effect of irbesartan on the development of diabetic nephropathy in patients with type 2 diabetes. *N Engl J Med* 2001; **345:** 870–8.
3. Brenner BM, *et al.* Effects of losartan on renal and cardiovascular outcomes in patients with type 2 diabetes and nephropathy. *N Engl J Med* 2001; **345:** 861–9.
4. Zandbergen AAM, *et al.* Effect of losartan on microalbuminuria in normotensive patients with type 2 diabetes mellitus: a randomized clinical trial. *Ann Intern Med* 2003; **139:** 90–6.
5. Mogensen CE, *et al.* Randomised controlled trial of dual blockade of renin-angiotensin system in patients with hypertension, microalbuminuria, and non-insulin dependent diabetes: the candesartan and lisinopril microalbuminuria (CALM) study. *BMJ* 2000; **321:** 1440–4.
6. Nakao N, *et al.* Combination treatment of angiotensin-II receptor blocker and angiotensin-converting-enzyme inhibitor in non-diabetic renal disease (COOPERATE): a randomised controlled trial. *Lancet* 2003; **361:** 117–24. Correction. *ibid.*; 1230.


**Migraine.** Angiotensin II receptor antagonists may reduce the incidence of headache. A randomised trial[1] in 60 patients with migraine suggested that candesartan might be effective for prophylaxis. However, there has been a report of migraine caused by an angiotensin II receptor antagonist (see under Adverse Effects, above).

1. Tronvik E, *et al.* Prophylactic treatment of migraine with an angiotensin II receptor blocker: a randomized controlled trial. *JAMA* 2003; **289:** 65–9.

**Uricosuric action.** Losartan has been found to increase urinary uric acid excretion and reduce serum uric acid concentrations in healthy subjects[1] and in hypertensive patients.[2,3] However, the effect is generally small and the clinical significance is not clear. Other angiotensin II receptor antagonists do not appear to have such an effect.[2,3]

1. Nakashima M, *et al.* Pilot study of the uricosuric effect of DuP-753, a new angiotensin II receptor antagonist, in healthy subjects. *Eur J Clin Pharmacol* 1992; **42:** 333–5.
2. Puig JG, *et al.* Effect of eprosartan and losartan on uric acid metabolism in patients with essential hypertension. *J Hypertens* 1999; **17:** 1033–9.
3. Würzner G, *et al.* Comparative effects of losartan and irbesartan on serum uric acid in hypertensive patients with hyperuricaemia and gout. *J Hypertens* 2001; **19:** 1855–60.

### Preparations

**Proprietary Preparations** (details are given in Part 3)
***Arg.:*** Cartan; Cozaarex; Enromic; Klosartan; Loctenk; Losacor; Niten; Paxon; Prelertan; Tacardia; Tenopres; ***Austral.:*** Cozaar; ***Austria:*** Cosaar; ***Belg.:*** Cozaar; Loortan; ***Braz.:*** Aradois; Corus; Cozaar; Lorsacor; Losartec; Losatal; Redupress; ***Canad.:*** Cozaar; ***Chile:*** Aratan; Corodin; Cozaar; Losapres; Sanipresin; Simperten; ***Denm.:*** Cozaar; ***Fin.:*** Cozaar; ***Fr.:*** Cozaar; ***Ger.:*** Lorzaar; ***Hong Kong:*** Cozaar; ***India:*** Covance; Losacar; Lozitan; ***Irl.:*** Cozaar; ***Israel:*** Ocsaar; ***Ital.:*** Lortaan; Losaprex; Neo-Lotan; ***Jpn:*** Nu-Lotan; ***Malaysia:*** Cozaar; ***Mex.:*** Cozaar; ***Neth.:*** Cozaar; ***Norw.:*** Cozaar; ***NZ:*** Cozaar; ***Port.:*** Cozaar; Lortaan; ***S.Afr.:*** Cozaar; ***Singapore:*** Cozaar; ***Spain:*** Cozaar; ***Swed.:*** Cozaar; ***Switz.:*** Cosaar; ***Thai.:*** Cozaar; ***UK:*** Cozaar; ***USA:*** Cozaar.

**Multi-ingredient:** ***Arg.:*** Cozaarex D; Losacor D; Niten D; Paxon-D; Tenopres D; ***Austria:*** Cosaar Plus; ***Belg.:*** Cozaar Plus; Loortan Plus; ***Braz.:*** Aradois H; Corus H; Hipress†; Hyzaar; Neopress; ***Canad.:*** Hyzaar; ***Chile:*** Aratan D; Corodin D; Hyzaar; Losapres-D; Sanipresin-D; Simperten-D; ***Denm.:*** Cozaar Comp; Fortzaar; ***Fin.:*** Cozaar Comp; ***Fr.:*** Fortzaar; Hyzaar; ***Ger.:*** Lorzaar plus; ***Hong Kong:*** Hyzaar; ***India:*** Losacar-H; Zaart-H; ***Irl.:*** Cozaar Comp; ***Israel:*** Ocsaar Plus; ***Ital.:*** Forzaar; Hizaar; Losazid; Neo-Lotan Plus; ***Malaysia:*** Fortzaar; Hyzaar; ***Mex.:*** Hyzaar; ***Neth.:*** Hyzaar; ***Norw.:*** Cozaar Comp; ***Port.:*** Cozaar Plus; Fortzaar; Lortaan Plus; ***S.Afr.:*** Cozaar Comp; Fortzaar; ***Singapore:*** Hyzaar; ***Spain:*** Cozaar Plus; Fortzaar; ***Swed.:*** Cozaar Comp; ***Switz.:*** Cosaar Plus; ***Thai.:*** Fortzaar; Hyzaar; ***UK:*** Cozaar Comp; ***USA:*** Hyzaar.

## Lovastatin *(BAN, USAN, rINN)*

L-154803; Lovastatina; Lovastatinum; MB-530B; 6α-Methylcompactin; Mevinolin; MK-803; Monacolin K; MSD-803. (3*R*,5*R*)-7-{(1*S*,2*S*,6*R*,8*S*,8a*R*)-1,2,6,7,8,8a-Hexahydro-2,6-dimethyl-8-[(*S*)-2-methylbutyryloxy]-1-naphthyl}-3-hydroxyheptan-5-olide.

$C_{24}H_{36}O_5$ = 404.5.

*CAS — 75330-75-5.*

*ATC — C10AA02.*

**Pharmacopoeias.** In *Eur.* (see p.vi) and *US.*

**Ph. Eur. 5.0** (Lovastatin). A white or almost white crystalline powder. Practically insoluble in water; sparingly soluble in dehydrated alcohol; soluble in acetone. Store under nitrogen at a temperature of 2° to 8°.

**USP 27** (Lovastatin). A white to off-white crystalline powder. Insoluble in water; sparingly soluble in alcohol; practically insoluble in petroleum spirit; freely soluble in chloroform; soluble in acetone, in acetonitrile, and in methyl alcohol. Store under nitrogen in airtight containers at a temperature not exceeding 8°.

### Adverse Effects and Precautions

As for Simvastatin, p.997.

**Incidence of adverse effects.** Adverse effects led to withdrawal of lovastatin in 21 of 745 patients receiving the drug for about 5 years.[1] They included asymptomatic elevation of hepatic aminotransferases in 10 patients, gastrointestinal symptoms in 3, rash in 2, myopathy in 2, myalgia in 1, arthralgia in 1, insomnia in 1, and weight gain in 1.

1. Lovastatin Study Groups. Lovastatin 5-year safety and efficacy study: Lovastatin Study Groups I through IV. *Arch Intern Med* 1993; **153:** 1079–87.

### Interactions

As for Simvastatin, p.998.

### Pharmacokinetics

Lovastatin is absorbed from the gastrointestinal tract and is hydrolysed in the liver to its active β-hydroxyacid form. Three other metabolites have also been isolated. Lovastatin undergoes extensive first-pass metabolism in the liver, its primary site of action, and less than 5% of the oral dose has been reported to reach the circulation. Lovastatin is metabolised by the cytochrome P450 isoenzyme CYP3A4. Peak plasma concentrations occur within 2 to 4 hours, and steady-state concentrations are achieved after 2 to 3 days with daily administration. Both lovastatin and its β-hydroxyacid metabolite are more than 95% bound to plasma proteins. It is mainly excreted in the bile; about 85% of a dose has been recovered from the faeces and about 10% from the urine. The half-life of the active metabolite is 1 to 2 hours.

◊ General reviews.

1. Desager J-P, Horsmans Y. Clinical pharmacokinetics of 3-hydroxy-3-methylglutaryl-coenzyme A reductase inhibitors. *Clin Pharmacokinet* 1996; **31:** 348–71.
2. Lennernäs H, Fager G. Pharmacodynamics and pharmacokinetics of the HMG-CoA reductase inhibitors: similarities and differences. *Clin Pharmacokinet* 1997; **32:** 403–25.

### Uses and Administration

Lovastatin, a 3-hydroxy-3-methylglutaryl coenzyme A (HMG-CoA) reductase inhibitor (a statin), is a lipid regulating drug with actions on plasma lipids similar to those of simvastatin (p.999).

Lovastatin is used to reduce cholesterol in the treatment of hyperlipidaemias (p.823), particularly in type IIa and IIb hyperlipoproteinaemias. It is also given prophylactically for both primary and secondary prevention of ischaemic heart disease.

Lovastatin is given in an initial dose of 10 to 20 mg daily in the evening with food, increased, if necessary, at intervals of 4 weeks or more to 80 mg daily in single or divided doses. Lower doses of lovastatin should be used in patients at risk of myopathy, including patients with severe renal impairment (see below) and those taking drugs that interact with lovastatin; an initial dose of 10 mg daily is recommended in patients taking ciclosporin, and the daily dose should not exceed 20 mg in patients taking ciclosporin, fibric acid derivatives, or nicotinic acid.

◊ General reviews.

1. Curran MP, Goa KL. Lovastatin extended release: a review of its use in the management of hypercholesterolaemia. *Drugs* 2003; **63:** 685–99.

**Administration in renal impairment.** Patients with renal impairment may be at increased risk of myopathy and doses of lovastatin above 20 mg daily should be used cautiously in patients with a creatinine clearance below 30 mL/minute.

**Adrenoleucodystrophy.** A preliminary study[1] has shown that lovastatin may be useful in the treatment of adrenoleucodystrophy (p.1707). Lovastatin reduced the plasma levels of very-long-chain fatty acids which are known to be elevated in patients with this rare metabolic disorder.

1. Pai GS, *et al.* Lovastatin therapy for X-linked adrenoleukodystrophy: clinical and biochemical observations on 12 patients. *Mol Genet Metab* 2000; **69:** 312–22.

### Preparations

***USP 27:*** Lovastatin Tablets.

**Proprietary Preparations** (details are given in Part 3)
***Arg.:*** Hipovastin; Loriter; Mevlor; Sivlor; ***Austria:*** Mevacor; ***Braz.:*** Lovasc†; Lovast; Lovaton; Mevacor; Minor; Neolipid; Reducol; ***Canad.:*** Mevacor; ***Chile:*** Colevix; Hiposterol; Lispor; Lovacol; Nij-Terol; Sanelor; ***Denm.:*** Lipivas†; Mevacor; ***Fin.:*** Lovacol; Mevacor; ***Ger.:*** Mevinacor; ***Gr.:*** Liferzit; Lipidless; Lovatex; Lovatop; Lowlipid; Medovascin; Mevacor; Mevastin; Mevinol; Misodomin; Nabicortin; Terveson; ***Hong Kong:*** Ellanco; Lofacol; Lomar; Medostatin; Mevacor; ***India:*** Pro-HDL; Rovacor; ***Israel:*** Lovalip; ***Malaysia:*** Lestric; Lovastin; Medostatin; Mevacor; ***Mex.:*** Dilucid; Mevacor; ***Norw.:*** Mevacor; ***Port.:*** Lipdaune; Lipus; Mevinacor; Mevlor; Tecnolip; ***Singapore:*** Elstatin; Lostatin; Medostatin; Rovacor; ***Spain:*** Aterkey; Colesvir; Lipofren; Liposcler; Mevacor; Mevasterol; Nergadan; Taucor; ***USA:*** Altocor; Mevacor.

**Multi-ingredient:** ***USA:*** Advicor.

## Low-molecular-weight Heparins

Depolymerised Heparins; Heparina Massae Molecularis Minoris; Heparinas de bajo peso molecular; LMW Heparins; Low-molecular-mass Heparins.

**Pharmacopoeias.** In *Eur.* (see p.vi).

**Ph. Eur. 5.0** (Heparins, Low-molecular Mass; Low-molecular-weight Heparins BP 2003). Salts of sulfated glucosaminoglycans having a mass-average molecular mass less than 8000. They are obtained by fractionation or depolymerisation of heparin of natural origin and display different chemical structures at the reducing or the non-reducing end of the polysaccharide chains.

The potency is not less than 70 units of anti-factor Xa activity per mg with reference to the dried substance and the ratio of anti-factor Xa activity to anti-factor IIa (antithrombin) activity is not less than 1.5.

A white or almost white hygroscopic powder. Freely soluble in water. A 1% solution in water has a pH of 5.5 to 8.0. Store in airtight containers.

### Units

The second International Standard for low-molecular-weight heparin was agreed in 2003 and is used to calibrate products for both anti-factor Xa and anti-factor IIa activities. Potency is expressed in terms of units of anti-factor Xa activity per mg and the ratio of anti-factor Xa to anti-factor IIa activity. This ratio differs for individual low-molecular-weight heparins and neither they nor unfractionated heparin can be used interchangeably unit for unit.

### Adverse Effects

As for Heparin, p.928.

**Effects on the adrenal glands.** Hyperkalaemia related to hypoaldosteronism has been reported in patients treated with low-molecular-weight heparins.[1-3] The UK Committee on Safety of Medicines suggests[4] that plasma-potassium concentrations should be monitored in all patients with risk factors for hyperkalaemia, particularly those receiving low-molecular-weight heparins for more than 7 days (see Heparin, p.928).

1. Levesque H, *et al.* Low molecular weight heparins and hypoaldosteronism. *BMJ* 1990; **300:** 1437–8.
2. Canova CR, *et al.* Effect of low-molecular-weight heparin on serum potassium. *Lancet* 1997; **349:** 1447–8.
3. Wiggam MI, Beringer TRO. Effect of low-molecular-weight heparin on serum concentrations of potassium. *Lancet* 1997; **350:** 292–3.
4. Committee on Safety of Medicines/Medicines Control Agency. Suppression of aldosterone secretion by heparin. *Current Problems* 1999; **25:** 6. Also available at: http://medicines.mhra.gov.uk/ourwork/monitorsafequalmed/currentproblems/cpvol25bsec2.htm (accessed 06/07/04)

**Effects on the blood.** It was hoped that, because of their higher ratio of anti-factor Xa to anti-thrombin activity compared with heparin, low-molecular-weight heparins might cause less bleeding while maintaining their antithrombotic activity. Some large studies[1,2] have suggested less bleeding with low-molecular-weight heparins than with unfractionated heparin. However, meta-analyses and reviews[3,4] have been unable to confirm a significant reduction in major haemorrhage in patients treated with low-molecular-weight heparins, compared with heparin, for venous thromboembolism, although they confirmed that low-molecular-weight heparins are not associated with an increase in risk.

Thrombocytopenia has also been reported with low-molecular-weight heparins[5-7] although in one study the incidence was less than with unfractionated heparin.[8]

There has also been a report of thrombocytosis in a patient receiving enoxaparin.[9]

1. Levine MN, *et al.* Prevention of deep vein thrombosis after elective hip surgery: a randomized trial comparing low molecular weight heparin with standard unfractionated heparin. *Ann Intern Med* 1991; **114:** 545–51.
2. Hull RD, *et al.* Subcutaneous low-molecular-weight heparin compared with continuous intravenous heparin in the treatment of proximal-vein thrombosis. *N Engl J Med* 1992; **326:** 975–82. Correction. *ibid.* **327:** 140.
3. Gould MK, *et al.* Low-molecular-weight heparins compared with unfractionated heparin for treatment of acute deep venous thrombosis: a meta-analysis of randomized, controlled trials. *Ann Intern Med* 1999; **130:** 800–809.
4. Levine MN, *et al.* Hemorrhagic complications of anticoagulant treatment. *Chest* 2001; **119** (suppl): 108S–121S.
5. Eichinger S, *et al.* Thrombocytopenia associated with low-molecular-weight heparin. *Lancet* 1991; **337:** 1425–6.
6. Lecompte T, *et al.* Thrombocytopenia associated with low-molecular-weight heparin. *Lancet* 1991; **338:** 1217.
7. Tardy B, *et al.* Thrombocytopenia associated with low-molecular-weight heparin. *Lancet* 1991; **338:** 1217.
8. Warkentin TE, *et al.* Heparin-induced thrombocytopenia in patients treated with low-molecular-weight heparin or unfractionated heparin. *N Engl J Med* 1995; **332:** 1330–5.
9. Rizzieri DA, *et al.* Thrombocytosis associated with low-molecular-weight heparin. *Ann Intern Med* 1996; **125:** 157.

**Effects on the skin.** Adverse effects of low-molecular-weight heparins on the skin have been reviewed[1] and are estimated to be rare. Most low-molecular-weight heparins have been implicated. Urticarial rash or immediate hypersensitivity has been reported (see below). Delayed hypersensitivity skin reactions have occurred mainly in women. These women were generally postmenopausal, pregnant, or in the postpartum period, suggesting a hormonal influence on pathogenesis. About half of these patients also had a history of allergy to unfractionated heparin.

Skin necrosis reactions are usually localised to the subcutaneous injection site, although distant lesions have also been reported.

1. Wütschert R, *et al.* Adverse skin reactions to low molecular weight heparins: frequency, management and prevention. *Drug Safety* 1999; **20:** 515–25.

**Hypersensitivity.** Reports of hypersensitivity reactions associated with low-molecular-weight heparins are rare. However, a patient being treated with enoxaparin 20 mg subcutaneously daily developed a widespread pruritic urticaria and swelling of lips and tongue after 3 days of treatment.[1] Antihistamines and prednisone given with enoxaparin failed to control the reaction and enoxaparin treatment was stopped after a further 3 days. Urticaria and angioedema rapidly resolved on withdrawal.

Delayed hypersensitivity skin reactions have also been reported (see above).

1. Odeh M, Oliven A. Urticaria and angioedema induced by low-molecular-weight heparin. *Lancet* 1992; **340:** 972–3.

### Treatment of Adverse Effects

Severe bleeding with low-molecular-weight heparins, usually caused by accidental overdosage, may be reduced by the slow intravenous administration of protamine sulfate (p.1051). The recommended doses of protamine sulfate are given in the individual monographs and should completely neutralise the antithrombin effect of the low-molecular-weight heparin but will only partially neutralise the anti-factor-Xa effect. Not more than 50 mg of protamine sulfate should be injected for any one dose.

## Precautions

As for Heparin, p.929.

Low-molecular-weight heparins should not be given to patients who have developed thrombocytopenia with heparin and who have a positive *in-vitro* platelet aggregation test (that is, cross-reactivity) with the particular low-molecular-weight heparin to be used.

**Spinal anaesthesia.** Spinal and epidural haematomas, sometimes leading to paralysis, have occurred in patients receiving low-molecular-weight heparin in association with spinal or epidural anaesthesia or analgesia (see p.929).

## Interactions

As for Heparin, p.929.

## Pharmacokinetics

Although the precise pharmacokinetic parameters of different low-molecular-weight heparins vary (see individual monographs), they generally have a greater bioavailability after subcutaneous injection and a longer half-life than heparin.

◊ References.

1. Kandrotas RJ. Heparin pharmacokinetics and pharmacodynamics. *Clin Pharmacokinet* 1992; **22:** 359–74.

## Uses and Administration

Low-molecular-weight heparins are salts of fragments of heparin produced by chemical or enzymatic depolymerisation of the heparin molecule. Commercially available low-molecular-weight heparins differ in their method of production, molecular-weight range, and degree of sulfation. Like heparin (p.929), these compounds enhance the action of antithrombin III but they are characterised by a higher ratio of anti-factor Xa to anti-factor IIa (antithrombin) activity than heparin. Low-molecular-weight heparins have less effect on platelet aggregation than heparin. They have no significant effect on blood coagulation tests such as activated partial thromboplastin time (APTT). Therapy may be monitored by measurement of plasma-anti-factor-Xa activity but monitoring is less frequently required than with heparin since low-molecular-weight heparins have a more predictable effect.

Low-molecular-weight heparins are used in the management of venous thromboembolism (deep-vein thrombosis and pulmonary embolism, p.839). They are used for prophylaxis, particularly during surgery, and for treatment of established thromboembolism. They are administered by subcutaneous injection once or twice daily. They are also given intravenously to prevent coagulation during haemodialysis and other extracorporeal circulatory procedures, and subcutaneously in the management of unstable angina (p.813).

Doses are expressed either in terms of the weight of low-molecular-weight heparin or in terms of units of anti-factor Xa activity. Since low-molecular-weight heparins differ in their relative inhibition of factor Xa and thrombin, doses, even when expressed in terms of anti-factor-Xa activity, cannot be equated. Different preparations of the same low-molecular-weight heparin may appear to have different doses depending on the reference preparation used.

◊ References.

1. Colvin BT, Barrowcliffe TW. The British Society for Haematology guidelines on the use and monitoring of heparin 1992: second revision. *J Clin Pathol* 1993; **46:** 97–103.
2. Green D, *et al.* Low molecular weight heparin: a critical analysis of clinical trials. *Pharmacol Rev* 1994; **46:** 89–109.
3. Nurmohamed MT, *et al.* Low molecular weight heparin(oid)s: clinical investigations and practical recommendations. *Drugs* 1997; **53:** 736–51.
4. Weitz JI. Low-molecular-weight heparins. *N Engl J Med* 1997; **337:** 688–98. Correction. *ibid.*: 1567.
5. Hirsh J, *et al.* Heparin and low-molecular-weight heparin: mechanisms of action, pharmacokinetics, dosing, monitoring, efficacy, and safety. *Chest* 2001; **119** (suppl): 64S–94S.

## Lubeluzole *(BAN, USAN, rINN)*

Lubeluzol; R-87926. (S)-1-{4-[1,3-Benzothiazol-2-yl(methyl)amino]piperidino}-3-(3,4-difluorophenoxy)propan-2-ol.
$C_{22}H_{25}F_2N_3O_2S$ = 433.5.
*CAS — 144665-07-6.*

### Profile

Lubeluzole is a neuroprotectant that has been investigated for ischaemic stroke, but results have been disappointing.

◊ References.

1. Gandolfo C, *et al.* Lubeluzole for acute ischaemic stroke. Available in The Cochrane Library; Issue 2. Chichester: John Wiley; 2004.

## Manidipine Hydrochloride *(rINNM)*

CV-4093; Franidipine Hydrochloride; Hidrocloruro de manidipino. 2-[4-(Diphenylmethyl)-1-piperazinyl]ethyl methyl (±)-1,4-dihydro-2,6-dimethyl-4-(m-nitrophenyl)-3,5-pyridinedicarboxylate dihydrochloride.
$C_{35}H_{38}N_4O_6$,2HCl = 683.6.
*CAS — 120092-68-4 (manidipine); 89226-75-5 (manidipine hydrochloride); 126229-12-7 (manidipine hydrochloride).*
*ATC — C08CA11.*

### Profile

Manidipine is a dihydropyridine calcium-channel blocker (see Nifedipine, p.966). It is given by mouth as the hydrochloride in the management of hypertension (p.825) in a usual dose of 10 to 20 mg once daily.

◊ Reviews.

1. Cheer SM, McClellan K. Manidipine: a review of its use in hypertension. *Drugs* 2001; **61:** 1777–99.

### Preparations

**Proprietary Preparations** (details are given in Part 3)
***Braz.:*** Manivasc; ***Ital.:*** Iperten; Vascoman; ***Jpn:*** Calslot; ***Thai.:*** Madiplot.

## Mannitol

Cordycepic Acid; E421; Manita; Manitol; Manna Sugar; Mannite; Mannitolum. D-Mannitol.
$C_6H_{14}O_6$ = 182.2.
*CAS — 69-65-8.*
*ATC — A06AD16; B05BC01; B05CX04.*

**Description.** Mannitol is a hexahydric alcohol related to mannose ($C_6H_{12}O_6$ = 180.2). It is isomeric with sorbitol.

**Pharmacopoeias.** In *Chin., Eur.* (see p.vi), *Int., Jpn, Pol., US,* and *Viet.*

**Ph. Eur. 5.0** (Mannitol). A white or almost white crystalline powder or free-flowing granules. It exhibits polymorphism. Freely soluble in water; very slightly soluble in alcohol.

**USP 27** (Mannitol). A white odourless crystalline powder or free-flowing granules with a sweet taste. Soluble 1 in 5.5 of water; very slightly soluble in alcohol; practically insoluble in ether; slightly soluble in pyridine; soluble in alkaline solutions.

**Incompatibility.** Mannitol should never be added to whole blood for transfusion or given through the same set by which blood is being infused. For details of the adverse effects of mannitol on red blood cells, see Effects on the Blood under Adverse Effects, below.

**Supersaturated solutions.** Supersaturated aqueous solutions are prepared with the aid of heat. Any crystals that form during storage of the injection should be dissolved by warming before use; this may be a particular problem with the 20 and 25% injections which are supersaturated. A 5.07% solution in water is iso-osmotic with serum.

### Adverse Effects

The most common adverse effect associated with mannitol therapy is fluid and electrolyte imbalance including circulatory overload and acidosis at high doses. The expansion of extracellular volume can precipitate pulmonary oedema and patients with diminished cardiac reserve are at special risk. The shift of fluid from the intracellular to extracellular compartment can cause tissue dehydration; dehydration of the brain, particularly in patients with renal failure, may give rise to CNS symptoms.

When given by mouth, mannitol causes diarrhoea. Intravenous infusion of mannitol has been associated with nausea, vomiting, thirst, headache, dizziness, chills, fever, tachycardia, chest pain, hyponatraemia, dehydration, blurred vision, urticaria, and hypotension or hypertension. Large doses have been associated rarely with acute renal failure. Hypersensitivity reactions have occurred.

Extravasation of the solution may cause oedema and skin necrosis; thrombophlebitis may occur.

**Effects on the blood.** Agglutination and irreversible crenation of erythrocytes occurred when blood was mixed with varying proportions of a 10% mannitol solution.[1] It was suggested that intravenous infusions should be carefully controlled and given at a slow rate. This observation could have particular relevance to patients with sickle-cell disease.[2,3] Although agglutination and crenation had been observed *in vitro*, dilutional effects would make *in-vivo* interaction with blood cells less likely.[4]

1. Roberts BE, Smith PH. Hazards of mannitol infusions. *Lancet* 1966; **ii:** 421–2.
2. Konotey-Ahulu FID. Hazards of mannitol infusions. *Lancet* 1966; **ii:** 591.
3. Roberts BE, Smith PH. Hazards of mannitol infusions. *Lancet* 1966; **ii:** 591.
4. Samson JH. Hazards of mannitol infusions. *Lancet* 1966; **ii:** 1191.

**Effects on the gastrointestinal tract.** Potentially explosive intracolonic concentrations of hydrogen gas have been measured in patients given mannitol before colonoscopy,[1,2] and cases of colonic explosion, including fatalities, have been reported in patients undergoing colonoscopic electrocautery, who had received mannitol bowel preparation. However, the risk of explosion was considered to be small when air or carbon dioxide insufflation and suction were used during the colonoscopy procedure.[2,3]
Colonic perforation and subsequent death has been attributed to the use of mannitol for the treatment of constipation.[4]

1. La Brooy SJ, *et al.* Potentially explosive colonic concentrations of hydrogen after bowel preparation with mannitol. *Lancet* 1981; **i:** 634–6.
2. Avgerinos A, *et al.* Bowel preparation and the risk of explosion during colonoscopic polypectomy. *Gut* 1984; **25:** 361–4.
3. Trotman I, Walt R. Mannitol and explosions. *Lancet* 1981; **i:** 848.
4. Moses FM. Colonic perforation due to oral mannitol. *JAMA* 1988; **260:** 640.

**Effects on the kidneys.** Focal osmotic nephrosis occurred in a patient who received mannitol 20% intravenously.[1]
Acute oliguric renal failure has been associated with the administration of large doses of mannitol to patients with previously normal renal function,[2-4] and acute renal failure developed[5] in a patient with diabetes mellitus complicated by nephropathy after he received 420 g of mannitol intravenously over 4 days.

1. Goodwin WE, Latta H. Focal osmotic nephrosis due to the therapeutic use of mannitol: a case of perirenal hematoma after renal biopsy. *J Urol (Baltimore)* 1970; **103:** 11–14.
2. Whelan TV, *et al.* Acute renal failure associated with mannitol intoxication. *Arch Intern Med* 1984; **144:** 2053–5.
3. Goldwasser P, Fotino S. Acute renal failure following massive mannitol infusion: appropriate response of tubuloglomerular feedback? *Arch Intern Med* 1984; **144:** 2214–16.
4. Rabetoy GM, *et al.* Where the kidney is concerned, how much mannitol is too much? *Ann Pharmacother* 1993; **27:** 25–8.
5. Matsumura M. Mannitol-induced toxicity in a diabetic patient receiving losartan. *Am J Med* 2001; **110:** 331.

**Overdosage.** Severe mannitol intoxication was reported in 8 patients with renal failure who had received large, and sometimes enormous, amounts of mannitol intravenously over 1 to 3 days.[1] These patients had CNS involvement out of proportion to uraemia, severe hyponatraemia, a large osmolality gap, and fluid overload. Six patients were treated with haemodialysis and this was considered to be more effective than peritoneal dialysis, which was used in 1 patient.

1. Borges HF, *et al.* Mannitol intoxication in patients with renal failure. *Arch Intern Med* 1982; **142:** 63–6.

### Precautions

Mannitol is contra-indicated in patients with pulmonary congestion or pulmonary oedema, intracranial bleeding (except during craniotomy), heart failure (in patients with diminished cardiac reserve, expansion of the extracellular fluid may lead to fulminating heart failure), and in patients with renal failure unless a test dose has produced a diuretic response (if urine flow is inadequate, expansion of the extracellular fluid may lead to acute water intoxication).

Mannitol should not be given with whole blood.

All patients given mannitol should be carefully observed for signs of fluid and electrolyte imbalance and renal function should be monitored.

### Pharmacokinetics

Only small amounts of mannitol are absorbed from the gastrointestinal tract. Following intravenous injection mannitol is excreted rapidly by the kidneys before any very significant metabolism can take place in the liver. Mannitol does not cross the blood-brain barrier or penetrate the eye. An elimination half-life of about 100 minutes has been reported.

### Uses and Administration

Mannitol is an osmotic agent. Although an isomer of sorbitol, it has little energy value, since it is largely eliminated from the body before any metabolism can take place.

Mannitol is mainly used, with adequate rehydration, to increase urine flow in patients with acute renal failure and to reduce raised intracranial pressure (p.833) and treat cerebral oedema. It is also used in the short-term management of glaucoma (p.1485), especially to reduce intra-ocular pressure prior to ophthalmic surgery, and to promote the excretion of toxic substances by forced diuresis.

Other indications include bladder irrigation during transurethral resection of the prostate in order to reduce haemolysis and oral administration as an osmotic laxative for bowel preparation. Mannitol is used as a diluent and excipient in pharmaceutical preparations and as a bulk sweetener.

When given parenterally, mannitol raises the osmotic pressure of the plasma thus drawing water out of body tissues and producing an osmotic diuresis. Reduction of CSF and intra-ocular fluid pressure occurs within 15 minutes of the start of a mannitol infusion and lasts for 3 to 8 hours after the infusion is discontinued; diuresis occurs after 1 to 3 hours.

When used as an osmotic diuretic, mannitol is administered by intravenous infusion. Careful monitoring of fluid balance, electrolytes, renal function, and vital signs is necessary during infusion to prevent fluid and electrolyte imbalance, including circulatory overload and tissue dehydration. Solutions containing more than 15% of mannitol may crystallise during storage, particularly at low temperatures; crystals may be redissolved by warming before use; the administration set should include a filter.

Mannitol may be used to treat patients in the oliguric phase of **renal failure** or those suspected of inadequate renal function after correction of plasma volume, provided a test dose of about 200 mg/kg given by rapid intravenous infusion of a 15 to 25% solution over 3 to 5 minutes produces a diuresis of at least 30 to 50 mL/hour during the next 2 to 3 hours; a second test dose is permitted if the response to the first is inadequate. The usual adult dose of mannitol ranges from 50 to 100 g in a 24 hour period, given by intravenous infusion of a 5 to 25% solution. The rate of administration is usually adjusted to maintain a urine flow of at least 30 to 50 mL/hour.

For children, a dose of 0.25 to 2 g/kg has been used.

The total dosage, the concentration, and the rate of administration depend on the fluid requirement, the urinary output, and the nature and severity of the condition being treated. Mannitol infusion has also been used to prevent acute renal failure during cardiovascular and other types of surgery, or following trauma.

To reduce **raised intracranial** or **intra-ocular pressure** mannitol may be given by intravenous infusion as a 15 to 25% solution in a dose of 0.25 to 2 g/kg over 30 to 60 minutes. Rebound increases in intracranial or intra-ocular pressure may occur but are less frequent than with urea.

During **transurethral prostatic resection** a 2.5 to 5% solution of mannitol has been used for irrigating the bladder.

**Ciguatera poisoning.** Ciguatera poisoning occurs as a result of the consumption of certain fish contaminated with ciguatoxin found throughout the Caribbean and Indopacific; it is increasingly seen in Europe, in travellers returning from these areas, or as a result of eating imported fish. Symptoms can be severe, including a bizarre reversal of hot and cold sensation. Some neurological symptoms, pruritus, arthralgia, and fatigue, may persist for years.[1] Treatment is usually symptomatic since there is no specific antidote. Dramatic reversal of neuromuscular symptoms with slower resolution of gastrointestinal upset has been reported following administration of mannitol 1 g/kg by intravenous infusion over 30 to 45 minutes in the acute phase of the illness.[2-4] Treatment with mannitol may also be beneficial up to a week after poisoning.[5] However, a double-blind trial[6] found mannitol to be no better than normal saline at relieving symptoms at 24 hours. Amitriptyline has been found on several occasions[7-9] to relieve neurological symptoms (dysaesthesias and paraesthesias) and pruritus. Gabapentin has also been reported to be of benefit.[10]


1. Lehane L. Ciguatera update. *Med J Aust* 2000; **172:** 176–9.
2. Palafox NA, *et al.* Successful treatment of ciguatera fish poisoning with intravenous mannitol. *JAMA* 1988; **259:** 2740–2.
3. Pearn JH, *et al.* Ciguatera and mannitol: experience with a new treatment regimen. *Med J Aust* 1989; **151:** 77–80.
4. Williamson J. Ciguatera and mannitol: a successful treatment. *Med J Aust* 1990; **153:** 306–7.
5. Fenner PJ, *et al.* A Queensland family with ciguatera after eating coral trout. *Med J Aust* 1997; **166:** 473–5.
6. Schnorf H, *et al.* Ciguatera fish poisoning: a double-blind randomized trial of mannitol therapy. *Neurology* 2002; **58:** 873–80.
7. Bowman PB. Amitriptyline and ciguatera. *Med J Aust* 1984; **140:** 802.
8. Davis RT, Villar LA. Symptomatic improvement with amitriptyline in ciguatera fish poisoning. *N Engl J Med* 1986; **315:** 65.
9. Calvert GM, *et al.* Treatment of ciguatera fish poisoning with amitriptyline and nifedipine. *J Toxicol Clin Toxicol* 1987; **25:** 423–8.
10. Perez CM, *et al.* Treatment of ciguatera poisoning with gabapentin. *N Engl J Med* 2001; **344:** 692–3.


**Gastrointestinal disorders.** BOWEL PREPARATION. Mannitol, 1000 mL of a 10% solution or 500 mL of 10 or 20% solution by mouth, has been used to prepare the bowel for surgical and diagnostic procedures.[1,2] The potential for formation of explosive gas in the bowel should be borne in mind (see under Adverse Effects, above).


1. Palmer KR, Khan AN. Oral mannitol: a simple and effective bowel preparation for barium enema. *BMJ* 1979; **2:** 1038.
2. Newstead GL, Morgan BP. Bowel preparation with mannitol. *Med J Aust* 1979; **2:** 582–3.


DIAGNOSIS AND TESTING. Mannitol has been used with lactulose[1,2] and with cellobiose[3,4] in the detection of abnormal small bowel permeability, particularly that occurring in coeliac disease. For further information on the use of differential sugar absorption tests, see Lactulose, p.1269.


1. Pearson ADJ, *et al.* The gluten challenge—biopsy v permeability. *Arch Dis Child* 1983; **58:** 653.
2. Cooper BT. Intestinal permeability in coeliac disease. *Lancet* 1983; **i:** 658–9.
3. Juby LD, *et al.* Cellobiose/mannitol sugar test—a sensitive tubeless test for coeliac disease: results on 1010 unselected patients. *Gut* 1989; **30:** 476–80.
4. Hodges S, *et al.* Cellobiose: mannitol differential permeability in small bowel disease. *Arch Dis Child* 1989; **64:** 853–5.


### Preparations

***BP 2003:*** Mannitol Intravenous Infusion;
***USP 27:*** Mannitol in Sodium Chloride Injection; Mannitol Injection.

**Proprietary Preparations** (details are given in Part 3)
***Austral.:*** Mede-Prep; Osmitrol; ***Austria:*** Osmofundin 20%; ***Canad.:*** Osmitrol; ***Fr.:*** Manicol†; ***Ger.:*** Mannit-Losung; Osmofundin 15% N; Osmosteril 20%; Thomaemannit; ***Ital.:*** Isotol; Mannistol; ***Mex.:*** Osmorol; ***NZ:*** Mede-Prep; Resectisol†; ***Port.:*** Osmofundina; ***Spain:*** Osmofundina Concentrada; ***Switz.:*** Mannite; ***Thai.:*** Maniton; ***USA:*** Osmitrol; Resectisol.

**Multi-ingredient:** ***Austria:*** Osmofundin 10%; Resectal; ***Chile:*** Gelsolets; ***Fin.:*** Somanol + Ethanol; ***Ger.:*** Freka-Drainjet Purisole; Osmofundin 10%†; Osmosteril 10%; ***Hong Kong:*** Lederscon†; ***Ital.:*** Levoplus; Naturalass; ***Port.:*** Purisole; Xarope de Macas Rainetas; ***Spain:*** Jorkil†; Osmofundina†; Salcedogen†; Salcemetic; Salmagne; ***Swed.:*** Somanol†; ***Switz.:*** Bigasan†; Cital; Purisole†.

## Mebutamate *(BAN, USAN, rINN)*

Mebutamato; W-583. 2-sec-Butyl-2-methyltrimethylene dicarbamate.

$C_{10}H_{20}N_2O_4$ = 232.3.
*CAS — 64-55-1.*
*ATC — N05BC04.*

### Profile

Mebutamate is a carbamate with general properties similar to those of meprobamate (p.706). It has been given by mouth as an adjunct in the treatment of hypertension.

### Preparations

**Proprietary Preparations** (details are given in Part 3)
***Ital.:*** Sigmafon†.

## Mebutizide *(rINN)*

Mebutizida. 6-Chloro-3-(1,2-dimethylbutyl)-3,4-dihydro-2*H*-1,2,4-benzothiadiazine-7-sulphonamide 1,1-dioxide.

$C_{13}H_{20}ClN_3O_4S_2$ = 381.9.
*CAS — 3568-00-1.*
*ATC — C03AA13.*

### Profile

Mebutizide is a thiazide diuretic (see Hydrochlorothiazide, p.933) that has been used in the treatment of oedema and hypertension.

### Preparations

**Proprietary Preparations** (details are given in Part 3)
***Belg.:*** Neoniagar†.
**Multi-ingredient:** ***Spain:*** Triniagar†.

## Mecamylamine Hydrochloride *(BANM, rINNM)*

Hidrocloruro de mecamilamina; Mecamine Hydrochloride. *N*-Methyl-2,3,3-trimethylbicyclo[2.2.1]hept-2-ylamine hydrochloride.

$C_{11}H_{21}N,HCl$ = 203.8.
*CAS — 60-40-2 (mecamylamine); 826-39-1 (mecamylamine hydrochloride).*
*ATC — C02BB01.*

**Pharmacopoeias.** In *US.*

**USP 27** (Mecamylamine Hydrochloride). Store in airtight containers.

### Adverse Effects, Treatment, and Precautions

As for Trimetaphan Camsilate, p.1017. The administration of mecamylamine may also cause tremor, convulsions, choreiform movements, insomnia, sedation, dysarthria, and mental aberrations.

### Pharmacokinetics

Mecamylamine hydrochloride is almost completely absorbed from the gastrointestinal tract. It crosses the placenta and the blood-brain barrier. About 50% of the dose is excreted unchanged in the urine over 24 hours, but the rate is diminished in alkaline urine.

### Uses and Administration

Mecamylamine hydrochloride is a ganglion blocker with actions similar to those of trimetaphan (p.1017). It is used in the management of hypertension (p.825), although other antihypertensives with fewer adverse effects are preferred.

The usual initial dosage is 2.5 mg twice daily by mouth, gradually increased or decreased, usually in steps of 2.5 mg at intervals of not less than 2 days, until a satisfactory response is obtained. The average maintenance dose is 25 mg daily in three divided doses. Tolerance may develop.

◊ Reviews.


1. Young JM, *et al.* Mecamylamine: new therapeutic uses and toxicity/risk profile. *Clin Ther* 2001; **23:** 532–65.


**Smoking cessation.** Mecamylamine acts centrally as a nicotinic antagonist and might be of some benefit in assisting withdrawal from smoking. Two studies[1,2] have shown that addition of oral mecamylamine therapy appeared to enhance the effectiveness of nicotine skin patches. Smoking cessation is discussed under Nicotine, p.1721.


1. Rose JE, *et al.* Mecamylamine combined with nicotine skin patch facilitates smoking cessation beyond nicotine patch treatment alone. *Clin Pharmacol Ther* 1994; **56:** 86–99.
2. Rose JE, *et al.* Nicotine-mecamylamine treatment for smoking cessation: the role of pre-cessation therapy. *Exp Clin Psychopharmacol* 1998; **6:** 331–43.


**Tourette's syndrome.** Mecamylamine has been tried[1-3] in the management of Tourette's syndrome (see under Tics, p.664) although results have been mixed.


1. Sanberg PR, *et al.* Treatment of Tourette's syndrome with mecamylamine. *Lancet* 1998; **352:** 705–6.
2. Silver AA, *et al.* Mecamylamine in Tourette's syndrome: a two-year retrospective case study. *J Child Adolesc Psychopharmacol* 2000; **10:** 59–68.
3. Silver AA, *et al.* Multicenter, double-blind, placebo-controlled study of mecamylamine monotherapy for Tourette's disorder. *J Am Acad Child Adolesc Psychiatry* 2001; **40:** 1103–10.


### Preparations

***USP 27:*** Mecamylamine Hydrochloride Tablets.

**Proprietary Preparations** (details are given in Part 3)
***USA:*** Inversine.

## Mefruside *(BAN, USAN, rINN)*

Bay-1500; FBA-1500; Mefrusida. 4-Chloro-$N^1$-methyl-$N^1$-(tetrahydro-2-methylfurfuryl)benzene-1,3-disulphonamide.

$C_{13}H_{19}ClN_2O_5S_2$ = 382.9.
*CAS — 7195-27-9.*
*ATC — C03BA05.*

**Pharmacopoeias.** In *Jpn.*

### Profile

Mefruside is a diuretic with properties similar to those of the thiazide diuretics (see Hydrochlorothiazide, p.933) even though it does not contain a thiazide ring system. It is used for oedema, including that associated with heart failure (p.820), and for hypertension (p.825).

Diuresis is initiated in about 2 to 4 hours and reaches a maximum between 6 and 12 hours.

In the treatment of oedema the usual dose is 25 to 50 mg daily by mouth, increasing if necessary to 75 to 100 mg. For long-term therapy a dose of 25 to 50 mg every second or third day is preferable.

In the treatment of hypertension the usual dose is 25 mg daily, either alone, or with other antihypertensives; initial doses of 25 to 50 mg daily have been recommended; alternate-day maintenance dosage may be used.

### Preparations

**Proprietary Preparations** (details are given in Part 3)
**Denm.:** Baycaron†; **Irl.:** Baycaron†; **Neth.:** Baycaron; **Norw.:** Baycaron†; **UK:** Baycaron†.
**Multi-ingredient: Ger.:** Bendigon N; duranifin Sali; Nifehexal Sali†; Sali-Adalat; Sali-Prent.

## Meglutol *(USAN, rINN)*

CB-337. 3-Hydroxy-3-methylglutaric acid.
$C_6H_{10}O_5$ = 162.1.
*CAS — 503-49-1.*
*ATC — C10AX05.*

### Profile

Meglutol is a lipid regulating drug used in the treatment of hyperlipidaemias (p.823). The usual dose is 1.5 to 3 g daily in divided doses by mouth.

### Preparations

**Proprietary Preparations** (details are given in Part 3)
**Ital.:** Mevalon.

## Melagatran *(rINN)*

H-319/68. N-[(R)-({(2S)-2-[(p-Amidinobenzyl)carbamoyl]-1-azetidinyl}carbonyl)cyclohexylmethyl]glycine.
$C_{22}H_{31}N_5O_4$ = 429.5.
*CAS — 159776-70-2.*
*ATC — B01AE04.*

## Ximelagatran *(USAN, rINN)*

H-376/95. Ethyl N-{(R)-cyclohexyl[((2S)-2-{[4-(hydroxycarbamimidoyl)benzyl]carbamoyl}-1-azetidinyl)carbonyl]methyl}glycinate.
$C_{24}H_{35}N_5O_5$ = 473.6.
*CAS — 192939-46-1.*
*ATC — B01AE05.*

### Profile

Melagatran, the active metabolite of ximelagatran, is a direct thrombin inhibitor that is under investigation as an anticoagulant in the management of venous thromboembolism and other thromboembolic disorders. It is given orally as ximelagatran or subcutaneously as melagatran.

◊ References.


1. Eriksson BI, *et al.* Ximelagatran and melagatran compared with dalteparin for prevention of venous thromboembolism after total hip or knee replacement: the METHRO II randomised trial. *Lancet* 2002; **360:** 1441–7.
2. Wallentin L, *et al.* Oral ximelagatran for secondary prophylaxis after myocardial infarction: the ESTEEM randomised controlled trial. *Lancet* 2003; **362:** 789–97.
3. Executive Steering Committee on behalf of the SPORTIF III Investigations. Stroke prevention with the oral direct thrombin inhibitor ximelagatran compared with warfarin in patients with non-valvular atrial fibrillation (SPORTIF III): randomised controlled trial. *Lancet* 2003; **362:** 1691–8.
4. Eriksson BI, *et al.* The direct thrombin inhibitor melagatran followed by oral ximelagatran compared with enoxaparin for the prevention of venous thromboembolism after total hip or knee replacement: the EXPRESS study. *J Thromb Haemost* 2003; **1:** 2490–6.


## Mephentermine Sulfate *(rINNM)*

Mephentermine Sulphate *(BANM)*; Mephentermini Sulfas; Mephetedrine Sulphate; Sulfato de Mefentermina; Sulfato de mefenterminа. N,α,α-Trimethylphenethylamine sulphate dihydrate.
$(C_{11}H_{17}N)_2,H_2SO_4,2H_2O$ = 460.6.
*CAS — 100-92-5 (mephentermine); 1212-72-2 (anhydrous mephentermine sulfate); 6190-60-9 (mephentermine sulfate dihydrate).*
*ATC — C01CA11.*

### Adverse Effects, Treatment, and Precautions

Mephentermine may produce CNS stimulation, especially in overdosage; anxiety, drowsiness, incoherence, hallucinations, and convulsions have been reported.

The hypertensive effects of mephentermine may be treated with an alpha blocker such as phentolamine mesilate.

For the adverse effects of sympathomimetics in general, and precautions to be observed, see Adrenaline, p.852.

### Interactions

For the interactions of sympathomimetics in general, see Adrenaline, p.853.

### Pharmacokinetics

Mephentermine acts in about 5 to 15 minutes following intramuscular injection and has a duration of action of up to about 4 hours; it acts almost immediately following intravenous injection with a duration of action of up to about 30 minutes. It is rapidly metabolised in the body by demethylation; hydroxylation may follow. It is excreted as unchanged drug and metabolites in the urine; excretion is more rapid in acidic urine.

### Uses and Administration

Mephentermine is a sympathomimetic (see Adrenaline, p.854) with mainly indirect effects on adrenergic receptors. It has alpha- and beta-adrenergic activity, and a slight stimulating effect on the CNS. It has an inotropic effect on the heart.

Mephentermine has been used to maintain blood pressure in hypotensive states, for example following spinal anaesthesia. It is given as the sulfate but doses are expressed in terms of the base; 21 mg of sulfate is approximately equivalent to 15 mg of base. Typical doses are up to 45 mg by slow intravenous injection, or 15 to 30 mg intramuscularly.

### Preparations

**Proprietary Preparations** (details are given in Part 3)
**India:** Mephentine; **USA:** Wyamine.
**Multi-ingredient: USA:** Emergent-Ez.

## Mepindolol Sulfate *(rINNM)*

LF-17895 (mepindolol); Mepindolol Sulphate *(BANM)*; SHE-222; Sulfato de mepindolol. 1-Isopropylamino-3-(2-methylindol-4-yloxy)propan-2-ol sulfate.
$(C_{15}H_{22}N_2O_2)_2,H_2SO_4$ = 622.8.
*CAS — 23694-81-7 (mepindolol); 56396-94-2 (mepindolol sulfate).*
*ATC — C07AA14.*

### Profile

Mepindolol, the methyl analogue of pindolol, is a non-cardioselective beta blocker (p.868). It is reported to possess intrinsic sympathomimetic activity.

Mepindolol is used by mouth as the sulfate in the management of various cardiovascular disorders in usual doses of 2.5 to 10 mg daily.

### Preparations

**Proprietary Preparations** (details are given in Part 3)
**Austria:** Corindolan†; **Ger.:** Corindolan; **Ital.:** Betagon†.
**Multi-ingredient: Ger.:** Corindocomb.

## Mersalyl Acid

Acidum Mersalylicum; Mersal. Acid; Mersálico, ácido; Mersalylum Acidum. A mixture of {3-[2-(carboxymethoxy)benzamido]-2-methoxypropyl}hydroxymercury and its anhydrides.
$C_{13}H_{17}HgNO_6$ = 483.9.
*CAS — 486-67-9.*
*ATC — C03BC01.*

## Mersalyl Sodium

Mersalyl *(pINN)*; Mersalilo. The sodium salt of mersalyl acid.
$C_{13}H_{16}HgNNaO_6$ = 505.8.
*CAS — 492-18-2.*
*ATC — C03BC01.*

### Profile

Mersalyl acid, in the form of its salts, is a powerful diuretic that acts on the renal tubules, increasing the excretion of sodium and chloride, in approximately equal amounts, and of water. Organic mercurial diuretics were widely used before the introduction of thiazide and other diuretics but have now been almost completely superseded by these orally active drugs, which are both potent and less toxic. The most frequently occurring adverse effects of mersalyl are stomatitis, gastric disturbance, vertigo, febrile reactions, and skin eruptions and irritation. Thrombocytopenia, neutropenia, and agranulocytosis have followed the use of mercurial diuretics. Intravenous injection may cause severe hypotension and cardiac arrhythmias and has been followed by sudden death.

Mersalyl acid was usually given by injection as the sodium salt with theophylline as this lessened the local irritant reaction and increased absorption. It was given by deep intramuscular injection after a test dose for hypersensitivity. Other organic mercurial diuretics include chlormerodrin, meralluride, mercaptomerin sodium, mercurophylline sodium, and merethoxylline procaine. They were mainly administered by intramuscular injection or, for those which were less irritant, subcutaneous injection.

## Metaraminol Tartrate *(BANM, rINNM)*

Hydroxynorephedrine Bitartrate; Metaradrine Bitartrate; Metaraminol Acid Tartrate; Metaraminol Bitartrate; Tartrato de metaraminol. (−)-2-Amino-1-(3-hydroxyphenyl)propan-1-ol hydrogen tartrate.
$C_9H_{13}NO_2,C_4H_6O_6$ = 317.3.
*CAS — 54-49-9 (metaraminol); 33402-03-8 (metaraminol tartrate).*
*ATC — C01CA09.*

**Pharmacopoeias.** In *Br., Chin.,* and *US.*

**BP 2003** (Metaraminol Tartrate). An odourless or almost odourless, white, crystalline powder. Freely soluble in water; sparingly soluble in alcohol; practically insoluble in chloroform and in ether. A 5% solution in water has a pH of 3.2 to 3.5.

**USP 27** (Metaraminol Bitartrate). A 5% solution in water has a pH of between 3.2 and 3.5. Store at a temperature of 25°, excursions permitted between 15° and 30°.

### Adverse Effects, Treatment, and Precautions

Metaraminol has a longer duration of action than adrenaline or noradrenaline and therefore an excessive vasopressor response may cause a prolonged rise in blood pressure. Tachycardia or other arrhythmias may also occur. Metaraminol may reduce placental perfusion and should be avoided during pregnancy.

The hypertensive effects of metaraminol may be treated with an alpha blocker such as phentolamine.

Tissue necrosis can occur as a result of accidental extravasation during intravenous injection. Infiltration with phentolamine may be beneficial if extravasation occurs.

For the adverse effects of sympathomimetics in general, and precautions to be observed, see Adrenaline, p.852.

### Interactions

For the interactions of sympathomimetics in general, see Adrenaline, p.853.

### Pharmacokinetics

Metaraminol acts about 10 minutes after intramuscular injection with a duration of action of up to about 1 hour. Effects are seen 1 to 2 minutes after intravenous injection with a duration of action of about 20 minutes.

### Uses and Administration

Metaraminol is a sympathomimetic (see Adrenaline, p.854) with direct and indirect effects on adrenergic receptors. It has alpha- and beta-adrenergic activity, the former being predominant. Metaraminol has an inotropic effect and acts as a peripheral vasoconstrictor, thus increasing cardiac output, peripheral resistance, and blood pressure. Coronary blood flow is increased and the heart rate slowed.

Metaraminol tartrate is used for its pressor action in **hypotensive states** such as those that may occur following spinal anaesthesia. Doses are expressed in terms of the base; metaraminol tartrate 9.5 mg is approximately equivalent to 5 mg of metaraminol. An intravenous infusion of 15 to 100 mg of metaraminol in 500 mL of glucose 5% or sodium chloride 0.9% may be used for maintaining the blood pressure, the rate of administration being adjusted according to blood pressure response. Higher concentrations have been given. As the maximum effects are not immediately apparent, at least 10 minutes should elapse before increasing the dose and the possibility of a cumulative effect should be borne in mind. In an emergency an initial dose of 0.5 to 5 mg may be given by direct intravenous injection followed by an intravenous infusion as above.

Metaraminol tartrate has also been given by intramuscular or subcutaneous injection for the prevention of hypotension in doses equivalent to 2 to 10 mg of metaraminol. Subcutaneous injection increases the risk of local tissue necrosis and sloughing.

**Priapism.** Metaraminol in low dosage and dilute solution, by intracavernosal injection, has been used successfully to treat priapism associated with a variety of conditions; these have included drug-induced priapism,[1] as a complication of chronic myeloid leukaemia,[2] associated with haemodialysis,[3] and during spinal block[4] or fentanyl-induced general anaesthesia.[4] It may be used to reverse the effects of alprostadil or papaverine given for the management of some types of erectile dysfunction. However, this use of metaraminol by intracavernosal injection has been associated with fatal hypertensive crisis (see also Alprostadil, p.1513).

Alternatives include the use of corporal aspiration followed by intracavernosal phenylephrine in low dosage and dilute solution in patients with low-flow priapism (due to decreased penile venous outflow);[5] in high-flow priapism (due to increased arterial inflow), which is less of an emergency, embolisation of the source of abnormal inflow is used. Surgery is usually favoured in low-flow priapism unresponsive to drug therapy. Phenylpropanolamine[5] and pseudoephedrine[6] have both been given by mouth as an alternative to phenylephrine or metaraminol injection. Intracavernosal irrigation with a dilute adrenaline solution or intracavernosal injection of etilefrine have been used for priapism caused by sickle-cell disease (see p.855); oral etilefrine has been used for prophylaxis.


1. Brindley GS. New treatment for priapism. *Lancet* 1984; **ii:** 220–1.

2. Stanners A, Colin-Jones D. Metaraminol for priapism. *Lancet* 1984; **ii:** 978.
3. Branger B, *et al.* Metaraminol for haemodialysis-associated priapism. *Lancet* 1985; **i:** 641.
4. Tsai SK, Hong CY. Intracavernosal metaraminol for treatment of intraoperative penile erection. *Postgrad Med J* 1990; **66:** 831–3.
5. Harmon WJ, Nehra A. Priapism: diagnosis and management. *Mayo Clin Proc* 1997; **72:** 350–5.
6. Millard RJ, *et al.* Risks of self-injection therapy for impotence. *Med J Aust* 1996; **165:** 117–18.


### Preparations

**BP 2003:** Metaraminol Injection;
**USP 27:** Metaraminol Bitartrate Injection.

**Proprietary Preparations** (details are given in Part 3)
**Arg.:** Fadamine; **Austral.:** Aramine; **Belg.:** Aramine†; **Braz.:** Aramin; **Gr.:** Aramine; **Hong Kong:** Aramine†; **Ital.:** Levicor†; **Norw.:** Aramine; **NZ:** Aramine; **Thai.:** Aramine; **UK:** Aramine†; **USA:** Aramine.

## Methazolamide *(BAN, rINN)*

Metazolamida. *N*-(4-Methyl-2-sulphamoyl-$\Delta^2$-1,3,4-thiadiazolin-5-ylidene)acetamide.

$C_5H_8N_4O_3S_2$ = 236.3.
*CAS — 554-57-4.*

**Pharmacopoeias.** In *US.*

**USP 27** (Methazolamide). A white or faintly yellow crystalline powder with a slight odour. Very slightly soluble in water and in alcohol; slightly soluble in acetone; soluble in dimethylformamide. Protect from light.

### Adverse Effects and Precautions

As for Acetazolamide, p.849.

◊ Cholestatic hepatitis with jaundice, rash, and subsequent pure red cell aplasia was associated with methazolamide in a patient.[1] Drug-induced hypersensitivity was suspected as the cause of the reaction.

1. Krivoy N, *et al.* Methazolamide-induced hepatitis and pure RBC aplasia. *Arch Intern Med* 1981; **141:** 1229–30.

### Pharmacokinetics

Methazolamide is absorbed from the gastrointestinal tract more slowly than acetazolamide. It has been reported not to be extensively bound to plasma protein, and to have a half-life of about 14 hours. About 15 to 30% of the dose is excreted in the urine; the fate of the remainder is unknown.

### Uses and Administration

Methazolamide is an inhibitor of carbonic anhydrase with actions similar to those of acetazolamide (p.850). It is used in the management of glaucoma (p.1485) in doses of 50 to 100 mg two or three times daily by mouth. Its action is less prompt but of longer duration than that of acetazolamide, lasting for 10 to 18 hours.

The diuretic activity of methazolamide is less pronounced than that of acetazolamide.

### Preparations

**USP 27:** Methazolamide Tablets.

**Proprietary Preparations** (details are given in Part 3)
**Arg.:** Glaumetax; **Austral.:** Neptazane†; **Canad.:** Neptazane; **Israel:** Neptazane; **Thai.:** Neptazane; **USA:** GlaucTabs†; MZM; Neptazane†.

## Methoxamine Hydrochloride *(BANM, rINNM)*

Hidrocloruro de metoxamina; Methoxamedrine Hydrochloride. 2-Amino-1-(2,5-dimethoxyphenyl)propan-1-ol hydrochloride.

$C_{11}H_{17}NO_3,HCl$ = 247.7.
*CAS — 390-28-3 (methoxamine); 61-16-5 (methoxamine hydrochloride).*
*ATC — C01CA10.*

**Pharmacopoeias.** In *Br.* and *Chin.*

**BP 2003** (Methoxamine Hydrochloride). Colourless crystals or white plate-like crystals or white crystalline powder; odourless or almost odourless. Freely soluble in water; soluble in alcohol; very slightly soluble in chloroform and in ether. A 2% solution in water has a pH of 4.0 to 6.0.

### Profile

Methoxamine is a sympathomimetic (see Adrenaline, p.854) with mainly direct effects on adrenergic receptors. It has alpha-adrenergic activity entirely; beta-adrenergic activity is not demonstrable and beta-adrenoceptor blockade has been postulated. Methoxamine hydrochloride has been used parenterally for its pressor action in the management of hypotensive states, particularly in anaesthesia, and also in the management of paroxysmal supraventricular tachycardia. It has also been used topically as a vasoconstrictor in the management of nasal congestion.

### Preparations

**BP 2003:** Methoxamine Injection.

**Proprietary Preparations** (details are given in Part 3)
**Canad.:** Vasoxyl†; **Irl.:** Vasoxine; **UK:** Vasoxine†; **USA:** Vasoxyl†.

## Methyclothiazide *(BAN, USAN, rINN)*

Meticlotiazida; NSC-110431. 6-Chloro-3-chloromethyl-3,4-dihydro-2-methyl-2*H*-1,2,4-benzothiadiazine-7-sulphonamide 1,1-dioxide.

$C_9H_{11}Cl_2N_3O_4S_2$ = 360.2.
*CAS — 135-07-9.*
*ATC — C03AA08.*

**Pharmacopoeias.** In *US.*

**USP 27** (Methyclothiazide). A white or practically white crystalline powder, odourless or with a slight odour. Very slightly soluble to practically insoluble in water and in chloroform; soluble 1 in 92.5 of alcohol and 1 in 2700 of ether; freely soluble in acetone and in pyridine; sparingly soluble in methyl alcohol; very slightly soluble in benzene.

### Profile

Methyclothiazide is a thiazide diuretic with properties similar to those of hydrochlorothiazide (see p.933). It is used for oedema, including that associated with heart failure (p.820), and for hypertension (p.825).

Diuresis starts in about 2 hours, reaches a peak at about 6 hours, and lasts for 24 hours or more.

In the treatment of oedema the usual initial dose is 2.5 to 5 mg by mouth daily, increasing to a maximum dose of 10 mg daily if necessary. In the treatment of hypertension the usual dose is 2.5 to 5 mg daily, either alone, or with other antihypertensives. Doses of up to 10 mg daily have been suggested, but this may not result in an increased hypotensive effect.

Children have been given a dose of 50 to 200 micrograms/kg daily.

### Preparations

**USP 27:** Methyclothiazide Tablets.

**Proprietary Preparations** (details are given in Part 3)
**Austral.:** Enduron†; **Hong Kong:** Enduron; **USA:** Aquatensen; Enduron.
**Multi-ingredient: Fr.:** Isobar; **Hong Kong:** Enduronyl; **Ital.:** Enduronil†; **USA:** Diutensen-R; Enduronyl†.

# Methyldopa *(BAN, USAN, rINN)*

Alpha-methyldopa; Methyldopum; Methyldopum Hydratum; Metildopa; MK-351. (–)-3-(3,4-Dihydroxyphenyl)-2-methyl-L-alanine sesquihydrate; (–)-2-Amino-2-(3,4-dihydroxybenzyl)propionic acid sesquihydrate.

$C_{10}H_{13}NO_4,1\frac{1}{2}H_2O$ = 238.2.
*CAS — 555-30-6 (anhydrous methyldopa); 41372-08-1 (methyldopa sesquihydrate).*
*ATC — C02AB01; C02AB02.*

**Pharmacopoeias.** In *Chin., Eur.* (see p.vi), *Int., Jpn,* and *US.*

**Ph. Eur. 5.0** (Methyldopa). Colourless or almost colourless crystals or a white to yellowish-white crystalline powder. Slightly soluble in water; very slightly soluble in alcohol; freely soluble in dilute mineral acids. Protect from light.

**USP 27** (Methyldopa). A white to yellowish-white odourless fine powder which may contain friable lumps. Sparingly soluble in water; slightly soluble in alcohol; practically insoluble in ether; very soluble in 3N hydrochloric acid. Protect from light.

## Methyldopate Hydrochloride *(BANM, USAN)*

Cloridrato de Metildopato; Hidrocloruro de metildopato. The hydrochloride of the ethyl ester of anhydrous methyldopa; Ethyl (–)-2-amino-2-(3,4-dihydroxybenzyl)propionate hydrochloride.

$C_{12}H_{17}NO_4,HCl$ = 275.7.
*CAS — 2544-09-4 (methyldopate); 2508-79-4 (methyldopate hydrochloride).*

**Pharmacopoeias.** In *Br.* and *US.*

**BP 2003** (Methyldopate Hydrochloride). A white or almost white, odourless or almost odourless, crystalline powder. Freely soluble in water, in alcohol, and in methyl alcohol; slightly soluble in chloroform; practically insoluble in ether. A 1% solution in water has a pH of 3.0 to 5.0. Protect from light.

**USP 27** (Methyldopate Hydrochloride). A white or almost white, odourless or almost odourless, crystalline powder. Freely soluble in water, in alcohol, and in methyl alcohol; slightly soluble in chloroform; practically insoluble in ether. A 1% solution in water has a pH of between 3.0 and 5.0. Store at a temperature of 25°, excursions permitted between 15° and 30°.

**Incompatibility.** A haze developed over 3 hours when methyldopate hydrochloride 1 mg/mL was mixed with amphotericin B 200 micrograms/mL in glucose; crystals were produced with methohexital sodium 200 micrograms/mL in sodium chloride, and a haze developed when they were mixed in glucose. A crystalline precipitate occurred with tetracycline hydrochloride 1 mg/mL in glucose, and with sulfadiazine sodium 4 mg/mL in glucose or sodium chloride.[1]

1. Riley BB. Incompatibilities in intravenous solutions. *J Hosp Pharm* 1970; **28:** 228–40.

### Adverse Effects

The adverse effects of methyldopa are mostly consequences of its pharmacological action. The incidence of adverse effects overall may be as high as 60% but most are transient or reversible. Drowsiness is common, especially initially and following an increase in dosage. Dizziness and lightheadedness may be associated with orthostatic hypotension; nausea, headache, weakness and fatigue, and decreased libido and impotence have also been reported quite frequently.

The mental and neurological effects of methyldopa have included impaired concentration and memory, mild psychoses, depression, disturbed sleep and nightmares, paraesthesias, Bell's palsy, involuntary choreoathetotic movements, and parkinsonism.

In addition to orthostatic hypotension, methyldopa is frequently associated with fluid retention and oedema, which responds to diuretics but may rarely progress to heart failure. Angina pectoris may be aggravated. Bradycardia, syncope, and prolonged carotid sinus hypersensitivity have been reported. Intravenous administration of methyldopate has been associated with a paradoxical rise in blood pressure.

Methyldopa may produce gastrointestinal disturbances including nausea and vomiting, diarrhoea, constipation, and rarely pancreatitis and colitis. A black or sore tongue, and inflammation of the salivary glands, have occurred, and dry mouth is quite common.

A positive Coombs' test may occur in 10 to 20% of all patients on prolonged therapy but only a small proportion develop haemolytic anaemia. Thrombocytopenia and leucopenia, notably granulocytopenia, have occurred and warrant prompt discontinuation. Other hypersensitivity effects have included myocarditis, fever, eosinophilia, and disturbances of liver function. Hepatitis may develop, particularly in the first 2 or 3 months of therapy, and is generally reversible on discontinuation, but fatal hepatic necrosis has occurred. Antinuclear antibodies may develop and cases of a lupus-like syndrome have been reported.

Other adverse effects that have been reported in patients receiving methyldopa include rashes, lichenoid and granulomatous eruptions, toxic epidermal necrolysis, a flu-like syndrome (of fever, myalgia, and mild arthralgia), nocturia, uraemia, nasal congestion, and retroperitoneal fibrosis. Hyperprolactinaemia may occur, with breast enlargement or gynaecomastia, galactorrhoea, and amenorrhoea.

Methyldopa may occasionally cause urine to darken on exposure to the air because of the breakdown of the drug or its metabolites.

◊ Reviews.

1. Furhoff A-K. Adverse reactions with methyldopa—a decade's reports. *Acta Med Scand* 1978; **203:** 425–8.
2. Lawson DH, *et al.* Adverse reactions to methyldopa with particular reference to hypotension. *Am Heart J* 1978; **96:** 572–9.

**Effects on the blood.** An analysis of drug-induced blood dyscrasias reported to the Swedish Adverse Drug Reaction Committee for the 10-year period 1966-75 showed that haemolytic anaemia attributable to methyldopa had been reported on 69 occasions and had caused 3 deaths. This represented the vast majority of all the reports of drug-induced haemolytic anaemia.[1] However, the actual incidence of haemolytic anaemia in patients receiving methyldopa is quite low; data from the Boston Collaborative Drug Surveillance Program indicated that only 2 of 1067 patients receiving methyldopa developed haemolytic anaemia,[2] an incidence of about 0.2%. The proportion of patients with a positive Coombs' test is much higher, being variously reported[3-5] at 10 to 20%. It has been suggested that the high incidence of autoantibody formation may be due to inhibition of suppressor T-cells by methyldopa[4] while the relatively low incidence of resultant haemolysis may be due to drug-associated impairment of the reticuloendothelial system which would normally clear the antibody-sensitised cells from the circulation.[5]

1. Böttiger LE, *et al.* Drug-induced blood dyscrasias. *Acta Med Scand* 1979; **205:** 457–61.
2. Lawson DH, *et al.* Adverse reactions to methyldopa with particular reference to hypotension. *Am Heart J* 1978; **96:** 572–9.
3. Carstairs K, *et al.* Methyldopa and haemolytic anaemia. *Lancet* 1966; **i:** 201.
4. Kirtland HH, *et al.* Methyldopa inhibition of suppressor-lymphocyte function: a proposed cause of autoimmune hemolytic anemia. *N Engl J Med* 1980; **302:** 825–32.
5. Kelton JG. Impaired reticuloendothelial function in patients treated with methyldopa. *N Engl J Med* 1985; **313:** 596–600.

**Effects on the gastrointestinal tract.** COLITIS. There has been a report of 6 cases of colitis associated with methyldopa.[1] An auto-immune mechanism was proposed.

1. Graham CF, *et al.* Acute colitis with methyldopa. *N Engl J Med* 1981; **304:** 1044–5.

DIARRHOEA. Severe chronic diarrhoea over a 2-year period in a 62-year-old woman was associated with methyldopa therapy. Diarrhoea stopped immediately after discontinuation of methyldopa.[1] In another case[2] progressively severe diarrhoea in an elderly senile patient, which had persisted for 7 years, stopped when methyldopa was withdrawn and recurred, after a delay, when the drug was resumed in a lower dose. Discontinuation of methyldopa resulted in complete freedom from diarrhoea and faecal incontinence within 7 days.

1. Quart BD, Guglielmo BJ. Prolonged diarrhea secondary to methyldopa therapy. *Drug Intell Clin Pharm* 1983; **17:** 462.
2. Gloth FM, Busby MJ. Methyldopa-induced diarrhea: a case of iatrogenic diarrhea leading to request for nursing home placement. *Am J Med* 1989; **87:** 480–1.

PANCREATITIS. Increases in serum- and urinary-amylase activity accompanied by fever and suggestive of pancreatitis were associated with methyldopa in 2 patients,[1] one of whom had symptoms of severe pancreatitis. Symptoms reappeared on rechallenge in both patients. A further report of acute pancreatitis in a patient who had recently begun methyldopa therapy (with a diuretic) also confirmed a recurrence of symptoms on rechallenge.[2] In contrast to the acute form, chronic pancreatitis is not generally attributable to drug use.[3] However, a case of florid chronic pancreatitis, with exocrine and endocrine insufficiency and heavy calcification over 30 months, associated with 2 periods of methyldopa treatment, has been reported.[4] Symptoms in this patient, who was also receiving a thiazide, included severe diabetic ketoacidosis.

1. van der Heide H, *et al.* Pancreatitis caused by methyldopa. *BMJ* 1981; **282:** 1930–1.
2. Anderson JR, *et al.* Drug-associated recurrent pancreatitis. *Dig Surg* 1985; **2:** 24–6.
3. Banergee AK, *et al.* Drug-induced acute pancreatitis. *Med Toxicol Adverse Drug Exp* 1989; **4:** 186–98.
4. Ramsay LE, *et al.* Methyldopa-induced chronic pancreatitis. *Practitioner* 1982; **226:** 1166–9.

**Effects on the heart.** Sudden death in a number of patients receiving methyldopa has been associated with myocarditis, often in association with hepatitis and pneumonitis.[1,2] The effect is thought to be due to hypersensitivity. Hypersensitivity myocarditis is generally marked by ECG changes, a slight rise in cardiac enzymes, cardiomegaly, and persistent sinus tachycardia, along with peripheral blood eosinophilia, and most patients will recover within days if the drug is withdrawn in time.[3]

1. Mullick FG, McAllister HA. Myocarditis associated with methyldopa therapy. *JAMA* 1977; **237:** 1699–1701. Correction. *ibid.*; **238:** 399.
2. Seeverens H, *et al.* Myocarditis and methyldopa. *Acta Med Scand* 1982; **211:** 233–5.
3. Anonymous. Myocarditis related to drug hypersensitivity. *Lancet* 1985; **ii:** 1165–6.

**Effects on the liver.** In a report of 6 cases of hepatitis in patients taking methyldopa, including a review of 77 cases from the literature,[1] most patients presented with symptoms including malaise, fatigue, anorexia, weight loss, nausea, and vomiting, and histopathological changes resembling those of viral hepatitis. Fever occurred in 28 of the 83 patients; rashes and eosinophilia occurred rarely. Symptoms usually began 1 to 4 weeks after the first dose of methyldopa. Clinically apparent jaundice occurred as early as 1 week and as late as 3 years after the initiation of therapy, although only 6 or 7 patients presented with jaundice later than 3 months. Liver damage was not dose-related and had features suggestive of an immunologically-mediated hypersensitivity reaction. The histological changes included chronic active hepatitis, massive fatal necrosis, and cirrhosis.

In a further analysis of 36 patients with liver damage due to methyldopa, hepatic injury tended to occur in 2 phases—acute and chronic.[2] Acute liver damage developed within a few months of starting treatment with methyldopa, and was considered to be an allergic reaction to methyldopa metabolites. The chronic form usually occurred at least a year after starting methyldopa, and was characterised by an accumulation of fat in the liver. Recovery after withdrawal of methyldopa was directly related to duration of exposure and degree of liver damage. There was also a suggestion of genetic predisposition, as acute methyldopa-induced liver damage occurred in 4 members of a family. Idiosyncratic metabolism of methyldopa in susceptible patients may be responsible for expression of an antigen on the surface of liver cells with which circulating antibodies react.[3]

See also Fever, below.

1. Rodman JS, *et al.* Methyldopa hepatitis: a report of six cases and review of the literature. *Am J Med* 1976; **60:** 941–8.
2. Sotaniemi EA, *et al.* Hepatic injury and drug metabolism in patients with alpha-methyldopa-induced liver damage. *Eur J Clin Pharmacol* 1977; **12:** 429–35.
3. Neuberger J, *et al.* Antibody mediated hepatocyte injury in methyldopa induced hepatotoxicity. *Gut* 1985; **26:** 1233–9.

**Effects on mental function.** Anecdotal reports have implicated methyldopa in the production of disturbances of mental acuity including inability to concentrate, an impaired calculating ability, and forgetfulness.[1-3] These have been confirmed to some extent by psychometric studies. Impaired verbal memory but not visual memory has been reported in 10 patients receiving methyldopa with a diuretic.[4] A crossover study in 16 patients also indicated impairment of cognitive function by methyldopa.[5]

1. Adler S. Methyldopa-induced decrease in mental activity. *JAMA* 1974; **230:** 1428–9.
2. Ghosh SK. Methyldopa and forgetfulness. *Lancet* 1976; **i:** 202–3.
3. Fernandez PG. Alpha methyldopa and forgetfulness. *Ann Intern Med* 1976; **85:** 128.
4. Solomon S, *et al.* Impairment of memory function by antihypertensive medication. *Arch Gen Psychiatry* 1983; **40:** 1109–12.
5. Johnson B, *et al.* Effects of methyldopa on psychometric performance. *J Clin Pharmacol* 1990; **30:** 1102–5.

DEPRESSION. Depression has been associated with methyldopa therapy, although the exact relationship is unclear.[1] One review[2] reported the incidence to be 3.6% and suggested that depression was more common in patients with a previous history.

1. Patten SB, Love EJ. Drug-induced depression. *Drug Safety* 1994; **10:** 203–19.
2. Paykel ES, *et al.* Psychiatric side effects of antihypertensive drugs other than reserpine. *J Clin Psychopharmacol* 1982; **2:** 14–39.

**Effects on the nervous system.** Involuntary choreoathetotic movements resembling those of Huntington's chorea began in a 59-year-old man with cerebrovascular disease following increase of his methyldopa dose from 1 to 1.5 g daily. He recovered when methyldopa therapy was withdrawn.[1] In another report methyldopa was associated with the development of bilateral choreiform movements in a patient without cerebrovascular disease but with chronic renal failure.[2]

1. Yamadori A, Albert ML. Involuntary movement disorder caused by methyldopa. *N Engl J Med* 1972; **286:** 610.
2. Neil EM, Waters AK. Generalized choreiform movements as a complication of methyldopa therapy in chronic renal failure. *Postgrad Med J* 1981; **57:** 732–3.

**Effects on sexual function.** Methyldopa has been associated with numerous cases of sexual dysfunction. In males failure to maintain erection, decreased libido, impaired ejaculation, and gynaecomastia have occurred, while in females decreased libido, painful breast enlargement, and delayed or absent orgasm have been reported.[1] The reported incidence varies and there is some evidence[2] that sexual dysfunction may be underreported: while only 2 of 30 men receiving methyldopa spontaneously reported erection failure the actual incidence on questioning was 16 of 30.

1. Stevenson JG, Umstead GS. Sexual dysfunction due to antihypertensive agents. *Drug Intell Clin Pharm* 1984; **18:** 113–21.
2. Alexander WD, Evans JI. Side effects of methyldopa. *BMJ* 1975; **2:** 501.

**Fever.** In a report of 78 cases of methyldopa-induced fever,[1] fever occurred 5 to 35 days after the first exposure to methyldopa in 77 patients and one day after recommencing methyldopa in the remaining patient. Rigors, headache, and myalgia were common accompanying symptoms, but eosinophilia and skin rashes were not seen. The majority of patients did not appear seriously ill, but 4 patients presented with symptoms of septic shock. Biochemical evidence of liver damage was found in 61% of patients but jaundice was uncommon. In the majority of patients, symptoms were relieved within 48 hours of the withdrawal of the drug.

1. Stanley P, Mijch A. Methyldopa: an often overlooked cause of fever and transient hepatocellular dysfunction. *Med J Aust* 1986; **144:** 603–5.

**Lupus erythematosus.** The incidence of antinuclear antibodies was 13% in 269 hypertensive patients taking methyldopa (irrespective of other medication), compared with 3.8% in 448 hypertensive patients not taking methyldopa.[1] Apart from the occasional case of methyldopa-induced lupus, however, patients did not appear to be at risk.

1. Wilson JD, *et al.* Antinuclear antibodies in patients receiving non-practolol beta-blockers. *BMJ* 1978; **1:** 14–16.

**Overdosage.** Ingestion of methyldopa 2.5 g produced coma, hypothermia, hypotension, bradycardia, and dry mouth in a 19-year-old man.[1] The serum-methyldopa concentration 10 hours after ingestion was 19.2 micrograms/mL compared with serum concentrations of about 2 micrograms/mL in patients receiving therapeutic doses of methyldopa. The patient recovered following treatment with intravenous fluids.

1. Shnaps Y, *et al.* Methyldopa poisoning. *J Toxicol Clin Toxicol* 1982; **19:** 501–3.

**Retroperitoneal fibrosis.** A 60-year-old patient developed retroperitoneal fibrosis and a positive direct Coombs' test associated with methyldopa given in a daily dose of 750 mg with bendroflumethiazide 2.5 mg for about 5 years.[1]

1. Iversen BM, *et al.* Retroperitoneal fibrosis during treatment with methyldopa. *Lancet* 1975; **ii:** 302–4.

## Treatment of Adverse Effects

Withdrawal of methyldopa or reduction in dosage causes the reversal of many side-effects. If overdosage occurs, patients who present within 1 hour may be given activated charcoal, or the stomach may be emptied by lavage. Treatment is largely symptomatic, but if necessary, intravenous fluid infusions may be given to promote urinary excretion, and vasopressors given cautiously. Atropine may be given for bradycardia. Severe hypotension may respond to placing the patient in the supine position with the feet raised.

Methyldopa is dialysable.

## Precautions

Methyldopa should be used with caution in patients with hepatic or renal impairment or with a history of haemolytic anaemia, liver disease, or depression. Care is also advisable in patients with parkinsonism. It should not be given to patients with active liver disease or depression and it is not recommended for phaeochromocytoma.

It is advisable to make periodic blood counts and to perform liver function tests at intervals during the first 6 to 12 weeks of treatment or if the patient develops an unexplained fever. Patients taking methyldopa may produce a positive response to a direct Coombs' test; if blood transfusion is required, prior knowledge of a positive direct Coombs' test reaction will aid cross-matching.

Methyldopa may cause sedation; if affected, patients should not drive or operate machinery.

**Breast feeding.** Methyldopa is distributed into breast milk in small amounts.[1] In a study[2] of 3 breast-feeding women, concentrations of free methyldopa in the breast milk were found to be between 19 and 30% of those in the plasma after a 500-mg dose. Detectable levels were found in the plasma of only 1 infant and adverse effects were seen in none. It was estimated that the amount of methyldopa a breast-fed infant would receive would be about 0.02% of the maternal dose. In another study[3] over a 3-month period no adverse effects were found in a breast-feeding infant whose mother was taking methyldopa, although the drug was detectable in the infant's urine. The American Academy of Pediatrics considers[4] that methyldopa is therefore usually compatible with breast feeding.

1. Jones HMR, Cummings AJ. A study of the transfer of α-methyldopa to the human foetus and newborn infant. *Br J Clin Pharmacol* 1978; **6:** 432–4.
2. White WB, *et al.* Alpha-methyldopa disposition in mothers with hypertension and in their breast-fed infants. *Clin Pharmacol Ther* 1985; **37:** 387–90.
3. Hauser GJ, *et al.* Effect of α-methyldopa excreted in human milk on the breast-fed infant. *Helv Paediatr Acta* 1985; **40:** 83–6.
4. American Academy of Pediatrics. The transfer of drugs and other chemicals into human milk. *Pediatrics* 2001; **108:** 776–89. Correction. *ibid*; 1029. Also available at: http://aappolicy.aappublications.org/cgi/content/full/pediatrics%3b108/3/776 (accessed 06/07/04)

**Porphyria.** Methyldopa has been associated with acute attacks of porphyria and is considered unsafe in porphyric patients.

**Pregnancy.** Methyldopa is commonly used in the management of hypertension occurring during pregnancy (p.825). There is little evidence of adverse effects on fetal development. However, methyldopa crosses the placenta[1] and reduced blood pressure has been reported in infants born to mothers receiving methyldopa.[2] There has also been a report of tremor in 7 infants associated with maternal methyldopa therapy during pregnancy.[3] Depressed noradrenaline concentrations in the CSF were noted in the 3 infants examined leading to successful treatment of the other 4 infants with atropine: tremor was abolished in 2 and substantially reduced in the other 2 infants.

1. Jones HMR, Cummings AJ. A study of the transfer of α-methyldopa to the human foetus and newborn infant. *Br J Clin Pharmacol* 1978; **6:** 432–4.
2. Whitelaw A. Maternal methyldopa treatment and neonatal blood pressure. *BMJ* 1981; **283:** 471.
3. Bódis J, *et al.* Methyldopa in pregnancy hypertension and the newborn. *Lancet* 1982; **ii:** 498–9.

## Interactions

The hypotensive effects of methyldopa are potentiated by diuretics, other antihypertensives, and drugs with hypotensive effects. However, there have been reports of paradoxical antagonism of the hypotensive effects by tricyclic antidepressants, antipsychotics, and beta blockers. Sympathomimetics may also antagonise the hypotensive effects.

There may be an interaction between methyldopa and MAOIs and care is required if they are given concomitantly. Caution is also needed with entacapone since it might inhibit the metabolism of methyldopa.

Patients receiving methyldopa may require lower doses of general anaesthetics.

**Alpha blockers.** Urinary incontinence occurred on concomitant administration of methyldopa and *phenoxybenzamine* in a patient who had undergone bilateral lumbar sympathectomy.[1]

1. Fernandez PG, *et al.* Urinary incontinence due to interaction of phenoxybenzamine and α-methyldopa. *Can Med Assoc J* 1981; **124:** 174–5.

**Antipsychotics.** Antipsychotics may enhance the hypotensive effects of methyldopa but a paradoxical increase in blood pressure has also been reported. A woman with systemic lupus erythematosus taking *trifluoperazine* up to 15 mg daily and prednisone up to 120 mg daily was given methyldopa up to 2 g and triamterene for high blood pressure.[1] Her blood pressure rose further to 200/140 mmHg. After discontinuation of trifluoperazine blood pressure returned to 160/100 mmHg.

In another report, 2 patients with essential hypertension who had been receiving methyldopa for 3 years and 18 months respectively developed symptoms of dementia within days of concurrent administration of *haloperidol* for anxiety.[2] In both patients the symptoms resolved rapidly on discontinuation of haloperidol.


1. Westervelt FB, Atuk NO. Methyldopa-induced hypertension. *JAMA* 1974; **227:** 557.
2. Thornton WE. Dementia induced by methyldopa with haloperidol. *N Engl J Med* 1976; **294:** 1222.


**Cephalosporins.** A pustular pruritic eruption occurred following administration of *cefazolin* to a patient receiving methyldopa.[1] A previous similar case has been reported in a patient receiving *cefradine* and methyldopa.


1. Stough D, *et al.* Pustular eruptions following administration of cefazolin: a possible interaction with methyldopa. *J Am Acad Dermatol* 1987; **16:** 1051–2.


**Digoxin.** Syncope associated with carotid sinus hypersensitivity has been reported to be possibly enhanced by methyldopa in a patient taking digoxin and chlortalidone.[1] In another report,[2] sinus bradycardia developed in 2 patients taking methyldopa and digoxin concomitantly.


1. Bauernfeind R, *et al.* Carotid sinus hypersensitivity with alpha methyldopa. *Ann Intern Med* 1978; **88:** 214–15.
2. Davis JC, *et al.* Sinus node dysfunction caused by methyldopa and digoxin. *JAMA* 1981; **245:** 1241–3.


**Iron.** Following results in healthy subjects that indicated that the absorption of methyldopa was reduced by 73% and 61% respectively when taken with a dose of *ferrous sulfate* or *ferrous gluconate*, 5 hypertensive patients receiving methyldopa were also given ferrous sulfate 325 mg three times daily for 2 weeks.[1] All patients experienced a rise in systolic pressure, and 4 had a rise in diastolic pressure, associated with ferrous sulfate administration, amounting to more than 15/10 mmHg in some patients after 2 weeks. Blood pressure fell again when the iron therapy was discontinued.


1. Campbell N, *et al.* Alteration of methyldopa absorption, metabolism, and blood pressure control caused by ferrous sulfate and ferrous gluconate. *Clin Pharmacol Ther* 1988; **43:** 381–6.


**Levodopa.** For reference to a mutual interaction between methyldopa and levodopa, see Antihypertensives, under Levodopa, Interactions, p.1208.

**Lithium.** For reference to the development of lithium toxicity on concurrent administration of methyldopa, see p.304.

**Sympathomimetics.** A 31-year-old man whose hypertension was well controlled with methyldopa and oxprenolol suffered a severe hypertensive episode when he took a preparation for a cold containing *phenylpropanolamine*.[1]


1. McLaren EH. Severe hypertension produced by interaction of phenylpropanolamine with methyldopa and oxprenolol. *BMJ* 1976; **2:** 283–4.


## Pharmacokinetics

Following oral administration methyldopa is variably and incompletely absorbed, apparently by an amino-acid active transport system. The mean bioavailability has been reported to be about 50%. It is extensively metabolised and is excreted in urine mainly as unchanged drug and the *O*-sulfate conjugate. It crosses the blood-brain barrier and is decarboxylated in the CNS to active alpha-methylnoradrenaline.

The elimination is biphasic with a half-life of about 1.7 hours in the initial phase; the second phase is more prolonged. Clearance is decreased and half-life prolonged in renal impairment. Plasma protein binding is reported to be minimal. Methyldopa crosses the placenta; small amounts are distributed into breast milk.

## Uses and Administration

Methyldopa is an antihypertensive that is thought to have a mainly central action. It is decarboxylated in the CNS to alpha-methylnoradrenaline, which is thought to stimulate $alpha_2$ adrenoceptors resulting in a reduction in sympathetic tone and a fall in blood pressure. It may also act as a false neurotransmitter, and have some inhibitory actions on plasma renin activity. Methyldopa reduces the tissue concentrations of dopamine, noradrenaline, adrenaline, and serotonin.

Methyldopa is used in the management of hypertension (p.825), although other drugs with fewer adverse effects are generally preferred. Methyldopa may, however, be the treatment of choice for hypertension in pregnancy. Oedema and tolerance sometimes associated with methyldopa therapy may be reduced when it is given with a thiazide diuretic.

Methyldopa is given by mouth as the sesquihydrate, but doses are usually expressed in terms of anhydrous methyldopa. Methyldopa sesquihydrate 1.13 g is approximately equivalent to 1 g of anhydrous methyldopa. For hypertensive crises, methyldopa has been given intravenously as methyldopate hydrochloride.

When methyldopa is given by mouth its effects reach a maximum in 4 to 6 hours following a single dose, although the maximum hypotensive effect may not occur until the second or third day of continuous treatment; some effect is usually apparent for 48 hours after withdrawal of methyldopa. When given intravenously the hypotensive effect may be obtained within 4 to 6 hours and last for 10 to 16 hours. It lowers the standing, and to a lesser extent the supine, blood pressure.

In **hypertension**, the usual initial adult dose by mouth is 250 mg of methyldopa two or three times daily for 2 days; this is then adjusted, not more frequently than every 2 days according to response, up to a usual maximum dose of 3 g daily. The usual maintenance dosage is 0.5 to 2 g of methyldopa daily. In the elderly an initial dose of 125 mg twice daily has been used; this dose may be increased gradually if necessary, but should not exceed 2 g daily.

An initial dose for children is 10 mg/kg daily in 2 to 4 divided doses, increased as necessary to a maximum of 65 mg/kg or 3 g daily, whichever is less.

### Preparations

***BP 2003:*** Methyldopa Tablets; Methyldopate Injection;
***USP 27:*** Methyldopa and Chlorothiazide Tablets; Methyldopa and Hydrochlorothiazide Tablets; Methyldopa Oral Suspension; Methyldopa Tablets; Methyldopate Hydrochloride Injection.

**Proprietary Preparations** (details are given in Part 3)
***Arg.:*** Aldomet; Dopagrand; Dopatral; ***Austral.:*** Aldomet; Aldopren†; Hydopa; Nudopa†; ***Austria:*** Aldometil; Presinol†; ***Belg.:*** Aldomet; ***Braz.:*** Aldomet; Aldotensin; Cardin†; Cardiodopa; Dopametil; Ductomet; Etildopanan; Kindomet; Metilcord; Tensioval; ***Canad.:*** Aldomet; Novo-Medopa†; Nu-Medopa; ***Chile:*** Aloset; ***Denm.:*** Aldomet; Dopamet†; ***Fr.:*** Aldomet; ***Ger.:*** Dopegyt; Presinol; Sembrina†; ***Gr.:*** Aldomet; ***Hong Kong:*** Aldomet; Dopamet; Dopegyt; ***India:*** Alphadopa; Dopagyt; ***Irl.:*** Aldomet; Meldopa; ***Israel:*** Aldomin; ***Ital.:*** Aldomet; Medopren; ***Malaysia:*** Aldomet; Dopamet; Dopegyt; ***Mex.:*** Aldomet; Amender; Biotenzol; Ehlindopa†; Hipten†; Medopal†; Prodop†; Pulsoton†; Selm†; Tenzone†; Toparal; Yuremetil D†; ***Neth.:*** Aldomet; Sembrina†; ***Norw.:*** Aldomet; Dopamet†; ***NZ:*** Aldomet†; Prodopa; ***Port.:*** Aldomet; ***S.Afr.:*** Aldomet; Hy-Po-Tone; Normopress; ***Singapore:*** Dopegyt; ***Spain:*** Aldomet; ***Swed.:*** Aldomet; ***Switz.:*** Aldomet; Dopamet†; ***Thai.:*** Aldomet; Dopamed; Dopasian; Dopegyt; Isomet; Medopa; Medopate†; Mefpa; Servidopa; Siamdopa; ***UK:*** Aldomet; Medomet†; Metalpha†; ***USA:*** Aldomet†.

**Multi-ingredient:** ***Arg.:*** Normatensil; ***Austria:*** Aldoretic; ***Braz.:*** Hydromet; ***Canad.:*** Aldoril†; Apo-Methazide; Novo-Doparil†; Supres; ***Irl.:*** Hydromet†; ***Ital.:*** Medozide; Saludopin; ***Port.:*** Aldoretic; ***S.Afr.:*** Aldoretic†; ***Swed.:*** Hydromet†; ***Switz.:*** Aldoretic†; ***USA:*** Aldoclor; Aldoril.

---

## Meticrane *(rINN)*

Meticrano; SD-17102. 6-Methylthiochroman-7-sulphonamide 1,1-dioxide.

$C_{10}H_{13}NO_4S_2$ = 275.3.
*CAS — 1084-65-7.*
*ATC — C03BA09.*

**Pharmacopoeias.** In *Jpn.*

### Profile

Meticrane is a thiazide diuretic (see Hydrochlorothiazide, p.933) that has been used in the treatment of hypertension.

---

## Metildigoxin *(BAN, rINN)*

Medigoxin; β-Methyl Digoxin; β-Methyldigoxin; Metildigoxina. 3β-[(*O*-2,6-Dideoxy-4-*O*-methyl-D-*ribo*-hexopyranosyl-(1→4)-*O*-2,6-dideoxy-D-*ribo*-hexopyranosyl-(1→4)-2,6-dideoxy-D-*ribo*-hexopyranosyl)oxy]-12β,14-dihydroxy-5β,14β-card-20(22)-enolide.

$C_{42}H_{66}O_{14}$ = 795.0.
*CAS — 30685-43-9.*
*ATC — C01AA08.*

**Pharmacopoeias.** In *Chin.* In *Jpn.* as $C_{42}H_{66}O_{14},\frac{1}{2}C_3H_6O$.

### Adverse Effects, Treatment, and Precautions

As for Digoxin, p.895.

### Interactions

As for Digoxin, p.896.

**Calcium-channel blockers.** For a report of an interaction between metildigoxin and *diltiazem*, see Calcium-channel Blockers, under Interactions of Digoxin, p.897.

### Pharmacokinetics

Metildigoxin is rapidly and almost completely absorbed from the gastrointestinal tract and at steady state has a half-life of 36 to 47.5 hours. Demethylation to digoxin occurs. About 60% of an oral or intravenous dose is excreted in the urine as unchanged drug and metabolites over 7 days.

**Hepatic impairment.** Hepatic demethylation of metildigoxin was reduced in 12 patients with cirrhosis of the liver compared with 12 healthy subjects. This resulted in a reduction in metildigoxin clearance, a smaller volume of distribution, and a significantly higher serum concentration.[1]


1. Rameis H, *et al.* Changes in metildigoxin pharmacokinetics in cirrhosis of the liver: a comparison with β-acetyldigoxin. *Int J Clin Pharmacol Ther Toxicol* 1984; **22:** 145–51.


**Renal impairment.** For reference to the pharmacokinetics of metildigoxin in patients with renal impairment, see under Uses and Administration, below.

### Uses and Administration

Metildigoxin is a cardiac glycoside with positive inotropic activity. It has actions similar to those of digoxin (p.898) and may be used in the treatment of some cardiac arrhythmias (p.816) and in heart failure (p.820).

The onset of action of metildigoxin is more rapid than that of digoxin. When metildigoxin is given by mouth an effect may appear within 5 to 20 minutes and a maximum effect on the myocardium may be seen in 15 to 30 minutes. The duration of action is similar to or a little longer than that of digoxin; therapeutic plasma concentrations are also similar. In stabilised patients a dose of 300 micrograms of metildigoxin is as effective as 500 micrograms of digoxin.

Metildigoxin may be given by mouth or intravenously. Initial doses of 150 to 600 micrograms daily by mouth may be given depending upon whether rapid or slow digitalisation is desired; digitalisation is usually performed over 2 to 4 days and the larger doses are given in divided daily doses. A daily dose of 400 micrograms intravenously for 3 days may also be employed. Maintenance therapy is continued with 50 to 300 micrograms daily by mouth in divided doses.

Dosage should be reduced in patients with renal impairment (see below).

**Administration in renal impairment.** Fairly good non-linear correlation was found between creatinine clearance and metildigoxin half-life in a study of 15 patients with chronic renal impairment, including 8 undergoing haemodialysis, and 4 patients with heart failure and unimpaired renal function. The mean elimination half-life was 5.62 days in patients undergoing dialysis (clearance essentially 0 mL/minute) and 3.41 days in the other patients with chronic renal impairment (clearance 15 to 50 mL/minute) compared with 1.49 days in patients with normal renal function (clearance 62 to 96 mL/minute). It was recommended that patients undergoing dialysis should be given 30 to 50% of the usual dose initially.[1] Other studies have suggested[2] that dose reduction may be necessary in renal impairment when creatinine clearance is below 50 mL/minute per 1.48 $m^2$.


1. Trovato GM, *et al.* Relationship between β-methyl-digoxin pharmacokinetics and degree of renal impairment. *Curr Ther Res* 1983; **33:** 158–64.
2. Tsutsumi K, *et al.* Pharmacokinetics of beta-methyldigoxin in subjects with normal and impaired renal function. *J Clin Pharmacol* 1993; **33:** 154–60.


### Preparations

**Proprietary Preparations** (details are given in Part 3)
***Austria:*** Lanitop; ***Belg.:*** Lanitop; ***Braz.:*** Lanitop; ***Ger.:*** Lanitop; ***Gr.:*** Lanitop; ***Hong Kong:*** Lanitop; ***Ital.:*** Cardiolan†; Lanitop; Miopat†; ***Port.:*** Lanitop; ***Spain:*** Lanirapid; ***Switz.:*** Lanitop.

---

## Metipranolol *(BAN, USAN, rINN)*

BMOI-004; Methypranolol; VUAB-6453 (SPOFA); VUFB-6453. 1-(4-Acetoxy-2,3,5-trimethylphenoxy)-3-isopropylaminopropan-2-ol; 4-(2-Hydroxy-3-isopropylaminopropoxy)-2,3,6-trimethylphenyl acetate.

$C_{17}H_{27}NO_4$ = 309.4.
*CAS — 22664-55-7.*
*ATC — S01ED04.*

NOTE. MPR is a code approved by the BP 2003 for use on single unit doses of eye drops containing metipranolol where the individual container may be too small to bear all the appropriate labelling information.

**Pharmacopoeias.** In *Br.*

**BP 2003** (Metipranolol). A white crystalline powder. Practically insoluble in water; soluble in alcohol, in acetone, and in methyl alcohol; dissolves in dilute mineral acids. The filtrate of a 2.5% suspension in water has a pH of 9.0 to 10.0. Protect from light.

### Adverse Effects, Treatment, and Precautions

As for Beta Blockers, p.869.

Conjunctivitis, conjunctival leucoplakia, transient stinging, as well as other ocular adverse effects have been reported with metipranolol eye drops. Granulomatous anterior uveitis has been reported rarely; the high incidence reported in the UK may have been associated with changes induced by radiation sterilisation of metipranolol eye drops in their final container, but this preparation is no longer available.

### Interactions

The interactions associated with beta blockers are discussed on p.870.

## Uses and Administration

Metipranolol is a non-cardioselective beta blocker (p.868). It is reported to be largely lacking in intrinsic sympathomimetic activity and membrane-stabilising properties.

Metipranolol is used to reduce raised intra-ocular pressure in the management of open-angle glaucoma and ocular hypertension (p.1485). Eye drops usually containing metipranolol 0.1 or 0.3% are used twice daily.

Metipranolol has also been used by mouth in the management of cardiovascular disorders.

## Preparations

**BP 2003:** Metipranolol Eye Drops.

**Proprietary Preparations** (details are given in Part 3)
***Austria:*** Beta-Ophtiole; ***Belg.:*** Beta-Ophtiole; ***Ger.:*** Betamann; ***Ital.:*** Turoptin; ***Malaysia:*** Beta-Ophtiole; ***Mon.:*** Betanol; ***Neth.:*** Beta-Ophtiole; ***Port.:*** Beta-Ophtiole; ***S.Afr.:*** Beta-Ophtiole; ***Singapore:*** Beta-Ophtiole; ***Switz.:*** Turoptin; ***Thai.:*** Beta-Ophtiole; ***USA:*** OptiPranolol.

**Multi-ingredient: *Austria:*** Betacarpin; Torrat†; ***Belg.:*** Normoglaucon; ***Ger.:*** Normoglaucon; Torrat; Tri-Torrat; ***Gr.:*** Beta Ophtiole; ***Hong Kong:*** Torrat; ***Ital.:*** Ripix; ***Malaysia:*** Normoglaucon; ***Neth.:*** Normoglaucon; ***Port.:*** Normoglaucon; ***Singapore:*** Normoglaucon; ***Switz.:*** Ripix; ***Thai.:*** Normoglaucon.

# Metirosine *(BAN, rINN)*

L-588357-0; Metirosina; Metyrosine *(USAN)*; MK-781. (−)-α-Methyl-L-tyrosine; 4-Hydroxy-α-methylphenylalanine.

$C_{10}H_{13}NO_3$ = 195.2.
*CAS — 672-87-7 (metirosine); 620-30-4 (racemetirosine).*
*ATC — C02KB01.*

NOTE. The term α-methyltyrosine (α-MPT; α-MT; α-methyl-*p*-tyrosine) is used below since although metirosine, the (−)-isomer, is the active form the manufacturers state that some racemate (racemetirosine; (±)-α-methyl-DL-tyrosine) is produced during synthesis but that the material supplied contains mainly (−)-isomer with a small amount of (+)-isomer.

The code name MK-781, applied to earlier investigational material, may have described a racemate or a preparation containing a smaller proportion of (−)-isomer than the product now available commercially.

Potency of the proprietary preparation (Demser) is expressed in terms of metirosine.

**Pharmacopoeias.** In *US.*

### Adverse Effects

Sedation occurs in almost all patients receiving α-methyltyrosine. Other adverse effects include extrapyramidal symptoms, such as trismus and frank parkinsonism; anxiety, depression, and psychic disturbances including hallucinations, disorientation, and confusion; and diarrhoea, which may be severe. Crystalluria, transient dysuria, and haematuria have been seen in a few patients. There have also been occasional reports of slight swelling of the breast, galactorrhoea, nasal congestion, decreased salivation, gastrointestinal disturbances, headache, impotence or failure of ejaculation, and hypersensitivity reactions. Eosinophilia, raised serum aspartate aminotransferase, and peripheral oedema have been reported rarely.

**Neuroleptic malignant syndrome.** Neuroleptic malignant syndrome occurred after the use of the dopamine-depleting drugs tetrabenazine and α-methyltyrosine in a patient with Huntington's chorea.[1]

1. Burke RE, *et al.* Neuroleptic malignant syndrome caused by dopamine-depleting drugs in a patient with Huntington disease. *Neurology* 1981; **31:** 1022–6.

### Precautions

To minimise the risk of crystalluria, patients receiving α-methyltyrosine should have a fluid intake sufficient to maintain a urine volume of at least 2 litres daily and their urine should be examined regularly for the presence of crystals.

α-Methyltyrosine has sedative effects and patients should be warned of the hazards of driving a motor vehicle or operating machinery while receiving the drug. Symptoms of psychic stimulation and insomnia may occur when α-methyltyrosine is withdrawn.

When α-methyltyrosine is used pre-operatively in patients with phaeochromocytoma, blood pressure and the ECG should be monitored continuously during surgery as the danger of hypertensive crises and arrhythmias is not eliminated. Concomitant alpha blockade (e.g. with phentolamine) may be required; a beta blocker or lidocaine may be needed for the management of arrhythmias. Blood volume must be maintained during and after surgery, particularly if an alpha blocker is used concurrently, in order to avoid hypotension.

### Interactions

The sedative effects of α-methyltyrosine may be potentiated by alcohol and other CNS depressants. Use with phenothiazines or haloperidol may exacerbate extrapyramidal effects.

### Pharmacokinetics

α-Methyltyrosine is well absorbed from the gastrointestinal tract and is excreted mainly unchanged by the kidneys. A plasma half-life of 3.4 to 7.2 hours has been reported. Less than 1% of a dose may be excreted as the metabolites α-methyldopa, α-methyldopamine, α-methylnoradrenaline, and α-methyltyramine.

### Uses and Administration

α-Methyltyrosine is an inhibitor of the enzyme tyrosine hydroxylase, and consequently of the synthesis of catecholamines. It is used to control the symptoms of excessive sympathetic stimulation in patients with phaeochromocytoma (p.831) and decreases the frequency and severity of hypertensive attacks and related symptoms in most patients. It may be given for pre-operative preparation, or for long-term management in those for whom surgery is contra-indicated or who have malignant phaeochromocytoma.

In the management of phaeochromocytoma, α-methyltyrosine is given by mouth in a dose of 250 mg four times daily, increased daily by 250 mg or 500 mg to a maximum of 4 g daily in divided doses. The optimum dose, achieved by monitoring clinical symptoms and catecholamine excretion, is usually in the range of 2 to 3 g daily and when used pre-operatively it should be given for at least 5 to 7 days before surgery. The concomitant use of alpha blockers may be necessary.

α-Methyltyrosine is not effective in controlling essential hypertension.

α-Methyltyrosine has also been tried in patients with schizophrenia.

### Preparations

**USP 27:** Metyrosine Capsules.

**Proprietary Preparations** (details are given in Part 3)
***UK:*** Demser†; ***USA:*** Demser.

# Metolazone *(BAN, USAN, rINN)*

Metolazona; SR-720-22. 7-Chloro-1,2,3,4-tetrahydro-2-methyl-4-oxo-3-o-tolylquinazoline-6-sulphonamide.

$C_{16}H_{16}ClN_3O_3S$ = 365.8.
*CAS — 17560-51-9.*
*ATC — C03BA08.*

**Pharmacopoeias.** In *US.*

**USP 27** (Metolazone). Store in airtight containers. Protect from light.

## Adverse Effects and Treatment

As for Hydrochlorothiazide, p.933. Metolazone has also been reported to cause palpitations, chest pain, and chills.

**Effects on the blood.** Profound neutropenia was observed in a 58-year-old woman within 10 days of starting treatment with metolazone.[1] Neutropenia persisted for a further 10 days after metolazone was withdrawn. No other haematological abnormalities were observed.

1. Donovan KL. Neutropenia and metolazone. *BMJ* 1989; **299:** 981.

**Effects on the nervous system.** Two patients experienced acute muscle cramps with impairment of consciousness and epileptiform movements after taking metolazone 5 mg (single dose) or 2.5 mg daily for 3 days.[1]

1. Fitzgerald MX, Brennan NJ. Muscle cramps, collapse, and seizures in two patients taking metolazone. *BMJ* 1976; **1:** 1381–2.

## Precautions

As for Hydrochlorothiazide, p.935.

## Interactions

As for Hydrochlorothiazide, p.935. Severe electrolyte disturbances may occur when metolazone and furosemide are used concurrently.

**ACE inhibitors.** Deterioration in renal function occurred in a 65-year-old woman when metolazone 5 mg [daily] was added to *captopril*, furosemide, spironolactone, and digoxin for heart failure.[1] An interaction between captopril and metolazone was suspected and both drugs were discontinued with a subsequent return to normal renal function. It was suggested that natriuresis and a fall in blood pressure caused by the diuretic may have compromised an already low renal perfusion pressure when autoregulatory mechanisms were blocked by captopril.

1. Hogg KJ, Hillis WS. Captopril/metolazone induced renal failure. *Lancet* 1986; **i:** 501–2.

**Antidiabetics.** Hypoglycaemia occurred in a patient with type 2 diabetes mellitus controlled with *glibenclamide* 40 hours after initiation of therapy with metolazone 5 mg daily.[1] Studies of protein binding *in vitro* did not reveal any evidence of displacement of glibenclamide from binding sites.

1. George S, *et al.* Possible protein binding displacement interaction between glibenclamide and metolazone. *Eur J Clin Pharmacol* 1990; **38:** 93–5.

**Ciclosporin.** An increase in serum-creatinine concentration in a renal transplant patient was attributed to a toxic drug interaction between metolazone and ciclosporin.[1] Serum-creatinine concentrations returned to pretreatment values when metolazone was discontinued.

1. Christensen P, Leski M. Nephrotoxic drug interaction between metolazone and cyclosporin. *BMJ* 1987; **294:** 578.

## Pharmacokinetics

Metolazone is slowly and incompletely absorbed from the gastrointestinal tract. An average of about 65% of a dose has been reported to be absorbed after oral administration in healthy subjects, and an average of about 40% in patients with cardiac disease. In some countries a formulation with enhanced bioavailability is available. About 95% of the drug is bound in the circulation: about 50 to 70% to the red blood cells and between 15 and 33% to plasma proteins. The half-life has been reported to be 8 to 10 hours in whole blood, and 4 to 5 hours in plasma, but the diuretic effect persists for up to 24 hours or more. About 70 to 80% of the amount of metolazone absorbed is excreted in the urine, of which 80 to 95% is excreted unchanged. The remainder is excreted in the bile and some enterohepatic circulation has been reported. Metolazone crosses the placenta and is distributed into breast milk.

◊ References.

1. Tilstone WJ, *et al.* Pharmacokinetics of metolazone in normal subjects and in patients with cardiac or renal failure. *Clin Pharmacol Ther* 1974; **16:** 322–9.

## Uses and Administration

Metolazone is a diuretic with actions and uses similar to those of the thiazide diuretics (see Hydrochlorothiazide, p.935) even though it does not contain a thiazide ring system. It is used for oedema, including that associated with heart failure (p.820), and for hypertension (p.825).

Unlike thiazides in general, metolazone is reported to be effective in patients with a glomerular filtration rate of less than 20 mL/minute. Diuresis starts in about 1 hour, reaches a peak in about 2 hours, and lasts for 12 to 24 hours depending on the dose.

In some countries a preparation is available with enhanced bioavailability which is effective in lower doses than conventional formulations. Doses given in *Martindale* refer to the conventional tablet formulation unless otherwise stated.

In the treatment of **oedema** the usual dose is 5 to 10 mg by mouth daily; in some cases doses of 20 mg or more may be required. No more than 80 mg should be given in any 24-hour period. In refractory cases, metolazone has been used with furosemide or other loop diuretics, but the electrolyte balance should be monitored closely.

In the treatment of **hypertension** the usual dose is 2.5 to 5 mg daily either alone, or with other antihypertensives. An initial dose of 1.25 mg has also been used. The dosage may be adjusted after 3 to 4 weeks according to response. A maintenance dose of 5 mg on alternate days may be used.

Formulations with enhanced bioavailability are given in doses of 0.5 to 1 mg daily in the treatment of hypertension. They are not bioequivalent to the conventional tablet formulation and should not be used interchangeably.

## Preparations

**USP 27:** Metolazone Tablets.

**Proprietary Preparations** (details are given in Part 3)
***Austria:*** Birobin†; ***Canad.:*** Zaroxolyn; ***Chile:*** Pavedal; ***Ger.:*** Zaroxolyn; ***Hong Kong:*** Zaroxolyn; ***Israel:*** Zaroxolyn; ***Ital.:*** Zaroxolyn; ***Mex.:*** Zaroxolyn†; ***Port.:*** Diulo; ***S.Afr.:*** Zaroxolyn; ***Spain:*** Diondel†; ***Swed.:*** Zaroxolyn†; ***Switz.:*** Zaroxolyne; ***UK:*** Metenix 5; ***USA:*** Mykrox; Zaroxolyn.

# Metoprolol *(BAN, USAN, rINN)*

(±)-1-Isopropylamino-3-[4-(2-methoxyethyl)phenoxy]propan-2-ol.

$C_{15}H_{25}NO_3$ = 267.4.
*CAS — 54163-88-1; 37350-58-6.*
*ATC — C07AB02.*

## Metoprolol Fumarate *(BANM, USAN, rINNM)*

CGP-2175C.

$(C_{15}H_{25}NO_3)_2,C_4H_4O_4$ = 650.8.
*CAS — 119637-66-0.*
*ATC — C07AB02.*

**Pharmacopoeias.** In *US.*

**USP 27** (Metoprolol Fumarate). A 10% solution in water has a pH of between 5.5 and 6.5. Store in airtight containers. Protect from light.

**Metoprolol Succinate** *(BANM, USAN, rINNM)*

Metoprololi Succinas.

$(C_{15}H_{25}NO_3)_2,C_4H_6O_4$ = 652.8.

*CAS — 98418-47-4.*

*ATC — C07AB02.*

**Pharmacopoeias.** In *Eur.* (see p.vi) and *US.*

**Ph. Eur. 5.0** (Metoprolol Succinate). A white crystalline powder. Freely soluble in water; soluble in methyl alcohol; slightly soluble in alcohol; very slightly soluble in ethyl acetate. A 2% solution in water has a pH of between 7.0 and 7.6. Protect from light.

**USP 27** (Metoprolol Succinate). A white to off-white powder. Freely soluble in water; soluble in methyl alcohol; sparingly soluble in alcohol; slightly soluble in isopropyl alcohol. A 6.5% solution in water has a pH of between 7.0 and 7.6. Store in airtight containers at controlled room temperature.

**Metoprolol Tartrate** *(BANM, USAN, rINNM)*

CGP-2175E; H-93/26; Metoprololi Tartras; Tartrato de metoprolol.

$(C_{15}H_{25}NO_3)_2,C_4H_6O_6$ = 684.8.

*CAS — 56392-17-7.*

*ATC — C07AB02.*

**Pharmacopoeias.** In *Chin., Eur.* (see p.vi) and *US.*

**Ph. Eur. 5.0** (Metoprolol Tartrate). A white crystalline powder or colourless crystals. It exhibits polymorphism. Very soluble in water; freely soluble in alcohol. A 2% solution in water has a pH of between 6.0 and 7.0. Protect from light.

**USP 27** (Metoprolol Tartrate). A white crystalline powder. Very soluble in water; freely soluble in alcohol, in chloroform, and in dichloromethane; slightly soluble in acetone; insoluble in ether. A 10% solution in water has a pH of between 6.0 and 7.0. Store in airtight containers at a temperature of 25°, excursions permitted between 15° and 30°. Protect from light.

**Stability.** Metoprolol tartrate 400 micrograms/mL in glucose 5% or sodium chloride 0.9% was stable for 36 hours when stored at 24° in PVC bags.[1]


1. Belliveau PP, *et al.* Stability of metoprolol tartrate in 5% dextrose injection or 0.9% sodium chloride injection. *Am J Hosp Pharm* 1993; **50:** 950–2.


## Adverse Effects, Treatment, and Precautions

As for Beta Blockers, p.869.

**Breast feeding.** Metoprolol is distributed into breast milk and studies[1-3] have shown that the concentration in milk is higher than that in plasma. However, the amount ingested by an infant is likely to be small, and in one study[3] the concentration of metoprolol in the infants' plasma was undetectable or very low. No adverse effects have been reported in breast-fed infants whose mothers were receiving metoprolol and the American Academy of Pediatrics considers[4] that it is therefore usually compatible with breast feeding.


1. Sandström B, Regårdh C-G. Metoprolol excretion into breast milk. *Br J Clin Pharmacol* 1980; **9:** 518–9.
2. Liedholm H, *et al.* Accumulation of atenolol and metoprolol in human breast milk. *Eur J Clin Pharmacol* 1981; **20:** 229–31.
3. Kulas J, *et al.* Atenolol and metoprolol: a comparison of their excretion into human breast milk. *Acta Obstet Gynecol Scand Suppl* 1984; **118:** 65–9.
4. American Academy of Pediatrics. The transfer of drugs and other chemicals into human milk. *Pediatrics* 2001; **108:** 776–89. Correction. *ibid.*; 1029. Also available at: http://aappolicy.aappublications.org/cgi/content/full/pediatrics%3b108/3/776 (accessed 06/07/04)


**Effects on hearing.** Loss of hearing in a patient receiving metoprolol appeared to be dose-related;[1] hearing gradually improved over several months once the drug was withdrawn.


1. Fäldt R, *et al.* β Blockers and loss of hearing. *BMJ* 1984; **289:** 1490–2.


**Effects on lipid metabolism.** Beta blockers may increase serum-triglyceride concentrations. For a report of acute pancreatitis provoked by severe hypertriglyceridaemia in a patient taking atenolol and metoprolol, see p.869.

**Effects on the liver.** Acute hepatitis associated with metoprolol has been reported in a 56-year-old woman.[1] The hepatotoxicity could not be explained by deficient oxidation of metoprolol; drug oxidation phenotyping showed she was an extensive metaboliser of debrisoquine and hence metoprolol.

For a discussion of the relationship between polymorphic oxidation of metoprolol and the incidence of adverse effects, see Metabolism, under Pharmacokinetics, below.


1. Larrey D, *et al.* Metoprolol-induced hepatitis: rechallenge and drug oxidation phenotyping. *Ann Intern Med* 1988; **108:** 67–8.


## Interactions

The interactions associated with beta blockers are discussed on p.870.

## Pharmacokinetics

Metoprolol is readily and completely absorbed from the gastrointestinal tract but is subject to considerable first-pass metabolism, with a bioavailability of about 50%. Peak plasma concentrations vary widely and occur about 1.5 to 2 hours after a single oral dose. It is moderately lipid-soluble.

Metoprolol is widely distributed; it crosses the blood-brain barrier and the placenta, and is distributed into breast milk. It is about 12% bound to plasma protein. It is extensively metabolised in the liver, predominantly by the cytochrome P450 isoenzyme CYP2D6, and undergoes oxidative deamination, *O*-dealkylation followed by oxidation, and aliphatic hydroxylation. The metabolites are excreted in the urine together with only small amounts of unchanged metoprolol. The rate of metabolism by CYP2D6 is determined by genetic polymorphism; the half-life of metoprolol in fast hydroxylators is stated to be 3 to 4 hours, whereas in poor hydroxylators it is about 7 hours.

**The elderly.** Several studies[1-3] indicate that age-related physiological changes have negligible effects on the pharmacokinetics of metoprolol.


1. Quarterman CP, *et al.* The effect of age on the pharmacokinetics of metoprolol and its metabolites. *Br J Clin Pharmacol* 1981; **11:** 287–94.
2. Regårdh CG, *et al.* Pharmacokinetics of metoprolol and its metabolite α-OH-metoprolol in healthy, non-smoking, elderly individuals. *Eur J Clin Pharmacol* 1983; **24:** 221–6.
3. Larsson M, *et al.* Pharmacokinetics of metoprolol in healthy, elderly, non-smoking individuals after a single dose and two weeks of treatment. *Eur J Clin Pharmacol* 1984; **27:** 217–22.


**Metabolism.** Metoprolol is metabolised by the cytochrome P450 isoenzyme CYP2D6 and therefore exhibits a debrisoquine-type genetic polymorphism with poor metabolisers of metoprolol also being poor metabolisers of debrisoquine.[1-3] However, the clinical relevance of the polymorphism has been questioned; one study[4] found no correlation between poor metaboliser status and increased incidence of adverse effects, whereas another study[5] found an increased frequency of poor metabolisers among patients who experienced adverse effects.

The subject may be further confused by variations in the phenotype between ethnic groups. Although the incidence of the poor metaboliser phenotype in whites of European origin is reported to be about 9%, a study in 138 Nigerians[6] failed to identify evidence of polymorphic metabolism, and the authors caution against extrapolation of data between different racial groups.


1. Lennard MS, *et al.* Defective metabolism of metoprolol in poor hydroxylators of debrisoquine. *Br J Clin Pharmacol* 1982; **14:** 301–3.
2. Lennard MS, *et al.* Oxidation phenotype—a major determinant of metoprolol metabolism and response. *N Engl J Med* 1982; **307:** 1558–60.
3. McGourty JC, *et al.* Metoprolol metabolism and debrisoquine oxidation polymorphism—population and family studies. *Br J Clin Pharmacol* 1985; **20:** 555–66.
4. Clark DWJ, *et al.* Adverse effects from metoprolol are not generally associated with oxidation status. *Br J Clin Pharmacol* 1984; **18:** 965–6.
5. Wuttke H, *et al.* Increased frequency of cytochrome P450 2D6 poor metabolizers among patients with metoprolol-associated adverse effects. *Clin Pharmacol Ther* 2002; **72:** 429–37.
6. Iyun AO, *et al.* Metoprolol and debrisoquin metabolism in Nigerians: lack of evidence for polymorphic oxidation. *Clin Pharmacol Ther* 1986; **40:** 387–94.


**Pregnancy.** The clearance of metoprolol was increased fourfold in 5 pregnant women during the last trimester, compared with that some months after delivery; this was probably due to enhanced hepatic metabolism in the pregnant state.[1]

The disposition of metoprolol was investigated in newborn infants of mothers treated with metoprolol 50 to 100 mg twice daily.[2] In 15 of the 17 neonates plasma-metoprolol concentrations increased in the first 2 to 5 hours of the postnatal period, then declined over the next 15 hours; 5 of these infants had no detectable metoprolol concentrations in the umbilical plasma. No infant demonstrated signs of beta blockade.


1. Högstedt S, *et al.* Increased oral clearance of metoprolol in pregnancy. *Eur J Clin Pharmacol* 1983; **24:** 217–20.
2. Lundborg P, *et al.* Disposition of metoprolol in the newborn. *Br J Clin Pharmacol* 1981; **12:** 598–600.


**Renal impairment.** A study[1] of the pharmacokinetics of metoprolol and its renally excreted metabolite α-hydroxymetoprolol in normal subjects and subjects with renal impairment showed that a single dose of a modified-release tablet of metoprolol produced similar plasma-metoprolol concentrations and values for the area under the concentration/time curve in both groups. Mean plasma concentrations of α-hydroxymetoprolol were increased two to threefold in subjects with renal impairment compared with normal subjects but such a rise was not considered likely to contribute to beta blockade.


1. Lloyd P, *et al.* The effect of impaired renal function on the pharmacokinetics of metoprolol after single administration of a 14/190 metoprolol OROS system. *Am Heart J* 1990; **120:** 478–82.


## Uses and Administration

Metoprolol is a cardioselective beta blocker (p.868). It is reported to lack intrinsic sympathomimetic activity and to have little or no membrane-stabilising activity.

It is used in the management of hypertension (p.825), angina pectoris (p.813), cardiac arrhythmias (p.816), myocardial infarction (p.828), and heart failure (p.820). It is also used in the management of hyperthyroidism (p.1594) and in the prophylactic treatment of migraine (p.464).

Metoprolol is given as the tartrate. The fumarate and succinate salts are used in some modified-release tablets but doses are usually expressed in terms of the tartrate; 95 mg of metoprolol fumarate or metoprolol succinate is approximately equivalent to 100 mg of metoprolol tartrate.

Reduced doses should be given to patients with hepatic impairment.

In **hypertension** metoprolol tartrate is usually given in an initial dose of 100 mg daily by mouth, increased weekly according to response to 400 mg daily; it may be taken as a single daily dose or twice daily. A usual maintenance dose is 100 to 200 mg daily. Some manufacturers recommend that the dose should be taken with or immediately following a meal.

The usual dose for **angina pectoris** is 50 to 100 mg two or three times daily by mouth.

In the treatment of **cardiac arrhythmias** the usual dose is 50 mg two or three times daily by mouth, increased if necessary up to 300 mg daily in divided doses.

For the emergency treatment of cardiac arrhythmias metoprolol tartrate may be given intravenously in an initial dose of up to 5 mg administered at a rate of 1 to 2 mg/minute; this may be repeated, if necessary, at intervals of 5 minutes to a total dose of 10 to 15 mg. When acute arrhythmias have been controlled, maintenance therapy may be started with doses not exceeding 50 mg three times daily by mouth 4 to 6 hours after intravenous therapy.

Arrhythmias may be prevented on induction of anaesthesia or controlled during anaesthesia, by the slow intravenous injection of 2 to 4 mg; further injections of 2 mg may be repeated as necessary to a maximum total dose of 10 mg.

Metoprolol is also used as an adjunct in the early management of acute **myocardial infarction.** Treatment should be given within 12 hours of the onset of chest pain; metoprolol tartrate 5 mg should be given intravenously at 2-minute intervals to a total of 15 mg, where tolerated. This should be followed, after 15 minutes, by the commencement of oral treatment, in patients who have received the full intravenous dose, with 50 mg every 6 hours for 2 days. In patients who have failed to tolerate the full intravenous dose a reduced oral dose should be given as, and when, their condition permits. Subsequent maintenance dosage is 100 mg given twice daily by mouth. In patients who did not receive metoprolol by intravenous injection as part of the early management of myocardial infarction, metoprolol 100 mg twice daily by mouth may be started once the clinical condition of the patient stabilises.

In the management of stable, symptomatic **heart failure** metoprolol succinate may be given as a modified-release preparation. The initial dose is the equivalent of metoprolol tartrate 12.5 to 25 mg once daily, increased as tolerated, at intervals of 2 weeks, to a maximum of 200 mg once daily.

As an adjunct in the treatment of **hyperthyroidism** metoprolol tartrate may be given in doses of 50 mg four times daily by mouth. Doses of 100 to 200 mg are given daily in divided doses for **migraine** prophylaxis.

◊ General references.


1. Plosker GL, Clissold SP. Controlled release metoprolol formulations: a review of their pharmacodynamic and pharmacokinetic properties, and therapeutic use in hypertension and ischaemic heart disease. *Drugs* 1992; **43:** 382–414.
2. Prakash A, Markham A. Metoprolol: a review of its use in chronic heart failure. *Drugs* 2000; **60:** 647–78.
3. Tangeman HJ, Patterson JH. Extended-release metoprolol succinate in chronic heart failure. *Ann Pharmacother* 2003; **37:** 701–10.


## Preparations

***BP 2003:*** Metoprolol Injection; Metoprolol Tartrate Tablets;
***USP 27:*** Metoprolol Succinate Extended-Release Tablets; Metoprolol

Tartrate and Hydrochlorothiazide Tablets; Metoprolol Tartrate Injection; Metoprolol Tartrate Tablets.

**Proprietary Preparations** (details are given in Part 3)

***Arg.:*** Beloc; Lopresor; ***Austral.:*** Betaloc; Lopresor; Metohexal; Metolol; Minax; Toprol; ***Austria:*** Beloc; Lanoc; Lopresor; Metohexal; Metolol†; MetoMed; Metopal; Metoros†; Metotyrol; Seloken; ***Belg.:*** Lopresor; Selo-Zok; Seloken; Slow-Lopresor; ***Braz.:*** Lopressor; Selo-Zok; Seloken; ***Canad.:*** Betaloc; Lopresor; Novo-Metoprol; Nu-Metop; ***Denm.:*** Dura-Zok; Mepronet; Metocar; Metozoc; Selo-Zok; Seloken; ***Fin.:*** Metblock; Metoprolin; Metozoc; Seloken; Seloken ZOC; Selopral; Spesicor; ***Fr.:*** Lopressor; Seloken; ***Ger.:*** Azumetop; Beloc; Beloc-Zok; Dignometoprol†; Jeprolol; Lopresor; Meprolol; Meto; Meto-Tablinen; Metobeta; Metodoc; Metodura; Metohexal; Metomerck; Metoprogamma; Prelis; Sigaprolol; ***Gr.:*** Lopresor; ***Hong Kong:*** Betaloc; Denex; Minax; Novo-Metoprol; Sefloc; ***India:*** Betaloc; Metolar; Selopres; ***Irl.:*** Betaloc; Betazok†; Lopresor; Metocor; Metop; Topromel†; ***Israel:*** Lopresor; Metopress; Neobloc; ***Ital.:*** Lopresor; Seloken; ***Jpn:*** Seloken; ***Malaysia:*** Beatrolol; Betaloc; Betatab; Denex; ***Mex.:*** Bioprol; Eurolol†; Kenaprol†; Leptoprol†; Letoprol†; Lopresor; Metopresol; Metozzard†; Proken M; Prolaken; Promiced; Prontol; Ritmolol; Selectadril; Seloken; Sermetrol; ***Neth.:*** Lopresor; Selokeen; ***Norw.:*** Metozoc; Selo-Zok; Seloken; ***NZ:*** Betaloc; Lopresor; Slow-Lopresor; ***Port.:*** Lopresor; ***S.Afr.:*** Lopresor; ***Singapore:*** Betaloc; Denex†; ***Spain:*** Beloken; Lopresor; Seloken†; ***Swed.:*** Seloken; Seloken ZOC; ***Switz.:*** Beloc COR; Beloc-Zok; Lopresor; Metopress; ***Thai.:*** Betaloc; Cardeloc; Cardoxone; Denex; Melol; Metoblock; Metolol; Minax; ***UK:*** Arbralene†; Betaloc; Lopresor; ***USA:*** Lopressor; Toprol XL.

**Multi-ingredient:** ***Arg.:*** Diubeloc; ***Austria:*** Beloc comp; Logimax; Metolol compositum†; Seloken retard Plus; Triloc; ***Belg.:*** Logimat; Logroton; Selozide; Zok-Zid; ***Braz.:*** Selopress; ***Denm.:*** Logimax; Zok-Zid; ***Fin.:*** Logimax; Selocomp ZOC; Seloken ZOC/ASA; ***Fr.:*** Logimax; Logroton; ***Ger.:*** Azumetop HCT; Belnif; Beloc comp†; Beloc-Zok comp; Meprolol Comp; Meto comp; Meto-comp†; meto-thiazid; Metobeta comp; Metodura comp; Metohexal comp; Metostad Comp; Mobloc; Prelis comp; Treloc; ***Hong Kong:*** Betaloc Comp; Logimax; ***Irl.:*** Co-Betaloc; ***Israel:*** Logimax; ***Ital.:*** Igroton-Lopresor; Selozide; ***Malaysia:*** Logroton; ***Mex.:*** Logimax; Selopres; ***Neth.:*** Logimax; Logroton†; Selokomb†; ***Norw.:*** Logimax†; ***Spain:*** Logimax; Selopresin; ***Swed.:*** Logimax; Seloken ZOC/ASA; ***Switz.:*** Logimax; Logroton; ***UK:*** Co-Betaloc; ***USA:*** Lopressor HCT.

---

### Mevastatin *(rINN)*

Compactin; CS-500; Mevastatina; ML-236B. (1*S*,7*S*,8*S*,8a*R*)-1,2,3,7,8,8a-Hexahydro-7-methyl-8-{2-[(2*R*,4*R*)-tetrahydro-4-hydroxy-6-oxo-2*H*-pyran-2-yl]ethyl}-1-naphthyl (*S*)-2-methylbutyrate.

$C_{23}H_{34}O_5$ = 390.5.

*CAS — 73573-88-3.*

#### Profile

Mevastatin, which has been isolated from *Penicillium citrinum*, is a lipid regulating drug. It is a 3-hydroxy-3-methylglutaryl coenzyme A (HMG-CoA) reductase inhibitor (a statin) (see Simvastatin, p.997) but is no longer used in clinical practice because of reports of toxicity in *animals*.

---

## Mexiletine Hydrochloride

*(BANM, USAN, rINNM)*

Kö-1173; Mexiletina, hidrocloruro de; Mexiletini Hydrochloridum. 1-Methyl-2-(2,6-xylyloxy)ethylamine hydrochloride.

$C_{11}H_{17}NO,HCl$ = 215.7.

*CAS — 31828-71-4 (mexiletine); 5370-01-4 (mexiletine hydrochloride).*

*ATC — C01BB02.*

**Pharmacopoeias.** In *Chin.*, *Eur.* (see p.vi), *Jpn*, and *US*.

**Ph. Eur. 5.0** (Mexiletine Hydrochloride). A white or almost white, crystalline powder. It exhibits polymorphism. Freely soluble in water and in methyl alcohol; sparingly soluble in dichloromethane. A 10% solution in water has a pH of 4.0 to 5.5.

**USP 27** (Mexiletine Hydrochloride). A white powder. Freely soluble in water and in dehydrated alcohol; practically insoluble in ether; slightly soluble in acetonitrile. A 10% solution in water has a pH of between 3.5 and 5.5. Store in airtight containers.

### Adverse Effects and Treatment

Mexiletine has a narrow therapeutic ratio; many adverse effects of mexiletine are dose-related and will respond to dosage reduction but may be severe enough to necessitate discontinuation of mexiletine and the institution of symptomatic and supportive therapy. Toxicity is commonly seen with oral or parenteral loading doses when plasma concentrations are high.

The most common adverse effects involve the gastrointestinal tract and CNS. Effects on the gastrointestinal tract include nausea, vomiting, constipation, and diarrhoea. Effects on the nervous system include tremor, confusion, lightheadedness, dizziness, blurred vision and other visual disturbances, sleep disturbances, and speech difficulties. The most frequent cardiovascular effects are hypotension, sinus bradycardia, atrioventricular dissociation, and atrial fibrillation. As with other antiarrhythmics mexiletine may exacerbate arrhythmias. Other adverse effects which have been reported include skin rashes, abnormal liver function tests, thrombocytopenia, positive antinuclear factor titres, and convulsions. The Stevens-Johnson syndrome has been reported rarely.

**Incidence of adverse effects.** In a study involving 100 patients with ventricular arrhythmias, mexiletine had to be discontinued in 49 patients due to intolerable adverse effects.[1] The most common of these affected the gastrointestinal system (27%) and included nausea (10%), vomiting (6%), heartburn (6%), and oesophageal spasm (3%). Intolerable effects on the CNS occurred in 10% of patients and these were most commonly tremor (4%), ataxia (2%), dyskinesia (1%), and tinnitus (1%). When mexiletine was used with another antiarrhythmic, the incidence of intolerable effects was 56%.

Tolerable adverse effects with mexiletine alone were transient and dose-dependent and occurred in 18% of patients. They most commonly affected the gastrointestinal tract. No irreversible adverse effects were reported and no proarrhythmic effects were seen.

1. Kerin NZ, *et al.* Mexiletine: long-term efficacy and side effects in patients with chronic drug-resistant potentially lethal ventricular arrhythmias. *Arch Intern Med* 1990; **150:** 381–4.

**Effects on the lungs.** Pulmonary fibrosis has been reported in an elderly patient receiving mexiletine; the manufacturer was aware of 3 other cases.[1]

1. Bero CJ, Rihn TL. Possible association of pulmonary fibrosis with mexiletine. *DICP Ann Pharmacother* 1991; **25:** 1329–31.

### Precautions

Mexiletine should be used with special caution in patients with sinus node dysfunction, conduction disorders, bradycardia, hypotension, cardiogenic shock, heart failure, or hepatic impairment. ECG and blood pressure monitoring should be carried out during treatment.

Absorption of mexiletine may be delayed after myocardial infarction.

**Breast feeding.** Mexiletine is distributed into human breast milk in higher concentrations than in maternal serum. A woman[1] who received 200 mg of mexiletine three times daily during the last trimester of pregnancy (see below), went on to breast feed the infant. Concentrations of mexiletine were measured in the maternal milk and serum and were found to be 0.6 and 0.3 micrograms/mL respectively on the second day postpartum, and 0.8 and 0.7 micrograms/mL respectively after 6 weeks. This represented a milk to serum ratio of 2.0 and 1.1 respectively. However, mexiletine was undetectable in the infant's serum on both occasions and no adverse effects were observed. In another report[2] a woman taking a similar dose of mexiletine for the last 5 months of her pregnancy also breast fed her infant. Twelve paired samples of maternal milk and blood were collected between the second and fifth day postpartum. The milk to plasma ratio varied between 0.78 and 1.89 with a mean of 1.45. It was considered unlikely that the infant would ingest more than 1.25 mg of mexiletine in any 24-hour period, and that this amount was not enough to cause adverse effects. Failure to feed was noted[3] in the first 17 days in an infant whose mother was receiving 750 mg daily of mexiletine and 50 mg daily of atenolol. After maternal education and formula supplementation an acceptable growth curve was established. Breast feeding continued until the infant was 3 months old, and no adverse effects were seen at 10 months. The American Academy of Pediatrics[4] therefore considers that mexiletine is usually compatible with breast feeding.

1. Timmis AD, *et al.* Mexiletine for control of ventricular dysrhythmias in pregnancy. *Lancet* 1980; **ii:** 647–8.
2. Lewis AM, *et al.* Mexiletine in human blood and breast milk. *Postgrad Med J* 1981; **57:** 546–7.
3. Lownes HE, Ives TJ. Mexiletine use in pregnancy and lactation. *Am J Obstet Gynecol* 1987; **157:** 446–7.
4. American Academy of Pediatrics. The transfer of drugs and other chemicals into human milk. *Pediatrics* 2001; **108:** 776–89. Correction. *ibid.*; 1029. Also available at: http://aappolicy.aappublications.org/cgi/content/full/pediatrics%3b108/3/776 (accessed 06/07/04)

**Pregnancy.** A normal infant was born to a woman given mexiletine with propranolol for the control of ventricular tachycardia during the third trimester of pregnancy.[1] During the first 6 hours after delivery the infant had a heart rate of only 90 beats/minute, probably due to the propranolol; it was normal thereafter. At delivery the serum concentration of mexiletine in mother and infant was the same.

1. Timmis AD, *et al.* Mexiletine for control of ventricular dysrhythmias in pregnancy. *Lancet* 1980; **ii:** 647–8.

### Interactions

Mexiletine undergoes extensive metabolism in the liver and interactions may occur with other drugs metabolised by the same enzymes. Plasma concentrations of mexiletine may be reduced by hepatic enzyme inducers such as phenytoin and rifampicin; increased plasma concentrations may occur with enzyme inhibitors.

Absorption of mexilitine may be delayed by drugs that slow gastric emptying such as opioid analgesics and atropine. The rate of absorption may be increased by metoclopramide; the extent of absorption is unaffected.

Drugs that acidify or alkalinise the urine enhance or reduce the rate of elimination of mexiletine, respectively.

There may be an increased risk of arrhythmias if mexiletine is used with other antiarrhythmics or with arrhythmogenic drugs.

Mexiletine has been reported to increase theophylline concentrations (p.801) and to precipitate lidocaine toxicity (p.1378).

◊ References.

1. Wing LMH, *et al.* The effect of metoclopramide and atropine on the absorption of orally administered mexiletine. *Br J Clin Pharmacol* 1980; **9:** 505–9.
2. Begg EJ, *et al.* Enhanced metabolism of mexiletine after phenytoin administration. *Br J Clin Pharmacol* 1982; **14:** 219–23.
3. Pentikäinen PJ, *et al.* Effect of rifampicin treatment on the kinetics of mexiletine. *Eur J Clin Pharmacol* 1982; **23:** 261–6.

### Pharmacokinetics

Mexiletine is readily and almost completely absorbed from the gastrointestinal tract, with a bioavailability of about 90%, although absorption may be delayed after myocardial infarction.

Mexiletine is metabolised in the liver to a number of metabolites; metabolism may involve cytochrome P450 isoenzymes CYP1A2, CYP2D6, and CYP3A4, and genetic polymorphism in relation to CYP2D6 has been identified. It is excreted in the urine, mainly in the form of its metabolites with about 10% excreted unchanged; the clearance of mexiletine is increased in acid urine.

Mexiletine is widely distributed throughout the body and is about 50 to 70% bound to plasma proteins. Mexiletine crosses the placenta and is distributed into breast milk. It has an elimination half-life of about 10 hours in healthy subjects but this may be prolonged in patients with heart disease, hepatic impairment, or severe renal impairment. Its therapeutic effect has been correlated with plasma concentrations of 0.5 to 2 micrograms/mL, but the margin between therapeutic and toxic concentrations is narrow, and severe toxicity may occur within this range.

◊ References.

1. Labbé L, Turgeon J. Clinical pharmacokinetics of mexiletine. *Clin Pharmacokinet* 1999; **37:** 361–84.

### Uses and Administration

Mexiletine is a class Ib antiarrhythmic (p.809) with actions similar to those of lidocaine (p.1379), to which it is structurally related. Unlike lidocaine it undergoes little hepatic first-pass metabolism and is suitable for oral administration.

Mexiletine is used for the treatment of ventricular **arrhythmias** (p.816).

It is given by mouth as the hydrochloride in an initial loading dose of 400 mg followed by 200 to 250 mg three or four times daily, starting 2 hours after the loading dose. Higher loading doses (for example, of 600 mg) may be necessary in patients after myocardial infarction to overcome delayed absorption, especially if they have received an opioid analgesic. The usual maintenance dosage of mexiletine is 600 to 900 mg daily in divided doses; doses up to 1200 mg daily may be given. Oral doses should be taken with food and swallowed with plenty of liquid to avoid oesophageal ulceration. Modified-release preparations have been used.

Mexiletine may be given by slow intravenous injection of the hydrochloride in doses of 100 to 250 mg at a rate of 25 mg/minute, followed by an infusion at a rate of 250 mg over 1 hour, 250 mg over the next 2 hours, and then at about 500 micrograms/minute for maintenance, according to response; when appropriate the patient may be transferred to oral therapy with doses of 200 to 250 mg of the hydrochloride three or four times daily. Alternatively, an initial intravenous dose of 200 mg at a rate of 25 mg/minute, may be followed by an oral dose of 400 mg on completion of the injection, with subsequent oral therapy as before.

Mexiletine has also been tried in the treatment of refractory neuropathic **pain** (see below).

◊ Reviews.

1. Monk JP, Brogden RN. Mexiletine: a review of its pharmacodynamic and pharmacokinetic properties, and therapeutic use in the treatment of arrhythmias. *Drugs* 1990; **40:** 374–411. Correction. *ibid.* 1991; **41:** 377.

**Administration in children.** The dose of mexiletine in children should be titrated according to the plasma concentration.[1] In a 2-week-old girl and a 20-month-old boy high oral doses of 25 and 15 mg/kg daily, respectively, were needed to produce therapeutic plasma concentrations and control of tachycardia.

1. Holt DW, *et al.* Paediatric use of mexiletine and disopyramide. *BMJ* 1979; **2:** 1476–7.

**Administration in the elderly.** The rate of absorption of mexiletine was slower in a group of 7 elderly subjects compared with 8 young subjects given mexiletine 100 mg by mouth, but the extent of absorption was probably not affected.[1] Elimination of mexiletine was not significantly different between the 2 groups and there was no pharmacokinetic basis for dosage modification of mexiletine in the elderly.

1. Grech-Bélanger O, *et al.* Pharmacokinetics of mexiletine in the elderly. *J Clin Pharmacol* 1989; **29:** 311–15.

**Administration in renal impairment.** The pharmacokinetics of mexiletine were not significantly modified in patients with chronic renal impairment when the creatinine clearance (CC) was above 10 mL/minute and these patients could be given usual doses of mexiletine.[1] However, in patients with a CC below 10 mL/minute the steady-state plasma concentration and half-life were increased and in these patients dosage should be adjusted according to plasma concentrations.

Continuous ambulatory peritoneal dialysis did not influence the clearance of mexiletine in a patient with chronic renal failure.[2]

1. El Allaf D, *et al.* Pharmacokinetics of mexiletine in renal insufficiency. *Br J Clin Pharmacol* 1982; **14:** 431–5.
2. Guay DRP, *et al.* Mexiletine clearance during peritoneal dialysis. *Br J Clin Pharmacol* 1985; **19:** 857–8.

**Pain.** Neuropathic pain is often insensitive to opioid analgesics and various drugs, including mexiletine, have been tried. Mexiletine has been tried in painful diabetic neuropathy (p.6) although results have been conflicting.[1-5] Two of the studies that reported no difference between treatment and placebo found that a subset of patients (those with stabbing or burning pain, heat sensations, and formication) appeared to benefit.[2,3]

Other painful states in which mexiletine has been reported to be of benefit include: Dercum's disease (a condition involving painful fatty deposits),[6] central post-stroke pain (thalamic pain syndrome)[7] (p.5), and severe scrotal and inguinal pain after radiation for prostate cancer.[8]

1. Dejgård A, *et al.* Mexiletine for treatment of chronic painful diabetic neuropathy. *Lancet* 1988; **i:** 9–11.
2. Stracke H, *et al.* Mexiletine in the treatment of diabetic neuropathy. *Diabetes Care* 1992; **15:** 1550–5.
3. Wright JM, *et al.* Mexiletine in the symptomatic treatment of diabetic peripheral neuropathy. *Ann Pharmacother* 1997; **31:** 29–34.
4. Oskarsson P, *et al.* Efficacy and safety of mexiletine in the treatment of painful diabetic neuropathy. *Diabetes Care* 1997; **20:** 1594–7.
5. Jarvis B, Coukell AJ. Mexiletine: a review of its therapeutic use in painful diabetic neuropathy. *Drugs* 1998; **56:** 691–707.
6. Petersen P, *et al.* Treating the pain of Dercum's disease. *BMJ* 1984; **288:** 1880.
7. Awerbuch GI, Sandyk R. Mexiletine for thalamic pain syndrome. *Int J Neurosci* 1990; **55:** 129–33.
8. Colclough G, *et al.* Mexiletine for chronic pain. *Lancet* 1993; **342:** 1484–5.

### Preparations

***BP 2003:*** Mexiletine Capsules; Mexiletine Injection;
***USP 27:*** Mexiletine Hydrochloride Capsules.

**Proprietary Preparations** (details are given in Part 3)
***Arg.:*** Mexitilen; ***Austral.:*** Mexitil; ***Austria:*** Mexitil; ***Belg.:*** Mexitil; ***Braz.:*** Mexitil; ***Canad.:*** Mexitil; ***Denm.:*** Mexitil†; ***Fin.:*** Mexitil; ***Fr.:*** Mexitil†; ***Ger.:*** Mexitil; ***Gr.:*** Mexitil; Myovek; ***Hong Kong:*** Mexitil; ***India:*** Mexitil; ***Irl.:*** Mexitil; ***Israel:*** Mexilen; ***Ital.:*** Mexitil; ***Mex.:*** Mexitil; ***Neth.:*** Mexitil†; ***Norw.:*** Mexitil†; ***NZ:*** Mexitil; ***S.Afr.:*** Mexitil; ***Spain:*** Mexitil; ***Swed.:*** Mexitil; ***Switz.:*** Mexitil†; ***Thai.:*** Mexitil; Ritalmex†; ***UK:*** Mexitil; ***USA:*** Mexitil.

## Mibefradil Hydrochloride *(BANM, rINNM)*

Hidrocloruro de mibefradil; Mibefradil Dihydrochloride *(USAN)*; Ro-40-5967 (mibefradil); Ro-40-5967/001 (mibefradil hydrochloride). (1*S*,2*S*)-(2-{[3-(2-Benzimidazolyl)propyl]methylamino}ethyl)-6-fluoro-1,2,3,4-tetrahydro-1-isopropyl-2-naphthyl methoxyacetate dihydrochloride.

$C_{29}H_{38}FN_3O_3,2HCl = 568.6.$

*CAS — 116644-53-2 (mibefradil); 116666-63-8 (mibefradil hydrochloride).*

*ATC — C08CX01.*

### Profile

Mibefradil is a calcium-channel blocker that acts principally on fast T-type calcium channels, unlike conventional calcium-channel blockers that act on slow L-type channels (see p.810). Mibefradil was introduced for the management of hypertension and angina pectoris but was withdrawn worldwide several months later due to increasing reports of serious interactions with a wide range of drugs.

## Midodrine Hydrochloride *(BANM, USAN, rINNM)*

Hidrocloruro de midodrina; ST-1085 (midodrine or midodrine hydrochloride); St. Peter-224. 2-Amino-*N*-(β-hydroxy-2,5-dimethoxyphenethyl)acetamide hydrochloride; (*RS*)-$N^1$-(β-Hydroxy-2,5-dimethoxyphenethyl)glycinamide hydrochloride.

$C_{12}H_{18}N_2O_4,HCl = 290.7.$

*CAS — 42794-76-3 (midodrine); 3092-17-9 (midodrine hydrochloride).*

*ATC — C01CA17.*

### Adverse Effects, Treatment, and Precautions

The most serious adverse effect of midodrine is supine hypertension. Paraesthesias, dysuria, pilomotor reaction (goose flesh), pruritus and rashes have been reported. The hypertensive effects of midodrine may be treated with an alpha blocker such as phentolamine.

For the adverse effects of sympathomimetics in general, and precautions to be observed, see Adrenaline, p.852.

### Interactions

For the interactions of sympathomimetics in general, see Adrenaline, p.853.

### Pharmacokinetics

Midodrine is well absorbed from the gastrointestinal tract and undergoes enzymatic hydrolysis in the systemic circulation to its active metabolite, deglymidodrine (desglymidodrine; ST-1059). Midodrine itself reaches its peak plasma concentrations about half an hour after a dose by mouth, and has a plasma half-life of about 25 minutes. The active metabolite reaches its peak plasma concentration about an hour after oral administration and has a terminal elimination half-life of about 3 hours. Deglymidodrine undergoes some further metabolism in the liver. Midodrine is primarily excreted in the urine as metabolites and a small amount of unchanged drug.

### Uses and Administration

Midodrine is a direct-acting sympathomimetic (see Adrenaline, p.854) with selective alpha-agonist activity; the main active moiety has been stated to be its major metabolite, deglymidodrine. It acts as a peripheral vasoconstrictor but has no direct cardiac stimulatory effects.

Midodrine hydrochloride is used in the treatment of hypotensive states (p.828) and in particular of orthostatic hypotension (p.1100). Alpha-agonist drugs such as midodrine have also been used as an adjunct in the management of urinary incontinence (p.476).

In **hypotensive states**, the usual initial dose of midodrine hydrochloride is 2.5 mg two or three times daily by mouth, adjusted gradually according to response; up to 10 mg three times daily may be required. The potential for supine hypertension is reduced by taking the last dose of the day at least 4 hours before bedtime.

A dose for **urinary incontinence** is 2.5 to 5 mg by mouth two or three times daily.

Midodrine hydrochloride can also be given in similar doses by slow intravenous injection. It has also been used in the treatment of **retrograde ejaculation** in a dose of 10 to 40 mg intravenously.

◊ References.

1. McClellan KJ, *et al.* Midodrine: a review of its therapeutic use in the management of orthostatic hypotension. *Drugs Aging* 1998; **12:** 76–86.

### Preparations

**Proprietary Preparations** (details are given in Part 3)
***Austria:*** Gutron; ***Canad.:*** Amatine; ***Chile:*** Gutron; ***Fr.:*** Gutron; ***Ger.:*** Gutron; ***Hong Kong:*** Gutron; ***Irl.:*** Midon; ***Israel:*** Gutron; ***Ital.:*** Gutron; ***Mex.:*** Gutron†; ***NZ:*** Gutron; ***Port.:*** Gutron; ***Singapore:*** Gutron; ***Switz.:*** Gutron; ***Thai.:*** Gutron; ***USA:*** ProAmatine.

## Milrinone *(BAN, USAN, rINN)*

Milrinona; Win-47203-2. 1,6-Dihydro-2-methyl-6-oxo[3,4′-bipyridine]-5-carbonitrile.

$C_{12}H_9N_3O = 211.2.$

*CAS — 78415-72-2.*

*ATC — C01CE02.*

**Pharmacopoeias.** In *US.*

**USP 27** (Milrinone). A white to tan, hygroscopic, crystalline solid. Practically insoluble in water, in chloroform, and in methyl alcohol; freely soluble in dimethyl sulfoxide. Store in airtight containers.

## Milrinone Lactate *(BANM, rINNM)*

Lactato de milrinona.

$C_{12}H_9N_3O,C_3H_6O_3 = 301.3.$

*ATC — C01CE02.*

**Incompatibility.** The UK manufacturer states that milrinone lactate injection is incompatible with furosemide and bumetanide, and it should not be diluted with sodium bicarbonate injection.

### Adverse Effects and Precautions

Prolonged oral treatment with milrinone has increased the mortality rate and milrinone is now only employed intravenously for short-term use.

Supraventricular and ventricular arrhythmias, hypotension, angina-like chest pain, and headache have been reported. Hypokalaemia, tremor, and thrombocytopenia may occur. For reference to a reduced incidence of arrhythmia but an increased risk of thrombocytopenia in *children* given milrinone see Administration in Children, below.

Milrinone should be used with caution in patients with severe obstructive aortic or pulmonary valvular disease or with hypertrophic cardiomyopathy. Since milrinone may facilitate conduction through the atrioventricular node it can increase the ventricular response rate in patients with atrial flutter or fibrillation. Digitalisation should be considered in these patients before milrinone therapy is started.

Blood pressure, heart rate, ECG, fluid and electrolyte balance, and renal function should be monitored during milrinone therapy.

Milrinone should be given in reduced doses to patients with renal impairment.

### Pharmacokinetics

Milrinone is rapidly and almost completely absorbed from the gastrointestinal tract, but is only given intravenously because of an increased mortality rate associated with prolonged administration via the oral route. It is about 70% bound to plasma proteins. Elimination occurs mainly via the urine; about 83% of a dose is excreted as unchanged drug. The elimination half-life is about 2.3 hours.

◊ General references.

1. Rocci ML, Wilson H. The pharmacokinetics and pharmacodynamics of newer inotropic agents. *Clin Pharmacokinet* 1987; **13:** 91–109. Correction. *ibid.* 1988; **14:** (contents page).

### Uses and Administration

Milrinone is a phosphodiesterase inhibitor similar to amrinone (p.863) with positive inotropic and vasodilator activity. It is, however, reported to have greater positive inotropic activity than amrinone. It is given intravenously, as the lactate, in the short-term management of severe heart failure unresponsive to other forms of therapy and in acute heart failure following cardiac surgery. In some longer-term studies milrinone was given by mouth, but an increased mortality rate was reported.

Doses of milrinone lactate are expressed in terms of the base; milrinone lactate 1.43 mg is approximately equivalent to 1 mg of milrinone. The initial loading dose is the equivalent of milrinone 50 micrograms/kg given over 10 minutes followed by a continuous maintenance infusion. The maintenance infusion may be titrated between 0.375 and 0.75 micrograms/kg per minute but a total daily dose of 1.13 mg/kg should not be exceeded.

Dosage should be reduced in patients with renal impairment (see below).

**Administration in children.** Pharmacokinetic studies[1,2] have suggested that steady-state plasma concentrations of milrinone are lower in children than in adults given similar doses, and that milrinone clearance is faster in children. It has been suggested[1] that in children an initial loading dose of 75 micrograms/kg should be administered, followed by maintenance infusions of 0.75 micrograms/kg per minute, increased to 1 microgram/kg per minute if required. An additional bolus dose of 25 micrograms/kg was recommended before each increase of 0.25 micrograms/kg per minute in infusion rate.

A study[3] of adverse effects in children given milrinone has suggested that arrhythmias are less common than in adults whereas thrombocytopenia is more common.

1. Lindsay CA, *et al.* Pharmacokinetics and pharmacodynamics of milrinone lactate in pediatric patients with septic shock. *J Pediatr* 1998; **132:** 329–34.
2. Ramamoorthy C, *et al.* Pharmacokinetics and side effects of milrinone in infants and children after open heart surgery. *Anesth Analg* 1998; **86:** 283–9.
3. Watson S, *et al.* Use of milrinone in the pediatric critical care unit. *Pediatrics* 1999; **104** (suppl): 681–2.

**Administration in renal impairment.** Doses of milrinone should be reduced in patients with renal impairment. The following doses for maintenance infusion are recommended based on creatinine clearance (CC):

- CC 50 mL/minute: 0.43 micrograms/kg per minute
- CC 40 mL/minute: 0.38 micrograms/kg per minute
- CC 30 mL/minute: 0.33 micrograms/kg per minute
- CC 20 mL/minute: 0.28 micrograms/kg per minute
- CC 10 mL/minute: 0.23 micrograms/kg per minute
- CC 5 mL/minute: 0.20 micrograms/kg per minute

**Heart failure.** Milrinone is one of several drugs that may be used in heart failure (p.820), but because of an increased mortality rate reported following long-term oral use it is usually only given intravenously for short-term management of heart failure unresponsive to other treatments. The PROMISE (Prospective Randomized Milrinone Survival Evaluation) study[1] showed that oral milrinone increased morbidity and mortality in patients with severe chronic heart failure. However, more recently, longer-term continuous intravenous administration for up to 8 weeks has been studied in patients awaiting heart transplantation and appeared to be well tolerated.[2] Intermittent use on several days a week has also been tried.[3]

In patients with acute exacerbation of heart failure, a prospective study[4] found no benefit from the routine use of short-term intravenous milrinone.


1. Packer M, *et al.* Effect of oral milrinone on mortality in severe chronic heart failure. *N Engl J Med* 1991; **325:** 1468–75.
2. Mehra MR, *et al.* Safety and clinical utility of long-term intravenous milrinone in advanced heart failure. *Am J Cardiol* 1997; **80:** 61–4.
3. Cesario D, *et al.* Beneficial effects of intermittent home administration of the inotrope/vasodilator milrinone in patients with end-stage congestive heart failure: a preliminary study. *Am Heart J* 1998; **135:** 121–9.
4. Cuffe MS, *et al.* Short-term intravenous milrinone for acute exacerbation of chronic heart failure: a randomized controlled trial. *JAMA* 2002; **287:** 1541–7.


### Preparations

**Proprietary Preparations** (details are given in Part 3)

***Arg.:*** Corotrope; ***Austral.:*** Primacor; ***Austria:*** Corotrop; ***Belg.:*** Corotrope; ***Braz.:*** Primacor; ***Canad.:*** Primacor; ***Fr.:*** Corotrope; ***Ger.:*** Corotrop; ***Gr.:*** Corotrope; ***Hong Kong:*** Primacor; ***Israel:*** Primacor; ***Jpn:*** Milrila; ***Malaysia:*** Primacor; ***Mex.:*** Primacor; ***Neth.:*** Corotrope; ***NZ:*** Primacor; ***Singapore:*** Primacor; ***Spain:*** Corotrope; ***Swed.:*** Corotrop; ***Switz.:*** Corotrop; ***Thai.:*** Primacor; ***UK:*** Primacor; ***USA:*** Primacor.

## Minoxidil *(BAN, USAN, rINN)*

Minoxidilum; U-10858. 2,6-Diamino-4-piperidinopyrimidine 1-oxide.

$C_9H_{15}N_5O$ = 209.2.

*CAS — 38304-91-5.*

*ATC — C02DC01; D11AX01.*

**Pharmacopoeias.** In *Chin., Eur.* (see p.vi), and *US.*

**Ph. Eur. 5.0** (Minoxidil). A white or almost white crystalline powder. Slightly soluble in water; soluble in methyl alcohol and in propylene glycol. Protect from light.

**USP 27** (Minoxidil). A white or off-white crystalline powder. Slightly soluble in water; soluble in alcohol and in propylene glycol; practically insoluble in acetone, in chloroform, in ethyl acetate, and in petroleum spirit; sparingly soluble in methyl alcohol.

### Adverse Effects and Treatment

Adverse effects commonly caused by minoxidil include reflex tachycardia, fluid retention accompanied by weight gain, oedema, and sometimes deterioration of existing heart failure and changes in the ECG. Hypertrichosis develops in up to 80% of patients within 3 to 6 weeks of the start of minoxidil therapy but is slowly reversible on discontinuation. Pericardial effusion, sometimes with associated tamponade, has been reported in about 3% of patients. Pericarditis may also occur. Minoxidil may aggravate or uncover angina pectoris. Other less frequent adverse effects include headache, nausea, gynaecomastia and breast tenderness, polymenorrhoea, allergic skin rashes, Stevens-Johnson syndrome, and thrombocytopenia.

Reflex tachycardia can be overcome by the concomitant administration of a beta blocker, or alternatively methyldopa, and a diuretic (usually a loop diuretic) is used to reduce fluid retention. If excessive hypotension occurs, an intravenous infusion of sodium chloride 0.9% can be given to maintain the blood pressure. If a pressor agent is necessary, drugs such as adrenaline, which can aggravate tachycardia, should be avoided; phenylephrine, angiotensinamide, vasopressin, or dopamine may be given if there is evidence of inadequate perfusion of a vital organ.

Topical application of minoxidil may be associated with contact dermatitis, pruritus, local burning, and flushing; sufficient may be absorbed to produce systemic adverse effects. Changes in hair colour or texture may occur.

◊ Two haemorrhagic lesions with Kaposi's features appeared on the forehead, an unusual location for HIV-associated Kaposi's sarcoma, in an HIV-positive patient who had applied topical minoxidil there for 3 months.[1] In another, healthy, patient an angioma of the scalp developed after 2 months of topical minoxidil therapy. The patient had had a similar lesion as a baby. Minoxidil may induce angiogenesis or may stimulate endothelial cells, fibroblasts, and muscle cells to proliferate. Care should be taken when minoxidil is applied to the skin of people who are predisposed to neo-angiogenesis, or who are HIV-positive.

For other effects of minoxidil on the skin following topical application, see below.


1. Pavlovitch JH, *et al.* Angiogenesis and minoxidil. *Lancet* 1990; **336:** 889.


**Effects on the eyes.** Bilateral optic neuritis and retinitis occurred in a patient during treatment with minoxidil for hypertension following a renal transplant.[1] The patient was also taking prednisolone and azathioprine.


1. Gombos GM. Bilateral optic neuritis following minoxidil administration. *Ann Ophthalmol* 1983; **15:** 259–61.


**Effects on the hair.** The hypertrichosis associated with minoxidil taken orally makes it unsuitable generally for use in women. As well as frequent hypertrichosis, there have been reports of changes in hair colour in patients receiving minoxidil.[1] In addition a case has been reported of increased hair loss, followed by subsequent regrowth of differently-coloured hair.[2] Substantial hair loss occurred in a female patient following withdrawal of minoxidil and she had to wear a wig.[3]

Severe hypertrichosis has also been reported in 5 of 56 women applying minoxidil 5% solution topically for androgenetic alopecia.[4] Facial, arm, and leg hypertrichosis were reported 2 to 3 months after starting treatment. Hypertrichosis had disappeared 5 months after discontinuation of minoxidil.


1. Traub YM, *et al.* Treatment of severe hypertension with minoxidil. *Isr J Med Sci* 1975; **11:** 991–8.
2. Ingles RM, Kahn T. Unusual hair changes with minoxidil therapy. *Int J Dermatol* 1983; **22:** 120–2.
3. Kidwai BJ, George M. Hair loss with minoxidil withdrawal. *Lancet* 1992; **340:** 609–10.
4. Peluso AM, *et al.* Diffuse hypertrichosis during treatment with 5% topical minoxidil. *Br J Dermatol* 1997; **136:** 118–20.


**Effects on skeletal muscle.** A polymyalgia syndrome, manifesting as fatigue, anorexia, weight loss, and severe pain in the shoulders and pelvic girdle was seen in 4 men using topical minoxidil.[1] All symptoms improved within 2 to 4 weeks of withdrawing the drug. In 2 of the patients rechallenge produced a relapse of the symptoms.


1. Colamarino R, *et al.* Polymyalgia and minoxidil. *Ann Intern Med* 1990; **113:** 256–7.


**Effects on the skin.** Although skin reactions to systemic minoxidil do not appear to be common, a case of classic Stevens-Johnson syndrome has been reported in a patient receiving minoxidil.[1] The syndrome responded to withdrawal and corticosteroid therapy; subsequent rechallenge provoked a recurrence. In another patient extensive erythematous weeping rash, with lesions consistent with actinic keratosis also appeared to be due to minoxidil; bullous lesions recurred on re-exposure.[2] Following topical application itching, scaling, flushing, and dermatitis have been the most common adverse effects; allergic contact dermatitis has been reported in rare instances.[3]

For other lesions associated with Kaposi's sarcoma and angioma and for effects on the hair, see above.


1. DiSantis DJ, Flanagan J. Minoxidil-induced Stevens-Johnson syndrome. *Arch Intern Med* 1981; **141:** 1515.
2. Ackerman BH, *et al.* Pruritic rash with actinic keratosis and impending exfoliation in a patient with hypertension managed with minoxidil. *Drug Intell Clin Pharm* 1988; **22:** 702–3.
3. Clissold SP, Heel RC. Topical minoxidil: a preliminary review of its pharmacodynamic properties and therapeutic efficacy in alopecia areata and alopecia androgenetica. *Drugs* 1987; **33:** 107–22.


### Precautions

Minoxidil is contra-indicated in phaeochromocytoma. It should be used with caution after a recent myocardial infarction, and in patients with pulmonary hypertension, angina pectoris, chronic heart failure, and significant renal impairment.

Topical application of minoxidil should be restricted to the scalp; it should not be applied to inflamed scalp skin or areas affected by psoriasis, severe sunburn, or severe excoriations, due to the risk of increased absorption. Patients being treated for hypertension should be monitored if topical minoxidil is used concurrently.

**AIDS.** For recommendations that topical minoxidil should be used with caution in HIV-positive patients, see under Adverse Effects, above.

**Breast feeding.** Study[1] of one breast-feeding mother showed that minoxidil was rapidly distributed into breast milk, achieving similar concentrations to those in the maternal plasma. No adverse effects were seen in the infant after 2 months and the American Academy of Pediatrics considers[2] that minoxidil is therefore usually compatible with breast feeding.


1. Valdivieso A, *et al.* Minoxidil in breast milk. *Ann Intern Med* 1985; **102:** 135.
2. American Academy of Pediatrics. The transfer of drugs and other chemicals into human milk. *Pediatrics* 2001; **108:** 776–89. Correction. *ibid.*; 1029. Also available at: http://aappolicy.aappublications.org/cgi/content/full/pediatrics%3b108/3/776 (accessed 06/07/04)


**Porphyria.** Minoxidil is considered to be unsafe in patients with porphyria because it has been shown to be porphyrinogenic in *animals* or *in-vitro* systems.

**Pregnancy.** A patient who took minoxidil, propranolol, and furosemide throughout pregnancy delivered a normal infant at 37 weeks. Pregnancy was uneventful.[1]


1. Valdivieso A, *et al.* Minoxidil in breast milk. *Ann Intern Med* 1985; **102:** 135.


### Interactions

The antihypertensive effect of minoxidil may be enhanced by use of other hypotensive drugs. Severe orthostatic hypotension may occur if minoxidil and sympathetic blocking drugs such as guanethidine or betanidine are given concurrently.

Topical minoxidil should not be used with other topical agents known to enhance absorption, such as corticosteroids, retinoids, or occlusive ointment bases.

### Pharmacokinetics

About 90% of an oral dose of minoxidil has been reported to be absorbed from the gastrointestinal tract. The plasma half-life is about 4.2 hours although the haemodynamic effect may persist for up to 75 hours, presumably due to accumulation at its site of action. Minoxidil is not bound to plasma proteins. It is distributed into breast milk. Minoxidil is extensively metabolised by the liver. It requires sulfation to become active, but the major metabolite is a glucuronide conjugate. Minoxidil is excreted predominantly in the urine mainly in the form of metabolites. Minoxidil and its metabolites are dialysable, although the pharmacological effect is not reversed.

Following topical application between 0.3 and 4.5% of the total applied dose of minoxidil is absorbed from intact scalp.

◊ References.


1. Pacifici GM, *et al.* Minoxidil sulphation in human liver and platelets: a study of interindividual variability. *Eur J Clin Pharmacol* 1993; **45:** 337–41.


### Uses and Administration

Minoxidil is an antihypertensive that acts predominantly by causing direct peripheral vasodilatation of the arterioles. It produces effects on the cardiovascular system similar to those of hydralazine (p.933). Minoxidil is administered by mouth for the treatment of severe hypertension unresponsive to standard therapy (p.825). When applied topically to the scalp minoxidil may stimulate hair growth to a limited extent and is used in the treatment of alopecia.

In the treatment of **hypertension** minoxidil is given with a beta blocker, or with methyldopa, to diminish the cardiac-accelerating effects, and with a diuretic, usually a loop diuretic, to control oedema. Following a single dose by mouth, the maximum hypotensive effect usually occurs after 2 to 3 hours, although the full effects may not occur until after 3 to 7 days of continuous treatment. An initial dose of 5 mg of minoxidil daily (or 2.5 mg daily in the elderly) is gradually increased at intervals of not less than 3 days to 40 or 50 mg daily according to response; in exceptional circumstances up to 100 mg daily has been given. If more rapid control of blood pressure is required, dosage adjustments may be made every 6 hours with careful monitoring. The daily dose may be given as a single dose or in 2 divided doses. For children, the initial dose is 200 micrograms/kg daily, increased in steps of 100 to 200 micrograms/kg at intervals of not less than 3 days, until control of blood pressure has been achieved or a maximum of 1 mg/kg or 50 mg daily has been reached. Reduced doses may be required in patients with renal impairment (see below).

In the treatment of **alopecia androgenetica** (male-pattern baldness) 1 mL of a 2% or 5% solution of minoxidil is applied twice daily to the scalp. The 5% solution is not recommended for women.

**Administration in renal impairment.** A study of the pharmacokinetics of minoxidil in patients with varying degrees of renal impairment found that the non-renal clearance was also impaired as renal function worsened.[1] Substantial accumulation of minoxidil might occur in these patients during multiple-dose therapy. It was advised that minoxidil therapy be initiated with smaller doses or a longer dose interval used in patients with renal impairment.


1. Halstenson CE, *et al.* Disposition of minoxidil in patients with various degrees of renal function. *J Clin Pharmacol* 1989; **29:** 798–802.


**Alopecia.** Although topical minoxidil clearly has some effect on hair growth in alopecia (p.1134), increases in pigmented non-vellus hair may be due to thickening and pigmentation of existing vellus rather than new growth.[1] As a result cosmetically acceptable hair growth may occur in less than 10% of patients with alopecia androgenetica (male-pattern baldness),[2-4] and fewer still among those with alopecia areata,[4] despite the fact that higher-strength 5% solutions have been tried in the latter condition.[4] One study indicated that topical minoxidil with 0.5% dithranol cream was more effective than either treatment alone in patients with alopecia areata.[5] The hair is lost again when treatment is stopped,[2-4] and even with continued use there is a waning of effect.[2,4] Minoxidil may be more effective in retarding the progression of male-pattern baldness than in reversing it,[1] and users are advised to abandon treatment if there is insufficient benefit after a year.[3]

A review of controlled trials, conducted mostly in men,[6] concluded that topical minoxidil 2% had only a minimal to modest effect on promoting hair regrowth in alopecia androgenetica and needed to be used indefinitely; some workers believed it to be more effective in females than in males, although another review of controlled studies in women[7] concluded that the effectiveness of minoxidil in female alopecia androgenetica was yet to be demonstrated and that larger trials were required. Minoxidil appeared to have no beneficial effect on alopecia areata.[6]


1. Katz HI. Topical minoxidil: review of efficacy and safety. *Cutis* 1989; **43:** 94–8.
2. de Groot AC, *et al.* Minoxidil: hope for the bald? *Lancet* 1987; **i:** 1019–22.
3. Shrank AB. Treating young men with hair loss. *BMJ* 1989; **298:** 847–8.
4. Anonymous. Topical minoxidil does little for baldness. *Drug Ther Bull* 1989; **27:** 74–5.
5. Fiedler VC, *et al.* Treatment-resistant alopecia areata. *Arch Dermatol* 1990; **126:** 756–9.
6. Anonymous. Topical minoxidil for baldness: a reappraisal. *Med Lett Drugs Ther* 1994; **36:** 9–10.
7. Wong WM, Seifert L. Minoxidil used in female alopecia. *Ann Pharmacother* 1994; **28:** 890–1.


CHEMOTHERAPY-INDUCED ALOPECIA. Minoxidil 2% solution was applied daily to the scalp of a boy with acute lymphoblastic leukaemia whose hair had failed to regrow satisfactorily following intensive chemotherapy.[1] Almost normal hair growth, achieved over a period of 9 months, was attributed to the application of minoxidil.

A small study[2] in women undergoing combination chemotherapy including doxorubicin found that topical minoxidil applied throughout the duration of antineoplastic therapy and for up to 4 months afterwards reduced the duration of alopecia by an average of 50 days.

Other methods for reducing chemotherapy-induced alopecia are described under the Treatment of Adverse Effects of Antineoplastics, p.496.


1. Vickers MA, Barton CJ. Minoxidil induced hair growth after leukaemia treatment? *Arch Dis Child* 1995; **73:** 184.
2. Duvic M, *et al.* A randomized trial of minoxidil in chemotherapy-induced alopecia. *J Am Acad Dermatol* 1996; **35:** 74–8.


### Preparations

***BP 2003:*** Minoxidil Scalp Application;
***USP 27:*** Minoxidil Tablets; Minoxidil Topical Solution.

**Proprietary Preparations** (details are given in Part 3)

***Arg.:*** Locemix; Macbirs Minoxidil; Toneon; Tricolocion; Tricoplus; Tricoxane; Ylox; ***Austral.:*** Loniten; Ralogaine†; Rogaine; ***Austria:*** Loniten; Moxiral; Regaine; Rogaine; ***Belg.:*** Lonnoten†; Neoxidil; Regaine; ***Braz.:*** Loniten; Minoxidine†; Neoxidil; Regaine; ***Canad.:*** Apo-Gain; Loniten; Minox; Minoxigaine†; Rogaine; ***Chile:*** Regaine; Tricoxane; ***Denm.:*** Regaine; ***Fin.:*** Minona†; Regaine; ***Fr.:*** Alopexy; Alostil; Lonoten; Neoxidil†; Regaine; Unipexil†; ***Ger.:*** Lonolox; Regaine; ***Gr.:*** Loniten; ***Hong Kong:*** Apo-Gain; Hairgrow; Headway; Loniten; Neoxidil; Regaine; ***Irl.:*** Loniten; Regaine; ***Israel:*** Apohair†; Hairgaine; Minoxi; Neoxidil; Regaine; ***Ital.:*** Aloxidil; Loniten; Minovital; Minoximen; Normoxidil; Regaine; Tricoxidil; ***Malaysia:*** Apo-Gain; Epokelan; Regaine; Regro; ***Mex.:*** Folcress; Neoxil†; Regaine; ***Neth.:*** Lonnoten; Regaine; ***Norw.:*** Regaine; ***NZ:*** Apo-Gain†; Headway; Loniten†; Rogaine; ***Port.:*** Biocrinal; Crinalsofex; Loniten; Mantai†; Minocalve; Minox; Regaine; Tricovivax; ***S.Afr.:*** Loniten; Regaine; ***Singapore:*** Loniten†; Minoxitrim; Neoxidil; Regaine; Regro; ***Spain:*** Dinaxil Capilar; Kapodin†; Kresse†; Lacovin; Loniten; Pilovital†; Regaine; Riteban; ***Swed.:*** Recrea; Regaine; ***Switz.:*** Alopexy; Loniten; Neocapil; Piloxil; Regaine; ***Thai.:*** Loniten; Minoxitrim; Modil; Neoxidil†; Noxidil; Nuhair; Regaine; Regrowth; ***UK:*** Loniten; Regaine; ***USA:*** Loniten; Rogaine.

**Multi-ingredient:** ***Arg.:*** Tricoplus Conef.

## Mivazerol *(rINN)*

UCB-22073.

*CAS — 125472-02-8.*

### Profile

Mivazerol is an alpha$_2$-adrenoceptor agonist that has been investigated for the prevention of perioperative complications resulting from myocardial ischaemia in patients with ischaemic heart disease undergoing non-cardiac surgery.

◊ References.


1. Oliver MF, *et al.* Effect of mivazerol on perioperative cardiac complications during non-cardiac surgery in patients with coronary heart disease: the European Mivazerol Trial (EMIT). *Anesthesiology* 1999; **91:** 951–61.


# Moexipril Hydrochloride

*(BANM, USAN, rINNM)*

CI-925; Hidrocloruro de moexipril; RS-10085-197; SPM-925. (3S-{2[R*(R*)],3R*})-2-(2-{[1-(Ethoxycarbonyl)-3-phenylpropyl]amino}-1-oxopropyl)-1,2,3,4-tetrahydro-6,7-dimethoxy-3-isoquinoline-carboxylic acid hydrochloride.

$C_{27}H_{34}N_2O_7$,HCl = 535.0.

*CAS — 103775-10-6 (moexipril); 82586-52-5 (moexipril hydrochloride).*

*ATC — C09AA13.*

### Adverse Effects, Treatment, and Precautions

As for ACE inhibitors, p.842.

### Interactions

As for ACE inhibitors, p.845.

### Pharmacokinetics

Moexipril acts as a prodrug of the diacid moexiprilat, its active metabolite. Following oral administration moexipril is rapidly but incompletely absorbed and is metabolised to moexiprilat in the gastrointestinal mucosa and liver. Absorption is reduced in the presence of food. The bioavailability of moexiprilat is about 13% following oral moexipril administration, and peak plasma concentrations of moexiprilat are reached in about 1.5 hours. Both moexipril and moexiprilat are moderately bound to plasma proteins. Moexipril is excreted predominantly in the urine as moexiprilat, unchanged drug, and other metabolites; some moexiprilat may also be excreted in the faeces. The functional elimination half-life of moexiprilat is about 12 hours.

### Uses and Administration

Moexipril is an ACE inhibitor (p.842). It is used in the treatment of hypertension (p.825).

Moexipril owes its activity to moexiprilat, to which it is converted after oral administration. The haemodynamic effects are seen about 1 hour after an oral dose and the maximum effect occurs after about 3 to 6 hours, although the full effect may not develop for 2 to 4 weeks during chronic dosing. Moexipril is given by mouth as the hydrochloride.

In the treatment of hypertension, the usual initial dose of moexipril hydrochloride is 7.5 mg once daily. Since there may be a precipitous fall in blood pressure in some patients when starting therapy with an ACE inhibitor, the first dose should preferably be given at bedtime. An initial dose of 3.75 mg once daily, given under close medical supervision, is suggested for patients who are receiving a *diuretic*; if possible the diuretic should be withdrawn 2 or 3 days before moexipril is started and resumed later if necessary. An initial dose of 3.75 mg once daily is also recommended for patients with renal or hepatic impairment and for the elderly.

The usual maintenance dose is 7.5 to 30 mg daily, which may be given in 2 divided doses if control is inadequate with a single dose.

◊ Reviews.


1. Brogden RN, Wiseman LR. Moexipril: a review of its use in the management of essential hypertension. *Drugs* 1998; **55:** 845–60.


**Administration in renal impairment.** In patients with renal impairment (creatinine clearance less than 40 mL/minute) an initial dose of moexipril hydrochloride 3.75 mg is given; in the USA it is required that the maximum dose in such patients should not exceed 15 mg daily.

### Preparations

**Proprietary Preparations** (details are given in Part 3)

***Denm.:*** Moex†; Perdix†; ***Fin.:*** Perdix†; ***Fr.:*** Moex; ***Ger.:*** Fempress; ***Hong Kong:*** Moex; ***Irl.:*** Perdix; ***Israel:*** Perdix; ***Ital.:*** Enulid; Femipres; Primoxil†; ***S.Afr.:*** Perdix; ***Swed.:*** Perdix†; ***Switz.:*** Fempress†; ***UK:*** Perdix; ***USA:*** Univasc.

**Multi-ingredient:** ***Ger.:*** Fempress Plus; ***Ital.:*** Femipres Plus; ***USA:*** Uniretic.

## Molsidomine *(BAN, USAN, rINN)*

CAS-276; Molsidomina; Morsydomine; SIN-10. N-Ethoxycarbonyl-3-morpholinosydnonimine.

$C_9H_{14}N_4O_4$ = 242.2.

*CAS — 25717-80-0.*

*ATC — C01DX12.*

### Profile

Molsidomine is a nitrovasodilator used in angina pectoris (p.813). It may also be used in heart failure (p.820) and following myocardial infarction (p.828).

Molsidomine is given by mouth in usual doses of 1 to 4 mg two to four times daily. Modified-release preparations are also available. It is also given intravenously in single doses of 2 to 4 mg and doses of 2 mg may be repeated at intervals of at least 2 hours if necessary; total doses of up to 40 mg daily have been given. Infusions may be employed at a rate of up to 3 mg/hour.

Molsidomine is metabolised to linsidomine (p.946), an active metabolite.

**Carcinogenicity.** Molsidomine tends to degrade into morpholine (even when protected from the light), a compound considered potentially carcinogenic. This finding led to the suspension of marketing of one molsidomine formulation;[1] an earlier temporary suspension was related to evidence of carcinogenicity in some *animals*, although this has not been confirmed in humans.


1. Anonymous. Corvaton Tropfen. *Dtsch Apotheker Ztg* 1989; **129** (49): VI.


**Myocardial infarction.** Although intravenous nitrates (glyceryl trinitrate or sodium nitroprusside) may be used in the management of acute myocardial infarction (p.828), molsidomine and its active metabolite linsidomine (a nitric oxide donor) had no effect on mortality.[1]


1. European Study of Prevention of Infarct with Molsidomine (ESPRIM) Group. The ESPRIM trial: short-term treatment of acute myocardial infarction with molsidomine. *Lancet* 1994; **344:** 91–7.


**Pharmacokinetics.** The pharmacokinetics of molsidomine have been reviewed.[1] Molsidomine is metabolised in the liver to linsidomine and other morpholine derivatives. Prolonged elimination half-lives of molsidomine and linsidomine due to reduced plasma clearance have been reported in patients with liver cirrhosis.[2]


1. Rosenkranz B, *et al.* Clinical pharmacokinetics of molsidomine. *Clin Pharmacokinet* 1996; **30:** 372–84.
2. Spreux-Varoquaux O, *et al.* Pharmacokinetics of molsidomine and its active metabolite, linsidomine, in patients with liver cirrhosis. *Br J Clin Pharmacol* 1991; **32:** 399–401.


### Preparations

**Proprietary Preparations** (details are given in Part 3)

***Arg.:*** Molsicor; Molsidaine; ***Austria:*** Molsicor; Molsidolat; Molsihexal; ***Belg.:*** Coruno; Corvatard; Corvaton; ***Fr.:*** Corvasal; Molsidirex†; ***Ger.:*** Corvaton; duracoron; Molsi-Azu; Molsi-Puren; Molsicor; Molsihexal; molsiket; ***Spain:*** Corpea; Molsidain; ***Switz.:*** Corsifar; Corvaton.

## Monteplase *(rINN)*

E-6010; Monteplasa.

$C_{2569}H_{3896}N_{746}O_{783}S_{39}$ = 59009.5.

*CAS — 156616-23-8.*

### Profile

Monteplase is a thrombolytic related to alteplase (p.857) used in acute myocardial infarction (p.828). The usual dose is 27 500 units/kg given by intravenous injection as soon as possible after the onset of symptoms.

◊ References.


1. Kawai C, *et al.* A prospective, randomized, double-blind multicenter trial of a single bolus injection of the novel modified t-PA E6010 in the treatment of acute myocardial infarction: comparison with native t-PA. *J Am Coll Cardiol* 1997; **29:** 1447–53.


### Preparations

**Proprietary Preparations** (details are given in Part 3)

***Jpn:*** Cleactor.

## Moracizine *(BAN, rINN)*

EN-313; Moricizine *(USAN)*. Ethyl [10-(3-morpholinopropionyl)phenothiazin-2-yl]carbamate.

$C_{22}H_{25}N_3O_4S$ = 427.5.

*CAS — 31883-05-3.*

*ATC — C01BG01.*

## Moracizine Hydrochloride (BANM, rINNM)

Hidrocloruro de moracizina.

$C_{22}H_{25}N_3O_4S,HCl = 464.0.$

*CAS — 29560-58-5.*

*ATC — C01BG01.*

**Pharmacopoeias.** In *US.*

**USP 27** (Moricizine Hydrochloride). A white to off-white crystalline powder. Soluble in water and in alcohol. Store in airtight containers.

### Adverse Effects

The most common adverse effects associated with moracizine affect the CNS and the gastrointestinal tract and include dizziness, headache, fatigue, nausea, and abdominal pain. Other adverse effects include dyspnoea, dry mouth, blurred vision, impotence, and urinary-tract disorders. There have been occasional reports of fever, thrombocytopenia, hepatic dysfunction, hypothermia, and skin rash.

Like other antiarrhythmics moracizine can provoke or worsen arrhythmias. This may range from an increase in the frequency of premature ventricular contractions to induction or worsening of ventricular tachycardia.

An increased mortality rate occurred when moracizine was tested in the control of asymptomatic ventricular arrhythmias in post-infarction patients (see Cardiac Arrhythmias under Uses and Administration, below).

**Effects on body temperature.** Fever with elevated creatine phosphokinase and hepatic transaminase concentrations was associated with moracizine in 2 patients.[1] The fever abated within 48 hours of withdrawing moracizine and recurred within 24 hours of rechallenge in both patients. Results suggested a similarity to the neuroleptic malignant syndrome which has been attributed to other phenothiazine derivatives.

1. Miura DS, *et al.* Ethmozine toxicity: fever of unknown origin. *J Clin Pharmacol* 1986; **26:** 153–5.

### Precautions

As for Flecainide Acetate, p.917.

### Interactions

Use of moracizine with other antiarrhythmics or arrhythmogenic drugs may increase the incidence of cardiac arrhythmias. Moracizine undergoes metabolism in the liver and its activity may be influenced by other drugs affecting the enzymes responsible for its metabolism; it is an enzyme inducer and may also affect the activity of other hepatically-metabolised drugs.

### Pharmacokinetics

Moracizine is readily and almost completely absorbed from the gastrointestinal tract. It undergoes significant first-pass hepatic metabolism so that the bioavailability after oral administration is about 38%. Moracizine is extensively metabolised and some of the numerous metabolites may be active. It induces its own metabolism; the plasma elimination half-life is about 2 hours after multiple doses. Although plasma concentrations are reduced with multiple dosing, clinical response is not affected. It is about 95% bound to plasma proteins. Moracizine is distributed into breast milk. About 56% of a dose is excreted in the faeces and about 39% in the urine.

◊ References.

1. Benedek IH, *et al.* Enzyme induction by moricizine: time course and extent in healthy subjects. *J Clin Pharmacol* 1994; **34:** 167–75.

### Uses and Administration

Moracizine is a phenothiazine compound with class I antiarrhythmic activity (p.809) but which does not readily fall into the subclasses a, b, or c. It is used as the hydrochloride in the treatment of serious symptomatic ventricular **arrhythmias**. Moracizine hydrochloride is given in a usual dose of 600 to 900 mg daily by mouth in 2 or 3 divided doses. Doses, which should be given initially in hospital, should be adjusted at intervals of not less than 3 days. If rapid control of life-threatening arrhythmias is essential an initial dose of 400 to 500 mg followed by 200 mg every 8 hours may be given. Doses should be reduced in patients with hepatic or renal impairment (see below).

◊ General reviews of moracizine published before[1-3] and after[4] the results of the Cardiac Arrhythmia Suppression Trial (CAST II), in which moracizine was associated with increased mortality (see Cardiac Arrhythmias, below).

1. Fitton A, Buckley MM-T. Moricizine: a review of its pharmacological properties, and therapeutic efficacy in cardiac arrhythmias. *Drugs* 1990; **40:** 138–67.
2. Carnes CA, Coyle JD. Moricizine: a novel antiarrhythmic agent. *DICP Ann Pharmacother* 1990; **24:** 745–53.
3. Mann HJ. Moricizine: a new class I antiarrhythmic. *Clin Pharm* 1990; **9:** 842–52.
4. Clyne CA, *et al.* Moricizine. *N Engl J Med* 1992; **327:** 255–60.

**Administration in hepatic or renal impairment.** Patients with hepatic or renal impairment should be started on a moracizine dosage of 600 mg or less daily and monitored closely before any adjustment of dose is made.

**Cardiac arrhythmias.** Although asymptomatic premature ventricular arrhythmias in subjects who have previously suffered a myocardial infarction are recognised as a risk factor for subsequent sudden cardiac death,[1] moracizine should not be used in such patients. A large multicentre study in the USA, the Cardiac Arrhythmia Suppression Trial (CAST),[2,3] found that encainide, flecainide, and moracizine,[4] were all associated with increased mortality. It is now accepted that these drugs should not be used prophylactically in post-infarction patients with asymptomatic arrhythmias.

Licensed indications for moracizine cover severe symptomatic ventricular arrhythmias (p.816).

1. Task Force of the Working Group on Arrhythmias of the European Society of Cardiology. CAST and beyond: implications of the cardiac arrhythmias suppression trial. *Circulation* 1990; **81:** 1123–7. Also published in *Eur Heart J* 1990; **11:** 194–9.
2. The Cardiac Arrhythmia Suppression Trial (CAST) Investigators. Preliminary report: effect of encainide and flecainide on mortality in a randomized trial of arrhythmia suppression after myocardial infarction. *N Engl J Med* 1989; **321:** 406–12.
3. Echt DS, *et al.* Mortality and morbidity in patients receiving encainide, flecainide, or placebo: the Cardiac Arrhythmia Suppression Trial. *N Engl J Med* 1991; **324:** 781–8.
4. The Cardiac Arrhythmia Suppression Trial II Investigators. Effect of the antiarrhythmic agent moricizine on survival after myocardial infarction. *N Engl J Med* 1992; **327:** 227–33.

### Preparations

***USP 27:*** Moricizine Hydrochloride Tablets.

**Proprietary Preparations** (details are given in Part 3)
***Irl.:*** Ethmozine†; ***UK:*** Ethmozine†; ***USA:*** Ethmozine.

## Moxisylyte Hydrochloride (BANM, rINNM)

Hidrocloruro de moxisilita; Moxisilita Clorhidrato; Thymoxamine Hydrochloride. 4-(2-Dimethylaminoethoxy)-5-isopropyl-2-methylphenyl acetate hydrochloride.

$C_{16}H_{25}NO_3,HCl = 315.8.$

*CAS — 54-32-0 (moxisylyte); 964-52-3 (moxisylyte hydrochloride).*

*ATC — C04AX10; G04BE06.*

NOTE. THY is a code approved by the BP 2003 for use on single unit doses of eye drops containing moxisylyte hydrochloride where the individual container may be too small to bear all the appropriate labelling information.

**Pharmacopoeias.** In *Br.*

**BP 2003** (Moxisylyte Hydrochloride). A white, odourless or almost odourless, crystalline powder. Freely soluble in water and in chloroform; soluble in alcohol; practically insoluble in ether and in petroleum spirit. A 5% solution in water has a pH of 4.5 to 5.5. Protect from light.

### Adverse Effects

Moxisylyte hydrochloride may cause nausea, diarrhoea, headache, vertigo, flushing of the skin, dry mouth, and nasal congestion. Hepatotoxicity has been reported. Overdosage may cause hypotension.

Transient ptosis has occurred occasionally following ophthalmic application. Prolonged erections or priapism have occurred rarely following intracavernosal injection and systemic effects may also occur.

**Effects on the liver.** Hepatic adverse reactions with moxisylyte first appeared in France following its use in benign prostatic hyperplasia, a condition in which relatively high doses were used (up to 480 mg daily compared with up to 320 mg daily for peripheral vascular disease). Since then the UK Committee on Safety of Medicines has received reports associated with lower doses.[1] Thirteen hepatic reactions, accounting for 17% of all reports of suspected adverse reactions to moxisylyte, had been received. These comprised 3 cases of hepatic function abnormalities, 3 of jaundice, 4 of cholestatic jaundice, 2 of hepatitis, and 1 of hepatitis with jaundice. In most cases the reaction occurred within 5 weeks of the start of treatment and resolved on drug withdrawal. In 9 cases the dosage of moxisylyte was known and varied from 80 to 320 mg daily with 7 patients receiving 160 mg or less daily.

1. Committee on Safety of Medicines/Medicines Control Agency. Hepatic reactions with thymoxamine (Opilon). *Current Problems* 1993; **19:** 11–12.

### Precautions

Moxisylyte hydrochloride should not be given to patients with active liver disease and should be given with care to patients with diabetes mellitus as it may theoretically decrease insulin requirements. Monitoring of liver function is recommended, especially if therapy is prolonged or if high doses are being used. Intracavernosal injection of moxisylyte is contra-indicated in patients with conditions that predispose to priapism.

### Interactions

Moxisylyte may enhance the effects of antihypertensives and the hypotensive effect of moxisylyte may be enhanced by tricyclic antidepressants.

### Uses and Administration

Moxisylyte is an alpha-adrenoceptor blocker with vasodilating activity. It is used by mouth in the treatment of peripheral vascular disease (p.831) and by intracavernosal injection in erectile dysfunction (p.1745).

Moxisylyte is given as the hydrochloride but the dose may be expressed in terms of the base. Moxisylyte hydrochloride 45.2 mg is approximately equivalent to 40 mg of moxisylyte.

In the management of **peripheral vascular disease**, the usual dose is the equivalent of 40 mg of moxisylyte four times daily by mouth increased if necessary to 80 mg four times daily. It should be withdrawn if there is no response in 2 weeks.

In the management of **erectile dysfunction**, moxisylyte is self-administered by intracavernosal injection The initial dose is 10 mg of moxisylyte hydrochloride; if this is unsuccessful a dose of 20 mg may be used. Moxisylyte should not be injected intracavernosally more than three times each week and there should be at least 24 hours between injections.

Moxisylyte has been used locally in the eye to reverse the mydriasis caused by phenylephrine and other sympathomimetics. It has also been used orally in benign prostatic hyperplasia, although such use has been associated with hepatotoxicity; the doses used in prostatic hyperplasia were generally higher than those in peripheral vascular disease.

◊ Reviews.

1. Marquer C, Bressolle F. Moxisylyte: a review of its pharmacodynamic and pharmacokinetic properties, and its therapeutic use in impotence. *Fundam Clin Pharmacol* 1998; **12:** 377–87.

### Preparations

***BP 2003:*** Moxisylyte Tablets.

**Proprietary Preparations** (details are given in Part 3)
***Fr.:*** Carlytene; Icavex; ***Irl.:*** Opilon; ***Ital.:*** Arlitene†; ***UK:*** Opilon.

## Moxonidine (BAN, USAN, rINN)

BDF-5895; BDF-5896; BE-5895; LY-326869; Moxonidina; Moxonidinum. 4-Chloro-5-(2-imidazolin-2-ylamino)-6-methoxy-2-methylpyrimidine.

$C_9H_{12}ClN_5O = 241.7.$

*CAS — 75438-57-2.*

*ATC — C02AC05.*

**Pharmacopoeias.** In *Eur.* (see p.vi).

**Ph. Eur. 5.0** (Moxonidine). A white or almost white powder. Very slightly soluble in water and in acetonitrile; slightly soluble in dichloromethane; sparingly soluble in methyl alcohol.

### Adverse Effects and Treatment

Moxonidine has similar adverse effects to clonidine (p.885) but causes less sedation. The incidence of dry mouth may also be lower.

### Precautions

Moxonidine should not be used in patients with conduction disorders, bradycardia, severe arrhythmias, severe heart failure, severe ischaemic heart disease, severe hepatic or renal impairment, or a history of angioedema. The manufacturer suggests that it should also be avoided in patients with intermittent claudication or Raynaud's disease, Parkinson's disease, epilepsy, glaucoma, and depression. Moxonidine is distributed into breast milk and should not be used during breast feeding.

Although rebound hypertension has not been reported following moxonidine withdrawal it should not be stopped abruptly but should be withdrawn gradually over 2 weeks. As for clonidine (p.886), in patients who are receiving a beta blocker concomitantly, the beta blocker should be stopped several days before moxonidine is withdrawn.

### Interactions

The hypotensive effect of moxonidine may be enhanced by other antihypertensives and drugs that cause hypotension. The effect of sedatives and hypnotics, including benzodiazepines, may be enhanced by moxonidine.

### Pharmacokinetics

Moxonidine is well absorbed following oral administration and has a bioavailability of about 88%. Peak plasma concentrations occur 0.5 to 3 hours after an oral dose. It is excreted almost entirely in the urine as unchanged drug and metabolites; about 50 to 75% of an oral dose is excreted as unchanged drug. The mean plasma elimination half-life is 2 to 3 hours and is prolonged in renal impairment. Moxonidine is about 7% bound to plasma proteins. It is distributed into breast milk.

### Uses and Administration

Moxonidine is a centrally acting antihypertensive structurally related to clonidine (p.885). It appears to act through stimulation of central imidazoline receptors to reduce sympathetic tone, and also has alpha$_2$-adrenoceptor agonist activity. It is used in the treatment of hypertension (p.825) and has also been investigated for heart failure (but see below).

In the treatment of hypertension, moxonidine is given by mouth in a usual initial dose of 200 micrograms once daily. The dose may be increased if necessary, after 3 weeks, to 400 micrograms daily as a single dose or in 2 divided doses, and after a further 3 weeks, to a maximum dose of 600 micrograms daily in 2 divided doses. The dose should be reduced in patients with renal impairment (see below).

◊ References.


1. Chrisp P, Faulds D. Moxonidine: a review of its pharmacology, and therapeutic use in essential hypertension. *Drugs* 1992; **44:** 993–1012.
2. Schachter M, *et al.* Safety and tolerability of moxonidine in the treatment of hypertension. *Drug Safety* 1998; **19:** 191–203.
3. Bousquet P, Feldman J. Drugs acting on imidazoline receptors: a review of their pharmacology, their use in blood pressure control and their potential interest in cardioprotection. *Drugs* 1999; **58:** 799–812.
4. Schachter M. Moxonidine. *Prescribers' J* 1999; **39:** 113–17.


**Administration in renal impairment.** In patients with moderate renal impairment (GFR 30 to 60 mL/minute) single doses of moxonidine should not exceed 200 micrograms and the daily dose should not exceed 400 micrograms; moxonidine should not be given in severe impairment (GFR less than 30 mL/minute).

**Heart failure.** Heart failure is usually treated with diuretics, ACE inhibitors, cardiac glycosides, and beta blockers (see p.820). Beta blockers are thought to act by suppressing the sympathetic nervous system, which is activated in heart failure. Centrally-acting antihypertensives such as moxonidine also suppress sympathetic activation and might therefore have a role in heart failure. A study[1] with moxonidine in patients with heart failure found that it reduced plasma-noradrenaline concentrations and increased left ventricular ejection fraction, but also led to an increase in adverse effects. A further study[2] was stopped early due to increased mortality in the group receiving moxonidine.


1. Swedberg K, *et al.* Effects of sustained-release moxonidine, an imidazoline agonist, on plasma norepinephrine in patients with chronic heart failure. *Circulation* 2002; **105:** 1797–1803.
2. Cohn JN, *et al.* Adverse mortality effect of central sympathetic inhibition with sustained-release moxonidine in patients with heart failure (MOXCON). *Eur J Heart Fail* 2003; **5:** 659–67.


## Preparations

**Proprietary Preparations** (details are given in Part 3)
***Austria:*** Normoxin; ***Belg.:*** Moxon; ***Braz.:*** Cynt; ***Denm.:*** Physiotens; ***Fin.:*** Physiotens; ***Fr.:*** Physiotens; ***Ger.:*** Cynt; Physiotens; ***Gr.:*** Cynt; Fisiotens; ***Neth.:*** Normatens; ***Norw.:*** Physiotens; ***S.Afr.:*** Physiotens; ***Singapore:*** Physiotens; ***Spain:*** Cynt†; Moxon; ***Swed.:*** Physiotens; ***Switz.:*** Physiotens; ***UK:*** Physiotens.

# Nadolol *(BAN, USAN, rINN)*

Nadololum; SQ-11725. (2*R*,3*S*)-5-(3-*tert*-Butylamino-2-hydroxypropoxy)-1,2,3,4-tetrahydronaphthalene-2,3-diol.

$C_{17}H_{27}NO_4$ = 309.4.

*CAS — 42200-33-9.*

*ATC — C07AA12.*

**Pharmacopoeias.** In *Eur.* (see p.vi), *Jpn*, and *US.*

**Ph. Eur. 5.0** (Nadolol). A white or almost white crystalline powder. Slightly soluble in water; freely soluble in alcohol; practically insoluble in acetone.

**USP 27** (Nadolol). A white or off-white, practically odourless, crystalline powder. Soluble in water at pH 2; slightly soluble in water at pH 7 to 10; freely soluble in alcohol and in methyl alcohol; insoluble in acetone, in ether, in petroleum spirit, in trichloroethane, and in benzene; slightly soluble in chloroform, in dichloromethane, and in isopropyl alcohol.

## Adverse Effects, Treatment, and Precautions

As for Beta Blockers, p.869.

**Breast feeding.** Nadolol is distributed into breast milk and concentrations in milk are higher than those in maternal plasma. In a study[1] in 12 lactating normotensive women given nadolol 80 mg daily by mouth for 5 days, the mean nadolol concentration in milk for the 24 hours after the last dose was 357 nanograms/mL; the equivalent mean serum-nadolol concentration was only 77 nanograms/mL. It was calculated that a 5-kg infant would therefore ingest about 2 to 7% of an equivalent adult dose. There have been no reports of adverse effects in breast-feeding infants whose mothers were receiving nadolol and the American Academy of Pediatrics considers[2] that it is therefore usually compatible with breast feeding.


1. Devlin RG, *et al.* Nadolol in human serum and breast milk. *Br J Clin Pharmacol* 1981; **12:** 393–6.
2. American Academy of Pediatrics. The transfer of drugs and other chemicals into human milk. *Pediatrics* 2001; **108:** 776–89. Correction. *ibid.*; 1029. Also available at: http://aappolicy.aappublications.org/cgi/content/full/pediatrics%3b108/3/776 (accessed 06/07/04)


**Hypersensitivity.** Hypersensitivity pneumonitis was associated with nadolol in a patient prescribed the drug for migraine.[1] Symptoms improved when nadolol was withdrawn.


1. Levy MB, *et al.* Nadolol and hypersensitivity pneumonitis. *Ann Intern Med* 1986; **105:** 806–7.


## Interactions

The interactions associated with beta blockers are discussed on p.870.

## Pharmacokinetics

Nadolol is incompletely absorbed from the gastrointestinal tract to give peak plasma concentrations about 3 or 4 hours after a dose. It has low lipid solubility. Nadolol is widely distributed and concentrations found in breast milk have been higher than those in serum. It is only about 30% bound to plasma proteins. It does not appear to be metabolised and is excreted mainly in the urine. The plasma half-life has been reported as ranging from about 12 to 24 hours. Nadolol is reported to be dialysable.

◊ In 4 patients with mild hypertension given nadolol 2 mg by mouth or intravenously, the elimination half-life from plasma was an average of 10 to 12 hours (a range of 5.9 to 12.2 hours following intravenous administration, and a range of 9.6 to 14.2 hours following oral administration). Calculations based on urinary excretion and plasma concentration data suggested that about 33% was absorbed after oral administration. There was evidence of biliary as well as urinary excretion since after intravenous administration about 73% was excreted in urine and 23% in faeces. Nadolol did not appear to be metabolised.[1] In a similar study of therapeutic oral doses, terminal half-lives ranging from 14 to 17 hours were reported for nadolol 80 mg given as a single dose and the same dose daily in a multiple dosage regimen.[2]


1. Dreyfuss J, *et al.* Metabolic studies in patients with nadolol: oral and intravenous administration. *J Clin Pharmacol* 1977; **17:** 300–7.
2. Dreyfuss J, *et al.* Pharmacokinetics of nadolol, a beta-receptor antagonist: administration of therapeutic single- and multiple-dosage regimens to hypertensive patients. *J Clin Pharmacol* 1979; **19:** 712–20.


**Children.** The pharmacokinetics of nadolol given intravenously and orally were studied in six children aged 3 months to 14 years.[1] The elimination half-lives for the two oldest children aged 10 and 14 years were 7.3 and 15.7 hours, respectively. These values are similar to those reported for adults whereas in the children 22 months of age or younger, shorter half-lives of 3.2 to 4.3 hours were found. The shorter half-lives were probably a result of a reduction in the total apparent volume of distribution of nadolol in the youngest children. Elimination rates were similar after either intravenous or oral administration.


1. Mehta AV, *et al.* Pharmacokinetics of nadolol in children with supraventricular tachycardia. *J Clin Pharmacol* 1992; **32:** 1023–7.


## Uses and Administration

Nadolol is a non-cardioselective beta blocker (p.868). It is reported to lack intrinsic sympathomimetic and membrane-stabilising activity. Nadolol is used in the management of hypertension (p.825), angina pectoris (p.813), and cardiac arrhythmias (p.816). It is also used in the management of hyperthyroidism (p.1594) and in the prophylactic treatment of migraine (p.464).

In the treatment of **hypertension**, nadolol is usually given in an initial dose of 40 to 80 mg once daily by mouth, increased weekly according to response to 240 mg or more daily.

In **angina pectoris**, the usual initial dose is 40 mg once daily, increased weekly according to response to usual doses of up to 160 mg daily; some patients may require up to 240 mg daily. Doses of 40 to 160 mg once daily have also been given for **cardiac arrhythmias**.

Doses of 40 to 160 mg once daily are used in **migraine** prophylaxis.

In the management of **hyperthyroidism**, doses of 80 to 160 mg once daily have been given; most patients are reported to require the higher dose.

Patients with renal impairment may require a reduction in dose (see below).

**Administration in renal impairment.** Patients with renal impairment may require a lower dose of nadolol or less frequent administration. One method of dose adjustment is to increase the dosage interval according to the patient's creatinine clearance (CC) as follows:

- CC between 31 and 50 mL/minute: give every 24 to 36 hours
- CC between 10 and 30 mL/minute: give every 24 to 48 hours
- CC less than 10 mL/minute: give every 40 to 60 hours.

## Preparations

***USP 27:*** Nadolol and Bendroflumethiazide Tablets; Nadolol Tablets.

**Proprietary Preparations** (details are given in Part 3)
***Arg.:*** Corgard; ***Austria:*** Solgol†; ***Belg.:*** Corgard; ***Braz.:*** Corgard; ***Canad.:*** Apo-Nadol; Corgard; ***Chile:*** Corgard; ***Fr.:*** Corgard; ***Ger.:*** Solgol; ***Hong Kong:*** Apo-Nadol; Corgard; ***Ital.:*** Corgard; ***Malaysia:*** Corgard; ***NZ:*** Corgard†; ***Port.:*** Anabet; ***S.Afr.:*** Corgard; ***Spain:*** Corgard; Solgol; ***Switz.:*** Corgard; ***UK:*** Corgard; ***USA:*** Corgard.

**Multi-ingredient:** ***Austria:*** Solgeretik†; ***Canad.:*** Corzide†; ***Ger.:*** Sotaziden N; ***S.Afr.:*** Corgaretic; ***Switz.:*** Corgaretic†; ***UK:*** Corgaretic†; ***USA:*** Corzide.

# Nadoxolol Hydrochloride *(rINNM)*

Hidrocloruro de nadoxolol; LL-1530. 3-Hydroxy-4-(1-naphthyloxy)butyramide oxime hydrochloride.

$C_{14}H_{16}N_2O_3$,HCl = 296.7.

*CAS — 54063-51-3 (nadoxolol); 35991-93-6 (nadoxolol hydrochloride).*

## Profile

Nadoxolol hydrochloride has been given by mouth as an antiarrhythmic.

## Preparations

**Proprietary Preparations** (details are given in Part 3)
***Fr.:*** Bradyl†.

# Nadroparin Calcium *(BAN, rINN)*

CY-216; Nadroparina cálcica; Nadroparinum Calcicum.

*ATC — B01AB06.*

**Pharmacopoeias.** In *Eur.* (see p.vi).

**Ph. Eur. 5.0** (Nadroparin Calcium). It is prepared by nitrous acid depolymerisation of heparin obtained from the intestinal mucosa of pigs. The majority of the components have a 2-*O*-sulfo-α-L-idopyranosuronic acid structure at the non-reducing end and a 6-*O*-sulfo-2,5-anhydro-D-mannitol structure at the reducing end of their chain. The mass-average molecular mass ranges between 3600 and 5000, with a characteristic value of 4300. The mass percentage of chains lower than 2000 is not more than 15%. The degree of sulfation is about 2 per disaccharide unit. The potency is not less than 95 units and not more than 130 units of anti-factor Xa activity per mg with reference to the dried substance, and the ratio of anti-factor Xa activity to anti-factor IIa (antithrombin) activity is between 2.5 and 4.0.

## Profile

Nadroparin calcium is a low-molecular-weight heparin (p.949) with anticoagulant properties. It is used in the treatment and prophylaxis of venous thromboembolism (p.839) and to prevent clotting during extracorporeal circulation. It is also used in the management of unstable angina (p.813).

Doses are expressed in terms of anti-factor Xa activity (anti-Xa units) although different values may be encountered in the literature depending upon the reference preparation used. For prophylaxis of venous thromboembolism during surgery, patients at moderate risk of thrombosis are given 2850 units of nadroparin calcium by subcutaneous injection daily for at least 7 days or until the patient is ambulant; the first dose is given 2 to 4 hours before the procedure. For patients at high risk of thrombosis the dose is adjusted according to body-weight. Usual doses are 38 units/kg 12 hours before surgery, 12 hours postoperatively and then daily until 3 days after the procedure; the dose is then increased by 50% to 57 units/kg daily. The total duration of treatment should be at least 10 days.

For the treatment of thromboembolism, nadroparin calcium is given in a dose of 85 units/kg by subcutaneous injection every 12 hours for up to 10 days. Alternatively, a dose of 171 units/kg is given once daily.

For prevention of clotting in the extracorporeal circulation during haemodialysis sessions lasting less than 4 hours, nadroparin calcium is administered into the arterial line of the circuit at the beginning of the dialysis session. The usual dose is 2850 units for patients weighing less than 50 kg, 3800 units for patients weighing 50 to 69 kg, and 5700 units for patients weighing 70 kg or more. Doses should be reduced in patients at high risk of haemorrhage.

In the management of unstable angina, nadroparin calcium is given subcutaneously in a dose of 86 units/kg every 12 hours, for about 6 days. An initial dose of 86 units/kg may be given intravenously. Low-dose aspirin should be given concomitantly.

◊ References.


1. Barradell LB, Buckley MM. Nadroparin calcium: a review of its pharmacology and clinical applications in the prevention and treatment of thromboembolic disorders. *Drugs* 1992; **44:** 858–88.


## Preparations

**Proprietary Preparations** (details are given in Part 3)
***Arg.:*** Fraxiparine; ***Austral.:*** Fraxiparine†; ***Austria:*** Fraxiparin; ***Belg.:*** Fraxiparine; ***Braz.:*** Fraxiparina; ***Canad.:*** Fraxiparine; ***Chile:*** Fraxiparine; ***Denm.:*** Fraxiparine†; ***Fin.:*** Fraxiparine†; ***Fr.:*** Fraxiparine; Fraxodi; ***Ger.:*** Fraxiparin; Fraxodi; ***Gr.:*** Fraxiparine; ***Hong Kong:*** Fraxiparine; ***Israel:*** Fraxiparine; ***Ital.:*** Fraxiparina; Seledie; Seleparina; ***Malaysia:*** Fraxiparine; ***Mex.:*** Fraxiparine; Fraxodi; ***Neth.:*** Fraxiparine; Fraxodi; ***Norw.:*** Fraxiparine; ***NZ:*** Fraxiparine; ***Port.:*** Fraxiparina; ***S.Afr.:*** Fraxiparine; ***Singapore:*** Fraxiparine; ***Spain:*** Fraxiparina; ***Swed.:*** Fraxiparine; ***Switz.:*** Fraxiforte; Fraxiparine; ***Thai.:*** Fraxiparine.

## Naftidrofuryl Oxalate *(BANM, rINNM)*

EU-1806; LS-121; Nafronyl Oxalate *(USAN)*; Naftidrofuryl Hydrogen Oxalate; Naftidrofuryli Hydrogenooxalas; Oxalato de naftidrofurilo. 2-Diethylaminoethyl 3-(1-naphthyl)-2-tetrahydrofurfurylpropionate hydrogen oxalate.

$C_{24}H_{33}NO_3,C_2H_2O_4$ = 473.6.

*CAS — 31329-57-4 (naftidrofuryl); 3200-06-4 (naftidrofuryl oxalate).*

*ATC — C04AX21.*

**Pharmacopoeias.** In *Eur.* (see p.vi).

**Ph. Eur. 5.0** (Naftidrofuryl Hydrogen Oxalate; Naftidrofuryl Oxalate BP 2003). A white or almost white powder. Freely soluble in water; freely soluble or soluble in alcohol; slightly or sparingly soluble in acetone.

### Adverse Effects

Naftidrofuryl oxalate given orally may cause nausea and epigastric pain. Rash has been reported occasionally. Hepatitis or hepatic failure has occurred rarely. Convulsions and depression of cardiac conduction may occur following overdosage. Following intravenous administration cardiac arrhythmias, hypotension, and convulsions have been reported and intravenous preparations have been withdrawn from the market (see below).

◊ In early 1995 the UK Committee on Safety of Medicines (CSM) published details of adverse reactions to naftidrofuryl.[1] Following parenteral administration of naftidrofuryl 47 reports of 79 reactions had been received, the most serious consequences being 9 cases of cardiac arrhythmias, 3 of convulsions, and 2 of hypotension. It was also noted that 2 fatal cases of cardiac arrest had occurred in Germany following bolus intravenous doses and it was stressed that the drug must not be given as a bolus but as a slow intravenous infusion. Additionally, 16 reports, including one fatality, of hepatitis or hepatic failure associated with oral naftidrofuryl had been received although this appeared to be a rare reaction.

Later in 1995, following a review conducted in the UK and Europe, it was announced by the CSM that intravenous naftidrofuryl was to be withdrawn.[2] It was considered that the risks of cardiac and neurological toxicity outweighed the benefits of intravenous administration in peripheral vascular disease. The oral form of naftidrofuryl would remain available.


1. Committee on Safety of Medicines/Medicines Control Agency. Adverse reactions with naftidrofuryl (Praxilene). *Current Problems* 1995; **21:** 2.
2. Committee on Safety of Medicines/Medicines Control Agency. Withdrawal of naftidrofuryl infusion (Praxilene Forte). *Current Problems* 1995; **21:** 7.


**Effects on the kidneys.** Calcium oxalate crystals in the renal tubules of 2 patients with acute renal failure[1] were associated with the high amounts of oxalate they had received when naftidrofuryl oxalate was administered intravenously.


1. Moesch C, *et al.* Renal intratubular crystallisation of calcium oxalate and naftidrofuryl oxalate. *Lancet* 1991; **338:** 1219–20.


### Uses and Administration

Naftidrofuryl oxalate is used as a vasodilator in the treatment of peripheral (p.831) and cerebral vascular disorders (p.820). It is also claimed to enhance cellular oxidative capacity thereby protecting cells against the results of ischaemia.

Naftidrofuryl oxalate is given by mouth in usual doses of 100 to 200 mg three times daily for peripheral vascular disorders and 100 mg three times daily for cerebrovascular disorders.

Naftidrofuryl oxalate has also been administered parenterally. However, intravenous administration has been associated with serious adverse effects (see above) and intravenous preparations have been withdrawn.

### Preparations

***BP 2003:*** Naftidrofuryl Capsules.

**Proprietary Preparations** (details are given in Part 3)
***Arg.:*** Iridus; ***Austria:*** Dusodril; Naftodril; ***Belg.:*** Praxilene; ***Braz.:*** Iridux†; ***Fr.:*** Di-Actane; Gevatran; Naftilux; Praxilene; ***Ger.:*** Artocoron; Azunaftil; Dusodril; Luctor†; Nafti; Naftilong; ***Hong Kong:*** Praxilene; ***Irl.:*** Praxilene; ***Ital.:*** Esedril†; Praxilene; ***Mex.:*** Iridus; ***Port.:*** Praxilene; ***Singapore:*** Praxilene; ***Spain:*** Praxilene; ***Switz.:*** Praxilene; Sodipryl retard; ***Thai.:*** Praxilene; ***UK:*** Praxilene; Stimlor†.

## Naftopidil *(rINN)*

BM-15275; KT-611. (±)-4-(o-Methoxyphenyl)-α-[(1-naphthyloxy)methyl]-1-piperazineethanol.

$C_{24}H_{28}N_2O_3$ = 392.5.

*CAS — 57149-07-2.*

### Profile

Naftopidil is a peripheral $alpha_1$-adrenoceptor blocker that is structurally related to urapidil (p.1018) and has similar general properties. It is under investigation in the management of hypertension, and in benign prostatic hyperplasia to relieve symptoms of urinary obstruction.

### Preparations

**Proprietary Preparations** (details are given in Part 3)
***Jpn:*** Avishot; Flivas.

## Nasaruplase *(rINN)*

Nasaruplasa; Prourokinase, Glycosylated. Prourokinase (enzyme-activating) (human clone pA3/pD2/pF1 protein moiety), glycosylated.

*CAS — 99821-44-0.*

NOTE. The term prourokinase has been used for both nasaruplase and saruplase (p.996).

## Nasaruplase Beta *(USAN, rINN)*

Abbott-74187; ABT-187. Prourokinase (enzyme-activating) human (clone pUK4/pUK18 protein moiety), glycosylated (murine cell line SP2/0).

*CAS — 136653-69-5.*

### Profile

Nasaruplase is a thrombolytic under investigation in acute ischaemic stroke.

◊ References.


1. Furlan A, *et al.* Intra-arterial prourokinase for acute ischemic stroke. The PROACT II study: a randomized controlled trial. *JAMA* 1999; **282:** 2003–11.


## Nateplase *(rINN)*

A mixture of *N*-[$N^2$-(*N*-glycyl-L-alanyl)-L-arginyl]plasminogen activator (human tissue-type 1-chain form, protein moiety), glycoform β (major component) and plasminogen activator (human tissue-type 1-chain form, protein moiety), glycoform β.

*CAS — 159445-63-3.*

### Profile

Nateplase is a thrombolytic related to alteplase (p.857) used in acute myocardial infarction (p.828). The usual dose is 300 000 units/kg, given by intravenous infusion as soon as possible after the onset of symptoms.

### Preparations

**Proprietary Preparations** (details are given in Part 3)
***Jpn:*** Milyzer.

## Natriuretic Peptides

Péptidos natriuréticos.

### Profile

Natriuretic peptides are endogenous substances that possess diuretic, natriuretic, and vasodilator properties. Three types are known. *Atrial natriuretic peptide* (ANP), also known as atrial natriuretic factor (ANF), atriopeptin, auriculin, or cardionatrin, is produced mainly in the cardiac atria, although another form, ularitide (urodilatin), is produced in the kidney. *Brain natriuretic peptide* (BNP, B-type natriuretic peptide) was originally isolated from brain tissue but is now known to be mainly produced by the cardiac ventricles. *C-type natriuretic peptide* (CNP) is produced by the endothelium and appears to act locally as a vasodilator but has little natriuretic effect.

Natriuretic peptides have an important physiological role in fluid and electrolyte homoeostasis and in the regulation of blood pressure, and they interact closely with other complex systems such as the renin-angiotensin-aldosterone cascade. Plasma concentrations of atrial natriuretic peptide and brain natriuretic peptide are altered in some pathological states and have been used as indicators of cardiac function. Natriuretic peptides that have been investigated for therapeutic use include anaritide, a synthetic form of atrial natriuretic peptide, and ularitide; both have been studied in acute renal failure. Recombinant forms of atrial natriuretic peptide (carperitide, p.880) and brain natriuretic peptide (nesiritide, p.964) are used in the management of acute heart failure.

The currently available natriuretic peptides have short half-lives and have to be given parenterally. Other approaches to manipulating their effects are under investigation and include the use of atriopeptidase inhibitors (neutral endopeptidase inhibitors; neutral metalloendopeptidase inhibitors), such as candoxatrilat (p.879) and ecadotril (sinorphan) to prolong the half-life of endogenous atrial natriuretic peptide. Compounds such as omapatrilat (p.976) that inhibit both neutral endopeptidase and angiotensin-converting enzyme are also being studied.

◊ References.


1. Tan ACITL, *et al.* Atrial natriuretic peptide: an overview of clinical pharmacology and pharmacokinetics. *Clin Pharmacokinet* 1993; **24:** 28–45.
2. Deutsch A, *et al.* Atrial natriuretic peptide and its potential role in pharmacotherapy. *J Clin Pharmacol* 1994; **34:** 1133–47.
3. Struthers AD. Ten years of natriuretic peptide research: a new dawn for their diagnostic and therapeutic use? *BMJ* 1994; **308:** 1615–19.
4. Richards AM. The renin-angiotensin-aldosterone system and the cardiac natriuretic peptides. *Heart* 1996; **76** (suppl 3): 36–44.
5. Wilkins MR, *et al.* The natriuretic-peptide family. *Lancet* 1997; **349:** 1307–10.
6. Allgren RL, *et al.* Anaritide in acute tubular necrosis. *N Engl J Med* 1997; **336:** 828–34.
7. Levin ER, *et al.* Natriuretic peptides. *N Engl J Med* 1998; **339:** 321–8.
8. O'Connor CM, *et al.* A randomized trial of ecadotril versus placebo in patients with mild to moderate heart failure: the U.S. ecadotril pilot safety study. *Am Heart J* 1999; **138:** 1140–8.
9. de Lemos JA, *et al.* B-type natriuretic peptide in cardiovascular disease. *Lancet* 2003; **362:** 316–22.


## Nebivolol *(BAN, USAN, rINN)*

R-65824. (1*RS*,1'*RS*)-1,1'-[(2*RS*,2'*SR*)-Bis(6-fluorochroman-2-yl)]-2,2'-iminodiethanol.

$C_{22}H_{25}F_2NO_4$ = 405.4.

*CAS — 99200-09-6; 118457-14-0.*

*ATC — C07AB12.*

## Nebivolol Hydrochloride *(BANM, rINNM)*

Hidrocloruro de nebivolol; R-67555.

$C_{22}H_{25}F_2NO_4,HCl$ = 441.9.

*CAS — 169293-50-9.*

*ATC — C07AB12.*

### Adverse Effects, Treatment, and Precautions

As for Beta Blockers, p.869. Nebivolol should not be used in patients with hepatic impairment.

### Interactions

The interactions associated with beta blockers are discussed on p.870.

### Pharmacokinetics

Nebivolol is rapidly absorbed following oral administration. It is extensively metabolised in the liver by alicyclic and aromatic hydroxylation, *N*-dealkylation, and glucuronidation; the hydroxy metabolites are reported to be active. The rate of aromatic hydroxylation by cytochrome P450 isoenzyme CYP2D6 is subject to genetic polymorphism and bioavailability and half-life vary widely. In fast metabolisers the elimination half-life of nebivolol is about 10 hours and of the hydroxy metabolites is about 24 hours. Peak plasma concentrations of unchanged drug plus active metabolites are 1.3 to 1.4 times higher in slow metabolisers and the half-lives of nebivolol and its hydroxy metabolites are prolonged.

Nebivolol is about 98% bound to plasma proteins. It is excreted in the urine and faeces, almost entirely as metabolites. Nebivolol is distributed into breast milk in *animals*.

### Uses and Administration

Nebivolol is a cardioselective beta blocker (p.868). It is also reported to have vasodilating activity but to lack intrinsic sympathomimetic and membrane-stabilising activity.

Nebivolol is used in the management of hypertension (p.825). It is given by mouth as the hydrochloride although doses are expressed in terms of the base; 5.45 mg of nebivolol hydrochloride is approximately equivalent to 5 mg of base. The usual dose is 5 mg of nebivolol daily. An initial dose of 2.5 mg daily is used in the elderly and in patients with renal impairment (see below).

◊ References.


1. McNeely W, Goa KL. Nebivolol in the management of essential hypertension: a review. *Drugs* 1999; **57:** 633–51. Correction. *ibid.:* 870.


**Administration in renal impairment.** The initial dose of nebivolol should be reduced to 2.5 mg once daily in patients with renal impairment, increased to 5 mg once daily for maintenance if required.

### Preparations

**Proprietary Preparations** (details are given in Part 3)
***Arg.:*** Nebilet; ***Belg.:*** Nobiten; ***Ger.:*** Nebilet; ***Gr.:*** Lobivon; ***Irl.:*** Nebilet; ***Ital.:*** Lobivon; Nebilox; ***Neth.:*** Nebilet; ***Port.:*** Nebilet; ***Singapore:*** Nebilet; ***Spain:*** Lobivon; Silostar; ***Switz.:*** Nebilet; ***UK:*** Nebilet.

## Nesiritide Citrate *(USAN, rINNM)*

$C_{143}H_{244}N_{50}O_{42}S_4,xC_6H_8O_7$.

*CAS — 124584-08-3 (nesiritide); 189032-40-4 (nesiritide citrate).*

*ATC — C01DX19.*

**Incompatibility.** The manufacturer states that nesiritide injection is physically and/or chemically incompatible with heparin, insulin, sodium etacrynate, bumetanide, enalaprilat, hydralazine, furosemide, and the preservative sodium metabisulfite. Nesiritide binds to heparin and should not be administered through heparin-coated central catheters.

### Adverse Effects and Precautions

The most common adverse effects of nesiritide relate to vasodilatation and include hypotension, headache, and dizziness. Nausea and vomiting, abdominal pain, back pain, angina pectoris, insomnia, and anxiety, have also been reported. Cardiac arrhythmias have occurred but may be associated with the underlying condition. If hypotension occurs the infusion of nesiritide should be stopped or the dose reduced and general supportive measures should be used; the hypotension may persist for several hours.

Nesiritide should not be used as primary therapy in patients with cardiogenic shock or with hypotension. It is not recommended in patients for whom vasodilators are inappropriate, such as those with significant valvular stenosis, restrictive or obstructive cardiomyopathy, constrictive pericarditis, or pericardial tamponade.

### Interactions

The risk of hypotension may be increased in patients receiving nesiritide with other drugs that lower blood pressure.

### Pharmacokinetics

Nesiritide is cleared from the circulation by 3 mechanisms: uptake into cells; proteolytic cleavage by endopeptidases; and excretion by the kidneys. It has a biphasic elimination, with a terminal elimination half-life of 18 minutes.

### Uses and Administration

Nesiritide is a recombinant brain natriuretic peptide (see p.964) used in the management of acutely decompensated heart failure (p.820). It is given intravenously as the citrate, but dosage is expressed in terms of the base. The initial dose of nesiritide is 2 micrograms/kg by intravenous injection over 1 minute, followed by a maintenance infusion of 10 nanograms/kg per minute.

◊ References.

1. Colucci WS, *et al.* Intravenous nesiritide, a natriuretic peptide, in the treatment of decompensated congestive heart failure. *N Engl J Med* 2000; **343:** 246–53. Correction. *ibid.*; 1504.
2. Publication Committee for the VMAC Investigators. Intravenous nesiritide vs nitroglycerin for treatment of decompensated congestive heart failure: a randomized controlled trial. *JAMA* 2002; **287:** 1531–40. Correction. *ibid.*; **288:** 577.
3. Burger AJ, *et al.* Effect of nesiritide (B-type natriuretic peptide) and dobutamine on ventricular arrhythmias in the treatment of patients with acutely decompensated congestive heart failure: the PRECEDENT study. *Am Heart J* 2002; **144:** 1102–8.
4. Vichiendilokkul A, *et al.* Nesiritide: a novel approach for acute heart failure. *Ann Pharmacother* 2003; **37:** 247–58.
5. Keating GM, Goa KL. Nesiritide: a review of its use in acute decompensated heart failure. *Drugs* 2003; **63:** 47–70.

### Preparations

**Proprietary Preparations** (details are given in Part 3)
***USA:*** Natrecor.

## Nicardipine Hydrochloride

*(BANM, USAN, rINNM)*

Hidrocloruro de nicardipino; RS-69216; RS-69216-XX-07-0; YC-93. 2-[Benzyl(methyl)amino]ethyl methyl 1,4-dihydro-2,6-dimethyl-4-(3-nitrophenyl)pyridine-3,5-dicarboxylate hydrochloride.

$C_{26}H_{29}N_3O_6$,HCl = 516.0.
*CAS — 55985-32-5 (nicardipine); 54527-84-3 (nicardipine hydrochloride).*
*ATC — C08CA04.*

**Pharmacopoeias.** In *Chin.* and *Jpn.*

**Incompatibility.** The manufacturers recommend that a solution containing nicardipine hydrochloride 100 micrograms/mL is used for intravenous infusion. Suitable diluents are solutions of glucose or sodium chloride. Sodium bicarbonate and lactated Ringer's are incompatible with nicardipine infusion. Nicardipine hydrochloride (1 mg/mL in glucose 5%) has also been reported[1] to be visually incompatible with furosemide, heparin, and thiopental.

1. Chiu MF, Schwartz ML. Visual compatibility of injectable drugs used in the intensive care unit. *Am J Health-Syst Pharm* 1997; **54:** 64–5.

### Adverse Effects, Treatment, and Precautions

As for dihydropyridine calcium-channel blockers (see Nifedipine, p.966).

### Interactions

As for dihydropyridine calcium-channel blockers (see Nifedipine, p.969).

### Pharmacokinetics

Nicardipine is rapidly and completely absorbed from the gastrointestinal tract but is subject to saturable first-pass hepatic metabolism. Bioavailability of about 35% has been reported following a 30-mg dose at steady state. The pharmacokinetics of nicardipine are non-linear due to the saturable first-pass hepatic metabolism and an increase in dose may produce a disproportionate increase in plasma concentration. There is also considerable interindividual variation in plasma-nicardipine concentrations. Nicardipine is more than 95% bound to plasma proteins. Nicardipine is extensively metabolised in the liver and is excreted in the urine and faeces, mainly as inactive metabolites. The terminal plasma half-life is about 8.6 hours, thus steady-state plasma concentrations are achieved after 2 to 3 days of dosing three times daily.

◊ References.

1. Graham DJM, *et al.* Pharmacokinetics of nicardipine following oral and intravenous administration in man. *Postgrad Med J* 1984; **60** (suppl 4): 7–10.
2. Graham DJM, *et al.* The metabolism and pharmacokinetics of nicardipine hydrochloride in man. *Br J Clin Pharmacol* 1985; **20:** 23S–28S.
3. Razak TA, *et al.* The effect of hepatic cirrhosis on the pharmacokinetics and blood pressure response to nicardipine. *Clin Pharmacol Ther* 1990; **47:** 463–9.
4. Porchet HC, Dayer P. Serum concentrations and effects of (±)-nicardipine compared with nifedipine in a population of healthy subjects. *Clin Pharmacol Ther* 1990; **48:** 155–60.

### Uses and Administration

Nicardipine is a dihydropyridine calcium-channel blocker with actions and uses similar to nifedipine (p.970). It is used in the management of hypertension (p.825) and angina pectoris (p.813).

Nicardipine hydrochloride is generally given by mouth although the intravenous route has been used for the short-term treatment of hypertension.

Oral doses of nicardipine hydrochloride are similar for both **hypertension** and **angina**. The initial dose is 20 mg by mouth three times daily and may be increased at intervals of at least 3 days until the required effect is achieved. The usual maintenance dose is 30 mg three times daily, but daily doses of between 60 and 120 mg in divided doses may be given. Modified-release preparations of nicardipine hydrochloride for administration twice daily are also available.

Nicardipine hydrochloride may be given by slow intravenous infusion as a 100 micrograms/mL solution in the short-term treatment of hypertension. An initial infusion rate of 5 mg/hour is recommended, increased, as necessary, up to a maximum of 15 mg/hour and subsequently reduced to 3 mg/hour.

Reduced doses of nicardipine hydrochloride and longer dosing intervals may be necessary in patients with hepatic or renal impairment (see below).

**Administration in children.** Intravenous infusion of nicardipine has been used in both infants and children for the management of hypertension. In studies[1-4] in children aged between 2 days and 17 years, initial doses ranged from 0.2 to 5 micrograms/kg per minute, with maintenance infusions of 0.15 to 6 micrograms/kg per minute. Adverse effects were rare; one study[4] reported adverse effects in 5 of 31 treatment courses, including tachycardia, flushing, palpitations, and hypotension. There has also been a report[5] of the successful use of intravenous infusion of nicardipine in 8 preterm infants (gestational age 28 to 36 weeks). Infusions were given at a dose of 0.5 to 2 micrograms/kg per minute and continued for periods of 3 to 36 days. No hypotension, oedema, or tachycardia were observed.

1. Treluyer JM, *et al.* Intravenous nicardipine in hypertensive children. *Eur J Pediatr* 1993; **152:** 712–4.
2. Sartori SC, *et al.* Intravenous nicardipine for treatment of systemic hypertension in children. *Pediatrics* 1999; **104** (suppl): 676–7.
3. Tobias JD. Nicardipine to control mean arterial pressure after cardiothoracic surgery in infants and children. *Am J Ther* 2001; **8:** 3–6.
4. Flynn JT, *et al.* Intravenous nicardipine for treatment of severe hypertension in children. *J Pediatr* 2001; **139:** 38–43.
5. Gouyon JB, *et al.* Intravenous nicardipine in hypertensive preterm infants. *Arch Dis Child* 1997; **76:** F126–F127.

**Administration in hepatic or renal impairment.** Reduced doses of nicardipine hydrochloride and longer dosing intervals may be necessary in patients with hepatic or renal impairment. The US manufacturers recommend an initial dose of 20 mg twice daily by mouth in patients with hepatic impairment.

**Cerebrovascular disorders.** Nicardipine has been reported to increase cerebral blood flow[1] and administration by various routes has been investigated for possible benefit in haemorrhagic[2-4] and ischaemic stroke[5,6] (p.836), although nimodipine (p.973) is the dihydropyridine calcium-channel blocker usually used. Nicardipine has also been tried[7] in patients with cerebrovascular insufficiency. However, studies have produced inconclusive results.

1. Savage I, James I. The effect of nicardipine hydrochloride on cerebral blood flow in normotensive volunteers. *Br J Clin Pharmacol* 1986; **21:** 591P–592P.
2. Rinkel GJE, *et al.* Calcium antagonists for aneurysmal subarachnoid haemorrhage. Available in The Cochrane Library; Issue 2. Chichester: John Wiley; 2004.
3. Suzuki M, *et al.* Intrathecal administration of nicardipine hydrochloride to prevent vasospasm in patients with subarachnoid hemorrhage. *Neurosurg Rev* 2001; **24:** 180–4.
4. Kasuya H, *et al.* Efficacy and safety of nicardipine prolonged-release implants for preventing vasospasm in humans. *Stroke* 2002; **33:** 1011–5.
5. Yao L, Ding D. Effect of nicardipine on somatosensory evoked potentials in patients with acute cerebral infarction. *J Neurol Neurosurg Psychiatry* 1990; **53:** 844–6.
6. Rosenbaum D, *et al.* Early treatment of ischemic stroke with a calcium antagonist. *Stroke* 1991; **22:** 437–41.
7. Silva APE, Diament CK. Nicardipine versus cinnarizine in cerebrovascular insufficiency. *Curr Ther Res* 1988; **43:** 888–99.

### Preparations

**Proprietary Preparations** (details are given in Part 3)
***Austria:*** Karden; ***Belg.:*** Rydene; ***Canad.:*** Cardene†; ***Fr.:*** Loxen; ***Ger.:*** Antagonil; ***Irl.:*** Cardene; ***Ital.:*** Bionicard; Cardioten; Cardip; Cordipina†; Cordisol; Lisanirc; Neucor; Nicant; Nicapress; Nicardal; Nicardium†; Nicarpin; Nicaven; Nimicor; Niven; Perdipina; Ranvil; Vasodin; Vasonorm†; ***Jpn:*** Perdipine; ***Malaysia:*** Cardepine; ***Mex.:*** Ridene†; ***Neth.:*** Cardene; ***Port.:*** Nerdipina; ***Singapore:*** Cardibloc; ***Spain:*** Dagan; Flusemide; Lecibral; Lincil; Lucenfal; Nerdipina; Vasonase; Vatrasin†; ***Thai.:*** Cardepine; Cenpine†; Nerdipine; ***UK:*** Cardene; ***USA:*** Cardene.

## Niceritrol *(BAN, rINN)*

PETN. Pentaerythritol tetranicotinate; 2,2-Bis(hydroxymethyl)propane-1,3-diol tetranicotinate.

$C_{29}H_{24}N_4O_8$ = 556.5.
*CAS — 5868-05-3.*
*ATC — C10AD01.*

NOTE. The synonym PETN has been applied to both niceritrol and pentaerithrityl tetranitrate.

**Pharmacopoeias.** In *Jpn.*

### Profile

Niceritrol, an ester of pentaerythritol and nicotinic acid, has general properties similar to those of nicotinic acid (p.1441), to which it is slowly hydrolysed. Niceritrol has been used as a lipid regulating drug in hyperlipidaemias and as a vasodilator in the treatment of peripheral vascular disease.

### Preparations

**Proprietary Preparations** (details are given in Part 3)
***Swed.:*** Perycit†.

## Nicofibrate Hydrochloride *(rINNM)*

Clofenpyride Hydrochloride; Hidrocloruro de nicofibrato. 3-Pyridylmethyl 2-(4-chlorophenoxy)-2-methylpropionate hydrochloride.

$C_{16}H_{16}ClNO_3$,HCl = 342.2.
*CAS — 31980-29-7 (nicofibrate); 17413-51-3 (nicofibrate hydrochloride).*

### Profile

Nicofibrate hydrochloride, a derivative of clofibrate (p.884) and nicotinic acid (p.1441), is a lipid regulating drug that has been used in the treatment of hyperlipidaemias.

### Preparations

**Proprietary Preparations** (details are given in Part 3)
***Spain:*** Arterium†.

## Nicorandil *(BAN, USAN, rINN)*

SG-75. N-[2-(Nitroxy)ethyl]-3-pyridinecarboxamide.

$C_8H_9N_3O_4$ = 211.2.
*CAS — 65141-46-0.*
*ATC — C01DX16.*

### Adverse Effects and Precautions

Adverse effects reported with nicorandil are headache which is usually transitory and occurring at the start of therapy, cutaneous vasodilatation and flushing, nausea, vomiting, dizziness, and weakness. Rarely reported effects include myalgia, skin rashes, and oral ulceration, and there have been very rare reports of angioedema and hepatic function abnormalities. A reduction in blood pressure and/or an increase in heart rate may occur with high doses.

Nicorandil is contra-indicated in patients with cardiogenic shock, left ventricular failure with low filling pressures, and hypotension. In patients with hypovolaemia, low systolic blood pressure, acute pulmonary oedema, or acute myocardial infarction with acute left ventricular failure and low filling pressures, nicorandil should preferably be avoided but may be used with caution.

◊ Postmarketing surveillance for nicorandil was carried out by prescription-event monitoring[1] of 13 620 patients, and showed that adverse reactions occurred in 175. The most frequent was headache, occurring in 58 patients, mainly in the first month of treatment. Unspecified side-effects occurred in 36 patients.

Other effects included dizziness (19), nausea (17), malaise (13), palpitations (8), flushing and vomiting (6 each), and lassitude (4). Rare side-effects included 3 cases each of angioedema and photosensitivity.

1. Dunn N, *et al.* Safety profile of nicorandil—prescription-event monitoring (PEM) study. *Pharmacoepidemiol Drug Safety* 1999; **8:** 197–205.

**Oral and anal ulceration.** Painful, large aphthous ulcers on the tongue and oral mucosa have been reported[1-3] in patients receiving nicorandil for angina. The ulcers were usually resistant to treatment but all healed when nicorandil was withdrawn. Colchicine or thalidomide treatment has improved ulcers associated with nicorandil in a few patients, but relapse occurred when the colchicine or thalidomide was stopped.[3] However, a large study[4] casts some doubt on the evidence for a causal link between nicorandil and oral ulceration, although it was suggested that this could be further investigated.

Anal ulceration has also been reported[5-7] in patients taking nicorandil. Healing of the ulcers occurred in those patients in whom nicorandil was withdrawn.

1. Cribier B, *et al.* Chronic buccal ulceration induced by nicorandil. *Br J Dermatol* 1998; **138:** 372–3.
2. Desruelles F, *et al.* Giant oral aphthous ulcers induced by nicorandil. *Br J Dermatol* 1998; **138:** 712–13.
3. Agbo-Godeau S, *et al.* Association of major aphthous ulcers and nicorandil. *Lancet* 1998; **352:** 1598–9.
4. Dunn N, *et al.* Safety profile of nicorandil—prescription-event monitoring (PEM) study. *Pharmacoepidemiol Drug Safety* 1999; **8:** 197–205.
5. Watson A, *et al.* Nicorandil associated anal ulceration. *Lancet* 2002; **360:** 546–7.
6. Vella M, Molloy RG. Nicorandil-associated anal ulceration. *Lancet* 2002; **360:** 1979.
7. Passeron T, *et al.* Chronic anal ulceration due to nicorandil. *Br J Dermatol* 2004; **150:** 394–6.

### Interactions

Nicorandil should not be used with sildenafil as the hypotensive effect of nicorandil may be significantly enhanced.

### Pharmacokinetics

Nicorandil is well absorbed from the gastrointestinal tract and maximum plasma concentrations are achieved 30 to 60 minutes after administration by mouth. Metabolism is mainly by denitration and about 20% of a dose is excreted in the urine mainly as metabolites. The elimination half-life is about 1 hour. Nicorandil is only slightly bound to plasma proteins.

### Uses and Administration

Nicorandil is a nitrate derivative of nicotinamide (p.1441) and acts as a vasodilator. It is a potassium-channel opener (p.812) providing vasodilatation of arterioles and large coronary arteries and its nitrate component produces venous vasodilatation through stimulation of guanylate cyclase. It thus reduces both preload and afterload, and improves coronary blood flow.

Nicorandil is used in angina pectoris (p.813). The usual initial dose by mouth is 10 mg twice daily (or 5 mg twice daily in patients susceptible to headache), increased as necessary to a maximum of 30 mg twice daily; the usual therapeutic dose is in the range of 10 to 20 mg twice daily.

◊ General references.

1. Frampton J, *et al.* Nicorandil: a review of its pharmacology and therapeutic efficacy in angina pectoris. *Drugs* 1992; **44:** 625–55.
2. Markham A, *et al.* Nicorandil: an updated review of its use in ischaemic heart disease with emphasis on its cardioprotective effects. *Drugs* 2000; **60:** 955–74.
3. Gomma AH, *et al.* Potassium channel openers in myocardial ischaemia: therapeutic potential of nicorandil. *Drugs* 2001; **12:** 1705–10.
4. Anonymous. Nicorandil for angina – an update. *Drug Ther Bull* 2003; **41:** 86–8.

**Ischaemic heart disease.** A large multicentred double-blind randomised placebo-controlled study[1] suggested that nicorandil, in addition to its anti-anginal effects, may have cardioprotective properties. The incidence of major coronary events, particularly unplanned admission for chest pain, was significantly reduced in patients with stable angina at high risk of future adverse events. Nicorandil may mimic the mechanism of ischaemic pre-conditioning, whereby a brief period of ischaemia makes the myocardium resistant to damage from a further episode,[2] but it is not clear how much this mechanism contributes to its effects.

1. The IONA Study Group. Effect of nicorandil on coronary events in patients with stable angina: the Impact Of Nicorandil in Angina (IONA) randomised trial. *Lancet* 2002; **359:** 1269–75. Correction. *ibid.*; **360:** 806.
2. Lesnefsky EJ. The IONA study: preparing the myocardium for ischaemia? *Lancet* 2002; **359:** 1262–3.

### Preparations

**Proprietary Preparations** (details are given in Part 3)
***Austral.:*** Ikorel; ***Austria:*** Dancor; ***Denm.:*** Angicor; ***Fr.:*** Adancor; Ikorel; ***India:*** Corflo; Zynicor; ***Irl.:*** Ikorel; ***Ital.:*** Andilex; ***Jpn:*** Sigmart; ***Neth.:*** Ikorel; ***NZ:*** Ikorel; ***Port.:*** Dancor; Nikoril; ***Spain:*** Dancor; ***Switz.:*** Dancor; ***UK:*** Ikorel.

## Nicotinyl Alcohol *(BAN, USAN)*

3-Hydroxymethylpyridine; Nicotinic Alcohol; Nicotinílico, alcohol; NSC-526046; NU-2121; 3-Pyridinemethanol; β-Pyridylcarbinol; Ro-1-5155. 3-Pyridylmethanol.

$C_6H_7NO = 109.1.$
*CAS — 100-55-0.*
*ATC — C04AC02; C10AD05.*

## Nicotinyl Alcohol Tartrate *(BANM)*

Alcohol nicotinílico, tartrato de; Nicotinyl Tartrate. 3-Pyridylmethanol hydrogen (2*R*,3*R*)-tartrate.

$C_6H_7NO,C_4H_6O_6 = 259.2.$
*CAS — 6164-87-0.*
*ATC — C04AC02; C10AD05.*

**Pharmacopoeias.** In *Br.*

**BP 2003** (Nicotinyl Alcohol Tartrate). A white or almost white, odourless or almost odourless, crystalline powder. Freely soluble in water; slightly soluble in alcohol; practically insoluble in chloroform and in ether. A 5% solution in water has a pH of 2.8 to 3.7.

### Profile

Nicotinyl alcohol is a vasodilator and lipid regulating drug with general properties similar to those of nicotinic acid (p.1441), to which it is partly hydrolysed.

Nicotinyl alcohol has been given by mouth, as the tartrate, in the management of peripheral vascular disease, and has also been used in Ménière's disease and in hyperlipidaemias.

### Preparations

***BP 2003:*** Nicotinyl Alcohol Tablets.

**Proprietary Preparations** (details are given in Part 3)
***Ger.:*** Radecol†.

**Multi-ingredient:** ***Austria:*** Thilocombin†; ***Braz.:*** Lipofacton; ***S.Afr.:*** Lipatent†.

## Nifedipine *(BAN, USAN, rINN)*

Bay-a-1040; Nifedipina; Nifedipino; Nifedipinum. Dimethyl 1,4-dihydro-2,6-dimethyl-4-(2-nitrophenyl)pyridine-3,5-dicarboxylate.

$C_{17}H_{18}N_2O_6 = 346.3.$
*CAS — 21829-25-4.*
*ATC — C08CA05.*

**Pharmacopoeias.** In *Chin., Eur.* (see p.vi), *Int., Jpn,* and *US.*

**Ph. Eur. 5.0** (Nifedipine). A yellow crystalline powder. Practically insoluble in water; sparingly soluble in dehydrated alcohol; freely soluble in acetone. When exposed to daylight or to certain wavelengths of artificial light it is converted to a nitrosophenylpyridine derivative, while exposure to ultraviolet light leads to formation of a nitrophenylpyridine derivative. Solutions should be prepared in the dark or under light of wavelength greater than 420 nm, immediately before use. Protect from light.

**USP 27** (Nifedipine). A yellow powder. Practically insoluble in water; soluble 1 in 10 of acetone. When exposed to daylight or to certain wavelengths of artificial light it is converted to a nitrosophenylpyridine derivative, while exposure to ultraviolet light leads to formation of a nitrophenylpyridine derivative. Store in airtight containers. Protect from light.

**Stability.** Yellow food colourings such as curcumin have been used[1] to slow photodegradation of nifedipine solutions. An extemporaneously prepared solution of nifedipine in a peppermint-flavoured vehicle was reported[2] to be stable for at least 35 days when stored in amber glass bottles.

1. Thoma K, Klimek R. Photostabilization of drugs in dosage forms without protection from packaging materials. *Int J Pharmaceutics* 1991; **67:** 169–75.
2. Dentinger PJ, *et al.* Stability of nifedipine in an extemporaneously compounded oral solution. *Am J Health-Syst Pharm* 2003; **60:** 1019–22.

### Adverse Effects

The most common adverse effects of nifedipine are associated with its vasodilator action and often diminish on continued therapy. They include dizziness, flushing, headache, hypotension, peripheral oedema, tachycardia, and palpitations. Nausea and other gastrointestinal disturbances, increased micturition frequency, lethargy, eye pain, visual disturbances, and mental depression have also occurred. A paradoxical increase in ischaemic chest pain may occur at the start of treatment and in a few patients excessive fall in blood pressure has led to cerebral or myocardial ischaemia or transient blindness.

There have been reports of rashes (including erythema multiforme), fever, and abnormalities in liver function, including cholestasis, due to hypersensitivity reactions. Gingival hyperplasia, myalgia, tremor, and impotence have been reported.

Overdosage may be associated with bradycardia and hypotension; hyperglycaemia, metabolic acidosis, and coma may also occur.

Nifedipine has been reported to be teratogenic in *animals.*

**Effects on mortality.** Since 1995 there have been reports and reviews that have implicated calcium-channel blockers (particularly short-acting nifedipine and high doses) in increasing cardiovascular[1] and overall mortality.[2] Possible links with cancer, haemorrhage, and depression and suicide are discussed separately (see Cancer Occurrence, Effects on the Blood, and Effects on Mental Function, below, respectively).

In response, the US National Heart, Lung, and Blood Institute issued a statement warning that short-acting nifedipine should be used with great caution (if at all), especially at higher doses, in the treatment of hypertension, angina, and myocardial infarction,[3] and in some countries short-acting nifedipine preparations have been withdrawn. However, there has been much debate and controversy over the reports that questioned the safety of calcium-channel blockers.[4-6]

A review by the WHO/ISH pointed out that much of the evidence for adverse effects comes from observational studies or small randomised studies and concluded that, as there was insufficient evidence to confirm either benefit or harm, recommendations on the management of angina, hypertension, and myocardial infarction should remain unchanged.[7] In addition, many of the studies that led to the negative reports employed the older short-acting calcium-channel blockers. The calcium-channel blockers used now are largely modified-release formulations of short half-life blockers or are calcium-channel blockers with long half-lives.

Since the WHO/ISH review was published, further studies have been completed that have generally failed to show any increase in mortality with calcium-channel blockers, although their effects on cardiovascular outcomes remain less clear. A placebo-controlled study (SYST-EUR) reported[8] a reduction in incidence of stroke and cardiovascular events in 4695 elderly patients treated with nitrendipine (and enalapril and hydrochlorothiazide in addition if necessary) for isolated systolic hypertension, while a retrospective cohort study[9] in post-myocardial infarction patients failed to show any increase in mortality after one year in those receiving calcium-channel blockers. A meta-analysis[10] of randomised trials comparing calcium-channel blockers with other antihypertensives in patients with hypertension suggested that calcium-channel blockers were associated with an increased risk of major cardiovascular events (except stroke) although all-cause mortality was not increased. However, the large, long-term, randomised Antihypertensive and Lipid-Lowering treatment to prevent Heart Attack Trial (ALLHAT)[11] found no difference between treatment with a calcium-channel blocker (amlodipine) and a diuretic (chlortalidone) for either cardiovascular outcomes or all-cause mortality.

1. Psaty BM, *et al.* The risk of myocardial infarction associated with antihypertensive drug therapies. *JAMA* 1995; **274:** 620–5.
2. Furberg CD, *et al.* Nifedipine: dose-related increase in mortality in patients with coronary heart disease. *Circulation* 1995; **92:** 1326–31.
3. McCarthy M. US NIH issues warning on nifedipine. *Lancet* 1995; **346:** 689–90.
4. Opie LH, Messerli FH. Nifedipine and mortality: grave defects in the dossier. *Circulation* 1995; **92:** 1068–72.
5. Grossman E, Messerli FH. Calcium antagonists in cardiovascular disease: a necessary controversy but an unnecessary panic. *Am J Med* 1997; **102:** 147–9.
6. Stanton AV. Calcium channel blockers. *BMJ* 1998; **316:** 1471–3.
7. Ad Hoc Subcommittee of the Liaison Committee of the World Health Organisation and the International Society of Hypertension. Effects of calcium antagonists on the risks of coronary heart disease, cancer and bleeding. *J Hypertens* 1997; **15:** 105–15.
8. Staessen JA, *et al.* Randomised double-blind comparison of placebo and active treatment for older patients with isolated systolic hypertension. *Lancet* 1997; **350:** 757–64. Correction. *ibid.*; 1636.
9. Jollis JG, *et al.* Calcium channel blockers and mortality in elderly patients with myocardial infarction. *Arch Intern Med* 1999; **159:** 2341–8.
10. Pahor M, *et al.* Health outcomes associated with calcium antagonists compared with other first-line antihypertensive therapies: a meta-analysis of randomised controlled trials. *Lancet* 2000; **356:** 1949–54.
11. The ALLHAT Officers and Coordinators for the ALLHAT Collaborative Research Group. Major outcomes in high-risk hypertensive patients randomized to angiotensin-converting enzyme inhibitor or calcium channel blocker vs diuretic: The Antihypertensive and Lipid-Lowering Treatment to Prevent Heart Attack Trial (ALLHAT). *JAMA* 2002; **288:** 2981–97. Correction. *ibid.*; **289:** 178.

**Cancer occurrence.** An observational study carried out between 1988 and 1992 suggested that calcium-channel blockers were associated with an increased risk of cancer.[1] Subsequent studies have failed to support this finding.[2-7] A review by the WHO/ISH concluded that there is no good evidence that calcium-channel blockers increase cancer risk,[8] and the biological basis for an effect of calcium-channel blockers on cancer risk has also been questioned.[9] The large, long-term, randomised Antihypertensive and Lipid-Lowering treatment to prevent Heart Attack Trial (ALLHAT)[10] found no increase in the incidence of cancer in patients receiving a calcium-channel blocker (amlodipine) compared with those receiving a diuretic (chlortalidone).

1. Pahor M, *et al.* Calcium-channel blockade and incidence of cancer in aged populations. *Lancet* 1996; **348:** 493–7.
2. Jick H, *et al.* Calcium-channel blockers and risk of cancer. *Lancet* 1997; **349:** 525–8.
3. Rosenberg L, *et al.* Calcium channel blockers and the risk of cancer. *JAMA* 1998; **279:** 1000–4.
4. Braun S, *et al.* Calcium channel blocking agents and risk of cancer in patients with coronary heart disease. *J Am Coll Cardiol* 1998; **31:** 804–8.
5. Sajadieh A, *et al.* Verapamil and risk of cancer in patients with coronary artery disease. *Am J Cardiol* 1999; **83:** 1419–22.
6. Meier CR, *et al.* Angiotensin-converting enzyme inhibitors, calcium channel blockers, and breast cancer. *Arch Intern Med* 2000; **160:** 349–53.

7. Cohen HJ, *et al.* Calcium channel blockers and cancer. *Am J Med* 2000; **108:** 210–15.
8. Ad Hoc Subcommittee of the Liaison Committee of the World Health Organisation and the International Society of Hypertension. Effects of calcium antagonists on the risks of coronary heart disease, cancer and bleeding. *J Hypertens* 1997; **15:** 105–15.
9. Mason RP. Calcium channel blockers, apoptosis and cancer: is there a biologic relationship? *J Am Coll Cardiol* 1999; **34:** 1857–66.
10. Major outcomes in high-risk hypertensive patients randomized to angiotensin-converting enzyme inhibitor or calcium channel blocker vs diuretic: The Antihypertensive and Lipid-Lowering Treatment to Prevent Heart Attack Trial (ALLHAT). *JAMA* 2002; **288:** 2981–97. Correction. *ibid.*; **289:** 178.

**Effects on the blood.** Treatment with nifedipine significantly reduces platelet aggregation *in vitro*[1] and results indicating inhibition of platelet function in healthy subjects receiving oral (but not intravenous) nifedipine have been reported.[2,3] Thus, concern has been expressed[4] that calcium-channel blockers may have the potential to produce haemorrhagic complications in surgical patients (specifically, those undergoing coronary bypass surgery). Major surgical bleeding was associated with nimodipine in patients undergoing cardiac valve replacement,[5] although it has been used in other situations apparently without an increased risk of bleeding.[6]

Conflicting results have been reported with regard to the risk of gastrointestinal bleeding. A prospective cohort study in 1636 elderly hypertensive patients,[7] and a subsequent case-control study,[8] reported that calcium-channel blockers were associated with an increased risk of gastrointestinal haemorrhage compared with beta blockers. However, it was suggested[9] that this may have been due to a protective effect of beta blockers rather than an adverse effect of calcium-channel blockers, and another study[10] also suggested that the risk of gastrointestinal bleeding was not materially increased by calcium-channel blockers.

Calcium-channel blockers have also been associated with a number of blood dyscrasias; there have been case reports of aplastic anaemia with nifedipine,[11] and of thrombocytopenia with amlodipine[12] and with diltiazem.[13,14]

1. Ośmiałwska Z, *et al.* Effect of nifedipine monotherapy on platelet aggregation in patients with untreated essential hypertension. *Eur J Clin Pharmacol* 1990; **39:** 403–4.
2. Winther K, *et al.* Dose-dependent effects of verapamil and nifedipine on in vivo platelet function in normal volunteers. *Eur J Clin Pharmacol* 1990; **39:** 291–3.
3. Walley TJ, *et al.* The effects of intravenous and oral nifedipine on ex vivo platelet function. *Eur J Clin Pharmacol* 1989; **37:** 449–52.
4. Becker RC, Alpert JS. The impact of medical therapy on hemorrhagic complications following coronary artery bypass grafting. *Arch Intern Med* 1990; **150:** 2016–21.
5. Wagenknecht LE, *et al.* Surgical bleeding: unexpected effect of a calcium antagonist. *BMJ* 1995; **310:** 776–7.
6. Öhman J and others. Surgical bleeding and calcium antagonists. *BMJ* 1995; **311:** 388–9. [Several letters.]
7. Pahor M, *et al.* Risk of gastrointestinal haemorrhage with calcium antagonists in hypertensive persons over 67 years old. *Lancet* 1996; **347:** 1061–5.
8. Kaplan RC, *et al.* Use of calcium channel blockers and risk of hospitalized gastrointestinal tract bleeding. *Arch Intern Med* 2000; **160:** 1849–55.
9. Suissa S, *et al.* Antihypertensive drugs and the risk of gastrointestinal bleeding. *Am J Med* 1998; **105:** 230–5.
10. Kelly JP, *et al.* Major upper gastrointestinal bleeding and the use of calcium channel blockers. *Lancet* 1999; **353:** 559.
11. Laporte J-R, *et al.* Fatal aplastic anaemia associated with nifedipine. *Lancet* 1998; **352:** 619–20.
12. Usalan C, *et al.* Severe thrombocytopenia associated with amlodipine treatment. *Ann Pharmacother* 1999; **33:** 1126–7.
13. Lehav M, Arav R. Diltiazem and thrombocytopenia. *Ann Intern Med* 1989; **110:** 327.
14. Michalets EL, Jackson DV. Diltiazem-associated thrombocytopenia. *Pharmacotherapy* 1997; **17:** 1345–8.

**Effects on the brain.** Cerebral ischaemia[1,2] has been reported in small numbers of patients given nifedipine.

1. Nobile-Orazio E, Sterzi R. Cerebral ischaemia after nifedipine treatment. *BMJ* 1981; **283:** 948.
2. Schwartz M, *et al.* Oral nifedipine in the treatment of hypertensive urgency: cerebrovascular accident following a single dose. *Arch Intern Med* 1990; **150:** 686–7.

**Effects on carbohydrate metabolism.** There are reports of deterioration of diabetes,[1] reduction in glucose tolerance,[2] and development of diabetes[1,3] in patients receiving treatment with nifedipine. Nifedipine has also been reported to increase plasma-glucose concentrations.[3,4] However, other reports and studies have found no change in glucose tolerance in either diabetic or non-diabetic patients taking nifedipine.[5-10]

See also Diabetes Mellitus under Precautions, below.

1. Bhatnagar SK, *et al.* Diabetogenic effects of nifedipine. *BMJ* 1984; **289:** 19.
2. Giugliano D, *et al.* Impairment of insulin secretion in man by nifedipine. *Eur J Clin Pharmacol* 1980; **18:** 395–8.
3. Zezulka AV, *et al.* Diabetogenic effects of nifedipine. *BMJ* 1984; **289:** 437–8.
4. Charles S, *et al.* Hyperglycaemic effect of nifedipine. *BMJ* 1981; **283:** 19–20.
5. Harrower ADB, Donnelly T. Hyperglycaemic effect of nifedipine. *BMJ* 1981; **283:** 796.
6. Greenwood RH. Hyperglycaemic effect of nifedipine. *BMJ* 1982; **284:** 50.
7. Abadie E, Passa P. Diabetogenic effects of nifedipine. *BMJ* 1984; **289:** 438.
8. Dante A. Nifedipine and fasting glycemia. *Ann Intern Med* 1986; **104:** 125–6.
9. Whitcroft I, *et al.* Calcium antagonists do not impair long-term glucose control in hypertensive non-insulin dependent diabetics (NIDDS). *Br J Clin Pharmacol* 1986; **22:** 208P.
10. Tentorio A, *et al.* Insulin secretion and glucose tolerance in non-insulin dependent diabetic patients after chronic nifedipine treatment. *Eur J Clin Pharmacol* 1989; **36:** 311–13.

**Effects on the ears.** There have been isolated reports[1] of tinnitus associated with several calcium-channel blockers including nifedipine, nicardipine, nitrendipine, diltiazem, verapamil, and cinnarizine.

1. Narváez M, *et al.* Tinnitus with calcium-channel blockers. *Lancet* 1994; **343:** 1229–30.

**Effects on the eyes.** Individual reports have implicated nifedipine in the development of transient retinal ischaemia and blindness,[1] and of periorbital oedema.[2] In a postmarketing survey painful or stinging eyes were more common in patients receiving nifedipine (178 of 757 evaluable) than in those given captopril (45 of 289), although the cause was uncertain.[3] Nifedipine has also been suggested as a risk factor in the development of cataract,[4,5] but the numbers involved in this analysis are small[6] and it is possible that the risk, if it exists,[7] relates to hypertension rather than nifedipine treatment.[6]

1. Pitlik S, *et al.* Transient retinal ischaemia induced by nifedipine. *BMJ* 1983; **287:** 1845–6.
2. Silverstone PH. Periorbital oedema caused by nifedipine. *BMJ* 1984; **288:** 1654.
3. Coulter DM. Eye pain with nifedipine and disturbance of taste with captopril: a mutually controlled study showing a method of postmarketing surveillance. *BMJ* 1988; **296:** 1086–8.
4. van Heyningen R, Harding JJ. Do aspirin-like analgesics protect against cataract? *Lancet* 1986; **i:** 1111–13.
5. Harding JJ, van Heyningen R. Drugs, including alcohol, that act as risk factors for cataract, and possible protection against cataract by aspirin-like analgesics and cyclopenthiazide. *Br J Ophthalmol* 1988; **72:** 809–14.
6. van Heyningen R, Harding JJ. Aspirin-like analgesics and cataract. *Lancet* 1986; **ii:** 283.
7. Kewitz H, *et al.* Aspirin and cataract. *Lancet* 1986; **ii:** 689.

**Effects on the heart.** The use of nifedipine has been associated with the development of various heart disorders in some patients. Complete heart block has been reported in an elderly patient who had previously developed heart block with verapamil,[1] and sudden circulatory collapse has been reported in 4 patients receiving nifedipine who underwent routine coronary bypass surgery.[2] One patient died despite all attempts at resuscitation.[2] However, probably the majority of reports have concerned the development or aggravation of cardiac ischaemia, up to and including frank myocardial infarction following administration of short-acting nifedipine.[3-6] Such cases appear to be chiefly associated with a too-rapid fall in blood pressure following the use of sublingual nifedipine for hypertensive urgencies or emergencies,[5,6] or occur in patients with a history of ischaemic heart disease.[3,4]

For discussion of the effects of calcium-channel blockers on cardiovascular mortality, see above.

1. Chopra DA, Maxwell RT. Complete heart block with low dose nifedipine. *BMJ* 1984; **288:** 760.
2. Goiti JJ. Calcium channel blocking agents and the heart. *BMJ* 1985; **291:** 1505.
3. Sia STB, *et al.* Aggravation of myocardial ischaemia by nifedipine. *Med J Aust* 1985; **142:** 48–50.
4. Boden WE, *et al.* Nifedipine-induced hypotension and myocardial ischemia in refractory angina pectoris. *JAMA* 1985; **253:** 1131–5.
5. O'Mailia JJ, *et al.* Nifedipine-associated myocardial ischemia or infarction in the treatment of hypertensive urgencies. *Ann Intern Med* 1987; **107:** 185–6.
6. Leavitt AD, Zweifler AJ. Nifedipine, hypotension, and myocardial injury. *Ann Intern Med* 1988; **108:** 305–6.

WITHDRAWAL. Exacerbation of coronary ischaemia and thrombosis of arteriovenous graft could have resulted from withdrawal of nifedipine in a patient.[1] Abrupt withdrawal of nisoldipine from 15 patients with stable angina pectoris after 6 weeks of therapy resulted in severe unstable angina in 2 patients and acute myocardial infarction in another.[2] It was postulated that the withdrawal effect could be due to an increase in sensitivity of vascular $\alpha_2$ adrenoceptors to circulating adrenaline.

1. Mysliwiec M, *et al.* Calcium antagonist withdrawal syndrome. *BMJ* 1983; **286:** 1898.
2. Mehta J, Lopez LM. Calcium-blocker withdrawal phenomenon: increase in affinity of alpha$_2$ adrenoceptors for agonist as a potential mechanism. *Am J Cardiol* 1986; **58:** 242–6.

**Effects on the kidneys.** Calcium-channel blockers may be of benefit in various forms of kidney disorder (see under Uses and Administration, below). However, reversible deterioration in renal function without any appreciable accompanying decline in systemic arterial blood pressure has been reported[1] in 4 patients with underlying renal insufficiency receiving nifedipine,[1] and in another report[2] nifedipine increased urinary protein excretion and exacerbated renal impairment in 14 type 2 diabetic patients.

Excessive diuresis occurred in a patient given nifedipine for angina pectoris,[3] and nocturia in 9 patients referred for prostatic surgery was also attributed to nifedipine.[4]

1. Diamond JR, *et al.* Nifedipine-induced renal dysfunction: alterations in renal hemodynamics. *Am J Med* 1984; **77:** 905–9.
2. Demarie BK, Bakris GL. Effects of different calcium antagonists on proteinuria associated with diabetes mellitus. *Ann Intern Med* 1990; **113:** 987–8.
3. Antonelli D, *et al.* Excessive nifedipine diuretic effect. *BMJ* 1984; **288:** 760.
4. Williams G, Donaldson RM. Nifedipine and nocturia. *Lancet* 1986; **i:** 738.

**Effects on the liver.** A number of cases of hepatitis, apparently due to a hypersensitivity reaction, and frequently accompanied by fever, sweating, chills, rigor, and arthritic symptoms, have been reported in patients receiving nifedipine.[1-4]

1. Rotmensch HH, *et al.* Lymphocyte sensitisation in nifedipine-induced hepatitis. *BMJ* 1980; **281:** 976–7.
2. Davidson AR. Lymphocyte sensitisation in nifedipine-induced hepatitis. *BMJ* 1980; **281:** 1354.
3. Abramson M, Littlejohn GO. Hepatic reactions to nifedipine. *Med J Aust* 1985; **142:** 47–8.
4. Shaw DR, *et al.* Nifedipine hepatitis. *Aust N Z J Med* 1987; **17:** 447–8.

**Effects on the menstrual cycle.** Menorrhagia in 2 women[1] and menstrual irregularity with heavy bleeding in another[2] have been reported in association with nifedipine treatment.

1. Rodger JC, Torrance TC. Can nifedipine provoke menorrhagia? *Lancet* 1983; **ii:** 460.
2. Singh G, *et al.* Can nifedipine provoke menorrhagia? *Lancet* 1983; **ii:** 1022.

**Effects on mental function.** Insomnia, hyperexcitability, pacing, agitation, and depression were reported[1] in a patient in association with nifedipine therapy. The symptoms disappeared within 2 days of withdrawal of nifedipine. Four further cases of major depression, which developed within a week of commencing nifedipine and resolved within a week of discontinuing the drug, have been reported.[2]

Although 2 epidemiological studies suggested that calcium-channel blockers may promote suicide,[3] a subsequent study[4] found no evidence of an association between depression and the use of calcium-channel blockers, and the number of suicides was low. Further studies[5,6] have also failed to find an increased risk of suicide with calcium-channel blockers compared with other antihypertensive drugs.

1. Ahmad S. Nifedipine-induced acute psychosis. *J Am Geriatr Soc* 1984; **32:** 408.
2. Hullett FJ, *et al.* Depression associated with nifedipine-induced calcium channel blockade. *Am J Psychiatry* 1988; **145:** 1277–9.
3. Lindberg G, *et al.* Use of calcium channel blockers and risk of suicide: ecological findings confirmed in population based cohort study. *BMJ* 1998; **316:** 741–5.
4. Dunn NR, *et al.* Cohort study on calcium channel blockers, other cardiovascular agents, and the prevalence of depression. *Br J Clin Pharmacol* 1999; **48:** 230–3.
5. Gasse C, *et al.* Risk of suicide among users of calcium channel blockers: population based, nested case-control study. *BMJ* 2000; **320:** 1251.
6. Sørensen HT, *et al.* Risk of suicide in users of beta-adrenoceptor blockers, calcium channel blockers and angiotensin converting enzyme inhibitors. *Br J Clin Pharmacol* 2001; **52:** 313–8.

**Effects on the mouth.** GINGIVAL HYPERPLASIA. A number of reports have implicated nifedipine in the development of gingival hyperplasia.[1-4] In most cases it has occurred about 1 to 6 months after starting therapy and has resolved following withdrawal of nifedipine. A patient who had taken nifedipine for 12 years developed gingival hyperplasia shortly after the dosage of nifedipine was increased.[5] Amlodipine has also induced gingival overgrowth.[6] A study involving 115 patients who had received nifedipine, diltiazem, or verapamil for at least 3 months indicated that gingival hyperplasia is an important adverse effect that may occur with calcium-channel blockers in general.[7] Dihydropyridine calcium-channel blockers were among the most common drugs associated with reports of gingival hyperplasia in the Australian Adverse Drug Reactions Advisory Committee database.[8]

1. Ramon Y, *et al.* Gingival hyperplasia caused by nifedipine—a preliminary report. *Int J Cardiol* 1984; **5:** 195–204.
2. van der Wall EE, *et al.* Gingival hyperplasia induced by nifedipine, an arterial vasodilating drug. *Oral Surg* 1985; **60:** 38–40.
3. Shaftic AA, *et al.* Nifedipine-induced gingival hyperplasia. *Drug Intell Clin Pharm* 1986; **20:** 602–5.
4. Jones CM. Gingival hyperplasia associated with nifedipine. *Br Dent J* 1986; **160:** 416–17.
5. Johnson RB. Nifedipine-induced gingival overgrowth. *Ann Pharmacother* 1997; **31:** 935.
6. Ellis JS, *et al.* Gingival sequestration of amlodipine and amlodipine-induced gingival overgrowth. *Lancet* 1993; **341:** 1102–3.
7. Steele RM, *et al.* Calcium antagonist-induced gingival hyperplasia. *Ann Intern Med* 1994; **120:** 663–4.
8. Adverse Drug Reactions Advisory Committee. Drug-induced gingival overgrowth. *Aust Adverse Drug React Bull* 1999; **18:** 6–7. Also available at: http://www.tga.gov.au/docs/html/aadrbltn/aadr9906.htm (accessed 06/07/04)

PAROTITIS. Acute swelling of the parotid glands occurred in a patient after sublingual administration of nifedipine.[1]

1. Bosch X, *et al.* Nifedipine-induced parotitis. *Lancet* 1986; **ii:** 467.

**Effects on the neuromuscular system.** Severe muscle cramps have been reported in a few patients taking nifedipine;[1,2] in one patient[2] the cramps were associated with widespread paraesthesia. Reversible myoclonic dystonia associated with nifedipine has been reported in a patient.[3] Severe rhabdomyolysis developed in a patient with a transplanted kidney who was receiving an intravenous infusion of nifedipine.[4] The patient recovered rapidly once the infusion was stopped. There has also been a report[5] of myopathy, myalgia, and arthralgia associated with amlodipine, and of arthralgia in a patient[6] receiving diltiazem.

Parkinsonism is a recognised adverse effect of flunarizine and cinnarizine, which have calcium-channel blocking properties (see p.434). It has also been reported with diltiazem (see p.900) and with amlodipine.[7,8]


1. Keidar S, *et al.* Muscle cramps during treatment with nifedipine. *BMJ* 1982; **285:** 1241–2.
2. Macdonald JB. Muscle cramps during treatment with nifedipine. *BMJ* 1982; **285:** 1744.
3. de Medina A, *et al.* Nifedipine and myoclonic dystonia. *Ann Intern Med* 1985; **104:** 125.
4. Horn S, *et al.* Severe rhabdomyolysis in a kidney-transplant recipient receiving intravenous nifedipine. *Lancet* 1995; **346:** 848–9.
5. Phillips BB, Muller BA. Severe neuromuscular complications possibly associated with amlodipine. *Ann Pharmacother* 1998; **32:** 1165–7.
6. Smith KM. Arthralgia associated with calcium-channel blockers. *Am J Health-Syst Pharm* 2000; **57:** 55–7.
7. Sempere AP, *et al.* Parkinsonism induced by amlodipine. *Mov Disord* 1995; **10:** 115–6.
8. Teive HA, *et al.* Parkinsonian syndrome induced by amlodipine: case report. *Mov Disord* 2002; **17:** 833–5.


**Effects on the peripheral circulation.** An erythromelalgia-like eruption occurred in a patient 8 weeks after starting therapy with nifedipine. Symptoms included severe burning pain and swelling in the feet and lower legs, which were fiery red, tender, and warm to the touch. Symptoms resolved in 2 days when nifedipine was discontinued.[1] Similar effects have been reported in other patients on nifedipine.[2-4] Erythromelalgia has also been reported with nicardipine.[5] This type of erythromelalgia may be termed secondary erythermalgia.[6]


1. Fisher JR, *et al.* Nifedipine and erythromelalgia. *Ann Intern Med* 1983; **98:** 671–2.
2. Grunwald Z. Painful edema, erythematous rash, and burning sensation due to nifedipine. *Drug Intell Clin Pharm* 1982; **16:** 492.
3. Brodmerkel GJ. Nifedipine and erythromelalgia. *Ann Intern Med* 1983; **99:** 415.
4. Sunahara JF, *et al.* Possible erythromelalgia-like syndrome associated with nifedipine in a patient with Raynaud's phenomenon. *Ann Pharmacother* 1996; **30:** 484–6.
5. Levesque H, *et al.* Erythromelalgia induced by nicardipine (inverse Raynaud's phenomenon?) *BMJ* 1989; **298:** 1252–3.
6. Drenth JPH, Michiels JJ. Three types of erythromelalgia. *BMJ* 1990; **301:** 454–5.


**Effects on the respiratory system.** There have been some reports of pulmonary oedema being precipitated by nifedipine therapy in patients with aortic stenosis.[1,2] Nifedipine has also been reported to exacerbate impaired tissue oxygenation in patients with cor pulmonale secondary to obstructive airways disease.[3]

For a report of exacerbation of laryngeal oedema, see under Hypersensitivity, below.


1. Gillmar DJ, Kark P. Pulmonary oedema precipitated by nifedipine. *BMJ* 1980; **280:** 1420–1.
2. Aderka D, Pinkhas J. Pulmonary oedema precipitated by nifedipine. *BMJ* 1984; **289:** 1272.
3. Kalra L, Bone MF. Nifedipine and impaired oxygenation in patients with chronic bronchitis and cor pulmonale. *Lancet* 1989; **i:** 1135–6.


**Effects on the skin.** The commonest skin reactions to nifedipine have been rash, pruritus, urticaria, alopecia, and exfoliative dermatitis;[1] there have been a few reports of erythema multiforme and the Stevens-Johnson syndrome.[1] Erythema multiforme occurred in a patient following substitution of amlodipine for nifedipine[2] and cross-sensitivity, manifest as a pruritic maculopapular rash, has been reported between amlodipine and diltiazem.[3] Generalised pruritus has been reported with amlodipine.[4] Other skin reactions that have been reported with nifedipine include severe photosensitivity reactions,[5] nonthrombocytopenic purpuric rashes,[6] and telangiectasias,[7] including photodistributed telangiectasias,[8] and pemphigoid nodularis.[9] Photodistributed telangiectasias have also been reported with amlodipine,[10,11] and in one case[10] recurred 3 years later. Amlodipine has also been associated[12] with a case of lichen planus.

For reference to erythromelalgia, see under Effects on the Peripheral Circulation, above.


1. Stern R, Khalsa JH. Cutaneous adverse reactions associated with calcium channel blockers. *Arch Intern Med* 1989; **149:** 829–32.
2. Bewley AP, *et al.* Erythema multiforme following substitution of amlodipine for nifedipine. *BMJ* 1993; **307:** 241.
3. Baker BA, Cacchione JG. Dermatologic cross-sensitivity between diltiazem and amlodipine. *Ann Pharmacother* 1994; **28:** 118–19.
4. Orme S, *et al.* Generalised pruritus associated with amlodipine. *BMJ* 1997; **315:** 463.
5. Thomas SE, Wood ML. Photosensitivity reactions associated with nifedipine. *BMJ* 1986; **292:** 992.
6. Oren R, *et al.* Nifedipine-induced nonthrombocytopenic purpura. *DICP Ann Pharmacother* 1989; **23:** 88.
7. Tsele E, Chu AC. Nifedipine and telangiectasias. *Lancet* 1992; **339:** 365–6.
8. Collins P, Ferguson J. Photodistributed nifedipine-induced facial telangiectasia. *Br J Dermatol* 1993; **129:** 630–3.
9. Ameen M, *et al.* Pemphigoid nodularis associated with nifedipine. *Br J Dermatol* 2000; **142:** 575–7.
10. Basarab T, *et al.* Calcium antagonist-induced photo-exposed telangiectasia. *Br J Dermatol* 1997; **136:** 974–5.
11. Grabczynska SA, Cowley N. Amlodipine induced-photosensitivity presenting as telangiectasia. *Br J Dermatol* 2000; **142:** 1255–6.
12. Swale VJ, McGregor JM. Amlodipine-associated lichen planus. *Br J Dermatol* 2001; **144:** 920–1.


**Effects on taste.** Although distortion of taste and smell has been reported in 2 patients taking nifedipine,[1] a large survey involving 922 patients receiving nifedipine and 343 taking captopril did not show any association of taste disturbances with nifedipine.[2]


1. Levenson JL, Kennedy K. Dysomia, dysgeusia, and nifedipine. *Ann Intern Med* 1985; **102:** 135–6.
2. Coulter DM. Eye pain with nifedipine and disturbance of taste with captopril: a mutually controlled study showing a method of postmarketing surveillance. *BMJ* 1988; **296:** 1086–8.


**Gynaecomastia.** Unilateral gynaecomastia developed in 3 men 4, 6, and 26 weeks after starting nifedipine therapy.[1]


1. Clyne CAC. Unilateral gynaecomastia and nifedipine. *BMJ* 1986; **292:** 380.


**Haemorrhage.** See Effects on the Blood, above.

**Hypersensitivity.** Nifedipine is associated with various hypersensitivity reactions including skin rashes and effects on the liver (see above).

Nifedipine, given sublingually, exacerbated laryngeal swelling that developed in a woman following the use of isosorbide dinitrate spray.[1]


1. Silfvast T, *et al.* Laryngeal oedema after isosorbide dinitrate spray and sublingual nifedipine. *BMJ* 1995; **311:** 232.


**Oedema.** Oedema of the feet and ankles is a common adverse effect of nifedipine and other dihydropyridine calcium-channel blockers. It occurs typically 2 or more weeks after starting treatment and is caused by pre-capillary arteriolar dilatation rather than fluid retention.[1] Evidence from a study in 10 diabetic subjects beginning nifedipine therapy, 5 of whom developed ankle oedema, suggested that nifedipine abolished the reflex vasoconstriction produced when the feet are below the level of the heart which is believed to prevent excessive fluid filtration into the tissues.[2]

The oedema may respond to simple measures such as elevation of the feet or to a reduction in dosage but if it persists the calcium-channel blocker should be withdrawn.[1]


1. Maclean D, MacConnachie AM. Selective side-effects: peripheral oedema with dihydropyridine calcium antagonists. *Prescribers' J* 1991; **31:** 4–6.
2. Williams SA, *et al.* Dependent oedema and attenuation of postural vasoconstriction associated with nifedipine therapy for hypertension in diabetic patients. *Eur J Clin Pharmacol* 1989; **37:** 333–5.


## Treatment of Adverse Effects

Activated charcoal may be given orally to adults or children who present within 1 hour of ingesting a potentially toxic overdose of nifedipine. Alternatively, gastric lavage may be considered in adults. Supportive and symptomatic care should be given. Hypotension may respond to placing the patient in the supine position with the feet raised and the administration of plasma expanders, although cardiac overload should be avoided. If hypotension is not corrected, calcium gluconate or calcium chloride should be given intravenously. Glucagon may also be used. If hypotension persists, intravenous administration of a sympathomimetic such as isoprenaline, dopamine, or noradrenaline may also be necessary. Bradycardia may be treated with atropine, isoprenaline, or cardiac pacing. Dialysis is not useful as nifedipine is highly protein bound. Plasmapheresis may be beneficial.

**Overdosage.** The management of calcium-channel blocker overdosage (see Treatment of Adverse Effects, above) has been reviewed.[1-4] Although the consequences and management of overdosage with all calcium-channel blockers are similar,[1] non-dihydropyridines may cause more severe effects and may require more aggressive treatment.[2]

Most reports of overdosage have been with verapamil,[3] although there have been a few published reports of nifedipine overdosage. In one, hypotension, tachycardia, and flushing, followed by hypokalaemia, were seen in a patient who took nifedipine 600 mg as modified-release tablets together with an overdose of paracetamol, but there was no evidence of heart block.[5] The patient was given calcium gluconate intravenously and subsequently activated charcoal and lactulose. Absorption of nifedipine was essentially complete 10 hours after ingestion. Potassium chloride was given by mouth to treat hypokalaemia and acetylcysteine was used to manage the paracetamol poisoning.

Third-degree atrioventricular block, progressing to asystole, developed in a 14-month-old child who ingested approximately 800 mg of nifedipine.[6] During cardiopulmonary resuscitation a total of 700 mg of calcium chloride was given, together with atropine, adrenaline, and sodium bicarbonate. The stomach was subsequently emptied by gastric lavage and activated charcoal given. The patient remained tachycardic and hypotensive, with evidence of pulmonary oedema and hyperglycaemia, and was given intravenous electrolytes and dopamine infusions and assisted ventilation, together with treatment to control subsequent tonic-clonic seizures. She eventually made an apparently complete recovery apart from a moderate speech delay.

Case reports[7,8] have suggested that administration of insulin infusion, with glucose if required to maintain normal blood-glucose concentrations, may be beneficial in patients in whom myocardial function fails to improve with conventional therapy.


1. Kenny J. Treating overdose with calcium channel blockers. *BMJ* 1994; **308:** 992–3.
2. Buckley NA, *et al.* Overdose with calcium channel blockers. *BMJ* 1994; **308:** 1639.
3. Howarth DM, *et al.* Calcium channel blocking drug overdose: an Australian series. *Hum Exp Toxicol* 1994; **13:** 161–6.
4. Salhanick SD, Shannon MW. Management of calcium channel antagonist overdose. *Drug Safety* 2003; **26:** 65–79.
5. Ferner RE, *et al.* Pharmacokinetics and toxic effects of nifedipine in massive overdose. *Hum Exp Toxicol* 1990; **9:** 309–11.
6. Wells TG, *et al.* Nifedipine poisoning in a child. *Pediatrics* 1990; **86:** 91–4.
7. Yuan TH, *et al.* Insulin-glucose as adjunctive therapy for severe calcium channel antagonist poisoning. *J Toxicol Clin Toxicol* 1999; **37:** 463–74.
8. Boyer EW, Shannon M. Treatment of calcium-channel-blocker intoxication with insulin infusion. *N Engl J Med* 2001; **344:** 1721–2.


## Precautions

Nifedipine should be used with caution in patients with hypotension, in patients whose cardiac reserve is poor, and in those with heart failure since deterioration of heart failure has been noted. Nifedipine should not be used in cardiogenic shock, in patients who have suffered a myocardial infarction in the previous 2 to 4 weeks, or in acute unstable angina. Nifedipine should not be used to treat an anginal attack in chronic stable angina. In patients with severe aortic stenosis nifedipine may increase the risk of developing heart failure. Sudden withdrawal of nifedipine might be associated with an exacerbation of angina. The dose may need to be reduced in patients with hepatic impairment.

Nifedipine should be discontinued in patients who experience ischaemic pain following its administration.

Nifedipine is reported to be teratogenic in *animals* and may inhibit labour, but it has been used in hypertension in pregnancy (see Hypertension, under Uses and Administration, below).

**Breast feeding.** Nifedipine is distributed into breast milk[1,2] but the amount present is probably too small to be harmful. There have been no reports of any clinical effects in breast-fed infants whose mothers were receiving nifedipine and the American Academy of Pediatrics therefore considers[3] that it is usually compatible with breast feeding.


1. Ehrenkranz RA, *et al.* Nifedipine transfer into human milk. *J Pediatr* 1989; **114:** 478–80.
2. Penny WJ, Lewis MJ. Nifedipine is excreted in human milk. *Eur J Clin Pharmacol* 1989; **36:** 427–8.
3. American Academy of Pediatrics. The transfer of drugs and other chemicals into human milk. *Pediatrics* 2001; **108:** 776–89. Correction. *ibid.*; 1029. Also available at: http://aappolicy.aappublications.org/cgi/content/full/pediatrics%3b108/3/776 (accessed 06/07/04)


**Diabetes mellitus.** Nifedipine may modify insulin and glucose responses (see Effects on Carbohydrate Metabolism under Adverse Effects, above) calling for adjustments in antidiabetic therapy. Also some studies have suggested that nifedipine may worsen proteinuria and renal dysfunction in diabetic patients with some degree of renal insufficiency,[1,2] but other studies, (see Kidney Disorders under Uses and Administration, below), have suggested that nifedipine treatment may prevent or retard the progression of albuminuria.

Some studies have suggested that patients with diabetes mellitus[3,4] or impaired glucose metabolism[5] may be more susceptible to adverse cardiovascular effects of calcium-channel blockers. The calcium-channel blockers used in these studies were nisoldipine, amlodipine, and isradipine (long-acting or intermediate-acting calcium-channel blockers). However, two of the studies[3,4] compared the calcium-channel blocker with an ACE inhibitor and it has been suggested that ACE inhibitors may have a protective effect in patients with diabetes that is additional to their antihypertensive action. Thus, ACE inhibitors may be particularly beneficial in these patients rather than calcium-channel blockers being particularly harmful.[6] Large randomised studies are underway that should provide further information.


1. Mimran A, *et al.* Contrasting effects of captopril and nifedipine in normotensive patients with incipient diabetic nephropathy. *J Hypertens* 1988; **6:** 919–23.
2. Demarie BK, Bakris GL. Effects of different calcium antagonists on proteinuria associated with diabetes mellitus. *Ann Intern Med* 1990; **113:** 987–8.
3. Estacio RO, *et al.* The effect of nisoldipine as compared with enalapril on cardiovascular outcomes in patients with non-insulin-dependent diabetes and hypertension. *N Engl J Med* 1998; **338:** 645–52. Correction. *ibid.*; **339:** 1339.
4. Tatti P, *et al.* Outcome results of the fosinopril versus amlodipine cardiovascular events randomized trial (FACET) in patients with hypertension and NIDDM. *Diabetes Care* 1998; **21:** 597–603.
5. Byington RP, *et al.* Isradipine, raised glycosylated haemoglobin, and risk of cardiovascular events. *Lancet* 1997; **350:** 1075–6.
6. Poulter NR. Calcium channel blockers and cardiovascular risk in diabetes. *Lancet* 1998; **351:** 1809–10.

**Interference with laboratory estimations.** Nifedipine may give falsely elevated spectrophotometric values of urinary vanillylmandelic acid; HPLC estimations are unaffected.

**Porphyria.** Nifedipine has been associated with acute attacks of porphyria and is considered unsafe in porphyric patients.

**Withdrawal.** Sudden withdrawal of nifedipine might be associated with an exacerbation of angina.

For a report of life-threatening coronary vasospasm occurring following withdrawal of nifedipine before a revascularisation procedure, see under Effects on the Heart, in Diltiazem, p.900.

## Interactions

Nifedipine may enhance the antihypertensive effects of other antihypertensive drugs such as beta blockers although the combination is generally well tolerated. Enhanced antihypertensive effects may also be seen with concomitant use of drugs such as aldesleukin and antipsychotics that cause hypotension. Nifedipine may modify insulin and glucose responses (see Effects on Carbohydrate Metabolism, above) and therefore diabetic patients may need to adjust their antidiabetic treatment when receiving nifedipine. Nifedipine is extensively metabolised in the liver by the cytochrome P450 isoenzyme CYP3A4, and interactions may occur with other drugs, such as quinidine, sharing the same metabolic pathway, and with enzyme inducers, such as carbamazepine, phenytoin, and rifampicin, and enzyme inhibitors, such as cimetidine and erythromycin.

**Alcohol.** A study involving 10 healthy subjects showed that the area under the concentration-time profile for nifedipine 20 mg by mouth was increased by 54% when taken with alcohol, and maximum pulse rate was achieved more rapidly, which was in line with *animal* and *in-vitro* studies suggesting that the metabolism of nifedipine is inhibited by alcohol.[1]

1. Qureshi S, *et al.* Nifedipine-alcohol interaction. *JAMA* 1990; **264:** 1660–1.

**Antiarrhythmics.** Nifedipine and *quinidine* probably have a common metabolic pathway in the liver and might be expected to interact if given concurrently. In one study,[1] quinidine appeared to inhibit nifedipine metabolism resulting in increased serum concentrations of nifedipine; quinidine concentrations were unchanged. However, conflicting effects on serum-quinidine concentrations have been reported, see p.993.

1. Bowles SK, *et al.* Evaluation of the pharmacokinetic and pharmacodynamic interaction between quinidine and nifedipine. *J Clin Pharmacol* 1993; **33:** 727–31.

**Antidiabetics.** See Diabetes Mellitus under Precautions and Effects on Carbohydrate Metabolism under Adverse Effects, above.

**Antiepileptics.** The effects of dihydropyridine calcium-channel blockers may be reduced by enzyme-inducing antiepileptics such as *carbamazepine, phenobarbital,* and *phenytoin.*[1-4] In contrast, *sodium valproate* has been reported to increase plasma-nimodipine concentrations.[3]

For reports of an interaction between dihydropyridines and *phenytoin* resulting in raised serum-phenytoin concentration, see p.374.

1. Capewell S, *et al.* Reduced felodipine bioavailability in patients taking anticonvulsants. *Lancet* 1988; **ii:** 480–2.
2. Schellens JHM, *et al.* Influence of enzyme induction and inhibition on the oxidation of nifedipine, sparteine, mephenytoin and antipyrine in humans as assessed by a "cocktail" study design. *J Pharmacol Exp Ther* 1989; **249:** 638–45.
3. Tartara A, *et al.* Differential effects of valproic acid and enzyme-inducing anticonvulsants on nimodipine pharmacokinetics in epileptic patients. *Br J Clin Pharmacol* 1991; **32:** 335–40.
4. Yasui-Furukori N, Tateishi T. Carbamazepine decreases antihypertensive effect of nilvadipine. *J Clin Pharmacol* 2002; **42:** 100–103.

**Antifungals.** Azole antifungals inhibit the cytochrome P450 enzyme system and may therefore interfere with metabolism of calcium-channel blockers. Two women who had been taking felodipine for about a year developed peripheral oedema a few days after starting treatment with *itraconazole.*[1] Plasma-felodipine concentrations were measured in one of the women before and during a subsequent course of itraconazole and increased considerably when the two drugs were used together. A similar interaction occurred when itraconazole therapy was started in a patient already taking nifedipine.[2] Potentiation of the effects of nifedipine by *fluconazole* has also been reported.[3]

1. Neuvonen PJ, Suhonen R. Itraconazole interacts with felodipine. *J Am Acad Dermatol* 1995; **33:** 134–5.
2. Tailor SAN, *et al.* Peripheral edema due to nifedipine-itraconazole interaction: a case report. *Arch Dermatol* 1996; **132:** 350–2.
3. Kremens B, *et al.* Loss of blood pressure control on withdrawal of fluconazole during nifedipine therapy. *Br J Clin Pharmacol* 1999; **47:** 707–8.

**Antihistamines.** Severe angina developed in a patient stabilised on nifedipine who took *terfenadine* 60 mg for seasonal allergy. The pain resolved within an hour or two.[1]

1. Falkenberg HM. Possible interaction report. *Can Pharm J* 1988; **121:** 294.

**Antineoplastics.** For reports of increased *vincristine* toxicity in children also receiving itraconazole and nifedipine concomitantly, see p.593.

**Beta blockers.** Although nifedipine is often used with beta blockers without untoward effects, heart failure has been reported in a few patients with angina who were given nifedipine and a beta blocker.[1,2] Severe hypotension has been reported in 1 of 15 angina patients given nifedipine and *atenolol*;[3] withdrawal of the beta blocker precipitated severe unstable angina in this patient. Severe hypotension in a patient was attributed to the use of nifedipine with *propranolol,* and was thought to have contributed to fatal myocardial infarction.[4]

1. Anastassiades CJ. Nifedipine and beta-blocker drugs. *BMJ* 1980; **281:** 1251–2.
2. Robson RH, Vishwanath MC. Nifedipine and beta-blockade as a cause of cardiac failure. *BMJ* 1982; **284:** 104.
3. Opie LH, White DA. Adverse interaction between nifedipine and β-blockade. *BMJ* 1980; **281:** 1462.
4. Staffurth JS, Emery P. Adverse interaction between nifedipine and beta-blockade. *BMJ* 1981; **282:** 225.

**Calcium-channel blockers.** Plasma concentrations of nifedipine were increased in a study in 6 healthy subjects when pretreated with *diltiazem*; the elimination half-life of nifedipine was prolonged from 2.54 hours to 3.40 hours after pretreatment with diltiazem 30 mg daily and to 3.47 hours after 90 mg daily. The effect was probably due to reduced hepatic metabolism of nifedipine.[1] Nifedipine and diltiazem are reported to be metabolised by the same hepatic enzyme and, conversely, pretreatment with nifedipine has resulted in increased concentrations of diltiazem.[2]

1. Tateishi T, *et al.* Dose dependent effect of diltiazem on the pharmacokinetics of nifedipine. *J Clin Pharmacol* 1989; **29:** 994–7.
2. Tateishi T, *et al.* The effect of nifedipine on the pharmacokinetics and dynamics of diltiazem: the preliminary study in normal volunteers. *J Clin Pharmacol* 1993; **33:** 738–40.

**Digoxin.** For the effect of nifedipine and other dihydropyridine calcium-channel blockers on digoxin, see p.897.

**Grapefruit juice.** Grapefruit juice inhibits the cytochrome P450 isoenzyme CYP3A4, particularly in the intestinal wall, and has been shown to increase markedly the bioavailability of orally-administered calcium-channel blockers;[1-3] calcium-channel blockers given intravenously appear to be unaffected.[4] The interaction may be less significant with calcium-channel blockers such as amlodipine that have a higher bioavailability,[5] but most calcium-channel blockers should not be taken orally at the same time as grapefruit juice.[6]

1. Bailey DG, *et al.* Interaction of citrus juices with felodipine and nifedipine. *Lancet* 1991; **337:** 268–9.
2. Bailey DG, *et al.* Effect of grapefruit juice and naringin on nisoldipine pharmacokinetics. *Clin Pharmacol Ther* 1993; **54:** 589–94.
3. Lundahl J, *et al.* Relationship between time of intake of grapefruit juice and its effect on pharmacokinetics and pharmacodynamics of felodipine in healthy subjects. *Eur J Clin Pharmacol* 1995; **49:** 61–7.
4. Rashid TJ, *et al.* Factors affecting the absolute bioavailability of nifedipine. *Br J Clin Pharmacol* 1995; **40:** 51–8.
5. Vincent J, *et al.* Lack of effect of grapefruit juice on the pharmacokinetics and pharmacodynamics of amlodipine. *Br J Clin Pharmacol* 2000; **50:** 455–63.
6. Committee on Safety of Medicines/Medicines Control Agency. Drug interactions with grapefruit juice. *Current Problems* 1997; **23:** 2. Also available at: http://www.mca.gov.uk/ourwork/monitorsafequalmed/currentproblems/volume23.htm (accessed 06/07/04)

**Histamine $H_2$-antagonists.** Pharmacokinetic studies have indicated that use of nifedipine with *cimetidine* can increase the bioavailability of nifedipine.[1-4] An increase in the area under the plasma concentration-time curve of between 77 and 92% has been reported.[2,3] Potentiation of the hypotensive effect of nifedipine by cimetidine was also shown in 7 hypertensive patients.[1] The mechanism of the interaction was thought to be due to inhibition of the cytochrome P450 system by cimetidine and thus inhibition of the metabolism of nifedipine.

*Ranitidine* was found to have little effect on the pharmacokinetics of nifedipine, although there was an increase in the bioavailability of nifedipine during ranitidine administration.[5] *Famotidine* has been reported not to interact with nifedipine.[6]

1. Kirch W, *et al.* Einfluß von cimetidin und ranitidin auf pharmakokinetik und antihypertensiven effekt von nifedipin. *Dtsch Med Wochenschr* 1983; **108:** 1757–61.
2. Renwick AG, *et al.* Factors affecting the pharmacokinetics of nifedipine. *Eur J Clin Pharmacol* 1987; **32:** 351–5.
3. Smith SR, *et al.* Ranitidine and cimetidine: drug interactions with single dose and steady-state nifedipine administration. *Br J Clin Pharmacol* 1987; **23:** 311–15.
4. Schwartz JB, *et al.* Effect of cimetidine or ranitidine administration on nifedipine pharmacokinetics and pharmacodynamics. *Clin Pharmacol Ther* 1988; **43:** 673–80.
5. Kirch W, *et al.* Ranitidine increases bioavailability of nifedipine. *Clin Pharmacol Ther* 1985; **37:** 204.
6. Kirch W, *et al.* Negative effects of famotidine on cardiac performance assessed by noninvasive hemodynamic measurements. *Gastroenterology* 1989; **96:** 1388–92.

**Immunosuppressants.** Flushing, paraesthesias, and rashes were reported in 2 patients given nifedipine 40 mg daily while taking *ciclosporin* for psoriasis.[1] A study in 8 psoriatic patients indicated that administration of nifedipine with ciclosporin resulted in reduced recovery of the principal metabolite of nifedipine, presumably because ciclosporin reduced nifedipine metabolism through competition for the cytochrome P450 metabolising enzymes.

For reference to the effects of calcium-channel blockers on ciclosporin concentrations in blood, see p.1355. For the possible protective effect of nifedipine against ciclosporin-induced nephrotoxicity, see Transplantation under Uses and Administration, below.

For the effect of nifedipine on *tacrolimus,* see p.1365.

1. McFadden JP, *et al.* Cyclosporin decreases nifedipine metabolism. *BMJ* 1989; **299:** 1224.

**Magnesium salts.** Profound hypotension has been reported in 2 women in whom a single dose of nifedipine 10 mg by mouth was added to treatment with magnesium sulfate infusion for pre-eclampsia; both women were also receiving methyldopa.[1] Neuromuscular blockade has been reported in 2 women following concomitant use of nifedipine and intravenous magnesium sulfate. In one woman receiving nifedipine as a tocolytic, symptoms of neuromuscular blockade occurred immediately on injection of magnesium sulfate and resolved within 25 minutes of stopping the injection.[2] In another woman who was receiving a magnesium sulfate infusion for pre-eclampsia, symptoms developed 30 minutes after the second of 2 doses of nifedipine had been given and improved following administration of calcium gluconate injection.[3]

1. Waisman GD, *et al.* Magnesium plus nifedipine: potentiation of hypotensive effect in pre-eclampsia? *Am J Obstet Gynecol* 1988; **159:** 308–9.
2. Snyder SW, Cardwell MS. Neuromuscular blockade with magnesium sulfate and nifedipine. *Am J Obstet Gynecol* 1989; **161:** 35–6.
3. Ben-Ami M, *et al.* The combination of magnesium sulphate and nifedipine: a cause of neuromuscular blockade. *Br J Obstet Gynaecol* 1994; **101:** 262–3.

**Melatonin.** Melatonin may cause a reduction in blood pressure and might be expected to have additive effects if given with antihypertensives. However, in a study[1] in hypertensive patients receiving nifedipine, administration of melatonin led to an increase in both blood pressure and heart rate.

1. Lusardi P, *et al.* Cardiovascular effects of melatonin in hypertensive patients well controlled by nifedipine: a 24-hour study. *Br J Clin Pharmacol* 2000; **49:** 423–7.

**Tobacco.** In a study of the effects of cigarette smoking and the treatment of angina with nifedipine, propranolol, or atenolol, smoking was shown to have direct and adverse effects on the heart and to interfere with the efficacy of all 3 anti-anginal drugs, with nifedipine being the most affected.[1]

1. Deanfield J, *et al.* Cigarette smoking and the treatment of angina with propranolol, atenolol, and nifedipine. *N Engl J Med* 1984; **310:** 951–4.

**Xanthines.** For the effect of nifedipine on *theophylline,* see p.802.

## Pharmacokinetics

Nifedipine is rapidly and almost completely absorbed from the gastrointestinal tract, but undergoes extensive hepatic first-pass metabolism. Bioavailability after oral administration of liquid-filled capsules is between 45 and 75%, but is lower for longer-acting formulations. Following administration by mouth peak blood concentrations are reported to occur after 30 minutes with liquid-filled capsules.

Nifedipine is about 92 to 98% bound to plasma proteins. It is distributed into breast milk. It is extensively metabolised in the liver and 70 to 80% of a dose is excreted in the urine almost entirely as inactive metabolites. The half-life is about 2 hours following intravenous administration or administration of liquid-filled capsules.

◊ General reviews.

1. Kelly JG, O'Malley K. Clinical pharmacokinetics of calcium antagonists: an update. *Clin Pharmacokinet* 1992; **22:** 416–33.

◊ The pharmacokinetics of nifedipine have been reviewed.[1] Studies have been complicated by the difficulty in preparing a stable intravenous formulation and the problems in developing a sufficiently sensitive and specific method of analysis. Nearly 100% of an oral dose of nifedipine is absorbed in the small intestine although the bioavailability from capsules is 45 to 68%. The rate of absorption from both oral and sublingual capsules varies widely among individuals: there has been a report that high plasma-nifedipine concentrations are achieved more rapidly if the capsule is bitten and swallowed than from standard oral and sublingual administration (but this is no longer recommended—see Hypertension, below). The absorption of nifedipine from tablets is slower than from capsules, with maximum plasma concentrations occurring at 1.6 to 4.2 hours compared with 0.5 to 2.17 hours, and absorption may still be occurring at 24 to 32 hours after administration.

Nifedipine undergoes almost complete hepatic oxidation to 3 pharmacologically inactive metabolites which are excreted in the urine. It has been reported that following oral administration 30 to 40% of the amount absorbed is metabolised during the first pass through the liver. The elimination half-life of nifedipine is apparently dependent upon the dosage form in which it is given, with half-lives of 6 to 11 hours, 2 to 3.4 hours, and 1.3 to 1.8 hours measured after oral tablet, oral capsule, and intravenous administration respectively. The total systemic clearance of nifedipine from plasma ranges from 27 to about 66 litres/hour. Renal impairment does not substantially alter nifedipine pharmacokinetics.

1. Sorkin EM, *et al.* Nifedipine: a review of its pharmacodynamic and pharmacokinetic properties, and therapeutic efficacy, in ischaemic heart disease, hypertension and related cardiovascular disorders. *Drugs* 1985; **30:** 182–274.

**Absorption.** Although studies have indicated that the absorption of nifedipine may be affected by administration with food the results appear to vary depending upon the preparation used. A reduction in peak plasma-nifedipine concentrations, and a delay in achieving them, was reported[1] when nifedipine *capsules* were given after a meal compared with 30 minutes before. In contrast, the bioavailability and maximum serum concentrations of nifedipine were markedly increased when a *modified-release tablet* (Adalat L) was given after a meal rather than fasting,[2] although another modified-release tablet (Slofedipine) showed delayed absorption when administered after food.[3] A further tablet formulation (Adalat OROS) was unaffected by food,[3] while a *modified-release capsule* containing uncoated and enteric-coated granules (Sepamit R) was reported to have essentially the same bioavailability when taken before or after a meal.[4]

1. Hirasawa K, *et al.* Effect of food ingestion on nifedipine absorption and haemodynamic response. *Eur J Clin Pharmacol* 1985; **28:** 105–7.
2. Ueno K, *et al.* Effect of food on nifedipine sustained-release preparation. *DICP Ann Pharmacother* 1989; **23:** 662–5.
3. Schug BS, *et al.* The effect of food on the pharmacokinetics of nifedipine in two slow release formulations: pronounced lag-time after a high fat breakfast. *Br J Clin Pharmacol* 2002; **53:** 582–8.
4. Ueno K, *et al.* Effect of a light breakfast on the bioavailability of sustained-release nifedipine. *DICP Ann Pharmacother* 1991; **25:** 317–19.

**Hepatic impairment.** The pharmacokinetics of nifedipine were found to be considerably altered in 7 patients with liver cirrhosis.[1] Systemic plasma clearance was substantially reduced and the elimination half-life was considerably longer than in healthy subjects. In addition, systemic availability of oral nifedipine was much higher in patients with cirrhosis and was complete in 3 patients with surgical portacaval shunt. Patients with liver cirrhosis seemed to be more sensitive to the effects of nifedipine on diastolic blood pressure and heart rate, and this could be explained by the higher free drug concentrations observed. It was concluded that lower doses of nifedipine may be required in patients with liver cirrhosis, and the patient's response should be closely monitored.

1. Kleinbloesem CH, *et al.* Nifedipine: kinetics and hemodynamic effects in patients with liver cirrhosis after intravenous and oral administration. *Clin Pharmacol Ther* 1986; **40:** 21–8.

**Interindividual variation.** A study in 53 Dutch subjects found a bimodal distribution of plasma concentrations of nifedipine following a single oral dose; it was proposed that the higher plasma concentrations in 17% of subjects represented a slow metaboliser phenotype, with the majority of the population being fast metabolisers.[1] Although further studies[2,3] in European populations have not confirmed these results, a study in 12 Mexican subjects supported the concept of polymorphic metabolism, with 5 fast and 7 slow metabolisers, a much higher proportion of slow metabolisers than in the European studies.[4] Studies have also reported a markedly increased area under the concentration-time curve in South Asian,[5,6] Mexican,[7] and Nigerian[8] subjects compared with Caucasians. The difference did not appear to be due to diet.[5,6] The initial dose of nifedipine might need to be lower in these ethnic groups. Another population study[9] found that clearance was slower in blacks compared with whites, and in men compared with women; alcohol ingestion and smoking both also reduced nifedipine clearance.

1. Kleinbloesem CH, *et al.* Variability in nifedipine pharmacokinetics and dynamics: a new oxidation polymorphism in man. *Biochem Pharmacol* 1984; **33:** 3721–4.
2. Renwick AG, *et al.* The pharmacokinetics of oral nifedipine—a population study. *Br J Clin Pharmacol* 1988; **25:** 701–8.
3. Lobo J, *et al.* The intra- and inter-subject variability of nifedipine pharmacokinetics in young volunteers. *Eur J Clin Pharmacol* 1986; **30:** 57–60.
4. Hoyo-Vadillo C, *et al.* Pharmacokinetics of nifedipine slow release tablet in Mexican subjects: further evidence for an oxidation polymorphism. *J Clin Pharmacol* 1989; **29:** 816–20.
5. Ahsan CH, *et al.* Ethnic differences in the pharmacokinetics of oral nifedipine. *Br J Clin Pharmacol* 1991; **31:** 399–403.
6. Ahsan CH, *et al.* The influences of dose and ethnic origins on the pharmacokinetics of nifedipine. *Clin Pharmacol Ther* 1993; **54:** 329–38.
7. Castañeda-Hernández G, *et al.* Interethnic variability in nifedipine disposition: reduced systemic plasma clearance in Mexican subjects. *Br J Clin Pharmacol* 1996; **41:** 433–4.
8. Sowunmi A, *et al.* Ethnic differences in nifedipine kinetics: comparisons between Nigerians, Caucasians and South Asians. *Br J Clin Pharmacol* 1995; **40:** 489–93.
9. Krecic-Shepard ME, *et al.* Race and sex influence clearance of nifedipine: results of a population study. *Clin Pharmacol Ther* 2000; **68:** 130–42.

## Uses and Administration

Nifedipine is a dihydropyridine calcium-channel blocker (p.810). It is a peripheral and coronary vasodilator, but, unlike the rate-limiting calcium-channel blockers verapamil or diltiazem, has little or no effect on cardiac conduction and negative inotropic activity is rarely seen at therapeutic doses. Administration of nifedipine results primarily in vasodilatation, with reduced peripheral resistance, blood pressure, and afterload, increased coronary blood flow, and a reflex increase in heart rate. This in turn results in an increase in myocardial oxygen supply and cardiac output. Nifedipine has no antiarrhythmic activity. Nicardipine and newer dihydropyridines such as amlodipine, felodipine, isradipine, and lacidipine may be even more selective than nifedipine for vascular smooth muscle. Nimodipine acts particularly on cerebral blood vessels. Most of the dihydropyridine calcium-channel blockers (nifedipine and lacidipine are exceptions) are chiral compounds used as racemic mixtures.

Nifedipine is used in the management of hypertension; in the management of angina pectoris (p.813), particularly when a vasospastic element is present, as in Prinzmetal's angina, but is not suitable for relief of an acute attack; and in the treatment of Raynaud's syndrome. Nifedipine has also been tried in numerous non-vascular disorders.

Nifedipine is usually given by mouth. It is available in a number of formulations. Liquid-filled capsules with a relatively rapid onset but short duration of action are administered three times daily. This short-acting preparation is not recommended for the management of hypertension (see below). There are also tablets and capsules with a slower onset and longer duration of action, enabling twice-daily administration; although these are often referred to by nomenclature implying extended or sustained release they should be distinguished from the true extended-release preparations available in some countries that allow administration once daily.

Doses of nifedipine are dependent upon the formulation used; they may need to be reduced in the elderly or those with impaired liver function.

For **hypertension** a long-acting preparation of nifedipine may be given in doses of 10 to 40 mg twice daily, or 20 to 90 mg once daily, depending on the preparation used.

For **angina pectoris**, nifedipine may be given as a long-acting preparation in a dose of 10 to 40 mg twice daily or 30 to 90 mg once daily, depending on the preparation. Alternatively, the liquid-filled capsules have been given in a dose of 5 to 20 mg three times daily, but longer-acting preparations are preferred.

Nifedipine has been administered by injection via a coronary catheter for the treatment of coronary spasm during coronary angiography and balloon angioplasty. Blood pressure and heart rate should be monitored carefully.

In the management of **Raynaud's syndrome**, nifedipine may be given as liquid-filled capsules in a dose of 5 to 20 mg three times daily.

◊ General reviews.

1. Fisher M, Grotta J. New uses for calcium channel blockers: therapeutic implications. *Drugs* 1993; **46:** 961–75.

**Administration in children.** Use of nifedipine capsules for acute hypertension is no longer recommended in adults because of the risk of severe adverse effects related to precipitous reductions in blood pressure (see Effects on Mortality under Adverse Effects, above). Although there have been reports of adverse effects in children,[1-3] they may be less susceptible than adults, and the use of nifedipine capsules may still be appropriate. A study[4] in 12 children aged 6 to 15 years with acute severe hypertension reported that sublingual nifedipine in a mean dose of 240 micrograms/kg (range 180 to 320 micrograms/kg) was safe and effective. A retrospective study[1] in 117 children found that nifedipine safely reduced blood pressure, and that precipitous declines only occurred with doses higher than 250 micrograms/kg, while another retrospective study[2] in 166 children found that nifedipine in a mean dose of 300 micrograms/kg (range 40 to 1300 micrograms/kg) was generally safe, although children with acute CNS injury were at higher risk of neurological adverse effects.

Other routes that have been used include rectal[5] and intranasal,[6] but these are less established.

1. Blaszak RT, *et al.* The use of short-acting nifedipine in pediatric patients with hypertension. *J Pediatr* 2001; **139:** 34–7.
2. Egger DW, *et al.* Evaluation of the safety of short-acting nifedipine in children with hypertension. *Pediatr Nephrol* 2002; **17:** 35–40.
3. Flynn JT. Nifedipine in the treatment of hypertension in children. *J Pediatr* 2002; **140:** 787–8.
4. Evans JHC, *et al.* Sublingual nifedipine in acute severe hypertension. *Arch Dis Child* 1988; **63:** 975–7.
5. Uchiyama M, Ogawa I. Rectal nifedipine in acute severe hypertension in young children. *Arch Dis Child* 1989; **64:** 632–3.
6. Lopez-Herce J, *et al.* Treatment of hypertensive crisis with intranasal nifedipine. *Crit Care Med* 1988; **9:** 914.

**Amaurosis fugax.** Relief of vasospasm might explain the efficacy of the calcium-channel blockers nifedipine and verapamil in a few patients with amaurosis fugax (see under Stroke, p.836) unresponsive to anticoagulants or antiplatelet drugs.[1]

1. Winterkorn JMS, *et al.* Brief report: treatment of vasospastic amaurosis fugax with calcium-channel blockers. *N Engl J Med* 1993; **329:** 396–8.

**Anal fissure.** Calcium antagonists, including oral and topical nifedipine, have been tried[1-4] in the treatment of chronic anal fissure (p.1390).

1. Antropoli C, *et al.* Nifedipine for local use in conservative treatment of anal fissures: preliminary results of a multicenter study. *Dis Colon Rectum* 1999; **42:** 1011–5.
2. Cook TA, *et al.* Oral nifedipine reduces resting anal pressure and heals chronic anal fissure. *Br J Surg* 1999; **86:** 1269–73.
3. Perrotti P, *et al.* Topical nifedipine with lidocaine ointment vs. active control for treatment of chronic anal fissure: results of a prospective, randomized, double-blind study. *Dis Colon Rectum* 2002; **45:** 1468–75.
4. Ezri T, Susmallian S. Topical nifedipine vs. topical glyceryl trinitrate for treatment of chronic anal fissure. *Dis Colon Rectum* 2003; **46:** 805–8.

**Atherosclerosis.** The use of drugs that interfere with atherogenesis (the development of atheromas) has been suggested as a means of reducing diseases associated with atherosclerosis (p.815). Calcium is thought to be necessary for several steps in atherogenesis and studies in *animals* have shown that calcium-channel blockers slow the development and progression of atherosclerotic lesions. However, studies in humans have been less convincing.[1] In a placebo-controlled study,[2] amlodipine had no demonstrable effect on angiographic progression of coronary atherosclerosis or the risk of major cardiovascular events although it was associated with fewer admissions to hospital for unstable angina and revascularisation. Similar results have been reported with nisoldipine.[3] In another study,[4] comparing lacidipine with a beta blocker, there was less progression of atherosclerosis in those receiving lacidipine and also a trend towards fewer cardiovascular events.

Calcium-channel blockers have also been tried in the prevention of restenosis following percutaneous coronary interventions. A meta-analysis[5] found that addition of calcium-channel blockers to standard therapy reduced the risk of restenosis and the occurrence of clinical events.

1. Borcherding SM, *et al.* Calcium-channel antagonists for prevention of atherosclerosis. *Ann Pharmacother* 1993; **27:** 61–7.
2. Pitt B, *et al.* Effect of amlodipine on the progression of atherosclerosis and the occurrence of clinical events. *Circulation* 2000; **102:** 1503–10.
3. Dens JA, *et al.* Long term effects of nisoldipine on the progression of coronary atherosclerosis and the occurrence of clinical events: the NICOLE study. *Heart* 2003; **89:** 887–92.
4. Zanchetti A, *et al.* Calcium antagonist lacidipine slows down progression of asymptomatic carotid atherosclerosis: principal results of the European Lacidipine Study on Atherosclerosis (ELSA), a randomized, double-blind, long-term trial. *Circulation* 2002; **106:** 2422–7.
5. Dens J, *et al.* An updated meta-analysis of calcium-channel blockers in the prevention of restenosis after coronary angioplasty. *Am Heart J* 2003; **145:** 404–8.

**Cardiomyopathies.** Calcium-channel blockers may have a role in some forms of cardiomyopathy (p.818). In *hypertrophic cardiomyopathy* verapamil is probably the calcium-channel blocker of choice (see p.1021). Nifedipine does not appear to reduce left ventricular outflow tract obstruction, and conflicting results have been demonstrated with respect to improvement in the diastolic function abnormality with this drug.[1] The use of calcium-channel blockers is not standard therapy in *dilated cardiomyopathy* although symptomatic improvement has been reported[2] with diltiazem.

1. Richardson PJ. Calcium antagonists in cardiomyopathy. *Br J Clin Pract* 1988; **42** (suppl 60): 33–7.
2. Figulla HR, *et al.* Diltiazem improves cardiac function and exercise capacity in patients with idiopathic dilated cardiomyopathy: results of the Diltiazem in Dilated Cardiomyopathy Trial. *Circulation* 1996; **94:** 346–52.

**Cough.** Nifedipine has been reported to reduce the severity of cough induced by captopril,[1] possibly by inhibiting prostaglandin synthesis. For further details on cough associated with ACE inhibitors, see p.843.

1. Fogari R, *et al.* Effects of nifedipine and indomethacin on cough induced by angiotensin-converting enzyme inhibitors: a double-blind, randomized, cross-over study. *J Cardiovasc Pharmacol* 1992; **19:** 670–3.

**Hiccup.** Hiccups (p.682) result from involuntary spasmodic contraction of the diaphragm. Intractable hiccups resolved completely with nifedipine 20 mg every 8 hours in a patient.[1] In a further 7 such patients,[2] nifedipine in doses of 20 to 80 mg daily stopped hiccups in 4 and improved them in another. Resolution of intractable hiccups has also been reported[3] in 2 patients given nimodipine; the drug was administered orally in one patient and intravenously in the other.

For the treatment of hiccups in palliative care the *British National Formulary* recommends a dose of 10 mg given three times daily.

1. Mukhopadhyay P, *et al.* Nifedipine for intractable hiccups. *N Engl J Med* 1986; **314:** 1256.

2. Lipps DC, *et al.* Nifedipine for intractable hiccups. *Neurology* 1990; **40:** 531–2.
3. Hernández JL, *et al.* Nimodipine treatment for intractable hiccups. *Am J Med* 1999; **106:** 600.

**High-altitude disorders.** Nifedipine lowers pulmonary artery pressure and is one of several drugs that are used in high-altitude disorders (p.822), success being reported for both the treatment[1,2] and prevention[2,3] of symptoms of pulmonary oedema. In a study conducted at 4559 m above sea-level[1] nifedipine 10 mg sublingually, then 20 mg as a modified-release dosage form was given to 6 subjects with symptoms of high-altitude pulmonary oedema. The sublingual dose was repeated if tolerated after 15 minutes and the subjects subsequently received modified-release nifedipine 20 mg every 6 hours while they remained at high altitude. Symptoms of high-altitude pulmonary oedema were relieved within 1 hour of beginning nifedipine and radiographic signs of oedema regressed during treatment despite remaining at high altitude for 36 hours and participating in mountaineering activities. Raised pulmonary arterial pressure was also reduced to control values by nifedipine. Successful treatment of pulmonary oedema in a climber at 6550 m has been described with doses of 20 mg every 8 hours for 36 hours and such doses also prevented the development of symptoms in 2 climbers who had taken nifedipine from the start of the climb.[2] Doses of 20 mg every 8 hours have been reported to allow rapid ascent to 4559 m without development of pulmonary oedema in 9 of 10 subjects who received nifedipine compared with 4 of 11 who received only placebo.[3] However, the point has been made that although it is reasonable that many climbers carry nifedipine in case of an attack, prophylactic nifedipine should not be considered an alternative to slow ascent and acclimatisation.[4]

1. Oelz O, *et al.* Nifedipine for high altitude pulmonary oedema. *Lancet* 1989; **ii:** 1241–4. Correction. *ibid.* 1991; **337:** 556.
2. Jamieson A, Kerr GW. Treatment of high-altitude pulmonary oedema. *Lancet* 1992; **340:** 1468.
3. Bärtsch P, *et al.* Prevention of high-altitude pulmonary oedema by nifedipine. *N Engl J Med* 1991; **325:** 1284–9.
4. A'Court CHD, *et al.* Doctor on a mountaineering expedition. *BMJ* 1995; **310:** 1248–52.

**Hyperinsulinaemic hypoglycaemia.** Nifedipine may have effects on blood-glucose levels due to inhibition of insulin release[1] (see Effects on Carbohydrate Metabolism, under Adverse Effects, above). There have been reports[1-4] of the successful use of nifedipine to increase blood-glucose levels in infants with hyperinsulinaemic hypoglycaemia, and it may have a role[5] as adjunctive therapy in such patients.

1. Lindley KJ, *et al.* Ionic control of beta cell function in nesidioblastosis: a possible therapeutic role for calcium channel blockade. *Arch Dis Child* 1996; **74:** 373–8.
2. Eichmann D, *et al.* Treatment of hyperinsulinaemic hypoglycaemia with nifedipine. *Eur J Pediatr* 1999; **158:** 204–6.
3. Bas F, *et al.* Successful therapy with calcium channel blocker (nifedipine) in persistent neonatal hyperinsulinemic hypoglycemia of infancy. *J Pediatr Endocrinol Metab* 1999; **12:** 873–8.
4. Shanbag P, *et al.* Persistent hyperinsulinemic hypoglycemia of infancy—successful therapy with nifedipine. *Indian J Pediatr* 2002; **69:** 271–2.
5. Aynsley-Green A, *et al.* Practical management of hyperinsulinism in infancy. *Arch Dis Child Fetal Neonatal Ed* 2000; **82:** F98–F107.

**Hypertension.** Although diuretics and beta blockers are generally considered to be first-line therapy in uncomplicated hypertension (p.825) calcium-channel blockers may be used as an alternative in selected patients. The use of short-acting calcium-channel blockers is not recommended since they may increase mortality (see under Adverse Effects, above) but meta-analyses[1] and large studies[2] using long-acting calcium-channel blockers have shown them to be as safe and effective as conventional first-line therapy. Combination therapy may be necessary in many patients and suitable combinations include a dihydropyridine calcium-channel blocker plus a beta blocker or an ACE inhibitor.

In **hypertensive crises**, where oral treatment is suitable, a calcium-channel blocker such as nifedipine has been widely used. Nifedipine has also been administered sublingually, or by biting the capsule and swallowing the contents,[3] but such use may cause dangerous hypotension and is no longer recommended. Some calcium-channel blockers, for example nicardipine, are available for intravenous administration and may be given when a parenteral antihypertensive drug is considered necessary. One study concluded that intravenous nicardipine was as effective as sodium nitroprusside in the treatment of postoperative hypertension.[4]

For **hypertension in pregnancy**, first-line treatment is usually methyldopa or a beta blocker but calcium-channel blockers may also be used. Nifedipine is reported to be teratogenic in *animals* and may inhibit labour, but it has been tried in a limited number of patients with pre-eclampsia. Although a high rate of caesarean deliveries, premature births, and small-for-date infants was reported[5] in patients given nifedipine as a second-line drug, assessment of the role of nifedipine is difficult because outcome is often poor in such severely compromised pregnancies.[6] Fetal nifedipine concentrations have been reported to be 75% of maternal values 2 to 3 hours after sublingual administration.[7] However, nifedipine in a single 20-mg oral dose lowered blood pressure without compromising blood flow in the fetus in 9 women in the third trimester with normal haemodynamics.[6] This is in line with other reports,[8] although there has also been a report[9] of severe hypotension and fetal distress following sublingual nifedipine administration. In a randomised controlled study,[10] nifedipine 10 to 30 mg sublingually followed by 10 mg as capsules by mouth every 6 hours increasing to 20 mg every 4 hours if necessary, was compared with hydralazine 12.5 mg intravenously as required followed by 20 to 30 mg by mouth every 6 hours, with added methyldopa if necessary. Both groups also received intravenous magnesium sulfate. Effective control of blood pressure was achieved in 23 of 24 patients given nifedipine compared with only 17 of 25 given hydralazine and 9 nifedipine patients achieved term delivery compared with only 2 of those receiving hydralazine. The average gestational age was greater in infants in the nifedipine group; hence these neonates weighed more and had fewer neonatal complications when compared with neonates from the hydralazine treated group.

1. Opie LH, Schall R. Evidence-based evaluation of calcium channel blockers for hypertension: equality of mortality and cardiovascular risk relative to conventional therapy. *J Am Coll Cardiol* 2002; **39:** 315–22. Correction. *ibid.*; 1409–10.
2. The ALLHAT Officers and Coordinators for the ALLHAT Collaborative Research Group. Major outcomes in high-risk hypertensive patients randomized to angiotensin-converting enzyme inhibitor or calcium channel blocker vs diuretic: The Antihypertensive and Lipid-Lowering Treatment to Prevent Heart Attack Trial (ALLHAT). *JAMA* 2002; **288:** 2981–97. Correction. *ibid.*; **289:** 178.
3. Gifford RW. Management of hypertensive crises. *JAMA* 1991; **266:** 829–35.
4. Halpern NA, *et al.* Postoperative hypertension: a multicenter, prospective, randomized comparison between intravenous nicardipine and sodium nitroprusside. *Crit Care Med* 1992; **20:** 1637–43.
5. Constantine G, *et al.* Nifedipine as a second line antihypertensive drug in pregnancy. *Br J Obstet Gynaecol* 1987; **94:** 1136–42.
6. Hanretty KP, *et al.* Effect of nifedipine on Doppler flow velocity waveforms in severe pre-eclampsia. *BMJ* 1989; **299:** 1205–6.
7. Pirhonen JP, *et al.* Single dose of nifedipine in normotensive pregnancy: nifedipine concentrations, hemodynamic responses, and uterine and fetal flow velocity waveforms. *Obstet Gynecol* 1990; **76:** 807–11.
8. Pirhonen JP, *et al.* Uterine and fetal flow velocity wave forms in hypertensive pregnancy: the effect of a single dose of nifedipine. *Obstet Gynecol* 1990; **76:** 37–41.
9. Impey L. Severe hypotension and fetal distress following sublingual administration of nifedipine to a patient with severe pregnancy induced hypertension at 33 weeks. *Br J Obstet Gynaecol* 1993; **100:** 959–61.
10. Fenakel K, *et al.* Nifedipine in the treatment of severe preeclampsia. *Obstet Gynecol* 1991; **77:** 331–7.

**Kidney disorders.** Although nifedipine may adversely affect renal function (see under Adverse Effects, above) there is evidence that calcium-channel blockers may be of benefit in various forms of kidney disorder. Proteinuria is an important indicator of glomerular kidney disease (p.1080) of various causes and the effects of calcium-channel blockers on proteinuria and renal dysfunction have been studied in a variety of patients. Results have been mixed,[1-5] and it is not clear whether any protective effect of calcium-channel blockers on renal function is only due to their antihypertensive action or whether they also have additional effects. The benefits of ACE inhibitors in kidney disorders are much better established (see p.847) and a study[6] in African American hypertensives was stopped early when treatment with ramipril was found to be superior to treatment with amlodipine.

Nifedipine has also been reported to protect against ciclosporin-induced nephrotoxicity in renal transplant patients (see Transplantation, below).

1. Demarie BK, Bakris GL. Effects of different calcium antagonists on proteinuria associated with diabetes mellitus. *Ann Intern Med* 1990; **113:** 987–8.
2. Melbourne Diabetic Nephropathy Study Group. Comparison between perindopril and nifedipine in hypertensive and normotensive diabetic patients with microalbuminuria. *BMJ* 1991; **302:** 210–16.
3. Reams G, *et al.* The effect of nifedipine GITS on renal function in hypertensive patients with renal insufficiency. *J Clin Pharmacol* 1991; **31:** 468–72.
4. Abbott K, *et al.* Effects of dihydropyridine calcium antagonists on albuminuria in patients with diabetes. *J Clin Pharmacol* 1996; **36:** 274–9.
5. Bouhanick B, *et al.* Equivalent effects of nicardipine and captopril on urinary albumin excretion of type 2, non-insulin-dependent diabetic subjects with mild to moderate hypertension. *Therapie* 1996; **51:** 41–7.
6. Agodoa LY, *et al.* Effect of ramipril vs amlodipine on renal outcomes in hypertensive nephrosclerosis: a randomized controlled trial. *JAMA* 2001; **285:** 2719–28.

**Migraine and cluster headache.** Drugs with calcium-channel blocking activity have been given in the management of headaches considered to have a vascular component such as migraine (p.464) and cluster headache (p.464).

In migraine prophylaxis, of those drugs with calcium-channel blocking activity studied, flunarizine (p.434) has the best documented efficacy, and verapamil may be useful. Other calcium-channel blockers such as diltiazem, nifedipine, and nimodipine have been tried, but results have been conflicting. Verapamil has also been used successfully in patients with hemiplegic migraine, both intravenously to abort attacks,[1,2] and orally for prophylaxis.[2]

Beneficial effects have been reported[3-5] with calcium-channel blockers in the prevention of cluster headache during cluster periods. Verapamil appears to have been the most widely used. In one double-blind study it was found to be of similar efficacy to lithium[6] and appeared to produce fewer adverse effects.

1. Ng TMH, *et al.* The effect of intravenous verapamil on cerebral hemodynamics in a migraine patient with hemiplegia. *Ann Pharmacother* 2000; **34:** 39–43.
2. Yu W, Horowitz SH. Treatment of sporadic hemiplegic migraine with calcium-channel blocker verapamil. *Neurology* 2003; **60:** 120–1.
3. Jónsdóttir M, *et al.* Efficacy, side effects and tolerance compared during headache treatment with three different calcium blockers. *Headache* 1987; **27:** 364–9.
4. Gabai IJ, Spierings ELH. Prophylactic treatment of cluster headache with verapamil. *Headache* 1989; **29:** 167–8.
5. Leone M, *et al.*. Verapamil in the prophylaxis of episodic cluster headache: a double-blind study versus placebo. *Neurology* 2000; **54:** 1382–5.
6. Bussone G, *et al.* Double blind comparison of lithium and verapamil in cluster headache prophylaxis. *Headache* 1990; **30:** 411–17.

**Oesophageal motility disorders.** Results from a number of studies have indicated that nifedipine, usually in doses of 10 to 20 mg sublingually, may be of benefit in patients with achalasia, reducing lower oesophageal sphincter pressure and producing some symptomatic improvement.[1-5] Nifedipine has a role when mechanical dilatation of the sphincter or surgery are not feasible (see Oesophageal Motility Disorders, p.1246).

1. Bortolotti M, Labò G. Clinical and manometric effects of nifedipine in patients with esophageal achalasia. *Gastroenterology* 1981; **80:** 39–44.
2. Gelfond M, *et al.* Isosorbide dinitrate and nifedipine treatment of achalasia: a clinical, manometric and radionuclide evaluation. *Gastroenterology* 1982; **83:** 963–9.
3. Traube M, *et al.* Effects of nifedipine in achalasia and in patients with high-amplitude peristaltic esophageal contractions. *JAMA* 1984; **252:** 1733–6.
4. Román FJ, *et al.* Effects of nifedipine in achalasia and patients with high-amplitude peristaltic esophageal contractions. *JAMA* 1985; **253:** 2046.
5. Coccia G, *et al.* Prospective clinical and manometric study comparing pneumatic dilatation and sublingual nifedipine in the treatment of oesophageal achalasia. *Gut* 1991; **32:** 604–6.

**Peripheral vascular disease.** Vasospastic arterial disease (p.831) is due to an inappropriate response to temperature, usually cold, when vasoconstriction and/or vasospasm occurs. The most important of these disorders is Raynaud's syndrome. Calcium-channel blockers have been of benefit in Raynaud's syndrome, but it is not entirely clear which of their pharmacological actions is responsible. The most widely used and studied is nifedipine. Evidence of subjective benefit has been seen both in primary idiopathic disease[1-4] and in Raynaud's phenomenon secondary to systemic sclerosis,[2,3,5,6] systemic lupus erythematosus,[2,3] rheumatoid arthritis,[3] and cancer chemotherapy.[7] Objective improvement as demonstrated by evidence of improved digital blood flow has been demonstrated in some[4,5,8,9] but not all[6] studies. Doses have varied; 10 mg of nifedipine twice daily initially, increased after a week to a maximum of 20 mg twice daily has been suggested,[10] but in many studies doses of up to 60 mg daily have been used, although side-effects have proved intolerable in some patients given such doses.[6] A modified-release preparation has also been used[11] and may reduce the incidence of adverse effects.

Nifedipine in doses of 20 to 60 mg daily has also been reported to be of benefit in the treatment of another vasospastic condition, chilblains, both for established chilblains and in the prevention of relapse.[12]

1. Roath S. Management of Raynaud's phenomenon: focus on newer treatments. *Drugs* 1989; **37:** 700–12.
2. Smith CD, McKendry RJR. Controlled trial of nifedipine in the treatment of Raynaud's phenomenon. *Lancet* 1982; **ii:** 1299–1301.
3. Kahan A, *et al.* Nifedipine for Raynaud's phenomenon. *Lancet* 1983; **i:** 131.
4. Gasser P. Reaction of capillary blood cell velocity in nailfold capillaries to nifedipine and ketanserin in patients with vasospastic disease. *J Int Med Res* 1991; **19:** 24–31.
5. Thomas RHM, *et al.* Nifedipine in the treatment of Raynaud's phenomenon in patients with systemic sclerosis. *Br J Dermatol* 1987; **117:** 237–41.
6. Rademaker M, *et al.* Comparison of intravenous infusions of iloprost and oral nifedipine in treatment of Raynaud's phenomenon in patients with systemic sclerosis: a double blind randomised study. *BMJ* 1989; **298:** 561–4.
7. Hantel A, *et al.* Nifedipine and oncologic Raynaud phenomenon. *Ann Intern Med* 1988; **108:** 767.
8. Nilsson H, *et al.* Treatment of digital vasospastic disease with the calcium-entry blocker nifedipine. *Acta Med Scand* 1984; **215:** 135–9.
9. Finch MB, *et al.* The peripheral vascular effects of nifedipine in Raynaud's disease. *Br J Clin Pharmacol* 1986; **21:** 100P–101P.
10. Grigg MH, Wolfe JHN. Raynaud's syndrome and similar conditions. *BMJ* 1991; **303:** 913–16.
11. Raynaud's Treatment Study Investigators. Comparison of sustained-release nifedipine and temperature biofeedback for treatment of primary Raynaud phenomenon: results from a randomized clinical trial with 1-year follow-up. *Arch Intern Med* 2000; **160:** 1101–8.
12. Rustin MHA, *et al.* The treatment of chilblains with nifedipine: the results of a pilot study, a double-blind placebo-controlled randomized study and a long-term open trial. *Br J Dermatol* 1989; **120:** 267–75.

**Phaeochromocytoma.** Pharmacological management of phaeochromocytoma (p.831) is principally achieved by alpha-adrenergic blockade and tachycardia may subsequently be controlled by cautious addition of a beta blocker. There have also been some reports[1-4] of the use of nifedipine to treat cardiovascular symptoms in adults and children with phaeochromocytoma.

1. Serfas D, *et al.* Phaeochromocytoma and hypertrophic cardiomyopathy: apparent suppression of symptoms and noradrenaline secretion by calcium-channel blockade. *Lancet* 1983; **ii:** 711–13.
2. Lenders JWM, *et al.* Treatment of a phaeochromocytoma of the urinary bladder with nifedipine. *BMJ* 1985; **290:** 1624–5.
3. Favre L, Vallotton MB. Nifedipine in pheochromocytoma. *Ann Intern Med* 1986; **104:** 125.
4. Deal JE, *et al.* Phaeochromocytoma—investigation and management of 10 cases. *Arch Dis Child* 1990; **65:** 269–74.

**Premature labour.** Although beta$_2$ agonists or magnesium are the drugs most commonly used as tocolytics to postpone premature labour (p.794), there is increasing interest in calcium-channel blockers such as nifedipine, either given alone or added to other tocolytics, as potential first-line drugs. Labour was successfully postponed in a patient given nifedipine 20 mg three times daily and terbutaline 5 mg 4-hourly by mouth.[1] Terbutaline 250 micrograms up to 4 times daily by subcutaneous injection was also occasionally necessary. Nifedipine was administered from the twenty-sixth week of pregnancy for 55 days. A normal, healthy infant was delivered in the thirty-sixth week of pregnancy. In a study[2] in 20 patients, nifedipine 30 mg initially, then 20 mg every 8 hours by mouth, was more effective in suppressing premature labour than ritodrine given intravenously or no treatment. However, a similar study[3] in 33 patients found nifedipine to be no more effective than ritodrine infusion, although associated with a lower incidence of adverse effects. Meta-analyses[4,5] have concluded that nifedipine is at least as effective as beta$_2$ agonists and is associated with fewer maternal adverse effects, and this was supported by the results of a further study[6] in 185 women using nifedipine in an initial dose of up to 40 mg followed by 60 to 160 mg daily. Similar results have been reported with nicardipine.[7]

1. Kaul AF, *et al.* The management of preterm labor with the calcium channel-blocking agent nifedipine combined with the β-mimetic terbutaline. *Drug Intell Clin Pharm* 1985; **19:** 369–71.
2. Read MD, Wellby DE. The use of a calcium antagonist (nifedipine) to suppress preterm labour. *Br J Obstet Gynaecol* 1986; **93:** 933–7.
3. Ferguson JE, *et al.* A comparison of tocolysis with nifedipine or ritodrine: analysis of efficacy and maternal, fetal, and neonatal outcome. *Am J Obstet Gynecol* 1990; **163:** 105–11.
4. Ray JG. Meta-analysis of nifedipine versus beta-sympathomimetic agents for tocolysis during preterm labour. *J Soc Obstet Gynaecol Can* 1998; **20:** 259–69.
5. Tsatsaris V, *et al.* Tocolysis with nifedipine or beta-adrenergic agonists: a meta-analysis. *Obstet Gynecol* 2001; **97:** 840–7.
6. Papatsonis DNM, *et al.* Nifedipine and ritodrine in the management of preterm labor: a randomized multicenter trial. *Obstet Gynecol* 1997; **90:** 230–4.
7. Jannet D, *et al.* Nicardipine versus salbutamol in the treatment of premature labor: a prospective randomized study. *Eur J Obstet Gynecol Reprod Biol* 1997; **73:** 11–16.

**Pulmonary hypertension.** Vasodilators have been tried in primary pulmonary hypertension (p.832) on the premise that pulmonary vasoconstriction is an important component of the condition. Calcium-channel blockers are the most widely-used. Improved survival over a 5-year period has been noted in a study in patients treated with high doses of calcium-channel blockers (nifedipine or diltiazem).[1] However, treatment failures have occurred with nifedipine, and at least one death has been reported shortly after starting therapy.[2] Other reports have also stressed the potentially deleterious effects of nifedipine (or other vasodilator) therapy in pulmonary hypertension. Increased dyspnoea and a fall in arterial $PO_2$ have been reported in a patient with primary pulmonary hypertension given nifedipine, probably due to preferential vasodilatation of underventilated hypoxic tissues resulting in an increased physiological shunt.[3] Invasive investigations, notably blood-gas monitoring, are therefore recommended when giving nifedipine to these patients[2,3] and it has been advised that an acute response test should be performed before embarking on long-term treatment.[1]

1. Rich S, *et al.* The effect of high doses of calcium-channel blockers on survival in primary pulmonary hypertension. *N Engl J Med* 1992; **327:** 76–81.
2. McLeod AA, Jewitt DE. Drug treatment of primary pulmonary hypertension. *Drugs* 1986; **31:** 177–84.
3. Krol RC, *et al.* Primary pulmonary hypotension, nifedipine, and hypoxemia. *Ann Intern Med* 1984; **100:** 163.

**Tardive dyskinesia.** Calcium-channel blockers have been tried in the treatment of tardive dyskinesia[1] (see under Extrapyramidal Disorders, p.677). However, results have been mixed and there is concern that, if their action is mediated through an antidopaminergic effect, they may only temporarily mask symptoms or exacerbate them in the long term.[1]

1. Cates M, *et al.* Are calcium-channel blockers effective in the treatment of tardive dyskinesia? *Ann Pharmacother* 1993; **27:** 191–6.

**Transplantation.** The main adverse effect of ciclosporin is reversible, dose-related nephrotoxicity. There is some evidence that nifedipine may be of value in protecting against this effect. Retrospective analysis[1] of 106 ciclosporin-treated renal transplant patients found that patients receiving nifedipine for hypertension had better graft function, despite having shorter graft duration and therefore requiring higher dosage of ciclosporin, than hypertensive patients receiving other drug treatment. Subsequent studies have similarly reported improved graft function[2] in patients receiving nifedipine and suggest that graft survival is also improved.[3,4] A nephroprotective effect has also been reported with nitrendipine,[5] felodipine,[6] isradipine,[7] and with the non-dihydropyridine diltiazem (see p.902), although a study[8] with nicardipine failed to demonstrate any improvement in graft function.

See also Kidney Disorders, above.

For a report of adverse effects attributed to reduced metabolism of nifedipine in patients taking ciclosporin, see Immunosuppressants, under Interactions, above.

1. Feehally J, *et al.* Does nifedipine ameliorate cyclosporin A nephrotoxicity? *BMJ* 1987; **295:** 310.
2. Shin GT, *et al.* Effect of nifedipine on renal allograft function and survival beyond one year. *Clin Nephrol* 1997; **47:** 33–6.
3. Weinrauch LA, *et al.* Role of calcium channel blockers in diabetic renal transplant patients: preliminary observations on protection from sepsis. *Clin Nephrol* 1995; **44:** 185–92.
4. Mehrens T, *et al.* The beneficial effects of calcium channel blockers on long-term kidney transplant survival are independent of blood-pressure reduction. *Clin Transplant* 2000; **14:** 257–61.
5. Rahn K-H, *et al.* Effect of nitrendipine on renal function in renal-transplant patients treated with cyclosporin: a randomised trial. *Lancet* 1999; **354:** 1415–20.
6. Madsen JK, *et al.* The effect of felodipine on renal function and blood pressure in cyclosporin-treated renal transplant recipients during the first three months after transplantation. *Nephrol Dial Transplant* 1998; **13:** 2327–34.
7. van Riemsdijk IC, *et al.* Addition of isradipine (Lomir) results in a better renal function after kidney transplantation: a double-blind, randomized, placebo-controlled, multi-center study. *Transplantation* 2000; **70:** 122–6.
8. Kessler M, *et al.* Influence of nicardipine on renal function and plasma cyclosporin in renal transplant patients. *Eur J Clin Pharmacol* 1989; **36:** 637–8.

**Urticaria.** Oral antihistamines are the main drugs used in the management of urticaria (p.1138). Addition of a calcium-channel blocker, such as nifedipine, has been suggested for patients unresponsive to treatment with oral antihistamines alone, but results have been mixed.[1,2]

1. Lawlor F, *et al.* Calcium antagonist in the treatment of symptomatic dermographism: low-dose and high-dose studies with nifedipine. *Dermatologica* 1988; **177:** 287–91.
2. Bressler RB, *et al.* Therapy of chronic idiopathic urticaria with nifedipine: demonstration of beneficial effect in a double-blinded, placebo-controlled, crossover trial. *J Allergy Clin Immunol* 1989; **83:** 756–63.

## Preparations

***BP 2003:*** Nifedipine Capsules;
***USP 27:*** Nifedipine Capsules; Nifedipine Extended-release Tablets.

**Proprietary Preparations** (details are given in Part 3)
***Arg.:*** Adalat; Nifecor; Nifed Sol; Nifedel; Nifelat; Prudencial; ***Austral.:*** Adalat; Adapine†; Nifecard; Nifehexal; Nyefax; ***Austria:*** Adalat; Buconif; Fedip; Majolat; Nifal; Nifebene; Nifecard; Nifehexal; Ospocard; ***Belg.:*** Adalat; Hypan; ***Braz.:*** Adalat; Adcor†; Biocord†; Cardalin; Cardiopina†; Dilaflux; Loncord; Neo Fedipina; Nifadil; Nifedax; Nifedin; Nifehexal; Normopres; Oxcord; ***Canad.:*** Adalat; Apo-Nifed; Novo-Nifedin; Nu-Nifed; ***Chile:*** Adalat; Carbloc; Cardicon; Coronovo; Nipress; Pabalat; Sulotil; ***Denm.:*** Adalat; Hexadilat; Nifecodan; Nycopin†; ***Fin.:*** Adalat; Nifangin; Nifdemin; Nifecor; ***Fr.:*** Adalate; Chronadalate; ***Ger.:*** Adalat; Aprical; Cisday†; Cordicant; Corinfar; Corotrend†; Dignokonstant; duranifin; Jedipin; Nife; nife uno; Nifeclair; Nifecor; Nifedipat; Nifehexal; Nifelat; Nifical; Nifreal†; Pidilat; ***Gr.:*** Adalat; Antiblut; Coracten; Flecor-N; Glopir; Macorel; Nefelid; Nifedicor; Viscard; ***Hong Kong:*** Adalat; Cardilate MR; Coracten; Fenamon; Nadipinia; Nifecard; Vidalat; Waridipin; ***India:*** Calcigard; Cardules; Depicor; Depin; Myogard; Nicardia; Nifedine; Nifelat; ***Irl.:*** Adalat; Nifed; Nifelease; Pinifed; Systepin; Vasofed; ***Israel:*** Aprical†; Megalat; Osmo-Adalat; Pressolat; ***Ital.:*** Adalat; Anifed†; Bionif; Citilat; Coral; Euxat; Fenidina; Nifedicor; Nifedicron; Nifedin; Nifesal; Nipin; ***Jpn:*** Adalat; ***Malaysia:*** Adalat; Adifen; Fenamon; ***Mex.:*** Adalat; Aldar†; Atenses; Cordilat; Corogal; Corotrend; Elocor†; Feniken†; Fusepina; Nifedigel†; Nifedipres; Nifezzard; ***Neth.:*** Adalat; ***Norw.:*** Adalat; Nycopin†; ***NZ:*** Adalat; Nyefax; ***Port.:*** Adalat; Medipina; Nifedate; Zenusin; ***S.Afr.:*** Adalat; Anginor†; Cardifen; Cardilat; Cipalat; Nifedalat; Vascard; Vasofed†; ***Singapore:*** Adalat; Apo-Nifed; Cordipin; Fenamon†; Nifecard; Nifedi-Denk; Nifelat; Vasdalat; ***Spain:*** Adalat; Cordilan†; Dari†; Dilcor; Pertensal; ***Swed.:*** Adalat; ***Switz.:*** Adalat; Aldipin; Cardipin; Corotrend; Ecodipine; nife-basan; Nifedicor; ***Thai.:*** Adalat; Calcigard; Coracten; Fenamon; Jedipin†; Nelapine; Nifecard; Nifelat; Nificard†; Nifiran; Nyefax; Servidipine†; Zenusin†; ***UAE:*** Cardiopine; ***UK:*** Adalat; Adipine; Angiopine; Calanif†; Calchan; Calcilat†; Cardilate MR; Coracten; Coroday; Fortipine; Hypolar Retard; Nifedipress; Nifopress; Nimodrel†; Slofedipine; Tensipine; Unipine XL†; ***USA:*** Adalat; Afeditab; Nifediac; Nifedical; Procardia.

**Multi-ingredient:** ***Arg.:*** Atel N; ***Austria:*** Beta-Adalat; Nif-Ten; Pontuc; ***Belg.:*** Beta-Adalat; Tenif; ***Braz.:*** Nifelat; ***Fin.:*** Beta-Adalat†; Nif-Ten; ***Fr.:*** Beta-Adalate; Tenordate; ***Ger.:*** AteNif beta; Belnif; Bresben; duranifin Sali; Nif-Ten; Nifatenol; Nifehexal Sali†; Pontuc†; Sali-Adalat; Tredalat; ***Hong Kong:*** Nif-Ten; ***India:*** Beta Nicardia; Cardules Plus; Depten; Nifetolol; Presolar; Tenofed; ***Irl.:*** Ate-Nife†; Beta-Adalat; Nif-Ten; ***Ital.:*** Mixer; Nif-Ten; ***Mex.:*** Plenacor; ***Neth.:*** Nif-Ten; ***Singapore:*** Nif-Ten; Nifetex; ***Switz.:*** Beta-Adalat; Nif-Atenil; Nif-Ten; ***UK:*** Beta-Adalat; Tenif.

---

# Nifekalant Hydrochloride *(rINNM)*

Hidrocloruro de nifekalant; MS-551. 6-[(2-{(2-Hydroxyethyl)[3-(*p*-nitrophenyl)propyl]amino}ethyl)amino]-1,3-dimethyluracil hydrochloride.

$C_{19}H_{27}N_5O_5,HCl$ = 441.9.

*CAS — 130636-43-0 (nifekalant); 130656-51-8 (nifekalant hydrochloride).*

## Profile

Nifekalant is a class III antiarrhythmic (p.809) used intravenously as the hydrochloride in the management of life-threatening ventricular arrhythmias (p.816). The usual dose is 300 micrograms/kg by intravenous injection over 5 minutes under continuous ECG monitoring; this may be followed by a maintenance dose of 400 micrograms/kg per hour by intravenous infusion if required, under ECG monitoring.

## Preparations

**Proprietary Preparations** (details are given in Part 3)
***Jpn:*** Shinbit.

---

# Nilvadipine *(USAN, rINN)*

CL-287389; FK-235; Nilvadipino; Nivadipine; SKF-102362. 5-Isopropyl 3-methyl 2-cyano-1,4-dihydro-6-methyl-4-(*m*-nitrophenyl)-3,5-pyridinedicarboxylate.

$C_{19}H_{19}N_3O_6$ = 385.4.

*CAS — 75530-68-6.*

*ATC — C08CA10.*

## Profile

Nilvadipine is a dihydropyridine calcium-channel blocker with general properties similar to those of nifedipine (p.966). It is used in the management of hypertension (p.825). Nilvadipine is given by mouth, usually as a modified-release preparation, in a dose of up to 16 mg daily.

◊ Reviews.

1. Brogden RN, McTavish D. Nilvadipine: a review of its pharmacodynamic and pharmacokinetic properties, therapeutic use in hypertension and potential in cerebrovascular disease and angina. *Drugs Aging* 1995; **6:** 150–71. Correction. *ibid.*; **7:** 116.

## Preparations

**Proprietary Preparations** (details are given in Part 3)
***Austria:*** Tensan; ***Denm.:*** Escor†; ***Fin.:*** Escor; ***Ger.:*** Escor; Nivadil; ***Hong Kong:*** Escor†; ***Irl.:*** Nivadil; ***Jpn:*** Nivadil; ***Port.:*** Nivadil; ***Switz.:*** Nivadil.

---

# Nimodipine *(BAN, USAN, rINN)*

Bay-e-9736; Nimodipino; Nimodipinum. Isopropyl 2-methoxyethyl 1,4-dihydro-2,6-dimethyl-4-(3-nitrophenyl)pyridine-3,5-dicarboxylate.

$C_{21}H_{26}N_2O_7$ = 418.4.

*CAS — 66085-59-4.*

*ATC — C08CA06.*

**Pharmacopoeias.** In *Eur.* (see p.vi) and *US.*

**Ph. Eur. 5.0** (Nimodipine). A light yellow or yellow crystalline powder. It exhibits polymorphism. Practically insoluble in water; sparingly soluble in dehydrated alcohol; freely soluble in ethyl acetate. Exposure to ultraviolet light leads to formation of a nitrophenylpyridine derivative. Solutions should be prepared in the dark or under light of wavelength greater than 420 nm, immediately before use. Protect from light.

**USP 27** (Nimodipine). A light yellow or yellow crystalline powder, affected by light. It exhibits polymorphism. Practically insoluble in water; sparingly soluble in alcohol; freely soluble in ethyl acetate. Store in airtight containers at a temperature of 25°, excursions permitted between 15° and 30°. Protect from light.

**Incompatibility.** The manufacturer states that solutions of nimodipine are incompatible with some plastics, including PVC, and that the only plastics suitable for use are polyethylene and polypropylene.

## Adverse Effects, Treatment, and Precautions

As for dihydropyridine calcium-channel blockers (see Nifedipine, p.966).

Nimodipine should be used with caution in patients with cerebral oedema or severely raised intracranial pressure.

**Effects on the heart.** Marked bradycardia developed in a patient with acute ischaemic stroke during treatment with nimodipine and was suspected to be related to the drug therapy.[1]

1. Fagan SC, Nacci N. Nimodipine and bradycardia in acute stroke—drug or disease? *DICP Ann Pharmacother* 1991; **25:** 247–9.

## Interactions

As for dihydropyridine calcium-channel blockers (see Nifedipine, p.969).

## Pharmacokinetics

Nimodipine is rapidly absorbed from the gastrointestinal tract after oral administration but undergoes extensive first-pass metabolism in the liver. The oral bioavailability is reported to be about 13%. Nimodipine is more than 95% bound to plasma proteins. It crosses the blood-brain barrier, but concentrations in CSF are lower than those in plasma. Nimodipine is extensively metabolised in the liver. It is excreted in faeces via the bile, and in urine, almost entirely as metabolites. The terminal elimination half-life is reported to be about 9 hours but the initial decline in plasma concentration is much more rapid, equivalent to a half-life of 1 to 2 hours.

## Uses and Administration

Nimodipine is a dihydropyridine calcium-channel blocker that has the general properties of nifedipine (p.970), but acts particularly on cerebral blood vessels. It is used in cerebrovascular disorders (see below), particularly in the prevention and treatment of ischaemic neurological deficits following aneurysmal subarachnoid haemorrhage.

To reduce the incidence and severity of neurological deficit following aneurysmal haemorrhage nimodipine is given by mouth in a dose of 60 mg every 4 hours. Treatment should begin within 4 days of onset of haemorrhage and should continue for 21 days. In patients with hepatic impairment the dose may be reduced (see below) and blood pressure should be closely monitored.

If cerebral ischaemia occurs or has already occurred, neurological deficit may be treated by intravenous infusion of nimodipine. It should be given via a bypass into a running intravenous infusion into a central vein. The initial dose should be nimodipine 1 mg/hour for 2 hours, increased (provided that no severe decrease in blood pressure occurs) to 2 mg/hour. The starting dose should be reduced to 500 micrograms/hour, or even lower if necessary, in patients weighing less than 70 kg and in those with unstable blood pressure; a similar reduction in dosage has been suggested in hepatic impairment, and blood pressure should be closely monitored. Treatment should be started as soon as possible and continued for at least 5 and no more than 14 days; if the patient has already received oral nimodipine, the total duration of nimodipine use should not exceed 21 days.

**Administration in hepatic impairment.** The clearance of nimodipine is reduced in patients with cirrhosis, and blood pressure should be closely monitored in such patients. The US manufacturer recommends that the oral dose of nimodipine should be halved to 30 mg every 4 hours in patients with hepatic cirrhosis. Some manufacturers have also suggested a reduction in the initial intravenous dose to 500 micrograms or less per hour.

**Cerebrovascular disorders.** Nimodipine is used orally and intravenously in the prevention and treatment of ischaemic neurological deficits caused by arterial vasospasm following aneurysmal subarachnoid haemorrhage (see Stroke, p.836), although the evidence for benefit following intravenous use is limited.[1] Nimodipine has also been used for traumatic subarachnoid haemorrhage.[2] In addition to dilating cerebral blood vessels and improving cerebral blood flow, nimodipine may also prevent or reverse ischaemic damage to the brain by limiting transcellular calcium influx.

These effects have led to the investigation of nimodipine in other conditions associated with cerebral ischaemia. Studies[3,4] of nimodipine given orally after ischaemic stroke have produced conflicting results. A meta-analysis[5] of controlled studies suggested that nimodipine is beneficial if given within 12 hours of stroke onset but a further study[6] failed to confirm these findings. In a controlled study[7] of 155 patients suffering a cardiac arrest, nimodipine was given by intravenous infusion for 24 hours. Nimodipine had no effect on overall survival, although it did improve survival of patients in whom advanced life support was delayed for more than 10 minutes after arrest. Nimodipine has also been tried in dementia (p.1484). Two multicentre studies[8] involving a total of 755 patients with dementia of vascular or degenerative origin given nimodipine for up to 6 months reported improvements in cognitive function and disability, and a systematic review[9] concluded that nimodipine could be of some benefit in patients with various forms of dementia.


1. Rinkel GJE, *et al.* Calcium antagonists for aneurysmal subarachnoid haemorrhage. Available in The Cochrane Library; Issue 2. Chichester: John Wiley; 2004.
2. Harders A, *et al.* Traumatic subarachnoid hemorrhage and its treatment with nimodipine. *J Neurosurg* 1996; **85:** 82–9.
3. Gelmers HJ, *et al.* A controlled trial of nimodipine in acute ischemic stroke. *N Engl J Med* 1988; **318:** 203–7.
4. Trust Study Group. Randomised, double-blind, placebo-controlled trial of nimodipine in acute stroke. *Lancet* 1990; **336:** 1205–9.
5. Mohr JP, *et al.* Meta-analysis of oral nimodipine trials in acute ischemic stroke. *Cerebrovasc Dis* 1994; **4:** 197–203.
6. Horn J, *et al.* Very Early Nimodipine Use in Stroke (VENUS): a randomized, double-blind, placebo-controlled trial. *Stroke* 2001; **32:** 461–5.
7. Roine RO, *et al.* Nimodipine after resuscitation from out-of-hospital ventricular fibrillation: a placebo-controlled, double-blind, randomized trial. *JAMA* 1990; **264:** 3171–7.
8. Parnetti L, *et al.* Nimodipine Study Group. Mental deterioration in old age: results of two multicenter, clinical trials with nimodipine. *Clin Ther* 1993; **15:** 394–406.
9. López-Arrieta J, Birks J. Nimodipine for primary degenerative, mixed and vascular dementia. Available in The Cochrane Library; Issue 2. Chichester: John Wiley; 2004.


**Migraine.** For reference to the use of calcium-channel blockers, including nimodipine, in the management of migraine, see under Nifedipine, p.971.

## Preparations

***BP 2003:*** Nimodipine Intravenous Infusion; Nimodipine Tablets.

**Proprietary Preparations** (details are given in Part 3)
***Arg.:*** AC Vascular; Acival; Ampina; Aniduv; Cebrofort; Cletonol; Eugerial; Finacilen; Macobal; Nimodilat; Nimotop; Nivas; Tenocard; ***Austral.:*** Nimotop; ***Austria:*** Nimotop; ***Belg.:*** Nimotop; ***Braz.:*** Eugerial; Nimotop; Nimovas; Noodipina; Norton; Oxigen; Vasodipina; ***Canad.:*** Nimotop; ***Chile:*** Brainal; Grifonimod; Neurogeron; Nimotop; Regental; Vasoflex; ***Denm.:*** Nimotop; ***Fin.:*** Nimotop; ***Fr.:*** Nimotop; ***Ger.:*** Nim; Nimotop; ***Gr.:*** Befimat; Curban; Figozant; Genovox; Myodipine; Nelbinex; Nimodil; Nimotop; Nortolan; Rosital; Stigmicarpin; Thrioniren; Vastripine; Ziremex; ***Hong Kong:*** Nimotop; ***India:*** Vasotop; ***Irl.:*** Nimotop; ***Israel:*** Nimotop; ***Ital.:*** Nimotop; Periplum; ***Malaysia:*** Nimotop; ***Mex.:*** Kenzolol; Nimotop; ***Neth.:*** Nimotop; ***Norw.:*** Nimotop; ***NZ:*** Nimotop; ***Port.:*** Brainox; Modina; Nimotop; Sobrepina; Trinalion; ***S.Afr.:*** Nimotop; ***Singapore:*** Nimotop; ***Spain:*** Admon; Brainal; Calnit; Kenesil; Modus; Nimotop; Remontal; ***Swed.:*** Nimotop; ***Switz.:*** Nimotop; ***Thai.:*** Nimotop; ***UK:*** Nimotop; ***USA:*** Nimotop.

**Multi-ingredient:** ***Arg.:*** Idesole Plus; Nimodilat Plus; Nimoreagin; Nivas Plus.

## Nipradilol *(rINN)*

K-351; Nipradolol. 8-[2-Hydroxy-3-(isopropylamino)propoxy]-3-chromanol 3-nitrate.

$C_{15}H_{22}N_2O_6$ = 326.3.
*CAS — 81486-22-8.*

### Profile

Nipradilol is a non-cardioselective beta blocker (p.868). It is also reported to have direct vasodilating activity. It is used in the management of glaucoma and ocular hypertension (p.1485); eye drops containing nipradilol 0.05% are instilled twice daily.

### Preparations

**Proprietary Preparations** (details are given in Part 3)
***Jpn:*** Hypadil.

## Nisoldipine *(BAN, USAN, rINN)*

Bay-k-5552; Nisoldipino. Isobutyl methyl 1,4-dihydro-2,6-dimethyl-4-(2-nitrophenyl)pyridine-3,5-dicarboxylate.

$C_{20}H_{24}N_2O_6$ = 388.4.
*CAS — 63675-72-9.*
*ATC — C08CA07.*

### Adverse Effects, Treatment, and Precautions

As for dihydropyridine calcium-channel blockers (see Nifedipine, p.966).

### Interactions

As for dihydropyridine calcium-channel blockers (see Nifedipine, p.969).

### Pharmacokinetics

Nisoldipine is well absorbed from the gastrointestinal tract after oral administration, but undergoes rapid and extensive first-pass metabolism in the gut wall and liver and bioavailability has been reported to be only about 4 to 8%. About 60 to 80% of an oral dose is excreted in the urine and the remainder in the faeces, mainly as metabolites. The terminal elimination half-life is about 7 to 12 hours. Nisoldipine is more than 99% bound to plasma proteins.

◊ A study[1] in 11 patients receiving nisoldipine 10 mg once or twice daily by mouth indicated that the pharmacokinetics of nisoldipine could best be described by an open 2-compartment model. Peak plasma concentrations occurred 1 hour after a single oral dose, and varied greatly between the patients. The mean plasma elimination half-life was 11.4 hours after a single dose and 14.0 hours after repeated dosing, which was longer than had been previously reported, perhaps reflecting the greater sensitivity of the assay.

In another study oral, but not intravenous, administration of nisoldipine increased liver blood flow in 10 healthy subjects and thus affected its own systemic availability.[2] Variations in liver blood flow may account for the interindividual variation in the pharmacokinetics of nisoldipine.


1. Ottosson A-M, *et al.* Analysis and pharmacokinetics of nisoldipine in hypertensive patients. *Curr Ther Res* 1989; **45:** 347–58.
2. van Harten J, *et al.* Variability in the pharmacokinetics of nisoldipine as caused by differences in liver blood flow response. *J Clin Pharmacol* 1989; **29:** 714–21.


### Uses and Administration

Nisoldipine is a dihydropyridine calcium-channel blocker with actions and uses similar to those of nifedipine (p.970). It is used in the management of hypertension (p.825) and angina pectoris (p.813).

Nisoldipine is given by mouth usually as a modified-release preparation. Absorption is affected by food and the modified-release preparation should be taken on an empty stomach; it should not be taken with high fat meals. Doses are similar for both hypertension and angina. The initial dose is 10 mg once daily and the usual maintenance dose is 20 to 40 mg once daily.

◊ Reviews.


1. Mitchell J, *et al.* Nisoldipine: a new dihydropyridine calcium-channel blocker. *J Clin Pharmacol* 1993; **33:** 46–52.
2. Plosker GL, Faulds D. Nisoldipine coat-core: a review of its pharmacology and therapeutic efficacy in hypertension. *Drugs* 1996; **52:** 232–53.
3. Langtry HD, Spencer CM. Nisoldipine coat-core; a review of its pharmacodynamic and pharmacokinetic properties and clinical efficacy in the management of ischaemic heart disease. *Drugs* 1997; **53:** 867–84.


### Preparations

**Proprietary Preparations** (details are given in Part 3)
***Arg.:*** Nisodipen; ***Austria:*** Syscor; ***Belg.:*** Sular; Syscor; ***Braz.:*** Syscor; ***Chile:*** Nivas; ***Fin.:*** Syscor; ***Ger.:*** Baymycard; ***Gr.:*** Syscor; ***Ital.:*** Syscor; Zadipina†; ***Mex.:*** Sular†; Syscor†; ***Neth.:*** Sular†; Syscor†; ***S.Afr.:*** Syscor; ***Spain:*** Cornel; Sular; Syscor; ***Swed.:*** Syscor†; ***Switz.:*** Syscor; ***UK:*** Syscor; ***USA:*** Sular.

## Nitrendipine *(BAN, USAN, rINN)*

Bay-e-5009; Nitrendipino; Nitrendipinum. Ethyl methyl 1,4-dihydro-2,6-dimethyl-4-(3-nitrophenyl)pyridine-3,5-dicarboxylate.

$C_{18}H_{20}N_2O_6$ = 360.4.
*CAS — 39562-70-4.*
*ATC — C08CA08.*

**Pharmacopoeias.** In *Chin.* and *Eur.* (see p.vi).

**Ph. Eur. 5.0** (Nitrendipine). A yellow crystalline powder. It exhibits polymorphism. Practically insoluble in water; sparingly soluble in dehydrated alcohol and in methyl alcohol; freely soluble in ethyl acetate. Exposure to ultraviolet light leads to formation of a nitrophenylpyridine derivative. Solutions should be prepared in the dark or under light of wavelength greater than 420 nm, immediately before use. Protect from light.

### Adverse Effects, Treatment, and Precautions

As for dihydropyridine calcium-channel blockers (see Nifedipine, p.966).

### Interactions

As for dihydropyridine calcium-channel blockers (see Nifedipine, p.969).

### Pharmacokinetics

Nitrendipine is reported to be well absorbed after oral administration but undergoes extensive first-pass metabolism; the absolute oral bioavailability is reported to range from about 10 to 20%, depending in part on the dosage form. Nitrendipine is about 98% bound to plasma proteins. It is extensively metabolised in the liver and is excreted as metabolites, mainly in urine, with small amounts in the faeces. Although early studies reported a terminal elimination half-life of about 2 to 4 hours, later studies, using more sensitive assay procedures, have recorded values between about 10 and 22 hours.

◊ References.


1. Soons PA, Breimer DD. Stereoselective pharmacokinetics of oral and intravenous nitrendipine in healthy male subjects. *Br J Clin Pharmacol* 1991; **32:** 11–16.


### Uses and Administration

Nitrendipine is a dihydropyridine calcium-channel blocker with actions similar to those of nifedipine (p.970). It is used in the treatment of hypertension (p.825).

The usual dose is 20 mg daily as a single dose by mouth or as 2 divided doses. The dose may be increased to 20 mg twice daily if necessary for the control of resistant hypertension. In the elderly, an initial dose of 10 mg daily should be used. The dose should also be reduced in hepatic impairment (see below).

◊ Reviews.


1. Santiago TM, Lopez LM. Nitrendipine: a new dihydropyridine calcium-channel antagonist for the treatment of hypertension. *DICP Ann Pharmacother* 1990; **24:** 167–75.


**Administration in hepatic impairment.** The initial dose of nitrendipine should be reduced to 5 to 10 mg once daily in patients with hepatic impairment.

### Preparations

**Proprietary Preparations** (details are given in Part 3)
***Arg.:*** Nirapel; Nitrendil; Tocrat; ***Austria:*** Baypress; ***Belg.:*** Baypress; ***Braz.:*** Caltren; Nitrencord; Nitrenpress†; ***Chile:*** Cardiazem; Grifonitren; Nitrendicor; Presabet; Tensofar; ***Denm.:*** Baypress; ***Fr.:*** Baypress; Nidrel; ***Ger.:*** Bayotensin; Nitre; Nitre-Puren; Nitregamma; Nitren; Nitren Lich; Nitrendepat; Nitrendidoc; Nitrendimerck; Nitrensal; Nitrepress; ***Gr.:*** Aroselin; Baypress; Crivion; G-Press; Leonitren; Lisba; Lostradyl; Nelconil; Nifecard; Potional; Pressodipin; Spidox; Tepanil; Ufocard; ***Hong Kong:*** Baypress; ***Ital.:*** Baypress; Deiten; ***Jpn:*** Baylotensin; ***Mex.:*** Baypress; ***Neth.:*** Baypress; ***Port.:*** Farnitran; Hiperdipina; Hipertenol; ***Spain:*** Balminil; Baypresol; Gericin; Monopress†; Niprina; Sub Tensin; Tensogradal; Trendinol; Vastensium; ***Switz.:*** Baypress; ***Thai.:*** Baypress; Ditrenil; Miniten.

**Multi-ingredient:** ***India:*** Cardif Beta; ***Spain:*** Eneas; Enit; Vipres; Zorail.

## Nitric Oxide *(USAN)*

Mononitrogen Monoxide; Nitrogen Monoxide; Nitrogenii Oxidum; OHM-11771; Óxido nítrico.

NO = 30.01.
*CAS — 10102-43-9.*
*ATC — R07AX01.*

**Pharmacopoeias.** In *Eur.* (see p.vi).

**Ph. Eur. 5.0** (Nitric Oxide). A colourless gas which turns brown when exposed to air. At 20° and at a pressure of 101 kPa, 1 volume dissolves in about 21 volumes of water. Store compressed at a pressure not exceeding 2.5 MPa measured at 15° in suitable containers.

## Adverse Effects

Inhaled nitric oxide may lead to the development of methaemoglobinaemia, particularly at higher doses. Although it is a selective pulmonary vasodilator, systemic hypotension may occur. Abrupt withdrawal of therapy may lead to a deterioration in oxygenation and the development of rebound pulmonary hypertension.

Nitrogen dioxide produced when nitric oxide combines with oxygen can cause acute lung injury; high concentrations of inhaled nitric oxide are directly irritant to the lungs.

◊ A potential complication of inhaled nitric oxide is methaemoglobinaemia but this is probably related to the dose; the risk does not appear to be increased during low-dose (20 ppm) therapy.[1] Another possible adverse event is an increased risk of bleeding due to inhibition of platelet aggregation.[2-5] Rebound pulmonary hypertension[6] and deterioration in oxygenation[7,8] have been reported in some children following withdrawal of nitric oxide therapy. Severe systemic hypotension has also been reported[9] following initiation of inhaled nitric oxide therapy in a neonate with severe left ventricular dysfunction. Pulmonary oedema has been associated with the use of nitric oxide in 2 patients with CREST syndrome, a form of systemic sclerosis.[10] Motor neurone disease in a patient with alcoholism has been partly attributed[11] to the use of nitric oxide for pulmonary hypertension.


1. Kinsella JP, Abman SH. Methaemoglobin during nitric oxide therapy with high-frequency ventilation. *Lancet* 1993; **342:** 615.
2. Högman M, *et al.* Bleeding time prolongation and NO inhalation. *Lancet* 1993; **341:** 1664–5.
3. Joannidis M, *et al.* Inhaled nitric oxide. *Lancet* 1996; **348:** 1448–9.
4. Cheung P-Y, *et al.* Inhaled nitric oxide and inhibition of platelet aggregation in critically ill neonates. *Lancet* 1998; **351:** 1181–2.
5. George TN, *et al.* The effect of inhaled nitric oxide therapy on bleeding time and platelet aggregation in neonates. *J Pediatr* 1998; **132:** 731–4.
6. Miller OI, *et al.* Rebound pulmonary hypertension on withdrawal from inhaled nitric oxide. *Lancet* 1995; **346:** 51–2.
7. Aly H, *et al.* Weaning strategy with inhaled nitric oxide treatment in persistent pulmonary hypertension of the newborn. *Arch Dis Child* 1997; **76:** F118–F122.
8. Davidson D, *et al.* Safety of withdrawing inhaled nitric oxide therapy in persistent pulmonary hypertension of the newborn. *Pediatrics* 1999; **104:** 231–6.
9. Henrichsen T, *et al.* Inhaled nitric oxide can cause severe systemic hypotension. *J Pediatr* 1996; **129:** 183.
10. Preston IR, *et al.* Pulmonary edema caused by inhaled nitric oxide therapy in two patients with pulmonary hypertension associated with the CREST syndrome. *Chest* 2002; **121:** 656–9.
11. Tsai GE, Gastfriend DR. Nitric oxide-induced motor neuron disease in a patient with alcoholism. *N Engl J Med* 1995; **332:** 1036.


## Precautions

Patients receiving inhaled nitric oxide should be monitored for methaemoglobinaemia and oxygenation. Inspired nitric oxide and nitrogen dioxide levels should also be monitored. Treatment should not be discontinued abruptly since rebound pulmonary hypertension and deterioration in oxygenation may occur.

The exposure of healthcare workers to nitric oxide and nitrogen dioxide should be limited.

◊ References.


1. Committee on Safety of Medicines/Medicines Control Agency. Inhaled nitric oxide. *Current Problems* 1996; **22:** 8.
2. Cuthbertson BH, *et al.* Use of inhaled nitric oxide in British intensive therapy units. *Br J Anaesth* 1997; **78:** 696–700.
3. Phillips ML, *et al.* Assessment of medical personnel exposure to nitrogen oxides during inhaled nitric oxide treatment of neonatal and pediatric patients. *Pediatrics* 1999; **104:** 1095–1100.


## Pharmacokinetics

Nitric oxide is absorbed systemically after inhalation but is rapidly inactivated by reaction with haemoglobin to form methaemoglobin and nitrate; it has a half-life of only a few seconds. It is excreted predominantly in the urine as nitrate.

## Uses and Administration

Nitric oxide is an endogenous chemical messenger that acts mainly by stimulating guanylate cyclase in smooth muscle to cause vasodilatation. It is also involved in platelet aggregation, neurotransmission, and the immune system, and possesses antimicrobial, antitumour, and antiviral activity.

Endogenous nitric oxide is synthesised from L-arginine and is now recognised to be the same substance as endothelium-derived relaxing factor (EDRF). Synthesis from L-arginine is by the enzyme, nitric oxide synthase. Three isoforms of this enzyme have been identified. Constitutive isoforms occur in endothelial cells (such as in vascular endothelium, platelets, and the heart) and neuronal cells (in some central and peripheral neurones). Small amounts of nitric oxide are regularly produced by these systems. In contrast, an inducible nitric oxide synthase isoform is expressed only after activation by external stimuli such as in infection or inflammation and larger amounts of nitric oxide are produced. This inducible nitric oxide synthase may be expressed in a wide range of cells, including macrophages and cells in vascular smooth muscle, the heart, gastrointestinal tract, and liver.

Inhaled nitric oxide is a highly selective pulmonary vasodilator. It is used in the management of term and near-term neonates with hypoxic respiratory failure associated with pulmonary hypertension. It is also used as a diagnostic tool to test acute vasoreactivity in patients with pulmonary hypertension of various aetiologies, and is being studied in a variety of other bronchopulmonary disorders and in different age groups.

In the management of hypoxic respiratory failure in neonates, nitric oxide is given by inhalation in a usual concentration of 20 ppm. Doses have been titrated above and below this concentration but due to the risk of methaemoglobinaemia, doses above 20 ppm are not generally recommended. The concentration should be reduced gradually before discontinuing nitric oxide treatment.

◊ General reviews.


1. Hart CM. Nitric oxide in adult lung disease. *Chest* 1999; **115:** 1407–17.
2. Vallance P, Chan N. Endothelial function and nitric oxide: clinical relevance. *Heart* 2001; **85:** 342–50.


◊ Inhaled nitric oxide is a potent and highly selective pulmonary vasodilator used in the management of persistent pulmonary hypertension of the newborn (below) and other conditions leading to hypoxic respiratory failure in neonates.

Nitric oxide is also under investigation in children and adults with acute respiratory distress syndrome (below), respiratory failure,[1] acute severe asthma,[2] primary pulmonary hypertension[3,4] including that in pregnancy,[5,6] and in pulmonary hypertension associated with a wide range of conditions including chronic obstructive pulmonary disease,[7] heart failure,[8] post-cardiac surgery,[9,10] and high-altitude disorders.[11] Nitric oxide is also being investigated[12] in sickle-cell crisis.


1. Dobyns EL, *et al.* Multicenter randomized controlled trial of the effects of inhaled nitric oxide therapy on gas exchange in children with acute hypoxemic respiratory failure. *J Pediatr* 1999; **134:** 406–12.
2. Nakagawa TA, *et al.* Life-threatening status asthmaticus treated with inhaled nitric oxide. *J Pediatr* 2000; **137:** 119–22.
3. Kinsella JP, *et al.* Selective and sustained pulmonary vasodilation with inhalational nitric oxide therapy in a child with idiopathic pulmonary hypertension. *J Pediatr* 1993; **122:** 803–6.
4. Goldman AP, *et al.* Is it time to consider domiciliary nitric oxide? *Lancet* 1995; **345:** 199–200.
5. Lam GK, *et al.* Inhaled nitric oxide for primary pulmonary hypertension in pregnancy. *Obstet Gynecol* 2001; **98:** 895–8.
6. Decoene C, *et al.* Use of inhaled nitric oxide for emergency Cesarean section in a woman with unexpected primary pulmonary hypertension. *Can J Anaesth* 2001; **48:** 584–7.
7. Vonbank K, *et al.* Controlled prospective randomised trial on the effects on pulmonary haemodynamics of the ambulatory long term use of nitric oxide and oxygen in patients with severe COPD. *Thorax* 2003; **58:** 289–93.
8. Matsumoto A, *et al.* Inhaled nitric oxide and exercise capacity in congestive heart failure. *Lancet* 1997; **349:** 999–1000. Correction. *ibid.*; **350:** 818.
9. Haydar A, *et al.* Inhaled nitric oxide for postoperative pulmonary hypertension in patients with congenital heart defects. *Lancet* 1992; **340:** 1545.
10. Miller OI, *et al.* Inhaled nitric oxide and prevention of pulmonary hypertension after congenital heart surgery: a randomised double-blind study. *Lancet* 2000; **356:** 1464–9.
11. Scherrer U, *et al.* Inhaled nitric oxide for high-altitude pulmonary edema. *N Engl J Med* 1996; **334:** 624–9.
12. Weiner DL, *et al.* Preliminary assessment of inhaled nitric oxide for acute vaso-occlusive crisis in pediatric patients with sickle cell disease. *JAMA* 2003; **289:** 1136–42.


**Acute respiratory distress syndrome.** Although inhalation of nitric oxide has been reported to improve oxygenation in patients with acute respiratory distress syndrome (p.1075), a meta-analysis[1] of its use in acute hypoxaemic respiratory failure (which included patients with acute respiratory distress syndrome) concluded that, while it may be useful in the short term, it appears to have no significant effect on mortality. However, other clinically relevant end-points could not be assessed because there was insufficient data. A further study[2] in patients with acute respiratory distress syndrome confirmed that nitric oxide improved oxygenation but had no substantial effect on duration of ventilation or on mortality.


1. Sokol J, *et al.* Inhaled nitric oxide for acute hypoxemic respiratory failure in children and adults. Available in The Cochrane Library; Issue 1. Chichester: John Wiley; 2004.
2. Taylor RW, *et al.* Low-dose inhaled nitric oxide in patients with acute lung injury: a randomized controlled trial. *JAMA* 2004; **291:** 1603–9.


**Respiratory disorders in neonates.** Inhaled nitric oxide is used in the management of hypoxic respiratory failure in term and near term neonates.[1-3] It has also been studied in premature neonates.

Most studies have been in neonates with persistent pulmonary hypertension of the newborn (p.832), although varying definitions have been used. A systematic review[4] of controlled studies in term and near-term neonates with hypoxic respiratory failure found that oxygenation was improved with inhaled nitric oxide, with a reduction in the need for extracorporeal membrane oxygenation, but no effect on mortality has been shown. Neonates with congenital diaphragmatic hernia, however, have not been shown to benefit,[5,6] and nitric oxide is not recommended in such patients.[4] Another study[7] suggested that the improvement in oxygenation may not be sustained, and that neonates with pulmonary hypoplasia and dysplasia are less sensitive to nitric oxide.

The dose of nitric oxide found to be effective in most studies has been from 20 to 80 ppm. However, since nitric oxide is associated with dose-related toxicity, lower doses (1 to 2 ppm) have also been studied. One study[8] found no significant difference between high and low doses, but another study[9] found that low doses did not improve oxygenation and diminished the response to subsequent higher doses.

Inhaled nitric oxide has also been reported to improve oxygenation in premature neonates with hypoxic respiratory failure. However, a systematic review[10] found insufficient evidence to support the use of nitric oxide in such infants, although there was possibly a reduction in the severity of chronic lung disease. A subsequent study[11] in premature infants with respiratory distress syndrome suggested that the incidence of chronic lung disease and death was reduced by nitric oxide. An open study[12] in very premature infants who had already developed chronic lung disease also found an improvement in oxygenation with nitric oxide therapy. There have been concerns that use of inhaled nitric oxide might adversely affect neurodevelopmental outcome more than conventional therapy, but this has not been confirmed in infants followed up for up to 2 years.[13,14] However, one study[15] has reported poor neurodevelopmental outcome in premature neonates who received nitric oxide treatment.


1. American Academy of Pediatrics Committee on Fetus and Newborn. Use of inhaled nitric oxide. *Pediatrics* 2000; **106:** 344–5.
2. Kinsella JP, Abman SH. Clinical approach to inhaled nitric oxide therapy in the newborn with hypoxemia. *J Pediatr* 2000; **136:** 717–26.
3. Hoehn T, Krause MF. Response to inhaled nitric oxide in premature and term neonates. *Drugs* 2001; **61:** 27–39.
4. Finer NN, Barrington KJ. Nitric oxide for respiratory failure in infants born at or near term. Available in The Cochrane Library; Issue 1. Chichester: John Wiley; 2004
5. Clark RH, *et al.* Low-dose nitric oxide therapy for persistent pulmonary hypertension of the newborn. *N Engl J Med* 2000; **342:** 469–74.
6. The Neonatal Inhaled Nitric Oxide Study Group. Inhaled nitric oxide and hypoxic respiratory failure in infants with congenital diaphragmatic hernia. *Pediatrics* 1997; **99:** 838–45.
7. Goldman AP, *et al.* Four patterns of response to inhaled nitric oxide for persistent pulmonary hypertension of the newborn. *Pediatrics* 1996; **98:** 706–13.
8. Finer NN, *et al.* Randomized, prospective study of low-dose versus high-dose inhaled nitric oxide in the neonate with hypoxic respiratory failure. *Pediatrics* 2001; **108:** 949–55.
9. Cornfield DN, *et al.* Randomized, controlled trial of low-dose inhaled nitric oxide in the treatment of term and near-term infants with respiratory failure and pulmonary hypertension. *Pediatrics* 1999; **104:** 1089–94.
10. Barrington KJ, Finer NN. Inhaled nitric oxide for respiratory failure in preterm infants. Available in The Cochrane Library; Issue 1. Chichester: John Wiley; 2004
11. Schreiber MD, *et al.* Inhaled nitric oxide in premature infants with the respiratory distress syndrome. *N Engl J Med* 2003; **349:** 2099–2107.
12. Clark PL, *et al.* Safety and efficacy of nitric oxide in chronic lung disease. *Arch Dis Child Fetal Neonatal Ed* 2002; **86:** F41–5.
13. Rosenberg AA, *et al.* Longitudinal follow-up of a cohort of newborn infants treated with inhaled nitric oxide for persistent pulmonary hypertension. *J Pediatr* 1997; **131:** 70–5.
14. The Neonatal Inhaled Nitric Oxide Study Group. Inhaled nitric oxide in term and near-term infants: neurodevelopmental follow-up of the Neonatal Inhaled Nitric Oxide Study Group (NINOS). *J Pediatr* 2000; **136:** 611–17.
15. Cheung P-Y, *et al.* The outcome of very low birth weight neonates (≤1500g) rescued by inhaled nitric oxide: neurodevelopment in early childhood. *J Pediatr* 1998; **133:** 735–9.


## Preparations

**Proprietary Preparations** (details are given in Part 3)
***Denm.:*** INOmax; ***Spain:*** INOmax; ***USA:*** INOmax.

# Noradrenaline *(BAN)*

Norepinephrine *(BAN, rINN)*; Norepinefrina; Norepirenamine. *(R)*-2-Amino-1-(3,4-dihydroxyphenyl)ethanol.

$C_8H_{11}NO_3$ = 169.2.

*CAS — 51-41-2.*

*ATC — C01CA03.*

**Pharmacopoeias.** *Jpn* includes the racemic form.

## Noradrenaline Acid Tartrate *(BANM)*

Norepinephrine Bitartrate *(USAN, rINNM)*; Arterenol Acid Tartrate; *l*-Arterenol Bitartrate; Bitartrato de norepinefrina; Levarterenol Acid Tartrate; Levarterenol Bitartrate; Levarterenoli

Bitartras; Noradrenaline Bitartrate; Noradrenaline Tartrate; Noradrenalini Tartras; Norepinephrine Acid Tartrate *(BANM)*; *l*-Norepinephrine Bitartrate.

$C_8H_{11}NO_3,C_4H_6O_6,H_2O = 337.3.$

*CAS — 51-40-1 (anhydrous noradrenaline acid tartrate); 69815-49-2 (noradrenaline acid tartrate monohydrate).*

*ATC — C01CA03.*

**Pharmacopoeias.** In *Chin., Eur.* (see p.vi), *Pol.,* and *US.*

**Ph. Eur. 5.0** (Noradrenaline Tartrate; Noradrenaline Acid Tartrate BP 2003; Norepinephrine Acid Tartrate BP 2003). A white or almost white crystalline powder. Freely soluble in water; slightly soluble in alcohol. Store in airtight containers, or preferably, in a sealed tube under vacuum or an inert gas. Protect from light.

**USP 27** (Norepinephrine Bitartrate). A white or faintly grey, odourless, crystalline powder. It slowly darkens on exposure to air and light. Soluble 1 in 2.5 of water and 1 in 300 of alcohol; practically insoluble in chloroform and in ether. Its solutions in water have a pH of about 3.5. Store in airtight containers at a temperature of 25°, excursions permitted between 15° and 30°. Protect from light.

**Incompatibility.** Noradrenaline acid tartrate is strongly acidic in solution, and would be expected to be incompatible with drugs having an alkaline pH. The manufacturers in the UK state that solutions are reportedly incompatible with alkalis and oxidising agents, barbiturates, chlorphenamine, chlorothiazide, nitrofurantoin, novobiocin, phenytoin, sodium bicarbonate, sodium iodide, and streptomycin. Incompatibility with insulin has also been reported.[1]

1. Yamashita SK, *et al.* Compatibility of selected critical care drugs during simulated Y-site administration. *Am J Health-Syst Pharm* 1996; **53:** 1048–51.

## Noradrenaline Hydrochloride *(BANM)*

Norepinephrine Hydrochloride *(BANM, rINNM)*; Hidrocloruro de norepinefrina; Noradrenalini Hydrochloridum.

$C_8H_{11}NO_3,HCl = 205.6.$

*CAS — 329-56-6.*

*ATC — C01CA03.*

**Pharmacopoeias.** In *Eur.* (see p.vi).

**Ph. Eur. 5.0** (Noradrenaline Hydrochloride; Norepinephrine Hydrochloride BP 2003). A white or brownish-white, crystalline powder. It becomes coloured on exposure to air and light. Very soluble in water; slightly soluble in alcohol. A 2% solution in water has a pH of 3.5 to 4.5. Store in airtight containers, or preferably, in a sealed tube under vacuum or an inert gas. Protect from light.

### Adverse Effects

Noradrenaline is an extremely potent peripheral vasoconstrictor and its potential adverse effects include hypertension (possibly associated with reflex bradycardia), headache, and peripheral ischaemia, which may be severe enough to result in gangrene of the extremities.

Noradrenaline is a severe tissue irritant and only very dilute solutions should be injected. The needle must be inserted well into the vein to avoid extravasation, otherwise severe phlebitis and sloughing may occur.

For the adverse effects of sympathomimetics in general, see Adrenaline, p.852.

◊ There has been a report[1] of severe headache, including a fatal cerebral haemorrhage, in dental patients who had received injections of lidocaine 2% with noradrenaline 1 in 25 000. It was suggested that a concentration of noradrenaline 1 in 25 000 was too high and could not be justified and that a concentration of 1 in 80 000 was to be preferred. However, in the UK the *Dental Practitioners' Formulary* states that noradrenaline should not be used as a vasoconstrictor in local anaesthetic solutions since it presents no advantages over adrenaline and carries additional hazard.

1. Boakes AJ, *et al.* Adverse reactions to local anaesthetic/vasoconstrictor preparations: a study of the cardiovascular responses to Xylestesin and Hostacain-with-Noradrenaline. *Br Dent J* 1972; **133:** 137–40.

### Treatment of Adverse Effects

The hypertensive effects of noradrenaline may be treated with an alpha blocker such as phentolamine. If extravasation occurs, infiltration with phentolamine (see p.982) as soon as possible, and certainly within 12 hours, may relieve pain and prevent tissue necrosis.

### Precautions

Noradrenaline must be avoided in the presence of hypertension and blood pressure and infusion rate must be monitored frequently. Noradrenaline-induced cardiac arrhythmias are more likely in patients with hypoxia or hypercapnia. Hypovolaemia should be corrected before starting noradrenaline infusion.

Noradrenaline may reduce placental perfusion throughout pregnancy and some consider that it and similar vasoconstrictor sympathomimetics are best avoided; also in late pregnancy noradrenaline provokes uterine contractions which can result in fetal asphyxia.

For the precautions to be observed with sympathomimetics in general, see Adrenaline, p.853.

### Interactions

For the interactions of the sympathomimetics in general, see Adrenaline, p.853.

### Pharmacokinetics

Like adrenaline (p.854), noradrenaline is inactive when given by mouth, and it is rapidly inactivated in the body by similar processes. When given intravenously it is extensively metabolised and only small amounts are excreted unchanged in the urine.

### Uses and Administration

The catecholamine, noradrenaline, is a direct-acting sympathomimetic (see Adrenaline, p.854) with pronounced effects on alpha-adrenergic receptors and less marked effects on beta-adrenergic receptors. It is a neurotransmitter, stored in granules in nerve axons, which is released at the terminations of post ganglionic adrenergic nerve fibres when they are stimulated; some is also present in the adrenal medulla from which it is liberated together with adrenaline. A major effect of noradrenaline is to raise systolic and diastolic blood pressure, which is accompanied by reflex slowing of the heart rate. This is a result of its alpha-stimulant effects which cause vasoconstriction, with reduced blood flow in the kidneys, liver, skin, and usually skeletal muscle. Noradrenaline causes the pregnant uterus to contract; high doses liberate glucose from the liver and have other hormonal effects similar to those of adrenaline. It produces little stimulation of the CNS. Beta-stimulant effects of noradrenaline have a positive inotropic action on the heart, but there is little bronchodilator effect.

Noradrenaline is used for the emergency restoration of blood pressure in acute hypotensive states such as shock (p.835). It has also been used in the management of cardiac arrest. Noradrenaline has been used in local anaesthesia to diminish the absorption and localise the effect of the local anaesthetic (p.1369) but adrenaline is now preferred (see also under Adverse Effects, above). Locally applied solutions have been used to control bleeding in upper gastrointestinal haemorrhage and similar disorders.

In **acute hypotensive states**, noradrenaline is used as the acid tartrate, or occasionally as the hydrochloride, but doses are expressed in terms of the base; noradrenaline acid tartrate 2 micrograms or noradrenaline hydrochloride 1.2 micrograms are approximately equivalent to 1 microgram of noradrenaline. It is given by intravenous infusion of a solution containing the equivalent of 4 micrograms of the base per mL in glucose 5%, or sodium chloride 0.9% and glucose 5%. To avoid tissue necrosis the infusion should be given through a central venous catheter or into a large vein high up in a limb, preferably the arm. Some sources have suggested that addition of phentolamine 5 to 10 mg/litre to the infusion may prevent sloughing, should extravasation occur, without affecting the vasopressor action. The infusion is usually given initially at a rate of 2 to 3 mL/minute (8 to 12 micrograms/minute) and adjusted according to the blood pressure response. Blood pressure is initially recorded every 2 minutes and the rate of infusion continuously monitored. The infusion must not be stopped suddenly but should be gradually withdrawn to avoid disastrous falls in blood pressure. The average maintenance dose is 0.5 to 1 mL/minute (2 to 4 micrograms/minute), but there is a wide variation and higher doses may be required. The concentration of the infusion may be altered according to clinical needs. Alternatively a solution containing the equivalent of 40 micrograms of the base per mL may be given at an initial rate of 0.16 to 0.33 mL/minute via a central venous catheter, using a syringe pump or drip counter.

### Preparations

***BP 2003:*** Noradrenaline Injection;

***USP 27:*** Norepinephrine Bitartrate Injection; Propoxycaine and Procaine Hydrochlorides and Norepinephrine Bitartrate Injection.

**Proprietary Preparations** (details are given in Part 3)

***Arg.:*** Fioritina; ***Austral.:*** Levophed; ***Belg.:*** Levophed; Norepine; ***Braz.:*** Levophed; ***Canad.:*** Levophed; ***Ger.:*** Arterenol; ***Gr.:*** Levophed; ***Hong Kong:*** Levophed; ***India:*** Adrenor; ***Irl.:*** Levophed; ***Israel:*** Levophed; ***Malaysia:*** Levophed; ***Mex.:*** Naprina†; Pridam; ***NZ:*** Levophed; ***Singapore:*** Levophed; ***Spain:*** Adrenor†; ***UK:*** Levophed†; ***USA:*** Levophed.

*Used as an adjunct in:* ***Austral.:*** Nurocain with Sympathin†; ***Austria:*** Neo-Xylestesin forte and Neo-Xylestesin special; Scandonest; ***Braz.:*** Scandinor†; Xylestesin; Xylocaina; ***Ger.:*** Anaesthol†; Meaverin "N" mit Noradrenaline†; Neo-Lidocaton†; Nor-Anaesthol†; Xylestesin-S; Xylestesin, Xylestesin-F; ***Ital.:*** Lident Andrenor; Xylonor; ***Port.:*** Xilonibsa; ***S.Afr.:*** Xylotox; ***Spain:*** Llorentecaina Noradrenal†; Stoma Anestesia Dental†; Xylonor Especial; ***Switz.:*** Scandonest; Xylestesin-F; Xylestesin-S "special"; Xylonor†; ***Thai.:*** Neo-Lidocaton; ***USA:*** Ravocaine and Novocain†.

## Norfenefrine Hydrochloride *(rINNM)*

Hidrocloruro de norfenefrina; Norphenylephrine Hydrochloride; *m*-Norsynephrine Hydrochloride; WV-569. 2-Amino-1-(3-hydroxyphenyl)ethanol hydrochloride.

$C_8H_{11}NO_2,HCl = 189.6.$

*CAS — 536-21-0 (norfenefrine); 15308-34-6 (norfenefrine hydrochloride).*

*ATC — C01CA05.*

NOTE. *m*-Octopamine has been used as a synonym for norfenefrine. Care should be taken to avoid confusion with *p*-octopamine, which is octopamine.

### Profile

Norfenefrine is a sympathomimetic (see Adrenaline, p.852) with predominantly alpha-adrenergic activity. It is used as the hydrochloride for its vasopressor effect in the treatment of hypotensive states (p.828). The usual dose is 15 mg three times daily by mouth, as a modified-release preparation, but doses of up to 45 mg three times daily have been given. Norfenefrine hydrochloride has also been given by injection.

### Preparations

**Proprietary Preparations** (details are given in Part 3)

***Austria:*** Novadral; ***Ger.:*** Energona†; Novadral; ***Mex.:*** AS Cor; ***Switz.:*** Novadral.

**Multi-ingredient:** ***Ger.:*** Adyston; Normotin-R; Ordinal Forte; ***Switz.:*** Ortho-Maren retard.

## Octodrine *(USAN, rINN)*

Octodrina; SKF-51. 1,5-Dimethylhexylamine.

$C_8H_{19}N = 129.2.$

*CAS — 543-82-8.*

### Profile

Octodrine is a sympathomimetic (see Adrenaline, p.852) with predominantly alpha-adrenergic activity. It is given by mouth as the camsilate, in combination with norfenefrine (p.975), in the treatment of hypotensive states. Octodrine phosphate has been used as an ingredient of preparations for obstructive airways disease.

### Preparations

**Proprietary Preparations** (details are given in Part 3)

**Multi-ingredient:** ***Austria:*** Ambredin; ***Ger.:*** Ordinal Forte.

## Olmesartan Medoxomil *(BAN, USAN, rINN)*

CS-866 (olmesartan medoxomil); RNH-6270 (olmesartan). (5-Methyl-2-oxo-1,3-dioxol-4-yl) methyl ester of 4-(1-Hydroxy-1-methylethyl)-2-propyl-1-{[2′-(1*H*-tetrazol-5-yl)[1,1′-biphenyl]-4-yl]methyl}-1*H*-imidazole-5-carboxylic acid.

$C_{29}H_{30}N_6O_6 = 558.6.$

*CAS — 144689-24-7 (olmesartan); 144689-63-4 (olmesartan medoxomil).*

NOTE. The name olmesartan has been applied to both the base and to the medoxomil ester.

### Adverse Effects and Precautions

As for Losartan Potassium, p.947.

### Interactions

As for Losartan Potassium, p.948.

### Pharmacokinetics

Olmesartan medoxomil is an ester prodrug that is hydrolysed during absorption from the gastrointestinal tract to the active form olmesartan. The absolute bioavailability is approximately 26%. Peak plasma concentrations of olmesartan occur about 1 to 2 hours after oral administration. Olmesartan is at least 99% bound to plasma proteins. It is excreted in the urine and the bile as olmesartan; about 35 to 50% of the absorbed dose is excreted in the urine and the remainder in the bile. The terminal elimination half-life is between 10 and 15 hours.

### Uses and Administration

Olmesartan is an angiotensin II receptor antagonist with actions similar to those of losartan (p.948). It is used in the management of hypertension (p.825).

Olmesartan is given by mouth as the ester prodrug olmesartan medoxomil. After an oral dose the hypotensive effect lasts for 24 hours. Most of the hypotensive effect is apparent within 2 weeks after initiating therapy and is maximal within about 8 weeks.

In hypertension, olmesartan medoxomil is given in a usual dose of 20 mg once daily, although in the UK an initial dose of 10 mg once daily is recommended. The dose may be increased to 40 mg once daily if required. In the UK, a maximum dose of 20 mg once daily is recommended for elderly patients and patients with renal impairment (see below).

◊ References.

1. Brunner HR. The new oral angiotensin II antagonist olmesartan medoxomil: a concise overview. *J Hum Hypertens* 2002; **16** (suppl 2): S13–S16.
2. Warner GT, Jarvis B. Olmesartan medoxomil. *Drugs* 2002; **62:** 1345–53. Correction. *ibid.*; 1852.
3. Gardner SF, Franks AM. Olmesartan medoxomil: the seventh angiotensin receptor antagonist. *Ann Pharmacother* 2003; **37:** 99–105.

**Administration in hepatic or renal impairment.** Olmesartan is excreted in both urine and bile and raised plasma concentrations have been noted in patients with renal or hepatic impairment. In the UK, olmesartan is contra-indicated in patients with hepatic impairment or with severe renal impairment and a maximum dose of 20 mg once daily is recommended in mild to moderate renal impairment (creatinine clearance 20 to 60 mL/minute).

### Preparations

**Proprietary Preparations** (details are given in Part 3)
***UK:*** Olmetec; ***USA:*** Benicar.
**Multi-ingredient:** ***USA:*** Benicar HCT.

---

## Olprinone Hydrochloride *(rINNM)*

Hidrocloruro de olprinona. 1,2-Dihydro-5-imidazo[1,2-*a*]pyridin-6-yl-6-methyl-2-oxonicotinonitrile hydrochloride.

$C_{14}H_{10}N_4O,HCl$ = 286.7.

*CAS — 106730-54-5 (olprinone); 119615-63-3 (olprinone hydrochloride).*

### Profile

Olprinone is a phosphodiesterase inhibitor with positive inotropic and vasodilator activity, used in acute heart failure (p.820). It is administered intravenously as the hydrochloride in an initial dose of 10 micrograms/kg given over 5 minutes, followed by a continuous infusion at a rate of 0.1 to 0.4 micrograms/kg per minute, according to response.

### Preparations

**Proprietary Preparations** (details are given in Part 3)
***Jpn:*** Coretec.

---

## Omapatrilat *(BAN, USAN, rINN)*

BMS-186716; BMS-186716-01; Omapatrilato. (4*S*,7*S*,10a*S*)-Octahydro-4-[(*S*)-α-mercaptohydrocinnamamido]-5-oxo-7*H*-pyrido[2,1-*b*][1,3]thiazepine-7-carboxylic acid.

$C_{19}H_{24}N_2O_4S_2$ = 408.5.

*CAS — 167305-00-2.*

### Profile

Omapatrilat is a vasopeptidase inhibitor. It inhibits both angiotensin-converting enzyme and neutral endopeptidase and is under investigation in the management of hypertension and heart failure. However, its use may be limited by severe angioedema.

◊ References.

1. Messerli FH, Nussberger J. Vasopeptidase inhibition and angiooedema. *Lancet* 2000; **356:** 608–9.
2. Rouleau JL, *et al.* Comparison of vasopeptidase inhibitor, omapatrilat, and lisinopril on exercise tolerance and morbidity in patients with heart failure: IMPRESS randomised trial. *Lancet* 2000; **356:** 615–20. Correction. *ibid.*; 1774.
3. Packer M, *et al.* Comparison of omapatrilat and enalapril in patients with chronic heart failure: the Omapatrilat Versus Enalapril Randomized Trial of Utility in Reducing Events (OVERTURE). *Circulation* 2002; **106:** 920–6.
4. Kostis JB, *et al.* Omapatrilat and enalapril in patients with hypertension: the Omapatrilat Cardiovascular Treatment vs. Enalapril (OCTAVE) trial. *Am J Hypertens* 2004; **17:** 103–11.

---

# Omega-3 Triglycerides

Ácidos grasos omega 3.

*ATC — C10AX06.*

## Docosahexaenoic Acid

DHA; Doconexent; Doconexento. Docosahexa-4,7,10,13,16,19-enoic acid.

$C_{22}H_{32}O_2$ = 328.5.

*CAS — 6217-54-5; 25167-62-8.*

NOTE. DHA is also used as a synonym for dihydroxyacetone.

## Eicosapentaenoic Acid

EPA; Icosapent; Icosapento. Eicosapenta-5,8,11,14,17-enoic acid.

$C_{20}H_{30}O_2$ = 302.5.

*CAS — 10417-94-4; 25378-27-2.*

NOTE. EPA is also used as a synonym for pheneturide.

## Omega-3 Acid Ethyl Esters

K-85; Omega-3 Acidorum Esteri Ethylici; Omega-3-acid Ethyl Esters *(USAN)*.

$C_{24}H_{36}O_2$; $C_{22}H_{34}O_2$.

*CAS — 81926-94-5 (docosahexaenoic acid ethyl ester); 86227-47-6 (eicosapentaenoic acid ethyl ester).*

**Pharmacopoeias.** In *Eur.* (see p.vi).

**Ph. Eur. 5.0** (Omega-3-Acid Ethyl Esters 60). A mixture of ethyl esters of omega-3 acids. They are obtained by transesterification of the body oil of fat fish species coming from families such as Engraulidae, Carangidae, Clupeidae, Osmeridae, Salmonidae, and Scombridae. The acids consist of alpha-linolenic acid, moroctic acid, eicosatetraenoic acid, eicosapentaenoic acid (timnodonic acid), heneicosapentaenoic acid, clupanodonic acid, and docosahexaenoic acid (cervonic acid). The total amount of omega-3 acid ethyl esters, eicosapentaenoic acid ethyl esters, and docosahexaenoic acid ethyl esters should be stated on the label. For a total omega-3 acid ethyl ester content of 55%, the amount of eicosapentaenoic acid ethyl esters and docosahexaenoic acid ethyl esters together is not less than 50% and the content of eicosapentaenoic acid ethyl esters is not less than 40%; for a total omega-3 acid ethyl ester content of 60%, the amount of eicosapentaenoic acid ethyl esters and docosahexaenoic acid ethyl esters together is not less than 50% and the content of docosahexaenoic acid ethyl esters is not less than 40%; and for a total omega-3 acid ethyl ester content of 65%, the amount of eicosapentaenoic acid ethyl esters and docosahexaenoic acid ethyl esters together is not less than 50%, the content of eicosapentaenoic acid ethyl esters is not less than 25%, and the content of docosahexaenoic acid ethyl esters is not less than 20%. Tocopherol may be added as an antoxidant.

A light yellow liquid with a slight fish-like odour. Practically insoluble in water; very soluble in acetone, in dehydrated alcohol, in heptane, and in methyl alcohol. Store in airtight containers under inert gas. Protect from light.

**Ph. Eur. 5.0** (Omega-3-Acid Ethyl Esters 90). A mixture of ethyl esters of omega-3 acids. They are obtained by transesterification of the body oil of fat fish species coming from families such as Engraulidae, Carangidae, Clupeidae, Osmeridae, Salmonidae, and Scombridae. The acids consist of alpha-linolenic acid, moroctic acid, eicosatetraenoic acid, eicosapentaenoic acid (timnodonic acid), heneicosapentaenoic acid, clupanodonic acid, and docosahexaenoic acid (cervonic acid). The total amount of omega-3 acid ethyl esters is not less than 90%, and that of both eicosapentaenoic acid ethyl esters and docosahexaenoic acid ethyl esters together is 80%; the content of eicosapentaenoic acid ethyl esters is not less than 40% and of docosahexaenoic acid ethyl esters is not less than 34%. Tocopherol may be added as an antoxidant.

A light yellow liquid with a slight fish-like odour. Practically insoluble in water; very soluble in acetone, in dehydrated alcohol, in heptane, and in methyl alcohol. Store in airtight containers under inert gas. Protect from light.

## Omega-3 Marine Triglycerides *(BAN)*

Triglicéridos marinos omega 3.

**Pharmacopoeias.** In *Eur.* (see p.vi) as Omega-3-Acid Triglycerides and Fish Oil, Rich in Omega-3-Acids. *Eur.* also includes Salmon Oil, Farmed.

**Ph. Eur. 5.0** (Omega-3-Acid Triglycerides; Omega-3 Acidorum Triglycerida). A mixture of mono-, di-, and triesters of omega-3 acids with glycerol, containing mainly triesters. They are obtained by esterification of concentrated and purified omega-3 acids with glycerol or by transesterification of the omega-3 acid ethyl esters with glycerol. The omega-3 acids are from the body oil of fatty fish species coming from families such as Engraulidae, Carangidae, Clupeidae, Osmeridae, Salmonidae, and Scombridae. The acids consist of alpha-linolenic acid, moroctic acid, eicosatetraenoic acid, eicosapentaenoic acid (timnodonic acid), heneicosapentaenoic acid, clupanodonic acid, and docosahexaenoic acid (cervonic acid). The total amount of omega-3 acids expressed as triglycerides is not less than 60% and that of both eicosapentaenoic acid and docosahexaenoic acid together, expressed as triglycerides, is not less than 45%. Tocopherol may be added as an antoxidant.

A pale yellow liquid. Practically insoluble in water; slightly soluble in dehydrated alcohol; very soluble in acetone and in heptane. Store in well-filled, airtight containers under inert gas. Protect from light.

**Ph. Eur. 5.0** (Fish Oil, Rich in Omega-3-Acids; Piscis Oleum Omega-3 Acidis Abundans). The purified, winterised, and deodorised fatty oil obtained from fish of the families Engraulidae, Carangidae, Clupeidae, Osmeridae, Scombridae, and Ammodytidae. The acids consist of alpha-linolenic acid, moroctic acid, eicosatetraenoic acid, eicosapentaenoic acid (timnodonic acid), heneicosapentaenoic acid, clupanodonic acid, and docosahexaenoic acid (cervonic acid). The minimum content, expressed as triglycerides, is eicosapentaenoic acid 13%, docosahexaenoic acid 9%, and total omega-3 acids 28%. Antoxidants may be added.

A pale yellow liquid. Practically insoluble in water; slightly soluble in dehydrated alcohol; very soluble in acetone and in heptane. Store in well-filled, airtight containers under inert gas. Protect from light.

**Ph. Eur. 5.0** (Salmon Oil, Farmed; Salmonis Domestici Oleum). The purified fatty oil obtained from fresh farmed *Salmo salar.* It contains 60 to 70% of docosahexaenoic acid (cervonic acid), 25 to 35% of eicosapentaenoic acid (timnodonic acid), and 40 to 55% of moroctic acid. The sum of eicosapentaenoic acid and docosahexaenoic acid, expressed as triglycerides, is 10.0 to 28.0%. Authorised antoxidants may be added. A pale pink liquid. Practically insoluble in water; slightly soluble in dehydrated alcohol; very soluble in acetone and in heptane. Store in well-filled airtight containers under an inert gas. Protect from light.

### Adverse Effects and Precautions

The most common adverse effects of omega-3 marine triglycerides and similar preparations are gastrointestinal disturbances, particularly at high doses, including nausea, eructation, vomiting, abdominal distension, diarrhoea, and constipation. There have been rare reports of acne and eczema. Moderate increases in hepatic transaminases have been reported in patients with hypertriglyceridaemia.

Preparations vary widely in concentration and purity. Some preparations contain significant amounts of vitamins A and D and long-term use could cause toxicity. There is a theoretical possibility of vitamin E deficiency with long-term use, although many preparations contain vitamin E as an antoxidant. Concern has been expressed over the high calorific value and cholesterol content of some preparations.

Omega-3 triglycerides have antithrombotic activity and should be given with caution to patients with haemorrhagic disorders or to those receiving anticoagulants or other drugs affecting coagulation. Hepatic function should be monitored in patients with hepatic impairment, particularly if receiving high doses. Caution may also be required in asthmatic patients sensitive to aspirin.

**Effects on the blood.** Omega-3 triglycerides have antithrombotic effects and may increase bleeding. In a study[1] in adolescents with familial hypercholesterolaemia, epistaxis occurred in 8 of 11 patients treated with a fish oil supplement; prolonged bleeding time was noted in 3 patients. However, in a study[2] in patients undergoing coronary artery bypass surgery, and who were also receiving warfarin or aspirin, fish oil supplementation had no effect on bleeding episodes or bleeding time.

1. Clarke JTR, *et al.* Increased incidence of epistaxis in adolescents with familial hypercholesterolemia treated with fish oil. *J Pediatr* 1990; **116:** 139–41.
2. Eritsland J, *et al.* Long-term effects of n-3 polyunsaturated fatty acids on haemostatic variables and bleeding episodes in patients with coronary artery disease. *Blood Coag Fibrinol* 1995; **6:** 17–22.

**Effects on glucose metabolism.** Although a deterioration in glycaemic control has been reported in both type 1 and type 2 diabetic patients taking omega-3 marine triglycerides and fish oil preparations, a meta-analysis[1] of studies in type 1 and type 2 diabetics, and a systematic review[2] of controlled studies in type 2 diabetics, both concluded that fish oils effectively lowered triglycerides without a deleterious effect on glycaemic control.

1. Friedberg CE, *et al.* Fish oil and glycemic control in diabetes: a meta-analysis. *Diabetes Care* 1998; **21:** 494–500.
2. Farmer A, *et al.* Fish oil in people with type 2 diabetes mellitus. Available in The Cochrane Library; Issue 2. Chichester: John Wiley; 2004.

### Uses and Administration

The omega-3 marine triglycerides contain triglycerides of the omega-3 fatty acids, particularly eicosapentaenoic acid and docosahexaenoic acid. These long-chain n-3 polyunsaturated fatty acids are precursors of eicosanoids in *fish* and when taken by man they compete with the precursor arachidonic acid. Their actions in man include a hypolipidaemic action (especially a reduction in plasma triglycerides), an anti-inflammatory action, and an antiplatelet effect.

Fish oils are a source of omega-3 triglycerides and preparations such as omega-3 marine triglycerides are used in patients with severe hypertriglyceridaemia (see Hyperlipidaemias, p.823) and for secondary prevention in patients who have had a myocardial infarction (below). They are also marketed as dietary supplements, and have been used in preparations for parenteral nutrition.

A wide range of preparations are available, with varying eicosapentaenoic acid and docosahexaenoic acid contents. Typical doses of fish oil by mouth for the treatment of hypertriglyceridaemia are 5 g twice daily of a preparation containing 17% eicosapentaenoic acid and 11.5% docosahexaenoic acid, or 2 to 4 g daily of a preparation containing 46% eicosapentaenoic acid and 38% docosahexaenoic acid. For the secondary prevention of myocardial infarction, 1 g daily of a preparation of omega-3 acid ethyl esters containing 46% eicosapentaenoic acid and 38% docosahexaenoic acid may be given.

**Action.** Fish oils and other omega-3 fatty acid preparations have been widely promoted as dietary supplements and a wide range of preparations of varying composition and potency is available. The interest in marine fish oils arose following observations that populations with a diet rich in marine fish oils generally have a low incidence of cardiovascular disease. In addition the incidence of asthma, psoriasis, and auto-immune diseases has been reported to be lower among Eskimos (Inuit) than in populations consuming a typical western diet, although the incidence of haemorrhagic stroke and epilepsy may be higher.

The omega-3 fatty acids eicosapentaenoic acid and docosahexaenoic acid are long-chain n-3 polyunsaturated fatty acids, which compete with arachidonic acid for inclusion in cyclo-oxygenase and lipoxygenase pathways. Their antithrombotic activity is attributed to effects on prostanoid synthesis, which promote vasodilatation, a reduction in platelet aggregation, increased bleeding time and decreased platelet counts. Their anti-inflammatory activity is attributed to effects on leukotriene synthesis. Omega-3 fatty acids also have hypolipidaemic activity, primarily reducing triglyceride concentrations by reducing very-low-density lipoproteins (VLDL). Other effects reported include an increase in erythrocyte deformability and a decrease in blood viscosity. A reduction in blood pressure has been reported[1,2] in patients with essential hypertension (p.825), and also in a small study[3] in heart transplant patients (p.1345).

Omega-3 fatty acids have been tried in a number of inflammatory and auto-immune disorders. Beneficial effects have been reported in rheumatoid arthritis[4] (p.9). Some studies have shown benefit in psoriasis (p.1137), both with oral[5,6] and with intravenous administration,[7,8] but other studies found neither the oral[9] nor the topical[10] route to be effective. Beneficial responses have also been reported in inflammatory bowel disease (p.1243), including Crohn's disease[11] and ulcerative colitis,[12] and in glomerular kidney disease[13-15] (p.1080). Although some studies[16] have shown a reduction in acute rejection following renal transplantation (p.1346), other studies[17] have found a lack of effect. Fish oils have also been tried in lung disorders, although systematic reviews have found no evidence of benefit in asthma[18] and only a limited benefit in cystic fibrosis.[19]

Omega-3 fatty acids have also been tried in a number of psychiatric disorders.[20]


1. Appel LJ, *et al.* Does supplementation of diet with 'fish oil' reduce blood pressure? A meta-analysis of controlled clinical trials. *Arch Intern Med* 1993; **153:** 1429–38.
2. Morris MC, *et al.* Does fish oil lower blood pressure? A meta-analysis of controlled trials. *Circulation* 1993; **88:** 523–33.
3. Holm T, *et al.* Omega-3 fatty acids improve blood pressure control and preserve renal function in hypertensive heart transplant recipients. *Eur Heart J* 2001; **22:** 428–36.
4. Cleland LG, *et al.* The role of fish oils in the treatment of rheumatoid arthritis. *Drugs* 2003; **63:** 845–53.
5. Gupta AK, *et al.* Double-blind, placebo-controlled study to evaluate the efficacy of fish oil and low-dose UVB in the treatment of psoriasis. *Br J Dermatol* 1989; **120:** 801–7.
6. Lassus A, *et al.* Effects of dietary supplementation with polyunsaturated ethyl ester lipids (Angiosen) in patients with psoriasis and psoriatic arthritis. *J Int Med Res* 1990; **18:** 68–73.
7. Grimminger F, *et al.* A double-blind, randomized, placebo-controlled trial of n-3 fatty acid based lipid infusion in acute, extended guttate psoriasis: rapid improvement of clinical manifestations and changes in neutrophil leukotriene profile. *Clin Investig* 1993; **71:** 634–43.
8. Mayser P, *et al.* n-3 Fatty acids in psoriasis. *Br J Nutr* 2002; **87** (Suppl 1): S77–S82.
9. Søyland E, *et al.* Effect of dietary supplementation with very-long-chain n-3 fatty acids in patients with psoriasis. *N Engl J Med* 1993; **328:** 1812–16.
10. Henneicke-von Zepelin H-H, *et al.* Highly purified omega-3-polyunsaturated fatty acids for topical treatment of psoriasis: results of a double-blind, placebo-controlled multicentre study. *Br J Dermatol* 1993; **129:** 713–17.
11. Belluzzi A, *et al.* Effect of an enteric-coated fish-oil preparation on relapses in Crohn's disease. *N Engl J Med* 1996; **334:** 1557–60.
12. Salomon P, *et al.* Treatment of ulcerative colitis with fish oil n-3-ω-fatty acid: an open trial. *J Clin Gastroenterol* 1990; **12:** 157–61.
13. Donadio JV, *et al.* A controlled trial of fish oil in IgA nephropathy. *N Engl J Med* 1994; **331:** 1194–9.
14. Donadio JV, *et al.* The long-term outcome of patients with IgA nephropathy treated with fish oil in a controlled trial. *J Am Soc Nephrol* 1999; **10:** 1772–7.
15. Donadio JV, *et al.* A randomized trial of high-dose compared with low-dose omega-3 fatty acids in severe IgA nephropathy. *J Am Soc Nephrol* 2001; **12:** 791–9.
16. Homan van der Heide JJ, *et al.* Effect of dietary fish oil on renal function and rejection in cyclosporine-treated recipients of renal transplants. *N Engl J Med* 1993; **329:** 769–73.
17. Hernández D, *et al.* Dietary fish oil does not influence acute rejection rate and graft survival after renal transplantation: a randomized placebo-controlled study. *Nephrol Dial Transplant* 2002; **17:** 897–904.
18. Thien FCK, *et al.* Dietary marine fatty acids (fish oil) for asthma in adults and children. Available in The Cochrane Library; Issue 2. Chichester: John Wiley; 2004.
19. Beckles Willson N, *et al.* Omega-3 fatty acids (from fish oils) for cystic fibrosis. Available in The Cochrane Library; Issue 2. Chichester: John Wiley; 2004.
20. Freeman MP. Omega-3 fatty acids in psychiatry: a review. *Ann Clin Psychiatry* 2000; **12:** 159–65.


**Cardiovascular risk reduction.** Lipid lowering therapy has an important role in patients at risk of cardiovascular disease (p.819) and there is some evidence of benefit with omega-3 fatty acids in secondary prevention of ischaemic heart disease.[1-3] Following myocardial infarction, long-term use of omega-3 fatty acid supplements reduced the risk of fatal cardiovascular events in a large group of Italian patients studied for 3.5 years.[4] Supplements taken for 2 years in another smaller study[5] had a modest beneficial effect on progression of coronary atherosclerosis, assessed by angiography, compared with placebo. Some,[6,7] but not other[8] studies have shown a decrease in coronary vessel restenosis after angioplasty. However, in a large long-term cohort study increased dietary intake of omega-3 fatty acids, as fish consumption, did not substantially reduce the risk of ischaemic heart disease in men who had initially been free of known cardiovascular disease,[9] although the risk of ischaemic stroke was reduced.[10] Another study[11] in women also found a reduction in the incidence of ischaemic stroke.


1. Carroll DN, Roth MT. Evidence for the cardioprotective effects of omega-3 fatty acids. *Ann Pharmacother* 2002; **36:** 1950–6.
2. Kris-Etherton PM, *et al.* Fish consumption, fish oil, omega-3 fatty acids, and cardiovascular disease. *Circulation* 2002; **106:** 2747–57. Correction. *ibid.* 2003; **107:** 512.
3. Din JN, *et al.* Omega 3 fatty acids and cardiovascular disease—fishing for a natural treatment. *BMJ* 2004; **328:** 30–5.
4. GISSI-Prevenzione Investigators. Dietary supplementation with n-3 polyunsaturated fatty acids and vitamin E after myocardial infarction: results of the GISSI-Prevenzione trial. *Lancet* 1999; **354:** 447–55. Correction. *ibid.* 2001; **357:** 642.
5. von Schacky C, *et al.* The effect of dietary ω-3 fatty acids on coronary atherosclerosis: a randomized, double-blind, placebo-controlled trial. *Ann Intern Med* 1999; **130:** 554–62.
6. Dehmer GJ, *et al.* Reduction in the rate of early restenosis after coronary angioplasty by a diet supplemented with n-3 fatty acids. *N Engl J Med* 1988; **319:** 733–40.
7. Gapinski JP, *et al.* Preventing restenosis with fish oils following coronary angioplasty: a meta-analysis. *Arch Intern Med* 1993; **153:** 1595–1601.
8. Reis GJ, *et al.* Randomised trial of fish oil for prevention of restenosis after coronary angioplasty. *Lancet* 1989; **ii:** 177–81.
9. Ascherio A, *et al.* Dietary intake of marine n-3 fatty acids, fish intake, and the risk of coronary disease among men. *N Engl J Med* 1995; **332:** 977–82.
10. He K, *et al.* Fish consumption and risk of stroke in men. *JAMA* 2002; **288:** 3130–6.
11. Iso H, *et al.* Intake of fish and omega-3 fatty acids and risk of stroke in women. *JAMA* 2001; **285:** 304–12.


## Preparations

**Proprietary Preparations** (details are given in Part 3)
***Arg.:*** Regulip; ***Austral.:*** Ethical Nutrients Maxepa†; Fishaphos†; Maxepa†; Natures Own Maxepa†; Natures Way Omega 3†; ***Austria:*** Eicosapen; Omegaven; ***Braz.:*** Votag; ***Chile:*** Epasan 30% Omega 3; Neuromins; Sanepa Forte; ***Denm.:*** Omegaven; ***Fr.:*** Maxepa; Mega 65†; Omega 3+†; Omegaven; ***Ger.:*** Bilatin Fischol†; Eicosan; Eicosapen; Lipiscor; Omegaven; ***Hong Kong:*** Lipomega; Maxepa†; ***Ital.:*** Esapent; Eskim; Fish Factor; Maxepa; Omegaven; Seacor; Triglicen†; Triolip; Triomar; ***Norw.:*** Omacor; ***Port.:*** Omegaven; ***Swed.:*** Omegaven; ***Switz.:*** Ameu; Eicosapen; Epacaps; Omega-3; Omegaven; Omesan†; ***Thai.:*** Omacor; ***UK:*** Best EPA†; Flowmega†; Gamma EPA†; Marinepa†; Maxepa; Omacor; Pure Omega; Triomar†; ***USA:*** Cardi-Omega 3; Maxepa; Promega; SuperEPA.

**Multi-ingredient:** ***Arg.:*** Cholesterol Reducing Plan; ***Austral.:*** APR Cream; Arthriforte†; Bioglan Arthri Plus†; Bioglan Maxepa†; Bioglan Zellulean with Escin†; Efacal†; Efalex; Efamarine; Epo + Maxepa + Vitamin E Herbal Plus Formula 8†; ER Cream; Ethical Nutrients Antioxidant Fish Oil Garlic Plus†; Himega; Lifechange Circulation Aid†; Lifesystem Herbal Plus Formula 9 Fatty Acids And Vitamin E†; Macro Maxepa†; Maxepa & EPO†; Maxepa Plus†; Naudicelle Marine†; Pre Natal†; Vita-Preg†; ***Braz.:*** Lipcor; Lisacol; ***Canad.:*** Efalex; ***Chile:*** Acnoxyl Jabon; ***Fr.:*** Bio-Marine Plus; Bionagrol Plus; Dioptec; Elteans; Omegacoeur; Phytophanere; Synerbiol; ***Hong Kong:*** Biomega-3; Himega; ***India:*** Cadvion; Maxepa; ***Ital.:*** Agedin Plus; Derman-Oil; Dermana Pasta; Fotrec DHA; Gammaplus; Ictom 3; Memoactive; Trofinerv; Trofinerv Antiox; Venactive; ***Malaysia:*** Adult Citrex Multivitamin + Ginseng + Omega 3; ***NZ:*** Efacal; Efalex; Efamarine; Efamax; ***Singapore:*** VitaEPA; VitaEPA Plus; ***UK:*** Efacal†; Efalex; Efamarine; Efatime†; Epopa†; Galmarin†; Gamma Marine†; Naudicelle Forte†; Naudicelle Plus†; Naudicelle SL†; Super GammaOil Marine†; ***USA:*** Marine Lipid Concentrate; Sea-Omega.

## Orbofiban Acetate *(USAN, rINNM)*

Acetato de orbofibrán; CS-511; SC-57099-B. *N*-[[(3*S*)-1-(*p*-Amidinophenyl)-2-oxo-3-pyrrolidinyl]carbamoyl]-β-alanine ethyl ester monoacetate quadrantihydrate.

$C_{17}H_{23}N_5O_4,C_2H_4O_2,\frac{1}{4}H_2O = 426.0.$

*CAS — 163250-90-6 (orbofiban); 165800-05-5 (orbofiban acetate).*

### Profile

Orbofiban is a glycoprotein IIb/IIIa-receptor antagonist. It has been investigated as an oral antiplatelet drug in unstable angina and myocardial infarction but has been associated with an increase in mortality.

◊ References.


1. Cannon CP, *et al.* Oral glycoprotein IIb/IIIa inhibition with orbofiban in patients with unstable coronary syndromes (OPUS-TIMI 16) trial. *Circulation* 2000; **102:** 149–56.


## Ouabain

Acocantherin; G-Strophanthin; Ouabaína; Ouabainum; Strophanthin-G; Strophanthinum; Strophanthoside-G; Uabaina; Ubaína. 3β-(α-L-Rhamnopyranosyloxy)-1β,5,11α,14,19-pentahydroxy-5β,14β-card-20(22)-enolide octahydrate.

$C_{29}H_{44}O_{12},8H_2O = 728.8.$

*CAS — 630-60-4 (anhydrous ouabain); 11018-89-6 (ouabain octahydrate).*

*ATC — C01AC01.*

**Pharmacopoeias.** In *Eur.* (see p.vi) and *Viet.*

**Ph. Eur. 5.0** (Ouabain). Colourless crystals or white, crystalline powder. Sparingly soluble in water and in dehydrated alcohol; practically insoluble in ethyl acetate. Protect from light.

### Profile

Ouabain is a cardiac glycoside with positive inotropic activity that is obtained from the seeds of *Strophanthus gratus* or from the wood of *Acokanthera schimperi* or *A. ouabaio* (Apocynaceae). It has general properties similar to those of digoxin (p.895) and may be used in the treatment of heart failure (p.820). Ouabain is given by mouth in a dose of up to 24 mg daily; it has also been given intravenously.

### Preparations

**Proprietary Preparations** (details are given in Part 3)
***Ger.:*** Strodival.

## Oxedrine *(BAN)*

Sinefrina; Sympaethaminum; Synephrine; *p*-Synephrine. (*RS*)-1-(4-Hydroxyphenyl)-2-(methylamino)ethanol.

$C_9H_{13}NO_2 = 167.2.$

*CAS — 94-07-5.*

*ATC — C01CA08; S01GA06.*

NOTE. *p*-Synephrine has been used as a synonym for oxedrine. Care should be taken to avoid confusion with *m*-synephrine, which is phenylephrine (p.1126).

## Oxedrine Hydrochloride *(BANM)*

Sinefrina, hidrocloruro de.

$C_9H_{13}NO_2,HCl = 203.7.$

*ATC — C01CA08; S01GA06.*

## Oxedrine Tartrate *(BANM)*

Aetaphen. Tartrat.; Aethaphenum Tartaricum; Oxedrini Tartras; Oxyphenylmethylaminoethanol Tartrate; Sinefrina Tartrato; Sinefrina, tartrato de; Synephrine Tartrate.

$(C_9H_{13}NO_2)_2,C_4H_6O_6 = 484.5.$

*CAS — 16589-24-5 (oxedrine tartrate); 67-04-9 (±oxedrine tartrate).*

*ATC — C01CA08; S01GA06.*

### Profile

Oxedrine is a sympathomimetic (see Adrenaline, p.852) given as the tartrate in the treatment of hypotensive states in doses of about 100 to 150 mg three times daily by mouth; it has also been given by subcutaneous, intramuscular, or intravenous injection.

Oxedrine is also used in eye drops as an ocular decongestant, usually as the tartrate in a concentration of 0.5% in combination preparations. The hydrochloride has also been used.

### Preparations

**Proprietary Preparations** (details are given in Part 3)
***Austria:*** Sympatol; ***Ger.:*** Sympatol†; ***Hong Kong:*** Ocuton; ***Ital.:*** Sympatol; ***Switz.:*** Sympalept.

**Multi-ingredient:** ***Austria:*** Dacrin; Pasuma-Dragees; ***Fr.:*** Antalyre; Dacryne; Dacryoboraline; Polyfra; Posine; Sedacollyre; Uvicol†; ***Ger.:*** Dacrin†; Ophtalmin†; Pasgensin†; Solupen-D†; ***Port.:*** Dacrine†; ***Switz.:*** Chibro-Boraline†; Dacrine†.

## Oxilofrine Hydrochloride *(rINNM)*

Hidrocloruro de oxilofrina; *p*-Hydroxyephedrine Hydrochloride; Methylsynephrine Hydrochloride; Oxyephedrine Hydrochloride. *erythro*-*p*-Hydroxy-α-[1-(methylamino)ethyl]benzyl alcohol hydrochloride.

$C_{10}H_{15}NO_2,HCl = 217.7.$

*CAS — 942-51-8.*

### Profile

Oxilofrine is a sympathomimetic related to ephedrine (p.1120). It is used as the hydrochloride in the treatment of hypotensive states in usual doses of 16 mg three times daily by mouth, although higher doses have been given. It has also been used in antitussive preparations.

### Preparations

**Proprietary Preparations** (details are given in Part 3)
***Austria:*** Carnigen; ***Ger.:*** Carnigen.

**Multi-ingredient:** ***Canad.:*** Cophylac†.

## Oxprenolol Hydrochloride

*(BANM, USAN, rINNM)*

Ba-39089; Hidrocloruro de oxprenolol; Oxprenololi Hydrochloridum; Oxyprenolol Hydrochloride. 1-(o-Allyloxyphenoxy)-3-isopropylaminopropan-2-ol hydrochloride.

$C_{15}H_{23}NO_3$,HCl = 301.8.

*CAS — 6452-71-7 (oxprenolol); 6452-73-9 (oxprenolol hydrochloride).*

*ATC — C07AA02.*

NOTE. Compounded preparations of oxprenolol hydrochloride may be represented by the following names:

- Co-prenozide (*BAN*)—oxprenolol hydrochloride 640 parts and cyclopenthiazide 1 part (w/w).

**Pharmacopoeias.** In *Eur.* (see p.vi), *Jpn, Pol.,* and *US. Chin.* includes the base.

**Ph. Eur. 5.0** (Oxprenolol Hydrochloride). A white or almost white, crystalline powder. Very soluble in water; freely soluble in alcohol. A 10% solution in water has a pH of 4.5 to 6.0. Protect from light.

**USP 27** (Oxprenolol Hydrochloride). A white crystalline powder. Freely soluble in water, in alcohol, and in chloroform; sparingly soluble in acetone; practically insoluble in ether. A 10% solution in water has a pH of 4.0 to 6.0.

### Adverse Effects, Treatment, and Precautions

As for Beta Blockers, p.869.

**Breast feeding.** Oxprenolol is distributed into breast milk but the amount likely to be ingested by an infant is small (see under Pharmacokinetics, below). No adverse effects have been reported in breast-fed infants whose mothers were receiving oxprenolol and the American Academy of Pediatrics considers[1] that it is therefore usually compatible with breast feeding.

1. American Academy of Pediatrics. The transfer of drugs and other chemicals into human milk. *Pediatrics* 2001; **108:** 776–89. Correction. *ibid*; 1029. Also available at: http://aappolicy.aappublications.org/cgi/content/full/pediatrics%3b108/3/776 (accessed 06/07/04)

**Hypersensitivity.** Oxprenolol-induced drug fever has been reported[1] in a patient and was confirmed by a challenge test.

1. Hasegawa K, *et al.* Drug fever due to oxprenolol. *BMJ* 1980; **281:** 27–8.

**Overdosage.** Rhabdomyolysis with myoglobinuria has been reported[1] as a complication of severe overdosage with oxprenolol.

1. Schofield PM, *et al.* Recovery after severe oxprenolol overdose complicated by rhabdomyolysis. *Hum Toxicol* 1985; **4:** 57–60.

### Interactions

The interactions associated with beta blockers are discussed on p.870.

### Pharmacokinetics

Oxprenolol is well absorbed from the gastrointestinal tract, but is subject to first-pass metabolism resulting in variable bioavailability (20 to 70%). Peak plasma concentrations have been reported to occur about 1 or 2 hours after a dose. Oxprenolol is about 80% bound to plasma proteins. It diffuses across the placenta and is present in breast milk. It is moderately lipid-soluble and crosses the blood-brain barrier. Oxprenolol is metabolised in the liver and almost entirely excreted in the urine. An elimination half-life of 1 to 2 hours has been reported.

**Pregnancy and breast feeding.** The placental transfer of oxprenolol and its passage into breast milk was studied[1] in 32 pregnant women receiving a preparation containing oxprenolol and dihydralazine (Trasipressol). At delivery the mean maternal plasma concentration was 0.386 nanomoles/mL compared with 0.071 and 0.081 nanomoles/mL in plasma from the umbilical artery and vein respectively. Oxprenolol plasma concentrations in the newborn ranged from 0 to 0.186 nanomoles/mL during the first 24 hours of life. The concentrations of oxprenolol in breast milk 3 to 6 days after delivery ranged from 0 to 1.342 nanomoles/mL, and the milk to plasma concentration ratio was 0.45:1. Based on the highest milk concentration observed it was calculated that a breast-fed infant could receive, at a maximum, a daily dose at least sixty times less than an average daily dose (240 mg daily) taken by a hypertensive adult. In another study[2] in 12 women receiving oxprenolol, mean milk to plasma concentration ratios were 0.21:1 to 0.43:1, depending on dose.

1. Sioufi A, *et al.* Oxprenolol placental transfer, plasma concentrations in newborns and passage into breast milk. *Br J Clin Pharmacol* 1984; **18:** 453–6.
2. Fidler J, *et al.* Excretion of oxprenolol and timolol in breast milk. *Br J Obstet Gynaecol* 1983; **90:** 961–5.

### Uses and Administration

Oxprenolol is a non-cardioselective beta blocker (p.868). It is reported to possess intrinsic sympathomimetic and membrane-stabilising activity.

Oxprenolol is used as the hydrochloride in the management of hypertension (p.825), angina pectoris (p.813), and cardiac arrhythmias (p.816). It is also used in anxiety disorders (p.663).

In **hypertension** oxprenolol hydrochloride is given by mouth in a usual dose of 80 to 160 mg daily in two or three divided doses. The dose may be increased at weekly or fortnightly intervals until a satisfactory response is achieved. The usual maximum dose is 320 mg daily although up to 480 mg daily has been given. Modified-release tablets may be given once daily in a dose of up to 320 mg.

The usual dose for **angina pectoris** is 80 to 160 mg daily in two or three divided doses with a usual maximum of 320 mg daily.

For **cardiac arrhythmias** a dose of 40 mg daily to not more than 240 mg daily in two or three divided doses may be used.

To relieve **anxiety** in stressful situations oxprenolol hydrochloride is given by mouth in usual doses of 40 to 80 mg daily, either as a single dose or in two divided doses.

### Preparations

***BP 2003:*** Oxprenolol Tablets;
***USP 27:*** Oxprenolol Hydrochloride Extended-release Tablets; Oxprenolol Hydrochloride Tablets.

**Proprietary Preparations** (details are given in Part 3)
***Austral.:*** Corbeton; ***Austria:*** Trasicor; ***Belg.:*** Trasicor†; ***Canad.:*** Slow-Trasicor; Trasicor; ***Denm.:*** Trasicor; ***Fr.:*** Trasicor; ***Ger.:*** Trasicor; ***Gr.:*** Trasicor; ***Irl.:*** Slow-Trasicor†; Trasicor†; ***Israel:*** Tevacor; Trasicor†; ***Neth.:*** Trasicor; ***NZ:*** Captol; Slow-Trasicor; Trasicor†; ***S.Afr.:*** Trasicor†; ***Spain:*** Trasicor; ***Switz.:*** Slow-Trasicor; Trasicor; ***UK:*** Slow-Trasicor; Trasicor.

**Multi-ingredient:** ***Austria:*** Trasitensin; Trepress; ***Fr.:*** Trasitensine; ***Ger.:*** Impresso; Trasitensin; Trepress; ***Irl.:*** Trasidrex†; ***Ital.:*** Trasitensin; ***S.Afr.:*** Trasidrex†; ***Spain:*** Trasitensin; ***Switz.:*** Slow-Trasitensine; Trasitensine†; Trepress†; ***UK:*** Trasidrex.

## Oxyfedrine Hydrochloride

*(BANM, rINNM)*

D-563; Hidrocloruro de oxifedrina; Oxifedrini Chloridum. L-3-(β-Hydroxy-α-methylphenethylamino)-3′-methoxypropiophenone hydrochloride.

$C_{19}H_{23}NO_3$,HCl = 349.9.

*CAS — 15687-41-9 (oxyfedrine); 16777-42-7 (oxyfedrine hydrochloride).*

*ATC — C01DX03.*

### Profile

Oxyfedrine hydrochloride has vasodilator properties and is used in angina pectoris (p.813), and myocardial infarction (p.828).

It is given in doses of 8 to 24 mg three times daily by mouth. It may also be given by slow intravenous injection or intravenous infusion. Oxyfedrine is metabolised to phenylpropanolamine (p.1127).

### Preparations

**Proprietary Preparations** (details are given in Part 3)
***Austria:*** Ildamen; ***Ger.:*** Ildamen; Myofedrin; ***Hong Kong:*** Ildamen†; ***India:*** Ildamen; ***Port.:*** Ildamen.

## Pamabrom

*(USAN)*

Pamabromo. 2-Amino-2-methylpropan-1-ol 8-bromotheophyllinate.

$C_4H_{11}NO,C_7H_7BrN_4O_2$ = 348.2.

*CAS — 606-04-2.*

**Pharmacopoeias.** In *US.*

### Profile

Pamabrom is a weak diuretic that has been used, with analgesics and antihistamines, for symptomatic relief of the premenstrual syndrome.

### Preparations

**Proprietary Preparations** (details are given in Part 3)
***USA:*** Maximum Strength Aqua-Ban.

**Multi-ingredient:** ***Canad.:*** Extra Strength Multi-Symptom PMS Relief; Midol PMS Extra Strength; Pamprin; Relievol PMS; Trendar PMS; Tylenol Menstrual; ***Chile:*** Kitadol Periodo Menstrual; Minfaden; Predual; Tapsin Periodo Menstrual; ***Malaysia:*** Panadol Menstrual; ***Singapore:*** Panadol Menstrual; ***USA:*** Bayer Select Maximum Strength Menstrual†; Fem-1; Lurline PMS; Midol Pre-Menstrual Syndrome; Midol Teen Formula; Painaid PMF Premenstrual Formula; Pamprin; Premsyn PMS; Womens Tylenol Multi-Symptom Menstrual Relief.

## Pamiteplase

*(rINN)*

YM-866. 275-L-Glutamic acid-(1–91)-(174–527)-plasminogen activator (human tissue-type protein moiety).

*CAS — 151912-42-4.*

### Profile

Pamiteplase is a thrombolytic related to alteplase (p.857) used in acute myocardial infarction. It is being investigated in ischaemic stroke.

### Preparations

**Proprietary Preparations** (details are given in Part 3)
***Jpn:*** Solinase.

## Pantethine

Pantetina. (R)-NN′-[Dithiobis(ethyleneiminocarbonylethylene)]-bis(2,4-dihydroxy-3,3-dimethylbutyramide).

$C_{22}H_{42}N_4O_8S_2$ = 554.7.

*CAS — 16816-67-4.*

*ATC — A11HA32.*

**Pharmacopoeias.** In *Jpn.*

### Profile

Pantethine is a component of coenzyme A. It is used as a lipid regulating drug in the treatment of hyperlipidaemias (p.823). The usual dose is 600 to 1200 mg daily by mouth in divided doses.

### Preparations

**Proprietary Preparations** (details are given in Part 3)
***Hong Kong:*** Pantomin; ***Ital.:*** Analip†; Lipodel†; Pantetina; ***Jpn:*** Pantosin; ***Spain:*** Atarone†; Liponet; Obliterol.

**Multi-ingredient:** ***Ital.:*** Carpantin.

## Pargyline Hydrochloride

*(BANM, USAN, rINNM)*

A-19120; Hidrocloruro de pargilina; MO-911; NSC-43798. N-Methyl-N-2-propynylbenzylamine hydrochloride; Benzylmethylprop-2-ynylamine hydrochloride.

$C_{11}H_{13}N$,HCl = 195.7.

*CAS — 555-57-7 (pargyline); 306-07-0 (pargyline hydrochloride).*

*ATC — C02KC01.*

### Profile

Pargyline hydrochloride is an MAOI (see Phenelzine Sulfate, p.312) that was formerly used in the treatment of moderate to severe hypertension.

## Parnaparin Sodium

*(BAN, rINN)*

OP-21-23; Parnaparina sódica; Parnaparinum Natricum.

*CAS — 9041-08-1.*

*ATC — B01AB07.*

**Pharmacopoeias.** In *Eur.* (see p.vi).

**Ph. Eur. 5.0** (Parnaparin Sodium). It is prepared by hydrogen peroxide and cupric salt depolymerisation of heparin obtained from the intestinal mucosa of pigs and cattle. The majority of the components have a 2-O-sulfo-α-L-idopyranosuronic acid structure at the non-reducing end and a 2-N,6-O-disulfo-D-glucosamine structure at the reducing end of their chain. The mass-average molecular mass ranges between 4000 and 6000, with a characteristic value of about 5000. The mass percentage of chains lower than 3000 is not more than 30%. The degree of sulfation is 2.0 to 2.6 per disaccharide unit. Potency is not less than 75 units and not more than 110 units of anti-factor Xa activity per mg with reference to the dried substance, and the ratio of anti-factor Xa activity to anti-factor IIa (antithrombin) activity is between 1.5 and 3.0.

### Profile

Parnaparin sodium is a low-molecular-weight heparin (p.949) with anticoagulant activity used in the prevention of postoperative venous thromboembolism (p.839); it has also been used in other thromboembolic disorders. For general surgical procedures it is given by subcutaneous injection in a dose of 3200 units 2 hours before the procedure, followed by 3200 units once daily for 7 days or until the patient is fully ambulant. For higher risk or orthopaedic patients a dose of 4250 units is given 12 hours before the procedure, followed by 4250 units 12 hours postoperatively and then once daily for 10 days.

◊ References.

1. Frampton JE, Faulds D. Parnaparin: a review of its pharmacology, and clinical application in the prevention and treatment of thromboembolic and other vascular disorders. *Drugs* 1994; **47:** 652–76.

### Preparations

**Proprietary Preparations** (details are given in Part 3)
***Arg.:*** Tromboparin; ***Ital.:*** Fluxum; Minidalton†; ***Mex.:*** Fluxum.

## Penbutolol Sulfate *(USAN, rINNM)*

Hoe-39-893d; Hoe-893d; Levopenbutolol Sulfate; Penbutolol Hemisulfate; Penbutolol Sulphate *(BANM)*; Penbutololi Sulfas; Sulfato de penbutolol. (*S*)-1-*tert*-Butylamino-3-(2-cyclopentylphenoxy)propan-2-ol hemisulfate.

$(C_{18}H_{29}NO_2)_2,H_2SO_4$ = 680.9.

*CAS — 38363-40-5 (penbutolol); 38363-32-5 (penbutolol sulfate).*

*ATC — C07AA23.*

**Pharmacopoeias.** In *Eur.* (see p.vi), *Jpn*, and *US*.

**Ph. Eur. 5.0** (Penbutolol Sulphate). A white or almost white, crystalline powder. Slightly soluble in water; practically insoluble in cyclohexane; soluble in methyl alcohol. Protect from light.

**USP 27** (Penbutolol Sulfate). A white to off-white, crystalline powder. Soluble in water and in methyl alcohol. Store in airtight containers. Protect from light.

### Adverse Effects, Treatment, and Precautions

As for Beta Blockers, p.869.

### Interactions

The interactions associated with beta blockers are discussed on p.870.

### Pharmacokinetics

Penbutolol is readily absorbed from the gastrointestinal tract and peak plasma concentrations occur about 1 to 3 hours after a dose. Penbutolol is 80 to 98% bound to plasma proteins. It has a high lipid solubility. It is extensively metabolised in the liver by hydroxylation and glucuronidation, the metabolites being excreted in the urine together with only small amounts of unchanged penbutolol. A plasma elimination half-life of about 20 hours has been reported.

**Renal impairment.** Glucuronidation was considered more prominent than hydroxylation in the metabolism of penbutolol and its activity was not altered in patients with renal impairment.[1]

1. Bernard N, *et al.* Pharmacokinetics of penbutolol and its metabolites in renal insufficiency. *Eur J Clin Pharmacol* 1985; **29:** 215–19.

### Uses and Administration

Penbutolol is a non-cardioselective beta blocker (p.868). It is reported to possess some intrinsic sympathomimetic activity but lacks membrane-stabilising properties.

Penbutolol is used as the sulfate in the management of hypertension (p.825). It may also be used in cardiac disorders such as angina pectoris (p.813).

In **hypertension** penbutolol sulfate is given in an initial dose of 20 mg daily by mouth; the dose may be increased if necessary to 40 to 80 mg daily. Maximum antihypertensive efficacy is reported to occur within 2 weeks in patients given a dose of 20 mg daily but about 4 weeks may be required for maximum effect in patients given 10 mg daily.

Penbutolol sulfate has also been used in similar doses in cardiac disorders such as **angina**.

◊ References.

1. Frishman WH, Covey S. Penbutolol and carteolol: two new beta-adrenergic blockers with partial agonism. *J Clin Pharmacol* 1990; **30:** 412–21.
2. Schlanz KD, Thomas RL. Penbutolol: a new beta-adrenergic blocking agent. *DICP Ann Pharmacother* 1990; **24:** 403–8.

### Preparations

***USP 27:*** Penbutolol Sulfate Tablets.

**Proprietary Preparations** (details are given in Part 3)
***Fr.:*** Betapressine†; ***Ger.:*** Betapressin; ***Mex.:*** Betapresin†; ***USA:*** Levatol.

**Multi-ingredient:** ***Austria:*** Normotensin†; ***Ger.:*** Betarelix; Betasemid.

## Pentaerithrityl Tetranitrate *(BAN, rINN)*

Erynite; Nitropentaerythrol; Nitropenthrite; Pentaerithrityli Tetranitras; Pentaerythritol Tetranitrate; Pentaerythritolum Tetranitricum; Pentanitrol; PETN; Tetranitrato de pentaeritritilo. 2,2-Bis(hydroxymethyl)propane-1,3-diol tetranitrate.

$C_5H_8N_4O_{12}$ = 316.1.

*CAS — 78-11-5.*

*ATC — C01DA05.*

NOTE. The synonym PETN has been applied to both nicetritol and pentaerithrityl tetranitrate.

**Pharmacopoeias.** In *Pol.*

*Chin.* and *Eur.* (see p.vi) includes as diluted pentaerithrityl tetranitrate.

**Ph. Eur. 5.0** (Pentaerithrityl Tetranitrate, Diluted). A mixture of pentaerithrityl tetranitrate with lactose monohydrate or mannitol. Its solubility depends on the diluent and its concentration. Protect from light and heat.

Undiluted pentaerithrityl tetranitrate is a white or slightly yellowish powder. Practically insoluble in water; slightly soluble in alcohol; soluble in acetone.

**Handling.** Undiluted pentaerithrityl tetranitrate can be exploded by percussion or excessive heat.

### Profile

Pentaerithrityl tetranitrate is a vasodilator with general properties similar to those of glyceryl trinitrate (p.923) but its duration of action is more prolonged.

It is used in angina pectoris (p.813) in usual oral doses of up to 240 mg daily, in divided doses, before a meal. It is also given as modified-release preparations.

Pentaerithrityl trinitrate, an active metabolite of pentaerithrityl tetranitrate, has also been used clinically under the name pentrinitrol.

### Preparations

**Proprietary Preparations** (details are given in Part 3)
***Canad.:*** Peritrate†; ***Fr.:*** Nitrodex; ***Ger.:*** Dilcoran; Nirason N; Pentalong; ***India:*** Peritrate; ***Irl.:*** Mycardol†; ***Ital.:*** Peritrate; ***Switz.:*** Nitrodex; ***Thai.:*** Peritrate.

**Multi-ingredient:** ***Austria:*** Spasmocor; ***Chile:*** Cardiosedantol; ***Ger.:*** Nitro-Crataegutt; Nitro-Obsidan; VisanoCor N.

## Pentifylline *(BAN, rINN)*

1-Hexyltheobromine; Pentifilina; SK7. 1-Hexyl-3,7-dimethylxanthine.

$C_{13}H_{20}N_4O_2$ = 264.3.

*CAS — 1028-33-7.*

*ATC — C04AD01.*

### Profile

Pentifylline is a xanthine derivative used as a vasodilator in the management of peripheral or cerebral vascular disorders.

### Preparations

**Proprietary Preparations** (details are given in Part 3)
***Ger.:*** Cosaldon.

**Multi-ingredient:** ***Austria:*** Cosaldon†; ***Ger.:*** Cosaldon A†; ***S.Afr.:*** Cosaldon.

## Pentosan Polysulfate Sodium *(BAN, USAN, rINN)*

Pentosan Polysulphate Sodium; Pentosano polisulfato de sodio; PZ-68; Sodium Pentosan Polysulphate; Sodium Xylanpolysulphate; SP-54.

*CAS — 37319-17-8; 116001-96-8.*

*ATC — C05BA04.*

**Description.** Pentosan polysulfate sodium is a mixture of linear polymers of β-1→4-linked xylose, usually sulfated at the 2- and 3-positions and occasionally (approximately 1 in every 4 residues) substituted at the 2-position with 4-*O*-methyl-α-D-glucuronic acid 2,3-*O*-sulfate. The average molecular weight lies between 4000 and 6000 with a total molecular weight range of 1000 to 40 000.

### Adverse Effects and Precautions

As for Heparin, p.928. Gastrointestinal disturbances may also occur.

### Uses and Administration

Pentosan polysulfate sodium is a heparinoid with anticoagulant and fibrinolytic properties; it may also have hypolipidaemic and anti-inflammatory effects. It is used in thromboembolic disorders, although its anticoagulant effect is less than that of heparin. It is also used in the management of interstitial cystitis (see below) and has been tried in a number of other conditions, including variant Creutzfeldt-Jakob disease. Pentosan polysulfate sodium has been administered orally, parenterally, and by topical application.

In the management of interstitial cystitis, pentosan polysulfate sodium is given orally in a dose of 100 mg three times daily.

**Cystitis.** Pentosan polysulfate sodium has been used in inflammatory conditions of the bladder, including interstitial cystitis (see under Uses and Administration of Dimethyl Sulfoxide, p.1473), and is postulated to act by enhancing the protective effect of mucins at the bladder surface. Studies have differed concerning its efficacy in the treatment of interstitial cystitis and an analysis[1] of placebo-controlled trials concluded that pentosan polysulfate sodium was more effective in treating pain, urgency, and frequency, but that the difference was small. Any benefit is usually apparent within 3 to 6 months of commencing treatment and only occurs in a minority of patients.[2] Pentosan polysulfate sodium was reported[3] to have minimal long-term efficacy in a group of patients with severe or refractory interstitial cystitis.

Administration of pentosan polysulfate sodium by mouth controlled haemorrhage in 5 patients with radiation cystitis.[4] An improvement in symptoms has also been reported[5] in an uncontrolled study of oral pentosan polysulfate sodium in men with chronic nonbacterial prostatitis.

1. Hwang P, *et al.* Efficacy of pentosan polysulfate in the treatment of interstitial cystitis: a meta-analysis. *Urology* 1997; **50:** 39–43.
2. Anonymous. Pentosan for interstitial cystitis. *Med Lett Drugs Ther* 1997; **39:** 56.
3. Jepsen JV, *et al.* Long-term experience with pentosanpolysulfate in interstitial cystitis. *Urology* 1998; **51:** 381–7.
4. Parsons CL. Successful management of radiation cystitis with sodium pentosanpolysulfate. *J Urol (Baltimore)* 1986; **136:** 813–14.
5. Nickel JC, *et al.* Pentosan polysulfate therapy for chronic nonbacterial prostatitis (chronic pelvic pain syndrome category II-IA): a prospective multicenter clinical trial. *Urology* 2000; **56:** 413–17.

### Preparations

**Proprietary Preparations** (details are given in Part 3)
***Arg.:*** Elmiron; ***Austral.:*** Elmiron; ***Austria:*** Polyanion; ***Canad.:*** Elmiron; ***Fr.:*** Hemoclar; ***Ger.:*** Fibrezym; ***Hong Kong:*** Elmiron; SP54; ***Ital.:*** Fibrase; ***Port.:*** Fibrocide; ***S.Afr.:*** Tavan-SP 54; ***Spain:*** Fibrocid†; Thrombocid; ***USA:*** Elmiron.

**Multi-ingredient:** ***Austria:*** Flexurat†; Thrombocid; ***Fr.:*** Collyrex†; Keratosane†; ***Ger.:*** Flexurat†; Thrombocid; ***Hong Kong:*** Anso; Thrombocid; ***Port.:*** Thrombocid; ***Spain:*** Anso; Plasmaclar†; ***Switz.:*** Thrombocid.

## Pentoxifylline *(BAN, USAN, rINN)*

BL-191; Oxpentifylline; Pentoxifilina; Pentoxifyllinum. 3,7-Dimethyl-1-(5-oxohexyl)xanthine.

$C_{13}H_{18}N_4O_3$ = 278.3.

*CAS — 6493-05-6.*

*ATC — C04AD03.*

**Pharmacopoeias.** In *Chin., Eur.* (see p.vi), and *US*.

**Ph. Eur. 5.0** (Pentoxifylline). A white or almost white crystalline powder. Soluble in water; sparingly soluble in alcohol; freely soluble in dichloromethane. Protect from light.

**USP 27** (Pentoxifylline). A white to almost white crystalline powder. Soluble in water; sparingly soluble in alcohol; freely soluble in chloroform and in methyl alcohol; slightly soluble in ether.

### Adverse Effects

Pentoxifylline can cause nausea, gastrointestinal disturbances, dizziness, and headache. Flushing, angina, palpitations, cardiac arrhythmias, and hypersensitivity reactions may also occur. Bleeding events have been reported rarely, usually in association with bleeding risk factors.

Overdosage with pentoxifylline may be associated with fever, faintness, flushing, hypotension, drowsiness, agitation, and seizures.

**Haemorrhage.** Three major bleeding episodes including 2 fatal cerebral haemorrhages were reported in a group of patients receiving pentoxifylline 400 mg three times daily together with acenocoumarol for intermittent claudication.[1] Gastrointestinal bleeding occurred in a 67-year-old patient with a history of duodenal ulcer following a single dose of pentoxifylline for optic neuropathy.[2]

1. APIC Study Group. Acenocoumarol and pentoxifylline in intermittent claudication: a controlled clinical study. *Angiology* 1989; **40:** 237–48.
2. Oren R, *et al.* Pentoxifylline-induced gastrointestinal bleeding. *DICP Ann Pharmacother* 1991; **25:** 315–16.

**Overdosage.** A 22-year-old woman who took pentoxifylline 4 to 6 g with suicidal intent experienced severe bradycardia and first- and second-degree atrioventricular block; other effects included nausea, vomiting, abdominal cramps, hypokalaemia, excitation, and insomnia.[1] She recovered after intensive supportive and symptomatic treatment.

1. Sznajder IJ, *et al.* First and second degree atrioventricular block in oxpentifylline overdose. *BMJ* 1984; **288:** 26.

### Precautions

Pentoxifylline should be avoided in cerebral haemorrhage, extensive retinal haemorrhage, severe cardiac arrhythmias, and acute myocardial infarction. It should be used with caution in patients with ischaemic heart disease or hypotension. The dose of pentoxifylline may need to be reduced in patients with hepatic or renal impairment (see under Uses and Administration, below).

**Porphyria.** Pentoxifylline is considered to be unsafe in patients with porphyria because it has been shown to be porphyrinogenic in *in-vitro* systems.

### Interactions

Pentoxifylline may potentiate the effect of antihypertensives. High parenteral doses of pentoxifylline may enhance the action of insulin and oral hypoglycaemics in diabetic patients. Pentoxifylline should not be given concomitantly with ketorolac as there is reported to be an increased risk of bleeding and/or prolongation of the prothrombin time. There may also be an increased risk of bleeding during concomitant use with meloxicam. Serum levels of theophylline may be raised by pentoxifylline.

### Pharmacokinetics

Pentoxifylline is readily absorbed from the gastrointestinal tract but undergoes first-pass hepatic metabolism. Some metabolites are active. The apparent plasma half-life of pentoxifylline is reported to be 0.4 to 0.8 hours; that of the metabolites varies from 1.0 to 1.6 hours. In 24 hours most of a dose is excreted in the urine, mainly as metabolites, and less than 4% is recovered in the faeces. Elimination of pentoxifylline is decreased in elderly patients and patients with hepatic disease. Pentoxifylline and its metabolites are distributed into breast milk.

◊ References.

1. Beermann B, *et al.* Kinetics of intravenous and oral pentoxifylline in healthy subjects. *Clin Pharmacol Ther* 1985; **37:** 25–8.
2. Witter FR, Smith RV. The excretion of pentoxifylline and its metabolites into human breast milk. *Am J Obstet Gynecol* 1985; **151:** 1094–7.
3. Smith RV, *et al.* Pharmacokinetics of orally administered pentoxifylline in humans. *J Pharm Sci* 1986; **75:** 47–52.
4. Rames A, *et al.* Pharmacokinetics of intravenous and oral pentoxifylline in healthy volunteers and in cirrhotic patients. *Clin Pharmacol Ther* 1990; **47:** 354–9.
5. Paap CM, *et al.* Multiple-dose pharmacokinetics of pentoxifylline and its metabolites during renal insufficiency. *Ann Pharmacother* 1996; **30:** 724–9.

## Uses and Administration

Pentoxifylline is a xanthine derivative used in the treatment of peripheral vascular disease (p.831). Although often classified as a vasodilator, its primary action seems to be a reduction in blood viscosity, probably by effects on erythrocyte deformability and platelet adhesion and aggregation. It is reported to increase blood flow to ischaemic tissues and improve tissue oxygenation in patients with peripheral vascular disease and to increase oxygen tension in the cerebral cortex and in the cerebrospinal fluid; it has been used in cerebrovascular disorders. Pentoxifylline also inhibits production of the cytokine, tumour necrosis factor alpha (TNFα), and this property is under investigation in a number of diseases (see below).

In the treatment of peripheral vascular disease the usual dose is 400 mg three times daily by mouth in a modified-release formulation; this may be reduced to 400 mg twice daily for maintenance or if adverse effects are troublesome. Doses should be taken with meals to reduce gastrointestinal disturbances. In severe hepatic or renal impairment, doses may need to be reduced (see below). Beneficial effects may not be evident until after 2 to 8 weeks of treatment. Pentoxifylline may also be administered parenterally.

◊ General references.

1. Ward A, Clissold SP. Pentoxifylline: a review of its pharmacodynamic and pharmacokinetic properties, and its therapeutic efficacy. *Drugs* 1987; **34:** 50–97.
2. Samlaska CP, Winfield EA. Pentoxifylline. *J Am Acad Dermatol* 1994; **30:** 603–21.

**Administration in hepatic and renal impairment.** The elimination half-life of pentoxifylline and its metabolites is significantly prolonged in patients with hepatic cirrhosis,[1] and some metabolites have a prolonged half-life in renal impairment.[2] The UK manufacturers state that in patients with severely impaired hepatic function the dose of pentoxifylline may need to be reduced, while accumulation may occur in patients with severe renal impairment (creatinine clearance less than 30 mL/minute) who receive more than 400 mg once or twice daily.

References.

1. Rames A, *et al.* Pharmacokinetics of intravenous and oral pentoxifylline in healthy volunteers and in cirrhotic patients. *Clin Pharmacol Ther* 1990; **47:** 354–9.
2. Paap CM, *et al.* Multiple-dose pharmacokinetics of pentoxifylline and its metabolites during renal insufficiency. *Ann Pharmacother* 1996; **30:** 724–9.

**Inhibition of tumour necrosis factor alpha.** Pentoxifylline inhibits production of tumour necrosis factor alpha (TNFα), a cytokine that is implicated in the pathogenesis of many diseases, and investigative work with pentoxifylline is being, or has been, carried out in many such disorders. Studies have been performed in patients with alcoholic hepatitis,[1] cardiomyopathy,[2] cerebral malaria,[3,4] diabetic nephropathy,[5] leishmaniasis,[6] leprosy,[7,8] membranous nephropathy,[9] severe sepsis or septic shock,[10] recurrent aphthous stomatitis,[11,12] and various vasculitic syndromes, including Behçet's syndrome.[13] Pentoxifylline has also been tried for improving graft survival in kidney transplantation.[14] For mention of a possible benefit in sarcoidosis, see p.1087. Although promising results have been reported in some of these studies, the place of pentoxifylline in the overall management of these disorders remains to be established.

1. Akriviadis E, *et al.* Pentoxifylline improves short-term survival in severe acute alcoholic hepatitis: a double-blind, placebo-controlled trial. *Gastroenterology* 2000; **119:** 1637–48.
2. Skudicky D, *et al.* Beneficial effects of pentoxifylline in patients with idiopathic dilated cardiomyopathy treated with angiotensin-converting enzyme inhibitors and carvedilol: results of a randomized study. *Circulation* 2001; **103:** 1083–8.
3. Di Perri, *et al.* Pentoxifylline as a supportive agent in the treatment of cerebral malaria in children. *J Infect Dis* 1995; **171:** 1317–22.
4. Looareesuwan S, *et al.* Pentoxifylline as an ancillary treatment for severe falciparum malaria in Thailand. *Am J Trop Med Hyg* 1998; **58:** 348–53.
5. Navarro JF, *et al.* Urinary protein excretion and serum tumor necrosis factor in diabetic patients with advanced renal failure: effects of pentoxifylline administration. *Am J Kidney Dis* 1999; **33:** 458–63.
6. Lessa HA, *et al.* Successful treatment of refractory mucosal leishmaniasis with pentoxifylline plus antimony. *Am J Trop Med Hyg* 2001; **65:** 87–9.
7. Nery JAC, *et al.* The use of pentoxifylline in the treatment of type 2 reactional episodes in leprosy. *Indian J Lepr* 2000; **72:** 457–67.
8. Dawlah ZM, *et al.* A phase 2 open trial of pentoxifylline for the treatment of leprosy reactions. *Int J Lepr Other Mycobact Dis* 2002; **70:** 38–43.
9. Ducloux D, *et al.* Use of pentoxifylline in membranous nephropathy. *Lancet* 2001; **357:** 1672–3.
10. Staubach K-H, *et al.* Effect of pentoxifylline in severe sepsis: results of a randomized, double-blind, placebo-controlled study. *Arch Surg* 1998; **133:** 94–100.
11. Pizarro A, *et al.* Treatment of recurrent aphthous stomatitis with pentoxifylline. *Br J Dermatol* 1995; **133:** 659–60.
12. Chandrasekhar J, *et al.* Oxypentifylline in the management of recurrent aphthous oral ulcers: an open clinical trial. *Oral Surg Oral Med Oral Pathol Oral Radiol Endod* 1999; **87:** 564–7.
13. Hisamatsu T, *et al.* Combination therapy including pentoxifylline for entero-Behçet's disease. *Bull Tokyo Dent Coll* 2001; **42:** 169–76.
14. Noel C, *et al.* Immunomodulatory effect of pentoxifylline during human allograft rejection: involvement of tumor necrosis factor α and adhesion molecules. *Transplantation* 2000; **69:** 1102–7.

**Venous leg ulcers.** A systematic review[1] of pentoxifylline used in the treatment of venous leg ulcers (p.1139) concluded that it was an effective adjunct to compression bandaging, and may be effective alone.

1. Jull AB, *et al.* Pentoxifylline for treating venous leg ulcers. Available in The Cochrane Library; Issue 2. Chichester: John Wiley; 2004.

## Preparations

*USP 27:* Pentoxifylline Extended-Release Tablets.

**Proprietary Preparations** (details are given in Part 3)

***Arg.:*** Dospan Pento; Pentolab; Previscan; Trental; ***Austral.:*** Trental; ***Austria:*** Haemodyn; Pentohexal; Pentomer; Pentoxi; Pentoximed; Trental; Vasonit; ***Belg.:*** Torental; ***Braz.:*** Chemopent; Pentox; Perental; Peripan; Trental; Vascer; ***Canad.:*** Trental; ***Chile:*** Trental; ***Denm.:*** Trental; ***Fin.:*** Artal; Pentoxin; Trental; ***Fr.:*** Pentoflux; Torental; ***Ger.:*** Agapurin; Azupentat; Claudicat; durapental; Pento; Pento-Puren; Pentohexal; Pentox; Pentoxy; Ralofekt; Rentylin; Trental; ***Hong Kong:*** Trental; ***India:*** Trental; ***Irl.:*** Trental; ***Israel:*** Oxopurin; Trental; ***Ital.:*** Trental; ***Malaysia:*** Trenlin; Trental; ***Mex.:*** Fixoten; Kentadin; Peridane; Sufisal; Trental; Vasofyl; ***Neth.:*** Trental; ***Norw.:*** Trental; ***NZ:*** Trental; ***Port.:*** Claudicat; Trental; ***S.Afr.:*** Trental; ***Singapore:*** Agapurin; Flexital†; Trenlin; Trental; ***Spain:*** Elorgan; Hemovas; Retimax; ***Switz.:*** Dinostral; Pentoxi; Trental; ***Thai.:*** Agapurin; Elastab; Flexital; Herden; Penlol; Sipental; Trental; ***UK:*** Trental; ***USA:*** Trental.

**Multi-ingredient:** ***Arg.:*** Ikatral Periferico.

## Perhexiline Maleate *(BANM, USAN, rINNM)*

Maleato de perhexilina; WSM-3978G. 2-(2,2-Dicyclohexylethyl)piperidine hydrogen maleate.

$C_{19}H_{35}N,C_4H_4O_4$ = 393.6.

*CAS — 6621-47-2 (perhexiline); 6724-53-4 (perhexiline maleate).*

*ATC — C08EX02.*

### Profile

Perhexiline maleate may be used in the long-term management of severe angina pectoris (p.813) in patients who have not responded to other anti-anginal drugs. Its mode of action is complex.

The usual initial dose is 100 mg daily by mouth, subsequently either increased or decreased, as necessary, at intervals of 2 to 4 weeks; it is generally recommended not to give more than 300 mg daily although doses of 400 mg daily have been necessary in some patients. The maintenance of plasma-perhexiline concentrations between 0.15 and 0.60 micrograms/mL has been recommended.

Perhexiline occasionally produces severe adverse effects including peripheral neuropathy affecting all four limbs with associated papilloedema, severe and occasionally fatal hepatic toxicity, and metabolic abnormalities with marked weight loss, hypertriglyceridaemia, and profound hypoglycaemia. It is contra-indicated in patients with hepatic or renal impairment. Perhexiline should be used with caution in diabetic patients. Hepatic metabolism of perhexiline is mediated by the cytochrome P450 isoenzyme CYP2D6. Therefore caution is advised if perhexiline is used with other drugs that inhibit or are metabolised by this enzyme, and perhexiline toxicity has been reported with SSRIs such as fluoxetine or paroxetine.

**Porphyria.** Perhexiline is considered to be unsafe in patients with porphyria because it has been shown to be porphyrinogenic in *animals* or *in-vitro* systems.

### Preparations

**Proprietary Preparations** (details are given in Part 3)

***Austral.:*** Pexid†; Pexsig; ***NZ:*** Pexsig.

# Perindopril *(BAN, USAN, rINN)*

McN-A-2833; S-9490. (2S,3aS,7aS)-1-{N-[(S)-1-Ethoxycarbonylbutyl]-L-alanyl}perhydroindole-2-carboxylic acid.

$C_{19}H_{32}N_2O_5$ = 368.5.

*CAS — 82834-16-0.*

*ATC — C09AA04.*

## Perindopril Erbumine *(BANM, USAN, rINNM)*

Erbumina de perindopril; McN-A-2833-109; Perindopril *tert*-Butylamine; S-9490-3.

$C_{19}H_{32}N_2O_5,C_4H_{11}N$ = 441.6.

*CAS — 107133-36-8.*

*ATC — C09AA04.*

**Pharmacopoeias.** In *Eur.* (see p.vi).

**Ph. Eur. 5.0** (Perindopril *tert*-Butylamine). A white or almost white, slightly hygroscopic, crystalline powder. It exhibits polymorphism. Freely soluble in water and in alcohol; sparingly soluble in dichloromethane. Store in airtight containers.

## Adverse Effects, Treatment, and Precautions

As for ACE inhibitors, p.842.

◊ In a postmarketing surveillance study[1] of 47 351 patients receiving perindopril for hypertension, no unexpected adverse effects were reported and serious reactions were rare; 1587 (6.3%) women and 782 (3.5%) men withdrew from therapy due to adverse effects.

Although a study[2] of perindopril administration to patients with stable chronic heart failure reported no significant first-dose hypotension, there has been a case report[3] of ischaemic stroke, possibly associated with hypotension, following a single dose of perindopril in a patient with post-infarction heart failure. Standard precautions as for other ACE inhibitors (p.844) should be followed when initiating perindopril therapy.

1. Speirs C, *et al.* Perindopril postmarketing surveillance: a 12 month study in 47 351 hypertensive patients. *Br J Clin Pharmacol* 1998; **46:** 63–70.
2. MacFadyen RJ, *et al.* Differences in first dose response to angiotensin converting enzyme inhibition in congestive heart failure: a placebo controlled study. *Br Heart J* 1991; **66:** 206–11.
3. Bagger JP. Adverse event with first-dose perindopril in congestive heart failure. *Lancet* 1997; **349:** 1671–2.

## Interactions

As for ACE inhibitors, p.845.

## Pharmacokinetics

Perindopril acts as a prodrug of the diacid perindoprilat, its active form. Following oral administration perindopril is rapidly absorbed with a bioavailability of about 65 to 75%. It is extensively metabolised, mainly in the liver, to perindoprilat and inactive metabolites including glucuronides. The presence of food is reported to reduce the conversion of perindopril to perindoprilat. Peak plasma concentrations of perindoprilat are achieved 3 to 4 hours after an oral dose of perindopril. Perindoprilat is about 10 to 20% bound to plasma proteins. Perindopril is excreted predominantly in the urine, as unchanged drug, as perindoprilat, and as other metabolites. The elimination of perindoprilat is biphasic with a distribution half-life of about 5 hours and an elimination half-life of 25 to 30 hours or longer, the latter half-life probably representing strong binding to angiotensin-converting enzyme. The excretion of perindoprilat is decreased in renal impairment. Both perindopril and perindoprilat are removed by dialysis.

◊ References.

1. Lecocq B, *et al.* Influence of food on the pharmacokinetics of perindopril and the time course of angiotensin-converting enzyme inhibition in serum. *Clin Pharmacol Ther* 1990; **47:** 397–402.
2. Verpooten GA, *et al.* Single dose pharmacokinetics of perindopril and its metabolites in hypertensive patients with various degrees of renal insufficiency. *Br J Clin Pharmacol* 1991; **32:** 187–92.
3. Sennesael J, *et al.* The pharmacokinetics of perindopril and its effects on serum angiotensin converting enzyme activity in hypertensive patients with chronic renal failure. *Br J Clin Pharmacol* 1992; **33:** 93–9.
4. Thiollet M, *et al.* The pharmacokinetics of perindopril in patients with liver cirrhosis. *Br J Clin Pharmacol* 1992; **33:** 326–8.
5. Guérin A, *et al.* The effect of haemodialysis on the pharmacokinetics of perindoprilat after long-term perindopril. *Eur J Clin Pharmacol* 1993; **44:** 183–7.

## Uses and Administration

Perindopril is an ACE inhibitor (p.842). It is used in the treatment of hypertension (p.825) and heart failure (p.820).

Perindopril is converted in the body into its active metabolite perindoprilat. ACE inhibition is reported to occur within 1 hour of a dose, to be at a maximum at about 4 to 8 hours, and to be maintained for 24 hours. Perindopril is given by mouth as the erbumine salt and should be taken before food.

In the treatment of **hypertension** perindopril erbumine is given in an initial dose of 4 mg once daily. Since there may be a precipitous fall in blood pressure in some patients when starting therapy with an ACE inhibitor, the first dose should preferably be given at bedtime. Hypotension is particularly likely in patients with renovascular hypertension, volume depletion, heart failure, or severe hypertension and such patients may be given a lower initial dose of 2 mg once daily. Patients taking diuretics should have the diuretic withdrawn 2 or 3 days before perindopril is started and resumed later if required; if this is not possible, an initial dose of 2 mg once daily may be given. An initial dose of 2 mg once daily may also be used in the elderly. The dose of perindopril may be increased according to response to a maximum of 8 mg daily. In the USA a maximum dose of 16 mg daily is allowed in uncomplicated hypertensive patients.

In the management of **heart failure**, severe first-dose hypotension on introduction of an ACE inhibitor is common in patients on loop diuretics, but their temporary withdrawal may cause rebound pulmonary oedema. Thus treatment should be initiated with a low dose under close medical supervision. Perindopril is given in an initial dose of 2 mg in the morning. The usual maintenance dose is 4 mg daily.

A reduction in dosage may be necessary in patients with impaired renal function (see below).

◊ References.

1. Todd PA, Fitton A. Perindopril: a review of its pharmacological properties and therapeutic use in cardiovascular disorders. *Drugs* 1991; **42:** 90–114.
2. Doyle AE, ed. Angiotensin-converting enzyme (ACE) inhibition: benefits beyond blood pressure control. *Am J Med* 1992; **92** (suppl 4B): 1S–107S.
3. Hurst M, Jarvis B. Perindopril: an updated review of its use in hypertension. *Drugs* 2001; **61** 867–96.
4. Simpson D, *et al.* Perindopril: in congestive heart failure. *Drugs* 2002; **62:** 1367–77.

**Administration in renal impairment.** The dose of perindopril should be reduced in patients with renal impairment. The UK manufacturer recommends the following doses:

- creatinine clearance (CC) between 30 and 60 mL/minute: 2 mg daily
- CC between 15 and 30 mL/minute: 2 mg on alternate days
- CC less than 15 mL/minute: 2 mg on dialysis days.

### Preparations

**Proprietary Preparations** (details are given in Part 3)
***Arg.:*** Coverene; ***Austral.:*** Coversyl; ***Austria:*** Coversum; ***Belg.:*** Coversyl; ***Braz.:*** Coversyl; ***Canad.:*** Coversyl; ***Chile:*** Coversyl; ***Denm.:*** Coversyl; ***Fin.:*** Coversyl; ***Fr.:*** Coversyl; ***Ger.:*** Coversum; ***Gr.:*** Coversyl; ***Hong Kong:*** Acertil; ***India:*** Coversyl; ***Irl.:*** Coversyl; ***Ital.:*** Coversyl; Procaptan; ***Jpn:*** Coversyl; ***Malaysia:*** Coversyl; ***Mex.:*** Coversyl; ***Neth.:*** Coversyl; ***NZ:*** Coversyl; ***Port.:*** Coversyl; ***S.Afr.:*** Coversyl; ***Singapore:*** Coversyl; ***Spain:*** Coversyl; ***Switz.:*** Coversum; ***Thai.:*** Coversyl; ***UK:*** Coversyl; ***USA:*** Aceon.

**Multi-ingredient:** ***Arg.:*** Preterax; ***Austral.:*** Coversyl Plus; ***Austria:*** Predonium; Preterax; ***Braz.:*** Preterax†; ***Fr.:*** Bipreterax; Preterax; ***Ger.:*** Coversum Combi; ***Hong Kong:*** Predonium; ***Irl.:*** Preterax; ***Ital.:*** Prelectal; Preterax; ***Neth.:*** Coversyl Plus; ***S.Afr.:*** Coversyl Plus; ***Singapore:*** Preterax; ***Switz.:*** Coversum Combi; ***UK:*** Coversyl Plus.

## Phenindione *(BAN, rINN)*

Fenindiona; Fenindione; Phenylindanedione; Phenylinium. 2-Phenylindan-1,3-dione.

$C_{15}H_{10}O_2$ = 222.2.
*CAS — 83-12-5.*
*ATC — B01AA02.*

**Pharmacopoeias.** In *Br.* and *Fr.*

**BP 2003** (Phenindione). Soft, odourless or almost odourless, white or creamy-white crystals. Very slightly soluble in water; slightly soluble in alcohol and in ether; freely soluble in chloroform. Solutions are yellow to red.

### Adverse Effects and Treatment

As for Warfarin Sodium, p.1022. However, phenindione and the other indanediones are generally more toxic than warfarin with hypersensitivity reactions involving many organs and sometimes resulting in death. Some of the reactions include skin rashes and exfoliative dermatitis, pyrexia, diarrhoea, vomiting, sore throat, liver and kidney damage, myocarditis, agranulocytosis, leucopenia, eosinophilia, and a leukaemoid syndrome.

Phenindione may discolour the urine pink or orange and this is independent of any haematuria. Taste disturbances have been reported.

**Effects on the gastrointestinal tract.** There have been cases of paralytic ileus, one fatal, associated with phenindione.[1,2]

1. Menon IS. Phenindione and paralytic ileus. *Lancet* 1966; **i:** 1421–2.
2. Nash AG. Phenindione and paralytic ileus. *Lancet* 1966; **ii:** 51–2.

### Precautions

As for Warfarin Sodium, p.1023.

Phenindione is not recommended in pregnancy.

**Breast feeding.** Phenindione is distributed into breast milk, with reported concentrations[1] of 1 to 5 micrograms/mL after a single dose of 50 or 75 mg. A woman receiving phenindione 50 mg each morning and 50 and 25 mg on alternate nights breast-fed her infant son,[2] who required a herniotomy at 5 weeks. After surgery he had an enormous scrotal haematoma and oozing from the wound, and was found to have extended prothrombin and partial thromboplastin times. The American Academy of Pediatrics therefore considers[3] that phenindione should be given with caution to breast-feeding mothers.

1. Goguel M, *et al.* Thérapeutique anticoagulante et allaitement: etude du passage de la phényl-2-dioxo, 1,3 indane dans le lait maternel. *Rev Fr Gynecol Obstet* 1970; **65:** 409–12.
2. Eckstein HB, Jack B. Breast-feeding and anticoagulant therapy. *Lancet* 1970; **i:** 672–3.
3. American Academy of Pediatrics. The transfer of drugs and other chemicals into human milk. *Pediatrics* 2001; **108:** 776–89. Correction. *ibid.*; 1029. Also available at: http://aappolicy.aappublications.org/cgi/content/full/pediatrics%3b108/3/776 (accessed 06/07/04)

### Interactions

The interactions associated with oral anticoagulants are described in detail under warfarin (p.1023). Specific references to interactions involving phenindione can be found there under the headings for the following drug groups: analgesics; antibacterials; antifungals; antiplatelets; anxiolytic sedatives; gastrointestinal drugs; lipid regulating drugs; and sex hormones.

### Pharmacokinetics

Phenindione is absorbed from the gastrointestinal tract. It diffuses across the placenta and is distributed into breast milk. Metabolites of phenindione excreted in the urine are responsible for any discoloration that may occur.

### Uses and Administration

Phenindione is an orally administered indanedione anticoagulant with actions similar to those of warfarin (p.1028). It is used in the management of thromboembolic disorders (p.837), but because of its higher incidence of severe adverse effects it is now rarely employed.

The usual initial dose of phenindione is 200 mg on the first day, 100 mg on the second day, and then maintenance doses of 50 to 150 mg daily according to coagulation tests.

### Preparations

***BP 2003:*** Phenindione Tablets.

**Proprietary Preparations** (details are given in Part 3)
***Austral.:*** Dindevan; ***Fr.:*** Pindione†; ***India:*** Dindevan; ***UK:*** Dindevan†.

## Phenoxybenzamine Hydrochloride

*(BANM, rINNM)*

Hidrocloruro de fenoxibenzamina; SKF-688A. Benzyl(2-chloroethyl)(1-methyl-2-phenoxyethyl)amine hydrochloride.

$C_{18}H_{22}ClNO,HCl$ = 340.3.
*CAS — 59-96-1 (phenoxybenzamine); 63-92-3 (phenoxybenzamine hydrochloride).*
*ATC — C04AX02.*

**Pharmacopoeias.** In *Br., Chin.,* and *US.*

**BP 2003** (Phenoxybenzamine Hydrochloride). A white or almost white, odourless or almost odourless, crystalline powder. Sparingly soluble in water; freely soluble in alcohol and in chloroform.

### Adverse Effects and Treatment

The adverse effects of phenoxybenzamine are primarily due to its alpha-adrenoceptor blocking activity. They include postural hypotension and dizziness, reflex tachycardia, nasal congestion, and miosis. Inhibition of ejaculation may occur. These effects may be minimised by using a low initial dose, and may diminish with continued administration, but the hypotensive effect can be exaggerated by exercise, heat, a large meal, or alcohol ingestion. Other side-effects include dry mouth, decreased sweating, drowsiness, fatigue, and confusion. Gastrointestinal effects are usually slight. When phenoxybenzamine is given intravenously, idiosyncratic profound hypotension can occur within a few minutes of starting the infusion. Convulsions have been reported after rapid intravenous infusion of phenoxybenzamine.

Severe hypotension may occur in overdose and treatment includes support of the circulation by postural measures and parenteral fluid volume replacement. Sympathomimetics are considered to be of little value, and adrenaline is contra-indicated since it also stimulates beta receptors causing increased hypotension and tachycardia. Sources differ as to the value of noradrenaline in overcoming alpha-receptor blockade.

Phenoxybenzamine has been shown to be mutagenic in *in vitro* tests and carcinogenic in *rodents.*

### Precautions

Phenoxybenzamine should be given with care to patients with heart failure, ischaemic heart disease, cerebrovascular disease, or renal impairment, and should be avoided if a fall in blood pressure would be dangerous. Phenoxybenzamine may aggravate the symptoms of respiratory infections.

When given intravenously, phenoxybenzamine hydrochloride should always be diluted and given by infusion. Intravenous fluids must always be given beforehand to ensure an adequate circulating blood volume and to prevent a precipitous fall in blood pressure. Care should be taken to avoid extravasation. Contamination of the skin should also be avoided since contact sensitisation may occur.

**Porphyria.** Phenoxybenzamine is considered to be unsafe in patients with porphyria because it has been shown to be porphyrinogenic in *in-vitro* systems.

### Interactions

Since phenoxybenzamine only blocks alpha receptors, leaving the beta receptors unopposed, concomitant use of drugs such as adrenaline that also stimulate beta receptors may enhance the cardiac-accelerating and hypotensive action of phenoxybenzamine.

### Pharmacokinetics

Phenoxybenzamine is incompletely and variably absorbed from the gastrointestinal tract. Following oral administration the onset of action is gradual over several hours and persists for 3 or 4 days following a single dose. The maximum effect is attained in about 1 hour after an intravenous dose. The plasma half-life after intravenous administration is about 24 hours. Phenoxybenzamine is metabolised in the liver and excreted in the urine and bile, but small amounts remain in the body for several days. The duration of action is thought to depend on the rate of synthesis of new alpha receptors following irreversible covalent bonding to existing alpha receptors by a reactive intermediate of phenoxybenzamine.

### Uses and Administration

Phenoxybenzamine is a powerful alpha-adrenoceptor blocker (p.809) with a prolonged duration of action; it binds covalently to alpha receptors in smooth muscle to produce an irreversible ('non-competitive') blockade. A single large dose of phenoxybenzamine can cause alpha-adrenoceptor blockade for 3 days or longer.

Phenoxybenzamine is used in the management of phaeochromocytoma (p.831). It has also been employed in severe shock (p.835) and in the treatment of urinary retention (p.476).

Phenoxybenzamine is used as the hydrochloride. It is given by mouth or by intravenous infusion as a dilute solution.

In **phaeochromocytoma** it is used to control the hypertension associated with excessive catecholamine release during the pre-operative period and in patients whose tumours are inoperable. A beta blocker may also be given to control tachycardia, but not before alpha blockade has completely suppressed the pressor effects of the phaeochromocytoma. The usual initial dose of phenoxybenzamine hydrochloride is 10 mg once or twice daily by mouth, increased gradually, according to the patient's response, to a usual dose of 1 to 2 mg/kg daily in 2 divided doses. It may be given intravenously for operative cover in patients with phaeochromocytoma in a daily dose of 1 mg/kg in 200 mL of sodium chloride 0.9% infused over at least 2 hours. A similar intravenous dose in 200 to 500 mL of sodium chloride 0.9% has been given in the management of severe **shock**.

For **urinary retention** due to neurogenic bladder a dose of 10 mg twice daily by mouth has been given.

### Preparations

***BP 2003:*** Phenoxybenzamine Capsules;
***USP 27:*** Phenoxybenzamine Hydrochloride Capsules.

**Proprietary Preparations** (details are given in Part 3)
***Austral.:*** Dibenyline; ***Austria:*** Dibenzyran; ***Belg.:*** Dibenyline†; ***Ger.:*** Dibenzyran; ***Gr.:*** Dibenyline; ***Hong Kong:*** Dibenyline; ***India:*** Fenoxene; ***Israel:*** Dibenyline; ***Neth.:*** Dibenyline; ***NZ:*** Dibenyline; ***UK:*** Dibenyline; ***USA:*** Dibenzyline.

## Phenprocoumon *(BAN, USAN, rINN)*

Fenprocomón; Phenylpropylhydroxycoumarin. 4-Hydroxy-3-(1-phenylpropyl)coumarin.

$C_{18}H_{16}O_3$ = 280.3.
*CAS — 435-97-2.*
*ATC — B01AA04.*

**Adverse Effects, Treatment, and Precautions**
As for Warfarin Sodium, p.1022.

**Effects on the liver.** A woman who had twice previously developed jaundice while taking phenprocoumon developed jaundice and parenchymal liver damage when, after some years, phenprocoumon was again given.[1] Two other cases of phenprocoumon-associated hepatitis have been reported.[2]

1. den Boer W, Loeliger EA. Phenprocoumon-induced jaundice. *Lancet* 1976; **i:** 912.
2. Slagboom G, Loeliger EA. Coumarin-associated hepatitis: report of two cases. *Arch Intern Med* 1980; **140:** 1028–9.

## Interactions

The interactions associated with oral anticoagulants are discussed in detail under warfarin (p.1023). Specific references to interactions involving phenprocoumon can be found there under the headings for the following drug groups: analgesics; antiarrhythmics; antidepressants; antidiabetics; antigout drugs; antineoplastics; gastrointestinal drugs; lipid regulating drugs; prostaglandins; and sex hormones.

## Pharmacokinetics

Phenprocoumon is readily absorbed from the gastrointestinal tract and is extensively bound to plasma proteins. A half-life of 5 to 6 days has been reported. It is excreted in the urine and faeces as conjugated hydroxy metabolites and parent compound. Phenprocoumon is given as a racemic mixture; the *S*-isomer is reported to be more potent. The stereo-isomers have different pharmacokinetics.

◊ References.

1. Husted S, Andreasen F. Individual variation in the response to phenprocoumon. *Eur J Clin Pharmacol* 1977; **11:** 351–8.
2. Toon S, *et al.* Metabolic fate of phenprocoumon in humans. *J Pharm Sci* 1985; **74:** 1037–40.

## Uses and Administration

Phenprocoumon is an orally administered coumarin anticoagulant with actions similar to those of warfarin (p.1028). It is used in the management of thromboembolic disorders (p.837). Initial doses of up to 9 mg on the first day followed by up to 6 mg on the second day are used. Maintenance doses are usually from 1.5 to 6 mg daily, depending on the response.

## Preparations

**Proprietary Preparations** (details are given in Part 3)
***Austria:*** Marcoumar; ***Belg.:*** Marcoumar; ***Braz.:*** Marcoumar; ***Denm.:*** Marcoumar; ***Ger.:*** Falithrom; Marcumar; marcuphen; Phenpro; ***Neth.:*** Marcoumar; ***Switz.:*** Marcoumar.

---

# Phentolamine Mesilate *(BANM, rINNM)*

Mesilato de fentolamina; Phentolamine Mesylate; Phentolamine Methanesulphonate; Phentolamini Mesilas. 3-[*N*-(2-Imidazolin-2-ylmethyl)-*p*-toluidino]phenol methanesulphonate.

$C_{17}H_{19}N_3O,CH_4SO_3$ = 377.5.

*CAS — 50-60-2 (phentolamine); 73-05-2 (phentolamine hydrochloride); 65-28-1 (phentolamine mesilate).*

*ATC — C04AB01; G04BE05.*

**Pharmacopoeias.** In *Chin., Eur.* (see p.vi), and *US.*

**Ph. Eur. 5.0** (Phentolamine Mesilate). A white, slightly hygroscopic, crystalline powder. Freely soluble in water and in alcohol; practically insoluble in dichloromethane. Store in airtight containers. Protect from light.

**USP 27** (Phentolamine Mesylate). A white or off-white, odourless crystalline powder. Soluble 1 in 1 of water, 1 in 4 of alcohol, and 1 in 700 of chloroform. Its solutions in water have a pH of about 5 and slowly deteriorate. Store in airtight containers at a temperature of 25°, excursions permitted between 15° and 30°. Protect from light.

## Adverse Effects and Treatment

The adverse effects of phentolamine are primarily due to its alpha-adrenoceptor blocking activity and include orthostatic hypotension and tachycardia. Myocardial infarction and cerebrovascular spasm or occlusion have been reported occasionally, usually in association with marked hypotension; flushing, sweating, and feelings of apprehension may accompany hypotensive episodes. Anginal pain and arrhythmias have been reported rarely. Nausea, vomiting, and diarrhoea may also occur. Other side-effects include weakness, dizziness, flushing, and nasal congestion. Hypoglycaemia has been reported following overdosage.

Severe hypotension may occur in overdosage although phentolamine has a short duration of action. Treatment may include support of the circulation by postural measures and parenteral fluid volume replacement. Noradrenaline may be administered cautiously to overcome alpha-adrenoceptor blockade. Adrenaline is contra-indicated since it also stimulates beta receptors causing increased hypotension and tachycardia.

When injected into the corpus cavernosum of the penis phentolamine has been associated with local pain; induration and fibrosis may occur with repeated use. Priapism has occurred.

## Precautions

Phentolamine should not generally be given to patients with angina pectoris or other evidence of ischaemic heart disease. Care should be taken in patients with peptic ulcer disease, which may be exacerbated.

## Interactions

Since phentolamine only blocks alpha receptors, use with drugs such as adrenaline may lead to severe hypotension and tachycardia due to unopposed beta-adrenoceptor stimulation.

## Pharmacokinetics

Following intravenous administration, the half-life of phentolamine has been reported to be 19 minutes. It is extensively metabolised and about 13% of an intravenous dose is excreted unchanged in the urine.

## Uses and Administration

Phentolamine is an alpha-adrenoceptor blocker (p.809) which also has a direct action on vascular smooth muscle. It produces vasodilatation, an increase in cardiac output, and has a positive inotropic effect, but is reported to have little effect on the blood pressure of patients with essential hypertension. The alpha-receptor blocking action is reversible ('competitive') and non-selective, and the duration of effect is relatively short.

Phentolamine is given in the management of hypertensive crises, particularly those due to excessive catecholamine release associated with surgery for phaeochromocytoma (p.831). It has been employed for the differential diagnosis of phaeochromocytoma, but has largely been superseded by estimations of catecholamines in blood and urine.

Phentolamine is also used to prevent or treat dermal necrosis and sloughing associated with the intravenous infusion or extravasation of noradrenaline. It has been used in the treatment of erectile dysfunction (p.1745).

Phentolamine is given by injection as the mesilate.

In patients with hypertensive crises during surgery for **phaeochromocytoma**, a dose of 2 to 5 mg of phentolamine mesilate is given intravenously and repeated if necessary; blood pressure should be monitored. A dose of 1 mg intravenously is used for children. The intramuscular route may be used pre-operatively and for diagnostic procedures.

For prevention of **dermal necrosis** during intravenous infusion of noradrenaline, 10 mg of phentolamine mesilate is added to each litre of solution containing noradrenaline. For treatment following extravasation of noradrenaline, 5 to 10 mg of phentolamine mesilate in 10 mL of sodium chloride 0.9% is injected into the affected area.

Injection of phentolamine mesilate, usually in association with papaverine, into the corpora cavernosa of the penis, has been used in the treatment of **erectile dysfunction**. Other approaches that have been used include administration by the oral route and intracavernosal use in combination with vasoactive intestinal polypeptide.

**Hyperhidrosis.** Hyperhidrosis (p.1136) is usually treated with topical aluminium salts or topical antimuscarinics, but intradermal botulinum A toxin or procedures such as endoscopic transthoracic sympathectomy may be needed in severe cases. Phentolamine has been tried as an alternative. Improvement in symptoms has been reported[1] in 2 patients with generalised hyperhidrosis given 100 mg of phentolamine mesilate by intravenous infusion over 6 hours. Improvement lasted for 2 to 3 months and the infusion was repeated, in 1 patient several times.

1. McCleane G. The use of intravenous phentolamine mesilate in the treatment of hyperhidrosis. *Br J Dermatol* 2002; **146:** 533–4.

**Pancreatic pain.** Pain due to pancreatitis (p.7) is usually treated with opioid analgesics. Long-term relief of pain has been reported in a patient with chronic pancreatitis following an intravenous infusion of phentolamine.[1]

1. McCleane GJ. Phentolamine abolishes the pain of chronic pancreatitis. *Br J Hosp Med* 1996; **55:** 521.

## Preparations

***BP 2003:*** Phentolamine Injection;
***USP 27:*** Phentolamine Mesylate for Injection.

**Proprietary Preparations** (details are given in Part 3)
***Arg.:*** Regitina; ***Austral.:*** Regitine; ***Belg.:*** Regitine; ***Braz.:*** Herivyl; Regitina; Vasomax†; ***Canad.:*** Rogitine; ***Denm.:*** Regitin; ***Gr.:*** Regitine; ***Hong Kong:*** Q-Tech†; ***Israel:*** Regitine; ***Mex.:*** Z-Max; ***Neth.:*** Regitine; ***NZ:*** Regitine; ***S.Afr.:*** Regitine; ***Switz.:*** Regitine; ***UK:*** Rogitine; ***USA:*** Regitine†.

**Multi-ingredient:** ***Austria:*** Androskat; ***Neth.:*** Androskat.

---

# Pholedrine Sulfate *(rINNM)*

Isodrine Sulphate; Pholedrine Sulphate *(BANM)*; Sulfato de foledrina; Sympropaminum (pholedrine). 4-(2-Methylaminopropyl)phenol sulfate.

$(C_{10}H_{15}NO)_2,H_2SO_4$ = 428.5.

*CAS — 370-14-9 (pholedrine); 6114-26-7 (pholedrine sulfate).*

## Profile

Pholedrine is a sympathomimetic (see Adrenaline, p.852) given by mouth as the sulfate in combination with other drugs in the treatment of hypotensive states. It is also an ingredient of preparations promoted for vascular disorders.

## Preparations

**Proprietary Preparations** (details are given in Part 3)
**Multi-ingredient:** ***Ger.:*** Adyston; Zellaforte N Plus; ***Spain:*** Venosan†; ***Switz.:*** Ortho-Maren retard; Venosan†.

---

# Phytosterol

Phytosterolum.

**Pharmacopoeias.** In *Eur.* (see p.vi).

**Ph. Eur. 5.0** (Phytosterol). A natural mixture of sterols obtained from plants of the genera *Hypoxis, Pinus,* and *Picea*. It contains not less than 70% β-sitosterol, calculated with reference to the dried substance. A white or almost white powder. Practically insoluble in water; soluble in tetrahydrofuran; sparingly soluble in ethyl acetate. Store in airtight containers. Protect from light.

## Sitosterol

β-Sitosterin; β-Sitosterol. Stigmast-5-en-3β-ol.

$C_{29}H_{50}O$ = 414.7.

*CAS — 83-46-5.*

## Profile

Phytosterols include plant sterols and their hydrogenation compounds, plant stanols (see Stanol Esters, p.1448). Sitosterol, one of the most common naturally occurring phytosterols, is used as a lipid regulating drug in the treatment of hyperlipidaemias (p.823). The usual dose is 3 to 6 g daily in divided doses by mouth. Sitosterol has been incorporated into margarine for use in the dietary management of hypercholesterolaemia.

It is also used in benign prostatic hyperplasia (p.1555) in usual initial doses of 20 mg three times daily by mouth reducing to 10 mg three times daily for long-term therapy.

◊ References.

1. Berges RR, *et al.* Randomised, placebo-controlled, double-blind clinical trial of β-sitosterol in patients with benign prostatic hyperplasia. *Lancet* 1995; **345:** 1529–32.
2. Klippel KF, *et al.* A multicentric, placebo-controlled, double-blind clinical trial of β-sitosterol (phytosterol) for the treatment of benign prostatic hyperplasia. *Br J Urol* 1997; **80:** 427–32.
3. Wilt TJ, *et al.* β-Sitosterol for the treatment of benign prostatic hyperplasia: a systematic review. *BJU Int* 1999; **83:** 976–83.
4. Wilt T, *et al.* Beta-sitosterols for benign prostatic hyperplasia. Available in The Cochrane Library; Issue 2. Chichester: John Wiley; 2004.

## Preparations

**Proprietary Preparations** (details are given in Part 3)
***Arg.:*** Prostacur; ***Austria:*** Harzol; ***Ger.:*** Azuprostat; Flemun; Harzol; Lipositt†; LP-Truw mono†; Prostasal; Sito-Lande; Triastonal; ***Thai.:*** Mebo; ***UAE:*** Mebo.

**Multi-ingredient:** ***Arg.:*** Cholesterol Reducing Plan; ***UK:*** Cholasitrol†; Kolestop; Lestrin; ***USA:*** Beta Prostate; Better Cholesterol; Better Prostate; Cholesterol Support; Prostate Support.

---

# Picotamide *(BAN)*

G-137; Picotamida; Picotamidum Monohydricum. 4-Methoxy-*N,N'*-bis(3-pyridinylmethyl)-1,3-benzenedicarboxamide monohydrate.

$C_{21}H_{20}N_4O_3,H_2O$ = 394.4.

*CAS — 32828-81-2 (anhydrous picotamide); 80530-63-8 (picotamide monohydrate).*

*ATC — B01AC03.*

**Pharmacopoeias.** In *Eur.* (see p.vi).

**Ph. Eur. 5.0** (Picotamide Monohydrate). A white or almost white, polymorphic, crystalline powder. Slightly soluble in water; soluble in dehydrated alcohol and in dichloromethane; dissolves in dilute mineral acids.

## Profile

Picotamide is a thromboxane synthase inhibitor and thromboxane receptor antagonist with antiplatelet activity. It is given by mouth in thromboembolic disorders (p.837) in initial doses of

900 to 1200 mg daily in divided doses, reducing to a maintenance dose of 300 to 600 mg daily.

**ACE inhibitor-induced cough.** Cough is a recognised adverse effect of ACE inhibitor administration and has been treated with a number of drugs (see p.843). Administration of picotamide led to the disappearance of cough in 8 of 9 patients receiving enalapril for hypertension,[1] suggesting that thromboxanes may be involved in the aetiology of ACE inhibitor-induced cough.

1. Malini PL, *et al.* Thromboxane antagonism and cough induced by angiotensin-converting-enzyme inhibitor. *Lancet* 1997; **350:** 15–18.

### Preparations

**Proprietary Preparations** (details are given in Part 3)
***Ital.:*** Plactidil.

## Pilsicainide Hydrochloride *(rINNM)*

Hidrocloruro de pilsicainida; SUN-1165. Tetrahydro-1*H*-pyrrolizine-7a(5*H*)-aceto-2′,6′-xylidide hydrochloride.

$C_{17}H_{24}N_2O,HCl = 308.8.$

*CAS — 88069-67-4 (pilsicainide); 88069-49-2 (pilsicainide hydrochloride).*

### Profile

Pilsicainide hydrochloride is an antiarrhythmic with class Ic activity (p.809).

◊ References.

1. Takabatake T, *et al.* Pharmacokinetics of SUN 1165, a new antiarrhythmic agent, in renal dysfunction. *Eur J Clin Pharmacol* 1991; **40:** 411–14.
2. Okishige K, *et al.* Pilsicainide for conversion and maintenance of sinus rhythm in chronic atrial fibrillation: a placebo-controlled, multicenter study. *Am Heart J* 2000; **140:** 437–44.
3. Kumagai K, *et al.* Single oral administration of pilsicainide versus infusion of disopyramide for termination of paroxysmal atrial fibrillation: a multicenter trial. *Pacing Clin Electrophysiol* 2000; **23:** 1880–2.

### Preparations

**Proprietary Preparations** (details are given in Part 3)
***Jpn:*** Sunrythm.

## Pimobendan *(USAN, rINN)*

Pimobendán; UDCG-115. 4,5-Dihydro-6-[2-(*p*-methyoxyphenyl)-5-benzimidazolyl]-5-methyl-3(2*H*)-pyridazinone.

$C_{19}H_{18}N_4O_2 = 334.4.$

*CAS — 74150-27-9; 118428-36-7.*

### Profile

Pimobendan is a phosphodiesterase inhibitor with calcium-sensitising properties. It has positive inotropic and vasodilator activity and is used as an adjunct to standard therapy in the management of heart failure (p.820). It is given orally in a dose of 1.25 to 2.5 mg twice daily.

Studies with other inotropic phosphodiesterase inhibitors have shown that their prolonged oral use can lead to an increased mortality rate.

◊ References.

1. Przechera M, *et al.* Pharmacokinetic profile and tolerability of pimobendan in patients with terminal renal insufficiency. *Eur J Clin Pharmacol* 1991; **40:** 107–11.
2. The Pimobendan in Congestive Heart Failure (PICO) Investigators. Effect of pimobendan on exercise capacity in patients with heart failure: main results from the Pimobendan in Congestive Heart Failure (PICO) trial. *Heart* 1996; **76:** 223–31.
3. Yoshikawa T, *et al.* Effectiveness of carvedilol alone versus carvedilol + pimobendan for severe congestive heart failure. *Am J Cardiol* 2000; **85:** 1495–7.
4. The EPOCH Study Group. Effects of pimobendan on adverse cardiac events and physical activities in patients with mild to moderate chronic heart failure: the effects of pimobendan on chronic heart failure study (EPOCH study). *Circ J* 2002; **66:** 149–57.

### Preparations

**Proprietary Preparations** (details are given in Part 3)
***Jpn:*** Acardi.

## Pinacidil *(USAN, rINN)*

P-1134. (±)-2-Cyano-1-(4-pyridyl)-3-(1,2,2-trimethylpropyl)guanidine.

$C_{13}H_{19}N_5 = 245.3.$

*CAS — 60560-33-0 (anhydrous pinacidil); 85371-64-8 (pinacidil monohydrate).*

*ATC — C02DG01.*

### Profile

Pinacidil is a potassium-channel opener (p.812) that produces direct peripheral vasodilatation of the arterioles. It has been used in the management of hypertension. It reduces blood pressure and peripheral resistance and produces fluid retention. Tachycardia and an increase in cardiac output occur mainly as a reflex response to the reduction in peripheral resistance.

◊ Reviews.

1. Friedel HA, Brogden RN. Pinacidil: a review of its pharmacodynamic and pharmacokinetic properties, and therapeutic potential in the treatment of hypertension. *Drugs* 1990; **39:** 929–67.

### Preparations

**Proprietary Preparations** (details are given in Part 3)
***Denm.:*** Pindac†.

## Pindolol *(BAN, USAN, rINN)*

LB-46; Pindololum; Prindolol; Prinodolol. 1-(Indol-4-yloxy)-3-isopropylaminopropan-2-ol.

$C_{14}H_{20}N_2O_2 = 248.3.$

*CAS — 13523-86-9.*

*ATC — C07AA03.*

**Pharmacopoeias.** In *Chin., Eur.* (see p.vi), *Jpn, Pol.,* and *US.*

**Ph. Eur. 5.0** (Pindolol). A white or almost white, crystalline powder. Practically insoluble in water; slightly soluble in methyl alcohol; dissolves in dilute mineral acids. Protect from light.

**USP 27** (Pindolol). A white to off-white, crystalline powder with a faint odour. Practically insoluble in water; very slightly soluble in chloroform; slightly soluble in methyl alcohol. Protect from light.

### Adverse Effects, Treatment, and Precautions

As for Beta Blockers, p.869.

**Effects on lipid metabolism.** Beta blockers can affect plasma-lipid concentrations, although these effects may be less pronounced with beta blockers having intrinsic sympathomimetic activity (p.869). Use of pindolol in patients with hypertension is not associated with any increases in total plasma-cholesterol concentrations or falls in high-density lipoprotein fraction.[1,2]

1. Hunter Hypertension Research Group. Effects of pindolol, or a pindolol/clopamide combination preparation, on plasma lipid levels in essential hypertension. *Med J Aust* 1989; **150:** 646–52.
2. Terént A, *et al.* Long-term effect of pindolol on lipids and lipoproteins in men with newly diagnosed hypertension. *Eur J Clin Pharmacol* 1989; **36:** 347–50.

**Tremor.** Fine tremor in the extremities of 5 patients during pindolol therapy was considered to have been due to its partial agonist activity.[1]

1. Hod H, *et al.* Pindolol-induced tremor. *Postgrad Med J* 1980; **56:** 346–7.

### Interactions

The interactions associated with beta blockers are discussed on p.870.

### Pharmacokinetics

Pindolol is almost completely absorbed from the gastrointestinal tract and peak plasma concentrations are obtained about 1 to 2 hours after an oral dose. It has a bioavailability of about 87%. About 40 to 60% is reported to be bound to plasma proteins. It is moderately lipid-soluble. Pindolol crosses the placenta and is distributed into breast milk. It is only partially metabolised in the liver and is excreted in the urine both unchanged and in the form of metabolites. A plasma elimination half-life of 3 to 4 hours has been reported in healthy adults. The half-life may be prolonged in elderly hypertensive patients and in patients with renal or hepatic impairment.

### Uses and Administration

Pindolol is a non-cardioselective beta blocker (p.868). It is reported to have intrinsic sympathomimetic activity but little membrane-stabilising activity.

Pindolol is used in the management of hypertension (p.825), angina pectoris (p.813), and other cardiovascular disorders. It is also used in glaucoma (p.1485).

In **hypertension** pindolol is usually given initially in a dosage of 5 mg two or three times daily, or 15 mg once daily, by mouth, subsequently increased according to response. The usual maintenance dose is 15 to 30 mg once daily, but up to 45 mg daily, as a single dose or in divided doses, may be required. Additional benefit is rarely obtained from doses higher than 45 mg daily, although doses up to 60 mg daily have been given.

The usual dose for **angina pectoris** is 2.5 to 5 mg up to three times daily; however, doses of up to 40 mg daily have been used.

Eye drops containing pindolol 1% are used in the management of **glaucoma.**

**Psychiatric disorders.** Pindolol has been studied[1-4] as an augmentation agent with serotonergic antidepressants in the treatment of refractory depression (p.279). Positive results have also been reported[5] with pindolol augmentation in a small study in patients with obsessive-compulsive disorder (p.663) resistant to paroxetine. Another study[6] found that pindolol augmentation of antipsychotic therapy reduced aggression in patients with schizophrenia (p.665).

1. Artigas F, *et al.* Pindolol induces a rapid improvement of depressed patients treated with serotonin reuptake inhibitors. *Arch Gen Psychiatry* 1994; **51:** 248–51.
2. Blier P, Bergeron R. Effectiveness of pindolol with selected antidepressant drugs in the treatment of major depression. *J Clin Psychopharmacol* 1995; **15:** 217–22.
3. Pérez V, *et al.* Randomised, double-blind, placebo-controlled trial of pindolol in combination with fluoxetine antidepressant treatment. *Lancet* 1997; **349:** 1594–7.
4. Maes M, *et al.* Pindolol and mianserin augment the antidepressant activity of fluoxetine in hospitalized major depressed patients, including those with treatment resistance. *J Clin Psychopharmacol* 1999; **19:** 177–82.
5. Dannon PN, *et al.* Pindolol augmentation in treatment-resistant obsessive compulsive disorder: a double-blind placebo controlled trial. *Eur Neuropsychopharmacol* 2000; **10:** 165–9.
6. Caspi N, *et al.* Pindolol augmentation in aggressive schizophrenic patients: a double-blind crossover randomized study. *Int Clin Psychopharmacol* 2001; **16:** 111–5.

### Preparations

***BP 2003:*** Pindolol Tablets;
***USP 27:*** Pindolol Tablets.

**Proprietary Preparations** (details are given in Part 3)
***Austral.:*** Barbloc; Visken; ***Austria:*** Visken; ***Belg.:*** Visken; ***Braz.:*** Visken; ***Canad.:*** Apo-Pindol; Novo-Pindol; Nu-Pindol; Visken; ***Denm.:*** Hexapindol; Visken; ***Fin.:*** Pindocor; Pinloc; Visken; ***Fr.:*** Visken; ***Ger.:*** durapindol; Glauco-Stulln; Pindoptan†; Pindoreal†; Visken; ***Gr.:*** Visken; ***Hong Kong:*** Visken; ***India:*** Visken; ***Irl.:*** Visken; ***Israel:*** Pinden; Visken†; ***Ital.:*** Visken; ***Mex.:*** Visken; ***Neth.:*** Visken; ***Norw.:*** Hexapindol†; ***NZ:*** Pindol; Visken†; Vypen†; ***S.Afr.:*** Visken†; ***Swed.:*** Hexapindol†; Visken; ***Switz.:*** Betapindol†; Viskene; ***Thai.:*** Pinsken†; ***UK:*** Visken; ***USA:*** Visken.

**Multi-ingredient:** ***Austria:*** Viskaldix; Viskenit; ***Belg.:*** Viskaldix; ***Braz.:*** Viskaldix; ***Canad.:*** Viskazide; ***Chile:*** Viskaldix; ***Fr.:*** Viskaldix; ***Ger.:*** Viskaldix; ***Irl.:*** Viskaldix; ***Malaysia:*** Viskaldix; ***Neth.:*** Viskaldix; ***NZ:*** Viskaldix†; ***Switz.:*** Viskaldix; ***Thai.:*** Viskaldix; ***UK:*** Viskaldix.

## Pipratecol *(rINN)*

711-SE. 1-(3,4-Dihydroxyphenyl)-2-[4-(2-methoxyphenyl)piperazin-1-yl]ethanol.

$C_{19}H_{24}N_2O_4 = 344.4.$

*CAS — 15534-05-1.*

### Profile

Pipratecol is a vasodilator that has been given in conjunction with raubasine (p.994) in the treatment of cerebrovascular disorders.

## Piretanide *(BAN, USAN, rINN)*

Hoe-118; Piretanida; Piretanidum; S73-4118. 4-Phenoxy-3-(pyrrolidin-1-yl)-5-sulphamoylbenzoic acid.

$C_{17}H_{18}N_2O_5S = 362.4.$

*CAS — 55837-27-9.*

*ATC — C03CA03.*

**Pharmacopoeias.** In *Eur.* (see p.vi).

**Ph. Eur. 5.0** (Piretanide). A yellowish-white to yellowish powder. It exhibits polymorphism. Very slightly soluble in water; sparingly soluble in dehydrated alcohol. Protect from light.

### Adverse Effects

As for Furosemide, p.919. Muscle cramps have been reported following high doses of piretanide.

### Precautions

Piretanide's precautions and contra-indications, which are dependent on its effects on fluid and electrolyte balance, are similar to those of the thiazide diuretics (see Hydrochlorothiazide, p.935). Patients with impaired micturition or prostatic hyperplasia may develop retention of urine with piretanide.

### Interactions

As for Furosemide, p.920.

### Pharmacokinetics

Piretanide has been reported to be almost completely absorbed following oral administration. It is extensively bound to plasma proteins, and is reported to have a half-life of about 1 hour after an oral dose.

◊ References.

1. Beermann B, Grind M. Clinical pharmacokinetics of some newer diuretics. *Clin Pharmacokinet* 1987; **13:** 254–66.

### Uses and Administration

Piretanide is a loop diuretic with actions and uses similar to those of furosemide (p.921). It is used for oedema, including that associated with heart failure (p.820), in doses of 3 to 6 mg daily by mouth. In the treatment of hypertension (p.825) it is given in a usual dose of 6 to 12 mg daily by mouth. The sodium salt is given by injection.

◊ References.

1. Clissold SP, Brogden RN. Piretanide: a preliminary review of its pharmacodynamic and pharmacokinetic properties, and therapeutic efficacy. *Drugs* 1985; **29:** 489–530.

### Preparations

**Proprietary Preparations** (details are given in Part 3)
***Austria:*** Arelix; ***Braz.:*** Arelix; ***Fr.:*** Eurelix; ***Ger.:*** Arelix; ***Irl.:*** Arelix; ***Ital.:*** Tauliz; ***Mex.:*** Diural; ***S.Afr.:*** Arelix; ***Spain:*** Perbilen; ***Switz.:*** Arelix.
**Multi-ingredient:** ***Austria:*** Trialix; ***Ger.:*** Arelix ACE; Aretensin; Betarelix; ***Irl.:*** Trialix; ***Ital.:*** Prilace; ***Switz.:*** Trialix.

## Pirifibrate *(rINN)*

EL-466; Pirifibrato. 6-Hydroxymethyl-2-pyridylmethyl 2-(4-chlorophenoxy)-2-methylpropionate.
$C_{17}H_{18}ClNO_4$ = 335.8.
*CAS — 55285-45-5.*

### Profile

Pirifibrate, a fibric acid derivative (see Bezafibrate, p.873), is a lipid regulating drug that has been used in the treatment of hyperlipidaemias.

### Preparations

**Proprietary Preparations** (details are given in Part 3)
***Spain:*** Bratenol†.

## Pirmenol Hydrochloride *(USAN, rINNM)*

CI-845; Hidrocloruro de pirmenol. (±)-*cis*-2,6-Dimethyl-α-phenyl-α-2-pyridyl-1-piperidinebutanol hydrochloride.
$C_{22}H_{30}N_2O,HCl$ = 374.9.
*CAS — 68252-19-7 (pirmenol); 61477-94-9 (pirmenol hydrochloride).*

### Profile

Pirmenol hydrochloride is an antiarrhythmic with class Ia activity (p.809).

◊ References.

1. Hampton EM, *et al.* Initial and long-term outpatient experience with pirmenol for control of ventricular arrhythmias. *Eur J Clin Pharmacol* 1986; **31:** 15–22.
2. Stringer KA, *et al.* Enhanced pirmenol elimination by rifampin. *J Clin Pharmacol* 1988; **28:** 1094–7.
3. Janiczek N, *et al.* Pharmacokinetics of pirmenol enantiomers and pharmacodynamics of pirmenol racemate in patients with premature ventricular contractions. *J Clin Pharmacol* 1997; **37:** 502–13.

## Pirozadil *(rINN)*

722-D. 2,6-Pyridinediyldimethylene bis(3,4,5-trimethoxybenzoate).
$C_{27}H_{29}NO_{10}$ = 527.5.
*CAS — 54110-25-7.*

### Profile

Pirozadil, a nicotinic acid derivative, is a lipid regulating drug that has been used in the treatment of hyperlipidaemias.

### Preparations

**Proprietary Preparations** (details are given in Part 3)
***Spain:*** Pemix†.

## Pitavastatin *(rINN)*

Itavastatin; Nisvastatin; NK-104. (3*R*,5*S*,6*E*)-7-[2-Cyclopropyl-4-(*p*-fluorophenyl)-3-quinolyl]-3,5-dihydroxy-6-heptenoic acid.
$C_{25}H_{24}FNO_4$ = 421.5.
*CAS — 147511-69-1 (pitavastatin); 147526-32-7 (pitavastatin calcium).*

### Profile

Pitavastatin, a hydroxymethylglutaryl coenzyme A (HMG-CoA) reductase inhibitor (a statin), is a lipid regulating drug with similar properties to simvastatin (p.997). It is used as the calcium salt in the treatment of hyperlipidaemias.

## Plasminogen *(BAN)*

Plasminógeno.
*CAS — 9001-91-6.*

### Profile

Plasminogen is the specific substance derived from plasma which, when activated to plasmin, has the property of lysing fibrinogen, fibrin, and some other proteins. Its role in the control of haemostasis is described further on p.735. Plasminogen has been investigated as a thrombolytic and has been used in combination with other blood products in wound-sealant preparations.

### Preparations

**Proprietary Preparations** (details are given in Part 3)
**Multi-ingredient:** ***Arg.:*** Tissucol Duo Quick; ***Austria:*** Tissucol; Tissucol Duo Quick; ***Canad.:*** Tisseel; ***Denm.:*** Tisseel Duo Quick; ***Fin.:*** Tisseel Duo Quick; ***Fr.:*** Tissucol; ***Ger.:*** Tissucol Duo S; Tissucol Fibrinkleber tiefgefroren†; Tissucol-Kit; ***Hong Kong:*** Tisseel; ***Israel:*** Tisseel; ***Spain:*** Tissucol Duo; ***Swed.:*** Tisseel Duo Quick; ***Switz.:*** Tissucol; Tissucol Duo S; ***UK:*** Tisseel.

## Policosanol

*CAS — 142583-61-7.*
*ATC — C10AX08.*

### Profile

Policosanol is a mixture of higher primary aliphatic alcohols isolated from sugar cane wax; the main component is octacosanol ($C_{28}H_{58}O$ = 410.8). Policosanol has been used in the treatment of hypercholesterolaemias.

◊ References.

1. Gouni-Berthold I, Berthold HK. Policosanol: clinical pharmacology and therapeutic significance of a new lipid-lowering agent. *Am Heart J* 2002; **143:** 356–65.
2. Pepping J. Policosanol. *Am J Health-Syst Pharm* 2003; **60:** 1112–5.

### Preparations

**Proprietary Preparations** (details are given in Part 3)
***Arg.:*** Lipex; ***Chile:*** PPG; ***Mex.:*** PPG-5†; ***USA:*** Cholestin.

## Polythiazide *(BAN, USAN, rINN)*

NSC-108161; P-2525; Politiazida. 6-Chloro-3,4-dihydro-2-methyl-3-(2,2,2-trifluoroethylthiomethyl)-2*H*-1,2,4-benzothiadiazine-7-sulphonamide 1,1-dioxide.
$C_{11}H_{13}ClF_3N_3O_4S_3$ = 439.9.
*CAS — 346-18-9.*
*ATC — C03AA05.*

**Pharmacopoeias.** In *Br.*

**BP 2003** (Polythiazide). A white or almost white, crystalline powder with an alliaceous odour. Practically insoluble in water and in chloroform; sparingly soluble in alcohol.

### Adverse Effects, Treatment, and Precautions

As for Hydrochlorothiazide, p.933.

### Interactions

As for Hydrochlorothiazide, p.935.

### Pharmacokinetics

Polythiazide is fairly readily absorbed from the gastrointestinal tract. The estimated plasma elimination half-life of about 26 hours. More than 80% may be bound to plasma proteins. It is excreted mainly in the urine as unchanged polythiazide and metabolites.

◊ References.

1. Hobbs DC, Twomey TM. Kinetics of polythiazide. *Clin Pharmacol Ther* 1978; **23:** 241–6.

### Uses and Administration

Polythiazide is a thiazide diuretic with actions and uses similar to those of hydrochlorothiazide (p.935). It is used for hypertension (p.825), and for oedema, including that associated with heart failure (p.820).

Diuresis is initiated within about 2 hours after administration, and lasts for 24 to 48 hours.

In the treatment of **hypertension** the usual dose is stated to be 2 to 4 mg daily, either alone or with other antihypertensives although doses of only 0.5 to 1 mg may be adequate. In the treatment of **oedema** the usual dose is 1 to 4 mg by mouth daily.

### Preparations

***BP 2003:*** Polythiazide Tablets.
**Proprietary Preparations** (details are given in Part 3)
***Belg.:*** Renese; ***Irl.:*** Nephril†; ***UK:*** Nephril†; ***USA:*** Renese†.
**Multi-ingredient:** ***Ger.:*** Polypress; ***USA:*** Minizide; Renese R.

## Potassium Canrenoate *(BANM, rINN)*

Aldadiene Potassium; Canrenoate Potassium *(USAN)*; Canrenoato de potasio; MF-465a; SC-14266. Potassium 17-hydroxy-3-oxo-17α-pregna-4,6-diene-21-carboxylate.
$C_{22}H_{29}KO_4$ = 396.6.
*CAS — 4138-96-9 (canrenoic acid); 2181-04-6 (potassium canrenoate).*
*ATC — C03DA02.*

**Pharmacopoeias.** In *Jpn.*

### Adverse Effects and Precautions

As for Spironolactone, p.1003. Irritation or pain may occur at the site of injection.

**Effects on endocrine function.** A lower incidence of gynaecomastia has been reported in patients with hepatic cirrhosis and ascites during use of potassium canrenoate than with equivalent doses of spironolactone,[1] and spironolactone-induced gynaecomastia disappeared when spironolactone was replaced by potassium canrenoate in a patient with hyperaldosteronism.[2] This suggests that metabolites other than canrenone (a common metabolite of both canrenoate and spironolactone thought to be responsible for their activity) or possibly spironolactone itself may be responsible for the anti-androgenic effects of spironolactone.[3,4]

1. Bellati G, Idéo G. Gynaecomastia after spironolactone and potassium canrenoate. *Lancet* 1986; **i:** 626.
2. Dupont A. Disappearance of spironolactone-induced gynaecomastia during treatment with potassium canrenoate. *Lancet* 1985; **ii:** 731.
3. Gardiner P. Spironolactone and potassium canrenoate metabolism. *Lancet* 1985; **ii:** 1432.
4. Overdiek JWPM, Merkus FWHM. Spironolactone metabolism and gynaecomastia. *Lancet* 1986; **i:** 1103.

### Interactions

As for Spironolactone, p.1004.

### Uses and Administration

Potassium canrenoate is a potassium-sparing diuretic with actions and uses similar to those of spironolactone (p.1004). Canrenone (p.879) is a metabolite common to both drugs, but its contribution to the pharmacological action is unclear. Potassium canrenoate is used in the treatment of refractory oedema associated with heart failure (p.820) or hepatic disease when an injectable aldosterone antagonist is required. It may be given in doses of 200 to 400 mg daily, increasing to 800 mg daily in exceptional cases; it is given by slow intravenous injection over a period of 2 to 3 minutes for each 200 mg or by intravenous infusion in glucose 5% or sodium chloride 0.9%.

### Preparations

**Proprietary Preparations** (details are given in Part 3)
***Austria:*** Aldactone; Osiren†; ***Belg.:*** Canrenol; Soldactone; ***Denm.:*** Soldactone†; ***Fin.:*** Soldactone†; ***Fr.:*** Soludactone; ***Ger.:*** Aldactone; Kalium-Can; Osyrol; ***Ital.:*** Diurek; Kanrenol; Luvion; Venactone; ***Neth.:*** Soldactone; ***Norw.:*** Soldactone; ***Swed.:*** Soldactone†; ***Switz.:*** Soldactone; Spiroctan†.
**Multi-ingredient:** ***Ital.:*** Kadiur.

## Prajmalium Bitartrate *(BAN, rINN)*

Bitartrato de prajmalio; GT-1012; NPAB; Prajmaline Bitartrate. *N*-Propylajmalinium hydrogen tartrate.
$C_{23}H_{33}N_2O_2,C_4H_5O_6$ = 518.6.
*CAS — 35080-11-6 (prajmalium); 2589-47-1 (prajmalium bitartrate).*
*ATC — C01BA08.*

### Adverse Effects and Precautions

As for Ajmaline, p.856.

**Effects on the liver.** Cholestatic jaundice associated with pruritus, chills, and eosinophilia[1] was attributed to an allergic reaction to prajmalium bitartrate in a patient 20 days after the start of treatment.

1. Rotmensch HH, *et al.* Cholestatic jaundice: an immune response to prajmalium bitartrate. *Postgrad Med J* 1980; **56:** 738–41.

**Effects on mental state.** Confusion and disorientation in time and place[1] occurred on 2 occasions in a 67-year-old man given prajmalium bitartrate 100 mg daily for the control of tachycardia; the confusion rapidly disappeared when prajmalium was withdrawn.

1. Lessing JB, Copperman IJ. Severe cerebral confusion produced by prajmalium bitartrate. *BMJ* 1977; **2:** 675.

### Uses and Administration

Prajmalium is a class I antiarrhythmic (p.809) and is the *N*-propyl derivative of ajmaline (p.856). It is given by mouth as the bitartrate in the management of supraventricular and ventricular arrhythmias (p.816) in initial doses of 60 to 80 mg daily. Maintenance doses of 20 to 40 mg daily in divided doses are used.

### Preparations

**Proprietary Preparations** (details are given in Part 3)
***Austria:*** Neo-Gilurytmal; ***Ger.:*** Neo-Gilurytmal; ***Israel:*** Neo-Gilurythmal; Neorythmin†; ***Ital.:*** Neo Aritmina†; ***Spain:*** Neo-Gilurytmal†.
**Multi-ingredient:** ***Spain:*** Cresophene.

## Pravastatin Sodium *(BANM, USAN, rINNM)*

CS-514; Eptastatin Sodium; 3β-Hydroxycompactin Sodium; Pravastatina sódica; Pravastatinum Natricum; SQ-31000. Sodium (3*R*,5*R*)-7-{(1*S*,2*S*,6*S*,8*S*,8a*R*)-1,2,6,7,8,8a-hexahydro-6-hydroxy-2-methyl-8-[(*S*)-2-methylbutyryloxy]-1-naphthyl}-3,5-dihydroxyheptanoate.
$C_{23}H_{35}O_7Na$ = 446.5.
*CAS — 81093-37-0 (pravastatin); 81131-70-6 (pravastatin sodium).*

**Pharmacopoeias.** In *Eur.* (see p.vi).

**Ph. Eur. 5.0** (Pravastatin Sodium). A white to yellowish-white, hygroscopic, powder or crystalline powder. Freely soluble in water and in methyl alcohol; soluble in dehydrated alcohol. A 5% solution in water has a pH of 7.2 to 9.0. Store in airtight containers.

### Adverse Effects and Precautions

As for Simvastatin, p.997.

### Interactions

The interactions of statins with other drugs are described under simvastatin (p.998). Pravastatin is not significantly metabolised by the cytochrome P450 enzyme system and does not have the same interactions with enzyme inhibitors as simvastatin, although caution has been advised when such combinations are used.

**Pharmacokinetics**

Pravastatin, unlike simvastatin or lovastatin, is active without the need for hydrolysis. It is rapidly but incompletely absorbed from the gastrointestinal tract and undergoes extensive first-pass metabolism in the liver, its primary site of action. The absolute bioavailability of pravastatin is 17%. Approximately 50% of the circulating drug is bound to plasma proteins. The plasma elimination half-life of pravastatin is 1.5 to 2 hours. About 70% of an oral dose of pravastatin is excreted in the faeces, as unabsorbed drug and via the bile, and about 20% is excreted in the urine.

◊ General reviews.

1. Quion JAV, Jones PH. Clinical pharmacokinetics of pravastatin. *Clin Pharmacokinet* 1994; **27:** 94–103.
2. Hatanaka T. Clinical pharmacokinetics of pravastatin: mechanisms of pharmacokinetic events. *Clin Pharmacokinet* 2000; **39:** 397–412.

## Uses and Administration

Pravastatin, a 3-hydroxy-3-methylglutaryl coenzyme A (HMG-CoA) reductase inhibitor (a statin), is a lipid regulating drug with actions on plasma lipids similar to those of simvastatin (p.999).

Pravastatin is used to reduce LDL-cholesterol, apolipoprotein B, and triglycerides, and to increase HDL-cholesterol in the treatment of hyperlipidaemias (p.823), including hypercholesterolaemias and combined (mixed) hyperlipidaemia (type IIa or IIb hyperlipoproteinaemias), hypertriglyceridaemia (type IV), and dysbetalipoproteinaemia (type III). It is also given prophylactically to hypercholesterolaemic patients for both primary and secondary prevention of ischaemic heart disease. It is also used in patients with a previous myocardial infarction or unstable angina to reduce the risk of stroke.

Pravastatin is given by mouth as the sodium salt in usual doses of 10 to 40 mg once daily at bedtime. The dose may be adjusted, according to response, at intervals of not less than 4 weeks, to a maximum dose of 80 mg daily. The initial dose should not exceed 10 mg daily in patients with severe renal or hepatic impairment and in patients receiving ciclosporin, and the dose should be increased with caution.

Children aged 8 to 13 years with heterozygous familial hypercholesterolaemia may be given pravastatin in a dose of 20 mg once daily. The dose for adolescents aged 14 to 18 years is 40 mg once daily.

◊ General reviews.

1. McTavish D, Sorkin EM. Pravastatin: a review of its pharmacological properties and therapeutic potential in hypercholesterolaemia. *Drugs* 1991; **42:** 65–89.
2. Haria M, McTavish D. Pravastatin: a reappraisal of its pharmacological properties and clinical effectiveness in the management of coronary heart disease. *Drugs* 1997; **53:** 299–336.

**Administration in renal or hepatic impairment.** Patients with severe renal or hepatic impairment should be given pravastatin sodium in an initial dose of 10 mg daily, and the dose should be increased with caution.

## Preparations

**Proprietary Preparations** (details are given in Part 3)
***Arg.:*** Pravacol; ***Austral.:*** Pravachol; ***Austria:*** Pravachol; Sanaprav; Selipran; ***Belg.:*** Prareduct; Pravasine; ***Braz.:*** Mevalotin; Pravacol; ***Canad.:*** Pravachol; ***Chile:*** Pravacol; ***Denm.:*** Pravachol; ***Fin.:*** Pravachol; ***Fr.:*** Elisor; Vasten; ***Ger.:*** Liprevil†; Mevalotin; Pravasin; ***Gr.:*** Maxudin; Pravachol; ***Hong Kong:*** Pravachol; ***India:*** Pravator; ***Irl.:*** Lipostat; ***Israel:*** Lipidal; Lipostat†; ***Ital.:*** Aplactin; Prasterol; Pravaselect; Sanaprav; Selectin; ***Jpn:*** Mevalotin; ***Malaysia:*** Pravachol; ***Mex.:*** Astin; Kenstatin; Kenvestin; Prascolend; Pravacol; Xipral; ***Neth.:*** Selektine; ***Norw.:*** Pravachol; ***NZ:*** Lipostat; ***Port.:*** Pravacol; Sanaprav; ***S.Afr.:*** Prava; ***Singapore:*** Pravachol; ***Spain:*** Bristacol; Lipemol; Liplat; Prareduct; ***Swed.:*** Pravachol; ***Switz.:*** Mevalotin; Selipran; ***Thai.:*** Mevalotin; ***UK:*** Lipostat; ***USA:*** Pravachol.

**Multi-ingredient:** ***USA:*** Pravigard PAC.

# Prazosin Hydrochloride

*(BANM, USAN, rINNM)*

CP-12299-1; Furazosin Hydrochloride; Hidrocloruro de prazosina; Prazosini Hydrochloridum. 2-[4-(2-Furoyl)piperazin-1-yl]-6,7-dimethoxyquinazolin-4-ylamine hydrochloride.

$C_{19}H_{21}N_5O_4,HCl = 419.9.$

*CAS — 19216-56-9 (prazosin); 19237-84-4 (prazosin hydrochloride).*

*ATC — C02CA01.*

**Pharmacopoeias.** In *Chin., Eur.* (see p.vi), and *US.*

**Ph. Eur. 5.0** (Prazosin Hydrochloride). A white or almost white powder. Very slightly soluble in water; slightly soluble in alcohol and in methyl alcohol; practically insoluble in acetone. Protect from light.

**USP 27** (Prazosin Hydrochloride). A white to tan powder. Slightly soluble in water, in dimethylacetamide, in dimethylformamide, and in methyl alcohol; very slightly soluble in alcohol; practically insoluble in acetone and in chloroform. Store in airtight containers. Protect from light.

## Adverse Effects

Prazosin hydrochloride can cause postural hypotension which may be severe and produce syncope following the initial dose; it may be preceded by tachycardia. This reaction can be avoided by starting treatment with a low dose, preferably at night (see Uses and Administration, below). The hypotensive effects may be exaggerated by exercise, heat, or alcohol ingestion.

The more common adverse effects include dizziness, drowsiness, headache, lack of energy, nausea, and palpitations, and may diminish with continued prazosin therapy or with a reduction in dosage. Other adverse effects include oedema, chest pain, dyspnoea, constipation, diarrhoea, vomiting, depression and nervousness, sleep disturbances, vertigo, hallucinations, paraesthesia, nasal congestion, epistaxis, dry mouth, urinary frequency and incontinence, reddened sclera, blurred vision, tinnitus, abnormal liver enzyme values, pancreatitis, arthralgia, alopecia, lichen planus, skin rashes, pruritus, and diaphoresis. Impotence and priapism have also been reported.

◊ General reviews.

1. Carruthers SG. Adverse effects of $\alpha_1$-adrenergic blocking drugs. *Drug Safety* 1994; **11:** 12–20.

**Effects on the cardiovascular system.** Postural hypotension, preceded by tachycardia and sometimes producing syncope, is an established adverse effect of prazosin following the initial dose. Sinus bradycardia was associated with prazosin in a patient who experienced light headedness following each daily dose.[1]

1. Ball J. Symptomatic sinus bradycardia due to prazosin. *Lancet* 1994; **343:** 121.

**Effects on the gastrointestinal tract.** Faecal incontinence in a 52-year-old man receiving prazosin was exacerbated by haemorrhoidectomy and appeared to be due to diminished resting anal tone, presumably because of smooth muscle relaxation secondary to alpha-adrenoceptor blockade.[1] Symptoms ceased almost immediately on discontinuing the drug.

1. Holmes SAV, *et al.* Faecal incontinence resulting from $\alpha_1$-adrenoceptor blockade. *Lancet* 1990; **336:** 685–6.

**Effects on mental function.** Psychiatric symptoms including confusion, paranoia, and hallucinations developed in 3 patients associated with prazosin treatment.[1] Two of the patients had chronic renal failure and the other had mild renal impairment. Acute psychosis has also been reported with doxazosin.[2]

1. Chin DKF, *et al.* Neuropsychiatric complications related to use of prazosin in patients with renal failure. *BMJ* 1986; **293:** 1347.
2. Evans M, *et al.* Drug induced psychosis with doxazosin. *BMJ* 1997; **314:** 1869.

**Hypersensitivity.** Urticaria and angioedema were attributed to prazosin in a 70-year-old woman.[1]

1. Ruzicka T, Ring J. Hypersensitivity to prazosin. *Lancet* 1983; **i:** 473–4.

**Lupus erythematosus.** One study has reported the formation of antinuclear antibodies in patients receiving prazosin,[1] but this is not in agreement with other reports,[2,3] and commentators consider the association unproven.[4] There is no evidence of the development of lupus erythematosus.[1]

1. Marshall AJ, *et al.* Positive antinuclear factor tests with prazosin. *BMJ* 1979; **1:** 165–6.
2. Wilson JD, *et al.* Antinuclear factor in patients on prazosin. *BMJ* 1979; **1:** 553–4.
3. Melkild A, Gaarder PI. Does prazosin induce formation of antinuclear factor? *BMJ* 1979; **1:** 620–1.
4. Kristensen BØ. Does prazosin induce formation of antinuclear factor? *BMJ* 1979; **1:** 621.

**Urinary incontinence.** There have been reports of urinary incontinence developing in patients receiving prazosin. Analysis[1] of 56 cases reported to the Australian Adverse Drug Reactions Advisory Committee indicated that typically symptoms appeared within 1 or 2 days of the start of therapy and persisted until the drug was withdrawn or the dose reduced. Both stress and urge incontinence occurred, sometimes in the same patient. Of the 56 patients, 51 were women and most were elderly. In a study[2] in women attending a hypertension clinic urinary incontinence was reported in 40.8% of 49 women receiving alpha blockers (prazosin, terazosin, or doxazosin) and in 16.3% of controls. Incontinence might be due to a reduction in urethral pressure induced by alpha-adrenoceptor blockade. Interestingly, faecal incontinence has also been reported with prazosin—see Effects on the Gastrointestinal Tract, above.

1. Mathew TH, *et al.* Urinary incontinence secondary to prazosin. *Med J Aust* 1988; **148:** 305–6.
2. Marshall HJ, Beevers DG. α-Adrenoceptor blocking drugs and female urinary incontinence: prevalence and reversibility. *Br J Clin Pharmacol* 1996; **42:** 507–9.

## Treatment of Adverse Effects

If overdosage with prazosin occurs activated charcoal should be given if the patient presents within 1 hour of ingestion. Severe hypotension may occur and treatment includes support of the circulation by postural measures and parenteral fluid volume replacement, and if necessary cautious intravenous infusion of a vasopressor. Prazosin is not removed by dialysis.

## Precautions

Treatment with prazosin should be introduced cautiously because of the risk of sudden collapse following the initial dose. Extra caution is necessary in patients with hepatic or renal impairment and in the elderly.

Prazosin is not recommended for the treatment of heart failure caused by mechanical obstruction, for example aortic or mitral valve stenosis, pulmonary embolism, and restrictive pericardial disease. It should be used with caution in patients with angina pectoris. Prazosin may cause drowsiness or dizziness; patients so affected should not drive or operate machinery.

**Cerebral haemorrhage.** Hypotension with disturbance of consciousness[1] occurred in 3 patients with recent cerebral haemorrhage following an initial dose of prazosin 500 micrograms.

1. Lin M-S, Hsieh W-J. Prazosin-induced first-dose phenomenon possibly associated with hemorrhagic stroke: a report of three cases. *Drug Intell Clin Pharm* 1987; **21:** 723–6.

**Tolerance.** Although prazosin may be of initial benefit in patients with chronic heart failure, some studies[1,2] have reported the development of tolerance to its haemodynamic effects on prolonged therapy. This may be partly due to upregulation of $alpha_1$ adrenoceptors.[3]

1. Packer M, *et al.* Role of the renin-angiotensin system in the development of hemodynamic and clinical tolerance to long-term prazosin therapy in patients with severe chronic heart failure. *J Am Coll Cardiol* 1986; **7:** 671–80.
2. Bayliss J, *et al.* Clinical importance of the renin-angiotensin system in chronic heart failure: double blind comparison of captopril and prazosin. *BMJ* 1985; **290:** 1861–5.
3. Kersting F, *et al.* Preliminary evidence for the mechanism underlying the development of tolerance to prazosin in congestive heart failure: the α-agonistic properties of dobutamine unmasked by prazosin treatment. *J Cardiovasc Pharmacol* 1993; **21:** 537–43.

## Interactions

The hypotensive effects of prazosin may be enhanced by use with diuretics and other antihypertensives, and by alcohol and other drugs that cause hypotension. The risk of first-dose hypotension may be particularly increased in patients receiving beta blockers or calcium-channel blockers.

**Analgesics.** *Indometacin* reduced prazosin-induced hypotension in 4 of 9 subjects.[1]

1. Rubin P, *et al.* Studies on the clinical pharmacology of prazosin II: the influence of indomethacin and of propranolol on the action and disposition of prazosin. *Br J Clin Pharmacol* 1980; **10:** 33–9.

**Antidepressants and antipsychotics.** A patient who was taking *amitriptyline* and *chlorpromazine* developed acute agitation on receiving prazosin.[1] The symptoms settled rapidly when prazosin was discontinued. Antidepressants and antipsychotics may enhance the hypotensive effect of prazosin and other alpha blockers.

1. Bolli P, Simpson FO. New vasodilator drugs for hypertension. *BMJ* 1974; **1:** 637.

**Calcium-channel blockers.** An enhanced hypotensive effect has been reported in normotensive subjects given prazosin and *verapamil* concurrently; the effect may be due in part to enhanced bioavailability of prazosin.[1] Markedly increased hypotensive responses have also been reported with combined use of prazosin and *nifedipine*,[2,3] although the validity of such reports has been questioned.[4]

1. Pasanisi F, *et al.* Combined alpha adrenoceptor antagonism and calcium channel blockade in normal subjects. *Clin Pharmacol Ther* 1984; **36:** 716–23.
2. Jee LD, Opie LH. Acute hypotensive response to nifedipine added to prazosin in treatment of hypertension. *BMJ* 1983; **287:** 1514.
3. Jee LD, Opie LH. Acute hypotensive response to nifedipine added to prazosin. *BMJ* 1984; **288:** 238–9.
4. Elliott HL, *et al.* Acute hypotensive response to nifedipine added to prazosin. *BMJ* 1984; **288:** 238.

**Digoxin.** For reference to the effect of prazosin on serum-digoxin concentrations, see under Digoxin, p.896.

### Pharmacokinetics

Prazosin is readily absorbed from the gastrointestinal tract with peak plasma concentrations occurring 1 to 3 hours after an oral dose. The bioavailability is variable and a range of 43 to 85% has been reported. Prazosin is highly bound to plasma proteins. It is extensively metabolised in the liver and some of the metabolites are reported to have hypotensive activity. It is excreted as the metabolites and 5 to 11% as unchanged prazosin mainly in the faeces via the bile. Less than 10% is excreted in the urine. Small amounts are distributed into breast milk. Its duration of action is longer than would be predicted from its relatively short plasma half-life of about 2 to 4 hours. Half-life is reported to be increased to about 7 hours in patients with heart failure.

**The elderly.** The bioavailability of prazosin was significantly reduced in the elderly, about 40% less unchanged drug reaching the systemic circulation compared with the young.[1] This was attributed to a reduction in the absorption from the gastrointestinal tract. The half-life was also prolonged in the elderly and this was associated with an increase in the volume of distribution at steady state. However, it was considered unlikely that these effects would have major clinical significance.

1. Rubin PC, *et al.* Prazosin disposition in young and elderly subjects. *Br J Clin Pharmacol* 1981; **12:** 401–4.

**Protein binding.** Although a study[1] found that prazosin was about 80 to 85% bound to serum albumin and only about 10 to 30% bound to $\alpha_1$-acid glycoprotein *in vitro*, potential interactions between the binding proteins *in vivo* were not taken into account; binding to $\alpha_1$-acid glycoprotein might be more significant in clinical practice. A subsequent study[2] indicated that variations in prazosin protein binding pre- and post-operatively were related to variations in concentration of the glycoprotein.

1. Brunner F, Müller WE. Prazosin binding to human $\alpha_1$-acid glycoprotein (orosomucoid), human serum albumin, and human serum: further characterisation of the 'single drug binding site' of orosomucoid. *J Pharm Pharmacol* 1985; **37:** 305–9.
2. Sager G, *et al.* Binding of prazosin and propranolol at variable $\alpha_1$-acid glycoprotein and albumin concentrations. *Br J Clin Pharmacol* 1989; **27:** 229–34.

### Uses and Administration

Prazosin is an alpha blocker (p.809) that acts by selective blockade of alpha$_1$-adrenoceptors. It is used in the management of hypertension (p.825), in Raynaud's syndrome (below), and to relieve symptoms of urinary obstruction in benign prostatic hyperplasia (p.1555). It has also been used in heart failure (p.820).

Prazosin produces peripheral dilatation of both arterioles and veins and reduction of peripheral resistance, usually without reflex tachycardia. It reduces both standing and supine blood pressure with a greater effect on the diastolic pressure. It is reported to have no effect on renal blood flow or glomerular filtration rate, and has little effect on cardiac output in hypertensive patients. In patients with heart failure, prazosin reduces both preload and afterload and produces an improvement in cardiac output, although tolerance may develop. In benign prostatic hyperplasia, prazosin may relieve the symptoms of urinary obstruction by reducing smooth muscle tone in the prostate and bladder neck.

Prazosin is given by mouth as the hydrochloride, but doses are usually expressed in terms of the base. Prazosin hydrochloride 1.1 mg is approximately equivalent to 1 mg of prazosin. Following oral administration the hypotensive effect is seen within 2 to 4 hours and persists for several hours. Full effects are seen after 4 to 6 weeks.

A low starting dose is given in the evening to lessen the risk of collapse which may occur in some patients after the first dose (see Adverse Effects, above). Doses may need to be reduced in the elderly and in patients with hepatic or renal impairment.

In **hypertension**, the usual initial dose in the UK is 500 micrograms two or three times daily for 3 to 7 days; if tolerated the dose may then be increased to 1 mg two or three times daily for a further 3 to 7 days, and thereafter gradually increased, according to the patient's response, to a usual maximum of 20 mg daily in divided doses. In the US the recommended starting dose is 1 mg two or three times daily and up to 40 mg daily in divided doses has been given; however, the usual maintenance dose is between 6 and 15 mg daily. Smaller doses may be required in patients also taking other antihypertensives. Modified-release preparations may allow once daily dosing.

In **Raynaud's syndrome** and in **benign prostatic hyperplasia** an initial dose of 500 micrograms twice daily may be given, increasing to a maintenance dose not exceeding 2 mg twice daily.

In **heart failure**, treatment has been started with 500 micrograms two to four times daily and increased gradually according to response; the usual maintenance dose has been 4 to 20 mg daily.

**Erectile dysfunction.** Prazosin has been administered transurethrally with alprostadil[1] in the management of erectile dysfunction (p.1745).

1. Peterson CA, *et al.* Erectile response to transurethral alprostadil, prazosin and alprostadil-prazosin combinations. *J Urol (Baltimore)* 1998; **159:** 1523–8.

**Familial Mediterranean fever.** Familial Mediterranean fever (p.416) is usually treated with prophylactic colchicine, but its use may be limited by adverse effects. A Japanese man who had suffered from attacks for 16 years was treated[1] with prazosin 3 mg daily. There were no further attacks for more than a year after starting treatment, but stopping prazosin resulted in a recurrence.

1. Kataoka H, *et al.* Treating familial Mediterranean fever with prazosin hydrochloride. *Ann Intern Med* 1998; **129:** 424–5.

**Muscle cramp.** Skeletal muscle cramp may occur during haemodialysis, possibly due to activation of the sympathetic nervous system. Prazosin was reported[1] to reduce the incidence of cramp in 4 of 5 patients with frequent haemodialysis-associated muscle cramp. However, the increased incidence of hypotension reported might limit its use for this indication.

1. Sidhom OA, *et al.* Low-dose prazosin in patients with muscle cramps during hemodialysis. *Clin Pharmacol Ther* 1994; **56:** 445–51.

**Peripheral vascular disease.** Alpha blockers, including prazosin, may be used in the management of Raynaud's syndrome (p.833). Studies of the benefits of prazosin have produced varying results. A short-term reduction in number and duration of attacks was reported in 5 of 7 patients given prazosin 2 mg daily but only 1 patient had complete relief from attacks and few could tolerate doses higher than 6 mg daily.[1] Improvements were not maintained during continued treatment for 2 months. Others[2,3] have reported benefit from prazosin 1 mg two or three times daily in the majority of patients, with one study suggesting greater benefit in Raynaud's disease (the primary, idiopathic form) than in secondary Raynaud's syndrome.[2] In a subsequent study, higher doses of prazosin (2 or 4 mg three times daily) were no more effective than 1 mg three times daily, and were associated with a significantly greater incidence of adverse effects.[4] A systematic review[5] concluded that prazosin was modestly effective in the treatment of Raynaud's syndrome secondary to scleroderma.

1. Nielsen SL, *et al.* Prazosin treatment of primary Raynaud's phenomenon. *Eur J Clin Pharmacol* 1983; **24:** 421–3.
2. Allegra C, *et al.* Pharmacological treatment of Raynaud's phenomenon: a new therapeutic approach. *Curr Ther Res* 1986; **40:** 303–11.
3. Wollersheim H, *et al.* Double-blind, placebo-controlled study of prazosin in Raynaud's phenomenon. *Clin Pharmacol Ther* 1986, **40:** 219–25.
4. Wollersheim H, Thien T. Dose-response study of prazosin in Raynaud's phenomenon: clinical effectiveness versus side effects. *J Clin Pharmacol* 1988; **28:** 1089–93.
5. Pope J, *et al.* Prazosin for Raynaud's phenomenon in progressive systemic sclerosis. Available in The Cochrane Library; Issue 2. Chichester: John Wiley; 2004.

**Post-traumatic stress disorder.** Post-traumatic stress disorder (p.664) is usually treated with psychotherapy or drugs such as SSRIs. Increased alpha$_1$-adrenergic receptor activity may be a contributory factor, and prazosin was reported[1] to produce a reduction in nightmares in all 5 patients with this condition taking part in a small 6-week open-label trial; a similar improvement was found in a retrospective study[2] of combat veterans with chronic treatment-resistant symptoms.

1. Taylor F, Raskind MA. The $\alpha_1$-adrenergic antagonist prazosin improves sleep and nightmares in civilian trauma posttraumatic stress disorder. *J Clin Psychopharmacol* 2002; **22:** 82–5.
2. Raskind MA, *et al.* Prazosin reduces nightmares in combat veterans with posttraumatic stress disorder. *J Clin Psychiatry* 2002; **63:** 565–8.

**Scorpion stings.** Stings from the Indian red scorpion (*Mesobuthus tamulus*) are potentially fatal. The scorpion venom is a potent sympathetic stimulator resulting in high circulating catecholamines, hypertension, arrhythmias, pulmonary oedema, and circulatory failure. The efficacy of antivenom is questionable and treatment for cardiotoxicity is supportive (see p.1638). Prazosin, given orally, appears to be beneficial and has been suggested[1] as first-line treatment, except in cases of severe pulmonary oedema.

1. Bawaskar HS, Bawaskar PH. Scorpion envenoming and the cardiovascular system. *Trop Doct* 1997; **27:** 6–9.

### Preparations

***BP 2003:*** Prazosin Tablets;
***USP 27:*** Prazosin Hydrochloride Capsules.

**Proprietary Preparations** (details are given in Part 3)
***Arg.:*** Decliten; Minipres; ***Austral.:*** Minipress; Mipraz†; Prasig; Pratsiol; Prazohexal; Pressin; ***Austria:*** Minipress; ***Belg.:*** Minipress; ***Braz.:*** Minipress; ***Canad.:*** Apo-Prazo; Minipress; Novo-Prazin; Nu-Prazo; ***Denm.:*** Hexapress; Peripress; Prazac; ***Fin.:*** Patsolin†; Peripress; Pratsiol; Prazocor†; ***Fr.:*** Alpress; Minipress; ***Ger.:*** Adversuten; duramipress; Eurex†; Minipress; ***Hong Kong:*** Apo-Prazo; Minipress; Mizosin; Pratsiol†; ***India:*** Minipress; ***Irl.:*** Hypovase; ***Israel:*** Hypotens; ***Jpn:*** Minipress; ***Malaysia:*** Atodel; Minipress; Minison; ***Mex.:*** Anapres; Europrazosin†; Minipres; Prabioquim†; Sinozzard; ***Neth.:*** Minipress; ***NZ:*** Hyprosin; Pratsiol; ***S.Afr.:*** Minipress; Pratsiol; ***Singapore:*** Minipress; ***Spain:*** Minipres; ***Switz.:*** Minipress; ***Thai.:*** Atodel; Lopress; Minima†; Minipress; Mysial†; Parabowl; Polypress; Pratsiol; Pressin; ***UK:*** Alphavase†; Hypovase; Kentovase; ***USA:*** Minipress.

**Multi-ingredient:** ***Ger.:*** Polypress; ***USA:*** Minizide.

## Prenalterol Hydrochloride *(BANM, USAN, rINNM)*

C-50005/A-Ba (racemate); CGP-7760B; H133/22; H-80/62 (racemate); Hidrocloruro de prenalterol. (*S*)-1-(4-Hydroxyphenoxy)-3-isopropylaminopropan-2-ol hydrochloride.

$C_{12}H_{19}NO_3,HCl = 261.7.$
*CAS — 57526-81-5 (prenalterol); 61260-05-7 (prenalterol hydrochloride).*
*ATC — C01CA13.*

### Profile

Prenalterol is a sympathomimetic (see Adrenaline, p.852) with stimulant effects on beta$_1$ adrenoceptors. It has an inotropic action on the heart with relatively little chronotropic effect. Prenalterol hydrochloride has been administered parenterally in the treatment of heart failure and shock. It has also been promoted for the reversal of beta blockade.

### Preparations

**Proprietary Preparations** (details are given in Part 3)
***Denm.:*** Hyprenan†; ***Norw.:*** Hyprenan†; ***Swed.:*** Hyprenan†.

## Probucol *(BAN, USAN, rINN)*

DH-581. 4,4′-(Isopropylidenedithio)bis(2,6-di-*tert*-butylphenol).

$C_{31}H_{48}O_2S_2 = 516.8.$
*CAS — 23288-49-5.*
*ATC — C10AX02.*

**Pharmacopoeias.** In *US.*

**USP 27** (Probucol). A white to off-white, crystalline powder. Insoluble in water; soluble in alcohol and in petroleum spirit; freely soluble in chloroform and in propyl alcohol. Protect from light.

### Adverse Effects and Precautions

The commonest adverse effects of probucol therapy are gastrointestinal disorders, with diarrhoea occurring in about 10% of patients; flatulence, abdominal pain, nausea, and vomiting may also occur. Hypersensitivity reactions including angioedema have been reported.

Fatal cardiac arrhythmias have been reported in *animals* and prolonged QT intervals in man. Probucol should be given with caution to patients with recent myocardial damage, severe ventricular arrhythmias, cardiovascular-associated syncope, hypokalaemia, or prolonged QT interval. The risk of arrhythmias may be increased in patients taking tricyclic antidepressants, class I or III antiarrhythmics, phenothiazines, or other drugs that prolong the QT interval.

◊ Adverse effects reported during a 1-year study involving 88 patients given probucol decreased after the first 3 months of therapy.[1] The most common was loose stools or diarrhoea; constipation was reported much less frequently. Other side-effects which occurred were flatulence, vertigo, dizziness, a different odour of the skin, and pruritus. No patient withdrew from the study because of side-effects.

1. McCaughan D. Nine years of treatment with probucol. *Artery* 1982; **10:** 56–70.

**Effects on the heart.** Modest prolongation of the QT interval has been reported with probucol in a number of studies.[1-3] Although serious cardiac arrhythmias were not noted in these studies, there have been individual reports[4,5] of potentially fatal polymorphic ventricular tachycardia (torsade de pointes) in patients with probucol-associated prolongation of the QT interval.

1. Troendle G, *et al.* Probucol and the QT interval. *Lancet* 1982; **i:** 1179.
2. Dujovne CA, *et al.* Electrocardiographic effects of probucol: a controlled prospective clinical trial. *Eur J Clin Pharmacol* 1984; **26:** 735–9.
3. Naukkarinen V, *et al.* Probucol-induced electrocardiographic changes in a five-year primary prevention of vascular diseases. *Curr Ther Res* 1989; **45:** 232–7.
4. Gohn DC, Simmons TW. Polymorphic ventricular tachycardia (torsade de pointes) associated with the use of probucol. *N Engl J Med* 1992; **326:** 1435–6.
5. Kajinami K, *et al.* Propranolol for probucol-induced QT prolongation with polymorphic ventricular tachycardia. *Lancet* 1993; **341:** 124–5.

### Interactions

The risk of arrhythmias in patients receiving probucol may be increased in those taking arrhythmogenic drugs concurrently (see Adverse Effects and Precautions, above).

**Ciclosporin.** For reference to the effect of probucol on ciclosporin concentrations, see p.1356.

### Pharmacokinetics

The absorption of probucol from the gastrointestinal tract is limited and variable, and is stated to be at a maximum if taken with food. Concentrations in blood rise slowly and reach steady state after 3 to 4 months of continuous treatment. Probucol accumulates in adipose tissue and concentrations fall only slowly, over several months, when treatment is withdrawn. Excretion is considered to be chiefly by the biliary system into the faeces.

### Uses and Administration

Probucol is a lipid regulating drug that has been used in the treatment of hyperlipidaemias (p.823), particularly type IIa hyperlipoproteinaemia. It lowers total plasma-cholesterol concentrations, mainly by reducing low-density lipoprotein (LDL)-cholesterol and high-density lipoprotein (HDL)-cholesterol concentrations. It has little effect on triglyceride or very-low-density lipoprotein (VLDL)-cholesterol concentrations. It may cause regression of xanthomas.

The usual dose by mouth is 500 mg twice daily, given with the morning and evening meals.

◊ Reviews.

1. Buckley MM-T, *et al.* Probucol: a reappraisal of its pharmacological properties and therapeutic use in hypercholesterolaemia. *Drugs* 1989; **37:** 761–800.
2. Zimetbaum P, *et al.* Probucol: pharmacology and clinical application. *J Clin Pharmacol* 1990; **30:** 3–9.

**Reperfusion and revascularisation procedures.** Restenosis commonly occurs following the use of percutaneous coronary revascularisation procedures (p.834) and various drugs have been tried for its prevention. Probucol has been reported to reduce the rate of restenosis after coronary angioplasty,[1] and to reduce the need for repeat interventions.[1,2]

1. Tardif J-C, *et al.* Probucol and multivitamins in the prevention of restenosis after coronary angioplasty. *N Engl J Med* 1997; **337:** 365–72.
2. Daida H, *et al.* Effect of probucol on repeat revascularization rate after percutaneous transluminal coronary angioplasty (from the Probucol Angioplasty Restenosis Trial [PART]). *Am J Cardiol* 2000; **86:** 550–2.

### Preparations

***USP 27:*** Probucol Tablets.

**Proprietary Preparations** (details are given in Part 3)
***Austral.:*** Lurselle†; ***Braz.:*** Lesterol†; ***Ger.:*** Lurselle†; ***Hong Kong:*** Lurselle†; ***Mex.:*** Colbuzer†; Lesterol†; Serterol; ***S.Afr.:*** Lurselle; ***Spain:*** Superlipid; ***Thai.:*** Lurselle.

## Procainamide Hydrochloride

*(BANM, rINNM)*

Hidrocloruro de procainimida; Novocainamidum; Procainamidi Chloridum; Procainamidi Hydrochloridum. 4-Amino-*N*-(2-diethylaminoethyl)benzamide hydrochloride.

$C_{13}H_{21}N_3O,HCl = 271.8.$

*CAS — 51-06-9 (procainamide); 614-39-1 (procainamide hydrochloride).*

*ATC — C01BA02.*

**Pharmacopoeias.** In *Chin., Eur.* (see p.vi), *Int., Jpn, Pol., US,* and *Viet.*

**Ph. Eur. 5.0** (Procainamide Hydrochloride). A white or very slightly yellow, hygroscopic, crystalline powder. Very soluble in water; freely soluble in alcohol; slightly soluble in acetone. A 10% solution in water has a pH of 5.6 to 6.3. Store in airtight containers. Protect from light.

**USP 27** (Procainamide Hydrochloride). A white to tan, odourless, crystalline powder. Very soluble in water; soluble in alcohol; slightly soluble in chloroform; very slightly soluble in ether and in benzene. A 10% solution in water has a pH of 5.0 to 6.5. Store in airtight containers at a temperature of 25°, excursions permitted between 15° and 30°.

**Stability.** Procainamide is more stable in neutral solutions such as sodium chloride, than in acidic solutions such as glucose, but patients requiring intravenous procainamide often have heart failure and cannot tolerate the sodium load associated with sodium chloride injections. The stability of procainamide in glucose 5% is improved by neutralising the glucose using sodium bicarbonate, or storing the admixture at 5°. The concentration of procainamide remained above 90% of the initial concentration for 24 hours if the glucose was first neutralised and this was considered more practical than refrigeration if extended stability was required.[1]

The compound formed by mixing procainamide hydrochloride with glucose 5% was shown to be a mixture of α- and β-glucosylamines[2] and about 10 to 15% of the procainamide was lost in this way after 10 hours at room temperature.

An oral liquid,[3] prepared from procainamide capsules, containing 5, 50, or 100 mg/mL of the hydrochloride was stable for at least 6 months when stored at 4° to 6°.

1. Raymond GG, *et al.* Stability of procainamide hydrochloride in neutralized 5% dextrose injection. *Am J Hosp Pharm* 1988; **45:** 2513–17.
2. Sianipar A, *et al.* Chemical incompatibility between procainamide hydrochloride and glucose following intravenous admixture. *J Pharm Pharmacol* 1994; **46:** 951–5.
3. Metras JI, *et al.* Stability of procainamide hydrochloride in an extemporaneously compounded oral liquid. *Am J Hosp Pharm* 1992; **49:** 1720–4.

### Adverse Effects

Cardiac effects occur particularly during intravenous administration of procainamide and in overdose. Rapid intravenous administration may result in severe hypotension, ventricular fibrillation, and asystole. High plasma concentrations are also associated with impaired cardiac conduction.

Hypersensitivity reactions to procainamide are common. Procainamide is a frequent cause of drug-induced systemic lupus erythematosus (SLE) and the incidence has been reported to be as high as 30% during long-term use. Antinuclear antibodies may be detected in a high proportion of patients, but they do not necessarily develop the symptoms of SLE, which include arthralgia, arthritis, myalgia, pleural effusion, pericarditis, and fever. Agranulocytosis, eosinophilia, neutropenia, thrombocytopenia, and haemolytic anaemia have been reported. Other symptoms of hypersensitivity not necessarily related to SLE may also occur including hepatomegaly, angioedema, skin rashes, pruritus, urticaria, flushing, and hypergammaglobulinaemia.

Anorexia, nausea, vomiting, a bitter taste, and diarrhoea are more common with higher oral doses. Effects on the CNS such as mental depression, dizziness, and psychosis with hallucinations, have been reported.

**Incidence of adverse effects.** Out of 488 hospitalised patients in the Boston Collaborative Drug Surveillance Program who had received procainamide, 45 experienced acute adverse effects attributed to the drug.[1] Life-threatening reactions included heart block in 3, tachyarrhythmias in 2, and bradycardia and/or hypotension in 2. Other reactions included gastrointestinal upsets in 19, pyrexia in 8, bradycardia and hypotension in 5, tachyarrhythmias in 3, heart block in 1, eosinophilia in 1, and urticaria in 1 patient.

1. Lawson DH, Jick H. Adverse reactions to procainamide. *Br J Clin Pharmacol* 1977; **4:** 507–11.

**Effects on the blood.** Adverse haematological effects reported during procainamide therapy include neutropenia,[1-3] agranulocytosis,[2-6] thrombocytopenia,[5] haemolytic anaemia,[7] and pancytopenia.[8] These disorders are usually reversible on withdrawing procainamide although some fatalities have been reported.[3,4] It has been suggested[2,6] that agranulocytosis or severe neutropenia is more likely in patients taking modified-release preparations, but others have found no difference in the incidence between modified-release and conventional-release preparations.[3] An increased risk of agranulocytosis with procainamide has been documented in one large study.[9] Although the precise estimate of excess risk could not be calculated, the order of magnitude was about 3 per million exposed for up to one week. This excess risk was low and of little relevance in the initial choice of therapy.

1. Riker J, *et al.* Bone marrow granulomas and neutropenia associated with procainamide. *Arch Intern Med* 1978; **138:** 1731–2.
2. Ellrodt AG, *et al.* Severe neutropenia associated with sustained-release procainamide. *Ann Intern Med* 1984; **100:** 197–201.
3. Meyers DG, *et al.* Severe neutropenia associated with procainamide: comparison of sustained release and conventional preparations. *Am Heart J* 1985; **109:** 1393–5.
4. Fleet S. Agranulocytosis, procainamide, and phenytoin. *Ann Intern Med* 1984; **100:** 616–17.
5. Christensen DJ, *et al.* Agranulocytosis, thrombocytopenia, and procainamide. *Ann Intern Med* 1984; **100:** 918.
6. Thompson JF, *et al.* Procainamide agranulocytosis: a case report and review of the literature. *Curr Ther Res* 1988; **44:** 872–81.
7. Kleinman S, *et al.* Positive direct antiglobulin tests and immune hemolytic anemia in patients receiving procainamide. *N Engl J Med* 1984; **311:** 809–12.
8. Bluming AZ, *et al.* Severe transient pancytopenia associated with procainamide ingestion. *JAMA* 1976; **236:** 2520–1.
9. Kelly JP, *et al.* Risks of agranulocytosis and aplastic anemia in relation to the use of cardiovascular drugs: The International Agranulocytosis and Aplastic Anemia Study. *Clin Pharmacol Ther* 1991; **49:** 330–41.

**Effects on the gastrointestinal tract.** Pseudo-obstruction of the bowel occurred in a diabetic patient when given procainamide both orally and intravenously. It was believed that the anticholinergic properties of procainamide, together with the diabetic state, contributed to the severe hypomotility of the gastrointestinal tract.[1]

1. Peterson AM, *et al.* Procainamide-induced pseudo-obstruction in a diabetic patient. *DICP Ann Pharmacother* 1991; **25:** 1334–5.

**Effects on the heart.** Procainamide has been associated with the development of torsade de pointes.[1,2] Elevated plasma concentrations of the major metabolite *N*-acetylprocainamide were present in 1 patient[1] and haemodialysis was used to reduce the plasma concentration and control the arrhythmia.

1. Nguyen KPV, *et al.* N-Acetylprocainamide, torsades de pointes, and hemodialysis. *Ann Intern Med* 1986; **104:** 283–4.
2. Habbab MA, El-Sherif N. Drug-induced torsades de pointes: role of early afterdepolarizations and dispersion of repolarization. *Am J Med* 1990; **89:** 241–6.

**Effects on the liver.** There have been reports of granulomatous hepatitis[1] and intrahepatic cholestasis[2,3] due to hypersensitivity reactions in patients taking procainamide. Fever and elevation of liver enzyme values also occurred. The reactions were reversible on withdrawing procainamide.

1. Rotmensch HH, *et al.* Granulomatous hepatitis: a hypersensitivity response to procainamide. *Ann Intern Med* 1978; **89:** 646–7.
2. Ahn C-S, Tow DE. Intrahepatic cholestasis due to hypersensitivity reaction to procainamide. *Arch Intern Med* 1990; **150:** 2589–90.
3. Chuang LC, *et al.* Possible case of procainamide-induced intrahepatic cholestatic jaundice. *Ann Pharmacother* 1993; **27:** 434–7.

**Effects on mental function.** Acute psychosis has been reported[1] in patients receiving therapy with procainamide.

1. Bizjak ED, *et al.* Procainamide-induced psychosis: a case report and review of the literature. *Ann Pharmacother* 1999; **33:** 948–51.

**Effects on the muscles.** Procainamide may affect neuromuscular transmission and there have been reports of severe generalised skeletal muscle weakness[1-3] in patients receiving procainamide. In 2 patients this was associated with respiratory failure[1,2] and developed shortly after starting therapy. Concentrations of procainamide and its *N*-acetyl metabolite exceeded the normal therapeutic ranges and rapid cycling peritoneal dialysis was used to remove the drug in 1 patient.[2] Adverse muscle symptoms are a feature of procainamide-induced lupus erythematosus (see below), but in such instances symptoms usually develop on long-term treatment.

1. Lewis CA, *et al.* Myopathy after short term administration of procainamide. *BMJ* 1986; **292:** 593–4.
2. Javaheri S, *et al.* Diaphragmatic paralysis. *Am J Med* 1989; **86:** 623–4.
3. Sayler DJ, DeJong DJ. Possible procainamide-induced myopathy. *DICP Ann Pharmacother* 1991; **25:** 436.

**Lupus erythematosus.** Procainamide is one of the most common causes of drug-induced lupus erythematosus.[1-3] Antinuclear antibodies are present in the majority of patients on long-term therapy but the clinical syndrome develops in only up to 30%. The development of antinuclear antibodies is more likely in slow acetylators than in rapid acetylators; also the antibodies appear earlier in slow acetylators.[4] The clinical syndrome may include fever, polyarthritis, arthralgia, myalgia, and pleuropulmonary and pericardial features, and is usually spontaneously reversible on withdrawal of procainamide.

1. Hughes GRV. Recent developments in drug-associated systemic lupus erythematosus. *Adverse Drug React Bull* 1987; (Apr.): 460–3.
2. Mitchell JA, *et al.* Immunotoxic side-effects of drug therapy. *Drug Safety* 1990; **5:** 168–78.
3. Price EJ, Venables PJW. Drug-induced lupus. *Drug Safety* 1995; **12:** 283–90.
4. Woosley RL, *et al.* Effect of acetylator phenotype on the rate at which procainamide induces antinuclear antibodies and the lupus syndrome. *N Engl J Med* 1978; **298:** 1157–9.

### Treatment of Adverse Effects

In overdosage treatment is largely symptomatic and supportive. Activated charcoal may be considered if the patient presents within 1 hour of ingestion. The ECG, blood pressure, and renal function should be monitored. Supportive measures include correction of hypotension, assisted ventilation, and electrical pacing. Haemodialysis or haemoperfusion increase the elimination of procainamide and *N*-acetylprocainamide.

Systemic lupus erythematosus will normally respond to withdrawal of procainamide but corticosteroids may be required.

**Dialysis.** There are reports of haemodialysis and haemoperfusion being effective in reducing concentrations of procainamide and *N*-acetylprocainamide.[1-3]

1. Atkinson AJ, *et al.* Hemodialysis for severe procainamide toxicity: clinical and pharmacokinetic observations. *Clin Pharmacol Ther* 1976; **20:** 585–92.
2. Braden GL, *et al.* Hemoperfusion for treatment of N-acetylprocainamide intoxication. *Ann Intern Med* 1986; **105:** 64–5.
3. Domoto DT, *et al.* Removal of toxic levels of N-acetylprocainamide with continuous arteriovenous hemofiltration or continuous arteriovenous hemodiafiltration. *Ann Intern Med* 1987; **106:** 550–2.

### Precautions

Procainamide is contra-indicated in patients with heart block or systemic lupus erythematosus, and should be used with caution in those with myocardial damage or severe organic heart disease. The *British National Formulary* considers that it should not be used in heart failure or hypotension. Patients with torsade de pointes may deteriorate if given procainamide. If procainamide is used to treat atrial tachycardia it may be necessary to pre-treat with digoxin. Procainamide should preferably not be used in patients with myasthenia gravis or digoxin toxicity. There may be cross-sensitivity between procaine and procainamide.

Accumulation of procainamide may occur in patients with heart failure or hepatic or renal impairment and dosage reduction may be necessary.

Blood counts and screening for lupus erythematosus and serum antinuclear factor should be carried out regularly during therapy.

Grave hypotension may follow intravenous administration of procainamide; it should be injected slowly under ECG control.

**Breast feeding.** There was evidence of accumulation of procainamide and N-acetylprocainamide in the breast milk of a woman taking procainamide 500 mg four times daily.[1] Milk and serum samples were obtained at three-hourly intervals for 15 hours. Mean serum concentrations of the drug and metabolite were found to be 1.1 and 1.6 micrograms/mL respectively; those in the milk were 5.4 and 3.5 micrograms/mL respectively. The mean milk:serum ratios were 4.3 (range 1.0 to 7.3) and 3.8 (range 1.0 to 6.2) respectively. However, it was considered that the amount ingested by the infant would not yield clinically significant serum concentrations. Although the manufacturer advises that procainamide should be avoided in breast-feeding women, there have been no reports of adverse effects in infants, and the American Academy of Pediatrics considers[2] that its use is therefore usually compatible with breast feeding.

1. Pittard WB, Glazier H. Procainamide excretion in human milk. *J Pediatr* 1983; **102:** 631–3.
2. American Academy of Pediatrics. The transfer of drugs and other chemicals into human milk. *Pediatrics* 2001; **108:** 776–89. Correction. *ibid.*; 1029. Also available at: http://aappolicy.aappublications.org/cgi/content/full/pediatrics%3b108/3/776 (accessed 06/07/04)

## Interactions

Procainamide may enhance the effects of antihypertensives, other antiarrhythmics and arrhythmogenic drugs, antimuscarinics, and neuromuscular blockers, and diminish those of parasympathomimetics, such as neostigmine. Procainamide is actively secreted by kidney tubules and interactions are possible with drugs secreted by the same pathway, such as cimetidine and trimethoprim.

**Alcohol.** The total body clearance of procainamide is increased by alcohol[1] and the elimination half-life reduced. The acetylation rate of procainamide is also increased resulting in a greater proportion of drug present as the active metabolite N-acetylprocainamide.

1. Olsen H, Mørland J. Ethanol-induced increase in procainamide acetylation in man. *Br J Clin Pharmacol* 1982; **13:** 203–8.

**Antacids.** Adsorption of procainamide by *antacids*[1] can reduce the bioavailability of procainamide and it is recommended that they are not administered together.

1. Al-Shora HI, *et al.* Interactions of procainamide, verapamil, guanethidine and hydralazine with adsorbent antacids and antidiarrhoeal mixtures. *Int J Pharmaceutics* 1988; **47:** 209–13.

**Antiarrhythmics.** *Amiodarone* given orally alters the pharmacokinetic properties of an intravenous dose of procainamide,[1] decreasing clearance and prolonging the plasma elimination half-life. The dosage of intravenous procainamide should be reduced by 20 to 30% during concurrent use.

1. Windle J, *et al.* Pharmacokinetic and electrophysiologic interactions of amiodarone and procainamide. *Clin Pharmacol Ther* 1987; **41:** 603–10.

**Antibacterials.** The renal clearance of procainamide and N-acetylprocainamide is reduced by *trimethoprim*[1] through competition for renal tubular secretion. Serum concentrations may be increased with a resulting increase in pharmacodynamic response.

1. Vlasses PH, *et al.* Trimethoprim decreases the renal clearance of procainamide and N-acetylprocainamide. *Clin Pharmacol Ther* 1986; **39:** 233.

**Histamine $H_2$-antagonists.** Histamine $H_2$-antagonists compete with other basic drugs for renal tubular secretion. *Cimetidine* reduces the renal clearance of procainamide and N-acetylprocainamide[1,2] and a dosage reduction may be necessary. Increases[3,4] and decreases[4] in renal and metabolic clearances of procainamide have occurred with *ranitidine*.

1. Christian CD, *et al.* Cimetidine inhibits renal procainamide clearance. *Clin Pharmacol Ther* 1984; **36:** 221–7.
2. Somogyi A, *et al.* Cimetidine-procainamide pharmacokinetic interaction in man: evidence of competition for tubular secretion of basic drugs. *Eur J Clin Pharmacol* 1983; **25:** 339–45.
3. Somogyi A, Bochner F. Dose and concentration dependent effect of ranitidine on procainamide disposition and renal clearance in man. *Br J Clin Pharmacol* 1984; **18:** 175–81.
4. Rocci ML, *et al.* Ranitidine-induced changes in the renal and hepatic clearances of procainamide are correlated. *J Pharmacol Exp Ther* 1989; **248:** 923–8.

## Pharmacokinetics

Procainamide is readily and almost completely absorbed from the gastrointestinal tract. It is widely distributed throughout the body and is only about 15 to 20% bound to plasma proteins. The therapeutic effect of procainamide has been correlated with plasma concentrations of about 3 to 10 micrograms/mL in most patients, progressively severe toxicity being noted at concentrations above 12 micrograms/mL.

Some procainamide undergoes acetylation in the liver to N-acetylprocainamide (acecainide, p.848). This metabolite also has antiarrhythmic properties. The rate of acetylation of procainamide is genetically determined, there being slow and fast acetylators. Procainamide also undergoes hydrolysis in plasma to para-aminobenzoic acid.

Procainamide is excreted in the urine following active renal secretion, 30 to 70% as unchanged procainamide, with the remainder as N-acetylprocainamide and other metabolites. The elimination half-life of procainamide is 2.5 to 5 hours and that of its acetyl metabolite 6 to 7 hours. N-Acetylprocainamide may represent a significant fraction of the total drug in the circulation.

Procainamide crosses the placental barrier and is distributed into breast milk.

◊ References.

1. Grasela TH, Sheiner LB. Population pharmacokinetics of procainamide from routine clinical data. *Clin Pharmacokinet* 1984; **9:** 545–54.

**Bioavailability.** Modified-release procainamide preparations have been shown[1] to produce similar steady-state serum concentrations of procainamide and N-acetylprocainamide when compared with equivalent total doses of immediate-release capsules. However, tablet matrices of a modified-release preparation have been recovered from the stools of a patient with diarrhoea[2] and 3.5 g of procainamide was recovered in these matrices over an 18-hour collection period; the patient had correspondingly low plasma-procainamide concentrations.

1. Vlasses PH, *et al.* Immediate-release and sustained-release procainamide: bioavailability at steady state in cardiac patients. *Ann Intern Med* 1983; **98:** 613–14.
2. Woosley RL, *et al.* Antiarrhythmic therapy: clinical pharmacology update. *J Clin Pharmacol* 1984; **24:** 295–305.

**The elderly.** Reduced renal clearance of procainamide has been reported in the elderly.[1]

1. Reidenberg MM, *et al.* Aging and renal clearance of procainamide and acetylprocainamide. *Clin Pharmacol Ther* 1980; **28:** 732–5.

**Hepatic impairment.** In 20 healthy subjects and 20 patients with chronic liver disease given a single 500-mg oral dose of procainamide hydrochloride about 64 and 33% respectively of the dose was excreted in the urine within 6 hours.[1] Decreased procainamide acetylation in the patients compared with the control group was not correlated with the severity of liver disease, whereas decreased procainamide hydrolysis and increased procainamide-derived aminobenzoic acid acetylation appeared to be related to the degree of hepatic impairment. It was suggested that the decrease in excretion of procainamide and its metabolites in the urine of the patients with liver disease could be due to an impairment in oral absorption since renal function was within the normal range but the variations in acetylation and hydrolysis were related to hepatic function.

1. du Souich P, Erill S. Metabolism of procainamide and p-aminobenzoic acid in patients with chronic liver disease. *Clin Pharmacol Ther* 1977; **22:** 588–95.

**Renal impairment.** Procainamide is excreted in the urine, largely as unchanged drug, and accumulation, especially of the active acetyl metabolite,[1] may occur in renal impairment. Haemodialysis and haemoperfusion increase the clearance of procainamide and N-acetylprocainamide (see Dialysis under Treatment of Adverse Effects, above).

1. Vlasses PH, *et al.* Lethal accumulation of procainamide metabolite in renal insufficiency. *Drug Intell Clin Pharm* 1984; **18:** 493–4.

## Uses and Administration

Procainamide hydrochloride is a class Ia antiarrhythmic (p.809); it has properties similar to those of quinidine (p.993).

Procainamide hydrochloride tends to be used for the short-term management of severe or symptomatic **arrhythmias** (p.816). It is used for the treatment of ventricular arrhythmias particularly those resistant to lidocaine and those following myocardial infarction. It may also be used for cardioversion and management of atrial fibrillation.

Therapeutic effect is generally associated with plasma concentrations of 3 to 10 micrograms/mL. The dose of procainamide hydrochloride required will depend on the age, renal and hepatic function, and underlying cardiac condition of the patient: an adult with normal renal function generally requires up to 50 mg/kg daily by mouth in divided doses every 3 to 6 hours. Higher doses may be necessary for atrial arrhythmias. A dose of 50 mg/kg daily by mouth in 4 divided doses has been used in children. Modified-release preparations are available.

In an emergency and under continuous ECG and blood pressure monitoring, procainamide hydrochloride may be given intravenously. The injection should be diluted in a 5% solution of glucose to permit better control of the speed of injection, and should be given in doses of 100 mg every 5 minutes at a rate not exceeding 50 mg/minute until the arrhythmia has been suppressed or a maximum dose of 1 g has been reached. A response may be obtained after 100 to 200 mg has been given and more than 500 or 600 mg is not generally required. Alternatively, procainamide hydrochloride may be given by continuous infusion of 500 to 600 mg over 25 to 30 minutes. Therapeutic plasma concentrations may then be maintained by giving an infusion in a 5% solution of glucose, at a rate of 2 to 6 mg/minute. When transferring to oral therapy, a period of about 3 to 4 hours should elapse between the last intravenous dose and the first oral dose.

Procainamide hydrochloride has also been given intramuscularly.

Procainamide hydrochloride may need to be given in reduced doses or at longer dosing intervals in the elderly and in patients with hepatic or renal impairment.

**Administration in children.** In a study in 5 children treated with procainamide for various cardiac arrhythmias the mean elimination half-life was found to be 1.7 hours, and the plasma clearance was higher than that reported in adults.[1] In contrast the total serum clearance of procainamide in 3 neonates with supraventricular tachycardia was found to be similar to that in adults and the mean elimination half-life was 5.3 hours.[2] A loading dose of 10 to 12 mg/kg intravenously was given followed by a continuous infusion of 20 to 75 micrograms/kg per minute.

1. Singh S, *et al.* Procainamide elimination kinetics in pediatric patients. *Clin Pharmacol Ther* 1982; **32:** 607–11.
2. Bryson SM, *et al.* Therapeutic monitoring and pharmacokinetic evaluation of procainamide in neonates. *DICP Ann Pharmacother* 1991; **25:** 68–71.

## Preparations

***BP 2003:*** Procainamide Injection; Procainamide Tablets;
***USP 27:*** Procainamide Hydrochloride Capsules; Procainamide Hydrochloride Extended-release Tablets; Procainamide Hydrochloride Injection; Procainamide Hydrochloride Tablets.

**Proprietary Preparations** (details are given in Part 3)
***Austral.:*** Pronestyl; ***Braz.:*** Procamide; ***Canad.:*** Procan; Pronestyl; ***Gr.:*** Pronestyl; ***Hong Kong:*** Pronestyl; ***India:*** Pronestyl; ***Irl.:*** Pronestyl; ***Israel:*** Pronestyl; ***Ital.:*** Procamide†; ***Neth.:*** Pronestyl; ***NZ:*** Pronestyl; ***S.Afr.:*** Pronestyl†; ***Spain:*** Biocoryl; ***Switz.:*** Pronestyl†; ***Thai.:*** Pronestyl†; ***UK:*** Pronestyl; ***USA:*** Procanbid; Pronestyl†.

# Propafenone Hydrochloride

*(BANM, USAN, rINNM)*

Fenopraine Hydrochloride; Hidrocloruro de propafenona; SA-79; WZ-884642; WZ-884643. 2′-(2-Hydroxy-3-propylamino-propoxy)-3-phenylpropiophenone hydrochloride.

$C_{21}H_{27}NO_3,HCl = 377.9.$

*CAS — 54063-53-5 (propafenone); 34183-22-7 (propafenone hydrochloride).*

*ATC — C01BC03.*

**Pharmacopoeias.** In *Chin.* and *US.*

**USP 27** (Propafenone Hydrochloride). A white powder. Soluble in hot water and in methyl alcohol; slightly soluble in alcohol and in chloroform; very slightly soluble in acetone; insoluble in ether and in toluene. A 0.5% solution in water has a pH of 5.0 to 6.2. Store in airtight containers at a temperature between 15° and 30°. Protect from light.

## Adverse Effects

Propafenone can cause disturbances in cardiac conduction which can result in bradycardia, heart block, and sinus arrest. It may aggravate heart failure and may cause hypotension. In common with other antiarrhythmics, propafenone may induce or worsen arrhythmias in some patients.

Among the most common adverse effects are gastrointestinal intolerance, dry mouth, a bitter or metallic taste, dizziness, blurred vision, headache, and fatigue. Convulsions, blood dyscrasias, liver disorders, lupus erythematosus, skin rashes, impotence, and increased breathlessness and worsening of asthma have also been reported.

**Effects on the heart.** Fatal exacerbation of ventricular tachycardia was associated with propafenone therapy in a 63-year-old man.[1]

1. Nathan AW, *et al.* Fatal ventricular tachycardia in association with propafenone, a new class IC antiarrhythmic agent. *Postgrad Med J* 1984; **60:** 155–6.

**Effects on the liver.** A review of liver injury secondary to propafenone therapy concluded that it is a rare occurrence and appears to be due to hepatocellular injury, cholestasis, or a combination.[1]

1. Spinler SA, *et al.* Propafenone-induced liver injury. *Ann Pharmacother* 1992; **26:** 926–8.

**Effects on mental function.** Delusions, hallucinations, and paranoia have been reported in an elderly patient following 2 doses of propafenone. The manufacturer had received reports of mania and psychosis.[1] Amnesia developed in a 61-year-old man 6 days after starting treatment with propafenone.[2] Symptoms resolved 6 to 7 hours after discontinuing the drug.

1. Robinson AJ. Paranoia after propafenone. *Pharm J* 1991; **247:** 556.
2. Jones RJ, *et al.* Probable propafenone-induced transient global amnesia. *Ann Pharmacother* 1995; **29:** 586–90.

**Effects on the nervous system.** Myoclonus has been reported in a patient receiving propafenone.[1] In another patient peripheral neuropathy developed 10 months after starting treatment but symptoms had resolved 6 months after stopping the drug.[2]

1. Chua TP, *et al.* Myoclonus associated with propafenone. *BMJ* 1994; **308:** 113.
2. Galasso PJ, *et al.* Propafenone-induced peripheral neuropathy. *Mayo Clin Proc* 1995; **70:** 469–72.

**Lupus erythematosus.** Symptoms of lupus erythematosus and raised antinuclear antibody titres were associated with propafenone therapy on 2 occasions in a 63-year-old woman.[1]

1. Guindo J, *et al.* Propafenone and a syndrome of the lupus erythematosus type. *Ann Intern Med* 1986; **104:** 589.

## Precautions

Propafenone is contra-indicated in patients with uncontrolled heart failure, conduction disturbances including heart block unless controlled by artificial pacing, cardiogenic shock (unless arrhythmia-induced), severe bradycardia, or pronounced hypotension. It may alter the endocardial pacing threshold and adjustment may be necessary in patients with pacemakers.

Propafenone's beta-blocking activity can exacerbate obstructive airways disease; it should be used with great caution in such patients and is contra-indicated in severe disease. Propafenone may aggravate myasthenia gravis and should be avoided in patients with this condition. Electrolyte disturbances should be corrected before initiating propafenone treatment. Propafenone should be used with caution in patients with hepatic or renal impairment.

**Pregnancy and breast feeding.** Experience in a patient given propafenone throughout the last trimester of pregnancy indicated that despite transplacental diffusion propafenone could safely be used at this time without harm to the fetus. Propafenone and its metabolite were detected in breast milk at concentrations considered to represent a markedly subtherapeutic dose to an infant.[1]

1. Libardoni M, *et al.* Transfer of propafenone and 5-OH-propafenone to foetal plasma and maternal milk. *Br J Clin Pharmacol* 1991; **32:** 527–8.

## Interactions

Propafenone is extensively metabolised by the cytochrome P450 enzyme system and plasma-propafenone concentrations may be reduced by inducers of this system such as rifampicin; enzyme inhibitors, such as cimetidine, quinidine, and HIV-protease inhibitors, may increase plasma-propafenone concentrations. Propafenone itself may alter the plasma concentrations of other drugs, possibly by interfering with their metabolism. Drugs affected include beta blockers, ciclosporin, desipramine, digoxin, theophylline, and warfarin. There may be an increased risk of arrhythmias if propafenone is given with other antiarrhythmics or arrhythmogenic drugs.

**Antiarrhythmics.** *Quinidine* inhibits the hepatic metabolism of propafenone and has raised plasma-propafenone concentrations in extensive metabolisers;[1] the plasma concentration of the active 5-hydroxy metabolite was reduced and that of the *N*-depropyl metabolite increased but there was no change in the clinical response.

1. Funck-Brentano C, *et al.* Genetically-determined interaction between propafenone and low dose quinidine: role of active metabolites in modulating net drug effect. *Br J Clin Pharmacol* 1989; **27:** 435–44.

**Antibacterials.** *Rifampicin* has lowered steady-state plasma concentrations of propafenone with the reappearance of arrhythmia.[1]

1. Castel JM, *et al.* Rifampicin lowers plasma concentrations of propafenone and its antiarrhythmic effect. *Br J Clin Pharmacol* 1990; **30:** 155–6.

**Histamine $H_2$-antagonists.** *Cimetidine* has been reported[1] to raise plasma-propafenone concentrations. The mean steady-state concentration increased by 22% but the wide interindividual variability meant this change was not significant.

1. Pritchett ELC, *et al.* Pharmacokinetic and pharmacodynamic interactions of propafenone and cimetidine. *J Clin Pharmacol* 1988; **28:** 619–24.

## Pharmacokinetics

Propafenone is readily and almost completely absorbed from the gastrointestinal tract. It is metabolised in the liver, largely by the cytochrome P450 isoenzyme CYP2D6. As a small proportion of the population lacks this enzyme, the extent of metabolism is genetically determined. In subjects with the extensive metaboliser phenotype there is extensive first-pass metabolism to two active metabolites, 5-hydroxypropafenone and *N*-depropylpropafenone, and to other minor inactive metabolites. In the small proportion of subjects with the slow metaboliser phenotype little or no 5-hydroxypropafenone is formed. The bioavailability of propafenone is dependent upon metaboliser phenotype but more importantly on dosage as the first-pass metabolism is saturable. In practice doses are high enough to compensate for differences in phenotype. Propafenone and its metabolites also undergo glucuronidation.

Propafenone is more than 95% protein bound.

Propafenone is excreted in the urine and faeces mainly in the form of conjugated metabolites. The elimination half-life is reported to be 2 to 10 hours in extensive metabolisers and 10 to 32 hours in slow metabolisers.

Propafenone crosses the placenta and is distributed into breast milk.

◊ General references.

1. Hii JTY, *et al.* Clinical pharmacokinetics of propafenone. *Clin Pharmacokinet* 1991; **21:** 1–10.

## Uses and Administration

Propafenone hydrochloride is a class Ic antiarrhythmic (p.809) with some negative inotropic and beta-adrenoceptor blocking activity. It is used in the management of supraventricular and ventricular **arrhythmias**.

The usual initial dose by mouth is 150 mg three times daily and this may be increased, if necessary, at intervals of 3 to 4 days up to a maximum of 300 mg three times daily. Patients weighing less than 70 kg should be given reduced doses; the elderly may also respond to reduced doses. Doses may need to be reduced in hepatic impairment (see below).

Propafenone hydrochloride has also been given by slow intravenous injection or by infusion.

◊ General references.

1. Bryson HM, *et al.* Propafenone: a reappraisal of its pharmacology, pharmacokinetics and therapeutic use in cardiac arrhythmias. *Drugs* 1993; **45:** 85–130.

**Administration in hepatic impairment.** Propafenone should be given with careful monitoring to patients with hepatic impairment, and the US manufacturer suggests that the dose should be only 20 to 30% of that given in normal hepatic function.

**Administration in renal impairment.** A study of the effect of renal function on disposition of propafenone found that renal impairment did not alter the pharmacokinetics of propafenone or 5-hydroxypropafenone.[1] Nevertheless, the manufacturers advise that caution is necessary if propafenone is given to patients with renal impairment.

1. Fromm MF, *et al.* Influence of renal function on the steady-state pharmacokinetics of the antiarrhythmic propafenone and its phase I and phase II metabolites. *Eur J Clin Pharmacol* 1995; **48:** 279–83.

**Cardiac arrhythmias.** Early reviews[1-4] showed propafenone, a class Ic antiarrhythmic, to be effective in a large variety of cardiac arrhythmias (p.816) including ventricular arrhythmias and supraventricular arrhythmias such as atrial flutter and atrial fibrillation. It has been used successfully to treat arrhythmias in children.[5,6] However, the results of the Cardiac Arrhythmia Suppression Trial (known as CAST), demonstrating that other class I antiarrhythmics (encainide, flecainide, and moracizine) were associated with an increased mortality rate when used for asymptomatic ventricular arrhythmias in post-infarction patients, led to many drugs of this class being restricted to severe or life-threatening ventricular arrhythmias; this restriction has also applied to propafenone in many countries although, in some, use in supraventricular arrhythmias is permitted. As well as having antiarrhythmic actions propafenone also has some beta-adrenoceptor blocking activity and this theoretically may be beneficial in post-infarction patients, but in the absence of data showing safety and efficacy of propafenone in this situation such use is not considered warranted.[4] A later review[7] acknowledged a general trend against the use of class Ic antiarrhythmics, including propafenone, in patients with nonsustained ventricular arrhythmias. Others[8,9] support its use in supraventricular arrhythmias, including as a single oral loading dose for recent-onset atrial fibrillation.[10,11]

1. Siddoway LA, Woosley RL. Propafenone: a promising new antiarrhythmic agent. *Cardiovasc Rev Rep* 1986; **7:** 153–5 and 158–9.
2. Harron DWG, Brogden RN. Propafenone: a review of its pharmacodynamic and pharmacokinetic properties, and therapeutic use in the treatment of arrhythmias. *Drugs* 1987; **34:** 617–47.
3. Chow MSS, *et al.* Propafenone: a new antiarrhythmic agent. *Clin Pharm* 1988; **7:** 869–77.
4. Funck-Brentano C, *et al.* Propafenone. *N Engl J Med* 1990; **322:** 518–25.
5. Heusch A, *et al.* Clinical experience with propafenone for cardiac arrhythmias in the young. *Eur Heart J* 1994; **15:** 1050–6.
6. Janoušek J, Paul T. Safety of oral propafenone in the treatment of arrhythmias in infants and children (European Retrospective Multicenter Study). *Am J Cardiol* 1998; **81:** 1121–4.
7. Capucci A, Boriani G. Propafenone in the treatment of cardiac arrhythmias: a risk-benefit appraisal. *Drug Safety* 1995; **12:** 55–72.
8. Kishore AGR, Camm AJ. Guidelines for the use of propafenone in treating supraventricular arrhythmias. *Drugs* 1995; **50:** 250–62.
9. Reimold SC, *et al.* Propafenone for the treatment of supraventricular tachycardia and atrial fibrillation: a meta-analysis. *Am J Cardiol* 1998; **82:** 66N–71N.
10. Khan IA. Single oral loading dose of propafenone for pharmacological cardioversion of recent-onset atrial fibrillation. *J Am Coll Cardiol* 2001; **37:** 542–7.
11. Boriani G, *et al.* Oral loading with propafenone for conversion of recent-onset atrial fibrillation: a review on in-hospital treatment. *Drugs* 2002; **62:** 415–23.

## Preparations

**Proprietary Preparations** (details are given in Part 3)
***Arg.:*** Normorytmin; ***Austria:*** Asonacor; Rhythmocor; Rytmonorma; ***Belg.:*** Rytmonorm; ***Braz.:*** Ritmonorm; ***Canad.:*** Rythmol; ***Chile:*** Ritmocor; Rytmonorm; ***Denm.:*** Rytmonorm; ***Fin.:*** Rytmonorm; ***Fr.:*** Rythmol; ***Ger.:*** Cuxafenon; Propafen†; Propamerck; Propastad†; Prorynorm†; Rytmo-Puren; Rytmogenat; Rytmonorm; Tachyfenon†; ***Gr.:*** Rythmonopm; ***Hong Kong:*** Rytmonorm; ***Irl.:*** Arythmol; ***Israel:*** Profex; Rythmex; ***Ital.:*** Fenorit; Rytmonorm; ***Malaysia:*** Rytmonorm; ***Mex.:*** Homopafen; Kenonat†; Nistaken; Norfenon; ***Neth.:*** Rytmonorm; ***NZ:*** Rytmonorm; ***Port.:*** Rytmonorm; ***S.Afr.:*** Rythmol; ***Singapore:*** Rytmonorm; ***Spain:*** Rytmonorm; ***Swed.:*** Rytmonorm; ***Switz.:*** Rytmonorm; ***Thai.:*** Rytmonorm; ***UK:*** Arythmol; ***USA:*** Rythmol.

## Propatylnitrate *(BAN, rINN)*

ETTN; Ettriol Trinitrate; Propatilnitrato; Propatyl Nitrate *(USAN)*; Trinettriol; Win-9317. 2-Ethyl-2-hydroxymethylpropane-1,3-diol trinitrate.

$C_6H_{11}N_3O_9$ = 269.2.
*CAS — 2921-92-8.*
*ATC — C01DA07.*

### Profile

Propatylnitrate is a vasodilator with general properties similar to those of glyceryl trinitrate (p.923) that has been used in angina pectoris.

### Preparations

**Proprietary Preparations** (details are given in Part 3)
***Braz.:*** Coronar; Sustrate.

## Propentofylline *(BAN, rINN)*

HWA-285; Propentofilina. 3-Methyl-1-(5-oxohexyl)-7-propylxanthine.

$C_{15}H_{22}N_4O_3$ = 306.4.
*CAS — 55242-55-2.*
*ATC — N06BC02.*

### Profile

Propentofylline is a xanthine derivative that has been investigated in cerebrovascular disorders including dementia. It is also used in veterinary medicine.

# Propranolol Hydrochloride

*(BANM, USAN, rINNM)*

AY-64043; Hidrocloruro de propranolol; ICI-45520; NSC-91523; Propranololi Hydrochloridum. (±)-1-Isopropylamino-3-(1-naphthyloxy)propan-2-ol hydrochloride.

$C_{16}H_{21}NO_2$,HCl = 295.8.
*CAS — 525-66-6 (propranolol); 13013-17-7 (propranolol); 318-98-9 (propranolol hydrochloride); 3506-09-0 (propranolol hydrochloride).*
*ATC — C07AA05.*

**Pharmacopoeias.** In *Chin., Eur.* (see p.vi), *Int., Jpn, Pol.,* and *US.*

**Ph. Eur. 5.0** (Propranolol Hydrochloride). A white or almost white powder. Soluble in water and in alcohol.

**USP 27** (Propranolol Hydrochloride). A white to off-white, odourless, crystalline powder. Soluble in water and in alcohol; slightly soluble in chloroform; practically insoluble in ether. Store at a temperature of 25°, excursions permitted between 15° and 30°.

**Stability.** In aqueous solutions propranolol decomposes with oxidation of the isopropylamine side-chain, accompanied by a reduction in pH and discoloration of the solution. Solutions are most stable at pH 3 and decompose rapidly when alkaline.

## Adverse Effects, Treatment, and Precautions

As for Beta Blockers, p.869.

**Breast feeding.** Propranolol is distributed into breast milk. A milk/plasma ratio range of 0.33 to 1.65 was reported in a study of 3 lactating women.[1] It was calculated that the maximum dose likely to be ingested by a breast-fed infant would be less than 0.1% of the maternal dose. Other small studies[2,3] have reported similar results. No adverse effects have been reported in breast-fed infants whose mothers were receiving propranolol and the American Academy of Pediatrics considers[4] that it is therefore usually compatible with breast feeding.


1. Smith MT, *et al.* Propranolol, propranolol glucuronide, and naphthoxylactic acid in breast milk and plasma. *Ther Drug Monit* 1983; **5:** 87–93.
2. Karlberg B, *et al.* Excretion of propranolol in human breast milk. *Acta Pharmacol Toxicol (Copenh)* 1974; **34:** 222–4.
3. Bauer JH, *et al.* Propranolol in human plasma and breast milk. *Am J Cardiol* 1979; **43:** 860–2.
4. American Academy of Pediatrics. The transfer of drugs and other chemicals into human milk. *Pediatrics* 2001; **108:** 776–89. Correction. *ibid.*; 1029. Also available at: http://aappolicy.aappublications.org/cgi/content/full/pediatrics%3b108/3/776 (accessed 06/07/04)


## Interactions

The interactions associated with beta blockers are discussed on p.870.

## Pharmacokinetics

Propranolol is almost completely absorbed from the gastrointestinal tract, but is subject to considerable hepatic tissue binding and first-pass metabolism. Peak plasma concentrations occur about 1 to 2 hours after an oral dose. Plasma concentrations vary greatly between individuals. Propranolol has high lipid solubility. It crosses the blood-brain barrier and the placenta, and is distributed into breast milk. Propranolol is about 90% bound to plasma proteins. It is metabolised in the liver and at least one of its metabolites (4-hydroxypropranolol) is considered to be biologically active, but the contribution of metabolites to its overall activity is uncertain. The metabolites and small amounts of unchanged drug are excreted in the urine. The plasma half-life of propranolol is about 3 to 6 hours. Propranolol is reported not to be significantly dialysable.

**Pregnancy.** A study in 6 pregnant patients (32 to 36 weeks' gestation) showed that the disposition of propranolol 120 mg by mouth and 10 mg intravenously was not altered in pregnancy compared with the postnatal period.[1] Another study[2] in 13 pregnant patients given propranolol to control hypertension demonstrated that the pharmacokinetics of propranolol and most of its major metabolites were not altered during pregnancy. Samples at term[3] in 10 of the women showed that propranolol and all of its known metabolites were present in maternal plasma, cord plasma, and neonatal plasma. At delivery plasma protein binding of propranolol was reported as 87.5% in maternal plasma and 67.2% in cord plasma. Similar results for maternal and cord plasma protein binding have been reported by others.[4]


1. O'Hare MFO, *et al.* Pharmacokinetics of propranolol during pregnancy. *Eur J Clin Pharmacol* 1984; **27:** 583–7.
2. Smith MT, *et al.* Chronic propranolol administration during pregnancy: maternal pharmacokinetics. *Eur J Clin Pharmacol* 1983; **25:** 481–90.
3. Smith MT, *et al.* Metabolism of propranolol in the human maternal-placental-foetal unit. *Eur J Clin Pharmacol* 1983; **24:** 727–32.
4. Wood M, Wood AJJ. Changes in plasma drug binding and $\alpha_1$-acid glycoprotein in mother and newborn infant. *Clin Pharmacol Ther* 1981; **29:** 522–6.


## Uses and Administration

Propranolol is a non-cardioselective beta blocker (p.868). It is reported to have membrane-stabilising properties, but does not possess intrinsic sympathomimetic activity.

Propranolol is used as the hydrochloride in the management of hypertension (p.825), phaeochromocytoma (p.831), angina pectoris (p.813), myocardial infarction (p.828), and cardiac arrhythmias (p.816). It is also used in hypertrophic cardiomyopathy (p.818). It is used to control symptoms of sympathetic overactivity in the management of hyperthyroidism (p.1594), anxiety disorders (p.663), and tremor (p.872). Other indications include the prophylaxis of migraine (p.464) and of upper gastrointestinal bleeding in patients with portal hypertension (see Variceal Haemorrhage under Monoethanolamine Oleate, p.1716).

Propranolol hydrochloride is usually given by mouth. In **hypertension** it is given in initial doses of 40 to 80 mg twice daily increased as required to a usual range of 160 to 320 mg daily; some patients may require up to 640 mg daily. Propranolol is *not* suitable for the emergency treatment of hypertension; it should not be given intravenously in hypertension.

In **phaeochromocytoma**, patients treated surgically may be given 60 mg daily on the 3 days before the operation, always with alpha blockade. If the tumour is inoperable prolonged treatment may be given with a daily dose of 30 mg.

In **angina**, initial doses of propranolol hydrochloride 40 mg given 2 or 3 times daily are increased as required to a usual range of 120 to 240 mg daily. Some patients may require up to 320 mg daily.

Propranolol hydrochloride is given within 5 to 21 days of **myocardial infarction** in doses of 40 mg given four times daily for 2 or 3 days followed by 80 mg twice daily. Another regimen is to give 180 to 240 mg daily in divided doses.

Propranolol may be given in doses of 30 to 160 mg daily in divided doses in the long-term management of **cardiac arrhythmias**. For the emergency treatment of cardiac arrhythmias, propranolol hydrochloride may be given by slow intravenous injection in a dose of 1 mg injected over a period of 1 minute, repeated if necessary every 2 minutes until a maximum total of 10 mg has been given in conscious patients and 5 mg in patients under anaesthesia. Patients receiving propranolol intravenously should be carefully monitored.

In **hypertrophic cardiomyopathy** the usual dose of propranolol hydrochloride is 10 to 40 mg given three or four times daily.

In **hyperthyroidism** propranolol hydrochloride is given in doses of 10 to 40 mg three or four times daily. If intravenous administration is necessary 1 mg is given over 1 minute, repeated at 2-minute intervals until a response is observed or to a maximum dose of 10 mg in conscious patients or 5 mg in patients under anaesthesia.

The dose for **anxiety** is 40 mg daily; this may be increased to 40 mg two or three times daily.

**Essential tremor** may be treated with 40 mg given two or three times daily; the dose can be increased at weekly intervals to 160 mg daily although doses up to 320 mg daily may be necessary.

An initial dose of 40 mg two or three times daily is used in **migraine** prophylaxis; the dose can be increased at weekly intervals up to 160 mg daily. Some patients have been given 240 mg daily.

In **portal hypertension,** propranolol hydrochloride should be given in initial doses of 40 mg twice daily; the dose may be increased as required up to 160 mg twice daily.

**Children.** Propranolol hydrochloride has been used in the treatment of hypertension in children in initial doses of 1 mg/kg daily in divided doses by mouth, increased as required to a usual range of 2 to 4 mg/kg daily in two divided doses. For arrhythmias, phaeochromocytoma, and hyperthyroidism, the dose is 250 to 500 micrograms/kg three or four times daily by mouth. Children requiring intravenous administration may be given 25 to 50 micrograms/kg injected slowly with appropriate monitoring; this dose may be repeated three or four times daily. Children under 12 years of age may be given 20 mg two or three times daily for the prophylaxis of migraine.

**Administration in hepatic impairment.** A study of the effects of cirrhosis on the disposition of propranolol during steady-state oral administration in 9 normal subjects and 7 with cirrhosis demonstrated a mean threefold increase in unbound propranolol concentrations in the blood in patients with cirrhosis when compared with the controls. Mean half-lives for the 2 groups were 11.2 and 4 hours respectively.[1] Another study of the pharmacokinetics of propranolol given as a single dose of a 20-mg tablet and as a 160-mg modified-release preparation daily for 7 days in 10 patients with cirrhosis and portal hypertension demonstrated higher plasma concentrations in patients with severe liver disease compared with those reported in normal controls.[2] Similar pharmacokinetic findings have been reported by others.[3]

In patients with severe liver disease, it has been suggested that propranolol therapy be started at a low dose such as 20 mg three times daily, or 80 mg of a modified-release preparation given once daily,[2] or 160 mg of a modified-release preparation given every other day.[3] Monitoring of beta blockade is essential; checking the heart rate[2] or exercise testing[3] have been suggested as suitable methods to assess the extent of beta blockade in patients with cirrhosis.


1. Wood AJJ, *et al.* The influence of cirrhosis on steady-state blood concentrations of unbound propranolol after oral administration. *Clin Pharmacokinet* 1978; **3:** 478–87.
2. Arthur MJP, *et al.* Pharmacology of propranolol in patients with cirrhosis and portal hypertension. *Gut* 1985; **26:** 14–19.
3. Calès P, *et al.* Pharmacodynamic and pharmacokinetic study of propranolol in patients with cirrhosis and portal hypertension. *Br J Clin Pharmacol* 1989; **27:** 763–70.


**Administration in renal impairment.** A study of the pharmacokinetics of propranolol in 11 patients with chronic renal insufficiency showed no impairment in the elimination kinetics of propranolol compared with 8 subjects with normal renal function.[1] Peak concentrations of propranolol reported in patients with chronic renal failure have been 2 to 3 times higher than those reported in patients receiving dialysis or normal subjects.[1,2] Additional studies indicate that there is no pharmacokinetic reason to amend the dosage of propranolol in patients with renal impairment.[3]

Findings from a study in 8 patients on haemodialysis include a slight elevation of propranolol-plasma concentrations, no elevation of plasma concentration of 4-hydroxypropranolol, but extremely high plasma concentrations of other propranolol metabolites.[4]


1. Lowenthal DT, *et al.* Pharmacokinetics of oral propranolol in chronic renal disease. *Clin Pharmacol Ther* 1974; **16:** 761–9.
2. Bianchetti G, *et al.* Pharmacokinetics and effects of propranolol in terminal uraemic patients and in patients undergoing regular dialysis treatment. *Clin Pharmacokinet* 1976; **1:** 373–84.
3. Wood AJJ, *et al.* Propranolol disposition in renal failure. *Br J Clin Pharmacol* 1980; **10:** 561–6.
4. Stone WJ, Walle T. Massive propranolol metabolite retention during maintenance hemodialysis. *Clin Pharmacol Ther* 1980; **28:** 449–55.


## Preparations

***BP 2003:*** Prolonged-release Propranolol Capsules; Propranolol Injection; Propranolol Tablets;
***USP 27:*** Propranolol Hydrochloride and Hydrochlorothiazide Extended-release Capsules; Propranolol Hydrochloride and Hydrochlorothiazide Tablets; Propranolol Hydrochloride Extended-release Capsules; Propranolol Hydrochloride Injection; Propranolol Hydrochloride Tablets.

**Proprietary Preparations** (details are given in Part 3)
***Arg.:*** Inderal; Pirimetan; Propalong; Propayerst; ***Austral.:*** Deralin; Inderal; ***Austria:*** Inderal; Proprahexal; ***Belg.:*** Inderal; ***Braz.:*** Antitensin; Betalevedim†; Inderal; Neo Propranol; Pradinolol; Propacor; Rebaten; Sanpronol; Uni Propralol; ***Canad.:*** Inderal; Novo-Pranol†; ***Chile:*** Coriodal; ***Denm.:*** Inderal; Propal; Propranet†; ***Fin.:*** Inderal; Propral; Ranoprin; ***Fr.:*** Adrexan; Avlocardyl; Hemipralon; ***Ger.:*** Beta-Tablinen; Dociton; Efektolol; Elbrol; Indobloc†; Obsidan; Propabloc; Prophylux; propra; Propra-ratiopharm; Propranur; ***Gr.:*** Inderal; ***Hong Kong:*** Angilol†; Antarol†; Becardin; Berkolol†; Hopranolol; Inderal; Inpanol; Palon; Prolol; Propa; ***India:*** Betabloc; Betaspan; Ciplar; Corbeta; Inderal; ***Irl.:*** Half Inderal; Inderal; Tiperal; ***Israel:*** Deralin; Inderal; Prolol; Slow Deralin; ***Ital.:*** Inderal; ***Malaysia:*** Inderal; Indon; Propanol; ***Mex.:*** Acifol; Europranolol†; Inderalici; Prochor†; Propalem; Propalen†; Propalgin†; Propol†; ***Neth.:*** Inderal; ***Norw.:*** Inderal; Pranolol; Pronovan†; ***NZ:*** Angilol†; Cardinol; ***Port.:*** Corpendol; Inderal; ***S.Afr.:*** Cardiblok†; Inderal; Nolol†; Prodorol; Pur-Bloka; ***Singapore:*** Inderal; Inpanol; ***Spain:*** Sumial; ***Swed.:*** Inderal; ***Switz.:*** Betaprol†; Inderal; ***Thai.:*** Atensin; Betalol; Betapress; Cardenol; Emforal; Inderal; Normpress; Palon; Perlol; Pralol; Prolol; Pronosil†; Servanolol†; Syntonol; ***UAE:*** Cardilol; ***UK:*** Angilol; Bedranol; Beta-Prograne; Betadur CR†; Cardinol†; Half Beta-Prograne; Half Betadur CR†; Half Inderal; Inderal; Syprol; ***USA:*** Inderal; InnoPran.

**Multi-ingredient:** ***Arg.:*** Propayerst Plus; ***Austria:*** Inderal compt†; Inderetic; ***Belg.:*** Inderetic; ***Braz.:*** Tenadren; ***Canad.:*** Inderide†; ***Ger.:*** Beta-Turfa; Betathiazid A†; Betathiazid†; Diutensat comp; Docidrazin; Docireticc; Dociteren; Manimon†; Nitro-Obsidan; Obsilazin N; Pertenso N; Propra comp; ***India:*** Beptazine; Beptazine-H; Ciplar-H; Corbetazine; ***Irl.:*** Inderetic†; ***Neth.:*** Inderetic; ***S.Afr.:*** Inderetic; ***Spain:*** Betadipresan; Betadipresan Diu; ***Switz.:*** Inderetic; ***UK:*** Inderetic†; Inderex†; ***USA:*** Inderide.

## Proroxan *(pINN)*

AY-24269 (proroxan hydrochloride). 1-(2,3-Dihydro-1,4-benzodioxin-6-yl)-3-(3-phenyl-1-pyrrolidinyl)-1-propanone.
$C_{21}H_{23}NO_3$ = 337.4.
*CAS — 33743-96-3 (proroxan); 33025-33-1 (proroxan hydrochloride).*

NOTE. Proroxan Hydrochloride is *USAN.*

### Profile

Proroxan is used as an antihypertensive.

## Proscillaridin *(BAN, USAN, rINN)*

2936; A-32686; Proscilaridina; Proscillaridin A; PSC-801. 14-Hydroxy-3β-(α-L-rhamnopyranosyloxy)-14β-bufa-4,20,22-trienolide.
$C_{30}H_{42}O_8$ = 530.6.
*CAS — 466-06-8.*
*ATC — C01AB01.*

### Profile

Proscillaridin is a cardiac glycoside obtained from *Drimia maritima* (Liliaceae). It is a positive inotrope with general properties similar to those of digoxin (p.895). It is reported to have a rapid onset and a short duration of action.

Proscillaridin is used in the treatment of heart failure (p.820). It is given by mouth in usual initial and maintenance doses of 1 to 1.5 mg daily; maintenance doses may range from 0.5 to 2.5 mg daily as required.

### Preparations

**Proprietary Preparations** (details are given in Part 3)
***Austral.:*** Talusin†; ***Austria:*** Caradrin†; ***Fin.:*** Talusin†; ***Ger.:*** Talusin; ***Switz.:*** Talusin†.
**Multi-ingredient:** ***Switz.:*** Theo-Talusin†.

## Quinapril Hydrochloride

*(BANM, USAN, rINNM)*

CI-906 (quinapril); Hidrocloruro de quinapril. (3S)-2-{N-[(S)-1-Ethoxycarbonyl-3-phenylpropyl]-L-alanyl}-1,2,3,4-tetrahydro-isoquinoline-3-carboxylic acid hydrochloride.
$C_{25}H_{30}N_2O_5,HCl = 475.0$.
*CAS — 85441-61-8 (quinapril); 82586-55-8 (quinapril hydrochloride).*
*ATC — C09AA06.*

**Pharmacopoeias.** In *US.*
**USP 27** (Quinapril Hydrochloride). A white to off-white powder, with a pink cast at times. Freely soluble in aqueous solvents.

### Adverse Effects, Treatment, and Precautions

As for ACE inhibitors, p.842.

**Breast feeding.** Following administration of a single dose of quinapril 20 mg to 6 lactating women, quinapril was detected in the breast milk in a milk to plasma ratio of 0.12; no quinaprilat was detected.[1] It was estimated that the dose received by the infant would only be about 1.6% of the maternal dose.

1. Begg EJ, *et al.* Quinapril and its metabolite quinaprilat in human milk. *Br J Clin Pharmacol* 2001; **51:** 478–81.

### Interactions

As for ACE inhibitors, p.845.

**Antibacterials.** Quinapril has been reported to reduce the absorption of *tetracyclines* due to the presence of magnesium carbonate in the tablet formulation.

### Pharmacokinetics

Quinapril acts as a prodrug of the diacid quinaprilat, its active metabolite. Following oral administration about 60% of a dose is absorbed. Quinapril is metabolised mainly in the liver to quinaprilat and inactive metabolites. Peak plasma concentrations of quinaprilat are achieved within 2 hours of an oral dose of quinapril. Quinaprilat is about 97% bound to plasma proteins. Following an oral dose, quinapril is excreted in the urine and faeces, as quinaprilat, other metabolites, and unchanged drug, with the urinary route predominating; up to 96% of an intravenous dose of quinaprilat is excreted in the urine. The effective half-life for accumulation of quinaprilat is approximately 3 hours following multiple doses of quinapril; a long terminal phase half-life of 25 hours may represent strong binding of quinaprilat to angiotensin-converting enzyme.

The pharmacokinetics of both quinapril and quinaprilat are affected by renal and hepatic impairment. Dialysis has little effect on the excretion of quinapril or quinaprilat.

Small amounts of quinapril are distributed into breast milk.

◊ References.

1. Begg EJ, *et al.* The pharmacokinetics and pharmacodynamics of quinapril and quinaprilat in renal impairment. *Br J Clin Pharmacol* 1990; **30:** 213–20.
2. Halstenson CE, *et al.* The pharmacokinetics of quinapril and its active metabolite, quinaprilat, in patients with various degrees of renal function. *J Clin Pharmacol* 1992; **32:** 344–50.
3. Wolter K, Fritschka E. Pharmacokinetics and pharmacodynamics of quinaprilat after low dose quinapril in patients with terminal renal failure. *Eur J Clin Pharmacol* 1993; **44** (suppl 1): S53–6.
4. Begg EJ, *et al.* The pharmacokinetics of quinapril and quinaprilat in patients with congestive heart failure. *Br J Clin Pharmacol* 1994; **37:** 302–4.
5. Squire IB, *et al.* Haemodynamic response and pharmacokinetics after the first dose of quinapril in patients with congestive heart failure. *Br J Clin Pharmacol* 1994; **38:** 117–23.
6. Breslin E, *et al.* A pharmacodynamic and pharmacokinetic comparison of intravenous quinaprilat and oral quinapril. *J Clin Pharmacol* 1996; **36:** 414–21.

### Uses and Administration

Quinapril is an ACE inhibitor (p.842). It is used in the treatment of hypertension (p.825) and heart failure (p.820).

Quinapril is converted in the body to its active metabolite quinaprilat. The haemodynamic effects are seen within 1 hour of a single dose by mouth and the maximum effect occurs after about 2 to 4 hours, although the full effect may not develop for 1 to 2 weeks during chronic administration. The haemodynamic action persists for about 24 hours, allowing once-daily dosing. Quinapril is given by mouth as the hydrochloride, but doses are expressed in terms of the base. Quinapril hydrochloride 10.8 mg is approximately equivalent to 10.0 mg of quinapril.

In the treatment of **hypertension** the initial dose is 10 mg of quinapril once daily. Since there may be a precipitous fall in blood pressure in some patients when starting therapy with an ACE inhibitor, the first dose should preferably be given at bedtime. An initial dose of 2.5 mg daily is recommended in the elderly, in patients with renal impairment, or in those receiving a *diuretic*; if possible, the diuretic should be withdrawn 2 or 3 days before quinapril is started and resumed later if necessary.

The usual maintenance dose is 20 to 40 mg daily, as a single dose or divided into 2 doses, although up to 80 mg daily has been given.

In the management of **heart failure**, severe first-dose hypotension on introduction of an ACE inhibitor is common in patients on loop diuretics, but their temporary withdrawal may cause rebound pulmonary oedema. Thus treatment should be initiated with a low dose under close medical supervision. Quinapril is given in an initial dose of 2.5 mg daily. Usual maintenance doses range from 10 to 20 mg daily, as a single dose or divided into 2 doses; up to 40 mg daily has been given.

Quinaprilat may be given intravenously in patients unable to take quinapril orally; usual doses range from 1.25 to 10 mg twice daily.

◊ Reviews.

1. Wadworth AN, Brogden RN. Quinapril: a review of its pharmacological properties, and therapeutic efficacy in cardiovascular disorders. *Drugs* 1991; **41:** 378–99.
2. Plosker GL, Sorkin EM. Quinapril: a reappraisal of its pharmacology and therapeutic efficacy in cardiovascular disorders. *Drugs* 1994; **48:** 227–52.
3. Culy CR, Jarvis B. Quinapril: a further update of its pharmacology and therapeutic use in cardiovascular disorders. *Drugs* 2002; **62:** 339–85.

### Preparations

***USP 27:*** Quinapril Tablets.

**Proprietary Preparations** (details are given in Part 3)
***Arg.:*** Accupril; ***Austral.:*** Accupril; Asig; ***Austria:*** Accupro; Continucor†; ***Belg.:*** Accupril; ***Braz.:*** Accupril; ***Canad.:*** Accupril; ***Chile:*** Accupril; ***Denm.:*** Accupro; ***Fin.:*** Accupro; ***Fr.:*** Acuitel; Korec; ***Ger.:*** Accupro; ***Gr.:*** Accupron; ***Hong Kong:*** Accupril; ***Irl.:*** Accupro; ***Ital.:*** Accuprin; Acequin; Quinazil; ***Jpn:*** Conan; ***Malaysia:*** Accupril; ***Mex.:*** Acupril; ***Neth.:*** Acupril; ***NZ:*** Accupril; ***Port.:*** Acupril; Vasocor; ***S.Afr.:*** Accupril; ***Singapore:*** Accupril; ***Spain:*** Acuprel; Acuretic; Ectren; Lidaltrin; ***Swed.:*** Accupro; ***Switz.:*** Accupro; ***Thai.:*** Accupril; ***UK:*** Accupro; ***USA:*** Accupril.

**Multi-ingredient:** ***Arg.:*** Accuretic; ***Austral.:*** Accuretic; ***Austria:*** Accuzide; ***Belg.:*** Accuretic; ***Braz.:*** Accuretic†; ***Canad.:*** Accuretic; ***Chile:*** Accuretic; ***Fin.:*** Accupro Comp; ***Fr.:*** Acuilix; Koretic; ***Ger.:*** Accuzide; ***Irl.:*** Accuretic; ***Ital.:*** Accuretic; Acequide; Quinazide; ***Neth.:*** Acuzide; ***NZ:*** Accuretic; ***Port.:*** Acuretic; ***S.Afr.:*** Accuretic; ***Spain:*** Bicetil; Lidaltrin Diu; ***Swed.:*** Accupro Comp; ***Switz.:*** Accuretic; ***UK:*** Accuretic; ***USA:*** Accuretic.

## Quinethazone

*(BAN, rINN)*

Chinethazonum; Quinetazona. 7-Chloro-2-ethyl-1,2,3,4-tetrahydro-4-oxoquinazoline-6-sulphonamide.
$C_{10}H_{12}ClN_3O_3S = 289.7$.
*CAS — 73-49-4.*
*ATC — C03BA02.*

### Profile

Quinethazone is a diuretic which is related chemically to metolazone and has properties similar to those of the thiazide diuretics (see Hydrochlorothiazide, p.933). It has been used for oedema, including that associated with heart failure, and for hypertension.

### Preparations

**Proprietary Preparations** (details are given in Part 3)
***USA:*** Hydromox†.

## Quinidine

*(BAN)*

Chinidinum; Quinidina. (8R,9S)-6′-Methoxycinchonan-9-ol; (+)-(αS)-α-(6-Methoxy-4-quinolyl)-α-[(2R,4S,5R)-(5-vinylquinuclidin-2-yl)]methanol.
$C_{20}H_{24}N_2O_2 = 324.4$.
*CAS — 56-54-2 (anhydrous quinidine); 63717-04-4 (quinidine dihydrate); 72402-50-7 (± quinidine).*
*ATC — C01BA01.*

**Description.** Quinidine is an isomer of quinine, obtained from the bark of species of *Cinchona* and their hybrids; it may also be obtained from *Remijia pedunculata*, or prepared from quinine. It may contain some hydroquinidine, a closely allied base with similar chemical, physical, and physiological properties.

### Quinidine Bisulfate

Quinidina, bisulfato de; Quinidine Bisulphate *(BANM)*.
$C_{20}H_{24}N_2O_2,H_2SO_4 = 422.5$.
*CAS — 747-45-5 (anhydrous quinidine bisulfate); 6151-39-9 (quinidine bisulfate tetrahydrate).*
*ATC — C01BA01.*

**Pharmacopoeias.** In *Br.*
**BP 2003** (Quinidine Bisulphate). Colourless, odourless or almost odourless, crystals. It contains not more than 15% of hydroquinidine bisulfate. Freely soluble in water and in alcohol; practically insoluble in ether. A 1% solution in water has a pH of 2.6 to 3.6. Protect from light.

### Quinidine Gluconate

*(BANM)*

Quinidina, gluconato de; Quinidinium Gluconate.
$C_{20}H_{24}N_2O_2,C_6H_{12}O_7 = 520.6$.
*CAS — 7054-25-3.*
*ATC — C01BA01.*

**Pharmacopoeias.** In *US.*
**USP 27** (Quinidine Gluconate). A white, odourless powder. It contains not more than 20% of hydroquinidine gluconate. Freely soluble in water; slightly soluble in alcohol. Store at a temperature of 25°, excursions permitted between 15° and 30°. Protect from light.

**Adsorption.** More than 40% of a dose of quinidine gluconate was lost when the drug was administered by intravenous infusion using a PVC infusion bag and tubing.[1]

1. Darbar D, *et al.* Loss of quinidine gluconate injection in a polyvinyl chloride infusion system. *Am J Health-Syst Pharm* 1996; **53:** 655–8.

### Quinidine Polygalacturonate

Quinidina, poligalacturonato de. Quinidine poly(D-galacturonate) hydrate.
$C_{20}H_{24}N_2O_2,(C_6H_{10}O_7)_x,xH_2O$.
*CAS — 27555-34-6 (anhydrous quinidine polygalacturonate); 65484-56-2 (quinidine polygalacturonate hydrate).*
*ATC — C01BA01.*

### Quinidine Sulfate

Chinidini Sulfas; Chinidinsulfate; Chinidinum Sulfuricum; Quinidina, sulfato de; Quinidine Sulphate *(BANM)*; Quinidini Sulfas.
$(C_{20}H_{24}N_2O_2)_2,H_2SO_4,2H_2O = 782.9$.
*CAS — 50-54-4 (anhydrous quinidine sulfate); 6591-63-5 (quinidine sulfate dihydrate).*
*ATC — C01BA01.*

**Pharmacopoeias.** In *Chin., Eur.* (see p.vi), *Int., Jpn, Pol.,* and *US.*
**Ph. Eur. 5.0** (Quinidine Sulphate). White or almost white, crystalline powder, or silky, colourless needles. It contains not more than 15% of hydroquinidine sulfate. Slightly soluble in water; soluble in boiling water and in alcohol; practically insoluble in acetone. A 1% solution in water has a pH of 6.0 to 6.8. Protect from light.
**USP 27** (Quinidine Sulphate). Fine, needle-like, white crystals, frequently cohering in masses, or a fine, white powder. It is odourless and darkens on exposure to light. It contains not more than 20% of hydroquinidine sulfate. Its solutions are neutral or alkaline to litmus. Soluble 1 in 100 of water, 1 in 10 of alcohol, and 1 in 15 of chloroform; insoluble in ether. Protect from light.

**Stability.** Quinidine sulfate was reported[1] to be stable for up to 60 days in a number of extemporaneously prepared oral liquid formulations.

1. Allen LV, Erickson MA. Stability of bethanechol chloride, pyrazinamide, quinidine sulfate, rifampin, and tetracycline hydrochloride in extemporaneously compounded oral liquids. *Am J Health-Syst Pharm* 1998; **55:** 1804–9.

### Adverse Effects and Treatment

Quinidine and its salts cause both cardiac and non-cardiac adverse effects. They commonly cause gastrointestinal irritation with nausea, vomiting, and diarrhoea. Hypersensitivity similar to that occurring with quinine may also occur and a test dose should be given to each patient (see Uses and Administration, below). Reactions include respiratory difficulties, urticaria, pruritus, skin rashes, purpura, thrombocytopenia and other blood dyscrasias, and, rarely, fever and anaphylaxis. Granulomatous hepatitis and a lupus-like syndrome have been reported.

Quinidine may give rise to cinchonism (see Quinine, p.460) with tinnitus, impaired hearing, visual disturbances, headache, confusion, vertigo, vomiting, and abdominal pain; it is usually associated with large doses, but may occur in idiosyncratic subjects given small doses.

Quinidine may induce hypotension; this is a special risk with intravenous administration. It may precipitate ventricular arrhythmias, including torsade de pointes.

In quinidine overdosage, the cardiac symptoms of intoxication predominate. Quinidine is cumulative in action and inappropriately high plasma concentrations may induce ECG changes, heart block, asystole, ventricular tachycardia, ventricular fibrillation, syncope, seizures, coma, and sometimes death. Treatment of adverse effects and overdosage is symptomatic and supportive. Activated charcoal may be considered if the patient presents within 1 hour of ingestion.

◊ A review of adverse effects associated with the class Ia antiarrhythmic drugs quinidine, disopyramide, and procainamide, and their clinical management.[1]

1. Kim SY, Benowitz NL. Poisoning due to class IA antiarrhythmic drugs quinidine, procainamide and disopyramide. *Drug Safety* 1990; **5:** 393–420.

**Effects on the blood.** Quinidine-induced thrombocytopenia is not uncommon and it is one of the best documented drugs known to cause drug-dependent thrombocytopenia. The reaction is considered to be a hypersensitivity reaction probably due to the binding of quinidine to the platelet surface causing production of autoantibodies and subsequent platelet lysis.[1] The antigenic constituent of the platelet membrane may be glycoprotein Ib although other surface glycoproteins have also been implicated.[2] Highly specific quinidine-dependent platelet antibodies have been found in the serum of patients with quinidine-induced thrombocytopenia;[3] the antibodies reacted with quinidine and the isomerically similar desmethoxy derivative cinchonine, but not with quinine. Once formed such antibodies may remain detectable for over 2 years.

A second mechanism has been proposed in which quinidine-autoantibody complexes are formed and then deposited on the platelet causing lysis.[2]

1. Mitchell JA, *et al.* Immunotoxic side-effects of drug therapy. *Drug Safety* 1990; **5:** 168–78.
2. Stricker RB, Shuman MA. Quinidine purpura: evidence that glycoprotein V is a target platelet antigen. *Blood* 1986; **67:** 1377–81.
3. Reid DM, Shulman NR. Drug purpura due to surreptitious quinidine intake. *Ann Intern Med* 1988; **108:** 206–8.

**Effects on the eyes.** Corneal deposits resembling those found in keratopathy developed in a patient who had been taking quinidine for 2 years.[1] Symptoms had improved and both corneas had cleared completely within 2 months of stopping the drug.

A small number of patients have also been identified[2] who developed uveitis during quinidine treatment.

1. Zaidman GW. Quinidine keratopathy. *Am J Ophthalmol* 1984; **97:** 247–9.
2. Fraunfelder FW, Rosenbaum JT. Drug-induced uveitis: incidence, prevention and treatment. *Drug Safety* 1997; **17:** 197–207.

**Effects on the joints.** Quinidine has been associated with the development of reversible, symmetrical polyarthritis in several patients.[1-3] No biochemical or immunological abnormalities were found and the reaction was considered to be distinct from quinidine-induced lupus erythematosus (see below). Symptoms resolved within 1 week of withdrawing quinidine.

1. Kertes P, Hunt D. Polyarthritis complicating quinidine treatment. *BMJ* 1982; **284:** 1373–4.
2. Cohen MG, *et al.* Two distinct quinidine-induced rheumatic syndromes. *Ann Intern Med* 1988; **108:** 369–71.
3. Naschitz JE, Yeshurun D. Quinidine and rheumatic syndromes. *Ann Intern Med* 1988; **109:** 248–9.

**Effects on the liver.** Hypersensitivity reactions involving the liver have been reported in about 2% of patients receiving quinidine.[1,2] The main clinical symptom is fever[1-3] but skin rash,[1-3] purpura,[2] and hepatomegaly[1] may also occur. Liver enzyme values are raised[1-4] and the platelet count may be reduced.[3] The reaction is reversible on withdrawing quinidine with fever resolving in about 48 hours and liver enzymes values returning to normal within about 2 weeks. Liver biopsy often shows granulomatous hepatitis,[1-3] but other inflammatory changes[2] and cholestatic jaundice[4] have been found.

1. Geltner D, *et al.* Quinidine hypersensitivity and liver involvement: a survey of 32 patients. *Gastroenterology* 1976; **70:** 650–2.
2. Knobler H, *et al.* Quinidine-induced hepatitis. *Arch Intern Med* 1986; **146:** 526–8.
3. Bramlet DA, *et al.* Granulomatous hepatitis as a manifestation of quinidine hypersensitivity. *Arch Intern Med* 1980; **140:** 395–7.
4. Hogan DB, *et al.* Unusual hepatotoxic reaction to quinidine. *Can Med Assoc J* 1984; **130:** 973.

**Effects on mental state.** Gradually progressive cerebral dysfunction characterised by intermittent confusion, agitation, restlessness, personality change, and paranoid features occurred in a 62-year-old man who had taken quinidine for about 15 years.[1] Within 24 hours of discontinuing quinidine there was a marked improvement and after 5 days he had returned to normal with no cognitive deficits. It was considered that quinidine had precipitated or exacerbated the functional psychosis.

1. Johnson AG, *et al.* A functional psychosis precipitated by quinidine. *Med J Aust* 1990; **153:** 47–9.

**Effects on the skin.** Skin reactions reported with quinidine include exacerbation of psoriasis,[1] blue-grey pigmentation,[2] and photosensitivity.[3] Purpuric bruising has occurred in a person who was subjected to inhalation of quinidine dust in the workplace.[4]

1. Harwell WB. Quinidine-induced psoriasis. *J Am Acad Dermatol* 1983; **9:** 278.
2. Mahler R, *et al.* Pigmentation induced by quinidine therapy. *Arch Dermatol* 1986; **122:** 1062–4.
3. Marx JL, *et al.* Quinidine photosensitivity. *Arch Dermatol* 1983; **119:** 39–43.
4. Salom IL. Purpura due to inhaled quinidine. *JAMA* 1991; **266:** 1220.

**Hypoglycaemia.** Mean plasma-insulin concentrations increased and mean plasma-glucose concentrations decreased in 8 healthy subjects and 10 patients with malaria given quinidine intravenously.[1] Profound hypoglycaemia occurred in 1 patient with cerebral malaria and acute renal failure. These effects were considered to be associated with stimulation of β-cell secretion of insulin by quinidine and it was concluded that hypoglycaemia may occur in any severely ill fasting patient given parenteral quinidine.

1. Phillips RE, *et al.* Hypoglycaemia and antimalarial drugs: quinidine and release of insulin. *BMJ* 1986; **292:** 1319–21.

**Lupus erythematosus.** There are several well-documented reports of quinidine-induced lupus erythematosus.[1-4] The syndrome involves polyarthritis with a positive antinuclear antibody test. Symptoms do not usually occur until several months after starting quinidine and resolve slowly on withdrawing the drug. A recurrence of lupus-like symptoms has occurred in patients with a previous reaction to procainamide.[2]

1. West SG, *et al.* Quinidine-induced lupus erythematosus. *Ann Intern Med* 1984; **100:** 840–2.
2. Amadio P, *et al.* Procainamide, quinidine, and lupus erythematosus. *Ann Intern Med* 1985; **102:** 419.
3. Lavie CJ, *et al.* Systemic lupus erythematosus (SLE) induced by quinidine. *Arch Intern Med* 1985; **145:** 446–8.
4. Cohen MG, *et al.* Two distinct quinidine-induced rheumatic syndromes. *Ann Intern Med* 1988; **108:** 369–71.

**Oesophageal stricture.** Oesophageal ulceration and stricture formation have been reported[1] in patients taking quinidine and reviews[1,2] suggest that quinidine is one of the most common causes of drug-induced oesophageal damage.

1. McCord GS, Clouse RE. Pill-induced esophageal strictures: clinical features and risk factors for development. *Am J Med* 1990; **88:** 512–18.
2. Jaspersen D. Drug-induced oesophageal disorders: pathogenesis, incidence, prevention and management. *Drug Safety* 2000; **22:** 237–49.

## Precautions

Quinidine is contra-indicated in patients with complete heart block. An initial test dose of quinidine should always be given to detect hypersensitivity; positive responders should not be given quinidine nor should patients who have previously experienced quinidine hypersensitivity. It should be used with extreme caution in patients with incomplete heart block or uncompensated heart failure and in those with myocarditis or severe myocardial damage. Care is also required in patients with myasthenia gravis as it can exacerbate the symptoms and may reduce the effectiveness of parasympathomimetic drugs. Antiarrhythmic therapy with quinidine should be initiated with extreme caution, if at all, during acute infections or fever as hypersensitivity reactions may be masked.

When quinidine is used to treat atrial flutter or fibrillation, the reduction in atrioventricular block may result in a very rapid ventricular rate. This can be avoided by prior digitalisation or by use of a rate-limiting calcium-channel blocker or beta blocker. However, quinidine is contra-indicated in digitalis overdosage as markedly increased plasma concentrations of digoxin may occur.

Reduced dosage should be considered for the elderly, for patients with hepatic or renal impairment, and on the occasions when it is used in heart failure.

**Breast feeding.** A woman[1] receiving 2.1 g quinidine daily throughout pregnancy had milk and serum concentrations measured 5 days after delivery. Concentrations were found to be 6.4 and 9.0 micrograms/mL respectively, giving a milk to serum ratio of 0.71. It was estimated that the amount of quinidine that would be ingested by an infant would be far below the therapeutic range for its weight. No adverse effects have been reported in infants and the American Academy of Pediatrics considers[2] that quinidine is therefore usually compatible with breast feeding.

1. Hill LM, Malkasian GD. The use of quinidine sulfate throughout pregnancy. *Obstet Gynecol* 1979; **54:** 366–8.
2. American Academy of Pediatrics. The transfer of drugs and other chemicals into human milk. *Pediatrics* 2001; **108:** 776–89. Correction. *ibid.*; 1029. Also available at: http://aappolicy.aappublications.org/cgi/content/full/pediatrics%3b108/3/776 (accessed 06/07/04)

**Pregnancy.** In a report[1] on the administration of quinidine sulfate to a woman throughout pregnancy, concentrations in the infant's serum at delivery were similar to the mother's although amniotic fluid concentrations were raised. The infant's weight, ECG, haemoglobin concentration, and platelet count were all found to be within normal limits.

1. Hill LM, Malkasian GD. The use of quinidine sulfate throughout pregnancy. *Obstet Gynecol* 1979; **54:** 366–8.

## Interactions

Quinidine is used with other antiarrhythmic drugs but caution is required with such combinations (see below). Use with other arrhythmogenic drugs should be avoided.

Quinidine is metabolised in the liver, mainly by the cytochrome P450 isoenzyme CYP3A4, and interactions may occur through inhibition or enhancement of hepatic metabolism. Rifampicin, phenobarbital, and phenytoin increase hepatic metabolism of quinidine and increased doses of quinidine may be needed if one of these drugs is added to quinidine therapy. The HIV-protease inhibitors nelfinavir and ritonavir may produce toxic concentrations of quinidine.

Urinary excretion of quinidine is dependent on urinary pH; drugs that increase urinary pH such as sodium bicarbonate, some antacids, and carbonic anhydrase inhibitors tend to increase the plasma concentration of quinidine since the proportion of nonionised drug in the urine is increased allowing greater renal tubular reabsorption.

As well as being affected by a range of drugs quinidine can in its turn affect other compounds which include oral anticoagulants, antihypertensives, antimuscarinics, beta blockers, digoxin, muscle relaxants, and parasympathomimetics. These interactions are discussed under the monographs for those drugs. Quinidine also inhibits the cytochrome P450 isoenzyme CYP2D6 and may affect drugs metabolised by this route.

**Antiarrhythmics.** *Amiodarone* may increase the plasma concentration of quinidine, increasing the risk of toxicity; prolongation of the QT interval with torsade de pointes has been reported.[1] This interaction is probably due to amiodarone inhibiting hepatic or renal clearance of quinidine or displacing quinidine from binding sites. If the two drugs are used together the dose of quinidine may need to be reduced and the patient should be closely monitored. *Verapamil* given intravenously has been reported[2] to cause severe hypotension in patients also receiving quinidine by mouth. Studies *in vitro* suggest this is due to the additive blockade of α-adrenergic receptors by both drugs and the simultaneous blockade of calcium channels by verapamil; verapamil may also increase the plasma concentration of quinidine. Quinidine may increase the plasma concentration of other antiarrhythmics when administered concomitantly (see Ajmaline, p.856, Digoxin, p.896, Disopyramide, p.904, Flecainide Acetate, p.917, and Propafenone Hydrochloride, p.989).

1. Lesko LJ. Pharmacokinetic drug interactions with amiodarone. *Clin Pharmacokinet* 1989; **17:** 130–40.
2. Maisel AS, *et al.* Hypotension after quinidine plus verapamil. *N Engl J Med* 1985; **312:** 167–70.

**Antibacterials.** *Erythromycin* might inhibit the hepatic metabolism of quinidine.[1]

1. Spinler SA, *et al.* Possible inhibition of hepatic metabolism of quinidine by erythromycin. *Clin Pharmacol Ther* 1995; **57:** 89–94.

**Antifungals.** *Ketoconazole* temporarily increased the plasma-quinidine concentration in a patient through reduced hepatic elimination.[1] Another antifungal that inhibits hepatic metabolism, *itraconazole*, has also been reported[2] to increase plasma-quinidine concentrations.

1. McNulty RM, *et al.* Transient increase in plasma quinidine concentrations during ketoconazole-quinidine therapy. *Clin Pharm* 1989; **8:** 222–5.
2. Kaukonen K-M, *et al.* Itraconazole increases plasma concentrations of quinidine. *Clin Pharmacol Ther* 1997; **62:** 510–17.

**Beta blockers.** Sinus bradycardia has been reported in a patient prescribed oral quinidine and *timolol* eye drops,[1] and orthostatic hypotension has occurred when quinidine was used with *aten-*

*olol.*[2] Use of quinidine or the beta blocker alone was well tolerated in each case with no adverse effects.

1. Dinai Y, *et al.* Bradycardia induced by interaction between quinidine and ophthalmic timolol. *Ann Intern Med* 1985; **103:** 890–1.
2. Manolis AS, Estes NAM. Orthostatic hypotension due to quinidine and atenolol. *Am J Med* 1987; **82:** 1083–4.

**Calcium-channel blockers.** *Nifedipine* has been reported[1] to reduce plasma-quinidine concentrations and increasing the dose of quinidine to up to 20 mg/kg failed to increase the plasma concentration. Withdrawal of nifedipine resulted in a doubling of the quinidine concentration. A pharmacokinetic and pharmacodynamic study in healthy subjects, however, failed to show that modified-release *felodipine* or nifedipine had any effect on quinidine disposition.[2] Another study in healthy subjects suggested that quinidine may inhibit nifedipine metabolism.[3] *Diltiazem* has also been reported[4] to decrease the clearance and increase the half-life of quinidine in healthy subjects, although it was noted that another study had failed to show any interaction.

For the effects of *verapamil* on quinidine, see Antiarrhythmics, above.

1. Green JA, *et al.* Nifedipine-quinidine interaction. *Clin Pharm* 1983; **2:** 461–5.
2. Bailey DG, *et al.* Quinidine interaction with nifedipine and felodipine: pharmacokinetic and pharmacodynamic evaluation. *Clin Pharmacol Ther* 1993; **53:** 354–9.
3. Bowles SK, *et al.* Evaluation of the pharmacokinetic and pharmacodynamic interaction between quinidine and nifedipine. *J Clin Pharmacol* 1993; **33:** 727–31.
4. Laganière S, *et al.* Pharmacokinetic and pharmacodynamic interactions between diltiazem and quinidine. *Clin Pharmacol Ther* 1996; **60:** 255–64.

**Diuretics.** *Carbonic anhydrase inhibitors* tend to increase plasma-quinidine concentrations due to increased renal tubular reabsorption of quinidine.

Administration of *amiloride* to 10 patients receiving quinidine produced arrhythmias in 4 of them.[1] It was suggested that additive sodium-channel blockade may be responsible.

1. Wang L, *et al.* Amiloride-quinidine interaction: adverse outcomes. *Clin Pharmacol Ther* 1994; **56:** 659–67.

**Histamine $H_2$-antagonists.** *Cimetidine* inhibits the hepatic metabolism of quinidine and increases in plasma concentration and half-life with a reduction in clearance have been reported.[1-3]

1. Hardy BG, *et al.* Effect of cimetidine on the pharmacokinetics and pharmacodynamics of quinidine. *Am J Cardiol* 1983; **52:** 172–5.
2. Kolb KW, *et al.* Effect of cimetidine on quinidine clearance. *Ther Drug Monit* 1984; **6:** 306–12.
3. MacKichan JJ, *et al.* Effect of cimetidine on quinidine bioavailability. *Biopharm Drug Dispos* 1989; **10:** 121–5.

## Pharmacokinetics

Quinidine is rapidly absorbed from the gastrointestinal tract, peak plasma concentrations being achieved about 1.5 hours after oral administration of quinidine sulfate and about 4 hours after quinidine gluconate; its bioavailability is variable, owing to first-pass metabolism in the liver.

Quinidine is metabolised in the liver, mainly by the cytochrome P450 isoenzyme CYP3A4, to a number of metabolites, at least some of which are pharmacologically active. It is excreted in the urine, mainly in the form of its metabolites. The proportion excreted unchanged is dependent on urinary pH; in acidic urine about 20% is excreted as unchanged quinidine but in alkaline urine this is reduced to about 5% due to increased renal tubular reabsorption.

Quinidine is widely distributed throughout the body and is 80 to 90% bound to plasma proteins including $\alpha_1$-acid glycoprotein. It has a plasma half-life of about 6 to 8 hours but this may show wide variation. Its therapeutic effect has been correlated with plasma concentrations of about 2 to 7 micrograms/mL. However, plasma concentrations can be misleading as, depending on the assay method, quinidine may not be differentiated from its metabolites. It has been suggested that with specific assays quinidine concentrations of 1 microgram or less per mL may be all that are required.

Quinidine crosses the placenta and is distributed into breast milk. Small amounts are removed by haemodialysis.

◊ Considerable intersubject and intrasubject variability in the pharmacokinetics of quinidine has been noted;[1] in one study the half-life ranged from about 1 to 16 hours regardless of whether the drug was administered as a tablet, capsule, oral solution, or intramuscular injection. There may also be considerable variations in absorption pharmacokinetic parameters depending upon the formulation and the salt used.[2,3] The effect of food on absorption is not clear.[4,5] The heart condition being treated or associated with the arrhythmia may alter quinidine's pharmacokinetics[6,7] as may the age of the patient.[8-10] Hepatic impairment may affect protein binding and prolong quinidine's half-life.[11] Protein binding increases in patients with renal impairment, although it returns to normal during dialysis procedures.[12] Accumulation of quinidine metabolites may occur in patients with renal dysfunction.[13-15]

1. Mason WD, *et al.* Comparative plasma concentrations of quinidine following administration of one intramuscular and three oral formulations to 13 human subjects. *J Pharm Sci* 1976; **65:** 1325–9.
2. Frigo GM, *et al.* Comparison of quinidine plasma concentration curves following oral administration of some short- and long-acting formulations. *Br J Clin Pharmacol* 1977; **4:** 449–54.
3. Mahon WA, *et al.* Comparative bioavailability study of three sustained release quinidine formulations. *Clin Pharmacokinet* 1987; **13:** 118–24.
4. Woo E, Greenblatt DJ. Effect of food on enteral absorption of quinidine. *Clin Pharmacol Ther* 1980; **27:** 188–93.
5. Martinez MN, *et al.* Effect of dietary fat content on the bioavailability of a sustained release quinidine gluconate tablet. *Biopharm Drug Dispos* 1990; **11:** 17–29.
6. Ueda CT, Dzindzio BS. Quinidine kinetics in congestive heart failure. *Clin Pharmacol Ther* 1978; **23:** 158–64.
7. Ueda CT, Dzindzio BS. Bioavailability of quinidine in congestive heart failure. *Br J Clin Pharmacol* 1981; **11:** 571–7.
8. Drayer DE, *et al.* Prevalence of high (3S)-3-hydroxyquinidine/quinidine ratios in serum, and clearance of quinidine in cardiac patients with age. *Clin Pharmacol Ther* 1980; **27:** 72–5.
9. Szefler SJ, *et al.* Rapid elimination of quinidine in pediatric patients. *Pediatrics* 1982; **70:** 370–5.
10. Pickoff AS, *et al.* Age-related differences in the protein binding of quinidine. *Dev Pharmacol Ther* 1981; **3:** 108–15.
11. Kessler KM, *et al.* Quinidine pharmacokinetics in patients with cirrhosis or receiving propranolol. *Am Heart J* 1978; **96:** 627–35.
12. Kessler KM, Perez GO. Decreased quinidine plasma protein binding during haemodialysis. *Clin Pharmacol Ther* 1981; **30:** 121–6.
13. Kessler KM, *et al.* Quinidine elimination in patients with congestive heart failure or poor renal function. *N Engl J Med* 1974; **290:** 706–9.
14. Drayer DE, *et al.* Steady-state serum levels of quinidine and active metabolites in cardiac patients with varying degrees of renal function. *Clin Pharmacol Ther* 1978; **24:** 31–9.
15. Hall K, *et al.* Clearance of quinidine during peritoneal dialysis. *Am Heart J* 1982; **104:** 646–7.

## Uses and Administration

Quinidine is a class Ia antiarrhythmic (p.809). It also has antimuscarinic and alpha-adrenoceptor blocking properties. Quinidine is used to maintain sinus rhythm after cardioversion of atrial fibrillation, and for the suppression of supraventricular and ventricular **arrhythmias**.

Quinidine is an isomer of quinine and may be used as an alternative to quinine in the treatment of **malaria** when quinine is not immediately available.

Quinidine is given by mouth as the sulfate and also as a range of salts including the bisulfate, the gluconate, and the polygalacturonate. Strengths of preparations and doses of quinidine salts used have been expressed in a variety of ways; as well as expressing in terms of the salt actually being employed, equivalences in terms of anhydrous quinidine base or quinidine sulfate dihydrate have commonly been used. Quinidine bisulfate (anhydrous) 260 mg, quinidine gluconate (anhydrous) 321 mg, quinidine sulfate (dihydrate) 241 mg, and quinidine sulfate (anhydrous) 230 mg are each approximately equivalent to 200 mg of quinidine (anhydrous).

For the management of cardiac arrhythmias, quinidine sulfate is given by mouth. An initial test dose of 200 mg should always be given to detect hypersensitivity. The usual dose is then 200 to 400 mg three or four times daily. Doses of up to 600 mg every 2 to 4 hours have been given for the treatment of supraventricular tachycardias to a maximum of 4 g daily; these higher doses should only be given with frequent monitoring of the ECG and plasma concentration.

Modified-release formulations are generally preferred as the plasma concentration profile is smoother and doses can be given at 8- to 12-hourly intervals.

Quinidine has been given intramuscularly or by slow intravenous injection, but absorption from the intramuscular route can be erratic and incomplete, and the intravenous route is associated with a risk of severe hypotension. Parenteral doses of quinidine gluconate are: intramuscularly, 600 mg initially then up to 400 mg repeated every 2 hours if necessary; by intravenous infusion 800 mg diluted to a volume of 50 mL with glucose 5% and given at a rate of 1 mL/minute with ECG and blood-pressure monitoring.

◊ General references.

1. Grace AA, Camm AJ. Quinidine. *N Engl J Med* 1998; **338:** 35–45.

**Cardiac arrhythmias.** Quinidine is a class Ia antiarrhythmic and has been used in the management of supraventricular and ventricular arrhythmias (p.816), but like other antiarrhythmics it may precipitate arrhythmias. The CAST (Cardiac Arrhythmia Suppression Trial) studies demonstrated that other class I antiarrhythmics (encainide, flecainide, and moracizine) were associated with an increased mortality rate when used for asymptomatic ventricular arrhythmias in post-infarction patients and led to many drugs of this class being restricted to severe or life-threatening arrhythmias. A meta-analysis of trials utilising quinidine was undertaken as it was believed this drug had gained in popularity after the adverse CAST results. This meta-analysis[1] suggested that quinidine was associated with at least as high a proportion of adverse events, such as death and early proarrhythmia, as the class Ic drugs flecainide and propafenone. It was, however, emphasised that these results do not necessarily apply to the use of quinidine for the treatment of life-threatening or sustained ventricular arrhythmias.

1. Morganroth J, Goin JE. Quinidine-related mortality in the short-to-medium-term treatment of ventricular arrhythmias: a meta-analysis. *Circulation* 1991; **84:** 1977–83.

**Congenital myasthenia.** Although quinidine may exacerbate the symptoms of myasthenia gravis and should be used with great caution in such patients, beneficial responses have been reported in patients with the slow-channel congenital myasthenic syndrome (see p.1489).

**Cramps.** Although quinidine would be expected to have similar efficacy to quinine in preventing nocturnal cramps, quinine is preferred due to its lower potential for cardiotoxicity.[1] For a discussion of the usual treatment of nocturnal cramp, see under Muscle Spasm, p.1386.

1. Beeley L. *BMJ* 1991; **302:** 33.

**Hiccup.** Quinidine is one of several drugs that have been tried in intractable hiccups. For details of a protocol for the control of hiccups see Chlorpromazine, p.682.

**Malaria.** Although quinidine might theoretically be superior to quinine as an antimalarial it is more likely to cause cardiac toxicity and hypersensitivity and WHO[1] has recommended that parenteral formulations of quinidine should only be used when parenteral quinine or artemisinin derivatives are not immediately available. In these situations intravenous infusions of quinidine could be used to initiate treatment for severe chloroquine-resistant malaria. Patients should be transferred to oral therapy with quinine as soon as possible to complete a 7-day course; alternatively a single oral treatment of pyrimethamine-sulfadoxine may be given.

In the USA, the Centers for Disease Control[2,3] have recommended parenteral quinidine gluconate as the drug of choice for the treatment of complicated falciparum malaria, but only because of the lack of availability of parenteral quinine.

Quinidine is given intravenously as the gluconate and doses have been expressed in terms of the base or salt; it should be given under close control, preferably with continuous ECG monitoring and frequent measurements of blood pressure. Regimens used include one[1,4] where the equivalent of 15 mg of the base per kg is infused over 4 hours as a loading dose followed by the equivalent of 7.5 mg of the base per kg every 8 hours as infusions over 4 hours; the patient should be transferred to an oral form of antimalarial as soon as possible. An alternative regimen[5] consists of a loading dose of 10 mg of quinidine gluconate per kg given by intravenous infusion over a period of 1 to 2 hours followed by a constant intravenous infusion of 20 micrograms/kg per minute for a maximum of 72 hours or until oral therapy with quinine can be instituted to complete a total 3-day course of treatment. It is generally recommended that loading doses should not be used if the patient has received quinine or quinidine within the previous 24 hours or mefloquine within the preceding 7 days.

The overall management of malaria is discussed in the chapter on Antimalarials, p.444.

1. WHO. *Management of severe malaria: a practical handbook.* Geneva: WHO, 2000.
2. Centers for Disease Control. Treatment with quinidine gluconate of persons with severe Plasmodium falciparum infection: discontinuation of parenteral quinine from CDC drug service. *MMWR* 1991; **40** (RR-4): 21–3. Also available at http://www.cdc.gov/mmwr/preview/mmwrhtml/00043932.htm (accessed 06/07/04)
3. Centers for Disease Control. Availability and use of parenteral quinidine gluconate for severe or complicated malaria. *MMWR* 2000; **49:** 1138–40.
4. Phillips RE, *et al.* Intravenous quinidine for the treatment of severe falciparum malaria: clinical pharmacokinetic studies. *N Engl J Med* 1985; **312:** 1273–8.
5. Miller KD, *et al.* Treatment of severe malaria in the United States with a continuous infusion of quinidine gluconate and exchange transfusion. *N Engl J Med* 1989; **321:** 65–70.

## Preparations

***BP 2003:*** Quinidine Sulphate Tablets;
***USP 27:*** Quinidine Gluconate Extended-release Tablets; Quinidine Gluconate Injection; Quinidine Sulfate Capsules; Quinidine Sulfate Extended-release Tablets; Quinidine Sulfate Tablets.

**Proprietary Preparations** (details are given in Part 3)
***Austral.:*** Kinidin; ***Belg.:*** Kinidine; ***Braz.:*** Natisedine†; Quinicardine; ***Canad.:*** Biquin; Cardioquin†; Natisedine†; Quinate†; Quinidex†; Quinobarb†; ***Denm.:*** Kinidin; ***Fin.:*** Kinidin†; Kiniduron; ***Fr.:*** Cardioquine†; Longacor†; Quinidurule†; ***Ger.:*** Optochinidin retard†; ***Gr.:*** Kinidin durules; Ydroquinidine Cooper; ***Hong Kong:*** Kinidin; ***Irl.:*** Kinidin; ***Israel:*** Quiniduran; ***Ital.:*** Chinteina; Longachin; Naticardina; Natisedina; Ritmocor; ***Mex.:*** Quineuron†; Quini; ***Neth.:*** Cardioquin; Kinidine; ***Norw.:*** Kinidin†; Systodin†; ***NZ:*** Kinidin†; ***S.Afr.:*** Quinaglute†; ***Spain:*** Cardioquine†; Longacor; Quinicardina†; ***Swed.:*** Kinidin; ***Switz.:*** Kinidin; Longacor; ***Thai.:*** Ki-

nidin†; *UK:* Kinidin; *USA:* Cardioquin†; Quinaglute†; Quinalan†; Quinidex; Quinora†.

**Multi-ingredient:** *Fr.:* Quinimax; *Ger.:* Cordichin.

## Ramipril *(BAN, USAN, rINN)*

Hoe-498; Ramiprilum. (2S,3aS,6aS)-1-{N-[(S)-1-Ethoxycarbonyl-3-phenylpropyl]L-alanyl}perhydrocyclopenta[*b*]pyrrole-2-carboxylic acid.

$C_{23}H_{32}N_2O_5$ = 416.5.

*CAS — 87333-19-5.*

*ATC — C09AA05.*

**Pharmacopoeias.** In *Eur.* (see p.vi) and *US.*

**Ph. Eur. 5.0** (Ramipril). A white or almost white, crystalline powder. Sparingly soluble in water; freely soluble in methyl alcohol. Protect from light.

**USP 27** (Ramipril). A white to almost white, crystalline powder. Sparingly soluble in water; freely soluble in methyl alcohol. Store in airtight containers.

### Adverse Effects, Treatment, and Precautions

As for ACE inhibitors, p.842.

### Interactions

As for ACE inhibitors, p.845.

### Pharmacokinetics

Ramipril acts as a prodrug of the diacid ramiprilat, its active metabolite. Following oral administration at least 50 to 60% is absorbed. Ramipril is metabolised in the liver to ramiprilat; other metabolites are inactive. Peak plasma concentrations of ramiprilat are achieved 2 to 4 hours after an oral dose of ramipril. Ramiprilat is about 56% bound to plasma proteins. Following oral administration ramipril is excreted primarily in the urine, as ramiprilat, other metabolites, and some unchanged drug. About 40% of an oral dose is excreted in the faeces; this may represent both biliary excretion and unabsorbed drug. The effective half-life for accumulation of ramiprilat is 13 to 17 hours following multiple doses of ramipril 5 to 10 mg, but is much longer for doses of 1.25 to 2.5 mg daily; the difference relates to the long terminal half-life associated with saturable binding to the angiotensin-converting enzyme. The clearance of ramiprilat is reduced in renal impairment.

◊ Reviews.


1. Meisel S, *et al.* Clinical pharmacokinetics of ramipril. *Clin Pharmacokinet* 1994; **26:** 7–15.
2. van Griensven JMT, *et al.* Pharmacokinetics, pharmacodynamics and bioavailability of the ACE inhibitor ramipril. *Eur J Clin Pharmacol* 1995; **47:** 513–8.
3. Fillastre JP, *et al.* Kinetics, safety, and efficacy of ramipril after long-term administration in hemodialyzed patients. *J Cardiovasc Pharmacol* 1996; **27:** 269–74.


### Uses and Administration

Ramipril is an ACE inhibitor (p.842). It is used in the treatment of hypertension (p.825), heart failure (p.820), and following myocardial infarction (p.828) to improve survival in patients with clinical evidence of heart failure. It is also used to reduce the risk of cardiovascular events in patients with certain risk factors (see Cardiovascular Risk Reduction, p.819).

Ramipril owes its activity to ramiprilat to which it is converted after oral administration. The haemodynamic effects are seen within 1 to 2 hours of a single oral dose and the maximum effect occurs after about 3 to 6 hours, although the full effect may not develop for several weeks during chronic dosing. The haemodynamic effect is maintained for at least 24 hours, allowing once-daily dosing.

In the treatment of **hypertension** an initial dose of 1.25 mg once daily is given by mouth. Since there may be a precipitous fall in blood pressure when starting therapy with an ACE inhibitor, the first dose should preferably be given at bedtime. Patients receiving diuretics should, if possible, have the diuretic discontinued 2 to 3 days before starting ramipril, and resumed later if necessary. The usual maintenance dose is 2.5 to 5 mg daily as a single dose, although up to 10 mg daily may be required. In the USA an initial dose of 2.5 mg once daily in hypertensive patients not receiving a diuretic and a maintenance dose of 2.5 to 20 mg daily, as a single dose or in two divided doses, have been suggested.

In the management of **heart failure**, severe first-dose hypotension on introduction of an ACE inhibitor is common in patients on loop diuretics, but their temporary withdrawal may cause rebound pulmonary oedema. Thus treatment should be initiated with a low dose under close medical supervision; high doses of diuretics should be reduced before starting ramipril. Ramipril is given in an initial dose of 1.25 mg once daily. The usual maximum dose is 10 mg daily; doses of 2.5 mg or more daily may be taken in 1 or 2 divided doses.

Following **myocardial infarction**, treatment with ramipril may be started in hospital 3 to 10 days after the infarction at a usual initial dose of 2.5 mg twice daily, increased after two days to 5 mg twice daily. The usual maintenance dose is 2.5 to 5 mg twice daily.

For the **prophylaxis of cardiovascular events** in patients considered to be at high risk, ramipril is given in an initial dose of 2.5 mg once daily. The dose should be increased, if tolerated, to 5 mg once daily after 1 week, then to the usual maintenance dose of 10 mg once daily after a further 3 weeks. In patients with hypertension or recent myocardial infarction it may also be given in divided doses.

A reduction in dosage of ramipril may be necessary in patients with impaired renal function (see below).

◊ References.


1. Todd PA, Benfield P. Ramipril: a review of its pharmacological properties and therapeutic efficacy in cardiovascular disorders. *Drugs* 1990; **39:** 110–35.
2. The Acute Infarction Ramipril Efficacy (AIRE) Study Investigators. Effect of ramipril on mortality and morbidity of survivors of acute myocardial infarction with clinical evidence of heart failure. *Lancet* 1993; **342:** 821–8.
3. Frampton JE, Peters DH. Ramipril: an updated review of its therapeutic use in essential hypertension and heart failure. *Drugs* 1995; **49:** 440–66.
4. The Heart Outcomes Prevention Evaluation Study Investigators. Effects of an angiotensin-converting-enzyme inhibitor, ramipril, on cardiovascular events in high-risk patients. *N Engl J Med* 2000; **342:** 145–53.
5. Warner GT, Perry CM. Ramipril: a review of its use in the prevention of cardiovascular outcomes. *Drugs* 2002; **62:** 1381–1405.
6. Vuong AD, Annis LG. Ramipril for the prevention and treatment of cardiovascular disease. *Ann Pharmacother* 2003; **37:** 412–19.


**Administration in renal impairment.** In patients with a creatinine clearance of less than 30 mL/minute, the initial dose of ramipril should not exceed 1.25 mg daily and the maintenance dose should not exceed 5 mg daily; for those with a creatinine clearance of less than 10 mL/minute, the maintenance dose should not exceed 2.5 mg daily.

### Preparations

**Proprietary Preparations** (details are given in Part 3)
***Arg.:*** Lostapres; Tritace; ***Austral.:*** Ramace; Tritace; ***Austria:*** Hypren; Tritace; ***Belg.:*** Ramace; Tritace; ***Braz.:*** Naprix; Triatec; ***Canad.:*** Altace; ***Chile:*** Ramipres; Triatec; ***Denm.:*** Ramace; Triatec; ***Fin.:*** Cardace; Ramace; ***Fr.:*** Triatec; ***Ger.:*** Delix; Vesdil; ***Gr.:*** Stiebenyl; Triatec; ***Hong Kong:*** Tritace; ***India:*** Cardace; ***Irl.:*** Tritace; ***Israel:*** Tritace; ***Ital.:*** Quark; Triatec; Unipril; ***Malaysia:*** Tritace; ***Mex.:*** Ramace; Tritace; ***Neth.:*** Tritace; ***Norw.:*** Triatec; ***Port.:*** Triatec; ***S.Afr.:*** Ramace; Tritace; ***Singapore:*** Tritace; ***Spain:*** Acovil; Carasel; ***Swed.:*** Pramace; Triatec; ***Switz.:*** Triatec; Vesdil; ***Thai.:*** Corpril; Tritace; ***UK:*** Tritace; ***USA:*** Altace.

**Multi-ingredient:** ***Arg.:*** Tritace-HCT; ***Austria:*** Hypren plus; Lasitace; Trialix; Triapin; Tritazide; Unimax; ***Belg.:*** Tritazide; ***Braz.:*** Naprix D; Triatec D; ***Denm.:*** Triatec Comp; ***Fin.:*** Cardace Comp; Unimax; ***Ger.:*** Arelix ACE; Aretensin; Delix plus; Delmuno; Unimax; Vesdil plus; ***Irl.:*** Trialix; ***Israel:*** Tritace Comp; ***Ital.:*** Idroquark; Prilace; Triatec HCT; Uniprildiur; ***Mex.:*** Tritazide; ***Neth.:*** Triapin; Tritazide; Unimax; ***Port.:*** Triatec Composto; ***S.Afr.:*** Tri-Plen; ***Spain:*** Unimest†; ***Swed.:*** Triatec Comp; ***Switz.:*** Trialix; Triatec Comp; Unimax; ***UK:*** Triapin.

## Ranolazine Hydrochloride *(USAN, rINNM)*

Hidrocloruro de ranolazina; RS-43285. (±)-4-[2-Hydroxy-3-(o-methoxyphenoxy)propyl]-1-piperazineaceto-2′,6′-xylidide dihydrochloride.

$C_{24}H_{33}N_3O_4,2HCl$ = 500.5.

*CAS — 95635-55-5 (ranolazine); 95635-56-6 (ranolazine hydrochloride).*

### Profile

Ranolazine hydrochloride is under investigation for use in angina pectoris.

◊ References.


1. McCormack JG, *et al.* Ranolazine: a novel metabolic modulator for the treatment of angina. *Gen Pharmacol* 1998; **30:** 639–45.
2. Pepine CJ, Wolff AA. A controlled trial with a novel anti-ischemic agent, ranolazine, in chronic stable angina pectoris that is responsive to conventional antianginal agents. *Am J Cardiol* 1999; **84:** 46–50.


## Raubasine

Ajmalicine; Alkaloid F; Raubasina; δ-Yohimbine. Methyl 16,17-didehydro-19α-methyl-18-oxayohimban-16-carboxylate.

$C_{21}H_{24}N_2O_3$ = 352.4.

*CAS — 483-04-5.*

### Profile

Raubasine is an alkaloid obtained from *Rauwolfia serpentina* (Apocynaceae). It is a vasodilator related chemically to reserpine (p.995) and has been given by mouth and by injection in peripheral and cerebral vascular disorders.

### Preparations

**Proprietary Preparations** (details are given in Part 3)
***Austria:*** Lamuran†; ***Ital.:*** Lamuran; ***S.Afr.:*** Melanex†.

**Multi-ingredient:** ***Austria:*** Defluina; ***Braz.:*** Vasofluina†; ***Fr.:*** Duxil; Iskedyl; ***Hong Kong:*** Duxaril; Iso Triraupin†; ***Port.:*** Duxil; Transoxyl; ***Singapore:*** Duxaril; ***Spain:*** Duxor; Iskedyl†; Isquebral†; Salvalion†; ***Thai.:*** Duxaril; Iso-Triraupin.

## Rauwolfia Serpentina

Chotachand; Rauvolfia; Rauwolfia; Rauwolfiae Radix; Rauwolfiawurzel.

*CAS — 8063-17-0 (rauwolfia).*

*ATC — C02AA04.*

**Pharmacopoeias.** In *Ger.* and *US.*

**USP 27** (Rauwolfia Serpentina). The dried roots of *Rauwolfia serpentina* (Apocynaceae). It contains not less than 0.15% of reserpine-rescinnamine group alkaloids calculated as reserpine. Store at 15° to 30° in a dry place.

### Profile

*Rauwolfia serpentina* contains numerous alkaloids, the most active as hypotensive agents being the ester alkaloids, reserpine and rescinnamine. Other alkaloids present have structures related to reserpic acid, but are not esterified, and include ajmaline (rauwolfine), ajmalinine, ajmalicine, isoajmaline (isoarauwolfine), serpentine, rauwolfinine, and sarpagine. The actions of rauwolfia serpentina are those of its alkaloids and it has been used for the same purposes as reserpine, p.995. It has been administered by mouth as the powdered whole root.

Rauwolfia vomitoria has also been used.

A crude form of rauwolfia serpentina has been used in India for centuries as preparations such as Sarpagandha, in the treatment of insomnia and certain forms of mental illness.

### Preparations

**USP 27:** Rauwolfia Serpentina Tablets.

**Proprietary Preparations** (details are given in Part 3)
***Ger.:*** Arte Rautin forte S†.

**Multi-ingredient:** ***Ger.:*** Hyperforat-forte; Raufuncton N†; Rauwoplant†; ***Spain:*** Diu Rauwiplus†; Rulun; ***USA:*** Rauzide.

## Remikiren *(rINN)*

Remikireno; Ro-42-5892. (αS)-α-[(αS)-α-[(*tert*-Butylsulfonyl)methyl]hydrocinnamamido]-N-[(1S,2R,3S)-1-(cyclohexylmethyl)-3-cyclopropyl-2,3-dihydroxypropyl]imidazole-4-propionamide.

$C_{33}H_{50}N_4O_6S$ = 630.8.

*CAS — 126222-34-2.*

*ATC — C09XA01.*

### Profile

Remikiren inhibits the actions of renin and thus prevents the conversion of angiotensinogen into angiotensin I. It is active by mouth and has been investigated in the management of hypertension and heart failure.

◊ A number of renin antagonists have been investigated as specific inhibitors of the renin-angiotensin system.[1,2] Remikiren is a nonpeptide that is active intravenously and orally, but it is reported to have a very low oral bioavailability.


1. Frishman WH, *et al.* Renin inhibition: a new approach to cardiovascular therapy. *J Clin Pharmacol* 1994; **34:** 873–80.
2. Rongen GA, *et al.* Clinical pharmacokinetics and efficacy of renin inhibitors. *Clin Pharmacokinet* 1995; **29:** 6–14.


## Rescinnamine *(BAN, rINN)*

Rescinamina. Methyl-O-(3,4,5-trimethoxycinnamoyl)reserpate.

$C_{35}H_{42}N_2O_9$ = 634.7.

*CAS — 24815-24-5.*

*ATC — C02AA01.*

### Profile

Rescinnamine is an ester alkaloid isolated from the root of *Rauwolfia serpentina* or *R. vomitoria.* It has properties similar to those described under reserpine (below) and has been used in the treatment of hypertension.

### Preparations

**Proprietary Preparations** (details are given in Part 3)

**Multi-ingredient:** ***Hong Kong:*** Iso Triraupin†; ***Spain:*** Diu Rauwiplus†; ***Thai.:*** Iso-Triraupin.

## Reserpine (BAN, rINN)

Reserpina; Reserpinum. Methyl 11,17α-dimethoxy-18β-(3,4,5-trimethoxybenzoyloxy)-3β,20α-yohimbane-16β-carboxylate; Methyl O-(3,4,5-trimethoxybenzoyl)reserpate.

$C_{33}H_{40}N_2O_9$ = 608.7.

*CAS — 50-55-5.*

*ATC — C02AA02.*

**Pharmacopoeias.** In *Chin., Eur.* (see p.vi), *Int., Jpn, Pol., US,* and *Viet.*

**Ph. Eur. 5.0** (Reserpine). It occurs as small, white to slightly yellow crystals or a crystalline powder. It darkens slowly on exposure to light. Practically insoluble in water; very slightly soluble in alcohol. Protect from light.

**USP 27** (Reserpine). A white or pale buff to slightly yellowish, odourless, crystalline powder. It darkens slowly on exposure to light, but more rapidly when in solution. Insoluble in water; soluble 1 in 1800 of alcohol and 1 in 6 of chloroform; freely soluble in acetic acid; very slightly soluble in ether; slightly soluble in benzene. Store in airtight containers at a temperature of 25°, excursions permitted between 15° and 30°. Protect from light.

**Stability.** Reserpine is unstable in the presence of alkalis, particularly when the drug is in solution.

### Adverse Effects

Adverse effects commonly include nasal congestion, headache and CNS symptoms including depression, drowsiness, dizziness, lethargy, nightmares, and symptoms of increased gastrointestinal tract motility including diarrhoea, abdominal cramps, and, at higher doses, increased gastric acid secretion. Respiratory distress, cyanosis, anorexia, and lethargy may occur in infants whose mothers have received reserpine prior to delivery.

Higher doses may cause flushing, bradycardia, severe depression which may lead to suicide, and extrapyramidal effects. Hypotension, coma, convulsions, respiratory depression and hypothermia also occur in overdosage. Hypotension is also more common in patients following a cerebrovascular accident.

Breast engorgement and galactorrhoea, gynaecomastia, increased prolactin concentrations, decreased libido, impotence, sodium retention, oedema, decreased or increased appetite, weight gain, miosis, dry mouth, sialorrhoea, dysuria, rashes, pruritus, and thrombocytopenic purpura have also been reported.

Reserpine has been shown to be tumorigenic in *rodents* following administration of large doses. Several reports have suggested an association between the ingestion of reserpine and the development of neoplasms of the breast (see below) but other surveys have failed to confirm the association.

**Neoplasms of the breast.** Although early studies suggested that the incidence of breast cancer was up to 3 to 4 times greater in hypertensive women treated with rauwolfia preparations than in control groups, analysis[1] of both prospective trials and case-control studies found only a low-grade association between use of rauwolfia preparations and risk of malignancy.

1. Grossman E, *et al.* Antihypertensive therapy and the risk of malignancies. *Eur Heart J* 2001; **22:** 1343–52.

### Treatment of Adverse Effects

Withdrawal of reserpine or reduction of the dosage causes the reversal of many adverse effects although mental disorders may persist for months and hypotensive effects may persist for weeks after the cessation of treatment. If overdosage occurs the stomach should be emptied by lavage. Activated charcoal may be considered within 1 hour of ingestion. Treatment is generally supportive and symptomatic. Severe hypotension may respond to placing the patient in the supine position with the feet raised. Direct-acting sympathomimetics may be effective for treatment of severe hypotension, but should be given with caution. The patient must be observed for at least 72 hours.

### Precautions

Reserpine should not be used in patients with depression or a history of depression, with active peptic ulcer disease or ulcerative colitis, or in patients with Parkinson's disease. It should also be avoided in phaeochromocytoma.

It should be used with caution in debilitated or elderly patients, and in the presence of cardiac arrhythmias, myocardial infarction, renal insufficiency, gallstones, epilepsy, or allergic conditions such as bronchial asthma.

Reserpine is contra-indicated in patients receiving ECT; if ECT is required in patients who have been taking reserpine an interval of at least 7 to 14 days should be allowed to elapse between the last dose of reserpine and the commencement of the shock treatment.

It is probably not necessary to discontinue treatment with reserpine during anaesthesia, although the effects of CNS depressants may be enhanced by reserpine.

### Interactions

Patients taking reserpine may be hypersensitive to adrenaline and other direct-acting sympathomimetics which should not be given except to antagonise reserpine. The effects of indirect-acting sympathomimetics such as ephedrine may be decreased by reserpine. The hypotensive effects of reserpine are enhanced by thiazide diuretics and other antihypertensives. Reserpine may cause excitation and hypertension in patients receiving MAOIs. Concurrent administration of digitalis or quinidine may cause cardiac arrhythmias. Reserpine may enhance the effects of CNS depressants.

### Pharmacokinetics

Reserpine is absorbed from the gastrointestinal tract with a reported bioavailability of 50%. It is extensively metabolised and is excreted slowly in the urine and faeces. In the first 4 days, about 8% has been reported to be excreted in the urine, mainly as metabolites, and about 60% in the faeces, mainly unchanged. Reserpine crosses the placenta and the blood-brain barrier and also appears in breast milk.

### Uses and Administration

Reserpine is an alkaloid obtained from the roots of certain species of *Rauwolfia* (Apocynaceae), mainly *Rauwolfia serpentina* and *R. vomitoria,* or by synthesis. The material obtained from natural sources may contain closely related alkaloids.

Reserpine is an antihypertensive drug that causes depletion of noradrenaline stores in peripheral sympathetic nerve terminals and depletion of catecholamine and serotonin stores in the brain, heart, and many other organs resulting in a reduction in blood pressure, bradycardia, and CNS depression. The hypotensive effect is mainly due to a reduction in cardiac output and a reduction in peripheral resistance. Cardiovascular reflexes are partially inhibited, but orthostatic hypotension is rarely a problem at the doses used in hypertension. When given by mouth the full effect is only reached after several weeks of continued treatment and persists for up to 6 weeks after treatment is discontinued.

Reserpine has been used in the management of hypertension (p.825) and in chronic psychoses (p.665) such as schizophrenia. It has also been tried in the treatment of Raynaud's syndrome (p.833).

In **hypertension**, reserpine may be given by mouth in an initial dose of up to 500 micrograms daily for about 2 weeks, subsequently reduced to the lowest dose necessary to maintain the response; some sources recommend an initial dose of 50 to 100 micrograms. A maintenance dose of about 100 to 250 micrograms daily may be adequate and 500 micrograms should not normally be exceeded. To reduce side-effects and tolerance smaller doses of reserpine may be used with a thiazide diuretic.

Reserpine has been used in chronic **psychoses** in daily doses of up to 1 mg.

### Preparations

***USP 27:*** Reserpine and Chlorothiazide Tablets; Reserpine and Hydrochlorothiazide Tablets; Reserpine Elixir; Reserpine Injection; Reserpine Tablets; Reserpine, Hydralazine Hydrochloride, and Hydrochlorothiazide Tablets.

**Proprietary Preparations** (details are given in Part 3)

***Braz.:*** Ortoserpina†; Rauserpin†; ***Port.:*** Serfinato; ***Thai.:*** Reserpina†.

**Multi-ingredient:** ***Arg.:*** Hygroton-Reserpina; Normatensil; ***Austria:*** Adelphan-Esidrex; Brinerdin; Darebon; Elfanex†; Pressimedin†; Resaltex†; Supergan†; Suprenoat†; ***Braz.:*** Adelfan-Esidrex; Higroton Reserpina; Id Sedin; Terbolan†; Vagoplex†; ***Canad.:*** Hydropres†; Ser-Ap-Es†; ***Fr.:*** Tensionorme; ***Ger.:*** Adelphan-Esidrix; Barotonal; Bendigon N; Briserin N; Darebon; Disalpin; Durotan; Modenol; Resaltex†; Tri-Thiazid Reserpin; Triniton; ***Hong Kong:*** Adelphane-Esidrex; Iso Triraupin†; ***India:*** Adelphane; Adelphane-Esidrex; ***Israel:*** Pressunic Compositum†; ***Ital.:*** Brinerdina; Igroton-Reserpina; ***Mex.:*** Higroton-Res; ***Port.:*** Brinerdine; ***S.Afr.:*** Brinerdin; Hygroton-Reserpine; Protensin-M; ***Spain:*** Adelfan-Esidrex; Brinerdina; Diu Rauwiplus†; Higrotona Reserpina; Resnedal†; Tensiocomplet; ***Switz.:*** Adelphan-Esidrex; Brinerdine; Hygroton-Reserpine; Pressimed†; ***Thai.:*** Bedin; Brinerdin; Hydrares; Hyperdine; Hypery; Iso-Triraupin; Medeserpine Co; Reser; Ser-Ap-Es; ***USA:*** Demi-Regroton; Diupres; Diutensen-R; Hydrap-ES; Hydro-Serp; Hydropres; Hydroserpine; Marpres; Metatensin; Regroton; Renese R; Salutensin; Ser-Ap-Es; Tri-Hydroserpine.

## Reteplase (BAN, USAN, rINN)

BM-06.022; Reteplasa; rPA. 173-L-Serine-174-L-tyrosine-175-L-glutamine-173–527-plasminogen activator (human tissue-type).

$C_{1736}H_{2653}N_{499}O_{522}S_{22}$ = 39571.1.

*CAS — 133652-38-7.*

*ATC — B01AD07.*

**Description.** Reteplase is a nonglycosylated protein produced by recombinant DNA technology. It consists of selected domains of human tissue plasminogen activator.

**Incompatibility.** Reteplase may precipitate out of solution if it is given with heparin in the same intravenous line.[1] Reteplase and heparin must therefore be given separately; if a single intravenous line is used it must be flushed thoroughly with sodium chloride 0.9% or with glucose 5% prior to, and following, reteplase injection.

1. Committee on Safety of Medicines/Medicines Control Agency. Reteplase (Rapilysin): incompatibility with heparin. *Current Problems* 2000; **26:** 5. Also available at: http://www.mca.gov.uk/ourwork/monitorsafequalmed/currentproblems/cpmay2000.pdf (accessed 06/07/04)

### Adverse Effects, Treatment, and Precautions

As for Streptokinase, p.1005. Allergic reactions may be less likely to occur with reteplase than with streptokinase.

### Interactions

As for Streptokinase, p.1007.

### Pharmacokinetics

Based on fibrinolytic activity, reteplase is reported to have an initial half-life of about 14 minutes and a terminal half-life of 1.6 hours in patients with myocardial infarction.

### Uses and Administration

Reteplase is a thrombolytic drug. It converts plasminogen to plasmin, a proteolytic enzyme which has fibrinolytic effects. The mechanisms of fibrinolysis are discussed further under Haemostasis and Fibrinolysis on p.735. Reteplase has some fibrin specificity (see p.812).

Reteplase is used similarly to streptokinase (p.1007) in acute myocardial infarction (p.828). It is given intravenously as soon as possible after the onset of symptoms. The dose is 10 units given by slow intravenous injection (but over not more than 2 minutes), and this dose of 10 units is repeated once, 30 minutes after the start of the first injection.

◊ General references.

1. Noble S, McTavish D. Reteplase: a review of its pharmacological properties and clinical efficacy in the management of acute myocardial infarction. *Drugs* 1996; **52:** 589–605.
2. Wooster MB, Luzier AB. Reteplase: a new thrombolytic for the treatment of acute myocardial infarction. *Ann Pharmacother* 1999; **33:** 318–24.
3. Llevadot J, *et al.* Bolus fibrinolytic therapy in acute myocardial infarction. *JAMA* 2001; **286:** 442–9.

**Catheters and cannulas.** Reteplase has been used[1] successfully to clear thrombi in central venous catheters. A single dose of 0.4 units of reteplase was given as a 1 unit/mL solution, further diluted to the volume required to fill the catheter. The minimum dwell time was 30 minutes and the solution was aspirated after treatment. A second dose of 0.4 units was given if necessary.

1. Owens L. Reteplase for clearance of occluded venous catheters. *Am J Health-Syst Pharm* 2002; **59:** 1638–40.

### Preparations

**Proprietary Preparations** (details are given in Part 3)

***Austral.:*** Rapilysin; ***Austria:*** Rapilysin; ***Belg.:*** Rapilysin; ***Canad.:*** Retavase; ***Denm.:*** Rapilysin; ***Fin.:*** Rapilysin; ***Fr.:*** Rapilysin; ***Ger.:*** Rapilysin; ***Gr.:*** Rapilysin; ***Irl.:*** Rapilysin; ***Ital.:*** Rapilysin; ***Neth.:*** Rapilysin; ***Norw.:*** Rapilysin; ***NZ:*** Rapilysin; ***Port.:*** Rapilysin; ***Spain:*** Rapilysin; ***Swed.:*** Rapilysin; ***Switz.:*** Rapilysin; ***UK:*** Rapilysin; ***USA:*** Retavase.

## Reviparin Sodium (BAN, rINN)

Reviparina sódica.

*CAS — 9041-08-1.*

*ATC — B01AB08.*

**Description.** Reviparin sodium is prepared by nitrous acid depolymerisation of heparin obtained from the intestinal mucosa of pigs. The majority of the components have a 2-*O*-sulfo-α-L-idopyranosuronic acid structure at the non-reducing end and a 6-*O*-sulfo-2,5-anhydro-D-mannitol structure at the reducing end of their chain. The mass-average molecular mass ranges between 3150 and 5150 with a characteristic value of about 4150. The degree of sulfation is about 2.1 per disaccharide unit.

### Units

As for Low-molecular-weight Heparins, p.949.

### Adverse Effects, Treatment, and Precautions

As for Low-molecular-weight Heparins, p.949.

Severe bleeding with reviparin sodium may be reduced by the slow intravenous injection of protamine sulfate; about 17.5 mg of protamine sulfate is stated to inhibit the effect of 1432 units of reviparin sodium.

### Interactions

As for Low-molecular-weight Heparins, p.950.

### Pharmacokinetics

Reviparin sodium is absorbed after subcutaneous administration with a bioavailability of about 95%. Peak plasma concentrations are reached after about 3 hours. Reviparin sodium is excreted mainly in the urine; the elimination half-life is about 3 hours.

### Uses and Administration

Reviparin sodium is a low-molecular-weight heparin (p.949) with anticoagulant activity. It is used in the prevention and treatment of venous thromboembolism (p.839) and has been used to prevent coagulation during haemodialysis.

Doses are expressed in terms of anti-factor Xa activity (anti-Xa units) although different values may be encountered in the literature depending upon the reference preparation used.

In the prophylaxis of venous thromboembolism during surgery, reviparin sodium is given subcutaneously in a dose of 1432 units once daily, with the first dose given 2 hours before surgery. Patients at high risk of thromboembolism may be given a dose of 3436 units once daily, beginning 12 hours before surgery. For treatment of thromboembolism, a dose of 71 units/kg is given subcutaneously twice daily.

◊ References.

1. The Columbus Investigators. Low-molecular-weight heparin in the treatment of patients with venous thromboembolism. *N Engl J Med* 1997; **337:** 657–62.
2. Breddin HK, *et al.* Effects of a low-molecular-weight heparin on thrombus regression and recurrent thromboembolism in patients with deep-vein thrombosis. *N Engl J Med* 2001; **344:** 626–31.
3. Wellington K, *et al.* Reviparin: a review of its efficacy in the prevention and treatment of venous thromboembolism. *Drugs* 2001; **61:** 1185–209.
4. Lassen MR, *et al.* Use of the low-molecular-weight heparin reviparin to prevent deep-vein thrombosis after leg injury requiring immobilization. *N Engl J Med* 2002; **347:** 726–30.

### Preparations

**Proprietary Preparations** (details are given in Part 3)
***Austria:*** Clivarin; ***Denm.:*** Clivarin; ***Fin.:*** Clivarin†; ***Fr.:*** Clivarine; ***Ger.:*** Clivarin; ***India:*** Clivarine; ***Ital.:*** Clivarina; ***Norw.:*** Clivarin†; ***Port.:*** Clivarin; ***Swed.:*** Clivarin†; ***UK:*** Clivarine.

## Rilmenidine Phosphate *(rINNM)*

Fosfato de rilmenidina; Oxaminozoline Phosphate; Rilmenidine Acid Phosphate; Rilmenidine Dihydrogen Phosphate; Rilmenidine Hydrogen Phosphate; Rilmenidini Dihydrogenophosphas; S-3341-3. 2-[(Dicyclopropylmethyl)amino]-2-oxazoline phosphate.

$C_{10}H_{16}N_2O,H_3PO_4$ = 278.2.

*CAS — 54187-04-1 (rilmenidine); 85409-38-7 (rilmenidine phosphate).*

*ATC — C02AC06.*

**Pharmacopoeias.** In *Eur.* (see p.vi).

**Ph. Eur. 5.0** (Rilmenidine Dihydrogen Phosphate). A white or almost white powder. Freely soluble in water; slightly soluble in alcohol; practically insoluble in dichloromethane.

### Profile

Rilmenidine is a centrally acting antihypertensive that appears to act through stimulation of central imidazoline receptors and also has alpha$_2$-adrenoceptor agonist activity. It has general properties similar to those of clonidine (p.885), but is reported to cause less sedation and central adverse effects. In the management of hypertension (p.825) it has been given as the phosphate, but doses are expressed in terms of the base. Rilmenidine phosphate 1.5 mg is approximately equivalent to 1 mg of rilmenidine. It is given in doses equivalent to 1 mg of base daily, as a single dose by mouth; this may be increased if necessary, after 1 month, to 2 mg daily in divided doses.

◊ References.

1. Bousquet P, Feldman J. Drugs acting on imidazoline receptors: a review of their pharmacology, their use in blood pressure control and their potential interest in cardioprotection. *Drugs* 1999; **58:** 799–812.
2. Reid JL. Rilmenidine: a clinical overview. *Am J Hypertens* 2000; **13:** 106S–111S.
3. Reid JL. Update on rilmenidine: clinical benefits. *Am J Hypertens* 2001; **14:** 322S–324S.

### Preparations

**Proprietary Preparations** (details are given in Part 3)
***Arg.:*** Hyperium; ***Austria:*** Iterium; ***Braz.:*** Hyperium; ***Fr.:*** Hyperium; ***Port.:*** Hyperium; ***Thai.:*** Hyperdix.

## Ronifibrate *(rINN)*

I-612; Ronifibrato. 3-Hydroxypropyl nicotinate 2-(4-chlorophenoxy)-2-methylpropionate.

$C_{19}H_{20}ClNO_5$ = 377.8.

*CAS — 42597-57-9.*

*ATC — C10AB07.*

### Profile

Ronifibrate, a derivative of clofibrate (p.884) and nicotinic acid (p.1441), is a lipid regulating drug that has been used in the treatment of hyperlipidaemias.

### Preparations

**Proprietary Preparations** (details are given in Part 3)
***Ital.:*** Cloprane†.

## Rosuvastatin Calcium *(BANM, USAN, rINNM)*

S-4522; ZD-4522 (rosuvastatin). (*E*)-(3*R*,5*S*)-7-{4-(4-Fluorophenyl)-6-isopropyl-2-[methyl(methylsulfonyl)amino]pyrimidin-5-yl}-3,5-dihydroxyhept-6-enoic acid calcium (2:1).

$(C_{22}H_{27}FN_3O_6S)_2Ca$ = 1001.1.

*CAS — 287714-41-4 (rosuvastatin); 147098-20-2 (rosuvastatin calcium).*

*ATC — C10AA07.*

### Adverse Effects and Precautions

As for Simvastatin, p.997.

### Interactions

The interactions of statins with other drugs are described under simvastatin, p.998. Rosuvastatin undergoes limited metabolism, principally by the cytochrome P450 isoenzyme CYP2C9, and may not have the same interactions with enzyme inhibitors as simvastatin. However, increased rosuvastatin plasma concentrations have been reported with ciclosporin and, to a lesser extent, with gemfibrozil, and such combinations should be avoided. If they must be given together, lower doses of rosuvastatin should be used (see Uses and Administration, below); in the UK, rosuvastatin is contra-indicated with ciclosporin.

### Pharmacokinetics

Rosuvastatin is incompletely absorbed from the gastrointestinal tract, with a bioavailability of about 20%. Peak plasma concentrations are achieved about 5 hours after an oral dose. It is taken up extensively by the liver, its primary site of action, and undergoes limited metabolism, mainly by the cytochrome P450 isoenzyme CYP2C9. It is about 90% bound to plasma proteins. The plasma elimination half-life of rosuvastatin is about 19 hours. Approximately 90% of an oral dose of rosuvastatin is excreted in the faeces, including absorbed and non-absorbed drug, and the remainder is excreted in the urine; about 5% of a dose is excreted unchanged in urine.

### Uses and Administration

Rosuvastatin, a hydroxymethylglutaryl coenzyme A (HMG-CoA) reductase inhibitor (a statin), is a lipid regulating drug with actions on plasma lipids similar to those of simvastatin (p.999). It is used to reduce LDL-cholesterol, apolipoprotein B, and triglycerides, and to increase HDL-cholesterol in the management of hyperlipidaemias (p.823), including primary hypercholesterolaemia (type IIa), mixed dyslipidaemia (type IIb), and hypertriglyceridaemia (type IV). It may also be used in patients with homozygous familial hypercholesterolaemia.

Rosuvastatin is given by mouth as the calcium salt, although doses are expressed in terms of the base; 10.4 mg of rosuvastatin calcium is equivalent to 10 mg of base.

In the UK, the initial dose is 10 mg once daily, increased after 4 weeks, if necessary, to 20 mg once daily. A maximum dose of 40 mg once daily may be given in severe hypercholesterolaemia, but should not be given to patients at high risk of myopathy, including those receiving fibrates; use with ciclosporin is contra-indicated.

In the USA, the usual initial dose is 10 mg once daily. However, a lower initial dose of 5 mg once daily is recommended for patients at risk of myopathy, whereas patients with marked hypercholesterolaemia, such as those with homozygous familial hypercholesterolaemia, may be started on 20 mg once daily. The dose should be adjusted after 2 to 4 weeks, to a maximum of 40 mg once daily. Patients receiving ciclosporin may be given a maximum of 5 mg once daily, and in those receiving gemfibrozil the maximum dose is 10 mg once daily.

The dose of rosuvastatin should be reduced in patients with renal impairment (see below).

◊ General reviews.

1. Chong PH, Yim BT. Rosuvastatin for the treatment of patients with hypercholesterolemia. *Ann Pharmacother* 2002; **36:** 93–101.
2. Carswell CI, *et al.* Rosuvastatin. *Drugs* 2002; **62:** 2075–85.
3. White CM. A review of the pharmacologic and pharmacokinetic aspects of rosuvastatin. *J Clin Pharmacol* 2002; **42:** 963–70.

**Administration in renal impairment.** Renal impairment increases the risk of myopathy in patients taking statins, and plasma-rosuvastatin concentrations are increased in patients with severe impairment. In the UK, rosuvastatin is contra-indicated in severe renal impairment (creatinine clearance less than 30 mL/minute) and a maximum dose of 20 mg is recommended in moderate impairment (creatinine clearance less than 60 mL/minute). In the USA, patients with severe impairment (creatinine clearance less than 30 mL/minute) may be given an initial dose of 5 mg once daily, increased to a maximum of 10 mg once daily.

### Preparations

**Proprietary Preparations** (details are given in Part 3)
***UK:*** Crestor; ***USA:*** Crestor.

## Saralasin Acetate *(BANM, USAN, rINNM)*

Acetato de sarasalina; P-113; The acetate of 1-Sar-8-Ala-angiotensin II. The hydrated acetate of Sar-Arg-Val-Tyr-Val-His-Pro-Ala; [1-(*N*-Methylglycine)-5-L-valine-8-L-alanine]-angiotensin II acetate hydrate.

$C_{42}H_{65}N_{13}O_{10},xCH_3COOH,xH_2O$ = 912.0 (saralasin).

*CAS — 34273-10-4 (saralasin); 54194-01-3 (anhydrous saralasin); 39698-78-7 (saralasin acetate hydrate).*

### Profile

Saralasin acetate is a competitive antagonist of angiotensin II and thus blocks its pressor action. It is also a partial agonist and causes a transient initial rise in blood pressure. Saralasin has a short half-life and has been used in the differential diagnosis of renovascular hypertension but its use has largely been superseded.

## Sarpogrelate Hydrochloride *(rINNM)*

Hidrocloruro de sarpogrelato; MCI-9042. (±)-2-(Dimethylamino)-1-{[*o*-(*m*-methoxyphenethyl)phenoxy]methyl}ethyl hydrogen succinate hydrochloride.

$C_{24}H_{31}NO_6,HCl$ = 466.0.

*CAS — 125926-17-2 (sarpogrelate); 135159-51-2 (sarpogrelate hydrochloride).*

### Profile

Sarpogrelate is a serotonin 5-HT$_2$-receptor antagonist used as an inhibitor of platelet aggregation in thromboembolic disorders. It is given for occlusive arterial disease (p.831) in doses of 100 mg of the hydrochloride, by mouth, three times daily.

### Preparations

**Proprietary Preparations** (details are given in Part 3)
***Jpn:*** Anplag.

## Saruplase *(BAN, rINN)*

Prourokinase, Non-glycosylated; Recombinant Human Single-Chain Urokinase-type Plasminogen Activator; Saruplasa; scuPA. Prourokinase (enzyme-activating) (human clone pUK4/pUK18), non-glycosylated.

$C_{2031}H_{3121}N_{585}O_{601}S_{31}$ = 46343.1.

*CAS — 99149-95-8.*

*ATC — B01AD08.*

NOTE. The term prourokinase has been used for both saruplase and nasaruplase (p.964).

### Profile

Saruplase is a thrombolytic drug. It is a urokinase-type plasminogen activator with a single chain structure prepared via recombinant DNA technology and is converted to urokinase (p.1018) in the body by plasmin. It also has some intrinsic plasminogen-activating properties. Saruplase has been investigated in acute myocardial infarction.

◊ References.

1. Tebbe U, *et al.* Randomized, double-blind study comparing saruplase with streptokinase therapy in acute myocardial infarction: the COMPASS equivalence trial. *J Am Coll Cardiol* 1998; **31:** 487–93.

## Sibrafiban *(BAN, USAN, rINN)*

G-7333; Ro-48-3657/001; Sibrafibán. Ethyl (*Z*)-[(1-{*N*-[(*p*-hydroxyamidino)benzoyl]-L-alanyl}-4-piperidyl)oxy] acetate.

$C_{20}H_{28}N_4O_6$ = 420.5.

*CAS — 172927-65-0.*

### Profile

Sibrafiban is a glycoprotein IIb/IIIa-receptor antagonist. It has been investigated as an oral antiplatelet drug in unstable angina and myocardial infarction but results have been disappointing.

◊ References.

1. Cannon CP, *et al.* Randomized trial of an oral platelet glycoprotein IIb/IIIa antagonist, sibrafiban, in patients after an acute coronary syndrome: results of the TIMI 12 trial. *Circulation* 1998; **97:** 340–9.

2. Newby LK. Long-term oral platelet glycoprotein IIb/IIIa receptor antagonism with sibrafiban after acute coronary syndromes: study design of the sibrafiban versus aspirin to yield maximum protection from ischemic heart events post-acute coronary syndromes (SYMPHONY) trial. *Am Heart J* 1999; **138:** 210–8.
3. The SYMPHONY Investigators. Comparison of sibrafiban with aspirin for prevention of cardiovascular events after acute coronary syndromes: a randomised trial. *Lancet* 2000; **355:** 337–45.
4. Second SYMPHONY Investigators. Randomized trial of aspirin, sibrafiban, or both for secondary prevention after acute coronary syndromes. *Circulation* 2001; **103:** 1727–33.

## Simfibrate *(rINN)*

CLY-503; Diclofibrate; Simfibrato. Trimethylene bis[2-(4-chlorophenoxy)-2-methylpropionate].

$C_{23}H_{26}Cl_2O_6$ = 469.4.
*CAS — 14929-11-4.*
*ATC — C10AB06.*

### Profile

Simfibrate, a fibric acid derivative (see Bezafibrate, p.873), is a lipid regulating drug that has been used in the treatment of hyperlipidaemias.

### Preparations

**Proprietary Preparations** (details are given in Part 3)
**Ital.:** Cholesolvin†.

## Simvastatin *(BAN, USAN, rINN)*

L-644128-000U; MK-733; Simvastatina; Simvastatinum; Synvinolin; Velastatin. (1*S*,3*R*,7*S*,8*S*,8a*R*)-1,2,3,7,8,8a-Hexahydro-3,7-dimethyl-8-{2-[(2*R*,4*R*)-tetrahydro-4-hydroxy-6-oxo-2*H*-pyran-2-yl]ethyl}-1-naphthyl 2,2-dimethylbutyrate.

$C_{25}H_{38}O_5$ = 418.6.
*CAS — 79902-63-9.*
*ATC — C10AA01.*

**Pharmacopoeias.** In *Eur.* (see p.vi) and *US*.

**Ph. Eur. 5.0** (Simvastatin). A white or almost white crystalline powder. Practically insoluble in water; freely soluble in alcohol; very soluble in dichloromethane. Store under nitrogen in airtight containers. Protect from light.

**USP 27** (Simvastatin). A white to off-white powder. Practically insoluble in water; freely soluble in alcohol, in chloroform, and in methyl alcohol; sparingly soluble in propylene glycol; very slightly soluble in petroleum spirit. Store under nitrogen.

### Adverse Effects

The commonest adverse effects of therapy with simvastatin and other statins are gastrointestinal disturbances. Other adverse effects reported include headache, skin rashes, dizziness, blurred vision, insomnia, and dysgeusia. Reversible increases in serum-aminotransferase concentrations may occur and liver function should be assessed before treatment is initiated and then monitored periodically until one year after the last elevation in dose. Hepatitis and pancreatitis have been reported. Hypersensitivity reactions including anaphylaxis and angioedema have also occurred. Myopathy, characterised by myalgia and muscle weakness and associated with increased creatine phosphokinase concentrations, has been reported, especially in patients taking statins concurrently with ciclosporin, fibric acid derivatives, or nicotinic acid. Rarely, rhabdomyolysis with acute renal failure may develop.

◊ General references.

1. Farmer JA, Torre-Amione G. Comparative tolerability of the HMG-CoA reductase inhibitors. *Drug Safety* 2000; **23:** 197–213.
2. Davidson MH. Safety profiles for the HMG-CoA reductase inhibitors: treatment and trust. *Drugs* 2001; **61:** 197–206.
3. Pasternak RC, *et al.* ACC/AHA/NHLBI clinical advisory on the use and safety of statins. *Circulation* 2002; **106:** 1024–8.

◊ In February 1992 the UK Committee on Safety of Medicines (CSM) briefly reviewed[1] the adverse effects that had been reported to it since simvastatin was made available in the UK in May 1989. There had been 257 000 prescriptions and 738 reports to the CSM. Abnormal hepatic function and myalgia were 2 of the most frequently reported reactions, with 36 and 48 reports respectively, including 5 reports of hepatitis and 2 of jaundice. Other muscle effects included 3 reports of myositis, 10 of myopathy, and 7 reports of asymptomatic increases in serum creatine kinase concentrations. Gastrointestinal adverse effects accounted for 20% of the reports; skin, neurological and musculoskeletal effects for 15% each; psychiatric effects for 10%; liver effects for 7%; and visual effects for 4%.

1. Committee on Safety of Medicines. Simvastatin. *Current Problems 33* 1992.

**Effects on the blood.** Thrombocytopenia has been reported rarely with statin therapy. Serious thrombocytopenic purpura in a patient taking simvastatin resolved when therapy was stopped,[1] although a causal role was not established. In another patient, thrombotic thrombocytopenic purpura occurred within 24 hours of taking the second dose of newly-initiated simvastatin therapy.[2] No other precipitating factor was apparent. There has also been a report of an immune thrombocytopenia attributed to atorvastatin.[3] Adverse haematological reactions had not been noted when the patient previously received simvastatin.

A case of haemolytic anaemia has been reported[4] in a patient taking lovastatin; no adverse effect was seen when the patient was given simvastatin.

1. Possamai G, *et al.* Thrombocytopenic purpura during therapy with simvastatin. *Haematologica* 1992; **77:** 357–8.
2. McCarthy LJ, *et al.* Thrombotic thrombocytopenic purpura and simvastatin. *Lancet* 1998; **352:** 1284–5.
3. González-Ponte ML, *et al.* Atorvastatin-induced severe thrombocytopenia. *Lancet* 1998; **352:** 1284.
4. Robbins MJ, *et al.* Lovastatin-induced hemolytic anemia; not a class-specific reaction. *Am J Med* 1995; **99:** 328–9.

**Effects on the eyes.** Studies in *animals* have suggested that some statins could cause cataracts. Although lens opacities were found in 13 of 101 patients taking lovastatin following an 18-week study,[1] no further deterioration was seen in 11 of these patients who continued to take lovastatin at follow-up after an average of 26 months from the start of treatment. Similarly, no differences were found in the development of lens opacities or in changes in visual acuity between patients treated with lovastatin for 48 weeks and patients taking placebo in a study of 8245 patients.[2] A large case-control study[3] found no evidence that use of therapeutic statin doses was associated with the development of cataracts, although the risk did appear to be increased in patients taking simvastatin and erythromycin concomitantly.

1. Hunninghake DB, *et al.* Lovastatin: follow-up ophthalmologic data. *JAMA* 1988; **259:** 354–5.
2. Laties AM, *et al.* The human lens after 48 weeks of treatment with lovastatin. *N Engl J Med* 1990; **323:** 683–4.
3. Schlienger RG, *et al.* Risk of cataract in patients treated with statins. *Arch Intern Med* 2001; **161:** 2021–6.

**Effects on the hair.** Since its introduction in Australia 16 cases of alopecia in association with the use of simvastatin had been reported to the Adverse Drug Reactions Advisory Committee.[1] Most cases involved either excessive hair loss or hair thinning, although 2 cases of hair loss in patches and 1 resembling alopecia areata were reported. Onset occurred between 3 days and 15 months of starting therapy. Progressive hair loss has also been reported[2] in a woman within 6 weeks of commencing atorvastatin; the hair regrew when atorvastatin was stopped but alopecia recurred when therapy was restarted 5 months later.

1. Anonymous. Simvastatin and alopecia. *Aust Adverse Drug React Bull* 1993; **12:** 7.
2. Segal AS. Alopecia associated with atorvastatin. *Am J Med* 2002; **113:** 171.

**Effects on the kidneys.** Proteinuria was reported in 10 patients taking simvastatin 40 mg daily.[1] The protein loss was of a pattern typical for increased glomerular permeability. In 2 patients proteinuria disappeared when simvastatin was withdrawn and recurred on its subsequent reintroduction.

Renal failure due to rhabdomyolysis has been reported rarely (see under Effects on Skeletal Muscle, below).

1. Deslypere JP, *et al.* Proteinuria as complication of simvastatin treatment. *Lancet* 1990; **336:** 1453.

**Effects on mental function.** A few cases have been reported of depressive symptoms developing in patients treated with pravastatin[1] or simvastatin.[2] The symptoms appeared during the first few weeks or months of treatment. However, a randomised placebo-controlled study[3] involving over 600 patients did not find that simvastatin treatment was associated with mood disturbances, while in the LIPID study[4] pravastatin had no effect on psychological well-being. A study[5] using lovastatin also found no effect on psychological well-being, although there was a small reduction in some measures of cognitive function.

For a suggestion that the risk of dementia may be reduced in patients taking statins, see under Uses, below.

1. Lechleitner M, *et al.* Depressive symptoms in hypercholesterolaemic patients treated with pravastatin. *Lancet* 1992; **340:** 910.
2. Duits N, Bos FM. Depressive symptoms and cholesterol-lowering drugs. *Lancet* 1993; **341:** 114.
3. Wardle J, *et al.* Randomised placebo controlled trial of effect on mood of lowering cholesterol concentration. *BMJ* 1996; **313:** 75–8.
4. Stewart RA, *et al.* Long-term assessment of psychological well-being in a randomized placebo-controlled trial of cholesterol reduction with pravastatin. *Arch Intern Med* 2000; **160:** 3144–52.
5. Muldoon MF, *et al.* Effects of lovastatin on cognitive function and psychological well-being. *Am J Med* 2000; **108:** 538–47.

**Effects on the nervous system.** A number of reports have suggested that peripheral neuropathy may be associated with statin treatment.[1] Up to 1993, the Australian Adverse Drug Reactions Advisory Committee had received 22 reports of paraesthesia associated with simvastatin.[2] Symptoms most frequently involved the face, scalp, tongue, and limbs and ranged from hypoaesthetic to hyperaesthetic sensations, although 4 cases of more serious neurological damage had also been reported. In a few cases symptoms occurred immediately on starting treatment while in others they appeared up to one year after initiating therapy. Symptoms disappeared shortly after treatment was withdrawn; in 5 cases symptoms recurred on rechallenge.

Further cases of motor and sensory neuropathy have been reported with simvastatin,[3,4] lovastatin,[4-6] fluvastatin (following lovastatin),[4] and pravastatin.[4,5] Patients had usually been taking the statin for several years before symptoms developed, and in most cases there was improvement following discontinuation, although several cases[4] appeared to be irreversible. In some patients symptoms recurred on rechallenge, either with the same[6] or with an alternative statin.[5] In 1 case[7] treated initially with lovastatin, symptoms recurred when treatment was changed sequentially to pravastatin, simvastatin, and atorvastatin, and also occurred with nicotinic acid. In many cases nerve conduction studies were carried out and revealed a mixed sensorimotor polyneuropathy. A case-control study[8] found that the risk of neuropathy was substantially increased in users of statins although the number of cases was small, and the authors concluded that the benefits of therapy generally outweighed the risks.

1. Backes JM, Howard PA. Association of HMG-CoA reductase inhibitors with neuropathy. *Ann Pharmacother* 2003; **37:** 274–8.
2. Anonymous. Paraesthesia and neuropathy with hypolipidaemic agents. *Aust Adverse Drug React Bull* 1993; **12:** 6.
3. Phan T, *et al.* Peripheral neuropathy associated with simvastatin. *J Neurol Neurosurg Psychiatry* 1995; **58:** 625–8.
4. Jeppesen U, *et al.* Statins and peripheral neuropathy. *Eur J Clin Pharmacol* 1999; **54:** 835–8.
5. Jacobs MB. HMG-CoA reductase inhibitor therapy and peripheral neuropathy. *Ann Intern Med* 1994; **120:** 970.
6. Ahmad S. Lovastatin and peripheral neuropathy. *Am Heart J* 1995; **130:** 1321.
7. Ziajka PE, *et al.* Peripheral neuropathy and lipid-lowering therapy. *South Med J* 1998; **91:** 667–8.
8. Gaist D, *et al.* Statins and risk of polyneuropathy: a case-control study. *Neurology* 2002; **58:** 1333–7.

**Effects on sexual function.** There have been reports of erectile dysfunction in some men receiving statins. Five men receiving simvastatin developed impotence,[1] which resolved when fluvastatin was substituted in 4 of them. In another case,[2] impotence occurred in a patient receiving lovastatin, and recurred when therapy was changed to pravastatin. The Australian Adverse Drug Reactions Advisory Committee[3] had received 28 reports of impotence associated with simvastatin, which had recurred on rechallenge in 4 cases. Others[4] suggest that simvastatin is unlikely to cause impotence, based on the number of men reporting impotence or sexual dysfunction during the Scandinavian Simvastatin Survival Study. However, a systematic review[5] including evidence from case reports, clinical trials, and reports to regulatory agencies, supported the conclusion that statins could cause erectile dysfunction.

There has also been a report[6] of a low sperm count in a patient receiving lovastatin.

1. Jackson G. Simvastatin and impotence. *BMJ* 1997; **315:** 31.
2. Halkin A, *et al.* HMG-CoA reductase inhibitor-induced impotence. *Ann Pharmacother* 1996; **30:** 192.
3. Australian Adverse Drug Reactions Advisory Committee. Simvastatin and adverse endocrine effects in men. *Aust Adverse Drug React Bull* 1995; **14:** 10. Also available at: http://www.tga.gov.au/docs/html/aadrbltn/v14n3.htm (accessed 06/07/04)
4. Pedersen TR, Færgeman O. Simvastatin seems unlikely to cause impotence. *BMJ* 1999; **318:** 192.
5. Rizvi K, *et al.* Do lipid-lowering drugs cause erectile dysfunction? A systematic review. *Fam Pract* 2002; **19:** 95–8.
6. Hildebrand RD, Hepperlen TW. Lovastatin and hypospermia. *Ann Intern Med* 1990; **112:** 549–50.

**Effects on skeletal muscle.** Muscle disorders including myositis and myopathy are well known to occur with statins.[1-6] Rhabdomyolysis, presenting as muscle pain with elevated creatine phosphokinase and myoglobinuria leading to renal failure, may also occur but appears to be rare. However, fatalities have been reported. Muscle toxicity is dose-related and the risk appears to be broadly similar with all of the currently-marketed statins;[5-7] the incidence with cerivastatin was found to be considerably higher and this led to its withdrawal worldwide in 2001 (see p.881). Patients with complex medical problems, including renal impairment and possibly endocrine disorders such as hypothyroidism, may be at increased risk of muscle toxicity; the risk is also increased by concomitant therapy with drugs that inhibit the cytochrome P450 enzyme system and increase plasma concentrations of statins (see Interactions, below). Fibrate lipid regulating drugs have also been associated with myopathy and the risk is increased if statins and fibrates are used together; however, combination therapy may have a role in patients with severe hyperlipidaemias although careful monitoring is necessary.[6,8] The UK Committee on Safety of Medicines[1] and a joint committee of the American College of Cardiology, American Heart Association, and National Heart, Lung and Blood Institute,[6] have both advised that patients treated with statins should consult their doctor if they develop muscle pain, tenderness, or weakness and that treatment should be stopped if muscle toxicity occurs or is suspected clinically or if creatine phosphokinase is markedly raised or progressively rising.

The mechanism by which statins cause muscle toxicity is not clear, but it has been suggested that depletion of ubidecarenone concentrations may be involved.[9] Muscle weakness and soreness in a patient taking lovastatin was relieved by the administration of ubidecarenone.[10]

Other muscular disorders that have been reported in patients receiving statins include an inflammatory myopathy resembling dermatomyositis in a woman treated for 5 months with pravastatin,[11] dermatomyositis in a patient receiving atorvastatin,[12] and ocular myasthenia in a patient receiving atorvastatin.[13]

1. Committee on Safety of Medicines/Medicines Control Agency. HMG CoA reductase inhibitors (statins) and myopathy. *Current Problems* 2002; **28:** 8–9. Also available at: http://www.mca.gov.uk/ourwork/monitorsafequalmed/currentproblems/cpoct2002.pdf (accessed 13/07/04)

2. Adverse Drug Reactions Advisory Committee (ADRAC). Fluvastatin and muscle disorders—a class effect. *Aust Adverse Drug React Bull* 1997; **16:** 3. Also available at: http://www.tga.gov.au/docs/html/aadrbltn/aadr9702.htm (accessed 06/07/04)
3. Ucar M, *et al.* HMG-CoA reductase inhibitors and myotoxicity. *Drug Safety* 2000; **22:** 441–57.
4. Omar MA, *et al.* Rhabdomyolysis and HMG-CoA reductase inhibitors. *Ann Pharmacother* 2001; **35:** 1096–1107.
5. Omar MA, Wilson JP. FDA adverse event reports on statin-associated rhabdomyolysis. *Ann Pharmacother* 2002; **36:** 288–95.
6. Pasternak RC, *et al.* ACC/AHA/NHLBI Clinical Advisory on the use and safety of statins. *Circulation* 2002; **106:** 1024–8.
7. Staffa JA, *et al.* Cerivastatin and reports of fatal rhabdomyolysis. *N Engl J Med* 2002; **346:** 539–540.
8. Shek A, Ferrill MJ. Statin-fibrate combination therapy. *Ann Pharmacother* 2001; **35:** 908–917.
9. Hargreaves IP, Heales S. Statins and myopathy. *Lancet* 2002; **359:** 711–2.
10. Walravens PA, *et al.* Lovastatin, isoprenes, and myopathy. *Lancet* 1989; **ii:** 1097–8.
11. Schalke BB, *et al.* Pravastatin-associated inflammatory myopathy. *N Engl J Med* 1992; **327:** 649–50.
12. Noël B, *et al.* Atorvastatin-induced dermatomyositis. *Am J Med* 2001; **110:** 670–1.
13. Parmar B, *et al.* Statins, fibrates, and ocular myasthenia. *Lancet* 2002; **360:** 717.

**Effects on sleep patterns.** Patients taking lovastatin have been reported to experience a reduction in the length of continuous sleep while no such effect was observed with pravastatin.[1] A similar sleep disturbance has been reported with simvastatin.[2] It was suggested that pravastatin might be less likely to affect sleep since it is hydrophilic and does not penetrate the brain easily. However, there have been conflicting reports: in other studies neither lovastatin,[3] pravastatin,[4] nor simvastatin,[3-5] had any adverse effect on sleep, but there have been further individual reports of sleep disturbances with lovastatin.[6,7]

1. Schaefer EJ. HMG-CoA reductase inhibitors for hypercholesterolemia. *N Engl J Med* 1988; **319:** 1222.
2. Barth JD, *et al.* Inhibitors of hydroxymethylglutaryl coenzyme A reductase for treating hypercholesterolaemia. *BMJ* 1990; **301:** 669.
3. Black DM, *et al.* Sleep disturbances and HMG CoA reductase inhibitors. *JAMA* 1990; **264:** 1105.
4. Eckernäs S-Å, *et al.* The effects of simvastatin and pravastatin on objective and subjective measures of nocturnal sleep: a comparison of two structurally different HMG CoA reductase inhibitors in patients with primary moderate hypercholesterolaemia. *Br J Clin Pharmacol* 1993; **35:** 284–9.
5. Keech AC, *et al.* Absence of effects of prolonged simvastatin therapy on nocturnal sleep in a large randomized placebo-controlled study. *Br J Clin Pharmacol* 1996; **42:** 483–90.
6. Rosenson RS, Goranson NL. Lovastatin-associated sleep and mood disturbances. *Am J Med* 1993; **95:** 548–9.
7. Sinzinger H, *et al.* Sleep disturbance and appetite loss after lovastatin. *Lancet* 1994; **343:** 973.

## Precautions

Statins should not be given to patients with active liver disease or unexplained persistently raised serum-aminotransferase concentrations. They should be avoided during pregnancy since there is a possibility that they could interfere with fetal sterol synthesis; there have been a few reports of congenital abnormalities associated with statins (but see Pregnancy, below). They should be discontinued if marked or persistent increases in serum-aminotransferase or creatine phosphokinase concentrations occur, or if myopathy is diagnosed.

Some statins, such as fluvastatin, pravastatin, rosuvastatin, and simvastatin, should be used with caution in patients with severe renal impairment.

**Children.** Bile-acid binding resins such as colestyramine have traditionally been used to treat heterozygous familial hyperlipidaemia in children and adolescents. Limited information suggests that statins are effective at lowering total cholesterol and low-density lipoprotein (LDL)-cholesterol in children older than 10 years.[1] However, there are concerns about the potential adverse effects of statins on growth and sexual development, because these patients require life-long therapy.[2] A placebo-controlled study[3] of lovastatin in 132 adolescent males reported significant reduction in LDL-cholesterol compared with placebo, but no significant differences between the groups in measures of growth and sexual maturation. However, patients were studied for one year only, and the authors acknowledge that further study is needed.

1. Duplaga BA. Treatment of childhood hypercholesterolemia with HMG-CoA reductase inhibitors. *Ann Pharmacother* 1999; **33:** 1224–7.
2. Rifkind BM, *et al.* When should patients with heterozygous familial hypercholesterolemia be treated? *JAMA* 1999; **281:** 180–1.
3. Stein EA, *et al.* Efficacy and safety of lovastatin in adolescent males with heterozygous familial hypercholesterolemia: a randomized controlled trial. *JAMA* 1999; **281:** 137–44.

**Porphyria.** Simvastatin is considered to be unsafe in patients with porphyria because it has been shown to be porphyrinogenic in *animals*.

**Pregnancy.** Statins are generally contra-indicated in pregnancy since there is a possibility that they might affect fetal sterol synthesis. Postmarketing surveillance identified 134 cases of unintentional exposure to lovastatin or simvastatin during pregnancy in which the outcome was known.[1] Although there were 9 reports of congenital anomalies these consisted of a spectrum of unrelated malformations and the frequency did not exceed that expected in the general population. It was therefore considered that these drugs did not adversely affect outcome of pregnancy.

1. Manson JM, *et al.* Postmarketing surveillance of lovastatin and simvastatin exposure during pregnancy. *Reprod Toxicol* 1996; **10:** 439–46.

## Interactions

The most serious consequence of drug interactions with simvastatin and other statins is the development of myopathy or rhabdomyolysis. Drugs that can cause myopathy when given alone increase the risk of myopathy with all statins; these drugs include fibric acid derivatives (fibrates or gemfibrozil), and nicotinic acid. The risk of myopathy is also increased by drugs that increase the plasma levels of statins by inhibiting their metabolism. Since the statins have different metabolic pathways, these interactions depend on the individual drug concerned. Simvastatin is metabolised by the cytochrome P450 isoenzyme CYP3A4, as are atorvastatin and lovastatin, and interactions may occur with drugs that inhibit this enzyme, including ciclosporin, itraconazole, ketoconazole, erythromycin, clarithromycin, HIV-protease inhibitors, nefazodone, amiodarone, and verapamil; there may also be a similar interaction with grapefruit juice. Fluvastatin is metabolised mainly by CYP2C9 and pravastatin is not significantly metabolised; interactions specific to these statins are discussed on p.918 and p.984, respectively.

Statins may also have effects on other drugs. Bleeding and increases in prothrombin time have been reported in patients taking simvastatin or other statins with coumarin anticoagulants.

◊ General reviews.

1. Garnett WR. Interactions with hydroxymethylglutaryl-coenzyme A reductase inhibitors. *Am J Health-Syst Pharm* 1995; **52:** 1639–45.
2. Williams D, Feely J. Pharmacokinetic-pharmacodynamic drug interactions with HMG-CoA reductase inhibitors. *Clin Pharmacokinet* 2002; **41:** 343–70.
3. Martin J, Krum H. Cytochrome P450 drug interactions within the HMG-CoA reductase inhibitor class: are they clinically relevant? *Drug Safety* 2003; **26:** 13–21.

**Antibacterials.** *Erythromycin* and other *macrolides* are inhibitors of the cytochrome P450 isoenzyme CYP3A4 and may increase plasma concentrations and the risk of myopathy with some statins. Increased plasma concentrations of simvastatin have been reported with concomitant erythromycin,[1] and increased plasma concentrations of atorvastatin have been found with erythromycin,[2] and *clarithromycin*,[3] but not with *azithromycin*.[3] There have been reports of myopathy or rhabdomyolysis in patients receiving simvastatin with clarithromycin,[4] and in patients receiving lovastatin with azithromycin,[5] clarithromycin,[5] or erythromycin.[6]

*Rifampicin*, an inducer of CYP2C9 and CYP3A4, may reduce the bioavailability of fluvastatin, and has also been reported[7] to reduce the plasma concentration of simvastatin.

There have been reports of rhabdomyolysis in patients receiving atorvastatin[8] or simvastatin[9] with *fusidic acid.*

1. Kantola T, *et al.* Erythromycin and verapamil considerably increase serum simvastatin and simvastatin acid concentrations. *Clin Pharmacol Ther* 1998; **64:** 177–82.
2. Siedlik PH, *et al.* Erythromycin coadministration increases plasma atorvastatin concentrations. *J Clin Pharmacol* 1999; **39:** 501–4.
3. Amsden GW, *et al.* A study of the interaction potential of azithromycin and clarithromycin with atorvastatin in healthy volunteers. *J Clin Pharmacol* 2002; **42:** 444–9.
4. Lee AJ, Maddix DS. Rhabdomyolysis secondary to a drug interaction between simvastatin and clarithromycin. *Ann Pharmacother* 2001; **35:** 26–31.
5. Grunden JW, Fisher KA. Lovastatin-induced rhabdomyolysis possibly associated with clarithromycin and azithromycin. *Ann Pharmacother* 1997; **31:** 859–63.
6. Ayanian JZ, *et al.* Lovastatin and rhabdomyolysis. *Ann Intern Med* 1988; **109:** 682–3.
7. Kyrklund C, *et al.* Rifampin greatly reduces plasma simvastatin and simvastatin acid concentrations. *Clin Pharmacol Ther* 2000; **68:** 592–7.
8. Wenisch C, *et al.* Acute rhabdomyolysis after atorvastatin and fusidic acid therapy. *Am J Med* 2000; **109:** 78.
9. Yuen SLS, McGarity B. Rhabdomyolysis secondary to interaction of fusidic acid and simvastatin. *Med J Aust* 2003; **179:** 172.

**Anticoagulants.** For reports of bleeding and increased prothrombin time in patients receiving oral anticoagulants with statins, see Lipid Regulating Drugs, p.1027.

**Antidepressants.** Myositis and rhabdomyolysis developed[1,2] in 2 patients receiving simvastatin when nefazodone was added to their therapy. A study[3] in healthy volunteers found that *hypericum* reduced the plasma concentration of simvastatin but had no effect on pravastatin.

1. Jacobson RH, *et al.* Myositis and rhabdomyolysis associated with concurrent use of simvastatin and nefazodone. *JAMA* 1997; **277:** 296.
2. Thompson M, Samuels S. Rhabdomyolysis with simvastatin and nefazodone. *Am J Psychiatry* 2002; **159:** 1607.
3. Sugimoto K-i, *et al.* Different effects of St John's Wort on the pharmacokinetics of simvastatin and pravastatin. *Clin Pharmacol Ther* 2001; **70:** 518–24.

**Antifungals.** *Itraconazole* and *ketoconazole* are inhibitors of the cytochrome P450 isoenzyme CYP3A4 and may increase plasma concentrations and the risk of myopathy with some statins. Raised plasma concentrations of simvastatin,[1,2] lovastatin,[3,4] and atorvastatin[5] have been reported with itraconazole, whereas the effect on pravastatin[1] or fluvastatin[4] appears to be minimal. Myopathy and rhabdomyolysis have been reported with simvastatin and itraconazole[2,6] or ketoconazole,[7] and with lovastatin and itraconazole.[8] *Fluconazole* inhibits CYP2C9 and has been reported[9] to increase the plasma concentration of fluvastatin. There has also been a report[10] of rhabdomyolysis in a patient taking fluconazole and simvastatin.

1. Neuvonen PJ, *et al.* Simvastatin but not pravastatin is very susceptible to interaction with the CYP3A4 inhibitor itraconazole. *Clin Pharmacol Ther* 1998; **63:** 332–41.
2. Segaert MF, *et al.* Drug-interaction-induced rhabdomyolysis. *Nephrol Dial Transplant* 1996; **11:** 1846–7.
3. Neuvonen PJ, Jalava K-M. Itraconazole drastically increases plasma concentrations of lovastatin and lovastatin acid. *Clin Pharmacol Ther* 1996; **60:** 54–61.
4. Kivistö KT, *et al.* Different effects of itraconazole on the pharmacokinetics of fluvastatin and lovastatin. *Br J Clin Pharmacol* 1998; **46:** 49–53.
5. Kantola T, *et al.* Effect of itraconazole on the pharmacokinetics of atorvastatin. *Clin Pharmacol Ther* 1998; **64:** 58–65.
6. Horn M. Coadministration of itraconazole with hypolipidemic agents may induce rhabdomyolysis in healthy individuals. *Arch Dermatol* 1996; **132:** 1254.
7. Gilad R, Lampl Y. Rhabdomyolysis induced by simvastatin and ketoconazole treatment. *Clin Neuropharmacol* 1999; **22:** 295–7.
8. Lees RS, Lees AM. Rhabdomyolysis from the coadministration of lovastatin and the antifungal agent itraconazole. *N Engl J Med* 1995; **333:** 664–5.
9. Kantola T, *et al.* Effect of fluconazole on plasma fluvastatin and pravastatin concentrations. *Eur J Clin Pharmacol* 2000; **56:** 225–9.
10. Shaukat A, *et al.* Simvastatin–fluconazole causing rhabdomyolysis. *Ann Pharmacother* 2003; **37:** 1032–5.

**Antivirals.** *HIV-protease inhibitors* are inhibitors of the cytochrome P450 isoenzyme CYP3A4 and may affect the metabolism of simvastatin and other statins. Studies have shown increased plasma concentrations of both simvastatin and atorvastatin with *nelfinavir*,[1] and with *ritonavir plus saquinavir*,[2] whereas the plasma concentration of pravastatin was reduced with ritonavir plus saquinavir.[2] Rhabdomyolysis has been reported[3] in a patient receiving simvastatin following the addition of ritonavir to her therapy.

There has also been a report[4] of rhabdomyolysis in a patient receiving atorvastatin with the non-nucleoside reverse transcriptase inhibitor *delavirdine*.

1. Hsyu P-H, *et al.* Pharmacokinetic interactions between nelfinavir and 3-hydroxy-3-methylglutaryl coenzyme A reductase inhibitors atorvastatin and simvastatin. *Antimicrob Agents Chemother* 2001; **45:** 3445–50.
2. Fichtenbaum CJ, *et al.* Pharmacokinetic interactions between protease inhibitors and statins in HIV seronegative volunteers: ACTG Study A5047. *AIDS* 2002; **16:** 569–77.
3. Cheng CH, *et al.* Rhabdomyolysis due to probable interaction between simvastatin and ritonavir. *Am J Health-Syst Pharm* 2002; **59:** 728–30.
4. Castro JG, Gutierrez L. Rhabdomyolysis with acute renal failure probably related to the interaction of atorvastatin and delavirdine. *Am J Med* 2002; **112:** 505.

**Calcium-channel blockers.** Calcium-channel blockers may increase plasma concentrations of some statins, probably by inhibition of the cytochrome P450 isoenzyme CYP3A4. Pharmacokinetic studies have reported increased plasma concentrations of simvastatin with *verapamil*,[1] and with *diltiazem*,[2] and of lovastatin with diltiazem;[3] the small increase with simvastatin and *lacidipine* was not considered clinically relevant.[4]

The interaction between statins and diltiazem has also been reported in patients. A retrospective study[5] found that the cholesterol-lowering effect of simvastatin was greater in patients who were also receiving diltiazem, and there have also been 2 reports[6,7] of rhabdomyolysis, associated with hepatitis in 1 case,[6] in patients receiving simvastatin and diltiazem together. Rhabdomyolysis and hepatitis have also been reported[8] in a patient receiving atorvastatin with diltiazem.

1. Kantola T, *et al.* Erythromycin and verapamil considerably increase serum simvastatin and simvastatin acid concentrations. *Clin Pharmacol Ther* 1998; **64:** 177–82.
2. Mousa O, *et al.* The interaction of diltiazem with simvastatin. *Clin Pharmacol Ther* 2000; **67:** 267–74.
3. Azie NE, *et al.* The interaction of diltiazem with lovastatin and pravastatin. *Clin Pharmacol Ther* 1998; **64:** 369–77.
4. Ziviani L, *et al.* The effects of lacidipine on the steady/state plasma concentrations of simvastatin in healthy subjects. *Br J Clin Pharmacol* 2001; **51:** 147–52.
5. Yeo KR, *et al.* Enhanced cholesterol reduction by simvastatin in diltiazem-treated patients. *Br J Clin Pharmacol* 1999; **48:** 610–615.
6. Kanathur N, *et al.* Simvastatin-diltiazem drug interaction resulting in rhabdomyolysis and hepatitis. *Tenn Med* 2001; **94:** 339–41.

7. Peces R, Pobes A. Rhabdomyolysis associated with concurrent use of simvastatin and diltiazem. *Nephron* 2001; **89:** 117–118.
8. Lewin JJ, *et al.* Rhabdomyolysis with concurrent atorvastatin and diltiazem. *Ann Pharmacother* 2002; **36:** 1546–9.

**Danazol.** Rhabdomyolysis has been reported[1] in a patient receiving lovastatin with a number of other drugs; it was considered that an interaction with danazol was the most likely cause.

1. Dallaire M, Chamberland M. Rhabdomyolyse sévère chez un patient recevant lovastatine, danazol et doxycycline. *Can Med Assoc J* 1994; **150:** 1991–4.

**Grapefruit juice.** Grapefruit juice inhibits the cytochrome P450 isoenzyme CYP3A4 and studies using concentrated grapefruit juice have reported increased plasma concentrations of simvastatin,[1] lovastatin,[2] and atorvastatin.[3] However, the clinical relevance of these interactions is not established; a study[4] using less concentrated grapefruit juice found a minimal effect on the activity of lovastatin, although the conclusions of this study have been criticised.[5]

1. Lilja JJ, *et al.* Grapefruit juice–simvastatin interaction: effect on serum concentrations of simvastatin, simvastatin acid, and HMG-CoA reductase inhibitors. *Clin Pharmacol Ther* 1998; **64:** 477–83.
2. Kantola T, *et al.* Grapefruit juice greatly increases serum concentrations of lovastatin and lovastatin acid. *Clin Pharmacol Ther* 1998; **63:** 397–402.
3. Lilja JJ, *et al.* Grapefruit juice increases serum concentrations of atorvastatin and has no effect on pravastatin. *Clin Pharmacol Ther* 1999; **66:** 118–27.
4. Rogers JD, *et al.* Grapefruit juice has minimal effects on plasma concentrations of lovastatin-derived 3-hydroxy-3-methylglutaryl coenzyme A reductase inhibitors. *Clin Pharmacol Ther* 1999; **66:** 358–66.
5. Bailey DG, Dresser GK. Grapefruit juice–lovastatin interaction. *Clin Pharmacol Ther* 2000; **67:** 690.

**Immunosuppressants.** Myopathy has been reported in patients receiving *ciclosporin*, and the risk may be increased when it is given with statins. There have been reports of myopathy and rhabdomyolysis in patients receiving simvastatin[1,2] or atorvastatin[3] with ciclosporin, and in patients receiving lovastatin[4-6] with various immunosuppressants, often including ciclosporin.

Ciclosporin has also been reported to increase the plasma concentrations of statins, including simvastatin,[7] atorvastatin,[8] fluvastatin,[9,10] lovastatin,[11] and pravastatin.[11,12] For the effects of statins on ciclosporin plasma concentrations, see p.1356.

1. Blaison G, *et al.* Rhabdomyolyse causée par la simvastatine chez un transplanté cardiaque sous ciclosporine. *Rev Med Interne* 1992; **13:** 61–3.
2. Meier C, *et al.* Rhabdomyolyse bei mit Simvastatin und Ciclosporin behandelten Patienten: Rolle der aktivität des Cytochrom-P450-Enzymsystems der Leber. *Schweiz Med Wochenschr* 1995; **125:** 1342–6.
3. Maltz HC, *et al.* Rhabdomyolysis associated with concomitant use of atorvastatin and cyclosporine. *Ann Pharmacother* 1999; **33:** 1176–9.
4. Norman DJ, *et al.* Myolysis and acute renal failure in a heart-transplant recipient receiving lovastatin. *N Engl J Med* 1988; **318:** 46–7.
5. East C, *et al.* Rhabdomyolysis in patients receiving lovastatin after cardiac transplantation. *N Engl J Med* 1988; **318:** 47–8.
6. Corpier CL, *et al.* Rhabdomyolysis and renal injury with lovastatin use: report of two cases in cardiac transplant recipients. *JAMA* 1988; **260:** 239–41.
7. Arnadottir M, *et al.* Plasma concentration profiles of simvastatin 3-hydroxy-3-methyl-glutaryl-coenzyme A reductase inhibitory activity in kidney transplant recipients with and without ciclosporin. *Nephron* 1993; **65:** 410–13.
8. Åsberg A, *et al.* Bilateral pharmacokinetic interaction between cyclosporine A and atorvastatin in renal transplant recipients. *Am J Transplant* 2001; **1:** 382–6.
9. Goldberg R, Roth D. Evaluation of fluvastatin in the treatment of hypercholesterolemia in renal transplant recipients taking cyclosporine. *Transplantation* 1996; **62:** 1559–64.
10. Park J-W, *et al.* Pharmacokinetics and pharmacodynamics of fluvastatin in heart transplant recipients taking cyclosporine A. *J Cardiovasc Pharmacol Ther* 2001; **6:** 351–61.
11. Olbricht C, *et al.* Accumulation of lovastatin, but not pravastatin, in the blood of cyclosporine-treated kidney graft patients after multiple doses. *Clin Pharmacol Ther* 1997; **62:** 311–21.
12. Regazzi MB, *et al.* Altered disposition of pravastatin following concomitant drug therapy with cyclosporin A in transplant recipients. *Transplant Proc* 1993; **25:** 2732–4.

**Lipid regulating drugs.** Myopathy and myositis are recognised adverse effects of both statins and fibric acid derivatives, including *fibrates* and *gemfibrozil*, and the risk is increased if they are given together. A similar effect has also been reported with *nicotinic acid*.[1] The interaction between gemfibrozil and statins may also have a pharmacokinetic basis; studies have shown increased plasma concentrations of lovastatin,[2] pravastatin,[3] and simvastatin[4] when given with gemfibrozil.

1. Reaven P, Witztum JL. Lovastatin, nicotinic acid, and rhabdomyolysis. *Ann Intern Med* 1988; **109:** 597–8.
2. Kyrklund C, *et al.* Plasma concentrations of active lovastatin acid are markedly increased by gemfibrozil but not by bezafibrate. *Clin Pharmacol Ther* 2001; **69:** 340–5.
3. Kyrklund C, *et al.* Gemfibrozil increases plasma pravastatin concentrations and reduces pravastatin renal clearance. *Clin Pharmacol Ther* 2003; **73:** 538–44.
4. Backman JT, *et al.* Plasma concentrations of active simvastatin acid are increased by gemfibrozil. *Clin Pharmacol Ther* 2000; **68:** 122–9.

**Thyroxine.** For reference to the effect of lovastatin in patients receiving levothyroxine, see Lipid Regulating Drugs, p.1601.

## Pharmacokinetics

Simvastatin is absorbed from the gastrointestinal tract and is hydrolysed to its active β-hydroxyacid form. Other active metabolites have been detected and a number of inactive metabolites are also formed. Simvastatin is a substrate for the cytochrome P450 isoenzyme CYP3A4 and undergoes extensive first-pass metabolism in the liver, its primary site of action. Less than 5% of the oral dose has been reported to reach the circulation as active metabolites. Both simvastatin and its β-hydroxyacid metabolite are about 95% bound to plasma proteins. Simvastatin is mainly excreted in the faeces via the bile as metabolites. About 10 to 15% is recovered in the urine, mainly in inactive forms. The half-life of the active β-hydroxyacid metabolite is 1.9 hours.

◊ General reviews.

1. Mauro VF. Clinical pharmacokinetics and practical applications of simvastatin. *Clin Pharmacokinet* 1993; **24:** 195–202.
2. Desager J-P, Horsmans Y. Clinical pharmacokinetics of 3-hydroxy-3-methylglutaryl-coenzyme A reductase inhibitors. *Clin Pharmacokinet* 1996; **31:** 348–71.
3. Lennernäs H, Fager G. Pharmacodynamics and pharmacokinetics of the HMG-CoA reductase inhibitors: similarities and differences. *Clin Pharmacokinet* 1997; **32:** 403–25.

## Uses and Administration

Simvastatin is a lipid regulating drug; it is a competitive inhibitor of 3-hydroxy-3-methylglutaryl coenzyme A reductase (HMG-CoA reductase), the rate-determining enzyme for cholesterol synthesis. Inhibition of HMG-CoA reductase leads to reduced cholesterol synthesis in the liver and lower intracellular cholesterol concentrations; this stimulates an increase in low-density-lipoprotein (LDL)-cholesterol receptors on hepatocyte membranes, thereby increasing the clearance of LDL from the circulation. HMG-CoA reductase inhibitors (also called statins) reduce total cholesterol, LDL-cholesterol, and very-low-density lipoprotein (VLDL)-cholesterol concentrations in plasma. They also tend to reduce triglycerides and to increase high-density lipoprotein (HDL)-cholesterol concentrations.

Simvastatin is used to reduce LDL-cholesterol, apolipoprotein B, and triglycerides, and to increase HDL-cholesterol in the treatment of hyperlipidaemias (p.823), including hypercholesterolaemias, combined (mixed) hyperlipidaemia (type IIa or IIb hyperlipoproteinaemias), hypertriglyceridaemia (type IV), and primary dysbetalipoproteinaemia (type III). Statins can be effective as adjunct therapy in patients with homozygous familial hypercholesterolaemia who have some LDL-receptor function. Simvastatin is also given prophylactically to hypercholesterolaemic patients with ischaemic heart disease.

Simvastatin is given by mouth in a usual initial dose of 10 to 20 mg in the evening; an initial dose of 40 mg may be used in patients who are at high cardiovascular risk. The dose may be adjusted at intervals of not less than 4 weeks up to a maximum of 80 mg once daily in the evening. Patients with homozygous familial hypercholesterolaemia may be treated with 40 mg once daily in the evening, or 80 mg daily in 3 divided doses of 20 mg, 20 mg, and an evening dose of 40 mg.

Children aged 10 to 17 years with familial heterozygous hypercholesterolaemia may be given an initial dose of 10 mg once daily, increased according to response, to a maximum dose of 40 mg once daily.

The dose of simvastatin should be reduced in patients at risk of myopathy, including patients with severe renal impairment (see below) and those taking drugs that interact with simvastatin; an initial dose of 5 mg once daily is recommended in patients taking ciclosporin, and the maximum dose should not exceed 10 mg once daily in those taking ciclosporin, gemfibrozil or other fibrates, or nicotinic acid, or 20 mg once daily in those taking amiodarone or verapamil.

◊ General reviews.

1. Mauro VF, MacDonald JL. Simvastatin: a review of its pharmacology and clinical use. *DICP Ann Pharmacother* 1991; **25:** 257–64.
2. Plosker GL, McTavish D. Simvastatin: a reappraisal of its pharmacology and therapeutic efficacy in hypercholesterolaemia. *Drugs* 1995; **50:** 334–63.
3. Schectman G, Hiatt J. Dose–response characteristics of cholesterol-lowering drug therapies: implications for treatment. *Ann Intern Med* 1996; **125:** 990–1000.
4. White CM. Pharmacological effects of HMG CoA reductase inhibitors other than lipoprotein modulation. *J Clin Pharmacol* 1999; **39:** 111–18.

**Action.** The effects of statins on plasma lipids are well established.[1-4] Their primary action is to increase the expression of low-density lipoprotein (LDL)-receptors in the liver, which occurs in response to inhibition of 3-hydroxy-3-methylglutaryl coenzyme A (HMG-CoA) reductase, the rate-limiting enzyme in cholesterol synthesis. This leads to increased clearance of LDL-cholesterol from the plasma, with a subsequent reduction in both LDL and total cholesterol. Triglycerides are also decreased, due to decreased synthesis of very-low-density lipoprotein (VLDL), while high-density lipoprotein (HDL)-cholesterol is either modestly increased or unchanged, leading to an improvement in the LDL:HDL ratio. Patients with homozygous familial hypercholesterolaemia have no functioning LDL-receptors and statins are therefore less effective; however, some statins have been shown to lower LDL-cholesterol in these patients, suggesting that inhibition of LDL synthesis also plays a role in their action.

Statins reduce cholesterol concentrations more effectively than bile-acid binding resins or fibrates, typically producing reductions in LDL-cholesterol of about 20 to 50%, depending on the statin used and the dose. Combination of statins with bile-acid binding resins further lowers LDL-cholesterol and may be beneficial in some patients; in some cases fibrates or nicotinic acid may also be required, although the risk of adverse effects needs to be considered.

Statins may also have a number of additional actions that contribute to their effects.[1-5] They have beneficial effects on endothelial function, which may be partly independent of their effect on lipids, and also appear to stabilise atherosclerotic plaques. A number of studies[6,7] have also shown that statins reduce concentrations of C-reactive protein, a marker of inflammation that is raised in atherosclerosis, although the clinical significance of this is not yet established.

1. Maron DJ, *et al.* Current perspectives on statins. *Circulation* 2000; **101:** 207–13.
2. Shepherd J. The statin era: in search of the ideal lipid regulating agent. *Heart* 2001; **85:** 259–64.
3. Chong PH, *et al.* Clinically relevant differences between the statins: implications for therapeutic selection. *Am J Med* 2001; **111:** 390–400.
4. Igel M, *et al.* Pharmacology of 3-hydroxy-3-methylglutaryl-coenzyme A reductase inhibitors (statins), including rosuvastatin and pitavastatin. *J Clin Pharmacol* 2002; **42:** 835–45.
5. Sotiriou CG, Cheng JWM. Beneficial effects of statins in coronary artery disease—beyond lowering cholesterol. *Ann Pharmacother* 2000; **34:** 1432–9.
6. Ridker PM, *et al.* Measurement of C-reactive protein for the targeting of statin therapy in the primary prevention of acute coronary events. *N Engl J Med* 2001; **344:** 1959–65.
7. Albert MA, *et al.* Effect of statin therapy on C-reactive protein levels: the pravastatin inflammation/CRP evaluation (PRINCE): a randomized trial and cohort study. *JAMA* 2001; **286:** 64–70.

**Administration in renal impairment.** Simvastatin does not undergo significant renal excretion and no dose modification is required in patients with mild or moderate renal impairment. However, patients with severe renal impairment may be at increased risk of myopathy and rhabdomyolysis; the recommended initial dose in such patients is 5 mg once daily and doses above 10 mg once daily should be used with caution.

**Cardiovascular risk reduction.** Hypercholesterolaemia is an established risk factor for the development of atherosclerotic cardiovascular disease, and lipid regulating drugs have an important role in cardiovascular risk reduction (p.819). The efficacy of statins in reducing cardiovascular events has been established in a wide range of patient groups for both primary and secondary prevention, and is believed to be a class effect, although outcome studies have not been performed for all the statins in every case.

Large, randomised studies have established the efficacy of simvastatin (4S[1]) and pravastatin (CARE,[2] LIPID[3]) for the prevention of further coronary events in patients with established ischaemic heart disease. Benefit has also been seen with fluvastatin,[4] including in patients also treated with percutaneous coronary interventions.[5] Some of the studies have also shown a reduction in the incidence of stroke,[6-8] and peripheral vascular disease.[6] A short-term study[9] with atorvastatin in patients with acute coronary syndromes has also shown a reduction in subsequent events, although cohort studies[10,11] of statin use in similar patients have shown mixed results.

Statins have also been tried for primary prevention of coronary events in patients at high risk. In WOSCOPS,[12] pravastatin reduced the incidence of myocardial infarction and death from cardiovascular causes in patients with moderate hypercholesterolaemia but no previous myocardial infarction, while in a similar study (AFCAPS/TexCAPS[13]), lovastatin reduced the risk of major coronary events in patients with average cholesterol concentrations and no evidence of atherosclerotic disease.

Reduction of blood lipid concentrations appears to be the primary mechanism by which statins act to reduce cardiovascular risk, although benefit has been seen in patients with both raised[1,4,12] and average[2,3,13,14] cholesterol concentrations. Most of the evidence for benefit has come from studies including mainly middle-aged men. Those studies that have included women[3,13,15,16] have suggested that there is a similar benefit, and analyses have also suggested that this is maintained in elderly patients.[15-18] The Heart Protection Study,[19] a large, randomised study of a fixed dose of simvastatin in high-risk patients (due to ischaemic heart disease, other occlusive arterial disease, or diabetes mellitus) confirmed that benefit was seen in a wide range of patients, including women and the elderly, irrespective of their initial cholesterol concentrations. Benefit has also been shown[20] for pravastatin in elderly patients at risk of cardiovascular disease.

Although other mechanisms may be involved, various studies have shown that reducing blood lipids with statins slows the progression of atherosclerosis.[21-23] However, neither fluvastatin[24] nor lovastatin[25] prevented restenosis following coronary angioplasty.


1. Scandinavian Simvastatin Survival Study Group. Randomised trial of cholesterol lowering in 4444 patients with coronary heart disease: the Scandinavian Simvastatin Survival Study (4S). *Lancet* 1994; **344:** 1383–9.
2. Sacks FM, *et al.* The effect of pravastatin on coronary events after myocardial infarction in patients with average cholesterol levels. *N Engl J Med* 1996; **335:** 1001–9.
3. The Long-Term Intervention with Pravastatin in Ischaemic Disease (LIPID) Study Group. Prevention of cardiovascular events and death with pravastatin in patients with coronary heart disease and a broad range of initial cholesterol levels. *N Engl J Med* 1998; **339:** 1349–57.
4. Riegger G, *et al.* The effect of fluvastatin on cardiac events in patients with symptomatic coronary artery disease during one year of treatment. *Atherosclerosis* 1999; **144:** 263–70.
5. Serruys PWJC, *et al.* Fluvastatin for prevention of cardiac events following successful first percutaneous coronary intervention: a randomized controlled trial. *JAMA* 2002; **287:** 3215–22.
6. Pedersen TR, *et al.* Effect of simvastatin on ischemic signs and symptoms in the Scandinavian Simvastatin Survival Study (4S). *Am J Cardiol* 1998; **81:** 333–5.
7. White HD, *et al.* Pravastatin therapy and the risk of stroke. *N Engl J Med* 2000; **343:** 317–26.
8. Plehn JF, *et al.* Reduction of stroke incidence after myocardial infarction with pravastatin: the Cholesterol and Recurrent Events (CARE) study. *Circulation* 1999; **99:** 216–23.
9. Schwartz GG, *et al.* Effects of atorvastatin on early recurrent ischemic events in acute coronary syndromes: the MIRACL study: a randomized controlled trial. *JAMA* 2001; **285:** 1711–18.
10. Stenestrand U, Wallentin L. Early statin treatment following acute myocardial infarction and 1-year survival. *JAMA* 2001; **285:** 430–6.
11. Newby LK, *et al.* Early statin initiation and outcomes in patients with acute coronary syndromes. *JAMA* 2002; **287:** 3087–95.
12. Shepherd J, *et al.* Prevention of coronary heart disease with pravastatin in men with hypercholesterolemia. *N Engl J Med* 1995; **333:** 1301–7.
13. Downs JR, *et al.* Primary prevention of acute coronary events with lovastatin in men and women with average cholesterol levels: results of AFCAPS/TexCAPS. *JAMA* 1998; **279:** 1615–22.
14. Sever PS, *et al.* Prevention of coronary and stroke events with atorvastatin in hypertensive patients who have average or lower-than-average cholesterol concentrations, in the Anglo-Scandinavian Cardiac Outcomes Trial--Lipid Lowering Arm (ASCOT-LLA): a multicentre randomised controlled trial. *Lancet* 2003; **361:** 1149–58.
15. Miettinen TA, *et al.* Cholesterol-lowering therapy in women and elderly patients with myocardial infarction or angina pectoris: findings from the Scandinavian Simvastatin Survival Study (4S). *Circulation* 1997; **96:** 4211–18.
16. Lewis SJ, *et al.* Effect of pravastatin on cardiovascular events in women after myocardial infarction: the Cholesterol and Recurrent Events (CARE) trial. *J Am Coll Cardiol* 1998; **32:** 140–6.
17. Lewis SJ, *et al.* Effect of pravastatin on cardiovascular events in older patients with myocardial infarction and cholesterol levels in the average range: results of the Cholesterol and Recurrent Events (CARE) trial. *Ann Intern Med* 1998; **129:** 681–9.
18. Hunt D, *et al.* Benefits of pravastatin on cardiovascular events and mortality in older patients with coronary heart disease are equal to or exceed those seen in younger patients: results from the LIPID trial. *Ann Intern Med* 2001; **134:** 931–40.
19. Heart Protection Study Collaborative Group. MRC/BHF Heart Protection Study of cholesterol lowering with simvastatin in 20 536 high-risk individuals: a randomised placebo-controlled trial. *Lancet* 2002; **360:** 7–22.
20. Shepherd J, *et al.* Pravastatin in elderly individuals at risk of vascular disease (PROSPER): a randomised controlled trial. *Lancet* 2002; **360:** 1623–30.
21. Furberg CD, *et al.* Effect of lovastatin on early carotid atherosclerosis and cardiovascular events. *Circulation* 1994; **90:** 1679–87.
22. MAAS Investigators. Effect of simvastatin on coronary atheroma: the Multicentre Anti-Atheroma Study (MAAS). *Lancet* 1994; **344:** 633–8. Correction. *ibid.*; 762.
23. Herd JA, *et al.* Effects of fluvastatin on coronary atherosclerosis in patients with mild to moderate cholesterol elevations (Lipoprotein and Coronary Atherosclerosis Study [LCAS]). *Am J Cardiol* 1997; **80:** 278–86.
24. Serruys PW, *et al.* A randomized placebo-controlled trial of fluvastatin for prevention of restenosis after successful coronary balloon angioplasty: final results of the fluvastatin angiographic restenosis (FLARE) trial. *Eur Heart J* 1999; **20:** 58–69.
25. Weintraub WS, *et al.* Lack of effect of lovastatin on restenosis after coronary angioplasty. *N Engl J Med* 1994; **331:** 1331–7.


**Dementia.** Epidemiological studies[1,2] have suggested that the risk of dementia is lower in patients who are taking statins. However, prospective, randomised trials are needed to determine their role, if any, in the prevention of dementia.


1. Wolozin B, *et al.* Decreased prevalence of Alzheimer disease associated with 3-hydroxy-3-methylglutaryl coenzyme A reductase inhibitors. *Arch Neurol* 2000; **57:** 1439–43.
2. Jick H, *et al.* Statins and the risk of dementia. *Lancet* 2000; **356:** 1627–31. Correction. *ibid.*; **357:** 562.


**Osteoporosis.** Statins appear to have effects on bone metabolism and preliminary studies[1,2] have suggested that some statins may increase bone mineral density. Several case-control studies[3-5] have also suggested that use of statins may protect against fractures. However, other studies[6-8] have failed to support this association, and prospective, randomised trials are needed[9] to confirm the role of statins in the management of osteoporosis (p.763).


1. Edwards CJ, *et al.* Oral statins and increased bone-mineral density in postmenopausal women. *Lancet* 2000; **355:** 2218–9.
2. Watanabe S, *et al.* Effects of 1-year treatment with fluvastatin or pravastatin on bone. *Am J Med* 2001; **110:** 584–7.
3. Chan KA, *et al.* Inhibitors of hydroxymethylglutaryl-coenzyme A reductase and risk of fracture among older women. *Lancet* 2000; **355:** 2185–8.
4. Meier CR, *et al.* HMG-CoA reductase inhibitors and the risk of fractures. *JAMA* 2000; **283:** 3205–10.
5. Wang PS, *et al.* HMG-CoA reductase inhibitors and the risk of hip fractures in elderly patients. *JAMA* 2000; **283:** 3211–16.
6. Reid IR, *et al.* Effect of pravastatin on frequency of fracture in the LIPID study: secondary analysis of a randomised controlled trial. *Lancet* 2001; **357:** 509–12.
7. van Staa T-P, *et al.* Use of statins and risk of fractures. *JAMA* 2001; **285:** 1850–55. Correction. *ibid.*; **286:** 674.
8. LaCroix AZ, *et al.* Statin use, clinical fracture, and bone density in postmenopausal women: results from the Women's Health Initiative Observational Study. *Ann Intern Med* 2003; **139:** 97–104.
9. Coons JC. Hydroxymethylglutaryl-coenzyme A reductase inhibitors in osteoporosis management. *Ann Pharmacother* 2002; **36:** 326–30.


## Preparations

**USP 27:** Simvastatin Tablets.

**Proprietary Preparations** (details are given in Part 3)
**Arg.:** Coledis; Labistatin; Lisac; Nivelipol; Redusterol; Tanavat; Vasotenal; Zocor; **Austral.:** Lipex; Zocor; **Austria:** Zocord; **Belg.:** Zocor; **Braz.:** Androlip; Clinfar; Lovacor; Mivalen; Revastin; Sinvascor; Sinvastacor; Sinvatrox; Vaslip; Zocor; **Canad.:** Zocor; **Chile:** Arterosan; Nimicor; Vasomed; Vasotenal; Zocor; **Denm.:** Zocor; **Fin.:** Corolin; Lipcut; Zocor; **Fr.:** Lodales; Zocor; **Ger.:** Denan; Zocor; **Gr.:** Kymazol; Lepur; Liporex; Normotherin; Zocor; **Hong Kong:** Zocor; **India:** Simvotin; **Irl.:** Zocor; **Israel:** Simovil; Simvacor; **Ital.:** Liponorm; Medipo; Sinvacor; Sivastin; Zocor; **Malaysia:** Covastin; Zocor; **Mex.:** Zocor; **Neth.:** Zocor; **Norw.:** Zocor; **NZ:** Lipex; Zocor†; **Port.:** Dislipina; Jabastatina; Lipaz; Simvacol; Sinpor; Sinvastil; Sumaclina; Zera; Zocor; **S.Afr.:** Zocor; **Singapore:** Zocor; **Spain:** Arudel; Belmalip; Colemin; Glutasey; Histop; Lipociden; Pantok; Simvasten; Teylor; Zocor; **Swed.:** Zocord; **Switz.:** Zocor; **Thai.:** Bestatin; Eucor; Simvor; Zimmex; Zocor; **UAE:** Simvast; **UK:** Simvador; Zocor; **USA:** Zocor.

**Multi-ingredient: Swed.:** Zocord/ASA.

## Sodium Apolate *(BAN, rINN)*

Apolato de sodio; Lyapolate Sodium *(USAN)*; Sodium Lyapolate. Poly(sodium ethylenesulphonate).

$(C_2H_3NaO_3S)_n$.
*CAS — 25053-27-4.*
*ATC — C05BA02.*

### Profile

Sodium apolate is a synthetic heparinoid anticoagulant. It has been used in the topical treatment of haematomas and superficial thromboses and for the relief of sprains and contusions.

### Preparations

**Proprietary Preparations** (details are given in Part 3)
**Multi-ingredient: Arg.:** Pergalen; **Braz.:** Pergalen†.

# Sodium Nitroprusside

Disodium (OC-6-22)-Pentakis(cyano-C)nitrosylferrate Dihydrate; Natrii Nitroprussias; Nitroprusiato sódico; Sodium Nitroferricyanide Dihydrate; Sodium Nitroprussiate. Sodium nitrosylpentacyanoferrate(III) dihydrate.

$Na_2Fe(CN)_5NO,2H_2O = 297.9.$
*CAS — 14402-89-2 (anhydrous sodium nitroprusside); 13755-38-9 (sodium nitroprusside dihydrate).*
*ATC — C02DD01.*

**Pharmacopoeias.** In *Chin., Eur.* (see p.vi), *Int.*, and *US.*

**Ph. Eur. 5.0** (Sodium Nitroprusside). Reddish-brown crystals or powder. Freely soluble in water; slightly soluble in alcohol. Protect from light.

**USP 27** (Sodium Nitroprusside). Reddish-brown, practically odourless crystals or powder. Freely soluble in water; slightly soluble in alcohol; very slightly soluble in chloroform; insoluble in benzene. Store in airtight containers at a temperature of 25°, excursions permitted between 15° and 30°. Protect from light.

**Incompatibility.** Sodium nitroprusside has been reported to be visually incompatible with cisatracurium besilate[1] and with levofloxacin[2] during simulated Y-site administration.


1. Trissel LA, *et al.* Compatibility of cisatracurium besylate with selected drugs during simulated Y-site administration. *Am J Health-Syst Pharm* 1997; **54:** 1735–41.
2. Saltsman CL, *et al.* Compatibility of levofloxacin with 34 medications during simulated Y-site administration. *Am J Health-Syst Pharm* 1999; **56:** 1458–9.


**Stability in solution.** Solutions of sodium nitroprusside decompose when exposed to light and must be protected during infusion by wrapping the container with aluminium foil or some other light-proof material. Nitroprusside will react with minute quantities of organic and inorganic substances forming highly coloured products. If this occurs the solution should be discarded. Solutions should not be used more than 24 hours after preparation.

The instability of sodium nitroprusside solutions has been the subject of considerable investigation. Although stated to be more stable in acid than in alkaline solution,[1] a later study[2] found that whereas the initial light-induced darkening of a 1% solution was independent of pH, further degradation leading to the development of a blue precipitate required an acid pH. If protected from light by wrapping in aluminium foil, sodium nitroprusside 50 or 100 micrograms/mL was found to be stable in 5% glucose, lactated Ringer's, and normal saline solutions for 48 hours.[3] In clinical practice the infusion container should be opaque or protected with foil, but an amber giving set may be used, to allow visual monitoring.[4,5]

Various substances have been reported to increase the stability of nitroprusside solutions, including dimethyl sulfoxide,[6] glycerol,[1] sodium citrate,[1] and other salts with anionic chelating potential such as sodium acetate or phosphate.[1] In contrast sodium bisulfite and the hydroxybenzoates are reported to reduce stability.[1]


1. Schumacher GE. Sodium nitroprusside injection. *Am J Hosp Pharm* 1966; **23:** 532.
2. Hargrave RE. Degradation of solutions of sodium nitroprusside. *J Hosp Pharm* 1974; **32:** 188–91.
3. Mahony C, *et al.* In vitro stability of sodium nitroprusside solutions for intravenous administration. *J Pharm Sci* 1984; **73:** 838–9.
4. Davidson SW, Lyall D. Sodium nitroprusside stability in light-protective administration sets. *Pharm J* 1987; **239:** 599–601.
5. Lyall D. Sodium nitroprusside stability. *Pharm J* 1988; **240:** 5.
6. Asker AF, Gragg R. Dimethyl sulfoxide as a photoprotective agent for sodium nitroprusside solutions. *Drug Dev Ind Pharm* 1983; **9:** 837–48.


## Adverse Effects

Sodium nitroprusside rapidly reduces blood pressure and is converted in the body to cyanide and then thiocyanate. Its adverse effects can be attributed mainly to excessive hypotension and excessive cyanide accumulation; thiocyanate toxicity may also occur, especially in patients with renal impairment. Intravenous infusion of sodium nitroprusside may produce nausea and vomiting, apprehension, headache, dizziness, restlessness, perspiration, palpitations, retrosternal discomfort, abdominal pain, and muscle twitching, but these effects may be reduced by slowing the rate of infusion.

An excessive amount of cyanide in plasma (more than 80 nanograms/mL), because of overdosage or depletion of endogenous thiosulfate (which converts cyanide to thiocyanate *in vivo*), may result in tachycardia, sweating, hyperventilation, arrhythmias, and profound metabolic acidosis. Metabolic acidosis may be the first sign of cyanide toxicity. Methaemoglobinaemia may also occur.

Adverse effects attributed to thiocyanate include tinnitus, miosis, and hyperreflexia; confusion, hallucinations, and convulsions have also been reported.

Other adverse effects include thrombocytopenia and phlebitis.

**Effects on the blood.** THROMBOCYTOPENIA. Platelet counts decreased in 7 of 8 patients with heart failure 1 to 6 hours after intravenous infusion of nitroprusside was started.[1] The counts began to return to normal 24 hours after the infusion was stopped.


1. Mehta P, *et al.* Nitroprusside lowers platelet count. *N Engl J Med* 1978; **299:** 1134.


**Effects on the gastrointestinal tract.** Five out of 38 patients who were given sodium nitroprusside intravenously for controlled hypotension during surgery developed symptoms of adynamic ileus postoperatively.[1] The symptoms could have been secondary to intestinal ischaemia due to diminished mesenteric arterial blood flow. However, other explanations have been proposed including sympathetic stimulation[2,3] or the concomitant use of opioid analgesics.[4]


1. Chen JW, *et al.* Adynamic ileus following induced hypotension. *JAMA* 1985; **253:** 633.
2. Gelman S. Adynamic ileus following induced hypotension. *JAMA* 1985; **254:** 1721.
3. Lampert BA. Adynamic ileus following induced hypotension. *JAMA* 1985; **254:** 1721.
4. Lemmo J, Karnes J. Adynamic ileus following induced hypotension. *JAMA* 1985; **254:** 1721.


**Effects on intracranial pressure.** A significant increase in intracranial pressure while the mean blood pressure was 90 or 80% of initial values was reported[1] in 14 normocapnic patients given an infusion of sodium nitroprusside to produce controlled hypotension prior to neurosurgery; values reverted towards normal at mean blood pressures of 70% of controls. A similar but insignificant trend occurred in 5 hypocapnic patients. In another report[2] a rise in intracranial pressure was noted following the use of nitroprusside in a patient with Reye's syndrome.


1. Turner JM, *et al.* Intracranial pressure changes in neurosurgical patients during hypotension induced with sodium nitroprusside or trimetaphan. *Br J Anaesth* 1977; **49:** 419–24.
2. Griswold WR, *et al.* Nitroprusside-induced intracranial hypertension. *JAMA* 1981; **246:** 2679–80.


**Phlebitis.** Acute transient phlebitis has occurred following sodium nitroprusside administration.[1]


1. Miller R, Stark DCC. Acute phlebitis from nitroprusside. *Anesthesiology* 1978; **49:** 372.


## Treatment of Adverse Effects

Adverse effects due to excessive hypotension may be treated by slowing or discontinuing the infusion.

For details of the treatment of cyanide poisoning see Hydrocyanic Acid, p.1506. Thiocyanate can be removed by dialysis.

### Precautions

Sodium nitroprusside should not be used in the presence of compensatory hypertension (for example, in arteriovenous shunts or coarctation of the aorta). It should be used with caution, if at all, in patients with hepatic impairment, and in patients with low plasma-cobalamin concentrations or Leber's optic atrophy. It should also be used with caution in patients with impaired renal or pulmonary function and with particular caution in patients with impaired cerebrovascular circulation. Thiocyanate, a metabolite of sodium nitroprusside, inhibits iodine binding and uptake and sodium nitroprusside should be used with caution in patients with hypothyroidism. The plasma-thiocyanate concentration should be monitored if treatment continues for more than 3 days and should not exceed 100 micrograms/mL although toxicity may be apparent at lower thiocyanate concentrations. Thiocyanate concentrations do not reflect cyanide toxicity and cyanide concentrations should also be monitored; the blood concentration of cyanide should not exceed 1 microgram/mL and the plasma concentration should not exceed 80 nanograms/mL. The acid-base balance should also be monitored. Care should be taken to ensure that extravasation does not occur. Sodium nitroprusside should not be withdrawn abruptly due to the risk of rebound effects.

**Aortic stenosis.** Vasodilators such as sodium nitroprusside are usually contra-indicated in conditions where cardiac outflow is obstructed since cardiac output cannot increase to compensate for the fall in blood pressure. However, a study[1] in patients with aortic stenosis and severe left ventricular dysfunction found that sodium nitroprusside was well tolerated and that it rapidly and markedly improved cardiac function.

1. Khot UN, *et al.* Nitroprusside in critically ill patients with left ventricular dysfunction and aortic stenosis. *N Engl J Med* 2003; **348:** 1756–63.

**Tachyphylaxis.** Tachyphylaxis to sodium nitroprusside was associated with high plasma concentrations of cyanide without metabolic acidosis in 3 patients undergoing hypotensive anaesthesia.[1]

1. Cottrell JE, *et al.* Nitroprusside tachyphylaxis without acidosis. *Anesthesiology* 1978; **49:** 141–2.

**Withdrawal.** Rebound haemodynamic changes, including hypertension and increased heart rate, occurred 10 to 30 minutes after discontinuation of intravenous sodium nitroprusside infusion in a study in 20 patients with heart failure.[1] The changes generally resolved spontaneously within 1 to 3 hours after drug withdrawal and produced only minimal exacerbation of symptoms in most patients, although 3 developed pulmonary oedema 20 to 30 minutes after stopping the nitroprusside infusion, requiring reinstitution of nitroprusside in 2 cases. A study[2] investigating a possible mechanism for this effect found that plasma-renin concentrations were increased during infusion of nitroprusside and remained elevated for 30 minutes after the infusion was stopped. It was suggested that this persistence of elevated plasma-renin concentrations after clearance of short-lived nitroprusside may be responsible for the rebound effects.

1. Packer M, *et al.* Rebound hemodynamic events after the abrupt withdrawal of nitroprusside in patients with severe chronic heart failure. *N Engl J Med* 1979; **301:** 1193–7.
2. Cottrell JE, *et al.* Rebound hypertension after sodium nitroprusside-induced hypotension. *Clin Pharmacol Ther* 1980; **27:** 32–6.

### Interactions

Enhanced hypotension should be expected if sodium nitroprusside is used with other antihypertensives or drugs that produce hypotension.

**Alteplase.** Sodium nitroprusside infusion prolonged the fibrinolytic activity of alteplase when given to *animals*; use of nitrovasodilators with alteplase may be responsible for the enhanced bleeding tendency seen in some patients on thrombolytic therapy.[1]

1. Korbut R, *et al.* Prolongation of fibrinolytic activity of tissue plasminogen activator by nitrovasodilators. *Lancet* 1990; **335:** 669.

### Pharmacokinetics

Sodium nitroprusside is rapidly metabolised to cyanide in erythrocytes and smooth muscle and, *in vivo*, this is followed by the release of nitric oxide, the active metabolite. Cyanide is further metabolised in the liver to thiocyanate, which is slowly excreted in the urine; this metabolism is mediated by the enzyme rhodanase and requires the presence of thiosulfate. The plasma half-life of thiocyanate is reported to be about 3 days, but may be much longer in patients with renal impairment.

◊ Reviews.

1. Schulz V. Clinical pharmacokinetics of nitroprusside, cyanide, thiosulphate and thiocyanate. *Clin Pharmacokinet* 1984; **9:** 239–51.

### Uses and Administration

Sodium nitroprusside is a short-acting hypotensive drug with a duration of action of 1 to 10 minutes. It produces peripheral vasodilatation and reduces peripheral resistance by a direct action on both veins and arterioles. It has been termed a nitrovasodilator because it releases nitric oxide *in vivo*. Its effects appear within a few seconds of intravenous infusion. Sodium nitroprusside is used in the treatment of hypertensive crises (p.825) and to produce controlled hypotension during general anaesthesia. It has also been used to reduce preload and afterload in severe heart failure (p.820) including that associated with myocardial infarction (p.828).

It is given by continuous intravenous infusion of a solution containing 50 to 200 micrograms/mL. A controlled infusion device must be used. The solution should be prepared immediately before use by dissolving sodium nitroprusside in glucose 5% and then diluting with glucose 5%; the solution must be protected from light during administration. Blood pressure should be monitored closely during administration and care should be taken to prevent extravasation. In general, treatment should not continue for more than 72 hours. If required for several days blood and plasma concentrations of cyanide should be monitored and should not exceed 1 microgram/mL and 0.08 micrograms/mL respectively; thiocyanate concentrations in serum should also be measured if infusion continues for more than 72 hours and should not exceed 100 micrograms/mL. Since rebound hypertension has been reported when sodium nitroprusside is withdrawn, the infusion should be tailed off gradually over 10 to 30 minutes.

For **hypertensive crises** in patients not receiving antihypertensive drugs, an initial dose of 0.3 to 1.5 micrograms/kg per minute may be given, increasing gradually under close supervision until the desired reduction in blood pressure is achieved. The average dose required to maintain the blood pressure 30 to 40% below the pretreatment diastolic blood pressure is 3 micrograms/kg per minute and the usual dose range is 0.5 to 6 micrograms/kg per minute. Lower doses should be used in patients already receiving other antihypertensives. The maximum recommended rate is about 8 micrograms/kg per minute in the UK, and 10 micrograms/kg per minute in the USA; infusions at these rates should be used for no longer than 10 minutes and should be stopped after 10 minutes if there is no response. If there is a response, sodium nitroprusside should ideally be given for only a few hours to avoid the risk of cyanide toxicity. Treatment with an oral antihypertensive should be introduced as soon as possible.

For the **induction of hypotension** during anaesthesia a maximum dose of 1.5 micrograms/kg per minute is recommended.

In **heart failure** an initial dose of 10 to 15 micrograms/minute has been used, increasing by increments of 10 to 15 micrograms/minute every 5 to 10 minutes according to response. The usual dosage range is 10 to 200 micrograms/minute and the dose should not exceed 280 micrograms/minute (or 4 micrograms/kg per minute).

Sodium nitroprusside has also been used as a reagent for detecting ketones in urine.

**Administration in children.** Although experience is more limited than with adults, sodium nitroprusside has been successfully used in infants and children. Continuous infusion of nitroprusside at a rate of 2 to 4 micrograms/kg per minute for 28 days was reported[1] in an 11-year-old child with refractory hypertension, without any signs of thiocyanate toxicity. In a series of 58 neonates with cardiovascular disorders or respiratory distress syndrome,[2] sodium nitroprusside was given in a usual initial dose of 250 to 500 nanograms/kg per minute, and the rate was then repeatedly doubled at intervals of 15 to 20 minutes until the desired effect was achieved, adverse effects supervened, or it was judged ineffective. The maximum rate did not exceed 6 micrograms/kg per minute. Infusion of sodium nitroprusside in doses of 0.5 to 8 micrograms/kg per minute to produce controlled reduction of blood pressure has also been reported[3] in 28 children with hypertensive crises; 16 had also received labetalol.[3]

1. Luderer JR, *et al.* Long-term administration of sodium nitroprusside in childhood. *J Pediatr* 1977; **91:** 490–1.
2. Benitz WE, *et al.* Use of sodium nitroprusside in neonates: efficacy and safety. *J Pediatr* 1985; **106:** 102–10.
3. Deal JE, *et al.* Management of hypertensive emergencies. *Arch Dis Child* 1992; **67:** 1089–92.

**Ergotamine poisoning.** For the use of sodium nitroprusside in the treatment of cyanosis of the extremities due to ergotamine overdosage, see p.467.

### Preparations

***BP 2003:*** Sodium Nitroprusside Intravenous Infusion;
***USP 27:*** Sodium Nitroprusside for Injection.

**Proprietary Preparations** (details are given in Part 3)
***Arg.:*** Doketrol; Niprusodio; Nitroprus; ***Braz.:*** Nipride; Nitropresabbott; Nitroprus; ***Canad.:*** Nipride†; ***Fr.:*** Nitriate; ***Ger.:*** Nipruss; ***Gr.:*** Nitriate; ***India:*** Sonide; ***Irl.:*** Nipride; ***Israel:*** Nipride†; Niprus; ***Jpn:*** Nitopro; ***Mex.:*** Nitan; ***S.Afr.:*** Hypoten; ***Spain:*** Nitroprussiat; ***USA:*** Nitropress.

## Sotalol Hydrochloride *(BANM, USAN, rINNM)*

Hidrocloruro de sotalol; MJ-1999; *d,l*-Sotalol Hydrochloride; Sotaloli Hydrochloridum. 4′-(1-Hydroxy-2-isopropylamino-ethyl)methanesulphonanilide hydrochloride.

$C_{12}H_{20}N_2O_3S,HCl$ = 308.8.

*CAS — 3930-20-9 (sotalol); 959-24-0 (sotalol hydrochloride).*

*ATC — C07AA07.*

**Pharmacopoeias.** In *Eur.* (see p.vi) and *US.*

**Ph. Eur. 5.0** (Sotalol Hydrochloride). A white or almost white powder. Freely soluble in water; soluble in alcohol; practically insoluble in dichloromethane. A 5% solution in water has a pH of 4.0 to 5.0. Protect from light.

**USP 27** (Sotalol Hydrochloride). A white to off-white powder. Freely soluble in water; soluble in alcohol; very slightly soluble in chloroform.

**Stability.** Suspensions of sotalol hydrochloride 5 mg/mL made using either commercially available or extemporaneously prepared vehicles were found[1] to be stable for up to 3 months when stored at 4° or 25°. Prolonged storage at 25° was not recommended, however, because of the risk of microbial growth.

1. Nahata MC, Morosco RS. Stability of sotalol in two liquid formulations at two temperatures. *Ann Pharmacother* 2003; **37:** 506–9.

### Adverse Effects, Treatment, and Precautions

As for Beta Blockers, p.869.

Torsade de pointes has been reported in patients given sotalol, usually due to prolongation of the QT interval. The QT interval should be monitored; extreme caution is required if the QT interval exceeds 0.50 seconds and sotalol should be discontinued or the dose reduced if the QT interval exceeds 0.55 seconds. As hypokalaemia or hypomagnesaemia may predispose patients to arrhythmias, serum-electrolyte concentrations should be monitored before and during treatment with sotalol.

Sotalol is contra-indicated in patients with renal impairment whose creatinine clearance is less than 10 mL/minute.

**Effects on the heart.** Atypical ventricular tachycardia ('torsade de pointes') has been reported in patients receiving sotalol and may be associated with prolongation of the QT interval.[1,2] Hypokalaemia may contribute to sotalol's proarrhythmic effect and was considered relevant in 8 of 12 patients who developed ventricular tachycardia when given sotalol in association with hydrochlorothiazide; 4 patients were also receiving other drugs known to prolong the QT interval.[3] A meta-analysis[4] of 22 clinical trials involving 3135 patients who had taken sotalol orally found women to be at increased risk of developing torsade de pointes. Torsade de pointes developed in 44 (1.9%) of 2336 men and in 33 (4.1%) of 799 women.

In 1 patient torsade de pointes was treated successfully with magnesium sulfate by intravenous infusion and withdrawal of sotalol.[5]

1. Kontopoulos A, *et al.* Sotalol-induced torsade de pointes. *Postgrad Med J* 1981; **57:** 321–3.
2. Krapf R, Gertsch M. Torsade de pointes induced by sotalol despite therapeutic plasma sotalol concentrations. *BMJ* 1985; **290:** 1784–5.
3. McKibbin JK, *et al.* Sotalol, hypokalaemia, syncope, and torsade de pointes. *Br Heart J* 1984; **541:** 157–62.

4. Lehmann MH, *et al.* Sex difference in risk of torsade de pointes with d,l-sotalol. *Circulation* 1996; **94:** 2534–41.
5. Arstall MA, *et al.* Sotalol-induced torsade de pointes: management with magnesium infusion. *Postgrad Med J* 1992; **68:** 289–90.

**Breast feeding.** Sotalol is distributed into breast milk and milk to serum ratios have been reported[1-3] to range from 2.2 to 8.8. In one report[2] it was calculated that a breast-fed infant might receive 20 to 23% of a maternal dose; however, no bradycardia was noted in the infant in this study. The American Academy of Pediatrics states[4] that there have been no reports of clinical effects in breast-fed infants whose mothers were receiving sotalol and that therefore it may be considered to be usually compatible with breast feeding.

1. O'Hare MF, *et al.* Sotalol as a hypotensive agent in pregnancy. *Br J Obstet Gynaecol* 1980; **87:** 814–20.
2. Hackett LP, *et al.* Excretion of sotalol in breast milk. *Br J Clin Pharmacol* 1990; **29:** 277–8.
3. Wagner X, *et al.* Coadministration of flecainide acetate and sotalol during pregnancy: lack of teratogenic effects, passage across the placenta, and excretion in human breast milk. *Am Heart J* 1990; **119:** 700–2.
4. American Academy of Pediatrics. The transfer of drugs and other chemicals into human milk. *Pediatrics* 2001; **108:** 776–89. Correction. *ibid.*; 1029. Also available at: http://aappolicy.aappublications.org/cgi/content/full/pediatrics%3b108/3/776 (accessed 06/07/04)

## Interactions

Sotalol should not be used with other drugs that prolong the QT interval due to the increased risk of precipitating ventricular arrhythmias. Thus sotalol should not be given with antiarrhythmics that prolong the QT interval (such as amiodarone, disopyramide, procainamide, or quinidine), phenothiazine antipsychotics, tricyclic antidepressants, certain antihistamines (astemizole or terfenadine), cisapride, erythromycin, halofantrine, pentamidine, sultopride, or vincamine. Also, sotalol should be given with great caution with drugs that cause electrolyte disturbances such as diuretics.

Other interactions associated with beta blockers are discussed on p.870.

## Pharmacokinetics

Sotalol is virtually completely absorbed from the gastrointestinal tract and peak plasma concentrations are obtained about 2 to 4 hours after a dose. The plasma elimination half-life is about 10 to 20 hours. Sotalol has low lipid solubility. Very little is metabolised and it is excreted unchanged in the urine. Binding to plasma proteins is reported to be low. It crosses the placenta and is distributed into breast milk where higher concentrations have been achieved than in maternal serum. Only small amounts are reported to cross the blood-brain barrier and enter the CSF. Sotalol is removed by dialysis.

◊ General references.

1. Singh BN, *et al.* Sotalol: a review of its pharmacodynamic and pharmacokinetic properties, and therapeutic use. *Drugs* 1987; **34:** 311–49.
2. Fitton A, Sorkin EM. Sotalol: an updated review of its pharmacological properties and therapeutic use in cardiac arrhythmias. *Drugs* 1993; **46:** 678–719.

**Pregnancy.** The systemic clearance of sotalol in 6 healthy women following an intravenous dose was significantly higher during pregnancy than in the postnatal period, and the mean elimination half-life shorter (6.6 versus 9.3 hours) although the latter difference was not significant.[1] Clearance following an oral dose was also higher during pregnancy than afterwards, but half-lives (10.9 versus 10.3 hours) and mean bioavailability were similar. The changes were probably due to alterations in renal function in the antenatal period.

In a study[2] of transplacental therapy, sotalol was found to cross the placenta easily and completely, with steady-state plasma concentrations similar in mother and fetus. Sotalol accumulated in the amniotic fluid but not in the fetus; it was not associated with fetal growth restriction.

1. O'Hare MF, *et al.* Pharmacokinetics of sotalol during pregnancy. *Eur J Clin Pharmacol* 1983; **24:** 521–4.
2. Oudijk MA, *et al.* Treatment of fetal tachycardia with sotalol: transplacental pharmacokinetics and pharmacodynamics. *J Am Coll Cardiol* 2003; **42:** 765–70.

**Stereo-isomers.** In a pharmacokinetic study, 6 subjects were given *d*-sotalol (dexsotalol; (+)-sotalol) in doses of 0.25 to 2 mg/kg by intravenous infusion and a single dose of 100 mg by mouth.[1] Results suggest that it has a linear pharmacokinetic profile over the doses studied. The oral absorption of *d*-sotalol was almost complete; peak concentrations were reached between 3 and 4 hours after oral administration. Unchanged *d*-sotalol was mainly excreted in the urine; an average of 75% of an intravenous dose was excreted in the urine within 48 hours. The elimination half-life averaged 7.2 and 7.5 hours following intravenous and oral administration respectively.

See Action under Uses and Administration, below for further information on the stereo-isomers of sotalol.

1. Poirier JM, *et al.* The pharmacokinetics of d-sotalol and d,l-sotalol in healthy volunteers. *Eur J Clin Pharmacol* 1990; **38:** 579–82.

## Uses and Administration

Sotalol is a non-cardioselective beta blocker (p.868). It is reported to lack both intrinsic sympathomimetic and membrane-stabilising properties. In addition to the class II antiarrhythmic activity of beta blockers, sotalol lengthens the duration of the action potential resulting in class III antiarrhythmic activity. For a classification and explanation of antiarrhythmic activity, see p.809.

Sotalol is used in the management of ventricular and supraventricular **arrhythmias** (p.816). It was also formerly used in the management of angina pectoris, hypertension, and myocardial infarction but, because of its proarrhythmic effect, it is no longer recommended for these indications. Its use in arrhythmias is restricted to severe disturbances. It should not be used in patients with asymptomatic ventricular arrhythmias.

Sotalol is usually given orally as the hydrochloride. Treatment should be started in hospital with suitable monitoring facilities. The QT interval is monitored before the start of treatment and whenever the dosage is adjusted (see Precautions above). Plasma-electrolyte concentrations and renal function should also be monitored. The dosage is individualised according to the response of the patient. Doses are increased gradually allowing 2 or 3 days between dosing increments. The initial dose of sotalol hydrochloride is 80 mg daily by mouth given as a single dose or in two divided doses; in the USA the recommended initial dose is 80 mg twice daily and this should not be increased for at least 3 days. Most patients respond to doses of 160 to 320 mg daily (usually given in two divided doses). Some patients may require doses as high as 640 mg daily.

Sotalol may be given intravenously as the hydrochloride to control acute arrhythmias, to substitute for oral therapy, and for programmed electrical stimulation. To control acute arrhythmias, a dose of 20 to 120 mg (500 to 1500 micrograms/kg) is given intravenously over 10 minutes. This dose may be repeated every six hours if necessary. To substitute for oral therapy an intravenous infusion of 200 to 500 micrograms/kg per hour may be used. The total daily dose should not exceed 640 mg. For programmed electrical stimulation (to test antiarrhythmic efficacy) an initial dose of 1.5 mg/kg is given over 10 to 20 minutes, followed by an intravenous infusion of 200 to 500 micrograms/kg per hour.

The dose should be reduced in patients with renal impairment (see below).

The use of sotalol as described above is as the racemic mixture; *d*-sotalol (dexsotalol; (+)-sotalol) has been investigated as an antiarrhythmic (see Action, below).

◊ General references.

1. Fitton A, Sorkin EM. Sotalol: an updated review of its pharmacological properties and therapeutic use in cardiac arrhythmias. *Drugs* 1993; **46:** 678–719.
2. Nappi JM, McCollam PL. Sotalol: a breakthrough antiarrhythmic? *Ann Pharmacother* 1993; **27:** 1359–68.
3. Zanetti LAF. Sotalol: a new class III antiarrhythmic agent. *Clin Pharm* 1993; **12:** 883–91.
4. Hohnloser SH, Woosley RL. Sotalol. *N Engl J Med* 1994; **331:** 31–8.

**Action.** Sotalol is used as the racemic mixture of the two stereoisomers, *d*-sotalol (dexsotalol; (+)-sotalol) and *l*-sotalol ((−)-sotalol). A comparison of the effects of *d*-sotalol and racemic sotalol in 6 healthy subjects[1] showed that the beta-blocking activity resided almost entirely in the *l*-isomer, while the effects on the QT interval, which are consistent with type III antiarrhythmic activity, appear to be due to both isomers. A study in 8 healthy subjects also showed a lack of beta blockade by *d*-sotalol.[2] This would suggest that the electrophysiological effects of sotalol are unrelated to its beta-blocking properties. *d*-Sotalol has been investigated as an antiarrhythmic.[3] However, a preliminary placebo-controlled study in patients with myocardial infarction at high risk of arrhythmia due to impaired left ventricular function was terminated early when increased mortality was seen in the treatment group.[4,5]

1. Johnston GD, *et al.* A comparison of the cardiovascular effects of (+)-sotalol and (±)-sotalol following intravenous administration in normal volunteers. *Br J Clin Pharmacol* 1985; **20:** 507–10.
2. Yasuda SU, *et al.* d-Sotalol reduces heart rate in vivo through a β-adrenergic receptor-independent mechanism. *Clin Pharmacol Ther* 1993; **53:** 436–42.
3. Advani SV, Singh BN. Pharmacodynamic, pharmacokinetic and antiarrhythmic properties of d-sotalol, the dextro-isomer of sotalol. *Drugs* 1995; **49:** 664–79.
4. Choo V. SWORD slashed. *Lancet* 1994; **344:** 1358.
5. Waldo AL, *et al.* Effect of d-sotalol on mortality in patients with left ventricular dysfunction after recent and remote myocardial infarction. *Lancet* 1996; **348:** 7–12. Correction. *ibid.*; 416.

**Administration in children.** Sotalol has been used to treat cardiac arrhythmias in children. In the UK, the Royal College of Paediatrics and Child Health suggests a dose of 1 to 4 mg/kg twice daily for children from 1 month to 12 years of age, with 2 or 3 days allowed between increments in dose; the US manufacturer recommends an initial dose of 30 mg/m² three times daily for children from 2 years of age, with at least 36 hours between increments.

In a retrospective review[1] of 62 children (aged from newborn to 17 years) with ventricular or supraventricular arrhythmias, sotalol at a dose ranging from 2 to 6 mg/kg daily was found to be effective in a large proportion of patients, with adverse effects seen in 6. In a study[2] of 13 children aged from 0.4 to 18.7 years with atrial flutter following surgery for congenital heart disease, conversion to sinus rhythm was achieved in 11; sotalol was given at an initial dose of 3 to 4 mg/kg daily in 2 divided doses, increasing to a maximum of 8 mg/kg daily. Sotalol has also been used[3] with flecainide for the treatment of supraventricular tachycardia refractory to either drug alone, in patients below 1 year of age. The doses used ranged from 100 to 250 mg/m² daily of sotalol and from 40 to 150 mg/m² daily of flecainide.

Sotalol has also been used transplacentally to treat fetal tachycardia. In a retrospective study[4] of 21 cases, with hydrops present in 9, sotalol was given to the mother at an initial dose of 80 to 160 mg twice daily. Sinus rhythm was established in 8 of 10 fetuses with atrial flutter, and it was suggested that sotalol may be considered a drug of first choice in this condition. However success was achieved in only 6 of 10 cases of supraventricular tachycardia and there were 3 deaths in this group, indicating that use of sotalol should be limited in the treatment of supraventricular tachycardia.

1. Çeliker A, *et al.* Sotalol in treatment of pediatric cardiac arrhythmias. *Pediatr Int* 2001; **43:** 624–30.
2. Beaufort-Krol GCM, Bink-Boelkens MTE. Effectiveness of sotalol for atrial flutter in children after surgery for congenital heart disease. *Am J Cardiol* 1997; **79:** 92–4.
3. Price JF, *et al.* Flecainide and sotalol: a new combination therapy for refractory supraventricular tachycardia in children <1 year of age. *J Am Coll Cardiol* 2002; **39:** 517–20.
4. Oudijk MA, *et al.* Sotalol in the treatment of fetal dysrhythmias. *Circulation* 2000; **101:** 2721–6.

**Administration in renal impairment.** Sotalol is excreted mainly by the renal route and elimination is therefore slower in patients with reduced renal function. The following dosage reductions based on creatinine clearance (CC) may be used for both the *oral* and *intravenous routes*:

- CC 30 to 60 mL/minute: half usual dose
- CC 10 to 30 mL/minute: quarter usual dose

*Alternatively*, when sotalol is given orally the dosage interval may be increased. At least 5 or 6 doses should be given before incremental dosage adjustments are made.

In a study of 10 hypertensive patients with varying degrees of renal impairment,[1] the apparent first-order elimination rate constant and plasma clearance of sotalol correlated with glomerular filtration rate. Another study[2] compared kinetics in patients with normal renal function, renal impairment, and renal failure. Elimination half-lives of 8.1 and 24.2 hours were reported in patients with creatinine clearance values above 39 mL/minute and between 8 and 38 mL/minute, respectively. It was suggested that an increase in the dosage interval to 48 or 72 hours may be necessary to compensate for longer half-lives. Caution is required when sotalol is used in patients on dialysis; a half-life of 33.9 hours was reported in patients with renal failure but this fell to 5.8 hours during dialysis which removed about 43% of sotalol.

1. Berglund G, *et al.* Pharmacokinetics of sotalol after chronic administration to patients with renal insufficiency. *Eur J Clin Pharmacol* 1980; **18:** 321–6.
2. Blair AD, *et al.* Sotalol kinetics in renal insufficiency. *Clin Pharmacol Ther* 1981; **29:** 457–63.

## Preparations

***BP 2003:*** Sotalol Injection; Sotalol Tablets;
***USP 27:*** Sotalol Hydrochloride Tablets.

**Proprietary Preparations** (details are given in Part 3)

***Arg.:*** Darob; Sotacor; ***Austral.:*** Cardol; Solavert; Sotab; Sotacor; Sotahexal; ***Austria:*** Darob; Sotacor; Sotahexal; Sotamed; Sotanorm; Sotastad; Sotatyrol; Ventricor; ***Belg.:*** Sotalex; ***Braz.:*** Cardionorm†; Sotacor; ***Canad.:*** Rylosol†; Sotacor; Sotamol†; ***Chile:*** Hipecor; ***Denm.:*** Dutacor; Sotabet; Sotacor; ***Fin.:*** Sotacor; Sotalin; ***Fr.:*** Sotalex; ***Ger.:*** CorSotalol; Darob; Favorex; Gilucor; Rentibloc; Sota; Sota Lich; Sota-Gry†; Sota-Puren; Sota-saar; Sotabeta; Sotagamma; Sotahexal; Sotalex; Sotalodoc; Sotaryt; Sotastad; Tachytalol†; ***Hong Kong:*** Sotacor; ***Irl.:*** Sotacor; Sotoger; ***Israel:*** Sotacor; ***Ital.:*** Betades†; Rytmobeta; Sotalex; ***Jpn:*** Sotacor; ***Malaysia:*** Sotacor; ***Mex.:*** Sotaper; ***Neth.:*** Sotacor; ***Norw.:*** Sotacor; ***NZ:*** Sotacor; ***Port.:*** Darob; ***S.Afr.:*** Sotacor; Sotahexal; ***Singapore:*** Sotacor; ***Spain:*** Sotapor; ***Swed.:*** Darob†; Sotabet; Sotacor; ***Switz.:*** Sotalex; ***Thai.:*** Sotacor†; ***UK:*** Beta-Cardone; Sotacor; ***USA:*** Betapace.

**Spirapril Hydrochloride** *(BANM, USAN, rINNM)*

Hidrocloruro de espirapril; Sch-33844; Spiraprili Hydrochloridum; TI-211-950. (S)-7-{N-[(S)-1-Ethoxycarbonyl-3-phenylpropyl]-L-alanyl}-1,4-dithia-7-azaspiro[4.4]nonane-8-carboxylic acid hydrochloride.

$C_{22}H_{30}N_2O_5S_2$,HCl = 503.1.

*CAS — 83647-97-6 (spirapril); 94841-17-5 (spirapril hydrochloride).*

*ATC — C09AA11.*

**Pharmacopoeias.** *Eur.* includes the monohydrate.

**Ph. Eur. 5.0** (Spirapril Hydrochloride Monohydrate). A white or almost white, fine crystalline powder. Very slightly soluble in water; slightly soluble in acetonitrile; practically insoluble in dichloromethane; soluble in methyl alcohol. Store in airtight containers. Protect from light.

## Profile

Spirapril is an ACE inhibitor (p.842) that is used in the management of hypertension (p.825). It owes its activity to the diacid spiraprilat, to which it is converted after oral administration. It is given by mouth as the hydrochloride in a usual maintenance dose of 6 mg once daily.

◊ References.


1. Noble S, Sorkin EM. Spirapril: a preliminary review of its pharmacology and therapeutic efficacy in the treatment of hypertension. *Drugs* 1995; **49:** 750–66.
2. Widimský J, *et al.* Czech and Slovak spirapril intervention study (CASSIS): a randomized, placebo and active-controlled, double-blind multicentre trial in patients with congestive heart failure. *Eur J Clin Pharmacol* 1995; **49:** 95–102.


## Preparations

**Proprietary Preparations** (details are given in Part 3)
***Austria:*** Quadropril; ***Ger.:*** Quadropril; ***Ital.:*** Renormax; Setrilan; ***Spain:*** Renormax; Renpress; ***Switz.:*** Cardiopril.

# Spironolactone *(BAN, rINN)*

Espironolactona; SC-9420; Spirolactone; Spironolactonum. 7α-Acetylthio-3-oxo-17α-pregn-4-ene-21,17β-carbolactone; (7α,17α)-7-(Acetylthio)-17-hydroxy-3-oxo-pregn-4-ene-21-carboxylic acid γ-lactone.

$C_{24}H_{32}O_4S$ = 416.6.

*CAS — 52-01-7.*

*ATC — C03DA01.*

NOTE. Compounded preparations of spironolactone may be represented by the following names:

- Co-flumactone (*BAN*)—spironolactone and hydroflumethiazide in equal parts (w/w)
- Co-spironozide (*PEN*)—spironolactone and hydrochlorothiazide.

**Pharmacopoeias.** In *Chin., Eur.* (see p.vi), *Int., Jpn, Pol.,* and *US.*

**Ph. Eur. 5.0** (Spironolactone). A white or yellowish-white powder. Practically insoluble in water; soluble in alcohol. It exhibits polymorphism. Protect from light.

**USP 27** (Spironolactone). A light cream-coloured to light tan, crystalline powder with a faint to mild mercaptan-like odour. Practically insoluble in water; soluble in alcohol and in ethyl acetate; freely soluble in chloroform and in benzene; slightly soluble in methyl alcohol and in fixed oils.

**Stability.** There was no appreciable loss of spironolactone from extemporaneously prepared suspensions of spironolactone, 2.5, 5 and 10 mg/mL, in a cherry syrup after storage for 2 weeks at 5° or 30° or at ambient room temperature under intense fluorescent light.[1] Degradation was less than 5% for samples stored for 4 weeks, but was more noticeable in suspensions with a higher initial concentration. There were no changes in colour or odour. Bacterial and fungal counts were well within acceptable limits after 4 weeks at 30°.


1. Mathur LK, Wickman A. Stability of extemporaneously compounded spironolactone suspensions. *Am J Hosp Pharm* 1989; **46:** 2040–2.


## Adverse Effects

Spironolactone may give rise to headache and drowsiness, and gastrointestinal disturbances, including cramp and diarrhoea. Ataxia, mental confusion, and skin rashes have been reported as adverse effects. Gynaecomastia is not uncommon and in rare cases breast enlargement may persist. Other endocrine disorders include hirsutism, deepening of the voice, menstrual irregularities, and impotence. Transient increases in blood-urea-nitrogen concentrations may occur and mild acidosis has been reported. Spironolactone has been demonstrated to cause tumours in *rats.*

Spironolactone may cause hyponatraemia and hyperkalaemia.

**Incidence of adverse effects.** A survey found that of 788 patients given spironolactone 164 developed adverse effects.[1] These included hyperkalaemia in 8.6%, dehydration in 3.4%, hyponatraemia in 2.4%, gastrointestinal disorders in 2.3%, neurological disorders in 2%, rash, and gynaecomastia. Hyperkalaemia was associated with renal impairment and the use of potassium supplements: only 2.8% of nonuraemic patients not receiving potassium chloride developed hyperkalaemia, while 42.1% of those with marked uraemia and treated with potassium chloride became hyperkalaemic.

In a study[2] of 54 patients (53 female, 1 male) taking spironolactone 200 mg daily for hirsutism or acne adverse effects were reported in 91%.[2] Menstrual disturbances occurred in 72% of patients, breast tenderness in 39%, dry skin in 39%, and breast enlargement in 24%. Other adverse effects included nausea and vomiting, dizziness, headache, drowsiness, and skin rashes. Two patients developed a chloasma-like pigmentation of the face. The gynaecological effects were reduced in patients taking oral contraceptives.


1. Greenblatt DJ, Koch-Weser J. Adverse reactions to spironolactone: a report from the Boston Collaborative Drug Surveillance Program. *JAMA* 1973; **225:** 40–3.
2. Hughes BR, Cunliffe WJ. Tolerance of spironolactone. *Br J Dermatol* 1988; **118:** 687–91.


**Carcinogenicity.** Breast cancer was reported in 5 patients taking spironolactone and hydrochlorothiazide for prolonged periods[1] although it was suggested[2] that the association with spironolactone therapy was unlikely to be causal.

Although the *rat* may not be an appropriate model for determining long-term safety in man,[3,4] evidence of carcinogenicity in this species prompted the UK Committee on Safety of Medicines to limit the product licences of spironolactone-containing products to exclude use in essential hypertension or idiopathic oedema.[5]


1. Loube SD, Quirk RA. Breast cancer associated with administration of spironolactone. *Lancet* 1975; **i:** 1428–9.
2. Jick H, Armstrong B. Breast cancer and spironolactone. *Lancet* 1975; **ii:** 368–9.
3. Lumb G, *et al.* Effects in animals of chronic administration of spironolactone—a review. *J Environ Pathol Toxicol* 1978; **i:** 641–60.
4. Wagner BM. Long-term toxicology studies of spironolactone in animals and comparison with potassium canrenoate. *J Drug Dev* 1987; **1** (suppl 2): 7–11.
5. Committee on Safety of Medicines. Spironolactone. *Current Problems* 1988; 21.


**Effects on the blood.** Agranulocytosis has been reported[1,2] in association with the administration of spironolactone.


1. Stricker BHC, Oei TT. Agranulocytosis caused by spironolactone. *BMJ* 1984; **289:** 731.
2. Whitling AM, *et al.* Spironolactone-induced agranulocytosis. *Ann Pharmacother* 1997; **31:** 582–5.


**Effects on electrolyte balance.** CALCIUM. A report[1] suggested that spironolactone may have a calcium-sparing effect, in addition to its well known potassium-sparing properties.


1. Puig JG, *et al.* Hydrochlorothiazide versus spironolactone: long-term metabolic modifications in patients with essential hypertension. *J Clin Pharmacol* 1991; **31:** 455–61.


POTASSIUM. There have been reports[1-3] of severe hyperkalaemia in patients taking spironolactone, including patients with renal impairment and those with a high potassium intake from either dietary sources or potassium supplements. In the Boston Collaborative Drug Surveillance Program[4] hyperkalaemia was reported in 42.1% of patients with uraemia taking spironolactone and receiving potassium supplements compared with 2.8% of those without uraemia and not receiving potassium supplements. Two deaths were attributed to hyperkalaemia in patients taking spironolactone and potassium chloride. Potassium supplements should be avoided in patients receiving spironolactone, and plasma-potassium concentrations should be carefully monitored in those with renal impairment.


1. Pongpaew C, *et al.* Hyperkalemic cardiac arrhythmia secondary to spironolactone. *Chest* 1973; **63:** 1023–5.
2. Udezue EO, Harrold BP. Hyperkalaemic paralysis due to spironolactone. *Postgrad Med J* 1980; **56:** 254–5.
3. O'Reilly PH, *et al.* Life-threatening hyperkalaemia after bladder decompression for high pressure chronic retention. *Lancet* 1987; **ii:** 859.
4. Greenblatt DJ, Koch-Weser J. Adverse reactions to spironolactone: a report from the Boston Collaborative Drug Surveillance Program. *JAMA* 1973; **225:** 40–3.


**Effects on endocrine function.** Spironolactone has been associated with disturbances of endocrine function. The most prominent in men is gynaecomastia which appears to be related to both dose and duration of treatment. Incidences of 62%[1] and 100%[2] have been reported. Gynaecomastia has also been accompanied by impotence.[3,4] The effects are generally reversible on discontinuing treatment. Reversal of male-pattern baldness has also been reported.[5]

In women symptoms include breast enlargement and tenderness.[6] The incidence of menstrual abnormalities may be high: unspecified disturbances have been reported in 33 of 53 women,[6] secondary amenorrhoea in 6 of 9,[7] and secondary and primary amenorrhoea in 1 and 2 patients, respectively.[8] The incidence of gynaecological disturbances has been found to be lower in women taking oral contraceptives.[6]

The mechanism of the effects of spironolactone on the endocrine system is unclear. Some workers[9] suggested that although spironolactone affects testosterone synthesis, the more likely explanation was its anti-androgenic action, and reduction in 17-hydroxylase activity. Others[10] found an alteration in the testosterone/oestrogen ratio due to an increase in testosterone clearance and increased peripheral conversion to estradiol. In addition, spironolactone is reported to inhibit binding of dihydrotestosterone to receptors.


1. Huffman DH, *et al.* Gynecomastia induced in normal males by spironolactone. *Clin Pharmacol Ther* 1978; **24:** 465–73.
2. Bellati G, Idéo G. Gynaecomastia after spironolactone and potassium canrenoate. *Lancet* 1986; **i:** 626.
3. Greenblatt DJ, Koch-Weser J. Gynecomastia and impotence complications of spironolactone therapy. *JAMA* 1973; **223:** 82.
4. Greenlaw C. Spironolactone induced gynecomastia: a case report. *Drug Intell Clin Pharm* 1977; **11:** 70–3.
5. Thomas PS. Hair: wanted and unwanted. *BMJ* 1986; **293:** 698.
6. Hughes BR, Cunliffe WJ. Tolerance of spironolactone. *Br J Dermatol* 1988; **118:** 687–91.
7. Levitt JI. Spironolactone therapy and amenorrhea. *JAMA* 1970; **211:** 2014–15.
8. Potter C, *et al.* Primary and secondary amenorrhea associated with spironolactone therapy in chronic liver disease. *J Pediatr* 1992; **121:** 141–3.
9. Loriaux DL, *et al.* Spironolactone and endocrine dysfunction. *Ann Intern Med* 1976; **85:** 630–6.
10. Rose LI, *et al.* Pathophysiology of spironolactone-induced gynecomastia. *Ann Intern Med* 1977; **87:** 398–403.


**Effects on lipid metabolism.** Unlike thiazide diuretics, spironolactone appeared not to increase serum-cholesterol concentrations in a study of 23 patients.[1]


1. Ames RP, Peacock PB. Serum cholesterol during treatment of hypertension with diuretic drugs. *Arch Intern Med* 1984; **144:** 710–14.


**Effects on the liver.** Hepatotoxicity characterised by cholestatic lesions has been reported in a patient receiving spironolactone.[1] Only one other published case of spironolactone-associated hepatic toxicity was known to the authors.


1. Renkes P, *et al.* Spironolactone and hepatic toxicity. *JAMA* 1995; **273:** 376–7.


**Effects on the skin.** Lichen-planus-like skin eruptions developed in a 62-year-old woman who was taking digoxin, propranolol, diazepam, spironolactone, and iron tablets.[1] Flares of the lichen-planus-like eruption seemed to be associated with administration of spironolactone and there was evidence of resolution when spironolactone was withdrawn. Cutaneous vasculitis was associated with spironolactone on 3 occasions in an 80-year-old man.[2] A chloasma-like pigmentation of the face was reported in 2 patients receiving spironolactone for hirsutism or acne.[3]


1. Downham TF. Spironolactone-induced lichen planus. *JAMA* 1978; **240:** 1138.
2. Phillips GWL, Williams AJ. Spironolactone induced vasculitis. *BMJ* 1984; **288:** 368.
3. Hughes BR, Cunliffe WJ. Tolerance of spironolactone. *Br J Dermatol* 1988; **118:** 687–91.


**Hypersensitivity.** Eosinophilia and a rash developed in 2 patients with alcoholic cirrhosis while taking spironolactone.[1]


1. Wathen CG, *et al.* Eosinophilia associated with spironolactone. *Lancet* 1986; **i:** 919–20.


## Precautions

Spironolactone should not be used in patients with hyperkalaemia or severe renal impairment. It should be used with care in patients who are at increased risk of developing hyperkalaemia; such patients include the elderly, those with diabetes mellitus, and those with some degree of renal or hepatic impairment. It should also be given with care to patients likely to develop acidosis. Serum electrolytes and blood-urea-nitrogen should be measured periodically.

**Breast feeding.** The concentration of canrenone was measured[1] in the serum and milk of a breast-feeding woman taking 25 mg of spironolactone four times daily. The milk to serum concentration ratios of canrenone at 2 and 14.5 hours after a dose of spironolactone were 0.72 and 0.51 respectively, and it was estimated that the amount of canrenone ingested by the infant would be 0.2% of the mother's daily dose of spironolactone. The serum potassium and sodium levels of the infant were in the normal range. The American Academy of Pediatrics[2] considers that spironolactone is therefore usually compatible with breast feeding.


1. Phelps DL, Karim A. Spironolactone: relationship between concentrations of dethioacetylated metabolite in human serum and milk. *J Pharm Sci* 1977; **66:** 1203.
2. American Academy of Pediatrics. The transfer of drugs and other chemicals into human milk. *Pediatrics* 2001; **108:** 776–89. Correction. *ibid.*; 1029. Also available at: http://aappolicy.aappublications.org/cgi/content/full/pediatrics%3b108/3/776 (accessed 06/07/04)


**Diabetes mellitus.** Severe hyperkalaemia was reported in a type 1 diabetic woman with hyporeninaemic hypoaldosteronism given spironolactone.[1]


1. Large DM, *et al.* Hyperkalaemia in diabetes mellitus—potential hazards of coexisting hyporeninaemic hypoaldosteronism. *Postgrad Med J* 1984; **60:** 370–3.


**Interference with laboratory estimations.** Spironolactone and canrenoate can interfere with some assays for plasma-digoxin concentrations.[1-3] However, spironolactone may also produce actual changes in digoxin concentrations (see p.897) and results of assays should be interpreted with caution.


1. Yosselson-Superstine S. Drug interferences with plasma assays in therapeutic drug monitoring. *Clin Pharmacokinet* 1984; **9:** 67–87.

2. Foukaridis GN. Influence of spironolactone and its metabolite canrenone on serum digoxin assays. *Ther Drug Monit* 1990; **12:** 82–4.
3. Steimer W, *et al.* Intoxication due to negative canrenone interference in digoxin drug monitoring. *Lancet* 1999; **354:** 1176–7.

**Porphyria.** Spironolactone has been associated with acute attacks of porphyria and is considered unsafe in porphyric patients.

## Interactions

There is an increased risk of hyperkalaemia if spironolactone is given with potassium supplements or with other potassium-sparing diuretics. Hyperkalaemia may also occur in patients receiving ACE inhibitors, angiotensin II receptor antagonists, NSAIDs, ciclosporin, or trilostane concomitantly. In patients receiving spironolactone with NSAIDs or ciclosporin the risk of nephrotoxicity may also be increased. Diuretics may reduce the excretion of lithium and increase the risk of lithium toxicity. Hyponatraemia may occur in patients receiving a potassium-sparing diuretic with a thiazide; this risk may be increased in patients receiving chlorpropamide. Spironolactone may reduce the ulcer-healing properties of carbenoxolone. As with other diuretics, spironolactone may enhance the effects of other antihypertensive drugs and may diminish vascular responses to noradrenaline.

**ACE inhibitors and angiotensin II receptor antagonists.** Severe hyperkalaemia has been reported in patients receiving spironolactone with ACE inhibitors or angiotensin II receptor antagonists and fatalities have occurred. In a study[1] of 44 patients taking such combinations for heart failure who were admitted to hospital with life-threatening hyperkalaemia, 37 required haemodialysis and 2 developed fatal complications. In another group[2] of 25 patients receiving spironolactone with ACE inhibitors who were admitted with severe hyperkalaemia, 2 died and 4 others developed severe cardiac arrhythmias. Advanced age, renal impairment or diabetes mellitus were risk factors for hyperkalaemia in both studies. It was suggested that combinations of spironolactone with ACE inhibitors or angiotensin II receptor antagonists should be used with caution in such patients and that they should not be given doses of spironolactone above 25 mg daily.

1. Wrenger E, *et al.* Interaction of spironolactone with ACE inhibitors or angiotensin receptor blockers: analysis of 44 cases. *BMJ* 2003; **327:** 147–9.
2. Schepkens H, *et al.* Life-threatening hyperkalemia during combined therapy with angiotensin-converting enzyme inhibitors and spironolactone: an analysis of 25 cases. *Am J Med* 2001; **110:** 438–41.

**Aspirin.** Aspirin has been shown to produce substantial reductions in sodium excretion[1] in healthy subjects taking spironolactone and to reduce the excretion of spironolactone's active metabolite, canrenone.[2] However, use of aspirin in hypertensive patients[3] did not alter the effect of spironolactone on blood pressure, serum electrolytes, blood urea nitrogen, or plasma-renin activity.

1. Tweeddale MG, Ogilvie RI. Antagonism of spironolactone-induced natriuresis by aspirin in man. *N Engl J Med* 1973; **289:** 198–200.
2. Ramsay LE, *et al.* Influence of acetylsalicylic acid on the renal handling of a spironolactone metabolite in healthy subjects. *Eur J Clin Pharmacol* 1976; **10:** 43–8.
3. Hollifield JW. Failure of aspirin to antagonize the antihypertensive effect of spironolactone in low-renin hypertension. *South Med J* 1976; **69:** 1034–6.

**Cardiac glycosides.** For discussions of the effects of spironolactone on *digoxin* and *digitoxin*, see p.897 and p.895, respectively. See also Interference with Laboratory Estimations, under Precautions, above.

**Mitotane.** For a report of the inhibition of the action of mitotane by spironolactone, see p.575.

**Warfarin.** For reference to the interaction between warfarin and spironolactone, see p.1026.

## Pharmacokinetics

Spironolactone is well absorbed from the gastrointestinal tract, with a bioavailability of about 90%. It is about 90% bound to plasma proteins.

Spironolactone is metabolised extensively to a number of metabolites including canrenone and the sulfur-containing 7α-thiomethylspirolactone, both of which are pharmacologically active. The major metabolite may be 7α-thiomethylspirolactone, although it is uncertain to what extent the actions of spironolactone are dependent on the parent compound or its metabolites.

Spironolactone is excreted mainly in the urine and also in the faeces, in the form of metabolites. Spironolactone or its metabolites may cross the placental barrier, and canrenone is distributed into breast milk.

◊ References.

1. Overdiek HWPM, Merkus FWHM. The metabolism and biopharmaceutics of spironolactone in man. *Rev Drug Metab Drug Interact* 1987; **5:** 273–302.
2. Gardiner P, *et al.* Spironolactone metabolism: steady-state serum levels of the sulfur-containing metabolites. *J Clin Pharmacol* 1989; **29:** 342–7.
3. Sungaila I, *et al.* Spironolactone pharmacokinetics and pharmacodynamics in patients with cirrhotic ascites. *Gastroenterology* 1992; **102:** 1680–5.

## Uses and Administration

Spironolactone, a steroid with a structure resembling that of the natural adrenocortical hormone aldosterone, acts on the distal portion of the renal tubule as a competitive antagonist of aldosterone. It acts as a potassium-sparing diuretic, increasing sodium and water excretion and reducing potassium excretion.

Spironolactone is reported to have a relatively slow onset of action, requiring 2 or 3 days for maximum effect, and a similarly slow diminishment of action over 2 or 3 days on discontinuation.

Spironolactone is used in the management of heart failure, both to treat refractory oedema and in lower doses as an adjunct to standard therapy (see below). It is also used for refractory oedema associated with cirrhosis of the liver (with or without ascites, p.815), or the nephrotic syndrome, and in ascites associated with malignancy. It is frequently given with the thiazides, furosemide, or similar diuretics, where it adds to their natriuretic but diminishes their kaliuretic effects, hence conserving potassium in those at risk from hypokalaemia. Diuretic-induced hypokalaemia and its management, including the role of potassium-sparing diuretics, is discussed under Effects on the Electrolyte Balance in the Adverse Effects of Hydrochlorothiazide, p.933. It has been used in the treatment of essential hypertension (in lower doses than for oedema), but in the UK is no longer recommended for use in either essential hypertension or idiopathic oedema; doubts have been expressed over its safety during long-term administration.

Spironolactone is also used in the diagnosis and treatment of primary hyperaldosteronism (below).

Other conditions in which spironolactone has been tried on the basis of its anti-androgenic properties include hirsutism, particularly in the polycystic ovary syndrome.

In the treatment of **oedema**, spironolactone is usually given in an initial dose of 100 mg daily by mouth, subsequently adjusted as necessary; some patients may require doses of up to 400 mg daily. In hepatic cirrhosis with ascites and oedema, patients with a urinary sodium/potassium ratio greater than 1 may be given an initial dose of spironolactone 100 mg daily while patients with a ratio of less than 1 may be given initial doses of 200 to 400 mg daily.

Spironolactone is given in doses of 400 mg daily in the presumptive diagnosis of primary **hyperaldosteronism**; in doses of 100 to 400 mg daily for the preoperative management of hyperaldosteronism; and in the lowest effective dosage for long-term maintenance therapy in the absence of surgery.

An initial dose of spironolactone for children is 1.5 to 3 mg/kg daily, in divided doses.

Potassium supplements should not be given with spironolactone.

◊ Reviews.

1. Skluth HA, Gums JG. Spironolactone: a re-examination. *DICP Ann Pharmacother* 1990; **24:** 52–9.
2. Doggrell SA, Brown L. The spironolactone renaissance. *Expert Opin Invest Drugs* 2001; **10:** 943–54.

**Acne.** Spironolactone has been used for its anti-androgenic properties in some cases of acne (p.1133) where standard therapy is unsuccessful. Beneficial responses to oral therapy have been reported in patients with acne from both open[1] and placebo-controlled[2,3] studies. Topical application has been tried[4,5] but response has been variable. It is possible that the vehicle may affect the response. In women, spironolactone may be useful when treatment with an oestrogen is contra-indicated.

1. Burke BM, Cunliffe WJ. Oral spironolactone therapy for female patients with acne, hirsutism or androgenic alopecia. *Br J Dermatol* 1985; **112:** 124–5.
2. Goodfellow A, *et al.* Oral spironolactone improves acne vulgaris and reduces sebum excretion. *Br J Dermatol* 1984; **111:** 209–14.
3. Muhlemann MF, *et al.* Oral spironolactone: an effective treatment for acne vulgaris in women. *Br J Dermatol* 1986; **115:** 227–32.
4. Messina M, *et al.* A new therapeutic approach to acne: an antiandrogen percutaneous treatment with spironolactone. *Curr Ther Res* 1983; **34:** 319–24.
5. Walton S, *et al.* Lack of effect of topical spironolactone on sebum excretion. *Br J Dermatol* 1986; **114:** 261–4.

**Bartter's syndrome.** Spironolactone may be used to reduce potassium wasting in patients with Bartter's syndrome (p.1220).

**Bronchopulmonary dysplasia.** Bronchopulmonary dysplasia (p.1077) is a major cause of chronic lung disease in infants. Treatment often involves the use of corticosteroids. Additional supportive therapy has included the use of diuretics such as furosemide (p.922); results with hydrochlorothiazide or spironolactone have been more ambiguous (p.936).

**Heart failure.** Drug therapy of heart failure (p.820) is based on the use of diuretics, ACE inhibitors, cardiac glycosides, beta blockers, and vasodilators. Spironolactone has been used as a diuretic for refractory oedema, but it also has an additional role as an aldosterone antagonist. Although the precise neurohormonal mechanisms leading to the development of heart failure are still not clear, there is evidence that raised levels of aldosterone may contribute to the pathophysiology.[1,2] ACE inhibitor therapy suppresses aldosterone production but this effect is not complete and spironolactone has therefore been studied in combination with ACE inhibitors. In the Randomized Aldactone Evaluation Study (RALES)[3] in patients with severe heart failure, addition of spironolactone in a dose of 25 to 50 mg daily to therapy with ACE inhibitors and loop diuretics reduced the risk of death or hospitalisation,[3] and the use of spironolactone should therefore be considered in such patients.[4,5] However, use of spironolactone with ACE inhibitors may lead to hyperkalaemia and careful monitoring of potassium concentrations is required,[6] (see above).

1. Struthers AD. Why does spironolactone improve mortality over and above an ACE inhibitor in chronic heart failure? *Br J Clin Pharmacol* 1999; **47:** 479–82.
2. Rocha R, Williams GH. Rationale for the use of aldosterone antagonists in congestive heart failure. *Drugs* 2002; **62:** 723–31.
3. Pitt B, *et al.* The effect of spironolactone on morbidity and mortality in patients with severe heart failure. *N Engl J Med* 1999; **341:** 709–17.
4. Packer M, Cohn JN, eds. Consensus recommendations for the management of chronic heart failure. *Am J Cardiol* 1999; **83** (suppl 2A): 1A–38A.
5. Scottish Intercollegiate Guidelines Network. Diagnosis and treatment of heart failure due to left ventricular systolic dysfunction (February 1999). Available at: http://www.show.scot.nhs.uk/sign/pdf/sign35.pdf (accessed 06/07/04)
6. Georges B, *et al.* Spironolactone and congestive heart-failure. *Lancet* 2000; **355:** 1369–70.

**High-altitude disorders.** Acetazolamide is generally the drug of choice for prophylaxis of high-altitude disorders (p.822). Anecdotal reports[1-4] and a small-scale double-blind study[5] suggested that spironolactone could be useful in preventing acute mountain sickness, although a deterioration in pulmonary function despite spironolactone prophylaxis has been noted in a patient.[6]

1. Currie TT, *et al.* Spironolactone and acute mountain sickness. *Med J Aust* 1976; **2:** 168–70.
2. Snell JA, Cordner EP. Spironolactone and acute mountain sickness. *Med J Aust* 1977; **1:** 828.
3. Turnbull G. Spironolactone prophylaxis in mountain sickness. *BMJ* 1980; **280:** 1453.
4. Rutter LD. Spironolactone prophylaxis in mountain sickness. *BMJ* 1980; **281:** 618.
5. Brown GV, *et al.* Spironolactone in acute mountain sickness. *Lancet* 1977; **i:** 855.
6. Meyers DH. Spironolactone prophylaxis of mountain sickness. *BMJ* 1980; **281:** 1569.

**Hirsutism.** Hirsutism (p.1545) is frequently treated with antiandrogens, usually cyproterone or spironolactone. Spironolactone in doses of 50 to 200 mg daily has produced both subjective and objective improvement in hirsutism in patients with idiopathic hirsutism or polycystic ovary syndrome.[1-4] It is preferably used with oral contraceptives,[5,6] to improve efficacy and menstrual irregularity and to avoid the risk of feminisation to a male fetus. Most studies have involved premenopausal women and it has been suggested[4,7] that spironolactone would be useful in women in whom cyproterone is contra-indicated or not tolerated. A randomised study (not placebo-controlled) found spironolactone 100 mg daily and cyproterone 100 mg daily to be equally effective,[8] while a meta-analysis[9] of the use of spironolactone in hirsutism concluded that it was significantly more effective than both cyproterone and finasteride for up to 12 months after treatment.

1. Cumming DC, *et al.* Treatment of hirsutism with spironolactone. *JAMA* 1982; **247:** 1295–8.
2. Burke BM, Cunliffe WJ. Oral spironolactone therapy for female patients with acne, hirsutism or androgenic alopecia. *Br J Dermatol* 1985; **112:** 124–5.
3. Evans DJ, Burke CW. Spironolactone in the treatment of idiopathic hirsutism and the polycystic ovary syndrome. *J R Soc Med* 1986; **79:** 451–3.
4. Barth JH, *et al.* Spironolactone therapy for hirsute women. *Br J Dermatol* 1988; **119** (suppl 33): 17.
5. Chapman MG, *et al.* Spironolactone in combination with an oral contraceptive: an alternative treatment for hirsutism. *Br J Obstet Gynaecol* 1985; **92:** 983–5.
6. Rittmaster RS. Hirsutism. *Lancet* 1997; **349:** 191–5.
7. West TET. Does spironolactone have a place in treating facial hirsutism in women? *BMJ* 1988; **296:** 1456.

8. O'Brien RC, *et al.* Comparison of sequential cyproterone acetate/estrogen versus spironolactone/oral contraceptive in the treatment of hirsutism. *J Clin Endocrinol Metab* 1991; **72:** 1008–13.
9. Farquhar C, *et al.* Spironolactone versus placebo or in combination with steroids for hirsutism and/or acne. Available in The Cochrane Library; Issue 2. Chichester: John Wiley; 2004.

**Hyperaldosteronism.** Hyperaldosteronism (aldosteronism) is a disorder characterised by mineralocorticoid excess due to high circulating levels of aldosterone. Mineralocorticoid excess due to other mineralocorticoids is rare. Primary hyperaldosteronism is usually caused by an aldosterone-producing adenoma (Conn's syndrome) or primary adrenal hyperplasia. Other causes include aldosterone-producing adrenal carcinoma, and glucocorticoid-suppressible hyperaldosteronism.

Secondary hyperaldosteronism is more common and results from conditions in which there is activation of the renin-angiotensin-aldosterone system, including diuretic therapy, and oedematous conditions such as heart failure, hepatic cirrhosis, and nephrotic syndrome. Bartter's syndrome (p.1220) also results in hyperaldosteronism.

Most patients with primary hyperaldosteronism are asymptomatic, although they may present with signs or symptoms of mineralocorticoid excess (p.1068). Diagnosis often follows the incidental discovery of hypokalaemia. Symptomatic hypokalaemia (p.1219) may develop in some patients, particularly those receiving diuretics.

Diagnosis is confirmed by the presence of raised plasma and urinary aldosterone concentrations. However, the concentrations may be affected by serum-potassium concentration, posture, and time of day, and interpretation may be difficult. The plasma aldosterone:renin ratio may also be measured. In primary hyperaldosteronism the aldosterone concentration is raised but renin is suppressed, although this does not necessarily prove the diagnosis; in secondary hyperaldosteronism both are raised. Radiological and nuclear imaging are useful for further differentiating between adenoma and hyperplasia.

Hyperaldosteronism due to an aldosterone-producing adenoma is usually treated surgically. The aldosterone antagonist spironolactone may be given pre-operatively to lower the blood pressure and normalise the serum potassium. In patients who are not suitable for surgery, long-term medical management involves spironolactone, initially in high doses but reduced to the lowest dose for maintenance. If spironolactone is not tolerated, amiloride may be used as an alternative, but high doses are required. Trilostane, an adrenal suppressant, has also been used to inhibit aldosterone synthesis.

In primary adrenal hyperplasia surgery is not usually effective and medical management with spironolactone or amiloride is required. Additional antihypertensive therapy may also be needed. Glucocorticoid-suppressible hyperaldosteronism, also known as familial hyperaldosteronism type I (FH-I), is a rare autosomal dominant form and may be treated with dexamethasone. However, this may not control the blood pressure and spironolactone or amiloride may be required in addition.

In secondary hyperaldosteronism the underlying condition should be treated, but spironolactone may be of benefit as part of the therapy.

References.

1. Ganguly A. Primary aldosteronism. *N Engl J Med* 1998; **339:** 1828–34.
2. Stewart PM. Mineralocorticoid hypertension. *Lancet* 1999; **353:** 1341–7.
3. Kaplan NM. Cautions over the current epidemic of primary aldosteronism. *Lancet* 2001; **357:** 953–4.
4. Fraser R, *et al.* Cautions over idiopathic aldosteronism. *Lancet* 2001; **358:** 332.

**Precocious puberty.** Spironolactone (as an anti-androgen) and testolactone were given to boys with familial precocious puberty (p.1318) for periods of up to 18 months. Rates of growth and bone maturation were restored to normal during combination therapy but not with either drug given alone.[1] However, after further treatment for 2 to 4.2 years there was a diminishing response manifested by the recurrence of clinical features of puberty and an increase in the bone maturation rate.[2] Addition of deslorelin appeared to restore the control of puberty,[2] and in a long-term study[3] growth rate remained normal for 6 years.

1. Laue L, *et al.* Treatment of familial male precocious puberty with spironolactone and testolactone. *N Engl J Med* 1989; **320:** 496–502.
2. Laue L, *et al.* Treatment of familial male precocious puberty with spironolactone, testolactone, and deslorelin. *J Clin Endocrinol Metab* 1993; **76:** 151–5.
3. Leschek EW, *et al.* Six-year results of spironolactone and testolactone treatment of familial male-limited precocious puberty with addition of deslorelin after central puberty onset. *J Clin Endocrinol Metab* 1999; **84:** 175–8.

**Premenstrual syndrome.** Spironolactone has been used for its diuretic and anti-androgenic properties in premenstrual syndrome (p.1551).

## Preparations

***BP 2003:*** Spironolactone Tablets;
***USP 27:*** Spironolactone and Hydrochlorothiazide Tablets; Spironolactone Tablets.

**Proprietary Preparations** (details are given in Part 3)
***Arg.:*** Aldactone; Osiren; ***Austral.:*** Aldactone; Spiractin; ***Austria:*** Aldactone; Aldopur; Deverol†; Osiren†; Spirobene; Spirohexal; Spirono; Spirox†; ***Belg.:*** Aldactone; Uractone†; ***Braz.:*** Aldactone; Espirolona; ***Canad.:*** Aldactone; Novo-Spiroton; ***Chile:*** Cardactona; ***Denm.:*** Hexalacton; Spilacnet†; Spirix; Spiron; ***Fin.:*** Aldactone; Spiresis; Spirix; ***Fr.:*** Aldactone; Flumach; Practon; Spiroctan; Spironone; ***Ger.:*** Aldactone; Aldopur†; Aquareduct; duraspiron; Jenaspiron; Osyrol; spiro; Spiro-Tablinen†; Spirobeta; Spirogamma; Spirono; verospiron; ***Gr.:*** Aldactone; Uridactone; ***Hong Kong:*** Aldactone; ***India:*** Aldactone; ***Irl.:*** Aldactone; Melactone†; ***Israel:*** Aldactone; Aldospirone; Spironol; ***Ital.:*** Aldactone; Spiroderm; Spirolang; Uractone; ***Mex.:*** Aldactone; Biolactona; Quimolactona; ***Neth.:*** Aldactone; ***Norw.:*** Aldactone; Spirix; Spiropal†; ***NZ:*** Aldactone; Spirotone; ***Port.:*** Aldactone; Aldonar; Nefrolactona; ***S.Afr.:*** Aldactone; Spiractin; ***Singapore:*** Aldactone; Spiridon†; Uractonum†; ***Spain:*** Aldactone; ***Swed.:*** Aldactone; Spirix; Spiroscand; ***Switz.:*** Aldactone; Primacton; Spiroctan†; Xenalon; ***Thai.:*** Aldactone; Altone; Berlactone; Pondactone; Spironex; ***UK:*** Aldactone; Laractone†; Spiretic†; Spirospare; ***USA:*** Aldactone.

**Multi-ingredient:** ***Arg.:*** Aldazida; Lasilacton; ***Austria:*** Aldactone Saltucin; Buti-Spirobene; Deverol mit Thiazid; Digi-Aldopur; Furo-Aldopur; Furo-Spirobene; Furolacton; Lasilacton; Sali-Aldopur; Spirono comp; Supracid; Suprenoat†; ***Belg.:*** Aldactazine; Uractazide†; ***Braz.:*** Aldazida; Lasilactona; ***Canad.:*** Aldactazide; Novo-Spirozine; ***Fr.:*** Aldactazine; Aldalix; Practazin; Prinactizide†; Spiroctazine; ***Ger.:*** Aldactone Saltucin; duraspiron-comp; Furo-Aldopur; Furorese Comp; Osyrol Lasix; Risicordin; Sali-Aldopur; Spiro comp; Spiro-D; Spironolacton Plus; Spironothiazid; Spirostada comp; ***India:*** Lasilactone; Spiromide; ***Irl.:*** Aldactide; ***Ital.:*** Aldactazide; Lasitone; Spiridazide; Spirofur; ***Mex.:*** Aldazida; Lasilacton; ***Port.:*** Aldactazine; Ondolen; ***S.Afr.:*** Aldazide; ***Spain:*** Aldactacine; Aldoleo; Miscidon; Resnedal†; Spirometon; ***Switz.:*** Aldozone; Furocombin; Furosemid comp†; Furospir; Lasilactone; Sali-Spiroctan†; Saluretin†; Spironothiazid†; Synureticum†; ***UK:*** Aldactide; Lasilactone; Spiro-Co†; ***USA:*** Aldactazide.

## Staphylokinase

Estafiloquinasa.

### Profile

Staphylokinase is a thrombolytic derived from *Staphylococcus aureus*. Recombinant and modified forms are under investigation for the treatment of thromboembolic disorders, including acute myocardial infarction.

◊ References.

1. Vanderschueren S, *et al.* Thrombolytic therapy of peripheral arterial occlusion with recombinant staphylokinase. *Circulation* 1995; **92:** 2050–57.
2. Vanderschueren S, *et al.* Randomized coronary patency trial of double-bolus recombinant staphylokinase versus front-loaded alteplase in acute myocardial infarction. *Am Heart J* 1997; **134:** 213–19.
3. Armstrong PW, *et al.* Collaborative angiographic patency trial of recombinant staphylokinase (CAPTORS II). *Am Heart J* 2003; **146:** 484–8.

## Streptokinase *(BAN, rINN)*

Estreptoquinasa; Plasminokinase; Streptokinasum.
*CAS — 9002-01-1.*
*ATC — B01AD01.*

**Pharmacopoeias.** *Eur.* (see p.vi) includes a bulk solution.
**Ph. Eur. 5.0** (Streptokinase Bulk Solution; Streptokinasi Solutio ad Praeparationem). A preparation of a protein obtained from culture filtrates of certain strains of haemolytic *Streptococcus* group C. It has the property of combining with human plasminogen to form plasminogen activator. The potency is not less than 96 000 international units per mg of protein. A clear, colourless liquid. pH 6.8 to 7.5. Store in sealed containers at a temperature of −20°. Protect from light.

**Stability.** The incorporation of albumin in commercial preparations of streptokinase has reduced the incidence of flocculation with streptokinase solutions. However, flocculation has occurred with small volumes prepared with sodium chloride 0.9% in sterilised glass containers apparently because of residual acid buffers that remain in empty evacuated containers following sterilisation.[1]

1. Thibault L. Streptokinase flocculation in evacuated glass bottles. *Am J Hosp Pharm* 1985; **42:** 278.

### Units

The potency of streptokinase is expressed in international units and preparations are assayed using the second International Standard (1989).

The Christensen unit is the quantity of streptokinase that will lyse a standard blood clot completely in 10 minutes and is equivalent to the international unit.

### Adverse Effects

In common with other thrombolytics streptokinase may cause haemorrhage, particularly from puncture sites; severe internal bleeding has occurred and may be difficult to control. Streptokinase is antigenic, and allergic reactions ranging from rashes to rarer anaphylactoid and serum-sickness-like symptoms have occurred. Fever, sometimes high, and associated symptoms such as chills and back or abdominal pain are quite frequent. Nausea and vomiting may occur. There have been a few reports of Guillain-Barré syndrome.

Streptokinase infusion may be associated with hypotension, both direct or as a result of reperfusion; bradycardia and arrhythmias may also occur due to reperfusion. The break-up of existing clots may occasionally produce emboli elsewhere; pulmonary embolism and acute renal failure due to cholesterol embolisation have been reported.

**Back pain.** Streptokinase infusion has been associated with the development of very severe low back pain, which resolves within a few minutes of stopping the infusion, and may be severe enough to warrant opioid analgesia.[1-4] The back pain may represent a hypersensitivity reaction. Providing that the pain is controlled and that dissecting aortic aneurysm is not suspected, it may still be possible to complete the streptokinase infusion.[4,5] Alternatively, immediate substitution with a different thrombolytic has been suggested.[6]

There have also been a few reports of low back pain associated with anistreplase infusion.[7,8]

1. Shah M, Taylor RT. Low back pain associated with streptokinase. *BMJ* 1990; **301:** 1219.
2. Dickinson RJ, Rosser A. Low back pain associated with streptokinase. *BMJ* 1991; **302:** 111–12.
3. Porter NJ, Nikoletatos K. Low back pain associated with streptokinase. *BMJ* 1991; **302:** 112.
4. Pinheiro RF, *et al.* Low back pain during streptokinase infusion. *Arq Bras Cardiol* 2002; **78:** 233–5.
5. Lear J, *et al.* Low back pain associated with streptokinase. *Lancet* 1992; **340:** 851.
6. Fishwick D, *et al.* Thrombolysis and low back pain. *BMJ* 1995; **310:** 504.
7. Hannaford P, Kay CR. Back pain and thrombolysis. *BMJ* 1992; **304:** 915.
8. Lear J, Rajapakse R. Low back pain associated with anistreplase. *BMJ* 1993; **306:** 896.

**Effects on the blood.** Although falls in the haemoglobin value of patients receiving thrombolytics are most likely to be due to blood loss from haemorrhage, there has been a report of a patient who had signs of haemolytic anaemia following intravenous infusion of streptokinase.[1] In a subsequent test *in vitro* the patient's serum caused strong agglutination of streptokinase-treated red blood cells, supporting the view that streptokinase was responsible for the haemolysis.

1. Mathiesen O, Grunnet N. Haemolysis after intravenous streptokinase. *Lancet* 1989; **i:** 1016–17.

**Effects on the eyes.** Acute uveitis[1,2] and iritis,[3,4] associated with transient renal impairment in one patient,[3] have followed treatment of myocardial infarction with intravenous streptokinase. In one case uveitis was associated with serum sickness[2] and in all of them hypersensitivity to streptokinase was suspected.

1. Kinshuck D. Bilateral hypopyon and streptokinase. *BMJ* 1992; **305:** 1332.
2. Proctor BD, Joondeph BC. Bilateral anterior uveitis: a feature of streptokinase-induced serum sickness. *N Engl J Med* 1994; **330:** 576–7.
3. Birnbaum Y, *et al.* Acute iritis and transient renal impairment following thrombolytic therapy for acute myocardial infarction. *Ann Pharmacother* 1993; **27:** 1539–40.
4. Gray MY, Lazarus JH. Iritis after treatment with streptokinase. *BMJ* 1994; **309:** 97.

**Effects on the kidneys.** Transient proteinuria has been reported following the administration of streptokinase. In some patients proteinuria and renal impairment have developed about 7 days after thrombolytic therapy and have been associated with a syndrome resembling serum sickness,[1,2] suggesting a delayed hypersensitivity reaction; a similar case in a patient receiving anistreplase was associated with Henoch-Schönlein-like vasculitis.[3] These delayed reactions should be distinguished from the transient and apparently self-limiting proteinuria that has been reported in some patients in the first 24 to 72 hours after beginning streptokinase.[4,5] Proteinuria within the first 24 hours has been attributed to deposition of an immune complex in the glomeruli,[6] although haemodynamic and neurohormonal changes associated with acute myocardial infarction may be responsible since proteinuria has occurred in patients not receiving thrombolytic therapy.[7,8]

Streptokinase infusion has also been associated with acute oliguric renal failure due to acute tubular necrosis, apparently as a result of hypotension during the infusion, in a patient with existing renovascular narrowing.[9] Interestingly, it has been pointed out that a variant streptokinase may be the pathogenic agent in glomerulonephritis occurring after *Streptococcus pyogenes* infection.[10]

Renal failure has developed as a consequence of streptokinase-induced cholesterol embolism, see under Embolism, below.

1. Payne ST, *et al.* Transient impairment of renal function after streptokinase therapy. *Lancet* 1989; **ii:** 1398.
2. Callan MFC, *et al.* Proteinuria and thrombolytic agents. *Lancet* 1990; **335:** 106.
3. Ali A, *et al.* Proteinuria and thrombolytic agents. *Lancet* 1990; **335:** 106–7.
4. Argent N, Adams PC. Proteinuria and thrombolytic agents. *Lancet* 1990; **335:** 106.
5. More RS, Peacock F. Haematuria and proteinuria after thrombolytic therapy. *Lancet* 1990; **336:** 1454.
6. Lynch M, *et al.* Proteinuria with streptokinase. *Lancet* 1993; **341:** 1024.
7. Pickett TM, Hilton PJ. Proteinuria and streptokinase. *Lancet* 1993; **341:** 1538.
8. von Eyben FE, *et al.* Albuminuria with or without streptokinase. *Lancet* 1993; **342:** 365–6.
9. Kalra PA, *et al.* Acute tubular necrosis induced by coronary thrombolytic therapy. *Postgrad Med J* 1991; **67:** 212.
10. Barnham M. Hypersensitivity and streptokinase. *Lancet* 1990; **335:** 535.

**Effects on the liver.** Raised serum-alanine aminotransferase values, and in some cases raised aspartate aminotransferase activity, were seen more frequently in 95 patients who received streptokinase than in 94 given placebo as part of a study in patients with myocardial infarction.[1] The mechanism for the raised aminotransferase activity was not clear; a concomitant rise in γ-glutamyltransferase activity and bilirubin concentration suggested an hepatic source.

For references to rupture of the liver occurring during treatment with streptokinase, see Haemorrhage, below.


1. Maclennan AC, *et al.* Activities of aminotransferases after treatment with streptokinase for acute myocardial infarction. *BMJ* 1990; **301:** 321–2.


**Effects on the nervous system.** There have been a few reports of Guillain-Barré syndrome following treatment with streptokinase.[1-4] Whether streptokinase was the cause is not certain although its antigenic properties do suggest that induction of an immunological reaction might be responsible.[3]

For discussion of cerebrovascular effects of streptokinase, see Haemorrhage, below.


1. Eden KV. Possible association of Guillain-Barré syndrome with thrombolytic therapy. *JAMA* 1983; **249:** 2020–1.
2. Leaf DA, *et al.* Streptokinase and the Guillain-Barré syndrome. *Ann Intern Med* 1984; **100:** 617.
3. Barnes D, Hughes RAC. Guillain-Barré syndrome after treatment with streptokinase. *BMJ* 1992; **304:** 1225.
4. Taylor BV, *et al.* Guillain-Barré syndrome complicating treatment with streptokinase. *Med J Aust* 1995; **162:** 214–15.


**Effects on the respiratory system.** Fatal acute respiratory distress syndrome occurred in a patient given streptokinase for pulmonary embolism.[1] It was suggested that streptokinase may have caused the pulmonary injury by altering vascular permeability due to generation of fibrinolytic products or via reperfusion oedema.


1. Martin TR, *et al.* Adult respiratory distress syndrome following thrombolytic therapy for pulmonary embolism. *Chest* 1983; **83:** 151–3.


**Effects on the skin.** Rashes may occur as an allergic reaction to streptokinase. For a report of skin necrosis possibly associated with cholesterol embolisation, see Embolism, below.

**Embolism.** Thrombolytic therapy has occasionally and paradoxically been associated with further embolism. This may be due to clots that break away from the thrombus being treated, or to cholesterol crystals released following removal of fibrin from atheromatous plaques by thrombolysis.

Fatal pulmonary embolism has been reported,[1] apparently due to breakaway from a deep-vein thrombus under treatment. However, comparative studies have suggested that there is no evidence of a higher rate of such complications with streptokinase than with heparin.[2] When they do occur a good clinical response is usually seen to continued streptokinase.[2] Complications due to multiple microemboli were reported[3] in 7 of 475 consecutive patients treated with streptokinase or anistreplase for acute myocardial infarction. The sites of embolism were the legs (in 4) and brain (in 3); one patient apparently had systemic effects with skin infarction and renal impairment. Five of the 7 patients died.

Cholesterol embolisation can have many clinical manifestations depending on the location of the emboli. A classic presentation is livedo reticularis, gangrenous lower extremities, and acute renal failure.[4,5] Symptoms may appear within a few hours of starting thrombolytic treatment,[6] although in some cases they may not become evident for several days.[7-10]


1. Hill LN. Streptokinase therapy and breakaway pulmonary emboli. *Am J Med* 1991; **90:** 411–12.
2. Rogers LQ, Lutcher CL. Streptokinase therapy and breakaway pulmonary emboli. *Am J Med* 1991; **90:** 412–13.
3. Stafford PJ, *et al.* Multiple microemboli after disintegration of clot during thrombolysis for acute myocardial infarction. *BMJ* 1989; **299:** 1310–12.
4. Blankenship JC. Cholesterol embolisation after thrombolytic therapy. *Drug Safety* 1996; **14:** 78–84.
5. Wong FKM, *et al.* Acute renal failure after streptokinase therapy in a patient with acute myocardial infarction. *Am J Kidney Dis* 1995; **26:** 508–10.
6. Pochmalicki G, *et al.* Cholesterol embolisation syndrome after thrombolytic therapy for myocardial infarction. *Lancet* 1992; **339:** 58–9.
7. Ridker PM, Michel T. Streptokinase therapy and cholesterol embolization. *Am J Med* 1989; **87:** 357–8.
8. Pirson Y, *et al.* Cholesterol embolism in a renal graft after treatment with streptokinase. *BMJ* 1988; **296:** 394–5.
9. Dass H, Fescharek R. Skin necrosis induced by streptokinase. *BMJ* 1994; **309:** 1513–14.
10. Penswick J, Wright AL. Skin necrosis induced by streptokinase. *BMJ* 1994; **309:** 378.


**Haemorrhage.** Haemorrhage is a common adverse effect of thrombolytic therapy, and the problem and its management have been reviewed.[1] Thrombolytics are used to lyse pathological thrombi, but can also produce a 'lytic state' due to depletion of the natural plasmin inhibitor $\alpha_2$-antiplasmin by excess plasmin production; they may also cause lysis of thrombi required for haemostasis.

Haemorrhage is a particular risk where there is existing or concomitant trauma. More than 70% of bleeding episodes occur at vascular puncture sites,[1] so invasive procedures should be avoided if possible; if catheterisation is considered essential meticulous care of the vascular puncture site is necessary. Bleeding or severe bruising in patients receiving thrombolytic therapy have also been associated with intramuscular injection of analgesics,[2] the use of an automatic blood-pressure measuring machine,[3] a pre-existing prosthetic abdominal aortic graft,[4] and recent dental extraction.[5] Other disease states may also contribute: haemospermia has been reported following thrombolysis in a patient with mild prostatic symptoms,[6] haemorrhagic bullae have been reported in a patient with lichen sclerosus et atrophicus,[7] and diabetic patients are at risk of retinal haemorrhage if they have diabetic retinopathy,[8] although any increase in risk seems to be small.[9] A review of the GUSTO-I Study[10] (40 903 patients) identified older age, low body-weight, female sex, and African ancestry as other factors that increased the risk of haemorrhage.

Intracranial haemorrhage leading to stroke is the most serious bleeding complication with thrombolytics, and has a high mortality. Assessment of data from national registries and large-scale trials has identified a number of risk factors for intracranial haemorrhage, including those mentioned above for overall haemorrhage, hypertension on admission, a history of stroke, and thrombolysis with current alteplase regimens.[11-14] The benefits and risks must be assessed for each patient and thrombolytic therapy should still be given to the elderly and to those with hypertension if the expected benefits are great. Intracranial haemorrhage is a particular concern with the use of thrombolytics for the treatment of ischaemic stroke. In the NINDS study, using alteplase, clinical outcome appeared to be improved despite an increased incidence of symptomatic intracerebral haemorrhage. Subgroup analysis[15] suggested that severe neurological deficit, brain oedema, and mass effect, before treatment, were risks associated with the increased incidence of haemorrhage.

Fibrin-specific thrombolytics such as alteplase were developed in the hope that they would have less systemic effect than fibrin-nonspecific thrombolytics such as streptokinase and therefore cause less bleeding. However, studies that have assessed comparative bleeding rates have failed to confirm this, although the use of adjunctive antithrombotics and different dose regimens makes comparison difficult. In GUSTO-I,[10] the bleeding rate with alteplase plus intravenous heparin was lower than with streptokinase plus intravenous heparin, but was similar to that with streptokinase plus subcutaneous heparin. However, the rate of intracranial haemorrhage was higher with alteplase.[16] In ASSENT-2,[17] which compared bolus administration of the highly fibrin-specific thrombolytic tenecteplase with front-loaded alteplase, tenecteplase produced fewer major non-cerebral bleeds than alteplase but the rates of intracranial haemorrhage were nearly identical. Although a meta-analysis[18] suggested that rates of intracranial haemorrhage may be higher with bolus thrombolytics, others have suggested that this may not be a problem with newer bolus regimens.[19]

Other bleeding complications reported with thrombolytics include rupture of the spleen[20,21] and liver,[22] and rupture of a follicle has been reported in a menstruating woman.[23] Rupture of the heart with fatal consequences has been reported, although thrombolytics do not appear to increase the overall risk of cardiac rupture following myocardial infarction,[24] except possibly for early rupture in women.[25]

Diffuse alveolar haemorrhage has been reported[26] in a patient treated with streptokinase after myocardial infarction. Intrapleural use was associated with life-threatening haemorrhage in empyema following cardiac surgery,[27] and with fatal haemorrhage in a case of aortic dissection misdiagnosed as empyema.[28]


1. Sane DC, *et al.* Bleeding during thrombolytic therapy for acute myocardial infarction: mechanisms and management. *Ann Intern Med* 1989; **111:** 1010–22.
2. Morris GC, Sterry MJG. [case report]. *BMJ* 1991; **302:** 246.
3. Gibson P. [case report]. *BMJ* 1991; **302:** 1412.
4. London NJM, *et al.* Systemic thrombolysis causing haemorrhage around a prosthetic abdominal aortic graft. *BMJ* 1993; **306:** 1530–1.
5. Lustig JP, *et al.* Thrombolytic therapy for acute myocardial infarction after oral surgery. *Oral Surg Oral Med Oral Pathol* 1993; **75:** 547–8.
6. Keeling PJ, Lawson CS. Haemospermia: a complication of thrombolytic therapy. *Br J Hosp Med* 1990; **44:** 244.
7. Dunn HM, Fulton RA. Haemorrhagic bullae in a patient with lichen sclerosus et atrophicus treated with streptokinase. *Heart* 1996; **76:** 448.
8. Caramelli B, *et al.* Retinal haemorrhage after thrombolytic therapy. *Lancet* 1991; **337:** 1356–7.
9. Ward H, Yudkin JS. Thrombolysis in patients with diabetes. *BMJ* 1995; **310:** 3–4.
10. Berkowitz SD, *et al.* Incidence and predictors of bleeding after contemporary thrombolytic therapy for myocardial infarction. *Circulation* 1997; **95:** 2508–16.
11. Simoons ML, *et al.* Individual risk assessment for intracranial haemorrhage during thrombolytic therapy. *Lancet* 1993; **342:** 1523–8.
12. Aylward PE, *et al.* Relation of increased arterial blood pressure to mortality and stroke in the context of contemporary thrombolytic therapy for acute myocardial infarction: a randomized trial. *Ann Intern Med* 1996; **125:** 891–900.
13. Bovill EG, *et al.* Hemorrhagic events during therapy with recombinant tissue plasminogen activator, heparin, and aspirin for unstable angina (Thrombolysis in Myocardial Ischemia, Phase IIIB trial). *Am J Cardiol* 1997; **79:** 391–6.
14. Gurwitz JH, *et al.* Risk for intracranial hemorrhage after tissue plasminogen activator treatment for acute myocardial infarction. *Ann Intern Med* 1998; **129:** 597–604.
15. The NINDS t-PA Stroke Study Group. Intracerebral hemorrhage after intravenous t-PA therapy for ischemic stroke. *Stroke* 1997; **28:** 2109–18.
16. Gore JM, *et al.* Stroke after thrombolysis: mortality and functional outcomes in the GUSTO-I trial. *Circulation* 1995; **92:** 2811–18.
17. Assessment of the Safety and Efficacy of a New Thrombolytic (ASSENT-2) Investigators. Single-bolus tenecteplase compared with front-loaded alteplase in acute myocardial infarction: the ASSENT-2 double-blind randomised trial. *Lancet* 1999; **354:** 716–22.
18. Mehta SR, *et al.* Risk of intracranial haemorrhage with bolus versus infusion thrombolytic therapy: a meta-analysis. *Lancet* 2000; **356:** 449–54.
19. Armstrong PW, *et al.* Bolus fibrinolysis: risk, benefit, and opportunities. *Circulation* 2001; **103:** 1171–3.
20. Wiener RS, Ong LS. Streptokinase and splenic rupture. *Am J Med* 1989; **86:** 249.
21. Blankenship JC, Indeck M. Spontaneous splenic rupture complicating anticoagulant or thrombolytic therapy. *Am J Med* 1993; **94:** 433–7.
22. Eklöf B, *et al.* Spontaneous rupture of liver and spleen with severe intra-abdominal bleeding during streptokinase treatment of deep venous thrombosis. *Vasa* 1977; **6:** 369–71.
23. Müller C-H, *et al.* Near-fatal intra-abdominal bleeding from a ruptured follicle during thrombolytic therapy. *Lancet* 1996; **347:** 1697.
24. Massel DR. How sound is the evidence that thrombolysis increases the risk of cardiac rupture? *Br Heart J* 1993; **69:** 284–7.
25. Becker RC, *et al.* Fatal cardiac rupture among patients treated with thrombolytic agents and adjunctive thrombin antagonists: observations from the Thrombolysis and Thrombin Inhibition in Myocardial Infarction 9 Study. *J Am Coll Cardiol* 1999; **33:** 479–87.
26. Yigla M, *et al.* Diffuse alveolar hemorrhage following thrombolytic therapy for acute myocardial infarction. *Respiration* 2000; **67:** 445–8.
27. Porter J, Banning AP. Intrapleural streptokinase. *Thorax* 1998; **53:** 720.
28. Srivastava P, *et al.* Fatal haemorrhage from aortic dissection following instillation of intrapleural streptokinase. *Scott Med J* 2000; **45:** 86–7.


**Hypersensitivity.** Streptokinase is a bacterial protein and has antigenic activity. The formation of streptokinase-neutralising antibodies may reduce the efficacy of subsequent doses and increase the risk of hypersensitivity reactions.

In a series of 25 patients given intravenous streptokinase for myocardial infarction, titres of streptokinase-neutralising antibodies rose from a mean neutralisation capacity of 0.16 million units before treatment to a mean of 25.54 million units 2 weeks after treatment, the highest individual titre being 93 million units. After 12 weeks the neutralisation capacity was still sufficient in 24 patients to have neutralised a standard 1.5-million unit dose of streptokinase. After 17 to 34 weeks titres were still high enough in 18 of 20 patients examined to neutralise at least half a standard dose.[1] As these results indicate, administration of standard doses of streptokinase within up to a year of a previous course may lead to reduced effect. Thus, the period in which it should not be repeated is usually between 5 days and 12 months post infarction (see Precautions, below). However, high titres of neutralising antibodies persisting for up to 7.5 years after administration of streptokinase have been reported.[2-4] Since readministration also increases the risk of hypersensitivity reactions, it has been suggested[2,5] that repeat courses should not be given within 4 or more years, and that if a repeat course is needed a non-antigenic thrombolytic such as alteplase or urokinase should be used until it is known whether or not high *in-vitro* titres affect efficacy. Increased titres of streptokinase-neutralising antibodies have also been measured in patients receiving topical streptokinase for wounds.[6]

Anistreplase also appears susceptible to neutralisation by streptokinase antibodies.[7]

Plasmacytosis,[8,9] serum-sickness,[8,10,11] rhabdomyolysis,[12] renal impairment (see Effects on the Kidneys, above), uveitis (see Effects on the Eyes, above), arthritis,[13] and anaphylaxis[14-17] have been reported in patients receiving streptokinase and are thought to represent hypersensitivity reactions, in some cases perhaps due to previous exposure to streptococcal antigens during infection. Back pain (see above) may also represent a hypersensitivity reaction. In some patients there may be a delay of between 1 and 10 days before appearance of the reaction.[18] The incidence of severe hypersensitivity reactions is probably fairly low, however; in the GISSI study anaphylaxis was reported in only 7 of 5860 patients although other hypersensitivity reactions leading to withdrawal of streptokinase were reported in 99 patients, with a further 42 such reactions after completion of the infusion.[15] Some episodes of apparent anaphylaxis seen with streptokinase administration may be fibrinolysin-mediated rather than antibody-antigen reactions. Administration of alteplase, which is considered non-antigenic, produced an anaphylactoid reaction in a patient who had a history of atopy.[19] Fibrinolysin, which activates complement cascade and the kinin system, is formed in quantity after the administration of a thrombolytic. In most patients these effects are clinically insignificant, but in those who are strongly atopic there is the possibility of precipitating an anaphylactoid reaction.


1. Jalihal S, Morris GK. Antistreptokinase titres after intravenous streptokinase. *Lancet* 1990; **335:** 184–5.
2. Elliott JM, *et al.* Neutralizing antibodies to streptokinase four years after intravenous thrombolytic therapy. *Am J Cardiol* 1993; **71:** 640–5.
3. Lee HS, *et al.* Raised levels of antistreptokinase antibody and neutralization titres from 4 days to 54 months after administration of streptokinase or anistreplase. *Eur Heart J* 1993; **14:** 84–9.
4. Squire IB, *et al.* Humoral and cellular immune responses up to 7.5 years after administration of streptokinase for acute myocardial infarction. *Eur Heart J* 1999; **20:** 1245–52.
5. Jennings K. Antibodies to streptokinase. *BMJ* 1996; **312:** 393–4.
6. Green C. Antistreptokinase titres after topical streptokinase. *Lancet* 1993; **341:** 1602–3.
7. Binette MJ, Agnone FA. Failure of APSAC thrombolysis. *Ann Intern Med* 1993; **119:** 637.
8. Straub PW, *et al.* Plasmozytose nach thrombolytischer Therapie mit Streptokinase. *Schweiz Med Wochenschr* 1974; **104:** 1891–2.

9. Chan NS, *et al.* Plasmacytosis and renal failure after readministration of streptokinase for threatened myocardial reinfarction. *BMJ* 1988; **297:** 717–18.
10. Payne ST, *et al.* Transient impairment of renal function after streptokinase therapy. *Lancet* 1989; **ii:** 1398.
11. Callan MFC, *et al.* Proteinuria and thrombolytic agents. *Lancet* 1990; **335:** 106.
12. Montgomery HE, *et al.* Rhabdomyolysis and multiple system organ failure with streptokinase. *BMJ* 1995; **311:** 1472.
13. Kelly MP, Bielawska C. Recurrence of a reactive arthritis following streptokinase therapy. *Postgrad Med J* 1991; **67:** 402.
14. McGrath KG, Patterson R. Anaphylactic reactivity to streptokinase. *JAMA* 1984; **252:** 1314–17.
15. Gruppo Italiano per lo Studio della Streptochinasi nell'Infarto Miocardico. Effectiveness of intravenous thrombolytic treatment in acute myocardial infarction. *Lancet* 1986; **i:** 397–401.
16. Bednarczyk EM, *et al.* Anaphylactic reaction to streptokinase with first exposure: case report and review of the literature. *DICP Ann Pharmacother* 1989; **23:** 869–72.
17. Tisdale JE, *et al.* Streptokinase-induced anaphylaxis. *DICP Ann Pharmacother* 1989; **23:** 984–7.
18. Seibert WJ, *et al.* Streptokinase morbidity—more common than previously recognised. *Aust N Z J Med* 1992; **22:** 129–33.
19. Purvis JA, *et al.* Anaphylactoid reaction after injection of alteplase. *Lancet* 1993; **341:** 966–7.

## Treatment of Adverse Effects

Allergic reactions may require treatment with antihistamines and corticosteroids, which have sometimes been given prophylactically. Anaphylaxis requires the administration of adrenaline (for further details, see Anaphylactic Shock, p.855).

Severe haemorrhage not controlled by local pressure requires discontinuation of the streptokinase infusion. Tranexamic acid, aminocaproic acid, or aprotinin may be of benefit. Packed red blood cells may be preferable to whole blood for replacement therapy; factor VIII preparations may also be given. Volume expansion may be necessary, but the use of dextrans should be avoided because of their platelet-inhibiting properties.

## Precautions

Streptokinase should be used with great care, if at all, in patients at increased risk of bleeding, or those in whom haemorrhage is likely to prove particularly dangerous. It should thus be avoided in patients with active internal bleeding or a recent history of peptic ulcer disease, oesophageal varices, ulcerative colitis or other bleeding gastrointestinal lesions, in patients with pancreatitis, in patients with subacute bacterial endocarditis, in patients with coagulation defects including those due to liver or kidney disease, or after recent surgery, childbirth, or trauma. It should not be given to patients at increased risk of cerebral bleeding including those with severe hypertension, haemorrhage or recent stroke, or to patients with cerebral neoplasm. It should not be given in pregnancy, particularly in the first 18 weeks because of the risk of placental separation and it has been suggested that it should not be used during heavy vaginal bleeding.

Invasive procedures, including intramuscular injections, should be avoided during, and immediately before and after, streptokinase therapy as they may increase the risk of bleeding; care should be taken when physically handling patients. Streptokinase should also be used with care in elderly patients. Patients with mitral stenosis associated with atrial fibrillation are more likely to have left heart thrombus which may lead to cerebral embolism following thrombolytic therapy. Although there is a theoretical risk of retinal bleeding in patients with diabetic retinopathy the benefits of treatment generally outweigh the risk.

Anti-streptokinase antibodies are formed following streptokinase use, with antibody titres rising abruptly after about 5 days. These antibodies may cause resistance or hypersensitivity to subsequent doses of streptokinase. Therefore, further doses of streptokinase should not be given in the period between 5 days and 12 months after the initial dose (even longer periods have been suggested, see Hypersensitivity, under Adverse Effects, above); if thrombolytic therapy is required in this period an alternative non-antigenic drug should be used. High titres of anti-streptokinase antibodies may also occur in patients following some streptococcal infections such as streptococcal pharyngitis or acute rheumatic fever or in those with acute glomerulonephritis secondary to streptococcal infections; in such patients there may be resistance to streptokinase or a reduced effect.

**Administration.** Overinfusion of streptokinase may occur if a drop-counting infusion pump is employed.[1] This arises as a result of flocculation of the streptokinase solution producing translucent fibres that affect the drop-forming mechanism so increasing the drop size.

For a comment on the incidence of flocculation in streptokinase solutions, see Stability, above.

1. Schad RF, Jennings RH. Overinfusions of streptokinase. *Am J Hosp Pharm* 1982; **39:** 1850.

**Aortic dissection.** A report of 4 cases of the inappropriate use of streptokinase in patients with aortic dissection misdiagnosed as myocardial infarction.[1] Thrombolytics are likely to extend aortic dissection and adversely affect the outcome. Of the 2 patients who died, one, who would have been suitable for early operation, died through the delay caused by impaired clotting. Although early intervention with thrombolytics may be of major benefit in acute myocardial infarction it is important that accurate differential diagnosis takes place to exclude conditions such as aortic dissection and prevent avoidable deaths.

For a report of fatal haemorrhage with streptokinase used in aortic dissection misdiagnosed as empyema, see Haemorrhage under Adverse Effects, above.

1. Butler J, *et al.* Streptokinase in acute aortic dissection. *BMJ* 1990; **300:** 517–19.

**Cardiopulmonary resuscitation.** Thrombolytics are not recommended after prolonged or traumatic cardiopulmonary resuscitation because of the risk of haemorrhage. However, studies[1,2] in patients who received cardiopulmonary resuscitation for cardiac arrest associated with acute myocardial infarction have suggested that thrombolytics are generally safe and that any increase in bleeding complications is outweighed by the benefits of thrombolysis.

1. Cross SJ, *et al.* Safety of thrombolysis in association with cardiopulmonary resuscitation. *BMJ* 1991; **303:** 1242.
2. Kurkciyan I, *et al.* Major bleeding complications after cardiopulmonary resuscitation: impact of thrombolytic treatment. *J Intern Med* 2003; **253:** 128–35.

**Pregnancy.** Thrombolytics are generally contra-indicated in pregnancy, although there are a few reports of their use which have been briefly reviewed.[1] In most cases, thrombolytics were given at 28 weeks of pregnancy or later to patients with deep-vein thrombosis, pulmonary embolism, or prosthetic valve thrombosis. There were some reports of favourable maternal and fetal outcomes although therapy was associated with maternal haemorrhage, including spontaneous abortion and minor vaginal bleeding, especially when given near the time of delivery. There was one report of placental abruption with fetal death.

1. Roth A, Elkayam U. Acute myocardial infarction associated with pregnancy. *Ann Intern Med* 1996; **125:** 751–62.

## Interactions

Oral anticoagulants, heparin, and antiplatelet drugs such as aspirin are often used with streptokinase, but may increase the risk of haemorrhage. The risk may also be increased with dextrans, and with other drugs that affect coagulation or platelet function.

◊ References.

1. Harder S, Klinkhardt U. Thrombolytics: drug interactions of clinical significance. *Drug Safety* 2000; **23:** 391–9.

## Pharmacokinetics

Streptokinase is rapidly cleared from the circulation following intravenous administration. Clearance is biphasic with the initial and more rapid phase being due to specific antibodies. A half-life of 23 minutes has been reported for the streptokinase-activator complex.

◊ References.

1. Grierson DS, Bjornsson TD. Pharmacokinetics of streptokinase in patients based on amidolytic activator complex activity. *Clin Pharmacol Ther* 1987; **41:** 304–13.
2. Gemmill JD, *et al.* A comparison of the pharmacokinetic properties of streptokinase and anistreplase in acute myocardial infarction. *Br J Clin Pharmacol* 1991; **31:** 143–7.

## Uses and Administration

Streptokinase is a thrombolytic drug derived from various streptococci. It rapidly activates endogenous plasminogen, indirectly by means of a streptokinase-plasminogen complex, to plasmin (see Fibrinolysin, p.916), which has fibrinolytic effects and can dissolve intravascular blood clots. The mechanisms of fibrinolysis are discussed further under Haemostasis and Fibrinolysis on p.735. Streptokinase affects circulating, unbound plasminogen as well as fibrin-bound plasminogen and thus may be termed a fibrin-nonspecific thrombolytic (see p.812).

Streptokinase is given by intravenous or sometimes intra-arterial infusion in the treatment of thromboembolic disorders such as myocardial infarction (p.828), peripheral arterial thromboembolism (below), and venous thromboembolism (deep-vein thrombosis and pulmonary embolism) (p.839). It has also been tried in ischaemic stroke (p.836), but this use is less well-established. Streptokinase may be used to clear cannulas and shunts and is used topically in conjunction with streptodornase to clear clots and purulent matter.

In acute **myocardial infarction** streptokinase is usually given intravenously as a single dose of 1.5 million units infused over 1 hour as soon as possible after the onset of symptoms. Streptokinase has also been given in a suitable dose by intracoronary infusion but coronary catheterisation with the aid of angiography is required, thus restricting administration to suitably equipped centres.

In the treatment of **pulmonary embolism** and other **arteriovenous occlusions** an initial loading dose of streptokinase, normally 250 000 units infused intravenously over 30 minutes, is given to overcome any resistance due to circulating antibodies. This is followed by infusion of a maintenance dose of 100 000 units/hour for 24 to 72 hours, depending on the condition to be treated; for central retinal thrombosis, 12 hours may be adequate. Treatment should be controlled by monitoring the thrombin clotting time, which should be maintained at 2 to 4 times normal values. Since thrombolytic activity rapidly fades when the infusion stops, streptokinase treatment is generally followed after 3 to 4 hours by intravenous heparin infusion, and then oral anticoagulation, to prevent re-occlusion.

Streptokinase, as a solution containing 250 000 units in 2 mL is used to clear occluded cannulas; 1000 units/mL, has been used to clear shunts of occluding thrombi.

◊ General references.

1. Fears R. Biochemical pharmacology and therapeutic aspects of thrombolytic agents. *Pharmacol Rev* 1990; **42:** 201–21.
2. Stringer KA. Beyond thrombolysis: other effects of thrombolytic drugs. *Ann Pharmacother* 1994; **28:** 752–6.
3. Ludlam CA, *et al.* Guidelines for the use of thrombolytic therapy. *Blood Coag Fibrinol* 1995; **6:** 273–85.

**Administration in children.** There are limited data on the use of systemic thrombolytic therapy for arterial or venous thromboembolism in children and various dosage regimens have been used, based on case studies. The most widely used drugs are streptokinase and alteplase. For streptokinase, the Sixth American College of Chest Physicians (ACCP) Consensus Conference on Antithrombotic Therapy[1] suggests a loading dose of 2000 units/kg to be given intravenously, followed by continuous infusion of 2000 units/kg per hour for 6 to 12 hours. In the UK, the Royal College of Paediatrics and Child Health (RCPCH) suggests a loading dose of 2500 to 4000 units/kg over 30 minutes, followed by infusion of 500 to 1000 units/kg per hour, continued until reperfusion occurs, up to a maximum of 3 days. The UK manufacturer states that the initial dose should be estimated by means of the streptokinase resistance test, and recommends a maintenance dose of 20 units per mL of blood volume per hour.

Alteplase may be preferred because of its fibrin specificity and low immunogenicity. The dose of alteplase suggested by the ACCP is 100 to 600 micrograms/kg per hour by continuous intravenous infusion over 6 hours, while the dose recommended by the RCPCH is 500 micrograms/kg per hour for no more than 3 hours. The use of alteplase to clear occluded catheters in children is discussed on p.857.

1. Monagle P, *et al.* Antithrombotic therapy in children. *Chest* 2001; **119** (suppl): 344S–370S.

**Empyema and pleural effusion.** Thoracic empyema is treated with antibacterials and pleural drainage. Efficient removal of fluid may be impaired by fibrinous clots within the pleural cavity. Intrapleural instillation of streptokinase (100 000 to 750 000 units in up to 100 mL of sodium chloride 0.9%) has been reported to be effective in small series of patients.[1-4] There have also been reports of the successful use of alteplase[5,6] and urokinase.[4,7] Intrapleural streptokinase has also been used successfully in a few patients with malignant multiloculated pleural effusion resistant to standard pleural drainage.[8]

Intrapericardial instillation of thrombolytics has been tried in a few patients with pericardial empyema to prevent the development of constrictive pericarditis.[9,10]

For reports of haemorrhage associated with intrapleural use of streptokinase, see Haemorrhage, under Adverse Effects, above.

1. Temes RT, *et al.* Intrapleural fibrinolytics in management of empyema thoracis. *Chest* 1996; **110:** 102–6.
2. Bouros D, *et al.* Role of streptokinase in the treatment of acute loculated parapneumonic pleural effusions and empyema. *Thorax* 1994; **49:** 852–5.
3. Davies RJO, *et al.* Randomised controlled trial of intrapleural streptokinase in community acquired pleural infection. *Thorax* 1997; **52:** 416–21.
4. Bouros D, *et al.* Intrapleural streptokinase versus urokinase in the treatment of complicated parapneumonic effusions: a prospective, double-blind study. *Am J Respir Crit Care Med* 1997; **155:** 291–5.

5. Bishop NB, *et al.* Alteplase in the treatment of complicated parapneumonic effusion: a case report. Abstract: *Pediatrics* 2003; **111:** 423. Full version: http://pediatrics.aappublications.org/cgi/reprint/111/2/e188 (accessed 16/06/04)
6. Walker CA, *et al.* Intrapleural alteplase in a patient with complicated pleural effusion. *Ann Pharmacother* 2003; **37:** 376–9.
7. Thomson AH, *et al.* Randomised trial of intrapleural urokinase in the treatment of childhood empyema. *Thorax* 2002; **57:** 343–7.
8. Davies CWH, *et al.* Intrapleural streptokinase in the management of malignant multiloculated pleural effusions. *Chest* 1999; **115:** 729–33.
9. Winkler W-B, *et al.* Treatment of exudative fibrinous pericarditis with intrapericardial urokinase. *Lancet* 1994; **344:** 1541–2.
10. Juneja R, *et al.* Intrapericardial streptokinase in purulent pericarditis. *Arch Dis Child* 1999; **80:** 275–7.

**Ischaemic heart disease.** Thrombolytics such as alteplase, streptokinase, and urokinase have an established role in the early management of acute myocardial infarction (p.828). Myocardial infarction is caused by coronary artery occlusion, usually due to thrombosis, and thrombolytics are given intravenously to break up the thrombus or clot and restore the patency of the coronary artery, thereby limiting infarct size and irreversible damage to the myocardium. Reduction of ECG abnormalities and modification of ventricular remodelling may also contribute to their effect. Other antithrombotics, in particular aspirin and heparin, are given as adjunctive therapy.

Several large studies have established that thrombolytics can preserve left ventricular function and improve short-term and 1-year mortality figures;[1,2] benefit has been maintained in 5-year[3] and 10-year[4,5] follow-up studies. Benefit is greatest with early treatment. Trials such as the GISSI-1 study[6] and the ISIS-2 study[7] helped to establish that mortality is reduced if thrombolytics are given within 6 hours of the onset of symptoms[8] and further studies provided evidence[9,10] that patients presenting within 12 hours should receive a thrombolytic. Use after 12 hours has been associated with an increase in adverse effects,[8] and is usually reserved for patients with evidence of ongoing ischaemia. Prehospital thrombolysis is feasible and reduces the time to thrombolytic administration and short-term mortality.[11] Five-year follow-up of one study[12] has suggested that there is also a beneficial effect on long-term mortality.

Choice of thrombolytic depends on factors such as cost, method of administration, and contra-indications. Although streptokinase has been the most widely used, several large studies have compared clinical benefit in terms of improved left ventricular function and mortality and have shown no difference between streptokinase and other thrombolytics, including saruplase,[13] the tissue plasminogen activator alteplase,[14] anistreplase,[15] and reteplase[16] in overall efficacy. In the GUSTO-I study,[17] accelerated or 'front loaded' alteplase (that is, rapid intravenous administration over 1½ hours rather than the conventional 3 hours) was more effective than streptokinase, although the study was criticised for not comparing like with like. On the other hand, alteplase might be associated with a greater risk of stroke than streptokinase.[18] Studies comparing bolus injections of reteplase with accelerated alteplase (GUSTO-III)[19] and tenecteplase with alteplase (ASSENT-2)[20] have also found no difference in mortality rate.

The overall effectiveness of thrombolytics is limited by persistent coronary occlusion, re-occlusion, and bleeding complications. Different thrombolytic administration regimens, such as bolus injections of reteplase, and combinations of thrombolytics, for example alteplase with streptokinase and alteplase with saruplase, have been investigated in attempts to improve patency rates. However, there has been concern that adverse effects may be higher with bolus administration. A study[21] comparing double-bolus administration of alteplase with accelerated alteplase was terminated early when excess deaths were found in the group receiving bolus injections, and a subsequent meta-analysis[22] found a higher incidence of intracranial haemorrhage associated with bolus administration of various thrombolytics.

Thrombolytics have also been tried in other acute coronary syndromes, including unstable angina and non-ST elevation myocardial infarction (p.813). Although small-scale studies reported some benefit the results were variable, and an overview[8] of trials in patients with suspected myocardial infarction, which included some patients with unstable angina, found that there was no mortality benefit in patients without ST elevation. In 2 studies that investigated alteplase (the TIMI-IIIB study[23] with 1473 patients) and anistreplase (the UNASEM study[24] involving 159 patients), thrombolysis failed to improve outcome and was associated with an excess of bleeding complications. Thrombolytic therapy is therefore not recommended for patients with unstable angina or non-ST elevation myocardial infarction.

1. Gruppo Italiano per lo Studio della Streptochinasi nell'Infarto Miocardico (GISSI). Long-term effects of intravenous thrombolysis in acute myocardial infarction: final report of the GISSI study. *Lancet* 1987; **ii:** 871–4.
2. Wilcox RG, *et al.* Effects of alteplase in acute myocardial infarction: 6-month results from the ASSET study. *Lancet* 1990; **335:** 1175–8.
3. Simoons ML, *et al.* Long-term benefit of early thrombolytic therapy in patients with acute myocardial infarction: 5 year follow-up of a trial conducted by the Interuniversity Cardiology Institute of the Netherlands. *J Am Coll Cardiol* 1989; **14:** 1609–15.
4. Baigent C, *et al.* ISIS-2: 10 year survival among patients with suspected acute myocardial infarction in randomised comparison of intravenous streptokinase, oral aspirin, both, or neither. *BMJ* 1998; **316:** 1337–43.
5. Franzosi MG, *et al.* Ten-year follow-up of the first megatrial testing thrombolytic therapy in patients with acute myocardial infarction: results of the Gruppo Italiano per lo Studio della Sopravvivenza nell'Infarto-1 Study. *Circulation* 1998; **98:** 2659–65.
6. Gruppo Italiano per lo Studio della Streptochinasi nell'Infarto Miocardico (GISSI). Effectiveness of intravenous thrombolytic treatment in acute myocardial infarction. *Lancet* 1986; **i:** 397–402.
7. Second International Study of Infarct Survival Collaborative Group. Randomised trial of intravenous streptokinase, oral aspirin, both, or neither among 17 187 cases of suspected acute myocardial infarction: ISIS-2. *Lancet* 1988; **ii:** 349–60.
8. Fibrinolytic Therapy Trialists' (FTT) Collaborative Group. Indications for fibrinolytic therapy in suspected acute myocardial infarction: collaborative overview of early mortality and major morbidity results from all randomised trials of more than 1000 patients. *Lancet* 1994; **343:** 311–22.
9. LATE Study Group. Late assessment of thrombolytic efficacy (LATE) study with alteplase 6–24 hours after onset of acute myocardial infarction. *Lancet* 1993; **342:** 759–66.
10. EMERAS (Estudio Multicéntrico Estreptoquinasa Repúblicas de América del Sur) Collaborative Group. Randomised trial of late thrombolysis in patients with suspected acute myocardial infarction. *Lancet* 1993; **342:** 767–72.
11. Morrison LJ, *et al.* Mortality and prehospital thrombolysis for acute myocardial infarction: a meta-analysis. *JAMA* 2000; **283:** 2686–92.
12. Rawles JM. Quantification of the benefit of earlier thrombolytic therapy: five-year results of the Grampian Region Early Anistreplase Trial (GREAT). *J Am Coll Cardiol* 1997; **30:** 1181–6.
13. PRIMI Trial Study Group. Randomised double-blind trial of recombinant pro-urokinase against streptokinase in acute myocardial infarction. *Lancet* 1989; **i:** 863–8.
14. GISSI-2 and International Study Group. Six-month survival in 20 891 patients with acute myocardial infarction randomized between alteplase and streptokinase with or without heparin. *Eur Heart J* 1992; **13:** 1692–7.
15. Third International Study of Infarct Survival Collaborative Group. ISIS-3: a randomised comparison of streptokinase vs tissue plasminogen activator vs anistreplase and of aspirin plus heparin vs aspirin alone among 41 299 cases of suspected acute myocardial infarction. *Lancet* 1992; **339:** 753–70.
16. International Joint Efficacy Comparison of Thrombolytics. Randomised, double-blind comparison of reteplase double-bolus administration with streptokinase in acute myocardial infarction (INJECT): trial to investigate equivalence. *Lancet* 1995; **346:** 329–36.
17. The GUSTO Investigators. An international randomized trial comparing four thrombolytic strategies for acute myocardial infarction. *N Engl J Med* 1993; **329:** 673–82.
18. Vaitkus PT, *et al.* Stroke complicating acute myocardial infarction: a meta-analysis of risk modification by anticoagulation and thrombolytic therapy. *Arch Intern Med* 1992; **152:** 2020–4.
19. The Global Use of Strategies to Open Occluded Coronary Arteries (GUSTO III) Investigators. A comparison of reteplase with alteplase for acute myocardial infarction. *N Engl J Med* 1997; **337:** 1118–23.
20. Assessment of the Safety and Efficacy of a New Thrombolytic (ASSENT-2) Investigators. Single-bolus tenecteplase compared with front-loaded alteplase in acute myocardial infarction: the ASSENT-2 double-blind randomised trial. *Lancet* 1999; **354:** 716–22.
21. The Continuous Infusion versus Double-Bolus Administration of Alteplase (COBALT) Investigators. A comparison of continuous infusion of alteplase with double-bolus administration for acute myocardial infarction. *N Engl J Med* 1997; **337:** 1124–30.
22. Mehta SR, *et al.* Risk of intracranial haemorrhage with bolus versus infusion thrombolytic therapy: a meta-analysis. *Lancet* 2000; **356:** 449–54.
23. The TIMI IIIB Investigators. Effects of tissue plasminogen activator and a comparison of early invasive and conservative strategies in unstable angina and non-Q-wave myocardial infarction: results of the TIMI IIIB trial. *Circulation* 1994; **89:** 1545–56.
24. Bär FW, *et al.* Thrombolysis in patients with unstable angina improves the angiographic but not the clinical outcome: results of UNASEM, a multicenter, randomized, placebo-controlled, clinical trial with anistreplase. *Circulation* 1992; **86:** 131–7.

**Intracardiac thrombosis.** In a study[1] of patients with left-sided prosthetic valve thrombosis, thrombolytic therapy was found to be more successful than surgery, especially in those who were critically ill. Streptokinase was the thrombolytic usually employed.

1. Lengyel M, Vándor L. The role of thrombolysis in the management of left-sided prosthetic valve thrombosis: a study of 85 cases diagnosed by transesophageal echocardiography. *J Heart Valve Dis* 2001; **10:** 636–49.

**Peripheral arterial thromboembolism.** Thrombolytics including streptokinase may be used in the management of peripheral arterial thromboembolism (p.830). Streptokinase has been injected intravenously or intra-arterially directly into the clot as an alternative to surgical treatment of the occlusion. It has also been infused intra-arterially to remove distal clots during surgery. The *intravenous* dose generally used is 250 000 units over 30 minutes followed by 100 000 units/hour. A lower dose of 5000 units/hour has been used *intra-arterially* directly into the clot[1] and for removal of distal clots during surgery streptokinase has been given intra-arterially in a dose of 100 000 units over 30 minutes or as five bolus doses of 20 000 units at 5-minute intervals.[2]

1. Anonymous. Non-coronary thrombolysis. *Lancet* 1990; **335:** 691–3.
2. Earnshaw JJ, Beard JD. Intraoperative use of thrombolytic agents. *BMJ* 1993; **307:** 638–9.

**Stroke.** Stroke is normally considered a contra-indication to the use of thrombolytics, and clearly they would be inappropriate in acute haemorrhagic stroke. However, when stroke is associated with thrombotic occlusion there is evidence, as with myocardial infarction, that a degree of neuronal recovery is possible if the occlusion is reversed sufficiently quickly, and thrombolytics may therefore have a role in some patients with acute ischaemic stroke.

Early studies with intravenous thrombolytics in acute *ischaemic stroke* suggested a reduction in early death, although subsequent randomised trials produced disappointing results, with the exception of one with alteplase given within 3 hours of the onset of stroke (NINDS—National Institute of Neurological Disorders and Stroke rt-PA Stroke Trial).[1] The studies using streptokinase—MAST-E (Multicentre Acute Stroke Trial-Europe),[2] ASK (Australian Streptokinase Trial),[3] and MAST-I (Multicentre Acute Stroke Trial-Italy)[4,5]—were terminated before completion because of adverse outcomes (intracranial bleeding and increased mortality) in the treatment groups, particularly in those receiving therapy more than 3 hours after stroke onset.[3] The study investigating alteplase given within 6 hours of the onset of symptoms (ECASS I—European Cooperative Acute Stroke Study)[6] reported that, although some patients might benefit, overall alteplase was associated with higher mortality rates and an increase in some intracranial bleeding (parenchymal haemorrhage). In the NINDS randomised study,[1] alteplase given within 3 hours of the onset of ischaemic stroke appeared to improve clinical outcome despite an increased incidence of symptomatic intracerebral haemorrhage. Patients treated with alteplase were more likely to have minimal or no disability 3 months following stroke,[1] and this benefit was maintained at 12 months.[7] However, there was no difference in mortality or rate of recurrence of stroke. A second ECASS study (ECASS II)[8] that hoped to confirm the early findings of the NINDS study failed to confirm a statistical benefit for alteplase over placebo and found no significant differences between patients who received alteplase within 3 hours or between 3 and 6 hours.

On the basis of the NINDS study, alteplase given within 3 hours of the onset of ischaemic stroke is now recommended for selected patients in most guidelines on stroke management.[9-12] Despite their own disappointing results, the ECASS II investigators reached a similar conclusion. However, these recommendations have been criticised.[13,14] It has been pointed out[15,16] that very few patients will be eligible for treatment with alteplase, since the time of onset of symptoms is often uncertain and in many patients more than 3 hours elapses before a definite diagnosis of ischaemic stroke is made. In addition, the NINDS study[1] excluded patients with severe stroke and those taking anticoagulants. The rationale for exclusion of patients with severe stroke is that haemorrhagic transformation is more likely to occur with large areas of infarction.[15] However, size of infarct is difficult to identify by CT scanning.[15] Anticoagulants or antiplatelets are also contra-indicated in the first 24 hours after administration of alteplase. The poor results obtained in studies using streptokinase have led to recommendations that streptokinase should be avoided in ischaemic stroke,[9,10] although an overview of thrombolytic studies[16] suggested that it may not be worse than alteplase and that the apparent hazards of streptokinase may be accounted for by differences in trial design (for example concomitant use of anticoagulants) and in patient population. Thus, while alteplase can be considered for those few patients meeting the entry criteria for the NINDS study, a systematic review[17] concluded that further large studies are required to establish more clearly the overall role of thrombolytics in acute ischaemic stroke. Studies of the use of alteplase outside the setting of a clinical trial have had mixed results.[18,19]

Intra-arterial administration of thrombolytics may have advantages over intravenous use and may be used in selected patients.[12] A study[20] with nasaruplase suggested that it was beneficial up to 6 hours after stroke due to middle cerebral artery occlusion, and use of intra-arterial thrombolytics may therefore be considered in such patients.[10] Intra-arterial urokinase and alteplase have been tried in basilar artery occlusion, but their use is not yet established.[9,21]

Intravenous thrombolytics have no role in the management of acute *haemorrhagic stroke*, but local administration has been used to facilitate the aspiration of haematomas in both intracerebral[22] and subarachnoid haemorrhage. Small studies with urokinase have shown benefit in patients with intraventricular haemorrhage.

1. The National Institute of Neurological Disorders and Stroke rt-PA Stroke Study Group. Tissue plasminogen activator for acute ischemic stroke. *N Engl J Med* 1995; **333:** 1581–7.
2. The Multicenter Acute Stroke Trial—Europe Study Group. Thrombolytic therapy with streptokinase in acute ischemic stroke. *N Engl J Med* 1996; **335:** 145–50.
3. Donnan GA, *et al.* Streptokinase for acute ischemic stroke with relationship to time of administration. *JAMA* 1996; **276:** 961–6.
4. Multicentre Acute Stroke Trial - Italy (MAST-I) Group. Randomised controlled trial of streptokinase, aspirin, and combination of both in treatment of acute ischaemic stroke. *Lancet* 1995; **346:** 1509–14.
5. Tognoni G, Roncaglioni MC. Dissent: an alternative interpretation of MAST-I. *Lancet* 1995; **346:** 1515.
6. Hacke W, *et al.* Intravenous thrombolysis with recombinant tissue plasminogen activator for acute hemispheric stroke: the European Cooperative Acute Stroke Study (ECASS). *JAMA* 1995; **274:** 1017–25.
7. Kwiatowski TG, *et al.* Effects of tissue plasminogen activator for acute ischemic stroke at one year. *N Engl J Med* 1999; **340:** 1781–7.
8. Hacke W, *et al.* Randomised double-blind placebo-controlled trial of thrombolytic therapy with intravenous alteplase in acute ischaemic stroke (ECASS II). *Lancet* 1998; **352:** 1245–51.
9. The European Stroke Initiative Executive Committee and the EUSI Writing Committee. European Stroke Initiative recommendations for stroke management – update 2003. *Cerebrovasc Dis* 2003; **16:** 311–37.
10. Adams HP, *et al.* Guidelines for the early management of patients with acute ischaemic stroke: a scientific statement from the Stroke Council of the American Stroke Association. *Stroke*

2003; **34:** 1056–83. Also available at: http://stroke.ahajournals.org/cgi/reprint/34/4/1056.pdf (accessed 06/07/04)
11. The American Heart Association in collaboration with the International Committee on Resuscitation (ILCOR). International guidelines 2000 for cardiopulmonary resuscitation and emergency cardiovascular care: a consensus on science. Part 7: the era of reperfusion. Section 2: acute stroke. *Circulation* 2000; **102** (suppl I): I204–I216. Also published in *Resuscitation* 2000; **46:** 239–52.
12. Albers GW, *et al.* Antithrombotic and thrombolytic therapy for ischemic stroke. *Chest* 2001; **119** (suppl): 300S–320S.
13. Caplan LR. Stroke thrombolysis—growing pains. *Mayo Clin Proc* 1997; **72:** 1090–2.
14. Caplan LR, *et al.* Should thrombolytic therapy be the first-line treatment for acute ischemic stroke? Thrombolysis—not a panacea for ischemic stroke. *N Engl J Med* 1997; **337:** 1309–10.
15. Muir KW. Thrombolysis for stroke: pushed out of the window? *Br J Clin Pharmacol* 1996; **42:** 681–2.
16. Wardlaw JM, *et al.* Systematic review of evidence on thrombolytic therapy for acute ischaemic stroke. *Lancet* 1997; **350:** 607–14.
17. Wardlaw JM, *et al.* Thrombolysis for acute ischaemic stroke. Available in The Cochrane Library; Issue 2. Chichester: John Wiley; 2004.
18. Albers GW, *et al.* Intravenous tissue-type plasminogen activator for treatment of acute stroke: the Standard Treatment with Alteplase to Reverse Stroke (STARS) Study. *JAMA* 2000; **283:** 1145–50.
19. Katzan IL, *et al.* Use of tissue-type plasminogen activator for acute ischemic stroke: the Cleveland area experience. *JAMA* 2000; **283:** 1151–8.
20. Furlan A, *et al.* Intra-arterial prourokinase for acute ischemic stroke. The PROACT II study: a randomized controlled trial. *JAMA* 1999; **282:** 2003–11.
21. Wijdicks EFM, *et al.* Intra-arterial thrombolysis in acute basilar artery thromboembolism: the initial Mayo Clinic experience. *Mayo Clin Proc* 1997; **72:** 1005–13.
22. Broderick JP, *et al.* Guidelines for the management of spontaneous intracerebral hemorrhage: a statement for healthcare professionals from a special writing group of the Stroke Council, American Heart Association. *Stroke* 1999; **30:** 905–15. Also available at: http://stroke.ahajournals.org/cgi/reprint/30/4/905.pdf (accessed 06/07/04)

### Preparations

***BP 2003:*** Streptokinase Injection.

**Proprietary Preparations** (details are given in Part 3)
***Austral.:*** Kabikinase†; Streptase; ***Austria:*** Kabikinase; Streptase; ***Belg.:*** Kabikinase†; Streptase†; ***Braz.:*** Kabikinase; Streptase; Streptonase; Unitinase; ***Canad.:*** Kabikinase†; Streptase; ***Chile:*** Streptase; ***Denm.:*** Kabikinase†; Streptase; ***Fin.:*** Kabikinase†; Streptase; ***Fr.:*** Kabikinase†; Streptase; ***Ger.:*** Kabikinase†; Streptase; ***Gr.:*** Streptase; ***Hong Kong:*** Kabikinase†; Streptase; ***India:*** Streptase; Zykinase; ***Irl.:*** Kabikinase†; Streptase; ***Israel:*** Kabikinase; Streptase; ***Ital.:*** Streptase; ***Malaysia:*** Streptase; ***Mex.:*** Kabikinase†; Streptase; ***Neth.:*** Kabikinase†; Streptase; ***Norw.:*** Kabikinase; Streptase; ***NZ:*** Kabikinase†; Streptase; ***Port.:*** Kabikinase†; Streptase; ***S.Afr.:*** Kabikinase†; Streptase; ***Singapore:*** Kabikinase†; Streptase†; ***Spain:*** Kabikinase; Streptase; ***Swed.:*** Kabikinase†; Streptase; ***Switz.:*** Kabikinase†; Streptase; ***Thai.:*** Kabikinase†; Streptase; ***UK:*** Kabikinase†; Streptase; ***USA:*** Kabikinase†; Streptase.

**Multi-ingredient:** ***Arg.:*** Varidasa; ***Austral.:*** Varidase; ***Austria:*** Varidase; ***Belg.:*** Varidase†; ***Denm.:*** Varidase; ***Fin.:*** Varidase; ***Ger.:*** Varidase; ***Irl.:*** Varidase; ***Israel:*** Varidase†; ***Ital.:*** Varidase; ***Mex.:*** Varidasa; ***Neth.:*** Varidase†; ***Norw.:*** Varidase†; ***NZ:*** Varidase†; ***Port.:*** Varidasa; ***S.Afr.:*** Varidase†; ***Spain:*** Ernodasa; Varibiotic†; Varidasa; ***Swed.:*** Varidase; ***UK:*** Varidase.

## Strophanthin-K

Estrofantina; Kombé Strophanthin; Strophanthin; Strophanthoside-K.
*CAS — 11005-63-3.*

NOTE. Do not confuse with K-strophanthin-α which is Cymarin.

**Pharmacopoeias.** In *Chin.*

### Profile

Strophanthin-K is a cardiac glycoside or a mixture of cardiac glycosides from strophanthus, the seeds of *Strophanthus kombe* (Apocynaceae) or other spp., adjusted by admixture with a suitable diluent such as lactose so as generally to possess 40% of the activity of anhydrous ouabain.

Strophanthin-K is a positive inotrope with general properties similar to those of digoxin (p.895). It is poorly absorbed from the gastrointestinal tract but may be given intravenously in doses of 125 to 500 micrograms daily in the management of heart failure (p.820).

### Preparations

**Proprietary Preparations** (details are given in Part 3)
***Austria:*** Laevostrophan†; ***Ger.:*** Kombetin†; ***Ital.:*** Kombetin†.

**Multi-ingredient:** ***Austria:*** Laevostrophan compositum†.

## Suleparoid *(rINNM)*

Heparan Sulfate; Heparan Sulphate; Heparitin Sulfate; Suleparoide.
*CAS — 9050-30-0 (suleparoid).*

## Suleparoid Sodium *(rINN)*

Heparan Sulfate Sodium; Sodium Heparitin Sulphate.
*CAS — 57459-72-0.*

### Profile

Suleparoid is a naturally occurring glycosaminoglycan given orally in the management of thromboembolic disorders; it is also used topically. Suleparoid sodium is a component of danaparoid sodium (p.891).

### Preparations

**Proprietary Preparations** (details are given in Part 3)
***Ital.:*** Aremin; Arteven; Clarema; Hemovasal; Iparen†; Leparan; Spatix; Tavidan; Tromir†; Tronan†; Vas; Vasorema; Vepar†.

**Multi-ingredient:** ***Ital.:*** Osmogel.

## Sulodexide *(rINN)*

KRX-101; Sulodexida. Glucurono-2-amino-2-deoxyglucoglucan sulphate.
*CAS — 57821-29-1.*
*ATC — B01AB11.*

### Profile

Sulodexide is a heparinoid consisting of a mixture of low-molecular-weight heparin and dermatan sulfate. It is used as a hypolipidaemic and antithrombotic and has been given orally and parenterally for peripheral vascular disease and cerebrovascular disease. It is also included in preparations used topically for local vascular inflammation and soft-tissue disorders. Sulodexide is also under investigation for the treatment of diabetic nephropathy.

◊ References.

1. Ofosu FA. Pharmacological actions of sulodexide. *Semin Thromb Hemost* 1998; **24:** 127–38.

### Preparations

**Proprietary Preparations** (details are given in Part 3)
***Braz.:*** Aterina†; ***Ital.:*** Clarens; Vessel Due F; ***Malaysia:*** Vessel Due F; ***Spain:*** Aterina; Luzone.

**Multi-ingredient:** ***Ital.:*** Dermoangiopan; Vessiflex.

## Talinolol *(rINN)*

(±)-1-{*p*-[3-(*tert*-Butylamino)-2-hydroxypropoxy]phenyl}-3-cyclohexylurea.
$C_{20}H_{33}N_3O_3$ = 363.5.
*CAS — 57460-41-0.*
*ATC — C07AB13.*

### Profile

Talinolol is a cardioselective beta blocker (p.868). It is given by mouth in the management of hypertension (p.825) and other cardiovascular disorders, in doses of up to 300 mg daily. It may also be given intravenously.

### Preparations

**Proprietary Preparations** (details are given in Part 3)
***Ger.:*** Cordanum.

# Tamsulosin Hydrochloride

*(BANM, USAN, rINNM)*

Amsulosin Hydrochloride; Hidrocloruro de tamsulosina; LY-253351; YM-617; R-(−)-YM-12617; YM-12617-1. (−)-(R)-5-(2-{[2-(*o*-Ethoxyphenoxy)ethyl]amino}-propyl)-2-methoxybenzenesulfonamide hydrochloride.
$C_{20}H_{28}N_2O_5S,HCl$ = 445.0.
*CAS — 106133-20-4 (tamsulosin); 106463-17-6 (tamsulosin hydrochloride).*
*ATC — G04CA02.*

## Adverse Effects, Treatment, and Precautions

As for Prazosin Hydrochloride, p.985. Because tamsulosin is selective for $\alpha_1$ receptors in the prostate the vasodilator effects may be less frequent. Tamsulosin may cause ejaculation abnormalities. It should be avoided in severe hepatic impairment.

## Interactions

As for Prazosin Hydrochloride, p.985.

## Pharmacokinetics

Tamsulosin is absorbed from the gastrointestinal tract and is almost completely bioavailable. The extent and rate of absorption are reduced by food. Following oral administration of an immediate-release preparation, peak plasma concentrations occur about 1 hour after a dose. Tamsulosin is about 99% bound to plasma proteins. It is metabolised slowly in the liver primarily by the cytochrome P450 isoenzymes CYP2D6 and CYP3A4; it is excreted mainly in the urine as metabolites and some unchanged drug. The plasma elimination half-life has been reported to be between 4 and 5.5 hours.

Some of the pharmacokinetic values cited above may be altered when tamsulosin is given as a modified-release preparation, the form in which it is usually used; for instance, peak plasma concentrations occur about 6 hours after a dose and the apparent elimination half-life may be 10 to 13 hours.

**Renal impairment.** Plasma-tamsulosin concentrations were reported to be increased in patients with renal impairment when compared with subjects with normal renal function.[1,2] However, plasma concentrations of unbound, pharmacologically active drug were similar in both groups and it was suggested that the raised total plasma concentrations were due to an increase in plasma protein binding.

1. Koiso K, *et al.* Pharmacokinetics of tamsulosin hydrochloride in patients with renal impairment: effects of $\alpha_1$-acid glycoprotein. *J Clin Pharmacol* 1996; **36:** 1029–38.
2. Wolzt M, *et al.* Pharmacokinetics of tamsulosin in subjects with normal and varying degrees of impaired renal function: an open-label single-dose and multiple-dose study. *Eur J Clin Pharmacol* 1998; **54:** 367–73.

## Uses and Administration

Tamsulosin is an alpha$_1$-adrenoceptor blocker (p.809) with actions similar to those of prazosin (p.986); it is reported to be more selective for the alpha$_{1A}$-adrenoceptor subtype, which accounts for approximately 70% of the $\alpha_1$ adrenoceptors in the prostate.. It is used in benign prostatic hyperplasia (p.1555) to relieve symptoms of urinary obstruction.

Tamsulosin is given by mouth as the hydrochloride. In benign prostatic hyperplasia it is administered in a modified-release formulation, in a dose of 400 micrograms once daily, after food at the same time each day. The US manufacturer states that the dose may be increased after 2 to 4 weeks, if necessary, to 800 micrograms once daily.

◊ Reviews.

1. Wilde MI, McTavish D. Tamsulosin: a review of its pharmacological properties and therapeutic potential in the management of symptomatic benign prostatic hyperplasia. *Drugs* 1996; **52:** 883–98.
2. Lee M. Tamsulosin for the treatment of benign prostatic hypertrophy. *Ann Pharmacother* 2000; **34:** 188–99.
3. Lyseng-Williamson KA, *et al.* Tamsulosin: an update of its role in the management of lower urinary tract symptoms. *Drugs* 2002; **62:** 135–67.

**Antidepressant-induced genito-urinary disorders.** Tamsulosin was used successfully[1] to treat urinary hesitancy observed in 6 male patients receiving reboxetine. Painful ejaculation associated with reboxetine was also treated successfully[2] in 2 men.

1. Demyttenaere K, *et al.* Tamsulosin as an effective treatment for reboxetine-associated urinary hesitancy. *Int Clin Psychopharmacol* 2001; **16:** 353–5.
2. Demyttenaere K, Huygens R. Painful ejaculation and urinary hesitancy in association with antidepressant therapy: relief with tamsulosin. *Eur Neuropsychopharmacol* 2002; **12:** 337–41.

### Preparations

**Proprietary Preparations** (details are given in Part 3)
***Arg.:*** Aclosan; Omnic; Reduprost; Secotex; ***Austral.:*** Flomax; ***Austria:*** Alna; Omix; ***Belg.:*** Omic; ***Braz.:*** Omnic; Secotex; ***Canad.:*** Flomax; ***Chile:*** Omnic; Prostall; Secotex; ***Denm.:*** Omnic; ***Fin.:*** Expros; Omnic; ***Fr.:*** Josir; Omix; ***Ger.:*** Alna; Omnic†; ***Gr.:*** Omnic; Pradif; ***Irl.:*** Omnic; ***Israel:*** Omnic; ***Ital.:*** Omnic; Pradif; ***Jpn:*** Harnal; ***Mex.:*** Secotex; ***Neth.:*** Omnic; ***Norw.:*** Omnic; ***NZ:*** Flomax; ***Port.:*** Omnic; Pradif; ***S.Afr.:*** Flomax; ***Spain:*** Omnic; Urolosin; ***Switz.:*** Pradif; ***Thai.:*** Harnal; ***UK:*** Flomax; ***USA:*** Flomax.

## Tasosartan *(BAN, USAN, rINN)*

ANA-756; Tasosartán; WAY-ANA-756. 5,8-Dihydro-2,4-dimethyl-8-[*p*-(*o*-1*H*-tetrazol-5-ylphenyl)benzyl]pyrido[2,3-*d*]pyrimidin-7(6*H*)-one.
$C_{23}H_{21}N_7O$ = 411.5.
*CAS — 145733-36-4.*
*ATC — C09CA05.*

### Profile

Tasosartan is an angiotensin II receptor antagonist that was investigated for the management of hypertension but development was discontinued due to hepatotoxicity.

◊ References.

1. Oparil S, *et al.* Tolerability profile of tasosartan, a long-acting angiotensin II $AT_1$ receptor blocker, in the treatment of patients with essential hypertension. *Curr Ther Res* 1997; **58:** 930–43.
2. Lacourcière Y, *et al.* A randomized, double-blind, placebo-controlled, parallel-group, multicenter trial of four doses of tasosartan in patients with essential hypertension. *Am J Hypertens* 1998; **11:** 454–61.
3. Neutel JM, *et al.* Efficacy and tolerability of tasosartan, a novel angiotensin II receptor blocker: results from a 10-week, double-blind, placebo-controlled, dose-titration study. *Am Heart J* 1999; **137:** 118–25.

### Teclothiazide Potassium *(BANM, rINNM)*

Teclotiazida potásica; Tetrachlormethiazide Potassium. 6-Chloro-3,4-dihydro-3-trichloromethyl-2*H*-1,2,4-benzothiadiazine-7-sulphonamide 1,1-dioxide potassium.

$C_8H_7Cl_4N_3O_4S_2,K = 454.2$.

*CAS — 4267-05-4 (teclothiazide); 5306-80-9 (teclothiazide potassium).*

#### Profile

Teclothiazide potassium is a thiazide diuretic (see Hydrochlorothiazide, p.933) used in the treatment of oedema.

#### Preparations

**Proprietary Preparations** (details are given in Part 3)
**Multi-ingredient:** ***Spain:*** Quimodril.

## Telmisartan *(BAN, USAN, rINN)*

BIBR-277; BIBR-277-SE; Telmisartán. 4′-{[4-Methyl-6-(1-methyl-2-benzimidazolyl)-2-propyl-1-benzimidazolyl]methyl}-2-biphenylcarboxylic acid.

$C_{33}H_{30}N_4O_2 = 514.6$.

*CAS — 144701-48-4.*

*ATC — C09CA07.*

#### Adverse Effects and Precautions

As for Losartan Potassium, p.947. Telmisartan should be used with caution in patients with hepatic impairment or biliary obstruction.

◊ References.

1. Michel MC, *et al.* Safety of telmisartan in patients with arterial hypertension : an open-label observational study. *Drug Safety* 2004; **27:** 335–44.

#### Interactions

As for Losartan Potassium, p.948.

**Digoxin.** Telmisartan may increase serum concentrations of digoxin (see Angiotensin II Receptor Antagonists under Interactions of Digoxin, p.896) but the interaction is probably not clinically significant.

#### Pharmacokinetics

Telmisartan is rapidly absorbed from the gastrointestinal tract; the absolute oral bioavailability is dose-dependent and is about 42% following a 40-mg dose and 58% following a 160-mg dose. Peak plasma concentrations of telmisartan are reached about 0.5 to 1 hour after an oral dose. Telmisartan is over 99% bound to plasma proteins. It is excreted almost entirely in the faeces via bile, mainly as unchanged drug. The terminal elimination half-life of telmisartan is about 24 hours.

◊ References.

1. Stangier J, *et al.* Absorption, metabolism, and excretion of intravenously and orally administered [$^{14}C$]telmisartan in healthy volunteers. *J Clin Pharmacol* 2000; **40:** 1312–22.

#### Uses and Administration

Telmisartan is an angiotensin II receptor antagonist with actions similar to those of losartan (p.948). It is used in the management of hypertension (p.825).

Telmisartan is given by mouth. After an oral dose the hypotensive effect peaks within 3 hours and persists for at least 24 hours. The maximum hypotensive effect is achieved within about 4 to 8 weeks after initiating therapy.

In hypertension, telmisartan is given in an initial dose of 40 mg once daily. This may be increased, if necessary, to a maximum dose of 80 mg once daily. Lower doses should be considered in patients with hepatic impairment (see below).

◊ Reviews.

1. McClellan KJ, Markham A. Telmisartan. *Drugs* 1998; **56:** 1039–44.
2. Sharpe M, *et al.* Telmisartan: a review of its use in hypertension. *Drugs* 2001; **61:** 1501–29.

**Administration in hepatic impairment.** Administration of telmisartan to patients with hepatic impairment resulted in an increase in bioavailability and a reduction in clearance compared with healthy volunteers.[1] Although telmisartan was well tolerated, it was suggested that lower doses should be considered in patients with hepatic impairment. In the UK telmisartan is contra-indicated in severe hepatic impairment and a maximum dose of 40 mg once daily is recommended for patients with mild to moderate impairment.

1. Stangier J, *et al.* Pharmacokinetics and safety of intravenous and oral telmisartan 20 mg and 120 mg in subjects with hepatic impairment compared with healthy volunteers. *J Clin Pharmacol* 2000; **40:** 1355–64.

#### Preparations

**Proprietary Preparations** (details are given in Part 3)
***Arg.:*** Gliosartan; Micardis; Pritor; ***Austral.:*** Micardis; Pritor; ***Belg.:*** Micardis; ***Braz.:*** Micardis; Pritor; ***Canad.:*** Micardis; ***Chile:*** Micardis; Pritoral; Samertan; ***Denm.:*** Micardis; ***Fin.:*** Micardis; ***Fr.:*** Micardis; Pritor; ***Ger.:*** Micardis; ***Gr.:*** Micardis; Pritor; ***Hong Kong:*** Micardis; ***Irl.:*** Micardis; ***Ital.:*** Micardis; Pritor; ***Malaysia:*** Micardis; ***Mex.:*** Micardis; ***Neth.:*** Micardis; ***Norw.:*** Micardis; ***Port.:*** Micardis; Pritor; ***S.Afr.:*** Micardis; ***Singapore:*** Micardis; ***Spain:*** Micardis; Pritor; ***Swed.:*** Micardis; ***Switz.:*** Micardis; ***Thai.:*** Micardis; ***UK:*** Micardis; ***USA:*** Micardis.
**Multi-ingredient:** ***Austral.:*** Micardis Plus; ***Canad.:*** Micardis Plus; ***Chile:*** Micardis Plus; ***Fr.:*** MicardisPlus; PritorPlus; ***Irl.:*** MicardisPlus; ***Port.:*** Micardis Plus; ***S.Afr.:*** Co-Micardis; ***Spain:*** Micardis Plus; Pritor Plus; ***UK:*** MicardisPlus; ***USA:*** Micardis HCT.

### Temocapril Hydrochloride *(BANM, USAN, rINNM)*

CS-622; Hidrocloruro de temocapril. (+)-(2S,6R)-6-{[(1S)-1-Ethoxycarbonyl-3-phenylpropyl]amino}tetrahydro-5-oxo-2-(2-thienyl)-1,4-thiazepine-4(5*H*)-acetic acid hydrochloride.

$C_{23}H_{28}N_2O_5S_2,HCl = 513.1$.

*CAS — 111902-57-9 (temocapril); 110221-44-8 (temocapril hydrochloride).*

*ATC — C09AA14.*

#### Profile

Temocapril is an ACE inhibitor (p.842) that is used in the treatment of hypertension (p.825). It owes its activity to the diacid temocaprilat to which it is converted after oral administration. It is given by mouth as the hydrochloride in a usual initial dose of 1 mg daily, increased to a maintenance dose of 2 to 4 mg daily as necessary.

◊ References.

1. Nakashima M, *et al.* Pharmacokinetics of temocapril hydrochloride, a novel angiotensin converting enzyme inhibitor, in renal insufficiency. *Eur J Clin Pharmacol* 1992; **43:** 657–9.
2. Oguchi H, *et al.* Pharmacokinetics of temocapril and enalapril in patients with various degrees of renal insufficiency. *Clin Pharmacokinet* 1993; **24:** 421–7.
3. Furuta S, *et al.* Pharmacokinetics of temocapril, an ACE inhibitor with preferential biliary excretion, in patients with impaired liver function. *Eur J Clin Pharmacol* 1993; **44:** 383–5.
4. Arakawa M, *et al.* Pharmacokinetics and pharmacodynamics of temocapril during repeated dosing in elderly hypertensive patients. *Eur J Clin Pharmacol* 2001; **56:** 775–9.

#### Preparations

**Proprietary Preparations** (details are given in Part 3)
***Austria:*** Acecor; ***Jpn:*** Acecol.

## Tenecteplase *(BAN, USAN, rINN)*

Tenecteplasa; TNK-tPA. [103-L-Asparagine-117-L-glutamine-296-L-alanine-297-L-alanine-298-L-alanine-299-L-alanine]plasminogen activator (human tissue-type).

*CAS — 191588-94-0.*

*ATC — B01AD11.*

**Description.** Tenecteplase is a 527 amino acid glycoprotein produced by recombinant DNA technology. It is a modified form of human tissue plasminogen activator.

#### Adverse Effects, Treatment, and Precautions

As for Streptokinase, p.1005

#### Interactions

As for Streptokinase, p.1007

#### Pharmacokinetics

Following intravenous injection in patients with acute myocardial infarction, tenecteplase has a biphasic clearance from plasma with an initial half-life of 20 to 24 minutes and a terminal phase half-life of 90 to 130 minutes. It is cleared mainly by hepatic metabolism.

◊ Reviews.

1. Tanswell P, *et al.* Pharmacokinetics and pharmacodynamics of tenecteplase in fibrinolytic therapy of acute myocardial infarction. *Clin Pharmacokinet* 2002; **41:** 1229–45.

#### Uses and Administration

Tenecteplase is a thrombolytic drug. It converts plasminogen to plasmin, a proteolytic enzyme which has fibrinolytic effects. The mechanisms of fibrinolysis are discussed further under Haemostasis and Fibrinolysis on p.735. Tenecteplase is a fibrin-specific thrombolytic (see p.812).

Tenecteplase is used similarly to streptokinase (p.1007) in acute myocardial infarction (p.828). It is given intravenously as a single bolus dose over 5 to 10 seconds as soon as possible after the onset of symptoms. The dose is based on body-weight and ranges from 30 mg in patients less than 60 kg to a maximum of 50 mg in those 90 kg or above.

◊ References.

1. Cannon CP, *et al.* TNK-tissue plasminogen activator compared with front-loaded alteplase in acute myocardial infarction: results of the TIMI 10B trial. *Circulation* 1998; **98:** 2805–14.
2. Assessment of the Safety and Efficacy of a New Thrombolytic (ASSENT-2) Investigators. Single-bolus tenecteplase compared with front-loaded alteplase in acute myocardial infarction: the ASSENT-2 double-blind randomised trial. *Lancet* 1999; **354:** 716–22.
3. Llevadot J, *et al.* Bolus fibrinolytic therapy in acute myocardial infarction. *JAMA* 2001; **286:** 442–9.
4. The Assessment of the Safety and Efficacy of a New Thrombolytic Regimen (ASSENT)-3 Investigators. Efficacy and safety of tenecteplase in combination with enoxaparin, abciximab, or unfractionated heparin: the ASSENT-3 randomised trial in acute myocardial infarction. *Lancet* 2001; **358:** 605–13.
5. Turcasso NM, Nappi JM. Tenecteplase for treatment of acute myocardial infarction. *Ann Pharmacother* 2001; **35:** 1233–40.

#### Preparations

**Proprietary Preparations** (details are given in Part 3)
***Austral.:*** Metalyse; ***Braz.:*** Metalyse; ***Denm.:*** Metalyse; ***Fin.:*** Metalyse; ***Fr.:*** Metalyse; ***Ger.:*** Metalyse; ***Gr.:*** Metalyse; ***Irl.:*** Metalyse; ***Norw.:*** Metalyse; ***NZ:*** Metalyse; ***Port.:*** Metalyse; ***S.Afr.:*** Metalyse; ***Spain:*** Metalyse; ***Swed.:*** Metalyse; ***Switz.:*** Metalyse; ***UK:*** Metalyse; ***USA:*** TNKase.

### Tenitramine

Tenitramina. *NNN′N′*-Tetrakis(2-hydroxyethyl)ethylenediamine tetranitrate.

$C_{10}H_{20}N_6O_{12} = 416.3$.

*CAS — 21946-79-2.*

*ATC — C01DA38.*

#### Profile

Tenitramine is a vasodilator with general properties similar to those of glyceryl trinitrate (p.923) and is used in angina pectoris (p.813). It is given in a dose of up to 10 mg by mouth for acute attacks and up to 10 mg every six hours for long-term management.

#### Preparations

**Proprietary Preparations** (details are given in Part 3)
***Braz.:*** Ditran†; ***Ital.:*** Tenitran.

### Teprotide *(BAN, USAN, rINN)*

$BPF_{9a}$; L-Pyroglutamyl-L-tryptophyl-L-prolyl-L-arginyl-L-prolyl-L-glutaminyl-L-isoleucyl-L-prolyl-L-proline; SQ-20881; Teprótido; 2-L-Tryptophan-3-de-L-leucine-4-de-L-proline-8-L-glutamine-bradykinin potentiator B. 5-oxo-Pro-Trp-Pro-Arg-Pro-Gln-Ile-Pro-Pro.

$C_{53}H_{76}N_{14}O_{12} = 1101.3$.

*CAS — 35115-60-7.*

#### Profile

Teprotide is a nonapeptide originally found in the venom of *Bothrops jararaca*, a South American pit-viper. It is an ACE inhibitor with a short duration of action and has been given parenterally as an investigational tool.

## Terazosin Hydrochloride

*(BANM, USAN, rINNM)*

Abbott-45975; Hidrocloruro de terazosina. 1-(4-Amino-6,7-dimethoxyquinazolin-2-yl)-4-(tetrahydro-2-furoyl)piperazine hydrochloride dihydrate; 6,7-Dimethoxy-2-[4-(tetrahydrofuran-2-carbonyl)piperazin-1-yl]quinazolin-4-ylamine hydrochloride dihydrate.

$C_{19}H_{25}N_5O_4,HCl,2H_2O = 459.9$.

*CAS — 63590-64-7 (terazosin); 63074-08-8 (anhydrous terazosin hydrochloride); 70024-40-7 (terazosin hydrochloride dihydrate).*

*ATC — G04CA03.*

**Pharmacopoeias.** In *US.*

**USP 27** (Terazosin Hydrochloride). A white to pale yellow, crystalline powder. soluble in water and in methyl alcohol; freely soluble in isotonic saline solution; slightly soluble in alcohol and in 0.1N hydrochloric acid; practically insoluble in acetone and in hexanes; very slightly soluble in chloroform. Store in airtight containers at a temperature between 20° and 25°.

#### Adverse Effects, Treatment, and Precautions

As for Prazosin Hydrochloride, p.985.

**Urinary incontinence.** For reference to urinary incontinence associated with terazosin, see under Adverse Effects of Prazosin Hydrochloride, p.985.

#### Interactions

As for Prazosin Hydrochloride, p.985.

#### Pharmacokinetics

Terazosin is rapidly and almost completely absorbed from the gastrointestinal tract after oral administration;

the bioavailability is reported to be about 90%. Peak plasma concentrations are achieved in about 1 hour. Terazosin is 90 to 94% protein bound. It is metabolised in the liver; one of the metabolites is reported to possess antihypertensive activity. The half-life in plasma is about 12 hours. Terazosin is excreted in faeces via the bile, and in the urine, as unchanged drug and metabolites.

### Uses and Administration

Terazosin is an alpha$_1$-adrenoceptor blocker (p.809) with actions similar to those of prazosin (p.986), but a longer duration of action.

It is used in the management of hypertension (p.825) and in benign prostatic hyperplasia (p.1555) to relieve symptoms of urinary obstruction.

Terazosin is given by mouth as the hydrochloride, but doses are usually expressed in terms of the base. Terazosin hydrochloride 1.2 mg is approximately equivalent to 1 mg of terazosin. Following oral administration its hypotensive effects are seen within 15 minutes and may last for up to 24 hours, permitting once daily dosage.

To avoid the risk of collapse which may occur in some patients after the first dose the initial dose for both hypertension and benign prostatic hyperplasia is 1 mg of terazosin at bedtime, increasing gradually at intervals of 7 days according to the patient's response. For **hypertension** the usual maintenance dose is 2 to 10 mg once daily and the usual maximum dose is 20 mg daily in a single dose or two divided doses. For **benign prostatic hyperplasia** the usual maintenance dose is 5 to 10 mg once daily.

◊ Reviews.


1. Titmarsh S, Monk JP. Terazosin: a review of its pharmacodynamic and pharmacokinetic properties, and therapeutic efficacy in essential hypertension. *Drugs* 1987; **33:** 461–77.
2. Achari R, Laddu A. Terazosin: a new alpha adrenoceptor blocking drug. *J Clin Pharmacol* 1992; **32:** 520–3.


### Preparations

**Proprietary Preparations** (details are given in Part 3)

***Arg.:*** Benaprost; Blavin; Eglidon; Flumarc; Fosfomik; Isontyn; ***Austral.:*** Hytrin; ***Austria:*** Uroflo; Vicard; ***Belg.:*** Hytrin; ***Braz.:*** Hytrin; ***Canad.:*** Hytrin; ***Chile:*** Adecur; Hytrin; ***Denm.:*** Sinalfa; ***Fr.:*** Dysalfa; Hytrine; ***Ger.:*** Flotrin; Heitrin; ***Gr.:*** Hytrin; ***Hong Kong:*** Hytrin; ***India:*** Hytrin; Olyster; ***Irl.:*** Hytrin; ***Israel:*** Hytrin; ***Ital.:*** Ezosina; Itrin; Terafluss; Teraprost; Unoprost; Urodie; ***Malaysia:*** Hytrin; ***Mex.:*** Adecur; Hytrin; ***Neth.:*** Hytrin; ***Norw.:*** Sinalfa; ***NZ:*** Hytrin; ***Port.:*** Hytrin; ***S.Afr.:*** Hytrin; ***Singapore:*** Hytrin; ***Spain:*** Deflox; Magnurol; Sutif; Tazusin; Teraumon; Zayasel; ***Swed.:*** Hytrinex; Sinalfa; ***Switz.:*** Hytrin BPH; ***Thai.:*** Hytrin; ***UK:*** Hytrin; ***USA:*** Hytrin.

---

## Tertatolol Hydrochloride *(BANM, rINNM)*

Hidrocloruro de tertatolol; S-2395 (tertatolol or tertatolol hydrochloride); SE-2395 (tertatolol or tertatolol hydrochloride). (±)-1-(*tert*-Butylamino)-3-(thiochroman-8-yloxy)propan-2-ol hydrochloride.

$C_{16}H_{25}NO_2S,HCl$ = 331.9.

*CAS — 34784-64-0 (tertatolol); 33580-30-2 (tertatolol hydrochloride).*

*ATC — C07AA16.*

### Profile

Tertatolol is a non-cardioselective beta blocker (p.868). It is reported to lack intrinsic sympathomimetic activity.

Tertatolol is given by mouth as the hydrochloride in the management of hypertension (p.825) in a dose of 5 mg once daily.

### Preparations

**Proprietary Preparations** (details are given in Part 3)

***Belg.:*** Artex†; ***Braz.:*** Artexal†; ***Denm.:*** Artexal; ***Fr.:*** Artex; ***Ger.:*** Prenalex†; ***Irl.:*** Artexal; ***Neth.:*** Artex; ***Port.:*** Artex.

---

## Tezosentan *(rINN)*

Tezosentán. *N*-[6-(2-Hydroxyethoxy)-5-(*o*-methoxyphenoxy)-2-[2-(1*H*-tetrazol-5-yl)-4-pyridyl]-4-pyrimidinyl]-5-isopropyl-2-pyridinesulfonamide.

$C_{27}H_{27}N_9O_6S$ = 605.6.

*CAS — 180384-57-0.*

### Profile

Tezosentan is an endothelin receptor antagonist under investigation for acute heart failure.

◊ References.


1. Torre-Amione G, *et al.* Hemodynamic effects of tezosentan, an intravenous dual endothelin receptor antagonist, in patients with class III to IV congestive heart failure. *Circulation* 2001; **103:** 973–80.
2. Tovar JM, Gums JG. Tezosentan in the treatment of acute heart failure. *Ann Pharmacother* 2003; **37:** 1877–83.


---

## Tiadenol *(rINN)*

LL-1558. 2,2′-(Decamethylenedithio)diethanol.

$C_{14}H_{30}O_2S_2$ = 294.5.

*CAS — 6964-20-1.*

*ATC — C10AX03.*

### Profile

Tiadenol is a lipid regulating drug used in the treatment of hyperlipidaemias (p.823). The usual dose is 1.2 to 2.4 g daily by mouth in divided doses.

### Preparations

**Proprietary Preparations** (details are given in Part 3)

***Fr.:*** Fonlipol; ***Ital.:*** Eulip†; Tiabrenolo†; Tiaden†; ***Spain:*** Endol†.

---

# Ticlopidine Hydrochloride

*(BANM, USAN, rINNM)*

4-C-32; 53-32C; Hidrocloruro de ticlopidina; Ticlopidini Hydrochloridum. 5-(2-Chlorobenzyl)-4,5,6,7-tetrahydrothieno[3,2-c]pyridine hydrochloride.

$C_{14}H_{14}ClNS,HCl$ = 300.2.

*CAS — 55142-85-3 (ticlopidine); 53885-35-1 (ticlopidine hydrochloride).*

*ATC — B01AC05.*

**Pharmacopoeias.** In *Eur.* (see p.vi) and *Jpn.*

**Ph. Eur. 5.0** (Ticlopidine Hydrochloride). A white or almost white, crystalline powder. Sparingly soluble in water and in dehydrated alcohol; very slightly soluble in ethyl acetate. A 2.5% solution in water has a pH of 3.5 to 4.0.

### Adverse Effects and Precautions

Gastrointestinal disturbances, skin rashes, and bleeding are the most commonly reported adverse effects associated with ticlopidine therapy. Blood dyscrasias, including neutropenia, thrombotic thrombocytopenic purpura, and aplastic anaemia, have also occurred. There have been reports of hepatitis and cholestatic jaundice. Blood-lipid concentrations may increase during long-term therapy.

Ticlopidine should not be administered to patients with haematopoietic disorders such as neutropenia or thrombocytopenia, haemorrhagic diathesis or other haemorrhagic disorders associated with a prolonged bleeding time, or conditions with an increased risk of bleeding such as peptic ulcer disease, acute cerebral haemorrhage, or severe liver dysfunction. Full blood counts should be performed before starting treatment and every 2 weeks during the first 3 months of therapy. If ticlopidine is discontinued during this period, a full blood count should be performed within 2 weeks of stopping treatment. Consideration should be given to stopping ticlopidine therapy 10 to 14 days before elective surgery.

**Effects on the blood.** Severe *neutropenia* or *agranulocytosis* may occur in about 1% of patients given ticlopidine[1] and fatal infection has been reported.[2] Neutropenia usually develops within the first three months of therapy and is reversible on discontinuation of ticlopidine, but there has been a report[3] of a delayed reaction that occurred 18 days after ticlopidine was discontinued. Isolated *thrombocytopenia* occurs in about 0.4% of patients and *thrombotic thrombocytopenic purpura*, sometimes fatal, has occurred.[1,4-7] Cases of thrombotic thrombocytopenic purpura and haemolytic uraemic syndrome have also been reported[8,9] with clopidogrel, although the association is less well established.[10] Conversely, good results have been achieved with ticlopidine as a treatment for thrombotic thrombocytopenic purpura,[11,12] but it should only be used with extreme caution.[13] Aplastic anaemia has occurred rarely with ticlopidine[1,14] and with clopidogrel.[15]


1. Love BB, *et al.* Adverse haematological effects of ticlopidine: prevention, recognition and management. *Drug Safety* 1998; **19:** 89–98.
2. Carlson JA, Maesner JE. Fatal neutropenia and thrombocytopenia associated with ticlopidine. *Ann Pharmacother* 1994; **28:** 1236–8.
3. Farver DK, Hansen LA. Delayed neutropenia with ticlopidine. *Ann Pharmacother* 1994; **28:** 1344–6.
4. Bennett CL, *et al.* Thrombotic thrombocytopenic purpura associated with ticlopidine: a review of 60 cases. *Ann Intern Med* 1998; **128:** 541–4.
5. Bennett CL, *et al.* Thrombotic thrombocytopenic purpura after stenting and ticlopidine. *Lancet* 1998; **352:** 1036–7.
6. Steinhubl SR, *et al.* Incidence and clinical course of thrombotic thrombocytopenic purpura due to ticlopidine following coronary stenting. *JAMA* 1999; **281:** 806–10.
7. Bennett CL, *et al.* Thrombotic thrombocytopenic purpura associated with ticlopidine in the setting of coronary artery stents and stroke prevention. *Arch Intern Med* 1999; **159:** 2524–8.
8. Bennett CL, *et al.* Thrombotic thrombocytopenic purpura associated with clopidogrel. *N Engl J Med* 2000; **342:** 1773–7.
9. Oomen PHN, *et al.* Hemolytic uremic syndrome in a patient treated with clopidogrel. *Ann Intern Med* 2000; **132:** 1006.
10. Hankey GJ. Clopidogrel and thrombotic thrombocytopenic purpura. *Lancet* 2000; **356:** 269–70.
11. Vianelli N, *et al.* Thrombotic thrombocytopenic purpura and ticlopidine. *Lancet* 1991; **337:** 1219.
12. Bobbio-Pallavicini E, *et al.* Antiplatelet agents in thrombotic thrombocytopenic purpura (TTP): results of a randomized multicenter trial by the Italian Cooperative Group for TTP. *Haematologica* 1997; **82:** 429–35.
13. Rock G, *et al.* Thrombotic thrombocytopenic purpura treatment in year 2000. *Haematologica* 2000; **85:** 410–19.
14. Yeh S-P, *et al.* Ticlopidine-associated aplastic anemia: a case report and review of literature. *Ann Hematol* 1998; **76:** 87–90.
15. Trivier J-M, *et al.* Fatal aplastic anaemia associated with clopidogrel. *Lancet* 2001; **357:** 446.


**Effects on the gastrointestinal tract.** Diarrhoea is a common side-effect of ticlopidine therapy; it usually occurs during the first few months of therapy and resolves within 1 to 2 weeks without stopping therapy. However, there has been a report[1] of diarrhoea and weight loss of 2 months duration that first presented 2 years after ticlopidine was started; diarrhoea resolved when ticlopidine was withdrawn.


1. Mansoor GA, Aziz K. Delayed chronic diarrhea and weight loss possibly due to ticlopidine therapy. *Ann Pharmacother* 1997; **31:** 870–2.


**Effects on the joints.** Acute arthritis associated with a diffuse rash developed in a patient shortly after starting treatment with ticlopidine.[1] Both the rash and the arthritis resolved following discontinuation, and it was suggested that a hypersensitivity reaction might be involved. One case of polyarthritis and 3 cases of arthralgia associated with ticlopidine had been reported to the UK Committee on Safety of Medicines up to March 2001. Two cases of acute arthritis have also been reported[2] with clopidogrel; symptoms developed 2 to 3 weeks after starting treatment and resolved following discontinuation.


1. Dakik HA, *et al.* Ticlopidine associated with acute arthritis. *BMJ* 2002; **324:** 27.
2. Garg A, *et al.* Clopidogrel associated with acute arthritis. *BMJ* 2000; **320:** 483.


**Effects on the kidneys.** A reversible deterioration in renal function has been reported in patients receiving ticlopidine following coronary stent implantation.[1,2] There has also been a report[3] of membranous nephropathy with nephrotic syndrome in a patient receiving clopidogrel.


1. Elsman P, Zijlstra F. Ticlopidine and renal function. *Lancet* 1996; **348:** 273–4.
2. Virdee M, *et al.* Ticlopidine and renal function. *Lancet* 1996; **348:** 1031–2.
3. Tholl U, *et al.* Clopidogrel and membranous nephropathy. *Lancet* 1999; **354:** 1443–4.


**Effects on the liver.** Cholestatic hepatitis has been reported in patients receiving ticlopidine and is usually reversible when ticlopidine is stopped.[1-3] However, there has been a report of persistent cholestasis following ticlopidine withdrawal.[4] A case of granulomatous hepatitis has also been reported.[5] Clopidogrel was substituted for ticlopidine in a patient who had developed raised liver enzymes during ticlopidine treatment;[6] liver enzyme values returned to normal during continued clopidogrel therapy. However, there has been a report[7] of hepatotoxicity with clopidogrel.


1. Cassidy LJ, *et al.* Probable ticlopidine-induced cholestatic hepatitis. *Ann Pharmacother* 1995; **29:** 30–2.
2. Pérez-Balsa AM, *et al.* Hepatotoxicity due to ticlopidine. *Ann Pharmacother* 1998; **32:** 1250–1.
3. Skurnik YD, *et al.* Ticlopidine-induced cholestatic hepatitis. *Ann Pharmacother* 2003; **37:** 371–5.
4. Colivicchi F, *et al.* Ticlopidine-induced chronic cholestatic hepatitis: a case report. *Curr Ther Res* 1994; **55:** 929–31.
5. Ruiz-Valverde P, *et al.* Ticlopidine-induced granulomatous hepatitis. *Ann Pharmacother* 1995; **29:** 633–4.
6. Zeolla MM, Carson JJ. Successful use of clopidogrel for cerebrovascular accident in a patient with suspected ticlopidine-induced hepatotoxicity. *Ann Pharmacother* 1999; **33:** 939–41.
7. Willens HJ. Clopidogrel-induced mixed hepatocellular and cholestatic liver injury. *Am J Ther* 2000; **7:** 317–8.


**Effects on the lungs.** Bronchiolitis obliterans-organising pneumonia developed in a 76-year-old woman receiving ticlopidine and prednisone for temporal arteritis.[1] The condition resolved over several months when ticlopidine was withdrawn.


1. Alonso-Martinez JL, *et al.* Bronchiolitis obliterans-organizing pneumonia caused by ticlopidine. *Ann Intern Med* 1998; **129:** 71–2.


### Interactions

Ticlopidine should be used with caution in patients receiving other drugs, such as anticoagulants and antiplatelets, that increase the risk of bleeding. Ticlopidine is an inhibitor of cytochrome P450, particularly the isoenzymes CYP2C19 and CYP2D6, and may inhibit the metabolism of other drugs that are metabolised by this route. The clearance of ticlopidine may be reduced by concomitant cimetidine therapy. Corticosteroids may antagonise the effect of ticlopidine on bleeding time.

**Anticoagulants.** Concomitant use of ticlopidine with anticoagulants may increase the risk of bleeding. However, ticlopidine has been reported to antagonise the effect of *acenocoumarol* (see Antiplatelets under Interactions of Warfarin, p.1026).

**Antiepileptics.** For a report of acute *phenytoin* toxicity in a well-stabilised patient following addition of ticlopidine, see p.374.

**Xanthines.** For reference to the effect of ticlopidine on *theophylline* half-life, see p.803.

## Pharmacokinetics

Ticlopidine is rapidly and almost completely absorbed from the gastrointestinal tract. It is about 98% bound to plasma proteins. The terminal half-life during chronic dosing is reported to be about 30 to 50 hours. Ticlopidine is extensively metabolised in the liver. About 60% of a dose is excreted in the urine as metabolites and 25% in the faeces.

◊ References.

1. Desager J-P. Clinical pharmacokinetics of ticlopidine. *Clin Pharmacokinet* 1994; **26:** 347–55.
2. Buur T, *et al.* Pharmacokinetics and effect of ticlopidine on platelet aggregation in subjects with normal and impaired renal function. *J Clin Pharmacol* 1997; **37:** 108–15.

## Uses and Administration

Ticlopidine hydrochloride is a thienopyridine antiplatelet drug used in thromboembolic disorders (p.837). It appears to act by inhibiting adenosine diphosphate-mediated platelet aggregation. It may be given prophylactically as an alternative to aspirin in patients at risk of thrombotic stroke (p.836) and in the management of intermittent claudication (see Peripheral Vascular Disease, p.831) and ischaemic heart disease. It is also licensed as an adjunct to aspirin for the prevention of subacute stent occlusion after intracoronary stenting (see Reperfusion and Revascularisation Procedures, p.834). Ticlopidine may also be used to prevent occlusion and platelet loss during extracorporeal circulatory procedures.

In the prevention of thrombotic **stroke**, and in **intermittent claudication**, ticlopidine hydrochloride is given in a dose of 250 mg twice daily by mouth, with meals. For the prevention of subacute stent occlusion after **intracoronary stenting** ticlopidine hydrochloride is given in a dose of 250 mg twice daily for 4 weeks, starting at the time of stent placement.

Regular haematological monitoring is required during ticlopidine therapy (see Adverse Effects and Precautions, above).

◊ References.

1. McTavish D, *et al.* Ticlopidine: an updated review of its pharmacology and therapeutic use in platelet-dependent disorders. *Drugs* 1990; **40:** 238–59.
2. Flores-Runk P, Raasch RH. Ticlopidine and antiplatelet therapy. *Ann Pharmacother* 1993; **27:** 1090–8.
3. Sharis PJ, *et al.* The antiplatelet effects of ticlopidine and clopidogrel. *Ann Intern Med* 1998; **129:** 394–405.

**Reperfusion and revascularisation procedures.** Coronary stents are being used increasingly to treat and prevent restenosis following angioplasty procedures. Thrombotic occlusion commonly complicates their use and patients have been aggressively treated with a combination of antiplatelet drugs and anticoagulants. Recent studies, however, suggest that antiplatelet treatment alone may be adequate if the stent has been positioned correctly and the risk of thrombosis is considered to be low.

In a study[1] comparing a combination of long-term aspirin with 4 weeks treatment with either ticlopidine or phenprocoumon, fewer cardiac events and fewer haemorrhagic complications occurred in the antiplatelet group. At 6-months follow-up,[2] however, there was no significant difference in rates of restenosis or repeat revascularisation between the groups. Similar short-term benefits have also been reported[3] in a study comparing antiplatelet with anticoagulant therapy for 6 weeks following coronary stenting. A larger study[4] also found antiplatelet therapy in the 30 days following coronary stent placement to be beneficial. The rate of stent thrombosis was reduced in the group treated with aspirin and ticlopidine compared with those treated with aspirin and warfarin or aspirin alone. However, the incidence of haemorrhagic complications was not significantly different for the ticlopidine and warfarin groups, but was significantly lower in the group treated with aspirin alone. An earlier small study[5] had suggested that aspirin alone may be as effective as ticlopidine with aspirin.

Shorter courses of ticlopidine for 2 weeks following intracoronary stent placement may reduce the risk of neutropenia caused by the drug without increasing the risk of stent thrombosis.[6]

Ticlopidine has also been reported[7] to improve the long-term patency of saphenous vein bypass grafts used to treat peripheral vascular disease in the legs.

1. Schömig A, *et al.* A randomized comparison of antiplatelet and anticoagulant therapy after the placement of coronary-artery stents. *N Engl J Med* 1996; **334:** 1084–9.
2. Kastrati A, *et al.* Restenosis after coronary stent placement and randomization to a 4-week combined antiplatelet or anticoagulant therapy: six-month angiographic follow-up of the Intracoronary Stenting and Antithrombotic Regimen (ISAR) trial. *Circulation* 1997; **96:** 462–7.
3. Bertrand ME, *et al.* Randomized multicenter comparison of conventional anticoagulation versus antiplatelet therapy in unplanned and elective coronary stenting: the Full Anticoagulation versus Aspirin and Ticlopidine (FANTASTIC) study. *Circulation* 1998; **98:** 1597–1603.
4. Leon MB, *et al.* A clinical trial comparing three antithrombotic-drug regimens after coronary-artery stenting. *N Engl J Med* 1998; **339:** 1665–71.
5. Hall P, *et al.* A randomized comparison of combined ticlopidine and aspirin therapy versus aspirin therapy alone after successful intravascular ultrasound-guided stent implantation. *Circulation* 1996; **93:** 215–22.
6. Berger PB, *et al.* Safety and efficacy of ticlopidine for only 2 weeks after successful intracoronary stent placement. *Circulation* 1999; **99:** 248–53.
7. Becquemin J-P. Effect of ticlopidine on the long-term patency of saphenous-vein bypass grafts in the legs. *N Engl J Med* 1997; **337:** 1726–31.

## Preparations

**Proprietary Preparations** (details are given in Part 3)
***Arg.:*** Dosier; Ticlid; Trombenal; ***Austral.:*** Ticlid; Tilodene; ***Austria:*** Thrombodine; Ticlodone; Tiklid; ***Belg.:*** Ticlid; ***Braz.:*** Plaket†; Ticlid; Ticlobal; ***Canad.:*** Ticlid; ***Chile:*** Ateroclar; Plaquetil; Ticlid; ***Fr.:*** Ticlid; Ticlomed; ***Ger.:*** Desiticlopidin; Tiklyd; ***Gr.:*** Anghostan-100; Etfariol; Neo Fulvigal; Neo-omnipen; Ruxicolan; Ticlid; Ticlodone; ***Hong Kong:*** Aplaket; Ticlid; ***India:*** Ticlop; Tikleen; Tyklid; ***Israel:*** Ticlidil; ***Ital.:*** Anagregal; Antigreg; Aplaket; Clox; Fluilast; Flupid; Klodin; Opteron; Parsilid; Ticlodone; Ticlogi; Ticloproge; Tiklid; ***Malaysia:*** Aplaket; Ticlid; ***Mex.:*** Ticlid; ***Norw.:*** Ticlid; ***NZ:*** Ticlid†; ***Port.:*** Aplaket; Betlife; Isaxion; Klodipin; Movin; Opidina; Plaquetal; Ticlodix; Ticlopat; Tiklyd; Trombopat; ***S.Afr.:*** Ticlid; ***Singapore:*** Antigreg; Aplaket; Tacron; Ticlid; Tipidin; ***Spain:*** Ticlodone; Tiklid; ***Swed.:*** Ticlid; ***Switz.:*** Ticlid†; ***Thai.:*** Aplaket; Ticdine; Ticlid; Tipidine; ***UK:*** Ticlid†; ***USA:*** Ticlid.

---

## Tienilic Acid *(BAN, rINN)*

Ácido tienílico; SKF-62698; Ticrynafen *(USAN)*. [2,3-Dichloro-4-(2-thenoyl)phenoxy]acetic acid.

$C_{13}H_8Cl_2O_4S$ = 331.2.
*CAS — 40180-04-9.*
*ATC — C03CC02.*

### Profile

Tienilic acid is a diuretic that was formerly used in the treatment of oedema and hypertension. It was withdrawn from the market because of reports of severe, sometimes fatal, liver damage.

---

# Timolol Maleate *(BANM, USAN, rINNM)*

Maleato de timolol; MK-950; Timololi Maleas. (*S*)-1-*tert*-Butylamino-3-(4-morpholino-1,2,5-thiadiazol-3-yloxy)propan-2-ol maleate.

$C_{13}H_{24}N_4O_3S,C_4H_4O_4$ = 432.5.
*CAS — 26839-75-8 (timolol); 91524-16-2 (timolol hemihydrate); 26921-17-5 (timolol maleate).*
*ATC — C07AA06; S01ED01.*

NOTE. TIM is a code approved by the BP 2003 for use on single unit doses of eye drops containing timolol maleate where the individual container may be too small to bear all the appropriate labelling information.

**Pharmacopoeias.** In *Chin., Eur.* (see p.vi), *Int.*, and *US.*

**Ph. Eur. 5.0** (Timolol Maleate). A white or almost white, crystalline powder or colourless crystals. Soluble in water and in alcohol. A 2% solution in water has a pH of 3.8 to 4.3. Protect from light.

**USP 27** (Timolol Maleate). A white to practically white, odourless or practically odourless powder. Soluble in water, in alcohol, and in methyl alcohol; sparingly soluble in chloroform and in propylene glycol; insoluble in cyclohexane and in ether. A 2% solution in water has a pH of 3.8 to 4.3.

## Adverse Effects, Treatment, and Precautions

As for Beta Blockers, p.869.

**Breast feeding.** Timolol is distributed into breast milk. Following instillation of timolol 0.5% eye drops twice daily, concentrations of timolol in breast milk of a lactating woman were approximately 6 times greater than those in serum, the values being 5.6 and 0.93 nanograms/mL respectively.[1] In a study[2] in patients receiving timolol 5 mg three times daily by mouth, the mean concentration in breast milk was 15.9 nanograms/mL, and the ratio of milk to plasma concentrations was 0.8; a similar ratio was found at higher doses, and the authors considered that the amount ingested by an infant would not be important. No adverse effects were reported in these studies and the American Academy of Pediatrics considers[3] that timolol is therefore usually compatible with breast feeding.

1. Lustgarten JS, Podos SM. Topical timolol and the nursing mother. *Arch Ophthalmol* 1983; **101:** 1381–2.
2. Fidler J, *et al.* Excretion of oxprenolol and timolol in breast milk. *Br J Obstet Gynaecol* 1983; **90:** 961–5.
3. American Academy of Pediatrics. The transfer of drugs and other chemicals into human milk. *Pediatrics* 2001; **108:** 776–89. Correction. *ibid*; 1029. Also available at: http://aappolicy.aappublications.org/cgi/content/full/pediatrics%3b108/3/776 (accessed 06/07/04)

## Interactions

The interactions associated with beta blockers are discussed on p.870.

## Pharmacokinetics

Timolol is almost completely absorbed from the gastrointestinal tract but is subject to moderate first-pass metabolism. Peak plasma concentrations occur about 1 to 2 hours after a dose. Timolol has low to moderate lipid solubility. Protein binding is reported to be low. It crosses the placenta and is distributed into breast milk. A plasma half-life of 4 hours has been reported. Timolol is extensively metabolised in the liver, the metabolites being excreted in the urine together with some unchanged timolol. Timolol is not removed by haemodialysis.

**Metabolism.** Studies[1-3] have shown that the metabolism of timolol is influenced by genetic polymorphism.

1. McGourty JC, *et al.* Pharmacokinetics and beta-blocking effects of timolol in poor and extensive metabolizers of debrisoquin. *Clin Pharmacol Ther* 1985; **38:** 409–13.
2. Lewis RV, *et al.* Timolol and atenolol: relationships between oxidation phenotype, pharmacokinetics and pharmacodynamics. *Br J Clin Pharmacol* 1985; **19:** 329–33.
3. Lennard MS, *et al.* Timolol metabolism and debrisoquine oxidation polymorphism: a population study. *Br J Clin Pharmacol* 1989; **27:** 429–34.

## Uses and Administration

Timolol is a non-cardioselective beta blocker (p.868). It is reported to lack intrinsic sympathomimetic and membrane-stabilising activity.

Timolol is used as the maleate in the management of glaucoma (p.1485), hypertension (p.825), angina pectoris (p.813), and myocardial infarction (p.828). It is also used in the prophylactic treatment of migraine (p.464). The hemihydrate is also used.

Eye drops containing timolol maleate or hemihydrate equivalent to 0.25 and 0.5% of timolol are instilled twice daily to reduce **raised intra-ocular pressure** in open-angle **glaucoma** and ocular hypertension. Once-daily instillation may suffice when the intra-ocular pressure has been controlled. Gel-forming eye drops are also available that are instilled once daily.

In **hypertension** timolol maleate is usually given in initial doses of 10 mg daily by mouth, increased according to response at intervals of 7 or more days. Usual maintenance doses are 10 to 40 mg daily, but doses up to 60 mg daily may be required in some patients; doses above 30 mg daily should be given in 2 equally divided doses.

In **angina pectoris** an initial dose of 5 mg two or three times daily has been recommended, increased at intervals of 3 or more days by no more than 10 mg daily initially and 15 mg daily subsequently, in divided doses. Most patients respond to 35 to 45 mg daily in divided doses, but some patients may require up to 60 mg daily.

In patients who have had a **myocardial infarction** timolol maleate is given in initial doses of 5 mg twice daily for 2 days, starting 7 to 28 days after infarction, and increased subsequently in the absence of any contra-indicating adverse effects, to 10 mg twice daily.

Doses of 10 to 20 mg daily of timolol maleate are used in the prophylaxis of **migraine**.

Reduced doses may be required in renal or hepatic impairment.

## Preparations

***BP 2003:*** Timolol Eye Drops; Timolol Tablets;
***USP 27:*** Timolol Maleate and Hydrochlorothiazide Tablets; Timolol Maleate Ophthalmic Solution; Timolol Maleate Tablets.

**Proprietary Preparations** (details are given in Part 3)
***Arg.:*** Glatim; Klonalol; Ofal; Plostim; Poentimol; Proflax; Protevis; Timed; Timoler; Timoptic; ***Austral.:*** Blocadren†; Optimol; Tenopt; Timoptol; Timoptol-XE; ***Austria:*** Blocadren; Dispatim; Ophtilan; Tim-Ophtal; Tima-

bak; Timax; Timoftal; Timohexal; Timoptic; **Belg.:** Blocadren; Timoptol; **Braz.:** Glautimol; Nyolol; Timabak†; Timoptol; **Canad.:** Apo-Timol; Apo-Timop; Beta-Tim†; Blocadren†; Novo-Timol; Tim-Ak; Timoptic; **Chile:** Glausolets; Nyolol; Timabak; Timop; Timoptol-XE; Tiof; **Denm.:** Aquanil; Oftamolol; Optimol; Timacar; Timosan; **Fin.:** Aquanil; Blocanol; Timosan; **Fr.:** Digaol; Nyogel; Nyolol; Ophtim; Timabak; Timacor; Timocomod; Timoptol; **Ger.:** Arutimol; Chibro-Timoptol; Dispatim; duratimol†; Nyogel; Tim-Ophtal; Timo-COMOD; Timo-Stulln; TimoEDO; Timohexal; Timomann; Timosine; **Gr.:** Flumetol; Glafemak; Lithimole; Nyolol; Temserin; Thilotim; Waucosin; Yesan; **Hong Kong:** Apo-Timop; Blocadren†; Cusimolol†; Glauco-Oph; Nyolol; Optimol; Timabak; Timoptol; **India:** Glucomol; Ocupres; Timolo; **Irl.:** Nyogel; Timoptol; **Israel:** Apotil†; Nyolol; Octil; Oftan†; Tiloptic; V-Optic; **Ital.:** Blocadren; Cusimolol; Droptimol; Nyogel; Oftimolo; Timolabak; Timolux; Timoptol; Timosoft; **Malaysia:** Cusimolol; Nyolol; Timoptol; **Mex.:** Blocadren†; Cusimolol†; Horex; Nyolol; Shemol; Timoptol; Timozzard; Tiof; **Mon.:** Gaoptol; **Neth.:** Blocadren†; Loptomit†; Timo-COMOD; Timoptol; **Norw.:** Aquanil; Betim†; Blocadren; Oftamolol; Oftan; Timosan; **NZ:** Apo-Timol†; Apo-Timop; Hypermol; Timoptol; **Port.:** Blocadren; Cusimolol; Nyogel; Nyolol; Timoglau; Timolen; Timoptol; **S.Afr.:** Blocadren†; Glaucosan; Timoptol; **Singapore:** Nyolol; Timabak; Timoptol; **Spain:** Cusimolol; Nyolol; Timoftol; Timogel; Unitimoftol†; **Swed.:** Aquanil; Blocadren; Optimol; Timosan; **Switz.:** Blocadren†; Nyolol; Oftan; Timisol; Timoptic; **Thai.:** Glauco-Oph; Nyolol; Oftan; Timo-Optal; Timodrop; Timoptol; Timosil; **UK:** Betim; Blocadren†; Glau-opt; Glaucol†; Nyogel; Timoptol; **USA:** Betimol; Blocadren; Timoptic.

**Multi-ingredient: Arg.:** Cosopt; Dorzoflax; Glaucocin; Glaucotensil; Glaucotensil TD; Moducren; Ofal P; Pilotim; Timed D; Timpilo; **Austral.:** Cosopt; Timpilo; Xalacom; **Austria:** Cosopt; Fotil; Moducrin; Timpilo; Timsopt; **Belg.:** Cosopt; Xalacom; **Braz.:** Cosopt; **Canad.:** Cosopt; Timolide; Timpilo; **Chile:** Cosopt; Dorsof T; Glaucotensil T; Latof-T; Xalacom; **Denm.:** Cosopt; Fotil; Timpilo; Xalcom; **Fin.:** Cosopt; Fotil; Timpilo; Xalcom; **Fr.:** Cosopt; Moducren; Timpilo; Xalacom; **Ger.:** Cosopt; Fotil; Moducrin; Timpilo; TP-Ophtal; Xalacom; **Gr.:** Cosopt; **Hong Kong:** Cosopt; Moducren; Timpilo; **Irl.:** Cosopt; Moducren; Prestim†; Xalacom; **Israel:** Cosopt; Timpilo; **Ital.:** Cosopt; Equiton; Glautimol; Pilobloc; Timicon; Xalacom; **Malaysia:** Timpilo; **Mex.:** Cosopt; Moducren†; Timpilo†; **Neth.:** Cosopt; Moducren†; Timpilo; Xalacom; **Norw.:** Cosopt; Fotil; Timpilo; Xalcom; **NZ:** Cosopt; Timpilo; **Port.:** Moducren; Timoglau Plus; Xalacom; **S.Afr.:** Cosopt; Moducren; Servatrin; **Singapore:** Cosopt; Timpilo; Xalacom; **Spain:** Xalacom; **Swed.:** Cosopt; Fotil; Timpilo; Xalcom; **Switz.:** Cosopt; Fotil; Moducren; Timpilo; Xalacom; **Thai.:** Cosopt; Fotil; **UK:** Cosopt; Moducren; Prestim; Xalacom; **USA:** Cosopt; Timolide.

## Tinzaparin Sodium *(BAN, USAN, rINN)*

Tinzaparina sódica; Tinzaparinum Natricum.

*CAS — 9041-08-1.*

*ATC — B01AB10.*

**Pharmacopoeias.** In *Eur.* (see p.vi).

**Ph. Eur. 5.0** (Tinzaparin Sodium). It is prepared by enzymatic depolymerisation, using heparinase from *Flavobacterium heparinum*, of heparin obtained from the intestinal mucosa of pigs. The majority of the components have a 2-*O*-sulfo-4-enepyranosuronic acid structure at the non-reducing end and a 2-*N*,6-*O*-disulfo-D-glucosamine structure at the reducing end of their chain. The mass-average molecular mass ranges between 5500 and 7500, with a characteristic value of about 6500. The mass percentage of chains lower than 2000 is not more than 10%. The degree of sulfation is 1.8 to 2.5 per disaccharide unit. The potency is not less than 70 units and not more than 120 units of anti-factor Xa activity per mg with reference to the dried substance and the ratio of anti-factor Xa activity to anti-factor IIa (antithrombin) activity is between 1.5 and 2.5.

### Units

As for Low-molecular-weight Heparins, p.949.

### Adverse Effects, Treatment, and Precautions

As for Low-molecular-weight Heparins, p.949.

Severe bleeding with tinzaparin sodium may be reduced by the slow intravenous injection of protamine sulfate; 1 mg of protamine sulfate is stated to inhibit the effects of 100 units of tinzaparin sodium.

### Interactions

As for Low-molecular-weight Heparins, p.950.

### Pharmacokinetics

Tinzaparin sodium is absorbed following subcutaneous injection with a bioavailability of about 90%. Peak plasma activity is reached within 4 to 6 hours. The elimination half-life is about 90 minutes but detectable anti-factor Xa activity persists for up to 24 hours.

### Uses and Administration

Tinzaparin sodium is a low-molecular-weight heparin (p.949) with anticoagulant properties. It is used in the treatment and prophylaxis of venous thromboembolism (p.839) and to prevent clotting during extracorporeal circulation.

For prophylaxis of **venous thromboembolism** during general surgical procedures 3500 units of tinzaparin sodium are given by subcutaneous injection 2 hours before the procedure, followed by 3500 units once daily for 7 to 10 days. In patients undergoing orthopaedic surgery a dose of 50 units/kg has been recommended; alternatively, a dose of 4500 units may be given 12 hours before surgery, followed by 4500 units once daily. For the treatment of venous thromboembolism tinzaparin sodium is given in a dose of 175 units/kg by subcutaneous injection once daily for at least 6 days and until adequate oral anticoagulation is established.

For prevention of clotting in the extracorporeal circulation during **haemodialysis**, tinzaparin sodium may be administered into the arterial side of the dialyser or intravenously. The dialyser may be primed with 500 to 1000 mL sodium chloride 0.9% containing 5000 units tinzaparin sodium/litre. For dialysis sessions lasting less than 4 hours a single dose of 2000 to 2500 units tinzaparin sodium is given; for longer sessions an initial dose of 2500 units is followed by an infusion of 750 units/hour.

◊ References.


1. Friedel HA, Balfour JA. Tinzaparin: a review of its pharmacology and clinical potential in the prevention and treatment of thrombo-embolic disorders. *Drugs* 1994; **48:** 638–60.
2. Neely JL, *et al.* Tinzaparin sodium: a low-molecular-weight heparin. *Am J Health-Syst Pharm* 2002; **59:** 1426–36.
3. Nutescu EA, *et al.* Tinzaparin: considerations for use in clinical practice. *Ann Pharmacother* 2003; **37:** 1831–40.


### Preparations

**Proprietary Preparations** (details are given in Part 3)
**Arg.:** Innohep; **Austria:** Logiparin†; **Belg.:** Innohep; **Canad.:** Innohep; **Denm.:** Innohep; **Fin.:** Innohep; **Fr.:** Innohep; **Ger.:** Innohep; **Gr.:** Innohep; **Hong Kong:** Innohep; **Irl.:** Innohep; **Israel:** Innohep; **Ital.:** Innohep†; **Malaysia:** Innohep; **Neth.:** Innohep; **Norw.:** Innohep; **NZ:** Innohep; **Port.:** Innohep; **Singapore:** Innohep; **Spain:** Innohep; **Swed.:** Innohep; **Thai.:** Innohep; **UK:** Innohep; **USA:** Innohep.

## Tioclomarol *(rINN)*

LM-550. 3-[5-Chloro-α-(4-chloro-β-hydroxyphenethyl)-2-thenyl]-4-hydroxycoumarin.

$C_{22}H_{16}Cl_2O_4S$ = 447.3.

*CAS — 22619-35-8.*

*ATC — B01AA11.*

### Profile

Tioclomarol is an orally administered coumarin anticoagulant with actions similar to those of warfarin (p.1022) that has been used in the management of thromboembolic disorders.

### Preparations

**Proprietary Preparations** (details are given in Part 3)
**Fr.:** Apegmone†.

## Tirilazad Mesilate *(BANM, rINNM)*

Mesilato de tirilazad; Tirilazad Mesylate *(USAN)*; U-74006F (tirilazad or tirilazad mesilate). 21-[4-(2,6-Di-1-pyrrolidinyl-4-pyrimidinyl)-1-piperazinyl]-16α-methylpregna-1,4,9(11)-triene-3,20-dione monomethanesulfonate hydrate.

$C_{38}H_{52}N_6O_2,CH_4O_3S,xH_2O$ = 721.0 (anhydrous).

*CAS — 110101-66-1 (tirilazad); 111793-42-1 (tirilazad mesilate); 149042-61-5 (tirilazad mesilate).*

*ATC — N07XX01.*

### Profile

Tirilazad, a lazaroid, is an inhibitor of lipid peroxidation thought to have a cytoprotective effect against radicals produced in response to tissue trauma. It may be used in the prevention of secondary tissue damage in subarachnoid haemorrhage (see Stroke, p.836). It is under investigation in spinal cord injuries (p.1088) and has also been investigated in head injuries and ischaemic stroke.

In subarachnoid haemorrhage the dose is 1.5 mg/kg of tirilazad mesilate by intravenous infusion every 6 hours for 8 to 10 days, starting within 48 hours of the onset of haemorrhage. Each dose should be infused over 10 to 30 minutes. This dosage regimen is only recommended for males; tirilazad clearance is higher in females than males and this dosage is ineffective in females.

◊ References.


1. Fleishaker JC, *et al.* Evaluation of the pharmacokinetics and tolerability of tirilazad mesylate, a 21-aminosteroid free radical scavenger: multiple-dose administration. *J Clin Pharmacol* 1993; **33:** 182–90.
2. Hulst LK, *et al.* Effect of age and gender on tirilazad pharmacokinetics in humans. *Clin Pharmacol Ther* 1994; **55:** 378–84.
3. Haley EC, *et al.* Phase II trial of tirilazad in aneurysmal subarachnoid haemorrhage: a report of the Cooperative Aneurysm Study. *J Neurosurg* 1995; **82:** 786–90.
4. Clark WM, *et al.* Lazaroids: CNS pharmacology and current research. *Drugs* 1995; **50:** 971–83.
5. Marshall LF, *et al.* A multicenter trial on the efficacy of using tirilazad mesylate in cases of head injury. *J Neurosurg* 1998; **89:** 519–25.
6. Fleishaker JC, *et al.* Hormonal effects on tirilazad clearance in women: assessment of the role of CYP3A. *J Clin Pharmacol* 1999; **39:** 260–7.
7. The Tirilazad International Steering Committee. Tirilazad for acute ischaemic stroke. Available in The Cochrane Library; Issue 2. Chichester: John Wiley; 2004.


### Preparations

**Proprietary Preparations** (details are given in Part 3)
**Austral.:** Freedox†; **Austria:** Freedox; **Belg.:** Freedox; **Denm.:** Freedox†; **Fin.:** Freedox†; **Norw.:** Freedox†; **S.Afr.:** Freedox; **Swed.:** Freedox†; **Switz.:** Freedox.

## Tirofiban Hydrochloride

*(BANM, USAN, rINNM)*

Hidrocloruro de tirofibán; L-700462; MK-383; MK-0383. *N*-(Butylsulfonyl)-4-[4-(4-piperidyl)butoxy]-L-phenylalanine hydrochloride monohydrate.

$C_{22}H_{36}N_2O_5S,HCl,H_2O$ = 495.1.

*CAS — 144494-65-5 (tirofiban); 142373-60-2 (anhydrous tirofiban hydrochloride); 150915-40-5 (tirofiban hydrochloride monohydrate);.*

*ATC — B01AC17.*

### Adverse Effects

Bleeding is the most common adverse effect of tirofiban. Other side-effects include nausea, headache, fever, rashes and other hypersensitivity reactions, and thrombocytopenia.

### Precautions

As for Abciximab, p.841.

### Pharmacokinetics

After stopping an infusion of tirofiban, the antiplatelet effect persists for about 4 to 8 hours. The plasma half-life is about 2 hours. Tirofiban is not highly bound to plasma proteins; the unbound fraction in plasma is about 35%. Tirofiban is eliminated largely unchanged in the urine, with some biliary excretion in the faeces. Tirofiban is removed by haemodialysis.

◊ Reviews.


1. Kondo K, Umemura K. Clinical pharmacokinetics of tirofiban, a nonpeptide glycoprotein IIb/IIIa receptor antagonist: comparison with the monoclonal antibody abciximab. *Clin Pharmacokinet* 2002; **41:** 187–95.


### Uses and Administration

Tirofiban hydrochloride is an antiplatelet drug that reversibly inhibits binding of fibrinogen to the glycoprotein IIb/IIIa receptors of platelets. It is given in combination with heparin and aspirin for the management of unstable angina, both in patients managed medically and in those undergoing percutaneous coronary procedures. Tirofiban is used as the hydrochloride, but the dose is expressed in terms of the base; 110 nanograms of tirofiban hydrochloride monohydrate is equivalent to 100 nanograms of tirofiban base.

Tirofiban is administered intravenously, at an initial rate of 400 nanograms/kg per minute for 30 minutes, and then continued at 100 nanograms/kg per minute. The recommended duration of treatment is at least 48 hours. Tirofiban infusion may be continued during coronary angiography, and should be maintained for 12 to 24 hours after angioplasty or atherectomy. The entire duration of treatment should not exceed 108 hours.

The dose of tirofiban should be reduced in patients with renal impairment (see below).

◊ General references.


1. McClellan KJ, Goa KL. Tirofiban: a review of its use in acute coronary syndromes. *Drugs* 1998; **56:** 1067–80.


**Administration in renal impairment.** Patients with renal impairment (creatinine clearance less than 30 mL/minute) should receive half the usual infusion dose of tirofiban.

**Ischaemic heart disease.** Patients with acute coronary syndromes may be treated either medically or with percutaneous coronary interventions such as angioplasty or stenting. Beneficial results have been reported in patients receiving tirofiban, in combination with heparin and aspirin, as an adjunct to medical or interventional therapy. A study[1] comparing tirofiban with heparin in the **medical management** of unstable angina (p.813) or non-Q-wave myocardial infarction reported an initial benefit, at 2 days, of reduced risk of refractory ischaemia, myocardial infarction, or death with tirofiban. This benefit was not maintained at 7 or 30 days following treatment, although a further analysis[2] found that the risk of death or myocardial infarction at

30 days was reduced in patients with raised troponin I concentrations who received tirofiban. In another study,[3] the combination of heparin and tirofiban also reduced the risk of refractory ischaemia, myocardial infarction, or death, compared with heparin alone, and benefit was maintained at 6 months. About half of these patients also underwent revascularisation procedures or surgery if required.

Tirofiban has also been studied in patients undergoing **interventional therapy** (angioplasty or atherectomy) within 72 hours of presentation with unstable angina or myocardial infarction.[4] Compared with heparin alone, tirofiban with heparin reduced the risk of death, non-fatal myocardial infarction, or repeat revascularisation at 2 and 7 days, but this benefit was not maintained at 30 days following treatment. Follow-up at 6 months showed no reduction in the incidence of restenosis. A further study[5] comparing tirofiban with abciximab in patients undergoing planned percutaneous intervention found that, after 30 days, tirofiban was less effective than abciximab in this setting. However, follow-up at 6 months[6] found that both drugs gave similar results.

1. The Platelet Receptor Inhibition in Ischemic Syndrome Management (PRISM) Study Investigators. A comparison of aspirin plus tirofiban with aspirin plus heparin for unstable angina. *N Engl J Med* 1998; **338:** 1498–1505.
2. Heeschen C, *et al.* Troponin concentrations for stratification of patients with acute coronary syndromes in relation to therapeutic efficacy of tirofiban. *Lancet* 1999; **354:** 1757–62.
3. The Platelet Receptor Inhibition in Ischemic Syndrome Management in Patients Limited by Unstable Signs and Symptoms (PRISM-PLUS) Study Investigators. Inhibition of the platelet glycoprotein IIb/IIIa receptor with tirofiban in unstable angina and non-Q-wave myocardial infarction. *N Engl J Med* 1998; **338:** 1488–97.
4. Gibson CM, *et al.* Six-month angiographic and clinical follow-up of patients prospectively randomized to receive either tirofiban or placebo during angioplasty in the RESTORE trial. *J Am Coll Cardiol* 1998; **32:** 28–34.
5. Topol EJ, *et al.* Comparison of two platelet glycoprotein IIb/IIIa inhibitors, tirofiban and abciximab, for the prevention of ischemic events with percutaneous coronary revascularization. *N Engl J Med* 2001; **344:** 1888–94.
6. Moliterno DJ, *et al.* Outcomes at 6 months for the direct comparison of tirofiban and abciximab during percutaneous coronary revascularisation with stent placement: the TARGET follow-up study. *Lancet* 2002; **360:** 355–60.

## Preparations

**Proprietary Preparations** (details are given in Part 3)

***Arg.:*** Agrastat; ***Austral.:*** Aggrastat; ***Austria:*** Aggrastat; ***Belg.:*** Aggrastat; ***Braz.:*** Agrastat; ***Canad.:*** Aggrastat; ***Denm.:*** Aggrastat; ***Fin.:*** Aggrastat; ***Fr.:*** Agrastat; ***Ger.:*** Aggrastat; ***Gr.:*** Aggrastat; ***Hong Kong:*** Aggrastat; ***Irl.:*** Aggrastat; ***Israel:*** Aggrastat; ***Ital.:*** Aggrastat; ***Malaysia:*** Aggrastat; ***Mex.:*** Aggrastat; ***Neth.:*** Aggrastat; ***Norw.:*** Aggrastat; ***NZ:*** Aggrastat; ***S.Afr.:*** Aggrastet; ***Singapore:*** Aggrastat; ***Spain:*** Agrastat; ***Swed.:*** Aggrastat; ***Switz.:*** Aggrastat; ***UK:*** Aggrastat; ***USA:*** Aggrastat.

---

# Tocainide *(BAN, USAN, rINN)*

W-36095. 2-Aminopropiono-2′,6′-xylidide.

$C_{11}H_{16}N_2O = 192.3$.

*CAS — 41708-72-9.*

*ATC — C01BB03.*

## Tocainide Hydrochloride *(BANM, rINNM)*

Hidrocloruro de tocainida.

$C_{11}H_{16}N_2O,HCl = 228.7$.

*CAS — 35891-93-1.*

*ATC — C01BB03.*

**Pharmacopoeias.** In *Chin.* and *US.*

**USP 27** (Tocainide Hydrochloride). A fine, white, odourless powder. Freely soluble in water and in alcohol; practically insoluble in chloroform and in ether.

## Adverse Effects

Tocainide causes severe haematological toxicity leading to neutropenia, agranulocytosis, thrombocytopenia, and aplastic anaemia; fatalities have occurred. Pulmonary toxicity has also proved fatal; patients have developed interstitial pneumonitis, pulmonary fibrosis, and other respiratory disorders.

The most common side-effects are dose-related CNS and gastrointestinal effects including tremor, dizziness, paraesthesia, lightheadedness, blurred vision, and nausea. These may occur particularly in the initial stages of therapy and may be transient. Other less frequent gastrointestinal side-effects include vomiting, anorexia, constipation, and diarrhoea. Various mental changes and ataxia have been reported.

Other adverse effects reported include skin rash, lupus erythematosus, sweating, tinnitus, taste disturbances, and liver disorders.

As with other antiarrhythmics, tocainide can cause various cardiac arrhythmias and disturbances of conduction. Bradycardia and hypotension may occur particularly after intravenous administration.

◊ The adverse effects associated with the class Ib antiarrhythmics tocainide, lidocaine, and mexiletine, have been reviewed,[1] with guidelines for the clinical management of toxicity.

1. Denaro CP, Benowitz NL. Poisoning due to class 1B antiarrhythmic drugs: lignocaine, mexiletine and tocainide. *Med Toxicol Adverse Drug Exp* 1989; **4:** 412–28.

**Effects on the blood.** Adverse haematological effects associated with tocainide are serious and have caused fatalities.[1-3] They include agranulocytosis, aplastic anaemia, thrombocytopenia, and neutropenia. The US manufacturer has reported that haematological reactions occur in up to 0.18% of patients and that the mortality rate of patients who develop agranulocytosis is 25%.

These haematological reactions usually occur in the first 12 weeks of treatment and it is therefore recommended that full blood counts are performed weekly during this time and monthly thereafter. Patients should be advised to report promptly any unusual bleeding or bruising, or signs of infection such as fever, sore throat, or chills. The seriousness of these adverse effects limits the use of tocainide.

1. Holmes GI, *et al.* Drug therapy: flecainide and tocainide. *N Engl J Med* 1987; **316:** 344.
2. Volosin K, *et al.* Tocainide associated agranulocytosis. *Am Heart J* 1985; **109:** 1392–3.
3. Morrill GB. Tocainide-induced aplastic anemia. *DICP Ann Pharmacother* 1989; **23:** 90–1.

**Effects on the liver.** Acute hepatocellular damage in one patient[1] and granulomatous hepatitis in another[2] have been associated with tocainide therapy.

1. Farquhar DL, Davidson NM. Possible hepatotoxicity of tocainide. *Scott Med J* 1984; **29:** 238.
2. Tucker LE. Tocainide-induced granulomatous hepatitis. *JAMA* 1986; **255:** 3362.

**Effects on the lungs.** Interstitial pneumonitis[1-3] and pulmonary fibrosis[4,5] have been reported in small numbers of patients receiving tocainide.

1. Perlow GM, *et al.* Tocainide-associated interstitial pneumonitis. *Ann Intern Med* 1981; **94:** 489.
2. Van Natta B, *et al.* Irreversible interstitial pneumonitis associated with tocainide therapy. *West J Med* 1988; **149:** 91–2.
3. Ahmad S. Tocainide: interstitial pneumonitis. *J Am Coll Cardiol* 1990; **15:** 1458.
4. Subauste CS, *et al.* Tocainide-induced pulmonary toxicity. *Illinois Med J* 1988; **174:** 287–9.
5. Feinberg L, *et al.* Pulmonary fibrosis associated with tocainide: report of a case with literature review. *Am Rev Respir Dis* 1990; **141:** 505–8.

**Effects on mental state.** Confusion, paranoia, and hallucinations have been reported[1-3] in a few patients receiving tocainide at recommended doses; all symptoms resolved on discontinuing tocainide. In one patient the reaction was confirmed by rechallenge with tocainide.

1. Currie P, Ramsdale DR. Paranoid psychosis induced by tocainide. *BMJ* 1984; **288:** 606–7.
2. Harrison DJ, Wathen CG. Paranoid psychosis induced by tocainide. *BMJ* 1984; **288:** 1010–11.
3. Clarke CWF, El-Mahdi EO. Confusion and paranoia associated with oral tocainide. *Postgrad Med J* 1985; **61:** 79–81.

**Effects on the skin.** The US FDA received 21 reports of severe dermatologic reactions associated with tocainide therapy during 1985 and 1986.[1] These included erythema multiforme, Stevens-Johnson syndrome, and exfoliative dermatitis. The reaction occurred within 3 weeks of starting tocainide in 67% of patients for whom the duration of treatment was given. Seventeen patients recovered on withdrawal of tocainide, 2 patients died, and the outcome was not available for 2 patients.

1. Arrowsmith JB, *et al.* Severe dermatologic reactions reported after treatment with tocainide. *Ann Intern Med* 1987; **107:** 693–6.

**Overdosage.** In overdosage with tocainide there may be convulsions, complete heart block, and asystole. Treatment is symptomatic and supportive. Haemodialysis and possibly charcoal haemoperfusion may be helpful. Treatment may need to be continued for a prolonged period due to tocainide's long half-life.

Fatal overdose occurred in a 70-year-old man after taking tocainide 16 g by mouth.[1] Postmortem tocainide concentrations were 384.8 micromol/mL in the blood and 2860 micromol/mL in the urine. Toxic effects included convulsions, complete heart block, multiple ventricular ectopic beats, profound hypotension, evidence of ischaemic cardiac changes, and multiple episodes of asystole which were eventually unresponsive to cardiac pacing.

1. Clarke CWF, El-Mahdi EO. Fatal oral tocainide overdosage. *BMJ* 1984; **288:** 760.

## Precautions

Tocainide should not be used in patients with second- or third-degree atrioventricular block in the absence of a pacemaker, or in patients with hypersensitivity to amide-type drugs. It should be used with caution in patients with uncompensated heart failure and in patients receiving other antiarrhythmics. Blood counts should be monitored weekly during the first 12 weeks of therapy and monthly thereafter. Tocainide should be given with caution to patients with hepatic or renal impairment. Hypokalaemia should be corrected before initiating tocainide therapy.

## Interactions

Tocainide is structurally related to lidocaine and concomitant use may produce additive CNS side-effects. Tocainide is metabolised in the liver and enzyme-inducing drugs may reduce the elimination half-life of tocainide.

Tocainide may have a modest inhibitory effect on theophylline metabolism (p.801).

**Antibacterials.** *Rifampicin* increased the total clearance and reduced the elimination half-life of tocainide in 8 healthy subjects,[1] probably due to an increase in hepatic metabolism of tocainide.

1. Rice TL, *et al.* Influence of rifampin on tocainide pharmacokinetics in humans. *Clin Pharm* 1989; **8:** 200–5.

**Histamine $H_2$-antagonists.** *Cimetidine* has been reported[1] to decrease the bioavailability of tocainide without affecting the renal clearance or half-life. The exact mechanism of the interaction could not be determined but may have been due to reduced absorption of tocainide secondary to a cimetidine-induced increase in gastrointestinal pH; however, no interaction was observed with *ranitidine*.

1. North DS, *et al.* The effect of histamine-2 receptor antagonists on tocainide pharmacokinetics. *J Clin Pharmacol* 1988; **28:** 640–3.

## Pharmacokinetics

Tocainide is readily and almost completely absorbed from the gastrointestinal tract. It is widely distributed throughout the body and is reported to be about 10% bound to plasma proteins.

Tocainide is metabolised to a number of apparently inactive metabolites and is excreted mainly in the urine, 30 to 50% as unchanged drug. It has an elimination half-life of about 10 to 20 hours; renal clearance is reduced in alkaline urine but acidification has no effect on excretion. Its therapeutic effect has been correlated with plasma concentrations of about 3 to 10 micrograms/mL.

## Uses and Administration

Tocainide is a class Ib antiarrhythmic (p.809) with actions similar to those of lidocaine (p.1379) to which it is structurally related. Unlike lidocaine, it undergoes negligible first-pass metabolism and can be given by mouth. Because of its toxicity (see Adverse Effects, above) tocainide is generally restricted to the treatment of life-threatening ventricular **arrhythmias** (p.816) that cannot be treated by other means.

For treatment of chronic arrhythmias tocainide hydrochloride is given by mouth at an initial dose of 400 mg every 8 hours, adjusted according to response. The usual maintenance dose is 1.2 to 1.8 g daily in 2 or 3 divided doses; doses above 2.4 g daily are not normally required. Treatment should be initiated in hospital under ECG monitoring. Doses may need to be reduced in patients with hepatic or renal impairment (see below). Tocainide hydrochloride was also formerly given intravenously for rapid control of acute arrhythmias.

◊ General references.

1. Holmes B, *et al.* Tocainide: a review of its pharmacological properties and therapeutic efficacy. *Drugs* 1983; **26:** 93–123.
2. Kutalek SP, *et al.* Tocainide: a new oral antiarrhythmic agent. *Ann Intern Med* 1985; **103:** 387–91.
3. Roden DM, Woosley RL. Tocainide. *N Engl J Med* 1986; **315:** 41–5.

**Administration in renal impairment.** Tocainide is mainly excreted in the urine, and in patients with renal impairment the elimination of tocainide is impaired and the half-life prolonged.[1,2] Alterations of urine pH can cause clinically significant alterations in tocainide excretion in patients with mild to moderate renal impairment.[2] It has been recommended[1] that the dose of tocainide should be reduced by 50% in patients with severe impairment; smaller reductions may be necessary in patients with less severe impairment.

Haemodialysis has been reported[1] to remove 25% of tocainide present in the body and a half-life of 8.5 hours was reported; patients may need a supplemental dose of tocainide following haemodialysis.

1. Wiegers U, *et al.* Pharmacokinetics of tocainide in patients with renal dysfunction and during haemodialysis. *Eur J Clin Pharmacol* 1983; **24:** 503–7.
2. Braun J, *et al.* Pharmacokinetics of tocainide in patients with severe renal failure. *Eur J Clin Pharmacol* 1985; **28:** 665–70.

### Preparations

***USP 27:*** Tocainide Hydrochloride Tablets.

**Proprietary Preparations** (details are given in Part 3)
***Canad.:*** Tonocard†; ***Ger.:*** Xylotocan; ***Hong Kong:*** Tonocard†; ***Neth.:*** Tonocard†; ***Swed.:*** Tonocard†; ***Thai.:*** Tonocard†; ***UK:*** Tonocard†; ***USA:*** Tonocard†.

## Tocoferil Nicotinate

Tocoferilo, nicotinato de; Tocopheryl Nicotinate; Vitamin E Nicotinate. (±)-α-Tocopherol nicotinate.

$C_{35}H_{53}NO_3$ = 535.8.

*CAS — 51898-34-1; 16676-75-8.*

**Pharmacopoeias.** In *Jpn.*

### Profile

Tocoferil nicotinate is a lipid regulating drug and a vasodilator. It is used in the treatment of hyperlipidaemias (p.823), and in peripheral (p.831) and cerebral vascular disorders (p.820). The usual dose is 100 to 200 mg three times daily by mouth.

### Preparations

**Proprietary Preparations** (details are given in Part 3)
***Hong Kong:*** Hijuven; ***Jpn:*** Juvela; ***Malaysia:*** Hijuven; ***Port.:*** Nicojuvel; Reoferol; ***Spain:*** Disclar†; Vitaber PP + E†; ***Thai.:*** Hijuven†.

**Multi-ingredient:** ***Arg.:*** Anaphase; ***Fr.:*** Anaphase; ***Ital.:*** Evitex; ***Spain:*** Evitex A E Fuerte.

## Tocofibrate *(rINN)*

Tocofibrato. 2,5,7,8-Tetramethyl-2-(4,8,12-trimethyltridecyl)-6-chromanyl 2-(4-chlorophenoxy)-2-methylpropionate.

$C_{39}H_{59}ClO_4$ = 627.3.

*CAS — 50465-39-9.*

### Profile

Tocofibrate, a fibric acid derivative (see Bezafibrate, p.873), is a lipid regulating drug that has been used in the treatment of hyperlipidaemias.

### Preparations

**Proprietary Preparations** (details are given in Part 3)
***Spain:*** Transferal†.

## Todralazine Hydrochloride *(BANM, pINNM)*

BT-621; CEPH; Ecarazine Hydrochloride; Hidrocloruro de todralazina. Ethyl 3-(phthalazin-1-yl)carbazate hydrochloride monohydrate.

$C_{11}H_{12}N_4O_2,HCl,H_2O$ = 286.7.

*CAS — 14679-73-3 (todralazine); 3778-76-5 (anhydrous todralazine hydrochloride).*

**Pharmacopoeias.** In *Jpn* and *Pol.*

### Profile

Todralazine hydrochloride is an antihypertensive structurally related to hydralazine (p.931) and with similar properties.

## Tolazoline Hydrochloride *(BANM, rINNM)*

Benzazoline Hydrochloride; Hidrocloruro de tolazolina; Tolazol. Hydrochlor.; Tolazolinium Chloratum. 2-Benzyl-2-imidazoline hydrochloride.

$C_{10}H_{12}N_2,HCl$ = 196.7.

*CAS — 59-98-3 (tolazoline); 59-97-2 (tolazoline hydrochloride).*

*ATC — C04AB02; M02AX02.*

**Pharmacopoeias.** In *Chin.* and *US.*

**USP 27** (Tolazoline Hydrochloride). A white to off-white, crystalline powder. Its solutions are slightly acid to litmus. Soluble 1 in less than 1 of water, 1 in 2 of alcohol, 1 in 3 of chloroform, and 1 in 10 000 of ether. Store at a temperature of 25°, excursions permitted between 15° and 30°.

### Adverse Effects

Side-effects of tolazoline include piloerection, headache, flushing, tachycardia, cardiac arrhythmias, tingling, chilliness, shivering, sweating, nausea, vomiting, diarrhoea, and epigastric pain. Orthostatic hypotension or marked hypertension may occur, especially with large doses. Tolazoline stimulates gastric acid and may exacerbate peptic ulcer disease. Oliguria, haematuria, myocardial infarction, gastrointestinal haemorrhage, thrombocytopenia and other blood dyscrasias have been reported.

Intra-arterial injection has been followed by a burning sensation in the limb.

**Effects in the neonate.** Hypochloraemic metabolic alkalosis,[1] acute renal failure,[2] and duodenal perforation[3] have been reported in neonates given tolazoline.

1. Adams JM, *et al.* Hypochloremic metabolic alkalosis following tolazoline-induced gastric hypersecretion. *Pediatrics* 1980; **65:** 298–300.
2. Trompeter RS, *et al.* Tolazoline and acute renal failure in the newborn. *Lancet* 1981; **i:** 1219.
3. Wilson RG, *et al.* Duodenal perforation associated with tolazoline. *Arch Dis Child* 1985; **60:** 878–9.

### Treatment of Adverse Effects

In the event of overdosage hypotension is best treated by keeping the patient recumbent with the head lowered. If necessary the circulation may be maintained by infusion of suitable electrolyte solutions. Hypotension may be treated with ephedrine. Adrenaline is not suitable for the reversal of hypotension induced by alpha blockers since it may exacerbate the hypotension by stimulating beta receptors.

### Precautions

Tolazoline should not be given to patients with ischaemic heart disease, hypotension, or after a cerebrovascular accident. Since tolazoline stimulates gastric secretion of hydrochloric acid, it should not be used in the presence of peptic ulcer disease. Pretreatment of infants with antacids may prevent gastrointestinal bleeding. Tolazoline should be used with caution in patients with mitral stenosis.

### Interactions

Tolazoline should not be used with drugs such as adrenaline since the hypotensive effect may be potentiated due to unopposed beta-adrenoceptor stimulation. Tolazoline may cause a disulfiram-like reaction if given with alcohol.

**Dopamine.** For the effect of tolazoline on dopamine, see p.907.

**Ranitidine.** Intravenous administration of ranitidine reversed the falls in pulmonary and systemic vascular resistances in 12 children who had been given tolazoline as a pulmonary vasodilator.[1]

1. Bush A, *et al.* Cardiovascular effects of tolazoline and ranitidine. *Arch Dis Child* 1987; **62:** 241–6.

### Pharmacokinetics

Tolazoline is absorbed from the gastrointestinal tract. It is more rapidly absorbed after intramuscular injection. A plasma half-life in neonates of 3 to 10 hours has been reported, although it may be as high as about 40 hours and is inversely related to urine output. Tolazoline is rapidly excreted in the urine, largely unchanged.

### Uses and Administration

Tolazoline hydrochloride is a vasodilator that has a direct dilator action on the peripheral blood vessels. It has some alpha-adrenoceptor blocking activity and also stimulates smooth muscle in the gastrointestinal tract, increases gastrointestinal secretion, can cause mydriasis, and has a stimulant effect on the heart.

Tolazoline hydrochloride is used intravenously to reduce pulmonary artery pressure in persistent pulmonary hypertension in newborn infants with persistent fetal circulation (see below). It has been used by mouth and by subcutaneous, intramuscular, intravenous, or slow intra-arterial injection in the treatment of peripheral vascular disease. It has also been given in some ophthalmic conditions.

**Pulmonary hypertension.** Tolazoline and other vasodilators have been tried in persistent pulmonary hypertension in the newborn (p.832) in an attempt to induce selective pulmonary vasodilatation and improve gas exchange. The response is variable and often unsuccessful due to concomitant systemic hypotension, a failure to achieve or sustain pulmonary vasodilatation, and adverse effects, and other therapies such as high-frequency oscillatory ventilation, extracorporeal membrane oxygenation, and inhaled nitric oxide are now more widely used.

The loading dose for pulmonary hypertension in neonates that has been recommended by the manufacturers is 1 to 2 mg/kg over 5 to 10 minutes by intravenous infusion; this is then followed by doses of up to 1 to 2 mg/kg per hour. Infants with reduced urine output may require lower maintenance doses. The high incidence of adverse effects has, however, led to several studies investigating the use of lower doses. One group suggested that a loading dose of 500 nanograms/kg given intravenously followed by a continuous infusion of 500 nanograms/kg per hour was more appropriate and safer than standard doses.[1] In a retrospective study[2] of extremely preterm infants (mean gestational age 24 weeks) with severe hypoxaemia (possibly attributable to persistent pulmonary hypertension), tolazoline was given as a slow bolus infusion, with most patients receiving a dose of 0.5 to 1 mg/kg; some required further doses.

Tolazoline has also been given via the endotracheal route,[3,4] although as tolazoline is acid in solution it may contribute to alveolar injury. In a study[4] of 12 neonates with gestational age ranging from 25 to 42 weeks, endotracheal tolazoline at doses from 1 to 2.5 mg/kg was found to cause no adverse systemic effects.

Some authorities[5] recommend a dose of 1 mg/kg by slow intravenous injection, followed by 200 micrograms/kg per hour by infusion if necessary; a suggested dose for endotracheal use is 200 micrograms/kg diluted in 0.5 to 1 mL of sodium chloride 0.9%.

1. Monin P, *et al.* Treatment of persistent fetal circulation syndrome of the newborn: comparison of different doses of tolazoline. *Eur J Clin Pharmacol* 1987; **31:** 569–73.
2. Nuntnarumit P, *et al.* Efficacy and safety of tolazoline for treatment of severe hypoxemia in extremely preterm infants. *Pediatrics* 2002; **109:** 852–6.
3. Welch JC, *et al.* Endotracheal tolazoline for severe persistent pulmonary hypertension of the newborn. *Br Heart J* 1995; **73:** 99–100.
4. Parida SK, *et al.* Endotracheal tolazoline administration in neonates with persistent pulmonary hypertension. *J Perinatol* 1997; **17:** 461–4.
5. Tolazoline. In: *Neonatal Formulary* 4. London: BMJ Books, 2003: 250.

### Preparations

***USP 27:*** Tolazoline Hydrochloride Injection.

**Proprietary Preparations** (details are given in Part 3)
***Austral.:*** Priscoline†; ***Austria:*** Vaso-Dilatan; ***Ger.:*** Priscol†; ***NZ:*** Priscoline†; ***USA:*** Priscoline†.

**Multi-ingredient:** ***Switz.:*** Lunadon.

## Torasemide *(BAN, rINN)*

AC-4464; BM-02015; Torasemida; Torsemide *(USAN)*. 1-Isopropyl-3-(4-*m*-toluidinopyridine-3-sulphonyl)urea.

$C_{16}H_{20}N_4O_3S$ = 348.4.

*CAS — 56211-40-6 (torasemide); 72810-59-4 (torasemide sodium).*

*ATC — C03CA04.*

**Pharmacopoeias.** In *US.*

**USP 27** (Torsemide). A white to off-white, crystalline powder. Practically insoluble in water and in ether; slightly soluble in alcohol, in methyl alcohol, in 0.1N sodium hydroxide, and in 0.1N hydrochloric acid; very slightly soluble in acetone and in chloroform.

### Adverse Effects and Precautions

As for Furosemide, p.919.

### Interactions

As for Furosemide, p.920.

### Pharmacokinetics

Torasemide is well absorbed from the gastrointestinal tract. Peak serum concentrations are achieved within 1 hour of oral administration. Torasemide is metabolised in the liver and inactive metabolites are excreted in the urine. The elimination half-life of torasemide is about 3.5 hours. Torasemide is extensively bound to plasma proteins. In patients with heart failure both hepatic and renal clearance are reduced. In patients with renal impairment, the renal clearance is reduced but total plasma clearance is not significantly altered.

◊ References.

1. Knauf H, Mutschler E. Clinical pharmacokinetics and pharmacodynamics of torasemide. *Clin Pharmacokinet* 1998; **34:** 1–24.

### Uses and Administration

Torasemide is a loop diuretic with actions similar to those of furosemide (p.921).

Torasemide is used for oedema associated with heart failure (p.820), including pulmonary oedema, and with renal and hepatic disorders. It is also used in the treatment of hypertension (p.825), either alone or with other antihypertensives.

Diuresis after oral use starts within 1 hour, reaches a maximum in about 1 to 2 hours, and lasts for up to 8 hours; after intravenous injection its effects are evident within 10 minutes but like oral use can last up to 8 hours.

In the treatment of **oedema** the usual dose is 5 mg once daily by mouth increased according to response to 20 mg once daily; doses of up to 40 mg daily have been required in some patients. Torasemide may also be given intravenously in usual doses of 10 to 20 mg daily. Higher intravenous doses may sometimes be necessary, especially in oedema of renal origin when an initial dose of 20 mg daily may be increased stepwise as necessary to a maximum of 200 mg daily, although doses should not exceed 40 mg daily in patients with hepatic cirrhosis.

In the treatment of **hypertension** torasemide is given in doses of 2.5 to 5 mg daily by mouth; sources in the USA have suggested that doses of up to 10 mg daily may be used although in the UK doses above 5 mg are considered unlikely to produce additional benefit.

◊ Reviews.

1. Blose JS, *et al.* Torsemide: a pyridine-sulfonylurea loop diuretic. *Ann Pharmacother* 1995; **29:** 396–402.
2. Dunn CJ, *et al.* Torasemide: an update of its pharmacological properties and therapeutic efficacy. *Drugs* 1995; **49:** 121–42.
3. Brater DC. Benefits and risks of torasemide in congestive heart failure and essential hypertension. *Drug Safety* 1996; **14:** 104–120.

### Preparations

**Proprietary Preparations** (details are given in Part 3)
***Austria:*** Unat; ***Belg.:*** Torrem; ***Canad.:*** Demadex†; ***Chile:*** Unat; ***Ger.:*** Torem; Unat; ***Hong Kong:*** Unat; ***Ital.:*** Diuremid; Diuresix; Toradiur; ***Jpn:***

Luprac; **Mex.:** Unat†; **S.Afr.:** Unat; **Spain:** Dilutol; Isodiur; Sutril; **Swed.:** Torem; **Switz.:** Torem; **UK:** Torem; **USA:** Demadex.

## Trandolapril *(BAN, rINN)*

RU-44570. Ethyl (2S,3aR,7aS)-1-{(S)-N-[(S)-1-carboxy-3-phenylpropyl]alanyl}hexahydro-2-indolinecarboxylate; (2S,3aR,7aS)-1-{N-[(S)-1-Ethoxycarbonyl-3-phenylpropyl]-L-alanyl}perhydroindole-2-carboxylic acid.

$C_{24}H_{34}N_2O_5$ = 430.5.

*CAS — 87679-37-6.*

*ATC — C09AA10.*

### Adverse Effects, Treatment, and Precautions

As for ACE inhibitors, p.842.

### Interactions

As for ACE inhibitors, p.845.

### Pharmacokinetics

Trandolapril acts as a prodrug of the diacid trandolaprilat, its active metabolite. Following oral administration of trandolapril the bioavailability of trandolaprilat is 40 to 60%. Trandolapril is metabolised in the liver to trandolaprilat and to some inactive metabolites. Peak plasma concentrations of trandolaprilat are achieved 4 to 6 hours after an oral dose of trandolapril. Trandolaprilat is more than 80% bound to plasma proteins. About 33% of an oral dose of trandolapril is excreted in the urine, mainly as trandolaprilat; the rest is excreted in the faeces. The effective half-life for accumulation of trandolaprilat is 16 to 24 hours following multiple doses of trandolapril.

Impaired renal function decreases the excretion of trandolaprilat. Trandolaprilat is removed by haemodialysis.

◊ References.


1. Bevan EG, *et al.* Effect of renal function on the pharmacokinetics and pharmacodynamics of trandolapril. *Br J Clin Pharmacol* 1993; **35:** 128–35.


### Uses and Administration

Trandolapril is an ACE inhibitor (p.842). It is used in the treatment of hypertension (p.825) and in left ventricular dysfunction following myocardial infarction (p.828).

Trandolapril owes its activity to trandolaprilat to which it is converted after oral administration. The haemodynamic effects are seen about 1 hour after an oral dose and the maximum effect occurs after 8 to 12 hours. The haemodynamic action lasts for at least 24 hours, allowing once-daily dosing.

In the treatment of **hypertension** the initial dose is 0.5 mg once daily by mouth. Since there may be a precipitous fall in blood pressure in some patients when starting therapy with an ACE inhibitor, the first dose should preferably be given at bedtime. In patients already receiving diuretic therapy, the diuretic should be discontinued, if possible, 2 to 3 days before starting trandolapril and resumed later if necessary. In patients with co-existing heart failure treatment with trandolapril should begin under close medical supervision. The usual maintenance dose for hypertension is 1 to 2 mg once daily, although up to 4 mg daily may be given, as a single dose or in 2 divided doses.

Following **myocardial infarction**, treatment with trandolapril may be started 3 days after the infarction in an initial dose of 0.5 mg once daily, gradually increased to a maximum of 4 mg once daily.

A reduction in dosage may be necessary in patients with renal impairment (see below).

◊ References.


1. Zannad F. Trandolapril: How does it differ from other angiotensin converting enzyme inhibitors? *Drugs* 1993; **46** (suppl 2): 172–82.
2. Wiseman LR, McTavish D. Trandolapril: a review of its pharmacodynamic and pharmacokinetic properties, and therapeutic use in essential hypertension. *Drugs* 1994; **48:** 71–90.
3. Køber L, *et al.* A clinical trial of the angiotensin-converting-enzyme inhibitor trandolapril in patients with left ventricular dysfunction after myocardial infarction. *N Engl J Med* 1995; **333:** 1670–6.
4. Peters DC, *et al.* Trandolapril: an update of its pharmacology and therapeutic use in cardiovascular disorders. *Drugs* 1998; **56:** 871–93.


**Administration in renal impairment.** The initial dose of trandolapril in patients with renal impairment should not exceed 0.5 mg daily. The UK manufacturer states that the maximum maintenance dose should be 2 mg daily in patients with a creatinine clearance of less than 10 mL/minute.

### Preparations

**Proprietary Preparations** (details are given in Part 3)
**Austral.:** Gopten; Odrik; **Austria:** Gopten; **Braz.:** Gopten; Odrik; **Canad.:** Mavik; **Denm.:** Gopten; Odrik; **Fin.:** Gopten; **Fr.:** Gopten; Odrik; **Ger.:** Gopten; Udrik; **Gr.:** Afenil; Odrik; **Irl.:** Gopten; Odrik; **Ital.:** Gopten; **Jpn:** Odric; Preran; **Mex.:** Gopten; **Neth.:** Gopten; **Norw.:** Gopten; **NZ:** Gopten; Odrik; **Port.:** Gopten; Odrik; **S.Afr.:** Gopten; **Spain:** Gopten; Odrik; **Swed.:** Gopten; **Switz.:** Gopten; **UK:** Gopten; Odrik; **USA:** Mavik.

**Multi-ingredient: Austria:** Tarka; **Braz.:** Tarka†; **Denm.:** Tarka; **Fin.:** Tarka; **Fr.:** Ocadrik; Tarka; **Ger.:** Tarka; Udramil; **Ital.:** Tarka; **Mex.:** Tarka; **Neth.:** Tarka; **S.Afr.:** Tarka; **Spain:** Tarka; Tricen; **Swed.:** Tarka; **Switz.:** Tarka; **UK:** Tarka; **USA:** Tarka.

## Trapidil *(BAN, rINN)*

AR-12008; Trapidilum. 7-Diethylamino-5-methyl-1,2,4-triazolo[1,5-*a*]pyrimidine.

$C_{10}H_{15}N_5$ = 205.3.

*CAS — 15421-84-8.*

*ATC — C01DX11.*

**Pharmacopoeias.** In *Eur.* (see p.vi) and *Jpn.*

**Ph. Eur. 5.0** (Trapidil). A white or almost white crystalline powder. Freely soluble in water; soluble in dehydrated alcohol and in dichloromethane. Protect from light.

### Profile

Trapidil is a vasodilator and an inhibitor of platelet aggregation. It is also an antagonist of platelet-derived growth factor. It is used in the management of ischaemic heart disease in doses of 300 to 400 mg daily, in divided doses, by mouth; doses of up to 600 mg daily may be used to prevent restenosis following angioplasty (see Reperfusion and Revascularisation Procedures, p.834). Ischaemic heart disease is discussed under Atherosclerosis (p.815) and the treatment of its clinical manifestations is described under Angina Pectoris (p.813) and Myocardial Infarction (p.828).

◊ References to anti-platelet activity.


1. Yasue H, *et al.* Effects of aspirin and trapidil on cardiovascular events after acute myocardial infarction: Japanese Antiplatelets Myocardial Infarction Study (JAMIS) Investigators. *Am J Cardiol* 1999; **83:** 1308–13.


◊ References to pharmacokinetics.


1. Harder S, *et al.* Pharmacokinetics of trapidil, an antagonist of platelet derived growth factor, in healthy subjects and in patients with liver cirrhosis. *Br J Clin Pharmacol* 1996; **42:** 443–9.


**Angioplasty and stenting.** Studies[1,2] have appeared to show that trapidil prevents restenosis after angioplasty. However, an investigation[3] into the use of trapidil after coronary stenting showed no benefit, and it was concluded that trapidil is not indicated for this purpose.


1. Okamoto S, *et al.* Effects of trapidil (triazolopyrimidine), a platelet-derived growth factor antagonist, in preventing restenosis after percutaneous transluminal coronary angioplasty. *Am Heart J* 1992; **123:** 1439–44.
2. Maresta A, *et al.* Trapidil (triazolopyrimidine), a platelet-derived growth factor antagonist, reduces restenosis after percutaneous transluminal coronary angioplasty: results of the randomized, double-blind STARC study. *Circulation* 1994; **90:** 2710–15.
3. Serruys PW, *et al.* The TRAPIST study: a multicentre randomized placebo controlled clinical trial of trapidil for prevention of restenosis after coronary stenting, measured by 3-D intravascular ultrasound. *Eur Heart J* 2001; **22:** 1938–47.


### Preparations

**Proprietary Preparations** (details are given in Part 3)
**Austria:** Rocornal; **Braz.:** Travisco; **Ger.:** Rocornal; **Ital.:** Avantrin; Travisco.

## Triamterene *(BAN, USAN, rINN)*

NSC-77625; SKF-8542; Triamtereno; Triamterenum; Trianterено. 6-Phenylpteridine-2,4,7-triamine; 2,4,7-Triamino-6-phenylpteridine.

$C_{12}H_{11}N_7$ = 253.3.

*CAS — 396-01-0.*

*ATC — C03DB02.*

NOTE. Compounded preparations of triamterene may be represented by the following names:

- Co-triamterzide (*BAN*)—triamterene 2 parts and hydrochlorothiazide 1 part (w/w)
- Co-triamterzide (*PEN*)—triamterene and hydrochlorothiazide.

**Pharmacopoeias.** In *Chin., Eur.* (see p.vi), *Jpn, Pol.,* and *US.*

**Ph. Eur. 5.0** (Triamterene). A yellow, crystalline powder. Very slightly soluble in water and in alcohol. Acidified solutions give a blue fluorescence. Protect from light.

**USP 27** (Triamterene). A yellow, odourless, crystalline powder. Practically insoluble in water, in chloroform, in ether, in benzene, and in dilute alkali hydroxides; very slightly soluble in alcohol, in acetic acid, and in dilute mineral acids; soluble 1 in 30 of formic acid and 1 in 85 of 2-methoxyethanol. Store in airtight containers. Protect from light.

### Adverse Effects

As for Amiloride Hydrochloride, p.858. Triamterene has also been reported to cause photosensitivity reactions, increases in uric acid concentrations, and blood dyscrasias. Renal calculi may occur in susceptible patients, and megaloblastic anaemia has been reported in patients with depleted folic acid stores such as those with hepatic cirrhosis. Reversible renal failure, due either to acute interstitial nephritis or to an interaction with NSAIDs (see under Interactions, below) has occurred.

**Incidence of adverse effects.** In a postmarketing surveillance study of 70 898 patients[1] taking triamterene with hydrochlorothiazide the most common adverse effects were fatigue, dizziness, and nausea. Adverse effects necessitated withdrawal in 8.1% of patients. A subgroup analysis of 21 731 patients[2] indicated that hyperkalaemia was more common in elderly patients and in those with diabetes mellitus.


1. Hollenberg NK, Mickiewicz CW. Postmarketing surveillance in 70,898 patients treated with a triamterene/hydrochlorothiazide combination (Maxzide). *Am J Cardiol* 1989; **63:** 37B–41B.
2. Hollenberg NK, Mickiewicz CW. Hyperkalemia in diabetes mellitus: effect of a triamterene-hydrochlorothiazide combination. *Arch Intern Med* 1989; **149:** 1327–30.


**Effects on the blood.** There have been case reports of pancytopenia associated with triamterene therapy.[1,2] Some patients had hepatic cirrhosis and the antifolate activity of triamterene was considered responsible.[2]


1. Castellano G, *et al.* Pancitopenia aguda y megaloblastosis medular durante el tratemiento con triamterene de la ascitis causada por cirrosis hepática: aportación de dos casos. *Gastroenterol Hepatol* 1983; **6:** 540–4.
2. Remacha A, *et al.* Triamterene-induced megaloblastosis: report of two new cases, and review of the literature. *Biol Clin Hematol* 1983; **5:** 127–34.


**Effects on the kidneys.** There have been a number of reports[1-4] of renal calculi containing triamterene or its metabolites, generally in patients also taking hydrochlorothiazide. An abnormal urinary sediment was described which was thought to represent precipitated triamterene.[5] These observations were expanded in a crossover study:[6] abnormal urinary sediment was seen in 14 of 26 patients taking triamterene but in none taking amiloride. Triamterene and its metabolites identified by others in 181 of 50 000 renal calculi.[7] Triamterene either formed the nucleus of the stone or was deposited with calcium oxalate or uric acid. One-third of the 181 stones were entirely or predominantly composed of triamterene and its metabolites and it was suggested that supersaturation of the urine with these substances could provide suitable nuclei for the crystallisation of calcium oxalate.[8] However, other workers were unable to demonstrate this and suggested that triamterene and its metabolites could become incorporated into the protein matrix of existing stones.[9] In addition, an epidemiological study[10] found no evidence that triamterene use was associated with an increased incidence of renal stones. Some authors[11] have therefore considered that there was not enough evidence to contra-indicate the drug in patients with a history of recurrent renal calculi.

Deposition of triamterene in the urine may also play a part in the development of interstitial nephritis, which was diagnosed in 4 patients also taking hydrochlorothiazide, over a period of 4 years.[6]

Triamterene has also been associated with transient decline in renal function and the development of renal failure.[12,13] Several mechanisms may be responsible including interstitial nephritis, intrarenal obstruction by crystalline deposits, and an interaction with NSAIDs (see under Interactions, below).[13] Elderly patients may be particularly at risk.[12]


1. Ettinger B, *et al.* Triamterene-induced nephrolithiasis. *Ann Intern Med* 1979; **91:** 745–6.
2. Socolow EL. Triamterene-induced nephrolithiasis. *Ann Intern Med* 1980; **92:** 437.
3. Gault MH, *et al.* Triamterene urolithiasis. *Can Med Assoc J* 1981; **124:** 1556–7.
4. Grunberg RW, Silberg SJ. Triamterene-induced nephrolithiasis. *JAMA* 1981; **245:** 2494–5.
5. Fairley KF, *et al.* Abnormal urinary sediment in patients on triamterene. *Lancet* 1983; **i:** 421–2.
6. Spence JD, *et al.* Effects of triamterene and amiloride on urinary sediment in hypertensive patients taking hydrochlorothiazide. *Lancet* 1985; **ii:** 73–5.
7. Ettinger B, *et al.* Triamterene nephrolithiasis. *JAMA* 1980; **244:** 2443–5.
8. White DJ, Nancollas GH. Triamterene and renal stone formation. *J Urol (Baltimore)* 1982; **127:** 593–7.
9. Werness PG, *et al.* Triamterene urolithiasis: solubility, pK, effect on crystal formation, and matrix binding of triamterene and its metabolites. *J Lab Clin Med* 1982; **99:** 254–62.
10. Jick H, *et al.* Triamterene and renal stones. *J Urol (Baltimore)* 1982; **127:** 224–5.
11. Woolfson RG, Mansell MA. Does triamterene cause renal calculi? *BMJ* 1991; **303:** 1217–18.

12. Lynn KL, *et al.* Renal failure with potassium-sparing diuretics. *N Z Med J* 1985; **98:** 629–33.
13. Sica DA, Gehr TWB. Triamterene and the kidney. *Nephron* 1989; **51:** 454–61.

**Effects on the skin.** Photodermatitis has been reported in a patient receiving triamterene.[1] Pseudoporphyria, possibly associated with exposure to sunlight, occurred in a patient with vitiligo during treatment with triamterene and hydrochlorothiazide.[2]

1. Fernández de Corres L, *et al.* Photodermatitis from triamterene. *Contact Dermatitis* 1987; **17:** 114–15.
2. Motley RJ. Pseudoporphyria due to Dyazide in a patient with vitiligo. *BMJ* 1990; **300:** 1468.

## Precautions

As for Amiloride Hydrochloride, p.858. Triamterene should also be given with caution to patients with hyperuricaemia or gout, or a history of renal calculi. Patients with depleted folic acid stores such as those with hepatic cirrhosis may be at increased risk of megaloblastic anaemia.

Triamterene may interfere with the fluorescent measurement of quinidine. It may slightly colour the urine blue.

## Interactions

As for Amiloride Hydrochloride, p.858.

**Digoxin.** For a report of the effect of triamterene on digoxin, see p.897.

**Dopaminergics.** For a report of increased *amantadine* toxicity associated with hydrochlorothiazide and triamterene, see p.1198.

**NSAIDs.** There have been several reports of renal failure in patients taking triamterene and NSAIDs.[1,2] Both types of drug are nephrotoxic and in combination the effect appears to be additive.[3-5] It has been suggested that the suppression of urinary prostaglandins by NSAIDs could potentiate the nephrotoxic effects of triamterene.[1]

NSAIDs may also antagonise the diuretic action of triamterene.[6]

1. Favre L, *et al.* Reversible acute renal failure from combined triamterene and indomethacin: a study in healthy subjects. *Ann Intern Med* 1982; **96:** 317–20.
2. Härkönen M, Ekblom-Kullberg S. Reversible deterioration of renal function after diclofenac in patient receiving triamterene. *BMJ* 1986; **293:** 698–9.
3. Bailey RR. Adverse renal reactions to non-steroidal anti-inflammatory drugs and potassium-sparing diuretics. *Adverse Drug React Bull* 1988; (Aug.): 492–5.
4. Lynn KL, *et al.* Renal failure with potassium-sparing diuretics. *N Z Med J* 1985; **98:** 629–33.
5. Sica DA, Gehr TWB. Triamterene and the kidney. *Nephron* 1989; **51:** 454–61.
6. Webster J. Interactions of NSAIDs with diuretics and β-blockers: mechanisms and clinical implications. *Drugs* 1985; **30:** 32–41.

## Pharmacokinetics

Triamterene is variably but fairly rapidly absorbed from the gastrointestinal tract. The bioavailability has been reported to be about 50%. The plasma half-life has been reported to be about 2 hours. It is estimated to be about 60% bound to plasma proteins. It is extensively metabolised and is mainly excreted in the urine in the form of metabolites with some unchanged triamterene. Triamterene crosses the placenta and may be distributed into breast milk.

◊ References.

1. Pruitt AW, *et al.* Variations in the fate of triamterene. *Clin Pharmacol Ther* 1977; **21:** 610–19.
2. Gundert-Remy U, *et al.* Plasma and urinary levels of triamterene and certain metabolites after oral administration to man. *Eur J Clin Pharmacol* 1979; **16:** 39–44.
3. Gilfrich HJ, *et al.* Pharmacokinetics of triamterene after iv administration to man: determination of bioavailability. *Eur J Clin Pharmacol* 1983; **25:** 237–41.
4. Sörgel F, *et al.* Oral triamterene disposition. *Clin Pharmacol Ther* 1985; **38:** 306–12.

**Hepatic impairment.** Triamterene clearance was markedly decreased in 7 patients with alcoholic cirrhosis and ascites.[1] The diuretic effect lasted for up to 48 hours in cirrhotic patients compared with 8 hours in healthy controls.

1. Villeneuve JP, *et al.* Triamterene kinetics and dynamics in cirrhosis. *Clin Pharmacol Ther* 1984; **35:** 831–7.

**Renal impairment.** Urinary excretion of triamterene and its metabolite, hydroxytriamterene sulfate, was significantly reduced in patients with renal impairment[1] and in the elderly whose renal function was reduced.[2] Accumulation of the active metabolite was possible in patients with renal impairment.[1]

1. Knauf H, *et al.* Delayed elimination of triamterene and its active metabolite in chronic renal failure. *Eur J Clin Pharmacol* 1983; **24:** 453–6.
2. Williams RL, *et al.* Absorption and disposition of two combination formulations of hydrochlorothiazide and triamterene: influence of age and renal function. *Clin Pharmacol Ther* 1986; **40:** 226–32.

## Uses and Administration

Triamterene is a weak diuretic with potassium-sparing properties which has actions and uses similar to those of amiloride (p.858). It produces a diuresis in about 2 to 4 hours, with a duration of 7 to 9 hours. The full therapeutic effect may be delayed until after several days of treatment.

Triamterene adds to the natriuretic but diminishes the kaliuretic effects of other diuretics. It is mainly used, as an adjunct to thiazide diuretics such as hydrochlorothiazide and loop diuretics such as furosemide, to conserve potassium in those at risk from hypokalaemia during the treatment of refractory oedema associated with hepatic cirrhosis, heart failure (p.820), and the nephrotic syndrome. It is also used with other diuretics in the treatment of hypertension (p.825).

When triamterene is given alone in the treatment of **oedema**, the dosage range is 150 to 250 mg daily by mouth; 100 mg twice daily, after breakfast and lunch, is considered to be the optimum dose, preferably on alternate days for maintenance therapy. More than 300 mg daily should not be given.

Smaller doses are used initially when other diuretics are also given. When used with hydrochlorothiazide, for example, in the treatment of **hypertension**, an initial dose of 50 mg of triamterene daily may be used.

Potassium supplements should not be given.

## Preparations

***BP 2003:*** Co-triamterzide Tablets; Triamterene Capsules;
***USP 27:*** Triamterene and Hydrochlorothiazide Capsules; Triamterene and Hydrochlorothiazide Tablets; Triamterene Capsules.

**Proprietary Preparations** (details are given in Part 3)
***Canad.:*** Dyrenium; ***Ger.:*** Jatropur†; ***Neth.:*** Dytac; ***Spain:*** Urocaudal†; ***Switz.:*** Dyrenium†; ***UK:*** Dytac; ***USA:*** Dyrenium.

**Multi-ingredient:** ***Austral.:*** Dyazide†; Hydrene; ***Austria:*** Confit; Diucomb†; Diurid†; Dytide H; Hydrotrix; Inderal comp†; Resaltex†; Salodiur; Triamteren comp; Triamteren/HCT; Triastad HCT; Trioral/HCT; ***Belg.:*** Diucomb; Dyta-Urese†; Dytenzide; Maxzide†; ***Braz.:*** Diurana; Iguassina; ***Canad.:*** Apo-Triazide; Dyazide†; Novo-Triamzide; Nu-Triazide; ***Chile:*** Hidroronol T; Uren; ***Fin.:*** Furesis comp; Uretren Comp; ***Fr.:*** Cycloteriam†; Isobar; Prestole; ***Ger.:*** Beta-Turfa; Betathiazid†; dehydro sanol tri; dehydro tri mite; Diu Venostasin; Diucomb; Diuretikum Verla; Diutensat; Diutensat comp; Dociteren; duradiuret; Dytide H; Esiteren†; Furesis comp†; Haemiton compositum; Hydrotrix; Hypertorr†; Jenateren comp; Manimon†; Neotri; Nephral; Propra comp; Resaltex†; Sali-Puren; Thiazid-comp; Tri-Thiazid; Tri-Thiazid Reserpin; Triampur compositum; Triamteren comp; Triamteren-H; Triamteren/HCT; Triarese; triazid; Turfa; Veratide; ***Hong Kong:*** Apo-Triazide; Dyazide; Triam-Co; Trizid†; ***Irl.:*** Dyazide; ***Ital.:*** Fluss 40; ***Malaysia:*** Apo-Triazide; ***Mex.:*** Dyazide; ***Neth.:*** Dyta-Urese; Dytenzide; ***NZ:*** Dyazide†; Triamizide; Trizid†; ***Port.:*** Dyazide; Triam-Tiazida R; ***S.Afr.:*** Dyazide; Loretic†; Renezide; ***Singapore:*** Apo-Triazide; Dyazide†; ***Spain:*** Salidur; Triniagar†; Urocaudal Tiazida†; ***Switz.:*** Diucomb†; Dyazide; Dyrenium compositum; Hydrotrix†; t/h-basan; ***Thai.:*** Dazid; Dinazide; Dyazide†; Dyterene; Skezide†; ***UK:*** Dyazide; Dytide; Frusene; Kalspare; Triamaxco; Triamco; ***USA:*** Dyazide; Maxzide.

---

## Trichlormethiazide *(rINN)*

Trichlormethiazidum; Triclormetiazida. 6-Chloro-3-dichloromethyl-3,4-dihydro-2*H*-1,2,4-benzothiadiazine-7-sulphonamide 1,1-dioxide.

$C_8H_8Cl_3N_3O_4S_2$ = 380.7.
*CAS — 133-67-5.*
*ATC — C03AA06.*

**Pharmacopoeias.** In *Jpn* and *US.*

**USP 27** (Trichlormethiazide). A white or practically white, crystalline powder, odourless or with a slight characteristic odour. Soluble 1 in 1100 of water, 1 in 48 of alcohol, 1 in 5000 of chloroform, 1 in about 4 of dimethylformamide, 1 in about 9 of dioxan, and 1 in 1400 of ether; freely soluble in acetone; soluble in methyl alcohol.

### Profile

Trichlormethiazide is a thiazide diuretic with properties similar to those of hydrochlorothiazide (p.933). It is used for oedema, including that associated with heart failure (p.820), and for hypertension (p.825).

Diuresis is initiated in about 2 hours, and lasts about 24 hours.

In the treatment of oedema the usual dose by mouth is 1 to 4 mg daily or intermittently. In the treatment of hypertension the usual dose is 2 to 4 mg daily, either alone, or with other antihypertensives. In some patients 1 mg daily may be adequate. In children over 6 months of age a dose of 70 micrograms/kg daily in one or two doses has been used.

### Preparations

***USP 27:*** Trichlormethiazide Tablets.

**Proprietary Preparations** (details are given in Part 3)
***USA:*** Diurese; Metahydrin; Naqua.

**Multi-ingredient:** ***Fin.:*** Uretren Comp; ***Ger.:*** Esmalorid; ***Spain:*** Rulun; ***USA:*** Metatensin.

---

## Triflusal *(BAN, rINN)*

Triflusalum; UR-1501. 2-Acetoxy-4-trifluoromethylbenzoic acid; *O*-Acetyl-4-(trifluoromethyl)salicylic acid.

$C_{10}H_7F_3O_4$ = 248.2.
*CAS — 322-79-2.*
*ATC — B01AC18.*

**Pharmacopoeias.** In *Eur.* (see p.vi).

**Ph. Eur. 5.0** (Triflusal). A white or almost white crystalline powder. Practically insoluble in water; very soluble in dehydrated alcohol; freely soluble in dichloromethane. Store in airtight containers at a temperature not exceeding 25°.

### Profile

Triflusal is an inhibitor of platelet aggregation used in the management of thromboembolic disorders (p.837) in usual doses of 300 to 900 mg daily by mouth.

◊ References.

1. McNeely W, Goa KL. Triflusal. *Drugs* 1998; **55:** 823–35.
2. Cruz-Fernández JM, *et al.* Randomized comparative trial of triflusal and aspirin following acute myocardial infarction. *Eur Heart J* 2000; **21:** 457–65.

### Preparations

**Proprietary Preparations** (details are given in Part 3)
***Braz.:*** Disgren; ***Chile:*** Logrosal; ***Gr.:*** Aflen; ***Ital.:*** Disgren†; Triflux; ***Mex.:*** Disgren; ***Port.:*** Tecnosal; ***Spain:*** Disgren.

---

## Trimetaphan Camsilate *(BAN, rINN)*

Cansilato de trimetafán; Méthioplégium; Trimetaphan Camphorsulphonate; Trimetaphan Camsylate; Trimetaphani Camsylas; Trimethaphan Camsylate. (+)-1,3-Dibenzylperhydro-2-oxothieno[1′,2′:1,2]thieno[3,4-*d*]-imidazol-5-ium 2-oxobornane-10-sulphonate; 4,6-Dibenzyl-4,6-diaza-1-thioniatricyclo-[6.3.0.0$^{3,7}$]undecan-5-one 2-oxobornane-10-sulphonate.

$C_{22}H_{25}N_2OS,C_{10}H_{15}O_4S$ = 596.8.
*CAS — 7187-66-8 (trimetaphan); 68-91-7 (trimetaphan camsilate).*
*ATC — C02BA01.*

**Incompatibility.** Trimetaphan is incompatible with thiopental sodium, gallamine triethiodide, iodides, bromides, and strongly alkaline solutions.

### Adverse Effects and Treatment

The adverse effects of trimetaphan are mainly due to ganglionic blockade. A reduction in gastrointestinal motility may result in constipation and, on prolonged administration, paralytic ileus. Urinary retention, cycloplegia, mydriasis, tachycardia, precipitation of angina, and gastrointestinal disturbances such as anorexia, nausea, or vomiting, may occur. Orthostatic hypotension may be severe. Rapid intravenous infusion at rates greater than 5 mg/minute can result in respiratory arrest. Other adverse effects include raised intra-ocular pressure, dry mouth, hypoglycaemia, hypokalaemia, fluid retention, weakness, urticaria, and itching. Trimetaphan crosses the placenta and can cause paralytic or meconium ileus in the neonate.

If severe hypotension occurs, administration of trimetaphan should be stopped and the patient positioned with the head lower than the feet. A vasopressor may be given cautiously if necessary.

**Effects on the eyes.** Although trimetaphan may increase intra-ocular pressure, a sudden and dramatic reduction of intra-ocular pressure to very low levels was noted in 5 patients undergoing surgery when the systolic blood pressure was reduced to 60 mmHg with trimetaphan infusion.[1]

1. Dias PLR, *et al.* Effect on the intraocular pressure of hypotensive anaesthesia with intravenous trimetaphan. *Br J Ophthalmol* 1982; **66:** 721–4.

### Precautions

Trimetaphan should be avoided in patients with asphyxia or respiratory insufficiency, uncorrected anaemia, shock or hypovolaemia, severe arteriosclerosis, severe ischaemic heart disease, or pyloric stenosis and should only be used with extreme caution in those with hepatic or renal impairment, degenerative disease of the CNS, Addison's disease, prostatic hyperplasia, glaucoma, cerebral or coronary vascular insufficiency, and diabetes. It should be used with care in elderly or debilitated patients and should be avoided in pregnancy. Owing to a histamine-liberating effect it should be used with caution in allergic subjects.

### Interactions

Trimetaphan should be used with caution in patients being treated with other antihypertensives, drugs that depress cardiac function, or muscle relaxants, and in those taking NSAIDs or corticosteroids. The hypotensive effect is enhanced by general and spinal anaesthetics. Adrenaline should not be infiltrated locally at the site of incision when trimetaphan is being given since this may antagonise the effect of trimetaphan.

**Neuromuscular blockers.** For a reference to possible potentiation of neuromuscular blockade by trimetaphan, see Ganglion Blockers, under Interactions of Atracurium, p.1401.

### Uses and Administration

Trimetaphan is a ganglion blocker which inhibits the transmission of nerve impulses in both sympathetic and parasympathetic ganglia. The sympathetic blockade produces peripheral vasodilatation. Trimetaphan also has a direct vasodilator effect on peripheral blood vessels. It is used for inducing controlled hypotension during surgical procedures although sodium nitroprusside is usually preferred. It acts rapidly to produce a hypotensive response which persists for about 10 to 15 minutes.

Trimetaphan camsilate is administered by slow intravenous infusion of a solution usually containing 1 mg/mL. The infusion is started at the rate of 3 to 4 mg/minute and then adjusted according to response. Blood pressure should be closely monitored and should be allowed to rise before wound closure.

Trimetaphan has also been used for the emergency treatment of hypertensive crises (p.825), especially in the presence of pulmonary oedema or acute dissecting aortic aneurysms, but sodium nitroprusside is often preferred.

## Trimetazidine Hydrochloride *(BANM, rINNM)*

Hidrocloruro de trimetazidina; Trimetazidine Dihydrochloride; Trimetazidini Dihydrochloridum; Trimetazine Hydrochloride. 1-(2,3,4-Trimethoxybenzyl)piperazine dihydrochloride.

$C_{14}H_{22}N_2O_3,2HCl$ = 339.3.

*CAS — 5011-34-7 (trimetazidine); 13171-25-0 (trimetazidine hydrochloride).*

*ATC — C01EB15.*

**Pharmacopoeias.** In *Eur.* (see p.vi) and *Jpn.*

**Ph. Eur. 5.0** (Trimetazidine Dihydrochloride; Trimetazidine Hydrochloride BP 2003). A slightly hygroscopic, white or almost white crystalline powder. Freely soluble in water; sparingly soluble in alcohol. Store in airtight containers.

### Profile

Trimetazidine hydrochloride is used in angina pectoris (p.813) and in ischaemia of neurosensorial tissues as in Ménière's disease (p.422); 40 to 60 mg is given daily by mouth in divided doses.

◊ References.

1. McClellan KJ, Plosker GL. Trimetazidine: a review of its use in stable angina pectoris and other coronary conditions. *Drugs* 1999; **58:** 143–57.

### Preparations

**Proprietary Preparations** (details are given in Part 3)
***Arg.:*** Vastarel; ***Braz.:*** Vastarel; ***Denm.:*** Vastarel; ***Fr.:*** Cardiazidine†; Centrophene; Oxygirex†; Vastarel; ***Gr.:*** Imovexil; Liomagen; Vastarel; ***Hong Kong:*** Vastarel; ***India:*** Flavedon; Metacard; ***Irl.:*** Vastarel; ***Ital.:*** Vastarel; ***Malaysia:*** Vastarel; ***Port.:*** Vastarel; ***Singapore:*** Vastarel; ***Spain:*** Idaptan; ***Thai.:*** Matenol; Vastarel; Vastinol.

## Tripamide *(USAN, rINN)*

ADR-033; E-614; Tripamida. 4-Chloro-*N*-(*endo*-hexahydro-4,7-methanoisoindolin-2-yl)-3-sulphamoylbenzamide.

$C_{16}H_{20}ClN_3O_3S$ = 369.9.

*CAS — 73803-48-2.*

### Profile

Tripamide is a diuretic structurally related to indapamide. It is used in the treatment of hypertension.

### Preparations

**Proprietary Preparations** (details are given in Part 3)
***Thai.:*** Normonal.

## Urapidil *(BAN, rINN)*

B-66256M. 6-[3-(4-*o*-Methoxyphenylpiperazin-1-yl)propylamino]-1,3-dimethyluracil.

$C_{20}H_{29}N_5O_3$ = 387.5.

*CAS — 34661-75-1.*

*ATC — C02CA06.*

## Urapidil Hydrochloride *(BANM, rINNM)*

Hidrocloruro de urapidil.

$C_{20}H_{29}N_5O_3,HCl$ = 423.9.

*CAS — 64887-14-5.*

*ATC — C02CA06.*

### Adverse Effects and Precautions

Urapidil is reported to be well-tolerated, with adverse effects generally transient and most frequent at the beginning of therapy. Dizziness, nausea, headache, fatigue, orthostatic hypotension, palpitations, nervousness, pruritus, and allergic skin reactions have been reported.

It should be used with care in elderly patients and those with severe hepatic impairment. Intravenous urapidil should not be used in patients with aortic stenosis.

**Urinary incontinence.** Enuresis was reported[1] to be associated with the use of urapidil in 2 elderly patients.

1. Jonville A-P, *et al.* Urapidil and enuresis. *Lancet* 1992; **339:** 688.

### Pharmacokinetics

Following oral administration urapidil is rapidly absorbed with a reported bioavailability of 70 to 80%. It is reported to be about 80% bound to plasma proteins. Urapidil is extensively metabolised in the liver, principally by hydroxylation, and excreted mostly in urine, as metabolites and 10 to 20% of unchanged drug. The elimination half-life is reported to be about 4.7 hours following oral administration as capsules and about 2.7 hours following intravenous administration.

◊ Reviews.

1. Kirsten R, *et al.* Clinical pharmacokinetics of urapidil. *Clin Pharmacokinet* 1988; **14:** 129–40.

### Uses and Administration

Urapidil is an antihypertensive drug that is reported to block peripheral alpha$_1$ adrenoceptors (see Alpha Blockers, p.809) and to have central actions. It produces a reduction in peripheral resistance and a fall in systolic and diastolic blood pressure, usually without reflex tachycardia.

Urapidil is used in the management of hypertension (p.825), including hypertensive crises.

Urapidil is given by mouth as the base and intravenously as the hydrochloride, but doses are usually expressed in terms of the base. Urapidil hydrochloride 10.94 mg is approximately equivalent to 10 mg of urapidil. Urapidil fumarate has also been given by mouth.

In hypertension doses of 30 to 90 mg are given twice daily by mouth. In hypertensive crises a suggested regimen is to give an initial dose of 25 mg by slow intravenous injection over 20 seconds, repeated if necessary, followed by a maintenance infusion of 9 to 30 mg/hour.

◊ Reviews.

1. Dooley M, Goa KL. Urapidil: a reappraisal of its use in the management of hypertension. *Drugs* 1998; **56:** 929–55.

### Preparations

**Proprietary Preparations** (details are given in Part 3)
***Austria:*** Ebrantil; ***Belg.:*** Ebrantil; ***Braz.:*** Ebrantil†; ***Fr.:*** Eupressyl; Mediatensyl; ***Ger.:*** Alpha-Depressan†; Ebrantil; ***Ital.:*** Ebrantil; ***Neth.:*** Ebrantil; ***Port.:*** Ebrantil; ***Spain:*** Elgadil; ***Switz.:*** Ebrantil.

## Urokinase *(BAN, USAN, rINN)*

Urokinasum; Uroquinasa.

*CAS — 9039-53-6.*

*ATC — B01AD04.*

**Pharmacopoeias.** In *Chin., Eur.* (see p.vi), and *Jpn.*

**Ph. Eur. 5.0** (Urokinase). An enzyme isolated from human urine that activates plasminogen. It consists of a mixture of low (33 000) and high (54 000) molecular mass forms, the high molecular mass form being predominant. The potency is not less than 70 000 international units per mg of protein. A white or almost white, amorphous powder. Soluble in water. Store in airtight containers at a temperature not exceeding 8°. Protect from light.

### Units

The potency of urokinase is expressed in international units. Preparations are assayed using the first International Reference Preparation (1968), a mixture of low-molecular-weight and high-molecular-weight urokinases. The first International Standard for high-molecular-weight urokinase was established in 1989 for use with preparations of this type of urokinase.

Potency used to be expressed in Ploug or Plough units or in CTA units, but these now appear to be obsolete.

### Adverse Effects, Treatment, and Precautions

As for Streptokinase, p.1005. Serious allergic reactions may be less likely to occur with urokinase than with streptokinase.

**Hypersensitivity.** Allergic reactions are considered to be less frequent with urokinase than with streptokinase. However, in a series of 6 patients who had previously been treated with streptokinase,[1] thrombolytic therapy with urokinase for recurrent myocardial infarction was associated with rigors in 4 patients, 2 of whom also developed bronchospasm. None of the patients had any history of atopy.

1. Matsis P, Mann S. Rigors and bronchospasm with urokinase after streptokinase. *Lancet* 1992; **340:** 1552.

**Transmission of infection.** Some preparations of urokinase are produced in cultures of human cells and there is a risk of transmission of infection associated with their use.

### Interactions

As for Streptokinase, p.1007.

### Pharmacokinetics

Following intravenous infusion urokinase is cleared rapidly from the circulation by the liver. A plasma half-life of up to 20 minutes has been reported.

### Uses and Administration

Urokinase is a thrombolytic drug. It directly converts plasminogen to plasmin, a proteolytic enzyme which has fibrinolytic effects. The mechanisms of fibrinolysis are discussed further under Haemostasis and Fibrinolysis on p.735. Urokinase affects circulating, unbound plasminogen as well as fibrin-bound plasminogen and thus may be termed a fibrin-nonspecific thrombolytic agent (see p.812).

Urokinase is used similarly to streptokinase (p.1007) in the management of pulmonary embolism (p.839). It has also been used in deep-vein thrombosis (p.839), acute myocardial infarction (p.828), peripheral arterial thromboembolism (p.830), and for clearing clots following haemorrhage within the eye. Like streptokinase it has also been used to clear cannulas and shunts of occluding thrombi.

In the treatment of **pulmonary embolism** urokinase is given by intravenous infusion in initial doses of 4400 units/kg over 10 minutes, followed by 4400 units/kg per hour for 12 hours.

### Preparations

**Proprietary Preparations** (details are given in Part 3)
***Austral.:*** Ukidan†; ***Austria:*** Abbokinase; Actosolv; Ukidan†; ***Belg.:*** Actosolv; ***Canad.:*** Abbokinase†; ***Denm.:*** Trombolysin†; ***Fr.:*** Actosolv†; ***Ger.:*** Actosolv†; Alphakinase†; Corase; rheotromb; ***Gr.:*** Urochinasi; ***Hong Kong:*** Ukidan†; ***India:*** Ukidan; ***Israel:*** Abbokinase; Actosolv†; Ukidan†; ***Ital.:*** Actosolv; Alfakinasi; Kisolv; Persolv Richter; Purochin†; Ukidan†; ***Port.:*** Ukidan; ***S.Afr.:*** Ukidan†; ***Spain:*** Abbokinase†; Uroquidan; ***Swed.:*** Abbokinase; Ukidan†; ***Switz.:*** Ukidan†; ***USA:*** Abbokinase.

## Valsartan *(BAN, USAN, rINN)*

CGP-48933; Valsartán. *N*-[*p*-(*o*-1*H*-Tetrazol-5-ylphenyl)benzyl]-*N*-valeryl-L-valine; *N*-Pentanoyl-*N*-[2′-(1*H*-tetrazol-5-yl)biphenyl-4-ylmethyl]-L-valine.

$C_{24}H_{29}N_5O_3$ = 435.5.

*CAS — 137862-53-4.*

*ATC — C09CA03.*

### Adverse Effects and Precautions

As for Losartan Potassium, p.947. Valsartan should be used with caution in patients with hepatic impairment, cirrhosis, or biliary obstruction.

### Interactions

As for Losartan Potassium, p.948. Increased mortality has been reported with valsartan in patients with heart failure also receiving both ACE inhibitors and beta blockers and it should not be used in such patients.

### Pharmacokinetics

Valsartan is rapidly absorbed following oral administration, with a bioavailability of about 23%. Peak plasma concentrations of valsartan occur 2 to 4 hours after an oral dose. It is between 94 and 97% bound to plasma proteins. Valsartan is not significantly metabolised and is excreted mainly via the bile as unchanged drug. The terminal elimination half-life is about 5 to 9 hours. Following an oral dose about 83% is excreted in the faeces and 13% in urine.

◊ References.

1. Brookman LJ, *et al.* Pharmacokinetics of valsartan in patients with liver disease. *Clin Pharmacol Ther* 1997; **62:** 272–8.

### Uses and Administration

Valsartan is an angiotensin II receptor antagonist with actions similar to those of losartan (p.948). It is used in the management of hypertension (p.825) and may also be used in patients with heart failure who are unable to tolerate ACE inhibitors (see under Losartan Potassium, p.948).

Valsartan is given by mouth. After an oral dose the hypotensive effect occurs within 2 hours, reaches a peak within 4 to 6 hours, and persists for over 24 hours. The maximum hypotensive effect is achieved within 2 to 4 weeks.

In **hypertension**, valsartan is given in an initial dose of 80 mg once daily. This may be increased, if necessary, to 160 mg once daily, although doses of up to 320 mg once daily have been used. A lower initial dose of 40 mg once daily may be used in elderly patients over 75 years, and in those with intravascular volume depletion; similar dosage reductions have been suggested in renal or hepatic impairment (but see below).

In **heart failure,** valsartan is given in an initial dose of 40 mg twice daily. The dose should be increased, as tolerated, to 160 mg twice daily.

◊ Reviews.

1. Markham A, Goa KL. Valsartan: a review of its pharmacology and therapeutic use in essential hypertension. *Drugs* 1997; **54:** 299–311.

**Administration in hepatic and renal impairment.** In the UK, product information recommends a lower initial dose of 40 mg daily in patients with moderate to severe renal impairment (creatinine clearance less than 20 mL/minute). A 40-mg initial dose is also recommended in patients with mild to moderate hepatic impairment with a maximum dose of 80 mg daily. In the USA, however, it is specifically stated that no dosage reduction is necessary in mild or moderate renal or hepatic impairment.

## Preparations

**Proprietary Preparations** (details are given in Part 3)
***Arg.:*** Diovan; Redutensil; ***Austria:*** Diovan; ***Belg.:*** Diovane; ***Braz.:*** Diovan; Tareg; ***Canad.:*** Diovan; ***Chile:*** Tareg; Vartalan; ***Denm.:*** Diovan; ***Fin.:*** Diovan; ***Fr.:*** Nisis; Tareg; ***Ger.:*** Diovan; Provas; ***Gr.:*** Diovan; ***Hong Kong:*** Diovan; ***Irl.:*** Diovan; ***Israel:*** Diovan; ***Ital.:*** Tareg; Valpression; ***Malaysia:*** Diovan; ***Mex.:*** Diovan; ***Neth.:*** Diovan; ***Norw.:*** Diovan; ***NZ:*** Diovan†; ***Port.:*** Diovan; Tareg; ***S.Afr.:*** Diovan; ***Singapore:*** Diovan; ***Spain:*** Diovan; Kalpress; Miten; Vals; ***Swed.:*** Diovan; ***Switz.:*** Diovan; ***Thai.:*** Diovan; ***UK:*** Diovan; ***USA:*** Diovan.

**Multi-ingredient:** ***Arg.:*** Diovan D; ***Austria:*** Co-Diovan; Valsartan/HCTZ; ***Belg.:*** Co-Diovane; ***Braz.:*** Cotareg; Diovan HCT; ***Canad.:*** Diovan HCT; ***Chile:*** Tareg-D; Vartalan D; ***Denm.:*** Diovan Comp; ***Fin.:*** Diovan Comp; ***Fr.:*** Cotareg; Nisisco; ***Ger.:*** Co-Diovan; Provas comp; ***Hong Kong:*** Co-Diovan; ***Irl.:*** Co-Diovan; ***Israel:*** Co-Diovan; ***Ital.:*** Combisartan; Cotareg; ***Malaysia:*** Co-Diovan; ***Mex.:*** Co-Diovan; Diovan HCT†; ***Neth.:*** Co-Diovan; ***Norw.:*** Diovan Comp; ***Port.:*** Co-Diovan; Co-Tareg; ***S.Afr.:*** Co-Diovan; ***Singapore:*** Co-Diovan; ***Spain:*** Co-Diovan; Co-Vals; Kalpress Plus; Miten Plus; ***Swed.:*** Diovan Comp; ***Switz.:*** Co-Diovan; ***Thai.:*** Co-Diovan; ***USA:*** Diovan HCT.

# Verapamil Hydrochloride

*(BANM, USAN, rINNM)*

CP-16533-1 (verapamil); D-365 (verapamil); Hidrocloruro de verapamilo; Iproveratril Hydrochloride; Verapamili Hydrochloridum. 5-[*N*-(3,4-Dimethoxyphenethyl)-*N*-methylamino]-2-(3,4-dimethoxyphenyl)-2-isopropylvaleronitrile hydrochloride.

$C_{27}H_{38}N_2O_4,HCl = 491.1.$

*CAS — 52-53-9 (verapamil); 152-11-4 (verapamil hydrochloride).*

*ATC — C08DA01.*

**Pharmacopoeias.** In *Chin., Eur.* (see p.vi), *Int., Jpn,* and *US.*

**Ph. Eur. 5.0** (Verapamil Hydrochloride). A white, crystalline powder. Soluble in water; sparingly soluble in alcohol; freely soluble in methyl alcohol. A 5% solution in water has a pH of 4.5 to 6.0. Protect from light.

**USP 27** (Verapamil Hydrochloride). A white or practically white, practically odourless, crystalline powder. Soluble in water; sparingly soluble in alcohol; freely soluble in chloroform; practically insoluble in ether. A 5% solution in water has a pH of 4.5 to 6.5. Store in airtight containers at a temperature of 25°, excursions permitted between 15° and 30°. Protect from light.

**Incompatibility.** Verapamil hydrochloride will precipitate in alkaline solutions. There have been reports of incompatibility with solutions of aminophylline,[1] nafcillin sodium,[2] and sodium bicarbonate.[3]

1. Johnson CE, *et al.* Compatibility of aminophylline and verapamil in intravenous admixtures. *Am J Hosp Pharm* 1989; **46:** 97–100.
2. Tucker R, Gentile JF. Precipitation of verapamil in an intravenous line. *Ann Intern Med* 1984; **101:** 880.
3. Cutie MR. Verapamil precipitation. *Ann Intern Med* 1983; **98:** 672.

## Adverse Effects

Treatment with verapamil is generally well tolerated, but adverse effects connected with verapamil's pharmacological effects on cardiac conduction can arise and may be particularly severe in patients with hypertrophic cardiomyopathies. Adverse effects on the heart include bradycardia, atrioventricular block, worsening heart failure, and transient asystole. These effects are more common with parenteral than with oral therapy.

The most troublesome non-cardiac adverse effect is constipation. Nausea may occur but is less frequently reported. Other adverse effects include hypotension, dizziness, flushing, headaches, fatigue, dyspnoea, and peripheral oedema. There have been reports of skin reactions and some cases of abnormal liver function and hepatotoxicity. Gingival hyperplasia has occurred. Gynaecomastia has been reported rarely.

In overdosage there may be severe cardiotoxicity and profound hypotension.

**Cancer occurrence.** See under Adverse Effects of Nifedipine, p.966.

**Effects on the cardiovascular system.** For discussion of the possibility that calcium-channel blockers might be associated with increased cardiovascular mortality, see Effects on Mortality, under Adverse Effects of Nifedipine, p.966.

Verapamil has vasodilating properties and negative inotropic activity and may cause adverse cardiovascular effects with worsening of arrhythmias. As discussed below under Precautions certain cardiac disorders put the patient at risk of severe toxicity.

Some references.

1. Radford D. Side effects of verapamil in infants. *Arch Dis Child* 1983; **58:** 465–6.
2. Perrot B, *et al.* Verapamil: a cause of sudden death in a patient with hypertrophic cardiomyopathy. *Br Heart J* 1984; **51:** 352–4.
3. Kirk CR, *et al.* Cardiovascular collapse after verapamil in supraventricular tachycardia. *Arch Dis Child* 1987; **62:** 1265–6.
4. Mohindra SK, Udeani GO. Long-acting verapamil and heart failure. *JAMA* 1989; **261:** 994.
5. Garratt C, *et al.* Degeneration of junctional tachycardia to pre-excited atrial fibrillation after intravenous verapamil. *Lancet* 1989; **ii:** 219.

**Effects on the ears.** There have been isolated reports[1] of tinnitus associated with several calcium-channel blockers including nifedipine, nicardipine, nitrendipine, diltiazem, verapamil, and cinnarizine.

1. Narváez M, *et al.* Tinnitus with calcium-channel blockers. *Lancet* 1994; **343:** 1229–30.

**Effects on the endocrine system.** There have been reports of a few patients developing elevated serum-prolactin concentrations during verapamil therapy;[1,2] one of these patients experienced galactorrhoea.[2]

Hyperglycaemia, metabolic acidosis, hyperkalaemia, and bradycardia have occurred[3] following a single dose of modified-release verapamil in a non-diabetic patient who had previously tolerated regular verapamil.

Verapamil has been reported not to affect the release of calcitonin,[4] thyroxine, tri-iodothyronine, thyrotrophin (TSH), follicle-stimulating hormone (FSH), luteinising hormone (LH), or testosterone when given by mouth;[1] however, intravenous administration has been reported to have an inhibitory effect on the release of FSH, LH, and TSH.[5]

1. Semple CG, *et al.* Calcium antagonists and endocrine status: lack of effect of oral verapamil on pituitary-testicular and pituitary-thyroid function. *Br J Clin Pharmacol* 1984; **17:** 179–82.
2. Gluskin LE, *et al.* Verapamil-induced hyperprolactinemia and galactorrhea. *Ann Intern Med* 1981; **95:** 66–7.
3. Roth A, *et al.* Slow-release verapamil and hyperglycemic metabolic acidosis. *Ann Intern Med* 1989; **110:** 171–2.
4. Amado JA, *et al.* No effect of verapamil on calcium stimulated calcitonin release. *Postgrad Med J* 1987; **63:** 23–4.
5. Barbarino A, De Marinis L. Calcium antagonists and hormone release II: effects of verapamil on basal, gonadotrophin-releasing hormone- and thyrotrophin-releasing hormone-induced pituitary hormone release in normal subjects. *J Clin Endocrinol Metab* 1980; **51:** 749–53.

**Effects on the liver.** Elevated serum concentrations of liver enzymes and bilirubin have been reported during verapamil therapy.[1-4] Clinical symptoms of hepatotoxicity such as abdominal pain, fever, darkened urine, and malaise have also occurred.[2-4] These reactions might have been due to a hypersensitivity reaction and were reversible on discontinuing verapamil.

1. Brodsky SJ, *et al.* Hepatotoxicity due to treatment with verapamil. *Ann Intern Med* 1981; **94:** 490–1.
2. Stern EH, *et al.* Possible hepatitis from verapamil. *N Engl J Med* 1982; **306:** 612–13.
3. Nash DT, Feer TD. Hepatic injury possibly induced by verapamil. *JAMA* 1983; **249:** 395–6.
4. Guarascio P, *et al.* Liver damage from verapamil. *BMJ* 1984; **288:** 362–3.

**Effects on the mouth.** Gingival hyperplasia[1] and oral mucosal injury[2] have been associated with verapamil therapy. A study involving 115 patients who had received nifedipine, diltiazem, or verapamil for at least 3 months indicated that gingival hyperplasia is an important side-effect that may occur with calcium-channel blockers in general.[3]

1. Pernu HE, *et al.* Verapamil-induced gingival overgrowth: a clinical, histologic, and biochemic approach. *J Oral Pathol Med* 1989; **18:** 422–5.
2. Guttenberg SA. Chemical injury of the oral mucosa from verapamil. *N Engl J Med* 1990; **323:** 615.
3. Steele RM, *et al.* Calcium antagonist-induced gingival hyperplasia. *Ann Intern Med* 1994; **120:** 663–4.

**Effects on the nervous system.** There has been a report[1] of 3 patients who complained of unusual perceptual symptoms, described as painful coldness and numbness or bursting feelings, especially in the legs, in association with oral verapamil.

1. Kumana CR, Mahon WA. Bizarre perceptual disorder of extremities in patients taking verapamil. *Lancet* 1981; **i:** 1324–5.

**Effects on the neuromuscular system.** A myoclonic, dystonic movement disorder was apparently induced by verapamil in a 70-year-old man.[1]

1. Hicks CB, Abraham K. Verapamil and myoclonic dystonia. *Ann Intern Med* 1985; **103:** 154.

**Effects on the peripheral circulation.** Persistent disabling burning pain and severe erythema and swelling of the feet occurred in a patient receiving verapamil;[1] it resolved when the drug was discontinued. The condition was diagnosed as secondary erythermalgia, a type of erythromelalgia secondary to a variety of diseases and to vasoactive drugs,[2] including the calcium-channel blocker nifedipine.[1]

1. Drenth JPH, *et al.* Verapamil-induced secondary erythermalgia. *Br J Dermatol* 1992; **127:** 292–4.
2. Drenth JPH, Michiels JJ. Three types of erythromelalgia. *BMJ* 1990; **301:** 454–5.

**Effects on the respiratory tract.** A patient with a history of bronchial asthma developed symptoms of acute asthma following administration of a modified-release verapamil preparation;[1] it was possible that excipients, notably alginate, may have been responsible for the reaction.

1. Ben-Noun L. Acute asthma associated with sustained-release verapamil. *Ann Pharmacother* 1997; **31:** 593–5.

**Effects on sexual function.** Impotence was associated with verapamil in 3 out of 14 men. In 1 patient normal sexual function returned when verapamil was discontinued and a recurrence of impotence was reported when it was re-instituted.[1]

1. King BD, *et al.* Impotence during therapy with verapamil. *Arch Intern Med* 1983; **143:** 1248–9.

**Effects on the skin and hair.** The commonest skin reactions to verapamil have been rash, pruritus, alopecia, and urticaria;[1] there have been a few reports of erythema multiforme, the Stevens-Johnson syndrome, and exfoliative dermatitis.[1] Hypertrichosis, over many parts of the body, has been reported in a male patient within about 1 month of starting verapamil therapy.[2] In a female patient who had been prematurely grey for about 40 years use of verapamil caused portions of the hair to regrow in its original natural black colour.[3]

1. Stern R, Khalsa JH. Cutaneous adverse reactions associated with calcium channel blockers. *Arch Intern Med* 1989; **149:** 829–32.
2. Sever PS. Hypertrichosis and verapamil. *Lancet* 1991; **338:** 1215–16.
3. Read GM. Verapamil and hair colour change. *Lancet* 1991; **338:** 1520.

**Extrapyramidal disorders.** Although calcium-channel blockers have been tried in the treatment of tardive dyskinesia (see under Uses of Nifedipine, p.972), verapamil has also been associated with the development of extrapyramidal effects. Tremor (postural and at rest) diagnosed as parkinsonism developed in a 70-year-old patient 4 months after starting treatment with verapamil. A 79-year-old patient developed symptoms including parkinsonism, rigidity, and bradykinesia 2 years after beginning verapamil therapy. Symptoms disappeared or improved considerably when verapamil was discontinued.[1]

1. Padrell MD, *et al.* Verapamil-induced parkinsonism. *Am J Med* 1995; **99:** 436.

**Haemorrhage.** See Effects on the Blood under Adverse Effects of Nifedipine, p.967.

**Overdosage.** Acute overdosage with verapamil generally produces cardiovascular symptoms[1-3] such as severe bradycardia, heart block, profound hypotension, and diminished peripheral perfusion with loss of peripheral pulses, cyanosis, and cold hands and feet. Overdosage may be fatal.[3] Haematemesis and gastric ulcers have been reported[4] following ingestion of verapamil 3.2 g.

Long-term treatment with verapamil 240 mg daily[5] in a patient with cirrhosis of the liver led to loss of consciousness, cardiogenic shock, cyanosis, hypotension, severe acidosis, hyperkalaemia, hypothermia, and renal failure. The patient recovered following treatment with high doses of dopamine, noradrenaline, sodium bicarbonate, and sodium chloride.

See also Treatment of Adverse Effects, below.

1. Perkins CM. Serious verapamil poisoning: treatment with intravenous calcium gluconate. *BMJ* 1978; **2:** 1127.
2. Crump BJ, *et al.* Lack of response to intravenous calcium in severe verapamil poisoning. *Lancet* 1982; **ii:** 939–40.
3. Orr GM, *et al.* Fatal verapamil overdose. *Lancet* 1982; **ii:** 1218–19.
4. Miller ARO, Ingamells CJ. Gastrointestinal haemorrhage associated with an overdose of verapamil. *BMJ* 1984; **288:** 1346.
5. Stehle G, *et al.* Cardiogenic shock associated with verapamil in a patient with liver cirrhosis. *Lancet* 1990; **336:** 1079.

## Treatment of Adverse Effects

In overdosage with verapamil by mouth activated charcoal may be given if the patient presents within 1 hour of ingestion; alternatively gastric lavage may be considered. Verapamil is not removed by dialysis. Treatment of cardiovascular effects is supportive and symptomatic. Intravenous infusion of calcium salts is recommended as a specific antagonist to verapamil and may reverse the haemodynamic and electrophysiological effects. A slow intravenous injection or an infusion of calcium gluconate in a dose of 10 to 20 mL of a 10% solution has been suggested; alternatively calcium chloride in a dose of 1 g may be used. If hypotension persists, intravenous administration of a sympathomimetic such as isoprenaline, dopamine, or noradrenaline may also be necessary. Bradycardia may be treated with atropine, isoprenaline, or cardiac pacing.

**Overdosage.** The usual management of verapamil overdosage is discussed under Treatment of Adverse Effects, above. Although the consequences and management of overdosage with all calcium-channel blockers are similar,[1] non-dihydropyridines such as verapamil may cause more severe effects and may require more aggressive treatment,[2] including thorough gastrointestinal decontamination and high doses of calcium intravenously.[3] The importance of these measures was also noted in a review of intoxication specifically with verapamil.[4] Other treatment of possible benefit in verapamil overdosage includes glucagon,[5] and the specific antidote fampridine.[6]

Overdosage with modified-release preparations of verapamil may result in prolonged toxicity of delayed onset.[7] Conventional-release preparations may also produce prolonged toxicity; elimination half-life was reported to be prolonged to 15 hours and peak plasma concentrations delayed to 6 to 7 hours in a 59-year-old man following ingestion of 2.4 g of verapamil.[8] Rate-limiting absorption at high doses was considered to be the cause. Pretreatment with calcium salts has been suggested[9] before intravenous administration of verapamil in patients for whom hypotension might result in serious adverse effects.


1. Kenny J. Treating overdose with calcium channel blockers. *BMJ* 1994; **308:** 992–3.
2. Buckley NA, *et al.* Overdose with calcium channel blockers. *BMJ* 1994; **308:** 1639.
3. Howarth DM, *et al.* Calcium channel blocking drug overdose: an Australian series. *Hum Exp Toxicol* 1994; **13:** 161–6.
4. Hofer CA, *et al.* Verapamil intoxication: a literature review of overdoses and discussions of therapeutic options. *Am J Med* 1993; **95:** 431–8.
5. White CM. A review of potential cardiovascular uses of intravenous glucagon administration. *J Clin Pharmacol* 1999; **39:** 442–7.
6. Stevens JJWM, Ghosh S. Overdose of calcium channel blockers. *BMJ* 1994; **309:** 193.
7. Barrow PM, *et al.* Overdose of sustained-release verapamil. *Br J Anaesth* 1994; **72:** 361–5.
8. Buckley CD, Aronson JK. Prolonged half-life of verapamil in a case of overdose: implications for therapy. *Br J Clin Pharmacol* 1995; **39:** 680–3.
9. Moser LR, *et al.* The use of calcium salts in the prevention and management of verapamil-induced hypotension. *Ann Pharmacother* 2000; **34:** 622–9.


## Precautions

Verapamil is contra-indicated in hypotension, in cardiogenic shock, in marked bradycardia, in second- or third-degree atrioventricular block, and in uncompensated heart failure. It is also contra-indicated in the sick-sinus syndrome unless a pacemaker is fitted. There is an increased incidence of adverse cardiac effects in patients with hypertrophic cardiomyopathy. In patients with atrial flutter or fibrillation and an accessory pathway with anterograde conduction, for example Wolff-Parkinson-White syndrome, verapamil may induce severe ventricular tachycardia and some authorities contra-indicate its use in such patients.

Special care is required in using verapamil as an antiarrhythmic in infants as they may be more susceptible to verapamil-induced arrhythmias.

Doses of verapamil should be reduced in patients with hepatic impairment.

Sudden withdrawal of verapamil might be associated with exacerbation of angina.

**Breast feeding.** Verapamil concentrations in breast milk similar to those found in plasma have been reported[1] in a woman taking verapamil 80 mg four times daily. The maximum concentration measured in breast milk was 300 nanograms/mL. However, the average concentration in milk in another woman[2] taking 80 mg three times daily was 23% of that in serum. The serum concentration of verapamil in the breast-fed child was 2.1 nanograms/mL during treatment and undetectable 38 hours after the last maternal dose. In another patient[3] taking the same dose, the average steady-state concentrations of verapamil and norverapamil in milk were, respectively, 60% and 16% of the concentration in plasma, with the ratio between milk and plasma varying during a dosage interval. It was estimated that the infant received less than 0.01% of the mother's dose, and no verapamil or norverapamil could be detected in the plasma of the infant. No adverse effects have been observed in breast-feeding infants, and the American Academy of Pediatrics considers[4] that verapamil is therefore usually compatible with breast feeding.


1. Inoue H, *et al.* Level of verapamil in human milk. *Eur J Clin Pharmacol* 1984; **26:** 657–8.
2. Andersen HJ. Excretion of verapamil in human milk. *Eur J Clin Pharmacol* 1983; **25:** 279–80.
3. Anderson P, *et al.* Verapamil and norverapamil in plasma and breast milk during breast feeding. *Eur J Clin Pharmacol* 1987; **31:** 625–7.
4. American Academy of Pediatrics. The transfer of drugs and other chemicals into human milk. *Pediatrics* 2001; **108:** 776–89. Correction. *ibid.*; 1029. Also available at: http://aappolicy.aappublications.org/cgi/content/full/pediatrics%3b108/3/776 (accessed 06/07/04)


**Muscular disorders.** Sudden respiratory failure was believed to have been precipitated by intravenous verapamil therapy in a patient with Duchenne's muscular dystrophy.[1]


1. Zalman F, *et al.* Acute respiratory failure following intravenous verapamil in Duchenne's muscular dystrophy. *Am Heart J* 1983; **105:** 510–11.


**Porphyria.** Verapamil has been associated with acute attacks of porphyria and is considered unsafe in porphyric patients.

**Wolff-Parkinson-White Syndrome.** Patients with atrial flutter or fibrillation in the presence of an accessory pathway such as Wolff-Parkinson-White syndrome may develop increased conduction across the anomalous pathway, precipitating ventricular tachycardia. Ventricular fibrillation and severe hypotension have been reported[1] following the administration of intravenous verapamil 5 to 10 mg to patients with the Wolff-Parkinson-White syndrome.


1. McGovern B, *et al.* Precipitation of cardiac arrest by verapamil in patients with Wolff-Parkinson-White syndrome. *Ann Intern Med* 1986; **104:** 791–4.


## Interactions

Verapamil should be used with caution with drugs that have antiarrhythmic or beta-blocking effects. The use of intravenous verapamil with a beta blocker is especially hazardous (see below). Verapamil is extensively metabolised in the liver and interactions may occur with drugs that inhibit or enhance hepatic metabolism. Grapefruit juice may cause increased plasma concentrations of verapamil. Verapamil can itself affect the pharmacokinetics of other drugs, particularly by inhibition of the cytochrome P450 isoenzyme CYP3A4 and by inhibition of P-glycoprotein. Increased plasma concentrations of many drugs, including carbamazepine, ciclosporin, digoxin, midazolam, simvastatin, and theophylline may occur, and the plasma concentration of alcohol may also be increased. For details of these interactions, see under the individual drug monographs.

**Analgesics.** For a possible interaction of verapamil with *aspirin*, see under Antiplatelets, below.

**Antiarrhythmics.** Cardiogenic shock and asystole has been described in 2 patients receiving *flecainide* when verapamil was added to their therapy.[1] Verapamil given intravenously has been reported to cause severe hypotension in patients also receiving *quinidine* by mouth.[2]


1. Buss J, *et al.* Asystole and cardiogenic shock due to combined treatment with verapamil and flecainide. *Lancet* 1992; **340:** 546.
2. Maisel AS, *et al.* Hypotension after quinidine plus verapamil: possible additive competition at alpha-adrenergic receptors. *N Engl J Med* 1985; **312:** 167–70.


**Antibacterials.** Acute verapamil toxicity manifested by complete heart block has been reported in a patient following the use of *ceftriaxone* and *clindamycin*.[1] Displacement of verapamil from binding sites was postulated as the probable mechanism of action. *Rifampicin* is an enzyme-inducing drug and has been reported[2,3] to reduce plasma-verapamil concentrations. A verapamil dose of 1.92 g was required to control supraventricular tachycardia in a patient also taking rifampicin[3] and when rifampicin was withdrawn the plasma-verapamil concentration 9 days later was almost four times higher. A patient taking propranolol and verapamil developed symptomatic bradycardia a few days after starting treatment with *clarithromycin* and on another occasion after starting treatment with *erythromycin*.[4] Inhibition of verapamil metabolism by the antibacterials was proposed as the mechanism for the interaction. A further case of severe hypotension and bradycardia has also been reported[5] in a patient shortly after beginning therapy with clarithromycin and verapamil. A case of complete heart block has been reported[6] in a patient aged 79 taking verapamil, one week after erythromycin was added to her therapy, probably due to mutual inhibition of hepatic metabolism of both drugs.


1. Kishore K, *et al.* Acute verapamil toxicity in a patient with chronic toxicity: possible interaction with ceftriaxone and clindamycin. *Ann Pharmacother* 1993; **27:** 877–80.
2. Rahn KH, *et al.* Reduction of bioavailability of verapamil by rifampin. *N Engl J Med* 1985; **312:** 920–1.
3. Barbarash RA. Verapamil-rifampin interaction. *Drug Intell Clin Pharm* 1985; **19:** 559–60.
4. Steenbergen JA, Stauffer VL. Potential macrolide interaction with verapamil. *Ann Pharmacother* 1998; **32:** 387–8.
5. Kaeser YA, *et al.* Severe hypotension and bradycardia associated with verapamil and clarithromycin. *Am J Health-Syst Pharm* 1998; **55:** 2417–18.
6. Goldschmidt N, *et al.* Compound cardiac toxicity of oral erythromycin and verapamil. *Ann Pharmacother* 2001; **35:** 1396–9.


**Antiepileptics.** *Phenobarbital* is a hepatic enzyme-inducing drug and has been reported[1] to increase the clearance of oral and intravenous verapamil and to reduce oral bioavailability in healthy subjects. Plasma protein binding of verapamil was also reduced. Dosage adjustment of verapamil may be needed in patients also taking phenobarbital. Marked reduction in verapamil concentrations has occurred with *phenytoin*.[2]


1. Rutledge DR, *et al.* Effects of chronic phenobarbital on verapamil disposition in humans. *J Pharmacol Exp Ther* 1988; **246:** 7–13.
2. Woodcock BG, *et al.* A reduction in verapamil concentrations with phenytoin. *N Engl J Med* 1991; **325:** 1179.


**Antiplatelets.** Calcium-channel blockers can inhibit platelet function (see Effects on the Blood under Adverse Effects of Nifedipine, p.967). Use of verapamil and *aspirin* in an 85-year-old man was considered to be the cause of ecchymoses and retroperitoneal bleeding that developed about 3 weeks after starting treatment with the combination.[1]


1. Verzino E, *et al.* Verapamil-aspirin interaction. *Ann Pharmacother* 1994; **28:** 536–7.


**Anxiolytics.** For the effect of verapamil on plasma-*buspirone* concentrations, see p.673.

**Beta blockers.** Oral verapamil and beta blockers have been used together in the treatment of angina and hypertension but both drugs have cardiodepressant activity and the combination, if used at all, must be used with extreme caution; bradycardia, heart block, and left ventricular failure have been reported.[1-4] Bradycardia has also been reported[5] in a patient treated with *timolol* eye drops and oral verapamil. Patients with severe ischaemic heart disease or heart failure are particularly at risk.[6] The risks are increased when verapamil is given intravenously and the interaction is especially hazardous when both verapamil and the beta blocker are given by this route. Treatment with beta blockers should be discontinued for at least 24 hours before administration of intravenous verapamil.[6]


1. Eisenberg JNH, Oakley GDG. Probable adverse interaction between oral metoprolol and verapamil. *Postgrad Med J* 1984; **60:** 705–6.
2. Hutchison SJ, *et al.* β blockers and verapamil: a cautionary tale. *BMJ* 1984; **289:** 659–60.
3. Findlay IN, *et al.* β blockers and verapamil: a cautionary tale. *BMJ* 1984; **289:** 1074.
4. McGourty JC, Silas JH. β blockers and verapamil: a cautionary tale. *BMJ* 1984; **289:** 1624.
5. Pringle SD, MacEwen CJ. Severe bradycardia due to interaction of timolol eye drops and verapamil. *BMJ* 1987; **294:** 155–6.
6. McInnes GT. Interactions that matter: calcium blockers. *Prescribers' J* 1988; **28:** 60–4.


**Calcium salts.** Calcium salts antagonise the pharmacological response to verapamil and are given intravenously to treat adverse effects of verapamil (see Treatment of Adverse Effects, above). Recurrence of atrial fibrillation has occurred[1] during maintenance verapamil treatment when calcium adipinate and calciferol were given by mouth.


1. Bar-Or D, Yoel G. Calcium and calciferol antagonise effect of verapamil in atrial fibrillation. *BMJ* 1981; **282:** 1585–6.


**Histamine $H_2$-antagonists.** Studies in healthy subjects using single doses of verapamil following pretreatment with *cimetidine* for up to 8 days have produced conflicting results. The pharmacokinetics of intravenous verapamil were unaltered by cimetidine in some studies,[1,2] but a 21% reduction in clearance and a 50% increase in the elimination half-life were also reported.[3] The pharmacokinetics of oral verapamil were unchanged in one study[2] but two others[1,4] reported a significant increase in bioavailability. Although one of these studies[1] found the interaction had no clinical effects, the other[4] reported an increased clinical effect in 5 of 6 subjects. The interaction with cimetidine appears to be stereoselective since the oral bioavailability of the *S*-enantiomer increased by 35% and that of the *R*-enantiomer by 15%.[4] The clinical significance of this interaction in patients and during long-term verapamil treatment is unknown, but cimetidine should be used with caution in patients receiving verapamil.


1. Smith MS, *et al.* Influence of cimetidine on verapamil kinetics and dynamics. *Clin Pharmacol Ther* 1984; **36:** 551–4.
2. Abernethy DR, *et al.* Lack of interaction between verapamil and cimetidine. *Clin Pharmacol Ther* 1985; **38:** 342–9.
3. Loi C-M, *et al.* Effect of cimetidine on verapamil disposition. *Clin Pharmacol Ther* 1985; **37:** 654–7.
4. Mikus G, *et al.* Interaction of verapamil and cimetidine: stereochemical aspects of drug metabolism, drug disposition and drug action. *J Pharmacol Exp Ther* 1990; **253:** 1042–8.


**Lithium.** Neurotoxicity has been reported in a patient receiving lithium following the addition of verapamil.[1] Serum-lithium concentrations were still inside the accepted therapeutic range and it was considered that the similar actions of lithium and verapamil on neurosecretory processes may have been responsible. Verapamil has also been reported to decrease serum-lithium concentrations.[2]


1. Price WA, Giannini AJ. Neurotoxicity caused by lithium-verapamil synergism. *J Clin Pharmacol* 1986; **26:** 717–19.
2. Weinrauch LA, *et al.* Decreased serum lithium during verapamil therapy. *Am Heart J* 1984; **108:** 1378–80.


## Pharmacokinetics

Verapamil is approximately 90% absorbed from the gastrointestinal tract, but is subject to very considerable first-pass metabolism in the liver and the bioavailability is only about 20%.

Verapamil exhibits bi- or tri-phasic elimination kinetics and is reported to have a terminal plasma half-life of 2 to 8 hours following a single oral dose or after intravenous administration. After repeated oral doses this increases to 4.5 to 12 hours. Verapamil acts within 5 minutes of intravenous administration and in 1 to 2 hours after oral administration; peak plasma concentrations occur 1 to 2 hours after an oral dose. There is considerable interindividual variation in plasma concentrations.

Verapamil is about 90% bound to plasma proteins. It is extensively metabolised in the liver to at least 12 metabolites of which norverapamil has been shown to have some activity. About 70% of a dose is excreted by the kidneys in the form of its metabolites but about 16% is excreted in the bile into the faeces. Less than 4% is excreted unchanged. Verapamil crosses the placenta and is distributed into breast milk.

◊ Reviews.


1. Hamann SR, *et al.* Clinical pharmacokinetics of verapamil. *Clin Pharmacokinet* 1984; **9:** 26–41.

2. Kelly JG, O'Malley K. Clinical pharmacokinetics of calcium antagonists: an update. *Clin Pharmacokinet* 1992; **22:** 416–33.
3. Kang D, *et al.* Population analyses of sustained-release verapamil in patients: effects of sex, race, and smoking. *Clin Pharmacol Ther* 2003; **73:** 31–40.

**The elderly.** Total verapamil clearance was found to be decreased in elderly (61 years of age or older) hypertensive patients compared with that in young patients, and the elimination half-life was prolonged.[1]

1. Abernethy DR, *et al.* Verapamil pharmacodynamics and disposition in young and elderly hypertensive patients: altered electrocardiographic and hypotensive responses. *Ann Intern Med* 1986; **105:** 329–36.

**Metabolism.** A study[1] has shown that both enantiomers of verapamil are predominantly metabolised by the cytochrome P450 isoenzymes CYP3A4, CYP3A5, and CYP2C8; these isoenzymes are also involved in the further metabolism of norverapamil. It was considered that CYP2C8 would play only a minor role in potential drug interactions.

1. Tracy TS, *et al.* Cytochrome P450 isoforms involved in metabolism of the enantiomers of verapamil and norverapamil. *Br J Clin Pharmacol* 1999; **47:** 545–52.

**Stereospecificity.** Verapamil is used as a racemic mixture. A series of studies have been carried out to determine whether differences in the pharmacokinetics of the *R*- and *S*-isomers of verapamil could account for observed differences in the plasma concentration-response curve following oral and intravenous administration. After intravenous administration, there were pronounced differences in the pharmacokinetics and protein binding of the 2 isomers;[1] the volume of distribution and total systemic clearance of *S*-verapamil were much higher than those of the *R*-isomer although the terminal half-life was similar. After oral administration of a mixture of *R*- and *S*-verapamil, plasma concentrations of the *R*-isomer were found to be substantially higher than those of the *S*-isomer[2] suggesting stereospecific first-pass hepatic metabolism. Following oral dosing total verapamil concentrations thus consist of a smaller proportion of the more potent *S*-isomer accounting for the apparent lower potency of verapamil when given orally. The proportion of *S*-isomer also depends on the oral formulation; modified-release formulations produce lower proportions of *S*-isomer in plasma than conventional formulations.[3] It has been shown[4] that *S*-verapamil is 3.3 times more potent than the racemic mixture and 11 times more potent than *R*-verapamil. Thus it was concluded that the cardiac effects of verapamil are related not to the total plasma-verapamil concentration but to the concentration of the *S*-isomer, and conventional plasma concentration monitoring will be of little value in establishing therapeutic plasma concentrations during multiple oral dosing.

1. Eichelbaum M, *et al.* Pharmacokinetics of (+)-, (−)- and (±)-verapamil after intravenous administration. *Br J Clin Pharmacol* 1984; **17:** 453–8.
2. Vogelgesang B, *et al.* Stereoselective first-pass metabolism of highly cleared drugs: studies of the bioavailability of L- and D-verapamil examined with a stable isotope technique. *Br J Clin Pharmacol* 1984; **18:** 733–40.
3. Karim A, Piergies A. Verapamil stereoisomerism: enantiomeric ratios in plasma dependent on peak concentrations, oral input rate, or both. *Clin Pharmacol Ther* 1995; **58:** 174–84.
4. Echizen H, *et al.* Effects of d,l-verapamil on atrioventricular conduction in relation to its stereoselective first-pass metabolism. *Clin Pharmacol Ther* 1985; **38:** 71–6.

## Uses and Administration

Verapamil is a calcium-channel blocker (p.810) and a class IV antiarrhythmic (p.809). Verapamil slows conduction through the atrioventricular node, and thus slows the increased ventricular response rate that occurs in atrial fibrillation and flutter. A decrease in both coronary and peripheral vascular resistance together with a sparing effect on myocardial intracellular oxygen consumption appear to be the modes of action in angina. The decrease in peripheral vascular resistance may explain the antihypertensive effect of verapamil. It is used in the control of supraventricular arrhythmias and in the management of angina pectoris and hypertension. It may also be used in the management of myocardial infarction.

Verapamil may be given intravenously or by mouth as the hydrochloride for the control of supraventricular **arrhythmias**. Intravenous injections should be given under continuous ECG monitoring. When given intravenously a dose of 5 to 10 mg is injected over a period of 2 to 3 minutes; if necessary, a further 5 mg may be injected 5 to 10 minutes after the first. In the USA a second dose of 10 mg given after 30 minutes if required is suggested. Children should be treated with great care; intravenous doses given over at least 2 minutes are: up to 1 year of age, 100 to 200 micrograms/kg; age 1 to 15 years, 100 to 300 micrograms/kg (to a maximum dose of 5 mg). The dose may be repeated after 30 minutes if necessary. Doses at the lower end of the range may be adequate and the injection should be stopped when a response has been obtained.

Oral doses for the treatment of supraventricular arrhythmias are 120 to 480 mg daily in 3 or 4 divided doses, according to the severity of the condition and the patient's response. Oral doses for children are: up to 2 years of age, 20 mg two or three times daily; 2 years and over, 40 to 120 mg two or three times daily according to age and response; great care is still required.

In the management of **angina pectoris,** verapamil hydrochloride is given by mouth in doses of 120 mg three times daily; some patients with angina of effort may respond to 80 mg three times daily, but this lower dose is not likely to be effective in angina at rest or Prinzmetal's variant angina. Modified-release preparations may be given in doses of up to 480 mg daily.

In **hypertension** the dose of verapamil hydrochloride is generally 160 mg twice daily by mouth with a range of 240 mg to 480 mg daily. Modified-release preparations may be given in similar daily doses. A dose of up to 10 mg/kg daily in divided doses may be used for children.

In the management of **myocardial infarction**, verapamil hydrochloride, as a modified-release oral preparation, may be started at least 1 week after acute infarction (in patients without heart failure) in a dose of 360 mg daily in divided doses.

Doses of verapamil should be reduced in patients with hepatic impairment (see below).

◊ General reviews.

1. Anonymous. Calcium antagonists for cardiovascular disease. *Drug Ther Bull* 1993; **31:** 81–4.
2. Fisher M, Grotta J. New uses for calcium channel blockers: therapeutic implications. *Drugs* 1993; **46:** 961–75.
3. Brogden RN, Benfield P. Verapamil: a review of its pharmacological properties and therapeutic use in coronary artery disease. *Drugs* 1996; **51:** 792–819.

**Administration in the elderly.** For a report that the pharmacokinetics of verapamil are altered in the elderly, see under Pharmacokinetics, above.

**Administration in hepatic impairment.** Doses of verapamil should be reduced to about one-third of the usual dose in patients with hepatic impairment.

In a study[1] of patients with liver cirrhosis steady-state plasma concentrations of verapamil were double those seen in patients with normal liver function following intravenous administration and 5 times the normal concentration when given by mouth, and it was suggested that verapamil dosage must be drastically reduced in these patients, especially when given orally. The elimination half-life was prolonged about fourfold following oral or intravenous administration and thus steady-state plasma concentration will not be reached in patients with liver cirrhosis until about 56 hours after therapy has started.

1. Somogyi A, *et al.* Pharmacokinetics, bioavailability and ECG response of verapamil in patients with liver cirrhosis. *Br J Clin Pharmacol* 1981; **12:** 51–60.

**Administration in renal impairment.** The pharmacokinetics and pharmacodynamic effects of verapamil are not significantly altered by renal impairment[1] and dosage adjustment is not considered to be necessary. The elimination of verapamil is not altered by haemodialysis,[1,2] haemofiltration,[2] or peritoneal dialysis[2] and no dosage supplement is required in patients undergoing these procedures.

1. Mooy J, *et al.* Pharmacokinetics of verapamil in patients with renal failure. *Eur J Clin Pharmacol* 1985; **28:** 405–10.
2. Beyerlein C, *et al.* Verapamil in antihypertensive treatment of patients on renal replacement therapy—clinical implications and pharmacokinetics. *Eur J Clin Pharmacol* 1990; **39** (suppl 1): S35–S37.

**Amaurosis fugax.** Verapamil and nifedipine were found to be effective[1] in a few patients with amaurosis fugax unresponsive to anticoagulants or antiplatelets, possibly due to relief of vasospasm.

1. Winterkorn JMS, *et al.* Brief report: treatment of vasospastic amaurosis fugax with calcium-channel blockers. *N Engl J Med* 1993; **329:** 396–8.

**Bipolar disorder.** Although lithium is the mainstay of therapy in bipolar disorder (p.278) it cannot be used in some patients because of undue toxicity, and is ineffective in others. Verapamil is one of several drugs that have been studied as an alternative.[1] Beneficial responses to verapamil at doses up to 480 mg daily have been reported,[2-4] although a review[5] concluded that there is limited support for its use.

1. Höschl C. Do calcium antagonists have a place in the treatment of mood disorders? *Drugs* 1991; **42:** 721–29.
2. Dubovsky SL, *et al.* Calcium antagonists in mania: a double-blind study of verapamil. *Psychiatry Res* 1986; **18:** 309–20.
3. Giannini AJ, *et al.* Verapamil and lithium in maintenance therapy of manic patients. *J Clin Pharmacol* 1987; **27:** 980–2.
4. Wisner KL, *et al.* Verapamil treatment for women with bipolar disorder. *Biol Psychiatry* 2002; **51:** 745–52.
5. Levy NA, Janicak PG. Calcium channel antagonists for the treatment of bipolar disorder. *Bipolar Disord* 2000; **2:** 108–19.

**Box jellyfish sting.** Stings by the box jellyfish (*Chironex fleckeri*) (p.1621) can be fatal due to the effects of the venom on the cardiovascular and respiratory systems and on the kidneys. Studies in *rodents* have reported a beneficial effect of intravenous verapamil in the treatment of box jellyfish envenomation. It has been suggested that intravenous verapamil be used in the acute management of patients with serious box jellyfish stings since it may reverse the cardiotoxic effects of the venom and allow more time for additional supportive care and for the antivenom to exert its action.[1]

1. Burnett JW. The use of verapamil to treat box-jellyfish stings. *Med J Aust* 1990; **153:** 363.

**Cardiac arrhythmias.** Verapamil may be used to control supraventricular arrhythmias such as atrial fibrillation and flutter and paroxysmal supraventricular tachycardia (p.816).

Verapamil has been given to the mother with digoxin for transplacental use in the management of fetal atrial flutter or supraventricular tachycardia.[1] Caution is necessary when verapamil is given to infants to treat arrhythmias, see Precautions, above.

1. Maxwell DJ, *et al.* Obstetric importance, diagnosis, and management of fetal tachycardias. *BMJ* 1988; **297:** 107–10.

**Cardiomyopathies.** Clinical trials have suggested that long-term administration of verapamil improves symptoms and exercise tolerance in many patients with *hypertrophic cardiomyopathy* and it may be considered for the treatment of those patients who continue to have disabling symptoms or who are unable to tolerate beta blockers.[1] However, in a crossover study exercise capacity was not improved by either verapamil or nadolol, although most patients preferred one or other of the drugs rather than placebo and quality of life did appear to be improved by verapamil.[2] The incidence of serious ventricular or supraventricular arrhythmias does not appear to be reduced by verapamil and caution is also required since patients with hypertrophic cardiomyopathy are especially susceptible to conduction disturbances associated with verapamil. This is because loss of the synchronised contribution of atrial contraction may cause diminished filling of the stiff left ventricle and result in hypotension.[1]

The use of calcium-channel blockers is not standard therapy in *dilated cardiomyopathy* and has resulted in clinical and haemodynamic deterioration.[3] However, symptomatic improvement has been reported with diltiazem over a 24-month period.

For a discussion of the management of cardiomyopathies in general, see p.818.

1. Lorell BH. Use of calcium channel blockers in hypertrophic cardiomyopathy. *Am J Med* 1985; **78** (suppl 2B): 43–54.
2. Gilligan DM, *et al.* A double-blind, placebo-controlled crossover trial of nadolol and verapamil in mild and moderately symptomatic hypertrophic cardiomyopathy. *J Am Coll Cardiol* 1993; **21:** 1672–9.
3. Richardson PJ. Calcium antagonists in cardiomyopathy. *Br J Clin Pract* 1988; **42** (suppl 60): 33–7.

**Kidney disorders.** Calcium-channel blockers may be of benefit in various forms of kidney disorder (see Nifedipine, p.971). Verapamil may also reduce the nephrotoxicity associated with certain drugs. For example, verapamil can prevent ciclosporin-induced deterioration in renal function (see under Transplantation, below) and may possibly reduce nephrotoxicity associated with the aminoglycoside gentamicin.[1]

1. Kazierad DJ, *et al.* The effect of verapamil on the nephrotoxic potential of gentamicin as measured by urinary enzyme excretion in healthy volunteers. *J Clin Pharmacol* 1995; **35:** 196–201.

**Malignant neoplasms.** Verapamil has been shown to reverse multidrug resistance to antineoplastics in cultured cells and in *animal* studies,[1] but studies in which verapamil was added to therapy for small cell lung cancer[2] or multiple myeloma[3] failed to demonstrate any benefit. See p.498 for a discussion of resistance to antineoplastics.

1. Ford JM, Hait WN. Pharmacology of drugs that alter multidrug resistance in cancer. *Pharmacol Rev* 1990; **42:** 155–99.
2. Milroy R, *et al.* A randomised clinical study of verapamil in addition to combination chemotherapy in small cell lung cancer. *Br J Cancer* 1993; **68:** 813–18.
3. Dalton WS, *et al.* A phase III randomized study of oral verapamil as a chemosensitizer to reverse drug resistance in patients with refractory myeloma: a Southwest Oncology Group Study. *Cancer* 1995; **75:** 815–20.

**Migraine.** For reference to the use of calcium-channel blockers, including verapamil, in the management of migraine and cluster headache, see under Nifedipine, p.971.

**Myocardial infarction.** Studies have not shown a reduction in mortality when calcium-channel blockers are given in the early phase of acute myocardial infarction (p.828). Results of the Danish Verapamil Infarction Trial (DAVIT I) suggested that early intervention (on admission to hospital) with verapamil might be harmful.[1] However, since myocardial stunning has been linked to intracellular calcium overload[2] there has been speculation that calcium-channel blockers might benefit patients about to undergo reperfusion. This is yet to be confirmed. Calcium-channel blockers are not routinely used in the long-term management of myocardial infarction although in selected patients without heart failure verapamil or diltiazem may be of some benefit. In the DAVIT II study[3] late intervention with verapamil (started in the second week after admission) reduced overall mortality, cardiac events, and re-infarction in such patients although another study[4] found only a benefit in re-infarction rate and not in overall mortality.


1. The Danish Study Group on Verapamil in Myocardial Infarction. The Danish studies on verapamil in acute myocardial infarction. *Br J Clin Pharmacol* 1986; **21:** 197S–204S.
2. Anonymous. Myocardial stunning. *Lancet* 1991; **337:** 585–6.
3. The Danish Study Group on Verapamil in Myocardial Infarction. Effect of verapamil on mortality and major events after acute myocardial infarction (the Danish Verapamil Infarction Trial II–DAVIT II). *Am J Cardiol* 1990; **66:** 779–85.
4. Rengo F, *et al.* A controlled trial of verapamil in patients after acute myocardial infarction: results of the calcium antagonist reinfarction Italian study (CRIS). *Am J Cardiol* 1996; **77:** 365–9.


**Transplantation.** Ciclosporin is widely used in transplantation to prevent rejection but its use is limited by its nephrotoxicity. A series of studies in renal[1] and heart or lung[2] transplant recipients suggested that verapamil can prevent ciclosporin-induced deterioration in renal function. Although the concentration of ciclosporin in blood was increased by verapamil, kidney function was improved. The incidence of transplant rejection was also reduced by verapamil. The beneficial effect of verapamil therapy on transplant outcome may be related to its ability to protect cells from ischaemia, selective vasodilatation of the afferent renal arterioles, elevation of plasma-ciclosporin concentrations, and inherent immunosuppressive properties. Concomitant use of verapamil also allows lower doses of ciclosporin to be employed.[2] However, caution is still required and careful monitoring of ciclosporin concentrations is needed.


1. Dawidson I, Rooth P. Improvement of cadaver renal transplantation outcomes with verapamil: a review. *Am J Med* 1991; **90** (suppl 5A): 37S–41S.
2. Chan C, *et al.* A randomized controlled trial of verapamil on cyclosporine nephrotoxicity in heart and lung transplant recipients. *Transplantation* 1997; **63:** 1435–40.


## Preparations

***BP 2003:*** Prolonged-release Verapamil Tablets; Verapamil Injection; Verapamil Tablets;
***USP 27:*** Verapamil Hydrochloride Extended-release Tablets; Verapamil Hydrochloride Injection; Verapamil Hydrochloride Tablets.

**Proprietary Preparations** (details are given in Part 3)

***Arg.:*** Isoptino; Veral; Verapal; ***Austral.:*** Anpec; Cordilox; Isoptin; Veracaps; Verahexal; ***Austria:*** Chronovera; Isoptin; Veraday; Verapabene; Verastad; Veratyrol; Verexamil†; ***Belg.:*** Isoptine; Lodixal; ***Braz.:*** Cordilat; Cronovera; Dilacard; Dilacor; Dilacoron; Neo Verpamil; Norvil†; Veracoron†; Veramil; Veraval; ***Canad.:*** Apo-Verap; Chronovera; Isoptin; Novo-Veramil; Nu-Verap; Verelan†; ***Chile:*** Cardiolen; Isoptina; Presocor; ***Denm.:*** Geangin; Hexasoptin; Isoptin; Veraloc; ***Fin.:*** Isoptin; Vermin; Verpacor†; Verpamil; ***Fr.:*** Arpamyl LP†; Isoptine; Novapamyl†; ***Ger.:*** Azupamil; Cardioprotect†; Dignover†; durasoptin; Falicard; Isoptin; Jenapamil; Praecicor†; Vera; Vera-Lich; Verabeta; Veragamma; Verahexal; Veramex; Veranorm; Verasal; Veroptinstada; ***Gr.:*** Elanver; Isoptin; ***Hong Kong:*** Akilen; Isoptin; ***India:*** Calaptin; Veramil; ***Irl.:*** Isoptin; Veramil; Verap; Verelan†; Verisop; ***Israel:*** Apoacor; Ikacor; Ikapress; Veracor; Verapress; ***Ital.:*** Cardinorm; Isoptin; Kata; Quasar†; Veraptin; ***Malaysia:*** Akilen; Anpec; Isoptin; Verpamil; Viratin; ***Mex.:*** Cronovera; Dilacoran; Euritmin†; Galenpamil†; Veraken†; Veralan†; ***Neth.:*** Chronovera; Isoptin; ***Norw.:*** Geangin†; Isoptin; Verakard; ***NZ:*** Civicor; Isoptin; Verpamil; ***Port.:*** Isoptin; ***S.Afr.:*** Calcicard; Iso-Card†; Isoptin; Ravamil; Vasomil; Verahexal; ***Singapore:*** Civicor†; Isoptin; Verpamil; ***Spain:*** Manidon; Redupres†; Veratensin†; ***Swed.:*** Isoptin; Veraloc†; ***Switz.:*** Corpamil; Flamon; Isoptin; Veracim†; Verapam; Verasifar†; ***Thai.:*** Caveril; Civicor; Isopamil; Isoptin; Vasopten†; Verapin; Vermine; ***UK:*** Angimon†; Cordilox; Ethimil†; Half Securon; Securon; Univer; Verapress; Vertab; Zolvera; ***USA:*** Calan; Covera; Isoptin; Verelan.

**Multi-ingredient:** ***Austria:*** Captocomp; Confit; Tarka; Veracapt; ***Braz.:*** Tarka†; ***Denm.:*** Tarka; ***Fin.:*** Tarka; ***Fr.:*** Ocadrik; Tarka; ***Ger.:*** Cordichin; Isoptin plus; Stenoptin; Tarka; Udramil; Veratide; ***Ital.:*** Tarka; ***Mex.:*** Tarka; ***Neth.:*** Tarka; ***S.Afr.:*** Tarka; ***Spain:*** Tarka; Tricen; ***Swed.:*** Tarka; ***Switz.:*** Tarka; ***UK:*** Tarka; ***USA:*** Tarka.

## Vesnarinone *(USAN, rINN)*

OPC-8212; Vesnarinona. 1-(1,2,3,4-Tetrahydro-2-oxo-6-quinolyl)-4-veratroylpiperazine.

$C_{22}H_{25}N_3O_4$ = 395.5.

*CAS — 81840-15-5.*

### Profile

Vesnarinone is a phosphodiesterase inhibitor with positive inotropic activity that has been tried by mouth in the management of heart failure.

◊ Studies with other inotropic phosphodiesterase inhibitors have shown that their prolonged oral use can lead to an increased mortality rate. In a multicentre study of vesnarinone,[1] doses of 120 mg daily resulted in increased mortality whereas 60 mg daily for 6 months was associated with lower morbidity and mortality. Reversible neutropenia occurred in 2.5% of the patients given 60 mg daily. However, in a subsequent larger study,[2] increased mortality was also reported with doses of 30 and 60 mg daily.


1. Feldman AM, *et al.* Effects of vesnarinone on morbidity and mortality in patients with heart failure. *N Engl J Med* 1993; **329:** 149–55.
2. Cohn JN, *et al.* A dose-dependent increase in mortality with vesnarinone among patients with severe heart failure. *N Engl J Med* 1998; **339:** 1810–16.


## Warfarin Sodium *(BANM, rINNM)*

Sodium Warfarin; Warfarina sódica; Warfarinum Natricum. The sodium salt of 4-hydroxy-3-(3-oxo-1-phenylbutyl)coumarin ; Sodium 2-oxo-3-[(1RS)-3-oxo-1-phenylbutyl]-2H-1-benzopyran-4-olate.

$C_{19}H_{15}NaO_4$ = 330.3.

*CAS — 81-81-2 (warfarin); 2610-86-8 (warfarin potassium); 129-06-6 (warfarin sodium).*

*ATC — B01AA03.*

NOTE. The use of the term warfarin sodium in *Martindale* should generally be taken to include the sodium clathrate. Until 1991 the BP, like the USP, allowed the use of either warfarin sodium or warfarin sodium clathrate in the definition of warfarin sodium.

**Pharmacopoeias.** In *Chin., Eur.* (see p.vi), *Int.*, and *US*.
*Chin., Int.*, and *US* permit either warfarin sodium or warfarin sodium clathrate. *Eur.* has a separate monograph for warfarin sodium clathrate (see below).
*Jpn* includes Warfarin Potassium.

**Ph. Eur. 5.0** (Warfarin Sodium). A white, hygroscopic powder. Very soluble in water and in alcohol; soluble in acetone; very slightly soluble in dichloromethane. A 1% solution in water has a pH of 7.6 to 8.6. Store in airtight containers. Protect from light.

**USP 27** (Warfarin Sodium). A white, odourless, amorphous solid or a crystalline clathrate which is discoloured by light. Very soluble in water; freely soluble in alcohol; very slightly soluble in chloroform and in ether. A 1% solution in water has a pH of 7.2 to 8.3. Protect from light.

**Adsorption.** Studies carried out for periods of 24 hours to 3 months found some adsorption of warfarin sodium by PVC when dissolved in 0.9% sodium chloride solution[1,2] or in 5% glucose solution.[3] In one of these studies,[1] adsorption was decreased by buffering the solution from its initial pH of 6.7 to a pH of 7.4. The second study[2] could demonstrate no adsorption onto polyethylene-lined or glass infusion containers.


1. Kowaluk EA, *et al.* Interactions between drugs and polyvinyl chloride infusion bags. *Am J Hosp Pharm* 1981; **38:** 1308–14.
2. Martens HJ, *et al.* Sorption of various drugs in polyvinyl chloride, glass, and polyethylene-lined infusion containers. *Am J Hosp Pharm* 1990; **47:** 369–73.
3. Moorhatch P, Chiou WL. Interactions between drugs and plastic intravenous fluid bags: part i: sorption studies on 17 drugs. *Am J Hosp Pharm* 1974; **31:** 72–8.


**Incompatibility.** Solutions of warfarin sodium have been reported to be incompatible with adrenaline hydrochloride, amikacin sulfate, metaraminol tartrate, oxytocin, promazine hydrochloride, and tetracycline hydrochloride. Visual incompatibility has been reported[1] with solutions of warfarin sodium mixed with solutions of aminophylline, bretylium tosilate, ceftazidime, cimetidine hydrochloride, ciprofloxacin lactate, dobutamine hydrochloride, esmolol hydrochloride, gentamicin sulfate, labetalol hydrochloride, metronidazole hydrochloride, or vancomycin hydrochloride. Haze was also reported after 24 hours with sodium chloride 0.9%.


1. Bahal SM, *et al.* Visual compatibility of warfarin sodium injection with selected medications and solutions. *Am J Health-Syst Pharm* 1997; **54:** 2599–2600.


## Warfarin Sodium Clathrate *(BANM)*

Warfarina sódica, clatrato de; Warfarinum Natricum Clathratum. The clathrate of warfarin sodium with isopropyl alcohol in the molecular proportions 2 to 1 respectively.

*ATC — B01AA03.*

NOTE. The use of the term warfarin sodium in *Martindale* should generally be taken to include the sodium clathrate. Until 1991 the BP, like the USP, allowed the use of either warfarin sodium or warfarin sodium clathrate in the definition of warfarin sodium.

**Pharmacopoeias.** In *Eur.* (see p.vi).
*Chin., Int.*, and *US* permit either warfarin sodium or warfarin sodium clathrate.

**Ph. Eur. 5.0** (Warfarin Sodium Clathrate). A white powder. Very soluble in water; freely soluble in alcohol; soluble in acetone; very slightly soluble in dichloromethane. A 1% solution in water has a pH of 7.6 to 8.6. Store in airtight containers. Protect from light.

Warfarin sodium clathrate contains approximately 92% of warfarin sodium.

## Adverse Effects

The major risk from warfarin therapy is of haemorrhage from almost any organ of the body with the consequent effects of haematomas as well as anaemia. Although good control of warfarin anticoagulation is essential in preventing haemorrhage, bleeding has occurred at therapeutic international normalised ratio (INR) values. In such cases the possibility of an underlying cause such as renal or alimentary tract disease should be investigated. Skin necrosis, and purple discoloration of the toes (due to cholesterol embolisation) have occasionally occurred. Hypersensitivity reactions are extremely rare. Other effects not necessarily associated with haemorrhage include alopecia, fever, nausea, vomiting, diarrhoea, skin reactions, jaundice, hepatic dysfunction, and pancreatitis.

Warfarin is a recognised teratogen. Given in the first trimester of pregnancy it can cause a fetal warfarin syndrome or warfarin embryopathy characterised by bone stippling (chondrodysplasia punctata) and nasal hypoplasia. CNS abnormalities may develop following use in any trimester but appear most likely after use in the second or third trimester. Use of warfarin during pregnancy has been associated with an increased rate of abortion and still-birth, although this may, in part, be the consequence of an underlying maternal condition. Use in the late stages of pregnancy is associated with fetal haemorrhage. Reported incidences of the above complications have varied; one estimate is that if a coumarin anticoagulant is taken during pregnancy, one-sixth of pregnancies will result in an abnormal liveborn infant, and one-sixth will result in abortion or still-birth.

**Effects on the blood.** The incidence and risk of haemorrhage during long-term oral anticoagulation has been studied in patients in clinical trials[1] and in population-based studies.[2-5] The risk of bleeding was generally higher with more intense anticoagulation and in the presence of other risk factors but the relationship with age was less clear. Some studies have shown higher rates of bleeding in elderly patients, but others have not; the risk of intracranial bleeding, however, does seem to be higher in the elderly.[1,5] Although cumulative risk of bleeding was related to duration of anticoagulation therapy, risk may be highest early in the course.[1]

Withdrawal of warfarin therapy may lead to rebound hypercoagulability and it has been suggested[6] that warfarin should be withdrawn gradually, although there is no clinical evidence to support this.

For the risk of corpus luteum haemorrhage or haematoma associated with ovulation in patients on oral anticoagulants, see under Precautions, below.


1. Levine MN, *et al.* Hemorrhagic complications of anticoagulant treatment. *Chest* 2001; **119** (suppl): 108S–121S.
2. Gitter MJ, *et al.* Bleeding and thromboembolism during anticoagulant therapy: a population-based study in Rochester, Minnesota. *Mayo Clin Proc* 1995; **70:** 725–33.
3. Fihn SD, *et al.* The risk for and severity of bleeding complications in elderly patients treated with warfarin. *Ann Intern Med* 1996; **124:** 970–9.
4. Palareti G, *et al.* Bleeding complications of oral anticoagulant treatment: an inception-cohort, prospective collaborative study (ISCOAT). *Lancet* 1996; **348:** 423–8.
5. Palareti G, *et al.* Oral anticoagulation treatment in the elderly: a nested, prospective, case-control study. *Arch Intern Med* 2000; **160:** 470–8.
6. Palareti G, Legnani C. Warfarin withdrawal: pharmacokinetic-pharmacodynamic considerations. *Clin Pharmacokinet* 1996; **30:** 300–13.


**Effects on the bones.** Vitamin K is involved in bone metabolism and vitamin K deficiency is associated with an increased risk of osteoporotic fractures. It has been suggested, therefore, that patients on long-term treatment with oral anticoagulants, which are vitamin K antagonists, may be at increased risk of osteoporosis and fractures. However, two large observational studies in older women have produced conflicting results. A prospective study[1] of both users and nonusers of warfarin found that warfarin was not associated with decrease in bone density or increase in fracture rates. A retrospective study[2] reported an association between long-term anticoagulant use and increased risk of vertebral and rib fractures, compared with the general population. Overall, however, the risk of any fracture was not significantly increased.


1. Jamal SA, *et al.* Warfarin use and risk for osteoporosis in elderly women. *Ann Intern Med* 1998; **128:** 829–32.
2. Caraballo PJ, *et al.* Long-term use of oral anticoagulants and the risk of fracture. *Arch Intern Med* 1999; **159:** 1750–6.


**Effects on the fetus.** Reviews of reported fetal complications after exposure to coumarin anticoagulants during pregnancy.


1. Hall JG, *et al.* Maternal and fetal sequelae of anticoagulation during pregnancy. *Am J Med* 1980; **68:** 122–40.
2. Chan WS, *et al.* Anticoagulation of pregnant women with mechanical heart valves: a systematic review of the literature. *Arch Intern Med* 2000; **160:** 191–6.
3. Ginsberg JS, *et al.* Use of antithrombotic agents during pregnancy. *Chest* 2001; **119** (suppl): 122S–131S.


**Effects on the liver.** There have been a few isolated reports of cholestatic liver damage in patients taking warfarin sodium.[1-3] In these cases hepatic injury resolved on withdrawal.


1. Rehnqvist N. Intrahepatic jaundice due to warfarin therapy. *Acta Med Scand* 1978; **204:** 335–6.
2. Jones DB, *et al.* Jaundice following warfarin therapy. *Postgrad Med J* 1980; **56:** 671.
3. Adler E, *et al.* Cholestatic hepatic injury related to warfarin exposure. *Arch Intern Med* 1986; **146:** 1837–9.


**Effects on sexual function.** There have been reports[1-3] of priapism in patients taking oral anticoagulants such as warfarin.


1. Baños JE, *et al.* Drug-induced priapism: its aetiology, incidence and treatment. *Med Toxicol* 1989; **4:** 46–58.

2. Daryanani S, Wilde JT. Priapism in a patient with protein C deficiency. *Clin Lab Haematol* 1997; **19:** 213–14.
3. Zimbelman J, *et al.* Unusual complications of warfarin therapy: skin necrosis and priapism. *J Pediatr* 2000; **137:** 266–8.

**Effects on the skin and hair.** Necrosis of skin and soft tissue associated with coumarin anticoagulant therapy has been reviewed.[1,2] Coumarin-induced necrosis occurs rarely and is characterised by a localised, painful skin lesion, initially erythematous or haemorrhagic in appearance, that becomes bullous and eventually culminates in gangrenous necrosis. Fatalities have occurred. Areas of increased subcutaneous fat such as breast, thigh, and buttocks have most often been involved. The aetiology appears to be thrombotic but the exact pathophysiology is not known. Patients with protein C deficiency appear to be at highest risk. Treatment with coumarin anticoagulants should be discontinued on appearance of skin lesions and vitamin K should be given to reverse their effect. Heparin should be administered to provide anticoagulation. Fresh frozen plasma or protein C concentrates may also have a role in reversing the condition. Surgical intervention is usually required if necrosis does develop.

Other skin reactions have also been reported with coumarins. Vasculitis affecting both legs developed in a 74-year-old woman a few weeks after starting treatment with acenocoumarol for deep-vein thrombosis and pulmonary embolism.[3] Acenocoumarol treatment was stopped and the skin lesions steadily improved over 15 days. However, the skin lesions reappeared a few hours after re-exposure to a single dose of acenocoumarol. The patient had also been taking amiodarone which may have contributed to the reaction.

Increased shedding of telogen hair has been stated to occur in patients given coumarin anticoagulants.[4]

1. Cole MS, *et al.* Coumarin necrosis—a review of the literature. *Surgery* 1988; **103:** 271–7.
2. Comp PC. Coumarin-induced skin necrosis: incidence, mechanisms, management and avoidance. *Drug Safety* 1993; **8:** 128–35.
3. Susano R, *et al.* Hypersensitivity vasculitis related to nicoumalone. *BMJ* 1993; **306:** 973.
4. Smith AG. Drug-induced disorders of hair and nails. *Adverse Drug React Bull* 1995 (173); 655–8.

## Treatment of Adverse Effects

The methods used to manage bleeding and/or excessive anticoagulation during warfarin therapy, or following warfarin overdosage, depend upon the degree of bleeding, the value of the international normalised ratio (INR), and the degree of thromboembolic risk.

If the INR is greater than 5.0 but there is no bleeding or only minor bleeding, warfarin should be temporarily withheld until the INR falls to below 5.0. In some cases where the INR is between 5.0 and 6.0 a reduction in warfarin dose, rather than withdrawal, may be sufficient. For an INR greater than 8.0 administration of phytomenadione (vitamin $K_1$) should also be considered if there are other risk factors for bleeding; typical doses of phytomenadione are 0.5 mg intravenously or up to 5 mg orally.

If there is any major bleeding warfarin should be stopped and phytomenadione 5 mg by slow intravenous injection given together with a concentrate of factors II, VII, IX, and X. The dose of concentrate should be calculated based on 50 units of factor IX/kg. If no concentrate is available fresh frozen plasma should be infused (about one litre for an adult), but may not be as effective. Higher doses of phytomenadione have been used (see Over-anticoagulation, p.1468) but it should be remembered that phytomenadione takes several hours to act and large doses may reduce the response to resumed therapy with anticoagulants for a week or more.

If bleeding occurs unexpectedly at therapeutic INR values, the possibility of an underlying cause such as renal or alimentary tract disease should be investigated.

See under Effects on the Skin and Hair, above, for the management of skin and soft tissue necrosis.

## Precautions

Warfarin should not be given to patients who are haemorrhaging. In general it should not be given to patients at serious risk of haemorrhage, although it has been used with very careful control; patients at risk include those with haemorrhagic blood disorders, peptic ulcer disease, severe wounds (including surgical wounds), cerebrovascular disorders, and bacterial endocarditis. Severe renal and hepatic impairment as well as severe hypertension are considered by some to be contra-indications. Pregnancy is also generally considered to be a contra-indication, especially in the first trimester and during the last few weeks of pregnancy (see Adverse Effects, above).

Many factors may affect anticoagulant control with warfarin. These include vitamin K status, thyroid status, renal function, bioavailability differences between warfarin preparations, factors affecting absorption of warfarin, and drug interactions. Such factors may be responsible for apparent resistance to warfarin and a few patients have displayed hereditary resistance. Dosage alterations should be guided by regular monitoring of oral anticoagulant therapy and clinical status. Patients should carry anticoagulant treatment booklets.

◊ A discussion of factors affecting the anticoagulant effect of warfarin sodium.[1]

1. Shetty HGM, *et al.* Clinical pharmacokinetic considerations in the control of oral anticoagulant therapy. *Clin Pharmacokinet* 1989; **16:** 238–53.

**Breast feeding.** Drug concentrations were measured[1] in the plasma and milk of 13 lactating women receiving between 2 and 12 mg of warfarin daily. Plasma concentrations varied from 1.6 to 8.5 micromoles/litre but none was detectable in the breast milk or in the plasma of the 7 infants who were breastfed (limit of detection 0.08 micromoles/litre). No anticoagulant effect was found in the 3 breast-fed infants tested. In another report[2] of 2 women (dose of warfarin not specified), no evidence of the drug was found in the milk of one mother, and no anticoagulant effect was found in either infant. The American Academy of Pediatrics considers[3] that warfarin is therefore usually compatible with breast feeding.

1. Orme ML'E, *et al.* May mothers given warfarin breast-feed their infants? *BMJ* 1977; **1:** 1564–5.
2. McKenna R, *et al.* Is warfarin sodium contraindicated in the lactating mother? *J Pediatr* 1983; **103:** 325–7.
3. American Academy of Pediatrics. The transfer of drugs and other chemicals into human milk. *Pediatrics* 2001; **108:** 776–89. Correction. *ibid.*; 1029. Also available at: http://aappolicy.aappublications.org/cgi/content/full/pediatrics%3b108/3/776 (accessed 06/07/04)

**Macular degeneration.** Intra-ocular haemorrhage leading to loss of vision has been reported[1,2] in patients with the neovascular form of age-related macular degeneration who were receiving warfarin, and caution has been advised[3] in such patients.

1. Tilanus MAD, *et al.* Relationship between anticoagulant medication and massive intraocular hemorrhage in age-related macular degeneration. *Graefes Arch Clin Exp Ophthalmol* 2000; **238:** 482–5.
2. Ung T, *et al.* Long term warfarin associated with bilateral blindness in a patient with atrial fibrillation and macular degeneration. *Heart* 2003; **89:** 985.
3. Kowal LM, Harper CA. Visual complications of warfarin. *Med J Aust* 2002; **176:** 351.

**Ovulation.** Corpus luteum haematoma or haemorrhage was associated with ovulation in 3 women being treated with coumarin anticoagulants.[1] It was suggested that suppression of ovulation be considered for women on anticoagulants during their fertile years, even if sterilisation had been performed.

See Sex Hormones under Interactions, below, for the effect of oral contraceptives on the activity of oral anticoagulants.

1. Bogers J-W, *et al.* Complications of anticoagulant therapy in ovulatory women. *Lancet* 1991; **337:** 618–19.

## Interactions

Many compounds interact with warfarin and other oral anticoagulants. Details of these interactions are given below for all oral anticoagulants with different groups of drugs; if the anticoagulant is other than warfarin, then its identity is specified. The major interactions are summarised in the tables, below. Readers should be aware that while interactions of a pharmacodynamic nature occurring with one anticoagulant may well apply to another, this is not necessarily the case with interactions of a pharmacokinetic nature.

An interaction may be due to increased or decreased anticoagulant metabolism; with warfarin some interacting drugs such as cimetidine, co-trimoxazole, or phenylbutazone have a selective effect on its stereoisomers. Altered absorption may sometimes play a part, as with colestyramine. Displacement of oral anticoagulants from plasma protein binding sites has been reported with many drugs, including some analgesics. Not all reports that have recorded an alteration in the pharmacokinetics of the anticoagulant have, however, shown a corresponding change in clinical response.

Interference with the coagulation process may be responsible for the increased risk of haemorrhage when aspirin, clofibrate, or thyroid hormones are used with anticoagulants. Many other compounds, such as asparaginase, some contrast media, epoprostenol, streptokinase, and urokinase also carry this risk; while interactions between these compounds and anticoagulants are not discussed further below, the possibility of an increased risk of haemorrhage should be considered when they are used together.

Where there is a risk of serious haemorrhage from an interaction, then use of the 2 drugs is best avoided. In other instances the anticoagulant activity should be carefully monitored so as to increase or decrease the anticoagulant dose as required. Critical periods are when patients stabilised on an anticoagulant start treatment with an interacting drug, or when patients stabilised on a regimen of an interacting drug and anticoagulant have the interacting drug withdrawn. Depending on the mechanism of the interaction, the clinical response to the interaction may be rapid or may take some days. Interactions involving displacement from plasma protein binding sites are often transient. Readers should also be aware that some interacting drugs do not produce predictable effects; there have for instance been reports of increased as well as decreased anticoagulant activity with disopyramide, phenytoin, quinidine, and oral contraceptives. Another problem occurs with dipyridamole; it can cause bleeding when given to patients taking anticoagulants but without any changes in the measures used for anticoagulant control.

◊ Reviews.

1. Harder S, Thürmann P. Clinically important drug interactions with anticoagulants: an update. *Clin Pharmacokinet* 1996; **30:** 416–44.

**Alcohol.** Alcohol has a variable effect on warfarin. Heavy regular drinkers may experience a diminished effect, perhaps through enzyme induction, although the effect of warfarin may be increased in the presence of liver impairment; acute ingestion has enhanced the effect of warfarin. A moderate alcohol intake is generally not considered to cause problems.

**Analgesics and NSAIDs.** All NSAIDs should be used with caution or not at all in patients on warfarin. Many NSAIDs inhibit platelet function to some extent and have an irritant effect on the gastrointestinal tract, so increasing the risk of haemorrhage. Furthermore, some NSAIDs increase the hypoprothrombinae-

Drugs generally recognised as diminishing the effects of oral anticoagulants are included in the following list. Further information on the interactions with these drugs and others where the interaction is not so well recognised is provided in the referenced section below.

| | |
|---|---|
| acetomenaphthone | ethchlorvynol |
| alcohol (chronic ingestion without liver impairment) | glutethimide |
| aminoglutethimide | griseofulvin |
| barbiturates | nafcillin |
| carbamazepine | phytomenadione |
| dichloralphenazone | rifampicin |

Drugs recognised or generally reported as enhancing oral anticoagulants are included in the following list. Further information on the interactions with these drugs and others where the interaction is not so well recognised is provided in the referenced section below.

| | |
|---|---|
| alcohol (acute ingestion or chronic ingestion with liver impairment) | etacrynic acid |
| allopurinol | ethylestrenol |
| amiodarone | fluconazole |
| aspirin | glucagon |
| cefamandole | itraconazole |
| chloramphenicol | ketoconazole |
| cimetidine | metronidazole |
| clofibrate | miconazole |
| cloral hydrate | norethandrolone |
| co-trimoxazole | NSAIDs |
| danazol | oxymetholone |
| dextropropoxyphene | quinidine |
| dextrothyroxine | stanozolol |
| dipyridamole | sulfinpyrazone |
| disulfiram | tamoxifen |
| erythromycin | thyroid agents |
| | tienilic acid |
| | triclofos sodium |

mic effect of warfarin, possibly by an intrinsic effect on coagulation or by displacement of warfarin from plasma protein-binding sites. Many studies have compared the relative displacing action of a range of NSAIDs *in vitro*, but such studies cannot easily be extrapolated to the clinical situation. Changes in plasma concentration of unbound warfarin resulting from displacement from plasma protein-binding sites are usually transient and are most likely to occur in the first few weeks after an NSAID is added to or withdrawn from warfarin therapy; monitoring of anticoagulant therapy is, therefore, most critical during this period.

High doses of *aspirin* and some other *salicylates* enhance the hypoprothrombinaemic effect of warfarin and should generally be avoided in patients on oral anticoagulant therapy. Low-dose aspirin with warfarin may have a role in some patients but the risk of gastrointestinal bleeding is increased. The possibility of an interaction with topical salicylates should also be considered.[1,2]

Use of *phenylbutazone* with warfarin has led to serious haemorrhage and should be avoided. Phenylbutazone affects the metabolism of the *R*- and *S*- isomers of warfarin in complex and different ways with the net effect of enhancing its anticoagulant activity.[3] Related drugs such as *oxyphenbutazone*, *azapropazone*,[4-6] and *feprazone*[7] behave similarly and should also be avoided.

For the following NSAIDs there are a few studies or isolated reports suggesting that they may enhance the hypoprothrombinaemic effect of warfarin or other specified oral anticoagulant: *diflunisal* (with acenocoumarol[8] or warfarin[9]), *flurbiprofen* (with acenocoumarol),[10] *indometacin*,[11,12] *ketoprofen*,[13] *meclofenamate sodium*,[14] *mefenamic acid*,[15] *piroxicam*, (with warfarin[16] or acenocoumarol[17]), *sulindac*,[18,19] *tiaprofenic acid* (with acenocoumarol),[20] and *tolmetin sodium*.[21] In many cases the result of concomitant therapy was an increased prothrombin time which may or may not be clinically significant; in other cases haemorrhage occurred. It should also be noted that for many of the above NSAIDs, perhaps particularly indometacin, there are studies (not cited) in which no enhancement of warfarin activity was found. NSAIDs with an apparently minimal effect on warfarin activity include *etodolac, ibuprofen*, and *naproxen*.

Although a study in healthy subjects indicated that there was no interaction between warfarin and *celecoxib*, a selective inhibitor of cyclo-oxygenase-2, there have been several reports[22-25] of an increase in the INR with concomitant therapy; bleeding has also been reported in some patients.[24] Increases in INR have also been reported in studies[25,26] of warfarin with *rofecoxib*; and there have also been reports of bleeding.[27]

In view of the above considerations, *paracetamol* is recommended as the general analgesic and antipyretic of choice in patients on oral anticoagulant therapy. However, caution should be observed since, although it has no effect on the gastric mucosa or on platelet function, some studies (with warfarin, anisindione, dicoumarol, or phenprocoumon)[28,29] and isolated reports[30] have found an increased risk of bleeding in patients taking regular doses of paracetamol while on an oral anticoagulant.

*Opioid analgesics* do not generally cause problems, although there have been reports of enhanced anticoagulant activity in patients receiving *tramadol* with warfarin[31] or phenprocoumon.[32] *Co-proxamol*, a combination of *dextropropoxyphene* and paracetamol, has increased the effect of warfarin.[33-35] *Co-codamol*, a combination of *codeine* and paracetamol, has also enhanced warfarin activity.[36]

Amongst other analgesics, *cinchophen* (with dicoumarol, ethyl biscoumacetate, or phenindione)[37] and *fenyramidol* (with warfarin, dicoumarol, or phenindione)[38] have been reported to enhance the activity of oral anticoagulants and there is the possibility of such an effect with *glafenine* (with phenprocoumon).[39] *Phenazone*, an inducer of enzyme metabolism, reduces plasma concentrations of warfarin and, in contrast with most other analgesics, may necessitate an increase in warfarin dosage.[40]


1. Chow WH, *et al.* Potentiation of warfarin anticoagulation by topical methylsalicylate ointment. *J R Soc Med* 1989; **82:** 501–2.
2. Littleton F. Warfarin and topical salicylates. *JAMA* 1990; **263:** 2888.
3. Banfield C, *et al.* Phenylbutazone-warfarin interaction in man: further stereochemical and metabolic considerations. *Br J Clin Pharmacol* 1983; **16:** 669–75.
4. Powell-Jackson PR. Interaction between azapropazone and warfarin. *BMJ* 1977; **1:** 1193–4.
5. Green AE, *et al.* Potentiation of warfarin by azapropazone. *BMJ* 1977; **1:** 1532.
6. Win N, Mitchell DC. Azapropazone and warfarin. *BMJ* 1991; **302:** 969–70.
7. Chierichetti S, *et al.* Comparison of feprazone and phenylbutazone interaction with warfarin in man. *Curr Ther Res* 1975; **18:** 568–72.
8. Tempero KF, *et al.* Diflunisal: a review of pharmacokinetic and pharmacodynamic properties, drug interactions, and special tolerability studies in humans. *Br J Clin Pharmacol* 1977; **4** (suppl 1): 31S–36S.
9. Serlin MJ, *et al.* The effect of diflunisal on the steady state pharmacodynamics and pharmacokinetics of warfarin. *Br J Clin Pharmacol* 1980; **9:** 287P–8P.
10. Stricker BHC, Delhez JL. Interaction between flurbiprofen and coumarins. *BMJ* 1982; **285:** 812–13.
11. Koch-Weser J. Hemorrhagic reactions and drug interactions in 500 warfarin-treated patients. *Clin Pharmacol Ther* 1973; **14:** 139.
12. Self TH, *et al.* Drug enhancement of warfarin activity. *Lancet* 1975; **ii:** 557–8.
13. Flessner MF. Prolongation of prothrombin time and severe gastrointestinal bleeding associated with combined use of warfarin and ketoprofen. *JAMA* 1988; **259:** 353.
14. Baragar FD, Smith TC. Drug interaction studies with sodium meclofenamate (Meclomen®). *Curr Ther Res* 1978; **23** (suppl 4): S51–S59.
15. Holmes EL. Experimental observations on flufenamic, mefenamic, and meclofenamic acids: IV: Toleration by normal human subjects. *Ann Phys Med* 1966; **9** (suppl): 36–49.
16. Rhodes RS, *et al.* A warfarin-piroxicam drug interaction. *Drug Intell Clin Pharm* 1985; **19:** 556–8.
17. Bonnabry P, *et al.* Stereoselective interaction between piroxicam and acenocoumarol. *Br J Clin Pharmacol* 1996; **41:** 525–30.
18. Carter SA. Potential effect of sulindac on response of prothrombin-time to oral anticoagulants. *Lancet* 1979; **ii:** 698–9.
19. Ross JRY, Beeley L. Sulindac, prothrombin time, and anticoagulants. *Lancet* 1979; **ii:** 1075.
20. Whittaker SJ, *et al.* A severe, potentially fatal, interaction between tiaprofenic acid and nicoumalone. *Br J Clin Pract* 1986; **40:** 440.
21. Koren JF, *et al.* Tolmetin-warfarin interaction. *Am J Med* 1987; **82:** 1278–9.
22. Mersfelder TL, Stewart LR. Warfarin and celecoxib interaction. *Ann Pharmacother* 2000; **34:** 325–7.
23. Haase KK, *et al.* Potential interaction between celecoxib and warfarin. *Ann Pharmacother* 2000; **34:** 666–7.
24. Adverse Drug Reactions Advisory Committee. Interaction of celecoxib and warfarin. *Aust Adverse Drug React Bull* 2001; **20:** 2.
25. Schaefer MG, *et al.* Interaction of rofecoxib and celecoxib with warfarin. *Am J Health-Syst Pharm* 2003; **60:** 1319–23.
26. Schwartz JI, *et al.* The effect of rofecoxib on the pharmacodynamics and pharmacokinetics of warfarin. *Clin Pharmacol Ther* 2000; **68:** 626–36.
27. Adverse Drug Reactions Advisory Committee (ADRAC). Interaction of rofecoxib with warfarin. *Aust Adverse Drug React Bull* 2002; **21:** 3.
28. Antlitz AM, *et al.* Potentiation of oral anticoagulant therapy by acetaminophen. *Curr Ther Res* 1968; **10:** 501–7.
29. Hylek EM, *et al.* Acetaminophen and other risk factors for excessive warfarin anticoagulation. *JAMA* 1998; **279:** 657–62.
30. Boeijinga JJ, *et al.* Interaction between paracetamol and coumarin anticoagulants. *Lancet* 1982; **i:** 506.
31. Scher ML, *et al.* Potential interaction between tramadol and warfarin. *Ann Pharmacother* 1997; **31:** 646–7.
32. Madsen H, *et al.* Interaction between tramadol and phenprocoumon. *Lancet* 1997; **350:** 637.
33. Orme M, *et al.* Warfarin and Distalgesic interaction. *BMJ* 1976; **1:** 200.
34. Jones RV. Warfarin and Distalgesic interaction. *BMJ* 1976; **1:** 460.
35. Smith R, *et al.* Propoxyphene and warfarin interaction. *Drug Intell Clin Pharm* 1984; **18:** 822.
36. Bartle WR, Blakely JA. Potentiation of warfarin anticoagulation by acetaminophen. *JAMA* 1991; **265:** 1260.
37. Jarnum S. Cinchophen and acetylsalicylic acid in anticoagulant treatment. *Scand J Clin Lab Invest* 1954; **6:** 91–3.
38. Carter SA. Potentiation of the effect of orally administered anticoagulants by phenyramidol hydrochloride. *N Engl J Med* 1965; **273:** 423–6.
39. Boeijinga JK, van der Vijgh WJF. Double blind study of the effect of glafenine (Glifanan®) on oral anticoagulant therapy with phenprocoumon (Marcumar®). *J Clin Pharmacol* 1977; **12:** 291–6.
40. Whitfield JB, *et al.* Changes in plasma γ-glutamyl transpeptidase activity associated with alterations in drug metabolism in man. *BMJ* 1973; **1:** 316–18.


**Antiarrhythmics.** *Amiodarone* has been shown in several studies to increase the activity of warfarin[1-5] and acenocoumarol,[6,7] probably through inhibition of metabolism. The potentiating effect of amiodarone has been reported to persist for up to 4 months after its withdrawal.[1] There is a report of phenprocoumon not being affected by amiodarone.[8] Isolated reports with *disopyramide*[9] and *quinidine*[10] have suggested that these drugs can enhance the anticoagulant effect of warfarin. In 7 patients on warfarin or dicoumarol treated with disopyramide or quinidine, however, all but one needed a small increase in the weekly anticoagulant dose suggesting that the antiarrhythmic had reduced the anticoagulant effect.[11] Since the effect was observed after conversion of atrial fibrillation to sinus rhythm an involvement of haemodynamic factors was postulated. Several studies (not cited) have failed to show an effect of quinidine on warfarin. There are also reports indicating that *propafenone*[12] and *moracizine*[13] can enhance warfarin.


1. Martinowitz U, *et al.* Interaction between warfarin sodium and amiodarone. *N Engl J Med* 1981; **304:** 671–2.
2. Almog S, *et al.* Mechanism of warfarin potentiation by amiodarone: dose—and concentration—dependent inhibition of warfarin elimination. *Eur J Clin Pharmacol* 1985; **28:** 257–61.
3. Watt AH, *et al.* Amiodarone reduces plasma warfarin clearance in man. *Br J Clin Pharmacol* 1985; **20:** 707–9.
4. O'Reilly RA, *et al.* Interaction of amiodarone with racemic warfarin and its separated enantiomorphs in humans. *Clin Pharmacol Ther* 1987; **42:** 290–4.
5. Kerin NZ, *et al.* The incidence, magnitude, and time course of the amiodarone-warfarin interaction. *Arch Intern Med* 1988; **148:** 1779–81.
6. Arboix M, *et al.* The potentiation of acenocoumarol anticoagulant effect by amiodarone. *Br J Clin Pharmacol* 1984; **18:** 355–60.
7. Richard C, *et al.* Prospective study of the potentiation of acenocoumarol by amiodarone. *Eur J Clin Pharmacol* 1985; **28:** 625–9.
8. Verstraete M, *et al.* Dissimilar effect of two anti-anginal drugs belonging to the benzofuran group on the action of coumarin derivatives. *Arch Int Pharmacodyn Ther* 1968; **176:** 33–41.
9. Haworth E, Burroughs AK. Disopyramide and warfarin interaction. *BMJ* 1977; **2:** 866–7.
10. Gazzaniga AB, Stewart DR. Possible quinidine-induced hemorrhage in a patient on warfarin sodium. *N Engl J Med* 1969; **280:** 711–12.
11. Sylvén C, Anderson P. Evidence that disopyramide does not interact with warfarin. *BMJ* 1983; **286:** 1181.
12. Kates RE, *et al.* Interaction between warfarin and propafenone in healthy volunteer subjects. *Clin Pharmacol Ther* 1987; **42:** 305–11.
13. Serpa MD, *et al.* Moricizine—warfarin: a possible drug interaction. *Ann Pharmacother* 1992; **26:** 127.


**Antibacterials.** Several antibacterials have been involved in interactions with warfarin. Only a few reports are of serious effects and it is unlikely that any of the drugs need to be contra-indicated with warfarin; careful control should suffice.

Most of the drugs enhance the effects of warfarin. Apart from possible effects on the metabolism or plasma-protein binding of warfarin, some antibacterials may interfere with platelet function or with the bacterial synthesis of vitamin K in the gastrointestinal tract and thus have an anticoagulant effect of their own. This is generally considered unlikely to be of clinical significance except, perhaps, in patients with an inadequate vitamin K intake. Fever itself may increase the catabolism of clotting factors and exaggerate a potential antibacterial-warfarin interaction.

There are several reports of an enhanced warfarin response with *co-trimoxazole*; stereospecific inhibition of warfarin metabolism is probably responsible.[1] The interaction is generally attributed to the *sulfamethoxazole* moiety and there are isolated reports suggesting that the activity of warfarin (or other specified oral anticoagulant) may be enhanced by other sulfonamides including *sulfafurazole*,[2] *sulfamethizole*,[3] and *sulfaphenazole* (with phenindione).[4]

There are several reports of potentiation of the effects of warfarin by *erythromycin* or its salts; inhibition of warfarin metabolism probably occurs. Although no clinically-significant increase in prothrombin time was found in 8 non-infected patients, the potential for an interaction was recognised.[5] An enhanced response to warfarin has also been reported with *azithromycin*[6,7] and with *roxithromycin*,[8] including reports of spontaneous bleeding with the latter. *Clarithromycin* may potentiate the effect of acenocoumarol[9] and of warfarin,[10] although other factors may also have been involved in this case.

*Cefamandole* has been reported to enhance the hypoprothrombinaemic response to warfarin.[11,12] Interference with vitamin K synthesis in the gastrointestinal tract and/or liver has been implicated. Related cephalosporins with an *N*-methylthiotetrazole side-chain such as *cefmetazole*, *cefmenoxime*, *cefoperazone*, and *latamoxef* may be expected to behave similarly although there appear to be no reports of an interaction. *Cefazolin*, which has a similar side-chain, may also enhance the effect of warfarin to some extent.[12]

There have been a few reports of increased activity of warfarin (or other specified oral anticoagulant) by quinolone antibacterials including *nalidixic acid* (with warfarin[13,14] or acenocoumarol[15]), *ciprofloxacin*,[16,17] *levofloxacin*,[18] *norfloxacin*,[19] and *ofloxacin*,[20,21] although for some of these there are also studies indicating no effect (not cited). *Enoxacin* has been reported to decrease the clearance of *R*-warfarin but not *S*-warfarin; no prolongation of prothrombin time occurred.[22]

There are isolated reports suggesting an enhanced effect of warfarin (or other specified oral anticoagulant) with *aminosalicylic acid*,[23] *benzylpenicillin*,[24] *chloramphenicol* (with dicoumarol),[25] *doxycycline*,[26] *isoniazid*,[27] and *neomycin*.[28] Prothrombin times might be prolonged by broad-spectrum antibacterials such as *ampicillin*, and there has been a report[29] of an increased INR and haematuria in a patient taking warfarin with amoxicillin and clavulanic acid. Manufacturers' warnings of potentiation of warfarin by *aztreonam*, *trimethoprim*, and *tetracyclines* other than doxycycline appear to have only a theoretical basis. *Metronidazole* is discussed under Antiprotozoals, below.

*Rifampicin* diminishes the effect of warfarin by induction of metabolising enzymes in the liver. There are several reports of a similar effect with *nafcillin*[30-32] and with *dicloxacillin sodium*.[33,34]


1. O'Reilly RA. Stereoselective interaction of trimethoprim-sulfamethoxazole with the separated enantiomorphs of racemic warfarin in man. *N Engl J Med* 1980; **302** 33–5.
2. Sioris LJ, *et al.* Potentiation of warfarin anticoagulation by sulfisoxazole. *Arch Intern Med* 1980; **140:** 546–7.
3. Lumholtz B, *et al.* Sulfamethizole-induced inhibition of diphenylhydantoin, tolbutamide, and warfarin metabolism. *Clin Pharmacol Ther* 1975; **17:** 731–4.
4. Varma DR, *et al.* Prothrombin response to phenindione during hypoalbuminaemia. *Br J Clin Pharmacol* 1975; **2:** 467–8.
5. Weibert RT, *et al.* Effect of erythromycin in patients receiving long-term warfarin therapy. *Clin Pharm* 1989; **8:** 210–14.
6. Lane G. Increased hypoprothrombinemic effect of warfarin possibly induced by azithromycin. *Ann Pharmacother* 1996; **30:** 884–5.
7. Woldtvedt BR, *et al.* Possible increased anticoagulation effect of warfarin induced by azithromycin. *Ann Pharmacother* 1998; **32:** 269–70.
8. Anonymous. Interaction of warfarin with macrolide antibiotics. *Aust Adverse Drug React Bull* 1995; **14:** 11.
9. Grau E, *et al.* Interaction between clarithromycin and oral anticoagulants. *Ann Pharmacother* 1996; **30:** 1495–6.
10. Recker MW, Kier KL. Potential interaction between clarithromycin and warfarin. *Ann Pharmacother* 1997; **31:** 996–8.
11. Angaran DM, *et al.* The influence of prophylactic antibiotics on the warfarin anticoagulation response in the postoperative prosthetic cardiac valve patient. *Ann Surg* 1984; **199:** 107–11.
12. Angaran DM, *et al.* The comparative influence of prophylactic antibiotics on the prothrombin response to warfarin in the postoperative prosthetic cardiac valve patient: cefamandole, cefazoline, vancomycin. *Ann Surg* 1987; **206:** 155–61.
13. Hoffbrand BI. Interaction of nalidixic acid and warfarin. *BMJ* 1974; **2:** 666.
14. Leor J, *et al.* Interaction between nalidixic acid and warfarin. *Ann Intern Med* 1987; **107:** 601.
15. Potasman I, Bassan H. Nicoumalone and nalidixic acid interaction. *Ann Intern Med* 1980; **92:** 571.
16. Mott FE, *et al.* Ciprofloxacin and warfarin. *Ann Intern Med* 1989; **111:** 542–3.
17. Kamada AK. Possible interaction between ciprofloxacin and warfarin. *DICP Ann Pharmacother* 1990; **24:** 27–8.

18. Jones CB, Fugate SE. Levofloxacin and warfarin interaction. *Ann Pharmacother* 2002; **36:** 1554–7.
19. Linville T, Matanin D. Norfloxacin and warfarin. *Ann Intern Med* 1989; **110:** 751–2.
20. Leor J, Matetzki S. Ofloxacin and warfarin. *Ann Intern Med* 1988; **109:** 761.
21. Baciewicz AM, *et al.* Interaction of ofloxacin and warfarin. *Ann Intern Med* 1993; **119:** 1223.
22. Toon S, *et al.* Enoxacin-warfarin interaction: pharmacokinetic and stereochemical aspects. *Clin Pharmacol Ther* 1987; **42:** 33–41.
23. Self TH. Interaction of warfarin and aminosalicylic acid. *JAMA* 1973; **223:** 1285.
24. Brown MA, *et al.* Interaction of penicillin-G and warfarin? *Can J Hosp Pharm* 1979; **32:** 18–19.
25. Christensen LK, Skovsted L. Inhibition of drug metabolism by chloramphenicol. *Lancet* 1969; **ii:** 1397–9.
26. Westfall LK, *et al.* Potentiation of warfarin by tetracycline. *Am J Hosp Pharm* 1980; **37:** 1620 and 1625.
27. Rosenthal AR, *et al.* Interaction of isoniazid and warfarin. *JAMA* 1977; **238:** 2177.
28. Udall JA. Drug interference with warfarin therapy. *Clin Med* 1970; **77** (Aug.): 20–5.
29. Davydov L, *et al.* Warfarin and amoxicillin/clavulanate drug interaction. *Ann Pharmacother* 2003; **37:** 367–70.
30. Qureshi GD, *et al.* Warfarin resistance with nafcillin therapy. *Ann Intern Med* 1984; **100:** 527–9.
31. Fraser GL, *et al.* Warfarin resistance associated with nafcillin therapy. *Am J Med* 1989; **87:** 237–8.
32. Davis RL, *et al.* Warfarin-nafcillin interaction. *J Pediatr* 1991; **118:** 300–3.
33. Krstenansky PM, *et al.* Effect of dicloxacillin sodium on the hypoprothrombinemic response to warfarin sodium. *Clin Pharm* 1987; **6:** 804–6.
34. Mailloux A, *et al.* Potential interaction between warfarin and dicloxacillin. *Ann Pharmacother* 1996; **30:** 1402–7.


**Antidepressants.** *Amitriptyline* and *nortriptyline* have been reported to prolong the half-life of dicoumarol in healthy subjects.[1,2] The few reports investigating the effect of tricyclic antidepressants on warfarin have not been able to conclude that a significant interaction exists. *Mianserin* and phenprocoumon have been reported not to interact.[3]

The *British National Formulary* considers that there is a possible risk of increased warfarin activity with *fluvoxamine* and other SSRIs. Increased warfarin activity has been reported in a few patients taking *fluoxetine*,[4] and in 1 patient taking fluvoxamine.[5] There has also been a report of increased anticoagulant activity in a patient taking acenocoumarol and *citalopram*.[6]

An increase in the dose of warfarin has been required by patients also taking *trazodone*.[7,8]


1. Vesell ES, *et al.* Impairment of drug metabolism in man by allopurinol and nortriptyline. *N Engl J Med* 1970; **283:** 1484–8.
2. Pond SM, *et al.* Effects of tricyclic antidepressants on drug metabolism. *Clin Pharmacol Ther* 1975; **18:** 191–9.
3. Kopera H, *et al.* Phenprocoumon requirement, whole blood coagulation time, bleeding time and plasma γ-GT in patients receiving mianserin. *Eur J Clin Pharmacol* 1978; **13:** 351–6.
4. Woolfrey S, *et al.* Fluoxetine-warfarin interaction. *BMJ* 1993; **307:** 241.
5. Limke KK, *et al.* Fluvoxamine interaction with warfarin. *Ann Pharmacother* 2002; **36:** 1890–2.
6. Borrás-Blasco J, *et al.* Probable interaction between citalopram and acenocoumarol. *Ann Pharmacother* 2002; **36:** 345.
7. Hardy J-L, Sirois A. Reduction of prothrombin and partial thromboplastin times with trazodone. *Can Med Assoc J* 1986; **135:** 1372.
8. Small NL, Giamonna KA. Interaction between warfarin and trazodone. *Ann Pharmacother* 2000; **34:** 734–6.


**Antidiabetics.** There have been a few early instances of *tolbutamide* enhancing the activity of dicoumarol.[1] However, this effect has not been seen in later studies involving dicoumarol,[1-3] warfarin,[2] and phenprocoumon,[4] although one study did find altered dicoumarol pharmacokinetics.[3] An absence of effect has been documented for phenprocoumon and *insulin*, *glibenclamide*, or *glibornuride*,[4] but there is a report of glibenclamide enhancing the effect of warfarin.[5]

There has been an isolated report of bleeding in a patient taking *phenformin* and warfarin.[6] *Metformin* has been reported to diminish phenprocoumon activity.[7]

An enhanced response to warfarin has been reported in a patient receiving *troglitazone*.[8]

Coumarin anticoagulants may increase the hypoglycaemic effect of *sulfonylureas* (see p.347).


1. Chaplin H, Cassell M. Studies on the possible relationship of tolbutamide to dicumarol in anticoagulant therapy. *Am J Med Sci* 1958; **235:** 706–16.
2. Poucher RL, Vecchio TJ. Absence of tolbutamide effect on anticoagulant therapy. *JAMA* 1966; **197:** 1069–70.
3. Jähnchen E, *et al.* Pharmacokinetic analysis of the interaction between dicoumarol and tolbutamide in man. *Eur J Clin Pharmacol* 1976; **10:** 349–56.
4. Heine P, *et al.* The influence of hypoglycaemic sulphonylureas on elimination and efficacy of phenprocoumon following a single oral dose in diabetic patients. *Eur J Clin Pharmacol* 1976; **10:** 31–6.
5. Jassal SV. *BMJ* 1991; **303:** 789.
6. Hamblin TJ. Interaction between warfarin and phenformin. *Lancet* 1971; **ii:** 1323.
7. Ohnhaus EE, *et al.* The influence of dimethylbiguanide on phenprocoumon elimination and its mode of action: a drug interaction study. *Klin Wochenschr* 1983; **61:** 851–8.
8. Plowman BK, Morreale AP. Possible troglitazone—warfarin interaction. *Am J Health-Syst Pharm* 1998; **55:** 1071.


**Antiepileptics.** Barbiturates such as *phenobarbital* and *primidone* diminish the activity of warfarin and other coumarins through increased metabolism. *Carbamazepine* is reported to have a similar effect.[1,2] Reports of the effect of *phenytoin* on anticoagulants do not provide a clear picture. There are reports of phenytoin enhancing the effects of warfarin[3,4] and a report of initial enhancement followed by decreased anticoagulant action.[5] Phenytoin has been reported to diminish the effect of dicoumarol.[6] Addition of *felbamate* has been reported[7] to necessitate a reduction in warfarin dosage in order to maintain a target INR. In another patient there was a transient increase in response to warfarin when *valproic acid* was started.[8] Valproate also inhibits platelet function and caution is required when it is given with warfarin.

For the effect of oral anticoagulants on phenytoin, see p.373.


1. Hansen JM, *et al.* Carbamazepine-induced acceleration of diphenylhydantoin and warfarin metabolism in man. *Clin Pharmacol Ther* 1971; **12:** 539–43.
2. Ross JRY, Beeley L. Interaction between carbamazepine and warfarin. *BMJ* 1980; **280:** 1415–16.
3. Nappi JM. Warfarin and phenytoin interaction. *Ann Intern Med* 1979; **90:** 852.
4. Panegyres PK, Rischbieth RH. Fatal phenytoin warfarin interaction. *Postgrad Med J* 1991; **67:** 98.
5. Levine M, Sheppard I. Biphasic interaction of phenytoin with warfarin. *Clin Pharm* 1984; **3:** 200–3.
6. Hansen JM, *et al.* Effect of diphenylhydantoin on the metabolism of dicoumarol in man. *Acta Med Scand* 1971; **189:** 15–19.
7. Tisdel KA, *et al.* Warfarin—felbamate interaction: first report. *Ann Pharmacother* 1994; **28:** 805.
8. Guthrie SK, *et al.* Hypothesized interaction between valproic acid and warfarin. *J Clin Psychopharmacol* 1995; **15:** 138–9.


**Antifungals.** *Griseofulvin* has been reported to diminish the activity of warfarin.[1-3] There are several reports indicating that *miconazole*, given either systemically or topically as the oral gel, may enhance the activity of oral anticoagulants (warfarin, ethyl biscoumacetate, acenocoumarol, phenindione, and tioclomarol).[4-11] Absorption of miconazole after intravaginal administration may have enhanced the activity of acenocoumarol in 2 patients;[12] it enhanced the activity of warfarin[13] in another. Studies in healthy subjects given a single warfarin dose[14,15] support case reports[16-18] suggesting that *fluconazole* may increase the anticoagulant activity of warfarin. There are isolated reports of the potentiation of warfarin by *itraconazole*[19] and *ketoconazole*.[20] There has been a case report of a reduction in the effect of warfarin by *terbinafine*,[21] although a study[22] in healthy subjects found no clinically significant interaction, and others[23] considered that no interaction usually occurs. A case of potentiation of warfarin by terbinafine has also been reported;[24] the authors speculate that concomitant cimetidine may have contributed to the interaction by increasing plasma-terbinafine concentrations.


1. Cullen SI, Catalano PM. Griseofulvin-warfarin antagonism. *JAMA* 1967; **199:** 582–3.
2. Udall JA. Drug interference with warfarin therapy. *Clin Med* 1970; **77** (Aug.): 20–5.
3. Okino K, Weibert RT. Warfarin-griseofulvin interaction. *Drug Intell Clin Pharm* 1986; **20:** 291–3.
4. Loupi E, *et al.* Interactions médicamenteuses et miconazole: a propos de 10 observations. *Therapie* 1982; **37:** 437–41.
5. Watson PG, *et al.* Drug interaction with coumarin derivative anticoagulants. *BMJ* 1982; **285:** 1045–6.
6. Colquhoun MC, *et al.* Interaction between warfarin and miconazole oral gel. *Lancet* 1987; **i:** 695–6.
7. Bailey GM, *et al.* Miconazole and warfarin interaction. *Pharm J* 1989; **242:** 183.
8. Ariyaratnam S, *et al.* Potentiation of warfarin anticoagulant activity by miconazole oral gel. *BMJ* 1997; **314:** 349.
9. Evans J, *et al.* Treating oral candidiasis: potentially fatal. *Br Dent J* 1997; **182:** 452.
10. Pemberton MN, *et al.* Derangement of warfarin anticoagulation by miconazole oral gel. *Br Dent J* 1998; **184:** 68–9.
11. Ortín M, *et al.* Miconazole oral gel enhances acenocoumarol anticoagulant activity: a report of three cases. *Ann Pharmacother* 1999; **33:** 175–7.
12. Lansdorp D, *et al.* Potentiation of acenocoumarol during vaginal administration of miconazole. *Br J Clin Pharmacol* 1999; **47:** 225–6.
13. Thirion DJG, Farquhar Zanetti LA. Potentiation of warfarin's hypoprothrombinemic effect with miconazole vaginal suppositories. *Pharmacotherapy* 2000; **20:** 98–9.
14. Lazar JD, Wilner KD. Drug interactions with fluconazole. *Rev Infect Dis* 1990; **12** (suppl 3): S327–S333.
15. Black DJ, *et al.* Warfarin–fluconazole II: a metabolically based drug interaction: in vivo studies. *Drug Metab Dispos* 1996; **24:** 422–8.
16. Seaton TL, *et al.* Possible potentiation of warfarin by fluconazole. *DICP Ann Pharmacother* 1990; **24:** 1177–8.
17. Gericke KR. Possible interaction between warfarin and fluconazole. *Pharmacotherapy* 1993; **13:** 508–9.
18. Baciewicz AM, *et al.* Fluconazole—warfarin interaction. *Ann Pharmacother* 1994; **28:** 1111.
19. Yeh J, *et al.* Potentiation of action of warfarin by itraconazole. *BMJ* 1990; **301:** 669.
20. Smith AG. Potentiation of oral anticoagulants by ketoconazole. *BMJ* 1984; **288:** 188–9. Correction. *ibid.*; 608.
21. Warwick JA, Corrall RJ. Serious interaction between warfarin and oral terbinafine. *BMJ* 1998; **316:** 440.
22. Guerret M, *et al.* Evaluation of effects of terbinafine on single oral dose pharmacokinetics and anticoagulant actions of warfarin in healthy volunteers. *Pharmacotherapy* 1997; **17:** 767–73.
23. Stockley IH. Terbinafine and warfarin mystery. *Pharm J* 1998; **260:** 408.
24. Gupta AK, Ross GS. Interaction between terbinafine and warfarin. *Dermatology* 1998; **196:** 266–7.


**Antigout drugs.** The two drugs in this group that have mostly been implicated in interactions with anticoagulants are allopurinol and sulfinpyrazone.

With *allopurinol* there are conflicting reports of patients experiencing no interaction or an enhanced anticoagulant effect with dicoumarol,[1] phenprocoumon,[2] or warfarin.[3,4]

Interactions with *sulfinpyrazone* have usually involved warfarin and, apart from a case of a mixed response,[5] have involved increased anticoagulant activity, sometimes with haemorrhage, so calling for careful control. It is still not clear how sulfinpyrazone exerts its effect, but studies point to a stereoselective effect on warfarin metabolism where the *S*-isomer's metabolic clearance is inhibited.[6] It should also be remembered that sulfinpyrazone affects platelets. Sulfinpyrazone has also enhanced the anticoagulant activity of acenocoumarol.[7] A significant interaction with phenprocoumon appears unlikely.[8]

*Probenecid* has accelerated the elimination of a single dose of phenprocoumon without effect on the prothrombin time.[9]

*Benziodarone* has been reported to enhance the effects of warfarin, diphenadione, ethyl biscoumacetate, and acenocoumarol, but not of dicoumarol, phenindione, or phenprocoumon.[10] A further study[11] confirmed that benziodarone could increase the half-life of ethyl biscoumacetate, but also found that the effect of phenprocoumon was enhanced. A study[12] of *benzbromarone*, which is structurally related to benziodarone, concluded that it enhanced the effect of warfarin by inhibition of the cytochrome P450 isoenzyme CYP2C9, leading to a stereoselective inhibition of the metabolism of warfarin.


1. Vesell ES, *et al.* Impairment of drug metabolism in man by allopurinol and nortriptyline. *N Engl J Med* 1970; **283:** 1484–8.
2. Jähnchen E, *et al.* Interaction of allopurinol with phenprocoumon in man. *Klin Wochenschr* 1977; **55:** 759–61.
3. Rawlins MD, Smith SE. Influence of allopurinol on drug metabolism in man. *Br J Pharmacol* 1973; **48:** 693–8.
4. Pond SM, *et al.* The effects of allopurinol and clofibrate on the elimination of coumarin anticoagulants in man. *Aust N Z J Med* 1975; **5:** 324–8.
5. Nenci GG, *et al.* Biphasic sulphinpyrazone-warfarin interaction. *BMJ* 1981; **282:** 1361–2.
6. Toon S, *et al.* The warfarin-sulfinpyrazone interaction: stereochemical considerations. *Clin Pharmacol Ther* 1986; **39:** 15–24.
7. Michot F, *et al.* Über die Beeinflussung der gerinnungshemmenden Wirkung von Acenocoumarol durch Sulfinpyrazon. *Schweiz Med Wochenschr* 1981; **111:** 255–60.
8. Heimark LD, *et al.* The effect of sulfinpyrazone on the disposition of pseudoracemic phenprocoumon in humans. *Clin Pharmacol Ther* 1987; **42:** 312–19.
9. Mönig H, *et al.* The effects of frusemide and probenecid on the pharmacokinetics of phenprocoumon. *Eur J Clin Pharmacol* 1990; **39:** 261–5.
10. Pyörälä K, *et al.* Benziodarone (Amplivix®) and anticoagulant therapy. *Acta Med Scand* 1963; **173:** 385–9.
11. Verstraete M, *et al.* Dissimilar effect of two anti-anginal drugs belonging to the benzofuran group on the action of coumarin derivatives. *Arch Int Pharmacodyn Ther* 1968; **176:** 33–41.
12. Takahashi H, *et al.* Potentiation of anticoagulant effect of warfarin caused by enantioselective metabolic inhibition by the uricosuric agent benzbromarone. *Clin Pharmacol Ther* 1999; **66:** 569–81.


**Antihistamines.** There has been a report[1] of a raised INR and severe epistaxis in a patient after the addition of *cetirizine* to long-term acenocoumarol.


1. Berod T, Mathiot I. Probable interaction between cetirizine and acenocoumarol. *Ann Pharmacother* 1997; **31:** 122.


**Antimalarials.** The ingestion of large amounts of tonic water by 2 patients necessitated a reduction in their warfarin dosage. The enhanced effect was attributed to the *quinine* content of the tonic water.[1] A woman stabilised on warfarin developed haematuria and a high prothrombin ratio after taking *proguanil* for malaria prophylaxis.[2]


1. Clark DJ. Clinical curio: warfarin and tonic water. *BMJ* 1983; **286:** 1258.
2. Armstrong G, *et al.* Warfarin potentiated by proguanil. *BMJ* 1991; **303:** 789.


**Antimuscarinics.** There have been 2 cases reported[1] of *tolterodine* enhancing the effect of warfarin. It was stated that the manufacturers of tolterodine were aware of 6 reports of a possible interaction with warfarin.


1. Colucci VJ, Rivey MP. Tolterodine–warfarin drug interaction. *Ann Pharmacother* 1999; **33:** 1173–6.


**Antineoplastics.** There have been several reports of interactions between warfarin and antineoplastics. No clear picture emerges from these reports which is not surprising considering that antineoplastics are often given in combination and that they can exert their own haematological effects. *Cyclophosphamide* for instance has been associated with an increase in warfarin's activity when given with *methotrexate* and *fluorouracil*,[1] but with a decrease when given with non-antineoplastic drugs.[2] An increase in the activity of warfarin and mucous membrane bleeding occurred in a patient who received 4 courses of fluorouracil and folic acid at weekly intervals.[3] The patient was also taking indometacin. Warfarin dosage had to be reduced in 5 patients who received fluorouracil-based antineoplastic regimens.[4] An increase in the effect of warfarin has been reported when given with fluorouracil and levamisole (see below). The manufacturers of *capecitabine* state that altered coagulation parameters and bleeding have been reported in patients taking capecitabine and warfarin or phenprocoumon. There have been 2 cases reported[5] where *trastuzumab* enhanced the effect of warfarin. *Etoposide* with *vindesine*[6] or with *carboplatin*,[7] *ifosfamide* with *mesna*,[8] and *tamoxifen*[9-11] have all produced an increased anticoagulant effect. *Aminoglutethimide* has led to decreased activity of warfarin or acenocoumarol,[12,13] probably due to increased warfarin metabolism. The manufacturers of the anti-androgen *flutamide* state that increases in prothrombin time have been reported after initiation of flutamide therapy in patients on long-term warfarin. *In vitro* data indicate a similar reaction is likely with *bicalutamide*. *Mercaptopurine*[14] and *mitotane*[15] have also decreased warfarin activity.


1. Seifter EJ, *et al.* Possible interactions between warfarin and antineoplastic drugs. *Cancer Treat Rep* 1985; **69:** 244–5.
2. Tashima CK. Cyclophosphamide effect on coumarin anticoagulation. *South Med J* 1979; **72:** 633–4.

3. Brown MC. Multisite mucous membrane bleeding due to a possible interaction between warfarin and 5-fluorouracil. *Pharmacotherapy* 1997; **17:** 631–3.
4. Kolesar JM, *et al.* Warfarin-5-FU interaction—a consecutive case series. *Pharmacotherapy* 1999; **19:** 1445–9.
5. Nissenblatt MJ, Karp GI. Bleeding risk with trastuzumab (Herceptin) treatment. *JAMA* 1999; **282:** 2299–2300.
6. Ward K, Bitran JD. Warfarin, etoposide, and vindesine interactions. *Cancer Treat Rep* 1984; **68:** 817–18.
7. Le AT, *et al.* Enhancement of warfarin response in a patient receiving etoposide and carboplatin chemotherapy. *Ann Pharmacother* 1997; **31:** 1006–8.
8. Hall G, *et al.* Intravenous infusions of ifosfamide/mesna and perturbation of warfarin anticoagulant control. *Postgrad Med J* 1990; **66:** 860–1.
9. Lodwick R, *et al.* Life threatening interaction between tamoxifen and warfarin. *BMJ* 1987; **295:** 1141.
10. Tenni P, *et al.* Life threatening interaction between tamoxifen and warfarin. *BMJ* 1989; **298:** 93.
11. Ritchie LD, Grant SMT. Tamoxifen-warfarin interaction: the Aberdeen hospitals drug file. *BMJ* 1989; **298:** 1253.
12. Lønning PE, *et al.* The influence of a graded dose schedule of aminoglutethimide on the disposition of the optical enantiomers of warfarin in patients with breast cancer. *Cancer Chemother Pharmacol* 1986; **17:** 177–81.
13. Bruning PF, Bonfrèr JGM. Aminoglutethimide and oral anticoagulant therapy. *Lancet* 1983; **ii:** 582.
14. Spiers ASD, Mibashan RS. Increased warfarin requirement during mercaptopurine therapy: a new drug interaction. *Lancet* 1974; **ii:** 221–2.
15. Cuddy PG, *et al.* Influence of mitotane on the hypoprothrombinemic effect of warfarin. *South Med J* 1986; **79:** 387–8.


**Antiplatelets.** The interaction between anticoagulants and *dipyridamole* is an oddity in that bleeding can occur without any alteration in prothrombin times; special care is therefore required as the usual method of monitoring the anticoagulant effect is of no value. This interaction has involved a small number of patients taking dipyridamole and warfarin or phenindione;[1] inhibition of platelet function by dipyridamole has been implicated. However, in general it does not appear to increase the risk of bleeding.[2]

Interestingly, in a group of patients receiving acenocoumarol for thromboprophylaxis, addition of *ticlopidine* was found to significantly increase acenocoumarol requirements.[3]

See also under Analgesics and NSAIDs (above).


1. Kalowski S, Kincaid-Smith P. Interaction of dipyridamole with anticoagulants in the treatment of glomerulonephritis. *Med J Aust* 1973; **2:** 164–6.
2. Levine MN, *et al.* Hemorrhagic complications of long-term anticoagulant therapy. *Chest* 1989; **95** (suppl): 26S–36S.
3. Salar A, *et al.* Ticlopidine antagonizes acenocoumarol treatment. *Thromb Haemost* 1997; **77:** 223–4.


**Antiprotozoals.** *Metronidazole* enhances the activity of warfarin[1,2] through selective inhibition of the metabolism of its *S*-isomer.[3]


1. Kazmier FJ. A significant interaction between metronidazole and warfarin. *Mayo Clin Proc* 1976; **51:** 782–4.
2. Dean RP, Talbert RL. Bleeding associated with concurrent warfarin and metronidazole therapy. *Drug Intell Clin Pharm* 1980; **14:** 864–6.
3. O'Reilly RA. The stereoselective interaction of warfarin and metronidazole in man. *N Engl J Med* 1976; **295:** 354–7.


**Antithyroid drugs.** See under Thyroid and Antithyroid Drugs, below.

**Antivirals.** Reductions in dosage of either warfarin[1] or acenocoumarol[2] were necessary in 2 patients receiving *interferon alfa* for hepatitis C. The interactions may have been due to decreased metabolism of the anticoagulant. A similar need for a reduced warfarin dose had also been noted in other patients taking *interferon alfa-2b* or *interferon beta*.[1] However, in a patient taking interferon alfa-2b with *ribavirin*,[3] the warfarin dose needed to be increased, probably due to the interaction between ribavirin and warfarin.

An enhanced response to warfarin has been reported[4] in a patient taking *saquinavir*. The mechanism may involve competitive inhibition of warfarin metabolism and might also occur with other HIV-protease inhibitors. However, a decreased response to warfarin seemed to be caused by *ritonavir* when it was added to the multidrug therapy of a patient.[5] Ritonavir has also been reported to decrease the response to acenocoumarol.[6]


1. Adachi Y, *et al.* Potentiation of warfarin by interferon. *BMJ* 1995; **311:** 292.
2. Serratrice J, *et al.* Interferon-alpha 2b interaction with acenocoumarol. *Am J Hematol* 1998; **57:** 89.
3. Schulman S. Inhibition of warfarin activity by ribavirin. *Ann Pharmacother* 2002; **36:** 72–4.
4. Darlington MR. Hypoprothrombinemia during concomitant therapy with warfarin and saquinavir. *Ann Pharmacother* 1997; **31:** 647.
5. Knoell KR, *et al.* Potential interaction involving warfarin and ritonavir. *Ann Pharmacother* 1998; **32:** 1299–1302.
6. Llibre JM, *et al.* Severe interaction between ritonavir and acenocoumarol. *Ann Pharmacother* 2002; **36:** 621–3.


**Anxiolytic sedatives, hypnotics, and antipsychotics.** *Barbiturates*, by inducing liver metabolism, can reduce the activity of anticoagulants; *glutethimide* has a similar action. The *benzodiazepines* on the other hand do not generally have any effect although there is the rare report of increased or decreased activity.

Although there is a report suggesting that *cloral hydrate* may decrease the effect of dicoumarol by enzyme induction,[1] other studies and experience indicate an increase in the anticoagulant activity of warfarin.[2-4] However, the increase is only transient and is probably the result of displacement of warfarin from plasma protein binding sites by the metabolite trichloroacetic acid.[2] *Triclofos sodium* appears to increase the activity of warfarin in a similar way.[5]

Reduced anticoagulant activity has been reported with *dichloralphenazone*,[6,7] *ethchlorvynol* (with dicoumarol),[8] and *haloperidol* (with phenindione).[9] Compounds such as *meprobamate* and *methaqualone* appear to have no effect on anticoagulants.


1. Cucinell SA, *et al.* The effect of chloral hydrate on bishydroxycoumarin metabolism: a fatal outcome. *JAMA* 1966; **197:** 366–8.
2. Sellers EM, Koch-Weser J. Kinetics and clinical importance of displacement of warfarin from albumin by acidic drugs. *Ann N Y Acad Sci* 1971; **179:** 213–25.
3. Boston Collaborative Drug Surveillance Program. Interaction between chloral hydrate and warfarin. *N Engl J Med* 1972; **286:** 53–5.
4. Udall JA. Warfarin-chloral hydrate interaction: pharmacological activity and clinical significance. *Ann Intern Med* 1974; **81:** 341–4.
5. Sellers EM, *et al.* Enhancement of warfarin-induced hypoprothrombinemia by triclofos. *Clin Pharmacol Ther* 1972; **13:** 911–15.
6. Breckenridge A, Orme M. Clinical implications of enzyme induction. *Ann N Y Acad Sci* 1971; **179:** 421–3.
7. Whitfield JB, *et al.* Changes in plasma α-glutamyl transpeptidase activity associated with alterations in drug metabolism in man. *BMJ* 1973; **1:** 316–18.
8. Johansson S-A. Apparent resistance to oral anticoagulant therapy and influence of hypnotics on some coagulation factors. *Acta Med Scand* 1968; **184:** 297–300.
9. Oakley DP, Lautch H. Haloperidol and anticoagulant treatment. *Lancet* 1963; **ii:** 1231.


**Beta blockers.** Possible potentiation of the effect of warfarin by *propranolol*[1] has been reported. Beta blockers, particularly those with a high lipid solubility such as propranolol, may inhibit the metabolism of warfarin.[2] However, although a number of studies have shown pharmacokinetic interactions between some beta blockers and oral anticoagulants, no effect on anticoagulant activity has been found.


1. Bax NDS, *et al.* Inhibition of drug metabolism by β-adrenoceptor antagonists. *Drugs* 1983; **25** (suppl 2): 121–6.
2. Mantero F, *et al.* Effect of atenolol and metoprolol on the anticoagulant activity of acenocoumarin. *Br J Clin Pharmacol* 1984; **17:** 94S–96S.


**Central stimulants.** While *methylphenidate* has been reported to increase the half-life of ethyl biscoumacetate,[1] it has also been reported to have no effect on the half-life or on the anticoagulant activity of ethyl biscoumacetate.[2] *Prolintane* also had no effect on ethyl biscoumacetate.[2]


1. Garrettson LK, *et al.* Methylphenidate interaction with both anticonvulsants and ethyl biscoumacetate: a new action of methylphenidate. *JAMA* 1969; **207:** 2053.
2. Hague DE, *et al.* The effect of methylphenidate and prolintane on the metabolism of ethyl biscoumacetate. *Clin Pharmacol Ther* 1971; **12:** 259–62.


**Corticosteroids and corticotropin.** There are several reports of corticosteroids or corticotropin either enhancing[1,2] or diminishing[3] the effects of anticoagulants. Matters are further confused by corticosteroids being associated with an increase in the coagulability of the blood. However, the extensive use of corticosteroids and anticoagulants, and very few reports of interaction, suggests that any problems are rare.


1. Van Cauwenberge H, Jaques LB. Haemorrhagic effect of ACTH with anticoagulants. *Can Med Assoc J* 1958; **79:** 536–40.
2. Costedoat-Chalumeau N, *et al.* Potentiation of vitamin K antagonists by high-dose intravenous methylprednisolone. *Ann Intern Med* 2000; **132:** 631–5.
3. Chatterjea JB, Salomon L. Antagonistic effect of ACTH and cortisone on the anticoagulant activity of ethyl biscoumacetate. *BMJ* 1954; **2:** 790–2.


**Cranberry.** Since 1999 the UK Committee on the Safety of Medicines (CSM)[1] had received 5 reports suggesting an interaction between warfarin and cranberry juice. In 3 patients the activity of warfarin had been potentiated and one of them had died. In the other patients the INR was either reduced or unstable. The CSM advised patients to limit or avoid drinking cranberry juice while taking warfarin.


1. Committee on Safety of Medicines/Medicines and Healthcare products Regulatory Agency. Possible interaction between warfarin and cranberry juice. *Current Problems* 2003; **29:** 8. Also available at: http://medicines.mhra.gov.uk/ourwork/monitorsafequalmed/currentproblems/cpsept2003.pdf (accessed 06/07/04)


**Dermatological drugs.** A patient's warfarin dose had to be increased when he started treatment with *etretinate*.[1]


1. Ostlere LS, *et al.* Reduced therapeutic effect of warfarin caused by etretinate. *Br J Dermatol* 1991; **124:** 505–10.


**Disulfiram.** Two reports suggesting that disulfiram enhances the activity of warfarin[1,2] were confirmed by a study in 8 healthy subjects.[3] Although inhibition of liver enzymes by disulfiram was considered responsible,[3] a later study[4] suggested that disulfiram acts directly on the liver to increase hypoprothrombinaemia. This interaction is complicated by the variable effects of alcohol on warfarin (see above). Special care is therefore called for when these drugs are used together.


1. Rothstein E. Warfarin effect enhanced by disulfiram. *JAMA* 1968; **206:** 1574–5.
2. Rothstein E. Warfarin effect enhanced by disulfiram (Antabuse). *JAMA* 1972; **221:** 1052–3.
3. O'Reilly RA. Interaction of sodium warfarin and disulfiram (Antabuse®) in man. *Ann Intern Med* 1973; **78:** 73–6.
4. O'Reilly RA. Dynamic interaction between disulfiram and separated enantiomorphs of racemic warfarin. *Clin Pharmacol Ther* 1981; **29:** 332–6.


**Diuretics.** There have been a number of studies on the effects of diuretics on anticoagulants. *Tienilic acid* produces the most serious interaction enhancing the activity of ethyl biscoumacetate,[1] acenocoumarol,[2] and warfarin[3] and has led to haemorrhage. *Etacrynic acid* has also been reported to enhance the activity of warfarin,[4] but reports do not show as severe an effect as with tienilic acid.

*Chlortalidone*[5] and *spironolactone*[6] have both been associated with a reduction in warfarin's activity in healthy subjects and it has been suggested that this might be a consequence of the diuresis concentrating the circulating clotting factors. However, *bumetanide*, *furosemide*, and the *thiazides* appear to have no effect on warfarin.


1. Detilleux M, *et al.* Potentialisation de l'effet des anticoagulants coumariniques par un nouveau diurétique, l'acide tiénilique. *Nouv Presse Med* 1976; **5:** 2395.
2. Grand A, *et al.* Potentialisation de l'action anticoagulante des anti-vitamines K par l'acide tiénilique. *Nouv Presse Med* 1977; **6:** 2691.
3. McLain DA, *et al.* Adverse reactions associated with ticrynafen use. *JAMA* 1980; **243:** 763–4.
4. Petrick RJ, *et al.* Interaction between warfarin and ethacrynic acid. *JAMA* 1975; **231:** 843–4.
5. O'Reilly RA, *et al.* Impact of aspirin and chlorthalidone on the pharmacodynamics of oral anticoagulant drugs in man. *Ann N Y Acad Sci* 1971; **179:** 173–86.
6. O'Reilly RA. Spironolactone and warfarin interaction. *Clin Pharmacol Ther* 1980; **27:** 198–201.


**Endothelin receptor antagonists.** A study in healthy volunteers[1] showed that bosentan decreased the anticoagulant effect of warfarin; a case report[2] confirmed this.


1. Weber C, *et al.* Effect of the endothelin-receptor antagonist bosentan on the pharmacokinetics and pharmacodynamics of warfarin. *J Clin Pharmacol* 1999; **39:** 847–54.
2. Murphey LM, Hood EH. Bosentan and warfarin interaction. *Ann Pharmacother* 2003; **37:** 1028–31.


**Gastrointestinal drugs.** Antacids may or may not interact with warfarin. *Bismuth carbonate* and *magnesium trisilicate* for example have been reported to reduce warfarin's absorption,[1] but *aluminium hydroxide* has been observed to have no effect on warfarin or dicoumarol.[2] *Psyllium*[3] and *magnesium hydroxide*[2] have also been reported to have no effect on warfarin, but the latter has increased the plasma concentrations of dicoumarol.[2]

There have been occasional reports of *sucralfate* diminishing the effect of warfarin.[4-6]

Histamine $H_2$-antagonists have been widely studied. There are several reports indicating that *cimetidine* can enhance the anticoagulant effect of warfarin and haemorrhage has occurred. A number of studies show that cimetidine can increase the plasma concentration and half-life of warfarin and that there is a selective inhibitory effect on the metabolism of its *R*-isomer.[7-10] Not all these studies have, however, found an increase in prothrombin time. The effect of cimetidine on warfarin appears to be dose-dependent[7] and to be subject to interindividual variation;[9,10] the need for careful monitoring of patients receiving both drugs is, therefore, evident. Limited evidence suggests that cimetidine has a similar effect on the metabolism of acenocoumarol[11,12] and phenindione[11] but not of phenprocoumon.[13] Studies with *ranitidine* have generally been unable to show an effect on the metabolism of warfarin,[10,14] although in one study warfarin clearance was reduced.[7] There is a case report suggesting that potentiation of warfarin by ranitidine may occasionally occur.[15]

One study has suggested that *omeprazole* could inhibit the metabolism of *R*-warfarin although a clinically significant effect on the activity of warfarin was unlikely.[16] No evidence of an interaction was found in a retrospective study[17] of patients on acenocoumarol who received omeprazole therapy. Similarly, *pantoprazole* appears to have no effect on the pharmacokinetics or pharmacodynamics of warfarin[18] or phenprocoumon.[19]

A marked increase in the effect of warfarin has been reported in a patient when *cisapride* was added.[20]

A reduction in the response to warfarin with development of venous thrombosis has been reported in a patient receiving *mesalazine*,[21] and in another patient receiving *sulfasalazine*.[22]


1. McElnay JC, *et al.* Interaction of warfarin with antacid constituents. *BMJ* 1978; **2:** 1166.
2. Ambre JJ, Fischer LJ. Effect of coadministration of aluminum and magnesium hydroxides on absorption of anticoagulants in man. *Clin Pharmacol Ther* 1973; **14:** 231–7.
3. Robinson DS, *et al.* Interaction of warfarin and nonsystemic gastrointestinal drugs. *Clin Pharmacol Ther* 1971; **12:** 491–5.
4. Mungall D, *et al.* Sucralfate and warfarin. *Ann Intern Med* 1983; **98:** 557.
5. Rey AM, Gums JG. Altered absorption of digoxin, sustained-release quinidine, and warfarin with sucralfate administration. *DICP Ann Pharmacother* 1991; **25:** 745–6.
6. Parrish RH, *et al.* Sucralfate-warfarin interaction. *Ann Pharmacother* 1992; **26:** 1015–16.
7. Desmond PV, *et al.* Decreased oral warfarin clearance after ranitidine and cimetidine. *Clin Pharmacol Ther* 1984; **35:** 338–41.
8. Choonara IA, *et al.* Stereoselective interaction between the R enantiomer of warfarin and cimetidine. *Br J Clin Pharmacol* 1986; **21:** 271–7.
9. Sax MJ, *et al.* Effect of two cimetidine regimens on prothrombin time and warfarin pharmacokinetics during long-term warfarin therapy. *Clin Pharm* 1987; **6:** 492–5.
10. Toon S, *et al.* Comparative effects of ranitidine and cimetidine on the pharmacokinetics and pharmacodynamics of warfarin in man. *Eur J Clin Pharmacol* 1987; **32:** 165–72.
11. Serlin MJ, *et al.* Cimetidine: interaction with oral anticoagulants in man. *Lancet* 1979; **ii:** 317–19.
12. Gill TS, *et al.* Cimetidine-nicoumalone interaction in man: stereochemical considerations. *Br J Clin Pharmacol* 1989; **27:** 469–74.

13. Harenberg J, *et al.* Cimetidine does not increase the anticoagulant effect of phenprocoumon. *Br J Clin Pharmacol* 1982; **14:** 292–3.
14. Serlin MJ, *et al.* Lack of effect of ranitidine on warfarin action. *Br J Clin Pharmacol* 1981; **12:** 791–4.
15. Baciewicz AM, Morgan PJ. Ranitidine-warfarin interaction. *Ann Intern Med* 1990; **112:** 76–7.
16. Sutfin T, *et al.* Stereoselective interaction of omeprazole with warfarin in healthy men. *Ther Drug Monit* 1989; **11:** 176–84.
17. Vreeburg EM, *et al.* Lack of effect of omeprazole on oral acenocoumarol anticoagulant therapy. *Scand J Gastroenterol* 1997; **32:** 991–4.
18. Duursema L, *et al.* Lack of effect of pantoprazole on the pharmacodynamics and pharmacokinetics of warfarin. *Br J Clin Pharmacol* 1995; **39:** 700–3.
19. Ehrlich A, *et al.* Lack of pharmacodynamic and pharmacokinetic interaction between pantoprazole and phenprocoumon in man. *Eur J Clin Pharmacol* 1996; **51:** 277–81.
20. Darlington MR. Hypoprothrombinemia induced by warfarin sodium and cisapride. *Am J Health-Syst Pharm* 1997; **54:** 320–1.
21. Marinella MA. Mesalamine and warfarin therapy resulting in decreased warfarin effect. *Ann Pharmacother* 1998; **32:** 841–2.
22. Teefy AM, *et al.* Warfarin resistance due to sulfasalazine. *Ann Pharmacother* 2000; **34:** 1265–8.

**Ginseng.** A reduction in the response to warfarin was reported[1] in a patient after taking a ginseng preparation. A study[2] in healthy volunteers also found a small reduction in response.

1. Janetzky K, Morreale AP. Probable interaction between warfarin and ginseng. *Am J Health-Syst Pharm* 1997; **54:** 692–3.
2. Yuan C-S, *et al.* American ginseng reduces warfarin's effect in healthy patients: a randomized, controlled trial. *Ann Intern Med* 2004; **141:** 23–7.

**Glucagon.** A dose-dependent enhancement of warfarin's anticoagulant activity has been reported with glucagon.[1]

1. Koch-Weser J. Potentiation by glucagon of the hypoprothrombinemic action of warfarin. *Ann Intern Med* 1970; **72:** 331–5.

**Hypericum.** Hypericum has been reported to reduce the anticoagulant effect of warfarin.[1]

1. Yue Q-Y, *et al.* Safety of St John's wort (Hypericum perforatum). *Lancet* 2000; **355:** 576–7.

**Immunosuppressants.** Severe bleeding occurred in a patient on long-term warfarin after discontinuing *azathioprine*,[1] while another patient[2] required an increased dose of warfarin when it was given with azathioprine.

There have been a few case reports of interaction between warfarin or acenocoumarol and *ciclosporin*, in which the dose of the anticoagulant or ciclosporin or both needed to be altered (see Anticoagulants under Interactions of Ciclosporin, p.1355).

There has been a report[3] of *leflunomide* enhancing the effects of warfarin, causing gross haematuria after the second dose; the patient's INR rose from 3.4 to 11. It was stated that the UK Committee on Safety of Medicines had received 4 reports of increased INR with leflunomide up to the end of 2002.

1. Singleton JD, Conyers L. Warfarin and azathioprine: an important drug interaction. *Am J Med* 1992; **92:** 217.
2. Rotenberg M, *et al.* Effect of azathioprine on the anticoagulant activity of warfarin. *Ann Pharmacother* 2000; **34:** 120–2.
3. Lim V, Pande I. Leflunomide can potentiate the anticoagulant effect of warfarin. *BMJ* 2002; **325:** 1333. Correction. *ibid.* 2003; **326:** 432.

**Leukotriene antagonists.** *Zafirlukast* is reported to decrease the clearance of *S*-warfarin.[1] The manufacturers of zafirlukast state that it probably inhibits the cytochrome P450 isoenzyme CYP2C9 which is involved in the metabolism of warfarin. Patients receiving warfarin may develop prolongation of the prothrombin time when zafirlukast is added and warfarin dosage should be adjusted accordingly.

A study[2] of *montelukast* and warfarin found no significant interaction between the two drugs.

1. Suttle AB, *et al.* Effect of zafirlukast on the pharmacokinetics of R- and S-warfarin in healthy men. *Clin Pharmacol Ther* 1997; **61:** 186.
2. Van Hecken, *et al.* Effect of montelukast on the pharmacokinetics and pharmacodynamics of warfarin in healthy volunteers. *J Clin Pharmacol* 1999; **39:** 495–500.

**Levamisole.** An increased INR has been reported[1] in a patient receiving chronic warfarin therapy after addition of *levamisole* and fluorouracil. Inhibition of warfarin metabolism was postulated as the mechanism responsible for the interaction. In a second patient, a similar reaction was reported[2] following administration of levamisole and fluorouracil and an episode of bleeding subsequently occurred after administration of levamisole alone.

1. Scarfe MA, Israel MK. Possible drug interaction between warfarin and combination of levamisole and fluorouracil. *Ann Pharmacother* 1994; **28:** 464–7.
2. Wehbe TW, Warth JA. A case of bleeding requiring hospitalization that was likely caused by an interaction between warfarin and levamisole. *Clin Pharmacol Ther* 1996; **59:** 360–2.

**Lipid regulating drugs.** *Clofibrate* can enhance the activity of warfarin, sometimes to the point of haemorrhage. The mechanism of this interaction is not clear, but it does not appear to be a pharmacokinetic effect. Similar enhancement of activity has been reported when clofibrate is given to patients taking dicoumarol or phenindione. *Bezafibrate* has been reported to enhance the effect of phenprocoumon[1] and warfarin,[2] and *fenofibrate*[3] and *gemfibrozil*[4] have been reported to enhance the effect of warfarin.

Hypoprothrombinaemia and bleeding has been reported in 2 patients on warfarin given *lovastatin*.[5] An increased response to warfarin has also been reported[6,7] in a number of patients receiving *fluvastatin*, and in a patient given *rosuvastatin*.[8] The manufacturers of *simvastatin* state that it has slightly enhanced the effect of coumarin anticoagulants. Simvastatin has been reported[9] to potentiate the effect of acenocoumarol in a patient. However, the INR in a patient on long-term warfarin remained stable on the addition of treatment with simvastatin.[10] The manufacturers of *pravastatin* have not observed any change in warfarin activity in patients given both drugs. However, there has been a report[11] of bleeding in a patient receiving fluindione when pravastatin was added. In a study[12] of 46 patients on warfarin who had been converted from pravastatin to *simvastatin*, the mean INR increased, but the median weekly warfarin dose did not differ significantly and no episodes of bleeding were reported.

*Dextrothyroxine* increases the anticoagulant effect of warfarin sodium[13,14] and dicoumarol.[15]

An opposite effect may occur with *colestyramine* which has reduced warfarin's serum concentration[16] and half-life[17] as well as its activity.[16,17] The mechanisms of this interaction include binding of warfarin to colestyramine and reduced absorption;[16] the enterohepatic recycling of warfarin may also be interrupted.[17] Phenprocoumon's activity has also been reduced by colestyramine.[18] It should be remembered, however, that colestyramine can also reduce vitamin K absorption, which may result in hypoprothrombinaemia and bleeding.

An increase in INR has been reported[19] in a patient taking *omega-3 triglycerides* (as fish oil) with warfarin.

*Benfluorex*[20] and *colestipol*[21] have been reported not to interact with phenprocoumon.

1. Zimmermann R, *et al.* The effect of bezafibrate on the fibrinolytic enzyme system and the drug interaction with racemic phenprocoumon. *Atherosclerosis* 1978; **29:** 477–85.
2. Beringer TRO. Warfarin potentiation with bezafibrate. *Postgrad Med J* 1997; **73:** 657–8.
3. Ascah KJ, *et al.* Interaction between fenofibrate and warfarin. *Ann Pharmacother* 1998; **32:** 765–8.
4. Ahmad S. Gemfibrozil interaction with warfarin sodium (Coumadin). *Chest* 1990; **98:** 1041–2.
5. Ahmad S. Lovastatin: warfarin interaction. *Arch Intern Med* 1990; **150:** 2407.
6. Trilli LE, *et al.* Potential interaction between warfarin and fluvastatin. *Ann Pharmacother* 1996; **30:** 1399–1402.
7. Kline SS, Harrell CC. Potential warfarin-fluvastatin interaction. *Ann Pharmacother* 1997; **31:** 790–1.
8. Barry M. Rosuvastatin–warfarin drug interaction. *Lancet* 2004; **363:** 328.
9. Grau E, *et al.* Simvastatin-oral anticoagulant interaction. *Lancet* 1996; **347:** 405–6.
10. Gaw A, Wosornu D. Simvastatin during warfarin therapy in hyperlipoproteinaemia. *Lancet* 1992; **340:** 979–80.
11. Trenque T, *et al.* Pravastatin: interaction with oral anticoagulant? *BMJ* 1996; **312:** 886.
12. Lin JC, *et al.* The effect of converting from pravastatin to simvastatin on the pharmacodynamics of warfarin. *J Clin Pharmacol* 1999; **39:** 86–90.
13. Owens JC, *et al.* Effect of sodium dextrothyroxine in patients receiving anticoagulants. *N Engl J Med* 1962; **266:** 76–9.
14. Solomon HM, Schrogie JJ. Change in receptor site affinity: a proposed explanation for the potentiating effect of D-thyroxine on the anticoagulant response to warfarin. *Clin Pharmacol Ther* 1967; **8:** 797–9.
15. Schrogie JJ, Solomon HM. The anticoagulant response to bishydroxycoumarin: II. The effect of D-thyroxine, clofibrate, and norethandrolone. *Clin Pharmacol Ther* 1967; **8:** 70–7.
16. Robinson DS, *et al.* Interaction of warfarin and nonsystemic gastrointestinal drugs. *Clin Pharmacol Ther* 1971; **12:** 491–5.
17. Jähnchen E, *et al.* Enhanced elimination of warfarin during treatment with cholestyramine. *Br J Clin Pharmacol* 1978; **5:** 437–40.
18. Meinertz T, *et al.* Interruption of the enterohepatic circulation of phenprocoumon by cholestyramine. *Clin Pharmacol Ther* 1977; **21:** 731–5.
19. Buckley MS, *et al.* Fish oil interaction with warfarin. *Ann Pharmacother* 2004; **38:** 50–3.
20. De Witte P, Brems HM. Co-administration of benfluorex with oral anticoagulant therapy. *Curr Med Res Opin* 1980; **6:** 478–80.
21. Harvengt C, Desager JP. Effect of colestipol, a new bile acid sequestrant, on the absorption of phenprocoumon in man. *Eur J Clin Pharmacol* 1973; **6:** 19–21.

**Pesticides.** Chlorinated insecticides diminished the activity of warfarin in a patient.[1]

1. Jeffery WH, *et al.* Loss of warfarin effect after occupational insecticide exposure. *JAMA* 1976; **236:** 2881–2.

**Piracetam.** Piracetam caused an increase in prothrombin time in a patient who had been stabilised on warfarin.[1]

1. Pan HYM, Ng RP. The effect of Nootropil in a patient on warfarin. *Eur J Clin Pharmacol* 1983; **24:** 711.

**Sex hormones.** There have been reports of steroids with anabolic or androgenic properties enhancing the activity of anticoagulants to the point of haemorrhage. Reports have covered *oxymetholone* and warfarin[1-3] or acenocoumarol;[4] *stanozolol* and warfarin[5,6] or dicoumarol;[7] *ethylestrenol* and phenindione;[8] *norethandrolone* and dicoumarol;[9] *methyltestosterone* and phenprocoumon;[10] and *danazol* and warfarin.[11-13] The mechanism of this interaction is not clear although it is considered that it is not caused by altered pharmacokinetics. Steroids with a 17-α-alkyl substituent appear to be most involved, but there has been a report of topically applied testosterone, which does not have such a substituent, enhancing warfarin.[14]

*Oral contraceptives* have also been implicated in interactions. However, while the effects of dicoumarol were diminished by a combined oral contraceptive,[15] those of acenocoumarol were enhanced by other preparations.[16] Combined oral contraceptives have increased the clearance of phenprocoumon without altering the anticoagulant effect.[17] There has also been a report[18] of a single course of *levonorgestrel* for emergency contraception increasing the effect of warfarin.

1. Robinson BHB, *et al.* Decreased anticoagulant tolerance with oxymetholone. *Lancet* 1971; **i:** 1356.
2. Longridge RGM, *et al.* Decreased anticoagulant tolerance with oxymetholone. *Lancet* 1971; **ii:** 90.
3. Edwards MS, Curtis JR. Decreased anticoagulant tolerance with oxymetholone. *Lancet* 1971; **ii:** 221.
4. de Oya JC, *et al.* Decreased anticoagulant tolerance with oxymetholone in paroxysmal nocturnal haemoglobinuria. *Lancet* 1971; **ii:** 259.
5. Acomb C, Shaw PW. A significant interaction between warfarin and stanozolol. *Pharm J* 1985; **234:** 73–4.
6. Shaw PW, Smith AM. Possible interaction of warfarin and stanozolol. *Clin Pharm* 1987; **6:** 500–2.
7. Howard W, *et al.* Anabolic steroids and anticoagulants. *BMJ* 1977; **1:** 1659–60.
8. Vere DW, Fearnley GR. Suspected interaction between phenindione and ethyloestrenol. *Lancet* 1968; **ii:** 281.
9. Schrogie JJ, Solomon HM. The anticoagulant response to bishydroxycoumarin: II. The effect of D-thyroxine, clofibrate, and norethandrolone. *Clin Pharmacol Ther* 1967; **8:** 70–7.
10. Husted S, *et al.* Increased sensitivity to phenprocoumon during methyltestosterone therapy. *Eur J Clin Pharmacol* 1976; **10:** 209–16.
11. Goulbourne IA, Macleod DAD. An interaction between danazol and warfarin: case report. *Br J Obstet Gynaecol* 1981; **88:** 950–1.
12. Meeks ML, *et al.* Danazol increases the anticoagulant effect of warfarin. *Ann Pharmacother* 1992; **26:** 641–2.
13. Booth CD. A drug interaction between danazol and warfarin. *Pharm J* 1993; **250:** 439–40.
14. Lorentz SMcQ, Weibert RT. Potentiation of warfarin anticoagulation by topical testosterone ointment. *Clin Pharm* 1985; **4:** 332–4.
15. Schrogie JJ, *et al.* Effect of oral contraceptives on vitamin K-dependent clotting activity. *Clin Pharmacol Ther* 1967; **8:** 670–5.
16. de Teresa E, *et al.* Interaction between anticoagulants and contraceptives: an unsuspected finding. *BMJ* 1979; **2:** 1260–1.
17. Mönig H, *et al.* Effect of oral contraceptive steroids on the pharmacokinetics of phenprocoumon. *Br J Clin Pharmacol* 1990; **30:** 115–18.
18. Ellison J, *et al.* Apparent interaction between warfarin and levonorgestrel used for emergency contraception. *BMJ* 2000; **321:** 1382.

**Thyroid and antithyroid drugs.** Since response to oral anticoagulants is dependent on thyroid status an interaction between oral anticoagulants and thyroid or antithyroid drugs might be expected. Thyroid compounds do enhance the activity of oral anticoagulants possibly by increased metabolism of clotting factors. Dextrothyroxine is discussed under Lipid Regulating Drugs, above. Antithyroid compounds have not, however, been reported to diminish the effect of anticoagulants and paradoxically *propylthiouracil* has been reported to have caused hypoprothrombinaemia (see Effects on the Blood, under Carbimazole, p.1596).

**Tobacco.** Although tobacco smoking may increase warfarin clearance,[1] an appreciable effect on anticoagulant activity appears unlikely.[1,2] However, there has been a report[3] of an increase in INR in a patient receiving warfarin when he stopped smoking.

1. Bachmann K, *et al.* Smoking and warfarin disposition. *Clin Pharmacol Ther* 1979; **25:** 309–15.
2. Weiner B, *et al.* Warfarin dosage following prosthetic valve replacement: effect of smoking history. *Drug Intell Clin Pharm* 1984; **18:** 904–6.
3. Colucci VJ, Knapp JF. Increase in international normalized ratio associated with smoking cessation. *Ann Pharmacother* 2001; **35:** 385–6.

**Ubidecarenone.** Decreased INR values and reduced effect of warfarin has been reported[1] in 3 patients given ubidecarenone.

1. Spigset O. Reduced effect of warfarin caused by ubidecarenone. *Lancet* 1994; **344:** 1372–3.

**Vaccines.** There have been a few reports of increased prothrombin time and bleeding in warfarin-stabilised patients after *influenza vaccination*. Studies investigating this possible interaction have found only a small or inconsistent increase in warfarin activity[1,2] or no effect.[3-5] One study suggested that influenza vaccine decreases rather than increases the prothrombin time.[6] In a group of patients on long-term acenocoumarol therapy, influenza vaccination had no effect on acenocoumarol activity.[7]

1. Kramer P, *et al.* Effect of influenza vaccine on warfarin anticoagulation. *Clin Pharmacol Ther* 1984; **35:** 416–18.
2. Weibert RT, *et al.* Effect of influenza vaccine in patients receiving long-term warfarin therapy. *Clin Pharm* 1986; **5:** 499–503.
3. Lipsky BA, *et al.* Influenza vaccination and warfarin anticoagulation. *Ann Intern Med* 1984; **100:** 835–7.
4. Scott AK, *et al.* Lack of effect of influenza vaccination on warfarin in healthy volunteers. *Br J Clin Pharmacol* 1985; **19:** 144P–145P.
5. Gomolin IH. Lack of effect of influenza vaccine on warfarin anticoagulation in the elderly. *Can Med Assoc J* 1986; **135:** 39–41.
6. Bussey HI, Saklad JJ. Effect of influenza vaccine on chronic warfarin therapy. *Drug Intell Clin Pharm* 1988; **22:** 198–201.
7. Souto JC, *et al.* Lack of effect of influenza vaccine on anticoagulation by acenocoumarol. *Ann Pharmacother* 1993; **27:** 365–8.

**Vitamins.** Since vitamin K reverses the effects of oral anticoagulants, it is not surprising that there have been reports of *acetomenaphthone* and *phytomenadione* reducing anticoagulant activity, or of foods or nutritional preparations containing vitamin K compounds doing the same.

Occasional reports of *ascorbic acid* reducing the activity of warfarin[1,2] have not been confirmed in subsequent studies.[3,4] There have also been isolated reports suggesting that *vitamin E* may enhance the activity of warfarin[5] or dicoumarol,[6] although no effect was found in a study[7] of patients receiving warfarin and vitamin E.

1. Rosenthal G. Interaction of ascorbic acid and warfarin. *JAMA* 1971; **215:** 1671.
2. Smith EC, *et al.* Interaction of ascorbic acid and warfarin. *JAMA* 1972; **221:** 1166.
3. Hume R, *et al.* Interaction of ascorbic acid and warfarin. *JAMA* 1972; **219:** 1479.

4. Feetam CL, *et al.* Lack of a clinically important interaction between warfarin and ascorbic acid. *Toxicol Appl Pharmacol* 1975; **31:** 544–7.
5. Corrigan JJ, Marcus FI. Coagulopathy associated with vitamin E ingestion. *JAMA* 1974; **230:** 1300–1.
6. Schrogie JJ. Coagulopathy and fat-soluble vitamins. *JAMA* 1975; **232:** 19.
7. Kim JM, White RH. Effect of vitamin E on the anticoagulant response to warfarin. *Am J Cardiol* 1996; **77:** 545–6.

## Pharmacokinetics

Warfarin sodium is readily absorbed from the gastrointestinal tract; it can also be absorbed through the skin. It is extensively bound to plasma proteins and its plasma half-life is about 37 hours. It crosses the placenta but does not occur in significant quantities in breast milk. Warfarin is used as a racemic mixture; the *S*-isomer is reported to be more potent. The *R*- and *S*-isomers are both metabolised in the liver, the *S*-isomer more rapidly than the *R*-isomer; the stereo-isomers may also be affected differently by other drugs (see Interactions, above). Metabolites, with negligible or no anticoagulant activity, are excreted in the urine following reabsorption from the bile.

◊ References.

1. Mungall DR, *et al.* Population pharmacokinetics of racemic warfarin in adult patients. *J Pharmacokinet Biopharm* 1985; **13:** 213–27.
2. Holford NHG. Clinical pharmacokinetics and pharmacodynamics of warfarin: understanding the dose-effect relationship. *Clin Pharmacokinet* 1986; **11:** 483–504.

## Uses and Administration

Warfarin is a coumarin anticoagulant used in the treatment and prophylaxis of thromboembolic disorders (p.837). It acts by depressing the hepatic vitamin K-dependent synthesis of coagulation factors II (prothrombin), VII, IX, and X, and of the anticoagulant protein C and its cofactor protein S. For an explanation of the coagulation cascade, see Haemostasis and Fibrinolysis, p.735. Since warfarin acts indirectly, it has no effect on existing clots. Also as the coagulation factors involved have half-lives ranging from 6 to 60 hours, several hours are required before an effect is observed. A therapeutic effect is usually apparent by 24 hours, but the peak effect may not be achieved until 2 or 3 days after a dose; the overall effect may last for 5 days.

Warfarin is used in the prevention and treatment of venous thromboembolism (deep-vein thrombosis and pulmonary embolism, p.839). If an immediate effect on blood coagulation is required, heparin should be given intravenously or subcutaneously to cover the first 2 to 3 days. Warfarin therapy may be initiated with or shortly after the initial heparin treatment. Warfarin is also used for the prevention of systemic thromboembolism and ischaemic stroke in some patients with atrial fibrillation (p.816), prosthetic heart valves (see Valvular Heart Disease, p.838), or who have suffered a myocardial infarction (p.828). It may also have a role in the prevention of myocardial infarction and in the management of stroke or transient ischaemic attacks (p.836). Antiplatelet drugs may be given concomitantly.

Some patients may show a hereditary resistance to warfarin. Warfarin is a potent rodenticide although resistance has been reported in *rats*.

**Administration and dosage.** Warfarin is equally effective either orally or intravenously, but is usually given by mouth. Dosage must be determined individually as discussed below under Control of Anticoagulant Therapy. When rapid anticoagulation is required, an initial dose of warfarin sodium 10 mg daily for 2 days may be used. However, in many cases an initial dose of 5 mg daily is adequate. Initial doses of less than 5 mg daily may be used in elderly patients and in those at increased risk of bleeding (see Precautions, above). Subsequent maintenance doses usually range from 3 to 9 mg daily. If necessary the same dose may be given by slow intravenous injection. Doses of warfarin sodium should be given at the same time each day. Theoretically, sudden discontinuation of warfarin may result in rebound hypercoagulability with risk of thrombosis. Therefore some clinicians tail off long-term treatment over several weeks but the need for this is unclear. Anticoagulant treatment booklets should be carried by patients.

Warfarin has also been given as the potassium salt; warfarin-deanol has been tried.

**Control of Oral Anticoagulant Therapy.** Treatment with oral anticoagulants must be monitored to ensure that the dose is providing the required effect on the vitamin-K-dependent clotting factors; too small a dose provides inadequate anticoagulation, too large a dose puts the patient at risk of haemorrhage. This monitoring is commonly carried out by checking the clotting property of the patient's plasma using a suitable preparation of thromboplastin and a source of calcium. The time taken for the clot to form due to the effect of the thromboplastin preparation on prothrombin is known as the prothrombin time (PT). The prothrombin time ratio (PTR) is the prothrombin time of the patient's plasma divided by that for a standard plasma sample.

So that there is some consistency in prothrombin time ratios measured at different times or at different laboratories, it is now common practice for the manufacturer or control laboratory to calibrate their batches of thromboplastin against the international reference preparation. This calibration produces an international sensitivity index (ISI) appropriate to that thromboplastin. The laboratory measuring the clotting capacity of a sample of plasma is thus able to convert the prothrombin time ratio to an international normalised ratio (INR) using the sensitivity index through the formula

$$INR = PTR^{(ISI)}$$

Thus a prothrombin time ratio of 2.0 obtained with a thromboplastin with a declared international sensitivity index of 1.5 would be converted to an international normalised ratio of 2.8. An international normalised ratio is therefore equivalent to a prothrombin time ratio carried out using the primary international reference preparation of thromboplastin.

This method of standardisation has taken over from methods involving use of a standard reagent such as the British or Manchester comparative thromboplastin. Preparations of thromboplastin derived from *rabbit* brain have superseded or are superseding those from human brain because of the dangers of viral transmission; a recombinant human form is also available.

Recommended target values or ranges of international normalised ratio for patients receiving anticoagulant treatment or cover for various conditions or procedures are given by the British Society for Haematology in the UK and the American College of Chest Physicians and the National Heart, Lung and Blood Institute in the USA. These are given in Table 5, below. An INR within 0.5 units of the target value in the UK is generally considered satisfactory. In the USA it is recommended that the INR be maintained at the mid-level of the range. An INR less than 2.0 generally represents inadequate anticoagulation and an INR above 4.5 represents greater risk of haemorrhage.

Measurements should be carried out before treatment and then daily or on alternate days in the early stages of treatment. Once the dose has been established and the patient well stabilised the measurement can be made at greater but regular intervals, for example every 8 weeks; allowances should be made for any events that might influence the activity of the anticoagulant.

◊ General references.

1. Harrington R, Ansell J. Risk-benefit assessment of anticoagulant therapy. *Drug Safety* 1991; **6:** 54–69.
2. Le DT, *et al.* The international normalized ratio (INR) for monitoring warfarin therapy: reliability and relation to other monitoring methods. *Ann Intern Med* 1994; **120:** 552–8.
3. Routledge PA. Practical prescribing: warfarin. *Prescribers' J* 1997; **37:** 173–9.
4. British Society for Haematology: British Committee for Standards in Haematology—Haemostasis and Thrombosis Task Force. Guidelines on oral anticoagulation: third edition. *Br J Haematol* 1998; **101:** 374–87. Also available at: http://www.bcshguidelines.com/pdf/bjh715.pdf (accessed 06/07/04)
5. Hardman SMC, Cowie MR. Anticoagulation in heart disease. *BMJ* 1999; **318:** 238–44.
6. Gage BF, *et al.* Management and dosing of warfarin therapy. *Am J Med* 2000; **109:** 481–8.
7. Hirsh J, *et al.* Oral anticoagulants: mechanism of action, clinical effectiveness, and optimal therapeutic range. *Chest* 2001; **119** (suppl): 8S–21S.
8. Ansell J, *et al.* Managing oral anticoagulant therapy. *Chest* 2001; **119** (suppl): 22S–38S.
9. Hirsh J, *et al.* American Heart Association/American College of Cardiology Foundation guide to warfarin therapy. *Circulation* 2003; **107:** 1692–1711. Also available at: http://circ.ahajournals.org/cgi/reprint/107/12/1692.pdf (accessed 06/07/04)

**Administration and dosage.** Algorithms and guidelines have been developed for the initiation of anticoagulant therapy, based on the method of Fennerty *et al.*[1] Although a loading dose of 10 mg daily for 2 days (depending on the INR) has been widely used, lower doses may be more appropriate. Studies[2-4] have compared warfarin loading doses of 5 and 10 mg and found that for both groups a therapeutic INR in the range of 2.0 to 3.0 was reached in most patients by day 5 of treatment.

In outpatient and community settings, when rapid anticoagulation is not necessary, loading doses may not be required. A low-dose regimen for elderly patients requiring anticoagulation prophylaxis has been described.[5] Warfarin was started at a dose of 2 mg daily for 2 weeks followed by weekly adjustment using an algorithm until the target INR was reached.

1. Fennerty A, *et al.* Flexible induction dose regimen for warfarin and prediction of maintenance dose. *BMJ* 1984; **288:** 1268–70.
2. Harrison L, *et al.* Comparison of 5-mg and 10-mg loading doses in initiation of warfarin therapy. *Ann Intern Med* 1997; **126:** 133–6.
3. Crowther MA, *et al.* Warfarin: less may be better. *Ann Intern Med* 1997; **127:** 333.
4. Crowther MA, *et al.* A randomized trial comparing 5-mg and 10-mg warfarin loading doses. *Arch Intern Med* 1999; **159:** 46–8.
5. Oates A, *et al.* A new regimen for starting warfarin therapy in out-patients. *Br J Clin Pharmacol* 1998; **46:** 157–61.

**Administration in infants and children.** Increasing numbers of infants and children are receiving anticoagulants for prophylaxis and treatment of thromboembolism. Doses of warfarin and therapeutic INR ranges have been adapted from adult therapy but cohort studies[1,2] of paediatric patients have found that warfarin requirements may be affected by a number of factors including age, and the use of infant formulas supplemented with vitamin K. Recommendations[3] for the use of oral anticoagulants in children have been published.

1. Tait RC, *et al.* Oral anticoagulation in paediatric patients: dose requirements and complications. *Arch Dis Child* 1996; **74:** 228–31.
2. Streif W, *et al.* Analysis of warfarin therapy in pediatric patients: a prospective cohort study of 319 patients. *Blood* 1999; **94:** 3007–14.
3. Monagle P, *et al.* Antithrombotic therapy in children. *Chest* 2001; **119** (suppl): 344S–370S.

**Table 5.** Recommended International Normalised Ratios (INR).

| | INR | Condition or procedure |
|---|---|---|
| UK | 2.5 | Pulmonary embolism; deep-vein thrombosis; recurrence of venous thromboembolism when no longer on warfarin; symptomatic inherited thrombophilia; atrial fibrillation; cardioversion; mural thrombus; cardiomyopathy. |
| | 3.5 | Recurrence of venous thromboembolism when on warfarin; antiphospholipid syndrome; mechanical prosthetic heart valves. |
| US | 2.0 to 3.0 | Prophylaxis of venous thromboembolism in high-risk surgical patients; treatment of venous thrombosis and pulmonary embolism; prophylaxis of systemic embolism in patients with atrial fibrillation, valvular heart disease, bioprosthetic heart valves, or acute myocardial infarction. |
| | 2.5 to 3.5 | Prophylaxis in patients with mechanical prosthetic heart valves; prevention of recurrent myocardial infarction. |

**Catheters and cannulas.** For mention of the use of oral anticoagulants to prevent thrombosis in patients with indwelling infusion devices, see Heparin Sodium, p.930.

**Connective tissue and muscular disorders.** Warfarin has been proposed to treat subcutaneous calcium deposition (calcinosis cutis) in patients with dermatomyositis, but its value is disputed, see Polymyositis and Dermatomyositis, p.1086.

### Preparations

**BP 2003:** Warfarin Tablets;
**USP 27:** Warfarin Sodium for Injection; Warfarin Sodium Tablets.

**Proprietary Preparations** (details are given in Part 3)
**Arg.:** Circuvit; Coumadin; **Austral.:** Coumadin; Marevan; **Belg.:** Marevan; **Braz.:** Marevan; **Canad.:** Coumadin; Warfilone†; **Chile:** Coumadin; **Denm.:** Marevan; **Fin.:** Marevan; **Fr.:** Coumadine; **Ger.:** Coumadin; **Gr.:** Marevan; Panwarfin; **India:** Uniwarfin; **Irl.:** Warfant; **Israel:** Coumadin; **Ital.:** Coumadin; **Malaysia:** Coumadin; Orfarin; **Mex.:** Romesa†; **Norw.:** Marevan; **NZ:** Coumadin; Marevan; **Port.:** Varfine; **S.Afr.:** Coumadin; **Singapore:** Coumadin; Marevan; **Spain:** Aldocumar; Tedicumar; **Swed.:** Waran; **Thai.:** Orfarin; **UK:** Marevan; **USA:** Coumadin; Jantoven.

---

## Xamoterol Fumarate *(BANM, USAN, rINNM)*

Fumarato de xamoterol; ICI-118587. N-{2-[2-Hydroxy-3-(4-hydroxyphenoxy)propylamino]ethyl}morpholine-4-carboxamide fumarate.

$(C_{16}H_{25}N_3O_5)_2,C_4H_4O_4$ = 794.8.
*CAS — 81801-12-9 (xamoterol); 90730-93-1 (xamoterol fumarate).*
*ATC — C01CX07.*

### Profile

Xamoterol is a beta-adrenoceptor partial agonist with a selective action on $beta_1$ receptors. As a partial agonist it exerts predominantly agonist activity at rest and under conditions of low sympathetic drive which results in improved ventricular function and increased cardiac output; during exercise and during conditions of increased sympathetic drive, such as that occurring in severe heart failure, xamoterol exerts beta-blocking activity. It therefore has the properties of both sympathomimetics (see Adrenaline, p.852) and beta blockers (see p.868).

Xamoterol has been used in the management of chronic mild heart failure but was associated with deterioration and an excess of deaths in those with more severe disease. It has also been used in orthostatic hypotension secondary to autonomic failure.

◊ References.


1. Anonymous. Xamoterol—more trouble than it's worth? *Drug Ther Bull* 1990; **28:** 53–4.
2. Anonymous. New evidence on xamoterol. *Lancet* 1990; **336:** 24.
3. The Xamoterol in Severe Heart Failure Study Group. Xamoterol in severe heart failure. *Lancet* 1990; **336:** 1–6.


### Preparations

**Proprietary Preparations** (details are given in Part 3)
**Belg.:** Corwin†; **UK:** Corwin†.

---

## Xantinol Nicotinate *(BAN, rINN)*

Nicotinato de xantinol; SK-331A; Xanthinol Niacinate *(USAN)*; Xanthinol Nicotinate. 7-{2-Hydroxy-3-[(2-hydroxyethyl)methylamino]propyl}theophylline nicotinate.

$C_{13}H_{21}N_5O_4,C_6H_5NO_2$ = 434.4.
*CAS — 437-74-1.*
*ATC — C04AD02.*

**Pharmacopoeias.** In *Pol.*

### Profile

Xantinol nicotinate is a vasodilator with general properties similar to those of nicotinic acid (p.1441), to which it is slowly hydrolysed. Xantinol nicotinate is used in the management of peripheral (p.831) and cerebral vascular disorders (p.820) and in hyperlipidaemias (p.823). Doses of up to 3 g daily may be given by mouth. It has also been given by intramuscular or slow intravenous injection.

### Preparations

**Proprietary Preparations** (details are given in Part 3)
**Austria:** Frigol; **Belg.:** Complamin†; **Canad.:** Complamin†; **Ger.:** Complamin; Complamin spezial; **India:** Complamina; **Ital.:** Complamin; Vedrin; **Neth.:** Complamin; **Swed.:** Complamin†; **Switz.:** Complamin.

**Multi-ingredient:** **Spain:** Plasmaclar†; Rulun.

---

## Xemilofiban Hydrochloride *(USAN, rINNM)*

Hidrocloruro de xemilofibán; SC-54684A. Ethyl (3S)-3-{3-[(p-amidinophenyl)carbamoyl]propionamido}-4-pentynoate monohydrochloride.

$C_{18}H_{22}N_4O_4,HCl$ = 394.9.
*CAS — 149820-74-6 (xemilofiban); 156586-91-3 (xemilofiban hydrochloride).*

### Profile

Xemilofiban is a glycoprotein IIb/IIIa-receptor antagonist. It has been investigated as an oral antiplatelet drug for the management of thromboembolic disorders such as unstable angina, and following angioplasty, but results have been disappointing.

◊ References.


1. O'Neill WW, *et al.* Long-term treatment with a platelet glycoprotein-receptor antagonist after percutaneous coronary revascularization. *N Engl J Med* 2000; **342:** 1316–24.


---

## Xipamide *(BAN, USAN, rINN)*

Be-1293; MJF-10938; Xipamida. 4-Chloro-5-sulphamoylsalicylo-2′,6′-xylidide; 5-(Aminosulphonyl)-4-chloro-N-(2,6-dimethylphenyl)-2-hydroxy-benzamide.

$C_{15}H_{15}ClN_2O_4S$ = 354.8.
*CAS — 14293-44-8.*
*ATC — C03BA10.*

### Adverse Effects, Treatment, and Precautions

As for Hydrochlorothiazide, p.933.

**Effects on electrolyte balance.** Although reductions in plasma-potassium concentrations with xipamide have been shown to be on average comparable with those produced by thiazide and loop diuretics at equipotent doses,[1] there have been several reports of marked hypokalaemia in individual patients. Asymptomatic hypokalaemia was reported in 4 of 5 patients[2] (serum-potassium concentrations of less than 3.4 mmol/litre) and in 3 of 13 patients[3] (serum-potassium concentrations of less than 3.0 mmol/litre). Severe hypokalaemia resulting in ventricular arrhythmias has been reported following xipamide alone[4] or in combination with indapamide.[5] Profound electrolyte disturbances with altered consciousness and ventricular extrasystoles occurred in a patient taking digoxin following the addition of xipamide for 10 days.[6] A case of hypokalaemic periodic paralysis associated with xipamide administration has also been reported.[7]


1. Prichard BNC, Brogden RN. Xipamide: a review of its pharmacodynamic and pharmacokinetic properties and therapeutic efficacy. *Drugs* 1985; **30:** 313–32.
2. Weissberg P, Kendall MJ. Hypokalaemia and xipamide. *BMJ* 1982; **284:** 975.
3. Raftery EB, *et al.* A study of the antihypertensive action of xipamide using ambulatory intra-arterial monitoring. *Br J Clin Pharmacol* 1981; **12:** 381–5.
4. Altmann P, Hamblin JJ. Ventricular fibrillation induced by xipamide. *BMJ* 1982; **284:** 494.
5. Boulton AJM, Hardisty CA. Ventricular arrhythmias precipitated by treatment with non-thiazide diuretics. *Practitioner* 1982; **226:** 125–8.
6. Bentley J. Hypokalaemia and xipamide. *BMJ* 1982; **284:** 975.
7. Boulton AJM, Hardisty CA. Hypokalaemic periodic paralysis precipitated by diuretic therapy and minor surgery. *Postgrad Med J* 1982; **58:** 106–7.


**Hepatic impairment.** For a recommendation that xipamide should be given with caution to patients with liver disease, see under Pharmacokinetics, below.

### Interactions

As for Hydrochlorothiazide, p.935.

### Pharmacokinetics

Xipamide has been reported to be well absorbed from the gastrointestinal tract. Absorption is fairly rapid with peak plasma concentrations occurring within 1 or 2 hours of oral administration. It is 99% bound to plasma proteins, and is excreted in the urine, partly unchanged and partly in the form of the glucuronide metabolite. It is reported to have a plasma half-life of about 5 to 8 hours. In patients with renal impairment excretion in the bile becomes more prominent.

◊ References.


1. Beermann B, Grind M. Clinical pharmacokinetics of some newer diuretics. *Clin Pharmacokinet* 1987; **13:** 254–66.


**Hepatic impairment.** Xipamide was present in the plasma and in ascitic fluid in patients with liver cirrhosis in proportion to the protein content of the respective compartments.[1] The amount of drug excreted into the urine was much greater in patients with liver disease than in healthy control subjects. This was attributed to a diminution in hepatic elimination, which could result in significant effects on the clinical response to xipamide. Thus patients with cholestasis could have an enhanced response to xipamide. On the other hand cirrhotic patients with the hepatorenal syndrome may be resistant to diuretics. Xipamide should be used with caution in patients with liver disease.


1. Knauf H, *et al.* Xipamide disposition in liver cirrhosis. *Clin Pharmacol Ther* 1990; **48:** 628–32.


**Renal impairment.** Following single oral and intravenous doses of xipamide 20 mg the drug appeared to be completely absorbed from the gastrointestinal tract.[1] The mean elimination half-life in healthy subjects was 7 hours and two-thirds of the clearance was by extrarenal routes. There was some accumulation in patients with chronic renal failure, with a calculated elimination half-life of 9 hours in end-stage renal disease.


1. Knauf H, Mutschler E. Pharmacodynamics and pharmacokinetics of xipamide in patients with normal and impaired kidney function. *Eur J Clin Pharmacol* 1984; **26:** 513–20.


### Uses and Administration

Xipamide is a diuretic, structurally related to indapamide, with actions and uses similar to those of the thiazide diuretics (see Hydrochlorothiazide, p.935). It is used for hypertension (p.825), and for oedema, including that associated with heart failure (p.820).

Diuresis is initiated in about 1 or 2 hours, reaches a peak at 4 to 6 hours, and lasts for about 12 hours.

In the treatment of **hypertension** the usual dose is 20 mg daily as a single morning dose, either alone, or with other antihypertensives. In some patients a dose of 10 mg daily may be adequate. In the treatment of **oedema** the usual initial dose is 40 mg by mouth daily, subsequently reduced to 20 mg daily, according to response; in resistant cases 80 mg daily may be required.

◊ References.


1. Prichard BNC, Brogden RN. Xipamide: a review of its pharmacodynamic and pharmacokinetic properties and therapeutic efficacy. *Drugs* 1985; **30:** 313–32.


### Preparations

**Proprietary Preparations** (details are given in Part 3)
**Austria:** Aquaphoril; **Belg.:** Diurexan†; **Fr.:** Chronexan†; Lumitens; **Ger.:** Aquaphor; **Hong Kong:** Diurexan†; **India:** Xipamid; **Irl.:** Diurexan†; **Ital.:** Aquafor; **Port.:** Diurexan; **S.Afr.:** Diurexan; **Spain:** Demiax; Diurex; **UK:** Diurexan.

**Multi-ingredient:** **Ger.:** Durotan; Neotri.

---

## Zofenopril Calcium *(BANM, USAN, rINNM)*

SQ-26991; Zofenopril cálcico. Calcium salt of (4S)-1-[(2S)-3-(Benzylthio)-2-methylpropionyl]-4-(phenylthio)-L-proline.

$C_{44}H_{44}CaN_2O_8S_4$ = 897.2.
*CAS — 81872-10-8 (zofenopril); 81938-43-4 (zofenopril calcium).*
*ATC — C09AA16.*

### Profile

Zofenopril is an ACE inhibitor (p.842) that is used in the management of hypertension (p.825) and myocardial infarction (p.828). It owes its activity to the active metabolite zofenoprilat (SQ-26333) to which it is converted after oral administration. It is given by mouth as the calcium salt in a usual maintenance dose of 30 to 60 mg daily, as a single dose or in two divided doses.

◊ References.


1. Ambrosioni E, *et al.* The effect of the angiotensin-converting-enzyme inhibitor zofenopril on mortality and morbidity after anterior myocardial infarction. *N Engl J Med* 1995; **332:** 80–5.
2. Borghi C, *et al.* Effects of the administration of an angiotensin-converting enzyme inhibitor during the acute phase of myocardial infarction in patients with arterial hypertension: SMILE study investigators: Survival of Myocardial Infarction Long-term Evaluation. *Am J Hypertens* 1999; **12:** 665–72.


### Preparations

**Proprietary Preparations** (details are given in Part 3)
**Fr.:** Zofenil; **Irl.:** Zofenil; **Ital.:** Bifril; Zantipres; Zopranol; **Swed.:** Bifril.

# Chelators Antidotes and Antagonists

The drugs included in this chapter act in a variety of ways to counter the toxic effects of exogenous and endogenous substances in the body. They are therefore used in the management of poisoning and overdosage, to protect against the toxicity of drugs such as antineoplastics, and in the management of metabolic disorders such as Wilson's disease where toxic substances accumulate. Some are antagonists, such as the opioid antagonist naloxone, that compete with the poison for receptor sites. Others inhibit the toxin by reacting with it to form less active or inactive complexes or by interfering with its metabolism; chelators are typical examples of the first group and methionine is an example of the second. Other compounds with a role in the treatment of specific types of poisoning include those such as atropine (p.476) that block essential receptors mediating the toxic effects, or those that reduce the rate of conversion of the poison to a more toxic compound, such as alcohol (p.1166) in methyl alcohol poisoning, or those that bypass the effect of the drug as happens with calcium folinate (p.1431) in methotrexate overdosage. Acetylcysteine (p.1112) is an antagonist used in paracetamol poisoning.

### Acute poisoning

In the management of suspected acute poisoning it is often impossible to determine the identity of the poison or the size of the dose received with any certainty. Moreover, specific antidotes and methods of elimination are available for relatively few poisons and the mainstay of treatment for patients with suspected acute poisoning is therefore supportive and symptomatic therapy; in many cases nothing further is required. Symptoms of acute poisoning are frequently non-specific, particularly in the early stages. Maintenance of the airway and ventilation is the most important initial measure; other treatment, for example for cardiovascular or neurological symptoms, may be added as appropriate. Patients who are unconscious may be given naloxone if opioid overdosage is suspected. Some centres also recommend the routine administration of glucose to all unconscious patients since hypoglycaemia may be a cause of unconsciousness; thiamine is given in addition since glucose may precipitate Wernicke's encephalopathy.

Specific antidotes are available for a number of poisons and are the primary treatment where there is severe poisoning with a known toxin. They may be life-saving in such cases but their use is not without hazard and in many situations they are not necessary; their use does not preclude relevant supportive treatment.

Measures to reduce or prevent the absorption of the poison are widely advocated. For inhalational poisoning the victim is removed from the source of poisoning. Some toxins, in particular pesticides, may be absorbed through the skin, and clothing should be removed and the skin thoroughly washed to avoid continued absorption. Caustic substances are removed from the skin or eyes with copious irrigation. Orally ingested poisons may be actively removed from the stomach by emesis or by gastric lavage, although these measures are of limited value (see under Ipecacuanha, p.1123). Activated charcoal may be administered to adsorb some poisons. Repeated doses may be of use to eliminate some substances even after systemic absorption has occurred.

Induction of emesis has been used in the home situation with an emetic agent such as syrup of ipecacuanha, but the practice is not generally recommended because there is no evidence that it reduces absorption and it may increase the risk of aspiration. If used at all, it should only be in fully conscious patients. Emesis should not be induced if the poison is corrosive or petroleum based, nor if the poison is removable by treatment with activated charcoal. Gastric lavage may occasionally be indicated for ingestion of non-caustic poisons that are not absorbed by activated charcoal, but only if less than one hour has elapsed since ingestion. Lavage should not be attempted if the airway is not adequately protected. Whole-bowel irrigation using a non-absorbable osmotic agent such as a macrogol has been used following ingestion of substances that pass beyond the stomach before being absorbed, such as iron preparations or enteric-coated or modified-release formulations. A single oral dose of activated charcoal is effective for a wide range of toxins, particularly if it is given within one hour of ingestion, although delayed use may still be beneficial particularly for modified-release preparations or for drugs which slow gastrointestinal transit time such as those with antimuscarinic properties; it is generally well tolerated, although vomiting is common and there is a risk of aspiration if the airway is not adequately protected.

Techniques intended to promote the elimination of poisons from the body, such as haemodialysis or haemoperfusion, are only of value for a limited number of poisons in a few severely poisoned patients; forced diuresis is generally no longer recommended. Repeated oral doses of activated charcoal may often be as effective as these more invasive methods.

Poisons Information Centres exist in many countries and should be consulted for more detailed information in specific situations.

## Activated Charcoal

Carbo Activatus; Carbón adsorbente; Decolorising Charcoal.

*CAS — 16291-96-6 (charcoal).*

*ATC — A07BA01.*

**Pharmacopoeias.** In *Chin., Eur.* (see p.vi), *Int., Jpn, Pol., US,* and *Viet.*

**Ph. Eur. 5.0** (Charcoal, Activated). It is obtained from vegetable matter by suitable carbonisation processes intended to confer a high adsorption power. A black, light powder free from grittiness. Practically insoluble in all usual solvents. It adsorbs not less than 40% of its own weight of phenazone, calculated with reference to the dried substance. Store in airtight containers.

**USP 27** (Activated Charcoal). The residue from the destructive distillation of various organic materials, treated to increase its adsorptive power. A fine, black, odourless, tasteless powder, free from gritty matter. The USP 27 has tests for adsorptive power in respect of alkaloids and dyes.

### Adverse Effects and Precautions

Activated charcoal is relatively non-toxic when given by mouth but gastrointestinal disturbances such as vomiting, constipation, or diarrhoea have been reported. It may colour the faeces black. Activated charcoal should be used with caution in patients at risk of gastrointestinal obstruction as it may reduce gastrointestinal motility.

Haemoperfusion with activated charcoal has produced various adverse effects including platelet aggregation, charcoal embolism, thrombocytopenia, haemorrhage, hypoglycaemia, hypocalcaemia, hypothermia, and hypotension.

Activated charcoal is best cleared from the stomach or avoided when specific oral antidotes such as methionine are used (see Interactions, below). As with any treatment given by mouth for poisoning the risk of aspiration should be considered in drowsy or comatose patients.

**Effects on the gastrointestinal tract.** Intestinal obstruction[1-4] or faecal impaction, in one case resulting in rectal ulceration,[5] has been reported following multiple oral doses of activated charcoal. Special care should be taken when treating overdoses of drugs with antimuscarinic activity, such as tricyclic antidepressants and phenothiazines.[2] Two cases of pseudo-obstruction, one of which was fatal, have also been reported[6] following the use of activated charcoal and sorbitol with opioid sedation for theophylline poisoning. Care should also be taken to prevent pulmonary aspiration (see below).


1. Watson WA, *et al.* Gastrointestinal obstruction associated with multiple-dose activated charcoal. *J Emerg Med* 1986; **4:** 401–7.
2. Anderson IM, Ware C. Syrup of ipecacuanha. *BMJ* 1987; **294:** 578.
3. Ray MJ, *et al.* Charcoal bezoar: small-bowel obstruction secondary to amitriptyline overdose therapy. *Dig Dis Sci* 1988; **33:** 106–7.
4. Atkinson SW, *et al.* Treatment with activated charcoal complicated by gastrointestinal obstruction requiring surgery. *BMJ* 1992; **305:** 563.
5. Mizutani T, *et al.* Rectal ulcer with massive haemorrhage due to activated charcoal treatment in oral organophosphate poisoning. *Hum Exp Toxicol* 1991; **10:** 385–6.
6. Longdon P, Henderson A. Intestinal pseudo-obstruction following the use of enteral charcoal and sorbitol and mechanical ventilation with papaveretum sedation for theophylline poisoning. *Drug Safety* 1992; **7:** 74–7.


**Effects on the lungs.** Pulmonary aspiration of activated charcoal, sometimes with fatal results, has been reported following oral administration for the treatment of acute poisoning.[1-4] Vomiting has been reported to be fairly common by some,[1,5] but not all,[6] correspondents after use of activated charcoal; the water load resulting from repeated administration of charcoal slurry could contribute to any nausea and vomiting[5] and the use of sorbitol-containing preparations may also contribute to the vomiting.[7] The use of a cuffed endotracheal tube has been recommended for any patient with impaired laryngeal reflexes to prevent aspiration.[4,8]


1. Hoffman JR. Charcoal for gastrointestinal clearance of drugs. *N Engl J Med* 1983; **308:** 157.
2. Harsch HH. Aspiration of activated charcoal. *N Engl J Med* 1986; **314:** 318.
3. Menzies DG, *et al.* Fatal pulmonary aspiration of oral activated charcoal. *BMJ* 1988; **297:** 459–60.
4. Rau NR, *et al.* Fatal pulmonary aspiration of oral activated charcoal. *BMJ* 1988; **297:** 918–19.
5. Danel V. Fatal pulmonary aspiration of oral activated charcoal. *BMJ* 1988; **297:** 684.
6. Levy G. Charcoal for gastrointestinal clearance of drugs. *N Engl J Med* 1983; **308:** 157.
7. McFarland AK, Chyka PA. Selection of activated charcoal products for the treatment of poisonings. *Ann Pharmacother* 1993; **27:** 358–61.
8. Power KJ. Fatal pulmonary aspiration of oral activated charcoal. *BMJ* 1988; **297:** 919.


### Interactions

Activated charcoal has the potential to reduce the absorption of many drugs from the gastrointestinal tract and simultaneous oral therapy should therefore be avoided. In the management of acute poisoning, concurrent medication should be given parenterally. Activated charcoal is best cleared from the stomach or avoided when a specific oral antidote such as methionine is given since adsorption of the antidote may decrease effectiveness.

### Uses and Administration

Activated charcoal can adsorb a wide range of plant and inorganic poisons and many drugs including salicylates, paracetamol, barbiturates, and tricyclic antidepressants; thus when given by mouth it reduces their systemic absorption from the gastrointestinal tract and is used in the treatment of acute oral poisoning. It is of no value in the treatment of poisoning by strong acids, alkalis, or other corrosive substances and its adsorptive capacity is too low to be of use in poisoning with iron salts, cyanides, lithium, malathion, clofenotane, and some organic solvents such as methyl alcohol or ethylene glycol. Adsorption characteristics can be influenced by charcoal's particle size, thus different responses may be obtained with different preparations.

Activated charcoal is given by mouth usually as a slurry in water. A usual adult dose for reduction of absorption is 50 g, but higher doses have been used. Children 1 to 12 years old may be given 25 to 50 g and infants under 1 year 1 g/kg. For maximum efficacy, activated charcoal should be administered as soon as possible (within 1 hour) after ingestion of the toxic compound. However, it may be effective several hours after poisoning with certain drugs that slow gastric emptying. In the case of drugs that undergo enterohepatic or enteroenteric recycling (e.g. phenobarbital and theophylline) *repeated doses* of activated charcoal are of value in enhancing faecal elimination. Adult doses for repeated administration in active elimination have varied but typically 50 g may be given every 4 hours or 25 g every 2 hours. Doses in children and infants are similar to those used above for reduction of absorption and may be given every 4 to 6 hours. Administration may also be via a nasogastric tube.

Mixtures such as 'universal antidote' that contained activated charcoal, magnesium oxide, and tannic acid should not be used; activated charcoal alone is more effective and tannic acid may cause hepatotoxicity.

In treatment of poisoning using charcoal haemoperfusion, activated charcoal is used to remove drugs from the bloodstream. It may be of value in acute severe poisoning by drugs such as the barbiturates, glutethimide, or theophylline when other intensive measures fail to improve the condition of the patient.

Activated charcoal is used in dressings for ulcers and suppurating wounds (p.1139) to reduce malodour and may improve the rate of healing.

Activated charcoal has been used as a marker of intestinal transit and has also been tried in the treatment of flatulence. Both activated charcoal and vegetable charcoal (wood charcoal; carbo ligni) are included in preparations for various gastrointestinal disorders.

Technical grades of activated charcoal have been used as purifying and decolorising agents, for the removal of residual gases in low-pressure apparatus, and in respirators as a protection against toxic gases.

**Administration.** Activated charcoal is most commonly given as a slurry in water but this is often found to be unpalatable because of the colour, gritty taste, lack of flavour, and difficulty in swallowing.[1] Efforts have therefore been made to improve its palatability, but studies *in vitro* or in healthy subjects indicated that some foods such as ice cream, milk, and cocoa might inhibit the adsorptive capacity of activated charcoal, whereas starches and jams appeared to have no effect.[2,3] Carmellose has improved palatability although it might also reduce adsorptive capacity.[4-6] Activated charcoal formulations containing sorbitol, carmellose sodium, or starch were more palatable and essentially equivalent to the aqueous slurry formulation in efficacy.[1] When chocolate syrup was used as a flavouring agent it had to be added just before administration as the sweetness and flavour disappeared after a few minutes of contact with the activated charcoal.[1] Saccharin sodium, sucrose, or sorbitol might be suitable flavours.[7] A survey[8] of commercially available ready-to-use charcoal preparations in the USA indicated that although differences did exist between the formulations, the clinical significance of such variations was unknown. The problems associated with sorbitol-containing products (see also under Poisoning, below) were highlighted and caution made against their use, especially for repeated-dose therapy.


1. Scholtz EC, *et al.* Evaluation of five activated charcoal formulations for inhibition of aspirin absorption and palatability in man. *Am J Hosp Pharm* 1978; **35:** 1355–9.
2. Levy G, *et al.* Inhibition by ice cream of the antidotal efficacy of activated charcoal. *Am J Hosp Pharm* 1975; **32:** 289–91.
3. De Neve R. Antidotal efficacy of activated charcoal in presence of jam, starch and milk. *Am J Hosp Pharm* 1976; **33:** 965–6.
4. Mathur LK, *et al.* Activated charcoal–carboxymethylcellulose gel formulation as an antidotal agent for orally ingested aspirin. *Am J Hosp Pharm* 1976; **33:** 717–19.
5. Manes M. Effect of carboxymethylcellulose on the adsorptive capacity of charcoal. *Am J Hosp Pharm* 1976; **33:** 1120, 1122.
6. Mathur LK, *et al.* Effect of carboxymethylcellulose on the adsorptive capacity of charcoal. *Am J Hosp Pharm* 1976; **33:** 1122.
7. Cooney DO. Palatability of sucrose-, sorbitol-, and saccharin-sweetened activated charcoal formulations. *Am J Hosp Pharm* 1980; **37:** 237–9.
8. McFarland AK, Chyka PA. Selection of activated charcoal products for the treatment of poisonings. *Ann Pharmacother* 1993; **27:** 358–61.


**Poisoning.** The management of acute poisoning is discussed on p.1030. The use of a *single oral dose* of activated charcoal has become a widespread method of preventing the absorption of ingested compounds and may be superior to gastric emptying. The American Academy of Clinical Toxicology (AACT) and the European Association of Poisons Centres and Clinical Toxicologists (EAPCCT) consider[1] that activated charcoal may be used if a patient presents within 1 hour of ingesting a potentially toxic amount of a poison known to be absorbed by charcoal. There are insufficient data to support general use beyond 1 hour after ingestion.[1,2] In addition, *multiple oral doses* of activated charcoal have been found to enhance the elimination of some drugs and toxic substances even after systemic absorption. Mechanisms by which activated charcoal may increase drug elimination from the body include interruption of the enterohepatic circulation of drugs excreted into the bile, reduction of the reabsorption of drugs which diffuse or are actively secreted into the intestines, and increased elimination of the drug via the gastrointestinal tract when given with a laxative to decrease gastrointestinal transit time, although the practice of using charcoal with a laxative has been questioned.[3-5] Repeated oral doses of activated charcoal may therefore be considered for compounds that undergo enterohepatic or enteroenteric circulation, have a small volume of distribution, are not extensively bound to plasma proteins, and have a low endogenous clearance. Following a review of the literature[5] the AACT and EAPCCT recommended that multiple doses of charcoal should be considered only if a patient has ingested a life-threatening amount of carbamazepine, dapsone, phenobarbital, quinine, or theophylline. Anecdotal reports and studies in acutely poisoned patients indicate that a technique of giving multiple doses of charcoal may offer an alternative to charcoal haemoperfusion or haemodialysis. However, while activated charcoal is generally well tolerated, major complications do occasionally occur, including pulmonary aspiration and bowel obstruction.[6] Also, use of multiple doses of charcoal preparations containing sorbitol or sodium bicarbonate can result in increased vomiting[7] or in electrolyte disturbances.[3,8,9]


1. Chyka PA, Seger D. American Academy of Clinical Toxicology; European Association of Poisons Centres and Clinical Toxicologists. Position statement: single-dose activated charcoal. *J Toxicol Clin Toxicol* 1997; **35:** 721–41.
2. Green R, *et al.* How long after drug ingestion is activated charcoal still effective? *J Toxicol Clin Toxicol* 2001; **39:** 601–5.
3. Neuvonen PJ, Olkkola KT. Oral activated charcoal in the treatment of intoxications: role of single and repeated doses. *Med Toxicol* 1988; **3:** 33–58.
4. Neuvonen PJ, Olkkola KT. Effect of purgatives on antidotal efficacy of oral activated charcoal. *Hum Toxicol* 1986; **5:** 255–63.
5. American Academy of Clinical Toxicology; European Association of Poisons Centres and Clinical Toxicologists. Position statement and practice guidelines on the use of multi-dose activated charcoal in the treatment of acute poisoning. *J Toxicol Clin Toxicol* 1999; **37:** 731–51.
6. Palatnick W, Tenenbein M. Activated charcoal in the treatment of drug overdose: an update. *Drug Safety* 1992; **7:** 3–7.
7. McFarland AK, Chyka PA. Selection of activated charcoal products for the treatment of poisonings. *Ann Pharmacother* 1993; **27:** 358–61.
8. McLuckie A, *et al.* Role of repeated doses of oral activated charcoal in the treatment of acute intoxications. *Anaesth Intensive Care* 1990; **18:** 375–84.
9. Tenenbein M. Multiple doses of activated charcoal: time for reappraisal? *Ann Emerg Med* 1991; **20:** 529–31.


HAEMOPERFUSION. Haemoperfusion involves the passage of blood through an adsorbent material such as activated charcoal or synthetic hydrophobic polystyrene resins that can retain certain drugs and toxic agents. Early problems with charcoal haemoperfusion such as charcoal embolism, marked thrombocytopenia, fibrinogen loss, and pyrogen reactions have been largely overcome by purification procedures and by coating the carbon with biocompatible polymers. However, transient falls in platelet count, leucocyte count, and circulatory concentrations of clotting factors, calcium, glucose, urea, creatinine, and urate have been reported during haemoperfusion. While there is no substitute for supportive measures, haemoperfusion can significantly reduce the body burden of certain compounds with a low volume of distribution within 4 to 6 hours in some severely poisoned patients; haemoperfusion is not effective for drugs or poisons with very large volumes of distribution.

**Porphyria.** Activated charcoal may be used as part of the management of erythropoietic protoporphyria, one of the non-acute porphyrias (p.1040). It acts as a sorbent in the gut lumen, interrupting the enterohepatic recycling of protoporphyrin. It has also been tried in a patient with photomutilation diagnosed as having congenital erythropoietic porphyria, a very rare porphyria.[1] Activated charcoal 30 g given by mouth every 3 hours for 36 hours reduced the plasma-porphyrin concentration to normal values by 20 hours and was more effective than colestyramine or transfusional therapy. After discontinuation of activated charcoal, plasma-porphyrin concentrations rose rapidly to near pretreatment levels within 10 days. Long-term treatment with oral charcoal over a 9-month period effected a clinical remission with low concentrations of plasma and skin porphyrin and an absence of photocutaneous activity. The optimal dose was determined to be 60 g three times daily. However, exacerbation following an initial period of remission has been reported in another patient[2] and total lack of efficacy in a third.[3]


1. Pimstone NR, *et al.* Therapeutic efficacy of oral charcoal in congenital erythropoietic porphyria. *N Engl J Med* 1987; **316:** 390–3.
2. Hift RJ, *et al.* The effect of oral activated charcoal on the course of congenital erythropoietic porphyria. *Br J Dermatol* 1993; **129:** 14–17.
3. Minder EI, *et al.* Lack of effect of oral charcoal in congenital erythropoietic porphyria. *N Engl J Med* 1994; **330:** 1092–4.


**Pruritus.** Activated charcoal has been tried in pruritus (p.1137) associated with renal failure. In a double-blind crossover study, administration of activated charcoal 6 g daily by mouth for 8 weeks was more effective than placebo in relieving generalised pruritus in 11 patients undergoing maintenance haemodialysis.[1]


1. Pederson JA, *et al.* Relief of idiopathic generalized pruritus in dialysis patients treated with activated oral charcoal. *Ann Intern Med* 1980; **93:** 446–8.


## Preparations

**Proprietary Preparations** (details are given in Part 3)

***Arg.:*** Mamograf; ***Austral.:*** Ad-Sorb; Carbosorb; Charcocaps†; Charcotabs†; Karbons†; ***Austria:*** Biocarbon; Kolemed; Norit; Norit-Carbomix; ***Belg.:*** Norit; Norit-Carbomix; ***Braz.:*** Neocarbon†; ***Canad.:*** Charac; Charcodote Aqueous; ***Fin.:*** Carbomix; ***Fr.:*** Actisorb†; Carbactive; Carbomix; Carbonet; Charbon de Belloc; Colocarb; Formocarbine; Splenocarbine; Toxicarb; ***Ger.:*** Kohle-Compretten; Kohle-Hevert; Kohle-Pulvis; Kohle-Tabletten; Ultracarbon; ***Gr.:*** Carbomix; Norit; ***Hong Kong:*** Charcodote; ***Irl.:*** Carbomix; Carbonet; ***Israel:*** Norit; ***Ital.:*** Carbomix; Neo Carbone Belloc†; ***Neth.:*** Norit; ***NZ:*** Carbosorb; ***Singapore:*** Aqueous Charcodote; Ultracarbon; ***Spain:*** Arkocapsulas Carbon Veg; Ultra Adsorb; ***Swed.:*** Carbomix; Kolsuspension; Medikol; ***Thai.:*** Ca-R-Bon; Ultracarbon; ***UK:*** Actidose-Aqua; Bragg's Medicinal Charcoal; Carbomix; Carbonet; Charcodote; Clinisorb; Liqui-Char†; Lyofoam C; Medicoal†; Modern Herbals Trapped Wind & Indigestion; ***USA:*** Actidose-Aqua; Charcoaid; Charcoal Plus; Charcocaps; Liqui-Char.

**Multi-ingredient:** ***Arg.:*** Carbogasol; Carbon Tabs; Diarrocalmol; Estreptocarbocaftiazol; Lefaenteril; Opocarbon; ***Austral.:*** Carboflex; Carbosorb S; No Gas†; ***Austria:*** Eucarbon; Intestinol; Sabatif; ***Belg.:*** Carbobel; Eucarbon†; ***Braz.:*** Carbo-Levedo†; Passicarbone†; ***Canad.:*** Charac Tol; Charcodote; ***Fr.:*** Acticarbine; Actisorb Plus; Carboflex; Carbolevure; Carbophagix†; Carbophos; Carbosylane; Carbosymag; Quinocarbine†; ***Ger.:*** Actisorb Silver; Hevert-Carmin symbio†; ***Hong Kong:*** Biscasil†; ***India:*** Distenil; Molzyme; Papytazyme; Unienzyme c MPS; ***Irl.:*** Actisorb Silver; ***Israel:*** Carbosylane; Charcodote; Eucarbon; Kaltocarb; Novicarbon; ***Ital.:*** Actisorb Plus; Carbondifer†; Carbone Composto; Carbonesia; Carbotiol†; Carboyoghurt; Curat†; Eucarbon; No-Gas; ***Malaysia:*** Eucarbon; ***Mex.:*** Acilin; ***NZ:*** Carbosorb S; ***Port.:*** Carboflex; ***S.Afr.:*** Rubilax; ***Switz.:*** Carbolevure; Carboticon; Eucarbon†; ***Thai.:*** Belacid; Bicobon; Biodan; Carbonpectate; Delta Charcoal; Papytazyme; Pepsitase; Polyenzyme-I; ***UK:*** Acidosis; Actisorb Silver; Carbellon; Papaya Plus†; ***USA:*** Actidose with Sorbitol; Flatulex; Poison Antidote Kit.

# Amifostine *(BAN, USAN, rINN)*

Amifostina; Ethiofos; Gammaphos; NSC-296961; WR-2721.
S-[2-(3-Aminopropylamino)ethyl] dihydrogen phosphorothioate.
$C_5H_{15}N_2O_3PS$ = 214.2.
*CAS — 20537-88-6 (amifostine); 63717-27-1 (amifostine monohydrate).*
*ATC — V03AF05.*

**Pharmacopoeias.** *US* includes the trihydrate.

**USP 27** (Amifostine). The trihydrate is a white crystalline powder. Freely soluble in water. pH of a 5% solution in water is between 6.5 and 7.5. Store in airtight containers at a temperature of 2° to 8°. Protect from light.

**Incompatibility.** Amifostine has been reported[1] to be physically incompatible with aciclovir sodium, amphotericin B, cefoperazone sodium, chlorpromazine hydrochloride, cisplatin, ganciclovir sodium, hydroxyzine hydrochloride, miconazole, minocycline hydrochloride, and prochlorperazine edisilate during simulated Y-site administration.


1. Trissel LA, Martinez JF. Compatibility of amifostine with selected drugs during simulated Y-site administration. *Am J Health-Syst Pharm* 1995; **52:** 2208–12.


## Adverse Effects, Treatment, and Precautions

Amifostine may cause a transient reduction, usually in systolic, or, less frequently, in diastolic blood pressure. However, more pronounced reductions in blood pressure may occur and transient loss of consciousness has been reported very rarely. To minimise hypotension, patients should be adequately hydrated before treatment with amifostine begins and should be in a supine position. Amifostine is contra-indicated in patients who are hypotensive or dehydrated. Patients taking antihypertensive drugs should discontinue treatment 24 hours before administration of amifostine. Arterial blood pressure must be monitored during the amifostine infusion and if systolic blood pressure decreases significantly, infusion must stop. It may be continued if blood pressure returns to normal within 5 minutes.

Nausea and vomiting are frequently reported and concurrent antiemetic therapy is recommended.

Amifostine reduces serum-calcium concentrations, although clinical hypocalcaemia has occurred only very rarely in patients who received multiple doses of amifostine within 24 hours. Serum-calcium concentrations should be monitored in patients at risk of hypocalcaemia.

Other side-effects include flushing, chills, somnolence, hiccups, and sneezing. Skin rashes may occur and there have been reports of more severe skin reactions including Stevens-Johnson syndrome and toxic epidermal necrolysis, in some cases resulting in fatality.

Administration of amifostine over a longer period than the recommended 15 minutes is associated with a higher incidence of side-effects.

**Effects on the skin.** Stevens-Johnson syndrome associated with the use of amifostine has been reported in 2 patients, in one case with additional toxic epidermal necrolysis.[1]


1. Lale Atahan I, *et al.* Two cases of Stevens-Johnson syndrome: toxic epidermal necrolysis possibly induced by amifostine during radiotherapy. *Br J Dermatol* 2000; **143:** 1072–3.


## Pharmacokinetics

Amifostine is rapidly cleared from the plasma following intravenous administration and is dephosphorylated by alkaline phosphatase to the active metabolite WR-1065, a free thiol compound. The elimination half-life of amifostine after a 15-minute infusion is less than 10 minutes. About 6% or less of a dose is excreted in the urine.

## Uses and Administration

Amifostine, an aminothiol compound, is a cytoprotective agent. It is converted in the body to its active metabolite WR-1065, which protects noncancerous cells against the toxic effects of antineoplastics and ionising radiation. It is used in patients with advanced ovarian cancer to reduce neutropenia-related infection associated with cyclophosphamide and cisplatin therapy and, in patients with advanced solid tumours of non-germ cell origin, to reduce the cumulative renal toxicity associated with repeated cisplatin administration. It is also used to reduce the incidence of xerostomia (dry mouth) in patients undergoing radiation therapy for head and neck cancer. Amifostine is under investigation in ameliorating the adverse effects of other antineoplastics.

In chemotherapy, amifostine is given by intravenous infusion over 15 minutes starting no more than 30 minutes before administration of antineoplastic therapy. The dose in adults is 910 mg/m$^2$ once daily. The dose should be reduced to 740 mg/m$^2$ in patients unable to tolerate the full dose. This lower dose of 740 mg/m$^2$ is also recommended for the reduction of renal toxicity of cisplatin if doses of cisplatin of less than 100 mg/m$^2$ are used.

In the prevention of xerostomia, amifostine is given in a dose of 200 mg/m$^2$ daily as a 3-minute intravenous infusion started 15 to 30 minutes before radiotherapy.

**Adjunct in antineoplastic therapy.** WR-1065, the active metabolite of amifostine, readily enters non-malignant cells where it deactivates cytotoxics such as alkylating and platinum-containing antineoplastics and protects against the effects of ionising radiation. The cytoprotective effects of amifostine are reported to be selective for normal cells and not to interfere with the cytotoxic effects of antineoplastics and radiation on malignant cells. Several factors contribute to this selectivity; malignant tumours contain less alkaline phosphatase than normal tissue and WR-1065 is less readily transported into malignant cells.

References.

1. Foster-Nora JA, Siden R. Amifostine for protection from antineoplastic drug toxicity. *Am J Health-Syst Pharm* 1997; **54:** 787–800.
2. Mabro M, *et al.* A risk-benefit assessment of amifostine in cytoprotection. *Drug Safety* 1999; **21:** 367–87.
3. Culy CR, Spencer CM. Amifostine: an update on its clinical status as a cytoprotectant in patients with cancer receiving chemotherapy or radiotherapy and its potential therapeutic application in myelodysplastic syndrome. *Drugs* 2001; **61:** 641–84.

## Preparations

**Proprietary Preparations** (details are given in Part 3)

***Arg.:*** Erifostine; Ethyol; ***Austral.:*** Ethyol; ***Belg.:*** Ethyol; ***Braz.:*** Ethyol; ***Canad.:*** Ethyol†; ***Chile:*** Ethyol; ***Denm.:*** Ethyol; ***Fin.:*** Ethyol; ***Fr.:*** Ethyol; ***Ger.:*** Ethyol; ***Gr.:*** Ethyol; ***Hong Kong:*** Ethyol; ***India:*** Amiphos; ***Israel:*** Ethyol; ***Ital.:*** Ethyol; ***Malaysia:*** Ethyol; ***Mex.:*** Ethyol; ***Neth.:*** Ethyol; ***NZ:*** Ethyol; ***Port.:*** Ethyol†; ***S.Afr.:*** Ethyol; ***Singapore:*** Ethyol; ***Spain:*** Ethyol; ***Swed.:*** Ethyol; ***Switz.:*** Ethyol; ***Thai.:*** Ethyol; ***UK:*** Ethyol†; ***USA:*** Ethyol.

# Ammonium Tetrathiomolybdate

Tetratiomolibdato de amonio.

$(NH_4)_2MoS_4$ = 260.3.

*CAS — 15060-55-6.*

## Profile

Ammonium tetrathiomolybdate is a chelator that aids the elimination of copper from the body. It is under investigation in the treatment of Wilson's disease.

**Wilson's disease.** Ammonium tetrathiomolybdate forms a complex with protein and copper. When it is taken with food it blocks the intestinal absorption of copper, and when given between meals it combines with albumin- and caeruloplasmin-bound copper. Ammonium tetrathiomolybdate is under investigation for the initial reduction of copper levels in patients with Wilson's disease (p.1049); it may be particularly suitable for patients with neurological symptoms.[1,2] Reversible bone marrow depression has been reported in 2 patients treated with ammonium tetrathiomolybdate.[3]

1. Brewer GJ, *et al.* Treatment of Wilson's disease with ammonium tetrathiomolybdate I: initial therapy in 17 neurologically affected patients. *Arch Neurol* 1994; **51:** 545–54.
2. Brewer GJ, *et al.* Treatment of Wilson disease with ammonium tetrathiomolybdate II: initial therapy in 33 neurologically affected patients and follow-up with zinc therapy. *Arch Neurol* 1996; **53:** 1017–25.
3. Harper PL, Walshe JM. Reversible pancytopenia secondary to treatment with tetrathiomolybdate. *Br J Haematol* 1986; **64:** 851–3.

# Amyl Nitrite

Amylis Nitris; Amylium Nitrosum; Azotito de Amilo; Isoamyl Nitrite; Isopentyl Nitrite; Nitrito de amilo; Pentanolis Nitris.

$C_5H_{11}NO_2$ = 117.1.

*ATC — V03AB22.*

**Pharmacopoeias.** In *Jpn* and *US.*

**USP 27** (Amyl Nitrite). A mixture of the nitrite esters of 3-methyl-1-butanol and 2-methyl-1-butanol. A clear, yellowish liquid having a peculiar, ethereal, fruity odour. It is very flammable. It is volatile even at low temperatures. B.p. about 96°. Practically insoluble in water; miscible with alcohol and with ether. Store in a cool place in airtight containers. Protect from light.

**Stability.** Amyl nitrite is liable to decompose with evolution of nitrogen, particularly if it has become acid in reaction.

## Adverse Effects, Treatment, and Precautions

Amyl nitrite inhalation commonly causes flushing, headache, and dizziness; nausea and vomiting, hypotension, restlessness, and tachycardia may also occur. Overdosage may result in cyanosis, syncope, dyspnoea, and muscular weakness, due to vasodilatation and methaemoglobinaemia. Methylthioninium chloride administration may be required for severe methaemoglobinaemia but should not be used if cyanide poisoning is suspected since cyanide may be displaced.

Amyl nitrite may increase intra-ocular and intracranial pressure and should be used with caution in patients with glaucoma, recent head trauma, or cerebral haemorrhage.

**Abuse.** Volatile nitrites (commonly known as 'poppers') have been abused, in the belief that they expand creativity, stimulate music appreciation, promote a sense of abandon in dancing, and intensify sexual experience.[1,2]

Inhalation of amyl, butyl, or isobutyl nitrite has caused headache, tachycardia, syncope, acute psychosis, increased intra-ocular pressure, transient hemiparesis, methaemoglobinaemia, coma, and, rarely, sudden death.[3]

Haemolytic anaemia has been reported in subjects after abuse of volatile nitrites;[4,5] in some subjects, Heinz body formation has been detected.[4] Methaemoglobinaemia has been reported following ingestion of volatile nitrites.[6-9] Symptoms are similar to those of hypoxia[8] and may be reversed by administration of methylthioninium chloride.[6-9]

Exposure to amyl nitrite inhalation has led to severe and extensive contact dermatitis around the face with secondary spread elsewhere on the body.[10]

1. Sigell LT, *et al.* Popping and snorting volatile nitrites: a current fad for getting high. *Am J Psychiatry* 1978; **135:** 1216–18.
2. Lockwood B. Poppers: volatile nitrite inhalants. *Pharm J* 1996; **257:** 154–5.
3. Anonymous. Treatment of acute drug abuse reactions. *Med Lett Drugs Ther* 1987; **29:** 83–6.
4. Romeril KR, Concannon AJ. Heinz body haemolytic anaemia after sniffing volatile nitrites. *Med J Aust* 1981; **1:** 302–3.
5. Brandes JC, *et al.* Amyl nitrite-induced hemolytic anemia. *Am J Med* 1989; **86:** 252–4.
6. Laaban JP, *et al.* Amyl nitrite poppers and methemoglobulinemia. *Ann Intern Med* 1985; **103:** 804–5.
7. Osterloh J, Olson K. Toxicities of alkyl nitrites. *Ann Intern Med* 1986; **104:** 727.
8. Pierce JMT, Nielsen MS. Acute acquired methaemoglobinaemia after amyl nitrite poisoning. *BMJ* 1989; **298:** 1566.
9. Forsyth RJ, Moulden A. Methaemoglobinaemia after ingestion of amyl nitrite. *Arch Dis Child* 1991; **66:** 152.
10. Bos JD, *et al.* Allergic contact dermatitis to amyl nitrite ('poppers'). *Contact Dermatitis* 1985; **12:** 109.

**Handling and storage.** Amyl nitrite is very flammable and must not be used where it may be ignited.

## Uses and Administration

Amyl nitrite is rapidly absorbed on inhalation and has been used in the immediate treatment of patients with definite cyanide poisoning (p.1506) to induce the formation of methaemoglobin, which combines with the cyanide to form non-toxic cyanmethaemoglobin. The value of such treatment has been questioned since only low levels of methaemoglobin are formed, but other mechanisms may also be important. A suggested procedure has been to administer amyl nitrite by inhalation for up to 30 seconds every minute until other measures can be instituted. It has also been suggested for use in the management of hydrogen sulfide poisoning (p.1236).

Amyl nitrite has an action similar to that of glyceryl trinitrate (p.924) and used to be given by inhalation for the relief of acute attacks of angina pectoris but is seldom used now.

Amyl nitrite is used in homoeopathic medicine.

## Preparations

***USP 27:*** Amyl Nitrite Inhalant.

**Proprietary Preparations** (details are given in Part 3)

***Multi-ingredient:*** ***S.Afr.:*** Tripac-Cyano; ***USA:*** Cyanide Antidote Package; Emergent-Ez.

# Asoxime Chloride

Asoxima, cloruro de; HI-6. 1-({[4-(Aminocarbonyl)pyridinio]methoxy}methyl)-2-[(hydroxyimino)methyl]pyridinium dichloride.

$C_{14}H_{16}Cl_2N_4O_3$ = 359.2.

*CAS — 34433-31-3.*

## Profile

Asoxime chloride is a cholinesterase reactivator that has been tried in the treatment of poisoning by organophosphorus pesticides and related compounds.

◊ References.

1. Jovanović D, *et al.* A case of unusual suicidal poisoning by the organophosphorus insecticide dimethoate. *Hum Exp Toxicol* 1990; **9:** 49–51.
2. Kušić R, *et al.* HI-6 in man: efficacy of the oxime in poisoning by organophosphorus insecticides. *Hum Exp Toxicol* 1991; **10:** 113–18.

# Atipamezole (BAN, USAN, rINN)

MPV-1248. 4-(2-Ethyl-2-indanyl)imidazole.

$C_{14}H_{16}N_2$ = 212.3.

*CAS — 104054-27-5.*

# Atipamezole Hydrochloride (BANM, rINNM)

Hidrocloruro de atipamezol.

$C_{14}H_{16}N_2,HCl$ = 248.8.

*CAS — 104075-48-1.*

## Profile

Atipamezole is a selective alpha$_2$-adrenergic receptor antagonist that is used as the hydrochloride in veterinary medicine to reverse the sedative effects of medetomidine.

# Calcium Polystyrene Sulfonate

Calcium Polystyrene Sulphonate; Poliestirenosulfonato cálcico.

*CAS — 37286-92-3.*

*ATC — V03AE01.*

**Pharmacopoeias.** In *Br.* and *Jpn.*

**BP 2003** (Calcium Polystyrene Sulphonate). A cream to light brown, fine powder. The calcium content is not less than 6.5% and not more than 9.5%, calculated with reference to the dried substance. Each g exchanges not less than 1.3 mmol and not more than 2.0 mmol of potassium, calculated with reference to the dried substance. Practically insoluble in water and in alcohol. Store in airtight containers.

## Adverse Effects and Precautions

As for Sodium Polystyrene Sulfonate, p.1053. Sorbitol should not be used with calcium polystyrene sulfonate due to the risk of colonic necrosis. Sodium overloading is not a problem with calcium polystyrene sulfonate, but calcium overloading and hypercalcaemia may occur. It should therefore be avoided in patients with conditions such as hyperparathyroidism, multiple myeloma, sarcoidosis, or metastatic carcinoma who may present with renal failure together with hypercalcaemia. Patients should be monitored for electrolyte disturbances, especially hypokalaemia and hypercalcaemia.

**Effects on the lungs.** An elderly man who died from cardiac arrest was found at necropsy to have bronchopneumonia associated with inhalation of calcium polystyrene sulfonate;[1] the resin had been given by mouth to treat hyperkalaemia.

1. Chaplin AJ, Millard PR. Calcium polystyrene sulphonate: an unusual cause of inhalation pneumonia. *BMJ* 1975; **3:** 77–8.

## Interactions

As for Sodium Polystyrene Sulfonate, p.1053. Calcium ions are released from the resin in the gastrointestinal tract and this may reduce the absorption of tetracycline given by mouth.

## Uses and Administration

Calcium polystyrene sulfonate, the calcium salt of sulfonated styrene polymer, is a cation-exchange resin that exchanges calcium ions for potassium ions and other cations in the gastrointestinal tract. It is used similarly to sodium polystyrene sulfonate (p.1053) to enhance potassium excretion in the treatment of hyperkalaemia (p.1219) and may be preferred to the sodium resin in patients who cannot tolerate an increase in their sodium load. It is estimated that 1 g of calcium polystyrene sulfonate could bind 1.3 to 2 mmol of potassium but it is unlikely that such figures could be achieved in practice.

It is given by mouth, in a dose of 15 g three or four times daily, as a suspension in water or syrup or as a sweetened paste. It should not be given in fruit juices that have a high potassium content. A dose for children is 1 g/kg daily in divided doses for acute hyperkalaemia, reduced to a maintenance dose of 500 mg/kg daily in divided doses; the oral route is not recommended for neonates.

When oral administration is difficult, calcium polystyrene sulfonate may be administered rectally as an enema. The usual daily dose is 30 g given as a suspension in 100 mL of 2% methylcellulose '450' and 100 mL of water and retained, if possible, for at least 9 hours. Initial therapy may constitute administration by both oral and rectal routes. Following retention of the enema the colon should be irrigated to remove the resin. Children and neonates may be given rectal doses similar to those suggested for children by mouth.

## Preparations

**Proprietary Preparations** (details are given in Part 3)
***Arg.:*** Resincalcio; RIC Calcio; ***Austral.:*** Calcium Resonium; ***Austria:*** CPS Pulver; Sorbisterit; ***Belg.:*** Kayexalate Calcium; ***Braz.:*** Sorcal; ***Canad.:*** Resonium Calcium; ***Denm.:*** Resonium Calcium; ***Fr.:*** Calcium-Sorbisterit†; ***Ger.:*** Anti-Kalium; Calcium Resonium; CPS Pulver; Elutit-Calcium; Sorbisterit; ***Gr.:*** Calcium Resonium; ***Hong Kong:*** Calcium Resonium; ***Irl.:*** Calcium Resonium; ***Jpn:*** Kalimate; ***Norw.:*** Resonium Calcium; ***NZ:*** Calcium Resonium; ***Port.:*** Resical; ***Spain:*** Resincalcio; ***Swed.:*** Resonium Calcium; ***Switz.:*** Sorbisterit; ***UK:*** Calcium Resonium.

## Deferiprone *(BAN, rINN)*

CP-20; Deferiprona; Dimethylhydroxypyridone; L1. 1,2-Dimethyl-3-hydroxypyrid-4-one; 3-Hydroxy-1,2-dimethyl-4-pyridone.

$C_7H_9NO_2$ = 139.2.
*CAS — 30652-11-0.*
*ATC — V03AC02.*

### Adverse Effects and Precautions

Deferiprone has been shown to cause neutropenia and should not be used in neutropenic patients; the neutrophil count should be monitored weekly and treatment should be stopped if neutropenia develops. Agranulocytosis has also occurred. Patients should be advised to seek immediate medical attention if symptoms indicative of infection such as fever, sore throat, or flu-like symptoms occur.

The patient's urine may have a reddish-brown discoloration.

Caution is advised in patients with hepatic or renal impairment.

◊ Concern has been expressed over the potential toxicity of deferiprone. Preclinical testing in *animals* revealed embryotoxicity, teratogenicity, organ atrophy, and haematological toxicity, and reversible neutropenia or agranulocytosis has been reported in patients. In addition, a case of fatal systemic lupus erythematosus has been reported although this could have been related to the patient's thalassaemia rather than to the drug. Other reported adverse effects include musculoskeletal and joint pain, gastrointestinal intolerance, transient liver enzyme abnormalities, and zinc deficiency.

References.

1. Kontoghiorghes GJ, *et al.* Benefits and risks of deferiprone in iron overload in thalassaemia and other conditions: comparison of epidemiological and therapeutic aspects with deferoxamine. *Drug Safety* 2003; **26:** 553–84.

### Uses and Administration

Deferiprone is an orally active iron chelator used in the treatment of iron overload in patients with thalassaemia for whom desferrioxamine is unsuitable. In adults and children over 6 years it may be given by mouth in doses of 25 mg/kg three times daily; dosage should be calculated to the nearest half tablet. Doses above 100 mg/kg daily are not recommended.

◊ Reviews.

1. Kontoghiorghes GJ, *et al.* Benefits and risks of deferiprone in iron overload in thalassaemia and other conditions: comparison of epidemiological and therapeutic aspects with deferoxamine. *Drug Safety* 2003; **26:** 553–84.

### Preparations

**Proprietary Preparations** (details are given in Part 3)
***Austral.:*** Ferriprox; ***Denm.:*** Ferriprox; ***Fr.:*** Ferriprox; ***Ger.:*** Ferriprox; ***Gr.:*** Ferriprox; Kelfer; ***Irl.:*** Ferriprox; ***Ital.:*** Ferriprox; ***Spain:*** Ferriprox; ***Swed.:*** Ferriprox; ***Switz.:*** Ferriprox; ***UK:*** Ferriprox.

## Desferrioxamine Mesilate *(BANM)*

Deferoxamine Mesilate *(pINNM)*; Ba-33112; Ba-29837 (desferrioxamine hydrochloride); Deferoxamine Mesylate *(USAN)*; Deferoxamini Mesilas; Desferrioxamine Mesylate; Desferrioxamine Methanesulphonate; Mesilato de deferoxamina; NSC-527604 (desferrioxamine). 30-Amino-3,14,25-trihydroxy-3,9,14,20,25-penta-azatriacontane-2,10,13,21,24-pentaone methanesulphonate; *N'*-{5-[(4-{[5-(Acetylhydroxyamino)pentyl]amino}-1,4-dioxobutyl)hydroxyamino]pentyl}-*N*-(5-aminopentyl)-*N*-hydroxybutanediamide monomethanesulphonate.

$C_{25}H_{48}N_6O_8,CH_3SO_3H$ = 656.8.
*CAS — 70-51-9 (desferrioxamine); 138-14-7 (desferrioxamine mesilate); 1950-39-6 (desferrioxamine hydrochloride).*
*ATC — V03AC01.*

**Pharmacopoeias.** In *Eur.* (see p.vi), *Int., Jpn,* and *US.*

**Ph. Eur. 5.0** (Deferoxamine Mesilate; Desferrioxamine Mesilate BP 2003). A white or almost white powder. Freely soluble in water; very slightly soluble in alcohol; slightly soluble in methyl alcohol. A freshly prepared 10% solution in water has a pH of 3.7 to 5.5. Store at 2° to 8°. Protect from light.

**USP 27** (Deferoxamine Mesylate). A white to off-white powder. Freely soluble in water; slightly soluble in methyl alcohol. pH of a 1% solution in water is between 4.0 and 6.0. Store in airtight containers.

**Incompatibility.** The manufacturers report that desferrioxamine solutions are incompatible with heparin.

### Adverse Effects and Treatment

Rapid intravenous injection of desferrioxamine may cause flushing, urticaria, hypotension, and shock. Local pain may occur with subcutaneous or intramuscular injections and pruritus, erythema, and swelling have occurred after prolonged subcutaneous administration. Gastrointestinal disorders, dysuria, fever, allergic skin rashes, tachycardia, cardiac arrhythmias, convulsions, and leg cramps have been reported. Visual disturbances, including retinal changes, and hearing loss may occur and may be reversible if desferrioxamine is withdrawn. Cataract formation has also been reported. Desferrioxamine therapy may retard growth in very young children.

◊ Reviews of the adverse effects of desferrioxamine.

1. Bentur Y, *et al.* Deferoxamine (desferrioxamine): new toxicities for an old drug. *Drug Safety* 1991; **6:** 37–46.

**Effects on the blood.** A patient with end-stage renal disease developed reversible thrombocytopenia on 3 separate occasions after intravenous infusions of desferrioxamine for dialysis osteomalacia.[1] Acute fatal aplastic anaemia occurred in a 16-year-old girl with thalassaemia following intravenous administration of high doses of desferrioxamine (80 mg/kg daily) for 20 days.[2]

1. Walker JA, *et al.* Thrombocytopenia associated with intravenous desferrioxamine. *Am J Kidney Dis* 1985; **6:** 254–6.
2. Sofroniadou K, *et al.* Acute bone marrow aplasia associated with intravenous administration of deferoxamine (desferrioxamine). *Drug Safety* 1990; **5:** 152–4.

**Effects on the ears and eyes.** Lens opacities, retinal pigmentary changes and other retinal abnormalities, and ocular disturbances including loss of colour vision, night blindness, decreased visual acuity, and field defects, have been reported in patients receiving long-term or high-dose treatment with desferrioxamine.[1-4] In assessments of patients on long-term therapy with desferrioxamine the incidence of symptomatic and asymptomatic ocular changes has varied from 2 of 52 patients[5] to 10 of 15 patients.[6]

Sensorineural hearing impairment has also been reported.[5,7-12] Tinnitus has been reported in a few patients.[11,13]

Both ophthalmic and auditory abnormalities can improve when desferrioxamine is withdrawn,[1,3,5-10] although sometimes the effects may be irreversible[14] or recovery may only be partial.[8,9]

Several mechanisms for desferrioxamine neurotoxicity have been suggested.[6,8,11,15-18]

1. Davies SC, *et al.* Ocular toxicity of high-dose intravenous desferrioxamine. *Lancet* 1983; **ii:** 181–4.
2. Simon P, *et al.* Desferrioxamine, ocular toxicity, and trace metals. *Lancet* 1983; **ii:** 512–13.
3. Borgna-Pignatti C, *et al.* Visual loss in patient on high-dose subcutaneous desferrioxamine. *Lancet* 1984; **i:** 681.
4. Rubinstein M, *et al.* Ocular toxicity of desferrioxamine. *Lancet* 1985; **i:** 817–18.
5. Cohen A, *et al.* Vision and hearing during deferoxamine therapy. *J Pediatr* 1990; **117:** 326–30.
6. De Virgiliis S, *et al.* Depletion of trace elements and acute ocular toxicity induced by desferrioxamine in patients with thalassaemia. *Arch Dis Child* 1988; **63:** 250–5.
7. Guerin A, *et al.* Acute deafness and desferrioxamine. *Lancet* 1985; **ii:** 39.
8. Olivieri NF, *et al.* Visual and auditory neurotoxicity in patients receiving subcutaneous deferoxamine infusions. *N Engl J Med* 1986; **314:** 869–73.
9. Barratt PS, Toogood IRG. Hearing loss attributed to desferrioxamine in patients with beta-thalassaemia major. *Med J Aust* 1987; **147:** 177–9.
10. Wonke B, *et al.* Reversal of desferrioxamine induced auditory neurotoxicity during treatment with Ca-DTPA. *Arch Dis Child* 1989; **64:** 77–82.
11. Porter JB, *et al.* Desferrioxamine ototoxicity: evaluation of risk factors in thalassaemic patients and guidelines for safe dosage. *Br J Haematol* 1989; **73:** 403–9.
12. Argiolu F, *et al.* Hearing impairment during deferoxamine therapy for thalassemia major. *J Pediatr* 1991; **118:** 826.
13. Marsh MN, *et al.* Tinnitus in a patient with beta-thalassaemia intermedia on long-term treatment with desferrioxamine. *Postgrad Med J* 1981; **57:** 582–4.
14. Bene C, *et al.* Irreversible ocular toxicity from single "challenge" dose of deferoxamine. *Clin Nephrol* 1989; **31:** 45–8.
15. Arden GB, *et al.* Ocular changes in patients undergoing long-term desferrioxamine treatment. *Br J Ophthalmol* 1984; **68:** 873–7.
16. Rahi AHS, *et al.* Ocular toxicity of desferrioxamine: light microscopic histochemical and ultrastructural findings. *Br J Ophthalmol* 1986; **70:** 373–81.
17. Pall H, *et al.* Ocular toxicity of desferrioxamine – an example of copper promoted auto-oxidative damage? *Br J Ophthalmol* 1989; **73:** 42–7.
18. Bentur Y, *et al.* Comparison of deferoxamine pharmacokinetics between asymptomatic thalassemic children and those exhibiting severe neurotoxicity. *Clin Pharmacol Ther* 1990; **47:** 478–82.

**Effects on growth rate.** Growth retardation has been noted in thalassaemic children undergoing desferrioxamine therapy.[1,2] Growth retardation was related to dose[1,2] and inversely related to iron stores.[1] It was greater in those who started receiving desferrioxamine at the start of transfusion therapy at about 9 months old than in those who started desferrioxamine once iron accumulation was established, after about 3 years. A sharp increase in growth velocity was reported in 15 patients with low ferritin levels after a 50% reduction in desferrioxamine dose.[1]

1. Piga A, *et al.* High-dose desferrioxamine as a cause of growth failure in thalassaemic patients. *Eur J Haematol* 1988; **40:** 380–1.
2. De Virgiliis S, *et al.* Deferoxamine-induced growth retardation in patients with thalassemia major. *J Pediatr* 1988; **113:** 661–9.

**Effects on the kidneys.** A 14-year-old boy with thalassaemia major and haemosiderosis developed acute renal insufficiency during intravenous infusion of desferrioxamine.[1] Acute decreases in renal function were reported in 3 patients following infusions of desferrioxamine.[2] Two of these patients had received 180 mg/kg daily and nephrotoxicity could have been related to these high doses,[3] although others reported reductions in glomerular filtration rates following regular doses.[4]

1. Batey R, *et al.* Acute renal insufficiency occurring during intravenous desferrioxamine therapy. *Scand J Haematol* 1979; **22:** 277–9.
2. Koren G, *et al.* Acute changes in renal function associated with deferoxamine therapy. *Am J Dis Child* 1989; **143:** 1077–80.
3. Li Volti S, *et al.* Acute changes in renal function associated with deferoxamine therapy. *Am J Dis Child* 1990; **144:** 1069–70.
4. Koren G, Bentur Y. Acute changes in renal function associated with deferoxamine. *Am J Dis Child* 1990; **144:** 1070.

**Effects on the lungs.** A pulmonary syndrome with tachypnoea, hypoxaemia, reduced pulmonary function, and radiographic evidence of diffuse interstitial pneumonia has been reported in patients receiving high doses of desferrioxamine intravenously.[1,2] It has been suggested that a hypersensitivity reaction was involved.[1,2]

Fatal acute respiratory distress syndrome has occurred in 4 patients; desferrioxamine infusions had been given for 65 to 92 hours. Pulmonary complications had not been noted in patients given desferrioxamine for less than 24 hours.[3] This report did, however, generate subsequent correspondence disagreeing with the view that prolonged use of desferrioxamine was the cause of the toxicity. Alternative explanations for the pulmonary injury included the use of doses above the daily maximum[4] as well as inadequate desferrioxamine therapy.[5]

1. Freedman MH, *et al.* Pulmonary syndrome in patients with thalassemia major receiving intravenous deferoxamine infusions. *Am J Dis Child* 1990; **144:** 565–9.
2. Scanderbeg AC, *et al.* Pulmonary syndrome and intravenous high-dose desferrioxamine. *Lancet* 1990; **336:** 1511.
3. Tenenbein M, *et al.* Pulmonary toxic effects of continuous desferrioxamine administration in acute iron poisoning. *Lancet* 1992; **339:** 699–701.
4. Macarol V, Yawalkar SJ. Desferrioxamine in acute iron poisoning. *Lancet* 1992; **339:** 1601.
5. Shannon M. Desferrioxamine in acute iron poisoning. *Lancet* 1992; **339:** 1601.

**Effects on the skin.** Desferrioxamine may be used in the management of porphyria cutanea tarda (see p.1040). However, lesions resembling porphyria cutanea tarda developed in 3 patients during long-term therapy with desferrioxamine for aluminium toxicity.[1] The lesions worsened on exposure to sun and resolved when desferrioxamine treatment was completed. It was also possible that the lesions were associated with aluminium accumulation. Alopecia was noted in 1 patient but an association with desferrioxamine therapy could not be established.

1. McCarthy JT, *et al.* Clinical experience with desferrioxamine in dialysis patients with aluminium toxicity. *Q J Med* 1990; **74:** 257–76.

**Hypersensitivity.** Individual cases of anaphylactoid reactions to desferrioxamine have been reported.[1,2] Rapid intravenous desensitisation was successful in 2 patients.[1,2] Effects on the lungs have also been attributed to hypersensitivity (see above).

1. Miller KB, *et al.* Rapid desensitisation for desferrioxamine anaphylactic reaction. *Lancet* 1981; **i:** 1059.
2. Bousquet J, *et al.* Rapid desensitisation for desferrioxamine anaphylactoid reactions. *Lancet* 1983; **ii:** 859–60.

**Treatment of adverse effects.** The adverse effects of desferrioxamine generally respond to dosage reduction. In acute overdosage desferrioxamine may be removed by haemodialysis.

Isoniazid, 50 or 100 mg with pyridoxine, suppressed intolerable adverse effects of desferrioxamine in a patient with Alzheimer's disease.[1] The adverse effects, anorexia and weight loss, were attributed to a toxic metabolite of desferrioxamine generated by the plasma monoamine oxidase enzyme system and isoniazid reduced the formation of this suspect metabolite.

1. Kruck TPA, *et al.* Suppression of deferoxamine mesylate treatment-induced side effects by coadministration of isoniazid in a patient with Alzheimer's disease subject to aluminum removal by ionspecific chelation. *Clin Pharmacol Ther* 1990; **48:** 439–46.

### Precautions

Desferrioxamine should be used with caution in patients with renal impairment since the metal complexes are excreted by the kidneys (in those with severe renal impairment dialysis increases elimination). The desferrioxamine-iron complex excreted by the kidneys may colour the urine reddish-brown.

Desferrioxamine may exacerbate aluminium-related encephalopathy and precipitate seizures. Prophylactic treatment with antiepileptics such as clonazepam has been suggested for patients judged to be at risk.

An increased susceptibility to infection, particularly with *Yersinia* species, has been reported in patients with iron overload treated with desferrioxamine. Severe fungal infections have also been reported, predominantly in patients undergoing dialysis. If infection is suspected, treatment with desferrioxamine should be stopped and appropriate antimicrobial treatment given. Skeletal fetal anomalies have occurred in *animals*.

The urinary excretion of iron should be regularly monitored during treatment and periodic ophthalmological and audiological examinations are recommended for patients on long-term therapy. Monitoring of cardiac function is also recommended for patients receiving combined treatment with ascorbic acid (see also under Interactions, below).

Inappropriately high dosage in children with low ferritin levels may retard growth and therefore regular checks on height and weight are recommended for children.

**Aluminium encephalopathy.** The precipitation of dialysis dementia with some fatal outcomes[1-3] has been associated with desferrioxamine therapy for aluminium overload in dialysis patients. Some workers[2] suggested that the effect could be dose related, but others[3] reported exacerbation of aluminium encephalopathy after the low dose of 500 mg twice weekly. Further authors[1] suggested that the onset of symptoms could be associated with high concentrations of aluminium seen after use of desferrioxamine, and recommended giving low doses (for example 10 mg/kg) immediately before dialysis in affected patients in conjunction with charcoal haemoperfusion to avoid high serum-aluminium concentrations.

1. Sherrard DJ, *et al.* Precipitation of dialysis dementia by deferoxamine treatment of aluminum related bone disease. *Am J Kidney Dis* 1988; **12:** 126–30.
2. McCauley J, Sorkin I. Exacerbation of aluminium encephalopathy after treatment with desferrioxamine. *Nephrol Dial Transplant* 1989; **4:** 110–14.
3. Lillevang ST, Pedersen FB. Exacerbation of aluminium encephalopathy after treatment with desferrioxamine. *Nephrol Dial Transplant* 1989; **4:** 676.

**Diagnostic tests.** Desferrioxamine could interfere with estimations of total iron-binding capacity.[1] It may also interfere with colorimetric iron assays.

Desferrioxamine may distort the results of gallium-67 imaging studies.

1. Bentur Y, *et al.* Misinterpretation of iron-binding capacity in the presence of deferoxamine. *J Pediatr* 1991; **118:** 139–42.

**Infection susceptibility.** *Yersinia enterocolitica* is one of the most iron-dependent of all microbes, but unlike most other aerobic bacteria, it produces no detectable iron-binding compounds, or siderophores.[1] Exogenous siderophores, such as desferrioxamine, may enable *Y. enterocolitica* to overcome this handicap[2] and the apparent increased susceptibility to yersiniosis in patients with severe iron overload may therefore be attributable at least in part to desferrioxamine therapy rather than just the increased availability of iron. Infections due to *Y. enterocolitica* (p.130) have been reported in patients receiving desferrioxamine for acute iron overdosage[3] or for chronic iron overload.[2,4-7] Severe infection with *Y. pseudotuberculosis* has also been reported in a thalassaemic patient on long-term desferrioxamine therapy.[8]

Treatment with desferrioxamine may also increase susceptibility to mucormycosis. Infections have occurred both in patients with iron overload disorders[9,10] and in those who do not have excessive iron stores.[11-13] A review[10] of 26 cases of mucormycosis in patients undergoing treatment revealed that 23 patients died; in 19 cases the diagnosis was only made at necropsy and only 9 patients received potentially effective treatment (surgery and/or amphotericin B). The organisms responsible were *Rhizopus* species in 13 cases and *Cunninghamella bertholletiae* in 3. In another review of 24 cases of mucormycosis in patients on dialysis,[14] at least 21 were receiving desferrioxamine; infection was fatal in 21 of the 24 patients.

In view of the serious nature of these infections it is important that they should be recognised and treated promptly. It has been suggested that a short course of a suitable antibacterial could be given as prophylaxis to young children from areas with a high incidence of yersiniosis who require treatment with desferrioxamine.[15]

1. Anonymous. Yersiniosis today. *Lancet* 1984; **i:** 84–5.
2. Robins-Browne RM, Prpic JK. Desferrioxamine and systemic yersiniosis. *Lancet* 1983; **ii:** 1372.
3. Melby K, *et al.* Septicaemia due to Yersinia enterocolitica after oral overdoses of iron. *BMJ* 1982; **285:** 467–8.
4. Scharnetzky M, *et al.* Prophylaxis of systemic yersinosis in thalassaemia major. *Lancet* 1984; **i:** 791.
5. Chiu HY, *et al.* Infection with Yersinia enterocolitica in patients with iron overload. *BMJ* 1986; **292:** 97.
6. Kelly D, *et al.* Yersinia and iron overload. *BMJ* 1986; **292:** 413.
7. Gallant T, *et al.* Yersinia sepsis in patients with iron overload treated with deferoxamine. *N Engl J Med* 1986; **314:** 1643.
8. Gordts B, *et al.* Yersinia pseudotuberculosis septicaemia in thalassaemia major. *Lancet* 1984; **i:** 41–2.
9. Sane A, *et al.* Deferoxamine treatment as a risk factor for zygomycete infection. *J Infect Dis* 1989; **159:** 151–2.
10. Daly AL, *et al.* Mucormycosis: association with deferoxamine therapy. *Am J Med* 1989; **87:** 468–71.
11. Goodill JJ, Abuelo JG. Mucormycosis–a new risk of deferoxamine therapy in dialysis patients with aluminum or iron overload? *N Engl J Med* 1987; **316:** 54.
12. Windus DW, *et al.* Fatal rhizopus infections in hemodialysis patients receiving deferoxamine. *Ann Intern Med* 1987; **107:** 678–80.
13. Boelaert JR, *et al.* Mucormycosis infections in dialysis patients. *Ann Intern Med* 1987; **107:** 782–3.
14. Boelaert JR, *et al.* Mucormycosis among patients on dialysis. *N Engl J Med* 1989; **321:** 190–1.
15. Hadjiminas JM. Yersiniosis in acutely iron-loaded children treated with desferrioxamine. *J Antimicrob Chemother* 1988; **21:** 680–1.

**Pregnancy.** Abnormalities in *animals* have been noted after the use of desferrioxamine in pregnancy. Thus the outcome after iron overdose during pregnancy was studied in 66 patients reported to the UK Teratology Information Service of whom 35 received desferrioxamine.[1] Seven infants of the 66 pregnancies had malformations (severe in only one) and all were associated with maternal overdoses after the first trimester and therefore could not be directly related to either iron or desferrioxamine. It was concluded that treatment of iron overdose with desferrioxamine should not be withheld solely on the grounds of pregnancy.

1. McElhatton PR, *et al.* Outcome of pregnancy following deliberate iron overdose by the mother. *Hum Exp Toxicol* 1993; **12:** 579.

## Interactions

Desferrioxamine is usually administered parenterally and thus drug interactions due to chelation with oral metal ions are not a problem.

**Ascorbic acid.** Ascorbic acid is often given in addition to desferrioxamine to patients with iron overload to achieve better iron excretion. However, early on in treatment when there is excess tissue iron there is some evidence that ascorbic acid may worsen the iron toxicity, particularly to the heart. Thus, ascorbic acid should not be given for the first month after starting desferrioxamine treatment.

**Phenothiazines.** Neurological symptoms including loss of consciousness occurred in 2 patients given *prochlorperazine* during desferrioxamine therapy.[1] Concomitant use should be avoided.

1. Blake DR, *et al.* Cerebral and ocular toxicity induced by desferrioxamine. *Q J Med* 1985; **56:** 345–55.

## Pharmacokinetics

Desferrioxamine mesilate is poorly absorbed from the gastrointestinal tract. Following parenteral administration, desferrioxamine forms chelates with metal ions and is also metabolised, primarily in the plasma. The iron-desferrioxamine chelate is excreted in the urine and bile. Desferrioxamine is absorbed during peritoneal dialysis if added to the dialysis fluid.

◊ References.

1. Summers MR, *et al.* Studies in desferrioxamine and ferrioxamine metabolism in normal and iron-loaded subjects. *Br J Haematol* 1979; **42:** 547–55.
2. Allain P, *et al.* Pharmacokinetics and renal elimination of desferrioxamine and ferrioxamine in healthy subjects and patients with haemochromatosis. *Br J Clin Pharmacol* 1987; **24:** 207–12.

## Uses and Administration

Desferrioxamine is a chelator that has a high affinity for ferric iron. When given by injection it forms a stable water-soluble iron-complex (ferrioxamine) that is readily excreted in the urine and in bile. Desferrioxamine appears to remove both free iron and bound iron from haemosiderin and ferritin but not from haemoglobin, transferrin, or cytochromes. It is estimated that 100 mg of desferrioxamine mesilate could bind about 8.5 mg of iron but it is unlikely that such a figure could be achieved in practice. Desferrioxamine also has an affinity for other trivalent metal ions including aluminium and theoretically 100 mg of the mesilate could bind 4.1 mg of aluminium.

Desferrioxamine increases the excretion of iron from the body and is used in conditions associated with chronic iron overload (such as the iron storage disorders haemochromatosis and haemosiderosis and after repeated transfusions as in thalassaemia) and in acute iron poisoning. It has been used as eye drops in the management of ocular siderosis and corneal rust stains. It is also used to reduce aluminium overload in patients with end-stage renal failure on maintenance dialysis.

Desferrioxamine is administered as the mesilate and may be given by subcutaneous or intravenous infusion, by intramuscular injection, or intraperitoneally. It may also be given orally in acute iron poisoning.

In the treatment of **chronic iron overload**, the dosage and route of administration should be determined for each patient by monitoring urinary iron excretion, with the aim of normalising serum-ferritin concentrations. Continuous subcutaneous infusions, preferably with the aid of a small portable infusion pump, are particularly convenient for ambulant patients and are more effective than intramuscular injections. Continuous intravenous infusion has been recommended for patients incapable of continuing subcutaneous infusions or for those with cardiac problems secondary to iron overload. An initial daily dose of desferrioxamine mesilate 500 mg may be given by subcutaneous infusion or intravenous infusion, increasing until a plateau of iron excretion is reached. The usual effective dose range is 20 to 60 mg/kg daily. Subcutaneous infusions are administered 3 to 7 times a week depending on the degree of iron overload and are given over 8 to 12 hours, or over 24 hours in some patients. When given by intramuscular injection the initial dose has been 0.5 to 1 g daily as 1 or 2 injections, but again the maintenance dose is determined by response. It has been suggested that in addition to intramuscular treatment, up to 2 g of desferrioxamine mesilate should be given by intravenous infusion for each unit of blood transfused, at a rate not more than 15 mg/kg per hour at the time of each blood transfusion. Desferrioxamine should be given separately from the blood. The co-administration of ascorbic acid supplements can enhance the excretion of iron, but, to reduce the risk of toxicity, should not be started until 1 month after starting desferrioxamine treatment (see under Interactions, above). Ascorbic acid is given in doses of up to 200 mg daily for adults or 50 to 100 mg daily for children; it also enhances iron absorption and should therefore be administered separately from food.

Desferrioxamine has been used as a *diagnostic test* for iron storage disease in patients with normal renal function by injecting 500 mg of the mesilate intramuscularly and estimating the excretion of iron in the urine collected over the next 6 hours; an excretion of more than 1 mg of iron by the patient under test is suggestive of iron storage disease and more than 1.5 mg can be regarded as pathological.

In the treatment of **acute iron poisoning**, the following doses and routes are suggested. In the UK, desferrioxamine mesilate 5 to 10 g in 50 to 100 mL of water has been given by mouth, or by stomach tube, to chelate any iron left in the stomach and prevent further absorption following gastric lavage. To eliminate iron already absorbed, desferrioxamine mesilate should be given intramuscularly or, if the patient is hypotensive or in shock, intravenously by slow infusion. The dose and route of parenteral administration should be adjusted according to the severity of the poisoning, preferably as indicated by the serum-iron concentration and total iron binding capacity, if available, although chelation therapy should be started in patients with significant symptoms without waiting for the results of blood concentrations. In the UK, the usual dose of desferrioxamine mesilate is 2 g in adults or 1 g in children by intramuscular injection. Alternatively, it may be given by slow intravenous infusion of up to 15 mg/kg per hour, reducing after 4 to 6 hours to provide a total dose not exceeding 80 mg/kg in 24 hours, although larger doses may be tolerated. In the USA, a recommended procedure is to give desferrioxamine mesilate 1 g initially by intramuscular injection followed by 500 mg every 4 hours for 2 doses. Subsequent doses of 500 mg may be administered every 4 to 12 hours to a maximum of 6 g in 24 hours. Alternatively, the same doses may be given by slow intravenous infusion at a rate of not more than 15 mg/kg per hour, but this route is only recommended for patients in a state of cardiovascular collapse.

In the treatment of **aluminium overload** in patients with end-stage renal failure, those undergoing maintenance haemodialysis or haemofiltration may be given desferrioxamine mesilate 5 mg/kg once a week by slow intravenous infusion during the last hour of a dialysis. In patients on peritoneal dialysis (CAPD or CCPD), desferrioxamine mesilate 5 mg/kg may be given once a week, by slow intravenous infusion, subcutaneously, intramuscularly, or intraperitoneally (the recommended route) before the final exchange of the day. For the *diagnosis* of aluminium overload, desferrioxamine mesilate 5 mg/kg is administered by slow intravenous infusion during the last hour of haemodialysis. An increase in serum-aluminium concentration above baseline of more than 150 nanograms/mL (measured at the start of the next dialysis session) suggests aluminium overload.

Eye drops containing desferrioxamine mesilate 10% have been used for the treatment of ocular siderosis and corneal rust stains.

**Administration.** Attempts have been made to overcome compliance problems with standard parenteral administration of desferrioxamine by developing oral,[1-3] rectal,[4] or intranasal[5] regimens. Although most regimens produced an increase in urinary iron excretion this was generally considered to be insufficient to be clinically useful, particularly in young children with low iron stores.[3] However, these alternative routes could be useful as an adjunct in selected patients.[1,5]

Greater success has been reported with daily intravenous infusion of desferrioxamine 6 to 12 g over 12 hours[6] or intermittent intravenous infusions in addition to subcutaneous administration[7] in patients poorly compliant with conventional subcutaneous therapy. No major disturbances in vision or hearing occurred in 8 patients undergoing intensive intravenous treatment for up to 24 months,[6] and established iron-induced heart disease in 2 of these patients improved. Twice-daily subcutaneous bolus injection has also been reported.[8]

Intraperitoneal administration of desferrioxamine may be used to reduce aluminium levels in patients receiving peritoneal dialysis for chronic renal failure. Good results have also been reported[9] in a patient with haemochromatosis complicated by cirrhosis and cardiomyopathy, in whom a chronic peritoneal dialysis catheter was used to control ascites and to administer desferrioxamine.

1. Callender ST, Weatherall DJ. Iron chelation with oral desferrioxamine. *Lancet* 1980; **ii:** 689.
2. Jacobs A, Chang Ting W. Iron chelation with oral desferrioxamine. *Lancet* 1980; **ii:** 794.
3. Kattamis C, *et al.* Oral desferrioxamine in young patients with thalassaemia. *Lancet* 1981; **i:** 51.
4. Kontoghiorghes G, *et al.* Desferrioxamine suppositories. *Lancet* 1983; **ii:** 454.
5. Gordon GS, *et al.* Intranasal administration of deferoxamine to iron overloaded patients. *Am J Med Sci* 1989; **297:** 280–4.
6. Cohen AR, *et al.* Rapid removal of excessive iron with daily, high-dose intravenous chelation therapy. *J Pediatr* 1989; **115:** 151–5.
7. Sabatino D. Rapid removal of excessive iron in thalassemia by high-dose intravenous chelation therapy. *J Pediatr* 1990; **116:** 157–8.
8. Borgna-Pignatti C, Cohen A. Evaluation of a new method of administration of the iron chelating agent deferoxamine. *J Pediatr* 1997; **130:** 86–8.
9. Swartz RD, Legault DJ. Long-term intraperitoneal deferoxamine for hemochromatosis. *Am J Med* 1996; **100:** 308–12.

**Aluminium overload.** Aluminium has been implicated in a number of disorders[1] including renal osteodystrophy, dialysis dementia, and Alzheimer's disease (see Dementia, p.1484). Patients with chronic renal failure may be exposed to aluminium from the use of aluminium-containing phosphate binders and from the high concentrations of aluminium sometimes found in tap water used to prepare dialysis fluids. Sources of aluminium in other patients include aluminium-containing antacids, preparations for total parenteral nutrition, contaminated albumin solutions, and environmental and industrial sources.[1] Further references to aluminium toxicity are included under Aluminium (see p.1652).

In patients with chronic renal failure the major sources of aluminium can be substantially reduced by the use of alternative phosphate binders (see Renal Osteodystrophy, p.764) and by reduction in the aluminium concentration of dialysis fluids by reverse osmosis and deionisation.[1] Desferrioxamine may also be used (but see Aluminium Encephalopathy, under Precautions, above, for a discussion of aluminium toxicity being exacerbated by desferrioxamine).

Desferrioxamine can greatly increase the removal of aluminium by adsorbent haemoperfusion or haemodialysis.[2] In the treatment of dialysis encephalopathy, desferrioxamine has been reported to have beneficial effects by mobilising and removing aluminium when administered in doses of up to 6 g once a week via the arterial line during the first 2 hours of haemodialysis.[3,4] In a study of 11 patients with dialysis encephalopathy 5 were treated with deionised or reverse-osmosis water alone and all died. The other 6 were treated similarly but were also given desferrioxamine 6 to 10 g intravenously each week at dialysis; 4 of these patients improved but 2 died of progressive dementia.[5]

Although the total amount of aluminium removed by desferrioxamine during peritoneal dialysis may be small compared with the amounts removed during haemodialysis, substantial improvement in early aluminium encephalopathy has been achieved in a patient on continuous ambulatory peritoneal dialysis by using intraperitoneal desferrioxamine.[6] In a study of 27 patients undergoing haemodialysis, but without clinical encephalopathy, impaired cerebral function associated with only mildly elevated plasma-aluminium concentrations was noted.[7] Use of desferrioxamine in 15 of these patients for 3 months improved psychomotor performance.

Desferrioxamine has produced rapid clinical improvement in patients with dialysis-related bone disease.[8-10] Reduction in the aluminium content of bone was reported in two studies involving 7 patients,[10] and 9 patients,[9] respectively. However, such findings were not replicated in a further 2 patients.[8] Measurement of plasma-aluminium concentrations 24 and 44 hours after administration of desferrioxamine 40 mg/kg has been used to diagnose aluminium-related osteodystrophy,[9,11] but a study[10] using a lower dose of desferrioxamine (28.5 mg/kg) and measuring plasma aluminium 5 hours later found similar increases in patients both with and without bone-aluminium accumulation.

Desferrioxamine therapy has also produced beneficial results in dialysis patients with anaemia[12-14] and has also been found to reverse aluminium-induced resistance to erythropoietin.[15,16]

Prurigo nodularis in chronic aluminium overload has responded to desferrioxamine with resolution of itch and skin lesions.[17]

Sustained low doses of desferrioxamine were found to slow the progression of the dementia of Alzheimer's disease in a study of 48 patients,[18] although these results have been questioned.[19,20]

1. Monteagudo FSE, *et al.* Recent developments in aluminium toxicology. *Med Toxicol* 1989; **4:** 1–16.
2. Chang TMS, Barre P. Effect of desferrioxamine on removal of aluminium and iron by coated charcoal haemoperfusion and haemodialysis. *Lancet* 1983; **ii:** 1051–3.
3. Ackrill P, *et al.* Successful removal of aluminium from patient with dialysis encephalopathy. *Lancet* 1980; **ii:** 692–3.
4. Arze RS, *et al.* Reversal of aluminium dialysis encephalopathy after desferrioxamine treatment. *Lancet* 1981; **ii:** 1116.
5. Milne FJ, *et al.* Low aluminium water, desferrioxamine, and dialysis encephalopathy. *Lancet* 1982; **ii:** 502.
6. Payton CD, *et al.* Successful treatment of aluminium encephalopathy by intraperitoneal desferrioxamine. *Lancet* 1984; **i:** 1132–3.
7. Altmann P, *et al.* Disturbance of cerebral function by aluminium in haemodialysis patients without overt aluminium toxicity. *Lancet* 1989; **ii:** 7–12.
8. Brown DJ, *et al.* Treatment of dialysis osteomalacia with desferrioxamine. *Lancet* 1982; **ii:** 343–5.
9. McCarthy JT, *et al.* Clinical experience with desferrioxamine in dialysis patients with aluminium toxicity. *Q J Med* 1990; **74:** 257–76.
10. Malluche HH, *et al.* The use of deferoxamine in the management of aluminum accumulation in bone in patients with renal failure. *N Engl J Med* 1984; **311:** 140–4.
11. Milliner DS, *et al.* Use of deferoxamine infusion test in the diagnosis of aluminium-related osteodystrophy. *Ann Intern Med* 1984; **101:** 775–80.
12. de la Serna F-J, *et al.* Improvement in the erythropoiesis of chronic haemodialysis patients with desferrioxamine. *Lancet* 1988; **i:** 1009–11.
13. Altmann P, *et al.* Aluminium chelation therapy in dialysis patients: evidence for inhibition of haemoglobin synthesis by low levels of aluminium. *Lancet* 1988; **i:** 1012–15.
14. Padovese P, *et al.* Desferrioxamine versus erythropoietin for treatment of dialysis anaemia. *Lancet* 1990; **335:** 1465.
15. Rosenlöf K, *et al.* Erythropoietin, aluminium, and anaemia in patients on haemodialysis. *Lancet* 1990; **335:** 247–9.
16. Zachée P, *et al.* Erythropoietin, aluminium, and anaemia in patients on haemodialysis. *Lancet* 1990; **335:** 1038–9.
17. Brown MA, *et al.* Prurigo nodularis and aluminium overload in maintenance haemodialysis. *Lancet* 1992; **340:** 48.
18. McLachlan DRC, *et al.* Intramuscular desferrioxamine in patients with Alzheimer's disease. *Lancet* 1991; **337:** 1304–8. Correction. *ibid.*: 1618.
19. Davies P. Desferrioxamine for Alzheimer's disease. *Lancet* 1991; **338:** 325.
20. Holleman DR, Goldstone JR. Desferrioxamine for Alzheimer's disease. *Lancet* 1991; **338:** 325.

**Iron overload.** Chronic iron overload can be caused by inappropriately increased gastrointestinal absorption, by grossly excessive oral intake over long periods, or by parenteral administration of iron, for example from transfused blood.[1] Excess iron is stored in the form of ferritin and haemosiderin. The term *haemosiderosis* is applied to the accumulation of haemosiderin in body tissues without associated tissue damage; *haemochromatosis* refers to a chronic disease state in which iron overload leads to tissue damage, predominantly in the heart, liver, and pancreas.[1-3] Primary or hereditary haemochromatosis is caused by a genetic defect in iron metabolism that results in excessive gastrointestinal absorption of iron. The treatment of choice for primary haemochromatosis is phlebotomy,[1-5] but chelation therapy may be needed in patients with anaemia, hypoproteinaemia, or severe cardiac disease.[1,3] Secondary or acquired haemochromatosis is commonly associated with chronic anaemias, in particular thalassaemia, in which excessive iron uptake due to disordered erythropoiesis and excess iron from repeated blood transfusions contribute to iron overload. In these patients the usual therapy is iron chelation with desferrioxamine (see below).

1. Halliday JW, Basset ML. Treatment of iron storage disorders. *Drugs* 1980; **20:** 2077–15.
2. Crawford DHG, Halliday JW. Current concepts in rational therapy for haemochromatosis. *Drugs* 1991; **41:** 875–82.
3. Kirking MH. Treatment of chronic iron overload. *Clin Pharm* 1991; **10:** 775–83.
4. Barton JC, *et al.* Management of hemochromatosis. *Ann Intern Med* 1998; **129:** 932–9.
5. Vautier G, *et al.* Hereditary haemochromatosis: detection and management. *Med J Aust* 2001; **175:** 418–21.

THALASSAEMIA. Patients homozygous for β-thalassaemia (p.735) have severe anaemia requiring regular blood transfusions. As a consequence of this treatment iron overload develops and the excessive deposition of iron in the myocardium usually results in these patients dying in their second or third decade from arrhythmias or cardiac failure. Desferrioxamine is used to retard the accumulation of iron, the greatest increase in iron excretion being seen in patients given the drug by continuous subcutaneous infusion rather than intramuscular bolus. Better iron excretion may be achieved if patients are given ascorbic acid 100 to 200 mg daily in addition to desferrioxamine (but see Interactions, above).

Desferrioxamine has been shown to improve survival in thalassaemic children given regular systemic therapy,[1-3] and there has also been some evidence that impaired organ function might improve with intensive desferrioxamine therapy. A reduction in liver-iron concentrations and an improvement in liver function was reported in some patients with transfusional iron overload treated with desferrioxamine 2 to 4 g by slow subcutaneous infusion over 12 hours on 6 nights a week.[4] However, in another study[5] improvement in the degree of hepatic fibrosis was seen after 3 to 5 years in only 2 of 7 patients given desferrioxamine up to 85 mg/kg daily by subcutaneous injection, despite reductions in iron concentrations. Beginning chelation therapy before puberty could help to ensure normal sexual development in patients with thalassaemia major.[6] Studies indicating that desferrioxamine treatment might preserve or possibly improve cardiac function impaired by iron overload in thalassaemic patients[7-9] have been supported by a decrease in mortality from cardiac disease since the introduction of desferrioxamine in Italy,[1] although it continues to be the main cause of death in patients with thalassaemia.[1,2] A further study[3] in patients with β-thalassaemia demonstrated a markedly improved prognosis for survival without cardiac disease in patients who began chelation therapy with desferrioxamine before iron loading was severe and in whom reduced serum-ferritin concentrations were maintained over a long period. Failure to prevent the accumulation of excess iron or to remove large stores of iron was associated with a poor prognosis at any age. Thus, it is considered advisable to begin chelation therapy as early as possible (in practice usually at 3 years of age when iron overload becomes significant) to try to prevent organ damage developing.

1. Zurlo MG, *et al.* Survival and causes of death in thalassaemia major. *Lancet* 1989; **ii:** 27–30.
2. Ehlers KH, *et al.* Prolonged survival in patients with beta-thalassemia major treated with deferoxamine. *J Pediatr* 1991; **118:** 540–5.
3. Olivieri NF, *et al.* Survival in medically treated patients with homozygous β-thalassemia. *N Engl J Med* 1994; **331:** 574–8.
4. Hoffbrand AV, *et al.* Improvement in status and liver function in patients with transfusional iron overload with long-term subcutaneous desferrioxamine. *Lancet* 1979; **i:** 947–9.
5. Maurer HS, *et al.* A prospective evaluation of iron chelation therapy in children with severe β-thalassemia: a six-year study. *Am J Dis Child* 1988; **142:** 287–92.
6. Bronspiegel-Weintrob N, *et al.* Effect of age at the start of iron chelation therapy on gonadal function in β-thalassemia major. *N Engl J Med* 1990; **323:** 713–19.
7. Freeman AP, *et al.* Early left ventricular dysfunction and chelation therapy in thalassemia major. *Ann Intern Med* 1983; **99:** 450–4.
8. Marcus RE, *et al.* Desferrioxamine to improve cardiac function in iron-overloaded patients with thalassaemia major. *Lancet* 1984; **i:** 392–3.
9. Wolfe L, *et al.* Prevention of cardiac disease by subcutaneous deferoxamine in patients with thalassemia major. *N Engl J Med* 1985; **312:** 1600–3.

**Iron poisoning.** Despite the frequency of acute poisoning with iron preparations, no universally accepted treatment protocol exists. It is often difficult to determine the amount of iron ingested, and assessment of clinical symptoms can be misleading since patients may exhibit mild symptoms despite having ingested potentially toxic quantities of iron. Measurement of the serum-iron concentration and the total iron-binding capacity (TIBC) is useful in assessing the severity of poisoning but may not be immediately available and may be misleading. The desferrioxamine challenge test entails giving desferrioxamine 50 mg/kg (to a maximum dose of 1 g) intramuscularly; if free iron is present, ferrioxamine will be excreted in the urine imparting a classic 'vin rosé' colour. However, the results can be difficult to interpret and a negative result does not rule out iron toxicity.

The initial stage of treatment entails removal of unabsorbed iron from the gastrointestinal tract by gastric lavage, with whole-bowel irrigation as a treatment option in patients suspected of ingesting modified-release preparations or those with radiographic evidence of unabsorbed tablets remaining after gastric lavage. The addition of desferrioxamine to the lavage fluid is controversial since there is little evidence of its efficacy and concern over possible toxic effects of ferrioxamine. Supportive care should be given as appropriate and may be all that is required in mild poisoning. Activated charcoal is not effective in iron poisoning.

Chelation therapy with desferrioxamine given intramuscularly or intravenously is indicated in patients with impaired consciousness, shock or hypotension; in those with other symptoms of severe poisoning, for example leucocytosis; in those in whom the serum-iron concentration exceeds the TIBC; in those with a positive desferrioxamine challenge test; and those with a serum-iron concentration above 350 micrograms per 100 mL if TIBC estimations are unavailable. In severe toxicity intravenous desferrioxamine is given immediately without waiting for the results of serum-iron measurements. There is no general agreement on the duration of chelation therapy; among the suggested end-points are the disappearance of the vin rosé coloration of the urine, 24 hours after the disappearance of coloration, and reduction of serum-iron concentrations to less than 100 micrograms per 100 mL.

General references.


1. Proudfoot AT, *et al.* Management of acute iron poisoning. *Med Toxicol* 1986; **1:** 83–100.
2. Engle JP, *et al.* Acute iron intoxication: treatment controversies. *Drug Intell Clin Pharm* 1987; **21:** 153–9.
3. Mann KV, *et al.* Management of acute iron overdose. *Clin Pharm* 1989; **8:** 428–40.


**Malaria.** Following the suggestion that iron-deficiency anaemia may offer some protection against infections (see Infections in the Precautions for Iron, p.1435), desferrioxamine was tried in a few patients with malaria.[1,2] Any antimalarial effect of desferrioxamine was thought to be as a result of chelation of parasite-associated iron rather than reduction in body-iron concentrations in the patient. Desferrioxamine given intravenously was reported[3] to shorten the time to regain consciousness in children with cerebral malaria receiving standard therapy with intravenous quinine and oral pyrimethamine-sulfadoxine. However, in another study[4] there was no evidence of a beneficial effect on mortality when desferrioxamine was added to an antimalarial treatment regimen that included a loading dose of quinine.


1. Gordeuk VR, *et al.* Iron chelation as a chemotherapeutic strategy for falciparum malaria. *Am J Trop Med Hyg* 1993; **48:** 193–7.
2. Thompson DF. Deferoxamine treatment of malaria. *Ann Pharmacother* 1994; **28:** 602–3.
3. Gordeuk V, *et al.* Effect of iron chelation therapy on recovery from deep coma, in children with cerebral malaria. *N Engl J Med* 1992; **327:** 1473–7.
4. Thuma PE, *et al.* Effect of iron chelation therapy on mortality in Zambian children with cerebral malaria. *Trans R Soc Trop Med Hyg* 1998; **92:** 214–18.


**Porphyria.** The management of various forms of porphyria is discussed on p.1040. Desferrioxamine may be used to reduce serum-iron concentrations in porphyria cutanea tarda if phlebotomy is contra-indicated. In a study of 25 patients with porphyria cutanea tarda,[1] subcutaneous infusion of desferrioxamine was found to be as effective as repeated phlebotomies in normalising porphyrin excretion and iron storage. Desferrioxamine was also used successfully to treat haemodialysis-related porphyria cutanea tarda in a 22-year-old man in whom venesection therapy was contra-indicated because of severe anaemia requiring multiple blood transfusion.[2] Each course of intravenous desferrioxamine therapy after the end of 3 haemodialysis sessions was accompanied by a marked decrease in plasma porphyrins, a sharp increase in haematocrit values, and a simultaneous improvement in skin lesions.


1. Rocchi E, *et al.* Iron removal therapy in porphyria cutanea tarda: phlebotomy versus slow subcutaneous desferrioxamine infusion. *Br J Dermatol* 1986; **114:** 621–9.
2. Praga M, *et al.* Treatment of hemodialysis-related porphyria cutanea tarda with deferoxamine. *N Engl J Med* 1987; **316:** 547–8.


### Preparations

***BP 2003:*** Desferrioxamine Injection;
***USP 27:*** Deferoxamine Mesylate for Injection.

**Proprietary Preparations** (details are given in Part 3)
***Arg.:*** Desferal; ***Austral.:*** Desferal; ***Austria:*** Desferal; ***Belg.:*** Desferal; ***Braz.:*** Desferal; ***Canad.:*** Desferal; ***Chile:*** Desferal; ***Denm.:*** Desferal; ***Fin.:*** Desferal; ***Fr.:*** Desferal; ***Ger.:*** Desferal; ***Gr.:*** Desferal; ***Hong Kong:*** Desferal; ***India:*** Desferal; ***Irl.:*** Desferal; ***Israel:*** Desferal; ***Ital.:*** Desferal; ***Malaysia:*** Desferal; ***Neth.:*** Desferal; ***Norw.:*** Desferal; ***NZ:*** Desferal; ***Port.:*** Desferal; ***S.Afr.:*** Desferal; ***Singapore:*** Desferal†; ***Spain:*** Desferin; ***Swed.:*** Desferal; ***Switz.:*** Desferal; ***Thai.:*** Desferal; ***UK:*** Desferal; ***USA:*** Desferal.

## Dexrazoxane *(BAN, USAN, rINN)*

ADR-529; Dexrazoxano; ICRF-187; NSC-169780. (+)-(S)-4,4′-Propylenebis(piperazine-2,6-dione).

$C_{11}H_{16}N_4O_4$ = 268.3.
*CAS — 24584-09-6.*
*ATC — V03AF02.*

### Adverse Effects and Precautions

Dexrazoxane may add to the bone-marrow depression caused by antineoplastics and frequent complete blood counts are recommended during concomitant therapy. Although dexrazoxane protects against the cardiotoxic effects of anthracyclines cardiac function should continue to be monitored when dexrazoxane is used. Pain on injection has been reported.

It has been recommended that dexrazoxane should only be given to patients who have received a cumulative dose of doxorubicin of 300 mg/m² and who require continued administration, since there is some evidence that dexrazoxane may reduce the efficacy of the antineoplastic regimen.

**Effects on the skin.** Severe cutaneous and subcutaneous necrosis has been reported[1] in a patient who received dexrazoxane by infusion into a peripheral forearm vein, followed by intravenous injection of doxorubicin at a different site in the same arm. Local pain occurred during the dexrazoxane infusion but there was no evidence of extravasation.


1. Lossos IS, Ben-Yehuda D. Cutaneous and subcutaneous necrosis following dexrazoxane-CHOP therapy. *Ann Pharmacother* 1999; **33:** 253–4.


### Pharmacokinetics

Dexrazoxane is mainly excreted in the urine as unchanged drug and metabolites. The elimination half-life is reported to be about 2 hours.

### Uses and Administration

Dexrazoxane is the (+)-enantiomorph of the antineoplastic drug razoxane (p.582) and is a cytoprotective agent that is used to reduce the cardiotoxicity of doxorubicin and other anthracyclines (see p.548). It is hydrolysed to an active metabolite that is similar to edetic acid. This chelates iron within the cells and appears to prevent the formation of the anthracycline-iron complex that is thought to be responsible for cardiotoxicity.

Dexrazoxane is used to reduce the incidence and severity of cardiomyopathy associated with doxorubicin in women with metastatic breast cancer who have received a cumulative dose of doxorubicin of 300 mg/m² and who require continued use. It is given as the hydrochloride, by slow intravenous injection or rapid intravenous infusion, starting within 30 minutes before doxorubicin administration. The dose is expressed as the base, calculated on a 10:1 ratio with doxorubicin; typically, 500 mg/m² of dexrazoxane is given for every 50 mg/m² of doxorubicin.

Dexrazoxane is also being investigated for use with doxorubicin in various other malignancies.

◊ References.


1. Wiseman LR, Spencer CM. Dexrazoxane: a review of its use as a cardioprotective agent in patients receiving anthracycline-based chemotherapy. *Drugs* 1998; **56:** 385–403.
2. Links M, Lewis C. Chemoprotectants: a review of their clinical pharmacology and therapeutic efficacy. *Drugs* 1999; **57:** 293–308.


### Preparations

**Proprietary Preparations** (details are given in Part 3)
***Austria:*** Cardioxane; ***Braz.:*** Cardioxane; ***Canad.:*** Zinecard; ***Chile:*** Cardioxane; ***Denm.:*** Cardioxane; ***Fr.:*** Cardioxane; ***Israel:*** Cardioxane; ***Ital.:*** Cardioxane; Eucardion†; ***Mex.:*** Cardioxane; ***USA:*** Zinecard.

## Dicobalt Edetate *(BAN, rINN)*

Cobalt Edetate; Cobalt EDTA; Cobalt Tetracemate; Edetato de dicobalto. Cobalt [ethylenediaminetetra-acetato(4—)-N,N′,O,O′]cobalt(II).

$C_{10}H_{12}Co_2N_2O_8$ = 406.1.
*CAS — 36499-65-7.*

### Adverse Effects and Precautions

Dicobalt edetate may cause hypotension, tachycardia, and vomiting. Anaphylactic reactions have occurred; oedema of the face and neck, sweating, chest pain, cardiac irregularities, and skin rashes have been reported.

The adverse effects of dicobalt edetate are more severe in the absence of cyanide. Therefore, dicobalt edetate should not be given unless cyanide poisoning is definitely confirmed and poisoning is moderate or severe, that is, when consciousness is impaired.

**Oedema.** A patient with cyanide toxicity developed severe facial and pulmonary oedema after treatment with dicobalt edetate.[1] It has been suggested that when dicobalt edetate is used, facilities for intubation and resuscitation should be immediately available.


1. Dodds C, McKnight C. Cyanide toxicity after immersion and the hazards of dicobalt edetate. *BMJ* 1985; **291:** 785–6.


### Uses and Administration

Dicobalt edetate is a chelator used in the treatment of acute cyanide poisoning (p.1506). Its use arises from the property of cobalt salts to form a relatively non-toxic stable ion-complex with cyanide. Owing to its toxicity, dicobalt edetate should be used only in confirmed cyanide poisoning and never as a precautionary measure. Cyanide poisoning must be treated as quickly as possible. A suggested dose is 300 mg given by intravenous injection, over about 1 minute, repeated if the response is inadequate; a further dose of 300 mg of dicobalt edetate may be given 5 minutes later if required. For less severe poisoning the injection should be given over 5 minutes. Each injection of dicobalt edetate may be followed immediately by 50 mL of glucose 50% intravenously to reduce toxicity, though the value of giving glucose has been questioned.

### Preparations

**Proprietary Preparations** (details are given in Part 3)
***Fr.:*** Kelocyanor; ***Gr.:*** Kelocyanor; ***Irl.:*** Kelocyanor†; ***UK:*** Kelocyanor†.

## Digoxin-specific Antibody Fragments

Digoxin Immune Fab (Ovine); F(ab); Fragmentos de anticuerpos específicos antidigoxina.
*ATC — V03AB24.*

### Adverse Effects and Precautions

Allergic reactions to digoxin-specific antibody fragments have been reported rarely. Patients known to be allergic to sheep protein and patients who have previously received digoxin-specific antibody fragments are likely to be at greater risk of developing an allergic reaction. Blood pressure, ECG, and potassium concentrations should be monitored closely during and after administration.

### Uses and Administration

Digoxin-specific antibody fragments are derived from antibodies produced in sheep immunised to digoxin. Digoxin has greater affinity for the antibodies than for tissue-binding sites, and the digoxin-antibody complex is then rapidly excreted in the urine. Digoxin-specific antibody fragments are generally restricted to the treatment of life-threatening digoxin or digitoxin intoxication in which conventional treatment is ineffective. Successful treatment of lanatoside C poisoning has also been reported.

It is estimated that 38 mg of antibody fragments could bind about 500 micrograms of digoxin or digitoxin and the dose calculation is based on this estimate and the body-load of digoxin (based on the amount ingested or ideally from the steady-state plasma concentration). Administration is by intravenous infusion over a 30-minute period. If cardiac arrest is imminent the dose may be given as a bolus. In the case of incomplete reversal or recurrence of toxicity a further dose can be given. In patients considered to be at high risk of an allergic response an intradermal or skin scratch test may be performed.

◊ Clinical studies and reviews of the use of digoxin-specific antibody fragments have confirmed their effectiveness in the treatment of severe digitalis toxicity in the majority of patients.[1-4] An initial response is usually seen within 30 minutes of the end of the infusion with a maximum response after 3 to 4 hours.[3] The main causes of treatment failure or partial response are incorrect diagnosis of digitalis intoxication, inadequate dosage of antibody fragments, and administration to patients already moribund.[3,4] Few adverse reactions have been attributed to the administration of digoxin-specific antibody fragments; a few cases of minor allergic reactions have been reported including erythema, facial swelling, urticaria, and rashes,[2,3] but no anaphylactic reactions have been reported.[1-4] Haemodynamic status normally improves, but withdrawal of the inotropic support provided by digoxin may produce a decline in cardiac function in some patients. There may be dramatic reductions in plasma potassium concentrations.

Treatment has been successful in patients with varying degrees of renal impairment.[2,3,5] Elimination of the antibody fragment-digoxin complex may be markedly delayed in severe renal impairment and prolonged monitoring may be required in such patients.[6] Measurement of free serum-digoxin concentrations may be useful.[7] Experience with digoxin-specific antibody fragments in a patient with chronic renal failure receiving haemodialysis has been reported.[8] The patient had a good clinical response but haemodialysis did not remove the antibody fragment-digoxin complex.

In patients with adequate renal function the half-life of the antibody fragment-digoxin complex has been reported[2] to be about 16 to 20 hours although longer half-lives have been reported.[9] It has been suggested[10] that the administration of digoxin-specific antibody fragments by infusion over 7 hours following an initial loading dose could be useful in ensuring adequate antibody concentrations are maintained to bind digoxin as it is released from tissue stores over a prolonged period.

Use of the antibody fragments has also been effective in children with severe digitalis intoxication.[11]

For reference to the use of digoxin-specific antibody fragments to treat poisoning due to common or yellow oleander, see Oleander, p.1723.


1. Smith TW, *et al.* Treatment of life-threatening digitalis intoxication with digoxin-specific Fab antibody fragments: experience in 26 cases. *N Engl J Med* 1982; **307:** 1357–62.
2. Wenger TL, *et al.* Treatment of 63 severely digitalis-toxic patients with digoxin-specific antibody fragments. *J Am Coll Cardiol* 1985; **5:** 118A–123A.
3. Stolshek BS, *et al.* The role of digoxin-specific antibodies in the treatment of digitalis poisoning. *Med Toxicol* 1988; **3:** 167–71.

4. Antman EM, *et al.* Treatment of 150 cases of life-threatening digitalis intoxication with digoxin-specific Fab antibody fragments: final report of a multicenter study. *Circulation* 1990; **81:** 1744–52.
5. Allen NM, *et al.* Clinical and pharmacokinetic profiles of digoxin immune Fab in four patients with renal impairment. *DICP Ann Pharmacother* 1991; **25:** 1315–20.
6. Ujhelyi MR, *et al.* Disposition of digoxin immune Fab in patients with kidney failure. *Clin Pharmacol Ther* 1993; **54:** 388–94.
7. Ujhelyi MR, Robert S. Pharmacokinetic aspects of digoxin-specific Fab therapy in the management of digitalis toxicity. *Clin Pharmacokinet* 1995; **28:** 483–93.
8. Clifton GD, *et al.* Free and total serum digoxin concentrations in a renal failure patient after treatment with digoxin immune Fab. *Clin Pharm* 1989; **8:** 441–5.
9. Gibb I, Parnham A. A star treatment for digoxin overdose? *BMJ* 1986; **293:** 1171–2.
10. Schaumann W, *et al.* Kinetics of the Fab fragments of digoxin antibodies and of bound digoxin in patients with severe digoxin intoxication. *Eur J Clin Pharmacol* 1986; **30:** 527–33.
11. Woolf AD, *et al.* The use of digoxin-specific Fab fragments for severe digitalis intoxication in children. *N Engl J Med* 1992; **326:** 1739–44.

### Preparations

**Proprietary Preparations** (details are given in Part 3)
***Austral.:*** Digibind; ***Austria:*** Digitalis Antidot; ***Belg.:*** Digitalis Antidot; ***Canad.:*** Digibind; ***Fr.:*** Digidot; ***Ger.:*** Digitalis Antidot; ***Gr.:*** Digibind; ***Hong Kong:*** Digitalis Antidote; ***Singapore:*** Digitalis Antidote†; ***Swed.:*** Digitalis Antidot; ***Switz.:*** Antidote Anti-Digitale BM†; ***UK:*** Digibind; ***USA:*** Digibind; DigiFab.

## Dimercaprol *(BAN, rINN)*

BAL; British Anti-Lewisite; Dimercaprolum. 2,3-Dimercaptopropan-1-ol.

$C_3H_8OS_2$ = 124.2.

*CAS — 59-52-9.*

*ATC — V03AB09.*

**Pharmacopoeias.** In *Chin., Eur.* (see p.vi), *Int., Jpn, US,* and *Viet.*

**Ph. Eur. 5.0** (Dimercaprol). A clear colourless or slightly yellow liquid. Soluble in water and in arachis oil; miscible with alcohol and with benzyl benzoate. Store at 2° to 8° in well-filled airtight containers. Protect from light.

**USP 27** (Dimercaprol). A colourless or practically colourless liquid, having a disagreeable, mercaptan-like odour. Soluble 1 in 20 of water; soluble in alcohol, in benzyl benzoate, and in methyl alcohol. Store at a temperature not exceeding 8° in airtight containers. Protect from light.

### Adverse Effects and Treatment

The most consistent side-effects produced by dimercaprol are hypertension and tachycardia. Other side-effects include nausea, vomiting, headache, burning sensation of the lips, mouth, throat, and eyes, lachrymation and salivation, tingling of the extremities, a sensation of constriction in the throat and chest, muscle pains and muscle spasm, rhinorrhoea, conjunctivitis, sweating, restlessness, and abdominal pain. Transient reductions in the leucocyte count have also been reported. Pain may occur at the injection site and sterile abscesses occasionally develop. In children, fever commonly occurs and persists during therapy.

Side-effects are dose-related, relatively frequent, and usually reversible. It has been suggested that oral administration of ephedrine sulfate 30 to 60 mg thirty minutes before each injection of dimercaprol may reduce side-effects; antihistamines may alleviate some of the symptoms.

### Precautions

Dimercaprol should be used with care in patients with hypertension or renal impairment. It should be discontinued, or continued with extreme caution, if acute renal insufficiency develops during therapy. Alkalinisation of the urine may protect the kidney during therapy by stabilising the dimercaprol-metal complex. Dimercaprol should not be used in patients with hepatic impairment unless due to arsenic poisoning. It should not be used in the treatment of poisoning due to cadmium, iron, or selenium as the dimercaprol-metal complexes formed are more toxic than the metals themselves.

**G6PD deficiency.** A report[1] of haemolysis during chelation therapy with dimercaprol and sodium calcium edetate for high blood-lead concentrations in 2 children with a deficiency of G6PD.

1. Janakiraman N, *et al.* Hemolysis during BAL chelation therapy for high blood lead levels in two G6PD deficient children. *Clin Pediatr (Phila)* 1978; **17:** 485–7.

### Interactions

Iron supplements should not be given during dimercaprol therapy as toxic dimercaprol-metal complexes are formed.

### Pharmacokinetics

After intramuscular injection, maximum blood concentrations of dimercaprol may be attained within 30 to 60 minutes. Dimercaprol is rapidly metabolised and the metabolites and dimercaprol-metal chelates are excreted in the urine and bile. Elimination is essentially complete within 4 hours of a single dose.

### Uses and Administration

Dimercaprol is a chelator used in the treatment of acute poisoning by arsenic (p.1657), gold (p.89), and mercury (p.1713); it may also be used in the treatment of poisoning by antimony, bismuth, and possibly thallium. It is also used, with sodium calcium edetate, in acute lead poisoning (p.1705).

The sulfhydryl groups on dimercaprol compete with endogenous sulfhydryl groups on proteins such as enzymes to combine with these metals; chelation by dimercaprol therefore prevents or reverses any inhibition of the sulfhydryl enzymes by the metal and the dimercaprol-metal complex formed is readily excreted by the kidney. Since the complex may dissociate, particularly at acid pH, or be oxidised, the aim of treatment is to provide an excess of dimercaprol in body fluids until the excretion of the metal is complete.

Dimercaprol should be administered by deep intramuscular injection and the injections should be given at different sites. Various dosage schedules are in use.

In the UK, a recommended schedule for adults is to give doses of 400 to 800 mg on the first day of treatment, 200 to 400 mg on the second and third days, and 100 to 200 mg on the fourth and subsequent days, all administered in divided doses. Within these dose ranges, the individual dose is determined by body-weight, severity of symptoms, and the causative agent. Single doses should not generally exceed 3 mg/kg but single doses of up to 5 mg/kg may be required initially in patients with severe acute poisoning. The dose for children is based on body-weight using a similar dose per kg as for adults. A minimum interval of 4 hours between doses appears to reduce side-effects.

In the USA, a recommended schedule for severe arsenical or gold poisoning is 3 mg/kg given at 4-hourly intervals throughout the first 2 days, 4 times on the third day, and twice on each of the next 10 days. Alternatively 3 mg/kg may be given every 4 hours on the first day, 2 mg/kg every 4 hours on the second day, 3 mg/kg every 6 hours on the third day, and 3 mg/kg every 12 hours on each of the next 10 days or until recovery. In milder cases, 2.5 mg/kg is given 4 times daily on each of the first 2 days, twice daily on the third day, and once daily on subsequent days for 10 days or until recovery. For mercury toxicity, 3 to 5 mg/kg is given every 4 hours for 2 days, then 2.5 to 3 mg/kg every 6 hours for 2 days, and then 2.5 to 3 mg/kg every 12 hours for 7 days.

Dimercaprol is also used with sodium calcium edetate (p.1052) in the treatment of lead poisoning. It can be of particular value in the treatment of acute lead encephalopathy and a suggested procedure is to give an initial dose of dimercaprol 4 mg/kg alone followed at 4-hourly intervals by dimercaprol 3 to 4 mg/kg with concomitant doses of sodium calcium edetate at a separate site; treatment may be maintained for 2 to 7 days depending on the clinical response.

### Preparations

***BP 2003:*** Dimercaprol Injection;
***USP 27:*** Dimercaprol Injection.

**Proprietary Preparations** (details are given in Part 3)
***Gr.:*** BAL.

### 4-Dimethylaminophenol Hydrochloride

Dimetamfenol Hydrochloride; 4-Dimetilaminofenol, hidrocloruro de; 4-DMAP.

$C_8H_{11}NO,HCl$ = 173.6.

*CAS — 619-60-3 (4-dimethylaminophenol); 5882-48-4 (4-dimethylaminophenol hydrochloride).*

*ATC — V03AB27.*

**Profile**

4-Dimethylaminophenol hydrochloride is reported to oxidise haemoglobin to methaemoglobin and has been used with sodium thiosulfate as an alternative to sodium nitrite (p.1052) in the treatment of cyanide poisoning. Doses of 3 to 4 mg/kg have been given intravenously.

◊ References.

1. Weger NP. Treatment of cyanide poisoning with 4-dimethylaminophenol (DMAP)–experimental and clinical overview. *Fundam Appl Toxicol* 1983; **3:** 387–96.

**Preparations**

**Proprietary Preparations** (details are given in Part 3)
***Ger.:*** 4-DMAP; ***Neth.:*** 4-DMAP.

### Diprenorphine Hydrochloride *(BANM, rINNM)*

Hidrocloruro de diprenorfina; M5050. (6R,7R,14S)-17-Cyclopropylmethyl-7,8-dihydro-7-(1-hydroxy-1-methylethyl)-6-*O*-methyl-6,14-ethano-17-normorphine hydrochloride; 2-[(−)-(5R,-6R,7R,14S)-9a-Cyclopropylmethyl-4,5-epoxy-3-hydroxy-6-methoxy-6,14-ethanomorphinan-7-yl]propan-2-ol hydrochloride.

$C_{26}H_{35}NO_4,HCl$ = 462.0.

*CAS — 14357-78-9 (diprenorphine); 16808-86-9 (diprenorphine hydrochloride).*

**Pharmacopoeias.** In *BP(Vet).*

**BP(Vet) 2003** (Diprenorphine Hydrochloride). A white or almost white crystalline powder. Sparingly soluble in water; slightly soluble in alcohol; very slightly soluble in chloroform; practically insoluble in ether. A 2% solution in water has a pH of 4.5 to 6.0. Protect from light.

**Profile**

Diprenorphine hydrochloride is an opioid antagonist used in veterinary medicine to reverse the effects of etorphine hydrochloride.

## Disodium Edetate *(BAN)*

Dinatrii Edetas; Disodium Edathamil; Disodium EDTA; Disodium Tetracemate; Edetate Disodium; Edetato disódico; Natrii Edetas; Sodium Versenate. Disodium dihydrogen ethylenediaminetetra-acetate dihydrate.

$C_{10}H_{14}N_2Na_2O_8,2H_2O$ = 372.2.

*CAS — 139-33-3 (anhydrous disodium edetate); 6381-92-6 (disodium edetate dihydrate).*

*ATC — S01XA05.*

NOTE. The term sodium edetate has been used in the literature for various sodium salts of edetic acid.

**Pharmacopoeias.** In *Eur.* (see p.vi), *Int., Jpn, Pol.,* and *US.*

**Ph. Eur. 5.0** (Disodium Edetate). A white, crystalline powder. Soluble in water; practically insoluble in alcohol. A 5% solution in water has a pH of 4.0 to 5.5. Protect from light.

**USP 27** (Edetate Disodium). A white crystalline powder. Soluble in water. pH of a 5% solution in water is between 4.0 and 6.0.

### Trisodium Edetate

Edetate Trisodium *(USAN)*; Edetato trisódico. Trisodium hydrogen ethylenediaminetetra-acetate.

$C_{10}H_{13}N_2Na_3O_8$ = 358.2.

*CAS — 150-38-9.*

*ATC — S01XA05.*

### Adverse Effects and Precautions

Disodium and trisodium edetate have similar adverse effects and precautions to sodium calcium edetate (p.1051) and, when used as pharmaceutical excipients, to edetic acid (p.1038).

Hypocalcaemia can occur if disodium or trisodium edetate is administered by intravenous infusion too rapidly or in too concentrated a solution and tetany, convulsions, respiratory arrest, and cardiac arrhythmias may result. Plasma-electrolyte concentrations, particularly of ionised calcium, should be monitored.

In addition, edetates should be used with caution in patients with tuberculosis, impaired cardiac function, or a history of seizures, and are contra-indicated in renal impairment.

The rate of infusion should be decreased if signs of muscle reactivity occur. The infusion should be discontinued if tetany occurs and should only be restarted cautiously after plasma ionised and total calcium concentrations indicate a need for further treatment and tetany has stopped.

## Interactions

Edetates chelate bivalent and trivalent metal ions and may affect the activity of drugs such as zinc insulin that contain such ions.

**Preservatives.** For reference to the inactivation of phenylmercuric salts by disodium edetate, see Phenylmercuric Nitrate, p.1189. For reports of edetates reducing the antimicrobial efficacy of thiomersal, see p.1194.

## Uses and Administration

Disodium and trisodium edetate are chelators with a high affinity for calcium, with which they form a stable, soluble complex that is readily excreted by the kidneys. They have been administered intravenously in the emergency treatment of hypercalcaemia (p.1218) and have been used to control digitalis-induced cardiac arrhythmias, although less toxic agents are generally preferred (p.895). They are also used to treat calcium deposits in the eye.

Disodium and trisodium edetate also chelate other polyvalent metals but, unlike sodium calcium edetate, which is saturated with calcium, they are not used for the treatment of heavy metal poisoning since hypocalcaemia rapidly develops.

In the treatment of hypercalcaemia, injections containing varying amounts of disodium and trisodium edetate are used. In the UK, the trisodium salt is generally used. A dose of up to 70 mg/kg daily has been suggested for adults; children may be given up to 60 mg/kg daily. It should be given by slow intravenous infusion over 2 to 3 hours and each gram of trisodium edetate should be diluted with 100 mL of glucose 5% or sodium chloride 0.9%. In the USA, disodium edetate is given in an adult dose of 50 mg/kg in 24 hours by slow intravenous infusion; the maximum daily dose is 3 g. Children may be given 40 to 70 mg/kg in 24 hours. The injection should be diluted with 500 mL of sodium chloride 0.9% or glucose 5% for adults or a concentration not greater than 3% for children, and infused over 3 hours or more, preferably 4 to 6 hours. The dosage may be repeated for a further 4 days followed by a two-day interval before subsequent courses of treatment. If necessary, up to fifteen doses may be given in total.

Disodium and trisodium edetate are used in the treatment of calcium deposits from calcium oxide or calcium hydroxide burns of the eye and in the treatment of calcified corneal opacities, either by topical application after removing the appropriate area of corneal epithelium or by iontophoresis. Irrigation has also been suggested for zinc chloride injury to the eye, but treatment may be ineffective unless started within 2 minutes. In the UK, a 0.4% solution of the trisodium salt is used for topical application to the eye; in the USA, a 0.35 to 1.85% solution of the disodium salt has been suggested.

Disodium and trisodium edetate are also used in cleaners for contact lenses and as antoxidant synergists in cosmetic and pharmaceutical preparations.

**Atherosclerosis.** Calcium is thought to be necessary for several steps in atherogenesis and removal of calcium from atherosclerotic plaques using a chelator such as disodium edetate has been tried in patients with atherosclerosis (p.815).[1] However, reports of beneficial clinical responses are largely anecdotal or from small, short-term, or uncontrolled clinical studies[1-3] and literature reviews[4,5] have concluded that in view of the potential toxicity of such treatment it should be considered obsolete. Furthermore, there is a report of fatal renal failure in a patient given such therapy.[6]


1. Grier MT, Meyers DG. So much writing, so little science: a review of 37 years of literature on edetate sodium chelation therapy. *Ann Pharmacother* 1993; **27:** 1504–9.
2. Rathmann KL, Golightly LK. Chelation therapy of atherosclerosis. *Drug Intell Clin Pharm* 1984; **18:** 1000–3.
3. Elihu N, *et al.* Chelation therapy in cardiovascular disease: ethylenediaminetetraacetic acid, deferoxamine, and dexrazoxane. *J Clin Pharmacol* 1998; **38:** 101–5.
4. Ernst E. Chelation therapy for peripheral arterial occlusive disease: a systematic review. *Circulation* 1997; **96:** 1031–3.
5. Ernst E. Chelation therapy for coronary heart disease: an overview of all clinical investigations. *Am Heart J* 2000; **140:** 139–41.
6. Magee R. Chelation treatment of atherosclerosis. *Med J Aust* 1985; **142:** 514–15.


## Preparations

***BP 2003:*** Trisodium Edetate Intravenous Infusion;
***USP 27:*** Edetate Disodium Injection.

**Proprietary Preparations** (details are given in Part 3)
***Fr.:*** Chelatran; ***Irl.:*** Limclair; ***UK:*** Limclair; ***USA:*** Disotate†; Endrate.

**Multi-ingredient: *Braz.:*** Flex-Care†; ***Ger.:*** Complete†; Duracare†; Oxysept†; ***Israel:*** Cleaner No 4†; ***Mex.:*** Adapettes; ***NZ:*** Conditioning Solution; ***UK:*** Uriflex G; Uriflex R.

# Ditiocarb Sodium *(rINN)*

DDTC; Dithiocarb Sodium; Ditiocarbo sódico; DTC; Sodium Diethyldithiocarbamate; U-14624.

$C_5H_{10}NNaS_2$ = 171.3.
*CAS — 148-18-5.*

## Profile

Ditiocarb sodium is a chelator that has been used in the destruction of cisplatin wastes and in nickel carbonyl poisoning. It also has immunomodulating properties and has been investigated in HIV infection. Disulfiram is rapidly metabolised to ditiocarb; for its further metabolism, see p.1682.

# Edetic Acid *(BAN, rINN)*

Ácido edético; Acidum Edeticum; Edathamil; EDTA; Tetracemic Acid. Ethylenediaminetetra-acetic acid.

$C_{10}H_{16}N_2O_8$ = 292.2.
*CAS — 60-00-4.*

**Pharmacopoeias.** In *Eur.* (see p.vi). Also in *USNF.*

**Ph. Eur. 5.0** (Edetic Acid). A white, crystalline powder or colourless crystals. Practically insoluble in water and in alcohol. It dissolves in dilute solutions of alkali hydroxides. Protect from light.

**USNF 22** (Edetic Acid). A white crystalline powder. Very slightly soluble in water; soluble in solutions of alkali hydroxides.

## Adverse Effects and Precautions

Edetic acid, used as a pharmaceutical excipient, is generally well tolerated. Adverse effects have been reported following inhalation of solutions containing edetic acid.

**Asthma.** Inhalation of an ipratropium nebuliser solution, that contained edetic acid as one of the preservatives, caused bronchoconstriction in 6 of 22 patients with asthma.[1] Inhalation of edetic acid alone produced dose-related bronchoconstriction that persisted for more than 1 hour.


1. Beasley CRW, *et al.* Bronchoconstrictor properties of preservatives in ipratropium bromide (Atrovent) nebuliser solution. *BMJ* 1987; **294:** 1197–8.


**Blood testing.** Edetic acid may induce platelet clumping in some specimens collected for blood-cell counting leading to diagnostic errors. The recognition of pseudothrombocytopenia resulting from the use of edetic acid as the anticoagulant in blood samples and the use of alternative anticoagulants have been discussed.[1,2]


1. Lombarts AJPF, de Kieviet W. Recognition and prevention of pseudothrombocytopenia and concomitant pseudoleukocytosis. *Am J Clin Pathol* 1988; **89:** 634–9.
2. Lippi U, *et al.* EDTA-induced platelet aggregation can be avoided by a new anticoagulant also suitable for automated complete blood count. *Haematologica* 1990; **75:** 38–41.


## Interactions

Edetic acid and its salts chelate polyvalent metal ions and may affect the activity of agents that contain such ions.

**Disinfectants.** Edetic acid has been reported to enhance the antimicrobial efficacy of some disinfectants such as *chloroxylenol* (p.1177). However, for a report of edetates reducing the antimicrobial efficacy of *thiomersal*, see p.1194.

## Uses

Edetic acid and its salts are chelators used in pharmaceutical manufacturing and as anticoagulants for blood taken for haematological investigations. Edetates have many industrial applications as chelators; for their use in medicine see Disodium Edetate, p.1038, and Sodium Calcium Edetate, p.1052.

**Gallstones.** Edetic acid has been suggested as a possible solvent for non-cholesterol gallstones (p.1761).

## Preparations

**Proprietary Preparations** (details are given in Part 3)

**Multi-ingredient: *Ital.:*** Conta-Lens Wetting†; ***USA:*** Summers Eve Post-Menstrual; Triv; Zonite.

# Flumazenil *(BAN, USAN, rINN)*

Flumazenilum; Flumazepil; Ro-15-1788; Ro-15-1788/000. Ethyl 8-fluoro-5,6-dihydro-5-methyl-6-oxo-4*H*-imidazo[1,5-*a*][1,4]benzodiazepine-3-carboxylate.

$C_{15}H_{14}FN_3O_3$ = 303.3.
*CAS — 78755-81-4.*
*ATC — V03AB25.*

**Pharmacopoeias.** In *Eur.* (see p.vi).

**Ph. Eur. 5.0** (Flumazenil). A white or almost white crystalline powder. Very slightly soluble in water; freely soluble in dichloromethane; sparingly soluble in methyl alcohol.

## Adverse Effects and Precautions

The adverse effects of flumazenil are generally due to the reversal of benzodiazepine effects and resemble benzodiazepine withdrawal symptoms (see p.690). Nausea, vomiting, dizziness, blurred vision, headache, and flushing may occur. Anxiety, fear, and agitation have been reported following too rapid reversal of sedation. There have been reports of seizures, especially in epileptics. Transient increases in blood pressure and heart rate have been observed. Patients who have received benzodiazepines for prolonged periods are particularly at risk of experiencing withdrawal symptoms and rapid injection of flumazenil should be avoided in such patients.

Because of its short duration of action, patients given flumazenil to reverse benzodiazepine-induced sedation should be kept under close observation; further doses of flumazenil may be necessary. Flumazenil is contra-indicated in patients who are receiving benzodiazepines to control potentially life-threatening conditions and should not be given to epileptic patients who have been receiving benzodiazepines for a prolonged period to control seizures.

In cases of mixed overdose, administration of flumazenil may unmask adverse effects of other psychotropic drugs. In particular, flumazenil should not be used in the presence of severe intoxication with tricyclic and related antidepressants.

Flumazenil should not be given to patients who have received neuromuscular blockers until the effects of neuromuscular blockade have fully cleared. Dosage should be adjusted individually. In high-risk or anxious patients, and after major surgery, it may be preferable to maintain some sedation during the early postoperative period. The risk of raising intracranial pressure in patients with head injuries needs to be borne in mind.

Careful titration of dosage is recommended in hepatic impairment.

◊ Cardiac arrhythmias,[1] sometimes preceded by tonic-clonic (grand mal) seizures[2,3] and occasionally fatal,[2] have been reported in several patients after the use of flumazenil for mixed overdoses with benzodiazepines and other psychotropics. Heart block has also been reported[4] after flumazenil use in a patient who had taken benzodiazepines, paracetamol, nifedipine, and atenolol. Death from refractory tonic-clonic seizures has been reported in a patient[5] after the use of flumazenil for a mixed overdose with a benzodiazepine and a tricyclic antidepressant.

Death from respiratory failure occurred in an 83-year-old woman after sedation with midazolam[6] despite flumazenil administration, although some[7] considered that this did not represent a failure by flumazenil to reverse the depressive effects on respiration of midazolam. Ventricular fibrillation followed by asystole and death has been reported in a patient given flumazenil during weaning from assisted ventilation (a period during which diazepam had been given).[8]


1. Short TG, *et al.* Ventricular arrhythmia precipitated by flumazenil. *BMJ* 1988; **296:** 1070–1.
2. Burr W, *et al.* Death after flumazenil. *BMJ* 1989; **298:** 1713.
3. Marchant B, *et al.* Flumazenil causing convulsions and ventricular tachycardia. *BMJ* 1989; **299:** 860.
4. Herd B, Clarke F. Complete heart block after flumazenil. *Hum Exp Toxicol* 1991; **10:** 289.
5. Haverkos GP, *et al.* Fatal seizures after flumazenil administration in a patient with mixed overdose. *Ann Pharmacother* 1994; **28:** 1347–9.
6. Lim AG. Death after flumazenil. *BMJ* 1989; **299:** 858–9. Correction. *ibid.*: 1531.
7. Birch BRP, Miller RA. Death after flumazenil? *BMJ* 1990; **300:** 467–8.
8. Katz Y, *et al.* Cardiac arrest associated with flumazenil. *BMJ* 1992; **304:** 1415.


**Effects on mental function.** A severe acute psychotic disorder, which developed during treatment with flumazenil in a patient with hepatic encephalopathy, resolved when flumazenil was discontinued.[1]


1. Seebach J, Jost R. Flumazenil-induced psychotic disorder in hepatic encephalopathy. *Lancet* 1992; **339:** 488–9.

## Pharmacokinetics

Flumazenil is well absorbed from the gastrointestinal tract but undergoes extensive first-pass hepatic metabolism and has a systemic bioavailability of about 20%. It is about 50% bound to plasma proteins. After intravenous administration it is extensively metabolised in the liver to the inactive carboxylic acid form, which is excreted predominantly in the urine. The elimination half-life is reported to be about 40 to 80 minutes. In patients with hepatic impairment the clearance of flumazenil is decreased with a resultant prolongation of half-life.

◊ References.


1. Klotz U, *et al.* Pharmacokinetics of the selective benzodiazepine antagonist Ro 15-1788 in man. *Eur J Clin Pharmacol* 1984; **27:** 115–17.
2. Roncari G, *et al.* Pharmacokinetics of the new benzodiazepine antagonist Ro 15-1788 in man following intravenous and oral administration. *Br J Clin Pharmacol* 1986; **22:** 421–8.
3. Breimer LTM, *et al.* Pharmacokinetics and EEG effects of flumazenil in volunteers. *Clin Pharmacokinet* 1991; **20:** 491–6.
4. Jones RDM, *et al.* Pharmacokinetics of flumazenil and midazolam. *Br J Anaesth* 1993; **70:** 286–92.
5. Roncari G, *et al.* Flumazenil kinetics in the elderly. *Eur J Clin Pharmacol* 1993; **45:** 585–7.


## Uses and Administration

Flumazenil is a benzodiazepine antagonist that acts competitively at CNS benzodiazepine receptors. It is used in anaesthesia and intensive care to reverse benzodiazepine-induced sedation; it may also be used to treat benzodiazepine overdosage (but see warnings in Precautions, above, and under Benzodiazepine Antagonism: Overdosage, below).

Flumazenil should be given by slow intravenous injection or infusion.

The usual initial dose for the reversal of benzodiazepine-induced sedation is 200 micrograms given over 15 seconds, followed at intervals of 60 seconds by further doses of 100 to 200 micrograms if required, to a maximum total dose of 1 mg or occasionally 2 mg (usual range, 0.3 to 1 mg). If drowsiness recurs an intravenous infusion may be used, at a rate of 100 to 400 micrograms per hour, adjusted according to response. Alternatively, further doses of up to 1 mg, in boluses of 200 micrograms as above, may be given at 20-minute intervals to a maximum of 3 mg in one hour. Patients at risk from the effects of benzodiazepine reversal, such as those dependent on benzodiazepines, should receive smaller bolus injections of 100 micrograms. A suggested dose for children is 10 micrograms/kg given intravenously over 15 seconds; repeated doses may be given after 45 seconds at 60-second intervals up to a maximum of 50 micrograms/kg or 1 mg, whichever is lower.

The usual initial dose for the management of benzodiazepine overdose is 200 micrograms given intravenously over 30 seconds. A further dose of 300 micrograms can be given after another 30 seconds and can be followed by doses of 500 micrograms at one-minute intervals if required, to a total dose of 3 mg or occasionally 5 mg. If a dose of up to 5 mg produces no response then further doses are unlikely to be effective. If symptoms of intoxication recur, repeated doses may be given at 20-minute intervals; not more than 1 mg should be given at any one time and not more than 3 mg in one hour. As before a slower rate of administration may be used for 'at risk' patients.

If signs of overstimulation occur during the use of flumazenil, then diazepam or midazolam may be given by slow intravenous injection.

◊ General references.


1. Brogden RN, Goa KL. Flumazenil: a reappraisal of its pharmacological properties and therapeutic efficacy as a benzodiazepine antagonist. *Drugs* 1991; **42:** 1061–89.
2. Hoffman EJ, Warren EW. Flumazenil: a benzodiazepine antagonist. *Clin Pharm* 1993; **12:** 641–56.
3. Krenzelok EP. Judicious use of flumazenil. *Clin Pharm* 1993; **12:** 691–2.


**Benzodiazepine antagonism.** Flumazenil is a specific benzodiazepine antagonist that binds competitively with benzodiazepine receptors. Flumazenil reverses the centrally mediated effects of benzodiazepines. Its effects are evident within a few minutes of intravenous administration, even after substantial doses of benzodiazepines, and last for up to 3 hours depending on the dose and on the characteristics of the benzodiazepine intoxication. In patients who have received benzodiazepines for prolonged periods, flumazenil may precipitate withdrawal symptoms.

SEDATION. Flumazenil reduces postoperative sedation and amnesia following induction or maintenance of general anaesthesia with benzodiazepines. However, use in some patients has increased analgesic requirements and some have experienced anxiety. Reversal of benzodiazepine sedation and amnesia may also be useful in some patients after minor surgery or diagnostic procedures. However, although flumazenil may antagonise the obvious effects of sedation, higher cognitive functions may still be impaired and the patient may be unfit to be discharged safely unaccompanied.[1] There is also a risk that sedation may recur if long-acting benzodiazepines have been used.[2-4] Patients who might benefit from sedation reversal include those at increased risk of postoperative complications, those in whom postoperative neurological evaluation would be beneficial, and those who are particularly sensitive to the effects of benzodiazepines.[2,3] Although experience with flumazenil in children is limited, it appears to be well tolerated and effective.[5] In an intensive care unit, flumazenil may assist in weaning sedated patients from mechanical ventilation and in extubation,[3,4,6,7] but multiple doses or an infusion may be required due to the short duration of action.[6]

OVERDOSAGE. Flumazenil may be used as an adjunct in the management of benzodiazepine overdose including overdose involving multiple agents. However, its use may unmask the effects of other intoxicants,[2-4,6-8] and since benzodiazepine overdose is rarely lethal and may even protect against the toxicity of other drugs, flumazenil should be used with great caution in mixed overdose, particularly when involving tricyclic antidepressants.[9] Repeated doses of flumazenil may be required to maintain consciousness depending on the benzodiazepine responsible and the magnitude of the overdose.


1. Sanders LD, *et al.* Reversal of benzodiazepine sedation with the antagonist flumazenil. *Br J Anaesth* 1991; **66:** 445–53.
2. Anonymous. Flumazenil. *Lancet* 1988; **ii:** 828–30.
3. Klotz U, Kanto J. Pharmacokinetics and clinical use of flumazenil (Ro 15-1788). *Clin Pharmacokinet* 1988; **14:** 1–12.
4. Karavokiros KAT, Tsipis GB. Flumazenil: a benzodiazepine antagonist. *DICP Ann Pharmacother* 1990; **24:** 976–81.
5. Shannon M, *et al.* Safety and efficacy of flumazenil in the reversal of benzodiazepine-induced conscious sedation. *J Pediatr* 1997; **131:** 582–6.
6. Amrein R, *et al.* Flumazenil in benzodiazepine antagonism: actions and clinical use in intoxications and anaesthesiology. *Med Toxicol* 1987; **2:** 411–29.
7. Anonymous. Flumazenil—the first benzodiazepine antagonist. *Drug Ther Bull* 1989; **27:** 39–40.
8. Weinbroum AA, *et al.* A risk-benefit assessment of flumazenil in the management of benzodiazepine overdose. *Drug Safety* 1997; **17:** 181–96.
9. Hoffman RS, Goldfrank LR. The poisoned patient with altered consciousness: controversies in the use of a 'coma cocktail'. *JAMA* 1995; **274:** 562–9.


**Hepatic encephalopathy.** Flumazenil has been tried in hepatic encephalopathy (p.1243) because of the suspected role of benzodiazepine-like agonists in the pathogenesis of the disorder.[1,2] However, benefits have generally been modest, and a meta-analysis[3] concluded that flumazenil did produce short-term improvement of hepatic encephalopathy but had no effect on recovery or survival; it might be considered for patients with chronic liver disease and hepatic encephalopathy but routine clinical use was not recommended.


1. Grimm G, *et al.* Improvement of hepatic encephalopathy treated with flumazenil. *Lancet* 1988; **ii:** 1392–4.
2. Basile AS, *et al.* The pathogenesis and treatment of hepatic encephalopathy: evidence for the involvement of benzodiazepine receptor ligands. *Pharmacol Rev* 1991; **43:** 27–71.
3. Als-Nielsen B, *et al.* Benzodiazepine receptor antagonists for hepatic encephalopathy. Available in The Cochrane Library; Issue 2. Chichester: John Wiley; 2004.


**Non-benzodiazepine antagonism.** Flumazenil blocks the effects of non-benzodiazepines, such as zopiclone and zolpidem, that act via the benzodiazepine receptor. In a double-blind study[1] in healthy subjects, flumazenil rapidly antagonised clinical sedation induced by zolpidem.


1. Patat A, *et al.* Flumazenil antagonizes the central effects of zolpidem, an imidazopyridine hypnotic. *Clin Pharmacol Ther* 1994; **56:** 430–6.


## Preparations

**Proprietary Preparations** (details are given in Part 3)
***Arg.:*** Fadaflumaz; Flumage; Flumanovag; Flumazen; Fluxifarm; Lanexat; ***Austral.:*** Anexate; ***Austria:*** Anexate; ***Belg.:*** Anexate; ***Braz.:*** Lanexat; ***Canad.:*** Anexate; ***Chile:*** Lanexat; ***Denm.:*** Lanexat; ***Fin.:*** Lanexat; ***Fr.:*** Anexate; ***Ger.:*** Anexate; ***Gr.:*** Anexate; ***Hong Kong:*** Anexate; ***Irl.:*** Anexate; ***Israel:*** Anexate; ***Ital.:*** Anexate; ***Mex.:*** Lanexat; ***Neth.:*** Anexate; ***Norw.:*** Anexate; ***NZ:*** Anexate; ***Port.:*** Anexate; ***S.Afr.:*** Anexate; ***Singapore:*** Anexate; ***Spain:*** Anexate; ***Swed.:*** Lanexat; ***Switz.:*** Anexate; ***Thai.:*** Anexate; ***UK:*** Anexate; ***USA:*** Romazicon.

## Fomepizole *(BAN, USAN, rINN)*

Fomepizol; 4-Methylpyrazole; 4-MP. 4-Methyl-1*H*-pyrazole.
$C_4H_6N_2$ = 82.10.
*CAS — 7554-65-6.*
*ATC — V03AB34.*

### Profile

Fomepizole is an inhibitor of alcohol dehydrogenase. It is used for the treatment of poisoning by ethylene glycol (p.1685) or methyl alcohol (p.1475), which are converted to toxic metabolites by alcohol dehydrogenase. Fomepizole is given in a loading dose of 15 mg/kg followed by 10 mg/kg every 12 hours for 4 doses, then 15 mg/kg every 12 hours until serum concentrations of ethylene glycol or methyl alcohol are less than 20 mg/100 mL. All doses should be given by intravenous infusion over 30 minutes.

◊ References.


1. Burns MJ, *et al.* Treatment of methanol poisoning with intravenous 4-methylpyrazole. *Ann Emerg Med* 1997; **30:** 829–32.
2. Baum CR, *et al.* Fomepizole treatment of ethylene glycol poisoning in an infant. *Pediatrics* 2000; **106:** 1489–91.
3. Brent J, *et al.* Fomepizole for the treatment of methanol poisoning. *N Engl J Med* 2001; **344:** 424–9.
4. Battistella M. Fomepizole as an antidote for ethylene glycol poisoning. *Ann Pharmacother* 2002; **36:** 1085–9.


### Preparations

**Proprietary Preparations** (details are given in Part 3)
***Canad.:*** Antizol; ***Israel:*** Antizol; ***UK:*** Antizol; ***USA:*** Antizol.

## Fuller's Earth

Terra Fullonica; Tierra de Fuller.
*CAS — 8031-18-3.*

### Profile

Fuller's earth consists largely of montmorillonite, a native hydrated aluminium silicate, with which very finely divided calcite (calcium carbonate) may be associated. It is an adsorbent which is used in dusting powders, toilet powders, and lotions. Fuller's earth of high adsorptive capacity is used in industry as a clarifying and filtering medium.

It has been used in the treatment of paraquat poisoning (p.1508). A 15% suspension is commonly used and an initial oral dose of about 100 g may be followed by further doses of about 50 g every 2 hours for 3 doses. Magnesium sulfate or mannitol may be given with the first dose to promote diarrhoea and empty the gut.

### Preparations

**Proprietary Preparations** (details are given in Part 3)
**Multi-ingredient:** ***Braz.:*** Camomila†.

## Glucagon *(BAN, rINN)*

Glucagón; Glucagonum; HGF. His-Ser-Gln-Gly-Thr-Phe-Thr-Ser-Asp-Tyr-Ser-Lys-Tyr-Leu-Asp-Ser-Arg-Arg-Ala-Gln-Asp-Phe-Val-Gln-Trp-Leu-Met-Asn-Thr.
$C_{153}H_{225}N_{43}O_{49}S$ = 3482.7.
*CAS — 16941-32-5.*
*ATC — H04AA01.*

**Pharmacopoeias.** In *Eur.* (see p.vi) and *US.*

**Ph. Eur. 5.0** (Glucagon). A polypeptide hormone obtained from beef or pork pancreas. A white or almost white powder. Practically insoluble in water and in most organic solvents; it dissolves in dilute mineral acids and in dilute solutions of alkali hydroxides. Store in airtight containers at a temperature below 8° and preferably at −20°.

**Ph. Eur. 5.0** (Glucagon, Human; Glucagonum Humanum). A polypeptide having the same structure as the hormone produced by the alpha cells of the human pancreas. It is produced by a method based on recombinant DNA technology. A white or almost white powder. Practically insoluble in water and in most organic solvents; soluble in dilute mineral acids and in dilute solutions of alkali hydroxides. Store in airtight containers at a temperature below −15°. Protect from light.

**USP 27** (Glucagon). A polypeptide hormone obtained from porcine and bovine pancreas glands. A fine, white or faintly coloured, practically odourless, crystalline powder. Soluble in dilute alkali and acid solutions; insoluble in most organic solvents. Store under nitrogen in airtight glass containers at a temperature of 2° to 8°.

### Adverse Effects

Nausea and vomiting may occur following administration of glucagon. Hypersensitivity reactions and hypokalaemia have also been reported.

### Precautions

Glucagon should generally not be given to patients with phaeochromocytoma since it can cause a release of catecholamines producing marked hypertension. Glucagon should be given with care to patients with insulinoma as it may induce hypoglycaemia due to its insulin-releasing effect. Glucagon was formerly used to diagnose phaeochromocytoma and insulinoma but this use has been largely abandoned. Caution is also required when it is being used as a diagnostic aid in diabetic patients or in elderly patients with heart disease.

Glucagon is not effective in patients with marked depletion of liver glycogen stores, as in starvation, adrenal insufficiency, alcohol-induced hypoglycaemia, or chronic hypoglycaemia.

## Interactions

**Warfarin.** For a report of glucagon enhancing the anticoagulant effect of warfarin, see p.1027.

## Pharmacokinetics

Glucagon has a plasma half-life of about 3 to 6 minutes. It is inactivated in the liver, kidneys, and plasma.

**Bioavailability.** In a study in healthy subjects and diabetic patients the bioavailability after intranasal administration of glucagon was about 30% of that following intramuscular administration.[1] However the apparent half-life after intramuscular injection was 28.6 and 31.4 minutes respectively in the two groups, 3 to 4 times longer than that after either intravenous or intranasal administration, possibly due to slow release of glucagon from the injection site. It was also recognised that the quicker onset of activity with the intranasal route might be of value in an emergency.

1. Pontiroli AE, *et al.* Pharmacokinetics of intranasal, intramuscular and intravenous glucagon in healthy subjects and diabetic patients. *Eur J Clin Pharmacol* 1993; **45:** 555–8.

## Uses and Administration

Glucagon is a polypeptide hormone that is produced by the alpha cells of the pancreatic islets of Langerhans. It is a hyperglycaemic which mobilises glucose by activating hepatic glycogenolysis. It can to a lesser extent stimulate the secretion of pancreatic insulin. Glucagon is given as the hydrochloride; doses are usually expressed as glucagon (note that 1 unit is equivalent to 1 mg of glucagon). Glucagon is used in the treatment of severe hypoglycaemic reactions when the patient cannot take glucose by mouth and intravenous glucose is not feasible. It is given by subcutaneous, intramuscular, or intravenous injection in a dose of 1 mg (or 500 micrograms in patients under about 25 kg bodyweight). If there is no response within 10 minutes, intravenous glucose should be given, although there is no contra-indication to repeating the dose of glucagon. Once the patient has responded sufficiently to take carbohydrate by mouth this should be given to restore liver glycogen stores and prevent secondary hypoglycaemia.

As glucagon reduces the motility of the gastrointestinal tract it is used as a diagnostic aid in gastrointestinal examinations. The route of administration and dose is dependent upon the diagnostic procedure. A dose of 1 to 2 mg administered intramuscularly has an onset of action of 4 to 15 minutes and a duration of effect of 10 to 40 minutes; 0.2 to 2 mg given intravenously produces an effect within 1 minute that lasts for 5 to 25 minutes.

Glucagon possesses positive cardiac inotropic activity but is not generally considered suitable for heart failure. However, as it can bypass blocked beta receptors, it is used in the treatment of beta-blocker overdosage, see Cardiovascular Effects, below.

Intranasal preparations have been studied.

**Administration.** References to intranasal administration of glucagon in healthy subjects and diabetics.

1. Freychet L, *et al.* Effect of intranasal glucagon on blood glucose levels in healthy subjects and hypoglycaemic patients with insulin-dependent diabetes. *Lancet* 1988; **i:** 1364–6.
2. Pontiroli AE, *et al.* Intranasal glucagon is a remedy for hypoglycemia: studies in healthy subjects and type I diabetic patients. *Diabetes Care* 1989; **12:** 604–8.
3. Pontiroli AE, *et al.* Nasal administration of glucagon and human calcitonin to healthy subjects: a comparison of powders and spray solutions and of different enhancing agents. *Eur J Clin Pharmacol* 1989; **37:** 427–30.
4. Hvidberg A, *et al.* Glucose recovery after intranasal glucagon during hypoglycaemia in man. *Eur J Clin Pharmacol* 1994; **46:** 15–17.
5. Teshima D, *et al.* Nasal glucagon delivery using microcrystalline cellulose in healthy volunteers. *Int J Pharm* 2002; **233:** 61–6.

**Cardiovascular effects.** Glucagon has chronotropic and inotropic effects due to its ability to raise cyclic AMP concentrations independently of a response to catecholamines. It is used in the management of beta-blocker overdosage (see p.870); doses of 2 to 10 mg (or 50 to 150 micrograms/kg in children) by intravenous injection, followed by an infusion of 50 micrograms/kg per hour, have been suggested.

Glucagon may be effective in the management of anaphylactic reactions to contrast media in patients receiving beta blockers.[1,2] A dramatic improvement in refractory hypotension during an anaphylactic reaction to contrast media was described in a 75-year-old man receiving beta blockers following intravenous administration of glucagon.[3]

While it is not regarded as standard treatment for overdosage with calcium-channel blockers, glucagon 10 mg intravenously has been reported to be beneficial.[4]

1. Lieber JJ. Risk for anaphylactoid reaction from contrast media. *Ann Intern Med* 1991; **115:** 985.
2. Lang DM, *et al.* Risk for anaphylactoid reaction from contrast media. *Ann Intern Med* 1991; **115:** 985.
3. Zaloga GP, *et al.* Glucagon reversal of hypotension in a case of anaphylactic shock. *Ann Intern Med* 1986; **105:** 65–6.
4. Walter FG, *et al.* Amelioration of nifedipine poisoning associated with glucagon therapy. *Ann Emerg Med* 1993; **22:** 1234–7.

**Diagnosis and testing.** Glucagon stimulates secretion of growth hormone and cortisol (hydrocortisone) and has been used both alone[1,2] and with a beta blocker[3,4] as a test of pituitary function. The test is contra-indicated in patients with heart block, asthma, heart failure, and diabetes mellitus,[4] and severe secondary hypoglycaemia and death has been reported in a 2-year-old child after a glucagon test for growth hormone secretion.[5] Reviews of growth hormone provocation tests[6-8] have discussed the merits of the glucagon test and compared it with others such as the insulin-tolerance test.

1. Milner RDG, Burns EC. Investigation of suspected growth hormone deficiency. *Arch Dis Child* 1982; **57:** 944–7.
2. Anonymous. Testing anterior pituitary function. *Lancet* 1986; **i:** 839–41.
3. Colle M, *et al.* Betaxolol and propranolol in glucagon stimulation of growth hormone. *Arch Dis Child* 1984; **59:** 670–2.
4. Abboud CF. Laboratory diagnosis of hypopituitarism. *Mayo Clin Proc* 1986; **61:** 35–48.
5. Shah A, *et al.* Hazards of pharmacologic tests of growth hormone secretion in childhood. *BMJ* 1992; **304:** 173–4.
6. Hindmarsh PC, Swift PGF. An assessment of growth hormone provocation tests. *Arch Dis Child* 1995; **72:** 362–8.
7. Gomez JM, *et al.* Growth hormone release after glucagon as a reliable test of growth hormone assessment in adults. *Clin Endocrinol (Oxf)* 2002; **56:** 329–34.
8. Abs R. Update on the diagnosis of GH deficiency in adults. *Eur J Endocrinol* 2003; **148:** S3–S8.

**Gastrointestinal disorders.** The relaxant effect of glucagon on smooth muscle has been used to stop hiccups caused by distension of the gallbladder[1] and to facilitate passage of swallowed foreign bodies and impacted food boluses which have become lodged in the lower oesophagus.[2,3] Glucagon has also been tried in the management of biliary colic.[4]

1. Gardner AMN. Glucagon stops hiccups. *BMJ* 1985; **290:** 822.
2. Cooke MW, Glucksman EE. Swallowed coins. *BMJ* 1991; **302:** 1607.
3. Farrugia M, *et al.* Radiological treatment of acute oesophageal food impaction. *Br J Hosp Med* 1995; **54:** 410–11.
4. Grossi E, *et al.* Different pharmacological approaches to the treatment of acute biliary colic. *Curr Ther Res* 1986; **40:** 876–82.

**Hypoglycaemia.** Hypoglycaemia most commonly occurs in diabetic patients, particularly those receiving insulin therapy. Other rare causes include alcohol ingestion and tumours such as insulinomas. Neonatal hypoglycaemia occurs in small-for-gestational-age infants or infants of diabetic mothers. Persistent or recurrent hypoglycaemia in neonates is usually due to an endocrine or metabolic disorder, such as nesidioblastosis.

Glucose is the treatment of choice for **acute** hypoglycaemia since it corrects the problem at source. Glucagon is generally used as an alternative to parenteral glucose in hypoglycaemic patients whose consciousness is impaired and who cannot therefore take glucose by mouth, or in other situations where glucose administration is not possible. Some have advocated the use of glucagon as a first-line treatment in patients requiring parenteral therapy since it is more convenient and easier to give than parenteral glucose.[1] However, this does not seem to be the general view. The action of glucagon relies upon the patient having adequate hepatic glycogen stores, which may not always be the case; for example, glycogen stores are depleted in patients with alcohol-induced hypoglycaemia or with insulinoma, and glucagon is not effective.

Hypoglycaemia in neonates is usually managed by adjusting the enteral feeds or by administration of parenteral glucose in symptomatic infants. Glucagon may be used if parenteral glucose is not effective or cannot be given.[2,3]

Continuous infusion of glucagon was reported to be effective in the management of hypoglycaemia in a patient with an extrapancreatic tumour.[4] **Intractable** hypoglycaemia (such as that resulting from excessive endogenous insulin production from islet cell tumours or hyperplasia) is usually treated with diazoxide (see p.894).

1. Gibbins RL. Treating hypoglycaemia in general practice. *BMJ* 1993; **306:** 600–1.
2. Carter PE, *et al.* Glucagon for hypoglycaemia in infants small for gestational age. *Arch Dis Child* 1988; **63:** 1264.
3. Williams AF. Hypoglycaemia of the newborn: a review. *Bull WHO* 1997; **75:** 261–90.
4. Samaan NA, *et al.* Successful treatment of hypoglycemia using glucagon in a patient with an extrapancreatic tumor. *Ann Intern Med* 1990; **113:** 404–6.

**Liver disorders.** For references to the use of glucagon with insulin in the treatment of liver disorders, see under Insulin, p.341.

## Preparations

***BP 2003:*** Glucagon Injection;
***USP 27:*** Glucagon for Injection.

**Proprietary Preparations** (details are given in Part 3)
***Arg.:*** GlucaGen; ***Austral.:*** GlucaGen; ***Austria:*** GlucaGen; ***Belg.:*** GlucaGen; ***Denm.:*** GlucaGen; ***Fin.:*** GlucaGen; ***Fr.:*** GlucaGen; ***Ger.:*** GlucaGen; ***Gr.:*** GlucaGen; ***Hong Kong:*** GlucaGen; ***India:*** GlucaGen; ***Irl.:*** GlucaGen; ***Israel:*** GlucaGen; ***Ital.:*** GlucaGen; ***Malaysia:*** GlucaGen; ***NZ:*** GlucaGen; ***Port.:*** GlucaGen; ***S.Afr.:*** GlucaGen; ***Singapore:*** GlucaGen; ***Switz.:*** GlucaGen; ***Thai.:*** GlucaGen†; ***UK:*** GlucaGen; ***USA:*** GlucaGen.

## Glutathione

Glutatión; GSH. *N*-(*N*-L-γ-Glutamyl-L-cysteinyl)glycine.
$C_{10}H_{17}N_3O_6S$ = 307.3.
*CAS — 70-18-8.*
*ATC — V03AB32.*

### Profile

Glutathione is an endogenous peptide with antioxidant and other metabolic functions. It has been used in the treatment of poisoning with a number of compounds including heavy metals. Glutathione sodium has been used similarly. Glutathione has also been tried in idiopathic pulmonary fibrosis and peripheral vascular disorders, and has been used in other conditions such as liver disorders, corneal disorders, eczema, and for mitigation of the adverse effects of antineoplastic therapy including the neurotoxicity of cisplatin and oxaliplatin.

**Antineoplastic toxicity.** Glutathione has been reported to reduce the incidence of neurotoxicity induced by cisplatin therapy. In a double-blind, randomised trial[1] in 50 patients receiving cisplatin for advanced gastric cancer, administration of glutathione significantly reduced the incidence of neuropathy assessed within one week of completing cisplatin therapy. There did not appear to be any reduction in cytotoxic activity. Similar benefit was observed in a randomised, double-blind, placebo-controlled trial involving 52 patients receiving oxaliplatin.[2]

1. Cascinu S, *et al.* Neuroprotective effect of reduced glutathione on cisplatin-based chemotherapy in advanced gastric cancer: a randomized double-blind placebo-controlled trial. *J Clin Oncol* 1995; **13:** 26–32.
2. Cascinu S, *et al.* Neuroprotective effect of reduced glutathione on oxaliplatin-based chemotherapy in advanced colorectal cancer: a randomized, double-blind, placebo-controlled trial. *J Clin Oncol* 2002; **20:** 3478–83.

**Lung disorders.** Glutathione is an important extracellular antioxidant in the lung and high concentrations are found in lung epithelial lining fluid. A deficiency of glutathione may contribute to the epithelial damage that occurs in cryptogenic fibrosing alveolitis (idiopathic pulmonary fibrosis). Preliminary studies have demonstrated beneficial biochemical results with glutathione delivered by aerosol in 10 patients with cryptogenic fibrosing alveolitis,[1] but no clinical effects have been reported.

1. Borok Z, *et al.* Effect of glutathione aerosol on oxidant-antioxidant imbalance in idiopathic pulmonary fibrosis. *Lancet* 1991; **338:** 215–16.

### Preparations

**Proprietary Preparations** (details are given in Part 3)
***Hong Kong:*** TAD; ***Ital.:*** Eudon; Glukot†; Glutamed†; Glutanil; Glutasan†; Gluthion; Glutoxil†; Ipatox; Maglut; Novatox†; Reglumax; Ridutox; Ribon; Scavenger; TAD; Tationil; Thioxene; ***Spain:*** Tition†; ***USA:*** Cachexon.

**Multi-ingredient:** ***Austral.:*** BSS Plus; ***Austria:*** BSS Plus; ***Belg.:*** BSS Plus†; ***Canad.:*** BSS Plus; ***Fr.:*** BSS Compose; ***Ger.:*** BSS Plus; ***Hong Kong:*** BSS Plus; ***Israel:*** BSS Plus; ***Malaysia:*** BSS Plus; ***Singapore:*** BSS Plus; ***Switz.:*** BSS Plus; ***Thai.:*** BSS Plus; ***UK:*** BSS Plus†; ***USA:*** B-Salt Forte†; BSS Plus.

## Haem Derivatives

Heme Derivatives; Hemo, derivados del grupo.
*ATC — B06AB01 (Haematin).*

### Profile

Haem is the iron protoporphyrin constituent of haemoglobin and is responsible for its colour and oxygen-carrying capacity. It is used in the management of porphyrias (below). Haem is administered intravenously as its derivatives, although there is some confusion over their terminology. The names haematin (hematin) and haemin (hemin) have been used interchangeably although chemically haematin is the hydroxy derivative, formed by the reaction of haemin and sodium carbonate in solution. The arginine salt (haem arginate; haemin arginate; heme arginate) is reported to be more stable.

Haem arginate is used alone or with tin-protoporphyrin (p.1756) in the treatment of acute intermittent porphyria. It is given by slow intravenous infusion in a dose of 3 mg/kg daily for 4 days, infused over at least 30 minutes.

Haematin is used intravenously for the amelioration of acute intermittent porphyria associated with the menstrual cycle in patients unresponsive to other therapy. It is given in a dose of 1 to 4 mg/kg daily for 3 to 14 days as an intravenous infusion over 10 to 15 minutes.

Phlebitis may occur after injection of haematin into small arm veins.

**Porphyrias.** The porphyrias are a group of inherited and acquired disorders of haem biosynthesis. Deficiencies occur in specific enzymes leading to the accumulation of different porphyrins and porphyrin precursors. They are generally classified as acute or non-acute, reflecting their clinical presentation, or as hepatic or erythropoietic, depending on the site of the enzyme defect. The three most common forms are acute intermittent porphyria, porphyria cutanea tarda, and erythropoietic protoporphyria.

ACUTE PORPHYRIAS. These are inherited disorders characterised by the accumulation of porphyrin precursors, leading to acute attacks of neurovisceral symptoms. The most common form is *acute intermittent porphyria* (acute hepatic porphyria); *variegate porphyria* and *hereditary coproporphyria* are generally less common forms in which there is accumulation of both porphyrin precursors and porphyrins, leading to acute attacks in conjunction with cutaneous symptoms similar to those seen in non-acute porphyrias (see below).

In acute porphyrias, the enzyme defect is not complete and only becomes apparent when demand for hepatic haem is increased by drugs, hormones, or nutritional factors. Attacks are rare before puberty and the disorder may remain latent in many patients. The presenting symptom is most commonly severe abdominal pain; other gastrointestinal symptoms such as nausea and vomiting also occur, along with autonomic effects including hypertension, tachycardia, sweating, pallor, and pyrexia. Convulsions may occur at the peak of an attack and may persist between attacks. Neuropathy leads to weakness and paralysis and may progress rapidly to respiratory distress. Psychiatric symptoms are also common, particularly agitation, anxiety, and behavioural disturbances. Attacks are usually precipitated by drugs, alcohol, steroid hormones, reduced caloric intake, or infection. They typically last for several days and are followed by complete recovery, although in some patients chronic abdominal pain may persist without other symptoms.

The primary management of an attack is to remove precipitants and to provide intensive support. *Symptomatic treatment* is complicated by the wide range of drugs that may precipitate porphyria. High doses of parenteral opioids may be required for pain and there is a danger of addiction occurring, particularly if attacks are frequent or if pain persists between attacks. Phenothiazines such as chlorpromazine are useful to control nausea and agitation and their sedative effect may also be beneficial. High doses of propranolol may be required for cardiovascular symptoms. Assisted ventilation may be necessary. Convulsions usually disappear as the attack resolves; management of patients who experience convulsions between attacks is a therapeutic problem since many antiepileptics are porphyrinogenic (see Porphyria, p.353). *Specific therapy* is aimed at suppressing the haem biosynthetic pathway. A high carbohydrate intake should be ensured in all patients to suppress precursor production; this is given orally to prevent fluid overload, but intravenous glucose may be required in patients who are vomiting. Haem is also effective; it is given as haematin or as haem arginate and tin-protoporphyrin may be used in conjunction. *Prevention* of attacks involves avoiding drugs that precipitate porphyria and maintaining an adequate carbohydrate intake. Gonadorelin analogues, such as buserelin, may have a role in preventing attacks related to the menstrual cycle.

NON-ACUTE PORPHYRIAS. These are characterised by the accumulation of porphyrins and usually present with cutaneous symptoms, although porphyrins also accumulate in the liver and liver damage commonly occurs. *Porphyria cutanea tarda* (cutaneous hepatic porphyria) is the most common form of porphyria. It is usually an acquired disorder and in most cases there is a history of moderate or heavy alcohol intake. There is usually a raised serum-iron concentration and oestrogen administration has also been implicated. The main clinical symptom is cutaneous photosensitivity leading to bullous dermatosis, pruritus, and skin fragility, in areas exposed to sunlight. *Management* involves protecting the skin from sunlight and trauma and avoiding causative agents such as alcohol and iron. Sunscreen preparations must be based on zinc oxide or titanium dioxide to be effective. Reduction of serum-iron concentrations by phlebotomy is effective in most patients and should be carried out at weekly intervals until remission occurs; desferrioxamine is an alternative method to aid iron excretion but is less effective. Chloroquine and hydroxychloroquine have also been used and may be effective where phlebotomy is contra-indicated; they appear to act by complexing with porphyrins and increasing their excretion, but low doses are necessary to avoid exacerbating the condition. Erythropoietin may be given in patients with renal failure who are too anaemic for phlebotomy and who cannot excrete chloroquine.

*Erythropoietic protoporphyria* is a less common non-acute porphyria and is an inherited disorder leading to accumulation of protoporphyrin. Symptoms are cutaneous and there is an acute reaction to sunlight leading to urticaria, pruritus, swelling, redness, and a severe burning sensation; liver damage may also occur. *Management* involves protection of the skin, as for porphyria cutanea tarda. Betacarotene produces benefit in most patients with photosensitivity and canthaxanthin may also be used. Haem administration, as haematin or haem arginate, may be beneficial in suppressing protoporphyrin production. Colestyramine and activated charcoal reduce protoporphyrin levels by interrupting enterohepatic recycling; they also bind other porphyrins and may have a role in rare forms of porphyria such as *congenital erythropoietic porphyria*.

References.


1. Todd DJ. Erythropoietic protoporphyria. *Br J Dermatol* 1994; **131:** 751–66.
2. Elder GH, *et al.* The acute porphyrias. *Lancet* 1997; **349:** 1613–17.
3. Gorchein A. Drug treatment in acute porphyria. *Br J Clin Pharmacol* 1997; **44:** 427–34.
4. Murphy GM. The cutaneous porphyrias: a review. *Br J Dermatol* 1999; **140:** 573–81.
5. Thadani H, *et al.* Diagnosis and management of porphyria. *BMJ* 2000; **320:** 1647–51.
6. Sarkany RPE. The management of porphyria cutanea tarda. *Clin Exp Dermatol* 2001; **26:** 225–32.


◊ References to haem derivatives in the management of porphyrias.


1. Herrick AL, *et al.* Controlled trial of haem arginate in acute hepatic porphyria. *Lancet* 1989; **i:** 1295–7.
2. Dover SB, *et al.* Haem-arginate plus tin-protoporphyrin for acute hepatic porphyria. *Lancet* 1991; **338:** 263.
3. Mustajoki P, Nordmann Y. Early administration of heme arginate for acute porphyric attacks. *Arch Intern Med* 1993; **153:** 2004–8.


## Preparations

**Proprietary Preparations** (details are given in Part 3)
***Austral.:*** Panhematin†; ***Fin.:*** Normosang; ***Fr.:*** Normosang; ***Ger.:*** Normosang†; ***Ital.:*** Normosang; ***Spain:*** Normosang; ***Swed.:*** Normosang; ***Switz.:*** Normosang; ***UK:*** Normosang; ***USA:*** Panhematin.

---

## Lofexidine Hydrochloride *(BANM, USAN, rINNM)*

Ba-168; Hidrocloruro de lofexidina; MDL-14042; MDL-14042A; RMI-14042A. 2-[1-(2,6-Dichlorophenoxy)ethyl]-2-imidazoline hydrochloride.

$C_{11}H_{12}Cl_2N_2O,HCl = 295.6.$

*CAS — 31036-80-3 (lofexidine); 21498-08-8 (lofexidine hydrochloride).*

*ATC — N07BC04.*

### Adverse Effects

Lofexidine has central alpha-adrenergic effects and may cause drowsiness, dryness of the mouth, throat, and nose, hypotension, and bradycardia. Symptoms of overdosage with lofexidine include sedation and coma.

Sudden withdrawal of lofexidine may produce rebound hypertension.

### Precautions

Lofexidine should be used with caution in patients with cerebrovascular disease, ischaemic heart disease including recent myocardial infarction, bradycardia, renal impairment, or a history of depression.

It may cause drowsiness and if affected, patients should not drive or operate machinery.

Withdrawal of lofexidine therapy should be gradual over 2 to 4 days or more to reduce the risk of rebound hypertension.

### Interactions

Lofexidine may enhance the central depressant effects of sedative agents including alcohol. Tricyclic antidepressants may reduce the efficacy of lofexidine.

### Uses and Administration

Lofexidine is an alpha$_2$-adrenoceptor agonist structurally related to clonidine (p.885). It has antihypertensive activity, but is used mainly in the control of opioid withdrawal symptoms.

In opioid withdrawal, lofexidine is given as the hydrochloride in an initial dose of 200 micrograms twice daily by mouth. The dose may be increased gradually by 200 to 400 micrograms daily to a maximum of 2.4 mg daily. After 7 to 10 days, or longer in some cases, treatment is withdrawn gradually over at least 2 to 4 days.

**Opioid dependence.** The use of lofexidine in the treatment of opioid dependence (p.71) has been reviewed.[1] It appears to be a useful addition to the range of treatments available, and may be more acceptable to patients than clonidine, though perhaps less acceptable than methadone.


1. Strang J, *et al.* Lofexidine for opiate detoxification: review of recent randomised and open controlled trials. *Am J Addict* 1999; **8:** 337–48.


### Preparations

**Proprietary Preparations** (details are given in Part 3)
***UK:*** Britlofex.

---

## Mesna *(BAN, USAN, rINN)*

D-7093; Mesnum; UCB-3983. Sodium 2-mercaptoethanesulphonate.

$C_2H_5NaO_3S_2 = 164.2.$

*CAS — 19767-45-4.*

*ATC — R05CB05; V03AF01.*

**Pharmacopoeias.** In *Eur.* (see p.vi).

**Ph. Eur. 5.0** (Mesna). A white or slightly yellow, hygroscopic, crystalline powder. Freely soluble in water; slightly soluble in alcohol; practically insoluble in cyclohexane. A 10% solution in water has a pH of 4.5 to 6.0. Store in airtight containers.

**Stability.** There was no evidence of degradation of mesna when stored in solution with ifosfamide in polyethylene infusion bags at room temperature for 7 hours[1] or in polypropylene syringes at room temperature or at 4° for 4 weeks.[2] However, in the latter study ifosfamide concentrations fell by about 3% after 7 days and 12% after 4 weeks at both temperatures.


1. Shaw IC, Rose JWP. Infusion of ifosphamide plus mesna. *Lancet* 1984; **i:** 1353–4.
2. Rowland CG, *et al.* Infusion of ifosfamide plus mesna. *Lancet* 1984; **ii:** 468.


### Adverse Effects and Precautions

Adverse effects which may occur after use of mesna include gastrointestinal effects, headache, fatigue, limb pains, depression, irritability, hypotension (but see below), tachycardia, and skin rash. Bronchospasm has been reported after administration by nebuliser.

Mesna may produce a false positive result in diagnostic tests for urinary ketones and may produce a false positive or false negative result in diagnostic tests for urinary erythrocytes.

**Effects on the blood pressure.** Severe hypertension occurred after use of mesna either alone or with ifosfamide.[1]


1. Gilleece MH, Davies JM. Mesna therapy and hypertension. *DICP Ann Pharmacother* 1991; **25:** 867.


**Effects on the nervous system.** For reports of severe encephalopathy in patients receiving mesna and ifosfamide, see p.561.

**Hypersensitivity.** Hypersensitivity reactions including rash, fever, nausea, facial and periorbital oedema, ulceration of mucous membranes, and tachycardia have been attributed to mesna.[1-4]


1. Lang E, Goos M. Hypersensitivity to mesna. *Lancet* 1985; **ii:** 329.
2. Seidel A, *et al.* Allergic reactions to mesna. *Lancet* 1991; **338:** 381.
3. Gross WL, *et al.* Allergic reactions to mesna. *Lancet* 1991; **338:** 381–2.
4. D'Cruz D, *et al.* Allergic reactions to mesna. *Lancet* 1991; **338:** 705–6.


### Pharmacokinetics

Mesna is rapidly excreted in the urine after oral or intravenous administration as the unchanged drug and as the metabolite mesna disulfide (dimesna). The half-lives of mesna and dimesna are reported to be about 20 minutes and 70 minutes respectively.

◊ References.


1. Burkert H, *et al.* Bioavailability of orally administered mesna. *Arzneimittelforschung* 1984; **34:** 1597–1600.
2. James CA, *et al.* Pharmacokinetics of intravenous and oral sodium 2-mercaptoethane sulphonate (mesna) in normal subjects. *Br J Clin Pharmacol* 1987; **23:** 561–8.
3. El-Yazigi A, *et al.* Pharmacokinetics of mesna and dimesna after simultaneous intravenous bolus and infusion administration in patients undergoing bone marrow transplantation. *J Clin Pharmacol* 1997; **37:** 618–24.


### Uses and Administration

Mesna is used for the prevention of urothelial toxicity in patients being treated with the antineoplastics ifosfamide or cyclophosphamide. In the kidney, dimesna, the inactive metabolite of mesna, is reduced to free mesna which has thiol groups that react with the metabolites of ifosfamide and cyclophosphamide, including acrolein, considered to be responsible for the toxic effects on the bladder.

The aim of mesna therapy is to ensure adequate levels of mesna in the urine throughout the period during which these toxic metabolites are present and the duration of mesna treatment should therefore equal that of the antineoplastic treatment plus the time taken for the concentration of antineoplastic metabolites in the urine to fall to non-toxic levels. Urinary output should be maintained and the urine monitored for haematuria and proteinuria throughout the treatment period. However, frequent emptying of the bladder should be avoided.

Mesna may be given intravenously or orally for the prevention of urothelial toxicity, the dosage and frequency depending on the antineoplastic regimen used. After oral administration, availability of mesna in urine is about 50% of that after intravenous administration and excretion in urine is delayed up to 2 hours and is more prolonged. The intravenous preparation may be given orally added to a flavoured drink; this mixture may be stored in a sealed container in a refrigerator for up to 24 hours. Alternatively, tablets are available.

**Intravenous bolus antineoplastic regimens.** If ifosfamide or cyclophosphamide is given as an intravenous bolus, the *intravenous dose of mesna* is 20% of the dose of the antineoplastic on a weight for weight basis given on 3 occasions over 15 to 30 minutes at intervals of 4 hours beginning at the same time as the antineoplastic injection; thus a total dose of mesna equivalent to 60% of the antineoplastic is given. This regimen is repeated each time the antineoplastic is used. The individual dose of mesna may be increased to 40% of the dose of the antineoplastic and given 4 times at intervals of 3 hours for children and patients at high risk of urotoxicity; in such cases the total dose of mesna is equivalent to 160% of the antineoplastic given. The *oral dose of mesna* is 40% of the dose of the antineoplastic given on 3 occasions at intervals of 4 hours beginning 2 hours before the antineoplastic injection; thus a total dose of mesna equivalent to 120% of the antineoplastic is given. Alternatively, the initial dose of mesna may be given *intravenously* (20% of the dose of the antineoplastic), followed by two *oral doses* (each 40% of the dose of the antineoplastic) given 2 and 6 hours after the intravenous dose. Any of these regimens may be used if **cyclophosphamide** is given **orally**.

**Intravenous infusion antineoplastic regimens.** If the antineoplastic is given as an intravenous infusion over 24 hours, an initial *intravenous injection* of mesna as 20% of the total antineoplastic dose is followed by 100% of the total dose by intravenous infusion concurrently over 24 hours, followed by 60% by intravenous infusion over a further 12 hours (total dose 180% of the antineoplastic). The final 12-hour infusion may be replaced either by 3 intravenous injections each of 20% of the antineoplastic dose at intervals of 4 hours, the first injection being given 4 hours after the infusion has been stopped, or by *oral mesna* given in 3 doses each of 40% of the antineoplastic dose, the first dose being given when the 24-hour infusion is stopped, and the second and third doses being given 2 and 6 hours later.

Mesna is also used as a mucolytic in the management of some respiratory-tract disorders. The usual daily dose is 0.6 to 1.2 g given by a nebuliser; it may also be given by direct endotracheal instillation.

◊ General references.

1. Schoenike SE, Dana WJ. Ifosfamide and mesna. *Clin Pharm* 1990; **9:** 179–91.

## Preparations

**Proprietary Preparations** (details are given in Part 3)
***Arg.:*** Delinar; Mesnex; Mestian; Neper; Uromitexan; Varimesna; ***Austral.:*** Uromitexan; ***Austria:*** Mistabron; Uromitexan; ***Belg.:*** Mistabron; Uromitexan; ***Braz.:*** Mesnil†; Mitexan; ***Canad.:*** Uromitexan; ***Chile:*** Mucofluid; Uromitexan; Uroprot; ***Denm.:*** Uromitexan; ***Fin.:*** Uromitexan; ***Fr.:*** Mucofluid; Uromitexan; ***Ger.:*** Mistabronco; Uromitexan; ***Hong Kong:*** Mistabron; Uromitexan; ***India:*** Uromitexan; ***Irl.:*** Uromitexan; ***Israel:*** Mexan; ***Ital.:*** Ausobronc†; Mucofluid; Mucolene; Uromitexan; ***Malaysia:*** Mistabron; Uromitexan; ***Mex.:*** Filesna†; Mesnil; Mesodal; Uromitexan; Uroprot; Ziken; ***Neth.:*** Mistabron; Uromitexan; ***Norw.:*** Uromitexan; ***NZ:*** Uromitexan; ***Port.:*** Uromitexan; ***S.Afr.:*** Mistabron; Uromitexan; ***Singapore:*** Mistabron; Uromitexan; ***Spain:*** Mucofluid; Uromitexan; ***Swed.:*** Uromitexan; ***Switz.:*** Mistabron; Uromitexan; ***Thai.:*** Mistabron; Uromitexan; ***UK:*** Uromitexan; ***USA:*** Mesnex.

**Multi-ingredient:** ***India:*** Holoxan Uromitexan.

# Methionine *(USAN, rINN)*

M; S-Methionine; L-Methionine; Methioninum; Metionina.
L-2-Amino-4-(methylthio)butyric acid.
$C_5H_{11}NO_2S$ = 149.2.
*CAS — 63-68-3.*
*ATC — V03AB26.*

**Pharmacopoeias.** In *Chin.*, *Eur.* (see p.vi), *Jpn*, *Pol.*, and *US*.

**Ph. Eur. 5.0** (Methionine). A white or almost white, crystalline powder or colourless crystals. Soluble in water; very slightly soluble in alcohol. A 2.5% solution in water has a pH of 5.5 to 6.5. Protect from light.

**USP 27** (Methionine). White crystals having a characteristic odour. Soluble in water, in warm dilute alcohol, and in dilute mineral acids; insoluble in dehydrated alcohol, in acetone, in ether, and in benzene. pH of a 1% solution in water is between 5.6 and 6.1.

## DL-Methionine

DL-Methioninum; DL-Metionina; Racemethionine *(USAN)*.
DL-2-Amino-4-(methylthio)butyric acid.
$C_5H_{11}NO_2S$ = 149.2.
*CAS — 59-51-8.*
*ATC — V03AB26.*

NOTE. The name methionine is often applied to DL-methionine. Compounded preparations of DL-methionine may be represented by the following names:

- Co-methiamol *x/y* (*BAN*)—where *x* and *y* are the strengths in milligrams of DL-methionine and paracetamol respectively.

**Pharmacopoeias.** In *Eur.* (see p.vi), *Int.*, and *Viet.*

**Ph. Eur. 5.0** (DL-Methionine). An almost white crystalline powder or small flakes. Sparingly soluble in water; very slightly soluble in alcohol; dissolves in dilute acids and in dilute solutions of alkali hydroxides. A 2% solution in water has a pH of 5.4 to 6.1. Protect from light.

## Adverse Effects and Precautions

Methionine may cause nausea, vomiting, drowsiness, and irritability. It should not be used in patients with acidosis. Methionine may aggravate hepatic encephalopathy in patients with established liver damage; it should be used with caution in patients with severe liver disease.

## Interactions

Orally administered methionine may be adsorbed by activated charcoal leading to a diminished effect of methionine if they are given together.

**Dopaminergics.** For the antagonism of the antiparkinsonian effect of *levodopa* by methionine, see Nutritional Agents, under Interactions of Levodopa, p.1208.

## Uses and Administration

L-Methionine is an essential amino acid and is therefore included in amino-acid solutions used for parenteral nutrition (p.1418).

Methionine also enhances the synthesis of glutathione and is used as an alternative to acetylcysteine in the treatment of paracetamol poisoning to prevent hepatotoxicity (see p.76). The literature relating to the use of methionine in paracetamol poisoning is, in general, imprecise as to the form of methionine used. In the UK, the usual dose of DL-methionine is 2.5 g by mouth every 4 hours for 4 doses starting less than 10 to 12 hours after ingestion of the paracetamol. Children under 6 years old may be given 1 g every 4 hours for 4 doses. Methionine has also been given intravenously. Preparations containing both methionine and paracetamol have been formulated for use in situations where overdosage may occur. However, the issue of whether methionine should be routinely added to paracetamol preparations is contentious for medical and ethical reasons.

Methionine has also been given orally to lower urinary pH and as an adjunct in the treatment of liver disorders.

## Preparations

**Proprietary Preparations** (details are given in Part 3)
***Arg.:*** Neutrodor; ***Austral.:*** Methnine; ***Austria:*** Acimethin; ***Ger.:*** Acimethin; Acimol; Methiotrans; Uromethin; ***Switz.:*** Acimethin; ***USA:*** M-Caps; Pedameth; Uracid.

**Multi-ingredient:** ***Austral.:*** Berberis Complex†; Liv-Detox†; ***Belg.:*** Verrulyse-Methionine†; ***Braz.:*** Aminotox; Anekron; Betaliver; Biofigado†; Biohepax; Colinvintol†; Enterofigon†; Epacrosil†; Eparex†; Epativan B6; Epocler; Eviepar†; Extrato Hepatico Composto; Extrato Hepatico Vitaminado; Figadobil†; Hecrosine B12†; Hepachofril†; Hepacitron†; Hepalin†; Hepasedan†; Hepationina†; Hepatocler†; Hepatotris; Hormo Hepatico; Infiltran B12†; Jecohepat†; Mesitol†; Metiocolin B12; Metiocolin Composto; Metionina Composta†; Necro B-6; Necrohepat†; Neofarmotox†; Panvitrop†; Regenom; Silimalon; Xantina B12; Xantinon B12; ***Canad.:*** Amino-Cerv; Selenium Plus; ***Fr.:*** Cysti-Z; Forcapil; Lobamine-Cysteine; Verrulyse-Methionine; ***Ger.:*** Hepalipon N†; Hepar-Pasc duo†; Hepar-Pasc N†; Lipovitan; ***Hong Kong:*** Bilsan; Lipochol; ***Ital.:*** Agedin Plus; Lozione Same AS†; Meziv; ***Mex.:*** Lipovitasi-Or; ***Port.:*** Drenomade†; Metionina†; ***S.Afr.:*** Hepavite; ***Spain:*** Dertrase; Epitelizante; ***Switz.:*** Lobamine-Cysteine†; Mechovit; ***Thai.:*** Bio-Vitas; Lipochol; Liporon; ***UK:*** Fat-Solv†; Lipotropic Factors; Paradote; ***USA:*** Amino-Cerv.

# Methylthioninium Chloride *(BAN, rINN)*

Azul de Metileno; Blu di Metilene; CI Basic Blue 9; Cloruro de metiltioninio; Colour Index No. 52015; Methylene Blue; Methylenii Caeruleum; Methylthioninii Chloridum; Schultz No. 1038; Tetramethylthionine Chloride Trihydrate. 3,7-Bis(dimethylamino)phenazathionium chloride trihydrate.
$C_{16}H_{18}ClN_3S,3H_2O$ = 373.9.
*CAS — 61-73-4 (anhydrous methylthioninium chloride); 7220-79-3 (methylthioninium chloride trihydrate).*
*ATC — V03AB17; V04CG05.*

NOTE. *Commercial methylthioninium chloride may consist of the double chloride of tetramethylthionine and zinc, and is not suitable for medicinal use.*

**Pharmacopoeias.** In *Chin.* and *US*; in *Eur.* (see p.vi) (as $xH_2O$); in *Int.* (as anhydrous or $3H_2O$).

**Ph. Eur. 5.0** (Methylthioninium Chloride). A dark blue, crystalline powder with a copper-coloured sheen, or green crystals with a bronze-coloured sheen. Soluble in water; slightly soluble in alcohol. Store in airtight containers. Protect from light.

**USP 27** (Methylene Blue). Dark green crystals or crystalline powder with a bronze-like lustre. Is odourless or practically so. Solutions in water or alcohol are deep blue in colour. Soluble 1 in 25 of water and 1 in 65 of alcohol; soluble in chloroform. Store at a temperature of 25°, excursions permitted between 15° and 30°.

## Adverse Effects and Precautions

After intravenous administration of high doses, methylthioninium chloride may cause nausea, vomiting, abdominal and chest pain, headache, dizziness, mental confusion, profuse sweating, dyspnoea, and hypertension; methaemoglobinaemia and haemolysis may occur. Haemolytic anaemia and hyperbilirubinaemia have been reported in newborn infants following intra-amniotic injection. Oral use may cause gastrointestinal disturbances and dysuria.

Methylthioninium chloride should not be injected subcutaneously as it has been associated with isolated cases of necrotic abscesses. It should not be given by intrathecal injection as neural damage has occurred. Methylthioninium chloride should be used with caution in patients with severe renal impairment and is contra-indicated in patients with G6PD deficiency (see Uses, below). Methylthioninium chloride is used to treat methaemoglobinaemia but in large doses it can itself produce methaemoglobinaemia and methaemoglobin concentration should therefore be closely monitored during treatment. Methylthioninium chloride should not be used to treat methaemoglobinaemia induced by sodium nitrite during the treatment of cyanide poisoning, since cyanide binding will be reduced with resultant increased toxicity. It has also been contra-indicated in methaemoglobinaemia due to chlorate poisoning because of the risk that the more toxic hypochlorite may be formed, although several authorities consider its use to treat methaemoglobinaemia in severe chlorate poisoning appropriate.

Methylthioninium chloride imparts a blue colour to saliva, urine, faeces, and skin, which may hinder a diagnosis of cyanosis.

**Aniline poisoning.** Methylthioninium chloride should be used with caution in the treatment of aniline-induced methaemoglobinaemia since it may precipitate Heinz body formation and haemolytic anaemia.[1] Methylthioninium chloride may reduce methaemoglobin concentrations, but repeated doses could aggravate haemolysis without further reducing methaemoglobinaemia.

1. Harvey JW, Keitt AS. Studies of the efficacy and potential hazards of methylene blue therapy in aniline-induced methaemoglobinaemia. *Br J Haematol* 1983; **54:** 29–41.

**Pregnancy.** Although intra-amniotic injection of methylthioninium chloride has been used to diagnose premature rupture of fetal membranes or to identify separate amniotic sacs in twin pregnancies, there have been several reports of haemolytic anaemia (Heinz-body anaemia) and hyperbilirubinaemia in neonates who had been exposed to methylthioninium chloride in the amniotic cavity.[1-5] In most cases, exchange transfusions and/or phototherapy were required to control the jaundice; in 1 case phototherapy led to a phototoxic reaction.[5] Some[3] have considered that the use of methylthioninium chloride for detecting premature rupture of the membranes should be avoided.

Multiple ileal occlusions have been reported in babies born to mothers who had twin pregnancies and who had received methylthioninium chloride by amniocentesis;[4,6,7] in some cases it was possible to determine that methylthioninium chloride had been injected into the amniotic sac of the affected twin. Analysis of data from the EUROCAT registries[8] for 1980 to 1988, which surveyed pregnancy outcomes in 11 countries, found a slightly higher risk of ileal and jejunal atresia or stenosis in twins regardless of whether they had received methylthioninium chloride, but the use of methylthioninium chloride was rare and no increased risk could be shown in babies exposed to it. A subsequent review[9] from the Centers for Disease Control and Prevention concluded that the epidemiological evidence for the teratogenicity of methylthioninium chloride was quite strong and advised that it should not be used midtrimester.

A further difficulty in using methylthioninium chloride by amniocentesis for the diagnosis of premature rupture of the membranes is that the resultant staining of the skin and mucous membranes of the neonate hinders assessment of hypoxia, including the use of pulse oximetry.[10]

1. Cowett RM, *et al.* Untoward neonatal effect of intraamniotic administration of methylene blue. *Obstet Gynecol* 1976; **48** (suppl): 74s–75s.
2. Serota FT, *et al.* The methylene-blue baby. *Lancet* 1979; **ii:** 1142–3.
3. Crooks J. Haemolytic jaundice in a neonate after intra-amniotic injection of methylene blue. *Arch Dis Child* 1982; **57:** 872–3.
4. Nicolini V, Monni G. Intestinal obstruction in babies exposed in utero to methylene blue. *Lancet* 1990; **336:** 1258–9.
5. Porat R, *et al.* Methylene blue-induced phototoxicity: an unrecognized complication. *Pediatrics* 1996; **97:** 717–21.
6. van der Pol JG, *et al.* Jejunal atresia related to the use of methylene blue in genetic amniocentesis in twins. *Br J Obstet Gynaecol* 1992; **99:** 141–3.
7. Lancaster PAL, *et al.* Intra-amniotic methylene blue and intestinal atresia in twins. *J Perinat Med* 1992; **20** (suppl 1): 262.

8. Dolk H. Methylene blue and atresia or stenosis of ileum and jejunum. *Lancet* 1991; **338:** 1021–2.
9. Cragan JD. Teratogen update: methylene blue. *Teratology* 1999; **60:** 42–8.
10. Troche BT. The methylene blue baby. *N Engl J Med* 1989; **320:** 1756–7.

## Pharmacokinetics

Methylthioninium chloride is absorbed from the gastrointestinal tract. It is believed to be reduced in the tissues to leucomethylene blue, which is slowly excreted, mainly in the urine, together with some unchanged drug.

## Uses and Administration

Methylthioninium chloride is a thiazine dye that is used in the treatment of methaemoglobinaemia; it is also used as an antiseptic and in diagnostic procedures.

In patients with methaemoglobinaemia, therapeutic doses of methylthioninium chloride can lower the levels of methaemoglobin in the red blood cells. It activates a normally dormant reductase enzyme system, which reduces the methylthioninium chloride to leucomethylene blue and in turn is able to reduce methaemoglobin to haemoglobin. However, in large doses methylthioninium chloride can itself produce methaemoglobinaemia and methaemoglobin concentration should therefore be closely monitored during treatment. Methylthioninium chloride is not effective for the treatment of methaemoglobinaemia in patients with G6PD deficiency as these patients have a diminished capacity to reduce methylthioninium chloride to leucomethylene blue; it is also potentially harmful as patients with G6PD deficiency are particularly susceptible to the haemolytic anaemias induced by methylthioninium chloride.

In the treatment of drug-induced methaemoglobinaemia, as in nitrite poisoning, methylthioninium chloride is given intravenously as a 1% solution in doses of 1 to 2 mg/kg injected over a period of several minutes. A repeat dose may be given after one hour if required. It may be of some value in inherited methaemoglobinaemia; doses of up to 300 mg daily by mouth have been used.

Methylthioninium chloride has a mildly antiseptic action and has been given by mouth in doses of 65 to 130 mg three times daily in minor urinary-tract infections and to prevent the formation of urinary oxalate stones. It is also included in some preparations intended for application to the eye, mouth and pharynx, and skin.

Methylthioninium chloride is also used as a bacteriological stain, as a dye in diagnostic procedures such as fistula detection and the diagnosis of ruptured amniotic membranes (but see Pregnancy under Adverse Effects and Precautions, above), and for the delineation of certain body tissues during surgery. The blue colour can be removed from the skin with hypochlorite solution. It was formerly used in a renal function test.

**Glutaricaciduria.** Methylthioninium chloride may be of benefit in glutaricaciduria. A response has been observed in one infant[1] with neonatal glutaricaciduria type II. Following the observation in one patient that ifosfamide neurotoxicity (encephalopathy) was associated with glutaricaciduria, methylthioninium chloride was used successfully in 3 patients to reverse or prevent ifosfamide neurotoxicity.[2,3] In glutaricaciduria, where there is, or is likely to be, an absence of electron-transferring flavoproteins, methylthioninium chloride may act as an electron acceptor.

1. Harpey J-P, *et al.* Methylene-blue for riboflavine-unresponsive glutaricaciduria type II. *Lancet* 1986; **i:** 391.
2. Küpfer A, *et al.* Prophylaxis and reversal of ifosfamide encephalopathy with methylene-blue. *Lancet* 1994; **343:** 763–4.
3. Zulian GB, *et al.* Methylene blue for ifosfamide-associated encephalopathy. *N Engl J Med* 1995; **332:** 1239–40.

**Ifosfamide encephalopathy.** See under Glutaricaciduria, above.

**Methaemoglobinaemia.** Methaemoglobinaemia is a rare disorder of the blood in which there is an increase in the proportion of haemoglobin present in the oxidised form. It may be inherited, due either to a deficiency of methaemoglobin reductase or to a structural abnormality of haemoglobin, or it may be acquired, usually secondary to exposure to agents that oxidise haemoglobin including nitrates and nitrites, sodium nitroprusside, dapsone, sulfonamides, phenacetin, and some local anaesthetics such as prilocaine. Administration of low doses over prolonged periods may lead to chronic methaemoglobinaemia whereas large doses may lead to an acute effect.

Methaemoglobinaemia has a profound effect on oxygen transport by the blood; there is an increase in oxygen affinity leading to reduced tissue delivery and varying degrees of cyanosis. The presence of symptoms depends upon the degree and rapidity of methaemoglobin formation. Chronic mild methaemoglobinaemia is generally well tolerated although patients may appear cyanotic. Acute methaemoglobinaemia, particularly where methaemoglobin levels exceed 20%, is associated with dyspnoea, headache, malaise, giddiness, and altered mental state; methaemoglobin levels above 50% may lead to vascular collapse, coma, and death.

Patients with inherited methaemoglobinaemia are usually asymptomatic but treatment may be given for cosmetic purposes to reduce the cyanotic skin colour. Patients with reductase deficiency generally respond to oral therapy with drugs that promote the reduction of methaemoglobin to haemoglobin, such as ascorbic acid, riboflavin, or methylthioninium chloride; methylthioninium chloride may also be given intravenously. Patients with structural abnormalities of haemoglobin do not respond. In acquired methaemoglobinaemia the causative agent should be identified and removed. Chronic or mild cases may not require treatment but acute symptomatic methaemoglobinaemia may be life-threatening and patients should be given intravenous methylthioninium chloride. Toxicity is uncommon with methylthioninium chloride but it should not be used for methaemoglobinaemia due to the use of nitrites for cyanide poisoning since increased toxicity may result (for debate about its use after chlorate poisoning, see Adverse Effects and Precautions, above). Severe methaemoglobinaemia may require exchange transfusion; exchange transfusion with haemodialysis is the treatment of choice in patients with acute methaemoglobinaemia and haemolysis. Ascorbic acid is not useful in the acute situation since it acts too slowly but it may be of benefit where maintenance therapy is required.

References.

1. Coleman MD, Coleman NA. Drug-induced methaemoglobinaemia: treatment issues. *Drug Safety* 1996; **14:** 394–405.

ADMINISTRATION. In acute methaemoglobinaemia, methylthioninium chloride is usually administered by intravenous bolus injection, but repeated doses may be needed. Methylthioninium chloride was administered by continuous intravenous infusion at a dose of 7.5 to 10 mg/hour for 43 hours to control methaemoglobinaemia following dapsone poisoning.[1] The patient had responded to two bolus doses of 100 mg but methaemoglobinaemia had subsequently increased again owing to the long half-life of dapsone. Additional therapy included repeated doses of activated charcoal. A dosing schedule for methylthioninium chloride of 1 to 2 mg/kg as a bolus followed by a continuous infusion at an initial rate of 100 to 150 micrograms/kg per hour was suggested.

1. Dawson AH, Whyte IM. Management of dapsone poisoning complicated by methaemoglobinaemia. *Med Toxicol Adverse Drug Exp* 1989; **4:** 387–92.

**Septic shock.** Nitric oxide may play a role in the hypotension that occurs in septicaemia (p.144). Methylthioninium chloride is a guanylate cyclase inhibitor and may block the vasodilator effects of nitric oxide. In an uncontrolled study[1] in 14 patients with septic shock, methylthioninium chloride increased arterial blood pressure, but cardiac output and tissue oxygenation did not improve; the study was not designed to show an effect on mortality. Improvement in blood pressure has also been reported[2] after use of methylthioninium chloride in 5 neonates with refractory hypotension assumed to be due to septic shock. However, nitric oxide is only one of many mediators that may be involved in septic shock and further studies are required to determine whether methylthioninium chloride has any effect on outcome.

1. Preiser J-C, *et al.* Methylene blue administration in septic shock: a clinical trial. *Crit Care Med* 1995; **23:** 259–64.
2. Driscoll W, *et al.* Effect of methylene blue on refractory neonatal hypotension. *J Pediatr* 1996; **129:** 904–8.

**Surgery.** References to the use of methylthioninium chloride to stain and identify the parathyroid glands before surgery.

1. Dudley NE. Methylene blue for rapid identification of the parathyroid. *BMJ* 1971; **3:** 680–1.
2. Rowntree T. Parathyroids—a personal series. *J R Soc Med* 1980; **73:** 14–18.
3. Bainbridge ET, Barnes AD. Some changing aspects of primary hyperparathyroidism. *Ann R Coll Surg Engl* 1983; **65:** 67–70.
4. Young AE. Intraoperative methods. *Br J Hosp Med* 1984; **31:** 198, 200–3.

## Preparations

***BP 2003:*** Methylthioninium Injection;
***USP 27:*** Methylene Blue Injection.

**Proprietary Preparations** (details are given in Part 3)
***Fr.:*** Collubleu†; Vitableu†; ***Mex.:*** Zumetil†; ***Spain:*** Azul Metile†; ***USA:*** Urolene Blue.

**Multi-ingredient:** ***Arg.:*** Lagrimas de Santa Lucia; Mictasol Azul; Muelita; Visubril; ***Austral.:*** Mackenzies Menthoids†; ***Austria:*** Methyment; ***Braz.:*** Acridin; Cezane†; Colyrazul†; Cystex; Oftazul†; Paludil†; Pilulas De Witt's; Sepurin; Urosalin†; Uroseptin†; Vislin; Visodin; Visolux†; ***Canad.:*** Blue Collyrium†; Collyre Bleu; ***Fr.:*** Antiseptique-Calmante†; Collyre Bleu; Mictasol Bleu†; Pastilles Monleon; Stilla†; ***Israel:*** Pronaestin; ***Ital.:*** Mictasol Bleu; Visustrin; ***NZ:*** De Witts Pills; ***Spain:*** Argentofenol; Centilux; Ojosbel Azul†; Tivitis; ***Switz.:*** Collyre Bleu Laiter; ***USA:*** Atrosept; Dolsed; MHP-A; MSP-Blu; Prosed/DS; Trac Tabs 2X; UAA; Urelle; Uretron; Uridon Modified; Urimar-T; Urimax; Urised; Uriseptic; Uritact; Uro Blue; Urogesic Blue; Utira.

## Milk Thistle

Carduus marianus; Silybum marianum.
*CAS — 84604-20-6.*

**Pharmacopoeias.** In *Eur.* (see p.vi). Also in *USNF.*

**Ph. Eur. 5.0** (Milk-Thistle Fruit). The mature fruit, devoid of the pappus, of *Silybum marianum*. It contains not less than 1.5% of silymarin expressed as silibinin (dried drug). Protect from light.

**USNF 22** (Milk Thistle). The dried ripe fruit of *Silybum marianum* (Asteraceae), the pappus having been removed. It contains not less than 2% of silymarin, calculated as silybin ($C_{25}H_{22}O_{10}$), on the dried basis. Store in airtight containers. Protect from light.

### Silibinin *(rINN)*

Silibinina; Silybin; Silybum Substance $E_6$. 3,5,7-Trihydroxy-2-[3-(4-hydroxy-3-methoxyphenyl)-2-(hydroxymethyl)-1,4-benzodioxan-6-yl]-4-chromanone.
$C_{25}H_{22}O_{10}$ = 482.4.
*CAS — 22888-70-6.*

NOTE. The name silymarin has also been used to denote silibinin.

### Silicristin *(rINN)*

Silicristina; Silychristin. 2-[2,3-Dihydro-7-hydroxy-2-(4-hydroxy-3-methoxyphenyl)-3-(hydroxymethyl)-5-benzofuranyl]-3,5,7-trihydroxy-4-chromanone.
$C_{25}H_{22}O_{10}$ = 482.4.
*CAS — 33889-69-9.*

### Silidianin *(rINN)*

Silidianina; Silydianin. (+)-2,3α,3aα,7a-Tetrahydro-7aα-hydroxy-8(R*)-(4-hydroxy-3-methoxyphenyl)-4-(3α,5,7-trihydroxy-4-oxo-2β-chromanyl)-3,6-methanobenzofuran-7(6αH)-one.
$C_{25}H_{22}O_{10}$ = 482.4.
*CAS — 29782-68-1.*

### Silymarin

Silimarina. A mixture of the isomers silibinin, silicristin, and silidianin.
*CAS — 65666-07-1.*
*ATC — A05BA03.*

### Profile

Silymarin is the active principle from the fruit of milk thistle (*Silybum marianum*; *Carduus marianus*). The principal components are the flavonolignans silibinin, silicristin, and silidianin of which silibinin is the major component.

Silymarin is claimed to be a free radical scavenger and has been used for the treatment of hepatic disorders. Silibinin has been used as the disodium dihemisuccinate salt in *Amanita phalloides* poisoning (p.1718). Silymarin is poorly water-soluble and has been given by mouth; disodium silibinin dihemisuccinate is water-soluble and has been given by intravenous injection. Silymarin in usual doses of up to 140 mg (equivalent to silibinin 60 mg) two or three times daily by mouth has been suggested for hepatic disorders. A dose of silibinin 20 mg/kg daily by intravenous infusion in 4 divided doses as the disodium dihemisuccinate has been suggested in *Amanita phalloides* poisoning.

**Amanita poisoning.** Silymarin and silibinin have been found to be effective in preventing hepatic damage following amanita poisoning.[1-3]

1. Vogel G. The anti-amanita effect of silymarin. In: Faulstich H, *et al.,* eds. *Amanita toxins and poisoning.* Baden-Baden: Verlag Gerhad Witzstrock, 1980: 180–7.
2. Lorenz D. Über die anwending von silibinin bei der knollenblätterpilzvergiftung. *Dtsch Arzt* 1982; **79:** 43–5.
3. Hruby K, *et al.* Chemotherapy of Amanita phalloides poisoning with intravenous silibinin. *Hum Toxicol* 1983; **2:** 183–90.

**Liver disorders.** References to the use of silymarin in patients with liver disorders.

1. Saller R, *et al.* The use of silymarin in the treatment of liver diseases. *Drugs* 2001; **61:** 2035–63.
2. Jacobs BP, *et al.* Milk thistle for the treatment of liver disease: a systematic review and meta-analysis. *Am J Med* 2002; **113:** 506–15.

## Preparations

***USNF 22:*** Milk Thistle Capsules; Milk Thistle Tablets.

**Proprietary Preparations** (details are given in Part 3)
***Arg.:*** Benevolus; Laragon; ***Austral.:*** Bioglan Liver-Vite†; Herbal Liver Formula†; Liver Tonic Capsules†; Prol†; Silymarin Phytosome†; ***Austria:*** Apihepar; Biogelat Leberschutz; Bornosan-Leberschutz; Hepa-Loges; Hepar Pasc Mono; Leberschutz; Legalon; Silyhexal; ***Belg.:*** Legalon; Legalon SIL; ***Braz.:*** Eleparon; Legalon; Siliver; ***Chile:*** Legalon; ***Fr.:*** Legalon; ***Ger.:*** Alepa; Ardeyhepan N; Carduus-monoplant†; Cefasilymarin; durasilymarin; Hegrimarin†; Heliplant†; Hepa-Loges; Hepa-Merz Sil; Hepaduran V; Hepar-Pasc; Heparano N†; Heparsyx N; Hepatorell†; Hepatos; Heplant; Legalon; Legalon SIL; Mariendistel Curarina; Phytohepar; Poikicholan; Probiophyt V†; Silibene; Silicur; Silimarit; Silmar; Silvaysan; Sily-Sabona; SX Carduus†; Vit-o-Mar†; ***Gr.:*** Legalon; ***Hong Kong:*** Legalon; ***India:*** Limarin; Silybon; ***Ital.:*** Eparsil†; Legalon; Locasil†; Marsil†; Silepar†; Silimarin; Silirex; Silliver; Trissil†; ***Mex.:*** Legalon; ***Neth.:*** Venoplant†; ***Port.:*** Legalon; ***S.Afr.:*** Legalon; ***Spain:*** Legalon; Legalon SIL; Silarine; Silimazu; ***Switz.:*** Legalon; Legalon SIL; ***Thai.:*** Legalon; Samarin.

**Multi-ingredient:** ***Arg.:*** Bibol Leloup; Hepadigenor; Quelodin F; ***Austral.:*** Antioxidant Forte Tablets†; Extralife Liva-Care†; Herbal Cleanse†; Lifesystem Herbal Formula 7 Liver Tonic†; Liver Tonic Herbal Formula 6†; Silybum Complex†; St Mary's Thistle Plus†; Super B Plus Liver Tonic†; T & T Antioxidant†; ***Austria:*** Aristochol†; Bakanasan Leber-Galle; Bio-Strath Leber-Galle; Hepabene; Pascopankreat†; Sanhelios Leber-Galle; Sidroga Leber-Galle-Tee; Tiroler Adler Leber- und Gallentee; Tiroler Adler

Schwedenbitter; **Braz.:** Silimalon; **Canad.:** Milk Thistle; Milk Thistle Formula; **Ger.:** Bilisan C3†; Bilisan Duo; Cefachol†; Cheiranthol; Cholhepan N; Cholosom-Tee; Doppelherz Magenstarkung†; Gallexier; Galloselect M; Hepar-Pasc duo†; Hepar-Pasc N†; Hepaticum-Medice H; Hepatofalk Planta N†; Heumann Leber- und Gallentee Solu-Hepar S; Heusin; Hevert-Gall S†; Iberogast; JuCholan S†; Legapas comp†; Marianon; Pankreaplex Neu; Pascohepan novo†; Pascopankreat novo; Presselin Hepaticum P; Schwohepan S; Vasesana-Vasoregulans†; Venacton; **Hong Kong:** Hepatofalk Planta; Simepar; **Ital.:** Castindia†; Epagest; Tarassaco (Specie Composta); Venoplus; **Malaysia:** Luckyhepa; Simepar; **Port.:** Cholagutt; Synchrorose; **Singapore:** Hepatofalk Planta; Noricaven; Simepar; **Spain:** Venoplant†; **Switz.:** Boldocynara; Demonatur Gouttes pour le foie et la bile; Iberogast; Phytomed Hepato; Simepar; Tisane hepatique et biliaire.

## Nalmefene *(BAN, USAN, pINN)*

6-Desoxy-6-methylene-naltrexone; JF-1; Nalmetrene; ORF-11676. 17-(Cyclopropylmethyl)-4,5α-epoxy-6-methylenemorphinan-3,14-diol; (5R)-9a-Cyclopropylmethyl-4,5-epoxy-6-methylenemorphinan-3,14-diol.

$C_{21}H_{25}NO_3$ = 339.4.

*CAS — 55096-26-9.*

### Nalmefene Hydrochloride *(BANM, pINNM)*

6-Desoxy-6-methylene-naltrexone hydrochloride; Hidrocloruro de nalmefeno; Nalmetrene Hydrochloride.

$C_{21}H_{25}NO_3,HCl$ = 375.9.

*CAS — 58895-64-0.*

### Adverse Effects

Nausea, vomiting, tachycardia, hypertension, fever, and dizziness have been reported with therapeutic doses of nalmefene. At higher doses or in patients later found to be physically dependent on opioids, symptoms suggestive of opioid withdrawal have been noted; these have included abdominal cramps, chills, dysphoria, myalgia, and joint pain.

### Precautions

As for Naloxone, p.1045.

Incremental doses of nalmefene should be given slowly in patients with renal impairment.

### Pharmacokinetics

Nalmefene is absorbed following oral administration, but bioavailability is not complete owing to significant first-pass metabolism. It is metabolised in the liver, mainly to the inactive glucuronide, and is excreted in the urine. Some of the dose is excreted in the faeces and it may undergo enterohepatic recycling. The plasma elimination half-life is reported to be about 10 hours.

◊ References.

1. Dixon R, *et al.* Nalmefene: intravenous safety and kinetics of a new opioid antagonist. *Clin Pharmacol Ther* 1986; **39:** 49–53.
2. Dixon R, *et al.* Nalmefene: safety and kinetics after single and multiple oral doses of a new opioid antagonist. *J Clin Pharmacol* 1987; **27:** 233–9.
3. Frye RF, *et al.* The effect of age on the pharmacokinetics of the opioid antagonist nalmefene. *Br J Clin Pharmacol* 1996; **42:** 301–6.
4. Frye RF, *et al.* Effects of liver disease on the disposition of the opioid antagonist nalmefene. *Clin Pharmacol Ther* 1997; **61:** 15–23.

### Uses and Administration

Nalmefene is a derivative of naltrexone and is a specific opioid antagonist with actions and uses similar to those of naloxone (p.1045), but with a longer duration of action. It is administered as the hydrochloride but doses are expressed in terms of the base. Nalmefene hydrochloride 111 micrograms is approximately equivalent to 100 micrograms of nalmefene. It is usually administered intravenously for a rapid onset of action; subcutaneous or intramuscular administration is also effective but has a slower onset. Nalmefene has also been given orally.

For the reversal of postoperative central depression due to the use of opioids, nalmefene is given intravenously, at a concentration of 100 micrograms/mL, in an initial dose of 250 nanograms/kg. Further doses of 250 nanograms/kg may be given at intervals of 2 to 5 minutes until the desired level of opioid reversal is reached; cumulative doses above 1 microgram/kg do not provide additional benefit. In patients with an increased cardiovascular risk a concentration of 50 micrograms/mL and doses and increments of 100 nanograms/kg are recommended.

In the management of known or suspected opioid overdosage, nalmefene is given intravenously at a concentration of 1 mg/mL. An initial dose of 500 micrograms per 70 kg is recommended, followed by a second dose of 1 mg per 70 kg after 2 to 5 minutes if necessary. If a total dose of 1.5 mg per 70 kg is not effective then additional doses are unlikely to have an effect. If the patient is suspected of being physically dependent on opioids an initial test dose of 100 micrograms per 70 kg is recommended; if there is no evidence of withdrawal symptoms within 2 minutes the usual dosage may be used.

Although nalmefene has a longer duration of action than naloxone, all patients should be closely observed and if respiratory depression does recur, the dose of nalmefene should be titrated as above to avoid over-reversal of opioid effects.

**Alcohol withdrawal and abstinence.** Nalmefene has been studied[1,2] as an alternative to naltrexone in the adjunctive management of patients with alcohol dependence (p.1166).

1. Mason BJ, *et al.* A double-blind, placebo-controlled pilot study to evaluate the efficacy and safety of oral nalmefene HCl for alcohol dependence. *Alcohol Clin Exp Res* 1994; **18:** 1162–7.
2. Mason BJ, *et al.* A double-blind, placebo-controlled study of oral nalmefene for alcohol dependence. *Arch Gen Psychiatry* 1999; **56:** 719–24.

**Pruritus.** It has been hypothesised that because central opioid receptors modulate itch, an opioid antagonist might block pruritus, and a number of opioid antagonists have been reported to be of benefit, although they are not part of the usual management of pruritus (p.1137).

Rapid improvement of severe pruritus was reported following a single oral dose of *nalmefene* 10 or 20 mg in a double-blind study of 80 patients with either chronic urticaria or atopic dermatitis.[1] Pruritus was almost completely eliminated in up to 60% of patients receiving nalmefene. Adverse effects occurred in 67% of patients and included dizziness or lightheadedness, fatigue, and nausea. In another study,[2] 14 patients with resistant pruritus secondary to cholestatic liver disease were treated with oral nalmefene for 2 to 26 months. The initial dose was 2 mg twice daily and the dose was increased gradually as necessary. Although 13 of the patients reported some amelioration of pruritus, 5 found that increasing doses were required to produce any benefit, and in 3 tolerance appeared to develop.

Continuous infusion of *naloxone* 200 nanograms/kg per minute was reported to reduce perception of pruritus and scratching activity in a double-blind study of 29 patients with pruritus due to cholestasis.[3] Although naloxone infusion is unlikely to have a role in the long-term management of this condition, longer acting oral opioid antagonists may be useful.

In a double-blind study in 15 haemodialysis patients with severe resistant pruritus, administration of *naltrexone* 50 mg daily by mouth significantly reduced pruritus scores. However, the long term safety and benefit in this situation was not known.[4]

1. Monroe EW. Efficacy and safety of nalmefene in patients with severe pruritus caused by chronic urticaria and atopic dermatitis. *J Am Acad Dermatol* 1989; **21:** 135–6.
2. Bergasa NV, *et al.* Open-label trial of oral nalmefene therapy for the pruritus of cholestasis. *Hepatology* 1998; **27:** 679–84.
3. Bergasa NV, *et al.* Effects of naloxone infusions in patients with the pruritus of cholestasis. *Ann Intern Med* 1995; **123:** 161–7.
4. Peer G, *et al.* Randomised crossover trial of naltrexone in uraemic pruritus. *Lancet* 1996; **348:** 1552–4.

### Preparations

**Proprietary Preparations** (details are given in Part 3)
**USA:** Revex.

## Nalorphine *(BAN, rINN)*

Nalorfina. (–)-(5R,6S)-9a-Allyl-4,5-epoxymorphin-7-en-3,6-diol; 17-Allyl-17-normorphine.

$C_{19}H_{21}NO_3$ = 311.4.

*CAS — 62-67-9.*

*ATC — V03AB02.*

### Nalorphine Hydrobromide *(BANM, rINNM)*

Hidrobromuro de nalorfina.

$C_{19}H_{21}NO_3,HBr$ = 392.3.

*ATC — V03AB02.*

**Pharmacopoeias.** In *Chin.*

### Nalorphine Hydrochloride *(BANM, rINNM)*

Hidrocloruro de nalorfina; Nalorphini Hydrochloridum; Nalorphinium Chloride.

$C_{19}H_{21}NO_3,HCl$ = 347.8.

*CAS — 57-29-4.*

*ATC — V03AB02.*

**Pharmacopoeias.** In *US.*

**USP 27** (Nalorphine Hydrochloride). Store in airtight containers at a temperature of 25°, excursions permitted between 15° and 30°. Protect from light.

### Adverse Effects and Precautions

Nalorphine may give rise to drowsiness, respiratory depression, miosis, dysphoria, and lethargy.

Nalorphine can induce an acute withdrawal syndrome in opioid-dependent patients.

### Uses and Administration

Nalorphine is an opioid antagonist with properties similar to those of naloxone (below); in addition it also possesses some agonist properties. It reverses severe opioid-induced respiratory depression but may exacerbate respiratory depression such as that induced by alcohol or other non-opioid central depressants.

Nalorphine has been used as the hydrobromide or hydrochloride in the treatment of opioid-induced respiratory depression. A dose of 5 to 10 mg has been given by intravenous injection, repeated every 10 to 15 minutes as necessary until respiration is restored, with a maximum total dosage of 40 mg. It has also been given intramuscularly.

### Preparations

**USP 27:** Nalorphine Hydrochloride Injection.

## Naloxone Hydrochloride

*(BANM, USAN, rINNM)*

N-Allylnoroxymorphone Hydrochloride; Cloridrato de Naloxona; EN-15304; Hidrocloruro de naloxona; Naloxoni Hydrochloridum. 17-Allyl-6-deoxy-7,8-dihydro-14-hydroxy-6-oxo-17-normorphine hydrochloride dihydrate; (–)-(5R,14S)-9a-Allyl-4,5-epoxy-3,14-dihydroxymorphinan-6-one hydrochloride dihydrate.

$C_{19}H_{21}NO_4,HCl,2H_2O$ = 399.9.

*CAS — 465-65-6 (naloxone); 357-08-4 (anhydrous naloxone hydrochloride); 51481-60-8 (naloxone hydrochloride dihydrate).*

*ATC — V03AB15.*

**Pharmacopoeias.** In *Chin., Eur.* (see p.vi), *Int., Jpn, Pol.,* and *US.* Forms specified may be anhydrous, dihydrate, or both.

**Ph. Eur. 5.0** (Naloxone Hydrochloride Dihydrate; Naloxone Hydrochloride BP 2003). It contains two molecules of water of hydration. A white or almost white, hygroscopic, crystalline powder. Freely soluble in water; soluble in alcohol; practically insoluble in toluene. Store in airtight containers. Protect from light.

**USP 27** (Naloxone Hydrochloride). It is anhydrous or contains two molecules of water of hydration. A white to slightly off-white powder. Soluble in water, in dilute acids, and in strong alkali; slightly soluble in alcohol; practically insoluble in chloroform and in ether. Its aqueous solution is acidic. Store in airtight containers at a temperature of 25°, excursions permitted between 15° and 30°. Protect from light.

**Incompatibility.** Infusions of naloxone hydrochloride should not be mixed with preparations containing bisulfite, metabisulfite, long-chain or high-molecular-weight anions, or solutions with an alkaline pH.

### Adverse Effects

Nausea and vomiting have occurred with naloxone. Some adverse effects may be associated with opioid withdrawal. There have been individual reports of hypotension, hypertension, cardiac arrhythmias, and pulmonary oedema, generally in patients given naloxone postoperatively. Seizures have also been reported infrequently.

◊ Hypertension,[1,2] pulmonary oedema,[3] and cardiac arrhythmias including ventricular tachycardia and fibrillation[4] have been reported after the postoperative use of naloxone, generally in patients with pre-existing heart disease undergoing cardiac surgery. However, pulmonary oedema, in 1 case fatal,[5] has also been reported in 2 healthy young men[5,6] given naloxone, although the role of naloxone in these cases has been questioned.[7]

Hypotension, bradycardia, and precipitation of focal seizures have been reported in patients given naloxone 4 mg/kg initially then a 24-hour infusion of 2 mg/kg per hour after acute stroke.[8]

Ventricular fibrillation has been observed in an opioid addict given naloxone to reverse the effects of diamorphine.[9] However, this patient was later shown to have hepatic cirrhosis and alcoholic cardiomyopathy and the National Poisons Information Service in London noted that it had never been informed of such a suspected adverse reaction despite being contacted in about 800 cases of opioid poisoning each year.[10] More recently, severe adverse effects were reported to have occurred in 6 of 453 subjects given naloxone to reverse diamorphine intoxication.[11] The effects were: asystole (1 case), generalised convulsions (3), pulmonary oedema (1), and violent behaviour (1).

1. Tanaka GY. Hypertensive reaction to naloxone. *JAMA* 1974; **228:** 25–6.
2. Azar I, Turndorf H. Severe hypertension and multiple atrial premature contractions following naloxone administration. *Anesth Analg* 1979; **58:** 524–5.
3. Flacke JW, *et al.* Acute pulmonary edema following naloxone reversal of high-dose morphine anesthesia. *Anesthesiology* 1977; **47:** 376–8.

4. Michaelis LL, *et al.* Ventricular irritability associated with the use of naloxone hydrochloride: two case reports and laboratory assessment of the effects of the drug on cardiac excitability. *Ann Thorac Surg* 1974; **18:** 608–14.
5. Wride SRN, *et al.* A fatal case of pulmonary oedema in a healthy young male following naloxone administration. *Anaesth Intensive Care* 1989; **17:** 374–7.
6. Taff RH. Pulmonary edema following naloxone administration in a patient without heart disease. *Anesthesiology* 1983; **59:** 576–7.
7. Allen T. No adverse reaction. *Ann Emerg Med* 1989; **18:** 116.
8. Barsan WG, *et al.* Use of high dose naloxone in acute stroke: possible side effects. *Crit Care Med* 1989; **17:** 762–7.
9. Cuss FM, *et al.* Cardiac arrest after reversal of effects of opiates with naloxone. *BMJ* 1984; **288:** 363–4.
10. Barret L, *et al.* Cardiac arrest following naloxone. *BMJ* 1984; **288:** 936.
11. Osterwalder JJ. Naloxone—for intoxications with intravenous heroin and heroin mixtures—harmless or hazardous? A prospective clinical study. *Clin Toxicol* 1996; **34:** 409–16.

## Precautions

Naloxone should be used with caution in patients physically dependent on opioids, or who have received large doses of opioids, as an acute withdrawal syndrome may be precipitated (see Dependence under Opioid Analgesics, p.71). Naloxone crosses the placenta and a withdrawal syndrome may be precipitated in newborn infants of opioid-dependent mothers.

Caution is required in patients with cardiac disease or those receiving cardiotoxic drugs.

The duration of action of some opioids exceeds that of naloxone; patients should therefore be carefully observed after administration in case of relapse.

## Pharmacokinetics

Naloxone is absorbed from the gastrointestinal tract but it is subject to considerable first-pass metabolism. It is metabolised in the liver, mainly by glucuronide conjugation, and excreted in the urine. It has a plasma half-life of about 1 hour after parenteral administration. Naloxone crosses the placenta.

**Pregnancy and the neonate.** A study in 30 mothers given a single intravenous dose of naloxone during the second stage of labour, indicated that naloxone rapidly crossed the placental barrier so that some therapeutic effect might be anticipated in most babies.[1] Placental transfer in 7 further mothers given naloxone intramuscularly was considered to be too variable for therapeutic purposes.

In 12 newborn infants given naloxone hydrochloride 35 or 70 micrograms intravenously via the umbilical vein, the mean plasma half-life of naloxone was 3.53 and 2.65 hours respectively.[2] These half-lives were 2 to 3 times longer than those reported for adults, possibly due to a diminished ability of the newborn to metabolise drugs by conjugation with glucuronic acid. Mean peak plasma concentrations of 8.2 nanograms/mL in those given 35 micrograms, and 13.7 nanograms/mL in those given 70 micrograms, were reached within 40 minutes of administration but this time was very variable, and in 5 infants peak plasma concentrations were reached within 5 minutes. When naloxone hydrochloride 200 micrograms was administered intramuscularly to 17 further newborn infants, peak concentrations of 7.4 to 34.6 nanograms/mL occurred at 0.5 to 2 hours.

1. Hibbard BM, *et al.* Placental transfer of naloxone. *Br J Anaesth* 1986; **58:** 45–8.
2. Moreland TA, *et al.* Naloxone pharmacokinetics in the newborn. *Br J Clin Pharmacol* 1980; **9:** 609–12.

## Uses and Administration

Naloxone is a specific opioid antagonist that acts competitively at opioid receptors. It is an effective antagonist of opioids that possess agonist or mixed agonist-antagonist activity although larger doses may be needed for compounds with the latter activity and for codeine, dextropropoxyphene, and methadone. It is used to reverse opioid central depression, including respiratory depression, induced by natural or synthetic opioids in the treatment of known or suspected opioid overdosage, postoperatively following the use of opioids during surgery, and in neonates after the administration of opioid analgesics to the mother during labour.

Naloxone hydrochloride is usually given intravenously for a rapid onset of action which occurs within 2 minutes. The onset of action is only slightly less rapid when it is given intramuscularly or subcutaneously; sublingual and endotracheal administration have also been suggested. The duration of action of naloxone is dependent on the dose and route of administration; it may be 1 to 4 hours or much shorter.

In the treatment of known or suspected **opioid overdosage**, the initial dose of naloxone hydrochloride is 0.4 to 2 mg given intravenously and repeated if necessary at intervals of 2 to 3 minutes. If no response has been observed after a total dose of 10 mg then the diagnosis of overdosage with drugs other than opioids should be considered. If the patient is suspected of being physically dependent on opioids the dose may be reduced to 100 to 200 micrograms to avoid precipitating withdrawal symptoms. In children, the usual initial dose is 10 micrograms/kg intravenously followed, if necessary, by a larger dose of 100 micrograms/kg (for an alternative children's dose suggested in the USA to treat opioid intoxication, see under Administration, below). In both adults and children, if the intravenous route is not feasible the intramuscular or subcutaneous route can be used.

Naloxone hydrochloride may also be used **postoperatively** to reverse central depression resulting from the use of opioids during surgery. A dose of 100 to 200 micrograms (1.5 to 3 micrograms/kg) may be given intravenously at intervals of at least 2 minutes, titrated for each patient in order to obtain an optimum respiratory response while maintaining adequate analgesia.

All patients receiving naloxone should be closely observed as the duration of action of some opioids exceeds that of naloxone and repeated doses by intravenous, intramuscular, or subcutaneous injection may be required. Alternatively, to sustain opioid antagonism, an intravenous infusion of naloxone hydrochloride has been suggested. Naloxone hydrochloride 4 micrograms/mL in sodium chloride 0.9% or glucose 5% may be infused at a rate titrated in accordance with the patient's response, both to the infusion and previous bolus injections; a rate of 400 to 800 micrograms per hour has been suggested.

Opioid-induced depression in **neonates** resulting from the administration of opioid analgesics to the mother during labour may be reversed by giving naloxone hydrochloride 10 micrograms/kg to the infant by intravenous, intramuscular, or subcutaneous injection, repeated at intervals of 2 to 3 minutes if necessary. Alternatively, a single intramuscular dose of about 60 micrograms/kg may be given at birth for a more prolonged action. Naloxone should be given with caution to the infants of opioid dependent mothers since withdrawal symptoms can result.

Some opioid analgesics have been formulated in combination with naloxone hydrochloride to reduce their potential for parenteral abuse. Naloxone hydrochloride has also been used cautiously in small doses to diagnose opioid dependence by precipitating the withdrawal syndrome (see below and under Naltrexone Hydrochloride, p.1046).

**Administration in infants and children.** The Committee on Drugs of the American Academy of Pediatrics[1,2] has recommended a dose for naloxone of 100 micrograms/kg by intramuscular, intravenous, or intratracheal administration for neonates, including premature infants, to the age of 5 years or 20 kg bodyweight for respiratory depression induced by opioids; absorption may be erratic after intramuscular use. Children over 5 years or 20 kg should be given a minimum of 2 mg. These doses may be repeated as necessary to maintain opioid reversal. The use of injections containing 20 micrograms/mL of naloxone hydrochloride are no longer recommended because of the fluid load involved at these doses, especially in small neonates.[1,3]

1. American Academy of Pediatrics. Emergency drug doses for infants and children and naloxone use in newborns: classification. *Pediatrics* 1989; **83:** 803.
2. Committee on Drugs. Drugs for pediatric emergencies. Abstract: *Pediatrics* 1998; **101:** e13. Full version: http://pediatrics.aappublications.org/cgi/content/full/101/1/e13 (accessed 26/06/04)
3. American Academy of Pediatrics. Naloxone dosage and route of administration for infants and children: addendum to emergency drug doses for infants and children. *Pediatrics* 1990; **86:** 484–5.

**Eating disorders.** Endogenous opioids may have a role in the pathophysiology of eating disorders,[1] thus opioid antagonists such as naloxone and naltrexone have been tried in their management. However, their role appears to be limited and they do not form part of the usual management of these conditions.

1. de Zwaan M, Mitchell JE. Opiate antagonists and eating behavior in humans: a review. *J Clin Pharmacol* 1992; **32**; 1060–72.

**Non-opioid overdosage.** Naloxone antagonises the action of exogenous and endogenous opioids. This may explain the varying responses reported to naloxone used in the treatment of overdosage with non-opioids, some of which may modulate endogenous opioids.

Naloxone was successfully used to reverse intoxication with *camylofin* in 2 infants.[1]

The response to naloxone in *clonidine* intoxication has been inconsistent. There have been reports of benefit in some patients,[2-7] while other studies have been unable to show any;[8,9] hypertension has been reported in some patients.[4,6,7]

1. Schvartsman S, *et al.* Camylofin intoxication reversed by naloxone. *Lancet* 1988; **ii:** 1246.
2. Kulig K, *et al.* Naloxone for treatment of clonidine overdose. *JAMA* 1982; **247:** 1697.
3. Niemann JT, *et al.* Reversal of clonidine toxicity by naloxone. *Ann Emerg Med* 1986; **15:** 1229–31.
4. Gremse DA, *et al.* Hypertension associated with naloxone treatment for clonidine poisoning. *J Pediatr* 1986; **108:** 776–8.
5. Wedin GP, Edwards JL. Clonidine poisoning treated with naloxone. *Am J Emerg Med* 1989; **7:** 343–4.
6. Fiser DH, *et al.* Critical care for clonidine poisoning in toddlers. *Crit Care Med* 1990; **18:** 1124–8.
7. Wiley JF, *et al.* Clonidine poisoning in young children. *J Pediatr* 1990; **116:** 654–8.
8. Rogers JF, Cubeddu LX. Naloxone does not antagonize the antihypertensive effect of clonidine in essential hypertension. *Clin Pharmacol Ther* 1983; **34:** 68–73.
9. Banner W, *et al.* Failure of naloxone to reverse clonidine toxic effect. *Am J Dis Child* 1983; **137:** 1170–1.

**Postoperative use.** Naloxone is used postoperatively to reverse central depression resulting from the use of opioids during surgery. However, it may antagonise the analgesic effects of the opioids in the control of postoperative pain, and the increasing use of short-acting intravenous opioid analgesics should reduce the need for its use. See also Reversal of Opioid Effects, below.

**Pruritus.** For reference to the use of opioid antagonists, including naloxone, in the management of pruritus, see under Nalmefene Hydrochloride, p.1044

**Reversal of opioid effects.** Naloxone has been reported to alleviate some of the adverse effects of opioids without loss of therapeutic efficacy. Naloxone reversed respiratory depression in a patient given intrathecal morphine,[1] and urinary retention in 3 patients after epidural morphine,[2] without reversing analgesia. Naloxone given intravenously has been shown to reverse the delay in gastric emptying induced by opioid analgesics in healthy subjects[3] and in women during labour.[4] Continuous intravenous infusion of naloxone reduced the incidence of adverse effects in patients receiving morphine by patient-controlled analgesia for postoperative pain.[5] Pain control was not compromised and the lower dose of naloxone used (250 nanograms/kg hourly as opposed to 1 microgram/kg hourly) appeared to have an opioid-sparing effect. In patients receiving long-term opioids, oral naloxone in a daily dose equivalent to 20 to 40% of the daily opioid dose relieved opioid-induced constipation without compromising analgesic control.[6,7] Doses equivalent to 10% or less of the opioid dose were ineffective.[8]

Other opioid antagonists that are under investigation for similar indications include methylnaltrexone.[9]

See also Postoperative Use, above.

1. Jones RDM, Jones JG. Intrathecal morphine: naloxone reverses respiratory depression but not analgesia. *BMJ* 1980; **281:** 645–6.
2. Rawal N, *et al.* Naloxone reversal of urinary retention after epidural morphine. *Lancet* 1981; **ii:** 1411.
3. Nimmo WS, *et al.* Reversal of narcotic-induced delay in gastric emptying and paracetamol absorption by naloxone. *BMJ* 1979; **2:** 1189.
4. Frame WT, *et al.* Effect of naloxone on gastric emptying during labour. *Br J Anaesth* 1984; **56:** 263–5.
5. Gan TJ, *et al.* Opioid-sparing effects of a low-dose infusion of naloxone in patient-administered morphine sulfate. *Anesthesiology* 1997; **87:** 1075–81.
6. Sykes NP. Oral naloxone in opioid-associated constipation. *Lancet* 1991; **337:** 1475.
7. Sykes NP. Oral naloxone in opioid-associated constipation. *Lancet* 1991; **338:** 582.
8. Robinson BA, *et al.* Oral naloxone in opioid-associated constipation. *Lancet* 1991; **338:** 581–2.
9. Foss JF. A review of the potential role of methylnaltrexone in opioid bowel dysfunction. *Am J Surg* 2001; **182:** (5A suppl): 19S–26S.

DIAGNOSTIC USE. Naloxone is used to reverse opioid effects in the diagnosis of opioid overdose, although some workers have recommended that administration should be restricted to those patients with clinical signs of opioid overdose.[1]

Naloxone has been given intravenously, to precipitate withdrawal symptoms in the diagnosis of opioid dependence; methods that do not induce acute withdrawal have also been investigated. One study[2] reported that pupillary dilatation in response to naloxone hydrochloride solution 1 mg/mL applied conjunctivally could distinguish patients with a physical dependence from non-dependent patients who had received opioids on a single occasion as pre-operative medication, but this response was not confirmed in another study[3] using naloxone 400 micrograms/mL solution. Furthermore, there has been a report[4] of withdrawal syndrome and pupillary dilatation in 4 opioid dependent subjects after instillation of naloxone solution 40 mg/mL.

1. Hoffman JR, *et al.* The empiric use of naloxone in patients with altered mental status: a reappraisal. *Ann Emerg Med* 1991; **20:** 246–52.
2. Creighton FJ, Ghodse AH. Naloxone applied to conjunctiva as a test for physical opiate dependence. *Lancet* 1989; **i:** 748–50.
3. Loimer N, *et al.* Conjunctival naloxone is no decision aid in opioid addiction. *Lancet* 1990; **335:** 1107–8.

4. Sanchez-Ramos JR, Senay EC. Ophthalmic naloxone elicits abstinence in opioid-dependent subjects. *Br J Addict* 1987; **82:** 313–15.

**Septic shock.** Naloxone has been shown to produce a rise in blood pressure in some cases of septic shock and may be useful as an adjunct in its treatment, although it has not been shown to improve patient survival. Moreover, the US manufacturers have noted that the optimal dose and duration of therapy with naloxone have not been established. In addition, the occurrence of adverse effects from naloxone dictates that caution should be exercised before its use in septic shock, particularly in patients with underlying pain or who have previously received opioids and may have developed opioid tolerance.

## Preparations

***BP 2003:*** Naloxone Injection; Neonatal Naloxone Injection;
***USP 27:*** Naloxone Hydrochloride Injection; Pentazocine and Naloxone Hydrochlorides Tablets.

**Proprietary Preparations** (details are given in Part 3)
***Arg.:*** Antiopiaz; Grayxona; Narcanti; ***Austral.:*** Narcan; ***Austria:*** Narcanti; ***Belg.:*** Narcan; ***Braz.:*** Narcan; ***Canad.:*** Narcan; ***Denm.:*** Narcanti; ***Fin.:*** Narcanti; ***Fr.:*** Nalone; Narcan; ***Ger.:*** Narcanti; ***Gr.:*** Narcan; ***Hong Kong:*** Mapin; Narcan; ***India:*** Narcotan; ***Irl.:*** Narcan; ***Israel:*** Narcan; ***Ital.:*** Narcan; ***Malaysia:*** Narcan; ***Mex.:*** Narcanti; ***Norw.:*** Narcanti; ***NZ:*** Narcan; ***Port.:*** Narcan; Naxan; Naxolan; ***S.Afr.:*** Narcan; Zynox†; ***Singapore:*** Narcan; ***Swed.:*** Narcanti; ***Switz.:*** Narcan; ***Thai.:*** Narcan; ***UK:*** Narcan; ***USA:*** Narcan.

**Multi-ingredient:** ***Israel:*** Rafazocine X†; ***USA:*** Suboxone.

*Used as an adjunct in:* ***Belg.:*** Valtran; ***Ger.:*** Andolor; Findol N; Gruntin Tropfen; Nalidin; Tili; Tili Comp; Tili-Puren; Tilicomp; Tilidalor; Tilidin comp; Tilidin N; Tilidin plus; Tilidin-saar; Tilidura; Tiligetic; Tilimerck; tilnalox; Valoron N; ***Israel:*** Talwin NX; ***NZ:*** Temgesic-nX†; ***USA:*** Talwin NX.

---

## Naltrexone *(BAN, USAN, rINN)*

(5*R*)-9a-Cyclopropylmethyl-3,14-dihydroxy-4,5-epoxymorphinan-6-one; 17-(Cyclopropylmethyl)-4,5α-epoxy-3,14-dihydroxymorphinan-6-one.

$C_{20}H_{23}NO_4$ = 341.4.
*CAS — 16590-41-3.*
*ATC — N07BB04.*

## Naltrexone Hydrochloride *(BANM, rINNM)*

EN-1639A; Hidrocloruro de naltrexona.

$C_{20}H_{23}NO_4,HCl$ = 377.9.
*CAS — 16676-29-2.*
*ATC — N07BB04.*

**Pharmacopoeias.** In *US.*

**USP 27** (Naltrexone Hydrochloride). Store in airtight containers.

### Adverse Effects

Difficulty in sleeping, loss of energy, anxiety, dysphoria, abdominal pain, nausea, vomiting, reduction in appetite, joint and muscle pain, and headache may occur with naltrexone. Other side-effects including dizziness, constipation, diarrhoea, skin rashes, and reduced potency and ejaculatory difficulties have also been reported. Some adverse effects may be associated with opioid withdrawal. Thrombocytopenic purpura has occurred rarely. High doses may cause hepatocellular injury.

**Effects on the liver.** Increased liver enzyme values were reported in 6 of 40 obese patients receiving naltrexone 50 or 100 mg daily for eight weeks.[1] Five of the 6 patients had minimally abnormal liver function before naltrexone was given and liver function tests returned to baseline values or better on discontinuing naltrexone.

Raised transaminase levels were noted in 5 of 26 obese patients after 3 weeks' treatment with naltrexone 300 mg daily; transaminase activity returned to normal when treatment was stopped.[2]

1. Atkinson RL, *et al.* Effects of long-term therapy with naltrexone on body weight in obesity. *Clin Pharmacol Ther* 1985; **38:** 419–22.
2. Mitchell JE. Naltrexone and hepatotoxicity. *Lancet* 1986; **i:** 1215.

### Precautions

Naltrexone should be avoided in patients receiving opioids therapeutically, or in those misusing them, as an acute withdrawal syndrome may be precipitated (see Dependence under Opioid Analgesics, p.71). Withdrawal symptoms may develop within 5 minutes and last up to 48 hours. Naltrexone should be discontinued at least 48 hours before elective surgery involving opioid analgesia. For further precautions when administering naltrexone as an adjunct in the treatment of opioid dependence, see under Uses and Administration, below.

When analgesia is required, larger doses than usual of opioids will be needed and there is an increased risk of respiratory depression and other adverse effects.

Naltrexone should be used with caution in patients with hepatic impairment and is contra-indicated in patients with acute hepatitis or hepatic failure. Regular monitoring of hepatic function has been recommended. Naltrexone should be given with caution to patients with renal impairment.

### Pharmacokinetics

Naltrexone is well absorbed from the gastrointestinal tract but is subject to considerable first-pass metabolism and may undergo enterohepatic recycling. It is extensively metabolised in the liver and the major metabolite, 6-β-naltrexol, may also possess weak opioid antagonist activity. Maximum plasma concentrations of naltrexone and 6-β-naltrexol are achieved in about 1 hour and naltrexone is about 20% bound to plasma proteins at therapeutic doses. The elimination half-life of naltrexone is approximately 4 hours and that of 6-β-naltrexol about 13 hours. Naltrexone and its metabolites are excreted mainly in the urine. Less than 1% of an oral dose of naltrexone is excreted unchanged.

### Uses and Administration

Naltrexone is a specific opioid antagonist with actions similar to those of naloxone (p.1045); however, it is more potent than naloxone and has a longer duration of action.

It is used as the hydrochloride as an aid to maintaining abstinence following opioid withdrawal in detoxified, formerly opioid-dependent patients. Naltrexone treatment should not be started until the patient has been detoxified and abstinent from opioids for at least 7 to 10 days because of the risk of acute withdrawal; abstinence should be verified by analysis of the patient's urine. A *naloxone challenge test* should then be performed to confirm the absence of opioid dependence, as follows: naloxone hydrochloride 200 micrograms is given intravenously and the patient observed for 30 seconds for evidence of withdrawal symptoms; if none occur, a further dose of 600 micrograms is given and the patient observed for 30 minutes. A confirmatory rechallenge with naloxone hydrochloride 1.6 mg intravenously may be considered if results are ambiguous. Sources in the USA suggest a naloxone challenge test with a single dose of 800 micrograms given subcutaneously as an alternative to the intravenous route.

Once a negative naloxone challenge test has been obtained, naltrexone hydrochloride is given by mouth to maintain abstinence. Treatment may be initiated with a dose of 25 mg. If no signs of opioid withdrawal occur subsequent doses may be increased to 50 mg daily. The usual maintenance dose of naltrexone hydrochloride is 350 mg weekly given as 50 mg daily, but the dosing interval may be lengthened to improve compliance; for example, doses of 100 mg on Monday and Wednesday and 150 mg on Friday may be effective and various other intermittent dosage regimens have been used. Patients should be carefully counselled and warned that attempts to overcome the opioid blockade with large doses of opioids could result in fatal opioid intoxication.

Naltrexone hydrochloride is also used as an adjunct in the management of alcohol dependence at a recommended dose of 50 mg daily.

**Alcohol withdrawal and abstinence.** Naltrexone may be of use as an adjunct to psychotherapy in maintaining abstinence after alcohol withdrawal in patients with alcohol dependence (p.1166). Short-term studies[1,2] of 12 weeks' duration indicate that it may be of benefit for reducing alcohol craving and the severity and number of relapses. Data on long-term efficacy are limited but some benefit may persist after withdrawal of treatment.[3] Reports[4] from patients who continued to drink during therapy suggest that naltrexone may reduce the pleasure associated with drinking, possibly by blocking the effect of endorphins released as a result of alcohol consumption.[5] It has been suggested[6] that naltrexone should be given for a minimum of 6 months because of the high relapse rates usually seen during the first 3 to 6 months after alcohol withdrawal. However, a multicentre, double-blind, placebo-controlled study,[7] in which naltrexone was given to each of 418 patients for either 3 months or 12 months with counselling, did not support the use of naltrexone for the treatment of chronic, severe alcohol dependence. Although naltrexone does not appear to be hepatotoxic at the dosage of 50 mg daily used for alcohol dependence, caution is recommended in patients with liver disease.[6] Use with disulfiram, which is potentially hepatotoxic, is not usually recommended.[5]

1. Volpicelli JR, *et al.* Naltrexone in the treatment of alcohol dependence. *Arch Gen Psychiatry* 1992; **49:** 876–80.
2. O'Malley SS, *et al.* Naltrexone and coping skills therapy for alcohol dependence: a controlled study. *Arch Gen Psychiatry* 1992; **49:** 881–7.
3. O'Malley SS, *et al.* Six-month follow-up of naltrexone and psychotherapy for alcohol dependence. *Arch Gen Psychiatry* 1996; **53:** 217–24.
4. Volpicelli JR, *et al.* Effect of naltrexone on alcohol "high" in alcoholics. *Am J Psychiatry* 1995; **152:** 613–15.
5. Anonymous. Naltrexone for alcohol dependence. *Med Lett Drugs Ther* 1995; **37:** 64–6.
6. Berg BJ, *et al.* A risk-benefit assessment of naltrexone in the treatment of alcohol dependence. *Drug Safety* 1996; **15:** 274–82.
7. Krystal JH, *et al.* Naltrexone in the treatment of alcohol dependence. *N Engl J Med* 2001; **345:** 1734–9.

**Opioid dependence.** MAINTENANCE. Naltrexone is a long-acting, non-addictive oral opioid antagonist. Although it can be effective in maintaining abstinence in opioid addicts following detoxification, compliance with therapy is difficult to maintain because although it blocks the euphoriant effects of opioids it does not block the craving for narcotics. It is thus most effective in highly motivated addicts with good sociological and psychological support to discourage impulsive use of opioids.

For a discussion of the management of opioid dependence, see p.71.

References.

1. Crabtree BL. Review of naltrexone, a long-acting opiate antagonist. *Clin Pharm* 1984; **3:** 273–80.
2. Anonymous. Naltrexone for opioid addiction. *Med Lett Drugs Ther* 1985; **27:** 11–12.
3. Ginzburg HM, MacDonald MG. The role of naltrexone in the management of drug abuse. *Med Toxicol* 1987; **2:** 83–92.
4. Gonzalez JP, Brogden RN. Naltrexone: a review of its pharmacodynamic and pharmacokinetic properties and therapeutic efficacy in the management of opioid dependence. *Drugs* 1988; **35:** 192–213.
5. Kirchmayer U, *et al.* Naltrexone maintenance treatment for opioid dependence. Available in The Cochrane Library; Issue 2. Chichester: John Wiley; 2004.

RAPID DETOXIFICATION. Use of clonidine with naltrexone enabled 38 of 40 opioid addicts to withdraw completely from long-term methadone therapy within 4 or 5 days.[1] Modification of the regimen allowed opioid withdrawal over 2 to 3 days.[2] The experimental technique of rapid detoxification with naltrexone while the patient is anaesthetised is controversial.

1. Charney DS, *et al.* The combined use of clonidine and naltrexone as a rapid, safe and effective treatment of abrupt withdrawal from methadone. *Am J Psychiatry* 1986; **143:** 831–7.
2. Brewer C, *et al.* Opioid withdrawal and naltrexone induction in 48–72 hours with minimal drop-out, using a modification of the naltrexone-clonidine technique. *Br J Psychiatry* 1988; **153:** 340–3.

**Pruritus.** For reference to the use of opioid antagonists, including naltrexone, in pruritus, see under Nalmefene Hydrochloride, p.1044.

## Preparations

***USP 27:*** Naltrexone Hydrochloride Tablets.

**Proprietary Preparations** (details are given in Part 3)
***Arg.:*** Revez; ***Austral.:*** Revia; ***Austria:*** Nemexin; Revia; ***Braz.:*** Antaxone†; Revia; ***Canad.:*** Revia; ***Chile:*** Nalerona; ***Denm.:*** Revia; ***Fin.:*** Revia; ***Fr.:*** Nalorex; Revia; ***Ger.:*** Nemexin; ***Gr.:*** Nalorex; ***Hong Kong:*** Revia; ***India:*** Nodict; ***Irl.:*** Nalorex; Revia; ***Israel:*** Revia; ***Ital.:*** Antaxone; Nalorex; Narcoral; ***Malaysia:*** Trexan; ***Mex.:*** Revia; ***Norw.:*** Revia; ***NZ:*** Revia; ***Port.:*** Antaxone; Basinal; Destoxican; Nalorex; ***S.Afr.:*** Revia; ***Singapore:*** Trexan; ***Spain:*** Antaxone; Celupan; Revia; ***Swed.:*** Revia; ***Switz.:*** Nemexin; ***Thai.:*** Revia; ***UK:*** Nalorex; ***USA:*** Depade; Revia; Trexan.

---

## Obidoxime Chloride *(USAN, rINN)*

Cloruro de obidoxima; LüH6. 1,1′-[Oxybis(methylene)]bis[4-(hydroxyimino)methyl]pyridinium dichloride.

$C_{14}H_{16}Cl_2N_4O_3$ = 359.2.
*CAS — 7683-36-5 (obidoxime); 114-90-9 (obidoxime chloride).*
*ATC — V03AB13.*

### Profile

Obidoxime chloride is a cholinesterase reactivator with similar actions and uses to pralidoxime (p.1050). It is given with atropine in the treatment of organophosphorus poisoning in a usual initial dose of 4 to 8 mg/kg by slow intravenous injection, followed by further infusion of 1 mg/kg per hour at intervals of 2 to 4 hours up to a usual total dose of 1 to 2 g.

◊ References.

1. Thiermann H, *et al.* Cholinesterase status, pharmacokinetics and laboratory findings during obidoxime therapy in organophosphate poisoned patients. *Hum Exp Toxicol* 1997; **16:** 473–80.

## Preparations

**Proprietary Preparations** (details are given in Part 3)
***Austria:*** Toxogonin; ***Chile:*** Toxogonin; ***Denm.:*** Toxogonin†; ***Ger.:*** Toxogonin; ***Neth.:*** Toxogonin; ***S.Afr.:*** Toxogonin; ***Swed.:*** Toxogonin; ***Switz.:*** Toxogonine.

---

## Penicillamine *(BAN, USAN, rINN)*

Penicilamina; D-Penicillamine; Penicillaminum. D-3,3-Dimethylcysteine; D-3-Mercaptovaline.

$C_5H_{11}NO_2S$ = 149.2.
*CAS — 52-67-5 (penicillamine); 2219-30-9 (penicillamine hydrochloride).*
*ATC — M01CC01.*

**Pharmacopoeias.** In *Chin., Eur.* (see p.vi), *Int., Pol.,* and *US.*

**Ph. Eur. 5.0** (Penicillamine). A white or almost white, crystalline powder. Freely soluble in water; slightly soluble in alcohol. A 1% solution in water has a pH of 4.5 to 5.5.

**USP 27** (Penicillamine). A white or practically white, crystalline powder having a slight characteristic odour. Freely soluble in water; slightly soluble in alcohol; insoluble in chloroform and in ether. pH of a 1% solution in water is between 4.5 and 5.5. Store in airtight containers.

### Adverse Effects and Treatment

Side-effects of penicillamine are frequent. Gastrointestinal disturbances including anorexia, nausea, and vomiting may occur; oral ulceration and stomatitis have been reported and impaired taste sensitivity is common.

Skin rashes occurring early in treatment are commonly allergic and may be associated with pruritus, urticaria, and fever; they are usually transient but temporary drug withdrawal and use of corticosteroids or antihistamines may be required. Lupus erythematosus and pemphigus have been reported. A Stevens-Johnson-like syndrome has been observed during penicillamine treatment.

Prolonged use of high doses may affect skin collagen and elastin, resulting in increased skin friability, eruptions resembling elastosis perforans serpiginosa, and a late rash or acquired epidermolysis bullosa (penicillamine dermatopathy) that may necessitate dosage reduction or discontinuation.

Haematological side-effects have included thrombocytopenia and, less frequently, leucopenia; these are usually reversible, but agranulocytosis and aplastic anaemia have occurred and fatalities have been reported. Haemolytic anaemia has also occurred.

Proteinuria occurs frequently and in some patients may progress to glomerulonephritis or nephrotic syndrome. Penicillamine-induced haematuria is rare but normally requires immediate discontinuation.

Other side-effects associated with penicillamine include Goodpasture's syndrome, bronchiolitis and pneumonitis, myasthenia gravis, polymyositis (rarely with cardiac involvement), intrahepatic cholestasis, and pancreatitis.

◊ References describing the range and incidence of adverse effects associated with of D-penicillamine.[1,2] The L- or DL-forms are much more toxic.[3]

1. Kean WF, *et al.* Efficacy and toxicity of D-penicillamine for rheumatoid disease in the elderly. *J Am Geriatr Soc* 1982; **30:** 94–100.
2. Steen VD, *et al.* The toxicity of D-penicillamine in systemic sclerosis. *Ann Intern Med* 1986; **104:** 699–705.
3. Kean WF, *et al.* Chirality in antirheumatic drugs. *Lancet* 1991; **338:** 1565–8.

**Effects on the blood.** Of the 18 deaths ascribed to penicillamine reported to the UK Committee on Safety of Medicines between January 1964 and December 1977, 14 were apparently due to blood disorders, at least 7 of them being marrow aplasias. The myelotoxicity of penicillamine was reviewed in 10 patients with confirmed or suspected marrow depression during penicillamine treatment for rheumatoid arthritis or scleroderma; 6 of these 10 patients died.[1]

An incidence of 12 to 27% of penicillamine-induced thrombocytopenia has been reported in patients with rheumatoid arthritis.[2] Thrombocytopenia appeared to be due to bone-marrow suppression and a reduced platelet-production rate.

There have been isolated reports[3-5] of thrombotic thrombocytopenic purpura attributed to the use of penicillamine with some fatalities.

For a brief discussion of the genetic factors influencing myelotoxicity, see under Genetic Factors, below.

1. Kay AGL. Myelotoxicity of D-penicillamine. *Ann Rheum Dis* 1979; **38:** 232–6.
2. Thomas D, *et al.* Thrombokinetics in patients with rheumatoid arthritis treated with D-penicillamine. *Ann Rheum Dis* 1984; **43:** 402–6.
3. Ahmed F, *et al.* Thrombohemolytic thrombocytopenic purpura during penicillamine therapy. *Arch Intern Med* 1978; **138:** 1292–3.
4. Speth PAJ, *et al.* Thrombotic thrombocytopenic purpura associated with D-penicillamine treatment in rheumatoid arthritis. *J Rheumatol* 1982; **9:** 812–13.
5. Trice JM, *et al.* Thrombotic thrombocytopenic purpura during penicillamine therapy in rheumatoid arthritis. *Arch Intern Med* 1983; **143:** 1487–8.

**Effects on the breasts.** Breast enlargement has been reported both in women[1-5] and in men[6] taking penicillamine and may be a rare adverse effect. In some patients breast enlargement was prolonged with poor resolution and others required surgery. Danazol has been used successfully to treat penicillamine-induced breast gigantism.[2-4]

1. Thew DCN, Stewart IM. D penicillamine and breast enlargement. *Ann Rheum Dis* 1980; **39:** 200.
2. Taylor PJ, *et al.* Successful treatment of D-penicillamine-induced breast gigantism with danazol. *BMJ* 1981; **282:** 362–3.
3. Rooney PJ, Cleland J. Successful treatment of D-penicillamine-induced breast gigantism with danazol. *BMJ* 1981; **282:** 1627–8.
4. Craig HR. Penicillamine induced mammary hyperplasia: report of a case and review of the literature. *J Rheumatol* 1988; **15:** 1294–7.
5. Tchebiner JZ. Breast enlargement induced by D-penicillamine. *Ann Pharmacother* 2002; **36:** 444–5.
6. Reid DM, *et al.* Reversible gynaecomastia associated with D-penicillamine in a man with rheumatoid arthritis. *BMJ* 1982; **285:** 1083–4.

**Effects on the gastrointestinal tract.** There have been isolated reports of acute colitis in patients taking penicillamine.[1,2] Ileal ulceration and stenosis in a patient with Wilson's disease was considered to be related to elastosis probably resulting from long-term penicillamine therapy.[3]

1. Hickling P, Fuller J. Penicillamine causing acute colitis. *BMJ* 1979; **2:** 367.
2. Grant GB. Penicillamine causing acute colitis. *BMJ* 1979; **2:** 555.
3. Wassef M, *et al.* Unusual digestive lesions in a patient with Wilson's disease treated with long-term penicillamine. *N Engl J Med* 1985; **313:** 49.

**Effects on the heart.** For reports of heart block, Stokes-Adams syndrome, and fatal myocarditis in patients taking penicillamine, see Polymyositis under Effects on the Muscles and the Neuromuscular System, below.

**Effects on the kidneys.** Proteinuria associated with penicillamine has usually occurred within 4 to 18 months of starting therapy, although onset can be later. A greater incidence has been found in patients with rheumatoid arthritis and cystinuria than in those with Wilson's disease. The severity of proteinuria varies; proteinuria of nephrotic proportions usually develops rapidly but resolves on drug withdrawal. Minimal change, mesangioproliferative, and membranous nephropathy have all been associated with penicillamine treatment and progressive glomerulonephritis has been observed in a few patients who had developed features of Goodpasture's syndrome.[1]

Although there is some evidence of a relationship between nephropathy and penicillamine dose and its rate of increase,[1] a study of 33 rheumatoid arthritis patients with penicillamine-induced nephropathy found no correlation with the dose or duration of treatment.[2] Appreciable proteinuria could still be detected 12 months after stopping penicillamine in 40% of these patients, but subsequently resolved in those whose proteinuria was solely related to penicillamine.

Penicillamine was successfully reintroduced and administered for at least 13 months in 5 patients with rheumatoid arthritis who had developed proteinuria during the first course of therapy. Proteinuria did not recur.[3]

Corticosteroids have been used in patients developing rapidly progressive glomerulonephritis[4] but may be unnecessary and potentially hazardous in patients who develop the nephrotic syndrome.[2]

For reports of Goodpasture's syndrome in patients taking penicillamine, see also under Effects on the Respiratory System, below.

For a brief discussion of the genetic factors influencing renal toxicity, see under Genetic Factors, below.

1. Anonymous. Penicillamine nephropathy. *BMJ* 1981; **282:** 761–2.
2. Hall CL, *et al.* Natural course of penicillamine nephropathy: a long term study of 33 patients. *BMJ* 1988; **296:** 1083–6.
3. Hill H, *et al.* Resumption of treatment with penicillamine after proteinuria. *Ann Rheum Dis* 1979; **38:** 229–31.
4. Ntoso KA, *et al.* Penicillamine-induced rapidly progressive glomerulonephritis in patients with progressive systemic sclerosis: successful treatment of two patients and a review of the literature. *Am J Kidney Dis* 1986; **8:** 159–63.

**Effects on the liver.** In a report of a patient with penicillamine-associated hepatotoxicity and a review of other reports,[1] the 9 patients considered all had liver function profiles consistent with intrahepatic cholestasis; 1 patient died of acute renal failure but the others improved rapidly after drug withdrawal.[1] In a later report,[2] a 72-year-old man with rheumatoid arthritis developed jaundice about 4 weeks after starting penicillamine therapy. Liver biopsy indicated a slight degree of cholangitis with eosinophils in the portal tracts and severe predominantly intrahepatocellular cholestasis. Jaundice cleared within 3 weeks of stopping penicillamine and liver enzyme values approached normal after 6 weeks. Monitoring of liver function and eosinophil counts in the early weeks of penicillamine therapy was recommended.[1]

1. Seibold JR, *et al.* Cholestasis associated with D-penicillamine therapy: case report and review of the literature. *Arthritis Rheum* 1981; **24:** 554–6.
2. Devogelaer JP, *et al.* A case of cholestatic hepatitis associated with D-penicillamine therapy for rheumatoid arthritis. *Int J Clin Pharmacol Res* 1985; **5:** 35–8.

**Effects on the muscles and the neuromuscular system.** Neuromyotonia[1] and profound sensory and motor neuropathy have been reported in patients taking penicillamine. Symptoms improved rapidly after the start of pyridoxine supplementation.[2] Low back pain with fever and rash developed in a patient during penicillamine therapy.[3] Fever and back pain recurred on rechallenge. It was suggested that an allergic mechanism was involved.

1. Reeback J, *et al.* Penicillamine-induced neuromyotonia. *BMJ* 1979; **1:** 1464–5.
2. Pool KD, *et al.* Penicillamine-induced neuropathy in rheumatoid arthritis. *Ann Intern Med* 1981; **95:** 457–8.
3. Bannwarth B, *et al.* Low back pain associated with penicillamine. *BMJ* 1991; **303:** 525.

MYASTHENIA. Myasthenia gravis is a well recognised, though uncommon, complication of long-term penicillamine therapy.[1] Symptoms are similar to those seen with spontaneous myasthenia gravis and include ptosis and diplopia, and generalised weakness, occasionally affecting the respiratory muscles.[1-3] The onset of symptoms usually occurs within 6 to 7 months but may be delayed for a number of years.[3] Myasthenic symptoms usually resolve spontaneously once penicillamine is withdrawn, but some patients require anticholinesterase therapy.[1-3] Acetylcholine receptor antibodies are found in about 75% of affected patients.[2,3] Patients with HLA antigens DRI and Bw35 may have a genetic predisposition to developing myasthenia.[4] Patients with auto-immune diseases may well display an increased susceptibility to drug-induced myasthenia.[3]

1. Delamere JP, *et al.* Penicillamine-induced myasthenia in rheumatoid arthritis: its clinical and genetic features. *Ann Rheum Dis* 1983; **42:** 500–4.
2. Carter H, *et al.* La myasthénie au cours du traitement de la polyarthrite rhumatoïde par la D-pénicillamine. *Therapie* 1984; **39:** 689–95.
3. Katz LJ, *et al.* Ocular myasthenia gravis after D-penicillamine administration. *Br J Ophthalmol* 1989; **73:** 1015–18.
4. Garlepp MJ, *et al.* HLA antigens and acetylcholine receptor antibodies in penicillamine induced myasthenia gravis. *BMJ* 1983; **286:** 338–40.

POLYMYOSITIS. Penicillamine therapy has been associated rarely with polymyositis and dermatomyositis,[1-6] usually reversible but in some cases fatal.[2] At least 2 deaths have resulted from myocarditis,[2] and complete heart block and severe Stokes-Adams attacks have been reported[4] in patients with polymyositis. It is possible that some patients may have a genetically determined susceptibility to this complication.[5]

1. Wojnarowska F. Dermatomyositis induced by penicillamine. *J R Soc Med* 1980; **73:** 885–6.
2. Doyle DR, *et al.* Fatal polymyositis in D-penicillamine-treated rheumatoid arthritis. *Ann Intern Med* 1983; **98:** 327–30.
3. Renier JC, *et al.* Polymyosite induite par la D-pénicillamine. *Therapie* 1984; **39:** 697–703.
4. Christensen PD, Sørensen KE. Penicillamine-induced polymyositis with complete heart block. *Eur Heart J* 1989; **10:** 1041–4.
5. Carroll GJ, *et al.* Penicillamine induced polymyositis and dermatomyositis. *J Rheumatol* 1987; **14:** 995–1001.
6. Aydintug AO, *et al.* Polymyositis complicating D-penicillamine treatment. *Postgrad Med J* 1991; **67:** 1018–20.

**Effects on the respiratory system.** Reports of pulmonary haemorrhage associated with progressive renal failure in individual patients treated with penicillamine have commonly been classified as Goodpasture's syndrome,[1,2] although an immune complex syndrome has been suggested.[3] There have been rare reports of obliterative bronchiolitis in patients with rheumatoid arthritis treated with penicillamine.[4-6]

1. Sternlieb I, *et al.* D-Penicillamine induced Goodpasture's syndrome in Wilson's disease. *Ann Intern Med* 1975; **82:** 673–6.
2. Gibson T, *et al.* Goodpasture syndrome and D-penicillamine. *Ann Intern Med* 1976; **84:** 100.
3. Turner-Warwick M. Adverse reactions affecting the lung: possible association with D-penicillamine. *J Rheumatol* 1981; **8** (suppl 7): 166–8.
4. Lyle WH. D-Penicillamine and fatal obliterative bronchiolitis. *BMJ* 1977; **1:** 105.
5. Epler GR, *et al.* Bronchiolitis and bronchitis in connective tissue disease: a possible relationship to the use of penicillamine. *JAMA* 1979; **242:** 528–32.
6. Murphy KC, *et al.* Obliterative bronchiolitis in two rheumatoid arthritis patients treated with penicillamine. *Arthritis Rheum* 1981; **24:** 557–60.

RHINITIS. Nasal blockage due to grossly oedematous nasal linings and severe disabling watery nasal discharge associated with penicillamine was reported in a 76-year-old patient.[1] The patient also developed a rash which was confirmed as pemphigus foliaceus. The rhinitis resolved promptly when penicillamine was discontinued, as did concurrent bilateral blepharitis.

1. Presley AP. Penicillamine induced rhinitis. *BMJ* 1988; **296:** 1332.

**Effects on the skin.** Penicillamine-induced skin lesions have been reviewed.[1] Reactions include those resulting from interference with collagen and elastin such as penicillamine dermatopathy, elastosis perforans serpiginosa, and cutis laxa; those associated with auto-immune mechanisms such as pemphigus, pemphigoid, lupus erythematosus, and dermatomyositis; and those classified as acute sensitivity reactions including macular or papular eruptions and urticaria. The effects on collagen and elastin (see below) tend to occur only after prolonged use of high doses, as in patients with Wilson's disease or cystinuria, whereas patients with diseases characterised by altered immune systems, such as rheumatoid arthritis, are more prone to develop the antibody-related adverse skin reactions. Acute hypersensitivity reactions tend to occur early in treatment, usually within the first 7 to 10 days, and appear not to be dose-related. Lichenoid reactions, stomatitis, nail changes, and adverse effects on hair have also occurred.

1. Levy RS, *et al.* Penicillamine: review and cutaneous manifestations. *J Am Acad Dermatol* 1983; **8:** 548–58.

INTERFERENCE WITH COLLAGEN AND ELASTIN. Long-term, high-dose treatment with penicillamine can interfere with elastin and collagen production giving rise to increased skin friability, haemorrhagic lesions, miliary papules, and excessive wrinkling and laxity of the skin.[1] Penicillamine dermatopathy, characterised by wrinkling and purpura over bony prominences, has been described.[2] In addition, lesions resembling pseudoxanthoma elasticum have been reported.[3,4] Abnormal elastic tissue has also been reported in patients taking low doses of penicillamine (less than 1 g daily), not only in the skin but also in joint capsules,[5] and elastosis perforans serpiginosa has been reported[6,7] in 2 patients receiving penicillamine. In all these cases, histological findings generally show damage to elastic fibres giving them a typical appearance described as 'lumpy-bumpy' or 'bramble-bush'.

For reports of cutis laxa in neonates, see under Pregnancy in Precautions, below.

1. Levy RS, *et al.* Penicillamine: review and cutaneous manifestations. *J Am Acad Dermatol* 1983; **8:** 548–58.
2. Sternlieb I, Scheinberg IH. Penicillamine therapy for hepatolenticular degeneration. *JAMA* 1964; **189:** 748–54.
3. Thomas RHM, *et al.* Pseudoxanthoma elasticum-like skin changes induced by penicillamine. *J R Soc Med* 1984; **77:** 794–8.
4. Bentley-Phillips B. Pseudoxanthoma elasticum-like skin changes induced by penicillamine. *J R Soc Med* 1985; **78:** 787.
5. Dalziel KL, *et al.* Elastic fibre damage induced by low-dose D-penicillamine. *Br J Dermatol* 1990; **123:** 305–12.

6. Sahn EE, *et al.* D-Penicillamine-induced elastosis perforans serpiginosa in a child with juvenile rheumatoid arthritis. *J Am Acad Dermatol* 1989; **20:** 979–88.
7. Hill VA, *et al.* Penicillamine-induced elastosis perforans serpiginosa and cutis laxa in Wilson's disease. *Br J Dermatol* 2000; **142:** 560–1.

LICHEN PLANUS. Observations in some patients reported in the 1980s led to the suggestion that penicillamine might exacerbate or unmask lichen planus.[1,2] However, there do not appear to have been subsequent reports.

1. Powell FC, Rogers RS. Primary biliary cirrhosis, penicillamine, and lichen planus. *Lancet* 1981; **ii:** 525.
2. Powell FC, *et al.* Lichen planus, primary biliary cirrhosis and penicillamine. *Br J Dermatol* 1982; **107:** 616.

PEMPHIGUS. Pemphigus vulgaris[1] and a number of variants including pemphigus foliaceus,[1] herpetiform pemphigus,[2] pemphigus erythematosus,[3] benign mucous membrane pemphigoid,[4] cicatricial pemphigoid,[5] and combined pemphigus and pemphigoid features[6] have been reported with penicillamine therapy.

1. Zone J, *et al.* Penicillamine-induced pemphigus. *JAMA* 1982; **247:** 2705–7.
2. Marsden RA, *et al.* Herpetiform pemphigus induced by penicillamine. *Br J Dermatol* 1977; **97:** 451–2.
3. de Jong MCJM, *et al.* Immunohistochemical findings in a patient with penicillamine pemphigus. *Br J Dermatol* 1980; **102;** 333–7.
4. Lever LR, Wojnarowska F. Benign mucous membrane pemphigoid and penicillamine. *Br J Dermatol* 1985; **113** (suppl 29): 88–9.
5. Shuttleworth D, Graham-Brown RAC. Cicatricial pemphigoid in a D-penicillamine treated patient with rheumatoid arthritis. *Br J Dermatol* 1985; **113** (suppl 29); 89–90.
6. Velthuis PJ, *et al.* Combined features of pemphigus and pemphigoid induced by penicillamine. *Br J Dermatol* 1985; **112:** 615–19.

PSORIASIFORM ERUPTIONS. Two patients with rheumatoid arthritis developed psoriasiform eruptions during penicillamine treatment.[1] In 1 patient the eruption resolved when penicillamine was stopped but worsened when treatment was restarted.

1. Forgie JC, Highet AS. Psoriasiform eruptions associated with penicillamine. *BMJ* 1987; **294:** 1101.

SYSTEMIC SCLEROSIS. Penicillamine has been used in the treatment of scleroderma and systemic sclerosis (see under Uses, below). However, systemic sclerosis-like lesions developed in a 14-year-old boy with Wilson's disease who had been treated with penicillamine for 11 years[1] and the suitability of penicillamine for this indication has therefore been questioned.

1. Miyagawa S, *et al.* Systemic sclerosis-like lesions during long-term penicillamine therapy for Wilson's disease. *Br J Dermatol* 1987; **116:** 95–100.

TOXIC EPIDERMAL NECROLYSIS. A 56-year-old woman developed agranulocytosis and toxic epidermal necrolysis 7 weeks after starting therapy with penicillamine 250 mg daily for primary biliary cirrhosis.[1]

1. Ward K, Weir DG. Life threatening agranulocytosis and toxic epidermal necrolysis during low dose penicillamine therapy. *Ir J Med Sci* 1981; **150:** 252–3.

**Genetic factors.** There is evidence that some patients may have a genetically determined increased susceptibility to the adverse effects of penicillamine. Several studies have suggested that rheumatoid arthritis patients with a poor capacity for producing sulfoxides may be more susceptible to the toxic effects of penicillamine.[1,2] The poor sulfoxidation capacity found in patients with primary biliary cirrhosis could partly explain their high incidence of adverse reactions to penicillamine,[3] although no association between penicillamine toxicity and sulfoxidation status was found in a study of 20 such patients.[4]

In addition to poor sulfoxidation, increased toxicity was noted in patients possessing the histocompatibility antigen HLA-DR3.[5] Other studies have shown associations between proteinuria and HLA antigens B8 and DR3,[6,7] myasthenia gravis and Bw35 and DR1,[8] thrombocytopenia and HLA antigens DR4,[6,7] A1,[6] and C4BQO,[6] and polymyositis or dermatomyositis and HLA antigens B18, B35, and DR4.[9] However, such associations are insufficiently strong and testing procedures too expensive to make testing sulfoxidation status or HLA-typing useful for identifying high-risk patients.[7,10]

1. Panayi GS, *et al.* Deficient sulphoxidation status and d-penicillamine toxicity. *Lancet* 1983; **i:** 414.
2. Emery P, *et al.* Sulphoxidation status of rheumatoid patients manifesting untoward reactions to chronic D-penicillamine therapy. *Br J Clin Pharmacol* 1984; **18:** 286P.
3. Olomu A, *et al.* Poor sulphoxidation in primary biliary cirrhosis. *Lancet* 1985; **i:** 1504.
4. Mitchison HC, *et al.* D-penicillamine-induced toxicity in primary biliary cirrhosis (PBC): the role of sulphoxidation status. *Gut* 1986; **27:** A622.
5. Emery P, *et al.* D-Penicillamine induced toxicity in rheumatoid arthritis: the role of sulphoxidation status and HLA-DR3. *J Rheumatol* 1984; **11:** 626–32.
6. Stockman A, *et al.* Genetic markers in rheumatoid arthritis: relationship to toxicity from D-penicillamine. *J Rheumatol* 1986; **13:** 269–73.
7. Moens HJB, *et al.* Longterm followup of treatment with D-penicillamine for rheumatoid arthritis: effectivity and toxicity in relation to HLA antigens. *J Rheumatol* 1987; **14:** 1115–19.
8. Garlepp MJ, *et al.* HLA antigens and acetylcholine receptor antibodies in penicillamine induced myasthenia gravis. *BMJ* 1983; **286:** 338–40.
9. Carroll GJ, *et al.* Penicillamine induced polymyositis and dermatomyositis. *J Rheumatol* 1987; **14:** 995–1001.
10. Hall CL. Penicillamine nephropathy. *BMJ* 1988; **297:** 137.

**Systemic lupus erythematosus.** A syndrome resembling lupus erythematosus developed in 6 women with long-standing severe rheumatoid arthritis while being treated with penicillamine;[1] these patients represented an approximate frequency of penicillamine-induced lupus erythematosus of 2%. All 6 had developed previous cutaneous reactions to gold therapy. A case of bullous systemic lupus erythematosus associated with penicillamine administration has also been reported.[2]

1. Chalmers A, *et al.* Systemic lupus erythematosus during penicillamine therapy for rheumatoid arthritis. *Ann Intern Med* 1982; **97:** 659–63.
2. Condon C, *et al.* Penicillamine-induced type II bullous systemic lupus erythematosus. *Br J Dermatol* 1997; **136:** 474–5.

## Precautions

Penicillamine is contra-indicated in patients with lupus erythematosus or a history of penicillamine-induced agranulocytosis, aplastic anaemia, or severe thrombocytopenia. It should be used with care in patients with mild renal impairment and is contra-indicated in patients with moderate or severe renal impairment.

Penicillamine should not be given with other drugs capable of causing similar serious haematological or renal adverse effects, for example gold salts, chloroquine or hydroxychloroquine, or immunosuppressive drugs. Penicillamine is a degradation product of penicillin and patients who are allergic to penicillin may react similarly to penicillamine but cross-sensitivity appears to be rare.

Patients need to be carefully monitored for adverse effects. In particular full blood counts and urinalysis should be carried out; one recommendation is to perform blood counts weekly or fortnightly, and urinalysis weekly, for the first 2 months of treatment and after any change in dosage, and monthly thereafter. Treatment should be withdrawn if there is a fall in white cell or platelet count, or if progressive or serious proteinuria or haematuria occur. Liver function tests at 6-monthly intervals have also been recommended and renal function should be monitored.

Pyridoxine 25 mg daily may be given to patients on long-term therapy, especially if they are on a restricted diet, since penicillamine increases the requirement for this vitamin.

Because of the effect of penicillamine on collagen and elastin and a possible delay in wound healing, it has been suggested that the dose should be reduced to 250 mg daily for 6 weeks before surgery and during the postoperative period until healing has taken place.

**Anaesthesia.** Penicillamine-induced myasthenia in a 57-year-old woman led to prolonged postoperative apnoea necessitating artificial ventilation.[1] The significance of this report in planning anaesthesia for patients with rheumatoid arthritis treated with penicillamine was discussed.

1. Fried MJ, Protheroe DT. D-Penicillamine induced myasthenia gravis: its relevance for the anaesthetist. *Br J Anaesth* 1986; **58:** 1191–3.

**Pregnancy.** Penicillamine teratogenicity has been reviewed.[1] Evidence of the embryotoxicity of maternal penicillamine exposure in *animal* studies has been confirmed in humans by 5 reports of cutis laxa in neonates of mothers who had taken penicillamine during pregnancy; 3 further reports of intra-uterine brain injury were less characteristic. Nevertheless most pregnancy outcomes were normal. No birth defects have been reported when penicillamine was discontinued in early pregnancy. Unless a safer therapy could be confirmed, penicillamine management of women with Wilson's disease should be continued throughout pregnancy since the benefits outweighed the risks. However, for conditions for which there were safer alternatives it would be prudent to discontinue penicillamine during pregnancy.

1. Rosa FW. Teratogen update: penicillamine. *Teratology* 1986; **33:** 127–31.

## Interactions

Penicillamine forms chelates with metal ions and oral absorption may be reduced by concomitant administration of iron and other metals, antacids, and food. Penicillamine should be taken on an empty stomach and it has been recommended that there should be an interval of at least 2 hours between taking penicillamine and iron supplements.

**Antacids or food.** In a single-dose study in 6 healthy subjects, penicillamine given by mouth immediately after food or a dose of an antacid mixture (aluminium hydroxide, magnesium hydroxide, and simeticone), resulted in plasma concentrations of penicillamine that were 52% and 66%, respectively, of those obtained after administration in a fasting state. Results suggested that the reduction in plasma-penicillamine concentrations was associated with decreased penicillamine absorption.[1] Another study[2] showed that the reduction of penicillamine plasma concentrations produced by aluminium- and magnesium-containing antacids did not occur with sodium bicarbonate, and thus the interaction was probably a result of chelation rather than a pH effect.

1. Osman MA, *et al.* Reduction in oral penicillamine absorption by food, antacid, and ferrous sulphate. *Clin Pharmacol Ther* 1983; **33:** 465–70.
2. Ifan A, Welling PG. Pharmacokinetics of oral 500 mg penicillamine: effect of antacids on absorption. *Biopharm Drug Dispos* 1986; **7:** 401–5.

**Diazepam.** For a report of exacerbation of intravenous diazepam-induced phlebitis by oral penicillamine, see under Diazepam, p.695.

**Gold.** There have been conflicting reports on the effect of previous gold therapy on the subsequent development of penicillamine toxicity in patients with rheumatoid arthritis.

A multicentre trial group[1] found no evidence of any interaction between gold and penicillamine but others[2] found that although the overall incidence of side-effects with penicillamine appeared unaffected by prior gold therapy, bone-marrow depression and rashes were more common in those patients previously treated with gold. Patients who had to stop gold therapy because of adverse effects were reported[3] to be more prone to develop major adverse effects to penicillamine and a study[4] indicated that patients who reacted adversely to gold were more likely to develop side-effects to penicillamine. The mean interval between finishing gold and beginning penicillamine in patients who developed identical adverse reactions to both drugs was found to be significantly shorter than in those who developed different side-effects or no side-effects;[4] this supported the theory that some adverse reactions to penicillamine might result from the mobilisation of gold previously stored in the tissues during gold therapy. An interval of at least 6 months between gold and penicillamine therapy in patients who had adverse reactions to gold was recommended. In contrast, others[5] found no evidence that the interval between gold and penicillamine therapy had any influence on the subsequent development of penicillamine toxicity. A genetic susceptibility in certain patients to react adversely to either drug was suggested. However, in a prospective study,[6] prior gold, penicillamine, or levamisole treatment had no influence on the subsequent efficacy or toxicity of any one of these alternative drugs.

There has been a report of gold therapy causing a recurrence of myasthenia that had previously occurred with penicillamine.[7]

1. Multi-centre Trial Group. Absence of toxic or therapeutic interaction between penicillamine and previously administered gold in a trial of penicillamine in rheumatoid disease. *Postgrad Med J* 1974; **50** (suppl 2): 77–8.
2. Webley M, Coomes EN. Is penicillamine therapy in rheumatoid arthritis influenced by previous treatment with gold? *BMJ* 1978; **2:** 91.
3. Hill H. Penicillamine and previous treatment with gold. *BMJ* 1978; **2:** 961.
4. Dodd MJ, *et al.* Adverse reactions to D-penicillamine after gold toxicity. *BMJ* 1980; **280:** 1498–1500.
5. Smith PJ, *et al.* Influence of previous gold toxicity on subsequent development of penicillamine toxicity. *BMJ* 1982; **285:** 595–6.
6. Steven MM, *et al.* Does the order of second-line treatment in rheumatoid arthritis matter? *BMJ* 1982; **284:** 79–81.
7. Moore AP, *et al.* Penicillamine induced myasthenia reactivated by gold. *BMJ* 1984; **288:** 192–3.

**Insulin.** Unexplained hypoglycaemia in 2 patients with type 1 diabetes occurred 6 to 8 weeks after penicillamine treatment for rheumatoid arthritis was started.[1] Both patients required a reduction in their insulin dose. A possible mechanism has been proposed.[2]

1. Elling P, Elling H. Penicillamine, captopril, and hypoglycemia. *Ann Intern Med* 1985; **103:** 644–5.
2. Becker RC, Martin RG. Penicillamine-induced insulin antibodies. *Ann Intern Med* 1986; **104:** 127–8.

**Iron.** Penicillamine plasma concentrations were reduced to 35% when penicillamine was administered after a dose of ferrous sulfate in healthy subjects.[1] Patients stabilised on penicillamine while on oral iron therapy were considered unlikely to respond fully to penicillamine and would be exposed to a large increase in penicillamine absorption with possible adverse reactions if the iron was stopped.[2]

1. Osman MA, *et al.* Reduction in oral penicillamine absorption by food, antacid, and ferrous sulfate. *Clin Pharmacol Ther* 1983; **33:** 465–70.
2. Harkness JAL, Blake DR. Penicillamine nephropathy and iron. *Lancet* 1982; **ii:** 1368–9.

**Probenecid.** Probenecid reduced the beneficial effects of penicillamine in cystinuria; co-administration in hyperuricaemic cystinuric patients was contra-indicated.[1]

1. Yu T-F, *et al.* Studies on the metabolism of D-penicillamine and its interaction with probenecid in cystinuria and rheumatoid arthritis. *J Rheumatol* 1984; **11:** 467–70.

## Pharmacokinetics

Penicillamine is readily absorbed from the gastrointestinal tract and reaches peak concentrations in the blood within 1 to 3 hours. It is reported to be more than 80% bound to plasma proteins. It is metabolised in the liver and excreted in the urine and faeces mainly as metabolites. Elimination is biphasic with an initial elimination half-life of about 1 to 3 hours followed by a slower phase, suggesting gradual release from tissues.

◊ Reviews.

1. Netter P, *et al.* Clinical pharmacokinetics of D-penicillamine. *Clin Pharmacokinet* 1987; **13:** 317–33.

## Uses and Administration

Penicillamine is a chelator that aids the elimination from the body of certain heavy-metal ions, including copper, lead, and mercury, by forming stable soluble complexes with them that are readily excreted by the kidney. It is used in the treatment of Wilson's disease (to promote the excretion of copper), in heavy-metal poisoning such as lead poisoning, in cystinuria (to reduce urinary concentrations of cystine), in severe active rheumatoid arthritis, and in chronic active hepatitis.

Penicillamine is given orally and should be taken on an empty stomach. A low initial dose increased gradually to the minimum optimal maintenance dosage may reduce the incidence of adverse effects as well as provide closer control of the condition being treated.

In the treatment of **Wilson's disease**, a dose of 1.5 to 2 g daily in divided doses may be given initially. The optimal dosage to achieve a negative copper balance should be determined initially by regular analysis of 24-hour urinary copper excretion and subsequently by monitoring free copper in the serum. A maintenance dose of 0.75 to 1 g daily may be adequate once remission is achieved and should be continued indefinitely; the UK manufacturers recommend that a maintenance dose of 2 g daily should not be continued for more than a year. In children, a suggested dose is up to 20 mg/kg daily (minimum 500 mg daily) in divided doses. A dose of 20 mg/kg daily is suggested for the elderly.

In the management of **lead poisoning**, penicillamine may be given in doses of 1 to 1.5 g daily in divided doses until urinary lead is stabilised at less than 500 micrograms/day. Children and the elderly may be given 20 mg/kg daily in divided doses.

In **cystinuria**, doses of penicillamine are adjusted according to cystine concentrations in the urine. For the *treatment* of cystinuria and cystine calculi, the dose is usually in the range of 1 to 4 g daily in divided doses; a suggested dose for children is 30 mg/kg daily in divided doses. For the *prevention* of cystine calculi, lower doses of 0.5 to 1 g at bedtime may be given. An adequate fluid intake is essential to maintain urine flow during penicillamine administration for cystinuria.

In the treatment of **severe active rheumatoid arthritis**, an initial dose of penicillamine 125 to 250 mg daily is increased gradually by the same amount at intervals of 4 to 12 weeks. Remission is usually achieved with maintenance doses of 500 to 750 mg daily in divided doses, but up to 1.5 g daily may be required. Improvement may not occur for several months; the USA manufacturers suggest that penicillamine should be discontinued if there is no response after treatment for 3 to 4 months with 1 to 1.5 g daily; in the UK, a trial for 12 months is suggested. After remission has been sustained for 6 months an attempt may be made gradually to reduce the dose by 125 to 250 mg daily every 3 months but relapse may occur. Lower doses may be required in the elderly who may be more susceptible to developing adverse effects. Initial doses of 125 mg daily are recommended, gradually increased to a maximum of 1 g daily if necessary. In children the maintenance dose is 15 to 20 mg/kg daily; a suggested initial dose is 2.5 to 5 mg/kg daily for one month increased gradually at 4-week intervals.

In the management of **chronic active hepatitis**, an initial dose of penicillamine 500 mg daily in divided doses may be given after liver function tests have indicated that the disease has been controlled by corticosteroids; the dose is gradually increased over 3 months to 1.25 g daily with a concurrent reduction in the corticosteroid dose.

Acetylpenicillamine has been used in mercury poisoning.

**Chronic active hepatitis.** Penicillamine has been tried in chronic active hepatitis (p.1078) as an alternative to prolonged corticosteroid maintenance therapy once control of the disease is achieved. The dose of penicillamine is increased over several months to a suitable maintenance dose with a concurrent reduction in the corticosteroid dose.

**Cystinuria.** Cystinuria is an inherited disorder of renal amino-acid excretion in which there is excessive excretion of cystine (cysteine disulfide), along with ornithine, lysine, and arginine. The low solubility of cystine leads to the formation of cystine stones in the kidney, resulting in pain, haematuria, renal obstruction, and infection. Treatment is primarily aimed at reducing the urinary concentration of cystine to below its solubility limit of 300 to 400 mg/litre at neutral pH. Patients with cystinuria excrete 400 to 1200 mg cystine daily and should be advised to drink at least 3 litres of water daily, including at night, to maintain a dilute urine. Cystine is more soluble in alkaline urine and urinary alkalinisers such as sodium bicarbonate, sodium citrate, or potassium citrate may be used; however, high doses are required and calcium stone formation may be promoted. In patients where these measures are ineffective or not tolerated, penicillamine may be used; it complexes with cysteine to form a more soluble mixed disulfide, therefore reducing cystine excretion, preventing cystine stone formation, and promoting the gradual dissolution of existing stones. Adverse effects are common and tiopronin, which has a similar action, may be used as an alternative. Surgical removal may be necessary for established stones but lithotripsy is not very effective.

**Lead poisoning.** Penicillamine may be used to treat asymptomatic lead intoxication and to achieve desirable lead-tissue levels in patients with symptomatic lead poisoning once they have received treatment with sodium calcium edetate and dimercaprol (see p.1705).

**Primary biliary cirrhosis.** Copper accumulation in the liver has been noted in patients with primary biliary cirrhosis (p.1761) and therapy with penicillamine to reduce liver-copper concentrations has been studied. Despite good preliminary results, most studies have found it to be ineffective and any benefit appears to be offset by the high incidence of side-effects.[1]

1. James OFW. D-Penicillamine for primary biliary cirrhosis. *Gut* 1985; **26:** 109–13.

**Retinopathy of prematurity.** Penicillamine has been investigated for the prophylaxis of retinopathy of prematurity (p.1466) in infants considered to be at risk, and a systematic review of 2 such studies considered that there was evidence for a reduced incidence of acute retinopathy.[1] Further studies were considered justified, with careful attention to possible adverse effects.

1. Phelps DL, *et al.* D-Penicillamine for preventing retinopathy of prematurity in preterm infants. Available in The Cochrane Library; Issue 2. Chichester: John Wiley; 2004.

**Rheumatoid arthritis.** *Rheumatoid arthritis* (p.9) and *juvenile idiopathic arthritis* (p.9) are generally treated using the same methods. Penicillamine is one of a diverse group of disease-modifying antirheumatic drugs that have been used in an attempt to suppress the rate of cartilage erosion or alter the course of the disease. However, early enthusiasm for penicillamine has been tempered by a high incidence of adverse effects.[1] During long-term therapy as many as 50% of patients taking penicillamine have been reported to withdraw from treatment because of adverse effects.[2] Low doses of penicillamine to reduce the incidence of adverse effects have been tried and while doses as low as 125 mg daily have been claimed to be effective in some patients with *rheumatoid arthritis*, a 36-week multicentre double-blind study[3] involving 225 patients concluded that a dose of penicillamine 500 mg daily was only slightly more effective than placebo. A dose of 125 mg daily was not significantly different from either the 500 mg dose or placebo. However, a 5-year open study[4] comparing penicillamine in doses up to 500 mg daily with hydroxychloroquine, sodium aurothiomalate, or auranofin in rheumatoid arthritis found penicillamine to be as effective as the other drugs and well tolerated, with 53% of the patients randomised to penicillamine still receiving it at 5 years, as opposed to about 30 to 35% of those randomised to other drugs.

In patients with *juvenile idiopathic arthritis* it has been suggested that gold therapy may be preferred to penicillamine.[5]

1. Suarez-Almazor ME, *et al.* Penicillamine for treating rheumatoid arthritis. Available in The Cochrane Library; Issue 2. Chichester: John Wiley; 2004.
2. Moens HJB, *et al.* Longterm followup of treatment with D-penicillamine for rheumatoid arthritis: effectivity and toxicity in relation to HLA antigens. *J Rheumatol* 1987; **14:** 1115–19.
3. Williams HJ, *et al.* Low-dose D-penicillamine therapy in rheumatoid arthritis: a controlled, double-blind clinical trial. *Arthritis Rheum* 1983; **26:** 581–92.
4. Jessop JD, *et al.* A long-term five-year randomized controlled trial of hydroxychloroquine, sodium aurothiomalate, auranofin and penicillamine in the treatment of patients with rheumatoid arthritis. *Br J Rheumatol* 1998; **37:** 992–1002.
5. Rosenberg AM. Advanced drug therapy for juvenile rheumatoid arthritis. *J Pediatr* 1989; **114:** 171–8.

**Scleroderma.** Despite the lack of conclusive evidence in its favour penicillamine, which affects the cross-linking of collagen,[1] has been widely thought to be of benefit in scleroderma (p.1348), and perhaps in some visceral manifestations of systemic sclerosis.[2,3] If used, treatment should probably be started early and continued for several years; therapy for 6 to 12 months may be required before any benefit is seen. A dose of 250 to 500 mg of penicillamine daily has been used.[2]

For a report of sclerodermatous lesions in a patient taking penicillamine for Wilson's disease, see Systemic Sclerosis, under Effects on the Skin, above.

1. Herbert CM, *et al.* Biosynthesis and maturation of skin collagen in scleroderma, and effect of D-penicillamine. *Lancet* 1974; **i:** 187–92.
2. Oliver GF, Winkelmann RK. The current treatment of scleroderma. *Drugs* 1989; **37:** 87–96.
3. Steen VD, *et al.* D-Penicillamine therapy in progressive systemic sclerosis (scleroderma): a retrospective analysis. *Ann Intern Med* 1982; **97:** 652–9.

**Wilson's disease.** Wilson's disease, or hepatolenticular degeneration, is a rare autosomal disorder of copper accumulation. Excretion of excess copper, which normally occurs via the bile, is impaired and total body copper progressively increases. The excess copper accumulates in the liver, brain, and other organs including the kidneys and corneas, and eventually causes tissue damage.

Effective treatment of Wilson's disease involves the use of copper-reducing drugs to establish a negative copper balance. This prevents deposition of more copper and also mobilises excess copper that has already been deposited making it available for excretion. Once negative copper balance has been achieved, maintenance treatment must be continued lifelong. Dietary restriction of copper is not generally considered to be an important part of the treatment of Wilson's disease, although patients may be advised to avoid copper-rich foods, such as liver and shellfish, during the first year of treatment and to restrict their consumption thereafter. Symptomatic recovery from copper overload occurs slowly, but is usually complete if treatment is started early enough, and a normal life expectancy can be achieved. However, once irreversible organ damage such as liver cirrhosis has occurred, treatment can only prevent further deterioration; those presenting with end-stage liver disease do not benefit from copper-reducing therapy, and liver transplantation is necessary (although successful medical treatment has been reported in children). The drugs used to reduce copper concentrations in the treatment of Wilson's disease are penicillamine, trientine, and zinc. Ammonium tetrathiomolybdate is under investigation.

*Penicillamine* reduces copper concentrations in several ways. Its main action is to chelate circulating copper, which is then excreted in the urine. In addition, penicillamine reduces the affinity of copper for proteins and polypeptides, allowing removal of copper from tissues. It also induces hepatic synthesis of metallothionein, a protein that combines with copper to form a non-toxic product. *Trientine* is a less potent copper chelator than penicillamine; it competes for copper bound to serum albumin and increases copper excretion. *Zinc* induces synthesis of metallothionein in the intestine so that absorption of copper from the gastrointestinal tract is blocked. It is usually given as the acetate as this form is less irritating to the stomach than the sulfate. *Ammonium tetrathiomolybdate* forms a complex with protein and copper. When it is given with food it blocks the intestinal absorption of copper, and when taken between meals it combines with albumin- and caeruloplasmin-bound copper.

CHOICE OF DRUG. Penicillamine is generally regarded as the drug of choice for the initial management of Wilson's disease as it produces a rapid reduction in copper levels. However, it may initially exacerbate neurological symptoms (possibly due to transiently increased brain and blood copper concentrations) and some practitioners therefore suggest starting with zinc; zinc is not suitable in those requiring rapid reduction of copper levels as it has a slow onset of action. Trientine, which may also exacerbate neurological symptoms, is used in patients intolerant of penicillamine. Ammonium tetrathiomolybdate is under investigation for the initial reduction of copper levels; it may be particularly suitable for patients with neurological symptoms.

Once a negative copper balance is achieved, maintenance therapy must be continued for life. Penicillamine, trientine, and zinc are all used for maintenance treatment. Patients taking penicillamine are also given pyridoxine to prevent deficiency (see under Precautions, above). The adverse effects of penicillamine may be a problem during long-term use and zinc, which has low toxicity, is often preferred. Zinc is also used in patients in the asymptomatic stage of the disease.

References.

1. Tankanow RM. Pathophysiology and treatment of Wilson's disease. *Clin Pharm* 1991; **10:** 839–49.
2. Stremmel W, *et al.* Wilson disease: clinical presentation, treatment, and survival. *Ann Intern Med* 1991; **115:** 720–6.
3. Brewer GJ. Practical recommendations and new therapies for Wilson's disease. *Drugs* 1995; **50:** 240–9.
4. Santos Silva EE, *et al.* Successful medical treatment of severely decompensated Wilson disease. *J Pediatr* 1996; **128:** 285–7.

## Preparations

***BP 2003:*** Penicillamine Tablets;
***USP 27:*** Penicillamine Capsules; Penicillamine Tablets.

**Proprietary Preparations** (details are given in Part 3)

***Arg.:*** Cuprimine; Cupripen; ***Austral.:*** D-Penamine; ***Austria:*** Artamin; ***Belg.:*** Kelatin; ***Braz.:*** Cuprimine; ***Canad.:*** Cuprimine; Depen; ***Denm.:*** Atamir; Rhumantin†; ***Fr.:*** Trolovol; ***Ger.:*** Metalcaptase; Trisorcin; Trolovol†; ***Hong Kong:*** Cuprimine; ***India:*** Cilamin; ***Irl.:*** Distamine; ***Israel:*** Cuprimine; ***Ital.:*** Pemine; ***Malaysia:*** Artamin; ***Mex.:*** Adalken; Sufortan; ***Neth.:*** Cuprimine†; Distamine†; Kelatin; ***Norw.:*** Cuprimine; ***NZ:*** D-Penamine†; Distamine; ***Port.:*** Kelatine; ***S.Afr.:*** Metalcaptase; ***Singapore:*** Artamin†; ***Spain:*** Cupripen; Sufortanon†; ***Swed.:*** Cuprimine†; ***Switz.:*** Mercaptyl; ***Thai.:*** Cuprimine; ***UK:*** Distamine; Pendramine†; ***USA:*** Cuprimine; Depen.

**Pentetic Acid** *(BAN, USAN, rINN)*

DTPA; ZK-43649. Diethylenetriamine-*NNN′N″N″*-penta-acetic acid.

$C_{14}H_{23}N_3O_{10}$ = 393.3.
*CAS — 67-43-6.*

**Pharmacopoeias.** In *US*.

**USP 27** (Pentetic Acid). A white odourless or almost odourless powder.

## Calcium Trisodium Pentetate *(BAN, rINN)*

Calcium Trisodium DTPA; NSC-34249; Pentetate Calcium Trisodium *(USAN)*; Pentetato cálcico trisódico; Trisodium Calcium Diethylenetriaminepentaacetate. Calcium trisodium nitrilodiethylenedinitrilopenta-acetate.

$C_{14}H_{18}CaN_3Na_3O_{10}$ = 497.4.
*CAS — 12111-24-9.*

### Profile

Pentetic acid and its salts are chelators with the general properties of the edetates (see Sodium Calcium Edetate, p.1051). Calcium trisodium pentetate is used in the treatment of poisoning by heavy metals and radioactive metals such as plutonium. Doses of 1 g daily have been given by intravenous infusion for 3 to 5 days. Further treatment may be given after an interval of 3 days.

Calcium pentetate has also been used.

Pentetates, labelled with metallic radionuclides, are used in nuclear medicine (see Indium-111, p.1523, and Technetium-99m, p.1525).

**Thalassaemia.** Calcium pentetate, 0.5 to 1 g by subcutaneous infusion on alternate days or for 5 days each week, was given to 5 patients with thalassaemia (p.735) in whom desferrioxamine had to be withdrawn because of high-tone deafness.[1] Calcium pentetate was as effective as desferrioxamine at increasing iron excretion. Hearing improved during treatment. Oral zinc supplements were necessary during treatment with calcium pentetate to maintain adequate plasma-zinc concentrations.

1. Wonke B, *et al.* Reversal of desferrioxamine induced auditory neurotoxicity during treatment with Ca-DTPA. *Arch Dis Child* 1989; **64:** 77–82.

### Preparations

**Proprietary Preparations** (details are given in Part 3)
***Braz.:*** TCK 6†; ***Ger.:*** Ditripentat-Heyl.

## Potassium Polystyrene Sulfonate

Poliestirenosulfonato potásico; Potassium Polystyrene Sulphonate.

*CAS — 9011-99-8.*
*ATC — V03AE01.*

### Profile

Potassium polystyrene sulfonate, the potassium salt of sulfonated styrene polymer, is a cation-exchange resin that exchanges potassium ions for calcium ions and other cations and has been used in the management of hypercalciuria and renal calculi.

### Preparations

**Proprietary Preparations** (details are given in Part 3)
***Ger.:*** Campanyl†.
**Multi-ingredient: *Ger.:*** Ujostabil.

# Pralidoxime *(BAN)*

Pralidoxima. 2-Hydroxyiminomethyl-1-methylpyridinium.

$C_7H_9N_2O$ = 137.2.
*CAS — 6735-59-7; 495-94-3.*
*ATC — V03AB04.*

## Pralidoxime Chloride *(BANM, USAN)*

2-Formyl-1-methylpyridinium Chloride Oxime; 2-PAM; 2-PAM Chloride; 2-PAMCl; Pralidoxima, cloruro de; 2-Pyridine Aldoxime Methochloride.

$C_7H_9ClN_2O$ = 172.6.
*CAS — 51-15-0.*
*ATC — V03AB04.*

**Pharmacopoeias.** In *US*.

**USP 27** (Pralidoxime Chloride). A white to pale yellow, odourless, crystalline powder. Freely soluble in water.

## Pralidoxime Iodide *(BANM, USAN, rINN)*

Ioduro de pralidoxima; NSC-7760; 2-PAM Iodide; 2-PAMI.

$C_7H_9IN_2O$ = 264.1.
*CAS — 94-63-3.*
*ATC — V03AB04.*

**Pharmacopoeias.** In *Chin.*

## Pralidoxime Mesilate

2-PAMM; Pralidoxima, mesilato de; Pralidoxime Mesylate *(BANM, USAN)*; Pralidoxime Methanesulphonate; P2S.

$C_7H_9N_2O,CH_3O_3S$ = 232.3.
*CAS — 154-97-2.*
*ATC — V03AB04.*

## Pralidoxime Metilsulfate

Pralidoxima, metilsulfato de; Pralidoxime Methylsulphate *(BANM)*.

$C_7H_9N_2O,CH_3SO_4$ = 248.3.
*CAS — 1200-55-1.*
*ATC — V03AB04.*

**Pharmacopoeias.** In *It.*

### Adverse Effects

Use of pralidoxime may be associated with drowsiness, dizziness, disturbances of vision, nausea, tachycardia, headache, hyperventilation, and muscular weakness. Tachycardia, laryngospasm, and muscle rigidity have been attributed to giving pralidoxime intravenously at too rapid a rate. Large doses of pralidoxime may cause transient neuromuscular blockade.

### Precautions

Pralidoxime should be used cautiously in patients with renal impairment; a reduction in dosage may be necessary. Caution is also required in giving pralidoxime to patients with myasthenia gravis as it may precipitate a myasthenic crisis. Pralidoxime should not be used to treat poisoning by carbamate pesticides.

When atropine and pralidoxime are given together, the signs of atropinisation may occur earlier than might be expected when atropine is used alone.

### Pharmacokinetics

Pralidoxime is not bound to plasma proteins, does not readily pass into the CNS, and is rapidly excreted in the urine partly unchanged and partly as a metabolite. The elimination half-life is about 1 to 3 hours.

◊ References.

1. Sidell FR, Groff WA. Intramuscular and intravenous administration of small doses of 2-pyridinium aldoxime methochloride to man. *J Pharm Sci* 1971; **60:** 1224–8.
2. Siddell FR, *et al.* Pralidoxime methanesulfonate: plasma levels and pharmacokinetics after oral administration to man. *J Pharm Sci* 1972; **61:** 1136–40.
3. Swartz RD, *et al.* Effects of heat and exercise on the elimination of pralidoxime in man. *Clin Pharmacol Ther* 1973; **14:** 83–9.

### Uses and Administration

Pralidoxime is a cholinesterase reactivator. It is used as an adjunct to, but *not* as a substitute for, atropine in the treatment of poisoning by certain cholinesterase inhibitors. Its main indication is in poisoning due to organophosphorus insecticides or related compounds (see p.1508). These compounds phosphorylate and consequently inactivate cholinesterase, causing acetylcholine accumulation and muscle paralysis. Pralidoxime acts principally to reactivate cholinesterase, restoring the enzymatic destruction of acetylcholine at the neuromuscular junction and relieving muscle paralysis. However, concomitant use of atropine is required to counteract directly the adverse effects of acetylcholine accumulation, particularly at the respiratory centre. Pralidoxime is not equally antagonistic to all organophosphorus anticholinesterases as reactivation is dependent on the nature of the phosphoryl group and the rate at which inhibition becomes irreversible. It is not effective in the treatment of poisoning due to phosphorus, inorganic phosphates, or organophosphates without anticholinesterase activity. It has usually been contra-indicated in the treatment of poisoning by carbamate insecticides (including carbaryl poisoning) as it may increase toxicity (see p.1501). The use of pralidoxime has been suggested for the treatment of overdosage by anticholinesterase drugs, including those used to treat myasthenia gravis such as neostigmine; however, it is only slightly effective and its use is not generally recommended.

Pralidoxime is usually given as the chloride or mesilate but the iodide and metilsulfate salts have also been used. Doses are expressed in terms of the salts.

Pralidoxime may be administered by slow intravenous injection over 5 to 10 minutes, by intravenous infusion over 15 to 30 minutes, or by subcutaneous or intramuscular injection; it has also been given orally.

In the treatment of **organophosphorus poisoning** pralidoxime should be given within 24 hours of poisoning to be fully effective as cholinesterase inactivation usually becomes irreversible after this time; however, patients with severe poisoning may occasionally respond up to 36 hours or longer after exposure. Injections of *atropine* should be given intravenously or intramuscularly and repeated as necessary until the patient shows signs of atropine toxicity; atropinisation should then be maintained for 48 hours or more. Large amounts of atropine may be required. See under Atropine Sulfate, p.478, for details of dosages. As soon as the effects of atropine become apparent, 1 to 2 g of *pralidoxime*, as the chloride, iodide, or mesilate, should be given intramuscularly or intravenously and repeated after 1 hour and then every 8 to 12 hours if necessary (alternatively, the *British National Formulary* recommends a dose of pralidoxime mesilate of 30 mg/kg given by slow intravenous injection, followed by 1 or 2 further doses if necessary, or by intravenous infusion at a rate of 8 mg/kg per hour). Another alternative, in severe poisoning, is the use of a continuous infusion of 200 to 500 mg/hour, titrated against response. A maximum dose of 12 g in 24 hours has been suggested. In children, pralidoxime mesilate 20 to 60 mg/kg may be given depending on the severity of poisoning and response to treatment. The dose of pralidoxime may need to be reduced in patients with renal impairment.

Treatment should preferably be monitored by the determination of blood-cholinesterase concentrations and clinical symptoms. Patients should be closely observed for at least 24 hours following resolution of symptoms.

Other oximes with cholinesterase-reactivating properties that have been used similarly include obidoxime chloride (p.1046), diacetyl monoxime, and trimedoxime bromide (TMB-4).

**Administration.** Pralidoxime was administered by continuous intravenous infusion in a dose of 9 to 19 mg/kg per hour immediately after a loading dose of 15 to 50 mg/kg to 7 children with symptomatic organophosphorus intoxication.[1] Continuous infusion for 18 to 60 hours was effective and well tolerated. In adults, rates of up to 500 mg/hour have been used for prolonged nicotinic symptoms.[2]

1. Farrar HC, *et al.* Use of continuous infusion of pralidoxime for treatment of organophosphate poisoning in children. *J Pediatr* 1990; **116:** 658–61.
2. Tush GM, Anstead MI. Pralidoxime continuous infusion in the treatment of organophosphate poisoning. *Ann Pharmacother* 1997; **31:** 441–4.

### Preparations

***USP 27:*** Pralidoxime Chloride for Injection.

**Proprietary Preparations** (details are given in Part 3)
***Arg.:*** Contrathion; ***Braz.:*** Contrathion; ***Canad.:*** Protopam; ***Fr.:*** Contrathion; ***Gr.:*** Contrathion; ***India:*** Neopam; ***Ital.:*** Contrathion; ***NZ:*** Pam; ***USA:*** Protopam.

# Protamine

Protamina.

*CAS — 9012-00-4.*
*ATC — V03AB14.*

## Protamine Hydrochloride *(BANM)*

Cloridrato de Protamina; Protamina, hidrocloruro de; Protamini Hydrochloridum.

*ATC — V03AB14.*

**Pharmacopoeias.** In *Eur.* (see p.vi).

**Ph. Eur. 5.0** (Protamine Hydrochloride). A mixture of the hydrochlorides of basic peptides prepared from the sperm or roe of suitable species of fish, usually from the families Clupeidae or Salmonidae. A white or almost white hygroscopic powder. Soluble in water; practically insoluble in alcohol. Store in airtight containers.

## Protamine Sulfate *(rINN)*

Protamine Sulphate *(BAN)*; Protamini Sulfas; Sulfato de Protamina; Sulfato de protamina.

*CAS — 9009-65-8.*
*ATC — V03AB14.*

**Pharmacopoeias.** In *Chin., Eur.* (see p.vi), *Int., Jpn*, and *US.*

**Ph. Eur. 5.0** (Protamine Sulphate). A mixture of the sulfates of basic peptides prepared from the sperm or roe of suitable species of fish, usually from the families Clupeidae or Salmonidae. A white or almost white hygroscopic powder. Sparingly soluble in water; practically insoluble in alcohol. Store in airtight containers.

**USP 27** (Protamine Sulfate). A purified mixture of simple protein principles obtained from the sperm or testes of suitable species of fish. Store at 2° to 8° in airtight containers.

## Adverse Effects and Precautions

Intravenous injections of protamine sulfate, particularly if given rapidly, may cause hypotension, bradycardia, and dyspnoea. A sensation of warmth, transitory flushing, nausea and vomiting, and lassitude may also occur.

Hypersensitivity reactions can occur; patients at risk include diabetics who have received protamine-insulin preparations, those who have previously undergone procedures such as coronary angioplasty or cardiopulmonary bypass surgery, those allergic to fish, and men who are infertile or who have had a vasectomy. Anaphylactoid reactions have been reported.

Protamine has an anticoagulant effect when administered in the absence of heparin.

When repeated doses of protamine are used to neutralise large doses of heparin, rebound bleeding which responds to further doses of protamine, may occur. Clotting parameters should be closely monitored in patients receiving such prolonged therapy.

◊ In a report on 4 patients given protamine sulfate after cardiac surgery to neutralise the effect of heparin, severe adverse reactions including marked hypotension, vascular collapse, and pulmonary oedema were described.[1] Previous reports of similar reactions to protamine were reviewed. A total of 17 patients had immediate anaphylactic reactions; in 1 patient a complement-dependent IgG antibody-mediated reaction had been demonstrated and 3 patients tested for allergy to protamine had positive skin tests. In 15 of these 17 patients there was evidence of previous exposure to protamine; those with a high risk of sensitisation included leucopheresis donors who had received the drug, diabetics using insulin containing protamine, and patients with fish allergy. Suspected reactions to protamine occurred in a further 10 patients after cardiac surgery. However, these reactions were characterised by severe vascular damage, manifested as noncardiogenic pulmonary oedema or persistent hypotension, and onset was delayed for 30 minutes to several hours. Evidence suggested that these reactions were not antibody mediated; only 2 of 7 evaluable patients had previous exposure. All patients required aggressive therapy.

In a review of the toxicity of protamine,[2] adverse cardiovascular responses were considered to be of 3 types: transient hypotension related to rapid drug administration, occasional anaphylactoid responses, and rarely, catastrophic pulmonary vasoconstriction.

1. Holland CL, *et al.* Adverse reactions to protamine sulfate following cardiac surgery. *Clin Cardiol* 1984; **7:** 157–62.
2. Horrow JC. Protamine: a review of its toxicity. *Anesth Analg* 1985; **64:** 348–61.

## Uses and Administration

Protamine is a basic protein that combines with heparin to form a stable inactive complex. Protamine is used to neutralise the anticoagulant action of heparin in the treatment of haemorrhage resulting from severe heparin or low-molecular-weight heparin overdosage. It is also used to neutralise the effect of heparin given before surgery and during extracorporeal circulation as in dialysis or cardiac surgery. Protamine is used in some insulin preparations to prolong the effects of insulin. Protamine is usually given as the sulfate, although the hydrochloride may also be used.

Protamine sulfate is given by slow intravenous injection over a period of about 10 minutes. The dose is dependent on the amount of heparin to be neutralised and ideally should be titrated against the coagulability of the patient's blood. Protamine sulfate has weak anticoagulating properties and if given in gross excess its anticoagulant action could be significant. As heparin is being continuously excreted the dose should be reduced if more than 15 minutes have elapsed since heparin administration; for example, if protamine sulfate is given 30 minutes after heparin the dose may be reduced to about one-half. Not more than 50 mg of protamine sulfate should be injected for any one dose; patients should be carefully monitored as further doses may be required. The Ph. Eur. 5.0 specifies that 1 mg of protamine sulfate precipitates not less than 100 units of heparin, but adds that this potency is based on a specific reference batch of heparin sodium. One UK manufacturer has stated that each mg of protamine sulfate will usually neutralise the anticoagulant effect of at least 80 international units of heparin (lung) or at least 100 international units of heparin (mucous). The US manufacturer has stated that each mg of protamine sulfate neutralises about 90 USP units of heparin (lung) or about 115 USP units of heparin (mucous).

Protamine neutralises the anti-thrombin activity of low-molecular-weight heparins but only partially neutralises the anti-factor-Xa effect; 1 mg of protamine sulfate is stated to inhibit the effects of:

- 71 units of bemiparin sodium
- 100 units of dalteparin sodium
- 1 mg (100 units) of enoxaparin sodium
- 82 units of reviparin sodium
- 100 units of tinzaparin sodium

Protamine hydrochloride may be used similarly.

**Haemorrhagic disorders.** Endogenous production of heparin-like substances may, rarely, be responsible for some bleeding disorders. Protamine could be useful as a diagnostic aid *in vitro* and could be administered intravenously to transiently control bleeding in such patients.[1,2]

1. Tefferi A, *et al.* Circulating heparin-like anticoagulants: report of five consecutive cases and a review. *Am J Med* 1990; **88:** 184–8.
2. Bayly PJM, Thick M. Reversal of post-reperfusion coagulopathy by protamine sulphate in orthotopic liver transplantation. *Br J Anaesth* 1994; **73:** 840–2.

## Preparations

***BP 2003:*** Protamine Sulphate Injection;
***USP 27:*** Protamine Sulfate for Injection; Protamine Sulfate Injection.

**Proprietary Preparations** (details are given in Part 3)
***Arg.:*** Denpru; ***Hong Kong:*** Prosulf; ***India:*** Prota; ***Israel:*** Prosulf; ***UK:*** Prosulf.

## Prussian Blue

Azul de Prusia; Berlin Blue; CI Pigment Blue 27; Colour Index No. 77510; Ferric Ferrocyanide; Ferric Hexacyanoferrate (II).

$Fe_4[Fe(CN)_6]_3$ = 859.2.
*CAS — 14038-43-8; 12240-15-2.*
*ATC — V03AB31.*

NOTE. The name Prussian Blue (CI Pigment Blue 27) is applied to both ferric hexacyanoferrate (II) and to potassium ferric hexacyanoferrate (II), $KFe[Fe(CN)_6]$ = 306.9 (Colour Index No. 77520).

### Profile

Prussian blue is used in the treatment of thallium poisoning (see p.1754). When given orally it forms a non-absorbable complex with thallium in the gastrointestinal tract which is excreted in the faeces. A suggested dose of Prussian blue is 10 g, or 125 mg/kg, twice daily by mouth or duodenal tube until the urinary excretion of thallium falls to 0.5 mg or less per 24 hours. It has been used similarly for the removal of radiocaesium from the body.

### Preparations

**Proprietary Preparations** (details are given in Part 3)
***Ger.:*** Antidotum Thallii-Heyl; Radiogardase-Cs; ***USA:*** Radiogardase.

## Sevelamer Hydrochloride *(BANM, USAN, rINNM)*

GT16-026A; Hidrocloruro de sevelámero. Allylamine polymer with 1-chloro-2,3-epoxypropane hydrochloride.

*CAS — 52757-95-6 (sevelamer); 182683-00-7 (sevelamer hydrochloride).*
*ATC — V03AE02.*

### Adverse Effects and Precautions

The most common adverse effects associated with sevelamer are diarrhoea, nausea and vomiting, constipation, headache, cough and other respiratory symptoms, dizziness, hypotension or hypertension, peripheral oedema, pain, and fever. Flatulence, pharyngitis, and skin rashes have also occurred. Patients with renal impairment may develop hypocalcaemia or hypercalcaemia, and serum-calcium concentrations should be monitored. Serum-chloride concentrations should also be monitored during treatment with sevelamer.

### Uses and Administration

Sevelamer hydrochloride is a phosphate binder used for hyperphosphataemia in patients with chronic renal failure on haemodialysis. The usual initial dose is 800 to 1600 mg of sevelamer hydrochloride three times daily with each meal, depending on the severity of hyperphosphataemia. Doses thereafter should be adjusted according to phosphate concentrations in the plasma.

◊ References.

1. Burke SK. Renagel®: reducing serum phosphorus in haemodialysis patients. *Hosp Med* 2000; **61:** 622–7.

### Preparations

**Proprietary Preparations** (details are given in Part 3)
***Canad.:*** Renagel; ***Denm.:*** Renagel; ***Fr.:*** Renagel; ***Ger.:*** Renagel; ***Gr.:*** Renagel; ***Irl.:*** Renagel; ***Israel:*** Renagel; ***Ital.:*** Renagel; ***Neth.:*** Renagel; ***Port.:*** Renagel; ***Spain:*** Renagel; ***Swed.:*** Renagel; ***UK:*** Renagel; ***USA:*** Renagel.

## Sodium Calcium Edetate *(BAN, rINN)*

Calcioedetato de sodio; Calcium Disodium Edathamil; Calcium Disodium Edetate; Calcium Disodium Ethylenediaminetetra-acetate; Calcium Disodium Versenate; Calcium EDTA; Disodium Calcium Tetracemate; E385; Edetate Calcium Disodium *(USAN)*; Natrii Calcii Edetas; Sodium Calciumedetate. The calcium chelate of disodium ethylenediaminetetra-acetate; Disodium[(ethylenedinitrilo)tetraacetato]calciate(2–) hydrate.

$C_{10}H_{12}CaN_2Na_2O_8,xH_2O$ = 374.3 (anhydrous).
*CAS — 23411-34-9 (sodium calcium edetate, hydrate); 62-33-9 (anhydrous sodium calcium edetate).*

**Pharmacopoeias.** In *Chin., Eur.* (see p.vi), *Int., Pol., US,* and *Viet.*

**Ph. Eur. 5.0** (Sodium Calcium Edetate). A white or almost white, hygroscopic, powder. Freely soluble in water; practically insoluble in alcohol. A 20% solution in water has a pH of 6.5 to 8.0. Store in airtight containers. Protect from light.

**USP 27** (Edetate Calcium Disodium). A mixture of the dihydrate and trihydrate, predominantly the dihydrate. White, slightly hygroscopic, odourless, crystalline powder or granules. Freely soluble in water. pH of a 20% solution in water is between 6.5 and 8.0. Store in airtight containers.

### Adverse Effects

Sodium calcium edetate is nephrotoxic and may cause renal tubular necrosis. Nausea and cramp may also occur. Thrombophlebitis has followed intravenous infusion and may be related to the concentration of the injection. Pain at the intramuscular injection site has been reported. Other side-effects that have been reported include fever, malaise, headache, myalgia, histamine-like responses such as sneezing, nasal congestion, and lachrymation, skin eruptions, transient hypotension, and ECG abnormalities.

Sodium calcium edetate chelates zinc within the body and zinc deficiency has been reported. Displacement of calcium from sodium calcium edetate may lead to hypercalcaemia.

**Effects on the kidneys.** Of 130 children with lead poisoning who received chelation therapy with sodium calcium edetate (25 mg/kg intramuscularly every 12 hours) and dimercaprol (3 mg/kg intramuscularly every 4 hours) for a total of 5 days, 21 developed clinical evidence of nephrotoxicity and in 4 severe oliguric acute renal failure began 1 or 2 days after chelation therapy was discontinued.[1] Nephrotoxicity was probably attributable to the use of sodium calcium edetate.

1. Moel DI, Kumar K. Reversible nephrotic reactions to a combined 2,3-dimercapto-1-propanol and calcium disodium ethylenediaminetetraacetic acid regimen in asymptomatic children with elevated blood lead levels. *Pediatrics* 1982; **70:** 259–62.

### Precautions

Sodium calcium edetate should be used with caution, if at all, in patients with renal impairment. Daily urinalysis to monitor proteinuria and haematuria and regular monitoring of renal function has been recommended.

Sodium calcium edetate can chelate several endogenous metals, including zinc, and may increase their excretion; therapy should be intermittent to prevent severe deficiency developing and monitoring of zinc levels may be required (see below).

Sodium calcium edetate should not be given orally in the treatment of lead poisoning as it has been suggested that absorption of lead may be increased as a result.

◊ Sodium calcium edetate 500 mg/m² was given by deep intramuscular injection every 12 hours for 5 days to 10 children with asymptomatic lead poisoning.[1] Blood-lead concentrations decreased to about 58% of the pretreatment values after 5 days and were essentially unchanged for up to 60 hours after the last dose. Sodium calcium edetate also produced a marked fall in the mean plasma-zinc concentration but this rebounded rapidly after the end of treatment. Mean urinary-lead excretion increased about 21-fold during the first 24 hours of therapy and urinary-zinc excretion increased about 17-fold. Sodium calcium edetate had little effect on the plasma concentrations or urinary excretion of copper. The results suggested that careful monitoring of zinc was required during treatment with sodium calcium edetate.

1. Thomas DJ, Chisolm JJ. Lead, zinc and copper decorporation during calcium disodium ethylenediamine tetraacetate treatment of lead-poisoned children. *J Pharmacol Exp Ther* 1986; **239:** 829–35.

### Pharmacokinetics

Sodium calcium edetate is poorly absorbed from the gastrointestinal tract. It distributes primarily to the extracellular fluid and does not penetrate cells. It is not significantly metabolised; after intravenous injection about 50% of a dose is excreted in the urine in 1 hour and over 95% in 24 hours.

### Uses and Administration

Sodium calcium edetate is the calcium chelate of disodium edetate and is a chelator used in the treatment of lead poisoning (see Lead, Treatment of Adverse Effects, p.1705). It mobilises lead from bone and tissues and aids elimination from the body by forming a stable, water-soluble, lead complex which is readily excreted by the kidneys. It may be used as a diagnostic test for lead poisoning but measurement of blood-lead concentrations is generally preferred.

Sodium calcium edetate is also a chelator of other heavy-metal polyvalent ions, including chromium. A cream containing sodium calcium edetate 10% has been used in the treatment of chrome ulcers and skin sensitivity reactions due to contact with heavy metals.

Edetates have been labelled with metallic radionuclides and used in nuclear medicine. Sodium calcium edetate is also used as a pharmaceutical excipient and as a food additive.

In the treatment of lead poisoning, sodium calcium edetate may be administered by intramuscular injection or by intravenous infusion. The intramuscular route may be preferred in patients with lead encephalopathy and increased intracranial pressure in whom excess fluids must be avoided, and also in children, who have an increased risk of incipient encephalopathy. Sodium calcium edetate may initially aggravate the symptoms of lead toxicity due to mobilisation of stored lead and it has often been given with dimercaprol (p.1037) in patients who are symptomatic; the first dose of dimercaprol should preferably be given at least 4 hours before the sodium calcium edetate.

For administration by intravenous infusion, 1 g of sodium calcium edetate should be diluted with 250 to 500 mL of glucose 5% or sodium chloride 0.9%; a concentration of 3% should not be exceeded. The infusion should be administered over a period of at least 1 hour with intervals of 8 to 12 hours between infusions. In the UK, the usual dose is 60 to 80 mg/kg daily given in two divided doses. In the USA, a dose of 1000 mg/m² daily in two divided doses is suggested for asymptomatic adults and children; a daily dose of 1500 mg/m² may be used in patients with symptomatic poisoning. Treatment is given for up to 5 days, repeated if necessary after an interval of at least 2 days. Any further treatment with sodium calcium edetate should then not be recommenced for at least 7 days.

Alternatively, the same daily dose of sodium calcium edetate may be given intramuscularly in 2 to 4 divided doses as a 20% solution. Intramuscular injection of sodium calcium edetate is painful and it is recommended that preservative-free procaine hydrochloride should be added to a concentration of 0.5 to 1.5% to minimise pain; alternatively, lidocaine may be added to a concentration of 0.5%.

As excretion is predominantly renal, an adequate urinary flow must be established and maintained during treatment. In patients with renal impairment, smaller and less frequent doses have been recommended.

### Preparations

***BP 2003:*** Sodium Calcium Edetate Intravenous Infusion;
***USP 27:*** Edetate Calcium Disodium Injection.

**Proprietary Preparations** (details are given in Part 3)
***Ger.:*** Calcium Vitis; ***Gr.:*** Ledclair; ***Irl.:*** Ledclair; ***Switz.:*** Chelintox; ***UK:*** Ledclair.

**Multi-ingredient: *Arg.:*** Calcium C.

## Sodium Cellulose Phosphate

Cellulose Sodium Phosphate *(USAN)*; Celulosa, fosfato sódico de.
*CAS — 9038-41-9; 68444-58-6.*
*ATC — V03AG01.*

**Pharmacopoeias.** In *US.*

**USP 27** (Cellulose Sodium Phosphate). It is prepared by the phosphorylation of alpha cellulose. A free-flowing, cream-coloured, odourless, powder. Insoluble in water, in dilute acids, and in most organic solvents. The pH of a filtrate of a 5% mixture in water is between 6.0 and 9.0. The inorganic bound phosphate content is not less than 31.0% and not more than 36.0%; the free phosphate content is not more than 3.5%; and the sodium content is not less than 9.5% and not more than 13.0%, all calculated on the dried basis. The calcium binding capacity, calculated on the dried basis, is not less than 1.8 mmol per g.

### Adverse Effects and Precautions

Diarrhoea and other gastrointestinal disturbances have been reported.

Sodium cellulose phosphate should not be administered to patients with primary or secondary hyperparathyroidism, hypomagnesaemia, hypocalcaemia, bone disease, or enteric hyperoxaluria. It should be administered cautiously to pregnant women and children, since they have high calcium requirements.

Patients should be monitored for electrolyte disturbances. Uptake of sodium and phosphate may increase and sodium cellulose phosphate should not be given to patients with renal failure or conditions requiring a restricted sodium intake such as heart failure. Theoretically, long-term treatment could result in calcium deficiency; regular monitoring of calcium and parathyroid hormone has therefore been recommended. Sodium cellulose phosphate is not a totally selective exchange resin and the intestinal absorption of other dietary cations may be reduced; magnesium deficiency has been reported but may be corrected by dosage reduction or oral magnesium supplements. Urinary excretion of oxalate may increase and dietary restriction of oxalate intake may be necessary.

◊ Potential complications of long-term sodium cellulose phosphate therapy include secondary hyperparathyroidism and bone disease; deficiency of magnesium, copper, zinc, and iron; and hyperoxaluria. A study in 18 patients[1] with absorptive hypercalciuria and recurrent renal stones indicated that these complications could largely be avoided if use was confined to those with absorptive hypercalciuria (hypercalciuria, intestinal hyperabsorption of calcium, and normal or suppressed parathyroid function), if the dose was adjusted so as not to reduce intestinal calcium absorption or urinary calcium subnormally (the optimal maintenance dose in most patients was 10 g daily), if oral magnesium supplements were provided, and if a moderate dietary restriction of calcium and oxalate was imposed. There was no evidence of zinc, copper, or iron deficiency.

1. Pak CYC. Clinical pharmacology of sodium cellulose phosphate. *J Clin Pharmacol* 1979; **19:** 451–7.

### Interactions

Sodium cellulose phosphate binds with calcium and other cations. Administration with calcium or magnesium salts, including cation-donating antacids or laxatives, may reduce the effectiveness of sodium cellulose phosphate. Magnesium supplements are often required in patients receiving sodium cellulose phosphate but should be administered at least one hour before or after any dose of the resin since the absorption of the magnesium may otherwise be impaired.

### Uses and Administration

Sodium cellulose phosphate, the sodium salt of the phosphate ester of cellulose, is a cation-exchange resin that exchanges sodium ions for calcium and other divalent cations. When given orally, it binds calcium ions within the stomach and intestine to form a non-absorbable complex which is excreted in the faeces. Theoretically a 5 g dose will bind about 350 mg calcium. It is used in the treatment of absorptive hypercalciuria and recurrent formation of calcium-containing renal calculi (p.936), usually with a low calcium diet. Sodium cellulose phosphate is also used in the treatment of hypercalcaemia associated with osteopetrosis, sarcoidosis, and vitamin D intoxication, and in idiopathic hypercalcaemia of infancy, although other more effective agents are usually used (see Vitamin D-mediated Hypercalcaemia p.1218).

The usual initial dose is 15 g daily by mouth in 3 divided doses with meals reducing to 10 g daily for maintenance. A suggested dose for children is 10 g daily (but see under Adverse Effects and Precautions, above). The powder may be taken dispersed in water or sprinkled onto food. Oral magnesium supplements equivalent to about 60 or 90 mg (about 2.4 or 3.6 mmol) of elemental magnesium twice daily have been recommended for patients taking daily doses of sodium cellulose phosphate 10 or 15 g respectively. The magnesium supplement should not be given simultaneously with sodium cellulose phosphate.

Sodium cellulose phosphate may also be used for the investigation of calcium absorption.

### Preparations

***USP 27:*** Cellulose Sodium Phosphate for Oral Suspension.

**Proprietary Preparations** (details are given in Part 3)
***Austral.:*** Calcisorb†; ***Belg.:*** Calcisorb†; ***Israel:*** Calcisorb; ***Neth.:*** Calcisorb; ***NZ:*** Calcisorb†; ***Spain:*** Anacalcit; ***UK:*** Calcisorb†; ***USA:*** Calcibind.

### Sodium Fytate *(rINNM)*

Fitato sódico; Phytate Sodium *(USAN)*; Sodium Phytate; SQ-9343.
The nonasodium salt of *myo*-inositol hexakis(dihydrogen phosphate); Sodium cyclohexanehexyl(hexaphosphate).
$C_6H_9Na_9O_{24}P_6$ = 857.9.
*CAS — 83-86-3 (fytic acid); 7205-52-9 (sodium fytate).*

**Profile**

Sodium fytate reacts with calcium in the gastrointestinal tract to form non-absorbable calcium fytate which is excreted in the faeces. Sodium fytate has been used in a similar manner to sodium cellulose phosphate (p.1052) to reduce the absorption of calcium from the gut in the treatment of hypercalciuria.

### Preparations

**Proprietary Preparations** (details are given in Part 3)
***Braz.:*** TCK 18†; ***Fr.:*** Phytat†.

**Multi-ingredient: *Ital.:*** Lightening; Phytic Acid.

## Sodium Nitrite

E250; Natrii Nitris; Natrium Nitrosum; Nitrito sódico.
$NaNO_2$ = 69.00.
*CAS — 7632-00-0.*
*ATC — V03AB08.*

**Pharmacopoeias.** In *Chin.*, *Eur.* (see p.vi), *Int.*, *Pol.*, and *US.*

**Ph. Eur. 5.0** (Sodium Nitrite). Hygroscopic, colourless crystals or mass or yellowish rods. Freely soluble in water; soluble in alcohol. Store in airtight containers.

**USP 27** (Sodium Nitrite). A white to slightly yellow, granular powder, or white or practically white, opaque, fused masses or sticks. It is deliquescent in air. Soluble 1 in 1.5 of water; sparingly soluble in alcohol. Its solutions are alkaline to litmus. Store in airtight containers at a temperature of 25°, excursions permitted between 15° and 30°.

### Adverse Effects

Sodium nitrite may cause nausea and vomiting, abdominal pain, dizziness, headache, flushing, cyanosis, tachypnoea, and dyspnoea; vasodilatation resulting in syncope, hypotension, and tachycardia may occur. Overdosage may result in cardiovascular collapse, coma, convulsions, and death. Ionised nitrites readily oxidise haemoglobin to methaemoglobin, causing methaemoglobinaemia.

Sodium nitrite is a precursor for the formation of nitrosamines many of which are carcinogenic in *animals*, but a relationship with human cancer has not been established.

**Methaemoglobinaemia.** Methaemoglobinaemia has been reported after the consumption of nitrite-contaminated meat.[1,2]

1. Walley T, Flanagan M. Nitrite-induced methaemoglobinaemia. *Postgrad Med J* 1987; **63:** 643–44.
2. Kennedy N, *et al.* Faulty sausage production causing methaemoglobinaemia. *Arch Dis Child* 1997; **76:** 367–8.

### Treatment of Adverse Effects

When toxicity results from the ingestion of nitrites, treatment is supportive and symptomatic; oxygen and methylthioninium chloride may be required for methaemoglobinaemia although methylthioninium chloride should not be administered if cyanide poisoning is suspected since cyanide may be displaced. Exchange transfusion may be considered when methaemoglobinaemia is severe.

### Uses and Administration

Sodium nitrite is used with sodium thiosulfate in the treatment of cyanide poisoning (p.1506). The sodium nitrite produces methaemoglobinaemia; it is postulated that the cyanide ions combine with the methaemoglobin to produce cyanmethaemoglobin, thus protecting cytochrome oxidase from the cyanide ions, although other mechanisms may have a significant role. As the cyanmethaemoglobin slowly dissociates, the cyanide is converted to relatively non-toxic thiocyanate and is excreted in the urine. Sodium thiosulfate provides an additional source of sulfur for this reaction and this accelerates the process.

The usual dosage regimen in adults is 300 mg of *sodium nitrite* (10 mL of a 3% solution) given by intravenous injection over 5 to 20 minutes followed by 12.5 g of *sodium thiosulfate* (50 mL of a 25% solution or 25 mL of a 50% solution) given intravenously over a period of about 10 minutes. A suggested dosage regimen in children is 0.13 to 0.33 mL/kg, or 6 to 8 mL/m$^2$, of a 3% solution of *sodium nitrite* (approximately 4 to 10 mg/kg) to a maximum of 10 mL, followed by 1.65 mL/kg, or 28 mL/m$^2$, of a 25% solution of *sodium thiosulfate* (412.5 mg/kg) to a maximum of 50 mL. The methaemoglobin concentration should not be allowed to exceed 30 to 40%. If symptoms of cyanide toxicity recur, some have suggested that the injections of nitrite and thiosulfate may be repeated after 30 minutes at half the initial doses.

Sodium nitrite has also been suggested in the treatment of hydrogen sulfide poisoning (see p.1236).

Sodium nitrite has been used as a rust inhibitor. It is also used as a preservative in foods such as cured meats but should not be used in food for infants under the age of 3 months due to the risk of methaemoglobinaemia. Potassium nitrite is also used as a food preservative.

### Preparations

***USP 27:*** Sodium Nitrite Injection.

**Proprietary Preparations** (details are given in Part 3)
***Austral.:*** O A R†.

**Multi-ingredient: *Canad.:*** Sporex†; ***Ital.:*** Benzogen Ferri†; Citrosil Alcolico Azzuro; Esoform Ferri Alcolico†; Esoform Ferri†; ***S.Afr.:*** Tripac-Cyano; ***USA:*** Cyanide Antidote Package.

## Sodium Polystyrene Sulfonate

Natrii Polystyrenesulfonas; Poliestirenosulfonato sódico; Sodium Polystyrene Sulphonate.

*CAS — 9003-59-2; 9080-79-9; 25704-18-1.*

*ATC — V03AE01.*

**Pharmacopoeias.** In *Eur.* (see p.vi), *Jpn*, and *US*.

**Ph. Eur. 5.0** (Sodium Polystyrene Sulphonate). An almost white to light brown powder. It contains 9.4 to 11.0% of sodium, calculated with reference to the dried substance. Each g exchanges 2.8 mmol to 3.4 mmol of potassium, calculated with reference to the dried substance. Practically insoluble in water, in alcohol, and in dichloromethane. Store in airtight containers.

**USP 27** (Sodium Polystyrene Sulfonate). A golden brown, fine, odourless powder containing not more than 10% of water. The sodium content is not less than 9.4% and not more than 11.5%, calculated on the anhydrous basis. Each g exchanges not less than 110 mg and not more than 135 mg of potassium, calculated on the anhydrous basis. Insoluble in water.

### Adverse Effects

Anorexia, nausea, vomiting, constipation, and occasionally diarrhoea may develop during treatment with sodium polystyrene sulfonate. Constipation may be severe; large doses in elderly patients and in children may result in faecal impaction and gastrointestinal concretions have occurred after oral administration to neonates. If necessary a mild laxative may be used to prevent or treat constipation; magnesium-containing laxatives should not be used (see Interactions, below).

Serious potassium deficiency can occur with sodium polystyrene sulfonate and signs of severe hypokalaemia may include irritability, confusion, ECG abnormalities, cardiac arrhythmias, and severe muscle weakness. Like other cation-exchange resins, sodium polystyrene sulfonate is not totally selective and its use may result in other electrolyte disturbances such as hypocalcaemia. Significant sodium retention may also occur, especially in patients with renal impairment, and may lead to heart failure.

**Effects on the gastrointestinal tract.** Colonic necrosis has been reported[1,2] in 6 patients following administration of sodium polystyrene sulfonate in sorbitol as enemas. The inclusion of sorbitol was considered to contribute to this effect,[1,2] although it was subsequently pointed out that colonic irrigation, as recommended by the manufacturer, had not been carried out to remove the residual resin.[3,4]

1. Lillemoe KD, *et al.* Intestinal necrosis due to sodium polystyrene (Kayexalate) in sorbitol enemas: clinical and experimental support for the hypothesis. *Surgery* 1987; **101:** 267–72.
2. Wootton FT, *et al.* Colonic necrosis with Kayexalate-sorbitol enemas after renal transplantation. *Ann Intern Med* 1989; **111:** 947–9.
3. Burnett RJ. Sodium polystyrene-sorbitol enemas. *Ann Intern Med* 1990; **112:** 311–12.
4. Shepard KV. Cleansing enemas after sodium polystyrene sulfonate enemas. *Ann Intern Med* 1990; **112:** 711.

**Effects on the lungs.** Particles of sodium polystyrene sulfonate were found at autopsy in the lungs of 3 patients who had taken the resin by mouth and were associated with acute bronchitis and bronchopneumonia in 2 and with early bronchitis in the third.[1] It was suggested that rectal administration of sodium polystyrene sulfonate may be preferable, but if administration by mouth is necessary the patient should be positioned carefully to facilitate ingestion of the resin and avoid aspiration.

1. Haupt HM, Hutchins GM. Sodium polystyrene sulfonate pneumonitis. *Arch Intern Med* 1982; **142:** 379–81.

### Precautions

Sodium polystyrene sulfonate should not be administered orally to neonates, and is contra-indicated by any route in neonates with reduced gut motility or in any patient with obstructive bowel disease. Care is also needed with rectal administration to neonates and children in order to avoid impaction of the resin. Treatment should be discontinued if clinically significant constipation develops. Sorbitol has been recommended for the prophylaxis and treatment of constipation (but see Effects on the Gastrointestinal Tract, above); magnesium-containing laxatives should not be used (see Interactions, below).

Patients receiving sodium polystyrene sulfonate should be monitored for electrolyte disturbances, especially hypokalaemia. Since serum concentrations may not always reflect intracellular potassium deficiency, symptoms of hypokalaemia should also be watched for and the decision to stop treatment assessed individually.

Use of sodium polystyrene sulfonate can result in sodium overloading and it should be used cautiously in patients with renal failure or conditions requiring a restricted sodium intake, such as heart failure and severe hypertension; calcium polystyrene sulfonate (p.1032) may be preferred in these patients.

The possible effects of sodium polystyrene sulfonate on serum electrolytes should be considered when diagnostic measurements are contemplated in patients receiving such treatment.

Following the administration of sodium polystyrene sulfonate retention enemas, the colon should be irrigated to ensure removal of the resin.

### Interactions

Sodium polystyrene sulfonate is not totally selective for potassium and may also bind other cations. Metabolic alkalosis has been reported in patients, particularly those with renal impairment, after the concomitant oral administration of sodium polystyrene sulfonate and cation-donating antacids and laxatives such as magnesium hydroxide, aluminium hydroxide, or calcium carbonate; binding of the cation by the resin prevents neutralisation of bicarbonate ions in the small intestine. The potassium-lowering effect of the resin will also be diminished.

Ion-exchange resins may also bind other drugs given concomitantly, reducing their absorption. For reference to such an effect with levothyroxine, see p.1601.

Hypokalaemia may exacerbate the adverse effects of digoxin and sodium polystyrene sulfonate should be used with caution in patients receiving cardiac glycosides.

### Uses and Administration

Sodium polystyrene sulfonate, the sodium salt of sulfonated styrene copolymer with divinylbenzene, is a cation-exchange resin which exchanges sodium ions for potassium ions and other cations in the gastrointestinal tract following oral or rectal administration. The exchanged resin is then excreted in the faeces. Each gram of resin exchanges about 3 mmol of potassium *in vitro*, and about 1 mmol *in vivo*.

Sodium polystyrene sulfonate is used to enhance potassium excretion in the treatment of hyperkalaemia, including that associated with anuria or severe oliguria (caution is required due to the sodium content). An effect may not be evident for several hours or longer, and in severe hyperkalaemia, where a rapid effect is required, other measures must also be considered (see p.1219).

Serum-electrolyte concentrations should be monitored throughout treatment and doses given according to response.

The usual oral dose is 15 g up to four times daily as a suspension in water or syrup or as a sweetened paste. It should not be given in fruit juices that have a high potassium content. A suggested dose for children is 1 g/kg daily by mouth in divided doses for acute hyperkalaemia, reduced to a maintenance dose of 500 mg/kg daily; the oral route is not recommended for neonates.

When oral administration is difficult, sodium polystyrene sulfonate may be administered rectally as an enema. The usual daily dose is 30 g given as a suspension in 100 mL of 2% methylcellulose '450' and 100 mL of water and retained, if possible, for at least 9 hours; higher doses, shorter retention times, and alternative vehicles have also been used. Following retention of the enema the colon should be irrigated to remove the resin. Initial therapy may constitute administration by both oral and rectal routes. Children and neonates may be given rectal doses similar to those suggested for children by mouth; particular care is needed with rectal administration in children as excessive dosage or inadequate dilution could result in impaction of resin.

Other polystyrene sulfonate resins include calcium polystyrene sulfonate (p.1032), which is used similarly to the sodium resin and potassium polystyrene sulfonate (p.1050), which is used in the treatment of hypercalciuria. Aluminium polystyrene sulfonate, ammonium polystyrene sulfonate, and magnesium polystyrene sulfonate have all occasionally been used.

### Preparations

***USP 27:*** Sodium Polystyrene Sulfonate Suspension.

**Proprietary Preparations** (details are given in Part 3)
***Austral.:*** Resonium A; ***Austria:*** Resonium A; ***Belg.:*** Kayexalate Sodium; ***Canad.:*** K-Exit; Kayexalate; ***Denm.:*** Resonium; ***Fin.:*** Resonium; ***Fr.:*** Kayexalate; ***Ger.:*** Elutit-Natrium; Resonium A; ***Gr.:*** Kayexalate; ***Hong Kong:*** Resonium A; ***Irl.:*** Resonium A; ***Israel:*** Kayexalate; ***Ital.:*** Kayexalate; ***Malaysia:*** Resonium A; ***Neth.:*** Resonium A; ***NZ:*** Resonium A; ***Port.:*** Resonium; ***S.Afr.:*** Kexelate; ***Singapore:*** Resinsodio; ***Spain:*** Resinsodio; ***Swed.:*** Resonium; ***Switz.:*** Resonium A; ***Thai.:*** Kayexalate; Resinsodio†; Resonium A; ***UK:*** Resonium A; ***USA:*** Kayexalate; Kionex; SPS.

**Multi-ingredient: *Ger.:*** Ujostabil.

## Sodium Thiosulfate

Disodium Thiosulfate Pentahydrate; Natrii Thiosulfas; Natrium Thiosulfuricum; Sodium Hyposulphite; Sodium Thiosulphate; Tiosulfato sódico.

$Na_2S_2O_3,5H_2O$ = 248.2.

*CAS — 7772-98-7 (anhydrous sodium thiosulfate); 10102-17-7 (sodium thiosulfate pentahydrate).*

*ATC — V03AB06.*

**Pharmacopoeias.** In *Chin., Eur.* (see p.vi), *Int., Jpn, Pol., US,* and *Viet.*

**Ph. Eur. 5.0** (Sodium Thiosulphate). Colourless transparent crystals; efflorescent in dry air. It dissolves in its own water of crystallisation at about 49°. Very soluble in water; practically insoluble in alcohol. A 10% solution in water has a pH of 6.0 to 8.4. Store in airtight containers.

**USP 27** (Sodium Thiosulfate). Large, colourless crystals, or a coarse, crystalline powder. Is deliquescent in moist air and effloresces in dry air at temperatures exceeding 33°. Soluble 1 in 0.5 of water; insoluble in alcohol. Its solutions are neutral or faintly alkaline to litmus. Store in airtight containers.

**Stability.** Solutions of sodium thiosulfate 50% stored in air developed cloudiness or a deposit after autoclaving.[1] Addition of sodium phosphate 0.5% or 1.2% improved stability but solutions became cloudy or developed a deposit after 12 and 6 weeks respectively at 25°. Solutions containing sodium bicarbonate 0.5% became cloudy or developed a deposit after 12 weeks at 25°. No significant improvement in stability was obtained when the concentration of sodium thiosulfate was reduced to 30% or 15%, or when the injection was sealed under nitrogen.

1. Anonymous. Sodium thiosulphate injection–effect of additives on stability. *PSGB Lab Rep* P/75/3 1975.

### Adverse Effects

Apart from osmotic disturbances sodium thiosulfate is relatively non-toxic. Large doses by mouth have a cathartic action.

### Interactions

◊ For reference to the inactivation of phenylmercuric salts by sodium thiosulfate, see Phenylmercuric Nitrate, p.1189.

### Pharmacokinetics

Sodium thiosulfate is poorly absorbed from the gastrointestinal tract. After intravenous injection it is distributed throughout the extracellular fluid and rapidly excreted in the urine.

◊ An intravenous infusion of sodium thiosulfate 12 g/m² was given over 6 hours to 8 patients receiving intraperitoneal antineoplastic therapy;[1] in 6 of the patients it was given to protect against the adverse effects of cisplatin. The thiosulfate was rapidly eliminated, 95% being excreted within 4 hours of stopping the infusion; on average only 28.5% of the dose was recovered unchanged in the urine. The mean plasma elimination half-life was 80 minutes.

1. Shea M, *et al.* Kinetics of sodium thiosulfate, a cisplatin neutralizer. *Clin Pharmacol Ther* 1984; **35:** 419–25.

### Uses and Administration

Sodium thiosulfate is used in the treatment of cyanide poisoning (p.1506). Sodium thiosulfate may be effective alone in less severe cases of cyanide poisoning, but it is often used after administration of sodium nitrite (p.1052).

Sodium thiosulfate acts as a sulfur-donating substrate for the enzyme rhodanese, which catalyses the conversion of cyanide to relatively non-toxic thiocyanate, and thus accelerates the detoxification of cyanide.

The usual dosage regimen in adults is 300 mg of *sodium nitrite* (10 mL of a 3% solution) given by intravenous injection over 5 to 20 minutes followed by 12.5 g of *sodium thiosulfate* (50 mL of a 25% solution or 25 mL of a 50% solution) given intravenously over a period of about 10 minutes. A suggested dosage regimen in children is 0.13 to 0.33 mL/kg, or 6 to 8 mL/m², of a 3% solution of *sodium nitrite* (about 4 to 10 mg/kg) to a maximum of 10 mL, followed by 1.65 mL/kg, or 28 mL/m², of a 25% solution of *sodium thiosulfate* (412.5 mg/kg) to a maximum of 50 mL. The methaemoglobin concentration should not be allowed to exceed 30 to 40%. If symptoms of cyanide toxicity recur, some have suggested that the injections of nitrite and thiosulfate may be repeated after 30 minutes at half the initial doses.

Sodium thiosulfate is used as an isotonic 4% solution in the management of extravasation of chlormethine and has been tried in the management of extravasation of some other antineoplastics (although this is a contentious area, see p.496).

Sodium thiosulfate has been used for its antifungal properties. Sodium thiosulfate and magnesium thiosulfate are included in mixed preparations for a variety of disorders.

**Antineoplastic toxicity.** Sodium thiosulfate may be used in the management of extravasation of chlormethine and some other antineoplastics (see p.496).

Sodium thiosulfate given by intravenous infusion has been reported to reduce the incidence of nephrotoxicity associated with intraperitoneal cisplatin (see under Adverse Effects in Cisplatin, p.538) and to reduce hearing loss associated with carboplatin (see Effects on the Ears, p.534).

**Bromate poisoning.** Sodium thiosulfate has been used in the treatment of bromate poisoning[1,2] although its clinical efficacy is unclear.[3] Sodium thiosulfate is thought to act by reducing bromate to the less toxic bromide ion, but evidence is lacking.[3] However, the high morbidity and mortality associated with bromate poisoning may justify the use of this relatively innocuous drug in some clinical circumstances.[4]

1. Lue JN, *et al.* Bromate poisoning from ingestion of professional hair-care neutralizer. *Clin Pharm* 1988; **7:** 66–70.
2. Lichtenberg R, *et al.* Bromate poisoning. *J Pediatr* 1989; **114:** 891–4.
3. McElwee NE, Kearney TE. Sodium thiosulfate unproven as bromate antidote. *Clin Pharm* 1988; **7:** 570, 572.
4. Johnson CE. Sodium thiosulfate unproven as bromate antidote. *Clin Pharm* 1988; **7:** 572.

### Preparations

***BP 2003:*** Sodium Thiosulphate Injection;
***USP 27:*** Sodium Thiosulfate Injection.

**Proprietary Preparations** (details are given in Part 3)
***Canad.:*** Consept Step 2†; ***Mex.:*** Hiposul†.

**Multi-ingredient:** ***Austria:*** Schwefelbad Dr Klopfer; ***Belg.:*** ITC†; ***Braz.:*** Desensibilizante Chauvin; Osmogenol†; TCK-1 Hematocis†; ***Canad.:*** Adasept; ***Fr.:*** Desintex; Desintex Infantile; Desintex-Choline; Rhino-Sulfuryl; Vagostabyl; ***Ger.:*** Corti Jaikal; Jaikal; Schwefelbad Dr Klopfer; Sulfuretten; ***Hong Kong:*** Colircusi Iodine-Thio-Calcic†; ***Ital.:*** Antimicotica Solforata; ***S.Afr.:*** Tripac-Cyano; ***Spain:*** Yodo Tio Calci†; ***Switz.:*** Thiorubrol†; ***USA:*** Cyanide Antidote Package; Tinver; Versiclear.

## Succimer *(BAN, USAN, rINN)*

DIM-SA; DMSA; Succímero. *meso*-2,3-Dimercaptosuccinic acid; (R*,S*)-2,3-Dimercapto-butanedioic acid.

$C_4H_6O_4S_2$ = 182.2.

*CAS — 304-55-2.*

**Pharmacopoeias.** In *Chin.*

### Adverse Effects and Precautions

Succimer may cause gastrointestinal disorders, skin rashes, increases in serum transaminase, flu-like symptoms, drowsiness, and dizziness. Mild to moderate neutropenia has been reported in some patients and regular full blood counts are recommended during therapy. Succimer should be used with caution in patients with renal impairment or a history of hepatic disease.

### Pharmacokinetics

Succimer is rapidly but incompletely absorbed after oral administration. It undergoes rapid and extensive metabolism and is excreted mainly in the urine with small amounts excreted in the bile and via the lungs.

◊ References.

1. Dart RC, *et al.* Pharmacokinetics of meso-2,3-dimercaptosuccinic acid in patients with lead poisoning and in healthy adults. *J Pediatr* 1994; **125:** 309–16.

### Uses and Administration

Succimer is a chelator structurally related to dimercaprol (p.1037). It forms water-soluble chelates with heavy metals and is used in the treatment of lead poisoning. It has also been used in the treatment of poisoning with arsenic or mercury.

Succimer, labelled with a radionuclide, is used in nuclear medicine.

In the treatment of lead poisoning, succimer is given by mouth in a suggested dose of 10 mg/kg or 350 mg/m² every 8 hours for 5 days then every 12 hours for an additional 14 days. The course of treatment may be repeated if necessary, usually after an interval of not less than 2 weeks.

**Lead poisoning.** The use of succimer in lead poisoning has been reviewed.[1,2] Although, in children, succimer is generally only indicated if blood-lead concentrations are greater than 45 micrograms/100 mL,[3] promising results have also been reported in those with lower concentrations.[4] A number of dosage regimens have been studied.[5] For the management of lead poisoning, see Lead, Treatment of Adverse Effects, p.1705.

1. Anonymous. Succimer—an oral drug for lead poisoning. *Med Lett Drugs Ther* 1991; **33:** 78.
2. Mann KV, Travers JD. Succimer, an oral lead chelator. *Clin Pharm* 1991; **10:** 914–22.
3. Rogan WJ, *et al.* The effect of chelation therapy with succimer on neuropsychological development in children exposed to lead. *N Engl J Med* 2001; **344:** 1421–6.
4. Besunder JB, *et al.* Short-term efficacy of oral dimercaptosuccinic acid in children with low to moderate lead intoxication. *Pediatrics* 1995; **96:** 683–7.
5. Farrar HC, *et al.* A comparison of two dosing regimens of succimer in children with chronic lead poisoning. *J Clin Pharmacol* 1999; **39:** 180–3.

**Mercury poisoning.** Extracorporeal infusion of succimer into the arterial blood line during haemodialysis, a procedure known as extracorporeal regional complexing haemodialysis, produced a substantial clearance of mercury in an anuric patient following intoxication with inorganic mercury.[1] Clearance was approximately ten times greater than that achieved with haemodialysis following intramuscular administration of dimercaprol. For the management of mercury poisoning, see Mercury, Treatment of Adverse Effects, p.1713.

1. Kostyniak PJ, *et al.* Extracorporeal regional complexing haemodialysis treatment of acute inorganic mercury intoxication. *Hum Toxicol* 1990; **9:** 137–41.

### Preparations

**Proprietary Preparations** (details are given in Part 3)
***Austria:*** Chemet†; ***Fr.:*** Succicaptal; ***USA:*** Chemet.

## Tiopronin *(rINN)*

Thiopronine; Tiopronina. *N*-(2-Mercaptopropionyl)glycine.

$C_5H_9NO_3S$ = 163.2.

*CAS — 1953-02-2.*

*ATC — R05CB12.*

### Adverse Effects and Precautions

Tiopronin has similar adverse effects and precautions to those of penicillamine (p.1046).

**Incidence of adverse effects.** In a study of 140 patients[1] with rheumatoid arthritis receiving long-term treatment with tiopronin, adverse effects necessitated withdrawal of treatment in 56 patients (40%). The majority of adverse effects occurred within the first 6 months of treatment. The most common were those affecting the skin and mucous membranes (46 patients) including stomatitis, pruritus, erythema, and 1 case of pemphigus. Proteinuria developed in 5 patients and nephrotic syndrome in 3. Haematological disorders developed in 13 patients. Gastrointestinal disorders and ageusia were also reported.

In another study of 74 patients[2] with rheumatoid arthritis adverse effects were reported in 32 patients (43%) and necessitated withdrawal in 24%. The most common adverse effects were ageusia (21%), mucocutaneous lesions (16%), and gastrointestinal disturbances (14%). Haematological disorders occurred in 5 patients and proteinuria in 3 patients.

In a comparative study in 200 patients,[3] treatment was withdrawn due to toxicity in 27% of patients taking tiopronin and 21% of patients treated with gold.

1. Sany J, *et al.* Etude de la tolérance à long terme de la thiopronine (Acadione) dans le traitement de la polyarthrite rhumatoïde: a propos de 140 cas personnels. *Rev Rhum* 1990; **57:** 105–11.
2. Ehrhart A, *et al.* Effets secondaires dus au traitement par la tiopronine de 74 polyarthrites rhumatoïdes. *Rev Rhum* 1991; **58:** 193–7.
3. Ferraccioli GF, *et al.* Long-term outcome with gold thiosulphate and tiopronin in 200 rheumatoid patients. *Clin Exp Rheumatol* 1989; **7:** 577–81.

**Effects on the blood.** Leucopenia or thrombocytopenia has been reported in 13 of 140 patients[1] and 5 of 74 patients[2] during long-term studies of tiopronin.

Isolated cases of agranulocytosis[3] and bone marrow aplasia[4] have been reported.

1. Sany J, *et al.* Etude de la tolérance à long terme de la thiopronine (Acadione) dans le traitement de la polyarthrite rhumatoïde: a propos de 140 cas personnels. *Rev Rhum* 1990; **57:** 105–11.
2. Ehrhart A, *et al.* Effets secondaires dus au traitement par la tiopronine de 74 polyarthrites rhumatoïdes. *Rev Rhum* 1991; **58:** 193–7.
3. Corda C, *et al.* Thiopronin-induced agranulocytosis. *Therapie* 1990; **45:** 161.
4. Taillan B, *et al.* Aplasie médullaire au cours d'une polyarthrite rhumatoïde traitée par tiopronine. *Rev Rhum* 1990; **57:** 443–4.

**Effects on the kidneys.** Proteinuria developed in 3 patients 4 to 14 months after starting treatment with tiopronin for cystinuria.[1] None of the patients had clinical symptoms of nephrotic syndrome. Renal biopsies in 2 patients demonstrated membranous glomerulonephritis. Proteinuria disappeared in all 3 patients 4 to 5 months after tiopronin was discontinued. However, there was histological evidence of irreversible changes and signs of progressive glomerular lesions in one patient.

Proteinuria was reported in 5 patients and nephrotic syndrome in 3 of 140 patients receiving tiopronin long term.[2]

1. Lindell A, *et al.* Membranous glomerulonephritis induced by 2-mercaptopropionylglycine (2-MPG). *Clin Nephrol* 1990; **34:** 108–15.
2. Sany J, *et al.* Etude de la tolérance à long terme de la thiopronine (Acadione) dans le traitement de la polyarthrite rhumatoïde: a propos de 140 cas personnels. *Rev Rhum* 1990; **57:** 105–11.

**Effects on the liver.** Acute liver damage often leading to jaundice has developed in patients given tiopronin; this has led to the Japanese authorities contra-indicating it in patients with a history of hypersensitivity and recommending that serial liver function tests be carried out during treatment.[1]

1. Anonymous. Tiopronin and liver damage. *WHO Drug Inf* 1989; **3:** 139.

**Effects on the skin.** Mucocutaneous lesions are among the most common adverse effects of tiopronin (see above). Lichenoid eruptions in a patient developed after 2 years of treatment with tiopronin and resolved when tiopronin was withdrawn.[1] Skin patch testing gave a positive response not only to tiopronin but also to penicillamine and captopril, neither of which the patient had taken. It was suggested that the lichenoid reaction was immunologically mediated and that the sulfhydryl group, which is common to all three compounds, could have been responsible.

Skin lesions resembling pemphigus have been reported in a few patients receiving tiopronin.[2,3] The lesions may improve when tiopronin is discontinued;[2] the remaining patients require treatment with a corticosteroid or other immunosuppressant drug, or both.[3]


1. Kurumaji Y, Miyazaki K. Tiopronine-induced lichenoid eruption in a patient with liver disease and positive patch test reaction to drugs with sulfhydryl group. *J Dermatol* 1990; **17:** 176–81.
2. Trotta F, *et al.* Thiopronine-induced pemphigus vulgaris in rheumatoid arthritis. *Scand J Rheumatol* 1984; **13:** 93–5.
3. Verdier-Sevrain S, *et al.* Thiopronine-induced herpetiform pemphigus: report of a case studied by immunoelectron microscopy and immunoblot analysis. *Br J Dermatol* 1994; **130:** 238–40.


## Pharmacokinetics

Tiopronin is absorbed from the gastrointestinal tract. Up to 48% of the dose is reported to be excreted in the urine during the first 4 hours and up to 78% by 72 hours.

◊ References.


1. Carlsson SM, *et al.* Pharmacokinetics of intravenous 2-mercaptopropionylglycine in man. *Eur J Clin Pharmacol* 1990; **38:** 499–503.
2. Carlsson MS, *et al.* Pharmacokinetics of oral tiopronin. *Eur J Clin Pharmacol* 1993; **45:** 79–84.


## Uses and Administration

Tiopronin is a sulfhydryl compound and chelator with properties similar to those of penicillamine (p.1049). It is given by mouth in the management of cystinuria, in conjunction with adequate hydration and alkalinisation of the urine, in usual doses of 0.8 to 1 g daily in divided doses, rising to 2 g daily if necessary. Tiopronin should be given on an empty stomach. Tiopronin is used in similar doses in rheumatoid arthritis. It has been tried in hepatic disorders, heavy-metal poisoning, and as a mucolytic in respiratory disorders, when it may be given by inhalation. It may also be given rectally or by intravenous or intramuscular injection.

The sodium salt has also been used.

**Cystinuria.** Tiopronin may be used as an alternative to penicillamine in the management of cystinuria (p.1049). In a multicentre study,[1] 66 patients with cystine nephrolithiasis were treated with tiopronin in doses of up to 2 g daily (mean 1.193 g); ongoing alkali therapy was continued and the same dietary and fluid regimens were maintained. Tiopronin significantly reduced urinary-cystine concentrations and the new stone formation rate. The adverse effects of tiopronin and penicillamine were compared in 49 patients who had been treated with penicillamine before starting the study. Both drugs had similar side-effects; 41 patients had side-effects to penicillamine, of which 34 required cessation of drug therapy, and 37 patients had side-effects to tiopronin, of which 15 required drug withdrawal. However, of the 34 patients who had to stop penicillamine therapy because of adverse effects, 22 were able to continue treatment with tiopronin. Of the 17 patients without a history of penicillamine therapy, 11 had adverse effects to tiopronin and 1 discontinued treatment because of proteinuria.


1. Pak CYC, *et al.* Management of cystine nephrolithiasis with alpha-mercaptopropionylglycine. *J Urol (Baltimore)* 1986; **136:** 1003–8.


**Lead poisoning.** Parenteral administration of tiopronin (30 g over a period of 10 days) to 27 men with symptoms of chronic lead poisoning had a beneficial effect on the biochemical indices of lead poisoning.[1] The mechanism of action was not clear since urinary lead excretion did not change. The usual treatment of lead poisoning is discussed on p.1705.


1. Candura F, *et al.* Sulphydryl compounds in lead poisoning. *Lancet* 1979; **i:** 330.


**Mucolytic activity.** Studies on the mucolytic activity of tiopronin.


1. Costantini D, *et al.* Evaluation of the therapeutic effectiveness of thiopronine in children with cystic fibrosis. *Curr Ther Res* 1982; **31:** 714–17.
2. Carratù L, *et al.* Clinico-functional and rheological research on mucolytic activity of thiopronine in chronic broncho-pneumopathies. *Curr Ther Res* 1982; **32:** 529–43.


**Rheumatoid arthritis.** Tiopronin has been reported to have activity comparable to that of gold salts[1] and penicillamine[2] in patients with rheumatoid disease, and could be tried cautiously to treat rheumatoid arthritis (p.9) in patients intolerant of penicillamine.


1. Ferraccioli GF, *et al.* Long-term outcome with gold thiosulphate and tiopronin in 200 rheumatoid patients. *Clin Exp Rheumatol* 1989; **7:** 577–81.
2. Sany J, *et al.* Etude de la tolérance à long terme de la thiopronine (Acadione) dans le traitement de la polyarthrite rhumatoïde: a propos de 140 cas personnels. *Rev Rhum* 1990; **57:** 105–11.


## Preparations

**Proprietary Preparations** (details are given in Part 3)
***Austral.:*** Thiola; ***Fr.:*** Acadione; ***Ger.:*** Captimer; ***Hong Kong:*** Thiola; ***Ital.:*** Mucolysin; Mucosyt; Thiola; Thiosol; ***Switz.:*** Mucolysin; ***USA:*** Thiola.

## Trientine Dihydrochloride *(BAN, rINNM)*

Dihidrocloruro de trientina; MK-0681; Trien Hydrochloride; Trientine Hydrochloride *(USAN)*; Triethylenetetramine Dihydrochloride. 2,2′-Ethylenedi-iminobis(ethylamine) dihydrochloride; *N,N′*-bis(2-Aminoethyl)-1,2-ethanediamine dihydrochloride.

$C_6H_{18}N_4,2HCl = 219.2.$

*CAS — 112-24-3 (trientine); 38260-01-4 (trientine dihydrochloride).*

**Pharmacopoeias.** In *US.*

**USP 27** (Trientine Hydrochloride). A white to pale yellow crystalline powder. Freely soluble in water; slightly soluble in alcohol; insoluble in chloroform and in ether; soluble in methyl alcohol. pH of a 1% solution in water is between 7.0 and 8.5. Store under an inert gas in airtight containers at 2° to 8°. Protect from light.

### Adverse Effects and Precautions

Trientine dihydrochloride may cause nausea. Iron deficiency may occur; if iron supplements are given an interval of at least 2 hours between the doses of trientine and iron has been recommended. Recurrence of symptoms of systemic lupus erythematosus has been reported in a patient who had previously reacted to penicillamine.

### Interactions

Chelation of trientine with metal ions in the diet or in mineral supplements may impair the absorption of both. Trientine should not be taken with mineral supplements and should be taken at least 1 hour apart from food, other drugs, or milk, to reduce the likelihood of absorption being affected. Iron supplements should be taken at least 2 hours before or after trientine.

### Uses and Administration

Trientine dihydrochloride is a copper chelator used in a similar way to penicillamine in the treatment of Wilson's disease (p.1049). It tends to be used in patients intolerant of penicillamine.

Trientine dihydrochloride is given orally, preferably on an empty stomach. In the USA, the usual initial dose in adults is 0.75 to 1.25 g daily in 2 to 4 divided doses increasing to a maximum of 2 g daily if required; daily doses of 1.2 to 2.4 g have been recommended in the UK. In children, the usual initial dose is 0.5 to 0.75 g daily increasing to a maximum of 1.5 g daily if required.

### Preparations

***USP 27:*** Trientine Hydrochloride Capsules.

**Proprietary Preparations** (details are given in Part 3)
***USA:*** Syprine.

## Unithiol

DMPS; Unitiol. Sodium 2,3-dimercaptopropanesulfonate.

$C_3H_7NaO_3S_3 = 210.3.$

*CAS — 4076-02-2.*

### Profile

Unithiol is a chelator structurally related to dimercaprol (p.1037). It is water soluble and reported to be less toxic than dimercaprol. Unithiol is used in the treatment of poisoning by heavy metals including arsenic, lead, inorganic and organic mercury compounds, and chromium. It may be less effective in cadmium poisoning.

Unithiol is given orally in doses of 100 mg three or four times daily in chronic poisoning. A dose of 1.2 to 2.4 g has been suggested in acute poisoning. It has also been given parenterally.

◊ Reviews.


1. Aposhian HV. DMSA and DMPS—water soluble antidotes for heavy metal poisoning. *Ann Rev Pharmacol Toxicol* 1983; **23:** 193–215.
2. Hruby K, Donner A. 2,3-Dimercapto-1-propanesulphonate in heavy metal poisoning. *Med Toxicol* 1987; **2:** 317–23.


**Lead poisoning.** Unithiol has been tried in chronic lead poisoning. In a study of 12 children[1] it reduced lead concentrations in blood but did not affect the concentrations of copper or zinc in plasma, although the urinary excretion of lead, copper, and zinc was increased during treatment.

The usual chelators used in the management of lead poisoning are discussed under Lead, Treatment of Adverse Effects, on p.1705.


1. Chisolm JJ, Thomas DJ. Use of 2,3-dimercaptopropane-1-sulfonate in treatment of lead poisoning in children. *J Pharmacol Exp Ther* 1985; **235:** 665–9.


**Mercury poisoning.** Unithiol 100 mg given twice daily by mouth for a maximum of 15 days enhanced urinary elimination of mercury in 7 patients with mercury poisoning.[1] The urinary elimination of copper and zinc was also increased in most patients and two developed skin rashes. Unithiol 50 mg per 10 kg body-weight by intramuscular injection three times daily, reducing to 50 mg per 10 kg once daily by the third day of treatment, effectively reduced the half-life of mercury in the blood following poisoning with methylmercury.[2]

There has also been a report of 4 weeks of intravenous treatment, followed by 3 weeks of oral treatment, with unithiol in the successful management of a patient with severe poisoning with mercuric chloride.[3]

For the management of mercury poisoning, see Mercury, Treatment of Adverse Effects, p.1713.


1. Mant TGK. Clinical studies with dimercaptopropane sulphonate in mercury poisoning. *Hum Toxicol* 1985; **4:** 346.
2. Clarkson TW, *et al.* Tests of efficacy of antidotes for removal of methylmercury in human poisoning during the Iraq outbreak. *J Pharmacol Exp Ther* 1981; **218:** 74–83.
3. Toet AE, *et al.* Mercury kinetics in a case of severe mercuric chloride poisoning treated with dimercapto-1-propane sulphonate (DMPS). *Hum Exp Toxicol* 1994; **13:** 11–16.


**Wilson's disease.** Unithiol 200 mg twice daily[1] was used successfully to maintain cupriuresis in a 13-year-old boy with Wilson's disease (see p.1049) after he developed systemic lupus during treatment with penicillamine and with trientine dihydrochloride. Unithiol was started in 2 similar patients[1] but both withdrew from treatment, one because of fever and a fall in leucocyte count following a test dose and the other because of intense nausea and taste impairment.


1. Walshe JM. Unithiol in Wilson's disease. *BMJ* 1985; **290:** 673–4.


### Preparations

**Proprietary Preparations** (details are given in Part 3)
***Ger.:*** Dimaval; Mercuval.

# Colouring Agents

Colouring agents have long been used in foods and cosmetics in an attempt to improve the appearance of the product or subject. They are also used in medicinal preparations with the aim of improving their acceptability to patients. This chapter describes the colouring agents used in medicines as well as some used in foods and cosmetics. Such uses are now widely controlled and this has resulted in restrictions on the extent to which colouring agents may be used. Matters of concern that have received considerable publicity include sensitivity reactions (see Tartrazine, p.1058) and hyperactive behaviour (see below).

Colouring agents can be broadly categorised into synthetic dyes and into natural agents (such as canthaxanthin, caramel, carmine, chlorophyll, cochineal, saffron, and turmeric, all of which are described in this chapter). Other compounds that may be used as cosmetic colours or food colours (and which are themselves natural pigments of foodstuffs) are anthocyanins (E163) and carotenoids. In this latter group are included bixin (E160b) and norbixin (E160b) which are obtained from annatto (E160b), capsanthin (E160c) which is an extract of paprika, carotenes (E160a) (see Betacarotene, p.1422), lycopene (E160d), beta-apo-8′-carotenal (E160e), and the ethyl ester of beta-apo-8′-carotenoic acid (E160f); lutein (E161b), like canthaxanthin, can be classified either as a carotenoid or as a xanthophyll.

Other agents described in *Martindale* that may be used as food colours include aluminium (p.1652), gold (p.1695), indigo carmine (p.1700), patent blue V (p.1729), riboflavin (p.1456), silver (p.1746), and titanium dioxide (p.1160).

**Hyperactivity.** The role of foods and food additives in hyperactive behaviour (p.1583) is not clear. In one double-blind placebo-controlled study,[1] children whose poor behaviour was attributed, by their parents, to the intake of food additives, were given oral challenges with food colours (amaranth, carmoisine, sunset yellow, and tartrazine) in doses far in excess of estimated normal daily intakes. Although the study investigators could measure a worsening of behavioural scores after the food colours, the parents did not note the difference between challenge and placebo periods. Another study[2] of similar design detected a dose-dependent association between tartrazine intake and behavioural changes (irritability, restlessness, and sleep disturbances). In a more recent study[3] improvement in hyperactive behaviour in 3-year-old children after withdrawal of artificial food colours and benzoate preservatives was detectable by parents but not by clinical assessment.


1. Pollock I, Warner JO. Effect of artificial food colours on childhood behaviour. *Arch Dis Child* 1990; **65:** 74–7.
2. Rowe KS, Rowe KJ. Synthetic food coloring and behavior: a dose response effect in a double-blind, placebo-controlled, repeated-measures study. *J Pediatr* 1994; **125:** 691–8.
3. Bateman B, *et al.* The effects of a double blind, placebo controlled, artificial food colourings and benzoate preservative challenge on hyperactivity in a general population sample of preschool children. *Arch Dis Child* 2004; **89:** 506–11.


## Allura Red AC

CI Food Red 17; Colour Index No. 16035; E129; FD & C Red No. 40; Rojo allura AC. Disodium 6-hydroxy-5-(6-methoxy-4-sulphonato-*m*-tolylazo)naphthalene-2-sulphonate.

$C_{18}H_{14}N_2Na_2O_8S_2$ = 496.4.
*CAS — 25956-17-6.*

### Profile

Allura red AC is used as a colouring agent in cosmetics and foodstuffs.

## Amaranth

Amaranto; Bordeaux S; CI Acid Red 27; CI Food Red 9; Colour Index No. 16185; E123. It consists mainly of trisodium 3-hydroxy-4-(4-sulphonato-1-naphthylazo)naphthalene-2,7-disulphonate.

$C_{20}H_{11}N_2Na_3O_{10}S_3$ = 604.5.
*CAS — 915-67-3.*

### Profile

Amaranth is used as a colouring agent in medicines, foodstuffs, and cosmetics.

**Carcinogenicity.** Although some evidence of carcinogenicity was found in early *animal* studies, subsequent work failed to confirm these findings and in the UK amaranth is considered suitable for use as a food colour.[1]


1. MAFF. Food advisory committee: final report on the review of the colouring matter in food regulations 1973. *FdAC/REP/4*. London: HMSO, 1987.


## Beetroot Red

Beet Red; E162; Rojo de remolacha.

### Profile

Beetroot red is obtained from the roots of red beets, *Beta vulgaris* var. *rubra* (Chenopodiaceae). The main colouring principle consists of betacyanins of which betanine is the main constituent. Beetroot red is used as a colouring agent for foodstuffs and cosmetics.

## Black PN

Brilliant Black BN; Brilliant Black PN; CI Food Black 1; Colour Index No. 28440; E151; Negro PN; Noir Brillant BN. It consists mainly of tetrasodium 4-acetamido-5-hydroxy-6-[7-sulphonato-4-(4-sulphonatophenylazo)-1-naphthylazo]naphthalene-1,7-disulphonate.

$C_{28}H_{17}N_5Na_4O_{14}S_4$ = 867.7.
*CAS — 2519-30-4.*

### Profile

Black PN is used as a colouring agent in medicines, cosmetics, and foods.

## Bordeaux B

Azorubrum; Burdeos B; CI Acid Red 17; Colour Index No. 16180. It consists mainly of disodium 3-hydroxy-4-(1-naphthylazo)naphthalene-2,7-disulphonate.

$C_{20}H_{12}N_2Na_2O_7S_2$ = 502.4.
*CAS — 5858-33-3.*

### Profile

Bordeaux B was formerly used as a colouring agent for medicines and foods but has been replaced by other colours.

## Brilliant Blue FCF

Azul brillante FCF; Blue EGS; CI Acid Blue 9; CI Food Blue 2; Colour Index No. 42090; E133; FD & C Blue No. 1; Patent Blue AC. Disodium 4′,4″-bis(*N*-ethyl-3-sulphonatobenzylamino)triphenylmethylium-2-sulphonate.

$C_{37}H_{34}N_2Na_2O_9S_3$ = 792.8.
*CAS — 3844-45-9.*

### Profile

Brilliant blue FCF is used as a colouring agent in medicines, cosmetics, and foodstuffs.

**Enteral feeds.** Blue colourings such as brilliant blue FCF have been added to enteral feeds to aid the detection of pulmonary aspiration but such use has been associated with toxic effects. Blue discoloration of the skin, initially attributed to cyanosis, has been reported[1] in a child who received a large quantity of brilliant blue FCF as a colouring in an enteral feed. Abnormal systemic absorption of the dye has also been reported[2] in 2 critically ill patients, both of whom subsequently died. As of September 2003 the FDA was aware of 20 cases of blue discoloration of body fluids and skin associated with the use of blue dyes, including 12 fatalities.[3] Most cases occurred in patients with a history of sepsis, suggesting that altered intestinal permeability could be a factor.


1. Zillich AJ, *et al.* Skin discoloration with blue food colouring. *Ann Pharmacother* 2000; **34:** 868–70.
2. Lucarelli MR, *et al.* Toxicity of Food Drug and Cosmetic Blue No. 1 dye in critically ill patients. *Chest* 2004; **125:** 793–5.
3. Anonymous. Blue discoloration and death from FD&C Blue No. 1. *WHO Drug Inf* 2003; **17:** 239–40.


### Preparations

**Proprietary Preparations** (details are given in Part 3)
**Multi-ingredient:** ***NZ:*** Electric Blue Headlice.

## Brown FK

Chocolate Brown FK; CI Food Brown 1; E154; Marrón FK. A mixture of 6 azo dyes: sodium 2′,4′-diaminoazobenzene-4-sulphonate; sodium 2′,4′-diamino-5′-methylazobenzene-4-sulphonate; disodium 4,4′-(4,6-diamino-1,3-phenylenebisazo) dibenzenesulphonate; disodium 4,4′-(2,4-diamino-1,3-phenylenebisazo) dibenzenesulphonate; disodium 4,4′-(2,4-diamino-5-methyl-1,3-phenylenebisazo) dibenzenesulphonate; trisodium 4,4′,4″-(2,4-diaminobenzene-1,3,5-triazo)tribenzenesulphonate.

*CAS — 8062-14-4.*

### Profile

Brown FK is used as a colouring agent for foodstuffs.

## Brown HT

Chocolate Brown HT; CI Food Brown 3; Colour Index No. 20285; E155; Marrón HT. Disodium 4,4′-(2,4-dihydroxy-5-hydroxymethyl-1,3-phenylenebisazo)di(naphthalene-1-sulphonate).

$C_{27}H_{18}N_4Na_2O_9S_2$ = 652.6.
*CAS — 4553-89-3.*

### Profile

Brown HT is used as a colouring agent for foodstuffs.

## Canthaxanthin

Cantaxantina; CI Food Orange 8; Colour Index No. 40850; E161(g). β,β-Carotene-4,4′-dione.

$C_{40}H_{52}O_2$ = 564.8.
*CAS — 514-78-3.*

### Profile

Canthaxanthin is a carotenoid but unlike betacarotene or β-apo-8′-carotenal it possesses no vitamin A activity. It has selected uses as a food colouring and is also given to salmon or trout to colour their flesh. It is also used in cosmetics.

Canthaxanthin has also been given by mouth to produce an artificial suntan, and as an adjunct to betacarotene in the management of erythropoietic protoporphyria (see Porphyrias under Haem Derivatives, p.1040). Such use has led to retinal deposits and in some cases to impairment of vision.

**Adverse effects.** Canthaxanthin has been associated with retinal changes involving accumulation of bright yellow particles around the macula ('gold speck' maculopathy), and alterations in eye function and visual deterioration have occurred.[1,2] Although these reports have related to oral use either for the production of an artificial tan by means of pigment deposition in the skin or for the medical treatment of erythropoietic protoporphyria, there has been concern about the use of canthaxanthin as a food colouring, and it was suggested that it should be restricted to use as a feed additive for farmed salmon and trout in order to produce a coloration of the fish flesh.[1] There has also been concern[2] about the potential for hepatotoxicity, following the results of long-term toxicity studies in *animals*. However, subsequent studies failed to confirm hepatotoxicity in humans and it is now allowed as a food colouring,[3] although its uses are restricted in some countries.

There has also been a report of fatal aplastic anaemia in a patient who took canthaxanthin in order to produce an artificial tan.[4]


1. MAFF. Food advisory committee: final report on the review of the colouring matter in food regulations 1973. *FdAC/REP/4*. London: HMSO, 1987.
2. FAO/WHO. Evaluation of certain food additives and contaminants: thirty-fifth report of the joint FAO/WHO expert committee on food additives. *WHO Tech Rep Ser 789* 1990.
3. FAO/WHO. Evaluation of certain food additives and contaminants: forty-fourth report of the joint FAO/WHO expert committee on food additives. *WHO Tech Rep Ser 859* 1995.
4. Bluhm R, *et al.* Aplastic anemia associated with canthaxanthin ingested for 'tanning' purposes. *JAMA* 1990; **264:** 1141–2.


### Preparations

**Proprietary Preparations** (details are given in Part 3)
***Arg.:*** Bronzearte.
**Multi-ingredient:** ***Arg.:*** Bronsul; Sol Bronce Vital; ***Fr.:*** Phenoro†; ***Switz.:*** Apotrin†.

## Caramel

Burnt Sugar; Caramelo; Sacch. Ust.; Saccharum Ustum.
*CAS — 8028-89-5.*

**Pharmacopoeias.** In *USNF.*

**USNF 22** (Caramel). A concentrated solution of the product obtained by heating sugar or glucose until the sweet taste is destroyed and a uniform dark brown mass results, a small amount of alkali or of alkaline carbonate or a trace of mineral acid being added while heating. It is a thick, dark brown liquid, having the characteristic odour of burnt sugar, and a pleasant bitter taste. One part dissolved in 1000 parts of water yields a clear solution having a distinct yellowish-orange colour. The colour of this solution is not changed and no precipitate is formed after exposure to sunlight for 6 hours. When spread as a thin layer on a glass plate, it appears homogeneous, reddish-brown, and transparent. Miscible with water; immiscible with ether, with chloroform, with acetone, with petroleum spirit, and with benzene; soluble in dilute alcohol up to 55%. Store in airtight containers.

**Profile**

Caramels are used as food colours to produce pale yellow to dark brown colours. They have no calorific value. They are complex mixtures of compounds prepared by heating carbohydrates (food-grade sweeteners consisting of glucose, fructose, or polymers of these) either alone or in the presence of acids or alkalis (food-grade citric or sulfuric acids or calcium, potassium, or sodium hydroxides, or mixtures of these). The caramels can be classified according to the reactants used in the manufacturing process:

Class I (E150a, plain caramel, spirit caramel, or caustic caramel); no ammonium or sulfite compounds are employed.

Class II (E150b or caustic sulfite caramel); sulfite compounds employed but not ammonium compounds.

Class III (E150c, ammonia caramel, or beer caramel); ammonium compounds employed but not sulfite compounds

Class IV (E150d, sulfite ammonia caramel, or soft-drink caramel); both ammonium and sulfite compounds employed.

Some caramels also have flavouring properties.

## Carmine

Carmín; CI Natural Red 4; Colour Index No. 75470; E120.

*CAS — 1390-65-4.*

**Profile**

Carmine is an aluminium lake of the colouring matter of cochineal. It contains carminic acid, an anthraquinone glycoside. Unless precautions are taken during manufacture and transport to prevent contamination, carmine may be infected with salmonella micro-organisms.

Carmine and some of its salts are used as colouring agents in medicines, foodstuffs, and cosmetics.

Carmine passes through the gastrointestinal tract unchanged and has been used as a faecal 'marker'.

**Hypersensitivity.** Extrinsic allergic alveolitis has been described (1 patient) due to occupational exposure to carmine used as a food additive.[1] Additionally, severe anaphylactic reactions have occurred following the ingestion of food[2,3] (2 patients) and drink[4] (1 patient) containing carmine as a colour.

1. Dietemann-Molard A, *et al.* Extrinsic allergic alveolitis secondary to carmine. *Lancet* 1991; **338:** 460.
2. Beaudouin E, *et al.* Food anaphylaxis following ingestion of carmine. *Ann Allergy Asthma Immunol* 1995; **74:** 427–30.
3. Baldwin JL, *et al.* Popsicle-induced anaphylaxis due to carmine dye allergy. *Ann Allergy Asthma Immunol* 1997; **79:** 415–19.
4. Kägi MK, *et al.* Campari-orange anaphylaxis due to carmine allergy. *Lancet* 1994; **344:** 60–1.

## Carmoisine

Azorubine; Carmoisina; CI Food Red 3; Colour Index No. 14720; E122. It consists mainly of disodium 4-hydroxy-3-(4-sulphonato-1-naphthylazo)naphthalene-1-sulphonate.

$C_{20}H_{12}N_2Na_2O_7S_2$ = 502.4.

*CAS — 3567-69-9.*

**Profile**

Carmoisine is used as a colouring agent in foods, medicines, and cosmetics.

## Chlorophyll

CI Natural Green 3; Clorofila; Colour Index No. 75810; E140 (chlorophylls or chlorophyllins).

*CAS — 479-61-8 (chlorophyll a); 519-62-0 (chlorophyll b).*

## Chlorophyllin Copper Complex Sodium

**Pharmacopoeias.** In *US.*

**USP 27** (Chlorophyllin Copper Complex Sodium). It contains sodium salts of copper-chelated chlorophyll derivatives, but no artificial colouring. Store in airtight containers. Protect from light.

**Profile**

Chlorophyll is a green colouring matter of plants that contains chlorophyll a ($C_{55}H_{72}MgN_4O_5$ = 893.5) and chlorophyll b ($C_{55}H_{70}MgN_4O_6$ = 907.5), two closely related substances. The only difference between the 2 chlorophylls is that a methyl side-chain in chlorophyll a is replaced by a formyl group in chlorophyll b.

*Oil-soluble chlorophyll derivatives.* Replacement of the magnesium atom in the chlorophylls by 2 hydrogen atoms using dilute mineral acids produces olive-green water-insoluble phaeophytins. Copper phaeophytins (sometimes called copper chlorophyll complex; E141) can be formed; these are more stable to acids and to light than the chlorophylls.

*Water-soluble chlorophyll derivatives.* When the chlorophylls are hydrolysed with alkali, phytyl alcohol and methyl alcohol are split off and green water-soluble chlorophyllins are formed as the potassium or sodium salts. Similar water-soluble compounds can be prepared in which the magnesium is replaced by copper to give copper chlorophyllin complex (E141).

Chlorophylls and chlorophyllins, as well as the copper complexes of these compounds, are employed principally as colouring agents, in foods, medicines, and cosmetics.

Chlorophyll is used as an external application in the treatment of wounds and ulcers. There is no clear evidence that it accelerates healing but it is considered to have a deodorant action. Chlorophyllin and copper chlorophyllin complex are used similarly.

**Preparations**

**Proprietary Preparations** (details are given in Part 3)
***Ger.:*** Anti-Geruchs†; ***USA:*** Chloresium; Derifil; Pals.

**Multi-ingredient:** ***Arg.:*** Fanaletas; Notoxin; Palan; ***Belg.:*** Ex'ail†; ***Braz.:*** Anapyon†; Broncopinol; Eucaliptan; Gargosedans†; Gargotrat†; Higienex†; Massageol; Mentolatun†; Mentozil†; Napiro†; Salimetin; Sanador†; Sanoclorofila†; ***Fr.:*** Ex'ail†; ***Ger.:*** Bagnisan med Heilbad†; Chlorophyl liquid "Schuh"; Chlorophyllin Salbe "Schuh"; Ginseng-Complex "Schuh"; Stomasal Med; ***Hong Kong:*** Crema-U†; ***Ital.:*** Dentovax†; ***Spain:*** Balneogel†; Odontocromil c Sulfamida; Vitavox Pastillas; ***Thai.:*** Sanaco; ***UK:*** Chlorophyll; ***USA:*** Panafil; Prophyllin.

## Cochineal

CI Natural Red 4; Coccionella; Coccus; Coccus Cacti; Cochinilla; Colour Index No. 75470; E120.

*CAS — 1343-78-8.*

**Pharmacopoeias.** In *Br.*

**BP 2003** (Cochineal). The dried female insect, *Dactylopius coccus* containing eggs and larvae. It has a characteristic odour. It complies with a test for contamination with *Escherichia coli* and salmonellae.

**Profile**

Cochineal, which is a source of carmine, is used as a red colouring agent in food, medicines, and cosmetics.

Cochineal is also used in homoeopathic medicine.

## Curcumin

Colour Index No. 75300; Curcumina; E100. 1,7-Bis(4-hydroxy-3-methoxyphenyl)hepta-1,6-diene-3,5-dione.

$C_{21}H_{20}O_6$ = 368.4.

**Profile**

Curcumin is the main colouring component of turmeric (p.1058). It is used as a colouring agent for foodstuffs and cosmetics.

## Eosin

CI Acid Red 87; Colour Index No. 45380; D & C Red No. 22; Eosin Y; Eosina; Éosine Disodique. The disodium salt of 2′,4′,5′,7′-tetrabromofluorescein .

$C_{20}H_6Br_4Na_2O_5$ = 691.9.

*CAS — 548-26-5; 17372-87-1.*

*ATC — D08AX02.*

**Pharmacopoeias.** In *Fr.*

**Profile**

Eosin has been incorporated in solution-tablets to give a distinctive colour to solutions prepared from them. It is also used in cosmetics.

## Erythrosine

CI Food Red 14; Colour Index No. 45430; E127; Eritrosina; Erythrosine BS; Erythrosine Sodium; FD & C Red No. 3. The monohydrate of the disodium salt of 2′,4′,5′,7′-tetraiodofluorescein .

$C_{20}H_6I_4Na_2O_5,H_2O$ = 897.9.

*CAS — 568-63-8 (anhydrous erythrosine sodium); 16423-68-0 (anhydrous erythrosine sodium); 49746-10-3 (erythrosine sodium monohydrate).*

**Profile**

Erythrosine is used as a colouring agent for medicines and foods. It is also used in cosmetics and as a disclosing agent for plaque on teeth.

◊ Although early *animal* studies had indicated that erythrosine might have an adverse effect on the thyroid gland, a review[1] of the evidence together with later studies, suggested that erythrosine was not genotoxic or mutagenic and was suitable for use as a food colour.

1. MAFF. Food advisory committee: final report on the review of the colouring matter in food regulations 1973. *FdAC/REP/4.* London: HMSO, 1987.

**Preparations**

**Proprietary Preparations** (details are given in Part 3)
***Arg.:*** Revelplac; ***Austral.:*** Disclo-Gel†; Disclo-Tabs†; ***UK:*** Ceplac†.

**Multi-ingredient:** ***Arg.:*** Revelplac 2001.

## Ferric Oxide

E172 (iron oxides or hydroxides); Óxido de hierro.

*CAS — 51274-00-1; 1309-37-1.*

**Pharmacopoeias.** *Chin.* includes red ferric oxide. *It.* includes both red and yellow ferric oxide. *USNF* allows the basic colours of red or yellow ferric oxide or mixtures of these.

**USNF 22** (Ferric Oxide). A powder exhibiting two basic colours (red and yellow), or other shades produced on blending the basic colours. Insoluble in water and in organic solvents; dissolves in hydrochloric acid upon warming, a small amount of insoluble residue usually remaining.

**Profile**

Ferric oxide is used for tinting pharmaceutical preparations and foodstuffs.

**Preparations**

**Proprietary Preparations** (details are given in Part 3)

**Multi-ingredient:** ***Port.:*** Filter Oil Free.

## Green S

Acid Brilliant Green BS; Acid Green S; CI Food Green 4; Colour Index No. 44090; E142; Lissamine Green; Verde S; Wool Green B. Sodium 1-[4-dimethylamino-α-(4-dimethyliminiocyclohexa-2,5-dienylidene)benzyl]-2-hydroxynaphthalene-3,6-disulphonate.

$C_{27}H_{25}N_2NaO_7S_2$ = 576.6.

*CAS — 3087-16-9.*

**Profile**

Green S is used as a colouring agent in medicines, cosmetics, and foodstuffs.

◊ Studies in *animals* indicated that there is some absorption of green S and caecal enlargement but it was considered that there is a very large margin of safety between the highest estimated human intake of green S of 130 micrograms daily and the level at which changes were seen in *animal* studies (500 mg/kg daily). It was recommended that the use of green S in food is acceptable.[1]

1. MAFF. Food advisory committee: final report on the review of the colouring matter in food regulations 1973. *FdAC/REP/4.* London: HMSO, 1987.

## Pigment Rubine

E180; Lithol Rubine BK; Litholrubine BK; Litolrubina BK.

**Profile**

Pigment rubine is used as a colouring agent for foodstuffs.

## Ponceau 4R

Brilliant Ponceau 4RC; Brilliant Scarlet; CI Food Red 7; Coccine Nouvelle; Cochineal Red A; Colour Index No. 16255; E124; Rojo de cochinilla A; Rouge Cochenille A. Trisodium 7-hydroxy-8-(4-sulphonato-1-naphthylazo)naphthalene-1,3-disulphonate.

$C_{20}H_{11}N_2Na_3O_{10}S_3$ = 604.5.

*CAS — 2611-82-7.*

**Profile**

Ponceau 4R is used as a colouring agent in medicines, cosmetics, and foods. Sensitivity reactions have been reported.

## Quinoline Yellow

Amarillo de quinoleína; Canary Yellow; CI Acid Yellow 3; CI Food Yellow 13; Colour Index No. 47005; E104; Jaune De Quinoléine. The sodium salts of a mixture of the mono- and disulfonic acids of quinophthalone or 2-(2-quinolyl)indanedione .

*CAS — 8004-92-0.*

NOTE. D & C yellow No. 10 is used as a synonym for quinoline yellow, but describes a mixture consisting mainly of the monosulfonic acid of quinophthalone.

**Profile**

Quinoline yellow is used as a colouring agent in medicines, cosmetics, and foodstuffs.

**Hypersensitivity.** A severe urticarial reaction[1] in a patient has been attributed to quinoline yellow.

1. Bell T. Colourants and drug reactions. *Lancet* 1991; **338:** 55–6.

## Raspberry

Framboise; Frambuesa; Fructus Rubi Idaei; Himbeer; Rubus Idaeus.

*CAS — 8027-46-1.*

**Profile**

Raspberry, the fresh ripe fruit of *Rubus idaeus* (Rosaceae), is used as a colouring and flavouring agent in medicines and foodstuffs.

### Preparations

**Proprietary Preparations** (details are given in Part 3)

**Multi-ingredient:** ***Fr.:*** IgeE.

## Red 2G

Acid Red 1; CI Food Red 10; Colour Index No. 18050; E128; Ext. D & C Red No. 11; Geranine 2G; Rojo 2G. Disodium 5-acetamido-4-hydroxy-3-phenylazonaphthalene-2,7-disulphonate.

$C_{18}H_{13}N_3Na_2O_8S_2$ = 509.4.

*CAS — 3734-67-6.*

### Profile

Red 2G is used as a colouring agent in medicines, cosmetics, and foods.

◊ There has been concern that red 2G might produce haemolysis in subjects deficient in G6PD, but investigations have not confirmed such a risk. However, red 2G might hydrolyse in acid solution to red 10B about which there is inadequate data. Therefore, it has been recommended[1] that red 2G should not be used in foods of high acidity that are subjected to a high temperature during processing and that the use of red 2G should be confined to certain meat products.

1. MAFF. Food advisory committee: final report on the review of the colouring matter in food regulations 1973. FdAC/REP/4. London: HMSO, 1987.

## Red Cherry

Cerasus; Cerise Rouge; Rojo cereza; Sour Cherry.

**Pharmacopoeias.** *USNF* includes cherry juice.

*Fr.* includes, under the title Griottier, cherry stalks from either the red (sour) cherry, *Prunus cerasus*, or from the sweet cherry, *P. avium*.

**USNF 22** (Cherry Juice). The liquid expressed from the fresh ripe fruit of *Prunus cerasus* (Rosaceae). It contains not less than 1.0% of malic acid. pH 3.0 to 4.0. Store in airtight containers. Protect from light.

### Profile

Red cherry is used as a colouring and flavouring agent.

### Preparations

***USNF 22:*** Cherry Syrup.

**Proprietary Preparations** (details are given in Part 3)

**Multi-ingredient:** ***Arg.:*** Vitamina C-Complex; ***Fr.:*** Evacrine.

## Red-Poppy Petal

Coquelicot; Klatschrose; Papaveris Rhoeados Flos; Pétalos de amapola; Rhoead. Pet.; Rhoeados Petalum.

**Pharmacopoeias.** In *Eur.* (see p.vi).

**Ph. Eur. 5.0** (Red Poppy Petals). The dried, whole or fragmented petals of *Papaver rhoeas*.

### Profile

Red-poppy petal has been used as a colouring agent. It is also included in several herbal preparations.

### Preparations

**Proprietary Preparations** (details are given in Part 3)

**Multi-ingredient:** ***Fr.:*** Actisane Nervosite†; Astressane†; Nocvalene; ***Ital.:*** Normalax†; Relaten†; ***Switz.:*** Baume; Melissa Tonic†; Tisane pectorale et antitussive.

## Red-Rose Petal

Fleur de Rose; Flos Rosae; Pétalos de rosa; Red Rose Petals; Ros. Pet.; Rosae Gallicae Petala; Rosae Petalum; Rose Rouge; Rosenblüte.

**Pharmacopoeias.** In *Fr.*

### Profile

Red-rose petal, the petals of the red or Provins rose, *Rosa gallica* (Rosaceae), has been employed as a colouring agent and for its mild astringent properties.

### Preparations

**Proprietary Preparations** (details are given in Part 3)

**Multi-ingredient:** ***Arg.:*** Expectosan Hierbas y Miel; ***Braz.:*** Broncmel†; ***Fr.:*** Ophtalmine; ***Ger.:*** Melrosum Hustensirup N†; ***Spain:*** Natusor Infenol.

## Saffron

Açafrão; Azafrán; CI Natural Yellow 6; Colour Index No. 75100; Croci Stigma; Crocus; Estigmas de Azafrán; Safran.

**Pharmacopoeias.** In *Chin.* and *Jpn.*

*Eur.* (see p.vi) includes Saffron for Homoeopathic Preparations.

**Ph. Eur. 5.0** (Saffron for Homoeopathic Preparations). The dried stigmas of *Crocus sativus* usually joined by the base to a short style. It has a characteristic, aromatic odour. Protect from light.

### Profile

Saffron consists of the dried stigmas and tops of the styles of *Crocus sativus* (Iridaceae), containing crocines, crocetins, and picrocrocine. Saffron is used as a food and cosmetic dye and flavouring agent. In some circles it is considered to be a food. It was once widely used for colouring medicines. Saffron has been included in preparations for teething pain. There have been reports of poisoning with saffron.

Saffron is also used in homoeopathic medicine.

### Preparations

**Proprietary Preparations** (details are given in Part 3)

**Multi-ingredient:** ***Austria:*** Zeller-Augenwasser; ***Belg.:*** Calmant Martou†; ***Ger.:*** Infi-tract; Schwedentrunk mit Ginseng†; Schwedentrunk†; ***Ital.:*** Fluxoten†; ***Spain:*** Dentol Topico; Dentomicin.

## Sunset Yellow FCF

Amarillo ocaso FCF; CI Food Yellow 3; Colour Index No. 15985; E110; FD & C Yellow No. 6; Jaune Orangé S; Jaune Soleil; Orange Yellow S. Disodium 6-hydroxy-5-(4-sulphonatophenylazo)naphthalene-2-sulphonate.

$C_{16}H_{10}N_2Na_2O_7S_2$ = 452.4.

*CAS — 2783-94-0.*

### Profile

Sunset yellow FCF is used as a colouring agent in foods, medicines, and cosmetics. Sensitivity reactions have been reported.

**Carcinogenicity.** Although some evidence of carcinogenicity was found in early *animal* studies subsequent work failed to confirm these findings and in the UK sunset yellow FCF is considered suitable for use as a food colour.[1]

1. MAFF. Food advisory committee: final report on the review of the colouring matter in food regulations 1973. *FdAC/REP/4.* London. HMSO, 1987.

**Hypersensitivity.** Hypersensitivity reactions including severe abdominal cramps[1] and Quincke's oedema[2] have been recorded in individual patients receiving medication that was coloured with sunset yellow FCF.

1. Gross PA, *et al.* Additive allergy: allergic gastroenteritis due to yellow dye #6. *Ann Intern Med* 1989; **111:** 87–8.
2. Lévesque H, *et al.* Reporting adverse drug reactions by proprietary name. *Lancet* 1991; **338:** 393.

## Tartrazine

CI Food Yellow 4; Colour Index No. 19140; E102; FD & C Yellow No. 5; Jaune Tartrique; Tartrazin.; Tartrazina; Tartrazol Yellow. It consists mainly of trisodium 5-hydroxy-1-(4-sulphonatophenyl)-4-(4-sulphonatophenylazo)pyrazole-3-carboxylate.

$C_{16}H_9N_4Na_3O_9S_2$ = 534.4.

*CAS — 1934-21-0.*

### Profile

Tartrazine is used as a colouring agent in foods, cosmetics, and medicines. Some patients may experience sensitivity reactions.

**Hypersensitivity.** There have been numerous reports of reactions to tartrazine and these cover angioedema, asthma, urticaria, and anaphylactic shock. Some of the reports have dealt with cross-sensitivity, especially with aspirin, although the connection with aspirin has been questioned.[1] A suggested incidence[2] of tartrazine sensitivity is 1 in 10 000. The mechanism of the reactions may not necessarily be immunological.[3]

In considering the reports of tartrazine sensitivity or intolerance the Food Advisory Committee in the UK[1] reported that similar evidence of intolerance might well be obtained for a variety of natural food ingredients if as many studies were conducted on them as on tartrazine. The Committee considered that tartrazine posed no more problems than other colours or food ingredients and recommended that the continued use of tartrazine in food is acceptable. However, use of tartrazine in medicines appears to be diminishing.

1. MAFF. Food advisory committee: final report on the review of the colouring matter in food regulations 1973. *FdAC/REP/4.* London: HMSO, 1987.
2. Anonymous. Tartrazine: a yellow hazard. *Drug Ther Bull* 1980; **18:** 53–5.
3. Murdoch RD, *et al.* Tartrazine induced histamine release in vivo in normal subjects. *J R Coll Physicians Lond* 1987; **21:** 257–61.

## Turmeric

CI Natural Yellow 3; Cúrcuma; Indian Saffron.

*CAS — 458-37-7.*

**Pharmacopoeias.** In *Chin.*

### Profile

Turmeric, the dried rhizome of *Curcuma longa* (Zingiberaceae), is used principally as a constituent of curry powders and other condiments. Turmeric and its main ingredient curcumin (p.1057) are used as yellow colouring agents in foods. Turmeric has also been used as an ingredient of preparations indicated for biliary and gastrointestinal disorders.

**Effects on the thyroid.** There has been some concern about the safety of turmeric oleoresin, an extract of turmeric, following reports of adverse thyroid changes in *pigs*.[1,2]

1. MAFF. Food advisory committee: final report on the review of the colouring matter in food regulations 1973. *FdAC/REP/4.* London: HMSO, 1987.
2. FAO/WHO. Evaluation of certain food additives and contaminants: thirty-fifth report of the joint FAO/WHO expert committee on food additives. *WHO Tech Rep Ser 789* 1990.

### Preparations

**Proprietary Preparations** (details are given in Part 3)

***Chile:*** Turmerik; ***Ger.:*** Choldestal; Meteophyt N†; Sergast.

**Multi-ingredient:** ***Austral.:*** Arthriforte†; Bioglan Joint Mobility†; Extralife Arthri-Care†; Extralife Liva-Care†; Herbal Digestive Formula†; ***Austria:*** Aktiv Leber- und Gallentee; Bakanasan Leber-Galle; Claim; Gallo Merz†; Kneipp Galle- und Leber-Tee; Neuners Krautertee Nr 17 - Leber-tee; Sanhelios Leber-Galle; Sanvita Leber-Galle; Spasmo Claim; ***Canad.:*** Milk Thistle; ***Fr.:*** Hepatoum; ***Ger.:*** Aristochol CC; Chol-Arbuz N; Cholagogum F; Cholagogum N; Cholosom Phyto N; Digest-Merz; Gallo Merz N; Gastrol S; Hepaticum-Medice H; Hevert-Gall S†; Horvilan N; Kneipp Galle- und Leber-Tee N†; Opobyl-phyto; spasmo gallo sanol; Steigal†; Ventracid N; ***Hong Kong:*** Hepatofalk Planta; Lipochol; ***Mex.:*** Ifuchol; ***Singapore:*** Artrex; ***Switz.:*** Stago†; ***UK:*** BackOsamine.

## Vegetable Carbon

Carbon Black; Carbón vegetal; E153; Vegetable Black.

NOTE. The name Carbon Black has also been used as a synonym for Channel Black, a colouring agent not used in food; care should be taken to avoid confusion between the two compounds.

### Profile

Vegetable carbon, which consists essentially of finely divided carbon, is produced by the carbonisation of vegetable material such as peat. It is used as a colouring agent for foodstuffs and cosmetics.

### Preparations

**Proprietary Preparations** (details are given in Part 3)

**Multi-ingredient:** ***Chile:*** Kordinol Compuesto.

## Yellow 2G

107; Acid Light Yellow 2G; Acid Yellow 17; Amarillo 2G; CI Food Yellow 5; Colour Index No. 18965. Disodium 2,5-dichloro-4-[5-hydroxy-3-methyl-4-(4-sulphonatophenylazo)pyrazol-1-yl]benzenesulphonate.

$C_{16}H_{10}Cl_2N_4Na_2O_7S_2$ = 551.3.

*CAS — 6359-98-4.*

### Profile

Yellow 2G is used as a colouring agent in cosmetics.

# Contrast Media

Contrast media are agents that enhance the images obtained from visualisation techniques such as radiography (X-ray imaging, including computed tomography), magnetic resonance imaging, or ultrasound imaging.

In **radiography**, contrast media may be used to increase the absorption of X-rays as they pass through the body, and this is described as *positive contrast*. A gas (air, oxygen, or carbon dioxide) may also be used for visualisation and this is referred to as *negative contrast*. When both gas and contrast medium are used concomitantly the procedure is called *double contrast*. Radiographic contrast media are described further below. Radiographic contrast media may also be used to enhance **computed tomography** images. Tomography is the procedure whereby a selected plane of the subject is visualised using X-rays.

**Magnetic resonance imaging** also provides sectional images. Contrast agents in magnetic resonance imaging (see below) enhance the images obtained from the absorption of radio waves by atomic nuclei.

In **ultrasound**, contrast agents enhance the images obtained from the reflection of sound waves by different tissues by providing gas-liquid interfaces (see below).

## Radiographic Contrast Media

Radiographic contrast media contain elements with high atomic numbers that absorb X-rays. The agents most commonly used are *iodinated organic compounds*, whose degree of opacity or radiodensity is directly proportional to their iodine content. *Barium sulfate* is a metal salt with a long established use as a contrast medium. Other heavy atoms have been investigated, but many, such as thorium dioxide and tantalum, were unsuitable due to acute or chronic toxicity.

The iodinated contrast media may be classified as either ionic or nonionic, and additionally as monomeric or dimeric.

The *ionic monomeric* media, such as the amidotrizoates, iodamide, and iopanoic acid, generally have very high osmolality when given in concentrations suitable for radiographic visualisation and the resulting hypertonic solutions are associated with a relatively high incidence of adverse effects. Since radiodensity depends solely upon the iodine concentration, and osmolality solely upon the number of particles present in a given weight of solvent, the osmolality of contrast medium solutions can be reduced for a given radiodensity by using an *ionic dimeric* medium, such as adipiodone or ioxaglic acid, that contains twice the number of iodine atoms in each molecule, or by using a *nonionic* medium that does not dissociate into cation and anion. Nonionic media may be *monomeric*, such as iohexol, iopamidol, iopromide, and ioversol, or *dimeric*, for example iotrolan. Thus the best ratio of radiodensity to osmolality is achieved with the nonionic dimeric media.

**Choice of radiographic contrast medium.** Radiographic techniques to visualise particular structures within the body depend upon the physical and chemical properties of the contrast medium used and upon the way in which it is administered. Some radiographic procedures and the specific contrast media used in them are described below. The likelihood of adverse effects is greater with the older iodinated ionic contrast media, especially in high risk patients (see below), and this also influences the choice of contrast medium.

For **urography** (visualisation of the kidneys and urinary tract) the molecule must be small and highly water-soluble, with low protein-binding, so that glomerular filtration is encouraged with subsequent passage through the urinary tract. For good visualisation high concentrations must be achieved in the urinary tract from the start, and this in turn means high plasma concentrations: contrast media for urography are thus invariably given by the intravenous route. Examples of ionic urographic media include the amidotrizoates, iotalamates, and metrizoates. These ionic monomeric media have a relatively high incidence of adverse effects, due in part to their high osmolality, and better tolerance may be achieved with compounds of lower osmolality, such as ionic dimeric media (ioxaglic acid) and nonionic media (iohexol, iopamidol, and iopromide).

The requirements for **angiography** (visualisation of the circulatory system) are similar to those for urography in that a water-soluble molecule is required that can be readily distributed through the blood vessels. In addition, the solution should be of low viscosity to facilitate rapid injection and of high radiodensity to counteract the diluting effects of the blood. There are no particular differences between requirements for visualisation of veins (**phlebography** or **venography**) and those for arteries (**arteriography**); however, for **angiocardiography** (visualisation of the heart and heart vessels), or **digital subtraction angiography** where movement of a bolus of contrast medium through the circulation is studied over a period of time, the heart may be exposed to higher-than-usual concentrations of contrast medium and low cardiotoxicity is particularly important. There has been a general trend towards the use of low osmolality media for all types of angiography, since greatly improved tolerance, and in particular less pain on injection, means that procedures can be carried out without general anaesthesia and with less risk of serious adverse effects. Examples of angiographic media include iodixanol, iohexol, iopamidol, iopromide, and ioversol.

For **gastrointestinal radiography** the principal requirements are that the contrast medium should not be absorbed but should form an even, homogeneous coat on the gastrointestinal mucosa, without interacting with gut secretions or producing misleading radiographic artifacts. The chief contrast medium for this purpose is barium sulfate, and much effort has been devoted to the production of suitable formulations to improve its coating properties and reduce the formation of bubbles, cracks, and other radiographic artifacts.

The requirements for **cholecystography** and **cholangiography** (visualisation of the gallbladder and biliary tract) depend to some degree on the intended route of administration. In order that the molecule should be preferentially excreted in the bile it should be sufficiently large for biliary excretion and must possess a free carboxy or other acidic group, since the biliary active transport mechanism is an anion transfer process. In addition, the molecule should be protected by virtue of its size or by protein binding from the more rapid renal excretion processes. However, the oral cholecystographic agents need to be absorbed from the gastrointestinal tract before they become effective, and this imposes a second, and to some extent conflicting, set of requirements. For optimal enteral absorption, molecules should be of relatively small size, sufficiently soluble in gastrointestinal fluids, and sufficiently lipophilic to pass the cell membranes of the mucosa. Examples of *oral* cholecystographic media include the iopodates, iocetamic acid, iopanoic acid, and sodium tyropanoate. These are relatively small, monomeric molecules and therefore they require conjugation with glucuronic acid within the body to achieve sufficient molecular weight for biliary excretion. They are often given after a fatty meal to enhance absorption and reduce the incidence of inadequate visualisation. The *intravenous* cholecystographic agents do not have to meet the above requirements for enteral absorption and are mostly larger, dimeric molecules that do not require conjugation. They are generally more effective than the oral media. Examples of intravenous cholecystographic media include salts of adipiodone and iotroxic acid.

For **myelography** (visualisation of the structures of the spinal cord) no special requirements other than good tolerance are necessary. Although visualisation was at one time achieved with oily media such as iofendylate these have now mostly been replaced with nonionic water-soluble media. These offer improved tolerance, better visualisation since they are miscible with cerebrospinal fluid, and, unlike the oil-based media, are removed from the subarachnoid space by normal pharmacokinetic mechanisms. Examples include iohexol and iopamidol.

**Arthrography** (visualisation of the joint capsule) may be performed with many different contrast media provided they are well-diluted before use.

**Bronchography** (examination of the bronchial tree) has been performed with oily or aqueous media, such as iopydol or iopydone, instilled through a catheter or bronchoscope to coat the airways.

For **hysterosalpingography** (visualisation of the uterus and fallopian tubes) a water-soluble contrast medium is required. Examples include iotrolan, ioxaglic acid, and metrizoic acid.

Very high radiodensity is required to obtain good visualisation of the lymphatic structures in radiography of the lymphatic system (**lymphography** or **lymphangiography**). In addition, water-soluble media rapidly leave the system and only particulate or water-insoluble media or very large molecules persist within the lymphatic vessels for any length of time. The medium that has been most frequently used is iodised oil. It gives good visualisation of that part of the lymphatic system between the point at which it is infused and the point at which it enters the general circulation, but it is not distributed throughout the whole lymphatic space and has the potential for a number of severe side-effects.

**Adverse effects.** The adverse effects of iodinated contrast media are described under Amidotrizoic Acid, p.1060. Many of the adverse effects[1,2] of iodinated ionic contrast media are associated with their high osmolality. The newer nonionic, low-osmolal contrast media have a lower incidence of adverse effects than the older ionic, high-osmolal agents.[1,3,4] There is evidence from studies in Australia[3] and Japan[4] suggesting that 'low-risk' patients given conventional ionic media are at greater risk of adverse effects than patients considered 'at-risk' who are given nonionic media.

Cost considerations mean that low-osmolal media tend to be reserved for patients considered to be at high risk of adverse effects (see Precautions under Amidotrizoic Acid, p.1060).


1. Thomsen HS, Bush WH. Adverse effects of contrast media: incidence, prevention and management. *Drug Safety* 1998; **19:** 313–24.
2. Ansell G. Adverse reactions profile: intravascular iodinated radiocontrast media. *Prescribers' J* 1993; **33:** 82–8.
3. Palmer FJ. The RACR Survey of intravenous contrast media reactions: final report. *Australas Radiol* 1988; **32:** 426–8.
4. Katayama H, *et al.* Adverse reactions to ionic and nonionic contrast media: a report from the Japanese Committee on the Safety of Contrast Media. *Radiology* 1990; **175:** 621–8.


HYPERSENSITIVITY. Anaphylactoid reactions to iodinated contrast media are more common with the ionic agents than the nonionic media of lower osmolality. Patients at increased risk are those with a history of asthma or allergy, drug hypersensitivity, adrenal suppression, heart disease, previous reaction to a contrast medium, and those receiving beta blockers or interleukin-2 therapy. In such patients, nonionic media are preferred. Discontinuation of beta blockers should be considered in patients with other risk factors.

Pretreatment with corticosteroids may be considered for preventing anaphylactoid reactions in high-risk patients and an antihistamine may be given. However, the value is uncertain.

References.


1. Greenberger PA, *et al.* Effects of beta-adrenergic and calcium antagonists on the development of anaphylactoid reactions from radiographic contrast media during cardiac angiography. *J Allergy Clin Immunol* 1987; **80:** 698–702.
2. Lang DM, *et al.* Increased risk for anaphylactoid reaction from contrast media in patients on β-adrenergic blockers or with asthma. *Ann Intern Med* 1991; **115:** 270–6.
3. Ansell G. Adverse reactions profile: intravascular iodinated radiocontrast media. *Prescribers' J* 1993; **33:** 82–8.
4. Wittbrodt ET, Spinler SA. Prevention of anaphylactoid reactions in high-risk patients receiving radiographic contrast media. *Ann Pharmacother* 1994; **28:** 236–41.
5. Sidhu PS, Dawson P. Corticosteroid prophylaxis in contrast examinations. *Br J Hosp Med* 1997; **58:** 304–6.


THROMBOEMBOLISM. Angiography is associated with a risk of thromboembolism. Contrast media have differing effects on coagulation, and choice of contrast medium may therefore affect this risk. Although nonionic media may be preferred in angiography due to their better tolerability, it has been suggested[1-4] that they may contribute to the risk of thromboembolism since they have less anticoagulant activity than the ionic contrast media. Mixing of blood and contrast media before injection may increase the risk of thromboembolism and should therefore be avoided.


1. Robertson HJ. Thrombogenic potential of nonionic contrast media. *Mayo Clin Proc* 1990; **65:** 603–4.
2. King BF. Thrombogenic potential of nonionic contrast media. *Mayo Clin Proc* 1990; **65:** 604.
3. Anonymous. Thromboembolism during angiography. *Lancet* 1992; **339:** 1576–8.
4. Esplugas E, *et al.* Comparative tolerability of contrast media used for coronary interventions. *Drug Safety* 2002; **25:** 1079–98.


## Magnetic Resonance Contrast Media

Magnetic resonance contrast media are paramagnetic or superparamagnetic agents that enhance the magnetic resonance image by interfering with the relaxation times of adjacent nuclei. Paramagnetic contrast media include the gadolinium complexes, such as gadodiamide, gadopentetic acid, and gadoteridol, and the manganese complex mangafodipir trisodium. Superparamagnetic contrast media include the iron compounds ferristene, ferucarbotran, ferumoxides, and ferumoxsil.

◊ References.


1. Armstrong P, Keevil SF. Magnetic resonance imaging—1: basic principles of image production. *BMJ* 1991; **303:** 35–40.
2. Armstrong P, Keevil SF. Magnetic resonance imaging—2: clinical uses. *BMJ* 1991; **303:** 105–9.
3. Edelman RR, Warach S. Magnetic resonance imaging (first of two parts). *N Engl J Med* 1993; **328:** 708–15.
4. Edelman RR, Warach S. Magnetic resonance imaging (second of two parts). *N Engl J Med* 1993; **328:** 785–91.


## Ultrasound Contrast Media

Contrast agents for use in ultrasound imaging are termed echocontrast agents or echo-enhancers. They include microbubbles of air encapsulated in albumin (p.741) or stabilised with galactose, or encapsulated fluorocarbons such as perflutren. Agitated saline injection may also be used.

◊ References.


1. Blomley H, Cosgrove D. Contrast agents in ultrasound. *Br J Hosp Med* 1996; **55:** 6–7.
2. Blomley MJK, *et al.* Microbubble contrast agents: a new era in ultrasound. *BMJ* 2001; **322:** 1222–5.
3. Stewart MJ. Contrast echocardiography. *Heart* 2003; **89:** 342–8.

## Adipiodone (BAN, rINN)

Adipiodona; Iodipamide. 3,3′-Adipoyldiaminobis(2,4,6-tri-iodobenzoic acid).

$C_{20}H_{14}I_6N_2O_6$ = 1139.8.
*CAS — 606-17-7.*
*ATC — V08AC04.*

**Description.** Adipiodone contains about 66.8% of I.

**Pharmacopoeias.** In *Chin.* and *US.*

**USP 27** (Iodipamide). A white, practically odourless, crystalline powder. Very slightly soluble in water, in chloroform, and in ether; slightly soluble in alcohol. Store at a temperature of 25°, excursions permitted between 15° and 30°.

## Meglumine Adipiodone (rINNM)

Adipiodona de meglumina; Adipiodone Meglumine (BANM); Dimeglumine Iodipamide; Iodipamide Meglumine; Meglumine Iodipamide. The di(N-methylglucamine) salt of adipiodone.

$C_{20}H_{14}I_6N_2O_6,(C_7H_{17}NO_5)_2$ = 1530.2.
*CAS — 3521-84-4.*
*ATC — V08AC04.*

**Description.** Meglumine adipiodone contains about 49.8% of I.

**Pharmacopoeias.** *US* includes only as an injection.

**Incompatibility.** Incompatibilities have been reported between meglumine adipiodone and some antihistamines.

### Adverse Effects, Treatment, and Precautions

See under the amidotrizoates, p.1060. The incidence of adverse effects may be increased following rapid administration.

Adipiodone may show some uricosuric activity.

**Effects on the liver.** Of 149 patients who received the dose of adipiodone recommended by the manufacturer 13 developed elevated serum aspartate aminotransferase (SGOT) values; of 126 who received twice the dose, 23 developed elevated values.[1] Hepatotoxicity has also been reported[2-4] on isolated occasions in patients given meglumine adipiodone.


1. Scholz FJ, *et al.* Hepatotoxicity in cholangiography. *JAMA* 1974; **229:** 1724.
2. Stillman AE. Hepatotoxic reaction to iodipamide meglumine injection. *JAMA* 1974; **228:** 1420–1.
3. Sutherland LR, *et al.* Meglumine iodipamide (Cholografin) hepatotoxicity. *Ann Intern Med* 1977; **86:** 437–9.
4. Imoto S. Meglumine hepatotoxicity. *Ann Intern Med* 1978; **88:** 129.


### Pharmacokinetics

Meglumine adipiodone is rapidly distributed in extracellular fluid following slow intravenous injection and is reported to be extensively bound to plasma proteins. It appears in the bile ducts within about 10 to 15 minutes after injection, with peak opacity at about 40 to 80 minutes, and reaches the gallbladder by about 1 hour, peak opacification occurring after about 2 hours. About 80 to 95% is excreted unchanged in the faeces; small amounts are excreted unchanged in urine. A terminal half-life of about 2 hours has been reported.

### Uses and Administration

Adipiodone is an iodinated ionic dimeric contrast medium that is used as its meglumine salt for cholecystography and cholangiography (p.1059).

It is administered by slow intravenous injection as a solution containing 52% of the meglumine salt over an average of 10 minutes; the usual dose of meglumine adipiodone used is about 10 g.

### Preparations

***BP 2003:*** Meglumine Iodipamide Injection;
***USP 27:*** Iodipamide Meglumine Injection.

**Proprietary Preparations** (details are given in Part 3)
***Belg.:*** Transbilix†; ***Canad.:*** Cholografin†; ***Fr.:*** Transbilix†; ***USA:*** Cholografin.

**Multi-ingredient:** ***Canad.:*** Sinografin†; ***USA:*** Sinografin.

## Amidotrizoic Acid (BAN, rINNM)

Acidum Amidotrizoicum; Amidotrizoico, ácido; Diatrizoic Acid (USAN); NSC-262168. 3,5-Diacetamido-2,4,6-tri-iodobenzoic acid.

$C_{11}H_9I_3N_2O_4,2H_2O$ = 649.9.
*CAS — 117-96-4 (anhydrous amidotrizoic acid); 50978-11-5 (amidotrizoic acid dihydrate).*
*ATC — V08AA01.*

**Description.** Amidotrizoic acid contains about 62% of I calculated on the anhydrous substance.

**Pharmacopoeias.** In *Chin., Eur.* (see p.vi), *Int., Jpn,* and *US.*

**Ph. Eur. 5.0** (Amidotrizoic Acid Dihydrate). A white or almost white, crystalline powder. Very slightly soluble in water and in alcohol; dissolves in dilute solutions of alkali hydroxides. Protect from light.

**USP 27** (Diatrizoic Acid). It is anhydrous or contains two molecules of water of hydration. A white, odourless, powder. Very slightly soluble in water and in alcohol; soluble in dimethylformamide and in alkali hydroxide solutions.

## Meglumine Amidotrizoate (BANM, rINNM)

Amidotrizoato de meglumina; Diatrizoate Meglumine; Meglumine Diatrizoate; Methylglucamine Diatrizoate. N-Methylglucamine 3,5-diacetamido-2,4,6-tri-iodobenzoate.

$C_{11}H_9I_3N_2O_4,C_7H_{17}NO_5$ = 809.1.
*CAS — 131-49-7.*
*ATC — V08AA01.*

**Description.** Meglumine amidotrizoate contains about 47.1% of I.

**Pharmacopoeias.** In *US.*

**USP 27** (Diatrizoate Meglumine). A white, odourless, powder. Freely soluble in water. Store at a temperature of 25°, excursions permitted between 15° and 30°.

## Sodium Amidotrizoate (BANM, rINN)

Amidotrizoato de sodio; Diatrizoate Sodium; Natrii Amidotrizoas; NSC-61815; Sodium Diatrizoate. Sodium 3,5-diacetamido-2,4,6-tri-iodobenzoate.

$C_{11}H_8I_3N_2NaO_4$ = 635.9.
*CAS — 737-31-5.*
*ATC — V08AA01.*

**Description.** Sodium amidotrizoate contains about 59.9% of I calculated on the anhydrous substance.

**Pharmacopoeias.** In *Eur.* (see p.vi), *Int., Pol.,* and *US.*
*Chin.* includes the injection.

**Ph. Eur. 5.0** (Sodium Amidotrizoate). A white or almost white powder. Freely soluble in water; slightly soluble in alcohol; practically insoluble in acetone. A 50% solution in water has a pH of 7.5 to 9.5. Protect from light.

**USP 27** (Diatrizoate Sodium). A white, odourless, powder. Soluble in water; slightly soluble in alcohol; practically insoluble in acetone and in ether.

**Incompatibility.** Incompatibilities of sodium amidotrizoate with some antihistamines have been reported.

### Adverse Effects and Treatment

Many of the effects of iodinated ionic monomeric contrast media can be attributed to the high osmolality, which is a feature of these agents; reducing the osmolality through altering the ionic or molecular profile produces a reduced incidence of adverse effects (see p.1059). The route and speed of administration, and the volume, concentration, and viscosity of the solution also affect the incidence of adverse effects. Most reactions occur within 5 to 10 minutes of injection, but they may be delayed.

Hyperthyroidism has been reported following administration of iodinated contrast media, presumably due to small amounts of iodine present as a contaminant or released by any breakdown of the medium in the body. For the effects of iodine on the thyroid gland, see p.1598.

When given by injection the amidotrizoates may cause nausea, a metallic taste, vomiting, flushing and sensations of heat, weakness, dizziness, headache, coughing, rhinitis, sweating, sneezing, lachrymation, visual disturbances, pruritus, salivary gland enlargement, pallor, tachycardia, bradycardia, transient ECG abnormalities, haemodynamic disturbances, and hypotension. Rarely, more severe adverse effects, including convulsions, paralysis, coma, rigors, ventricular fibrillation, pulmonary oedema, circulatory failure, and cardiac arrest have occurred. Occasionally anaphylactoid or hypersensitivity reactions occur; dyspnoea, bronchospasm, angioedema, and severe urticaria have been reported, and reactions have sometimes been fatal. Injection of amidotrizoates into the CNS produces severe neurotoxicity.

Deaths have also been recorded due to acute renal failure, which may follow intravenous administration, particularly in dehydrated patients and patients with other predisposing factors (see also under Effects on the Kidneys, and Precautions, below).

Pain may occur at the injection site; extravasation may be followed by tissue damage, thrombophlebitis, thrombosis, venospasm, and embolism.

Fibrinolysis and a possible depressant effect on blood coagulation factors has been reported. Disseminated intravascular coagulation has occurred. Meglumine salts are reportedly better tolerated and produce less pain on injection than sodium salts, but the sodium salts may be associated with a lower incidence of arrhythmias. As a result, the sodium and meglumine salts are often given in combination to minimise adverse effects.

Mild diarrhoea may follow the oral or rectal use of sodium and meglumine amidotrizoates for gastrointestinal examinations. The accidental aspiration of solutions of these salts has caused fatal pulmonary oedema.

Adverse effects are treated symptomatically and adequate resuscitative facilities should be available when radiographic procedures are to be employed.

**Effects on the blood.** Reports of amidotrizoates adversely affecting the blood.


1. Catterall JR, *et al.* Intravascular haemolysis with acute renal failure after angiocardiography. *BMJ* 1981; **282:** 779–80.
2. Shojania AM. Immune-mediated thrombocytopenia due to an iodinated contrast medium (diatrizoate). *Can Med Assoc J* 1985; **133:** 123.
3. Fairley S, Ihle BU. Thrombotic microangiopathy and acute renal failure associated with arteriography. *BMJ* 1986; **293:** 922–3.


**Effects on the kidneys.** Contrast media may be associated with renal toxicity.[1-3] Estimates of the incidence of nephrotoxicity vary widely, but the figure is probably less than 1% of all patients receiving contrast media and does not appear to differ significantly with ionic or nonionic media; use of high-osmolality agents may increase the risk.[4,5] In the majority of patients who develop contrast-medium-induced renal impairment the condition develops within about 24 hours of the procedure, is asymptomatic, and resolves completely within about 10 days. However, the condition may occasionally be severe, producing oliguria and renal failure that requires dialysis; fatalities have occurred.

The mechanism of nephrotoxicity is not well understood and it seems probable that more than one type of lesion may contribute to the overall incidence of toxicity. Possible mechanisms are tubular necrosis (including that due to anaphylaxis or cardiovascular collapse), traumatic occlusion of the renal arteries, cholesterol embolism, and obstruction of the tubules by protein casts (as in patients with multiple myeloma).

Risk factors include pre-existing renal impairment, especially in patients with diabetes mellitus, and conditions where there is reduced renal blood flow, such as heart failure and dehydration. Old age, repeated administration (over a short period of time), multiple myeloma, and pre-existing hepatic impairment have also been proposed as risk factors.

Various methods have been tried to prevent contrast medium-induced nephropathy in high-risk patients.[4,6] Hydration before and after the procedure is of established benefit, but the benefits of other interventions are less clear. Positive results have been reported with acetylcysteine[7] and with fenoldopam,[8] although a larger randomised trial failed to confirm any benefit with fenoldopam.[9] Some benefit has also been found with haemofiltration started before the procedure,[10] but not with haemodialysis immediately after the procedure.[11]


1. Brezis M, Epstein FH. A closer look at radiocontrast-induced nephropathy. *N Engl J Med* 1989; **320:** 179–81.
2. Parfrey PS, *et al.* Contrast material-induced renal failure in patients with diabetes mellitus, renal insufficiency, or both. *N Engl J Med* 1989; **320:** 143–9.
3. Schwab SJ, *et al.* Contrast nephrotoxicity: a randomized controlled trial of a nonionic and an ionic radiographic contrast agent. *N Engl J Med* 1989; **320:** 149–53.
4. Esplugas E, *et al.* Comparative tolerability of contrast media used for coronary interventions. *Drug Safety* 2002; **25:** 1079–98.
5. Rudnick MR, Goldfarb S. Pathogenesis of contrast-induced nephropathy: experimental and clinical observations with an emphasis on the role of osmolality. *Rev Cardiovasc Med* 2003; **4** (suppl 5): S28–S33.
6. Lepor NE. A review of pharmacologic interventions to prevent contrast-induced nephropathy. *Rev Cardiovasc Med* 2003; **4** (suppl 5): S34–S42.
7. Birck R, *et al.* Acetylcysteine for prevention of contrast nephropathy: meta-analysis. *Lancet* 2003; **362:** 598–603.
8. Chu VL, Cheng JWM. Fenoldopam in the prevention of contrast media-induced acute renal failure. *Ann Pharmacother* 2001; **35:** 1278–82. Correction. *ibid.*; 1677.
9. Stone GW, *et al.* Fenoldopam mesylate for the prevention of contrast-induced nephropathy: a randomized controlled trial. *JAMA* 2003; **290:** 2284–91.
10. Marenzi G, *et al.* The prevention of radiocontrast-agent-induced nephropathy by hemofiltration. *N Engl J Med* 2003; **349:** 1333–40.
11. Vogt B, *et al.* Prophylactic hemodialysis after radiocontrast media in patients with renal insufficiency is potentially harmful. *Am J Med* 2001; **111:** 692–8.


### Precautions

The amidotrizoates and similar contrast media should be administered with great caution to patients with asthma or a history of allergy and should be avoided in patients with known hypersensitivity to contrast media or to iodine. An intravenous injection of 0.5 to 1 mL of contrast medium has been given as a test for sensitivity before administration of the main dose but it does not predict hypersensitivity with certainty and severe reactions and fatalities have followed the test dose. Pretreatment with corticosteroids may be considered in patients considered 'at risk' but its value is uncertain (see Hypersensitivity under Adverse Effects of Radiographic Contrast Media, p.1059). An antihistamine may be given with the corticosteroid.

Caution is needed in patients with severe hepatic or renal impairment or others who may be at increased risk of renal failure; dehydrated patients should have their fluid and electrolyte balance corrected before contrast medium administration. Patients with multiple myeloma may be at particular risk if dehydrated, since precipitation of protein in the renal tubules may lead to anuria and fatal renal failure.

An increased risk of adverse effects has also been reported in patients with severe hypertension, advanced cardiac disease, phaeochromocytoma, sickle-cell disease, or hyperthyroidism. Debilitated, severely ill, very old, or very young patients are also at risk.

Certain problems may be associated with particular radiographic techniques. Administration of amidotrizoates or similar hypertonic media into the CNS, e.g. for myelography, should be avoided, and use for cerebral angiography or computed tomography of the brain is contra-indicated in patients with subarachnoid haemorrhage. All intravascular use requires caution in patients with occlusive vascular disorders. These media should not be given for hysterosalpingography in the presence of infection or inflammation of the pelvic cavity, nor during menstruation or in pregnancy (but all abdominal radiography should be avoided in any case during pregnancy because of the risks of radiation to the fetus).

Iodine-containing contrast media may interfere with thyroid function tests. There may also be interference with blood coagulation tests and certain urine tests.

**Breast feeding.** No adverse effects have been observed in breast-feeding infants whose mothers were receiving amidotrizoates and the American Academy of Pediatrics considers[1] that they are therefore usually compatible with breast feeding.

1. American Academy of Pediatrics. The transfer of drugs and other chemicals into human milk. *Pediatrics* 2001; **108:** 776–89. Correction. *ibid.*; 1029. Also available at: http://aappolicy.aappublications.org/cgi/content/full/pediatrics%3b108/3/776 (accessed 05/07/04)

**Neonates.** The use of meglumine amidotrizoate might have contributed to the death, with bowel necrosis, perforation, and peritonitis, of 2 infants with meconium ileus.[1]

1. Leonidas JC, *et al.* Possible adverse effects of methylglucamine diatrizoate compounds on the bowel of newborn infants with meconium ileus. *Radiology* 1976; **121:** 693–6.

### Pharmacokinetics

Amidotrizoates are very poorly absorbed from the gastrointestinal tract. Amidotrizoates in the circulation are not significantly bound to plasma proteins. If renal function is not impaired, unchanged amidotrizoate is rapidly excreted by glomerular filtration; over 95% of an intravascular dose is reported to be excreted in urine within 24 hours, and about 1 to 2% of a dose may be excreted in faeces. Trace amounts may be detected in other body fluids including tears and saliva. Faecal excretion may increase to 10 to 50% in severe renal impairment. The half-life of amidotrizoates has been reported to be 30 to 60 minutes, which can increase to 20 to 140 hours in severe renal impairment. They are removed by haemodialysis and peritoneal dialysis.

The amidotrizoates cross the placenta and have been reported to be present in breast milk.

### Uses and Administration

The amidotrizoates are iodinated ionic monomeric contrast media (p.1059). Both the sodium and the meglumine salt have been widely used in diagnostic radiography including computed tomography (p.1059), but a mixture of both is often preferred to minimise side-effects.

The amidotrizoates are used in an extensive range of procedures. The route of administration and the dose employed depend on the type of procedure and the degree and extent of contrast required. They may be given by many routes including the oral, intravenous, intramuscular, subcutaneous, intra-arterial, intra-articular, and intra-osseous. For some procedures, they may be injected into the gallbladder, biliary ducts, or spleen.

Solutions of amidotrizoates have also been given as an enema in the treatment of uncomplicated meconium ileus.

Calcium amidotrizoate and lysine amidotrizoate have also been used as contrast media.

### Preparations

***BP 2003:*** Meglumine Amidotrizoate Injection; Sodium Amidotrizoate Injection;
***USP 27:*** Diatrizoate Meglumine and Diatrizoate Sodium Injection; Diatrizoate Meglumine and Diatrizoate Sodium Solution; Diatrizoate Meglumine Injection; Diatrizoate Sodium Injection; Diatrizoate Sodium Solution.

**Proprietary Preparations** (details are given in Part 3)
***Arg.:*** Angiografina; Densopax; Hypaque 60%; Hypaque 76%; MD-76; MD-Gastroview; Plenigraf; Tomoray; Triyosom; Urografina; Urovisona; ***Austral.:*** Angiografin; Gastrografin; MD-60; MD-76; MD-Gastroview; Urografin; ***Austria:*** Gastrografin; Peritrast†; Urografin; Urovison†; ***Belg.:*** Urografine; ***Braz.:*** Hypaque; Pielograf†; Plenigraf†; Relievt†; Trazograf†; Urografina†; ***Canad.:*** Gastrografin†; Hypaque; Hypaque-M; MD-76; Reno-M†; Renografin†; ***Chile:*** Angiovist; Hypaque 60%; Hypaque 76%; Pielograf; Reliev; Reliev 76%; ***Denm.:*** Urografin; Urografin Meglumin; ***Fin.:*** Gastrografin; ***Fr.:*** Gastrografine; Radioselectan; ***Ger.:*** Angiografin†; Ethibloc; Gastrografin; Gastrolux; Peritrast; Peritrast comp; Peritrast-Infusio 160/32%; Peritrast-Infusio 180/31%; Peritrast-Oral CT; Peritrast-Oral-GI; Peritrast-RE; Urografin†; Urolux Retro; Urovison; ***Gr.:*** Gastrografin; ***India:*** Urografin; ***Israel:*** Urografin; ***Ital.:*** Gastrografin; Selectografin†; ***Neth.:*** Angiografin; Gastrografin; Urografin; Urovison; ***Norw.:*** Gastrografin; ***NZ:*** Gastrografin; Urografin; ***Port.:*** Gastrografina; Urografina†; ***S.Afr.:*** Angiografin†; Gastrografin; Urografin; ***Spain:*** Gastrografin; Pielograf; Plenigraf; Radialar 280; Trazograf; Uro Angiografin; Urografin; ***Swed.:*** Gastrografin; Urografin; ***Switz.:*** Ethibloc†; Gastrografin; Urografin; ***UK:*** Gastrografin; Hypaque; Urografin 150, 325, and 370; ***USA:*** Cystografin; Gastrografin; Hypaque; Hypaque-M, Hypaque-76; MD-76; MD-Gastroview; Reno-M; Renografin.

**Multi-ingredient:** ***Braz.:*** Hypaque-M; ***Canad.:*** Sinografin†; ***USA:*** Sinografin.

## Barium Sulfate

Barii Sulfas; Barii Sulphas; Barium Sulfuricum; Barium Sulphate; Baryum (Sulfate de); Sulfato de bario.

$BaSO_4$ = 233.4.
*CAS — 7727-43-7.*

**Pharmacopoeias.** In *Chin., Eur.* (see p.vi), *Int., Jpn, Pol., US,* and *Viet.*

**Ph. Eur. 5.0** (Barium Sulphate). A fine, heavy, white powder, free from gritty particles. Practically insoluble in water and in organic solvents; very slightly soluble in acids and in solutions of alkali hydroxides.

**USP 27** (Barium Sulfate). A fine, white, odourless, bulky powder, free from grittiness. Practically insoluble in water, in organic solvents, and in solutions of acids and of alkalis. pH of a 10% w/w aqueous suspension is between 3.5 and 10.0.

### Adverse Effects

Because barium sulfate is almost insoluble it lacks the severe toxicity characteristic of the barium ion; deaths have occurred following the administration of the more soluble barium sulfide in error for the sulfate.

Constipation may occur after oral or rectal barium sulfate; impaction, obstruction, and appendicitis have occurred. Surgical removal of faecaliths has sometimes been necessary. Cramping or diarrhoea have also been reported. Venous intravasation has led to the formation of emboli; deaths have occurred. Perforation of the bowel has led to peritonitis, adhesions, granulomas, and a high mortality rate.

ECG abnormalities have occurred during the use of barium sulfate enemas.

Accidental aspiration into the lungs has led to pneumonitis or granuloma formation.

**Hypersensitivity.** A survey of hypersensitivity reactions to barium preparations found that although barium is inert many of the additives used in formulation have the potential to cause reactions.[1] Of 106 reactions reported or found in the literature, 61% involved the skin and only 8% the respiratory tract; unconsciousness was reported in 8% of cases. In view of the frequency of use of barium preparations, such adverse reactions must be very rare, but radiologists should be aware that they may be somewhat more common than is usually appreciated. A number of severe reactions associated with the use of barium enemas supplied with an inflatable latex cuff may have been due to leaching of components from the latex.[2]

1. Janower ML. Hypersensitivity reactions after barium studies of the upper and lower gastrointestinal tract. *Radiology* 1986; **161:** 139–40.
2. Nightingale SL. Severe adverse reactions to barium enema procedures. *JAMA* 1990; **264:** 2863.

### Precautions

Barium sulfate should not be given to patients with intestinal obstruction and care is needed in those with conditions such as pyloric stenosis or lesions that may predispose to obstruction. Adequate hydration should be ensured after the procedure to prevent severe constipation.

It is contra-indicated in patients with gastrointestinal perforation, and should be avoided, particularly when given rectally, in those at risk of perforation, such as patients with acute ulcerative colitis or diverticulitis and following rectal or colonic biopsy, sigmoidoscopy, or radiotherapy.

### Uses and Administration

Barium sulfate is used as a contrast medium for X-ray examination of the gastrointestinal tract involving single- or double-contrast techniques or computed tomography (p.1059).

The dose of barium sulfate is dependent upon the type of examination and technique employed. For examination of the oesophagus, up to 150 mL of a 50 to 200% w/v suspension may be given by mouth. For examination of the stomach and duodenum, up to 300 mL of a 30 to 200% w/v suspension may be given by mouth. For examination of the small intestine, 100 to 300 mL of a 30 to 150% w/v suspension may be given by mouth. For examination of the colon, 200 mL to 2 litres of a 20 to 130% w/v suspension may be given as an enema.

For double-contrast examination, gas can be introduced into the gastrointestinal tract by using suspensions of barium sulfate containing carbon dioxide; separate gas-producing preparations based on sodium bicarbonate are also available. Air administered via a tube may be used as an alternative to carbon dioxide.

◊ Reviews.

1. Nolan DJ, Traill ZC. The current role of the barium examination of the small intestine. *Clin Radiol* 1997; **52:** 809–20.
2. Mendelson RM. The role of the barium enema in the diagnosis of colorectal neoplasia. *Australas Radiol* 1998; **42:** 191–6.
3. de Zwart IM, *et al.* Barium enema and endoscopy for the detection of colorectal neoplasia: sensitivity, specificity, complications and its determinants. *Clin Radiol* 2001; **56:** 401–9.
4. Rubesin SE, Maglinte DD. Double-contrast barium enema technique. *Radiol Clin North Am* 2003; **41:** 365–76.

**Intussusception.** Contrast media enemas and ultrasound are both used in the diagnosis of intussusception, a condition in infants where part of the intestine prolapses into the lumen of an adjacent part causing an obstruction.[1] However, some consider ultrasound to be superior for diagnosis and reserve enemas for the therapeutic reduction of intussusception. Reduction is achieved as a result of the hydrostatic pressure of the enema pushing the intestine back into its natural position. Although there is extensive experience using barium enemas for reduction some centres prefer to use water-soluble contrast media so as to minimise the risk of chemical peritonitis if perforation of the bowel occurs. Other agents used instead of barium for reduction include air enemas or ultrasound guided saline enemas, both of which avoid or reduce radiographic exposure. Surgery is indicated when enema therapy fails or is considered unsuitable.

1. del-Pozo G, *et al.* Intussusception in children: current concepts in diagnosis and enema reduction. *Radiographics* 1999; **19:** 299–319.

### Preparations

***BP 2003:*** Barium Sulphate for Suspension; Barium Sulphate Oral Suspension;
***USP 27:*** Barium Sulfate for Suspension; Barium Sulfate Paste; Barium Sulfate Suspension; Barium Sulfate Tablets.

**Proprietary Preparations** (details are given in Part 3)
***Arg.:*** Barigraf; Bariofarma; Barosperse; E-Z-Cat; Entero VU; Gastropaque; Novopac; Opti-Up; Scheribar; Tixobar; Top-Cat; ***Austral.:*** Medebar; Medescan; Tixobar†; ***Austria:*** Barilux; Prontobario; Scannotrast; ***Belg.:*** E-Z-Paque; Micropaque; Polibar; ***Braz.:*** Bariogel†; Bariotest†; Baropac†; Celobar; Duplobar†; Neobar†; Telebar†; ***Canad.:*** E-Z-Cat†; Ultra-R†; Unibar†; ***Chile:*** Barigraf; ***Denm.:*** Micropaque; Microtrast; Mixobar; ***Fin.:*** Mixobar; ***Fr.:*** Micropaque; Microtrast; ***Ger.:*** Barilux; Micropaque; Microtrast; ***Gr.:*** Micropaque; Unibaryt-R; ***Israel:*** E-Z-HD; Polibar ACB; ***Ital.:*** Mixobar; Prontobario; TAC Esofago; ***Neth.:*** Micropaque†; ***Norw.:*** Mixobar; ***NZ:*** Medebar; ***Port.:*** Duogas†; E-Z-Cat; E-Z-HD; Gastrobario; Micropaque; Microtrast; Polibar; Prontobario†; ***Spain:*** Barigraf; Barigraf Tac†; Bario Dif; Bario Llorente; Bariopacin†; Disperbarium; Justebarin†; Micropaque; ***Swed.:*** Barytgen†; Mixobar; ***Switz.:*** CAT-Barium (E-Z-CAT); Microbar-Colon†; Microbar-HD (E-Z-HD); Micropaque; Polibar ACB; ***UK:*** Baritop; E-Z-Cat; E-Z-HD; E-Z-Paque; Polibar; Polibar Rapid; Polibar Viscous†; ***USA:*** Anatrast; Baricon; Baro-cat; Barosperse; Enecat†; Entrobar; Epi-C; Flo-Coat; HD 200 Plus; HD 85; Liquipake; Prepcat; Tomocat; Tonopaque.

**Multi-ingredient:** ***Switz.:*** Calcipulpe†; Endomethasone†.

## Ferristene *(BAN, USAN)*

Ferristeno.

$C_8H_{11}NO_3S,(Fe_2O_3)_{0.725}$.
*CAS — 155773-56-1.*
*ATC — V08CB02.*

**Description.** Ferristene consists of iron ferrite crystals carried on monosized spheres of cross-linked poly(ammonium styrenesulfonate). Ferristene contains about 23.4% of Fe.

### Adverse Effects and Precautions

Nausea, vomiting, and constipation or loose stools may occur. Ferristene should not be used in patients with gastrointestinal obstruction or perforation and should be used with care in patients prone to developing these conditions.

### Uses and Administration

Ferristene is a superparamagnetic agent that has been used orally for contrast enhancement in magnetic resonance imaging (p.1059) of the abdomen.

### Preparations

**Proprietary Preparations** (details are given in Part 3)
***Austria:*** Abdoscan†; ***Denm.:*** Abdoscan†; ***Fin.:*** Abdoscan†; ***Ger.:*** Abdoscan†; ***Norw.:*** Abdoscan†; ***Spain:*** Abdoscan†; ***Swed.:*** Abdoscan†; ***Switz.:*** Abdoscan†; ***UK:*** Abdoscan†.

## Ferucarbotran *(BAN, USAN)*

ZK-132281. Superparamagnetic iron oxide particles coated with carboxydextran.

### Profile

Ferucarbotran is a superparamagnetic contrast medium used for contrast enhancement in magnetic resonance imaging of the liver. It is given intravenously as a solution containing 28 mg/mL of iron. The usual dose is 0.9 mL for patients weighing less than 60 kg and 1.4 mL for patients weighing 60 kg and over.

### Preparations

**Proprietary Preparations** (details are given in Part 3)
***Austral.:*** Resovist; ***Fin.:*** Resovist; ***Ger.:*** Resovist; ***Port.:*** Resovist; ***Swed.:*** Resovist; ***Switz.:*** Resovist.

## Ferumoxides *(BAN, USAN)*

AMI-25; Ferumóxidos.

$(Fe_2O_3)_m(FeO)_n$.
*CAS — 119683-68-0.*

### Profile

Ferumoxides is a superparamagnetic agent used intravenously for contrast enhancement in magnetic resonance imaging (p.1059) of the liver. The usual dose, expressed in terms of iron, is up to 0.84 mg/kg, given in 100 mL of glucose 5% over at least 30 minutes.

### Preparations

***USP 27:*** Ferumoxides Injection.

**Proprietary Preparations** (details are given in Part 3)
***Arg.:*** Feridex; ***Austria:*** Endorem; ***Belg.:*** Endorem; ***Denm.:*** Endorem; ***Fin.:*** Endorem; ***Fr.:*** Endorem; ***Ger.:*** Endorem; ***Gr.:*** Endorem; ***Israel:*** Feridex; ***Ital.:*** Endorem; ***Jpn:*** Feridex; ***Neth.:*** Endorem†; ***Norw.:*** Endorem; ***Port.:*** Endorem; ***Spain:*** Endorem; ***Swed.:*** Endorem; ***Switz.:*** Endorem; ***USA:*** Feridex.

## Ferumoxsil *(BAN, USAN)*

AMI-121.
*ATC — V08CB01.*

### Profile

Ferumoxsil is a superparamagnetic agent used for contrast enhancement in magnetic resonance imaging (p.1059) of the gastrointestinal tract. It is usually given orally in a dose of 600 to 900 mL of a suspension containing 0.175 mg/mL of iron. A dose of 300 to 600 mL is used rectally.

### Preparations

***USP 27:*** Ferumoxsil Oral Suspension.

**Proprietary Preparations** (details are given in Part 3)
***Austria:*** Lumirem; ***Denm.:*** Lumirem; ***Fin.:*** Lumirem; ***Fr.:*** Lumirem; ***Ger.:*** Lumirem; ***Ital.:*** Lumirem; ***Neth.:*** Lumirem†; ***Port.:*** Lumirem; ***Swed.:*** Lumirem; ***Switz.:*** Lumirem†.

## Gadobenic Acid (BAN, rINN)

Ácido gadobénico; B-19036; Gd-BOPTA. [2-(Benzyloxymethyl)-6-(carboxylatomethyl-κO)-3,9-bis(carboxymethyl-κO)-3,6,9-triazaundecanedioato-$\kappa^3N^{3,6,9}\kappa^2O^{1,11}$] gadolinium (III).

$C_{22}H_{28}GdN_3O_{11}$ = 667.7.
*CAS — 113662-23-0.*
*ATC — V08CA08.*

## Meglumine Gadobenate (BANM, rINNM)

B-19036/7; Gadobenate Dimeglumine *(USAN)*; Gadobenato de meglumina. Dihydrogen [(±)-4-carboxy-5,8,11-tris(carboxymethyl)-1-phenyl-2-oxa-5,8,11-triaza-tridecan-13-oato(5-)]gadolinate(2-) compound with 1-deoxy-1-(methylamino)-D-glucitol (1:2).

$C_{22}H_{28}GdN_3O_{11},2C_7H_{17}NO_5$ = 1058.1.
*CAS — 127000-20-8.*
*ATC — V08CA08.*

### Profile

Gadobenic acid is an ionic paramagnetic agent used, as meglumine gadobenate, for contrast enhancement in magnetic resonance imaging (p.1059) of the liver and CNS.

Meglumine gadobenate is available as a solution containing 529 mg/mL (0.5 mmol/mL). The usual dose is 0.1 mL/kg (0.05 mmol/kg) intravenously for imaging of the liver, and 0.2 mL/kg (0.1 mmol/kg) intravenously for imaging of the brain or spine.

### Preparations

**Proprietary Preparations** (details are given in Part 3)
***Austria:*** MultiHance; ***Belg.:*** MultiHance; ***Denm.:*** MultiHance; ***Fin.:*** MultiHance; ***Fr.:*** MultiHance; ***Ger.:*** MultiHance; ***Gr.:*** Multi Hance; ***Irl.:*** MultiHance; Myocet; ***Ital.:*** MultiHance; ***Neth.:*** MultiHance; ***Port.:*** MultiHance; ***Swed.:*** MultiHance; ***UK:*** MultiHance.

## Gadobutrol (rINN)

{10-[(1*RS*,2*SR*)-2,3-Dihydroxy-1-(hydroxymethyl)propyl]-1,4,7,10-tetraazacyclododecane-1,4,7-triacetato(3-)}gadolinium.

$C_{18}H_{31}GdN_4O_9$ = 604.7.
*CAS — 138071-82-6.*
*ATC — V08CA09.*

### Profile

Gadobutrol is a nonionic paramagnetic agent used for contrast enhancement in magnetic resonance imaging (p.1059) of cranial and spinal structures and in magnetic resonance angiography.

Gadobutrol is available as solutions containing 302.5 mg/mL (0.5 mmol/mL) or 605 mg/mL (1 mmol/mL). The usual dose in adults is the equivalent of 0.1 mmol/kg intravenously for imaging of the CNS, and 0.1 to 0.3 mmol/kg for angiography.

### Preparations

**Proprietary Preparations** (details are given in Part 3)
***Austral.:*** Gadovist; ***Austria:*** Gadovist; ***Denm.:*** Gadovist; ***Fin.:*** Gadovist; ***Ger.:*** Gadovist; ***Ital.:*** Gadovist; ***Norw.:*** Gadovist; ***Port.:*** Gadovist; ***S.Afr.:*** Gadovist; ***Spain:*** Gadograf; Gadovist; ***Swed.:*** Gadovist; ***Switz.:*** Gadovist; ***UK:*** Gadovist.

## Gadodiamide (BAN, USAN, rINN)

Gadodiamida; GdDTPA-BMA; S-041. [*N*,*N*-Bis(2-{(carboxymethyl)[(methylcarbamoyl)methyl]amino}ethyl)glycinato(3-)]gadolinium; a complex of gadolinium with diethylenetriamine pentaacetic acid bismethylamide.

$C_{16}H_{26}GdN_5O_8$ = 573.7.
*CAS — 131410-48-5 (anhydrous gadodiamide); 122795-43-1 (gadodiamide hydrate).*
*ATC — V08CA03.*

**Pharmacopoeias.** In *US.*

**USP 27** (Gadodiamide). A white, odourless, powder. Freely soluble in water and in methyl alcohol; soluble in alcohol; slightly soluble in acetone and in chloroform. Store in airtight containers.

### Adverse Effects and Precautions

As for Gadopentetic Acid, below.

**Effects on the pancreas.** There has been a report[1] of acute pancreatitis developing in a patient shortly after injection of gadodiamide for hepatic imaging.

1. Terzi C, Sökmen S. Acute pancreatitis induced by magnetic-resonance-imaging contrast agent. *Lancet* 1999; **354:** 1789–90. Correction. *ibid.* 2000; **355:** 660.

**Interference with diagnostic tests.** Gadodiamide may interfere with colorimetric methods for measuring serum calcium concentrations, and severe pseudohypocalcaemia has been reported[1] following the use of gadodiamide.

1. Doorenbos CJ, *et al.* Severe pseudohypocalcemia after gadolinium-enhanced magnetic resonance angiography. *N Engl J Med* 2003; **349:** 817–18.

### Pharmacokinetics

Gadodiamide is rapidly distributed into extracellular fluid. About 96% of a dose is excreted unchanged in the urine within 24 hours. An elimination half-life of about 70 minutes has been reported. Gadodiamide is not bound to plasma proteins.

### Uses and Administration

Gadodiamide is a nonionic paramagnetic agent used for contrast enhancement in magnetic resonance imaging (p.1059) of cranial and spinal structures and of the whole body, and in angiography.

Gadodiamide is available as a solution containing 287 mg/mL (0.5 mmol/mL). The usual dose in adults is 0.2 mL/kg (0.1 mmol/kg) intravenously. The dose may be increased to up to 0.6 mL/kg (0.3 mmol/kg) for whole body imaging and for angiography, but doses of greater than 60 mL are not usually required.

### Preparations

***USP 27:*** Gadodiamide Injection.

**Proprietary Preparations** (details are given in Part 3)
***Arg.:*** Omniscan; ***Austral.:*** Omniscan; ***Austria:*** Omniscan; ***Belg.:*** Omniscan†; ***Braz.:*** Omniscan; ***Canad.:*** Omniscan; ***Chile:*** Omniscan; ***Denm.:*** Omniscan; ***Fin.:*** Omniscan; ***Fr.:*** Omniscan; ***Ger.:*** Omniscan; ***Gr.:*** Omniscan; ***Israel:*** Omniscan; ***Ital.:*** Omniscan; ***Jpn:*** Omniscan; ***Norw.:*** Omniscan; ***NZ:*** Omniscan; ***Spain:*** Omniscan; ***Swed.:*** Omniscan; ***Switz.:*** Omniscan; ***UK:*** Omniscan; ***USA:*** Omniscan.

## Gadopentetic Acid (BAN, rINN)

Ácido gadopentético; Gadolinium-DTPA. {*N'*,*N''*-Bis(carboxymethyl)-*N'*,*N''*-[(acetato)iminodiethylene]diglycinato-*O*,*O'*,*O''*,*N*,*N'*,*N''*}gadolinium(3+); a complex of gadolinium with diethylenetriamine penta-acetic acid.

$C_{14}H_{20}GdN_3O_{10}$ = 547.6.
*CAS — 80529-93-7.*
*ATC — V08CA01.*

## Meglumine Gadopentetate (BANM, rINNM)

Dimeglumine Gadopentetate; Gadopentetate Dimeglumine *(USAN)*; Gadopentetate Meglumine; Gadopentetato de meglumina; SH-L-451-A. The di(*N*-methylglucamine) salt of gadopentetic acid.

$C_{14}H_{20}GdN_3O_{10},(C_7H_{17}NO_5)_2$ = 938.0.
*CAS — 86050-77-3.*
*ATC — V08CA01.*

**Pharmacopoeias.** *US* includes only as an injection.

### Adverse Effects

There may be headache, nausea, vomiting, and transient sensations of heat or cold or taste disturbances following injection of gadopentetate. Rarely, convulsions, hypotension, allergic or anaphylactoid reactions, and shock may occur. Paraesthesias, dizziness, and localised pain have also been reported. Transient elevations of serum iron and bilirubin values have been observed.

◊ General references.

1. Nelson KL, *et al.* Clinical safety of gadopentetate dimeglumine. *Radiology* 1995; **196:** 439–43.

**Hypersensitivity.** Anaphylactic shock has been reported[1] in a patient after intravenous meglumine gadopentetate. The patient had a history of pollen allergy and had experienced anaphylactic shock when given an iodine-based contrast agent intravenously 2 months earlier.

1. Tardy B, *et al.* Anaphylactic shock induced by intravenous gadopentetate dimeglumine. *Lancet* 1992; **339:** 494.

### Precautions

Gadopentetate should be given with care to patients with severe renal impairment, epilepsy, hypotension, or a history of hypersensitivity, asthma, or other allergic respiratory disorders. Care should be taken to avoid extravasation. Gadopentetate may interfere with tests of serum iron or bilirubin concentrations.

**Breast feeding.** No adverse effects have been observed in breast-feeding infants whose mothers were receiving gadopentetic acid and the American Academy of Pediatrics considers[1] that it is therefore usually compatible with breast feeding.

1. American Academy of Pediatrics. The transfer of drugs and other chemicals into human milk. *Pediatrics* 2001; **108:** 776–89. Correction. *ibid.*; 1029. Also available at: http://aappolicy.aappublications.org/cgi/content/full/pediatrics%3b108/3/776 (accessed 05/07/04)

**Myasthenia gravis.** Acute deterioration of myasthenia gravis has been reported[1] in a patient after imaging of the brain using gadopentetate.

1. Nordenbo AM, Somnier FE. Acute deterioration of myasthenia gravis after intravenous administration of gadolinium-DTPA. *Lancet* 1992; **340:** 1168.

### Pharmacokinetics

Gadopentetate is rapidly distributed into the extracellular space following intravenous injection. An elimination half-life of 1.6 hours has been reported. It is not metabolised and about 90% of a dose is excreted in the urine within 24 hours. A small amount is distributed into breast milk. Gadopentetate is removed by haemodialysis.

### Uses and Administration

Gadopentetic acid is an ionic paramagnetic agent used, as meglumine gadopentetate, for contrast enhancement in magnetic resonance imaging (p.1059) of cranial and spinal structures, of the whole body, and of the gastrointestinal tract; it may also be used for the evaluation of renal function.

Meglumine gadopentetate is used intravenously for cranial, spinal, and whole body imaging as a solution containing 469.01 mg/mL (0.5 mmol/mL). The usual dose in adults, children, and neonates is 0.2 mL/kg (0.1 mmol/kg) intravenously. For cranial and spinal imaging, a further dose of 0.2 mL/kg (0.1 mmol/kg) may be given within 30 minutes if necessary; in adults this second dose may be 0.4 mL/kg (0.2 mmol/kg). For whole body imaging in adults and children over 2 years, a dose of 0.4 mL/kg (0.2 mmol/kg) may be needed in some cases to produce adequate contrast and in special circumstances a dose of 0.6 mL/kg (0.3 mmol/kg) may be used in adults.

Meglumine gadopentetate is administered orally and rectally for gastrointestinal imaging. A solution containing 9.38 mg/mL is diluted before use (100 mL with 900 mL of water) and doses in the range of 100 to 1000 mL of this diluted solution are used in adults depending upon the organ or tissue being investigated.

### Preparations

***USP 27:*** Gadopentetate Dimeglumine Injection.

**Proprietary Preparations** (details are given in Part 3)
***Arg.:*** Magnevist; Opacite; Viewgam; ***Austral.:*** Magnevist; ***Austria:*** Magnevist; ***Belg.:*** Magnevist; ***Braz.:*** Magnevistan†; ***Canad.:*** Magnevist; ***Chile:*** Magnevistan; ***Denm.:*** Magnevist; ***Fin.:*** Magnevist; ***Fr.:*** Magnevist; ***Ger.:*** Magnevist; ***Gr.:*** Magnevist; ***Ital.:*** Magnevist; ***Neth.:*** Magnevist; ***Norw.:*** Magnevist; ***NZ:*** Magnevist; ***Port.:*** Magnevist; ***S.Afr.:*** Magnevist; ***Spain:*** Magnevist; Magnograf; ***Swed.:*** Magnevist; ***Switz.:*** Magnevist; ***UK:*** Magnevist; ***USA:*** Magnevist.

## Gadoteric Acid (BAN, rINN)

Ácido gadotérico; ZK-112004. Hydrogen [1,4,7,10-tetraazacyclododecane-1,4,7,10-tetraaceto(4–)]gadolinate(1–); Hydrogen [1,4,7,10-tetrakis(carboxylatomethyl)-1,4,7,10-tetra-azacyclododecane-$\kappa^4N$]gadolinate(1–).

$C_{16}H_{25}GdN_4O_8$ = 558.6.
*CAS — 72573-82-1.*
*ATC — V08CA02.*

## Meglumine Gadoterate (BANM, rINNM)

Gadoterate Meglumine; Gadoterato de meglumina.
*ATC — V08CA02.*

### Profile

Gadoteric acid is an ionic paramagnetic contrast medium with actions similar to those of gadopentetic acid (above). It is used, as meglumine gadoterate, for contrast enhancement in magnetic resonance imaging (p.1059) of cranial and spinal structures, of the liver, and of the whole body, and in magnetic resonance angiography.

Meglumine gadoterate is available as a solution containing 377 mg/mL (0.5 mmol/mL). The usual dose in adults and children is 0.2 mL/kg (0.1 mmol/kg) by intravenous injection. A second dose of up to 0.4 mL/kg (0.2 mmol/kg) may be given if necessary.

### Preparations

**Proprietary Preparations** (details are given in Part 3)
***Arg.:*** Dotarem; ***Austral.:*** Dotarem; ***Austria:*** Dotarem; ***Belg.:*** Dotarem; ***Braz.:*** Dotarem; ***Chile:*** Dotarem; ***Denm.:*** Dotarem; ***Fin.:*** Dotarem; ***Fr.:*** Dotarem; ***Gr.:*** Dotarem; ***Israel:*** Dotarem; ***Ital.:*** Dotarem; ***Neth.:*** Dotarem†; ***Norw.:*** Dotarem; ***Port.:*** Dotarem; ***Spain:*** Dotarem; ***Swed.:*** Dotarem; ***Switz.:*** Dotarem.

## Gadoteridol (BAN, USAN, rINN)

SQ-32692. (±)-[10-(2-Hydroxypropyl)-1,4,7,10-tetraazacyclododecane-1,4,7-triacetato(3–)]gadolinium.

$C_{17}H_{29}GdN_4O_7$ = 558.7.
*CAS — 120066-54-8.*
*ATC — V08CA04.*

**Pharmacopoeias.** In *US.*

**USP 27** (Gadoteridol). A white to off-white, odourless, crystalline powder. Freely soluble in water and in methyl alcohol; soluble in isopropyl alcohol. Store in airtight containers. Protect from light.

### Adverse Effects and Precautions

As for Gadopentetic Acid, above.

**Hypersensitivity.** Vasovagal response and anaphylactoid reaction has been reported during intravenous use of gadoteridol.[1]

1. Shellock FG, *et al.* Adverse reaction to intravenous gadoteridol. *Radiology* 1993; **189:** 151–2.

### Pharmacokinetics

About 94% of a dose of gadoteridol is excreted unchanged in the urine within 24 hours. An elimination half-life of about 1.57 hours has been reported.

### Uses and Administration

Gadoteridol is a nonionic paramagnetic agent used for contrast enhancement in magnetic resonance imaging (p.1059) of cranial and spinal structures and of the whole body.

Gadoteridol is available as a solution containing 279.3 mg/mL (0.5 mmol/mL). The usual adult dose is 0.2 mL/kg (0.1 mmol/kg) intravenously; an additional dose of up to 0.4 mL/kg (0.2 mmol/kg) may be given approximately 30 minutes after the first if necessary. A single dose of 0.2 mL/kg (0.1 mmol/kg) is used in children from 6 months of age.

### Preparations

***USP 27:*** Gadoteridol Injection.

**Proprietary Preparations** (details are given in Part 3)
***Austral.:*** Prohance; ***Austria:*** Prohance; ***Belg.:*** Prohance; ***Canad.:*** Prohance†; ***Denm.:*** Prohance; ***Fin.:*** Prohance; ***Fr.:*** Prohance; ***Ger.:*** Pro-

hance; **Irl.:** Prohance; **Ital.:** Prohance; **Jpn:** Prohance; **Neth.:** Prohance; **Norw.:** Prohance; **Spain:** Prohance; **Swed.:** Prohance; **Switz.:** Prohance; **UK:** Prohance; **USA:** Prohance.

## Gadoversetamide *(BAN, USAN, rINN)*

MP-1177. {N,N-Bis[2-({(carboxymethyl)[(2-methoxyethyl)carbamoyl]methyl}amino)ethyl]glycinato(3-)}gadolinium.

$C_{20}H_{34}GdN_5O_{10}$ = 661.8.
*CAS — 131069-91-5.*
*ATC — V08CA06.*

**Pharmacopoeias.** In *US.*

**USP 27** (Gadoversetamide). A white odourless powder. Freely soluble in water. Store in airtight containers. Protect from light.

### Profile

Gadoversetamide is a nonionic paramagnetic agent used for contrast enhancement in magnetic resonance imaging (p.1059) of cranial and spinal structures and of the whole body.

Gadoversetamide is available as a solution containing 331 mg/mL (0.5 mmol/mL). The usual dose in adults is 0.2 mL/kg (0.1 mmol/kg) intravenously.

### Preparations

***USP 27:*** Gadoversetamide Injection.

**Proprietary Preparations** (details are given in Part 3)
***Austral.:*** Optimark; ***Braz.:*** Optimark†.

## Gadoxetic Acid *(rINN)*

Gd-EOB-DTPA. Dihydrogen [N-{(2S)-2-[bis(carboxymethyl)amino]-3-(p-ethoxyphenyl)propyl}-N-{2-[bis(carboxymethyl)amino]ethyl}glycinato(5-)]gadolinate(2-).

$C_{23}H_{30}GdN_3O_{11}$ = 681.7.
*CAS — 135326-11-3 (gadoxetic acid); 135326-22-6 (gadoxetate disodium).*

### Profile

Gadoxetic acid is a paramagnetic contrast medium used as the disodium salt for contrast enhancement in magnetic resonance imaging of the liver.

### Preparations

**Proprietary Preparations** (details are given in Part 3)
***Swed.:*** Primovist.

## Galactose *(USAN)*

D-Galactopyranose; Galactosa; D-Galactose; Galactosum.

$C_6H_{12}O_6$ = 180.2.
*CAS — 59-23-4 (D-galactose); 3646-73-9 (α-D-galactose).*
*ATC — V04CE01.*

**Pharmacopoeias.** In *Eur.* (see p.vi).

**Ph. Eur. 5.0** (Galactose). A white, crystalline or finely granulated powder. Freely soluble or soluble in water; very slightly soluble in alcohol.

### Profile

Galactose is a naturally occurring monosaccharide used as an ultrasound contrast medium (p.1059). It is administered intravenously or transcervically as a microbubble-microparticle suspension to enhance ultrasound images of the heart or female genital tract, respectively. Palmitic acid may be included to stabilise the microbubbles.

The clearance of galactose given intravenously has been used as a measure of liver function.

### Preparations

**Proprietary Preparations** (details are given in Part 3)
***Arg.:*** Levovist; ***Austral.:*** Levovist; ***Austria:*** Echovist; Levovist; Ombravist; ***Braz.:*** Ecovist†; Levovist†; ***Canad.:*** Echovist; Levovist; ***Denm.:*** Echovist†; Levovist; ***Fin.:*** Echovist; Levovist; ***Fr.:*** Echovist; Levovist; ***Ger.:*** Echovist; Levovist; ***Israel:*** Echovist; Levovist†; ***Ital.:*** Levovist; ***Neth.:*** Echovist; Levovist; ***Norw.:*** Echovist†; Levovist; ***NZ:*** Echovist†; Levovist†; ***Port.:*** Levovist; ***S.Afr.:*** Echovist†; ***Spain:*** Levograf; Levovist; ***Swed.:*** Echovist; Levovist; ***Switz.:*** Echovist†; Levovist; ***UK:*** Echovist; Levovist.

**Multi-ingredient: *Gr.:*** L-Vist.

## Iobitridol *(BAN, rINN)*

N,N′-Bis(2,3-dihydroxypropyl)-5-[2-(hydroxymethyl)hydracrylamido]-2,4,6-triiodo-N,N′-dimethylisophthalamide; N,N′-Bis(2,3-dihydroxypropyl)-5-(3-hydroxy-2-hydroxymethylpropionamido)-2,4,6-tri-iodo-N,N′-dimethylisophthalamide.

$C_{20}H_{28}I_3N_3O_9$ = 835.2.
*CAS — 136949-58-1.*
*ATC — V08AB11.*

### Profile

Iobitridol is an iodinated nonionic monomeric contrast medium used parenterally for a wide range of radiographic diagnostic procedures (p.1059).

### Preparations

**Proprietary Preparations** (details are given in Part 3)
***Arg.:*** Xenetix; ***Austria:*** Xenetix; ***Belg.:*** Xenetix; ***Braz.:*** Henetix; ***Chile:*** Xenetix; ***Denm.:*** Xenetix; ***Fin.:*** Xenetix; ***Fr.:*** Xenetix; ***Ger.:*** Xenetix; ***Gr.:*** Xenetix; ***Israel:*** Xenetix; ***Ital.:*** Xenetix; ***Neth.:*** Xenetix†; ***Norw.:*** Xenetix; ***Port.:*** Xenetix; ***Spain:*** Xenetix; ***Swed.:*** Xenetix; ***Switz.:*** Xenetix.

## Iocetamic Acid *(BAN, USAN, pINN)*

Ácido iocetámico; DRC-1201; MP-620. N-Acetyl-N-(3-amino-2,4,6-tri-iodophenyl)-2-methyl-β-alanine; 2-[N-(3-Amino-2,4,6-tri-iodophenyl)acetamidomethyl]-propionic acid.

$C_{12}H_{13}I_3N_2O_3$ = 614.0.
*CAS — 16034-77-8.*
*ATC — V08AC07.*

**Description.** Iocetamic acid contains about 62% of I.

### Adverse Effects and Precautions

As for Iopanoic Acid, p.1065.

### Pharmacokinetics

Iocetamic acid is variably absorbed from the gastrointestinal tract. It is conjugated in the liver with glucuronic acid, and is excreted in the bile and concentrated in the gallbladder; about 62% of a dose is excreted in the urine within 48 hours.

### Uses and Administration

Iocetamic acid is an iodinated ionic monomeric contrast medium that has been used mainly for cholecystography (p.1059).

### Preparations

**Proprietary Preparations** (details are given in Part 3)
***Braz.:*** Colebrina†; ***Neth.:*** Cholebrine; ***Swed.:*** Cholebrin†.

## Iodamide *(BAN, USAN, rINN)*

Ametriodinic Acid; B-4130; Iodamida; SH-926. α,5-Diacetamido-2,4,6-tri-iodo-m-toluic acid; 3-Acetamido-5-acetamidomethyl-2,4,6-tri-iodobenzoic acid.

$C_{12}H_{11}I_3N_2O_4$ = 627.9.
*CAS — 440-58-4.*
*ATC — V08AA03.*

**Description.** Iodamide contains about 60.6% of I.

**Pharmacopoeias.** In *Jpn.*

## Meglumine Iodamide *(BANM, rINNM)*

Iodamida de meglumina; Iodamide Meglumine *(USAN)*. The N-methylglucamine salt of iodamide.

$C_{12}H_{11}I_3N_2O_4,C_7H_{17}NO_5$ = 823.2.
*CAS — 18656-21-8.*
*ATC — V08AA03.*

**Description.** Meglumine iodamide contains about 46.3% of I.

## Sodium Iodamide *(BANM, rINNM)*

Iodamida sódica; Iodamide Sodium.

$C_{12}H_{10}I_3N_2NaO_4$ = 649.9.
*CAS — 10098-82-5.*
*ATC — V08AA03.*

**Description.** Sodium iodamide contains about 58.6% of I.

### Profile

Iodamide is an iodinated ionic monomeric contrast medium given by intravenous or local administration in a variety of radiographic diagnostic procedures (p.1059).

It is usually given as a 24 to 65% solution of the meglumine salt, as an approximately 53% solution of the sodium salt, or as a mixture of the sodium and meglumine salts. The dose varies according to the procedure and route of administration. The meglumine salt has also been used for contrast enhancement in computed tomography of the brain.

### Preparations

**Proprietary Preparations** (details are given in Part 3)
***Austria:*** Uromiro; ***Braz.:*** Uromiron†; ***Ital.:*** Isteropac ER; Opacist ER; Uromiro 24%, 36%, and 300; Uromiro 300 Sodico; Uromiro 340 and 420; ***Port.:*** Uromiro†; ***Switz.:*** Isteropac; Opacist ER; Uromiro.

## Iodised Oil

Aceite yodado; Ethiodized Oil.

*CAS — 8001-40-9 (iodised oil); 8008-53-5 (ethiodized oil injection).*

**Description.** Iodised oil is an iodine addition product of the ethyl esters of the fatty acids obtained from poppy-seed oil. It contains about 35 to 39% of combined iodine.

**Incompatibility.** Because of its solvent action on polystyrene, iodised oil injection should not be administered in plastic syringes made with polystyrene.

### Adverse Effects and Precautions

The risk of hypersensitivity reactions or iodism is greater after the use of iodised oil than after water-soluble iodinated contrast media such as the amidotrizoates. Pulmonary oil embolism is reported to be relatively frequent following lymphography but is not usually severe; however, hypotension, tachycardia, and pulmonary oedema and infarction may occur rarely and deaths have been reported in patients with pulmonary disease. Chemical pneumonitis, oedema, granuloma formation, and goitre have occurred.

Great care should be taken to avoid vascular structures, because of the danger of oil embolism; it should not therefore be used in areas affected by haemorrhage or local trauma. Iodised oil should be used with care in patients with thyroid dysfunction or a history of allergic reactions. The use of iodised oil may interfere with thyroid-function tests for several months.

◊ The use of oily contrast media for hysterosalpingography has been associated with serious adverse effects, including tubal occlusion, and it has been suggested[1] that such use is dangerous and unnecessary.

1. Wright FW, Stallworthy J. Female sterility produced by investigation. *BMJ* 1973; **3:** 632.

### Pharmacokinetics

Iodised oil may persist in the body for several weeks or months. It is only slowly absorbed from most body sites, although absorption from the peritoneal cavity is stated to be relatively rapid. It is reported to be slowly metabolised to fatty acids and iodine.

### Uses and Administration

Iodised oil is an iodinated contrast medium that is used mainly for lymphography although it has also been used in various other radiographic diagnostic procedures (p.1059). It has been used for hysterosalpingography but water-soluble agents are preferred. The dose is dependent upon the procedure. The fluid injection of iodised oil is unsuitable for use in bronchography.

Because it is slowly metabolised to release iodine, iodised oil is used in the management of iodine deficiency (p.1599).

**Malignant neoplasms.** Injection of iodised oil into the hepatic artery is followed by selective and long-lasting retention within hepatic carcinomas and used with computed tomography is considered to be more sensitive than other imaging techniques.[1] The sensitivity of this method also enables the imaging of very small satellite nodules, which if undetected are responsible for high early rates of recurrence after resection. Iodised oil has also been used to provide targeted delivery of lipophilic antineoplastics or radioactive iodine to hepatic[1-4] or breast tumours.[5]

1. Anonymous. Lipiodol computed tomography for small hepatocellular carcinomas. *Lancet* 1991; **337:** 333–4.
2. Novell R, *et al.* Ablation of recurrent primary liver cancer using $^{131}$I-lipiodol. *Postgrad Med J* 1991; **67:** 393–5.
3. Group d'Etude et de Traitement du Carcinome Hépatocellulaire. A comparison of Lipiodol chemoembolization and conservative treatment for unresectable hepatocellular carcinoma. *N Engl J Med* 1995; **332:** 1256–61.
4. Lau WY, *et al.* Adjuvant intra-arterial iodine-131-labelled lipiodol for resectable hepatocellular carcinoma: a prospective randomised trial. *Lancet* 1999; **353:** 797–801.
5. Novell JR, *et al.* Targeted therapy for recurrent breast carcinoma with regional 'Lipiodol'/epirubicin infusion. *Lancet* 1990; **336:** 1383.

### Preparations

***BP 2003:*** Iodised Oil Fluid Injection;
***USP 27:*** Ethiodized Oil Injection.

**Proprietary Preparations** (details are given in Part 3)
***Arg.:*** Lipiodol; ***Austral.:*** Lipiodol; ***Austria:*** Lipiodol; ***Belg.:*** Lipiodol; ***Braz.:*** Lipiodol†; ***Chile:*** Lipiodol; ***Denm.:*** Lipiodol; ***Fr.:*** Lipiodol; ***Ger.:*** Lipiodol; ***Gr.:*** Lipiodol; ***Israel:*** Lipiodol; ***Ital.:*** Lipiodol; ***Neth.:*** Lipiodol†; ***Norw.:*** Lipiodol; ***NZ:*** Lipiodol; ***Port.:*** Lipiodol; ***UK:*** Lipiodol; ***USA:*** Ethiodol.

## Iodixanol *(BAN, USAN, rINN)*

2-5410-3A. 5,5′-[(2-Hydroxytrimethylene)bis(acetylimino)]bis[N,N′-bis(2,3-dihydroxypropyl)-2,4,6-triiodoisophthalamide].

$C_{35}H_{44}I_6N_6O_{15}$ = 1550.2.
*CAS — 92339-11-2.*
*ATC — V08AB09.*

**Description.** Iodixanol contains about 49.1% of I.

**Pharmacopoeias.** In *US.*

**USP 27** (Iodixanol). A white to off-white, amorphous, odourless, hygroscopic powder. Freely soluble in water. Store at a temperature of 25°, excursions permitted between 15° and 30°. Protect from light.

### Adverse Effects, Treatment, and Precautions

See under the amidotrizoates, p.1060.

### Pharmacokinetics

Iodixanol is rapidly distributed into extracellular fluid following intravenous injection. It is not bound to plasma proteins. It is not metabolised and about 97% of a dose is excreted in the urine within 24 hours. A terminal elimination half-life of about 2 hours has been reported. Iodixanol is removed by dialysis.

### Uses and Administration

Iodixanol is an iodinated nonionic dimeric contrast medium that is used for angiography, urography, and other procedures, and for contrast enhancement during computed tomography (p.1059).

Iodixanol is given by injection as a solution usually containing between 30.5 and 65.2% of iodixanol (equivalent to between 150 and 320 mg/mL of iodine). The dose and strength used vary according to the procedure and route of injection.

◊ References.

1. Spencer CM, Goa KL. Iodixanol: a review of its pharmacodynamic and pharmacokinetic properties and diagnostic use as an x-ray contrast medium. *Drugs* 1996; **52:** 899–927.

## Preparations

***USP 27:*** Iodixanol Injection.

**Proprietary Preparations** (details are given in Part 3)
***Austral.:*** Visipaque; ***Austria:*** Visipaque; ***Belg.:*** Visipaque†; ***Canad.:*** Visipaque; ***Chile:*** Visipaque; ***Denm.:*** Visipaque; ***Fin.:*** Visipaque; ***Fr.:*** Visipaque; ***Ger.:*** Visipaque; ***Gr.:*** Visipaque; ***Israel:*** Visipaque; ***Ital.:*** Visipaque; ***Neth.:*** Visipaque†; ***Norw.:*** Visipaque; ***NZ:*** Visipaque; ***Spain:*** Visipaque; ***Swed.:*** Visipaque; ***Switz.:*** Visipaque; ***UK:*** Visipaque; ***USA:*** Visipaque.

---

## Iodoxamic Acid *(BAN, USAN, rINN)*

Ácido iodoxámico; B-10610; SQ-21982. 3,3′-(4,7,10,13-Tetraoxahexadecanedioyldiamino)bis(2,4,6-tri-iodobenzoic acid).
$C_{26}H_{26}I_6N_2O_{10}$ = 1287.9.
*CAS — 31127-82-9.*
*ATC — V08AC01.*

**Description.** Iodoxamic acid contains about 59.1% of I.

## Meglumine Iodoxamate *(BANM, rINNM)*

Dimeglumine Iodoxamate; Iodoxamate Meglumine *(USAN)*; Iodoxamato de meglumina. The di(*N*-methylglucamine) salt of iodoxamic acid.
$C_{26}H_{26}I_6N_2O_{10},(C_7H_{17}NO_5)_2$ = 1678.3.
*CAS — 51764-33-1.*
*ATC — V08AC01.*

**Description.** Meglumine iodoxamate contains about 45.4% of I.

### Profile

Iodoxamic acid is an iodinated ionic dimeric contrast medium that has been used as the meglumine salt for cholecystography and cholangiography (p.1059).

### Preparations

**Proprietary Preparations** (details are given in Part 3)
***Irl.:*** Endobil†.

---

## Iofendylate *(BAN, rINN)*

Ethyl Iodophenylundecylate; Iodophendylate; Iofendilato; Iophendylate. A mixture of stereoisomers of ethyl 10-(4-iodophenyl)undecanoate.
$C_{19}H_{29}IO_2$ = 416.3.
*CAS — 99-79-6; 1320-11-2.*
*ATC — V08AD04.*

**Description.** Iofendylate contains about 30.5% of I.

**Pharmacopoeias.** In *Chin.* and *US.*

**USP 27** (Iophendylate). A colourless to pale yellow, viscous liquid, darkening on long exposure to air. Is odourless or has a faintly ethereal odour. Very slightly soluble in water; freely soluble in alcohol, in chloroform, in ether, and in benzene. Store in airtight containers at a temperature of 25°, excursions permitted between 15° and 30°. Protect from light.

**Incompatibility.** Polystyrene was soluble in iofendylate and syringes made from polystyrene were rapidly attacked.[1] Syringes made from polypropylene appeared to be unaffected.

1. Irving JD, Reynolds PV. Disposable syringe danger. *Lancet* 1966; **i:** 362.

### Profile

Iofendylate is an iodinated ionic monomeric contrast medium that was formerly used mainly for myelography (p.1059); it was also formerly used for examination of the third and fourth ventricles, and to visualise the fetus in the amniotic sac prior to intrauterine blood transfusion. However, serious adverse effects including allergy, arachnoiditis, and aseptic meningitis have occurred with its use and it has been superseded by nonionic media such as iohexol (p.1064). Residues of iofendylate remaining years after myelography have been associated with adverse effects.

### Preparations

***BP 2003:*** Iofendylate Injection;
***USP 27:*** Iophendylate Injection.

---

## Ioglicic Acid *(BAN, USAN, rINN)*

Ácido ioglícico; SH-H-200-AB. 5-Acetamido-2,4,6-tri-iodo-*N*-(methylcarbamoylmethyl)isophthalamic acid.
$C_{13}H_{12}I_3N_3O_5$ = 671.0.
*CAS — 49755-67-1.*
*ATC — V08AA06.*

**Description.** Ioglicic acid contains about 56.7% of I.

## Meglumine Ioglicate *(BANM, rINNM)*

Ioglicate Meglumine; Ioglicato de meglumina. The *N*-methylglucamine salt of ioglicic acid.
$C_{13}H_{12}I_3N_3O_5,C_7H_{17}NO_5$ = 866.2.
*ATC — V08AA06.*

**Description.** Meglumine ioglicate contains about 44.0% of I.

## Sodium Ioglicate *(BANM, rINNM)*

Ioglicate Sodium; Ioglicato sódico.
$C_{13}H_{11}I_3N_3NaO_5$ = 692.9.
*ATC — V08AA06.*

**Description.** Sodium ioglicate contains about 54.9% of I.

### Profile

Ioglicic acid is an iodinated ionic monomeric contrast medium that has been given by injection, as the meglumine and sodium salts, for urography, angiography, and related procedures (p.1059).

### Preparations

**Proprietary Preparations** (details are given in Part 3)
***Austria:*** Rayvist 180†; ***Braz.:*** Biligrama†; ***Switz.:*** Rayvist†.

---

## Iohexol *(BAN, USAN, rINN)*

Iohexolum; Win-39424. *N,N′*-Bis(2,3-dihydroxypropyl)-5-[*N*-(2,3-dihydroxypropyl)acetamido]-2,4,6-tri-iodoisophthalamide.
$C_{19}H_{26}I_3N_3O_9$ = 821.1.
*CAS — 66108-95-0.*
*ATC — V08AB02.*

**Description.** Iohexol contains about 46.4% of I.

**Pharmacopoeias.** In *Eur.* (see p.vi), *Int.*, and *US.*

**Ph. Eur. 5.0** (Iohexol). A white or greyish-white, hygroscopic powder. Very soluble in water; practically insoluble in dichloromethane; freely soluble in methyl alcohol. Store in airtight containers. Protect from light.

**USP 27** (Iohexol). A white to off-white, hygroscopic, odourless powder. Very soluble in water and in methyl alcohol; practically insoluble or insoluble in chloroform and in ether. Store at a temperature of 25°, excursions permitted between 15° and 30°. Protect from light.

### Adverse Effects and Precautions

See under the amidotrizoates, p.1060.

Additional neurological adverse effects may occur when iodinated nonionic contrast media such as iohexol are used for myelography. These include severe headache, backache, neck stiffness, dizziness, and leg or sciatic-type pain. Convulsions, aseptic meningitis, and mild and transitory perceptual aberrations, such as visual and speech disturbances, and confusion, may occur occasionally; rarely, more severe mental disturbances have occurred. Urinary retention has also been reported.

**Breast feeding.** No adverse effects have been observed in breast-feeding infants whose mothers were receiving iohexol and the American Academy of Pediatrics considers[1] that it is therefore usually compatible with breast feeding.

1. American Academy of Pediatrics. The transfer of drugs and other chemicals into human milk. *Pediatrics* 2001; **108:** 776–89. Correction. *ibid.*; 1029. Also available at: http://aappolicy.aappublications.org/cgi/content/full/pediatrics%3b108/3/776 (accessed 05/07/04)

**Effects on the nervous system.** Encephalopathy developed in a 48-year-old man with sciatica within 9 hours of iohexol for lumbar myelography but had largely resolved 48 hours after the myelogram; complete resolution took 4 days.[1] However, recovery was slow in a patient who developed paraplegia and areflexia in the legs after a similar procedure. Five months later the patient still complained of paraesthesia in her legs and could not stand without support.[2]

1. Donaghy M, *et al.* Encephalopathy after iohexol myelography. *Lancet* 1985; **ii:** 887.
2. Noda K, *et al.* Prolonged paraplegia after iohexol myelography. *Lancet* 1991; **337:** 681.

### Pharmacokinetics

Following intravascular use, 90% or more of iohexol is eliminated unchanged in the urine within 24 hours. An elimination half-life of approximately 2 hours in patients with normal renal function has been reported. Protein binding in blood is reported to be very low.

**Pregnancy.** Contrast material was detected[1] in the intestines of twin neonates who were born 17 hours after iohexol was given to their mother for angiography, suggesting that transplacental transfer had taken place.

1. Moon AJ, *et al.* Transplacental passage of iohexol. *J Pediatr* 2000; **136:** 548–9.

### Uses and Administration

Iohexol is an iodinated nonionic monomeric contrast medium that is used by injection and locally for a wide range of diagnostic procedures including myelography, angiography, urography, arthrography, and visualisation of the gastrointestinal tract and body cavities (p.1059). Iohexol is also used to produce contrast enhancement during computed tomography.

Iohexol is usually available as solutions containing 30.2 to 75.5% of iohexol (equivalent to 140 to 350 mg/mL of iodine) and the dose and strength used vary according to the procedure and the route of administration.

### Preparations

***USP 27:*** Iohexol Injection.

**Proprietary Preparations** (details are given in Part 3)
***Arg.:*** Omnipaque; ***Austral.:*** Omnipaque; ***Austria:*** Accupaque; Omnipaque; ***Belg.:*** Omnipaque†; ***Braz.:*** Omnipaque; ***Canad.:*** Omnipaque; ***Chile:*** Omnipaque; ***Denm.:*** Omnipaque; ***Fin.:*** Omnipaque; ***Fr.:*** Omnipaque; ***Ger.:*** Accupaque; Omnipaque; ***Gr.:*** Omnipaque; ***India:*** Radiopaque; ***Israel:*** Omnipaque; ***Ital.:*** Omnipaque; ***Norw.:*** Omnipaque; ***NZ:*** Omnipaque; ***Spain:*** Omnigraf; Omnipaque; Omnitrast; ***Swed.:*** Omnipaque; ***Switz.:*** Accupaque; Omnipaque; ***UK:*** Omnipaque; ***USA:*** Omnipaque.

---

## Iomeprol *(BAN, USAN, rINN)*

*N,N′*-Bis(2,3-dihydroxypropyl)-2,4,6-triiodo-5-(*N*-methylglycolamido)-isophthalamide.
$C_{17}H_{22}I_3N_3O_8$ = 777.1.
*CAS — 78649-41-9.*
*ATC — V08AB10.*

**Description.** Iomeprol contains about 49% of I.

### Profile

Iomeprol is an iodinated nonionic monomeric contrast medium that is used for a wide range of radiographic procedures (p.1059) including myelography, angiography, urography, and arthrography. It is also used to produce contrast enhancement during computed tomography.

Iomeprol is usually available as solutions containing 30.62 to 81.65% of iomeprol (equivalent to 150 to 400 mg/mL of iodine) and the dose and strength used vary according to the procedure and the route of administration.

◊ Reviews.

1. Dooley M, Jarvis B. Iomeprol: a review of its use as a contrast medium. *Drugs* 2000; **59:** 1169–86.

### Preparations

**Proprietary Preparations** (details are given in Part 3)
***Austral.:*** Iomeron; ***Austria:*** Iomeron; ***Belg.:*** Iomeron; ***Denm.:*** Iomeron; ***Fin.:*** Iomeron; ***Fr.:*** Iomeron; ***Ger.:*** Imeron; ***Gr.:*** Iomeron; ***Irl.:*** Iomeron; ***Israel:*** Iomeron; ***Ital.:*** Iomeron; ***Jpn:*** Iomeron; ***Neth.:*** Iomeron; ***Norw.:*** Iomeron; ***NZ:*** Iomeron; ***Port.:*** Iomeron; ***Spain:*** Iomeron; ***Swed.:*** Iomeron; ***Switz.:*** Iomeron; ***UK:*** Iomeron.

---

## Iopamidol *(BAN, USAN, rINN)*

B-15000; Iopamidolum; SQ-13396. (*S*)-*N,N′*-Bis[2-hydroxy-1-(hydroxymethyl)ethyl]-2,4,6-tri-iodo-5-lactamidoisophthalamide.
$C_{17}H_{22}I_3N_3O_8$ = 777.1.
*CAS — 60166-93-0; 62883-00-5.*
*ATC — V08AB04.*

**Description.** Iopamidol contains about 49% of I.

**Pharmacopoeias.** In *Eur.* (see p.vi), *Jpn*, and *US.*

**Ph. Eur. 5.0** (Iopamidol). A white or almost white powder. Freely soluble in water; practically insoluble in alcohol and in dichloromethane; very slightly soluble in methyl alcohol. Protect from light.

**USP 27** (Iopamidol). A white to off-white, practically odourless, powder. Very soluble in water; practically insoluble in alcohol and in chloroform; sparingly soluble in methyl alcohol. Store at a temperature of 25°, excursions permitted between 15° and 30°. Protect from light.

### Adverse Effects and Precautions

As for the amidotrizoates, p.1060. For the adverse effects relating to the use of nonionic contrast media such as iopamidol for myelography, see under Iohexol, p.1064; specific references are given below.

**Effects on the nervous system.** Reports of serious neurological sequelae to lumbar myelography with iopamidol.

1. Wallers K, *et al.* Severe meningeal irritation after intrathecal injection of iopamidol. *BMJ* 1985; **291:** 1688.
2. Robinson C, Fon G. Adverse reaction to iopamidol. *Med J Aust* 1986; **144:** 553.
3. Bell JA, McIlwaine GG. Postmyelographic lateral rectus palsy associated with iopamidol. *BMJ* 1990; **300:** 1343–4.
4. Mallat Z, *et al.* Aseptic meningoencephalitis after iopamidol myelography. *Lancet* 1991; **338:** 252.
5. Bain PG, *et al.* Paraplegia after iopamidol myelography. *Lancet* 1991; **338:** 252–3.

### Uses and Administration

Iopamidol is an iodinated nonionic monomeric contrast medium used by injection for a variety of radiographic procedures including angiography, arthrography, myelography, and urography (p.1059). Iopamidol is also used for contrast enhancement during computed tomography.

Iopamidol is usually available as solutions containing 26.1 to 75.5% of iopamidol (equivalent to 128 to 370 mg/mL of iodine) and the dose and strength used vary according to the procedure and route of administration.

Iopamidol has also been given orally or by enema for visualisation of the gastrointestinal tract.

### Preparations

***USP 27:*** Iopamidol Injection.

**Proprietary Preparations** (details are given in Part 3)
***Arg.:*** Hemoray; Iopamiron; ***Austral.:*** Isovue; ***Austria:*** Gastromiro; Jopamiro; Scanlux; ***Braz.:*** Iopamiron†; ***Canad.:*** Isovue†; ***Chile:*** Radiomiron; ***Denm.:*** Iopamiro; ***Fin.:*** Iopamiro†; ***Fr.:*** Iopamiron; ***Ger.:*** Solutrast; Unilux; ***Gr.:*** Iopamiro 200, 300, and 370; ***Irl.:*** Gastromiro; Niopam; ***Israel:*** Gastromiro; Iopamiro; ***Ital.:*** Gastromiro; Iopamiro; ***Norw.:*** Iopamiro; ***NZ:*** Iopamiro; ***Port.:*** Gastromiro; Iopamiro; ***Spain:*** Iopamiro; ***Swed.:*** Iopamiro; ***Switz.:*** Iopamiro; ***UK:*** Gastromiro; Niopam; Scanlux; ***USA:*** Isovue.

---

## Iopanoic Acid *(BAN, rINN)*

Ácido iopanoico; Acidum Iopanoicum; Iodopanoic Acid. 2-(3-Amino-2,4,6-tri-iodobenzyl)butyric acid.

$C_{11}H_{12}I_3NO_2$ = 570.9.
*CAS — 96-83-3.*
*ATC — V08AC06.*

**Description.** Iopanoic acid contains about 66.7% of I.

**Pharmacopoeias.** In *Chin., Eur.* (see p.vi), *Int.*, and *US.*

**Ph. Eur. 5.0** (Iopanoic Acid). A white or yellowish-white powder. Practically insoluble in water; soluble in dehydrated alcohol and in methyl alcohol; dissolves in dilute solutions of alkali hydroxides. Protect from light.

**USP 27** (Iopanoic Acid). A cream-coloured powder, with a faint characteristic odour. Insoluble in water; soluble in alcohol, in chloroform, in ether, and in solutions of alkali hydroxides and carbonates. Store in airtight containers. Protect from light.

### Adverse Effects

Gastrointestinal disturbances such as nausea, vomiting, abdominal cramp, and diarrhoea are reported to occur in up to 40% of patients but are usually mild and transient. Mild stinging or burning on micturition, and skin rashes and flushing have occurred occasionally. Acute renal failure, thrombocytopenia, and hypersensitivity reactions have been reported.

Iopanoic acid has potent uricosuric and anticholinesterase effects.

### Precautions

Iopanoic acid is contra-indicated in severe hepatic or renal disease; doses higher than 3 g should not be given to patients with renal impairment. It should not be used in the presence of acute gastrointestinal disorders that may impair absorption. It should be used with caution in patients with a history of hypersensitivity to iodine or to other contrast media, severe hyperthyroidism, hyperuricaemia, or cholangitis. Because of its cholinergic action, premedication with atropine has been suggested in some countries for patients with coronary heart disease. Iodine-containing contrast media may interfere with thyroid-function tests and with some blood and urine tests.

**Breast feeding.** No adverse effects have been observed in breast-feeding infants whose mothers were receiving iopanoic acid and the American Academy of Pediatrics considers[1] that it is therefore usually compatible with breast feeding.

1. American Academy of Pediatrics. The transfer of drugs and other chemicals into human milk. *Pediatrics* 2001; **108:** 776–89. Correction. *ibid.*; 1029. Also available at: http://aappolicy.aappublications.org/cgi/content/full/pediatrics%3b108/3/776 (accessed 05/07/04)

### Pharmacokinetics

Iopanoic acid is variably absorbed from the gastrointestinal tract and is strongly and extensively bound to plasma proteins. It is conjugated in the liver to the glucuronide and excreted largely in the bile and the remainder (about one-third of the dose) in the urine. It appears in the gallbladder about 4 hours after a dose is taken and maximum concentrations occur after about 17 hours. About 50% of a dose is excreted in 24 hours, but elevated protein-bound iodine concentrations may persist for several months.

### Uses and Administration

Iopanoic acid is an iodinated ionic monomeric contrast medium used for cholecystography and cholangiography (p.1059). Usual doses of 3 g are given by mouth with plenty of water about 10 to 14 hours before X-ray examination. For repeat examinations an additional 3 g may be given on the same day. Alternatively, repeat examination may be carried out after an interval of 5 to 7 days with a single 6 g dose. No more than 6 g of iopanoic acid should be taken during any 24-hour period, and doses over 3 g should be avoided in renal impairment. Adequate visualisation is achieved in the majority of patients with a single dose.

### Preparations

***BP 2003:*** Iopanoic Acid Tablets;
***USP 27:*** Iopanoic Acid Tablets.

**Proprietary Preparations** (details are given in Part 3)
***Arg.:*** Colesom; ***Austral.:*** Telepaque†; ***Braz.:*** Telepaque†; ***Canad.:*** Telepaque†; ***Ital.:*** Cistobil; ***Spain:*** Colegraf; Neocontrast†; ***Switz.:*** Cistobil†; ***USA:*** Telepaque.

## Iopentol *(BAN, USAN, rINN)*

Compound 5411. *N,N'*-Bis(2,3-dihydroxypropyl)-5-[*N*-(2-hydroxy-3-methoxypropyl)acetamido]-2,4,6-tri-iodoisophthalamide.

$C_{20}H_{28}I_3N_3O_9$ = 835.2.
*CAS — 89797-00-2.*
*ATC — V08AB08.*

**Description.** Iopentol contains about 45.6% of I.

### Profile

Iopentol is an iodinated nonionic monomeric contrast medium that is used for a variety of radiographic procedures including enhancement of computed tomography (p.1059).

### Preparations

**Proprietary Preparations** (details are given in Part 3)
***Austria:*** Imagopaque; ***Fin.:*** Imagopaque†; ***Fr.:*** Ivepaque; ***Ger.:*** Imagopaque; ***Gr.:*** Imagopaque; ***Ital.:*** Imagopaque; ***Norw.:*** Imagopaque†; ***Spain:*** Imagopaque; ***Switz.:*** Imagopaque.

## Iopodic Acid *(BANM, rINNM)*

Iopódico, ácido; Ipodic Acid. 3-(3-Dimethylaminomethyleneamino-2,4,6-tri-iodophenyl)propionic acid.

$C_{12}H_{13}I_3N_2O_2$ = 598.0.
*CAS — 5587-89-3.*
*ATC — V08AC08; V08AC10.*

## Calcium Iopodate *(BANM, rINNM)*

Calcium Ipodate; Iopodato cálcico; Ipodate Calcium. Calcium 3-(3-dimethylaminomethyleneamino-2,4,6-tri-iodophenyl)propionate.

$(C_{12}H_{12}I_3N_2O_2)_2Ca$ = 1234.0.
*CAS — 1151-11-7.*
*ATC — V08AC10.*

**Description.** Calcium iopodate contains about 61.7% of I.

## Sodium Iopodate *(BAN, rINN)*

Iopodato de sodio; Ipodate Sodium *(USAN)*; NSC-106962; Sodium Ipodate. Sodium 3-(3-dimethylaminomethyleneamino-2,4,6-tri-iodophenyl)propionate.

$C_{12}H_{12}I_3N_2NaO_2$ = 619.9.
*CAS — 1221-56-3.*
*ATC — V08AC08.*

**Description.** Sodium iopodate contains about 61.4% of I.

**Pharmacopoeias.** In *US.*

**USP 27** (Ipodate Sodium). A fine, white or off-white, odourless, crystalline powder. Soluble 1 in less than 1 of water, 1 in 2 of alcohol, 1 in 2 of dimethylacetamide, and 1 in 3.5 of dimethylformamide and of dimethyl sulfoxide; very slightly soluble in chloroform; freely soluble in methyl alcohol. Store in airtight containers.

### Adverse Effects and Precautions

As for Iopanoic Acid, above. Effects on the gastrointestinal tract may be less with iopodate salts than with iopanoic acid.

### Pharmacokinetics

The iopodate salts are absorbed from the gastrointestinal tract following oral or rectal administration, and almost completely metabolised. Protein binding to plasma proteins is reported to be high. Elimination is by the renal and hepatic routes; about half of an oral dose is stated to be excreted in the urine within 24 hours.

### Uses and Administration

Iopodic acid is an iodinated ionic monomeric contrast medium given by mouth as the sodium salt for cholecystography and cholangiography (p.1059). Following administration, optimal visualisation of the bile ducts usually occurs after 1 to 3 hours and that of the gallbladder after 10 to 12 hours.

For routine cholecystography sodium iopodate is given by mouth in a dose of 3 g in the evening, 10 to 12 hours before the examination; in fractionated oral cholecystography this may be followed by a second similar dose the following day, 3 hours before examination. In rapid cholecystography a single dose of 3 or 6 g may be given.

For cholangiography, a single dose of 6 g may be given.

The calcium salt has been used similarly.

### Preparations

***USP 27:*** Ipodate Sodium Capsules.

**Proprietary Preparations** (details are given in Part 3)
***Austria:*** Biloptin†; ***Ger.:*** Biloptin†; ***Port.:*** Biloptin†; ***S.Afr.:*** Biloptin†; ***Switz.:*** Biloptin†; ***UK:*** Biloptin; Solu-Biloptin; ***USA:*** Oragrafin†.

## Iopromide *(BAN, USAN, rINN)*

Iopromida; ZK-35760. *N,N'*-Bis(2,3-dihydroxypropyl)-2,4,6-tri-iodo-5-(2-methoxyacetamido)-*N*-methylisophthalamide.

$C_{18}H_{24}I_3N_3O_8$ = 791.1.
*CAS — 73334-07-3.*
*ATC — V08AB05.*

**Description.** Iopromide contains about 48.1% of I.

**Pharmacopoeias.** In *US.*

**USP 27** (Iopromide). A white to slightly yellow powder. Freely soluble in water and in dimethyl sulfoxide; practically insoluble in alcohol, in acetone, and in ether. Protect from light.

### Adverse Effects and Precautions

See under the amidotrizoates, p.1060.

### Uses and Administration

Iopromide is an iodinated nonionic monomeric contrast medium that is used for angiography, urography, arthrography, and the visualisation of body cavities (p.1059). It is also used for contrast enhancement during computed tomography, and to check functioning of a dialysis shunt.

Iopromide is given locally and by injection. It is usually available as solutions containing 31.2 to 76.9% of iopromide (equivalent to 150 to 370 mg/mL of iodine) and the dose and strength used vary according to the procedure and route of administration.

### Preparations

***USP 27:*** Iopromide Injection.

**Proprietary Preparations** (details are given in Part 3)
***Arg.:*** Clarograf; ***Austral.:*** Ultravist; ***Austria:*** Ultravist; ***Belg.:*** Ultravist; ***Canad.:*** Ultravist; ***Denm.:*** Ultravist; ***Fin.:*** Ultravist; ***Fr.:*** Ultravist; ***Ger.:*** Ultravist; ***Gr.:*** Ultravist; ***Israel:*** Ultravist; ***Ital.:*** Ultravist; ***Jpn:*** Proscope; ***Neth.:*** Ultravist; ***Norw.:*** Ultravist; ***NZ:*** Ultravist; ***Port.:*** Ultravist; ***S.Afr.:*** Ultravist; ***Spain:*** Clarograf; Ultravist; ***Swed.:*** Ultravist; ***Switz.:*** Ultravist; ***UK:*** Ultravist; ***USA:*** Ultravist.

## Iopydol *(BAN, USAN)*

Iopidol. 1-(2,3-Dihydroxypropyl)-3,5-di-iodo-4-pyridone.

$C_8H_9I_2NO_3$ = 421.0.
*CAS — 5579-92-0.*
*ATC — V08AD02.*

**Description.** Iopydol contains about 60.3% of I.

### Profile

Iopydol is an iodinated contrast medium that has been used with iopydone for bronchography (p.1059).

### Preparations

**Proprietary Preparations** (details are given in Part 3)
**Multi-ingredient:** ***Braz.:*** Hytrast†.

## Iopydone *(BAN, USAN)*

Iopidona. 3,5-Di-iodo-4-pyridone.

$C_5H_3I_2NO$ = 346.9.
*CAS — 5579-93-1.*

**Description.** Iopydone contains about 73.2% of I.

### Profile

Iopydone is an iodinated contrast medium that has been used with iopydol for bronchography (p.1059).

### Preparations

**Proprietary Preparations** (details are given in Part 3)
**Multi-ingredient:** ***Braz.:*** Hytrast†.

## Iotalamic Acid *(BAN, rINN)*

Ácido iotalámico; Iothalamic Acid *(USAN)*; Methalamic Acid; MI-216. 5-Acetamido-2,4,6-tri-iodo-*N*-methylisophthalamic acid.

$C_{11}H_9I_3N_2O_4$ = 613.9.
*CAS — 2276-90-6.*
*ATC — V08AA04.*

**Description.** Iotalamic acid contains about 62% of I.

**Pharmacopoeias.** In *Chin., Eur.* (see p.vi), *Jpn*, and *US.*

**Ph. Eur. 5.0** (Iotalamic Acid). A white or almost white powder. Slightly soluble in water and in alcohol; dissolves in dilute solutions of alkali hydroxides. Protect from light.

**USP 27** (Iothalamic Acid). A white, odourless, powder. Slightly soluble in water and in alcohol; soluble in solutions of alkali hydroxides. Store at a temperature of 25°, excursions permitted between 15° and 30°.

## Meglumine Iotalamate *(BANM, rINNM)*

Iotalamato de meglumina; Iothalamate Meglumine; Meglumine Iothalamate. The *N*-methylglucamine salt of iotalamic acid.

$C_{11}H_9I_3N_2O_4,C_7H_{17}NO_5$ = 809.1.
*CAS — 13087-53-1.*
*ATC — V08AA04.*

**Description.** Meglumine iotalamate contains about 47.1% of I.

**Pharmacopoeias.** *US* includes only as various injections.

## Sodium Iotalamate *(BANM, rINNM)*

Iotalamato de sodio; Iothalamate Sodium; Sodium Iothalamate.

$C_{11}H_8I_3N_2NaO_4$ = 635.9.
*CAS — 17692-74-9; 1225-20-3.*
*ATC — V08AA04.*

**Description.** Sodium iotalamate contains about 59.9% of I.

**Pharmacopoeias.** *US* includes only as various injections.

### Adverse Effects, Treatment, and Precautions

As for the amidotrizoates, p.1060.

**Incidence of adverse effects.** In 40 patients who underwent phlebography with 60% meglumine iotalamate minor adverse reactions were common despite the use of saline flushing and muscle contraction to clear the veins after examination.[1] The commonest effect was pain at the site of injection, or in the calf and foot; 15 patients of those who had pain in the calf or foot were found to have venous thrombosis. Serious complications to phlebography appear to be rare but can cause serious morbidity; examination of 200 case notes and a retrospective study involving 3060 patients revealed 4 cases of necrosis in the skin of the foot and gangrene of the foot in 2.

1. Thomas ML, MacDonald LM. Complications of ascending phlebography of the leg. *BMJ* 1978; **ii:** 317–18.

### Pharmacokinetics

Following intravascular use the iotalamates are rapidly distributed; suitable concentrations for urography reach the urinary tract within 3 to 8 minutes of a bolus intravenous injection. Protein binding of both the sodium and meglumine salts is reported to be low. The iotalamates are eliminated by the kidneys. In patients with normal renal function more than 90% of the dose injected is excreted in urine within 24 hours. Small amounts are reported to be excreted via the bile in the faeces. The iotalamates are removed by peritoneal dialysis and haemodialysis.

### Uses and Administration

Iotalamic acid is an iodinated ionic monomeric contrast medium with actions similar to the amidotrizoates (p.1061). It is given locally and by injection for a wide range of radiographic procedures, including angiography, arthrography, cholangiography, urography, and for contrast enhancement during computed tomography (p.1059); oral or rectal administration has been used to visualise the gastrointestinal tract.

Iotalamic acid is usually available as solutions containing up to 80% of sodium iotalamate or up to 60% of meglumine iotalamate. The dose and strength used vary according to the procedure and route of administration. A mixture of the two salts is often preferred to minimise adverse effects.

Iotalamates are not suitable for injection into the subarachnoid space.

### Preparations

***USP 27:*** Iothalamate Meglumine and Iothalamate Sodium Injection; Iothalamate Meglumine Injection; Iothalamate Sodium Injection.

**Proprietary Preparations** (details are given in Part 3)
***Arg.:*** Conray; Cysto-Conray; ***Austral.:*** Conray 280; Conray 420†; ***Braz.:*** Conray†; Vascoray†; ***Canad.:*** Conray; Cysto-Conray; ***Ger.:*** Conray 30; Conray 60; Conray 70†; Conray FL†; ***Ital.:*** Angio-Conray†; Conray; ***UK:*** Conray; ***USA:*** Conray; Cysto-Conray; Vascoray†.

## Iotrolan *(BAN, USAN, rINN)*

Iotrol; Iotrolán; Iotrolum; ZK-39482. *N,N',N'',N'''*-Tetrakis(2,3-dihydroxy-1-hydroxymethylpropyl)-2,2',4,4',6,6'-hexaiodo-5,5'-(*N,N'*-dimethylmalonyldi-imino)di-isophthalamide.
$C_{37}H_{48}I_6N_6O_{18}$ = 1626.2.
*CAS — 79770-24-4.*
*ATC — V08AB06.*

**Description.** Iotrolan contains about 46.8% of I.

### Adverse Effects and Precautions

As for the amidotrizoates, p.1060. For the adverse effects relating to the use of nonionic contrast media such as iotrolan for myelography, see under Iohexol, p.1064.

### Uses and Administration

Iotrolan is an iodinated nonionic dimeric contrast medium that is given locally or by injection for a wide range of diagnostic procedures, including myelography, lymphography, arthrography, hysterosalpingography, cholangiopancreatography, and for visualisation of the mammary ducts and the gastrointestinal tract (p.1059). It is also used for contrast enhancement during computed tomography.

Iotrolan is usually available as solutions containing 51.3% or 64.1% of iotrolan (equivalent to 240 mg/mL or 300 mg/mL of iodine, respectively) and the dose and strength used vary according to the procedure and route of administration.

### Preparations

**Proprietary Preparations** (details are given in Part 3)
***Austral.:*** Isovist; ***Austria:*** Isovist; ***Canad.:*** Osmovist; ***Denm.:*** Isovist; ***Fin.:*** Isovist; ***Ger.:*** Isovist; ***Ital.:*** Isovist†; ***Neth.:*** Isovist; ***Norw.:*** Isovist†; ***NZ:*** Isovist; ***Port.:*** Iotrovist†; ***S.Afr.:*** Isovist; ***Swed.:*** Isovist†; ***Switz.:*** Isovist; ***UK:*** Isovist.

## Iotroxic Acid *(BAN, USAN, rINN)*

Ácido iotróxico; SH-213AB. 3,3'-(3,6,9-Trioxaundecanedioyldi-imino)bis(2,4,6-tri-iodobenzoic acid).
$C_{22}H_{18}I_6N_2O_9$ = 1215.8.
*CAS — 51022-74-3.*
*ATC — V08AC02.*

**Description.** Iotroxic acid contains about 62.6% of I.

**Pharmacopoeias.** In *Int.* and *Jpn.*

## Meglumine Iotroxate *(BANM, rINNM)*

Dimeglumine Iotroxate; Iotroxate Meglumine; Iotroxato de meglumina; Meglumine Iotroxinate. The di(*N*-methylglucamine)salt of iotroxic acid.
$C_{22}H_{18}I_6N_2O_9,2C_7H_{17}NO_5$ = 1606.2.
*CAS — 68890-05-1.*
*ATC — V08AC02.*

**Description.** Meglumine iotroxate contains about 47.4% of I.

### Adverse Effects, Treatment, and Precautions

See under the amidotrizoates, p.1060.

### Uses and Administration

Iotroxic acid is an iodinated ionic dimeric contrast medium that is used intravenously as the meglumine salt for cholecystography and cholangiography (p.1059).

Meglumine iotroxate is given by intravenous infusion in a dose equivalent to about 5 g of iodine usually as a 10.5% solution. The infusion should be administered over not less than 15 minutes.

### Preparations

**Proprietary Preparations** (details are given in Part 3)
***Austral.:*** Biliscopin; ***Austria:*** Biliscopin; ***Braz.:*** Biliscopin†; ***Ger.:*** Biliscopin; ***NZ:*** Biliscopin; ***Spain:*** Bilisegrol; ***Swed.:*** Biliscopin; ***Switz.:*** Biliscopin; ***UK:*** Biliscopin.

## Ioversol *(BAN, USAN, rINN)*

MP-328. *N,N'*-Bis(2,3-dihydroxypropyl)-5-[*N*-(2-hydroxyethyl)-glycolamido]-2,4,6-tri-iodoisophthalamide.
$C_{18}H_{24}I_3N_3O_9$ = 807.1.
*CAS — 87771-40-2.*
*ATC — V08AB07.*

**Description.** Ioversol contains about 47.2% of I.

**Pharmacopoeias.** In *US.*

**USP 27** (Ioversol). Store at a temperature of 25°, excursions permitted between 15° and 30°.

### Adverse Effects, Treatment, and Precautions

See under the amidotrizoates, p.1060.

### Uses and Administration

Ioversol is an iodinated nonionic monomeric contrast medium that is used by injection in angiography and urography (p.1059). It is also used for contrast enhancement during computed tomography. It is usually available as a solution containing 34 to 74% (equivalent to 160 to 350 mg/mL of iodine). The dose and strength used vary according to the procedure and route of administration.

### Preparations

***USP 27:*** Ioversol Injection.

**Proprietary Preparations** (details are given in Part 3)
***Arg.:*** Optiray; ***Austral.:*** Optiray; ***Austria:*** Optiray; ***Belg.:*** Optiject; Optiray; ***Braz.:*** Optiray†; ***Canad.:*** Optiray; ***Denm.:*** Optiray; ***Fin.:*** Optiray; ***Fr.:*** Optiject; Optiray; ***Ger.:*** Optiray; ***Israel:*** Optiray; ***Ital.:*** Optiray; ***Port.:*** Optiray; ***Spain:*** Optiray; ***Swed.:*** Optiray; ***Switz.:*** Optiray; ***USA:*** Optiray.

## Ioxaglic Acid *(BAN, USAN, rINN)*

Ácido ioxáglico; Acidum Ioxaglicum; P-286. *N*-(2-Hydroxyethyl)-2,4,6-tri-iodo-5-[2',4',6'-tri-iodo-3'-(*N*-methylacetamido)-5'-methylcarbamoylhippuramido]isophthalamic acid.
$C_{24}H_{21}I_6N_5O_8$ = 1268.9.
*CAS — 59017-64-0.*
*ATC — V08AB03.*

**Description.** Ioxaglic acid contains about 60% of I.

**Pharmacopoeias.** In *Eur.* (see p.vi) and *US.*

**Ph. Eur. 5.0** (Ioxaglic Acid). A white or almost white hygroscopic powder. Very slightly soluble in water and in dichloromethane; slightly soluble in alcohol. It dissolves in dilute solutions of alkali hydroxides. Store in airtight containers. Protect from light.

**USP 27** (Ioxaglic Acid). Store at a temperature of 25°, excursions permitted between 15° and 30°.

## Meglumine Ioxaglate *(BANM, rINNM)*

Ioxaglate Meglumine *(USAN)*; Ioxaglato de meglumina; MP-302 (with sodium ioxaglate). The *N*-methylglucamine salt of ioxaglic acid.
$C_{24}H_{21}I_6N_5O_8,C_7H_{17}NO_5$ = 1464.1.
*CAS — 59018-13-2.*
*ATC — V08AB03.*

**Description.** Meglumine ioxaglate contains about 52% of I.

## Sodium Ioxaglate *(BANM, rINNM)*

Ioxaglate Sodium *(USAN)*; Ioxaglato sódico; MP-302 (with meglumine ioxaglate).
$C_{24}H_{20}I_6N_5NaO_8$ = 1290.9.
*CAS — 67992-58-9.*
*ATC — V08AB03.*

**Description.** Sodium ioxaglate contains about 59% of I.

### Adverse Effects, Treatment, and Precautions

See under the amidotrizoates, p.1060.

### Pharmacokinetics

Following intravascular use, ioxaglates are rapidly distributed throughout the extracellular fluid. Protein binding is reported to be very low. About 90% of a dose is excreted unchanged in the urine within 24 hours. An elimination half-life of about 90 minutes has been reported, which may be prolonged in renal impairment. Ioxaglates cross the placenta and are distributed into breast milk. They are removed by haemodialysis and peritoneal dialysis.

### Uses and Administration

Ioxaglic acid is an iodinated ionic dimeric contrast medium that is given locally and by injection as a combined solution of its meglumine and sodium salts for a wide range of diagnostic procedures, including angiography, arthrography, hysterosalpingography, and urography (p.1059). It is also used for contrast enhancement during computed tomography.

The dose and strength used depend upon the procedure and route of administration. Commonly used solutions contain 39.3% of meglumine ioxaglate and 19.6% of sodium ioxaglate (equivalent to 320 mg/mL of iodine) or 24.6% of meglumine ioxaglate and 12.3% of sodium ioxaglate (equivalent to 200 mg/mL of iodine).

Ioxaglate is unsuitable for myelography and should not be given by the subarachnoid or epidural routes.

### Preparations

***USP 27:*** Ioxaglate Meglumine and Ioxaglate Sodium Injection.

**Proprietary Preparations** (details are given in Part 3)
***Arg.:*** Hexabrix; ***Austral.:*** Hexabrix; ***Austria:*** Hexabrix; ***Belg.:*** Hexabrix; ***Braz.:*** Hexabrix; ***Canad.:*** Hexabrix; ***Chile:*** Hexabrix; ***Denm.:*** Hexabrix; ***Fin.:*** Hexabrix; ***Fr.:*** Hexabrix; ***Ger.:*** Hexabrix; ***Gr.:*** Hexabrix; ***Israel:*** Hexabrix; ***Ital.:*** Hexabrix; ***Neth.:*** Hexabrix†; ***Norw.:*** Hexabrix; ***NZ:*** Hexabrix; ***Port.:*** Hexabrix; ***Spain:*** Hexabrix; ***Swed.:*** Hexabrix; ***Switz.:*** Hexabrix; ***UK:*** Hexabrix; ***USA:*** Hexabrix.

## Ioxilan *(USAN, rINN)*

Ioxilán. *N*-(2,3-Dihydroxypropyl)-5-[*N*-(2,3-dihydroxypropyl)-acetamido]-*N'*-(2-hydroxyethyl)-2,4,6-triidoisophthalamide.
$C_{18}H_{24}I_3N_3O_8$ = 791.1.
*CAS — 107793-72-6.*
*ATC — V08AB12.*

**Description.** Ioxilan contains about 48.1% of I.

**Pharmacopoeias.** In *US.*

**USP 27** (Ioxilan). A white to off-white, practically odourless, powder. Soluble in water and in methyl alcohol. pH of a 10% solution in water is between 5.0 and 7.5. Store at a temperature of 25°, excursions permitted between 15° and 30°. Protect from light.

### Profile

Ioxilan is an iodinated nonionic monomeric contrast medium used for various radiographic procedures including enhancement of computed tomography (p.1059). It is given by injection.

### Preparations

***USP 27:*** Ioxilan Injection.

**Proprietary Preparations** (details are given in Part 3)
***Braz.:*** Oxilan†.

## Ioxitalamic Acid *(rINN)*

Ácido ioxitalámico; AG-58107; Ioxithalamic Acid. 5-Acetamido-*N*-(2-hydroxyethyl)-2,4,6-tri-iodoisophthalamic acid.
$C_{12}H_{11}I_3N_2O_5$ = 643.9.
*CAS — 28179-44-4.*
*ATC — V08AA05.*

**Description.** Ioxitalamic acid contains about 59.1% of I.

**Pharmacopoeias.** In *Fr.*

## Meglumine Ioxitalamate *(rINNM)*

Ioxitalamate Meglumine; Ioxitalamato de meglumina. The *N*-methylglucamine salt of ioxitalamic acid.
$C_{12}H_{11}I_3N_2O_5,C_7H_{17}NO_5$ = 839.2.
*CAS — 29288-99-1.*
*ATC — V08AA05.*

**Description.** Meglumine ioxitalamate contains about 45.4% of I.

## Sodium Ioxitalamate *(rINNM)*

Ioxitalamate Sodium; Ioxitalamato sódico.
$C_{12}H_{10}I_3N_2NaO_5$ = 665.9.
*CAS — 33954-26-6.*
*ATC — V08AA05.*

**Description.** Sodium ioxitalamate contains about 57.2% of I.

### Profile

Ioxitalamic acid is an iodinated ionic monomeric contrast medium with actions similar to those of the amidotrizoates (p.1060). It is used as its meglumine and sodium salts locally and by injection for a wide range of diagnostic procedures, including angiography, cholangiography, hysterosalpingography, and urography (p.1059). It may be given by mouth or rectally for visualisation of the gastrointestinal tract. It is also used for contrast enhancement during computed tomography.

Monoethanolamine ioxitalamate has also been used.

### Preparations

**Proprietary Preparations** (details are given in Part 3)
***Arg.:*** Telebrix 38; Telebrix Coronario; Telebrix Hystero; ***Belg.:*** Telebrix; Telebrix Gastro; Telebrix Hystero; ***Braz.:*** Telebrix 30†; Telebrix 35; Telebrix 38†; Telebrix Coronar†; Telebrix Hystero; Telebrix TC†; Vasobrix†; Vasurix Polividona†; ***Canad.:*** Telebrix; ***Chile:*** Telebrix 30; Telebrix 35; ***Denm.:*** Telebrix†; ***Fr.:*** Telebrix 12; Telebrix 30; Telebrix 35; Telebrix Gastro; Telebrix Hystero; ***Ger.:*** Telebrix Gastro; Telebrix N 180 and 300; ***Gr.:*** Telebrix Gastro; Telebrix Hystero; ***Israel:*** Telebrix; Telebrix Gastro; ***Ital.:*** Telebrix 30†; Telebrix 38†; ***Neth.:*** Telebrix 12†; Telebrix 30†; Telebrix 350†; Telebrix Gastro†; Telebrix Polyvidone†; ***Port.:*** Telebrix 12; Telebrix 30; Telebrix 35; Telebrix 350†; Telebrix Gastro; Telebrix Hystero; ***Switz.:*** Telebrix 12; Telebrix 30; Telebrix 35; Telebrix Gastro.

## Mangafodipir Trisodium *(BANM, USAN, rINNM)*

Mangafodipir trisódico; MnDPDP (mangafodipir); S-095 (mangafodipir); Win-59010; Win-59010-2 (mangafodipir). Trisodium trihydrogen (*OC*-6-13)-{[*N,N*'-ethylenebis(*N*-{[3-hydroxy-5-(hydroxymethyl)-2-methyl-4-pyridyl]methyl}glycine) 5,5'-bis(phosphato)](8-)} manganate(6-); Trisodium trihydrogen (*OC*-6-13)-*N,N*'-ethane-1,2-diylbis{N-[2-methyl-3-oxido-κO-5-(phosphonatooxymethyl)-4-pyridylmethyl]glycinato(*O,N*)}manganate(II).

$C_{22}H_{27}MnN_4Na_3O_{14}P_2$ = 757.3.

*CAS — 155319-91-8 (mangafodipir); 140678-14-4 (mangafodipir trisodium).*

*ATC — V08CA05.*

**Pharmacopoeias.** In *US.*

**USP 27** (Mangafodipir Trisodium). Pale yellow crystals or crystalline powder. Freely soluble in water; very slightly soluble in alcohol and in acetone; slightly soluble in chloroform; sparingly soluble in methyl alcohol. pH of a 1% solution in water is between 5.5 and 7.0. Store at a temperature of 25°, excursions permitted between 15° and 30°.

### Profile

Mangafodipir trisodium is a paramagnetic agent used intravenously for contrast enhancement in magnetic resonance imaging (p.1059) of the liver and pancreas.

Mangafodipir trisodium is available as a solution containing 7.57 mg/mL (10 micromol/mL). The usual dose in adults is 0.5 mL/kg (5 micromol/kg) given by intravenous infusion at a rate of 2 to 3 mL/minute for imaging of the liver and 4 to 6 mL/minute for imaging of the pancreas.

### Preparations

***USP 27:*** Mangafodipir Trisodium Injection.

**Proprietary Preparations** (details are given in Part 3)

***Austria:*** Teslascan; ***Belg.:*** Teslascan†; ***Denm.:*** Teslascan; ***Fin.:*** Teslascan; ***Fr.:*** Teslascan; ***Ger.:*** Teslascan; ***Gr.:*** Teslascan; ***Ital.:*** Teslascan; ***Norw.:*** Teslascan; ***NZ:*** Teslascan; ***Spain:*** Teslascan; ***Swed.:*** Teslascan; ***Switz.:*** Teslascan; ***UK:*** Teslascan; ***USA:*** Teslascan.

---

## Metrizamide *(BAN, USAN, rINN)*

Metrizamida; Win-39103. 2-[3-Acetamido-2,4,6-tri-iodo-5-(*N*-methylacetamido)benzamido]-2-deoxy-D-glucose.

$C_{18}H_{22}I_3N_3O_8$ = 789.1.

*CAS — 31112-62-6 (metrizamide); 55134-11-7 (metrizamide, glucopyranose form).*

*ATC — V08AB01.*

**Description.** Metrizamide contains about 48.2% of I.

### Adverse Effects and Precautions

As for the amidotrizoates, p.1060. For the adverse effects relating to the use of nonionic contrast media such as metrizamide for myelography, see under Iohexol, p.1064.

**Breast feeding.** No adverse effects have been observed in breast-feeding infants whose mothers were receiving metrizamide and the American Academy of Pediatrics considers[1] that it is therefore usually compatible with breast feeding.

1. American Academy of Pediatrics. The transfer of drugs and other chemicals into human milk. *Pediatrics* 2001; **108:** 776–89. Correction. *ibid.*; 1029. Also available at: http://aappolicy.aappublications.org/cgi/content/full/pediatrics%3b108/3/776 (accessed 05/07/04)

### Pharmacokinetics

Following intrathecal administration metrizamide diffuses upwards through the CSF and enters the extracellular fluid of the brain. Most of a dose is eliminated from the CSF within several hours. It enters the blood and is eliminated primarily in urine; in patients with normal renal function 60% or more of an intrathecal dose is excreted in urine within 48 hours. Small amounts are excreted in bile. Metrizamide is not significantly bound to plasma proteins. It has been reported to be distributed into breast milk.

### Uses and Administration

Metrizamide is an iodinated nonionic monomeric contrast medium that has been used in myelography, angiography, intravenous urography, and arthrography (p.1059), and also for contrast enhancement during computed tomography.

---

## Metrizoic Acid *(BANM, rINNM)*

Metrizoico, ácido. 3-Acetamido-2,4,6-tri-iodo-5-(*N*-methylacetamido)benzoic acid.

$C_{12}H_{11}I_3N_2O_4$ = 627.9.

*CAS — 1949-45-7.*

*ATC — V08AA02.*

**Description.** Metrizoic acid contains about 60.6% of I.

## Meglumine Metrizoate *(BANM, rINNM)*

Metrizoate Meglumine; Metrizoato de meglumina. The *N*-methylglucamine salt of metrizoic acid.

$C_{12}H_{11}I_3N_2O_4,C_7H_{17}NO_5$ = 823.2.

*CAS — 7241-11-4.*

*ATC — V08AA02.*

**Description.** Meglumine metrizoate contains about 46.3% of I.

## Sodium Metrizoate *(BAN, rINN)*

Metrizoate Sodium *(USAN)*; Metrizoato de sodio; NSC-107431.

$C_{12}H_{10}I_3N_2NaO_4$ = 649.9.

*CAS — 7225-61-8.*

*ATC — V08AA02.*

**Description.** Sodium metrizoate contains about 58.6% of I.

### Profile

Metrizoic acid is an iodinated ionic monomeric contrast medium with actions similar to those of the amidotrizoates (p.1060). It has been used as the meglumine and sodium salts, often together with calcium metrizoate and magnesium metrizoate, for a variety of diagnostic procedures including angiography, cholangiography, and hysterosalpingography (p.1059).

**Breast feeding.** No adverse effects have been observed in breast-feeding infants whose mothers were receiving metrizoate and the American Academy of Pediatrics considers[1] that it is therefore usually compatible with breast feeding.

1. American Academy of Pediatrics. The transfer of drugs and other chemicals into human milk. *Pediatrics* 2001; **108:** 776–89. Correction. *ibid.*; 1029. Also available at: http://aappolicy.aappublications.org/cgi/content/full/pediatrics%3b108/3/776 (accessed 05/07/04)

### Preparations

**Proprietary Preparations** (details are given in Part 3)

***Denm.:*** Isopaque†; ***Norw.:*** Isopaque Cysto†; ***Swed.:*** Isopaque Cysto†; ***UK:*** Isopaque Cysto.

---

## Perflenapent *(USAN, rINN)*

Dodecafluoropentane.

$C_5F_{12}$ = 288.0.

*CAS — 678-26-2.*

*ATC — V08DA03.*

### Profile

Perflenapent is a fluorocarbon ultrasound contrast medium (p.1059) used with perflisopent (below) for echocardiography.

◊ References.

1. Robbin ML, Eisenfeld AJ. Perflenapent emulsion: a US contrast agent for diagnostic radiology—multicenter, double-blind comparison with a placebo. *Radiology* 1998; **207:** 717–22.

---

## Perflexane *(USAN, rINN)*

Tetradecafluorohexane.

$C_6F_{14}$ = 338.0.

*CAS — 355-42-0.*

### Profile

Perflexane is a fluorocarbon ultrasound contrast medium that has been used as lipid-coated microspheres for echocardiography.

### Preparations

**Proprietary Preparations** (details are given in Part 3)

***USA:*** Imagent.

---

## Perflisopent *(USAN, rINN)*

Nonafluoro-2-(trifluoromethyl)butane.

$C_5F_{12}$ = 288.0.

*CAS — 594-91-2.*

### Profile

Perflisopent is a fluorocarbon ultrasound contrast medium (p.1059) used with perflenapent (above) for echocardiography.

---

## Perflutren *(USAN, rINN)*

DMP-115; FS-069; MRX-115; Perfluoropropane. Octafluoropropane.

$C_3F_8$ = 188.0.

*CAS — 76-19-7.*

### Profile

Perflutren is a fluorocarbon ultrasound contrast medium used as albumin- or lipid-coated microspheres for echocardiography.

### Preparations

***USP 27:*** Perflutren Protein-Type A Microspheres for Injection.

**Proprietary Preparations** (details are given in Part 3)

***Arg.:*** Optison; ***Austria:*** Optison†; ***Denm.:*** Optison; ***Ger.:*** Optison†; ***Port.:*** Optison†; ***Spain:*** Optison; ***Swed.:*** Optison; ***USA:*** Definity; Optison.

---

## Propyliodone *(rINN)*

Propiliodona; Propyliodonum. Propyl 1,4-dihydro-3,5-di-iodo-4-oxo-1-pyridylacetate.

$C_{10}H_{11}I_2NO_3$ = 447.0.

*CAS — 587-61-1.*

*ATC — V08AD03.*

**Description.** Propyliodone contains about 56.8% of I.

**Pharmacopoeias.** In *Int.* and *US.*

**USP 27** (Propyliodone). A white or almost white, crystalline powder. Is odourless or has a faint odour. Practically insoluble in water; soluble in alcohol, in acetone, and in ether. Store in airtight containers at a temperature of 25°, excursions permitted between 15° and 30°. Protect from light.

### Adverse Effects

Propyliodone may cause transient pyrexia, sometimes associated with malaise and aching of the joints, especially with the aqueous suspension, lasting 48 hours and sometimes accompanied by coughing. In a few cases, dyspnoea, atelectasis, or pneumonia have occurred. Hypersensitivity reactions may occur rarely.

### Precautions

Propyliodone should be used with great care where there is hypersensitivity to iodine and is contra-indicated in patients with severe heart disease. It should also be used with caution in patients with asthma, bronchiectasis, or pulmonary emphysema, or in whom pulmonary function is otherwise reduced. If bilateral examination of the bronchial tract is necessary in such patients an interval of several days should elapse between the examinations. Use of an excessive volume or too-rapid administration may result in lobar collapse.

Iodine-containing contrast media may interfere with thyroid-function tests.

### Pharmacokinetics

After instillation into the lungs some propyliodone may be expectorated and swallowed but the remainder is absorbed into the blood. It is rapidly hydrolysed and is excreted in the urine as di-iodopyridone acetate. Approximately 50% of the dose is reported to be eliminated in the urine within 3 days.

### Uses and Administration

Propyliodone is an iodinated contrast medium that has been used for bronchography (p.1059) as either a 50% aqueous suspension or as a 60% oily suspension.

### Preparations

***USP 27:*** Propyliodone Injectable Oil Suspension.

**Proprietary Preparations** (details are given in Part 3)

***Israel:*** Dionosil.

---

## Sodium Tyropanoate *(BAN, rINN)*

NSC-107434; Tiropanoato de sodio; Tyropanoate Sodium *(USAN)*; Win-8851-2. Sodium 2-(3-butyramido-2,4,6-tri-iodobenzyl)butyrate.

$C_{15}H_{17}I_3NNaO_3$ = 663.0.

*CAS — 27293-82-9 (tyropanoic acid); 7246-21-1 (sodium tyropanoate).*

**Description.** Sodium tyropanoate contains about 57.4% of I.

### Profile

Sodium tyropanoate is an iodinated ionic monomeric contrast medium with actions similar to those of iopanoic acid (p.1065) and has been used for cholecystography and cholangiography (p.1059).

### Preparations

**Proprietary Preparations** (details are given in Part 3)

***USA:*** Bilopaque†.

---

## Sulfur Hexafluoride *(USAN)*

BRI; Sulphur Fluoride; Sulphur Hexafluoride.

$F_6S$ = 146.1.

*CAS — 2551-62-4.*

*ATC — V08DA05.*

### Profile

Sulfur hexafluoride is used as an ultrasound contrast medium for imaging of blood vessels. It is given intravenously as a microbubble suspension containing 45 micrograms/mL, in a usual dose of 2.4 mL, repeated once if necessary.

Sulfur hexafluoride has also been used as an adjunct in eye surgery for retinal detachment.

### Preparations

**Proprietary Preparations** (details are given in Part 3)

***Belg.:*** SonoVue; ***Denm.:*** SonoVue; ***Ital.:*** SonoVue; ***Neth.:*** SonoVue; ***Norw.:*** SonoVue; ***Port.:*** SonoVue; ***Swed.:*** SonoVue.

# Corticosteroids

Adverse Effects of Corticosteroids and their Treatment, p.1068
Withdrawal of Corticosteroids, p.1070
Precautions for Corticosteroids, p.1071
Interactions of Corticosteroids, p.1072
Pharmacokinetics of Corticosteroids, p.1073
Uses and Administration of Corticosteroids, p.1073
Administration, p.1074
Diurnal effect, p.1074
Epidural route, p.1074
Inhalational therapy, p.1074
Intra-articular route, p.1074
Surgery, p.1074
Topical application, p.1074
Acute respiratory distress syndrome, p.1075
Adrenal hyperplasia, congenital, p.1075
Adrenocortical insufficiency, p.1075
AIDS, p.1076
Alopecia, p.1076
Anaemias, p.1076
Anaphylactic shock, p.1076
Aspiration syndromes, p.1076
Asthma, p.1076
Behçet's syndrome, p.1076
Bell's palsy, p.1076
Bites and stings, p.1077
Bone cysts, p.1077
Brain injury, p.1077
Bronchiolitis, p.1077
Bronchopulmonary dysplasia, p.1077
Cachexia, p.1077
Cerebral oedema, p.1078
Chronic active hepatitis, p.1078
Chronic obstructive pulmonary disease, p.1078
Churg-Strauss syndrome, p.1078
Cogan's syndrome, p.1078
Congenital adrenal hyperplasia, p.1078
Corneal graft rejection, p.1079
Croup, p.1079
Cystic fibrosis, p.1079
Deafness, p.1079
Dermatomyositis, p.1079
Diffuse parenchymal lung disease, p.1079
Eczema, p.1080
Epidermolysis bullosa, p.1080
Epilepsy, p.1080
Erythema multiforme, p.1080
Giant cell arteritis, p.1080
Glomerular kidney disease, p.1080
Graves' ophthalmopathy, p.1081
Haemangioma, p.1081
Headache, p.1081
Herpes infections, p.1081
Hypercalcaemia, p.1081
Hypersensitivity vasculitis, p.1081
Idiopathic thrombocytopenic purpura, p.1082
Infections, p.1083
Infectious mononucleosis, p.1083
Inflammatory bowel disease, p.1083
Leishmaniasis, p.1083
Leprosy, p.1083
Lichen, p.1083
Liver disorders, p.1083
Male infertility, p.1083
Malignant neoplasms, p.1083
Meningitis, p.1083
Mouth ulceration, p.1083
Multiple sclerosis, p.1083
Muscular dystrophies, p.1083
Myasthenia gravis, p.1084
Nasal polyps, p.1084
Nausea and vomiting, p.1084
Neonatal intraventricular haemorrhage, p.1084
Neonatal respiratory distress syndrome, p.1084
Optic neuropathies, p.1085
Organ and tissue transplantation, p.1085
Osteoarthritis, p.1085
Osteopetrosis, p.1085
Pain, p.1085
Pancreatitis, p.1085
Pemphigus and pemphigoid, p.1085
Pneumocystis carinii pneumonia, p.1085
Polyarteritis nodosa and microscopic polyangiitis, p.1085
Polychondritis, p.1086
Polymyalgia rheumatica, p.1086
Polymyositis and dermatomyositis, p.1086
Polyneuropathies, p.1086
Postoperative ocular inflammation, p.1087
Pregnancy, p.1087
Psoriasis, p.1087
Pyoderma gangrenosum, p.1087
Respiratory disorders, p.1087
Retinal vasculitis, p.1087
Rheumatoid arthritis, p.1087
Rhinitis, p.1087
Sarcoidosis, p.1087
Sciatica, p.1088
Scleritis, p.1088
Seborrhoeic dermatitis, p.1088
Septic shock, p.1088
Sickle-cell disease, p.1088
Skin disorders, p.1088
Soft-tissue rheumatism, p.1088
Spinal cord injury, p.1088
Spondyloarthropathies, p.1088
Systemic lupus erythematosus, p.1088
Takayasu's arteritis, p.1089
Tuberculosis, p.1089
Urticaria and angioedema, p.1090
Uveitis, p.1090
Vasculitic syndromes, p.1090
Vitiligo, p.1090
Wegener's granulomatosis, p.1090

The adrenal cortex synthesises both corticosteroids, based on a 21-carbon nucleus, and some sex hormones, primarily androgens, based on a 19-carbon nucleus. The corticosteroids are traditionally divided into those with predominantly glucocorticoid actions, of which cortisol (hydrocortisone) is the most important endogenous example, and those that are primarily mineralocorticoid, of which aldosterone is much the most important.

The endogenous glucocorticoids are under regulatory control from the hypothalamus and pituitary, via the releasing hormones corticorelin (p.1321) and corticotropin or ACTH (p.1322). In return the glucocorticoids act to inhibit production and release of these releasing hormones by a negative feedback mechanism. The system is known collectively as the hypothalamic-pituitary-adrenal (HPA) axis. Aldosterone secretion, by contrast, is under the control of the renin-angiotensin system.

The main **mineralocorticoid** actions are on fluid and electrolyte balance. They enhance sodium reabsorption in the kidney and hence expand the extracellular fluid volume, and they enhance renal excretion of potassium and $H^+$.

The **glucocorticoid** actions are wide-ranging. They have potent anti-inflammatory and immunosuppressive effects, at least partly through inhibition of the release of various cytokines, and it is primarily these that are made use of clinically (see p.1073). They also have profound metabolic effects: blood glucose concentrations are maintained or increased by a decrease in peripheral glucose utilization and an increase in gluconeogenesis; glycogen deposition, protein breakdown, and lipolysis are increased, and effects on calcium uptake and excretion lead to a decrease in body calcium stores. Glucocorticoids facilitate the action of many other active endogenous substances, and affect the function of cardiovascular system, kidneys, skeletal muscle and CNS.

Many synthetic congeners and derivatives of the corticosteroids are available. The main corticosteroids used systemically are hydroxy compounds (alcohols). They are relatively insoluble in water and the sodium salt of the phosphate or succinate ester is generally used to provide water-soluble forms for injections or solutions. Such esters are readily hydrolysed in the body.

Various structure-activity relationships are understood for the corticosteroids and have been made use of in the development of new compounds. The presence of a hydroxyl group at position 11 seems to be essential for glucocorticoid activity, while a hydroxyl at position 21 is required for mineralocorticoid activity. Fluorination at position 9 enhances both mineralocorticoid and glucocorticoid activity. Substitution at carbon 16 (as in betamethasone, dexamethasone, or triamcinolone) virtually eliminates mineralocorticoid activity. Esterification of corticosteroids at the 17 or 21 positions with fatty acids generally increases the topical activity. The formation of cyclic acetonides at the 16 and 17 positions further increases topical anti-inflammatory activity, usually without increasing systemic glucocorticoid activity.

In the medical and pharmacological literature the names of unesterified corticosteroids have frequently been used indiscriminately for both the unesterified and esterified forms and it is not always apparent to which form reference is being made. The unesterified form is sometimes qualified by the phrase 'free alcohol'.

## Adverse Effects of Corticosteroids and their Treatment

The adverse effects of corticosteroids may result from unwanted mineralocorticoid or glucocorticoid actions, or from inhibition of the hypothalamic-pituitary-adrenal axis.

**Mineralocorticoid** adverse effects are manifest in the retention of sodium and water, with oedema and hypertension, and in the increased excretion of potassium with the possibility of hypokalaemic alkalosis. In susceptible patients, cardiac failure may be induced. Disturbances of electrolyte balance are common with the naturally occurring corticosteroids, such as cortisone and hydrocortisone, but are less frequent with many synthetic glucocorticoids, which have little or no mineralocorticoid activity.

Adverse **glucocorticoid** effects lead to mobilisation of calcium and phosphorus, with osteoporosis and spontaneous fractures; muscle wasting and nitrogen depletion; and hyperglycaemia with accentuation or precipitation of the diabetic state. The insulin requirements of diabetic patients are increased. Increased appetite is often reported.

Impaired tissue repair and immune function can lead to delayed wound healing, and increased susceptibility to infection. Increased susceptibility to all kinds of infection, including septicaemia, tuberculosis, fungal infections, and viral infections, has been reported in patients on corticosteroid therapy. Infections may also be masked by the anti-inflammatory, analgesic, and antipyretic effects of glucocorticoids. The increased severity of varicella and measles may lead to a fatal outcome in non-immune patients receiving systemic corticosteroid therapy.

Other adverse effects include menstrual irregularities, amenorrhoea, hyperhidrosis, skin thinning, ocular changes including development of glaucoma and cataract, mental and neurological disturbances, benign intracranial hypertension, acute pancreatitis, and avascular necrosis of bone. An increase in the coagulability of the blood may lead to thromboembolic complications. Peptic ulceration has been reported but reviews of the literature do not always agree that corticosteroids are responsible for an increased incidence.

The negative feedback effects of glucocorticoids on the hypothalamic-pituitary-adrenal (HPA) axis may lead to adrenal atrophy, in some cases after therapy for as little as 7 days. This produces secondary adrenocortical insufficiency, which may become manifest following overly rapid withdrawal of treatment or be precipitated by some stress such as infection or trauma. Patients vary considerably in the degree and duration of adrenal suppression following a given course of corticosteroid, but adrenal atrophy may persist for months or years, and withdrawal should be gradual in those who have been treated for any length of time (see also Withdrawal, below). High doses of corticosteroids given during pregnancy may cause fetal or neonatal adrenal suppression. Although the precise mechanism is uncertain, growth retardation may follow the use of even relatively small doses of corticosteroids in children.

Large doses of corticosteroids, or of corticotropin, may produce Cushingoid symptoms typical of hyperactivity of the adrenal cortex, with moon-face, sometimes with hirsutism, buffalo hump, flushing, increased bruising, ecchymoses, striae, and acne (see also Cushing's Syndrome, p.1313). Rapid intravenous administration of large doses of corticosteroids may cause cardiovascular collapse.

Hypersensitivity reactions have occurred with corticosteroids, mainly when administered topically.

Adverse effects occur, in general, fairly equally with all systemic corticosteroid preparations and their incidence rises steeply if dosage increases much above physiological values, traditionally considered to be about 7.5 mg daily of prednisolone or its equivalent (see Uses and Administration, below, for equivalent doses of other corticosteroids). Short courses at high dosage for emergencies appear to cause fewer side-effects than prolonged courses with lower doses.

Most topically applied (including inhaled) corticosteroids may, under certain circumstances, be absorbed in sufficient amounts to produce systemic effects. The topical application of corticosteroid preparations to the eyes has produced corneal ulcers, raised intra-ocular pressure, and reduced visual function. Application of corticosteroids to the skin has led to loss of skin collagen and subcutaneous atrophy; local hypopigmentation of deeply pigmented skins has been reported following both the intradermal injection and topical application of potent corticosteroids. Dryness, irritation, epistaxis, and rarely ulceration or perforation of the nasal septum have followed intranasal use; smell and taste disturbances may also occur. Hoarseness and candidiasis of the mouth or throat may occur in patients receiving inhaled corticosteroids.

Intrathecal administration (including inadvertent intrathecal administration after attempted epidural injection) has been associated with arachnoiditis.

Adverse effects should be treated symptomatically, with the corticosteroid dosage reduced or slowly withdrawn where possible.

**Adrenal suppression.** The inhibition of hypothalamic-pituitary-adrenocortical function associated with corticosteroid use may persist for a year or more after treatment is withdrawn and may cause acute adrenocortical insufficiency with circulatory collapse during stress. The degree of suppression depends on a number of factors, including length of treatment, time of day of administration, type of corticosteroid preparation used, route of administration, dose administered, and dosing interval. In general, suppression of secretion of adrenocorticotrophic hormone and atrophy of the adrenal gland become progressively more definite as doses of corticosteroid exceed physiological amounts (see Uses and Administration, below), and as the duration of therapy increases (significant suppression is likely in patients receiving more than 3 weeks of therapy). It is less when the corticosteroid is given as a single dose in the morning, and even less if this morning dose is given on alternate days or less frequently. In patients taking high enough doses of corticosteroids to suppress the adrenals the dose should be increased during any form of stress (for example, illness or surgery); similarly those treated with such doses within the last 2 or 3 months should be restarted on therapy. Where the interval since treatment is greater than 3 months, resumption of treatment depends on clinical assessment of signs of adrenocortical insufficiency.

To avoid precipitating acute adrenocortical insufficiency, withdrawal of corticosteroid treatment should be carried out gradually, differing regimens being used according to the disease being treated and the duration of therapy. Examples of withdrawal regimens that have been used are described under Withdrawal, below.

Adrenal suppression may occur after very short courses of high-dose therapy and since many patients undergoing such therapy will be under continuing stress when the drugs are stopped, gradual withdrawal of corticosteroids over 5 to 7 days is preferable.

It should also be remembered that corticosteroid-induced adrenal suppression has been associated not only with systemic therapy, but has followed topical application of corticosteroid preparations, particularly those containing potent corticosteroids. Some degree of adrenal suppression is also associated with the use of high dose inhalants and nasal preparations, and has followed the topical application of eye drops and eye ointments.

**Effects on bones and joints.** Corticosteroid-induced **avascular necrosis** of bone is an uncommon but disabling complication of therapy.[1-3] The incidence may vary in patients with different disease states; alcoholics, and patients with connective tissue disease (especially systemic lupus erythematosus) may have increased susceptibility.[3,4] There may be a relationship with corticosteroid dose: even short courses of high-dose corticosteroids may be associated with its development.[1-3] Avascular necrosis has also been associated with topical application of corticosteroids.[5]

Corticosteroids may also produce **osteoporosis.** A review[6] of data obtained from studies published between 1970 and 1990 established that osteoporosis is a common consequence of long-term treatment with corticosteroids, occurring in about 50% of patients. Bone loss is more rapid during the early stages of therapy and is most rapid in areas of the skeleton containing the greatest proportion of trabecular bone such as the spine, hip, distal radius, pelvis, and ribs.

Reviews and guidelines[7-9] on the prevention and management of corticosteroid-induced osteoporosis suggest that the dose should be minimised, as oral doses above 7.5 mg of prednisolone or prednisone (or the equivalent) daily are associated with more significant bone loss and increased fracture risk.[10] Alternate-day therapy, although desirable for its reduced effect on the hypothalamic-pituitary-adrenal axis, does not reduce the risk of bone loss. It should be borne in mind that long-term use of inhaled corticosteroids may also reduce bone mineral density. Patients should maintain an adequate intake of calcium and vitamin D, should take regular exercise, and avoid smoking and excessive alcohol intake. HRT has been advocated in postmenopausal women but recent re-evaluation of the risks and benefits of HRT may render this option unattractive. Bisphosphonates may be used in high-risk patients as they are effective at preventing and treating corticosteroid-induced bone loss[11] and may reduce fracture rates.[8,9] There is some evidence to suggest that calcitonin has a beneficial effect on bone mass, and it may be considered as an alternative when bisphosphonates cannot be used. Fluoride has been studied in corticosteroid-induced osteoporosis, but although it was found to increase bone density, there is concern about the resultant bone structure and a possible increase in fracture rates. There are reports of benefit from anabolic therapy, but evidence is limited. A thiazide diuretic may be helpful in controlling hypercalciuria in patients not receiving calcitriol.[8] Whether some corticosteroids have reduced effects on the bone is unclear.[9]


1. Nixon JE. Early diagnosis and treatment of steroid induced avascular necrosis of bone. *BMJ* 1984; **288:** 741–4.
2. Anonymous. Transplant osteonecrosis. *Lancet* 1985; **i:** 965–6.
3. Capell H. Selected side-effects: 5. steroid therapy and osteonecrosis. *Prescribers' J* 1992; **32:** 32–4.
4. Knight A. Images in clinical medicine: corticosteroid osteonecrosis. *N Engl J Med* 1995; **333:** 130.
5. McLean CJ, *et al.* Cataracts, glaucoma, and femoral avascular necrosis caused by topical corticosteroid ointment. *Lancet* 1995; **345:** 330.
6. Lukert BP, Raisz LG. Glucocorticoid-induced osteoporosis: pathogenesis and management. *Ann Intern Med* 1990; **112:** 352–64.
7. American College of Rheumatology Ad Hoc Committee on Glucocorticoid-Induced Osteoporosis. Recommendations for the prevention and treatment of glucocorticoid-induced osteoporosis. *Arthritis Rheum* 2001; **44:** 1496–1503.
8. Adachi JD, Papaioannou A. Corticosteroid-induced osteoporosis: detection and management. *Drug Safety* 2001; **24:** 607–24.
9. Bone and Tooth Society, National Osteoporosis Society, and Royal College of Physicians. Glucocorticoid-induced osteoporosis: guidelines for prevention and treatment (December 2002). Available at: http://www.rcplondon.ac.uk/pubs/books/glucocorticoid/index.asp (accessed 27/04/04)
10. van Staa, *et al.* Oral corticosteroids and fracture risk: relationship to daily and cumulative doses. *Rheumatology (Oxford)* 2000; **39:** 1383–9.
11. Homik J, *et al.* Bisphosphonates for steroid induced osteoporosis. Available in The Cochrane Library; Issue 1. Chichester: John Wiley; 2004.


**Effects on carbohydrate and protein metabolism.** Corticosteroids produce glucose intolerance[1-4] and protein catabolism.[5,6] Although mainly associated with systemic use, there is a report of deterioration in diabetic control associated with high-dose inhaled corticosteroid treatment.[7]


1. Landy HJ, *et al.* The effect of chronic steroid therapy on glucose tolerance in pregnancy. *Am J Obstet Gynecol* 1988; **159:** 612–15.
2. O'Byrne S, Feely J. Effects of drugs on glucose tolerance in non-insulin-dependent diabetics (part I). *Drugs* 1990; **40:** 6–18.
3. Bruno A, *et al.* Serum glucose, insulin and C-peptide response to oral glucose after intravenous administration of hydrocortisone and methylprednisolone in man. *Eur J Clin Pharmacol* 1994; **46:** 411–5.
4. Hurel SJ, Taylor R. Drugs and glucose tolerance. *Adverse Drug React Bull* 1995; (Oct.): 659–62.
5. Brownlee KG, *et al.* Catabolic effect of dexamethasone in the preterm baby. *Arch Dis Child* 1992; **67:** 1–4.
6. Van Goudoever JB, *et al.* Effect of dexamethasone on protein metabolism in infants with bronchopulmonary dysplasia. *J Pediatr* 1994; **124:** 112–18.
7. Faul JL, *et al.* High dose inhaled corticosteroids and dose dependent loss of diabetic control *BMJ* 1998; **317:** 1491.


**Effects on the cerebrovascular system.** Despite being used in high doses to treat benign intracranial hypertension, corticosteroids may also occasionally cause this disorder. Children receiving long-term therapy are mainly affected, an increase in dosage often being responsible. Symptoms usually subside when dosage is reduced.[1]


1. Gibberd B. Drug-induced benign intracranial hypertension. *Prescribers' J* 1991; **31:** 118–21.


**Effects on the eyes.** During ophthalmic use of corticosteroids about one-third of patients will develop **raised intra-ocular pressure**, usually within a few weeks of treatment with potent corticosteroids, or within months with weaker ones.[1] The effects on children are variable, but they may be at risk of a greater and more rapid response to ophthalmic corticosteroids.[1] Raised intra-ocular pressure and glaucoma can also be caused by topical administration of corticosteroids to the face, particularly with prolonged use.[2] There is evidence of an increased risk in patients receiving prolonged high-dose inhaled corticosteroids.[3] Increases in intra-ocular pressure appear to be less common with systemic corticosteroids,[4] but a study in elderly patients demonstrated that the risk of raised intra-ocular pressure or open-angle glaucoma increased with the dose and duration of oral use.[5]

Topical administration of corticosteroids to patients with bacterial, fungal, or viral **eye infection** can alleviate the symptoms but allow the infection to develop.[1,6] In ocular herpes simplex infection there is the risk of corneal ulceration and scarring that may lead to loss of vision.

**Cataract formation** is associated with systemic corticosteroid use. It has also been reported following ophthalmic[1,4] and topical[2,7] administration. There is evidence that cataract formation may also be associated with prolonged use of high-dose inhaled corticosteroids.[8-10] The intranasal use of corticosteroids, however, does not appear to increase the risk.[11] It has been suggested that the lens in children might be more sensitive than in adults, but this may be due to the large doses of corticosteroids, relative to body size, given orally in these cases. Evidence of an increased risk in children from inhaled corticosteroids is limited, but is probably outweighed by the benefits of asthma control.[12]

Systemic corticosteroid use has also been associated with damage to the retinal pigment epithelial barrier, predisposing the patient to serous **retinal detachment**.[13]


1. McGhee CNJ, *et al.* Locally administered ocular corticosteroids: benefits and risks. *Drug Safety* 2002; **25:** 33–55.
2. McLean CJ, *et al.* Cataracts, glaucoma, and femoral avascular necrosis caused by topical corticosteroid ointment. *Lancet* 1995; **345:** 330.
3. Garbe E, *et al.* Inhaled and nasal glucocorticoids and the risks of ocular hypertension or open-angle glaucoma. *JAMA* 1997; **277:** 722–7.
4. Butcher JM, *et al.* Bilateral cataracts and glaucoma induced by long term use of steroid eye drops. *BMJ* 1994; **309:** 43.
5. Garbe E, *et al.* Risk of ocular hypertension or open-angle glaucoma in elderly patients on oral glucocorticoids. *Lancet* 1997; **350:** 979–82.
6. Baratz KH, Hattenhauer MG. Indiscriminate use of corticosteroid-containing eyedrops. *Mayo Clin Proc* 1999; **74:** 362–6.
7. Costagliola C, *et al.* Cataracts associated with long-term topical steroids. *Br J Dermatol* 1989; **120:** 472–3.
8. Cumming RG, *et al.* Use of inhaled corticosteroids and the risk of cataracts. *N Engl J Med* 1997; **337:** 8–14.
9. Garbe E, *et al.* Association of inhaled corticosteroid use with cataract extraction in elderly patients. *JAMA* 1998; **280:** 539–43. Correction. *ibid.*; 1830.
10. Smeeth L, *et al.* A population based case-control study of cataract and inhaled corticosteroids. *Br J Ophthalmol* 2003; **87:** 1247–51.
11. Derby L, Maier WC. Risk of cataract among users of intranasal corticosteroids. *J Allergy Clin Immunol* 2000; **105:** 912–16.
12. Cumming RG, Mitchell P. Inhaled corticosteroids and cataract: prevalence, prevention and management. *Drug Safety* 1999; **20:** 77–84.
13. Polak BCP, *et al.* Diffuse retinal pigment epitheliopathy complicating systemic corticosteroid treatment. *Br J Ophthalmol* 1995; **79:** 922–5.


**Effects on the gastrointestinal tract.** It has long been considered that treatment with corticosteroids might lead to peptic ulcers. Some years ago a review of the data then available suggested that since an ulcer developed in 1% of control patients not receiving corticosteroids, the 2% incidence for patients receiving corticosteroids did not warrant the prophylactic use of anti-ulcer drugs in all patients.[1] Others have found little evidence of an increased risk of peptic ulcer produced by corticosteroids alone although there is some increased risk when using them with NSAIDs.[2] A later cohort study[3] found a modest increase in risk of gastrointestinal bleeding with current use of corticosteroids, which increased when NSAIDs were also used. It has been suggested that it might be prudent to avoid such combination therapy whenever possible.[4]

Doubt has therefore been cast on the prophylactic value of anti-ulcer therapy given with corticosteroids.[1,3] If an ulcer does develop and there is good reason to continue treatment then corticosteroids may be continued along with some form of ulcer therapy.[1]

There have been several reports of corticosteroids being associated with gastrointestinal perforation.[6-9] There is a risk that the anti-inflammatory properties of corticosteroids may mask the signs of perforation and delay diagnosis with potentially fatal results.


1. Spiro HM. Is the steroid ulcer a myth? *N Engl J Med* 1983; **309:** 45–7.
2. Piper JM, *et al.* Corticosteroid use and peptic ulcer disease: role of nonsteroidal anti-inflammatory drugs. *Ann Intern Med* 1991; **114:** 735–40.
3. Nielsen GL, *et al.* Risk of hospitalization resulting from upper gastrointestinal bleeding among patients taking corticosteroids: a register-based cohort study. *Am J Med* 2001; **111:** 541–5.
4. Guslandi M, Tittobello A. Steroid ulcers: a myth revisited. *BMJ* 1992; **304:** 655–6.

5. Marcus P, McCauley DL. Steroid therapy and $H_2$-receptor antagonists: pharmacoeconomic implications. *Clin Pharmacol Ther* 1997; **61:** 503–8.
6. Arsura EL. Corticosteroid-associated perforation of colonic diverticula. *Arch Intern Med* 1990; **150:** 1337–8.
7. Ng PC, *et al.* Gastroduodenal perforation in preterm babies treated with dexamethasone for bronchopulmonary dysplasia. *Arch Dis Child* 1991; **66:** 1164–6.
8. O'Neil EA, *et al.* Dexamethasone treatment during ventilator dependency: possible life threatening gastrointestinal complications. *Arch Dis Child* 1992; **67:** 10–11.
9. Epstein A, *et al.* Perforation of colon diverticula during corticosteroid therapy for pemphigus vulgaris. *Ann Pharmacother* 1993; **27:** 979–80.

**Effects on growth.** Corticosteroids impair normal growth in children when given systemically,[1-3] and although alternate day therapy may reduce the effect on growth it does not abolish it. There has been some concern about possible effects of inhaled corticosteroids on growth.[1,4] Some studies have not found an effect of inhaled corticosteroids on growth if doses are modest, even when treatment is prolonged.[1,5,6] Others have found that inhaled corticosteroids, particularly in high doses, do have some effect on growth parameters,[5,7-10] but it is unclear whether this has long-term effects on the child's ultimate height, and the alternative in children requiring such high-dose therapy is likely to be an oral corticosteroid, with its consequent effects. Some studies,[11,12] in children with mild to moderate asthma, have suggested that a small reduction in growth velocity may occur in the first year of treatment, but that it then normalises and adult height is not adversely affected. Nonetheless, in the light of the increasing number of studies suggesting some effects of inhaled or intranasal corticosteroids on growth the FDA has required the inclusion of a warning in US labelling that such products may slow growth rates. For a suggestion that inhalation of a single dose of budesonide in the morning had less effect on growth than twice daily dosage, see Administration, p.1094.

1. Allen DB, *et al.* A meta-analysis of the effect of oral and inhaled corticosteroids on growth. *J Allergy Clin Immunol* 1994; **93:** 967–76.
2. Lai H-C, *et al.* Risk of persistent growth impairment after alternate-day prednisone treatment in children with cystic fibrosis. *N Engl J Med* 2000; **342:** 851–9.
3. Mushtaq T, Ahmed SF. The impact of corticosteroids on growth and bone health. *Arch Dis Child* 2002; **87:** 93–6.
4. Hanania NA, *et al.* Adverse effects of inhaled corticosteroids. *Am J Med* 1995; **98:** 196–208.
5. Wolthers OD, Pedersen S. Controlled study of linear growth in asthmatic children during treatment with inhaled glucocorticosteroids. *Pediatrics* 1992; **89:** 839–42.
6. Volovitz B, *et al.* Growth and pituitary-adrenal function in children with severe asthma treated with inhaled budesonide. *N Engl J Med* 1993; **329:** 1703–8.
7. Wolthers OD, Pedersen S. Short term growth during treatment with inhaled fluticasone propionate and beclomethasone dipropionate. *Arch Dis Child* 1993; **68:** 673–6.
8. Todd G, *et al.* Growth and adrenal suppression in asthmatic children treated with high-dose fluticasone propionate. *Lancet* 1996; **348:** 27–9.
9. McCowan C, *et al.* Effect of asthma and its treatment on growth: four year follow up of cohort of children from general practices in Tayside, Scotland. *BMJ* 1998; **316:** 668–72.
10. Sharek PJ, Bergman DA. The effect of inhaled steroids on the linear growth of children with asthma: a meta-analysis. Abstract: *Pediatrics* 2000; **106:** 129. Full version: http://pediatrics.aappublications.org/cgi/content/full/106/1/e8 (accessed 27/04/04)
11. The Childhood Asthma Management Program Research Group. Long-term effects of budesonide or nedocromil in children with asthma. *N Engl J Med* 2000; **343:** 1054–63.
12. Agertoft L, Pedersen S. Effect of long-term treatment with inhaled budesonide on adult height in children with asthma. *N Engl J Med* 2000; **343:** 1064–9.

**Effects on immune response.** Owing to their immunosuppressant effect administration of corticosteroids in doses greater than those required for physiological replacement therapy is associated with increased susceptibility to infection, aggravation of existing infection, and activation of latent infection. An additional problem is that the anti-inflammatory effect of corticosteroids may mask symptoms until the infection has progressed to an advanced stage; the altered response of the body may also permit the bizarre spread of infections, frequently in aberrant forms, such as disseminated parasitic infections. The risk is greater in patients receiving high doses, or associated therapy with other immunosuppressants such as cytotoxic drugs, and in those who are already debilitated. Children receiving high doses of corticosteroids are at special risk from childhood diseases, such as chickenpox, but vaccination with living organisms is contra-indicated since infection may be induced (killed vaccines or toxoids can be given but the response may be reduced).

This increased susceptibility to infection and masking of symptoms may also be caused by topical or local corticosteroid therapy. Thus, topical application to the skin has led to unusual changes such as atypical ringworm infection. Fungal infections (particularly candidiasis), generally restricted to the mouth and throat, are associated with corticosteroid inhalations. Severe damage to the eye has followed the ocular use of corticosteroids in herpetic infections, and a generalised spread of herpes infection may follow application to the mouth in the presence of herpes infection.

Conversely, the effect of corticosteroids on the symptoms and course of some infections may be life-saving (see Uses and Administration, below). Before embarking on a long-term course of corticosteroid therapy general measures for the reduction of risk of infection include a diligent search for active or quiescent infection and, where appropriate, prevention or eradication of the infection before starting, or concurrent administration of chemoprophylaxis during corticosteroid treatment.

**Effects on lipid metabolism.** Glucocorticoids have potent effects on lipid metabolism, facilitating the effects of growth hormone and endogenous stimulants of lipolysis. As a result they increase both high- and low-density lipoprotein cholesterol concentrations in the blood.

On prolonged administration glucocorticoids also have a dramatic effect on body fat distribution, resulting in the characteristic Cushingoid appearance of moon face, and increased fat at the back of the neck and supraclavicular area.

**Effects on mental state.** Mental disturbances caused by corticosteroids include depression, mania, euphoria, and delirium.[1] The risk of adverse effects appears to be dose-related, but there are reports of cases associated with very low dosages. Impairment of memory has been associated with pulsed intravenous methylprednisolone.[2]

1. Patten SB, Neutel CI. Corticosteroid-induced adverse psychiatric effects: incidence, diagnosis and management. *Drug Safety* 2000; **22:** 111–22.
2. Oliveri RL, *et al.* Pulsed methylprednisolone induces a reversible impairment of memory in patients with relapsing-remitting multiple sclerosis. *Acta Neurol Scand* 1998; **97:** 366–9.

**Effects on the neonate.** Various adverse effects have been reported in premature neonates given corticosteroids, see under Dexamethasone, p.1097.

**Effects on the nervous system.** Paraesthesia, usually localised to the perineum, has been associated with intravenous administration of dexamethasone sodium phosphate[1-4] and hydrocortisone sodium phosphate,[5] but not with hydrocortisone sodium succinate.[5] Descriptions of this reaction include itching, burning, tingling, and severe pain. It can begin within seconds of giving the injection, and clear within minutes of stopping administration. This reaction appears to be caused by the corticosteroid phosphate ester itself, and clears in the time it takes for the drug to be hydrolysed. It has been suggested that the reaction can be abolished or avoided by giving the drug as a dilute solution, over at least 5 to 15 minutes.[2-4]

Epidural lipomatosis (fat deposition around the spinal cord) is a rare complication of systemic corticosteroids.[6] It has been associated with both high daily doses (more than 30 mg prednisone daily) and lower doses given over several years. The onset of symptoms is usually gradual, ranging from 6 months to more than 20 years after beginning corticosteroid use. Spinal cord compression causes back pain radiating to the lower limbs, and severe neurological complications can develop. The lipomatosis may regress or disappear after the corticosteroid is discontinued or the dose is lowered, but patients with myelopathy or rapidly progressive neurological deficit may need emergency surgery.

1. Czerwinski AW, *et al.* Effects of a single, large, intravenous injection of dexamethasone. *Clin Pharmacol Ther* 1972; **13:** 638–42.
2. Allan SG, Leonard RCF. Dexamethasone antiemesis and side-effects. *Lancet* 1986; **i:** 1035.
3. Neff SPW, *et al.* Excruciating perineal pain after intravenous dexamethasone. *Anaesth Intensive Care* 2002; **30:** 370–1.
4. Perron G, *et al.* Perineal pruritus after iv dexamethasone administration. *Can J Anesth* 2003; **50:** 749–50.
5. Novak E, *et al.* Anorectal pruritus after intravenous hydrocortisone sodium succinate and sodium phosphate. *Clin Pharmacol Ther* 1976; **20:** 109–12.
6. Hierholzer J, *et al.* Epidural lipomatosis: case report and literature review. *Neuroradiology* 1996; **38:** 343–8.

**Effects on the pancreas.** Acute pancreatitis has been associated with corticosteroid use,[1-3] although evidence supporting the association has been challenged on a number of grounds, both clinical and experimental.[2]

1. Nakashima Y, Howard JM. Drug-induced acute pancreatitis. *Surg Gynecol Obstet* 1977; **145:** 105–9.
2. Banerjee AK, *et al.* Drug-induced acute pancreatitis: a critical review. *Med Toxicol Adverse Drug Exp* 1989; **4:** 186–98.
3. Felig DM, Topazian M. Corticosteroid-induced pancreatitis. *Ann Intern Med* 1996; **124:** 1016.

**Effects on the skin.** Topical corticosteroids are associated with a number of local adverse effects on the skin, principally due to their antiproliferative effects on keratinocytes and fibroblasts (leading to skin thinning and atrophy), and to possible interference with the skin flora (leading to increased risk of superinfection or opportunistic infection).[1] Skin thinning is more likely if corticosteroids are applied under occlusion (this is especially true of halogenated corticosteroids, which are more resistant to inactivation by enzymes in the epidermis). Striae, which occur usually in intertriginous areas such as axillae and groin where skin is thin, moist, and occluded, are the most readily appreciable manifestation of skin atrophy, and are irreversible, unlike more minor degrees of atrophy. Other local adverse effects include telangiectasias and purpura.[1] Acneform pustules at the site of application have occurred.

The balance between benefit and the likelihood of local or systemic adverse effects following topical application of corticosteroids will depend on the chemical structure of the drug (i.e. its lipophilicity and resistance to enzymic degradation), the formulation of the vehicle, the way in which it is applied, and the nature of the skin to be treated.[1]

Skin thinning and purpura have also been reported in patients receiving inhaled corticosteroids.[2,3] There have been a few case reports of eczematous and erythematous lesions of the face and body, and urticaria, following inhalation or intranasal use.[4]

The adverse skin effects arising from systemic corticosteroids also include striae and skin thinning as well as acneform eruptions. Somewhat counter-intuitively a case-control study has suggested an increased risk of Stevens-Johnson syndrome or toxic epidermal necrolysis in patients receiving corticosteroids, particularly in the period shortly after beginning therapy.[5]

1. Mori M, *et al.* Topical corticosteroids and unwanted local effects: improving the benefit/risk ratio. *Drug Safety* 1994; **10:** 406–12.
2. Shuttleworth D, *et al.* Inhaled corticosteroids and skin thinning. *Br J Dermatol* 1990; **122:** 268.
3. Capewell S, *et al.* Purpura and dermal thinning associated with high dose inhaled corticosteroids. *BMJ* 1990; **300:** 1548–51.
4. Isaksson M. Skin reactions to inhaled corticosteroids: incidence, avoidance and management. *Drug Safety* 2001; **24:** 369–73.
5. Roujeau J-C, *et al.* Medication use and the risk of Stevens-Johnson syndrome or toxic epidermal necrolysis. *N Engl J Med* 1995; **333:** 1600–7.

**Effects on the voice.** Dysphonia is associated with inhaled corticosteroids.[1] Although oropharyngeal candidiasis and dysphonia may occur at the same time, many patients with dysphonia do not have candidiasis, and the two conditions do not appear to be directly related. The cause of this dysphonia has not been fully explained, but clinical investigations have found changes including bowing of the vocal cords due to bilateral adductor myopathy, mucosal changes, and supraglottic hyperfunction.

1. Lavy JA, *et al.* Dysphonia associated with inhaled steroids. *J Voice* 2000; **14:** 581–8.

**Hypersensitivity and anaphylaxis.** There have been occasional reports of hypersensitivity reactions, and sometimes anaphylaxis, caused by corticosteroids.[1] Reactions have occurred with any route, although the topical route is mainly involved. It has been observed that the incidence of hypersensitivity is increasing[2] and it has been suggested that a lack of response in chronic eczema might be due to a reaction to the corticosteroid treatment.[2] Fluorinated corticosteroids may be less likely to induce a contact hypersensitivity reaction than non-fluorinated compounds.[3]

1. Kamm GL, Hagmeyer KO. Allergic-type reactions to corticosteroids. *Ann Pharmacother* 1999; **33:** 451–60.
2. Dooms-Goossens A. Sensitivity to corticosteroids: consequences for anti-inflammatory therapy. *Drug Safety* 1995; **13:** 123–9.
3. Thomson KF, *et al.* The prevalence of corticosteroid allergy in two U.K. centres: prescribing implications. *Br J Dermatol* 1999; **141:** 863–6.

**Tumour lysis syndrome.** There have been reports of corticosteroid-induced tumour lysis syndrome.[1-3]

1. Sparano J, *et al.* Increasing recognition of corticosteroid-induced tumour lysis syndrome in non-Hodgkin's lymphoma. *Cancer* 1990; **65:** 1072–3.
2. Smith RE, Stoiber TR. Acute tumor lysis syndrome in prolymphocytic leukemia. *Am J Med* 1990; **88:** 547–8.
3. Haller C, Dhadly M. The tumor lysis syndrome. *Ann Intern Med* 1991; **114:** 808–9.

## Withdrawal of Corticosteroids

The use of pharmacological doses of corticosteroids suppresses the endogenous secretion of corticotropin by the anterior pituitary, with the result that the adrenal cortex becomes atrophied. Sudden withdrawal or reduction in dosage, or an increase in corticosteroid requirements associated with the stress of infection or accidental or surgical trauma, may then precipitate acute adrenocortical insufficiency; deaths have followed the abrupt withdrawal of corticosteroids. Adrenocortical insufficiency has also occurred following the effective reduction in systemic corticosteroid concentrations produced by overly rapid transfer from oral to inhaled corticosteroid therapy. For the emergency treatment of acute adrenocortical insufficiency caused by abrupt withdrawal of corticosteroids, see Adrenocortical Insufficiency, p.1075.

In some instances, withdrawal symptoms may involve or resemble a clinical relapse of the disease for which the patient has been undergoing treatment. Other effects that may occur during withdrawal or change of corticosteroid therapy include fever, myalgia, arthralgia, weight loss, benign intracranial hypertension with headache and vomiting, and papilloedema caused by cerebral oedema. Latent rhinitis or eczema may be unmasked.

Duration of treatment and dosage are important factors in determining suppression of the pituitary-adrenal response to stress on cessation of corticosteroid treatment, and individual liability to suppression is also important.

Following short courses at moderate doses it may be appropriate to withdraw corticosteroids without tapering the dose (see below). However, after high-dose or prolonged therapy, withdrawal should be gradual, the rate depending upon the individual patient's response, the dose, the disease being treated, and the duration of therapy. Recommendations for initial reduction, stated in terms of prednisolone, have varied from as little as steps of 1 mg monthly to 2.5 to 5 mg every 2 to 7 days. Provided the disease is unlikely to relapse the dose of systemic corticosteroid may be reduced rapidly to physiological values; dose reduction should then be slower to allow recovery of pituitary-adrenal function. Symptoms attributable to over-rapid withdrawal should be countered by resuming a higher dose and continuing the reduction at a slower rate. The administration of corticotropin does not help to re-establish adrenal responsiveness.

This gradual withdrawal of corticosteroid therapy permits a return of adrenal function adequate for daily needs, but years may sometimes be required for the return of function necessary to meet the stress of infection, surgery, or trauma. On such occasions patients with a history of recent corticosteroid withdrawal should be protected by means of supplementary corticosteroid therapy as described under Precautions, below.

◊ The UK Committee on Safety of Medicines recommends that moderate dosage with corticosteroids (up to 40 mg daily of prednisolone, or equivalent), for up to 3 weeks, may be stopped without tapering provided that the original disease is unlikely to relapse, although prophylactic cover may be required for any stress within a week of finishing the course.[1] However, it should be borne in mind that individuals vary widely in their response to corticosteroids and their ability to tolerate withdrawal. Gradual withdrawal should be considered, even after shorter courses, if higher doses are given, or in patients with other risk factors for adrenocortical insufficiency, including those who have had repeated courses of systemic corticosteroids, those who receive a course within one year of finishing long-term corticosteroid therapy, or those who regularly take doses in the evening, when their suppressive effect is greater. Withdrawal should not be abrupt in any patient who receives systemic corticosteroids for more than 3 weeks.[1]

How dose reduction is carried out depends largely on the likelihood of relapse of the original disease. If this is unlikely, the dose of systemic corticosteroid may be reduced rapidly to physiological values (traditionally considered to be 7.5 mg of prednisolone daily or equivalent). It should then be reduced more slowly to allow the hypothalamic-pituitary-adrenal axis to recover.[1] Where disease relapse is a possibility even the initial reduction may need to be more cautious. Long-term treatment may require withdrawal over many months (such as a reduction of 1 mg in the daily dose of prednisolone every 3 to 4 weeks).

In reviews of the inhibition of hypothalamic-pituitary-adrenocortical function associated with corticosteroid administration, further regimens for corticosteroid withdrawal are described.[2-4] For example, patients who have been treated for weeks or months may have their daily dose of prednisolone reduced by 2.5 to 5 mg every 2 or 3 days, or, for those on longer-term treatment, the reduction may be more gradual at a rate of 2.5 mg every 1 to 3 weeks and possibly less. When the dose has reached 10 mg daily decrements may be made with 1-mg tablets. Another approach may be to convert daily therapy gradually into alternate-day therapy by progressively reducing the amount of corticosteroid received on every second day, and once alternate-day therapy is established the dose may be further reduced until, for example, a dose of 1 mg on alternate days for one week is attained.


1. Committee on Safety of Medicines/Medicines Control Agency. Withdrawal of systemic corticosteroids. *Current Problems* 1998; **24:** 5–7. Also available at: http://www.mca.gov.uk/ourwork/monitorsafequalmed/currentproblems/volume24may.htm (accessed 27/04/04)
2. Anonymous. Corticosteroids and hypothalamic-pituitary-adrenocortical function. *BMJ* 1980; **280:** 813–14.
3. Helfer EL, Rose LI. Corticosteroids and adrenal suppression: characterising and avoiding the problem. *Drugs* 1989; **38:** 838–45.
4. Page RC. How to wean a patient off corticosteroids. *Prescribers' J* 1997; **37:** 11–16.


## Precautions for Corticosteroids

Systemic corticosteroids should be used with great caution in the presence of heart failure, recent myocardial infarction, or hypertension, in patients with diabetes mellitus, epilepsy (but see below for use in infantile seizures), glaucoma, hypothyroidism, hepatic failure, osteoporosis, peptic ulceration, psychoses or severe affective disorders, and renal impairment. Children may be at increased risk of some adverse effects; in addition, corticosteroids may cause growth retardation, and prolonged administration is rarely justified. The elderly too may be at greater risk from adverse effects.

Corticosteroids are usually contra-indicated in the presence of acute infections uncontrolled by appropriate antimicrobial therapy. Similarly, patients already receiving corticosteroids are more susceptible to infection, the symptoms of which, moreover, may be masked until an advanced stage has been reached. Patients with active or doubtfully quiescent tuberculosis should not be given corticosteroids except, very rarely, as adjuncts to treatment with antitubercular drugs. Patients with quiescent tuberculosis should be observed closely and should receive chemoprophylaxis if corticosteroid therapy is prolonged.

The risks of chickenpox and probably of severe herpes zoster are increased in non-immune patients receiving therapeutic doses of systemic corticosteroids, and patients should avoid close personal contact with either infection. Passive immunisation is recommended for non-immune patients who do come into contact with chickenpox. Similar precautions apply to measles. Live vaccines should not be given to patients receiving high-dose systemic corticosteroid therapy nor for at least 3 months afterwards; killed vaccines or toxoids may be given although the response may be attenuated.

During prolonged courses of corticosteroid therapy, patients should be examined regularly. Sodium intake may need to be reduced and calcium and potassium supplements may be necessary. Monitoring of the fluid intake and output, and daily weight records may give early warning of fluid retention. Back pain may signify osteoporosis. Children are at special risk from raised intracranial pressure. Patients should carry cards (and preferably also wear bracelets) giving full details of their corticosteroid therapy; they and their relatives should be fully conversant with the implications of their therapy and the precautions to be taken.

Measures to compensate for the adrenals' inability to respond to stress (see Withdrawal, above) include increasing the dose to cover minor intercurrent illnesses or trauma such as surgery (with intramuscular administration to cover vomiting). For details of dosages used, see Uses and Administration, below.

Rapid intravenous injection of massive doses of corticosteroids may sometimes cause cardiovascular collapse and injections should therefore be given slowly or by infusion.

Many drugs have been reported to interfere with certain assay procedures for corticosteroids in body fluids and corticosteroids themselves may interfere with or alter the results of assays for some endogenous substances or drugs.

The risk of systemic absorption should always be considered when applying corticosteroids topically. They should not be applied with an occlusive dressing to large areas of the body. Long-term topical use is best avoided, especially in children. Also they should not be used for the treatment of ulcerative conditions, nor of rosacea, and should not be used indiscriminately for pruritus. Occasionally they may be used with the addition of a suitable antimicrobial substance in the treatment of infected skin but there is a risk of sensitivity reactions occurring.

Height should be monitored in children receiving prolonged therapy with inhaled or nasal corticosteroids. High doses of inhaled corticosteroids should preferably be inhaled using large-volume spacer devices to reduce oropharyngeal deposition and hence the incidence of candidiasis; rinsing the mouth with water after inhalation may also be helpful. In addition the use of spacer devices may reduce systemic absorption (see also Inhalation Therapy, under Uses and Administration, below). Paradoxical bronchospasm has occurred with inhaled corticosteroids and may require discontinuation of therapy, although if mild it may be prevented by inhalation of a beta$_2$ adrenoceptor agonist, or by transfer from an aerosol to a dry powder formulation.

Caution is required when corticosteroids are used locally to treat eye disorders (see below).

**Contraception.** There are some isolated case reports of contraceptive failure in women using intra-uterine devices and receiving corticosteroid therapy.[1-3]


1. Zerner J, *et al.* Failure of an intrauterine device concurrent with administration of corticosteroids. *Fertil Steril* 1976; **27:** 1467–8.
2. Inkeles DM, Hansen RI. Unexpected pregnancy in a woman using an intrauterine device and receiving steroid therapy. *Ann Ophthalmol* 1982; **14:** 975.
3. Buhler M, Papiernik E. Successive pregnancies in women fitted with intrauterine devices who take anti-inflammatory drugs. *Lancet* 1983; **i:** 483.


**Eye disorders.** Topical corticosteroids have transformed the management of inflammatory disease of the anterior segment of the eye and it should be noted that while their proper use may be sight-saving their inappropriate use is potentially blinding.[1] The dangers include the conversion of a simple dendritic herpes simplex epithelial lesion into an extensive amoeboid ulcer with the likelihood of permanent corneal scarring and loss of vision and also the risk of potentiation of bacterial and fungal infections. Other dangers include the development of open-angle glaucoma and cataracts. Topical corticosteroids are used by ophthalmologists in herpes simplex keratitis but always under appropriate antiviral cover and their use requires considerable experience. They should never be given for an undiagnosed red eye and many consultant ophthalmic surgeons believe that general practitioners should never initiate therapy without an ophthalmic opinion.

Further studies and discussions on the inappropriate use of corticosteroids to treat eye disorders are listed below.[2-10]


1. St Clair Roberts D. Steroids, the eye, and general practitioners. *BMJ* 1986; **292:** 1414–15.
2. Lavin MJ, Rose GE. Use of steroid eye drops in general practice. *BMJ* 1986; **292:** 1448–50.
3. Claoué CMP, Stevenson KE. Incidence of inappropriate treatment of herpes simplex keratitis with topical steroids. *BMJ* 1986; **292:** 1450–1.
4. Livingstone A. Steroids, the eye, and general practitioners. *BMJ* 1986; **292:** 1737.
5. Lawrence M. Steroids, the eye, and general practitioners. *BMJ* 1986; **292:** 1737–8.
6. Trevor-Roper P. Steroids, the eye, and general practitioners. *BMJ* 1986; **292:** 1738.
7. Jay B. Steroids, the eye, and general practitioners. *BMJ* 1986; **293:** 205.
8. Rose GE, Lavin MJ. Steroids, the eye, and general practitioners. *BMJ* 1986; **293:** 205.
9. O'Day DM. Corticosteroids: an unresolved debate. *Ophthalmology* 1991; **98:** 845–6.
10. Stern GA, Buttross M. Use of corticosteroids in combination with antimicrobial drugs in the treatment of infectious corneal disease. *Ophthalmology* 1991; **98:** 847–53.


**Intranasal administration.** There have been cases of Cushing's syndrome associated with inappropriately prolonged use of corticosteroid nasal drops in children.[1,2] Such drops should not be prescribed on a repeat prescription basis; where treatment is contemplated for more than 6 weeks appropriate monitoring has been recommended. See also Adrenal Suppression, under Adverse Effects, above.


1. Findlay CA, *et al.* Childhood Cushing's syndrome induced by betamethasone nose drops, and repeat prescriptions. *BMJ* 1998; **317:** 739–40.
2. Perry RJ, *et al.* Cushing's syndrome, growth impairment, and occult adrenal suppression associated with intranasal steroids. *Arch Dis Child* 2002; **87:** 45–8.


**Porphyria.** Corticosteroids are generally considered to be safe in patients with porphyria although there is conflicting evidence of porphyrinogenicity. In a review[1] of drug-induced porphyrias it was noted that a report suggesting that corticosteroids may have a role in treating the acute attack together with many reports attesting to their safety, contrasted with their repeated incrimination as the offending agent in producing such episodes. It was considered that as corticosteroids may be life-saving, they should be used if really indicated.


1. Moore MR, Disler PB. Drug-induction of the acute porphyrias. *Adverse Drug React Acute Poisoning Rev* 1983; **2:** 149–89.


**Pregnancy.** Studies have shown that corticosteroid use in pregnant women did not have adverse effects on the fetus in terms of psychological development[1] or growth and general health factors.[2] However, there has been an isolated report[3] wherein the topical administration of triamcinolone to a pregnant woman for treatment of eczema was considered to have caused fetal growth retardation. In another study[4] of 11 women with placenta praevia given intramuscular betamethasone 12 mg repeated 24 hours later, there were 2 cases of constriction of the ductus arteriosus; neither case was severe.

Early studies in *animals* demonstrated an increase in fetal cleft palate following maternal ingestion of high corticosteroid doses, and cortisone has been used widely as a tool for the investigation of mechanisms responsible for cleft lip and palate. With doses used in clinical practice, however, the risk appears to be low. In an analysis of several hundred cases reported in the literature[5] it was concluded that the incidence of cleft palate in exposed children was slightly higher than in a random sample, but that in the small selected group studied, this higher incidence might be fallacious. Although an increased incidence of malformations in the children of asthmatic mothers given prednisolone 2.5 to 30 mg daily during pregnancy was noted,[6] others[7] have suggested that the outcome might have been worse in untreated asthmatic mothers. Moreover, no significant increase in the risk of fetal or maternal complications was found in a study of asthmatic mothers given prednisolone 2.5 to 20 mg daily.[8] Subsequently, no evidence of a teratogenic effect for corticosteroids was noted in a comparison of the maternal drug histories of the mothers of 764 infants born with anomalies of the CNS and 764 controls,[9] and in another study[10] there were no striking differences in birthweight and frequency of 'small for dates' infants born to mothers who received systemic corticosteroids during pregnancy for pemphigoid gestationis and those who did not.

Fears concerning the use of corticosteroids during late pregnancy relate to their direct adverse effects on the fetus. These involve the known side-effects of corticosteroids, such as increased risk of infection and adrenal insufficiency. No such adverse effects were noted in the infants of 70 exposed pregnancies,[8] although there have been individual reports.[11,12] The potential dangers of maternal diabetogenic effects have been demonstrated in a study of metabolic changes induced in diabetic women by salbutamol (used in the prevention of premature labour) which could be exacerbated by concomitant use of dexamethasone (to promote maturation of the fetal lung) with consequent danger to the fetus.[13]

A review[14] by the UK Committee on Safety of Medicines concluded that there was no convincing evidence that corticosteroids caused an increased incidence of congenital abnormality. Prolonged or repeated use during pregnancy did increase the risk of intra-uterine growth retardation but this did not seem to be a problem following short-term treatment. It was noted that the ability of different corticosteroids to cross the placenta varied very markedly.


1. Schmand B, *et al.* Psychological development of children who were treated antenatally with corticosteroids to prevent respiratory distress syndrome. *Pediatrics* 1990; **86:** 58–64.
2. Doyle LW, *et al.* Antenatal steroid therapy and 5-year outcome of extremely low birth weight infants. *Obstet Gynecol* 1989; **73:** 743–6.
3. Katz VL, *et al.* Severe symmetric intrauterine growth retardation associated with the topical use of triamcinolone. *Am J Obstet Gynecol* 1990; **162:** 396–7.
4. Wasserstrum N, *et al.* Betamethasone and the human fetal ductus arteriosus. *Obstet Gynecol* 1989; **74:** 897–900.
5. Popert AJ. Pregnancy and adrenocortical hormones: some aspects of their interaction in rheumatic diseases. *BMJ* 1962; **1:** 967–72.
6. Warrell DW, Taylor R. Outcome for the foetus of mothers receiving prednisolone during pregnancy. *Lancet* 1968; **i:** 117–18.
7. Scott JK. Foetal risk with maternal prednisolone. *Lancet* 1968; **i:** 208.
8. Schatz M, *et al.* Corticosteroid therapy for the pregnant asthmatic patient. *JAMA* 1975; **233:** 804–7.
9. Winship KA, *et al.* Maternal drug histories and central nervous system anomalies. *Arch Dis Child* 1984; **59:** 1052–60.
10. Holmes RC, Black MM. The fetal prognosis in pemphigoid gestationis (herpes gestationis). *Br J Dermatol* 1984; **110:** 67–72.
11. Grajwer LA, *et al.* Neonatal subclinical adrenal insufficiency: result of maternal steroid therapy. *JAMA* 1977; **238:** 1279–80.
12. Evans TJ, *et al.* Congenital cytomegalovirus infection after maternal renal transplantation. *Lancet* 1975; **i:** 1359–60.
13. Gündoğdu AS, *et al.* Comparison of hormonal and metabolic effects of salbutamol infusion in normal subjects and insulin-requiring diabetics. *Lancet* 1979; **ii:** 1317–21.
14. Committee on Safety of Medicines/Medicines Control Agency. Systemic corticosteroids in pregnancy and lactation. *Current Problems* 1998; **24:** 9. Also available at: http://www.mca.gov.uk/ourwork/monitorsafequalmed/currentproblems/volume24may.htm (accessed 27/04/04)


**Septic shock.** Some manufacturers recommend that corticosteroids should not be given to patients with septic shock and references to the controversial use of high-dose corticosteroids are given under Septic Shock, in Uses and Administration, below.

**Sickle-cell disease.** Sickle-cell crisis was reported to have been precipitated by corticosteroids in 2 patients with sickle C disease.[1] The crises in these patients were considered to have started with ischaemic necrosis of the bone marrow leading to fat embolism, cerebral hypoxia, and coma.

For mention of the use of corticosteroids in sickle-cell crisis, see under Sickle-cell Disease, in Uses and Administration, below.


1. Huang JC, *et al.* Sickling crisis, fat embolism, and coma after steroids. *Lancet* 1994; **344:** 951–2.


**Tooth erosion.** The increased incidence of tooth erosion seen in patients with asthma might be related to the pH of inhaled powder (but not aerosol) formulations.[1] Beclometasone dipropionate and fluticasone had pHs of 4.76 as powder formulations, whereas the pHs of the aerosols were well above the pH of 5.5 at which tooth substance begins to dissolve. Budesonide was less acidic in its powder formulation (pH 6.47).


1. O'Sullivan EA, Curzon MEJ. Drug treatments for asthma may cause erosive tooth damage. *BMJ* 1998; **317:** 820.


**Varicella.** A number of cases of fatal or near fatal chickenpox have been reported in patients receiving corticosteroids.[1-3] Although mostly associated with systemic use, severe disseminated varicella and staphylococcal pericarditis have been reported in an infant following a single application of a potent topical corticosteroid cream.[4] Guidelines issued by the UK Committee on Safety of Medicines (CSM) state that all patients taking systemic corticosteroids for purposes other than replacement, and who have not had chickenpox, should be regarded as being at risk of severe chickenpox, irrespective of the dose or duration of treatment.[2,5] Passive immunisation with varicella-zoster immunoglobulin should be given to non-immune patients who are receiving corticosteroids, or who have received them within the last 3 months, if they are exposed to chickenpox. Passive immunisation should preferably be given within 3 days and not later than 10 days from exposure.[2] The CSM considered that there was no good evidence that topical, inhaled, or rectal corticosteroids were associated with an increased risk of severe chickenpox.


1. Rice P, *et al.* Near fatal chickenpox during prednisolone treatment. *BMJ* 1994; **309:** 1069–70.
2. Committee on Safety of Medicines/Medicines Control Agency. Severe chickenpox associated with systemic corticosteroids. *Current Problems* 1994; **20:** 1–2.
3. Dowell SF, Breese JS. Severe varicella associated with steroid use. *Pediatrics* 1993; **92:** 223–8.
4. Brumund MR, *et al.* Disseminated varicella and staphylococcal pericarditis after topical steroids. *J Pediatr* 1997; **131:** 162–3.
5. Ellender D, *et al.* Severe chickenpox during treatment with corticosteroids. *BMJ* 1995; **310:** 327.


## Interactions of Corticosteroids

Concurrent use of barbiturates, carbamazepine, phenytoin, primidone, or rifampicin may enhance the metabolism and reduce the effects of systemic corticosteroids. Conversely oral contraceptives or ritonavir may increase plasma concentrations of corticosteroids. Use of corticosteroids with potassium-depleting diuretics, such as thiazides or furosemide, may cause excessive potassium loss. There is also an increased risk of hypokalaemia with concurrent amphotericin B or bronchodilator therapy with xanthines or beta$_2$ agonists. There may be an increased incidence of gastrointestinal bleeding and ulceration when corticosteroids are given with NSAIDs. Response to anticoagulants may be altered by corticosteroids and requirements of antidiabetic drugs and antihypertensives may be increased. Corticosteroids may decrease serum concentrations of salicylates and may decrease the effect of anticholinesterases in myasthenia gravis.

**Analgesics.** For the effect of corticosteroids on *salicylates,* see Aspirin, Interactions, p.17.

**Antibacterials.** *Rifampicin* reduces the activity of corticosteroids[1-8] by accelerating their metabolism, and a similar effect would be expected with other rifamycins. There is limited evidence that the macrolide antibacterials *troleandomycin,*[9-11] and perhaps *erythromycin,*[12] may inhibit the metabolism of methylprednisolone, but not of prednisolone.[10] Dosage reduction should be made as necessary if troleandomycin and methylprednisolone are used concurrently. There is no evidence of a clinically significant interaction between these macrolides and other corticosteroids.

For reference to corticosteroids lowering plasma concentrations of *isoniazid* and enhancing its renal clearance, see p.223.


1. Edwards OM, *et al.* Changes in cortisol metabolism following rifampicin therapy. *Lancet* 1974; **ii:** 549–51.
2. Maisey DN, *et al.* Rifampicin and cortisone replacement therapy. *Lancet* 1974; **ii:** 896–7.
3. Steenbergen GJ, Pfaltzgraff RE. Treatment of neuritis in borderline leprosy with rifampicin and corticosteroids—a pilot trial. *Lepr Rev* 1975; **46:** 115–18.
4. Buffington GA, *et al.* Interaction of rifampin and glucocorticoids: adverse effect on renal allograft function. *JAMA* 1976; **236:** 1958–60.
5. Hendrickse W, *et al.* Rifampicin-induced non-responsiveness to corticosteroid treatment in nephrotic syndrome. *BMJ* 1979; **1:** 306.
6. van Marle W, *et al.* Concurrent steroid and rifampicin therapy. *BMJ* 1979; **1:** 1020.
7. Jopline WH, Pettit JHS. Interaction between rifampicin, steroids and oral contraceptives. *Lepr Rev* 1979; **50:** 331–2.
8. McAllister WAC, *et al.* Rifampicin reduces effectiveness and bioavailability of prednisolone. *BMJ* 1983; **286:** 923–5.
9. Szefler SJ, *et al.* The effect of troleandomycin on methylprednisolone elimination. *J Allergy Clin Immunol* 1980; **66:** 447–51.
10. Szefler SJ, *et al.* Steroid-specific and anticonvulsant interaction aspects of troleandomycin-steroid therapy. *J Allergy Clin Immunol* 1982; **69:** 455–60.
11. Kamada AK, *et al.* Glucocorticoid reduction with troleandomycin in chronic severe asthmatic children: implication for future trials and clinical application. *J Allergy Clin Immunol* 1992; **89:** 285.
12. LaForce CF, *et al.* Inhibition of methylprednisolone elimination in the presence of erythromycin therapy. *J Allergy Clin Immunol* 1983; **72:** 34–9.


**Anticoagulants.** For the various effects of corticosteroids on anticoagulants, see under Warfarin Sodium, p.1026.

**Antiepileptics.** Reduced efficacy of corticosteroids has been noted in asthmatic, arthritic, renal transplant, and other patients who also received *phenytoin* or *phenobarbital,*[1-3] and the clearance of corticosteroids has also been reported to be markedly increased by *carbamazepine.*[3] Induction of microsomal liver enzymes by the antiepileptic, resulting in enhanced metabolism of the corticosteroid is believed to be the underlying mechanism. Different corticosteroids appear to be affected to different degrees, but the disease state, doses, and other determinants such as diet, sex, and other drugs used may also be contributory factors. An increase in the dosage of the corticosteroids may be necessary in order to maintain the desired therapeutic response.[1]


1. Brooks SM, *et al.* Adverse effects of phenobarbital on corticosteroid metabolism in patients with bronchial asthma. *N Engl J Med* 1972; **286:** 1125–8.
2. Nation RL, *et al.* Pharmacokinetic drug interactions with phenytoin (part II). *Clin Pharmacokinet* 1990; **18:** 131–50.
3. Bartoszek M, *et al.* Prednisolone and methylprednisolone kinetics in children receiving anticonvulsant therapy. *Clin Pharmacol Ther* 1987; **42:** 424–32.


**Antifungals.** *Ketoconazole*[1,2] and *itraconazole*[3,4] increase serum-methylprednisolone concentrations and enhance methylprednisolone's adrenal suppressive effects. A 50% reduction in intravenous methylprednisolone dose was suggested during ketoconazole therapy.[2] A similar effect was not evident with oral prednisone[4,5] although some workers[6] found that ketoconazole reduced the total clearance of prednisolone given intravenously and of prednisone given by mouth. Itraconazole can also reduce the clearance of dexamethasone; in a study[7] of 8 healthy subjects, the area under the concentration-time curve (AUC) for both intravenous and oral dexamethasone was increased about 3.5-fold, and the morning plasma-cortisol concentration was suppressed for at least 2 days longer. A study[8] of healthy subjects found that ketoconazole increased the AUC for oral budesonide more than sixfold when they were given together, but only about fourfold when the doses were given 12 hours apart. Systemic exposure to inhaled budesonide is increased by itraconazole, which probably reduces the metabolism of budesonide.[9] Adrenal suppression was found in 11 of 25 patients with cystic fibrosis who were treated with this combination; one patient developed Cushing's syndrome.[10] A similar interaction may have been the cause of significant adrenal suppression in a patient with cystic fibrosis who was treated with itraconazole and inhaled fluticasone propionate.[11]


1. Glynn AM, *et al.* Effects of ketoconazole on methylprednisolone pharmacokinetics and cortisol secretion. *Clin Pharmacol Ther* 1986; **39:** 654–9.
2. Kandrotas RJ, *et al.* Ketoconazole effects on methylprednisolone disposition and their joint suppression of endogenous cortisol. *Clin Pharmacol Ther* 1987; **42:** 465–70.
3. Varis T, *et al.* Plasma concentrations and effects of oral methylprednisolone are considerably increased by itraconazole. *Clin Pharmacol Ther* 1998; **64:** 363–8.
4. Lebrun-Vignes B, *et al.* Effect of itraconazole on the pharmacokinetics of prednisolone and methylprednisolone and cortisol secretion in healthy subjects. *Br J Clin Pharmacol* 2001; **51:** 443–50.
5. Ludwig EA, *et al.* Steroid-specific effects of ketoconazole on corticosteroid disposition: unaltered prednisolone elimination. *DICP Ann Pharmacother* 1989; **23:** 858–61.
6. Zürcher RM, *et al.* Impact of ketoconazole on the metabolism of prednisolone. *Clin Pharmacol Ther* 1989; **45:** 366–72.
7. Varis T, *et al.* The cytochrome P450 3A4 inhibitor itraconazole markedly increases the plasma concentrations of dexamethasone and enhances its adrenal-suppressant effect. *Clin Pharmacol Ther* 2000; **68:** 487–94.
8. Seidegård J. Reduction of the inhibitory effect of ketoconazole on budesonide pharmacokinetics by separation of their time of administration. *Clin Pharmacol Ther* 2000; **68:** 13–17.
9. Raaska K, *et al.* Plasma concentrations of inhaled budesonide and its effects on plasma cortisol are increased by the cytochrome P4503A4 inhibitor itraconazole. *Clin Pharmacol Ther* 2002; **72:** 362–9.
10. Skov M, *et al.* Iatrogenic adrenal insufficiency as a side-effect of combined treatment of itraconazole and budesonide. *Eur Respir J* 2002; **20:** 127–33.
11. Parmar JS, *et al.* Profound adrenal suppression secondary to treatment with low dose inhaled steroids and itraconazole in allergic bronchopulmonary aspergillosis in cystic fibrosis. *Thorax* 2002; **57:** 749–50.


**Antineoplastics.** For reference to single doses of prednisone inhibiting the activation of *cyclophosphamide* (but longer-term treatment increasing its activation), see Cyclophosphamide, p.541.

**Antivirals.** For a possible effect of corticosteroids on the metabolism of HIV-protease inhibitors, see p.639.

*Ritonavir* can greatly increase plasma concentrations of fluticasone, through inhibition of cytochrome P450 isoenzyme CYP3A4, leading to systemic corticosteroid effects including Cushing's syndrome and adrenal suppression.[1]


1. GlaxoSmithKline, Canada. Important safety information regarding a drug interaction between fluticasone propionate (Flonase®/Flovent®/Advair®) and ritonavir (Norvir®/Kaletra®), 22 January 2004. Available at: http://www.hc-sc.gc.ca/hpfb-dgpsa/tpd-dpt/fluticasone_propionate-ritonavir_hpc_e.html (accessed 04/02/04)


**Calcium-channel blockers.** Studies in healthy subjects have found that *diltiazem* reduces the clearance of methylprednisolone.[1,2]


1. Varis T, *et al.* Diltiazem and mibefradil increase the plasma concentrations and greatly enhance the adrenal-suppressant effect of oral methylprednisolone. *Clin Pharmacol Ther* 2000; **67:** 215–21.
2. Booker BM, *et al.* Pharmacokinetic and pharmacodynamic interactions between diltiazem and methylprednisolone in healthy volunteers. *Clin Pharmacol Ther* 2002; **72:** 370–82.


**Gastrointestinal drugs.** *Aprepitant* increased plasma concentrations of dexamethasone and methylprednisolone in a pharmacokinetic study.[1] The manufacturers of aprepitant recommend that the usual dose of oral dexamethasone be reduced by 50%, and the dose of methylprednisolone by approximately 25% when given intravenously, and by 50% when given orally. For the appropriate regimen when these drugs are given together for nausea and vomiting, see p.1251.


1. McCrea JB, *et al.* Effects of the neurokinin$_1$ receptor antagonist aprepitant on the pharmacokinetics of dexamethasone and methylprednisolone. *Clin Pharmacol Ther* 2003; **74:** 17–24.


**Immunosuppressants.** It has been suggested that mutual inhibition of metabolism occurs between *ciclosporin* and corticosteroids, and may increase the plasma concentrations of either drug.[1,2] A review[3] cited studies supporting this conclusion but also mentioned studies that showed that ciclosporin did not significantly decrease clearance of prednisolone[4] and that corticosteroids either did not change, or decreased, ciclosporin concentrations.[5,6] Some of these conflicting results may be due to differences in the methods used to measure ciclosporin concentrations.


1. Ost L. Effects of cyclosporin on prednisolone metabolism. *Lancet* 1984; **i:** 451.
2. Klintmalm G, Säwe J. High dose methylprednisolone increases plasma cyclosporin levels in renal transplant recipients. *Lancet* 1984; **i:** 731.

3. Yee GC, McGuire TR. Pharmacokinetic drug interactions with cyclosporin (part II). *Clin Pharmacokinet* 1990; **19:** 400–15.
4. Frey FJ, *et al.* Evidence that cyclosporine does not affect the metabolism of prednisolone after renal transplantation. *Transplantation* 1987; **43:** 494–8.
5. Ptachcinski RJ, *et al.* Cyclosporine - high-dose steroid interaction in renal transplant recipients: assessment by HPLC. *Transplant Proc* 1987; **19:** 1728–9.
6. Hricik DE, *et al.* Association of the absence of steroid therapy with increased cyclosporine blood levels in renal transplant recipients. *Transplantation* 1990; **49:** 221–3.

**Leukotriene antagonists.** Severe peripheral oedema occurred in a patient treated with *montelukast* and prednisone for asthma, but not when either drug was used alone.[1] Montelukast may have potentiated sodium and fluid retention caused by the corticosteroid.

1. Geller M. Marked peripheral edema associated with montelukast and prednisone. *Ann Intern Med* 2000; **132:** 924.

**Lipid regulating drugs.** Giving *colestipol* to a patient with hypopituitarism taking oral hydrocortisone maintenance therapy resulted in headaches, ataxia, and lethargy.[1] Mental status returned to normal within hours of an intravenous dose of hydrocortisone 100 mg, and colestipol was subsequently withdrawn uneventfully.

1. Nekl KE, Aron DC. Hydrocortisone-colestipol interaction. *Ann Pharmacother* 1993; **27:** 980–1.

**Neuromuscular blockers.** For reference to corticosteroids antagonising the effects of *competitive neuromuscular blockers*, see under Atracurium, p.1401.

**Sex hormones.** There have been reviews[1,2] discussing several reports of an enhanced effect of corticosteroids in women also receiving *oestrogens* or *oral contraceptives* and commenting that the dose of corticosteroids in some cases may need to be reduced. There is some evidence that budesonide may be less affected by concurrent use of oral contraceptives than prednisolone.[3]

1. Shenfield GM. Drug interactions with oral contraceptive preparations. *Med J Aust* 1986; **144:** 205–10.
2. Back DJ, Orme ML'E. Pharmacokinetic drug interactions with oral contraceptives. *Clin Pharmacokinet* 1990; **18:** 472–84.
3. Seidegård J, *et al.* Effect of an oral contraceptive on the plasma levels of budesonide and prednisolone and the influence on plasma cortisol. *Clin Pharmacol Ther* 2000; **67:** 373–81.

**Smoking.** There was a report of an appreciable and consistent increase in plasma corticosteroids after cigarette smoking.[1] However, a review concerning the clinical importance of smoking and drug interactions[2] concluded that in the majority of examples, including corticosteroids, there was little evidence of a recognisable hazard from the interaction.

1. Kershbaum A, *et al.* Effect of smoking and nicotine on adrenocortical secretion. *JAMA* 1968; **203:** 275–8.
2. D'Arcy PF. Tobacco smoking and drugs: a clinically important interaction? *Drug Intell Clin Pharm* 1984; **18:** 302–7.

**Sympathomimetics.** Studies in 21 asthmatic patients suggested that the plasma half-life of dexamethasone was decreased by *ephedrine*.[1] More importantly use of corticosteroids with *beta*$_2$ *agonists* may potentiate any hypokalaemic effects.[2]

1. Brooks SM, *et al.* The effects of ephedrine and theophylline on dexamethasone metabolism in bronchial asthma. *J Clin Pharmacol* 1977; **17:** 308–18.
2. Committee on Safety of Medicines. $\beta_2$ agonists, xanthines and hypokalaemia. *Current Problems 28* 1990.

**Thalidomide.** In a double-blind crossover study of thalidomide in the treatment of severe chronic erythema nodosum leprosum,[1] the dose of prednisolone necessary to suppress symptoms was considerably reduced in 9 of 10 patients while they were receiving thalidomide; there has been a comment[2] that prednisolone should not be given with thalidomide.

For reference to a possible interaction between thalidomide and dexamethasone, see Effects on the Skin under Adverse Effects of Thalidomide, p.1753.

1. Waters MFR. An internally-controlled double blind trial of thalidomide in severe erythema nodosum leprosum. *Lepr Rev* 1971; **42:** 26–42.
2. WHO, Regional Office for the Western Pacific. Final report on the first regional working group on leprosy, Manila, Philippines, 7–12 December, 1978. *Lepr Rev* 1979; **50:** 326–9.

**Xanthines.** For the effect of corticosteroids on *theophylline*, see p.802.

## Pharmacokinetics of Corticosteroids

Corticosteroids are, in general, readily absorbed from the gastrointestinal tract. They are also absorbed from sites of local administration. When used topically, particularly under an occlusive dressing or when the skin is broken, or as a rectal enema, sufficient corticosteroid may be absorbed to give systemic effects; this is also a possibility with other local routes of administration such as inhalation. Water-soluble forms of corticosteroids are given by intravenous injection for a rapid response; more prolonged effects are achieved using lipid-soluble forms of corticosteroids by intramuscular injection.

Corticosteroids are rapidly distributed to all body tissues. They cross the placenta to varying degrees and may be distributed in small amounts into breast milk. Most corticosteroids in the circulation are extensively bound to plasma proteins, mainly to globulin and less so to albumin. The corticosteroid-binding globulin (transcortin) has high affinity but low binding capacity, while albumin has low affinity but large binding capacity. The synthetic corticosteroids are less extensively protein bound than hydrocortisone (cortisol). They also tend to have longer half-lives.

Corticosteroids are metabolised mainly in the liver but also in other tissues, and are excreted in the urine. The slower metabolism of the synthetic corticosteroids with their lower protein-binding affinity may account for their increased potency compared with the natural corticosteroids.

◊ Reviews.

1. Begg EJ, *et al.* The pharmacokinetics of corticosteroid agents. *Med J Aust* 1987; **146:** 37–41.
2. McGhee CNJ. Pharmacokinetics of ophthalmic corticosteroids. *Br J Ophthalmol* 1992; **76:** 681–4.
3. Jusko WJ. Pharmacokinetics and receptor-mediated pharmacodynamics of corticosteroids. *Toxicology* 1995; **102:** 189–96.
4. Derendorf H, *et al.* Pharmacokinetics and pharmacodynamics of inhaled corticosteroids. *J Allergy Clin Immunol* 1998; **101** (suppl 2): S440–6.

## Uses and Administration of Corticosteroids

The corticosteroids are used in physiological doses for replacement therapy in adrenal insufficiency. Pharmacological doses are used when palliative anti-inflammatory or immunosuppressant effects are required. Before instituting therapy the benefits and risks of corticosteroids should be considered; where appropriate, local rather than systemic therapy should be used. The lowest effective dose should be used for the shortest possible time; high doses may be needed for life-threatening situations.

The effects of different corticosteroids vary qualitatively as well as quantitatively, and it may not be possible to substitute one for another in equal therapeutic amounts without provoking side-effects. Thus, whereas cortisone and hydrocortisone have very appreciable mineralocorticoid (or sodium-retaining) properties relative to their glucocorticoid (or anti-inflammatory) properties, prednisolone and prednisone have considerably less, and others, such as betamethasone and dexamethasone, have none or virtually none. In contrast, the mineralocorticoid properties of fludrocortisone are so pronounced that its glucocorticoid effects are considered to have no clinical significance.

As a rough guide, the approximate **equivalent doses** of the main corticosteroids in terms of their glucocorticoid (or anti-inflammatory) properties alone, are:

- betamethasone 0.75 mg
- cortisone acetate 25 mg
- dexamethasone 0.75 mg
- hydrocortisone 20 mg
- methylprednisolone 4 mg
- prednisolone 5 mg
- prednisone 5 mg
- triamcinolone 4 mg

The mineralocorticoid properties of corticosteroids (see p.1068) are rarely used. Exceptions include the treatment of primary adrenocortical insufficiency, in which both mineralocorticoid and glucocorticoid replacement is necessary, usually in the form of fludrocortisone with hydrocortisone (for details, see p.1075). The mineralocorticoid properties of fludrocortisone are also used to maintain blood pressure in patients with orthostatic hypotension (see p.1100).

The anti-inflammatory and immunosuppressant glucocorticoid properties of corticosteroids (see p.1068) are used to suppress the clinical manifestations of disease in a wide range of disorders considered to have inflammatory or immunological components. For these purposes, the synthetic analogues with their considerably reduced mineralocorticoid properties linked with enhanced glucocorticoid properties, are preferred. Despite the existence of very powerful synthetic glucocorticoids with virtually no mineralocorticoid activity, the hazards of inappropriately high glucocorticoid therapy are such that the less powerful prednisolone and prednisone are the glucocorticoids of choice for most conditions, since they allow for a greater margin of safety. There is little to choose between prednisolone and prednisone; prednisolone is usually recommended in the UK since it exists in a metabolically active form, whereas prednisone is inactive and must be converted into its active form by the liver; hence, particularly in some liver disorders, bioavailability of prednisone is less reliable (but see under Precautions of Prednisolone, p.1108).

Because the therapeutic effects of corticosteroids seem to be of longer duration than the metabolic effects, intermittent treatment with corticosteroids has been used to allow the metabolic rhythm of the body to become re-established while maintaining the therapeutic effects. Regimens of intermittent therapy have usually consisted of short courses of treatment or of the use of single doses on alternate days. Such alternate-day therapy, however, is only appropriate for corticosteroids with a relatively short duration of action and small mineralocorticoid effect, such as prednisolone, and only in certain disease states. Corticosteroids are also given in single daily doses at times coinciding with maximum or minimum output of the adrenal cortex in order to obtain the desired effect on the adrenals (see Administration, below).

Doses of corticosteroids higher than those required for physiological replacement will eventually lead to some degree of adrenal suppression, the extent depending on the dose given, and the route, frequency, time, and duration of administration. The adrenal glands are traditionally considered to have a daily output equivalent to about 20 mg of hydrocortisone (cortisol), but individual blood-cortisol concentrations may vary widely, and can increase up to tenfold or more during stress. Therefore, during periods of stress or trauma, such as during and after surgery and when suffering from infections, the corticosteroid dosage of patients must be increased. In patients on long-term corticosteroid therapy undergoing surgery this is usually provided by parenteral hydrocortisone; graduated regimens tailored to the severity of surgery (see p.1104) are now preferred to the former high-dose standard regimens tapered over 5 days, whose use has been questioned (see Surgery, under Administration, below).

Although the empirical use of a corticosteroid is appropriate in a life-threatening situation, generally it is advisable not to begin corticosteroid therapy until a definite diagnosis has been made, for otherwise symptoms may be masked to such an extent that a true diagnosis becomes extremely difficult to make and the disease may reach an advanced stage before detection.

**Systemic therapy** is indicated in a wide variety of conditions. Where possible the oral route is preferred but parenteral administration may be used if the disease is severe or an emergency arises. Intravenous therapy is generally employed for intensive emergency treatment as the onset of action is relatively fast although intramuscular injections, often formulated as longer-acting depot preparations, may also be used to provide subsequent cover. Examples of conditions treated with systemic corticosteroids include:

- as an adjunct to adrenaline in life-threatening allergic reactions such as angioedema or anaphylaxis (see p.855)
- some blood disorders, including auto-immune haemolytic anaemia (p.733) and idiopathic thrombocytopenic purpura (p.1082)
- selected connective tissue and muscle disorders, such as Behçet's syndrome (p.1076), polymyalgia rheumatica (p.1086), polymyositis (p.1086), systemic lupus erythematosus (p.1088), and the vasculitic syndromes (p.1090)
- some inflammatory eye disorders, particularly those affecting the posterior chamber
- inflammatory gastrointestinal disorders, such as Crohn's disease and ulcerative colitis, although administration by the rectal route may be preferred in some circumstances (see p.1243)
- infections accompanied by a severe inflammatory component provided that appropriate anti-infective drugs are also given and that the benefits of corticosteroid therapy outweigh the possible risk of disseminated infection; examples of conditions where corticosteroid may be considered

include helminthic infections, the Jarisch-Herxheimer reaction, and tuberculous meningitis (p.1089)
- selected kidney disorders including lupus nephritis (p.1088) and various glomerular disorders (p.1080)
- selected liver disorders, including auto-immune chronic active hepatitis (p.1078)
- some neurological disorders such as infantile seizures and subacute demyelinating polyneuropathy; also in cerebral oedema (p.1078), including that associated with malignancy
- some respiratory disorders, such as asthma (see p.777, although inhaled corticosteroids are preferred to oral therapy for prophylaxis), diffuse parenchymal lung disease (p.1079), pulmonary sarcoid (p.1087), and neonatal respiratory distress syndrome (p.1084)
- some cases of rheumatoid arthritis, where recent evidence suggests there may be value in early treatment of active disease (see p.1087)
- severe skin disorders such as pemphigus and pemphigoid (p.1137)

Glucocorticoids are also used with antineoplastics in regimens for the management of malignant disease. They are also given to reduce immune responses after organ transplantations, often with other immunosuppressants (see p.1344).

Corticosteroids are not now considered useful in patients with aspiration syndromes, stroke, or septic shock.

**Intra-articular injection**, in the absence of infection and with full aseptic precautions, may be used, for example, in the treatment of rheumatoid arthritis (p.9), osteoarthritis (p.9), and ankylosing spondylitis (see Spondyloarthropathies, p.11). Either hydrocortisone acetate or one of the esters of the synthetic corticosteroids is used. It should be noted that there have been several reports of joint damage after the intra-articular injection of corticosteroids into load-bearing joints.

**Topical application** often produces dramatic suppression of skin diseases in which inflammation is a prominent feature, such as eczema, seborrhoeic dermatitis, and some forms of psoriasis. However, the disease may return or be exacerbated when corticosteroids are withdrawn and this appears to be a particular problem in some of the forms of psoriasis. Occasionally, corticosteroids may be used with the addition of a suitable antimicrobial, such as neomycin, in the treatment of infected skin. For comments on the topical application of preparations containing a corticosteroid and neomycin, see Adverse Effects of Neomycin, p.235.

**Intralesional injection** sometimes hastens the resolution of chronic skin lesions such as lichen planus, alopecia areata, and keloids.

**Topical application to the eye** in inflammatory and traumatic disorders has led to dramatic results, but the occurrence of herpetic and fungal infections of the cornea and other serious complications are considerable obstacles, and eye drops containing corticosteroids should be used under strict ophthalmic supervision with regular checks of intra-ocular pressure. Care is also required when corticosteroids are given by **subconjunctival injection** in inflammatory eye disorders.

**Ear drops** containing corticosteroids are used in the treatment of otitis externa (see p.138).

**Inhalational therapy** is widely used in the prophylaxis of asthma (see p.777).

**Nasal application** is used in the prophylaxis and treatment of allergic and non-allergic rhinitis (see p.422).

**Rectal administration**, by either suppository or enema, may be used for some corticosteroids, notably in the treatment of inflammatory bowel disease (p.1243).

## Administration

**Diurnal effect.** The diurnal rhythm of the adrenal cortex leads to about 70% of the daily secretion being made between midnight and 9 am.[1] In the treatment of adrenal cortical hyperplasia a dose of hydrocortisone given at night will be nearly twice as suppressive as the same dose given during the day. However, in treating allergic or collagen disease when suppression of adrenal cortical activity is best avoided a dose of hydrocortisone at about 8 am is indicated. When reducing corticosteroid dosage after treatment, a single dose given at 8 am will be most beneficial and will not inhibit corticotropin secretion. Also, for similar reasons,[2] when used for replacement therapy corticosteroids are given in unequal doses during the day (two-thirds of the daily dose in the morning, and one-third at night).


1. Demos CH, *et al.* A modified (once a day) corticosteroid dosage regimen. *Clin Pharmacol Ther* 1964; **5:** 721–7.
2. Aronson JK. Chronopharmacology: reflections on time and a new text. *Lancet* 1990; **335:** 1515–16.


**Epidural route.** Reviews[1,2] of the epidural use of corticosteroids in sciatica concluded that reported clinical complications were uncommon but that their role is unclear. Another study[3] suggested that although epidural injection of methylprednisolone acetate produced short-term improvement in pain and sensory deficit, treatment resulted in no functional benefit and did not reduce the need for surgery.

It should be noted that inadvertent intrathecal injection of corticosteroids has resulted in severe neurological complications.


1. Bogduk N, Cherry D. Epidural corticosteroid agents for sciatica. *Med J Aust* 1985; **143:** 402–6.
2. Tonkovich-Quaranta LA, Winkler SR. Use of epidural corticosteroids in low back pain. *Ann Pharmacother* 2000; **34:** 1165–72. Correction. *ibid.*; 1489.
3. Carette S, *et al.* Epidural corticosteroid injections for sciatica due to herniated nucleus pulposus. *N Engl J Med* 1997; **336:** 1634–40.


**Inhalational therapy.** Corticosteroids are given by inhalation, particularly in the maintenance therapy of asthma, in order to deliver the drug directly to the lungs, at smaller doses than are needed orally, and minimise systemic adverse effects. Different inhaled corticosteroids differ in their potency, though there is little evidence of a difference in efficacy at recommended doses.[1] Of those widely available by inhalation, flunisolide is less potent than beclometasone while budesonide is considered more potent, and fluticasone more potent still. (However, a general practice study in New Zealand has suggested that budesonide is less potent than beclometasone.[2]) The ability to use fewer inhalations with more potent drugs might enhance compliance.[1] For inhaled corticosteroids to be effective in the prophylaxis of asthma they must be taken regularly and patient compliance is important.

Efficient delivery to the bronchial tree is crucial and a number of different devices are available for administration, including pressurised aerosol inhalers, breath-actuated aerosol inhalers, and dry powder inhalers. These devices appear to be equally effective for the delivery of corticosteroids.[3] However, many patients, especially children, find that inhalation is made much easier by fitting a spacer device to the inhaler.[4] Such a device is recommended when high doses are to be inhaled, to prevent oropharyngeal deposition and subsequent systemic absorption. However, the type of spacer used and the method of use may dramatically alter the amount of drug available for inhalation. The drug should be introduced into the spacer by single actuations, each followed by inhalation, with the delay between actuation of the inhaler and inhalation from the spacer kept to a minimum. In some spacers static electricity accumulates, and the build up of charge reduces drug delivery: this can be controlled by washing and drying the spacer in air once a month. Considerable differences in the dose delivered to the airways may also be seen between different types of nebuliser, and between nebulisers and spacer devices.[5]

Changes in formulation of the propellant, to remove chlorofluorocarbons, may also affect drug availability; it is reported to be increased, requiring dose reduction with some formulations.[6]

It should be borne in mind that apparent differences in the dose supplied from inhaler devices in different countries may in some cases be artefacts, due to variations in the way the dose is measured or expressed. In the UK, for example, the dose supplied from a metered-dose inhaler is generally quoted as the amount released into the mouthpiece from the valve. In the USA, however, doses may be stated in terms of the amount of drug emitted from the mouthpiece, which due to drug deposition will be slightly less than the amount released from the valve.


1. Kelly HW. Comparison of inhaled corticosteroids. *Ann Pharmacother* 1998; **32:** 220–32.
2. Pethica BD, *et al.* Comparison of potency of inhaled beclomethasone and budesonide in New Zealand: retrospective study of computerised general practice records. *BMJ* 1998; **317:** 986–90.
3. Brocklebank D, *et al.* Systematic review of clinical effectiveness of pressurised metered dose inhalers versus other hand held inhaler devices for delivering corticosteroids in asthma. *BMJ* 2001; **323:** 896–900.
4. O'Callaghan C, Barry PW. How to choose delivery devices for asthma. *Arch Dis Child* 2000; **82:** 185–7.
5. O'Callaghan C, Barry P. Delivering inhaled corticosteroids to patients. *BMJ* 1999; **318:** 410–11.
6. Newman SP. Deposition and effects of inhaled corticosteroids. *Clin Pharmacokinet* 2003; **42:** 529–44.


**Intra-articular route.** Intra-articular and periarticular injection of corticosteroids is an established treatment for a variety of joint and soft-tissue lesions.[1-3] Pain and inflammation associated with rheumatoid and juvenile idiopathic arthritis, crystal arthropathies such as gout, and osteoarthritis can be alleviated by injection of a suitable corticosteroid, and in some cases the benefits may be quite prolonged. The longer-acting esters methylprednisolone acetate, triamcinolone acetonide, and triamcinolone hexacetonide are generally preferred. In some cases these may be combined with a local anaesthetic and a short-acting soluble corticosteroid for more rapid relief and to reduce the risk of a post-injection flare.

The risks associated with this technique have been reviewed.[4] Accurate injection technique is essential, and vigorous skin cleansing and an aseptic technique are required to avoid the introduction of infection into the joint; pre-existing joint infection is a contra-indication to corticosteroid injection. Intra-articular injections may be repeated if necessary but it has been suggested that a single joint should not be injected more than 3 or 4 times a year.

Periarticular injection is also used in various soft tissue disorders such as bursitis, capsulitis (painful shoulder syndromes), epicondylitis, tenosynovitis, and carpal tunnel syndrome. Particular care is required to avoid injection directly into a tendon, as this may cause the tendon to rupture. A shorter-acting corticosteroid such as hydrocortisone acetate may be more suitable for extra-articular lesions.


1. Anonymous. Articular and periarticular corticosteroid injections. *Drug Ther Bull* 1995; **33:** 67–70.
2. Caldwell JR. Intra-articular corticosteroids: guide to selection and indications for use. *Drugs* 1996; **52:** 507–14.
3. Pullar T. Routes of drug administration: intra-articular route. *Prescribers' J* 1998; **38:** 123–6.
4. Hunter JA, Blyth TH. A risk-benefit assessment of intra-articular corticosteroids in rheumatic disorders. *Drug Safety* 1999; **21:** 353–65.


**Surgery.** In the light of what was known in 1994 about the adrenal stress response to surgery, a discussion on the appropriate glucocorticoid supplementation for patients receiving corticosteroids who undergo surgery concluded that some recommendations were excessive.[1] (At this time in the UK recommended regimens consisted of the equivalent of 100 mg of hydrocortisone, usually as the sodium succinate, intravenously or intramuscularly before surgery, repeated every 8 hours, with the dose being tapered over 5 days to 20 or 30 mg daily.) It was suggested that for minor surgery 25 mg of hydrocortisone or its equivalent pre-operatively was adequate; where surgical stress was likely to be moderate, 50 to 75 mg of hydrocortisone or its equivalent daily in divided doses for 1 to 2 days was suggested. For major surgical stress, a target of 100 to 150 mg of hydrocortisone or its equivalent should be given daily in divided doses for 2 to 3 days, although less might be given if the patient's pre-operative glucocorticoid dose was low. It was also considered that the practice of gradually reducing postoperative coverage over several days was not supported by evidence except in cases of high-dose glucocorticoid use for prolonged periods.

Another review[2] of this subject also concluded that for minor surgery, 25 mg of hydrocortisone, or the patient's usual dose of corticosteroid, given pre-operatively, was appropriate. However, the authors argued that for surgery causing greater stress, it was preferable to avoid the increases in plasma-cortisol associated with intermittent bolus doses. They suggested that for moderate surgery an intravenous dose of hydrocortisone 25 mg at induction should be followed by an infusion of 100 mg over 24 hours; for major surgery the infusion should be continued for 48 to 72 hours following surgery. The usual oral corticosteroid dose may be resumed once these infusions have been completed, providing the postoperative course is uncomplicated and gastrointestinal function has returned.

For currently recommended regimens see p.1104.


1. Salem M, *et al.* Perioperative glucocorticoid coverage: a reassessment 42 years after emergence of a problem. *Ann Surg* 1994; **219:** 416–25.
2. Nicholson G, *et al.* Peri-operative steroid supplementation. *Anaesthesia* 1998; **53:** 1091–1104.


**Topical application.** Guidelines[1,2] for the correct use of topical corticosteroids recommend that an appropriately potent preparation to bring the skin disorder under control should be used. Some recommend use of the lowest potency that will control the disorder, while others have advocated starting treatment with a more potent preparation, treatment may then be continued with a less potent preparation and with less frequent application, once control is obtained. The most potent topical corticosteroids are generally reserved for recalcitrant dermatoses. Once the skin has healed, treatment should be tailed off. Particular care is necessary in the use of topical corticosteroids in children, and the more potent preparations are contra-indicated in infants under 1 year of age, although potent preparations may be needed briefly in older children. It has been suggested that a 'steroid holiday' of at least 2 weeks be considered in children after each 2 or 3 weeks of daily topical therapy to allow thinned epidermis to restore itself and maintain its barrier function.[3]

Care is also necessary in applying corticosteroids to certain anatomical sites such as the face and flexures; some advocate using only hydrocortisone 0.5 or 1% on the face. Advice should be given that topical corticosteroids should be applied sparingly in thin layers, by smoothing gently into the skin preferably after a bath, and that no benefit is gained from more frequent than twice daily application or by vigorous rubbing.

In a study to determine the requirement of topical corticosteroids,[4] 16 adult patients with eczema were treated with a variety of topical preparations until substantial clearing had occurred (up to 10 days). Results indicated that the mean requirement of preparation, regardless of potency or vehicle, was 6.86 g/m². Using this value the calculated quantities of topical corticosteroid to the nearest 5 g required for twice daily application for one week for the whole body, arms and legs only, and trunk only respectively were as follows:

- 6 months of age, 35 g, 20 g, and 15 g
- 1 year, 45 g, 25 g, and 15 g
- 4 years, 60 g, 35 g, and 20 g
- 8 years, 90 g, 50 g, and 35 g
- 12 years, 120 g, 65 g, and 45 g
- 16 years, 155 g, 85 g, and 55 g
- adult (70-kg male), 170 g, 90 g, and 60 g

Calculated quantities for the same application schedule for an adult (70-kg male) for individual portions of the body were:

- face and neck, 10 g
- one arm, 15 g
- one leg, 30 g
- hands and feet, 10 g

Table 1 below, is a guide to the potency of topical corticosteroids. There may be some degree of overlap between these groups and, not surprisingly, there are minor variations to this classification. For example, some authorities consider fluocinolone acetonide 0.2% to be potent rather than very potent and halcinonide 0.1% to be potent rather than very potent.

It has been suggested, however, that the advent of nonfluorinated double esters such as hydrocortisone and methylprednisolone aceponates, or prednicarbate, has resulted in corticosteroids whose topical anti-inflammatory potency is not as closely related to their potential atrophic effects on skin, and that a classification taking both into account would be desirable.[5,6]


1. Miller JA, Munro DD. Topical corticosteroids: clinical pharmacology and therapeutic use. *Drugs* 1980; **19:** 119–34.
2. Savin JA. Some guidelines to the use of topical corticosteroids. *BMJ* 1985; **290:** 1607–8.
3. Hepburn D, *et al.* Topical steroid holiday. *Pediatrics* 1995; **95:** 455.
4. Maurice PDL, Saihan EM. Topical steroid requirement in inflammatory skin conditions. *Br J Clin Pract* 1985; **39:** 441–2.
5. Mori M, *et al.* Topical corticosteroids and unwanted local effects: improving the benefit/risk ratio. *Drug Safety* 1994; **10:** 406–12.
6. Schäfer-Korting M, *et al.* Topical glucocorticoids with improved risk-benefit ratio: rationale of a new concept. *Drug Safety* 1996; **14:** 375–85.


## Acute respiratory distress syndrome

Acute respiratory distress syndrome (ARDS) is characterised by areas of lung damage leading to decreased pulmonary compliance, pulmonary oedema associated with increased capillary and alveolar permeability, and refractory hypoxaemia. Diffuse pulmonary infiltrates are seen on radiography, and patients exhibit dyspnoea, tachypnoea, or both. Diagnosis is primarily clinical, and there has been some disagreement as to what should be included in the syndrome;[1] it is now seen as forming the most severe end of a spectrum of symptoms due to lung inflammation and increased permeability known as acute lung injury.[1-3] ARDS is sometimes considered to refer to 'adult respiratory distress syndrome' but it is not confined to adult patients.[1,2]

ARDS may be caused by a variety of pulmonary or systemic insults but is particularly frequent in patients with sepsis; because of an association with failure of other organs it has been suggested that it represents the pulmonary component of multiple organ failure syndrome.[4] A wide variety of inflammatory mediators have been implicated in its pathogenesis but evidence suggests that recruitment of neutrophils by interleukins plays an important role.[1]

**Management**. Therapy for ARDS is essentially supportive. Mechanical ventilation is necessary in most cases, and circulatory support may require fluids, cardiac inotropes, and vasodilators. Optimum management may include diuretics and fluid restriction provided that cardiac output and oxygen delivery are maintained.[5] Because of the association with sepsis antibacterial therapy may be important, but studies of anti-endotoxin antibodies have produced disappointing results.[3] Improvements in supportive care and mechanical ventilation are considered to have reduced the mortality rate.[1,6]

Numerous drugs have been proposed for the management of ARDS, but, although case reports are often encouraging, none has been conclusively shown to improve mortality in controlled trials. Corticosteroids do not appear to reduce acute mortality,[3,4] although they may be tried in the later phases of the syndrome (5 or more days from onset) to try to prevent fibroproliferative lung changes.[1,7,8] Good results have been reported with inhaled epoprostenol,[9,10] but these results await confirmation from larger controlled studies.

There is evidence that ketoconazole may prevent development of ARDS in patients considered at risk,[11,12] but it does not appear to be effective as a treatment for ARDS or acute lung injury.[13] Among the drugs which have proved disappointing are acetylcysteine,[14,15] alprostadil,[16,17] pulmonary surfactants[18-20] (although some investigation is ongoing[6,8]), and nitric oxide[21] (which may, however, improve oxygenation to some degree).

A high-fat, low-carbohydrate diet has been advocated for patients with ARDS. Supplementation with eicosapentaenoic acid and gamolenic acid has been reported to benefit oxygenation, but with no significant effect on mortality.[6,8]


1. Ware LB, Matthay MA. The acute respiratory distress syndrome. *N Engl J Med* 2000; **342:** 1334–49. Correction. *ibid.*; **343:** 520.
2. Bernard GR, *et al.* The American-European Consensus Conference on ARDS: definitions, mechanisms, relevant outcomes, and clinical trial coordination. *Am J Respir Crit Care Med* 1994; **149:** 818–24.
3. Bigatello LM, Zapol WM. New approaches to acute lung injury. *Br J Anaesth* 1996; **77:** 99–109.
4. Weinberger SE. Recent advances in pulmonary medicine (part 2). *N Engl J Med* 1993; **328:** 1462–70.
5. Elsasser S, *et al.* Adjunctive drug treatment in severe hypoxic respiratory failure. *Drugs* 1999; **58:** 429–46.
6. Hite RD, Morris PE. Acute respiratory distress syndrome: pharmacological treatment options in development. *Drugs* 2001; **61:** 897–907.
7. Meduri GU, *et al.* Effect of prolonged methylprednisolone therapy in unresolving acute respiratory distress syndrome: a randomized controlled trial. *JAMA* 1998; **280:** 159–65.
8. Cranshaw J, *et al.* The pulmonary physician in critical care 9: non-ventilatory strategies in ARDS. *Thorax* 2002; **57:** 823–9.
9. Walmrath D, *et al.* Aerosolised prostacyclin in adult respiratory distress syndrome. *Lancet* 1993; **342:** 961–2.
10. Walmrath D, *et al.* Direct comparison of inhaled nitric oxide and aerosolized prostacyclin in acute respiratory distress syndrome. *Am J Respir Crit Care Med* 1996; **153:** 991–6.
11. Yu M, Tomasa G. A double-blind, prospective, randomized trial of ketoconazole, a thromboxane synthetase inhibitor, in the prophylaxis of the adult respiratory distress syndrome. *Crit Care Med* 1993; **21:** 1635–42.
12. Sinuff T, *et al.* Development, implementation, and evaluation of a ketoconazole practice guideline for ARDS prophylaxis. *J Crit Care* 1999; **14:** 1–6.
13. The ARDS Network Authors. Ketoconazole for early treatment of acute lung injury and acute respiratory distress syndrome: a randomized controlled trial. *JAMA* 2000; **283:** 1995–2002.
14. Jepsen S, *et al.* Antioxidant treatment with N-acetylcysteine during adult respiratory distress syndrome: a prospective, randomized, placebo-controlled study. *Crit Care Med* 1992; **20:** 918–23.
15. Domenighetti G, *et al.* Treatment with N-acetylcysteine during acute respiratory distress syndrome: a randomized, double-blind, placebo-controlled clinical study. *J Crit Care* 1997; **12:** 177–82.
16. Bone RC, *et al.* Randomized double-blind, multicenter study of prostaglandin $E_1$ in patients with the adult respiratory distress syndrome. *Chest* 1989; **96:** 114–19.
17. Abraham E, *et al.* Liposomal prostaglandin $E_1$, in acute respiratory distress syndrome: a placebo-controlled, randomized, double-blind, multicenter clinical trial. *Crit Care Med* 1996; **24:** 10–15.
18. Haslam PL, *et al.* Surfactant replacement therapy in late-stage adult respiratory distress syndrome. *Lancet* 1994; **343:** 1009–11.
19. Weg JG, *et al.* Safety and potential efficacy of an aerosolized surfactant in human sepsis-induced adult respiratory distress syndrome. *JAMA* 1994; **272:** 1433–8.
20. Anzueto A, *et al.* Aerosolized surfactant in adults with sepsis-induced acute respiratory distress syndrome. *N Engl J Med* 1996; **334:** 1417–21.
21. Sokol J, *et al.* Inhaled nitric oxide for acute hypoxemic respiratory failure in children and adults. Available in The Cochrane Library; Issue 1. Chichester: John Wiley; 2004.


## Adrenal hyperplasia, congenital

See Congenital Adrenal Hyperplasia, below.

## Adrenocortical insufficiency

The major function of the adrenal cortex is the production of glucocorticoid and mineralocorticoid hormones, of which cortisol (hydrocortisone) and aldosterone respectively are the most important. Glucocorticoid production is

**Table 1.** Guide to potencies of topical corticosteroids.

| Very potent | Potent | Moderately potent | Mild |
|---|---|---|---|
| Clobetasol propionate 0.05% | Amcinonide 0.1% | Alclometasone dipropionate 0.05% | Fluocinolone acetonide 0.0025% |
| Diflucortolone valerate 0.3% | Beclometasone dipropionate 0.025% | Betamethasone valerate 0.025% | Hydrocortisone 0.5% and 1% |
| Fluocinolone acetonide 0.2% | Betamethasone benzoate 0.025% | Clobetasone butyrate 0.05% | Hydrocortisone acetate 1% |
| Halcinonide 0.1% | Betamethasone dipropionate 0.05% | Desoximetasone 0.05% | Methylprednisolone acetate 0.25% |
| Ulobetasol propionate 0.05% | Betamethasone valerate 0.1% | Fludroxycortide 0.0125% | |
| | Budesonide 0.025% | Flumetasone pivalate 0.02% | |
| | Desonide 0.05% | Fluocinolone acetonide 0.00625% and 0.01% | |
| | Desoximetasone 0.25% | Fluocortin butyl 0.75% | |
| | Diflorasone diacetate 0.05% | Fluocortolone preparations (caproate with pivalate, each 0.1% and caproate with either free alcohol or pivalate, each 0.25%) | |
| | Diflucortolone valerate 0.1% | | |
| | Fluclorolone acetonide 0.025% | Hydrocortisone aceponate 0.1% | |
| | Fluocinolone acetonide 0.025% | Hydrocortisone buteprate 0.1% | |
| | Fluocinonide 0.05% | Prednicarbate 0.25% | |
| | Fluprednidene acetate 0.1% | | |
| | Fluticasone propionate 0.005% and 0.05% | | |
| | Hydrocortisone butyrate 0.1% | | |
| | Methyprednisolone aceponate 0.1% | | |
| | Mometasone furoate 0.1% | | |
| | Triamcinolone acetonide 0.1% | | |

regulated by the hypothalamic-pituitary-adrenal axis, being stimulated by the release of ACTH (adrenocorticotrophic hormone; corticotropin) from the pituitary, while mineralocorticoid production is primarily controlled by the renin-angiotensin system.

Adrenocortical insufficiency is defined as inadequate production of endogenous corticosteroids. It may be primary (Addison's disease), due to destruction of the adrenal cortex; or secondary, due to hypothalamic or pituitary disease, or corticosteroid therapy which suppresses ACTH release.[1] Diagnosis can be difficult, even with the aid of hormone tests such as the tetracosactide stimulation test.[2]

Clinical manifestations of adrenocortical insufficiency are usually seen once about 90% of the adrenal cortex is destroyed. Weight loss, anorexia, weakness, and fatigue may be accompanied by gastrointestinal symptoms such as abdominal pain, nausea, vomiting, and diarrhoea, as well as electrolyte abnormalities (hyponatraemia, hyperkalaemia), salt craving, and orthostatic hypotension. In acute cases, abdominal pain and rigidity, fever, volume depletion, hypotension, and shock may occur. Hyperpigmentation, especially of skin creases, exposed areas, and scars is a distinguishing feature of primary, but not secondary, insufficiency. Hypoglycaemia is more likely in secondary deficiency due to lack of growth hormone, and failure of other pituitary hormones usually accompanies secondary adrenocortical insufficiency.

**Treatment for acute insufficiency** should be with intravenous hydrocortisone as the sodium succinate, sodium phosphate or other readily soluble ester: the usual dose is the equivalent of 100 mg every 6 to 8 hours for 24 hours. Volume depletion, dehydration, hypotension and hypoglycaemia should be corrected with intravenous saline and glucose, and precipitating factors, such as infection, should be dealt with appropriately. Provided no complications occur, the dosage of hydrocortisone can be tapered over 4 or 5 days to maintenance therapy by mouth.

For chronic insufficiency the usual dosage of **maintenance** or **replacement therapy** is hydrocortisone 20 to 30 mg by mouth, preferably divided unequally, e.g. 30 mg as 20 mg in the morning and 10 mg in the evening, in an attempt to mimic the natural pattern of secretion. Other corticosteroids have been used, including cortisone acetate, prednisolone, prednisone, and dexamethasone, but offer no advantage over hydrocortisone. Patients with primary insufficiency also require additional mineralocorticoid replacement with fludrocortisone, usually in a dose of 100 micrograms daily. Mineralocorticoid replacement is not usually necessary in secondary insufficiency. There has been some evidence of benefit from studies of adjunctive oral administration of prasterone, another steroidal compound secreted by the adrenal glands, in patients with primary or secondary adrenal insufficiency.

**Corticosteroid cover.** An increase in replacement therapy is required during periods of stress. In mild infection, a doubling of the maintenance dose of hydrocortisone may be appropriate but for major infection, or severe stress such as surgery, parenteral therapy is required. It is generally considered safer to overestimate rather than underestimate the appropriate cover. For regimens used to provide cover in patients with secondary insufficiency due to corticosteroid therapy see Uses and Administration of Hydrocortisone, p.1104.

1. Arlt W, Allolio B. Adrenal insufficiency. *Lancet* 2003; **361:** 1881–93.
2. Dorin RI, *et al.* Diagnosis of adrenal insufficiency. *Ann Intern Med* 2003; **139:** 194–204.

## AIDS

For the use of corticosteroids in AIDS patients with *Pneumocystis carinii* pneumonia, see p.1085.

## Alopecia

The management of alopecia (p.1134) is often difficult. In alopecia areata intralesional corticosteroids, most commonly triamcinolone, will induce hair growth although they are not suitable when more than 50% of the scalp is involved.[1] Regrowth is confined to the site of injection and therefore patchy, although soon concealed by spontaneous growth from uninjected regions. Some atrophy of the scalp is inevitable. Topical corticosteroids are mostly reported to be ineffective although some consider them beneficial; the use of systemic corticosteroids is controversial, given their adverse effects and a lack of evidence that they alter the long-term prognosis.

1. Meidan VM, Touitou E. Treatments for androgenetic alopecia and alopecia areata: current options and future prospects. *Drugs* 2001; **61:** 53–69.

## Anaemias

For the use of corticosteroids in haemolytic anaemias, including cold haemagglutinin disease, see p.733.

## Anaphylactic shock

For the use of corticosteroids in the management of anaphylactic shock, see p.855. Intravenous corticosteroids are given following initial treatment with adrenaline as part of the management of anaphylaxis; their effects are delayed, and they are not suited for immediate relief, but early use may help prevent deterioration after primary treatment has been given.

## Aspiration syndromes

For a review of the management of aspiration syndromes, including reference to the probable lack of value of corticosteroids, see p.1240.

## Asthma

The cornerstones of current asthma therapy, as discussed in more detail on p.777, are the beta$_2$-adrenoceptor agonists and the corticosteroids. Drug therapy for **chronic asthma** is managed by a stepwise approach. Patients requiring only occasional relief from symptoms may be managed with an inhaled short-acting beta$_2$ agonist as required. An inhaled corticosteroid such as beclometasone dipropionate, budesonide, or fluticasone may be added to therapy if symptomatic relief is needed more than two or three times a week but regular use is important since corticosteroids take several hours to exert an effect in asthma. If control is still inadequate, a long-acting beta$_2$ agonist is added. The dose of inhaled corticosteroid may be increased if further control is needed, and other additional therapies include anti-leukotrienes or theophylline. Severe asthma requires regular bronchodilator therapy as well as high-dose inhaled corticosteroids, while in the most severe cases, regular oral corticosteroids may also be required. A short 'rescue' course of oral corticosteroid may be needed at any stage for an acute exacerbation. Corticosteroids should be used cautiously in children because of possible adverse effects on growth.

**Acute severe asthma** (status asthmaticus) is potentially life-threatening and is treated with inhaled oxygen and beta$_2$ agonists, as well as systemic corticosteroids; inhaled ipratropium bromide, and intravenous magnesium sulfate, xanthine, or beta$_2$ agonist may need to be added. Once lung function is stabilised the patient can be discharged on a regimen of oral and inhaled corticosteroids, and bronchodilators.

## Behçet's syndrome

Behçet's syndrome (or Behçet's disease) is a recurrent multifocal disorder most prevalent in the Far East and countries of the Mediterranean and Middle East.

The clinical features include oral and genital ulceration, skin lesions, arthritis, vasculitis leading to thromboembolic disorders and aneurysms, ocular lesions (including uveitis, hypopyon, and iridocyclitis leading eventually to blindness), and CNS involvement (meningomyelitis, dementia, extrapyramidal symptoms, and paralysis, sometimes fatal). Gastrointestinal disturbances and involvement of other body systems have been reported. However, the complete gamut of symptoms is unlikely in a single patient, and the disease has been classified into mucocutaneous, arthritic, neurological, and ocular forms depending on the predominant symptoms. Diagnosis can be difficult, but oral ulceration, together with recurrent genital ulceration, ocular involvement, and skin lesions or a positive pathergy test are considered the major diagnostic criteria.[1,2]

Treatment of Behçet's syndrome is essentially symptomatic and empirical. Controlled studies are mostly lacking, which has hindered meta-analysis.[3] Where possible topical treatment of **mucocutaneous** lesions should be attempted before embarking on systemic therapy. Topical application of a potent corticosteroid, such as triamcinolone acetonide, or a tetracycline solution may be tried for oral ulceration.[1,2] Genital ulcers can be treated topically with betamethasone ointment.[2] Sucralfate suspension used topically has also been reported to be effective in oral and genital ulceration,[4] and topical mesalazine has been tried.[5] Systemically, colchicine is reportedly beneficial in the treatment of mucocutaneous lesions,[1,2] although a small meta-analysis failed to find any evidence of benefit from colchicine treatment.[3] Systemic corticosteroids are advocated for severe mucocutaneous disease;[4] oral prednisolone has been given for erythema nodosum.[1,2] Thalidomide is also effective for mucocutaneous symptoms,[2,4] although relapses occur on cessation of therapy. Other drugs with reported efficacy for mucocutaneous symptoms include azathioprine,[4] benzathine benzylpenicillin (sometimes with colchicine),[4] dapsone,[1,2,4] interferon alfa,[4] levamisole,[4] pentoxifylline,[1] and rebamipide.[4]

The use of NSAIDs in the treatment of **arthritis** in patients with Behçet's disease is controversial,[4] although indometacin is used.[2] Colchicine is also used,[2,4] and sulfasalazine may be beneficial in patients who do not respond to NSAIDs.[1] Corticosteroids used with azathioprine are effective,[2,4] as are interferon alfa,[1,2,4] and benzathine benzylpenicillin.[3]

Short courses of intravenous methylprednisolone or high-dose oral prednisolone with subsequent tapering are used in the acute phase of **neurological** involvement, and may be followed by chlorambucil, cyclophosphamide, or methotrexate.[2] Chronic CNS disease is generally resistant to therapy.[2]

**Ocular** involvement in Behçet's disease leads to blindness in about a quarter of patients.[1,2] For acute attacks of anterior uveitis, topical mydriatics such as tropicamide, or corticosteroid drops may be sufficient. Local injections of corticosteroids are used to treat acute attacks of posterior uveitis, and systemic administration may also be required.[2] Oral corticosteroid therapy does not improve visual prognosis, however, and may lead to secondary retinal thrombosis or cataracts;[2] good evidence of its benefit is lacking.[3] Colchicine is used for prophylaxis of both anterior and posterior uveitis;[2] ciclosporin is considered more effective at controlling acute ocular attacks[1] but its efficacy appears to gradually decline.[2,4] Other drugs deemed effective in preventing ocular inflammation include azathioprine,[1-4] chlorambucil,[2,4] and cyclophosphamide.[2,4] There are reports of benefit with benzathine benzylpenicillin, interferon alfa, levamisole, methotrexate, pentoxifylline, sulfasalazine, and thalidomide.[4] Tacrolimus has also been beneficial in cases of refractory uveitis.[1,4] Combinations of the above drugs are also used, such as corticosteroids with immunosuppressants, or corticosteroids with cytotoxics.[4]

In patients with **vasculitis**, arteritis is treated with systemic corticosteroids and cyclophosphamide, either orally or pulsed monthly boluses.[1,2] Deep-vein thrombosis has been treated with anticoagulants, such as warfarin or heparin, but caution is advised in those with pulmonary arteritis because of the risk of potentially fatal haemoptysis,[2] and their use is generally not recommended.[1,4] Aspirin is used with immunosuppressants, particularly azathioprine.[4] Stanozolol is also used to treat the vascular symptoms of Behçet's disease.

Corticosteroids and sulfasalazine are the main drugs used for **gastrointestinal** lesions;[2] thalidomide has also been beneficial.[1]

Infliximab has been found to reduce acute ocular inflammation,[6] and heal gastrointestinal ulceration,[7] as well as concomitant manifestations of Behçet's disease, and trials are ongoing.[6]

1. Kaklamani VG, *et al.* Behçet's disease. *Semin Arthritis Rheum* 1998; **27:** 197–217.
2. Sakane T, *et al.* Behçet's disease. *N Engl J Med* 1999; **341:** 1284–91.
3. Saenz A, *et al.* Pharmacotherapy for Behçet's syndrome. Available in The Cochrane Library; Issue 1. Chichester: John Wiley; 2004.
4. Kaklamani VG, Kaklamanis PG. Treatment of Behçet's disease—an update. *Semin Arthritis Rheum* 2001; **30:** 299–312. Correction. *ibid.*; **31:** 69.
5. Ranzi T, *et al.* Successful treatment of genital and oral ulceration in Behcet's disease with topical 5-aminosalicylic acid (5-ASA). *Br J Dermatol* 1989; **120:** 471–2.
6. Sfikakis PP, *et al.* Effect of infliximab on sight-threatening panuveitis in Behçet's disease. *Lancet* 2001; **358:** 295–6.
7. Travis SPL, *et al.* Treatment of intestinal Behçet's syndrome with chimeric tumour necrosis factor α antibody. *Gut* 2001; **49:** 725–8.

## Bell's palsy

Bell's palsy is a condition that may be caused[1] by herpes simplex virus 1. It affects the facial nerves and results in facial muscle weakness and paralysis. It is often accompanied by pain and lachrymation. Untreated, over 80% of all patients recover completely or almost so, while in a smaller number facial weakness persists; complete failure of motor recovery is very rare.

Corticosteroids dramatically relieve the pain of Bell's palsy,[2] and their use in treatment is widely accepted.[3] The suggested dose of prednisone for adults is 1 mg/kg daily by mouth in divided doses morning and evening; if the paralysis remains incomplete after 5 or 6 days the prednisone is gradually withdrawn over the next 5 days but if the paralysis is complete the initial dosage should be continued for another 10 days and then gradually withdrawn.[2] However, the benefits of corticosteroids in this condition have never been established by a large controlled trial,[4,5] although a systematic review of 4 small studies suggested an increased rate of complete recovery with corticosteroid treatment.[6] There is some suggestion that addition of aciclovir or valaciclovir to corticosteroid treatment may improve outcome,[3,7] although again substantive evidence is lacking.[8]

1. Murakami S, *et al.* Bell palsy and herpes simplex virus: identification of viral DNA in endoneurial fluid and muscle. *Ann Intern Med* 1996; **124:** 27–30.
2. Adour KK. Current concepts in neurology: diagnosis and management of facial paralysis. *N Engl J Med* 1982; **307:** 348–51.
3. Knox GW. Treatment controversies in Bell palsy. *Arch Otolaryngol Head Neck Surg* 1998; **124:** 821–3.
4. Karis R. Facial paralysis. *N Engl J Med* 1982; **307:** 1647.
5. Staal A, *et al.* Facial paralysis. *N Engl J Med* 1982; **307:** 1647.
6. Williamson IG, Whelan TR. The clinical problem of Bell's palsy: is treatment with steroids effective? *Br J Gen Pract* 1996; **46:** 743–7.
7. Axelsson S, *et al.* Outcome of treatment with valacyclovir and prednisone in patients with Bell's palsy. *Ann Otol Rhinol Laryngol* 2003; **112:** 197–201.
8. Sipe J, Dunn L. Aciclovir for Bell's palsy (Idiopathic facial paralysis). Available in The Cochrane Library; Issue 1. Chichester: John Wiley; 2004.

## Bites and stings

Corticosteroids (prednisone 100 mg daily) have been recommended for the stabilisation of erythrocyte membranes in the management of systemic envenomation by the brown recluse spider (*Loxosceles reclusa*).[1] They have also been given following stings by some species of scorpion, although their value is not certain.[1] Corticosteroids are considered to have no place in snake venom poisoning.[2] Topical corticosteroids may be useful for mild itching of healing skin after some types of jelly fish sting, while systemic corticosteroids have been used for delayed hypersensitivity reactions.[3]

1. Binder LS. Acute arthropod envenomation: incidence, clinical features and management. *Med Toxicol Adverse Drug Exp* 1989; **4:** 163–73.
2. Nelson BK. Snake envenomation: incidence, clinical presentation and management. *Med Toxicol* 1989; **4:** 17–31.
3. Fenner PJ, Williamson JA. Worldwide deaths and severe envenomation from jelly fish stings. *Med J Aust* 1996; **165:** 658–61.

## Bone cysts

Intralesional corticosteroid injection (usually methylprednisolone) has been used as an alternative to surgical or other methods for the treatment of bone cysts.[1-6] An early report indicated that methylprednisolone acetate 40 to 200 mg injected into unicameral bone cysts under brief general anaesthesia stimulated bone formation to obliterate the cyst or promoted sufficient healing to prevent further fractures.[1] A single injection was sufficient for healing in 10 to 25% of cysts; only rarely were more than 4 injections needed. Treatment of an aneurysmal bone cyst with methylprednisolone and calcitonin has also been reported.[7] (Systemic corticosteroids are, of course, generally associated with bone loss rather than bone formation—see Effects on Bones and Joints, p.1069).

1. Weinert CR. Administering steroids in unicameral bone cysts. *West J Med* 1989; **150:** 684–5.
2. Rud B, *et al.* Simple bone cysts in children treated with methylprednisolone acetate. *Orthopedics* 1991; **14:** 185–7.
3. Goel AR, *et al.* Unicameral bone cysts: treatment with methylprednisone acetate injections. *J Foot Ankle Surg* 1994; **33:** 6–15.
4. Parsch K, *et al.* Die juvenile Knochenzyste: Stellenwert und Therapieergebnisse der Kortisoninjektion. *Orthopade* 1995; **24:** 65–72.
5. Hashemi-Nejad A, Cole WG. Incomplete healing of simple bone cysts after steroid injections. *J Bone Joint Surg Br* 1997; **79:** 727–30.
6. Journeau P, Ciotlos D. Place de l'embrochage centro-médullaire et de l'injection de corticoïdes dans le traitement des kystes osseux essentiels de l'enfant. *Rev Chir Orthop Reparatrice Appar Mot* 2003; **89:** 333–7.
7. Gladden ML, *et al.* Aneurysmal bone cyst of the first cervical vertebrae in a child treated with percutaneous intralesional injection of calcitonin and methylprednisolone: a case report. *Spine* 2000; **25:** 527–30.

## Brain injury

See Spinal Cord Injury, p.1088.

## Bronchiolitis

Acute bronchiolitis is usually caused by respiratory syncytial virus (RSV) infection (p.625) in children, and may contribute to the subsequent development of asthma. Supportive therapy, where necessary, may involve the use of oxygen and bronchodilators (see also p.794). Numerous studies have failed to show a benefit from corticosteroid therapy, and it has generally been considered that corticosteroids have no role in the management of the condition. Although one study did find that oral prednisolone might be of benefit,[1] it was suggested that the results might be due to inclusion of children with asthma among the study population.[2] However, a subsequent meta-analysis also showed that systemic corticosteroids could be of benefit.[3] Inhaled corticosteroids seem to be of little value.[4]

1. van Woensel JBM, *et al.* Randomised double blind placebo controlled trial of prednisolone in children admitted to hospital with respiratory syncytial virus bronchiolitis. *Thorax* 1997; **52:** 634–7.
2. Milner AD. The role of corticosteroids in bronchiolitis and croup. *Thorax* 1997; **52:** 595–7.
3. Garrison MM, *et al.* Systemic corticosteroids in infant bronchiolitis: a meta-analysis. Abstract: *Pediatrics* 2000; **105:** 849. Full version: http://pediatrics.aappublications.org/cgi/content/full/105/4/e44 (accessed 27/04/04)
4. Richter H, Seddon P. Early nebulized budesonide in the treatment of bronchiolitis and the prevention of postbronchiolitic wheezing. *J Pediatr* 1998; **132:** 849–53.

## Bronchopulmonary dysplasia

Bronchopulmonary dysplasia is the major cause of chronic lung disease (defined as the need for supplementary oxygen more than 28 days after birth) in neonates. It is considered to comprise 4 radiographically distinct stages, of which stage 1 is effectively indistinguishable from neonatal respiratory distress syndrome (see p.1084), with which it is usually associated. A 'bubbly' appearance of the lung is seen in radiographs of advanced disease. Bronchopulmonary dysplasia is invariably associated with prolonged mechanical ventilation, but it is uncertain whether it plays a causative role, or whether the disease develops anyway in infants with respiratory failure severe enough to need prolonged ventilation.[1]

**Treatment.** Corticosteroids,[2-9] usually in the form of intravenous dexamethasone, have been widely used in premature infants with bronchopulmonary dysplasia, or who are considered to be at high risk of it (the borderline between treatment and prophylaxis in studies in these mechanically ventilated infants is not always clear[6]). Dexamethasone has been reported to improve pulmonary outcome, allowing more rapid weaning from mechanical ventilation, and in some studies was reported to improve neurological outcome as well.[3] However, some investigators consider its benefits in the long term inadequately established,[6,8,10] and there remains some concern about possible adverse effects, especially on long-term development.[11,12] One meta-analysis suggests that use is associated with a high incidence of cerebral palsy and neurodevelopmental impairment, and should be abandoned.[13] UK guidelines[14] issued in 1998, and awaiting update, noted that many studies have favoured an initial dose of 500 micrograms/kg daily intravenously, tapered over a period of days to weeks, but it is not always clear if this is expressed in terms of the base or one of its esters,[15] and in any case regimens have varied between studies. Despite suggestions that beginning therapy shortly after birth might minimise lung injury, evidence suggests that early therapy offers no advantage,[10,16] and may be more hazardous.[10,12,17-19] Meta-analysis has suggested that while beginning dexamethasone at any time between birth and 14 days of age reduced the risk of chronic lung disease, mortality was only reduced in the group who began treatment between 7 and 14 days of age.[20] However, a subsequent systematic review concluded that the benefits of therapy started between 7 to 14 days may not outweigh the adverse effects.[18] Inhaled corticosteroids have also been investigated. A systematic review did not demonstrate any reduction in the incidence of chronic lung disease but inhaled therapy was associated with less need for systemic corticosteroids.[21] Another systematic review of controlled studies found that inhaled corticosteroids may improve the rate of extubation in infants.[22]

Additional therapy is essentially supportive, including fluid restriction, nutritional supplementation, bronchodilators, and diuretics. Routine use of bronchodilators for prevention of bronchopulmonary dysplasia is not recommended, and studies of use in treatment are limited.[1] The 1998 UK guidelines considered that diuretics were indicated for episodes of associated cardiac failure but their long-term value was uncertain; if used, consideration should be given to a calcium-sparing regimen.[14] Improved pulmonary status has been reported with furosemide in established dysplasia,[23,24] although routine or sustained use cannot be recommended at present. Results with hydrochlorothiazide and spironolactone are more ambiguous.[25,26] Anaemia in infants with bronchopulmonary dysplasia has benefited from erythropoietin.[27] Although vitamin A deficiency has been implicated in the pathogenesis of bronchopulmonary dysplasia, trials of vitamin A supplementation have produced conflicting results. However, differences in patient population, postnatal therapies, and dosage of vitamin A could explain these results,[28] and some recommend supplementation to reduce the incidence of chronic lung disease.[1,28] Despite promising preliminary results,[29] treatment with alpha$_1$-proteinase inhibitor has not been shown to reduce the incidence of chronic lung disease.[1] Similarly, although there is evidence suggesting that early administration of sudismase may reduce development of chronic lung disease (but not bronchopulmonary dysplasia),[30] routine use is not recommended.[1]

1. Shah PS. Current perspectives on the prevention and management of chronic lung disease in preterm infants. *Pediatr Drugs* 2003; **5:** 463–80.
2. Mammel MC, *et al.* Controlled trial of dexamethasone therapy in infants with bronchopulmonary dysplasia. *Lancet* 1983; **i:** 1356–8.
3. Cummings JJ, *et al.* A controlled trial of dexamethasone therapy in preterm infants with bronchopulmonary dysplasia. *N Engl J Med* 1989; **320:** 1505–10.
4. Kazzi NJ, *et al.* Dexamethasone effects on the hospital course of infants with bronchopulmonary dysplasia who are dependent on artificial ventilation. *Pediatrics* 1990; **86:** 722–7.
5. Collaborative Dexamethasone Trial Group. Dexamethasone therapy in neonatal chronic lung disease: an international placebo-controlled trial. *Pediatrics* 1991; **88:** 421–7.
6. Kari MA, *et al.* Dexamethasone treatment in preterm infants at risk for bronchopulmonary dysplasia. *Arch Dis Child* 1993; **68:** 566–9.
7. Durand M, *et al.* Effects of early dexamethasone therapy on pulmonary mechanics and chronic lung disease in very low birth weight infants: a randomized, controlled trial. *Pediatrics* 1995; **95:** 584–90.
8. Jones R, *et al.* Controlled trial of dexamethasone in neonatal chronic lung disease: a 3-year follow-up. *Pediatrics* 1995; **96:** 897–906.
9. Rastogi A, *et al.* A controlled trial of dexamethasone to prevent bronchopulmonary dysplasia in surfactant-treated infants. *Pediatrics* 1996; **98:** 204–10.
10. Papile L-A, *et al.* A multicenter trial of two dexamethasone regimens in ventilator-dependent premature infants. *N Engl J Med* 1998; **338:** 1112–18.
11. Greenough A. Gains and losses from dexamethasone for neonatal chronic lung disease. *Lancet* 1998; **352:** 835–6.
12. American Academy of Pediatrics Committee on Fetus and Newborn, Canadian Paediatric Society Fetus and Newborn Committee. Postnatal corticosteroids to treat or prevent chronic lung disease in preterm infants. *Pediatrics* 2002; **109:** 330–8. Also available at: http://aappolicy.aappublications.org/cgi/content/full/pediatrics;109/2/330 (accessed 27/04/04)
13. Barrington KJ. The adverse neuro-developmental effects of postnatal steroids in the preterm infant: a systematic review of RCTs. Available at: http://www.biomedcentral.com/1471-2431/1/1 (accessed 27/04/04)
14. Report of the second working group of the British Association of Perinatal Medicine. Guidelines for good practice in the management of neonatal respiratory distress syndrome. Guideline produced in November 1998, not valid beyond 2002. Available at: http://www.bapm.org/documents/publications/rds.pdf (accessed 27/04/04)
15. Jones RAK, Grant AM. The "dose" question. *Pediatrics* 1992; **90:** 781.
16. Tapia JL, *et al.* The effect of early dexamethasone administration on bronchopulmonary dysplasia in preterm infants with respiratory distress syndrome. *J Pediatr* 1998; **132:** 48–52.
17. Halliday HL, *et al.* Early postnatal (<96 hours) corticosteroids for preventing chronic lung disease in preterm infants. Available in The Cochrane Library; Issue 1. Chichester: John Wiley; 2004.
18. Halliday HL, *et al.* Moderately early (7-14 days) postnatal corticosteroids for preventing chronic lung disease in preterm infants. Available in The Cochrane Library; Issue 1. Chichester: John Wiley; 2004.
19. The Vermont Oxford Network Steroid Study Group. Early postnatal dexamethasone therapy for the prevention of chronic lung disease. *Pediatrics* 2001; **108:** 741–8.
20. Bhuta T, Ohlsson A. Systematic review and meta-analysis of early postnatal dexamethasone for prevention of chronic lung disease. *Arch Dis Child Fetal Neonatal Ed* 1998; **79:** F26–F33.
21. Shah V, *et al.* Early administration of inhaled corticosteroids for preventing chronic lung disease in ventilated very low birth weight preterm neonates. Available in The Cochrane Library; Issue 1. Chichester: John Wiley; 2004.
22. Lister P, *et al.* Inhaled steroids for neonatal chronic lung disease. Available in The Cochrane Library; Issue 1. Chichester: John Wiley; 2004.
23. Brion LP, *et al.* Aerosolized diuretics for preterm infants with (or developing) chronic lung disease. Available in The Cochrane Library; Issue 1. Chichester: John Wiley; 2004.
24. Brion LP, Primhak RA. Intravenous or enteral loop diuretics for preterm infants with (or developing) chronic lung disease. Available in The Cochrane Library; Issue 1. Chichester: John Wiley; 2004.
25. Engelhardt B, *et al.* Effect of spironolactone-hydrochlorothiazide on lung function in infants with chronic bronchopulmonary dysplasia. *J Pediatr* 1989; **114:** 619–24.
26. Albersheim SG, *et al.* Randomized, double-blind, controlled trial of long-term diuretic therapy for bronchopulmonary dysplasia. *J Pediatr* 1989; **115:** 615–20.
27. Ohls RK, *et al.* A randomized double-blind, placebo-controlled trial of recombinant erythropoietin in treatment of the anemia of bronchopulmonary dysplasia. *J Pediatr* 1993; **123:** 996–1000.
28. Shenai JP. Vitamin A supplementation in very low birth weight neonates: rationale and evidence. *Pediatrics* 1999; **104:** 1369–74.
29. Stiskal JA, *et al.* $\alpha_1$-Proteinase inhibitor therapy for the prevention of chronic lung disease of prematurity: a randomized, controlled trial. *Pediatrics* 1998; **101:** 89–94.
30. Davis JM, *et al.* Pulmonary outcome at 1 year corrected age in premature infants treated at birth with recombinant human CuZn superoxide dismutase. *Pediatrics* 2003; **111:** 469–76.

## Cachexia

For mention of the use of corticosteroids in cancer-related cachexia see p.1558.

### Cerebral oedema

Corticosteroids (usually dexamethasone) play an important role in the treatment of cerebral oedema caused by malignancy and dexamethasone is advocated for the cerebral oedema associated with high-altitude disorders (see p.822). Corticosteroids have also been used for the management of raised intracranial pressure in patients with head injuries or stroke, but despite earlier small studies showing them to be beneficial in some patients, more recent evidence shows that survival and neurological outcome is not improved in these conditions. Current opinion is that corticosteroids are not useful in head injuries (see also Spinal Cord Injury, p.1088) or stroke, and that their adverse effects may outweigh any possible benefit. The management of raised intracranial pressure and the usual drugs used to treat it are discussed on p.833.

References.


1. Jeevaratnam DR, Menon DK. Survey of intensive care of severely head injured patients in the United Kingdom. *BMJ* 1996; **312:** 944–7.
2. Roberts I, *et al.* Absence of evidence for the effectiveness of five interventions routinely used in the intensive care management of severe head injury: a systematic review. *J Neurol Neurosurg Psychiatry* 1998; **65:** 729–33.
3. Roberts I. The CRASH trial: the first large-scale, randomised, controlled trial in head injury. *Crit Care* 2001; **5:** 292–3.
4. Alderson P, Roberts I. Corticosteroids for acute traumatic brain injury. Available in The Cochrane Library; Issue 1. Chichester: John Wiley; 2004.
5. Qizilbash N, *et al.* Corticosteroids for acute ischaemic stroke. Available in The Cochrane Library; Issue 1. Chichester: John Wiley; 2004.


### Chronic active hepatitis

Chronic hepatitis is characterised by liver cell necrosis and inflammation that persists for more than 6 to 12 months. Probably the most serious form is chronic active hepatitis in which inflammatory infiltrates (mononuclear and plasma cells) are found within and around the portal areas, with piecemeal necrosis of adjacent liver cells, and in severe cases bands of necrotic tissue between portal tracts or to the central vein (bridging necrosis). Symptoms are essentially non-specific and include fatigue, malaise, fever, anorexia, jaundice, and raised serum aminotransferase values; biopsy is required for accurate diagnosis. The causes of chronic active hepatitis vary and may include: infection with hepatitis viruses; adverse effects of drugs such as isoniazid, methyldopa, or nitrofurantoin; or, particularly in women, an apparently idiopathic form, auto-immune hepatitis.

Treatment with corticosteroids is widely used in patients with auto-immune hepatitis.[1,2] A moderate initial dose of 20 to 30 mg of prednisolone or prednisone daily by mouth or a higher dose of 60 mg daily may be used,[3-5] and is then slowly tapered over several months to the minimum required for maintenance. Daily maintenance therapy appears more effective than alternate day regimens. Patients who respond (as shown by a return of serum aminotransferase values to the normal or near normal range and a reduction in the inflammatory processes on biopsy) usually require prolonged treatment; although some patients remain in remission for months to years after withdrawal, relapse generally occurs, and therapy should be reinstated when the disease becomes active again.[1]

Combined treatment including azathioprine is frequently given and may be the preferred initial treatment in some patients;[4,5] such treatment is at least as effective as a corticosteroid alone,[2] can produce[6,7] and maintain[8,9] remission, and permits a reduction in corticosteroid dosage in a group of patients who will require long-term drug treatment.[1] There has been some dispute about the value of azathioprine alone, but combined therapy has generally been found to be superior.[6] However, azathioprine has been used alone in high doses to maintain remission.[5,9]

In contrast to the fairly extensive experience with azathioprine, ciclosporin is little used in this condition; once started it appears to be required indefinitely.[4] It may be an alternative in severe disease where corticosteroids alone or with azathioprine cannot suffice. Mycophenolate mofetil may offer an alternative to azathioprine.[5] Some investigators have also used cyclophosphamide successfully,[3] and tacrolimus has been reported to be of benefit.[10]

Penicillamine has been tried as an alternative to prolonged use of corticosteroid maintenance therapy, the dose of penicillamine being gradually increased over several months to a suitable maintenance dose as the dosage of corticosteroid is tapered off.

It is generally agreed that immunosuppression is not suitable in patients with viral chronic active hepatitis.[1,11] However, combination therapy has been reported to produce benefit in patients positive for HBsAg,[6] and it has been reported[12] that patients with chronic active hepatitis of unknown cause, at least some of whom may have hepatitis C,[11] respond as well to corticosteroids or combined therapy as patients with proven auto-immune disease.


1. Krawitt EL. Autoimmune hepatitis. *N Engl J Med* 1996; **334:** 897–903.
2. Stavinoha MW, Soloway RD. Current therapy of chronic liver disease. *Drugs* 1990; **39:** 814–40.
3. Meyer zum Büschenfelde K-H, Lohse AW. Autoimmune hepatitis. *N Engl J Med* 1995; **333:** 1004–5.
4. Czaja AJ. Drug therapy in the management of type 1 autoimmune hepatitis. *Drugs* 1999; **57:** 49–68.
5. Al-Khalidi JA, Czaja AJ. Current concepts in the diagnosis, pathogenesis, and treatment of autoimmune hepatitis. *Mayo Clin Proc* 2001; **76:** 1237–52.
6. Giusti G, *et al.* Immunosuppressive therapy in chronic active hepatitis (CAH): a multicentric retrospective study on 867 patients. *Hepatogastroenterology* 1984; **31:** 24–9.
7. Vegnente A, *et al.* Duration of chronic active hepatitis and the development of cirrhosis. *Arch Dis Child* 1984; **59:** 330–5.
8. Stellon AJ, *et al.* Randomised controlled trial of azathioprine withdrawal in autoimmune chronic active hepatitis. *Lancet* 1985; **i:** 668–70.
9. Johnson PJ, *et al.* Azathioprine for long-term maintenance of remission in autoimmune hepatitis. *N Engl J Med* 1995; **333:** 958–63.
10. Van Thiel DH, *et al.* Tacrolimus: a potential new treatment for autoimmune chronic active hepatitis: results of an open-label preliminary trial. *Am J Gastroenterol* 1995; **90:** 771–6.
11. Gitnick G. Cryptogenic versus autoimmune chronic hepatitis: to split or to lump? *Mayo Clin Proc* 1990; **65:** 119–21.
12. Czaja AJ, *et al.* Clinical features and prognostic implications of severe corticosteroid-treated cryptogenic chronic active hepatitis. *Mayo Clin Proc* 1990; **65:** 23–30.


### Chronic obstructive pulmonary disease

Corticosteroids play some part in the symptomatic and palliative management of chronic obstructive pulmonary disease (COPD—p.779), although there is controversy as to their value. Most patients do not respond to corticosteroids but in about 10% of those receiving maximal bronchodilator therapy a short course of oral corticosteroid therapy can improve airflow further. In these patients maintenance therapy may be given, preferably by inhalation. However, whether corticosteroids slow the deterioration rate and improve long-term outcome in COPD, regardless of corticosteroid responsiveness, remains to be confirmed. Some studies have suggested that inhaled corticosteroids might reduce the number of acute exacerbations and slow the decline in lung function,[1-3] whereas others found no, or limited, benefit.[4-7] Some commentators have therefore cautioned against the routine use of corticosteroids in patients with COPD;[8] certain subgroups of patients, however, may benefit from corticosteroid therapy,[8,9] and a systematic review[10] concluded that inhaled corticosteroids were beneficial in reducing COPD exacerbation rates.

A large randomised trial[11] found that combination therapy with fluticasone and salmeterol reduced exacerbation rate compared with placebo, and improved lung function significantly more than treatment with either drug alone.

Short courses of systemic corticosteroids are commonly used for acute exacerbations of COPD, despite limited evidence of clinical benefit. However, a systematic review[12] concluded that the benefit from corticosteroid therapy is evident within the first day and lasts for at least 5 days of therapy, although there is no evidence suggesting advantage to courses for longer than 2 weeks. Dose-dependent deleterious effects on bone mineral density may occur.


1. Paggiaro PL, *et al.* Multicentre randomised placebo-controlled trial of inhaled fluticasone propionate in patients with chronic obstructive pulmonary disease. *Lancet* 1998; **351:** 773–80.
2. Burge PS, *et al.* Randomised, double blind, placebo controlled study of fluticasone propionate in patients with moderate to severe chronic obstructive pulmonary disease: the ISOLDE trial. *BMJ* 2000; **320:** 1297–1303.
3. van Grunsven PM, *et al.* Long term effects of inhaled corticosteroids in chronic obstructive pulmonary disease: a meta-analysis. *Thorax* 1999; **54:** 7–14.
4. Pauwels RA, *et al.* Long-term treatment with inhaled budesonide in persons with mild chronic obstructive pulmonary disease who continue smoking. *N Engl J Med* 1999; **340:** 1948–53.
5. Bourbeau J, *et al.* Randomised controlled trial of inhaled corticosteroids in patients with chronic obstructive pulmonary disease. *Thorax* 1998; **53:** 477–82.
6. Vestbo J, *et al.* Long-term effect of inhaled budesonide in mild and moderate chronic obstructive pulmonary disease: a randomised controlled trial. *Lancet* 1999; **353:** 1819–23.
7. The Lung Health Study Research Group. Effect of inhaled triamcinolone on the decline in pulmonary function in chronic obstructive pulmonary disease. *N Engl J Med* 2000; **343:** 1902–9.
8. Bonay M, *et al.* Benefits and risks of inhaled corticosteroids in chronic obstructive pulmonary disease. *Drug Safety* 2002; **25:** 57–71.
9. Burge S. Should inhaled corticosteroids be used in the long term treatment of chronic obstructive pulmonary disease? *Drugs* 2001; **61:** 1535–44.
10. Alsaeedi A, *et al.* The effects of inhaled corticosteroids in chronic obstructive pulmonary disease: a systematic review of randomized placebo-controlled trials. *Am J Med* 2002; **113:** 59–65.
11. Calverley P, *et al.* Combined salmeterol and fluticasone in the treatment of chronic obstructive pulmonary disease: a randomised controlled trial. *Lancet* 2003; **361:** 449–56. Correction. *ibid.*; 1660.
12. Singh JM, *et al.* Corticosteroid therapy for patients with acute exacerbations of chronic obstructive pulmonary disease: a systematic review. *Arch Intern Med* 2002; **162:** 2527–36.


### Churg-Strauss syndrome

The Churg-Strauss syndrome is sometimes classified with polyarteritis nodosa (see p.1085), although, unlike the latter, pulmonary manifestations are relatively common in Churg-Strauss syndrome. Patients commonly have a history of allergic disease (rhinitis, sinusitis, and asthma), and intractable asthma and eosinophilia together with granulomatous vasculitis characterise the syndrome.

Treatment is similar to that of polyarteritis nodosa, being based on systemic corticosteroids and, where necessary, cyclophosphamide.[1-4] When cyclophosphamide is used, intravenous pulse therapy is often preferred to continuous oral administration,[2,3] as it has been shown to reduce adverse effects and allows for a lower total dose.[3,4] Substitution of cyclophosphamide with azathioprine or mycophenolate mofetil after 4 to 6 months can also allow for reduced overall doses of cyclophosphamide to be given,[3,4] although azathioprine is not as effective as cyclophosphamide for primary treatment.[4] In patients with haemorrhagic cystitis, there is some suggestion that mycophenolate mofetil may be more effective than azathioprine.[4] Interferon alfa may also be of benefit.[3,5] In patients refractory to corticosteroids and cyclophosphamide, there are reports of benefit with antilymphocyte immunoglobulins or intravenous immunoglobulins.[4]


1. Guillevin L, *et al.* Treatment of polyarteritis nodosa and Churg-Strauss syndrome: a meta-analysis of 3 prospective controlled trials including 182 patients over 12 years. *Ann Med Interne (Paris)* 1992; **143:** 405–16.
2. Guillevin L, Lhote F. Classification and management of necrotising vasculitides. *Drugs* 1997; **53:** 805–16.
3. Noth I, *et al.* Churg-Strauss syndrome. *Lancet* 2003; **361:** 587–94.
4. Conron M, Beynon HLC. Churg-Strauss syndrome. *Thorax* 2000; **55:** 870–7.
5. Tatsis E, *et al.* Interferon-α treatment of four patients with the Churg-Strauss syndrome. *Ann Intern Med* 1998; **129:** 370–4.


### Cogan's syndrome

Corticosteroids are useful in the treatment of Cogan's syndrome, a condition characterised by non-syphilitic interstitial keratitis and audiovestibular symptoms including deafness.[1-3] The deafness, although often irreversible, may respond to systemic corticosteroids initiated within 2 weeks of onset of symptoms (prednisolone or prednisone, at least 1.5 mg/kg daily for 2 weeks is advised) and ocular involvement benefits from topical corticosteroid therapy (e.g. prednisolone 1% at a rate of 1 drop every hour for 1 to 2 weeks).[3] Improvement in ocular symptoms has also been seen with sodium cromoglicate eye drops.[4] For patients with severe Cogan's syndrome including large-vessel vasculitis, corticosteroids have been used in conjunction with other immunosuppressants such as azathioprine, ciclosporin and cyclophosphamide.[5] Methotrexate has also been tried.[6]


1. Anonymous. Cogan's syndrome. *Lancet* 1991; **337:** 1011–12.
2. Vollertsen RS, *et al.* Cogan's syndrome: 18 cases and a review of the literature. *Mayo Clin Proc* 1986; **61:** 344–61.
3. St Clair EW, McCallum RM. Cogan's syndrome. *Curr Opin Rheumatol* 1999; **11:** 47–52.
4. Carter F, Nabarro J. Cromoglycate for Cogan's syndrome. *Lancet* 1987; **i:** 858.
5. Allen NB, *et al.* Use of immunosuppressive agents in the treatment of severe ocular and vascular manifestations of Cogan's syndrome. *Am J Med* 1990; **88:** 296–301.
6. Riente L, *et al.* Efficacy of methotrexate in Cogan's syndrome. *J Rheumatol* 1996; **23:** 1830–1.


### Congenital adrenal hyperplasia

Congenital adrenal hyperplasia comprises a heterogeneous group of disorders due to inherited defects of steroid synthesis in the adrenal gland, the most frequent of which are defects involving 21-hydroxylase or 11-β-hydroxylase. Defective enzyme production blocks the formation of cortisol and aldosterone; the pituitary produces increased amounts of ACTH in an attempt to compensate, but this results in excessive adrenal androgen production. Presentation varies from virilisation and abnormal genital formation at birth to mild cryptic forms that may be detected only later in life. Salt-losing forms (due to lack of aldosterone or the accumulation of precursors with antagonist activity) may lead to hyperkalaemia, acidosis, and dehydration. Patients with 11-β-hydroxylase defect are also prone to hypertension.

Neonates with **salt-losing forms** of congenital adrenal hyperplasia require urgent treatment. Treatment usually consists of a mineralocorticoid, fludrocortisone, and a glucocorticoid (usually hydrocortisone) in regimens similar to those for adrenocortical insufficiency (see p.1075).[1-4] Saline infusion or addition of salt to the feed is required initially.

Even where salt-losing symptoms are not overt or marked, control is reportedly better with a mineralocorticoid added to therapy, rather than with hydrocortisone alone,[4] and it has been recommended that children with salt-losing congenital adrenal hyperplasia should continue to receive combined therapy at least until adult life.[1] Careful titration of dosage is important to avoid growth retardation and toxicity, and potent synthetic glucocorticoids such as betamethasone and dexamethasone may be inappropriate in infants and children with the condition, even in the non-salt-losing form. An alternative approach is the use of flutamide and testolactone to block androgenic effects, together with a reduced dose of hydrocortisone.[4,5] However, studies suggest that normal growth is possible with regular glucocorticoid therapy.[6,7]

Patients with **non-salt-losing congenital adrenal hyperplasia** may be adequately managed with glucocorticoids alone, and in mild late-onset forms a single dose daily in the late evening (when its suppressive effect on ACTH production is greatest) may be sufficient. In adults who do not require mineralocorticoid treatment betamethasone or dexamethasone may be useful because of their lack of mineralocorticoid actions.

Surgical correction may be necessary in females with masculinised external genitalia. Administration of a glucocorticoid to pregnant women whose offspring are considered at risk has been tried in an attempt to prevent virilisation:[3] dexamethasone is preferred to hydrocortisone because of a lack of placental degradation.[4]


1. Griffiths KD, *et al.* Plasma renin activity in the management of congenital adrenal hyperplasia. *Arch Dis Child* 1984; **59:** 360–5.
2. Young MC, Hughes IA. Response to treatment of congenital adrenal hyperplasia in infancy. *Arch Dis Child* 1990; **65:** 441–4.
3. American Academy of Pediatrics. Technical report: congenital adrenal hyperplasia. *Pediatrics* 2000; **106:** 1511–18. Correction. *ibid.* 2001; **107:** 1450.
4. Speiser PW, White PC. Congenital adrenal hyperplasia. *N Engl J Med* 2003; **349:** 776–88.
5. Merke DP, Cutler GB. New approaches to the treatment of congenital adrenal hyperplasia. *JAMA* 1997; **277:** 1073–6.
6. Rivkees SA, Crawford JD. Dexamethasone treatment of virilizing congenital adrenal hyperplasia: the ability to achieve normal growth. *Pediatrics* 2000; **106:** 767–73.
7. Eugster EA, *et al.* Height outcome in congenital adrenal hyperplasia caused by 21-hydroxylase deficiency: a meta-analysis. *J Pediatr* 2001; **138:** 26–32.


## Corneal graft rejection

Corticosteroids are the mainstay of postoperative prophylaxis and treatment of corneal graft rejection.[1] Topical and subconjunctival corticosteroids are widely used, but in acute rejection episodes involving the endothelium systemic therapy is usually necessary. A single 500-mg intravenous pulse of methylprednisolone appears to be as effective as up to 2 weeks' treatment with oral prednisolone 60 to 80 mg daily for the management of severe endothelial rejection.[2] However, another trial found that addition of a single intravenous pulse of 500 mg methylprednisolone to local corticosteroid treatment with betamethasone and dexamethasone gave no benefit over local therapy alone.[3]

In high-risk patients corticosteroids alone provide insufficient immunosuppression and systemic ciclosporin is occasionally used.[1,4] Mycophenolate mofetil appears to be as effective as ciclosporin in preventing acute rejection following high-risk corneal transplantation.[4] Topical ciclosporin has also been investigated.[5]

For discussions of the role of corticosteroids in other forms of organ and tissue grafting, see Organ and Tissue Transplantation, p.1344.


1. Hill JC. Immunosuppression in corneal transplantation. *Eye* 1995; **9:** 247–53.
2. Hill JC, *et al.* Corticosteroids in corneal graft rejection: oral versus single pulse therapy. *Ophthalmology* 1991; **98:** 329–33.
3. Hudde T, *et al.* Randomised controlled trial of corticosteroid regimens in endothelial corneal allograft rejection. *Br J Ophthalmol* 1999; **83:** 1348–52.
4. Reis A, *et al.* Mycophenolate mofetil versus cyclosporin A in high risk keratoplasty patients: a prospectively randomised clinical trial. *Br J Ophthalmol* 1999; **83:** 1268–71.
5. Zhao J-C, Jin X-Y. Local therapy of corneal allograft rejection with cyclosporine. *Am J Ophthalmol* 1995; **19:** 189–94.


## Croup

Croup is an acute childhood syndrome of upper respiratory tract inflammation (laryngotracheobronchitis) associated with viral infection, usually by parainfluenza virus although other viruses may also produce the syndrome. It is characterised by harsh, barking cough, stridor, and hoarseness, most usually occurring at night.[1,2]

Traditional home management has revolved around the inhalation of steam, despite a lack of evidence for effectiveness, but symptoms may be sufficiently alarming to result in presentation to a hospital.

In severe croup there is clear evidence that treatment with a systemic corticosteroid reduces symptoms and decreases the need for intubation.[3-5] Oral dexamethasone is as effective as intramuscular administration,[6] and while dexamethasone 600 micrograms/kg is commonly prescribed, lower doses of 300 micrograms/kg and 150 micrograms/kg appear to be equally effective.[2] Nebulised budesonide has also been reported to be effective,[7-9] and of similar efficacy to inhalation of nebulised adrenaline.[10] However despite the theoretical attraction of this route, studies have failed to find any significant difference in effectiveness between nebulised budesonide 2 mg and oral dexamethasone 600 micrograms/kg,[11] or combination therapy with both,[12] and another study found 600 micrograms/kg of dexamethasone given intramuscularly to be more effective than 4 mg of nebulised budesonide.[13] In contrast, others have found that addition of nebulised budesonide to oral dexamethasone produced more rapid improvement than the latter alone.[14] Studies have also shown a significant benefit from corticosteroids in children with mild to moderate croup,[11,15,16] and although the use of such potent drugs in children with a mild, largely self-limiting condition has been questioned,[17] a review of the risks and benefits concluded that oral dexamethasone 150 micrograms/kg, or nebulised budesonide 2 mg were the treatment of choice in mild to moderate croup while oral prednisolone 1 mg/kg should be given for croup requiring intubation.[1] However, nebulised adrenaline is probably the drug of choice where rapid relief of obstructive symptoms is required.[2] Heliox, a mixture of helium and oxygen, may be used as adjunctive therapy to glucocorticoids, for short-term treatment of refractory croup.[2]


1. Yates RW, Doull IJM. A risk-benefit assessment of corticosteroids in the management of croup. *Drug Safety* 1997; **16:** 48–55.
2. Brown JC. The management of croup. *Br Med Bull* 2002; **61:** 189–202.
3. Kairys SW, *et al.* Steroid treatment of laryngotracheitis: a meta-analysis of the evidence from randomized trials. *Pediatrics* 1989; **83:** 683–93.
4. Freezer NJ, *et al.* Steroids in croup: do they increase the incidence of successful extubation? *Anaesth Intensive Care* 1990; **18:** 224–8.
5. Geelhoed GC. Sixteen years of croup in a Western Australian teaching hospital: effects of routine steroid treatment. *Ann Emerg Med* 1996; **28:** 621–6.
6. Rittichier KK, Ledwith CA. Outpatient treatment of moderate croup with dexamethasone: intramuscular versus oral dosing. *Pediatrics* 2000; **106:** 1344–8.
7. Klassen TP, *et al.* Nebulized budesonide for children with mild-to-moderate croup. *N Engl J Med* 1994; **331:** 285–9.
8. Husby S, *et al.* Treatment of croup with nebulised steroid (budesonide): a double blind, placebo controlled study. *Arch Dis Child* 1993; **68:** 352–5.
9. Godden CW, *et al.* Double blind placebo controlled trial of nebulised budesonide for croup. *Arch Dis Child* 1997; **76:** 155–8.
10. Fitzgerald D, *et al.* Nebulized budesonide is as effective as nebulized adrenaline in moderately severe croup. *Pediatrics* 1996; **97:** 722–5.
11. Geelhoed GC, MacDonald WBG. Oral and inhaled steroids in croup: a randomized placebo-controlled trial. *Pediatr Pulmonol* 1995; **20:** 355–61.
12. Klassen TP, *et al.* Nebulized budesonide and oral dexamethasone for treatment of croup: a randomized controlled trial. *JAMA* 1998; **279:** 1629–32.
13. Johnson DW, *et al.* A comparison of nebulised budesonide, intramuscular dexamethasone, and placebo for moderately severe croup. *N Engl J Med* 1998; **339:** 498–503.
14. Klassen TP, *et al.* The efficacy of nebulized budesonide in dexamethasone-treated outpatients with croup. *Pediatrics* 1996; **97:** 463–6.
15. Geelhoed GC, *et al.* Efficacy of a small single dose of oral dexamethasone for outpatient croup: a double blind placebo controlled clinical trial. *BMJ* 1996; **313:** 140–2.
16. Russell K, *et al.* Glucocorticoids for croup. Available in The Cochrane Library; Issue 1. Chichester: John Wiley; 2004.
17. Macfarlane PI, Suri S. Steroids in the management of croup. *BMJ* 1996; **312:** 510.


## Cystic fibrosis

Corticosteroids have been used by mouth or by inhalation in the management of the inflammatory response of the lungs in cystic fibrosis (see p.123).

## Deafness

For references to the use of corticosteroids in the treatment of deafness associated with Cogan's syndrome, see above.

## Dermatomyositis

For references to the treatment of dermatomyositis with corticosteroids, see Polymyositis and Dermatomyositis, p.1086.

## Diffuse parenchymal lung disease

Diffuse parenchymal lung disease (DPLD; interstitial lung disease) represents a large and heterogeneous group of inflammatory disorders that have in common a thickening of the interstitial walls between alveoli. In some cases, particularly in the early stages, this is due to accumulation of inflammatory cells in the interstitium, and control of inflammation can reverse the changes; however, when fibrotic changes to the alveolar walls take place these are usually irreversible. The causes of chronic DPLD are numerous and include pneumoconioses due to inhalation of inorganic dusts (as in asbestosis and silicosis); extrinsic allergic alveolitis due to inhalation of, usually, organic antigens (as in farmers' lung, bird fanciers' lung, and many similar occupational disorders); cryptogenic fibrosing alveolitis (idiopathic pulmonary fibrosis); adverse effects of drugs such as bleomycin; sarcoidosis; lung disease associated with collagen vascular disorders such as rheumatoid arthritis and systemic lupus erythematosus, or with the vasculitides; histiocytic syndromes; and pulmonary eosinophilic syndromes. Cryptogenic fibrosing alveolitis (below) and sarcoidosis (p.1087) are probably the most common chronic DPLDs.[1]

The symptoms of DPLD are usually insidious and non-specific, and may include dyspnoea of varying severity, usually first noticed on exertion, cough, and fatigue; fine crackling sounds (rales) on breathing and finger clubbing occur in some forms. If the disease progresses, respiratory failure becomes more severe, and eventually may prove fatal.

Where a causative agent can be identified, initial treatment is to prevent exposure but where inflammation persists, or where the causation is uncertain, corticosteroids are the mainstay of treatment (despite a lack of controlled trials for efficacy),[2] in an attempt to control inflammation and preserve as much normal tissue as possible. The management of cryptogenic fibrosing alveolitis is discussed in more detail below.

**Cryptogenic fibrosing alveolitis** (idiopathic pulmonary fibrosis) is a form of DPLD of uncertain origin, associated with alveolitis and thickening of the interstitial walls by oedema, cellular exudate, and fibrosis. The clinical course is variable but the mean survival is only 3 to 5 years.[3] Cryptogenic fibrosing alveolitis itself appears to represent a spectrum of disorders; some have advocated that usual interstitial pneumonia (the most common form) should be distinguished from forms such as non-specific or desquamative interstitial pneumonia, or cryptogenic organising pneumonia (bronchiolitis obliterans organising pneumonia), which may respond better to corticosteroid therapy.[4-8]

The British[1] and American[8] Thoracic Societies have recommended that where therapy is considered appropriate initial treatment should be with oral prednisone or prednisolone 500 micrograms/kg plus azathioprine. Azathioprine may be used alone where corticosteroid therapy is problematic, or cyclophosphamide may be given with the corticosteroid if azathioprine is not tolerated. About 50% of patients with cryptogenic fibrosing alveolitis show a symptomatic response to corticosteroids and about 25% show an improvement in lung function.[1] However, in the absence of placebo-controlled trials there is no clear evidence that treatment improves survival.[1,7] Survival does seem to be improved following treatment with corticosteroids plus azathioprine, compared with corticosteroids alone.[1] It should also be borne in mind that patients defined as having cryptogenic fibrosing alveolitis are a heterogeneous group, with some forms appearing to respond better to treatment than others, which makes comparison of studies difficult.[5] If the condition stabilises, the dose of corticosteroid may be reduced gradually for maintenance. Corticosteroid therapy is usually continued lifelong; attempts at withdrawal should be gradual and cautious. Relapse or clinical deterioration may warrant an increased dose of corticosteroid, or addition of an immunosuppressant.[8]

A variety of other drugs have been tried in patients with cryptogenic fibrosing alveolitis;[1,5,8,9] responses have been reported in a few patients given ciclosporin or penicillamine, and there is some evidence suggesting that colchicine may be as effective as a corticosteroid. Toxicity has limited the use of chlorambucil and methotrexate.[8] Other drugs under investigation include interferon gamma and pirfenidone.[5]

In patients in whom other options fail, lung transplantation (p.1347) should be considered.[1,5,8,9]


1. British Thoracic Society. The diagnosis, assessment and treatment of diffuse parenchymal lung disease in adults. *Thorax* 1999; **54:** (suppl 1): S1–S30. Also available at: http://www.brit-thoracic.org.uk/docs/Parenchymaltext.pdf (accessed 27/04/04)

2. Johnston IDA, *et al.* British Thoracic Society study of cryptogenic fibrosing alveolitis: current presentation and initial management. *Thorax* 1997; **52:** 38–44.
3. Chan-Yeung M, Müller NL. Cryptogenic fibrosing alveolitis. *Lancet* 1997; **350:** 651–6.
4. Ryu JH, *et al.* Idiopathic pulmonary fibrosis: current concepts. *Mayo Clin Proc* 1998; **73:** 1085–1101.
5. Gross TJ, Hunninghake GW. Idiopathic pulmonary fibrosis. *N Engl J Med* 2001; **345:** 517–25.
6. Cordier J-F. Update on cryptogenic organising pneumonia (idiopathic bronchiolitis obliterans organising pneumonia). *Swiss Med Wkly* 2002; **132:** 588–91.
7. Richeldi L, *et al.* Corticosteroids for idiopathic pulmonary fibrosis. Available in The Cochrane Library; Issue 1. Chichester: John Wiley; 2004.
8. American Thoracic Society. Idiopathic pulmonary fibrosis: diagnosis and treatment: international consensus statement. *Am J Respir Crit Care Med* 2000; **161:** 646–64. Also available at: http://www.thoracic.org/adobe/statements/idiopathic1-19.pdf (accessed 27/04/04)
9. Nicod LP. Recognition and treatment of idiopathic pulmonary fibrosis. *Drugs* 1998; **55:** 555–62.


## Eczema

Several treatments may be used in the management of atopic eczema (p.1135) but topical corticosteroids are the mainstay. The least potent preparation that is effective should be used, combined with regular use of an emollient; in mild to moderate disease the topical corticosteroid is only given for 1 to 2 weeks at a time. Most patients with mild to moderate eczema respond to treatment with a mildly potent preparation such as 1% hydrocortisone ointment. For older children and adults with refractory disease, a more potent topical corticosteroid should be considered for long enough to bring the disease under control, followed by a weaker preparation as the condition improves.

The use of systemic corticosteroids is a treatment of last resort in resistant severe eczema, usually for short periods to control the disease, and very rarely for maintenance.

## Epidermolysis bullosa

High-dose oral corticosteroids may be tried to control blistering in severe forms of epidermolysis bullosa (p.1135).

## Epilepsy

Corticosteroids and corticotropin have been commonly used to treat **infantile spasms,**[1] which are generally unresponsive to conventional antiepileptics. One study[2] indicated that high-dose corticotropin was preferable to prednisone. However, as discussed on p.349, corticotropin and corticosteroids are associated with frequent and severe adverse effects, and some now prefer newer antiepileptics such as vigabatrin.

It has been suggested that high doses of corticosteroids may produce a response in epilepsia partialis continua (a form of **status epilepticus**) refractory to standard antiepileptics (see p.352).


1. Robinson RO. Seizures and steroids. *Arch Dis Child* 1985; **60:** 94–5.
2. Baram TZ, *et al.* High-dose corticotropin (ACTH) versus prednisone for infantile spasms: a prospective, randomized, blinded study. *Pediatrics* 1996; **97:** 375–9.


## Erythema multiforme

In the management of erythema multiforme (p.1135) systemic corticosteroids may be considered in severe reactions but there has been controversy about their value.

## Giant cell arteritis

Giant cell arteritis (temporal arteritis; cranial arteritis) is a vasculitic disorder that is frequently associated with polymyalgia rheumatica (p.1086). It occurs mainly in persons over 50 years of age of European, particularly Scandinavian, extraction and is more common in women than men. It is characterised by inflammatory, granulomatous lesions with giant mononuclear cell infiltrates affecting large and medium sized arteries, particularly those supplying the neck and extracranial structures of head and arms. Symptoms vary but may include headache, scalp tenderness, claudication of the jaw, swelling and absence of pulse in the temporal artery, fever, weight loss, malaise, anaemia, visual disturbances, and irreversible blindness. About a third of all patients also exhibit polymyalgia rheumatica.

Treatment is with corticosteroids,[1-7] and early diagnosis and treatment is desirable to reduce the risk of sudden blindness. Most regimens have involved high initial doses of corticosteroid to control the disease followed by reduction to a maintenance dose, but both initial and maintenance doses have varied considerably. Prednisone or prednisolone 40 to 60 mg daily by mouth initially is generally considered adequate in uncomplicated cases without visual symptoms;[1,4-6] this can then be reduced gradually according to the patient's response. Some, however, recommend[3] lower initial doses of about 20 mg daily. While it is suggested that patients presenting with visual symptoms should receive 80 mg daily or 1 mg/kg daily of prednisone or prednisolone,[3,7] some ophthalmologists[8] recommend that all patients with giant cell arteritis receive these doses, as visual loss may be sudden and profound. Initial 1-g doses of pulsed intravenous methylprednisolone have also been used.[2,5,8]

Maintenance treatment is usually required and while a small number require indefinite treatment, most patients should be able to discontinue treatment within 5 years; however, relapses are not uncommon.[7]

Because of the need for prolonged corticosteroid therapy, side-effects are common,[7] and their management difficult. Azathioprine has been added to corticosteroid therapy for its modest 'steroid-sparing' effect,[9] whereas results with methotrexate have been conflicting.[4,6,10] Other immunosuppressants have been tried,[4,6] but are not routinely used. Dapsone has been reported to be of benefit, but its use is limited by haematological toxicity.[4]

The prognosis is excellent in adequately-treated patients, as the life expectancy of patients with giant cell arteritis is the same as the general population.[11]


1. Swannell AJ. Polymyalgia rheumatica and temporal arteritis: diagnosis and management. *BMJ* 1997; **314:** 1329–32.
2. Gurwood AS, Malloy KA. Giant cell arteritis. *Clin Exp Optom* 2002; **85:** 19–26.
3. Wilke WS. What is the appropriate initial dose of corticosteroids to treat giant cell arteritis? *Cleve Clin J Med* 2000; **67:** 546–8.
4. Barilla-LaBarca M-L, *et al.* Polymyalgia rheumatica/temporal arteritis: recent advances. *Curr Rheumatol Rep* 2002; **4:** 39–46.
5. Salvarani C, *et al.* Polymyalgia rheumatica and giant-cell arteritis. *N Engl J Med* 2002; **347:** 261–71.
6. Weyand CM, Goronzy JJ. Giant-cell arteritis and polymyalgia rheumatica. *Ann Intern Med* 2003; **139:** 505–15.
7. Buch MH, Bird HA. Polymyalgia rheumatica and giant cell arteritis. In: Snaith ML, ed. *ABC of rheumatology.* 3rd ed. London: BMJ Books, 2004: 75–9.
8. Ferris J, Lamb R. Polymyalgia rheumatica and giant cell arteritis. *BMJ* 1995; **311:** 455.
9. De Silva M, Hazleman BL. Azathioprine in giant cell arteritis/polymyalgia rheumatica: a double blind study. *Ann Rheum Dis* 1986; **45:** 136–8.
10. Hernández-García C, *et al.* Methotrexate treatment in the management of giant cell arteritis. *Scand J Rheumatol* 1994; **23:** 295–8.
11. Matteson EL, *et al.* Long-term survival of patients with giant cell arteritis in the American College of Rheumatology giant cell arteritis classification criteria cohort. *Am J Med* 1996; **100:** 193–6.


## Glomerular kidney disease

Glomerular disease accounts for a considerable proportion of all kidney disease. Various forms of primary glomerular disease (glomerulopathy) are known, and are discussed below; in addition, numerous systemic diseases (connective tissue disorders such as systemic lupus erythematosus as well as malignancy and conditions such as diabetes), may result in secondary glomerular disorders. Despite the various potential causes it is thought that many of these diseases act by common immunological mechanisms to damage the glomerulus, either by accumulation of antigen-antibody complexes (immune-complex nephritis) or more rarely by the formation of antibodies to the glomerular basement membrane (anti-GBM nephritis).

Since the kidney can respond in only a limited number of ways to glomerular damage, certain common presentations are seen regardless of aetiology, including **acute glomerulonephritis** (acute nephritis syndrome), which is marked by haematuria and proteinuria of abrupt onset, usually with renal impairment (a decrease in glomerular filtration rate), salt and water retention, and hypertension; and the **nephrotic syndrome**, which is marked by severe proteinuria, hypoalbuminaemia, and oedema. Other, less dramatic presentations of glomerular disease are asymptomatic proteinuria or microscopic haematuria; alternatively, glomerular disease may be one of the many potential causes of chronic renal failure. Appropriate management of these conditions depends to a considerable extent on the underlying disease.

• MANAGEMENT OF PRIMARY GLOMERULAR DISEASE.

**Minimal change nephropathy** (MCN; minimal change disease). This condition occurs mainly in children, the highest incidence being at 2 to 4 years, and is the main cause of childhood nephrotic syndrome. It also accounts for about 20% of adult cases of nephrotic syndrome.[1] It is treated with a corticosteroid. Regimens vary somewhat but a suggested regimen for adults has been 60 mg prednisolone daily by mouth for 4 days, reduced to 40 mg daily until remission occurs (which in 90% of patients will be within 3 weeks) and then tapered off.[1] In children, initial doses of 60 mg/m$^2$ of prednisolone or prednisone daily have been used,[2] which may be given for 4 weeks before switching to 40 mg/m$^2$ given on alternate days for a further 4 weeks, and then tapered off.[3] Lower relapse rates have been reported with 60 mg/m$^2$ prednisone given daily for 6 weeks, followed by 40 mg/m$^2$ on alternate days for 6 weeks; this 12-week course may be preferable to the standard 8-week course.[2] A modification to the children's dose is to give 60 mg/m$^2$ of prednisolone daily until there is a response when the dose is reduced to 40 mg/m$^2$ on alternate days for the next 4 weeks. If there is no response within 4 weeks' treatment with the 60 mg/m$^2$ dose then the drug should be withdrawn and the child considered to be corticosteroid resistant.[4] A systematic review of treatment regimens found that children with their first episode of nephropathy should be treated with prednisone for at least 3 months, and possibly up to 7, to reduce the risk of relapse.[5]

Relapse is common and occurs in about 60% of cases; relapses usually respond to a further course of corticosteroids, but if a third relapse occurs cyclophosphamide 2 to 3 mg/kg daily for 8 to 12 weeks may be added to a course of corticosteroid therapy.[1,2] Deflazacort may also be effective in corticosteroid-sensitive patients who do not respond to prednisone.[5] Cytotoxics or immunosuppressants are reserved for frequently relapsing or corticosteroid-dependent cases because of their potential for severe toxicity, including carcinogenesis; cyclophosphamide appears to be preferred to chlorambucil because it is perceived as entailing a somewhat lower risk, although both are effective.[2,6] Ciclosporin has been used long-term to achieve and maintain remission, although renal biopsies are advised to screen for nephrotoxicity.[2,6] Levamisole has also been reported to be of benefit.[2,6]

**Focal glomerulosclerosis**. Focal glomerulosclerosis is a sclerosing lesion affecting parts of the glomeruli which occurs in some patients who otherwise have symptoms characteristic of minimal change nephropathy, and some authorities do not regard it as a distinct disease. It is common in abusers of diamorphine and has also been linked with the nephropathy that can occur in patients with AIDS. Treatment is similar to that for minimal change nephropathy but only about 20% of cases respond to corticosteroids; addition of a cytotoxic immunosuppressant such as cyclophosphamide may improve the prospect of remission. Responses to ciclosporin have been seen in both adults and children with corticosteroid-resistant disease.[2,7] Prolonged treatment may be necessary and relapse is common when ciclosporin is discontinued.[6] Tacrolimus has been reported to be successful after ciclosporin failure,[2,7] and mycophenolate mofetil has been tried with conflicting results.[7] High-dose pulsed methylprednisolone, given in a tapering schedule over 6 years, has been reported to show high response rates in focal glomerulosclerosis.[2] In patients who fail to respond, progression to renal failure may occur over several years, but renal transplantation may not be helpful as disease can recur in the transplanted kidney.

**Membranous nephropathy** (membranous glomerulonephritis). This is a disease predominately of adults, in whom it is the single most important cause of the nephrotic syndrome, accounting for about 50% of cases. It is characterised by diffuse thickening of the glomerular basement membrane following subepithelial deposition of immune complexes. The course of disease is variable and often slow, with some spontaneous remissions, which makes the benefits of treatment difficult to demonstrate and the use of potentially toxic drugs difficult to justify. Cyclophosphamide or chlorambucil combined with a corticosteroid appear to produce some clinical improvement, and stabilisation of progressive disease but corticosteroids alone do not appear to be of benefit.[8,9] Ciclosporin is an alternative but therapy may need to be continued for 6 months or more before remission occurs.[8,9] Other immunosuppressants under investigation in this condition include mycophenolate mofetil[9] and rituximab. Recent studies have also emphasised the control of blood pressure and proteinuria using ACE inhibitors and angiotensin II receptor antagonists.[9]

**Mesangiocapillary glomerulonephritis** (MCGN; membranoproliferative glomerulonephritis; MPGN). Mesangiocapillary glomerulonephritis comprises 2 separate diseases, known as type I and type II, which both occur in children and young adults and usually result in nephrotic syndrome, although about 20% of cases present with acute glomerulonephritis. Both forms show proliferation of mesangial cells and thickening of glomerular walls with formation of deposits (in type I disease due to immune complexes) in capillary walls and basement membranes. There is no established treatment regimen: some improvement or stabilisation of renal function may occur with corticosteroids and cytotoxic immunosuppressants, but about half of all patients develop end-stage renal failure within 15 to 20 years (type I disease) or 6 to 10 years (type II disease). Antiplatelet drugs and anticoagulants have also been tried but as with other therapies there is little evidence of benefit, and some centres do not recommend any specific therapy, although prednisolone and cyclophosphamide may be offered to those with a rapidly progressive course.[10]

**IgA nephropathy** (Berger's disease) is the commonest cause of primary glomerular disease, and is most common in young men. It results in focal, segmental proliferative glomerulonephritis associated with mesangial formation of immune deposits largely composed of IgA. The usual presentation is acute glomerulonephritis with gross haematuria, often during or just after viral upper-respiratory-tract infection. Some patients develop rapidly progressive disease similar to idiopathic rapidly progressive glomerulonephritis, with renal failure within 6 months, but in many others the syndrome is benign, and requires only observation. No form of therapy has been unequivocally shown to be of value, but control of associated hypertension, usually with ACE inhibitors, is considered important. Corticosteroids and cytotoxic immunosuppressants may be tried in severe rapidly progressive disease.[11-15] Promising results have been seen with the use of n-3 fatty acids from fish oil, and there are also reports of benefit with normal immunoglobulin, and mycophenolate mofetil.[14]

**Idiopathic rapidly progressive glomerulonephritis** (RPGN). Although rapidly progressive glomerulonephritis (crescentic glomerulonephritis) may be a feature of other forms of glomerular disease such as IgA nephropathy (see above) or Goodpasture's syndrome (see below) it also occurs in an idiopathic form. The disease is characterised by the formation of glomerular crescents associated with leakage of fibrin from damaged capillaries, and loss of renal function is very rapid, sometimes with renal failure within weeks. Oral corticosteroids are of little value alone, but pulsed intravenous methylprednisolone followed by oral prednisone or prednisone and cyclophosphamide over several months has produced some impressive responses;[16,17] an alternative is the use of intensive plasma exchange together with a corticosteroid and cytotoxic immunosuppressants.[18] Controlled trials of these therapies are mostly lacking, although a small prospective study[19] found lymphocytapheresis to be more effective than pulsed methylprednisolone as an addition to prednisolone and cyclophosphamide therapy for reduction of glomerular injury.

**Goodpasture's syndrome**. Goodpasture's syndrome is a form of anti-GBM nephritis in which rapidly progressive glomerulonephritis is accompanied by pulmonary haemorrhage (because the antibody responsible for the renal symptoms also reacts with the membranes of the alveoli). It is a disease predominately of young males. Pulmonary haemorrhage responds to high dose oral prednisolone or prednisone, or pulsed intravenous methylprednisolone, but corticosteroids are of little value in controlling renal lesions, which requires vigorous plasma exchange therapy with corticosteroids and cyclophosphamide on a daily or alternate day basis for several weeks, until antibody is no longer detectable and disease progression has halted; it is important to begin therapy before renal damage becomes irreversible.[20]

• MANAGEMENT OF SECONDARY GLOMERULAR DISEASE.

**Post-infectious glomerulonephritis**. The classical form of post-infectious glomerulonephritis is post-streptococcal glomerulonephritis, which produces an immune-complex-mediated acute glomerulonephritis, but glomerular disease may follow other bacterial infections, as well as protozoal infections such as malaria (malaria-associated nephrotic syndrome is familiar in endemic regions) and viral infections such as AIDS (see Focal Glomerulosclerosis, above). In most cases no additional treatment beyond appropriate management of infection and general supportive care is warranted, and corticosteroids and cytotoxic immunosuppressants are not generally used and may in some cases be harmful.[21] Nonetheless, delayed progressive renal disease may occur in a minority of patients, and has prompted efforts to treat.[20]

**Other secondary glomerulopathies**. Where glomerular disease is secondary to other diseases (connective tissue disorders such as systemic lupus erythematosus, the vasculitides, Henoch-Schönlein purpura, thrombotic thrombocytopenic purpura, or others such as rheumatoid arthritis, amyloidosis, neoplasia, sickle-cell disease, gout, or diabetes mellitus) most treatment is directed at the underlying disease. In addition, symptomatic management such as the use of sodium restriction for the oedema of nephrotic syndrome may be appropriate; diuretics should be used cautiously because of the risk of hypovolaemia.[22] Proteinuria of various causes may respond to the use of ACE inhibitors or NSAIDs,[1,22] although care is required in patients with renal artery stenosis or renal failure respectively. Associated hypertension and hypercholesterolaemia should be treated, and anticoagulants such as heparin may be required for associated coagulation disorders.[22] Renal toxicity can arise from various drug treatments and this should also be treated symptomatically.


1. Boulton-Jones M. Management of nephrotic syndrome. *Prescribers' J* 1993; **33:** 96–102. Correction. *ibid.*; 176.
2. Eddy AA, Symons JM. Nephrotic syndrome in childhood. *Lancet* 2003; **362:** 629–39.
3. Hogg RJ, *et al.* Evaluation and management of proteinuria and nephrotic syndrome in children: recommendations from a pediatric nephrology panel established at the National Kidney Foundation conference on proteinuria, albuminuria, risk, assessment, detection, and elimination (PARADE). *Pediatrics* 2000; **105:** 1242–9.
4. Report of a Workshop by the British Association for Paediatric Nephrology and Research Unit, Royal College of Physicians. Consensus statement on management and audit potential for steroid responsive nephrotic syndrome. *Arch Dis Child* 1994; **70:** 151–7.
5. Hodson EM, *et al.* Corticosteroid therapy for nephrotic syndrome in children. Available in The Cochrane Library; Issue 1. Chichester: John Wiley; 2004.
6. Abeyagunawardena A, *et al.* Immunosuppressive therapy of childhood idiopathic nephrotic syndrome. *Expert Opin Pharmacother* 2002; **3:** 513–19.
7. Ponticelli C, Passerini P. Alternative treatments for focal and segmental glomerular sclerosis. *Clin Nephrol* 2001; **55:** 345–8.
8. Ponticelli C, Passerini P. Treatment of membranous nephropathy. *Nephrol Dial Transplant* 2001; **16** (suppl 5): 8–10.
9. Kincaid-Smith P. Pharmacological management of membranous nephropathy. *Curr Opin Nephrol Hypertens* 2002; **11:** 149–54.
10. Mason PD, Pusey CD. Glomerulonephritis: diagnosis and treatment. *BMJ* 1994; **309:** 1557–63. Correction. *ibid.* 1995; **310:** 116.
11. Goumenos D, *et al.* Can immunosuppressive drugs slow the progression of IgA nephropathy? *Nephrol Dial Transplant* 1995; **10:** 1173–81.
12. Faedda R, *et al.* Immunosuppressive treatment of Berger's disease. *Clin Pharmacol Ther* 1996; **60:** 561–7.
13. Kobayashi Y, *et al.* Steroid therapy during the early stage of progressive IgA nephropathy: a 10-year follow-up study. *Nephron* 1996; **72:** 237–42.
14. Donadio JV, Grande JP. IgA nephropathy. *N Engl J Med* 2002; **347:** 738–48.
15. Pozzi C, *et al.* Corticosteroids in IgA nephropathy: a randomised controlled trial. *Lancet* 1999; **353:** 883–7.
16. Bolton WK, Sturgill BC. Methylprednisolone therapy for acute crescentic rapidly progressive glomerulonephritis. *Am J Nephrol* 1989; **9:** 368–75.
17. Bruns FJ, *et al.* Long-term follow-up of aggressively treated idiopathic rapidly progressive glomerulonephritis. *Am J Med* 1989; **86:** 400–6.
18. Gianviti A, *et al.* Retrospective study of plasma exchange in patients with idiopathic rapidly progressive glomerulonephritis and vasculitis. *Arch Dis Child* 1996; **75:** 186–90.
19. Furuta T, *et al.* Lymphocytapheresis to treat rapidly progressive glomerulonephritis: a randomised comparison with steroid-pulse treatment. *Lancet* 1998; **352:** 203–4.
20. Couser WG. Glomerulonephritis. *Lancet* 1999; **353:** 1509–15.
21. Adeniyi A, *et al.* A controlled trial of cyclophosphamide and azathioprine in Nigerian children with the nephrotic syndrome and poorly selective proteinuria. *Arch Dis Child* 1979; **54:** 204–7.
22. Robinson RF, *et al.* Management of nephrotic syndrome in children. *Pharmacotherapy* 2003; **23:** 1021–36.


## Graves' ophthalmopathy

Patients with moderate to severe ophthalmopathy as a result of hyperthyroidism (p.1594) may be treated with high-dose systemic corticosteroids or with orbital radiotherapy, which appear to be equally effective. Both therapies may also be combined. Giving a corticosteroid with radioiodine therapy may prevent transient exacerbation of Graves' ophthalmopathy.[1]


1. Bartalena L, *et al.* Relation between therapy for hyperthyroidism and the course of Graves' ophthalmopathy. *N Engl J Med* 1998; **338:** 73–8.


## Haemangioma

Haemangiomas are benign vascular neoplasms of the skin that may enlarge dramatically before regressing spontaneously. Although no treatment is normally required, occasional complications due to ocular or visceral involvement, or associated thrombocytopenia due to platelet trapping (the Kasabach-Merritt syndrome), may merit treatment, generally with corticosteroids. Oral prednisone or prednisolone is usually given; intravenous high-dose methylprednisolone has been used for life-threatening haemangiomas.[1] Response is variable.[1-3] Another common technique is intralesional injection of a mixture of triamcinolone with betamethasone.[4] There has been a report of 2 infants responding to vincristine after corticosteroids had failed.[5] Interferon alfa has been used for corticosteroid-refractory lesions.[1] Phototherapy with a pulsed dye laser has also been reported to be effective;[6] a randomised trial of this method found no benefit compared with observation only,[7] but treatment is still recommended by some[8] for problematic lesions.


1. Drolet BA, *et al.* Hemangiomas in children. *N Engl J Med* 1999; **341:** 173–81.
2. Enjolras O, *et al.* Management of alarming hemangiomas in infancy: a review of 25 cases. *Pediatrics* 1990; **85:** 491–8.
3. Sadan N, Wolach B. Treatment of hemangiomas of infants with high doses of prednisone. *J Pediatr* 1996; **128:** 141–6.
4. Yap E-Y, *et al.* Periocular capillary hemangioma: a review for pediatricians and family physicians. *Mayo Clin Proc* 1998; **73:** 753–9.
5. Payarols JP, *et al.* Treatment of life-threatening infantile hemangiomas with vincristine. *N Engl J Med* 1995; **333:** 69.
6. Barlow RJ, *et al.* Treatment of proliferative haemangiomas with the 585 nm pulsed dye laser. *Br J Dermatol* 1996; **34:** 700–4.
7. Batta K, *et al.* Randomised controlled study of early pulsed dye laser treatment of uncomplicated childhood haemangiomas: results of a 1-year analysis. *Lancet* 2002; **360:** 521–7.
8. Hohenleutner U, Landthaler M. Laser treatment of childhood haemangioma: progress or not? *Lancet* 2002; **360:** 502–3.


## Headache

Corticosteroids have a limited role in the management of some types of headache. Although their long-term use is not considered desirable, short courses of prednisolone or prednisone in doses of 20 to 40 mg daily can be an effective alternative to standard drugs such as ergotamine in the prevention of cluster headache attacks during cluster periods (p.464). Corticosteroids have also been used for the emergency treatment of prolonged severe attacks of migraine (status migrainosus) (p.464) refractory to other drugs.

## Herpes infections

Although corticosteroids alone are contra-indicated for most forms of ocular herpes simplex infection (p.620), which should be treated with a topical antiviral such as aciclovir, a combination of corticosteroid and antiviral may be useful in some cases. For mention of the use of corticosteroids in Bell's palsy, which may be associated with herpes simplex virus, see p.1076, and for discussion of their role in postherpetic neuralgia, see p.7.

## Hypercalcaemia

For a description of the treatment of hypercalcaemia, including the specific role of corticosteroids, see p.1218.

## Hypersensitivity vasculitis

Hypersensitivity vasculitis is usually associated with an antigenic stimulus, either exogenous (e.g. a drug[1] or microbe), or endogenous (e.g. an immune complex associated with connective tissue disease). The term covers a heterogeneous group of disorders, many of which are associated with some underlying disease process (including infections, malignant neoplasms and disorders such as rheumatoid arthritis or systemic lupus erythematosus), as well as vasculitis of less clear aetiology such as Henoch-Schönlein purpura, a disease typically seen in prepubertal males. There is a suggestion that such a broad grouping is inappropriate, and that the term 'hypersensitivity vasculitis' should not be used;[2] however, at present it continues to be employed in the literature.

Hypersensitivity vasculitis is characterised by small vessel involvement (arterioles and venules), particularly of the skin, and skin manifestations such as purpura, rashes, and urticaria predominate. Neutrophil debris is typically present around the vessel (**leucocytoclastic vasculitis**). However other organ systems may also be involved: in **Henoch-Schönlein purpura**, the skin lesions are associated with arthralgia, abdominal pain and other gastrointestinal symptoms, and glomerulonephritis.[3] Although not always immediately apparent, renal impairment may be delayed, and progress to end-stage renal failure.[4]

The prognosis is typically much better in hypersensitivity vasculitis than in the other major vasculitic syndromes, and most cases resolve spontaneously. Where a recognised antigenic stimulus is present it should be removed if possible, e.g. by withdrawal of a drug[1] or by appropriate therapy of infection. Hypersensitivity vasculitis generally responds less well to conventional drug therapy than other vasculitic syndromes. Nonetheless, where disease persists or results in organ dysfunction, a corticosteroid should be given, typically prednisone or prednisolone 60 mg, or 1 mg/kg by mouth daily, tapered rapidly until therapy can be discontinued. Plasmapheresis has also been used, but the use of cytotoxic immunosuppressants is less well established. However azathioprine[4] and cyclophosphamide[5] have been used successfully with corticosteroids. Anecdotal reports of excellent responses to dapsone in Henoch-Schönlein purpura exist.[6] Other drugs that have been tried include danazol,[7] pentoxifylline,[8] the latter sometimes in conjunction with dapsone,[8] and normal immunoglobulin.[9]


1. ten Holder SM, *et al.* Cutaneous and systemic manifestations of drug-induced vasculitis. *Ann Pharmacother* 2002; **36:** 130–47.
2. Jennette JC, *et al.* Nomenclature of systemic vasculitides: proposal of an international consensus conference. *Arthritis Rheum* 1994; **37:** 187–92.
3. Tizard EJ. Henoch-Schönlein purpura. *Arch Dis Child* 1999; **80:** 380–3.
4. Foster BJ, *et al.* Effective therapy for severe Henoch-Schonlein purpura nephritis with prednisone and azathioprine: a clinical and histopathologic study. *J Pediatr* 2000; **136:** 370–5.
5. Worm M, *et al.* Hypocomplementaemic urticarial vasculitis: successful treatment with cyclophosphamide-dexamethasone pulse therapy. *Br J Dermatol* 1998; **139:** 704–7.
6. Hoffbrand BI. Dapsone in Henoch-Schönlein purpura—worth a trial. *Postgrad Med J* 1991; **67:** 961–2.
7. Lee YJ, *et al.* Danazol for Henoch-Schönlein purpura. *Ann Intern Med* 1993; **118:** 827.
8. Nürnberg W, *et al.* Synergistic effects of pentoxifylline and dapsone in leucocytoclastic vasculitis. *Lancet* 1994; **343:** 491.
9. Rostoker G, *et al.* High-dose immunoglobulin therapy for severe IgA nephropathy and Henoch-Schönlein purpura. *Ann Intern Med* 1994; **120:** 476–84.


### Idiopathic thrombocytopenic purpura

Idiopathic thrombocytopenic purpura (ITP; sometimes referred to as auto-immune thrombocytopenic purpura[1]) is an auto-immune bleeding disorder characterised by the development of antibodies to the body's own platelets, with consequent sequestration and destruction of platelets. Both acute and chronic forms are seen; the acute form, which is usually self-limiting and follows viral or other infection, is the usual form in children, whereas chronic and sometimes more serious disease is more likely in adults, particularly young or middle-aged women. Patients develop petechiae, ecchymoses, and epistaxis, and women may develop menorrhagia; death due to haemorrhage is not unknown.

**Treatment**. For both adults and children with mild thrombocytopenia (counts of 20 000 to 30 000 cells/mm$^3$ or more) and no severe bruising or haemorrhage, no treatment is required.[2-7] American guidelines[7] recommend treatment for children with platelet counts below 10 000 cells/mm$^3$ and minor bruising; British guidelines[6] recommend that clinical severity also be considered before treating, as even pronounced bruising does not necessarily indicate a serious bleeding risk. In many cases the platelet count will return to normal or remain in a safe range despite the lack of therapy, and spontaneous remission can occur, even after a period of years.[8]

Where treatment is required in chronic disease, corticosteroids are the mainstay of therapy in adults.[9,10] Prednisolone or prednisone 1 mg/kg daily is used, usually for 2 to 4 weeks,[6,7] and then tapered down.[6] Most responses occur within the first 3 weeks, but there is no consensus as to appropriate duration of treatment.[5,10] Response rates vary widely, but most patients will relapse when the drug is withdrawn.[6] Good responses have also been reported with the use of high-dose oral or intravenous methylprednisolone for 3 to 7 days.[11-14] This has also been tried in children with the acute form[15] although controlled studies in children[16] and adults[17] found intravenous normal immunoglobulin to be more effective. Pulsed high-dose dexamethasone at 40 mg daily for 4 days has produced promising results,[3,18,19] although it is not clear how great the benefits will be in children.[20-22]

Use of corticosteroids for acute or chronic ITP in children is in any case controversial. Some consider low daily doses of prednisolone (250 micrograms/kg daily for 21 days) to be effective, while others have used high doses (prednisone 4 mg/kg daily for 7 days, then tapered).[6,7] Generally, lower doses of prednisone or prednisolone 1 to 2 mg/kg daily should not be used for longer than 2 to 3 weeks in children with ITP, and higher doses of 4 mg/kg daily are to be used for a maximum of 4 to 7 days, and tapered off as necessary.[6,7] Some centres consider that corticosteroids are of at best temporary benefit in children.[23]

In patients with chronic disease and symptoms of bleeding who fail to respond to first-line therapy, splenectomy should be considered.[2,3,5-7,9,23] About 70% of patients will respond but the operative and postoperative risks (notably of sepsis) must be considered, particularly in children.

Responses can also be achieved with intravenous normal immunoglobulin, which in practice is often preferred to corticosteroids for initial drug therapy of acute ITP in children.[4,24] Although the effect may be transient, an increase in platelet count is achievable with doses of 400 mg/kg daily for 5 days;[6,7] single doses of 800 mg/kg or 1 g/kg are equally effective. Response is often achievable even in patients refractory to other therapies,[2,3] but treatment must be repeated periodically. It is perhaps most useful when acute symptoms supervene, because of its rapid activity, and it is recommended that it be reserved for patients with acute severe bleeding, as pre-operative prophylaxis in patients with severe thrombocytopenia, or for patients with bleeding symptoms refractory to corticosteroids.[2,3,6,7] A response to normal immunoglobulin has been reported to be a good predictor of benefit from splenectomy.[25,26] An alternative to normal immunoglobulin in rhesus-positive patients may be the use of anti-D immunoglobulin,[4,5,27] although there are conflicting views as to its effectiveness,[9,27-31] and it has been associated with haemoglobinuria and haemoglobinaemia.[32]

Various other second-line drugs have been tried in the minority of patients with refractory chronic disease, but few have been well evaluated. Generally,[33-36] but not universally,[37] good results have been reported with danazol, particularly in older patients. It may have advantages for long-term maintenance, and is a potential alternative to splenectomy, at least in selected patients.[35,36] It can be used as a 'steroid-sparing' drug, permitting reduction in corticosteroid maintenance doses.[5,35] Dapsone may also elicit responses in patients with chronic ITP, but is less effective in severe cases.[6]

Antineoplastic and immunosuppressive drugs have been tried in refractory disease, but their potential toxicity has meant that they have often been reserved for older patients, as a treatment of last resort. Cyclophosphamide 1 to 2 mg/kg or azathioprine 1 to 4 mg/kg have been given daily by mouth[5] to adults; responses to cyclophosphamide generally occur within 8 weeks but for azathioprine several months' treatment is generally necessary before response can be assessed.[3,6] High-dose cyclophosphamide has also been tried in refractory, life-threatening disease.[3] Although some patients have responded to intravenous injection of vincristine, responses have tended to be partial and inadequate, and somewhat better results have been achieved with infusions of platelets incubated with vinblastine or vincristine to encourage binding and permit selective drug delivery to the macrophages responsible for platelet destruction.[38-40] Although the developers of this technique have reported long-lasting remission in 38% of patients,[40] enthusiasm elsewhere appears to be muted.[5,41] Combination chemotherapy (cyclophosphamide and prednisone plus vincristine, vincristine and procarbazine, or etoposide) has produced prolonged remission in a few patients,[3,42,43] but such aggressive treatment would be difficult to justify in most cases. Ciclosporin may be a reasonable salvage treatment in refractory ITP,[44] and mycophenolate mofetil has been reported to be of benefit in small numbers of patients.[6] Rituximab[45] may also be a useful alternative, and alemtuzumab has been well tolerated.[6]

Other reports of benefit exist for colchicine,[46-48] heparin,[49] and ascorbic acid,[50] the latter having at least the advantage that it is relatively non-toxic, but such therapies remain experimental.

Thrombopoietin may offer a future new approach to treatment.[5,51]

Tranexamic acid may be helpful in the symptomatic management of menorrhagia, although hysterectomy is occasionally necessary.

**In pregnancy**. Particular problems arise in the management of ITP in pregnancy, since antiplatelet antibodies can cross the placenta and produce thrombocytopenia in the fetus. The risk is greater when disease exists before pregnancy than when it develops in the course of pregnancy.

If therapy is considered necessary the mother may be given corticosteroids or normal immunoglobulin, with platelet infusions for more serious, unresponsive symptoms.[6,7] Treatment may be required for the neonate[5] if there are complications or the platelet count falls below 30 000 cells/mm$^3$. The risk of intracranial haemorrhage is not necessarily reduced by caesarean section,[5] and the mode of delivery should be determined by obstetric indications.[6]


1. Karpatkin S. Autoimmune (idiopathic) thrombocytopenic purpura. *Lancet* 1997; **349:** 1531–6.
2. Gillis S. The thrombocytopenic purpuras: recognition and management. *Drugs* 1996; **51:** 942–53.
3. McMillan R. Therapy for adults with refractory chronic immune thrombocytopenic purpura. *Ann Intern Med* 1997; **126:** 307–14.
4. Bolton-Maggs PHB. Idiopathic thrombocytopenic purpura. *Arch Dis Child* 2000; **83:** 220–2.
5. Cines DB, Blanchette VS. Immune thrombocytopenic purpura. *N Engl J Med* 2002; **346:** 995–1008. Correction. *ibid.*; 1923.
6. British Committee for Standards in Haematology General Haematology Task Force. Guidelines for the investigation and management of idiopathic thrombocytopenic purpura in adults, children and in pregnancy. *Br J Haematol* 2003; **120:** 574–96. Also available at: http://www.bcshguidelines.com/pdf/BJH574.pdf (accessed 27/04/04)
7. George JN, *et al.* Idiopathic thrombocytopenic purpura: a practice guideline developed by explicit methods for the American Society of Hematology. *Blood* 1996; **88:** 3–40. Also available at: http://www.hematology.org/practice/idiopathic.cfm (accessed 27/04/04)
8. Tait RC, Evans DIK. Late spontaneous recovery of chronic thrombocytopenia. *Arch Dis Child* 1993; **68:** 680–1.
9. Stasi R, *et al.* Long-term observation of 208 adults with chronic idiopathic thrombocytopenic purpura. *Am J Med* 1995; **98:** 436–42.
10. George JN, Vesely SK. Immune thrombocytopenic purpura—let the treatment fit the patient. *N Engl J Med* 2003; **349:** 903–5.
11. Özsoylu Ş, *et al.* Megadose methylprednisolone for chronic idiopathic thrombocytopenic purpura. *Lancet* 1990; **336:** 1078–9.
12. Akoğlu T, *et al.* Megadose methylprednisolone pulse therapy in adult idiopathic thrombocytopenic purpura. *Lancet* 1991; **337:** 56.
13. Özsoylu S. Mega-dose methylprednisolone for chronic idiopathic thrombocytopenic purpura. *Lancet* 1991; **337:** 1611–12.
14. Alpdoğan Ö, *et al.* Efficacy of high-dose methylprednisolone as a first-line therapy in adult patients with idiopathic thrombocytopenic purpura. *Br J Haematol* 1998; **103:** 1061–3.
15. Albayrak D, *et al.* Acute immune thrombocytopenic purpura: a comparative study of very high oral doses of methylprednisolone and intravenously administered immune globulin. *J Pediatr* 1994; **125:** 1004–7.
16. Rosthøj S, *et al.* Randomized trial comparing intravenous immunoglobulin with methylprednisolone pulse therapy in acute idiopathic thrombocytopenic purpura. *Acta Paediatr* 1996; **85:** 910–15.
17. Godeau B, *et al.* Intravenous immunoglobulin or high-dose methylprednisolone, with or without oral prednisone, for adults with untreated severe autoimmune thrombocytopenic purpura: a randomised, multicentre trial. *Lancet* 2002; **359:** 23–9.
18. Andersen JC. Response of resistant idiopathic thrombocytopenic purpura to pulsed high-dose dexamethasone therapy. *N Engl J Med* 1994; **330:** 1560–4.
19. Cheng Y, *et al.* Initial treatment of immune thrombocytopenic purpura with high-dose dexamethasone. *N Engl J Med* 2003; **349:** 831–6.
20. Adams DM, *et al.* High-dose oral dexamethasone therapy for chronic childhood idiopathic thrombocytopenic purpura. *J Pediatr* 1996; **128:** 281–3.
21. Borgna-Pignatti C, *et al.* A trial of high-dose dexamethasone therapy for chronic idiopathic thrombocytopenic purpura in childhood. *J Pediatr* 1997; **130:** 13–16.
22. Kühne T, *et al.* Platelet and immune responses to oral cyclic dexamethasone therapy in childhood chronic immune thrombocytopenic purpura. *J Pediatr* 1997; **130:** 17–24.
23. Reid MM. Chronic idiopathic thrombocytopenic purpura: incidence, treatment, and outcome. *Arch Dis Child* 1995; **72:** 125–8.
24. Bolton-Maggs PHB, Moon I. Assessment of UK practice for management of acute childhood idiopathic thrombocytopenic purpura against published guidelines. *Lancet* 1997; **350:** 620–3.
25. Law C, *et al.* High-dose intravenous immune globulin and the response to splenectomy in patients with idiopathic thrombocytopenic purpura. *N Engl J Med* 1997; **336:** 1494–8.
26. Holt D, *et al.* Response to intravenous immunoglobulin predicts splenectomy response in children with immune thrombocytopenic purpura. *Pediatrics* 2003; **111:** 87–90.
27. Anonymous. Rho(D) immune globulin iv for prevention of Rh isoimmunization and for treatment of ITP. *Med Lett Drugs Ther* 1996; **38:** 6–8.
28. Blanchette V, *et al.* Randomised trial of intravenous immunoglobulin G, intravenous anti-D, and oral prednisone in childhood acute immune thrombocytopenic purpura. *Lancet* 1994; **344:** 703–7.
29. Andrew M, *et al.* A multicenter study of the treatment of childhood chronic idiopathic thrombocytopenic purpura with anti-D. *J Pediatr* 1992; **120:** 522–7.
30. Zunich KM, *et al.* Intravenous anti-D immunoglobulin for childhood acute immune thrombocytopenic purpura. *Lancet* 1995; **346:** 1363–4.
31. Blanchette V, Wang E. Intravenous anti-D immunoglobulin for childhood acute immune thrombocytopenic purpura. *Lancet* 1995; **346:** 1364–5.
32. Gaines AR. Acute onset hemoglobinemia and/or hemoglobinuria and sequelae following $Rh_o$(D) immune globulin intravenous administration in immune thrombocytopenic purpura patients. *Blood* 2000; **95:** 2523–9.
33. Buelli M, *et al.* Danazol for the treatment of idiopathic thrombocytopenic purpura. *Acta Haematol (Basel)* 1985; **74:** 97–8.
34. Mylvaganam R, *et al.* Very low dose danazol in idiopathic thrombocytopenic purpura and its role as an immune modulator. *Am J Med Sci* 1989; **298:** 215–20.
35. Ahn YS, *et al.* Long-term danazol therapy in autoimmune thrombocytopenia: unmaintained remission and age-dependent response in women. *Ann Intern Med* 1989; **111:** 723–9.
36. Edelmann DZ, *et al.* Danazol in non-splenectomized patients with refractory idiopathic thrombocytopenic purpura. *Postgrad Med J* 1990; **66:** 827–30.
37. McVerry BA, *et al.* The use of danazol in the management of chronic immune thrombocytopenic purpura. *Br J Haematol* 1985; **61:** 145–8.
38. Ahn YS, *et al.* The treatment of idiopathic thrombocytopenia with vinblastine-loaded platelets. *N Engl J Med* 1978; **298:** 1101–7.
39. Agnelli G, *et al.* Vinca-loaded platelets. *N Engl J Med* 1984; **311:** 599.
40. Ahn YS, *et al.* Vinca-loaded platelets. *N Engl J Med* 1984; **311:** 599–600.
41. Rosse WF. Whatever happened to vinca-loaded platelets? *N Engl J Med* 1984; **310:** 1051–2.
42. Figueroa M, *et al.* Combination chemotherapy in refractory immune thrombocytopenic purpura. *N Engl J Med* 1993; **328:** 1226–9.
43. McMillan R. Long-term outcomes after treatment for refractory immune thrombocytopenic purpura. *N Engl J Med* 2001; **344:** 1402–3.
44. Emilia G, *et al.* Long-term salvage therapy with cyclosporin A in refractory idiopathic thrombocytopenic purpura. *Blood* 2002; **99:** 1482–5.
45. Stasi R, *et al.* Rituximab chimeric anti-CD20 monoclonal antibody treatment for adults with chronic idiopathic thrombocytopenic purpura. *Blood* 2001; **98:** 952–7.
46. Strother SV, *et al.* Colchicine therapy for refractory idiopathic thrombocytopenic purpura. *Arch Intern Med* 1984; **144:** 2198–2200.

47. Jim RTS. Therapeutic use of colchicine in thrombocytopenia. *Hawaii Med J* 1986; **45:** 221–6.
48. Baker RI, Manoharan A. Colchicine therapy for idiopathic thrombocytopenic purpura—an inexpensive alternative. *Aust N Z J Med* 1989; **19:** 412–13.
49. Shen ZX, *et al.* Thrombocytopoietic effect of heparin given in chronic immune thrombocytopenic purpura. *Lancet* 1995; **346:** 220–1.
50. Cohen HA, *et al.* Treatment of chronic idiopathic thrombocytopenic purpura with ascorbate. *Clin Pediatr (Phila)* 1993: **32:** 300–2.
51. Schick BP. Hope for treatment of thrombocytopenia. *N Engl J Med* 1994; **331:** 875–6.

#### Infections

Although long-term corticosteroid therapy has an adverse effect on the body's response to infection (see Effects on Immune Response, under Adverse Effects, p.1070), the judicious use of corticosteroids, usually on a short-term basis, with appropriate anti-infective drugs, may have a beneficial effect on the symptoms of selected acute infections, and may on occasions be life-saving. Guidelines have been published concerning a number of infections and whether corticosteroids should be used or not.[1]

For further comment on the use of corticosteroids in ocular herpes infections, infectious mononucleosis, leishmaniasis, leprosy, meningitis, *Pneumocystis carinii* pneumonia in AIDS patients, septic shock, and tuberculosis, see under the relevant headings in this section.

1. McGowan JE, *et al.* Report by the Working Group on Steroid Use, Antimicrobial Agents Committee, Infectious Diseases Society of America: Guidelines for the use of systemic glucocorticoids in the management of selected infections. *J Infect Dis* 1992; **165:** 1–13.

#### Infectious mononucleosis

In a short discussion on the use of corticosteroids in infectious mononucleosis (glandular fever—see Epstein-Barr Virus Infections, p.620) it was considered that although all cases would respond promptly to therapy, only patients with an unduly prolonged infection and those with an exceptionally severe sore throat that interferes with either respiratory function or eating should be treated with a corticosteroid.[1] Most experts would use corticosteroids in patients with severe thrombocytopenia, haemolytic anaemia, encephalitis, pericarditis, or myocarditis associated with infection by the Epstein-Barr virus. Doses of prednisone may be 80 mg daily initially, decreasing gradually and withdrawn after 14 days. Prednisone is very safe in infectious mononucleosis but the theoretical risk of impairing immunity is a concern as there might be an increased risk of Epstein-Barr virus-related tumours in later life.[1] Others have also expressed a relatively negative view of the value of corticosteroids.[2]

1. Sheagren JN. Corticosteroids for treatment of mononucleosis and aphthous stomatitis. *JAMA* 1986; **256:** 1051.
2. McGowan JE, *et al.* Report by the Working Group on Steroid Use, Antimicrobial Agents Committee, Infectious Diseases Society of America: Guidelines for the use of systemic glucocorticoids in the management of selected infections. *J Infect Dis* 1992; **165:** 1–13.

#### Inflammatory bowel disease

Together with aminosalicylates, the corticosteroids form the mainstay of treatment for active ulcerative colitis and Crohn's disease (see Inflammatory Bowel Disease, p.1243). In moderate to severe acute disease systemic corticosteroids are indicated for initial management, either orally or in the most severe cases intravenously. Doses are high initially and are gradually reduced as symptoms resolve. In patients with disease confined to the distal colon or rectum, local topical therapy with suppositories or enemas of corticosteroids are appropriate. Oral or rectal formulations of poorly absorbed or rapidly metabolised corticosteroids such as beclometasone, budesonide, or tixocortol have been developed in the hope of producing local improvement without systemic effects.

#### Leishmaniasis

Corticosteroids may be required to control severe inflammation in patients with mucocutaneous leishmaniasis (p.597), although pentavalent antimony is usually the drug used for initial treatment.

#### Leprosy

Type I lepra (reversal) reactions in patients with leprosy (p.133) frequently respond to high-dose corticosteroids (for example 40 to 60 mg of prednisolone daily) started immediately and given for several days.[1] Doses may be reduced over several weeks or months. Corticosteroids may also be used for type II reactions.

Corticosteroid treatment of nerve function impairment should be started within 6 months of onset, as the earlier that treatment is started, the more likely it is that function will be restored. A standardised regimen in which the usual adult dose was 40 mg daily of prednisolone for 4 weeks, tapered over the following 12 weeks, has been successfully used in the field management of acute nerve function impairment,[2] as has a regimen consisting of 30 mg of prednisone for 2 weeks tapered down with a minimum duration of 10 weeks.[3]

1. WHO. WHO expert committee on leprosy. *WHO Tech Rep Ser 874* 1998.
2. Croft RP, *et al.* Field treatment of acute nerve function impairment in leprosy using a standardized corticosteroid regimen—first year's experience with 100 patients. *Lepr Rev* 1997; **68:** 316–25.
3. Bernink EHM, Voskens JEJ. Study on the detection of leprosy reactions and the effect of prednisone on various nerves, Indonesia. *Lepr Rev* 1997; **68:** 225–32.

#### Lichen

Lichen planus (p.1136) is generally controlled with corticosteroids applied topically, or occasionally, injected intralesionally; systemic corticosteroids (usually prednisone or prednisolone) are used for severe erosive lichen planus.[1,2] Prednisone has generally been used in oral doses of 30 to 60 mg daily, for courses of 4 to 6 weeks.[1] Shorter courses may be of value: prednisolone (30 mg daily for 10 days) was reported to be effective and safe for mild or moderately severe lichen planus.[3]

The use of topically applied corticosteroids in the treatment of lichen sclerosus (p.1136) has been discussed.[4,5] Relief from vulvar pruritus is obtained in most cases with a potent corticosteroid preparation, such as clobetasol propionate, applied twice daily for up to 3 months before tapering the dose.[4]

1. Cribier B, *et al.* Treatment of lichen planus: an evidence-based medicine analysis of efficacy. *Arch Dermatol* 1998; **134:** 1521–30.
2. Edwards L. Vulvar lichen planus. *Arch Dermatol* 1989; **125:** 1677–80.
3. Kellett JK, Ead RD. Treatment of lichen planus with a short course of oral prednisolone. *Br J Dermatol* 1990; **123:** 550–1.
4. Powell JJ, Wojnarowska F. Lichen sclerosus. *Lancet* 1999; **353:** 1777–83.
5. Neill SM, *et al.* Guidelines for the management of lichen sclerosus. *Br J Dermatol* 2002; **147:** 640–9.

#### Liver disorders

Corticosteroids are considered to be useful in chronic active hepatitis (p.1078). There is some disagreement over the benefit from corticosteroid therapy in alcoholic liver disease with hepatic encephalopathy,[1-4] and they do not appear to be of benefit in acute hepatic failure.[5] Corticosteroid therapy may however be of benefit in sclerosing cholangitis.[6]

No treatment has proven unequivocally successful in the management of primary biliary cirrhosis (p.1761). Corticosteroids are one of a number of drugs for which reports of benefit exist, but their use has been restricted as they may exacerbate bone disease.

1. Imperiale TF, McCullough AJ. Do corticosteroids reduce mortality from alcoholic hepatitis? A meta-analysis of the randomized trials. *Ann Intern Med* 1990; **113:** 299–307.
2. Ramond M-J, *et al.* A randomized trial of prednisolone in patients with severe alcoholic hepatitis. *N Engl J Med* 1992; **326:** 507–12.
3. Wrona SA, Tankanow RM. Corticosteroids in the management of alcoholic hepatitis. *Am J Hosp Pharm* 1994; **51:** 347–53.
4. Christensen E, Gluud C. Glucocorticoids are ineffective in alcoholic hepatitis: a meta-analysis adjusting for confounding variables. *Gut* 1995; **37:** 113–18.
5. Caraceni P, Van Thiel DH. Acute liver failure. *Lancet* 1995; **345:** 163–9.
6. Lindor KD, *et al.* Advances in primary sclerosing cholangitis. *Am J Med* 1990; **89:** 73–80.

#### Male infertility

Immunosuppressive treatment with corticosteroids is given for male infertility (p.1316) due to low-grade auto-immune orchitis.[1] Examples of regimens after which pregnancy has been successfully achieved in female partners include oral methylprednisolone 96 mg daily for 7 days beginning on day 21 of the partner's menstrual cycle[2] and oral prednisolone 20 mg twice daily on days 1 to 10 of the partner's menstrual cycle plus 5 mg on days 11 and 12.[3] However, there is a lack of evidence from substantial controlled trials of benefit from corticosteroid therapy in men with auto-immune causes of infertility.

1. Haidl G, Schill W-B. Guidelines for drug treatment of male infertility. *Drugs* 1991; **41:** 60–8.
2. Shulman JF, Shulman S. Methylprednisolone treatment of immunologic infertility in the male. *Fertil Steril* 1982; **38:** 591–9.
3. Hendry WF, *et al.* Comparison of prednisolone and placebo in subfertile men with antibodies to spermatozoa. *Lancet* 1990; **335:** 85–8.

#### Malignant neoplasms

Corticosteroids are extensively prescribed in malignant disease for the relief of pain, nerve compression, or raised intracranial pressure; to alleviate dyspnoea, effusion, or hypercalcaemia; to counteract adverse effects of other therapies such as antineoplastic-induced nausea and vomiting or radiation-induced inflammation; and in the management of cachexia and to improve mood and sense of well-being.[1] In addition they form an important part of multidrug anticancer regimens used for various haematological malignancies such as acute lymphoblastic leukaemia (p.506) and Hodgkin's disease (p.509). In contrast, it has been postulated that the use of corticosteroids in patients with solid, non-haematological tumours might induce resistance in cancer cells to cytotoxic therapy, and increase the risk of treatment failure, although clinical evidence for this is lacking.[2]

1. Twycross R. The risks and benefits of corticosteroids in advanced cancer. *Drug Safety* 1994; **11:** 163–78.
2. Rutz HP. Effects of corticosteroid use on treatment of solid tumours. *Lancet* 2002; **360:** 1969–70.

#### Meningitis

Corticosteroids may be given as adjuncts to antibacterial therapy in bacterial meningitis (p.134), in the hope of moderating any neurological sequelae; there is some evidence that dexamethasone, especially if given early, may reduce the risk of deafness in children and reduce mortality in adults.

#### Mouth ulceration

Local treatment of mouth ulcers (p.1245) often involves a topical corticosteroid for symptomatic relief. Systemic corticosteroids have occasionally been given where there is severe underlying disease.

#### Multiple sclerosis

Corticosteroids are often used in the management of multiple sclerosis (p.646). Corticosteroid therapy reduces the duration of the relapse and accelerates recovery, but it is not known whether it alters the course of the disease in the long term.[1,2] Methylprednisolone has superseded corticotropin and prednisolone as the drug of choice. Methylprednisolone is usually given intravenously in high doses (typically 1 g daily) for 3 to 5 days, sometimes followed by a tapering dose of oral prednisolone. Doses of up to 2 g of methylprednisolone daily have been tried.[3] In patients with acute optic neuritis (frequently the first manifestation of multiple sclerosis), methylprednisolone delayed the onset of other symptoms of multiple sclerosis[4] although the effect was not sustained beyond 2 years.[5] Beneficial responses have also been reported with oral methylprednisolone at doses including 500 mg once daily for 5 days followed by a tapering dose over 10 days[6] and 48 mg once daily for 7 days followed by a tapering dose over 14 days.[7]

In patients with primary progressive disease, the benefits of short-course methylprednisolone lasted no longer than 3 months[8] although, in patients with secondary progressive disease, a preliminary study has suggested that progression may be delayed by intermittent high-dose methylprednisolone therapy.[9]

1. Rudick RA, *et al.* Management of multiple sclerosis. *N Engl Med J* 1997; **337:** 1604–11.
2. Filippini G, *et al.* Corticosteroids or ACTH for acute exacerbations in multiple sclerosis. Available in The Cochrane Library; Issue 1. Chichester: John Wiley; 2004.
3. Oliveri RL, *et al.* Randomized trial comparing two different high doses of methylprednisolone in MS: a clinical and MRI study. *Neurology* 1998; **50:** 1833–6.
4. Beck RW, *et al.* The effect of corticosteroids for acute optic neuritis on the subsequent development of multiple sclerosis. *N Engl J Med* 1993; **329:** 1764–9.
5. Beck RW, *et al.* The optic neuritis treatment trial: three-year follow-up results. *Arch Ophthalmol* 1995; **113:** 136–7.
6. Sellebjerg F, *et al.* Double-blind, randomized, placebo-controlled study of oral, high-dose methylprednisolone in attacks of MS. *Neurology* 1998; **51:** 529–34.
7. Barnes D, *et al.* Randomised trial of oral and intravenous methylprednisolone in acute relapses of multiple sclerosis. *Lancet* 1997; **349:** 902–6.
8. Cazzato G, *et al.* Double-blind, placebo-controlled, randomized, crossover trial of high-dose methylprednisolone in patients with chronic progressive form of multiple sclerosis. *Eur Neurol* 1995; **35:** 193–8.
9. Goodkin DE, *et al.* A phase II study of IV methylprednisolone in secondary-progressive multiple sclerosis. *Neurology* 1998; **51:** 239–45.

#### Muscular dystrophies

Muscular dystrophies are a range of inherited myopathies in which there is progressive degeneration of muscle fibres and associated muscle weakness. They may be classified according to the mode of inheritance. The most common type is the fatal recessive X-linked **Duchenne muscular dystrophy** (DMD) in which there is a deficiency in the structural muscle protein dystrophin. There is no effective therapy that affects the ultimate outcome of the various muscular dystrophies. Management is mainly through the use of physiotherapy, supports, and surgery. Drug treatment has been tried for symptomatic management, but generally the number of patients studied has been small. However, prednisone given in doses of up to 2 mg/kg daily has been effective in increasing muscle strength in children and slowing the progression of Duchenne muscular dystrophy;[1-5] improvement does not appear to be sustained to the same degree with alternate day therapy.[4] Benefit has also been seen with deflazacort.[6] It has been suggested that the failure of azathioprine to produce any beneficial effect when used alone or added to prednisone treatment might indicate that prednisone's effectiveness is not due to immunosuppression.[5] There have also been reports of benefit in small numbers of patients given ciclosporin or oxandrolone; evidence to support the use of most other drugs (e.g. allopurinol) is either conflicting or unconvincing. Future prospects for treatment include gene therapy, haematopoietic stem-cell therapy, or upregulation of proteins related to dystrophin that might ameliorate the dystrophy.[7]


1. DeSilva S, *et al.* Prednisone treatment in Duchenne muscular dystrophy: long-term benefit. *Arch Neurol* 1987; **44:** 818–22.
2. Mendell JR, *et al.* Randomized double-blind six-month trial of prednisone in Duchenne's muscular dystrophy. *N Engl J Med* 1989; **320:** 1592–7.
3. Griggs RC, *et al.* Prednisone in Duchenne dystrophy: a randomized, controlled trial defining the time course and dose response. *Arch Neurol* 1991; **48:** 383–8.
4. Fenichel GM, *et al.* A comparison of daily and alternate-day prednisone therapy in the treatment of Duchenne muscular dystrophy. *Arch Neurol* 1991; **48:** 575–9.
5. Griggs RC, *et al.* Duchenne dystrophy: randomized, controlled trial of prednisone (18 months) and azathioprine (12 months). *Neurology* 1993; **43:** 520–7.
6. Bigger WD, *et al.* Deflazacort treatment of Duchenne muscular dystrophy. *J Pediatr* 2001; **138:** 45–50.
7. Emery AEH. The muscular dystrophies. *Lancet* 2002; **359:** 687–95.


### Myasthenia gravis

Corticosteroids are the main immunosuppressants used in the management of myasthenia gravis (p.1486).

### Nasal polyps

Nasal polyps are outgrowths of the nasal mucosa, typically pale, smooth, translucent, and round or pear-shaped.[1,2] They are often associated with a history of rhinitis or asthma; the triad of nasal polyps, asthma, and hypersensitivity to aspirin may occur. Patients typically present with obstruction, loss of smell, and often rhinorrhoea and postnasal drip.

Corticosteroids are extremely effective in reducing polyp size, either by intranasal[3] or systemic administration. In the former case beginning with betamethasone sodium phosphate nasal drops, and subsequently maintaining the reduction with an intranasal spray such as beclometasone, budesonide, or fluticasone, has been suggested.[1] Alternatively prednisone, prednisolone, or dexamethasone can be given by mouth: suggested regimens have included prednisone 60 mg daily, tapered over 10 or 14 days and followed by intranasal corticosteroids,[2] or dexamethasone 12, 8, and 4 mg daily, each for 3 days.[1] Surgery may be necessary where there is marked obstruction, and most patients require it at some point,[1] although polyps usually recur. Pre-operative administration of systemic corticosteroids may help reduce recurrence.[2] Continued use of topical corticosteroids may reduce the frequency of relapses.[3]


1. Lund VJ. Diagnosis and treatment of nasal polyps. *BMJ* 1995; **311:** 1411–14.
2. Slavin RG. Nasal polyps and sinusitis. *JAMA* 1997; **278:** 1849–54.
3. Badia L, Lund V. Topical corticosteroids in nasal polyposis. *Drugs* 2001; **61:** 573–8.


### Nausea and vomiting

Corticosteroids, usually in the form of dexamethasone, play an important role in antiemetic regimens (see p.1245) used to combat the effects of moderately to severely emetogenic cancer chemotherapy: they have been shown to enhance the effects of both metoclopramide- and 5-$HT_3$ antagonist-based regimens. Dexamethasone is probably the best established treatment for delayed emesis at present. A study of corticosteroid treatment in refractory hyperemesis gravidarum showed improvements in appetite, weight gain, and well-being, and suggested that corticosteroids might improve nausea and vomiting but was too small to provide conclusive evidence.[1]


1. Nelson-Piercy C, *et al.* Randomised, double-blind, placebo-controlled trial of corticosteroids for the treatment of hyperemesis gravidarum. *Br J Obstet Gynaecol* 2001; **108:** 9–15.


### Neonatal intraventricular haemorrhage

For the suggestion that antenatal corticosteroids may reduce the incidence of intraventricular haemorrhage in neonates, see p.740.

### Neonatal respiratory distress syndrome

Neonatal respiratory distress syndrome is a condition of increasing respiratory distress occurring at, or shortly after, birth. It is marked by cyanosis, tachypnoea, expiratory grunting and sternal retraction. Symptoms increase in severity with progressive collapse of the lung (atelectasis), leakage of plasma into alveolar spaces, and the formation of hyaline membranes, until death occurs or slow recovery takes place from about the 2nd to 4th day. The syndrome affects primarily premature infants and its incidence increases with the degree of prematurity; severe problems are most likely in those delivered before 30 weeks' gestation. Symptoms are thought to be at least partly due to inadequate amounts of surfactant in the premature lung resulting in high internal surface tension and increased risk of alveolar collapse, but in very immature infants other factors, possibly including impaired sodium and fluid absorption from the lung, may play a role.[1]

**Treatment**. The optimum treatment is prevention, and the 1998 UK guidelines[2] (awaiting update) recommend the administration of betamethasone 12 mg daily by intramuscular injection for 2 days to women in whom delivery before 34 weeks of gestation is likely. Similar recommendations apply elsewhere. In the USA, for example, antenatal corticosteroid treatment (with betamethasone or dexamethasone) is recommended for women between 24 and 34 weeks of pregnancy who show signs of premature delivery.[3] Betamethasone may be preferable to dexamethasone, as the latter appears to have a deleterious effect on neurodevelopment.[4] An overview of studies of antenatal corticosteroid therapy suggests that it may reduce the risk of respiratory distress syndrome by about 50% overall;[5] the risk of death, and of periventricular haemorrhage and necrotising enterocolitis is also reduced. Whether repeat courses should be considered is uncertain,[6] although the practice has become widespread; it has been recommended that they be restricted to patients in clinical trials.[4,7] While repeat doses of corticosteroids may reduce the development of severe respiratory distress syndrome, especially among neonates of less than 28 weeks' gestation, weekly courses of betamethasone or dexamethasone did not reduce neonatal morbidity compared with a single course of treatment.[8] Delaying delivery with a tocolytic (see Premature Labour, p.794) may be considered to increase the time available for management with antenatal corticosteroids.[2] Reported benefit from adding protirelin to antenatal corticosteroids has not been borne out by 2 large multicentre studies.[9-11] The earlier of these studies actually found neonatal outcome and maternal morbidity to be worse in those who also received protirelin,[9,10] but this conclusion has been questioned.[12,13]

In infants born with the syndrome rapid supportive care is required, which may include correction of metabolic acidosis, circulatory support, oxygen supplementation, and assisted ventilation, although there is a lack of consensus about the most appropriate method for these.[2] It has been suggested that ventilation using a helium-oxygen mixture gives better results than a nitrogen-oxygen mix.[14] Another alternative is the use of partial liquid ventilation with the fluorocarbon compound perflubron.[15] Meta-analysis suggests that inhaled nitric oxide improves outcomes in infants born at or near term who are hypoxaemic,[16] but evidence of benefit in preterm infants has not been shown.[17] The majority of infants survive the acute episode with careful management, although associated complications may subsequently develop, including bronchopulmonary dysplasia (p.1077), retinopathy of prematurity (p.1466), and cerebral palsy. There is evidence that supplementation with inositol can significantly reduce the incidence of adverse outcomes in preterm infants.[18]

Since deficiency of surfactant is considered to play an important role in the neonatal respiratory distress syndrome, the use of surfactant replacement therapy has been intensively investigated, and is now accepted as reducing the risk of death from the disease and the development of pneumothorax and other lung complications.[2,19,20] Both natural and synthetic surfactants have been used and although both are effective there is some evidence that results are better with the preparations of natural origin.[21-23] Natural surfactants of differing origins may also vary in their properties: poractant,[24] or calfactant,[25] have both been reported to give better responses than beractant. Surfactant is given as a suspension by endotracheal tube directly into the infant's lung, although other means of administration, such as nebulisers, have been investigated. Most surfactants are given in recommended doses of 100 to 200 mg/kg phospholipids. Repeat doses may be given if necessary, and a meta-analysis[26] of data from two randomised controlled trials using preparations of natural surfactant extract in neonates with established disease found a more favourable clinical outcome, including a decreased risk of pneumothorax, with multiple rather than single doses. However, in clinical practice the number of doses and the dosage interval varies. One large study[27] found that a dose of 100 mg/kg, repeated twice, was as effective as 200 mg/kg followed by up to four further doses of 100 mg/kg. Another found that 3 doses, given at 12-hour intervals with the first dose shortly after birth were more effective than the first dose alone in improving physiological findings and mortality rates in low birth-weight infants.[28] One large multicentre randomised controlled trial[29] investigated the difference between giving repeat doses of a surfactant (calfactant) at a low threshold of respiratory support, as recommended by the manufacturer, versus a higher threshold. The conclusion was that efficacy was not compromised by delaying surfactant re-treatment in infants with uncomplicated respiratory distress syndrome until they had reached a higher level of respiratory support than is currently recommended, but infants with complications should continue to be treated by the currently recommended low-threshold strategy.

There has been debate whether 'prophylactic' early therapy, given immediately after birth to all infants deemed at risk of the syndrome, or delayed therapy given 2 or more hours after birth to intubated infants who have developed symptoms, is the more appropriate,[30] but the large OSIRIS study,[31] and later systematic reviews,[32,33] found in favour of early intervention, and this strategy is recommended in the 1998 UK guidelines.[2]


1. Barker PM, *et al.* Decreased sodium ion absorption across nasal epithelium of very premature infants with respiratory distress syndrome. *J Pediatr* 1997; **130:** 373–7.
2. Report of the second working group of the British Association of Perinatal Medicine. Guidelines for good practice in the management of neonatal respiratory distress syndrome. Guideline produced in November 1998, not valid beyond 2002. Available at: http://www.bapm.org/documents/publications/rds.pdf (accessed 27/04/04)
3. NIH Consensus Development Panel on the Effect of Corticosteroids for Fetal Maturation on Perinatal Outcomes. Effect of corticosteroids for fetal maturation on perinatal outcomes. *JAMA* 1995; **273:** 413–18.
4. Lawson EE. Antenatal corticosteroids—too much of a good thing? *JAMA* 2001; **286:** 1628–30.
5. Crowley PA. Antenatal corticosteroid therapy: a meta-analysis of the randomized trials, 1972 to 1994. *Am J Obstet Gynecol* 1995; **173:** 322–35.
6. Crowther CA, Harding J. Repeat doses of prenatal corticosteroids for women at risk of preterm birth for preventing neonatal respiratory disease. Available in The Cochrane Library; Issue 1. Chichester: John Wiley; 2004.
7. National Institutes of Health. Consensus development conference statement—antenatal corticosteroids revisited: repeat courses. Available at: http://consensus.nih.gov/cons/112/112_statement.htm (accessed 27/04/04)
8. Guinn DA, *et al.* Single vs weekly courses of antenatal corticosteroids for women at risk of preterm delivery: a randomized controlled trial. *JAMA* 2001; **286:** 1581–7.
9. ACTOBAT Study Group. Australian collaborative trial of antenatal thyrotropin-releasing hormone (ACTOBAT) for prevention of neonatal respiratory disease. *Lancet* 1995; **345:** 877–82.
10. Crowther CA, *et al.* Australian Collaborative Trial of antenatal thyrotropin-releasing hormone: adverse effects at 12-month follow-up. *Pediatrics* 1997; **99:** 311–17.
11. Ballard RA, *et al.* Antenatal thyrotropin-releasing hormone to prevent lung disease in preterm infants. *N Engl J Med* 1998; **338:** 493–8.
12. Moya FR, Maturana A. Thyrotropin-releasing hormone for prevention of neonatal respiration disease. *Lancet* 1995; **345:** 1572–3.
13. McCormick MC. The credibility of the ACTOBAT follow-up study. *Pediatrics* 1997; **99:** 476–8.
14. Elleau C, *et al.* Helium-oxygen mixture in respiratory distress syndrome: a double-blind study. *J Pediatr* 1993; **122:** 132–6.
15. Leach CL, *et al.* Partial liquid ventilation with perflubron in premature infants with severe respiratory distress syndrome. *N Engl J Med* 1996; **335:** 761–7.
16. Finer NN, Barrington KJ. Nitric oxide for respiratory failure in infants born at or near term. Available in The Cochrane Library; Issue 1. Chichester: John Wiley; 2004.
17. Barrington KJ, Finer NN. Inhaled nitric oxide for respiratory failure in preterm infants. Available in The Cochrane Library; Issue 1. Chichester: John Wiley; 2004.
18. Howlett A, Ohlsson A. Inositol for respiratory distress syndrome in preterm infants. Available in The Cochrane Library; Issue 1. Chichester: John Wiley; 2004.
19. Schwartz RM, *et al.* Effect of surfactant on morbidity, mortality, and resource use in newborn infants weighing 500 to 1500 g. *N Engl J Med* 1994; **330:** 1476–80.

20. Walti H, Monset-Couchard M. A risk-benefit assessment of natural and synthetic exogenous surfactants in the management of neonatal respiratory distress syndrome. *Drug Safety* 1998; **18:** 321–37.
21. Halliday HL. Natural vs synthetic surfactants in neonatal respiratory distress syndrome. *Drugs* 1996; **51:** 226–37.
22. Hudak ML, *et al.* A multicenter randomized, masked comparison trial of natural versus synthetic surfactant for the treatment of respiratory distress syndrome. *J Pediatr* 1996; **128:** 396–406.
23. Soll RF, Blanco F. Natural surfactant extract versus synthetic surfactant for neonatal respiratory distress syndrome. Available in The Cochrane Library; Issue 1. Chichester: John Wiley; 2004.
24. Speer CP, *et al.* Randomised clinical trial of two treatment regimens of natural surfactant preparations in neonatal respiratory distress syndrome. *Arch Dis Child* 1995; **72:** F8–F13.
25. Bloom BT, *et al.* Randomized double-blind multicenter trial of Survanta (SURV) and Infasurf (IS). *Pediatr Res* 1994; **35:** 326.
26. Soll RF. Multiple versus single dose natural surfactant extract for severe neonatal respiratory distress syndrome. Available in The Cochrane Library; Issue 1. Chichester: John Wiley; 2004.
27. Halliday HL, *et al.* Multicentre randomised trial comparing high and low dose surfactant regimens for the treatment of respiratory distress syndrome (the Curosurf 4 trial). *Arch Dis Child* 1993; **69:** 276–80.
28. Corbet A, *et al.* Double-blind, randomized trial of one versus three prophylactic doses of synthetic surfactant in 826 neonates weighing 700 to 1100 grams: effects on mortality rate. *J Pediatr* 1995; **126:** 969–78.
29. Kattwinkel J, *et al.* High- versus low-threshold surfactant retreatment for neonatal respiratory distress syndrome. *Pediatrics* 2000; **106:** 282–8.
30. Dunn MS. Surfactant replacement therapy: prophylaxis or treatment? *Pediatrics* 1993; **92:** 148–50.
31. The OSIRIS Collaborative Group (Open Study of Infants at high risk of or with Respiratory Insufficiency—the role of surfactant). Early versus delayed neonatal administration of a synthetic surfactant—the judgement of OSIRIS. *Lancet* 1992; **340:** 1363–9.
32. Morley CJ. Systematic review of prophylactic vs rescue surfactant. *Arch Dis Child* 1997; **77:** F70–4.
33. Yost CC, Soll RF. Early versus delayed selective surfactant treatment for neonatal respiratory distress syndrome. Available in The Cochrane Library; Issue 1. Chichester: John Wiley; 2004.

### Optic neuropathies

Causes of optic neuropathies are diverse, and they may be classified by their aetiology.[1,2] Ischaemic optic neuropathies, of which the acute anterior form is most common, may be caused by vasculitic syndromes (p.1090) such as giant cell arteritis (p.1080).[3] Inflammatory optic neuropathies (optic neuritis) may be caused by infectious disease, immune-mediated disorders such as Behçet's disease (p.1076), sarcoidosis (p.1087), or demyelination of the optic nerve such as occurs with multiple sclerosis (p.646).[4,5] Other causes include hereditary disorders, trauma, or compression. Vitamin or nutritional deficiency (often due to alcohol abuse) or toxicity (due to drugs such as amiodarone, digoxin, or isoniazid) may also lead to optic neuropathy.[1,2] Clinical features such as pattern of visual field loss and pain can aid diagnosis.[2]

Management will depend on the type of neuropathy and any underlying disease. Improvement in vision was reported in patients with auto-immune optic neuropathy following 5 to 7 days of treatment with high doses of intravenous methylprednisolone (1 to 2 g daily) or oral prednisolone (80 to 400 mg daily).[6] In some patients, recurrent visual loss required repeated high-dose intravenous methylprednisolone, an increase in oral prednisolone dosage, or additional immunosuppressants, but in many patients visual benefits were maintained even when treatment was withdrawn. Visual recovery has also been reported in patients with optic neuritis of unknown aetiology receiving intravenous methylprednisolone 250 or 500 mg every 6 hours for 3 to 7 days.[7] One study has found oral prednisone alone (1 mg/kg daily for 14 days) to be ineffective whereas intravenous methylprednisolone (1 g daily for 3 days) followed by oral prednisone (1 mg/kg daily for 11 days) was beneficial in the treatment of acute optic neuritis.[8] A review of corticosteroid use in optic neuritis concluded that high-dose oral or parenteral methylprednisolone, or corticotropin, were of value in the treatment of acute disease. However, their long-term benefit could not be determined.[9]

1. Van Stavern GP, Newman NJ. Optic neuropathies: an overview. *Ophthalmol Clin North Am* 2001; **14:** 61–71.
2. Purvin VA. Optic neuropathies for the neurologist. *Semin Neurol* 2000; **20:** 97–110.
3. Arnold AC. Ischemic optic neuropathies. *Ophthalmol Clin North Am* 2001; **14:** 83–98.
4. Eggenberger ER. Inflammatory optic neuropathies. *Ophthalmol Clin North Am* 2001; **14:** 73–82.
5. Hickman SJ, *et al.* Management of acute optic neuritis. *Lancet* 2002; **360:** 1953–62.
6. Kupersmith MJ, *et al.* Autoimmune optic neuropathy: evaluation and treatment. *J Neurol Neurosurg Psychiatry* 1988; **51:** 1381–6.
7. Spoor TC, Rockwell DL. Treatment of optic neuritis with intravenous megadose corticosteroids: a consecutive series. *Ophthalmology* 1988; **95:** 131–4.
8. Beck RW, *et al.* A randomized, controlled trial of corticosteroids in the treatment of acute optic neuritis. *N Engl J Med* 1992; **326:** 581–8.
9. Kaufman DI, *et al.* Practice parameter: the role of corticosteroids in the management of acute monosymptomatic optic neuritis: report of the quality standards subcommittee of the American Academy of Neurology. *Neurology* 2000; **54:** 2039–44.

### Organ and tissue transplantation

For a discussion of organ and tissue transplantation, including the role of corticosteroids, see, p.1344.

### Osteoarthritis

Systemic corticosteroids are not considered to have a place in the management of osteoarthritis (p.9); however, intra-articular or peri-articular injection, although controversial, may be of some help in patients with localised inflammation. Such injections should be given only infrequently and as adjunctive therapy.

### Osteopetrosis

Osteopetrosis is a rare set of heterogeneous disorders characterised by an increase in bone density, generally due to a failure of the osteoclasts to resorb mineralised bone. In the severe infantile malignant form there is reduction in the bone marrow space, leading to anaemia, hepatosplenomegaly, and nerve compression that may produce blindness and deafness; early death often results. The adult form is benign; patients typically present with fractures, back and bone pain, but no haematological abnormalities, and generally have a full life expectancy.[1]

Bone marrow transplantation may be curative for the infantile malignant form if a suitable donor can be found.[1,2] Corticosteroids are used palliatively. Benefit has been reported in 3 of 4 children treated with prednisone 1 mg/kg daily by mouth, together with phosphate supplements and a low-calcium diet.[3] Some patients have also benefited from the use of high-dose calcitriol, again with a low-calcium diet.[4]

Another study, in 14 patients, found that treatment with interferon gamma-1b increased bone resorption.[5] In 11 who received this treatment for 18 months there was stabilisation or improvement in clinical condition and a reduction in the frequency of serious infection.

1. Kocher MS, Kasser JR. Osteopetrosis. *Am J Orthop* 2003; **32:** 222–8.
2. Gerritsen EJ, *et al.* Bone marrow transplantation for autosomal recessive osteopetrosis: a report from the Working Party on Inborn Errors of the European Bone Marrow Transplantation Group. *J Pediatr* 1994; **125:** 896–902.
3. Dorantes LM, *et al.* Juvenile osteopetrosis: effects on blood and bone of prednisone and a low calcium, high phosphate diet. *Arch Dis Child* 1986; **61:** 666–70.
4. Key LL, Ries WL. Osteopetrosis: the pharmaco-physiologic basis of therapy. *Clin Orthop* 1993; **294:** 85–9.
5. Key LL, *et al.* Long-term treatment of osteopetrosis with recombinant human interferon gamma. *N Engl J Med* 1995; **332:** 1594–9.

### Pain

Corticosteroids have produced improvement, often substantial, in neuropathic pain, including pain due to nerve damage and sympathetically maintained pain, and are widely used in conditions such as chronic low back pain and cancer pain. Dexamethasone, methylprednisolone, and prednisolone have been used for pain management, sometimes in the form of long-acting depot injections administered locally. The exact mechanism of action of corticosteroids in analgesia is not clear but may involve relief of pressure on nervous tissue by reduction of inflammation and oedema.

For discussions of pain and its management, see p.2.

### Pancreatitis

Corticosteroids are generally contra-indicated for pancreatitis (p.1726), but a response has been reported[1,2] in patients with acute episodes caused by sarcoidosis (p.1087).

1. McCormick PA, *et al.* Pancreatitis in sarcoidosis. *BMJ* 1985; **290:** 1472–3.
2. Limaye AP, *et al.* Sarcoidosis associated with recurrent pancreatitis. *South Med J* 1997; **90:** 431–3.

### Pemphigus and pemphigoid

Systemic corticosteroids are the mainstay of management of pemphigus and pemphigoid (p.1137). Initially, high doses are used to control blistering, and up to 400 mg of prednisolone daily has been suggested, although most dermatologists attempt to keep the dose below 120 mg daily. Adjuvant therapy such as azathioprine, cyclophosphamide, or gold may be given.[1] Maintenance treatment must be individualised, but in general the dose of prednisolone should be reduced by 50% every 2 to 3 weeks. Once the dose has been lowered to 80 mg daily it is desirable to convert gradually to alternate-day therapy. During this period topical therapy with potent corticosteroids is useful, and is also a valuable first-line treatment for early relapses. A combined corticosteroid-antibacterial preparation reduces the chance of infection. For mucosal lesions corticosteroids may be applied topically, sucked as lozenges, or possibly inhaled. High dose oral prednisolone and oral cyclophosphamide also relieve inflammation in patients with ocular cicatricial pemphigoid, although they may not completely prevent cicatrisation.[2]

With the aim of reducing adverse effects, corticosteroids have been given in lower initial doses by mouth (prednisolone 45 to 60 mg daily)[3] or by intravenous pulse therapy (dexamethasone 136 mg given over 1 to 2 hours daily for 3 days, repeated at least monthly, with intravenous cyclophosphamide 500 mg infused on day 1);[4] pemphigus responded to both of these regimens.

Bullous pemphigoid is probably best treated with high potency corticosteroids applied topically;[5] a large randomised trial[6] found that topical application of 40 g of clobetasol propionate cream 0.05% daily was superior to oral prednisone 500 micrograms/kg daily for moderate disease and 1 mg/kg daily for severe disease.

1. Carson PJ, *et al.* Influence of treatment on the clinical course of pemphigus vulgaris. *J Am Acad Dermatol* 1996; **34:** 645–52.
2. Elder MJ, *et al.* Role of cyclophosphamide and high dose steroid in ocular cicatricial pemphigoid. *Br J Ophthalmol* 1995; **79:** 264–6.
3. Ratnam KV, *et al.* Pemphigus therapy with oral prednisolone regimens. *Int J Dermatol* 1990; **29:** 363–7.
4. Kaur S, Kanwar AJ. Dexamethasone–cyclophosphamide pulse therapy in pemphigus. *Int J Dermatol* 1990; **29:** 371–4.
5. Stern RS. Bullous pemphigoid therapy—think globally, act locally. *N Engl J Med* 2002; **346:** 364–7.
6. Joly P, *et al.* A comparison of oral and topical corticosteroids in patients with bullous pemphigoid. *N Engl J Med* 2002; **346:** 321–7.

### Pneumocystis carinii pneumonia

The management of *Pneumocystis carinii* pneumonia (p.389) is primarily with either co-trimoxazole or pentamidine. In patients with moderate or severe attacks, adjuvant therapy with high-dose oral or intravenous corticosteroids reduces both the risk of respiratory failure and the risk of death.[1,2] Concerns about the potential for further immunosuppression with such adjuvant therapy in patients with HIV infection[3] do not seem to have been borne out: a comparative study noted no increase in mortality or the risk of developing other opportunistic infections.[4]

1. Miller RF, *et al.* Pneumocystis carinii infection: current treatment and prevention. *J Antimicrob Chemother* 1996; **37** (suppl B): 33–53.
2. Bye MR, *et al.* Markedly reduced mortality associated with corticosteroid therapy of Pneumocystis carinii pneumonia in children with acquired immunodeficiency syndrome. *Arch Pediatr Adolesc Med* 1994; **148:** 638–41.
3. Nelson MR, *et al.* Treatment with corticosteroids—a risk factor for the development of clinical cytomegalovirus disease in AIDS. *AIDS* 1993; **7:** 375–8.
4. Gallant JE, *et al.* The effect of adjunctive corticosteroids for the treatment of Pneumocystis carinii pneumonia on mortality and subsequent complications. *Chest* 1998; **114:** 1258–63.

### Polyarteritis nodosa and microscopic polyangiitis

Polyarteritis nodosa is considered the prototype of systemic necrotising vasculitis. It may occur at any age but is more common in white patients and in men. It is characterised by inflammation throughout the arterial wall with fibrinoid necrosis of the arterial media, particularly in medium-sized vessels, partial occlusion of the vessel due to proliferation of the intima (possibly leading to thrombosis and infarction), fibrosis, and the formation of aneurysms. Microscopic polyangiitis, in which small vessels are primarily involved, with frequent renal and pulmonary involvement, has been seen as part of the spectrum of polyarteritis nodosa but is now considered an entity in its own right, although patients may have features of both. Antineutrophil cytoplasmic antibodies (ANCA) are common in patients with microscopic polyangiitis, which has many similarities to Wegener's granulomatosis (p.1090), but not in classic polyarteritis nodosa.

Symptoms depend on the vessels affected but most patients have fever, weight loss, myalgia, and arthralgia. Those associated with gastrointestinal involvement include mouth ulceration, diarrhoea, visceral pain, haemorrhage, or sometimes infarction of the bowel, while involvement of liver can lead to hepatomegaly or hepatic necrosis and pancreatic involvement may simulate pancreatitis. Renal involvement may present as acute glomerulonephritis and renal failure or as nephrotic syndrome; like pulmonary involvement it is a feature particularly of microscopic polyangiitis, and associated with a poor prognosis. Skin lesions, peripheral neuropathies, alterations in mental function, convulsions, episcleritis or scleritis and retinal vasculitis, ischaemic heart disease, heart failure, Raynaud's phenomenon, and hypertension are among other potential symptoms. If untreated, death, usually due to renal or cardiac involvement, occurs in about 90% of patients within 5 years.

Classic polyarteritis nodosa may respond to treatment with a corticosteroid given alone, typically prednisone or prednisolone in a dose of 40 to 60 mg daily; however, although the benefits of adding a cytotoxic to the regimen have been queried,[1,2] a combined regimen with cyclophosphamide is often preferred.[1,3,4] In patients with microscopic polyangiitis a combined regimen is recommended. One suggested regimen is prednisone or prednisolone 1 mg/kg together with cyclophosphamide 2 mg/kg, both daily by mouth, for initial induction of remission.[5] Pulsed intravenous methylprednisolone has also been used at initiation, followed by a tapering dose of corticosteroid. There is a trend towards the use of shorter courses of cyclophosphamide, and to the use of intravenous pulsed cyclophosphamide rather than oral administration, in an attempt to reduce adverse effects.[5,6] Treatment with corticosteroids and cyclophosphamide should not exceed 1 year.[6] Azathioprine has been substituted for cyclophosphamide to maintain remission, and mycophenolate mofetil has been tried in a few patients as an alternative to cyclophosphamide in combination therapy after initial induction.[7]

A monoclonal anti-CD4 antibody, alemtuzumab, has produced benefit in a patient with a systemic vasculitis (not identified as polyarteritis nodosa) refractory to standard therapy[8] and it may be that monoclonal antibodies will prove useful in this disease; results in microscopic polyangiitis are encouraging (see below). Polyarteritis nodosa may be associated with hepatitis B infection; the vasculitis responds in most cases to treatment with antiviral drugs and plasma exchange.[3,6]

Alemtuzumab and other anti-CD4 monoclonal antibodies have been used successfully in patients with microscopic polyangiitis unresponsive to conventional treatment.[9] Another therapy that has been tried in this group, but with ambiguous results, is high dose intravenous normal immunoglobulin.[5]

Vasodilators such as calcium-channel blockers, inhibitors of platelet activation, or drugs that improve blood flow may be useful to improve local ischaemia.[10] Skin lesions in a patient with cutaneous polyarteritis nodosa have reportedly responded to oral pentoxifylline.[11]


1. Taylor HG, Samanta A. Treatment of vasculitis. *Br J Clin Pharmacol* 1993; **35:** 93–104.
2. Conn DL. Role of cyclophosphamide in treatment of polyarteritis nodosa? *J Rheumatol* 1991; **18:** 489–90.
3. Guillevin L, *et al.* Treatment of polyarteritis nodosa and Churg-Strauss syndrome: a meta-analysis of 3 prospective controlled trials including 182 patients over 12 years. *Ann Med Interne (Paris)* 1992; **143:** 405–16.
4. Guillevin L, *et al.* Longterm follow up after treatment of polyarteritis nodosa and Churg-Strauss angiitis with comparison of steroids, plasma exchange and cyclophosphamide to steroids and plasma exchange: a prospective randomized trial of 71 patients. *J Rheumatol* 1991; **18:** 567–74.
5. Savage COS, *et al.* Primary systemic vasculitis. *Lancet* 1997; **349:** 553–8.
6. Guillevin L, Lhote F. Treatment of systemic vasculitides. *Adv Nephrol Necker Hosp* 1999; **29:** 35–52.
7. Nowack R, *et al.* Mycophenolate mofetil for systemic vasculitis and IgA nephropathy. *Lancet* 1997; **349:** 774.
8. Mathieson PW, *et al.* Monoclonal-antibody therapy in systemic vasculitis. *N Engl J Med* 1990; **323:** 250–4.
9. Lockwood CM, *et al.* Long-term remission of intractable systemic vasculitis with monoclonal antibody therapy. *Lancet* 1993; **341:** 1620–2.
10. Conn DL. Update on systemic necrotizing vasculitis *Mayo Clin Proc* 1989; **64:** 535–43.
11. Calderón MJ, *et al.* Successful treatment of cutaneous PAN with pentoxifylline. *Br J Dermatol* 1993; **128:** 706–7.


### Polychondritis

Relapsing polychondritis is a rare systemic disease that results in inflammation and destruction of cartilage in various parts of the body, most seriously in the respiratory system (e.g. nose, larynx, and trachea). Airway narrowing and obstruction due to loss of cartilaginous support results, and may be complicated by pneumonia; fatalities have resulted. Cardiovascular involvement, ocular manifestations, skin disorders, and renal disease may occur; it may also be associated with other diseases such as the vasculitic syndromes. Mild inflammation is usually treated with dapsone, colchicine, or NSAIDs. Relatively high doses of corticosteroid may improve symptoms in active disease, but do not appear to retard progression. Acute airway obstruction is treated with high-dose intravenous pulse corticosteroids.[1] Methotrexate[2] or azathioprine[1] may be of value in reducing corticosteroid requirements. CD4 antibodies[3,4] have also been tried in refractory disease.


1. Letko E, *et al.* Relapsing polychondritis: a clinical review. *Semin Arthritis Rheum* 2002; **31:** 384–95.
2. Trentham DE, Le CH. Relapsing polychondritis. *Ann Intern Med* 1998; **129:** 114–22.
3. van der Lubbe PA, *et al.* Anti-CD4 monoclonal antibody for relapsing polychondritis. *Lancet* 1991; **337:** 1349.
4. Choy EHS, *et al.* Chimaeric anti-CD4 monoclonal antibody for relapsing polychondritis. *Lancet* 1991; **338:** 450.


### Polymyalgia rheumatica

Polymyalgia rheumatica is a rheumatic disorder of uncertain aetiology. It occurs mainly in persons over 50 years of age of European, especially Scandinavian, extraction and is more common in women than in men. The disease is characterised by myalgia and severe morning stiffness in the neck and shoulder girdle and in the hips and pelvic girdle, which may spread in more advanced cases to the muscles of the thighs, chest, and arms. Stiffness and pain are worse after periods of inactivity. There may be some joint involvement; other symptoms include fatigue, weight loss, and fever, and anaemia and raised erythrocyte sedimentation rate are seen. In some patients polymyalgia rheumatica is associated with giant cell arteritis (p.1080).

**Treatment.** Although NSAIDs may improve the symptoms of polymyalgia rheumatica they do not control the disease process, and corticosteroids are preferred;[1-5] in particular, corticosteroid therapy is essential where giant cell arteritis is present.

The usual initial dose is prednisolone or prednisone 10 to 20 mg daily by mouth, depending on the severity of symptoms; higher doses are needed where giant cell arteritis is also present, particularly if there are ophthalmic symptoms.[4,6] After 1 to 2 months a reduction in dosage is usually possible provided symptoms are well controlled. Dosage reduction should be gradual;[4,5] mean maintenance dose at one year is about 6 mg daily.[1,5]

Maintenance therapy may need to be prolonged. Although about a third to a half of all patients may be able to have corticosteroids withdrawn within about 2 years,[2] maintenance can be required for considerably longer periods.[5] Intramuscular methylprednisolone has also been found to be effective in polymyalgia rheumatica; because the cumulative dose with prolonged therapy is lower it has been suggested that this has advantages over the use of oral corticosteroids.[7] Intravenous pulse methylprednisolone has also been used.[5] Relapse is not uncommon and is most likely within one year of corticosteroid withdrawal.[2,3,5] It may be associated with arteritic symptoms, but arteritic relapses are unusual in patients whose original presentation was pure polymyalgia.[2] Methotrexate or azathioprine may be used for their corticosteroid-sparing effect in patients in whom withdrawal is difficult.[2-4]


1. Kyle V. Polymyalgia rheumatica. *Prescribers' J* 1997; **37:** 138–44.
2. Swannell AJ. Polymyalgia rheumatica and temporal arteritis: diagnosis and management. *BMJ* 1997; **314:** 1329–32.
3. Zilko PJ. Polymyalgia rheumatica and giant cell arteritis. *Med J Aust* 1996; **165:** 438–42.
4. Salvarani C, *et al.* Polymyalgia rheumatica. *Lancet* 1997; **350:** 43–7.
5. Gran JT. Current therapy of polymyalgia rheumatica. *Scand J Rheumatol* 1999; **28:** 269–72.
6. Buch MH, Bird HA. Polymyalgia rheumatica and giant cell arteritis. In: Snaith ML, ed. *ABC of rheumatology.* 3rd ed. London: BMJ Books, 2004: 75–9.
7. Dasgupta B, *et al.* An initially double-blind controlled 96 week trial of depot methylprednisolone against oral prednisolone in the treatment of polymyalgia rheumatica. *Br J Rheumatol* 1998; **37:** 189–95.


### Polymyositis and dermatomyositis

The term polymyositis has been used to describe several types of rare idiopathic inflammatory muscle disorders (myopathies).

The cardinal symptom of polymyositis is symmetrical progressive muscle weakness, usually starting in the shoulder girdle and neck, and pelvic girdle. Onset is usually gradual over a period of months, and accompanied by mild pain and tenderness, although more rapidly evolving disease with intense muscle pain is known. With progression, weakness may prevent the patient from moving their limbs, and muscle atrophy and contracture can develop. Dysphagia, pulmonary aspiration, and hypoventilation may occur, and some patients develop fibrosing alveolitis; pulmonary involvement, especially aspiration pneumonia, can be fatal. ECG abnormalities, usually asymptomatic, are common, and some patients develop Raynaud's syndrome. Primary disease may be associated with skin rashes, in which case it is known as dermatomyositis. Purplish scaly rashes on knees, elbows, and knuckles, and a characteristic purplish ('heliotrope') coloration and oedema of the eyelids may occur. A childhood form known as juvenile dermatomyositis exists, in which additional signs include vasculitis and subcutaneous calcium deposition (calcinosis cutis), and gastrointestinal haemorrhage and perforation may occur.

**Treatment.** Patients with active disease require bed rest, with the head elevated in patients at risk of aspiration. Physiotherapy to maintain muscle tone and avoid the development of contractures may be required.

Initial drug therapy is based on corticosteroids.[1-4] The usual choice is oral prednisone or prednisolone 40 to 60 mg or more, or 1 to 2 mg/kg daily. This usually produces improvement within 1 to 2 months. The dose may then be gradually tapered off to the minimum required for disease control;[1-3] some patients with well controlled disease may be satisfactorily maintained on an alternate-day regimen.[2,3] In patients with severe disease or extramuscular manifestations such as lung involvement, pulse intravenous methylprednisolone may be preferred initially, to gain more rapid disease control.[1,2,4] Maintenance therapy may need to be prolonged and a reduction in corticosteroid dosage to the minimum is therefore desirable, but too early or too rapid a reduction may lead to relapse.

Up to 30% of patients do not respond to corticosteroids,[2] or develop unacceptable adverse effects, and in these cases the second-line drugs are cytotoxic immunosuppressants.[1-3] There is considerable experience with the use of methotrexate, by mouth, subcutaneously, intramuscularly, or intravenously, usually at weekly intervals; it may be used with corticosteroids, permitting a reduction in corticosteroid dose. Azathioprine may also be given with corticosteroids, again permitting a reduction in corticosteroid dosage, and the combination has also been shown to be superior to a corticosteroid alone for long-term maintenance (although this was only apparent after more than a year of therapy).[5] There is some evidence that methotrexate may be superior to azathioprine in patients unresponsive to prednisone alone.[6] Combining methotrexate and azathioprine has also been suggested.[2,4]

Some consider that corticosteroid therapy should be combined with a cytotoxic immunosuppressant such as azathioprine or methotrexate from the outset of treatment.

The role of other drugs is less well defined. Cyclophosphamide may be of use in patients with lung disease,[1,3] while chlorambucil and tacrolimus have produced benefit in individual cases but have not been formally assessed.[4] There have been reports of ciclosporin producing a response in refractory disease.[2,4] Normal immunoglobulin has also produced responses; it is usually reserved for refractory cases, or as an add-on therapy in patients inadequately controlled on corticosteroids and immunosuppressants, or for whom immunosuppressants are contra-indicated.[2,3] Promising results have been obtained with fludarabine[1] and mycophenolate mofetil;[2,3] there are preliminary reports of success with etanercept, and infliximab, and interferon beta has been investigated.[2]

Cutaneous symptoms in patients with dermatomyositis do not always respond satisfactorily to corticosteroids, but hydroxychloroquine is reputed to be of benefit in patients with rash,[7] probably due to a photoprotective effect.[8] Calcinosis, which can cause considerable morbidity, is particularly difficult to treat but some cases have responded to treatment with aluminium hydroxide, alendronate, diltiazem, or magnesium sulfate.[4] Warfarin therapy has been used,[9,10] but its value for calcinosis is disputed.[11]


1. Oddis CV. Current approach to the treatment of polymyositis and dermatomyositis. *Curr Opin Rheumatol* 2000; **12:** 492–7.
2. Mastaglia FL, *et al.* Inflammatory myopathies: clinical, diagnostic and therapeutic aspects. *Muscle Nerve* 2003; **27:** 407–25.
3. Dalakas MC. Therapeutic approaches in patients with inflammatory myopathies. *Semin Neurol* 2003; **23:** 199–206.
4. Reed AM, Lopez M. Juvenile dermatomyositis: recognition and treatment. *Pediatr Drugs* 2002; **4:** 315–21.
5. Bunch TW. Prednisone and azathioprine for polymyositis: long-term followup. *Arthritis Rheum* 1981; **24:** 45–8.
6. Joffe MM, *et al.* Drug therapy of the idiopathic inflammatory myopathies: predictors of response to prednisone, azathioprine, and methotrexate and a comparison of their efficacy. *Am J Med* 1993; **94:** 379–87.
7. Woo TY, *et al.* Cutaneous lesions of dermatomyositis are improved by hydroxychloroquine. *J Am Acad Dermatol* 1984; **10:** 592–600.
8. Cox NH. Amyopathic dermatomyositis, photosensitivity and hydroxychloroquine. *Br J Dermatol* 1995; **132:** 1016–17.
9. Berger RG, Hadler NM. Treatment of calcinosis universalis secondary to dermatomyositis or scleroderma with low dose warfarin. *Arthritis Rheum* 1983; **26** (suppl): S11.
10. Martinez-Cordero E, *et al.* Calcinosis in childhood dermatomyositis. *Clin Exp Rheumatol* 1990; **8:** 198–200.
11. Ansell B. Is there a treatment for the calcinosis of juvenile dermatomyositis? *Br J Rheumatol* 1990; **29:** 263.


### Polyneuropathies

Ten patients with subacute demyelinating polyneuropathy obtained a beneficial response to corticosteroid therapy.[1] In one patient the response was initially slight, but became dramatic when azathioprine was added. Prednisone was given in initial single daily doses of 40 to 150 mg, until definite clinical improvement was obtained, and followed by a single-dose alternate-day regimen. Corticosteroids are generally considered to be of little use in Guillain-Barré syndrome (p.1630), which usually occurs due to an acute inflammatory polyradiculoneuropathy.[2] In chronic inflammatory demyelinating polyradiculoneuropathy

(CIDP), corticosteroids are reported to be beneficial,[1,3] although a review[3] found weak evidence to support this. Subacute demyelinating neuropathy appeared to be a distinct and clinically identifiable entity in which corticosteroid therapy is indicated.[1]

1. Oh SJ. Subacute demyelinating polyneuropathy responding to corticosteroid treatment. *Arch Neurol* 1978; **35:** 509–16.
2. Hughes RAC, van der Meché FGA. Corticosteroids for Guillain-Barré syndrome. Available in The Cochrane Library; Issue 1. Chichester: John Wiley; 2004.
3. Mehndiratta MM, Hughes RAC. Corticosteroids for chronic inflammatory demyelinating polyradiculoneuropathy. Available in The Cochrane Library; Issue 1. Chichester: John Wiley; 2004.

### Postoperative ocular inflammation

Corticosteroid eye drops are used to control the inflammatory response commonly observed following cataract surgery; prednisolone is usually used but dexamethasone may be necessary if the inflammation is severe.

Corticosteroids should only be used with care and for short periods for topical control of postoperative ocular inflammation, as discussed on p.70.

### Pregnancy

Although some adverse effects have been recorded and certain precautions need to be observed, the use of corticosteroids during pregnancy (see under Precautions, p.1071) is appropriate to promote fetal maturation where there is a risk of premature delivery (see Neonatal Respiratory Distress Syndrome, above). In addition, in those maternal conditions serious enough to require systemic corticosteroids the risk to both mother and offspring of discontinuing therapy is often greater than that of corticosteroid use during pregnancy.

### Psoriasis

Reviews of psoriasis (p.1137) and its management[1-4] include topical corticosteroids among first-line treatments. Combination therapy using corticosteroids with other topical treatments, such as calcipotriol or tazarotene, may be used to reduce adverse effects and improve efficacy of both drugs.[5]

Intralesional injection of corticosteroids has been used for small, localised, recalcitrant plaques of psoriasis but caution is required to avoid skin atrophy or depigmentation.[1]

Systemic corticosteroids are not generally recommended, but have been used for short periods in extreme or rare cases; there is a risk of systemic adverse effects and of rebound psoriasis occurring on stopping therapy.[2]

Topical corticosteroids remain the mainstay of treatment in scalp psoriasis, although long-term treatment is not recommended; the more potent corticosteroids are reserved for adult use.[6]

1. Menter A, Barker JNWN. Psoriasis in practice. *Lancet* 1991; **338:** 231–4.
2. British Association of Dermatologists. Clinical guidelines: psoriasis. Available at: http://www.bad.org.uk/doctors/guidelines/psoriasis.asp (accessed 27/04/04)
3. Linden KG, Weinstein GD. Psoriasis: current perspectives with an emphasis on treatment. *Am J Med* 1999; **107:** 595–605.
4. Peters BP, *et al.* Pathophysiology and treatment of psoriasis. *Am J Health-Syst Pharm* 2000; **57:** 645–62.
5. Trozak DJ. Topical corticosteroid therapy in psoriasis vulgaris: update and new strategies. *Cutis* 1999; **64:** 315–18.
6. van der Vleuten CJM, van de Kerkhof PCM. Management of scalp psoriasis: guidelines for corticosteroid use in combination treatment. *Drugs* 2001; **61:** 1593–8.

### Pyoderma gangrenosum

A systemic corticosteroid is one of the treatments that has been tried in pyoderma gangrenosum (p.1138). Six of eight patients with severe refractory pyoderma gangrenosum responded favourably to treatment with high-dose systemic corticosteroid pulse therapy;[1] none had serious complications. However, pulse therapy needs very careful use and monitoring, as it is not without adverse effects.[2]

Healing of superficial granulomatous pyoderma has occurred following intralesional injection of triamcinolone,[3,4] oral administration of prednisolone,[3,4] and following long-term topical corticosteroids.[4]

1. Prystowsky JH, *et al.* Present status of pyoderma gangrenosum: review of 21 cases. *Arch Dermatol* 1989; **125:** 57–64.
2. Callen JP. Pyoderma gangrenosum. *Lancet* 1998; **351:** 581–5.
3. Quimby SR, *et al.* Superficial granulomatous pyoderma: clinicopathologic spectrum. *Mayo Clin Proc* 1989; **64:** 37–43.
4. Hardwick N, Cerio R. Superficial granulomatous pyoderma: a report of two cases. *Br J Dermatol* 1993; **129:** 718–22.

### Respiratory disorders

Although corticosteroids have been used in the management of many forms of respiratory disorder, this use has frequently been on an empirical and uncontrolled basis, and evidence of benefit is often somewhat mixed. Thus, while an established role exists for corticosteroids in the management of asthma (p.777), the antenatal prevention of neonatal respiratory distress syndrome (p.1084), and probably in croup (p.1079) they are no longer used in aspiration syndromes (p.1240) and their role in diffuse parenchymal lung disorders (see p.1079 and under Sarcoidosis, below) and in acute respiratory distress syndrome (p.1075) is uncertain. Other disorders in which they have been tried with varying success include bronchiolitis (p.1077), chronic obstructive pulmonary disease (see p.1078), fat embolism syndrome,[1] acute eosinophilic pneumonia[2] and pulmonary eosinophilia,[3] diffuse alveolar haemorrhage,[4] and 'ice hockey lung' (due to nitrogen dioxide).[5]

1. Van Besouw J-P, Hinds CJ. Fat embolism syndrome. *Br J Hosp Med* 1989; **42:** 304–11.
2. Anonymous. Acute eosinophilic pneumonia. *Lancet* 1990; **335:** 947.
3. Anonymous. Pulmonary eosinophilia. *Lancet* 1990; **335:** 512.
4. Metcalf JP, *et al.* Corticosteroids as adjunctive therapy for diffuse alveolar hemorrhage associated with bone marrow transplantation. *Am J Med* 1994; **96:** 327–34.
5. Anonymous. Ice hockey lung: $NO_2$ poisoning. *Lancet* 1990; **335:** 1191.

### Retinal vasculitis

In the treatment of retinal vasculitis, corticosteroids are the most useful drugs for the management of inflammation and its sequelae when vision is compromised.[1] For uniocular disease treatment with orbital floor injection of corticosteroids such as methylprednisolone acetate may be possible. For bilateral disease systemic therapy is required, with additional immunosuppressant cover if relapse occurs despite high-dose corticosteroid therapy.

1. Anonymous. Retinal vasculitis. *Lancet* 1989; **i:** 823–4.

### Rheumatoid arthritis

Although a mainstay of treatment in juvenile idiopathic arthritis (p.9), the use of corticosteroids in adult rheumatoid arthritis (p.9) is controversial. Systemic corticosteroids can suppress symptoms of the disease, but their value is limited by their adverse effects and they have usually been reserved for severe rapidly progressing disease unresponsive to therapy with NSAIDs and disease-modifying antirheumatic drugs (DMARDs). They may also be used temporarily to control disease activity during initiation of therapy with DMARDs, or in disease accompanied by severe extra-articular effects. However, recent results indicate that there may be advantages to the early use of low doses of corticosteroids in active disease. Intra-articular injection of corticosteroids may be used when an acute flare affects one or two individual joints but should be given infrequently.

References.

1. Gotzsche PC, Johansen HK. Short-term low-dose corticosteroids vs placebo and nonsteroidal antiinflammatory drugs in rheumatoid arthritis. Available in The Cochrane Library; Issue 1. Chichester: John Wiley; 2004.
2. Criswell LA, *et al.* Moderate-term, low-dose corticosteroids for rheumatoid arthritis. Available in The Cochrane Library; Issue 1. Chichester: John Wiley; 2004.
3. Cleary AG, *et al.* Intra-articular corticosteroid injections in juvenile idiopathic arthritis. *Arch Dis Child* 2003; **88:** 192–6.

### Rhinitis

For a brief description of rhinitis and a discussion of its management including the use of corticosteroids, see p.422. Reviews[1,2] including a systematic review,[1] found that intranasal corticosteroids produced greater relief of the nasal symptoms of allergic rhinitis than oral antihistamines, and there was no difference between the two treatments in relief of eye symptoms.

1. Weiner JM, *et al.* Intranasal corticosteroids versus oral $H_1$ receptor antagonists in allergic rhinitis: systematic review of randomised controlled trials. *BMJ* 1998; **317:** 1624–9.
2. Nielsen LP, *et al.* Intranasal corticosteroids for allergic rhinitis: superior relief? *Drugs* 2001; **61:** 1563–79.

### Sarcoidosis

Sarcoidosis is a disorder involving the development of multiple granulomas in a variety of organs, which may subsequently resolve or progress to chronic fibrosis.[1] The disease is frequently asymptomatic, and since it usually regresses spontaneously estimating the incidence is difficult, but it appears to vary considerably in different countries. It is most often seen in young adults and is slightly more common in female than male and in black than white patients.

Almost any organ can be affected, but manifestations in lymph nodes, lungs, skin, joints, and eyes are common. Lymphadenopathy, some decrease in pulmonary function, dyspnoea, and cough may mark lung and lymph node involvement. Skin manifestations include erythema nodosum, macular or papular lesions due to granuloma formation in the skin, and violaceous plaques on fingers, nose, ears, and cheeks known as lupus pernio. Arthropathy, with painful joint swellings, may be associated with erythema nodosum and fever in acute presentations; bone lesions are most common in fingers and toes. Involvement of the nervous system may be particularly difficult to diagnose because of its protean manifestations. Involvement of the eyes is usually manifest as uveitis although other symptoms include keratoconjunctivitis sicca. Symptomatic disease involving the gastrointestinal tract, liver, pancreas, heart, or kidneys is rare, although asymptomatic involvement may occur.

In addition to symptoms directly due to the disease, sarcoidosis is often associated with hypercalcaemia (p.1218) and hypersensitivity to the effects of vitamin D. Other biochemical abnormalities include raised serum concentrations of angiotensin-converting enzyme (ACE), and there are abnormalities of some aspects of immune function.

Diagnosis of sarcoidosis is problematic because of its multiple manifestations and the fact that it is so often clinically silent. It is often detected by accident, when radiography is performed for other reasons, but biopsy is often needed to help confirm the disease. The Kveim test, in which an antigen derived from patients with sarcoidosis (see p.1703) is given intradermally and produces a delayed reaction in patients with the disease, is now rarely used because of its perceived lack of precision, although some still consider it useful.[2]

**Treatment.** Asymptomatic disease requires no therapy, and since spontaneous remission can occur, corticosteroids, which are the usual therapy,[1] are generally reserved for patients in whom the disease affects the function of a vital organ or for patients with hypercalcaemia. NSAIDs alone may be adequate to control the fever and arthropathy of acute disease. Where corticosteroids are called for a typical regimen is prednisolone or prednisone 30 to 40 mg daily by mouth, the dose being reduced after several weeks as the patient improves.[3-5] Therapy should be continued (at the minimum effective maintenance dose) for 12 to 18 months before any attempt is made to withdraw it.[3] Alternate-day administration has been suggested, with 40 mg every other day as initial therapy,[6] and 5 to 10 mg every other day as maintenance.[7] There is some evidence[8] that relapse may be more likely following withdrawal of corticosteroids than in patients who do not receive corticosteroid therapy, but this may simply reflect the natural course of disease in this group. There also remains some dispute about the value of oral corticosteroids in pulmonary disease: although they are useful in the short term their long-term benefits are more uncertain.[9] Inhaled corticosteroids have also been investigated in pulmonary sarcoidosis; they appear less reliable than oral therapy for primary treatment, but may have a role as maintenance therapy.[5,10] In patients with ocular disease corticosteroid drops and ointment are used for anterior uveitis; resistant cases, or patients with posterior uveitis, require systemic corticosteroids.[1] Skin lesions usually respond to corticosteroids but the high doses that may be required for suppression of lupus pernio may produce changes in appearance as disfiguring as the disease.[3]

Other drugs have occasionally been used in sarcoidosis but are very much second-line. In patients in whom corticosteroids are not effective or not tolerated cytotoxic immunosuppressants have been given, with variable results.[1,3,5,7] Methotrexate has perhaps been most useful, having been found to be effective in low doses (up to 15 mg weekly) by mouth in refractory disease;[1,11] corticosteroid-sparing effects may be evident after 6 months.[7] Azathioprine has been used for severe refractory cases.[5] Results with ciclosporin have been variable,[7] although there are reports of response in refractory skin lesions and optic neuropathy.[1] Toxicity and concerns about carcinogenesis limit the use of chlorambucil and cyclophosphamide.[1,5] The antimalarials have also been tried as adjuncts or alternatives to corticosteroid therapy,[5] and may be useful for skin disease and hypercalcaemia.[7] Potential ocular toxicity is a concern, however, and although hydroxychloroquine may be less oculotoxic than chloroquine,[7] regular ophthalmological assessment is recommended.[5] Other reports of benefit in cutaneous sarcoidosis have involved allopurinol,[12] thalidomide,[13] and tranilast,[14] while there is report of response to melatonin in 2 patients with refractory sarcoidosis.[15] Infliximab and pentoxifylline have also shown promising results.[7]

1. Newman LS, *et al.* Sarcoidosis. *N Engl J Med* 1997; **336:** 1224–34. Correction. *ibid.*; **337:** 139.

2. Zajicek JP, *et al.* Central nervous system sarcoidosis—diagnosis and management. *Q J Med* 1999; **92:** 103–17.
3. Muthiah MM, Macfarlane JT. Current concepts in the management of sarcoidosis. *Drugs* 1990; **40:** 231–7.
4. Judson MA. An approach to the treatment of pulmonary sarcoidosis with corticosteroids: the six phases of treatment. *Chest* 1999; **115:** 1158–65.
5. Gibson GJ. Sarcoidosis: old and new treatments. *Thorax* 2001; **56:** 336–9.
6. DeRemee RA. Sarcoidosis. *Mayo Clin Proc* 1995; **70:** 177–81.
7. Baughman RP, *et al.* Sarcoidosis. *Lancet* 2003; **361:** 1111–18.
8. Gottlieb JE, *et al.* Outcome in sarcoidosis: the relationship of relapse to corticosteroid therapy. *Chest* 1997; **111:** 623–31.
9. Paramothayan NS, Jones PW. Corticosteroids for pulmonary sarcoidosis. Available in The Cochrane Library; Issue 1. Chichester: John Wiley; 2004.
10. British Thoracic Society. The diagnosis, assessment and treatment of diffuse parenchymal lung disease in adults. *Thorax* 1999; **54** (suppl 1): S1–S30. Also available at: http://www.brit-thoracic.org.uk/docs/Parenchymaltext.pdf (accessed 27/04/04)
11. Baughman RP, Lower EE. A clinical approach to the use of methotrexate for sarcoidosis. *Thorax* 1999; **54:** 742–6.
12. Brechtel B, *et al.* Allopurinol: a therapeutic alternative for disseminated cutaneous sarcoidosis. *Br J Dermatol* 1996; **135:** 307–9.
13. Baughman RP, *et al.* Thalidomide for chronic sarcoidosis. *Chest* 2002; **122:** 227–32.
14. Yamada H, *et al.* Treatment of cutaneous sarcoidosis with tranilast. *J Dermatol* 1995; **22:** 149–52.
15. Cagnoni ML, *et al.* Melatonin for treatment of chronic refractory sarcoidosis. *Lancet* 1995; **346:** 1229–30.

## Sciatica

For mention of the use of epidural corticosteroid injections to treat sciatica, and doubts about the extent of benefit, see Administration, Epidural Route, p.1074.

## Scleritis

Scleritis and episcleritis are inflammatory diseases of the sclera often associated with various systemic diseases. Episcleritis tends to be a benign superficial condition but treatment can be difficult and it tends to recur. The use of topical corticosteroids and topical NSAIDs are sometimes of temporary benefit. Scleritis is a rarer more deep-seated inflammation. Initial treatment of non-necrotising scleritis is with NSAIDs; high dose systemic corticosteroids (usually prednisone or prednisolone 60 to 80 mg by mouth daily) have been used successfully in many patients unresponsive to NSAIDs.[1,2] If necessary, to reduce any attendant adverse effects, corticosteroids have been given by orbital floor injection (methylprednisolone acetate 40 mg)[1] or at a reduced systemic dosage with an additional immunosuppressant such as ciclosporin, methotrexate, cyclophosphamide, or azathioprine.[3] Immunosuppressants may also be of value alone in severe or unresponsive disease.[4] It has been suggested that immunosuppressant therapy should be the initial choice in necrotising scleritis, as therapeutic failure is very common with less aggressive regimens.[4]

1. Hakin KN, *et al.* Use of orbital floor steroids in the management of patients with uniocular non-necrotising scleritis. *Br J Ophthalmol* 1991; **75:** 337–9.
2. Hakin KN, *et al.* Use of cyclosporin in the management of steroid-dependent non-necrotising scleritis. *Br J Ophthalmol* 1991; **75:** 340–1.
3. Jabs DA, *et al.* Guidelines for the use of immunosuppressive drugs in patients with ocular inflammatory disorders: recommendations of an expert panel. *Am J Ophthalmol* 2000; **130:** 492–513.
4. Sainz de la Maza M, *et al.* An analysis of therapeutic decision for scleritis. *Ophthalmology* 1993; **100:** 1372–6.

## Seborrhoeic dermatitis

Topical corticosteroids are used, together with an antifungal imidazole, in the management of seborrhoeic dermatitis (p.1138).

## Septic shock

The role of corticosteroids in septic shock (p.144) has been controversial. Early studies reported both beneficial[1] and detrimental[2] effects, but corticosteroids were considered ineffective[2,3] and likely to worsen secondary infection.[4-7] More recently, supplemental corticosteroids have been suggested to be beneficial in patients with established septic shock who exhibit adrenal insufficiency.[8] However, results have raised further controversy, and their routine use in septic shock is not recommended.[9]

1. Sprung CL, *et al.* The effects of high-dose corticosteroids in patients with septic shock: a prospective, controlled study. *N Engl J Med* 1984; **311:** 1137–43.
2. Bone RC, *et al.* A controlled clinical trial of high-dose methylprednisolone in the treatment of severe sepsis and septic shock. *N Engl J Med* 1987; **317:** 653–8.
3. The Veterans Administration Systemic Sepsis Cooperative Study Group. Effect of high-dose glucocorticoid therapy on mortality in patients with clinical signs of systemic sepsis. *N Engl J Med* 1987; **317:** 659–65.
4. Anonymous. No evidence that corticosteroids help in septic shock. *Drug Ther Bull* 1990; **28:** 74–5.
5. Rackow EC, Astiz ME. Pathophysiology and treatment of septic shock. *JAMA* 1991; **266:** 548–54.
6. Cohen J, Glauser MP. Septic shock: treatment. *Lancet* 1991; **338:** 736–9.
7. McGowan JE, *et al.* Report by the Working Group on Steroid Use, Antimicrobial Agents Committee, Infectious Diseases Society of America: Guidelines for the use of systemic glucocorticoids in the management of selected infections. *J Infect Dis* 1992; **165:** 1–13.
8. Cooper MS, Stewart PM. Corticosteroid insufficiency in acutely ill patients. *N Engl J Med* 2003; **348:** 727–34.
9. Bernard G. The International Sepsis Forum's controversies in sepsis: corticosteroids should not be routinely used to treat septic shock. *Crit Care* 2002; **6:** 384–6.

## Sickle-cell disease

A study[1] has suggested that a short course of high-dose methylprednisolone might be a useful adjunct in controlling pain in sickle-cell crisis (p.8). However, the use of corticosteroids in sickle-cell disease is problematic; apart from the usual adverse effects, including the risk of exacerbating underlying infection, corticosteroid therapy has been reported to provoke sickle-cell crisis in patients with sickle C disease—see under Precautions, p.1072.

1. Griffin TC, *et al.* High-dose intravenous methylprednisolone therapy for pain in children and adolescents with sickle cell disease. *N Engl J Med* 1994; **330:** 733–7.

## Skin disorders

For some guidelines to the use of topical application of corticosteroids in skin disorders, see under Administration, p.1074. For discussion of the use of corticosteroids in individual skin disorders see under the relevant headings in this section.

## Soft-tissue rheumatism

Soft-tissue rheumatism (p.11) includes a number of conditions affecting tendons, ligaments, muscles, fascia, and joint capsules; some lesions may respond to local injections of corticosteroid, often given with a local anaesthetic. In the treatment of shoulder pain, intra-articular injection of triamcinolone acetonide was considered to be superior to physiotherapy for reducing pain in the short-term.[1] Injection of corticosteroids below the point where the clavicle joins the shoulder blade may be superior to placebo for rotator cuff disease, as may intra-articular injection for adhesive capsulitis.[2] However, there is concern over accuracy of needle placement, and little overall evidence to guide treatment.[2,3] Similarly, in lateral epicondylitis (tennis elbow), local injections of triamcinolone acetonide with local anaesthetic improved short-term outcomes such as pain and disability, although long-term results favoured physiotherapy.[4] Evidence appears to support the use of corticosteroids such as betamethasone and methylprednisolone, with local anaesthetic, in trigger finger.[3] In contrast, no benefit has been demonstrated in Achilles' tendinopathy.[3] In carpal tunnel syndrome, injection of methylprednisolone with local anaesthetic proximal to the carpal tunnel resulted in long-term improvement.[5] Concerns have been expressed about the lack of trials to support the use of corticosteroids,[2,3] and some have suggested that in tendinopathies, they be reserved for chronic injuries, and that short- or moderate-acting, soluble preparations be used.[3] Tendon rupture after local corticosteroid injection may occur.[3]

See also Administration, Intra-articular Route, p.1074

1. van der Windt DAWM, *et al.* Effectiveness of corticosteroid injections versus physiotherapy for treatment of painful stiff shoulder in primary care: randomised trial. *BMJ* 1998; **317:** 1292–6.
2. Buchbinder R, *et al.* Corticosteroid injections for shoulder pain. Available in The Cochrane Library; Issue 1. Chichester: John Wiley; 2004.
3. Speed CA. Corticosteroid injections in tendon lesions. *BMJ* 2001; **323:** 382–6.
4. Smidt N, *et al.* Corticosteroid injections, physiotherapy, or a wait-and-see policy for lateral epicondylitis: a randomised controlled trial. *Lancet* 2002; **359:** 657–62.
5. Dammers JWHH, *et al.* Injection with methylprednisolone proximal to the carpal tunnel: randomised double blind trial. *BMJ* 1999; **319:** 884–6.

## Spinal cord injury

Results of a multicentre placebo-controlled study in the USA[1] indicated that high-dose intravenous corticosteroids resulted in improvements in neurological function if given within 8 hours of spinal cord injury. Methylprednisolone was given in an initial dose of 30 mg/kg followed by 5.4 mg/kg per hour for 23 hours. A subsequent study found that although this regimen was adequate if begun within 3 hours of injury, better results were obtained by continuing methylprednisolone for 48 hours in patients in whom therapy commenced 3 to 8 hours after injury.[2,3] The lazaroid tirilazad, given for 48 hours, had some benefit in this study, although it was less effective than 48 hours' treatment with methylprednisolone in the doses used. In contrast, a systematic review found that high-dose methylprednisolone did not improve neurological function in patients, and might potentially have a deleterious effect.[4]

There is little evidence that corticosteroids or tirilazad are of any value in acute traumatic brain injury.[5-7]

1. Bracken MB, *et al.* A randomized, controlled trial of methylprednisolone or naloxone in the treatment of acute spinal-cord injury: results of the Second National Acute Spinal Cord Injury Study. *N Engl J Med* 1990; **322:** 1405–11.
2. Bracken MB, *et al.* Administration of methylprednisolone for 24 or 48 hours or tirilazad mesylate for 48 hours in the treatment of acute spinal cord injury: results of the third National Acute Spinal Cord Injury Randomized Controlled Trial. *JAMA* 1997; **277:** 1597–1604.
3. Bracken MB, *et al.* Methylprednisolone or tirilazad mesylate administration after acute spinal cord injury: 1-year follow up. Results of the third National Acute Spinal Cord Injury randomized controlled trial. *J Neurosurg* 1998; **89:** 699–706.
4. Short DJ, *et al.* High dose methylprednisolone in the management of acute spinal cord injury—a systematic review from a clinical perspective. *Spinal Cord* 2000; **38:** 273–86.
5. Newell DW, *et al.* Corticosteroids in acute traumatic brain injury. *BMJ* 1998; **316:** 396.
6. Alderson P, Roberts I. Corticosteroids for acute traumatic brain injury. Available in The Cochrane Library; Issue 1. Chichester: John Wiley; 2004.
7. Roberts I. Aminosteroids for acute traumatic brain injury. Available in The Cochrane Library; Issue 1. Chichester: John Wiley; 2004.

## Spondyloarthropathies

Intra-articular injections of corticosteroids have been given in ankylosing spondylitis (see Spondyloarthropathies, p.11).

## Systemic lupus erythematosus

Systemic lupus erythematosus (SLE) is an auto-immune disease of complex aetiology characterised by autoantibodies that participate in the mediation of tissue damage affecting joints, skin, kidney, CNS, and other organs. It is far more common in women than in men, the evidence suggesting that male hormones have a protective effect, and peak onset is usually in women in their 20s and 30s.

The commonest symptom in patients with SLE is arthralgia or arthritis; fatigue, fever, weight loss, rashes (characteristically a so-called 'butterfly rash' on the cheeks and bridge of the nose), CNS involvement including personality changes, anaemia, nephritis, and pulmonary symptoms (notably pleurisy) are also frequent, while other symptoms include myalgia, alopecia, Raynaud's syndrome, convulsions, coma, stroke, pneumonitis, pericarditis, myocarditis with tachycardia, leucopenia, thrombocytopenia, coagulation disorders (both thrombosis and haemorrhage), hepatomegaly, splenomegaly, and lymphadenopathy. Thrombotic symptoms and recurrent miscarriage may represent an 'antiphospholipid antibody syndrome' due to antibodies against phospholipids, which occurs in about a third of all patients with SLE but may also occur independently.[1]

**Management**. SLE is characterised by exacerbation and remission so individualised management with careful monitoring and appropriate and timely symptomatic treatment is required. Treatment is largely empirical and there have been few controlled studies.

In addition to any specific treatment, patients require emotional support, extensive rest, and avoidance where possible of stimuli that may provoke disease exacerbation, including ultraviolet light, certain drugs or foods rich in psoralens, infections, and psychological stress.

Mild disease may require no treatment, or may be managed simply with NSAIDs for muscular and joint symptoms.[2] In more severe, but non-life-threatening disease chloroquine or, more often, hydroxychloroquine is effective, particularly for cutaneous and joint manifestations,[3,4] although disease flare may occur on withdrawal.[5] Retinoids such as acitretin have also been shown to be of use in some patients.[6]

Many patients require treatment with corticosteroids at some point, although in such patients they can be a major cause of morbidity.[3,7] It is usual to use a corticosteroid when treatment with NSAIDs or antimalarials has failed, or when life or vital organs are threatened.[2] They are usually given in high doses (1 mg/kg or more of prednisone or prednisolone daily, sometimes preceded by a course of intravenous methylprednisolone)[2] for life-threatening manifestations such as high fever, severe thrombocytopenia, coma, seizures, or involvement of a major organ such as the kidney (see also Lupus Nephritis, below). Non-life-threatening symptoms that fail to respond to other measures will usually respond to lower corticosteroid doses (not more than 500 micrograms/kg daily of prednisolone or prednisone).[2] Once a response is achieved the dose should be tapered to the lowest required to control symptoms, sometimes in the form of alternate-day dosage, although disease may relapse.[2] Complete withdrawal is optimal, although some patients may need long-term maintenance on about 5 mg daily.[2] One study found that raising the maintenance corticosteroid dose temporarily to counteract any increases in the concentration of antibodies to double-stranded DNA may reduce the number of relapses,[8] but the design and conclusions of this study are open to criticism.

Prolonged corticosteroid therapy, particularly at the higher doses, is associated with adverse effects such as aseptic bone necrosis and an increased susceptibility to infection, and other drugs have been added to corticosteroid therapy in an attempt to lower the corticosteroid dose but maintain disease control. In particular the immunosuppressant azathioprine has been used for its corticosteroid-sparing effect.[2] Oral or intravenous pulse cyclophosphamide has been used with some success to treat severe organ involvement although toxicity may be of concern.[2,3] Low-dose weekly methotrexate may also be helpful in patients with cutaneous or joint involvement.[9] The antimalarials may also be combined with corticosteroid therapy, and in addition to a corticosteroid-sparing effect there is a suggestion that hydroxychloroquine may counter the adverse effects of corticosteroids on serum-lipid profiles.[2,10] Prasterone is under investigation for the treatment of severe disease.[11] Thalidomide has been investigated for treating cutaneous manifestations of SLE.[12]

Thrombotic symptoms due to antiphospholipid antibodies require adequate long-term anticoagulation with warfarin or low-dose aspirin, and it should be borne in mind that stroke and related CNS symptoms will not respond to corticosteroids. In patients with other severe CNS symptoms that fail to respond to corticosteroids intravenous cyclophosphamide may be helpful,[13,14] but response is unpredictable. Intravenous immunoglobulin has been used as an adjunct in CNS lupus, although its role is unclear; it may also be used in the management of thrombocytopenic symptoms.[15]

In patients with severe and potentially fatal symptoms plasma exchange may provide temporary benefit by removing circulating antibodies.

**Lupus nephritis.** Renal disease is probably the best studied symptom of SLE. Almost all patients develop some renal involvement,[16] with clinical nephritis in up to 50%.[17,18] Usual manifestations of renal disease include hypertension, oedema, proteinuria or frank nephrotic syndrome, and oliguria; more severe disease is usually associated with focal or diffuse proliferative glomerulonephritis on biopsy.[17,18]

Patients with active disease (worsening renal function, proteinuria, and urinary sediment) require aggressive treatment to prevent irreversible renal damage. It is generally accepted that the use of a cytotoxic immunosuppressant with a corticosteroid is more effective than the use of corticosteroids alone in controlling nephritis and the risk of end-stage renal failure,[16,17] although corticosteroids alone may be used for less severe disease.[15]

One suggested outline for treatment in severe active disease is to begin with pulsed intravenous methylprednisolone as 3 doses of 1g daily, or prednisone or prednisolone by mouth (initially 0.5 to 1 mg/kg daily, gradually reduced) accompanied if necessary by cyclophosphamide or azathioprine.[18] An alternative approach is to begin therapy with intermittent intravenous cyclophosphamide,[19] which appears to be more effective than pulsed methylprednisolone[20,21] and then to maintain patients with low-dose oral prednisone plus pulsed intravenous cyclophosphamide. Azathioprine may be a useful alternative for patients who cannot tolerate cyclophosphamide;[17,18] it may be used as maintenance after cyclophosphamide induction in an attempt to reduce toxicity.[16,18] Ciclosporin has also been investigated, with preliminary results suggestive of benefit,[22,23] but has been viewed with caution because of its nephrotoxicity.[17,18] Mycophenolate mofetil has shown promising results;[24] abetimus is under investigation,[17] and other drugs that have been reported to be of benefit include intravenous immunoglobulins,[17] cladribine, and fludarabine.[16] Autologous haematopoietic stem-cell transplantation (p.1344) is considered feasible in SLE.[17,25]

**Pregnancy.** Although symptoms of SLE do not appear to be exacerbated in most patients during pregnancy,[26,27] it is considered advisable that pregnancy be deferred until the disease is in remission or controlled by therapy, since complications are more likely in active disease.[12,26] Cyclophosphamide or methotrexate are contra-indicated in pregnancy because of the risk of teratogenesis but corticosteroids, azathioprine, and hydroxychloroquine may be used if necessary:[2-4,28] the risks of miscarriage, still-birth, growth retardation, or preterm delivery due to the disease are considered greater than the risks to the fetus of continued therapy. The use of low-dose aspirin (75 mg daily) has been recommended in women with renal involvement or a history of pre-eclampsia or fetal growth retardation;[28] in women with antiphospholipid antibodies, low-dose aspirin together with subcutaneous heparin or low-molecular-weight heparin markedly improves the live birth rate.[1,12,29] The use of high-dose prednisone, with or without aspirin, to suppress antiphospholipid antibodies, while reportedly effective in some women with bad obstetric histories,[30,31] has been found by others to be of no benefit,[32] and is associated with unacceptable maternal morbidity.[33] Warfarin prophylaxis, which appears effective in other patients with the antiphospholipid antibody syndrome,[34] is unsuited to pregnant women because of the teratogenic effects of warfarin.[35]

Postpartum exacerbation is well recognised,[26,28] and some workers favour prophylactic corticosteroid cover during the puerperium. A small proportion of neonates born to mothers with lupus exhibit a neonatal lupus syndrome,[36] manifesting most seriously as heart block which may require a permanent pacemaker.


1. Levine JS, *et al.* The antiphospholipid syndrome. *N Engl J Med* 2002; **346:** 752–63.
2. Anonymous. Systemic lupus erythematosus. *Drug Ther Bull* 1996; **34:** 20–3.
3. Lian T-Y, Gordon C. Systemic lupus erythematosus, antiphospholipid antibody syndrome, and other lupus-like syndromes. In: Snaith ML, ed. *ABC of rheumatology.* 3rd ed. London: BMJ Publishing Group, 2004: 80–6.
4. Borden MB, Parke AL. Antimalarial drugs in systemic lupus erythematosus: use in pregnancy. *Drug Safety* 2001; **24:** 1055–63.
5. The Canadian Hydroxychloroquine Study Group. A randomized study of the effect of withdrawing hydroxychloroquine sulfate in systemic lupus erythematosus. *N Engl J Med* 1991; **324:** 150–4.
6. Ruzicka T, *et al.* Treatment of cutaneous lupus erythematosus with acitretin and hydroxychloroquine. *Br J Dermatol* 1992; **127:** 513–18.
7. Mills JA. Systemic lupus erythematosus. *N Engl J Med* 1994; **330:** 1871–9.
8. Bootsma H, *et al.* Prevention of relapses in systemic lupus erythematosus. *Lancet* 1995; **345:** 1595–9. Correction. *ibid.*; **346:** 516.
9. Sato EI. Methotrexate therapy in systemic lupus erythematosus. *Lupus* 2001; **10:** 162–4.
10. Hodis HN, *et al.* The lipid, lipoprotein, and apolipoprotein effects of hydroxychloroquine in patients with systemic lupus erythematosus. *J Rheumatol* 1993; **20:** 661–5.
11. van Vollenhoven RF. Dehydroepiandrosterone in systemic lupus erythematosus. *Rheum Dis Clin North Am* 2000; **26:** 349–62.
12. Ruiz-Irastorza G, *et al.* Systemic lupus erythematosus. *Lancet* 2001; **357:** 1027–32.
13. Fricchione GL, *et al.* Electroconvulsive therapy and cyclophosphamide in combination for severe neuropsychiatric lupus with catatonia. *Am J Med* 1990; **88:** 442–3.
14. Neuwelt CM, *et al.* Role of intravenous cyclophosphamide in the treatment of severe neuropsychiatric systemic lupus erythematosus. *Am J Med* 1995; **98:** 32–41.
15. Boumpas DT, *et al.* Systemic lupus erythematosus: emerging concepts. Part 1. *Ann Intern Med* 1995; **122:** 940–50.
16. Hejaili FF, *et al.* Treatment of lupus nephritis. *Drugs* 2003; **63:** 257–74.
17. Kuiper-Geertsma DG, Derksen RHWM. Newer drugs for the treatment of lupus nephritis. *Drugs* 2003; **63:** 167–80.
18. Anonymous. Treat lupus nephritis according to disease presentation. *Drugs Ther Perspect* 1999; **14:** 6–9.
19. Austin HA, *et al.* Therapy of lupus nephritis: controlled trial of prednisone and cytotoxic drugs. *N Engl J Med* 1986; **314:** 614–19.
20. Boumpas DT, *et al.* Controlled trial of pulse methylprednisolone versus two regimens of pulse cyclophosphamide in severe lupus nephritis. *Lancet* 1992; **340:** 741–5.
21. Gourley MF, *et al.* Methylprednisolone and cyclophosphamide, alone or in combination, in patients with lupus nephritis: a randomized, controlled trial. *Ann Intern Med* 1996; **125:** 549–57.
22. Fu LW, *et al.* Clinical efficacy of cyclosporin A Neoral in the treatment of paediatric lupus nephritis with heavy proteinuria. *Br J Rheumatol* 1998; **37:** 217–21.
23. Tam LS, *et al.* Long-term treatment of lupus nephritis with cyclosporin A. *Q J Med* 1998; **91:** 573–80.
24. Chan TM, *et al.* Efficacy of mycophenolate mofetil in patients with diffuse proliferative lupus nephritis. *N Engl J Med* 2000; **343:** 1156–62.
25. Traynor AE, *et al.* Treatment of severe systemic lupus erythematosus with high-dose chemotherapy and haemopoietic stem-cell transplantation: a phase I study. *Lancet* 2000; **356:** 701–7.
26. Anonymous. Systemic lupus erythematosus in pregnancy. *Lancet* 1991; **338:** 87–8.
27. Yell JA, Burge SM. The effect of hormonal changes on cutaneous disease in lupus erythematosus. *Br J Dermatol* 1993; **129:** 18–22.
28. Hunt BJ, Lakasing L. Management of pre-existing disorders in pregnancy: connective-tissue disorders. *Prescribers' J* 1997; **37:** 54–60.
29. Rai R, *et al.* Randomised controlled trial of aspirin and aspirin plus heparin in pregnant women with recurrent miscarriage associated with phospholipid antibodies (or antiphospholipid antibodies). *BMJ* 1997; **314:** 253–7.
30. Lubbe WF, *et al.* Fetal survival after prednisone suppression of maternal lupus-anticoagulant. *Lancet* 1983; **i:** 1361–3.
31. Branch DW, *et al.* Obstetric complications associated with the lupus anticoagulant. *N Engl J Med* 1985; **313:** 1322–6.
32. Laskin CA, *et al.* Prednisone and aspirin in women with autoantibodies and unexplained recurrent fetal loss. *N Engl J Med* 1997; **337:** 148–53.
33. Greaves M. Antiphospholipid antibodies and thrombosis. *Lancet* 1999; **353:** 1348–53.
34. Khamashta MA, *et al.* The management of thrombosis in the antiphospholipid-antibody syndrome. *N Engl J Med* 1995; **332:** 993–7.
35. Lockshin MD. Answers to the antiphospholipid-antibody syndrome? *N Engl J Med* 1995; **332:** 1025–7.
36. Anonymous. Neonatal lupus syndrome. *Lancet* 1987; **ii:** 489–90.


## Takayasu's arteritis

Takayasu's arteritis is a vasculitis of the aorta and its branches seen particularly in young women and in Oriental patients. It is characterised by vasculitis followed by fibrosis, leading to stenosis or occlusion of the vessel. Symptoms vary depending on the anatomical site, but include constitutional symptoms such as fever, malaise, and arthralgia, syncope, dyspnoea, palpitations, loss of pulses, intermittent claudication, and visual disturbances.

Active inflammatory disease may respond to corticosteroids: doses of 1 mg/kg daily of prednisone or prednisolone, tapered after one month in patients who respond, have been suggested.[1,2] In patients who do not respond, azathioprine, cyclophosphamide, or methotrexate have been added, although opinions vary as to the necessity of cytotoxic agents in these patients.[1-3] Ciclosporin[4] and mycophenolate mofetil[5] have also been used. Widely varying estimates of mortality and aggressiveness exist for Takayasu's arteritis, and in the absence of large controlled studies it is difficult to assess the benefits of drug therapy. The course may be very prolonged, and minimising the maintenance dosage (e.g. by alternate-day corticosteroid therapy) is important to avoid adverse effects.[6]

Surgical reconstruction of affected vessels has been carried out in patients at risk of ischaemic compromise.[7] Angioplasty has been tried.


1. Shelhamer JH, *et al.* Takayasu's arteritis and its therapy. *Ann Intern Med* 1985; **103:** 121–6.
2. Sabbadini MG, *et al.* Takayasu's arteritis: therapeutic strategies. *J Nephrol* 2001; **14:** 525–31.
3. Hall S, Hunder GG. Treatment of Takayasu's arteritis. *Ann Intern Med* 1986; **104:** 288.
4. Horigome H, *et al.* Treatment of glucocorticoid-dependent Takayasu's arteritis with cyclosporin. *Med J Aust* 1999; **170:** 566.
5. Daina E, *et al.* Mycophenolate mofetil for the treatment of Takayasu arteritis: report of three cases. *Ann Intern Med* 1999; **130:** 422–6.
6. Taylor HG, Samanta A. Treatment of vasculitis. *Br J Clin Pharmacol* 1993; **35:** 93–104.
7. Kerr GS, *et al.* Takayasu arteritis. *Ann Intern Med* 1994; **120:** 919–29.


## Tuberculosis

The use of corticosteroids in tuberculosis (p.150) is controversial.[1-3] They should never be given to patients with active disease without protective chemotherapy cover, and must be used with caution in patients with dormant disease as it may be reactivated. Use of corticosteroids in pulmonary tuberculosis is to be avoided except in life-threatening disease. WHO suggests that corticosteroids may be useful adjuvants to antituberculous therapy in selected conditions including tuberculous meningitis, pericarditis, pleural effusion, or laryngitis, or tuberculosis of the renal tract, adrenocortical insufficiency due to adrenal gland tuberculosis, massive lymph node enlargement, or to control drug hypersensitivity. They are also likely to be of benefit in patients with HIV infection and the above conditions.[4] Similar recommendations are made by the British Thoracic Society.[5] However, systematic reviews of tuberculous pleurisy,[6] pericarditis,[7] and meningitis[8] have concluded that there is insufficient evidence to support the use of corticosteroids in these conditions.


1. Horne NW, ed. *Modern drug treatment of tuberculosis.* 7th ed. London: The Chest, Heart and Stroke Association, 1990.
2. McGowan JE, *et al.* Report by the Working Group on Steroid Use, Antimicrobial Agents Committee, Infectious Diseases Society of America: Guidelines for the use of systemic glucocorticoids in the management of selected infections. *J Infect Dis* 1992; **165:** 1–13.
3. Alzeer AH, FitzGerald JM. Corticosteroids and tuberculosis: risks and use as adjunct therapy. *Tubercle Lung Dis* 1993; **74:** 6–11.
4. WHO. *TB/HIV: a clinical manual.* Geneva: WHO, 1996.
5. Joint Tuberculosis Committee of the British Thoracic Society. Chemotherapy and management of tuberculosis in the United Kingdom: recommendations 1998. *Thorax* 1998; **53:** 536–48. Also available at: http://www.brit-thoracic.org.uk/docs/Chemotherapy.pdf (accessed 27/04/04)
6. Matchaba PT, Volmink J. Steroids for treating tuberculous pleurisy. Available in The Cochrane Library; Issue 1. Chichester: John Wiley; 2004.
7. Mayosi BM, *et al.* Interventions for treating tuberculous pericarditis. Available in The Cochrane Library; Issue 1. Chichester: John Wiley; 2004.
8. Prasad K, *et al.* Steroids for treating tuberculous meningitis. Available in The Cochrane Library; Issue 1. Chichester: John Wiley; 2004.

### Urticaria and angioedema

Oral antihistamines are the mainstay of treatment for urticaria (p.1138). Severe attacks refractory to standard therapy may require a short course of oral corticosteroid therapy.

When angioedema affecting the larynx (laryngeal oedema) is present, the patients should be treated with adrenaline as an allergic emergency (see Anaphylactic Shock, p.855).

### Uveitis

Uveitis is inflammation of the uveal tract of the eye, which comprises the choroid, ciliary body, and the iris. It is usually idiopathic but may be secondary to infection, allergy, or inflammatory disorders with an auto-immune component.

In anterior uveitis, also referred to as iridocyclitis, there is inflammation of the iris (iritis) and the ciliary body (cyclitis). It tends to be acute and self-limiting and is likely to be associated with infection. The iris becomes spongy and hyperaemic and exudates may result in adhesions between the iris and the lens (posterior synechiae). Chronic anterior uveitis is associated with formation of cataracts and glaucoma. Posterior uveitis can be acute or chronic and may just affect the choroid (choroiditis) or may also involve the retina (chorioretinitis). It is more likely to be an auto-immune condition.

The treatment of uveitis has been reviewed.[1-3]

Corticosteroids given topically and, when necessary, systemically are the mainstay of treatment for acute anterior uveitis.[4] Cycloplegics and mydriatics such as atropine, cyclopentolate, and homatropine are used adjunctively to rest the ciliary body and iris, diminish hyperaemia, and to prevent the formation of posterior synechiae. Antibacterials should be used to treat any infection. In children with chronic anterior uveitis associated with juvenile idiopathic arthritis, corticosteroids are supplemented with chronic use of an oral NSAID if inflammation persists after 90 days of treatment and attempted corticosteroid withdrawal.[5] In the 30% or so of cases that do not respond to corticosteroids and NSAIDs, low-dose weekly methotrexate (with folic acid supplements daily) is advocated, with other immunosuppressants being substituted or used adjunctively when methotrexate fails or is not tolerated.

Treatment of posterior uveitis is less satisfactory than that of acute anterior uveitis since gross damage to the retina often occurs before the condition can be controlled. Corticosteroids are usually required given either as periocular injections or as high-dose systemic therapy.[4] A suggested protocol[2] involves the use of high-dose systemic corticosteroids to control active disease; long-term control is then maintained primarily with low-dose ciclosporin, corticosteroids being tapered to a low dose or eventually withdrawn. Certain patients may require an additional immunosuppressant, usually azathioprine, although methotrexate, cyclophosphamide, or chlorambucil may be considered. Other immunosuppressants being studied include tacrolimus, and there are reports of improvement with mycophenolate mofetil.[4]

Visual impairment in chronic uveitis is often the result of macular oedema and is not necessarily prevented by immunosuppressants. Short-term treatment with acetazolamide is considered to have produced some encouraging results in reducing chronic uveitic macular oedema but its long-term efficacy or efficacy with low-dose corticosteroids remains to be determined.[6] Although systemic and topical NSAIDs have been shown to reduce cystoid macular oedema in post cataract extraction (see Postoperative Inflammatory Ocular Disorders, p.70) their role in the treatment of macular oedema associated with uveitis is less clear.


1. Anglade E, Whitcup SM. The diagnosis and management of uveitis. *Drugs* 1995; **49:** 213–23.
2. Dick AD, *et al.* Immunosuppressive therapy for chronic uveitis: optimising therapy with steroids and cyclosporin A. *Br J Ophthalmol* 1997; **81:** 1107–12.
3. McCluskey PJ, *et al.* Management of chronic uveitis. *BMJ* 2000; **320:** 555–8.
4. Jabs DA, *et al.* Guidelines for the use of immunosuppressive drugs in patients with ocular inflammatory disorders: recommendations of an expert panel. *Am J Ophthalmol* 2000; **130:** 492–513.
5. Nguyen QD, Foster S. Saving the vision of children with juvenile rheumatoid arthritis-associated uveitis. *JAMA* 1998; **280:** 1133–4.
6. Dick AD. The treatment of chronic uveitic macular oedema: is immunosuppression enough? *Br J Ophthalmol* 1994; **78:** 1–2.


### Vasculitic syndromes

Vasculitis may be defined as inflammation of the blood vessel wall, and the term has been applied in describing a wide range of diseases involving blood vessels of various sizes and types. Vasculitis may occur as part of a systemic disease such as rheumatoid arthritis or systemic lupus erythematosus, or may itself be the primary disorder, and symptoms may vary from superficial cutaneous disease, with purpura and urticaria, to progressive and fatal systemic vasculitides such as Wegener's granulomatosis. In some forms of vasculitis, such as giant cell arteritis, mononuclear giant cells may be seen, while in granulomatous vasculitis the mononuclear cells form granulomata adjacent to the damaged vessel wall. Necrotising vasculitis is used to describe inflammation associated with necrosis of the media, the middle part of the vessel wall, while polyarteritis implies inflammation of the full thickness of an arterial wall.

Because of the heterogeneous nature of this group of diseases and the degree of overlap which exists between some of them, and between them and other diseases, classification has been difficult. Classification has often been based on the size of the affected vessel, as well as the presence or absence of granulomata and antineutrophil cytoplasmic antibodies (ANCA), and whether the vasculitis is primary or secondary. Of the major primary vasculitic syndromes, giant cell arteritis (p.1080) and Takayasu's arteritis (p.1089) are examples of large vessel disease; classic polyarteritis nodosa (p.1085) affects medium-sized vessels; Churg-Strauss syndrome (p.1078), microscopic polyangiitis (p.1085), and Wegener's granulomatosis (below) are diseases of small or medium-sized vessels; the so-called 'hypersensitivity vasculitides', including Henoch-Schönlein purpura, are small vessel diseases (p.1081), though usually limited in extent.

Treatment depends on the type of vasculitis, its severity, and prognosis. Treatment of the systemic vasculitides has revolved around corticosteroids and cyclophosphamide; other cytotoxic immunosuppressants, normal immunoglobulins, NSAIDs, anticoagulants, dapsone, and colchicine have been tried in various forms of disease.

### Vitiligo

Topical corticosteroids are sometimes effective in inducing repigmentation in patients with vitiligo (p.1137 under Pigmentation Disorders).

### Wegener's granulomatosis

Wegener's granulomatosis is a form of granulomatous vasculitis that occurs more frequently in men and in white patients. It is characterised by necrotising vasculitis of small arteries and veins, accompanied by granuloma formation, and affecting particularly the respiratory tract and kidneys. It is usually associated with antineutrophil cytoplasmic antibodies (ANCA). Symptoms include rhinorrhoea, sinusitis, cough and dyspnoea (signs of pulmonary infiltration which is seen in the majority of patients at presentation); renal manifestations include haematuria, proteinuria, uraemia, and oedema of the lower limbs due to a focal glomerulonephritis which can progress to crescentic glomerulonephritis and rapidly progressive renal failure. Other organ systems may be involved, with effects similar to those of microscopic polyangiitis (see p.1085). If untreated, the disease is fatal.

Treatment is with a combination regimen based on cyclophosphamide with a corticosteroid. A standard regimen has been low-dose (1 to 2 mg/kg daily) oral cyclophosphamide, together with prednisolone or prednisone 1 mg/kg daily by mouth initially, subsequently tapered to an alternate-day regimen and eventually discontinued.[1-3] Cyclophosphamide is usually continued for at least a year before considering gradual discontinuation but there is a trend in Europe towards the use of shorter courses of cyclophosphamide.[4] Standard treatment regimens produce improvement or remissions in about 90% of patients.[1,5] Relapses may subsequently occur in about half, and require re-treatment; prompt intensification of treatment when serum ANCA concentrations begin to rise may avert relapse.[6] There is evidence from one controlled study that addition of co-trimoxazole to maintenance regimens reduces the incidence of relapse,[7] although another suggested that it might actually increase the risk of relapse.[8]

Despite the success of regimens based on low-dose oral cyclophosphamide there is considerable concern about their toxicity, particularly since prolonged use may be necessary. Intermittent high-dose intravenous ('pulse') cyclophosphamide has been suggested as an alternative to the oral regimen with fewer adverse effects,[9] but results in practice seem to have been variable.[10,11] Regimens similar to the standard regimen, but substituting azathioprine for cyclophosphamide once remission is achieved (usually after 3 to 6 months) and continuing with low-dose corticosteroids concomitantly have been used.[12] Other drugs, such as methotrexate, have been tried and addition of low-dose weekly methotrexate to a corticosteroid may be a possible treatment option.[8,13-15] Ciclosporin has been reported to reverse acute renal failure in 2 patients with Wegener's granulomatosis, as well as controlling fulminant symptoms unresponsive to cyclophosphamide and corticosteroids in one of them,[16] but others have found ciclosporin plus a corticosteroid to be ineffective in suppressing disease activity.[17] Etoposide[18] and infliximab[19] have also been successfully used to induce remission in cyclophosphamide-resistant disease. Other drugs that have been investigated include high-dose intravenous immunoglobulin,[20] and mycophenolate mofetil,[21] while anti-CD4 monoclonal antibodies have proved useful in patients with microscopic polyangiitis, which has some similarities to Wegener's granulomatosis, but the role of such investigational regimens remains to be determined.


1. Fauci AS, *et al.* Wegener's granulomatosis: prospective clinical and therapeutic experience with 85 patients for 21 years. *Ann Intern Med* 1983; **98:** 76–85.
2. Hoffman GS, *et al.* Wegener granulomatosis: an analysis of 158 patients. *Ann Intern Med* 1992; **116:** 488–98.
3. Langford CA, Hoffman GS. Wegener's granulomatosis. *Thorax* 1999; **54:** 629–37.
4. Savage COS, *et al.* Primary systemic vasculitis. *Lancet* 1997; **349:** 553–8.
5. Rottem M, *et al.* Wegener granulomatosis in children and adolescents: clinical presentation and outcome. *J Pediatr* 1993 **122:** 26–31.
6. Tervaert JWC, *et al.* Prevention of relapses in Wegener's granulomatosis by treatment based on antineutrophil cytoplasmic antibody titre. *Lancet* 1990; **336:** 709–11.
7. Stegeman CA, *et al.* Trimethoprim-sulfamethoxazole (co-trimoxazole) for the prevention of relapses of Wegener's granulomatosis. *N Engl J Med* 1996; **335:** 16–20.
8. de Groot K, *et al.* Therapy for the maintenance of remission in sixty-five patients with generalized Wegener's granulomatosis: methotrexate versus trimethoprim/sulfamethoxazole. *Arthritis Rheum* 1996; **39:** 2052–61.
9. Cupps TR. Cyclophosphamide: to pulse or not to pulse? *Am J Med* 1990; **89:** 399–402.
10. Hoffman GS, *et al.* Treatment of Wegener's granulomatosis with intermittent high-dose intravenous cyclophosphamide. *Am J Med* 1990; **89:** 403–10.
11. Reinhold-Keller E, *et al.* Influence of disease manifestation and antineutrophil cytoplasmic antibody titre on the response to pulse cyclophosphamide therapy in patients with Wegener's granulomatosis. *Arthritis Rheum* 1994; **37:** 919–24.
12. Jayne D, *et al.* A randomized trial of maintenance therapy for vasculitis associated with antineutrophil cytoplasmic autoantibodies. *N Engl J Med* 2003; **349:** 36–44.
13. Sneller MC. Wegener's granulomatosis. *JAMA* 1995; **273:** 1288–91.
14. Gottlieb BS, *et al.* Methotrexate treatment of Wegener granulomatosis in children. *J Pediatr* 1996; **129:** 604–7.
15. Langford CA, *et al.* Use of a cyclophosphamide-induction methotrexate-maintenance regimen for the treatment of Wegener's granulomatosis: extended follow-up and rate of relapse. *Am J Med* 2003; **114:** 463–9.
16. Gremmel F, *et al.* Cyclosporin in Wegener granulomatosis. *Ann Intern Med* 1988; **108:** 491.
17. Inoue K-I, *et al.* Successful treatment with combination therapy of cyclophosphamide and cyclosporin for late recurrence of Wegener granulomatosis. *Arch Intern Med* 2000; **160:** 393–4.
18. D'Cruz D, *et al.* Response of cyclophosphamide-resistant Wegener's granulomatosis to etoposide. *Lancet* 1992; **340:** 425–6.
19. Lamprecht P, *et al.* Effectiveness of TNF-α blockade with infliximab in refractory Wegener's granulomatosis. *Rheumatology (Oxford)* 2002; **41:** 1303–7.
20. Jayne DRW, *et al.* Treatment of systemic vasculitis with pooled intravenous immunoglobulin. *Lancet* 1991; **337:** 1137–9.
21. Nowack R, *et al.* Mycophenolate mofetil for systemic vasculitis and IgA nephropathy. *Lancet* 1997; **349:** 774.


## Alclometasone Dipropionate *(BANM, USAN, rINNM)*

Dipropionato de alclometasona; Sch-22219. 7α-Chloro-11β,17α,21-trihydroxy-16α-methylpregna-1,4-diene-3,20-dione 17,21-dipropionate.

$C_{28}H_{37}ClO_7$ = 521.0.

*CAS — 67452-97-5 (alclometasone); 66734-13-2 (alclometasone dipropionate).*

*ATC — D07AB10; S01BA10.*

**Pharmacopoeias.** In *US.*

**USP 27** (Alclometasone Dipropionate). Store in airtight containers.

### Profile

Alclometasone dipropionate is a corticosteroid used topically for its glucocorticoid activity (p.1068) in the treatment of various skin disorders. It is usually employed as a cream or ointment containing 0.05%.

When applied topically, particularly to large areas, when the skin is broken, or under occlusive dressings, corticosteroids may be absorbed in sufficient amounts to cause systemic effects (p.1068). The effects of topical corticosteroids on the skin are described on p.1070. For recommendations concerning the correct use of corticosteroids on the skin, and a rough guide to the clinical potencies of topical corticosteroids, see p.1074.

### Preparations

**USP 27:** Alclometasone Dipropionate Cream; Alclometasone Dipropionate Ointment.

**Proprietary Preparations** (details are given in Part 3)

***Austral.:*** Logoderm; ***Chile:*** Logoderm; ***Denm.:*** Legederm; ***Fin.:*** Legederm; ***Fr.:*** Aclosone†; ***Ger.:*** Delonal; ***Gr.:*** Lomesone; ***Hong Kong:*** Perderm; ***Irl.:*** Modrasone; ***Ital.:*** Legederm; ***Malaysia:*** Perderm; ***Mex.:*** Logoderm; ***Neth.:*** Aclosone; ***NZ:*** Logoderm; ***Port.:*** Miloderme; ***S.Afr.:*** Aclosone†; ***Singapore:*** Perderm; ***Swed.:*** Legederm; ***Switz.:*** Delonal; ***UK:*** Modrasone; ***USA:*** Aclovate.

## Aldosterone *(BAN, rINN)*

Aldosterona; Electrocortin. 11β,18-Epoxy-18,21-dihydroxypregn-4-ene-3,20-dione.

$C_{21}H_{28}O_5$ = 360.4.

*CAS — 52-39-1.*

*ATC — H02AA01.*

### Adverse Effects

Aldosterone has very pronounced mineralocorticoid actions and little effect on carbohydrate metabolism. It may therefore exhibit the mineralocorticoid adverse effects described for the corticosteroids in general (p.1068).

### Uses and Administration

Aldosterone is the main mineralocorticoid (p.1068) secreted by the adrenal cortex. It has no significant glucocorticoid (anti-inflammatory) properties.

Aldosterone has been given by intramuscular or intravenous injection, in association with a glucocorticoid, in the treatment of primary adrenocortical insufficiency (p.1075) but synthetic mineralocorticoids such as fludrocortisone (p.1100), which can be given by mouth, are usually preferred. It has also been used as the sodium succinate.

### Preparations

**Proprietary Preparations** (details are given in Part 3)

**Multi-ingredient:** ***Ital.:*** Sinsurrene†.

## Amcinonide *(BAN, USAN, rINN)*

Amcinónida; Amcinopol; CL-34699. 16α,17α-Cyclopentylidenedioxy-9α-fluoro-11β,21-dihydroxypregna-1,4-diene-3,20-dione 21-acetate.

$C_{28}H_{35}FO_7$ = 502.6.

*CAS — 51022-69-6.*

*ATC — D07AC11.*

**Pharmacopoeias.** In *US.*

### Profile

Amcinonide is a corticosteroid used topically for its glucocorticoid activity (p.1068) in the treatment of various skin disorders. It is usually used as a cream, lotion, or ointment containing 0.1%.

When applied topically, particularly to large areas, when the skin is broken, or under occlusive dressings, corticosteroids may be absorbed in sufficient amounts to cause systemic effects (p.1068). The effects of topical corticosteroids on the skin are described on p.1070. For recommendations concerning the correct use of corticosteroids on the skin, and a rough guide to the clinical potencies of topical corticosteroids, see p.1074.

### Preparations

**USP 27:** Amcinonide Cream; Amcinonide Ointment.

**Proprietary Preparations** (details are given in Part 3)

***Belg.:*** Amicla; ***Canad.:*** Cyclocort; ***Fr.:*** Penticort; ***Ger.:*** Amciderm; ***Ital.:*** Amcinil†; ***Mex.:*** Visderm; ***Thai.:*** Amciderm; Visderm; ***USA:*** Cyclocort.

**Multi-ingredient:** ***Fr.:*** Penticort Neomycine†.

# Beclometasone Dipropionate

*(BANM, rINNM)*

Beclometasoni Dipropionas; Beclomethasone Dipropionate *(USAN)*; 9α-Chloro-16β-methylprednisolone Dipropionate; Dipropionato de beclometasona; Sch-18020W. 9α-Chloro-11β,17α,21-trihydroxy-16β-methylpregna-1,4-diene-3,20-dione 17,21-dipropionate.

$C_{28}H_{37}ClO_7$ = 521.0.

*CAS — 4419-39-0 (beclometasone); 5534-09-8 (beclometasone dipropionate).*

*ATC — A07EA07; D07AC15; R01AD01; R03BA01.*

**Pharmacopoeias.** In *Chin., Eur.* (see p.vi), *Int.*, and *Jpn.*

*US* allows either the anhydrous or monohydrate form. *Br.* includes a separate monograph for the monohydrate.

**Ph. Eur. 5.0** (Beclometasone Dipropionate). A white or almost white, crystalline powder. Practically insoluble in water; sparingly soluble in alcohol; freely soluble in acetone. Protect from light.

**BP 2003** (Beclometasone Dipropionate Monohydrate). A white or almost white, crystalline powder. It exhibits polymorphism. Practically insoluble in water; sparingly soluble in alcohol; freely soluble in acetone and in chloroform. Protect from light.

**USP 27** (Beclomethasone Dipropionate). It is anhydrous or contains one molecule of water of hydration. A white to cream white, odourless powder. Very slightly soluble in water; freely soluble in alcohol and in acetone; very soluble in chloroform.

## Adverse Effects, Treatment, Withdrawal, and Precautions

As for corticosteroids in general (p.1068).

Adrenal suppression may occur in some patients treated with high-dose long-term inhalation therapy for asthma. It has been stated that in the majority of patients no significant suppression is likely to occur when total daily doses of less than 1.5 mg are used (but see Adrenal Suppression, below).

When applied topically, particularly to large areas, when the skin is broken, or under occlusive dressings, corticosteroids may be absorbed in sufficient amounts to cause systemic effects. Systemic absorption may also follow nasal administration, particularly if high doses are used or treatment is prolonged.

**Adrenal suppression.** The problem of adrenal suppression with corticosteroids is discussed on p.1069. Listed below are some references and correspondence concerning adrenal suppression due to beclometasone inhalation therapy,[1-8] in some cases occurring with doses below 1.5 mg daily.[6] However, one study found that function of the hypothalamic-pituitary-adrenal axis remained normal in most patients at beclometasone doses below 3 mg daily.[9]


1. Grant IWB, Crompton GK. Becloforte inhaler. *BMJ* 1983; **286:** 644–5.
2. Slessor IM. Becloforte inhaler. *BMJ* 1983; **286:** 645.
3. Ebden P, Davies BH. High-dose corticosteroid inhalers for asthma. *Lancet* 1984; **ii:** 576.
4. Law CM, *et al.* Nocturnal adrenal suppression in asthmatic children taking inhaled beclomethasone dipropionate. *Lancet* 1986; **i:** 942–4.
5. Brown HM. Nocturnal adrenal suppression in children inhaling beclomethasone dipropionate. *Lancet* 1986; **i:** 1269.
6. Maxwell DL, Webb J. Adverse effects of inhaled corticosteroids. *BMJ* 1989; **298:** 827–8.
7. Priftis K, *et al.* Adrenal function in asthma. *Arch Dis Child* 1990; **65:** 838–40.
8. Tabachnik E, Zadik Z. Diurnal cortisol secretion during therapy with inhaled beclomethasone dipropionate in children with asthma. *J Pediatr* 1991; **118:** 294–7.
9. Brown PH, *et al.* Large volume spacer devices and the influence of high dose beclomethasone dipropionate on hypothalamo-pituitary-adrenal axis function. *Thorax* 1993; **48:** 233–8.


**Candidiasis.** Results of a study involving 229 asthmatic children indicated that the presence of a sore throat or a hoarse voice was not related to the presence of *Candida* or to treatment with inhaled beclometasone.[1] The occurrence of only one clinical case of oral candidiasis in 129 of the children receiving beclometasone confirmed previous observations that it is an uncommon finding in children compared with the reported incidence of between 4.5 and 13% in adults. The incidence of colonisation with *Candida* was greater in those children who received corticosteroids than in those who did not but was not affected by either the dose or type of inhaler used.


1. Shaw NJ, Edmunds AT. Inhaled beclomethasone and oral candidiasis. *Arch Dis Child* 1986; **61:** 788–90.


**Effects on the bones.** The adverse effects of corticosteroids in general on bones are discussed on p.1069.

Studies in healthy subjects have shown that inhaled beclometasone dipropionate can suppress bone metabolism.[1-3] These studies measured biochemical markers such as serum-osteocalcin concentrations, serum alkaline phosphatase activity, and urinary hydroxyproline-creatinine ratio, over short periods of time. Another study found that markers of collagen turnover, but not osteocalcin, were reduced by beclometasone or budesonide 800 micrograms daily in mildly asthmatic children.[4] Results are difficult to interpret since osteocalcin concentrations are reduced in patients with asthma regardless of treatment,[5] and it is uncertain whether significant bone loss does occur in practice. One 12-month study[6] in adults with asthma found that biochemical markers showed suppressed bone formation from inhaled beclometasone, and that there was some loss of bone mineral density from the hip. This study also found that fluticasone, in equivalent therapeutic doses, may have less adverse effect on bone. Another, smaller, study[7] found no adverse effects from beclometasone or fluticasone on bone mass or metabolism. In a study[8] of asthmatic children, comparing those treated with inhaled budesonide with those who received no corticosteroids, an average daily dose of about 500 micrograms budesonide for 3 to 6 years did not adversely affect bone density and mineral measures.


1. Pouw EM, *et al.* Beclomethasone inhalation decreases serum osteocalcin concentrations. *BMJ* 1991; **302:** 627–8.
2. Ali N, *et al.* Beclomethasone and osteocalcin. *BMJ* 1991; **302:** 1080.
3. Teelucksingh S, *et al.* Inhaled corticosteroids, bone formation and osteocalcin. *Lancet* 1991; **338:** 60–1.
4. Birkebæk NH, *et al.* Bone and collagen turnover during treatment with inhaled dry powder budesonide and beclomethasone dipropionate. *Arch Dis Child* 1995; **73:** 524–7.
5. König P, *et al.* Bone metabolism in children with asthma treated with inhaled beclomethasone dipropionate. *J Pediatr* 1993; **122:** 219–26.
6. Pauwels RA, *et al.* Safety and efficacy of fluticasone and beclomethasone in moderate to severe asthma. *Am J Respir Crit Care Med* 1998; **157:** 827–32.
7. Medici TC, *et al.* Effect of one year treatment with inhaled fluticasone propionate or beclomethasone dipropionate on bone density and bone metabolism: a randomised parallel group study in adult asthmatic subjects. *Thorax* 2000; **55:** 375–82.
8. Agertoft L, Pedersen S. Bone mineral density in children with asthma receiving long-term treatment with inhaled budesonide. *Am J Respir Crit Care Med* 1998; **157:** 178–83.


**Effects on growth.** Meta-analysis of 3 eligible studies (out of 92 examined) concluded that inhaled beclometasone therapy at a dose of 400 micrograms daily may cause a 1.54 cm/year decrease in growth in children with mild to moderate asthma.[1] The long-term effects of treatment are unknown, and therefore it is not clear whether catch-up growth will occur upon cessation of therapy. The lowest possible dose of corticosteroid therapy should be used in asthma, and growth should be monitored.[1] There is also evidence[2] that long-term intranasal beclometasone for the treatment of allergic rhinitis can slow growth in children; the effect on final height is unknown. For further details of the effects of corticosteroids on growth, see p.1070.


1. Sharek PJ, *et al.* Beclomethasone for asthma in children: effects on linear growth. Available in The Cochrane Library; Issue 1. Chichester: John Wiley; 2004.
2. Skoner DP, *et al.* Detection of growth suppression in children during treatment with intranasal beclomethasone dipropionate. Abstract: *Pediatrics* 2000; **105:** 415–16. Full version: http://pediatrics.aappublications.org/cgi/content/full/105/2/e23 (accessed 27/04/04)


**Effects on the lungs.** Pulmonary eosinophilia has occurred in patients treated with inhaled beclometasone.[1-4]


1. Paterson IC, *et al.* Pulmonary eosinophilia after substitution of aerosol for oral corticosteroid therapy. *Br J Dis Chest* 1975; **69:** 217–22.
2. Hudgel DW, Spector SL. Pulmonary infiltration with eosinophilia: recurrence in an asthmatic patient treated with beclomethasone dipropionate. *Chest* 1977; **72:** 359–60.
3. Klotz LR, *et al.* The use of beclomethasone dipropionate inhaler complicated by the development of an eosinophilic pneumonia reaction. *Ann Allergy* 1977; **39:** 133–6.
4. Mollura JL, *et al.* Pulmonary eosinophilia in a patient receiving beclomethasone dipropionate aerosol. *Ann Allergy* 1979; **42:** 326–9.


**Hypersensitivity.** There have been reports of asthmatic reactions to beclometasone dipropionate inhalations, possibly associated with materials used in their formulation, or with the containers.


1. Maddern PJ, *et al.* Adverse reaction after aerosol inhalation. *Med J Aust* 1978; **1:** 274.
2. Godin J, Malo JL. Acute bronchoconstriction caused by Becovent and not Vanceril. *Clin Allergy* 1979; **9:** 585–9.
3. Clark RJ. Exacerbation of asthma after nebulised beclomethasone dipropionate. *Lancet* 1986; **ii:** 574–5.
4. Beasley R, *et al.* Benzalkonium chloride and bronchoconstriction. *Lancet* 1986; **ii:** 1227.


**Reformulation.** Reformulation of some metered-dose inhalers to use a chlorofluorocarbon (CFC)-free propellant has resulted in a change of efficacy. One CFC-free product (*Qvar, UK*) is reported to be effective at about half the dose[1] required with the standard product (see Uses and Administration, below) and the UK Committee on Safety of Medicines has issued a reminder of the need for dosage reduction when converting from the conventional formulation to this product.[2] This dose reduction does not apply to all CFC-free formulations of beclometasone. However, an open-label, crossover study in healthy volunteers also found higher beclometasone plasma concentrations following the use of another brand (*Beclozone, Eire*) of CFC-free product.[3]


1. Davies RJ, *et al.* Hydrofluoroalkane-134a beclomethasone dipropionate extrafine aerosol provides equivalent asthma control to chlorofluorocarbon beclomethasone dipropionate at approximately half the total daily dose. *Respir Med* 1998; **92** (suppl): 23–31.
2. Committee on Safety of Medicines/Medicines Control Agency. Dose of CFC-free inhaled beclomethasone (Qvar). *Current Problems* 1999; **25:** 5–6. Also available at: http://www.mca.gov.uk/ourwork/monitorsafequalmed/currentproblems/volume25mar.htm (accessed 27/04/04)
3. Lipworth BJ, Jackson CM. Pharmacokinetics of chlorofluorocarbon and hydrofluoroalkane metered-dose inhaler formulations of beclomethasone dipropionate. *Br J Clin Pharmacol* 1999; **48:** 866–8.


## Interactions

The interactions of corticosteroids in general are described on p.1072.

## Pharmacokinetics

For a brief outline of the pharmacokinetics of corticosteroids, see p.1073. Beclometasone is stated to be readily absorbed from sites of local application, and rapidly distributed to all body tissues. It is metabolised principally in the liver, but also in other tissues including gastrointestinal tract and lung; enzymatic hydrolysis rapidly produces the monopropionate (which has some glucocorticoid activity), and, more slowly, the free alcohol, which is virtually devoid of activity. Only a small proportion of an absorbed dose is excreted in urine, the remainder being excreted in the faeces mainly as metabolites.

## Uses and Administration

Beclometasone dipropionate is a corticosteroid with mainly glucocorticoid activity (p.1068) that is stated to exert a topical effect on the lungs without significant systemic activity at recommended doses (but see Adrenal Suppression under Adverse Effects, above). It is used by inhalation, generally from a metered-dose aerosol, for the prophylaxis of asthma (see below).

A wide variety of formulations is now available, with differing dosage regimens, and the appropriate product literature should be consulted before starting therapy or changing to another formulation. Furthermore in the UK the doses of beclometasone dipropionate for asthma and rhinitis are expressed in units of 50 micrograms or multiples thereof (dose supplied into the mouthpiece per actuation) whereas in the USA the dose-unit is 42 micrograms or multiples thereof (dose emitted from the mouthpiece); recommended doses therefore appear somewhat lower in the USA than the UK doses given below, although in practical terms there is probably no difference.

In the UK the adult dosage of the **conventional aerosol** and some dry powder inhalers is usually 400 micrograms daily, inhaled in 2 to 4 divided doses for maintenance treatment; if necessary, 600 to 800 micrograms may be inhaled daily initially, subsequently adjusted according to the patient's response. In patients with severe asthma or in those showing only a partial response to standard inhalation doses, high-dose inhalation therapy may be considered; doses of 1 mg daily (250 micrograms four times daily or 500 micrograms twice daily) may be used and may be increased to 1.5 to 2 mg daily (500 micrograms three or four times daily) if necessary; a maximum of 2 mg daily should not be exceeded. In children, 50 or 100 micrograms may be inhaled 2 to 4 times daily according to the response or alternatively, 100 or 200 micrograms may be inhaled twice daily.

Although beclometasone dipropionate is generally inhaled in aerosol form, **inhalation capsules** or **discs** containing powder for inhalation are available for patients who experience difficulty in using the aerosol. Owing to differences in the relative bioavailability to the lungs a 100-microgram dose from an inhalation capsule or disc is approximately equivalent in activity to a 50-microgram dose from a conventional aerosol. Recommended maintenance doses of beclometasone dipropionate from inhalation capsules or discs are therefore *higher*: 200 micrograms inhaled 3 or 4 times daily or 400 micrograms inhaled twice daily for adults, and 100 micrograms inhaled 2 to 4 times daily or 200 micrograms inhaled twice daily for children. Up to 800 micrograms twice daily may be inhaled if necessary in adults requiring high-dose therapy.

In some countries beclometasone dipropionate is now available as a **CFC-free aerosol**. Because of changes in particle size the dose required from some such inhalers may be *lower* than that from a conventional aerosol: typical UK doses for one product (*Qvar*) range from 100 to 200 micrograms daily in mild asthma to 400 to 800 micrograms daily in severe asthma, given as 2 divided doses.

Inhalation of **nebulised** beclometasone dipropionate has also been used in the management of asthma in children.

Beclometasone dipropionate is also used as a **nasal spray** in the prophylaxis and treatment of allergic and non-allergic rhinitis (p.422). Usual doses are 100 micrograms in each nostril twice daily or 50 micrograms in each nostril 3 or 4 times daily; a total of 400 micrograms daily should not generally be exceeded. A dose of 50 micrograms in each nostril twice daily may be sufficient for prophylaxis. The nasal spray is also used in the prevention of recurrence of nasal polyps following surgical removal (p.1084).

Beclometasone dipropionate is also used **topically** in the treatment of various skin disorders. It is generally applied as a cream or ointment containing 0.025%. Beclometasone salicylate has also been used topically. For recommendations concerning the correct use of corticosteroids on the skin, and a rough guide to the clinical potencies of topical corticosteroids, see p.1074.

**Adenoidal hypertrophy.** Although normally managed by surgery (or if less severe simply by symptomatic relief) adenoidal hypertrophy in children was reported to respond to aqueous nasal beclometasone 336 micrograms daily in an 8-week crossover study.[1] Improvements in adenoidal obstruction and symptom scores were enhanced in a subsequent 16-week follow-on study using 168 micrograms daily. Another similar study,[2] of an initial 4-week crossover period followed by 24 weeks of open-label treatment, found symptomatic improvements in about half of the patients, and at 100 weeks there was a decrease in the rate of adenotonsillectomy in children who had responded to beclometasone compared with nonresponders.

1. Demain JG, Goetz DW. Pediatric adenoidal hypertrophy and nasal airway obstruction: reduction with aqueous nasal beclomethasone. *Pediatrics* 1995; **95:** 355–64.
2. Criscuoli G, *et al.* Frequency of surgery among children who have adenotonsillar hypertrophy and improve after treatment with nasal beclomethasone. Abstract: *Pediatrics* 2003; **111:** 663. Full version: http://pediatrics.aappublications.org/cgi/content/full/111/3/e236 (accessed 27/04/04)

**Asthma.** Corticosteroids and beta$_2$-adrenoceptor agonists form the cornerstone of the management of asthma (p.777). Patients requiring only occasional relief from symptoms may be managed with an inhaled short-acting beta$_2$ agonist, and an inhaled corticosteroid such as beclometasone is added if symptomatic relief is needed more than once daily. The dose of inhaled corticosteroid is increased in more severe asthma, often together with the addition of other drugs.

High-dose regimens may pose problems of compliance if beclometasone must be inhaled several times daily. However, one study[1] found once-daily inhalation to be as effective as the same dose divided into 2 daily inhalations in short-term control of moderate asthma. Also there have been doubts that increasing the dose of inhaled beclometasone brings about increased benefits,[2] but guidelines and clinical practice suggest that improved control can often be achieved by increasing the dose. A systematic review[3] noted that while there was little evidence of an effect of dose titration, evidence was lacking in patients with more severe disease (who are more likely to be given high-dose therapy), and studies were needed to resolve the question.

Inhalation of beclometasone dipropionate as a nebulised solution has been found to be useful in the management of severe asthma in children aged 2 years or under previously unresponsive to other drugs.[4] Nebulised beclometasone dipropionate was also effective in the management of recurrent episodes of bronchopulmonary obstruction following bronchiolitis in children under 2 years of age.[5] However, in other reports nebulised beclometasone dipropionate, although more effective than saline in preschool children, produced a response less than that usually observed with inhalation of beclometasone from an aerosol or capsules,[6] or no benefit at all.[7] This may have been due to beclometasone somehow failing to reach the lungs.[8] In pre-school children able to use a spacer device with a metered aerosol, intermittent therapy with high-dose beclometasone dipropionate, given at the first sign of symptoms, reduced the severity of acute episodic asthma.[9]

1. Gagnon M, *et al.* Comparative safety and efficacy of single or twice daily administration of inhaled beclomethasone in moderate asthma. *Chest* 1994; **105:** 1732–7.
2. Boe J, *et al.* High-dose inhaled steroids in asthmatics: moderate efficacy gain and suppression of the hypothalamic-pituitary-adrenal axis. *Eur Respir J* 1994; **7:** 2179–84.
3. Adams NP, *et al.* Inhaled beclomethasone versus placebo for chronic asthma. Available in The Cochrane Library; Issue 1. Chichester: John Wiley; 2004.
4. Pedersen W, Prahl P. Jet-nebulized beclomethasone dipropionate in the management of bronchial asthma: topical steroids for asthmatic children younger than 4 years. *Allergy* 1987; **42:** 272–5.
5. Carlsen KH, *et al.* Nebulised beclomethasone dipropionate in recurrent obstructive episodes after acute bronchiolitis. *Arch Dis Child* 1988; **63:** 1428–33.
6. Storr J, *et al.* Nebulised beclomethasone dipropionate in preschool asthma. *Arch Dis Child* 1986; **61:** 270–3.
7. Webb MSC, *et al.* Nebulised beclomethasone dipropionate suspension. *Arch Dis Child* 1986; **61:** 1108–10.
8. Clarke SW. Nebulised beclomethasone dipropionate suspension: commentary. *Arch Dis Child* 1986; **61:** 1110.
9. Wilson NM, Silverman M. Treatment of acute, episodic asthma in preschool children using intermittent high dose inhaled steroids at home. *Arch Dis Child* 1990; **65:** 407–10.

**Chronic obstructive pulmonary disease.** For discussion of the value of inhaled corticosteroids in chronic obstructive pulmonary disease, including reference to the use of beclometasone, see p.1078.

**Cough.** In children with recurrent cough (p.1112) inhalation of beclometasone 200 micrograms twice daily from a conventional aerosol or salbutamol 200 micrograms twice daily had no effect on cough frequency or severity.[1]

1. Chang AB, *et al.* A randomised, placebo controlled trial of inhaled salbutamol and beclomethasone for recurrent cough. *Arch Dis Child* 1998; **79:** 6–11.

**Graft-versus-host disease.** Beclometasone is under investigation for its topical effect in the treatment of intestinal graft-versus-host disease (GVHD). A study[1] in patients with acute intestinal GVHD after bone marrow transplantation (see Haematopoietic Stem Cell Transplantation, p.1344) found that addition of oral beclometasone to prednisolone therapy was associated with a greater proportion of durable responses after 30 days.

1. McDonald GB, *et al.* Oral beclomethasone dipropionate for treatment of intestinal graft-versus-host disease: a randomized, controlled trial. *Gastroenterology* 1998; **115:** 28–35.

**Inflammatory bowel disease.** Beclometasone 500 micrograms given nightly as an enema was as effective as betamethasone 5 mg enemas in the treatment of acute attacks of distal ulcerative colitis.[1] Although betamethasone produced slightly superior histological improvement and faster disappearance of blood from the stools, systemic adverse effects observed with betamethasone therapy were absent in patients treated with beclometasone.

A comparison of beclometasone dipropionate enemas (3 mg) with prednisolone sodium phosphate enemas (30 mg) found them to be equally effective.[2] The incidence of adverse effects in both groups was low.

For a review of the management of inflammatory bowel disease, including the role of corticosteroids, see p.1243.

1. Halpern Z, *et al.* A controlled trial of beclomethasone versus betamethasone enemas in distal ulcerative colitis. *J Clin Gastroenterol* 1991; **13:** 38–41.
2. Campieri M, *et al.* Beclomethasone dipropionate enemas versus prednisolone sodium phosphate enemas in the treatment of distal ulcerative colitis. *Aliment Pharmacol Ther* 1998; **121:** 361–6.

## Preparations

***BP 2003:*** Beclometasone Cream; Beclometasone Nasal Spray; Beclometasone Ointment; Beclometasone Pressurised Inhalation.

**Proprietary Preparations** (details are given in Part 3)

***Arg.:*** Airbeclosona; Egosona; Menaderm Simple; Propavent; Qvar; Rinosol; ***Austral.:*** Aldecin; Becloforte; Beconase; Becotide; Qvar; Respocort†; ***Austria:*** Beclomet; Beconase; Becotide; Metosan; ***Belg.:*** Aldecin†; Beclophar; Beconase; Becotide; Qvar; ***Braz.:*** Aldecina†; Beclosol; Clenil; Miflasona; ***Canad.:*** Beclodisk†; Becloforte†; Beclovent†; Beconase†; Gen-Beclo; Propaderm; Qvar; Rivanase; Vancenase†; Vanceril†; ***Chile:*** Beclosema; Beclovent; Beconase; Destap; Filair; Flumates; Xiten; ***Denm.:*** AeroBec; Aldecin†; Andion†; Becloforte†; Beclomet; Becocent†; Beconase; Becotide†; ***Fin.:*** AeroBec; Beclomet; Beclonasal; Beconase; Becotide; ***Fr.:*** Asmabec; Beclo-Rhino; Beclojet; Beclone; Beconase; Becotide; Bemedrex; Ecobec; Miflasone; Nexxair; Prolair; Qvar; Rhinirex†; Spir; ***Ger.:*** AeroBec; Beclo Siozwo; Beclomet; Beclorhinol; Becloturmant; Beconase Aquosum; Bronchocort; Junik; ratioAllerg; Rhinivict; Sanasthmax; Sanasthmyl; Ventolair; Viarox; ***Gr.:*** Becotide; Clenil "Forte Jet"; Respocort; Rinosol; ***Hong Kong:*** Aldecin; Atomase†; Beclazone; Beclo Asma; Becloforte; Becodisks; Beconase; Becotide; Clenil†; Nasobec†; Qvar; Rino Clenil†; ***India:*** Beclate; ***Irl.:*** AeroBec; Asmabec; Beclazone; Beclo-Rhino; Becodisks; Beconase; Becotide; Nasobec; Qvar; ***Israel:*** Becloforte; Beconase; Becotide; Rhinocort; Viarex; ***Ital.:*** Becotide; Becotide A; Bronco-Turbinal; Cleniderm†; Clenil; Clenilexx; Clipper; Menaderm Simplex; Prontinal; Rino Clenil; Topster; Turbinal; ***Jpn:*** Rhinocort; Salcoat; ***Malaysia:*** Atomase; Becloforte; Beclomet; Beconase; Becotide; Qvar; ***Mex.:*** AeroBec†; Beconase; Becotide; ***Neth.:*** AeroBec; Becloforte; Beconase; Becotide; Qvar; ***Norw.:*** AeroBec; Beclomet; Becotide; ***NZ:*** Alanase; Aldecin†; Atomase; Atomide†; Beclazone; Becloforte†; Becodisk†; Beconase Hayfever; Becotide†; Miflasone; Qvar; Respocort; Sinase†; ***Port.:*** Aldecina; Beclotaide; Beconase; ***S.Afr.:*** AeroBec; Anceron; Beceze; Beclate; Becloforte; Becodisks; Beconase; Becotide; Clenil; Cycloson; Nobec; Qvar; Rinaze†; Ventnaze; Ventzone†; Viarox; ***Singapore:*** Atomase; Beclazone; Beclo Asma; Becloforte; Beclomet; Beconase†; Becotide; Clenil; Decomit; Qvar; Rino Clenil; ***Spain:*** Asmabec; Beclo Asma; Beclo Rino; Becloforte; Beclomet; Beclosona; Beconase; Becotide; Betsuril; Broncivent; Decasona; Dereme; Dermisone Beclo†; Menaderm Simple; Novahaler†; Qvar; Recto Menaderm NF; ***Swed.:*** Beclomet; Becotide; ***Switz.:*** AeroBec; Aldecin†; Becloforte; Beclomet; Becodisk; Beconase; Beconasol; Becotide; ***Thai.:*** Atomase; Becloforte; Beclomet; Becodisk; Beconase; Becotide; Clenil; ***UAE:*** Beclohale; ***UK:*** AeroBec; Asmabec; Beceze; Beclazone; Beclo Aqua†; Becloforte; Beclogen; Becodisks; Beconase; Becotide; Filair; Hayfever Relief; Nasal Spray for Hayfever†; Nasal-Bec; Nasobec; Propaderm; Pulvinal Beclometasone Dipropionate; Qvar; Vivabec; Zonivent†; ***USA:*** Beclovent; Beconase; Qvar; Vancenase†; Vanceril†.

**Multi-ingredient: *Arg.:*** Beclasma; Biotaer Nebulizable; Salbutol Beclo; Ventide; ***Austria:*** Ventide; ***Braz.:*** Aerotide; Beclotamol†; Clenil Compositum; ***Chile:*** Aero-Plus; Aerosoma; Asmavent-B; Beclasma; Belomet; Broncoterol-B; Butotal B; Herolan Aerosol; Ventide; ***Hong Kong:*** Ventide; ***India:*** Aerocort; Anovate; Beclate-C; Beclate-N; Cloben-G; Ecodax; Stecort-NM; ***Ital.:*** Clenil Compositum; Menaderm; Ventolin Flogo; ***Mex.:*** Ventide; ***Singapore:*** Clenil Compositum; Ventide; ***Spain:*** Butosol; Menaderm Clio; Menaderm Neomicina; Menaderm Otologico; Recto Menaderm†; ***Switz.:*** Beclonarin; ***Thai.:*** Clenil Compositum; Ventide; ***UK:*** Ventide†.

---

## Bendacort

AF-2071; Cortazac; Hydrocortisone Bendazac.

$C_{37}H_{42}N_2O_7$ = 626.7.

*CAS — 53716-43-1.*

### Profile

Bendacort is the 21-ester of hydrocortisone with bendazac (p.20). It has been applied topically for its glucocorticoid activity (p.1068) in the management of various skin disorders.

## Betamethasone *(BAN, USAN, rINN)*

Betadexamethasone; Betametasona; Betamethasonum; Flubenisolone; Flubenisolonum; 9α-Fluoro-16β-methylprednisolone; β-Methasone; NSC-39470; Sch-4831. 9α-Fluoro-11β,17α,21-trihydroxy-16β-methylpregna-1,4-diene-3,20-dione.

$C_{22}H_{29}FO_5$ = 392.5.
*CAS — 378-44-9.*
*ATC — A07EA04; C05AA05; D07AC01; H02AB01; R01AD06; R03BA04; S01BA06; S02BA07; S03BA03.*

**Pharmacopoeias.** In *Chin., Eur.* (see p.vi), *Int., Jpn,* and *US.*

**Ph. Eur. 5.0** (Betamethasone). A white or almost white, crystalline powder. Practically insoluble in water; sparingly soluble in dehydrated alcohol; very slightly soluble in dichloromethane. Protect from light.

**USP 27** (Betamethasone). A white to practically white, odourless, crystalline powder. Soluble 1 in 5300 of water, 1 in 65 of alcohol, 1 in 15 of warm alcohol, 1 in 325 of chloroform, and 1 in 3 of methyl alcohol; sparingly soluble in acetone and in dioxan; very slightly soluble in ether. Store in airtight containers at a temperature between 2° and 30°.

### Betamethasone Acetate *(BANM, rINNM)*

Acetato de betametasona; Betamethasoni Acetas. Betamethasone 21-acetate.

$C_{24}H_{31}FO_6$ = 434.5.
*CAS — 987-24-6.*
*ATC — A07EA04; C05AA05; D07AC01; H02AB01; R01AD06; R03BA04; S01BA06; S02BA07; S03BA03.*

**Pharmacopoeias.** In *Eur.* (see p.vi) and *US.*

**Ph. Eur. 5.0** (Betamethasone Acetate). A white or almost white, crystalline powder. Practically insoluble in water; soluble in alcohol and in dichloromethane; freely soluble in acetone. It shows polymorphism. Protect from light.

**USP 27** (Betamethasone Acetate). A white to creamy-white, odourless powder. Soluble 1 in 2000 of water, 1 in 9 of alcohol, and 1 in 16 of chloroform; freely soluble in acetone. Store in airtight containers at a temperature between 2° and 30°.

### Betamethasone Benzoate *(BANM, USAN, rINNM)*

Benzoato de betametasona; W-5975. Betamethasone 17α-benzoate.

$C_{29}H_{33}FO_6$ = 496.6.
*CAS — 22298-29-9.*
*ATC — A07EA04; C05AA05; D07AC01; H02AB01; R01AD06; R03BA04; S01BA06; S02BA07; S03BA03.*

**Pharmacopoeias.** In *US.*

**USP 27** (Betamethasone Benzoate). A white to practically white, practically odourless, powder. Insoluble in water; soluble in alcohol, in chloroform, and in methyl alcohol. Store in airtight containers at a temperature between 2° and 30°.

### Betamethasone Dipropionate *(BANM, USAN, rINNM)*

Betamethasoni Dipropionas; Dipropionato de betametasona; Sch-11460. Betamethasone 17α,21-dipropionate.

$C_{28}H_{37}FO_7$ = 504.6.
*CAS — 5593-20-4.*
*ATC — A07EA04; C05AA05; D07AC01; H02AB01; R01AD06; R03BA04; S01BA06; S02BA07; S03BA03.*

NOTE. Compounded preparations of betamethasone dipropionate may be represented by the following names:

- Co-climasone *(PEN)*—clotrimazole and betamethasone dipropionate.

**Pharmacopoeias.** In *Eur.* (see p.vi), *Jpn,* and *US.*

**Ph. Eur. 5.0** (Betamethasone Dipropionate). A white or almost white, crystalline powder. Practically insoluble in water; sparingly soluble in alcohol; freely soluble in acetone and in dichloromethane. Protect from light.

**USP 27** (Betamethasone Dipropionate). A white to creamwhite, odourless powder. Insoluble in water; sparingly soluble in alcohol; freely soluble in acetone and in chloroform. Store in airtight containers at a temperature of 25°, excursions permitted between 15° and 30°.

### Betamethasone Sodium Phosphate *(BANM, rINNM)*

Betamethasone Disodium Phosphate; Betamethasoni Natrii Phosphas; Fosfato sódico de betametasona. Betamethasone 21-(disodium phosphate).

$C_{22}H_{28}FNa_2O_8P$ = 516.4.
*CAS — 360-63-4 (betamethasone phosphate); 151-73-5 (betamethasone sodium phosphate).*
*ATC — A07EA04; C05AA05; D07AC01; H02AB01; R01AD06; R03BA04; S01BA06; S02BA07; S03BA03.*

NOTE. BET is a code approved by the BP 2003 for use on single unit doses of eye drops containing betamethasone sodium phosphate where the individual container may be too small to bear all the appropriate labelling information.

**Pharmacopoeias.** In *Eur.* (see p.vi), *Jpn,* and *US.*

**Ph. Eur. 5.0** (Betamethasone Sodium Phosphate). A white or almost white, very hygroscopic, powder. Freely soluble in water; slightly soluble in alcohol; practically insoluble in dichloromethane. A 1% solution in water has a pH of 7.5 to 9.0. Store in airtight containers. Protect from light.

**USP 27** (Betamethasone Sodium Phosphate). A white to practically white, odourless, hygroscopic, powder. Soluble 1 in 2 of water and 1 in 470 of alcohol; freely soluble in methyl alcohol; practically insoluble in acetone and in chloroform. Store in airtight containers.

### Betamethasone Valerate *(BANM, USAN, rINNM)*

Betamethasoni Valeras; Valerato de betametasona. Betamethasone 17α-valerate.

$C_{27}H_{37}FO_6$ = 476.6.
*CAS — 2152-44-5.*
*ATC — A07EA04; C05AA05; D07AC01; H02AB01; R01AD06; R03BA04; S01BA06; S02BA07; S03BA03.*

**Pharmacopoeias.** In *Eur.* (see p.vi), *Int., Jpn, US,* and *Viet.*

**Ph. Eur. 5.0** (Betamethasone Valerate). A white or almost white, crystalline powder. Practically insoluble in water; soluble in alcohol; freely soluble in acetone and in dichloromethane. Protect from light.

**USP 27** (Betamethasone Valerate). A white to practically white, odourless, powder. Practically insoluble in water; soluble 1 in 16 of alcohol, 1 in less than 10 of chloroform, and 1 in 400 of ether; freely soluble in acetone; slightly soluble in benzene. Store in airtight containers.

## Adverse Effects, Treatment, Withdrawal, and Precautions

As for corticosteroids in general (see p.1068).

Betamethasone has little or no effects on sodium and water retention.

When applied topically, particularly to large areas, when the skin is broken, or under occlusive dressings, or when given intranasally, corticosteroids may be absorbed in sufficient amounts to cause systemic effects. Prolonged application to the eye of preparations containing corticosteroids has caused raised intra-ocular pressure and reduced visual function.

**Anosmia.** Complete anosmia was reported in 2 patients after the use of nasal drops containing betamethasone and neomycin sulfate[1] and, in one patient, showed no sign of resolving 1 year later. The reaction was thought to be due to the preservative thiomersal present in the drops, although it was noted that neomycin could exert a toxic effect on the olfactory mucosa and that there have been several reports of anosmia associated with the use of betamethasone alone.

1. Whittet HB, *et al.* Anosmia due to nasal administration of corticosteroid. *BMJ* 1991; **303:** 651.

## Interactions

The interactions of corticosteroids in general are described on p.1072.

## Pharmacokinetics

For a brief outline of the pharmacokinetics of corticosteroids, see p.1073. Betamethasone crosses the placenta.

## Uses and Administration

Betamethasone is a corticosteroid with mainly glucocorticoid activity (p.1068); the anti-inflammatory activity of 750 micrograms of betamethasone is equivalent to about 5 mg of prednisolone. It has been used, either in the form of the free alcohol or in one of the esterified forms, in the treatment of conditions for which corticosteroid therapy is indicated (p.1073), except adrenal-deficiency states for which hydrocortisone with supplementary fludrocortisone is preferred. Its virtual lack of mineralocorticoid properties makes betamethasone particularly suitable for treating conditions in which water retention would be a disadvantage.

The dose is usually expressed in terms of the base, and the following are each approximately equivalent to 1 mg of betamethasone:

- betamethasone acetate 1.1 mg
- betamethasone benzoate 1.3 mg
- betamethasone dipropionate 1.3 mg
- betamethasone sodium phosphate 1.3 mg
- betamethasone valerate 1.2 mg

For administration by mouth betamethasone or betamethasone sodium phosphate is used; the usual dose, expressed in terms of betamethasone, ranges from 0.5 to 5 mg daily.

For parenteral administration the sodium phosphate ester may be given intravenously by injection or infusion or intramuscularly by injection in doses equivalent to 4 to 20 mg of betamethasone. It may also be given by local injection into soft tissues in doses equivalent to 4 to 8 mg of betamethasone. Doses in children, as a slow intravenous injection, are, in infants aged up to 1 year the equivalent of 1 mg of betamethasone; children aged 1 to 5 years, 2 mg; 6 to 12 years, 4 mg. Doses may be repeated 3 or 4 times in 24 hours if necessary, depending on the condition being treated and the clinical response. The sodium phosphate ester is also sometimes used with the acetate or dipropionate esters, which have a slower and more prolonged action.

Betamethasone sodium phosphate is also used in the topical treatment of allergic and inflammatory conditions of the eyes, ears, or nose, usually as drops or ointment containing 0.1%.

For topical application in the treatment of various skin disorders the dipropionate and valerate esters of betamethasone are extensively used; the usual concentrations available are the equivalent of 0.05% of betamethasone as the dipropionate, and 0.025 or 0.1% as the valerate. For recommendations concerning the correct use of corticosteroids on the skin, and a rough guide to the clinical potencies of topical corticosteroids, see p.1074.

Betamethasone valerate has also been used by inhalation for the prophylaxis of asthma.

Other esters of betamethasone which have occasionally been used include the benzoate, butyrate propionate, phosphate, salicylate (cortobenzolone), and valero-acetate.

Betamethasone adamantoate has been used in veterinary practice.

**Haemangioma.** For reference to the use of a mixture of betamethasone and triamcinolone for the intralesional injection of haemangiomas, see p.1081.

**Inflammatory bowel disease.** For a comparison of betamethasone and beclometasone enemas in the treatment of ulcerative colitis, see under Beclometasone, p.1092. Corticosteroids are one of the mainstays of treatment of inflammatory bowel disease, the general management of which is discussed on p.1243.

## Preparations

***BP 2003:*** Betamethasone and Clioquinol Cream; Betamethasone and Clioquinol Ointment; Betamethasone Eye Drops; Betamethasone Injection; Betamethasone Sodium Phosphate Tablets; Betamethasone Tablets; Betamethasone Valerate Cream; Betamethasone Valerate Lotion; Betamethasone Valerate Ointment; Betamethasone Valerate Scalp Application; ***USP 27:*** Betamethasone Benzoate Gel; Betamethasone Cream; Betamethasone Dipropionate Cream; Betamethasone Dipropionate Lotion; Betamethasone Dipropionate Ointment; Betamethasone Dipropionate Topical Aerosol; Betamethasone Sodium Phosphate and Betamethasone Acetate Injectable Suspension; Betamethasone Sodium Phosphate Injection; Betamethasone Syrup; Betamethasone Tablets; Betamethasone Valerate Cream; Betamethasone Valerate Lotion; Betamethasone Valerate Ointment; Clotrimazole and Betamethasone Dipropionate Cream.

**Proprietary Preparations** (details are given in Part 3)
***Arg.:*** Beta Adenil; Betacort; Betasone-G; Betasone-G 12 Horas; Betnovate; Blacor; Butasona; Butasona RL; Celestone; Celestone Cronodose; Cevicort; Corteroid; Corteroid Retard; Cortiderma; Cronocorteroid; Cronolevel; Deltalaf; Dermizol; Diprocel; Diprosone; Maxisona; Quiacort; Transderma B; Valederm; ***Austral.:*** Antroquoril; Betnovate; Celestone Chronodose; Celestone M; Celestone V; Cortival; Diprosone; Eleuphrat; ***Austria:*** Betnesol; Betnovate; Celestan; Diproderm; Diproforte; Diprophos; Solu-Celestan; ***Belg.:*** Betnelan-V; Betnesol†; Celestone; Celestone Chronodose; Diprolene; Diprosone; ***Braz.:*** Alersan; Bebyderm†; Beclonato; Benevat; Beta Long†; Betaderm; Betametagen; Betaprospan; Betaspan; Betnelan; Betnovate; Betrat B; Betsona; Celestan; Celestone; Celestone Soluspan; Dermobet†; Dermoval; Dermovate†; Diprobeta; Diprosone; Diprospan; Duoflam; Epidermil†; Sensitex; Valbet; ***Canad.:*** Beben†; Betacort†; Betaderm; Betaject; Betnesol; Betnovate†; Celestoderm; Celestone Soluspan; Celestone†; Diprolene Glycol; Diprosone; Ectosone; Occlucort†; Prevex B; Rivasone†; Rolene†; Rosone†; Taro-Sone; Topilene; Topisone; Valisone; ***Chile:*** Betnovate; Cidoten; Cidoten Rapilento; Cidoten V; Coritex; Cremirit; Cronolevel; Dacam; Dacam RL; Diprolene; Diprospan; Disopranil; Konicortil; Labosona; Oftasona P; Spel; ***Denm.:*** Betnovat; Betoid†; Bettamousse; Celeston; Diproderm; Diprolen; Diprospan; ***Fin.:*** Bemetson; Betapred; Betnovat; Bettamousse†; Celestoderm; Celeston Chronodose; Diproderm; Diprolen; ***Fr.:*** Betnes
Betneval; Celestene; Celestene Chronodose; Celestoderm; Dipr
Diprosone; ***Ger.:*** Bemon; Beta-Stulln; Beta-Wolff; BetaCreme; P
Betam-Ophtal; BetaSalbe; Betnesol; Betnesol-V; Celestamin
Depot; Celestan solubile; Celestan-V; Cordes Beta; Dir
Diprosone Depot; Euvaderm†; Lygal E Creme†; Pe
Betnovate; Celestene; Celestoderm-V; Flogoz
Movithiol; Osmoran; Propioform; Sanor
Betasone; Betazone; Betnovate; Cel
Diprocel; Diprosone; Diprospan; F
Betnelan; Betnesol; Topicasone
Betnesol; Betnovate; Betta
nesol; Betnovate; Bet
dose; Dicorten; Dir
Beta 21; Betamesol,
Cronodose; Diprosc
sone; Besone; Beta; B
derm-V; Celestone; De
Diprospan; Setrosone; U
stone; Celestone Solusp
Diprospan; ***Neth.:*** Betnelan,
stone Chronodose; Diprolene

Bettamousse; Celeston; Diproderm; ***NZ:*** Beta; Betnesol†; Betnovate; Bivate; Celestone Chronodose; Diprolene; Diprosone; ***Port.:*** Betnasol; Betnovate; Celesdepot; Celestone; Cilestoderme; Dibetop; Diprofos; Diprosone; Soluderme; Vabeta; ***S.Afr.:*** Betanoid; Betnesol; Betnovate; Celestoderm-V; Celestone; Celestone Soluspan; Diprolene; Diprosone; Lenasone; Lenovate; Persivate; Repivate; Steromien; Topivate; ***Singapore:*** Beprogel; Beprosone; Besone; Betacorten; Betasone; Betnovate; Celestoderm-V; Celestone†; Derzid; Dibetasol; Diprocel; Diprosone; Diprospan; Medobeta†; Uniflex; ***Spain:*** Betamatil†; Betnovate; Bettamousse; Celestoderm; Celestoderm-V; Celestone; Celestone Cronodose; Diproderm; ***Swed.:*** Betapred; Betnovat; Betoid†; Bettamousse; Celeston; Celeston bifas; Celeston valerat; Diproderm; Diprolen; ***Switz.:*** Betnesol; Betnovate; Celestoderm-V; Celestone; Celestone Chronodose; Diprolene; Diprosone; ***Thai.:*** Bennasone; Beprosone; Besone; Bessasone; Beta; Betameth; Bethasone; Betnovate; Betosone; Bipro; Celestoderm-V†; Celestone†; Derzid; Diprobet; Diprosone; Diprospan; Diprotop; Prevex B; Sebo; Valbet; Valerbet; ***UAE:*** Betasone; ***UK:*** Betacap; Betnelan; Betnesol; Betnovate; Betnovate RD (Ready Diluted); Bettamousse; Diprosone; Vista-Methasone; ***USA:*** Alphatrex; Beta-Val; Betatrex†; Cel-U-Jec; Celestone; Celestone Soluspan; Diprolene; Diprosone; Luxiq; Maxivate; Teladar; Valisone.

**Multi-ingredient:** ***Arg.:*** Adenil; Algio Nervomax Fuerte; Antiflogol; Antihemorroidal; Bacticort; Bacticort Complex; Becortin; Betnovate Antihemorroidal; Betnovate-C; Betnovate-N; Blokium B12; Celestamine; Celestamine-L; Cevaderm; Ciprocort L; Clarityne Cort; Confor-Tar; Corteroid Gesic; Cortispec; Cortistamin L; Cortistamin NF; Denvercrem; Dermizol G; Dermizol Trio; Dermosona; Dermovit; Dioxaflex B12; Diprogenta; Diprosalic; Eubetal Biotic; Factor Dermico; Fucicort; Fusimed B; Gelbiotic Plus; Gentasol; Hifamonil Crema; Histamino Corteroid L; Lisaler Beta; Lotricomb; Macril; Maxisalic; Mencogrin; Micomazol B; Miklogen; Negalerg; Neo-Mudapenil; Nularef Cort; Oxa B12; Quadriderm; Quadriderm CD; Quiacort G; Quiacort G Plus; Sinaler B; Sirotamicin BG; Sorsis Beta; Triplex; Vesalion B12; Virobron B12 NF; Vitacortil; Xedenol B12; ***Austral.:*** Celestone VG; ***Austria:*** Betnesol-N; Betnovate-C; Betnovate-N; Celestamin; Diprogenta; Diprosalic; ***Belg.:*** Betnelan-VC; Betnelan-VN†; Diprophos; Diprosalic; Fucicort; Garasone; Lotriderm; ***Braz.:*** Betazol Cort; Betazon†; Betnovate-N; Betnovate-Q; Candicort; Celestamil; Celestamine; Cetobeta; Cetocort; Cremederme; Dermosalic; Dipro AS; Diprogenta; Diprosalic; Garasone; Gentacort; Microbiogen†; Novacort; Oto Betnovate; Poliderms; Quadriderm; Quadrikin; Quadrilon; Quadriplus; Reumix†; Tetraderm; ***Canad.:*** Diprogen; Diprosalic; Garasone; Lotriderm; Valisone-G; ***Chile:*** B-Laboterol; Betnovate-N; Cam; Celestamine; Cestop B; Clofexan; Clotrimin-B; Cobefen; Contralmor; Creminem-B; Deucoaler; Diproquin; Diprosalic; Diprospan G; Donomix; Fucicort; Gentasone; Gotalgic; Labosalic; Labosona G; Labosona N; Locrim; Lotriderm; Mixgen; Novadrel; Novarnela; Oftagen Compuesto; Oftasona N; Otandrol; Otazol; Oticum; Otolisan; Plexus; Prodel B; Vilterm; ***Denm.:*** Betnovat med Chinoform; Betnovat Rektal; Celeston med Chinoform; Clotrason; Daivobet; Diproform†; Diprosalic; Fucicort; ***Fin.:*** Betnovat Comp; Betnovat-C; Celestoderm cum Chinoform; Celestoderm cum Garamycin; Diprosalic; Fucicort; ***Fr.:*** Betnesalic; Betneval-Neomycine; Celestamine; Diprosalic; Diprosept; Diprosone Neomycine; Diprostene; Gentasone†; ***Ger.:*** Betadermic; Betagentam; Betamethason Plus; Betnesalic†; Celestamine; Daivobet; Diprogenta; Diprosalic; Euvaderm N†; Euvaderm†; Fucicort; Lotricomb; Lygal E Tinktur; Soderm Plus; Sulmycin mit Celestan-V; Terracortril N; ***Gr.:*** Celestone Chronodose; Fucicort; Propiochrone; Propiosalic; ***Hong Kong:*** Allersan; Bechlomin; Beclomin; Betnesalic; Betnovate-C; Betnovate-N; Celestamine; Celestoderm-V with Garamycin; Celestoderm-V with Neomycin†; Dexmin; Diprogenta; Diprosalic; Fucicort; Garasone; Lozopin; Quadriderm; Synbetamine; Triderm; ***India:*** Betamil-M; Betnesol-N; Betnesol-N Nasal; Betnor; Betnovate-C; Betnovate-GM; Betnovate-M; Betnovate-N; Betnovate-S; Genticyn B Eye/Ear; Quiss; Surfaz-SN; Topicasone with Neomycin; Valbet; ***Irl.:*** Betnesol-N; Betnovate-C; Betnovate-N; Diprosalic; Dovobet; Fucibet; Lotriderm; Vista-Methasone N†; ***Israel:*** Betacorten-G; Betnesol-N; Betnovate-C; Betnovate-N; Celestoderm-V with Garamycin†; Diprogenta; Diprosalic; Fucicort; Triderm; ***Ital.:*** Alfaflor; Apsor†; Beben Clorossina; Betabioptal; Betafloroto; Biorinil; Brumeton Colloidale S; Deltavagin; Dermatar; Diproform; Diprogenta†; Diprosalic; Ecoval con Neomicina; Eubetal Antibiotico; Eubetal†; Fluororinil; Fucicort; Gentalyn Beta; Micutrin Beta; Psorinase; Rinojet; Stranoval; Viobeta†; Visublefarite; Visumetazone Antibiotico; Visumidriatic Antiflogistico†; ***Malaysia:*** Beavate N; Beprogent; Beprosalic; Besone-N; Betacin; Betagen; Betnesol-N; Betnovate-N; Celestoderm-V with Garamycin; Dermal C; Dermal G; Dermal SA; Dermasole N; Diprogenta; Fobancort; Fucicort; Garasone; Germacort; Joysun; Triderm-C; Uniflex-N; ***Mex.:*** Artridol; Celestamine; Celestamine NS; Celestamine-F; Claricort; Clio-Betnovate; Diprosalic; Diprosone G; Diprosone Y; Fucicort; Garamicina-V; Garasone; Gelmicin; Genrex-B†; Miclobet; Quadriderm NF; Triderm; ***Neth.:*** Celestoderm met Neomycine; Celestoform; Diprosalic; ***Norw.:*** Betnovat med Chinoform; Daivobet; Diprosalic; ***NZ:*** Betnesol Aqueous; Betnesol-N†; Betnovate-C; Diprosalic; Fucicort; Lotricomb; Ultrazon N†; ***Port.:*** Betnovate-C; Betnovate-N; Dibetop Q; Diprogenta; Diprosalic; Epione; Flotiran; Fucicort; Psodermil; Quadriderme; ***S.Afr.:*** Betanoid N; Betnesol-N; Betnovate-C; Betnovate-N; Celestamine; Celestoderm-V with Garamycin; Diprogenta; Diprosalic; Garasone; Lotriderm; Quadriderm; ***Singapore:*** B-Tasone-G; Beprogent; Beprosalic; Besone-N; Betnovate-C†; Betnovate-GM†; Betnovate-M†; Betnovate-N†; Bufencon; Celestoderm-V with Garamycin; Celestoderm-V with Neomycin; Clotrasone; Combiderm; Conazole; Diprogenta; Diprosalic; Fobancort; Fucicort; Garasone; Gentrisone; Neoderm; Quadriderm; Tri-Micon; Triderm; Uniflex-N†; ***Spain:*** Alergical; Beta Micoter; Betamatil con Neomicina†; Betamida; Betartrinovo†; Bronsal; Celesemine; Celestoderm Gentamicina; Celestone S; Clotrasone; Cuatroderm; Daivobet; Diprogenta; Diprosalic; Fucibet; Nasotic Oto†; Resorborina; [illegible]lane†; Visublefarite†; ***Swed.:*** Betnovat med Chinoform; Betnovat med [illegible]omycin; Celeston valerat comp; Celeston valerat med chinoform; Ce[illegible]n valerat med gentamicin; Daivobet; Diprosalic; ***Switz.:*** Betnesalic; [illegible]vate-C; Betnovate-N; Celestamine; Diprogenta; Diprophos; Dipro[illegible]cicort; Ophtasone; Quadriderm; Triderm; ***Thai.:*** Benn†; Bepro[illegible]sone-N; Beta-C; Beta-Dipo; Beta-N; Beta-S; Betama-EN; Beta[illegible]ethasone-N; Betnesalic; Betnovate-C; Betnovate-N; Betosalic; [illegible]E; Canasone; Canazol-BE; Celestoderm-V with Neomycin†; [illegible]erzid-C; Diprogenta; Diprosalic; Fucicort; Fungiderm-B; Gy[illegible]driderm†; Topaben-N; Twina; Valbet-N; ***UAE:*** Futasone; [illegible]K: Betnesol-N; Betnovate Rectal Ointment†; Betnovate-[illegible] Diprosalic; Dovobet; Fucibet; Lotriderm†; Vipsogal†; [illegible] ***USA:*** Lotrisone.

## Budesonide *(BAN, USAN, rINN)*

Budesónida; Budesonidum; S-1320. An epimeric mixture of the α- and β-propyl forms of 16α,17α-butylidenedioxy-11β,21-dihydroxypregna-1,4-diene-3,20-dione.

$C_{25}H_{34}O_6$ = 430.5.

*CAS — 51333-22-3 (11β,16α); 51372-29-3 (11β,16α(R)); 51372-28-2 (11β,16α(S)).*

*ATC — A07EA06; D07AC09; H02AB16; R01AD05; R03BA02.*

**Pharmacopoeias.** In *Eur.* (see p.vi) and *Pol.*

**Ph. Eur. 5.0** (Budesonide). A white or almost white, crystalline powder. Practically insoluble in water; sparingly soluble in alcohol; freely soluble in dichloromethane.

### Adverse Effects, Treatment, Withdrawal, and Precautions

As for corticosteroids in general (see p.1068).

Inhalation of high doses of budesonide is associated with some adrenal suppression. Systemic absorption may follow nasal administration, particularly if high doses are used or treatment is prolonged. The dose of oral budesonide may need to be reduced in hepatic impairment (see also Administration in Hepatic Impairment, below).

When applied topically, particularly to large areas, when the skin is broken, or under occlusive dressings, or when given intranasally, corticosteroids may be absorbed in sufficient amounts to cause systemic effects.

**Effects on the bones.** For mention of the effects of inhaled budesonide on markers of collagen turnover and bone density in asthmatic children, see under Adverse Effects of Beclometasone, p.1091. For the suggestion that inhalation once-daily in the morning may have less marked effects on growth and collagen turnover than twice-daily inhalation, see Administration, below.

**Effects on the nervous system.** Psychotic behaviour has been reported following use of inhaled budesonide.[1-3]


1. Lewis LD, Cochrane GM. Psychosis in a child inhaling budesonide. *Lancet* 1983; **ii:** 634.
2. Meyboom RHB, de Graff-Breederveld N. Budesonide and psychic side effects. *Ann Intern Med* 1988; **109:** 683.
3. Connett G, Lenney W. Inhaled budesonide and behavioural disturbances. *Lancet* 1991; **338:** 634–5.


**Hypersensitivity.** Contact dermatitis has been reported to topical or intranasal budesonide.[1] An anaphylactoid reaction occurred 5 minutes after the first dose of oral budesonide in a patient who had previously reacted in a similar way to mesalazine.[2]


1. Quintiliani R. Hypersensitivity and adverse reactions associated with the use of newer intranasal corticosteroids for allergic rhinitis. *Curr Ther Res* 1996; **57:** 478–88.
2. Heeringa M, *et al.* Anaphylactic-like reaction associated with oral budesonide. *BMJ* 2000; **321:** 927.


### Interactions

The interactions of corticosteroids in general are described on p.1072.

### Pharmacokinetics

For a brief outline of the pharmacokinetics of corticosteroids, see p.1073. Budesonide is rapidly and almost completely absorbed following administration by mouth, but has poor systemic availability (about 10%) due to extensive first-pass metabolism in the liver, mainly by the cytochrome P450 isoenzyme CYP3A4. The major metabolites, 6-β-hydroxybudesonide and 16-α-hydroxyprednisolone have less than 1% of the glucocorticoid activity of unchanged budesonide. Budesonide is reported to have a terminal half-life of about 2 to 4 hours.

◊ Reviews.


1. Donnelly R, Seale JP. Clinical pharmacokinetics of inhaled budesonide. *Clin Pharmacokinet* 2001; **40:** 427–40.


### Uses and Administration

Budesonide is a corticosteroid with mainly glucocorticoid activity (p.1068). It is used by inhalation in the management of asthma, in usual doses of 400 micrograms daily in 2 divided doses from a metered-dose aerosol; in severe asthma the dosage may be increased up to a total of 1.6 mg daily, and guidelines for the management of asthma permit up to 2 mg daily (see p.777). Maintenance doses may be less than 400 micrograms daily but should not be below 200 micrograms daily. A dose for children is 50 to 400 micrograms inhaled twice daily. Budesonide is also available for the management of asthma in the form of a dry powder inhaler; doses are 200 to 800 micrograms daily, as 2 divided doses or a single daily dose; up to 800 micrograms twice daily may be given to adults if necessary. Patients for whom administration of budesonide from a pressurised inhaler or dry powder formulation is unsatisfactory may use a nebulised solution. The usual adult dosage by this method is 1 to 2 mg inhaled twice daily. This may be increased if asthma is severe. Maintenance doses are 0.5 to 1 mg inhaled twice daily. For children between 3 months and 12 years of age, an initial dose is 0.5 to 1 mg twice daily with a maintenance dose of 0.25 to 0.5 mg twice daily.

Budesonide is also given by inhalation as a nebulised solution in the management of childhood croup (p.1079). The usual dose is 2 mg, as a single inhaled dose or 2 doses of 1 mg, given 30 minutes apart.

Budesonide is used topically in the treatment of various skin disorders, as a cream or ointment containing 0.025%. For recommendations concerning the correct use of corticosteroids on the skin, and a rough guide to the clinical potencies of topical corticosteroids, see p.1074.

Budesonide is also used as a nasal spray for the prophylaxis and treatment of rhinitis (p.422), and in the management of nasal polyps (p.1084). In the UK it is used for rhinitis in a usual initial dose of 200 micrograms into each nostril once daily, subsequently reduced to the lowest dose adequate to control symptoms which may be 100 micrograms into each nostril daily. Alternatively, the initial dose may be 100 micrograms into each nostril twice daily. The latter dose is given for up to 3 months in the treatment of nasal polyps. In the USA and some other countries the intranasal dose may be expressed in multiples of 32 micrograms, which is the quantity of budesonide delivered from the nasal adaptor. When given from a nasal inhaler an initial dose of 128 micrograms daily in each nostril, reduced once control is established, is recommended in adults and children over 6 years of age. An alternative regimen, beginning with 32 micrograms daily in each nostril and increasing as necessary up to a maximum of 128 micrograms daily in each nostril for adults or half this amount in children, is recommended when the dose is given as an aqueous nasal spray.

Local formulations of budesonide are used in the management of inflammatory bowel disease (see below). In mild to moderate Crohn's disease affecting the ileum or ascending colon it is given by mouth as modified-release capsules intended for a topical effect on the gastrointestinal tract. The recommended dose is 9 mg daily for up to 8 weeks. The dosage should be reduced 2 to 4 weeks before discontinuing therapy. There is some absorption of budesonide from the gastrointestinal tract, and the dose may need to be reduced in patients with hepatic impairment, especially those with cirrhosis (see also Administration in Hepatic Impairment, below). An enema solution containing 0.002% is also available; it is given at bedtime for 4 weeks in the treatment of ulcerative colitis at a dose of 2 mg.

◊ General references.


1. Brogden RN, McTavish D. Budesonide: an updated review of its pharmacological properties, and therapeutic efficacy in asthma and rhinitis. *Drugs* 1992; **44:** 375–407 and 1012.
2. Hvizdos KM, Jarvis B. Budesonide inhalation suspension: a review of its use in infants, children and adults with inflammatory respiratory disorders. *Drugs* 2000; **60:** 1141–78.


**Administration.** INHALATIONAL ROUTE. One study in 6 children aged up to 30 months found that about 75% of the nominal dose of nebulised budesonide was deposited in the nebuliser system,[1] while a study in 126 older children indicated that maintenance doses of budesonide could be halved when the dose was given by dry powder inhaler rather than nebuliser, without any loss of asthma control.[2] Although oropharyngeal deposition is thought to play a role in the systemic effects of inhaled corticosteroids, another study[3] indicated that only about 20% of the systemically available drug appeared to be derived from oropharyngeal deposition following inhalation from a dry powder inhaler.

There is evidence that the timing of inhaled therapy might influence some systemic effects. A study[4] in children with mild asthma found that 800 micrograms of budesonide inhaled in the morning had less effect on measurements of short-term growth and collagen turnover than inhalation of 400 micrograms twice daily.

1. Carlsen KCL, *et al.* How much nebulised budesonide reaches infants and toddlers? *Arch Dis Child* 1992; **67:** 1077–9.
2. Agertoft L, Pedersen S. Importance of the inhalation device on the effect of budesonide. *Arch Dis Child* 1993; **69:** 130–3.
3. Pedersen S, *et al.* The influence of orally deposited budesonide on the systemic availability of budesonide after inhalation from a Turbuhaler. *Br J Clin Pharmacol* 1993; **36:** 211–14.
4. Heuck C, *et al.* Adverse effects of inhaled budesonide (800 micrograms) on growth and collagen turnover in children with asthma: a double-blind comparison of once-daily versus twice-daily administration. *J Pediatr* 1998; **133:** 608–12.

**Administration in hepatic impairment.** In a study[1] of patients with primary biliary cirrhosis the clearance of oral budesonide was significantly reduced in those with cirrhosis (stage IV) compared with milder disease (stage I/II). Elevated budesonide concentrations were sufficient to suppress cortisol production, and believed to be associated with the development of portal vein thrombosis in 2 cirrhotic patients.

1. Hempfling W, *et al.* Pharmacokinetics and pharmacodynamic action of budesonide in early- and late-stage primary biliary cirrhosis. *Hepatology* 2003; **38:** 196–202.

**Asthma.** References to the use of budesonide in asthma.[1-4]

1. Baker JW, *et al.* A multiple-dosing, placebo-controlled study of budesonide inhalation suspension given once or twice daily for treatment of persistent asthma in young children and infants. *Pediatrics* 1999; **103:** 414–21.
2. The Childhood Asthma Management Program Research Group. Long-term effects of budesonide or nedocromil in children with asthma. *N Engl J Med* 2000; **343:** 1054–63.
3. Leflein JG, *et al.* Nebulized budesonide inhalation suspension compared with cromolyn sodium nebulizer solution for asthma in young children: results of a randomized outcomes trial. *Pediatrics* 2002; **109:** 866–72.
4. Pauwels RA, *et al.* Early intervention with budesonide in mild persistent asthma: a randomised, double-blind trial. *Lancet* 2003; **361:** 1071–6.

**Chronic obstructive pulmonary disease.** For discussion of the value of inhaled corticosteroids in chronic obstructive pulmonary disease, including reference to the use of budesonide, see p.1078.

**Collagenous colitis.** Budesonide has been used in a few small controlled studies[1-3] of the management of collagenous colitis (p.1240). Treatment courses given orally for 6 or 8 weeks were found to improve symptoms and histology, but long-term efficacy has not been established, and a high rate of relapse after stopping treatment was reported in one study.[3]

1. Baert F, *et al.* Budesonide in collagenous colitis: a double-blind placebo-controlled trial with histologic follow-up. *Gastroenterology* 2002; **122:** 20–5.
2. Miehlke S, *et al.* Budesonide treatment for collagenous colitis: a randomized, double-blind, placebo-controlled, multicenter trial. *Gastroenterology* 2002; **123:** 978–84.
3. Bonderup OK, *et al.* Budesonide treatment of collagenous colitis: a randomised, double blind, placebo controlled trial with morphometric analysis. *Gut* 2003; **52:** 248–51.

**Cystic fibrosis.** Cystic fibrosis (p.123) is associated with bronchial hyper-responsiveness; a small study[1] has suggested that inhalation of budesonide 1.6 mg daily for 6 weeks improves hyper-responsiveness slightly and leads to improvement in cough and dyspnoea. A larger study[2] of budesonide given for two successive 3-month treatment periods found improved hyper-responsiveness and a trend towards slower decline in lung function.

1. Van Haren EHJ, *et al.* The effects of the inhaled corticosteroid budesonide on lung function and bronchial hyperresponsiveness in adult patients with cystic fibrosis. *Respir Med* 1995; **89:** 209–14.
2. Bisgaard H, *et al.* Controlled trial of inhaled budesonide in patients with cystic fibrosis and chronic bronchopulmonary Pseudomonas aeruginosa infection. *Am J Respir Crit Care Med* 1997; **156:** 1190–6.

**Inflammatory bowel disease.** Budesonide has been given as an enema for the treatment of distal ulcerative colitis, in which context its potency and low systemic availability are advantageous.[1] It is available as a modified-release oral dosage form for the management of active Crohn's disease.[1,2] It has also been investigated for its potential in delaying relapse in quiescent disease,[3-5] although any benefit appears short-term, and a systematic review[6] concluded that oral modified-release budesonide was not effective in preventing relapse during 12 months of treatment. Similarly, oral budesonide was ineffective in preventing postoperative recurrence after resection for Crohn's disease.[7] Oral budesonide has also been tried as an alternative to conventional systemic corticosteroids in ulcerative colitis.[8]

For a discussion of inflammatory bowel disease, see p.1243.

1. Spencer CM, McTavish D. Budesonide: a review of its pharmacological properties and therapeutic efficacy in inflammatory bowel disease. *Drugs* 1995; **50:** 854–72.
2. McKeage K, Goa KL. Budesonide (Entocort® EC capsules): a review of its therapeutic use in the management of active Crohn's disease in adults. *Drugs* 2002; **62:** 2263–82.
3. Greenberg GR, *et al.* Oral budesonide as maintenance treatment for Crohn's disease: a placebo-controlled dose-ranging study. *Gastroenterology* 1996; **110:** 45–51.
4. Löfberg R, *et al.* Budesonide prolongs time to relapse in ileal and ileocaecal Crohn's disease: a placebo controlled one year study. *Gut* 1996; **39:** 82–6.
5. Gross V, *et al.* Low dose oral pH modified release budesonide for maintenance of steroid induced remission in Crohn's disease. *Gut* 1998; **42:** 493–6.
6. Simms L, Steinhart AH. Budesonide for maintenance of remission in Crohn's disease. Available in The Cochrane Library; Issue 1. Chichester: John Wiley; 2004.
7. Hellers G, *et al.* Oral budesonide for prevention of postsurgical recurrence in Crohn's disease. *Gastroenterology* 1999; **116:** 294–300.
8. Keller R, *et al.* Oral budesonide therapy for steroid-dependent ulcerative colitis: a pilot trial. *Aliment Pharmacol Ther* 1997; **11:** 1047–52.

## Preparations

**Proprietary Preparations** (details are given in Part 3)

***Arg.:*** Budefarma; Budeson; Cuteral; Despex; Entocort; Hypersol B; Kerpet; Nastizol Hidrospray; Neumotex; Proetzonide; Pulmo Lisoflam; Rino-B; Spirocort; ***Austral.:*** Budamax; Entocort; Pulmicort; Rhinocort; ***Austria:*** Budo-san; Entocort; Miflonide; Predermid; Pulmicort; Rhinocort; Rhinocortol; ***Belg.:*** Budenofalk; Entocort; Miflonide; Preferid†; Pulmicort; Rhinocort; ***Braz.:*** Budecort; Busonid; Cortasm†; Entocort; Miflonide; Pulmicort; ***Canad.:*** Entocort; Pulmicort; Rhinocort; ***Chile:*** Aero-Bud; Aerovial; Budenofalk; Clebudan; Entocort; Inflammide; Pulmicort; ***Denm.:*** Entocort; Miflonide; Rhinocort; Rhinosol; Spirocort; ***Fin.:*** Cortivent; Entocort; Pulmicort; Rhinocort; ***Fr.:*** Entocort; Pulmicort; Rhinocort; ***Ger.:*** Benosid; Bronchocux†; Budapp; Budecort; Budefat; Budenofalk; Budepur E†; Budes; Budon; Entocort; Miflonide; Novopulmon; Pulmicort; Respicort; ***Gr.:*** Astrocast; Biosonide; Budecol; Budenofalk; Budesan; Dedostryl; Esonide; Ixor; Obeciroi; Obusonid; Olfosonide; Olyspal; Pulmicort; Resata; Rhinoside; Sonidal; Udesospray; Vericort; Vinecort; ***Hong Kong:*** Budenofalk; Eltair†; Entocort; Pulmicort; Rhinocort; ***India:*** Pulmicort; Rhinocort; ***Irl.:*** Entocort; Preferid†; Pulmicort; Rhinocort; ***Israel:*** Budeson; Budicort; Entocort; Nasocort; Pulmotide; ***Ital.:*** Aircort; Bidien; Desonax; Eltair; Enterocir; Entocir; Miflonide; Preferid; Pulmaxan; Rhinocort; Spirocort; ***Malaysia:*** Eltair; Inflammide; Pulmicort; Rhinocort; ***Mex.:*** Entocort; Numark; Pulmicort; Rhinocort; ***Neth.:*** Entocort; Pulmicort; Rhinocort; ***Norw.:*** Entocort; Preferid†; Pulmicort; Rhinocort; ***NZ:*** Butacort; Eltair; Entocort; Hayclear†; Pulmicort; Rhinocort†; ***Port.:*** Entocort; Miflonide; Pulmicort; ***S.Afr.:*** Budeflam; Entocord; Inflacor; Inflammide; Inflanaze; Pulmicort; Rhinocort; ***Singapore:*** Eltair; Entocort; Inflammide; Pulmicort; Rhinocort; ***Spain:*** Demotest; Entocord; Miflonide; Neo Rinactive; Olfex; Pulmicort; Pulmictan; Rhinocort; Ribujet; Ribusol†; ***Swed.:*** Entocort; Pulmicort; Rhinocort; ***Switz.:*** Budenofalk; Entocort; Miflonide; Preferid†; Pulmicort; Rhinocort; ***Thai.:*** Budecort; Eltair; Inflammide; Pulmicort; Rhinocort; ***UAE:*** Sonidar; ***UK:*** Budenofalk; Entocort; Pulmicort; Rhinocort; ***USA:*** Entocort; Pulmicort; Rhinocort.

**Multi-ingredient:** ***Arg.:*** Neumoterol; Symbicort; ***Austral.:*** Symbicort; ***Austria:*** Symbicort; ***Belg.:*** Symbicort; ***Braz.:*** Foraseq; Symbicort; ***Chile:*** Symbicort; ***Denm.:*** Symbicort; ***Fin.:*** Symbicort; ***Fr.:*** Symbicort; ***Ger.:*** Symbicort; ***Hong Kong:*** Symbicort; ***India:*** Foracort; ***Irl.:*** Symbicort; ***Israel:*** Symbicort; ***Ital.:*** Assieme; Sinestic; Symbicort; ***Neth.:*** Symbicort; ***Norw.:*** Symbicort; ***NZ:*** Symbicort; ***Port.:*** Assieme; Symbicort; ***Singapore:*** Symbicort; ***Spain:*** Symbicort; ***Swed.:*** Symbicort; ***Switz.:*** Symbicort; ***Thai.:*** Symbicort; ***UK:*** Symbicort.

## Ciclesonide *(USAN, rINN)*

RPR-251526. (*R*)-11β,16α,17,21-Tetrahydroxypregna-1,4-diene-3,20-dione cyclic 16,17-acetal with cyclohexanecarboxaldehyde, 21-isobutyrate.

$C_{32}H_{44}O_7$ = 540.7.

*CAS — 126544-47-6; 141845-82-1.*

*ATC — R03BA08.*

### Profile

Ciclesonide is a corticosteroid with glucocorticoid activity (p.1068) that is inhaled in the treatment of asthma. It is also under investigation for the treatment of allergic rhinitis.

◊ References.

1. Schmidt BM, *et al.* The new topical steroid ciclesonide is effective in the treatment of allergic rhinitis. *J Clin Pharmacol* 1999; **39:** 1062–9.
2. Postma DS, *et al.* Treatment of asthma by the inhaled corticosteroid ciclesonide given either in the morning or evening. *Eur Respir J* 2001; **17:** 1083–8.
3. Rohatagi S, *et al.* Population pharmacokinetics and pharmacodynamics of ciclesonide. *J Clin Pharmacol* 2003; **43:** 365–78.

### Preparations

**Proprietary Preparations** (details are given in Part 3)

***Austral.:*** Alvesco.

## Ciprocinonide *(USAN, rINN)*

Ciprocinonida; RS-2386. (6α,11β,16α)-21-[(cyclopropylcarbonyl)oxy]-6,9-difluoro-11-hydroxy-16,17-[(1-methylethylidene)-bis(oxy)]-pregna-1,4-diene-3,20-dione.

$C_{28}H_{34}F_2O_7$ = 520.6.

*CAS — 58524-83-7.*

### Profile

Ciprocinonide is a derivative of fluocinolone acetonide (p.1101) that has been applied topically in combination with fluocinonide and procinonide in the management of various skin disorders.

### Preparations

**Proprietary Preparations** (details are given in Part 3)

**Multi-ingredient:** ***Canad.:*** Trisyn†.

## Clobetasol Propionate *(BANM, USAN, rINNM)*

CCI-4725; GR-2/925; Propionato de clobetasol. 21-Chloro-9α-fluoro-11β,17α-dihydroxy-16β-methylpregna-1,4-diene-3,20-dione 17-propionate.

$C_{25}H_{32}ClFO_5$ = 467.0.

*CAS — 25122-41-2 (clobetasol); 25122-46-7 (clobetasol propionate).*

*ATC — D07AD01.*

**Pharmacopoeias.** In *Br., Chin.,* and *US.*

**BP 2003** (Clobetasol Propionate). A white or almost white, crystalline powder. Practically insoluble in water; sparingly soluble in alcohol; freely soluble in acetone and in dichloromethane. Protect from light.

**USP 27** (Clobetasol Propionate). A white to cream crystalline powder. Practically insoluble in water; sparingly soluble in dehydrated alcohol; soluble in acetone, in chloroform, in dimethyl sulfoxide, in dioxan, and in methyl alcohol; slightly soluble in benzene and in ether. Store in airtight containers. Protect from light.

### Profile

Clobetasol propionate is a corticosteroid used topically for its glucocorticoid activity (p.1068) in the treatment of various skin disorders. It is usually employed as a cream, ointment, or scalp application containing 0.05%.

When applied topically, particularly to large areas, when the skin is broken, or under occlusive dressings, corticosteroids may be absorbed in sufficient amounts to cause systemic effects (p.1068). The effects of topical corticosteroids on the skin are described on p.1070. For recommendations concerning the correct use of corticosteroids on the skin, and a rough guide to the clinical potencies of topical corticosteroids, see p.1074.

### Preparations

***BP 2003:*** Clobetasol Cream; Clobetasol Ointment;

***USP 27:*** Clobetasol Propionate Cream; Clobetasol Propionate Ointment; Clobetasol Propionate Topical Solution.

**Proprietary Preparations** (details are given in Part 3)

***Arg.:*** Cantril; Clobesol; Dermadex; Ribatra; Salac; ***Austria:*** Dermovate; ***Belg.:*** Dermovate; ***Braz.:*** Clob-X; Clobesol; Cortalen C; Dermacare; Propiosol; Psorex; Psorin; Therapsor†; ***Canad.:*** Dermasone; Dermovate; ***Chile:*** Alticort; Clodavan; Cortopic; Dermovate; Koniderm; Lobevat; Xinder; ***Denm.:*** Dermovat; ***Fin.:*** Dermovat; ***Fr.:*** Dermoval; ***Ger.:*** Clobegalen; Dermoxin; Dermoxinale; Karison; ***Gr.:*** Butavate; Rubocord; ***Hong Kong:*** Clobasol; Dermasone; Dermovate; Medodermone; Uniderm; ***India:*** Lobate; Tenovate; Topifort; ***Irl.:*** Dermovate; ***Israel:*** Dermovate; ***Ital.:*** Clobesol; ***Malaysia:*** Betasol; Clobet; Cloderm; Dermapro; Dermosol; Dermovate; Lobesol; Univate; ***Mex.:*** Dermatovate; Lobevat; ***Neth.:*** Dermovate; ***Norw.:*** Dermovat; ***NZ:*** Dermol; Dermovate†; ***Port.:*** Dermovate; ***S.Afr.:*** Dermovate; Dovate; Xenovate; ***Singapore:*** Clobeson; Cloderm; Dermosol; Dermovate; Dhabesol; Medodermone†; Uniderm; Univate; ***Spain:*** Clovate; Decloban; ***Swed.:*** Dermovat; ***Switz.:*** Dermovate; ***Thai.:*** Betasol; Clinoderm; Clobasone; Clobet; Clobetate; Clonovate; Dermasil; Dermovate; Medodermone; P-vate; Stivate; ***UAE:*** Gamavate; ***UK:*** Dermovate; ***USA:*** Clobex; Cormax; Embeline; Olux; Temovate.

**Multi-ingredient:** ***Arg.:*** Clobeplus; Clobesol LA; Dermadex NN; ***India:*** Lobate-G; Lobate-GM; Lobate-M; Tenovate G; Tenovate M; ***Port.:*** Dermovate-NN; ***Switz.:*** Dermovate-NN; ***UK:*** Dermovate-NN.

## Clobetasone Butyrate *(BANM, USAN, rINNM)*

Butirato de clobetasona; CCI-5537; Clobetasoni Butyras; GR-2/1214. 21-Chloro-9α-fluoro-17α-hydroxy-16β-methylpregna-1,4-diene-3,11,20-trione 17-butyrate.

$C_{26}H_{32}ClFO_5$ = 479.0.

*CAS — 54063-32-0 (clobetasone); 25122-57-0 (clobetasone butyrate).*

*ATC — D07AB01; S01BA09.*

**Pharmacopoeias.** In *Eur.* (see p.vi).

**Ph. Eur. 5.0** (Clobetasone Butyrate). A white or almost white powder. Practically insoluble in water; slightly soluble in alcohol; freely soluble in acetone and in dichloromethane. Protect from light.

### Profile

Clobetasone butyrate is a corticosteroid used topically for its glucocorticoid activity (p.1068) in the treatment of various skin disorders. It is usually employed as a cream or ointment containing 0.05%. When applied topically, particularly to large areas, when the skin is broken, or under occlusive dressings, corticosteroids may be absorbed in sufficient amounts to cause systemic effects (p.1068). The effects of topical corticosteroids on the skin are described on p.1070. For recommendations concerning the correct use of corticosteroids on the skin, and a rough guide to the clinical potencies of topical corticosteroids, see p.1074.

Clobetasone butyrate is also used for inflammatory eye disorders, as eye drops containing 0.1%. Prolonged application to the eye of preparations containing corticosteroids has caused raised intra-ocular pressure and reduced visual function.

### Preparations

***BP 2003:*** Clobetasone Cream; Clobetasone Ointment.

**Proprietary Preparations** (details are given in Part 3)

***Arg.:*** Eumovate; ***Austria:*** Emovate; ***Belg.:*** Eumovate; ***Braz.:*** Eumovate; ***Canad.:*** Eumovate; ***Chile:*** Eumovate; ***Denm.:*** Emovat; ***Fin.:*** Emovat; ***Ger.:*** Emovate; ***Gr.:*** Rettavate; ***Hong Kong:*** Eumovate; ***India:*** Eumosone; ***Irl.:*** Eumovate; ***Israel:*** Eucorten; Eumovate; ***Ital.:*** Clobet; Eumovate; Visucloben; ***Malaysia:*** Cortoftal; Eumovate; Euvaderm; ***Neth.:*** Emovate; ***Norw.:*** Cloptison; ***NZ:*** Eumovate; ***Port.:*** Emovate; ***S.Afr.:*** Eumovate; ***Singapore:*** Amisol; Eumovate; ***Spain:*** Cortoftal; Emovate; ***Swed.:*** Emovat; ***Switz.:*** Cloptison†; Emovate; ***Thai.:*** Eumovate; ***UK:*** Cloburate†; Eumovate.

**Multi-ingredient:** ***Arg.:*** Cloptison-N; ***Israel:*** Cicloderm-C; ***Ital.:*** Visucloben Antibiotico; Visucloben Decongestionante; ***Switz.:*** Cloptison-N†; ***UK:*** Trimovate.

## Clocortolone Pivalate *(USAN, rINNM)*

CL-68; Pivalato de clocortolona; SH-863. 9α-Chloro-6α-fluoro-11β,21-dihydroxy-16α-methylpregna-1,4-diene-3,20-dione 21-pivalate.

$C_{27}H_{36}ClFO_5$ = 495.0.

*CAS — 4828-27-7 (clocortolone); 34097-16-0 (clocortolone pivalate).*

*ATC — D07AB21.*

**Pharmacopoeias.** In *US.*

**USP 27** (Clocortolone Pivalate). A white to yellowish-white, odourless powder. Sparingly soluble in alcohol; soluble in acetone; freely soluble in chloroform and in dioxan; slightly soluble in ether and in benzene. Store in airtight containers. Protect from light.

### Profile

Clocortolone pivalate is a corticosteroid used topically for its glucocorticoid activity (p.1068), as a 0.1% cream or ointment, in the treatment of various skin disorders. Clocortolone caproate has been used in combination with the pivalate.

When applied topically, particularly to large areas, where the skin is broken, or under occlusive dressings, corticosteroids may be absorbed in sufficient amounts to cause systemic effects (p.1068). The effects of topical corticosteroids on the skin are described on p.1070. For recommendations concerning the correct use of corticosteroids on the skin, see p.1074.

### Preparations

*USP 27:* Clocortolone Pivalate Cream.

**Proprietary Preparations** (details are given in Part 3)
***Austria:*** Glimbal; ***USA:*** Cloderm.

**Multi-ingredient:** ***Ger.:*** Corto-Tavegil; Crino-Kaban N; Kaban; Kabanimat; Procto-Kaban.

## Cloprednol *(BAN, USAN, rINN)*

RS-4691. 6-Chloro-11β,17α,21-trihydroxypregna-1,4,6-triene-3,20-dione.

$C_{21}H_{25}ClO_5$ = 392.9.

*CAS — 5251-34-3.*

*ATC — H02AB14.*

### Profile

Cloprednol is a corticosteroid with mainly glucocorticoid activity (p.1068); the anti-inflammatory activity of 2.5 mg of cloprednol is equivalent to about 5 mg of prednisolone. Cloprednol is given by mouth in various disorders for which corticosteroid therapy is helpful (p.1073), in usual doses ranging from 1.25 to 12.5 mg daily.

### Preparations

**Proprietary Preparations** (details are given in Part 3)
***Ger.:*** Syntestan; ***Ital.:*** Cloradryn†; ***Mex.:*** Novacort†.

## Cortisone Acetate *(BANM, rINNM)*

Acetato de cortisona; Compound E Acetate; Cortisoni Acetas; 11-Dehydro-17-hydroxycorticosterone Acetate. 17α,21-Dihydroxypregn-4-ene-3,11,20-trione 21-acetate.

$C_{23}H_{30}O_6$ = 402.5.

*CAS — 53-06-5 (cortisone); 50-04-4 (cortisone acetate).*

*ATC — H02AB10; S01BA03.*

**Pharmacopoeias.** In *Chin., Eur.* (see p.vi), *Jpn, Pol., US,* and *Viet.*

**Ph. Eur. 5.0** (Cortisone Acetate). A white or almost white, crystalline powder. It shows polymorphism. Practically insoluble in water; slightly soluble in alcohol and in methyl alcohol; sparingly soluble in acetone; freely soluble in dichloromethane; soluble in dioxan. Protect from light.

**USP 27** (Cortisone Acetate). A white or practically white, odourless, crystalline powder. Insoluble in water; soluble 1 in 350 of alcohol, 1 in 75 of acetone, 1 in 4 of chloroform, and 1 in 30 of dioxan. Store at a temperature of 25°, excursions permitted between 15° and 30°.

### Adverse Effects, Treatment, Withdrawal, and Precautions

As for corticosteroids in general (see p.1068).

### Interactions

The interactions of corticosteroids in general are described on p.1072.

### Pharmacokinetics

For a brief outline of the pharmacokinetics of corticosteroids, see p.1073.

Cortisone acetate is readily absorbed from the gastrointestinal tract and the cortisone is rapidly converted in the liver to its active metabolite, hydrocortisone (cortisol). The biological half-life of cortisone itself is only about 30 minutes. Absorption of cortisone acetate from intramuscular sites is considerably slower than following oral administration.

### Uses and Administration

Cortisone is a corticosteroid secreted by the adrenal cortex. It has glucocorticoid activity (p.1068), as well as appreciable mineralocorticoid activity; 25 mg of cortisone acetate is equivalent in anti-inflammatory activity to about 5 mg of prednisolone.

Cortisone acetate is rapidly effective when given by mouth, and more slowly by intramuscular injection.

Cortisone acetate has been used mainly for replacement therapy in adrenocortical insufficiency (p.1075), but hydrocortisone (p.1103) is generally preferred since cortisone itself is inactive and must be converted by the liver to hydrocortisone, its active metabolite; hence, in some liver disorders the activity of cortisone may be less reliable. Doses of cortisone acetate by mouth for replacement therapy are 12.5 to 37.5 mg daily in divided doses, together with fludrocortisone if additional mineralocorticoid activity is required.

Cortisone acetate has been used in the treatment of many of the allergic and inflammatory disorders for which corticosteroid therapy is helpful (p.1073) but prednisolone or other synthetic glucocorticoids are generally preferred. Doses of cortisone acetate employed have generally ranged from about 25 to 300 mg daily by mouth or by intramuscular injection.

### Preparations

*BP 2003:* Cortisone Tablets;
*USP 27:* Cortisone Acetate Injectable Suspension; Cortisone Acetate Tablets.

**Proprietary Preparations** (details are given in Part 3)
***Austral.:*** Cortate; ***Austria:*** Cortone†; ***Belg.:*** Adreson; ***Canad.:*** Cortone; ***Ital.:*** Cortone; ***Norw.:*** Cortone†; ***S.Afr.:*** Cortogen; ***Spain:*** Altesona†; ***Swed.:*** Cortal†; Cortone†; ***UK:*** Cortisyl; ***USA:*** Cortone.

**Multi-ingredient:** ***Braz.:*** Corciclen; ***Ital.:*** Dutimelan†; ***Spain:*** Antiblefarica†; Blefarida; Gingilone; ***Switz.:*** Septicortin†.

## Cortivazol *(USAN, pINN)*

H-3625; MK-650; NSC-80998. 11β,17α,21-Trihydroxy-6,16α-dimethyl-2′-phenyl-2′H-pregna-2,4,6-trieno[3,2-c]pyrazol-20-one 21-acetate.

$C_{32}H_{38}N_2O_5$ = 530.7.

*CAS — 1110-40-3.*

*ATC — H02AB17.*

### Profile

Cortivazol is a corticosteroid with mainly glucocorticoid activity (p.1068); 300 micrograms of cortivazol is equivalent in anti-inflammatory activity to about 5 mg of prednisolone. It is given in the treatment of musculoskeletal and joint disorders by intra-articular, periarticular, or epidural injection in doses of about 1.25 to 3.75 mg, according to the size of the joint, usually at intervals of 1 to 3 weeks. It has also been given by mouth.

### Preparations

**Proprietary Preparations** (details are given in Part 3)
***Fr.:*** Altim.

## Deflazacort *(BAN, USAN, rINN)*

Azacort; DL-458-IT; L-5458; MDL-458; Oxazacort. 11β,21-Dihydroxy-2′-methyl-5′βH-pregna-1,4-dieno[17,16-d]oxazole-3,20-dione 21-acetate.

$C_{25}H_{31}NO_6$ = 441.5.

*CAS — 14484-47-0.*

*ATC — H02AB13.*

### Profile

Deflazacort is a corticosteroid with mainly glucocorticoid activity (p.1068); 6 mg of deflazacort is reportedly equivalent in anti-inflammatory activity to about 5 mg of prednisolone (but see Action, below).

Deflazacort is used for its anti-inflammatory and immunosuppressant properties in conditions responsive to corticosteroid therapy (p.1073). It is given by mouth in initial doses of up to 120 mg daily; usual maintenance doses are 3 to 18 mg daily. Doses of 0.25 to 1.5 mg/kg daily have been used in children.

◊ References.

1. Markham A, Bryson HM. Deflazacort: a review of its pharmacological properties and therapeutic efficacy. *Drugs* 1995; **50:** 317–33.

**Action.** Although it has been suggested that deflazacort produces fewer adverse effects than some conventional corticosteroids such as prednisolone, a study in healthy subjects found that the ratio of efficacy for deflazacort compared with prednisolone was higher than the 1.2 : 1 previously assumed,[1] implying that lower effective doses of deflazacort had been used in such comparisons. A review[2] of clinical trials of patients treated with deflazacort concluded that it was slightly less potent than prednisolone, and that many of the data on adverse effects were inconsistent. All systemic corticosteroids may produce clinically significant adverse reactions (see also p.1068) which are primarily dependent on dose and duration of use.

1. Babadjanova G, *et al.* Comparison of the pharmacodynamic effects of deflazacort and prednisolone in healthy subjects. *Eur J Clin Pharmacol* 1996; **51:** 53–7.
2. Anonymous. Deflazacort – an alternative to prednisolone? *Drug Ther Bull* 1999; **37:** 57–8.

### Preparations

**Proprietary Preparations** (details are given in Part 3)
***Arg.:*** Azacortid; Flamirex; ***Austria:*** Lantadin; ***Braz.:*** Calcort; Cortax; Deflanil; Denacen; ***Chile:*** Azacortid; Dezartal; ***Ger.:*** Calcort; ***Irl.:*** Calcort; ***Ital.:*** Deflan; Flantadin; ***Mex.:*** Calcort; ***Port.:*** Rosilan; ***Spain:*** Dezacor; Zamene; ***Switz.:*** Calcort; ***UK:*** Calcort.

## Deprodone *(BAN, rINN)*

Deprodona; Desolone; RD-20000 (propionate). 11β,17α-Dihydroxypregna-1,4-diene-3,20-dione.

$C_{21}H_{28}O_4$ = 344.4.

*CAS — 20423-99-8 (deprodone); 20424-00-4 (deprodone propionate).*

### Profile

Deprodone is a corticosteroid that has been used topically as the propionate.

## Desonide *(BAN, USAN, rINN)*

D-2083; Desfluorotriamcinolone Acetonide; Desonida; 16-Hydroxyprednisolone 16,17-Acetonide; Prednacinolone Acetonide. 11β,21-Dihydroxy-16α,17α-isopropylidenedioxypregna-1,4-diene-3,20-dione.

$C_{24}H_{32}O_6$ = 416.5.

*CAS — 638-94-8.*

*ATC — D07AB08; S01BA11.*

### Profile

Desonide is a corticosteroid used topically for its glucocorticoid activity (p.1068) in the treatment of various skin disorders. It is usually used as a cream, ointment, or lotion containing 0.05%. The pivalate and the sodium phosphate esters have also been used.

When applied topically, particularly to large areas, when the skin is broken, or under occlusive dressings, corticosteroids may be absorbed in sufficient amounts to cause systemic effects (p.1068). The effects of topical corticosteroids on the skin are described on p.1070. For recommendations concerning the correct use of corticosteroids on the skin, and a rough guide to the clinical potencies of topical corticosteroids, see p.1074.

### Preparations

**Proprietary Preparations** (details are given in Part 3)
***Arg.:*** Desoplus; DesOwen; Esteronide; Locatop; Prenacid; ***Austral.:*** DesOwen; ***Belg.:*** Sterax; ***Braz.:*** Desonol; DesOwen; Epidex†; Steronide; ***Canad.:*** Desocort; Tridesilon†; ***Chile:*** DesOwen; Sterax; ***Fin.:*** Apolar; ***Fr.:*** Locapred; Locatop; Tridesonit; ***Ger.:*** Sterax†; ***Hong Kong:*** DesOwen; ***India:*** DesOwen; ***Ital.:*** PR 100†; Prenacid; Reticus; Sterades; ***Mex.:*** DesOwen; ***Norw.:*** Apolar; ***NZ:*** DesOwen†; ***Port.:*** Locapred; Zotinar; ***Singapore:*** DesOwen; ***Swed.:*** Apolar; ***Switz.:*** Locapred; Locatop; Sterax; ***USA:*** DesOwen; LoKara; Tridesilon.

**Multi-ingredient:** ***Fr.:*** Cirkan a la Prednacinolone; ***Ital.:*** PR 100-Clorestidina†; ***Norw.:*** Apolar med dekvalon; ***Port.:*** Zotinar-N; ***USA:*** Tridesilon.

## Desoximetasone *(BAN, USAN, rINN)*

A-41-304; Desoximetasona; Desoxymethasone; Hoe-304; R-2113. 9α-Fluoro-11β,21-dihydroxy-16α-methylpregna-1,4-diene-3,20-dione.

$C_{22}H_{29}FO_4$ = 376.5.

*CAS — 382-67-2.*

*ATC — D07AC03.*

**Pharmacopoeias.** In *US.*

**USP 27** (Desoximetasone). A white to practically white, odourless, crystalline powder. Insoluble in water; freely soluble in alcohol, in acetone, and in chloroform.

### Profile

Desoximetasone is a corticosteroid used topically for its glucocorticoid activity (p.1068) in the treatment of various skin disorders. It is usually employed as a cream, gel, lotion, or ointment; concentrations used range from 0.05 to 0.25%.

When applied topically, particularly to large areas, when the skin is broken, or under occlusive dressings, corticosteroids may be absorbed in sufficient amounts to cause systemic effects (p.1068). The effects of topical corticosteroids on the skin are described on p.1070. For recommendations concerning the correct use of corticosteroids on the skin, and a rough guide to the clinical potencies of topical corticosteroids, see p.1074.

**Adverse effects.** A photosensitivity reaction occurred in a patient treated for psoriasis with topical desoximetasone; rechallenge led to a recurrence.[1] The patient was also receiving propranolol hydrochloride.

1. Stierstorfer MB, Baughman RD. Photosensitivity to desoximetasone emollient cream. *Arch Dermatol* 1988; **124:** 1870–1.

### Preparations

*USP 27:* Desoximetasone Cream; Desoximetasone Gel; Desoximetasone Ointment.

**Proprietary Preparations** (details are given in Part 3)
***Austria:*** Topisolon; ***Braz.:*** Esperson; ***Canad.:*** Desoxi; Topicort; ***Denm.:*** Ibaril; ***Fin.:*** Ibaril; ***Fr.:*** Topicorte†; ***Ger.:*** Topisolon; ***Hong Kong:*** Esperson†; ***Irl.:*** Topisolon; ***Israel:*** Desicort; ***Ital.:*** Flubason; ***Neth.:*** Ibaril; Topicorte; ***Norw.:*** Ibaril; ***Singapore:*** Topicorte†; ***Spain:*** Flubason; ***Swed.:*** Ibaril; ***Switz.:*** Topisolon; ***Thai.:*** Esperson; Topicorte; ***UK:*** Stiedex LP; ***USA:*** Topicort.

**Multi-ingredient:** ***Austria:*** Topisolon mit Salicylsaure; ***Braz.:*** Esperson N; ***Denm.:*** Ibaril med salicylsyre; ***Fr.:*** Topifram†; ***Ger.:*** Topisolon; ***Norw.:*** Ibaril med salicylsyre; ***Singapore:*** Topifram†; ***Swed.:*** Ibaril med salicylsyra; ***Thai.:*** Topifram; ***UK:*** Stiedex.

### Desoxycortone Acetate (BANM, rINNM)

Acetato de desoxicortona; Cortin; Decortone Acetate; 11-Deoxycorticosterone Acetate; Deoxycortone Acetate; Desoxycorticosterone Acetate; Desoxycortoni Acetas. 21-Hydroxypregn-4-ene-3,20-dione 21-acetate.

$C_{23}H_{32}O_4$ = 372.5.
*CAS — 64-85-7 (desoxycortone); 56-47-3 (desoxycortone acetate).*
*ATC — H02AA03.*

**Pharmacopoeias.** In *Eur.* (see p.vi), *Pol.*, and *US.*

**Ph. Eur. 5.0** (Desoxycortone Acetate). A white or almost white, crystalline powder or colourless crystals. Practically insoluble in water; sparingly soluble in alcohol; soluble in acetone; freely soluble in dichloromethane; slightly soluble in propylene glycol and in fatty oils. Protect from light.

**USP 27** (Desoxycorticosterone Acetate). A white or creamy-white, odourless, crystalline powder. Practically insoluble in water; sparingly soluble in alcohol, in acetone, and in dioxan; slightly soluble in vegetable oils. Store at a temperature of 25°, excursions permitted between 15° and 30°. Protect from light.

### Desoxycortone Pivalate (BANM, rINNM)

Deoxycorticosterone Pivalate; Deoxycorticosterone Trimethylacetate; Deoxycortone Pivalate; Deoxycortone Trimethylacetate; Desoxycorticosterone Pivalate; Desoxycorticosterone Trimethylacetate; Pivalato de desoxicortona. 21-Hydroxypregn-4-ene-3,20-dione 21-pivalate.

$C_{26}H_{38}O_4$ = 414.6.
*CAS — 808-48-0.*
*ATC — H02AA03.*

**Pharmacopoeias.** In *US* for veterinary use only.

**USP 27** (Desoxycorticosterone Pivalate). Store at a temperature of 25°, excursions permitted between 15° and 30°. Protect from light.

#### Profile

Desoxycortone is a corticosteroid secreted by the adrenal cortex and has primarily mineralocorticoid activity (p.1068). It has no significant glucocorticoid action.

Desoxycortone acetate has been used in the treatment of adrenocortical insufficiency (p.1075) as an adjunct to cortisone or hydrocortisone. For this purpose, however, fludrocortisone given by mouth is now usually preferred.

Desoxycortone acetate is given by intramuscular injection as an oily solution, in doses of up to 10 mg once or twice daily.

Desoxycortone has also been administered as its enantate, phenylpropionate, and sodium hemisuccinate esters. Desoxycortone pivalate is used in veterinary medicine.

#### Preparations

*USP 27:* Desoxycorticosterone Acetate Injection; Desoxycorticosterone Acetate Pellets.

**Proprietary Preparations** (details are given in Part 3)
***Austria:*** Cortiron†; ***Fr.:*** Syncortyl; ***Ital.:*** Cortiron; ***Switz.:*** Cortisteron.
**Multi-ingredient:** ***Braz.:*** Cortobion†; ***Ital.:*** Sinsurrene†.

## Dexamethasone (BAN, rINN)

Desamethasone; Dexametasona; Dexametasone; Dexamethasonum; 9α-Fluoro-16α-methylprednisolone; Hexadecadrol. 9α-Fluoro-11β,17α,21-trihydroxy-16α-methylpregna-1,4-diene-3,20-dione.

$C_{22}H_{29}FO_5$ = 392.5.
*CAS — 50-02-2.*
*ATC — A01AC02; C05AA09; D07AB19; H02AB02; R01AD03; S01BA01; S02BA06; S03BA01.*

**Pharmacopoeias.** In *Chin., Eur.* (see p.vi), *Int., Jpn, Pol., US,* and *Viet.*

**Ph. Eur. 5.0** (Dexamethasone). A white or almost white, crystalline powder. Practically insoluble in water; sparingly soluble in dehydrated alcohol; slightly soluble in dichloromethane. Protect from light.

**USP 27** (Dexamethasone). A white to practically white, odourless, crystalline powder. Practically insoluble in water; sparingly soluble in alcohol, in acetone, in dioxan, and in methyl alcohol; slightly soluble in chloroform; very slightly soluble in ether.

### Dexamethasone Acetate (BANM, USAN, rINNM)

Acetato de dexametasona; Dexamethasoni Acetas. Dexamethasone 21-acetate.

$C_{24}H_{31}FO_6$ = 434.5.
*CAS — 1177-87-3 (anhydrous dexamethasone acetate); 55812-90-3 (dexamethasone acetate monohydrate).*
*ATC — A01AC02; C05AA09; D07AB19; H02AB02; R01AD03; S01BA01; S02BA06; S03BA01.*

**Pharmacopoeias.** In *Chin., Eur.* (see p.vi), and *Viet.*
*Int.* and *US* allow the anhydrous form or the monohydrate.

**Ph. Eur. 5.0** (Dexamethasone Acetate). A white or almost white, crystalline powder. It shows polymorphism. Practically insoluble in water; freely soluble in alcohol and in acetone; slightly soluble in dichloromethane. Protect from light.

**USP 27** (Dexamethasone Acetate). It contains one molecule of water of hydration or is anhydrous. A clear, white to off-white, odourless powder. Practically insoluble in water; freely soluble in acetone, in dioxan, and in methyl alcohol. Store at a temperature of 25°, excursions permitted between 15° and 30°.

### Dexamethasone Isonicotinate (BANM, rINNM)

Isonicotinato de dexametasona. Dexamethasone 21-isonicotinate.

$C_{28}H_{32}FNO_6$ = 497.6.
*CAS — 2265-64-7.*
*ATC — A01AC02; C05AA09; D07AB19; H02AB02; R01AD03; S01BA01; S02BA06; S03BA01.*

### Dexamethasone Phosphate (BANM, rINNM)

Fosfato de dexametasona. Dexamethasone 21-(dihydrogen phosphate).

$C_{22}H_{30}FO_8P$ = 472.4.
*CAS — 312-93-6.*
*ATC — A01AC02; C05AA09; D07AB19; H02AB02; R01AD03; S01BA01; S02BA06; S03BA01.*

### Dexamethasone Sodium Metasulfobenzoate (rINNM)

Dexamethasone Sodium Metasulphobenzoate (BANM); Metasulfobenzoato sódico de dexametasona. Dexamethasone 21-(sodium *m*-sulphobenzoate).

$C_{29}H_{32}FNaO_9S$ = 598.6.
*CAS — 3936-02-5.*
*ATC — A01AC02; C05AA09; D07AB19; H02AB02; R01AD03; S01BA01; S02BA06; S03BA01.*

### Dexamethasone Sodium Phosphate (BANM, rINNM)

Dexamethasone Phosphate Sodium; Dexamethasoni Natrii Phosphas; Fosfato sódico de dexametasona; Sodium Dexamethasone Phosphate. Dexamethasone 21-(disodium orthophosphate).

$C_{22}H_{28}FNa_2O_8P$ = 516.4.
*CAS — 2392-39-4.*
*ATC — A01AC02; C05AA09; D07AB19; H02AB02; R01AD03; S01BA01; S02BA06; S03BA01.*

NOTE. DSP is a code approved by the BP 2003 for use on single unit doses of eye drops containing dexamethasone sodium phosphate where the individual container may be too small to bear all the appropriate labelling information.

**Pharmacopoeias.** In *Chin., Eur.* (see p.vi), *Int., US,* and *Viet.*

**Ph. Eur. 5.0** (Dexamethasone Sodium Phosphate). A white or almost white, very hygroscopic, powder. It exhibits polymorphism. Freely soluble in water; slightly soluble in alcohol; practically insoluble in dichloromethane. A 1% solution in water has a pH of 7.5 to 9.5. Store in airtight containers. Protect from light.

**USP 27** (Dexamethasone Sodium Phosphate). A white or slightly yellow, crystalline powder. Is odourless or has a slight odour of alcohol, and is exceedingly hygroscopic. Soluble 1 in 2 of water; slightly soluble in alcohol; insoluble in chloroform and in ether; very slightly soluble in dioxan. pH of a 1% solution in water is between 7.5 and 10.5. Store in airtight containers.

#### Adverse Effects, Treatment, Withdrawal, and Precautions

As for corticosteroids in general (see p.1068).

Dexamethasone has little or no effect on sodium and water retention.

When applied topically, particularly to large areas, when the skin is broken, or under occlusive dressings, or when given intranasally, corticosteroids may be absorbed in sufficient amounts to cause systemic effects. Prolonged application to the eye of preparations containing corticosteroids has caused raised intra-ocular pressure and reduced visual function.

**Effects on the nervous system.** Paraesthesia, usually localised to the perineum, has been associated with the intravenous use of dexamethasone sodium phosphate (see p.1070).

**Neonates.** The adverse effects of corticosteroids on the fetus are discussed on p.1071.

Adverse effects noted in premature neonates with bronchopulmonary dysplasia receiving dexamethasone treatment to enable weaning from assisted ventilation have included hypertension[1-4] often accompanied by bradycardia,[1,2] gastroduodenal perforation,[4-6] ulceration and thinning of the gastric wall,[5] development of a catabolic state,[4,7] renal calcification,[8,9] and transient myocardial hypertrophy.[10-13] There is some evidence of a suppressive effect on motor activity and spontaneous movement.[14] It has been postulated that neonatal dexamethasone may both increase[15] and decrease[16] retinopathy of prematurity; its true effect is uncertain.[17]

There is also a concern that longer term development of the child may be adversely affected.[18,19] Although data are scanty, a meta-analysis[20] has concluded that postnatal use of corticosteroids to treat or prevent bronchopulmonary dysplasia is associated with dramatic increases in the incidence of cerebral palsy and neurodevelopmental impairment, and suggested that such use should be abandoned.

Pulsed administration may reduce the adverse effects but may also reduce efficacy.[21]


1. Ohlsson A, Heyman E. Dexamethasone-induced bradycardia. *Lancet* 1988; **ii:** 1074.
2. Puntis JWL, *et al.* Dexamethasone-induced bradycardia. *Lancet* 1988; **ii:** 1372.
3. Marinelli KA, *et al.* Effects of dexamethasone on blood pressure in premature infants with bronchopulmonary dysplasia. *J Pediatr* 1997; **130:** 594–602.
4. Stark AR, *et al.* Adverse effects of early dexamethasone treatment in extremely-low-birth-weight infants. *N Engl J Med* 2001; **344:** 95–101.
5. Ng PC, *et al.* Gastroduodenal perforation in preterm babies treated with dexamethasone for bronchopulmonary dysplasia. *Arch Dis Child* 1991; **66:** 1164–6.
6. Smith H, Sinha S. Gastrointestinal complications associated with dexamethasone treatment. *Arch Dis Child* 1992; **67:** 667.
7. Macdonald PD, *et al.* A catabolic state in dexamethasone treatment of bronchopulmonary dysplasia. *Arch Dis Child* 1990; **65:** 560–1.
8. Kamitsuka MD, Peloquin D. Renal calcification after dexamethasone in infants with bronchopulmonary dysplasia. *Lancet* 1991; **337:** 626.
9. Narendra A, *et al.* Nephrocalcinosis in preterm babies. *Arch Dis Child Fetal Neonatal Ed* 2001; **85:** F207–F213.
10. Werner JC, *et al.* Hypertrophic cardiomyopathy associated with dexamethasone therapy for bronchopulmonary dysplasia. *J Pediatr* 1992; **120:** 286–91.
11. Bensky AS, *et al.* Cardiac effects of dexamethasone in very low birth weight infants. *Pediatrics* 1996; **97:** 818–21.
12. Skelton R, *et al.* Cardiac effects of short course dexamethasone in preterm infants. *Arch Dis Child* 1998; **78:** F133–F137.
13. Zecca E, *et al.* Cardiac adverse effects of early dexamethasone treatment in preterm infants: a randomized clinical trial. *J Clin Pharmacol* 2001; **41:** 1075–81.
14. Bos AF, *et al.* Qualitative assessment of general movements in high-risk preterm infants with chronic lung-disease requiring dexamethasone therapy. *J Pediatr* 1998; **132:** 300–6.
15. Batton DG, *et al.* Severe retinopathy of prematurity and steroid exposure. *Pediatrics* 1992; **90:** 534–6.
16. Sobel DB, Philip AGS. Prolonged dexamethasone therapy reduces the incidence of cryotherapy for retinopathy of prematurity in infants of less than 1 kilogram birth weight with bronchopulmonary dysplasia. *Pediatrics* 1992; **90:** 529–33.
17. Ehrenkranz RA. Steroids, chronic lung disease, and retinopathy of prematurity. *Pediatrics* 1992; **90:** 646–7.
18. Greenough A. Gains and losses from dexamethasone for neonatal chronic lung disease. *Lancet* 1998; **352:** 835–6.
19. Shinwell ES, *et al.* Early postnatal dexamethasone treatment and increased incidence of cerebral palsy. *Arch Dis Child Fetal Neonatal Ed* 2000; **83:** F177–F181.
20. Barrington KJ. The adverse neuro-developmental effects of postnatal steroids in the preterm infant: a systematic review of RCTs. *BMC Pediatr* 2001; **1:** 1. Available at: http://www.biomedcentral.com/1471-2431/1/1 (accessed 27/04/04)
21. Bloomfield FH, *et al.* Side effects of 2 different dexamethasone courses for preterm infants at risk of chronic lung disease: a randomized trial. *J Pediatr* 1998; **133:** 395–400.


#### Interactions

The interactions of corticosteroids in general are described on p.1072.

**Antiepileptics.** As described on p.374, dexamethasone may decrease or increase plasma concentrations of phenytoin. Like other enzyme-inducing drugs, phenytoin also has the potential to increase the metabolism of dexamethasone.

#### Pharmacokinetics

For a brief outline of the pharmacokinetics of corticosteroids, see p.1073.

Dexamethasone is readily absorbed from the gastrointestinal tract. Its biological half-life in plasma is about 190 minutes. Binding of dexamethasone to plasma proteins is about 77%, which is less than for most other corticosteroids. Up to 65% of a dose is excreted in urine within 24 hours. Clearance in premature neonates is reported to be proportional to gestational age, with a reduced elimination rate in the most premature. It readily crosses the placenta with minimal inactivation.

#### Uses and Administration

Dexamethasone is a corticosteroid with mainly glucocorticoid activity (p.1068); 750 micrograms of dexamethasone is equivalent in anti-inflammatory activity to about 5 mg of prednisolone.

It has been used, either in the form of the free alcohol or in one of the esterified forms, in the treatment of conditions for which corticosteroid therapy is indicated (p.1073), except adrenocortical insufficiency for which hydrocortisone with supplementary fludrocortisone is preferred. Its lack of mineralocorticoid properties makes dexamethasone particularly suitable for treating conditions where water retention would be a disadvantage.

The dose may be expressed in terms of the base, and the following are each approximately equivalent to 1 mg of dexamethasone:

- dexamethasone acetate 1.1 mg
- dexamethasone isonicotinate 1.3 mg
- dexamethasone phosphate 1.2 mg
- dexamethasone sodium metasulfobenzoate 1.5 mg
- dexamethasone sodium phosphate 1.3 mg

Dexamethasone sodium phosphate 1.1 mg is approximately equivalent to 1 mg of dexamethasone phosphate.

For administration **by mouth** dexamethasone is given in usual doses of 0.5 to 10 mg daily. Dexamethasone is also used by mouth in the dexamethasone suppression tests for the diagnosis of Cushing's syndrome (for further details see under Diagnosis and Testing, below).

For **parenteral administration** in **intensive therapy** or in **emergencies**, the sodium phosphate ester may be given intravenously by injection or infusion or intramuscularly by injection; doses are sometimes expressed in terms of the free alcohol, the phosphate, or the sodium phosphate and confusion has sometimes arisen in the literature because of these variations. Initial doses used, expressed in terms of dexamethasone phosphate, range from about 0.5 to 24 mg daily (about 0.4 to 20 mg of dexamethasone). Intravenous doses equivalent to 2 to 6 mg/kg of dexamethasone phosphate given slowly over a minimum period of several minutes have been suggested for the treatment of severe shock. These high doses may be repeated within 2 to 6 hours and this treatment should be continued only until the patient's condition is stable and usually for no longer than 48 to 72 hours. Alternatively, the initial intravenous injection may be followed by a continuous intravenous infusion of 3 mg/kg per 24 hours.

Dexamethasone sodium phosphate is also used in the treatment of **cerebral oedema** caused by malignancy. An initial intravenous dose equivalent to 10 mg of dexamethasone phosphate is usually given followed by 4 mg intramuscularly every 6 hours; a response is usually obtained after 12 to 24 hours and dosage may be reduced after 2 to 4 days, and gradually discontinued over 5 to 7 days. A much higher dosage schedule has also been suggested for use in acute life-threatening cerebral oedema; initial doses equivalent to 50 mg of dexamethasone phosphate have been given intravenously on the first day together with 8 mg intravenously every 2 hours reduced gradually over 7 to 13 days. A maintenance dose of 2 mg two or three times daily has been used in patients with recurrent or inoperable neoplasms.

The sodium phosphate ester is given by **intra-articular, intralesional**, or **soft-tissue injection**. For intra-articular injection doses equivalent to 0.8 to 4 mg of dexamethasone phosphate are employed depending upon the size of the joint. For soft-tissue injection doses of 2 to 6 mg are used. Injections are repeated every 3 to 5 days to every 2 to 3 weeks.

Dexamethasone acetate may be given by **intramuscular injection** in conditions where corticosteroid treatment is indicated but a prompt response of short duration is not required; doses are equivalent to 8 to 16 mg of dexamethasone, repeated, if necessary, every 1 to 3 weeks. The acetate may also be given locally by **intra-articular** or **soft-tissue injection** in doses equivalent to 4 to 16 mg of dexamethasone, repeated, if necessary, every 1 to 3 weeks, or by intralesional injection in doses equivalent to 0.8 to 1.6 mg.

For **ophthalmic disorders** or for topical application in the treatment of various skin disorders, either dexamethasone or its esters may be used; concentrations are often expressed in terms of dexamethasone or dexamethasone phosphate and are commonly 0.05 to 0.1% for eye or ear drops and ointments and 0.1% for topical skin preparations. For recommendations concerning the correct use of corticosteroids on the skin, and a rough guide to the clinical potencies of topical corticosteroids, see p.1074.

For allergic rhinitis and other allergic or inflammatory **nasal conditions** (p.422), a nasal spray containing dexamethasone isonicotinate is available; the acetate, phosphate, sodium phosphate, and sodium metasulfobenzoate have also been used.

Dexamethasone is given intravenously and orally for the prevention of **nausea and vomiting** induced by cancer chemotherapy (see below).

Other esters of dexamethasone that have occasionally been used include the hemisuccinate, linoleate, palmitate, pivalate, propionate, sodium succinate, tebutate, and valerate.

The phenpropionate and troxundate esters have been used in veterinary medicine.

**Alcohol withdrawal syndrome.** Dexamethasone was reported to be effective in a patient with benzodiazepine-resistant delirium tremens[1] and resolved symptoms of alcohol withdrawal syndrome resistant to other treatments in another 110 patients.[2] However, a subsequent small study found no evidence that dexamethasone was effective.[3]

1. Fischer DK, *et al.* Efficacy of dexamethasone in benzodiazepine-resistant delirium tremens. *Lancet* 1988; **i:** 1340–1.
2. Pol S, *et al.* Dexamethasone for alcohol withdrawal. *Ann Intern Med* 1991; **114:** 705–6.
3. Adinoff B, Pols B. Dexamethasone in the treatment of the alcohol withdrawal syndrome. *Am J Drug Alcohol Abuse* 1997; **23:** 615–22.

**Amyloidosis.** For mention of the use of dexamethasone in patients with amyloidosis, see p.567.

**Blood disorders.** High-dose pulsed dexamethasone therapy has been found useful in some patients with idiopathic thrombocytopenic purpura (p.1082), although results have been variable in children.

**Cerebral oedema.** Corticosteroids, usually dexamethasone, play an important role in the treatment of cerebral oedema in malignancy (see Raised Intracranial Pressure, p.833), and dexamethasone is advocated for the cerebral oedema associated with high-altitude disorders (see below).

**Congenital adrenal hyperplasia.** Because of its lack of mineralocorticoid properties, dexamethasone has little advantage in the salt-losing form of congenital adrenal hyperplasia (p.1078), in which mineralocorticoid therapy must be given, and its potency means that dose titration to avoid toxicity can be difficult in infants and children, even with the non-salt-losing form. However, it may be useful in adults with forms of the syndrome that do not require mineralocorticoid replacement. It has also been given antenatally to the mother to prevent virilisation of female fetuses.

**Diagnosis and testing.** CUSHING'S SYNDROME. Dexamethasone has been used to differentiate Cushing's disease (adrenal hyperplasia caused by defects of pituitary origin) from other forms of Cushing's syndrome (caused by ectopic ACTH secretion from non-pituitary tumours or by cortisol secretion from adrenal tumours). The dexamethasone suppression test as first proposed[1] involved the administration of dexamethasone in low doses of 500 micrograms four times daily by mouth for 8 doses followed by higher doses of 2 mg again four times daily for 8 doses. In the low-dose tests the urinary excretion of cortisol and 17-hydroxycorticosteroids is suppressed in healthy persons but not in patients and in the high-dose tests the excretion is still not suppressed in those with Cushing's syndrome but is partially suppressed in those with Cushing's disease. Because this test usually involves patients being admitted to hospital for urine collection over a number of days and because false-negative responses are reported to be fairly frequent, more rapid and reliable tests have been sought. The low-dose test plus measurement of serum-cortisol concentrations and the excretion of free cortisol in urine over 24 hours has been suggested[2] to be a reliable method for screening for Cushing's syndrome. In the UK a single dose of 1 mg of dexamethasone given at night is often used and is considered sufficient to inhibit corticotropin secretion for 24 hours in most subjects. In another variation[3] a single dose of dexamethasone 8 mg has been given at night and plasma-cortisol concentrations measured the next day; this test (known as the overnight high-dose dexamethasone suppression test) has again been said to be a practical and reliable alternative for the differential diagnosis of Cushing's syndrome.

Further variations in the dexamethasone suppression test have included administration of a continuous intravenous infusion of dexamethasone at a rate of 1 mg/hour for 7 hours, with hourly measurement of blood-cortisol concentrations.[4] Initial results indicate that this variation produces a lower number of false-positive diagnoses than the test using oral dexamethasone. Other alternatives are a combined low-dose dexamethasone suppression test and corticotropin-releasing hormone (corticorelin) test,[5] or combination of a dexamethasone suppression test with a metyrapone test.[6]

A review[7] of diagnostic tests for Cushing's syndrome has outlined both the advantages and disadvantages of tests using dexamethasone. The authors suggested that where there is suspicion of Cushing's syndrome, the overnight low-dose dexamethasone suppression test may be used as part of a range of measures, and that the dexamethasone-corticorelin test may be useful when there are equivocal results from initial screening. In the differentiation of ACTH-dependent and ACTH-independent forms of Cushing's syndrome, they suggested that the high-dose dexamethasone suppression test cannot be recommended because of poor specificity.

For further discussion of the various methods used for the diagnosis of Cushing's syndrome and details of its management, see p.1313.

1. Liddle GW. Tests of pituitary-adrenal suppressibility in the diagnosis of Cushing's syndrome. *J Clin Endocrinol Metab* 1960; **20:** 1539–60.
2. Kennedy L, *et al.* Serum cortisol concentrations during low dose dexamethasone suppression test to screen for Cushing's syndrome. *BMJ* 1984; **289:** 1188–91.
3. Tyrrell JB, *et al.* An overnight high-dose dexamethasone suppression test for rapid differential diagnosis of Cushing's syndrome. *Ann Intern Med* 1986; **104:** 180–6.
4. Biemond P, *et al.* Continuous dexamethasone infusion for seven hours in patients with the Cushing syndrome: a superior differential diagnostic test. *Ann Intern Med* 1990; **112:** 738–42.
5. Yanovski JA, *et al.* Corticotropin-releasing hormone stimulation following low-dose dexamethasone administration: a new test to distinguish Cushing's syndrome from pseudo-Cushing's states. *JAMA* 1993; **269:** 2232–8.
6. Avgerinos PC, *et al.* The metyrapone and dexamethasone suppression tests for the differential diagnosis of the adrenocorticotropin-dependent Cushing syndrome: a comparison. *Ann Intern Med* 1994; **121:** 318–27.
7. Raff H, Findling JW. A physiologic approach to diagnosis of the Cushing syndrome. *Ann Intern Med* 2003; **138:** 980–91.

DEPRESSION. The Health and Public Policy Committee of the American College of Physicians noted that the dexamethasone suppression test for depression (p.279) was based on the premise that endogenously depressed patients have shown pituitary-adrenal axis abnormalities but had been found to have a low sensitivity for detecting depression. It was of unproven value and was not recommended as a screening test.[1]

1. Young M, Schwartz JS. The dexamethasone suppression test for the detection, diagnosis, and management of depression. *Ann Intern Med* 1984; **100:** 307–8.

**High-altitude disorders.** Dexamethasone is effective in the prevention of symptoms of acute mountain sickness (p.822), for which mild cerebral oedema may be a contributing factor, but it is not generally considered suitable for routine prophylaxis because of concern about its adverse effects. In the treatment of acute severe mountain sickness, which may involve the development of pulmonary and cerebral oedema, the mandatory treatment is immediate descent, and drug therapy is primarily adjunctive, to facilitate descent or maintain the patient until descent is possible. Under these circumstances dexamethasone and oxygen form the mainstays of treatment.

References.

1. Ferrazzini G, *et al.* Successful treatment of acute mountain sickness with dexamethasone. *BMJ* 1987; **294:** 1380–2.
2. Ellsworth AJ, *et al.* A randomized trial of dexamethasone and acetazolamide for acute mountain sickness prophylaxis. *Am J Med* 1987; **83:** 1024–30.
3. Montgomery AB, *et al.* Effects of dexamethasone on the incidence of acute mountain sickness at two intermediate altitudes. *JAMA* 1989; **261:** 734–6.
4. Levine BD, *et al.* Dexamethasone in the treatment of acute mountain sickness. *N Engl J Med* 1989; **321:** 1707–13.
5. Keller H-R, *et al.* Simulated descent v dexamethasone in treatment of acute mountain sickness: a randomised trial. *BMJ* 1995; **310:** 1232–5.
6. Dumont L, *et al.* Efficacy and harm of pharmacological prevention of acute mountain sickness: quantitative systematic review. *BMJ* 2000; **321:** 267–72.

**Hirsutism.** Unbound testosterone concentrations were consistently elevated in 32 hirsute women; when concentrations were suppressed to normal by dexamethasone 0.5 to 1 mg at night hirsutism was generally improved or ceased to progress after 8 to 10 months of treatment.[1] Other studies have shown only a modest improvement[2] or no improvement at all[3] in hirsutism when treated with dexamethasone. Addition of dexamethasone to anti-androgen therapy appeared to prolong the duration of remission in a later study.[4]

The mainstay of drug treatment for hirsutism tends to be an anti-androgen such as cyproterone or spironolactone (p.1545). Although low dose corticosteroids can suppress adrenal androgen production, careful consideration of the risks and benefits is advisable, especially since therapy for hirsutism may have to be given long-term.

1. Paulson JD, *et al.* Free testosterone concentration in serum: elevation is the hallmark of hirsutism. *Am J Obstet Gynecol* 1977; **128:** 851–7.
2. Carmina E, Lobo RA. Peripheral androgen blockade versus glandular androgen suppression in the treatment of hirsutism. *Obstet Gynecol* 1991; **78:** 845.
3. Rittmaster RS, Thompson DL. Effect of leuprolide and dexamethasone on hair growth and hormone levels in hirsute women: the relative importance of the ovary and the adrenal in the pathogenesis of hirsutism. *J Clin Endocrinol Metab* 1990; **70:** 1096–1102.
4. Carmina E, Lobo RA. The addition of dexamethasone to antiandrogen therapy for hirsutism prolongs the duration of remission. *Fertil Steril* 1998; **69:** 1075–9.

**Malaria.** Corticosteroids, especially dexamethasone, have been used in cerebral malaria (p.444) in the belief that their anti-inflammatory effect would reduce cerebral oedema. However, studies have shown that cerebral oedema does not play a significant role in the pathophysiology of cerebral malaria and, indeed, double-blind studies using both moderate doses (2 mg/kg) and high doses (11 mg/kg) of dexamethasone intravenously over 48 hours found no reduction in death rates. Thus it is now considered that corticosteroids have no place in the treatment of cerebral malaria.[1]

1. Prasad K, Garner P. Steroids for treating cerebral malaria. Available in The Cochrane Library; Issue 1. Chichester: John Wiley; 2004.

**Malignant neoplasms.** Dexamethasone has been used in some regimens for the treatment of malignancy, for example in acute lymphoblastic leukaemia (p.506) and multiple myeloma (p.511).

**Meningitis.** The role of corticosteroids in the adjuvant treatment of bacterial meningitis (p.134) has been the subject of considerable debate.[1,2] However, a systematic review[3] has concluded that there is evidence of benefit, particularly in reducing deafness in children, and in reducing mortality in adults. It has been suggested[3] that a 4-day regimen of dexamethasone be given, preferably before or with the first dose of antibacterial.

1. Molyneux EM, *et al.* Dexamethasone treatment in childhood bacterial meningitis in Malawi: a randomised controlled trial. *Lancet* 2002; **360:** 211–18.
2. de Gans J, van de Beek D. Dexamethasone in adults with bacterial meningitis. *N Engl J Med* 2002; **347:** 1549–56.
3. van de Beek D, *et al.* Corticosteroids in acute bacterial meningitis. Available in The Cochrane Library; Issue 1. Chichester: John Wiley; 2004.

**Nausea and vomiting.** Dexamethasone has antiemetic properties, particularly against acute and delayed vomiting induced by cancer chemotherapy[1] (p.1245). It may be used alone for prevention of acute symptoms associated with moderately-emetogenic treatment and is combined with a 5-$HT_3$ antagonist for highly-emetogenic treatment. Typical dosage regimens have been dexamethasone 4 to 8 mg by mouth immediately before moderately-emetogenic chemotherapy and 20 mg by intravenous injection for more severely emetogenic chemotherapy. Dexamethasone is the drug of choice for prevention of delayed symptoms, given alone or in combination with other antiemetics. A typical dose is 8 mg twice daily by mouth for 2 to 4 days. Dexamethasone is also effective for the prevention of postoperative nausea and vomiting.[2]

1. Ioannidis JPA, *et al.* Contribution of dexamethasone to control of chemotherapy-induced nausea and vomiting: a meta-analysis of randomized evidence. *J Clin Oncol* 2000; **18:** 3409–22.
2. Henzi I, *et al.* Dexamethasone for the prevention of postoperative nausea and vomiting: a quantitative systematic review. *Anesth Analg* 2000; **90:** 186–94.

**Opportunistic mycobacterial infections.** Dexamethasone in doses of 1 to 4 mg daily was associated with weight gain, reduction in fever, and an improved sense of well-being in 5 patients with HIV and disseminated *Mycobacterium avium* complex infection.[1] Combination antimycobacterial therapy for opportunistic mycobacterial infections (p.137) was also given. Similar results have been noted by others.[2]

1. Wormser GP, *et al.* Low-dose dexamethasone as adjunctive therapy for disseminated Mycobacterium avium complex infections in AIDS patients. *Antimicrob Agents Chemother* 1994; **38:** 2215–17.
2. Dorman SE, *et al.* Adjunctive corticosteroid therapy for patients whose treatment for disseminated Mycobacterium avium complex infection has failed. *Clin Infect Dis* 1998; **26:** 682–6.

**Respiratory disorders.** Corticosteroids such as dexamethasone have been given antenatally to mothers at risk of premature delivery in order to hasten fetal lung maturation and help prevent *neonatal respiratory distress syndrome* (p.1084) and *bronchopulmonary dysplasia* (p.1077). Neonatal dexamethasone has been reported to improve pulmonary outcome and assist weaning from mechanical ventilation in infants that have developed bronchopulmonary dysplasia.

Dexamethasone is also one of the drugs of choice for the management of severe *croup* (see p.1079). However, as with other corticosteroids (p.1077) it appears to be of little value in *bronchiolitis*.[1,2]

1. Roosevelt G, *et al.* Dexamethasone in bronchiolitis: a randomised controlled trial. *Lancet* 1996; **348:** 292–5.
2. Klassen TP, *et al.* Dexamethasone in salbutamol-treated inpatients with acute bronchiolitis: a randomized controlled trial. *J Pediatr* 1997; **130:** 191–6.

**Retinopathy of prematurity.** For a suggestion that antenatal dexamethasone might be helpful in the prophylaxis of retinopathy of prematurity, see p.1466. For mention of the uncertain effect of neonatal dexamethasone on retinopathy of prematurity, see under Adverse Effects above.

**Status epilepticus.** Dexamethasone is used in some patients with status epilepticus (for example when associated with cerebral neoplasms) as mentioned on p.352.

## Preparations

***BP 2003:*** Dexamethasone Sodium Phosphate Injection; Dexamethasone Tablets;
***USP 27:*** Dexamethasone Acetate Injectable Suspension; Dexamethasone Elixir; Dexamethasone Gel; Dexamethasone Ophthalmic Suspension; Dexamethasone Oral Solution; Dexamethasone Sodium Phosphate Cream; Dexamethasone Sodium Phosphate Inhalation Aerosol; Dexamethasone Sodium Phosphate Injection; Dexamethasone Sodium Phosphate Ophthalmic Ointment; Dexamethasone Sodium Phosphate Ophthalmic Solution; Dexamethasone Tablets; Dexamethasone Topical Aerosol; Neomycin and Polymyxin B Sulfates and Dexamethasone Ophthalmic Ointment; Neomycin and Polymyxin B Sulfates and Dexamethasone Ophthalmic Suspension; Neomycin Sulfate and Dexamethasone Sodium Phosphate Cream; Neomycin Sulfate and Dexamethasone Sodium Phosphate Ophthalmic Ointment; Neomycin Sulfate and Dexamethasone Sodium Phosphate Ophthalmic Solution; Tobramycin and Dexamethasone Ophthalmic Ointment; Tobramycin and Dexamethasone Ophthalmic Suspension.

**Proprietary Preparations** (details are given in Part 3)
***Arg.:*** Decadron; Degabina; Dexafarm; Dexalergin; Dexameral; Duo Decadron; Fadametasona; Gotabiotic D; Isopto Maxidex; Lormine; Nexadron; Sedesterol; Trofinan; ***Austral.:*** Decadron†; Dexmethsone; Maxidex; ***Austria:*** Dexabene; Fortecortin; ***Belg.:*** Aacidexam; Decadron; Maxidex; Oradexon; ***Braz.:*** Decadron; Decadronal; Deflaren; Dexadermil; Dexaflan; Dexameson; Dexametax†; Dexametonal; Dexaminor; Dexanil; Dexason; Dexazen; Dexazona; Dextasona; Maxidex; Minidex; Neodex; Topidexa; Uni Dexametason; ***Canad.:*** Decadron; Dexasone; Diodex; Hexadrol; Maxidex; ***Chile:*** Maxidex; Oradexon; ***Denm.:*** Decadron; Maxidex; ***Fin.:*** Decadron; Oftan Dexa; Oradexon; ***Fr.:*** Cebedex†; Decadron†; Dectancyl; Desocort; Maxidex; Soludecadron†; ***Ger.:*** afpred-DEXA; Anemul mono†; Auxiloson; Cortidexason; Cortisumman; Decadron Phosphat†; Dexa; Dexa in der Ophtiole†; Dexa Loscon mono; Dexa-Allvoran; Dexa-Brachialin N†; dexa-clinit; Dexa-Effekton; Dexa-ratiopharm; Dexa-Rhinospray M; Dexa-sine; Dexabene; DexaEDO; Dexaflam N; Dexaflam†; Dexagalen†; Dexagel; Dexahexal; Dexamonozon; Dexamonozon N; Dexapos; Fortecortin; Isopto Dex; Lipotalon; Predni-F-Tablinen†; Solupen N; Solutio Cordes Dexa N; Spersadex; Totocortin; Tuttozem N†; ***Gr.:*** Clenil; Decadron; Dexacollyre; Iriniozol; Maxidex; Oradexon; Soldesanil; Thilodexine; Thiloxedine; ***Hong Kong:*** Decadron†; Dexalocal†; Dexamed; Dexasone; Dexmethsone; Limethason†; Maxidex; Spersadex; ***India:*** Decdan; Dexona; Millicortenol; Wymesone; ***Irl.:*** Decadron; Maxidex; ***Israel:*** Dexacort; Maxidex; Sterodex; ***Ital.:*** Decadron; Dermadex; Desalark†; Eta Cortilen†; Luxazone; Megacort; Soldesam; Visumetazone; ***Jpn:*** Limethason; ***Malaysia:*** Cortidax; Decadron; Decan; Dexalone; Dexaltin; Dexasone; Limethason; Maxidex; ***Mex.:*** Adrecort; Alin; Azona†; Beamoken A†; Bexine; Cortidex; Cryometasona; Decadron; Decadronal; Decorex; Dexagrin; Dexatam†; Dexicar; Dexona†; Dibasona; Indarzona-N; Metax; Mexona†; Polideltaxin; Reusan†; Taprodex; Taxyl; ***Neth.:*** Decadron; Dexa-POS†; Oradexon; ***Norw.:*** Decadron; Isopto Maxidex; Spersadex; ***NZ:*** Decadron†; Maxidex; ***Port.:*** Decadron; Dexaval; Oradexon; Ronic; ***S.Afr.:*** Decadron; Decasone; Maxidex; Oradexon; Spersadex; ***Singapore:*** Dexaltin; Dexamed†; Dexasone; Erladexone; Limethason; Maxidex; Mexasone; ***Spain:*** Dalamon Inyectable; Decadran†; Fortecortin; Maxidex; ***Swed.:*** Decadron; Dexacortal; Isopto Maxidex; Opnol; ***Switz.:*** Decadron; Dexa-Helvacort†; Dexacortin; Dexalocal; Fortecortin; Maxidex; Mephamesone; Millicortene; Oradexon†; Spersadex; ***Thai.:*** Decadron; Dexa; Dexa ANB; Dexa-P; Dexacortisone†; Dexaltin; Dexano; Dexasone; Dexon; Dexthasol; Dexton; Limethason; Oradexon; ***UK:*** Decadron; Dexsol; Maxidex; ***USA:*** Aeroseb-Dex; Ak-Dex†; Dalalone; Decadron; Decaject†; Decaspray; Dexacort†; Dexameth; Dexasone; DexPak; Hexadrol; Maxidex; Solurex.

**Multi-ingredient:** ***Arg.:*** Alergi; Belbar; Bio Cabal; Bioptic DX; Biotaer Ultrason Nebulizable; Ciprocort; Cortaler Novo; Decadron con Neomicina; Dexa Aminoflin; Dexa Teosona; Dexa-Rhinospray N; Dexabion; Dexafurazon; Dexalergin; Dexaprof D; Dexatopic; Empecid Cort; Factoneye; Flexicamin B12; Flogiatrin B12; Fluoropoen; Gotabiotic F; Isoptomax; Larsen; Linfol; Mefenix Relax; Melasmax; Naxo TV; Neodexa Plus; Neoftalm Dexa; Neosona; Nexadron Compuesto; Nipiol; Paraflex Plus; Polioftal; Proetztotal; Provisual Compuesto; Radina Dex; Sincerum Biotic; Sincerum Biotic L; Sindrolen; Solocalm Plus; Tobradex; Toflamixina Plus; Vixidone; Vixidone T; Xao-Dex; ***Austral.:*** Otodex; Sofradex; ***Austria:*** Ambene; Dexagenta; Dexasalyl; Doxiproct mit Dexamethason; Endomethazone†; Multodrin; Rheumesser; Tobradex; Uromont; ***Belg.:*** De Icin; De Icol; Decadron avec Neomycine†; Dexa-Rhinospray; Maxitrol; Neodexon†; Percutalgine; Polaronil†; Polydexa; Tobradex; ***Braz.:*** Baycuten; Biamotil-D; Cianotrat-Dexa; Cilodex; Decadron Nasal; Decadron Oftalmico; Dermazon†; Dermogen†; Dexa-Citoneurin; Dexa-Cronobe; Dexa-Neuriberi; Dexa-Vastrictol†; Dexaclor; Dexacloran†; Dexacobal; Dexacort; Dexador; Dexadoze; Dexafenicol; Dexagil; Dexalgen; Dexamytrex; Dexaneurin; Dexanevral; Dexanil; Dexavison; Dexazona; Duo-Decadron; Emistin; Fenidex; Gynax-N; Hidrocin; Maxitrol; Metcort; Neocortin; Neodex; Oftcor†; Orlamix†; Otofenicol-D; Rinosbon; Tobracort; Tobradex; Trivagel N; Vagitrin-N; Vibetrat Dexa†; Vitatonus Dexa; ***Canad.:*** Dioptrol; Maxitrol; NeoDecadron†; Sofracort; Tobradex; ***Chile:*** Baycuten; Ciprodex; Grifoftal-D; Maxitrol; Poentobral Plus; Spersadex Comp; Telugren Plus; Tobradex; Tobrin-D; Todexona; Tribesona; Xolof D; ***Denm.:*** Decadron med Neomycin; Sofradex; Spersadex Comp; ***Fin.:*** Dexatopic†; Maxitrol; Oftan Dexa-Chlora; Otomize†; Sofradex; ***Fr.:*** Auricularum; Cebedexacol; Chibro-Cadron; Corticetine; Dexagrane; Frakidex; Framyxone; Maxidrol; Percutalgine; Polydexa; Polydexa a la Phenylephrine†; Ster-Dex; Tobradex; ***Ger.:*** Baycuten; Chibro-Cadron†; Corti Biciron N; Cortidexason comp; Corto-Tavegil; Dexa Biciron; Dexa Polyspectran; Dexa-Gentamicin; Dexa-Phlogont L; Dexa-Rhinospray N†; Dexa-Siozwo; Dexacrinin†; Dexamytrex; Dexasalyl†; Dispadex comp; Duodexa N; Ell-Cranell dexa; Ell-Cranell†; Isopto Max; Lokalison-antimikrobiell Creme N; Magopsor†; Millicorten-Vioform†; Nystalocal; Otobacid N; Rheumasit; Rhinoguttae Dexamethasoni cum Naphazolino; Solupen-D†; Spersadex Comp; Spersadexolin; Supertendin 2000 N; Supertendin-Depot; Ultra-Demoplas; Uro-Stilloson; ***Hong Kong:*** Chloram-D; Colircusi Gentadexa†; Decadron with Neomycin†; Dexa-Polyspectran†; Dexasalyl†; Dexoph; Dextracin; Frakidex; Maxitrol; Neo-Dex (Improved); Oftalmolosa Cusi de Icol†; Parasone; Sofradex; Spersadex Comp; Spersadexoline; Tobradex; Trabit†; ***India:*** Decdan-N; Dexona Eye/Ear; Dexosyn-C; Dexosyn-N; Millicorten-Vioform; Mycidex; Ocupol-D; Pyrimon; Sofracort; Sofradex; Sofradex-F; Tobazon; ***Irl.:*** Dexa-Rhinaspray Duo; Dexa-Rhinaspray†; Maxitrol; Otomize; Sofradex; ***Israel:*** Adexone; Auricularum; Desoren; Dethamycin; Dethaphrine; Dex-Otic; Dexamycin; Dexefrin; Maxitrol; Otomize; Polycutan; Tarocidin D; Tevacutan; ***Ital.:*** Antimicotico†; Cloradex; Corti-Arscolloid; Desalfa; Desamix Effe; Desamix-Neomicina; Dexoline; Doxiproct; Eta Biocortilen; Eta Biocortilen VC; Fluorobioptal†; Kanazone†; Lasoproct†; Luxazone Eparina; Nasicortin†; Neo Cortofen; Rinedrone†; Tobradex; Visumetazone Antistaminico; Visumetazone Decongestionante; ***Malaysia:*** Baycuten N; De Icol; Dexa-Gentamicin; Dexamytrex Ophtiole; Dextracin; Gentadexa; Maxitrol; Neo-Deca; Sofradex; Spersadex Comp; Spersadexoline; Tobradex; ***Mex.:*** Alin Nasal; Alin Oftalmico; Baycuten N; Biodexan; Decadron con Neomicina; Decadron con Nistatina; Dexabion; Dexafrin; Dexamicin; Dexne; Dexsul; Exafenil; Gotadex; Kodakon; Levodexan; Levofenil; Maxitrol; Neobacigrin; Neuralin; Obrydex; Soldrin; Tiamidexal; Tobradex; Trazidex; Vengesic; Zolidime; ***Neth.:*** Decadron met neomycine; Dexagenta-POS†; Dexamytrex; Dexatopic†; Sofradex; ***Norw.:*** Maxitrol; Sofradex; Spersadex med kloramfenikol; ***NZ:*** Maxitrol; Sofradex; Tobradex; ***Port.:*** Baycuten; Decadron com Neomicina; Dexamytrex; Dexaval A; Dexaval N; Dexaval O; Dexaval V; Frakidex; Gentadexa; Polydexa; ***S.Afr.:*** Covomycin-D; Maxitrol; Sofradex; Spersadex Comp; Spersadexoline; Tobradex; ***Singapore:*** Dexamytrex; Dextracin; Frakidex; Maxitrol; Neo-Deca†; Neo-Dex (Improved)†; Polydexa; Sofradex; Spersadex Comp; Spersadexoline; Tobradex; ***Spain:*** Amplidermis; Broncoformo Muco Dexa; Cloram Hemidexa; Cresophene; Dalamon; Decadran Neomicina; Dexa Fenic†; Dexa Tavegil; Dexa Vasoc†; Dexafenicol†; Dexam Constric; Gentadexa; Hem Anth; Hongosan; Icol; Inzitan; Liquipom Dexa Antib; Liquipom Dexa Const†; Liquipom Dexamida†; Maxitrol; Neodexa; Neurocatavin Dexa; Neurodavur Plus; Oftalmol Dexa†; Oftalmotrim Dexa; Otix; Oto Vitna; Percutalin†; Phonal; Resorborina; Rino Dexa; Rinoblanco Dexa Antibio†; Sabanotropico; Sedofarin; Talkosona†; Tobradex; Vasodexa; ***Swed.:*** Decadron cum neomycin; Sofradex†; ***Switz.:*** Antikeloides Creme; Chronocorte; Corticetine; Cresophene; Dexacortin-K; Dexalocal-F; Dexasalyl; Dexolan; Doxiproct Plus; Frakidex; Maxitrol; Nystalocal; Otospray; Pigmanorm; Polydexa; Pulpomixine†; Sebo-Psor; Sofradex; Spersadex Comp; Spersadexoline; Tobradex; ***Thai.:*** Archidex; Cadexcin-N; Decadron with Neomycin; Dex-Otic†; Dexacin; Dexamytrex; Dexasil; Dexoph; Dexylin; Eyedex; Maxitrol; Neo-Optal; Neodex; Opsardex; Percutalgine; Sofradex; Spersadexoline; Tobradex; Trabit; ***UK:*** Dexa-Rhinaspray Duo; Maxitrol; Otomize; Sofradex; Tobradex; ***USA:*** Ak-Neo-Dex; Ak-Trol; Ciprodex; Dexacidin; Dexacine; Dexasporin; Maxitrol; Neo-Dexameth; NeoDecadron; Neodexasone; Neopolydex; Ocu-Trol; Poly-Dex; Tobradex.

## Dichlorisone Acetate *(rINNM)*

Acetato de diclorisona; Diclorisone Acetate. 9α,11β-Dichloro-17α,21-dihydroxypregna-1,4-diene-3,20-dione 21-acetate.

$C_{23}H_{28}Cl_2O_5$ = 455.4.
*CAS — 7008-26-6 (dichlorisone); 79-61-8 (dichlorisone acetate).*

### Profile

Dichlorisone acetate is a corticosteroid used topically for its glucocorticoid activity (p.1068) in the treatment of various skin disorders. It is usually employed as a cream or ointment containing 0.25 to 1%.

When applied topically, particularly to large areas, when the skin is broken, or under occlusive dressings, corticosteroids may be absorbed in sufficient amounts to cause systemic effects (see p.1068). The effects of topical corticosteroids on the skin are described on p.1070. For recommendations concerning the correct use of corticosteroids on the skin, see p.1074.

### Preparations

**Proprietary Preparations** (details are given in Part 3)
***Spain:*** Dermaren; Dicloderm Forte.

## Diflorasone Diacetate *(BANM, USAN, rINNM)*

Diacetato de diflorasona; U-34865. 6α,9α-Difluoro-11β,17α,21-trihydroxy-16β-methylpregna-1,4-diene-3,20-dione 17,21-diacetate.

$C_{26}H_{32}F_2O_7$ = 494.5.
*CAS — 2557-49-5 (diflorasone); 33564-31-7 (diflorasone diacetate).*
*ATC — D07AC10.*

**Pharmacopoeias.** In *US.*

**USP 27** (Diflorasone Diacetate). A white to pale yellow, crystalline powder. Insoluble in water; soluble in acetone and in methyl alcohol; very slightly soluble in ether; sparingly soluble in ethyl acetate; slightly soluble in toluene. Store in airtight containers.

### Profile

Diflorasone diacetate is a corticosteroid used topically for its glucocorticoid activity (p.1068) in the treatment of various skin disorders. It is usually employed as a cream or ointment containing 0.05%.

When applied topically, particularly to large areas, when the skin is broken, or under occlusive dressings, corticosteroids may be absorbed in sufficient amounts to cause systemic effects (p.1068). The effects of topical corticosteroids on the skin are described on p.1070. For recommendations concerning the correct use of corticosteroids on the skin, and a rough guide to the clinical potencies of topical corticosteroids, see p.1074.

### Preparations

***USP 27:*** Diflorasone Diacetate Cream; Diflorasone Diacetate Ointment.

**Proprietary Preparations** (details are given in Part 3)
***Canad.:*** Florone†; ***Ger.:*** Florone; ***Ital.:*** Dermaflor; Sterodelta†; ***Spain:*** Murode; ***USA:*** ApexiCon; Florone; Maxiflor; Psorcon.

**Multi-ingredient:** ***Arg.:*** Filoderma; Filoderma Plus; Griseocrem; Novo Bacticort; Novo Bacticort Complex.

## Diflucortolone *(BAN, USAN, rINN)*

6α,9α-Difluoro-11β,21-dihydroxy-16α-methylpregna-1,4-diene-3,20-dione.

$C_{22}H_{28}F_2O_4$ = 394.5.
*CAS — 2607-06-9.*
*ATC — D07AC06.*

## Diflucortolone Pivalate *(BANM, USAN)*

SH-968. Diflucortolone 21-pivalate.

$C_{27}H_{36}F_2O_5$ = 478.6.
*CAS — 15845-96-2.*
*ATC — D07AC06.*

## Diflucortolone Valerate *(BANM, rINNM)*

Valerato de diflucortolona. Diflucortolone 21-valerate.

$C_{27}H_{36}F_2O_5$ = 478.6.
*CAS — 59198-70-8.*
*ATC — D07AC06.*

**Pharmacopoeias.** In *Br.*

**BP 2003** (Diflucortolone Valerate). A white to creamy white crystalline powder. Practically insoluble in water; freely soluble in dichloromethane and in dioxan; sparingly soluble in ether; slightly soluble in methyl alcohol. Protect from light.

### Profile

Diflucortolone is a corticosteroid used topically for its glucocorticoid activity (p.1068) in the treatment of various skin disorders. It is usually employed as a cream or ointment containing 0.1 or 0.3% of the valerate.

When applied topically, particularly to large areas, when the skin is broken, or under occlusive dressings, corticosteroids may be absorbed in sufficient amounts to cause systemic effects (p.1068). The effects of topical corticosteroids on the skin are described on p.1070. For recommendations concerning the correct use of corticosteroids on the skin, and a rough guide to the clinical potencies of topical corticosteroids, see p.1074.

### Preparations

***BP 2003:*** Diflucortolone Cream; Diflucortolone Oily Cream; Diflucortolone Ointment.

**Proprietary Preparations** (details are given in Part 3)
***Arg.:*** Nerisona; ***Austria:*** Neriforte; Nerisona; ***Belg.:*** Nerisona; ***Braz.:*** Nerisona; ***Canad.:*** Nerisone; ***Denm.:*** Nerisona; ***Fr.:*** Nerisone; ***Ger.:*** Nerisona; ***Hong Kong:*** Nerisone; ***Israel:*** Neriderm; ***Ital.:*** Cortical; Dermaval; Dervin; Dicortal; Flu-Cortanest; Nerisona; Temetex; ***Malaysia:*** Nerisone; ***Mex.:*** Nerisona; ***Neth.:*** Nerisona; ***NZ:*** Nerisone; ***Port.:*** Nerisona; ***S.Afr.:*** Nerisone; ***Singapore:*** Nerisone; ***Spain:*** Claral; ***Switz.:*** Nerisona; ***UK:*** Nerisone.

**Multi-ingredient:** ***Arg.:*** Nerisona C; Scheriderm; ***Austria:*** Neriquinol†; Travocort; ***Belg.:*** Travocort; ***Braz.:*** Bi-Nerisona; ***Canad.:*** Nerisalic; ***Chile:*** Bi-Nerisona; ***Fr.:*** Nerisalic; Nerisone C; ***Ger.:*** Nerisona C; Travocort; ***Gr.:*** Travocort; ***Hong Kong:*** Nerisone C; Travocort; ***Irl.:*** Travocort; ***Israel:*** Isocort; Multiderm; ***Ital.:*** Corti-Fluoral; Dermaflogil; Dermobios†; Impetex; Nerisona C; Travocort; ***Malaysia:*** Isoradin; Travocort; ***Mex.:*** Bi-Nerisona; Scheriderm; ***NZ:*** Nerisone C; ***Port.:*** Nerisona C; Travocort; ***S.Afr.:*** Travocort; ***Singapore:*** Nerisone C; Travocort; ***Spain:*** Claral Plus; ***Switz.:*** Travocort; ***Thai.:*** Travocort.

## Difluprednate *(USAN, rINN)*

CM-9155; Difluprednato; W-6309. 6α,9α-Difluoro-11β,17α,21-trihydroxypregna-1,4-diene-3,20-dione 21-acetate 17-butyrate.
$C_{27}H_{34}F_2O_7$ = 508.6.
*CAS — 23674-86-4.*
*ATC — D07AC19.*

### Profile

Difluprednate is a corticosteroid used topically for its glucocorticoid activity (p.1068) in the treatment of various skin disorders. It is usually employed as a cream, gel, or ointment; concentrations used range from 0.02 to 0.05%.

When applied topically, particularly to large areas, when the skin is broken, or under occlusive dressings, corticosteroids may be absorbed in sufficient amounts to cause systemic effects (p.1068). The effects of topical corticosteroids on the skin are described on p.1070. For recommendations concerning the correct use of corticosteroids on the skin, see p.1074.

### Preparations

**Proprietary Preparations** (details are given in Part 3)
***Fr.:*** Epitopic; ***Jpn:*** Myser.

## Fluclorolone Acetonide *(BAN, rINN)*

Acetónido de fluclorolona; Flucloronide *(USAN)*; RS-2252. 9α,11β-Dichloro-6α-fluoro-21-hydroxy-16α,17α-isopropylidenedioxypregna-1,4-diene-3,20-dione.
$C_{24}H_{29}Cl_2FO_5$ = 487.4.
*CAS — 3693-39-8.*
*ATC — D07AC02.*

### Profile

Fluclorolone acetonide is a corticosteroid used topically for its glucocorticoid activity (p.1068) in the treatment of various skin disorders. It is usually employed as a cream or ointment containing 0.2%.

When applied topically, particularly to large areas, when the skin is broken, or under occlusive dressings, corticosteroids may be absorbed in sufficient amounts to cause systemic effects (p.1068). The effects of topical corticosteroids on the skin are described on p.1070. For recommendations concerning the correct use of corticosteroids on the skin, and a rough guide to the clinical potencies of topical corticosteroids, see p.1074.

### Preparations

**Proprietary Preparations** (details are given in Part 3)
***Spain:*** Cutanit.

# Fludrocortisone Acetate *(BANM, rINNM)*

Acetato de fludrocortisona; Fludrocortisoni Acetas; 9α-Fluorohydrocortisone 21-Acetate. 9α-Fluoro-11β,17α,21-trihydroxypregn-4-ene-3,20-dione 21-acetate.
$C_{23}H_{31}FO_6$ = 422.5.
*CAS — 127-31-1 (fludrocortisone); 514-36-3 (fludrocortisone acetate).*
*ATC — H02AA02.*

**Pharmacopoeias.** In *Chin., Eur.* (see p.vi), *Int., Pol.,* and *US.*

**Ph. Eur. 5.0** (Fludrocortisone Acetate). A white or almost white, crystalline powder. Practically insoluble in water; sparingly soluble in dehydrated alcohol.

**USP 27** (Fludrocortisone Acetate). White to pale yellow, odourless or practically odourless, hygroscopic, crystals or crystalline powder. Insoluble in water; sparingly soluble in alcohol and in chloroform; slightly soluble in ether. Protect from light.

## Adverse Effects, Treatment, Withdrawal, and Precautions

Fludrocortisone acetate has glucocorticoid actions about 10 times as potent as hydrocortisone and mineralocorticoid effects more than 100 times as potent. Adverse effects are mainly those due to mineralocorticoid activity, as described on p.1068.

When applied topically, particularly to large areas, when the skin is broken, or under occlusive dressings, corticosteroids may be absorbed in sufficient amounts to cause systemic effects. Prolonged application to the eye of preparations containing corticosteroids has caused raised intra-ocular pressure and reduced visual function.

## Interactions

The interactions of corticosteroids in general are described on p.1072.

## Pharmacokinetics

For a brief outline of the pharmacokinetics of corticosteroids, see p.1073.

Fludrocortisone is readily absorbed from the gastrointestinal tract. The plasma half-life is about 3.5 hours or more, but fludrocortisone exhibits a more prolonged biological half-life of 18 to 36 hours.

## Uses and Administration

Fludrocortisone is a corticosteroid with glucocorticoid and highly potent mineralocorticoid activity (p.1068).

Fludrocortisone acetate is given by mouth to provide mineralocorticoid replacement in primary adrenocortical insufficiency (p.1075), together with glucocorticoids. It is used in a dose range of 50 to 300 micrograms daily.

Fludrocortisone acetate may also be given concomitantly with glucocorticoid therapy in doses of up to 200 micrograms daily in the salt-losing form of congenital adrenal hyperplasia (p.1078).

It is also given by mouth in the management of severe orthostatic hypotension (see below).

Fludrocortisone acetate is applied topically to the skin, eye, and ear for its glucocorticoid actions in the treatment of various disorders. It is used as an ingredient of cream, lotion, ointment, gel, or drops, usually in a concentration of 0.1%. For recommendations concerning the correct use of corticosteroids on the skin, see p.1074.

**Administration.** A study of fludrocortisone requirements in 10 patients with Addison's disease indicated that dosage was often inadequate.[1] Nine were initially on fludrocortisone 50 to 100 micrograms daily in addition to cortisone or hydrocortisone; 5 were also taking levothyroxine for an associated auto-immune thyroid disease; one, who had detectable levels of aldosterone, was not initially receiving fludrocortisone. All the patients had evidence of sodium and water depletion and initiation of fludrocortisone 300 micrograms daily, with downwards adjustments, demonstrated that most patients required 200 micrograms daily. Two patients elected to remain on 300 micrograms daily, but in most this dose caused pronounced sodium and water retention. The patient with detectable aldosterone levels required 50 micrograms daily. Eight of the 10 patients felt better on the higher fludrocortisone doses while 2 felt no change.

1. Smith SJ, *et al.* Evidence that patients with Addison's disease are undertreated with fludrocortisone. *Lancet* 1984; **i:** 11–14.

**Neurally mediated hypotension.** Fludrocortisone is reported to be one of the standard drugs used in the management of neurally mediated hypotension (see p.828).

**Orthostatic hypotension.** Orthostatic (postural) hypotension[1-6] is a fall in blood pressure that occurs upon rising abruptly to an erect position, although it may also occur following a period of prolonged standing. Characteristic symptoms include lightheadedness, dizziness, blurred vision, weakness in the limbs, and syncope.

The causes of orthostatic hypotension are wide-ranging and include autonomic dysfunction, such as in the Shy-Drager syndrome, diabetes mellitus, and Parkinson's disease, circulating volume depletion, phaeochromocytoma, and Addison's disease. Orthostatic hypotension may also occur following a period of prolonged bed rest or following meals.

Orthostatic hypotension may result from the adverse effects of a range of drugs, such as antihypertensives, diuretics, tricyclic antidepressants, phenothiazines, and MAOIs.

In mild cases **nonpharmacological treatment** alone may be adequate. This includes increasing salt intake if not contra-indicated, maintaining adequate hydration, the use of elastic stockings to improve venous return and increase cardiac output, and elevating the head of the bed to reduce early morning symptoms. Drug-induced orthostatic hypotension should be treated by withdrawing the drug or by dose reduction.

**Pharmacological treatment**. No pharmacological treatment is entirely satisfactory: responses and tolerance vary greatly between patients. Fludrocortisone acetate is usually tried first; it increases sodium retention and thus plasma volume. Most reports indicate some response in about 80% of patients, but hypokalaemia, fluid retention, and supine hypertension may limit its use. In patients who fail to respond adequately an NSAID (usually indometacin) may be tried, alone or with fludrocortisone. In patients with overt autonomic failure a beta blocker with some partial agonist activity, such as xamoterol or pindolol, may be tried although they are potentially dangerous.

Sympathomimetics may be useful in some patients with autonomic failure; the direct acting drugs such as phenylephrine or midodrine are usually more consistently effective than the indirect such as ephedrine, but even so, responses tend to vary with the degree of denervation. Ambulatory noradrenaline infusion therapy is under investigation for severe refractory orthostatic hypotension. Patients with central neurological abnormalities may respond to desmopressin, while drugs such as ergotamine or dihydroergotamine may be useful for resistant disease.

Other drugs that have been tried include metoclopramide, which may be useful for autonomic symptoms in patients with diabetes mellitus, fluoxetine, octreotide, yohimbine, clonidine, and in patients with concurrent anaemia, erythropoietin. Caffeine has been tried in postprandial hypotension but its value in all but the mildest cases is dubious.[5] The use of MAOIs (which given alone can induce orthostatic hypotension) with a sympathomimetic to induce a pressor reaction is controversial. Most of these drugs have potentially serious adverse effects and few are well evaluated.

1. Ahmad RAS, Watson RDS. Treatment of postural hypotension: a review. *Drugs* 1990; **39:** 74–85.
2. Tonkin AL, Wing LMH. Hypotension: assessment and management. *Med J Aust* 1990; **153:** 474–85.
3. Schoenberger JA. Drug-induced orthostatic hypotension. *Drug Safety* 1991; **6:** 402–7.
4. Stumpf JL, Mitrzyk B. Management of orthostatic hypotension. *Am J Hosp Pharm* 1994; **51:** 648–60.
5. Mathias CJ. Orthostatic hypotension. *Prescribers' J* 1995; **35:** 124–32.
6. Frishman WH, *et al.* Drug treatment of orthostatic hypotension and vasovagal syncope. *Heart Dis* 2003; **5:** 49–64.

### Preparations

***BP 2003:*** Fludrocortisone Tablets;
***USP 27:*** Fludrocortisone Acetate Tablets.

**Proprietary Preparations** (details are given in Part 3)
***Arg.:*** Lonikan; ***Austral.:*** Florinef; ***Austria:*** Astonin H; ***Braz.:*** Florinefe; ***Canad.:*** Florinef; ***Chile:*** Florinef; ***Denm.:*** Florinef; ***Fin.:*** Florinef; ***Ger.:*** Astonin H; ***Gr.:*** Florinef; ***Hong Kong:*** Florinef; ***Irl.:*** Florinef; ***Israel:*** Florinef; ***Malaysia:*** Florinef; ***Neth.:*** Florinef; ***Norw.:*** Florinef; ***NZ:*** Florinef; ***S.Afr.:*** Florinef; ***Singapore:*** Florinef; ***Spain:*** Astonin; ***Swed.:*** Florinef; ***Switz.:*** Florinef; ***Thai.:*** Florinef; ***UK:*** Florinef; ***USA:*** Florinef.

**Multi-ingredient:** ***Belg.:*** Panotile; ***Braz.:*** Oto-Ped†; Otodol; Panotil; Rinofluimucil; ***Fr.:*** Panotile; ***Ger.:*** Panotile N; ***Neth.:*** Panotile; ***Spain:*** Fludronef; Panotile; ***Switz.:*** Panotile; ***Thai.:*** Otosamthong.

## Fludroxycortide *(BAN, rINN)*

33379; Fludroxicortida; Fluorandrenolone; 6α-Fluoro-16α-hydroxyhydrocortisone 16,17-Acetonide; Flurandrenolide *(USAN)*; Flurandrenolone. 6α-Fluoro-11β,21-dihydroxy-16α,17α-isopropylidenedioxypregn-4-ene-3,20-dione.
$C_{24}H_{33}FO_6$ = 436.5.
*CAS — 1524-88-5.*
*ATC — D07AC07.*

**Pharmacopoeias.** In *US.*

**USP 27** (Flurandrenolide). A white to off-white, fluffy, odourless, crystalline powder. Practically insoluble in water and in ether; soluble 1 in 72 of alcohol, 1 in 10 of chloroform, and 1 in 25 of methyl alcohol. Store in airtight containers at a temperature not exceeding 8°. Protect from light.

### Profile

Fludroxycortide is a corticosteroid used topically for its glucocorticoid activity (p.1068) in the treatment of various skin disorders. It is usually employed as a cream or ointment containing 0.0125% or a lotion containing 0.05%. It is also used as an adhesive polyethylene tape impregnated with fludroxycortide 4 micrograms/cm$^2$.

When applied topically, particularly to large areas, when the skin is broken, or under occlusive dressings, corticosteroids may be absorbed in sufficient amounts to cause systemic effects (p.1068). The effects of topical corticosteroids on the skin are described on p.1070. For recommendations concerning the correct use of corticosteroids on the skin, and a rough guide to the clinical potencies of topical corticosteroids, see p.1074.

### Preparations

*USP 27:* Flurandrenolide Cream; Flurandrenolide Lotion; Flurandrenolide Ointment; Flurandrenolide Tape; Neomycin Sulfate and Flurandrenolide Cream; Neomycin Sulfate and Flurandrenolide Lotion; Neomycin Sulfate and Flurandrenolide Ointment.

**Proprietary Preparations** (details are given in Part 3)
***Braz.:*** Drenison; ***Canad.:*** Drenison†; ***Ger.:*** Sermaka†; ***Irl.:*** Haelan†; ***Spain:*** Drenison†; ***UK:*** Haelan; ***USA:*** Cordran.

**Multi-ingredient:** ***Braz.:*** Dreniformio; Drenison N; ***Hong Kong:*** Drenison N†; ***Spain:*** Drenison Neomicina†.

## Flumetasone Pivalate *(BANM, rINNM)*

Flumetasoni Pivalas; Flumethasone Pivalate *(USAN)*; Flumethasone Trimethylacetate; NSC-107680; Pivalato de flumetasona. Flumethasone 21-pivalate.

$C_{27}H_{36}F_2O_6$ = 494.6.
*CAS — 2002-29-1.*
*ATC — D07AB03.*

**Pharmacopoeias.** In *Eur.* (see p.vi), *Pol.*, and *US.*

**Ph. Eur. 5.0** (Flumetasone Pivalate). A white or almost white, crystalline powder. It shows polymorphism. Practically insoluble in water; slightly soluble in alcohol and in dichloromethane; sparingly soluble in acetone. Protect from light.

**USP 27** (Flumethasone Pivalate). A white to off-white crystalline powder. Insoluble in water; soluble 1 in 89 of alcohol, 1 in 350 of chloroform, and 1 in 2800 of ether; slightly soluble in methyl alcohol; very slightly soluble in dichloromethane. Store in airtight containers. Protect from light.

### Profile

Flumetasone pivalate is a corticosteroid used topically for its glucocorticoid activity (p.1068) in the treatment of various skin disorders. It is usually employed as a 0.02% cream, ointment, or lotion. When applied topically, particularly to large areas, when the skin is broken, or under occlusive dressings, corticosteroids may be absorbed in sufficient amounts to cause systemic effects (p.1068). The effects of topical corticosteroids on the skin are described on p.1070. For recommendations concerning the correct use of corticosteroids on the skin, and a rough guide to the clinical potencies of topical corticosteroids, see p.1074.

Flumetasone pivalate is also used in ear drops in a concentration of 0.02% with clioquinol 1%.

### Preparations

*USP 27:* Flumethasone Pivalate Cream.

**Proprietary Preparations** (details are given in Part 3)
***Belg.:*** Locacortene†; ***Canad.:*** Locacorten†; ***Ger.:*** Cerson; Locacorten; ***Israel:*** Locacorten†; ***Ital.:*** Locorten; ***Neth.:*** Locacorten; ***Spain:*** Locortene†; ***Switz.:*** Locacorten.

**Multi-ingredient:** ***Arg.:*** Locorten Vioformo; Salena; Tresite F; ***Austral.:*** Locacorten Vioform; ***Austria:*** Locacorten mit Neomycin; Locacorten Tar; Locacorten Vioform; Locasalen; ***Belg.:*** Locacortene Tar†; Locacortene Vioforme†; Locasalen†; ***Braz.:*** Locorten Neomicina; Locorten Vioformio; Losalen; ***Canad.:*** Locacorten Vioform; ***Denm.:*** Locacorten med Salicylsyre†; Locacorten Vioform; ***Fin.:*** Locacorten Vioform; ***Fr.:*** Locacortene Vioforme†; Locacortene†; Locasalene†; Psocortene†; ***Ger.:*** Locacorten Vioform; Locasalen; Lorinden T; ***Gr.:*** Locasalene; ***Hong Kong:*** Locacorten Tar; Locasalen; ***Israel:*** Locacorten Tar†; Locacorten with Neomycin; Locasalen†; Topicorten V; Topicorten-Tar; Topisalen; ***Ital.:*** Locorten; Locorten Vioformio; Losalen; Vasosterone Oto; ***Neth.:*** Locacorten Vioform; Locasalen; ***Norw.:*** Locacorten Vioform†; ***NZ:*** Locorten Vioform; ***Port.:*** Locorten Vioformio; Losalen; ***S.Afr.:*** Locacorten Vioform; ***Singapore:*** Locasalen†; ***Spain:*** Locortene Vioformo†; Losalen; ***Swed.:*** Locacorten Vioform; ***Switz.:*** Locacorten Tar†; Locacorten Triclosan†; Locasalen; ***Thai.:*** Flumasalen; Locasalen; ***UK:*** Locorten Vioform.

## Flunisolide *(BAN, USAN, rINN)*

Flunisolida; RS-3999; RS-1320 (flunisolide acetate). 6α-Fluoro-11β,21-dihydroxy-16α,17α-isopropylidenedioxypregna-1,4-diene-3,20-dione.

$C_{24}H_{31}FO_6$ = 434.5.
*CAS — 3385-03-3 (flunisolide); 77326-96-6 (flunisolide hemihydrate); 4533-89-5 (flunisolide acetate).*
*ATC — R01AD04; R03BA03.*

**Pharmacopoeias.** In *US* which specifies the hemihydrate.

**USP 27** (Flunisolide). A white to creamy-white crystalline powder. Practically insoluble in water; soluble in acetone; sparingly soluble in chloroform; slightly soluble in methyl alcohol.

### Adverse Effects, Treatment, Withdrawal, and Precautions

As for corticosteroids in general (see p.1068).

### Interactions

The interactions of corticosteroids in general are described on p.1072.

### Pharmacokinetics

For a brief outline of the pharmacokinetics of corticosteroids, see p.1073. Flunisolide is reported to undergo extensive first-pass metabolism, with only 20% of the dose available systemically if it is given by mouth. The major metabolite, 6β-hydroxyflunisolide has some glucocorticoid activity; it has a half-life of about 4 hours. Only small amounts of flunisolide are absorbed following intranasal administration.

◊ References.

1. Chaplin MD, *et al.* Flunisolide metabolism and dynamics of a metabolite. *Clin Pharmacol Ther* 1980; **27:** 402–13.
2. Möllmann H, *et al.* Pharmacokinetic/pharmacodynamic evaluation of systemic effects of flunisolide after inhalation. *J Clin Pharmacol* 1997; **37:** 893–903.

### Uses and Administration

Flunisolide is a corticosteroid with glucocorticoid activity (p.1068) used as a nasal spray for the prophylaxis and treatment of allergic rhinitis (p.422). It is used in a usual initial dose of 50 micrograms into each nostril two or three times daily, subsequently reduced to the lowest dose adequate to control symptoms which may be as little as 25 micrograms into each nostril daily. Children over 5 years of age may be given 25 micrograms into each nostril up to three times daily. In the USA a dose of 50 micrograms into each nostril twice daily has also been permitted in children.

Flunisolide is also used by inhalation from a metered-dose aerosol in the management of asthma (p.777). The usual adult dosage is 500 micrograms inhaled twice daily. In severe asthma the dosage may be increased but should not exceed a total of 2 mg daily. A dose for children over 6 years of age is 500 micrograms inhaled twice daily.

### Preparations

*USP 27:* Flunisolide Nasal Solution.

**Proprietary Preparations** (details are given in Part 3)
***Arg.:*** Flunitec; ***Austria:*** Pulmilide; Syntaris†; ***Belg.:*** Broncort†; Syntaris; ***Braz.:*** Flunitec†; ***Canad.:*** Bronalide†; Rhinalar; ***Denm.:*** Flunitec†; Locasyn; ***Fr.:*** Bronilide†; Nasalide; ***Ger.:*** Inhacort; Syntaris; ***Gr.:*** Bronalide; ***Hong Kong:*** Rhinalar†; ***Irl.:*** Syntaris; ***Israel:*** Flunase; ***Ital.:*** Aerflu; Aerolid; Asmaflu; Careflu; Citiflux; Doricoflu; Euroflu; Fluminex; Flunigar; Flunitop; Gibiflu; Inalcort; Lunibron; Lunis; Nebulcort; Nereflun; Nisolid; Pantasol; Pulmist; Syntaris; Ventoflu; ***Neth.:*** Syntaris; ***Norw.:*** Flunitec†; Lokilan; ***Port.:*** Paftec†; ***S.Afr.:*** Syntaris†; ***Swed.:*** Lokilan Nasal†; ***Switz.:*** Broncort; Syntaris; ***UK:*** Syntaris; ***USA:*** AeroBid; Nasalide†; Nasarel.

**Multi-ingredient:** ***Ital.:*** Plenaer.

## Fluocinolone Acetonide *(BANM, USAN, rINN)*

Acetónido de fluocinolona; 6α,9α-Difluoro-16α-hydroxyprednisolone Acetonide; Fluocinoloni Acetonidum; NSC-92339. 6α,9α-Difluoro-11β,21-dihydroxy-16α,17α-isopropylidenedioxypregna-1,4-diene-3,20-dione.

$C_{24}H_{30}F_2O_6$ = 452.5.
*CAS — 67-73-2.*
*ATC — C05AA10; D07AC04.*

**Pharmacopoeias.** In *Eur.* (see p.vi), *Jpn, Pol.*, and *Viet. Br.* and *Viet.* have a separate monograph for the dihydrate; *US* allows either the anhydrous form or the dihydrate.

**Ph. Eur. 5.0** (Fluocinolone Acetonide). A white or almost white, crystalline powder. It exhibits polymorphism. Practically insoluble in water; soluble in dehydrated alcohol and in acetone. Protect from light.

**BP 2003** (Fluocinolone Acetonide Dihydrate). A white or almost white, crystalline powder. Practically insoluble in water and in hexane; soluble in dehydrated alcohol; freely soluble in acetone; sparingly soluble in dichloromethane and in methyl alcohol. Protect from light.

**USP 27** (Fluocinolone Acetonide). It is anhydrous or contains two molecules of water of hydration. A white or practically white, odourless, crystalline powder. Insoluble in water; soluble 1 in 45 of alcohol, 1 in 25 of chloroform, and 1 in 350 of ether; soluble in methyl alcohol.

### Profile

Fluocinolone acetonide is a corticosteroid used topically for its glucocorticoid activity (p.1068) in the treatment of various skin disorders. It is usually employed as a cream, gel, lotion, ointment, or scalp application; usual concentrations used range from 0.0025 to 0.025%. When applied topically, particularly to large areas, when the skin is broken, or under occlusive dressings, corticosteroids may be absorbed in sufficient amounts to cause systemic effects (p.1068). The effects of topical corticosteroids on the skin are described on p.1070. For recommendations concerning the correct use of corticosteroids on the skin, and a rough guide to the clinical potencies of topical corticosteroids, see p.1074.

Fluocinolone acetonide is also used topically in combination with an antibacterial in the treatment of infective inflammatory eye, ear, and nose disorders.

**Formulation.** The potency of fluocinolone acetonide varied with the formulation in a study[1] involving different Synalar topical preparations, the gel, ointment, and cream. The cream was the most potent followed by the gel, and then the ointment. A comparison of topical vasoconstrictor activity (used as an index of potency) unexpectedly found that the commercial dilutions of the cream (containing 0.00625% and 0.0025%) were indistinguishable in their effects from the full-strength (0.025%) cream.

1. Gao HY, Li Wan Po A. Topical formulations of fluocinolone acetonide: are creams, gels and ointments bioequivalent and does dilution affect activity? *Eur J Clin Pharmacol* 1994; **46:** 71–5.

### Preparations

*BP 2003:* Fluocinolone Cream; Fluocinolone Ointment;
*USP 27:* Fluocinolone Acetonide Cream; Fluocinolone Acetonide Ointment; Fluocinolone Acetonide Topical Solution; Neomycin Sulfate and Fluocinolone Acetonide Cream.

**Proprietary Preparations** (details are given in Part 3)
***Arg.:*** Flulone; ***Austria:*** Synalar; ***Belg.:*** Synalar; ***Braz.:*** Synalar†; ***Canad.:*** Capex; Fluoderm; Synalar; ***Chile:*** Adermina; ***Denm.:*** Synalar; ***Fr.:*** Synalar; ***Ger.:*** Flucinar; Jellin; Jellisoft; ***Gr.:*** Synalar Simple; ***Hong Kong:*** Cinotec; Flunolone-V; Synalar; ***India:*** Flucort; Flucort-H; Luci; ***Irl.:*** Synalar; ***Israel:*** Dermalar; ***Ital.:*** Alfa-Fluorone†; Alfabios†; Atoactive; Boniderma†; Cortamide; Dermobeta; Dermolin; Esacinone; Fluomix Same; Fluovitef; Fluvean; Localyn; Localyn SV; Neoderm Ginecologico†; Omniderm; Sterolone; Ultraderm; ***Malaysia:*** Synalar; ***Mex.:*** Cortilona; Cremisona; Flucin†; Fusalar; Synalar; ***Norw.:*** Synalar; ***NZ:*** Synalar; ***Port.:*** Oto-Synalar N; Synalar; ***S.Afr.:*** Cortoderm; Synalar†; ***Singapore:*** Flunolone-V; Synalar†; ***Spain:*** Alvadermo Fuerte†; Anatopic†; Co Fluocin Fuerte; Cortiespec; Fluocid Forte; Fluocortan†; Fluodermo Fuerte; Flusolgen; Gelidina; Oxidermiol Fuerte†; Synalar; Synalar Rectal Simple; ***Swed.:*** Synalar; ***Switz.:*** Synalar; ***Thai.:*** Fluciderm; Flunolone-V; Supralan; Synalar; ***UK:*** Synalar; ***USA:*** Capex; Derma-Smoothe/FS; Fluonid; Flurosyn; Synalar; Synemol.

**Multi-ingredient:** ***Arg.:*** Adop-Tar; ***Austria:*** Myco-Synalar; Procto-Synalar; Synalar N; ***Belg.:*** Procto-Synalar; Synalar Bi-Otic; ***Braz.:*** Dermobel; Dermoxin; Elotin; Fluo-Fenicol†; Fluo-Vaso; Gotas Ototilan†; Histalerg†; Neocinolon; Otauril†; Otocort; Otolone†; Otomixyn; Otosynalar; ***Chile:*** Otoseptil; ***Denm.:*** Synalar med Chinoform; ***Fr.:*** Antibio-Synalar; Synalar Neomycine†; ***Ger.:*** Jellin polyvalent; Jellin-Neomycin; Jellisoft-Neomycin†; Procto-Jellin; ***Gr.:*** Procto Synalar; ***Hong Kong:*** Aplosyn-Otic; Flunolone; Fluonid-N; Synalar N; Synco-CFN; ***India:*** Eczo-Wokadine; Flucort-C; Flucort-MZ; Flucort-N; Flucreme NM; Zole-F; ***Irl.:*** Synalar C; Synalar N; ***Ital.:*** Alfa-Fluorone†; Cortanest Plus; Doricum; Lauromicina; Localyn; Localyn-Neomicina; Mecloderm F; Meclutin; Nefluan; Proctolyn; ***Malaysia:*** Fluonid-N; Synalar N; ***Mex.:*** Cetoquina Y; Cortilona Compuesta; Ercal†; Flunal; Flunal-Neo; Fluo Grin; Lasalar-Y; Luzolona Y; Promibasol-Plus; Synalar C; Synalar N; Synalar Neo; Synalar O; Synalar Oftalmico; Vagitrol-V; ***Neth.:*** Synalar Bi-Otic; ***Norw.:*** Synalar med Chinoform; ***Port.:*** Synalar Rectal; ***S.Afr.:*** Synalar C†; Synalar N†; ***Singapore:*** Flunolone; Synalar C†; Synalar N†; ***Spain:*** Abrasone; Abrasone Rectal; Aceoto Plus; Alergical; Artrodesmol Extra; Bazalin; Cetraxal Plus; Cexidal Otico; Creanolona; Flodermol; Fluo Fenic; Fluo Vasoc†; Intradermo Cort Ant Fung; Midacina; Myco-Synalar†; Neo Analsona; Neo-Synalar†; Otomidrin; Poxider†; Synalar Nasal; Synalar Neomicina; Synalar Otico; Synalar Rectal; Synobel; Ultramicina Plus; Vinciseptil Otico; ***Switz.:*** Myco-Synalar; Procto-Synalar N; Procto†; Synalar N; ***Thai.:*** Fluciderm-N; Flunolone; Fluonid-N; Gental-F; Supralan-N; Synalar N; ***UK:*** Synalar C; Synalar N; ***USA:*** Tri-Luma.

## Fluocinonide *(BAN, USAN, rINN)*

Fluocinolide; Fluocinolone Acetonide 21-Acetate; Fluocinónida; NSC-101791. 6α,9α-Difluoro-11β,21-dihydroxy-16α,17α-isopropylidenedioxypregna-1,4-diene-3,20-dione 21-acetate.

$C_{26}H_{32}F_2O_7$ = 494.5.
*CAS — 356-12-7.*
*ATC — C05AA11; D07AC08.*

**Pharmacopoeias.** In *Br., Chin., Jpn,* and *US.*

**BP 2003** (Fluocinonide). A white or almost white, crystalline powder. Practically insoluble in water; slightly soluble in dehydrated alcohol and in chloroform. Protect from light.

**USP 27** (Fluocinonide). A white to cream-coloured, crystalline powder having not more than a slight odour. Practically insoluble in water; slightly soluble in alcohol, in methyl alcohol, and in dioxan; sparingly soluble in acetone and in chloroform; very slightly soluble in ether.

### Profile

Fluocinonide is a corticosteroid used topically for its glucocorticoid activity (p.1068) in the treatment of various skin disorders. It is usually employed as a cream, gel, lotion, ointment, or scalp application containing 0.05%.

When applied topically, particularly to large areas, when the skin is broken, or under occlusive dressings, corticosteroids may be absorbed in sufficient amounts to cause systemic effects (p.1068). The effects of topical corticosteroids on the skin are described on p.1070. For recommendations concerning the correct use of corticosteroids on the skin, and a rough guide to the clinical potencies of topical corticosteroids, see p.1074.

### Preparations

*BP 2003:* Fluocinonide Cream; Fluocinonide Ointment;
*USP 27:* Fluocinonide Cream; Fluocinonide Gel; Fluocinonide Ointment; Fluocinonide Topical Solution.

**Proprietary Preparations** (details are given in Part 3)
***Austria:*** Topsym; Topsymin F; ***Belg.:*** Lidex; ***Canad.:*** Lidemol; Lidex; Lyderm; Lydonide; Tiamol; Topsyn; ***Denm.:*** Metosyn; ***Fr.:*** Topsyne†; ***Ger.:*** Topsym; ***Gr.:*** Lidex; ***Hong Kong:*** Novoter†; ***Irl.:*** Metosyn†; ***Ital.:*** Flu-21; Topsyn; ***Mex.:*** Gelisyn†; Topsyn; ***Neth.:*** Topsyne; ***Norw.:*** Metosyn; ***Singapore:*** Lidex; Metosyn†; ***Spain:*** Cusigel†; Klariderm; Novoter; ***Switz.:*** Korticoid†; Topsym; Topsymin; ***UK:*** Metosyn; ***USA:*** Lidex.

**Multi-ingredient:** ***Austria:*** Topsym polyvalent; ***Canad.:*** Trisyn†; ***Fr.:*** Topsyne Neomycine†; ***Ger.:*** Jelliproct; Topsym polyvalent; ***Hong Kong:*** Novoter Gentamicin†; ***Israel:*** Comagis; ***Mex.:*** Topsyn-Y; ***Spain:*** Novoter Gentamicina; ***Switz.:*** Korticoid polyvalent†; Topsym polyvalent; ***UK:*** Vipsogal†.

### Fluocortin Butyl *(BAN, USAN, rINN)*

Butil éster de la fluocortina; SH-K-203. Butyl 6α-fluoro-11β-hydroxy-16α-methyl-3,20-dioxopregna-1,4-dien-21-oate.

$C_{26}H_{35}FO_5$ = 446.6.

*CAS — 33124-50-4 (fluocortin); 41767-29-7 (fluocortin butyl).*

*ATC — D07AB04.*

#### Profile

Fluocortin butyl is a corticosteroid that has been used topically for its glucocorticoid activity (p.1068) in the treatment of various skin disorders. It is usually employed as a cream or ointment containing 0.75%. When applied topically, particularly to large areas, when the skin is broken, or under occlusive dressings, or intranasally, corticosteroids may be absorbed in sufficient amounts to cause systemic effects (p.1068). The effects of topical corticosteroids on the skin are described on p.1070. For recommendations concerning the correct use of corticosteroids on the skin, and a rough guide to the clinical potencies of topical corticosteroids, see p.1074.

Fluocortin butyl has also been used in the form of a dry powder nasal inhalation for the management of allergic rhinitis.

#### Preparations

**Proprietary Preparations** (details are given in Part 3)
***Belg.:*** Varlane; ***Ger.:*** Lenen†; Vaspit; ***Ital.:*** Vaspit; ***Spain:*** Vaspit.
**Multi-ingredient: *Ger.:*** Bi-Vaspit.

### Fluocortolone *(BAN, USAN, rINN)*

Fluocortolona; 6α-Fluoro-16α-methyl-1-dehydrocorticosterone; SH-742. 6α-Fluoro-11β,21-dihydroxy-16α-methylpregna-1,4-diene-3,20-dione.

$C_{22}H_{29}FO_4$ = 376.5.

*CAS — 152-97-6.*

*ATC — C05AA08; D07AC05; H02AB03.*

### Fluocortolone Caproate *(USAN, rINNM)*

Caproato de fluocortolona; Fluocortolone Hexanoate *(BANM)*; SH-770. Fluocortolone 21-hexanoate.

$C_{28}H_{39}FO_5$ = 474.6.

*CAS — 303-40-2.*

*ATC — C05AA08; D07AC05; H02AB03.*

**Pharmacopoeias.** In *Br.*

**BP 2003** (Fluocortolone Hexanoate). A white or creamy-white, odourless or almost odourless, crystalline powder. It exhibits polymorphism. Practically insoluble in water and in ether; very slightly soluble in alcohol and in methyl alcohol; slightly soluble in acetone and in dioxan; sparingly soluble in chloroform. Protect from light.

### Fluocortolone Pivalate *(BANM, rINNM)*

Fluocortolone Trimethylacetate; Fluocortoloni Pivalas; Pivalato de fluocortolona. Fluocortolone 21-pivalate.

$C_{27}H_{37}FO_5$ = 460.6.

*CAS — 29205-06-9.*

*ATC — C05AA08; D07AC05; H02AB03.*

**Pharmacopoeias.** In *Eur.* (see p.vi).

**Ph. Eur. 5.0** (Fluocortolone Pivalate). A white or almost white crystalline powder. Practically insoluble in water; sparingly soluble in alcohol; freely soluble in dichloromethane and in dioxan. Protect from light.

#### Profile

Fluocortolone and its esters are corticosteroids mainly used topically for their glucocorticoid activity (p.1068) in the treatment of various skin disorders. They are usually employed as a cream or ointment; concentrations usually used are 0.25% of the caproate with 0.25% of either the free alcohol or pivalate ester. The pivalate and caproate esters have also been used together in ointments or suppositories for the treatment of anorectal disorders.

When applied topically, particularly to large areas, when the skin is broken, or under occlusive dressings, corticosteroids may be absorbed in sufficient amounts to cause systemic effects (p.1068). The effects of topical corticosteroids on the skin are described on p.1070. For recommendations concerning the correct use of corticosteroids on the skin, and a rough guide to the clinical potencies of topical corticosteroids, see p.1074.

Fluocortolone free alcohol is sometimes given by mouth for its systemic effects in conditions for which corticosteroids are indicated (p.1073), in usual doses of 5 to 100 mg daily.

#### Preparations

***BP 2003:*** Fluocortolone Cream.

**Proprietary Preparations** (details are given in Part 3)
***Arg.:*** Ultracur S; ***Austria:*** Ultralan; ***Chile:*** Ultralan; ***Ger.:*** Ultralan; ***Hong Kong:*** Ultralan; ***Israel:*** Ultralan; ***Ital.:*** Ultralan; ***Mex.:*** Ultralan; ***Neth.:*** Ultralan; ***Spain:*** Ultralan M.

**Multi-ingredient: *Arg.:*** Ultraproct; ***Austral.:*** Ultraproct; ***Austria:*** Pilison; Ultralan; Ultraproct; ***Belg.:*** Ultraproct; ***Braz.:*** Ultraproct; ***Chile:*** Ultraproct; ***Denm.:*** Doloproct; Doloproct Comp; ***Fin.:*** Neoproct; ***Fr.:*** Myco-Ultralan†; Ultralan; Ultraproct; ***Ger.:*** Doloproct; Ultralan; Ultralan-crinale†; Ultraproct; ***Hong Kong:*** Ultraproct; ***Irl.:*** Ultraproct; ***Ital.:*** Ultralan; Ultraproct; ***Mex.:*** Ultraproct; ***NZ:*** Ultraproct; ***Port.:*** Ultraproct; ***Switz.:*** Ultralan†; Ultraproct†; ***UK:*** Ultralanum Plain; Ultraproct.

### Fluorometholone *(BAN, rINN)*

Fluorometolona. 9α-Fluoro-11β,17α-dihydroxy-6α-methylpregna-1,4-diene-3,20-dione.

$C_{22}H_{29}FO_4$ = 376.5.

*CAS — 426-13-1.*

*ATC — C05AA06; D07AB06; S01BA07.*

**Pharmacopoeias.** In *Br., Jpn,* and *US.*

**BP 2003** (Fluorometholone). A white to yellowish white, crystalline powder. Practically insoluble in water; slightly soluble in dehydrated alcohol and in ether.

**USP 27** (Fluorometholone). A white to yellowish-white, odourless, crystalline powder. Practically insoluble in water; soluble 1 in 200 of alcohol and 1 in 2200 of chloroform; very slightly soluble in ether. Store in airtight containers. Protect from light.

### Fluorometholone Acetate *(BANM, USAN, rINNM)*

Acetato de fluorometolona; U-17323. Fluorometholone 17-acetate.

$C_{24}H_{31}FO_5$ = 418.5.

*CAS — 3801-06-7.*

*ATC — C05AA06; D07AB06; S01BA07.*

#### Profile

Fluorometholone is a corticosteroid employed for its glucocorticoid activity (p.1068), usually as eye drops containing 0.1%, in the treatment of allergic and inflammatory conditions of the eye. Fluorometholone acetate is used similarly.

Fluorometholone is also used topically in the treatment of various skin disorders.

Prolonged application to the eye of preparations containing corticosteroids has caused raised intra-ocular pressure and reduced visual function. When applied topically, particularly to large areas, when the skin is broken, or under occlusive dressings, corticosteroids may be absorbed in sufficient amounts to cause systemic effects (p.1068). The effects of topical corticosteroids on the skin are described on p.1070. For recommendations concerning the correct use of corticosteroids on the skin, see p.1074.

#### Preparations

***BP 2003:*** Fluorometholone Eye Drops;
***USP 27:*** Fluorometholone Cream; Fluorometholone Ophthalmic Suspension; Neomycin Sulfate and Fluorometholone Ointment; Tobramycin and Fluorometholone Acetate Ophthalmic Suspension.

**Proprietary Preparations** (details are given in Part 3)
***Arg.:*** Flarex; FML; ***Austral.:*** Flarex; Flucon; FML; ***Austria:*** Flarex; ***Belg.:*** Flucon; FML; ***Braz.:*** Florate; Flumex; ***Canad.:*** Flarex; FML; ***Chile:*** Aflarex; Fluforte; ***Denm.:*** Flurolon; ***Fin.:*** FML; ***Fr.:*** Flucon; ***Ger.:*** Efflumidex; Fluoro-Ophtal; Fluoropos; Isopto Flucon; ***Gr.:*** Flucon; Fluxinam; FML; ***Hong Kong:*** Flucon; Flumetholon; FML; ***India:*** Flosef; ***Irl.:*** FML; ***Israel:*** Flarex; FML; ***Ital.:*** Flarex; Fluaton; Flumetol Semplice; ***Malaysia:*** FML; ***Mex.:*** Flarex†; Fluforte; Flumetol NF; FML†; ***NZ:*** Flarex†; Flucon; FML; ***Port.:*** Flurop; FML; ***S.Afr.:*** Flucon; FML; ***Singapore:*** FML; ***Spain:*** FML; Isopto Flucon; ***Switz.:*** Flarex†; FML; ***Thai.:*** Flarex; Flu Oph; Flucon; FML; ***UK:*** FML; ***USA:*** Eflone; Flarex; Fluor-Op; FML.

**Multi-ingredient: *Arg.:*** Efemolina; FML Neo; Larsimal; ***Braz.:*** Flumex N; Infectoflam†; ***Chile:*** Fluforte N; ***Ger.:*** Cibaflam; Efemolin; Efflumycin; ***Hong Kong:*** Efemoline; Infectoflam†; ***Israel:*** FML Neo†; ***Ital.:*** Efemoline; Flumetol; Flumetol Antibiotico; Gentacort; ***Malaysia:*** Efemoline; Infectoflam; ***Mex.:*** Fluforte N; ***NZ:*** Tobrasone†; ***Port.:*** FML Neo; Neo-Preocil; ***S.Afr.:*** Efemoline; FML Neo; ***Singapore:*** Efemoline; Infectoflam; ***Spain:*** Bexicortil; Cortisdin Urea; Flugen; Fluorvas; FML Neo†; ***Switz.:*** Efemoline; FML Neo; Infectoflam; ***Thai.:*** Efemoline; FML Neo; Infectoflam; ***UK:*** FML Neo Liquifilm†; ***USA:*** FML-S.

### Fluprednidene Acetate *(BANM, rINNM)*

Acetato de fluprednideno; Fluprednylidene 21-Acetate. 9α-Fluoro-11β,17α,21-trihydroxy-16-methylenepregna-1,4-diene-3,20-dione 21-acetate.

$C_{24}H_{29}FO_6$ = 432.5.

*CAS — 2193-87-5 (fluprednidene); 1255-35-2 (fluprednidene acetate).*

*ATC — D07AB07.*

#### Profile

Fluprednidene acetate is a corticosteroid used topically for its glucocorticoid activity (p.1068) in the treatment of various skin disorders. It is usually employed as a cream, lotion, or ointment containing 0.1%.

When applied topically, particularly to large areas, when the skin is broken, or under occlusive dressings, corticosteroids may be absorbed in sufficient amounts to cause systemic effects (p.1068). The effects of topical corticosteroids on the skin are described on p.1070. For recommendations concerning the correct use of corticosteroids on the skin, and a rough guide to the clinical potencies of topical corticosteroids, see p.1074.

#### Preparations

**Proprietary Preparations** (details are given in Part 3)
***Austria:*** Decoderm; ***Belg.:*** Decoderm; ***Denm.:*** Corticoderm†; ***Ger.:*** Decoderm; ***Neth.:*** Decoderm†; ***Norw.:*** Corticoderm†; ***Spain:*** Decoderm†; ***Swed.:*** Corticoderm; ***Switz.:*** Decoderm.

**Multi-ingredient: *Arg.:*** Tri-Emcortina; ***Austria:*** Decoderm compositum; Decoderm trivalent; Sali-Decoderm†; ***Belg.:*** Decoderm Comp; ***Braz.:*** Emecort; Pan-Emecort; ***Ger.:*** Candio-Hermal Plus; Crinohermal fem; Decoderm Comp; Decoderm tri; Sali-Decoderm; Vobaderm; ***Gr.:*** Micogen; Verdal; ***Spain:*** Decoderm Trivalente†; ***Switz.:*** Decoderm bivalent; ***Thai.:*** Supracortin 3.

### Fluprednisolone *(BAN, USAN, rINN)*

6α-Fluoroprednisolone; Fluprednisolona; NSC-47439; U-7800. 6α-Fluoro-11β,17α,21-trihydroxypregna-1,4-diene-3,20-dione.

$C_{21}H_{27}FO_5$ = 378.4.

*CAS — 53-34-9 (fluprednisolone); 23257-44-5 (fluprednisolone valerate).*

#### Profile

Fluprednisolone is a corticosteroid with mainly glucocorticoid activity (p.1068); 2 mg of fluprednisolone is roughly equivalent in anti-inflammatory activity to 5 mg of prednisolone. It has been given by mouth in the management of a variety of conditions requiring systemic glucocorticoid therapy (p.1073).

## Fluticasone Propionate

*(BANM, USAN, rINNM)*

CCI-18781; Fluticasoni Propionas; Propionato de fluticasona. S-Fluoromethyl 6α,9α-difluoro-11β,17α-dihydroxy-16α-methyl-3-oxoandrosta-1,4-diene-17β-carbothioate 17-propionate.

$C_{25}H_{31}F_3O_5S$ = 500.6.

*CAS — 80474-14-2.*

*ATC — D07AC17; R01AD08; R03BA05.*

**Pharmacopoeias.** In *Eur.* (see p.vi).

**Ph. Eur. 5.0** (Fluticasone Propionate). A white or almost white powder. Practically insoluble in water; slightly soluble in alcohol; sparingly soluble in dichloromethane. Protect from light.

### Adverse Effects, Treatment, Withdrawal, and Precautions

As for corticosteroids in general (see p.1068). Hypersensitivity reactions have occurred. Eosinophilic conditions, including Churg-Strauss syndrome, have been reported rarely, in most cases following a transfer from oral corticosteroid therapy.

When applied topically, particularly to large areas, when the skin is broken, or under occlusive dressings, corticosteroids may be absorbed in sufficient amounts to cause systemic effects. Inhalation or nasal administration of large amounts of fluticasone propionate may produce systemic effects also (see below).

**Adrenal suppression.** Despite the fact that inhaled fluticasone is generally thought to lack systemic effects at therapeutic doses, a study in 25 healthy subjects[1] indicated that fluticasone propionate as single inhaled doses of 250, 500, and 1000 micrograms did produce a reduction in plasma cortisol, indicating suppression of the hypothalamic-pituitary-adrenal axis to some degree. Others have also found evidence of adrenal suppression with fluticasone,[2-5] particularly at high doses, and the effect may be more marked with repeated than with single doses.[4,6,7] A number of cases of adrenal crisis have been associated with high-dose inhaled fluticasone.[8,9]

1. Grahnén A, *et al.* An assessment of the systemic activity of single doses of inhaled fluticasone propionate in healthy volunteers. *Br J Clin Pharmacol* 1994; **38:** 521–5.
2. Clark DJ, *et al.* Comparative systemic bioactivity of inhaled budesonide and fluticasone propionate in asthmatic children. *Br J Clin Pharmacol* 1996; **42:** 264P.
3. Rohatagi S, *et al.* Dynamic modeling of cortisol reduction after inhaled administration of fluticasone propionate. *J Clin Pharmacol* 1996; **36:** 938–41.
4. Clark DJ, Lipworth BJ. Adrenal suppression with chronic dosing of fluticasone propionate compared with budesonide in adult asthmatic patients. *Thorax* 1997; **52:** 55–8.
5. Eid N, *et al.* Decreased morning serum cortisol levels in children with asthma treated with inhaled fluticasone propionate. *Pediatrics* 2002; **109:** 217–21.
6. Lönnebo A, *et al.* An assessment of the systemic effects of single and repeated doses of inhaled fluticasone propionate and inhaled budesonide in healthy volunteers. *Eur J Clin Pharmacol* 1996; **49:** 459–63.
7. Wilson AM, *et al.* Adrenal suppression with high doses of inhaled fluticasone propionate and triamcinolone acetonide in healthy voluteers. *Eur J Clin Pharmacol* 1997; **53:** 33–7.
8. Todd GRG, *et al.* Survey of adrenal crisis associated with inhaled corticosteroids in the United Kingdom. *Arch Dis Child* 2002; **87:** 457–61.
9. Adverse Drug Reactions Advisory Committee (ADRAC). Fluticasone and adrenal crisis. *Aust Adverse Drug React Bull* 2003; **22:** 6. Also available at: http://www.tga.health.gov.au/adr/aadrb/aadr0304.htm (accessed 06/05/04)

**Aspergillosis.** The fungal infection aspergillosis has been reported in patients receiving inhaled[1,2] and intranasal[3] fluticasone.

1. Fairfax AJ, *et al.* Laryngeal aspergillosis following high dose inhaled fluticasone therapy for asthma. *Thorax* 1999; **54:** 860–1.
2. Leav BA, *et al.* Invasive pulmonary aspergillosis associated with high-dose inhaled fluticasone. *N Engl J Med* 2000; **343:** 586.
3. Bratton RL, *et al.* Aspergillosis related to long-term nasal corticosteroid use. *Mayo Clin Proc* 2002; **77:** 1353–7.

**Effects on the bones.** For studies of the effects on bone of inhaled fluticasone, compared with beclometasone, see p.1091.

### Interactions

The interactions of corticosteroids in general are described on p.1072.

## Pharmacokinetics

For a brief outline of the pharmacokinetics of corticosteroids, see p.1073.

Fluticasone propionate is poorly absorbed from the gastrointestinal tract and undergoes extensive first-pass metabolism; oral bioavailability is reported to be only about 1%.

◊ References.


1. Mackie AE, *et al.* Pharmacokinetics of intravenous fluticasone propionate in healthy subjects. *Br J Clin Pharmacol* 1996; **41:** 539–42.
2. van Boxtel CJ, Sheffer AL, eds. The pharmacokinetics of fluticasone propionate. *Clin Pharmacokinet* 2000; **39** (suppl): 1–54.
3. Daley-Yates PT, Baker RC. Systemic bioavailability of fluticasone propionate administered as nasal drops and aqueous nasal spray formulations. *Br J Clin Pharmacol* 2001; **51:** 103–5.


## Uses and Administration

Fluticasone propionate is a corticosteroid with mainly glucocorticoid activity (p.1068).

Fluticasone propionate is stated to exert a topical effect on the lungs without significant systemic effects at usual doses, due to its low systemic bioavailability (but see Adrenal Suppression, above). It is used by powder or aerosol inhalation for the prophylaxis of asthma. Initial doses in the UK range from 100 to 250 micrograms twice daily in mild asthma up to 1 mg twice daily in severe asthma, adjusted according to response. Children over 4 years of age may be given initial doses of 50 to 100 micrograms twice daily, increased to 200 micrograms twice daily if necessary. The drug may also be given via a nebuliser in severe chronic asthma. Usual adult doses are 0.5 to 2 mg twice daily.

Fluticasone propionate is also available in some countries as a powder or aerosol inhalation for the treatment of chronic obstructive pulmonary disease, when it is given in doses of 500 micrograms twice daily.

Fluticasone propionate is administered by nasal spray in the prophylaxis and treatment of allergic rhinitis. The usual dose is 100 micrograms into each nostril once daily, increased if necessary to 100 micrograms into each nostril twice daily. Children over 4 years of age may be given half these doses. Fluticasone propionate drops are used in the treatment of nasal polyps. A total dose of 400 micrograms should be instilled once or twice daily for at least 4 to 6 weeks.

It is applied topically in the treatment of various skin disorders. Creams and ointments containing 0.05% and 0.005% respectively are available. For recommendations concerning the correct use of corticosteroids on the skin, see p.1074.

**Asthma.** Corticosteroids and beta$_2$-adrenoceptor agonists form the cornerstone of the management of asthma (p.777). Patients requiring only occasional relief from symptoms may be managed with an inhaled short-acting beta$_2$ agonist, and an inhaled corticosteroid such as fluticasone is added if symptomatic relief is needed more than once daily. The dose of inhaled corticosteroid is increased in more severe asthma, often together with the addition of other drugs.

Some references to the use of fluticasone propionate for asthma are given below,[1-9] including one to a study indicating that increasing the dose of inhaled fluticasone did not produce increased benefit.[1]


1. Boe J, *et al.* High-dose inhaled steroids in asthmatics: moderate efficacy gain and suppression of the hypothalamic-pituitary-adrenal (HPA) axis. *Eur Respir J* 1994; **7:** 2179–84.
2. Jarvis B, Faulds D. Inhaled fluticasone propionate: a review of its therapeutic efficacy at dosages ≤ 500 micrograms/day in adults and adolescents with mild to moderate asthma. *Drugs* 1999; **57:** 769–803.
3. Bisgaard H, *et al.* The effect of inhaled fluticasone propionate in the treatment of young asthmatic children: a dose comparison study. *Am J Respir Crit Care Med* 1999; **160:** 126–31.
4. Markham A, Jarvis B. Inhaled salmeterol/fluticasone propionate combination: a review of its use in persistent asthma. *Drugs* 2000; **60:** 1207–33.
5. ZuWallack R, *et al.* Long-term efficacy and safety of fluticasone propionate powder administered once or twice daily via inhaler to patients with moderate asthma. *Chest* 2000; **118:** 303–312.
6. Holt S, *et al.* Dose-response relation of inhaled fluticasone propionate in adolescents and adults with asthma: meta-analysis. *BMJ* 2001; **323:** 253–6.
7. Adams N, *et al.* Inhaled fluticasone propionate for chronic asthma. Available in The Cochrane Library; Issue 1. Chichester: John Wiley; 2004.
8. Adams N, *et al.* Inhaled fluticasone at different doses for chronic asthma. Available in The Cochrane Library; Issue 1. Chichester: John Wiley; 2004.
9. Adams N, *et al.* Fluticasone versus beclomethasone or budesonide for chronic asthma. Available in The Cochrane Library; Issue 1. Chichester: John Wiley; 2004.


**Chronic obstructive pulmonary disease.** For discussion of the value of inhaled corticosteroids in chronic obstructive pulmonary disease, including reference to the use of fluticasone, see p.1078.

**Inflammatory bowel disease.** Fluticasone propionate, given by mouth, has produced variable results in the treatment of Crohn's disease[1] and ulcerative colitis;[2,3] some benefit was also reported in coeliac disease.[4] The dose was 5 mg four times daily but some consider[2] higher doses necessary.

For a review of the management of inflammatory bowel disease, including the role of corticosteroids, see p.1243.


1. Carpani de Kaski M, *et al.* Fluticasone propionate in Crohn's disease. *Gut* 1991; **32:** 657–61.
2. Hawthorne AB, *et al.* Double blind trial of oral fluticasone propionate v prednisolone in the treatment of active ulcerative colitis. *Gut* 1993; **34:** 125–8.
3. Angus P, *et al.* Oral fluticasone propionate in active distal ulcerative colitis. *Gut* 1992; **33:** 711–14.
4. Mitchison HC, *et al.* A pilot study of fluticasone propionate in untreated coeliac disease. *Gut* 1991; **32:** 260–5.


**Nasal polyps.** For discussion of the value of corticosteroids in the treatment of nasal polyps, including reference to the use of fluticasone, see p.1084.

**Rhinitis.** For a discussion of the management of rhinitis, including the use of corticosteroids, see p.422. Some further references to the use of fluticasone in rhinitis are given below.


1. Wiseman LR, Benfield P. Intranasal fluticasone propionate: a reappraisal of its pharmacology and clinical efficacy in the treatment of rhinitis. *Drugs* 1997; **53:** 885–907.


### Preparations

***BP 2003:*** Fluticasone Cream; Fluticasone Ointment.

**Proprietary Preparations** (details are given in Part 3)
***Arg.:*** Cutivate; Flixonase; Flixotide; ***Austral.:*** Beconase Allergy; Flixotide; ***Austria:*** Cutivate; Flixonase; Flixotide; ***Belg.:*** Cutivate; Flixonase; Flixotide; ***Braz.:*** Flixonase; Flixotide; Flutivate; ***Canad.:*** Flonase; Flovent; ***Chile:*** Albeoler; Brexonase; Brexovent; Flixonase; Flixotide; Flusona; Flutivate; Raffonin; ***Denm.:*** Cutivat; Flixonase; Flixotide; ***Fin.:*** Flixonase; Flixotide; ***Fr.:*** Flixonase; Flixotide; Flixovate; ***Ger.:*** Atemur; Flutide; Flutivate; ***Gr.:*** Flixotide; ***Hong Kong:*** Cutivate; Flixonase; Flixotide; ***India:*** Flohale; Zoflut; ***Irl.:*** Flixonase; Flixotide; ***Israel:*** Allegro; Cutivate; Flixonase; Flixotide; ***Ital.:*** Flixoderm; Flixonase; Flixotide; Fluspiral; Seretide; ***Malaysia:*** Cutivate; Flixonase; Flixotide; ***Mex.:*** Cutivate; Flixonase; Flixotide; ***Neth.:*** Cutivate; Flixonase; Flixotide; ***Norw.:*** Flutide; Flutivate; ***NZ:*** Flixonase; Flixotide; ***Port.:*** Asmatil; Asmo-Lavi; Brisovent; Cutivate; Eustidil; Flixotaide; Flutaide; Rontilona; Ubizol; ***S.Afr.:*** Cutivate; Flixonase; Flixotide; ***Singapore:*** Cutivate; Flixonase; Flixotide; ***Spain:*** Cutivate†; Drolasona; Flixonase; Flixotide; Fluinol; Flusonal; Inalacor; Rinosone; Rontilona; Trialona; ***Swed.:*** Flutide; Flutivate; ***Switz.:*** Axotide; Cutivate; Flutinase; ***Thai.:*** Flixonase; Flixotide; ***UAE:*** Potencort; ***UK:*** Cutivate; Flixonase; Flixotide; ***USA:*** Cutivate; Flonase; Flovent.

**Multi-ingredient:** ***Arg.:*** Seretide; ***Austral.:*** Seretide; ***Austria:*** Seretide; Viani; ***Belg.:*** Seretide; ***Braz.:*** Seretide; ***Canad.:*** Advair; ***Chile:*** Brexotide; Seretide; ***Denm.:*** Seretide; ***Fin.:*** Seretide; ***Fr.:*** Seretide; ***Ger.:*** Atmadisc; Viani; ***Gr.:*** Seretide; Viani; ***Hong Kong:*** Seretide; ***India:*** Seroflo; ***Irl.:*** Seretide; ***Israel:*** Seretide; ***Ital.:*** Aliflus; ***Malaysia:*** Seretide; ***Mex.:*** Seretide; ***Neth.:*** Seretide; ***Norw.:*** Seretide; ***Port.:*** Brisomax; Maizar; Seretaide; ***S.Afr.:*** Seretide; ***Singapore:*** Seretide; ***Spain:*** Anasma; Inaladuo; Plusvent; Seretide; ***Swed.:*** Seretide; ***Switz.:*** Seretide; ***Thai.:*** Seretide; ***UK:*** Seretide; ***USA:*** Advair.

## Formocortal *(BAN, USAN, rINN)*

FI-6341; Fluoroformylon. 3-(2-Chloroethoxy)-9α-fluoro-11β,21-dihydroxy-16α,17α-isopropylidenedioxy-20-oxopregna-3,5-diene-6-carbaldehyde 21-acetate.

$C_{29}H_{38}ClFO_8$ = 569.1.
*CAS — 2825-60-7.*
*ATC — S01BA12.*

### Profile

Formocortal is a corticosteroid that is used for its glucocorticoid activity (see p.1068) in the treatment of inflammatory eye disorders as eye drops and eye ointments containing 0.05%.

Prolonged application to the eye of preparations containing corticosteroids has caused raised intra-ocular pressure and reduced visual function.

### Preparations

**Proprietary Preparations** (details are given in Part 3)
***Ital.:*** Formoftil.

**Multi-ingredient:** ***Ital.:*** Formomicin.

## Halcinonide *(BAN, USAN, rINN)*

Alcinonide; Halcinónida; SQ-18566. 21-Chloro-9α-fluoro-11β-hydroxy-16α,17α-isopropylidenedioxypregn-4-ene-3,20-dione.

$C_{24}H_{32}ClFO_5$ = 455.0.
*CAS — 3093-35-4.*
*ATC — D07AD02.*

**Pharmacopoeias.** In *Chin.* and *US.*

**USP 27** (Halcinonide). A white to off-white, odourless, crystalline powder. Insoluble in water and in hexanes; slightly soluble in alcohol and in ether; soluble in acetone and in chloroform.

### Profile

Halcinonide is a corticosteroid used topically for its glucocorticoid activity (p.1068) in the treatment of various skin disorders. It is usually employed as a 0.1% cream, lotion, or ointment.

When applied topically, particularly to large areas, when the skin is broken, or under occlusive dressings, corticosteroids may be absorbed in sufficient amounts to cause systemic effects (p.1068). The effects of topical corticosteroids on the skin are described on p.1070. For recommendations concerning the correct use of corticosteroids on the skin, and a rough guide to the clinical potencies of topical corticosteroids, see p.1074.

### Preparations

***USP 27:*** Halcinonide Cream; Halcinonide Ointment; Halcinonide Topical Solution.

**Proprietary Preparations** (details are given in Part 3)
***Austral.:*** Halciderm†; ***Austria:*** Halog; ***Braz.:*** Halog; ***Canad.:*** Halog; ***Fr.:*** Halog†; ***Ger.:*** Halog; ***Hong Kong:*** Halog; ***India:*** Cortilate; ***Ital.:*** Halciderm; ***Mex.:*** Dermalog; ***Norw.:*** Halog†; ***Spain:*** Halog; ***Switz.:*** Betacortone; ***UK:*** Halciderm; ***USA:*** Halog.

**Multi-ingredient:** ***Braz.:*** Halcicomb†; ***Fr.:*** Halog Neomycine†; ***Ger.:*** Halog Tri; ***India:*** Cobederm-H; ***Ital.:*** Anfocort; Halciderm; Halciderm Combi; ***Mex.:*** Dermalog-C; ***Switz.:*** Betacortone; Betacortone S.

## Halometasone *(rINN)*

C-48401-Ba; Halometasona; Halomethasone. 2-Chloro-6α,9-difluoro-11β,17,21-trihydroxy-16α-methylpregna-1,4-diene-3,20-dione.

$C_{22}H_{27}ClF_2O_5$ = 444.9.
*CAS — 50629-82-8.*
*ATC — D07AC12.*

### Profile

Halometasone is a corticosteroid used topically for its glucocorticoid activity (p.1068) in the treatment of various skin disorders. It is usually employed as a cream or ointment containing 0.05% of halometasone monohydrate.

When applied topically, particularly to large areas, when the skin is broken, or under occlusive dressings, corticosteroids may be absorbed in sufficient amounts to cause systemic effects (p.1068). The effects of topical corticosteroids on the skin are described on p.1070. For recommendations concerning the correct use of corticosteroids on the skin, see p.1074.

### Preparations

**Proprietary Preparations** (details are given in Part 3)
***Austria:*** Sicorten; ***Belg.:*** Sicorten†; ***Ger.:*** Sicorten; ***Hong Kong:*** Sicorten; ***Israel:*** Sicorten†; ***Neth.:*** Sicorten; ***Port.:*** Sicorten; ***Spain:*** Sicorten; ***Switz.:*** Sicorten.

**Multi-ingredient:** ***Ger.:*** Sicorten Plus; ***Hong Kong:*** Sicorten Plus; ***Israel:*** Sicorten Plus; ***Port.:*** Sicorten Plus; ***Spain:*** Sicorten Plus; ***Switz.:*** Sicorten Plus.

## Hydrocortamate Hydrochloride *(rINNM)*

Ethamicort; Hidrocloruro de hidrocortamato; Hydrocortisone Diethylaminoacetate Hydrochloride. 11β,17α,21-Trihydroxypregn-4-ene-3,20-dione 21-diethylaminoacetate hydrochloride.

$C_{27}H_{41}NO_6$,HCl = 512.1.
*CAS — 76-47-1 (hydrocortamate); 125-03-1 (hydrocortamate hydrochloride).*

### Profile

Hydrocortamate hydrochloride is a corticosteroid that has been used topically for its glucocorticoid activity (p.1068) in the treatment of various skin disorders.

### Preparations

**Proprietary Preparations** (details are given in Part 3)
**Multi-ingredient:** ***Ital.:*** Cortanest†.

# Hydrocortisone *(BAN, rINN)*

Anti-inflammatory Hormone; Compound F; Cortisol; Hidrocortisona; Hydrocortisonum; 17-Hydroxycorticosterone; NSC-10483. 11β,17α,21-Trihydroxypregn-4-ene-3,20-dione.

$C_{21}H_{30}O_5$ = 362.5.
*CAS — 50-23-7.*
*ATC — A01AC03; A07EA02; C05AA01; D07AA02; H02AB09; S01BA02; S02BA01.*

**Pharmacopoeias.** In *Chin., Eur.* (see p.vi), *Int., Jpn, Pol.,* and *US.*

**Ph. Eur. 5.0** (Hydrocortisone). A white or almost white, crystalline powder. It shows polymorphism. Practically insoluble in water; sparingly soluble in alcohol and in acetone; slightly soluble in dichloromethane. Protect from light.

**USP 27** (Hydrocortisone). A white to practically white, odourless, crystalline powder. Very slightly soluble in water and in ether; soluble 1 in 40 of alcohol and 1 in 80 of acetone; slightly soluble in chloroform. Store at a temperature of 25°, excursions permitted between 15° and 30°.

## Hydrocortisone Acetate *(BANM, rINNM)*

Acetato de hidrocortisona; Cortisol Acetate; Hydrocortisoni Acetas. Hydrocortisone 21-acetate.

$C_{23}H_{32}O_6$ = 404.5.
*CAS — 50-03-3.*
*ATC — A01AC03; A07EA02; C05AA01; D07AA02; H02AB09; S01BA02; S02BA01.*

NOTE. HCOR is a code approved by the BP 2003 for use on single unit doses of eye drops containing hydrocortisone acetate where the individual container may be too small to bear all the appropriate labelling information.

**Pharmacopoeias.** In *Chin., Eur.* (see p.vi), *Int., Jpn, Pol., US,* and *Viet.*

**Ph. Eur. 5.0** (Hydrocortisone Acetate). A white or almost white, crystalline powder. Practically insoluble in water; slightly soluble in dehydrated alcohol and in dichloromethane. Protect from light.

**USP 27** (Hydrocortisone Acetate). A white to practically white, odourless, crystalline powder. Insoluble in water; soluble 1 in 230 of alcohol and 1 in 200 of chloroform.

### Hydrocortisone Buteprate *(BANM, rINNM)*

Hydrocortisone Butyrate Propionate; Hydrocortisone Probutate *(USAN)*; TS-408. Hydrocortisone 17-butyrate 21-propionate.

$C_{28}H_{40}O_7$ = 488.6.
*CAS — 72590-77-3.*
*ATC — D07AB11.*

### Hydrocortisone Butyrate *(BANM, USAN, rINNM)*

Butirato de hidrocortisona; Cortisol Butyrate. Hydrocortisone 17α-butyrate.

$C_{25}H_{36}O_6$ = 432.5.
*CAS — 13609-67-1.*
*ATC — D07AB02.*

**Pharmacopoeias.** In *Chin., Jpn,* and *US.*

**USP 27** (Hydrocortisone Butyrate). A white to practically white, practically odourless crystalline powder. Practically insoluble in water; soluble in alcohol, in acetone, and in methyl alcohol; freely soluble in chloroform; slightly soluble in ether.

### Hydrocortisone Cipionate *(BANM, rINNM)*

Cipionato de hidrocortisona; Cortisol Cypionate; Hydrocortisone Cyclopentylpropionate; Hydrocortisone Cypionate. Hydrocortisone 21-(3-cyclopentylpropionate).

$C_{29}H_{42}O_6$ = 486.6.
*CAS — 508-99-6.*
*ATC — A01AC03; A07EA02; C05AA01; D07AA02; H02AB09; S01BA02; S02BA01.*

### Hydrocortisone Hydrogen Succinate *(BANM, rINNM)*

Cortisol Hemisuccinate; Hidrogenosuccinato de hidrocortisona; Hydrocortisone Hemisuccinate; Hydrocortisone Succinate; Hydrocortisoni Hydrogenosuccinas. Hydrocortisone 21-(hydrogen succinate).

$C_{25}H_{34}O_8$ = 462.5.
*CAS — 2203-97-6 (anhydrous hydrocortisone hydrogen succinate); 83784-20-7 (hydrocortisone hydrogen succinate monohydrate).*
*ATC — A01AC03; A07EA02; C05AA01; D07AA02; H02AB09; S01BA02; S02BA01.*

**Pharmacopoeias.** In *Eur.* (see p.vi) and *Jpn. US* allows the anhydrous form or the monohydrate.

**Ph. Eur. 5.0** (Hydrocortisone Hydrogen Succinate). A white or almost white, hygroscopic powder. Practically insoluble in water; freely soluble in dehydrated alcohol and in acetone; dissolves in dilute solutions of alkali carbonates and alkali hydroxides. Store in airtight containers. Protect from light.

**USP 27** (Hydrocortisone Hemisuccinate). It contains one molecule of water of hydration or is anhydrous. Store in airtight containers.

### Hydrocortisone Sodium Phosphate *(BANM, rINNM)*

Cortisol Sodium Phosphate; Fosfato sódico de hidrocortisona. Hydrocortisone 21-(disodium orthophosphate).

$C_{21}H_{29}Na_2O_8P$ = 486.4.
*CAS — 6000-74-4.*
*ATC — A01AC03; A07EA02; C05AA01; D07AA02; H02AB09; S01BA02; S02BA01.*

**Pharmacopoeias.** In *Br., Jpn,* and *US.*

**BP 2003** (Hydrocortisone Sodium Phosphate). A white or almost white, hygroscopic powder. Freely soluble in water; practically insoluble in dehydrated alcohol and in chloroform. A 0.5% solution in water has a pH of 7.5 to 9.0. Protect from light.

**USP 27** (Hydrocortisone Sodium Phosphate). A white to light yellow, odourless or practically odourless, exceedingly hygroscopic, powder. Soluble 1 in 1.5 of water; slightly soluble in alcohol; practically insoluble in chloroform, in dioxan, and in ether. Store in airtight containers.

### Hydrocortisone Sodium Succinate *(BANM, rINNM)*

Cortisol Sodium Succinate; Succinato sódico de hidrocortisona. Hydrocortisone 21-(sodium succinate).

$C_{25}H_{33}NaO_8$ = 484.5.
*CAS — 125-04-2.*
*ATC — A01AC03; A07EA02; C05AA01; D07AA02; H02AB09; S01BA02; S02BA01.*

**Pharmacopoeias.** In *Int., It., Jpn., Pol.,* and *US.*

**USP 27** (Hydrocortisone Sodium Succinate). A white or nearly white, odourless, hygroscopic, amorphous solid. Very soluble in water and in alcohol; very slightly soluble in acetone; insoluble in chloroform. Store in airtight containers. Protect from light.

### Hydrocortisone Valerate *(BANM, USAN, rINNM)*

Cortisol Valerate; Valerato de hidrocortisona. Hydrocortisone 17-valerate.

$C_{26}H_{38}O_6$ = 446.6.
*CAS — 57524-89-7.*
*ATC — A01AC03; A07EA02; C05AA01; D07AA02; H02AB09; S01BA02; S02BA01.*

**Pharmacopoeias.** In *US.*

## Adverse Effects, Treatment, Withdrawal, and Precautions

As for corticosteroids in general (see p.1068).

When applied topically, particularly to large areas, when the skin is broken, or under occlusive dressings, corticosteroids may be absorbed in sufficient amounts to cause systemic effects. Prolonged application to the eye of preparations containing corticosteroids has caused raised intra-ocular pressure and reduced visual function.

**Effects on fluid and electrolyte balance.** A report of marked hypokalaemia and hypomagnesaemia associated with high-dose intravenous hydrocortisone therapy in an alcoholic patient with suspected immune thrombocytopenia.[1] Cardiac arrhythmias developed, and prolonged infusion of magnesium and potassium was required to restore normal plasma concentrations.

1. Ramsahoye BH, *et al.* The mineralocorticoid effects of high dose hydrocortisone. *BMJ* 1995; **310:** 656–7.

**Effects on the nervous system.** For reports and comments on paraesthesia or perineal irritation associated with hydrocortisone sodium phosphate given intravenously, see p.1070.

**Hypersensitivity and anaphylaxis.** References to hypersensitivity reactions and anaphylaxis associated with the intravenous administration of hydrocortisone;[1-6] topical application can also result in hypersensitivity.[7]

1. Chan CS, *et al.* Hydrocortisone-induced anaphylaxis. *Med J Aust* 1984; **141:** 444–6.
2. Seale JP. Anaphylactoid reaction to hydrocortisone. *Med J Aust* 1984; **141:** 446.
3. Corallo CE, Sosnin M. Bronchospasm, tachycardia following intravenous hydrocortisone. *Aust J Hosp Pharm* 1985; **15:** 103–4.
4. Al Mahdy H, Hall M. Anaphylaxis and hydrocortisone. *Ann Intern Med* 1988; **108:** 487–8.
5. Fulcher DA, Katelaris CH. Anaphylactoid reaction to intravenous hydrocortisone sodium succinate: a case report and literature review. *Med J Aust* 1991; **154:** 210–14.
6. Kawane H. Anaphylactoid reaction to intravenous hydrocortisone sodium succinate. *Med J Aust* 1991; **154:** 782.
7. Wilkinson SM, *et al.* Hydrocortisone: an important cutaneous allergen. *Lancet* 1991; **337:** 761–2.

## Interactions

The interactions of corticosteroids in general are described on p.1072.

## Pharmacokinetics

For a brief account of the pharmacokinetics of corticosteroids, see p.1073.

Hydrocortisone is readily absorbed from the gastrointestinal tract and peak blood concentrations are attained in about an hour. The plasma half-life is about 100 minutes. It is more than 90% bound to plasma proteins. Following intramuscular injection, the absorption of the water-soluble sodium phosphate and sodium succinate esters is rapid, while absorption of hydrocortisone free alcohol and its lipid-soluble esters is slower. Absorption of hydrocortisone acetate after intra-articular or soft-tissue injection is also slow. Hydrocortisone is absorbed through the skin, particularly in denuded areas.

Hydrocortisone is metabolised in the liver and most body tissues to hydrogenated and degraded forms such as tetrahydrocortisone and tetrahydrocortisol. These are excreted in the urine, mainly conjugated as glucuronides, together with a very small proportion of unchanged hydrocortisone. Hydrocortisone readily crosses the placenta.

## Uses and Administration

Hydrocortisone is a corticosteroid with both glucocorticoid and to a lesser extent mineralocorticoid activity (p.1068). As cortisol it is the most important of the predominantly glucocorticoid steroids secreted by the adrenal cortex. Hydrocortisone is used, usually with a more potent mineralocorticoid, for replacement therapy in adrenocortical insufficiency (p.1075). It may also be used for its glucocorticoid properties in other conditions for which corticosteroid therapy is indicated (p.1073) but drugs with fewer mineralocorticoid effects tend to be preferred for the long-term systemic therapy of auto-immune and inflammatory disease.

The dose may be expressed in terms of the base, and the following are each approximately equivalent to 100 mg of hydrocortisone:

- hydrocortisone acetate 112 mg
- hydrocortisone buteprate 135 mg
- hydrocortisone butyrate 119 mg
- hydrocortisone cipionate 134 mg
- hydrocortisone hydrogen succinate 128 mg
- hydrocortisone sodium phosphate 134 mg
- hydrocortisone sodium succinate 134 mg
- hydrocortisone valerate 123 mg

However, esterification generally alters potency and compounds with equivalent hydrocortisone content may not have equivalent clinical effect.

For administration by mouth hydrocortisone free alcohol is usually used; the cipionate ester is used in some formulations.

For **replacement therapy** in acute or chronic adrenocortical insufficiency the normal requirement is 20 to 30 mg daily (usually taken in 2 doses, the larger in the morning and the smaller in the early evening, to mimic the circadian rhythm of the body). Additional sodium chloride may be required if there is defective aldosterone secretion, but mineralocorticoid activity is usually supplemented by fludrocortisone acetate orally. Similar regimens have also been used to correct glucocorticoid deficiency in the salt-losing form of congenital adrenal hyperplasia (p.1078).

Hydrocortisone may be given **intravenously**, by slow injection or infusion, in the form of a water-soluble derivative such as hydrocortisone sodium succinate or hydrocortisone sodium phosphate when a rapid effect is required in **emergencies**: such conditions are acute adrenocortical insufficiency caused by Addisonian or post-adrenalectomy crises, by the abrupt accidental withdrawal of therapy in corticosteroid-treated patients, or by the inability of the adrenal glands to cope with increased stress in such patients; certain allergic emergencies such as anaphylaxis; acute severe asthma (status asthmaticus—see also p.777); and shock. The usual dose is the equivalent of 100 to 500 mg of hydrocortisone, repeated 3 or 4 times in 24 hours, according to the severity of the condition and the patient's response. Children up to 1 year of age may be given 25 mg, those aged 1 to 5 years 50 mg, and those aged 6 to 12 years 100 mg. Fluids and electrolytes should be given as necessary to correct any associated metabolic disorder. Similar doses to those specified above may also be given **intramuscularly** but the response is likely to be less rapid than that observed following intravenous administration. Corticosteroids are considered to be of secondary value in anaphylactic shock because of their relatively slow onset of action, but intravenous hydrocortisone may be a useful adjunct to adrenaline to prevent further deterioration in severely affected patients.

In patients with adrenal deficiency states supplementary corticosteroid therapy may be necessary during some **surgical operations** and hydrocortisone sodium succinate or sodium phosphate may be given intramuscularly or intravenously before surgery. Various regimens have been proposed (see also Surgery, p.1074). In patients taking more than 10 mg of prednisolone or its equivalent by mouth daily, the *British National Formulary* recommends the following regimen:

- *minor surgery under general anaesthesia*, either the usual oral corticosteroid dose on the morning of surgery *or* hydrocortisone 25 to 50 mg (usually as the sodium succinate) intravenously at induction; the usual oral corticosteroid dose is recommenced after surgery
- *moderate or major surgery*, the usual oral corticosteroid dose on the morning of surgery, *plus* hydrocortisone 25 to 50 mg intravenously at induction, and followed by similar doses of hydrocortisone 3 times daily, for 24 hours after moderate surgery and

48 to 72 hours after major surgery; the usual corticosteroid dose is resumed once hydrocortisone injections are stopped.

For **local injection** into soft tissues hydrocortisone is usually used in the form of the sodium phosphate or sodium succinate esters; doses in terms of hydrocortisone are usually 100 to 200 mg. For intra-articular injection hydrocortisone acetate is usually used in doses of 5 to 50 mg depending upon the size of the joint.

For **topical application** in the treatment of various skin disorders hydrocortisone and the acetate, buteprate, butyrate, and valerate esters are normally employed in creams, ointments, or lotions. Concentrations usually used have ranged from 0.1 to 2.5%. Although it is considered that hydrocortisone has fewer side-effects on the skin and is less liable to cause adrenal suppression than the more potent topical corticosteroids (see p.1074 for a rough guide to the clinical potencies of topical corticosteroids), it should be borne in mind, that this property may be considerably modified both by the type of formulation or vehicle used and by the type of esterification present; other factors that may also influence the degree of absorption include the site of application, use of an occlusive dressing, the degree of skin damage, and the size of the area to which the preparation is applied.

Hydrocortisone or its esters are also available in a variety of other dosage forms including those for ophthalmic, aural, dental, and rectal application, for use in allergic and inflammatory disorders.

Other esters of hydrocortisone that have occasionally been used include the aceponate, glycyrrhetinate, and propionate. Esters such as the aceponate may show modified topical activity.

## Preparations

***BP 2003:*** Hydrocortisone Acetate and Neomycin Ear Drops; Hydrocortisone Acetate and Neomycin Eye Drops; Hydrocortisone Acetate and Neomycin Eye Ointment; Hydrocortisone Acetate Cream; Hydrocortisone Acetate Injection; Hydrocortisone Acetate Ointment; Hydrocortisone and Clioquinol Cream; Hydrocortisone and Clioquinol Ointment; Hydrocortisone and Neomycin Cream; Hydrocortisone Cream; Hydrocortisone Ointment; Hydrocortisone Oromucosal Tablets; Hydrocortisone Sodium Phosphate Injection; Hydrocortisone Sodium Succinate Injection;
***USP 27:*** Chloramphenicol and Hydrocortisone Acetate for Ophthalmic Suspension; Chloramphenicol, Polymyxin B Sulfate, and Hydrocortisone Acetate Ophthalmic Ointment; Clioquinol and Hydrocortisone Cream; Clioquinol and Hydrocortisone Ointment; Colistin and Neomycin Sulfates and Hydrocortisone Acetate Otic Suspension; Hydrocortisone Acetate Cream; Hydrocortisone Acetate Injectable Suspension; Hydrocortisone Acetate Lotion; Hydrocortisone Acetate Ointment; Hydrocortisone Acetate Ophthalmic Ointment; Hydrocortisone Acetate Ophthalmic Suspension; Hydrocortisone and Acetic Acid Otic Solution; Hydrocortisone Butyrate Cream; Hydrocortisone Cream; Hydrocortisone Gel; Hydrocortisone Injectable Suspension; Hydrocortisone Lotion; Hydrocortisone Ointment; Hydrocortisone Rectal Suspension; Hydrocortisone Sodium Phosphate Injection; Hydrocortisone Sodium Succinate for Injection; Hydrocortisone Tablets; Hydrocortisone Valerate Cream; Hydrocortisone Valerate Ointment; Neomycin and Polymyxin B Sulfates and Hydrocortisone Acetate Cream; Neomycin and Polymyxin B Sulfates and Hydrocortisone Acetate Ophthalmic Suspension; Neomycin and Polymyxin B Sulfates and Hydrocortisone Ophthalmic Suspension; Neomycin and Polymyxin B Sulfates and Hydrocortisone Otic Solution; Neomycin and Polymyxin B Sulfates and Hydrocortisone Otic Suspension; Neomycin and Polymyxin B Sulfates, Bacitracin Zinc, and Hydrocortisone Acetate Ophthalmic Ointment; Neomycin and Polymyxin B Sulfates, Bacitracin Zinc, and Hydrocortisone Ointment; Neomycin and Polymyxin B Sulfates, Bacitracin Zinc, and Hydrocortisone Ophthalmic Ointment; Neomycin and Polymyxin B Sulfates, Bacitracin, and Hydrocortisone Acetate Ointment; Neomycin and Polymyxin B Sulfates, Bacitracin, and Hydrocortisone Acetate Ophthalmic Ointment; Neomycin and Polymyxin B Sulfates, Gramicidin, and Hydrocortisone Acetate Cream; Neomycin Sulfate and Hydrocortisone Acetate Cream; Neomycin Sulfate and Hydrocortisone Acetate Lotion; Neomycin Sulfate and Hydrocortisone Acetate Ointment; Neomycin Sulfate and Hydrocortisone Acetate Ophthalmic Ointment; Neomycin Sulfate and Hydrocortisone Acetate Ophthalmic Suspension; Neomycin Sulfate and Hydrocortisone Cream; Neomycin Sulfate and Hydrocortisone Ointment; Neomycin Sulfate and Hydrocortisone Otic Suspension; Oxytetracycline Hydrochloride and Hydrocortisone Acetate Ophthalmic Suspension; Oxytetracycline Hydrochloride and Hydrocortisone Ointment; Polymyxin B Sulfate and Hydrocortisone Otic Solution.

**Proprietary Preparations** (details are given in Part 3)

***Arg.:*** Alfacort; Anusol-HC; Cortenem; Efficort; Fridalit; Hidrotisona; Medrocil; Microsona; Oralsone; Schericur; Sirotamicin HC; Stiefcortil; Transderma H; ***Austral.:*** Colifoam; Cortaid; Cortef; Cortic; Derm-Aid; Egocort; Hycor; Hysone; Nordicort†; Sigmacort; Siguent Hycor; Solu-Cortef; Squibb-HC†; ***Austria:*** Colifoam; Ekzemsalbe F; Hydrocortone; Hydroderm; Locoidon; Retef; Schericur†; ***Belg.:*** Buccalsone; Colifoam†; Cortril; Cremicort-H; Locoid; Pannocort; Solu-Cortef; ***Braz.:*** Berlison; Cortisonal; Cortiston; Flebocortid†; Hidrocol†; Hidyn H; Locoid; Nutracort; Solu-Cortef; Stiefcortil; Therasona†; Westcort; ***Canad.:*** A-Hydrocort; Aquacort†; Barriere-HC; Claritin Skin Itch Relief; Cortacet; Cortamed†; Cortate; Cortef; Cortenema; Corticreme†; Cortifoam; Cortiment†; Cortoderm; Dermarest Dricort Anti-Itch; Emo-Cort; Hycort; Hyderm; Hydrosone; HydroVal; Lanacort†; Novo-Hydrocort; Prevex HC; Rectocort†; Sarna HC; Solu-Cortef; Texacort†; Westcort; ***Chile:*** Aquanil HC; Calmurid; Efficort; Hipoge; Lacticare-HC; Locoid; Nutralona; Pandel; Solu-Cortef; Vitulpas; ***Denm.:*** Colifoam; Dermil†; Locoid; Mildison; Solu-Cortef; Uniderm; ***Fin.:*** Apocort; Bucort; Colifoam; Cortril†; Dermacort†; Kyypakkaus; Locoid; Mildison†; Nutracort; Solu-Cortef; Uniderm†; ***Fr.:*** Aphilan; Colofoam; Cortapaisyl; Dermaspraid Demangeaison; Dermaspray demangeaison†; Dermofenac; Efficort; Hydracort; Locoid; Mitocortyl; Proctocort; ***Ger.:*** Alfason; Colifoam; Dermallerg; Dermo Posterisan; Ebenol; Fenistil; Ficortril; Glycocortison; Hydro-Wolff; Hydrocort; Hydrocort Mild†; Hydrocutan; Hydrocutan mild; Hydroderm HC; Hydrogalen; Laticort; Latimit†; Munitren H; Pandel; Posterine Corte; ratioAllerg; Remederm HC; Retef†; Sagittacortin†; Sanatison Mono; Soventol HC; Systral Hydrocort; velopural; ***Gr.:*** Colifoam; Filocot; Nutracort; Solu-Cortef; ***Hong Kong:*** Corticreme†; Efficort; Egocort; Hycortin; Hytisone; Lacticare-HC; Rectocort†; Solu-Cortef; ***India:*** Wycort; ***Irl.:*** Colifoam; Corlan; Cortopin; Dioderm; Hc45; Hydrocortisyl; Hydrocortone; Locoid; Mildison; Solu-Cortef; ***Israel:*** Colifoam†; Cortifoam; Cortizone; Efficort; Hydrocort†; Lanacort; Solu-Cortef; ***Ital.:*** Colifoam; Cortaid; Cortidro; Cortop; Dermirit; Dermocortal; Efficort; Flebocortid; Foille Insetti; Idracemi; Lanacort; Lenirit; Locoidon; Novocortal†; Paro†; Rapicort†; Sintotrat; Solu-Cortef; ***Malaysia:*** Derm-Aid; Dhacort; Efficort; Egocort; Hydrocort; Solu-Cortef; ***Mex.:*** Aquanil HC; Efficort; Fadol; Flebocortid; Flemex†; Lacticare-HC; Locoid; Nositrol; Nutracort; Vicortin†; Westcort; ***Neth.:*** Buccalsone; Hydro-Adreson†; Locoid; Mildison; Solu-Cortef; ***Norw.:*** Apocortal†; Colifoam; Locoid; Mildison; Solu-Cortef; ***NZ:*** BK HC†; Colifoam; Cortaid†; Derm-Aid; DP Hydrocortisone; Egocort; Lemnis Fatty Cream HC; Locoid; Mildison; Skincalm; Solu-Cortef; ***Port.:*** Colifoam; Dermimade Hidrocortisona; Hidalone; Hydrocortone; Lactisona; Locoid; Pandel; Pandermil; Solu-Cortef; ***S.Afr.:*** Biocort†; Colifoam; Covocort; Cutaderm; Dilucort; Locoid; Mylocort; Procutan; Solu-Cortef; Stopitch; ***Singapore:*** Derm-Aid; Dhacort; Efficort; Egocort; Hydro-Adreson†; Hydrocort; Solu-Cortef; ***Spain:*** Actocortina; Aftasone; Ceneo; Derminovag†; Dermosa Hidrocortisona; Hemorrane; Hidroaltesona; Hidrocisdin; Lactisona; Oralsone; Picosyl†; Scalpicin Capilar; Schericur; Suniderma; Supralef†; ***Swed.:*** Colifoam; Ficortril; Locoid; Locoid Crelo; Mildison; Solu-Cortef; Uniderm; ***Switz.:*** Alfacortone; Colifoam†; Glycocortisone H; Hydrocortone; Locoid; Sanadermil; Solu-Cortef; ***Thai.:*** Hydro-Adreson†; Hytisone; Prevex HC; Solu-Cortef; ***UAE:*** Alfacort; ***UK:*** Colifoam; Corlan; Cortopin; Cortropin; Dermacort; Dioderm; Efcortelan; Efcortesol; Exe-Cort; Hc45; Hydrocortistab; Hydrocortone; Jungle Formula Sting Relief Cream†; Lanacort; Locoid; Mildison; Solu-Cortef; Zenoxone; ***USA:*** A-Hydrocort; Acticort; Ala-Cort; Anucort-HC; Anusol-HC; Aquanil HC; Bactine; CaldeCort; Carmol HC; Cetacort; Cort-Dome; Cortaid; Cortef; Cortef Feminine Itch; Cortenema; Corticaine; Cortifoam; Cortizone; Dermarest Dri-Cort; Dermol HC; Dermolate; EarSol-HC; Gynecort; Hemril-HC; Hi-Cor; Hycort; Hydrocortone; HydroSkin; HydroTex†; Hytone; Lacticare-HC; Lanacort; Locoid; Massengill Medicated; Neutrogena T/Scalp; Nutracort; Orabase HCA; Pandel; Penecort; Procort; Proctocort; Proctocream HC 2.5%; Recort Plus; S-T Cort†; Solu-Cortef; Synacort; Tegrin-HC; Texacort; Westcort.

**Multi-ingredient: *Arg.:*** Aeromicrosona C; Alercortil; Antibiocort; Anusol Duo; Anusol Duo S; Atomoderma Plus; Bexon; Biocortin; Cipro HC; Ciprocort; Ciriax Otic; Cristalomicina; Derivoco; Dermoperative; Disel Hidrocortisona; Epiprocto; Gramicortil; Griseoplus; Hidrocortin; Hipoglos con Hidrocortisona; Irigal; Lactiderm HC; Masivol Urea; Micozol Compuesto; Microsona C; Microsona Otica; Neo Pelvicillin; Otex HC; Oto Biotaer; Otocipro; Otoseptil; Otosporin; Otosporin L; Procto-Ikatral; Prurisedan Biotic; Quemicetina con Hidrocortisona; Start NP; Terra-Cortril Nistatina; Tridermal; Triefect; Vagicural; Xyloprocto; ***Austral.:*** Chlorocort†; Ciproxin HC; Hydroform; Hydrozole; Proctosedyl; Rectinol HC; Resolve Plus; Xyloproct; ***Austria:*** Calmurid HC; Ciproxin HC; Cortison Kemicetin; Daktacort†; Endomethazone†; Hydoftal; Hydrocortimycin; Hydrodexan†; Ichtho-Cortin; Otosporin; Systrason†; Tropoderm; ***Belg.:*** Alphaderm†; Daktacort; Eoline; Fucidin Hydrocortisone†; Onctose a l'Hydrocortisone†; Otosporin; Pimafucort†; Sulfo-Selenium†; Terra-Cortril; Xyloproct†; ***Braz.:*** Anusol-HC; Cipro HC; Dermilan†; Elocort†; Furazolon†; Gingilone; Hemodotti; Hermodotti†; Hidrocorte; Hidroneo; Hipoglos Oftalmico†; Infladerm†; Nitrolerg; Otosporin; Terra-Cortril; Terra-Cortril com Polimixina B†; Vioformio-Hidrocortisona; Xyloproct; ***Canad.:*** Actinac†; Anodan-HC; Anugesic-HC; Anusol-HC; Anuzinc HC; Anuzinc HC Plus; Calmurid HC†; Cipro HC; Cortimyxin; Cortisporin; Diospor HC†; Fucidin H; Hemcort HC; Neo-Cortef; Ophthocort†; Pentamycetin-HC; PMS-Egozinc-HC; Pramox HC; Proctodan-HC; Proctofoam-HC; Proctomyxin; Proctosedyl; Proctosone; Rectogel HC; Rivasol HC; Ti-U-Lac HC†; Uremol-HC; Vioform-Hydrocortisone; VoSoL HC; ***Chile:*** Cortifenol H; Fucidin H; ***Denm.:*** Brentacort; Ciflox; Fucidin-Hydrocortison; Locoidol; Proctosedyl; ***Fin.:*** Ciproxin-Hydrocortison; Daktacort; Duocort; Fucidin-Hydrocortison; Locoidol; Pantyson; Pimafucort; Proctosedyl; Sibicort; Terra-Cortril; Terra-Cortril P; Trosycort; Xyloproct; ***Fr.:*** Anti-Hemorroidaires†; Bacicoline; Cortibiotique†; Daktacort†; Dermocalm†; Locoide N†; Madecassol Neomycine Hydrocortisone; Onctose Hydrocortisone†; Framycine Hydrocortisone†; ***Ger.:*** Antiprurit; Calmurid HC†; Canesten HC; Corti Jaikal; Corti-Flexiole†; Eksalb†; Farco-Tril; Fucidine plus; Hydrodexan; Ichthocortin; Novifort; Nubral 4 HC†; Nystaderm comp; Otosporin†; Pantocrinale†; Pigmanorm; Pimafucort†; Polyspectran HC; Posterisan Forte; Terracortril; Topoderm N†; ***Gr.:*** Daktodor; Fucidin H; Terra-Cortril; ***Hong Kong:*** Anusol-HC†; Canesten HC; Cipro HC; Corticin; Cortiphenol H; Cortison Kemicetine†; Daktacort; Fucidin H; Hemcort HC; Hydro-Funga; Otosporin; Posterisan Forte; Proctosedyl; Proctosone; Protozone†; Xyloproct; ***India:*** Bell Diono Resolvent; Bell Resolvent; Cortison Kemicetine; Cortola-m; Cortoquinol; Crotorax-HC; Daktacort; Efcorlin; Furacin-S; Genticyn HC; Keralin; Medithane; Multifungin H; Neosporin-H; Pino-Cort; Proctosedyl; Shield; Wycort c Neomycin; ***Irl.:*** Actinac†; Alphaderm; Alphosyl HC; Anugesic-HC; Anusol-HC; Calmurid HC; Canesten HC; Daktacort; Eurax-Hydrocortisone; Fucidin H; Gentisone HC; Hydrocal†; Locoid C; Neo-Cortef†; Nystaform-HC; Otosporin; Perinal; Proctofoam-HC; Proctosedyl; Quinocort; Terra-Cortril Nystatin†; Terra-Cortril†; Timodine; Vioform-Hydrocortisone; Xyloproct; ***Israel:*** Alphosyl HC; Benzantine H; Calmurid HC; Ciproxin HC; Daktacort; Epifoam; Fucidin H; Hycocin; Hycomycin; Hydroagisten; Otosporin†; Panthisone; Perinal; Proctofoam-HC; Proctosedyl†; Proctozorin-N; Xyloproct; ***Ital.:*** Argisone; Cort-Inal; Cortison Chemicetina; Emorril; Fucidin H; Idracemi Eparina†; Idrocet; Idroneomicil; Kinogen; Mictasone; Mixotone; Mobilat; Nasomixin; Nevacort; Pomata Midy HC†; Prepacort H; Preparazione Antiemorroidaria; Proctidol; Proctofoam-HC; Proctosedyl; Proctosoll; Reumacort; Scalpicin; Sedalen Cort; Sinsurrene†; Vasosterone Antibiotico; Vasosterone Collirio; Xyloproct†; ***Malaysia:*** Becacort; Candacort; Daktacort; Decocort; Fucidin H; H-C; Neo-Hydro; Pocin H; Proctosedyl; Setarin H; Ucort; Xyloproct; Zaricort; ***Mex.:*** Biotarson N; Cortisporin; Daktacort; Hidrofenil; Hidropolicin; Otolone; Soldrin; Sulfa Hidro; Ultracortin; Vioformo-Cort; Xyloproct; ***Neth.:*** Alphacortison†; Bacicoline-B; Calmurid HC; Daktacort; Otosporin; Proctosedyl; Terra-Cortril Gel Steraject met polymyxine-B; Terra-Cortril met polymyxine-B; Xyloproct†; ***Norw.:*** Daktacort; Fucidin-Hydrocortison; Locoidol; Proctosedyl; Terra-Cortril; Terra-Cortril Polymyxin B; Xyloproct; ***NZ:*** Ciproxin HC; Coly-Mycin S Otic†; Daktacort; DP Lotion - HC; Fungocort; Locoid C; Micreme H; Pimafucort; Proctosedyl; Xyloproct; ***Port.:*** Alphosyl HC†; Anucet; Clorcorticil; Corticil T; Cortigripe; Daktacort; Davimicina; Fucidine H; Leuco Hubber; Locoid C; Otolys†; Otosporin†; Pimafucort; Proctonostrum; ***S.Afr.:*** Anusol-HC†; Calmurid HC; Ciprobay HC; Daktacort; Fucidin H; Nasomixin; Neoderm; Otosporin; Proctofoam; Proctosedyl; Quinoderm-H†; Terra-Cortril; Viocort; ***Singapore:*** Canesten HC; Ciprobay HC; Cortaid with Aloe; Daktacort; Decocort; Fucidin H; Otosporin†; Proctosedyl; Xyloproct†; Zaricort; ***Spain:*** Aftajuventus; Aftasone B C; Alantomicina Complex†; Anginovag; Antiblef Eczem†; Antihemorroidal; Bacisporin; Brentan; Cilinafosal Hidrocort; Ciproxina; Cohortan; Cohortan Antibiotico†; Cohortan†; Cortenema; Cortison Chemicet Topica; Dermo Hubber; Detraine; Edifaringen; Euraxil Hidrocort†; Fucidine H†; Grietalgen Hidrocort; Halibut Hidrocortisona; Hemodren Compuesto; Hepro; Hidroc Cloranf†; Hidroc Neomic†; Leuco Hubber; Milrosina Nistatina; Neo Bacitrin Hidrocortis†; Neo Hubber; Neo Visage†; Oftalmo†; Oto Difusor†; Oto Neomicin Calm†; Oto Vitna; Otosporin; Roberfarin; Terra-Cortril; Tisuderma; Tyroneomicin†; ***Swed.:*** Calmuril-Hydrokortison†; Cortimyk; Daktacort; Fenuril-Hydrokortison; Fucidin-Hydrocortison; Proctosedyl; Terracortril; Terracortril med polymyxin B; Xyloproct; ***Switz.:*** Calmurid HC; Ciproxin HC; Cortifluid N; Cortimycine; Daktacort; Dermacalm-d; Endomethasone†; Fucidin H; Haemocortin; Hydrocortisone comp; Neo-Hydro; Otosporin; Rocanal Permanent Gangrene†; Septomixine; Terracortril; ***Thai.:*** Antergan; Daktacort; Dermasol; Doproct; Fucidin H; Ladocort; Neo-Hytisone†; Otosporin; Proctosedyl; Xyloproct†; ***UK:*** Actinac; Alphaderm; Alphosyl HC; Anugesic-HC; Anusol-HC, Plus HC; Calmurid HC; Canesten HC; Daktacort; Daktacort HC; Econacort; Eurax-Hydrocortisone; Fucidin H; Gentisone HC; Germoloids HC; Gregoderm; Locoid C; Neo-Cortef†; Nystaform-HC; Otosporin; Perinal; Proctocream HC†; Proctofoam-HC; Proctosedyl; Quinocort†; Terra-Cortril; Terra-Cortril Nystatin†; Timodine; Uniroid-HC; Vioform-Hydrocortisone; Xyloproct; ***USA:*** 1 + 1-F; AA-HC Otic†; Acetasol HC; Ak-Spore HC†; Analpram-HC; AnaMantle HC; AntibiOtic†; Anumed HC; Cipro HC; Coly-Mycin S Otic; Corque; Cortane-B; Cortatrigen; Cortic; Corticaine; Cortimycin; Cortisporin; Cortisporin-TC; Cyotic; Dermtex HC with Aloe; Ear-Eze; Emergent-Ez; Enzone; Epifoam; Fungoid HC; HC Derma-Pax; Hysone; LazerSporin-C; LidaMantle HC; Neotricin HC; Octicair; Oti-Med; Otic-Care; OtiTricin; Otobiotic; Otocort; Otomar-HC; Otomycin-HPN; Otosporin; Pedi-Cort V†; Pediotic; Pramosone; Proctofoam-HC; Terra-Cortril; Tri-Otic; UAD-Otic; Vanoxide-HC; VoSoL HC; Vytone; Zone-A; Zoto-HC.

---

## Isoflupredone Acetate *(BANM, USAN, rINNM)*

Acetato de isoflupredona; 9α-Fluoroprednisolone Acetate; U-6013. 9α-Fluoro-11β,17α,21-trihydroxypregna-1,4-diene-3,20-dione 21-acetate.

$C_{23}H_{29}FO_6$ = 420.5.

*CAS — 338-95-4 (isoflupredone); 338-98-7 (isoflupredone acetate).*

**Pharmacopoeias.** In *US* for veterinary use only.

**USP 27** (Isoflupredone Acetate). Protect from light.

### Profile

Isoflupredone acetate is a corticosteroid that has been used for its topical glucocorticoid activity (p.1068) in allergic rhinitis.

Isoflupredone is also employed in veterinary medicine.

### Preparations

**Proprietary Preparations** (details are given in Part 3)

**Multi-ingredient: *Israel:*** Proaf.

---

## Loteprednol Etabonate *(BANM, USAN, rINNM)*

CDDD-5604; HGP-1; Loteprednol, etabonato de; Loteprednol Ethyl Carbonate; P-5604. (11β,17α)-17-[(Ethoxycarbonyl)oxy]-11-hydroxy-3-oxoandrosta-1,4-diene-17-carboxylic acid chloromethyl ester.

$C_{24}H_{31}ClO_7$ = 467.0.

*CAS — 129260-79-3 (loteprednol); 82034-46-6 (loteprednol etabonate).*

### Profile

Loteprednol etabonate is a corticosteroid used for its glucocorticoid activity (p.1068) in the topical management of inflammatory and allergic disorders of the eye. It is usually used as eye drops containing 0.2 or 0.5%.

Prolonged application to the eye of preparations containing corticosteroids has caused raised intra-ocular pressure and reduced visual function.

◊ References.

1. Noble S, Goa KL. Loteprednol etabonate: clinical potential in the management of ocular inflammation. *BioDrugs* 1998; **10:** 329–39.

### Preparations

**Proprietary Preparations** (details are given in Part 3)

***Arg.:*** Lotemax; Lotesoft; ***Braz.:*** Alrex†; Loteprol†; ***USA:*** Alrex; Lotemax.

---

## Mazipredone *(rINN)*

11β,17-Dihydroxy-21-(4-methyl-1-piperazinyl)pregna-1,4-diene-3,20-dione.

$C_{26}H_{38}N_2O_4$ = 442.6.

*CAS — 13085-08-0.*

### Profile

Mazipredone is a corticosteroid used topically for its glucocorticoid activity (p.1068). It is used as the hydrochloride in combination with miconazole in the treatment of fungal infections of the skin.

When applied topically, particularly to large areas, when the skin is broken, or under occlusive dressings, corticosteroids may be absorbed in sufficient amounts to cause systemic effects (p.1068). The effects of topical corticosteroids on the skin are described on p.1070.

### Medrysone (USAN, pINN)

11β-Hydroxy-6α-methylprogesterone; Medrisona; NSC-63278; U-8471. 11β-Hydroxy-6α-methylpregn-4-ene-3,20-dione.

$C_{22}H_{32}O_3$ = 344.5.

*CAS — 2668-66-8.*

*ATC — S01BA08.*

#### Profile

Medrysone is a corticosteroid used for its glucocorticoid activity (see p.1068) in the topical treatment of allergic and inflammatory conditions of the eye. It is usually given as 1% eye drops.

Prolonged application to the eye of preparations containing corticosteroids has caused raised intra-ocular pressure and reduced visual function.

#### Preparations

**Proprietary Preparations** (details are given in Part 3)
***Austral.:*** HMS†; ***Ger.:*** Spectramedryn†; ***Port.:*** Medrisocil; ***Spain:*** Liquipom Medrisone†; ***Switz.:*** HMS†; ***USA:*** HMS.

**Multi-ingredient:** ***Ital.:*** Medramil†; ***Spain:*** Mirantal†.

### Meprednisone (USAN, rINN)

Meprednisona; 16β-Methylprednisone; NSC-527579; Sch-4358. 17α,21-Dihydroxy-16β-methylpregna-1,4-diene-3,11,20-trione.

$C_{22}H_{28}O_5$ = 372.5.

*CAS — 1247-42-3.*

*ATC — H02AB15.*

**Pharmacopoeias.** In *US.*

**USP 27** (Meprednisone). Store in airtight containers at a temperature not exceeding 40°. Protect from light.

#### Profile

Meprednisone is a corticosteroid with mainly glucocorticoid activity (p.1068). It has been given by mouth as either the free alcohol or the acetate and by injection as the sodium hemisuccinate.

#### Preparations

**Proprietary Preparations** (details are given in Part 3)
***Arg.:*** Cortipyren B; Deltisona B.

## Methylprednisolone (BAN, rINN)

6α-Methylprednisolone; Methylprednisolonum; Metilprednisolona; NSC-19987. 11β,17α,21-Trihydroxy-6α-methylpregna-1,4-diene-3,20-dione.

$C_{22}H_{30}O_5$ = 374.5.

*CAS — 83-43-2.*

*ATC — D07AA01; H02AB04.*

**Pharmacopoeias.** In *Eur.* (see p.vi), *Jpn,* and *US.*

**Ph. Eur. 5.0** (Methylprednisolone). A white or almost white, crystalline powder. It shows polymorphism. Practically insoluble in water; sparingly soluble in alcohol; slightly soluble in acetone and in dichloromethane. Protect from light.

**USP 27** (Methylprednisolone). A white to practically white, odourless, crystalline powder. Practically insoluble in water; soluble 1 in 100 of alcohol, and in 1 in 800 of chloroform and of ether; slightly soluble in acetone; sparingly soluble in dioxan and in methyl alcohol. Store in airtight containers. Protect from light.

### Methylprednisolone Acetate (BANM, rINNM)

Acetato de metilprednisolona; Methylprednisoloni Acetas. Methylprednisolone 21-acetate.

$C_{24}H_{32}O_6$ = 416.5.

*CAS — 53-36-1.*

*ATC — D07AA01; H02AB04.*

**Pharmacopoeias.** In *Eur.* (see p.vi) and *US.*

**Ph. Eur. 5.0** (Methylprednisolone Acetate). A white or almost white, crystalline powder. Practically insoluble in water; sparingly soluble in alcohol and in acetone. Protect from light.

**USP 27** (Methylprednisolone Acetate). A white or practically white, odourless, crystalline powder. Soluble 1 in 1500 of water, 1 in 400 of alcohol, 1 in 250 of chloroform, and 1 in 1500 of ether; sparingly soluble in acetone and in methyl alcohol; soluble in dioxan. Store in airtight containers at a temperature of 25°, excursions permitted between 15° and 30°. Protect from light.

### Methylprednisolone Hydrogen Succinate

(BANM, rINNM)

Hidrogenosuccinato de metilprednisolona; Methylprednisolone Hemisuccinate; Methylprednisoloni Hydrogenosuccinas. Methylprednisolone 21-(hydrogen succinate).

$C_{26}H_{34}O_8$ = 474.5.

*CAS — 2921-57-5.*

*ATC — D07AA01; H02AB04.*

**Pharmacopoeias.** In *Eur.* (see p.vi) and *US.*

**Ph. Eur. 5.0** (Methylprednisolone Hydrogen Succinate). A white or almost white, hygroscopic powder. Practically insoluble in water; slightly soluble in dehydrated alcohol and in acetone; dissolves in dilute solutions of alkali hydroxides. Store in airtight containers. Protect from light.

**USP 27** (Methylprednisolone Hemisuccinate). A white or nearly white, odourless or nearly odourless, hygroscopic solid. Very slightly soluble in water; freely soluble in alcohol; soluble in acetone. Store in airtight containers.

### Methylprednisolone Sodium Succinate

(BANM, rINNM)

Methylprednisolone Sodium Hemisuccinate; Succinato sódico de metilprednisolona. Methylprednisolone 21-(sodium succinate).

$C_{26}H_{33}NaO_8$ = 496.5.

*CAS — 2375-03-3.*

*ATC — D07AA01; H02AB04.*

**Pharmacopoeias.** In *US.*

**USP 27** (Methylprednisolone Sodium Succinate). A white or nearly white, odourless, hygroscopic, amorphous solid. Soluble 1 in 1.5 of water and 1 in 12 of alcohol; very slightly soluble in acetone; insoluble in chloroform and in ether. Store in airtight containers. Protect from light.

**Stability.** Methylprednisolone sodium succinate injection (*Solu-Medrol, USA*) was considered to be stable for 7 days when diluted in water for injection and stored in glass vials at 4°. When stored under similar conditions at 22°, it was considered to be stable for 24 hours.[1] The manufacturers state that the prepared solution should be stored at 20 to 25° and used within 48 hours of mixing.

1. Nahata MC, *et al.* Stability of diluted methylprednisolone sodium succinate injection at two temperatures. *Am J Hosp Pharm* 1994; **51:** 2157–9.

### Adverse Effects, Treatment, Withdrawal, and Precautions

As for corticosteroids in general (see p.1068). Rapid intravenous administration of large doses has been associated with cardiovascular collapse.

Methylprednisolone may be slightly less likely than prednisolone to cause sodium and water retention.

When applied topically, particularly to large areas, when the skin is broken, or under occlusive dressings, corticosteroids may be absorbed in sufficient amounts to cause systemic effects.

◊ References to various adverse effects associated with intravenous administration of methylprednisolone in high-dose pulse therapy[1-11] and to adverse effects following intra-articular[12,13] and intranasal injection.[14] Epidural administration (or more particularly inadvertent intrathecal administration during attempted epidural placement) may be associated with serious adverse effects including arachnoiditis and aseptic meningitis, although the degree of risk is uncertain.[15]

1. Newmark KJ, *et al.* Acute arthralgia following high-dose intravenous methylprednisolone therapy. *Lancet* 1974; **ii:** 229.
2. Bailey RR, Armour P. Acute arthralgia after high-dose intravenous methylprednisolone. *Lancet* 1974; **ii:** 1014.
3. Bennett WM, Strong D. Arthralgia after high-dose steroids. *Lancet* 1975; **i:** 332.
4. Moses RE, *et al.* Fatal arrhythmia after pulse methylprednisolone therapy. *Ann Intern Med* 1981; **95:** 781–2.
5. Oto A, *et al.* Methylprednisolone pulse therapy and peritonitis. *Ann Intern Med* 1983; **99:** 282.
6. Suchman AL, *et al.* Seizure after pulse therapy with methyl prednisolone. *Arthritis Rheum* 1983; **26:** 117.
7. Ayoub WT, *et al.* Central nervous system manifestations after pulse therapy for systemic lupus erythematosus. *Arthritis Rheum* 1983; **26:** 809–10.
8. Williams AJ, *et al.* Disseminated aspergillosis in high dose steroid therapy. *Lancet* 1983; **i:** 1222.
9. Barrett DF. Pulse methylprednisolone therapy. *Lancet* 1983; **ii:** 800.
10. Baethge BA, Lidsky MD. Intractable hiccups associated with high-dose intravenous methylprednisolone therapy. *Ann Intern Med* 1986; **104:** 58–9.
11. Gardiner PVG, Griffiths ID. Sudden death after treatment with pulsed methylprednisolone. *BMJ* 1990; **300:** 125.
12. Black DM, Filak AT. Hyperglycemia with non-insulin-dependent diabetes following intraarticular steroid injection. *J Fam Pract* 1989; **28:** 462–3.
13. Pollock B, *et al.* Chronic urticaria associated with intra-articular methylprednisolone. *Br J Dermatol* 2001; **144:** 1228–30.
14. Johns KJ, Chandra SR. Visual loss following intranasal corticosteroid injection. *JAMA* 1989; **261:** 2413.
15. Rodgers PT, Connelly JF. Epidural administration of methylprednisolone for back pain. *Am J Hosp Pharm* 1994; **51:** 2789–90.

### Interactions

The interactions of corticosteroids in general are described on p.1072.

### Pharmacokinetics

For a brief outline of the pharmacokinetics of corticosteroids, see p.1073.

Methylprednisolone is fairly rapidly distributed following oral administration, with a plasma half-life of 3.5 hours or more. The tissue half-life is reported to range from 18 to 36 hours.

Methylprednisolone acetate is absorbed from joints over a week but is more slowly absorbed following deep intramuscular injection. The sodium succinate ester is rapidly absorbed following intramuscular administration, with peak plasma concentrations obtained in 2 hours.

Methylprednisolone crosses the placenta.

◊ References.

1. Tornatore KM, *et al.* Repeated assessment of methylprednisolone pharmacokinetics during chronic immunosuppression in renal transplant recipients. *Ann Pharmacother* 1995; **29:** 120–4.
2. Rohatagi S, *et al.* Pharmacokinetics of methylprednisolone and prednisolone after single and multiple oral administration. *J Clin Pharmacol* 1997; **37:** 916–25.

### Uses and Administration

Methylprednisolone is a corticosteroid with mainly glucocorticoid activity (p.1068); 4 mg of methylprednisolone is equivalent in anti-inflammatory activity to about 5 mg of prednisolone.

It is used, either in the form of the free alcohol or in one of the esterified forms, in the treatment of conditions for which corticosteroid therapy is indicated (see p.1073) except adrenocortical-deficiency states, for which hydrocortisone with supplementary fludrocortisone is preferred.

The dose is usually expressed in terms of the base, and the following are each approximately equivalent to 40 mg of methylprednisolone:

- methylprednisolone acetate 44 mg
- methylprednisolone hydrogen succinate 51 mg
- methylprednisolone sodium succinate 53 mg

For administration by mouth, methylprednisolone is usually given in an initial dosage range of 4 to 48 mg daily but higher initial doses of up to 100 mg or more daily may be used in acute severe disease.

For parenteral administration in intensive or emergency therapy, methylprednisolone sodium succinate may be given by intramuscular or intravenous injection or by intravenous infusion. The intravenous route is preferred for its more rapid effect in emergency therapy. The usual initial intramuscular or intravenous dose ranges from the equivalent of 10 to 500 mg of methylprednisolone daily. Large intravenous doses (over 250 mg) should normally be given slowly over at least 30 minutes; doses up to 250 mg should be given over at least 5 minutes. High doses should generally not be given for prolonged periods; emergency treatment should only be used until the patient is stabilised. High doses given intermittently for a limited period have sometimes been known as 'pulse therapy' (see Administration, below) and in graft rejection (see Organ and Tissue Transplantation, p.1344) up to 1 g has been given daily for up to 3 days. In intensive therapy of acute spinal cord injury (p.1088) initial doses of the equivalent of up to 30 mg/kg of methylprednisolone have been given by bolus intravenous injection over 15 minutes and followed, after a 45-minute pause, by intravenous infusion of 5.4 mg/kg per hour over 24 hours or longer. For slow intravenous infusion methylprednisolone sodium succinate is dissolved in an appropriate volume of glucose 5% or sodium chloride 0.9% or sodium chloride 0.9% and glucose 5%.

Parenteral doses in children have varied considerably, depending on the condition: a range of 1 to 30 mg/kg of methylprednisolone daily has been given by the intravenous or intramuscular routes. A total dose of 1 g daily should not normally be exceeded.

Methylprednisolone acetate may be given by intramuscular injection for a prolonged systemic effect, the dose varying from 40 mg every 2 weeks to 120 mg weekly.

For intra-articular injection and for injection into soft tissues methylprednisolone acetate as an aqueous suspension is used. The dose by intra-articular injection varies from 4 to 80 mg according to the size of the affected joint. The acetate may also be given by intralesional injection in doses of 20 to 60 mg.

For use in the treatment of various skin disorders methylprednisolone acetate may be applied topically, usually in concentrations of 0.25 to 1%. The aceponate, which may exhibit modified topical activity, has also been applied as a 0.1% cream, lotion, or ointment. For recommendations concerning the correct use of corticosteroids on the skin, and a rough guide to the clinical potencies of topical corticosteroids, see p.1074.

Other esters of methylprednisolone that have occasionally been used include the cipionate and the suleptanate.

◊ General references.


1. Cronstein BN. Clinical use of methylprednisolone sodium succinate: a review. *Curr Ther Res* 1995; **56:** 1–15.


**Administration.** For short-term intensive therapy or in certain emergency situations a technique of corticosteroid administration known as 'pulse therapy' has been employed. Methylprednisolone has often been used in this manner. Typically, high doses of about 1 g intravenously have been given, daily or on alternate days or weekly, for a limited number of doses; the most common regimen appears to be 1 g daily for 3 days.

**Blood disorders.** Methylprednisolone is one of the corticosteroids that have been used in the management of haemangioma (p.1081) and the Kasabach-Merritt syndrome.[1] There are also reports of benefit from very high-dose therapy in a few patients with refractory primary acquired pure red cell aplasia,[2] or aplasia due to Blackfan-Diamond anaemia.[3]


1. Özsoylu Ş, *et al.* Megadose methylprednisolone therapy for Kasabach-Merritt syndrome. *J Pediatr* 1996; **129:** 947.
2. Kadikoylu G, *et al.* High-dose methylprednisolone therapy in pure red cell aplasia. *Ann Pharmacother* 2002; **36:** 55–8.
3. Bernini JC, *et al.* High-dose intravenous methylprednisolone therapy for patients with Diamond-Blackfan anemia refractory to conventional doses of prednisone. *J Pediatr* 1995; **127:** 654–9.


IDIOPATHIC THROMBOCYTOPENIC PURPURA. High-dose intravenous methylprednisolone may be used as part of the emergency management of acute idiopathic thrombocytopenic purpura (p.1082), for example when major acute bleeding or intracranial haemorrhage supervene. There is some evidence that methylprednisolone is less effective than normal immunoglobulins. Methylprednisolone has also been used by mouth or intravenously in the management of the chronic form, although prednisolone or prednisone are more frequently used for oral therapy and good controlled trials are scanty.

References.


1. von dem Borne AEGKR, *et al.* High dose intravenous methylprednisolone or high dose intravenous gammaglobulin for autoimmune thrombocytopenia. *BMJ* 1988; **296:** 249–50.
2. Özsoylu S, *et al.* Megadose methylprednisolone for chronic idiopathic thrombocytopenic purpura. *Lancet* 1990; **336:** 1078–9.
3. Akoğlu T, *et al.* Megadose methylprednisolone pulse therapy in adult idiopathic thrombocytopenic purpura. *Lancet* 1991; **337:** 56.
4. Özsoylu S. Mega-dose methylprednisolone for chronic idiopathic thrombocytopenic purpura. *Lancet* 1991; **337:** 1611–12.
5. Rosthøj S, *et al.* Randomized trial comparing intravenous immunoglobulin with methylprednisolone pulse therapy in acute idiopathic thrombocytopenic purpura. *Acta Paediatr* 1996; **85:** 910–15.
6. Alpdoğan Ö, *et al.* Efficacy of high-dose methylprednisolone as a first-line therapy in adult patients with idiopathic thrombocytopenic purpura. *Br J Haematol* 1998; **103:** 1061–3.
7. Godeau B, *et al.* Intravenous immunoglobulin or high-dose methylprednisolone, with or without oral prednisone, for adults with untreated severe autoimmune thrombocytopenic purpura: a randomised, multicentre trial. *Lancet* 2002; **359:** 23–9.


**Rheumatoid arthritis.** Methylprednisolone administered in intravenous pulses has been reported[1-7] to be effective in the treatment of rheumatoid arthritis (p.9) including juvenile idiopathic arthritis. Some studies have shown this treatment to be of greatest benefit when given with a disease-modifying antirheumatic drug (DMARD),[1,2,4] although others showed the addition of methylprednisolone to existing therapy to have no extra benefit.[6] A comparatively low dose of 100 mg was found to be as effective as 1000 mg in one study.[3] Monthly administration of methylprednisolone by deep intramuscular injection was also an effective adjunct to gold therapy.[8]

A preliminary study in children has found intravenous pulses of methylprednisolone 30 mg/kg to be effective treatment for systemic flares of juvenile idiopathic arthritis.[7]


1. Walters HT, Cawley MID. Combined suppressive drug treatment in severe refractory rheumatoid disease: an analysis of the relative effects of parenteral methylprednisolone, cyclophosphamide and sodium aurothiomalate. *Ann Rheum Dis* 1988; **47:** 924–9.
2. Smith MD, *et al.* The clinical and immunological effects of pulse methylprednisolone therapy in rheumatoid arthritis I: clinical effects. *J Rheumatol* 1988; **15:** 229–32.
3. Igelhart IW, *et al.* Intravenous pulsed steroids in rheumatoid arthritis: a comparative dose study. *J Rheumatol* 1990; **17:** 159–62.
4. Smith MD, *et al.* Pulse methylprednisolone therapy in rheumatoid arthritis: unproved therapy, unjustified therapy, or effective adjunctive treatment? *Ann Rheum Dis* 1990; **49:** 265–7.
5. Kapisinszky N, Keszthelyi B. High dose intravenous methylprednisolone pulse therapy in patients with rheumatoid arthritis. *Ann Rheum Dis* 1990; **49:** 567–8.
6. Hansen TM, *et al.* Double blind placebo controlled trial of pulse treatment with methylprednisolone combined with disease modifying drugs in rheumatoid arthritis. *BMJ* 1990; **301:** 268–70.
7. Adebajo AO, Hall MA. The use of intravenous pulsed methylprednisolone in the treatment of systemic-onset juvenile chronic arthritis. *Br J Rheumatol* 1998; **37:** 1240–2.
8. Corkill MM, *et al.* Intramuscular depot methylprednisolone induction of chrysotherapy in rheumatoid arthritis: a 24-week randomized controlled trial. *Br J Rheumatol* 1990; **29:** 274–9.


## Preparations

***BP 2003:*** Methylprednisolone Acetate Injection; Methylprednisolone Tablets;
***USP 27:*** Methylprednisolone Acetate Cream; Methylprednisolone Acetate Injectable Suspension; Methylprednisolone Sodium Succinate for Injection; Methylprednisolone Tablets; Neomycin Sulfate and Methylprednisolone Acetate Cream.

**Proprietary Preparations** (details are given in Part 3)
***Arg.:*** Advantan; Cipridanol; Corticel; Cortisolona; Solu-Medrol; ***Austral.:*** Advantan; Depo-Medrol; Depo-Nisolone; Medrol; Solu-Medrol; ***Austria:*** Advantan; Depo-Medrol; Solu-Medrol; Urbason; ***Belg.:*** Advantan; Depo-Medrol; Medrol; Solu-Medrol; ***Braz.:*** Advantan; Alergolon; Depo-Medrol; Predmetil; Solu-Medrol; ***Canad.:*** Depo-Medrol; Medrol; Medrol Veriderm†; Solu-Medrol; ***Chile:*** Depo-Medrol; Medrol; Solu-Medrol; ***Denm.:*** Depo-Medrol; Medrol; Solu-Medrol; ***Fin.:*** Advantan; Depo-Medrol; Medrol; Solomet; Solu-Medrol; ***Fr.:*** Depo-Medrol; Medrol; Solu-Medrol; ***Ger.:*** Advantan; Depo-Medrate; Medrate; Metypred; Metysolon; Predni M; Urbason; ***Gr.:*** Advantan; Depo-Medrol; Medrol; Solu-Medrol; ***Hong Kong:*** Advantan; Depo-Medrol; Medrol; Solu-Medrol; ***India:*** Solu-Medrol; Unidrol; ***Irl.:*** Depo-Medrone; Medrone†; Solu-Medrone; ***Israel:*** A-Methapred; Depo-Medrol; Medrol; Solu-Medrol; Vanderm; ***Ital.:*** Advantan; Asmacortone; Avancort; Depo-Medrol; Emmetipi†; Esametone; Firmacort†; Medrol; Metilbetasone Solubile; Solu-Medrol; Supresol; Urbason; ***Malaysia:*** Depo-Medrol; Solu-Medrol; ***Mex.:*** Advantan; Cryosolona; Depo-Medrol; Metisona†; Prednilem; Radilem; Solsolona†; Solu-Medrol; ***Neth.:*** Depo-Medrol; Medrol; Solu-Medrol; ***Norw.:*** Depo-Medrol; Medrol; Solu-Medrol; ***NZ:*** Advantan; Depo-Medrol; Medrol; Solu-Medrol; ***Port.:*** Advantan; Depo-Medrol; Medrol; Metilpren; Solu-Medrol; ***S.Afr.:*** Advantan; Depo-Medrol; Medrol; Metypresol†; Solu-Medrol; ***Singapore:*** Solu-Medrol; ***Spain:*** Adventan; Depo Moderin; Lexxema; Solu-Moderin; Urbason; ***Swed.:*** Depo-Medrol; Medrol; Solu-Medrol; ***Switz.:*** Advantan; Depo-Medrol; Medrol; Solu-Medrol; Urbason†; ***Thai.:*** Depo-Medrol; Solu-Medrol; ***UK:*** Depo-Medrone; Medrone; Solu-Medrone; ***USA:*** A-Methapred; depMedalone; Depo-Medrol; Depoject†; Depopred; Duralone†; M-Prednisol†; Medralone†; Medrol; Solu-Medrol.

**Multi-ingredient: *Austral.:*** Neo-Medrol; ***Austria:*** Depo-Medrol mit Lidocain; ***Belg.:*** Depo-Medrol + Lidocaine; ***Canad.:*** Depo-Medrol with Lidocaine; Medrol Acne Lotion; Neo-Medrol Acne; Neo-Medrol Veriderm; ***Fin.:*** Depo-Medrol cum Lidocain; Neo-Medrol comp; Solomet c bupivacain hydrochlorid; ***Hong Kong:*** Depo-Medrol with Lidocaine; Neo-Medrol Acne; ***Irl.:*** Depo-Medrone with Lidocaine; Neo-Medrone†; ***Israel:*** Depo-Medrol with Lidocaine; Neo-Medrol; ***Ital.:*** Depo-Medrol + Lidocaina; Medrol Lozione Antiacne; Neo-Medrol Veriderm; ***Malaysia:*** Neo-Medrol; ***Neth.:*** Depo-Medrol + Lidocaine; ***Norw.:*** Depo-Medrol cum Lidocain; ***NZ:*** Depo-Medrol with Lidocaine; ***Port.:*** Depo-Medrol com Lidocaina; ***S.Afr.:*** Depo-Medrol with Lidocaine; Neo-Medrol; ***Singapore:*** Neo-Medrol; ***Spain:*** Moderin Acne; Neo Moderin†; ***Swed.:*** Depo-Medrol cum Lidokain; ***Switz.:*** Depo-Medrol Lidocaine; ***Thai.:*** Depo-Medrol with Lidocaine; Neo-Medrol; ***UK:*** Depo-Medrone with Lidocaine.

---

## Mometasone Furoate *(BANM, USAN, rINNM)*

Furoato de mometasona; Mometasoni Furoas; Sch-32088.
9α,21-Dichloro-11β,17-dihydroxy-16α-methylpregna-1,4-diene-3,20-dione 17-(2-furoate).

$C_{27}H_{30}Cl_2O_6$ = 521.4.

*CAS — 105102-22-5 (mometasone); 83919-23-7 (mometasone furoate).*

*ATC — D07AC13; R01AD09; R03BA07.*

**Pharmacopoeias.** In *Eur.* (see p.vi) and *US.*

**Ph. Eur. 5.0** (Mometasone Furoate). A white or almost white powder. Practically insoluble in water; slightly soluble in alcohol; soluble in acetone and in dichloromethane.

**USP 27** (Mometasone Furoate). A white to off-white powder. Soluble in acetone and in dichloromethane.

### Profile

Mometasone furoate is a corticosteroid used topically for its glucocorticoid activity (see p.1068) in the treatment of various skin disorders. It is usually employed as a cream, ointment, or lotion containing 0.1%.

It is also given as a nasal suspension of mometasone furoate 0.05%, as the monohydrate, in the treatment and prophylaxis of the symptoms of allergic rhinitis (p.422); the usual adult dose is the equivalent of 100 micrograms of mometasone furoate in each nostril once daily, increased if necessary to 200 micrograms in each nostril daily. Once symptoms are controlled a dose of 50 micrograms in each nostril daily may be effective for maintenance. In the UK, the dose for children aged between 6 and 11 years is the equivalent of 50 micrograms in each nostril once daily. In the USA, similar doses may be given to treat allergic rhinitis in children from 2 years of age.

Mometasone furoate is used by dry powder inhaler for the prophylaxis of asthma (p.777). An initial dose for mild to moderate asthma is 400 micrograms once daily. The dose may be adjusted to a maintenance dose of 200 micrograms inhaled once or twice daily. In severe asthma an initial dose of 400 micrograms twice daily is used, then titrated to the lowest effective dose once symptoms are controlled.

When applied topically, particularly to large areas, when the skin is broken, or under occlusive dressings, or when given intranasally, corticosteroids may be absorbed in sufficient amounts to cause systemic effects (see p.1068). The effects of topical corticosteroids on the skin are described on p.1070. For recommendations concerning the correct use of corticosteroids on the skin, see p.1074.

◊ References.


1. Prakash A, Benfield P. Topical mometasone: a review of its pharmacological properties and therapeutic use in the treatment of dermatological disorders. *Drugs* 1998; **55:** 145–63.
2. Onrust SV, Lamb HM. Mometasone furoate: a review of its intranasal use in allergic rhinitis. *Drugs* 1998; **56:** 725–45.
3. Meltzer EO, *et al.* A dose-ranging study of mometasone furoate aqueous nasal spray in children with seasonal allergic rhinitis. *J Allergy Clin Immunol* 1999; **104:** 107–14.
4. Meltzer EO, *et al.* Added relief in the treatment of acute recurrent sinusitis with adjunctive mometasone furoate nasal spray. *J Allergy Clin Immunol* 2000; **106:** 630–7.
5. Sharpe M, Jarvis B. Inhaled mometasone furoate: a review of its use in adults and adolescents with persistent asthma. *Drugs* 2001; **61:** 1325–50.
6. O'Connor B, *et al.* Dose-ranging study of mometasone furoate dry powder inhaler in the treatment of moderate persistent asthma using fluticasone propionate as an active comparator. *Ann Allergy Asthma Immunol* 2001; **86:** 397–404.


### Preparations

***USP 27:*** Mometasone Furoate Cream; Mometasone Furoate Ointment; Mometasone Furoate Topical Solution.

**Proprietary Preparations** (details are given in Part 3)
***Arg.:*** Elocon; Metason; Nasonex; Novasone; Uniclar; ***Austral.:*** AllerMax; Elocon; Nasonex; Novasone; ***Austria:*** Elocon; Nasonex; ***Belg.:*** Elocom; Nasonex; ***Braz.:*** Elocom; Nasonex; ***Canad.:*** Elocom; Nasonex; ***Chile:*** Dermenet; Dermosona; Elocom; Flogocort; Lisoder; Nasonex; Rinoval; Uniclar; ***Denm.:*** Elocon; Nasonex; ***Fin.:*** Elocon; Nasonex; ***Fr.:*** Nasonex; ***Ger.:*** Ecural; Nasonex; ***Gr.:*** Elocon; ***Hong Kong:*** Elomet; Nasonex; ***India:*** Elocon; Metaspray; ***Irl.:*** Elocon; Nasonex; ***Israel:*** Elocom; Nasonex; ***Ital.:*** Altosone; Elocon; Nasonex; Rinelon; Uniclar; ***Malaysia:*** Elomet; Nasonex; ***Mex.:*** Elica; Elomet; Rinelon; Uniclar; ***Neth.:*** Elocon; Nasonex; ***Norw.:*** Elocon; Nasonex; ***NZ:*** Elocon; ***Port.:*** Elocom; Nasomet; ***S.Afr.:*** Elica; Elocon; Nasonex; Rinelon; ***Singapore:*** Elomet; Nasonex; ***Spain:*** Elica; Elocom; Nasonex; Rinelon; ***Swed.:*** Elocon; Nasonex; ***Switz.:*** Elocom; Nasonex; ***Thai.:*** Elomet; Nasonex; Rinelon; ***UK:*** Asmanex; Elocon; Nasonex; ***USA:*** Elocon; Nasonex.

**Multi-ingredient: *Arg.:*** Elosalic; ***Braz.:*** Elosalic†; ***Chile:*** Velosalic; ***Hong Kong:*** Elosalic; ***S.Afr.:*** Elosalic; ***Swed.:*** Elosalic; ***Thai.:*** Elosalic.

---

## Paramethasone Acetate *(BANM, USAN, rINNM)*

Acetato de parametasona; 6α-Fluoro-16α-methylprednisolone 21-Acetate. 6α-Fluoro-11β,17α,21-trihydroxy-16α-methylpregna-1,4-diene-3,20-dione 21-acetate.

$C_{24}H_{31}FO_6$ = 434.5.

*CAS — 53-33-8 (paramethasone); 1597-82-6 (paramethasone acetate).*

*ATC — H02AB05.*

**Pharmacopoeias.** In *Fr.* and *US.*

**USP 27** (Paramethasone Acetate). A white to creamy-white, fluffy, odourless, crystalline powder. Insoluble in water; soluble 1 in 50 of chloroform and 1 in 40 of methyl alcohol; soluble in ether. Store in airtight containers.

### Profile

Paramethasone acetate is a corticosteroid that has been used systemically for its predominantly glucocorticoid activity (p.1068); 2 mg of paramethasone is equivalent in anti-inflammatory activity to about 5 mg of prednisolone. The disodium phosphate has also been used.

### Preparations

***USP 27:*** Paramethasone Acetate Tablets.

**Proprietary Preparations** (details are given in Part 3)
***Fr.:*** Dilar†; ***Mex.:*** Dilar; ***Spain:*** Cortidene.

**Multi-ingredient: *Mex.:*** Dilarmine; ***Spain:*** Triniol†.

---

## Prednicarbate *(BAN, USAN, rINN)*

Hoe-777; Prednicarbato; Prednicarbatum; S-77-0777.
11β,17,21-Trihydroxypregna-1,4-diene-3,20-dione 17-(ethyl carbonate) 21-propionate.

$C_{27}H_{36}O_8$ = 488.6.

*CAS — 73771-04-7.*

*ATC — D07AC18.*

**Pharmacopoeias.** In *Eur.* (see p.vi).

**Ph. Eur. 5.0** (Prednicarbate). A white or almost white, crystalline powder. It shows polymorphism. Practically insoluble in water; freely soluble in alcohol and in acetone; sparingly soluble in propylene glycol. Protect from light.

### Profile

Prednicarbate is a corticosteroid used topically for its glucocorticoid activity (see p.1068) in the treatment of various skin disorders. It has usually been employed as a cream, ointment, or lotion, containing 0.1 to 0.25%.

When applied topically, particularly to large areas, when the skin is broken, or under occlusive dressings, corticosteroids may be absorbed in sufficient amounts to cause systemic effects (see p.1068). The effects of topical corticosteroids on the skin are described on p.1070. For recommendations concerning the correct use of corticosteroids on the skin, and a rough guide to the clinical potencies of topical corticosteroids, see p.1074.

◊ References.


1. Schäfer-Korting M, *et al.* Prednicarbate activity and benefit/risk ratio in relation to other topical glucocorticoids. *Clin Pharmacol Ther* 1993; **54:** 448–56.


### Preparations

**Proprietary Preparations** (details are given in Part 3)
***Arg.:*** Primaderm; ***Austria:*** Prednitop; ***Braz.:*** Dermatop; Invex; ***Chile:*** Dermatop; ***Ger.:*** Dermatop; ***Ital.:*** Dermatop; ***Spain:*** Batmen; Peitel; ***Switz.:*** Prednitop; ***Thai.:*** Dermatop; ***USA:*** Dermatop.

---

## Prednisolone *(BAN, rINN)*

1,2-Dehydrohydrocortisone; Deltahydrocortisone; $\Delta^1$-Hydrocortisone; Metacortandralone; NSC-9120; Prednisolona; Prednisolonum. 11β,17α,21-Trihydroxypregna-1,4-diene-3,20-dione.
$C_{21}H_{28}O_5$ = 360.4.
*CAS — 50-24-8 (anhydrous prednisolone); 52438-85-4 (prednisolone sesquihydrate).*
*ATC — A07EA01; C05AA04; D07AA03; H02AB06; R01AD02; S01BA04; S02BA03; S03BA02.*

**Pharmacopoeias.** In *Chin., Eur.* (see p.vi), *Int., Jpn, Pol.*, and *Viet.*
*US* allows the anhydrous form or the sesquihydrate.
**Ph. Eur. 5.0** (Prednisolone). A white or almost white, hygroscopic, crystalline powder. It shows polymorphism. Very slightly soluble in water; soluble in alcohol and in methyl alcohol; sparingly soluble in acetone; slightly soluble in dichloromethane. Store in airtight containers. Protect from light.
**USP 27** (Prednisolone). It is anhydrous or contains one and one-half molecules of water of hydration. A white to practically white, odourless, crystalline powder. Very slightly soluble in water; soluble 1 in 30 of alcohol, 1 in 50 of acetone, and 1 in 180 of chloroform; soluble in dioxan and in methyl alcohol.

### Prednisolone Acetate *(BANM, rINNM)*

Acetato de prednisolona; Prednisoloni Acetas. Prednisolone 21-acetate.
$C_{23}H_{30}O_6$ = 402.5.
*CAS — 52-21-1.*
*ATC — A07EA01; C05AA04; D07AA03; H02AB06; R01AD02; S01BA04; S02BA03; S03BA02.*

**Pharmacopoeias.** In *Chin., Eur.* (see p.vi), *Int., Jpn, Pol.*, and *US.*
**Ph. Eur. 5.0** (Prednisolone Acetate). A white or almost white, crystalline powder. Practically insoluble in water; slightly soluble in alcohol and in dichloromethane. Protect from light.
**USP 27** (Prednisolone Acetate). A white to practically white, odourless, crystalline powder. Practically insoluble in water; soluble 1 in 120 of alcohol; slightly soluble in acetone and in chloroform. Store at a temperature of 25°, excursions permitted between 15° and 30°.

### Prednisolone Caproate *(rINNM)*

Caproato de prednisolona; Prednisolone Hexanoate *(BANM)*. Prednisolone 21-hexanoate.
$C_{27}H_{38}O_6$ = 458.6.
*ATC — A07EA01; C05AA04; D07AA03; H02AB06; R01AD02; S01BA04; S02BA03; S03BA02.*

### Prednisolone Hydrogen Succinate *(BANM, rINNM)*

Hidrogenosuccinato de prednisolona; Prednisolone Hemisuccinate. Prednisolone 21-(hydrogen succinate).
$C_{25}H_{32}O_8$ = 460.5.
*CAS — 2920-86-7.*
*ATC — A07EA01; C05AA04; D07AA03; H02AB06; R01AD02; S01BA04; S02BA03; S03BA02.*

**Pharmacopoeias.** In *Jpn* and *US.*
**USP 27** (Prednisolone Hemisuccinate). A fine, creamy-white, practically odourless, powder with friable lumps. Soluble 1 in 4170 of water, 1 in 6.3 of alcohol, 1 in 1064 of chloroform, and 1 in 248 of ether; soluble in acetone. Store in airtight containers.

### Prednisolone Metasulfobenzoate Sodium *(rINNM)*

Metasulfobenzoato sódico de prednisolona; Prednisolone Metasulphobenzoate Sodium *(BANM)*; Prednisolone Sodium Metasulphobenzoate; R-812. Prednisolone 21-(sodium *m*-sulphobenzoate).
$C_{28}H_{31}NaO_9S$ = 566.6.
*CAS — 630-67-1.*
*ATC — A07EA01; C05AA04; D07AA03; H02AB06; R01AD02; S01BA04; S02BA03; S03BA02.*

### Prednisolone Pivalate *(BANM, rINNM)*

Pivalato de prednisolona; Prednisolone Trimethylacetate; Prednisoloni Pivalas. Prednisolone 21-pivalate.
$C_{26}H_{36}O_6$ = 444.6.
*CAS — 1107-99-9.*
*ATC — A07EA01; C05AA04; D07AA03; H02AB06; R01AD02; S01BA04; S02BA03; S03BA02.*

**Pharmacopoeias.** In *Eur.* (see p.vi) and *Pol.*
**Ph. Eur. 5.0** (Prednisolone Pivalate). A white, or almost white, crystalline powder. Practically insoluble in water; slightly soluble in alcohol; soluble in dichloromethane. Protect from light.

### Prednisolone Sodium Phosphate *(BANM, rINNM)*

Fosfato sódico de prednisolona; Prednisoloni Natrii Phosphas. Prednisolone 21-(disodium orthophosphate).
$C_{21}H_{27}Na_2O_8P$ = 484.4.
*CAS — 125-02-0.*
*ATC — A07EA01; C05AA04; D07AA03; H02AB06; R01AD02; S01BA04; S02BA03; S03BA02.*

NOTE. PRED is a code approved by the BP 2003 for use on single unit doses of eye drops containing prednisolone sodium phosphate where the individual container may be too small to bear all the appropriate labelling information.

**Pharmacopoeias.** In *Eur.* (see p.vi), *Int.*, and *US.*
**Ph. Eur. 5.0** (Prednisolone Sodium Phosphate). A white or almost white, hygroscopic, crystalline powder. Freely soluble in water; very slightly soluble in alcohol. A 5% solution in water has a pH of 7.5 to 9.0. Protect from light.
**USP 27** (Prednisolone Sodium Phosphate). A white or slightly yellow friable granules or powder. Is odourless or has a slight odour. Is slightly hygroscopic. Soluble 1 in 4 of water and 1 in 13 of methyl alcohol; slightly soluble in alcohol and in chloroform; very slightly soluble in acetone and in dioxan. pH of a 1% solution in water is between 7.5 and 10.5. Store in airtight containers.

### Prednisolone Sodium Succinate *(BANM, rINNM)*

Prednisolone Sodium Hemisuccinate; Succinato sódico de prednisolona. 11β,17α,21-Trihydroxypregna-1,4-diene-3,20-dione 21-(sodium succinate).
$C_{25}H_{31}NaO_8$ = 482.5.
*CAS — 1715-33-9.*
*ATC — A07EA01; C05AA04; D07AA03; H02AB06; R01AD02; S01BA04; S02BA03; S03BA02.*

**Pharmacopoeias.** *US* includes Prednisolone Sodium Succinate for Injection.
**USP 27** (Prednisolone Sodium Succinate for Injection). A creamy white powder with friable lumps, having a slight odour.

### Prednisolone Steaglate *(BAN, rINN)*

Esteaglato de prednisolona. Prednisolone 21-stearoylglycolate.
$C_{41}H_{64}O_8$ = 684.9.
*CAS — 5060-55-9.*
*ATC — A07EA01; C05AA04; D07AA03; H02AB06; R01AD02; S01BA04; S02BA03; S03BA02.*

### Prednisolone Tebutate *(BANM, rINNM)*

Prednisolone Butylacetate; Prednisolone 21-*tert*-Butylacetate; Prednisolone Tertiary-butylacetate; Tebutato de prednisolona. Prednisolone 21-(3,3-dimethylbutyrate).
$C_{27}H_{38}O_6,H_2O$ = 476.6.
*CAS — 7681-14-3 (anhydrous prednisolone tebutate).*
*ATC — A07EA01; C05AA04; D07AA03; H02AB06; R01AD02; S01BA04; S02BA03; S03BA02.*

**Pharmacopoeias.** In *US.*
**USP 27** (Prednisolone Tebutate). A white to slightly yellow, hygroscopic, free-flowing powder, which may show some soft lumps. Is odourless or has not more than a moderate characteristic odour. Very slightly soluble in water; sparingly soluble in alcohol and in methyl alcohol; soluble in acetone; freely soluble in chloroform and in dioxan. Store in airtight containers sealed under nitrogen at a temperature not exceeding 8°.

## Adverse Effects, Treatment, Withdrawal, and Precautions

As for corticosteroids in general (see p.1068).

Owing to its less pronounced mineralocorticoid activity prednisolone is less likely than cortisone or hydrocortisone to cause sodium retention, electrolyte imbalance, and oedema. Prolonged application to the eye of preparations containing corticosteroids has caused raised intra-ocular pressure and reduced visual function.

**Breast feeding.** Concentrations of prednisone and prednisolone in breast milk from one lactating woman 120 minutes after prednisone 10 mg by mouth were found to be 26.7 nanograms and 1.6 nanograms/mL respectively.[1] In 7 similar women given a single 5-mg dose of tritium-labelled prednisolone by mouth, a mean of 0.14% of the radioactivity from the dose was recovered per litre of milk during the following 48 to 61 hours.[2] In a study of 3 women, only about 0.025% of a single intravenous dose of prednisolone phosphate 50 mg was recovered in breast milk over 6 hours.[3] During maintenance therapy with prednisolone in daily doses of 10 to 80 mg in 6 lactating women, the milk to serum concentration ratio of prednisolone ranged from 0.2, for doses of 30 mg or more, to 0.1 for lower doses.[4] The authors estimated that the breast-fed infant would receive less than 0.1% of the maternal dose of prednisolone, and that this would be a negligible addition to the infant's endogenous cortisol production. They also concluded that exposure could be minimised by breast feeding at least 4 hours after the dose.

A review[5] by the UK Committee on Safety of Medicines remarked that prednisolone was distributed into breast milk in small amounts and recommended that infants of mothers receiving 40 mg or more daily should be monitored for signs of adrenal suppression. The American Academy of Pediatrics considers[6] that the use of prednisone or prednisolone is usually compatible with breast feeding.

1. Katz FH, Duncan BE. Entry of prednisone into human milk. *N Engl J Med* 1975; **293:** 1154.
2. McKenzie SA, *et al.* Secretion of prednisolone into breast milk. *Arch Dis Child* 1975; **50:** 894–6.
3. Greenberger PA, *et al.* Pharmacokinetics of prednisolone transfer to breast milk. *Clin Pharmacol Ther* 1993; **53:** 324–8.
4. Öst L, *et al.* Prednisolone excretion in human milk. *J Pediatr* 1985; **106:** 1008–11.
5. Committee on Safety of Medicines/Medicines Control Agency. Systemic corticosteroids in pregnancy and lactation. *Current Problems* 1998; **24:** 9. Also available at: http://www.mca.gov.uk/ourwork/monitorsafequalmed/currentproblems/volume24may.htm (accessed 27/04/04)
6. American Academy of Pediatrics. The transfer of drugs and other chemicals into human milk. *Pediatrics* 2001; **108:** 776–89. Correction. *ibid.*; 1029. Also available at: http://aappolicy.aappublications.org/cgi/content/full/pediatrics%3b108/3/776 (accessed 27/04/04)

**Hepatic impairment.** Conversion of prednisone to prednisolone has been reported to be impaired in chronic active liver disease.[1,2] However, although plasma-prednisolone concentrations were found to be more predictable after administration of prednisolone than of prednisone to a group of healthy subjects,[3] no difference was noted in patients with chronic active hepatitis, in whom impaired elimination of prednisolone compensated for any impaired conversion of prednisone. A review of the pharmacokinetics of prednisone and prednisolone[4] concluded that fear of inadequate conversion of prednisone into prednisolone was not justified.

1. Powell LW, Axelsen E. Corticosteroids in liver disease: studies on the biological conversion of prednisone to prednisolone and plasma protein binding. *Gut* 1972; **13:** 690–6.
2. Madsbad S, *et al.* Impaired conversion of prednisone to prednisolone in patients with liver cirrhosis. *Gut* 1980; **21:** 52–6.
3. Davis M, *et al.* Prednisone or prednisolone for the treatment of chronic active hepatitis? A comparison of plasma availability. *Br J Clin Pharmacol* 1978; **5:** 501–5.
4. Frey BM, Frey FJ. Clinical pharmacokinetics of prednisone and prednisolone. *Clin Pharmacokinet* 1990; **19:** 126–46.

**Inflammatory bowel disease.** Symptoms recurred in a patient with Crohn's disease on changing from conventional to enteric-coated tablets of prednisolone.[1] This was not an isolated occurrence in the authors' unit, and it was advocated that only non-enteric-coated prednisolone tablets should be used in Crohn's disease, and that the enteric-coated form be used with caution in any condition characterised by diarrhoea or a rapid transit time.

1. Beattie RM, Walker-Smith JA. Use of enteric coated prednisolone in Crohn's disease. *Arch Dis Child* 1994; **71:** 282.

## Interactions

The interactions of corticosteroids in general are described on p.1072.

## Pharmacokinetics

For a brief outline of the pharmacokinetics of corticosteroids, see p.1073.

Prednisolone and prednisone are both readily absorbed from the gastrointestinal tract, but whereas prednisolone already exists in a metabolically active form, prednisone must be converted in the liver to its active metabolite, prednisolone. In general, this conversion is rapid so this difference is of little consequence when seen in the light of intersubject variation in the pharmacokinetics of prednisolone itself; bioavailability also depends on the dissolution rates of the tablet formulations. As discussed under Hepatic Impairment, above, reduced corticosteroid concentrations when giving prednisone to patients with liver disease do not seem to be a problem in practice. Following intramuscular administration the sodium phosphate ester of prednisolone is rapidly absorbed whereas the acetate, in the suspension form, is only slowly absorbed.

Peak plasma concentrations of prednisolone are obtained 1 or 2 hours after a dose by mouth, and it has a usual plasma half-life of 2 to 4 hours. Its initial absorption, but not its overall bioavailability, is affected by food.

Prednisolone is extensively bound to plasma proteins, although less so than hydrocortisone (cortisol). The volume of distribution, and also the clearance are reported to increase with an increase from low to moderate doses; at very high doses, clearance appears to become saturated.

Prednisolone is excreted in the urine as free and conjugated metabolites, together with an appreciable proportion of unchanged prednisolone. Prednisolone is largely inactivated as it crosses the placenta; small amounts are excreted in breast milk.

Prednisolone has a biological half-life lasting several hours, intermediate between those of hydrocortisone (cortisol) and the longer-acting glucocorticoids, such as dexamethasone. It is this intermediate duration of action that makes it suitable for the alternate-day administration regimens which have been found to reduce the risk of adrenocortical insufficiency, yet provide adequate corticosteroid coverage in some disorders.

◊ General reviews of the pharmacokinetics of prednisolone[1,2] and some references to its pharmacokinetics in healthy subjects[3] and in various disease states.[4-8]


1. Begg EJ, *et al*. The pharmacokinetics of corticosteroid agents. *Med J Aust* 1987; **146:** 37–41.
2. Frey BM, Frey FJ. Clinical pharmacokinetics of prednisone and prednisolone. *Clin Pharmacokinet* 1990; **19:** 126–46.
3. Rohatagi S, *et al*. Pharmacokinetics of methylprednisolone and prednisolone after single and multiple oral administration. *J Clin Pharmacol* 1997; **37:** 916–25.
4. Berghouse LM, *et al*. Plasma prednisolone levels during intravenous therapy in acute colitis. *Gut* 1982; **23:** 980–3.
5. Shaffer JA, *et al*. Absorption of prednisolone in patients with Crohn's disease. *Gut* 1983; **24:** 182–6.
6. Reece PA, *et al*. Prednisolone protein binding in renal transplant patients. *Br J Clin Pharmacol* 1985; **20:** 159–62.
7. Frey FJ, *et al*. Altered metabolism and decreased efficacy of prednisolone and prednisone in patients with hyperthyroidism. *Clin Pharmacol Ther* 1988; **44:** 510–21.
8. Miller PFW, *et al*. Pharmacokinetics of prednisolone in children with nephrosis. *Arch Dis Child* 1990; **65:** 196–200.


### Uses and Administration

Prednisolone is a corticosteroid with mainly glucocorticoid activity (p.1068); 5 mg of prednisolone is equivalent in anti-inflammatory activity to about 25 mg of cortisone acetate. In general, prednisolone, either in the form of the free alcohol or in one of the esterified forms, is the drug of choice in the UK for conditions in which routine systemic corticosteroid therapy is indicated (see p.1073), except adrenocortical-deficiency states for which hydrocortisone with supplementary fludrocortisone is preferred. The more potent pituitary-suppressant properties of a glucocorticoid such as dexamethasone may, however, be required for the diagnosis and management of conditions associated with adrenal hyperplasia.

The dose may be expressed in terms of the base, and the following are each approximately equivalent to 100 mg of prednisolone:

- prednisolone acetate 110 mg
- prednisolone caproate 127 mg
- prednisolone hydrogen succinate 128 mg
- prednisolone metasulfobenzoate sodium 157 mg
- prednisolone pivalate 123 mg
- prednisolone sodium phosphate 135 mg
- prednisolone sodium succinate 134 mg
- prednisolone steaglate 190 mg
- prednisolone tebutate 132 mg

For administration by mouth prednisolone is usually used although prednisolone sodium phosphate or prednisolone steaglate are also employed; the usual dose, expressed in terms of prednisolone, is about 2.5 to 60 mg daily in divided doses, as a single daily dose after breakfast, or as a double dose on alternate days. Alternate-day early-morning dosage regimens produce less suppression of the hypothalamic-pituitary axis but may not always provide adequate control. Enteric-coated tablets of prednisolone are also available (for the view that these should not be used in patients with inflammatory bowel disease, see above).

For parenteral administration the sodium phosphate ester is normally used and may be given intravenously by injection or infusion or intramuscularly by injection; doses appear to have been variously expressed in terms of prednisolone, prednisolone phosphate, or prednisolone sodium phosphate but are generally within the range of 4 to 60 mg daily. An aqueous suspension of prednisolone acetate is also used intramuscularly for a prolonged effect, in doses of 25 to 100 mg once or twice weekly. The sodium succinate ester has also been given parenterally.

For intra-articular injection the acetate, sodium phosphate, and tebutate esters are used. Suggested doses are 5 to 25 mg of prednisolone acetate, 2 to 30 mg of prednisolone phosphate (for the sodium phosphate ester), and 4 to 40 mg of prednisolone tebutate. The sodium phosphate and tebutate esters are also given by intralesional injection and by injection into soft tissue.

Prednisolone acetate and prednisolone sodium phosphate are also used in the topical treatment of allergic and inflammatory conditions of the eyes or ears, usually as drops containing 0.5 or 1%. Prednisolone has also been used topically as the free alcohol and as the hemisuccinate, pivalate, and metasulfobenzoate sodium esters.

For rectal use prednisolone metasulfobenzoate sodium or prednisolone sodium phosphate are often employed. Retention enemas containing the equivalent of 20 mg of prednisolone per 100 mL, rectal foam containing the equivalent of 20 mg of prednisolone per dose, or suppositories containing the equivalent of 5 mg of prednisolone are available. Prednisolone has also been used rectally as the free alcohol and as the acetate and caproate esters.

Other esters of prednisolone that have occasionally been used include the farnesil, palmitate, and sodium tetrahydrophthalate.

### Preparations

***BP 2003:*** Enteric-coated Prednisolone Tablets; Prednisolone Enema; Prednisolone Sodium Phosphate Eye Drops; Prednisolone Tablets;
***USP 27:*** Chloramphenicol and Prednisolone Ophthalmic Ointment; Gentamicin and Prednisolone Acetate Ophthalmic Ointment; Neomycin and Polymyxin B Sulfates and Prednisolone Acetate Ophthalmic Suspension; Neomycin Sulfate and Prednisolone Acetate Ointment; Neomycin Sulfate and Prednisolone Acetate Ophthalmic Ointment; Neomycin Sulfate and Prednisolone Acetate Ophthalmic Suspension; Neomycin Sulfate and Prednisolone Sodium Phosphate Ophthalmic Ointment; Neomycin Sulfate, Sulfacetamide Sodium, and Prednisolone Acetate Ophthalmic Ointment; Prednisolone Acetate Injectable Suspension; Prednisolone Acetate Ophthalmic Suspension; Prednisolone Cream; Prednisolone Sodium Phosphate Injection; Prednisolone Sodium Phosphate Ophthalmic Solution; Prednisolone Sodium Succinate for Injection; Prednisolone Syrup; Prednisolone Tablets; Prednisolone Tebutate Injectable Suspension; Sulfacetamide Sodium and Prednisolone Acetate Ophthalmic Ointment; Sulfacetamide Sodium and Prednisolone Acetate Ophthalmic Suspension.

**Proprietary Preparations** (details are given in Part 3)
***Arg.:*** Cortizul; ***Austral.:*** Panafcortelone; Predmix; Predsol; Redipred; Solone; Sterofrin; ***Austria:*** Aprednislon; Kuhlprednon; Prednihexal; Rectopred; Solu-Dacortin; Ultracortenol; ***Belg.:*** Deltacortril; Pred Forte; Prednicortelone; Solu-Dacortine; ***Braz.:*** Pred Fort; Pred Mild; Predsim; Prelone; ***Canad.:*** Diopred; Inflamase; Ophtho-Tate; Pediapred; Pred Forte; Pred Mild; ***Chile:*** Pred Forte; Pred Mild; Predsolets; Preventan; ***Denm.:*** Pred-Clysma; Predniment†; Ultracortenol; ***Fin.:*** Di-Adreson-F; Pred Forte; Predniment†; Ultracortenol; ***Fr.:*** Hydrocortancyl; Solucort†; Solupred; ***Ger.:*** Decaprednil†; Decortin H; Dermosolon; Dontisolon D; duraprednisolon; hefasolon; Infectocortikrupp; Inflanefran; Klismacort; Linola-H N; Linola-H-Fett N; Lygal Kopftinktur N; Prectal; Prednabene; Predni; Predni H; Predni-Ophtal; Predni-POS; Prednigalen; Prednihexal; Prednisolut; Solu-Decortin-H; Ultracortenol; ***Gr.:*** Adelcort; Adelone; Deltacortril; Prezolon; ***Hong Kong:*** Dhasolone; Di-Adreson-F; Panafcortelone; Pred Forte; Pred Mild; Predenema†; Predfoam†; Prelone; Sintisone†; Ultracortenol; ***India:*** Wysolone; ***Irl.:*** Deltacortril; Pred Forte; Pred Mild; Predenema; Predfoam; Prednesol; Predsol; ***Israel:*** Pred Forte; Prelone; Ultracorten H†; Ultracortenol; ***Ital.:*** Meticortelone; Soludacortin; ***Jpn:*** Farnerate; Farnezone; ***Malaysia:*** Dhasolone; Pred Forte; Pred Mild; Setsolone; Sterosone; ***Mex.:*** Delta-Diona†; Fisopred; Pred; Prednefrin SF; Sophipren; ***Neth.:*** Di-Adreson-F; Ultracortenol; ***Norw.:*** Pred-Clysma; Ultracortenol; ***NZ:*** Pred Forte; Pred Mild; Predsol†; Redipred; ***Port.:*** Frisolona; Lepicortinolo; Predniocil; Sintisone; Solu-Dacortina; ***S.Afr.:*** Capsoid; Lenisolone; Meticortelone; Pred Mild; Predsol; Prelone; ***Singapore:*** Dhasolone; Pred; Walesolone; Xepasone; ***Spain:*** Dacortin H; Estilsona; Pred Forte; Solu-Dacortin H†; ***Swed.:*** Precortalon aquosum; Pred-Clysma; Ultracortenol; ***Switz.:*** Corti-Clyss; Hexacortone; Pred Forte; Pred Mild; Predni-Helvacort†; Solu-Dacortine; Spiricort; Ultracortene-H; Ultracortenol; ***Thai.:*** Di-Adreson-F; Inf-Oph; Opredsone; Polypred; Pred Forte; Pred Mild; Predisole; Prednersone; Prednisil; Prenilone†; ***UAE:*** Gupisone; ***UK:*** Deltacortril; Deltastab; Precortisyl; Pred Forte; Predenema; Predfoam; Prednesol†; Predsol; ***USA:*** Ak-Pred; Delta-Cortef; Econopred; Hydeltrasol; Inflamase; Key-Pred; Key-Pred-SP; Orapred; Pediapred; Pred; Pred Forte; Pred Mild; Pred-Phosphate; Predalone; Predcor; Prednisol; Prelone.

**Multi-ingredient:** ***Arg.:*** Bactio Rhin Prednisolona; Blefamide; Cortizul; Delta Tomanil B12; Esodar; Neocortizul; Oftalmoflogol; Otidrops; Prednefrin; Prednifarma; Rucaten Prednisolona; Scheriproct; ***Austral.:*** Blephamide†; Prednefrin; Scheriproct; ***Austria:*** Alpicort; Blephamide†; Delta-Hadensa; Phoscortil; Scheriproct; ***Belg.:*** Cetapred†; Hemosedan; Isopto Cetapred†; Predmycin P; Scheriproct; Sofrasolone; Viscocort†; ***Braz.:*** Asmosterona†; Colutoide; Dermicin†; Fonergin; Isopto Cetapred; Polimixina B Composto†; Polipred; Predmicin; Prenefrin†; Proctium†; Reumazine†; Rifocort; Rinisone; ***Canad.:*** Blephamide; Dioptimyd; Metimyd†; Vasocidin; ***Chile:*** Banedif Oftalmico con Prednisolona; Blefamide; Gemitin con Prednisolona; Pred G; Scheriproct; Sintoftona; ***Fin.:*** Scheriproct; Septison; ***Fr.:*** Colicort†; Cortisal; Deliproct; Derinox; Desocort†; Deturgylone; Tergynan†; ***Ger.:*** Adeptolon†; Alferm; Alpicort; Alpicort F; Anumedin; Aquapred; Berlicetin; Bismolan H Corti; Blefcon†; Blephamide; Corti-Dynexan; Dexa-Phlogont L; Imazol comp; Inflanegent; Leioderm P; Linola-H-compositum N; Linoladiol-H N; NeyChondrin N (Revitorgan-Dilutionen N Nr 68); NeyNormin N (Revitorgan-Dilutionen N Nr 65); NeyTumorin N (Revitorgan-Dilutionen N Nr 66); Prednitracin†; Scheriproct; Thesit P†; Ultra-Demoplas; Virunguent P; ***Gr.:*** Scheriproct Neo; ***Hong Kong:*** Blephamide; Chlomy-P; Cortison Kemicetine†; Prednitracin; ***India:*** Atrisolon; Otek-AC; Perfocyn; Polyderm; ***Irl.:*** Scheriproct; ***Israel:*** Aflumycin; Blephamide; Prednistyle†; Threolone; ***Ital.:*** Bio-Delta Cortilen; Deltamidrina; Dutimelan†; Solprene; ***Malaysia:*** Blephamide; ***Mex.:*** Artrilan; Blefamide SF; Blefamide SOP; Deltamid; Metimyd; Obrypre; Premid; Scheriproct; ***Norw.:*** Scheriproct; ***NZ:*** Blephamide; ***Port.:*** Anacal; Blifamol†; Conjunctilone-S; Flogiftalmina; Meocil; Mobilat; Neo-Davisolona; Predniderma; Predniftalmina; Scheriproct; Vitasma; ***S.Afr.:*** Blephamide†; Pred G†; Scheriproct; ***Singapore:*** Blephamide; Predmycin-P; ***Spain:*** Alergical; Antigrietun; Kanapomada†; Lidrone†; Nasopomada; Otonina; Poly Pred; Predni Azuleno; Proctium; Rinobanedif; Rinovel; Ruscus; Scheriproct; Teolixir Compositum; ***Swed.:*** Blefcon†; Metimyd†; Scheriproct N; ***Switz.:*** Alpicort F; Alpicort†; Blephamide; Calpred; Deri-nox†; Imacort; Locaseptil-Neo; Mycinopred; Nystacortone; Pred G†; Prednitracin; Premandol; Scheriproct; ***Thai.:*** Denson; Farakil; Levoptin; Mysolone-N; Neopred; Neozolone; Otosil†; Pred Oph; Predex; Predmycin; Prednisil; Prednisil-N; Scheriproct; Unipred; ***UK:*** Predsol-N; Scheriproct; ***USA:*** Ak-Cide†; Blephamide; Cetapred†; Isopto Cetapred†; Metimyd; Poly-Pred; Pred G; Sulfamide; Vasocidin; Vasocine†.

## Prednisone *(BAN, rINN)*

$\Delta^1$-Cortisone; 1,2-Dehydrocortisone; Deltacortisone; Deltadehydrocortisone; Metacortandracin; NSC-10023; Prednisona; Prednisonum. 17α,21-Dihydroxypregna-1,4-diene-3,11,20-trione.

$C_{21}H_{26}O_5$ = 358.4.

*CAS — 53-03-2.*

*ATC — A07EA03; H02AB07.*

**Pharmacopoeias.** In *Eur.* (see p.vi). *US* allows the anhydrous form or the monohydrate.

**Ph. Eur. 5.0** (Prednisone). A white or almost white, crystalline powder. It shows polymorphism. Practically insoluble in water; slightly soluble in alcohol and in dichloromethane. Protect from light.

**USP 27** (Prednisone). It contains one molecule of water of hydration or is anhydrous. A white to practically white, odourless, crystalline powder. Very slightly soluble in water; soluble 1 in 150 of alcohol and 1 in 200 of chloroform; slightly soluble in dioxan and in methyl alcohol.

### Prednisone Acetate *(BANM, rINNM)*

Acetato de prednisona. Prednisone 21-acetate.

$C_{23}H_{28}O_6$ = 400.5.

*CAS — 125-10-0.*

*ATC — A07EA03; H02AB07.*

**Pharmacopoeias.** In *Chin.* and *Pol.*

### Profile

Prednisone is a biologically inert corticosteroid that is converted to the predominantly glucocorticoid corticosteroid prednisolone in the liver. It has the same chemical relationship to prednisolone as cortisone has to hydrocortisone. The indications and dosage of prednisone for oral use are exactly the same as those for prednisolone (see p.1109, and the chapter introduction, p.1073).

In the UK prednisolone has historically been preferred to prednisone, on the grounds that it does not require conversion to the active substance, but in practice this is rarely significant (see Hepatic Impairment, under Prednisolone, p.1108), and in some countries, such as the USA, prednisone is the drug of choice for many of the conditions in which routine systemic corticosteroid therapy is indicated.

### Preparations

***USP 27:*** Prednisone Oral Solution; Prednisone Tablets.

**Proprietary Preparations** (details are given in Part 3)
***Arg.:*** Meticorten; Prednipirine; Prenisonal; ***Austral.:*** Panafcort; Sone; ***Belg.:*** Prednicort; ***Braz.:*** Artinizona; Corticorten; Meticorten; Precortil; Predicorten; Predval; ***Canad.:*** Deltasone†; Winpred; ***Chile:*** Bersen; Cortiprex; Meticorten; Procion; ***Fr.:*** Cortancyl; ***Ger.:*** Decortin; Predni Tablinen; Rectodelt; ***Hong Kong:*** Deltasone†; ***Israel:*** Prednitone; ***Ital.:*** Deltacortene; ***Mex.:*** Meprosona-F; Meticorten; Nosipren; Ofisolona; Predicor; Prednidib; Premagnol; Promifen†; ***NZ:*** Deltasone†; ***Port.:*** Meticorten; ***S.Afr.:*** Meticorten; Panafcort; Predeltin; Pulmison; ***Spain:*** Dacortin; ***Swed.:*** Deltison; ***USA:*** Deltasone; Liquid Pred; Meticorten; Panasol-S; Sterapred.

**Multi-ingredient:** ***Arg.:*** Peganix; ***Austria:*** Fluorex Plus; Oleomycetin-Prednison; ***Canad.:*** Metreton†; ***Chile:*** Alerzona; ***Ger.:*** Oleomycetin-Prednison; ***Mex.:*** Pre Clor; ***Port.:*** Ciclobiotico; ***Spain:*** Coliriocilina Prednisona; Fiacin; Kanafosal Predni; Prednis Neomic.

## Prednylidene *(BAN, rINN)*

16-Methyleneprednisolone; Prednilideno. 11β,17α,21-Trihydroxy-16-methylenepregna-1,4-diene-3,20-dione.

$C_{22}H_{28}O_5$ = 372.5.

*CAS — 599-33-7.*

*ATC — H02AB11.*

### Profile

Prednylidene is a corticosteroid that has been used for its glucocorticoid activity similarly to prednisolone (see p.1108). It has been given by mouth as the free alcohol and by injection as the diethylaminoacetate hydrochloride.

### Preparations

**Proprietary Preparations** (details are given in Part 3)
***Ger.:*** Decortilen.

## Procinonide (USAN, rINN)

Procinonida; RS-2362. (6α,11β,16α)-6,9-Difluoro-11-hydroxy-16,17-[(1-methylethylidene)bis(oxy)]-21-(1-oxopropoxy)-pregna-1,4-diene-3,20-dione.

$C_{27}H_{34}F_2O_7$ = 508.6.
*CAS — 58497-00-0.*

### Profile

Procinonide is a derivative of fluocinolone acetonide (p.1101) that has been applied topically in combination with fluocinonide and ciprocinonide in the management of various skin disorders.

### Preparations

**Proprietary Preparations** (details are given in Part 3)
**Multi-ingredient: *Canad.:*** Trisyn†.

## Rimexolone (BAN, USAN, rINN)

Org-6216; Rimexolona; Trimexolone. 11β-Hydroxy-16α,17α-dimethyl-17β-propionylandrosta-1,4-dien-3-one.

$C_{24}H_{34}O_3$ = 370.5.
*CAS — 49697-38-3.*
*ATC — H02AB12; S01BA13.*

**Pharmacopoeias.** In *US.*
**USP 27** (Rimexolone). A white to off-white powder. Freely soluble in chloroform; sparingly soluble in methyl alcohol.

### Profile

Rimexolone is a corticosteroid applied topically to the eye for its glucocorticoid activity (see p.1068) in the treatment of inflammatory eye disorders including uveitis (p.1090) and postoperative inflammation. It is used as a 1% suspension.

Prolonged application to the eye of preparations containing corticosteroids has caused raised intra-ocular pressure and reduced visual function.

### Preparations

*USP 27:* Rimexolone Ophthalmic Suspension.

**Proprietary Preparations** (details are given in Part 3)
***Austria:*** Vexol; ***Belg.:*** Vexolon; ***Braz.:*** Vexol; ***Canad.:*** Vexol; ***Denm.:*** Vexol; ***Fin.:*** Vexol; ***Fr.:*** Vexol; ***Ger.:*** Rimexel; Vexol; ***Gr.:*** Vexol; ***Hong Kong:*** Vexol; ***Irl.:*** Vexol; ***Ital.:*** Vexol; ***Mex.:*** Vexol; ***Norw.:*** Vexol; ***Port.:*** Vexol; ***Spain:*** Vexol†; ***Swed.:*** Vexol; ***Switz.:*** Vexol; ***UK:*** Vexol; ***USA:*** Vexol.

## Suprarenal Cortex

Corteza suprarrenal.

### Profile

Suprarenal cortex contains a number of steroid compounds the most active of which are corticosterone, dehydrocorticosterone, hydrocortisone, cortisone, and aldosterone. It has been prepared from the adrenal glands of oxen. Suprarenal cortex was formerly used intramuscularly for the treatment of adrenocortical insufficiency but it has been superseded by hydrocortisone and other corticosteroids (see p.1075).

Suprarenal cortex is an ingredient of a wide range of preparations, often together with other organ extracts or vitamins, promoted for indications ranging from asthenia to liver disorders.

### Preparations

**Proprietary Preparations** (details are given in Part 3)
***Austria:*** Cortiglanden†; ***Fr.:*** Cortine Naturelle†; ***Spain:*** Pleocortex†.

**Multi-ingredient: *Austria:*** Flexurat†; Mobilat; ***Belg.:*** Mobilat; ***Braz.:*** Broncopinol; Mobilat; Suprasten; ***Canad.:*** Heracline; Revitonus C; ***Chile:*** Mobilat; ***Fin.:*** Mobilat; ***Ger.:*** Arthrodeformat P; Flexurat†; Mobilat; ***Hong Kong:*** Mobilat; ***Singapore:*** Mobilat; ***Spain:*** Neurocatavin Dexa; Pleocortex B6†; Rubrocortin; ***Switz.:*** Mobilat†; ***Thai.:*** Mobilat.

## Tixocortol Pivalate (BANM, USAN, rINNM)

JO-1016; Pivalato de tixocortol. 11β,17α-Dihydroxy-21-mercaptopregn-4-ene-3,20-dione 21-pivalate.

$C_{26}H_{38}O_5S$ = 462.6.
*CAS — 61951-99-3 (tixocortol); 55560-96-8 (tixocortol pivalate).*
*ATC — A07EA05; R01AD07.*

### Profile

Tixocortol pivalate is a corticosteroid with mainly glucocorticoid activity (p.1068). It is used as buccal, nasal, throat, and rectal preparations. It is reported to undergo rapid first-pass metabolism, primarily in the liver, and to have minimal systemic effect.

### Preparations

**Proprietary Preparations** (details are given in Part 3)
***Belg.:*** Rhinovalon; ***Canad.:*** Rectovalone†; ***Fr.:*** Pivalone; Rectovalone†; ***Neth.:*** Rectovalone†; ***Singapore:*** Pivalone; ***Spain:*** Rectovalone†; Tiovalone; ***Switz.:*** Pivalone.

**Multi-ingredient: *Belg.:*** Rhinovalon Neomycine; ***Fr.:*** Dontopivalone†; Oropivalone Bacitracine; Pivalone Neomycine†; Thiovalone; ***Singapore:*** Pivalone Neomycin; ***Switz.:*** Oro-Pivalone; Pivalone compositum.

## Triamcinolone (BAN, rINN)

9α-Fluoro-16α-hydroxyprednisolone; Fluoxiprednisolonum; Triamcinolona; Triamcinolonum. 9α-Fluoro-11β,16α,17α,21-tetrahydroxypregna-1,4-diene-3,20-dione.

$C_{21}H_{27}FO_6$ = 394.4.
*CAS — 124-94-7.*
*ATC — A01AC01; D07AB09; H02AB08; R01AD11; R03BA06; S01BA05.*

**Pharmacopoeias.** In *Chin., Eur.* (see p.vi), *Jpn, Pol.,* and *US.*
**Ph. Eur. 5.0** (Triamcinolone). A white or almost white, crystalline powder. It shows polymorphism. Practically insoluble in water and in dichloromethane; slightly soluble in methyl alcohol. Protect from light.
**USP 27** (Triamcinolone). A white or practically white, odourless, crystalline powder. Very slightly soluble in water, in chloroform, and in ether; slightly soluble in alcohol and in methyl alcohol.

## Triamcinolone Acetonide (BANM, rINNM)

Acetónido de triamcinolona; Triamcinoloni Acetonidum. 9α-Fluoro-11β,21-dihydroxy-16α,17α-isopropylidenedioxypregna-1,4-diene-3,20-dione.

$C_{24}H_{31}FO_6$ = 434.5.
*CAS — 76-25-5.*
*ATC — A01AC01; D07AB09; H02AB08; R01AD11; R03BA06; S01BA05.*

**Pharmacopoeias.** In *Chin., Eur.* (see p.vi), *Jpn, Pol.,* and *US. Chin.* also includes Triamcinolone Acetonide Acetate.
**Ph. Eur. 5.0** (Triamcinolone Acetonide). A white or almost white, crystalline powder. It shows polymorphism. Practically insoluble in water; sparingly soluble in alcohol. Protect from light.
**USP 27** (Triamcinolone Acetonide). A white to cream-coloured crystalline powder, having not more than a slight odour. Practically insoluble in water; sparingly soluble in dehydrated alcohol, in chloroform, and in methyl alcohol. Store at a temperature of 25°, excursions permitted between 15° and 30°.

## Triamcinolone Acetonide Sodium Phosphate (BANM, USAN, rINNM)

CL-61965; CL-106359. Triamcinolone acetonide 21-disodium phosphate.

$C_{24}H_{30}FNa_2O_9P$ = 558.4.
*CAS — 1997-15-5.*
*ATC — A01AC01; D07AB09; H02AB08; R01AD11; R03BA06; S01BA05.*

## Triamcinolone Diacetate (BANM, rINNM)

Diacetato de triamcinolona. Triamcinolone 16α,21-diacetate.

$C_{25}H_{31}FO_8$ = 478.5.
*CAS — 67-78-7.*
*ATC — A01AC01; D07AB09; H02AB08; R01AD11; R03BA06; S01BA05.*

**Pharmacopoeias.** In *US.*
**USP 27** (Triamcinolone Diacetate). A fine, white to off-white, crystalline powder, having not more than a slight odour. Practically insoluble in water; soluble 1 in 13 of alcohol, 1 in 80 of chloroform, and 1 in 40 of methyl alcohol; slightly soluble in ether.

## Triamcinolone Hexacetonide (BAN, USAN, rINN)

CL-34433; Hexacetónido de triamcinolona; TATBA; Triamcinolone Acetonide 21-(3,3-Dimethylbutyrate); Triamcinoloni Hexacetonidum. 9α-Fluoro-11β,21-dihydroxy-16α,17α-isopropylidenedioxypregna-1,4-diene-3,20-dione 21-(3,3-dimethylbutyrate).

$C_{30}H_{41}FO_7$ = 532.6.
*CAS — 5611-51-8.*
*ATC — A01AC01; D07AB09; H02AB08; R01AD11; R03BA06; S01BA05.*

**Pharmacopoeias.** In *Eur.* (see p.vi) and *US.*
**Ph. Eur. 5.0** (Triamcinolone Hexacetonide). A white or almost white, crystalline powder. Practically insoluble in water; sparingly soluble in dehydrated alcohol and in methyl alcohol. Protect from light.
**USP 27** (Triamcinolone Hexacetonide). A white to cream-coloured powder. Practically insoluble in water; soluble in chloroform; slightly soluble in methyl alcohol.

### Adverse Effects, Treatment, Withdrawal, and Precautions

As for corticosteroids in general (see p.1068). High doses of triamcinolone may have a greater tendency to produce proximal myopathy. Its effects on sodium and water retention are less than those of prednisolone.

When applied topically, particularly to large areas, when the skin is broken, or under occlusive dressings, or when given intranasally, corticosteroids may be absorbed in sufficient amounts to cause systemic effects.

**Hypersensitivity.** Local reactions to topical triamcinolone preparations have been attributed to the content of ethylenediamine.[1,2] However, there have also been reports of anaphylactic shock following intra-articular[3] or intramuscular[4] injection of triamcinolone acetonide.

1. Wright S, Harman RRM. Ethylenediamine and piperazine sensitivity. *BMJ* 1983; **287:** 463–4.
2. Freeman S. Allergy to Kenacomb cream. *Med J Aust* 1986; **145:** 361.
3. Larsson L. Anaphylactic shock after ia administration of triamcinolone acetonide in a 35-year-old female. *Scand J Rheumatol* 1989; **18:** 441–2.
4. Gonzalo FE, *et al.* Anaphylactic shock caused by triamcinolone acetonide. *Ann Pharmacother* 1994; **28:** 1310.

### Interactions

The interactions of corticosteroids in general are described on p.1072.

### Pharmacokinetics

For a brief outline of the pharmacokinetics of corticosteroids, see p.1073.

Triamcinolone is reported to have a half-life in plasma of about 2 to over 5 hours. It is bound to plasma albumin to a much smaller extent than hydrocortisone.

The acetonide, diacetate, and hexacetonide esters of triamcinolone are only very slowly absorbed from injection sites.

Triamcinolone crosses the placenta.

◊ References to the pharmacokinetics of triamcinolone and its esters.

1. Möllmann H, *et al.* Pharmacokinetics of triamcinolone acetonide and its phosphate ester. *Eur J Clin Pharmacol* 1985; **29:** 85–9.
2. Derendorf H, *et al.*. Pharmacokinetics and pharmacodynamics of glucocorticoid suspensions after intra-articular administration. *Clin Pharmacol Ther* 1986; **39:** 313–17.
3. Derendorf H, *et al.* Pharmacokinetics of triamcinolone acetonide after intravenous, oral, and inhaled administration. *J Clin Pharmacol* 1995; **35:** 302–5.
4. Argenti D, *et al.* A mass balance study to evaluate the biotransformation and excretion of [$^{14}$C]-triamcinolone acetonide following oral administration. *J Clin Pharmacol* 2000; **40:** 770–80.

### Uses and Administration

Triamcinolone is a corticosteroid with mainly glucocorticoid activity (p.1068); 4 mg of triamcinolone is equivalent in anti-inflammatory activity to about 5 mg of prednisolone. It is used, either in the form of the free alcohol or in one of the esterified forms, in the treatment of conditions for which corticosteroid therapy is indicated (see p.1073), except adrenocortical insufficiency for which hydrocortisone with supplementary fludrocortisone is preferred.

For administration by mouth triamcinolone is used in doses of 4 to 48 mg daily although daily doses over 32 mg are seldom indicated.

For parenteral administration the acetonide or diacetate esters are used in doses of about 40 mg by intramuscular injection. They are usually given as suspensions to provide a prolonged systemic effect. A dose of 40 to 100 mg of the acetonide may provide symptomatic control throughout the pollen season for hay fever sufferers (but see Rhinitis, below); for the diacetate, a 40-mg dose is administered weekly.

For intra-articular injection triamcinolone acetonide, diacetate, and hexacetonide have all been used. Doses for these esters have been in the range of 2.5 to 40 mg, 3 to 48 mg, and 2 to 30 mg respectively, depending upon the size of the joint injected.

For topical application in the treatment of various skin disorders triamcinolone acetonide is used, usually in creams, lotions, or ointments containing 0.1% although concentrations ranging from 0.025 to 0.5% have been employed. Several topical preparations also contain an antimicrobial drug. For recommendations concerning the correct use of corticosteroids on the skin, and a rough guide to the clinical potencies of topical corticosteroids, see p.1074.

Triamcinolone esters are also commonly used by intralesional or intradermal injection in the treatment of some inflammatory skin disorders such as keloids. Suggested doses for the various esters have been:

- acetonide: 1 to 3 mg per site with no more than 5 mg injected into any one site or not more than 30 mg in total if several sites of injection are used

- diacetate: a total of 5 mg in divided doses into small lesions or up to a total of 48 mg in divided doses into large lesions with no more than 12.5 mg injected into any one site or 25 mg injected into any one lesion
- hexacetonide: up to 500 micrograms per square inch (about 80 micrograms/$cm^2$) of affected skin.

Triamcinolone acetonide is also used by inhalation for the control of asthma in a usual dose of about 200 micrograms by metered-dose inhaler three or four times daily; the dose should not exceed 1600 micrograms daily.

In the prophylaxis and treatment of allergic rhinitis triamcinolone acetonide may be administered by a nasal spray in a usual initial dose of 2 sprays (110 micrograms) into each nostril once daily, reduced to 1 spray (55 micrograms) when control is achieved.

Other esters of triamcinolone that have occasionally been used include the acetonide dipotassium phosphate, acetonide hemisuccinate, aminobenzal benzamidoisobutyrate, and benetonide. Flupamesone (triamcinolone acetonide metembonate) has also been used.

**Asthma.** Intramuscular triamcinolone acetonide has been reported to be more effective than oral low-dose prednisone in controlling exacerbations in patients with severe, chronic, life-threatening asthma,[1] although this conclusion is controversial.[2-7] Corticosteroids and beta$_2$-adrenoceptor agonists form the cornerstone of the management of asthma (p.777). Inhaled corticosteroids are added to therapy with a short-acting beta$_2$ agonist if symptom relief with the latter is needed more than once daily, although corticosteroids with reduced systemic activity are generally preferred to triamcinolone. Systemic corticosteroids are reserved for the most severe cases, and for the management of acute severe asthma attacks (status asthmaticus).


1. Ogirala RG, *et al.* High-dose intramuscular triamcinolone in severe, chronic, life-threatening asthma. *N Engl J Med* 1991; **324:** 589–9. Correction. *ibid.*; 1380.
2. Salmeron S, *et al.* Intramuscular triamcinolone in severe asthma. *N Engl J Med* 1991; **325:** 429–30.
3. Nicholas SS. Intramuscular triamcinolone in severe asthma. *N Engl J Med* 1991; **325:** 430.
4. Kidney JC, *et al.* Intramuscular triamcinolone in severe asthma. *N Engl J Med* 1991; **325:** 430.
5. Capewell S, McLeod DT. Intramuscular triamcinolone in severe asthma. *N Engl J Med* 1991; **325:** 430.
6. Ogirala RG, *et al.* Intramuscular triamcinolone in severe asthma. *N Engl J Med* 1991; **325:** 431.
7. Capewell S, McLeod D. Injected corticosteroids in refractory asthma. *Lancet* 1991; **338:** 1075–6.


**Chronic obstructive pulmonary disease.** For discussion of the value of inhaled corticosteroids in chronic obstructive pulmonary disease, including reference to the use of triamcinolone acetonide, see p.1078.

**Haemangioma.** For reference to the use of a mixture of triamcinolone and betamethasone for intralesional injection of haemangioma, see p.1081.

**Rhinitis.** Triamcinolone is used[1,2] in the management of allergic rhinitis (p.422). However, the use of depot injections of triamcinolone to manage seasonal allergic rhinitis has been deemed unacceptable by some.[3]


1. Jeal W, Faulds D. Triamcinolone acetonide: a review of its pharmacological properties and therapeutic efficacy in the management of allergic rhinitis. *Drugs* 1997; **53:** 257–80.
2. Gawchik SM, Saccar CL. A risk-benefit assessment of intranasal triamcinolone acetonide in allergic rhinitis. *Drug Safety* 2000; **23:** 309–22.
3. Anonymous. Any place for depot triamcinolone in hay fever? *Drug Ther Bull* 1999; **37:** 17–18.


## Preparations

***BP 2003:*** Triamcinolone Acetonide Injection; Triamcinolone Cream; Triamcinolone Hexacetonide Injection; Triamcinolone Ointment; Triamcinolone Oromucosal Paste; Triamcinolone Tablets;
***USP 27:*** Neomycin Sulfate and Triamcinolone Acetonide Cream; Neomycin Sulfate and Triamcinolone Acetonide Ophthalmic Ointment; Nystatin and Triamcinolone Acetonide Cream; Nystatin and Triamcinolone Acetonide Ointment; Nystatin, Neomycin Sulfate, Gramicidin, and Triamcinolone Acetonide Cream; Nystatin, Neomycin Sulfate, Gramicidin, and Triamcinolone Acetonide Ointment; Triamcinolone Acetonide Cream; Triamcinolone Acetonide Dental Paste; Triamcinolone Acetonide Injectable Suspension; Triamcinolone Acetonide Lotion; Triamcinolone Acetonide Ointment; Triamcinolone Acetonide Topical Aerosol; Triamcinolone Diacetate Injectable Suspension; Triamcinolone Diacetate Syrup; Triamcinolone Hexacetonide Injectable Suspension; Triamcinolone Tablets.

**Proprietary Preparations** (details are given in Part 3)

***Arg.:*** Fortcinolona; Glytop; Kenacort; Kenacort-A; Ledercort; Nasacort; Rezamid D, Rezamid F, Rezamid M; Triamciterap; Triampoen; ***Austral.:*** Aristocort; Kenacort-A; Kenalog in Orabase; Kenalone†; Nasacort AQ†; ***Austria:*** Delphicort; Lederspan†; Nasacort; Solu-Volon A; Volon; Volon A; ***Belg.:*** Albicort; Delphi; Kenacort; Kenacort Solubile†; Kenacort-A; Ledercort; Lederspan†; ***Braz.:*** Azmacort; Nasacort; Omcilon A Orabase; Theracort†; Triancil; ***Canad.:*** Aristocort; Aristospan; Azmacort†; Kenalog; Kenalog in Orabase; Nasacort; Oracort; Scheinpharm Triamcine-A†; Triaderm; ***Chile:*** Kenacort-A; Nasacort; ***Denm.:*** Kenalog; Lederspan†; Nasacort; ***Fin.:*** Aftab; Kenacort-T; Lederspan†; Nasacort; ***Fr.:*** Hexatrione; Kenacort; Nasacort; ***Ger.:*** Aftab†; Arutrin; Berlicort; Delphicort; Delphimix; Extracort†; Kenalog; Kortikoid-ratiopharm; Lederlon; Nasacort; Rhinisan; Tri-Anemul†; Triam; TriamCreme; Triamgalen; Triamhexal; TriamSalbe; Volon; Volon A; Volonimat; Volonimat N; ***Hong Kong:*** Aristocort; Denkacort; Dermacort; Kemzid; Kenacort-A; Kenalog in Orabase; Nasacort; Stacort-A†; ***India:*** Kenacort; Ledercort; Tess; ***Irl.:*** Adcortyl; Adcortyl in Orabase; Kenalog; Lederspan†; Nasacort; ***Israel:*** Adcortyl; Kenalog; Kenalog in Orabase; Oracort; Sterocort; Steronase Aq; ***Ital.:*** Aftab; Ipercortis; Kenacort; Ledercort; Nasacort; Triamvirgi; ***Jpn:*** Aftach; ***Malaysia:*** Dermacort; Kenacort-A; Kenaderm; Kenalog in Orabase; Nasacort AQ; Orrepaste; Shincort; Trim; ***Mex.:*** Kenacort; Kenalog Dental; Nasacort; Triamsicort; Zamacort; ***Neth.:*** Albicort; Delphi†; Kenacort-A; Ledercort†; Lederspan†; Nasacort; ***Norw.:*** Kenacort-T; Lederspan; Nasacort; ***NZ:*** Aristocort; Kenacort-A; Kenalog in Orabase; Nasacort†; Oracort; ***Port.:*** Aftach; ***S.Afr.:*** Kenalog in Orabase; Ledercort†; Lederspan†; Nasacor; ***Singapore:*** Dermacort; Kemzid; Kenacort-A; Kenalog in Orabase; Nasacort; Oramedy; Orrepaste; Shincort; Triam; Trinolone; ***Spain:*** Flutenal; Kenalog in Orabase; Ledercort†; Nasacort; Proctosteroid; Trigon Depot; ***Swed.:*** Kenacort-T; Lederspan†; Nasacort; ***Switz.:*** Kenacort; Kenacort-A; Kenacort-A Solubile; Ledercort; Nasacort; Triamcort; ***Thai.:*** Aristocort; Facort; Ftorocort; Generlog; Kanolone; Kela; Kemzid; Kenacort; Kenalog in Orabase; Keno; Laver; Manolone; Metoral; Milanolone; Nasacort; Oracort†; Oral-T; Orcilone; Risto; Shincort; Simacort; Tacinol; Topilone; Tramsilione; Triama; Trilosil; Trim; Trimasone†; Unif; Vacinolone; ***UK:*** Adcortyl; Adcortyl in Orabase; Kenalog; Ledercort†; Lederspan†; Nasacort; ***USA:*** Amcort; Aristocort; Aristospan; Atolone; Azmacort; Delta-Tritex; Flutex; Kenacort†; Kenaject†; Kenalog; Kenalog in Orabase; Kenonel; Nasacort; Oralone Dental; Tac; Tri-Kort; Tri-Nasal; Triacet; Triam; Triam-A; Triamonide; Triderm; Trilog; Trilone; Tristoject†.

**Multi-ingredient:** ***Arg.:*** Bagovit A Plus; Biotaer Nasal; Exfolium; Kenacomb; Ledercort con Neomicina; Mantus; Rezamid; Salicort; Sorsis; ***Austral.:*** Kenacomb; Otocomb Otic; ***Austria:*** Aureocort; Ledermix; Mycostatin V; Neo-Delphicort; Pevisone; Steros-Anal; Trilon; Volon A antibiotikahaltig; Volon A Tinktur; Volon A-Zinklotion; ***Belg.:*** Albicort Compositum†; Albicort Oticum†; Mycolog; Pevisone; Trianal; ***Braz.:*** Londerm-N; Neolon-D; Omcilon A M; Omcilon A†; Onciplus; ***Canad.:*** Kenacomb; Triacomb; Viaderm-KC; ***Denm.:*** Kenacutan; Kenalog Comp med Mycostatin; Kenalog Comp†; Kenalog med Salicylsyre; Ledermix; Pevisone; ***Fin.:*** Aureocort†; Kenacort-T comp†; Pevisone; ***Fr.:*** Cidermex; Corticotulle Lumiere; Kenalcol; Localone; Mycolog; Pevisone; ***Ger.:*** Ampho-Moronal V L†; Ampho-Moronal V†; Aureodelf; Corticotulle Lumiere; Epipevisone; Extracort Rhin sine†; Extracort Tinktur; Moronal V; mykoproct sine; Polcortolon TC; Steros-Anal; Ultexiv†; Volon A antibiotikahaltig N; Volon A Tinktur N; Volon A-Rhin; Volon A-Schuttelmix; Volonimat Plus N; ***Gr.:*** Olamyc; Pevison; ***Hong Kong:*** Anso; Clotrinolon; Kenacomb; Oragesic; Pevisone; Tri-Gel; Triacomb; Triaformo†; Triditol-G; ***India:*** Kenacomb; Kenalog-S; Ledercort-N; ***Irl.:*** Audicort; Aureocort†; Kenacomb; Ledermix†; ***Israel:*** Dermacombin; Kenacomb; Ledermix; Oracort E; Pevisone; ***Ital.:*** Assocort; Aureocort; Dirahist; Kataval; Neo-Audiocort†; Pevisone; ***Malaysia:*** Ecocort; Econazine; Kenacomb; Oral-Aid; Pevisone; ***Mex.:*** Kenacomb; ***Neth.:*** Albicort Compositum; Kenalog; Mycolog; Trianal; ***Norw.:*** Kenacort-T comp; Kenacutan; Pevisone; ***NZ:*** Kenacomb; Kenoid†; ***Port.:*** Kenacomb; Localone; Pevisone; ***S.Afr.:*** Kenacomb; Ledermix†; Pevisone; Trialone; ***Singapore:*** Ecocort; Econazine; Kenacomb; Oral-Aid; Pevisone; ***Spain:*** Aldo Otico; Aldoderma; Anasilpiel; Anso; Cemalyt; Cremsol; Flutenal Gentamicina; Flutenal Sali; Interderm; Nesfare; Positon; Trigon Rectal; Trigon Topico; ***Swed.:*** Kenacombin Novum; Kenacort-T comp; Kenacutan; Pevisone; ***Switz.:*** Kenacort-A; Ledermix; Mycolog; Pevisone; ***Thai.:*** Dermacombin; Ecoderm; Fungisil-T; KA-Cilone; Kelaplus; Kenacomb; Pevisone; Tara-Plus; Timi; Trilosil N†; Trimicon; ***UAE:*** Panderm; ***UK:*** Adcortyl with Graneodin†; Audicort; Aureocort; Ledermix; Nystadermal†; Pevaryl TC†; Tri-Adcortyl; ***USA:*** Myco-Biotic II; Myco-Triacet II; Mycogen II; Mycolog-II; Myconel; Mytrex†; NGT; Tri-Statin II.

---

## Ulobetasol Propionate *(rINNM)*

BMY-30056; CGP-14458; 6-α-Fluoroclobetasol Propionate; Halobetasol Propionate *(USAN)*; Propionato de ulobetasol. 21-Chloro-6α,9-difluoro-11β,17-dihydroxy-16β-methylpregna-1,4-diene-3,20-dione 17-propionate.

$C_{25}H_{31}ClF_2O_5$ = 485.0.

*CAS — 98651-66-2 (ulobetasol); 66852-54-8 (ulobetasol propionate).*

*ATC — D07AC21.*

### Profile

Ulobetasol propionate is a corticosteroid that is used topically for its glucocorticoid activity (p.1068) in the treatment of various skin disorders. It is usually employed as a cream or ointment containing 0.05%.

When applied topically, particularly to large areas, when the skin is broken, or under occlusive dressings, corticosteroids may be absorbed in sufficient amounts to cause systemic effects (p.1068). The effects of topical corticosteroids on the skin are described on p.1070. For recommendations concerning the correct use of corticosteroids on the skin, and a rough guide to the clinical potencies of topical corticosteroids, see p.1074.

### Preparations

**Proprietary Preparations** (details are given in Part 3)

***Austria:*** Miracorten†; ***Canad.:*** Ultravate; ***Switz.:*** Miracorten†; ***USA:*** Ultravate.

---

# Cough Suppressants Expectorants Mucolytics and Nasal Decongestants

This chapter describes drugs that are used mainly as cough suppressants, expectorants, or mucolytics, and also those sympathomimetics primarily used for the relief of nasal congestion. Other drugs used in cough include antihistamines (p.419), bronchodilators (p.475 and p.777), and local anaesthetics (p.1367). Compounds with a demulcent action such as glycerol (p.1694) and sucrose (p.1450) are also used, as are various hydrating inhalations.

**Cough suppressants** have either a central or a peripheral action on the cough reflex or a combination of both. Centrally acting cough suppressants increase the threshold of the cough centre in the brain to incoming stimuli whereas those acting peripherally decrease the sensitivity of the receptors in the respiratory tract. Some drugs have an indirect peripheral mechanism of action and may alter mucociliary factors, exert a local analgesic or anaesthetic action on the receptors, protect the receptors from irritant stimuli, or act as bronchodilators.

Those centrally acting cough suppressants structurally related to morphine that are included in this chapter, such as dextromethorphan, have little or no analgesic action. Those that also have an important analgesic action, such as codeine or diamorphine, are described in the chapter on Analgesics, p.1.

**Expectorants** are considered to increase the volume of secretions in the respiratory tract thereby facilitating their removal by ciliary action and coughing. Some, such as small doses of ipecacuanha and squill, ammonium salts, some volatile oils, and various iodide compounds are traditionally believed to achieve this by a reflex irritant effect on the gastric mucosa.

**Mucolytics** alter the structure of mucus to decrease its viscosity thereby facilitating its removal by ciliary action or expectoration.

Acetylcysteine, carbocisteine, mecysteine, and stepronin all have thiol groups; if this group is free, as in acetylcysteine, it may be substituted for disulfide bonds in mucus and therefore break the mucus chains. However, drugs such as carbocisteine with 'protected' thiol groups cannot act by this mechanism and their exact mode of action is unclear. Thiol groups are also involved in the mechanism of action of some of these drugs when they are used in the treatment of poisoning.

Deoxyribonucleases such as dornase alfa act as mucolytics by hydrolysing the accumulated extracellular DNA from decaying neutrophils that contributes to the viscous respiratory secretions of cystic fibrosis.

**Sympathomimetics** described in this chapter may be used systemically (e.g. phenylephrine, p.1126) or locally (e.g. naphazoline, p.1124), for their alpha agonist actions to produce vasoconstriction of the nasal mucosa, thus relieving congestion. Others (e.g. ephedrine, p.1120) have both alpha and beta agonist actions. The beta agonist actions confer upon them bronchodilating properties, but they have been superseded as bronchodilators by the more selective beta$_2$ agonists such as salbutamol (p.791). The value of bronchodilators in non-asthmatic cough has not been confirmed.

### Cough

Cough is an important physiological protective mechanism, but may also occur as a symptom of an underlying disorder such as asthma, gastro-oesophageal reflux disease, and postnasal drip. Treatment of the disorder often alleviates the cough, but there are times when symptomatic treatment is appropriate. The treatment chosen depends on whether the cough is productive or non-productive.

A **non-productive cough** such as that often seen with the common cold serves no useful purpose for the patient, and cough suppressants may provide some relief, particularly if given at night.

- Of the commonly used *cough suppressants*, pholcodine and dextromethorphan are considered to have fewer adverse effects than codeine. However, there is little evidence that these drugs are effective in severe cough. Codeine or similar opioids are not generally recommended as cough suppressants in children, and should be avoided altogether in those under 1 year of age.
- *Sedating antihistamines* such as diphenhydramine are frequently used as cough suppressants in compound preparations. Suggested mechanisms of action have included reduction in cholinergic nerve transmission, or cough suppression as a result of their sedative effects. Antihistamines reduce nasal secretions and may be of value in treating cough caused by postnasal drip, particularly if associated with allergic rhinitis (see p.422). However, they should not be used to treat a productive cough because they may cause formation of viscid mucus plugs. Their sedative effects are a disadvantage for daytime use but may be a short-term advantage for night coughs.
- *Demulcents* probably act as indirect peripherally acting cough suppressants by providing a protective coating over sensory receptors in the pharynx. Demulcents include glycerol, honey, liquorice, and sucrose syrups.

A potent cough suppressant such as morphine is needed for the relief of **intractable cough** in terminal illness. The use of such a potent opioid is not otherwise considered appropriate for cough.

- *Local anaesthetics* such as lidocaine or bupivacaine have been inhaled in severe intractable cough, including cough caused by malignant neoplasms. Cough suppression is produced by an indirect peripheral action on sensory receptors, but as all protective pulmonary reflexes may be lost and bronchospasm may be induced, such treatment should be used with care. There may also be temporary loss of the swallowing reflex.

A **productive cough** is characterised by the presence of sputum and may be associated with conditions such as chronic bronchitis, bronchiectasis, or cystic fibrosis. Cough suppressants are inappropriate, since the cough serves the purpose of clearing the airways, but expectorants have been used on the grounds that increasing the volume of secretions in the respiratory tract facilitates removal by ciliary action and coughing. However, clinical evidence of efficacy is lacking, and many authorities consider expectorants to be of no value other than as a placebo.

- Commonly used *expectorants* include ammonium salts, guaifenesin, ipecacuanha, and sodium citrate. Iodides have also been used but there has been concern over their safety for prolonged administration in respiratory disorders and because of their potential for thyroid suppression; in particular, it has been recommended that they should not be given to children, adolescents, pregnant women, or patients with goitre.
- *Mucolytics* have been shown to affect sputum viscosity and structure and patients have reported alleviation of their symptoms, but no consistent improvement has been demonstrated in lung function. Commonly used mucolytics include acetylcysteine, bromhexine, carbocisteine, and mecysteine. Dornase alfa is also available, in particular for patients with cystic fibrosis. In theory mucolytics may disrupt the gastric mucosal barrier and caution has been recommended in patients with a history of peptic ulcer disease.
- *Hydrating agents* liquefy mucus and also have a demulcent effect. Hydration may be achieved simply by inhaled warm moist air. The addition of substances such as menthol, benzoin, or volatile oils is unlikely to provide any additional benefit but may encourage the use of such inhalations. Inhaled aerosols of water, sodium bicarbonate, sodium chloride, surfactants such as tyloxapol, and proteolytic enzymes such as chymotrypsin and trypsin, have also been used for their reported hydrating or mucolytic effects on respiratory secretions.

Cough may sometimes be associated with **bronchospasm** in patients with asthma.

- *Bronchodilators* such as salbutamol (a beta$_2$ agonist) or ipratropium (an antimuscarinic) alleviate cough associated with bronchospasm. However, they are not generally considered of benefit in other forms of cough, and hence are not recommended for use in non-asthmatic patients.

**Cough and cold preparations** containing various combinations of cough suppressants and expectorants, together with sympathomimetics, antihistamines, or analgesics are available. Some combinations, such as a cough suppressant and an expectorant, are illogical and have little evidence to support their efficacy. As with many combinations, doses of individual drugs may be inadequate or inappropriate, and the large number of ingredients may expose the patient to unnecessary adverse effects.

References.


1. Fuller RW, Jackson DM. Physiology and treatment of cough. *Thorax* 1990; **45:** 425–30.
2. Pratter MR, *et al.* An algorithmic approach to chronic cough. *Ann Intern Med* 1993; **119:** 977–83.
3. Irwin RS, *et al.* Appropriate use of antitussives and protussives: a practical review. *Drugs* 1993; **46:** 80–91.
4. Irwin RS, *et al.* Managing cough as a defense mechanism and as a symptom: a consensus panel report of the American College of Chest Physicians. *Chest* 1998; **114** (suppl): 133S–181S.
5. Anonymous. Cough medications in children. *Drug Ther Bull* 1999; **37:** 19–21.
6. Irwin RS, Madison JM. The diagnosis and treatment of cough. *N Engl J Med* 2000; **343:** 1715–21.
7. Morice AH, Kastelik JA. Chronic cough in adults. *Thorax* 2003; **58:** 901–7.
8. de Jongste JC, Shields MD. Chronic cough in children. *Thorax* 2003; **58:** 998–1003.
9. Fontana GA, Pistolesi M. Chronic cough and gastro-oesophageal reflux. *Thorax* 2003; **58:** 1092–5.
10. Dicpinigaitis PV. Cough in asthma and eosinophilic bronchitis. *Thorax* 2004; **59:** 71–2.
11. Schroeder K, Fahey T. Over-the-counter medications for acute cough in children and adults in ambulatory settings. Available in The Cochrane Library; Issue 2. Chichester: John Wiley; 2004.


### Nasal congestion

Nasal congestion is frequently a symptom of conditions such as rhinitis (p.422), treatment of which can include the use of antihistamines, sympathomimetics, corticosteroids, antimuscarinics, and cromoglicate or nedocromil.

*Sympathomimetics* are also widely used as nasal decongestants to provide symptomatic relief of the common cold (p.618). They are used for the vasoconstriction produced by their alpha-adrenergic effects; redistribution of local blood flow reduces oedema of the nasal mucosa, thus improving ventilation, drainage, and nasal stuffiness. Sympathomimetics such as ephedrine, phenylephrine, naphazoline, oxymetazoline, and xylometazoline can be used topically as nasal drops or sprays. Those such as pseudoephedrine are given by mouth.

Topical use may lead to rebound congestion, particularly if prolonged, as vasodilatation becomes prominent and the effects of vasoconstriction subside. Use is therefore restricted to periods of not more than 7 consecutive days. Administration by mouth is not associated with such rebound congestion, but is more likely to be associated with systemic side-effects and a higher risk of drug interactions. A systematic review found no difference in efficacy between oral and topical decongestants from the limited evidence available.[1]

The benefits of *antihistamines* in nasal congestion other than that associated with allergic rhinitis are doubtful, particularly by topical application.

Inhalations of warm moist air are also useful in the treatment of nasal congestion associated with the common cold. As in the case of cough (see above) the addition of substances such as menthol, benzoin, or volatile oils may encourage the use of such inhalations.


1. Taverner D, *et al.* Nasal decongestants for the common cold. Available in The Cochrane Library; Issue 2. Chichester: John Wiley; 2004.


## Acetylcysteine *(BAN, USAN, rINN)*

5052; Acetilcisteína; Acetylcysteinum; NSC-111180. *N*-Acetyl-L-cysteine.

$C_5H_9NO_3S$ = 163.2.

*CAS — 616-91-1.*

*ATC — R05CB01; S01XA08; V03AB23.*

**Pharmacopoeias.** In *Chin., Eur.* (see p.vi), and *US.*

**Ph. Eur. 5.0** (Acetylcysteine). A white, crystalline powder or colourless crystals. Freely soluble in water and in alcohol; practically insoluble in dichloromethane. A 1% solution in water has a pH of 2.0 to 2.8. Protect from light.

**USP 27** (Acetylcysteine). A white crystalline powder having a slight acetic odour. Soluble 1 in 5 of water and 1 in 4 of alcohol; practically insoluble in chloroform and in ether. pH of a 1% solution in water is between 2.0 and 2.8. Store in airtight containers.

**Incompatibility.** Acetylcysteine is incompatible with some metals, including iron and copper, with rubber, and with oxygen and oxidising substances. Some antimicrobials including amphotericin B, ampicillin sodium, erythromycin lactobionate, and some tetracyclines are either physically incompatible with, or may be inactivated on mixture with, acetylcysteine.

**Stability.** A change in colour of solutions of acetylcysteine to light purple does not indicate significant impairment of safety or efficacy.

## Acetylcysteine Sodium *(BANM, rINNM)*

$C_5H_8NNaO_3S$ = 185.2.
*CAS — 19542-74-6.*
*ATC — R05CB01; S01XA08; V03AB23.*

## Adverse Effects

Hypersensitivity reactions have been reported in patients receiving acetylcysteine, including bronchospasm, angioedema, rashes and pruritus; hypotension, or occasionally hypertension, may occur. Other adverse effects reported with acetylcysteine include flushing, nausea and vomiting, fever, syncope, sweating, arthralgia, blurred vision, disturbances of liver function, acidosis, convulsions, and cardiac or respiratory arrest. Haemoptysis, rhinorrhoea, and stomatitis have been associated with inhalation of acetylcysteine.

**Hypersensitivity.** The most common symptoms of patients experiencing **anaphylactoid** reactions after the intravenous use of acetylcysteine in the treatment of paracetamol poisoning are rash and pruritus; other features have included flushing, nausea or vomiting, angioedema, tachycardia, bronchospasm, hypotension, and hypertension;[1,2] ECG abnormalities associated with an anaphylactoid reaction have also been reported in a patient.[3] Anaphylactoid reactions to intravenous acetylcysteine appear to be dose-related.[4] One group estimated that when acetylcysteine was given correctly the **frequency** of the anaphylactoid response was between 0.3 and 3%, whereas 11 of 15 patients who had received an overdose had an anaphylactoid reaction.[5] Intradermal testing and study of plasma-acetylcysteine concentrations in patients who developed reactions to acetylcysteine suggests a 'pseudo-allergic' rather than an immunological reaction,[6,7] although symptoms consistent with a serum sickness-like illness developed after exposure to acetylcysteine in one patient.[8] It has been suggested that generalised reactions to acetylcysteine can be **treated** with intravenous injection of an antihistamine;[4,9] infusion of acetylcysteine should be temporarily stopped but can usually be restarted at a slower rate without further reaction.

Symptoms after **overdosage** with acetylcysteine have been more severe. Hypotension appears to be especially prominent;[5] additional symptoms have included respiratory depression, haemolysis, disseminated intravascular coagulation, and renal failure, but some of these may have been due to paracetamol poisoning.[1] Death occurred in 3 patients who received an overdose of acetylcysteine while being treated for paracetamol poisoning,[1,10] but in 2 of them the role of acetylcysteine in this outcome was unclear.


1. Mant TGK, *et al.* Adverse reactions to acetylcysteine and effects of overdose. *BMJ* 1984; **289:** 217–19.
2. Dawson AH, *et al.* Adverse reactions to N-acetylcysteine during treatment for paracetamol poisoning. *Med J Aust* 1989; **150:** 329–31.
3. Bonfiglio MF, *et al.* Anaphylactoid reaction to intravenous acetylcysteine associated with electrocardiographic abnormalities. *Ann Pharmacother* 1992; **26:** 22–5.
4. Bailey B, McGuigan MA. Management of anaphylactoid reactions to intravenous N-acetylcysteine. *Ann Emerg Med* 1998; **31:** 710–15.
5. Sunman W, *et al.* Anaphylactoid response to intravenous acetylcysteine. *Lancet* 1992; **339:** 1231–2.
6. Bateman DN, *et al.* Adverse reactions to N-acetylcysteine. *Hum Toxicol* 1984; **3:** 393–8.
7. Donovan JW, *et al.* Adverse reactions of N-acetylcysteine and their relation to plasma levels. *Vet Hum Toxicol* 1987; **29:** 470.
8. Mohammed S, *et al.* Serum sickness-like illness associated with N-acetylcysteine therapy. *Ann Pharmacother* 1994; **28:** 285.
9. Bateman DN. Adverse reactions to antidotes. *Adverse Drug React Bull* 1988; (Dec.): 496–9.
10. Anonymous. Death after N-acetylcysteine. *Lancet* 1984; **i:** 1421.


## Precautions

Acetylcysteine should be used with caution in asthmatic patients. It should also be used with caution in patients with a history of peptic ulcer disease, both because drug-induced nausea and vomiting may increase the risk of gastrointestinal haemorrhage in patients predisposed to the condition, and because of a theoretical risk that mucolytics may disrupt the gastric mucosal barrier.

**Asthma.** Reports of bronchospasm precipitated in two asthmatic patients[1] and severe asthma and respiratory arrest in another[2] after intravenous treatment with acetylcysteine. The increased risk does not justify delaying or witholding acetylcysteine in asthmatic patients with paracetamol poisoning, but consideration might be given to initial intravenous infusion over 30 to 60 minutes rather than the conventional 15 minutes.[3]


1. Ho SW-C, Beilin LJ. Asthma associated with N-acetylcysteine infusion and paracetamol poisoning: report of two cases. *BMJ* 1983; **287:** 876–7.
2. Reynard K, *et al.* Respiratory arrest after N-acetylcysteine for paracetamol overdose. *Lancet* 1992; **340:** 675.
3. Schmidt LE, Dalhoff K. Risk factors in the development of adverse reactions to N-acetylcysteine in patients with paracetamol poisoning. *Br J Clin Pharmacol* 2001; **51:** 87–91.


**Hepatic impairment.** The total clearance of acetylcysteine in patients with cirrhosis was found to be markedly impaired, and the elimination half-life almost twice that of healthy controls.[1] Since some of the more serious adverse effects of acetylcysteine occur when plasma concentrations are high, the authors considered that increased vigilance for untoward anaphylactoid reactions and other adverse effects was necessary in patients with cirrhosis receiving acetylcysteine, and further studies to determine the optimum dosage regimen in such patients were required.


1. Jones AL, *et al.* Pharmacokinetics of N-acetylcysteine are altered in patients with chronic liver disease. *Aliment Pharmacol Ther* 1997; **11:** 787–91.


## Pharmacokinetics

◊ Acetylcysteine is rapidly absorbed from the gastrointestinal tract and peak plasma concentrations occur about 0.5 to 1 hour after oral administration of doses of 200 to 600 mg.[1] Some studies indicate dose-dependent pharmacokinetics with peak concentrations, the time taken to reach peak concentrations, and bioavailability increasing with increasing doses.[2] Acetylcysteine may be present in plasma as the parent compound or as various oxidised metabolites such as *N*-acetylcystine, *N,N*-diacetylcystine, and cysteine either free or bound to plasma proteins by labile disulfide bonds or as a fraction incorporated into protein peptide chains.[3] In a study about 50% was in a covalently protein-bound form 4 hours after administration.[4] Oral bioavailability is low and mean values have ranged from 4 to 10% depending on whether total acetylcysteine or just the reduced forms are measured.[4,5] It has been suggested that acetylcysteine's low oral bioavailability may be due to metabolism in the gut wall and first-pass metabolism in the liver.[4,5] Renal clearance may account for about 30% of total body clearance.[5] Following intravenous administration mean terminal half-lives have been calculated to be 1.95 and 5.58 hours for reduced and total acetylcysteine, respectively; the terminal half-life of total acetylcysteine was 6.25 hours after oral administration.[4]

For reference to altered pharmacokinetics in patients with hepatic impairment, see above.


1. Holdiness MR. Clinical pharmacokinetics of N-acetylcysteine. *Clin Pharmacokinet* 1991; **20:** 123–34.
2. Borgström L, Kågedal B. Dose dependent pharmacokinetics of N-acetylcysteine after oral dosing to man. *Biopharm Drug Dispos* 1990; **11:** 131–6.
3. De Caro L, *et al.* Pharmacokinetics and bioavailability of oral acetylcysteine in healthy volunteers. *Arzneimittelforschung* 1989; **39:** 383–6.
4. Olsson B, *et al.* Pharmacokinetics and bioavailability of reduced and oxidized N-acetylcysteine. *Eur J Clin Pharmacol* 1988; **34:** 77–82.
5. Borgström L, *et al.* Pharmacokinetics of N-acetylcysteine in man. *Eur J Clin Pharmacol* 1986; **31:** 217–22.


## Uses and Administration

Acetylcysteine is a mucolytic that reduces the viscosity of secretions probably by the splitting of disulfide bonds in mucoproteins. This action is greatest at a pH of 7 to 9 and the pH may have been adjusted in commercial preparations with sodium hydroxide. It is sometimes stated that acetylcysteine sodium is used, although the dose is expressed in terms of acetylcysteine.

Acetylcysteine is also able to promote the detoxification of an intermediate paracetamol metabolite, and has a key role in the management of paracetamol overdosage.

Acetylcysteine is used for its **mucolytic** activity in respiratory disorders associated with acute cough. Administration can be by nebulisation of 3 to 5 mL of a 20% solution or 6 to 10 mL of a 10% solution through a face mask or mouthpiece 3 or 4 times daily. If necessary 1 to 10 mL of a 20% solution or 2 to 20 mL of a 10% solution may be given by nebulisation every 2 to 6 hours. It can also be given by direct endotracheal instillation of 1 to 2 mL of a 10 to 20% solution as often as every hour. Mechanical suction of the liquefied secretions may be necessary, and nebulisers containing iron, copper, or rubber components should not be used.

Acetylcysteine has been given by mouth in doses of 200 mg two or three times daily as granules or effervescent tablets dissolved in water. Children aged 1 month to 2 years may be given 100 mg twice daily, and those aged 2 to 7 years 200 mg twice daily.

In the treatment of **dry eye** (p.1576) associated with abnormal mucus production, acetylcysteine, usually as a 5% solution with hypromellose, is administered topically 3 or 4 times daily. Higher concentrations have been used in some centres.

Acetylcysteine is given by intravenous infusion or by mouth in the treatment of **paracetamol poisoning**.

- If given intravenously: 150 mg/kg of acetylcysteine in 200 mL of glucose 5% is given initially over 15 minutes, followed by infusion of 50 mg/kg in 500 mL of glucose 5% over the next 4 hours and then 100 mg/kg in one litre of glucose 5% over the next 16 hours. Sodium chloride 0.9% may be used where glucose 5% is unsuitable. The volume of intravenous fluids should be modified for children.
- If given by mouth: an initial dose of 140 mg/kg as a 5% solution is followed by 70 mg/kg every 4 hours for an additional 17 doses.

Acetylcysteine is reported to be most effective when administered within 8 hours of paracetamol overdosage, with the protective effect diminishing after this time. However, later initiation of treatment with acetylcysteine (up to and beyond 24 hours) may still be of benefit (see also below).

**Aspergillosis.** Although it is not one of the standard therapies discussed on p.386, local instillation of acetylcysteine into the cavity containing the fungus ball has been used to treat aspergilloma.[1] There is some evidence *in vitro* that acetylcysteine has inhibitory properties against *Aspergillus* and *Fusarium* spp.[2]


1. Kauffman CA. Quandary about treatment of aspergillomas persists. *Lancet* 1996; **347:** 1640.
2. De Lucca AJ, *et al.* N-Acetylcysteine inhibits germination of conidia and growth of Aspergillus spp. and Fusarium spp. *Antimicrob Agents Chemother* 1996; **40:** 1274–6.


**Burns.** Children with inhalation injury (see Burns, p.1134) who were treated with aerosolised heparin 5000 units alternating with 3 mL of 20% acetylcysteine solution, inhaled every 2 hours for the first 7 days after injury, appeared to have significantly reduced mortality and reintubation rates compared with historical controls.[1]


1. Desai MH, *et al.* Reduction in mortality in pediatric patients with inhalation injury with aerosolized heparin/N-acetylcystine [sic] therapy. *J Burn Care Rehabil* 1998; **19:** 210–12. Correction. *ibid.* 1999; **20:** 49.


**Cystic fibrosis.** Mucolytics such as acetylcysteine are generally not considered[1] to be effective in treating the pulmonary manifestations of cystic fibrosis (p.123).

Meconium ileus equivalent (bowel obstruction due to abnormally viscid contents of the terminal ileum and right colon[2]) in patients with cystic fibrosis has largely disappeared with the use of pancreatic enzymes but may occur when insufficient doses are given;[3] mild cases may be treated with acetylcysteine.[3] Doses of 10 mL of a 20% solution of acetylcysteine have been given by mouth 4 times daily with 100 mL of a 10% solution of acetylcysteine administered as an enema up to 4 times daily depending on the degree of the obstruction.[2]


1. Duijvestijn YC, Brand PL. Systematic review of N-acetylcysteine in cystic fibrosis. *Acta Paediatr* 1999; **88:** 38–41.
2. Hanly JG, Fitzgerald MX. Meconium ileus equivalent in older patients with cystic fibrosis. *BMJ* 1983; **286:** 1411–13.
3. David TJ. Cystic fibrosis. *Arch Dis Child* 1990; **65:** 152–7.


**HIV infection and AIDS.** The cysteine-containing peptide glutathione is involved in intracellular defence mechanisms, and it has been shown that low glutathione concentrations are associated with poorer survival in HIV-infected patients.[1] Since acetylcysteine can replenish glutathione, it has been suggested[2,3] that it may have a role in the treatment of AIDS (p.621). *In-vitro* studies indicate that acetylcysteine can suppress HIV expression,[4,5] and there has been a suggestion from observational data that acetylcysteine supplements can improve survival in HIV-infected individuals.[1] However, an attempt to use acetylcysteine supplementation to reduce the frequency of adverse reactions to co-trimoxazole in HIV-infected patients was not successful.[6]


1. Herzenberg LA, *et al.* Glutathione deficiency is associated with impaired survival in HIV disease. *Proc Natl Acad Sci U S A* 1997; **94:** 1967–72.
2. Staal FJT, *et al.* Glutathione deficiency and human immunodeficiency virus infection. *Lancet* 1992; **339:** 909–12.
3. Roederer M, *et al.* N-acetylcysteine: potential for AIDS therapy. *Pharmacology* 1993; **46:** 121–9.
4. Roederer M, *et al.* Cytokine-stimulated human immunodeficiency virus replication is inhibited by N-acetyl-L-cysteine. *Proc Natl Acad Sci U S A* 1990; **87:** 4884–8.
5. Kalebic T, *et al.* Suppression of human immunodeficiency virus expression in chronically infected monocytic cells by glutathione, glutathione ester, and N-acetylcysteine. *Proc Natl Acad Sci U S A* 1991; **88:** 986–90.
6. Åkerlund B, *et al.* N-acetylcysteine treatment and the risk of toxic reactions to trimethoprim-sulphamethoxazole in primary Pneumocystis carinii prophylaxis in HIV-infected patients. *J Infect* 1997; **35:** 143–7.


**Kidney disorders.** Acetylcysteine has been reported to improve kidney function in patients with the hepatorenal syndrome and may offer a potential bridging therapy in such patients awaiting liver transplantation.[1] It has also been of benefit in the prevention of contrast media-induced nephrotoxicity in patients with chronic renal impairment.[2]


1. Holt S, *et al.* Improvement in renal function in hepatorenal syndrome with N-acetylcysteine. *Lancet* 1999; **353:** 294–5.
2. Birck R, *et al.* Acetylcysteine for prevention of contrast nephropathy: meta-analysis. *Lancet* 2003; **362:** 598–603.


**Liver disorders.** Although benefit has been reported from studies of acetylcysteine in acute liver failure[1] (alone or with epoprostenol[2]), and some have suggested that it may be useful in preventing tissue hypoxia in patients with acute liver failure receiving vasopressors,[3] trials have mainly been small and clinical outcomes are not well studied.[1] It does not appear to be of benefit in patients undergoing orthotopic liver transplantation.[4,5]

For reference to use in the hepatorenal syndrome, see under Kidney Disorders, above. For use in paracetamol-induced liver damage see Overdosage, under Paracetamol, p.76.


1. Sklar GE, Subramaniam M. Acetylcysteine treatment for non-acetaminophen-induced acute liver failure. *Ann Pharmacother* 2004; **38:** 498–501.
2. Harrison PM, *et al.* Improvement by acetylcysteine of hemodynamics and oxygen transport in fulminant hepatic failure. *N Engl J Med* 1991; **324:** 1852–7.
3. Caraceni P, Van Thiel DH. Acute liver failure. *Lancet* 1995; **345:** 163–9.
4. Bromley PN, *et al.* Effects of intraoperative N-acetylcysteine in orthotopic liver transplantation. *Br J Anaesth* 1995; **75:** 352–4.
5. Steib A, *et al.* Does N-acetylcysteine improve hemodynamics and graft function in liver transplantation? *Liver Transpl Surg* 1998; **4:** 152–7.


**Myocardial infarction.** Some studies suggest that addition of intravenous acetylcysteine to thrombolytic therapy in patients with acute myocardial infarction (p.828) may be of benefit.[1,2] The growing evidence of the value of acetylcysteine as an adjunct in patients with or at risk of myocardial infarction has been reviewed.[3,4]


1. Arstall MA, *et al.* N-Acetylcysteine in combination with nitroglycerin and streptokinase for the treatment of evolving acute myocardial infarction: safety and biochemical effects. *Circulation* 1995; **92:** 2855–62.
2. Šochman J, *et al.* Infarct size limitation: acute N-acetylcysteine defense (ISLAND trial): preliminary analysis and report after the first 30 patients. *Clin Cardiol* 1996; **19:** 94–100.
3. Marchetti G, *et al.* Use of N-acetylcysteine in the management of coronary artery diseases. *Cardiologia* 1999; **44:** 633–7.
4. Sochman J. N-acetylcysteine in acute cardiology: 10 years later: what do we know and what would we like to know?! *J Am Coll Cardiol* 2002; **39:** 1422–8.


**Nitrate tolerance.** Acetylcysteine appears to be able to potentiate the peripheral and coronary effects of glyceryl trinitrate.[1,2] While some studies[3-6] suggest that it can reverse tolerance to nitrates in patients with coronary heart disease or heart failure, others have failed to demonstrate any benefit,[7] although there may be a specific subgroup of responders.[6] The various attempts at overcoming nitrate tolerance are discussed on p.924.


1. Horowitz JD, *et al.* Combined use of nitroglycerin and N-acetylcysteine in the management of unstable angina pectoris. *Circulation* 1988; **77:** 787–94.
2. Elkayam U. Tolerance to organic nitrates: evidence, mechanisms, clinical relevance, and strategies for prevention. *Ann Intern Med* 1991; **114:** 667–77.
3. Packer M, *et al.* Prevention and reversal of nitrate tolerance in patients with congestive heart failure. *N Engl J Med* 1987; **317:** 799–804.
4. May DC, *et al.* In vivo induction and reversal of nitroglycerin tolerance in human coronary arteries. *N Engl J Med* 1987; **317:** 805–9.
5. Boesgaard S, *et al.* Preventive administration of intravenous N-acetylcysteine and development of tolerance to isosorbide dinitrate in patients with angina pectoris. *Circulation* 1992; **85:** 143–9.
6. Pizzulli L, *et al.* N-acetylcysteine attenuates nitroglycerin tolerance in patients with angina pectoris and normal left ventricular function. *Am J Cardiol* 1997; **79:** 28–33.
7. Hogan JC, *et al.* Chronic administration of N-acetylcysteine fails to prevent nitrate tolerance in patients with stable angina pectoris. *Br J Clin Pharmacol* 1990; **30:** 573–7.


**Poisoning and toxicity.** Acetylcysteine has been studied for the potential treatment of many forms of toxicity,[1] but only treatment of acute paracetamol poisoning is widely accepted.


1. Chyka PA, *et al.* Utility of acetylcysteine in treating poisonings and adverse drug reactions. *Drug Safety* 2000; **22:** 123–48.


CARBON TETRACHLORIDE. The treatment of carbon tetrachloride poisoning is discussed on p.1472. Reports suggest that prompt intravenous therapy with acetylcysteine may help to minimise hepatorenal damage in acute poisoning with carbon tetrachloride.[1,2] It could be used in addition to supportive therapy when the initial dosage regimen should be that used for paracetamol poisoning but as carbon tetrachloride has a much longer half-life than paracetamol, the duration of treatment may need to be increased.[3]


1. Ruprah M, *et al.* Acute carbon tetrachloride poisoning in 19 patients: implications for diagnosis and treatment. *Lancet* 1985; **i:** 1027–9.
2. Mathieson PW, *et al.* Survival after massive ingestion of carbon tetrachloride treated by intravenous infusion of acetylcysteine. *Hum Toxicol* 1985; **4:** 627–31.
3. Meredith TJ, *et al.* Diagnosis and treatment of acute poisoning with volatile substances. *Hum Toxicol* 1989; **8:** 277–86.


PARACETAMOL. Acetylcysteine is the antidote of choice for paracetamol overdosage (see p.76). The intravenous route is favoured in the UK, despite possible anaphylactic reaction, mainly because of concerns over the effects of vomiting and activated charcoal on oral absorption.[1] In the USA the oral route has conventionally been used, despite the unpleasant odour and taste of acetylcysteine solutions, with no evident reduction in effect by charcoal.[2] The intravenous route is now also licensed in the USA.


1. Vale JA, Proudfoot AT. Paracetamol (acetaminophen) poisoning. *Lancet* 1995; **346:** 547–52.
2. Bowden CA, Krenzelok EP. Clinical applications of commonly used contemporary antidotes: a US perspective. *Drug Safety* 1997; **16:** 9–47.


**Respiratory disorders.** Acetylcysteine has been used as a mucolytic in a variety of respiratory disorders associated with productive cough (p.1112). Although there is controversy over the benefits of mucolytics in treating chronic bronchitis, there is some evidence that they may reduce exacerbations (see p.779).

Repeated bronchoalveolar lavage with heparin and acetylcysteine to remove proteinaceous material in patients with alveolar proteinosis may prolong survival.[1] (For the use of aerosolised heparin and acetylcysteine to treat inhalation injury see Burns, above.) Administration of acetylcysteine by nebulisation has relieved severe recurrent atelectasis during mechanical ventilation in premature infants.[2] It has been suggested that intravenous acetylcysteine might also be of use in acute respiratory distress syndrome (ARDS—p.1075),[3] possibly due to its action as a free radical scavenger,[3,4] but controlled studies in established ARDS failed to show benefit.[5,6]

See above for the use of acetylcysteine in the management of cystic fibrosis.


1. Morrison HM, Stockley RA. The many uses of bronchoalveolar lavage. *BMJ* 1988; **296:** 1758.
2. Amir J, *et al.* Acetylcysteine for severe atelectasis in premature infants. *Clin Pharm* 1985; **4:** 255.
3. Bernard GR. Potential of N-acetylcysteine as treatment for the adult respiratory distress syndrome. *Eur Respir J* 1990; **3** (suppl 11): 496S–498S.
4. Skolnick A. Inflammation-mediator blockers may be weapons against sepsis syndrome. *JAMA* 1990; **263:** 930–1.
5. Jepsen S, *et al.* Antioxidant treatment with N-acetylcysteine during adult respiratory distress syndrome: a prospective, randomized, placebo-controlled study. *Crit Care Med* 1992; **20:** 918–23.
6. Domenighetti G, *et al.* Treatment with N-acetylcysteine during acute respiratory distress syndrome: a randomized, double-blind, placebo-controlled clinical study. *J Crit Care* 1997; **12:** 177–82.


## Preparations

***BP 2003:*** Acetylcysteine Injection;
***USP 27:*** Acetylcysteine and Isoproterenol Hydrochloride Inhalation Solution; Acetylcysteine Solution.

**Proprietary Preparations** (details are given in Part 3)
***Arg.:*** ACC; Acemuk; Fluimucil; Lubrisec; ***Austral.:*** Mucomyst; Parvolex; ***Austria:*** ACC; Aeromuc; Aerosolv; Bisolrapid; Bronchohexal; Broncho-plus; Cimelin; Cimexyl; Fluimucil; Husten ACC; Lysomucil; Mucobene; Mucomyst; Pulmovent; Siccoral; Solvomed†; ***Belg.:*** Lysodrop; Lysomucil; Lysox; Mucolair†; Mucolator†; Mucomyst; Pectomucil; ***Braz.:*** Bromuc; Flucistein; Fluimucil; Fluimucil Solucao Nasal†; Notoxid†; ***Canad.:*** Mucomyst; Parvolex; ***Chile:*** Mucolitico; ***Denm.:*** Alcur; Granon; Hostop†; Mucolysin; Mucomyst; ***Fin.:*** Mucomyst; Mucoporetta; ***Fr.:*** Broncoclar; Codotussyl Expectorant; Exomuc; Fluimucil; Genac; Humex Expectorant; Mucolator; Mucomyst; Mucospire; Solmucol; Tixair; ***Ger.:*** ACC; Acemuc; Acetabs; Acetyst; Atse; Azubronchin; Bisolvon NAC†; Bromuc; Broncho-Fips†; Durabronchal; Fluimucil; Jenacysteine†; Larylin NAC Husten-Loser†; Mentopin†; Muciteran; Muco Sanigen; Mucocedyl; Mucret; Myxofat; NAC; Optipect†; Phamuc; Pulmicret; Sigamucil†; Siran; Stas Akut†; Tussiverlan†; Vitenur†; ***Gr.:*** Elicor; Mucomyst; Parvolex; Trebon; Trebon-N; ***Hong Kong:*** Fluimucil; Hidonac; Mucolator; Parvolex; Solmucol; ***India:*** Mucomix; ***Irl.:*** Alveolex†; Parvolex; ***Israel:*** Agisolvan†; Mucodex†; Mucomyst; Siran; ***Ital.:*** Altersol; Brunac; Fluimucil; Hidonac; Mucisol; Mucofial; Mucoxan; Solmucol; Tirocular; Ultraflu; ***Malaysia:*** Acypront; Mucolator; Parvolex; ***Mon.:*** Euronac; ***Neth.:*** Bisolbruis; Dampo Mucopect†; Fluimucil; Libronchin; Mucocil; Mucomyst; ***Norw.:*** Bronkyl; Mucomyst; ***NZ:*** Parvolex; ***Port.:*** Fluimucil; Tirocular; ***S.Afr.:*** ACC; Parvolex; Solmucol; ***Singapore:*** Fluimucil; Mucoza; Solmucol; ***Spain:*** Fluimucil; Flumil; Flumil Antidoto; Locomucil; Solmucol; ***Swed.:*** Mucomyst; Viskoferm; ***Switz.:*** ACC; Acemucol; Bisolapid; Demolibral; Dynamucil; Ecomucyl; Fluimucil; L-Cimexyl; Muco-Mepha; Mucofluid; Mucostop; Neo Expectan†; NeoCitran Expectorant; Robitussin Expectorant; Secresol†; Solmucol; ***Thai.:*** Acetin; Flemex-AC; Flucil; Fluimucil; Mucil; Mucocil; Mucotic; Mucoza; Mysoven; NAC; ***UK:*** Parvolex; ***USA:*** Acetadote; Mucomyst; Mucosil.

**Multi-ingredient:** ***Arg.:*** Fluimucil Biotic; ***Braz.:*** Fluimucil Biotic†; Rinofluimucil; ***Fr.:*** Rhinofluimucil; ***Ger.:*** Rinofluimucil-S; ***Hong Kong:*** Rinofluimucil; ***Irl.:*** Ilube; ***Ital.:*** Rinofluimucil; ***Spain:*** Flumil Antibiotico; Rinofluimucil†; Rinoflumil; ***Switz.:*** Rinofluimucil; Solmucaine; Solmucalm; ***Thai.:*** Fluimucil Antibiotic; Rinofluimucil; ***UK:*** Ilube.

---

## Acetyldihydrocodeine Hydrochloride

Acetildihidrocodeína, hidrocloruro de. 4,5-Epoxy-3-methoxy-9a-methylmorphinan-6-yl acetate hydrochloride.

$C_{20}H_{25}NO_4,HCl = 379.9.$
*CAS — 3861-72-1 (acetyldihydrocodeine).*

### Profile

Acetyldihydrocodeine hydrochloride is an opioid derivative related to dihydrocodeine (p.34). It is used as a centrally acting cough suppressant for non-productive cough (p.1112) and has been given by mouth in a usual daily dose of 20 to 50 mg; no more than 20 mg should be taken as a single dose.

### Preparations

**Proprietary Preparations** (details are given in Part 3)
***Belg.:*** Acetylcodone.

---

## Alloclamide Hydrochloride *(rINNM)*

CE-264; Hidrocloruro de aloclamida. 2-Allyloxy-4-chloro-N-(2-diethylaminoethyl)benzamide hydrochloride.

$C_{16}H_{23}ClN_2O_2,HCl = 347.3.$
*CAS — 5486-77-1 (alloclamide); 5107-01-7 (alloclamide hydrochloride).*

### Profile

Alloclamide hydrochloride is a cough suppressant.

### Preparations

**Proprietary Preparations** (details are given in Part 3)
**Multi-ingredient:** ***Spain:*** Tuselin Expectorante†.

---

## Ambroxol Hydrochloride *(BANM, rINNM)*

Ambroxoli Hydrochloridum; Hidrocloruro de ambroxol; NA-872 (ambroxol). *trans*-4-(2-Amino-3,5-dibromobenzylamino)cyclohexanol hydrochloride.

$C_{13}H_{18}Br_2N_2O,HCl = 414.6.$
*CAS — 18683-91-5 (ambroxol); 15942-05-9 (ambroxol hydrochloride); 23828-92-4 (ambroxol hydrochloride).*
*ATC — R05CB06.*

**Pharmacopoeias.** In *Eur.* (see p.vi).

**Ph. Eur. 5.0** (Ambroxol Hydrochloride). A white or yellowish crystalline powder. Sparingly soluble in water; practically insoluble in dichloromethane; soluble in methyl alcohol. A 1% solution in water has a pH of 4.5 to 6.0. Protect from light.

### Profile

Ambroxol is a metabolite of bromhexine (p.1115) and is used similarly as a mucolytic. It is given in a usual daily dose of 60 to 120 mg of the hydrochloride by mouth, in 2 or 3 divided doses. Ambroxol has also been given by inhalation, injection, or rectally.

Ambroxol acefyllinate (acebrofylline) has been used similarly.

**Adverse effects.** HYPERSENSITIVITY. A report[1] of contact allergy to ambroxol, but not bromhexine.


1. Mancuso G, Berdondini RM. Contact allergy to ambroxol. *Contact Dermatitis* 1989; **20:** 154.


**Pharmacokinetics.** References to pharmacokinetic studies of ambroxol.


1. Hammer R, *et al.* Speziesvergleich in Pharmakokinetik und Metabolismus von NA 872 Cl Ambroxol bei Ratte, Kaninchen, Hund und Mensch. *Arzneimittelforschung* 1978; **28:** 899–903.
2. Jauch R, *et al.* Ambroxol, Untersuchungen zum Stoffwechsel beim Menschen und zum quantitativen Nachweis in biologischen Proben. *Arzneimittelforschung* 1978; **28:** 904–11.
3. Vergin H, *et al.* Untersuchungen zur Pharmakokinetik und Bioäquivalenz unterscheidlicher Darreichungsformen von Ambroxol. *Arzneimittelforschung* 1985; **35:** 1591–5.


**Respiratory disorders.** Ambroxol has been tried in a variety of respiratory disorders: mixed results[1-3] were obtained when used in chronic bronchitis (p.779); it was ineffective[4] when given to mothers for the prophylaxis of neonatal respiratory distress syndrome (p.1084), although it may be of modest benefit in the early treatment of established disease in infants.[5,6]

Inhalation of ambroxol aerosol has also produced beneficial effects in a patient with alveolar proteinosis who refused alveolar lavage.[7]

For the use of mucolytics in productive cough see p.1112.


1. Olivieri D, *et al.* Ambroxol for the prevention of chronic exacerbations: long-term multicenter trial: protective effect of ambroxol against winter semester exacerbations: a double-blind study versus placebo. *Respiration* 1987; **51** (suppl 1): 42–51.
2. Guyatt GH, *et al.* A controlled trial of ambroxol in chronic bronchitis. *Chest* 1987; **92:** 618–20.
3. Alcozer G, *et al.* Prevention of chronic bronchitis exacerbations with ambroxol (Mucosolvan Retard): an open, long-term, multicenter study in 5,635 patients. *Respiration* 1989; **55** (suppl 1): 84–96.
4. Dani C, *et al.* Antenatal ambroxol treatment does not prevent the respiratory distress syndrome in premature infants. *Eur J Pediatr* 1997; **156:** 392–3.
5. Wauer RR, *et al.* Randomized double blind trial of Ambroxol for the treatment of respiratory distress syndrome. *Eur J Pediatr* 1992; **151:** 357–63.
6. Schmalisch G, *et al.* Changes in pulmonary function in preterm infants recovering from RDS following early treatment with ambroxol: results of a randomized trial. *Pediatr Pulmonol* 1999; **27:** 104–12.
7. Diaz JP, *et al.* Response to surfactant activator (ambroxol) in alveolar proteinosis. *Lancet* 1984; **i:** 1023.


**Uricosuric action.** A study[1] was carried out in 48 young male healthy subjects to examine the uricosuric effect of ambroxol. The minimum effective dose for lowering plasma-uric acid concentrations was found to be between 250 and 500 mg daily given in 2 divided doses. Although these doses are much higher than those used to treat bronchopulmonary disease, doses as high as 1 g daily were well tolerated.


1. Oosterhuis B, *et al.* Dose-dependent uricosuric effect of ambroxol. *Eur J Clin Pharmacol* 1993; **44:** 237–41.


### Preparations

**Proprietary Preparations** (details are given in Part 3)
***Arg.:*** Ambril; Apracur Expectorante; Cortos; Dogistin; Graneodin Expectorante; Mucomex; Mucosolvon; Tabcin Expectorante; Tavinex Expectorante; Tavinex Expectotabs; ***Austria:*** Ambrobene; Ambrohexal; Ambrolan; Ambrolos; Broxol; Mucosolvan; Sekretovit; ***Belg.:*** Surbronc; ***Braz.:*** Ambroten; Ambroxolvan†; Anabron; Benatoss†; Benetoss†; Brismucol; Broncoflux; Brondilat; Expectuss; Fluibron; Fluidin; Fluxol; Mucibron; Mucoclean; Mucolin; Mucosolvan; Mucoxolan; Neossolvan; Probec; Surfactil; ***Chile:*** Bronchopront; Broncot; Fluibron; Fluomit; Milbron; Mintamox; Mucosolvan; Muxol; Tocalm; ***Fr.:*** Muxol; Surbronc; ***Ger.:*** Ambril; Ambro; Ambro-Puren; Ambrobeta; Ambrodoc; Ambrohexal; Ambroinfant; Ambrolos; Ambropp; Antussan†; Bisolvon AM†; Bronchopront; Bronchowern; Contac Husten-Trunk†; Dignobroxol†; duramucal; Expit; Farmabroxol†; frenopect; Jenabroxol†; Larylin Husten-Heissgetrank†; Larylin Husten-Loser Pastillen; Larylin Husten-Loser Saft; Lindoxyl; Mibrox†; Muco-Aspecton; Muco-Fips†; Muco-Tablinen†; Mucobroxol; Mucophlogat; Mucosolvan; Mucotablin†; Neo-Bronchol; Nymix Mucolytikum†; Padiamuc; Pect Hustenloser†; Sigabroxol; stas-Hustenloser; Tussot†; ***Gr.:*** Abrolen; Afrodor; Amboral; Ambrobion; Ambromyc; Anavix;

Aprinol; Bunafon; Ebertuss; Effercet; Fluibrox; Grenovix; Hivotex; Kriolen; Lextarol; Mavixan; Mucolin; Mucosolvan; Nibren; Olbenorm; Provixen-N; Puntol; Respirol; Stefolant; Strubelin; Tevoril; Tussefar; Zyrantol; ***Hong Kong:*** Amxol; Bronchopront; Max; Medovent; Mucosolvan; ***India:*** Acocontin; Acolyt; ***Ital.:*** Ambromucil; Amobronc; Atus; Broncomnes; Broxol; Fluibron; Fluixol; Lisopulm; Muciclar; Mucobron; Mucosolvan; Secretil; Surfactal; Surfolase; Tauxolo; Viscomucil; ***Jpn:*** Mucosolvan; ***Malaysia:*** Amxol; Axol; Mucosolvan; Shinoxol; ***Mex.:*** Ambodil†; Ambrofur; Ambrowel†; Amocol; Balsibron; Bionoxol; Brismucol; Brogal; Bronolban; Brosolan; Broxofar; Broxol; Broxolan†; Ebromin; Exabrol; Expeflen; Fantrodol; Ital-Ultra; Loexom; Minisol†; Mucibron; Mucosolvan; Mucovibrol; Mucovibrol T; Mucoxol; Muxol; Oxoway†; Prospec†; Randex; Rimoxol; Sekretovit; Septacin; Softixol; Solpat; Tradexol; Trimexine; Tunitol-BX; Tusibron†; Viaxol; Weiscal; ***Port.:*** Benflux; Bromax; Bronchopront; Broncoliber; Drenoxol; Fluidox; Fluidrenol; Hipotosse; Mucodrenol; Mucosolvan; Surfolase; Tusolven; ***Singapore:*** Amxol; Axol; Bronchopront; Flubiron†; Max; Mucosolvan; Shinoxol; ***Spain:*** Ambrolitic; Dinobroxol; Motosol; Mucibron; Mucosan; Naxpa; ***Switz.:*** Fluibron; Mucabrox; Mucosolvon; ***Thai.:*** Ambrol; Ambrolytic; Ambrox; Ambroxan; Amxol; Bronchopront; Broncol; Broxol; Broxsa; Max; Medovent; Misovan; Movent; Mucodic; Mucolan; Mucolid; Mucomed; Mucopec; Mucosolvan; Mucoxine-F; Mucozan; Musocan; Nucobrox; Polibroxol; Posecus†; Simusol.

**Multi-ingredient: *Arg.:*** Amoxi Respiratorio; Amoxidal Respiratorio; Amoxidal Respiratorio Duo; Amoxigrand Bronquial; Amoxipenil Bronquial; Amoxitenk Respiratorio; Aseptobron Respiratorio; Bronco Biotaer; Bronquisedan; Bronquisedan Mucolitico; Cefacar Mucolitico; Cefacilina Bronquial; Gentiabron; Letondal; Muco Cortos; Muco Dosodos; Muco Dosodos Biotic; Mucoprednibron; Mucosolvon Compositum; No-Tos Biotic; Nobactam Bronquial; Oxibron NF; Oximar Respiratorio; Trexirol NF; ***Austria:*** Mucospas; Mucotectan†; ***Braz.:*** Penetro; ***Chile:*** Ambrotos; ***Ger.:*** Ambrodoxy; Ambroxol AL comp; Ambroxol comp; Amdox-Puren; Azudoxat comp; Broncho-Euphyllin; Doxam; Doximucol; Doxy Comp; Doxy Lindoxyl; Doxy Plus; Doxy-duramucal†; Doxy-Wolff Mucolyt; Doxysolvat; Jenabroxol comp; Mucotectan†; Sagittamuc†; Sigamuc; Spasmo-Mucosolvan; Terelit; ***India:*** Kofarest; ***Mex.:*** Acimox-Ex; Aeroflux; Aminoefedrison NF; Balsibron-C; Brogal Compositum; Brogal-T; Brosolan-C; Broxofar Compuesto; Broxol Plus; Cibronal; Coricidin Expec; Dexol; Ebromin-P; Epicol NF; Gimabrol; Histiacil NF; Mucosolvan Compositum; Mucovibrol C; Pentibroxil; Pentrexyl Expec; Rombox; Sekretovit Amoxi; Sekretovit Ex; Septacin Amoxi; Septacin Ex; Tenalif; ***Port.:*** Clembroxol†; Mucospas; Ventoliber.

## Amidefrine Mesilate *(BANM, rINN)*

5190; Amidephrine Mesylate *(USAN)*; Mesilato de amidefrina; MJ-5190. 3-(1-Hydroxy-2-methylaminoethyl)methanesulphonanilide methanesulphonate.

$C_{10}H_{16}N_2O_3S,CH_4O_3S$ = 340.4.
*CAS — 3354-67-4 (amidefrine); 1421-68-7 (amidefrine mesilate).*

### Profile

Amidefrine mesilate is a sympathomimetic with alpha-adrenergic activity similar to that of phenylephrine (p.1126). It is used for its vasoconstrictor properties in the local treatment of nasal congestion.

### Preparations

**Proprietary Preparations** (details are given in Part 3)
***Austria:*** Fentrinol.

## Ammonium Acetate

Amonio, acetato de.

$CH_3CO_2NH_4$ = 77.08.
*CAS — 631-61-8 (ammonium acetate); 8013-61-4 (ammonium acetate solution).*

**Pharmacopoeias.** *Br.* includes Strong Ammonium Acetate Solution.

## Ammonium Bicarbonate *(BAN)*

Ammonii Hydrogenocarbonas; Amonio, bicarbonato de; E503. Ammonium hydrogen carbonate.

$NH_4HCO_3$ = 79.06.
*CAS — 1066-33-7.*

**Pharmacopoeias.** In *Eur.* (see p.vi).

**Ph. Eur. 5.0** (Ammonium Hydrogen Carbonate; Ammonium Bicarbonate BP 2003). A fine, white, slightly hygroscopic, crystalline powder or white crystals. It volatilises rapidly at 60°; volatilisation takes place slowly at ambient temperatures if slightly moist. It is in a state of equilibrium with ammonium carbamate. Freely soluble in water; practically insoluble in alcohol. Store in airtight containers.

The BP 2003 directs that when Ammonium Carbonate is prescribed or demanded Ammonium Bicarbonate shall be dispensed or supplied.

## Ammonium Carbonate

Amonio, carbonato de; Carbonato de Amonio; E503.

*CAS — 8000-73-5.*

**Pharmacopoeias.** In *Fr.* Also in *USNF.*

**BP 2003.** The BP directs that Ammonium Bicarbonate shall be dispensed or supplied when Ammonium Carbonate is prescribed or demanded.

**USNF 22** (Ammonium Carbonate). A white powder, or hard, white or translucent masses having a strong odour of ammonia, without empyreuma. It consists of ammonium bicarbonate and ammonium carbamate, in varying proportions. It yields 30 to 34% of $NH_3$. On exposure to air it loses ammonia and carbon dioxide, becoming opaque, and is finally converted into friable porous lumps or a white powder of ammonium bicarbonate. Soluble 1 in 4 of water. It is decomposed by hot water. Its solutions are alkaline to litmus. Store in airtight containers at a temperature not exceeding 30°. Protect from light.

## Ammonium Chloride

510; Ammonii Chloridum; Ammonium Chloratum; Amonio, cloruro de; Cloruro de Amonio; Muriate of Ammonia; Sal Ammoniac.

$NH_4Cl$ = 53.49.
*CAS — 12125-02-9.*
*ATC — B05XA04; G04BA01.*

**Pharmacopoeias.** In *Chin., Eur.* (see p.vi), *Pol., US,* and *Viet.*

**Ph. Eur. 5.0** (Ammonium Chloride). A white, crystalline powder or colourless crystals. Freely soluble in water.

**USP 27** (Ammonium Chloride). Colourless crystals or white, fine or course, crystalline powder. Is somewhat hygroscopic. Freely soluble in water and in glycerol, and even more so in boiling water; sparingly soluble in alcohol. pH of a 5% solution in water is between 4.6 and 6.0. Store in airtight containers.

### Adverse Effects and Treatment

Ammonium salts are irritant to the gastric mucosa and may produce nausea and vomiting particularly in large doses. Large doses of ammonium chloride may cause a profound acidosis and hypokalaemia which should be treated symptomatically. Intravenous administration of ammonium chloride may cause pain and irritation at the site of injection, which may be decreased by slowing the rate of infusion.

Excessive doses of ammonium salts, particularly if administered by rapid intravenous injection, may give rise to hepatic encephalopathy due to the inability of the liver to convert the increased load of ammonium ions to urea.

### Precautions

Ammonium salts are contra-indicated in patients with hepatic or renal impairment.

### Pharmacokinetics

Ammonium chloride is absorbed from the gastrointestinal tract. The ammonium ion is converted into urea in the liver; the anion thus liberated into the blood and extracellular fluid causes a metabolic acidosis and decreases the pH of the urine; this is followed by transient diuresis.

### Uses and Administration

Ammonium chloride is used as an expectorant in productive cough (p.1112). Other ammonium salts which have been used similarly include the acetate, bicarbonate, camphorate, carbonate, citrate (p.1654), and glycyrrhizinate.

The administration of ammonium chloride produces a transient diuresis and acidosis. It may be used in the treatment of severe metabolic alkalosis (p.1217). Each g of ammonium chloride represents 18.69 mmol of chloride. It is usually given as a 1 to 2% solution by slow intravenous infusion, in a dosage depending on the severity of the alkalosis. A concentrated solution of ammonium chloride may be diluted by sodium chloride injection.

Ammonium chloride may also be used to maintain the urine at an acid pH in the treatment of some urinary-tract disorders, or in forced acid diuresis procedures to aid the excretion of basic drugs, such as amfetamines, in severe cases of overdosage. It is usually given by mouth, often as enteric-coated tablets, in a dose of 1 to 2 g every four to six hours, although higher doses have been used in forced acid diuresis procedures.

Ammonium chloride has been promoted for self administration as a diuretic, for example in premenstrual water retention; a dose of 650 mg three times daily for up to 6 days has been suggested, but such use is generally considered inappropriate.

### Preparations

***BP 2003:*** Ammonium Chloride Mixture; Aromatic Ammonia Solution; Aromatic Ammonia Spirit; Strong Ammonium Acetate Solution; White Liniment;
***USP 27:*** Ammonium Chloride Delayed-release Tablets; Ammonium Chloride Injection; Aromatic Ammonia Spirit; Potassium Gluconate, Potassium Citrate, and Ammonium Chloride Oral Solution.

**Proprietary Preparations** (details are given in Part 3)
***Austral.:*** Nyal Bronchitis; ***Fr.:*** Chlorammonic; ***Ger.:*** Extin N; ***Spain:*** Apir Cloruro Amonico†; ***Switz.:*** Chloramon.

**Multi-ingredient:** numerous preparations are listed in Part 3.

## Benproperine *(rINN)*

ASA-158/5 (benproperine phosphate); Benproperina. 1-[2-(2-Benzylphenoxy)-1-methylethyl]piperidine.

$C_{21}H_{27}NO$ = 309.4.
*CAS — 2156-27-6.*
*ATC — R05DB02.*

**Pharmacopoeias.** *Chin.* includes the phosphate.

### Profile

Benproperine is used as a cough suppressant in non-productive cough (p.1112). It is reported to have a peripheral and central action and has been given by mouth in usual doses of 25 to 50 mg two to four times daily as the embonate or the phosphate.

### Preparations

**Proprietary Preparations** (details are given in Part 3)
***Ger.:*** Tussafug; ***Hong Kong:*** Cofrel; ***Jpn:*** Flaveric; ***Switz.:*** Tussafug†.

## Benzonatate *(BAN, rINN)*

Benzonatato; Benzononatine; KM-65. 3,6,9,12,15,18,21,24,27-Nonaoxaoctacosyl 4-butylaminobenzoate.

$C_{13}H_{18}NO_2(OCH_2CH_2)_nOCH_3$, where *n* has an average value of 8.
*CAS — 104-31-4 (where n = 8).*
*ATC — R05DB01.*

**Pharmacopoeias.** In *US.*

**USP 27** (Benzonatate). A clear, pale yellow, viscous liquid having a faint characteristic odour. Soluble 1 in less than 1 of water, of alcohol, of chloroform, and of ether; freely soluble in benzene. Store in airtight containers. Protect from light.

### Adverse Effects

Headache, dizziness, gastrointestinal disturbances, nasal congestion, hypersensitivity, pruritus, and skin rash have been reported. There may be drowsiness. Benzonatate has local anaesthetic properties and can produce numbness of the mouth, tongue, and pharynx. CNS stimulation and convulsions, followed by CNS depression, may occur in overdosage.

### Uses and Administration

Benzonatate is a cough suppressant used in non-productive cough (p.1112); it is stated to act peripherally. It is related to tetracaine (p.1385) and has a local anaesthetic action on mucosa. It is given by mouth in a dose of 100 mg three times daily; up to 600 mg daily in divided doses may be given if necessary. Benzonatate is reported to act within about 20 minutes and its effects are reported to last for 3 to 8 hours.

### Preparations

***USP 27:*** Benzonatate Capsules.

**Proprietary Preparations** (details are given in Part 3)
***Mex.:*** Alzomed-F; Beknol†; Benzonal; Bloktus†; Capsicof†; D-Tato†; Lemtosid; Nactol; Novapsyl; Pebegal; Tesalon; Tesopen; Texoven; Tusehli†; Tusical; Tusitato; Tuzzil; Velpro; ***USA:*** Tessalon.

## Bibenzonium Bromide *(BAN, rINN)*

Bromuro de bibenzonio; Diphenetholine Bromide; ES-132. [2-(1,2-Diphenylethoxy)ethyl]trimethylammonium bromide.

$C_{19}H_{26}BrNO$ = 364.3.
*CAS — 59866-76-1 (bibenzonium); 15585-70-3 (bibenzonium bromide).*
*ATC — R05DB12.*

### Profile

Bibenzonium bromide is a cough suppressant used in non-productive cough (p.1112) which is stated to have a central action. It has been given by mouth in a usual dose of 30 to 60 mg two or three times daily.

### Preparations

**Proprietary Preparations** (details are given in Part 3)
***Austria:*** Lysbex; ***Port.:*** Tussis†.

## Bromhexine *(BAN, rINN)*

Bromexina; Bromhexina. 2-Amino-3,5-dibromobenzyl(cyclohexyl)methylamine.

$C_{14}H_{20}Br_2N_2$ = 376.1.
*CAS — 3572-43-8.*
*ATC — R05CB02.*

## Bromhexine Hydrochloride *(BANM, USAN, rINNM)*

Bromhexini Hydrochloridum; Cloridrato de Bromexina; Hidrocloruro de bromhexina; NA-274.

$C_{14}H_{20}Br_2N_2,HCl$ = 412.6.
*CAS — 611-75-6.*
*ATC — R05CB02.*

**Pharmacopoeias.** In *Chin., Eur.* (see p.vi), *Jpn,* and *Pol.*

**Ph. Eur. 5.0** (Bromhexine Hydrochloride). A white or almost white crystalline powder. It exhibits polymorphism. Very slightly soluble in water; slightly soluble in alcohol and in dichloromethane. Protect from light.

### Adverse Effects

Gastrointestinal side-effects may occur occasionally with bromhexine and a transient rise in serum aminotransferase values has been reported. Other reported adverse effects include headache, dizziness, sweating, and skin rashes. Inhalation of bromhexine has occasionally produced cough or bronchospasm in susceptible subjects.

### Precautions

Since mucolytics may disrupt the gastric mucosal barrier bromhexine should be used with care in patients with a history of peptic ulcer disease. Care is also advisable in asthmatic patients. Clearance of bromhexine or its metabolites may be reduced in patients with severe hepatic or renal impairment.

### Pharmacokinetics

Bromhexine hydrochloride is rapidly absorbed from the gastrointestinal tract and undergoes extensive first-pass metabolism in the liver: its oral bioavailability is stated to be only about 20%. It is widely distributed to body tissues. About 85 to 90% of a dose is excreted in the urine mainly as metabolites. Ambroxol (p.1114) is a metabolite of bromhexine. Bromhexine is highly bound to plasma proteins. It has a terminal elimination half-life of up to about 12 hours. Bromhexine crosses the blood-brain barrier and small amounts cross the placenta.

◊ Administration of bromhexine hydrochloride by mouth to healthy subjects produced peak plasma concentrations after about 1 hour.[1] Only small amounts were excreted unchanged in the urine with a half-life of about 6.5 hours.

1. Bechgaard E, Nielsen A. Bioavailability of bromhexine tablets and preliminary pharmacokinetics in humans. *Biopharm Drug Dispos* 1982; **3:** 337–44.

## Uses and Administration

Bromhexine is a mucolytic used in the treatment of respiratory disorders associated with productive cough (p.1112). Bromhexine is usually given by mouth in a dose of 8 to 16 mg of the hydrochloride three times daily. It has also been given by deep intramuscular or slow intravenous injection or inhaled as an aerosol solution.

Bromhexine has also been used orally and topically in the treatment of dry eye associated with abnormal mucus production (see below).

**Dry eye.** Bromhexine has been used orally in the treatment of dry eye (p.1576) in Sjögren's syndrome but results have been conflicting,[1-3] and it appears to have no effect on tear secretion in healthy subjects.[4] It has also been tried topically.

1. Frost-Larsen K, *et al.* Sjögren's syndrome treated with bromhexine: a randomised clinical study. *BMJ* 1978; **1:** 1579–81.
2. Tapper-Jones LM, *et al.* Sjögren's syndrome treated with bromhexine: a reassessment. *BMJ* 1980; **280:** 1356.
3. Prause JU, *et al.* Lacrimal and salivary secretion in Sjögren's syndrome: the effect of systemic treatment with bromhexine. *Acta Ophthalmol (Copenh)* 1984; **62:** 489–97.
4. Avisar R, *et al.* Oral bromhexine has no effect on tear secretion in healthy subjects. *Ann Pharmacother* 1996; **30:** 1498.

**Respiratory-tract infection.** USE WITH AN ANTIBACTERIAL. Bromhexine has been shown to enhance the penetration of erythromycin into bronchial secretions.[1] Although bromhexine is used as an adjuvant in the treatment of respiratory infections, few controlled studies appear to have been conducted to determine if any additional benefit is obtained. However, some studies have found improved responses with cefalexin[2] and amoxicillin.[3]

1. Bergogne-Berezin E, *et al.* Etude de l'influence d'un agent mucolytique (bromhexine) sur le passage de l'érythromycine dans les sécrétions bronchiques. *Therapie* 1979; **34:** 705–11.
2. Boraldi F, Palmieri B. Antibiotic and mucolytic therapy in elderly patients with different cases of bronchopulmonary diseases. *Curr Ther Res* 1983; **33:** 686–91.
3. Roa CC, Dantes RB. Clinical effectiveness of a combination of bromhexine and amoxicillin in lower respiratory tract infection: a randomized controlled trial. *Arzneimittelforschung* 1995; **45:** 267–72.

### Preparations

**Proprietary Preparations** (details are given in Part 3)
***Arg.:*** Amiorel; Aseptobron Expectorante; Balsasulf; Bisolvon; Bromexidryl; Broncocalmine; Bronquisedan Elixir; Catarrosine; Lorbi; Namir; Nastizol Expectorante; No-Tos Mucolitico; Pulmosan; Toscalmin; ***Austral.:*** Bisolvon Chesty; Dur-Elix†; Duro-Tuss Mucolytic Cough Liquid; ***Austria:*** Bisolvon; ***Belg.:*** Bisolvon; Bromex; ***Braz.:*** Bisolvon; ***Chile:*** Bisolvon; Flumed; ***Denm.:*** Bisolvon; Viscolyt; ***Fin.:*** Bisolvon; Medipekt; Mucovin; ***Fr.:*** Bisolvon; ***Ger.:*** Aparsonin N; Bisolvon; Hustentabs; Lubrirhin†; Omniapharm; ***Gr.:*** Bisolvon; Bolisegna; Bromiramin; Bronchotussine; ***Hong Kong:*** Asthmaxine; Bisolvon; Bromoson; Bromxine; Exolit; Mucolix†; Vasican; ***Irl.:*** Bisolvon; ***Israel:*** Movex; Solvex; ***Ital.:*** Bisolvon; Broncokin; ***Malaysia:*** Beacolytic; Bislan; Bisolvon; Bromxine; Ekxine; Hexolvon; Vasican; ***Mex.:*** Bisolvon; Dibroxin; Dizolvin; Normoflex; Tesacof; ***Neth.:*** Bisolvon; Darolan Slijmplossende†; Famel Broomhexine; ***Norw.:*** Bisolvon; ***NZ:*** Bisolvon Chesty; Duro-Tuss Mucolytic; ***Port.:*** Bisolvon; Lisomucin; Tosseque; ***S.Afr.:*** Bisolvon; Bronkese; Dur-Elix†; ***Singapore:*** Bislan; Bisolvon; Bromxine; Broxine; Exolit†; Mucosol; Vasican; ***Spain:*** Bisolvon; ***Swed.:*** Bisolvon; ***Switz.:*** Bisolvon; Hustosol; Metasolvens†; Solvolin†; ***Thai.:*** Asovon; Axistal; Behexine; Bislan†; Bisoltab; Bisolvon; Bomexin; Bromex; Bromoson; Bromso; Bromxin; Bromxine; Bronclear; Disol; Dutross; Exolit; Ida; Manovon; Mihexine; Mucine; Mucola; Mucoxin; Ohexine; Romulin; Tromadil; ***UAE:*** Mucolyte.

**Multi-ingredient:** numerous preparations are listed in Part 3.

---

## Brovanexine Hydrochloride *(rINNM)*

Hidrocloruro de brovanexina. 4-(Acetyloxy)-*N*-[2,4-dibromo-6-[(cyclohexylmethylamino)methyl]phenyl]-3-methoxybenzamide monohydrochloride.

$C_{24}H_{29}Br_2ClN_2O_4$ = 604.8.

*CAS — 54340-61-3 (brovanexine); 54340-60-2 (brovanexine hydrochloride).*

### Profile

Brovanexine is a derivative of bromhexine (above) and is given orally as the hydrochloride, usually as an adjunct to antibacterials in preparations for the treatment of respiratory-tract infections.

### Preparations

**Proprietary Preparations** (details are given in Part 3)
***Braz.:*** Bronquimucil; ***Port.:*** Bronquimucil; Pulmo-San; ***Spain:*** Broncimucil.

**Multi-ingredient:** ***Arg.:*** Trifamox Bronquial; ***Spain:*** Amoxidel Bronquial†; Bronquimucil; Eupen Bronquial.

---

## Butamirate Citrate *(BANM, USAN, rINNM)*

Abbott-36581; Butamyrate Citrate; Citrato de butamirato; HH-197. 2-(2-Diethylaminoethoxy)ethyl 2-phenylbutyrate dihydrogen citrate.

$C_{18}H_{29}NO_3,C_6H_8O_7$ = 499.6.

*CAS — 18109-80-3 (butamirate); 18109-81-4 (butamirate citrate).*

*ATC — R05DB13.*

### Profile

Butamirate citrate is a cough suppressant used in non-productive cough (p.1112) and stated to have a central action. The usual dose is up to 30 mg daily in 3 or 4 divided doses by mouth; some countries permit up to 90 mg daily in divided doses. Modified-release tablets containing 50 mg have been given 2 or 3 times daily.

### Preparations

**Proprietary Preparations** (details are given in Part 3)
***Arg.:*** Dosodos; Talasa NF; Tossec; ***Belg.:*** Quintex; Quintex Pediatrique; Sinecod; ***Braz.:*** Besedan; ***Gr.:*** Antis; Betavix; Butamir; Chemisolv; Chributan; Codexine-R; Codimin; Cyne; Devix; Drosten; Leogumil; Novamir; Oaxen; Pandigal; Pintal; Roctylan; Safarol; Sinecod; Stilex; ***Ital.:*** Butiran; Lenistar; Sinecod Tosse Sedativo; ***Port.:*** Sinecod; ***Switz.:*** Demotussol; NeoCitran Antitussif; Sinecod; ***Thai.:*** Sinecod.

**Multi-ingredient:** ***Arg.:*** Muco Dosodos; Muco Dosodos Biotic; ***Braz.:*** Novotussan; ***Switz.:*** Hicoseen†.

---

## Butetamate Citrate *(BANM, rINNM)*

Butethamate Citrate; Butethamate Dihydrogen Citrate; Citrato de butetamato. 2-Diethylaminoethyl 2-phenylbutyrate citrate.

$C_{16}H_{25}NO_2,C_6H_8O_7$ = 455.5.

*CAS — 14007-64-8 (butetamate); 13900-12-4 (butetamate citrate).*

### Profile

Butetamate citrate is reported to be an antispasmodic and bronchodilator and has been used alone or in combination preparations for the symptomatic treatment of coughs and other associated respiratory-tract disorders.

### Preparations

**Proprietary Preparations** (details are given in Part 3)
***Arg.:*** Heliphenicol; ***Irl.:*** CAM†.

**Multi-ingredient:** ***Arg.:*** Febrigrip; Kiper; Muco Cortos; Mucoprednibron; Pulmocler; Refenax Jarabe; Tabcin Antigripal; ***Austria:*** Coldadolin; Influbene; Panax†; ***Switz.:*** Bronchotussine; Dragees contre la toux no 536†.

---

## Calcium Iodide

Ioduro cálcico.

$CaI_2$ = 293.9.

*CAS — 10102-68-8.*

### Profile

Calcium iodide has been used by mouth in expectorant mixtures. The limitations of iodides as expectorants are discussed under Cough, p.1112. The actions of the iodides are discussed under Iodine (p.1598).

### Preparations

**Proprietary Preparations** (details are given in Part 3)

**Multi-ingredient:** ***Arg.:*** Zantril; ***USA:*** Calcidrine; Norisodrine with Calcium Iodide.

---

## Caramiphen Edisilate *(BANM, rINNM)*

Caramiphen Edisylate; Edisilato de caramifeno. 2-Diethylaminoethyl 1-phenylcyclopentane-1-carboxylate ethane-1,2-disulphonate.

$C_{38}H_{60}N_2O_{10}S_2$ = 769.0.

*CAS — 77-22-5 (caramiphen); 125-86-0 (caramiphen edisilate); 125-85-9 (caramiphen hydrochloride).*

### Profile

Caramiphen is a centrally acting cough suppressant that has been used as the edisilate in combination preparations for coughs (p.1112). Caramiphen hydrochloride was originally used similarly to trihexyphenidyl (p.490) for its antimuscarinic actions.

### Preparations

**Proprietary Preparations** (details are given in Part 3)

**Multi-ingredient:** ***USA:*** Ordrine AT Extended-Release†; Rescaps-D SR†; Tuss-Allergine Modified TD†; Tussogest Extended-Release†.

---

# Carbocisteine *(BAN, rINN)*

AHR-3053; Carbocisteína; Carbocisteinum; Carbocysteine (USAN); LJ-206. S-Carboxymethyl-L-cysteine.

$C_5H_9NO_4S$ = 179.2.

*CAS — 2387-59-9; 638-23-3 (carbocisteine, L-form).*

*ATC — R05CB03.*

**Pharmacopoeias.** In *Chin., Eur.* (see p.vi), *Jpn*, and *Pol.*

**Ph. Eur. 5.0** (Carbocisteine). A white crystalline powder. Practically insoluble in water and in alcohol; dissolves in dilute mineral acids and in dilute solutions of alkali hydroxides. A 1% suspension in water has a pH of 2.8 to 3.0. Protect from light.

**Incompatibility.** The UK manufacturer states that mixing carbocisteine with pholcodine linctus causes precipitation of carbocisteine from solution but no information is given on whether this incompatibility is with the pholcodine or some component of the formulation used.

## Carbocisteine Sodium *(BANM, rINNM)*

Carbocisteína sódica; Carbocysteine Sodium.

*CAS — 49673-84-9 (carbocisteine sodium, L-form).*

*ATC — R05CB03.*

## Adverse Effects and Precautions

Nausea and gastric discomfort, gastrointestinal bleeding, and skin rash have occasionally occurred with carbocisteine.

Since mucolytics may disrupt the gastric mucosal barrier carbocisteine should be used with caution in patients with a history of peptic ulcer disease.

**Effects on endocrine function.** Transient hypothyroidism associated with the use of carbocisteine developed in a patient with compromised thyroid function.[1]

1. Wiersinga WM. Antithyroid action of carbocisteine. *BMJ* 1986; **293:** 106.

## Pharmacokinetics

Carbocisteine is rapidly and well absorbed from the gastrointestinal tract with peak plasma concentrations occurring 90 to 120 minutes after an oral dose. It appears to penetrate into lung tissue and respiratory mucus. Carbocisteine is excreted in the urine as unchanged drug and metabolites. Acetylation, decarboxylation, and sulfoxidation have been identified as the major metabolic pathways. Sulfoxidation may be governed by genetic polymorphism.

◊ References.

1. Karim EFIA, *et al.* An investigation of the metabolism of S-carboxymethyl-L-cysteine in man using a novel HPLC-ECD method. *Eur J Drug Metab Pharmacokinet* 1988; **13:** 253–6.
2. Brockmoller J, *et al.* Evaluation of proposed sulphoxidation pathways of carbocysteine in man by HPLC quantification. *Eur J Clin Pharmacol* 1991; **40:** 387–92.
3. Steventon GB. Diurnal variation in the metabolism of S-carboxymethyl-L-cysteine in humans. *Drug Metab Dispos* 1999; **27:** 1092–7.

## Uses and Administration

Carbocisteine is used for its mucolytic activity in respiratory disorders associated with productive cough (p.1112). It is given by mouth in a dose of 750 mg three times daily, reduced by one-third when a response is obtained. Children aged 2 to 5 years may be given 62.5 to 125 mg four times daily and those aged 6 to 12 years 250 mg three times daily. Carbocisteine is also given by mouth as the sodium or lysine salts.

**Chronic obstructive pulmonary disease.** The value of mucolytic therapy in bronchitis (p.779) is controversial. Two studies have reported some improvements in lung function in patients with chronic bronchitis given carbocisteine for up to 6 months,[1,2] but it appeared to have no effect on the number of acute exacerbations.[1] However, a later multicentre study (using the lysine salt) did report a reduction in the number of acute exacerbations.[3] Carbocisteine may also produce some beneficial effects on sputum rheology.[2,4]

1. Grillage M, Barnard-Jones K. Long-term oral carbocisteine therapy in patients with chronic bronchitis: a double blind trial with placebo control. *Br J Clin Pract* 1985; **39:** 395–8.
2. Aylward M, *et al.* Clinical evaluation of carbocisteine (Mucolex) in the treatment of patients with chronic bronchitis: a double-blind trial with placebo control. *Clin Trials J* 1985; **22:** 36–44.
3. Allegra L, *et al.* Prevention of acute exacerbations of chronic obstructive bronchitis with carbocysteine lysine salt monohydrate: a multicenter, double-blind, placebo-controlled trial. *Respiration* 1996; **63:** 174–80.
4. Braga PC, *et al.* Identification of subpopulations of bronchitic patients for suitable therapy by a dynamic rheological test. *Int J Clin Pharmacol Res* 1989; **IX:** 175–82.

### Preparations

**Proprietary Preparations** (details are given in Part 3)
***Arg.:*** Mucolitic; ***Belg.:*** Bronchathiol; Muco Rhinathiol; Mucosteine; Pulmoclase†; Romilar Mucolyticum; Siroxyl; ***Braz.:*** Carbocin; Carbofan; Certuss; Fluitoss; Fluizan; Lisomuc†; Mucocil†; Mucocistein; Mucodestrol†; Mucofan; Mucoflux; Mucolisil; Mucolitic; Mucolix†; Mucomax†; Mucotoss; Tossimel†; ***Chile:*** Coldin; ***Fin.:*** Pulmoclase†; Reodyn; Toclapekt; ***Fr.:*** Actifed Expectorant; Bronchathiol; Bronchocyst†; Bronchokod; Bronchyteine†; Broncoclar; Broncorinol Expectorant; Bronkirex; Codotussyl Expectorant; Dimotapp Expectorant; Drill Expectorant; Ergix; Fluditec; Fluvic; Hexafluid†; Humex Expectorant; Medibronc†; Muciclar; Mucotrophir†; Pectojuvene†; Pectosan Expectorant; Pneumoclar†; Rhinathiol; Sirop des Vosges Expectorant; Solutricine Expectorant; Toclase Expectorant; Tussilene; ***Ger.:*** Mucopront; Sedotussin muco; Transbronchin; ***Gr.:*** Allstam; Chilvax; Ectofus; Estival; Mucorem; Mucothiol; Pulmoclase; Santamex-Expectorant; ***Hong Kong:*** Mucodyne†; Mucospect; Rhinathiol; Solmux; ***Irl.:*** Exputex; Mucodyne; Mucogen; Mucolex; Pulmoclase; Vis-

colex; **Israel:** Mical; Mucolit; Mucomed; **Ital.:** Broncomucil; Bronx; Carbocit; Fluifort; Lisil†; Lisomucil; Mucocis; Mucojet; Mucolase; Mucostar; Mucotreis; Polifluidil; Polimucil; Reomucil; Sinecod Tosse Fluidificante; Solfomucil†; Solucis; Superthiol†; Tossefluid; **Jpn:** Mucodyne; **Malaysia:** Kastipron; Mucopront; Rhinathiol; SCMC; **Mex.:** Loviscol†; Mucolin; **Neth.:** Dampo Solvopect; Mucodyne; Pulmoclase†; Rami Slijmoplossende; Rhinathiol†; **Port.:** Drill Mucolitico; Finatux; Mucolex; Mucorhinathiol Mucoral; Pulmiben; Pulmoclase; **S.Afr.:** Acuphlem†; Arcanacysteine†; Betaphlem; Bronchette; Carbospect†; Co-Flem; Corbar M†; Flemex; Flemgo; Flemlite; Ilvispect†; Lessmusec; Medphlem†; Mucocaps; Mucoflem; Mucoless; Mucolinct†; Mucosirop; Mucospect; **Singapore:** Mucopront; Rhinathiol; SCMC; **Spain:** Actithiol; Anatac; Fluidin Mucolitico NF; Mucovital; Pectodrill; Pectox; Viscoteina; **Switz.:** Mephathiol; Mucogeran; Mucoseptal†; Pectox†; Rhinathiol; Tussantiol; **Thai.:** Bocytin; Exflem; Flemex; Mucolex; Mucopront; Muflex; Pectox†; Rhinathiol; Rhinex; Solmux; **UK:** Mucodyne.

**Multi-ingredient:** **Arg.:** Mucolitic Antitusivo; Polimucil; **Fr.:** Acnaveen†; Rhinathiol Promethazine; **Hong Kong:** Rhinathiol Promethazine; **India:** Caceff; Carbomox; Moxycarb; **Ital.:** Broncofluid; Keraflex; Libexin Mucolitico; Sebaveen†; **Malaysia:** Rhinathiol Promethazine; SCMC Promethazine; **Mex.:** Caltusine; Mucolin A; **Port.:** Acnaveen†; Bronquial; Niflux; Sebaveen†; **Singapore:** Rhinathiol Promethazine†; **Spain:** Actithiol Antihist; Amoxtiol†; Bronquicisteina; Eduprim Mucolitico; Pectoral Funk Antitus†; Pectox Ampicilina†; Tilfilin†; Tuselin Expectorante†; **Switz.:** Broncatar†; Rhinathiol Promethazine; Triofan.

## Clobutinol Hydrochloride *(rINNM)*

Hidrocloruro de clobutinol; KAT-256. 2-(4-Chlorobenzyl)-3-(dimethylaminomethyl)butan-2-ol hydrochloride.

$C_{14}H_{22}ClNO,HCl = 292.2$.

*CAS — 14860-49-2 (clobutinol); 1215-83-4 (clobutinol hydrochloride).*

*ATC — R05DB03.*

### Profile

Clobutinol hydrochloride is a centrally acting cough suppressant for non-productive cough (p.1112) given by mouth in doses of 40 to 80 mg three times daily; doses of 20 mg have been given by subcutaneous, intramuscular, or intravenous injection.

### Preparations

**Proprietary Preparations** (details are given in Part 3)

**Arg.:** Silomat; **Austria:** Silomat; **Belg.:** Silomat; **Braz.:** Silomat; **Chile:** Broncodual; Clobatos; Cloval; Pulbronc Simple; Silomat; **Fin.:** Mixtus; Silomat; **Fr.:** Silomat; **Ger.:** Mentopin Hustenstiller†; Nullatuss; Rofatuss; Silomat; stas-Hustenstiller N; Tussamed†; Tussed; **Gr.:** Silomat; **Ital.:** Silomat-Fher; **Malaysia:** Silomat; **Port.:** Silomat; **Singapore:** Silomat; **Thai.:** Silomat.

**Multi-ingredient:** **Arg.:** Bronquisedan; Bronquisedan Mucolitico; **Braz.:** Hytos Plus; Silomat Plus; **Chile:** Broncodual Compuesto; Cloval Compuesto; Pulbronc; Solvanol; Tusabron; Vapoflu; **Fr.:** Silomat; **S.Afr.:** Silomat DA; **Thai.:** Silomat Compositum†; **UAE:** Orcinol.

## Clofedanol Hydrochloride *(BANM, rINNM)*

Chlophedianol Hydrochloride *(USAN)*; Hidrocloruro de clofedanol; SL-501. 2-Chloro-α-(2-dimethylaminoethyl)benzyl alcohol hydrochloride.

$C_{17}H_{20}ClNO,HCl = 326.3$.

*CAS — 791-35-5 (clofedanol); 511-13-7 (clofedanol hydrochloride).*

*ATC — R05DB10.*

**Pharmacopoeias.** In *Jpn.*

### Profile

Clofedanol hydrochloride is a centrally acting cough suppressant for non-productive cough (p.1112) that has been given by mouth in doses of 25 to 30 mg three or four times daily.

### Preparations

**Proprietary Preparations** (details are given in Part 3)

**Canad.:** Ulone; **Hong Kong:** Coldrin; **Singapore:** Coldrin; **Spain:** Gentos.

**Multi-ingredient:** **Arg.:** Bronco Biotaer; Causalon Bronquial; Cofron; Gentiabron; Neo-Tosel; Notozen; Pectoral Hebert; Predual; Selectus FN; **Chile:** Bauxol; Brontal; Cofron; Diadicon; Kolibel; Mucobrol; **Spain:** Xibornol Prodes†.

## Clonazoline Hydrochloride *(rINNM)*

Hidrocloruro de clonazolina. 2-[(4-Chloro-1-naphthyl)methyl]-2-imidazoline hydrochloride.

$C_{14}H_{13}ClN_2,HCl = 281.2$.

*CAS — 17692-28-3 (clonazoline); 23593-08-0 (clonazoline hydrochloride).*

### Profile

Clonazoline hydrochloride is a sympathomimetic with effects similar to those of naphazoline (p.1125) used for its vasoconstrictor activity in the local treatment of nasal congestion (p.1112)

### Preparations

**Proprietary Preparations** (details are given in Part 3)

**Multi-ingredient:** **Ital.:** Localyn.

## Cloperastine Fendizoate *(rINNM)*

Cloperastine Hydroxyphenylbenzoyl Benzoic Acid; Cloperastine Phendizoate; Fendizoato de cloperastina. 1-{2-[(p-Chloro-α-phenylbenzyl)oxy]ethyl}piperidine fendizoate.

$C_{20}H_{24}ClNO,C_{20}H_{14}O_4 = 648.2$.

*CAS — 3703-76-2 (cloperastine); 85187-37-7 (cloperastine fendizoate).*

*ATC — R05DB21.*

## Cloperastine Hydrochloride *(rINNM)*

Hidrocloruro de cloperastina.

$C_{20}H_{24}ClNO,HCl = 366.3$.

*CAS — 14984-68-0.*

*ATC — R05DB21.*

**Pharmacopoeias.** In *Jpn.*

### Profile

Cloperastine is primarily a centrally acting cough suppressant used for non-productive cough (p.1112). It also has some antihistaminic action. The hydrochloride has been given by mouth as tablets in usual doses of 10 to 20 mg three times daily. Cloperastine fendizoate is used in oral liquid preparations in equivalent doses. Cloperastine fendizoate 17.7 mg is approximately equivalent to 10 mg of cloperastine hydrochloride.

### Preparations

**Proprietary Preparations** (details are given in Part 3)

**Belg.:** Novotossil; Sekin; **Braz.:** Seki; **Hong Kong:** Costop†; **Ital.:** Cloel; Clofend; Mitituss; Nitossil; Politosse; Privituss; Quik; Risoltuss†; Seki; **Jpn:** Hustazol; **Malaysia:** Copastin; **Spain:** Flutox; Sekisan.

**Multi-ingredient:** **Thai.:** Hustazol-C.

## Cocillana

Grape Bark; Guapi Bark; Huapi Bark.

*CAS — 1398-77-2.*

### Profile

Cocillana is used as an expectorant similarly to ipecacuanha (p.1122). It has been used in large doses as an emetic.

### Preparations

**Proprietary Preparations** (details are given in Part 3)

**Multi-ingredient:** **Braz.:** Elixir de Marinheiro†; **Canad.:** Alsidrine; Bronchosyl†; Sirop Cocillana Codeine; **Fin.:** Codesan Comp; Codesan N; **Hong Kong:** Cocillana Compound; Mefedra-N; **Ital.:** Broncosedina; **S.Afr.:** Cocillana Co; Corbar; **Swed.:** Cocillana-Etyfin.

## Coltsfoot

Coughwort; Fárfara; Huflattich; Tussilage.

**Pharmacopoeias.** *Chin.* and *Fr.* include Coltsfoot Flower.

### Profile

The leaves and flowers of coltsfoot (*Tussilago farfara*) have been used for their demulcent and supposed expectorant properties in the treatment of cough and other mild respiratory disorders. However, there has been some concern about potential hepatotoxicity and carcinogenicity due to the content of pyrrolizidine alkaloids.

◊ A review[1] of the actions and uses of coltsfoot pointed out that given the potential risks of its use long-term or in pregnancy, and the availability of other demulcent herbs, the use of coltsfoot preparations to treat throat irritations can no longer be considered appropriate.

1. Berry M. Coltsfoot. *Pharm J* 1996; **256:** 234–5.

### Preparations

**Proprietary Preparations** (details are given in Part 3)

**Multi-ingredient:** **Arg.:** Arceligasol; Negacne; **Fr.:** Mediflor Tisane Pectorale d'Alsace†; **Ital.:** Lozione Same Urto; **Spain:** Llantusil; **UK:** Antibron; Chesty Cough Relief.

## Creosote

Creasote; Creosota; Creosotal (creosote carbonate); Wood Creosote.

*CAS — 8021-39-4 (creosote); 8001-59-0 (creosote carbonate).*

*ATC — R05CA08.*

**Pharmacopoeias.** In *Jpn.*

### Profile

Creosote is a liquid consisting of a mixture of guaiacol, cresol, and other phenols obtained from wood tar. It possesses disinfectant properties and has been used as an expectorant. It has also been used as the carbonate and as lactocreosote.

Adverse effects are similar to those of Phenol, p.1188.

Commercial creosote used for timber preservation is obtained from coal tar.

### Preparations

**Proprietary Preparations** (details are given in Part 3)

**Multi-ingredient:** **Austral.:** Compound Inhalation of Menthol†; **Austria:** Famel cum Codein; Famel cum Ephedrin; **Braz.:** Calmante Creosotado†; Rhum Creosotado; **India:** Pulmo-Cod (C & G); **Ital.:** Creosoto Composto; Famel; **Neth.:** Famel†; **Port.:** Creodermol†; **Spain:** Dentikrisos; Sanaden Reforzado†; **Switz.:** Famel; **UK:** Catarrh Pastilles†; Famel Original; Potter's Catarrh Pastilles; Potters Strong Bronchial Catarrh Pastilles.

## Dembrexine *(BAN, rINN)*

Dembrexina; Dembroxol. *trans*-4-[(3,5-Dibromosalicyl)amino]cyclohexanol.

$C_{13}H_{17}Br_2NO_2 = 379.1$.

*CAS — 83200-09-3 (dembrexine); 52702-51-9 (dembrexine hydrochloride).*

### Profile

Dembrexine is a mucolytic used as the hydrochloride in veterinary medicine.

# Dextromethorphan *(BAN, pINN)*

Dextrometorfano. (+)-3-Methoxy-9a-methylmorphinan; (9S,13S,-14S)-6,18-Dideoxy-7,8-dihydro-3-O-methylmorphine.

$C_{18}H_{25}NO = 271.4$.

*CAS — 125-71-3.*

*ATC — R05DA09.*

**Pharmacopoeias.** In *US.*

**USP 27** (Dextromethorphan). A practically white to slightly yellow, odourless, crystalline powder. Practically insoluble in water; freely soluble in chloroform. Store in airtight containers.

## Dextromethorphan Hydrobromide *(BANM, pINNM)*

Dextromethorphani Hydrobromidum; Hidrobromuro de dextrometorfano. Dextromethorphan hydrobromide monohydrate.

$C_{18}H_{25}NO,HBr,H_2O = 370.3$.

*CAS — 125-69-9 (anhydrous dextromethorphan hydrobromide); 6700-34-1 (dextromethorphan hydrobromide monohydrate).*

*ATC — R05DA09.*

**Pharmacopoeias.** In *Eur.* (see p.vi), *Int., Jpn, Pol., US,* and *Viet.*

**Ph. Eur. 5.0** (Dextromethorphan Hydrobromide). An almost white, crystalline powder. Sparingly soluble in water; freely soluble in alcohol. Protect from light.

**USP 27** (Dextromethorphan Hydrobromide). Practically white crystals or crystalline powder having a faint odour. Soluble 1 in 65 of water; freely soluble in alcohol and in chloroform; insoluble in ether. pH of a 1% solution in water is between 5.2 and 6.5. Store in airtight containers.

## Adverse Effects and Treatment

Adverse effects with dextromethorphan appear to be rare and may include dizziness and gastrointestinal disturbances. Excitation, confusion, and respiratory depression may occur after overdosage. Dextromethorphan has been subject to abuse, but there is little evidence of dependence of the morphine type.

◊ General references.

1. Bem JL, Peck R. Dextromethorphan: an overview of safety issues. *Drug Safety* 1992; **7:** 190–9.

**Effects on the skin.** A fixed-drug reaction developed in a patient after ingestion of dextromethorphan 30 mg.[1] Oral provocation with dextromethorphan produced a positive reaction but the results of topical application tests were negative.

1. Stubb S, Reitamo S. Fixed-drug eruption due to dextromethorphan. *Arch Dermatol* 1990; **126:** 970–1.

**Overdosage.** There have been reports[1-6] of overdosage or accidental poisoning (usually in children) due to dextromethorphan, including rare fatalities. Naloxone may be effective in reversing toxicity. Extrapyramidal reactions were seen in a child who ingested dextromethorphan.[6] Overdosage has also been associated with abuse (see below).

1. Shaul WL, *et al.* Dextromethorphan toxicity: reversal by naloxone. *Pediatrics* 1977; **59:** 117–19.
2. Katona B, Wason S. Dextromethorphan danger. *N Engl J Med* 1986; **314:** 993.
3. Rammer L, *et al.* Fatal intoxication by dextromethorphan: a report on two cases. *Forensic Sci Int* 1988; **37:** 233–6.
4. Schneider SM, *et al.* Dextromethorphan poisoning reversed by naloxone. *Am J Emerg Med* 1991; **9:** 237–8.
5. Pender ES, Parks BR. Toxicity with dextromethorphan-containing preparations: a literature review and report of two additional cases. *Pediatr Emerg Care* 1991; **7:** 163–5.
6. Warden CR, *et al.* Dystonic reaction associated with dextromethorphan ingestion in a toddler. *Pediatr Emerg Care* 1997; **13:** 214–15.

## Precautions

Dextromethorphan should not be given to patients at risk of developing respiratory failure. Caution is needed in patients with a history of asthma and it should not be given during an acute attack.

**Abuse.** Dextromethorphan has been abused[1-9], alone or in combination with other drugs in over-the-counter preparations or as a powder sold under the name DXM.

1. Fleming PM. Dependence on dextromethorphan hydrobromide. *BMJ* 1986; **293:** 597.

2. Orrell MW, Campbell PG. Dependence on dextromethorphan hydrobromide. *BMJ* 1986; **293:** 1242–3.
3. Walker J, Yatham LN. Benylin (dextromethorphan) abuse and mania. *BMJ* 1993; **306:** 896.
4. Wolfe TR, Caravati EM. Massive dextromethorphan ingestion and abuse. *Am J Emerg Med* 1995; **13:** 174–6.
5. Nordt SP. DXM: a new drug of abuse? *Ann Emerg Med* 1998; **31:** 794–5.
6. Cranston JW, Yoast R. Abuse of dextromethorphan. *Arch Fam Med* 1999; **8:** 99–100.
7. Price LH, Lebel J. Dextromethorphan-induced psychosis. *Am J Psychiatry* 2000; **157:** 304.
8. Noonan WC, *et al.* Dextromethorphan abuse among youth. *Arch Fam Med* 2000; **9:** 791–2.
9. Banerji S, Anderson IB. Abuse of Coricidin HBP cough and cold tablets: episodes recorded by a poison center. *Am J Health-Syst Pharm* 2001; **58:** 1811–14.

**Children.** For doubts about the use of dextromethorphan as an antitussive in children see Cough, under Uses and Administration, below.

## Interactions

Severe and sometimes fatal reactions have been reported following use of dextromethorphan in patients receiving MAOIs. Dextromethorphan is primarily metabolised by the cytochrome P450 isoenzyme CYP2D6; the possibility of interactions with inhibitors of this enzyme, including amiodarone, fluoxetine, haloperidol, paroxetine, propafenone, quinidine, and thioridazine, should be borne in mind.

**Antiarrhythmics.** *Quinidine* can increase serum concentrations of dextromethorphan markedly, and some patients have experienced symptoms of dextromethorphan toxicity when the two drugs have been used together.[1] *Amiodarone* also appears to be able to increase serum concentrations of dextromethorphan.[2]

1. Zhang Y, *et al.* Dextromethorphan: enhancing its systemic availability by way of low-dose quinidine-mediated inhibition of cytochrome P4502D6. *Clin Pharmacol Ther* 1992; **51:** 647–55.
2. Funck-Brentano C, *et al.* Influence of amiodarone on genetically determined drug metabolism in humans. *Clin Pharmacol Ther* 1991; **50:** 259–66.

**Antidepressants.** A patient receiving *fluoxetine* experienced visual hallucinations after she began taking dextromethorphan.[1] The hallucinations were similar to those she had had 12 years earlier with lysergide. She had previously taken dextromethorphan alone without any adverse reactions. A serotonin syndrome (p.313) has been reported in a patient who took a cold-remedy containing dextromethorphan while receiving *paroxetine*.[2]

1. Achamallah NS. Visual hallucinations after combining fluoxetine and dextromethorphan. *Am J Psychiatry* 1992; **149:** 1406.
2. Skop BP, *et al.* The serotonin syndrome associated with paroxetine, an over-the-counter cold remedy, and vascular disease. *Am J Emerg Med* 1994; **12:** 642–4.

## Pharmacokinetics

Dextromethorphan is rapidly absorbed from the gastrointestinal tract. It is metabolised in the liver and excreted in the urine as unchanged dextromethorphan and demethylated metabolites including dextrorphan (p.1679), which has some cough suppressant activity.

◊ The *O*-demethylation of dextromethorphan and the hydroxylation of debrisoquine are under common polymorphic control, involving the cytochrome P450 isoenzyme CYP2D6, and dextromethorphan has been used as an alternative to debrisoquine for the phenotyping of oxidative metabolism.[1,2] Non-invasive determinations can be made using samples of urine or saliva.[3,4] Dextromethorphan has also been suggested as a tool to investigate *N*-demethylation, an alternate metabolic pathway for this drug.[5]

1. Belec L, *et al.* Extensive oxidative metabolism of dextromethorphan in patients with almitrine neuropathy. *Br J Clin Pharmacol* 1989; **27:** 387–90.
2. Streetman DS, *et al.* Dose dependency of dextromethorphan for cytochrome P450 2D6 (CYP2D6) phenotyping. *Clin Pharmacol Ther* 1999; **66:** 535–41.
3. Hildebrand M, *et al.* Determination of dextromethorphan metabolizer phenotype in healthy volunteers. *Eur J Clin Pharmacol* 1989; **36:** 315–18.
4. Hou Z-Y, *et al.* Salivary analysis for determination of dextromethorphan metabolic phenotype. *Clin Pharmacol Ther* 1991; **49:** 410–19.
5. Jones DR, *et al.* Determination of cytochrome P450 3A4/5 activity in vivo with dextromethorphan N-demethylation. *Clin Pharmacol Ther* 1996; **60:** 374–84.

## Uses and Administration

Dextromethorphan hydrobromide is a cough suppressant used for the relief of non-productive cough; it has a central action on the cough centre in the medulla. It is also an antagonist of *N*-methyl-D-aspartate (NMDA) receptors. Although structurally related to morphine, dextromethorphan has no classical analgesic properties (but see Pain below) and little sedative activity.

Dextromethorphan hydrobromide is reported to act within half an hour of administration by mouth and to exert an effect for up to 6 hours. It is given by mouth in doses of 10 to 20 mg every 4 hours, or 30 mg every 6 to 8 hours, to a usual maximum of 120 mg in 24 hours. Children aged 6 to 12 years may be given 5 to 10 mg every 4 hours or 15 mg every 6 to 8 hours to a maximum of 60 mg in 24 hours, and children aged 2 to 6 years 2.5 to 5 mg every 4 hours, or 7.5 mg every 6 to 8 hours, to a maximum of 30 mg in 24 hours. (But see also Cough, below.)

Dextromethorphan polistirex (a dextromethorphan and sulfonated diethenylbenzene-ethenylbenzene copolymer complex) is used in modified-release oral preparations. The dosage of dextromethorphan polistirex, expressed as dextromethorphan hydrobromide, is the equivalent of 60 mg every 12 hours; children aged 6 to 12 years may be given 30 mg every 12 hours; children aged 2 to 6 years may be given 15 mg every 12 hours.

Dextrorphan (p.1679), the *O*-demethylated metabolite of dextromethorphan, also has cough suppressant properties.

**Cough.** Equal doses of dextromethorphan hydrobromide and codeine phosphate were of similar efficacy in reducing the frequency of chronic cough (p.1112) in a double-blind crossover study in adults, but dextromethorphan had a greater effect than codeine on cough intensity.[1] However, these drugs were little more effective than placebo in suppressing night-time cough in children.[2,3] The American Academy of Pediatrics has commented[4] that there is no good evidence for the antitussive efficacy of dextromethorphan in children, that dosage guidelines are derived from (possibly inappropriate) extrapolation from effects in adults, and that adverse effects have been reported.

There is also some evidence that genetic polymorphism in the cytochrome P450 isoenzyme CYP2D6, and hence variations in metabolism, may have a significant influence on the antitussive efficacy of dextromethorphan.[5]

1. Matthys H, *et al.* Dextromethorphan and codeine: objective assessment of antitussive activity in patients with chronic cough. *J Int Med Res* 1983; **11:** 92–100.
2. Gadomski A, Horton L. The need for rational therapeutics in the use of cough and cold medicine in infants. *Pediatrics* 1992; **89:** 774–6.
3. Taylor JA, *et al.* Efficacy of cough suppressants in children. *J Pediatr* 1993; **122:** 799–802.
4. American Academy of Pediatrics Committee on Drugs. Use of codeine- and dextromethorphan-containing cough remedies in children. *Pediatrics* 1997; **99:** 918–20.
5. Wright CE, *et al.* CYP2D6 polymorphism and the anti-tussive effect of dextromethorphan in man. *Thorax* 1997; **52** (suppl 6): A73.

**Neurological disorders.** Dextromethorphan appears to have anticonvulsant activity and may have neuroprotective effects in cerebral ischaemia.[1] These effects may be related to its activity as an antagonist of *N*-methyl-D-aspartate (NMDA) receptors or to interaction with σ-receptors. It has been studied in Parkinson's disease for treatment[2] or for management of levodopa-induced dyskinesias,[3] and for its potential protective action in stroke (p.836) and acute brain injury. Dextromethorphan has also been studied for the management of amyotrophic lateral sclerosis (see Motor Neurone Disease, p.1739) but has not been found to be of benefit.[4-6] Its NMDA-antagonist properties have also been investigated for the treatment[7,8] of nonketotic hyperglycinaemia (see under Strychnine, p.1750).

1. Tortella FC, *et al.* Dextromethorphan and neuromodulation: old drug coughs up new activities. *Trends Pharmacol Sci* 1989; **10:** 501–7.
2. Bonuccelli U, *et al.* Dextromethorphan and parkinsonism. *Lancet* 1992; **340:** 53.
3. Verhagen Metman L, *et al.* Dextromethorphan improves levodopa-induced dyskinesias in Parkinson's disease. *Neurology* 1998; **51:** 203–6.
4. Askmark H, *et al.* A pilot trial of dextromethorphan in amyotrophic lateral sclerosis. *J Neurol Neurosurg Psychiatry* 1993; **56:** 197–200.
5. Blin O, *et al.* A controlled one-year trial of dextromethorphan in amyotrophic lateral sclerosis. *Clin Neuropharmacol* 1996; **19:** 189–92.
6. Gredal O, *et al.* A clinical trial of dextromethorphan in amyotrophic lateral sclerosis. *Acta Neurol Scand* 1997; **96:** 8–13.
7. Alemzadeh R, *et al.* Efficacy of low-dose dextromethorphan in the treatment of nonketotic hyperglycinemia. *Pediatrics* 1996; **97:** 924–6.
8. Hamosh A, *et al.* Long-term use of high-dose benzoate and dextromethorphan for the treatment of nonketotic hyperglycinemia. *J Pediatr* 1998; **132:** 709–13.

**Pain.** Dextromethorphan has a potential role in the blockade of pain. It has been investigated[1-3] in the management of neuropathic pain with promising results in diabetic neuropathy (p.6), although pain was not reduced in postherpetic neuralgia (p.7). High doses of dextromethorphan may be needed for an effect. However, a review[4] concluded that there were insufficient data to justify the use of dextromethorphan in diabetic neuropathy and further well-controlled trials were needed.

Dextromethorphan given pre-operatively and for 48 hours post-operatively at the highest tolerable dose did not reduce postoperative pain (p.4) immediately after oral surgery,[5] but did reduce pain after 48 hours, suggesting that NMDA receptor antagonists such as dextromethorphan might be useful pharmacologic interventions to reduce hyperalgesia or mitigate chronic pain. Dextromethorphan given as an adjunct to analgesics also demonstrated a morphine-sparing effect in adults 48 hours after hysterectomy,[6] but pre-operative administration to adults undergoing laparotomy,[7] or children scheduled for adenotonsillectomy,[8] did not improve postoperative pain at 24 hours.

1. Nelson KA, *et al.* High-dose oral dextromethorphan versus placebo in painful diabetic neuropathy and postherpetic neuralgia. *Neurology* 1997; **48:** 1212–18.
2. Sang CN, *et al.* Dextromethorphan and memantine in painful diabetic neuropathy and postherpetic neuralgia: efficacy and dose-response trials. *Anesthesiology* 2002; **96:** 1053–61.
3. Carlsson KC, *et al.* Analgesic effect of dextromethorphan in neuropathic pain. *Acta Anaesthesiol Scand* 2004; **48:** 328–36.
4. Criner TM, Perdun CS. Dextromethorphan and diabetic neuropathy. *Ann Pharmacother* 1999; **33:** 1221–3.
5. Gordon SM, *et al.* Antihyperalgesic effect of the N-methyl-D-aspartate receptor antagonist dextromethorphan in the oral surgery model. *J Clin Pharmacol* 1999; **39:** 139–46.
6. Henderson DJ, *et al.* Perioperative dextromethorphan reduces postoperative pain after hysterectomy. *Anesth Analg* 1999; **89:** 399–402.
7. Grace RF, *et al.* Preoperative dextromethorphan reduces intraoperative but not postoperative morphine requirements after laparotomy. *Anesth Analg* 1998; **87:** 1135–8.
8. Rose JB, *et al.* Preoperative oral dextromethorphan does not reduce pain or analgesic consumption in children after adenotonsillectomy. *Anesth Analg* 1999; **88:** 749–53.

## Preparations

***USP 27:*** Acetaminophen, Dextromethorphan Hydrobromide, Doxylamine Succinate, and Pseudoephedrine Hydrochloride Oral Solution; Dextromethorphan Hydrobromide Syrup; Guaifenesin, Pseudoephedrine Hydrochloride, and Dextromethorphan Hydrobromide Capsules; Pseudoephedrine Hydrochloride, Carbinoxamine Maleate, and Dextromethorphan Hydrobromide Oral Solution.

**Proprietary Preparations** (details are given in Part 3)
***Arg.:*** Dextrotos; Romilar; ***Austral.:*** Benadryl for the Family Dry Forte; Bisolvon Dry; Dexi-Tuss; Nucosef DM; Robitussin DX; Robitussin Honey Cough Syrup; Strepsils Cough Relief; Tussinol for Dry Coughs; ***Austria:*** Prontodex; Wick Formel 44; Wick Formel 44 Plus Hustenstiller; ***Belg.:*** Actifed; Akindex†; Benylin Antitussivum†; Bronchosedal; Dexir; Humex; Nortussine Mono; Romilar Antitussivum; Touxium†; Tussipect; Tussiphane†; Tusso Rhinathiol; Vicks Vaposyrup Antitussif; ***Canad.:*** Balminil DM; Benylin DM; Broncho-Grippol-DM; Bronchopan DM; Buckley's DM; Calmylin #1; Centratuss DM†; Cough Suppressant Syrup DM†; Cough Syrup DM; Cough Syrup†; Delsym; DM Cough Syrup; DM Sans Sucre; Drixoral Cough†; Drixoral†; Formula 44; Koffex DM; Koffex†; Novahistex DM†; Novahistine DM†; Pharmilin-DM; Pharminil DM; Robitussin Childrens Cough DM; Robitussin Honey Cough DM; Sedatuss DM; Sirop DM†; Sucrets Cough Control; Syrup DM; Triaminic Cough; Triaminic DM; Tussin Antitussive; ***Chile:*** Tusminal; ***Denm.:*** Dexofan; ***Fin.:*** Lagun; Resilar; ***Fr.:*** Akindex; Atuxane†; Bronchytuc†; Capsyl†; Codotussyl Toux Seche; Dexir; Drill toux seche; Ergix; Nodex; Pulmodexane; Rhinathiol Toux Seche†; Sebrane†; Taritux†; Tussidane; Tuxium; Vicks Toux Seche; ***Ger.:*** Arpha Hustensirup; Em-eukal forte N; Hustenstiller; NeoTussan; Tuss Hustenstiller; Wick Formel 44 Husten-Stiller; Wick Formel 44 plus Husten-Pastillen S; Wick Kinder Formel 44 Husten-Stiller†; ***Hong Kong:*** Balminil DM; Pusiran; Robitussin Maximum Strength Cough; Robitussin Paediatric Cough; Tussils; ***India:*** Alex Cough; Lastuss; ***Irl.:*** Benylin Non-Drowsy Dry Cough; Delsym; Robitussin Dry Cough; ***Israel:*** Cough Control Sucrets†; Tarodex; ***Ital.:*** Aricodiltosse; Bechilar; Bronchenolo; Fluprim Tosse†; Formitrol; Honeytuss; Lisomucil Tosse Sedativo; Metorfan; Neo Borocillina Tosse Sciroppo; Sanabronchiol; Tossoral; Tussycalm; Valatux†; Vicks Tosse Pastiglie; Vicks Tosse Sedativo; ***Malaysia:*** Dexcophan; Metofen Forte; Nospan; Pusiran; Tussils; Upha Dextrophan; ***Mex.:*** Atassol; Athos; Balbek; Balsedrina; Bekfan†; Bekidiba Dex; Bioquidan; Brocolan; Debequin; Delsym†; Dontuxin†; Formula S†; Garde Jarabe; Mebran†; Megal Simple; Neo-Ulcoid; Neopulmonier; Numonyl D; Protan†; Romilar†; Tartrina†; Versan†; ***Neth.:*** Dampo bij droge hoest; Darolan Hoestprikkeldempende†; Rami-Dextromethorphan; Vicks Vaposiroop; Vicks Vapotab; ***NZ:*** Benadryl Dry Forte; Robitussin DX; Strepsils Cough; Strepsils Dry Cough; ***Port.:*** Akindex†; Diacol; Drill Tosse Seca; Rhinathiol Tosse Seca†; ***S.Afr.:*** Benylin Dry Cough; Benylin Solid†; ***Singapore:*** Nospan; Pusiran; Tussidex; Tussils; ***Spain:*** Benylin Antitusivo; Cinfatos; Formulatus; Frenatus; Ilvitus; Pastillas Dr Andreu; Robitussin DM Antitusivo; Romilar; Siepex†; Streptuss; TIP†; Tosfriol†; Tosrhimatiol; Tusitinas; Tusorama; Tussidrill; Valdatos†; ***Swed.:*** Tussidyl†; ***Switz.:*** Astho-Med; Bexine; Calmerphan-L; Calmerphan†; Calmesine; Dextrocalmine†; Emedrin N; Pulmofor; Toux seche; Vicks Formule 44 Calmine; ***Thai.:*** Cortuss; Dec; Detuss†; Dex; Dextroral; Polydex; Pusiran; Romilar; Tusco; Tussils; ***UAE:*** Sedofan P; ***UK:*** Adult Dry Cough; Benylin Dry Coughs Non-Drowsy; Contac Coughcaps†; Covonia for Children†; Dry Cough Syrup; Franolyn Sedative†; Nirolex for Dry Coughs†; Robitussin for Dry Coughs; Robitussin Junior†; Strepsils Cough†; Vicks Vaposyrup for Dry Coughs; ***USA:*** Benylin Adult; Benylin DM†; Benylin Pediatric; Creo-Terpin; Delsym; DexAlone; Diabe-Tuss DM; Hold DM; Pertussin†; Robitussin Cough Calmers†; Robitussin Pediatric; Scot-Tussin DM Cough Chasers; Silphen DM; Simply Cough; St. Joseph Cough Suppressant†; Sucrets 4-Hour Cough†; Sucrets Cough Control†; Suppress†; Trocal; Vicks 44 Cough Relief; Vicks Dry Hacking Cough†.

**Multi-ingredient:** numerous preparations are listed in Part 3.

---

## Dimemorfan Phosphate *(rINNM)*

AT-17; Fosfato de dimemorfano. (+)-3,9a-Dimethylmorphinan phosphate.

$C_{18}H_{25}N,H_3PO_4$ = 353.4.

*CAS — 36309-01-0 (dimemorfan); 36304-84-4 (dimemorfan phosphate).*

*ATC — R05DA11.*

**Pharmacopoeias.** In *Jpn*.

### Profile

Dimemorfan phosphate is a centrally acting cough suppressant used for non-productive cough (p.1112). It is given by mouth in doses of 10 to 20 mg three or four times daily.

### Preparations

**Proprietary Preparations** (details are given in Part 3)
***Ital.:*** Gentus†; Tusben; ***Spain:*** Dastosin.

## Dimethoxanate Hydrochloride *(BANM, rINNM)*

Hidrocloruro de dimetoxanato. 2-(2-Dimethylaminoethoxy)-ethyl phenothiazine-10-carboxylate hydrochloride.

$C_{19}H_{22}N_2O_3S,HCl$ = 394.9.

*CAS — 477-93-0 (dimethoxanate); 518-63-8 (dimethoxanate hydrochloride).*

### Profile

Dimethoxanate hydrochloride is a centrally acting cough suppressant used for non-productive cough (p.1112). It is given by mouth in usual doses of 37.5 mg three or four times daily.

### Preparations

**Proprietary Preparations** (details are given in Part 3)
***Belg.:*** Cotrane.

## Dioxethedrin Hydrochloride *(rINNM)*

Dioxethedrine Hydrochloride; Hidrocloruro de dioxetedrina. α-(1-Ethylaminoethyl)protocatechuyl alcohol hydrochloride.

$C_{11}H_{17}NO_3,HCl$ = 247.7.

*CAS — 497-75-6 (dioxethedrin).*

### Profile

Dioxethedrin hydrochloride is a sympathomimetic that has been used with antitussives in preparations intended for the relief of coughs and associated respiratory-tract disorders.

### Preparations

**Proprietary Preparations** (details are given in Part 3)
**Multi-ingredient:** ***Fr.:*** Quintopan Enfant†.

## Domiodol *(USAN, pINN)*

MG-13608. 2-Iodomethyl-1,3-dioxolan-4-ylmethanol.

$C_5H_9IO_3$ = 244.0.

*CAS — 61869-07-6.*

*ATC — R05CB08.*

### Profile

Domiodol has been used for its mucolytic properties in the relief of productive cough (p.1112).

The actions of the iodides are discussed under Iodine, p.1598.

### Preparations

**Proprietary Preparations** (details are given in Part 3)
***Ital.:*** Mucolitico Maggioni†.

# Dornase Alfa *(BAN, USAN, rINN)*

Deoxyribonuclease; Desoxyribonuclease; DNase I; Dornasa alfa; rhDNase. Deoxyribonuclease I (human recombinant).

$C_{1321}H_{1995}N_{339}O_{396}S_9$ = 29249.6.

*CAS — 143831-71-4; 132053-08-8.*

*ATC — B06AA10; R05CB13.*

**Description.** Dornase alfa is a recombinant enzyme having the same amino acid sequence and glycosylation pattern as human deoxyribonuclease I.

### Adverse Effects

Common adverse effects with dornase alfa aerosol include pharyngitis, hoarseness of the voice, and chest pain. Occasionally laryngitis, conjunctivitis, and skin rashes and urticaria have been reported. There may be a transient decline in pulmonary function on beginning therapy with dornase alfa.

### Uses and Administration

Dornase alfa acts as a mucolytic by hydrolysing DNA that has accumulated in sputum from decaying neutrophils. It is used as a nebulised solution in patients with cystic fibrosis; in the UK its indication is limited to patients with a forced vital capacity greater than 40% of predicted value and to patients over 5 years of age, but in the USA it may also be given for advanced disease (FVC less than 40%) and to younger children. The usual dose is 2500 units (2.5 mg) of dornase alfa given once daily via a jet nebuliser. This dose may be given twice daily to patients over 21 years of age.

Bovine deoxyribonuclease has been used similarly. It has also been used topically, often with fibrinolysin, as a debriding agent in a variety of inflammatory and infected lesions. Bovine deoxyribonuclease has also been given by injection.

**Administration in children.** Although in some countries dornase alfa is not recommended for use in children under 5 years of age, a study[1] to assess the delivery of dornase alfa to the lungs of children with cystic fibrosis aged between 3 months and 5 years, showed that the amounts present in the lower airways were comparable to those in older children. It also appeared to be safe in these younger patients during the 2-week study period.

1. Wagener JS, *et al.* Aerosol delivery and safety of recombinant human deoxyribonuclease in young children with cystic fibrosis: a bronchoscopic study. *J Pediatr* 1998; **133:** 486–91.

**Asthma.** There are reports of the use of dornase alfa to liquefy mucus plugs and relieve an attack of acute severe asthma (p.777) in children.[1-3]

1. Greally P. Human recombinant DNase for mucus plugging in status asthmaticus. *Lancet* 1995; **346:** 1423–4.
2. Patel A, *et al.* Intratracheal recombinant human deoxyribonuclease in acute life-threatening asthma refractory to conventional treatment. *Br J Anaesth* 2000; **84:** 505–7.
3. Durward A, *et al.* Resolution of mucus plugging and atelectasis after intratracheal rhDNase therapy in a mechanically ventilated child with refractory status asthmaticus. *Crit Care Med* 2000; **28:** 560–2.

**Chronic obstructive pulmonary disease.** A large phase III study in patients hospitalised for acute exacerbations of chronic bronchitis (p.779) was halted prematurely because of a non-significant trend to increased mortality in patients given dornase alfa.[1]

1. Hudson TJ. Dornase in treatment of chronic bronchitis. *Ann Pharmacother* 1996; **30:** 674–5.

**Cystic fibrosis.** There is good evidence that inhalation therapy with dornase alfa can produce modest but useful improvement in lung function in some patients with cystic fibrosis (p.123). Most studies have concentrated on patients with mild or moderate disease (forced vital capacity at least 40% of the predicted value) in whom $FEV_1$ and forced vital capacity have shown improvements generally of the order of 5 to 10%,[1-3] and in whom more prolonged therapy (24 weeks) has been shown to reduce the risk of exacerbations of respiratory infections, and hence the need for intravenous antibiotic therapy.[3] There is also evidence that benefit may occur in patients with more severe disease.[4] A systematic review[5] of studies concluded that there is evidence to show that dornase alfa therapy over a 1-month period is associated with improved lung function. Furthermore, a randomised, multicentre, placebo-controlled study[6] in children showed that dornase alfa maintained lung function and reduced the risk of exacerbations over a period of 96 weeks. However, only a minority of patients, perhaps about one-third,[7] benefit from the drug, and at present there is no way of identifying those who will respond other than by a therapeutic trial.[8,9]

Given the high cost of therapy, which is not entirely recouped by savings in acute care, there has been some controversy about the appropriate use of dornase alfa:[10-13] it seems to be generally felt that it should be reserved for specialist use in cystic fibrosis clinics, but that patients should not be denied a trial where appropriate. Most responders with mild to moderate impairment of lung function will show improvements within 2 weeks, although in more severely affected patients a 6-week trial is advocated.[8]

1. Ramsey BW, *et al.* Efficacy and safety of short-term administration of aerosolized recombinant human deoxyribonuclease in patients with cystic fibrosis. *Am Rev Respir Dis* 1993; **148:** 145–51.
2. Ranasinha C, *et al.* Efficacy and safety of short-term administration of aerosolised recombinant human DNase I in adults with stable stage cystic fibrosis. *Lancet* 1993; **342:** 199–202.
3. Fuchs H, *et al.* Effect of aerosolized recombinant human DNase on exacerbations of respiratory symptoms and on pulmonary function in patients with cystic fibrosis. *N Engl J Med* 1994; **331:** 637–42.
4. McCoy K, *et al.* Effects of 12-week administration of dornase alfa in patients with advanced cystic fibrosis lung disease. *Chest* 1996; **110:** 889–95.
5. Jones AP, *et al.* Recombinant human deoxyribonuclease for cystic fibrosis. Available in the Cochrane Library; Issue 2. Chichester: John Wiley; 2004.
6. Quan JM, *et al.* A two-year randomized, placebo-controlled trial of dornase alfa in young patients with cystic fibrosis with mild lung function abnormalities. *J Pediatr* 2001; **139:** 813–20.
7. Davis PB. Evolution of therapy for cystic fibrosis. *N Engl J Med* 1994; **331:** 672–3.
8. Conway SP, Littlewood JM. rhDNase in cystic fibrosis. *Br J Hosp Med* 1997; **57:** 371–2.
9. Ledson MJ, *et al.* Targeting of dornase alpha therapy in adult cystic fibrosis. *J R Soc Med* 1998; **91:** 360–4.
10. Anonymous. Dornase alfa for cystic fibrosis. *Drug Ther Bull* 1995; **33:** 15–16.
11. Spencer D, Weller P. Dornase-alfa for cystic fibrosis. *Lancet* 1995; **345:** 1307.
12. Bush A, *et al.* Dornase alfa for cystic fibrosis. *BMJ* 1995; **310:** 1533.
13. Robert G, *et al.* Dornase alfa for cystic fibrosis. *BMJ* 1995; **311:** 813.

### Preparations

**Proprietary Preparations** (details are given in Part 3)
***Arg.:*** Pulmozyme; ***Austral.:*** Pulmozyme; ***Austria:*** Pulmozyme; ***Belg.:*** Pulmozyme; ***Braz.:*** Pulmozyme; ***Canad.:*** Pulmozyme; ***Chile:*** Viscozyme; ***Denm.:*** Pulmozyme; ***Fin.:*** Pulmozyme; ***Fr.:*** Pulmozyme; ***Ger.:*** Pulmozyme; ***Gr.:*** Pulmozyme; ***Irl.:*** Pulmozyme; ***Israel:*** Pulmozyme; ***Ital.:*** Pulmozyme; ***Mex.:*** Pulmozyme; ***Neth.:*** Pulmozyme; ***Norw.:*** Pulmozyme; ***NZ:*** Pulmozyme; ***Port.:*** Pulmozyme; ***S.Afr.:*** Pulmozyme; ***Spain:*** Pulmozyme; ***Swed.:*** Pulmozyme; ***Switz.:*** Pulmozyme; ***UK:*** Pulmozyme; ***USA:*** Pulmozyme.

**Multi-ingredient:** ***Arg.:*** Clorfibrase; ***Austria:*** Fibrolan; ***Braz.:*** Cauterex; Dermofibrin C; Fibrabene; Fibrase; Gino-Cauterex; Gino-Fibrase; Procutan; ***Canad.:*** Elase-Chloromycetin†; Elase†; ***Chile:*** Elase; ***Fr.:*** Elase; ***Ger.:*** Fibrolan; ***Ital.:*** Derinase Plus†; Elase; ***Malaysia:*** Elase; ***Mex.:*** Fibrase; Fibrase SA; Ridasa; ***Neth.:*** Elase; ***Spain:*** Parkelase Chloromycetin†; Parkelase†; ***Switz.:*** Fibrolan.

## Dropropizine *(BAN, rINN)*

Dropropizina; UCB-1967. 3-(4-Phenylpiperazin-1-yl)propane-1,2-diol.

$C_{13}H_{20}N_2O_2$ = 236.3.

*CAS — 17692-31-8.*

*ATC — R05DB19.*

## Levodropropizine *(BAN, rINN)*

DF-526; Levdropropizine; Levodropropizina; Levodropropizinum. The (−)-(*S*)-isomer of dropropizine.

$C_{13}H_{20}N_2O_2$ = 236.3.

*CAS — 99291-25-5.*

*ATC — R05DB27.*

**Pharmacopoeias.** In *Eur.* (see p.vii).

**Ph. Eur. 5.0** (Levodropropizine). A white or almost white powder. Slightly soluble in water and in alcohol; freely soluble in dilute acetic acid and in methyl alcohol. A 2.5% solution in water has a pH of 9.2 to 10.2. Protect from light.

### Profile

Dropropizine is a cough suppressant reported to have a peripheral action in non-productive cough (p.1112). It is given by mouth in a dose of 30 mg three or four times daily. Levodropropizine, the (−)-(*S*)-isomer of dropropizine, is claimed to produce fewer CNS effects and is used similarly by mouth in a dose of 60 mg up to three times daily.

◊ References.

1. Catena E, Daffonchio L. Efficacy and tolerability of levodropropizine in adult patients with non-productive cough: comparison with dextromethorphan. *Pulm Pharmacol Ther* 1997; **10:** 89–96.

### Preparations

**Proprietary Preparations** (details are given in Part 3)
***Arg.:*** Perlatos; ***Belg.:*** Catabex; Levotuss†; ***Braz.:*** Antux; Atossion; Ecos; Eritos; Flextoss; Neotoss; Tussiflex D; Vibral; Zyplo; ***Chile:*** Broncard; ***Ger.:*** Larylin Husten-Stiller; Larylin Hustensirup N†; ***Gr.:*** Levotuss; ***Ital.:*** Danka; Domutussina; Levotuss; Rapitux; Ribex Tosse; Salvituss; ***Mex.:*** Troferit; Zyplo; ***Port.:*** Catabina; ***Singapore:*** Levopront; ***Spain:*** Levotuss; Tautoss; Tusofren†; ***Thai.:*** Levopront.

**Multi-ingredient:** ***Belg.:*** Catabex Expectorans; ***Braz.:*** Notuss; ***Ital.:*** Elisir Terpina; Guaiacalcium Complex; Ribexen con Espettorante; Tiocalmina; Tussamag Complex; ***Port.:*** Catabina Expectorante.

## Elecampane

Alant; Aunée; Helenio; Inula.

**Pharmacopoeias.** In *Chin.* (which also includes various other species of *Inula*) and *Fr.*

### Profile

Elecampane is the root of *Inula helenium* (Compositae). It has been used in herbal preparations for the treatment of cough for its supposed expectorant and cough suppressant properties. It is also used as a flavouring in foods and alcoholic beverages.

Elecampane contains sesquiterpene lactones including alantolactone (alant camphor; elecampane camphor; inula camphor; helenin), which was formerly employed in the treatment of worm infections, and has also been an ingredient of some cough preparations.

### Preparations

**Proprietary Preparations** (details are given in Part 3)
**Multi-ingredient:** ***Belg.:*** Euphon; ***Fr.:*** Marrubene Codethyline†; Mediflor Tisane Digestive No 3; Mediflor Tisane Hepatique No 5; Tisanes de l'Abbe Hamon no 15†; Tossarel†; ***Ger.:*** Leber-Galle-Tropfen 83; ***Spain:*** Bronpul; Natusor Asmaten; Natusor Broncopul; ***Switz.:*** Boldoflorine†; Hederix; ***UK:*** Catarrh-eeze; Cough-eeze†; Horehound and Aniseed Cough Mixture; Vegetable Cough Remover.

## Ephedra

Efedra; Ma-huang.

**Pharmacopoeias.** In *Chin., Ger.,* and *Jpn.*

*Chin.* also includes the roots of *Ephedra sinica* or *E. intermedia.*

### Profile

Ephedra consists of the dried young branches of *Ephedra sinica, E. equisetina,* and *E. gerardiana* (including *E. nebrodensis*) (Ephedraceae), containing not less than 1.25% of alkaloids, calculated as ephedrine.

The action of ephedra is due to the presence of ephedrine (p.1120) and pseudoephedrine (p.1129). It has been used chiefly as a source of these alkaloids. The FDA has banned the sale of ephedra-containing dietary supplements in the USA.

◊ For reference to the adverse effects of herbal products containing ephedra see under Abuse in Ephedrine, below.

### Preparations

**Proprietary Preparations** (details are given in Part 3)
**Multi-ingredient:** ***Canad.:*** Herbal Cold Relief; ***Ger.:*** Cardibisana; Cefadrin; Repursan ST†.

## Ephedrine (BAN)

Efedrina; Ephedrina; (−)-Ephedrine; Ephedrinum. (1R,2S)-2-Methylamino-1-phenylpropan-1-ol.

$C_{10}H_{15}NO$ = 165.2.

*CAS — 299-42-3 (anhydrous ephedrine); 50906-05-3 (ephedrine hemihydrate).*

*ATC — R01AA03; R01AB05; R03CA02; S01FB02.*

**Description.** Ephedrine is an alkaloid obtained from species of *Ephedra*, or prepared synthetically. It may exist in a hemihydrate form or as the anhydrous substance.

**Pharmacopoeias.** In *Eur.* (see p.vi), *Int.*, and *US*, which have specifications, in either the same monograph or in separate monographs, for the anhydrous form and for the hemihydrate.

**Ph. Eur. 5.0** (Ephedrine, Anhydrous). A white, crystalline powder or colourless crystals. Soluble in water; very soluble in alcohol. It melts at about 36°. Protect from light.

**Ph. Eur. 5.0** (Ephedrine Hemihydrate; Ephedrine BP 2003). A white, crystalline powder or colourless crystals. Soluble in water; very soluble in alcohol. It melts at about 42°, determined without previous drying. Protect from light.

**USP 27** (Ephedrine). It is anhydrous or contains not more than one-half molecule of water of hydration. It is an unctuous, practically colourless solid or white crystals or granules. It gradually decomposes on exposure to light. M.p. between 33° and 40°, the variability being the result of differences in the moisture content, anhydrous ephedrine having a lower melting-point than the hemihydrate. Soluble 1 in 20 of water and 1 in 0.2 of alcohol; soluble in chloroform and in ether; moderately and slowly soluble in liquid paraffin, the solution becoming turbid if the ephedrine contains more than about 1% of water. Its solutions are alkaline to litmus. Store in airtight containers at a temperature not exceeding 8°. Protect from light.

## Ephedrine Hydrochloride (BANM)

Efedrina, hidrocloruro de; Ephedrinae Hydrochloridum; Ephedrine Chloride; Ephedrini Hydrochloridum; Ephedrinium Chloratum; *l*-Ephedrinum Hydrochloricum.

$C_{10}H_{15}NO,HCl$ = 201.7.

*CAS — 50-98-6.*

*ATC — R01AA03; R01AB05; R03CA02; S01FB02.*

**Pharmacopoeias.** In *Chin.*, *Eur.* (see p.vi), *Int.*, *Jpn*, *Pol.*, *US*, and *Viet.*

*Eur.* also includes the racemic form.

**Ph. Eur. 5.0** (Ephedrine Hydrochloride). A white, crystalline powder or colourless crystals. Freely soluble in water; soluble in alcohol. It melts at about 219°. Protect from light.

**Ph. Eur. 5.0** (Ephedrine Hydrochloride, Racemic; Racephedrine Hydrochloride BP 2003). A white, crystalline powder or colourless crystals. Freely soluble in water; soluble in alcohol; practically insoluble in ether. It melts at about 188°. Protect from light.

**USP 27** (Ephedrine Hydrochloride). Fine, white, odourless crystals or powder. Soluble 1 in 3 of water and 1 in 14 of alcohol; insoluble in ether. Protect from light.

## Ephedrine Sulfate

Efedrina, sulfato de; Ephedrine Sulphate (BANM).

$(C_{10}H_{15}NO)_2,H_2SO_4$ = 428.5.

*CAS — 134-72-5.*

*ATC — R01AA03; R01AB05; R03CA02; S01FB02.*

**Pharmacopoeias.** In *Int.* and *US*.

**USP 27** (Ephedrine Sulfate). Fine, white, odourless crystals or powder. It darkens on exposure to light. Soluble 1 in 1.3 of water and 1 in 90 of alcohol. Protect from light.

## Adverse Effects

For the adverse effects of sympathomimetics in general, see under Adrenaline, p.852. The commonest adverse effects of ephedrine are tachycardia, anxiety, restlessness, and insomnia. Tremor, dry mouth, impaired circulation to the extremities, hypertension, and cardiac arrhythmias may also occur.

Ephedrine may be used in labour to maintain blood pressure during spinal anaesthesia but can cause fetal tachycardia.

Paranoid psychosis, delusions, and hallucinations may also follow ephedrine overdosage. Prolonged administration has no cumulative effect, but tolerance with dependence has been reported.

◊ For a discussion of the toxicity reported from the self-administration of ephedrine-containing dietary supplements or herbal stimulants, see under Abuse, below.

## Precautions

For the precautions to be observed with sympathomimetics in general, see under Adrenaline, p.853. Ephedrine should be given with care to patients with hyperthyroidism, diabetes mellitus, ischaemic heart disease, hypertension, renal impairment, or angle-closure glaucoma. In patients with prostatic enlargement, ephedrine may increase difficulty with micturition.

Irritability and disturbed sleep have been reported in breast-fed infants.

**Abuse.** Although illicit use of ephedrine is primarily in the manufacture of street stimulants such as metamfetamine (p.1589), there is increasing evidence of the abuse of ephedrine preparations in some countries,[1] and the public health and social problems associated with its abuse appear to be significant, particularly in certain African countries. Ephedrine is also sold as a street substitute for 'Ecstasy' (Methylenedioxyamfetamine, p.1589).

Adverse effects reported with illicit ephedrine use include cardiovascular toxicity[2,3] and chest pain.[4]

There is controversy over the abuse liability of over-the-counter (OTC) stimulants such as ephedrine:[5] some studies have indicated that ephedrine is, overall, a relatively weak reinforcer whereas others have suggested that the abuse potential may be high. Examination of the characteristics of 5 patients who had been taking ephedrine-containing OTC preparations in high doses for periods ranging from 8 months to 2 years, emphasised the reinforcing and, therefore, addictive potential of ephedrine; similar observations were made for 2 patients who had ingested phenylpropanolamine long term, combined with pseudoephedrine in one of these cases. The authors suggested that, for most people, OTC preparations containing weaker sympathomimetics will not be reinforcing at the recommended doses. However, these cases strengthen the research findings that high-dose use of an OTC stimulant increases its potency, and thus its effects become more like amfetamine (p.1584).

Toxicity has also been reported[6] from the self-administration of ephedrine-containing dietary supplements or herbal stimulants, usually based on ephedra (ma-huang) and marketed for a variety of purposes including weight loss and as an alternative to illegal drugs of abuse. Not all cases of ephedrine toxicity have arisen as a result of overt abuse but rather because of inadequate labelling of content and dosage instructions on some unlicensed products. The use of ephedra-containing dietary supplements is now banned in some countries including the USA.[7]

Adverse effects from ingestion of ephedrine-containing OTC preparations, including herbal products (usually in high doses and/or long term) have included coronary artery thrombosis, myocardial infarction, seizures,[8] psychotic reactions,[9] nephrolithiasis,[10,11] and myocarditis;[12] a number of fatalities have been reported. Frank dependence has been reported in female weightlifters following long-term use of high doses.[13]

For a report of urinary calculi developing in a patient who had ingested a preparation containing guaifenesin and ephedrine, see under Guaifenesin, p.1122.


1. WHO. Recommendations from the Expert Committee on Drug Dependence. *WHO Drug Inf* 1998; **12:** 227–9.
2. Cockings JGL, Brown MA. Ephedrine abuse causing acute myocardial infarction. *Med J Aust* 1997; **167:** 199–200.
3. Zahn KA, *et al.* Cardiovascular toxicity after ingestion of "herbal ecstacy" [sic]. *J Emerg Med* 1999; **17:** 289–91.
4. James LP, *et al.* Sympathomimetic drug use in adolescents presenting to a pediatric emergency department with chest pain. *J Toxicol Clin Toxicol* 1998; **36:** 321–8.
5. Tinsley JA, Watkins DD. Over-the-counter stimulants: abuse and addiction. *Mayo Clin Proc* 1998; **73:** 977–82.
6. Haller CA, Benowitz NL. Adverse cardiovascular and central nervous system events associated with dietary supplements containing ephedra alkaloids. *N Engl J Med* 2000; **343:** 1833–8.
7. US Food and Drug Administration. FDA issues regulation prohibiting sale of dietary supplements containing ephedrine alkaloids and reiterates its advice that consumers stop using these products (issued 6 February 2004). Available at: http://www.cfsan.fda.gov/~lrd/fpephed6.html (accessed 01/07/04)
8. Anonymous. Adverse events associated with ephedrine-containing products—Texas, December 1993-September 1995. *JAMA* 1996; **276:** 1711–12.
9. Doyle H, Kargin M. Herbal stimulant containing ephedrine has also caused psychosis. *BMJ* 1996; **313:** 756.
10. Powell T, *et al.* Ma-huang strikes again: ephedrine nephrolithiasis. *Am J Kidney Dis* 1998; **32:** 153–9.
11. Blau JJ. Ephedrine nephrolithiasis associated with chronic ephedrine abuse. *J Urol (Baltimore)* 1998; **160:** 825.
12. Zaacks SM, *et al.* Hypersensitivity myocarditis associated with ephedra use. *J Toxicol Clin Toxicol* 1999; **37:** 485–9.
13. Gruber AJ, Pope HG. Ephedrine abuse among 36 female weightlifters. *Am J Addict* 1998; **7:** 256–61.


## Interactions

For the interactions of the sympathomimetics in general, see under Adrenaline, p.853. Ephedrine may cause a hypertensive crisis in patients receiving an MAOI (including an RIMA); the possibility of such an interaction following intranasal use of ephedrine should also be borne in mind. See also under Phenelzine (p.314) and Moclobemide (p.308). Ephedrine should be avoided or used with care in patients undergoing anaesthesia with cyclopropane, halothane, or other volatile anaesthetics. An increased risk of arrhythmias may occur if given to patients receiving cardiac glycosides, quinidine, or tricyclic antidepressants, and there is an increased risk of vasoconstrictor or pressor effects in patients receiving ergot alkaloids or oxytocin.

## Pharmacokinetics

Ephedrine is readily and completely absorbed from the gastrointestinal tract. It is largely excreted unchanged in the urine, together with small amounts of metabolites produced by hepatic metabolism. Ephedrine has been variously reported to have a plasma half-life ranging from 3 to 6 hours depending on urinary pH; elimination is enhanced and half-life accordingly shorter in acid urine.

◊ References.


1. Welling PG, *et al.* Urinary excretion of ephedrine in man without pH control following oral administration of three commercial ephedrine sulfate preparations. *J Pharm Sci* 1971; **60:** 1629–34.
2. Sever PS, *et al.* The metabolism of (−)-ephedrine in man. *Eur J Clin Pharmacol* 1975; **9:** 193–8.
3. Pickup ME, *et al.* The pharmacokinetics of ephedrine after oral dosage in asthmatics receiving acute and chronic treatment. *Br J Clin Pharmacol* 1976; **3:** 123–34.


## Uses and Administration

Ephedrine is a sympathomimetic (see Adrenaline, p.854) with direct and indirect effects on adrenergic receptors. It has alpha- and beta-adrenergic activity and has pronounced stimulating effects on the CNS. It has a more prolonged though less potent action than adrenaline. In therapeutic doses it raises the blood pressure by increasing cardiac output and also by inducing peripheral vasoconstriction. Tachycardia may occur but is less frequent than with adrenaline. Ephedrine also causes bronchodilatation, reduces intestinal tone and motility, relaxes the bladder wall while contracting the sphincter muscle but relaxes the detrusor muscle of the bladder and usually reduces the activity of the uterus. It has a stimulant action on the respiratory centre. It dilates the pupil but does not affect the light reflexes. After ephedrine has been used for a short while, tachyphylaxis may develop.

Ephedrine salts are used, either alone or in combination preparations, in the symptomatic relief of nasal congestion (p.1112). They may be given by mouth or topically as nasal drops or sprays. Ephedrine salts have sometimes been used in motion sickness in combination preparations with hyoscine or an antihistamine and have been tried for postoperative nausea and vomiting (p.1245).

Ephedrine salts have been given parenterally to combat a fall in blood pressure during spinal or epidural anaesthesia. Ephedrine is of little value in hypotensive crises due to shock, circulatory collapse, or haemorrhage. It is no longer generally advocated for orthostatic hypotension.

Ephedrine salts have been used as bronchodilators, but the more $beta_2$-selective sympathomimetics, such as salbutamol, are now preferred.

Other uses of ephedrine salts include diabetic neuropathic oedema, in which they may provide marked relief. They have also been used in micturition disorders.

Nasal drops or sprays usually containing ephedrine 0.5 or 1% are used in the treatment of *nasal congestion*; the 0.5% strength may also be used for infants and young children. Ephedrine salts can also be given by oral inhalation.

To *reverse hypotension induced by spinal or epidural anaesthesia*, a solution containing ephedrine hydrochloride 3 mg/mL is given by slow intravenous injection in doses of 3 to 6 mg (or at most 9 mg) repeated every 3 to 4 minutes as required; the maximum total dose is 30 mg. Ephedrine salts have also been given by intramuscular or subcutaneous injection.

The *British National Formulary* suggests a dose of 30 to 60 mg of ephedrine hydrochloride three times daily by mouth in the treatment of *diabetic neuropathic oedema*.

Several other salts of ephedrine have been given including the camsilate, the levulinate, and the tannate. Racephedrine hydrochloride has also been used.

**Micturition disorders.** Ephedrine salts have been used in nocturnal enuresis, although other treatments are usually preferred, and have been tried in patients with stress incontinence but the value of such treatment is not clear.

**Spinal anaesthesia.** Parenteral sympathomimetics such as ephedrine and phenylephrine have been advocated for the correction of hypotension associated with local anaesthesia. The risk of hypotension with spinal or epidural block is greater than many other forms of nerve block (see Adverse Effects of Central Block, p.1367). Ephedrine has been used[1,2] although not always successfully[3] for the correction of such hypotension. It has also been used prophylactically,[4] although adequate hydration of the patient beforehand is more important in minimising hypotension.

1. Hall PA, *et al.* Spinal anaesthesia for Caesarean section: comparison of infusions of phenylephrine and ephedrine. *Br J Anaesth* 1994; **73:** 471–4.
2. Thomas DG, *et al.* Randomized trial of bolus phenylephrine or ephedrine for maintenance of arterial pressure during spinal anaesthesia for Caesarean section. *Br J Anaesth* 1996; **76:** 61–5.
3. Critchley LAH, *et al.* Hypotension during subarachnoid anaesthesia: haemodynamic effects of ephedrine. *Br J Anaesth* 1995; **74:** 373–8.
4. Sternlo J-E, *et al.* Prophylactic im ephedrine in bupivacaine spinal anaesthesia. *Br J Anaesth* 1995; **74:** 517–20.

### Preparations

***BP 2003:*** Ephedrine Elixir; Ephedrine Hydrochloride Tablets; Ephedrine Nasal Drops;
***USP 27:*** Ephedrine Sulfate Capsules; Ephedrine Sulfate Injection; Ephedrine Sulfate Nasal Solution; Ephedrine Sulfate Syrup; Theophylline, Ephedrine Hydrochloride, and Phenobarbital Tablets.

**Proprietary Preparations** (details are given in Part 3)
***Arg.:*** Muchan; ***Belg.:*** Ephedronguent; ***Chile:*** Efedrosan; ***Gr.:*** Neo Rhinovit; Rhinolex; ***Mex.:*** Ephed 20th†; Tendrin; ***UK:*** CAM; ***USA:*** Kondon's Nasal; Pretz-D.
**Multi-ingredient:** numerous preparations are listed in Part 3.

## Eprazinone Hydrochloride *(rINNM)*

CE-746; Hidrocloruro de eprazinona. 3-[4-(β-Ethoxyphenethyl)piperazin-1-yl]-2-methylpropiophenone dihydrochloride.
$C_{24}H_{32}N_2O_2,2HCl = 453.4.$
*CAS — 10402-90-1 (eprazinone); 10402-53-6 (eprazinone hydrochloride).*
*ATC — R05CB04.*

### Profile

Eprazinone hydrochloride has been variously described as having mucolytic or expectorant properties (p.1112) as well as a direct relaxant action on bronchial smooth muscle. It is given by mouth in doses of 50 to 100 mg three times daily. It has also been administered rectally.

**Effects on the skin.** Skin eruptions have been associated with the oral administration of eprazinone.[1]

1. Faber M, *et al.* Eprazinonexanthem mit subkornealer Pustelbildung. *Hautarzt* 1984; **35:** 200–3.

**Overdosage.** Symptoms in two 22-month-old children who received an overdose of 800 mg of eprazinone included somnolence, ataxia, and seizures.[1]

1. Merigot P, *et al.* Les convulsions avec trois antitussifs dérivés substitués de la pipérazine: (zipéprol, éprazinone, éprozinol). *Ann Pediatr (Paris)* 1985; **32:** 504–11.

### Preparations

**Proprietary Preparations** (details are given in Part 3)
***Austria:*** Eftapan; ***Belg.:*** Isilung; ***Fr.:*** Mucitux†; ***Ger.:*** Eftapan.
**Multi-ingredient:** ***Austria:*** Eftapan Tetra.

## Eprozinol Hydrochloride *(rINNM)*

Hidrocloruro de eprozinol. 3-[4-(β-Methoxyphenethyl)piperazin-1-yl]-1-phenylpropan-1-ol dihydrochloride.
$C_{22}H_{30}N_2O_2,2HCl = 427.4.$
*CAS — 32665-36-4 (eprozinol).*
*ATC — R03DX02.*

### Profile

Eprozinol hydrochloride has been given by mouth for its mucolytic or expectorant properties.

**Adverse effects.** Convulsions and coma were reported in a 19-year-old patient following administration of eprozinol.[1]

1. Merigot P, *et al.* Les convulsions avec trois antitussifs dérivés substitués de la pipérazine: (zipéprol, éprazinone, éprozinol). *Ann Pediatr (Paris)* 1985; **32:** 504–11.

### Preparations

**Proprietary Preparations** (details are given in Part 3)
***Fr.:*** Eupneron.

## Erdosteine *(rINN)*

Erdosteína. (±)-({[(Tetrahydro-2-oxo-3-thienyl)carbamoyl]methyl}thio)acetic acid.
$C_8H_{11}NO_4S_2 = 249.3.$
*CAS — 84611-23-4.*
*ATC — R05CB15.*

### Profile

Erdosteine is a mucolytic that is used in the treatment of disorders of the respiratory tract characterised by productive cough (p.1112) It is given by mouth in doses of 300 mg twice daily.

**Chronic obstructive pulmonary disease.** Erdosteine has been used[1,2] in the management of chronic obstructive pulmonary disease (p.779) but the value of mucolytics in this disorder is controversial.

1. Dechant KL, Noble S. Erdosteine. *Drugs* 1996; **52:** 875–81.
2. Marchioni CF, *et al.* Evaluation of efficacy and safety of erdosteine in patients affected by chronic bronchitis during an infective exacerbation phase and receiving amoxycillin as basic treatment (ECOBES, European Chronic Obstructive Bronchitis Erdosteine Study). *Int J Clin Pharmacol Ther* 1995; **33:** 612–18.

### Preparations

**Proprietary Preparations** (details are given in Part 3)
***Arg.:*** Amuctol; Fluidasa; ***Belg.:*** Mucothera; ***Braz.:*** Erdotin; Flusten; ***Chile:*** Biopulmin; ***Fin.:*** Erdopect; ***Fr.:*** Edirel; Vectrine; ***Ital.:*** Erdotin; ***Mex.:*** Dostein; Esteclin; ***Switz.:*** Mucofor.
**Multi-ingredient:** ***Mex.:*** Esteclin Bac.

## Eriodictyon

Hierba santa; Mountain Balm; Yerba Santa.
*CAS — 8013-08-9.*

### Profile

Eriodictyon consists of the dried leaves of *Eriodictyon californicum* (Hydrophyllaceae). It has been used as an expectorant. It has also been used in the treatment of dry mouth and to mask the taste of bitter drugs.

### Preparations

**Proprietary Preparations** (details are given in Part 3)
***Canad.:*** Mouth Kote; ***Hong Kong:*** Pretz.
**Multi-ingredient:** ***Ital.:*** Broncosedina; ***USA:*** Feminease.

## Etafedrine Hydrochloride *(BANM, USAN, rINNM)*

Ethylephedrine Hydrochloride; Hidrocloruro de etafedrina. (−)-2-(Ethylmethylamino)-1-phenylpropan-1-ol hydrochloride.
$C_{12}H_{19}NO,HCl = 229.7.$
*CAS — 7681-79-0 (etafedrine); 48141-64-6 ((−)-etafedrine); 5591-29-7 (etafedrine hydrochloride).*

### Profile

Etafedrine hydrochloride is a sympathomimetic related to ephedrine (p.1120). It is used for its bronchodilator effects in combination preparations for the relief of cough and associated respiratory-tract disorders.

### Preparations

**Proprietary Preparations** (details are given in Part 3)
**Multi-ingredient:** ***Braz.:*** Bronco-Ped†; Broncolex; EMS Expectorante; Revenil; Revenil Dospan; Revenil Expectorante†; ***Canad.:*** Calmydone; Dalmacol; Mercodol with Decapryn†; ***S.Afr.:*** Nethaprin Dospan; Nethaprin Expectorant; ***Thai.:*** Brondil.

## Ethyl Cysteine Hydrochloride

Etilcisteína, hidrocloruro de. Ethyl L-2-amino-3-mercaptopropionate hydrochloride.
$C_5H_{11}NO_2S,HCl = 185.7.$
*CAS — 3411-58-3 (ethyl cysteine); 868-59-7 (ethyl cysteine hydrochloride).*

**Pharmacopoeias.** In *Jpn.*

### Profile

Ethyl cysteine hydrochloride is a mucolytic that has been used in the treatment of disorders of the respiratory tract associated with productive cough.

## Ethyl Orthoformate

Ether de Kay; Triethoxymethane; Trietoximetano. Triethyl orthoformate.
$C_7H_{16}O_3 = 148.2.$
*CAS — 122-51-0.*

**Pharmacopoeias.** In *Fr.*

### Profile

Ethyl orthoformate is a cough suppressant (see p.1112). It is reported to be a respiratory antispasmodic and has been administered by mouth or rectally.

### Preparations

**Proprietary Preparations** (details are given in Part 3)
**Multi-ingredient:** ***Switz.:*** Rectoquintyl-Promethazine†; Rectoquintyl†.

## Fedrilate *(rINN)*

Fedrilato; Fedrilatum; UCB-3928. 1-Methyl-3-morpholinopropyl perhydro-4-phenylpyran-4-carboxylate.
$C_{20}H_{29}NO_4 = 347.4.$
*CAS — 23271-74-1.*
*ATC — R05DB14.*

### Profile

Fedrilate is a cough suppressant used by mouth for non-productive cough.

### Preparations

**Proprietary Preparations** (details are given in Part 3)
***Braz.:*** Gotas Binelli; Sedatoss†; ***S.Afr.:*** Corbar S†.

## Fenoxazoline Hydrochloride *(rINNM)*

Hidrocloruro de fenoxazolina. 2-(2-Isopropylphenoxymethyl)-2-imidazoline hydrochloride.
$C_{13}H_{18}N_2O,HCl = 254.8.$
*CAS — 4846-91-7 (fenoxazoline); 21370-21-8 (fenoxazoline hydrochloride).*
*ATC — R01AA12.*

### Profile

Fenoxazoline hydrochloride is a sympathomimetic with effects similar to those of naphazoline (p.1124) that has been used topically for its vasoconstrictor properties in the symptomatic treatment of nasal congestion.

### Preparations

**Proprietary Preparations** (details are given in Part 3)
***Arg.:*** Nebulicina; ***Braz.:*** Aturgyl.

## Fominoben Hydrochloride *(rINNM)*

Hidrocloruro de fominobén; PB-89. 3′-Chloro-2′-[*N*-methyl-*N*-(morpholinocarbonylmethyl)aminomethyl]benzanilide hydrochloride.
$C_{21}H_{24}ClN_3O_3,HCl = 438.3.$
*CAS — 18053-31-1 (fominoben); 24600-36-0 (fominoben hydrochloride).*

### Profile

Fominoben hydrochloride is a centrally acting cough suppressant (see p.1112) that is also reported to have respiratory stimulant properties. It is given in doses of 160 mg up to three times daily by mouth; it has also been given by slow intravenous injection.

### Preparations

**Proprietary Preparations** (details are given in Part 3)
***Mex.:*** Noleptan; ***Spain:*** Tosifar.

## Fudosteine *(rINN)*

SS-320A. (−)-3-[(3-Hydroxypropyl)thio]-L-alanine.
$C_6H_{13}NO_3S = 179.2.$
*CAS — 13189-98-5.*

### Profile

Fudosteine is an expectorant given orally in a dose of 400 mg three times daily.

### Preparations

**Proprietary Preparations** (details are given in Part 3)
***Jpn:*** Cleanal.

## Glaucine

Boldine Dimethyl Ether; DL-832 (*dl*-glaucine phosphate); Glaucina; *dl*-Glaucine; MDL-832 (*dl*-glaucine phosphate). DL-1,2,9,10-Tetramethoxyaporphine.
$C_{21}H_{25}NO_4 = 355.4.$
*CAS — 5630-11-5 (dl-glaucine); 73239-87-9 (dl-glaucine phosphate); 475-81-0 (d-glaucine); 5996-06-5 (d-glaucine hydrobromide).*

### Profile

Glaucine is a centrally acting cough suppressant used in non-productive cough (p.1112) which has been studied as the phosphate. *d*-Glaucine has been used as the hydrobromide and the hydrochloride as a cough suppressant in eastern Europe. It has been obtained from *Glaucium flavum* (Papaveraceae).

◊ References.

1. Redpath JBS, Pleuvry BJ. Double-blind comparison of the respiratory and sedative effects of codeine phosphate and (±)-glaucine phosphate in human volunteers. *Br J Clin Pharmacol* 1982; **14:** 555–8.
2. Rühle KH, *et al.* Objective evaluation of dextromethorphan and glaucine as antitussive agents. *Br J Clin Pharmacol* 1984; **17:** 521–4.
3. Gastpar H, *et al.*. Efficacy and tolerability of glaucine as an antitussive agent. *Curr Med Res Opin* 1984; **9:** 21–7.
4. Cortijo J, *et al.* Bronchodilator and anti-inflammatory activities of glaucine: in vitro studies in human airway smooth muscle and polymorphonuclear leukocytes. *Br J Pharmacol* 1999; **127:** 1641–51.

## Guacetisal *(rINN)*

Acetylsalicylic Acid Guaiacol Ester. *o*-Methoxyphenyl salicylate acetate.
$C_{16}H_{14}O_5 = 286.3.$
*CAS — 55482-89-8.*
*ATC — N02BA14.*

### Profile

Guacetisal has been used in respiratory disorders as an expectorant (see p.1112). It has also been used as an antipyretic to reduce fever (p.8). It has been administered by mouth and rectally.

### Preparations

**Proprietary Preparations** (details are given in Part 3)
***Ital.:*** Guaiaspir†; Guajabronc†; Prontomucil.

## Guaiacol

Guajacol; Guayacol; Methyl Catechol.

*CAS — 90-05-1 (guaiacol); 553-17-3 (guaiacol carbonate); 60296-02-8 (calcium guaiacolglycolate); 4112-89-4 (guaiacol phenylacetate).*

**Pharmacopoeias.** In *Fr.* and *Swiss. Fr.* also includes guaiacol carbonate.

### Profile

Guaiacol has disinfectant properties and has been used as an expectorant for productive cough (p.1112). The main constituent of guaiacol is 2-methoxyphenol, $CH_3O.C_6H_4.OH$ = 124.1.

Adverse effects are similar to those of phenol (p.1188).

A wide range of salts and derivatives of guaiacol have been used similarly including the carbonate, cinnamate, ethylglycolate, calcium and sodium glycolates, phenylacetate, and phenylbutyrate. See also Guaifenesin, p.1122 and Sulfogaiacol, p.1131.

### Preparations

**Proprietary Preparations** (details are given in Part 3)
***Ger.:*** Anastil†.

**Multi-ingredient: *Arg.:*** Aseptobron; Atomo Desinflamante Familiar; ***Belg.:*** Baume Dalet†; Eucalyptine Pholcodine Le Brun; ***Braz.:*** Axol†; Bac Septin Balsamico†; Canfomenol†; Durapen Balsamico†; Egotussano; Eucalyptine†; Massubal†; Ozonyl; Transpulmin; Transpulmin Balsamo; Tripulmin Balsamico; Tripulmin†; Yatropan†; ***Canad.:*** Analgesic Balm†; Creo-Rectal; Demo-Cineol; Dentalgar†; Gouttes Dentaires†; Omni-Tuss; Pastilles Valda†; Sedatuss†; Valda; ***Fr.:*** Baume Dalet†; Bi-Qui-Nol†; Bronchorectine au Citral; Campho-Pneumine†; Essence Algerienne; Gaiarsol†; Pulmo Bailly; Pulmoserum; Rectophedrol†; Sirop Boin†; Valda; ***Ger.:*** Dalet Med Balsam; ***Hong Kong:*** Biocalyptol; Valda; ***Irl.:*** Pulmo Bailly†; Valda; ***Ital.:*** Eugenol-Guaiacolo Composto; Fosfoguaiacol; Lactocol; Lipobalsamo; Resina Carbolica Dentilin†; ***Mex.:*** Eucalin; Guayalin-Plus; Yadegal Compuesto; ***Mon.:*** Bronchodermine; ***Port.:*** Analgil; Valda; ***Spain:*** Bronco Aseptilex Fuerte; Bronco Aseptilex†; Bronquimar Vit A†; Bronquimar†; Edusan Fte Rectal†; Eucalyptospirine; Eucalyptospirine Lact†; Maboterpen†; Pulmo Grey Balsam†; Tos Mai; ***Switz.:*** Liberol†; Rectoseptal-Neo Pholcodine†; Spirogel†; ***UK:*** Dragon Balm; Pulmo Bailly; ***USA:*** Methagual.

## Guaietolin *(rINN)*

Glycerylguethol; Glyguetol; Guayetolina. 3-(2-Ethoxyphenoxy)propane-1,2-diol.

$C_{11}H_{16}O_4$ = 212.2.

*CAS — 63834-83-3.*

### Profile

Guaietolin is an analogue of guaifenesin which is used as an expectorant (see p.1112). It has been given by mouth in doses of 300 to 600 mg two or three times daily.

### Preparations

**Proprietary Preparations** (details are given in Part 3)
***Fr.:*** Guethural.

## Guaifenesin *(BAN, USAN, rINN)*

Glyceryl Guaiacolate; Glycerylguayacolum; Guaiacol Glycerol Ether; Guaiacyl Glyceryl Ether; Guaifenesina; Guaifenesinum; Guaiphenesin; Guajacolum Glycerolatum. (RS)-3-(2-Methoxyphenoxy)propane-1,2-diol.

$C_{10}H_{14}O_4$ = 198.2.

*CAS — 93-14-1.*

*ATC — R05CA03.*

**Pharmacopoeias.** In *Eur.* (see p.vi), *Jpn*, and *US*.

**Ph. Eur. 5.0** (Guaifenesin). A white or almost white, crystalline powder. Sparingly soluble in water; soluble in alcohol.

**USP 27** (Guaifenesin). A white to slightly grey crystalline powder. May have a slight characteristic odour. Soluble 1 in 60 to 70 of water; soluble in alcohol, in chloroform, and in propylene glycol; sparingly soluble in glycerol. Store in airtight containers.

### Adverse Effects and Precautions

Gastrointestinal discomfort, nausea, and vomiting have occasionally been reported with guaifenesin, particularly in very large doses.

**Abuse.** Urinary calculi have been reported in patients consuming large quantities of over-the-counter preparations containing guaifenesin.[1,2] Spectroscopic analysis[1] revealed that the stones were composed of a calcium salt of beta-(2-methoxyphenoxy)-lactic acid, which is a metabolite of guaifenesin. Small quantities of ephedrine were also present in the stones of one of several patients who had ingested preparations containing a combination of guaifenesin and ephedrine.[2]

1. Pickens CL, *et al.* Abuse of guaifenesin-containing medications generates an excess of a carboxylate salt of beta-(2-methoxyphenoxy)-lactic acid, a guaifenesin metabolite, and results in urolithiasis. *Urology* 1999; **54:** 23–7.
2. Assimos DG, *et al.* Guaifenesin- and ephedrine-induced stones. *J Endourol* 1999; **13:** 665–7.

**Porphyria.** Guaifenesin is considered to be unsafe in patients with porphyria because it has been shown to be porphyrinogenic in *animals*.

### Pharmacokinetics

Guaifenesin is absorbed from the gastrointestinal tract. It is metabolised and then excreted in the urine.

### Uses and Administration

Guaifenesin is reported to increase the volume and reduce the viscosity of tenacious sputum and is used as an expectorant for productive cough. It is given by mouth in doses of 200 to 400 mg every 4 hours. Modified-release preparations, given every 12 hours, are also available. Children may be given the following doses every 4 hours by mouth, depending on age:

- 6 to 12 years, 100 to 200 mg
- 2 to 6 years, 50 to 100 mg
- 6 months to 2 years, 25 to 50 mg

Guaifenesin has been used similarly as the calcium salt.

**Respiratory disorders.** An FDA review of preparations available 'over-the-counter' concluded that guaifenesin was an effective expectorant.[1] The use of expectorants for productive cough is discussed on p.1112.

1. Thomas J. Guaiphenesin—an old drug now found to be effective. *Aust J Pharm* 1990; **71:** 101–3.

### Preparations

**USP 27:** Dyphylline and Guaifenesin Elixir; Dyphylline and Guaifenesin Tablets; Guaifenesin and Codeine Phosphate Syrup; Guaifenesin and Pseudoephedrine Hydrochloride Capsules; Guaifenesin Capsules; Guaifenesin Syrup; Guaifenesin Tablets; Guaifenesin, Pseudoephedrine Hydrochloride, and Dextromethorphan Hydrobromide Capsules; Theophylline and Guaifenesin Capsules; Theophylline and Guaifenesin Oral Solution.

**Proprietary Preparations** (details are given in Part 3)
***Arg.:*** Omega 100 Bronquial; Plenum; Robitussin; Vick 44 Exp; ***Austral.:*** Lemsip Chesty Cough†; Robitussin EX; Vicks Cough Syrup for Chesty Coughs; ***Austria:*** Guafen; Myoscain; Resyl; Wick Formel 44 Plus Husten-loser; ***Belg.:*** Vicks Vaposyrup Expectorant; ***Braz.:*** Vick Xarope; ***Canad.:*** Balminil Expectorant; Benylin-E; Calmylin Expectorant; Cough Syrup Expectorant; Expectorant Cough Formula; Expectorant Cough Syrup; Expectorant Syrup†; Extra Strength Cough Syrup Expectorant; Koffex Expectorant; Robitussin; Sirop Expectorant; Tussin Expectorant; Vicks Chest Congestion Relief; ***Fin.:*** Tintus; ***Fr.:*** Vicks Expectorant; ***Ger.:*** Fagusan†; Wick Formel 44 Husten-Loser; Wick Kinder Formel 44 Husten-Loser†; ***Hong Kong:*** Breacol; Excough; Robitussin Expectorant; Uni-Colex; ***Irl.:*** Benylin Childrens Chesty Coughs; Robitussin Chesty Cough; Tixylix Chesty Cough; ***Israel:*** Bronchocal†; Resyl; Robitussin; Vitussin; ***Ital.:*** Broncovanil; Idropulmina†; Resyl; Vicks Tosse Fluidificante; ***Malaysia:*** Fuston; ***Mex.:*** 44 Exp; Formula E†; Robitussin; Tukol; ***NZ:*** Actifed CC Chesty; Lemsip Chesty Cough; Robitussin EX; ***S.Afr.:*** Actospect; Expelinct; ***Singapore:*** Breacol; Robitussin; ***Spain:*** Fluidin†; Formulaexpec; Lactocol Expectorante†; Robitussin; ***Swed.:*** Resyl; ***Switz.:*** Bronchol; Resyl; Vicks Formule 44 Expectine; ***Thai.:*** Robitussin; Tussa; ***UK:*** Adult Chesty Cough Non Drowsy; Benylin Childrens Chesty Coughs; Boots Chesty Cough Syrup 1 Year Plus; Do-Do Expectorant Linctus†; Expectorant Cough Syrup; Expulin Chesty Cough†; Famel Expectorant†; Hill's Balsam Chesty Cough; Jackson's All Fours; Jackson's Bronchial Balsam; Nurse Sykes Balsam†; Owbridges for Chesty Coughs†; Robitussin for Chesty Coughs; Tixylix Chesty Cough; Venos for Kids; Vicks Vaposyrup for Chesty Coughs; ***USA:*** Allfen; Anti-Tuss; Breonesin†; Diabetic Tussin EX†; Duratuss G†; Fenesin; Ganidin NR; Gee-Gee†; Genatuss†; Glyate†; Glycotuss; Glytuss†; Guaifenex G; Guaifenex LA; Guiatuss; Halotussin; Humavent; Hytuss; Liquibid; Monafed†; Mucinex; Muco-Fen; Muco-Fen-LA†; Mytussin†; Naldecon Senior EX†; Organidin NR; Pneumomist†; Refenesen; Respa-GF†; Robitussin; Scot-Tussin Expectorant; Siltussin; Sinumist-SR†; Touro Ex; Tusibron; Uni-tussin†.

**Multi-ingredient:** numerous preparations are listed in Part 3.

## Guaimesal *(rINN)*

(±)-2-(*o*-Methoxyphenoxy)-2-methyl-1,3-benzodioxan-4-one.

$C_{16}H_{14}O_5$ = 286.3.

*CAS — 81674-79-5.*

### Profile

Guaimesal is reported to have expectorant and antipyretic properties and has been given by mouth as an adjunct in the treatment of respiratory-tract disorders. It has also been administered rectally in suppositories.

### Preparations

**Proprietary Preparations** (details are given in Part 3)
***Ital.:*** Bronteril†.

## Guethol

Guetol. 2-Ethoxyphenol.

$C_8H_{10}O_2$ = 138.2.

*CAS — 94-71-3.*

### Profile

Guethol has been used as the carbonate as an expectorant for productive cough (p.1112); the nicotinate has also been used in respiratory-tract disorders.

### Preparations

**Proprietary Preparations** (details are given in Part 3)
**Multi-ingredient: *Fr.:*** Bronchospray†.

## Helicidine

Helicidina; Helixinum.

### Profile

Helicidine is a mucoglycoprotein from the snail *Helix pomatia* that has been used as a cough suppressant.

◊ References.

1. Pons F, *et al.* L'effect bronchorelaxant de l'helicidine, un extrait d'Helix pomatia, fait intervenir une liberation de prostaglandine E2. *Pathol Biol (Paris)* 1999; **47:** 73–80.

### Preparations

**Proprietary Preparations** (details are given in Part 3)
**Multi-ingredient: *Ger.:*** Original Schneckensirup.

## Indanazoline Hydrochloride *(rINNM)*

Hidrocloruro de indanazolina.

$C_{12}H_{15}N_3,HCl$ = 237.7.

*CAS — 56601-85-5.*

### Profile

Indanazoline is a sympathomimetic with effects similar to those of naphazoline (p.1124). It has been used as the hydrochloride for its vasoconstrictor effect in the management of nasal congestion (p.1112). It has been given as nasal drops, a nasal gel, or a nasal spray in a concentration equivalent to indanazoline 0.1%.

### Preparations

**Proprietary Preparations** (details are given in Part 3)
***Ger.:*** Farial.

## Iodinated Glycerol *(BAN, USAN)*

Glicerol iodado; Iodopropylidene Glycerol.

$C_6H_{11}IO_3$ = 258.1.

*CAS — 5634-39-9.*

### Profile

Iodinated glycerol, a methyl derivative of domiodol (p.1119), is an isomeric mixture of iodinated dimers of glycerol. It has been used as an expectorant. The limitations of iodides as expectorants are discussed under Cough on p.1112. The actions of iodides and iodine compounds are discussed under Iodine p.1598. Prolonged use of iodinated glycerol has been associated with hypothyroidism and severe skin eruptions; gastrointestinal disturbances and hypersensitivity reactions have also occurred. Malignant neoplasms have developed in *animals* given iodinated glycerol.

**Chronic obstructive pulmonary disease.** Studies[1-3] of the use of iodinated glycerol in patients with chronic bronchitis have produced conflicting results. The use of mucolytics or expectorants in chronic obstructive pulmonary disease (p.779) is controversial.

1. Petty TL. The National Mucolytic Study: results of a randomized, double-blind, placebo-controlled study of iodinated glycerol in chronic obstructive bronchitis. *Chest* 1990; **97:** 75–83.
2. Repsher LH. Treatment of stable chronic bronchitis with iodinated glycerol: a double-blind, placebo-controlled trial. *J Clin Pharmacol* 1993; **33:** 856–60.
3. Rubin BK, *et al.* Iodinated glycerol has no effect on pulmonary function, symptom score, or sputum properties in patients with stable chronic bronchitis. *Chest* 1996; **109:** 348–52.

**Effects on the thyroid gland.** Thyroid dysfunction (both hyperthyroidism and hypothyroidism) has developed after giving iodinated glycerol to previously euthyroid patients. It was recommended that baseline thyroid function tests should be carried out before starting treatment with iodinated glycerol;[1] it should be withdrawn if abnormal results are obtained during use.

1. Gittoes NJL, Franklyn JA. Drug-induced thyroid disorders. *Drug Safety* 1995; **13:** 46–55.

### Preparations

**Proprietary Preparations** (details are given in Part 3)
***USA:*** Iophen; Par Glycerol; R-Gen.

**Multi-ingredient: *Ital.:*** Golamed Oral†; Mucantil†; ***Spain:*** Mucorama TS†; Mucorama†.

# Ipecacuanha

Ipecac; Ipecacuana; Ipecacuanha Root; Ipecacuanhae Radix.

*CAS — 8012-96-2.*

*ATC — R05CA04; V03AB01.*

**Pharmacopoeias.** In *Eur.* (see p.vi), *Int.*, *Jpn*, *Pol.*, and *US*.
*Eur.*, *Jpn*, and *US* also include a monograph for Prepared Ipecacuanha or a similar standardised form.

**Ph. Eur. 5.0** (Ipecacuanha Root; Ipecacuanha BP 2003). It consists of the fragmented and dried underground organs of *Cephaelis ipecacuanha* known as Matto Grosso ipecacuanha, or of *C. acuminata* known as Costa Rica ipecacuanha, or a mixture of both species. It contains not less than 2.0% of total alkaloids, calculated as emetine. It has a slight odour. Store in airtight containers. Protect from light.

The BP 2003 directs that when Ipecacuanha, Ipecacuanha Root, or Powdered Ipecacuanha is prescribed or demanded, Prepared Ipecacuanha shall be dispensed or supplied.

**Ph. Eur. 5.0** (Ipecacuanha, Prepared; Ipecacuanhae Pulvis Normatus). It is ipecacuanha root powder adjusted to an alkaloidal content of 1.9 to 2.1% of total alkaloids, calculated as emetine. Store in airtight containers. Protect from light.

**USP 27** (Ipecac). The dried rhizome and roots of *Cephaelis acuminata* or of *C. ipecacuanha* (Rubiaceae). It yields not less than 2% of ether-soluble alkaloids of which not less than 90% is emetine and cephaeline; the content of cephaeline varies from an amount equal to, to an amount not more than 2.5 times, that of emetine.

**USP 27** (Powdered Ipecac). It contains 1.9 to 2.1% of ether-soluble alkaloids, with emetine and cephaeline content as for Ipecacuanha. It is pale brown, weak yellow, or light olive-grey powder that should be stored in airtight containers.

## Adverse Effects

Large doses of ipecacuanha have an irritant effect on the gastrointestinal tract, and persistent bloody vomiting or bloody diarrhoea may occur. Mucosal erosions of the entire gastrointestinal tract have been reported. The absorption of emetine, which is most likely if vomiting does not occur after the administration of emetic doses of ipecacuanha, may give rise to adverse effects on the heart, such as conduction abnormalities or myocardial infarction. These, combined with dehydration due to vomiting may cause vasomotor collapse followed by death.

There have been several reports of chronic abuse of ipecacuanha to induce vomiting in eating disorders; cardiotoxicity and myopathy have occurred and may be a result of accumulation of emetine.

There have also been several reports of ipecacuanha poisoning due to the unwitting substitution of Ipecac Fluidextract (a former USP preparation) for Ipecac Syrup (USP); the fluidextract was about 14 times the strength of the syrup.

◊ References.

1. Manno BR, Manno JE. Toxicology of ipecac: a review. *Clin Toxicol* 1977; **10:** 221–42.

**Hypersensitivity.** Allergy, characterised by rhinitis, conjunctivitis, and chest tightness, has occurred due to inhalation of ipecacuanha dust in packers of ipecacuanha tablets.[1]

1. Luczynska CM, *et al.* Occupational allergy due to inhalation of ipecacuanha dust. *Clin Allergy* 1984; **14:** 169–75.

**Vomiting.** Prolonged vomiting has been reported in 17% of patients given ipecacuanha in the treatment of poisoning and may lead to gastric rupture, Mallory-Weiss tears of the oesophagogastric junction, cerebrovascular events, and pneumomediastinum and pneumoperitoneum.[1]

1. Bateman DN. Adverse reactions to antidotes. *Adverse Drug React Bull* 1988; **133:** (Dec.): 496–9.

## Treatment of Adverse Effects

After acute overdose of ipecacuanha, activated charcoal is given to delay absorption followed if necessary by gastric lavage. Prolonged vomiting may be controlled by the injection of antiemetics. Fluid and electrolyte imbalance should be corrected and facilities should be available to correct any cardiac effects and subsequent shock.

After the withdrawal of ipecacuanha following chronic abuse, recovery may be prolonged due to the slow elimination of emetine.

## Precautions

The use of emetics is now rarely favoured; in particular, ipecacuanha should not be used as an emetic in patients who are unconscious or whose condition otherwise increases the risk of aspiration, nor in patients who have taken substances, such as corrosive compounds or petroleum products, that might be especially dangerous if aspirated. Ipecacuanha should not be given to patients in shock or to those at risk from seizures either as a result of their condition or from compounds, such as strychnine, that have been ingested. Patients with cardiovascular disorders are at risk if ipecacuanha is absorbed.

**Abuse.** Ipecac Syrup has been abused by patients with eating disorders to induce vomiting.[1] Adverse effects of repeated vomiting, such as metabolic complications, aspiration pneumonitis, parotid enlargement, dental abnormalities, and oesophagitis or haematemesis due to mucosal lacerations (the Mallory-Weiss syndrome) may be observed. Cardiotoxicity may occur and fatalities have been reported including one patient who had ingested 90 to 120 mL of ipecac syrup daily for 3 months.[2] It has been suggested that cardiac effects and myopathy following the prolonged abuse of Ipecac Syrup may be due to the long-term accumulation of emetine[3,4] but some have expressed doubts.[5]

Cardiomyopathy has also been reported in children given ipecacuanha to produce factitious illness (Munchausen's syndrome by proxy);[6,7] fatalities have occurred.

1. Harris RT. Bulimarexia and related serious eating disorders with medical complications. *Ann Intern Med* 1983; **99:** 800–7.
2. Adler AG, *et al.* Death resulting from ipecac syrup poisoning. *JAMA* 1980; **243:** 1927–8.
3. Palmer EP, Guay AT. Reversible myopathy secondary to abuse of ipecac in patients with major eating disorders. *N Engl J Med* 1985; **313:** 1457–9.
4. Pope HG, *et al.* The epidemiology of ipecac abuse. *N Engl J Med* 1986; **314:** 245–6.
5. Isner JM. Effects of ipecac on the heart. *N Engl J Med* 1986; **314:** 1253.
6. Goebel J, *et al.* Cardiomyopathy from ipecac administration in Munchausen syndrome by proxy. *Pediatrics* 1993; **92:** 601–3.
7. Schneider DJ, *et al.* Clinical and pathologic aspects of cardiomyopathy from ipecac administration in Munchausen's syndrome by proxy. *Pediatrics* 1996; **97:** 902–6.

## Interactions

The action of ipecacuanha may be delayed or diminished if it is given with or after charcoal; antiemetics may also diminish its effect.

**Food.** Concomitant administration of milk had been believed to impair the emetic efficacy of ipecacuanha but there was no significant difference in the time to onset of vomiting, the duration of vomiting, or the number of episodes in 250 children who were given ipecac syrup with milk compared with 250 given ipecac syrup with clear fluids.[1]

1. Klein-Schwartz W, *et al.* The effect of milk on ipecac-induced emesis. *J Toxicol Clin Toxicol* 1991; **29:** 505–11.

## Uses and Administration

Ipecacuanha has been used as an **expectorant** in productive cough (p.1112) in doses of up to about 1.4 mg of total alkaloids.

Ipecacuanha may also be used in larger doses as an **emetic** but is of very limited value (see below). Vomiting usually occurs within 30 minutes of administration by mouth of an emetic dose due to an irritant effect on the gastrointestinal tract and a central action on the chemoreceptor trigger zone. Doses are usually followed by a copious drink of water or fruit juice; in young children this may be given before the dose. Adults have been given doses of 21 to 42 mg of total alkaloids; children aged 6 months to 1 year have been given 7 to 14 mg of total alkaloids and older children 21 mg. Each 5 mL of Paediatric Ipecacuanha Emetic Mixture (BP 2003) or of Ipecac Syrup (USP 27) supplies 7 mg of total alkaloids. Doses may be repeated once only after 20 to 30 minutes if emesis has not occurred.

Ipecacuanha (Ipeca) is used in homoeopathic medicine.

**Emesis induction in acute poisoning.** Standard practice in the management of acute poisoning (p.1030) has varied widely, with different procedures favoured at different times and in different countries. However, measures to reduce absorption of the toxic substance, such as stomach emptying, have often been advocated.

Two techniques of stomach emptying have been very widely employed: gastric lavage; and emesis induction, with ipecacuanha as the emetic of choice. Neither technique is without hazard and the dangers of attempting to empty the stomach have to be balanced against the toxicity of the ingested poison. If the patient presents late or the risk of toxicity is small, then gastric emptying is unnecessary.

- **Gastric lavage** is not recommended in the routine management of poisoned patients[1] because there is little evidence from experimental studies that it improves the clinical outcome and it may cause significant morbidity. *It should only be considered if a potentially life-threatening amount of toxic substance has been ingested within the preceding hour.* There is significant danger of aspiration of stomach contents associated with the procedure and it should only be attempted in fully conscious patients with good airway protective reflexes, unless other means are undertaken to protect the airway. Gastric lavage is also contra-indicated if corrosive or petroleum products have been ingested. There is also a risk that the procedure may propel stomach contents beyond the pylorus and thus enhance absorption in some cases.[2]
- Induction of **emesis** with ipecacuanha has often been advocated for use in children, in whom gastric lavage may be particularly traumatic; it has also been used in adults. However, like gastric lavage, its routine use is not recommended in the management of poisoned patients[3] because there is no clear evidence from clinical studies that it improves the outcome; clinically significant absorption may not be prevented even if it is administered within 1 hour of the ingested poison. It may also delay the administration or reduce the effectiveness of activated charcoal or oral antidotes. Ipecacuanha should not be administered to patients with compromised airway relexes, nor following ingestion of corrosive or petroleum products. In addition it should be avoided in debilitated or elderly patients, or those with medical conditions that may be compromised by induction of emesis. *It may be considered if a potentially life-threatening amount of toxic substance has been ingested within the preceding hour, and if gastric lavage or administration of activated charcoal are deemed inappropriate.*

Because of the limitations of both methods of gastric emptying, a number of studies have addressed the question of whether either is appropriate. Such studies have indicated that the use of activated charcoal alone to prevent absorption, without gastric emptying, is as effective as a combination of both methods.[4-6]

1. American Academy of Clinical Toxicology, European Association of Poisons Centres and Clinical Toxicologists. Position statement: gastric lavage. *Clin Toxicol* 1997; **35:** 711–19.
2. Saetta JP, *et al.* Gastric emptying procedures in the self-poisoned patient: are we forcing gastric content beyond the pylorus? *J R Soc Med* 1991; **84:** 274–6.
3. American Academy of Clinical Toxicology, European Association of Poisons Centres and Clinical Toxicologists. Position statement: ipecac syrup. *Clin Toxicol* 1997; **35:** 699–709.
4. Albertson TE, *et al.* Superiority of activated charcoal alone compared with ipecac and activated charcoal in the treatment of acute toxic ingestions. *Ann Emerg Med* 1989; **18:** 56–9.
5. Merigian KS, *et al.* Prospective evaluation of gastric emptying in the self-poisoned patient. *Am J Emerg Med* 1990; **8:** 479–83.
6. Pond SM, *et al.* Gastric emptying in acute overdose: a prospective randomised controlled trial. *Med J Aust* 1995; **163:** 345–9.

## Preparations

***BP 2003:*** Paediatric Ipecacuanha Emetic Mixture;
***Ph. Eur.:*** Ipecacuanha Liquid Extract, Standardised; Ipecacuanha Tincture, Standardised;
***USP 27:*** Ipecac Syrup.

**Proprietary Preparations** (details are given in Part 3)
***Austria:*** Ipetitrin; ***Fin.:*** Ipeca; ***Gr.:*** Ipecavom; ***Switz.:*** Orpec†; ***UK:*** Jacksons Little Healers.

**Multi-ingredient:** ***Arg.:*** Cobenzil Compuesto; No-Tos Infantil; ***Belg.:*** Folcodex†; Phenergan Expectorant†; Solucamphre†; ***Braz.:*** Agrimel†; Expec; Expectomel; Fenergan Expectorante; Iodesin; Iodobec†; Iodopulmin†; Ipecol; KI-Expectorante; Melagriao†; Pectoss†; Pilulas Ross; Tosseina†; Tussol†; Tussucalman†; Xarope Comp Mel e Agriao†; Xarope Grindelia de Oliveira Junior†; ***Canad.:*** Bronchisaft†; ***Fr.:*** Elixir Contre La Toux Weleda†; Humex; Sirop Pectoral adulte†; ***Hong Kong:*** Pectoral; ***Irl.:*** Ipesil†; Venos Honey & Lemon; ***Israel:*** Doveri; Laxative Comp; Promethazine Expectorants; Prothiazine Expectorant; ***Neth.:*** Abdijsiroop (Akker-Siroop)†; ***Port.:*** Fluidin Adulto†; Fluidin Antiasmatico†; ***S.Afr.:*** Linctus Tussi Infans; ***Spain:*** Alofedina; Buco Regis; Encialina; Fenergan Expectorante; Pectoral Brum†; Toscal Compuesto†; Toscal†; Tuselin Expectorante†; ***Switz.:*** Aloinophen†; Bromocod N; Bronchalin†; Bronchofluid†; Cimex Sirop contre la toux†; Demo elixir pectoral N; Demo gouttes contre la toux†; Demo pates pectorales†; Demo sirop contre la toux†; Gouttes contre la toux "S"; Neo-Codion N; Pastilles pectorales Demo N; Phenergan Expectorant†; Sirop antitussif Wyss a base de codeine†; Sirop Wyss contre la toux†; Spedro†; Thymodrosin†; ***Thai.:*** Diolin†; ***UK:*** Allens Dry Tickly Cough; Allens Pine & Honey; Asthma & Catarrh Relief; Beehive Balsam; Bronchial Mixture†; Buttercup Infant Cough Syrup; Buttercup Syrup (Blackcurrant flavour)†; Buttercup Syrup (Honey and Lemon flavour); Cough-eeze†; ES Bronchial Mixture†; Galloway's Cough Syrup; Hill's Balsam Chesty Cough for Children; Hill's Balsam Chesty Cough Pastilles; Hill's Balsam Extra Strong; Honey & Molasses; Jackson's Troublesome Coughs; Kilkof; Lockets Medicated Linctus; Modern Herbals Cough Mixture; Potters Children's Cough Pastilles; Vegetable Cough Remover; ***USA:*** Poison Antidote Kit; Quelidrine; Tusquelin†.

## Isoaminile *(BAN, rINN)*

Isoaminilo. 4-Dimethylamino-2-isopropyl-2-phenylpentanonitrile.

$C_{16}H_{24}N_2$ = 244.4.
*CAS — 77-51-0.*
*ATC — R05DB04.*

## Isoaminile Citrate *(BANM, rINNM)*

Citrato de isoaminilo. 4-Dimethylamino-2-isopropyl-2-phenylvaleronitrile dihydrogen citrate.

$C_{16}H_{24}N_2,C_6H_8O_7$ = 436.5.
*CAS — 126-10-3; 28416-66-2.*
*ATC — R05DB04.*

### Profile

Isoaminile is a centrally acting cough suppressant that has actions and uses similar to dextromethorphan hydrobromide (p.1117). Isoaminile has usually been given by mouth as the citrate but the cyclamate has also been used.

### Preparations

**Proprietary Preparations** (details are given in Part 3)
***Austria:*** Peracon†; ***Gr.:*** Peracon; ***S.Afr.:*** Peracon.

**Multi-ingredient:** ***S.Afr.:*** Peracon Expectorant.

## Letosteine *(pINN)*

Letosteína. 2-[2-(Ethoxycarbonylmethylthio)ethyl]thiazolidine-4-carboxylic acid.

$C_{10}H_{17}NO_4S_2$ = 279.4.
*CAS — 53943-88-7.*
*ATC — R05CB09.*

### Profile

Letosteine is a mucolytic that has been used in the treatment of respiratory disorders associated with productive cough (p.1112) in a dose of 50 mg by mouth two or three times daily.

### Preparations

**Proprietary Preparations** (details are given in Part 3)
***Fr.:*** Viscotiol†; ***Ital.:*** Letofort†; Viscotiol†; ***Spain:*** Broluidan.

## Levmetamfetamine (USAN, rINN)

*l*-Deoxyephedrine; L-Desoxyephedrine; Lesoxyephedrine; Levometanfetamina; *l*-Methamphetamine; *l*-Methylamphetamine. (R)-N,α-Dimethylbenzeneethanamine; (−)-(R)-N,α-Dimethylphenethylamine.

$C_{10}H_{15}N = 149.2$.

*CAS — 33817-09-3.*

**Pharmacopoeias.** In *US.*

**USP 27** (Levmetamfetamine). A clear, practically colourless, liquid. Store in airtight containers. Protect from light.

### Profile

Levmetamfetamine is the *laevo* isomer of metamfetamine (p.1589) and is used topically in the treatment of nasal congestion (p.1112).

### Preparations

**Proprietary Preparations** (details are given in Part 3)
***USA:*** Vicks Vapor Inhaler.

## Levopropoxyphene Napsilate (BANM, rINNM)

29866; Levopropoxyphene Napsylate (USAN); Napsilato de levopropoxifeno. (1R,2S)-1-Benzyl-3-dimethylamino-2-methyl-1-phenylpropyl propionate naphthalene-2-sulphonate monohydrate.

$C_{22}H_{29}NO_2,C_{10}H_8O_3S,H_2O = 565.7$.

*CAS — 2338-37-6 (levopropoxyphene); 5714-90-9 (anhydrous levopropoxyphene napsilate); 55557-30-7 (levopropoxyphene napsilate monohydrate).*

### Profile

Levopropoxyphene napsilate has been used as a centrally acting cough suppressant for non-productive cough (p.1112). Unlike the dextro-isomer, dextropropoxyphene, levopropoxyphene has little or no analgesic activity. It has also been given as the dibudinate.

## Marrubium

Andornkraut; Herba Marrubii; Marrubio; White Horehound.

**Pharmacopoeias.** In *Fr.*

### Profile

Marrubium is the flower or leaf of *Marrubium vulgare* (Labiatae). It has been used for its supposed expectorant properties in herbal preparations for the treatment of cough. It has also been used as a flavouring.

### Preparations

**Proprietary Preparations** (details are given in Part 3)
***Ger.:*** Angocin Bronchialtropfen.

**Multi-ingredient:** ***Austral.:*** Verbascum Complex†; ***Austria:*** Asthmatee EF-EM-ES; Gallen- und Lebertee EF-EM-ES; Neuners Krautertee Nr 28 - zur Unterstutzung der Tatigkeit der Galle; Neuners Krautertee Nr 7 - Bronchial- und Lungentee; St Radegunder Leber-Galle-Tee; ***Canad.:*** Herbal Throat; Swiss Herb Cough Drops; ***Chile:*** Fucus Compuesto; ***Fr.:*** Elixir Contre La Toux Weleda†; Marrubene Codethyline†; Tisanes de l'Abbe Hamon no 15†; Tossarel†; ***Ital.:*** Broncosedina; ***Spain:*** Natusor Asmaten; Natusor Broncopul; Stomosan†; ***Switz.:*** Hederix; ***UK:*** Allens Chesty Cough; Asthma & Catarrh Relief; Catarrh Tablets†; Catarrh-eeze; Catarrh†; Chest Mixture; Cough-eeze†; Herb and Honey Cough Elixir; Honey & Molasses; Horehound and Aniseed Cough Mixture; Modern Herbals Cough Mixture; Vegetable Cough Remover.

## Mecysteine Hydrochloride (BANM, rINNM)

Hidrocloruro de mecisteína; Methyl Cysteine Hydrochloride; Methylcysteine Hydrochloride. Methyl L-2-amino-3-mercaptopropionate hydrochloride.

$C_4H_9NO_2S,HCl = 171.6$.

*CAS — 2485-62-3 (mecysteine); 18598-63-5 (mecysteine hydrochloride); 5714-80-7 (mecysteine hydrochloride).*

### Adverse Effects and Precautions

Nausea and heartburn have occasionally been reported. Since mucolytics may disrupt the gastric mucosal barrier mecysteine hydrochloride should be used with caution in patients with a history of peptic ulcer disease.

### Uses and Administration

Mecysteine hydrochloride is used as a mucolytic in respiratory disorders associated with productive cough (p.1112). It is given by mouth in a usual dose of 200 mg three times daily before meals reduced to 200 mg twice daily after 6 weeks. A rapid clinical effect can be achieved by giving 200 mg four times daily for the first 2 days. Children over 5 years of age may be given 100 mg three times daily. It has also been administered by inhalation.

**Respiratory disorders.** Mecysteine hydrochloride given by mouth has reduced symptoms of cough in patients with chronic bronchitis or other respiratory disorders, but its effect on sputum production and pulmonary function has been variable.[1,2] The use of mucolytics in chronic obstructive pulmonary disease (p.779) is controversial.

1. Aylward M, *et al.* Clinical therapeutic evaluation of methyl-cysteine hydrochloride in patients with chronic obstructive bronchitis: a balanced double-blind trial with placebo control. *Curr Med Res Opin* 1978; **5:** 461–71.
2. Sahay JN, *et al.* The effect of methyl cysteine (Visclair) in respiratory diseases: a pilot study. *Clin Trials J* 1982; **19:** 137–43.

### Preparations

**Proprietary Preparations** (details are given in Part 3)
***Irl.:*** Visclair; ***UK:*** Visclair.

**Multi-ingredient:** ***Ital.:*** Donatiol.

## Menglytate (rINN)

Menglitato; Menthol Ethylglycolate. *p*-Menth-3-yl ethoxyacetate.

$C_{14}H_{26}O_3 = 242.4$.

*CAS — 579-94-2.*

### Profile

Menglytate is an ingredient of a number of preparations promoted for the treatment of cough.

### Preparations

**Proprietary Preparations** (details are given in Part 3)

**Multi-ingredient:** ***Austria:*** Expigen; ***Ital.:*** Coryfin C; Neo Borocillina Balsamica.

## Methoxyphenamine Hydrochloride (BANM, rINNM)

Hidrocloruro de metoxifenamina; Methoxiphenadrin Hydrochloride; Mexyphamine Hydrochloride. 2-Methoxy-Nα-dimethylphenethylamine hydrochloride.

$C_{11}H_{17}NO,HCl = 215.7$.

*CAS — 93-30-1 (methoxyphenamine); 5588-10-3 (methoxyphenamine hydrochloride).*

*ATC — R03CB02.*

### Profile

Methoxyphenamine is a sympathomimetic with effects similar to those of ephedrine (p.1120), given by mouth as the hydrochloride. It has been used as a bronchodilator and in combination preparations for the relief of cough and nasal congestion.

### Preparations

**Proprietary Preparations** (details are given in Part 3)

**Multi-ingredient:** ***Belg.:*** Orthoxicol†; ***Braz.:*** Cheracap†; Sedagripe†; ***Chile:*** Cheracol; ***Hong Kong:*** Asmeton; ***Irl.:*** Casacol; ***Mex.:*** Cheracol; ***S.Afr.:*** Orthoxicol†; ***Thai.:*** Asmeton.

## Methyl Dacisteine (rINNM)

Dacisteína de metilo; EL-1035 (dacisteine); Methyl Diacetylcysteinate. Methyl *N,S*-diacetyl-L-cysteinate.

$C_8H_{13}NO_4S = 219.3$.

*CAS — 18725-37-6 (dacisteine); 19547-88-7 (methyl dacisteine).*

### Profile

Like acetylcysteine (p.1112), methyl dacisteine has been used as a mucolytic in respiratory disorders associated with productive cough (p.1112). It has been given by mouth in a usual dose of 600 mg daily, divided into 3 or 4 doses.

### Preparations

**Proprietary Preparations** (details are given in Part 3)
***Fr.:*** Mucothiol; ***Ital.:*** Mucothiol.

## Methylephedrine Hydrochloride (BANM)

Metilefedrina, hidrocloruro de. 2-Dimethylamino-1-phenylpropan-1-ol hydrochloride.

$C_{11}H_{17}NO,HCl = 215.7$.

*CAS — 552-79-4 ((−)-methylephedrine); 1201-56-5 ((±)-methylephedrine); 38455-90-2 ((−)-methylephedrine hydrochloride); 942-46-1 ((±)-methylephedrine hydrochloride); 18760-80-0 ((±)-methylephedrine hydrochloride).*

**Pharmacopoeias.** *Jpn* includes the (±)-form, *dl*-Methylephedrine Hydrochloride.

### Profile

Methylephedrine hydrochloride is a sympathomimetic with effects similar to those of ephedrine (p.1120). It has been used as a bronchodilator and is given by mouth in combination preparations for the relief of cough and nasal congestion.

### Preparations

**Proprietary Preparations** (details are given in Part 3)

**Multi-ingredient:** ***Austria:*** Tussoretardin; ***Hong Kong:*** Codaewon; ***S.Afr.:*** Ilvico; ***Switz.:*** Tossamine plus; ***Thai.:*** Coughmin; Hustazol-C; Methorcon.

## Metizoline Hydrochloride (BANM, USAN, rINNM)

EX-10-781; Hidrocloruro de metizolina; Metyzoline Hydrochloride; RMI-10482A. 2-(2-Methylbenzo[*b*]thienylmethyl)-2-imidazoline hydrochloride.

$C_{13}H_{14}N_2S,HCl = 266.8$.

*CAS — 17692-22-7 (metizoline); 5090-37-9 (metizoline hydrochloride).*

*ATC — R01AA10.*

### Profile

Metizoline hydrochloride is a sympathomimetic with effects similar to those of naphazoline (p.1124) that has been used for its vasoconstrictor activity in the treatment of nasal congestion.

### Preparations

**Proprietary Preparations** (details are given in Part 3)
***Ital.:*** Eunasin†.

## Morclofone (rINN)

Dimeclofenone; Morclofona; Morclophon. 4′-Chloro-3,5-dimethoxy-4-(2-morpholinoethoxy)benzophenone.

$C_{21}H_{24}ClNO_5 = 405.9$.

*CAS — 31848-01-8 (morclofone); 31848-02-9 (morclofone hydrochloride).*

*ATC — R05DB25.*

### Profile

Morclofone is a centrally acting cough suppressant used for non-productive cough (p.1112) by mouth in usual doses of 150 mg four or five times daily. It has also been given as the hydrochloride.

### Preparations

**Proprietary Preparations** (details are given in Part 3)
***Ital.:*** Plausitin; ***Mex.:*** Plausital†; ***Switz.:*** Nitux.

# Naphazoline (BAN, rINN)

Nafazolina. 2-(1-Naphthylmethyl)-2-imidazoline.

$C_{14}H_{14}N_2 = 210.3$.

*CAS — 835-31-4.*

*ATC — R01AA08; R01AB02; S01GA01.*

## Naphazoline Hydrochloride (BANM, rINNM)

Hidrocloruro de nafazolina; Naphazolini Hydrochloridum.

$C_{14}H_{14}N_2,HCl = 246.7$.

*CAS — 550-99-2.*

*ATC — R01AA08; R01AB02; S01GA01.*

**Pharmacopoeias.** In *Chin., Eur.* (see p.vi), *Jpn,* and *US.*

**Ph. Eur. 5.0** (Naphazoline Hydrochloride). A white or almost white, crystalline powder. Freely soluble in water; soluble in alcohol. Protect from light.

**USP 27** (Naphazoline Hydrochloride). A white, odourless, crystalline powder. Freely soluble in water and in alcohol; very slightly soluble in chloroform; practically insoluble in ether. pH of a 1% solution in water is between 5.0 and 6.6. Store in airtight containers. Protect from light.

## Naphazoline Nitrate (BANM, rINNM)

Naphazolini Nitras; Naphazolinium Nitricum; Naphthizinum; Nitrato de nafazolina.

$C_{14}H_{14}N_2,HNO_3 = 273.3$.

*CAS — 5144-52-5.*

*ATC — R01AA08; R01AB02; S01GA01.*

**Pharmacopoeias.** In *Eur.* (see p.vi), *Jpn, Pol.,* and *Viet.*

**Ph. Eur. 5.0** (Naphazoline Nitrate). A white or almost white, crystalline powder. Sparingly soluble in water; soluble in alcohol. A 1% solution in water has a pH of 5.0 to 6.5. Protect from light.

## Adverse Effects, Treatment, and Precautions

After local use of naphazoline transient irritation may occur. Rebound congestion may occur after frequent or prolonged use. Systemic effects, including nausea, headache, and dizziness have occurred after topical use. Overdosage or accidental administration by mouth may cause CNS depression with marked reduction of body temperature and bradycardia, sweating, drowsiness, and coma, particularly in children; it should be used with great caution, if at all, in infants and young children. Use of naphazoline in the eye may liberate pigment granules from the iris, especially when given in high doses to elderly patients. Hypertension may be followed by rebound hypotension. Treatment of side-effects is symptomatic.

For the adverse effects of sympathomimetics in general, and precautions for their use, see under Adrenaline, p.852.

**Effects on the eyes.** For mention of conjunctivitis induced by ophthalmic decongestant preparations containing naphazoline, see under Phenylephrine, p.1127.

## Interactions

Since naphazoline is absorbed through the nasal mucosa interactions may follow topical application. The *British National Formulary* considers that all sympathomimetic nasal decongestants may cause a hypertensive crisis if used during treatment with an MAOI. For the interactions of sympathomimetics in general, see under Adrenaline, p.853.

## Pharmacokinetics

Systemic absorption has been reported following topical application of solutions of naphazoline. It is not used systemically, but it is readily absorbed from the gastrointestinal tract.

## Uses and Administration

Naphazoline is a sympathomimetic (see Adrenaline, p.854) with marked alpha-adrenergic activity. It is a vasoconstrictor with a rapid and prolonged action in reducing swelling and congestion when applied to mucous membranes.

Naphazoline and its salts are used for the symptomatic relief of nasal congestion (p.1112). Solutions containing 0.05 to 0.1% of the hydrochloride or the nitrate may be applied topically as nasal drops or a spray usually up to once every 6 hours. Children aged 7 years and over have used a preparation containing 0.05%.

Solutions containing up to 0.1% of naphazoline hydrochloride have been instilled into the eye as a conjunctival decongestant (see Conjunctivitis, p.421).

Naphazoline has been used as a vasoconstrictor with local anaesthetics.

Naphazoline acetate has also been used in nasal preparations.

## Preparations

***USP 27:*** Naphazoline Hydrochloride and Pheniramine Maleate Ophthalmic Solution; Naphazoline Hydrochloride Nasal Solution; Naphazoline Hydrochloride Ophthalmic Solution.

**Proprietary Preparations** (details are given in Part 3)

***Arg.:*** Bactio Rhin; Dazolin; Disel; Gotabiotic D; Gotinal; Mirasan; Mirus-S; Privina; Rhinal; ***Austral.:*** Albalon; Clear Eyes; Naphcon; Optazine; ***Austria:*** Aconex; Coldan; Isoftal; Privin; Rhinon; Rhinoperd; ***Belg.:*** Albalon; Deltarhinol-Mono; Neusinol; Priciasol; Vasocedine; ***Braz.:*** Claroft; Narialt†; Naridex†; Narix; Nazicol; Neosoro; Privina; Rino Resfenol†; Rinoklin†; Rinos-A; Rinox Adulto†; ***Canad.:*** Ak-Con; Albalon; Allergy Drops; Clear Eyes; Diopticon; Naphcon Forte; Red Away; Rhino-Mex-N†; RO-Naphz†; Vasocon; ***Chile:*** Albasol; Clarimir; Red Off; Vi-Claro; ***Denm.:*** Antistina-Privin; ***Ger.:*** Idril N sine; Piniol Nasenspray; Piniol†; Privin; Proculin; Rhinex; Tele-Stulln; Vistalbalon†; ***Gr.:*** Coldan; ***Hong Kong:*** Albalon; ***India:*** Clearine; ***Israel:*** Naphasal; Naphcon Forte; ***Ital.:*** Collirio Alfa; Desamin Same; Imidazyl; Imizol†; Iridina Due; Lucisan†; Naftazolina; Pupilla; Rinazina; Rino Naftazolina; Video-Mill; Virginiana Gocce Verdi; ***Malaysia:*** Albalon; ***Mex.:*** Afazol; Alphadinal; Oftazil†; ***NZ:*** Albalon; Clear Eyes; Naphcon; ***Port.:*** Murine†; ***S.Afr.:*** Albalon†; Murine Clear Eyes; ***Singapore:*** Antistin-Privin; ***Spain:*** Alfa; Miraclar; Vasoconstrictor Pensa; ***Swed.:*** Rimidol; ***Switz.:*** Albalon; Minha; ***Thai.:*** Albalon; Naphcon; ***UK:*** Murine; ***USA:*** Ak-Con; Albalon; All Clear; Allerest; Allergy Drops; Allersol†; Clear Eyes; Comfort Eye Drops; Degest; Nafazair; Napha Forte; Naphcon; Privine; Vasocon.

**Multi-ingredient:** ***Arg.:*** Alercortil; Alvo Nasal; Antibiocort; Bactio Rhin Prednisolona; Biotaer Nasal; Dexafurazon; Dexalergin; Disel Hidrocortisona; Drynisan; Factioneye; Fadanasal; Gramicortil; Hyalcrom; Mira Klonal; Mirus; Nasojol; Nasomicina; Neo-Currino; Neodexa Plus; Neoefodil; Neosona; Nexadron Compuesto; Panoptic; Provacsin Nasal; Refenax Colirio; Refenax Gotas Nasales; Rinoflax AG M; Rinogel; Suavithiol; Vistacloran; ***Austral.:*** Albalon-A; Antistine-Privine; In A Wink†; Naphcon-A; Optrex; Visine Allergy with Antihistamine; ***Austria:*** Coldistan; Coldophthal; Histophtal†; Luuf-Nasenspray; Ophtaguttal; Rectosan†; Rhinodrin; Rhinon; Rhinoperd comp; ***Belg.:*** Diphenhydramine Constrictor; Neofenox; Sofraline; Sofrasolone; Zincfrin Antihistaminicum; ***Braz.:*** Adnax†; Albassol†; Alergotox Nasal†; Borato de Sodio†; Claril; Colirio Blumen†; Colirio Legrand; Colirio Moura Brasil†; Colirio Teuto; Colirio Vimat†; Colyrazul†; Conidrin; Dexa-Vastrictol†; Fluo-Vaso; Hemodotti; Hermodotti†; Hidrocin; Inhadrina†; Lerin; Mentodrin†; Naricin†; Naridrin; Naso Instil†; Nasopan†; Nazobel; Nazobio; Nazotiran†; Neo Quimica Colirio; Nitrileno; Nitronasal†; Novo Rino; Oftazul†; Penetran†; Rhinodex†; Rhinosept; Rinatrol†; Rinisone; Rinocron†; Rinosite; Rinozin†; Sinus†; Sinustrat Vasoconstritor; Solucao Nasal de Nafazolina†; Sorine Adulto; Vastrictol†; Visiplex; Visolon†; Visual; Zincolok; ***Canad.:*** Albalon-A; Blue Collyrium†; Collyre Bleu; Cooper AR†; Diopticon A; Naphcon-A; Onrectal; Opcon-A; Rhino-Mex†; Vasocon-A; Zincfrin-A; ***Chile:*** Albasol A; Clarimir F; Dessolets; Miral; Mirus; Naphcon-A; Naphtears; Novo-Tears; Oculosan; Oftalirio; Red Off Plus; ***Denm.:*** Sesal; ***Fin.:*** Antistin-Privin; Zincfrin-A; ***Fr.:*** Collyre Bleu; Derinox; Frazoline†; Soframycine Naphazoline†; ***Ger.:*** Antistin-Privin; Diabenyl-Rhinex; duraultra; Konjunktival Thilo; Oculosan N; Ophtalmin†; Ophtopur-N†; Rhinoguttae Dexamethasoni cum Naphazolino; Rhinosovil; Siozwo; Solupen-D†; Stipo; ***Gr.:*** Oculosan; Septobore; Zabysept; ***Hong Kong:*** Konjunktival; Naphcon-A; Oculosan; ***India:*** Andre; Andre-I-Kul; Betnesol-N Nasal; Efcorlin; Fenox; Nazalin; Ocurest; Ocurest-AH; Ocurest-Z; Proto-Boric; ***Israel:*** Alnase; Antistin-Privin; Diphenazol; Nazodin; Nodryl; Optryl; Phenyphrine-Azol; Proaf; ***Ital.:*** Alfaflor; Antisettico Astringente Sedativo; Antistin-Privina; Citroftalmina VC†; Collirio Alfa Antistaminico; Corizzina; Deltarinolo; Fenox†; Fotofil; Genalfa; Idroneomicil; Imidazyl Antistaminico; Indaco; Iristamina; Nafcon A; Oftalmil; Oftalzina†; Pupilla Antistaminico; Rinocidina; Rinofomentil; Rinospray†; Rinovit Nube†; Zinc-Imizol; ***Malaysia:*** Alergoftal; Naphcon-A; Oculosan; ***Mex.:*** Afazol Z; Biotarson O; Colirio Sulvi; Naphacel; Oftalirio; Soltrictor con Lagrifilm; Solutina; ***NZ:*** Albalon-A; Betnesol Aqueous; Clear Eyes ACR; Degest 2; Naphcon-A†; Optrex Red-Eye Relief; Visine Allergy with Antihistamine; ***Port.:*** Alergiftalmina; Colircusi Anestesico; Gramixina†; Naso-Prieulina; ***S.Afr.:*** Albalon-A; Antistin-Privin; Covomycin; Covosan; ENT; Fenox†; Nasdro; Oculosan; Universal Nasal Drops†; Wink†; ***Singapore:*** Alergoftal†; Flucur; Naphcon-A; ***Spain:*** Alergoftal; Centilux; Clo Zinc†; Cloram Zinc; Coliriocilina Adren Astr; Dexa Vasoc†; Epistaxol; Euboral; Fluo Vasoc†; Kanafosal; Kanafosal Predni; Lidrone†; Oftalmol Dexa†; Oftalmol Ocular; Ojosbel; Ojosbel Azul†; Rinovel; Vasocon Ant†; Vasoconstr†; Zolina; ***Swed.:*** Antasten-Privin; ***Switz.:*** Antistin-Privin; Collyre Alpha; Collyre Bleu Laiter; Derinox†; Gouttes nasales N; Oculosan; Optazine†; ***Thai.:*** Levoptin; Naphcon-A; Oculosan; ***UK:*** Eye Dew; Optrex Clear Eyes; ***USA:*** 4-Way Fast Acting; Antazoline-V; Clear Eyes ACR; Maximum Strength Allergy Drops; Nafazair A; Naphazoline Plus; Naphcon-A; Naphoptic-A; Ocuhist; Opcon-A; VasoClear; VasoClear A; Vasocon-A.

*Used as an adjunct in:* ***Fr.:*** Xylocaine; ***Spain:*** Anest Compuesto†; Anestesico.

## Neltenexine *(rINN)*

Neltenexina. 4′,6′-Dibromo-α-[(*trans*-4-hydroxycyclohexyl)amino]-2-thiophene-carboxy-*o*-toluidide.

$C_{18}H_{20}Br_2N_2O_2S$ = 488.2.
*CAS — 99453-84-6.*
*ATC — R05CB14.*

### Profile

Neltenexine is a mucolytic that has been used in patients with respiratory disorders associated with productive cough (p.1112). It has been given by mouth as the monohydrate, in usual doses of 37.4 mg three times daily. Neltenexine has also been given rectally as the hydrochloride.

### Preparations

**Proprietary Preparations** (details are given in Part 3)
***Ital.:*** Alveoten; Muco4; Tenoxol.

## Nepinalone *(rINN)*

Nepinalona. (±)-3,4-Dihydro-1-methyl-1-(2-piperidinoethyl)-2(1*H*)-napthalenone.

$C_{18}H_{25}NO$ = 271.4.
*CAS — 22443-11-4.*
*ATC — R05DB26.*

### Profile

Nepinalone has been used as the hydrochloride as a cough suppressant in non-productive cough (p.1112). Doses of nepinalone hydrochloride 10 mg have been given three times daily by mouth.

### Preparations

**Proprietary Preparations** (details are given in Part 3)
***Ital.:*** Nepituss; Placatus; Tussolvina.

## Nicocodine *(BAN, rINN)*

Nicocodina. 6-Nicotinoylcodeine; 3-*O*-Methyl-6-*O*-nicotinoylmorphine.

$C_{24}H_{24}N_2O_4$ = 404.5.
*CAS — 3688-66-2.*

### Profile

Nicocodine is an opioid related to codeine (p.27). It has been used as the hydrochloride for its central cough suppressant effects in non-productive cough (p.1112). Nicocodine hydrochloride is given by mouth in doses of 5 to 7.5 mg up to three times daily.

### Preparations

**Proprietary Preparations** (details are given in Part 3)
***Austria:*** Tusscodin.

## Normethadone Hydrochloride *(BANM, rINNM)*

Desmethylmethadone Hydrochloride; Hidrocloruro de normetadona; Hoechst-10582 (normethadone); Phenyldimazone Hydrochloride. 6-Dimethylamino-4,4-diphenylhexan-3-one hydrochloride.

$C_{20}H_{25}NO,HCl$ = 331.9.
*CAS — 467-85-6 (normethadone); 847-84-7 (normethadone hydrochloride).*
*ATC — R05DA06.*

### Profile

Normethadone is closely related to methadone (p.57). The hydrochloride has been given by mouth as a cough suppressant in non-productive cough.

### Preparations

**Proprietary Preparations** (details are given in Part 3)
**Multi-ingredient:** ***Canad.:*** Cophylac†.

## Noscapine *(BAN, rINN)*

Narcotine; L-α-Narcotine; Noscapina; Noscapinum; NSC-5366. (3*S*)-6,7-Dimethoxy-3-[(5*R*)-5,6,7,8-tetrahydro-4-methoxy-6-methyl-1,3-dioxolo[4,5-*g*]isoquinolin-5-yl]phthalide.

$C_{22}H_{23}NO_7$ = 413.4.
*CAS — 128-62-1.*
*ATC — R05DA07.*

**Description.** Noscapine is an alkaloid obtained from opium.

**Pharmacopoeias.** In *Chin., Eur.* (see p.vi), *Int., Jpn,* and *US.*

**Ph. Eur. 5.0** (Noscapine). A white, crystalline powder or colourless crystals. Practically insoluble in water at 20°, very slightly soluble at 100°; slightly soluble in alcohol; soluble in acetone; dissolves in strong acids although the base may be precipitated on dilution with water. Protect from light.

**USP 27** (Noscapine). A fine, white or practically white, crystalline powder. Practically insoluble in water; slightly soluble in alcohol and in ether; soluble in acetone; freely soluble in chloroform.

## Noscapine Camsilate

Camphoscapine; Noscapina, camsilato de; Noscapine Camsylate. Noscapine camphor-10-sulphonate.

$C_{22}H_{23}NO_7,C_{10}H_{16}O_4S$ = 645.7.
*CAS — 25333-79-3.*
*ATC — R05DA07.*

## Noscapine Hydrochloride *(BANM, rINNM)*

Hidrocloruro de noscapina; Narcotine Hydrochloride; Noscapini Hydrochloridum; Noscapinium Chloride.

$C_{22}H_{23}NO_7,HCl,H_2O$ = 467.9.
*CAS — 912-60-7 (anhydrous noscapine hydrochloride).*
*ATC — R05DA07.*

**Pharmacopoeias.** In *Eur.* (see p.vi) and *Int.* (both with $H_2O$); in *Jpn* (with $xH_2O$).

**Ph. Eur. 5.0** (Noscapine Hydrochloride). A white, hygroscopic, crystalline powder or colourless crystals. Freely soluble in water and in alcohol. Aqueous solutions are faintly acid; the base may be precipitated when the solutions are allowed to stand. A 2% solution in water has a pH of not less than 3.0. Protect from light.

### Adverse Effects and Precautions

As for Dextromethorphan, p.1117. Hypersensitivity reactions have been reported.

**Breast feeding.** Maximum concentrations of noscapine in the breast milk of 8 women given 100 or 150 mg of noscapine ranged[1] from 11 to 83 nanograms/mL. It was estimated that breast-fed infants of mothers receiving noscapine 50 mg three times daily would ingest at most 300 nanograms/kg of noscapine, an amount considered unlikely to be a hazard. No adverse effects have been observed in breast-feeding infants whose mothers were receiving noscapine, and the American Academy of Pediatrics[2] considers that it is therefore usually compatible with breast feeding.

1. Olsson B, *et al.* Excretion of noscapine in human breast milk. *Eur J Clin Pharmacol* 1986; **30:** 213–15.
2. American Academy of Pediatrics. The transfer of drugs and other chemicals into human milk. *Pediatrics* 2001; **108:** 776–89. Correction. *ibid.*; 1029. Also available at: http://aappolicy.aappublications.org/cgi/content/full/pediatrics%3b108/3/776 (accessed 01/07/04)

**Pregnancy.** The UK Committee on Safety of Medicines stood by their recommendation[1] that products containing noscapine should be contra-indicated in women of child-bearing potential (because of potential mutagenic effects[2]), after criticism that the decision was based solely on the results of *in-vitro* work.[3]

1. Asscher AW, Fowler LK. Papaveretum in women of childbearing potential. *BMJ* 1991; **303:** 648.
2. Committee on Safety of Medicines. Genotoxicity of papaveretum and noscapine. *Current Problems 31* 1991.
3. Allen S, *et al.* Papaveretum in women of child bearing potential. *BMJ* 1991; **303:** 647.

### Interactions

Noscapine should not be given with alcohol or other CNS depressants.

### Pharmacokinetics

◊ References to the pharmacokinetics of noscapine.

1. Karlsson MO, *et al.* Pharmacokinetics of oral noscapine. *Eur J Clin Pharmacol* 1990; **39:** 275–9.
2. Karlsson MO, Dahlström B. Serum protein binding of noscapine: influence of a reversible hydrolysis. *J Pharm Pharmacol* 1990; **42:** 140–3.

### Uses and Administration

Noscapine is a centrally acting cough suppressant that has actions and uses similar to those of dextromethorphan (p.1118). It is given by mouth in a dose of up to 50 mg three times daily. It has also been given as the ascorbate, camsilate, embonate, and the hydrochloride, and also administered rectally.

### Preparations

**Proprietary Preparations** (details are given in Part 3)
***Belg.:*** Nosca-Mereprine; Noscaflex; ***Chile:*** Factos; ***Ger.:*** Capval; ***Neth.:*** Finipect†; Libronchin Prikkelhoest; ***S.Afr.:*** Nitepax; ***Spain:*** Tuscalman; ***Swed.:*** Nipaxon; ***Switz.:*** Tussanil N.

**Multi-ingredient:** ***Arg.:*** Graneodin N; Jarabe Bago; Saltos; Vi-Balsabron; ***Austria:*** Pneumopect†; Tuscalman; ***Belg.:*** Noscaflex; Rosils; ***Braz.:*** Broncotussan†; Expectussin†; Ipecol; ***Chile:*** AB Antitusivo; Captus; Congestex; Cotibin Flu; Freshmel Tos; Graneodin N; Graneodin-Tos; Gripexin

Limonada Caliente; Gripexin Nueva Formula Compuesto; Kitadol Flu; Kitadol Flu Noche; Pectoserum; Tapsin Compuesto; Tapsin Compuesto con Clorfenamina; Tapsin Compuesto Dia/Noche Plus; **Fin.:** Codesan N; Posivil; **Fr.:** Broncho-Tulisan Eucalyptol†; Tussisedal; **Hong Kong:** Asmeton; Coldrex; Mefedra-N; Panadol Cold and Flu; **India:** Coscopin; Coscopin Plus; **Ital.:** Difmetus Compositum†; Ribelfan†; Tuscalman†; **Swed.:** Spasmofen; **Switz.:** Brosoline-Rectocaps; Demotussil; Hederix; No Grip†; Noscorex; Spasmosol; Tossamine; Tossamine plus; Tuscalman; Tussanil Compositum; **Thai.:** Asmeton.

## Oxeladin Citrate *(BANM, rINNM)*

Hidrocloruro de oxeladina; Oxeladini Hydrogenocitras. 2-(2-Diethylaminoethoxy)ethyl 2-ethyl-2-phenylbutyrate dihydrogen citrate.

$C_{20}H_{33}NO_3,C_6H_8O_7$ = 527.6.

*CAS — 468-61-1 (oxeladin); 52432-72-1 (oxeladin citrate).*

*ATC — R05DB09.*

**Pharmacopoeias.** In *Eur.* (see p.vi).

**Ph. Eur. 5.0** (Oxeladin Hydrogen Citrate). A white or almost white, crystalline powder. It exhibits polymorphism. Freely soluble in water; slightly to very slightly soluble in ethyl acetate.

### Profile

Oxeladin citrate has been given by mouth as a centrally acting cough suppressant for non-productive cough (p.1112). Up to 50 mg daily in divided doses has been given by mouth. Higher doses of up to 120 mg daily have been given as a modified-release preparation.

### Preparations

**Proprietary Preparations** (details are given in Part 3)
**Arg.:** Elitos; Frenotos; Nadetos; **Fr.:** Paxeladine; **Norw.:** Pectamol†.

**Multi-ingredient:** **Arg.:** Aseptobron Bromexina; Aseptobron C; Frenotos Muc; **Braz.:** Novotussan; Tetrabronco†; Tetratoss†; Tossivitan; Transpulmin; Transpulmin Xarope; Tripulmin; **Fr.:** Paxeladine Noctee†; **Ital.:** Tussiflex†; **Mex.:** Fluxedan; Tenalif.

## Oxolamine *(rINN)*

683-M; Oxolamina. 5-[2-(Diethylamino)ethyl]-3-phenyl-1,2,4-oxadiazole.

$C_{14}H_{19}N_3O$ = 245.3.

*CAS — 959-14-8.*

*ATC — R05DB07.*

## Oxolamine Citrate *(rINNM)*

AF-438; Citrato de oxolamina; SKF-9976.

$C_{14}H_{19}N_3O,C_6H_8O_7$ = 437.4.

*CAS — 1949-20-8.*

*ATC — R05DB07.*

## Oxolamine Phosphate *(rINNM)*

Fosfato de oxolamina.

*CAS — 1949-19-5.*

*ATC — R05DB07.*

### Profile

Oxolamine is a cough suppressant with a predominantly peripheral action that has been used for non-productive cough (p.1112). It has been given as the citrate or phosphate in usual doses of 100 to 200 mg three times daily. It has also been given as the tannate.

Hallucinations in children have been reported after its use.

◊ References.

1. McEwen J, *et al.* Hallucinations in children caused by oxolamine citrate. *Med J Aust* 1989; **150:** 449–52.

### Preparations

**Proprietary Preparations** (details are given in Part 3)
**Chile:** Numosol; Perebron; Respibron; Tulox; **Israel:** Symphocal; **Ital.:** Gantrimex; Perebron; Tussibron; **Mex.:** Aledron; Bredon; Cideox†; Contuxin†; Eumol†; Exalamin†; Fartoxol; Kentosanil†; Oxathos; Oxobron; Oxolam†; Oxomar; Oxomifer†; Oxoquin†; Toxal; Tukson†; Tusol†; **Spain:** Perebron†.

**Multi-ingredient:** **Ital.:** Uniplus; Upsa Plus†; **Mex.:** Caltusine; **Spain:** Bequipecto†; Dimayon†; Pectoral Funk Antitus†.

# Oxymetazoline Hydrochloride

*(BANM, USAN, rINNM)*

H-990; Hidrocloruro de oximetazolina; Oxymetazolini Hydrochloridum; Sch-9384.

$C_{16}H_{24}N_2O,HCl$ = 296.8.

*CAS — 2315-02-8.*

*ATC — R01AA05; R01AB07; S01GA04.*

**Pharmacopoeias.** In *Eur.* (see p.vi) and *US.*

**Ph. Eur. 5.0** (Oxymetazoline Hydrochloride). A white or almost white, crystalline powder. Freely soluble in water and in alcohol.

**USP 27** (Oxymetazoline Hydrochloride). A white to practically white, fine, hygroscopic, crystalline powder. Soluble 1 in 6.7 of water, 1 in 3.6 of alcohol, and 1 in 862 of chloroform; practically insoluble in ether and in benzene. pH of a 5% solution in water is between 4.0 and 6.5. Store in airtight containers.

## Adverse Effects and Precautions

As for Naphazoline, p.1124.

After local use of oxymetazoline transient irritation may occur. Rebound congestion may occur after frequent or prolonged nasal use. Systemic effects have occurred after local administration.

**Porphyria.** Oxymetazoline has been associated with acute attacks of porphyria and is considered unsafe in porphyric patients.

## Interactions

Since oxymetazoline is absorbed through the mucosa interactions may follow topical application. The *British National Formulary* considers that all sympathomimetic nasal decongestants may cause a hypertensive crisis if used during treatment with an MAOI. For the interactions of sympathomimetics in general, see under Adrenaline, p.853.

## Uses and Administration

Oxymetazoline is a direct-acting sympathomimetic (see Adrenaline, p.854) with marked alpha-adrenergic activity. It is a vasoconstrictor which reduces swelling and congestion when applied to mucous membranes. It acts within a few minutes and the effect lasts for up to 12 hours. It is used as the hydrochloride for the symptomatic relief of nasal congestion (p.1112). In adults and children over 6 years, a 0.05% solution of oxymetazoline hydrochloride is applied topically as nasal drops or a spray, usually twice daily to each nostril as required.

A 0.025% solution of oxymetazoline hydrochloride may be instilled into the eye every 6 hours when necessary as a conjunctival decongestant in adults and children over 6 years (see Conjunctivitis, p.421).

## Preparations

**USP 27:** Oxymetazoline Hydrochloride Nasal Solution; Oxymetazoline Hydrochloride Ophthalmic Solution.

**Proprietary Preparations** (details are given in Part 3)
**Arg.:** Apracur Nasal; Dristan Nasal; Isly; Lidl; Vick Sinex; Yusin; **Austral.:** Chemists Own Decongestant Nasal Spray; Dimetapp 12 Hour Nasal; Drixine Nasal; Logicin Rapid Relief; Ordov Sinudec†; **Austria:** Nasivin; **Belg.:** Nesivine; Vicks Sinex; **Braz.:** Afrin; Desfrin; Freenal; Nasivin; Oxilin†; Rino Spray†; **Canad.:** Claritin Allergic Congestion Relief; Claritin Eye Allergy Relief; Decongestant Nasal Mist; Dristan; Drixoral; Long Lasting Nasal Mist; Nafrine; Ocuclear†; Vicks Sinex; Visine Workplace; **Chile:** Iliadin; Isly; **Denm.:** Drixin; Iliadin; Nezeril†; **Fin.:** Dristan†; Nezeril†; Vicks Sinex; **Fr.:** Aturgyl; **Ger.:** Em-eukal Mono; Larylin Nasenspray N†; Nasivin gegen Schnupfen; Nasivin Sanft; Nasivinetten gegen Schnupfen; Vistoxyn; Wick Sinex; **Hong Kong:** Afrin; Duration; Iliadin; Logicin Rapid Relief; Nezeril; Oxylin; **India:** Nasivion; Sinarest; Sinarest-PD; **Irl.:** Dristan; Vicks Sinex†; **Israel:** Alrin; Nasivin; Oxylin†; Rhinoclir; Sinulen; **Ital.:** Actifed Nasale; Coricidin; Nasivin†; Oxilin; Rino Calyptol; **Malaysia:** Afrin; Iliadin; **Mex.:** Afrin; Fracidin; Iliadin; Ocuclear; Oxylin; Sinex; Visine AD; **Neth.:** Dampo†; Nasivin; Vicks Sinex; **Norw.:** Iliadin; Rhinox; **NZ:** At-Eze; Drixine; **Port.:** Alerjon; Bisolspray; Nasarox; Nasex; Neozine; Oxylin; Rinerge; Robinaz†; **S.Afr.:** Drixine; Iliadin; Oxylin; Sparkling White Eye Drops; **Singapore:** Afrin; Iliadin; Nazolin; Oxylin†; **Spain:** Alerfrin; Antirrinum; Corilisina; Descongestan†; Egarone Oximetazolina†; Idasal Nebulizador; Ilvinax; Inalintra†; Nasolina†; Nasovalda†; Nebulicina; Oftinal; Respibien; Respir; Rinocorin†; Rinodif†; Utabon; **Swed.:** Iliadin; Nasin; Nezeril; Zolin; **Switz.:** Nasivine; Nasivinettes; Vistoxyn; **Thai.:** Iliadin; Nasil†; Oxylin†; Oxymet; **UAE:** Nasivin; **UK:** Afrazine; Dristan†; Nasivin; Vicks Sinex; **USA:** 4-Way Long Lasting; Afrin; Allerest 12 Hour Nasal; Cheracol Nasal†; Chlorphed-LA; Dristan 12-hr Nasal Decongestant Spray; Dristan Long Lasting; Duramist Plus; Duration; Genasal; Nasal Relief; Nasal Spray; Neo-Synephrine 12 Hour; Nostrilla; NTZ Long Acting Nasal; Ocuclear; Twice-A-Day; Vicks Sinex 12-Hour; Visine LR.

**Multi-ingredient:** **Arg.:** Panoxi; **Austral.:** Euky Bear Nasex†; Extra-life Nasex; Nasex†; Vasylox; Vicks Sinex; **Austria:** Wick Sinex; **Braz.:** Narizima Adulto†; **Fr.:** Deturgylone; **Israel:** Sinaf; **Ital.:** Nasicortin†; Triaminic; Vicks Sinex; **NZ:** Vicks Sinex; **S.Afr.:** Nazene; **Spain:** Egarone; Orto Nasal†; Respir Balsamico†; Seniospray; Vicks Spray; **Switz.:** Vicks Sinex.

## Pentoxyverine *(BAN, rINN)*

Carbetapentane; Pentoxiverina. 2-[2-(Diethylamino)ethoxy]-ethyl 1-phenylcyclopentanecarboxylate.

$C_{20}H_{31}NO_3$ = 333.5.

*CAS — 77-23-6.*

*ATC — R05DB05.*

## Pentoxyverine Citrate *(BANM, rINNM)*

Carbetapentane Citrate; Citrato de pentoxiverina; Pentoxyverine Hydrogen Citrate; Pentoxyverini Hydrogenocitras; UCB-2543.

$C_{20}H_{31}NO_3,C_6H_8O_7$ = 525.6.

*CAS — 23142-01-0.*

*ATC — R05DB05.*

**Pharmacopoeias.** In *Chin., Eur.* (see p.vi), and *Jpn.*

**Ph. Eur. 5.0** (Pentoxyverine Hydrogen Citrate; Pentoxyverine Citrate BP 2003). A white or almost white crystalline powder. M.p. about 93°. Freely soluble in water and in methyl alcohol; soluble in alcohol and in dichloromethane; very soluble in glacial acetic acid. A 10% solution in water has a pH of 3.3 to 3.7. Protect from light.

## Pentoxyverine Hydrochloride *(BANM)*

Pentoxiverina, hidrocloruro de.

$C_{20}H_{31}NO_3,HCl$ = 369.9.

*CAS — 1045-21-2.*

*ATC — R05DB05.*

### Profile

Pentoxyverine is a centrally acting cough suppressant used for non-productive cough (p.1112). Up to 200 mg daily of the citrate has been given by mouth in divided doses. The hydrochloride and the tannate are also given by mouth. The base has been administered rectally.

### Preparations

**Proprietary Preparations** (details are given in Part 3)
**Austral.:** Nyal Dry Cough; **Austria:** Atenos; Sedotussin; **Belg.:** Balsoclase Antitussivum; Tuclase; **Denm.:** Toclase; **Fin.:** Toclase; **Fr.:** Merol†; Pectosan Toux Seche; Sirop Pectoral Vicks†; Toclase Toux Seche; **Ger.:** Pertix-Solo-N, Pertix-T, Pertix-Z, and Pertix-L; Sedotussin; **Hong Kong:** Toclase; **Ital.:** Tuclase; **Neth.:** Balsoclase; Tuclase; **Norw.:** Toclase; **Port.:** Toclase†; **Swed.:** Toclase; **Thai.:** Toclase.

**Multi-ingredient:** **Arg.:** Bio Grip Plus; Rynatus; Wilpan; Wilpan C; **Austral.:** Vicks Cough Syrup†; **Austria:** Tussoretardin; **Belg.:** Balsoclase Expectorans; Balsoclase†; **Braz.:** Alergo Glucalbet; Coficold-Ped†; Coldrin; Fluviral†; Gegrip; Resprin; **Canad.:** Vicks Cough Syrup†; **Fin.:** Toclase Expectorant; **Ger.:** Sedotussin Expectorans†; Sedotussin plus; **Hong Kong:** Vida Cough; **Neth.:** Balsoclase Compositum†; Balsoclase-E; **Switz.:** Sedotussin; **Thai.:** PD Cough†; **USA:** C-Tanna 12D; Cophene-X†; Rentamine Pediatric; Ry-Tuss; Rynatuss; Tannic-12; Tri-Tannate Plus Pediatric; Tuss-Tan; Tussi-12; Tussi-12 D; Tussi-12D S; Tussizone; Xiratuss.

# Phenylephrine *(BAN, rINN)*

Fenilefrina; Phenylephrinum; *m*-Synephrine. (*1R*)-1-(3-Hydroxyphenyl)-2-methylaminoethanol.

$C_9H_{13}NO_2$ = 167.2.

*CAS — 59-42-7.*

*ATC — C01CA06; R01AA04; R01AB01; R01BA03; S01FB01; S01GA05.*

NOTE. Synephrine has been used as a synonym for oxedrine (p.977). Care should be taken to avoid confusion with phenylephrine (*m*-synephrine).

**Pharmacopoeias.** In *Eur.* (see p.vi).

**Ph. Eur. 5.0** (Phenylephrine). A white or almost white crystalline powder. Slightly soluble in water and in alcohol; sparingly soluble in methyl alcohol. It dissolves in dilute mineral acids and in solutions of alkali hydroxides. Store in airtight containers. Protect from light.

## Phenylephrine Acid Tartrate

Fenilefrina, bitartrato de; Phenylephrine Bitartrate; Phenylephrine Tartrate *(BANM)*.

$C_9H_{13}NO_2,C_4H_6O_6$ = 317.3.

*CAS — 13998-27-1.*

*ATC — C01CA06; R01AA04; R01AB01; R01BA03; S01FB01; S01GA05.*

## Phenylephrine Hydrochloride *(BANM, rINNM)*

Hidrocloruro de fenilefrina; Mesatonum; Metaoxedrini Chloridum; Phenylephrini Hydrochloridum.

$C_9H_{13}NO_2,HCl$ = 203.7.

*CAS — 61-76-7.*

*ATC — C01CA06; R01AA04; R01AB01; R01BA03; S01FB01; S01GA05.*

NOTE. PHNL is a code approved by the BP 2003 for use on single unit doses of eye drops containing phenylephrine hydrochloride where the individual container may be too small to bear all the appropriate labelling information. PHNCYC is a similar code approved for eye drops containing phenylephrine hydrochloride and cyclopentolate hydrochloride.

**Pharmacopoeias.** In *Chin., Eur.* (see p.vi), *Jpn, Pol.,* and *US.*

**Ph. Eur. 5.0** (Phenylephrine Hydrochloride). A white or almost white, crystalline powder. Freely soluble in water and in alcohol.

**USP 27** (Phenylephrine Hydrochloride). White or practically white, odourless, crystals. Freely soluble in water and in alcohol. Store in airtight containers at a temperature of 25°, excursions permitted between 15° and 30°. Protect from light.

**Incompatibility.** Phenylephrine is stated to be incompatible with the local anaesthetic butacaine.

## Adverse Effects and Precautions

For the adverse effects of sympathomimetics in general, and precautions for their use, see under Adrenaline, p.852. Phenylephrine has a longer duration of action than noradrenaline and an excessive vasopressor response may cause a prolonged rise in blood pressure. It induces tachycardia or reflex bradycardia and should therefore be avoided in severe hyperthyroidism and used with caution in severe ischaemic heart disease.

Since phenylephrine is absorbed through the mucosa systemic effects may follow application to the eyes or the nasal mucosa. In particular, phenylephrine 10% eye drops should be avoided or only used with extreme caution in infants and the elderly since they can have powerful systemic effects.

Use of phenylephrine in the eye may liberate pigment granules from the iris, especially when given in high doses to elderly patients. Ophthalmic solutions of phenylephrine are contra-indicated in patients with angle-closure glaucoma. Corneal clouding may occur if corneal epithelium has been denuded or damaged.

Excessive or prolonged use of phenylephrine nasal drops can lead to rebound congestion.

Phenylephrine hydrochloride is irritant and may cause local discomfort at the site of application; extravasation of the injection may even cause local tissue necrosis.

**Effects on the cardiovascular system.** Systemic side-effects have occurred following the use of phenylephrine as eye drops (particularly at a strength of 10%), or nasal drops.

Hypertension[1] and hypertension with pulmonary oedema[2] have been described in infants after the use of phenylephrine 10% eye drops, and hypertension has occurred in an infant after phenylephrine was also given intranasally with pseudoephedrine orally.[3] The specific problem of eye drops and neonatal blood pressure has also been reviewed.[4] Hypertension with arrhythmias has been reported in an 8-year-old child[5] and in an adult[6] after phenylephrine 10% eye drops had been used. Details have also been published on a series of 32 patients who experienced systemic cardiovascular reactions after the administration of phenylephrine 10% solutions to the eye.[7] Severe cardiovascular adverse reactions have also been reported to the use of phenylephrine as topical 10% ocular[8] or 0.25% nasal[9] pledgets.

Although the incidence of such reactions seems low,[10] the use of lower concentrations[1,7] and caution in susceptible patients such as those with cardiovascular disorders or the elderly,[7] have been advocated. A reduction in the eye-drop volume has been found to produce adequate mydriasis and may reduce systemic absorption and the risk of adverse cardiovascular effects.[11,12]


1. Borromeo-McGrail V, *et al.* Systemic hypertension following ocular administration of 10% phenylephrine in the neonate. *Pediatrics* 1973; **51:** 1032–6.
2. Matthews TG, *et al.* Eye-drop induced hypertension. *Lancet* 1977; **ii:** 827.
3. Saken R, *et al.* Drug-induced hypertension in infancy. *J Pediatr* 1979; **95:** 1077–9.
4. Anonymous. Babies' blood pressure raised by eye drops. *BMJ* 1974; **1:** 2–3.
5. Vaughan RW. Ventricular arrhythmias after topical vasoconstrictors. *Anesth Analg* 1973; **52:** 161–5.
6. Lai Y-K. Adverse effect of intraoperative phenylephrine 10%: case report. *Br J Ophthalmol* 1989; **73:** 468–9.
7. Fraunfelder FT, Scafidi AF. Possible adverse effects from topical ocular 10% phenylephrine. *Am J Ophthalmol* 1978; **85:** 447–53.
8. Fraunfelder FW, *et al.* Adverse systemic effects from pledgets of topical ocular phenylephrine 10%. *Am J Ophthalmol* 2002; **134:** 624–5.
9. Hecker RB, *et al.* Myocardial ischemia and stunning induced by topical intranasal phenylephrine pledgets. *Mil Med* 1997; **162:** 832–5.
10. Brown MM, *et al.* Lack of side effects from topically administered 10% phenylephrine eyedrops: a controlled study. *Arch Ophthalmol* 1980; **98:** 487–9.
11. Craig EW, Griffiths PG. Effect on mydriasis of modifying the volume of phenylephrine drops. *Br J Ophthalmol* 1991; **75:** 222–3.
12. Wheatcroft S, *et al.* Reduction in mydriatic drop size in premature infants. *Br J Ophthalmol* 1993; **77:** 364–5.


**Effects on the eyes.** Acute and chronic conjunctivitis has been reported[1] following use of over-the-counter ophthalmic decongestant preparations of phenylephrine, naphazoline, or tetryzoline. The conjunctival inflammation took several weeks to resolve in some cases. Dermatoconjunctivitis[2] has also been reported following use of phenylephrine eye drops.


1. Soparkar CN, *et al.* Acute and chronic conjunctivitis due to over-the-counter ophthalmic decongestants. *Arch Ophthalmol* 1997; **115:** 34–8.
2. Moreno-Ancillo A, *et al.* Allergic contact reactions due to phenylephrine hydrochloride in eyedrops. *Ann Allergy Asthma Immunol* 1997; **78:** 569–72.


**Effects on mental function.** Hallucinations and paranoid delusions have been reported[1] in a patient following excessive use of a nasal spray containing phenylephrine 0.5%. Mania has also followed the use of high doses by mouth.[2]


1. Snow SS, *et al.* Nasal spray 'addiction' and psychosis: a case report. *Br J Psychiatry* 1980; **136:** 297–9.
2. Waters BGH, Lapierre YD. Secondary mania associated with sympathomimetic drug use. *Am J Psychiatry* 1981; **138:** 837–40.


**Hypersensitivity.** Cross-sensitivity to phenylephrine has been reported in a patient hypersensitive to pseudoephedrine.[1] See also under Effects on the Eyes, above.


1. Buzo-Sanchez G, *et al.* Stereoisomeric cutaneous hypersensitivity. *Ann Pharmacother* 1997; **31:** 1091.


## Interactions

For the interactions of sympathomimetics in general, see under Adrenaline, p.853.

Phenylephrine is less liable than adrenaline or noradrenaline to induce ventricular fibrillation if used as a pressor agent during anaesthesia with inhalational anaesthetics such as cyclopropane and halothane; nevertheless, caution is necessary. Since phenylephrine is absorbed through the mucosa, interactions may also follow topical application, particularly in patients receiving an MAOI (including an RIMA). See also under Phenelzine (p.314) and Moclobemide (p.308).

**Cardiovascular drugs.** Hypertensive reactions have been reported in a patient stabilised on *debrisoquine* when given phenylephrine orally,[1] in patients receiving *reserpine* or *guanethidine* when given phenylephrine eye drops,[2] and a fatal reaction occurred in a patient receiving *propranolol* and *hydrochlorothiazide* also after the instillation of phenylephrine eye drops.[3]


1. Aminu J, *et al.* Interaction between debrisoquine and phenylephrine. *Lancet* 1970; **ii:** 935–6.
2. Kim JM, *et al.* Hypertensive reactions to phenylephrine eyedrops in patients with sympathetic denervation. *Am J Ophthalmol* 1978; **85:** 862–8.
3. Cass E, *et al.* Hazards of phenylephrine topical medication in persons taking propranolol. *Can Med Assoc J* 1979; **120:** 1261–2.


## Pharmacokinetics

Phenylephrine has low oral bioavailability owing to irregular absorption and first-pass metabolism by monoamine oxidase in the gut and liver. When injected subcutaneously or intramuscularly it takes 10 to 15 minutes to act; subcutaneous and intramuscular injections are effective for up to about 1 hour and up to about 2 hours, respectively. Intravenous injections are effective for about 20 minutes.

Systemic absorption follows topical application.

## Uses and Administration

Phenylephrine hydrochloride is a sympathomimetic (see Adrenaline, p.854) with mainly direct effects on adrenergic receptors. It has predominantly alpha-adrenergic activity and is without significant stimulating effects on the CNS at usual doses. Its pressor activity is weaker than that of noradrenaline (p.975) but of longer duration. After injection it produces peripheral vasoconstriction and increased arterial pressure; it also causes reflex bradycardia. It reduces blood flow to the skin and to the kidneys.

Phenylephrine and its salts are most commonly used, either topically or by mouth, for the symptomatic relief of **nasal congestion** (p.1112). They are frequently included in preparations intended for the relief of cough and cold symptoms. For nasal congestion, a 0.25 to 1% solution may be instilled as nasal drops or a spray into each nostril every 4 hours as required, or phenylephrine hydrochloride may be given by mouth in doses up to 20 mg every four hours.

In ophthalmology, phenylephrine hydrochloride is used as a **mydriatic** (p.476) in concentrations of up to 10%; generally solutions containing 2.5 or 10% are employed but systemic absorption can occur (see Effects on the Cardiovascular System, above) and the 10% strength, in particular, should be used with caution. The mydriatic effect can last several hours. Solutions stronger than 2% may cause intense irritation and a local anaesthetic other than butacaine (which is incompatible) should be instilled into the eye a few minutes beforehand.

Ocular solutions containing lower concentrations (usually 0.12% phenylephrine hydrochloride) are used as a **conjunctival decongestant** (see Conjunctivitis, p.421).

Phenylephrine has been used parenterally in the treatment of hypotensive states, such as those encountered during circulatory failure or spinal anaesthesia. For **hypotension**, an initial dose of phenylephrine hydrochloride 2 to 5 mg may be given as a 1% solution subcutaneously or intramuscularly with further doses of 1 to 10 mg if necessary, according to response. A dose of 100 to 500 micrograms by slow intravenous injection as a 0.1% solution, repeated as necessary after at least 15 minutes, has also been employed. In severe hypotensive states, 10 mg in 500 mL of glucose 5% or sodium chloride 0.9% has been infused intravenously, initially at a rate of up to 180 micrograms/minute, reduced, according to the response, to 30 to 60 micrograms/minute. Phenylephrine has also been used in orthostatic hypotension (p.1100).

Phenylephrine hydrochloride has been given by intravenous injection to stop **paroxysmal supraventricular tachycardia** but other drugs are preferred (see Cardiac Arrhythmias, p.816). The initial dose is usually not greater than 500 micrograms given as a 0.1% solution with subsequent doses gradually increased up to 1 mg if necessary.

Phenylephrine hydrochloride has been used for its vasoconstrictor action as an **adjunct** to local anaesthetics.

Phenylephrine has also been used as the acid tartrate to prolong the bronchodilator effects of isoprenaline when administered by inhalation. However, isoprenaline is now little used by this route.

Phenylephrine tannate has also been used.

**Faecal incontinence.** Topical application of phenylephrine gel has been shown to increase resting anal tone[1] and has been investigated in patients with faecal incontinence. Although application of a 10% gel did not appear to be of clinical benefit in a double-blind crossover study in 36 patients with faecal incontinence caused by internal sphincter dysfunction,[2] continence was improved in another small study in patients with ileoanal pouches.[3]


1. Cheetham MJ, *et al.* Topical phenylephrine increases anal canal resting pressure in patients with faecal incontinence. *Gut* 2001; **48:** 356–9.
2. Carapeti EA, *et al.* Randomized controlled trial of topical phenylephrine in the treatment of faecal incontinence. *Br J Surg* 2000; **87:** 38–42.
3. Carapeti EA, *et al.* Randomized, controlled trial of topical phenylephrine for fecal incontinence in patients after ileoanal pouch construction. *Dis Colon Rectum* 2000; **43:** 1059–63.


**Priapism.** For reference to phenylephrine in low dosage and dilute solution being given by intracavernosal injection to reverse priapism, see under Alprostadil, p.1513.

## Preparations

**BP 2003:** Phenylephrine Eye Drops; Phenylephrine Injection;
**USP 27:** Antipyrine, Benzocaine, and Phenylephrine Hydrochloride Otic Solution; Isoproterenol Hydrochloride and Phenylephrine Bitartrate Inhalation Aerosol; Phenylephrine Hydrochloride Injection; Phenylephrine Hydrochloride Nasal Jelly; Phenylephrine Hydrochloride Nasal Solution; Phenylephrine Hydrochloride Ophthalmic Solution.

**Proprietary Preparations** (details are given in Part 3)
***Arg.:*** Fadalefrina; Mydfrin; Poen Efrina; Prefrin; ***Austral.:*** Albalon Relief; Isopto Frin; Neo-Synephrine; Nyal Decongestant; Nyal Sinus Relief; Prefrin; Visopt; ***Austria:*** Prefrin†; Visadron; ***Belg.:*** Isopto Frin†; Neo-Synephrine†; Visadron; ***Braz.:*** Neo-Sinefrina†; ***Canad.:*** Ak-Dilate; Dionephrine; Mydfrin; Neo-Synephrine; Novahistine†; Prefrin; ***Chile:*** Mydfrin; ***Fin.:*** Oftan Metaoksedrin; ***Fr.:*** Auristan; Neosynephrine; ***Ger.:*** Neo-Mydrial; Neosynephrin-POS; Visadron; Vistosan†; ***Hong Kong:*** Analux†; Mydfrin; Prefrin; ***India:*** Drosyn; Pupiletto; ***Irl.:*** Isopto Frin; ***Israel:*** Af-Taf; Efrin; Neo-Synephrine; Prefrin; ***Ital.:*** Isonefrine; Neo-Synephrine; Ribex Nasale; Visadron; ***Malaysia:*** Analux; Isopto Frin; Mydfrin; Prefrin; ***Mex.:*** Lefrine; Rinolan; Weiscalina; ***Neth.:*** Boradrine†; Visadron†; ***NZ:*** Albalon Relief; Isopto Frin; Neosynephrine; Prefrin; ***Port.:*** Davinefrina; Humoxal†; Neo-Sinefrina; Visadron; ***S.Afr.:*** I-Glo; Naphensyl; Prefrin; ***Singapore:*** Analux†; Isopto Frin; Mydfrin; Prefrin; ***Spain:*** ADA; Analux; Boraline; Disneumon Pernasal; Mirazul; Neo Lacrim†; Pulverizador Nasal†; Rin Up; Visadron; Vistafrin; ***Swed.:*** Neo-Synephrine†; ***Switz.:*** Gouttes nasales; Rexophtal N; ***UK:*** Boots Decongestant Capsules; Fenox; Isopto Frin†; Non-Drowsy Sudafed Congestion Relief; ***USA:*** AH-chew D; Ak-Dilate; Ak-Nefrin†; Children's Nostril; Eye Drops Extra†; Mydfrin; Neo-Synephrine; Neofrin; Nostril; Ocu-Phrin; Phenoptic; Prefrin; Rectacaine; Relief; Rhinall; Sinex.

**Multi-ingredient:** numerous preparations are listed in Part 3.

*Used as an adjunct in:* ***Braz.:*** Anestesico.

# Phenylpropanolamine *(BAN, rINN)*

Fenilpropanolamina; (±)-Norephedrine. (*1RS,2SR*)-2-Amino-1-phenylpropan-1-ol.

$C_9H_{13}NO$ = 151.2.

*CAS — 14838-15-4.*

*ATC — R01BA01.*

## Phenylpropanolamine Hydrochloride

*(BANM, rINNM)*

Hidrocloruro de fenilpropanolamina; Mydriatin; Phenylpropanolamini Hydrochloridum.

$C_9H_{13}NO,HCl$ = 187.7.

*CAS — 154-41-6.*

*ATC — R01BA01.*

**Pharmacopoeias.** In *Eur.* (see p.vi) and *US.*

*US* also includes phenylpropanolamine bitartrate.

**Ph. Eur. 5.0** (Phenylpropanolamine Hydrochloride). A white or almost white, crystalline powder. Freely soluble in water and in alcohol; practically insoluble in dichloromethane.

**USP 27** (Phenylpropanolamine Hydrochloride). A white crystalline powder, having a slight aromatic odour. Soluble 1 in 1.1 of water, 1 in 7.4 of alcohol, and 1 in 4100 of chloroform; insoluble in ether. pH of a 3% solution in water is between 4.2 and 5.5. Store in airtight containers. Protect from light.

## Adverse Effects and Precautions

As for Ephedrine, p.1120.

Severe hypertensive episodes have followed phenylpropanolamine ingestion (see below). As with other indirect-acting sympathomimetics, tolerance to the therapeutic effects of phenylpropanolamine has been reported with prolonged administration.

◊ An extensive and detailed review[1] of adverse effects attributed to phenylpropanolamine noted in 1990 that many of the adverse drug reactions reported in Europe described an alteration of mental status whereas those in North America were more often compatible with hypertension. The author suggested that this might be due to a difference in the isomers present in phenylpropanolamine preparations, based on earlier reports that *d*-norpseudoephedrine, the most potent of several isomeric forms as a stimulant of the CNS, was present in European preparations of phenylpropanolamine. However, later investigation suggests that currently the racemic mixture (±)-norephedrine (*d,l*-norephedrine) is the isomeric form present in commercial preparations in both Europe and the USA.[2]

The original review[1] concentrated on North American cases. The majority of products available were decongestants or cough or cold remedies; a small number were promoted as diet aids.

The data suggested that over-the-counter (OTC) products were more likely to be associated with an adverse reaction than a prescription medication; this may be because such OTC products were more likely to be overused and to be considered innocuous by the patient. It was also likely that drug interactions (below) rather than 'true overdosages' were involved in many of the adverse events, particularly as many OTC preparations contain other ingredients. (See also under Abuse of Ephedrine, p.1120, for further discussion about the consequences of use of OTC preparations containing sympathomimetics, including phenylpropanolamine.)

The adverse reactions varied widely ranging from headache and elevated blood pressure to cardiopulmonary arrest, intracranial haemorrhage, and death. Mild reactions included blurred vision, dizziness, anxiety, agitation, tremor, confusion, and hypersensitivity reaction. Severe reactions included hypertensive crisis with hypertensive encephalopathy, seizures, arrhythmias, psychosis, and acute tubular necrosis. One unifying theme of many of the severe cases was that high blood pressure or symptoms suggestive of this were the presenting feature; an acute, persistent, severe headache was also noted in many cases.

It was pointed out that overall phenylpropanolamine was relatively safe. Although billions of doses were consumed annually, few cases of adverse drug reactions had been reported.

It was believed that certain groups may be at particular risk of adverse reactions to phenylpropanolamine: persons with elevated blood pressure, overweight persons (who are likely to be both hypertensive and to use diet aids), patients with eating disorders (who tend to abuse substances including diet aids), and the elderly (who may be multiple drug takers and likely to be hypertensive and at risk already of a stroke).

Subsequently, following a large case-control study in the USA which found an increased risk of haemorrhagic stroke associated with the use of preparations containing phenylpropanolamine (and in particular in women who used phenylpropanolamine as an appetite suppressant),[3] the FDA took steps to remove phenylpropanolamine from all drug products in the USA and requested that it no longer be marketed. Products containing phenylpropanolamine have also been withdrawn in some other countries. However, this study has been criticised[4,5] on the basis that it provided no evidence of an increased risk with the amount of phenylpropanolamine normally present in decongestant preparations. The UK Committee on Safety of Medicines[6] considered that the evidence of a link between UK products containing phenylpropanolamine and haemorrhagic stroke was weak (phenylpropanolamine is not licensed as an appetite suppressant in the UK and the maximum recommended dose of 100 mg daily was lower than the 150 mg daily recommended in the USA). It was therefore suggested by UK commentators that use of licensed doses, with appropriate precautions, posed no additional risk.[2] However, subsequently, UK preparations containing phenylpropanolamine have either been reformulated (mainly with pseudoephedrine) or withdrawn by the manufacturers.

1. Lake CR, *et al.* Adverse drug effects attributed to phenylpropanolamine: a review of 142 case reports. *Am J Med* 1990; **89:** 195–208.
2. Moffatt T, *et al.* Phenylpropanolamine: putting the record straight. *Pharm J* 2000; **265:** 817.
3. Kernan WN, *et al.* Phenylpropanolamine and the risk of hemorrhagic stroke. *N Engl J Med* 2000; **343:** 1826–32.
4. Ernst ME, Hartz A. Phenylpropanolamine and hemorrhagic stroke. *N Engl J Med* 2001; **344:** 1094.
5. Wolowich WR, *et al.* Phenylpropanolamine and hemorrhagic stroke. *N Engl J Med* 2001; **344:** 1094–5.
6. Committee on Safety of Medicines/Medicines Control Agency. Phenylpropanolamine and haemorrhagic stroke. *Current Problems* 2001; **27:** 5–6. Also available at: http://www.mca.gov.uk/ourwork/monitorsafequalmed/currentproblems/cpfeb2001.pdf (accessed 01/07/04)

## Interactions

For the interactions of sympathomimetics in general, see under Adrenaline, p.853. For a comment that drug interactions were likely to have been involved in many adverse events associated with phenylpropanolamine see under Adverse Effects and Precautions, above. Hypertensive crisis is a particular risk in patients receiving MAOIs.

**Amantadine.** Severe psychosis has been reported[1] in a woman taking amantadine and phenylpropanolamine together.

1. Stroe AE, *et al.* Psychotic episode related to phenylpropanolamine and amantadine in a healthy female. *Gen Hosp Psychiatry* 1995; **17:** 457–8.

**Antipsychotics.** A 27-year-old woman with schizophrenia and T-wave abnormality of the heart, who had responded to *thioridazine* 100 mg daily with procyclidine 2.5 mg twice daily, died from ventricular fibrillation within 2 hours of taking a single dose of a preparation reported to contain chlorphenamine maleate 4 mg with phenylpropanolamine hydrochloride 50 mg (Contac C), concurrently with thioridazine.[1]

1. Chouinard G, *et al.* Death attributed to ventricular arrhythmia induced by thioridazine in combination with a single Contac C capsule. *Can Med Assoc J* 1978; **119:** 729–31.

**Antivirals.** Hypertensive crisis developed in a patient taking an over-the-counter nasal decongestant preparation containing phenylpropanolamine and clemastine concomitantly with a triple-drug HIV prophylactic regimen 3 days after *stavudine* was substituted for *zidovudine*;[1] the other antivirals in the regimen were *indinavir* and *lamivudine*.

1. Khurana V, *et al.* Hypertensive crisis secondary to phenylpropanolamine interacting with triple-drug therapy for HIV prophylaxis. *Am J Med* 1999; **106:** 118–19.

**Bromocriptine.** For a report of hypertension and life-threatening complications following concomitant use of phenylpropanolamine and bromocriptine, see p.1202.

**NSAIDs.** A 27-year-old woman who had been taking D-phenylpropanolamine [sic] 85 mg daily for some months, experienced severe hypertension when she also took *indometacin* 25 mg. It was considered that the inhibition of prostaglandin synthesis by indometacin might have caused enhancement of the sympathomimetic effect of phenylpropanolamine.[1]

1. Lee KY, *et al.* Severe hypertension after ingestion of an appetite suppressant (phenylpropanolamine) with indomethacin. *Lancet* 1979; **i:** 1110–11.

## Pharmacokinetics

Phenylpropanolamine is readily and completely absorbed from the gastrointestinal tract, peak plasma concentrations being achieved about 1 or 2 hours after oral doses. It undergoes some metabolism in the liver, to an active hydroxylated metabolite, but up to 80 to 90% of a dose is excreted unchanged in the urine within 24 hours. The half-life has been reported to be about 3 to 5 hours.

◊ References.

1. Scherzinger SS, *et al.* Steady state pharmacokinetics and dose-proportionality of phenylpropanolamine in healthy subjects. *J Clin Pharmacol* 1990; **30:** 372–7.
2. Simons FER, *et al.* Pharmacokinetics of the orally administered decongestants pseudoephedrine and phenylpropanolamine in children. *J Pediatr* 1996; **129:** 729–34.

## Uses and Administration

Phenylpropanolamine is a largely indirect-acting sympathomimetic (see Adrenaline, p.854) with an action similar to that of ephedrine (p.1120) but less active as a CNS stimulant.

Phenylpropanolamine has been given by mouth as the hydrochloride for the symptomatic treatment of nasal congestion (p.1112). It is frequently used in combination preparations for the relief of cough and cold symptoms.

In the management of nasal congestion, phenylpropanolamine hydrochloride has been given in doses of up to 50 mg twice daily by mouth as modified-release preparations.

Other uses of phenylpropanolamine have included the control of urinary incontinence in some patients (see p.476). It has also been given in the management of some forms of priapism (see under Metaraminol, p.952). Phenylpropanolamine has been used to suppress appetite in the management of obesity (p.1583) but the use of stimulants is no longer recommended.

Phenylpropanolamine polistirex (a phenylpropanolamine and sulfonated diethenylbenzene-ethenylbenzene copolymer complex) has also been used, as have phenylpropanolamine bitartrate and phenylpropanolamine sulfate.

## Preparations

**USP 27:** Chlorpheniramine Maleate and Phenylpropanolamine Hydrochloride Extended-release Capsules; Chlorpheniramine Maleate and Phenylpropanolamine Hydrochloride Extended-release Tablets; Phenylpropanolamine Hydrochloride Capsules; Phenylpropanolamine Hydrochloride Extended-release Capsules; Phenylpropanolamine Hydrochloride Extended-release Tablets; Phenylpropanolamine Hydrochloride Oral Solution; Phenylpropanolamine Hydrochloride Tablets.

**Proprietary Preparations** (details are given in Part 3)

***Fin.:*** Rinexin; ***Ger.:*** Fasupond†; Recatol mono; ***Hong Kong:*** Slimomin†; ***Norw.:*** Monydrin†; Rinexin; ***S.Afr.:*** Restaslim; ***Swed.:*** Monydrin†; Rinexin; ***Switz.:*** Capton Diet†; Dexatrim†; Kontexin; Merex; Slim Caps; ***Thai.:*** Fansia†; ***USA:*** Acutrim†; Appedrine†; Control†; Dexatrim†; Just One Per Day†; Phenoxine†; Phenyldrine†; Propagest†; Spray-U-Thin†; Unitrol†.

**Multi-ingredient:** numerous preparations are listed in Part 3.

# Pholcodine *(BAN, rINN)*

Folcodina; Pholcodinum. 3-*O*-(2-Morpholinoethyl)morphine monohydrate.

$C_{23}H_{30}N_2O_4,H_2O = 416.5.$

*CAS — 509-67-1 (anhydrous pholcodine).*

*ATC — R05DA08.*

**Pharmacopoeias.** In *Chin.* and *Eur.* (see p.vi).

**Ph. Eur. 5.0** (Pholcodine). A white or almost white crystalline powder or colourless crystals. Sparingly soluble in water; freely soluble in alcohol and in acetone; dissolves in dilute mineral acids.

## Adverse Effects and Precautions

As for Dextromethorphan, p.1117. Constipation or drowsiness have been reported occasionally.

## Interactions

Use of pholcodine with alcohol or other CNS depressants may increase the effects on the CNS.

## Uses and Administration

Pholcodine is a centrally acting cough suppressant that has actions and uses similar to those of dextromethorphan (p.1118). It is given by mouth in a usual dose of 5 to 10 mg three or four times daily; children over 5 years of age may be given 2.5 to 5 mg three or four times daily and children 1 to 5 years, 2 to 2.5 mg three times daily. The citrate has also been used. Pholcodine polistirex (a pholcodine and sulfonated diethenylbenzene-ethenylbenzene copolymer complex) is used in modified-release preparations.

## Preparations

**BP 2003:** Pholcodine Linctus; Strong Pholcodine Linctus.

**Proprietary Preparations** (details are given in Part 3)

***Austral.:*** Actifed CC Dry; Actuss; Duro-Tuss; Logicin Cough Suppressant†; Nyal Plus+ Dry Cough; Ordov Dry Tickly Cough†; Pholtrate†; Tussinol; ***Fin.:*** Tuxi; ***Fr.:*** Biocalyptol; Broncorinol toux seche; Codotussyl Toux Seche; Humex; Respilene; Rhinathiol Toux Seche Pholcodine; Sirop Des Vosges Toux Seche; ***Hong Kong:*** Duro-Tuss; Uni-Pholco; ***Irl.:*** Expulin Dry Cough; Pholcolin; ***Malaysia:*** Dhacodine; Duro-Tuss; ***Norw.:*** Tuxi; ***NZ:*** Actifed CC Dry; Duro-Tuss; Pharmacycare Cough†; ***S.Afr.:*** Pholcolinct; ***Singapore:*** Duro-Tuss; ***Spain:*** Trophires; ***UK:*** Benylin Childrens Dry Coughs; Boots Dry Cough Syrup 1 Year Plus; Evaphol†; Expulin Dry Cough†; Galenphol; Hill's Balsam Dry Cough; Pavacol-D; Tixylix Daytime.

**Multi-ingredient:** ***Austral.:*** Chemists Own Kiddicol; Difflam Anti-inflammatory Cough Lozenges; Duro-Tuss Cough Lozenges; Duro-Tuss Decongestant; Duro-Tuss Expectorant; Phensedyl; Tixylix Nightime; ***Belg.:*** Broncal†; Bronchalene†; Broncho-pectoralis; Eucalyptine Pholcodine Le Brun; Folcodex†; Folex; Pholco-Mereprine; ***Fr.:*** Broncalene; Clarix; Denoral; Dimetane; Eucalyptine Pholcodine†; Hexapneumine; Isomyrtine; Pholcodyl†; Pholcones†; Polery; Pulmosodyl†; Quintopan Enfant†; Trophires; ***Hong Kong:*** Biocalyptol; Denoral†; Duro-Tuss Decongestant; Duro-Tuss Expectorant; Hexapneumine; Tixylix Nightime†; Tripe P; ***India:*** Tixylix; ***Irl.:*** Expulin; Expulin Childrens Cough; Tixylix†; ***Malaysia:*** Tixylix; ***Norw.:*** Tuxidrin†; ***NZ:*** Difflam Cough; Duro-Tuss Decongestant; Duro-Tuss Expectorant; Duro-Tuss Lozenges; Phensedyl Dry Family Cough; Tixylix; ***S.Afr.:*** Contra-Coff†; Docsed; Folcofen; Pholtex; Procof; Respinol Compound; Tixylix; ***Singapore:*** 3P; Delix†; Duro-Tuss Decongestant; Duro-Tuss Expectorant; ***Spain:*** Caltoson Balsamico; ***Switz.:*** Pecto-Baby; Phol-Tussil; Phol-Tux; Rectoseptal-Neo Pholcodine†; Tussiplex; ***UK:*** Boots Nightime Cough Syrup 1 Year Plus; Cold Relief Daytime†; Cold Relief Night-Time†; Day & Night Nurse; Day Cold Comfort†; Day Nurse; Expulin Childrens Cough†; Expulin†; Night Cold Comfort†; Nirolex Day Cold & Flu; Nirolex Night Cold & Flu; Phensedyl Plus†; Tixylix Cough & Cold; Tixylix Night-Time.

## Pipazetate (BAN, rINN)

D-254; Pipazethate (USAN); SKF-70230-A; SQ-15874. 2-(2-Piperidinoethoxy)ethyl pyrido[3,2-*b*][1,4]benzothiazine-10-carboxylate.

$C_{21}H_{25}N_3O_3S$ = 399.5.
*ATC — R05DB11.*

## Pipazetate Hydrochloride (BANM, rINNM)

Hidrocloruro de pipazetato; Pipazethate Hydrochloride; Piperestazine Hydrochloride.

$C_{21}H_{25}N_3O_3S,HCl$ = 436.0.
*CAS — 6056-11-7 (pipazetate hydrochloride).*
*ATC — R05DB11.*

### Profile

Pipazetate hydrochloride is a centrally acting cough suppressant which also has some peripheral actions in non-productive cough (p.1112). It has been given by mouth and rectally.

**Overdosage.** A healthy 4-year-old child became somnolent and agitated, with convulsions, followed by coma, after swallowing an unknown number of tablets containing pipazetate; cardiac arrhythmias also developed.[1] Fatal toxicity has also been reported in children.[2,3]

1. da Silva OA, Lopez M. Pipazethate—acute childhood poisoning. *Clin Toxicol* 1977; **11:** 455–8.
2. Bonavita V, *et al.* Accidental lethal pipazethate poisoning in a child. *Z Rechtsmed* 1982; **89:** 145–8.
3. Soto E, *et al.* Pipazethate lethality in a baby. *Vet Hum Toxicol* 1993; **35:** 41.

### Preparations

**Proprietary Preparations** (details are given in Part 3)
***Austria:*** Selvigon†; ***Braz.:*** Selvigon; ***Ger.:*** Selvigon Hustensaft†; ***Ital.:*** Selvjgon; ***Mex.:*** Selvigon; ***Thai.:*** Transpulmin.

## Poppy Capsule

Dormideiras; Fruit du Pavot; Fruto de adormidera; Mohnfrucht; Papaveris Capsula; Poppy Heads.

**Pharmacopoeias.** In *Chin.*

### Profile

Poppy capsule consists of dried fruits of *Papaver somniferum* (Papaveraceae), collected before dehiscence has occurred, containing very small amounts of morphine with traces of other opium alkaloids. It is mildly sedative and has been used as a liquid extract or syrup in cough mixtures.

### Preparations

**Proprietary Preparations** (details are given in Part 3)
**Multi-ingredient:** ***Belg.:*** Tisane Pectorale†; Tisane pour Dormir†; ***Braz.:*** Malvodon; Pectoss†; ***Fr.:*** Mediflor Tisane Pectorale d'Alsace†.

## Prednazoline (rINN)

Prednazolina; Prednisolone-Fenoxazoline Compound. 11β,17α,-21-Trihydroxypregna-1,4-diene-3,20-dione 21-(dihydrogen phosphate) compound with 2-(2-isopropylphenoxymethyl)-2-imidazoline.

$C_{21}H_{29}O_8P,C_{13}H_{18}N_2O$ = 658.7.
*CAS — 6693-90-9.*

### Profile

Prednazoline has the general properties of prednisolone (p.1108) and of fenoxazoline (p.1121) and has been used locally in the form of a nasal spray in the treatment of pharyngitis, rhinitis, and sinusitis.

### Preparations

**Proprietary Preparations** (details are given in Part 3)
***Braz.:*** Oto-Rinil†.

## Prenoxdiazine Hydrochloride (rINNM)

Hidrocloruro de prenoxdiazina; HK-256; Prenoxdiazin Hydrochloride. 3-(2,2-Diphenylethyl)-5-(2-piperidinoethyl)-1,2,4-oxadiazole hydrochloride.

$C_{23}H_{27}N_3O,HCl$ = 397.9.
*CAS — 47543-65-7 (prenoxdiazine); 37671-82-2 (prenoxdiazine hibenzate); 982-43-4 (prenoxdiazine hydrochloride).*
*ATC — R05DB18.*

### Profile

Prenoxdiazine hydrochloride is a peripherally acting cough suppressant for non-productive cough (p.1112) that has been given by mouth. Prenoxdiazine hibenzate has also been used.

### Preparations

**Proprietary Preparations** (details are given in Part 3)
***India:*** Libexin; ***Switz.:*** Libexine†; Mephatussine†; Mephaxine†.

**Multi-ingredient:** ***Ital.:*** Broncofluid; Libexin Mucolitico; ***Switz.:*** Libexine Compositum†; Mephatussine Compositum†; Mephaxine Compositum†.

## Promolate (rINN)

Morphethylbutyne. 2-Morpholinoethyl 2-methyl-2-phenoxypropionate.

$C_{16}H_{23}NO_4$ = 293.4.
*CAS — 3615-74-5.*

### Profile

Promolate is a cough suppressant that has been given rectally.

### Preparations

**Proprietary Preparations** (details are given in Part 3)
***Chile:*** Atusil.

# Pseudoephedrine (BAN, rINN)

*d*-Ψ-Ephedrine; *d*-Isoephedrine; Pseudoefedrina. (+)-(1*S*,2*S*)-2-Methylamino-1-phenylpropan-1-ol.

$C_{10}H_{15}NO$ = 165.2.
*CAS — 90-82-4.*
*ATC — R01BA02.*

**Description.** Pseudoephedrine is an alkaloid obtained from *Ephedra* spp.

## Pseudoephedrine Hydrochloride (BANM, USAN, rINNM)

Hidrocloruro de pseudoefedrina; Pseudoephedrini Hydrochloridum.

$C_{10}H_{15}NO,HCl$ = 201.7.
*CAS — 345-78-8.*
*ATC — R01BA02.*

**Pharmacopoeias.** In *Chin., Eur.* (see p.vi), and *US.*

**Ph. Eur. 5.0** (Pseudoephedrine Hydrochloride). A white or almost white, crystalline powder or colourless crystals. Freely soluble in water and in alcohol; sparingly soluble in dichloromethane. Protect from light.

**USP 27** (Pseudoephedrine Hydrochloride). A fine, white to off-white crystalline powder, having a faint characteristic odour. Soluble 1 in 0.5 of water, 1 in 3.6 of alcohol, 1 in 91 of chloroform, and 1 in 7000 of ether. pH of a 5% solution in water is between 4.6 and 6.0. Store in airtight containers. Protect from light.

## Pseudoephedrine Sulfate (USAN, rINNM)

Pseudoephedrine Sulphate (BANM); Sch-4855; Sulfato de pseudoefedrina.

$(C_{10}H_{15}NO)_2,H_2SO_4$ = 428.5.
*CAS — 7460-12-0.*
*ATC — R01BA02.*

**Pharmacopoeias.** In *US.*

**USP 27** (Pseudoephedrine Sulfate). Odourless, white crystals or crystalline powder. Freely soluble in alcohol. pH of a 5% solution in water is between 5.0 and 6.5. Store in airtight containers. Protect from light.

## Adverse Effects and Precautions

As for Ephedrine, p.1120. The commonest adverse effects of pseudoephedrine include tachycardia, anxiety, restlessness, and insomnia; skin rashes and urinary retention have occasionally occurred. Hallucinations have been reported rarely, particularly in children.

**Abuse.** Acute psychosis and visual and tactile hallucinations have been reported[1] in an 18-year-old male following intravenous misuse of pseudoephedrine hydrochloride.

For reference to toxic effects following long-term use of over-the-counter preparations containing sympathomimetics, including pseudoephedrine, see under Ephedrine, p.1120.

1. Sullivan G. Acute psychosis following intravenous abuse of pseudoephedrine: a case report. *J Psychopharmacol* 1996; **10:** 324–5.

**Breast feeding.** The American Academy of Pediatrics[1] states that, although usually compatible with breast feeding, preparations used by breast-feeding mothers that contain pseudoephedrine with dexbrompheniramine maleate have resulted in crying, irritability, and poor sleep patterns in the infant.

The concentrations of pseudoephedrine and triprolidine in plasma and breast milk of 3 lactating mothers for up to 48 hours after ingestion of a preparation containing pseudoephedrine hydrochloride 60 mg with triprolidine hydrochloride 2.5 mg have been studied.[2] Concentrations of pseudoephedrine in milk were consistently higher than in plasma; the half-life in both fluids was between 4.2 and 7.0 hours. Assuming a generous milk secretion of 500 mL over 12 hours it was calculated that the excreted dose was the equivalent of 250 to 330 micrograms of pseudoephedrine base, or 0.5 to 0.7% of the dose ingested by the mothers. Triprolidine did not appear to be concentrated in breast milk. The amounts of pseudoephedrine and triprolidine distributed into breast milk were probably not high enough to warrant cessation of breast feeding.

1. American Academy of Pediatrics. The transfer of drugs and other chemicals into human milk. *Pediatrics* 2001; **108:** 776–89. Correction. *ibid.*; 1029. Also available at: http://aappolicy.aappublications.org/cgi/content/full/pediatrics%3b108/3/776 (accessed 01/07/04)
2. Findlay JWA, *et al.* Pseudoephedrine and triprolidine in plasma and breast milk of nursing mothers. *Br J Clin Pharmacol* 1984; **18:** 901–6.

**Convulsions.** A child who suffered a generalised seizure after ingesting a large quantity of pseudoephedrine hydrochloride tablets was believed to be the first report of convulsions associated with overdose of a preparation containing the drug as a single ingredient.[1]

1. Clark RF, Curry SC. Pseudoephedrine dangers. *Pediatrics* 1990; **85:** 389–90.

**Effects on the gastrointestinal tract.** Ischaemic colitis has been reported[1,2] after acute or chronic use of pseudoephedrine in combination cold and allergy preparations.

1. Dowd J, *et al.* Ischemic colitis associated with pseudoephedrine: four cases. *Am J Gastroenterol* 1999; **94:** 2430–4.
2. Lichtenstein GR, Yee NS. Ischemic colitis associated with decongestant use. *Ann Intern Med* 2000; **132:** 682.

**Effects on mental function.** Adverse mental effects (particularly in children) have been associated with combination preparations containing pseudoephedrine.[1-5] See also under Abuse, above.

1. Leighton KM. Paranoid psychosis after abuse of Actifed. *BMJ* 1982; **284:** 789–90.
2. Sankey RJ, *et al.* Visual hallucinations in children receiving decongestants. *BMJ* 1984; **288:** 1369.
3. Stokes MA. Visual hallucinations in children receiving decongestants. *BMJ* 1984; **288:** 1540.
4. Roberge RJ, *et al.* Dextromethorphan and pseudoephedrine-induced agitated psychosis and ataxia: case report. *J Emerg Med* 1999; **17:** 285–8.
5. Soutullo CA, *et al.* Psychosis associated with pseudoephedrine and dextromethorphan. *J Am Acad Child Adolesc Psychiatry* 1999; **38:** 1471–2.

**Effects on the skin.** Recurrent pseudo-scarlatina has been described in a female patient and attributed, on some occasions at least, to ingestion of pseudoephedrine.[1] Further fixed drug eruptions associated with pseudoephedrine have been reported.[2-4] In another woman, an erythematous macular rash developed 5½ hours after a challenge dose of pseudoephedrine 60 mg by mouth; other symptoms, which mimicked the effects of toxic shock syndrome, included nausea and vomiting, fever, orthostatic hypotension, light-headedness, fatigue, and desquamation of the skin on her palms and soles.[3] However, considering the frequent use of pseudoephedrine in over-the-counter medications, associated drug eruptions generally appear to be rare.[2]

1. Taylor BJ, Duffill MB. *Br J Dermatol* 1988; **118:** 827–9.
2. Camisa C. Fixed drug reactions to pseudoephedrine hydrochloride. *Br J Dermatol* 1989; **120:** 857–8.
3. Cavanah DK, Ballas ZK. Pseudoephedrine reaction presenting as recurrent toxic shock syndrome. *Ann Intern Med* 1993; **119:** 302–3.
4. Hauken M. Fixed drug eruption and pseudoephedrine. *Ann Intern Med* 1994; **120:** 442.

**Tolerance.** In 34 healthy males given pseudoephedrine 120 or 150 mg twice daily for 7 days, as a modified-release preparation, mean plasma concentrations were about 450 or 510 nanograms/mL, respectively. Side-effects (dry mouth, anorexia, insomnia, anxiety, tension, restlessness, tachycardia, palpitations) were common; there was some evidence of tachyphylaxis.[1]

1. Dickerson J, *et al.* Dose tolerance and pharmacokinetic studies of L(+) pseudoephedrine capsules in man. *Eur J Clin Pharmacol* 1978; **14:** 253–9.

## Interactions

As for Ephedrine, p.1120. Pseudoephedrine may cause a hypertensive crisis in patients receiving an MAOI (including an RIMA). For additional warnings see under phenelzine (p.314) and moclobemide (p.308).

**Antacids.** The absorption rate of pseudoephedrine hydrochloride was increased by *aluminium hydroxide* mixture but was decreased by *kaolin*; in the latter case adsorption may have competed with absorption.[1]

1. Lucarotti RL, *et al.* Enhanced pseudoephedrine absorption by concurrent administration of aluminium hydroxide gel in humans. *J Pharm Sci* 1972; **61:** 903–5.

**Vaccines.** A 21-year-old mildly obese man taking pseudoephedrine in an over-the-counter formulation for weight loss collapsed and died with a core temperature of 42.2° while exercising, shortly after inoculation with *Japanese encephalitis vaccine* and *typhoid vaccine*.[1] The combined effects of the pseudoephedrine, activity, and the pyrogenic action of the vaccines appeared to have contributed to failure of the thermoregulatory system.

1. Franklin QJ. Sudden death after typhoid and Japanese encephalitis vaccination in a young male taking pseudoephedrine. *Mil Med* 1999; **164:** 157–9.

## Pharmacokinetics

Pseudoephedrine is readily absorbed from the gastrointestinal tract. It is largely excreted unchanged in the urine together with small amounts of its hepatic metabolite. It has a half-life of about 5 to 8 hours; elimination is enhanced and half-life accordingly shorter in acid urine. Small amounts are distributed into breast milk.

◊ References.

1. Kuntzman RG, *et al.* The influence of urinary pH on the plasma half-life of pseudoephedrine in man and dog and a sensitive assay for its determination in human plasma. *Clin Pharmacol Ther* 1971; **12:** 62–7.
2. Lai CM, *et al.* Urinary excretion of chlorpheniramine and pseudoephedrine in humans. *J Pharm Sci* 1979; **68:** 1243–6.
3. Yacobi A, *et al.* Evaluation of sustained-action chlorpheniramine-pseudoephedrine dosage form in humans. *J Pharm Sci* 1980; **69:** 1077–81.
4. Simons FER, *et al.* Pharmacokinetics of the orally administered decongestants pseudoephedrine and phenylpropanolamine in children. *J Pediatr* 1996; **129:** 729–34.

## Uses and Administration

Pseudoephedrine is a direct- and indirect-acting sympathomimetic (see Adrenaline, p.854). It is a stereoisomer of ephedrine (p.1120) and has a similar action, but has been stated to have less pressor activity and fewer CNS effects.

Pseudoephedrine and its salts are given by mouth for the symptomatic relief of nasal congestion (p.1112). They are commonly combined with other ingredients in preparations intended for the relief of cough and cold symptoms.

Pseudoephedrine hydrochloride or sulfate are generally given in doses of 60 mg three or four times daily by mouth. Suggested oral doses for children are: 2 to 5 years, 15 mg three or four times daily; 6 to 12 years, 30 mg three or four times daily. Modified-release preparations are also available; a usual adult dose is 120 mg every 12 hours or 240 mg every 24 hours.

Other uses of pseudoephedrine include the control of urinary incontinence (p.476) in some patients. It has also been given in the management of some forms of priapism (see under Metaraminol, p.952).

Pseudoephedrine polistirex (a pseudoephedrine and sulfonated diethenylbenzene-ethenylbenzene copolymer complex) has also been used, as has pseudoephedrine tannate.

**Barotrauma.** Results from a controlled trial[1] suggest that pseudoephedrine administered to adults at least 30 minutes before flying appears to decrease the incidence of ear pain associated with pressure changes.[1] However, a similar decrease in risk was not noted in children.[2]

1. Jones JS, *et al.* A double-blind comparison between oral pseudoephedrine and topical oxymetazoline in the prevention of barotrauma during air travel. *Am J Emerg Med* 1998; **16:** 262–4.
2. Buchanan BJ, *et al.* Pseudoephedrine and air travel-associated ear pain in children. *Arch Pediatr Adolesc Med* 1999; **153:** 466–8.

## Preparations

***BP 2003:*** Pseudoephedrine Tablets;
***USP 27:*** Acetaminophen and Pseudoephedrine Hydrochloride Tablets; Acetaminophen, Dextromethorphan Hydrobromide, Doxylamine Succinate, and Pseudoephedrine Hydrochloride Oral Solution; Acetaminophen, Diphenhydramine Hydrochloride, and Pseudoephedrine Hydrochloride Tablets; Chlorpheniramine Maleate and Pseudoephedrine Hydrochloride Extended-release Capsules; Chlorpheniramine Maleate and Pseudoephedrine Hydrochloride Oral Solution; Dexbrompheniramine Maleate and Pseudoephedrine Sulfate Oral Solution; Diphenhydramine and Pseudoephedrine Capsules; Guaifenesin and Pseudoephedrine Hydrochloride Capsules; Guaifenesin, Pseudoephedrine Hydrochloride, and Dextromethorphan Hydrobromide Capsules; Ibuprofen and Pseudoephedrine Hydrochloride Tablets; Pseudoephedrine Hydrochloride Extended-Release Capsules; Pseudoephedrine Hydrochloride Extended-release Tablets; Pseudoephedrine Hydrochloride Syrup; Pseudoephedrine Hydrochloride Tablets; Pseudoephedrine Hydrochloride, Carbinoxamine Maleate, and Dextromethorphan Hydrobromide Oral Solution; Triprolidine and Pseudoephedrine Hydrochlorides Syrup; Triprolidine and Pseudoephedrine Hydrochlorides Tablets.

**Proprietary Preparations** (details are given in Part 3)
***Arg.:*** Mex; ***Austral.:*** Chemists Own Sinus Relief; Demazin Sinus; Dimetapp Sinus; Logicin Sinus; Nyal Plus+ Decongestant; Sudafed; Sudafed Sinus & Nasal Decongestant†; ***Belg.:*** Nasa-12†; Rinomar; Vasocedine Pseudoephedrine; ***Canad.:*** Balminil Decongestant†; Congest Aid; Congest-Eze; Contac Cold Nondrowsy; Decongestant Tablets; Drixoral ND; Eltor; Maxenal†; Nasal & Sinus Relief; Plus Sinus†; Pseudofrin; Robidrine†; Sudafed Decongestant; Sudodrin†; Tantafed; Triaminic Allergy Congestion; Triaminic Pediatric Drops; ***Chile:*** Asafen Nueva Formula; ***Fr.:*** Drill rhinites†; Ephedroides; Sudafed; ***Hong Kong:*** Balminil Decongestant†; Logicin Sinus; Sudafed†; ***India:*** Sudafed; ***Irl.:*** Galpseud†; Sudafed; ***Israel:*** Afalpi Tiptipot; Otrinol†; Sinufed; Sinufed Kid Day; Tarophed; ***Ital.:*** Narixan; ***Mex.:*** Dofedrin; Dofen†; Suboffen; Sudafed; ***NZ:*** Dimetapp Sinus; Sudafed 12 Hour Relief; Sudafed for Children; Sudafed Sinus & Nasal Decongestant; Sudomyl; ***Port.:*** Sudafed; ***S.Afr.:*** Acunaso†; Adco-Sufedrin; Demazin Decongestant; Drilix; Drixora†; Flutex Decon-S; Monofed; Sinumed; Sudafed; Symptofed; ***Singapore:*** Sudafed; ***Switz.:*** Otrinol; ***Thai.:*** Pseudono†; Sudosian; ***UAE:*** Sedofan II; ***UK:*** Bronalin Decongestant†; Contac Non Drowsy; Decongestant Tablets†; Galsud; Meltus Decongestant; Non-Drowsy Sudafed Decongestant; ***USA:*** Afrin; Allermed; Cenafed; Childrens Sudafed Nasal Decongestant; Congestaid; Congestion Relief†; Decofed; DeFed; Dimetapp Decongestant; Dorcol Children's Decongestant; Drixoral Non-Drowsy Formula; Dynafed Pseudo†; Efidac 24 Pseudoepehdrine; Genaphed; Halofed; Kid Kare Pediatric Nasal Decongestant; Medi-First Sinus Decongestant; Mini Pseudo; PediaCare Infant's Decongestant; Pseudo; Pseudo-Gest; Seudotabs; Silfedrine; Simply Stuffy; Sinustop Pro; Sudafed; Triaminic AM Decongestant Formula; Triaminic Infant Oral Decongestant.

**Multi-ingredient:** numerous preparations are listed in Part 3.

## Senega Root

Polígala Raíz; Polygalae Radix; Raíz de polígala; Rattlesnake Root; Seneca Snakeroot; Senega.

*CAS — 1260-04-4 (polygalic acid).*
*ATC — R05CA06.*

**Pharmacopoeias.** In *Eur.* (see p.vi) and *Jpn.*
*Jpn* also describes the powdered root.

**Ph. Eur. 5.0** (Senega Root). The dried and usually fragmented root and root crown of *Polygala senega* or certain closely related species of *Polygala* or a mixture of these. It has a faint, sweet odour, slightly rancid or reminiscent of methyl salicylate. Protect from light and humidity.

### Profile

Senega root has been used as an expectorant in preparations given by mouth for respiratory-tract disorders.

*Polygala amara* is a related species that is used similarly.

### Preparations

**Proprietary Preparations** (details are given in Part 3)

**Multi-ingredient:** ***Arg.:*** Hebert Caramelos; Ixana; No-Tos Adultos; No-Tos Infantil; Pectobron; ***Austral.:*** Asa Tones†; Senagar; Senega and Ammonia†; ***Austria:*** Anitos; Breston; Bronchiplant; Bronchiplant light; Luuf Krauter-Hustensaft; Tussimont; ***Belg.:*** Tux; ***Braz.:*** Broncmel†; Expectomel; Limao Bravo†; Mel de Jatahy†; Melagriao†; Pectal; Xarope Comp Mel e Agriao†; ***Canad.:*** Bronchial; Bronchozone; Sirop Cocillana Codeine; Wampole Bronchial Cough Syrup; ***Fr.:*** Desbly†; Neo-Codion; Sirop Pectoral adulte†; ***Ger.:*** Asthma 6-N; ***Hong Kong:*** Cocillana Compound; Mefedra-N; Mist Expect Stim; Pectoral; ***Port.:*** Calmarum; Fluidin Antiasmatico†; Fluidin Infantil†; Stodal; ***Spain:*** Broncovital; Combitorax†; Pastillas Pectoral Kely; Pulmofasa; Pulmofasa Antihist†; ***Swed.:*** Cocillana-Etyfin; ***Switz.:*** Bronchofluid N; Bronchofluid†; Expectoran Codein; Foral; Hederix; Liberol Pastilles contre la toux; Liberol Sirop contre la toux; Makatussin forte†; Makatussin†; Pastilles pectorales formule 541†; Pectocalmine; Pectoral N; Phol-Tux; Sirop antitussif Wyss a base de codeine†; Sirop Wyss contre la toux†; ***UK:*** Antibron; Chest Mixture; Chesty Cough Relief; ES Bronchial Mixture†; Tickly Cough & Sore Throat Relief.

## Sobrerol

Ciclidrol; Cyclidrol; Sobrerolo. *p*-Menth-6-ene-2,8-diol.

$C_{10}H_{18}O_2$ = 170.2.
*CAS — 498-71-5.*
*ATC — R05CB07.*

**Pharmacopoeias.** In *It.*

### Profile

Sobrerol is a mucolytic that has been used in respiratory disorders characterised by productive cough (p.1112). Doses of up to 800 mg have been given by mouth daily in divided doses. Sobrerol has also been given by injection, inhalation, or rectally.

**Pharmacokinetics.** The pharmacokinetics of sobrerol after oral or intravenous administration has been studied in patients with acute exacerbations of chronic bronchitis.[1] Sobrerol was rapidly absorbed from the gastrointestinal tract and rapidly distributed. Following intravenous and oral administration, 13 and 23% of the dose respectively was excreted in the urine as unchanged drug, glucuronidated sobrerol, and hydrated carvone. Sobrerol was shown to accumulate in bronchial mucus.

1. Braga PC, *et al.* Pharmacokinetics of sobrerol in chronic bronchitis: comparison of serum and bronchial mucus levels. *Eur J Clin Pharmacol* 1983; **24:** 209–15.

**Respiratory disorders.** References.

1. Bellussi L, *et al.* Evaluation of the efficacy and safety of sobrerol granules in patients suffering from chronic rhinosinusitis. *J Int Med Res* 1990; **18:** 454–9.
2. Azzollini E, *et al.* Sobrerol (Sobrepim®) administered dropwise to children with acute hypersecretory bronchopulmonary disease: a controlled trial v bromhexine. *Clin Trials J* 1990; **27:** 241–9.

### Preparations

**Proprietary Preparations** (details are given in Part 3)
***Braz.:*** Sobrepin; ***Hong Kong:*** Mucoflux; ***Ital.:*** Sobrepin; Sopulmin; ***Malaysia:*** Mucoflux; ***Port.:*** Broncopulmo; Mucodox; Mucolavi; ***Singapore:*** Mucoflux; ***Spain:*** Sobrepin; ***Thai.:*** Mucoflux.

**Multi-ingredient:** ***Arg.:*** Polimucil; ***Ital.:*** Fluental; ***Port.:*** Bronquial; Niflux.

## Sodium Dibunate *(BAN, rINN)*

Dibunato de sodio; L-1633. Sodium 2,6-di-*tert*-butylnaphthalene-1-sulphonate.

$C_{18}H_{23}NaO_3S$ = 342.4.
*CAS — 14992-59-7 (sodium dibunate).*
*ATC — R05DB16.*

### Profile

Sodium dibunate is a cough suppressant given by mouth in non-productive cough (p.1112). It is claimed to have central and peripheral actions. Chlorcyclizine dibunate (naftoclizine) has also been administered by mouth or rectally.

### Preparations

**Proprietary Preparations** (details are given in Part 3)
***Port.:*** Becantex†; ***Thai.:*** Becantex.

**Multi-ingredient:** ***Belg.:*** Becantex†; ***Braz.:*** Becantosse†; Beclase†; Cessatosse†; Coquevit†; Glotil†; Gotas Nican; Naquinto†; Natoss†; Pectal; Pinosil†; Plactosse†; Pulmoverina; Tossedrin†; Tossefedrin†; Tossefin†; Tussodina; Xarope das Criancas†; ***Canad.:*** Balminil Suppositories; ***Chile:*** Dibunafon; ***Ger.:*** Cito-Guakalin; Ephepect-Blocker-Pastillen N; ***Ital.:*** Sedobex†; ***Mex.:*** Neobrontyl; Tasakal; ***Thai.:*** Coughmin.

## Squill

Bulbo de Escila; Cebolla Albarrana; Cila; Escila; Meerzwiebel; Scilla; Scillae Bulbus; Scille; White Squill.

**Pharmacopoeias.** In *Br.* and *Ger.*

**BP 2003** (Squill). The dried sliced bulb of *Drimia maritima* with the membranous outer scales removed, and containing not less than 68% of alcohol (60%)-soluble extractive. Store at a temperature not exceeding 25° in a dry place.

## Indian Squill

Escila india; Urginea.

**Pharmacopoeias.** In *Br.*

**BP 2003** (Indian Squill). The bulb of *Drimia indica*, with the outer membranous scales removed, usually sliced and dried. Store at a temperature not exceeding 25° in a dry place.

### Adverse Effects, Treatment, and Precautions

The adverse effects of squill and Indian squill in large doses include nausea, vomiting, and diarrhoea. As squill and Indian squill contain cardiac glycosides they can cause similar adverse effects to digoxin (p.895).

**Abuse.** Reports of cardiac glycoside toxicity and myopathy associated with the abuse of linctuses which have contained opiates and squill.[1-5]

1. Kennedy M. Cardiac glycoside toxicity: an unusual manifestation of drug addiction. *Med J Aust* 1981; **2:** 686–9.
2. Kilpatrick C, *et al.* Myopathy with myasthenic features possibly induced by codeine linctus. *Med J Aust* 1982; **2:** 410.
3. Seow SSW. Abuse of APF linctus codeine and cardiac glycoside toxicity. *Med J Aust* 1984; **140:** 54.
4. Thurston D, Taylor K. Gee's Linctus. *Pharm J* 1984; **233:** 63.
5. Smith W, *et al.* Wenckebach's phenomenon induced by cough linctus. *BMJ* 1986; **292:** 868.

### Uses and Administration

Squill and Indian squill are used as expectorants in productive cough (p.1112) and have been given as the oxymel, elixir, tincture, or vinegar. Preparations containing squill are used in some countries in the treatment of cardiovascular disorders.

Red squill has been used as a rodenticide (p.1509).

◊ A history[1] of the use of squill.

1. Court WE. Squill – energetic diuretic. *Pharm J* 1985; **235:** 194–7.

### Preparations

***BP 2003:*** Squill Liquid Extract; Squill Oxymel.

**Proprietary Preparations** (details are given in Part 3)
***Ger.:*** Digitalysat Scilla-Digitaloid; Scillase N.

**Multi-ingredient:** ***Canad.:*** Bronco Asmol; Sirop Cocillana Codeine; ***Ger.:*** Cefascillan†; Cor-loges; Cor-Vel N†; Hevert-Entwasserungs-Tee†; Miroton; Miroton N; Nephrisan P; Raufuncton N†; Szillosan forte†; ***Hong Kong:*** Cocillana Compound; Mefedra-N; Mist Expect Stim; ***Irl.:*** Ipesil†; ***S.Afr.:*** Cocillana Co; Contra-Coff†; Linctus Tussi Infans; ***UK:*** Allens Chesty Cough; Balm of Gilead; Bronchial Mixture†; Buttercup Syrup; Catarrh Pastilles†; Catarrh Tablets†; Chest Mixture; Collins Elixir Pastilles†; Covonia Mentholated; ES Bronchial Mixture†; Galloway's Cough Syrup; Honey & Molasses; Lobelia Compound†; Modern Herbals Cough Mixture; Potters Children's Cough Pastilles; Potters Gees Linctus; Sanderson's Throat Specific.

## Stepronin *(rINN)*

Esteprónina; 2-(α-Thenoylthio)-propionylglycine; Tiofacic. *N*-(2-Mercaptopropionyl)glycine 2-thiophenecarboxylate.

$C_{10}H_{11}NO_4S_2$ = 273.3.
*CAS — 72324-18-6 (stepronin); 78126-10-0 (stepronin sodium).*
*ATC — R05CB11.*

### Profile

Stepronin has been reported to have mucolytic actions in productive cough (p.1112), and has also been used in the treatment of liver disorders. It is reported to be metabolised to tiopronin (p.1054). Stepronin has been mainly used as the sodium and lysinate salts.

### Preparations

**Proprietary Preparations** (details are given in Part 3)
***Ital.:*** Broncoplus†; Masor†; Mucodil†; Tioten†.

## Sulfogaiacol *(rINN)*

Kalium Guajacolsulfonicum; Potassium Guaiacolsulfonate; Potassium Guaiacolsulphonate; Sulfoguayacol. Potassium hydroxymethoxybenzenesulphonate hemihydrate.

$C_7H_7KO_5S,\frac{1}{2}H_2O$ = 251.3.

*CAS — 1321-14-8 (anhydrous sulfogaiacol); 78247-49-1 (sulfogaiacol hemihydrate).*

**Pharmacopoeias.** In *Pol.* and *US.* Also in *Fr.* and *Jpn*, both of which do not specify the hemihydrate.

**USP 27** (Potassium Guaiacolsulfonate). Protect from light.

### Profile

Sulfogaiacol is used as an expectorant for productive cough (p.1112). Calcium guaiacolsulfonate has been used similarly.

### Preparations

**Proprietary Preparations** (details are given in Part 3)
***Austria:*** Pectosorin; ***Ital.:*** Tioguaialina; ***Mex.:*** Broncoserum.

**Multi-ingredient:** ***Arg.:*** Medex Rub; No-Tos Infantil; Pectobron; Pectoral Pagliano; Polipectol; ***Austria:*** Asthma-Hilfe; Pneumopan; ***Belg.:*** Broncal†; Broncho-pectoralis; Bronchobel†; Eucalyptine Pholcodine Le Brun; Eucalytux; Folcodex†; Neo-Codion†; Phenergan Expectorant†; Pholco-Mereprine; ***Braz.:*** Benzomel; Broncofisin; Broncotussan†; Bronkotrat; Cessatosse†; Expectil; Fenergan Expectorante; Frenotossil†; Iodetal; Iodeto de Potassio; Ipecol; Mel de Jatahy†; Pinosil†; Pulmonix; Pulmoverina; Telbon†; Thiodeol†; Tossefin†; Trifedrin; Tussodina; Tussucalman†; Xarope de Iodeto de Potassio†; Xarope de Limao Bravo†; Xarope de Lobelia Composto†; Xarope Sao Joao; Xpe SPC; ***Canad.:*** Ambenyl†; Phenergan Expectorant with Codeine†; Phenergan Expectorant†; Phenergan VC Expectorant with Codeine†; Phenergan VC Expectorant†; ***Fr.:*** Bronpax†; Camphodionyl; Ephydion; Eucalyptine Le Brun; Germose; Neo-Codion; Passedyl; Pectosan†; Pneumaseptic†; Quintopan Enfant†; Sirop Pectoral adulte†; Sirop Pectoral enfant†; Thiosedal†; ***Ger.:*** Pulmocordio forte†; ***Hong Kong:*** Bendracol; ***India:*** Neogadine SG; Pulmo-Cod (C & G); ***Israel:*** Cod-Guaiacol; Oxacatin; Promethazine Expectorants; Tusophedrine; ***Ital.:*** Balsamina Kroner; Balsatux; Broncal; Bronchenolo; Bronchiase; Bronco-Dex†; Donalg; Guaiacalcium Complex; Ingro†; Polised; Pulmarin; Sciroppo Berta; Stenobronchial; Tauglicolo; Tiocalmina; Tiocosol; Tionamil; Tussanyl; ***Mex.:*** Pulmovital; ***Port.:*** Calmarum; Lesil†; Xarope Antigripal; ***Spain:*** Bronco Medical; Broncovir; Broncovital; Brota Rectal Bals; Etermol†; Fenergan Expectorante; Maboterpen†; Pastillas Pectoral Kely; Pazbronquial; Pectoral Brum†; Pulmofasa; Pulmofasa Antihist†; ***Switz.:*** Neo-Codion N; Phol-Tux; Saintbois; ***Thai.:*** Bisolvon EX; Bromso-Ex; Expiran†; Hustazol-C; Med-Mucolo; ***USA:*** Cophene-X†; Cypex; De-Chlor NX; Entuss Expectorant; Humibid; Humibid DM; Hy-KXP; Hydron EX; Hydron KGS; KGS-PE; Lemotussin-DM; Marcof; Protuss; Protuss-D; Tusquelin†.

## Telmesteine *(rINN)*

Telmesteína. (−)-3-Ethyl hydrogen (*R*)-3,4-thiazolidinedicarboxylate.

$C_7H_{11}NO_4S$ = 205.2.

*CAS — 122946-43-4.*

### Profile

Telmesteine has been used as a mucolytic (p.1112) in the treatment of respiratory-tract disorders in doses of 300 mg two or three times daily.

### Preparations

**Proprietary Preparations** (details are given in Part 3)
***Ital.:*** Muconorm; Reolase.

## Terpin Hydrate *(BANM)*

Terpene Hydrate; Terpina, hidrato de; Terpinol. *p*-Menthane-1,8-diol monohydrate; 4-Hydroxy-α,α,4-trimethylcyclohexanemethanol monohydrate.

$C_{10}H_{20}O_2,H_2O$ = 190.3.

*CAS — 80-53-5 (anhydrous terpin); 2451-01-6 (terpin monohydrate).*

**Pharmacopoeias.** In *Fr., Swiss, US,* and *Viet.*

**USP 27** (Terpin Hydrate). Colourless lustrous crystals or white powder with a slight odour. It effloresces in dry air. Soluble 1 in 200 of water, 1 in 35 of boiling water, 1 in 13 of alcohol, 1 in 3 of boiling alcohol, and 1 in 140 of chloroform and of ether. A hot 1% solution is neutral to litmus. Store in airtight containers.

**Stability.** If crystals form in terpin hydrate elixir, they may be redissolved by warming the closed container of solution in warm water and then gently shaking it.

### Profile

Terpin hydrate has been stated to increase bronchial secretion directly and has been given by mouth as an expectorant in productive cough (p.1112).

Nausea, vomiting, or abdominal pain may follow the ingestion of terpin hydrate on an empty stomach.

Terpin hydrochloride has also been used.

### Preparations

***USP 27:*** Terpin Hydrate and Codeine Elixir; Terpin Hydrate Elixir.

**Proprietary Preparations** (details are given in Part 3)
***Fr.:*** Pectotussyl†; Terpine des Monts-Dore†.

**Multi-ingredient:** ***Belg.:*** Balsoclase†; Tri-Cold†; ***Braz.:*** Cortagrip D†; Ozonyl; Pyocoline†; Tetrapulmo; ***Canad.:*** Pastilles Valda†; Valda; ***Chile:*** Broncodeina; ***Fin.:*** Toclase Expectorant; ***Fr.:*** Bronchorectine au Citral; Bronpax†; Marrubene Codethyline†; Pulmofluide Simple; Pulmoll; Terpine Gonnon†; Terpone; Tossarel†; ***Ger.:*** Ozothin; Sedotussin Expectorans†; ***Hong Kong:*** Bendracol; Codoplex; Coldrex; Panadol Cold and Flu; ***Ital.:*** Elisir Terpina; Neo Borocillina Balsamica; Tionamil; Tussiflex†; ***Neth.:*** Balsoclase Compositum†; ***Port.:*** Codoforme†; Fluidin Nocturno†; Recto Bronco Tosse†; ***Spain:*** Pastillas Pectoral Kely; Terponil; ***Switz.:*** Bromocod N; Libexine Compositum†; Mephatussine Compositum†; Mephaxine Compositum†; Rectoseptal-Neo bismuthe; Rectoseptal-Neo Pholcodine†; Rectoseptal-Neo simple; Sedotussin; Spedro†; ***Thai.:*** Antust; D-Coate; Dexpin; Dextro BS; Dimophen†; Fartussin; Med-Guaiphan; Mila-Tercon; Rocal; Seco; Stocof; Terco-C; Terco-D; ***UK:*** Original Cabdrivers Expectorant.

## Tetryzoline Hydrochloride *(BANM, rINNM)*

Hidrocloruro de tetrizolina; Tetrahydrozoline Hydrochloride. 2-(1,2,3,4-Tetrahydro-1-naphthyl)-2-imidazoline hydrochloride.

$C_{13}H_{16}N_2,HCl$ = 236.7.

*CAS — 84-22-0 (tetryzoline); 522-48-5 (tetryzoline hydrochloride).*

*ATC — R01AA06; R01AB03; S01GA02.*

**Pharmacopoeias.** In *US.*

**USP 27** (Tetrahydrozoline Hydrochloride). A white odourless solid. Soluble 1 in 3.5 of water and 1 in 7.5 of alcohol; very slightly soluble in chloroform; practically insoluble in ether. Store in airtight containers.

### Profile

Tetryzoline is a sympathomimetic with effects similar to those of naphazoline (p.1124). It is used as the hydrochloride for its vasoconstrictor effect in the symptomatic relief of nasal congestion (p.1112). A 0.1% solution is instilled into each nostril as nasal drops or a spray as necessary, although not more often than every 3 hours. Children aged 2 to 6 years of age may be given 2 or 3 drops of a 0.05% solution in each nostril as necessary, although again not more often than every 3 hours.

Solutions of tetryzoline hydrochloride containing 0.05% are used as a conjunctival decongestant (see Conjunctivitis, p.421).

Other salts of tetryzoline including the nitrate, phosphate, and sulfate have been used similarly.

**Effects on the eyes.** For mention of conjunctivitis induced by ophthalmic decongestant preparations containing tetryzoline, see under Phenylephrine, p.1127.

### Preparations

***USP 27:*** Tetrahydrozoline Hydrochloride Nasal Solution; Tetrahydrozoline Hydrochloride Ophthalmic Solution.

**Proprietary Preparations** (details are given in Part 3)
***Arg.:*** Bano Ocular; Octilia; Ocudiafan; ***Austral.:*** Murine Sore Eyes; Optazine Fresh; Visine Original; ***Belg.:*** Visine†; ***Canad.:*** Eye Drops; RO-Eye Drops†; Visine; ***Chile:*** Murine Plus; Visional Gotas; ***Denm.:*** Tyzine; ***Fin.:*** Oftan Starine; Visine; ***Fr.:*** Constrilia; ***Ger.:*** Berberil N; Caltheon; Diabenyl T; Exrhinin†; Ophtalmin N; Rhinopront; Sanopinwern T; Tetrilin; Tyzine; Vasopos N; Vidiseptal EDO Sine†; Yxin; ***Gr.:*** Visine; ***Hong Kong:*** Optizoline; Visine Original; ***India:*** Visine; ***Israel:*** Azoline; Stilla; V-Zoline; Visine; ***Ital.:*** Demetil; Octilia; Stilla Decongestionante; Vasorinil; Visine; ***Malaysia:*** Visine; ***Mex.:*** Ischemol†; ***NZ:*** Visine; ***Port.:*** Edolzine†; Visine; ***Singapore:*** Octilia; Visine; ***Spain:*** Azulina; Vispring; ***Switz.:*** Rhinopront Top; Tyzine†; Visine; ***Thai.:*** Visine; ***USA:*** Eye Drops; Eye-Zine; Eyesine†; Geneye Extra; Mallazine; Optigene 3; Tetrasine; Tyzine; Visine Original.

**Multi-ingredient:** ***Arg.:*** Antiflogol; Biocortin; Efemolina; Larsimal; Provisual Compuesto; Visubril; ***Austral.:*** In A Wink Allergy†; Visine Advanced Relief; Visine Allergy†; Visine Revive†; ***Braz.:*** Fenidex; Mirabel; Vislin; Visodin; Visolux†; ***Canad.:*** Collyrium†; Visine Allergy; Visine Moisturizing; ***Chile:*** Spersallerg; ***Ger.:*** Allergopos N; Efemolin; Spersadexolin; Spersallerg; ***Hong Kong:*** Colircusi Gentadexa†; Efemoline; Eye Mo 36†; Spersadexoline; Spersallerg; Visine Allergy Relief; Visine Moisturizing; ***Israel:*** Visine AC; ***Ital.:*** Biorinil; Cromozil; Dexoline; Efemoline; Eta Biocortilen VC; Flumetol; Ischemol A; Medramil†; Tetramil; Vasosterone; Vasosterone Antibiotico; Vasosterone Collirio; Visublefarite; Visucloben Decongestionante; Visumetazone Antibiotico; Visumetazone Decongestionante; Visumicina†; Visustrin; ***Malaysia:*** Efemoline; Gentadexa; Murine Plus; Spersadexoline; Spersallerg; ***Mex.:*** Visine Extra; ***Norw.:*** Spersallerg; ***NZ:*** Revive†; Visine Advanced Relief; ***Port.:*** Gentadexa; Medrivas Antibiotico; Medrivas†; ***S.Afr.:*** Efemoline; Gemini; Oculoforte; Safyr Bleu Antihistamine; Spersadexoline; Spersallerg; ***Singapore:*** Efemoline; Spersadexoline; Spersallerg; ***Spain:*** Dexam Constric; Fluorvas; Gentadexa; Gentavasor†; Medrivas; Medrivas Antib; Tivitis; Vasodexa; Visublefarite†; ***Switz.:*** Collypan; Efemoline; Oculosan forte†; Spersadexoline; Spersallerg; ***Thai.:*** Antazallerge; Efemoline; Histaoph; Mano; Opsa-His; Opsil-A; Spersadexoline; Spersallerg; ***USA:*** Advanced Relief Visine; Collyrium Fresh; Murine Plus; Tetrasine Extra; Visine Allergy Relief; Visine Moisturizing.

## Thebacon Hydrochloride *(BANM, rINNM)*

Acethydrocodone Hydrochloride; Acetyldihydrocodeinone Hydrochloride; Dihydrocodeinone Enol Acetate Hydrochloride; Hidrocloruro de tebacón. 6-*O*-Acetyl-7,8-dihydro-3-*O*-methyl-6,7-didehydromorphine hydrochloride; (−)-(5*R*)-4,5-Epoxy-3-methoxy-9a-methylmorphin-6-en-6-yl acetate hydrochloride.

$C_{20}H_{23}NO_4,HCl$ = 377.9.

*CAS — 466-90-0 (thebacon); 20236-82-2 (thebacon hydrochloride).*

*ATC — R05DA10.*

### Profile

Thebacon hydrochloride is a centrally acting cough suppressant used for non-productive cough (p.1112). It has actions similar to those of codeine (p.27) but is stated to be approximately 4 times more potent. It is given by mouth in a usual daily dose of 10 mg in divided doses; the maximum daily dose should not exceed 20 mg.

### Preparations

**Proprietary Preparations** (details are given in Part 3)
***Belg.:*** Acedicone.

## Tipepidine Hibenzate *(rINNM)*

AT-327 (tipepidine); CR-662 (tipepidine); Hibenzato de tipepidina; Tipepidine Hibenzate. 3-[Di(2-thienyl)methylene]-1-methylpiperidine 2-(4-hydroxybenzoyl)benzoate.

$C_{15}H_{17}NS_2,C_{14}H_{10}O_4$ = 517.7.

*CAS — 5169-78-8 (tipepidine); 31139-87-4 (tipepidine hibenzate).*

*ATC — R05DB24.*

**Pharmacopoeias.** In *Jpn.*

### Profile

Tipepidine hibenzate is a cough suppressant used for non-productive cough (p.1112) which is claimed also to have an expectorant action. It is given by mouth as the hibenzate but doses are expressed as the citrate; tipepidine hibenzate 22.2 mg is approximately equivalent to 20 mg of tipepidine citrate. A usual dose is the equivalent of 20 to 40 mg of the citrate 3 times daily.

**Epileptogenic effect.** Generalised convulsions associated with therapeutic oral doses of tipepidine hibenzate have occurred in some patients.[1]

1. Cuomo RM. On the possible convulsive activity of an antitussive piperidinic derivative ('tipepidina ibenzato') in man. *Acta Neurol (Napoli)* 1982; **37:** 110–16.

### Preparations

**Proprietary Preparations** (details are given in Part 3)
***Jpn:*** Asverin.

**Multi-ingredient:** ***Arg.:*** Di-Neumobron.

## Tolu Balsam

Bálsamo de tolú; Balsamum Tolutanum; Baume de Tolu.

*CAS — 9000-64-0; 8017-09-2.*

**Pharmacopoeias.** In *Eur.* (see p.vi) and *US.*

**Ph. Eur. 5.0** (Tolu Balsam). Oleoresin obtained from the trunk of *Myroxylon balsamum* var. *balsamum*. It contains 25 to 50% of free or combined acids, expressed as cinnamic acid, calculated with reference to the dried drug. It occurs as a hard, friable, brownish to reddish-brown mass; thin fragments are brownish-yellow when examined against the light. It has an odour reminiscent of vanillin. Practically insoluble in water and in petroleum spirit; very soluble or freely soluble in alcohol. Do not store in powdered form.

**USP 27** (Tolu Balsam). A balsam obtained from *Myroxylon balsamum* (Leguminosae). It is a brown or yellowish-brown plastic solid transparent in thin layers and brittle when old, dried, or exposed to cold temperatures. It has a pleasant aromatic odour, resembling that of vanilla. Practically insoluble in water and in petroleum spirit; soluble in alcohol, in chloroform, and in ether, sometimes with slight residue or turbidity. Store at a temperature not exceeding 40° in airtight containers.

### Profile

Tolu balsam is considered to have very mild antiseptic properties and some expectorant action but is mainly used in the form of a syrup to flavour cough mixtures. However, Tolu Syrup (BP 2003) no longer contains tolu balsam but is based on cinnamic acid (p.1177).

### Preparations

***BPC 1954:*** Compound Iodoform Paint;
***USNF 22:*** Tolu Balsam Syrup; Tolu Balsam Tincture;
***USP 27:*** Compound Benzoin Tincture.

**Proprietary Preparations** (details are given in Part 3)

**Multi-ingredient:** ***Arg.:*** Cobenzil Compuesto; No-Tos Adultos; No-Tos Infantil; Pastillas Medex; Pectobron; Polipectol; Refenax Caramelos Expectorantes; ***Austral.:*** Camphor Linctus Compound†; ***Belg.:*** Folcodex†; Tux; ***Braz.:*** Agrimel†; Broncofisin; Calmante Creosotado†; Calmatoss; Codelasa†; Expectomel; Frenotosse; Frenotossil†; Glycon; Inalobel†; Infantoss; Inhalante Yatropan; Iodetal; Ipecol; Mel de Jatahy†; Melagriao†; Peitoral Angico Pelotense; Pulmoformil†; Pulmonix; Tossanil†; Vick Pastilhas†; Xarope de Caraguata; Xarope Sao Joao; Yatropan†; ***Canad.:*** Bronco Asmol; Rophelin; ***Chile:*** Elitos Et; Fitotos; Flemex Jat; Jarabe Palto Compuesto Con Miel; Notosil; Pulmosina; Sedotus; ***Fr.:*** Broncalene Nourisson; Bronpax†; Dinacode; Dinacode avec codeine; Gaiarsol†; Hexapneumine; Pastilles Medicinales Vicks; Pastilles Monleon; Pates Pectorales†; Phytotux; Pulmonase†; Pulmosodyl†; Sirop Pectoral adulte†; Sirop Pectoral enfant†; Terpine Gonnon†; Theralene Pectoral Nourrisson; Tussipax; ***Hong Kong:*** Baby Cough with Antihistamine; Hexapneumine; ***Ital.:*** Stenobronchial; ***Mex.:*** Epicol; ***Port.:*** Lesil†; Stodal; ***S.Afr.:*** Linctus Tussi Infans; ***Spain:*** Bactopumon; Bronco Sergo†; Broncomicin Bals†; Bronquidiazina CR; Maboterpen†; Mentobox†; Pastillas Antisep Garg M; Pectoral Brum†; Pulmofasa; Pulmofasa Antihist†; Toscal Compuesto†; Toscal†; Tosdiazina; ***Switz.:*** Baume; Cimex Sirop contre la toux†; Demo pates pectorales†; Demo sirop contre la toux†; Dinacode N; Euphon N; Ipeca; Neo-Codion N; Neo-DP; Pastilles pectorales Demo N; Pectocalmine Junior N; Phol-Tussil; Saintbois; Sano Tuss; Sirop pectoral DP1†; Sirop pectoral DP2, DP3†; ***Thai.:*** Baby Cough Syrup; Baby Cough with Antihistamine; ***UK:*** Allens Chesty Cough; Chesty Cough Relief; Modern Herbals Cold & Congestion; Sanderson's Throat Specific; ***USA:*** Vicks Menthol Cough Drops.

## Tramazoline Hydrochloride *(BANM, USAN, rINNM)*

Hidrocloruro de tramazolina; Tramazolini Hydrochloridum. 2-(5,6,7,8-Tetrahydro-1-naphthylamino)-2-imidazoline hydrochloride monohydrate.

$C_{13}H_{17}N_3,HCl,H_2O$ = 269.8.

*CAS — 1082-57-1 (tramazoline); 3715-90-0 (tramazoline hydrochloride).*

*ATC — R01AA09.*

**Pharmacopoeias.** In *Eur.* (see p.vi).

**Ph. Eur. 5.0** (Tramazoline Hydrochloride Monohydrate). A white or almost white crystalline powder. Soluble in water and in alcohol. A 5% solution in water has a pH of 4.9 to 6.3.

### Profile

Tramazoline hydrochloride is a sympathomimetic with effects similar to those of naphazoline (p.1124). It is used to provide symptomatic relief of nasal congestion (p.1112). Tramazoline hydrochloride is given as a 0.1264% solution, instilled into each nostril as nasal drops or a spray three to four times daily.

Solutions of tramazoline hydrochloride containing 0.0632% have also been used in eye drops as a conjunctival decongestant (see Conjunctivitis, p.421).

### Preparations

**Proprietary Preparations** (details are given in Part 3)

***Austral.:*** Spray-Tish; ***Austria:*** Rinorix; ***Belg.:*** Rhinospray; ***Ger.:*** Biciron; Ellatun; Rhinospray; ***Ital.:*** Rinogutt Spray-Fher; ***Neth.:*** Bisolnasal; ***Port.:*** Rhinospray; ***Spain:*** Rhinospray.

**Multi-ingredient:** ***Arg.:*** Dexa-Rhinospray N; ***Austria:*** Rhinospray Plus; ***Belg.:*** Dexa-Rhinospray; ***Ger.:*** Dexa Biciron; Dexa-Rhinospray N†; Oxy Biciron; Rhinospray Plus; ***Irl.:*** Dexa-Rhinaspray Duo; Dexa-Rhinaspray†; ***Ital.:*** Rinogutt Antiallergico Spray; Rinogutt Eucalipto-Fher; ***Spain:*** Rhinospray Antialergico; ***UK:*** Dexa-Rhinaspray Duo.

## Tuaminoheptane Sulfate *(rINNM)*

Sulfato de tuaminoheptano; Tuaminoheptane Sulphate *(BANM)*.

$(C_7H_{17}N)_2,H_2SO_4 = 328.5$.

*CAS — 6411-75-2.*

*ATC — R01AA11; R01AB08.*

### Profile

Tuaminoheptane is a volatile sympathomimetic (see Adrenaline, p.854) that has been used as the sulfate for the symptomatic relief of nasal congestion. Tuaminoheptane has also been employed in the form of the carbonate.

### Preparations

**Proprietary Preparations** (details are given in Part 3)

**Multi-ingredient:** ***Braz.:*** Rinofluimucil; ***Fr.:*** Rhinofluimucil; ***Ger.:*** Rinofluimucil-S; ***Hong Kong:*** Rinofluimucil; ***Ital.:*** Otomicetina†; Rinofluimucil; ***Spain:*** Rinofluimucil†; Rinoflumil; ***Switz.:*** Rinofluimucil; ***Thai.:*** Rinofluimucil.

## Tymazoline Hydrochloride *(BANM)*

2-Thymyloxymethyl-2-imidazoline Hydrochloride; Timazolina, hidrocloruro de. 2-(2-Isopropyl-5-methylphenoxymethyl)-2-imidazoline hydrochloride.

$C_{14}H_{20}N_2O,HCl = 268.8$.

*CAS — 24243-97-8 (tymazoline); 28120-03-8 (tymazoline hydrochloride).*

*ATC — R01AA13.*

**Pharmacopoeias.** In *Pol.*

### Profile

Tymazoline is a sympathomimetic that has been used as the hydrochloride similarly to naphazoline (p.1124) for its local vasoconstrictor effect in the symptomatic relief of nasal congestion (p.1112).

### Preparations

**Proprietary Preparations** (details are given in Part 3)

***Thai.:*** Pernazene.

## Xylometazoline Hydrochloride

*(BANM, rINNM)*

Hidrocloruro de xilometazolina; Xylometazolini Hydrochloridum. 2-(4-tert-Butyl-2,6-dimethylbenzyl)-2-imidazoline hydrochloride.

$C_{16}H_{24}N_2,HCl = 280.8$.

*CAS — 526-36-3 (xylometazoline); 1218-35-5 (xylometazoline hydrochloride).*

*ATC — R01AA07; R01AB06; S01GA03.*

**Pharmacopoeias.** In *Eur.* (see p.vi), *Pol.*, and *US.*

**Ph. Eur. 5.0** (Xylometazoline Hydrochloride). A white or almost white, crystalline powder. Freely soluble in water, in alcohol, and in methyl alcohol. Protect from light.

**USP 27** (Xylometazoline Hydrochloride). A white to off-white, odourless, crystalline powder. Soluble 1 in 35 of water; freely soluble in alcohol; sparingly soluble in chloroform; practically insoluble in ether and in benzene. pH of a 5% solution in water is between 5.0 and 6.6. Store in airtight containers. Protect from light.

### Adverse Effects and Precautions

As for Naphazoline, p.1124.

### Interactions

Since xylometazoline is absorbed through the mucosa interactions may follow topical application. The *British National Formulary* considers that all sympathomimetic nasal decongestants may cause a hypertensive crisis if used during treatment with an MAOI. For the interactions of sympathomimetics in general, see under Adrenaline, p.853.

### Uses and Administration

Xylometazoline is a direct-acting sympathomimetic (see Adrenaline, p.854) with marked alpha-adrenergic activity. It is a vasoconstrictor which reduces swelling and congestion when applied to mucous membranes. The effect begins within 5 to 10 minutes of application and lasts for up to 10 hours.

Xylometazoline is used as the hydrochloride for the symptomatic relief of nasal congestion (p.1112). A 0.1% solution of xylometazoline hydrochloride is applied topically as nasal drops or a spray into each nostril two or three times daily. A 0.05% solution is used once or twice daily for children under 12 years of age but is not recommended for infants of less than 3 months of age; 1 or 2 drops of the solution are instilled into each nostril.

A 0.1% solution of xylometazoline hydrochloride has also been instilled into the eye as a conjunctival decongestant (see Conjunctivitis, p.421).

### Preparations

***BP 2003:*** Xylometazoline Nasal Drops;
***USP 27:*** Xylometazoline Hydrochloride Nasal Solution.

**Proprietary Preparations** (details are given in Part 3)

***Arg.:*** Nastizol; Otrivina; ***Austral.:*** Otrivin; ***Austria:*** Olynth; Otrivin; ***Belg.:*** Nasa Rhinathiol; Nasasinutab; Otrivine Anti-Rhinitis; Rhinidine; ***Braz.:*** Orlaxyl; Otrivina; ***Canad.:*** Certified Decongestant; Decongest; Decongestant Nasal Spray; Decongestant Nose Drops; Nasal Decongestant; Otrivin; Vaporisateur Nasal Decongestionnant†; ***Denm.:*** Otrivin; Passagen; Zymelin; ***Fin.:*** Nasolin; Otrivin; ***Ger.:*** Balkis; Dorenasin†; Gelonasal; Imidin K; Imidin N; Mentopin Nasenspray; Nasan; Nasengel; Nasengel AL; Nasenspray AL; Nasenspray E; Nasenspray K; Nasentropfen AL; Nasentropfen E; Nasentropfen K; Olynth; Otalgicin†; Otriven; Otriven gegen Schnupfen; Rapako xylo; Rhino-stas†; schnupfen endrine; Snup; stas Nasentropfen, Nasenspray; ViviRhin S†; Xylo; Xylo Siozwo; Xylo-COMOD; ***Gr.:*** Otrivin; ***Hong Kong:*** Decongest†; Otrivin; Xyloma; ***India:*** Decon; Otrivin; ***Irl.:*** Otrivine; ***Israel:*** Kalaf†; Nazalet; Otrivin; Xylovit; ***Ital.:*** Neo Rinoleina; Otrivin; Respiro; ***Malaysia:*** Otrivin; ***Neth.:*** Otrivin; ***Norw.:*** Otrivin; Zymelin; ***NZ:*** Otrivine; ***Port.:*** Otrivina; ***S.Afr.:*** Otrivin; Sinutab†; ***Singapore:*** Otrivin; ***Spain:*** Amidrin; Desconasal†; Otrivin; Rationasal†; Rinoblanco; ***Swed.:*** Nasoferm; Otrivin; ***Switz.:*** Nasben; Olynth; Otrivin; Rhinostop; Rhume; Rinosedin; ***Thai.:*** Otrivin; ***UAE:*** Xylolin; ***UK:*** Non-Drowsy Sudafed Decongestant Nasal Spray; Otradrops; Otraspray; Otrivine; Tixycolds Cold and Allergy; ***USA:*** Otrivin.

**Multi-ingredient:** ***Austral.:*** Allergy Eyes†; Murine Allergy†; ***Belg.:*** Lomusol plus Xylometazoline†; ***Canad.:*** Ophtrivin-A†; ***Chile:*** Bacitopic Compuesto; Nasomin; Rinobanedif; ***Denm.:*** Kombicrom†; Otrivin Menthol; ***Fin.:*** Otrivin Menthol; ***Ger.:*** Lomupren compositum; Nasic; Vividrin comp†; ***Hong Kong:*** Rynacrom Compound†; ***Irl.:*** Otrivine-Antistin; Rynacrom Compound†; ***Israel:*** Aforinol; ***Ital.:*** Inalar; Nasalemed†; Rinos†; Tririnol†; ***Malaysia:*** Rynacrom Compound; ***Neth.:*** Otrivin Menthol; ***NZ:*** Otrivine Menthol; Otrivine-Antistin; ***Port.:*** Rynacrom Composto†; ***Singapore:*** Rynacrom Compound†; ***Spain:*** Rinoblanco Dexa Antibio†; ***Swed.:*** Otrivin Menthol; ***Switz.:*** Lomusol-X; Muco-Trin; Triofan; ***Thai.:*** Rynacrom Compound; ***UK:*** Otrivine-Antistin; Rynacrom Allergy†; Rynacrom Compound.

## Zipeprol Hydrochloride *(rINNM)*

CERM-3024; Hidrocloruro de zipeprol. α-(α-Methoxybenzyl)-4-(β-methoxyphenethyl)-1-piperazineethanol dihydrochloride.

$C_{23}H_{32}N_2O_3,2HCl = 457.4$.

*CAS — 34758-83-3 (zipeprol); 34758-84-4 (zipeprol hydrochloride).*

*ATC — R05DB15.*

### Profile

Zipeprol is a centrally acting cough suppressant which is stated to have a peripheral action on bronchial spasm. It has been given as the hydrochloride, typically in a dose range of 150 to 300 mg daily in divided doses. There have been reports of abuse and overdosage producing neurological symptoms.

**Abuse and overdosage.** Severe neurological symptoms have been reported in young adults following habitual abuse of zipeprol for euphoria. Patients have presented with generalised seizures, followed by coma.[1] One patient who ingested 750 mg of zipeprol [over twice the maximum daily dose] had several opisthotonic crises and developed cerebral oedema.[2] Symptoms of overdosage in children have included restlessness, somnolence, ataxia, choreic movements, forced deviation of the head and eyes, generalised seizures, respiratory depression, and coma.[1,3] Fatalities have been reported.

Dependence and withdrawal symptoms similar to those produced by opioids have been reported.[4] WHO has assessed zipeprol to have a moderate potential for dependence and liability for abuse.[5] Although zipeprol is a weak opioid agonist at high doses its toxicity and hallucinogenic and other psychotropic effects constitute a significant element in its abuse, and the public health and social problems associated with such abuse were considered substantial.

1. Moroni C, *et al.* Overdosage of zipeprol, a non-opioid antitussive agent. *Lancet* 1984; **i:** 45.
2. Perraro F, Beorchia A. Convulsions and cerebral oedema associated with zipeprol abuse. *Lancet* 1984; **i:** 45–6.
3. Merigot P, *et al.* Les convulsions avec trois antitussifs dérivés substitués dé la pipérazine (zipéprol, éprazinone, éprozinol). *Ann Pediatr (Paris)* 1985; **32:** 504–11.
4. Mallaret MP, *et al.* Zipeprol: primary dependence in an unaddicted patient. *Ann Pharmacother* 1995; **29:** 540.
5. WHO. WHO expert committee on drug dependence: twenty-ninth report. *WHO Tech Rep Ser 856* 1995.

### Preparations

**Proprietary Preparations** (details are given in Part 3)

***Chile:*** Frenotos; ***Gr.:*** Dovavixin; Duo-Extolen; Jactuss; ***Mex.:*** Respilene; Tusigen; ***Port.:*** Respiral†; ***Switz.:*** Mirsol†.

# Dermatological Drugs and Sunscreens

Acne, p.1133
Alopecia, p.1134
Burns, p.1134
Darier's disease, p.1134
Dermatitis herpetiformis, p.1134
Drug-induced skin reactions, p.1134
Eczema, p.1135
Epidermolysis bullosa, p.1135
Erythema multiforme, p.1135
Hyperhidrosis, p.1136
Ichthyosis, p.1136
Keratinisation disorders, p.1136
Lichen planus, p.1136
Lichen sclerosus, p.1136
Light-induced skin reactions, p.1136
Pemphigus and pemphigoid, p.1137
Pigmentation disorders, p.1137
Pruritus, p.1137
Psoriasis, p.1137
Pyoderma gangrenosum, p.1138
Rosacea, p.1138
Seborrhoeic dermatitis, p.1138
Toxic epidermal necrolysis, p.1138
Urticaria and angioedema, p.1138
Warts, p.1139
Wounds and ulcers, p.1139

The skin is subject to a very wide range of lesions. Some may be characteristic of specific systemic diseases and fade as the disease regresses. Some are caused by specific local infections and are best treated by the appropriate antimicrobial (see Skin Infections in the chapters Antibacterials, p.146, and Antifungals, p.390). The skin is also subject to damage from environmental hazards. Excessive or prolonged exposure to solar radiation is associated with degenerative changes in the skin (premature ageing of the skin or photoageing), actinic (solar) keratoses (which are risk factors or precursors of skin cancers), and malignant neoplasms of the skin (see p.522). Many skin disorders are side-effects of therapeutic and other agents, ranging from mild hypersensitivity to the life-threatening Stevens-Johnson syndrome or toxic epidermal necrolysis (see Drug-induced Skin Reactions, below). There also remains a wide range of skin disorders whose aetiology is poorly understood.

The distribution and morphological description of the skin lesion (its shape, colour, and surface characteristics) are important in the diagnosis of skin disorders. There are many terms used to describe skin lesions:

- abscess–a collection of pus in a cavity
- bulla (or blister)–a fluid-filled circumscribed lesion larger than 0.5 cm in diameter
- comedo–a plug of keratin and sebum in a pilosebaceous follicle
- ecchymosis–an extravasation of blood into the skin
- erythema–red coloration due to vascular dilatation
- fissure–a slit through the whole thickness of the skin
- horn–a thickening of the skin that is taller than it is broad
- keratosis–a horny thickening of the skin
- lichenification–hard, thickened skin with increased markings
- macule–an area of altered colour or texture with no elevation above the surface of the surrounding skin
- nodule–a dome-shaped or spherical-shaped, solid lesion, usually more than 0.5 cm in diameter and depth
- papilloma–a nipple-like mass
- papule–a raised solid lesion, usually less than 0.5 cm in diameter
- petechia–a pinhead-sized macule of blood in the skin
- plaque–a raised, flat-topped, circumscribed lesion, usually larger than 2 cm in diameter but with no substantial depth
- purpura–a macule of blood in the skin, larger than a petechia
- pustule–an accumulation of pus in the skin
- scale–a flat plate or flake of stratum corneum
- stria–a streak-like, linear, atrophic lesion, pink, purple, or white in colour
- telangiectasia–a visible dilatation of small cutaneous blood vessels
- vesicle–a fluid-filled circumscribed lesion less than 0.5 cm in diameter
- wheal–an elevated, white, compressible area of oedema often surrounded by a red flare.

This chapter describes some drugs used in the management of skin disorders and the treatment of some of the commoner conditions. Treatment may include topical and/or systemic drug therapy, although the pharmacology of many of the drugs used in dermatology is poorly understood. Physical methods such as cryotherapy, UV radiation, radiotherapy, and surgery also have a role.

Drugs with a traditional place in the treatment of skin disorders include coal tar, dithranol, ichthammol, and urea, as well as *keratolytics* such as benzoyl peroxide and salicylic acid. *Photosensitisers* such as the psoralen methoxsalen, vitamin D analogues such as calcipotriol, and the vitamin A analogues (retinoids) such as acitretin, isotretinoin, and tretinoin have an important role in certain skin disorders. Recently, *immunosuppressants* such as alefacept and efalizumab have been approved for use in psoriasis and pimecrolimus for eczema. Other immunosuppressants used in dermatology are included in the section beginning on p.1344. Perhaps the most important immunosuppressant and anti-inflammatory drugs used in skin disorders are, however, the corticosteroids (see p.1068).

Drugs with primarily a *protective* function include calamine, starch, talc, titanium dioxide, and zinc oxide. Some drugs, for example ammonium lactate and sodium pidolate, have *humectant* properties and are used in topical moisturising preparations.

Drugs used to *increase pigmentation* include dihydroxyacetone, methoxsalen, and trioxysalen. Those used to *reduce pigmentation* include hydroquinone, mequinol, and monobenzone.

Other substances used to *protect against sunlight* are the sunscreens. These are of 2 types: *chemical* (absorbent or organic) agents that because of their chromophore groups absorb a particular range of wavelengths within the UV spectrum and *physical* (reflective or inorganic) agents that are opaque and reflect both UVA and UVB radiation. A classification of the chemical sunscreens included in this chapter is given in Table 1, below. Trolamine salicylate (p.95) is a chemical sunscreen that is also used as a topical analgesic. Physical sunscreens include titanium dioxide (p.1160) and zinc oxide (p.1163). Many of the available products combine sunscreens from the different groups in order to widen the protection afforded. Other agents used as physical sunscreens include calcium carbonate, kaolin, magnesium oxide, red veterinary petroleum, and talc.

**Table 1.** Chemical sunscreens.

| UVA absorbers | UVB absorbers |
|---|---|
| **Anthranilates** | **Aminobenzoates** |
| Meradimate | Aminobenzoic acid |
| **Camphorsulfonic acid derivatives** | Lisadimate |
| Ecamsule | Padimate |
| **Dibenzoylmethanes** | Padimate O |
| Avobenzone | Roxadimate |
| Dibenzoylmethane | **Camphor derivatives** |
| Isopropyldibenzoylmethane | Enzacamene |
| **UVA and UVB absorbers** | **Cinnamates** |
| **Benzophenones** | Amiloxate |
| Benzophenone-6 | Cinoxate |
| Dioxybenzone | Octinoxate |
| Mexenone | Octocrilene |
| Oxybenzone | **Salicylates** |
| Sulisobenzone | Homosalate |
| | Octisalate |

For drugs that are applied topically, the vehicle and formulation may be as important as the active drug. Indeed, some cream and ointment bases are used alone for their protective or emollient properties, while adverse effects of topical preparations are sometimes attributed to constituents of the vehicle such as stabilisers and preservatives. The *choice of formulation* depends on the skin condition being treated and the area affected. Lotions and gels are useful for hairy areas. Creams (oil-in-water emulsions) have cooling and emollient effects, are readily absorbed by the skin, and are used for acute and exudative conditions. Ointments (water-in-oil emulsions) are more occlusive than creams and are particularly suitable for chronic dry lesions. Pastes (powder incorporated in an ointment basis) are less occlusive than ointments and are useful for their protective properties and for their use on circumscribed lesions. Other less frequently used formulations include applications, collodions, and dusting powders. Typical quantities of preparations required per week for twice daily application to specific areas of an adult are given in Table 2, below.

**Table 2.** Typical quantities of preparations required per week for twice daily application to an adult.

| | Creams and Ointments | Lotions |
|---|---|---|
| Face | 15 to 30 g | 100 mL |
| Both hands | 25 to 50 g | 200 mL |
| Scalp | 50 to 100 g | 200 mL |
| Both arms or both legs | 100 to 200 g | 200 mL |
| Trunk | 400 g | 500 mL |
| Groins and genitalia | 15 to 25 g | 100 mL |

NOTE. These quantities do *not* apply to corticosteroid preparations.

## Acne

Acne is a disorder of the pilosebaceous follicle; common features include increased sebum production, follicular keratinisation, colonisation by *Propionibacterium acnes*, and localised inflammation. Mild acne is characterised by open or closed comedones (blackheads and whiteheads), some of the latter developing into inflamed lesions such as papules and pustules. In moderate acne, the papules and pustules are more widespread, and there may be mild scarring. Severe acne is characterised by the presence of nodular abscesses or cysts in addition to widespread pustules and papules, and may lead to extensive scarring.

The most common form of acne is acne vulgaris. It is common in teenagers and while by their mid-20s the majority of cases have resolved, a few people still require treatment in their 30s and 40s. Skin areas typically affected are the face, shoulders, upper chest, and back. Acne may also occur in late middle age and in the elderly (late onset acne) and in infants (infantile acne). Certain drugs, including androgens, corticosteroids, corticotropin, hormonal contraceptives containing androgenic progestogens such as levonorgestrel, isoniazid, lithium, methoxsalen, and some antiepileptics may produce an acneform rash, as may substances such as tars, oils, and oily cosmetics.

Treatment aims to reduce the bacterial population of the pilosebaceous follicles, reduce the rate of sebum production, reduce inflammation, and remove the keratinised layer blocking the follicles. Drugs used include keratolytics, retinoids, and antibacterials. If topical preparations are not effective, oral preparations may be required. Response to therapy is commonly slow and long-term treatment is usually necessary.[1-6]

**Mild acne** is treated topically, in particular with benzoyl peroxide, retinoids, or antibacterials. Abrasives have been used but their effectiveness is doubtful, and preparations based on sulfur or salicylic acid are considered by some to be obsolete; the effectiveness of degreasing agents has also been questioned. Topical corticosteroids, despite their presence in some compound preparations, should not be used.

Benzoyl peroxide has an antimicrobial action and mild keratolytic properties, and both comedones and inflammation generally respond well. It is probably the most widely used first-line drug. Azelaic acid is an alternative to benzoyl peroxide that may cause less local irritation. Both have been used in combination with other topical agents.

Topical retinoids are an alternative to benzoyl peroxide and some dermatologists consider them to be the treatment of choice for mild to moderate comedonal acne. Isotretinoin and tretinoin appear to be equally effective when used topically; tazarotene is a recently-introduced retinoid for topical use and adapalene, a naphthoic acid derivative, may also be used. Topical retinoids and antibacterials may be particularly effective if used together, since antibacterials are more effective for inflammation and retinoids for comedones; retinoids may also be alternated with benzoyl peroxide.

Topical antibacterials may be used particularly for inflammatory acne, following ineffective or poorly tolerated benzoyl peroxide application. Tetracycline, clindamycin, and erythromycin are generally available as solutions for topical use, and appear to be roughly equivalent in efficacy. However, development of resistance by the skin flora is an increasing problem. Combination therapy with benzoyl peroxide and erythromycin may help to prevent the selection of resistant mutants; alternatively, short intervening courses of benzoyl peroxide or azelaic acid during antibacterial therapy may help to eliminate any resistant bacteria that have been selected. It has also been recommended:[7]

- that courses of topical antibacterials be continued for no longer than necessary (although treatment should be used for at least 6 months)
- that the same drug be used if further treatment is required
- that concomitant treatment with different oral and topical drugs or rotation be avoided.

Nicotinamide is also used topically in mild to moderate acne.

**Moderate acne** is best treated with oral antibacterials. Topical drugs may also be used as adjunctive anticomedonal treatment. Of the oral antibacterials tetracyclines appear to be the drugs of first choice. Tetracycline, doxycycline, lymecycline, or oxytetracycline may be used. Minocycline has also been reported to be effective; however, it may cause skin pigmentation and may be associated rarely with immunologically mediated reactions. Alternatives to the tetracyclines include erythromycin, co-trimoxazole, and trimethoprim. All oral antibacterials have to be used for at least 3 months; the maximal response is thought to occur after 3 to 6 months, although in some cases treatment for 2 or more years may be necessary. Again, resistance may be a problem particularly with erythromycin.

Women with moderate acne who also require oral contraception may be treated additionally with a combined oral contraceptive containing a non-androgenic progestogen.

**Severe acne** is usually treated with oral isotretinoin. Where it cannot be used, high doses of oral antibacterials may be considered. In women with hormonal disturbances, the anti-androgen cyproterone with ethinylestradiol (available as a combination preparation) or a combined (non-androgenic) contraceptive may be effective as adjunctive treatment. Spironolactone used for its anti-androgenic properties has been advocated for women in whom oestrogens are contra-indicated. Colchicine is being investigated in acne resistant to antibacterial treatment.

Topical drugs, particularly antibacterials, described above under mild acne, may be used as adjunctive treatment.

There is evidence to suggest that photodynamic therapy with a photosensitiser, such as 5-aminolevulinic acid, may be beneficial in acne.


1. Leyden JJ. Therapy for acne vulgaris. *N Engl J Med* 1997; **336:** 1156–62.
2. Livingstone C. Acne. *Pharm J* 1997; **259:** 725–7.
3. Brown SK, Shalita AR. Acne vulgaris. *Lancet* 1998; **351:** 1871–6.
4. Krowchuk DP. Treating acne: a practical guide. *Med Clin North Am* 2000; **84:** 811–28.
5. Webster GF. Acne vulgaris. *BMJ* 2002; **325:** 475–9.
6. Gollnick H. Current concepts of the pathogenesis of acne: implications for drug treatment. *Drugs* 2003; **63:** 1579–96.
7. Eady EA, *et al.* Antibiotic resistant propionibacteria in acne: need for policies to modify antibiotic usage. *BMJ* 1993; **306:** 555–6.


## Alopecia

Alopecia (hair loss) has many causes. The most common form, male-pattern alopecia, is androgen-related. Alopecia may also be congenital, be associated with systemic disorders, severe emotional and physical stress, or skin disorders, or be due to nutritional deficiencies. Some drugs may cause alopecia; examples include antineoplastics (see p.496), beta blockers, diazoxide, heparin, verapamil, and warfarin. In some cases there is destruction of the hair follicles (scarring) resulting in permanent hair loss. If the hair follicles remain intact (nonscarring alopecia) then treatment of the underlying condition or removal of the suspected drug may produce hair regrowth. Drug treatment may be tried in alopecia areata and male-pattern alopecia, although it is often unsuccessful.

**Alopecia areata** is an auto-immune disorder in which there is a loss of hair in sharply defined areas of skin that normally bear hair. The affected area can vary in size from about 1 $cm^2$ to the whole scalp (alopecia totalis) or all body hair (alopecia universalis).

Small or isolated patches of alopecia areata may not need treatment and in many patients hair regrows within a few months. If loss of hair becomes a problem cosmetically, treatment may be offered but is often not totally satisfactory. Several treatment options have been tried.[1,2] Intralesional corticosteroids stimulate hair regrowth at the site of injection and may be of benefit for limited patchy hair loss. Oral pulsed or continuous corticosteroids may be used in severe progressive cases. Potent topical corticosteroids, topical dithranol, and minoxidil lotion may also be used, although their efficacy is debatable. Contact immunotherapy with diphencyprone has shown benefit in patients with extensive patchy hair loss, alopecia totalis and universalis. Photochemotherapy with ultraviolet A radiation (PUVA) with either systemic or topical psoralens such as methoxsalen has been tried, but potentially serious side-effects and limited efficacy restrict its use.

**Male-pattern alopecia** (androgenetic alopecia or male-pattern baldness)[1,3,4] involves recession of the hairline in the frontal region of the scalp or loss of hair at the vertex. It is usually associated with increasing age in men. A similar pattern of hair loss occurs in women with elevated androgen concentrations; hair loss associated with increasing age in women with normal androgen concentrations is usually much more diffuse. Topical minoxidil is more effective in male-pattern alopecia than it is in the areata forms of alopecia, but is still, at best, only modestly effective. Because of the role of androgens in this condition anti-androgens and 5α-reductase inhibitors may also be tried. The 5α-reductase inhibitor finasteride has been shown to be of benefit in men with male-pattern alopecia, but is restricted to use in males.


1. Price VH. Treatment of hair loss. *N Engl J Med* 1999; **341:** 964–73.
2. MacDonald Hull SP, *et al.* Guidelines for the management of alopecia areata. *Br J Dermatol* 2003; **149:** 692–9.
3. Bergfeld WF. Androgenetic alopecia: an autosomal dominant disorder. *Am J Med* 1995; **98** (suppl 1A): 95S–98S.
4. Sinclair R. Male pattern androgenetic alopecia. *BMJ* 1998; **317:** 865–9.


## Burns

Burns may be caused by chemicals or heat. Initial treatment of burns is irrigation with cold water for 10 to 15 minutes. This limits the skin damage in burns caused by heat and removes the causative agent in chemical burns. Sodium bicarbonate solution is then used on acid burns and acetic acid solution on alkaline burns. The extent of a burn injury is described by area and depth. The affected body-surface can be calculated, and the depth of the burn may be classified as superficial (first-degree); partial thickness (second-degree), which may be further classified as superficial or deep partial thickness; or full thickness (third-degree). The major problems associated with burns are hypovolaemic shock, inhalation injury, metabolic abnormalities, and infection.

- After a burn, fluid accumulates rapidly in the wound area due to increased permeability of the microcirculation and this loss of fluid from the circulation may produce hypovolaemic shock (p.835) if burns involve at least 15 to 20% of the body-surface.
- Inhalation injury producing airway oedema is mainly a result of exposure to toxic gases. Endotracheal intubation is required until the oedema subsides. Oxygen therapy is used, and nebulised beta$_2$ agonists may be given to treat bronchospasm. Inhalation of heparin and acetylcysteine may be of benefit in reducing pulmonary failure.
- Hypermetabolism and marked catabolism can result from major burn injury. Protein breakdown and loss causes muscle wasting and weakness, impaired wound healing and skin breakdown, and impaired immunity. Other effects of metabolic disturbances include an increase in liver fat and hepatomegaly, osteopenia, tachycardia and increased myocardial oxygen consumption. Enteral feeding (p.1418) to match nutrient requirements is essential for metabolic management. Other treatments that have been tried to reduce net catabolism include the amino acids arginine and glutamine, and drugs with anabolic effects including oxandrolone and somatropin (for concerns about the latter use see p.1329).
- Prevention of infection is an important part of burn wound management. Micro-organisms proliferate rapidly in burn wounds, especially those severe enough to impair immune function and sepsis remains the major fatal complication of burns. Burn wounds should be cleansed with normal saline (see Wounds and Ulcers, below). This may be all that is required for very minor burn wounds; a non-adherent dressing, such as paraffin tulle, may be used if necessary. Topical antibacterials, such as sulfadiazine silver, silver nitrate, and mafenide acetate, may be applied as required. Sodium hypochlorite (Dakin's solution) may also be of value, although opinions differ as to its usefulness. Removal of devitalised tissue is also an essential element of management. Infections require aggressive systemic treatment (see under Skin Infections, p.146).

Full thickness burn wounds require skin grafting. This is performed as soon as possible after stabilisation of the patient. Skin grafting may also be considered for deep partial thickness wounds. If the area to be grafted is very extensive, the grafting procedure may have to be in stages (at intervals of about a week) as sufficient autologous skin becomes available. Alternatively, temporary skin substitutes may be used to supplement autologous skin and allow wound closure in one stage.

References.


1. Monafo WW. Initial management of burns. *N Engl J Med* 1996; **335:** 1581–6.
2. Clarke J. Burns. *Br Med Bull* 1999; **55:** 885–94.
3. Ramzy PI, *et al.* Thermal injury. *Crit Care Clin* 1999; **15:** 333–52.
4. Demling RH, Seigne P. Metabolic management of patients with severe burns. *World J Surg* 2000; **24:** 673–80.
5. Murphy KD, *et al.* Current pharmacotherapy for the treatment of severe burns. *Expert Opin Pharmacother* 2003; **4:** 369–84.


## Darier's disease

Darier's disease (keratosis follicularis) is an uncommon inherited keratinisation disorder (see below) and is characterised by groups of horny papules over the body. These may become irritated and/or infected, exudative, and crusted. Severity varies greatly; mild disease may require the use of emollients only. More severe cases are treated by topical application of keratolytics such as salicylic acid or topical retinoids such as isotretinoin, tretinoin, or tazarotene. Treatment with oral retinoids (acitretin, etretinate, or isotretinoin) may be needed and has been combined with topical retinoids. Ciclosporin and topical fluorouracil have also been tried.

References.


1. Burge S. Management of Darier's disease. *Clin Exp Dermatol* 1999; **24:** 53–6.


## Dermatitis herpetiformis

Dermatitis herpetiformis is a rare blistering disorder of the subepidermal tissue in which the vesicles and papules are intensely irritant and pruritic. The knees, elbows, buttocks, shoulders, and scalp are areas typically affected. The disease presents usually during early to middle adult life and is a chronic condition, although there may be periods of remission that last several months. In many patients there is also a mild gastrointestinal absorptive defect characterised by gluten hypersensitivity (gluten enteropathy). Skin lesions can be suppressed by dapsone; the sulfonamides sulfamethoxypyridazine or sulfapyridine have been used as alternatives to dapsone.[1-3] A gluten-free diet may improve both gastrointestinal symptoms and the skin disorder.[2,4]


1. Fine J-D. Management of acquired bullous skin diseases. *N Engl J Med* 1995; **333:** 1475–84.
2. Fry L. Dermatitis herpetiformis. *Baillieres Clin Gastroenterol* 1995; **9:** 371–93.
3. Garioch JJ. Dermatitis herpetiformis and its management. *Prescribers' J* 1996; **36:** 141–5.
4. Garioch JJ, *et al.* 25 years' experience of a gluten-free diet in the treatment of dermatitis herpetiformis. *Br J Dermatol* 1994; **131:** 541–5.


## Drug-induced skin reactions

Drugs are a frequent cause of adverse skin reactions. The skin reaction may mimic a spontaneously occurring skin disorder and is therefore included in the differential diagnosis of most skin diseases. Alternatively, the drug may produce quite specific changes. The reaction can develop after the first dose or after a period of sensitisation. Pigmentation changes or effects on hair may take some months to become apparent. Drug-induced nail changes have also been reported.

Reactions range from mild rashes to severe life-threatening reactions including angioedema with urticaria, Stevens-Johnson syndrome, and toxic epidermal necrolysis. Other serious skin reactions include hypersensitivity syndromes, serum sickness, and vasculitis.

**Stevens-Johnson syndrome** (see also Erythema Multiforme, below) is a severe, blistering skin reaction also affecting the mucous membranes of the oropharynx, eyes, and genitalia and accompanied sometimes by fever, pain, and malaise. **Toxic epidermal necrolysis** (Lyell's syndrome or scalded skin syndrome) as described below, is a more severe form of the reaction where considerable amounts of the epidermis may be shed. Sulfonamides, carbamazepine, and allopurinol are among the many drugs that have been associated with both these reactions.

**Hypersensitivity syndrome** is a severe, idiosyncratic reaction which includes rash and fever, and often hepatitis, arthralgias, lymphadenopathy, and haematological abnormalities. It tends to have a relatively late and slow onset. Some antiepileptics and sulfonamides cause this syndrome, as well as allopurinol, dapsone, and gold salts. **Serum sickness** is manifest as rash, fever, arthralgia and arthritis and typically develops 8 to 14 days after administration of serum preparations and vaccines. **Vasculitic reactions** may occur 7 to 21 days after beginning therapy with drugs such as allopurinol, penicillins, and sulfonamides (see Hypersensitivity Vasculitis, p.1081). The vasculitis usually affects small vessels of the lower extremities producing purpura, although it can also affect vessels in the kidney, liver, and gastrointestinal tract, in which case it may be life-threatening.

**Maculopapular exanthematic eruptions** are probably the most frequent drug-induced skin reaction. Drugs commonly causing these rashes include carbamazepine, chlorpromazine, nitrofurantoin, penicillins, and sulfonamides. **Urticaria** (below) is also frequently drug-induced. **Photosensitivity** rashes where the skin reaction is confined to light-exposed areas may be phototoxic or photoallergic in nature. Phototoxic reactions occur in many patients and are dose-dependent, while photoallergic reactions affect only a few individuals. Amiodarone produces a phototoxic reaction in many patients. Some drugs cause **pigmentary changes** (see Pigmentation Disorders, below). Chlorpromazine can cause both photosensitivity and pigmentary changes. **Acneform eruptions** may be produced by a number of drugs (see Acne, above). Some drugs produce skin reactions resembling **pemphigus** and **pemphigoid** (see below). Most of the drugs implicated contain a thiol group or metabolism of the drug generates a thiol group. Examples include captopril, penicillamine, penicillins, piroxicam, and rifampicin. **Fixed-drug eruptions** are inflammatory patches that appear at the same sites each time the drug is taken, and may occur with many drugs including dapsone, sulfonamides, and tetracycline.

Drug-induced **nail changes** include onychomadesis, nail fragility, onycholysis, paronychia, pigmentation, and vascular changes. The effect is usually transient and disappears with drug withdrawal. Drugs reported to cause nail changes include antineoplastics, psoralens, retinoids, tetracyclines, and zidovudine.

The majority of drug-induced adverse skin reactions are mild. However, severe reactions necessitate rapid withdrawal of the suspected drug. In some cases, this may mean stopping several drugs. In most cases the skin reaction will be resolved by symptomatic treatment. Readministration of the offending drug may establish whether the skin eruption is drug-induced, although reactions may be more severe and therefore rechallenge should not be performed after a serious reaction.

General references.


1. Smith AG. Important cutaneous adverse drug reactions. *Adverse Drug React Bull* 1994; **167:** 631–4.
2. Roujeau JC, Stern RS. Severe adverse cutaneous reactions to drugs. *N Engl J Med* 1994; **331:** 1272–85.
3. Wolkenstein P, Revuz J. Drug-induced severe skin reactions: incidence, management and prevention. *Drug Safety* 1995; **13:** 56–68.
4. Lee A, Thomson J. Drug-induced skin reactions. *Pharm J* 1999; **262:** 357–62.
5. Piraccini BM, Tosti A. Drug-induced nail disorders: incidence, management and prognosis. *Drug Safety* 1999; **21:** 187–201.
6. Anonymous. Drug-induced cutaneous photosensitivity: some drugs warrant routine precautions. *Prescrire Int* 2000; **9:** 117–22.
7. ten Holder SM, *et al.* Cutaneous and systemic manifestations of drug-induced vasculitis. *Ann Pharmacother* 2002; **36:** 130–47.


## Eczema

Eczema (often used synonymously with dermatitis) refers to a variety of skin conditions characterised by epidermal inflammation and itching. The areas of skin affected vary in the different types of eczema, but the skin lesions share certain common features. In acute eczema the skin is typically red and inflamed with papules, vesicles, and blisters. In chronic eczema the skin may show the same features but be more dry, scaly, pigmented, and thickened. Eczema may be categorised as exogenous (including allergic, irritant, and photosensitivity eczema) or endogenous (such as atopic, discoid/nummular, gravitational, and seborrhoeic eczema), but there may be multiple causes of eczema, both endogenous and exogenous, in an individual patient. Two of the most common forms of eczema are atopic eczema and seborrhoeic dermatitis (below).

Atopic eczema predominantly affects infants and children although adults may also suffer. The skin is itchy and there is a chronic or relapsing dermatitis in which the face and neck and flexures of the elbows and knees are involved most often and are excoriated and lichenified.

General principles for the management of **atopic eczema** may also be applied to other eczematous skin disorders. Cure of atopic eczema is said to be unrealistic, but good control can be achieved with proper management. The objective of treatment should be to reduce signs and symptoms, to prevent or reduce recurrences, and to provide long-term management by preventing exacerbation. Guidelines have been issued by the Primary Care Dermatology Society with the British Association of Dermatologists[1] and by the International Consensus Conference on Atopic Dermatitis (ICCAD II).[2] The management of eczema has also been reviewed.[3]

**First-line treatment**.

- Regular bathing using soap substitutes is important to *cleanse and hydrate* the skin; soaps and detergents should be avoided as these remove the natural lipid from the skin. Suitable bath oils should be used to maintain skin hydration. Emollients should be applied liberally to the whole body at least twice daily, especially after bathing, and more frequently throughout the day to hands and face.
- Patients should be educated on the *avoidance of trigger factors*. These may include irritants, microbes, and psychological or allergic factors.

**Acute control** of pruritus and inflammation.

- Intermittent topical *corticosteroids* are the mainstay of treatment and are used for up to a week to manage acute flares of atopic eczema. Treatment for up to 6 weeks may be needed for initial control of chronic eczema. To minimise potential side-effects the minimum strength preparation to control the disease should be used, and the age of patient, site of eczema, and extent of disease should be considered when selecting the appropriate preparation. Very potent preparations should be used in children only under specialist supervision.
- Topical *calcineurin inhibitors* (pimecrolimus or tacrolimus) may be used as alternative therapy. Pimecrolimus is indicated for mild to moderate disease and tacrolimus for moderate to severe eczema. The main side-effect is burning at the site of application. Once the condition settles the patient should revert to treatment with emollients.

**Maintenance therapy**.

- For persistent disease or frequent flares, topical calcineurin inhibitors are effective and should be used at the earliest sign of recurrence. While these drugs prevent disease progression they do not have the adverse effects of corticosteroids and consequently may be used on all body areas (including sensitive areas like the face, eyelids, and neck) for extended periods. Studies so far suggest that these new drugs are safe in the short term. However, they do suppress T lymphocytes and although systemic absorption is minimal there may be a possibility of immunosuppression, skin cancers, or bacterial infection.
- Topical corticosteroids may be used intermittently for acute exacerbations. Once the patient is back in remission emollients should be continued.
- *Coal tar* preparations may be used occasionally for chronic atopic eczema, and *ichthammol* may be used as an ointment or paste bandages for chronic lichenified eczema.

**Adjunctive therapy**.

- Overt bacterial, fungal, or viral infections should be treated with an appropriate systemic drug (see Skin Infections under Antibacterials, p.146, and under Antifungals, p.390). Topical preparations are generally not used as they should be restricted to limited areas and patients with eczema often have widespread infections.
- A sedating *antihistamine* may be used short term for severe pruritus associated with relapse or at night-time if scratching disturbs sleep or occurs while asleep. Non-sedating antihistamines are generally ineffective in eczema but may be of benefit in atopic dermatitis and concomitant urticaria.

Patients whose eczema fails to respond to these first-line treatments, even under specialist supervision, require further measures.

**Severe refractory disease**.

- *Phototherapy* with ultraviolet A or B, or in combination, may be useful, and phototherapy using a psoralen (generally methoxsalen) with ultraviolet A (PUVA) may be used in severe, widespread disease. However, potential long term effects such as premature ageing of the skin and skin malignancy need to be considered.
- Therapy with *more potent topical and oral corticosteroids* may be considered for short periods of time. In general, only mild corticosteroids (such as 1% hydrocortisone) should be used on the face and in flexures as absorption is increased in these areas.
- Various *other drugs* have been tried in resistant eczema. Azathioprine, ciclosporin, or methotrexate may be tried in selected patients. Systemic corticosteroids are rarely indicated.

Evening primrose oil and borage oil have also been tried although evidence in favour of a useful therapeutic effect is poor. Other drugs at an experimental stage include interferons, mycophenolate mofetil, and thymopentin. There has been much interest in the use of complementary and alternative therapies and herbal medicines, but serious adverse effects have occasionally occurred and although encouraging results have been reported the degree of benefit is still uncertain.[4,5]


1. Primary Care Dermatology Society & British Association of Dermatologists. Guidelines for the management of atopic eczema, 2003. Available at: http://www.bad.org.uk/doctors/service/primary/eczema.pdf (accessed 16/06/04)
2. Ellis C, *et al.* International consensus conference on atopic dermatitis II (ICCAD II): clinical update and current treatment strategies. *Br J Dermatol* 2003; **148** (suppl 63): 3–10.
3. Leung DYM, Bieber T. Atopic dermatitis. *Lancet* 2003; **361:** 151–60.
4. Armstrong NC, Ernst E. The treatment of eczema with Chinese herbs: a systematic review of randomized clinical trials. *Br J Clin Pharmacol* 1999; **48:** 262–4.
5. Zuckerman GB, Bielory L. Complementary and alternative medicine herbal therapies for atopic disorders. *Am J Med* 2002; **113** (suppl 9A): 47S–51S.


## Epidermolysis bullosa

Epidermolysis bullosa consists of a group of similar congenital disorders characterised by severe blistering of the skin. Sometimes the mucosae, especially of the mouth and oesophagus, are also affected. The blistering may be caused by various structural and metabolic defects and occurs at different levels in the skin in the different forms (simple, junctional, and dystrophic). Blistering can follow even minor trauma or can arise spontaneously. In some patients blistering and scarring can cause marked tissue loss of the affected areas and the most severe forms are fatal in early infancy due to infection of the blisters. Milder forms may be managed by avoiding trauma and keeping blisters clean and dry, but there is no truly effective treatment for the severe forms. High-dose oral corticosteroids may be needed. Phenytoin has been tried, but was unsuccessful in a controlled study. Thalidomide has also been tried.

There is also an acquired form of the disease, epidermolysis bullosa acquisita, and it too is difficult to treat;[1] corticosteroids and immunosuppressants may be tried. Individual patients have responded to high-dose intravenous immunoglobulins or extracorporeal photochemotherapy (oral methoxsalen followed by removal of blood and UV irradiation of leucocytes outside the body before reinfusion).[2,3] There is a case report of successful treatment with basiliximab (an interleukin-2 receptor antibody).[4]


1. Fine J-D. Management of acquired bullous skin diseases. *N Engl J Med* 1995; **333:** 1475–84.
2. Miller JL, *et al.* Remission of severe epidermolysis bullosa acquisita induced by extracorporeal photochemotherapy. *Br J Dermatol* 1995; **133:** 467–71.
3. Gordon KB, *et al.* Treatment of refractory epidermolysis bullosa acquisita with extracorporeal photochemotherapy. *Br J Dermatol* 1997; **136:** 415–20.
4. Haufs MG, Haneke E. Epidermolysis bullosa acquisita treated with basiliximab, an interleukin-2 receptor antibody. *Acta Derm Venereol (Stockh)* 2001; **81:** 72.


## Erythema multiforme

Erythema multiforme is an inflammatory reaction of the skin characterised by maculopapular lesions that may become annular and blister. Areas typically affected are the hands, forearms, elbows, knees, and feet. It is usually associated with a precipitating trigger such as infection (notably herpes simplex infection); it may also be associated with drug use, neoplastic disease, or collagen or inflammatory diseases. In severe forms there is also blistering of the mucous membranes (usually of the mouth). There is some overlap in the descriptions of erythema multiforme, Stevens-Johnson syndrome, and toxic epidermal necrolysis, and attempts have been made to classify them into distinct categories.[1,2] Erythema multiforme occurs predominantly after infections, whereas the Stevens-Johnson syndrome is mainly a drug-induced reaction and seems to be part of a spectrum of skin reactions, with life-threatening toxic epidermal necrolysis being the more severe form (see Drug-induced Skin Reactions, above).

As erythema multiforme is usually an acute reaction of relatively short duration, symptomatic treatment as for burns (see above) may be all that is required. If severe reactions occur systemic corticosteroids may be considered, although there has been controversy about their value. Erythema multiforme may become a recurrent disorder in some patients and various drugs have been tried for treatment and prophylaxis.[3] Aciclovir, given in short courses or continuously, has been used particularly when herpes simplex infection appeared to be a trigger factor. Other drugs that have been tried for recurrent erythema multiforme include dapsone, hydroxychloroquine, mepacrine, azathioprine, and thalidomide.

1. Assier H, *et al.* Erythema multiforme with mucous membrane involvement and Stevens-Johnson syndrome are clinically different disorders with distinct causes. *Arch Dermatol* 1995; **131:** 539–43.
2. Forman R, *et al.* Erythema multiforme, Stevens-Johnson syndrome and toxic epidermal necrolysis in children: a review of 10 years' experience. *Drug Safety* 2002; **25:** 965–72.
3. Schofield JK, *et al.* Recurrent erythema multiforme: clinical features and treatment in a large series of patients. *Br J Dermatol* 1993; **128:** 542–5.

## Hyperhidrosis

Hyperhidrosis (excessive sweating) can affect the hands, feet, and axillae. No cause can usually be established although it may be secondary to an underlying endocrinological or inflammatory disorder.[1]

Drug therapy should be tried initially but is often ineffective in severe cases. Aluminium salts, such as aluminium chloride or aluminium chlorohydrate in alcoholic solvents applied topically, may be successful in milder forms. Topical antimuscarinics such as diphemanil metilsulfate, glycopyrronium bromide, or hyoscine hydrobromide may also provide some relief. Side-effects of antimuscarinics given by mouth generally preclude such use, although oral propantheline bromide has been used successfully to control excessive sweating in a few patients with spinal cord injuries. An intravenous infusion of phentolamine mesilate may be effective in some patients with generalised hyperhidrosis.[2] Intradermal injection of botulinum A toxin is used in patients with severe resistant hyperhidrosis; the subcutaneous route has also been tried.[3] Formaldehyde and glutaral solutions have been used topically for hyperhidrosis affecting the feet but are not very effective and are not usually recommended.

When drug therapy fails to provide adequate relief surgery may be attempted.[1,3] Subcutaneous curettage or excision of skin bearing the eccrine glands has been employed but minimally invasive techniques, notably endoscopic transthoracic sympathectomy, are now available; the latter offers a simple and effective management for severe localised upper limb hyperhidrosis.

1. Quraishy MS, Giddings AEB. Treating hyperhidrosis. *BMJ* 1993; **306:** 1221–2.
2. McCleane G. The use of intravenous phentolamine mesilate in the treatment of hyperhidrosis. *Br J Dermatol* 2002; **146:** 533–4.
3. Collin J, Whatling P. Treating hyperhidrosis. *BMJ* 2000; **320:** 1221–2.

## Ichthyosis

Ichthyosis is a term used for generalised noninflammatory dry scaling or keratinisation disorders (see below). There are several different forms of ichthyosis and severity and incidence varies. They are generally inherited disorders. Emollients, including urea, are used to provide relief to the dry skin by coating the skin surface with an oily film thus preventing evaporation of water. If scaling is more severe topical keratolytics such as salicylic acid or urea are used. Topical retinoids such as tazarotene may be tried. In the severest forms of ichthyosis oral retinoids may be necessary. Acitretin, etretinate, and isotretinoin have all been used. A few patients have responded to topical calcipotriol or tacrolimus, but systemic absorption may be a problem.

References.

1. Shwayder T. Ichthyosis in a nutshell. *Pediatr Rev* 1999; **20:** 5–12.
2. Rubeiz N, Kibbi AG. Management of ichthyosis in infants and children. *Clin Dermatol* 2003; **21:** 325–8.

## Keratinisation disorders

Keratinisation is the process whereby basal epidermal cells are transformed into dead cells of the stratum corneum from where they are shed. The process takes about fourteen days and shedding normally balances production so that the thickness of the stratum corneum does not alter. Keratinisation disorders (keratoses) are characterised by reduced shedding and the formation of scale at the skin surface. A scale is an aggregate of horn cells that have failed to separate horizontally and hyperkeratosis is an exaggeration of this failure in which there is also a vertical build up of the horn cells. Keratinisation disorders include Darier's disease and ichthyosis (see above). Certain inflammatory skin disorders, such as psoriasis (see below), also show enhanced epidermal proliferation.

## Lichen planus

Lichen planus is an inflammatory skin disorder with itchy papular lesions arising usually on the extremities. The nails and oral or buccal mucosa, and rarely the genital mucosa, may also be affected. Its cause is uncertain although sufferers have a higher incidence of auto-immune disease than normal. Some drugs can produce lichenoid reactions; examples include mepacrine, methyldopa, penicillamine, and sodium aurothiomalate.

Evidence for the various treatments that have been tried is mostly scanty.[1,2] In most patients lichen planus remits spontaneously and, if mild and localised, little or no treatment is needed. For more generalised mild disease topical corticosteroids may be useful for relieving pruritus and intralesional corticosteroids can be used for hypertrophic and hyperkeratotic lesions.[3,4] Mucosal lesions are usually asymptomatic and require no treatment; symptomatic mucosal lesions may be treated with corticosteroid pastes or lozenges. Ciclosporin mouthwashes have been tried for oral mucosal lesions, with variable results. In severe forms systemic therapy may be necessary. Corticosteroids, ciclosporin, and retinoids such as acitretin, etretinate, and isotretinoin have been successfully used by mouth. Other treatments tried have included griseofulvin, antimalarials such as chloroquine or hydroxychloroquine, enoxaparin, topical tacrolimus, and oral photochemotherapy with PUVA.

1. Cribier B, *et al.* Treatment of lichen planus: an evidence-based medicine analysis of efficacy. *Arch Dermatol* 1998; **134:** 1521–30.
2. Chan ES-Y, *et al.* Interventions for treating oral lichen planus. Available in The Cochrane Library; Issue 2. Chichester: John Wiley, 2004.
3. Anonymous. Treatment of oral lichen planus. *Lancet* 1990; **336:** 913–14.
4. Oliver GF, Winkelmann RK. Treatment of lichen planus. *Drugs* 1993; **45:** 56–65.

## Lichen sclerosus

Lichen sclerosus is a chronic inflammatory skin condition that most commonly occurs in women, but is also seen in men and children. It affects the anogenital area, causing itching, soreness, urinary, and sexual problems. Extragenital lesions may occur, but do not usually itch, and some patients may show no symptoms at all.[1,2] Lichen sclerosus runs a relapsing and remitting course and complications include secondary infection, most commonly with *Candida*, physical scarring, and vulvodynia. The most common complication seen in male patients is phimosis. Although the exact cause of the disease is unknown, there appears to be a strong association with auto-immune disorders and genetic factors have also been implicated. There is also an association between lichen sclerosus and squamous cell and verrucous carcinoma.[2,3]

Management of lichen sclerosus includes the control of symptoms, prevention and treatment of complications, and the early detection of malignancies.[3] Topical potent corticosteroids such as clobetasol proprionate or betamethasone dipropionate 0.05% have been shown to be safe and effective for both genital and extragenital disease. Intralesional triamcinolone was found to be effective in a small trial. The benefit and safety of other topical treatments, such as tacrolimus, retinoids, testosterone, and progesterone are not clear. Systemic retinoids may be useful in complicated disease that is not responding to topical corticosteroids. There have been reports of benefit for treatment with PUVA or stanazolol. Laser and photodynamic therapy have also been used with some success. Surgical intervention is only indicated for complications of scarring or the development of malignancy.[2,3]

1. Powell JJ, Wojnarowska F. Lichen sclerosus. *Lancet* 1999; **353:** 1777–83.
2. Neill SM, *et al.* Guidelines for the management of lichen sclerosus. *Br J Dermatol* 2002; **147:** 640–9. Also available at: http://www.bad.org.uk/doctors/guidelines/Lichen_Sclerosis.pdf [sic] (accessed 16/06/04)
3. Tasker GL, Wojnarowska F. Lichen sclerosus. *Clin Exp Dermatol* 2003; **28:** 128–33.

## Light-induced skin reactions

Light, although essential for many biological functions, may cause a variety of disorders, particularly due to the ultraviolet portion of the solar spectrum.

**Ultraviolet (UV) light** has different properties according to its wavelength.

- UVA (wavelengths 320 to 400 nm) produces immediate direct tanning of the skin with little erythema although it does contribute to the long-term harmful effects of photoageing and cancers.
- UVB (wavelengths 290 to 320 nm) is about 1000 times stronger than UVA in producing erythema and is that part of the sun's spectrum that is responsible for producing sunburn and it too contributes to long-term effects. UVB also produces tanning by indirect pigmentation.
- UVC (wavelengths 200 to 290 nm) produces erythema without tanning. The earth's surface is usually screened by the ozone layer from UVC radiation although UVC may be emitted by artificial sources such as bactericidal lamps and industrial welding arcs.

In normal healthy individuals **exposure to sunlight** (including reflected light from snow, white sand, or water) causes an increase in pigmentation (tanning). This is an adaptive mechanism to protect the skin from uv radiation. However, excessive exposure to strong sunlight causes erythema and sunburn, which is an inflammatory response to the damage caused by uv radiation. Immediate tanning may occur resulting from the oxidation of melanin precursors in the uppermost layers of the skin. There may also be a delayed and indirect pigmentation due to the formation of new melanin. The ability of an individual to form a tan is genetically predetermined. Melanin provides some protection against further exposure, but the main protection is provided by thickening of the corneous layer.

Excessive and prolonged exposure to intense sunlight may lead to degenerative changes in the skin (premature ageing of the skin or photoageing), actinic (solar) keratoses (which are risk factors or precursors of skin cancers), immunosuppression, and some skin cancers such as basal cell or squamous cell carcinomas and malignant melanomas (see Malignant Neoplasms of the Skin, p.522).

In some persons even brief exposure to sunlight can result in **light-induced disorders** of the skin. *Polymorphic light eruption* is a hypersensitivity reaction characterised by pruritic erythematous lesions that develop some hours after exposure to sunlight. *Chronic actinic dermatitis* is manifested by a persistent eczematous eruption that usually only affects the exposed areas although in a small number of patients the whole skin can be affected. Photosensitivity can also be produced by drugs given either systemically or applied topically (see Drug-induced Skin Reactions, p.1134). Such photosensitivity can be either phototoxic or photoallergic in nature. In *phototoxicity*, tissues are damaged when the drug is energised by absorbing radiation. In *photoallergy*, a hypersensitivity reaction is produced when the drug is chemically altered after exposure to light. Photosensitivity reactions have sometimes occurred to the sunscreens intended to prevent them. Other conditions that can be exacerbated by sunlight include the *cutaneous porphyrias (p.1040), lupus erythematosus (p.1088), solar urticaria, xeroderma pigmentosum*, and sometimes *herpes labialis* (p.620). In many of these cases the photosensitivity is particularly associated with the longer UVA wavelengths.

**Protection** against sunlight is therefore beneficial, both in healthy people to prevent skin damage, and in patients with the disorders mentioned above. Protection may also be necessary in patients with *hypopigmentation disorders* such as vitiligo (see Pigmentation Disorders, below) or albinism, and medical personnel exposed to ultraviolet bactericidal lamps may need protection against the whole of the UV spectrum.

This may be achieved by appropriate dress and through the use of **sunscreens** applied to the skin. Sunscreens may be of chemical or physical types (see above) and many products combine sunscreens of different types to maximise protection. It may be difficult to formulate physical sunscreens in cosmetically acceptable ways.

The efficacy of a particular sunscreen preparation is often expressed as its **sun protection factor (SPF)**. This is a ratio of the time required for irradiation to produce minimal perceptible erythema (minimal erythemal dose; MED) with the skin protected with the sunscreen compared with the MED without protection, for a standard 2 $mg/cm^2$ dose of sunscreen. Thus the SPF is predominantly an indication of efficacy against UVB light. Various systems have been suggested for classifying the relative efficacies of sunscreens against UVA light but none appears, as yet, to be universally accepted. The efficacy of a sunscreen is also highly dependent upon its correct application.

References.


1. Rosen CF. Photoprotection. *Semin Cutan Med Surg* 1999; **18:** 307–14.
2. Lenane P, Murphy GM. Sunscreens and the photodermatoses. *J Dermatol Treat* 2001; **12:** 53–7.
3. Millard TP, Hawk JL. Photosensitivity disorders: cause, effect and management. *Am J Clin Dermatol* 2002; **3:** 239–46.
4. Moore DE. Drug-induced cutaneous photosensitivity: incidence, mechanism, prevention and management. *Drug Safety* 2002; **25:** 345–72.
5. Ferguson J. Diagnosis and treatment of the common idiopathic photodermatoses. *Australas J Dermatol* 2003; **44:** 90–6.
6. Ting WW, *et al.* Practical and experimental consideration of sun protection in dermatology. *Int J Dermatol* 2003; **42:** 505–13.
7. Rosen CF. Topical and systemic photoprotection. *Dermatol Ther* 2003; **16:** 8–15.
8. Tutrone WD, *et al.* Polymorphic light eruption. *Dermatol Ther* 2003; **16:** 28–39.
9. Wolf P. Lichtschutzmittel: Wirkung gegen Hautkrebs und Lichtalterung. *Hautarzt* 2003; **54:** 839–44.
10. Stern RS. Treatment of photoaging. *N Engl J Med* 2004; **350:** 1526–34.


### Pemphigus and pemphigoid

Pemphigus and pemphigoid are rare, disabling, and severe or potentially fatal blistering skin diseases. They are distinct disorders although both have an auto-immune basis.

- There are several types of pemphigus. In pemphigus vulgaris, the most common type, the blistering is intraepidermal and can occur anywhere on the skin surface or on the mucous membranes. It is a chronic, progressive disorder requiring prolonged treatment.
- Pemphigoid is also known as bullous pemphigoid and occurs mainly in elderly persons. The blistering is subepidermal and affects the skin but rarely the mucous membranes. Pemphigoid is usually a self-limiting disorder and treatment can often be stopped after a couple of years.
- Cicatricial pemphigoid (mucous membrane pemphigoid) is a rare form that affects mainly the oral mucosa and conjunctiva, and may affect other mucosae, causing scarring.

The treatment of the blistering in both pemphigus and pemphigoid follows a similar pattern. Wet dressings and general treatment as for burns (see above) are commonly used. Systemic corticosteroids are given to control the blistering and high doses initially are usually required. The doses suggested have varied enormously; the usual range is equivalent to about 60 to 100 mg daily of prednisolone by mouth although up to 400 mg daily has been suggested. However, there is some controversy about the appropriate dosage for initial therapy, since one study has indicated that the highest doses are associated with a poorer prognosis.[1] Maintenance therapy with corticosteroids at lower oral doses or topically may then follow. Intralesional corticosteroids may be useful for isolated lesions. Pulsed intravenous corticosteroids may be considered for severe or refractory disease, particularly if there has been no response to high oral doses. There is also some evidence[2] to show that a potent topical corticosteroid (clobetasol propionate) can be at least as effective as oral prednisolone in moderate to severe bullous pemphigoid. Blistering of the oral mucous membranes may be treated with corticosteroid lozenges, and dinoprostone has also been reported to be effective.

Various therapies have been used as adjuncts or occasionally as alternatives to treatment with corticosteroids.[3-11] However, due to the rarity of the diseases, few controlled studies have been performed. Immunosuppressive therapy, usually with azathioprine, cyclophosphamide, or methotrexate, may be combined with a corticosteroid to improve disease control and permit a reduction in corticosteroid dosage. Mycophenolate mofetil has been used similarly in small numbers of patients. Intramuscular gold therapy has also been used. However, it has been suggested that evidence for the corticosteroid-sparing effect of these drugs is lacking, and that they should be reserved for patients who cannot tolerate corticosteroids or in whom corticosteroids are contra-indicated.[4] Ciclosporin has been tried in a few patients with refractory pemphigus, with some apparent benefit, and high-dose intravenous immunoglobulin has been given to permit reduction of corticosteroid therapy to maintenance doses in pemphigus and pemphigoid. Some patients with bullous pemphigoid respond to dapsone. Plasmapheresis (plasma exchange) may be tried in severe, unresponsive pemphigus.

There have also been a number of reports suggesting that a tetracycline (often minocycline) alone or with nicotinamide, may be useful in controlling the lesions of various types of pemphigus and pemphigoid. They may be tried in patients with mild to moderated disease.[10,11]


1. Mourellou O, *et al.* The treatment of pemphigus vulgaris: experience with 48 patients seen over an 11-year period. *Br J Dermatol* 1995; **133:** 83–7.
2. Joly P, *et al.* A comparison of oral and topical corticosteroids in patients with bullous pemphigoid. *N Engl J Med* 2002; **346:** 321–7.
3. Fine J-D. Management of acquired bullous skin diseases. *N Engl J Med* 1995; **333:** 1475–84.
4. Bystryn J-C, Steinman NM. The adjuvant therapy of pemphigus: an update. *Arch Dermatol* 1996; **132:** 203–12.
5. Carson PJ, *et al.* Influence of treatment on the clinical course of pemphigus vulgaris. *J Am Acad Dermatol* 1996; **34:** 645–52.
6. Stanley JR. Therapy of pemphigus vulgaris. *Arch Dermatol* 1999; **135:** 76–8.
7. Scully C, *et al.* Pemphigus vulgaris: the manifestations and long-term management of 55 patients with oral lesions. *Br J Dermatol* 1999; **140:** 84–9.
8. Nousari HC, Anhalt GJ. Pemphigus and bullous pemphigoid. *Lancet* 1999; **354:** 667–72.
9. Yancey KB, Egan CA. Pemphigoid: clinical, histologic, immunopathologic, and therapeutic considerations. *JAMA* 2000; **284:** 350–6.
10. Wojnarowska F, *et al.* Guidelines for the management of bullous pemphigoid. *Br J Dermatol* 2002; **147:** 214–21. Also available at: http://www.bad.org.uk/doctors/guidelines/Bullous_Pemphigoid.pdf (accessed 16/06/04)
11. Harman KE, *et al.* Guidelines for the management of pemphigus vulgaris. *Br J Dermatol* 2003; **149:** 926–37. Also available at: http://www.bad.org.uk/doctors/guidelines/Pemphigus_Vulgaris.pdf (accessed 16/06/04)


### Pigmentation disorders

The pigment melanin is produced in melanocytes in the basal layer of the epidermis. It is a complex polymer synthesised from the amino acid, dihydroxyphenylalanine. Melanin production is under pituitary control but is also influenced by other endocrine secretions.

Decreased pigmentation (hypopigmentation) and excessive pigmentation (hyperpigmentation) can occur and may be either generalised or localised.

Albinism is a rare inherited disorder that can cause generalised **hypopigmentation**. Affected individuals are extremely sensitive to solar irradiation and must use sunscreens regularly.

A common form of localised hypopigmentation is **vitiligo**. Sharply defined areas of depigmentation are seen and may remain localised or spread so that total depigmentation eventually occurs. There is no totally effective treatment, although some therapies may offer a degree of benefit. Oral or topical photochemotherapy with psoralens (PUVA) is currently considered to be the best treatment.[1-3] Topical corticosteroids are sometimes effective at inducing repigmentation.[4,5] Dihydroxyacetone produces a brown staining of the skin that may be cosmetically acceptable. Experimental drug therapy for re-inducing pigment has included UVA light therapy with either khellin or phenylalanine; oral levamisole, alone or with topical corticosteroids, has also been reported to be of benefit. UVB phototherapy has also been tried and some consider it to be superior to the use of UVA.[4,5] Transplantation of autologous cultured melanocytes, ultrathin epidermal sheets, or basal cell layer suspension may be beneficial in some forms of vitiligo. Transplantation is not suitable for progressive, widespread vitiligo vulgaris.[5,6] If the vitiligo affects a large proportion of the body (more than 50%), and if PUVA is ineffective at inducing repigmentation, an option is to consider inducing depigmentation in the remaining normal skin in order to match the lighter vitiligous areas. Permanent depigmentation may be induced by monobenzone, but patients must subsequently use topical sunscreens in order to avoid damage caused by solar exposure. Hydroquinone produces less permanent depigmentation; exposure to sunlight reverses the effect and sunscreens are used to maintain the benefit.

**Hyperpigmentation** can be caused by increased amounts of melanin, or by other substances such as iron in the skin. Generalised hyperpigmentation may be seen in Addison's disease, acanthosis nigricans, and primary haemochromatosis; other causes may include cirrhosis, chronic renal failure, and glycogen storage disease. Darkening of the skin can also occur in patients taking certain drugs due to a deposition of the drug-melanin complex in the skin. Notable examples include amiodarone, minocycline, and phenothiazines. Localised hyperpigmentation is seen in chloasma (melasma) in which there is facial involvement and is encountered most commonly in pregnancy. A number of compounds have been used basically as bleaching agents in hyperpigmentary disorders, and of these hydroquinone has been used most often;[7] monobenzone is not recommended. A beneficial response to topical tretinoin and azelaic acid in patients with chloasma has been described. Laser therapy, or the use of chemical peels, has also been tried.[7]


1. Antoniou C, Katsambas A. Guidelines for the treatment of vitiligo. *Drugs* 1992; **43:** 490–8.
2. British Photodermatology Group. British Photodermatology Group guidelines for PUVA. *Br J Dermatol* 1994; **130:** 246–55.
3. Drake LA, *et al.* Guidelines of care for vitiligo. *J Am Acad Dermatol* 1996; **35:** 620–6.
4. Njoo MD, *et al.* Nonsurgical repigmentation therapies in vitiligo: meta-analysis of the literature. *Arch Dermatol* 1998; **134:** 1532–40.
5. Hartmann A, *et al.* Hypopigmentary skin disorders: current treatment options and future directions. *Drugs* 2004; **64:** 89–107.
6. Olsson MJ, Juhlin L. Long-term follow-up of leucoderma patients treated with transplants of autologous cultured melanocytes, ultrathin epidermal sheets and basal cell layer suspension. *Br J Dermatol* 2002; **147:** 893–904.
7. Grimes PE. Melasma: etiologic and therapeutic considerations. *Arch Dermatol* 1995; **131:** 1453–7.


### Pruritus

Pruritus (itching) is a common and distressing symptom of many skin disorders but may also be due to systemic causes such as obstructive jaundice, chronic renal disease, endocrine disease, certain malignancies, and of drug hypersensitivity reactions. The exact pathophysiology of itching is unclear, and different inflammatory mediators may be associated with itching in different disorders; the CNS is also thought to play a role in the perception of itch.

Pruritus should be considered as symptomatic of the underlying disorder and treatment should focus on the removal of the offending trigger. However, symptomatic treatment of pruritus may also be necessary.

Emollients may be useful where dry skin is a contributory factor, and may be applied for **topical** management of pruritus in otherwise healthy elderly people. Calamine and crotamiton are often used topically, despite some uncertainty about their value, as are preparations containing phenol or agents such as menthol that cause capillary dilatation with a subsequent sensation of cold and analgesia. Topical capsaicin has also been used and topical corticosteroids may be used to relieve pruritus when there is associated inflammation. Local anaesthetics or antihistamines are only marginally effective for topical use and can very occasionally cause sensitisation. However, lauromacrogol 400 has proved of benefit. Doxepin, a tricyclic antidepressant with very potent antihistaminic activity, has been used topically for the relief of pruritus associated with dermatitis, although its efficacy is questioned by some.

Sedating antihistamines given **by mouth** are commonly used to relieve more generalised pruritus and are used to control the severe itching associated with dermatoses such as atopic eczema (see above). Bile-acid binding resins, such as colestyramine, are used to relieve pruritus associated with the deposition in dermal tissue of excess bile acids in patients with partial biliary obstruction, primary biliary cirrhosis, or intrahepatic cholestasis of pregnancy. There are reports of cholestatic pruritus also responding to ondansetron although results from controlled trials have been mixed. Pruritus caused by obstetric cholestasis has been treated with ursodeoxycholic acid, which also corrects the associated biochemical abnormalities. Central opioid receptors modulate itch and opioid antagonists such as nalmefene and naltrexone have been reported to relieve pruritus. Many other drugs, including cimetidine and propofol, have been of benefit in some patients. Paroxetine has been useful in some patients with cancer-related pruritus, but the effect tended to wear off after several weeks. PUVA (see under Methoxsalen, p.1153) may be helpful in some pruritic skin conditions including aquagenic pruritus.

References.


1. Charlesworth EN, Beltrani VS. Pruritic dermatoses: overview of etiology and therapy. *Am J Med* 2002; **113** (suppl 9A): 25S–33S.
2. Jenkins JK, Boothby LA. Treatment of itching associated with intrahepatic cholestasis of pregnancy. *Ann Pharmacother* 2002; **36:** 1462–5.
3. Yosipovitch G, *et al.* Itch. *Lancet* 2003; **361:** 690–4.
4. Twycross R, *et al.* Itch: scratching more than the surface. *Q J Med* 2003; **96:** 7–26.


### Psoriasis

Psoriasis is a chronic inflammatory skin disorder characterised by enhanced epidermal proliferation leading to erythema, scaling, and thickening of the skin. It appears to be a T-cell mediated auto-immune disease. There are several types of psoriasis including guttate, flexural, pustular, and erythrodermic, but chronic plaque psoriasis (psoriasis vulgaris) is the most common form. In chronic plaque psoriasis the areas most commonly affected are the extensor sides of the knees, elbows, and hands, and the scalp and sacrum. There is no cure and treatment is designed to induce a remission or suppress disease to a tolerable level.

The treatment of psoriasis has been the subject of a number of reviews.[1-6]

**Topical drugs** are the treatment of first choice for chronic plaque psoriasis. Mild conditions may be managed with the use of emollients alone but dithranol, coal tar, or calcipotriol are the usual active treatments for mild to moderate forms. Patients unresponsive to one topical drug may respond to another and alternatives should be tried before considering more aggressive management. Topical drugs are often used in combination.

- Although effective, dithranol stains the skin and clothes and as it is irritant careful adjustment of the strength and duration of application needs to be made. It has traditionally been applied overnight in the form of ointments or pastes but newer short-contact regimens and creams are more suitable for home therapy.
- Coal tar is used either as crude extracts or refined products and although the refined products may be more aesthetically acceptable they may also be less effective.
- Salicylic acid enhances the rate of loss of surface scale and is included in many combination preparations with dithranol or coal tar.
- Calcipotriol and tacalcitol are vitamin D analogues, that have the advantage of being odourless and nonstaining. Maxacalcitol is another vitamin D analogue under investigation.
- Topical corticosteroids are also effective but they may lead to dermal atrophy, tachyphylaxis, systemic toxicity, and may precipitate unstable and pustular psoriasis. They are reported to be the most widely used treatment in the USA.[1]
- A topical retinoid, tazarotene is also effective in psoriasis but significant irritation can limit its use and it should be avoided in pruritic psoriasis.

Guttate psoriasis is strongly associated with streptococcal infection and patients may require antimicrobial treatment but firm evidence of a beneficial effect on the skin lesions[7] (or indeed of any intervention for guttate psoriasis[8]) is lacking.

**Phototherapy** with UVB light (290 to 320 nm) is effective used alone for chronic plaque or guttate psoriasis but also enhances the effectiveness of calcipotriol, coal tar, or dithranol. Studies have indicated that the therapeutic wavelengths are in the region of 311 to 313 nm. Consequently, narrowband UVB lamps (TL-01) have been developed to emit a spectrum that peaks at 311 nm.

**Photochemotherapy (PUVA)** involves the use of oral or topical psoralens such as methoxsalen with UVA light and is generally considered to be the treatment of first choice for psoriasis that is resistant to topical therapies. Guidelines for PUVA have been published.[9,10] Psoralens have also been used with UVB light. Commercially available sunbeds, which emit UVA light, are not recommended as they are rarely effective and induce skin ageing and fragility.

Psoriasis refractory to topical therapy and PUVA may respond to **systemic drugs**. Systemic treatment may also be indicated for extensive chronic plaque psoriasis in elderly or infirm patients, for generalised pustular or erythrodermic psoriasis, or for severe psoriatic arthritis (see Spondyloarthropathies, p.11).

Immunosuppressants such as methotrexate are useful for severe refractory psoriasis, the aim of treatment being to bring psoriasis under control, enabling a return to other modes of treatment rather than to induce remission. Ciclosporin is also used in severe refractory psoriasis and may be used either to induce a remission or in low-dose maintenance therapy to prevent relapse. Tacrolimus is under investigation for both oral and topical use, and azathioprine has been tried. With the recognition that psoriasis is an auto-immune disease, immunomodulating drugs have been developed with an aim to provide selective immunotherapy, by either targeting T-cells or by cytokine modulation. Alefacept and efalizumab inhibit T-cell activation and show similar efficacy in the treatment of psoriasis. Cytokine modulating therapy includes blocking the action of tumour necrosis factor with either etanercept or infliximab and both have been found to be effective for psoriasis skin lesions and psoriatic arthritis.[4,11,12]

Retinoids such as acitretin are also effective, and use with PUVA may allow a reduction in doses and associated toxicity for each therapy. Generalised pustular and palmoplantar pustular psoriasis are particularly responsive to acitretin.

Hydroxycarbamide, fumarates, tioguanine, and sulfasalazine have also been tried. Many anecdotal reports note improvement of psoriasis when patients are given drug therapy for other concomitant disease. The value of such drugs can be difficult to establish particularly due to the chronic relapsing and recurring nature of psoriasis.


1. Linden KG, Weinstein GD. Psoriasis: current perspectives with an emphasis on treatment. *Am J Med* 1999; **107:** 595–605.
2. Peters BP, *et al.* Pathophysiology and treatment of psoriasis. *Am J Health-Syst Pharm* 2000; **57:** 645–62.
3. Griffiths CEM, *et al.* A systematic review of treatments for severe psoriasis. *Health Technol Assess* 2000; **4:** 1–125. Also available at: http://www.ncchta.org/fullmono/mon440.pdf (accessed 16/06/04)
4. Lebwohl M. Psoriasis. *Lancet* 2003; **361:** 1197–1204.
5. Callen JP, *et al.* AAD consensus statement on psoriasis therapies. *J Am Acad Dermatol* 2003; **49:** 897–9.
6. British Association of Dermatologists. Clinical guidelines - psoriasis. Available at: http://www.bad.org.uk/doctors/guidelines/psoriasis.asp (accessed 16/06/04)
7. Owen CM, *et al.* Antistreptococcal interventions for guttate and chronic plaque psoriasis. Available in The Cochrane Library; Issue 2. Chichester: John Wiley; 2004.
8. Chalmers RJG, *et al.* Interventions for guttate psoriasis. Available in The Cochrane Library; Issue 2. Chichester: John Wiley; 2004.
9. British Photodermatology Group. British Photodermatology Group guidelines for PUVA. *Br J Dermatol* 1994; **130:** 246–55.
10. Halpern SM, *et al.* Guidelines for topical PUVA: a report of a workshop of the British Photodermatology Group. *Br J Dermatol* 2000; **142:** 22–31.
Also available at: http://www.bad.org.uk/doctors/guidelines/Topical_Puva_Therapy.pdf (accessed 16/06/04)
11. Kirby B, Griffiths CEM. Novel immune-based therapies for psoriasis. *Br J Dermatol* 2002; **146:** 546–51.
12. Griffiths CEM. Immunotherapy for psoriasis: from serendipity to selectivity. *Lancet* 2002; **359:** 279–80.


## Pyoderma gangrenosum

Pyoderma gangrenosum is a rare serious ulcerative skin disorder often associated with systemic diseases such as inflammatory bowel disease, rheumatoid arthritis, or myeloproliferative disorders. Initially an acutely inflamed nodule is present which progresses very rapidly to large ulcers. Any area of the body may be involved, but the face, legs, and buttocks are frequent sites.

Treatment essentially consists of cleansing and dressings for the ulcers and appropriate therapy for any underlying disease. When necessary high doses of systemic corticosteroids have been given. There have also been reports in small numbers of patients of benefit with sulfasalazine, dapsone, azathioprine, ciclosporin, tacrolimus, thalidomide, infliximab, colchicine, and nicotine chewing gum.

A related but less severe form of the disease, superficial granulomatous pyoderma, has responded to intralesional or oral corticosteroids.

General references.


1. Callen JP. Pyoderma gangrenosum. *Lancet* 1998; **351:** 581–5.


## Rosacea

Rosacea is a chronic condition affecting the face; rarely, the trunk and limbs may be affected. Phases of this disorder include flushing episodes, persistent erythema and telangiectasia, an inflammatory papulopustular phase, and in advanced cases rhinophyma (nasal hypertrophy and deformity). Ocular involvement is also common and can cause conjunctivitis, keratitis, styes, and chalazia.[1-3] The precise cause of rosacea remains unclear. It has been suggested that *Helicobacter pylori* in the gastrointestinal tract may cause flushing by inducing the production of endogenous vasodilators, and that *Demodex folliculorum*, a mite found in human follicles, may have a role in papulopustular rosacea.[3]

The inflammatory episodes of rosacea (papules, swelling, and pustules) are responsive to treatment, but the underlying erythema and telangiectasia usually persist.

- Episodes of flushing may be limited by avoiding trigger factors such as alcoholic and hot drinks, and spicy foods.[1] Patients should use soap-free cleansers and high factor sunscreens.[1,3] In severe cases clonidine or a beta blocker such as atenolol, has been used.[3]
- Persistent erythema may be improved by *H. pylori* eradication (see Peptic Ulcer Disease, p.1246) but the effectiveness of such therapy has not been established.[3]
- Papulopustular rosacea is usually controlled effectively by oral antibacterials.[1,3] Tetracyclines (doxycycline, minocycline, oxytetracycline, tetracycline) have been widely used, but clarithromycin, erythromycin, and metronidazole are suitable alternatives. Improvement occurs over several weeks, and long-term treatment may be necessary. Systemic isotretinoin is also effective, but it is generally reserved for severe or resistant cases of rosacea.

Topical therapies, particularly metronidazole and azelaic acid,[3,4] provide effective alternatives to oral drugs. Other topical therapies that may be useful include tetracyclines, clindamycin, erythromycin, retinoids, or imidazole antifungals such as ketoconazole.[1] Where infestations of *D. folliculorum* are suspected of aggravating the condition, topical treatments such as benzyl benzoate, crotamiton, or permethrin may be tried. There are also anecdotal reports of the successful treatment of demodicidosis with oral ivermectin. Topical corticosteroids should not be used because they exacerbate rosacea.

- Rhinophyma requires conventional or laser surgery;[1,3] isotretinoin may be used for a few months pre-operatively to shrink the bulbous portions.[1]

Non-drug therapies that have been advocated include facial massage;[1] however, as for many of the drug therapies[4] controlled studies are lacking. Laser therapy has been used to obliterate telangiectasia.[1,3]


1. Jansen T, Plewig G. Rosacea: classification and treatment. *J R Soc Med* 1997; **90:** 144–50.
2. Wilkin J, *et al.* Standard classification of rosacea: report of the National Rosacea Society Expert Committee on the Classification and Staging of Rosacea. *J Am Acad Dermatol* 2002; **46:** 584–7.
3. Rebora A. The management of rosacea. *Am J Clin Dermatol* 2002; **3:** 489–96.
4. van Zuuren EJ, *et al.* Interventions for rosacea. Available in The Cochrane Library; Issue 2. Chichester: John Wiley; 2004.


## Seborrhoeic dermatitis

Seborrhoeic dermatitis is a common eczematous skin disorder (see Eczema above) in which erythematous pruritic patches of skin may become either scaly or exudative and crusted. Scaling lesions are the type most commonly observed. In some cases, known as seborrhoeic folliculitis, there may also be follicular papules or pustules. Seborrhoeic dermatitis occurs in regions of the body where sebaceous glands are plentiful, such as the scalp, face, and chest, although the condition is not associated with increased sebum production. The cause of seborrhoeic dermatitis is unknown, although it might be related to overgrowth with *Malassezia ovalis* (*Pityrosporum ovale*), a normal commensal yeast.

Treatment is suppressive rather than curative. Topical preparations containing antifungals such as ciclopirox olamine, terbinafine, or an imidazole (bifonazole, ketoconazole, miconazole), usually with hydrocortisone, are the main drugs used. If unsuccessful, keratolytics such as salicylic acid or tars may be used. Topical macrolactam immunosuppressants such as pimecrolimus and tacrolimus are being investigated as alternate therapy. Shampoos containing ketoconazole, pyrithione zinc, or selenium sulfide are commonly used for scalp involvement. Topical lithium succinate has been tried.

Dandruff due to normal shedding of scalp skin (pityriasis capitis) is treated similarly to seborrhoeic dermatitis of the scalp.

Reviews.


1. Gupta AK, Bluhm R. Seborrheic dermatitis. *J Eur Acad Dermatol Venereol* 2004; **18:** 13–26.


## Toxic epidermal necrolysis

Toxic epidermal necrolysis (Lyell's syndrome or scalded skin syndrome) is usually a drug-induced skin reaction (above). It has been described as a severe form of Stevens-Johnson syndrome, or as the most severe form of erythema multiforme (above), although such classifications have been debated. It generally begins with lesions of the mucous membranes of the oropharynx, eyes, and genitalia, and fever and pain. Subsequently, a macular rash, blisters, or diffuse erythema develop, and affected skin may detach irregularly, sometimes in large sheets. Toxic epidermal necrolysis is managed similarly to burns (above), but specific treatments have not been established. The use of systemic corticosteroids is controversial because of a higher risk of infection. Other treatments that have been tried with some reports of benefit include plasmapheresis, intravenous immunoglobulin, cyclophosphamide, ciclosporin, and infliximab.

References.


1. Becker DS. Toxic epidermal necrolysis. *Lancet* 1998; **351:** 1417–20.
2. Spies M, *et al.* Treatment of extensive toxic epidermal necrolysis in children. *Pediatrics* 2001; **108:** 1162–8.
3. Fischer M, *et al.* Antitumour necrosis factor-α antibodies (infliximab) in the treatment of a patient with toxic epidermal necrolysis. *Br J Dermatol* 2002; **146:** 707–8.
4. Majumdar S, *et al.* Interventions for toxic epidermal necrolysis. Available in The Cochrane Library; Issue 2. Chichester: John Wiley; 2004.


## Urticaria and angioedema

Urticaria and angioedema are conditions caused by the release of inflammatory mediators from mast cells and basophils. **Urticaria** (also known as nettlerash or hives) is characterised by circumscribed, elevated, erythematous, and usually pruritic areas of oedema (wheals) involving the superficial portion of the dermis. Individual lesions arise suddenly, often within a few minutes, and may last up to 24 hours. In severe, acute urticaria, wheals may cover most of the skin surface. In chronic urticaria (continuous or recurrent lesions over at least 6 weeks) only a few wheals may develop each day. When subcutaneous or submucosal tissues are involved, causing swelling of the eyelids, lips, tongue, larynx, or genitalia, the condition is called **angioedema**.

Although urticaria may be caused by an allergy, it often has a non-allergic mechanism. Urticaria occurs as an adverse effect of many drugs, for example aspirin and many antibacterials. Other types of urticaria include dermographism (linear wheal formation on scratching or stroking) and cholinergic urticaria (evoked by such triggers as exercise, heat, and emotion and characterised by small papulous wheals surrounded by an erythematous flare). In idiopathic anaphylaxis, patients experience attacks of urticaria or angioedema, sometimes with bronchospasm, hypotension, or syncope.[1]

The **management** of urticaria and angioedema has been reviewed.[2-7] Avoidance of unnecessary exposure to known allergens or triggers is of prime importance in the management of urticaria, although in the majority of chronic cases no trigger factor can be found. Severe, acute urticaria or angioedema requires urgent treatment as for anaphylaxis (p.855).

Topical treatment of urticaria is rarely effective except for mild cases. Calamine, menthol, and crotamiton have cooling or antipruritic effects. Topical corticosteroids are of no value; topical antihistamines are not very effective and carry a slight risk of sensitisation.

Most patients with urticaria derive some benefit from oral antihistamines, especially in the relief of pruritus. A non-sedating antihistamine is the first line of treatment. Sedating antihistamines are useful at bedtime. If such antihistamines ($H_1$-antagonists) are only partly successful, combination with an $H_2$-antagonist may be tried; cimetidine or ranitidine, administered alone or with an $H_1$-antagonist, have shown benefit in certain types of urticaria, especially those associated with cold or angioedema. The routine use of $H_2$-antagonists in urticaria is controversial, but in practice their addition to conventional treatment can be tried in resistant cases. Little additional benefit has been found with combination therapy in dermographic urticaria.[8]

The tricyclic antidepressant doxepin has $H_1$- and $H_2$-antagonist properties and has sometimes been effective in patients with urticaria.

Leukotriene antagonists such as montelukast and zafirlukast have been shown to be effective in chronic urticaria, but there is no evidence that they have additional effect once maximum $H_1$ - and $H_2$-receptor blockade has been reached.[7]

Addition of a sympathomimetic such as terbutaline or a calcium-channel blocker such as nifedipine has also been suggested for patients unresponsive to treatment with an $H_1$-antagonist alone, but results have varied.

A short course of an oral corticosteroid may be indicated for patients refractory to other measures. It has been suggested that chronic urticaria may be associated with thyroid auto-immunity and that levothyroxine therapy may be of benefit in patients with antithyroid antibodies. A number of other drugs including danazol, stanozolol, dapsone, sulfasalazine, ciclosporin, and intravenous immunoglobulin have reportedly produced benefit in limited numbers of patients, but such therapies are largely used empirically.

Patients with frequent attacks of idiopathic anaphylaxis have benefited from prophylaxis with a corticosteroid and antihistamine, sometimes with a beta agonist.[9]

1. Patterson R, Harris KE. Idiopathic anaphylaxis. *Allergy Asthma Proc* 1999; **20:** 311–15.
2. Ormerod AD. Urticaria: recognition, causes, and treatment. *Drugs* 1994; **48:** 717–30.
3. Greaves MW. Chronic urticaria. *N Engl J Med* 1995; **332:** 1767–72.
4. Greaves MW, Sabroe RA. Allergy and the skin: urticaria. *BMJ* 1998; **316:** 1147–50.
5. Greaves M. Management of urticaria. *Hosp Med* 2000; **61:** 463–9.
6. Grattan C, *et al.* Management and diagnostic guidelines for urticaria and angio-oedema. *Br J Dermatol* 2001; **144:** 708–14.
7. Kaplan AP. Chronic urticaria and angioedema. *N Engl J Med* 2002; **346:** 175–9.
8. Sharpe GR, Shuster S. In dermographic urticaria $H_2$ receptor antagonists have a small but therapeutically irrelevant additional effect compared with $H_1$ antagonists alone. *Br J Dermatol* 1993; **129:** 575–9.
9. Wong S, *et al.* Outcome of prophylactic therapy for idiopathic anaphylaxis. *Ann Intern Med* 1991; **114:** 133–6.

## Warts

Warts are caused by human papillomaviruses. The lesions present in several different forms and can affect any skin site although the hands, feet, and anogenital areas are most frequently affected. Plantar warts on the soles of the feet are sometimes called verrucas. Anogenital warts are known as condylomata acuminata. Warts do disappear spontaneously but as they may not do so for months or years patients often seek treatment.

There is no specific antiviral therapy against the human papillomavirus.[1-7] Treatment usually relies on some form of local tissue destruction.

- Non-pharmacological techniques include surgical excision, electrocauterisation, or laser therapy. Photodynamic therapy using 5-aminolevulinic acid has also been investigated. Cryotherapy (tissue freezing) may be performed with liquid nitrogen or solid carbon dioxide.
- Chemical destruction with acids (acetic acid, lactic acid, nitric acid, salicylic acid, or trichloroacetic acid), silver nitrate, formaldehyde or glutaral, or podophyllum resin or its derivatives (podophyllotoxin) is another option. Podophyllum resin or podophyllotoxin are often used for anogenital warts.
- Intralesional injection of cytotoxics such as bleomycin or fluorouracil also destroys the wart and may be used in severe or resistant cases. Fluorouracil may also be applied topically.

Other treatments based on less destructive mechanisms have also been used.

- Tretinoin has been tried topically for its effect on epidermal growth.
- Imiquimod is an immune response modifier that is used topically to treat anogenital warts. There is also some evidence to suggest that it is effective for other cutaneous warts. Other drugs with immunomodulatory effects, such as cimetidine, have been tried in a few patients. There are also small studies of treatment with diphencyprone, a contact sensitiser.
- Interferons have antiviral, antiproliferative, and immunomodulatory actions and have thus been investigated in the management of warts; some studies, especially those involving intralesional administration, have demonstrated benefit.

Early investigational data suggests that vaccines for the treatment and prophylaxis of genital human papillomavirus infection may be safe and effective.

1. Anonymous. Tackling warts on the hands and feet. *Drug Ther Bull* 1998; **36:** 22–4.
2. Verbov J. How to manage warts. *Arch Dis Child* 1999; **80:** 97–9.
3. von Krogh G, *et al.* European course on HPV associated pathology: guidelines for primary care physicians for the diagnosis and management of anogenital warts. *Sex Transm Infect* 2000; **76:** 162–8.
4. Sterling JC, *et al.* Guidelines for the management of cutaneous warts. *Br J Dermatol* 2001; **144:** 4–11.
5. Wiley DJ, *et al.* External genital warts: diagnosis, treatment, and prevention. *Clin Infect Dis* 2002; **35** (suppl 2): S210–S224.
6. Centers for Disease Control. Sexually transmitted diseases treatment guidelines 2002. *MMWR* 2002; **51** (RR-6): 1–80. Also available at: http://www.cdc.gov/mmwr/PDF/rr/rr5106.pdf (accessed 16/06/04)
7. Gibbs S, *et al.* Local treatments for cutaneous warts. Available in The Cochrane Library; Issue 2. Chichester: John Wiley; 2004.

## Wounds and ulcers

Wounds (physical injuries of the skin and underlying structures) may be the result of mechanical trauma, burns, or chemical injury. Ulcers are often the result of various underlying disorders. Among the commonest types, *decubitus ulcers* (bedsores, pressure sores) occur in patients with extended immobility when prolonged pressure on the skin over a bony prominence produces localised ischaemia. *Leg ulcers* may result from venous incompetence (venous ulcers) or be ischaemic in origin (arterial ulcers), while patients with peripheral neuropathy, such as diabetics or those with leprosy, may develop *neuropathic ulcers* due to repetitive inadvertent injury. Wounds or ulcers may be described as superficial, partial thickness, or full thickness. Superficial wounds are limited to epithelial tissue and heal rapidly by regeneration of epithelial cells. Partial thickness wounds involve the dermis and include some blood vessel damage, and therefore wound repair is a longer process. Full thickness wounds extend at least to subcutaneous fat, and healing requires synthesis of new connective tissue.

Healing mechanisms are essentially the same regardless of the cause of the damage:

- immediate haemostatic processes involve formation of a platelet plug and fibrin clot, as described under Haemostasis and Fibrinolysis, p.735
- the early granulation and re-epithelialisation phase takes place up to about 21 days after injury depending on wound size and site. Platelet-derived growth factors stimulate fibroblasts to produce granulation tissue, comprising a collagen matrix well-supplied with capillary vessels, and growth of epidermal cells leading to re-epithelialisation of the wound surface
- during the final dermal repair and remodelling phase the collagen matrix undergoes strengthening and there is a reduction in vascularity. This phase can continue for up to 2 years after injury.

Several factors are important for efficient wound healing. Adequate supplies of nutrients, especially vitamin C and zinc (which are often given as supplements) and oxygen are needed. A good blood supply is thus essential. Clinical infection, either systemic or local, due to contamination by environmental microbes, causes tissue damage and delays healing. The process of wound repair requires many cellular and acellular factors, such as platelets and growth factors, and deficiencies in these may also be responsible for delayed healing. Thus, the patient's age, systemic conditions, concomitant drugs, nutritional status, and congenital deficiencies all influence the rate of healing.

Local **wound management** includes cleansing, removal of exudate, and prevention of microbial contamination. Choice of wound treatment preparation will depend on the size, location, type, and cause of the wound, on the presence of infection, and on the particular stage of healing.

Wound **cleansing** is required to remove any dirt or foreign bodies and to **remove exudate** and slough (pus and necrotic tissue). This helps to prevent infection and aids healing. Commonly used cleansing solutions are sodium chloride 0.9%, hypochlorite, hydrogen peroxide, povidone-iodine, and chlorhexidine. However, some antiseptics and hypochlorites might be associated with delayed wound healing, especially with prolonged use, as they delay collagen production and cause inflammation. Also, many antiseptics are inactivated by organic material. Sodium chloride solution may be all that is required for routine cleansing of non-infected wounds.

Many of the cleansing solutions also help to remove slough. Other wound management preparations more specifically directed at removing slough include dextranomer, hydrogels, hydrocolloids, and enzyme preparations such as a mixture of streptokinase and streptodornase. Dextranomer, hydrogels, and hydrocolloids cause debridement by their occlusive, rehydrating properties. Surgical debridement is a fast and efficient way of removing necrotic tissue. Larval therapy (the use of live sterile maggots of *Lucilia sericata*, the common greenbottle fly) has also been effective for debridement of infected or necrotic wounds, including diabetic foot ulceration.

Wounds may produce large volumes of exudate as a result of inflammatory reactions, especially during the first few days. Hydrocolloid and alginate preparations and foam dressings are effective moisture absorbers.

All wounds are colonised by bacteria to some extent and there is no evidence that this superficial **infection** affects healing. However, infection with *Pseudomonas aeruginosa* may delay healing and sulfadiazine silver is used especially in burns. Acetic acid has also been used. Infections are treated systemically if there are indications of clinical infection such as sudden pain, cellulitis, and increased discharge; systemic management of bacterial skin infections is described on p.146.

Wound **dressings** and packing preparations help to protect the wound and provide the correct environment for wound healing. Some also help by absorbing exudate. Superficial wounds usually only require a low-adherent dressing. Alginates may be used for exuding wounds. Traditional dry dressings such as cotton wool, gauze, and lint are not used for partial or full thickness cavity wounds since they shed fibres, adhere to the wound, and cause wound dehydration. Hydrogels, hydrocolloids, polysaccharides, cadexomer-iodine, alginates, and foam dressings are all effective cavity wound preparations. Hyaluronic acid is incorporated into some dressings to promote wound healing.

Activated charcoal is very effective at reducing offensive odours from **malodorous wounds**, as are sugar (sucrose) pastes. Sucrose may exert its antibacterial effect by competing for water present in the cells of bacteria. Metronidazole is active against anaerobic bacteria that are associated with the pungent smell and is used topically for deodorising malodorous tumours. Metronidazole is not generally used on wounds because of the risk of inducing resistance but it is sometimes used to deodorise malodorous venous leg ulcers or decubitus ulcers.

In addition to the use of wound preparations, there may be other measures that aid healing of specific wounds or ulcers. Some wounds may require skin grafting. Skin substitutes, and growth factors, such as becaplermin, molgramostim, trafermin, and urogastrone, are being used or developed for non-healing ulcers and wounds. Topical phenytoin has produced some encouraging results in promoting the healing of various types of ulcers. Measures that aid the return of fluid from the leg, such as flexing the ankles, elevation, and use of compression bandages are beneficial in **venous ulcers**. The bioflavonoids, given orally, may improve venous insufficiency and therefore also aid healing. Systemic drugs that improve the supply of oxygen to tissues, for example pentoxifylline, may be useful in ischaemic and venous ulcers. Topical and systemic ketanserin has been investigated in a few patients and may be beneficial in wounds and ulcers where there is impaired blood flow. Vascular surgery may be necessary in the management of some ulcers caused by ischaemia. In **decubitus ulcers**, relief of pressure is the most important measure in management. The management of **burns** and **chemical burns** is described above.

General references.


1. Vohra RK, McCollum CN. Pressure sores. *BMJ* 1994; **309:** 853–7.
2. Douglas WS, Simpson NB. Guidelines for the management of chronic venous leg ulceration: report of a multidisciplinary workshop. *Br J Dermatol* 1995; **132:** 446–52.
3. Smith DM. Pressure ulcers in the nursing home. *Ann Intern Med* 1995; **123:** 433–42.
4. Cooke ED, Nicolaides AN. Management of leg ulcers. *Prescribers' J* 1997; **37:** 61–8.
5. Angle N, Bergan JJ. Chronic venous ulcer. *BMJ* 1997; **314:** 1019–23.
6. Warren K, Bennett G. Wound care. *Prescribers' J* 1998; **38:** 115–22.
7. Grey JE, Harding KG. The chronic non-healing wound: how to make it better. *Hosp Med* 1998; **59:** 557–63.
8. Orlando PL. Pressure ulcer management in the geriatric patient. *Ann Pharmacother* 1998; **32:** 1221–7.
9. Anonymous. Leg ulcers. In: Buxton PK, ed. *ABC of Dermatology.* 4th ed. London: BMJ Publishing Group, 2003: 43–6.
10. Thomas S, *et al.* Maggots are useful in treating infected or necrotic wounds. *BMJ* 1999; **318:** 807–8.
11. Singer AJ, Clark RAF. Cutaneous wound healing. *N Engl J Med* 1999; **341:** 738–46.
12. Morgan DA. Wound management products in the drug tariff. *Pharm J* 1999; **263:** 820–5.
13. London NJM, Donnelly R. ABC of arterial and venous disease: ulcerated lower limb. *BMJ* 2000; **320:** 1589–91.
14. Harding KG, *et al.* Healing chronic wounds. *BMJ* 2002; **324:** 160–3.
15. de Araujo T, *et al.* Managing the patient with venous ulcers. *Ann Intern Med* 2003; **138:** 326–34.


## Abrasive Agents

Abrasivos.

## Aluminium Oxide

Aluminii Oxidum; Óxido de aluminio.

$Al_2O_3$ = 102.0.
*CAS — 1344-28-1.*
*ATC — D10AX04.*

**Pharmacopoeias.** *Eur.* (see p.vi) includes the hydrated form.

**Ph. Eur. 5.0** (Aluminium Oxide, Hydrated). It contains the equivalent of 47 to 60% of $Al_2O_3$. A white, amorphous powder. Practically insoluble in water; it dissolves in dilute mineral acids and in solutions of alkali hydroxides. Store in airtight containers at a temperature below 30°.

## Pumice

Lapis Pumicis; Piedra pómez; Pierre Ponce Granulée; Pumex; Pumex Granulatus; Pumice Stone.

*CAS — 1332-09-8.*

**Pharmacopoeias.** In *US.*

**USP 27** (Pumice). Pumice is a substance of volcanic origin consisting chiefly of complex silicates of aluminium, potassium, and sodium. Odourless, very light, hard, rough, porous greyish masses or gritty, greyish powder. It is stable in air. Practically insoluble in water and not attacked by acids. Three grades of powdered pumice are recognised:

- superfine (=pumice flour)—not less than 97% passes through a No. 200 [US] sieve
- fine—not less than 95% passes through a No. 150 sieve and not more than 75% through a No. 200 sieve
- coarse—not less than 95% passes through a No. 60 sieve and not more than 5% through a No. 200 sieve

### Profile

Abrasive agents such as fused synthetic aluminium oxide or powdered pumice have been used either as adjuncts in the treatment of acne (despite doubts about their value—see p.1133) or for the removal of hard skin. Pumice has also been used as a dental abrasive and as a filtering medium. Other agents used as abrasives for acne include polyethylene granules.

### Preparations

**Proprietary Preparations** (details are given in Part 3)

***Arg.:*** Ionax Scrub; ***Austral.:*** Brasivol†; Ionax Scrub†; ***Braz.:*** Ionax Scrub; ***Canad.:*** Brasivol†; ***Chile:*** Ionax Scrub; ***Fr.:*** Brasivol; Ionax Scrub; ***Ger.:*** Brasivil†; ***Hong Kong:*** Brasivol; Ionax Scrub; ***Irl.:*** Brasivol; Ionax Scrub; ***Singapore:*** Ionax Scrub; ***Thai.:*** Ionax Scrub†; ***UK:*** Brasivol; Ionax Scrub†; ***USA:*** Ionax Scrub.

**Multi-ingredient:** ***Canad.:*** Pernox; ***Ital.:*** Gastrodue; Neo Zeta-Foot†; ***Malaysia:*** Belcid; ***Mex.:*** Dermobras; Ionax Scrub; ***S.Afr.:*** Magagel†; Pedimed; ***Switz.:*** Cliniderm; ***Thai.:*** Belcid; ***USA:*** Pernox; Zanfel.

## Acitretin *(BAN, USAN, rINN)*

Acitretina; Acitretinum; Etretin; Ro-10-1670; Ro-10-1670/000. *(all-trans)*-9-(4-Methoxy-2,3,6-trimethylphenyl)-3,7-dimethyl-2,4,6,8-nonatetraenoic acid; (2*E*,4*E*,6*E*,8*E*)-9-(4-Methoxy-2,3,6-trimethylphenyl)-3,7-dimethylnona-2,4,6,8-tetraenoic acid.

$C_{21}H_{26}O_3$ = 326.4.
*CAS — 55079-83-9.*
*ATC — D05BB02.*

**Pharmacopoeias.** In *Eur.* (see p.vi).

**Ph. Eur. 5.0** (Acitretin). A yellow or greenish-yellow, crystalline powder. Practically insoluble in water; slightly soluble in alcohol and in acetone; very slightly soluble in cyclohexane; sparingly soluble in tetrahydrofuran. It is sensitive to air, heat, and light, especially in solution. Store at 2° to 8° in airtight containers. Protect from light. It is recommended that the contents of an opened container be used as soon as possible and any unused part be protected by an atmosphere of inert gas.

### Adverse Effects and Precautions

As for Isotretinoin, p.1148.

Acitretin has a relatively short half-life, but etretinate, which has a much longer half-life, has been detected in the plasma of some patients receiving acitretin. Recommendations vary slightly in different countries but pregnancy should be avoided for at least 2 to 3 years after treatment has been withdrawn (see also under Pregnancy, below) and patients should not donate blood for at least 1 to 3 years after cessation of therapy. Female patients should avoid alcohol during treatment with acitretin and for 2 months after stopping treatment (see under Interactions, below).

**Breast feeding.** Acitretin was distributed into the breast milk of a women treated with oral acitretin for psoriasis. Although the estimated amount of acitretin that would be consumed by a breast-fed infant was only 1.5% of the maternal dose, the authors considered that the toxic potential of acitretin to the infant justified its avoidance. In this case, the infant was not breast-fed during acitretin therapy.[1] The manufacturers also recommend that breast-feeding women should not be given acitretin. The American Academy of Pediatrics, however, has found no mention of clinical effect on the infant, and considers the maternal use of acitretin to be usually compatible with breast feeding.[2]

1. Rollman O, Pihl-Lundin I. Acitretin excretion into human breast milk. *Acta Derm Venereol (Stockh)* 1990; **70:** 487–90.
2. American Academy of Pediatrics. The transfer of drugs and other chemicals into human milk. *Pediatrics* 2001; **108:** 776–89. Correction. *ibid.*; 1029. Also available at: http://aappolicy.aappublications.org/cgi/content/full/pediatrics%3b108/3/776 (accessed 16/06/04)

**Effects on the musculoskeletal system.** For reference to severe myopathy occurring during therapy with acitretin, see under Isotretinoin, p.1149.

**Effects on the skin.** For mention of the phototoxic potential of acitretin, see under Isotretinoin, p.1150.

**Pregnancy.** In the UK the manufacturers of acitretin recommend that pregnancy should be avoided for at least 2 years (3 years in the USA) after withdrawal of therapy since etretinate, which is teratogenic and has a much longer half-life than acitretin, has been detected in the plasma of some patients receiving acitretin. It has been pointed out that plasma-etretinate concentrations are a poor indication of total body stores; one study[1] has indicated that there may be substantial concentrations of etretinate in the fatty tissues of women who have received acitretin.

1. Sturkenboom MCJM, *et al.* Inability to detect plasma etretinate and acitretin is a poor predictor of the absence of these teratogens in tissue after stopping acitretin treatment. *Br J Clin Pharmacol* 1994; **38:** 229–35.

### Interactions

As for Isotretinoin, p.1150.

Etretinate has been detected in the plasma of some patients receiving acitretin and acitretin is also a metabolite of etretinate; therefore interactions associated with etretinate (see p.1147) may also apply to acitretin. Concurrent ingestion of acitretin and alcohol has been associated with etretinate formation.

For discussion of the potential interactions of retinoids with hormonal contraceptives, and the effect this might have on contraceptive choice during retinoid treatment, see p.1534.

### Pharmacokinetics

Acitretin is absorbed from the gastrointestinal tract and peak plasma concentrations have been obtained 1 to 6 hours after oral administration. Oral bioavailability may be increased by administration with food. Acitretin is highly bound to plasma proteins. It is metabolised to 13-*cis*-acitretin. Etretinate (p.1147) has also been detected in the plasma of some patients following administration of acitretin. The elimination half-life of acitretin is approximately 2 days but account should always be taken of the fact that the half-life of etretinate is much longer, being about 120 days. Acitretin is excreted in bile and urine, and is distributed into breast milk.

◊ General references.

1. Larsen FG, *et al.* Pharmacokinetics and therapeutic efficacy of retinoids in skin diseases. *Clin Pharmacokinet* 1992; **23:** 42–61.

**Renal impairment.** The pharmacokinetics of acitretin are reported to be altered in patients with chronic renal failure but neither acitretin nor its 13-*cis* metabolite are removed by haemodialysis.[1]

1. Stuck AE, *et al.* Pharmacokinetics of acitretin and its 13-cis metabolite in patients on haemodialysis. *Br J Clin Pharmacol* 1989; **27:** 301–4.

### Uses and Administration

Acitretin is a retinoid. It is a metabolite of etretinate (p.1147). Acitretin is used by mouth in the treatment of severe psoriasis resistant to other forms of therapy, palmo-plantar pustular psoriasis, and in severe congenital ichthyosis and Darier's disease (keratosis follicularis).

In the UK, it is given in an initial daily dose of 25 or 30 mg with food for 2 to 4 weeks; in the USA initial doses up to 50 mg daily are permitted. The daily dosage is adjusted thereafter according to clinical response and adverse effects; optimal results are usually obtained with 25 to 50 mg given daily for a further 6 to 8 weeks but some patients may require up to 75 mg daily. For the treatment of Darier's disease a starting dose of 10 mg may be appropriate, adjusted thereafter according to response. In Darier's disease and congenital ichthyosis treatment may be required for more than 3 months but a daily dosage of 50 mg should not be exceeded. In the UK, the manufacturer recommends that continuous treatment should not last longer than 6 months for any indication.

Acitretin is not generally considered suitable for use in children, but if deemed necessary a dose of 500 micrograms/kg daily or occasionally up to 1 mg/kg daily has been suggested, but the maximum daily dose should not exceed 35 mg.

**Administration in children.** Acitretin is not generally considered suitable for use in children. However, a review of its use in 29 children with severe inherited disorders of keratinisation[1] reported that acitretin is an effective and safe treatment in children provided that the minimal effective dose is used and that side-effects are carefully monitored.

1. Lacour M, *et al.* An appraisal of acitretin therapy in children with inherited disorders of keratinization. *Br J Dermatol* 1996; **134:** 1023–9.

**Eye disorders.** A case report indicated that acitretin, given for psoriasis at an initial dose of 30 mg/day for one month and then reduced to 20 mg/day, improved corneal opacities in a patient with chronic tuberculosis-related interstitial keratitis.[1]

1. Labetoulle M, *et al.* Rapid improvement of chronic interstitial keratitis with acitretin. *Br J Ophthalmol* 2002; **86:** 1445–6.

**Skin disorders.** Acitretin is used alone or with PUVA or UVB in psoriasis[1] (p.1137). Studies have shown that use with PUVA or UVB light may increase efficacy and allow a reduction in the exposure to radiation required. It is also used in keratinisation disorders such as severe forms of ichthyosis[2,3] (p.1136) and Darier's disease (keratosis follicularis)[4] (p.1134). Benefit has been reported in various other skin disorders.[5-15]

1. Gollnick HPM. Oral retinoids—efficacy and toxicity in psoriasis. *Br J Dermatol* 1996; **135** (suppl 49): 6–17.
2. Bruckner-Tuderman L, *et al.* Acitretin in the symptomatic therapy for severe recessive X-linked ichthyosis. *Arch Dermatol* 1988; **124:** 529–32.
3. Steijlen PM, *et al.* Acitretin in the treatment of lamellar ichthyosis. *Br J Dermatol* 1994; **130:** 211–14.
4. van Dooren-Greebe RJ, *et al.* Acitretin monotherapy in Darier's disease. *Br J Dermatol* 1989; **121:** 375–9.

5. Lassus A, Geiger J-M. Acitretin and etretinate in the treatment of palmoplantar pustulosis: a double-blind comparative trial. *Br J Dermatol* 1988; **119:** 755–9.
6. Ruzicka T, *et al.* Efficiency of acitretin in the treatment of cutaneous lupus erythematosus. *Arch Dermatol* 1988; **124:** 897–902.
7. Laurberg G, *et al.* Treatment of lichen planus with acitretin: a double-blind, placebo-controlled study in 65 patients. *J Am Acad Dermatol* 1991; **24:** 434–7.
8. Ruzicka T, *et al.* Treatment of cutaneous lupus erythematosus with acitretin and hydroxychloroquine. *Br J Dermatol* 1992; **127:** 513–18.
9. Lucker GPH, *et al.* Treatment of palmoplantar lichen nitidus with acitretin. *Br J Dermatol* 1994; **130:** 791–3.
10. Yuan Z-f, *et al.* Use of acitretin for the skin complications in renal transplant recipients. *N Z Med J* 1995; **108:** 255–6.
11. McKenna DB, Murphy GM. Skin cancer chemoprophylaxis in renal transplant recipients: 5 years of experience using low-dose acitretin. *Br J Dermatol* 1999; **140:** 656–60.
12. Kirby B, Watson R. Pityriasis rubra pilaris treated with acitretin and narrow-band ultraviolet B (Re-TL-01). *Br J Dermatol* 2000; **142:** 376–7.
13. Herbst RA, *et al.* Combined ultraviolet A1 radiation and acitretin therapy as a treatment option for pityriasis rubra pilaris. *Br J Dermatol* 2000; **142:** 574–5.
14. Avermaete A, *et al.* Keratosis lichenoides chronica: characteristics and response to acitretin. *Br J Dermatol* 2001; **144:** 422–4.
15. Ruiz-Genao DP, *et al.* A case of IgA pemphigus successfully treated with acitretin. *Br J Dermatol* 2002; **147:** 1040–2.

### Preparations

**Proprietary Preparations** (details are given in Part 3)
***Arg.:*** Neotigason; ***Austral.:*** Neotigason; ***Austria:*** Neotigason; ***Belg.:*** Neotigason; ***Braz.:*** Neotigason; ***Canad.:*** Soriatane; ***Chile:*** Neotigason; ***Denm.:*** Neotigason; ***Fin.:*** Neotigason; ***Fr.:*** Soriatane; ***Ger.:*** Neotigason; ***Gr.:*** Neotigason; ***Hong Kong:*** Neotigason; ***Irl.:*** Neotigason; ***Israel:*** Neotigason; ***Ital.:*** Neotigason; ***Mex.:*** Neotigason; ***Neth.:*** Neotigason; ***Norw.:*** Neotigason; ***NZ:*** Neotigason; ***Port.:*** Neotigason; ***S.Afr.:*** Neotigason; ***Singapore:*** Neotigason; ***Spain:*** Neotigason; ***Swed.:*** Neotigason; ***Switz.:*** Neotigason; ***Thai.:*** Neotigason; ***UK:*** Neotigason; ***USA:*** Soriatane.

## Adapalene *(BAN, USAN, rINN)*

Adapaleno; CD-271. 6-[3-(1-Adamantyl)-4-methoxyphenyl]-2-naphthoic acid.

$C_{28}H_{28}O_3$ = 412.5.
*CAS — 106685-40-9.*
*ATC — D10AD03.*

### Adverse Effects

Adapalene is a skin irritant. Topical application may cause transitory stinging and a feeling of warmth at the site of application.

### Precautions

As for Tretinoin, p.1161.

**Pregnancy.** Anophthalmia and agenesis of the optic chiasma were found in a fetus following termination of pregnancy in a woman who had applied adapalene 0.1% topically for the month before pregnancy until 13 weeks' gestation.[1]

1. Autret E, *et al.* Anophthalmia and agenesis of optic chiasma associated with adapalene gel in early pregnancy. *Lancet* 1997; **350:** 339.

### Uses and Administration

Adapalene is a naphthoic acid derivative and retinoid analogue with actions similar to those of tretinoin (p.1161). Adapalene is used in topical treatment of mild to moderate acne (p.1133) where comedones, papules, and pustules predominate.

Adapalene is applied once daily at night as a 0.1% solution, cream, or gel to skin that has been cleansed and dried. Some patients may require less frequent applications. Other topical preparations that may cause irritation should not be used concurrently. If treatment with topical antibacterials or benzoyl peroxide is required, these should be applied with an interval of 12 hours between application of adapalene.

There may be apparent exacerbations of the acne during early treatment and a therapeutic response may not be evident for 8 to 12 weeks.

◊ References.

1. Brogden RN, Goa KL. Adapalene: a review of its pharmacological properties and clinical potential in the management of mild to moderate acne. *Drugs* 1997; **53:** 511–19.

### Preparations

**Proprietary Preparations** (details are given in Part 3)
***Arg.:*** Differin; ***Austral.:*** Differin; ***Austria:*** Differin; ***Belg.:*** Differin; ***Braz.:*** Differin; ***Canad.:*** Differin; ***Chile:*** Differin; ***Denm.:*** Redap; ***Fin.:*** Differin; ***Fr.:*** Differine; ***Ger.:*** Differin; ***Gr.:*** Adaferin; ***Hong Kong:*** Differin; ***India:*** Adaferin; ***Irl.:*** Differin; ***Israel:*** Adaferin; ***Ital.:*** Differin; ***Malaysia:*** Differin; ***Mex.:*** Adaferin; ***Norw.:*** Differin; ***NZ:*** Differin; ***Port.:*** Differin; ***S.Afr.:*** Differin; ***Singapore:*** Differin; ***Spain:*** Differine; ***Swed.:*** Differin; ***Switz.:*** Differin; ***Thai.:*** Differin; ***UK:*** Differin; ***USA:*** Differin.

## Alcloxa *(USAN, rINN)*

ALCA; Aluminium Chlorhydroxyallantoinate; RC-173. Chlorotetrahydroxy[(2-hydroxy-5-oxo-2-imidazolin-4-yl)ureato]dialuminium.

$C_4H_9Al_2ClN_4O_7$ = 314.6.
*CAS — 1317-25-5.*

### Profile

Alcloxa is an astringent and keratolytic related to allantoin (below). It is present in multi-ingredient preparations intended for various skin and gastrointestinal disorders.

### Preparations

**Proprietary Preparations** (details are given in Part 3)
***Arg.:*** Babysan.

**Multi-ingredient:** ***Fr.:*** Ulfon†; ***Ital.:*** Aseptil†; ***Malaysia:*** Neo-Medrol; ***NZ:*** Acnederm; ***Singapore:*** Neo-Medrol; ***Thai.:*** Neo-Medrol; ***UK:*** Dermidex.

## Aldioxa *(USAN, rINN)*

ALDA; Aluminium Dihydroxyallantoinate; Dihydroxyaluminum Allantoinate; RC-172. Dihydroxy[(2-hydroxy-5-oxo-2-imidazolin-4-yl)ureato]aluminium.

$C_4H_7AlN_4O_5$ = 218.1.
*CAS — 5579-81-7.*

**Pharmacopoeias.** In *Jpn.*

### Profile

Aldioxa is an astringent and keratolytic related to allantoin (below). It is present in multi-ingredient preparations intended for various skin and gastrointestinal disorders.

### Preparations

**Proprietary Preparations** (details are given in Part 3)

**Multi-ingredient:** ***Arg.:*** ZeaSorb; ***Austral.:*** ZeaSorb; ***Canad.:*** ZeaSorb; ***Chile:*** ZeaSorb; ***Fr.:*** Ulfon†; ZeaSorb; ***Ger.:*** ZeaSorb†; ***Irl.:*** ZeaSorb; ***Israel:*** Aronal Forte; ***Ital.:*** Rikospray; ***Malaysia:*** ZeaSorb; ***Mex.:*** Dentsiblen; ***Singapore:*** ZeaSorb; ***Thai.:*** ZeaSorb; ***UK:*** Cetanorm; ZeaSorb.

## Alefacept *(BAN, USAN, rINN)*

BG-9273; BG-9712; LFA3TIP; Recombinant Human LFA-3/$IgG_1$ Fusion Protein. A dimer of 1-92 antigen LFA-3 (human) fusion protein with human immunoglobulin G1 (hinge-$C_H2$-$C_H3$ γ1-chain).

*CAS — 222535-22-0.*
*ATC — L04AA15.*

### Adverse Effects and Precautions

Chills are common on intravenous administration. Other adverse effects are cough, dizziness, injection site pain and inflammation, myalgia, nausea, pharyngitis, and pruritus. More serious adverse reactions are cardiovascular events (including coronary artery disorder and myocardial infarction), hypersensitivity reactions, lymphopenia, and serious infections requiring hospitalisation. Like other drugs with immunosuppressant actions, alefacept may increase the risk of malignancies, particularly basal or squamous cell cancers of the skin. It should not be given to patients with a history of malignancy.

Alefacept should also not be given to patients with pre-existing serious infections, and should be discontinued if these develop. Its use should be considered carefully in patients with a history of infection.

Alefacept induces a dose-dependent reduction in circulating CD4+ and CD8+ T-lymphocyte counts. CD4+ T-lymphocyte counts should be monitored before starting therapy and then weekly during the 12-week treatment period. Treatment should not be started in patients with a CD4+ T-lymphocyte count below normal, doses should be withheld if the counts are below 250 cells/microlitre and treatment stopped if the counts remain below this level for one month.

Therapy should be stopped immediately, and appropriate treatment given, in patients who experience anaphylaxis or serious hypersensitivity; it should not be restarted.

### Uses and Administration

Alefacept is a recombinant human fusion protein that binds to CD2 on memory T-lymphocytes, preventing their activation and reducing their number. It used in the management of moderate to severe chronic plaque psoriasis (p.1137) and is given in a dose of 7.5 mg once weekly by intravenous injection, or 15 mg once weekly by intramuscular injection, for 12 weeks. A second 12-week course may be given if necessary, starting not less than 12 weeks after the completion of the first.

◊ General references.

1. Ellis CN, Krueger GG. Treatment of chronic plaque psoriasis by selective targeting of memory effector T lymphocytes. *N Engl J Med* 2001; **345:** 248–55.
2. Krueger GG, *et al.* A randomized, double-blind, placebo-controlled phase III study evaluating efficacy and tolerability of 2 courses of alefacept in patients with chronic plaque psoriasis. *J Am Acad Dermatol* 2002; **47:** 821–33.
3. Krueger GG, Ellis CN. Alefacept therapy produces remission for patients with chronic plaque psoriasis. *Br J Dermatol* 2003; **148:** 784–8.
4. Lebwohl M, *et al.* An international, randomized, double-blind, placebo-controlled phase 3 trial of intramuscular alefacept in patients with chronic plaque psoriasis. *Arch Dermatol* 2003; **139:** 719–27.

### Preparations

**Proprietary Preparations** (details are given in Part 3)
***USA:*** Amevive.

## Allantoin *(BAN, USAN)*

Alantoína; Glyoxyldiureide. 5-Ureidohydantoin; 5-Ureidoimidazolidine-2,4-dione; 2,5-Dioxoimidazolidin-4-ylurea.

$C_4H_6N_4O_3$ = 158.1.
*CAS — 97-59-6.*

**Pharmacopoeias.** In *Eur.* (see p.vi) and *US.*

**Ph. Eur. 5.0** (Allantoin). A white crystalline powder. Slightly soluble in water; very slightly soluble in alcohol.

**USP 27** (Allantoin). A white crystalline powder. Slightly soluble in water; very slightly soluble in alcohol.

### Profile

Allantoin is an astringent and keratolytic. It is present in multi-ingredient preparations intended for various skin disorders and is also used for its astringent properties in preparations for the treatment of haemorrhoids and other anorectal disorders.

**Psoriasis.** In the USA the FDA decided that allantoin should be removed from lotions indicated for psoriasis as it was considered to be ineffective.[1]

1. Anonymous. Nonprescription drug review gains momentum. *WHO Drug Inf* 1991; **5:** 62.

### Preparations

**Proprietary Preparations** (details are given in Part 3)
***Canad.:*** Soothex; ***India:*** Masse Cream.

**Multi-ingredient:** ***Arg.:*** Afonisan; Atomoderma A-E; Bushi; Contractubex; Cremsor N; Esmedent con Fluor; Lactocrem Bebe; Medic; Mencogrin; Mencogrin AP; Pastillas Lorbi; Pastillas Medex; Quem Plus; Sorsis; ***Austral.:*** Acne & Pimple Gel; Alphosyl; Blistex Medicated Lip Ointment†; ER Cream; Hemocane; Macro Natural Vitamin E Cream; Medi Creme†; Medi Pulv†; Paxyl; SoloSite; Solyptol; VR; ***Austria:*** Alphosyl; Contractubex; Rheumex; Sunsan-Heillotion; Ulcurilen; ***Belg.:*** Alphosyl†; ***Braz.:*** Babyglos†; Gargotrat†; Lactrex; Nixoderm†; Senol; Tratoderm†; Vitaderme†; ***Canad.:*** Actinac†; Alphosyl†; Blistex Lip Ointment; Bye Bye Burn†; Le Stick a Levres; Phenoris; Tanac; ***Chile:*** Dermaglos; Dermaglos Plus; Lactrex; Pancrit; Sanoderm; ***Fin.:*** Alphosyl†; ***Fr.:*** Alpha 5 DS; Alphosyl; Aveenoderm†; Cicatryl; Genola†; Hydracuivre; Provictol; ***Ger.:*** Brand- und Wund-Gel Eu Rho; Contractubex; Ellsurex; Essaven Tri-Complex; Haemo-Exhirud; Hydro Cordes; Leukona-Wundsalbe; Lipo Cordes; Magopsor†; Poloris†; Psoriasis-Salbe M†; Psoriasis-Salbe S; Retterspitz Gelee†; Retterspitz Heilsalbe†; Ulcurilen N; Wund- und Brand-Gel Eu Rho†; ***Hong Kong:*** Blistex Lip Ointment; Burn Cream; Contractubex; Egoderm; Medicreme; Medipulv; Pyodontyl; ***India:*** New Eye Lotion; Shield; ***Irl.:*** Actinac†; Alphosyl; Alphosyl HC; ***Israel:*** Alphosyl; Alphosyl HC; Comfrey Plus; Pitrisan; Proctozorin-N; Rekasitin; ***Ital.:*** Afloginet†; Alphosyle; Angstrom Viso; Balta-Crin Tar; Centella Complex; Cerox; Ginoxil Ecoschiuma; Herbatar Plus†; Herbatar†; Keraflex; Orostick†; Sensigel; Sensiquell; Xerial; ***Malaysia:*** Egoderm; ***Mex.:*** Antaderm; Dealan; Glossderm; Hipoglos Plus; Sebryl; Sebryl Plus; ***NZ:*** Egoderm; Egopsoryl TA; Medipulv; ***Port.:*** Alphosyl HC†; Alphosyl†; Aveenocream†; Aveenoderm†; Hidratoderme; Tegrin†; ***S.Afr.:*** Alphosyl; Arola Rosebalm; Masse†; ***Singapore:*** Egoderm; ***Spain:*** Alantomicina Complex†; Alphosyl; Amplidermis; Antigrietun; Balneogel†; Cortenema; Egarone; Hepro; Polaramine Topico; ***Swed.:*** Alphosyl; ***Switz.:*** Alphastria; Alphosyl; Alumagall; Contractubex; Dolorex Neo†; Gorgonium; Hepathrombine; Kelimed; Leniderm; Lyman; Optrex compresses; Sportium; Teerol-H†; Unatol; ***Thai.:*** Opplin; ***UK:*** Actinac; Alphosyl HC; Alphosyl†; Anodesyn; Modantis†; Sunspot†; Vesagex Heelbalm; ***USA:*** Alasulf; Blistex; Blistex Lip Balm; Deltavac; DIT1-2; Dr Dermi-Heal; Herpecin-L; Ionax Astringent; Orabase Lip; Tanac; Tanac Dual Core.

## Aloe Vera

Áloe.

### Profile

Aloe vera gel is a mucilaginous preparation obtained from the leaves of *Aloe vera* (=*A. barbadensis*). It does not include the sap of *Aloe vera,* which contains anthraquinones, and should not be confused with aloes (p.1248).

◊ Aloe vera is widely used in cosmetics and toiletries for a reported moisturising and revitalising action. There are also claims for the beneficial and even curative properties of aloe vera gel in the treatment of conditions such as acne, psoriasis, burns, wounds, arthritis, diabetes, hyperlipidaemia, peptic ulcer, and genital herpes.[1,2] Evidence to support these claims is lacking.

1. Marshall JM. Aloe vera gel: what is the evidence? *Pharm J* 1990; **244:** 360–2.
2. Vogler BK, Ernst E. Aloe vera: a systematic review of its clinical effectiveness. *Br J Gen Pract* 1999; **49:** 823–8.

### Preparations

**Proprietary Preparations** (details are given in Part 3)
***Arg.:*** Capson; ***Braz.:*** Probeks; ***Fr.:*** Veraskin; ***Ital.:*** Epitaloe; ***NZ:*** Solarcaine Aloe Vera; ***UK:*** Forehead-C†.

**Multi-ingredient:** ***Arg.:*** Acuaderm; Aloebel; Aristaloe; Brunavera; Eurocolor Post Solar; Europrotec Post Solar; Herbaccion Nutriderm; KW; Mucobase; Negacne; Pedicrem; Puraloe; Sadeltan F; Talowin; Yuyo; ***Austral.:*** Aloe Vera Plus†; Psor-Asist; Rapaid Rash-Relief; ***Braz.:*** Derm'attive Solaire; ***Chile:*** Ac-Sal; Solarcaine Aloe Vera Gel; ***Fr.:*** Alra; Rhinodoron; ***Ital.:*** Capso; Ektrofil; Ginoxil Ecoschiuma; Vulnopur; ***Malaysia:*** Boots Antenatal Massage Cream; Neo-Healar; ***NZ:*** Chap Stick; Odor Eze; ***Port.:*** Alkagin; Antiacneicos Ac-Sal; Disoderme†; Equilibrium Creme

Anti-transpirante†; Multi-Mam Compressas; **Singapore:** Cortaid with Aloe; Desitin Creamy; **UK:** Solarcaine†; **USA:** Aloe Grande; Dermtex HC with Aloe; Entertainer's Secret; Hawaiian Tropic Cool Aloe with I.C.E.; Hemorid For Women; Maximum Strength Flexall 454; Nasal-Ease; Solarcaine Aloe Extra Burn Relief.

## Aluminium Chloride

Aluminii Chloridum Hexahydricum; Aluminio, cloruro de; Aluminium Chloratum; Aluminum Chloride; Cloreto de Aluminio; Cloruro de Aluminio. Aluminium chloride hexahydrate.

$AlCl_3,6H_2O$ = 241.4.

*CAS — 7446-70-0 (anhydrous aluminium chloride); 7784-13-6 (aluminium chloride hexahydrate).*

*ATC — D10AX01.*

**Pharmacopoeias.** In *Eur.* (see p.vi) and *US.*

**Ph. Eur. 5.0** (Aluminium Chloride Hexahydrate). A deliquescent, white or slightly yellow, crystalline powder or colourless crystals. Very soluble in water; freely soluble in alcohol; soluble in glycerol. Store in airtight containers.

**USP 27** (Aluminium Chloride). Deliquescent, white or yellowish-white, practically odourless, crystalline powder. Its solutions are acid to litmus. Soluble 1 in 0.9 of water and 1 in 4 alcohol; soluble in glycerol. Store in airtight containers.

### Adverse Effects

Aluminium chloride may cause irritation especially if applied to damp skin; this is attributed to the formation of hydrochloric acid.

### Uses and Administration

Aluminium chloride has astringent properties and is used in a 20% alcoholic solution as an antiperspirant in the treatment of hyperhidrosis (p.1136). It is applied to dry skin usually at bedtime and is washed off in the morning before the sweat glands are fully active.

◊ References.

1. Scholes KT, *et al.* Axillary hyperhidrosis treated with alcoholic solution of aluminium chloride hexahydrate. *BMJ* 1978; **2:** 84–5.

### Preparations

***BP 2003:*** Aluminium Chloride Solution.

**Proprietary Preparations** (details are given in Part 3)
**Arg.:** Alumpak; Anhidrot; **Austral.:** Driclor; Odaban; **Chile:** Drysol; **Fr.:** Driclor; **Ger.:** Alubron-Saar†; Gargarisma zum Gurgeln; Mallebrin Konzentrat; **Hong Kong:** Driclor; **Irl.:** Anhydrol Forte; Driclor; **Israel:** Anhydrol Forte; **Malaysia:** Driclor; **Mex.:** Prespir; **NZ:** Hidrosol; **Port.:** Anidrosan†; **Singapore:** Driclor; **Switz.:** Etiaxil; Racestyptine; **UK:** Anhydrol Forte; Driclor; Odaban; **USA:** Drysol.

**Multi-ingredient: Arg.:** Carnot Topico; **Austria:** Racestyptin†; **Chile:** Hidrofugal; Hidrofugal Forte; Xerac AC; **Switz.:** Racestyptine†; **USA:** Stypto-Caine; Xerac AC.

## Aluminium Chlorohydrate

Aluminio, clorohidróxido de; Aluminium Chlorhydrate; Aluminium Chloride Hydroxide Hydrate; Aluminum Chlorhydroxide; Aluminum Chloride Hydroxide Hydrate; Aluminum Chlorohydrate *(USAN)*; Aluminum Hydroxychloride; Basic Aluminium Chloride.

$Al_2(OH)_5Cl,xH_2O$.

*CAS — 1327-41-9 (anhydrous aluminium chlorohydrate).*

*ATC — D09AA08; M05BX02.*

**Pharmacopoeias.** In *US.*

*US* also includes a range of compounds based on aluminium chlorohydrate. These are:

- aluminium dichlorohydrate and sesquichlorohydrate
- the polyethylene glycol (macrogol) complexes and propylene glycol complexes of aluminium chlorohydrex, aluminium dichlorohydrex, and aluminium sesquichlorohydrex
- the tri-, tetra-, penta-, and octachlorohydrates of aluminium zirconium and their respective glycine derivatives.

**USP 27** (Aluminum Chlorohydrate). A 15% w/w solution in water has a pH of 3.0 to 5.0

### Profile

Aluminium chlorohydrate is used similarly to aluminium chloride in hyperhidrosis (p.1136). Single-ingredient products for hyperhidrosis generally have a concentration in the range of 10 to 25%.

Aluminium chlorohydrate is also included in a variety of dermatological preparations for its astringent and antiperspirant properties.

### Preparations

***USP 27:*** Aluminum Chlorohydrate Solution; Aluminum Dichlorohydrate Solution; Aluminum Sesquichlorohydrate Solution; Aluminum Zirconium Octachlorohydrex Gly Solution; Aluminum Zirconium Pentachlorohydrate Solution; Aluminum Zirconium Pentachlorohydrex Gly Solution; Aluminum Zirconium Tetrachlorohydrate Solution; Aluminum Zirconium Tetrachlorohydrex Gly Solution; Aluminum Zirconium Trichlorohydrate Solution; Aluminum Zirconium Trichlorohydrex Gly Solution.

**Proprietary Preparations** (details are given in Part 3)
**Arg.:** Bromhistop; Daewo; Normoskin; Sodorant; **Canad.:** Roll-On; Scholl Dry Antiperspirant Foot Spray; **Chile:** Hansaplast Footcare; Hidrofugal; **Fr.:** pM; Spirial; **Ger.:** Phosphonorm; Primamed†; **Israel:** Aloxan Derma; **Ital.:** Spirial; **Mex.:** Drysol; Skin Dry; **Mon.:** Dermagor; **NZ:** Neat Effect; Neat Feat; Neat One; Neat Touch; **Port.:** Dermagor-Antitranspirante; Lambda; **Switz.:** Alopon; Gelsica; Phosphonorm; Sansudor; **UK:** Chiron Barrier Cream; **USA:** Bromi-Lotion.

**Multi-ingredient: Arg.:** Neobitiol Compuesto; Sodorant; Ublosid; **Austral.:** Nappy-Mate†; Neo-Medrol; **Austria:** Sulgan 99; **Canad.:** Athletes Foot Antifungal†; Medrol Acne Lotion; Neo-Medrol Acne; **Chile:** Hidrofugal; Hidrofugal Forte; Lady Fittig; **Fin.:** Neo-Medrol comp; **Ger.:** Ansudor; Epipak; **Hong Kong:** Neo-Medrol Acne; **Irl.:** Neo-Medrone†; **Israel:** Fungimon; Neo-Medrol; Pedisol; **Ital.:** Medrol Lozione Antiacne; **Port.:** Equilibrium Creme Anti-transpirante†; **S.Afr.:** Neo-Medrol; **Spain:** Hongosan; Moderin Acne; **USA:** Ostiderm; Pedi-Pro.

## Amiloxate *(USAN, rINN)*

Amiloxato; E-1000; Isoamyl *p*-Methoxycinnamate. Isopentyl *p*-methoxycinnamate.

$C_{15}H_{20}O_3$ = 248.3.

*CAS — 71617-10-2.*

**Pharmacopoeias.** In *US.*

**USP 27** (Amiloxate). Store in airtight containers.

### Profile

Amiloxate, a substituted cinnamate, is a sunscreen (see p.1133) with actions similar to those of octinoxate (p.1154).

### Preparations

**Proprietary Preparations**
Some preparations are listed in Part 3.

## Aminobenzoic Acid

Acidum 4-Aminobenzoicum; Amben; Aminobenzoico, ácido; PAB; PABA; Pabacidum; Para-aminobenzoic Acid; Vitamin H′. 4-Aminobenzoic acid.

$C_7H_7NO_2$ = 137.1.

*CAS — 150-13-0.*

*ATC — D02BA01.*

**Pharmacopoeias.** In *Eur.* (see p.vi) and *US.*

**Ph. Eur. 5.0** (4-Aminobenzoic Acid; Aminobenzoic Acid BP 2003). White or slightly yellow crystalline powder. Slightly soluble in water; freely soluble in alcohol; it dissolves in dilute solutions of alkali hydroxides. Protect from light.

**USP 27** (Aminobenzoic Acid). White or slightly yellow, odourless crystals or crystalline powder. It discolours on exposure to air or light. Slightly soluble in water and in chloroform; freely soluble in alcohol and in solutions of alkali hydroxides or carbonates; sparingly soluble in ether. Store in airtight containers. Protect from light.

### Adverse Effects

Contact and photocontact allergic dermatitis has been reported after the topical use of aminobenzoate sunscreens.

◊ Adverse skin reactions have been reported following the topical use[1-6] of aminobenzoic acid or its esters. Skin reactions (vitiligo) have also been reported following the oral administration of aminobenzoic acid[7] and the adverse effects associated with the former use of high oral doses for various conditions have been highlighted.[8]

1. Parrish JA, *et al.* Facial irritation due to sunscreen products. *Arch Dermatol* 1975; **111:** 525.
2. Mathias CGT, *et al.* Allergic contact photodermatitis to para-aminobenzoic acid. *Arch Dermatol* 1978; **114:** 1665–6.
3. Horio T, Higuchi T. Photocontact dermatitis from p-aminobenzoic acid. *Dermatologica* 1978; **156:** 124–8.
4. Marmelzat J, Rapaport MJ. Photodermatitis with PABA. *Contact Dermatitis* 1980; **6:** 230–1.
5. Thune P. Contact and photocontact allergy to sunscreens. *Photodermatology* 1984; **1:** 5–9.
6. English JSC, *et al.* Sensitivity to sunscreens. *Contact Dermatitis* 1987; **17:** 159–62.
7. Hughes CG. Oral PABA and vitiligo. *J Am Acad Dermatol* 1983; **9:** 770.
8. Worobec S, LaChine A. Dangers of orally administered para-aminobenzoic acid. *JAMA* 1984; **251:** 2348.

### Precautions

Aminobenzoate sunscreens should not be used by those with a history of photosensitivity or hypersensitivity reactions to chemically related drugs such as sulfonamides, thiazide diuretics, and certain local anaesthetics, particularly benzocaine.

Aminobenzoic acid may stain clothing.

### Pharmacokinetics

If given by mouth, aminobenzoic acid is absorbed from the gastrointestinal tract. It is metabolised in the liver and excreted in the urine as unchanged drug and metabolites.

### Uses and Administration

Aminobenzoic acid is used by topical application as a sunscreen (see p.1133). Aminobenzoic acid and its derivatives effectively absorb light throughout the UVB range but absorb little or no UVA light (for definitions, see p.1136). Aminobenzoate sunscreens may therefore be used to prevent sunburn, but are unlikely to prevent drug-related or other photosensitivity reactions associated with UVA light; combination with a benzophenone may give some added protection against such photosensitivity.

Aminobenzoic acid has sometimes been included as a member of the vitamin-B group, but deficiency of aminobenzoic acid in man or animals has not been demonstrated.

Aminobenzoic acid has been used with bentiromide (p.1659) in the PABA or BTPABA test of pancreatic function.

### Preparations

***USP 27:*** Aminobenzoic Acid Gel; Aminobenzoic Acid Topical Solution.

**Proprietary Preparations**
Some preparations are listed in Part 3.

## Ammonium Lactate *(USAN)*

BMS-186091; Lactato de amonio.

$C_3H_9NO_3$ = 107.1.

*CAS — 52003-58-4.*

### Profile

Ammonium lactate is a humectant applied as a cream or lotion containing 12% lactic acid neutralised with ammonium hydroxide. It is used in the treatment of dry scaly conditions of the skin including ichthyosis.

### Preparations

**Proprietary Preparations** (details are given in Part 3)
**Arg.:** Lactrex; **Braz.:** Lac-Hydrin; **Canad.:** Lac-Hydrin; **Chile:** Kerapil; Topilact 12; **Fr.:** Kerapil; Lactagel†; **Ital.:** Keratotal†; **Mex.:** Lac-Hydrin†; **NZ:** Lac-Hydrin; Lanate; **USA:** Amlactin; Lac-Hydrin; LAC-Lotion.

**Multi-ingredient: Arg.:** Clobeplus; Clobesol LA; Lactiderm; Lactiderm HC; Lacto-Cev Zn; Urecrem Hidro; **Chile:** Ichtyosoft; Kpl; Lactrex; **Fr.:** Ichtyosoft; Keralac Plus; Keraliss 14†; Lactar†; Zeniac; Zeniac LP; Zeniac LP Fort; **Ital.:** Alfa Acid; Herbatar Plus†; **Port.:** Lactonico.

## Avobenzone *(USAN, rINN)*

Avobenzona; Butylmethoxydibenzoylmethane; 4-*tert*-Butyl-4′-methoxydibenzoylmethane; Parsol 1789. 1-(*p*-*tert*-Butylphenyl)-3-(*p*-methoxyphenyl)-1,3-propanedione; 1-[4-(1,1-dimethylethyl)phenyl]-3-(4-methoxyphenyl)-1,3-propanedione.

$C_{20}H_{22}O_3$ = 310.4.

*CAS — 70356-09-1.*

**Pharmacopoeias.** In *US.*

**USP 27** (Avobenzone). M.p. 81° to 86°. Store in airtight containers. Protect from light.

### Profile

Avobenzone is a substituted dibenzoylmethane used by topical application as a sunscreen (see p.1133). Dibenzoylmethanes absorb light in the UVA range (for definitions, see p.1136) and may therefore be used with other sunscreens that absorb UVB light to prevent sunburn; they will also provide some protection against drug-related or other photosensitivity reactions associated with UVA light.

Contact and photocontact allergic dermatitis has occasionally been reported following the topical use of dibenzoylmethane sunscreens.

### Preparations

**Proprietary Preparations**
Numerous preparations are listed in Part 3.

## Azelaic Acid *(USAN, rINN)*

Ácido azelaico; Anchoic acid; Lepargylic acid; ZK-62498. Nonanedioic acid; Heptane-1,7-dicarboxylic acid.

$C_9H_{16}O_4$ = 188.2.

*CAS — 123-99-9.*

*ATC — D10AX03.*

### Adverse Effects and Precautions

Topical application of azelaic acid may produce a transient skin irritation that disappears on continued treatment. In a few patients the irritation may persist, requiring reduced frequency of application or temporary suspension of treatment. There have been rare reports of hypopigmentation and photosensitivity. Azelaic acid should not be applied to the eyes, mouth, or other mucous membranes.

### Uses and Administration

Azelaic acid inhibits the growth of *Propionibacterium* spp. and reduces keratinisation. It is used in the topical treatment of mild to moderate inflammatory acne (p.1133) and for the inflammatory papules and pustules of mild to moderate rosacea (p.1138). It has also been tried in hyperpigmentary skin disorders such as melasma, and in malignant melanoma.

In the treatment of **acne** azelaic acid is applied twice daily for up to 6 months as a 20% cream. Improvement usually occurs within four weeks.

For the treatment of mild to moderate **rosacea**, a 15% gel should be applied to the affected area twice daily for a period of up to 12 weeks.

◊ References.


1. Fitton A, Goa KL. Azelaic acid: a review of its pharmacological properties and therapeutic efficacy in acne and hyperpigmentary skin disorders. *Drugs* 1991; **41:** 780–98.
2. Breathnach AS. Melanin hyperpigmentation of skin: melasma, topical treatment with azelaic acid, and other therapies. *Cutis* 1996; **57** (suppl): 36–45.
3. Thiboutot D, *et al.* Efficacy and safety of azelaic acid (15%) gel as a new treatment for papulopustular rosacea: results from two vehicle-controlled, randomized phase III studies. *J Am Acad Dermatol* 2003; **48:** 836–45.
4. Elewski BE, *et al.* A comparison of 15% azelaic acid gel and 0.75% metronidazole gel in the topical treatment of papulopustular rosacea: results of a randomized trial. *Arch Dermatol* 2003; **139:** 1444–50.


## Preparations

**Proprietary Preparations** (details are given in Part 3)
***Arg.:*** Cutacelan; ***Austral.:*** Skinoren; ***Austria:*** Skinoren; ***Belg.:*** Skinoren; ***Braz.:*** Azelan; Dermizan; ***Denm.:*** Skinoren; ***Fin.:*** Skinoren; ***Fr.:*** Skinoren†; ***Ger.:*** Skinoren; ***Gr.:*** Alenzantyl; Azelderm; Cevigen; Exazen; Forcilen; Kenedril; Noreskin; Opilet; Prevolac; Skinoren; Sonalent; Zelicrema; ***Hong Kong:*** Skinoren; ***Israel:*** Skinoderm; ***Ital.:*** Acnezaic; Azelcream†; Neocutis; Skinoren; ***Malaysia:*** Skinoren; ***Mex.:*** Cutacelan; ***Norw.:*** Skinoren; ***NZ:*** Skinoren; ***Port.:*** Skinoren; ***S.Afr.:*** Skinoren; ***Singapore:*** Skinoren; ***Spain:*** Skinoren; Zeliderm; ***Swed.:*** Skinoren; ***Switz.:*** Skinoren; ***Thai.:*** Skinoren; ***UK:*** Skinoren; ***USA:*** Azelex; Finacea; Finevin.

**Multi-ingredient: *Ital.:*** Zeroac; ***NZ:*** Acnederm.

---

## Becaplermin *(BAN, USAN, rINN)*

Becaplermina; RWJ-60235. Recombinant human platelet-derived growth factor B.

*CAS — 165101-51-9.*
*ATC — D03AX06.*

### Profile

Becaplermin is a platelet-derived growth factor that enhances the formation of granulation tissue and promotes wound healing (p.1139). Becaplermin is applied topically as a 0.01% gel in the management of neuropathic diabetic skin ulcers (see Diabetic Complications, p.326). It is applied once daily, covered by a moist saline gauze dressing, for up to 20 weeks.

◊ References.


1. Anonymous. Platelet-derived growth factor for diabetic ulcers. *Med Lett Drugs Ther* 1998; **40:** 73–4.
2. Wieman TJ, *et al.* Efficacy and safety of a topical gel formulation of recombinant human platelet-derived growth factor-BB (becaplermin) in patients with chronic neuropathic diabetic ulcers: a phase III randomized placebo-controlled double-blind study. *Diabetes Care* 1998; **21:** 822–7.
3. Smiell JM, *et al.* Efficacy and safety of becaplermin (recombinant human platelet-derived growth factor-BB) in patients with nonhealing, lower extremity diabetic ulcers: a combined analysis of four randomized studies. *Wound Repair Regen* 1999; **7:** 335–46.


### Preparations

**Proprietary Preparations** (details are given in Part 3)
***Canad.:*** Regranex; ***Fr.:*** Regranex; ***Ger.:*** Regranex; ***Israel:*** Regranex; ***Mex.:*** Regranex; ***Neth.:*** Regranex; ***Singapore:*** Regranex†; ***Swed.:*** Regranex†; ***Switz.:*** Regranex; ***UK:*** Regranex; ***USA:*** Regranex.

---

## Bentoquatam *(USAN)*

Quaternium 18-bentonite.

*CAS — 1340-69-8.*

### Profile

Bentoquatam, described as an organoclay compound, is a barrier preparation that is applied topically as a 5% lotion to prevent allergic contact dermatitis caused by poison ivy, poison oak, or poison sumac. The lotion is applied in a sufficient quantity to form a visible coating 15 minutes before possible contact with the plants. If continued protection is required the lotion may be re-applied every 4 hours or at any time if the visible coating is removed.

### Preparations

**Proprietary Preparations** (details are given in Part 3)
***USA:*** Ivy Block.

---

## Benzophenone-6

6-Benzofenona. 2,2′-Dihydroxy-4,4′-dimethoxybenzophenone.

$C_{15}H_{14}O_5$ = 274.3.
*CAS — 131-54-4.*

### Profile

Benzophenone-6 is a sunscreen (see p.1133) with actions similar to those of oxybenzone (p.1155). It is effective against UVB and some UVA light (for definitions, see p.1136).

### Preparations

**Proprietary Preparations**
Some preparations are listed in Part 3.

---

## Benzoyl Peroxide *(USAN)*

Benzoylis Peroxidum; NSC-675; Peróxido de benzoílo. Dibenzoyl peroxide.

$C_{14}H_{10}O_4$ = 242.2.
*CAS — 94-36-0 (anhydrous benzoyl peroxide).*
*ATC — D10AE01.*

**Pharmacopoeias.** In *Chin., Eur.* (see p.vi), *Int.*, and *US.*

**Ph. Eur. 5.0** (Benzoyl Peroxide, Hydrous). It contains not less than 70% and not more than 77% of anhydrous benzoyl peroxide and not less than 20% of water. It rapidly loses water on exposure to air and may explode if the water content is too low. A white amorphous or granular powder. Practically insoluble in water; slightly soluble in alcohol; soluble in acetone; soluble in dichloromethane with separation of water. Store at 2° to 8° in a container that has been treated to reduce static charges and that has a device for the release of excess pressure. Unused material should not be returned to its original container but should be destroyed by the addition of sodium hydroxide solution (10%). Destruction can be considered to be complete if the addition of a crystal of potassium iodide does not result in the release of free iodine after acidification with dilute hydrochloric acid. Protect from light.

**USP 27** (Hydrous Benzoyl Peroxide). It contains not less than 65% and not more than 82% of anhydrous benzoyl peroxide with a water content of about 26%. The hydrous form is a white granular powder with a characteristic odour. Sparingly soluble in water and in alcohol; soluble in acetone, in chloroform, and in ether. Store in the original container, treated to reduce static charges. Unused material should not be returned to its original container but should be destroyed by the addition of sodium hydroxide solution (10%). Destruction can be considered to be complete if the addition of a crystal of potassium iodide does not result in the release of free iodine.

### Adverse Effects and Precautions

Topical application of benzoyl peroxide may produce skin irritation, particularly on beginning treatment. In some patients the irritation may require reduced frequency of application or temporary suspension of treatment. Skin dryness, peeling, rash, and transient local oedema may also occur. Contact sensitisation has been reported in some patients using preparations containing benzoyl peroxide. Caution is required when applying it near the eyes, the mouth and other mucous membranes, and to the neck and other sensitive areas. Patients should be alerted to benzoyl peroxide's bleaching property.

**Body odour.** A report of an unusual unpleasant body odour in a patient attributed to the topical use of benzoyl peroxide.[1]


1. Molberg P. Body odor from topical benzoyl peroxide. *N Engl J Med* 1981; **304:** 1366.


**Carcinogenicity.** There has been concern at the implications of some *animal* studies showing benzoyl peroxide to possess some tumour-promoting activity.[1] However, a retrospective survey in Canada concluded that there was no indication that the normal use of benzoyl peroxide in the treatment of acne was associated with an increased risk of facial cancer.[2]


1. Jones GRN. Skin cancer: risk to individuals using the tumour promoter benzoyl peroxide for acne treatment. *Hum Toxicol* 1985; **4:** 75–8.
2. Hogan DJ, *et al.* A study of acne treatments as risk factors for skin cancer of the head and neck. *Br J Dermatol* 1991; **125:** 343–8.


**Handling.** Benzoyl peroxide may explode if subjected to grinding, percussion, or heat. Hydrous benzoyl peroxide containing water to reduce the risk of explosion may still explode if exposed to temperatures higher than 60° or cause fires in the presence of reducing substances.

**Hypersensitivity.** Benzoyl peroxide appears to induce contact hypersensitivity quite often when used to treat leg ulcers,[1] but it is unclear how often this occurs when used in the treatment of acne.[2] Patch testing[3,4] in some studies suggests that up to 76% of patients may be hypersensitive to benzoyl peroxide but this does not appear to correlate with the clinical irritation produced during treatment, which usually resolves on continued use, or with the reported incidence of hypersensitivity.[2,4] In one study 25% of patients were considered to be hypersensitive from patch testing but only 2 of 44 patients developed clinical hypersensitivity.[4] Another study involving 204 patients with acne found that the incidence of false-positive irritant skin reactions to benzoyl peroxide was about 15% but only 1% of the patients had true allergic reactions to the drug on further testing.[5] However, there has been concern that hypersensitivity to benzoyl peroxide may be mistaken for irritation or worsening of the acne.[3]


1. Vena GA, *et al.* Contact dermatitis to benzoyl peroxide. *Contact Dermatitis* 1982; **8:** 338.
2. Cunliffe WJ, Burke B. Benzoyl peroxide: lack of sensitization. *Acta Derm Venereol (Stockh)* 1982; **62:** 458–9.
3. Leyden JJ, Kligman AM. Contact sensitization to benzoyl peroxide. *Contact Dermatitis* 1977; **3:** 273–5.
4. Rietschel RL, Duncan SH. Benzoyl peroxide reactions in an acne study group. *Contact Dermatitis* 1982; **8:** 323–6.
5. Balato N, *et al.* Acne and allergic contact dermatitis. *Contact Dermatitis* 1996; **34:** 68–9.


### Pharmacokinetics

◊ Work *in vitro* and in *animals*[1] suggests that although there is some absorption of benzoyl peroxide following topical application, any absorbed drug appears to be metabolised in the skin to benzoic acid and rapidly excreted in the urine.


1. Yeung D, *et al.* Benzoyl peroxide: percutaneous penetration and metabolic disposition II: effect of concentration. *J Am Acad Dermatol* 1983; **9:** 920–4.


### Uses and Administration

Benzoyl peroxide has mild keratolytic properties. Its antimicrobial action is probably due to its oxidising effect and activity has been reported against *Staphylococcus epidermidis* and *Propionibacterium acnes*. It is used mainly in the treatment of acne (below), in topical preparations usually containing 2.5 to 10%, sometimes with other antimicrobials. It has been used similarly in the treatment of fungal skin infections (p.390), such as tinea pedis although other drugs are usually preferred. A 20% lotion has been applied every 8 to 12 hours in the treatment of decubitus or stasis ulcers. Strengths are expressed as anhydrous benzoyl peroxide although it is employed in a hydrous form for safety (see Pharmacopoeial Description, above).

Benzoyl peroxide is also used as a bleaching agent in the food industry and as a catalyst in the plastics industry.

**Acne.** Benzoyl peroxide applied topically in concentrations of up to 10% is probably the most widely used first-line drug in the management of mild acne (p.1133). Early studies in *animals* found benzoyl peroxide to be sebosuppressive[1] but later studies demonstrated that sebum excretion rises during the first few months of treatment,[2,3] probably due to the comedolytic action of benzoyl peroxide, and remains at a stable level thereafter. Benzoyl peroxide has been shown to have a significant inhibitory effect on skin microflora, with reductions in surface and follicular micro-organisms within 48 hours of beginning treatment, but clinical improvement took several more days to appear.[4] Benzoyl peroxide has also been used in combination therapy with topical erythromycin when it has been reported to be helpful in preventing the selection of antibacterial resistance.[5,6]


1. Gloor M, *et al.* Cytokinetic studies on the sebo-suppressive effect of drugs using the example of benzoyl peroxide. *Arch Dermatol Res* 1980; **267:** 97–9.
2. Cunliffe WJ, *et al.* Topical benzoyl peroxide increases the sebum excretion rate in patients with acne. *Br J Dermatol* 1983; **109:** 577–9.
3. Pierard-Franchimont C, *et al.* Topical benzoyl peroxide increases the sebum excretion rate. *Br J Dermatol* 1984; **110:** 506.
4. Bojar RA, *et al.* The short-term treatment of acne vulgaris with benzoyl peroxide: effects on the surface and follicular cutaneous microflora. *Br J Dermatol* 1995; **132:** 204–8.
5. Eady EA, *et al.* Effects of benzoyl peroxide and erythromycin alone and in combination against antibiotic-sensitive and -resistant skin bacteria from acne patients. *Br J Dermatol* 1994; **131:** 331–6.
6. Eady EA, *et al.* The effects of acne treatment with a combination of benzoyl peroxide and erythromycin on skin carriage of erythromycin-resistant propionibacteria. *Br J Dermatol* 1996; **134:** 107–13.


### Preparations

***BP 2003:*** Benzoyl Peroxide Cream; Benzoyl Peroxide Gel; Benzoyl Peroxide Lotion; Potassium Hydroxyquinoline Sulphate and Benzoyl Peroxide Cream;
***USP 27:*** Benzoyl Peroxide Gel; Benzoyl Peroxide Lotion; Erythromycin and Benzoyl Peroxide Topical Gel.

**Proprietary Preparations** (details are given in Part 3)
***Arg.:*** Acnesan; Benzihex; Eclaran; Ecnagel PB; Paracne; PB Gel; Solugel; Tiltis; Vixiderm E; ***Austral.:*** Benzac; Brevoxyl; Clearasil Ultra; Neutrogena Acne Mask†; Oxy; PanOxyl; ***Austria:*** Akneroxid; Benzaknen; Brevoxyl; PanOxyl; Scherogel; Ultra-Clear-A-Med†; ***Belg.:*** Akneroxid; Benzac; Pangel; Scherogel†; Tinagel†; ***Braz.:*** Acnesan†; Benzac-AC; Benzac†; Benzagel†; PanOxyl; Solugel; ***Canad.:*** Acetoxyl; Benoxyl; Benzac; Benzagel; Clean & Clear Persa; Clearasil B.P. Plus; Dermacne†; Dermoxyl; Desquam-X; $H_2$Oxyl†; Johnsons Clean & Clear Persa Gel; Loroxide†; Neostrata Astringent Acne Treatment; Neostrata Blemish Spot; Neutrogena Acne Mask; Neutrogena On The Spot Acne Treatment; Oxy; Oxyderm; PanOxyl; Solugel; ***Chile:*** Benzac; Pansulfox; Peroxiben Plus; Pirobac; Solugel; ***Denm.:*** Basiron†; ***Fin.:*** Basiron; Brevoxyl; PanOxyl†; ***Fr.:*** Brevoxyl; Cutacnyl; Eclaran; Effacne; Pannogel; PanOxyl; ***Ger.:*** Aknederm Oxid; Aknefugoxid; Akneroxid; Benzaknen; Benzoyt; Benzperox; Brevoxyl; Cordes BPO; Dercome; Klinoxid; Marduk; Oxy Fissan†; Oxy†; PanOxyl; Sanoxit; Scherogel; ***Gr.:*** Benzac-W; Brevoxyl; ***Hong Kong:*** Acnacyl; Antopar†; Benzac-AC; Brevoxyl; Oxy; PanOxyl; ***India:*** Persol; ***Irl.:*** Acnecide; Benoxyl†; Brevoxyl; PanOxyl; ***Israel:*** Acne Derm; Acne Mask; Benzac-AC; Clearex Cover Up; Oxy; Oxy Sensitive; PanOxyl; ***Ital.:*** Benoxid; Benzac; Benzomix†; Clearasil Ultra†; PanOxyl; Reloxyl; Scherogel†; ***Malaysia:*** Akneroxid; Benzac-AC; Brevoxyl; PanOxyl; ***Mex.:*** Benoxyl; Benzac; Benzaderm; Clearasil Plus†; Oxy†; PanOxyl†; Solugel; ***Neth.:*** Akneroxid; Benzac; ***Norw.:*** Basiron; Brevoxyl; PanOxyl; ***NZ:*** Benoxyl†; Benzac; Brevoxyl; Clearasil Ultra; PanOxyl; ***Port.:*** Benacne; Benoxygel; Benzac; Eclaran; PanOxyl; ***S.Afr.:*** Benoxyl; Benzac-AC; PanOxyl; ***Singapore:*** Acnacyl; Akneroxid; Benzac; Brevoxyl; PanOxyl; ***Spain:*** Aldoacne†; Benoxygel; Clearamed†; Oxiderma; PanOxyl; Peroxacne; Peroxiben; Solucel; Stop Espinilla Normaderm; ***Swed.:*** Basiron; Bexid; Brevoxyl; Stioxyl; ***Switz.:*** Acnefuge; Akneroxid; Aknex; Basiron; Benzac; Desanden†; Effacne; Ledoxid Acne†; Lubexyl; PanOxyl; ***Thai.:*** Acnexyl; Benzac; Brevoxyl; PanOxyl; ***UK:*** Acnecide†; Benoxyl†; Brevoxyl; Clearasil Max 10†; Mediclear†; Nericur†; Oxy; PanOxyl; ***USA:*** Ambi 10; Benoxyl†; Benzac; Benzagel†; Benzashave†; Blemerase†; Brevoxyl; Clear By Design†; Clearasil;

Clinac BPO; Del Aqua; Desquam; Exact†; Fostex; Loroxide†; Neutrogena Acne Mask†; Oxy; PanOxyl; Peroxin†; Persa-Gel†; Triaz; Vanoxide†.

**Multi-ingredient:** ***Arg.:*** Benzamycin; Erimicin; Kitacne PB; Peroximicina; ***Austria:*** Acne Plus; Acnidazil†; ***Belg.:*** Acnidazil†; Benzamycin; ***Braz.:*** Acnase; Acnosil†; Akirol; Benzac Eritromicina; Nixoderm†; ***Canad.:*** Benzamycin; Persol†; Sulfoxyl†; ***Chile:*** Benzamycin; ***Denm.:*** Acnidazil†; ***Ger.:*** Acne Plus; Acnidazil†; ***Hong Kong:*** Benzamycin; ***India:*** Persol Forte; ***Irl.:*** Benzamycin; Quinoderm; ***Israel:*** Benzamycin; ***Ital.:*** Acnidazil; Delta 80; Delta 80 Plus; Katoxyn; ***Mex.:*** Benzamycin; ***Neth.:*** Acnecure; Acnidazil; ***S.Afr.:*** Acneclear; Acnidazil; Benzamycine; Quinoderm; Quinoderm-H†; ***Singapore:*** Benzamycin; ***Switz.:*** Acne Creme Plus; Quinoderm†; ***UK:*** Acnidazil†; Benzamycin; Duac Once Daily; Quinoderm; Quinoped†; ***USA:*** BenzaClin; Benzamycin; Duac; Sulfoxyl; Vanoxide-HC.

## Calamine

Calamina; Prepared Calamine.

**Pharmacopoeias.** In *Br., Chin., Int.,* and *US.*

**BP 2003** (Calamine). It is a basic zinc carbonate coloured with ferric oxide. It is an amorphous, impalpable, pink or reddish-brown powder, the colour depending on the variety and amount of ferric oxide present and the process by which it is incorporated. Practically insoluble in water; it dissolves with effervescence in hydrochloric acid.

**USP 27** (Calamine). It is zinc oxide with a small proportion of ferric oxide. A pink, odourless, fine powder. Insoluble in water; practically completely soluble in mineral acids.

### Profile

Calamine has mild astringent and antipruritic actions and is used as a dusting powder, cream, lotion, or ointment in a variety of skin conditions although its value is uncertain.

### Preparations

***BP 2003:*** Aqueous Calamine Cream; Calamine and Coal Tar Ointment; Calamine Lotion; Calamine Ointment;
***USP 27:*** Calamine Lotion; Phenolated Calamine Lotion.

**Proprietary Preparations** (details are given in Part 3)
***Spain:*** Talquistina; ***USA:*** Calamox†.

**Multi-ingredient:** ***Arg.:*** Acuaderm; Caladryl; Calcusan; Pinklot; Piracalamina; Pruripelen; Prurisedan; Urtikalma; ***Austral.:*** Animine†; Calaband; Caladryl†; Calamine Lotion†; Dermalife Plus; Quinaband; ***Braz.:*** Caladerm; Caladryl; Calamina; Calamina Composta; Calmapele†; Dermamina; Dermdryl; Solardril Composto; ***Canad.:*** Aveeno Anti-Itch; Caladryl; Calamine Antihistamine; Noivy†; ***Chile:*** Ivarest; ***Fr.:*** Gel de Calamine; Pruriced; ***Hong Kong:*** Cadramine-V; Caladryl; Calamine-D; Improved Versal†; ***India:*** Caladryl; Siloderm; ***Irl.:*** Caladryl†; Hydrocal†; RBC; Vasogen; ***Israel:*** Baby Paste + Chamomile; Calamine Lotion; Calatrim; Calatrim cum Sulphur; Kamiltract Baby†; ***Ital.:*** Mavipiu; ***Malaysia:*** Dermoplex Calamine; ***Neth.:*** Caladryl; ***NZ:*** Am-O-Lin; Dermalife Plus†; Lacto Calamine; Ungvita†; ***Port.:*** Benaderma com Calamina; Caladryl; Pruridermase; Solpic; ***S.Afr.:*** Biohist; Caladryl; Calasthetic; Histamed; Lacto Calamine; ***Spain:*** Caladryl; Poliglicol Anti Acne†; Talco Antihistam Calber†; Talquisar†; ***Thai.:*** Ancamin; Cadinyl; Cadramine; Caladerm; Caladryl; Calanol; Calapro; Caldramine†; Lanol; M-D; ***UK:*** Calaband; Lacto Calamine; Quinaband; RBC; Swarm; Vasogen; ***USA:*** Aveeno Anti-Itch†; Caladryl; Calamatum†; Calamycin; Dome-Paste; Ivarest; RA Lotion; Resinol†; Rhuli Spray†.

## Calcipotriol *(BAN, rINN)*

Calcipotriene *(USAN)*; MC-903. (5Z,7E,22E,24S)-24-Cyclopropyl-9,10-secochola-5,7,10(19),22-tetraene-1α,3β,24-triol.

$C_{27}H_{40}O_3$ = 412.6.

*CAS — 112828-00-9; 112965-21-6.*

*ATC — D05AX02.*

### Adverse Effects and Precautions

The most frequent adverse effect associated with calcipotriol is skin irritation and it should not therefore be applied to the facial area. Symptoms may include burning, itching, erythema, and dry skin, but discontinuation of therapy is seldom necessary. Aggravation of psoriasis may occur. Hypercalcaemia that is rapidly reversible on withdrawal has occurred during treatment with calcipotriol and it should not be used in patients with disorders of calcium metabolism. Other rare adverse effects may include skin atrophy and photosensitivity.

**Effects on calcium homoeostasis.** Calcipotriol is a vitamin D derivative and therefore has the potential to cause hypercalcaemia and hypercalciuria. Up to December 1993, when about 150 000 patients in the UK had been treated with calcipotriol, the UK Committee on Safety of Medicines had received 6 reports of hypercalcaemia and 2 of hypercalciuria.[1] Three of the patients with hypercalcaemia either had used doses in excess of the recommended maximum (see Uses and Administration, below) or had pustular or exfoliative psoriasis. Hypercalcaemia and hypercalciuria were reversible on withdrawal of calcipotriol. A study[2] investigating the effect of calcipotriol on urine calcium excretion found that use of the maximum recommended dose for 4 weeks produced increased urine calcium excretion, and the authors suggested that patients requiring the maximum dose of calcipotriol should be monitored for hypercalciuria before and during treatment. A review[3] of the effects of vitamin D analogues on calcium homoeostasis concluded that patients with unstable psoriasis are at particular risk of toxicity from calcipotriol and that measurement of urine calcium excretion is a more sensitive indicator of toxicity than serum-calcium concentrations.

1. Committee on Safety of Medicines/Medicines Control Agency. Dovonex ointment (calcipotriol). *Current Problems* 1994; **20:** 3.
2. Berth-Jones J, *et al.* Urine calcium excretion during treatment of psoriasis with topical calcipotriol. *Br J Dermatol* 1993; **129:** 411–14.
3. Bourke JF, *et al.* Vitamin D analogues in psoriasis: effects on systemic calcium homeostasis. *Br J Dermatol* 1996; **135:** 347–54.

**Hyperpigmentation.** Hyperpigmentation occurred at the site of calcipotriol application in 2 patients following use with PUVA-bath therapy for psoriasis.[1] The effect persisted for at least 4 and 5 months respectively, in these patients.

1. Gläser R, *et al.* Hyperpigmentation due to topical calcipotriol and photochemotherapy in two psoriatic patients. *Br J Dermatol* 1998; **139:** 148–51.

### Uses and Administration

Calcipotriol is a vitamin $D_3$ derivative. *In vitro* it appears to induce differentiation and to suppress proliferation of keratinocytes.

Calcipotriol is used in a cream or ointment for the management of plaque psoriasis and as a solution in the management of scalp psoriasis; the concentration of calcipotriol used is 0.005%. In adults, applications should be made once or twice daily. No more than 100 g of cream or ointment, or 60 mL of scalp solution, should be applied in one week. If both are used, the limit is 60 g of cream or ointment with 30 mL of scalp solution, or 30 g of cream or ointment with 60 mL of scalp solution.

In children, the cream or ointment may be applied twice daily. The maximum applied in one week should be 50 g in children aged 6 to 12 years and 75 g in children more than 12 years of age.

**Skin disorders.** Topical drugs are the treatment of first choice for *chronic plaque psoriasis* (p.1137). Calcipotriol, dithranol, and coal tar are commonly used for mild to moderate forms of the disorder. Calcipotriol has been shown to be effective[1,2] and has the advantages of being odourless and nonstaining. Its efficacy in children[3] and during long-term[4] use has also been demonstrated. A study comparing calcipotriol ointment with coal tar for chronic plaque psoriasis[5] found rapid improvement within the first 2 weeks of treatment with calcipotriol, whereas improvement with tar occurred only after 4 weeks. When solutions of calcipotriol and betamethasone were compared for mild to moderate scalp psoriasis,[6] calcipotriol produced a satisfactory response, but betamethasone was more effective and was associated with less irritation of the scalp and face. In a study of patients with nail psoriasis about half received benefit from calcipotriol ointment over a 3 to 5 month treatment period.[7] This result was similar to that found for patients treated with betamethasone and salicylic acid ointment. Combination of calcipotriol with other antipsoriatic drugs may be beneficial; combination with betamethasone was more effective than treatment with calcipotriol alone in two studies[8,9] and in another,[10] addition of calcipotriol to treatment with acitretin improved efficacy. Calcipotriol applied before either broad or narrowband ultraviolet B treatment has been shown to have an UVB-sparing effect and hence may decrease the risk of skin cancers.[11] However, because of the potential for the vehicle of topical calcipotriol preparations to block UV irradiation, they should be applied at least 2 hours before irradiation.[12] A 2-week course of high-dose calcipotriol (up to 360 g of 0.005% ointment weekly) has been used for inpatient treatment of extensive psoriasis, followed by the usual recommended dose (up to 100 g weekly) for residual psoriasis.[13] Asymptomatic hypercalcaemia and hypercalciuria occurred in some patients; the monitoring of calcium homoeostasis is mandatory (see Effects on Calcium Homoeostasis, above). Relapse occurred in most patients within one year.

Beneficial results with calcipotriol have also been reported in *pityriasis rubra pilaris,*[14] *congenital ichthyoses,*[15] *acrodermatitis continua of Hallopeau,*[16] and *confluent and reticulated papillomatosis.*[17] A small open study[18] has indicated that topical calcipotriol may be effective in the treatment of oral leucoplakia (see under Bleomycin, p.531).

1. Murdoch D, Clissold SP. Calcipotriol: a review of its pharmacological properties and therapeutic use in psoriasis vulgaris. *Drugs* 1992; **43:** 415–29.
2. Ashcroft DM, *et al.* Systematic review of comparative efficacy and tolerability of calcipotriol in treating chronic plaque psoriasis. *BMJ* 2000; **320:** 963–7.
3. Darley CR, *et al.* Safety and efficacy of calcipotriol ointment (Dovonex®) in treating children with psoriasis vulgaris. *Br J Dermatol* 1996; **135:** 390–3.
4. Ellis JP, *et al.* Long-term treatment of chronic plaque psoriasis with calcipotriol ointment in patients unresponsive to short-contact dithranol. *Eur J Clin Res* 1995; **7:** 247–57.
5. Tham SN, *et al.* A comparative study of calcipotriol ointment and tar in chronic plaque psoriasis. *Br J Dermatol* 1994; **131:** 673–7.
6. Klaber MR, *et al.* Comparative effects of calcipotriol solution (50 micrograms/mL) and betamethasone 17-valerate solution (1 mg/mL) in the treatment of scalp psoriasis. *Br J Dermatol* 1994; **131:** 678–83.
7. Tosti A, *et al.* Calcipotriol ointment in nail psoriasis: a controlled double-blind comparison with betamethasone dipropionate and salicylic acid. *Br J Dermatol* 1998; **139:** 655–9.
8. Ruzicka T, Lorenz B. Comparison of calcipotriol monotherapy and a combination of calcipotriol and betamethasone valerate after 2 weeks' treatment with calcipotriol in the topical therapy of psoriasis vulgaris: a multicentre, double-blind, randomized study. *Br J Dermatol* 1998; **138:** 254–8.
9. Guenther L, *et al.* Efficacy and safety of a new combination of calcipotriol and betamethasone dipropionate (once or twice daily) compared to calcipotriol (twice daily) in the treatment of psoriasis vulgaris: a randomized, double-blind, vehicle-controlled clinical trial. *Br J Dermatol* 2002; **147:** 316–23.
10. van de Kerkhof PCM, *et al.* The effect of addition of calcipotriol ointment (50 micrograms/g) to acitretin therapy in psoriasis. *Br J Dermatol* 1998; **138:** 84–9.
11. Woo WK, McKenna KE. Combination TL01 ultraviolet B phototherapy and topical calcipotriol for psoriasis: a prospective randomized placebo-controlled clinical trial. *Br J Dermatol* 2003; **149:** 146–50.
12. De Rie MA, *et al.* Calcipotriol ointment and cream or their vehicles applied immediately before irradiation inhibit ultraviolet B-induced erythema. *Br J Dermatol* 2000; **142:** 1160–5.
13. Bleiker TO, *et al.* Long-term outcome of severe chronic plaque psoriasis following treatment with high-dose topical calcipotriol. *Br J Dermatol* 1998; **139:** 285–6.
14. van de Kerkhof PCM, Steijlen PM. Topical treatment of pityriasis rubra pilaris with calcipotriol. *Br J Dermatol* 1994; **130:** 675–8.
15. Lucker GPH, *et al.* Effect of topical calcipotriol on congenital ichthyoses. *Br J Dermatol* 1994; **131:** 546–50.
16. Mozzanica N, Cattaneo A. The clinical effect of topical calcipotriol in acrodermatitis continua of Hallopeau. *Br J Dermatol* 1998; **138:** 556.
17. Güleç AT, Seçkin D. Confluent and reticulated papillomatosis: treatment with topical calcipotriol. *Br J Dermatol* 1999; **141:** 1150–1.
18. Femiano F, *et al.* Oral leukoplakia: open trial of topical therapy with calcipotriol compared with tretinoin. *Int J Oral Maxillofac Surg* 2001; **30:** 402–6.

### Preparations

**Proprietary Preparations** (details are given in Part 3)
***Arg.:*** Daivonex; Dermocal; ***Austral.:*** Daivonex; ***Austria:*** Psorcutan; ***Belg.:*** Daivonex; ***Braz.:*** Daivonex; ***Canad.:*** Dovonex; ***Chile:*** Daivonex; ***Denm.:*** Daivonex; ***Fin.:*** Daivonex; ***Fr.:*** Daivonex; ***Ger.:*** Psorcutan; ***Gr.:*** Dovonex; ***Hong Kong:*** Daivonex; ***Irl.:*** Dovonex; ***Israel:*** Daivonex; ***Ital.:*** Daivonex; Psorcutan; ***Jpn:*** Dovonex; ***Malaysia:*** Daivonex; ***Mex.:*** Daivonex; ***Neth.:*** Daivonex; ***Norw.:*** Daivonex; ***NZ:*** Daivonex; ***Port.:*** Daivonex; ***S.Afr.:*** Dovonex; ***Singapore:*** Daivonex; ***Spain:*** Daivonex; ***Swed.:*** Daivonex; ***Switz.:*** Daivonex; ***Thai.:*** Daivonex; ***UK:*** Dovonex; ***USA:*** Dovonex.

**Multi-ingredient:** ***Denm.:*** Daivobet; ***Ger.:*** Daivobet; ***Irl.:*** Dovobet; ***Norw.:*** Daivobet; ***Spain:*** Daivobet; ***Swed.:*** Daivobet; ***UK:*** Dovobet.

## Centella

Centellae Asiaticae Herba; Herba Centellae; Hydrocotyle; Indian Pennywort.

*CAS — 18449-41-7 (madecassic acid); 464-92-6 (asiatic acid); 16830-15-2 (asiaticoside).*

**Pharmacopoeias.** In *Chin.* and *Eur.* (see p.vi).

**Ph. Eur. 5.0** (Centella). The dried, fragmented aerial parts of *Centella asiatica*. It contains not less than 6% of total triterpenoid derivatives, expressed as asiaticoside, calculated with reference to dried drug. Protect from light.

### Profile

Centella contains madecassic acid, asiatic acid, and asiaticoside. It has been used topically and by mouth in the management of wounds, ulcers, and keloid scars. Contact dermatitis has been reported.

The names gotu kola, gotu cola, and gota kola are used for *Centella asiatica* (*=Hydrocotyle asiatica*) in herbal medicine. Centella is also used in homoeopathic medicine.

◊ References.

1. Santucci B, *et al.* Contact dermatitis due to Centelase®. *Contact Dermatitis* 1985; **13:** 39.

### Preparations

**Proprietary Preparations** (details are given in Part 3)
***Arg.:*** Gotu Kola; Pertusan; Remiderm; ***Austria:*** Collaven†; Madecassol; ***Belg.:*** Madecassol; ***Braz.:*** Celumax†; Centella-Vit; ***Canad.:*** Cothilyne†; ***Chile:*** Celulase; Celulase Plus; Centabel; Escar T; Madecassol; ***Fr.:*** Madecassol; Madecassol Tulgras; ***Ital.:*** Centellase; ***Mex.:*** Madecassol; ***Port.:*** Madecassol; ***Singapore:*** Centellase; Centica; ***Spain:*** Blastoestimulina; ***Switz.:*** Madecassol†; ***Thai.:*** Madecassol.

**Multi-ingredient:** ***Arg.:*** Centella Queen Complex; Centella Queen Reductora; Clevosan; Enlinea; Garcinol Max; Ginal Cent; Ginkan; Redudiet; Vagicural Plus; Venoful; ***Austral.:*** Extralife Leg-Care†; ***Braz.:*** Composto Anticelulitico†; Composto Emagrecedor; Derm'attive; Emagrevit; ***Chile:*** Celulase Con Neomicina; Dermaglos Plus; Escar T-Neomicina; Madecassol Neomicina; ***Fr.:*** Calmiphase; Fadiamone; Madecassol Neomycine Hydrocortisone; ***Ital.:*** Angioton; Capill; Centella Complex; Centeril H; Dermilia Flebozin; Emmenoiasi; Fluiven†; Neomyrt Plus; Osmogel; Pik-Gel†; Varicofit; Venactive; ***Mex.:*** Madecassol C; Madecassol N; ***Mon.:*** Akildia; ***Port.:*** Antiestrias; Equilibrium Creme Anti-transpirante†; ***Spain:*** Blastoestimulina; Cemalyt; Nesfare.

## Cerous Nitrate

Cerium Nitrate; Nitrato de cerio.

$Ce(NO_3)_3$ = 326.1.

*CAS — 10108-73-3.*

### Profile

Cerous nitrate has been used topically, mainly with sulfadiazine silver, in the treatment of burns.

◊ References.


1. Scheidegger D, *et al.* Survival in major burn injuries treated by one bathing in cerium nitrate. *Burns* 1992; **18:** 296–300.
2. Boeckx W, *et al.* Effect of cerium nitrate-silver sulphadiazine on deep dermal burns: a histological hypothesis. *Burns* 1992; **18:** 456–62.
3. Ross DA, *et al.* The use of cerium nitrate-silver sulphadiazine as a topical burns dressing. *Br J Plast Surg* 1993; **46:** 582–4.
4. Koller J, Orsag M. Our experience with the use of cerium sulphadiazine in the treatment of extensive burns. *Acta Chir Plast* 1998; **40:** 73–5.


## Preparations

**Proprietary Preparations** (details are given in Part 3)

**Multi-ingredient:** ***Arg.:*** Sulfatral-Cerio; ***Belg.:*** Flammacerium; ***Braz.:*** Dermacerium†; ***Fr.:*** Flammacerium; ***Israel:*** Flammacerium†; ***Neth.:*** Flammacerium; ***UK:*** Flammacerium.

## Cinoxate *(USAN, rINN)*

Cinoxato. 2-Ethoxyethyl *p*-methoxycinnamate.

$C_{14}H_{18}O_4$ = 250.3.

*CAS — 104-28-9.*

### Profile

Cinoxate, a substituted cinnamate, is a sunscreen (see p.1133) with actions similar to those of octinoxate (p.1154). It is effective against UVB light (for definitions, see p.1136).

### Preparations

**Proprietary Preparations**

Some preparations are listed in Part 3.

## Crilanomer *(rINN)*

Acrylonitrile-starch Copolymer; Crilanómero; ZK-94006. A starch polymer with acrylonitrile.

*CAS — 37291-07-9.*

*ATC — D03AX09.*

### Profile

Crilanomer is a starch copolymer used as a hydrogel wound dressing in the management of wounds.

### Preparations

**Proprietary Preparations** (details are given in Part 3)

***Austral.:*** Intrasite; ***S.Afr.:*** Intrasite.

## Crotamiton *(BAN, rINN)*

Crotam; Crotamitón; Crotamitonum. *N*-Ethyl-*N*-*o*-tolylcrotonamide; *N*-Ethylcrotono-*o*-toluidide; *N*-Ethyl-*N*-(2-methylphenyl)-2-butenamide.

$C_{13}H_{17}NO$ = 203.3.

*CAS — 483-63-6.*

**Pharmacopoeias.** In *Chin., Eur.* (see p.vi), and *US.*

**Ph. Eur. 5.0** (Crotamiton). A colourless or pale yellow oily liquid. It solidifies partly or completely at low temperatures. It is predominantly the (*E*)-isomer, with not more than 15% of the (*Z*)-isomer. Slightly soluble in water; miscible with alcohol. Protect from light.

**USP 27** (Crotamiton). A colourless to slightly yellowish oil with a faint amine-like odour. It is a mixture of *cis-* and *trans-*isomers. Soluble in alcohol and in methyl alcohol. Store in airtight containers. Protect from light.

### Adverse Effects and Precautions

Applied topically, crotamiton occasionally causes irritation. There have been rare reports of hypersensitivity reactions. Crotamiton should not be used in the presence of acute exudative dermatitis. It should not be applied near the eyes, mouth, or other mucous membranes or on excoriated skin.

Ingestion of crotamiton may cause burning and irritation of oral, oesophageal, and gastric mucosa with nausea, vomiting, and abdominal pain.

**Overdosage.** A 23-year-old woman developed tonic-clonic seizures, requiring treatment with diazepam, after ingestion of a crotamiton emulsion.[1] Other hospital treatment included gastric lavage, activated charcoal, and metoclopramide. Crotamiton was detected in serum at a concentration of 34 micrograms/mL and was also detectable with several metabolites in the urine. Reference was also made to a report of a 2½-month-old child who had developed pallor and cyanosis after excessive dermal application of a crotamiton cream.


1. Meredith TJ, *et al.* Crotamiton overdose. *Hum Exp Toxicol* 1990; **9:** 57.


### Uses and Administration

Crotamiton is used as an antipruritic (p.1137), although its value is considered uncertain (see also below). It is applied as a 10% cream or lotion 2 or 3 times daily; children aged less than 3 years may receive one application daily.

Crotamiton has also been used as an acaricide in the treatment of scabies but other more effective drugs are usually preferred (p.1499). The 10% cream or lotion is applied, after first bathing and drying, to the whole of the body surface below the chin, particular attention being paid to body folds and creases. A second application should be applied 24 hours later but it may need to be used once daily up to a total of 5 days to be effective.

**Pruritus.** A double-blind study in 31 patients[1] found that 10% crotamiton lotion was no more effective an antipruritic than its vehicle.


1. Smith EB, *et al.* Crotamiton lotion in pruritus. *Int J Dermatol* 1984; **23:** 684–5.


### Preparations

***BP 2003:*** Crotamiton Cream; Crotamiton Lotion;

***USP 27:*** Crotamiton Cream.

**Proprietary Preparations** (details are given in Part 3)

***Austral.:*** Eurax; ***Austria:*** Eurax; ***Belg.:*** Eurax; ***Canad.:*** Eurax; ***Chile:*** Eurax; ***Fr.:*** Eurax; ***Ger.:*** Crotamitex; Eraxil; Euraxil†; ***Hong Kong:*** Eurax; ***India:*** Crotorax; ***Irl.:*** Eurax; ***Israel:*** Eurax; Scabicin; ***Ital.:*** Eurax; ***Malaysia:*** Eurax; Moz-Bite; ***Mex.:*** Eurax; ***Norw.:*** Eurax; ***NZ:*** Eurax; ***Port.:*** Eurax; Scabicin; ***S.Afr.:*** Eurax; ***Singapore:*** Eurax; Moz-Bite; ***Spain:*** Euraxil; ***Switz.:*** Eurax; ***UK:*** Eurax; ***USA:*** Eurax.

**Multi-ingredient:** ***Arg.:*** Anastim con RTH; ***Fr.:*** Acarcid; ***India:*** Crotorax-HC; ***Irl.:*** Eurax-Hydrocortisone; ***Israel:*** Duo-Scabil; ***Malaysia:*** H-C; ***Spain:*** Euraxil Hidrocort†; ***UK:*** Eurax-Hydrocortisone.

## Dextranomer *(BAN, rINN)*

Dextranómero. Dextran cross-linked with epichlorohydrin (1-chloro-2,3-epoxypropane); Dextran 2,3-dihydroxypropyl 2-hydroxy-1,3-propanediyl ether.

*CAS — 56087-11-7.*

*ATC — D03AX02.*

### Precautions

Dextranomer should not be used in deep wounds or cavities from which its removal cannot be assured, nor should it be used on dry wounds. Care should be exercised when paste formulations of dextranomer are used near the eyes.

Spillage may render surfaces very slippery.

◊ Implantation studies in *animals* indicated that entrapment of dextranomer beads in wounds was unlikely to initiate granuloma formation or chronic inflammation.[1] Most beads were apparently unchanged 3 years after implantation.


1. Falk J, Tollerz G. Chronic tissue response to implantation of Debrisan®: an experimental study. *Clin Ther* 1977; **1:** 185–91.


### Uses and Administration

The action of dextranomer depends upon its ability to absorb up to 4 times its weight of fluid, including dissolved and suspended material of molecular weight up to about 5000.

Dextranomer is used for the cleansing of exudative and infected burns (p.1134), wounds and ulcers (p.1139), and for preparation for skin grafting.

The wound is cleansed with sterile water or saline and allowed to remain wet; dextranomer in the form of spherical beads is sprinkled on to a depth of at least 3 to 6 mm and covered with a sterile dressing. Occlusive dressings are not recommended as they may lead to maceration around the wound. The dextranomer can be renewed up to 5 times daily (usually once or twice daily), before the layer has become saturated with exudate; the old layer is washed off with a stream of sterile water or saline before renewal. All dextranomer must be removed before skin grafting. Dextranomer may also be applied as a paste (either ready-made or prepared by mixing 4 parts of the dextranomer beads with 1 part glycerol) or as a paste-containing absorbent pad that need only be changed twice daily to every 2 days according to the rate of wound exudation.

### Preparations

**Proprietary Preparations** (details are given in Part 3)

***Austria:*** Debrisorb; ***Belg.:*** Debrisan; ***Canad.:*** Debrisan†; ***Fr.:*** Debrisan†; ***Ger.:*** Debrisorb; ***Hong Kong:*** Debrisan; ***Irl.:*** Debrisan; ***Israel:*** Debrisan†; ***Ital.:*** Debrisan; ***Mex.:*** Debrisan; ***Neth.:*** Debrisan†; ***S.Afr.:*** Debrisan†; ***Swed.:*** Debrisan†; ***Switz.:*** Debrisan†; ***UK:*** Debrisan; ***USA:*** Debrisan.

## Dibenzoylmethane

Dibenzoilmetano. 1,3-Diphenyl-1,3-propanedione.

$C_{15}H_{12}O_2$ = 224.3.

*CAS — 120-46-7.*

### Profile

Dibenzoylmethane is a sunscreen (see p.1133) with actions similar to those of avobenzone (p.1142). It absorbs UVA light (for definitions, see p.1136).

### Preparations

**Proprietary Preparations**

Some preparations are listed in Part 3.

## Dihydroxyacetone

DHA; Dihidroxiacetona; Ketotriose. 1,3-Dihydroxypropan-2-one.

$C_3H_6O_3$ = 90.08.

*CAS — 96-26-4.*

**Pharmacopoeias.** In *US.*

**USP 27** (Dihydroxyacetone). A white to off-white crystalline powder. The monomeric form is freely soluble in water, in alcohol, and in ether; the dimeric form is freely soluble in water, soluble in alcohol, and sparingly soluble in ether. A 5% solution in water has a pH between 4.0 and 6.0. Store at a temperature of 8° to 15° in airtight containers.

### Adverse Effects and Precautions

Skin irritation from dihydroxyacetone occurs rarely; rashes and allergic dermatitis have been reported. Contact with eyes, abraded skin, and clothing should be avoided.

### Uses and Administration

Application to the skin of preparations containing dihydroxyacetone slowly produces a brown coloration similar to that caused by exposure to the sun, probably due to a reaction with the amino acids of the skin.

A single application may give rise to a patchy appearance; progressive darkening of the skin results from repeated use until a point is reached when the maximum effect is achieved. If the treatment is stopped the colour starts to fade after about 2 days and disappears completely within 8 to 14 days as the external epidermal cells are lost by normal attrition.

Preparations usually contain 5% of dihydroxyacetone and have been used to camouflage vitiligo (see Pigmentation Disorders, p.1137) or to produce an artificial suntan. Some preparations include sunscreens since the pigmentation produced gives no protection against sunburn.

### Preparations

**Proprietary Preparations** (details are given in Part 3)

***Arg.:*** Autohelios; Eurocolor Sin Sol; Leche Autobronceadora; Lelco sin Sol; ***Austral.:*** Le Tan Fast Extra Dark†; Le Tan Fast Self Tan†; Vitadye; ***Chile:*** Fotoprotectores; Leche Autobronceadora Cara Y Cuerpo; Neutrogena Bronceador; Sans Soleil Skin Ceuticals; ***Malaysia:*** Vitadye; ***USA:*** Chromelin Complexion Blender.

**Multi-ingredient:** ***Austral.:*** Le Tan Fast Plus†; ***USA:*** QT.

## Dioxybenzone *(USAN, rINN)*

Benzophenone-8; Dioxibenzona; NSC-56769. 2,2′-Dihydroxy-4-methoxybenzophenone.

$C_{14}H_{12}O_4$ = 244.2.

*CAS — 131-53-3.*

**Pharmacopoeias.** In *US.*

**USP 27** (Dioxybenzone). A yellow powder. Practically insoluble in water; freely soluble in alcohol and in toluene. Store in airtight containers. Protect from light.

### Profile

Dioxybenzone, a substituted benzophenone, is a sunscreen (see p.1133) with actions similar to those of oxybenzone (p.1155). It is effective against UVB and some UVA light (for definitions, see p.1136).

### Preparations

***USP 27:*** Dioxybenzone and Oxybenzone Cream.

**Proprietary Preparations**

Some preparations are listed in Prt 3.

## Diphencyprone

Difenciprona. 2,3-Diphenylcyclopropenone-1.

$C_{15}H_{10}O$ = 206.2.

*CAS — 886-38-4.*

### Profile

Diphencyprone has been applied as a contact sensitiser for the treatment of alopecia. It has also been tried in warts.

**Adverse effects.** Diphencyprone is considered to lack serious adverse effects but some patients may not be able to tolerate the induced hypersensitivity reaction and there have been reports of generalised urticaria following the use of diphencyprone.[1,2] Allergy to diphencyprone has been reported in medical and nursing staff in spite of taking protective precautions during its application.[3] One patient who received diphencyprone treatment for warts developed a widespread pruritic rash and palpitations due to ventricular extrasystoles.[2] Vitiligo has also been reported in patients treated with diphencyprone[4-6] and it has been suggested that this might be due to unmasking of subclinical vitiligo.[4,5] Erythema multiforme-like eruptions were associated with the topical application of diphencyprone in 3 patients.[7]


1. Tosti A, *et al.* Contact urticaria during topical immunotherapy. *Contact Dermatitis* 1989; **21:** 196–7.
2. Lane PR, Hogan DJ. Diphencyprone. *J Am Acad Dermatol* 1988; **19:** 364–5.
3. Shah M, *et al.* Hazards in the use of diphencyprone. *Br J Dermatol* 1996; **134:** 1151–65.
4. Hatzis J, *et al.* Vitiligo as a reaction to topical treatment with diphencyprone. *Dermatologica* 1988; **177:** 146–8.
5. Duhra P, Foulds IS. Persistent vitiligo induced by diphencyprone. *Br J Dermatol* 1990; **123:** 415–16.
6. Henderson CA, Ilchyshyn A. Vitiligo complicating diphencyprone sensitization therapy for alopecia universalis. *Br J Dermatol* 1995; **133:** 496–7.
7. Perret CM, *et al.* Erythema multiforme-like eruptions: a rare side effect of topical immunotherapy with diphenylcyclopropenone. *Dermatologica* 1990; **180:** 5–7.


**Alopecia.** Diphencyprone has been used with varying degrees of success in the treatment of various forms of alopecia (p.1134) including areata, totalis, and universalis.[1-6] While some workers have achieved good results in adults[1,2,4] and children[5,7] others have obtained little benefit using diphencyprone.[3] Induction of a delayed (type IV) hypersensitivity reaction after application of diphencyprone appears to be an integral part of successful treatment.[8] Sensitisation has been achieved by applying a 2% solution of diphencyprone in acetone to a small area of scalp but this may be repeated if necessary beneath plastic occlusion if adequate sensitisation is not produced.[4] Thereafter, weaker concentrations of 0.01 to 2% are applied and gradually increased in strength to produce erythema and pruritus for 36 hours post-therapy; treatment is repeated weekly. Only one side of the scalp is treated until the optimum concentration is found, in order to prevent a widespread adverse reaction. One group of patients who achieved total regrowth of hair were able to discontinue treatment with diphencyprone for a mean of 15 months without relapse[9] and another group maintained satisfactory hair growth for a mean follow-up period of 19.8 months.[10]

1. MacDonald Hull S, Norris JF. Diphencyprone in the treatment of long-standing alopecia areata. *Br J Dermatol* 1988; **119:** 367–74.
2. Monk B, Williams HC. Topical diphencyprone therapy in alopecia totalis. *Br J Dermatol* 1988; **119** (suppl 33): 16.
3. Ashworth J, *et al.* Allergic and irritant contact dermatitis compared in the treatment of alopecia totalis and universalis: a comparison of the value of topical diphencyprone and tretinoin gel. *Br J Dermatol* 1989; **120:** 397–401.
4. MacDonald Hull S, Cunliffe WJ. Successful treatment of alopecia areata using the contact allergen diphencyprone. *Br J Dermatol* 1991; **124:** 212–13.
5. MacDonald Hull S, *et al.* Alopecia areata in children: response to treatment with diphencyprone. *Br J Dermatol* 1991; **125:** 164–8.
6. Hoting E, Boehm A. Therapy of alopecia areata with diphencyprone. *Br J Dermatol* 1992; **127:** 625–9.
7. Schuttelaar M-L, *et al.* Alopecia areata in children: treatment with diphencyprone. *Br J Dermatol* 1996; **135:** 581–5.
8. MacDonald Hull S, *et al.* Alopecia areata treated with diphencyprone: is an allergic response necessary? *Br J Dermatol* 1990; **122:** 716–17.
9. van der Steen PHM, *et al.* Topical immunotherapy for alopecia areata: re-evaluation of 139 cases after an additional follow-up period of 19 months. *Dermatology* 1992; **184:** 198–201.
10. Gordon PM, *et al.* Topical diphencyprone for alopecia areata: evaluation of 48 cases after 30 months' follow-up. *Br J Dermatol* 1996; **134:** 869–71.

**Warts.** Diphencyprone has been tried in the treatment of recalcitrant warts. The successful treatment of digital or plantar warts in 42 of 60 patients has been described.[1] The patients were initially sensitised with a 2% topical solution of diphencyprone, then the warts treated with solutions ranging from 0.01 to 6%.

1. Buckley DA, *et al.* Recalcitrant viral warts treated by diphencyprone immunotherapy. *Br J Dermatol* 1999; **141:** 292–6.

## Dipyrithione *(USAN, rINN)*

Dipiritiona; OMDS. 2,2′-Dithiodipyridine 1,1′-dioxide.

$C_{10}H_8N_2O_2S_2$ = 252.3.

*CAS — 3696-28-4.*

### Profile

Dipyrithione is reported to have antibacterial and antifungal properties and is included in preparations for the treatment of dandruff.

### Preparations

**Proprietary Preparations** (details are given in Part 3)

**Multi-ingredient:** ***Switz.:*** Crimanex.

## Dithiosalicylic Acid

Ditiosalicílico, ácido. 2-Hydroxybenzenecarbodithioic acid.

$C_7H_6OS_2$ = 170.3.

*CAS — 527-89-9.*

### Profile

Dithiosalicylic acid has been used in multi-ingredient preparations used topically for the treatment of acne and seborrhoeic dermatitis.

### Preparations

**Proprietary Preparations** (details are given in Part 3)

**Multi-ingredient:** ***Ital.:*** Sacnel.

## Dithranol *(BAN, rINN)*

Anthralin; Dioxyanthranol; Dithranolum; Ditranol. 1,8-Dihydroxyanthrone; 1,8-Dihydroxy-9(10*H*)-anthracenone.

$C_{14}H_{10}O_3$ = 226.2.

*CAS — 1143-38-0 (dithranol); 16203-97-7 (dithranol triacetate).*

*ATC — D05AC01.*

**Pharmacopoeias.** In *Chin.*, *Eur.* (see p.vi), *Int.*, and *US.*

**Ph. Eur. 5.0** (Dithranol). A yellow or brownish-yellow, crystalline powder. Practically insoluble in water; slightly soluble in alcohol; sparingly soluble in acetone; soluble in dichloromethane; dissolves in dilute solutions of alkali hydroxides. Protect from light.

**USP 27** (Anthralin). A yellowish-brown, odourless, crystalline powder. Insoluble in water; slightly soluble in alcohol, in ether, and in glacial acetic acid; soluble in acetone, in chloroform, in benzene, and in solutions of alkali hydroxides. The filtrate from a suspension in water is neutral to litmus. Store at a temperature of 8° to 15° in airtight containers. Protect from light.

**Stability.** The stability of dithranol has been studied in a number of bases and vehicles.[1,2] The weaker preparations of dithranol may be less stable.[1] Salicylic acid is included in dithranol preparations as an antoxidant and its inclusion in pastes also containing zinc oxide prevents their discoloration due to the inactivation of dithranol by zinc oxide.[3] However, zinc oxide or starch can be omitted from dithranol pastes without loss of effectiveness provided stiffness is maintained.[3] Addition of ascorbic or oxalic acid may improve dithranol's stability in 'Unguentum Merck' but salicylic acid appears to be ineffective.[1] The effect of salicylic acid on the instability of dithranol in yellow soft paraffin is variable[1,2] and its inclusion has been questioned as it can be irritant and percutaneous absorption can be significant.[1] Dithranol is relatively stable in white soft paraffin.[1]

The application of any type of heat and contact with metal spatulas should be avoided during the manufacture of dithranol pastes[4] and if milling facilities are not available dithranol can be incorporated into Lassar's paste by dissolving it first in chloroform.[3]

1. Green PG, *et al.* The stability of dithranol in various bases. *Br J Dermatol* 1985; **113** (suppl 29): 26.
2. Lee RLH. Stability of dithranol (anthralin) in various vehicles. *Aust J Hosp Pharm* 1987; **17:** 254–8.
3. Comaish S, *et al.* Factors affecting the clearance of psoriasis with dithranol (anthralin). *Br J Dermatol* 1971; **84:** 282–9.
4. *PSGB Lab Report P/79/1* 1979.

### Adverse Effects and Precautions

Dithranol may cause a burning sensation especially on perilesional skin. Patients with fair skin may be more sensitive than those with dark skin. It is irritant to the eyes and mucous membranes. Use on the face, skin flexures, and genitals should be avoided. Hands should be washed after use.

Dithranol should not be used for acute or pustular psoriasis or on inflamed skin. It stains skin, hair, some fabrics, plastics, and enamel. Staining of bathroom ware may be less of a problem with creams than ointments. Stains on skin and hair slowly disappear on cessation of treatment.

**Handling.** Dithranol is a powerful irritant and should be kept away from the eyes and tender parts of the skin.

### Uses and Administration

Dithranol is used in the treatment of subacute and chronic psoriasis, usually in one of two ways.

*Conventional treatment* is commonly started with an ointment or paste containing 0.1% dithranol (0.05% in very fair patients) applied for a few hours; the strength is gradually increased as necessary to 0.5%, occasionally to 1%, and the duration of contact extended to overnight periods or longer. The preparation is sparingly and accurately applied to the lesions only. If, on initial treatment, lesions spread or excessive irritation occurs, the concentration of dithranol or the frequency of application should be reduced; if necessary, treatment should be stopped. After each treatment period the patient should bathe or shower to remove any residual dithranol.

For *short-contact therapy* dithranol is usually applied in a soft basis to the lesions for up to 60 minutes daily, before being washed off. As with conventional treatment the strength used is gradually increased from 0.1 to 2% but strengths up to 5% have been used. Surrounding unaffected skin may be protected by white soft paraffin.

Treatment for psoriasis should be continued until the skin is entirely clear. Intermittent courses may be needed to maintain the response. Treatment schedules often involve coal tar and UV irradiation (preferably UVB) before the application of dithranol (see below). Salicylic acid is included in many topical preparations of dithranol.

A cream containing dithranol triacetate 1% has been used similarly to dithranol in conventional treatment of psoriasis.

**Alopecia.** Dithranol cream (0.5 to 1%) applied for 20 to 60 minutes to the scalp and then washed off, has been found to be of benefit in the treatment of alopecia areata (p.1134). However, at least 6 months of treatment may be required for a cosmetically acceptable result.[1] The response rate has, however, been difficult to evaluate because of the small number of reports, and although it has been widely prescribed for limited patchy alopecia areata, some guidelines conclude that there is no convincing evidence of efficacy.[2]

1. Meidan VM, Touitou E. Treatments for androgenetic alopecia and alopecia areata: current options and future prospects. *Drugs* 2001; **61:** 53–69.
2. MacDonald Hull SP, *et al.* Guidelines for the management of alopecia areata. *Br J Dermatol* 2003; **149:** 692–9. Also available at: http://www.bad.org.uk/doctors/guidelines/Alopecia_Areata.pdf (accessed 16/06/04)

**Psoriasis.** Dithranol used alone or with coal tar, (with or without ultraviolet light), continues to be one of the drugs of first-line treatment for psoriasis (p.1137). It is particularly suited to the treatment of stable chronic plaque psoriasis but unlike coal tar, is irritant to healthy skin and care is required to ensure that it is only applied to lesions. Treatment with dithranol is therefore more feasible when the plaques are large, or few in number. Concomitant use of coal tar may help to reduce the irritant effects of dithranol without affecting efficacy. Traditional treatment with dithranol is time consuming and more suitable for use on hospital inpatients. Dithranol formulated in stiff preparations such as Lassar's paste to minimise spreading to perilesional skin is left on overnight covered with a suitable dressing and washed off the next day. Treatment is usually started with a concentration of 0.1% (0.05% in fair-skinned patients) and gradually increased according to the response and irritation produced. Cream formulations may be less effective but are more suitable for domestic use. Short-contact therapy in which concentrations of up to 5% of dithranol are applied daily for up to 1 hour is more suitable for use on an outpatient basis and there appears to be little reduction in efficacy; irritation and staining may also be reduced.

Dithranol is also used with UVB phototherapy and there have been many modifications of the original Ingram's regimen in which dithranol is applied after bathing in a tar bath and exposure to ultraviolet light. Inpatient stays of up to 3 weeks may be required but long periods of remission can be obtained.

### Preparations

***BP 2003:*** Dithranol Cream; Dithranol Ointment; Dithranol Paste; ***USP 27:*** Anthralin Cream; Anthralin Ointment.

**Proprietary Preparations** (details are given in Part 3)

***Austral.:*** Dithrocream; Micanol; ***Austria:*** Micanol; ***Belg.:*** Micanol; ***Braz.:*** Antranol†; ***Canad.:*** Anthraforte; Anthranol; Anthrascalp; Micanol; ***Denm.:*** Micanol; ***Fin.:*** Micanol; ***Ger.:*** Micanol; ***Hong Kong:*** Micanol; ***Irl.:*** Dithrocream; Micanol; ***Israel:*** Dithrocream; Micanol; ***Ital.:*** Psoriderm; Timicolid; ***Mex.:*** Anthranol†; ***Neth.:*** Psoricreme; ***Norw.:*** Micanol; ***NZ:*** Micanol; ***Port.:*** Desmoline†; Micanol†; ***Singapore:*** Micanol†; ***Spain:*** Anthranol†; Micanol; ***Swed.:*** Micanol; ***Thai.:*** Micanol; ***UK:*** Dithrocream; Micanol; ***USA:*** Anthra-Derm; Dritho-Scalp; Drithocreme; Psoriatec.

**Multi-ingredient:** ***Austral.:*** Dithrasal; ***Austria:*** Anthraderm; ***Fr.:*** Anaxeryl; ***Ger.:*** Psoradexan; Psoralon MT; ***India:*** Derobin Skin; ***Irl.:*** Psoradrate†; ***Singapore:*** Dithrasal; ***Spain:*** Lapices Epiderm Metadier; Psorantral†; ***Switz.:*** Psoradexan†; ***UK:*** Psorin.

## Ecamsule *(USAN, rINN)*

Mexoryl SX. (±)-(3*E*,3′*E*)-3,3′-(*p*-Phenylenedimethylidyne)bis[2-oxo-10-bornanesulfonic acid]; Terephthalylidene-3,3′-dicamphor-10,10′-disulfonic acid.

$C_{28}H_{34}O_8S_2$ = 562.7.

*CAS — 92761-26-7.*

### Profile

Ecamsule, a camphorsulfonic acid derivative, is used as a sunscreen (see p.1133). It is effective against UVA light (for definitions, see p.1136).

### Preparations

**Proprietary Preparations**

Some preparations are listed in Part 3.

## Efalizumab *(USAN, rINN)*

Anti-CD11a; hu1124.

*CAS — 214745-43-4.*

*ATC — L04AA21.*

### Adverse Effects and Precautions

The most common adverse affects associated with efalizumab are chills, fever, headache, myalgia, and nausea. These reactions are dose-related in both incidence and severity and usually occur within two days following the first two injections. Other adverse effects include acne, flu-like symptoms, and an elevation in alkaline phosphatase concentrations. More serious adverse effects of efalizumab include arthritis, interstitial pneumonitis, hypersensitivity reactions, a worsening of psoriasis or development of variant forms, and thrombocytopenia. As a result of immunosuppression, patients given efalizumab are at increased risk of infection, and may be at increased risk of developing malignancies. It should not be given to patients with pre-existing serious infection and should be used with care in patients with a history of infection or malignancy.

Assessment of the platelet count is advised before starting therapy and monthly during early treatment. Frequency of monitoring may be decreased with ongoing treatment. Acellular, live, and live-attenuated vaccines should not be given during efalizumab treatment.

Treatment should be discontinued in patients who develop hypersensitivity reactions, and should not be resumed.

## Uses and Administration

Efalizumab is a humanised monoclonal antibody that binds to human CD11a on leucocytes to inhibit the activation of T-lymphocytes. It is used for the treatment of chronic moderate to severe plaque psoriasis (p.1137) and is considered to be suppressive therapy as continued therapy is required to maintain the initial response. Efalizumab is given by subcutaneous injection. The initial dose is 700 micrograms/kg, followed by a weekly dose of 1 mg/kg; a single dose should not exceed 200 mg.

◊ References.


1. Lebwohl M, *et al.* A novel targeted T-cell modulator, efalizumab, for plaque psoriasis. *N Engl J Med* 2003; **349:** 2004–13.
2. Gordon KB, *et al.* Efalizumab for patients with moderate to severe plaque psoriasis: a randomized controlled trial. *JAMA* 2003; **290:** 3037–80. Correction. *ibid.* 2004; **291:** 1070.


### Preparations

**Proprietary Preparations** (details are given in Part 3)
***USA:*** Raptiva.

---

## Ensulizole *(USAN, rINN)*

Ensulizol; Phenylbenzimidazole Sulphonic Acid. 2-Phenyl-1H-benzimidazole-5-sulphonic acid.

$C_{13}H_{10}N_2O_3S$ = 274.3.
*CAS — 27503-81-7.*

**Pharmacopoeias.** In *US.*

**USP 27** (Ensulizole). A white to ivory-coloured, odourless powder. Practically insoluble in water and in oily solvents; soluble in alcohol; its salts are freely soluble in water. Store in airtight containers at a temperature of 8° to 15°.

### Profile

Ensulizole is used topically as a sunscreen (see p.1133).

### Preparations

**Proprietary Preparations**
Some preparations are listed in Part 3.

---

## Enzacamene *(USAN, rINN)*

Enzacameno; Methyl Benzylidene Camphor; 3-(4-Methylbenzylidene)bornan-2-one; 3-(4-Methylbenzylidene)camphor. 1,7,7-Trimethyl-3-[(4-methylphenyl)methylene]bicyclo[2.2.1]heptan-2-one.

$C_{18}H_{22}O$ = 254.4.
*CAS — 36861-47-9 (D,L-form); 38102-62-4 (form unspecified).*

**Pharmacopoeias.** In *US.*

**USP 27** (Enzacamene). A white, fine crystalline powder. M.p. between 66° and 68°. Practically insoluble in water; freely soluble in alcohol; very soluble in chloroform. Store in airtight containers.

### Profile

Enzacamene is a camphor derivative used as a sunscreen (see p.1133). It is effective against UVB light (for definitions, see p.1136).

### Preparations

**Proprietary Preparations**
Numerous preparations are listed in Part 3.

---

## Ethyl Lactate

Lactato de etilo.

$C_5H_{10}O_3$ = 118.1.
*CAS — 97-64-3.*

### Profile

Ethyl lactate has been applied topically in the treatment of acne vulgaris. It is reported to lower the pH within the skin thereby exerting a bactericidal effect.

Ethyl lactate is also used in the flavouring of foods.

---

## Etretinate *(BAN, USAN, rINN)*

Etretinato; Ro-10-9359. Ethyl 3-methoxy-15-apo-φ-caroten-15-oate; Ethyl (*all-trans*)-9-(4-methoxy-2,3,6-trimethylphenyl)-3,7-dimethylnona-2,4,6,8-tetra-enoate.

$C_{23}H_{30}O_3$ = 354.5.
*CAS — 54350-48-0.*
*ATC — D05BB01.*

### Adverse Effects and Precautions

As for Isotretinoin, p.1148.

Donation of blood should be avoided for at least 2 years after cessation of treatment. The period of time during which pregnancy must be avoided following cessation of treatment has not been determined; detectable plasma-etretinate concentrations have been reported nearly 3 years after stopping treatment.

◊ In addition to the references cited below under the various headings, further references to the adverse effects of etretinate can be found in Isotretinoin, p.1149, under Effects on the Blood, Eyes, Liver, Musculoskeletal System, Serum Lipids, and the Skin as well as under Vasculitic Syndromes.

**Carcinogenicity.** A report of 2 patients developing lymphomas while receiving etretinate[1] prompted a report of 3 other malignancies in patients taking etretinate.[2]


1. Woll PJ, *et al.* Lymphoma in patients taking etretinate. *Lancet* 1987; **ii:** 563–4.
2. Harrison PV. Retinoids and malignancy. *Lancet* 1987; **ii:** 801.


**Effects on the cardiovascular system.** The Italian Ministry of Health recommended[1] that the ECG, blood lipids, and clotting factors should be monitored before, and throughout, treatment with etretinate as there had been rare suspected cases of myocardial ischaemia and infarction.


1. Anonymous. Reports from regulatory agencies: etretinate. *WHO Drug Inf* 1987; **1:** 29.


**Effects on the kidneys.** A report of impaired renal function associated with etretinate in a patient.[1] It was noted that in manufacturer-sponsored studies the mean serum-creatinine concentration had been raised in patients receiving etretinate.


1. Horber FF, *et al.* Impaired renal function and hypercalcaemia associated with etretinate. *Lancet* 1984; **ii:** 1093.


**Oedema.** A report of generalised oedema following treatment with etretinate.[1] Five other cases had been reported in the literature and rechallenge in 4 patients had provoked a recurrence.


1. Allan S, Christmas T. Severe edema associated with etretinate. *J Am Acad Dermatol* 1988; **19:** 140.


### Interactions

As for Isotretinoin, p.1150.

**Methotrexate.** The risk of developing hepatotoxicity may be increased when etretinate is used with methotrexate (see Retinoids, p.571).

**Oral contraceptives.** For discussion of the potential interactions of retinoids with hormonal contraceptives, and the effect this might have on contraceptive choice during retinoid treatment, see p.1534.

**Warfarin.** Etretinate has been reported to reduce the therapeutic efficacy of warfarin (see p.1026).

### Pharmacokinetics

The mean bioavailability of etretinate is about 40% following oral doses but there is a large interindividual variation. Absorption can be increased if taken with milk or fatty food. Etretinate undergoes significant first-pass metabolism and plasma concentrations of the active carboxylic acid metabolite, acitretin (p.1140), may be detected before those of the parent drug; acitretin may itself be metabolised to etretinate (p.1140). Both etretinate and acitretin are extensively bound to plasma protein. Etretinate appears to accumulate in adipose tissue after repeated dosing and has a prolonged elimination half-life of about 120 days; detectable serum concentrations have been observed up to 3 years after the discontinuation of therapy. Up to 75% of a dose is excreted in the faeces mainly as unchanged drug. Etretinate is also excreted in the urine as metabolites. Etretinate crosses the placenta and is distributed into breast milk.

◊ References.


1. Brazzell RK, Colburn WA. Pharmacokinetics of the retinoids isotretinoin and etretinate. *J Am Acad Dermatol* 1982; **6:** 643–51.
2. Rollman O, Vahlquist A. Retinoid concentrations in skin, serum and adipose tissue of patients treated with etretinate. *Br J Dermatol* 1983; **109:** 439–47.
3. Colburn WA, *et al.* Effect of meals on the kinetics of etretinate. *J Clin Pharmacol* 1985; **25:** 583–9.
4. Lucek RW, Colburn WA. Clinical pharmacokinetics of the retinoids. *Clin Pharmacokinet* 1985; **10:** 38–62.
5. DiGiovanna JJ, *et al.* Etretinate: persistent serum levels after long-term therapy. *Arch Dermatol* 1989; **125:** 246–51.


### Uses and Administration

Etretinate is a retinoid and is a derivative of tretinoin (p.1161). It has been given by mouth for the treatment of severe, extensive psoriasis that has not responded to other treatment, especially generalised and palmo-plantar pustular psoriasis. It has also been used in severe congenital ichthyosis, severe Darier's disease (keratosis follicularis) as well as other disorders of keratinisation, and oral lichen planus. Acitretin (p.1140) is now preferred to etretinate.

Therapy generally started at doses of 0.75 to 1 mg/kg daily in divided doses by mouth. A maximum dose of 1.5 mg/kg daily should not be exceeded (some sources have suggested a maximum of 75 mg daily). Erythrodermic psoriasis may respond to lower initial doses of 250 micrograms/kg daily, increased at weekly intervals by 250 micrograms/kg daily until optimal response occurs. Following the initial response, generally after 8 to 16 weeks of therapy, maintenance doses of 500 to 750 micrograms/kg daily have been given. Therapy should be discontinued once lesions have sufficiently resolved.

### Preparations

**Proprietary Preparations** (details are given in Part 3)
***Braz.:*** Tigason†; ***Ital.:*** Tigason†; ***Jpn:*** Tigason; ***USA:*** Tegison†.

---

## Fumaric Acid

Allomalenic Acid; Boletic Acid; E297; Fumárico, ácido. *trans*-Butenedioic acid.

$C_2H_2(CO_2H)_2$ = 116.1.
*CAS — 110-17-8 (fumaric acid); 624-49-7 (dimethyl fumarate).*
*ATC — D05AX01.*

**Pharmacopoeias.** In *Pol.* Also in *USNF.*

**USNF 22** (Fumaric Acid). White, odourless granules or crystalline powder. Slightly soluble in water and in ether; soluble in alcohol; very slightly soluble in chloroform.

### Profile

Fumaric acid and some of its derivatives have been used in the treatment of psoriasis and other skin disorders.

Fumaric acid is also used as an acidifier and flavouring agent in foods.

**Skin disorders.** Fumaric acid, its sodium salts, and derivatives such as dimethyl fumarate, monoethyl fumarate (ethyl hydrogen fumarate), and octil hydrogen fumarate have been used, both topically and systemically, in the treatment of psoriasis (p.1137) and other skin disorders. Dimethyl fumarate appears to be the most active compound given orally but combination with various salts of monoethyl fumarate has been claimed to improve efficacy.[1-6] However, there have been reports of acute renal failure associated with treatment and the German Federal Office of Health has expressed the opinion that the available evidence did not establish the value of fumaric acid derivatives in psoriasis or other skin disorders.[7] A subsequent retrospective analysis of 41 patients who received fumaric acid esters orally, for between 1 and 14 years, suggested that they might be effective. Reported adverse effects were generally mild, with only 1 case of elevated serum creatinine; however, lymphocytopenia was noted in 76% of patients and treatment consequently stopped in 4 patients.[8] Other adverse effects with oral therapy have included disturbances of liver function,[3,9] gastrointestinal effects,[2-4,9,10] and flushing.[2-4,9,10] There has been a report of exanthema in a patient receiving dimethylfumarate for lichen planus.[11]


1. van Loenen AC, *et al.* Fumaarzuurtherapie: van fictie tot werkelijkheid? *Pharm Weekbl* 1989; **124:** 894–900.
2. Kolbach DN, Nieboer C. Fumaric acid therapy in psoriasis: a long-term retrospective study on the effect of fumaric acid combination (FAC-EC) therapy and dimethyl-fumaric acid ester (DMFAE) monotherapy. *Br J Dermatol* 1990; **123:** 534–5.
3. Nugteren-Huying WM, *et al.* Fumaric acid therapy for psoriasis: a randomized, double-blind, placebo-controlled study. *J Am Acad Dermatol* 1990; **22:** 311–12.
4. Altmeyer PJ, *et al.* Antipsoriatic effect of fumaric acid derivatives: results of a multicenter double-blind study in 100 patients. *J Am Acad Dermatol* 1994; **30:** 977–81.
5. Mrowietz U, *et al.* Treatment of severe psoriasis with fumaric acid esters: scientific background and guidelines for therapeutic use. *Br J Dermatol* 1999; **141:** 424–9.
6. Ständer H, *et al.* Efficacy of fumaric acid ester monotherapy in psoriasis pustulosa palmoplantaris. *Br J Dermatol* 2003; **149:** 220–2.
7. Anonymous. Fumaric acid derivatives and nephrotoxicity. *WHO Drug Inf* 1990; **4:** 28.
8. Hoefnagel JJ, *et al.* Long-term safety aspects of systemic therapy with fumaric acid esters in severe psoriasis. *Br J Dermatol* 2003; **149:** 363–9.
9. Nieboer C, *et al.* Systemic therapy with fumaric acid derivates: new possibilities in the treatment of psoriasis. *J Am Acad Dermatol* 1989; **20:** 601–8.
10. Mrowietz U, *et al.* Treatment of psoriasis with fumaric acid esters: results of a prospective multicentre study. *Br J Dermatol* 1998; **138:** 456–60.
11. Guenther CH, *et al.* Macular exanthema due to fumaric acid esters. *Ann Pharmacother* 2003; **37:** 234–6.


### Preparations

**Proprietary Preparations** (details are given in Part 3)
***Ger.:*** Psoriasis-Solution; Psoriasis-Tabletten.

**Multi-ingredient:** ***Austral.:*** Pro-PS†; ***Ger.:*** Fumaderm; Psoriasis-Bad; Psoriasis-Salbe M†; Psoriasis-Salbe S.

---

## Glycolic Acid

Glicólico, ácido; Hydroxyacetic Acid. Hydroxyethanoic acid.

$C_2H_4O_3$ = 76.05.

### Profile

Glycolic acid is an organic acid that has been used in topical preparations for hyperpigmentation and photodamaged skin.

### Preparations

**Proprietary Preparations** (details are given in Part 3)
***Arg.:*** Alfabase 8; ***Canad.:*** Neostrata; Reversa; ***Chile:*** Alastik; Neosolets; Teen Derm; ***Hong Kong:*** Glyderm; ***Ital.:*** Neostrata; Revitalizing; ***Malaysia:*** Glyderm; ***Mex.:*** Glicoderm; Nova Derm; ***Singapore:*** Glyderm.

**Multi-ingredient:** ***Arg.:*** Effalpha; Hydragenic; Keracnyl; Melacler; Negacne; Neoquin; Neoquin Forte; Neostrata; Neostrata Gel Despigmentante; ***Austral.:*** Neostrata†; ***Canad.:*** Biobase-G; Dilusol AHA; Neostrata AHA Blemish; Neostrata AHA Daytime; Neostrata AHA Smoothing and Moisturizing; Reversa AHA HQ†; Reversa UV; Viquin Forte; ***Chile:*** Alastik; D 4; Neostrata; Neutrogena Healthy Skin; Neutrogena Limpiadora; Primacy C+AHA; Ureadin Forte; ***Fr.:*** Alpha 5 DS; Hyfac Plus; Item Alphakeptol; Keracnyl; Nightpeel; ***Hong Kong:*** Glyquin; ***Ital.:*** Acnesan; Lightening; NeoCeuticals Spot Treatment; Phytic Acid; Same-Seb Beta; Sebacnol; ***Mex.:*** Nova Derm; ***Port.:*** Bioclin Sebo Care; Eutrofic Forte Gel Despigmentante†; Hyfac AHA†; Ureadin 30; Ureadin Forte; ***Singapore:*** AHA Skin Lightening Gel†; Glyquin; ***USA:*** Glyquin-XM.

### Homosalate *(USAN, rINN)*

Homomenthyl Salicylate; Homosalato. 3,3,5-Trimethylcyclohexyl salicylate.
$C_{16}H_{22}O_3$ = 262.3.
*CAS — 118-56-9.*

**Pharmacopoeias.** In *US.*

**USP 27** (Homosalate). Store in airtight containers.

#### Profile

Homosalate, a substituted salicylate, is a sunscreen (see p.1133) with actions similar to those of octisalate (p.1154). It is effective against UVB light (for definitions, see p.1136).

#### Preparations

**Proprietary Preparations**
Numerous preparations are listed in Part 3.

## Hydroquinone

Hidroquinona; Hydrochinonum; Quinol. 1,4-Benzenediol.
$C_6H_6O_2$ = 110.1.
*CAS — 123-31-9.*
*ATC — D11AX11.*

NOTE. Do not confuse with Hydroquinine (p.1699).

**Pharmacopoeias.** In *US.*

**USP 27** (Hydroquinone). Fine white needles which darken on exposure to light and air. Soluble 1 in 17 of water, 1 in 4 of alcohol, 1 in 51 of chloroform, and 1 in 16.5 of ether. Store in airtight containers. Protect from light.

#### Adverse Effects, Treatment, and Precautions

Topical hydroquinone may cause transient erythema and a mild burning sensation. High concentrations or prolonged use may produce hyperpigmentation especially on areas of skin exposed to sunlight. Occasionally hypersensitivity has occurred and some recommend skin testing before use. Hydroquinone should not be applied to abraded or sunburnt skin. It should not be used to bleach eyelashes or eyebrows and contact with the eyes should be avoided as it may produce staining and corneal opacities. The systemic effects of hydroquinone and their treatment are similar to those of phenol (see p.1188) but tremors and convulsions may also occur.

**Effects on the liver.** Toxic hepatitis in a radiographer was attributed to occupational exposure to hydroquinone fumes from the developing medium used in the darkroom.[1] However, it has been pointed out[2] that hydroquinone is not volatile under normal conditions of use and that surveillance of 879 people engaged in the manufacture and use of hydroquinone from 1942 to 1990 found no association between toxic hepatitis and hydroquinone exposure.

1. Nowak AK, *et al.* Darkroom hepatitis after exposure to hydroquinone. *Lancet* 1995; **345:** 1187.
2. O'Donaghue JL, *et al.* Hydroquinone and hepatitis. *Lancet* 1995; **346:** 1427–8.

**Effects on the skin.** The incidence of exogenous ochronosis (blue-black hyperpigmentation) in a survey of black South African patients was found to be 15% in males and 42% in females with 69% of affected individuals admitting to using hydroquinone-containing preparations.[1] This was considered to be more consistent with a toxic side-effect of a drug with a low therapeutic index, rather than an idiosyncratic reaction. The data revealed that even preparations with hydroquinone 2% or less with a sunscreen produced ochronosis. Ochronosis usually became apparent after about 6 months of use and, once established, was probably irreversible. Patients may initially use skin lighteners for cosmetic purposes but once ochronosis develops they may fall into the 'skin lightener trap' as they use other hydroquinone preparations to remove the disfigurement.[1] The problems caused by over-the-counter skin-lightening creams in countries such as the UK have also been highlighted.[2] Reversible brown discoloration of the nails has also been reported following the use of skin lighteners containing hydroquinone.[3]

1. Hardwick N, *et al.* Exogenous ochronosis: an epidemiological study. *Br J Dermatol* 1989; **120:** 229–38.
2. Williams H. Skin lightening creams containing hydroquinone. *BMJ* 1992; **305:** 903–4.
3. Mann RJ, Harman RRM. Nail staining due to hydroquinone skin-lightening creams. *Br J Dermatol* 1983; **108:** 363–5.

#### Uses and Administration

Hydroquinone increases melanin excretion from melanocytes and may also prevent its production. Hydroquinone is used topically as a depigmenting agent for the skin in hyperpigmentation conditions (p.1137) such as chloasma (melasma), freckles, and lentigines (small macules that resemble freckles). Concentrations of 2 to 4% are commonly used; higher concentrations may be very irritant and increase the risk of ochronosis. It may be several weeks before any effect is apparent but depigmentation may last for 2 to 6 months after discontinuation. Application of hydroquinone should be discontinued if there is no improvement after 2 months. Hydroquinone should be applied twice daily only to intact skin which should be protected from sunlight to reduce repigmentation. Hydroquinone preparations often include a sunscreen or a sunblocking basis.

Hydroquinone is also used as an antoxidant for ether and in photographic developers.

#### Preparations

***USP 27:*** Hydroquinone Cream; Hydroquinone Topical Solution.

**Proprietary Preparations** (details are given in Part 3)
***Arg.:*** Claripel; ***Braz.:*** Clariderm†; Claripel; Solaquin; ***Canad.:*** African Gold; Banishing Cream; Eldopaque; Eldoquin; Esoterica Regular; Esoterica Unscented; Jouvence†; Lustra; Nadinola; Neostrata AHA HQ; Porcelana Nighttime Formula; Ultraquin Plain; ***Chile:*** Etnoderm; ***Fr.:*** Aida†; Creme des 3 Fleurs d'Orient†; ***Hong Kong:*** Eldopaque; Eldoquin; Solaquin; ***Ital.:*** Discromil†; Epocler†; ***Malaysia:*** Eldopaque; Eldoquin; ***Mex.:*** Crema Blanca; Eldopaque; Eldoquin; Hidroquin; Melanex; ***NZ:*** Eldoquin; ***Singapore:*** Aida†; Eldopaque; Eldoquin; Melanex†; Melanox†; Polyquin; Solaquin; ***Spain:*** Hidroquilaude; Licostrata; Melanasa; Nadona; Pigmentasa; ***UK:*** Eldopaque; Eldoquin; Esoterica†; Solaquin; ***USA:*** Claripel; Eldopaque; Eldoquin; EpiQuin; Esoterica Regular; Lustra; Melanex†; Solaquin.

**Multi-ingredient:** ***Arg.:*** Melacler; Melasmax; Neoceuticals Crema Despigmentante de Dia; Neoquin; Neoquin Forte; Neostrata Gel Despigmentante; Solaquin Forte; ***Austral.:*** Superfade†; ***Canad.:*** Esoterica; Lustra-AF; Porcelana Daytime Formula; Reversa AHA HQ†; Skinicles†; Solaquin Forte; Ultraquin; Viquin Forte; ***Chile:*** Alastik; Clasifel; D 4; Neostrata; Trio-D; ***Fr.:*** Melanex Duo†; ***Ger.:*** Pigmanorm; ***Hong Kong:*** Glyquin; ***Malaysia:*** Solaquin Forte; ***Mex.:*** Clasifel; Nova Derm; Quinoret; Solaquin; ***Port.:*** Eutrofic Forte Gel Despigmentante†; Melanex Duo†; ***Singapore:*** AHA Skin Lightening Gel†; Glyquin; High Potency Lightening Serum†; ***Switz.:*** Pigmanorm; ***USA:*** Ambi Skin Tone†; Esoterica Facial and Sunscreen; Glyquin-XM; Solaquin Forte; Tri-Luma.

### Ichthammol *(BAN)*

Ammonii Sulfogyrodalas; Ammonio Sulfoittiolato; Ammonium Bithiolicum; Ammonium Bitumenosulfonicum; Ammonium Bituminosulphonate; Ammonium Ichthosulphonate; Ammonium Sulfobituminosum; Ammonium Sulpho-Ichthyolate; Bithiolate Ammonique; Bithyol; Bituminol; Ichthammolum; Ichthosulphol; Ichthyol; Ichthyolammonium; Ictiol.
*CAS — 8029-68-3.*

**Pharmacopoeias.** In *Chin., Eur.* (see p.vi), *Jpn, Pol.,* and *US.*

**Ph. Eur. 5.0** (Ichthammol). A dense blackish-brown liquid. It is obtained by distillation of certain bituminous schists, sulfonation of the distillate, and neutralisation of the product with ammonia. It contains not less than 4.5% and not more than 7.0% of total ammonia, not less than 10.5% of organically combined sulfur, calculated with reference to the dried substance, and not more than 20% of the total sulfur in the form of sulfates.

Miscible with water and with glycerol; slightly soluble in alcohol, in fatty oils, and in liquid paraffin; forms homogeneous mixtures with wool fat and soft paraffin.

**USP 27** (Ichthammol). A reddish-brown to brownish-black viscous fluid with a strong characteristic empyreumatic odour. It is obtained by the destructive distillation of a bituminous schist, sulfonation of the distillate, and neutralisation of the product with ammonia. It yields not less than 10.0% of total sulfur and not less than 2.5% of ammonia. Miscible with water, with glycerol, and with fixed oils and fats. Partially soluble in alcohol and in ether.

**Incompatibility.** Ichthammol is incompatible with wool alcohols.

#### Profile

Ichthammol has slight bacteriostatic properties and is used in a wide range of topical preparations, for a variety of skin disorders; it has also been used in suppositories for anorectal disorders. Ichthammol is often used with zinc oxide in medicated bandages for chronic lichenified eczema (p.1135). Ichthammol may be slightly irritant to the skin and there have been rare reports of hypersensitivity.

Light Ammonium Bituminosulfonate (Ammoniumbituminosulfonat Hell) is produced from the light distillate fraction of shale oil.

Ammoniumsulfobitol, an ammonium bituminosulfonate similar to ichthammol but with a low sulfur content, is commercially available as Tumenol Ammonium.

#### Preparations

***BP 2003:*** Zinc and Ichthammol Cream;
***USP 27:*** Ichthammol Ointment.

**Proprietary Preparations** (details are given in Part 3)
***Austral.:*** Egoderm; ***Austria:*** Ichtho-Bad; Ichtholan; Ichtopur; ***Fr.:*** Gelictar; ***Ger.:*** Ichtho-Bad; Ichtholan; Ichtholan spezial; Ichthyol; Schwarze-Salbe†; Thiobitum; ***Switz.:*** Ichtho-Bad; Ichtholan.

**Multi-ingredient:** ***Arg.:*** Cicatrina; ***Austral.:*** Acnederm†; Egoderm; Icthaband; ***Austria:*** Aknemycin compositum; Delta-Hadensa; Hadensa; Ichth-Oestren; Inotyol; ***Belg.:*** Inotyol; Zinc-Ichtyol†; ***Canad.:*** Boil Ease; Ictholin†; ***Denm.:*** Inotyol; ***Fin.:*** Hadensa; ***Fr.:*** Anaxeryl; Gelictar Fort; Inotyol; Node DS; Oxythyol; Phytolithe; Provictol; ***Ger.:*** Aknemycin; Hoemarin Derma†; Rheumichthol Bad†; ***Hong Kong:*** Acnederm; Egoderm; ***Israel:*** Aknemycin; Inotyol; ***Ital.:*** Antiemorroidali; Bal Tar†; Dermatar; Ichthopaste; Inotyol; Tricoderm F; ***Malaysia:*** Acnederm; Egoderm; ***Norw.:*** Inotyol; ***NZ:*** Acnederm; Egoderm; ***Port.:*** Banholeum Composto; Efluvium Anti-caspa; Efluvium Anti-seborreico; Oleoban Composto; Pansebase Composto; Secpel Composto; ***S.Afr.:*** Antipeol; ***Singapore:*** Acnederm; Egoderm; ***Spain:*** Hadensa; Ictiomen; Lamnotyl; Queratil†; ***Swed.:*** Inotyol; ***Switz.:*** Aknemycin; Bain extra-doux dermatologique Nouvelle Formule; Furodermal; Furodermil†; Phlogidermil†; Riccomycine†; Riccovitan; ***UK:*** Antipeol; Ichthopaste; Icthaband; St James Balm; ***USA:*** Boil Ease; Boyol Salve; Medicone Derma.

### Ictasol *(USAN)*

Ichthyol-Natrium Hell; Light Sodium Bituminosulphonate; Natrium Sulfobituminosum Decoloratum.
$C_{28}H_{36}Na_2O_6S_3$ = 610.8.
*CAS — 12542-33-5; 1340-06-3.*

#### Profile

Ictasol is a sodium bituminosulfonate produced from the light distillate fraction of shale oil. Sodium bituminosulfonate is obtained by the destructive distillation of certain bituminous schists, sulfonation of the distillate, and neutralisation of the product with sodium hydroxide.

Ictasol has similar properties to ichthammol (above) and is used in a wide range of preparations for a variety of skin disorders.

#### Preparations

**Proprietary Preparations** (details are given in Part 3)
***Austria:*** Ichthraletten; Lavichthol; Solutio Cordes†; ***Ger.:*** Aknichthol Creme; Crino Cordes N; Dermichthol; Ichthoderm; Ichtholan T; Ichthosin; Ichthraletten; Leukichtan; Solutio Cordes.

**Multi-ingredient:** ***Austria:*** Aknichthol; Crino Cordes; Ichthalgan forte; Ichtho-Bellol; Ichtho-Cadmin†; Ichtho-Cortin; Leukichtan; Pelvichthol†; ***Chile:*** Ichtyosoft; ***Fr.:*** Ichtyosoft; Sebosquam†; ***Ger.:*** Aknederm Neu; Aknichthol N; Ichthalgan; Ichtho-Bellol; Ichtho-Bellol compositum S; Ichthocortin; Ichthoseptal; Pelvichthol N; ***Switz.:*** Aknichthol N.

### Isopropyldibenzoylmethane

Isopropildibenzoilmetano. 1-[4-(1-Methylethyl)phenyl]-3-phenyl-1,3-propanedione.
$C_{18}H_{18}O_2$ = 266.3.
*CAS — 63250-25-9.*

#### Profile

Isopropyldibenzoylmethane, a substituted dibenzoylmethane, is a sunscreen (see p.1133) with actions similar to those of avobenzone (p.1142). It absorbs UVA light (for definitions, see p.1136).

#### Preparations

**Proprietary Preparations**
Some preparations are listed in Part 3.

## Isotretinoin *(BAN, USAN, rINN)*

Isotretinoína; Isotretinoinum; 13-*cis*-Retinoic Acid; Ro-4-3780. (13*Z*)-15-Apo-β-caroten-15-oic acid; (2*Z*,4*E*,6*E*,8*E*)-3,7-Dimethyl-9-(2,6,6-trimethylcyclohex-1-enyl)nona-2,4,6,8-tetraenoic acid.
$C_{20}H_{28}O_2$ = 300.4.
*CAS — 4759-48-2.*
*ATC — D10AD04; D10BA01.*

**Pharmacopoeias.** In *Chin., Eur.* (see p.vi), *Pol.,* and *US.*

**Ph. Eur. 5.0** (Isotretinoin). A yellow or light orange, crystalline powder. Practically insoluble in water; slightly soluble in alcohol; soluble in dichloromethane. It is sensitive to air, heat, and light, especially in solution. Store in airtight containers at a temperature not exceeding 25°. Protect from light. It is recommended that the contents of an opened container be used as soon as possible and that any unused part be protected by an atmosphere of an inert gas.

**USP 27** (Isotretinoin). Yellow crystals. Practically insoluble in water; sparingly soluble in alcohol, in isopropyl alcohol, and in macrogol 400; soluble in chloroform. Store in airtight containers under an atmosphere of an inert gas. Protect from light.

#### Adverse Effects

The adverse effects of isotretinoin and other oral retinoids are similar to those of vitamin A (see p.1451) and are generally reversible and dose-related. The most common are dryness of the mucous membranes and of the skin with scaling, fragility, and erythema, especially of the face, cheilitis, pruritus, epistaxis, conjunctivitis, dry sore mouth, and palmo-plantar exfoliation. Corneal opacities, dry eyes, visual disturbances, skeletal hyperostosis, and musculoskeletal symptoms may also occur. Elevation of serum triglycerides, hepatic enzymes, erythrocyte sedimentation rate, and blood glucose have been reported. Pancreatitis may occur, in particular in patients with high triglyceride concentrations. Other effects have included hair thinning (occasionally irreversible), photosensitivity, changes in skin pigmentation, paronychia, gastrointestinal symptoms, jaundice or hepatitis, headache, drowsiness, sweating, mood changes, psychotic symptoms, depression, suicidal behaviour, benign intracranial hypertension, seizures, vasculitis, hypersensitivity reactions including anaphylaxis, and an association with skin infections and an inflammatory bowel syndrome.

Isotretinoin and other retinoids are teratogenic.

When isotretinoin is applied topically the adverse effects are similar to those of tretinoin (see p.1161).

◊ General references.


1. David M, *et al.* Adverse effects of retinoids. *Med Toxicol* 1988; **3:** 273–88.
2. Mills CM, Marks R. Adverse reactions to oral retinoids: an update. *Drug Safety* 1993; **9:** 280–90.
3. Keefe M. Adverse reactions profile: retinoids. *Prescribers' J* 1995; **35:** 71–6.


**Effects on the blood.** Thrombocytopenia has been reported in 2 patients receiving etretinate and in a patient treated with isotretinoin.[1] A further case reports the development of thrombocytopenia after three and a half months' treatment with isotretinoin.[2] There has also been a report of agranulocytosis associated with isotretinoin therapy in a 16-year-old boy.[3]


1. Naldi L, *et al.* Etretinate therapy and thrombocytopenia. *Br J Dermatol* 1991; **124:** 395.
2. Moeller KE, Touma SC. Prolonged thrombocytopenia associated with isotretinoin. *Ann Pharmacother* 2003; **37:** 1622–4.
3. Waisman M. Agranulocytosis from isotretinoin. *J Am Acad Dermatol* 1988; **18:** 395–6.


**Effects on the eyes.** Corneal opacities and papilloedema are among the more serious effects of isotretinoin on the eye but they are usually reversible if therapy is discontinued; papilloedema can result from benign intracranial hypertension[1,2] and patients receiving concomitant treatment with tetracyclines are particularly at risk.[2] Oral retinoids appear to interfere with retinal function[3] and there have been reports of alterations in colour sense,[4] poor night vision, and photophobia.[5] However, a 1-year follow-up failed to find any evidence of ocular toxicity attributable to etretinate in patients who had received long-term treatment and one patient who had toxic optic neuropathy due to methotrexate was able to continue treatment with etretinate.[6] A unilateral subconjunctival haemorrhage occurred during a 16-week course of isotretinoin in a patient being treated for acne.[7] An analysis[8] of 1741 spontaneous reports of ocular adverse effects concluded that there was a certain association between isotretinoin and abnormal meibomian gland secretion and gland atrophy, blepharoconjunctivitis, corneal opacities, decreased dark adaptation, decreased vision, increased tear osmolarity, keratitis, myopia, ocular discomfort and decreased tolerance to contact lenses, photophobia, and ocular sicca. There was also a probable association with reversible decreased colour vision and permanent loss of dark adaptation.

Ectropion has been associated with etretinate therapy in a patient.[9]


1. Fraunfelder FT, *et al.* Adverse ocular reactions possibly associated with isotretinoin. *Am J Ophthalmol* 1985; **100:** 534–7.
2. Gibberd B. Drug-induced benign intracranial hypertension. *Prescribers' J* 1991; **31:** 118–21.
3. Brown RD, Grattan CEH. Visual toxicity of synthetic retinoids. *Br J Ophthalmol* 1989; **73:** 286–8.
4. Weber U, *et al.* Abnormal retinal function associated with long-term etretinate? *Lancet* 1988; **i:** 235–6.
5. Weleber RG, *et al.* Abnormal retinal function associated with isotretinoin therapy for acne. *Arch Ophthalmol* 1986; **104:** 831–7.
6. Pitts JF, *et al.* Etretinate and visual function: a 1-year follow-up study. *Br J Dermatol* 1991; **125:** 53–5.
7. Azurdia RM, Sharpe GR. Isotretinoin treatment for acne vulgaris and its cutaneous and ocular side-effects. *Br J Dermatol* 1999; **141:** 947.
8. Fraunfelder FT, *et al.* Ocular side effects possibly associated with isotretinoin usage. *Am J Ophthalmol* 2001; **132:** 299–305.
9. Brenner S, *et al.* Ectropion: an adverse effect of etretinate therapy for psoriasis. *DICP Ann Pharmacother* 1990; **24:** 1007.


**Effects on the liver.** Transient slight elevations of serum concentrations of liver enzymes are common with etretinate, but there have been few reports of acute hepatitis[1,2] or cholestatic jaundice.[3] In one patient, acute hepatitis progressed to chronic active hepatitis, despite cessation of etretinate therapy[4] but studies of serial liver biopsies from patients receiving long-term etretinate have failed to show any significant chronic liver damage.[5-7] The manufacturers have reported instances of hepatic fibrosis, necrosis, and/or cirrhosis.

An overview considered that some form of hepatotoxicity may be seen in up to 20% of patients treated with etretinate and significant liver disease in 1%.[8]

Isotretinoin may also cause mild elevations of liver enzymes and the manufacturers state that jaundice and hepatitis have occurred rarely. There is also a report of fatty liver.[9]


1. Foged EK, Jacobsen FK. Side effects due to RO 10-9359 (Tigason). *Dermatologica* 1982; **164:** 395–403.
2. Weiss VC, *et al.* Hepatotoxic reactions in a patient treated with etretinate. *Arch Dermatol* 1984; **120:** 104–6.
3. Gavish D, *et al.* Cholestatic jaundice, an unusual side effect of etretinate. *J Am Acad Dermatol* 1985; **13:** 669–70.
4. Weiss VC, *et al.* Chronic active hepatitis associated with etretinate therapy. *Br J Dermatol* 1985; **112:** 591–7.
5. Glazer SD, *et al.* Ultrastructural survey and tissue analysis of human livers after a 6-month course of etretinate. *J Am Acad Dermatol* 1984; **10:** 632–8.
6. Foged E, *et al.* Histologic changes in the liver during etretinate treatment. *J Am Acad Dermatol* 1984; **11:** 580–3.
7. Roenigk HH, *et al.* Serial liver biopsies in psoriatic patients receiving long-term etretinate. *Br J Dermatol* 1985; **112:** 77–81.
8. Boyd AS. An overview of the retinoids. *Am J Med* 1989; **86:** 568–74.
9. Taylor AEM, Mitchison H. Fatty liver following isotretinoin therapy. *Br J Dermatol* 1991; **124:** 505–6.


**Effects on mental function.** Case reports provide evidence of depression, psychotic symptoms, suicide, and suicide attempts occurring as idiosyncratic adverse effects of isotretinoin. However, the high background prevalence of psychiatric illness among adolescents in general, and among patients with acne, are potentially confounding factors. Retrospective studies have not demonstrated a clear cause and effect mechanism and prospective trials have been limited by sample size. In the absence of better evidence, monitoring for depression and other psychiatric effects has been advised for all patients receiving isotretinoin.[1-5]

Two cases of sustained dreaming have also been reported. After 2 to 3 weeks of oral isotretinoin, both patients reported changes in their dreaming pattern with a feeling that they had been 'dreaming all night'. The dreams persisted for 4 to 5 weeks after which they subsided despite continued isotretinoin therapy.[6]


1. Jick SS, *et al.* Isotretinoin use and risk of depression, psychotic symptoms, suicide, and attempted suicide. *Arch Dermatol* 2000; **136:** 1231–6.
2. Anonymous. Is Accutane really dangerous? *Med Lett Drugs Ther* 2002; **44:** 82.
3. Enders SJ, Enders JM. Isotretinoin and psychiatric illness in adolescents and young adults. *Ann Pharmacother* 2003; **37:** 1124–7.
4. Ng CH, Schweitzer I. The association between depression and isotretinoin use in acne. *Aust N Z J Psychiatry* 2003; **37:** 78–84.
5. Anonymous. Acne, isotretinoin and depression. *Drug Ther Bull* 2003; **41:** 76–8.
6. Gupta MA, Gupta AK. Isotretinoin use and reports of sustained dreaming. *Br J Dermatol* 2001; **144:** 919–20.


**Effects on the musculoskeletal system.** An ossification disorder resembling diffuse skeletal hyperostosis, with myalgia, arthralgia, and stiffness, was first reported in patients who had taken large doses of isotretinoin for prolonged periods.[1] Premature closure of the epiphyses in a child treated with isotretinoin has also been described.[2] A later report found radiographic evidence of extraspinal tendon and ligament calcification in patients who had received long-term therapy with etretinate[3] and there were reports of spinal hyperostosis[4] and one of spinal cord compression.[5] Some were unable to find radiographic skeletal changes after 6 to 18 months of treatment with etretinate[6] but others[7] found that hyperostosis was fairly common in patients taking moderately prolonged therapy and recommended that radiological examinations should be carried out every 12 months in patients taking etretinate. However, there was no clear association between these effects and the total dose or duration of treatment. Another study found evidence of changes after 4 months in patients who had taken isotretinoin 1 mg/kg daily and recommended that radiological examinations should be made every 6 months in patients receiving isotretinoin for more than a year.[8] However, a further study found that although 12% of patients receiving isotretinoin 500 micrograms/kg had evidence of hyperostoses this was not clinically significant in any patient.[9] It has been suggested that monitoring beyond the treatment period might be unnecessary as calcifications and hyperostosis in patients who had received isotretinoin for 3 years had neither progressed nor improved 10 to 24 months after the end of treatment; additionally no new hyperostoses had developed during that period.[10] Of 25 patients treated with acitretin for a mean of 5 years one had abnormal calcification thought to be caused by the drug;[11] therapy with acitretin was continued with no further side-effects. The authors recommended radiological examinations after twelve months of treatment and then every second year. A study in 135 patients[12] who had received oral retinoids for a mean of 30 months could establish no relationship between spinal abnormalities and prolonged oral retinoid treatment and the authors suggested that spinal abnormalities only occur sporadically in predisposed patients.

There have also been individual reports of hypercalciuria[7] or hypercalcaemia[13-15] associated with oral retinoid therapy. Oral retinoids may also cause muscle damage;[16,17] myositis has been reported with tretinoin[18] and severe myopathy with acitretin.[19]


1. Pittsley RA, Yoder FW. Retinoid hyperostosis: skeletal toxicity associated with long-term administration of 13-cis-retinoic acid for refractory ichthyosis. *N Engl J Med* 1983; **308:** 1012–14.
2. Milstone LM, *et al.* Premature epiphyseal closure in a child receiving oral 13-cis-retinoic acid. *J Am Acad Dermatol* 1982; **7:** 663–6.
3. DiGiovanna JJ, *et al.* Extraspinal tendon and ligament calcification associated with long-term therapy with etretinate. *N Engl J Med* 1986; **315:** 1177–82.
4. Archer CB, *et al.* Spinal hyperostosis and etretinate. *Lancet* 1987; **i:** 741.
5. Tfelt-Hansen P, *et al.* Spinal cord compression after long-term etretinate. *Lancet* 1989; **ii:** 325–6.
6. Gilbert M, *et al.* Lack of skeletal radiographic changes during short-term etretinate therapy for psoriasis. *Dermatologica* 1986; **172:** 160–3.
7. Wilson DJ, *et al.* Skeletal hyperostosis and extraosseous calcification in patients receiving long-term etretinate (Tigason). *Br J Dermatol* 1988; **119:** 597–607.
8. Török L, *et al.* Bone-scintigraphic examinations in patients treated with retinoids: a prospective study. *Br J Dermatol* 1989; **120:** 31–6.
9. Carey BM, *et al.* Skeletal toxicity with isotretinoin therapy: a clinico-radiological evaluation. *Br J Dermatol* 1988; **119:** 609–14.
10. Tangrea JA, *et al.* Isotretinoin and the axial skeleton. *Lancet* 1992; **340:** 495–6.
11. Mørk N-J, *et al.* Skeletal side-effects of 5 years' acitretin treatment. *Br J Dermatol* 1996; **134:** 1156–7.
12. Van Dooren-Greebe RJ, *et al.* Prolonged treatment with oral retinoids in adults: no influence on the frequency and severity of spinal abnormalities. *Br J Dermatol* 1996; **134:** 71–6.
13. Valentic JP, *et al.* Hypercalcemia associated with oral isotretinoin in the treatment of severe acne. *JAMA* 1983; **250:** 1899–1900.
14. Horber FF, *et al.* Impaired renal function and hypercalcaemia associated with etretinate. *Lancet* 1984; **ii:** 1093.
15. Akiyama H, *et al.* Hypercalcaemia due to all-trans retinoic acid. *Lancet* 1992; **339:** 308–9.
16. Hodak E, *et al.* Muscle damage induced by isotretinoin. *BMJ* 1986; **293:** 425–6.
17. David M, *et al.* Electromyographic abnormalities in patients undergoing long-term therapy with etretinate. *J Am Acad Dermatol* 1988; **19:** 273–5.
18. Miranda N, *et al.* Myositis with tretinoin. *Lancet* 1994; **334:** 1096.
19. Lister RK, *et al.* Acitretin-induced myopathy. *Br J Dermatol* 1996; **134:** 989–90.


**Effects on the respiratory system.** There have been reports of exercise-induced wheezing,[1] eosinophilic pleural effusion,[2] and worsening asthma[3,4] associated with isotretinoin therapy. The US manufacturers have records of adverse effects on the lung including worsening asthma, recurrent pneumothorax, interstitial fibrosis, and pulmonary granuloma.[5] A study of healthy subjects confirmed that lung function tests could deteriorate after treatment with isotretinoin.[5]


1. Fisher DA. Exercise-induced bronchoconstriction related to isotretinoin therapy. *J Am Acad Dermatol* 1985; **13:** 524.
2. Bunker CB, *et al.* Isotretinoin and eosinophilic pleural effusion. *Lancet* 1989; **i:** 435–6.
3. Sabroe RA, *et al.* Bronchospasm induced by isotretinoin. *BMJ* 1996; **312:** 886.
4. Kapur N, *et al.* Exacerbation of asthma by isotretinoin. *Br J Dermatol* 2000; **142:** 388–9.
5. Bunker CB, *et al.* Isotretinoin and the lung. *Br J Dermatol* 1991; **125** (suppl 38): 29.


**Effects on serum lipids.** The oral retinoids induce dose-dependent changes in serum lipids. There can be increases in very-low-density-lipoprotein cholesterol with smaller increases in low-density-lipoprotein cholesterol and reductions in high-density-lipoprotein cholesterol.[1,2] These effects appear to be unrelated to age or sex. They occur early during treatment and are usually reversible within a few weeks of discontinuation. Overall, the effect of isotretinoin is much greater than that of etretinate. Although the total cholesterol and triglyceride concentrations may remain within normal limits, types IIb and IV hyperlipidaemias are not uncommon among patients receiving oral retinoids. Pancreatitis may be associated with hypertriglyceridaemia in patients treated with isotretinoin.[3]

Retinoids should be used with caution in patients with pre-existing hypertriglyceridaemia or in those at risk of developing hypertriglyceridaemia.[1] Use of fish oil containing eicosapentaenoic acid has been reported to attenuate retinoid-induced increases in serum-cholesterol and serum-triglyceride concentrations.[2,4]


1. Henkin Y, *et al.* Secondary dyslipidemia: inadvertent effects of drugs in clinical practice. *JAMA* 1992; **267:** 961–8.
2. Mantel-Teeuwisse AK, *et al.* Drug-induced lipid changes: a review of the unintended effects of some commonly used drugs on serum lipid levels. *Drug Safety* 2001; **24:** 443–56.
3. Flynn WJ, *et al.* Pancreatitis associated with isotretinoin-induced hypertriglyceridemia. *Ann Intern Med* 1987; **107:** 63.
4. Marsden JR. Effect of dietary fish oil on hyperlipidaemia due to isotretinoin and etretinate. *Hum Toxicol* 1987; **6:** 219–22.


**Effects on sexual function.** Ejaculatory failure has been reported in 3 men to be associated with isotretinoin treatment.[1] A possible mechanism could be an effect on the goblet cells of the seminal vesicles, an effect similar to the general reduction in body secretions which leads to dry mucous membranes.


1. Coleman R, MacDonald D. Effects of isotretinoin on male reproductive system. *Lancet* 1994; **344:** 198.


**Effects on the skin, hair, and nails.** Apart from the more common effects of oral retinoids on the skin and hair (see Adverse Effects, above), there have been isolated reports of granulomatous lesions,[1-3] precipitation or exacerbation of erythroderma,[4,5] palmo-plantar eruptions,[6] prurigo-like eruptions,[7] scalp folliculitis,[8] pyoderma gangrenosum,[8,9] palmo-plantar stickiness,[10] curling hair,[11] and chloasma (melasma).[12] There has been a report of fatal toxic epidermal necrolysis associated with etretinate.[13] Acne fulminans has been reported as a complication of isotretinoin treatment[14] although there have also been cases of acne fulminans being treated successfully with isotretinoin.[15] For other reports of acne fulminans and eruptions associated with vasculitic syndromes, see below. Skin erosion following wax depilation has been reported in patients receiving retinoids (see Skin Fragility under Precautions, below).

Oral retinoids have been associated with paronychia and other forms[16] of nail dystrophy.


1. Lane PR, Hogan DJ. Granulomatous lesions appearing during isotretinoin therapy. *Can Med Assoc J* 1984; **130:** 550.
2. Williamson DM, Greenwood R. Multiple pyogenic granulomata occurring during etretinate therapy. *Br J Dermatol* 1983; **109:** 615–17.
3. Kanoh H, *et al.* Granulomatous nodule on vocal cord possibly induced by etretinate therapy. *Br J Dermatol* 2000; **142:** 1258–60.
4. Wantzin GL, Thomsen K. A new cutaneous side effect of isotretinoin. *J Am Acad Dermatol* 1985; **13:** 665.
5. Levin J, Almeyda J. Erythroderma due to etretinate. *Br J Dermatol* 1985; **112:** 373.
6. David M, *et al.* Palmoplantar eruption associated with etretinate therapy. *Acta Derm Venereol (Stockh)* 1986; **66:** 87–9.
7. Boer J, Smeenk G. Nodular prurigo-like eruptions induced by etretinate. *Br J Dermatol* 1987; **116:** 271–4.

8. Hughes BR, Cunliffe WJ. Development of folliculitis and pyoderma gangrenosum in association with abdominal pain in a patient following treatment with isotretinoin. *Br J Dermatol* 1990; **122:** 683–7.
9. Gangaram HB, *et al.* Pyoderma gangrenosum following treatment with isotretinoin. *Br J Dermatol* 1997; **136:** 636–7.
10. Penneys NS, Hernandez D. A sticky problem with etretinate. *N Engl J Med* 1991; **325:** 521.
11. van der Pijl JW, *et al.* Isotretinoin and azathioprine: a synergy that makes hair curl? *Lancet* 1996; **348:** 622–3.
12. Burke H, Carmichael AJ. Reversible melasma associated with isotretinoin. *Br J Dermatol* 1996; **135:** 862.
13. McIvor A. Fatal toxic epidermal necrolysis associated with etretinate. *BMJ* 1992; **304:** 548.
14. Huston NR, Mules R. Acne fulminans with severe myalgia precipitated by isotretinoin therapy. *N Z Med J* 1985; **36:** 821.
15. Darley CR, *et al.* Acne fulminans with arthritis in identical twins treated with isotretinoin. *J R Soc Med* 1984; **77:** 328–30.
16. Dharmagunawardena B, Charles-Holmes R. Median canaliform dystrophy following isotretinoin therapy. *Br J Dermatol* 1997; **137:** 658–9.

PHOTOTOXICITY. *In vitro* photohaemolysis studies demonstrated that tretinoin and isotretinoin have a phototoxic potential while etretinate has none.[1] However, acitretin, the major metabolite of etretinate, had a phototoxic potential greater than that of tretinoin. The apparently low incidence of photosensitivity suggested that an idiosyncrasy is responsible. Patients should use appropriate photoprotection against UVA and UVB light.

1. Ferguson J, Johnson BE. Photosensitivity due to retinoids: clinical and laboratory studies. *Br J Dermatol* 1986; **115:** 275–83.

**Effects on taste.** Almost complete loss of taste has been reported in a patient given isotretinoin 600 micrograms/kg daily by mouth for 20 weeks.[1] Sense of taste returned about 6 months after isotretinoin was discontinued. Up to September 1994 the UK Committee on Safety of Medicines knew of 5 cases of taste changes, including 4 reports of loss of taste.

1. Halpern SM, *et al.* Loss of taste associated with isotretinoin. *Br J Dermatol* 1996; **134:** 378.

**Overdosage.** Apart from vague abdominal discomfort there were no other symptoms or significant abnormalities in a 15-year-old who was treated with gastric lavage 1.5 hours after ingestion of 350 mg of isotretinoin.[1] There was a similar outcome in the 2 other cases of isotretinoin overdosage reported in the literature.

1. Hepburn NC. Deliberate self-poisoning with isotretinoin. *Br J Dermatol* 1990; **122:** 840–1.

**Vasculitic syndromes.** The manufacturer of isotretinoin and etretinate has received isolated reports of vasculitis associated with the use of these oral retinoids; Wegener's granulomatosis has also been reported after the use of isotretinoin.[1,2] The precise mechanism underlying these effects is unknown; in some patients there may have been a direct toxic effect as symptoms developed shortly after the start of treatment, in other patients the onset was long-delayed and in some may have been triggered by the incidental use of antibacterials. Erythema nodosum and acne fulminans associated with circulating immune complexes had previously been reported after the use of isotretinoin.[3]

1. Dwyer JM, *et al.* Vasculitis and retinoids. *Lancet* 1989; **ii:** 494–6.
2. Anonymous. Retinoids and necrotizing vasculitis. *WHO Drug Inf* 1989; **3:** 187.
3. Kellett JK, *et al.* Erythema nodosum and circulating immune complexes in acne fulminans after treatment with isotretinoin. *BMJ* 1985; **290:** 820.

## Precautions

Isotretinoin and other oral retinoids are teratogenic and therefore contra-indicated in pregnant patients. It is advisable for female patients to commence using contraceptive measures one month before starting isotretinoin treatment. Pregnancy should be excluded before starting therapy and avoided during treatment and for 1 month after treatment has been withdrawn. Patients receiving isotretinoin should not donate blood during, or for 1 month after cessation of therapy. *Pregnancy or blood donation must be avoided for much longer periods in patients taking acitretin or etretinate.* Isotretinoin is contra-indicated in patients with hepatic and renal impairment, hyperlipidaemias, hypervitaminosis A, and in breast-feeding mothers. Isotretinoin should be used with care in patients with a history of depression and patients receiving isotretinoin should be monitored for signs of depressive illness.

Liver function and fasting blood lipids should be measured at the start of therapy, after the first month (or every 1 to 2 weeks for the first 2 months for acitretin), and thereafter as appropriate. Blood glucose should be monitored throughout treatment in patients who either have, or are predisposed to, diabetes mellitus. Some recommend routine radiological evaluation in patients receiving long-term therapy (see under Effects on the Musculoskeletal System, above). Patients may experience a reduced tolerance to contact lenses.

Excessive exposure to sunlight and UV light should be avoided.

When applied topically the precautions described under tretinoin (see p.1161) should be adopted.

**Pregnancy.** The problem of prescribing oral retinoids to women of child-bearing potential has been discussed.[1,2] Intra-uterine exposure to isotretinoin has caused spontaneous abortion and a characteristic pattern of fetal malformations involving craniofacial, cardiac, thymic, and CNS structures.[3,4] Some infants have also shown subnormal intelligence and other neuropsychological impairments.[5] The risk of malformation appears to be high at all therapeutic doses of isotretinoin even when the duration of exposure is short.[6] Despite warnings on the use of retinoids during pregnancy and the need for adequate contraception in women of child-bearing potential, and other strict guidelines on their use, intra-uterine exposure to retinoids has still occurred.[7,8]

Isotretinoin has a relatively short half-life and it has been recommended that conception should be avoided for at least one month after the end of treatment. A survey of women who conceived after the use of isotretinoin (64% within one month of discontinuation of treatment) suggested that the incidence of spontaneous abortion or congenital malformations was no greater than in the general population.[9]

However, patients taking oral retinoids with longer half-lives must avoid conception for much longer periods; at least 2 years (3 years in the US) is recommended if patients are taking acitretin although the period of time for patients taking etretinate has not been established. Malformations similar to those associated with isotretinoin have been reported in infants conceived within 2 years of stopping etretinate.[10-12]

Unless otherwise contra-indicated, oral combined contraceptives have been recommended as the contraceptive method of choice for women undergoing retinoid treatment.[13] The concomitant use of another form of contraception, such as a barrier method, is also recommended.[2,8] For further information on the use of hormonal contraceptives with retinoids, see p.1534.

1. Mitchell AA. Oral retinoids: what should the prescriber know about their teratogenic hazards among women of child-bearing potential? *Drug Safety* 1992; **7:** 79–85.
2. Chan A, *et al.* Oral retinoids and pregnancy. *Med J Aust* 1996; **165:** 164–7.
3. Lammer EJ, *et al.* Retinoic acid embryopathy. *N Engl J Med* 1985; **313:** 837–41.
4. Rosa F. Isotretinoin dose and teratogenicity. *Lancet* 1987; **ii:** 1154.
5. Adams J. High incidence of intellectual deficits in 5-year-old children exposed to isotretinoin 'in utero'. *Teratology* 1990; **41:** 614.
6. Dai WS, *et al.* Epidemiology of isotretinoin exposure during pregnancy. *J Am Acad Dermatol* 1992; **26:** 599–606.
7. Stern RS. When a uniquely effective drug is teratogenic: the case of isotretinoin. *N Engl J Med* 1989; **320:** 1007–9.
8. Atanackovic G, Koren G. Fetal exposure to oral isotretinoin: failure to comply with the Pregnancy Prevention Program. *Can Med Assoc J* 1999; **160:** 1719–20.
9. Dai WS, *et al.* Safety of pregnancy after discontinuation of isotretinoin. *Arch Dermatol* 1989; **125:** 362–5.
10. Grote W, *et al.* Malformation of fetus conceived 4 months after termination of maternal etretinate treatment. *Lancet* 1985; **i:** 1276.
11. Lammer EJ. Embryopathy in infant conceived one year after termination of maternal etretinate. *Lancet* 1988; **ii:** 1080–1.
12. Geiger J-M, *et al.* Teratogenic risk with etretinate and acitretin treatment. *Dermatology* 1994; **189:** 109–16.
13. Lehucher Ceyrac D, *et al.* Retinoids and contraception. *Dermatology* 1992; **184:** 161–70.

**Skin fragility.** Wax depilation should be avoided in patients receiving retinoids since they cause increased skin fragility and facial and leg erosions have occurred.[1-3] The UK manufacturers also recommend that wax depilation should be avoided for at least 6 months after isotretinoin treatment because of the risk of scarring and dermatitis, and that aggressive dermabrasion should be avoided for a period of 5 to 6 months after treatment because of the risk of hypertrophic scarring in atypical areas.

1. Egido Romo M. Isotretinoin and wax epilation. *Br J Dermatol* 1991; **124:** 393.
2. Holmes SC, Thomson J. Isotretinoin and skin fragility. *Br J Dermatol* 1995; **132:** 165.
3. Woollons A, Price ML. Roaccutane and wax epilation: a cautionary tale. *Br J Dermatol* 1997; **137:** 839–40.

## Interactions

Use of isotretinoin with vitamin A (including dietary supplements) should be avoided because of additive toxic effects. Tetracyclines should be avoided as their use with isotretinoin has been associated with the development of benign intracranial hypertension.

**Carbamazepine.** For the effect of isotretinoin on carbamazepine, see p.356.

**Oral contraceptives.** For discussion of the potential interactions of retinoids with hormonal contraceptives, and the effect this might have on contraceptive choice during retinoid treatment, see p.1534.

## Pharmacokinetics

Isotretinoin is absorbed from the gastrointestinal tract and absorption may be increased by food. Minimal systemic absorption occurs following topical application. Peak plasma concentrations occur 1 to 4 hours after oral doses. Oral bioavailability is low, possibly due to metabolism in the gut wall and first-pass metabolism in the liver. Isotretinoin is highly bound to plasma proteins. It is metabolised in the liver to its major metabolite 4-oxo-isotretinoin; there is also some isomerisation of isotretinoin to tretinoin. Isotretinoin, tretinoin, and their metabolites undergo enterohepatic recycling. The terminal elimination half-life of isotretinoin is 10 to 20 hours, while that of the 4-oxo metabolite may be up to 50 hours; return to physiological levels of retinoids takes about 2 weeks after stopping therapy. Equal amounts of a dose appear in the faeces, mainly as unchanged drug, and in the urine as metabolites.

Isotretinoin crosses the placenta.

◊ References.

1. Colburn WA, *et al.* Food increases the bioavailability of isotretinoin. *J Clin Pharmacol* 1983; **23:** 534–9.
2. Lucek RW, Colburn WA. Clinical pharmacokinetics of the retinoids. *Clin Pharmacokinet* 1985; **10:** 38–62.
3. Kraft JC, *et al.* Embryonic retinoid concentrations after maternal intake of isotretinoin. *N Engl J Med* 1989; **321:** 262.
4. Larsen FG, *et al.* Pharmacokinetics and therapeutic efficacy of retinoids in skin diseases. *Clin Pharmacokinet* 1992; **23:** 42–61.
5. Chen C, *et al.* Negligible systemic absorption of topical isotretinoin cream: implications for teratogenicity. *J Clin Pharmacol* 1997; **37:** 279–84.
6. Nulman I, *et al.* Steady-state pharmacokinetics of isotretinoin and its 4-oxo metabolite: implications for fetal safety. *J Clin Pharmacol* 1998; **38:** 926–30.

## Uses and Administration

Isotretinoin is a retinoid. It is the *cis* configuration of tretinoin (p.1161), which is the acid form of vitamin A (p.1451). Isotretinoin is given by mouth for the treatment of severe acne (below) that has not responded to other measures; it is also applied topically in milder forms of acne. It is not indicated for uncomplicated adolescent acne. Isotretinoin has also been tried in a number of other skin disorders and in some forms of neoplastic disease.

In the UK and a number of other countries the initial oral dose of isotretinoin for acne is 500 micrograms/kg daily, although in the USA initial doses of up to 1 mg/kg daily are permitted. The dose is given with food once daily or in two divided doses and adjusted if necessary after 4 weeks up to 1 mg/kg daily according to response and side-effects. Patients intolerant to the initial dose may be able to continue treatment at 100 to 200 micrograms/kg daily. Doses up to 2 mg/kg daily are permitted in the USA and some other countries for patients whose disease is very severe or primarily on the body instead of the face.

Acute exacerbation of acne is occasionally seen during the initial period, but usually subsides within 7 to 10 days on continued treatment. Treatment should continue for 12 to 20 weeks or until the total cyst count has decreased by over 70%. Improvement may continue for several months after cessation of treatment; prolonged remissions can occur.

It is recommended that repeat courses should not normally be given but occasionally they may be required. However, since acne may continue to improve after discontinuation of isotretinoin, there must be at least a 2-month drug-free period before starting repeat treatment.

For the topical treatment of acne a gel containing 0.05% of isotretinoin is applied sparingly once or twice daily. A therapeutic response may not be evident for 6 to 8 weeks.

◊ General reviews.

1. Orfanos CE, *et al.* Current use and future potential role of retinoids in dermatology. *Drugs* 1997; **53:** 358–88.

◊ Apart from its established role in the treatment of acne (below), isotretinoin has been used in other skin disorders including the keratinisation disorders Darier's disease[1] (p.1134) and ichthyosis (p.1136); lichen planus (p.1136); rosacea[2] (p.1138); and some malignant neoplasms (below).

1. Burge SM, Buxton PK. Topical isotretinoin in Darier's disease. *Br J Dermatol* 1995; **133:** 924–8.
2. Ertl GA, *et al.* A comparison of the efficacy of topical tretinoin and low-dose oral isotretinoin in rosacea. *Arch Dermatol* 1994; **130:** 319–24.

**Acne.** The retinoids play an important role in the treatment of acne (p.1133). Severe conglobate and nodulocystic acne unresponsive to other therapy including systemic antibacterials is the main indication for oral isotretinoin therapy. Isotretinoin produces a dose-related reduction in sebum excretion with a subsequent reduction in levels of *Propionibacterium acnes*, inflammation, and cyst formation.[1] A skin reaction with the appearance of papulopustules frequently occurs after 2 to 4 weeks of therapy but this rapidly clears with continued treatment. Although sebum excretion may approach pretreatment levels after discontinuation of therapy most patients remain free of their disease after a single course and long-term remissions lasting months or years have been obtained.[2,3] Men under 25 appear to be more prone to relapse than older men or women.[4] To avoid relapse long-term therapy to a cumulative dose of 120 to 150 mg/kg is required.[2,3] Improvement may continue for several months after withdrawal and at least 2 months should elapse before determining whether further treatment is necessary. About 10% of patients relapse and may require further treatment with antibacterials; repeat courses of isotretinoin are not usually recommended but may occasionally be required. There is evidence to suggest that patients who repeatedly relapse after stopping standard isotretinoin therapy may benefit from continuous use of very low doses of isotretinoin, such as 250 or 500 micrograms/kg per day taken every 4th week for 6 months, 100 micrograms/kg per day, or a single dose of 20 mg once or twice a week.[5] Use of isotretinoin with antibacterials or anti-androgens does not markedly improve efficacy but if concomitant antibacterial therapy is contemplated then erythromycin is preferred as use with tetracyclines can produce benign intracranial hypertension. Isotretinoin has also been used for the treatment of acne associated with immunosuppressive therapy in transplant recipients.[6,7] Variable results have been obtained when using isotretinoin topically[8,9] and it appears to interact with the epidermis in a different manner to other retinoids.[10]

Although isotretinoin is not licensed for the treatment of prepubertal acne because of the risk of adverse effects including early epiphyseal closure, it has been tried orally in a few children with toddler-age nodulocystic acne.[11]


1. Jones DH. The role and mechanism of action of 13-cis-retinoic acid in the treatment of severe (nodulocystic) acne. *Pharmacol Ther* 1989; **40:** 91–106.
2. Layton AM, *et al.* Isotretinoin for acne vulgaris—10 years later: a safe and successful treatment. *Br J Dermatol* 1993; **129:** 292–6.
3. Lehucher-Ceyrac D, Weber-Buisset MJ. Isotretinoin and acne in practice: a prospective analysis of 188 cases over 9 years. *Dermatology* 1993; **186:** 123–8.
4. Orfanos CE, *et al.* The retinoids: a review of their clinical pharmacology and therapeutic use. *Drugs* 1987; **34:** 459–503.
5. Palmer RA, *et al.* 'Microdose' isotretinoin. *Br J Dermatol* 2000; **143:** 205–6.
6. Tam M, Cooper A. The use of isotretinoin in a renal transplant patient with acne. *Br J Dermatol* 1987; **116:** 463.
7. Bunker CB, *et al.* Isotretinoin treatment of severe acne in post-transplant patients taking cyclosporine. *J Am Acad Dermatol* 1990; **22:** 693–4.
8. Harms M, *et al.* Isotretinoin ineffective topically. *Lancet* 1985; **i:** 398.
9. Chalker DK, *et al.* Efficacy of topical isotretinoin 0.05% gel in acne vulgaris: results of a multicenter, double-blind investigation. *J Am Acad Dermatol* 1987; **17:** 251–4.
10. Hirschel-Scholz S, *et al.* Isotretinoin differs from other synthetic retinoids in its modulation of human cellular retinoic acid binding protein (CRABP). *Br J Dermatol* 1989; **120:** 639–44.
11. Mengesha YM, Hansen RC. Toddler-age nodulocystic acne. *J Pediatr* 1999; **134:** 644–8.


**Malignant neoplasms.** Retinoids such as isotretinoin have been studied in the treatment of various neoplastic or preneoplastic disorders. Encouraging results were reported in a pilot study[1] of isotretinoin in juvenile chronic myelogenous leukaemia. [Note that oral tretinoin (p.1161) is used in acute promyelocytic leukaemia.]

Benefit has been noted in patients with T-cell lymphomas, including mycosis fungoides[2-4] (p.511), although in patients with advanced disease[5] treated with isotretinoin rather than acitretin (which had been used in some of the previous successes) no benefit, and even deterioration, occurred. The comment[6] was also made that the two retinoids do not share a similar therapeutic profile.

There is some evidence that retinoids may be useful in preventing the development of cutaneous squamous cell carcinoma in high-risk individuals (p.522). Retinoids may be useful for the prevention of second primary tumours after treatment for squamous cell carcinoma of the head and neck (p.517).[7] There has also been some interest in the use of retinoids, given orally or topically, in the management of leucoplakia (see under Bleomycin, p.531). However, despite reports of beneficial response,[8,9] relapse frequently occurs on stopping retinoid therapy.[10] Retinoids have also shown some promise as chemoprevention in other neoplasms.[11]


1. Castleberry RP, *et al.* A pilot study of isotretinoin in the treatment of juvenile chronic myelogenous leukaemia. *N Engl J Med* 1994; **331:** 1680–4.
2. Thomsen K, *et al.* Retinoids plus PUVA (RePUVA) and PUVA in mycosis fungoides, plaque stage: a report from the Scandinavian Mycosis Fungoides Group. *Acta Derm Venereol (Stockh)* 1989; **69:** 536–8.
3. Knobler RM, *et al.* Treatment of cutaneous T cell lymphoma with a combination of low-dose interferon alfa-2b and retinoids. *J Am Acad Dermatol* 1991; **24:** 247–52.
4. French LE, *et al.* Remission of cutaneous T-cell lymphoma with combined calcitriol and acitretin. *Lancet* 1994: **344:** 686–7.
5. Thomsen K. Cutaneous T-cell lymphoma and calcitriol and isotretinoin treatment. *Lancet* 1995; **345:** 1583.
6. French LE, Saurat J-H. Treatment of cutaneous T-cell lymphoma by retinoids and calcitriol. *Lancet* 1995; **346:** 376.
7. Hong WK, *et al.* Prevention of second primary tumors with isotretinoin in squamous-cell carcinoma of the head and neck. *N Engl J Med* 1990; **323:** 795–801.
8. Lippman SM, *et al.* Comparison of low-dose isotretinoin with beta carotene to prevent oral carcinogenesis. *N Engl J Med* 1993; **328:** 15–20.
9. Epstein JB, Gorsky M. Topical application of vitamin A to oral leukoplakia: a clinical case series. *Cancer* 1999; **86:** 921–7.
10. Gorsky M, Epstein JB. The effect of retinoids on premalignant oral lesions: focus on topical therapy. *Cancer* 2002; **95:** 1258–64.
11. De Palo G, Formelli F. Risks and benefits of retinoids in the chemoprevention of cancer. *Drug Safety* 1995; **13:** 245–56.


## Preparations

***BP 2003:*** Isotretinoin Capsules; Isotretinoin Gel;
***USP 27:*** Isotretinoin Capsules.

**Proprietary Preparations** (details are given in Part 3)
***Arg.:*** Isotrex; Roaccutan; ***Austral.:*** Accure; Isohexal; Isotrex; Oratane; Roaccutane; ***Austria:*** Roaccutan; ***Belg.:*** Roaccutane; ***Braz.:*** Isoacne; Isotrex; Roacutan; ***Canad.:*** Accutane; Isotrex; ***Chile:*** Isotrex Gel; Lisacne; Roacnetan; ***Denm.:*** Accutin; Isotrex; Roaccutan; ***Fin.:*** Roaccutan; ***Fr.:*** Curacne; Isotrex†; Procuta; Roaccutane; ***Ger.:*** Isotrex; Roaccutan; ***Gr.:*** Roaccutan; Stiefotrex; Tretin; ***Hong Kong:*** Isotrex; Oratane; Roaccutane; ***Irl.:*** Isotrex; Roaccutane; ***Israel:*** Curatane; Isotrex; Roaccutane; ***Ital.:*** Isotrex; Roaccutan; ***Malaysia:*** Isotrex; ***Mex.:*** Isotrex; Roaccutan; ***Neth.:*** Roaccutane; ***NZ:*** Isotrex; Oratane; Roaccutane; ***Port.:*** Isotrex; Roaccutan; ***S.Afr.:*** Isotrex; Roaccutane; ***Singapore:*** Isotrex; Nimegen; Oratane; Roaccutane; ***Spain:*** Isotrex; Roacutan; ***Switz.:*** Liderma; Roaccutane; ***Thai.:*** Isotrex; Roaccutane; ***UK:*** Isotrex; Roaccutane; ***USA:*** Accutane; Amnesteem; Claravis; Sotret.

**Multi-ingredient:** ***Austria:*** Isotrex; Isotrexin; ***Braz.:*** Isotrexin; Isotrexol; ***Chile:*** Piplex; ***Fr.:*** Antibiotrex; ***Ger.:*** Isotrexin; ***Irl.:*** Isotrexin; ***Ital.:*** Isotrexin; ***Port.:*** Isotrexin; ***Spain:*** Isotrex Eritromicina; ***UK:*** Isotrexin.

## Keluamid

Keluamida.

### Profile

Keluamid has been used in topical preparations for the treatment of seborrhoeic dermatitis and other scaling skin disorders.

### Preparations

**Proprietary Preparations** (details are given in Part 3)
***Arg.:*** Kelual; ***Fr.:*** Kelual.

**Multi-ingredient:** ***Arg.:*** Kelual Zinc; ***Fr.:*** Kelual Zinc; Sabal†.

## Kojic Acid

5-Hydroxy-2-hydroxymethyl-4-pyrone.
$C_6H_6O_4$ = 142.1.
*CAS — 501-30-4.*

### Profile

Kojic acid is reported to inhibit melanin production and is used in topical preparations for the treatment of hyperpigmentation disorders (p.1137).

◊ References.


1. Lim JT. Treatment of melasma using kojic acid in a gel containing hydroquinone and glycolic acid. *Dermatol Surg* 1999; **25:** 282–4.


### Preparations

**Proprietary Preparations** (details are given in Part 3)
**Multi-ingredient:** ***Arg.:*** Melasoft; Neoquin; ***Chile:*** Alastik; D 4; Neostrata; Primacy Phyto +; ***Port.:*** Despigmentante; Fade Cream; ***Singapore:*** AHA Skin Lightening Gel†; High Potency Lightening Serum†.

## Lisadimate *(USAN, rINN)*

Glyceryl Aminobenzoate; Glyceryl PABA; Lisadimato. Glyceryl 1-(4-aminobenzoate).
$C_{10}H_{13}NO_4$ = 211.2.
*CAS — 136-44-7.*

### Profile

Lisadimate is a sunscreen (see p.1133) with actions similar to those of aminobenzoic acid (p.1142). It is effective against UVB light (for definitions, see p.1136).

### Preparations

**Proprietary Preparations**
Some preparations are listed in Part 3.

## Lithium Succinate

Succinato de litio.
$C_4H_6O_4.xLi$.
*CAS — 16090-09-8.*
*ATC — D11AX04.*

### Profile

Lithium succinate is reported to have anti-inflammatory properties and is used as an 8% cream or ointment, usually with zinc sulfate. It is applied twice daily initially in the treatment of seborrhoeic dermatitis (p.1138). It should be used with caution in patients with psoriasis as it may exacerbate their condition.

◊ References.


1. Gould DJ, *et al.* A double-blind, placebo-controlled, multicenter trial of lithium succinate ointment in the treatment of seborrheic dermatitis. *J Am Acad Dermatol* 1992; **26:** 452–7.
2. Cuelenaere C, *et al.* Use of topical lithium succinate in the treatment of seborrhoeic dermatitis. *Dermatology* 1992; **184:** 194–7.
3. Langtry JA, *et al.* Topical lithium succinate ointment (Efalith) in the treatment of AIDS-related seborrhoeic dermatitis. *Clin Exp Dermatol* 1997; **22:** 216–19.


### Preparations

**Proprietary Preparations** (details are given in Part 3)
**Multi-ingredient:** ***Arg.:*** Litiofarm; ***Austria:*** Efalith; ***Ger.:*** Efadermin; ***Irl.:*** Efalith; ***NZ:*** Efalith†; ***Switz.:*** Efalith; ***UK:*** Efalith†.

## Maggots

Larvas; Sterile Larvae.

### Profile

Maggots used in wound management are the live sterile larvae of *Lucilia sericata*, the common greenbottle fly. Larval therapy (sometimes called biosurgery) may be used for debridement of infected or necrotic wounds (p.1139), including diabetic foot ulcers. Maggots produce a mixture of proteolytic enzymes that breaks down the necrotic tissue while leaving the healthy tissue unharmed, and kill or prevent the growth of micro-organisms, particularly Gram-positive bacteria. The movement of the maggots also appears to stimulate the growth of granulation tissue.

The maggots are applied to the surface of the wound and kept in place with dressings for up to 3 days. They are removed with the dressing, and the wound is irrigated with sodium chloride solution; any remaining maggots are removed with forceps.

Maggots should not be applied to wounds that have a tendency to bleed easily, or that communicate with a body cavity or any internal organ. Pain has been reported with larval therapy and some patients may require analgesics.

◊ References.


1. Thomas S, *et al.* Maggots are useful in treating infected or necrotic wounds. *BMJ* 1999; **318:** 807–8.
2. Courtenay M, *et al.* Larva therapy in wound management. *J R Soc Med* 2000; **93:** 72–4.
3. Jukema GN, *et al.* Amputation-sparing treatment by nature: "surgical" maggots revisited. *Clin Infect Dis* 2002; **35:** 1566–71.


### Preparations

**Proprietary Preparations** (details are given in Part 3)
***UK:*** LarvE.

## Mequinol *(USAN, rINN)*

BMS-181158; *p*-Guaiacol; 4-HA; HQMME; Hydroquinone Monomethyl Ether; *p*-Hydroxyanisole; Hydroxyquinone Methyl Ether. 4-Methoxyphenol.
$C_7H_8O_2$ = 124.1.
*CAS — 150-76-5.*
*ATC — D11AX06.*

### Profile

Mequinol is used similarly to hydroquinone (p.1148), in concentrations of up to 20%, in the treatment of hyperpigmentation (see Pigmentation Disorders, p.1137). It has also been investigated in the treatment of melanoma.

**Adverse effects.** A report of severe reversible irregular hypopigmentation of the hands, arms, neck, and legs in a West Indian woman who applied a bleaching wax containing mequinol for 2 to 3 months to lighten the colour of her skin.[1]


1. Boyle J, Kennedy CTC. British cosmetic regulations inadequate. *BMJ* 1984; **288:** 1998–9.


**Pigmentation disorders.** References.


1. Fleischer AB, *et al.* The combination of 2% 4-hydroxyanisole (mequinol) and 0.01% tretinoin is effective in improving the appearance of solar lentigines and related hyperpigmented lesions in two double-blind multicenter clinical studies. *J Am Acad Dermatol* 2000; **42:** 459–67.
2. Njoo MD, *et al.* Depigmentation therapy in vitiligo universalis with topical 4-methoxyphenol and the Q-switched ruby laser. *J Am Acad Dermatol* 2000; **42:** 760–9.


### Preparations

**Proprietary Preparations** (details are given in Part 3)
***Austria:*** Leucobasal; ***Braz.:*** Leucodin; ***Fr.:*** Any; Clairodermyl†; Creme des 3 Fleurs d'Orient†; Leucodinine B; ***Gr.:*** Leucodinin-M; ***Spain:*** Novo Dermoquinona†; ***Switz.:*** Leucobasal†.

**Multi-ingredient:** ***USA:*** Solage.

## Meradimate *(USAN, rINN)*

Menthyl O-Aminobenzoate; Menthyl Anthranilate; Meradimato. 5-Methyl-2-(1-methylethyl)-cyclohexyl 2-aminobenzoate.
$C_{17}H_{25}NO_2$ = 275.4.
*CAS — 134-09-8.*

**Pharmacopoeias.** In *US.*

**USP 27** (Meradimate). Store in airtight containers.

### Profile

Meradimate is used as a sunscreen (see p.1133). It is effective against UVA light (for definitions, see p.1136).

### Preparations

**Proprietary Preparations**
Some preparations are listed in Part 3.

## Ammoniated Mercury

Aminomercuric Chloride; Hydrargyri Aminochloridum; Hydrargyrum Amidochloratum; Hydrargyrum Ammoniatum; Hydrargyrum Praecipitatum Album; Mercuric Ammonium Chloride; Mercurio amoniacal; Mercury Amide Chloride; Mercury Aminochloride; White Precipitate.

$NH_2HgCl$ = 252.1.

*CAS — 10124-48-8.*

NOTE. 'White Precipitate' has also been used as a name for Precipitated Mercurous Chloride.

**Pharmacopoeias.** In *US.*

**USP 27** (Ammoniated Mercury). A white amorphous powder or pulverulent pieces; odourless. It is stable in air, but darkens on exposure to light. Insoluble in water and in alcohol; readily soluble in warm hydrochloric, nitric, and acetic acids. Protect from light.

### Profile

Ammoniated mercury was formerly used topically in the treatment of skin infections and psoriasis but the use of such mercurial preparations is generally deprecated. Frequent or prolonged application to large areas or to broken skin or mucous membranes can cause mercury poisoning (see p.1713) and use on infants has produced acrodynia (pink disease). Ammoniated mercury is also a potent sensitiser and can produce allergic reactions.

**Effects on the kidneys.** Of 60 patients who were found to have nephrotic syndrome, 32 had used skin-lightening creams containing 5 to 10% of ammoniated mercury.[1] Concentrations of mercury in the urine of these patients were up to 250 nanograms/mL compared with a usual upper limit of 80 nanograms/mL. Of 26 patients followed up for up to 2 years, 13 had no remission or response to treatment; 6 of these had used skin lighteners.


1. Barr RD, *et al.* Nephrotic syndrome in adult Africans in Nairobi. *BMJ* 1972; **2:** 131–4.


### Preparations

**Proprietary Preparations** (details are given in Part 3)

**Multi-ingredient:** ***USA:*** Emersal†; Unguentum Bossi†.

## Mesulphen *(BAN)*

Mesulfen *(pINN)*; Dimethyldiphenylene Disulphide; Dimethylthianthrene; Mesulfeno. It consists mainly of 2,7-dimethylthianthrene.

$C_{14}H_{12}S_2$ = 244.4.

*CAS — 135-58-0.*

*ATC — D10AB05; P03AA03.*

**Pharmacopoeias.** *Jpn* includes thianthol, a mixture of 2,7-dimethylthianthrene and ditolyl disulfide.

### Profile

Mesulphen has been used as a parasiticide and antipruritic in a range of skin disorders including acne, scabies, and seborrhoea. Sensitivity to mesulphen has occasionally been reported.

### Preparations

**Proprietary Preparations** (details are given in Part 3)

***Ger.:*** Citemul S; ***Switz.:*** Soufrol.

**Multi-ingredient:** ***India:*** Polyderm.

## Methoxsalen *(BAN)*

Ammoidin; 8-Methoxypsoralen; Metoxaleno; Xanthotoxin. 9-Methoxyfuro[3,2-g]chromen-7-one; 9-Methoxy-7*H*-furo[3,2-g][1]benzopyran-7-one.

$C_{12}H_8O_4$ = 216.2.

*CAS — 298-81-7.*

*ATC — D05AD02; D05BA02.*

**Pharmacopoeias.** In *Jpn* and *US.*

**USP 27** (Methoxsalen). White to cream-coloured, odourless, fluffy, needle-like crystals. Practically insoluble in water; sparingly soluble in boiling water and in ether; soluble in boiling alcohol, in acetone, in acetic acid, in propylene glycol, and in benzene; freely soluble in chloroform. Protect from light.

### Adverse Effects

Methoxsalen given orally commonly causes nausea and less frequently mental effects including insomnia, nervousness, and depression.

Photochemotherapy or PUVA (see under Uses and Administration, below) may cause pruritus and mild transient erythema. Other effects include oedema, dizziness, headache, vesiculation, bulla formation, onycholysis, acneform eruption, and severe skin pain. Overexposure to sunlight or UVA radiation may produce severe burns in patients being treated with psoralens. PUVA can produce premature ageing of the skin. Hypertrichosis and pigmentation alterations of skin or nails have also been reported. PUVA may be associated with an increased risk of malignant neoplasms of the skin.

**Carcinogenicity.** See under Effects on the Blood and Effects on the Skin, below.

**Effects on the blood.** There have been isolated reports of leukaemia[1-3] or a preleukaemic condition[4] developing after PUVA therapy.


1. Hansen NE. Development of acute myeloid leukaemia in a patient with psoriasis treated with oral 8-methoxypsoralen and longwave ultraviolet light. *Scand J Haematol* 1979; **22:** 57–60.
2. Sheehan-Dare RA, *et al.* Transformation of myelodysplasia to acute myeloid leukaemia during psoralen photochemotherapy (PUVA) treatment of psoriasis. *Acta Derm Venereol (Stockh)* 1989; **69:** 262–4.
3. Kwong YL, *et al.* Acute myeloid leukemia following psoralen with ultraviolet A therapy: a fluorescence in situ hybridization study. *Cancer Genet Cytogenet* 1997; **99:** 11–13.
4. Wagner J, *et al.* Preleukaemia (haemopoietic dysplasia) developing in a patient with psoriasis treated with 8-methoxypsoralen and ultraviolet light (PUVA) treatment. *Scand J Haematol* 1978; **21:** 299–304.


**Effects on the eyes.** Free methoxsalen has been detected in the lens of the eye for at least 12 hours after oral administration.[1] It may become integrated into the structure of the lens if there is exposure to UV light, promoting cataract formation in patients who fail to wear suitable eye protection for 12 to 24 hours after methoxsalen ingestion.[2] However, provided that eye protection is used there appears to be no significant dose-dependent increase in the risk of cataract formation, although a higher risk of developing nuclear sclerosis and posterior subcapsular opacities has been noted in patients who have received more than 100 treatments.[3] Other ocular effects include dose-related transient visual-field defects reported in 3 patients receiving PUVA therapy.[4] Psoralens may also increase the sensitivity of the retina to visible light.[5]


1. Lerman S, *et al.* Potential ocular complications from PUVA therapy and their prevention. *J Invest Dermatol* 1980; **74:** 197–9.
2. Woo TY, *et al.* Lenticular psoralen photoproducts and cataracts of a PUVA-treated psoriatic patient. *Arch Dermatol* 1985; **121:** 1307–8.
3. Stern RS, *et al.* Ocular findings in patients treated with PUVA. *J Invest Dermatol* 1985; **85:** 269–73.
4. Fenton DA, Wilkinson JD. Dose-related visual-field defects in patients receiving PUVA therapy. *Lancet* 1983; **i:** 1106.
5. Souêtre E, *et al.* 5-Methoxypsoralen increases the sensitivity of the retina to light in humans. *Eur J Clin Pharmacol* 1989; **36:** 59–61.


**Effects on the hair.** Hypertrichosis was noticed in 15 of 23 female patients receiving PUVA therapy compared with 2 of 14 patients treated with UVA alone.[1]


1. Rampen FHJ. Hypertrichosis in PUVA-treated patients. *Br J Dermatol* 1983; **109:** 657–60.


**Effects on the immune system.** PUVA therapy appears to have immunosuppressive effects and inhibits lymphocytes, polymorphonuclear leucocytes, and Langerhans' cells.[1-3] It is capable of inducing antinuclear antibody formation and a syndrome similar to systemic lupus syndrome has developed during treatment.[4,5] An immunological basis has also been suspected for the development of nephrotic syndrome in one patient who received PUVA therapy.[6]

See also Hypersensitivity, below.


1. Farber EM, *et al.* Long-term risks of psoralen and UV-A therapy for psoriasis. *Arch Dermatol* 1983; **119:** 426–31.
2. Morison WL, *et al.* Abnormal lymphocyte function following long-term PUVA therapy for psoriasis. *Br J Dermatol* 1983; **108:** 445–50.
3. Chang A, *et al.* PUVA and UVB inhibit the intra-epidermal accumulation of polymorphonuclear leukocytes. *Br J Dermatol* 1988; **119:** 281–7.
4. Bruze M, *et al.* Fatal connective tissue disease with antinuclear antibodies following PUVA therapy. *Acta Derm Venereol (Stockh)* 1984; **64:** 157–60.
5. Bruze M, Ljunggren B. Antinuclear antibodies appearing during PUVA therapy. *Acta Derm Venereol (Stockh)* 1985; **65:** 31–6.
6. Lam Thuon Mine LTK, *et al.* Nephrotic syndrome after treatment with psoralens and ultraviolet A. *BMJ* 1983; **287:** 94–5.


**Effects on the skin.** MALIGNANT NEOPLASMS. Squamous cell carcinoma, basal cell carcinoma, keratoacanthoma, actinic keratosis, Bowen's disease, and malignant melanoma have all been reported during or after cessation of PUVA.[1-3] There have been several large long-term follow-up studies to assess the risk of **non-melanoma** skin cancer in patients receiving PUVA therapy. Early studies from Europe found no clear evidence that PUVA was independently carcinogenic but did find that previous treatment with arsenic, methotrexate, or ionising radiation increased the incidence of skin tumours.[4] Studies from the USA have found an increase in the incidence of basal cell carcinoma and squamous cell carcinoma independent of other treatment,[5] which was dose-related in some studies.[6] Male genitalia appeared to be particularly susceptible.[7] It has been suggested that the differences between the findings might be due to the fact that in Europe higher and fewer doses are used and the median total dose employed may be only 29% of that used in the USA.[8] However, more recent studies from northern Europe have also found a dose-related increase in the risk of developing squamous cell carcinomas.[9-11] One small series suggested that about 50% of the recipients of high-dose PUVA went on to develop squamous cell carcinomas or premalignant lesions.[12] While some European workers have findings that confirm the increased susceptibility of the male genitalia[13] others have failed to find any such evidence.[14,15] A few patients have gone on to develop metastatic disease.[16,17]

There are anecdotal reports of **malignant melanomas** occurring in patients who had received PUVA. A prospective study[18] study in 1380 patients with psoriasis who were first treated with PUVA in 1975 or 1976 found that the risk of melanoma increases about 15 years after the first treatment with PUVA and that the risk was increased especially in patients who had received 250 treatments or more. The authors suggested that long-term PUVA should therefore be used with caution, especially in younger patients. However, a similar follow-up study[11] of 4799 patients treated with PUVA found no increase in the risk for malignant melanoma. Comparing their findings with the earlier study, the authors suggested that the results might differ because one-fifth of their cohort had received bath PUVA in which lower UVA doses are used. The comment has also been made[19] that patients receiving long-term therapy should be followed up carefully and that such therapy should not be used in patients at risk for melanoma.

A study[20] of follow-up data on patients who had received trioxysalen bath PUVA did not find an increase in risk of developing either squamous cell carcinoma or malignant melanoma, but the authors suggested that further study is needed to determine the carcinogenicity of trioxysalen PUVA.

There has also been a suggestion that PUVA may increase the risk of some internal cancers.[10] For mention of a possible association with leukaemia see Effects on the Blood, above.


1. Reshad H, *et al.* Cutaneous carcinoma in psoriatic patients treated with PUVA. *Br J Dermatol* 1984; **110:** 299–305.
2. Kemmett D, *et al.* Nodular malignant melanoma and multiple squamous cell carcinomas in a patient treated by photochemotherapy for psoriasis. *BMJ* 1984; **289:** 1498.
3. Suurmond D, *et al.* Skin cancer and PUVA maintenance therapy for psoriasis. *Br J Dermatol* 1985; **113:** 485–6.
4. Henseler T, *et al.* Skin tumors in the European PUVA study. *J Am Acad Dermatol* 1987; **16:** 108–16.
5. Forman AB, *et al.* Long-term follow-up of skin cancer in the PUVA-48 cooperative study. *Arch Dermatol* 1989; **125:** 515–19.
6. Stern RS, *et al.* Non-melanoma skin cancer occurring in patients treated with PUVA five to ten years after first treatment. *J Invest Dermatol* 1988; **91:** 120–4.
7. Stern RS, *et al.* Genital tumors among men with psoriasis exposed to psoralens and ultraviolet A radiation (PUVA) and ultraviolet B radiation. *N Engl J Med* 1990; **322:** 1093–7.
8. Moseley H, Ferguson J. Photochemotherapy: a reappraisal of its use in dermatology. *Drugs* 1989; **38:** 822–37.
9. Bruynzeel I, *et al.* 'High single-dose' European PUVA regimen also causes an excess of non-melanoma skin cancer. *Br J Dermatol* 1991; **124:** 49–55.
10. Lindelöf B, *et al.* PUVA and cancer: a large-scale epidemiological study. *Lancet* 1991; **338:** 91–3.
11. Lindelöf B, *et al.* PUVA and cancer risk: the Swedish follow-up study. *Br J Dermatol* 1999; **141:** 108–12.
12. Lever LR, Farr PM. Skin cancers or premalignant lesions occur in half of high-dose PUVA patients. *Br J Dermatol* 1994; **131:** 215–19.
13. Perkins W, *et al.* Cutaneous malignancy in males treated with photochemotherapy. *Lancet* 1990; **336:** 1248.
14. Wolff K, Hönigsmann H. Genital carcinomas in psoriasis patients treated with photochemotherapy. *Lancet* 1991; **337:** 439.
15. Aubin F, *et al.* Genital squamous cell carcinoma in men treated by photochemotherapy: a cancer registry-based study from 1978 to 1998. *Br J Dermatol* 2001; **144:** 1204–6.
16. Lewis FM, *et al.* Metastatic squamous-cell carcinoma in patient receiving PUVA. *Lancet* 1994; **344:** 1157.
17. Stern RS. Metastatic squamous cell cancer after psoralen photochemotherapy. *Lancet* 1994; **344:** 1644–5.
18. Stern RS, *et al.* Malignant melanoma in patients treated for psoriasis with methoxsalen (psoralen) and ultraviolet A radiation (PUVA). *N Engl J Med* 1997; **336:** 1041–5.
19. Wolff K. Should PUVA be abandoned? *N Engl J Med* 1997; **336:** 1090–1.
20. Hannuksela-Svahn A, *et al.* Trioxsalen bath PUVA did not increase the risk of squamous cell skin carcinoma and cutaneous malignant melanoma in a joint analysis of 944 Swedish and Finnish patients with psoriasis. *Br J Dermatol* 1999; **141:** 497–501.


NON-MALIGNANT SKIN DISORDERS. Toxic pustuloderma, marked by erythema and superficial pustular lesions, has been reported in a patient given PUVA therapy for mycosis fungoides.[1] Another effect sometimes associated with PUVA is severe skin pain;[2,3] the pain may respond to treatment with topical capsaicin.[3] Long-term PUVA treatment accelerates ageing of the skin.[4]


1. Yip J, *et al.* Toxic pustuloderma due to PUVA treatment. *Br J Dermatol* 1991; **125:** 401–2.
2. Burrows NP, *et al.* PUVA-induced skin pain. *Br J Dermatol* 1993; **129:** 504.
3. Burrows NP, Norris PG. Treatment of PUVA-induced skin pain with capsaicin. *Br J Dermatol* 1994; **131:** 584–5.
4. Sator P-G, *et al.* Objective assessment of photoageing effects using high-frequency ultrasound in PUVA-treated psoriasis patients. *Br J Dermatol* 2002; **147:** 291–8.


**Hypersensitivity.** Hypersensitivity reactions to methoxsalen and PUVA therapy occur rarely but there have been reports of drug-induced fever,[1] bronchoconstriction,[2] and contact dermatitis.[3] A case of anaphylaxis has also been attributed to 5-methoxypsoralen.[4]


1. Tóth Kása I, Dobozy A. Drug fever caused by PUVA treatment. *Acta Derm Venereol (Stockh)* 1985; **65:** 557–8.
2. Ramsay B, Marks JM. Bronchoconstriction due to 8-methoxypsoralen. *Br J Dermatol* 1988; **119:** 83–6.
3. Takashima A, *et al.* Allergic contact and photocontact dermatitis due to psoralens in patients with psoriasis treated with topical PUVA. *Br J Dermatol* 1991; **124:** 37–42.
4. Lagat FJ, *et al.* Anaphylaxis to 5-methoxypsoralen during photochemotherapy. *Br J Dermatol* 2001; **145:** 821–2.

### Precautions

Methoxsalen should not be given to patients with diseases associated with light sensitivity such as porphyria, although it is used with care to decrease some patients' sensitivity to sunlight. Other contra-indications include aphakia, melanoma or a history of melanoma, and invasive squamous cell carcinoma. It is generally recommended that PUVA therapy should not be used in children. Methoxsalen should be used with caution in patients with hepatic insufficiency.

Patients should not sunbathe for 24 hours before and 48 hours after PUVA treatment. They should avoid exposure to sun, even through glass or cloud cover for at least 8 hours after methoxsalen ingestion and should wear wrap-around UVA absorbing glasses for 24 hours after ingestion. Photosensitivity is more prolonged after topical application and treated skin should be protected from exposure to sunlight for at least 12 to 48 hours. It has been recommended that patients undergo an ophthalmic examination, and that measurements of anti-nuclear antibody titre and hepatic function be carried out before, and at intervals after, starting therapy. Unless specific treatment is required male genitalia should be shielded during PUVA therapy. Patients should also receive regular examinations for signs of premalignant or malignant skin lesions.

**Porphyria.** Methoxsalen should not be given to patients with porphyria.

### Interactions

Methoxsalen should be used with caution with other drugs also known to cause photosensitivity. It inhibits the action of cytochrome P450 isoenzyme CYP2A6, and may increase plasma concentrations of drugs metabolised via this enzyme.

**Food.** Some foods, for example, celery, parsnip, and parsley, contain psoralens and consumption of large quantities may increase the risk of phototoxicity with methoxsalen. A patient[1] who had consumed a large quantity of celery soup the evening before and two hours before undergoing PUVA therapy for atopic eczema developed severe phototoxicity following the treatment which was attributed to the additive effects of methoxsalen and psoralens contained in the celery.

1. Boffa MJ, *et al.* Celery soup causing severe phototoxicity during PUVA therapy. *Br J Dermatol* 1996; **135:** 334.

**Phenytoin.** Failure of PUVA treatment due to abnormally low serum concentrations of methoxsalen in a patient with epilepsy was probably a result of induction of hepatic enzymes by phenytoin.[1]

1. Staberg B, Hueg B. Interaction between 8-methoxypsoralen and phenytoin. *Acta Derm Venereol (Stockh)* 1985; **65:** 553–5.

### Pharmacokinetics

When taken by mouth methoxsalen is well but variably absorbed from the gastrointestinal tract and there is considerable interindividual variation in peak serum concentrations. Depending on the oral formulation used increased photosensitivity is present 1 hour after a dose, reaches a peak at about 1 to 4 hours, and disappears after about 8 hours. Methoxsalen is highly protein bound. It appears to be preferentially taken up by epidermal cells. It also diffuses into the lens of the eye. Methoxsalen is almost completely metabolised. About 95% of a dose is excreted in the urine within 24 hours. The photosensitising action of methoxsalen may persist for several days after topical application. The erythema induced by oral or topical PUVA is usually delayed and peaks after 2 to 3 days.

◊ References.

1. de Wolff FA, Thomas TV. Clinical pharmacokinetics of methoxsalen and other psoralens. *Clin Pharmacokinet* 1986; **11:** 62–75.

### Uses and Administration

Methoxsalen, a psoralen, is a constituent of the fruits of *Ammi majus*. It is a photosensitiser markedly increasing skin reactivity to long-wavelength ultraviolet radiation (320 to 400 nm), an effect used in photochemotherapy or PUVA [psoralen (P) and high-intensity long-wavelength UVA irradiation]. In the presence of UVA methoxsalen bonds with DNA, inhibiting DNA synthesis and cell division, and can lead to cell injury. Recovery from the cell injury may be followed by increased melanisation of the epidermis. Methoxsalen may also increase pigmentation by an action on melanocytes.

PUVA is used to treat idiopathic vitiligo and severe, recalcitrant, disabling psoriasis not adequately responsive to conventional topical therapy. It may also be useful in selected cases of atopic eczema and polymorphic light eruptions and may be used in T-cell lymphomas such as mycosis fungoides.

Methoxsalen is given orally or applied topically in PUVA regimens. Differing oral dosage forms of methoxsalen may exhibit significantly varying bioavailabilities and times to onset of photosensitisation. The UVA exposure dose should generally be based on prior measurement of the minimal phototoxic dose although it can be calculated with regard to the skin type of the patient if phototoxic dose testing cannot be carried out.

- To repigment **vitiliginous** areas, methoxsalen is given in a dose of up to 600 micrograms/kg *by mouth* 2 to 4 hours before measured periods of exposure to UVA twice a week, at least 48 hours apart.
- Methoxsalen may also be applied *topically* to repigment small, well-defined vitiliginous lesions. Preparations containing up to 1% have been used but dilution to 0.1 or 0.01% may be necessary to avoid adverse cutaneous effects. The surrounding skin should be protected by an opaque sunscreen. Some suggest that the treated area should be exposed to UVA immediately after application while others recommend waiting up to 2 hours. After exposure the lesions should be washed and protected from light; protection may be necessary for up to 48 hours or longer. Treatment is repeated usually once weekly. Significant repigmentation may not appear until after 6 to 9 months of treatment.
- For the treatment of **psoriasis** a similar schedule is used to that outlined above for vitiligo. A dose of up to about 600 micrograms/kg *by mouth* 2 hours before UVA is usually given twice a week although increased frequencies, but with at least 48-hour intervals between doses, have been suggested. If there is no response or only minimal response after the fifteenth PUVA treatment some suggest that the dosage may be increased, once only, by 10 mg for the remainder of the course of treatment.
- Methoxsalen may also be used *topically* with UVA exposure for the treatment of psoriasis. For direct application to affected areas of skin a preparation containing approximately 0.15% (or diluted to 0.015% if necessary to avoid adverse cutaneous effects) is applied 15 minutes before UVA exposure. Alternatively the patient may take a whole-body bath for 15 minutes in a methoxsalen solution, followed immediately by UVA exposure. UK guidelines (see also below) suggest a typical concentration of methoxsalen 2.6 mg/litre for such solutions although higher concentrations (up to about 3.7 mg/litre) have been used. Hand and foot soaks may be used to treat only those affected areas; a solution containing methoxsalen 3 mg/litre may be used with the affected areas immersed for 15 minutes followed by a delay of 30 minutes before UVA exposure. Baths or soaks are generally given twice a week.

Psoralen itself has also been used.

**Administration.** The dose of methoxsalen is usually calculated on the basis of body-weight. This method of dose calculation produces a considerable difference between the doses received by heavy and light patients. A study in 41 patients with psoriasis[1] suggested that using methoxsalen 25 mg/m$^2$ gave more consistent plasma concentrations and may reduce the potential for burning in heavy patients and prevent underdosing in light patients undergoing PUVA therapy.

1. Sakuntabhai A, *et al.* Calculation of 8-methoxypsoralen dose according to body surface area in PUVA treatment. *Br J Dermatol* 1995; **133:** 919–23.

**PUVA.** PUVA combines psoralens with ultraviolet A irradiation. The psoralens may be given directly to the patient, either orally or topically, and the patient is then exposed to UVA. In extracorporeal PUVA (extracorporeal photochemotherapy; photopheresis), an oral dose of psoralen is administered, after which the patient's leucocytes are isolated, exposed to UVA extracorporeally, and then reinfused. In another method of photopheresis that is under investigation, methoxsalen is added directly to leucocytes that have already been removed from the patient. The mixture is then treated with UVA extracorporeally after which it is returned to the patient; the total dose of methoxsalen used by this method is lower than that used orally. PUVA has been used in a wide range of disorders including skin disorders, mycosis fungoides, and organ and tissue transplant rejection (below).

MYCOSIS FUNGOIDES. PUVA therapy is used in the treatment of the manifestations of cutaneous mycosis fungoides and Sèzary syndrome, two forms of cutaneous T-cell lymphoma (see p.511). Extracorporeal PUVA therapy (photopheresis; see above) has also been used,[1-4] particularly for disease with erythrodermic features.

1. Duvic M, *et al.* Photopheresis therapy for cutaneous T-cell lymphoma. *J Am Acad Dermatol* 1996; **35:** 573–9.
2. Zic JA, *et al.* Long-term follow-up of patients with cutaneous T-cell lymphoma treated with extracorporeal photochemotherapy. *J Am Acad Dermatol* 1996; **35:** 935–45.
3. Zic JA, *et al.* The North American experience with photopheresis. *Ther Apher* 1999; **3:** 50–62.
4. Rubegni P, *et al.* Extracorporeal photochemotherapy in long-term treatment of early stage cutaneous T-cell lymphoma. *Br J Dermatol* 2000; **143:** 894–6.

ORGAN AND TISSUE TRANSPLANTATION. PUVA and extracorporeal PUVA therapy (photopheresis; see above) have been tried in patients with graft-versus-host disease[1-3] and to prevent rejection in cardiac[4] and other solid organ transplantation.[2]

1. Konstantinow A, *et al.* Chronic graft-versus-host disease: successful treatment with extracorporeal photochemotherapy: a follow-up. *Br J Dermatol* 1996; **135:** 1007–8.
2. Zic JA, *et al.* The North American experience with photopheresis. *Ther Apher* 1999; **3:** 50–62.
3. Kunz M, *et al.* Treatment of severe erythrodermic acute graft-versus-host disease with photochemotherapy. *Br J Dermatol* 2001; **144:** 901–2.
4. Barr ML, *et al.* Photopheresis for the prevention of rejection in cardiac transplantation. *N Engl J Med* 1998; **339:** 1744–51.

SKIN DISORDERS. PUVA has been used in a wide range of skin disorders and guidelines have been published by the British Photodermatology Group,[1,2] which are summarised as follows:

- Indications for PUVA in chronic plaque **psoriasis** include severe extensive psoriasis unresponsive to conventional topical therapies, relapse within 3 to 6 months of successful topical treatment, or patient refusal of topical treatment if UVB phototherapy has failed (see p.1137 for a discussion of the various treatments of psoriasis). Initial UVA exposure should preferably be determined on the basis of prior measurement of the minimal phototoxic dose rather than on the skin type. Increases in UVA irradiation are then calculated as a percentage of previous doses.

  Methoxsalen in a dose of 600 micrograms/kg by mouth given 2 hours before UVA exposure is the widely accepted standard regimen. Alternatively, 5-methoxypsoralen 1.2 mg/kg, again 2 hours before UVA exposure, can be given and appears to be almost free of the adverse reactions such as nausea, pruritus, and erythema induced by methoxsalen. However, until the clinical efficacy of 5-methoxypsoralen has been clearly demonstrated, methoxsalen should remain the psoralen of choice for most clinical situations.

  Alternatives to oral PUVA are baths or soaks using methoxsalen or trioxysalen. For whole-body bathing a concentration of methoxsalen 2.6 mg/litre is typically utilised with the patient bathing for 15 minutes followed by immediate exposure to UVA. For hand and foot soaks a concentration of methoxsalen 3 mg/litre is used with the affected area immersed for 15 minutes followed by a delay of 30 minutes before UVA exposure. For trioxysalen a concentration of about 330 micrograms/litre is used for a 15-minute whole-body bath or hand and foot soak followed by immediate UVA exposure for whole-body therapy, or a 30 minute delay before hand and foot UVA exposure. Whole-body baths or hand and foot soaks are given twice each week.

  Methoxsalen may also be applied topically to the affected areas. A concentration of about 0.15% (or 0.015% if erythema occurs) is used in an emulsion, or 0.005% in an aqueous gel, and applied 15 minutes before UVA exposure. PUVA treatment should be discontinued as soon as clearance is achieved and maintenance PUVA after routine clearance should be avoided.

  A combination of PUVA with acitretin (300 to 700 micrograms/kg by mouth) or etretinate (0.5 to 1 mg/kg by mouth) may be considered in patients who have reached 50 treatment sessions or relapsed within 6 months of PUVA. PUVA and methotrexate are effective for severe psoriasis but should be reserved for such cases because of the possible increased risk of skin cancer

- Oral PUVA twice weekly with methoxsalen 600 micrograms/kg or 5-methoxypsoralen 1.2 mg/kg has been effective in many patients with **vitiligo** (see Pigmentation Disorders, p.1137). If patches are large and well demarcated topical application of methoxsalen 0.15% may be preferable
- In **mycosis fungoides** PUVA is an effective symptomatic treatment for early disease and a useful adjunct for late-stage disease but optimal regimens have not been established (see above)

- PUVA is effective for atopic **eczema** (p.1135) but clearance is less certain than for psoriasis, twice the number of treatments may be needed, and relapse is more frequent. It should therefore be reserved for severe disease unresponsive to conventional treatments. Optimal regimens have not been established
- In **polymorphic light eruptions** PUVA is effective in up to 90% of patients but is only indicated in those who are frequently or severely affected despite the regular use of high-protection broad-spectrum sunscreens. Several arbitrary regimens are in use
- Variable results have also been reported in a variety of other disorders but data has been insufficient to establish precise guidelines. Such disorders include actinic prurigo, alopecia areata, aquagenic pruritus, chronic actinic dermatitis, granuloma annulare, lichen planus, nodular prurigo, pityriasis lichenoides, localised scleroderma, solar urticaria, and urticaria pigmentosa. In most cases relapse occurs in the absence of maintenance therapy and PUVA should usually only be tried as a last resort.

Extracorporeal PUVA has been tried in patients with severe epidermolysis bullosa acquisita,[3,4] and scleroderma.[5]


1. British Photodermatology Group. British Photodermatology Group guidelines for PUVA. *Br J Dermatol* 1994; **130:** 246–55.
2. Halpern SM, *et al.* Guidelines for topical PUVA: a report of a workshop of the British Photodermatology Group. *Br J Dermatol* 2000; **142:** 22–31. Also available at: http://www.bad.org.uk/doctors/guidelines/Topical_PUVA_Therapy.pdf (accessed 25/05/04)
3. Miller JL, *et al.* Remission of severe epidermolysis bullosa acquisita induced by extracorporeal photochemotherapy. *Br J Dermatol* 1995; **133:** 467–71.
4. Gordon KB, *et al.* Treatment of refractory epidermolysis bullosa acquisita with extracorporeal photochemotherapy. *Br J Dermatol* 1997; **136:** 415–20.
5. Zic JA, *et al.* The North American experience with photopheresis. *Ther Apher* 1999; **3:** 50–62.


## Preparations

***USP 27:*** Methoxsalen Capsules; Methoxsalen Topical Solution.

**Proprietary Preparations** (details are given in Part 3)
***Austral.:*** Oxsoralen; Pentaderm; ***Austria:*** Oxsoralen; ***Belg.:*** Mopsoralen; Oxsoralon†; ***Canad.:*** Oxsoralen; Ultramop; ***Denm.:*** Geroxalen; ***Fr.:*** Meladinine; ***Ger.:*** Meladinine; ***Gr.:*** Melaoline; ***Hong Kong:*** Oxsoralen; ***India:*** Macsoralen; Manaderm; Melanocyl; ***Irl.:*** Deltasoralen; ***Israel:*** Oxsoralen†; ***Ital.:*** Oxsoralen; ***Malaysia:*** Meladinine; Oxsoralen; ***Mex.:*** Dermox; Meladinina; Oxsoralen; ***Neth.:*** Geroxalen; Meladinine; Oxsoralen; ***Norw.:*** Geroxalen; ***NZ:*** Oxsoralen; ***S.Afr.:*** Oxsoralen; ***Singapore:*** Oxsoralen; ***Spain:*** Novo Melanidina†; Oxsoralen; ***Switz.:*** Meladinine; ***Thai.:*** Meladinine; ***UK:*** Puvasoralen; ***USA:*** Oxsoralen; Uvadex.

**Multi-ingredient:** ***India:*** Melanocyl.

## 5-Methoxypsoralen

Bergapten; 5-Metoxipsoraleno. 4-Methoxy-7*H*-furo[3,2-*g*]chromen-7-one.

$C_{12}H_8O_4$ = 216.2.
*CAS — 484-20-8.*
*ATC — D05BA03.*

### Profile

5-Methoxypsoralen is a photosensitiser with actions similar to those of methoxsalen (above). It may be given by mouth in the PUVA therapy (see under Methoxsalen, p.1153) of psoriasis and vitiligo.

5-Methoxypsoralen is included in some cosmetic suntan preparations to enhance tanning but because of its potential phototoxicity this is considered unwise by some authorities. Photosensitivity caused by 5-methoxypsoralen is sometimes known as Berloque dermatitis.

5-Methoxypsoralen is an ingredient of bergamot oil (p.1659).

◊ References.


1. McNeely W, Goa KL. 5-Methoxypsoralen: a review of its effects in psoriasis and vitiligo. *Drugs* 1998; **56:** 667–90.


**Hypersensitivity.** For mention of anaphylaxis associated with the use of 5-methoxypsoralen, see Hypersensitivity, under Adverse Effects of Methoxsalen, p.1152.

### Preparations

**Proprietary Preparations** (details are given in Part 3)
***Austria:*** Geralen; ***Fr.:*** Psoraderm 5; ***Switz.:*** Psoraderm 5†.

## Methyl Anthranilate

Methyl 2-aminobenzoate.

$C_8H_9NO_2$ = 151.2.
*CAS — 134-20-3.*

### Profile

Methyl anthranilate has been used in sunscreen preparations. It is a constituent of several essential oils.

### Preparations

**Proprietary Preparations**
Some preparations are listed in Part3.

## Mexenone *(BAN, pINN)*

Benzophenone-10; Mexenona. 2-Hydroxy-4-methoxy-4'-methylbenzophenone.

$C_{15}H_{14}O_3$ = 242.3.
*CAS — 1641-17-4.*

**Pharmacopoeias.** In *Br.*

**BP 2003** (Mexenone). A pale yellow odourless or almost odourless crystalline powder. Practically insoluble in water; sparingly soluble in alcohol; freely soluble in acetone.

### Profile

Mexenone, a substituted benzophenone, is a sunscreen (see p.1133) with actions similar to those of oxybenzone (p.1155). It is effective against UVB and some UVA light (for definitions, see p.1136)

### Preparations

***BP 2003:*** Mexenone Cream.

**Proprietary Preparations**
Some preparations are listed in Part 3.

## Monobenzone *(rINN)*

Hydroquinone Monobenzyl Ether; Monobenzona. 4-Benzyloxyphenol.

$C_{13}H_{12}O_2$ = 200.2.
*CAS — 103-16-2.*
*ATC — D11AX13.*

**Pharmacopoeias.** In *US.*

**USP 27** (Monobenzone). Store at a temperature not exceeding 30° in airtight containers. Protect from light.

### Adverse Effects and Precautions

Monobenzone may cause skin irritation and sensitisation. In some patients this is transient and the drug need not be withdrawn. In others, an eczematous sensitisation may occur. Excessive depigmentation may occur even beyond the areas under treatment and may produce unsightly patches.

Monobenzone can produce permanent depigmentation and should not be used as a substitute for hydroquinone.

### Interactions

**Agalsidase.** For the recommendation that monobenzone not be used with agalsidase alfa or beta, see p.1651.

### Uses and Administration

Monobenzone has actions similar to those of hydroquinone (p.1148) but in some patients it also produces extensive and selective destruction of melanocytes. It is used locally for final, permanent depigmentation of normal skin in extensive vitiligo (see Pigmentation Disorders, p.1137). Monobenzone is not recommended for freckling, chloasma, or hyperpigmentation following skin inflammation or due to photosensitisation after the use of certain perfumes. It has no effect on melanomas or pigmented naevi.

For vitiligo monobenzone is applied in the form of a cream containing up to 20% to the affected parts two or three times daily until a satisfactory response is obtained, and thereafter as necessary, usually about twice weekly. Excessive exposure to sunlight should be avoided during treatment. The results are variable. Depigmentation only becomes apparent when the preformed melanin pigments have been lost with the normal sloughing of the stratum corneum and this may take several months. If, however, no improvement is noted after 4 months, treatment should be abandoned.

### Preparations

***USP 27:*** Monobenzone Cream.

**Proprietary Preparations**
Some preparations are listed in Part 3.

## Monochloroacetic Acid

Chloroacetic Acid.

$C_2H_3O_2Cl$ = 94.5.
*CAS — 79-11-8.*

### Profile

Preparations containing 50% of monochloroacetic acid are used as a caustic for the removal of plantar warts (p.1139).

### Preparations

**Proprietary Preparations** (details are given in Part 3)
***Austria:*** Warzenmittel; ***Ger.:*** Acetocaustin; ***Switz.:*** Acetocaustine.

## Motretinide *(USAN, rINN)*

Motretinida; Ro-11-1430. (*all-trans*)-*N*-Ethyl-9-(4-methoxy-2,3,6-trimethylphenyl)-3,7-dimethyl-2,4,6,8-nonatetraenamide.

$C_{23}H_{31}NO_2$ = 353.5.
*CAS — 56281-36-8.*
*ATC — D10AD05.*

### Profile

Motretinide is a retinoid structurally related to acitretin (p.1140). Motretinide is used topically in the treatment of acne (p.1133). It is applied in preparations containing 0.1%.

### Preparations

**Proprietary Preparations** (details are given in Part 3)
***Switz.:*** Tasmaderm.

## Octil Triazone

Octyl Triazone. 2,4,6-Trianilino-*p*-(carbo-2'-ethylhexyl-1'-oxy)-1,3,5-triazine.

$C_{48}H_{66}N_6O_6$ = 823.1.
*CAS — 88122-99-0.*

### Profile

Octil triazone is used as a sunscreen (p.1133). It is effective against UVB light (for definitions, see p.1136).

### Preparations

**Proprietary Preparations**
Some preparations are listed in Part 3.

## Octinoxate *(USAN, rINN)*

Octinoxato; Octyl methoxycinnamate; Parsol MCX. 2-Ethylhexyl-*p*-methoxycinnamate.

$C_{18}H_{26}O_3$ = 290.4.
*CAS — 5466-77-3.*
*ATC — D02BA02.*

**Pharmacopoeias.** In *US.*

**USP 27** (Octinoxate). Pale yellow oil. Insoluble in water. Store in airtight containers at a temperature of 8° to 15°.

### Profile

Octinoxate, a substituted cinnamate, is used by topical application as a sunscreen (see p.1133). Cinnamate sunscreens effectively absorb light throughout the UVB range but absorb little or no UVA light (for definitions, see p.1136). Cinnamate sunscreens may therefore be used to prevent sunburn but are unlikely to prevent drug-related or other photosensitivity reactions associated with UVA light; combination with a benzophenone may give some added protection against such photosensitivity. Cinnamates may occasionally produce photosensitivity reactions.

### Preparations

**Proprietary Preparations**
Numerous preparations are listed in Part 3.

## Octisalate *(USAN, rINN)*

Octisalato; Octyl Salicylate. 2-Ethylhexyl salicylate.

$C_{15}H_{22}O_3$ = 250.3.
*CAS — 118-60-5.*

**Pharmacopoeias.** In *US.*

**USP 27** (Octisalate). Store in airtight containers.

### Profile

Octisalate is a substituted salicylate used by topical application as a sunscreen (see p.1133). Salicylates effectively absorb light throughout the UVB range but absorb little or no UVA light (for definitions, see p.1136). Salicylate sunscreens may therefore be used to prevent sunburn, but are unlikely to prevent drug-related or other photosensitivity reactions associated with UVA light; combination with a benzophenone may give some added protection.

Salicylates may occasionally produce photosensitivity reactions.

### Preparations

**Proprietary Preparations**
Numerous preparations are listed in Part 3.

## Octocrilene *(rINN)*

2-Ethylhexyl α-cyano-β-phenylcinnamate; Octocrileno; Octocrylene *(USAN)*. 2-Ethylhexyl 2-cyano-3,3-diphenylacrylate.

$C_{24}H_{27}NO_2$ = 361.5.
*CAS — 6197-30-4.*

**Pharmacopoeias.** In *US.*

**USP 27** (Octocrylene). Store in airtight containers.

### Profile

Octocrilene, a substituted cinnamate, is a sunscreen (see p.1133) with actions similar to those of octinoxate (p.1154). It is effective against UVB light (for definitions, see p.1136).

### Preparations

**Proprietary Preparations**
Numerous preparations are listed in Part 3.

## Oxybenzone *(USAN, rINN)*

Benzophenone-3; Oxibenzona. 2-Hydroxy-4-methoxybenzophenone.

$C_{14}H_{12}O_3$ = 228.2.
*CAS — 131-57-7.*

**Pharmacopoeias.** In *US.*

**USP 27** (Oxybenzone). A pale yellow powder. Practically insoluble in water; freely soluble in alcohol and in toluene. Store in airtight containers. Protect from light.

### Profile

Oxybenzone is a substituted benzophenone used by topical application as a sunscreen (see p.1133). Benzophenones effectively absorb light throughout the UVB range (wavelengths 290 to 320 nm) and also absorb some UVA light with wavelengths of 320 to about 360 nm and some UVC light with wavelengths of about 250 to 290 nm (for definitions, see p.1136). Benzophenones may therefore be used to prevent sunburn and may also provide some protection against drug-related or other photosensitivity reactions associated with UVA light; in practice they are usually combined with a sunscreen from another group.

Contact and photocontact allergic dermatitis has occasionally been reported following the topical administration of benzophenone sunscreens.

**Hypersensitivity.** References to allergic and photoallergic reactions in a few patients using oxybenzone sunscreens.[1-4]

1. Thompson G, *et al.* Allergic contact dermatitis from sunscreen preparations complicating photodermatitis. *Arch Dermatol* 1977; **113:** 1252–3.
2. Thune P. Contact and photocontact allergy to sunscreens. *Photodermatology* 1984; **1:** 5–9.
3. Knoler E, *et al.* Photoallergy to benzophenone. *Arch Dermatol* 1989; **125:** 801–4.
4. Collins P, Ferguson J. Photoallergic contact dermatitis to oxybenzone. *Br J Dermatol* 1994; **131:** 124–9.

### Preparations

***USP 27:*** Dioxybenzone and Oxybenzone Cream.

**Proprietary Preparations**
Numerous preparations are listed in Part 3.

## Padimate *(BAN, rINN)*

Amyl Dimethylaminobenzoate; Isoamyl Dimethylaminobenzoate; Padimate A *(USAN)*; Padimato. A mixture of pentyl, isopentyl, and 2-methylbutyl 4-dimethylaminobenzoates.

$C_{14}H_{21}NO_2$ = 235.3.
*CAS — 14779-78-3 (pentyl 4-dimethylaminobenzoate); 21245-01-2 (isopentyl 4-dimethylaminobenzoate).*

### Profile

Padimate, a substituted aminobenzoate, is a sunscreen (p.1133) with actions similar to those of aminobenzoic acid (p.1142). It is effective against UVB light (for definitions, see p.1136).

### Preparations

**Proprietary Preparations**
Some preparations are listed in Part 3.

## Padimate O *(BANM, USAN)*

Octyl Dimethyl PABA; Padimato O. 2-Ethylhexyl 4-(dimethylamino)benzoate.

$C_{17}H_{27}NO_2$ = 277.4.
*CAS — 21245-02-3.*

**Pharmacopoeias.** In *US.*

**USP 27** (Padimate O). A light yellow, mobile liquid with a faint aromatic odour. Practically insoluble in water, in glycerol, and in propylene glycol; soluble in alcohol, in isopropyl alcohol, and in liquid paraffin. Store in airtight containers. Protect from light.

### Profile

Padimate O, a substituted aminobenzoate, is a sunscreen (see p.1133) with actions similar to those of aminobenzoic acid (p.1142). It is effective against UVB light (for definitions, see p.1136).

**Hypersensitivity.** References to contact or photocontact allergy to padimate O.

1. Weller P, Freeman S. Photocontact allergy to octyldimethyl PABA. *Australas J Dermatol* 1984; **25:** 73–6.
2. Thune P. Contact and photocontact allergy to sunscreens. *Photodermatology* 1984; **1:** 5–9.
3. English JSC, *et al.* Sensitivity to sunscreens. *Contact Dermatitis* 1987; **17:** 159–62.

### Preparations

***USP 27:*** Padimate O Lotion.

**Proprietary Preparations**
Numerous preparations are listed in Part 3.

## Pimecrolimus *(BAN, USAN, rINN)*

SDZ-ASM-981.
(3S,4R,5S,8R,9E,12S,14S,15R,16S,18R,19R,26aS)-3-{(E)-2-[(1R,3R,4S)-4-Chloro-3-methoxycyclohexyl]-1-methylvinyl}-8-ethyl-5,6,8,11,12,13,14,15,16,17,18,19,24,25,26,26a-hexadecahydro-5,19-dihydroxy-14,16-dimethoxy-4,10,12,18-tetramethyl-15,19-epoxy-3H-pyrido[2,1-c][1,4]oxaazacyclotricosine-1,7,20,21(4H,23H)-tetrone.

$C_{43}H_{68}ClNO_{11}$ = 810.5.
*CAS — 137071-32-0.*
*ATC — D11AX15.*

### Profile

Pimecrolimus is a macrolactam ascomycin derivative related to tacrolimus (p.1363) and with similar anti-inflammatory and immunosuppressant actions. It is used for short-term and intermittent long-term treatment of mild to moderate atopic eczema (p.1135) in non-immunocompromised patients over the age of two years. Pimecrolimus is applied twice daily as a 1% cream.

The most frequent adverse effects of pimecrolimus are a burning sensation, irritation, pruritus, erythema, and skin infections, at the application site.

Oral forms of pimecrolimus are also being investigated for the treatment of psoriasis and atopic eczema.

◊ Reviews.

1. Wellington K, Jarvis B. Topical pimecrolimus: a review of its clinical potential in the management of atopic dermatitis. *Drugs* 2002; **62:** 817–40.
2. Anonymous. Topical pimecrolimus (Elidel) for treatment of atopic dermatitis. *Med Lett Drugs Ther* 2002; **44:** 48–50.
3. Anonymous. Pimecrolimus cream for atopic dermatitis. *Drug Ther Bull* 2003; **41:** 33–6.

**Administration in infants.** A 6-week, double-blind, randomised study of 186 infants between the age of 3 and 23 months, followed by a 20-week open-label phase, demonstrated that 1% pimecrolimus cream, applied twice daily was both safe and effective in mild to moderate atopic eczema.[1] The manufacturers, however, do not recommend its use in patients under 2 years of age as the effect of pimecrolimus cream on the developing immune system in infants is unknown.

1. Ho VC, *et al.* Safety and efficacy of nonsteroid pimecrolimus cream 1% in the treatment of atopic dermatitis in infants. *J Pediatr* 2003; **142:** 155–62.

### Preparations

**Proprietary Preparations** (details are given in Part 3)
***NZ:*** Elidel; ***UK:*** Elidel; ***USA:*** Elidel.

## Piroctone Olamine *(USAN, rINNM)*

Piroctona olamina. 1-Hydroxy-4-methyl-6-(2,4,4-trimethylpentyl)-2(1H)-pyridone compound with 2-aminoethanol (1:1).

$C_{14}H_{23}NO_2,C_2H_7NO$ = 298.4.
*CAS — 50650-76-5 (piroctone); 68890-66-4 (piroctone olamine).*

### Profile

Piroctone olamine has been used in shampoos for the treatment of dandruff.

### Preparations

**Proprietary Preparations** (details are given in Part 3)
***Arg.:*** Lovilia; Megacistin G; Plusgel; ***Austral.:*** Neoceuticals Therapeutic Shampoo†; ***Fr.:*** Cystel Antipelliculaire; ***Irl.:*** Saliker; ***Ital.:*** Olamin P.

**Multi-ingredient:** ***Arg.:*** Aspergun; Micocert; Pitiriax; Pityval; Saliker; Tersoderm Anticaspa; ***Braz.:*** Ortosol P; Saliker; ***Chile:*** Foltene Research Anticaspa; Neostrata; ***Fr.:*** Alpha 5 DS; Biolan Tar†; Epiphane; Hyfac Plus; Ionax P; Item Alphakeptol; Liperol; Node DS; Node P; Pityker; Pityval; Saliker; Squaphane; T/Gel†; ***Ital.:*** Biothymus DS; Genisol; Nonak; Shamday Antiforfora; Tricoderm F; ***Port.:*** Alpha Septol†; Alphakeptol; Bioclin Sebo Care; Hyfac AHA†; Hyfac†; Ionil P; Peliphane†; Savorix T†; Squaphane†; ***Spain:*** Ionax P.

# Podophyllum

American Mandrake; May Apple Root; Podófilo; Podoph.; Podophyllum Rhizome.

*CAS — 568-53-6 (α-peltatin); 518-29-6 (β-peltatin).*

**Pharmacopoeias.** In *US.*

**USP 27** (Podophyllum). The dried rhizomes and roots of *Podophyllum peltatum* (Berberidaceae). It yields not less than 5% of resin. It has a slight odour.

## Indian Podophyllum

Ind. Podoph.; Indian Podophyllum Rhizome; Podófilo indio.

**Description.** The dried fruits or rhizomes and roots of *Podophyllum hexandrum (P. emodi)* (Berberidaceae).

## Podophyllum Resin

Podofilino; Podoph. Resin; Podophylli Resina; Podophyllin.

*CAS — 8050-60-0.*

**Pharmacopoeias.** In *Int., Swiss,* and *US* (all from podophyllum only). In *Br.* from Indian podophyllum.

**BP 2003** (Podophyllum Resin). The resin obtained from the rhizomes and roots of *Podophyllum hexandrum (P. emodi).* It contains not less than 50% of total aryltetralin lignans, calculated as podophyllotoxin.

An amorphous powder, varying in colour from light brown to greenish-yellow or brownish-grey masses, with a characteristic odour; caustic. On exposure to light or to temperatures above 25° it becomes darker in colour.

Partly soluble in hot water but precipitated again on cooling; partly soluble in chloroform, in ether, and in dilute ammonia solution. Protect from light.

**USP 27** (Podophyllum Resin). The powdered mixture of resins extracted from podophyllum (the rhizomes and roots of *Podophyllum peltatum*) by percolation with alcohol and subsequent precipitation with acidified water. It contains not less than 40% and not more than 50% of hexane-insoluble matter.

An amorphous caustic powder, varying in colour from light brown to greenish-yellow. On exposure to light or to temperatures above 25° it becomes darker in colour. Soluble in alcohol with a slight opalescence; partially soluble in chloroform and in ether. A solution in alcohol is acid to litmus. Store in airtight containers. Protect from light.

## Podophyllotoxin *(BAN)*

Podofilotoxina; Podofilox *(USAN)*. (5R,5aR,8aR,9R)-5,5a,6,8,8a,9-Hexahydro-9-hydroxy-5-(3,4,5-trimethoxyphenyl)furo[3′4′:6,7]naphtho[2,3-d]-1,3-dioxol-6-one.

$C_{22}H_{22}O_8$ = 414.4.
*CAS — 518-28-5.*
*ATC — D06BB04.*

### Adverse Effects

Podophyllum is very irritant, especially to the eyes and mucous membranes. It can also cause severe systemic toxicity after ingestion or topical application, which is usually reversible but has been fatal. Symptoms of toxicity include nausea, vomiting, abdominal pain, and diarrhoea; there may be thrombocytopenia, leucopenia, renal failure, and hepatotoxicity. Central effects are delayed in onset and prolonged in duration and include acute psychotic reactions, hallucinations, confusion, dizziness, stupor, ataxia, hypotonia, seizures, and coma. EEG changes may persist for several days. Peripheral and autonomic neuropathies develop later and may result in paraesthesias, reduced reflexes, muscle weakness, tachycardia, apnoea, orthostatic hypotension, paralytic ileus, and urinary retention. Neuropathy may improve but full recovery is unusual.

**Carcinogenicity.** A report of the transformation of a condyloma acuminatum into an invasive squamous cell carcinoma after treatment with podophyllum 25% in alcohol.[1]

1. Svindland HB. Malignant transformation of condyloma acuminatum after treatment with podophyllin. *Eur J Sex Transm Dis* 1984; **1:** 165–7.

**Poisoning.** Reports and reviews of podophyllum toxicity.[1-7] A few of the cases followed consumption of herbal preparations containing podophyllum or the related plant bajiaolian (*Dysosma pleianthum*). Death has occurred following ingestion of 10 g of podophyllum.

1. Cassidy DE, *et al.* Podophyllum toxicity: a report of a fatal case and a review of the literature. *J Toxicol Clin Toxicol* 1982; **19:** 35–44.
2. Dobb GJ, Edis RH. Coma and neuropathy after ingestion of herbal laxative containing podophyllin. *Med J Aust* 1984; **140:** 495–6.
3. Holdright DR, Jahangiri M. Accidental poisoning with podophyllin. *Hum Exp Toxicol* 1990; **9:** 55–6.
4. Tomczak RL, Hake DH. Near fatal systemic toxicity from local injection of podophyllin for pedal verrucae treatment. *J Foot Surg* 1992; **31:** 36–42.
5. Kao W-F, *et al.* Podophyllotoxin intoxication: toxic effect of bajiaolian in herbal therapeutics. *Hum Exp Toxicol* 1992; **11:** 480–7.
6. Chan TYK, Critchley JAJH. Usage and adverse effects of Chinese herbal medicines. *Hum Exp Toxicol* 1996; **15:** 5–12.
7. Chu CC, *et al.* Sensory neuropathy due to bajiaolian (podophyllotoxin) intoxication. *Eur Neurol* 2000; **44:** 121–3.

### Precautions

Podophyllum should not be used during pregnancy or breast feeding or in children.

The risk of systemic toxicity after topical application is increased by the treatment of large areas with excessive amounts for prolonged periods, by the treatment of friable, bleeding, or recently biopsied warts, and by inadvertent application to normal skin or mucous membranes.

**Handling.** Podophyllum resin is strongly irritant to the skin, eyes, and mucous membranes and requires careful handling.

### Uses and Administration

Podophyllum resin has an antimitotic action and is used principally as a topical treatment for anogenital warts (condylomata acuminata). It is applied as a 15% (Indian podophyllum) or up to a 25% solution (American podophyllum) in alcohol or compound benzoin tincture, left on the warts for 1 to 6 hours, and then washed off. This procedure is carried out once a week and, if unsuccessful after about 6 weeks, an alternative treatment should be tried. A preparation containing podophyllotoxin 0.5% in alcohol or alcoholic gel, or a 0.15% podophyllotoxin cream is used similarly. They are applied twice daily for 3 days but not washed off. Treatment may be repeated at weekly intervals for up to a total of 5 weeks of treatment. Podophyllum resin has been used on external genital, perianal, and intrameatal warts, but should not be used on cervical or urethral warts. Only a small area or number of warts should be treated at any one time. Care must be taken to avoid application to healthy tissue. Podophyllum resin is also used with other keratolytics for the removal of plantar warts.

When taken by mouth podophyllum resin has a drastic purging action and it is highly irritant to the intestinal mucosa and produces violent peristalsis. It has been superseded by less toxic laxatives.

Podophyllum has been used in homoeopathic medicine.

**Anogenital warts.** Podophyllum preparations are one of the treatment choices for anogenital warts caused by human papillomavirus infection (condylomata acuminata) (p.1139).

Paints containing 10% or 25% of podophyllum resin appear to be equally effective for the treatment of external anogenital warts.[1] However, preparations containing podophyllotoxin 0.5%, the major active constituent of podophyllum resin, appear to be initially more effective[2] and unlike podophyllum, may be suitable for self-treatment in both men and women.[3,4]

1. Simmons PD. Podophyllin 10% and 25% in the treatment of anogenital warts: a comparative double-blind study. *Br J Vener Dis* 1981; **57:** 208–9.
2. Anonymous. Painting penile warts. *Drug Ther Bull* 1990; **28:** 63–4.
3. Beutner KR, *et al.* Patient-applied podofilox for treatment of genital warts. *Lancet* 1989; **i:** 831–4.
4. Greenberg MD, *et al.* A double-blind, randomized trial of 0.5% podofilox and placebo for the treatment of genital warts in women. *Obstet Gynecol* 1991; **77:** 735–9.

### Preparations

***BP 2003:*** Compound Podophyllin Paint;
***USP 27:*** Podophyllum Resin Topical Solution.

**Proprietary Preparations** (details are given in Part 3)
***Arg.:*** Podoxin; ***Austral.:*** Condyline; Wartec; ***Austria:*** Condylox; ***Belg.:*** Condyline†; ***Braz.:*** Wartec; ***Canad.:*** Condyline; Podofilm; Wartec; ***Chile:*** Wartec; ***Denm.:*** Condyline; Wartec; ***Fin.:*** Condyline; Wartec; ***Fr.:*** Condyline; Wartec; ***Ger.:*** Condylox; Wartec; ***Gr.:*** Podofilox; Wartec; ***Hong Kong:*** Podofilm†; Wartec; ***Irl.:*** Condyline; Warticon; ***Israel:*** Condylox; ***Ital.:*** Condyline; Wartec; ***Mex.:*** Condil†; Papilo Lisin†; Podofilia; Vipodo; ***Neth.:*** Condyline; ***Norw.:*** Condyline; Wartec; ***NZ:*** Condyline; Wartec; ***Port.:*** Condyline†; ***S.Afr.:*** Wartec; ***Singapore:*** Podofilm†; Wartec; ***Spain:*** Condelone†; Wartec; ***Swed.:*** Condyline; Wartec; ***Switz.:*** Condyline; Warix; ***UK:*** Condyline; Warticon; ***USA:*** Condylox; Pod-Ben-25; Podocon; Podofin.

**Multi-ingredient:** ***Arg.:*** Calculina; ***Austral.:*** Posalfilin; ***Belg.:*** Sanicolax†; ***Braz.:*** Steitonit†; ***Canad.:*** Canthacur-PS; Cantharone Plus; ***Ger.:*** Unguentum lymphaticum; ***Hong Kong:*** Posalfilin; ***Irl.:*** Posalfilin; ***Malaysia:*** Posalfilin; ***NZ:*** Posalfilin; ***Port.:*** Cholagutt; ***S.Afr.:*** Posalfilin; ***Singapore:*** Posalfilin; ***Spain:*** Alofedina; Laxo Vian†; ***UK:*** Posalfilin.

## Polyphloroglucinol Phosphate

Polifloroglucinol, fosfato de; Polyphloroglucin Phosphate. Poly-[benzene-1,3,5-triol mono(dihydrogen phosphate)].

$(C_6H_7O_6P)_n$.

*CAS — 51202-77-8.*

### Profile

Polyphloroglucinol phosphate has an inhibitory effect on hyaluronidase and has been applied topically in the treatment of wounds and pruritic skin disorders.

### Preparations

**Proprietary Preparations** (details are given in Part 3)
***Austria:*** Dealyd.

## Polyprenoic Acid

E-5166; Poliprenoico, ácido; Polyprenic Acid. (*all-E*)-3,7,11,15-Tetramethyl-2,4,6,10,14-hexadecapentaenoic acid.

$C_{20}H_{30}O_2$ = 302.5.

*CAS — 81485-25-8.*

### Profile

Polyprenoic acid is a retinoid that has been tried in psoriasis and keratoderma and is being studied in the treatment of liver cancers.

◊ References.

1. Muto Y, *et al.* Prevention of second primary tumors by an acyclic retinoid, polyprenoic acid, in patients with hepatocellular carcinoma. *N Engl J Med* 1996; **334:** 1561–7.
2. Muto Y, *et al.* Prevention of second primary tumors by an acyclic retinoid in patients with hepatocellular carcinoma. *N Engl J Med* 1999; **340:** 1046–7.

## Prezatide Copper Acetate *(USAN, rINN)*

Acetato de prezatida cúprica; PC-1020 (prezatide copper). Hydrogen [$N^2$-(*N*-glycyl-L-histidyl)-L-lysinato][$N^2$-(*N*-glycyl-L-histidyl)-L-lysinato(2−)]cuprate(1−) diacetate.

$C_{28}H_{46}CuN_{12}O_8,2C_2H_4O_2$ = 862.4.

*CAS — 130120-57-9.*

### Profile

Prezatide copper acetate is a copper-containing tripeptide that is used as a wound-healing agent and has been investigated in inflammatory bowel disease.

### Preparations

**Proprietary Preparations** (details are given in Part 3)
***Braz.:*** Prezatim; ***Mex.:*** lamin; ***USA:*** lamin Hydrating Gel.

## Pyrithione Zinc *(BAN, USAN, rINN)*

Piritiona cíncica; Zinc 2-Pyridinethiol 1-Oxide; Zinc Pyridinethione. Bis[1-hydroxypyridine-2(1*H*)-thionato]zinc.

$C_{10}H_8N_2O_2S_2Zn$ = 317.7.

*CAS — 13463-41-7.*

*ATC — D11AX12.*

### Profile

Pyrithione zinc has bacteriostatic and fungistatic properties. It is used similarly to selenium sulfide (p.1157) in usual concentrations of 1 to 2% in the control of seborrhoeic dermatitis and dandruff (p.1138). It is an ingredient of some proprietary shampoos. It has also been used in the treatment of pityriasis versicolor.

Pyrithione magnesium has also been used.

**Effects on the nervous system.** Peripheral neuritis with paraesthesia and muscle weakness in a patient was associated with the prolonged use of a shampoo containing pyrithione zinc 2%.[1] The muscle weakness had disappeared 3 months after stopping the shampoo and 2 years later the paraesthesia had improved by about 75%.

Studies in *animals* had found signs of neurotoxicity following oral administration of pyrithione zinc but whereas absorption following topical application was found to be 13% for pyrithione sodium it was less than 1% for pyrithione zinc.[2]

1. Beck JE. Zinc pyrithione and peripheral neuritis. *Lancet* 1978; **i:** 444.
2. Parekh CK. Zinc pyrithione and peripheral neuritis. *Lancet* 1978, **i:** 940.

### Preparations

**Proprietary Preparations** (details are given in Part 3)
***Arg.:*** Aeroseb; Amenite Cap; Antiminth; Dermazinc; Min Huil; Skin-Cap; ZNP; ***Austral.:*** Dan-Gard; Dandruff Control Pert 2 in 1†; ***Austria:*** Desquaman; ***Canad.:*** Advance; Anti-Dandruff Shampoo†; Avant Garde Shampoo†; Avon Techniques Anti-Dandruff†; Brylcreem Anti-Dandruff; Dan-Gard; Dandruff Shampoo plus Conditioner; Dandruff Treatment Shampoo; Hair & Scalp; Head & Shoulders; Keep Clear Anti-Dandruff Shampoo†; Lander Dandruff Control; No-Name Dandruff Treatment†; Out of Africa; Pert Plus; Redken Solve Acid Balance†; Satinique Anti-Dandruff; Scott Dandruff Shampoo; Sebulon; Shaklee Dandruff Control; Shampooing Anti-Pelliculaire; Solve Dandruff; Techniques Anti-Dandruff; ZNP; ZP 11; ***Chile:*** DHS Zinc; Skin Cap; ZNP; ***Denm.:*** Skaelud; ***Fr.:*** Hermal†; Provegol; Shampooing Traitant Antipelliculaire; ZNP; ***Ger.:*** De-squaman N; ***Gr.:*** Daohair-S; ***Hong Kong:*** Hair & Scalp†; ***Israel:*** Desquaman; ***Ital.:*** Rivescal ZPT; Shampoo SDE Zinc; ZNP; ***Mex.:*** Skin Cap†; ZNP; ***Port.:*** Desquaman†; ZP Dermil; ***Spain:*** Zincation; ***USA:*** DHS Zinc; Head & Shoulders; Skin Cure; Theraplex Z†; Zincon; ZNP.

**Multi-ingredient:** ***Arg.:*** Aeroseb; Hairplus; Molnia; Neo Moldava; ***Austral.:*** Fongitar; ***Canad.:*** Dan-Tar Plus; Multi-Tar Plus; Polytar AF; X-Seb Plus; Z-Plus; ***Fr.:*** Item Alphakeptol; Node DS; Node P; ***Hong Kong:*** Fongitar; Multi-Tar; ***Ital.:*** Aminotril†; Biothymus DS; Fongitar†; Kevis; Omadine†; ***NZ:*** Fongitar; ***Port.:*** All Pecium; Alpha Septol†; Alphakeptol; Fongitar; Hyfac†; ***Singapore:*** Fongitar; pHisoHex Reformulated; ***Spain:*** Zincation Plus; ***Switz.:*** Crinotar†; Sebo Shampooing; Sebo-Soufrol; Soufrol ZNP†; Squa-med; ***Thai.:*** Fongitar; ***UK:*** Polytar AF; ***USA:*** X-Seb Plus.

## Pyrogallol

Pirogálico, ácido; Pyrogallic Acid. Benzene-1,2,3-triol.

$C_6H_6O_3$ = 126.1.

*CAS — 87-66-1.*

**Pharmacopoeias.** In *Fr.* and *Pol.*

### Profile

Pyrogallol was formerly used topically in the treatment of psoriasis and parasitic skin diseases, but application over large areas or denuded surfaces is dangerous and may produce systemic effects similar to phenol poisoning (see p.1188); methaemoglobinaemia, haemolysis, and kidney damage may also occur.

Pyrogallol stains the skin and hair black.

### Preparations

**Proprietary Preparations** (details are given in Part 3)
***USA:*** Pyrogallic.

## Pyroxylin *(rINN)*

Algodão-Pólvora; Cellulose Nitrate; Colloxylinum; Fulmicoton; Gossypium Collodium; Kollodiumwolle; Piroxilina; Pyroxylinum; Soluble Guncotton.

*CAS — 9004-70-0.*

**Pharmacopoeias.** In *Br., Jpn, Pol.,* and *US.*

**BP 2003** (Pyroxylin). A nitrated cellulose obtained by the action of a mixture of nitric and sulfuric acids on wood pulp or cotton linters that have been freed from fatty matter. It must be damped with not less than 25% of isopropyl alcohol or of industrial methylated spirit. White or almost white cuboid granules or fibrous material resembling absorbent cotton but harsher to the touch and more powdery. It is highly flammable. Soluble in acetone and in glacial acetic acid. Store in well-closed containers, loosely packed, protected from light, and at a temperature not exceeding 15°, remote from fire. The container should be suitably designed to disrupt should the internal pressure reach or exceed 1400 kPa. The amount of damping fluid must not be allowed to fall below 25% w/w; should this happen, the material should be either re-wetted or used immediately for the preparation of Collodion.

**USP 27** (Pyroxylin). Pyroxylin is obtained by the action of a mixture of nitric and sulfuric acids on cotton and consists chiefly of cellulose tetranitrate $(C_{12}H_{16}N_4O_{18})_n$. It occurs as a light yellow, matted mass of filaments resembling raw cotton but harsher to the touch. It is highly flammable. Store loosely packed, protected from light. When kept in well-closed containers and exposed to light, it decomposes with the evolution of nitrous vapours, leaving a carbonaceous residue.

### Profile

Pyroxylin is used in the preparation of collodions which are applied to the skin for the protection of small cuts and abrasions. Collodions are also used as vehicles for the application of drugs when prolonged local action is required.

**Handling.** Dry pyroxylin is explosive and sensitive to ignition by impact or friction and should be handled carefully.

### Preparations

***BP 2003:*** Collodion; Flexible Collodion;
***USP 27:*** Collodion; Flexible Collodion.

**Proprietary Preparations** (details are given in Part 3)
**Multi-ingredient:** ***UK:*** Dispello.

## Resorcinol

*m*-Dihydroxybenzene; Dioxybenzolum; Resorcin; Resorcinolum. Benzene-1,3-diol.

$C_6H_6O_2$ = 110.1.

*CAS — 108-46-3.*

*ATC — D10AX02; S01AX06.*

**Pharmacopoeias.** In *Chin., Eur.* (see p.vi), *Pol.,* and *US.*

**Ph. Eur. 5.0** (Resorcinol). Colourless or slightly pinkish-grey crystals or crystalline powder. M.p. 109° to 112°. It becomes red on exposure to air and light. Very soluble in water and in alcohol. Protect from light.

**USP 27** (Resorcinol). White or practically white, needle-shaped crystals or powder with a faint characteristic odour. M.p. 109° to 111°. It acquires a pink tint on exposure to air and light. Soluble 1 in 1 of water and of alcohol; slightly soluble in chloroform; freely soluble in ether and in glycerol. A 5% solution in water is neutral or acid to litmus. Protect from light.

**Incompatibility.** Resorcinol is incompatible with ferric salts.

## Resorcinol Monoacetate

Resorcin Acetate; Resorcinol, monoacetato de. 3-Acetoxyphenol.

$C_8H_8O_3$ = 152.1.

*CAS — 102-29-4.*

*ATC — D10AX02; S01AX06.*

**Pharmacopoeias.** In *US.*

**USP 27** (Resorcinol Monoacetate). A pale yellow or amber, viscous liquid with a faint characteristic odour. Sparingly soluble in water; soluble in alcohol and in most organic solvents. A saturated solution in water is acid to litmus. Store in airtight containers. Protect from light.

### Adverse Effects, Treatment, and Precautions

Resorcinol is a mild irritant and may result in skin sensitisation. It should not be applied to large areas of the body, for prolonged periods, or in high concentrations, especially in children, as it is absorbed through intact skin as well as broken skin and may interfere with thyroid function or produce methaemoglobinaemia. Resorcinol may produce hyperpigmentation in patients with dark skins and may darken light-coloured hair. Systemic toxic effects of resorcinol are similar to those of phenol and are treated similarly (see p.1188) but convulsions may occur more frequently.

**Abnormal coloration.** Resorcinol could cause green discoloration of the urine.[1]

1. Karlstrand J. The pharmacist and the ostomate. *J Am Pharm Assoc* 1977; **NS17:** 735–8.

### Uses and Administration

Resorcinol has keratolytic properties and has been used, usually with sulfur, in topical preparations for the treatment of acne (p.1133) and seborrhoeic skin conditions (p.1138), although other treatments are generally preferred.

Resorcinol has also been used in preparations for the treatment of anorectal disorders often complexed with bismuth compounds (see Haemorrhoids, p.1243).

Resorcinol monoacetate has been used similarly but may provide a milder action with a longer duration.

**Dentistry.** Resorcinol powder added incrementally to a few drops of formaldehyde 40% solution to saturation and polymerised using 1 or 2 drops of sodium hydroxide 10% solution produces a hard red material known as "Russian Red". This resin has been used in dentistry in Eastern Europe, Russia, and China. Zinc oxide or barium sulfate is often added to the mixture before polymerisation to make it radio-opaque.[1]

1. Schwandt NW, Gound TG. Resorcinol-formaldehyde resin "Russina Red" endodontic therapy. *J Endod* 2003; **29:** 435–7.

### Preparations

**BPC 1973:** Magenta Paint;
**USP 27:** Carbol-Fuchsin Topical Solution; Compound Resorcinol Ointment; Resorcinol and Sulfur Lotion.

**Proprietary Preparations** (details are given in Part 3)
**Chile:** Dermobarrina; **Mex.:** Astriderm†; **USA:** Castel.

**Multi-ingredient:** **Arg.:** Acnomel; Acnoxin; Callicida; Coltix; Cutidermin; Ecnagel; Ecnagel E; Farmigras; Histidanol; Nemegel; Pinklot; **Austral.:** Acne & Pimple Gel; Egomycol†; Eskamel; Seborrol†; **Austria:** Apotheker Bauer's Huhneraugentinktur; Wisamt; **Belg.:** Synthol†; **Braz.:** Clearasil†; Cravo-Espin†; Pantevit; **Canad.:** Acne-Aid†; Acnomel Acne Mask†; Acnomel†; Clearasil Acne Cream; Clearskin 2 Tinted Blemish†; Lanacane Medicated Cream; Mazon Medicated Cream; Sebo Concept D/A†; Vagisil; **Chile:** Acnaid; Antiacne; Dermac Crema; **Fr.:** Anaxeryl; Bain de Bouche Lipha; Eau Precieuse; Gelictar Fort; Nestosyl; Osmotol; Squaphane; Synthol; **Ger.:** Jaikal; Wisamt N; **Hong Kong:** Acne-Aid; Seborrol†; **Irl.:** Anugesic-HC; Anusol-HC; **Israel:** Acnex; Pitrisan; Vagisil†; **Ital.:** Anusol; Blefarolin; Fucsina Fenica; Labocaina; Rinantipiol; **Malaysia:** Acne-Aid; **Mex.:** Crema Axel; Dermac; **NZ:** Egomycol; Lanacane; Seborrol; **Port.:** Edoltar; Resodermil; Squaphane†; **S.Afr.:** Anugesic; Anusol-HC†; **Singapore:** Acne-Aid; Anusol; **Spain:** Acnisdin; Acnosan†; Anti-Acne†; Dermomycose Liquido; Milrosina; Poliglicol Anti Acne†; Resorborina; **Switz.:** Clabin; Euproctol; Lotio decapans; **Thai.:** Anusol; **UK:** Eskamel; **USA:** Acnomel; Bensulfoid; Bicozene; Castaderm; Dermarest; Fungi-Nail; Heal Aid Plus; RA Lotion; Resinol†; Rezamid; Sulforcin; Vagisil.

---

## Roxadimate *(USAN, rINN)*

Ethyl Dihydroxypropyl PABA; Roxadimato. Ethyl (±)-4-[bis(2-hydroxypropyl)amino]benzoate.

$C_{15}H_{23}NO_4$ = 281.3.
*CAS — 58882-17-0.*

### Profile

Roxadimate, a substituted aminobenzoate, is a sunscreen (see p.1133) with actions similar to those of aminobenzoic acid (p.1142). It is effective against UVB light (for definitions, see p.1136).

### Preparations

**Proprietary Preparations**
Some preparations are listed in Part 3.

---

## Salicylic Acid

Acido Ortóxibenzoico; Acidum Salicylicum; Salicílico, ácido; Salizylsäure. 2-Hydroxybenzoic acid.

$C_7H_6O_3$ = 138.1.
*CAS — 69-72-7.*
*ATC — D01AE12; S01BC08.*

**Pharmacopoeias.** In *Chin., Eur.* (see p.vi), *Int., Jpn, Pol., US,* and *Viet.*

**Ph. Eur. 5.0** (Salicylic Acid). White or colourless acicular crystals or a white crystalline powder. Slightly soluble in water; freely soluble in alcohol; sparingly soluble in dichloromethane. Protect from light.

**USP 27** (Salicylic Acid). White crystals, usually in fine needles or a white, fluffy, crystalline powder. The synthetic form is white and odourless but if prepared from natural methyl salicylate it may have a slightly yellow or pink tint, and a faint, mint-like odour. Soluble 1 in 460 of water, 1 in 15 of boiling water, 1 in 3 of alcohol, 1 in 45 of chloroform, 1 in 3 of ether, and 1 in 135 of benzene.

### Adverse Effects and Precautions

Salicylic acid is a mild irritant and application of salicylic acid preparations to the skin may cause dermatitis. It is readily absorbed through the skin and symptoms of acute systemic salicylate poisoning (see Aspirin, p.15) have been reported after excessive use; deaths have occurred, mainly in children. To minimise absorption following topical application salicylic acid should not be used for prolonged periods, in high concentrations, on large areas of the body, or on inflamed or broken skin. Contact with mouth, eyes, and other mucous membranes should be avoided. It should also be used with care on the extremities of patients with impaired peripheral circulation or diabetes; caution has also been suggested for the use of caustic preparations in patients with significant peripheral neuropathy.

**PUVA.** There has been a report that application of 2% salicylic acid in a cream base before phototherapy delayed or reduced the clearance of psoriatic lesions when compared with the use of the base alone.[1] It was suggested that salicylic acid might have been acting as a photoprotective agent[1] but a later study[2] failed to confirm this. However, emulsifying ointment was found to have such an effect and it was recommended that it should not be used before phototherapy or in phototesting procedures.[2]


1. Kristensen B, Kristensen O. Salicylic acid and ultraviolet B for psoriasis. *Lancet* 1989; **ii:** 1109–10.
2. Cox NH, Sharpe G. Emollients, salicylic acid, and ultraviolet erythema. *Lancet* 1990; **335:** 53–4.


### Uses and Administration

Salicylic acid has **keratolytic** properties and is applied topically in the treatment of hyperkeratotic and scaling skin conditions such as dandruff and seborrhoeic dermatitis (p.1138), ichthyosis (p.1136), psoriasis (p.1137), and acne (p.1133). Initially a concentration of about 2% is used, increased to about 6% if necessary, though a wider range of concentrations has been used. It is often used with other drugs, notably coal tar.

Preparations containing up to 60% salicylic acid have been used as a **caustic** for the removal of plantar warts (p.1139), corns, or calluses.

Salicylic acid also possesses **fungicidal** properties and is used topically in the treatment of dermatophyte skin infections (see p.390); propyl salicylate and bromosalicylic acid have been used similarly.

Zinc salicylate has been used similarly to salicylic acid in the treatment of seborrhoeic dermatitis and acne.

### Preparations

**BP 2003:** Coal Tar and Salicylic Acid Ointment; Compound Benzoic Acid Ointment; Dithranol Paste; Salicylic Acid Collodion; Salicylic Acid Ointment; Zinc and Salicylic Acid Paste;
**BPC 1973:** Salicylic Acid and Sulphur Ointment;
**USP 27:** Benzoic and Salicylic Acids Ointment; Salicylic Acid Collodion; Salicylic Acid Gel; Salicylic Acid Plaster; Salicylic Acid Topical Foam; Zinc Oxide and Salicylic Acid Paste.

**Proprietary Preparations** (details are given in Part 3)
**Arg.:** Callicida; Desconphar; Duofilm; Duoforte; Kertyol; Koal; Neo A-V; Salpad; Verrutopic AS; Verrutrix; Verruxane; **Austral.:** Clear Away; Clearasil Medicated Wipes; Duofilm; Egozite Cradle Cap; Ionil; Johnsons Clean & Clear Skin Balancing Moisturiser†; Salact†; Sunspot; **Austria:** Dermi-cyl Schrunden; Squamasol†; **Belg.:** Sicombyl; **Braz.:** A Curitybina; Clean & Clear Gel Secativo; Clean & Clear Hidratante; Clean & Clear Locao Adstringente; Clean & Clear Sabonete Liquido Refrescante; Curakalos†; Denorex Daily; Denorex Plus; Duoforte; Ionil Plus†; Ionil-T Plus†; Ionil†; Neutrogena Antiacne; Salipads; Verrux†; **Canad.:** Acnex; Anti-Acne Control Formula; Anti-Acne Spot Treatment; Band-Aid Corn Remover; Blemish Control; Callus Salve†; Carnation; Clean & Clear Deep Cleaning Astringent; Clean & Clear Invsible Blemish; Clear Away†; Clear Pore†; Clearasil Cleanser; Clearasil Clearstick; Clearasil Pads; Clearasil Stay Clear; Clearskin 2 Medicated Wash†; Clearskin 2 Triple Action†; Clearskin Acne Defense Stick; Clearskin Cleansing; Clearskin Medicated Wash; Clearskin Overnight Acne Treatment; Clinique Acne Spot Treatment; Compound W; Compound W Plus; Duofilm; Duoforte; Fostex Medicated Cleansing†; Freezone; Herbal Essence Anti-Dandruff; Ionil†; Johnsons Clean & Clear Dual Action Moisturizer; Johnsons Clean & Clear Pore Prep; Keralyt†; Moscot†; Mudd Acne†; Neostrata AHA Astringent Acne; Neutrogena Acne Wash; Neutrogena Clear Pore; Neutrogena Healthy Scalp Anti-Dandruff; Neutrogena Skin Cleaning; Neutrogena T/Gel Therapeutic; Nova Perfecting Lotion†; Noxema 2-in-1; Occlusal; Off-Ezy; Oil-Free Acne Wash†; Oxy Clean Pore†; Oxy Control†; Oxy Daily Cleaning Pads; Oxy Deep Pore; Oxy Finishing Toner; Oxy Medicated Pads; Oxy Night Watch†; P & S; Propa PH; Salac†; Salseb; Scholl 2-Drop Corn Remedy; Scholl Callus Remover; Scholl Clear Away; Scholl Corn Remover; Scholl Corn Salve†; Scholl Corn, Callus Plaster Preparation†; Scholl One Step; Scholl Wart Remover†; Scholl Zino; Sebcur; Soluver; Soluver Plus; Ten-O-Six†; Trans-Plantar; Trans-Ver-Sal; Wart Remover†; X-Seb; **Chile:** DHS Sal; Duoplant Gel; Eucerin; Mediklin; Neutrogena Acondicionador Neutar Gel; Neutrogena Gel Control Brillo; Neutrogena Linea Acne; Trans-Plantar; Trans-Ver-Sal; **Denm.:** Salicyl; **Fr.:** A-Derma Pain Salicylique; Ciella; Clear Pore†; Coricide le Diable; Disques Coricides; Feuille de Saule; Kertyol; Pansements Coricides; Pommade Mo Cochon; S/Gel†; Sanitos; Septisol†; Transvercid; Verrucosal†; **Ger.:** Aknefug-liquid; Cornina Hornhaut†; Cornina Huhneraugen†; Efasit N†; Gehwol Schalpaste; Guttaplast; Hansaplast Hornhaut-Pflaster; Hansaplast Huhneraugen-Pflaster; Humopin N; Lygal Kopfsalbe N; Psorimed; Schrundensalbe Dermi-cyl; Sophtal-POS N; Squamasol; Urgo Activ Huhneraugenpflaster; Verrucid; **Gr.:** Gallifugo; **Hong Kong:** Egozite Cradle Cap; Oxy Balance†; **Irl.:** Acnisal; Compound W; Freezone†; Occlusal; Psorimed; Saliker; Vericaps; **Israel:** Clearex; Salikaren; Scholl Corn/Callous Removers; **Ital.:** Keranon; Neutrogena Anti-Acne†; Salicil; Sebium K2†; Trans-Ver-Sal; **Malaysia:** Egozite Cradle Cap; **Mex.:** Clearasil Pads†; Duoplant; Excelsior; Ionil; Ionil Plus; Trans-Ver-Sal; **Neth.:** Formule W; **NZ:** Clear Away†; Duofilm; Egozite Cradle Cap; **Port.:** Psorimed; Verrufilm; Verucid; **Spain:** Callicida Globodermis†; Callicida Gras; Callicida Salve; Callofin; Cornina; Unguento Morry; Urgocall; Verrupatch; Verruplan; **Swed.:** Salsyvase; **Switz.:** Verrufilm; **UK:** Acnisal; Carnation; Clearasil Double Action Pads; Clearasil Nightclear†; Compound V†; Compound W; Occlusal; Pickles Foot Ointment; Scholl Callus Removal; Scholl Corn Removal; Scholl Verucca Removal; SCR; Snufflebabe Cradle Cap; Verrugon; Verucca Removal System†; Wartex; **USA:** Clearasil Clearstick; Compound W; Dr Scholl's Callus Removers; Dr Scholl's Clear Away; Dr Scholl's Corn Removers; Dr Scholl's Corn/Callus Remover; Dr Scholl's Wart Remover; Duofilm; Duoplant; Fostex Acne Medication Cleansing; Freezone; Gordofilm; Hydrisalic; Ionil; Ionil Plus; Keralyt; Mediplast; MG217 Sal-Acid; Mosco; Occlusal; Off-Ezy; Oxy Night Watch; P & S; Panscol; PropapH; Psor-a-set; Sal-Acid; Sal-Plant; Salac; Salactic Film; Sebucare; Stri-Dex Clear; Trans-Ver-Sal AdultPatch; Trans-Ver-Sal PediaPatch; Trans-Ver-Sal PlantarPatch; Wart Remover; Wart-Off; X-Seb.

**Multi-ingredient:** Numerous preparations are listed in Part3.

---

## Salnacedin *(USAN, rINN)*

*N*-Acetyl-L-cysteine salicylate.

$C_{12}H_{13}NO_5S$ = 283.3.
*CAS — 87573-01-1.*

### Profile

Salnacedin has anti-inflammatory and keratolytic properties and is applied topically in the treatment of seborrhoeic dermatitis and acne.

### Preparations

**Proprietary Preparations** (details are given in Part 3)
**Port.:** Encaskin Creme; Encaskin Detergente; **Switz:** Encaskin Cream; Encaskin Liquid Detergent.

---

## Sebacic Acid

Sebácico, ácido. Decanedioic acid; Octane-1,8-dicarboxylic acid.

$C_{10}H_{18}O_4$ = 202.2.
*CAS — 111-20-6.*

### Profile

Sebacic acid is an emollient included in preparations used to protect damaged skin.

Diisopropyl sebacate ($C_{16}H_{30}O_4$ = 286.4) has been used in skin moisturising preparations.

### Preparations

**Proprietary Preparations** (details are given in Part 3)
**Multi-ingredient:** **Port.:** Pirrolfungin.

---

## Selenium Sulfide

Selenii Disulfidum; Selenium Disulphide; Selenium Sulphide; Sulfuro de selenio.

$SeS_2$ = 143.1.
*CAS — 7488-56-4.*
*ATC — D01AE13.*

**Pharmacopoeias.** In *Chin., Eur.* (see p.vi), *Int.,* and *US.*

**Ph. Eur. 5.0** (Selenium Disulphide; Selenium Sulphide BP 2003). A bright orange to reddish-brown powder. Practically insoluble in water.

**USP 27** (Selenium Sulfide). A bright orange to reddish-brown powder with not more than a faint odour. Practically insoluble in water and in organic solvents; soluble 1 in 161 of chloroform and 1 in 1667 of ether.

### Adverse Effects and Treatment

Topical application of selenium sulfide can produce irritation of the conjunctiva, scalp, and skin, especially in the genital area and skin folds. Oiliness or dryness of scalp or hair, hair discoloration, and hair loss have been reported.

Selenium sulfide can be highly toxic when taken by mouth. Only traces of selenium sulfide are absorbed through intact skin but prolonged use on broken skin has resulted in systemic toxicity.

Treatment of poisoning is symptomatic.

**Systemic toxicity.** A woman with excoriated eruptions on her scalp developed weakness, anorexia, abdominal pain, vomiting, tremors, sweating, a metallic taste in her mouth, and a garlic-like smell on her breath after using a shampoo containing selenium sulfide 2 or 3 times weekly for 8 months.[1] All symptoms subsided 10 days after withdrawal of the shampoo.


1. Ransone JW, *et al.* Selenium sulfide intoxication. *N Engl J Med* 1961; **264:** 384–5.


### Precautions

To minimise absorption selenium sulfide should not be applied to mucous membranes, inflamed or broken skin, or to extensive areas of the skin. Contact with the eyes should be avoided. Selenium sulfide may discolour metals.

Selenium sulfide shampoos should not be used within 48 hours of applying hair colours or permanent waving preparations.

### Uses and Administration

Selenium sulfide has antifungal and antiseborrhoeic properties. It is used as a shampoo in the treatment of dandruff (pityriasis capitis) and seborrhoeic dermatitis of the scalp (p.1138). Five to 10 mL of a suspension containing 2.5% of selenium sulfide is applied to the wet scalp; the hair is rinsed and the application repeated; the suspension should remain in contact with the scalp for 2 to 3 minutes each time. The hair should be well rinsed after the treatment and all traces of the suspension removed from the hands and nails. Applications are usually made twice weekly for 2 weeks, then once weekly for 2 weeks and then only when necessary. Shampoos containing 1% are also used.

Selenium sulfide is also used as a 2.5% lotion in the treatment of pityriasis versicolor (see Skin Infections, p.390). The lotion may be applied to the affected areas with a small amount of water and allowed to remain for 10 minutes before thorough rinsing. This procedure is repeated once daily for about 7 days. Alternatively undiluted 2.5% lotion has been applied at bedtime and washed off in the morning on 3 separate occasions at 3-day intervals.

Selenium sulfide has also been used as an adjunct to the systemic treatment of tinea capitis (see Dermatophytoses under Skin Infections, p.390).

### Preparations

***BP 2003:*** Selenium Sulphide Scalp Application;
***USP 27:*** Selenium Sulfide Lotion.

**Proprietary Preparations** (details are given in Part 3)
***Arg.:*** Selegel; Selsun; ***Austral.:*** Selsun; ***Austria:*** Selsun; Selukos†; STOI-X; ***Belg.:*** Selsun; ***Braz.:*** Caspacil; Selsun†; ***Canad.:*** Selsun; Versel; ***Chile:*** Selsun; ***Denm.:*** Selenol; Selsun; ***Fin.:*** Selsun; Selukos; ***Fr.:*** Selegel; Selsun; ***Ger.:*** Selsun; Selukos; ***Gr.:*** Selsun; ***Hong Kong:*** Selsun; ***Irl.:*** Lenium†; Selsun; ***Israel:*** Sebosel; Selsun; ***Ital.:*** Selsun Blu; ***Malaysia:*** Selsun; ***Neth.:*** Selsun-R; ***Norw.:*** Selsun; Selukos; ***NZ:*** Selsun; ***Port.:*** Selenix; Selsun†; ***S.Afr.:*** Selsun; ***Spain:*** Abbottselsun; Bioselenium; Caspiselenio; ***Swed.:*** Selsun; Selukos; ***Switz.:*** Selsun; ***Thai.:*** Sebosel; Selsun; ***UK:*** Lenium†; Selsun; ***USA:*** Exsel; Head & Shoulders Intensive Treatment; Selsun.

**Multi-ingredient:** ***Belg.:*** Sulfo-Selenium†; ***Canad.:*** Selsun with Provitamin $B_5$; ***Ger.:*** Ellsurex; ***Ital.:*** Node Tar†; Selsun Plus; ***Spain:*** Sebumselen; Sulfiselen†; ***Switz.:*** Ektoselene.

## Skin Substitutes

Sustitutos de la piel.

### Profile

Biological and semisynthetic materials have been developed for use as temporary dressings in burns, ulcers, and other injuries associated with skin loss. The rationale is to prevent fluid and heat loss, to reduce infection, to protect exposed structures, to reduce pain, and to prepare the site for grafting (see Burns, p.1134).

Denatured porcine and bovine skin, consisting of the dermal and/or epidermal layers, have been used. More recently bioengineered human skin equivalents have been produced which more closely mimic human skin, as well as a human, living dermal replacement product.

◊ References.


1. Muhart M, *et al.* Bioengineered skin. *Lancet* 1997; **350:** 1142.
2. Purdue GF, *et al.* A multicenter clinical trial of a biosynthetic skin replacement, Dermagraft-TC, compared with cryopreserved human cadaver skin for temporary coverage of excised burn wounds. *J Burn Care Rehabil* 1997; **18:** 52–7.
3. Freedlander E. New forms of skin grafting: from the laboratory to the clinic. *Hosp Med* 1998; **59:** 484–7.
4. Demling RH, DeSanti L. Management of partial thickness facial burns (comparison of topical antibiotics and bio-engineered skin substitutes). *Burns* 1999; **25:** 256–61.
5. Noordenbos J, *et al.* Safety and efficacy of TransCyte for the treatment of partial-thickness burns. *J Burn Care Rehabil* 1999; **20:** 275–81.
6. Falanga V, Sabolinski M. A bilayered living skin construct (APLIGRAF) accelerates complete closure of hard-to-heal venous ulcers. *Wound Repair Regen* 1999; **7:** 201–7.
7. Marston WA, *et al.* The efficacy and safety of Dermagraft in improving the healing of chronic diabetic foot ulcers: results of a prospective randomized trial. *Diabetes Care* 2003; **26:** 1701–5.


### Preparations

**Proprietary Preparations** (details are given in Part 3)
***Arg.:*** Pel Cupron; ***UK:*** Corethium†; Dermagraft; TransCyte; ***USA:*** Apligraf; Dermagraft; Orcel; TransCyte.

**Multi-ingredient:** ***Arg.:*** Kytinon; Kytinon ABC.

## Sodium Pidolate *(pINNM)*

NaPCA; Pidolato sódico; Sodium Pyroglutamate; Sodium Pyrrolidone Carboxylate. Sodium 5-oxopyrrolidine-2-carboxylate.

$C_5H_7NNaO_3$ = 152.1.

*CAS — 28874-51-3 (DL-sodium pidolate); 54571-67-4 (L-sodium pidolate).*

### Profile

Sodium pidolate is used as a humectant. It is applied topically as a cream or lotion, often in multi-ingredient preparations, in the treatment of dry skin disorders.

### Preparations

**Proprietary Preparations** (details are given in Part 3)

**Multi-ingredient:** ***Arg.:*** Lacticare; ***Austral.:*** Dermadrate; DermaVeen Moisturising†; DermaVeen Shower & Bath†; ***Braz.:*** Lacticare; ***Canad.:*** Lacticare; ***Chile:*** Lacticare; ***Fr.:*** Hydracuivre; Lacticare; ***Hong Kong:*** Lacticare; ***Irl.:*** Hydromol; Lacticare; ***Ital.:*** Angstrom Viso; ***Malaysia:*** Lacticare; ***Mex.:*** Lacticare; ***NZ:*** Dermadrate; ***Port.:*** Hidro-Lact†; Hyseke†; ***Singapore:*** Dermadrate; DermaVeen Shower & Bath; Lacticare; ***Thai.:*** Lacticare; ***UK:*** Hydromol; Lacticare.

## Squaric Acid Dibutylester

Éster dibutílico del ácido escuárico; Quadratic Acid Dibutylester. The dibutyl ester of 3,4-dihydroxy-3-cyclobutene-1,2-dione; 3,4-Dibutoxy-3-cyclobutene-1,2-dione; .

$C_{12}H_{18}O_4$ = 226.3.

*CAS — 2892-62-8 (squaric acid dibutylester); 2892-51-5 (squaric acid).*

### Profile

Squaric acid dibutylester has been tried similarly to diphencyprone (p.1145) as a contact sensitiser in the treatment of alopecia. It has also been tried in warts.

◊ References.


1. Van der Steen PHM, *et al.* Topical immunotherapy for alopecia areata: re-evaluation of 139 cases after an additional follow-up period of 19 months. *Dermatology* 1992; **184:** 198–201.
2. Tosti A, *et al.* Long-term results of topical immunotherapy in children with alopecia totalis or alopecia universalis. *J Am Acad Dermatol* 1996; **35:** 199–201.
3. Micali G, *et al.* Treatment of alopecia areata with squaric acid dibutylester. *Int J Dermatol* 1996; **35:** 52–6.
4. Lee AN, Mallory SB. Contact immunotherapy with squaric acid dibutylester for the treatment of recalcitrant warts. *J Am Acad Dermatol* 1999; **41:** 595–9.


## Sulfur

Azufre; Enxôfre; Schwefel; Soufre; Sulphur.

S = 32.065.

*CAS — 7704-34-9.*

*ATC — D10AB02.*

**Pharmacopoeias.** In *Chin., Eur.* (see p.vi), *Jpn, Pol.,* and *US.* Some have monographs for Precipitated Sulfur (Milk of Sulfur), Sublimed Sulfur (Flowers of Sulfur), or both. Some specify it is only for external use.

**Ph. Eur. 5.0** (Sulphur for External Use). A yellow powder. The size of most of the particles is not greater than 20 micrometres and that of almost all the particles is not greater than 40 micrometres. Practically insoluble in water; soluble in carbon disulfide; slightly soluble in vegetable oils. Protect from light.

**USP 27** (Precipitated Sulfur). A very fine, pale yellow, odourless, amorphous or microcrystalline powder. Practically insoluble in water; very slightly soluble in alcohol; slowly and usually incompletely soluble 1 in 2 of carbon disulfide; soluble 1 in 100 of olive oil.

**USP 27** (Sublimed Sulfur). A fine, yellow, crystalline powder with a faint odour. Practically insoluble in water and in alcohol; sparingly soluble in olive oil.

### Adverse Effects and Precautions

Topical application of sulfur can cause skin irritation and dermatitis has been reported following repeated application. Contact with the eyes, mouth, and other mucous membranes should be avoided. Contact with sulfur can discolour certain metals such as silver, and concomitant application of sulfur and topical mercurial compounds can lead to the generation of hydrogen sulfide which has a foul odour and may stain the skin black.

**Handling.** Sulfur has been used for the illicit preparation of explosives or fireworks; care is required with its supply.

### Uses and Administration

Sulfur is a keratolytic, a mild antiseptic, a mild antifungal, and a parasiticide.

Colloidal sulfur has a smaller particle size than either precipitated or sublimed sulfur. It is sulfur in an aqueous medium containing a colloid such as albumin or gelatin.

Sulfur has been widely used in lotions, creams, or ointments, usually in combination with other agents, in concentrations of up to 10% in the treatment of acne, dandruff, seborrhoeic conditions, scabies, and superficial fungal infections, although there are more convenient and effective preparations.

Lotions of precipitated sulfur with lead acetate have been used to darken grey hair.

Sulfur was also formerly used as a mild irritant laxative.

Sulfur is used in homoeopathic medicine.

◊ General references.


1. Lin AN, *et al.* Sulfur revisited. *J Am Acad Dermatol* 1988; **18:** 553–8.


### Preparations

***BPC 1973:*** Salicylic Acid and Sulphur Ointment;
***USP 27:*** Resorcinol and Sulfur Lotion; Sulfur Ointment.

**Proprietary Preparations** (details are given in Part 3)
***Arg.:*** Macbirs; Merbenloc; Suffisance; Suldiamin; ***Braz.:*** Sabonete Sulfuroso; ***Canad.:*** Acne Blemish Cream†; Postacne; Pureness Blemish Control†; ***Ger.:*** Schwefel-Diasporal†; Sulfopino; ***Ital.:*** Acqua di Sirmione; Eudermal Sapone Allo Zolfo pH 5†; Misurid; Nosebo†; Veriderm†; ***Mex.:*** Azuder†; ***USA:*** Acne Lotion 10; Liquimat; Sastid; Sulfoam; Sulmasque.

**Multi-ingredient:** Numerous preparations are listed in Part3.

## Sulfurated Lime

Cal sulfurada; Calcium Sulphide; Calx Sulphurata; Sulphurated Lime.

*CAS — 8028-82-8 (sulfurated lime solution).*

### Profile

Sulfurated lime is a mixture containing calcium sulfate and not less than 50% of calcium sulfide (CaS), prepared by heating calcium sulfate. Sulfurated lime solution (Vleminckx's solution) is an aqueous solution containing calcium polysulfides and calcium thiosulfate prepared by boiling sublimed sulfur with calcium hydroxide in water.

Sulfurated lime has been used topically as sulfurated lime solution for acne, scabies, seborrhoeic dermatitis, and pustular infections such as boils and carbuncles. A similar solution known as 'lime-sulphur' is used as a fungicide in horticulture.

An impure grade of calcium sulfide (Hepar Sulphuris; Hepar Sulph.) is used in homoeopathic medicine.

NOTE. The titles Hepar Sulfuris and Hepar Sulph are also applied to Sulfurated Potash (see below).

## Sulfurated Potash

Foie de Soufre; Hepar Sulfuris; Kalii Sulfidum; Liver of Sulphur; Potasa sulfurada; Potassa Sulphurata; Schwefelleber; Sulphurated Potash.

*CAS — 39365-88-3.*

NOTE. The title Hepar Sulphuris is used in homoeopathic medicine for an impure grade of calcium sulfide—see Sulfurated Lime, above.

**Pharmacopoeias.** In *US.*

**USP 27** (Sulfurated Potash). A mixture composed chiefly of potassium polysulfides and potassium thiosulfate, containing not less than 12.8% of sulfur as sulfide. Irregular, liver-brown pieces when freshly made, changing to greenish-yellow. It has an odour of hydrogen sulfide. Soluble 1 in 2 of water, usually leaving a slight residue. Alcohol dissolves only the sulfides. A 10% solution is light brown in colour and alkaline to litmus. Store in small, airtight containers.

**Incompatibility.** Sulfurated potash is incompatible with acids.

### Profile

Sulfurated potash has been used in the treatment of acne and other skin disorders usually in the form of a lotion with zinc sulfate.

Sulfurated potash is used in homoeopathic medicine when it is known as Hepar Sulph.

### Preparations

***USP 27:*** White Lotion.

**Proprietary Preparations** (details are given in Part 3)
***Ger.:*** Schwefelbad-Saar†.

**Multi-ingredient:** ***Austria:*** Leukona-Sulfomoor-Bad.

## Sulisobenzone *(USAN, rINN)*

Benzophenone-4; NSC-60584; Sulisobenzona. 5-Benzoyl-4-hydroxy-2-methoxybenzenesulphonic acid.

$C_{14}H_{12}O_6S$ = 308.3.

*CAS — 4065-45-6.*

**Pharmacopoeias.** In *US.*

**USP 27** (Sulisobenzone). Light tan powder. M.p. about 145°. Freely soluble in water, in alcohol, and in methyl alcohol; sparingly soluble in ethyl acetate. Store in airtight containers. Protect from light.

### Profile

Sulisobenzone, a substituted benzophenone, is a sunscreen (see p.1133) with actions similar to those of oxybenzone (p.1155). It is effective against UVB and some UVA light (for definitions, see p.1136).

### Preparations

**Proprietary Preparations**
Some preparations are listed in Part 3.

## Tacalcitol *(BAN, rINN)*

1α,24-Dihydroxycholecalciferol; 1α,24-Dihydroxyvitamin $D_3$. (+)-(5Z,7E,24R)-9,10-Secocholesta-5,7,10(19)-triene-1α,3β,24-triol monohydrate.

$C_{27}H_{44}O_3,H_2O$ = 434.7.

*CAS — 57333-96-7 (anhydrous tacalcitol); 93129-94-3 (tacalcitol monohydrate).*

*ATC — D05AX04.*

### Adverse Effects and Precautions

As for Calcipotriol, p.1144. Paraesthesia may also occur. Tacalcitol may be applied to the face, but care should be taken to avoid the eyes. Tacalcitol may be degraded by UV radiation (see Uses and Administration, below).

### Uses and Administration

Tacalcitol is a vitamin $D_3$ derivative. *In vitro* it appears to induce differentiation and to suppress proliferation of keratinocytes.

Tacalcitol is applied topically in the management of plaque psoriasis (p.1137). It is used as the monohydrate, but the concentration is expressed in terms of the base; 4.17 micrograms of tacalcitol monohydrate is approximately equivalent to 4 micrograms of tacalcitol. It is applied as an ointment containing the equivalent of tacalcitol 4 micrograms/g (0.0004%). Applications are made once daily, preferably at bedtime, and no more than 10 g of ointment should be applied each day. Duration of treatment depends on the severity of the lesions; continuous and intermittent treatments for up to 12 months have been used.

Tacalcitol may be degraded by UV radiation and therefore if combined with UV therapy, the radiation should be given in the morning and tacalcitol applied at bedtime.

◊ References.


1. Peters DC, Balfour JA. Tacalcitol. *Drugs* 1997; **54:** 265–71.

2. Gollnick H, Menke T. Current experience with tacalcitol ointment in the treatment of psoriasis. *Curr Med Res Opin* 1998; **14:** 213–18.
3. Harrison PV. Topical tacalcitol treatment for psoriasis. *Hosp Med* 2000; **61:** 402–5.
4. Van de Kerkhof PCM, *et al.* Long-term efficacy and safety of tacalcitol ointment in patients with chronic plaque psoriasis. *Br J Dermatol* 2002; **146:** 414–22.


### Preparations

**Proprietary Preparations** (details are given in Part 3)
***Arg.:*** Bonalfa; ***Austria:*** Curatoderm; ***Belg.:*** Curatoderm; ***Chile:*** Bonalfa; ***Fr.:*** Apsor; ***Ger.:*** Curatoderm; ***Israel:*** Curatoderm; ***Ital.:*** Vellutan; ***Jpn:*** Bonalfa; ***Mex.:*** Bonalfa; ***Port.:*** Bonalfa; ***Spain:*** Bonalfa; ***Switz.:*** Curatoderm; ***UK:*** Curatoderm.

## Purified Talc

E553(b); Powdered Talc; Purified French Chalk; Talc; Talco purificado; Talcum; Talcum Purificatum.

*CAS — 14807-96-6.*

**Pharmacopoeias.** In *Chin., Eur.* (see p.vi), *Int., Jpn, Pol., US,* and *Viet.*

**Ph. Eur. 5.0** (Talc; Purified Talc BP 2003). A powdered, selected, natural, hydrated, magnesium silicate. Pure talc has the formula $Mg_3Si_4O_{10}(OH)_2$; it may contain varying amounts of associated minerals. A light, homogeneous, white or almost white powder, greasy and non-abrasive to the touch. It should be free from asbestos. Practically insoluble in water, in alcohol, and in dilute solutions of acids and of alkali hydroxides.

**USP 27** (Talc). A native hydrous magnesium silicate containing a small proportion of aluminium silicate. A very fine, white or greyish-white, unctuous crystalline powder, which adheres readily to the skin, and is free from grittiness.

### Adverse Effects and Precautions

Contamination of wounds or body cavities with talc is liable to cause granulomas and it should not be used for dusting surgical gloves.

Inhalation of talc can cause respiratory irritation; prolonged exposure may produce pneumoconiosis.

Talc is liable to be heavily contaminated with bacteria, including *Clostridium tetani, Cl. welchii,* and *Bacillus anthracis.* When used in dusting powders or to treat pneumothorax and pleural effusions, it should be sterilised.

**Abuse.** Pulmonary granulomas occurring after intravenous or intranasal drug abuse have been associated with the presence of talc as a filler in the abused preparations.[1,2]


1. Schwartz IS, Bosken C. Pulmonary vascular talc granulomatosis. *JAMA* 1986; **256:** 2584.
2. Johnson DC, *et al.* Foreign body pulmonary granulomas in an abuser of nasally inhaled drugs. *Pediatrics* 1991; **88:** 159–61.


**Carcinogenicity.** A review by a working group of the International Agency for Research on Cancer concluded that there was inadequate evidence to confirm whether purified talc was carcinogenic in humans but there was sufficient evidence to confirm that talc containing asbestiform fibres was carcinogenic to man.[1] There have been suggestions of a link between the use of talc and ovarian cancer[2] but although a case-controlled study suggested an approximate doubling of the risk among women after perineal use of talc the working group noted that information was not available on the asbestos content of the talcs.[1]


1. IARC/WHO. Silica and some silicates. *IARC monographs on the evaluation of the carcinogenic risk of chemicals to humans volume 42* 1987.
2. Longo DL, Young RC. Cosmetic talc and ovarian cancer. *Lancet* 1979; **ii:** 349–51.


**Effects on the lungs.** Inhalation of talc can cause respiratory irritation. Acute respiratory failure developed in 4 of 338 patients who underwent pleurodesis for benign or malignant effusions using insufflated talc with thoracoscopy.[1] Three of the 4 patients died. Talc crystals were found in the bronchoalveolar lavage of all 4 patients and on necropsy of one patient talc crystals were found in almost every organ.

For other effects on the lungs, see under Abuse, above and Infant Skin Care, below.


1. Campos JRM, *et al.* Respiratory failure due to insufflated talc. *Lancet* 1997; **349:** 251–2.


**Infant skin care.** The routine use of non-medicated powders in the skin care of infants can be hazardous and their use should be discouraged.[1,2] Talc acts as a pulmonary irritant and inhalation of baby-powders by infants has caused severe respiratory difficulties and several deaths have been reported. Careful respiratory monitoring is indicated in children suspected of inhaling talcum powder as the onset of symptoms may be delayed for several hours.[1] There have also been reports of umbilical granulomas resulting from contamination of umbilical stumps with talcum powder used for skin care.[2]


1. Pairaudeau PW, *et al.* Inhalation of baby powder: an unappreciated hazard. *BMJ* 1991; **302:** 1200–1.
2. Sparrow SA, Hallam LA. Talc granulomas. *BMJ* 1991; **303:** 58.


### Uses and Administration

Purified talc is used in massage and as a dusting powder to allay irritation and prevent chafing. It is usually mixed with starch, to increase absorption of moisture, and zinc oxide. Talc used in dusting powders or as talc poudrage should be sterilised. Purified talc is used as a lubricant and diluent in making tablets and capsules and to clarify liquids.

Talc may be used as a sclerosant for malignant effusions and for recurrent spontaneous pneumothorax (see below).

**Pleural effusions.** Talc is used as a sclerosant to achieve pleurodesis in the management of benign and malignant pleural effusions (p.512) and recurrent spontaneous pneumothorax.[1-4] It is generally administered into the pleural space as a slurry via intercostal tube, or by insufflation at thoracoscopy. Most reports have used a dose of 2 to 5 g, but it has been given in doses ranging from 1 to 10 g. The most common side-effects associated with this use of talc are pain and fever. Other reported effects have included local infection and empyema, cardiovascular complications, and respiratory failure (see also Effects on the Lungs, above).


1. Kennedy L, Sahn SA. Talc pleurodesis for the treatment of pneumothorax and pleural effusion. *Chest* 1994; **106:** 1215–22.
2. de Campos JRM, *et al.* Thoracoscopy talc poudrage: a 15 year experience. *Chest* 2001; **119:** 801–6.
3. Antunes G, *et al.* BTS guidelines for the management of malignant pleural effusions. *Thorax* 2003; **58** (suppl 2): ii29–ii38. Also available at: http://www.brit-thoracic.org.uk/docs/PleuralDiseaseMalignantPE.pdf (accessed 16/06/04)
4. Henry M, *et al.* BTS guidelines for the management of spontaneous pneumothorax. *Thorax* 2003; **58** (suppl 2): ii39–ii52. Also available at: http://www.brit-thoracic.org.uk/docs/PleuralDiseaseSpontaneous.pdf (accessed 16/06/04)


### Preparations

***BP 2003:*** Talc Dusting Powder.

**Proprietary Preparations** (details are given in Part 3)
***USA:*** Sclerosol.

**Multi-ingredient:** ***Arg.:*** Dr Selby; ***Austral.:*** ZSC; ***Austria:*** Cutimix; Herposicc; Prurimix; Rombay; ***Belg.:*** Aloplastine; Baseler Haussalbe†; ***Braz.:*** Pasta d'Agua; Pomaderme; Talco Alivio; ***Canad.:*** Bebia†; ***Chile:*** Hansaplast Footcare; ***Fr.:*** Aloplastine; ***Israel:*** Pedisol; ***Mex.:*** Hipoglos Plus; ***NZ:*** Grans Remedy; Odor Eze; ***Port.:*** Cuidaderma; ***Spain:*** Amniolina; Ictiomen; Pomada Infantil Vera; Talco Antihistam Calber†; Talquis Cusi†; Talquissar†; Tegunal†; ***USA:*** Columbia Antiseptic Powder; ZBT†.

## Tars and Tar Oils

Breas y aceites de brea.

### Birch Tar Oil

Aceite de brea de abedul; Birkenteer; Goudron de Bouleau; Oleum Betulae Albae; Oleum Betulae Empyreumaticum; Oleum Betulae Pyrolignеum; Oleum Rusci; Pix Betulae; Pyroleum Betulae.

**Description.** Birch tar oil is obtained by the destructive distillation of the wood and bark of the silver birch, *Betula verrucosa* (*B. pendula*; *B. alba*), and the birch, *B. pubescens* (Betulaceae); the distillate is allowed to stand and the oily upper layer separated from the residual tar.

### Cade Oil

Alquitrán de Enebro; Brea de enebro; Goudron de Cade; Juniper Tar; Juniper Tar Oil; Kadeöl; Oleum Cadinum; Oleum Juniperi Empyreumaticum; Pix Cadi; Pix Juniperi; Pix Oxycedri; Pyroleum Juniperi; Pyroleum Oxycedri; Wacholderteer.

**Description.** Cade oil contains guaiacol, ethylguaiacol, creosol, and cadinene.

**Pharmacopoeias.** In *US.*

**USP 27** (Juniper Tar). The empyreumatic volatile oil obtained from the woody portions of *Juniperus oxycedrus* (Pinaceae). It is a dark brown, clear, thick liquid with a tarry odour. Very slightly soluble in water; soluble 1 in 9 of alcohol; soluble 1 in 3 of ether leaving only a slight flocculent residue; partially soluble in petroleum spirit; miscible with amyl alcohol, with chloroform, and with glacial acetic acid. Store in airtight containers at a temperature not exceeding 40°. Protect from light.

### Coal Tar

Alcatrão Mineral; Alquitrán de Hulla; Brea de hulla; Crude Coal Tar; Goudron de Houille; Oleum Lithanthracis; Pix Carbon.; Pix Carbonis; Pix Lithanthracis; Pix Mineralis; Pyroleum Lithanthracis; Steinkohlenteer.

**Description.** Prepared coal tar is commercial coal tar heated at 50° for 1 hour.

Alcoholic solutions of coal tar or prepared coal tar prepared with the aid of polysorbate have been referred to as Liquor Picis Carbonis and Liquor Carbonis Detergens.

**Pharmacopoeias.** In *Br., Fr., Int.,* and *US.*

**BP 2003** (Coal Tar). A product obtained by the destructive distillation of bituminous coal at a temperature of about 1000°. A nearly black, viscous liquid with a strong characteristic penetrating odour. On exposure to air it gradually becomes more viscous. It burns in air with a luminous sooty flame. Slightly soluble in water; partly soluble in absolute alcohol, in chloroform, in ether, and in volatile oils. A saturated solution is alkaline to litmus.

**USP 27** (Coal Tar). The tar obtained by the destructive distillation of bituminous coal at temperatures in the range of 900° to 1100°. It may be processed further either by extraction with alcohol and suitable dispersing agents and maceration times or by fractional distillation with or without the use of suitable organic solvents.

A nearly black, viscous liquid with a characteristic naphthalene-like odour. Slightly soluble in water to which it imparts an alkaline reaction; partially soluble in alcohol, in acetone, in carbon disulfide, in chloroform, in ether, in methyl alcohol, and in petroleum spirit; more soluble in benzene; almost completely soluble in nitrobenzene. Store in airtight containers.

### Tar

Alquitrán Vegetal; Brea de Pino; Brea vegetal; Goudron Végétal; Nadelholzteer; Pine Tar; Pix Abietinarum; Pix Liquida; Pix Pini; Pyroleum Pini; Wood Tar.

**Pharmacopoeias.** In *Br.*

**BP 2003** (Tar). A bituminous liquid obtained from the wood of various trees of the family Pinaceae by destructive distillation. It is known in commerce as Stockholm Tar. A dark brown or nearly black semi-liquid with a characteristic empyreumatic odour; it is heavier than water. Soluble in alcohol (90%), in chloroform, in ether, and in fixed and volatile oils. The aqueous liquid obtained by shaking 1 g with 20 mL of water for 5 minutes is acidic to litmus paper.

**Storage.** When stored for some time tar separates into a layer which is granular in character due to minute crystallisation of catechol, resin acids, etc. and a surface layer of a syrupy consistence.

### Adverse Effects and Precautions

Tars and tar oils may cause irritation and acne-like eruptions of the skin and should not be applied to inflamed or broken skin. They should be used with caution on the face, skin flexures, or on the genitalia. Hypersensitivity reactions are rare but wood tars are more likely to cause sensitisation than coal tar. However, unlike wood tars, coal tar has a photosensitising action. Preparations of refined tar products appear to be less likely than crude tars to stain the skin, hair, and clothing.

Depending on their composition the systemic effects of tars and tar oils are similar to those for phenol (see p.1188).

**Carcinogenicity.** Although an increased risk of skin carcinoma was found[1] in 59 patients with psoriasis who had had very high exposures to tar and/or UV radiation, no such evidence was apparent[2] in 260 patients followed for a mean of 20 years and long-term topical tar therapy alone was not associated with an increase in malignancy in 719 patients.[3] Relatively high systemic absorption of polycyclic aromatic hydrocarbons, which are potential carcinogens, has, however, been reported after use of a coal-tar shampoo.[4]


1. Stern RS, *et al.* Skin carcinoma in patients with psoriasis treated with topical tar and artificial ultraviolet radiation. *Lancet* 1980; **i:** 732–5.
2. Pittelkow MR, *et al.* Skin cancer in patients with psoriasis treated with coal tar. *Arch Dermatol* 1981; **117:** 465–8.
3. Jones SK, *et al.* Further evidence of the safety of tar in the management of psoriasis. *Br J Dermatol* 1985; **113:** 97–101.
4. van Schooten F-J, *et al.* Dermal uptake of polycyclic aromatic hydrocarbons after hairwash with coal-tar shampoo. *Lancet* 1994; **344:** 1505–6.


**Extemporaneous preparation.** Concern about the possible carcinogenic potential of coal tar (see above) led the Health and Safety Executive in the UK to recommend that chemical gloves, as opposed to disposable surgeon's gloves, should be worn during the extemporaneous preparation of formulations containing coal tar.[1]


1. Anonymous. Chemical protection gloves recommended for coal tar ointments. *Pharm J* 1997; **259:** 757.


### Uses and Administration

Tars and tar oils can reduce the thickness of the epidermis. They are antipruritic and may be weakly antiseptic. They are used topically in eczema (p.1135), psoriasis (below), dandruff, seborrhoeic dermatitis (p.1138), and other skin disorders. Coal tar preparations have largely replaced the use of wood tars. Ultraviolet (UVB) light increases the efficacy of coal tar in the treatment of psoriasis.

Some wood tars, including creosote (p.1117) have been used in expectorant preparations. Tar has also been used in homoeopathic medicine.

**Nonprescription use.** Following its review of products for safety and efficacy the FDA ruled that cade oil or tar should not be used in nonprescription shampoos[1] and that tar should no longer be included in nonprescription expectorants.[2]

1. Anonymous. Nonprescription drug review gains momentum. *WHO Drug Inf* 1991; **5:** 62.
2. Anonymous. FDA announces standards for nonprescription sleep-aid products and expectorants. *Clin Pharm* 1989; **8:** 388.

**Psoriasis.** Coal tar has long been employed in the treatment of psoriasis (p.1137), and used alone or with dithranol and/or ultraviolet light it continues to be a first-line option, although its use is declining. It is particularly suited to the treatment of stable chronic plaque psoriasis. Its mode of action is unknown but it is considered to have antiproliferative and anti-inflammatory activity, producing a reduction in the thickness of viable epidermis. Crude tar preparations are rather messy and unpleasant; refined products may be more aesthetically acceptable and less likely to stain skin, hair, and clothing although some consider them to be less effective.

Treatments usually start with concentrations equivalent to 0.5 to 1% of crude coal tar with the concentration being increased as necessary every few days up to a maximum of 10%. The higher strength preparations may be required for the management of thicker patches of psoriasis. Coal tar may not clear psoriasis as fast as other agents but extended periods of remission can be obtained with its use. The Goeckerman regimen utilises the enhanced efficacy obtained when coal tar is applied before exposure to ultraviolet (UVB) light. The mechanism for this effect is not known but it does not appear to be due to the photosensitising action of coal tar. In most regimens the coal tar is applied 2 hours before exposure to UVB light. In Ingram's regimen and its modifications the use of coal tar and UVB light is followed by topical treatment with dithranol. It has been suggested that the irritant effects of dithranol treatment are reduced by concomitant treatment with coal tar without loss of efficacy.

References.

1. Rotstein H, Baker C. The treatment of psoriasis. *Med J Aust* 1990; **152:** 153–64.
2. Menter A, Barker JNWN. Psoriasis in practice. *Lancet* 1991; **338:** 231–4.
3. Foreman MI, *et al.* Isoquinoline is a possible anti-psoriatic agent in coal tar. *Br J Dermatol* 1985; **112:** 323–8.
4. Arnold WP. Tar. *Clin Dermatol* 1997; **15:** 739–44.
5. British Association of Dermatologists. Clinical guidelines - psoriasis. Available at: http://www.bad.org.uk/doctors/guidelines/psoriasis.asp (accessed 16/06/04)

## Preparations

***BP 2003:*** Calamine and Coal Tar Ointment; Coal Tar and Salicylic Acid Ointment; Coal Tar and Zinc Ointment; Coal Tar Paste; Coal Tar Solution; Strong Coal Tar Solution; Zinc and Coal Tar Paste;
***USP 27:*** Coal Tar Ointment; Coal Tar Topical Solution; Compound Resorcinol Ointment.

**Proprietary Preparations** (details are given in Part 3)
***Arg.:*** Alcoderm; Alcontar; Fijacid; Ionil-T Plus; Soriacur; Sorial; Supertar; Sutrico Tar; Targel; ***Austral.:*** Alpha Keri Tar†; Alphosyl; Exorex; Ionil-T Plus; Linotar; Neutrogena T/Gel†; Pinetarsol; Psorigel; ***Austria:*** Exorex; ***Braz.:*** Neutrogen TGel†; Tarflex; Theratar†; ***Canad.:*** Balnetar; Doak-Oil; Estar; Ionil-T Plus†; Ionil-T†; Mazon Medicated Soap; Neutrogena T/Gel; Pentrax; Psoriasol†; Psorigel†; Robatar†; Spectro Tar; Tar Doak†; Targel; Tarseb; Tegrin†; Tersa-Tar; Zetar; ***Chile:*** DHS Tar Gel; Neutrogena Shampoo Neutar; Psorigel; Tarmed; Tigel IRM; ***Denm.:*** Basotar; ***Fr.:*** Caditar; Cosmetar-S†; Ramet Cade†; ***Ger.:*** Basiter; Berniter; Hoepixin Bad N; Pixfix†; Tarmed; Teer-Linola-Fett; ***Gr.:*** Ionil; Tarmed; ***Hong Kong:*** Pinetarsol; Psorigel†; Tersatar†; Zetar; ***Irl.:*** Baltar†; Clinitar†; Exorex; Pentrax; Psoriderm; Psorigel†; ***Israel:*** Alphosyl 2 in 1; Denorex; T/Gel; ***Ital.:*** Konor; Meditar†; Polytar†; Shampoo SDE Tar; Tarmed†; ***Malaysia:*** Pinetarsol; ***Mex.:*** Ionil-T Plus; Shampoo Tersa-Tar; Tarmed; ***Norw.:*** Soraderm; ***NZ:*** Pinetarsol; Psoriacreme†; Psorigel; ***Port.:*** Tarmed; ***S.Afr.:*** Exarex; Linotar; Psorigel†; ***Singapore:*** Pinetarsol; ***Spain:*** Alfitar; Alphosyl; Piroxgel; Psoriasdin; Tar Isdin Champu; Tarmed; Tejel; ***Switz.:*** Teerol†; ***UK:*** Alphosyl 2 in 1; Carbo-Dome; Clinitar; Exorex; Pentrax; Psoriderm; T/Gel; ***USA:*** Advanced Formula Tegrin†; AquaTar†; Balnetar; Creamy Tar; Cutar†; DHS Tar; Doctar†; Duplex T†; Estar; Fototar; Iocon†; Ionil-T Plus; MG217 Medicated; Neutrogena T/Derm†; Neutrogena T/Gel; Oxipor VHC; Pentrax; Pentrax Gold†; Polytar; Psorigel; Taraphilic; Tegrin; Tegrin Medicated†; Theraplex T†; Zetar.

**Multi-ingredient:** ***Arg.:*** Acnetrol; Adop-Tar; Aeroseb; Champuacid; Cicatrol; Confor-Tar; Cremsor N; Eurocoal; Farm-X; Ionil-T; Laurinol Plus; Medic; Mencogrin; Mencogrin AP; Oilalfo; Sequals G; Sorsis; Sorsis Beta; ***Austral.:*** Alpha Keri Tar†; Alphosyl; Eczema Cream; Egopsoryl TA; ER Cream; Fongitar; Ionil-T; Neutrogena T/Sal†; Pinetarsol; Polytar; Psor-Asist; Sebitar; Tarband; ***Austria:*** Alphosyl; Alpicort; Balneum mit Teer; Locacorten Tar; ***Belg.:*** Alphosyl†; Locacortene Tar†; ***Braz.:*** Codelasa†; Dai Nathat†; Hebrin; Ionil-T†; Kabala†; Polytar; Xarope Sao Joao; ***Canad.:*** Alphosyl†; Boil Ease; Dan-Tar Plus; Denorex; Mazon Medicated Cream; Mazon Medicated Shampoo; Medi-Dan; Multi-Tar Plus; Oxipor; P & S Plus; Polytar; Polytar AF; Sebcur/T; Sebutone; SJ Liniment; Spectro Tar; Sterex; Tardan; Targel SA; X-Seb T; X-Seb T Plus; X-Tar; ***Chile:*** Denorex Herbal; Ionil-T; Tarytar; ***Fin.:*** Alphosyl†; ***Fr.:*** Alphosyl; Biolan Tar†; Coaltar Saponine le Beuf†; Cystel Shampooing Antiseborrheique; Epiphane; Ionax T†; Item Alphacade; Laccoderme a l'huile de cade; Lactar†; Node DS; Node P; Phytolithe; Psocortene†; S-Coaltar†; Sebosquam†; Squaphane; ***Ger.:*** Dexacrinin†; Discmigon†; Hoepixin N†; Lorinden T; Poloris†; Polytar†; Psoriasis-Salbe M†; Psorigerb N; ***Hong Kong:*** 2-4-2; Cocois; Egopsoryl TA; Fongitar; Gelcotar†; Ionil-T; Locacorten Tar; Multi-Tar; Polytar; Polytar Emollient; Polytar Plus†; Sebitar; ***India:*** Derobin Skin; ***Irl.:*** Alphosyl; Alphosyl HC; Balneum with Tar†; Capasal; Cocois; Denorex; Gelcotar; Genisol†; Ionil-T; Polytar; Polytar Emollient; Polytar Plus†; Pragmatar; ***Israel:*** Alphosyl; Alphosyl HC; Capasal; CT Ointment; CT Pommade; CT Shampoo; Locacorten Tar†; Polytar; Topicorten-Tar; ***Ital.:*** Alphosyle; Balta-Crin Tar; Fongitar†; Herbatar Plus†; Herbatar†; Ionil-T†; Node Tar†; Pentrax†; Rivescal Tar; Soluzione Composta Alcoolica Saponosa di Coaltar†; ***Malaysia:*** Cocois; Egopsoryl TA; Polytar; Sebitar; ***Mex.:*** Antaderm; Dariseb; Dealan; Ionil-T; Polytar; Sebryl; Sebryl Plus; ***Neth.:*** Denorex; ***NZ:*** Cocois; Egopsoryl TA; Fongitar; Ionil-T; Polytar; Polytar Emollient; Polytar Plus; Sebitar; ***Port.:*** Alpha Cade; Alphosyl HC†; Alphosyl†; Edoltar; Fongitar; Ionax T†; Polytar; Squaphane†; Sucadermil; Tegrin†; ***S.Afr.:*** Alphosyl; Polytar; ***Singapore:*** Denorex; Egopsoryl TA; Fongitar; Ionil-T; Polytar; Sebitar; Sebutone†; ***Spain:*** Alphosyl; Bazalin; Emolytar; Ionil; Ionil Champu; Polytar; Quinortar; Tar Isdin Plus; Tarisdin†; Zincation Plus; ***Swed.:*** Alphosyl; ***Switz.:*** Alphosyl; Bain extra-doux dermatologique†; Crinotar†; Jonil T†; Locacorten Tar†; Teerol-H†; ***Thai.:*** Fongitar; Ionil-T; Polytar; ***UK:*** Alphosyl HC; Alphosyl†; Capasal; Cocois; Coltapaste†; Denorex†; Gelcosal†; Gelcotar†; Ionil-T†; Polytar AF; Polytar Emollient; Polytar Liquid; Polytar Plus; Pragmatar; Psorin; Snowfire; Tarband†; Varicose Ointment; ***USA:*** Boil Ease; Denorex†; Ionil-T; Medotar; Neutrogena T/Sal; P & S Plus†; Sal-Oil-T; Sebex-T; SLT; Tarlene; Tarsum; Unguentum Bossi†; X-Seb T; X-Seb T Plus.

## Tazarotene *(BAN, USAN, rINN)*

AGN-190168; Tazaroteno. Ethyl 6-[(4,4-dimethylthiochroman-6-yl)ethynyl]nicotinate.
$C_{21}H_{21}NO_2S$ = 351.5.
*CAS — 118292-40-3.*
*ATC — D05AX05.*

### Adverse Effects and Precautions

As for Tretinoin, p.1161.

Systemic absorption is low, and the most frequent adverse effects with tazarotene are on the skin; the incidence of adverse events appears to be concentration related.

*Animal* studies have indicated that tazarotene is fetotoxic and teratogenic, and manufacturers recommend that tazarotene should not be used during pregnancy or in women planning a pregnancy. Similarly, tazarotene should not be used, or used with caution, during breast feeding, as *animal* data indicate that it may be distributed into breast milk.

**Effects on the skin.** A 57-year-old man with diabetes and recalcitrant psoriasis on the trunk and limbs developed acute dermatitis[1] in the genital area two weeks after starting treatment with topical tazarotene 0.1%. The affected areas became ulcerated over the next few days. It was suspected that accidental contact with the tazarotene that had been applied to the truncal psoriasis was responsible.

1. Wollina U. Genital ulcers in a psoriasis patient using topical tazarotene. *Br J Dermatol* 1998; **138:** 713–14.

### Uses and Administration

Tazarotene is a retinoid used for the topical treatment of mild to moderate acne and plaque psoriasis. Tazarotene is a prodrug that is de-esterified in the skin to its active form, tazarotenic acid. The mode of action of tazarotenic acid in acne and psoriasis is unknown but it appears to modulate cell proliferation and differentiation.

In the treatment of **psoriasis**, tazarotene 0.05% cream or gel is used initially and increased to 0.1% if necessary. It is applied once daily in the evening. In the UK tazarotene is licensed for use in patients with psoriasis affecting up to 10% of the body surface; in the USA, it may be used on psoriasis involving up to 20% of the body surface.

In the treatment of **acne**, tazarotene is applied as a 0.1% gel or cream once daily in the evening.

There may be exacerbation of acne during early treatment or of psoriasis at any time during treatment. The treatment period is usually up to 12 weeks, although tazarotene has been used for up to 12 months in the treatment of psoriasis.

A 0.1% cream is used in the topical treatment of certain signs of **photodamage** (facial fine wrinkling, mottled hypo- and hyperpigmentation, and benign facial lentigines). It is applied once daily at bedtime to lightly cover the entire face.

◊ Reviews.

1. Foster RH, *et al.* Tazarotene. *Drugs* 1998; **55:** 705–11.
2. Tang-Liu DD-S, *et al.* Clinical pharmacokinetics and drug metabolism of tazarotene: a novel topical treatment for acne and psoriasis. *Clin Pharmacokinet* 1999; **37:** 273–87.

**Skin disorders.** Tazarotene is used for the topical treatment of mild to moderate acne (p.1133) and plaque psoriasis[1] (p.1137). Some benefit has been reported in keratinisation disorders such as Darier's disease[2] (p.1134) and congenital ichthyosis[3] (p.1136). Benefit has also been reported for psoriasis of the nails.[4]

1. Anonymous. Tazarotene—a topical retinoid for psoriasis. *Drug Ther Bull* 1999; **37:** 47–8.
2. Oster-Schmidt C. The treatment of Darier's disease with topical tazarotene. *Br J Dermatol* 1999; **141:** 603–4.
3. Hofmann B, *et al.* Effect of topical tazarotene in the treatment of congenital ichthyosis. *Br J Dermatol* 1999; **141:** 642–6.
4. Bianchi L, *et al.* Tazarotene 0.1% gel for psoriasis of the fingernails and toenails: an open, prospective study. *Br J Dermatol* 2003; **149:** 207–9.

### Preparations

**Proprietary Preparations** (details are given in Part 3)
***Austria:*** Zorac; ***Braz.:*** Zorac; ***Canad.:*** Tazorac; ***Fin.:*** Zorac; ***Fr.:*** Zorac; ***Ger.:*** Zorac; ***Gr.:*** Zorac; ***Irl.:*** Zorac; ***Ital.:*** Suretin†; Zorac; ***S.Afr.:*** Zorak; ***Spain:*** Zorac; ***Swed.:*** Zorac; ***Switz.:*** Zorac; ***UK:*** Zorac; ***USA:*** Avage; Tazorac.

## Thioglycollic Acid

Tioglicólico, ácido. Mercaptoacetic acid.
$C_2H_4O_2S$ = 92.12.
*CAS — 68-11-1.*

## Calcium Thioglycollate

Calcium Mercaptoacetate; Tioglicolato cálcico. Calcium mercaptoacetate trihydrate.
$C_2H_2CaO_2S,3H_2O$ = 184.2.
*CAS — 814-71-1.*

### Profile

Thioglycollic acid is used, usually as the calcium salt, in depilatory preparations. Thioglycollates are also used in hair waving or straightening products with potassium bromate as the neutraliser. There have been reports of skin reactions associated with the use of thioglycollates.

## Tioxolone *(BAN, rINN)*

OL-110; Thioxolone; Tioxolona. 6-Hydroxy-1,3-benzoxathiol-2-one; 4-Hydroxy-1,3-benzoxathiol-2-one.
$C_7H_4O_3S$ = 168.2.
*CAS — 4991-65-5.*
*ATC — D10AB03.*

**Pharmacopoeias.** In *Pol.*

### Profile

Tioxolone has been used topically in the treatment of various skin and scalp disorders.

### Preparations

**Proprietary Preparations** (details are given in Part 3)
**Multi-ingredient:** ***Ger.:*** Loscon.

## Titanium Dioxide

CI Pigment White 6; Colour Index No. 77891; Dióxido de titanio; E171; Titanii Dioxidum; Titanium Oxide.
$TiO_2$ = 79.87.
*CAS — 13463-67-7.*

**Pharmacopoeias.** In *Chin., Eur.* (see p.vi), *Jpn,* and *US.*

**Ph. Eur. 5.0** (Titanium Dioxide). A white or almost white powder. Practically insoluble in water; it does not dissolve in dilute mineral acids but dissolves slowly in hot concentrated sulfuric acid.

**USP 27** (Titanium Dioxide). A white odourless powder. Insoluble in water, in hydrochloric acid, in nitric acid, and in 2N sulfuric acid; dissolves in hot sulfuric acid and in hydrofluoric acid; it is rendered soluble by fusion with potassium bisulfate or with alkali hydroxides or carbonates. A 10% suspension in water is neutral to litmus.

### Profile

Titanium dioxide has an action on the skin similar to that of zinc oxide (p.1163) and has similar uses. Titanium peroxide and titanium salicylate are used with titanium dioxide for napkin rash. Titanium dioxide reflects ultraviolet light and is used as a physical sunscreen (see p.1133). It is also an ingredient of some cosmetics. It is used to pigment and opacify hard gelatin capsules and tablet coatings and as a delustring agent for regenerated cellulose and other man-made fibres. Specially purified grades may be used in food colours.

### Preparations

***BP 2003:*** Titanium Ointment.

**Proprietary Preparations** (details are given in Part 3)
***Arg.:*** Eurocolor; Europrotec P; Lelco Bebe; Refrane Gel; Skin Sol P; ***Austral.:*** Sunsense Low Irritant†; UV Triplegard Low Allergenic†; UV Triplegard Sensitive Skin; ***Canad.:*** Baby Block; Life Brand Natural Source†; Marcelle Protective Block; Natural Defense†; Neutrogena Sensitive Skin; Neutrogena Sunblocker†; Presun; Shiseido Skincare Day Protective; Special Defense Sun Block†; Sunblock†; True Illusion†; ***Chile:*** Eucerin Solar; Fotocrem-P; Neutrogena Bloqueador Solar Piel Sensible; ***Fr.:*** Anthelios T†; Uriage Ecran Total Mineral†; ***Ger.:*** Haemo-Exhirud Bufexamac; ***Hong Kong:*** Sunsense Low Irritant; ***Malaysia:*** Sunsense Low Irritant; ***Mex.:*** Blancaler; ***NZ:*** Hamilton Sunscreen; ***Port.:*** Dermagor Ecran Solar†; ***Singapore:*** Sunsense Low Irritant; ***UK:*** Coppertone Sunstick†; ***USA:*** Hawaiian Tropic Protective Tanning; Neutrogena Chemical-Free; TI Baby Natural; TI Screen Natural.

**Multi-ingredient:** Numerous preparations are listed in Part 3.

## Trafermin *(USAN, rINN)*

CAB-2001. 2-155-Basic fibroblast growth factor (human clone λKB7/λHFL1 precursor reduced).
*CAS — 131094-16-1.*

### Profile

Trafermin is a human recombinant basic fibroblast growth factor (b-FGF) that promotes tissue granulation and the formation of new blood vessels. It is used as a topical liquid spray for the treatment of burns and intractable skin ulcers.

## Tretinoin *(BAN, USAN, rINN)*

NSC-122758; Retinoic Acid; Tretinoína; Tretinoinum; Vitamin A Acid. *all-trans*-Retinoic acid; 15-Apo-β-caroten-15-oic acid; 3,7-Dimethyl-9-(2,6,6-trimethylcyclohex-1-enyl)nona-2,4,6,8-*all-trans*-tetraenoic acid.

$C_{20}H_{28}O_2$ = 300.4.

*CAS — 302-79-4.*

*ATC — D10AD01; L01XX14.*

**Pharmacopoeias.** In *Chin., Eur.* (see p.vi), *Pol.*, and *US.*

**Ph. Eur. 5.0** (Tretinoin). A yellow or light orange crystalline powder. Practically insoluble in water; slightly soluble in alcohol; soluble in dichloromethane. It is sensitive to light, heat, and air, especially in solution. Store in airtight containers at a temperature not exceeding 25°. Protect from light. The contents of an opened container should be used as soon as possible and any unused portion should be protected by an atmosphere of an inert gas.

**USP 27** (Tretinoin). A yellow to light-orange crystalline powder. Insoluble in water; slightly soluble in alcohol and in chloroform. Store in airtight containers, preferably under an atmosphere of an inert gas. Protect from light.

### Adverse Effects

Tretinoin is a skin irritant. Topical application may cause transitory stinging and a feeling of warmth and in normal use it produces some erythema and peeling similar to that of mild sunburn. Sensitive individuals may experience oedema, blistering, and crusting of the skin. Excessive application can cause severe erythema, peeling, and discomfort with no increase in efficacy. Photosensitivity may occur. Temporary hypopigmentation and hyperpigmentation have been reported.

Oral administration of tretinoin may produce similar adverse effects to those of isotretinoin (see p.1148). Adverse cardiovascular effects have also been reported; the most common were arrhythmias, flushing, hypotension, hypertension, and heart failure. Less common events were cardiac arrest, myocardial infarction, cardiomegaly, heart murmur, ischaemia, stroke, myocarditis, pericarditis, pulmonary hypertension, and secondary cardiomyopathy. A potentially life-threatening 'retinoic acid syndrome' (see below) has been described following oral use.

**Carcinogenicity.** Studies in *mice* suggested that tretinoin could enhance photocarcinogenesis.[1] However, other studies refuted this[2] and evidence indicates that topical tretinoin is not carcinogenic in humans.


1. Epstein JH. Chemicals and photocarcinogenesis. *Australas J Dermatol* 1977; **18:** 57–61.
2. Epstein JH. All-trans-retinoic acid and cutaneous cancers. *J Am Acad Dermatol* 1986; **15:** 772–8.


**Effects on the endocrine system.** Symptoms typical of the premenstrual syndrome followed by vaginal bleeding in a 64-year-old woman were reported to be associated with the topical application of tretinoin[1] but others doubted a causal relationship.[2]


1. Meurehg CC, Xóchitl Amelio P. Vaginal bleeding and tretinoin cream. *Ann Intern Med* 1990; **113:** 483.
2. Worobec SM, *et al.* Topical tretinoin and vaginal bleeding. *Ann Intern Med* 1991, **114:** 97.


**Effects on the musculoskeletal system.** For a report of myositis occurring in a patient receiving oral tretinoin, see Isotretinoin, p.1149.

**Effects on the nervous system.** Oral retinoids may produce neurotoxic adverse effects. Children seem to be particularly sensitive to the CNS effects of tretinoin.[1,2] Neurotoxicity (ataxia, dysarthria, and headache) has been reported in a woman with liver impairment using topical tretinoin 0.025% for acne.[3]


1. Warrell RP, *et al.* Acute promyelocytic leukemia. *N Engl J Med* 1993; **329:** 177–89.
2. Mahmoud HH, *et al.* Tretinoin toxicity in children with acute promyelocytic leukaemia. *Lancet* 1993; **342:** 1394–5.
3. Bernstein AL, Leventhal-Rochon JL. Neurotoxicity related to the use of topical tretinoin (Retin-A). *Ann Intern Med* 1996; **124:** 227–8.


**Retinoic acid syndrome.** A syndrome consisting primarily of fever and respiratory distress developed in 9 of 35 patients between 2 and 21 days after starting induction therapy with oral tretinoin for suspected acute promyelocytic leukaemia.[1] Other symptoms included weight gain, oedema of the lower extremities, pleural or pericardial effusions, and episodic hypotension. Symptoms were life-threatening in 5 patients, 3 of whom subsequently died of multi-system failure. Leucocytosis was frequently, although not invariably, associated with development of the syndrome. Experience showed that early treatment with high-dose corticosteroids should be given to these patients irrespective of the leucocyte count.

A review[2] of this syndrome, known as the 'retinoic acid syndrome', reported that it occurs in about 25% of patients with acute promyelocytic leukaemia treated with tretinoin and that the median time to onset is 10 to 12 days after the start of treatment; the severity of the syndrome varies greatly. A high leucocyte count at diagnosis or a rapidly-increasing count on initiation of therapy increase the likelihood of the syndrome occurring. Close monitoring of leucocyte counts and clinical signs is recommended with the initiation of high-dose intravenous corticosteroids, and possibly the use of antineoplastic drugs, if symptoms appear or the leucocyte count increases rapidly.

A similar syndrome has also been reported in patients with acute promyelocytic leukaemia treated with arsenic trioxide (see p.1657).


1. Frankel SR, *et al.* The "retinoic acid syndrome" in acute promyelocytic leukemia. *Ann Intern Med* 1992; **117:** 292–6.
2. Fenaux P, De Botton S. Retinoic acid syndrome: recognition, prevention and management. *Drug Safety* 1998; **18:** 273–9.


### Precautions

Tretinoin is contra-indicated in pregnancy and in breast-feeding mothers.

Contact of tretinoin with the eyes, mouth, or other mucous surfaces should be avoided. It should not be applied to eczematous, sunburnt, or abraded skin and the effects of other topical treatment, especially with keratolytics, should be allowed to subside before topical use of tretinoin. Exposure to UV light and excessive exposure to sunlight should be avoided.

Absorption does not seem to occur to any great extent with topical use. When tretinoin is given by mouth the precautions described under isotretinoin (see p.1150) should be adopted.

**Pregnancy.** Although there have been isolated reports[1-4] of congenital abnormalities in infants born to mothers who used tretinoin 0.05% topically before and during pregnancy, studies involving a total of 309 women[5,6] showed no increased risk for major congenital disorders in infants who had been exposed in the first trimester.


1. Camera G, Pregliasco P. Ear malformation in baby born to mother using tretinoin cream. *Lancet* 1992; **339:** 687.
2. Lipson AH, *et al.* Multiple congenital defects associated with maternal use of topical tretinoin. *Lancet* 1993; **341:** 1352–3.
3. Navarre-Belhassen C, *et al.* Multiple congenital malformations associated with topical tretinoin. *Ann Pharmacother* 1998; **32:** 505–6.
4. Colley SMJ, *et al.* Topical tretinoin and fetal malformations. *Med J Aust* 1998; **168:** 467.
5. Jick SS, *et al.* First trimester topical tretinoin and congenital disorders. *Lancet* 1993; **341:** 1181–2.
6. Shapiro L, *et al.* Safety of first-trimester exposure to topical tretinoin: prospective cohort study. *Lancet* 1997; **350:** 1143–4.


**Skin fragility.** As with other retinoids (see Isotretinoin, p.1150) the use of depilatory products should be avoided in patients treated with tretinoin. Erosions of the skin occurred in 2 patients after the use of wax depilation on facial areas also being treated topically with tretinoin.[1]


1. Goldberg NS, Zalka AD. Retin-A and wax epilation. *Arch Dermatol* 1989; **125:** 1717.


### Interactions

As for Isotretinoin, p.1150.

Tretinoin is metabolised by the hepatic cytochrome P450 isoenzyme system, therefore there is a potential for interaction between oral tretinoin and inhibitors or inducers of these enzymes.

**Minoxidil.** Percutaneous absorption of minoxidil is enhanced by tretinoin as a result of increased stratum corneum permeability.[1]


1. Ferry JJ, *et al.* Influence of tretinoin on the percutaneous absorption of minoxidil from an aqueous topical solution. *Clin Pharmacol Ther* 1990; **47:** 439–46.


### Pharmacokinetics

After oral doses tretinoin is well absorbed from the gastrointestinal tract, and peak plasma concentrations are obtained after 1 to 2 hours. Oral bioavailability is about 50%. Tretinoin is highly bound to plasma proteins. It undergoes metabolism in the liver by the cytochrome P450 isoenzyme system. Metabolites include isotretinoin, 4-oxo-*trans*-retinoic acid, and 4-oxo-*cis*-retinoic acid. The terminal elimination half-life of tretinoin is 0.5 to 2 hours. Tretinoin is excreted in the bile and the urine. There is some evidence that tretinoin induces its own metabolism.

◊ References.


1. Regazzi MB, *et al.* Clinical pharmacokinetics of tretinoin. *Clin Pharmacokinet* 1997; **32:** 382–402.


### Uses and Administration

Tretinoin is a retinoid and is the acid form of vitamin A (p.1451).

Tretinoin is used primarily in the topical treatment of **acne vulgaris** when comedones, papules, and pustules predominate. It appears to stimulate mitosis and turnover of follicular epithelial cells and reduce their cohesiveness thereby facilitating the extrusion of existing comedones and preventing the formation of new ones. It also appears to have a thinning effect on the stratum corneum. Tretinoin is applied as a cream, gel, or alcoholic solution, usually containing 0.01 to 0.1%. The skin should be cleansed to remove excessive oiliness and dried 15 to 30 minutes before applying tretinoin lightly, once or twice daily according to response and irritation; some patients may require less frequent applications. Other topical preparations (including skin moisturisers) should not be applied at the same time as tretinoin is applied, and caution is required if other local irritants are used concurrently. There may be apparent exacerbations of the acne during early treatment and a therapeutic response may not be evident for 6 to 8 weeks. When the condition has resolved maintenance therapy should be less frequent.

Preparations containing 0.02 or 0.05% tretinoin are available for the treatment of mottled hyperpigmentation, roughness, and fine wrinkling of **photodamaged skin**. It is applied once daily at night. Effects may not be seen until about 6 months after starting treatment.

Tretinoin is also used to induce remission in acute promyelocytic **leukaemia**. A daily dose of 45 mg/m² is given by mouth in 2 divided doses. Treatment is continued until complete remission occurs or 90 days of treatment have been given.

◊ General reviews.


1. Orfanos CE, *et al.* Current use and future potential role of retinoids in dermatology. *Drugs* 1997; **53:** 358–88.


**Malignant neoplasms.** Tretinoin differentiation therapy has become the established treatment for acute promyelocytic leukaemia (APL), a subtype of acute myeloid leukaemia (p.506). Tretinoin is effective in APL because the characteristic chromosomal abnormalities result in an abnormal retinoic acid receptor. When given by *mouth*, it has produced complete remissions in more than 90% of patients.[1] However the duration of remission is short unless consolidation, usually with an anthracycline- and cytarabine-based regimen, is given concurrently or subsequently. The combination of tretinoin followed by chemotherapy has been shown to result in improved survival compared with chemotherapy alone.[2,3] Prolonged maintenance therapy including intermittent tretinoin also appears to reduce the rate of relapse.[3] Although benefit has been reported with continuous tretinoin maintenance this is generally considered to lead to resistance.[4] A life-threatening syndrome has developed in some patients who have received oral tretinoin for APL (see Retinoic Acid Syndrome, under Adverse Effects, above). Children seem particularly sensitive to the adverse effects of oral tretinoin on the CNS (see also under Adverse Effects, above). A lipid-based *intravenous* formulation of tretinoin is under investigation for the treatment of APL.

Tretinoin has also been tried for the *topical* treatment of various neoplastic and related **skin disorders**. Some beneficial effects have been reported in the treatment of actinic keratoses, basal cell carcinoma, metastatic melanoma, and dysplastic naevi.[5-7] It also appears to be of use for the treatment of warts and solar keratoses in organ transplant recipients.[8]

There has been some interest in the use of retinoids in the management of oral leucoplakia (see Malignant Neoplasms, under Isotretinoin, p.1151).


1. Gillis JC, Goa KL. Tretinoin: a review of its pharmacodynamic and pharmacokinetic properties and use in the management of acute promyelocytic leukaemia. *Drugs* 1995; **50:** 897–923.
2. Tallman MS, *et al.* Acute promyelocytic leukemia: evolving therapeutic strategies. *Blood* 2002; **99:** 759–67.
3. Tallman MS, Nabhan C. Management of acute promyelocytic leukemia. *Curr Oncol Rep* 2002; **4:** 381–9.
4. Fenaux P, *et al.* A randomized comparison of all transretinoic acid (ATRA) followed by chemotherapy and ATRA plus chemotherapy and the role of maintenance therapy in newly diagnosed acute promyelocytic leukemia. *Blood* 1999; **94:** 1192–1200.
5. Meyskens FL, *et al.* Role of topical tretinoin in melanoma and dysplastic nevi. *J Am Acad Dermatol* 1986; **15:** 822–5.
6. Peck GL. Topical tretinoin in actinic keratosis and basal cell carcinoma. *J Am Acad Dermatol* 1986; **15:** 829–35.
7. Edwards L, Jaffe P. The effect of topical tretinoin on dysplastic nevi: a preliminary trial. *Arch Dermatol* 1990; **126:** 494–9.
8. Euvrard S, *et al.* Topical retinoids for warts and keratoses in transplant recipients. *Lancet* 1992; **340:** 48–9.


**Skin disorders.** Topical treatment with tretinoin has been tried with varying success in a wide range of cutaneous conditions. Its use in acne (p.1133) is well established. Some benefit has also been reported in rosacea[1] (p.1138), in keratinisation disorders such as Darier's disease (p.1134), in pigmentation disorders (p.1137) such as chloasma,[2] and in some neoplastic disorders (above).

A number of studies suggest that tretinoin can reverse some of the skin changes associated with chronic exposure to sunlight.[3-12] However, the effects seen during treatment are transient and the skin reverts to its pretreatment state once application stops.[13] One study found that several changes taken as indicative of an antiphoto-ageing effect, such as thickening of the skin and epidermis and an increase in the blood supply were not specific to topically applied retinoids and could equally be produced by the use of an abrasive preparation.[14]


1. Ertl GA, *et al.* A comparison of the efficacy of topical tretinoin and low-dose oral isotretinoin in rosacea. *Arch Dermatol* 1994; **130:** 319–24.
2. Griffiths CEM, *et al.* Topical tretinoin (retinoic acid) improves melasma: a vehicle-controlled, clinical trial. *Br J Dermatol* 1993; **129:** 415–21.
3. Weiss JS, *et al.* Topical tretinoin improves photoaged skin: a double-blind vehicle-controlled study. *JAMA* 1988; **259:** 527–32.
4. Leyden JJ, *et al.* Treatment of photodamaged facial skin with topical tretinoin. *J Am Acad Dermatol* 1989; **21:** 638–44.
5. Lever L, *et al.* Topical retinoic acid for treatment of solar damage. *Br J Dermatol* 1990; **122:** 91–8.
6. Berardesca E, *et al.* In vivo tretinoin-induced changes in skin mechanical properties. *Br J Dermatol* 1990; **122:** 525–9.
7. Woodley DT, *et al.* Treatment of photoaged skin with topical tretinoin increases epidermal-dermal anchoring fibrils: a preliminary report. *JAMA* 1990; **263:** 3057–9.
8. Weinstein GD, *et al.* Topical tretinoin for treatment of photodamaged skin: a multicenter study. *Arch Dermatol* 1991; **127:** 659–65.
9. Rafal ES. Topical tretinoin (retinoic acid) treatment for liver spots associated with photodamage. *N Engl J Med* 1992; **326:** 368–74.
10. Griffiths CEM, *et al.* Restoration of collagen formation in photodamaged human skin by tretinoin (retinoic acid). *N Engl J Med* 1993; **329:** 530–5.
11. Popp C, *et al.* Pretreatment of photoaged forearm skin with topical tretinoin accelerates healing of full-thickness wounds. *Br J Dermatol* 1995; **132:** 46–53.
12. Gilchrest BA. A review of skin ageing and its medical therapy. *Br J Dermatol* 1996; **135:** 867–75.
13. Anonymous. Tretinoin for sun-aged skin. *Drug Ther Bull* 1996; **34:** 55–6.
14. Marks R, *et al.* The effects of an abrasive agent on normal skin and on photoaged skin in comparison with topical tretinoin. *Br J Dermatol* 1990; **123:** 457–66.


## Preparations

***BP 2003:*** Tretinoin Gel; Tretinoin Solution;
***USP 27:*** Tretinoin Cream; Tretinoin Gel; Tretinoin Topical Solution.

**Proprietary Preparations** (details are given in Part 3)
***Arg.:*** A Acido; Dorpiel; Eurotretin; Lotioblanc; Neotretin; Niterey; Retacnyl; Retin-A; Tretinoderm; Vesanoid; Vitanol-A; ***Austral.:*** Retin-A; Re-Trieve; Stieva-A; Vesanoid; ***Austria:*** Eudyna; Retin-A; Vesanoid; ***Belg.:*** Retinova†; Vesanoid; ***Braz.:*** Dermoretin†; Retacnyl; Retin-A; Retinova; Vesanoid; Vitanol-A; ***Canad.:*** Rejuva-A; Renova; Retin-A; Retisol-A; Stieva-A; Vesanoid; Vitinoin†; ***Chile:*** Dermodan; Retacnyl; Retin-A; Stieva-A; Vesanoid; ***Fin.:*** Avitcid; Vesanoid; ***Fr.:*** Aberel†; Effederm; Kerlocal†; Ketrel; Locacid; Retacnyl; Retin-A; Retinova; Retitop†; Tretinoine Kefrane†; Vesanoid; ***Ger.:*** Airol; Cordes VAS; Epi-Aberel†; Eudyna†; Vesanoid; ***Gr.:*** Airol; Vesanoid; ***Hong Kong:*** Acta; Alten; Eudyna†; Locacid; Retacnyl; Retin-A; Stieva-A; Vesanoid; Vitamin A Acid; ***India:*** Eudyna; ***Irl.:*** Retin-A; ***Israel:*** Airol; Locacid; Retavit; Retin-A; Vesanoid; ***Ital.:*** Airol; Retin-A; Vesanoid; ***Malaysia:*** Alten; Retacnyl; Retin-A; Stieva-A; Tretinon; ***Mex.:*** A-Plex†; Airol†; Arretin; Eudyna†; Reacel-A; Ret-A-Pres†; Retacnyl; Retin-A; Stieva-A; Tretinon†; Vesanoid; ***Neth.:*** Acid A Vit†; Vesanoid; ***Norw.:*** Aberela; Vesanoid†; ***NZ:*** Retin-A; Retinova; Vesanoid; ***Port.:*** Ketrel; Locacid; Retin-A; Vesanoid; Vitacid; ***S.Afr.:*** Ilotycin-A; Renova; Retacnyl; Retin-A; Vesanoid; ***Singapore:*** Acta†; Airol†; Alten†; Eudyna†; Retacnyl; Retin-A; Stieva-A; Vesanoid; ***Spain:*** Dermojuventus; Retinova; Retirides; Vitanol; ***Swed.:*** Aberela; Retinova; Vesanoid†; ***Switz.:*** Airol; Retin-A; Vesanoid; ***Thai.:*** A-Tinic; Renova; Retacnyl; Retin-A; Stieva-A; ***UK:*** Acticin†; Retin-A; Retinova; Vesanoid; ***USA:*** Altinac†; Avita; Renova; Retin-A; Vesanoid.

**Multi-ingredient:** ***Arg.:*** Hidrosam T; Kitacne AR; Melasmax; Puraloe; Tratacne; ***Austria:*** Keratosis forte; ***Canad.:*** Stievamycin; ***Chile:*** Stievamycin; ***Fin.:*** Wicaran; ***Fr.:*** Antibio-Aberel†; Erylik; ***Ger.:*** Aknemycin Plus; Balisa VAS; Carbamid + VAS; Clinesfar; Pigmanorm; Ureotop + VAS; ***Hong Kong:*** Dermabaz; Erylik; ***Israel:*** Aknemycin Plus; ***Ital.:*** Apsor†; Psorinase; ***Malaysia:*** Aknemycin Plus; ***Mex.:*** Stievamycin; ***Singapore:*** Aknemycin Plus; ***Spain:*** Acnisdin Retinoico; Loderm Retinoico; ***Switz.:*** Carbamide + VAS; Pigmanorm; Sebo-Psor; Tretinoine†; Verra-med; ***UK:*** Aknemycin Plus; ***USA:*** Solage; Tri-Luma.

## Trichloroacetic Acid

Acidum Trichloraceticum; Trichloracetic Acid; Trichloressigsäure; Tricloroacético, ácido.

$C_2HCl_3O_2$ = 163.4.
*CAS — 76-03-9.*

**Pharmacopoeias.** In *Eur.* (see p.vi) and *Pol.*

**Ph. Eur. 5.0** (Trichloroacetic Acid). A very deliquescent white crystalline mass or colourless crystals. Very soluble in water, in alcohol, and in dichloromethane. Store in airtight containers.

### Adverse Effects and Treatment

As for Hydrochloric Acid, p.1699.

### Uses and Administration

Trichloroacetic acid is caustic and astringent. It is used as a quick escharotic for warts. It is applied as a strong solution, prepared by adding 10% by weight of water [e.g. trichloroacetic acid 10 g plus water 1 g]; the surrounding parts are usually protected. It has also been used for the removal of tattoos and in cosmetic surgery for chemical peeling of the skin.

**Tattoo removal.** References to the use of trichloroacetic acid in the removal of tattoos.


1. Hall-Smith P, Bennett J. Tattoos: a lasting regret. *BMJ* 1991; **303:** 397.


**Warts.** References to the use of trichloroacetic acid in the treatment of genital warts (p.1139).


1. Godley MJ, *et al.* Cryotherapy compared with trichloroacetic acid in treating genital warts. *Genitourin Med* 1987; **63:** 390–2.
2. Davis AJ, Emans SJ. Human papilloma virus infection in the pediatric and adolescent patient. *J Pediatr* 1989; **115:** 1–9.
3. Boothby RA, *et al.* Single application treatment of human papillomavirus infection of the cervix and vagina with trichloroacetic acid: a randomized trial. *Obstet Gynecol* 1990; **76:** 278–80.


### Preparations

**Proprietary Preparations** (details are given in Part 3)
***Hong Kong:*** AccuPeel; ***Ital.:*** Averuk Bruciaporri†; CL tre; Porriver†; Verrupor; ***Singapore:*** AccuPeel; ***USA:*** Tri-Chlor.

**Multi-ingredient:** ***Spain:*** Callicida Brum.

## Trioxysalen *(rINN)*

NSC-71047; 4,5′,8-Trimethylpsoralen; Trioxisaleno; Trioxsalen (*USAN*). 2,5,9-Trimethyl-7*H*-furo[3,2-g][1]benzopyran-7-one.

$C_{14}H_{12}O_3$ = 228.2.
*CAS — 3902-71-4.*
*ATC — D05AD01; D05BA01.*

**Pharmacopoeias.** In *US.*

**USP 27** (Trioxsalen). A white to off-white or greyish, odourless, crystalline solid. Practically insoluble in water; soluble 1 in 1150 of alcohol, 1 in 84 of chloroform, 1 in 43 of dichloromethane, and 1 in 100 of methyl isobutyl ketone. Protect from light.

### Profile

Trioxysalen, a psoralen, is a photosensitiser used similarly to methoxsalen in photochemotherapy or PUVA therapy (p.1153). Trioxysalen is used in idiopathic vitiligo to enhance pigmentation or increase the tolerance to sunlight in selected patients. In vitiligo a dose of 10 mg daily is given by mouth 2 to 4 hours before exposure to sunlight or ultraviolet radiation; prolonged therapy may be necessary. To increase tolerance to sunlight a dose of 10 mg daily is given 2 hours before exposure; treatment should not be continued for longer than 14 days.

Trioxysalen may also be used topically in the PUVA treatment of psoriasis.

◊ References.


1. Snellman E, Rantanen T. Concentration-dependent phototoxicity in trimethylpsoralen bath psoralen ultraviolet A. *Br J Dermatol* 2001; **144:** 490–4.


### Preparations

***USP 27:*** Trioxsalen Tablets.

**Proprietary Preparations** (details are given in Part 3)
***Arg.:*** Trisoralen; ***Canad.:*** Trisoralen†; ***Fin.:*** Tripsor; ***Hong Kong:*** Puvadin; Trisoralen†; ***India:*** Neosoralen; ***Ital.:*** Trisoralen†; ***Malaysia:*** Puvadin; ***USA:*** Trisoralen†.

## Urea

Carbamide; E927b; Ureia; Ureum. Carbonic acid diamide.

$NH_2.CO.NH_2$ = 60.06.
*CAS — 57-13-6.*
*ATC — B05BC02; D02AE01.*

**Pharmacopoeias.** In *Chin., Eur.* (see p.vi), *Jpn, Pol.,* and *US.*

**Ph. Eur. 5.0** (Urea). Transparent, slightly hygroscopic, crystals or a white crystalline powder. Very soluble in water; soluble in alcohol; practically insoluble in dichloromethane. Store in airtight containers.

**USP 27** (Urea). Colourless or white, practically odourless, prismatic crystals, or white crystalline powder or pellets. May gradually develop a slight odour of ammonia on prolonged standing. Soluble 1 in 1.5 of water, 1 in 10 of alcohol, and 1 in 1 of boiling alcohol; practically insoluble in chloroform and in ether. Solutions are neutral to litmus. Store at a temperature of 25°, excursions permitted between 15° and 30°.

**Incompatibility.** Urea can cause haemolysis when mixed with blood and should never be added to whole blood for transfusion or given through the same set by which blood is being infused.

### Adverse Effects and Precautions

As for Mannitol, p.950.

Urea is reported to be more irritant than mannitol, and intravenous administration may cause venous thrombosis or phlebitis at the site of injection; extravasation may cause sloughing or necrosis. Only large veins should be used for infusion, and urea should not be infused into veins of the lower limbs of elderly subjects. Extreme care is essential to prevent accidental extravasation of urea infusions.

Rapid intravenous injection of solutions of urea can cause haemolysis; the risk is reduced by using glucose or invert sugar solutions as diluent. Urea should not be administered with whole blood.

Topical applications may be irritant to sensitive skin.

**Infants and neonates.** High plasma-urea concentrations have been reported[1,2] in neonates following topical application of emollient creams containing urea. Since there was no evidence of dehydration[2,3] absorption of urea through the skin was the likely cause. Raised plasma-urea concentrations have been reported[4] in infants with erythematous skin conditions who had not been treated with urea cream and this was attributed to dehydration due to increased insensible water loss through the damaged skin.


1. Beverley DW, Wheeler D. High plasma urea concentrations in collodion babies. *Arch Dis Child* 1986; **61:** 696–8.
2. Oudesluys-Murphy AM, van Leeuwen M. High plasma urea concentrations in collodion babies. *Arch Dis Child* 1987; **62:** 212.
3. Beverley DW, Wheeler D. High plasma urea concentration in babies with lamellar ichthyosis. *Arch Dis Child* 1986; **61:** 1245–6.
4. Garty BZ. High plasma urea concentration in babies with lamellar ichthyosis. *Arch Dis Child* 1986; **61:** 1245.


**Pregnancy.** There have been reports of women suffering coagulopathy associated with urea administered for termination of pregnancy.[1,2]


1. Grundy MFB, Craven ER. Consumption coagulopathy after intra-amniotic urea. *BMJ* 1976; **2:** 677–8.
2. Burkman RT, *et al.* Coagulopathy with midtrimester induced abortion: association with hyperosmolar urea administration. *Am J Obstet Gynecol* 1977; **127:** 533–6.


### Pharmacokinetics

Urea is fairly rapidly absorbed from the gastrointestinal tract but causes gastrointestinal irritation. Urea is distributed into extracellular and intracellular fluids including lymph, bile, CSF, and blood. It is reported to cross the placenta, and penetrate the eye. It is excreted unchanged in the urine.

### Uses and Administration

Urea promotes hydration and is mainly applied topically in the treatment of ichthyosis and hyperkeratotic skin disorders (p.1136). Used intravenously it has osmotic diuretic properties similar to mannitol (p.951) and has been used in the treatment of acute increases in intracranial pressure (p.833), due to cerebral oedema, and to decrease intra-ocular pressure in acute glaucoma (p.1485), but has been largely superseded by mannitol. Urea has also been given intra-amniotically for the termination of pregnancy (p.1512).

When applied topically urea has hydrating and keratolytic properties. In the management of ichthyosis and other dry skin disorders it is applied in creams or lotions containing 5 to 25% urea. A preparation containing 40% may be used for nail destruction.

For the reduction of raised intracranial or intra-ocular pressure, urea is given intravenously, as an infusion of a 30% solution in glucose 5 to 10% or invert sugar 10%, at a rate not exceeding 4 mL/minute, in a dose of 0.5 to 1.5 g/kg to a maximum of 120 g daily. For children under 2 years a dose of 100 mg/kg has been suggested. Rebound increases in intracranial and intra-ocular pressure may occur after about 12 hours.

Solutions of urea 40 to 50% have been given by intra-amniotic injection for the termination of pregnancy.

Urea labelled with carbon-13 (p.1667) is used in the *in vivo* diagnosis of *Helicobacter pylori* infection (see Peptic Ulcer Disease, p.1246). The test involves collecting a breath sample before and after oral ingestion of a single dose of $^{13}$C-urea. *H. pylori* produces urease which hydrolyses the urea to carbon dioxide and ammonia; therefore, an excess of carbon-13-labelled carbon dioxide in the sample, compared with a baseline sample, indicates infection. Doses of $^{13}$C-urea include 50 mg, 75 mg, or 100 mg depending on the kit being used. Urea labelled with the radionuclide carbon-14 is also used in a urea breath test for *H. pylori* detection.

### Preparations

***BP 2003:*** Urea Cream;
***USP 27:*** Urea for Injection.

**Proprietary Preparations** (details are given in Part 3)
***Arg.:*** Hidroplus; Lociherp; Nutralcon; Ureadin; Urecrem; ***Austral.:*** Aquacare; Hamilton Dry Skin; Nutraplus; Urecare; Urederm; ***Austria:*** Basodexan†; Nubral; ***Braz.:*** Hidrapel; Nutraplus; ***Canad.:*** Dermaflex; Ti-U-Lac; Ultra Mide; Uree; Uremol; Urisec; Velvelan†; ***Chile:*** Ayr-5; Hyderm; Nutraplus; Ureadin 10 and 20; ***Fin.:*** Fenuril; ***Fr.:*** Anti-Dessechement; Charlieu Topic; Ictyoderm; Nutraplus; Urecrem†; ***Ger.:*** Balisa; Basodexan; Elacutan; Eucerin Salbe; Hyanit N†; Laceran†; Linola Urea; Nubral; Onychomal; Penaderm†; Rubio N†; Sebexol cum urea; Ureotop; ***Hong Kong:*** Carmol; Euderm; Nutraplus; Urederm; ***Irl.:*** Aquadrate; Nutraplus; ***Ital.:*** Dermal Care; ***Malaysia:*** Balneum Intensiv; Euderm; Nutraplus; UO; Urecare; ***Mex.:*** Derma Keri; Dermoplast; Nutraplus; ***Neth.:*** Alphadrate†; ***NZ:*** Aquacare; Nutraplus; ***Port.:*** Eucerin Pele Seca; Laceran†; Rebladerm; Ureadin 10 and 20; ***S.Afr.:*** Eulactol†; ***Singapore:*** Balneum In-

tensiv; Euderm; Nutraplus; Urecare; **Spain:** Nutraplus; **Swed.:** Canoderm; Caress; Fenuril; Karbaderm; Karbasal; Monilen; **Switz.:** Eucerin peau seche; Excipial U; Linola Urea; Nutraplus; Vita-Merfen Soins dermatologiques; **Thai.:** Balneum Intensiv; **UK:** Aquadrate; Nutraplus; **USA:** Aquacare; Carmol; Gormel; Lanaphilic; Nutraplus; Ultra Mide; Ureacin; Ureaphil; Vanamide.

**Multi-ingredient:** **Arg.:** Acilac; Akerat; Aloebel; Cremisona; Cremsor N; Hidrolac; Lactiderm; Lactiderm HC; Lactocrem; Masivol Urea; Onixol; Sadeltan F; Urecrem Hidro; **Austral.:** Aussie Tan Skin Moisturiser†; Calmurid; Curaderm; Dermadrate; Psor-Asist; SP Cream; **Austria:** Aleot; Calmurid; Calmurid comp; Calmurid HC; Fungiderm comp; Hydrodexan†; Ichth-Oestren; Keratosis; Keratosis forte; Mirfulan; Optiderm†; **Belg.:** Alphaderm†; Calmurid; **Braz.:** Colpanist†; Donnagel; Emoderm†; Oticerim; Oto-Biotic; Sedauric†; Tricolpex; Vagi Biotic†; Vagi-Sulfa; **Canad.:** Amino-Cerv; Calmurid HC†; Calmurid†; Hydrophil; Kerasal; Ti-U-Lac HC†; Uremol-HC; **Chile:** Akerat; Mycosporan Onycoset; Ureadin Forte; Ureadin Pediatrics; **Denm.:** Mycospor Carbamid†; **Fin.:** Calmuril; Wicaran; Wicarba; Wicnecarb; Wicnevit; **Fr.:** Akerat; Amycor Onychoset; Charlieu Topicrem; Keratosane†; Liperol; Nightpeel; Provictol; **Ger.:** Balisa VAS; Brand- u. Wundgel-Medice N; Calmurid; Calmurid HC†; Carbamid + VAS; Fungidexan; Grune Salbe "Schmidt" N†; Hydrodexan; Kelofibrase; Mirfulan; Mycospor Nagelset; Nubral 4; Nubral 4 HC†; Nubral Forte; Oestrugol N; Optiderm; Psoradexan; Psorigerb N; Remederm; Ureata S; Ureotop + VAS; **Hong Kong:** Balneum Intensiv; Balneum Intensiv Plus; **India:** Cotaryl; **Irl.:** Alphaderm; Calmurid; Calmurid HC; Psoradrate†; **Israel:** Agispor Onychoset; Calmurid; Calmurid HC; Derma-Care; Keratospor; U-Lactin Foot Cream; U-Lactin Forte; **Ital.:** Eudermico; Keraflex; Optiderm; Verunec; Xerial; **Malaysia:** Balneum Intensiv Plus; Ucort; **Mex.:** Eucerin Piel Seca/Reseca; Mycospor Onicoset; **Neth.:** Alphacortison†; Calmurid; Calmurid HC; Symbial; **Norw.:** Mycospor Carbamid†; **NZ:** Calmurid; Dermadrate; **Port.:** Calmurid; Carmitol; Creme Laser Hidrante; Hidratoderme; Mycospor; Optiderme†; U Lactin; Ureadin 10 Plus; Ureadin 30; Ureadin Facial; Ureadin Forte; Ureadin Maos; **S.Afr.:** Calmurid HC; Covancaine; **Singapore:** Balneum Intensiv Plus; Dermadrate; Topicrem; **Spain:** Cortisdin Urea; Kanapomada†; Mycospor Onicoset; **Swed.:** Calmuril; Calmuril-Hydrokortison†; Fenuril-Hydrokortison; Mycosporan Karbamid†; **Switz.:** Acne Gel; Antikeloides Creme; Betacortone; Calmurid; Calmurid HC; Carbamide + VAS; Carbamide Creme; Kerasal; Klyx Magnum; Optiderm; Psoradexan†; Sebo Creme; Sebo-Psor; Squa-med; Tretinoine†; Turexan Capilla; Turexan Lotion; **Thai.:** Balneum Intensiv Plus; Gynestin; **UK:** Alphaderm; Antipeol; Balneum Plus; Calmurid; Calmurid HC; Cymex; E45 Itch Relief; St James Balm; Vesagex Heelbalm; **USA:** Accuzyme; Amino-Cerv; Dayto Sulf†; Ethezyme; Gladase; Panafil; Panafil-White; Rosula.

---

## Xenysalate Hydrochloride *(BANM, rINNM)*

Biphenamine Hydrochloride *(USAN)*; Hidrocloruro de xenisalato. 2-Diethylaminoethyl 3-phenylsalicylate hydrochloride; 2-Diethylaminoethyl 2-hydroxy-3-phenylbenzoate hydrochloride.

$C_{19}H_{23}NO_3,HCl = 349.9.$

*CAS — 3572-52-9 (xenysalate); 5560-62-3 (xenysalate hydrochloride).*

*ATC — D11AC09.*

### Profile

Xenysalate hydrochloride has antibacterial and antifungal properties and has been used for the control of seborrhoeic dermatitis of the scalp.

### Preparations

**Proprietary Preparations** (details are given in Part 3)

**Fr.:** Sebaklen†.

---

## Zinc Carbonate *(USAN)*

Zinc, carbonato de.

$ZnCO_3 = 125.4.$

*CAS — 3486-35-9.*

## Basic Zinc Carbonate

Zinc, carbonato básico de.

NOTE. The names zinc carbonate, hydrated zinc carbonate, zinc subcarbonate, and zinc carbonate hydroxide have all been applied to basic zinc carbonate of varying composition occurring naturally or produced by the reaction of a soluble zinc salt with sodium carbonate.

**Pharmacopoeias.** In *US.*

**USP 27** (Zinc Carbonate). It corresponds to $3Zn(OH)_2.2ZnCO_3$ containing the equivalent of not less than 70% ZnO. Store in airtight containers.

### Profile

Zinc carbonate is mildly astringent and protective to the skin and is used topically, mainly in the form of calamine (p.1144), in a variety of skin conditions. In the USA the name calamine is used for zinc oxide (rather than zinc carbonate) with a small proportion of ferric oxide.

### Preparations

**Proprietary Preparations** (details are given in Part 3)

**Multi-ingredient:** **Fr.:** Pygmal; **Spain:** Neo Visage†.

---

## Zinc Oxide

Blanc de Zinc; Flores de Zinc; Zinc, óxido de; Zinci Oxidum; Zinci Oxydum; Zincum Oxydatum.

$ZnO = 81.41.$

*CAS — 1314-13-2.*

NOTE. 'Zinc White' is a commercial form of zinc oxide for use as a pigment.

**Pharmacopoeias.** In *Chin., Eur.* (see p.vi), *Int., Jpn, Pol., US,* and *Viet.*

**Ph. Eur. 5.0** (Zinc Oxide). A white or faintly yellowish-white, soft, amorphous powder, free from gritty particles. Practically insoluble in water and in alcohol; it dissolves in dilute mineral acids.

**USP 27** (Zinc Oxide). A white or yellowish-white, odourless, amorphous, very fine powder, free from grittiness. It gradually absorbs carbon dioxide from air. Insoluble in water and in alcohol; soluble in dilute acids.

**Incompatibility.** Black discoloration has been reported when zinc oxide and glycerol are in contact in the presence of light.

### Profile

Zinc oxide is mildly astringent and is used topically as a soothing and protective application in eczema and slight excoriations, in wounds, and for haemorrhoids. It is also used with coal tar (p.1159) or ichthammol (p.1148) in the treatment of eczema. Zinc oxide reflects ultraviolet radiation and is used as a physical sunscreen (see p.1133).

In the USA the name calamine is used for zinc oxide with a small proportion of ferric oxide.

Zinc oxide is used as the basis for the production of a number of dental cements. Mixed with phosphoric acid it forms a hard material composed largely of zinc phosphate; mixed with clove oil or eugenol, it is used as temporary dental filling.

For further details of zinc and its salts, see p.1469.

**Complications of dental use.** Solitary aspergillosis of the maxillary sinus in 29 of 30 patients was associated with zinc oxide from overfilled teeth.[1] Treatment consisted of removal of the fungal ball containing the zinc oxide; no antifungal treatment was necessary. Zinc oxide has been shown to accelerate the growth of *Aspergillus fumigatus.*

1. Beck-Mannagetta J, *et al.* Solitary aspergillosis of maxillary sinus, a complication of dental treatment. *Lancet* 1983; **ii:** 1260.

### Preparations

**BP 2003:** Aqueous Calamine Cream; Calamine and Coal Tar Ointment; Calamine Lotion; Coal Tar and Zinc Ointment; Coal Tar Paste; Compound Aluminium Paste; Compound Zinc Paste; Dithranol Paste; Hexachlorophene Dusting Powder; Zinc and Castor Oil Ointment; Zinc and Coal Tar Paste; Zinc and Ichthammol Cream; Zinc and Salicylic Acid Paste; Zinc Cream; Zinc Ointment;

**USP 27:** Calamine Lotion; Coal Tar Ointment; Compound Resorcinol Ointment; Zinc Oxide and Salicylic Acid Paste; Zinc Oxide Ointment; Zinc Oxide Paste.

**Proprietary Preparations** (details are given in Part 3)

**Arg.:** Balmex; Caladaryl Panal; Pasta Dermic; Sinamida-D; Zincoxid; **Austral.:** Curash Anti-Rash; Curash Medicated†; Prickly Heat Powder†; Ungvita; Zinc Cream White†; Zincaband; Zink'N'Swim†; **Canad.:** Aveeno Diaper Rash; Babys Own Ointment; Diaper Rash; Egozinc; Herisan†; Infazinc; Johnson's Diaper Rash; Johnson's Medicated; Neoderm†; Pate d'Unna†; Prevex Diaper Rash Cream†; Triple Care Cream; Woodward's Diaper Rash; Zinaderm; Zincoderm; Zincofax; **Denm.:** Zipzoc; **Fin.:** Zipzoc; **Fr.:** Babygella; Lanofene†; Oxyplastine; Senophile; Veinopress A3 and A4; **Ger.:** Cutaninfant; Desitin; Fissan-Zinkschuttelmixtur; Labiosan; Pinal S; Robuvalen; St. Jakobs-Balsam Mono; Weiche Zinkpaste†; Zinkorell†; Zinkpaste; Zinksalbe Dialon; **Hong Kong:** Desitin Daily Care; **India:** Belle Cream; **Irl.:** Coltapaste†; Viscopaste; Zipzoc; **Israel:** Dyprotex; Lotio Zinc; Lotio Zinci; Zinc Lotion; **Ital.:** Delicate Skin Pasta; Gelocast; Gelostretch; Milsana; Oz; Triderm Zeta; Varicex; Viscopaste PB7; Zinco All' Acqua; Zincoderm; Zincotape†; Zincotex†; **Mex.:** Dermo Lassar†; Lassarmex†; Pasta De Lassar; Rosatil BB; **Neth.:** Zinkolie; Zinkzalf; **Port.:** Lassadermil; Oleo Dermosina Simples; Zincoderma; **S.Afr.:** Johnson's Baby Nappy Rash Ointment†; Vernleigh Baby Cream; Viscopaste PB7†; **Spain:** Anticongestiva; **Swed.:** Zincaband†; Zipzoc Salvstrumpa; **Switz.:** Oxyplastine; Zincream; **Thai.:** Nappy-Hippo; Spectraban; **UAE:** Proskin; **UK:** Steripaste; Viscopaste PB7; Zincaband; Zipzoc; **USA:** Borofax; Diaparene Diaper Rash; Dr Smiths; Nupercainal; Triple Paste; Tronolane.

**Multi-ingredient:** numerous perparations are listed in Part 3.

---

## Zinc Phenolsulfonate

Zinc, fenosulfonato de; Zinc 4-Hydroxybenzenesulphonate. Zinc *p*-hydroxybenzenesulphonate; Zinc Phenolsulphonate.

$C_{12}H_{10}O_8S_2Zn = 411.7.$

*CAS — 127-82-2.*

### Profile

Zinc phenolsulfonate has astringent properties and has been used in multi-ingredient preparations applied topically for the treatment of a variety of disorders.

### Preparations

**Proprietary Preparations** (details are given in Part 3)

**Multi-ingredient:** **Arg.:** Gineseptina; **Austral.:** BFI†; **Braz.:** Lerin; Neo Quimica Colirio; **Ital.:** Antisettico Astringente Sedativo; Citroftalmina VC†; Citroftalmina†; Oftalmil; **Switz.:** Medi-Kord†; **USA:** BFI.

---

# Disinfectants and Preservatives

Contact lens care, p.1164
Disinfection in Creutzfeldt-Jakob disease, p.1164
Disinfection of endoscopes, p.1164
Disinfection in hepatitis and HIV infection, p.1165
Disinfection of water, p.1165
Injection site and catheter care, p.1165
Wound disinfection, p.1165

This chapter describes those antimicrobial agents that are used for chemical methods of disinfection, antisepsis, preservation, and sterilisation. There is some overlap between these procedures and some agents may be used as both disinfectants and preservatives. Iodine (p.1598), not in this chapter, is also used for its disinfectant properties.

**Definition of terms.** There is often confusion between the terms disinfectant and antiseptic.

- The term **disinfectant** is applied to a chemical agent that destroys or inhibits the growth of pathogenic micro-organisms in the non-sporing or vegetative state; disinfectants do not necessarily kill all micro-organisms, but reduce them to a level that is harmful neither to health nor the quality of perishable goods. The term is applicable to agents used to treat inanimate objects and materials and may also be applied to agents used to treat the skin and other body membranes and cavities
- An **antiseptic** is a disinfectant which is used on skin and other living tissues thereby limiting or preventing infection
- **Sterilisation** is the total removal or destruction of all living micro-organisms; a few disinfectants (such as ethylene oxide) are capable of producing sterility under suitable conditions but, in general, sterility is produced by heat or radiation methods, with filtration being used for some heat-labile materials. Sterilisation by heating with a bactericide is no longer a recommended practice
- A **preservative** is one of a number of chemical agents which are included in preparations to prevent deterioration from oxidation **(antoxidants)** or to kill or inhibit the growth of micro-organisms inadvertently introduced during manufacture or use **(antimicrobial preservatives)**.

**Use of disinfectants.** Disinfectants are used in hospitals, industrial establishments, public buildings, on farms, and in the home for control and prevention of infection.

The choice of disinfectant depends on the purpose for which it is used and the likely contaminating organisms. In addition to vegetative bacteria, many common disinfectants could be expected to kill some fungi and lipid-containing viruses. Gram-negative bacteria, mycobacteria, and bacterial spores are generally more resistant to disinfectants, and some disinfectants are less effective against non-lipid enveloped viruses, for example the enteroviruses including polio and coxsackie. Prions are generally resistant to many disinfectants (see Disinfection in Creutzfeldt-Jakob Disease, below). Other factors affecting the effectiveness of disinfectants include the contact time, concentration of the disinfectant, the pH of the system, the number and accessibility of the contaminating micro-organisms, and the presence of interfering substances including lipids, organic matter, rubber, and plastics. Aqueous solutions of disinfectants, particularly quaternary ammonium compounds (such as benzalkonium chloride and cetrimide), chlorhexidine, and phenols, may be susceptible to contamination with micro-organisms. To reduce this risk many preparations are provided for clinical use in a sterile form for single use.

**Use of preservatives.** Antimicrobial preservatives are used in sterile preparations such as eye drops and multidose injections to maintain sterility during use. They may also be added to aqueous injections that cannot be sterilised in their final containers and have to be prepared using aseptic precautions, unless the volume to be injected as a single dose exceeds 15 mL. Antimicrobial preservatives are also used in cosmetics, foods, and non-sterile pharmaceutical products such as oral liquids and creams to prevent microbial spoilage. They should not be used indiscriminately. Preparations that should *not* contain preservatives include those for injection into the CSF, eye, or heart. Generally, the antimicrobial preservatives that may be added to foods, animal feeding stuffs, and cosmetics are controlled.

Preservatives used as antoxidants may be classified in 3 groups:

- *true antoxidants*, or anti-oxygens, which probably inhibit oxidation by reacting with free radicals blocking the chain reaction. Examples are the alkyl gallates, butylated hydroxyanisole, butylated hydroxytoluene, nordihydroguaiaretic acid, and the tocopherols (see Vitamin E Substances, p.1464).
- *reducing agents*, which are substances having a lower redox potential than the drug or adjuvants which they are intended to protect and are therefore more readily oxidised. Reducing agents may act also by reacting with free radicals. Examples are ascorbic acid (p.1460) and the potassium and sodium salts of sulfurous acid (see Sulfites and Sulfur Dioxide)
- *antoxidant synergists*, which usually have little antoxidant effect themselves but probably enhance the action of antoxidants in the first group by reacting with heavy-metal ions which catalyse oxidation. Examples of synergists are citric acid (p.1673), edetic acid and its salts (p.1038), lecithin (p.1706), and tartaric acid (p.1752).

◊ General references and guidelines for the use of disinfectants.

1. BMA. *A code of practice for sterilisation of instruments and control of cross-infection.* London: BMA, 1989.
2. Ayliffe GAJ, *et al. Hospital-acquired infection: principles and prevention.* London: Wright, 1990.
3. Ayliffe GAJ, *et al. Chemical disinfection in hospitals.* 2nd ed. London: PHLS, 1993.
4. Rutala WA. APIC guideline for selection and use of disinfectants. *Am J Infect Control* 1996; **24:** 313–42.
5. Russell AD, *et al. Principles and practice of disinfection, preservation, and sterilization.* 3rd ed. Oxford: Blackwell, 1999.
6. DoH. Standard principle for preventing hospital-acquired infections. *J Hosp Infect* 2001; **47** (suppl): S21–S37.

## Contact lens care

Wearers of contact lenses are at increased risk of corneal infections. Factors that predispose the cornea to infection include surface abrasions that may occur during normal wear, accidental trauma during insertion of a lens, and anoxia. In addition, the lens may provide a medium for introducing pathogens into the eye, especially if handling, cleaning, and disinfecting procedures are not adhered to. The most common pathogens are bacteria, in particular *Pseudomonas aeruginosa, Serratia marcescens, Staphylococcus aureus, Staph. epidermidis,* and *Streptococcus pneumoniae.* Fungi rarely cause lens-related keratitis, although contamination of soft (hydrogel) lenses has been reported. *Acanthamoeba* can cause rare but serious corneal infections (p.595) mainly associated with soft contact lens wear; these protozoa are resistant to some commonly used disinfection systems and can colonise lens storage cases.

Lens care systems for rigid lenses typically entail cleansing and disinfection stages. Daily cleansing with solutions containing surfactants and sometimes mild abrasives can substantially reduce microbial contamination as well as removing organic material which can compromise the activity of the disinfection stage. Cleansing solutions frequently contain substances that are irritant to the eye and should be removed by rinsing and soaking the lens. Soaking solutions also maintain lens hydration, disinfect the lens, and prevent contamination during storage. Although not intended for use in the eye, soaking solutions should be non-irritant. Commonly used disinfectants include benzalkonium chloride and chlorhexidine. Thiomersal is also used but has been associated with a high incidence of hypersensitivity reactions. Wetting or rewetting solutions are used to improve the comfort of the lens and, since they are applied to the eye, must be non-irritant. They commonly contain hypromellose, hyetellose, polyvinyl alcohol, or povidone, although a simple sodium chloride 0.9% solution may be used.

Soft contact lenses contain a high proportion of water and are liable to absorb substances from solution. For this reason some disinfectants, notably benzalkonium chloride, are not suitable for inclusion in solutions for soft lenses. Soft lenses may be disinfected by heating in a suitable unit, usually in isotonic saline solution, but this can shorten the life of the lens by denaturing the polymer or causing deposits of denatured protein, minerals, or preservatives from the saline solution. Stabilised hydrogen peroxide is suitable for cold disinfection of soft lenses and is particularly useful for preventing *Acanthamoeba* infections. However, it is irritant to the cornea and must be neutralised before the lens is inserted into the eye. Other disinfectants for soft lenses may include chlorhexidine and polihexanide. Cleansers for soft lenses may contain surfactants or enzymes such as papain or pancreatin which remove protein deposits.

## Disinfection in Creutzfeldt-Jakob disease

Creutzfeldt-Jakob disease is a transmissible spongiform encephalopathy believed to be caused by infection of the nervous system with prions. The agent causing Creutzfeldt-Jakob disease (CJD) is resistant to many disinfection procedures including dry heat, ultraviolet irradiation, alcohols, ethylene oxide, eusol, formaldehyde, glutaral, hydrogen peroxide, iodine or iodophores, peracetic acid, phenolics, and propiolactone. Although no sterilisation procedure can be guaranteed to be completely effective under all circumstances, a method recommended in the UK[1] is immersion in sodium hypochlorite (providing 20 000 ppm available chlorine) for 1 hour. Alternatives are autoclaving at 134° to 137° for a single cycle of 18 minutes, or 6 successive cycles of 3 minutes each, or immersion in 1M sodium hydroxide for 1 hour; however these methods are known not to be completely effective. Neurosurgical and ophthalmic instruments should be destroyed by incineration if used in patients with confirmed or suspected CJD. Recommendations for disinfection and sterilisation in CJD have also been published in the USA.[2]

1. Advisory Committee on Dangerous Pathogens, Spongiform Encephalopathy Advisory Committee. *Transmissible spongiform encephalopathy agents: safe working and the prevention of infection.* London: Department of Health, 2003.
Also available at: http://www.dh.gov.uk/PolicyAndGuidance/HealthAndSocialCareTopics/CJD/CJDGeneralInformation/CJDGeneralArticle/fs/en?CONTENT_ID=4031067&chk=4gOe2r (accessed 09/06/04)
2. Rutala WA, Weber DJ. Creutzfeldt-Jakob disease: recommendations for disinfection and sterilization. *Clin Infect Dis* 2001; **32:** 1348–56.

## Disinfection of endoscopes

Whenever possible, medical equipment that comes into intimate contact with the body should be heat sterilised, but some equipment, notably endoscopes, will not withstand high temperatures. Low-temperature steam and formaldehyde or ethylene oxide will achieve sterilisation, but may not be practical in a clinical setting. Satisfactory chemical disinfection of endoscopes and other heat-sensitive instruments relies on initial thorough cleansing of the instrument and choice of an appropriate disinfectant which should be rapidly active against a wide range of pathogens including vegetative bacteria, bacterial spores, mycobacteria, and viruses. The disinfectant should not damage the instrument or discolour the optical components, and it should not leave a toxic residue. It is usually necessary to rinse the instrument with sterile water or alcohol after disinfection.[1,2]

Glutaral 2% is commonly used.[1] To achieve sterilisation, immersion in glutaral 2% for 3 hours is necessary, but high-level disinfection, achieved by immersion for 20 minutes, is usually considered adequate for most endoscopes.[1,3,4] Immersion for a minimum of 20 minutes is required for elimination of tubercle bacilli, but immersion for 4 minutes may be adequate for gastroscopes, except those for use on immunocompromised patients. For specific information relating to HIV and hepatitis viruses, see below.

A disadvantage of glutaral is that it is irritant and may cause sensitisation. In addition, glutaral-resistant strains of *M. chelonae* have been isolated from endoscope disinfecting equipment.[5] Alternative disinfectants include peracetic acid, chlorine dioxide, *o*-phthaldialdehyde, and superoxidised water (hypochlorous acid).[4,6,7] Other alternatives include peroxygen compounds, quaternary ammonium compounds, glucoprotamine, electrolysed acid water, succinic dialdehyde, povidone-iodine, and alcohol 70%.[1,4,6-9] However, peracetic acid and chlorine dioxide produce irritant fumes, peroxygen-containing compounds and quaternary ammonium compounds have questionable activity against mycobacteria and viruses, and alcohol and povidone-iodine have a number of practical limitations.[4,10]

1. Ayliffe GAJ, *et al. Chemical disinfection in hospitals.* 2nd ed. London: PHLS, 1993.
2. Ryan CK, Potter GD. Disinfectant colitis: rinse as well as you wash. *J Clin Gastroenterol* 1995; **21:** 6–9.
3. American Society for Gastrointestinal Endoscopy. Multi-society guideline for reprocessing flexible gastrointestinal endoscopes. *Gastrointest Endosc* 2003; **58:** 1–8.

4. British Society of Gastroenterology Working Party. Cleaning and disinfection of equipment for gastrointestinal endoscopy. *Gut* 1998; **42:** 585–93. Also available at: http://www.bsg.org.uk/pdf_word_docs/glutaraldehyde.doc (accessed 14/06/04)
5. Griffiths PA, *et al.* Glutaraldehyde-resistant Mycobacterium chelonae from endoscope washer disinfectors. *J Appl Microbiol* 1997; **82:** 519–26.
6. British Society of Gastroenterology. BSG Working Party Report 2003. BSG guidelines for decontamination of equipment for gastrointestinal endoscopy. Available at: http://www.bsg.org.uk/pdf_word_docs/disinfection.doc (accessed 14/06/04)
7. Rey J-F, *et al.* ESGE (European Society of Gastrointestinal Endoscopy); ESGENA (European Society of Gastrointestinal Endoscopy Nurses and Associates). ESGE/ESGENA technical note on cleaning and disinfection. *Endoscopy* 2003; **35:** 869–77. Also available at: http://www.esge.com/downloads/pdfs/guidelines/technical_note_on_cleaning_and_disinfection.pdf (accessed 14/06/04)
8. Axon ATR, Cotton PB. Endoscopy and infection. *Gut* 1983; **24:** 1064–6.
9. Fraise AP. Disinfection in endoscopy. *Lancet* 1995; **346:** 787–8.
10. Ridgway GL. Decontamination of fibreoptic endoscopes. *J Hosp Infect* 1985; **6:** 363–8.

#### Disinfection in hepatitis and HIV infection

Hepatitis viruses and HIV are susceptible to heat and the methods recommended for sterilisation of equipment in the UK[1] are conventional procedures using moist or dry heat. Heat-labile articles and surfaces may undergo chemical disinfection but only in the absence of a satisfactory alternative. Although various publications have claimed efficacy against HIV for a wide range of disinfectants and detergents, the evidence for some claims is equivocal.

Fresh aqueous solutions of sodium hypochlorite or sodium dichloroisocyanurate are recommended for general surface disinfection. If contaminated by blood, the concentration must be equivalent to 10 000 ppm of available chlorine. For non-corrosive disinfection of delicate items such as fibreoptic endoscopes, freshly activated alkaline glutaral 2% may be used following thorough washing. If a sterile body cavity will be entered the endoscope must be immersed for a minimum of 3 hours; otherwise a minimum of 30 minutes is sufficient, or 1 hour if the presence of *Mycobacterium tuberculosis* is suspected.

1. DoH. *UK Health Departments guidance for clinical health care workers: protection against infection with blood-borne viruses: recommendations of the expert advisory group on AIDS and the advisory group on hepatitis* [undated]. Available at: http://www.dh.gov.uk/assetRoot/04/01/44/74/04014474.pdf (accessed 09/06/04)

#### Disinfection of water

Travellers to regions of the world where water is not disinfected at source should be advised to boil or chemically sterilise water for drinking, cleaning teeth, and washing fruit and vegetables.[1] Chlorine-releasing disinfectants including tosylchloramide sodium, halazone, sodium dichloroisocyanurate, and sodium hypochlorite are commonly used. Iodine-releasing disinfectants such as tetraglycine hydroperiodide or iodine itself are also sometimes used. Organic material suspended in the water may reduce the available halogen concentration, and cloudy water should be filtered or allowed to settle and decanted before treatment. Emergency treatment of drinking water with lemon juice has been suggested during epidemics of waterborne gastro-enteritis.[2] Chlorine-releasing disinfectants are also used for recreational and therapeutic bathing pools, often in combination with ozone.[3]

Legionnaires' disease (p.133) is commonly transmitted via cooling water in air conditioning systems or hot water supplies. Hyperchlorination has been attempted to eradicate the organism from contaminated water sources but has been largely ineffective[4,5] and is no longer recommended. Other disadvantages of using chlorine-based systems at these temperatures and concentrations are corrosion of the plumbing system[5] and the production of potentially carcinogenic byproducts.[6] Effective disinfection can be achieved by raising the water temperature, ultraviolet light, and copper-silver ionisation.

1. Backer H. Water disinfections for international and wilderness travelers. *Clin Infect Dis* 2002; **34:** 355–64.
2. D'Aquino M, Teves SA. Lemon juice as a natural biocide for disinfecting drinking water. *Bull Pan Am Health Organ* 1994; **28:** 324–30.
3. Dadswell JV. Managing swimming, spa, and other pools to prevent infection. *Commun Dis Rep* 1996; **6** (review 2): R37–R40.
4. Kurtz JB, *et al.* Legionella pneumophila in cooling water systems: report of a survey of cooling towers in London and a pilot trial of selected biocides. *J Hyg (Camb)* 1982; **88:** 369–81.
5. Helms CM, *et al.* Legionnaires' disease associated with a hospital water system: a five-year progress report on continuous hyperchlorination. *JAMA* 1988; **259:** 2423–7.
6. Morris RD, *et al.* Chlorination, chlorination by-products, and cancer: a meta-analysis. *Am J Public Health* 1992; **82:** 955–63.

#### Injection site and catheter care

The need to disinfect the skin before injection is controversial.[1] Routine skin preparation of the injection site by swabbing with antiseptic has been reported to be both ineffective and unnecessary.[2,3] Central venous and arterial catheters, however, require the application of strict aseptic technique and injection site antisepsis to reduce the chance of infection.[4] Disinfection of catheter insertion sites with aqueous chlorhexidine 2% has been reported to be associated with fewer local and systemic infections than site preparation with either 10% povidone-iodine solution or 70% isopropyl alcohol,[5] although this has been challenged.[6] A subsequent study reported lower rates of catheter colonisation and catheter-related infection with an alcoholic solution of chlorhexidine 0.25% and benzalkonium chloride 0.025% than with povidone-iodine 10%.[7] In a study in preterm infants, technique had greater influence on bacterial counts at injection sites than the antiseptic used; chlorhexidine 0.5% in isopropyl alcohol and aqueous povidone-iodine 10% were equally effective, but cleansing with alcoholic chlorhexidine for 30 seconds or for two 10-second periods was more effective than cleansing for 5 or 10 seconds.[8]

The use of catheters impregnated with antiseptics or antibacterials has also been studied. Catheters impregnated with chlorhexidine and sulfadiazine silver do appear to be effective in reducing both catheter colonisation and related bloodstream infection in high-risk patients.[9] Central venous catheters impregnated with minocycline and rifampicin have been reported to be associated with a lower infection rate than those impregnated with chlorhexidine and sulfadiazine silver.[10]

Guidelines have been produced for the prevention of infection associated with both peripheral intravascular and central venous catheterisation.[11-13]

1. Ayliffe GAJ, *et al. Chemical disinfection in hospitals.* 2nd ed. London: PHLS, 1993.
2. Dann TC. Routine skin preparation before injection: an unnecessary procedure. *Lancet* 1969; **ii:** 96–8.
3. Liauw J, Archer GJ. Swabaholics? *Lancet* 1995; **345:** 1648.
4. Shepherd A, Williams N. Care of long-term central venous catheters. *Br J Hosp Med* 1994; **51:** 598–602.
5. Maki DG, *et al.* Prospective randomised trial of povidone-iodine, alcohol, and chlorhexidine for prevention of infection associated with central venous and arterial catheters. *Lancet* 1991; **338:** 339–43.
6. Segura M, Sitges-Serra A. Intravenous catheter sites and sepsis. *Lancet* 1991; **338:** 1218.
7. Mimoz O, *et al.* Prospective, randomized trial of two antiseptic solutions for prevention of central venous or arterial catheter colonization and infection in intensive care unit patients. *Crit Care Med* 1996; **24:** 1818–23.
8. Malathi I, *et al.* Skin disinfection in preterm infants. *Arch Dis Child* 1993; **69:** 312–16.
9. Veenstra DL, *et al.* Efficacy of antiseptic-impregnated central venous catheters in preventing catheter-related bloodstream infection: a meta-analysis. *JAMA* 1999; **281:** 261–7.
10. Darouiche RO, *et al.* A comparison of two antimicrobial-impregnated central venous catheters. *N Engl J Med* 1999; **340:** 1–8.
11. DoH. Guidelines for preventing infections associated with the insertion and maintenance of central venous catheters. *J Hosp Infect* 2001; **47**(suppl): S47–S67.
12. O'Grady NP, *et al.* Guidelines for the prevention of intravascular catheter-related infections. *Clin Infect Dis* 2002; **35:** 1281–1307. Also available at: http://www.cdc.gov/mmwr/preview/mmwrhtml/rr5110a1.htm (accessed 09/06/04)
13. National Institute for Clinical Excellence. Infection control: prevention of healthcare-associated infections in primary and community care (June 2003). Section 5: central venous catheterisation. Available at: http://www.nice.org.uk/pdf/Infection_control_fullguideline.pdf (accessed 09/06/04)

#### Wound disinfection

Antiseptic preparations are widely used to treat or prevent superficial infections, but their usefulness on broken skin and wounds has been questioned.[1] Antiseptic solutions are commonly used to clean wounds (p.1139) but are of doubtful value. Chlorine-releasing antiseptic solutions are generally regarded as irritant and although there is little direct evidence in patients there is concern that they may delay wound healing. Cetrimide,[2] tosylchloramide sodium,[3] hydrogen peroxide 3%,[4] iodophores,[4] and sodium hypochlorite solutions[2] are all reported to be cytotoxic *in vitro* or in *animal* models. Long-term or repeated use of these antiseptics for wound toilet should probably be avoided. Chlorhexidine is relatively non-toxic.[2,3]

1. Brown CD, Zitelli JA. A review of topical agents for wounds and methods of wounding: guidelines for wound management. *J Dermatol Surg Oncol* 1993; **19:** 732–7.
2. Thomas S, Hay NP. Wound cleansing. *Pharm J* 1985; **2:** 206.
3. Brennan SS, *et al.* Antiseptic toxicity in wounds healing by secondary intention. *J Hosp Infect* 1986; **8:** 263–7.
4. Lineweaver W, *et al.* Topical antimicrobial toxicity. *Arch Surg* 1985; **120:** 267–70.

## Acridine Derivatives

Acridina, derivados.

**Description.** Acridine derivatives are a group of quinoline antimicrobial dyes structurally related to acridine.

### Acriflavinium Chloride *(rINN)*

Acriflavine; Acriflavine Hydrochloride; Acriflavinii Dichloridum; Cloruro de acriflavinio. A mixture of 3,6-diamino-10-methylacridinium chloride hydrochloride and 3,6-diaminoacridine dihydrochloride.

*CAS — 8063-24-9; 65589-70-0.*
*ATC — R02AA13.*

**Pharmacopoeias.** In *Swiss.*

### Acriflavinium Monochloride

Acriflavinii Monochloridum; Euflavina; Euflavine; Neutral Acriflavine; Neutroflavin. A mixture of 3,6-diamino-10-methylacridinium chloride and 3,6-diaminoacridine monohydrochloride. The latter is usually present to the extent of between 30 and 40%.

*CAS — 68518-47-8.*
*ATC — D08AA03.*

**Pharmacopoeias.** In *Eur.* (see p.vi).

**Ph. Eur. 5.0** (Acriflavinium Monochloride). A reddish-brown, hygroscopic powder. Freely soluble in water; sparingly soluble in alcohol; very slightly soluble in dichloromethane. A 2% solution in water has a pH of 4.5 to 7.5. Store in airtight containers. Protect from light.

### Aminoacridine Hydrochloride *(BANM, rINNM)*

Aminacrine Hydrochloride *(USAN)*; Hidrocloruro de aminoacridina; NSC-7571. 9-Aminoacridine hydrochloride monohydrate.

$C_{13}H_{10}N_2,HCl,H_2O$ = 248.7.
*CAS — 90-45-9 (aminoacridine); 134-50-9 (anhydrous aminoacridine hydrochloride).*
*ATC — D08AA02.*

### Ethacridine Lactate *(BANM, rINNM)*

Acrinol; Aethacridinium Lacticum; Ethacridini Lactas; Lactato de etacridina; Lactoacridine. 6,9-Diamino-2-ethoxyacridine lactate.

$C_{15}H_{15}N_3O,C_3H_6O_3$ = 343.4.
*CAS — 442-16-0 (ethacridine); 1837-57-6 (ethacridine lactate); 6402-23-9 (ethacridine lactate monohydrate).*
*ATC — B05CA08; D08AA01.*

**Pharmacopoeias.** In *Pol.* and *Swiss.*

*Chin., Eur.* (see p.vi), and *Jpn* describe the monohydrate.

**Ph. Eur. 5.0** (Ethacridine Lactate Monohydrate). A yellow crystalline powder. Sparingly soluble in water; very slightly soluble in alcohol; practically insoluble in dichloromethane. A 2% solution in water has a pH of 5.5 to 7.0. Protect from light.

### Proflavine Hemisulfate

Proflavine Hemisulphate *(pINNM)*; Hemisulfato de proflavina; Neutral Proflavine Sulphate. 3,6-Diaminoacridine sulphate dihydrate.

$(C_{13}H_{11}N_3)_2,H_2SO_4,2H_2O$ = 552.6.
*CAS — 92-62-6 (proflavine).*

#### Profile

The acridine derivatives are slow-acting antiseptics. They are bacteriostatic against many Gram-positive bacteria but less effective against Gram-negative bacteria. They are ineffective against spores. Their activity is increased in alkaline solutions and is not reduced by tissue fluids.

The acridine derivatives have been used for the treatment of infected wounds or burns and for skin disinfection, although they have been largely superseded by other antiseptics or suitable antibacterials. Prolonged treatment may delay healing. They have also been used for the local treatment of ear, oropharyngeal, and genito-urinary infections.

Aminoacridine is reported to be non-staining and is used as the hydrochloride as eye drops in the treatment and prophylaxis of superficial eye infections.

Ethacridine lactate is included in some preparations for the treatment of diarrhoea. It has also been given by extra-amniotic injection for the termination of pregnancy (p.1512) but other methods are usually preferred.

Hypersensitivity to acridine derivatives has been reported.

#### Preparations

***BPC 1973:*** Proflavine Cream.

**Proprietary Preparations** (details are given in Part 3)
***Austral.:*** Aminopt; ***Ger.:*** Metifex; Neochinosol; Panflavin†; Rivanol; Urocridin†; Uroseptol; ***India:*** Emcredil; Vecredil; ***Singapore:*** Dettol†.

**Multi-ingredient: *Arg.:*** Carnot Topico; Nene Dent; Otocuril; ***Austral.:*** Medijel; ***Austria:*** Dermowund; Tebege-Tannin†; ***Braz.:*** Acridin; Cezane†; Cystex; Senol; ***Chile:*** Molca; ***Fr.:*** Chromargon; Pyorex; ***Ger.:*** Anaesthesin-Rivanol; Nordapanin N; Otolitan N mit Rivanol; Tannacomp; ***Hong Kong:*** Burn Cream; Medijel; ***India:*** Anaebell; Emscab; ***Israel:*** Medijel; ***Malaysia:*** Burnol Plus; Medijel; ***NZ:*** Medijel; ***S.Afr.:*** Achromide; AMS†; Daromide; Masse†; Vagarsol; ***Singapore:*** Burnol Plus; Medijel; ***Spain:*** Antigrietun; Hepro; ***Switz.:*** Anginol†; Euproctol N; Flavangin†; Haemocortin; Haemolan; Tyrothricin; ***Thai.:*** Burnol Plus; Flavinol; ***UK:*** Medijel; ***USA:*** Alasulf; Deltavac; DIT1-2.

# Alcohol

Aethanolum; Alcool; Ethanol; Ethanolum; Ethyl Alcohol.
$C_2H_5OH$ = 46.07.
*CAS — 64-17-5.*
*ATC — D08AX08; V03AB16; V03AZ01.*

**Pharmacopoeias.** Various strengths are included in *Br., Chin., Eur.* (see p.vi), *Int., Jpn, Pol., US,* and *Viet.* Also in *USNF.*
In *Martindale* the term alcohol is used for alcohol 95 or 96% v/v.
**Ph. Eur. 5.0** (Ethanol, Anhydrous; Ethanolum Anhydricum; Ethanol BP 2003). It contains not less than 99.5% v/v or 99.2% w/w of $C_2H_5OH$ at 20°. A colourless, clear, volatile, flammable, hygroscopic liquid; it burns with a blue, smokeless flame. B.p. about 78°. Miscible with water and with dichloromethane. Protect from light.
The BP 2003 gives Absolute Alcohol and Dehydrated Alcohol as approved synonyms.
**Ph. Eur. 5.0** (Ethanol (96 per cent)). It contains not less than 95.1% v/v or 92.6% w/w and not more than 96.9% v/v or 95.2% w/w of $C_2H_5OH$ at 20°, and water. A colourless, clear, volatile, flammable, hygroscopic liquid; it burns with a blue, smokeless flame. B.p. about 78°. Miscible with water and with dichloromethane. Protect from light.
The BP 2003 gives Alcohol (96 per cent) as an approved synonym.
**BP 2003** (Dilute Ethanols). The monograph describes several dilute alcohols containing between 20 and 90% v/v of $C_2H_5OH$, and one of these, ethanol (90%), is also known as rectified spirit.
**USP 27** (Alcohol). It contains not less than 92.3% w/w or 94.9% v/v and not more than 93.8% w/w or 96.0% v/v of $C_2H_5OH$ at 15.56°. A clear, colourless, mobile, volatile liquid with a characteristic odour and burning taste; readily flammable. B.p. about 78°. Miscible with water and with almost all other organic solvents. Store away from fire in airtight containers.
**USP 27** (Dehydrated Alcohol). It contains not less than 99.5% v/v or 99.2% w/w of $C_2H_5OH$ (sp. gr. not more than 0.7962 at 15.56°). Store away from fire in airtight containers.
**USNF 22** (Diluted Alcohol). It contains 48.4 to 49.5% v/v or 41 to 42% w/w of $C_2H_5OH$. Store away from fire in airtight containers.

**Alcoholic strength.** This is expressed as a percentage by volume of alcohol. It was previously often expressed in terms of *proof spirit.* Proof spirit contained about 57.1% v/v or 49.2% w/w of $C_2H_5OH$, and was defined as 'that which at the temperature of 51°F weighs exactly twelve-thirteenths of an equal measure of distilled water'. Spirit of such a strength that 100 volumes contained as much ethyl alcohol as 160 volumes of proof spirit was described as '60 OP' (over proof). Spirit of which 100 volumes contained as much alcohol as 40 volumes of proof spirit was described as '60 UP' (under proof).

An alternative method of indicating spirit strength was used on the labels of alcoholic beverages in the UK when the strength was given as a number of degrees, proof spirit being taken as 100°. In the USA alcoholic strength is expressed in degrees, the value of which is equal to twice the percentage by volume. Thus 70° proof (old UK system) is equivalent to 40% v/v, and therefore to 80° proof (USA system).

## Adverse Effects

Adverse effects of alcohol arise chiefly from the intake of alcoholic beverages. The concentration of alcohol in the blood producing a state of intoxication varies between individuals. At low to moderate concentrations, alcohol acts as an apparent stimulant; depression of cortical function causes loss of judgement, emotional lability, visual impairment, slurred speech, and ataxia. Hangover effects may include nausea, headache, dizziness, and tremor. Alcohol depresses medullary action; lethargy, amnesia, hypothermia, hypoglycaemia (especially in children), stupor, coma, respiratory depression, cardiomyopathy, hypertension or hypotension, and cardiovascular collapse may occur. The median lethal blood-alcohol concentration is generally estimated to be about 400 to 500 mg per 100 mL. Death may occur at lower blood-alcohol concentrations due to inhalation of vomit during unconsciousness.

Chronic excessive consumption of alcohol may cause damage to many organs, particularly the brain and the liver. Brain damage may lead to Wernicke-Korsakoff syndrome. Fat deposits may occur in the liver and there may be a reduction in various blood-cell counts. Nutritional diseases may occur due to inadequate diet. High alcohol consumption has been associated with pancreatitis, and an increased risk of cardiovascular disease, although some consider that moderate consumption might have a protective effect against ischaemic heart disease.

Alcohol consumption has also been associated with an increased risk of some types of cancer.

The term '**alcoholism**' may be used to denote dependence on alcohol, which is of the barbiturate-alcohol type (see Amobarbital, p.670) and usually involves tolerance to other sedatives and anaesthetics. Following prolonged periods of excessive alcohol consumption, a drop in blood-alcohol concentration may precipitate a withdrawal syndrome characterised by tremor, agitation, feelings of dread, nausea, vomiting, and sweating; hallucinations, seizures, and delirium tremens may also develop.

A **fetal alcohol syndrome** has been identified in which infants born to some alcoholic mothers have characteristic features and abnormalities. There have been some reports of the syndrome and other adverse effects on the fetus being associated with moderate alcohol intake in pregnancy; it is generally suggested that alcohol is best avoided during pregnancy.

Frequent application of alcohol to the skin produces irritation and dry skin.

◊ Reviews of the adverse effects of alcohol.


1. Adinoff B, *et al.* Acute ethanol poisoning and the ethanol withdrawal syndrome. *Med Toxicol* 1988; **3:** 172–96.
2. Charness ME, *et al.* Ethanol and the nervous system. *N Engl J Med* 1989; **321:** 442–54.
3. Edwards G, Peters TJ, eds. Alcohol and alcohol problems. *Br Med Bull* 1994; **50:** 1–230.
4. Lieber CS. Medical disorders of alcoholism. *N Engl J Med* 1995; **333:** 1058–65.
5. Sherlock S. Alcoholic liver disease. *Lancet* 1995; **345:** 227–9.
6. Cowie MR. Alcohol and the heart. *Br J Hosp Med* 1997; **57:** 457–60.
7. Hills KS, Westaby D. Alcohol and the liver. *Br J Hosp Med* 1997; **57:** 517–21.
8. Scheepers BDM. Alcohol and the brain. *Br J Hosp Med* 1997; **57:** 548–51.
9. Marshall EJ, Alan F. Psychiatric problems associated with alcohol misuse and dependence. *Br J Hosp Med* 1997; **58:** 44–6.
10. O'Connor PG, Schottenfeld RS. Patients with alcohol problems. *N Engl J Med* 1998; **338:** 592–601.
11. Dunn N, Cook CCH. Psychiatric aspects of alcohol misuse. *Hosp Med* 1999; **60:** 169–72.
12. Riedel F, *et al.* Alcohol-related diseases of the mouth and throat. *Best Pract Res Clin Gastroenterol* 2003; **17:** 543–55.
13. Salaspuro MP. Alcohol consumption and cancer of the gastrointestinal tract. *Best Pract Res Clin Gastroenterol* 2003; **17:** 679–94.


**Effects on the skin.** A 70% solution of alcohol, containing povidone-iodine, caused partial thickness chemical burns beneath tourniquets in 3 young children.[1] Other adverse effects on the skin reported with the topical application of alcohols have included necrosis following skin cleansing of preterm neonates with methylated spirits[2,3] and haemorrhagic skin necrosis due to the alcohol content of chlorhexidine in spirit used as a disinfectant in umbilical artery catheterisation in preterm infants.[4]

See also Children, under Adverse Effects of Isopropyl Alcohol, p.1184.


1. Dickinson JC, Bailey BN. Chemical burns beneath tourniquets. *BMJ* 1988; **297:** 1513.
2. Harpin V, Rutter N. Percutaneous alcohol absorption and skin necrosis in a preterm infant. *Arch Dis Child* 1982; **57:** 477–9.
3. Murch S, Costelloe K. Hyperosmolality related to propylene glycol in an infant. *BMJ* 1990; **301:** 389.
4. Al-Jawad ST. Percutaneous alcohol absorption and skin necrosis in a preterm infant. *Arch Dis Child* 1983; **58:** 395–6.


## Treatment of Adverse Effects

In acute poisoning the patient should be kept warm and given supportive and symptomatic care. The use of intravenous infusions of fructose to treat severe alcohol poisoning is not recommended as metabolic disturbances may occur. Haemodialysis is of value in severe alcoholic poisoning.

The management of the alcohol withdrawal syndrome and long-term abstinence following withdrawal are discussed below.

**Alcohol withdrawal and abstinence.** The alcohol withdrawal syndrome presents in the early stages as a classical hyperadrenergic state with tremor, tachycardia, sweating, and hypertension. Sometimes this is accompanied by mild disorientation, anxiety, impaired concentration, depression, agitation, and gastrointestinal symptoms. Insomnia, nightmares, and transient hallucinations can also be present. The condition may be self-limiting without the need for therapeutic intervention or it may progress to the severe and potentially fatal condition of delirium tremens (DTs), often characterised by delirium, disorientation, and hallucinations. In some cases generalised tonic-clonic seizures occur within 24 hours of alcohol withdrawal and are followed by delirium tremens.

**Withdrawal.** The general management of the alcohol withdrawal syndrome has been the subject of many reviews and discussions.[1-15] In most cases symptoms do not require treatment and disappear within a few days, but more severe cases may require managed withdrawal from alcohol to avoid complications.

Sedatives are commonly used to reduce the symptoms of alcohol withdrawal and, if given promptly, can prevent progression to seizures and delirium tremens. *Benzodiazepines* are usually the drugs of first choice. Longer-acting drugs such as chlordiazepoxide or diazepam may be more effective against withdrawal seizures and provide smoother withdrawal, while shorter-acting ones such as lorazepam or oxazepam have a smaller risk of producing oversedation and may be more suitable for use in the elderly and, since they do not rely on hepatic enzymes for their metabolism, for patients with liver disease. Benzodiazepines should be given in short courses only to prevent the development of dependence. Some advocate that benzodiazepine dosage should be adjusted according to the severity of symptoms with special care being paid to patients with a history of withdrawal seizures, comorbid conditions, or those using sedative or hypnotic medication. This reduces the amount of drug required and the duration of treatment but entails regular monitoring by trained nursing staff. For mild to moderate symptoms, standard anxiolytic or muscle-relaxing oral doses of benzodiazepines may be sufficient. For severe symptoms, or for the treatment of delirium tremens, higher doses and use of the intravenous route may be required. *Clomethiazole* appears to be an effective alternative to the benzodiazepines (but see p.683); although widely used in Europe, it is not available in the USA. Some centres use phenobarbital but *barbiturates* are generally not recommended for the treatment of alcohol withdrawal syndrome.

*Antipsychotics* are not usually recommended for use in the control of symptoms of alcohol withdrawal since they do not reduce delirium tremens and some may reduce the seizure threshold. However, they might be considered for use as adjuncts in patients requiring treatment of marked agitation or hallucinations.

The generalised tonic-clonic seizures associated with alcohol withdrawal are usually self-limiting and patients who experience only one or two seizures do not usually require any specific treatment beyond continuing therapy with benzodiazepines or clomethiazole. For recurrent seizures or status epilepticus (p.352) diazepam may be given intravenously. Other types of seizure may be associated with head trauma or pre-existing seizure disorders (p.349) and should be treated accordingly. Other *antiepileptics* such as carbamazepine have been tried in the treatment of alcohol withdrawal seizures and may be of use as adjuncts in controlling other symptoms of alcohol withdrawal syndrome. As benzodiazepines are effective in preventing withdrawal seizures, other prophylactic drugs are not usually indicated.

*Beta blockers* can reduce symptoms of autonomic overactivity such as tachycardia, hypertension, tremor, and agitation but because they can mask these symptoms of withdrawal and do not prevent the development of more serious complications they should not be used alone. Some beta blockers such as propranolol that penetrate the CNS may produce CNS effects that complicate therapy. The alpha$_2$-adrenoceptor agonist *clonidine* may be of similar benefit as an adjunct.

*Other drugs* that have been reported to be of benefit in alcohol withdrawal syndrome include nitrous oxide and gamma-hydroxybutyric acid.

It is essential that in all cases of alcohol withdrawal syndrome hypoglycaemia, dehydration, electrolyte disturbances (in particular magnesium), and vitamin deficiencies be corrected. It is usually recommended that all patients should be given thiamine because of their increased risk of developing Wernicke's encephalopathy (p.1455). It should be noted that intravenous administration of glucose solutions before thiamine may precipitate Wernicke's encephalopathy in thiamine-deficient patients. However, hydration should be undertaken with care as alcoholics may be more prone to develop cerebral oedema, the management of which is discussed under Raised Intracranial Pressure on p.833.

**Abstinence.** Once the initial acute withdrawal of alcohol is achieved treatment may be required to maintain long-term abstinence. Pharmacotherapy should only be used as an adjunct to psychotherapy and supportive care. Drugs used to modify alcohol seeking behaviour either sensitise the patient to alcohol (aversive drugs) or reduce or alleviate the craving for alcohol. The main ones used for aversive therapy are *disulfiram* and *calcium carbimide.* A patient who ingests alcohol after taking an adequate dose of one of these drugs will experience a severe and unpleasant reaction (p.1681). However, the deterrent value of aversive drugs, and their potential toxicity, has long been a matter of debate. Such treatment is likely to be of little use unless it is undertaken with the willing cooperation of the patient and is used with psychotherapy, and even then there is no evidence that it has any effect on the long-term course of alcoholism.

Of those drugs that have been reported to reduce alcohol craving *acamprosate* and *naltrexone* have been the most promising as adjuncts for management of alcohol dependence and have been shown to improve abstinence and reduce relapse rates. Whether benefit is maintained long-term after treatment is stopped is unclear. *Other drugs* tried with varying benefit include tiapride, gamma-hydroxybutyric acid, and bromocriptine.


1. McMicken DB, Freedland ES. Alcohol-related seizures: pathophysiology, differential diagnosis, evaluation, and treatment. *Emerg Med Clin North Am* 1994; **12:** 1057–79.
2. Lohr RH. Treatment of alcohol withdrawal in hospitalized patients. *Mayo Clin Proc* 1995; **70:** 777–82.
3. Erstad BL, Cotugno CL. Management of alcohol withdrawal. *Am J Health-Syst Pharm* 1995; **52:** 697–709.

4. Hall W, Zador D. The alcohol withdrawal syndrome. *Lancet* 1997; **349:** 1897–1900.
5. Mayo-Smith MF. American Society of Addiction Medicine Working Group on Pharmacological Management of Alcohol Withdrawal. Pharmacological management of alcohol withdrawal: a meta-analysis and evidence-based practice guideline. *JAMA* 1997; **278:** 144–51.
6. Saitz R, O'Malley SS. Pharmacotherapies for alcohol abuse: withdrawal and treatment. *Med Clin North Am* 1997; **81:** 881–907.
7. O'Connor PG, Schottenfeld RS. Patients with alcohol problems. *N Engl J Med* 1998; **338:** 592–602.
8. Tinsley JA, *et al.* Developments in the treatment of alcoholism. *Mayo Clin Proc* 1998; **73:** 857–63.
9. Schaffer A, Naraiyo CA. Recommended drug treatment strategies for the alcoholic patient. *Drugs* 1998; **56:** 571–85.
10. Naik PC, Brownell LW. Treatment of psychiatric aspects of alcohol misuse. *Hosp Med* 1999; **60:** 173–7.
11. Garbutt JC, *et al.* Pharmacological treatment of alcohol dependence: a review of the evidence. *JAMA* 1999; **281:** 1318–25.
12. Swift RM. Drug therapy for alcohol dependence. *N Engl J Med* 1999; **340:** 1482–90.
13. Kraemer KL, *et al.* Managing alcohol withdrawal in the elderly. *Drugs Aging* 1999; **14:** 409–25.
14. Myrick H, *et al.* New developments in the pharmacotherapy of alcohol dependence. *Am J Addict* 2001; **10** (suppl): 3–15.
15. Kosten TR, O'Connor PG. Management of drug and alcohol withdrawal. *N Engl J Med* 2003; **348:** 1786–95.

## Precautions

Women and the elderly may be more susceptible to the adverse effects of alcohol ingestion. Alcohol may aggravate peptic ulcer disease or hepatic impairment. Ingestion of alcohol during pregnancy or breast feeding is not advisable. Excessive alcohol intake should be avoided, especially in patients with diabetes mellitus or epilepsy. In chronic alcoholics there may be tolerance to the effects of other CNS depressants including general anaesthetics.

All processes requiring judgement and coordination are affected by alcohol and these include the driving of any form of transport and the operating of machinery. It is an offence in many countries for motorists to drive when the blood-alcohol concentration is above a stated value. The alcohol concentration in urine and expired air can be used to estimate the blood-alcohol concentration.

It should be remembered that alcohol may be present in a number of pharmaceutical preparations such as elixirs and mouthwashes, and that children may be particularly susceptible to its hypoglycaemic effects.

**Breast feeding.** The American Academy of Pediatrics[1] states that, although usually compatible with breast feeding, ingestion of large amounts of alcohol by breast-feeding mother may cause drowsiness, diaphoresis, deep sleep, weakness, decrease in linear growth, and abnormal weight gain in the infant; maternal ingestion of 1 g/kg or more daily decreases the milk ejection reflex.

1. American Academy of Pediatrics. The transfer of drugs and other chemicals into human milk. *Pediatrics* 2001; **108:** 776–89. Correction. *ibid.*; 1029. Also available at: http://aappolicy.aappublications.org/cgi/content/full/pediatrics%3b108/3/776 (accessed 09/06/04)

**Porphyria.** Alcohol has been associated with acute attacks of porphyria and is considered unsafe in porphyric patients.

## Interactions

Reports of interactions between alcohol and other drugs are not consistent, possibly because acute alcohol intake may inhibit drug metabolism while chronic alcohol intake may enhance the induction of drug-metabolising enzymes in the liver. Alcoholic beverages containing tyramine may cause reactions when taken by patients receiving MAOIs. Alcohol may enhance the acute effects of CNS depressants, such as hypnotics, antihistamines, opioid analgesics, antiepileptics, antidepressants, antipsychotics, and sedatives. Unpleasant reactions, similar to those occurring with disulfiram (p.1681), may occur when alcohol is taken with chlorpropamide, mepacrine, metronidazole and other nitroimidazoles, the nitrofuran derivatives furazolidone and nifuratel, procarbazine, or some cephalosporins.

Alcohol may cause hypoglycaemic reactions in patients receiving sulfonylurea antidiabetics or insulin, and may cause orthostatic hypotension in patients taking drugs with a vasodilator action. It may enhance the hypotensive effects of antihypertensives and has also increased the sedative effect of indoramin. Alcohol may increase gastric bleeding caused by analgesics and may have a variable effect on oral anticoagulants. It may decrease the antidiuretic effect of vasopressin.

◊ Reviews.

1. McInnes GT. Interactions that matter: alcohol. *Prescribers' J* 1985; **25:** 87–90.
2. Lieber CS. Interaction of alcohol with other drugs and nutrients: implications for the therapy of alcoholic liver disease. *Drugs* 1990; **40** (suppl 3): 23–44.
3. Fraser AG. Pharmacokinetic interactions between alcohol and other drugs. *Clin Pharmacokinet* 1997; **33:** 79–90.

**Cycloserine.** Increased blood-alcohol concentrations have been reported in patients receiving cycloserine.[1]

1. Glass F, *et al.* Beobachtungen und untersuchungen über die gemeinsame wirkung von alkohol und D-cycloserin. *Arzneimittelforschung* 1965; **15:** 684–8.

**$H_2$-antagonists.** The existence of an interaction between $H_2$-antagonists and alcohol is controversial and has not been established. While some studies suggest that *cimetidine*[1-3] and *nizatidine*[3] can increase peak blood-alcohol concentrations the effects of *ranitidine*[2,4] have been variable; *famotidine* appears to have no significant effect.[2] Later studies report that any interaction between $H_2$-antagonists and alcohol is minor and unlikely to be of clinical importance.[5-8]

1. Caballeria J, *et al.* Effects of cimetidine on gastric alcohol dehydrogenase activity and blood ethanol levels. *Gastroenterology* 1989; **96:** 388–92.
2. DiPadova C, *et al.* Effects of ranitidine on blood alcohol levels after ethanol ingestion: comparison with other $H_2$-receptor antagonists. *JAMA* 1992; **267:** 83–6.
3. Holt S, *et al.* Evidence for an interaction between alcohol and certain $H_2$ receptor antagonists. *Gut* 1991; **32:** A1220.
4. Toon S, *et al.* Lack of effect of high dose ranitidine on the postprandial pharmacokinetics of alcohol. *Gut* 1992; **33** (suppl): S10.
5. Raufman J-P, *et al.* Histamine-2 receptor antagonists do not alter serum ethanol levels in fed, nonalcoholic men. *Ann Intern Med* 1993; **118:** 488–94.
6. Levitt MD. Do histamine-2 receptor antagonists influence the metabolism of ethanol? *Ann Intern Med* 1993; **118:** 564–5.
7. Kleine M-W, Ertl D. Comparative trial in volunteers to investigate possible ethanol-ranitidine interaction. *Ann Pharmacother* 1993; **27:** 841–5.
8. Gugler R. $H_2$-antagonists and alcohol: do they interact? *Drug Safety* 1994; **10:** 271–80.

**Paracetamol.** The effects of paracetamol poisoning may be exacerbated by chronic alcohol consumption (see p.76).

**Verapamil.** When verapamil has been taken with alcohol there has been a reported increase in peak blood-alcohol concentrations of approximately 17%.[1] Such an interaction may extend the toxic effects of alcohol and raise its blood concentration above the legal limit for driving.[2]

1. Schumock G, *et al.* Verapamil inhibits ethanol elimination. *Pharmacotherapy* 1989; **9:** 184–5.
2. Anonymous. Does verapamil increase the effects of alcohol? *Pharm J* 1990; **244:** 14.

## Pharmacokinetics

Alcohol is rapidly absorbed from the gastrointestinal tract and is distributed throughout the body fluids. It readily crosses the placenta. Alcohol vapour can be absorbed through the lungs. Absorption through intact skin is said to be negligible.

The rate of absorption of alcohol from the gastrointestinal tract may be modified by such factors as the presence of food, the concentration of alcohol, and the period of time during which it is ingested. Some alcohol is reported to be metabolised by the gastric mucosa.

Alcohol is mainly metabolised in the liver; it is converted by alcohol dehydrogenase to acetaldehyde and is then further oxidised to acetate. A hepatic microsomal oxidising system is also involved. About 90 to 98% of alcohol is oxidised and the remainder is excreted unchanged by the kidneys and the lungs. It also appears in breast milk, sweat, and other secretions.

The rate of metabolism may be accelerated following repeated excessive intake and by certain substances including insulin.

◊ Reviews.

1. Holford NHG. Clinical pharmacokinetics of ethanol. *Clin Pharmacokinet* 1987; **13:** 273–92.

## Uses and Administration

Alcohol has bactericidal activity and is used to disinfect skin before injection, venepuncture, or surgical procedures. It is also used to disinfect hands and clean surfaces. A concentration of 70%, often as methylated spirits (p.1185), is commonly used for disinfection. Alcohol should not be used for disinfection of surgical or dental instruments because of its low efficacy against bacterial spores.

Alcohol also has anhidrotic, rubefacient, and astringent and haemostatic properties. It is sometimes used for its skin-cooling properties and to harden the skin. It is an ingredient of several topical preparations used for skin disorders.

Alcohol is widely used as a solvent and preservative in pharmaceutical preparations.

Alcohol may be used as a neurolytic in the management of severe and chronic pain.

Alcohol is given intravenously in the treatment of acute poisoning from ethylene glycol (p.1685) and methyl alcohol (p.1475).

Alcohol is also used in sclerotherapy.

**Pain.** The use of alcohol as a neurolytic to produce destructive nerve block (p.1369) has produced variable results, and some consider the risk of complications outweighs the benefits. However, alcohol has been injected into the pituitary gland for relief of severe pain of the head and neck;[1,2] doses of 1 mL of absolute alcohol have been used.[1] It may be useful in coeliac plexus block, and has been injected into the muscle sheath to relieve painful muscle spasms in patients with multiple sclerosis.[1] Alcohol 50 to 100% may be used for peripheral or central nerve block in terminally ill patients with pain that does not respond to drug therapy;[3] the block produced by alcohol may occasionally last up to 2 years, even longer than that produced by phenol.

Intrathecal injection of alcohol has also been used for the intractable pain of spasticity (p.1386).

1. Lloyd JW. Use of anaesthesia: the anaesthetist and the pain clinic. *BMJ* 1980; **281:** 432–4.
2. Lipton S. Pain relief in active patients with cancer: the early use of nerve blocks improves the quality of life. *BMJ* 1989; **298:** 37–8.
3. Hardy, PAJ. The role of the pain clinic in the management of the terminally ill. *Br J Hosp Med* 1990; **43:** 142–6.

**Sclerotherapy.** Alcohol has been used successfully as a sclerosant in a variety of conditions including aldosterone-producing adenoma,[1] parathyroid adenomas,[2] thyroid nodules,[3,4] advanced rectal cancer,[5] hepatocellular carcinoma,[6,7] dysphagia associated with oesophogastric cancer,[8,9] hepatic cyst,[10] and gallbladder obstruction.[11] It has also been used in the sclerotherapy of oesophageal varices[12,13] although the safety of this procedure has been questioned following a report of complications developing in 13 of 17 patients, 2 of whom died.[14] Other conditions in which alcohol has been used include bleeding from ruptured hepatomas[15] and in peptic ulcer disease,[16] and obstructive cardiomyopathies[17] resistant to usual treatment.

Other sclerosants used in oesophageal varices are discussed on p.1716.

1. Mathias CJ, *et al.* Therapeutic venous infarction of an aldosterone producing adenoma (Conn's tumour). *BMJ* 1984; **288:** 1416–17.
2. Verges B, *et al.* Percutaneous ethanol injection of parathyroid adenomas in primary hyperparathyroidism. *Lancet* 1991; **337:** 1421–2.
3. Monzani F, *et al.* Autonomous thyroid nodule and percutaneous ethanol injection. *Lancet* 1991; **337:** 743.
4. Bennedbaek FN, Hegedüs L. Alcohol sclerotherapy for benign solitary solid cold thyroid nodules. *Lancet* 1995; **346:** 1227.
5. Payne-James J, *et al.* Advanced rectal cancer. *BMJ* 1990; **300:** 746.
6. Sheu J-C, *et al.* Intratumor injection of absolute ethanol under ultrasound guidance for the treatment of small hepatocellular carcinoma. *Hepatogastroenterology* 1987; **34:** 255–61.
7. Salmi A. Percutaneous alcohol injection of hepatocellular carcinoma. *Ann Intern Med* 1989; **110:** 494.
8. Payne-James JJ, *et al.* Use of ethanol-induced tumor necrosis to palliate dysphagia in patients with esophagogastric cancer. *Gastrointest Endosc* 1990; **36:** 43–6.
9. Stanners AJ, *et al.* Alcohol injection for palliation of malignant oesophageal disease. *Lancet* 1993; **341:** 767.
10. Bean WJ, Rodan BA. Hepatic cysts: treatment with alcohol. *Am J Roentg* 1985; **144:** 237–41.
11. Asfar S, *et al.* Percutaneous sclerosis of gallbladder. *Lancet* 1989; **ii:** 387.
12. Sarin SK, *et al.* Endoscopic sclerotherapy using absolute alcohol. *Gut* 1985; **26:** 120–4.
13. Hassall E, *et al.* Sclerotherapy for extrahepatic portal hypertension in childhood. *J Pediatr* 1989; **115:** 69–74.
14. Bhargava DK, *et al.* Endoscopic sclerotherapy using absolute alcohol. *Gut* 1986; **27:** 1518.
15. Chung SCS, *et al.* Injection of alcohol to control bleeding from ruptured hepatomas. *BMJ* 1990; **301:** 421.
16. Lin HJ, *et al.* Heat probe thermocoagulation and pure alcohol injection in massive peptic ulcer haemorrhage: a prospective, randomised controlled trial. *Gut* 1990; **31:** 753–7.
17. Sigwart U. Non-surgical myocardial reduction for hypertrophic obstructive cardiomyopathy. *Lancet* 1995; **346:** 211–14.

## Preparations

***USP 27:*** Alcohol in Dextrose Injection; Dehydrated Alcohol Injection; Rubbing Alcohol.

**Proprietary Preparations** (details are given in Part 3)

***Austral.:*** Microshield Antimicrobial Hand Gel; ***Canad.:*** Skin So Soft Antibacterial; ***Fr.:*** Curethyl†; Pharmadose alcool; ***Ger.:*** AHD 2000; Amphisept E; Fugaten; Manusept HD; Sterillium Virugard; ***Spain:*** Alcohten†; ***Switz.:*** Amphisept; ***USA:*** Alcare; Kleen-Handz.

**Multi-ingredient:** ***Austral.:*** Dermatech Liquid; Johnsons Clean & Clear Invisible Blemish Treatment†; Johnsons Clean & Clear Oil Controlling Toner†; Microshield Handrub; Microshield Tincture; ***Austria:*** Apotheker Bauer's Franzbranntwein-Gel; Cleanomed; Dodesept; Dodesept Gefarbt; Dodesept N; Skinsept; Skinsept mucosa; ***Belg.:*** Solution Antiseptique; ***Braz.:*** Pelmic†; ***Canad.:*** Biobase; Biobase-G; Chase Kolik Gripe Water; Clearasil Medicated Cleanser†; Clearasil Sensitive Skin Cleanser†; Clearskin 2 Overnight Acne Treatment†; Cold Sore Lotion†; Dilusol; Dilusol AHA; Duonalc-E; Franzbranns; Green Antiseptic Mouthwash & Gargle; Mouthwash Antiseptic & Gargle; MRX; Sans-Acne; Sea Breeze†; ***Chile:*** Abboderm; Acnoxyl Locion Tonica; Alcolex; Listerine; Listermint Con Fluor; Xerac AC; ***Fin.:*** Otiborin; Somanol + Ethanol; ***Fr.:*** Chlorispray; Frekaderm†; Novospray†; Parogencyl gencives fragilisees; Pulvispray†; **Ger.:** Aerodesin; Antifect†; Bacillol; Bacillol AF; Betaseptic; Desderman N; Franzbranntwein mit Fichtennadelol; Freka-Derm; Freka-Nol; Freka-Sept 80; Hospidermin; Hospisept; Incidin Spezial; Incidur Spray; Klosterfrau Franzbranntwein; Klosterfrau Franzbranntwein Latschenkiefer; Kneipp Fichtennadel Franzbranntwein†; Kneipp Latschenkiefer Franzbranntwein†; Mikrozid†; Mucasept-A; Promanum N; Pursept A†; Riwa Franzbranntwein; Skinman Intensiv†; Skinsept G; Skinsept mucosa; Softa Man; Softasept N; Spitacid; **India:** Daslin; Dettolin; **Israel:** Oxy Clean Medicated; Salisol; Septadine; Spirit Salicyl; **Ital.:** Bemonalcool; Cedril Strumenti†; Citromed 80 and 85; Citromed Chirurgico; Citrosil Alcolico Azzuro; Citrosil Alcolico Bruno; Citrosil Alcolico Incolore; Citrosteril Strumenti; Clorexan Ferri; Eso Ferri Alcolico; Esoalcolico Incolore; Esoform Alcolico; Esoform Ferri Alcolico†; Forbrand; Formedico; Incidin Spezial; Incidur Spray; Jodieci; Melsept Spray; Neomedil; Panseptil; Resina Carbolica Dentilin†; Sekumatic; Simpottantacinque; Softa Man; Soluzione Composta Alcoolica Saponosa di Coaltar†; **Mon.:** Akila spray†; **Spain:** Alcohcan†; Alcohocel; Alcohol Benzalconio; Alcohol Cetil; Alcohol Cetilpi Cuve; Alcohol CL Benz; Alcohol Poten; Alcohol Potenciado; Alcohol Reforzado†; Alcohol Sanit Cuve†; Alcopac Reforzado†; Analgesico Ut Asens Fn†; Beta Alcanforado; Beta Romero; Embrocacion Gras; Farmalcohol; Licor Amoniacal†; Linimento Naion; Menalcol; Mercrotona; Morde X; Salvesept†; **Switz.:** Adro-derm†; Betaseptic; Desitur; Frekaderm; Promanum N; Sclerovein; Softasept N; **UK:** Brushtox†; Clearasil Pore Cleansing Lotion; Medi-Tissue†; Medi-Wipe; Oxy Cleanser; Oxy Duo Pads; Primahex†; Spectrum; **USA:** Banadyne-3; Clearasil Double Clear; Clearasil Double Textured Pads; EarSol†; Lipmagik; Massengill; Massengill Disposable; Maximum Strength Anbesol; Orasol; Stri-Dex Pads; Xerac AC.

## Alkyl Gallates

Galatos de alquilo.

### Dodecyl Gallate

Dodecylis Gallas; E312; Galato de dodecilo; Lauryl Gallate; Laurylum Gallicum. Dodecyl 3,4,5-trihydroxybenzoate.

$C_{19}H_{30}O_5$ = 338.4.

*CAS — 1166-52-5.*

**Pharmacopoeias.** In *Eur.* (see p.vi).

**Ph. Eur. 5.0** (Dodecyl Gallate). A white or almost white crystalline powder. M.p. about 96°. Very slightly soluble or practically insoluble in water; freely soluble in alcohol; slightly soluble in dichloromethane. Store in nonmetallic containers. Protect from light.

### Ethyl Gallate

Galato de etilo. Ethyl 3,4,5-trihydroxybenzoate.

$C_9H_{10}O_5$ = 198.2.

*CAS — 831-61-8.*

**Pharmacopoeias.** In *Br.*

**BP 2003** (Ethyl Gallate). A white to creamy-white, odourless or almost odourless, crystalline powder. Slightly soluble in water; freely soluble in alcohol and in ether; practically insoluble in arachis oil. Protect from light. Avoid contact with metals.

### Octil Gallate

E311; Galato de octilo; Octyl Gallate; Octylis Gallas. Octyl 3,4,5-trihydroxybenzoate.

$C_{15}H_{22}O_5$ = 282.3.

*CAS — 1034-01-1.*

**Pharmacopoeias.** In *Eur.* (see p.vi).

**Ph. Eur. 5.0** (Octyl Gallate). A white or almost white crystalline powder. Practically insoluble in water and in dichloromethane; freely soluble in alcohol. Store in nonmetallic containers. Protect from light.

### Propyl Gallate

E310; Galato de propilo; Propylis Gallas; Propylum Gallicum. Propyl 3,4,5-trihydroxybenzoate.

$C_{10}H_{12}O_5$ = 212.2.

*CAS — 121-79-9.*

**Pharmacopoeias.** In *Eur.* (see p.vi) and *Pol.* Also in *USNF.*

**Ph. Eur. 5.0** (Propyl Gallate). A white or almost white, crystalline powder. Very slightly soluble in water; freely soluble in alcohol; dissolves in dilute solutions of alkali hydroxides. Protect from light.

**USNF 22** (Propyl Gallate). A white crystalline powder with a slight characteristic odour. Slightly soluble in water; freely soluble in alcohol. Store in airtight containers. Avoid contact with metals. Protect from light.

#### Adverse Effects and Precautions

The alkyl gallates may cause contact sensitivity and skin reactions.

**Effects on the blood.** Methaemoglobinaemia associated with the antioxidants (butylated hydroxyanisole, butylated hydroxytoluene, and propyl gallate) used to preserve the oil in a soybean infant feed formula has been reported.[1] Propyl gallate was suspected of being the most likely cause because its chemical structure is similar to pyrogallol, a methaemoglobinaemia inducer.


1. Nitzan M, *et al.* Infantile methemoglobinemia caused by food additives. *Clin Toxicol* 1979; **15:** 273–80.


#### Uses

The alkyl esters of gallic acid (3,4,5-trihydroxybenzoic acid) have antoxidant properties and are used as preservatives in pharmaceuticals and cosmetics. Alkyl gallates are also used as antoxidants in foods and are useful in preventing deterioration and rancidity of fats and oils. They are used in concentrations of 0.001 to 0.1%.

To improve acceptability and efficacy, the alkyl gallates are frequently used with other antoxidants such as butylated hydroxyanisole or butylated hydroxytoluene and with sequestrants and synergists such as citric acid.

The alkyl gallates have also been reported to have limited antimicrobial activity.

## Aminoquinuride Hydrochloride *(rINNM)*

Hidrocloruro de aminoquinurida. 1,3-Bis(4-amino-2-methyl-6-quinolyl)urea dihydrochloride.

$C_{21}H_{20}N_6O,2HCl$ = 445.3.

*CAS — 3811-56-1 (aminoquinuride); 5424-37-3 (aminoquinuride hydrochloride).*

#### Profile

Aminoquinuride hydrochloride is an antiseptic that has been used in topical preparations for the treatment of mouth and skin disorders.

#### Preparations

**Proprietary Preparations** (details are given in Part 3)

**Multi-ingredient:** ***Austria:*** Herviros; ***Ger.:*** Herviros; ***Hong Kong:*** Herviros†.

## Amylmetacresol *(BAN, rINN)*

Amilmetacresol. 6-Pentyl-*m*-cresol; 5-Methyl-2-pentylphenol.

$C_{12}H_{18}O$ = 178.3.

*CAS — 1300-94-3.*

**Pharmacopoeias.** In *Br.*

**BP 2003** (Amylmetacresol). A clear or almost clear liquid or a solid crystalline mass with a characteristic odour, colourless or slightly yellow when freshly prepared; it darkens on keeping. F.p. about 22°. Practically insoluble in water; soluble in alcohol, in ether, and in fixed and volatile oils. Protect from light.

#### Profile

Amylmetacresol is a phenolic antiseptic used chiefly as an ingredient of lozenges in the treatment of minor infections of the mouth and throat.

#### Preparations

**Proprietary Preparations** (details are given in Part 3)

***Canad.:*** Strepsils 1†; ***Ital.:*** Benagol Collutorio†; ***UK:*** Antiseptic Throat Lozenges; Throaties Anti-Bacterial Pastilles.

**Multi-ingredient:** ***Austral.:*** Sore Throat Chewing Gum†; Strepsils; Strepsils Plus; ***Austria:*** Coldangin; Neo-Angin; ***Belg.:*** Strepsils; Strepsils + Lidocaine; Strepsils Menthol; Strepsils Vit C; ***Canad.:*** Strepsils; ***Denm.:*** Strepsils; ***Fin.:*** Strepsils; Strepsils Menthol; ***Fr.:*** Strepsils; Strepsils Lidocaine; Strepsils Miel-Citron; Strepsils Vitamine C; Strepsilspray Lidocaine; ***Ger.:*** Neo-Angin N; ***Hong Kong:*** Strepsils; Strepsils Dual Action; ***Irl.:*** Strepsils; Strepsils Dual Action; Strepsils Vitamin C; ***Israel:*** Strepsils; Strepsils Plus; Strepsils with Vitamin C; ***Ital.:*** Benagol; Benagol Mentolo-Eucaliptolo; Benagol Vitamina C; ***Malaysia:*** Strepsils; Strepsils Dual Action; ***Neth.:*** Strepsils; Strepsils Menthol en Eucalyptus; Strepsils Sinaasappel en Vitamine C; ***NZ:*** Strepsils; Strepsils Plus Anaesthetic; Strepsils with Vitamin C; ***S.Afr.:*** Strepsils; Strepsils Eucalyptus Menthol; Strepsils Orange-C; Strepsils Plus; Strepsils Soothing Honey & Lemon†; ***Singapore:*** Floxil†; Strepsils; Strepsils Dual Action; ***Spain:*** Strepsils; Strepsils con Anestesico; Strepsils con Vitamina C; ***Swed.:*** Strepsils†; ***Switz.:*** Neo-Angin au miel et citron; Neo-Angin avec vitamin C exempt de sucre; Neo-Angin exempt de sucre; ***Thai.:*** Strepsils Plus Anaesthetic; Strepsils Plus Vit C; Strepsils Sugar Free; ***UK:*** Antiseptic Lozenges†; Mac†; Strepsils; Strepsils Pain Relief Plus†; Strepsils with Vitamin C.

## Ascorbyl Palmitate

Ascorbilo, palmitato de; Ascorbylis Palmitas; Vitamin C Palmitate. L-Ascorbic acid 6-hexadecanoate; L-Ascorbic acid 6-palmitate; 3-Oxo-L-gulofuranolactone 6-palmitate.

$C_{22}H_{38}O_7$ = 414.5.

*CAS — 137-66-6.*

NOTE. The code E304 is used for fatty acid esters of ascorbic acid, which include ascorbyl palmitate.

**Pharmacopoeias.** In *Eur.* (see p.vi). Also in *USNF.*

**Ph. Eur. 5.0** (Ascorbyl Palmitate). A white or yellowish-white powder. Practically insoluble in water; freely soluble in alcohol and in methyl alcohol; practically insoluble in dichloromethane and in fatty oils. Store at 8° to 15° in airtight containers. Protect from light.

**USNF 22** (Ascorbyl Palmitate). A white to yellowish-white powder with a characteristic odour. Very slightly soluble in water, in chloroform, in ether, and in vegetable oils; soluble 1 in 125 of alcohol. Store at 8° to 15° in airtight containers.

#### Profile

Ascorbyl palmitate is an antioxidant used as a preservative in pharmaceutical products and foods. It is often used with alpha tocopherol (p.1464), and this combination shows marked synergy.

#### Preparations

**Proprietary Preparations** (details are given in Part 3)

**Multi-ingredient:** ***Hong Kong:*** Proflavanol; ***Port.:*** Thiospot.

## Benzalkonium Chloride *(BAN, rINN)*

Benzalconio Cloruro; Benzalkonii Chloridum; Benzalkonium Chloratum; Cloreto de Benzalconio; Cloruro de benzalconio.

*CAS — 8001-54-5.*

*ATC — D08AJ01; D09AA11; R02AA16.*

**Pharmacopoeias.** In *Chin., Eur.* (see p.vi), *Int., Jpn,* and *Pol.* Also in *USNF.* Some pharmacopoeias also have a monograph for a solution.

*Chin.* also includes benzalkonium bromide.

**Ph. Eur. 5.0** (Benzalkonium Chloride). A mixture of alkylbenzyldimethylammonium chlorides, the alkyl groups having chain lengths of $C_8$ to $C_{18}$. It contains not less than 95% and not more than 104% of alkylbenzyldimethylammonium chlorides, calculated as $C_{22}H_{40}ClN$ with reference to the anhydrous substance. A white or yellowish-white powder, or gelatinous yellowish-white pieces, hygroscopic and soapy to the touch. It forms a clear molten mass on heating. It contains not more than 10% of water. Very soluble in water and in alcohol. An aqueous solution froths copiously when shaken.

**USNF 22** (Benzalkonium Chloride). A mixture of alkylbenzyldimethylammonium chlorides of the general formula $[C_6H_5.CH_2.N(CH_3)_2.R]Cl$, in which R represents a mixture of the alkyls having chain lengths from $C_8$ to $C_{16}$. It contains not less than 40% of the $C_{12}H_{25}$ compound, calculated on the anhydrous substance, not less than 20% of the $C_{14}H_{29}$ compound, and not less than 70% of the 2 compounds together.

A white or yellowish-white, thick gel, or gelatinous pieces with a mild aromatic odour. It contains not more than 15% of water. Very soluble in water and in alcohol; the anhydrous form is soluble 1 in 100 of ether and 1 in 6 of benzene. A solution in water is usually slightly alkaline and foams strongly when shaken. Store in airtight containers.

**Incompatibility.** Benzalkonium chloride is incompatible with soaps and other anionic surfactants, citrates, iodides, nitrates, permanganates, salicylates, silver salts, and tartrates. Incompatibilities have been demonstrated with ingredients of some commercial rubber mixes or plastics. Incompatibilities have also been reported with other substances including aluminium, cotton dressings, fluorescein sodium, hydrogen peroxide, kaolin, hydrous wool fat, and some sulfonamides.

### Adverse Effects, Treatment, and Precautions

As for Cetrimide, p.1172.

**Catheters and cannulas.** For reference to benzalkonium chloride used in the manufacturing process of heparin-bonded catheters interfering with determination of serum concentrations of sodium and potassium, see under Precautions for Heparin, p.929.

**Effects on the eyes.** Benzalkonium chloride is one of the most disruptive ophthalmic additives to the stability of the lipid film and to corneal epithelial membranes; it has been shown to be toxic to the eyes of *rabbits* but less so to the eyes of humans.[1] Toxicity experiments have tended to be carried out using relatively high concentrations of benzalkonium chloride[2] but deleterious effects on the tear film and corneoconjunctival surface have been noted in patients receiving regular long-term treatment for glaucoma with eye drops preserved with benzalkonium chloride in usual concentrations.[3,4] However, the use of preservatives in eye drops should generally be avoided and the formulation of such preparations in single-dose containers is desirable.[1,2] Benzalkonium chloride is not suitable for use in solutions for storing and washing hydrophilic soft contact lenses, as it can bind to the lenses and may later produce ocular toxicity when the lenses are worn.[5]

Corneal toxicity has also been reported in patients inadvertently exposed to benzalkonium chloride as a preservative in viscoelastic material during cataract surgery.[6]


1. Burstein NL. The effects of topical drugs and preservatives on the tears and corneal epithelium in dry eye. *Trans Ophthalmol Soc U K* 1985; **104:** 402–9.
2. Burstein NL. Corneal cytotoxicity of topically applied drugs, vehicles and preservatives. *Surv Ophthalmol* 1980; **25:** 15–30.
3. Herreras JM, *et al.* Ocular surface alteration after long-term treatment with an antiglaucomatous drug. *Ophthalmology* 1992; **99:** 1082–8.
4. Kuppens EVMJ, *et al.* Effect of timolol with and without preservative on the basal tear turnover in glaucoma. *Br J Ophthalmol* 1995; **79:** 339–42.
5. Gasset AR. Benzalkonium chloride toxicity to the human cornea. *Am J Ophthalmol* 1977; **84:** 169–71.
6. Eleftheriadis H, *et al.* Corneal toxicity secondary to inadvertent use of benzalkonium chloride preserved viscoelastic material in cataract surgery. *Br J Ophthalmol* 2002; **86:** 299–305.


**Effects on the respiratory tract.** Hypersensitivity to benzalkonium chloride, used as a preservative in nasal drops, was confirmed in a patient by a challenge that produced nasal congestion and irritation of the eyes and throat lasting 48 hours.[1] Benzalkonium chloride used as a preservative in nebulised solutions of anti-asthma drugs has been reported to cause dose-related bronchoconstriction especially in asthmatic patients,[2] and has been associated with the precipitation of respiratory arrest.[3]


1. Hillerdal G. Adverse reaction to locally applied preservatives in nose drops. *ORL J Otorhinolaryngol Relat Spec* 1985; **47:** 278–9.

2. Committee on Drugs, American Academy of Pediatrics. "Inactive" ingredients in pharmaceutical products: update. *Pediatrics* 1997; **99:** 268–78.
3. Boucher M, *et al.* Possible association of benzalkonium chloride in nebulizer solutions with respiratory arrest. *Ann Pharmacother* 1992; **26:** 772–4.

## Interactions

Benzalkonium chloride is not suitable for eye drops containing local anaesthetics as it accelerates their dehydrating effect.

## Uses and Administration

Benzalkonium chloride is a quaternary ammonium antiseptic and disinfectant with actions and uses similar to those of the other cationic surfactants (see Cetrimide, p.1172). It is also used as an antimicrobial preservative for pharmaceutical products. Benzalkonium bromide and benzalkonium saccharinate have also been used.

Solutions of benzalkonium chloride 0.01 to 0.1% are used for cleansing skin, mucous membranes, and wounds. More dilute solutions of 0.005% are suitable for irrigation of deep wounds. A 0.02 to 0.05% solution has been used as a vaginal douche. An aqueous solution containing 0.005 to 0.02% has been used for irrigation of the bladder and urethra and a 0.0025 to 0.005% solution for retention lavage of the bladder.

Creams containing benzalkonium chloride are used in the treatment of napkin rash and other dermatoses.

A 0.2 to 0.5% solution has been used as a shampoo in seborrhoeic dermatitis.

Lozenges containing benzalkonium chloride are used for the treatment of superficial infections of the mouth and throat.

A 0.005 to 0.02% solution of benzalkonium chloride is used as a preservative for some eye drops. Because some rubbers are incompatible with benzalkonium chloride silicone rubber teats should be used on eye drop containers unless the suitability has been established. Benzalkonium chloride is used for disinfecting rigid contact lenses (p.1164) but is unsuitable as a preservative in solutions for washing and storing hydrophilic soft contact lenses (see also Effects on the Eyes, above).

Benzalkonium chloride is also used as a spermicide.

Solutions of 0.13% are used for disinfection and storage of surgical instruments, sometimes with the addition of sodium nitrite to inhibit rust.

**Action.** The antibacterial effect of benzalkonium chloride 0.003% was enhanced by 0.175% of benzyl alcohol, phenylpropanol, or phenethyl alcohol.[1] For the use of phenethyl alcohol with benzalkonium chloride as a preservative for ophthalmic solutions, see Phenethyl Alcohol, p.1188.

1. Richards RME, McBride RJ. Enhancement of benzalkonium chloride and chlorhexidine acetate activity against Pseudomonas aeruginosa by aromatic alcohols. *J Pharm Sci* 1973; **62:** 2035–7.

**Catheter-related sepsis.** Benzalkonium chloride has been investigated[1,2] for incorporation into catheters to reduce catheter-related sepsis (p.1165).

1. Tebbs SE, Elliott TSJ. A novel, antimicrobial central venous catheter impregnated with benzalkonium chloride. *J Antimicrob Chemother* 1993; **31:** 261–71.
2. Moss HA, *et al.* A central venous catheter coated with benzalkonium chloride for the prevention of catheter-related microbial colonization. *Eur J Anaesthesiol* 2000; **17:** 680–7.

## Preparations

***USNF 22:*** Benzalkonium Chloride Solution.

**Proprietary Preparations** (details are given in Part 3)

***Arg.:*** Benzalcream; Hidratant; Pharmatex; Usnicon; ***Austral.:*** Bepanthen; Dettol Antiseptic Spray; ***Belg.:*** Cedium; Pansteryl†; ***Braz.:*** Bacterian; Fluimucil Solucao Nasal†; Merthiolate†; ***Canad.:*** Antiseptic Skin Cream; Arkonsol†; Zephiran†; ***Chile:*** Germosept; ***Fr.:*** Comprimes Gynecologiques Pharmatex†; Flexogyne†; Humex; Pharmatex; Sparaplaie; ***Ger.:*** Baktonium; Laudamonium; Lysoform Killavon; Quartamon Med†; Rheila Stringiet N†; ***Irl.:*** Dettol Fresh; Roccal†; ***Israel:*** Pharmatex; ***Ital.:*** Alfa C; Amuclean; Benalcon; Bergagyn; Bluesteril; Ceroxmed Steril†; Citrosil; Citrosteril Ambiente; Citrosteril Deterferri; Colli†; Collirium Geymonat†; Contusil†; Detergil; Dimanin R; DiMill; Diseptil; Disintyl; Display; Distasil; Disteril; Eso Deterferri; Eso Ferri; Esoform Deterferri†; Esosan; Esosan Casa; Germicidin; Geyderm†; Helis; Hygienist Pavimenti e Piastrelle; Iridina Light; Lacribase; Lozione Vittoria; Neo-Desogen; Norica; Polisan; Sanaform; Sangen; SaniSteril Deterferri; Saquat; Sguardi; Sincosan†; Sirigen; Steramin; Steramina G; Stilla Delicato; Streptosil L PMC; Ten-Quat; Video-Light; Zefirol†; ***Mex.:*** Lubrizal; Merthiolate; ***NZ:*** Dettol; Dettol Fresh; Virasolve; ***Port.:*** Pharmatex; ***Spain:*** Armil; Benzalc†; Crema Contracepti Lanzas; Mini Ovulo Lanzas; Novamina†; ***Thai.:*** Pose-Bac; Zephirol†; ***UK:*** Bradosol; Dettol Antiseptic Wash; Dettol Fresh; ***USA:*** Bacti-Cleanse; Benza; Mycocide NS; Ony-Clear; Zephiran.

**Multi-ingredient: *Arg.:*** Antisepthic Hexil; Crema de Ordene; Eurocoal; Muelita; Neo Coltirot; Oilalfo; Polviderm NF; Soquette; ***Austral.:*** Animine†; Clean Skin Face Wash†; Gum-Ese†; Mycil Healthy Feet; Oilatum Plus; Paxyl; Solyptol; TAGG†; Virasolve; ***Austria:*** Aleot; Cutasept; Dequonal; Dermaspray; Dorithricin; Dr Schmidgall Halsweh; Halset plus Dexpanthenol; Limexx; Nasimild†; Tonsicur†; Tyrothricin comp; ***Belg.:*** Akinspray; Dermaspray; ***Braz.:*** Belagin; Belglos†; Cetrilan†; Colpanist†; Colpatrin; Colpist; Colpistar; Colpistatin; Dermol; Dinill; Donnagel; Drapolene; Ginestatin; Ginometrim†; Nestosyl†; Pomada Minancora; Rhinodex†; Rinosoro; Rinotil†; Sorine Adulto; Sorine Infantil; Soro Nasal; Soronal†; Vagi Biotic†; Visolon†; ***Canad.:*** Aseptone Quat†; Bactine; Family Medic First Aid Treatment; Medi-Dan; Medi-Quik†; Orajel Mouth Aid; Protectaid; Sporex†; Tanac; ***Chile:*** Dermobarrina; Medisept; Orajel Compuesto; ***Fr.:*** Acarcid; Biseptine; Dermaspraid Antiseptique; Dermobacter; Euvanol†; Frekaderm†; Humex; Kenalcol; Mercryl; Pharmatex; Rhinofluimucil; ***Ger.:*** Baccalin; Bacillocid rasant; Bacillocid Spezial†; Baktobod N†; Baktobod†; Cutasept; Dequonal; Dorithricin Original; Dynexan Mundgel; Freka-Derm; Freka-Sept 80; Gingicain D; Hexaquart L; Hexaquart S; Incidin Extra; Incidin extra N; Incidin perfekt; Incidur Spray; Indulfan plus†; Inova; Kohrsolin FF; Korsolex Extra; Korsolex FF; Lysetol Med; Mikrobac; Neo-Angin†; Quatohex; Sekusept Extra N; Sekusept forte; Septolit; Skinman Soft; Terralin†; Ultrasol-F; Ultrasol-S†; ***Gr.:*** Beta Ophtiole; Olamyc; ***Hong Kong:*** Dermojela; Drapolene; Mycil; Oilatum Plus; Protectaid; Virasolve; ***India:*** Rashfree; ***Irl.:*** Conotrane; Drapolene; Emulsiderm; Mycil; Oilatum Junior Flare-Up†; Oilatum Plus; Torbetol; ***Israel:*** Emulsiderm; Garonsept; ***Ital.:*** Agipiu; Alfa-Fluorone†; AZ 15; Barrycidal; Bemonalcool; Benzogen Ferri†; Betaform Habitat†; Cedril Strumenti†; Cedril†; Cepacol†; Cerox; Citromed 80 and 85; Citromed Chirurgico; Citromedics Pronto; Citrosil Alcolico Azzuro; Citrosil Alcolico Bruno; Citrosil Alcolico Incolore; Citrosil Nubesan; Citrosteril Impronte; Citrosteril Pronto; Citrosteril Strumenti; Collyria; Conta-Lens Wetting†; Dentaton Antisettico†; Eso Ferri Alcolico; Eso Ferri Alcolico Plus; Eso S 80; Esoalcolico Incolore; Esoform 92; Esoform Alcolico; Esoform Ferri Alcolico†; Esoform Ferri†; Esosan Pronto; Germozero Dermo; Germozero Plus; Hamamilla; Herbe; Incidin Spezial; Incidur Spray; Indulfan; Ipragocce; Linea F; Lycia Luminique; Mediplus; Neo Emocicatrol; Neomedil; Norica; Odongi; Oradyne-Z†; Pupilla Light; Rexichlor; Sangen Casa; SaniSteril Strumenti Alcolico; Sekusept Extra N; Silvana†; Simp; Simpottantacinque; Sterosan; Tirs; Zincometil; ***Malaysia:*** Drapolene; Oilatum Plus Antibacterial; ***Mex.:*** Glossderm; Sutin; ***Mon.:*** Akila spray†; ***NZ:*** Oilatum Plus; ***S.Afr.:*** Oilatum Plus; ***Singapore:*** Dettol†; Dorithricin; Drapolene; Oilatum Plus; QV Flare Up; ***Spain:*** Aftajuventus; Alcohcan†; Alcohol Benzalconio; Alcohol CL Benz; Alcohol Potenciado; Alcohol Reforzado†; Alcopac Reforzado†; Avril; Curine; Dermo Halibut Infantil; Desinvag; Egarone; Ginejuvent; Gradin Del D Andreu; Hemostatico Antisep Asen†; Lindemil; Mercryl Plus; Odamida; Otogen Calmante; Pental Forte; Phonal; Pomada Heridas; Resorborina; Sebumselen; Talkosona†; Topicaina†; Tulgrasum Cicatrizante; Vaselatum; ***Switz.:*** Cutasept; Dequonal; Frekaderm; Jonil T†; ***Thai.:*** Drapolene; Gynecon; Gynoco; Gynova; Gyracon; Napilene; Nystin; Oilatum Plus; Sanaco; ***UK:*** Beechams Max Strength Sore Throat Relief; Beechams Throat-Plus; Bumps 'n Falls†; Cetanorm; Conotrane; Dermol; Dettol; Drapolene; Emulsiderm; Germolene; Germoloids; Medi-Tissue†; Mycil; Neo Baby Cream; Oilatum Junior Flare-Up; Oilatum Plus; Protectaid; Sunspot†; ***USA:*** Bactine Antiseptic; Bactine Pain Relieving Cleansing; Cetylcide II; Medi-Quik; Orajel Mouth Aid; Oxyzal; Tanac; Tanac Dual Core; Vagi-Gard Medicated Cream; Zonite.

---

# Benzethonium Chloride *(BAN, rINN)*

Benzethonii Chloridum; Cloruro de bencetonio; Diisobutylphenoxyethoxyethyldimethylbenzylammonium chloride. Benzyldimethyl(2-{2-[4-(1,1,3,3-tetramethylbutyl)phenoxy]ethoxy}ethyl)ammonium chloride.

$C_{27}H_{42}ClNO_2$ = 448.1.
*CAS — 121-54-0.*
*ATC — R02AA09.*

**Pharmacopoeias.** In *Eur.* (see p.vi), *Jpn,* and *US.*

**Ph. Eur. 5.0** (Benzethonium Chloride). A white or yellowish-white powder. Very soluble in water and in alcohol; freely soluble in dichloromethane. An aqueous solution froths copiously when shaken. Protect from light.

**USP 27** (Benzethonium Chloride). White crystals with a mild odour. Soluble 1 in less than 1 of water, of alcohol, and of chloroform, and 1 in 6000 of ether. A 1% solution in water is slightly alkaline to litmus. Store in airtight containers. Protect from light.

**Incompatibility.** Benzethonium chloride is incompatible with soaps and other anionic surfactants.

## Profile

Benzethonium chloride is a quaternary ammonium antiseptic with actions and uses similar to those of other cationic surfactants (see Cetrimide, p.1172). It has also been used as a vaginal spermicide.

◊ Benzethonium chloride, which produced mild skin irritation at a concentration of 5% but not lower, was not considered to be a sensitiser, and was considered to be safe at a concentration of 0.5% in cosmetics applied to the skin and at a maximum concentration of 0.02% in cosmetics used in the eye area.[1]

1. The Expert Panel of the American College of Toxicology. Final report on the safety assessment of benzethonium chloride and methylbenzethonium chloride. *J Am Coll Toxicol* 1985; **4:** 65–106.

## Preparations

***USP 27:*** Benzethonium Chloride Concentrate; Benzethonium Chloride Tincture; Benzethonium Chloride Topical Solution.

**Proprietary Preparations** (details are given in Part 3)

***Canad.:*** Clearskin Antibacterial; Skin Cleanser & Deodorizer; ***S.Afr.:*** Johnson's Antiseptic Powder†.

**Multi-ingredient: *Arg.:*** Butimerin; Solumerin; ***Austral.:*** Summers Eve Feminine†; ***Belg.:*** Neo-Golaseptine; ***Braz.:*** Acitra†; Andolba; Hipodex; Otosulf†; Solemil†; Spray Anti-Septico; ***Canad.:*** Antiseptic Skin Cream; Buro Derm†; Dermoplast†; Lipsorex; MRX; Protecto; Skin Shield†; VoSoL; VoSoL HC; ***Chile:*** Aucusik; Dermaglos; Dermaglos Plus; Molca; ***Ger.:*** Brand- u. Wundgel-Medice N; ***Hong Kong:*** Cemaquin; ***Ital.:*** Barrycidal; Borossigeno Plus Stomatologico†; Cedril Strumenti†; Cedril†; Neo Topico Giusto†; Sangen Casa; ***NZ:*** VoSoL; ***Spain:*** Alcohol Poten; Eupnol; Halibut; Halibut Hidrocortisona; Isdinex; Tegunal†; ***Switz.:*** Angidine; Cemaquin; Rhinocure Simplex†; Rhinocure†; Tyrocombine; Tyrothricine + Gramicidine; ***Thai.:*** Iwazin; Sigatricin; ***USA:*** AA-HC Otic†; Acetasol; Acetasol HC; Aerocaine; Aerotherm†; Americaine First Aid; Skin Shield; Vagisil; VoSoL; VoSoL HC.

---

# Benzoates

Benzoatos.

## Benzoic Acid

Acidum Benzoicum; Benzoesäure; Benzoico, ácido; Dracylic Acid; E210.

$C_6H_5.CO_2H$ = 122.1.
*CAS — 65-85-0.*

**Pharmacopoeias.** In *Chin., Eur.* (see p.vi), *Int., Jpn, Pol., US,* and *Viet.*

**Ph. Eur. 5.0** (Benzoic Acid). A white, crystalline powder or colourless crystals, odourless or with a very slight characteristic odour. Slightly soluble in water; soluble in boiling water; freely soluble in alcohol and in fatty oils. M.p. 121° to 124°.

**USP 27** (Benzoic Acid). White crystals, scales, or needles, with a slight characteristic odour. Soluble 1 in 300 of water, 1 in 3 of alcohol, 1 in 5 of chloroform, and 1 in 3 of ether; freely volatile in steam. Congealing range 121° to 123°.

**Incompatibility.** The incompatibilities of benzoic acid are described under Sodium Benzoate, below.

## Sodium Benzoate

Benzoato sódico; E211; Natrii Benzoas; Natrium Benzoicum; Sodii Benzoas.

$C_6H_5.CO_2Na$ = 144.1.
*CAS — 532-32-1.*

**Pharmacopoeias.** In *Chin., Eur.* (see p.vi), *Jpn, Pol.,* and *Viet.* Also in *USNF.*

**Ph. Eur. 5.0** (Sodium Benzoate). A white, slightly hygroscopic, crystalline or granular powder or flakes. Freely soluble in water; sparingly soluble in alcohol (90% v/v).

**USNF 22** (Sodium Benzoate). A white, odourless or practically odourless, granular or crystalline powder. Soluble 1 in 2 of water, 1 in 75 of alcohol, and 1 in 50 of alcohol 90%.

**Incompatibility.** Benzoic acid and its salts are incompatible with quaternary compounds, calcium salts, ferric salts, and salts of heavy metals. Their activity is also diminished by nonionic surfactants or due to absorption by kaolin. They are relatively inactive above a pH of about 5.

## Adverse Effects and Precautions

The benzoates can cause hypersensitivity reactions, but there have also been reports of non-immunological contact urticaria. The acid can be irritant to skin, eyes, and mucous membranes.

Infants given large doses of sodium benzoate have suffered vomiting. Symptoms of overdosage reported in this group have been restricted to vomiting and irritability.

Premature infants have been reported to be at risk of metabolic acidosis and kernicterus.

**Hypersensitivity.** Respiratory reactions to benzoates may occur, especially in patients susceptible to aspirin-induced asthma.[1,2] Urticarial reactions have also been associated with these compounds,[3,4] though at a lower incidence[5] and they can be non-immunological.[6] However, these reports have to be balanced against a controlled study[7] that showed no difference in the incidence of urticaria or atopic symptoms between patients given benzoic acid and those given lactose placebo.

Anaphylactoid reactions have been reported in 2 patients.[8,9]

Erythema multiforme has been observed in several patients.[10]

1. Rosenhall L. Evaluation of intolerance to analgesics, preservatives and food colorants with challenge tests. *Eur J Respir Dis* 1982; **63:** 410–19.
2. Settipane GA. Aspirin and allergic diseases: a review. *Am J Med* 1983; **74** (suppl): 102–9.
3. Michaëlsson G, Juhlin L. Urticaria induced by preservatives and dye additives in food and drugs. *Br J Dermatol* 1973; **88:** 525–32.
4. Warin RP, Smith RJ. Challenge test battery in chronic urticaria. *Br J Dermatol* 1976; **94:** 401–6.
5. Wüthrich B, Fabro L. Acetysalicylsäure-und lebensmitteladditiva-intoleranz bei urtikaria, asthma bronchiale und chronischer rhinopathie. *Schweiz Med Wochenschr* 1981; **III:** 1445–50.
6. Nethercott JR, *et al.* Airborne contact urticaria due to sodium benzoate in a pharmaceutical manufacturing plant. *J Occup Med* 1984; **26:** 734–6.
7. Lahti A, Hannuksela M. Is Benzoic acid really harmful in cases of atopy and urticaria? *Lancet* 1981; **ii:** 1055.
8. Moneret-Vautrin DA, *et al.* Anaphylactoid reaction to general anaesthesia: a case of intolerance to sodium benzoate. *Anaesth Intensive Care* 1982; **10:** 156–7.
9. Michils A, *et al.* Anaphylaxis with sodium benzoate. *Lancet* 1991; **337:** 1424–5.
10. Lewis MAO, *et al.* Recurrent erythema multiforme: a possible role of foodstuffs. *Br Dent J* 1989; **166:** 371–3.

**Neonates.** Serious metabolic disturbances in premature neonates given intravenous fluids with benzyl alcohol as a preservative have been attributed to the accumulation of benzoic acid, a metabolite of benzyl alcohol (see p.1170). This risk led to the recommendation that Caffeine and Sodium Benzoate Injection (USP), which has been given as a respiratory stimulant, should not be used in neonates.[1]

Benzoates can also displace bound bilirubin from albumin putting neonates at risk of kernicterus.[2] However, sodium benzoate has been tried in the treatment of some neonatal metabolic disorders (see Uses and Administration, below).


1. Edwards RC, Voegeli CJ. Inadvisability of using caffeine and sodium benzoate in neonates. *Am J Hosp Pharm* 1984; **41:** 658.
2. Schiff D, *et al.* Fixed drug combinations and the displacement of bilirubin from albumin. *Pediatrics* 1971: **48:** 139–41.


## Pharmacokinetics

The benzoates are absorbed from the gastrointestinal tract and conjugated with glycine in the liver to form hippuric acid, which is rapidly excreted in the urine.

**Neonates.** References.


1. Green TP, *et al.* Disposition of sodium benzoate in newborn infants with hyperammonemia. *J Pediatr* 1983; **102:** 785–90.


## Uses and Administration

Benzoates have antibacterial and antifungal properties. Their antimicrobial activity is due to the undissociated benzoic acid and is therefore pH-dependent. They are relatively inactive above a pH of about 5.

Benzoates are used as preservatives in pharmaceutical formulations including oral preparations; benzoic acid and sodium benzoate are typically used in concentrations of up to 0.2% and 0.5%, respectively. They are used as preservatives in foods, (and are also present naturally in some foods), and at similar concentrations in cosmetics.

Benzoic acid 6% with salicylic acid 3%, as Compound Benzoic Acid Ointment (BP 2003) (Whitfield's Ointment) has a long history of use as an antifungal (see Skin Infections, p.390). Benzoic acid has also been used in desloughing preparations and has been given as a urinary antiseptic.

An injection of caffeine and sodium benzoate has been used as a CNS stimulant, but see above for a caution against its use in neonates.

Sodium benzoate is used as part of the treatment of hyperammonaemia that occurs in inborn errors of the urea cycle. It has also been reported to be effective in reducing plasma-glycine concentrations in nonketotic hyperglycinaemia (p.1750), although it may not be effective in preventing mental retardation.

Sodium benzoate is a common ingredient of cough preparations.

**Hyperammonaemia.** The dose of sodium benzoate used for treatment of hyperammonaemia (p.1421) has generally been 250 mg/kg daily by intravenous infusion.[1-3] A similar dose may be given in divided doses by mouth for maintenance.


1. Maestri NE, *et al.* Long-term survival of patients with argininosuccinate synthetase deficiency. *J Pediatr* 1995; **127:** 929–35.
2. Maestri NE, *et al.* Long-term treatment of girls with ornithine transcarbamylase deficiency. *N Engl J Med* 1996; **335:** 855–9.
3. Zammarchi E, *et al.* Neonatal onset of hyperornithinemia-hyperammonemia-homocitrullinuria syndrome with favorable outcome. *J Pediatr* 1997; **131:** 440–3.


## Preparations

***BP 2003:*** Benzoic Acid Solution; Compound Benzoic Acid Ointment; Tolu-flavour Solution;
***USP 27:*** Benzoic and Salicylic Acids Ointment; Caffeine and Sodium Benzoate Injection.

**Proprietary Preparations** (details are given in Part 3)
***Mex.:*** Colufase.

**Multi-ingredient:** ***Arg.:*** Fungicida; Ixana; No-Tos Adultos; No-Tos Infantil; Pectobron; Pectoral Pagliano; Refenax Jarabe; Solvex Liquido Fungicida; ***Austral.:*** Egomycol†; Whitfields (Benzoic Acid Compound) Ointment†; ***Austria:*** Acerbine; Aplexil†; Expigen; Mycopol; ***Belg.:*** Bronchobel†; Colimax; Kamfeine; Normogastryl†; Pholco-Mereprine; Rectoplexil†; Toplexil; Tux; ***Braz.:*** Benzomel; Bronquidex; Bronquiogem; Cessatosse†; Codelasa†; Colagolen†; Dermicon; Dermofytol†; Dermycose; Eaca Balsamico; Efedronal†; Egotussano; Expec; Expectobron; Frenotosse; Fungodermol†; Gotas Nican; Iodermol†; Iodesin; Iodeto de Potassio; Iodobec†; Iodopulmin†; Iol; Ipecol; KI-Expectorante; Limao Bravo†; Locao Mancha Branca†; Mel de Jatahy†; Mentoval†; Micocid†; Micotiazol; Micotissim†; Micotox†; Micoz; Mictarin†; Natoss†; Pectoss†; Peitoral Angico Pelotense; Penetro; Pinosil†; Plactosse†; Po Antisseptico; Pulmoforte†; Pulmoverina; Rhum Creosotado; Solucao ABC†; Sudonol†; Tiratosse†; Tolusil†; Toplexil; Tossanil†; Tosseina†; Traqueobron†; Tussodina; Tussol†; Tussucalman†; Tuzo†; Xarope das Criancas†; Xarope de Caraguata; Xarope de Limao Bravo†; Xarope Peitoral de Ameixa Composto; Xarope Sao Joao; Xarope Valda†; Xpe SPC; ***Canad.:*** Mouthrinse†; MRX; Plax; Sea Breeze†; ***Chile:*** Broncodeina; Caristop; Dibunafon; Gotas Nican; Gruben; Listerine; Pectoral Pasteur; Pectoserum; Pulmagol; Summer's Eve Hierbas; Summer's Eve Vinagre y Agua; ***Denm.:*** Pectyl; Throat†; ***Fr.:*** Asthmalgine†; Broncalene; Broncalene Nourisson; Bronpax†; Codotussyl Maux de Gorge; Dermacide; Dimetane Expectorant Enfant; Dinacode; Dinacode avec codeine; Ephydion; Fluocaril blancheur; Germose; Gynescal†; Marrubene Codethyline†; Neo-Codion; Ozothine; Paregorique; Passedyl; Pneumaseptic†; Pulmocod†; Pulmofluide Simple; Pulmonase†; Pulmosodyl†; Quintopan; Rhinamide; Silomat; Sirop Pectoral adulte†; Sirop Pectoral enfant†; Tossarel†; ***Ger.:*** Sagrosept; ***Hong Kong:*** Fungifax; ***India:*** Keralin; Mycoderm; Pragmatar; ***Israel:*** Oxacatin; Phytoderm Compositum; Pitrisan; Spirit Whitfield; Toplexil; Tussophedrine; Whitfield Plus†; ***Ital.:*** Borocaina; Dentinale; Neo Borocillina; Paracodina; Sedobex†; Sedocalcio; Tiocosol; Tionamil; ***Malaysia:*** Nixoderm; ***Mex.:*** Pulmovital; ***Mon.:*** Glyco-Thymoline; ***Neth.:*** Toplexil; ***NZ:*** Egomycol; Listerine; Listerine Tartar Control; ***Port.:*** Broncodiazina; Bronquiasmol; Calmarum; Codeisan†; Codoforme†; Drenoflux†; Fluidin Adulto†; Fluidin Antiasmatico†; Fluidin Infantil†; Lactucol†; Micaveen†; ***S.Afr.:*** Aserbine; ***Singapore:*** Whitfield; ***Spain:*** Acerbiol; Bronco Sergo†; Broncoformo Muco Dexa; Broncomicin Bals†; Broncovital; Bronquidiazina CR; Bronquimar; Etermol Antitusivo; Maboterpen†; Mentobox†; Neumopectolina; Pastillas Pectoral Kely; Pazbronquial; Pectoral Brum†; Pulmo Menal; Pulmofasa; Pulmofasa Antihist†; Tos Mai; ***Switz.:*** Acerbine; Bronchalin†; Demo pates pectorales†; Dinacode N; Foral; Nasobol; Neo-DP; Nican; Phol-Tussil; Phol-Tux; Saintbois; Sirop pectoral DP1†; Sirop pectoral DP2, DP3†; Spedro†; Toplexil; ***UK:*** Aserbine; Eczema Ointment; Hemocane; Melissin†; Potters Gees Linctus; Sanderson's Throat Specific; Toepedo; ***USA:*** Atrosept; Bensal HP; Cystex; Dolsed; Feminique; MHP-A; Prosed/DS; Summers Eve Disposable; Trac Tabs 2X; UAA; Ucephan; Uridon Modified; Urised; Uriseptic; Uritact.

## Benzododecinium Bromide

Benzododecinio, bromuro de; Lauralkonium Bromide; Lauryldimethylbenzylammonium Bromide. Benzyldodecyldimethylammonium bromide.

$C_{21}H_{38}BrN$ = 384.4.
*CAS — 10328-35-5 (benzododecinium); 7281-04-1 (benzododecinium bromide).*
*ATC — D09AA05.*

**Pharmacopoeias.** In *Fr.*

## Benzododecinium Chloride *(rINN)*

Lauralkonium Chloride. Benzyldodecyldimethylammonium chloride.

$C_{21}H_{38}ClN$ = 340.0.
*CAS — 139-07-1.*
*ATC — D09AA05.*

### Profile

Benzododecinium bromide is a quaternary ammonium antiseptic with properties similar to those of other cationic surfactants (see Cetrimide, p.1172). It is used in mouthwashes and nasal sprays and solutions for the treatment of minor infections. It has also been used as a spermicide. Benzododecinium chloride has also been used.

### Preparations

**Proprietary Preparations** (details are given in Part 3)
***Fr.:*** Rhinedrine.

**Multi-ingredient:** ***Fr.:*** Fluorhinose†; Genola†; Prorhinel; Sedacollyre; ***Ital.:*** Larilon†; ***Switz.:*** Kemerhinose; Prorhinel.

## Benzoxiquine *(USAN, rINN)*

NSC-3951. 8-Quinolinol benzoate (ester).

$C_{16}H_{11}NO_2$ = 249.3.
*CAS — 86-75-9.*

### Profile

Benzoxiquine is an antiseptic that has been included in multi-ingredient preparations used topically for the treatment of fungal infections. The salicylate has also been used.

### Preparations

**Proprietary Preparations** (details are given in Part 3)
**Multi-ingredient:** ***Ital.:*** Antimicotico†.

## Benzoxonium Chloride *(rINN)*

Cloruro de benzoxonio. Benzyldodecylbis(2-hydroxyethyl)ammonium chloride.

$C_{23}H_{42}ClNO_2$ = 400.0.
*CAS — 19379-90-9.*
*ATC — A01AB14; D08AJ05.*

### Profile

Benzoxonium chloride is a quaternary ammonium antiseptic used for disinfection of the skin and mucous membranes. It is also used for instrument disinfection.

### Preparations

**Proprietary Preparations** (details are given in Part 3)
***Belg.:*** Orofar; ***Chile:*** Bialcol; ***Gr.:*** Orocil; ***Ital.:*** Bactofen; Bialcol; Sinecod Bocca†.

**Multi-ingredient:** ***Belg.:*** Orofar Lidocaine; ***Chile:*** Alcolex; ***Ger.:*** Lemocin Flexibels†; Loscon; ***Israel:*** Merphen; Vita-Merfen NF; ***Port.:*** Orofar; ***Spain:*** Cohortan Antibiotico†; Cohortan†; ***Switz.:*** Mebucalets f; Merfen; Orofar; Vita-Merfen; ***Thai.:*** Orofar†.

# Benzyl Alcohol *(rINN)*

Alcohol bencílico; Alcohol Benzylicus; Alcool Benzylique; Benzenemethanol; Phenylcarbinol; Phenylmethanol.

$C_6H_5.CH_2OH$ = 108.1.
*CAS — 100-51-6.*

**Pharmacopoeias.** In *Chin., Eur.* (see p.vi), *Int., Jpn,* and *Pol.* Also in *USNF.*

**Ph. Eur. 5.0** (Benzyl Alcohol). A clear colourless, oily liquid. Soluble in water; miscible with alcohol, with fatty and essential oils. Store under nitrogen in airtight containers at a temperature of 2° to 8°. Protect from light.

**USNF 22** (Benzyl Alcohol). A clear, colourless, oily liquid. Sparingly soluble in water; freely soluble in alcohol (50%); miscible with alcohol, with chloroform, and with ether. It is neutral to litmus. Store in airtight containers. Protect from light.

**Incompatibility.** Benzyl alcohol is incompatible with oxidising agents and strong acids. The antimicrobial activity may be reduced by nonionic surfactants and benzyl alcohol may be lost from solutions stored in polyethylene containers.

**Stability.** Benzyl alcohol oxidises to produce benzaldehyde and benzoic acid and oxidation may take place slowly on exposure to air. Benzaldehyde may also be produced on autoclaving.

## Adverse Effects and Precautions

There have been a few reports of hypersensitivity reactions to benzyl alcohol when used as a preservative.

The pure alcohol is irritant and requires handling with care; ingestion or inhalation can cause nausea, vomiting, diarrhoea, headache, vertigo, and CNS depression. However, concentrations of benzyl alcohol normally used for preservation are not associated with such effects.

There have been some instances of neurotoxic effects in patients given intrathecal injections that contained benzyl alcohol.

A fatal toxic syndrome in premature infants was attributed to benzyl alcohol present as a preservative in solutions used to flush intravenous catheters. This has led to restriction on the use of benzyl alcohol in neonates and young children, see below.

**Effects on the lungs.** Severe bronchitis and haemoptysis was reported in a patient with obstructive pulmonary disease who, over a period of 2 years, had inhaled salbutamol nebuliser solution diluted with a bacteriostatic sodium chloride solution containing benzyl alcohol.[1]


1. Reynolds RD. Nebulizer bronchitis induced by bacteriostatic saline. *JAMA* 1990; **264:** 35.


**Effects on the nervous system.** Rapid development of flaccid areflexic paraplegia, total anaesthesia below the groin, and radicular abdominal pain occurred in a 64-year-old man after a lumbar intrathecal injection of cytarabine that contained 1.5% benzyl alcohol.[1] The patient recovered fully after 100 mL of CSF was replaced with sodium chloride 0.9% and 40 mg of methylprednisolone. Intrathecal injections of cytarabine dissolved in sterile distilled water before and after the episode of paraplegia caused no neurologic symptoms. On reviewing 20 other cases of paraparesis associated with methotrexate or cytarabine intrathecal injections, benzyl alcohol had been used as a preservative in 7. Of the 7, 4 developed neurotoxicity immediately; in the other 3 it did not develop until 6 to 48 hours after administration. The duration varied. One patient did not improve, one made a partial recovery, a third took 6 weeks to recover, another took 5 days; yet 2 patients recovered within 1½ to 2½ hours while the final patient experienced only transient effects.


1. Hahn AF, *et al.* Paraparesis following intrathecal chemotherapy. *Neurology* 1983; **33:** 1032–8.


**Hypersensitivity.** Some reports of hypersensitivity reactions to benzyl alcohol.


1. Grant JA, *et al.* Unsuspected benzyl alcohol hypersensitivity. *N Engl J Med* 1982; **306:** 108.
2. Shmunes E. Allergic dermatitis to benzyl alcohol in an injectable solution. *Arch Dermatol* 1984; **120:** 1200–1.
3. Wilson JP, *et al.* Parenteral benzyl alcohol-induced hypersensitivity reaction. *Drug Intell Clin Pharm* 1986; **20:** 689–91.


**Neonates.** During 1981 and 1982 reports were published from 2 centres in the USA[1-3] of 20 deaths in low-birth-weight neonates attributed to the use of benzyl alcohol as a preservative in solutions used to flush their umbilical catheters and in some cases also to dilute their medication. The neonates suffered a toxic syndrome whose features included metabolic acidosis, symptoms of progressive encephalopathy, intracranial haemorrhage, and respiratory depression with gasping.

These deaths prompted the FDA[4] to recommend that benzyl alcohol should not be used in such flushing solutions; sodium chloride injection 0.9% without preservative should be used instead. The FDA had also advised against the use of benzyl alcohol or any preservative in fluids being used for the dilution or reconstitution of medicines for the newborn.

Those reporting the deaths[2,3] considered that the toxic syndrome could have been caused by the accumulation of the benzoic acid metabolite of benzyl alcohol, which could not be handled effectively by the immature liver; given the very low weight of the neonates they would have been receiving a high dose of benzyl alcohol. In commenting on the problem, the American Academy of Pediatrics[5] agreed that the FDA's warning was warranted, but pointed out that there was no evidence from controlled studies to confirm that benzyl alcohol was responsible.


1. Gershanik JJ, *et al.* The gasping syndrome: benzyl alcohol (BA) poisoning? *Clin Res* 1981; **29:** 895A.
2. Brown WJ, *et al.* Fatal benzyl alcohol poisoning in a neonatal intensive care unit. *Lancet* 1982; **i:** 1250.

3. Gershanik J, *et al.* The gasping syndrome and benzyl alcohol poisoning. *N Engl J Med* 1982; **307:** 1384–8.
4. Anonymous. Benzyl alcohol may be toxic to newborns. *FDA Drug Bull* 1982; **12:** 10–11.
5. American Academy of Pediatrics. Benzyl alcohol: toxic agent in neonatal use. *Pediatrics* 1983; **72:** 356–7.

## Pharmacokinetics

Benzyl alcohol is metabolised to benzoic acid. This is conjugated with glycine in the liver to form hippuric acid which is excreted in the urine. Benzaldehyde and benzoic acid are degradation products *in vitro*.

## Uses

Benzyl alcohol is used as an antimicrobial preservative. It is bacteriostatic mainly against Gram-positive organisms and some fungi. It is used in a range of pharmaceutical preparations in concentrations up to 2%. Concentrations of 5% or more are employed when it is used as a solubiliser. Benzyl alcohol is used as a preservative in foods and cosmetics. It is also used as a disinfectant at a concentration of 10%.

In addition to its antiseptic properties, diluted benzyl alcohol possesses weak local anaesthetic and antipruritic activity.

## Preparations

**Proprietary Preparations** (details are given in Part 3)
***Canad.:*** Babys Own Teething Gel; Zilactin; ***USA:*** Zilactin.

**Multi-ingredient:** ***Austral.:*** Coso†; Soothe'n Heal†; ***Austria:*** Dermaspray; ***Belg.:*** Dermaspray; ***Canad.:*** Foille†; ***Chile:*** Aucusik; Medikem; Medisept; ***Denm.:*** Doloproct Comp; ***Fr.:*** Biseptine; Codotussyl Maux de Gorge; Dermaspraid Antiseptique; Pastilles Medicinales Vicks; ***Ger.:*** Spitacid; ***Irl.:*** Sudocrem†; ***Israel:*** Otomycin; ***Ital.:*** Borocaina; Foille Scottature; Foille Sole; ***Port.:*** Friax†; ***Singapore:*** Saak; ***Spain:*** Acerbiol; Pastillas Antisep Garg M; ***UK:*** Sudocrem; ***USA:*** Anusol; Cepacol Throat; Itch-X; MouthKote O/R; Oragesic; Rhuli Gel†; Super Ivy Dry; Topic.

*Used as an adjunct in:* ***Jpn:*** Panpurol.

---

## Biclotymol *(rINN)*

Biclotimol. 2,2′-Methylenebis(6-chlorothymole).
$C_{21}H_{26}Cl_2O_2$ = 381.3.
*CAS — 15686-33-6.*

### Profile

Biclotymol is a phenolic antiseptic that is used in lozenges and sprays for mouth and throat infections. It is also an ingredient of cough preparations.

### Preparations

**Proprietary Preparations** (details are given in Part 3)
***Fr.:*** Hexaspray; Humex; Rhinathiol; Sagadreps; ***Hong Kong:*** Hexaspray.

**Multi-ingredient:** ***Fr.:*** Hexalyse; Hexapneumine; ***Hong Kong:*** Hexalyse; Hexapneumine.

---

## Brilliant Green

CI Basic Green 1; Colour Index No. 42040; Diamond Green G; Emerald Green; Ethyl Green; Malachite Green G; Solid Green; Verde brillante; Viride Nitens. 4-(4-Diethylaminobenzhydrylidene)cyclohexa-2,5-dien-1-ylidenediethylammonium hydrogen sulphate.
$C_{27}H_{34}N_2O_4S$ = 482.6.
*CAS — 633-03-4.*

NOTE. The name Emerald Green has also been used for copper acetoarsenite.

### Profile

Brilliant green is a triphenylmethane antiseptic dye with actions similar to those of methylrosanilinium chloride (p.1186). Its activity is greatly reduced in the presence of serum.

A gel containing brilliant green 0.5% with lactic acid was formerly used in the treatment of skin ulcers.

An alcoholic solution of brilliant green 0.5% and methylrosanilinium chloride 0.5% (Bonney's Blue) was formerly used for disinfecting the skin, but concern over evidence of *animal* carcinogenicity with methylrosanilinium chloride has led to the decline of such paints. A solution of the two disinfectants has been used for marking incisions before surgery.

There have been occasional reports of sensitivity to brilliant green.

**Adverse effects.** For a report of necrotic skin reactions following application of a 1% solution of brilliant green to stripped skin, see under the Adverse Effects of Methylrosanilinium Chloride, p.1186.

---

## Bromchlorophen

Bromchlorophene; Bromochlorophane; Bromoclorofeno. 2,2′-Methylenebis[6-bromo-4-chlorophenol].
$C_{13}H_8Br_2Cl_2O_2$ = 426.9.
*CAS — 15435-29-7.*

### Profile

Bromchlorophen is a halogenated bisphenol antiseptic more active against Gram-positive than Gram-negative bacteria. It is used for disinfection of the hands and skin.

### Preparations

**Proprietary Preparations** (details are given in Part 3)
**Multi-ingredient:** ***Ger.:*** Dibromol.

---

## Bromsalans

Bromosalicilanilidas.
*CAS — 55830-61-0.*

**Description.** Bromsalans are a series of brominated salicylanilides that possess antimicrobial activity.

## Dibromsalan *(USAN, pINN)*

Dibromsalán; NSC-20527. 4′,5-Dibromosalicylanilide; 5-Bromo-*N*-(4-bromophenyl)-2-hydroxybenzamide.
$C_{13}H_9Br_2NO_2$ = 371.0.
*CAS — 87-12-7.*

## Metabromsalan *(USAN, pINN)*

Metabromsalán; NSC-526280. 3,5-Dibromosalicylanilide; 3,5-Dibromo-2-hydroxy-*N*-phenylbenzamide.
$C_{13}H_9Br_2NO_2$ = 371.0.
*CAS — 2577-72-2.*

## Tribromsalan *(BAN, USAN, rINN)*

ET-394; NSC-20526; TBS; Tribromsalán. 3,4′,5-Tribromosalicylanilide; 3,5-Dibromo-*N*-(4-bromophenyl)-2-hydroxybenzamide.
$C_{13}H_8Br_3NO_2$ = 449.9.
*CAS — 87-10-5.*

### Profile

Bromsalans have antibacterial and antifungal activity and have been used in medicated soaps, but there have been many reports of photosensitivity arising from this use.

### Preparations

**Proprietary Preparations** (details are given in Part 3)
***Ital.:*** Bergamon Sapone.

---

## Bronopol *(BAN, rINN)*

2-Bromo-2-nitropropane-1,3-diol.
$C_3H_6BrNO_4$ = 200.0.
*CAS — 52-51-7.*

**Pharmacopoeias.** In *Br.* and *Pol.*

**BP 2003** (Bronopol). White or almost white crystals or crystalline powder, odourless or almost odourless. Freely soluble in water and in alcohol; slightly soluble in glycerol and in liquid paraffin. A 1% solution in water has a pH of 5.0 to 7.0. Protect from light.

**Incompatibility.** The activity of bronopol can be diminished by sodium metabisulfite, sodium thiosulfate, cysteine hydrochloride, and compounds with a thiol group. Incompatibility with unprotected aluminium affects packaging.

**Stability.** The stability of bronopol is affected by increases in temperature and by increases in pH above 8.

Creams and shampoos containing bronopol 0.01% as a preservative were found to contain free nitrite and, as a result of amines present in the preparations, nitrosamines.[1] It was recommended that nitrosamine formation could be reduced in preparations containing amines and bronopol by limiting the bronopol concentration to 0.01% and inclusion of alpha tocopherol 0.2% or butylated hydroxytoluene 0.05%.

1. Dunnett PC, Telling GM. Study of the fate of bronopol and the effects of antioxidants on N-nitrosamine formation in shampoos and skin creams. *Int J Cosmet Sci* 1984; **6:** 241–7.

### Adverse Effects

Bronopol may be irritant when applied topically.

### Pharmacokinetics

Bronopol is absorbed following topical administration.

### Uses

Bronopol is active against a wide range of bacteria, including *Pseudomonas aeruginosa*, but is less active against moulds and yeasts. Bronopol is used as a preservative in shampoos, cosmetics, and both topical and oral pharmaceutical preparations; concentrations in pharmaceutical preparations range from 0.01 to 0.1%, with the usual concentration being 0.02%.

---

## Butylated Hydroxyanisole *(BAN)*

BHA; Butilhidroxianisol; Butilidrossianisolo; Butylhydroxyanisole; Butylhydroxyanisolum; E320. 2-*tert*-Butyl-4-methoxyphenol; 2-(1,1-dimethylethyl)-4-methoxyphenol.
$C_{11}H_{16}O_2$ = 180.2.
*CAS — 25013-16-5.*

**Pharmacopoeias.** In *Eur.* (see p.vi), *Int.*, and *Pol.* Also in *USNF.*

**Ph. Eur. 5.0** (Butylhydroxyanisole; Butylated Hydroxyanisole BP 2003). A white, yellowish, or slightly pinkish, crystalline powder. It contains not more than 10% of 3-(1,1-dimethylethyl)-4-methoxyphenol. Practically insoluble in water; freely soluble in alcohol and in fatty oils; very soluble in dichloromethane; it dissolves in dilute solutions of alkali hydroxides. Protect from light.

**USNF 22** (Butylated Hydroxyanisole). A white, or slightly yellow, waxy solid with a faint characteristic odour. Insoluble in water; soluble 1 in 4 of alcohol, 1 in 2 of chloroform, and 1 in 1.2 of ether; freely soluble in propylene glycol.

**Incompatibility.** Butylated hydroxyanisole is incompatible with oxidising agents and ferric salts. Traces of metals can cause loss of activity.

### Adverse Effects

Butylated hydroxyanisole can be irritant to the eyes, skin, and mucous membranes and can cause depigmentation. There are reports of delayed (type IV) hypersensitivity reactions and non-immunogenic skin reactions.

**Effects on the blood.** For a report of methaemoglobinaemia associated with the antoxidants (butylated hydroxyanisole, butylated hydroxytoluene, and propyl gallate) used to preserve the oil in a soybean infant feed, see under Adverse Effects in Alkyl Gallates (p.1168).

### Pharmacokinetics

Butylated hydroxyanisole is absorbed from the gastrointestinal tract, then metabolised and conjugated, and excreted in the urine; less than 1% is excreted in the urine as unchanged drug within 24 hours of ingestion.

### Uses

Butylated hydroxyanisole is an antoxidant with some antimicrobial activity. It is used as a preservative in cosmetics and foods as well as pharmaceutical preparations, particularly to delay or prevent oxidative rancidity of fats and oils in concentrations of up to 0.02%; higher concentrations have been used for essential oils. It is also used to prevent the loss of activity of oil-soluble vitamins.

Commercial supplies of butylated hydroxyanisole used in food technology consist of mixtures of the 2-*tert* and 3-*tert* isomers.

To improve efficacy, butylated hydroxyanisole is frequently used with other antoxidants such as butylated hydroxytoluene or an alkyl gallate and with sequestrants or synergists such as citric acid.

**Use in food.** In the UK the Food Advisory Committee has recommended that the use of butylated hydroxyanisole and butylated hydroxytoluene should no longer be permitted as additives for infant formulas as they are no longer required for the economic manufacture of vitamin A and vitamin A esters.[1]

1. MAFF. Food Advisory Committee: report on the review of the use of additives in foods specially prepared for infants and young children. *FdAC/REP/12.* London: HMSO, 1992.

---

## Butylated Hydroxytoluene *(BAN)*

BHT; Butilhidroxitolueno; Butylhydroxitoluenum; Butylhydroxytoluene; E321. 2,6-Di-*tert*-butyl-*p*-cresol.
$C_{15}H_{24}O$ = 220.4.
*CAS — 128-37-0.*

**Pharmacopoeias.** In *Eur.* (see p.vi), *Int.*, and *Pol.* Also in *USNF.*

**Ph. Eur. 5.0** (Butylhydroxytoluene; Butylated Hydroxytoluene BP 2003). A white or yellowish-white, crystalline powder. F.p. 69° to 70°. Practically insoluble in water; freely soluble in alcohol and in vegetable oils; very soluble in acetone.

**USNF 22** (Butylated Hydroxytoluene). A white crystalline solid with a faint characteristic odour. Insoluble in water and in propylene glycol; soluble 1 in 4 of alcohol and 1 in 1.1 of chloroform and of ether.

**Incompatibility.** Butylated hydroxytoluene is incompatible with oxidising agents and ferric salts. Traces of metals can cause loss of activity.

### Adverse Effects

As for Butylated Hydroxyanisole, p.1171.

**Effects on the blood.** For a report of methaemoglobinaemia associated with the antoxidants (butylated hydroxyanisole, butylated hydroxytoluene, and propyl gallate) used to preserve the oil in a soybean infant feed formula, see under Adverse Effects in Alkyl Gallates, p.1168.

**Poisoning.** A 22-year-old woman experienced severe epigastric cramping, nausea and vomiting, and generalised weakness, followed by dizziness, confusion, and a brief loss of consciousness after ingesting 4 g of butylated hydroxytoluene. She recovered following conservative treatment which was given 2 days later. The antoxidant had been taken as an unauthorised remedy for genital herpes simplex.[1]

1. Shlian DM, Goldstone J. Toxicity of butylated hydroxytoluene. *N Engl J Med* 1986; **314:** 648–9.

### Pharmacokinetics

Butylated hydroxytoluene is readily absorbed from the gastrointestinal tract. It is excreted in the urine mainly as glucuronide conjugates of oxidation products.

### Uses

Butylated hydroxytoluene is an antoxidant with uses similar to those of Butylated Hydroxyanisole, p.1171.

### Preparations

**Proprietary Preparations** (details are given in Part 3)

**Multi-ingredient:** ***Arg.:*** Deca-Scab.

## Cadexomer-Iodine *(BAN)*

Cadexomer Iodine *(USAN)*; Cadexómero yodado. 2-Hydroxymethylene cross-linked (1→4)-α-D-glucan carboxymethyl ether containing iodine.

*CAS — 94820-09-4.*
*ATC — D03AX01.*

### Adverse Effects and Precautions

As for Povidone-Iodine, p.1190. Some patients have experienced stinging and erythema following application of cadexomer-iodine to their ulcers. Free iodine is released during exposure of cadexomer-iodine preparations to wound exudate and absorption of iodine may occur. Prolonged treatment with cadexomer-iodine should be used with caution in patients with thyroid disorders.

### Uses and Administration

Cadexomer-iodine, like povidone-iodine (p.1191), is an iodophore that releases iodine. It is used for its absorbent and antiseptic properties in the management of venous leg ulcers and pressure sores. It is applied as a powder, ointment, or paste containing iodine 0.9%; sufficient powder or ointment should be applied to form a layer about 3 mm thick. Treatment should not usually be continued for more than 3 months.

### Preparations

**Proprietary Preparations** (details are given in Part 3)

***Austral.:*** Iodoflex†; Iodosorb; ***Austria:*** Iodosorb; ***Canad.:*** Iodosorb; ***Denm.:*** Iodosorb; ***Fin.:*** Iodosorb; ***Ger.:*** Iodosorb; ***Irl.:*** Iodoflex; ***Ital.:*** Iodosorb; ***Singapore:*** Iodoflex; Iodosorb; ***Spain:*** Iodosorb; ***Swed.:*** Iodosorb; ***Switz.:*** Iodosorb; ***UK:*** Iodoflex; Iodosorb.

## Cetalkonium Chloride *(BAN, USAN, rINN)*

Cloruro de cetalconio; NSC-32942. Benzylhexadecyldimethylammonium chloride.

$C_{25}H_{46}ClN$ = 396.1.
*CAS — 122-18-9.*

### Profile

Cetalkonium chloride is a quaternary ammonium antiseptic with actions and uses similar to those of other cationic surfactants (see Cetrimide, p.1172). It is used in a variety of topical preparations in the treatment of minor infections of the mouth and throat. It has also been used in the treatment of eye infections. Cetalkonium bromide has also been used.

### Preparations

**Proprietary Preparations** (details are given in Part 3)

**Multi-ingredient:** ***Arg.:*** Pansoral; ***Austral.:*** Bonjela; ***Austria:*** Mundisal; ***Braz.:*** Pondicilina; ***Canad.:*** Bionet; Emercol†; ***Fr.:*** Pansoral; ***Ger.:*** Mundisal; ***Hong Kong:*** Bonjela; ***Irl.:*** Bonjela; ***Israel:*** Bonjela; ***Malaysia:*** Bonjela; ***NZ:*** Bonjela; ***Port.:*** Bucagel; ***S.Afr.:*** AAA; Bonjela; ***Singapore:*** Bonjela; ***Switz.:*** Mundisal; Pansoral†; ***Thai.:*** Bonjela; ***UK:*** Bonjela; Bonjela Teething Gel; ***USA:*** Babee.

## Cethexonium Bromide

Cetexonio, bromuro de. Hexadecyl(2-hydroxycyclohexyl)dimethylammonium bromide.

$C_{24}H_{50}BrNO$ = 448.6.
*CAS — 6810-42-0 (cethexonium); 1794-74-7 (cethexonium bromide); 58703-78-9 (cethexonium chloride).*

NOTE. Cethexonium Chloride is *rINN*.

### Profile

Cethexonium bromide is a quaternary ammonium antiseptic with properties similar to those of other cationic surfactants (see Cetrimide, p.1172). It is used in preparations for the local treatment of minor infections of the eye, nose, and throat.

### Preparations

**Proprietary Preparations** (details are given in Part 3)

***Fr.:*** Biocidan; ***Mon.:*** Bactyl.

**Multi-ingredient:** ***Fr.:*** Biocidan.

# Cetrimide *(BAN, rINN)*

Cetrimida; Cetrimidum.

*CAS — 1119-97-7 (trimethyltetradecylammonium bromide); 1119-94-4 (dodecyltrimethylammonium bromide); 8044-71-1 (cetrimide).*
*ATC — D08AJ04; D11AC01.*

NOTE. The name cetrimonium bromide was often formerly used for cetrimide. Cetrimonium bromide is hexadecyltrimethylammonium bromide (see below).

**Pharmacopoeias.** In *Eur.* (see p.vi) and *Int.*

*Br.* also includes strong cetrimide solution.

**Ph. Eur. 5.0** (Cetrimide). It consists of trimethyltetradecylammonium bromide and may contain smaller amounts of dodecyltrimethylammonium bromide and hexadecyltrimethylammonium bromide (= cetrimonium bromide, p.1173). A white or almost white, voluminous, free-flowing powder. Freely soluble in water and in alcohol. A 2.0% solution in water froths copiously when shaken.

**BP 2003** (Strong Cetrimide Solution). It is an aqueous solution of cetrimide. It contains 20 to 40% w/v of cetrimide, calculated as $C_{17}H_{38}BrN$ and up to 10% alcohol or isopropyl alcohol, or both; alcohol may be replaced by industrial methylated spirit. It may be perfumed and may contain colouring matter. Store at a temperature above 15°.

**Incompatibility.** Cetrimide is incompatible with soaps and other anionic surfactants, bentonite, iodine, phenylmercuric nitrate, and alkali hydroxides. Aqueous solutions react with metals.

### Adverse Effects and Treatment

At the concentrations used on the skin, solutions of cetrimide and other quaternary compounds do not generally cause irritation, but some patients become hypersensitive to cetrimide after repeated applications. Cetrimide powder is reported to be irritant. There have been rare reports of burns with concentrated solutions of cetrimide.

If ingested, cetrimide and other quaternary ammonium compounds cause nausea and vomiting; strong solutions may cause oesophageal damage and necrosis. They have depolarising muscle relaxant properties and toxic symptoms include dyspnoea and cyanosis due to paralysis of the respiratory muscles, possibly leading to asphyxia. CNS depression (sometimes preceded by excitement and convulsions), hypotension, coma, and death may also occur. Accidental intra-uterine or intravenous administration may cause haemolysis.

Treatment of poisoning is symptomatic; demulcents and diluents may be given if necessary but emesis should be avoided, particularly if concentrated solutions have been ingested. Activated charcoal may be considered if the patient presents within an hour of ingestion. CNS stimulants and cholinesterase inhibitors are reported not to reverse paralysis due to cetrimide intoxication although sympathomimetics have been tried. Corticosteroids may reduce oropharyngeal oedema.

**Effects following cyst irrigation.** Adverse effects following irrigation with cetrimide solutions in the treatment of hydatid cysts have included chemical peritonitis,[1] methaemoglobinaemia with cyanosis,[2] and metabolic acidosis.[3]

1. Gilchrist DS. Chemical peritonitis after cetrimide washout in hydatid-cyst surgery. *Lancet* 1979; **ii:** 1374.
2. Baraka A, *et al.* Cetrimide-induced methaemoglobinaemia after surgical excision of hydatid cyst. *Lancet* 1980; **ii:** 88–9.
3. Momblano P, *et al.* Metabolic acidosis induced by cetrimonium bromide. *Lancet* 1984; **ii:** 1045.

**Poisoning.** The fatal dose of quaternary ammonium compounds was estimated to be 1 to 3 g.[1]

1. Arena JM. Poisonings and other health hazards associated with use of detergents. *JAMA* 1964; **190:** 56–8.

### Precautions

Prolonged and repeated applications of cetrimide to the skin are inadvisable as hypersensitivity may occur. Contact with the eyes, brain, meninges, and middle ear should be avoided. Cetrimide should not be used in body cavities or as an enema.

Quaternary ammonium compounds are not reliable for sterilising surgical instruments and heat-labile articles. The antimicrobial activity of quaternary ammonium compounds may be reduced through absorption, or through combination with organic matter, or by reducing pH.

Solutions of quaternary ammonium compounds should not be used for disinfection of soft contact lenses.

Aqueous solutions of cetrimide or other quaternary ammonium disinfectants may be susceptible to contamination with micro-organisms. To reduce this risk, a sterilised preparation should be used or, where necessary, solutions must be freshly prepared at the recommended concentration and appropriate measures should be taken to prevent contamination during storage or dilution.

**Handling.** Cetrimide powder is irritant; it has been recommended that the nose and mouth should be protected by a mask when working with the powder[1] and eyes should be protected by goggles.

1. Jacobs JY. Work hazards from drug handling. *Pharm J* 1984; **233:** 195–6.

### Uses and Administration

Cetrimide is a quaternary ammonium antiseptic with actions and uses typical of cationic surfactants. These surfactants dissociate in aqueous solution into a relatively large and complex cation that is responsible for the surface activity and a smaller inactive anion. In addition to emulsifying and detergent properties, quaternary ammonium compounds have bactericidal activity against Gram-positive and, at a higher concentration, against some Gram-negative bacteria. Some *Pseudomonas* spp. are particularly resistant as are strains of *Mycobacterium tuberculosis*. They are ineffective against bacterial spores, have variable antifungal activity, and are effective against some viruses.

Quaternary ammonium compounds are most effective in neutral or slightly alkaline solution and their bactericidal activity is appreciably reduced in acid media; their activity is enhanced by alcohols.

Like other quaternary ammonium compounds, notably benzalkonium chloride (p.1168), cetrimide has been employed for cleansing skin, wounds (but see under Wound Disinfection, p.1165), and burns. For these purposes it has been used as a 0.1 to 1.0% aqueous solution, generally prepared by dilution of a more concentrated solution, or as a cream containing 0.5%. However, a mixture of cetrimide with chlorhexidine (p.1173) has often been preferred to cetrimide alone. This combination is also used in a lotion for acne (p.1133).

Solutions containing up to 10% of cetrimide have been used as shampoos to remove the scales in seborrhoeic dermatitis (p.1138).

Cetrimide solution 0.5 or 1% has been used as a scolicide to irrigate hydatid cysts during surgery (see Echinococcosis, p.98) but systemic adverse effects have been reported (see above).

Cetrimide and benzalkonium chloride are also used as preservatives in cosmetics and pharmaceutical formulations including eye drops and in disinfecting solutions for hard contact lenses; neither compound should be used for disinfection of soft contact lenses.

Cetrimide is also present in some emulsifying preparations such as Cetrimide Emulsifying Ointment (BP 2003).

### Preparations

***BP 2003:*** Cetrimide Cream; Cetrimide Emulsifying Ointment; Cetrimide Solution.

**Proprietary Preparations** (details are given in Part 3)

***Arg.:*** Boucren; Sorbicet; ***Austral.:*** Acnederm Wash†; ***Canad.:*** Resdan†; Savlon†; ***Fr.:*** Cetavlon; Septisept†; ***Irl.:*** Cetavlex; Vesagex; ***Israel:*** Capillon†; ***Malaysia:*** Acnederm Wash; Cetavlex; Dermoplex Antiseptic; ***Neth.:*** Cetavlon†; ***Port.:*** Cetavlex†; ***S.Afr.:*** Cetavlon†; Wound-A-Sept†; ***Singapore:*** Acnederm Wash; Cetavlex†; ***Spain:*** Cetavlon; ***UK:*** Bactrian†; Bansor; Cetavlex; Cradocap†; Medi-Prep; Medicaid; Richmond Antiseptic Cream; Vesagex.

**Multi-ingredient:** ***Arg.:*** Jabonacid; Otidrops; Otoclean Gotas Oticas; Sincerum; ***Austral.:*** Curacleanse; Dermocaine†; Dimethicream; Hamilton Skin Repair; Hibicet†; Medi Creme†; Microshield Antiseptic; Pro-PS†; Savlon Antiseptic; Soov Bite; Soov Burn; Soov Cream; ***Austria:*** Lemocin; Xylonor; ***Belg.:*** Lemocin; ***Braz.:*** Cetrilan†; ***Canad.:*** Savlodil; Savlon†; ***Fr.:*** Broncorinol rhinites; Buccawalter†; Rectoquotane; ***Hong Kong:*** Borraginol-N; Drapolene; Hamilton Skin Repair; Hibicet Hospital Concentrate; Medicreme; Soov Bite; Tri-Gel; ***India:*** Iteol-3; Scabine; Siloderm; ***Irl.:*** Ceanel; Drapolene; Hibicet; RBC; Savlon; Siopel; Torbetol; ***Israel:*** Cetrin; Dermaor†; Savior; Septacare; Tisept; Travasept; ***Ital.:*** Baxidin; Cetrexidin; Cetrisan; Clotramid; Cuprosodio; Farvicett; Germozero Hospital†; Hibicet†; Hibizene; Iketoncid†; Panseptil; Steridol; ***Malaysia:*** Burnol Plus; Drapolene; Hibicet; Soov Bite; ***Neth.:*** Hibicet concentraat†; Hibicet verdunning†; ***NZ:*** Acnederm Foaming Wash; Acnederm Wash; Dermocaine†; Hairscience Conditioner; Hibicet†; Karicare Barrier Cream; Medicreme; Savlon; Soov Bite; Soov Burn; Soov Cream; ***Port.:*** Friax†; Savlon†; ***S.Afr.:*** Benzet; Burnocaine†; Ceanel†; Hibicet; Medituss; Orocaine†; Savlon†; Siopel†; Trochain; Virobis; ***Singapore:*** Burnol Plus; Drapolene; Hibicet Hospital Concentrate†; Savlon; Soov Bite; Soov Cream; ***Spain:*** Lidrone†; ***Thai.:*** Bacard; Burnol Plus; Chlorhex-C; Dekka; Drapolene; Frebac; Hibicet; Inhibac; Napilene; Sepdine; Septone; ***UK:*** Ceanel; Cetanorm; Cymex; Dermidex; Drapolene; Hibicet; Lypsyl Cold Sore Gel; Modantis†; Neo Baby Cream; Quinoderm Antibacterial Face Wash; Savlon Antiseptic Cream; Savlon Antiseptic Liquid; Siopel; Steripod Chlorhexidine Gluconate with Cetrimide; Tisept; Torbetol; Travasept; ***USA:*** Scadan.

### Cetrimonium Bromide *(rINN)*

Bromuro de cetrimonio; Cetyltrimethylammonium Bromide; CTAB. Hexadecyltrimethylammonium bromide.

$C_{19}H_{42}BrN$ = 364.4.

*CAS — 6899-10-1 (cetrimonium); 57-09-0 (cetrimonium bromide).*

*ATC — D08AJ02; R02AA17.*

NOTE. The name cetrimonium bromide was formerly applied to cetrimide (see above).

**Pharmacopoeias.** In *USNF.*

**USNF 22** (Cetrimonium Bromide). A white to creamy white, voluminous, free-flowing powder, with a characteristic faint odour. Freely soluble in water and in alcohol; practically insoluble in ether. Protect from moisture. Store at a temperature not exceeding 40°. Do not allow to freeze.

### Cetrimonium Chloride *(BAN)*

Hexadecyltrimethylammonium chloride.

$C_{19}H_{42}ClN$ = 320.0.

*CAS — 112-02-7.*

#### Profile

Cetrimonium bromide is a quaternary ammonium antiseptic with actions and uses similar to those of other cationic surfactants (see Cetrimide, p.1172). Cetrimonium chloride and cetrimonium tosilate are also used.

#### Preparations

**Proprietary Preparations** (details are given in Part 3)
***Belg.:*** Aseptiderm†; ***Braz.:*** Tiracaspa; ***Ital.:*** Golaval; Neo-Intol†; Senol; Sterilene; ***Switz.:*** Turisan.

**Multi-ingredient:** ***Arg.:*** Bagociletas sin Anestesia; Bagoderm; Salvicutan; ***Austria:*** Xylestesin; ***Belg.:*** Cetavlex; HAC†; Hacdil-S†; ***Braz.:*** Amigdalol; Drapolene; Laringex; Leucocida; ***Canad.:*** Bye Bye Burn†; Clearasil Sensitive Skin Cleanser†; ***Fr.:*** Eryteal†; Nostril; ***Ger.:*** Lemocin; Xylestesin Pumpspray; ***Israel:*** Lemocin; ***Ital.:*** Aflogine†; Golamixin; Leucorsan†; Xylonor; ***Spain:*** Diformiltricina; Hongosan; Topicaina†; Xylonor; ***Switz.:*** Desitur; Largal ultra†; Lemocin; Septivon N; Turexan Capilla; Xylestesin; Xylonor.

---

### Cetylpyridinium Chloride *(BAN, rINN)*

Cetylpyridinii Chloridum; Cloruro de cetilpiridinio. 1-Hexadecylpyridinium chloride monohydrate.

$C_{21}H_{38}ClN,H_2O$ = 358.0.

*CAS — 7773-52-6 (cetylpyridinium); 123-03-5 (anhydrous cetylpyridinium chloride); 6004-24-6 (cetylpyridinium chloride, monohydrate).*

*ATC — B05CA01; D08AJ03; D09AA07; R02AA06.*

**Pharmacopoeias.** In *Eur.* (see p.vi) and *US.*

**Ph. Eur. 5.0** (Cetylpyridinium Chloride). A white powder, slightly soapy to the touch. Soluble in water, frothing copiously when shaken; soluble in alcohol.

**USP 27** (Cetylpyridinium Chloride). A white powder with a slight characteristic odour. Soluble 1 in 4.5 of water and of chloroform, and 1 in 2.5 of alcohol; slightly soluble in ether and in benzene.

**Incompatibility.** Cetylpyridinium chloride is incompatible with soaps and other anionic surfactants.

#### Profile

Cetylpyridinium chloride is a quaternary pyridinium antiseptic with actions and uses similar to those of other cationic surfactants (see Cetrimide, p.1172). It is used chiefly as lozenges or solutions for the treatment of minor infections of the mouth and throat. It is also used topically for the treatment of skin and eye infections.

#### Preparations

***USP 27:*** Cetylpyridinium Chloride Lozenges; Cetylpyridinium Chloride Topical Solution.

**Proprietary Preparations** (details are given in Part 3)
***Austral.:*** Cepacol Antibacterial; Cepacol Mint†; Cepacol Regular†; Lemsip Lozenges†; ***Austria:*** Dobendan; Halset; ***Braz.:*** Gargocetil; Gurgol†; ***Canad.:*** Cepacol; Emereze Plus†; Mouthwash; Rince Bouche Antiseptique; Throat Lozenges; ***Chile:*** Freesept; ***Fr.:*** Cetylyre; Novoptine; ***Ger.:*** Dobendan; Frubizin†; ***Hong Kong:*** Cepacol; ***Irl.:*** Merocets; ***Israel:*** Gargaron†; ***Ital.:*** Alsol†; Bat; Borocaina Gola; Bronchenolo; Cetilsan; Citromed Soap; Exil; Farin Gola; Geyderm Sepsi†; Golacetin; Herbagola†; Honeygola; Johnson's Penaten Crema Disinfettante†; Neo Cepacol Pastiglie; Neo Coricidin Gola; Neo Formitrol; Periogard Plus; Ragaden; Sterinet†; ***Mex.:*** Cepadyne†; ***Norw.:*** Pyrisept; ***NZ:*** Cepacol; Lemsip Throat Lozenges; ***Port.:*** Septoral†; ***S.Afr.:*** Cepacol; Universal Throat Lollies†; ***Singapore:*** Cepacol; ***Spain:*** Angifonil; ***Thai.:*** Cepacol; Orasept; ***UK:*** Listermint; Merocets; ***USA:*** Cepacol Mouthwash; Scope.

**Multi-ingredient:** ***Arg.:*** Collubiazol; Desenfriol Caramelos; Oral-B Enjuague Bucal; Solumerin; ***Austral.:*** Cepacaine; Cepacol Antibacterial; Cepacol Cough +; Cepacol Plus with Anaesthetic; Difflam Anti-inflammatory Cough Lozenges; Difflam Lozenges; Difflam Mouth Gel; Duro-Tuss Cough Lozenges; Gentlees†; Seda-Gel; ***Austria:*** Coldistan; Dentinox; Paididont; Tetesept; ***Braz.:*** Alergotox Pastilhas†; Cepacaina; Cetildrops; Dentalivio; Eucament†; Fenotricin†; Filogargan†; Forsalil†; Gargotrat†; Glytoss†; Limao Bravo; Limao Bravo com Vitamina C; Malvol†; Malvona; Neopiridin; Pondicilina; Proplax†; Psiu; Sanil Menta Bucal†; Sanilin†; Tonsildrops†; Xarope Valda†; Xarope Vick†; ***Canad.:*** Balminil Lozenges†; Cepacol Citrus; Cepacol with Fluoride; Emercol†; Emercreme No 4†; Green Antiseptic Mouthwash & Gargle; Kank-A; Mouthrinse†; Mouthwash & Gargle†; Mouthwash Mint/Peppermint†; Oral Plan; Oral-B Anti-Bacterial with Fluoride; Scope†; Throat Lozenges; ***Chile:*** Halita; Kank-Eze; Pancrit; Perio-Aid c Cloruro de Cetilpiridinio; ***Fin.:*** Bafucin; ***Fr.:*** Alodont; Broncorinol maux de gorge; ***Ger.:*** Bioget; Brand- und Wund-Gel Eu Rho; Broncho-Tyrosolvetten; Dolo-Dobendan; Dori†; Em-eukal; Frubienzym; Frubizin Forte; Imposit N†; Nordathricin N; Psilo-Balsam N†; stas Halsschmerz-Tabletten†; Trachiform; Tyrosolvetten; Tyrosolvetten-C; Tyrosur; Wick Sulagil; Wund- und Brand-Gel Eu Rho†; ***Hong Kong:*** Dentinox Teething Gel; Pharynx; Setronges; ***Irl.:*** Anbesol; Listermint with Fluoride†; Merocaine; Vicks Original Cough Syrup for Chesty Coughs†; ***Israel:*** Cepadont; Kank-A; ***Ital.:*** Bo-Gum†; Cepral†; Delta 80; Delta 80 Plus; Farmagola; Ginvapast; Gola Action; Neo Cepacol Collutorio†; Neo-Stomygen; Oral-B Collutorio per la Protezione di Denti e Gengive; Oraseptic Gola†; Orosanyl; Ridiodent; Rikospray; Rinosil†; Stomygen; ***Malaysia:*** Dentinox Teething Gel; Difflam Anti-inflammatory Lozenges (with Antibacterial); Difflam Mouth Gel; Pharynx; Setronges; ***Mex.:*** Mentalgina; ***Neth.:*** Agre-Gola; ***Norw.:*** Aselli; ***NZ:*** Cepacaine; Cepacol Anaesthetic; Cepacol Cough Discs; Difflam Anti-inflammatory Antibacterial Lozenges†; Difflam Cough; Difflam Mouth Gel; Duro-Tuss Lozenges; Lenactin†; ***Port.:*** Bioflu-or Sensitive; Dropcina; Mebocaina; ***S.Afr.:*** Cepacaine; Cepacol; Cepacol Cough Discs; Cetoxol†; Colphen; Endcol Lozenges; Medi-Kain; Medi-Keel A; Vagarsol; ***Singapore:*** Dentinox Teething Gel; Difflam Mouth Gel; Pharynx; ***Spain:*** Alcohocel; Alcohol Cetil; Alcohol Cetilpi Cuve; Alcohol Sanit Cuve†; Babysiton; Dequadin Complex†; Farmalcohol; Pastillas Antisep Garg L; Pastillas Antisep Garg M; Silidermil; Vicks Formula 44; Xylonibsa†; ***Swed.:*** Bafucin; ***Switz.:*** Alodont; Angina MCC; Anginazol; Flavangin†; Hextriletten; Lidazon; Maux de gorge; Mebucaine; Nasex; Neo-Angin Lido; Novomint N†; Otothricinol; Vicks Formel 44†; ***Thai.:*** Sentril; Sore Mouth Gel; ***UAE:*** B-Cool; New B-Cool; ***UK:*** Adult Meltus for Chesty Coughs & Catarrh†; Allens Dry Tickly Cough; Anbesol; Calgel; De Witt's Lozenges†; Dentinox Teething Gel; Kilkof; Listermint with Fluoride; Macleans Mouthguard; Meltus Expectorant; Meltus Junior Expectorant; Merocaine; Merocets Plus; Oragard†; Rinstead; Rinstead Teething Gel†; Vicks Expectorant†; Woodwards Teething Gel; ***USA:*** Cepacol Anesthetic; Cepacol Maximum Strength Sore Throat; Cepacol Regular Strength; Cepacol Throat; Cylex; Massengill Disposable; MouthKote O/R; MouthKote P/R; Orajel Mouth Aid.

---

## Chlorhexidine *(BAN, rINN)*

Clorhexidina.

*CAS — 55-56-1.*

*ATC — A01AB03; B05CA02; D08AC02; D09AA12; R02AA05; S01AX09; S02AA09; S03AA04.*

### Chlorhexidine Acetate *(BANM, rINNM)*

Acetato de clorhexidina; Chlorhexidine Diacetate; Chlorhexidini Diacetas. 1,1′-Hexamethylenebis[5-(4-chlorophenyl)biguanide] diacetate.

$C_{22}H_{30}Cl_2N_{10},2C_2H_4O_2$ = 625.6.

*CAS — 56-95-1.*

*ATC — A01AB03; B05CA02; D08AC02; D09AA12; R02AA05; S01AX09; S02AA09; S03AA04.*

**Pharmacopoeias.** In *Chin., Eur.* (see p.vi), *Int.,* and *Pol.*

**Ph. Eur. 5.0** (Chlorhexidine Diacetate). A white or almost white, microcrystalline powder. Sparingly soluble in water; soluble in alcohol; slightly soluble in glycerol and in propylene glycol.

**Incompatibility.** The incompatibilities of chlorhexidine salts are discussed under Chlorhexidine Hydrochloride, below.

**Stability.** The stability of chlorhexidine salts is discussed under Chlorhexidine Hydrochloride, below.

### Chlorhexidine Gluconate *(BANM, USAN, rINNM)*

Chlorhexidine Digluconate; Gluconato de clorhexidina. 1,1′-Hexamethylenebis[5-(4-chlorophenyl)biguanide] digluconate.

$C_{22}H_{30}Cl_2N_{10},2C_6H_{12}O_7$ = 897.8.

*CAS — 18472-51-0.*

*ATC — A01AB03; B05CA02; D08AC02; D09AA12; R02AA05; S01AX09; S02AA09; S03AA04.*

**Pharmacopoeias.** *Chin., Eur.* (see p.vi), *Pol.,* and *US* include a solution which contains 19 to 21% of chlorhexidine gluconate.

**Ph. Eur. 5.0** (Chlorhexidine Digluconate Solution; Chlorhexidini Digluconatis Solutio; Chlorhexidine Gluconate Solution BP 2003). An aqueous solution which contains not less than 190 g/litre and not more than 210 g/litre of chlorhexidine gluconate. An almost colourless or pale-yellowish liquid. Miscible with water, with not more than 5 parts of alcohol, and with not more than 3 parts of acetone. A 5% v/v dilution in water has a pH of 5.5 to 7.0. Protect from light.

**USP 27** (Chlorhexidine Gluconate Solution). An aqueous solution which contains not less than 19% and not more than 21% of chlorhexidine gluconate. An almost colourless or pale yellow, clear liquid. Miscible with water and with glacial acetic acid; miscible with five times its volume of dehydrated alcohol and with three times its volume of acetone; further addition of dehydrated alcohol or of acetone yields a white turbidity. A 5% v/v dilution in water has a pH of 5.5 to 7.0. Store in airtight containers. Protect from light.

**Incompatibility.** The incompatibilities of chlorhexidine salts are discussed under Chlorhexidine Hydrochloride, below.

**Stability.** The stability of chlorhexidine salts is discussed under Chlorhexidine Hydrochloride, below.

**Sterilisation.** Dilutions of commercial concentrated solutions may be sterilised by autoclaving.

### Chlorhexidine Hydrochloride *(BANM, USAN, rINNM)*

AY-5312; Chlorhexidine Dihydrochloride; Chlorhexidini Dihydrochloridum; Hidrocloruro de clorhexidina. 1,1′-Hexamethylenebis[5-(4-chlorophenyl)biguanide] dihydrochloride.

$C_{22}H_{30}Cl_2N_{10},2HCl$ = 578.4.

*CAS — 3697-42-5.*

*ATC — A01AB03; B05CA02; D08AC02; D09AA12; R02AA05; S01AX09; S02AA09; S03AA04.*

**Pharmacopoeias.** In *Eur.* (see p.vi), *Int.,* and *Jpn.*

**Ph. Eur. 5.0** (Chlorhexidine Dihydrochloride; Chlorhexidine Hydrochloride BP 2003). A white or almost white, crystalline powder. Sparingly soluble in water and in propylene glycol; very slightly soluble in alcohol.

**Incompatibility.** Chlorhexidine salts are incompatible with soaps and other anionic materials. Activity may be reduced in the presence of suspending agents such as alginates and tragacanth, insoluble powders such as kaolin, and insoluble compounds of calcium, magnesium, and zinc. Chlorhexidine acetate is incompatible with potassium iodide. At a concentration of 0.05%, chlorhexidine salts are incompatible with borates, bicarbonates, carbonates, chlorides, citrates, nitrates, phosphates, and sulfates, forming salts of low solubility which may precipitate out of solution. At dilutions of 0.01% or more, these salts are generally soluble. Insoluble salts may form in hard water. Chlorhexidine salts are inactivated by cork.

References to incompatibilities of chlorhexidine with suspending agents and insoluble solids.[1-3]


1. McCarthy TJ. The influence of insoluble powders on preservatives in solution. *J Mond Pharm* 1969; **12:** 321–8.
2. Yousef RT, *et al.* Effect of some pharmaceutical materials on the bactericidal activities of preservatives. *Can J Pharm Sci* 1973; **8:** 54–6.
3. McCarthy TJ, Myburgh JA. The effect of tragacanth gel on preservative activity. *Pharm Weekbl* 1974; **109:** 265–8.


**Stability.** Chlorhexidine and its salts are stable at normal storage temperatures but when heated may decompose with the production of trace amounts of 4-chloroaniline. Chlorhexidine hydrochloride is less readily decomposed than chlorhexidine acetate and may be heated at 150° for 1 hour without appreciable production of 4-chloroaniline. Aqueous solutions of chlorhexidine salts decompose with the formation of trace amounts of 4-chloroaniline. This decomposition is increased by heating and alkaline pH.

## Adverse Effects and Treatment

Skin sensitivity to chlorhexidine has occasionally been reported. Strong solutions may cause irritation of the conjunctiva and other sensitive tissues. The use of chlorhexidine dental gel and mouthwash has been associated with reversible discoloration of the tongue, teeth, and silicate or composite dental restorations. Transient taste disturbances and a burning sensation of the tongue may occur on initial use. Oral desquamation and occasional parotid gland swelling have been reported with the mouthwash. If desquamation occurs, 50% dilution of the mouthwash with water and less vigorous rinsing may allow continued use.

The main consequence of ingestion is mucosal irritation and systemic toxicity is rare (see Poisoning, below). Haemolysis has been reported following accidental intravenous administration. Gastric lavage with demulcents has been suggested for acute ingestion.

**Effects on the eyes.** Report of 4 cases of corneal damage due to contact with chlorhexidine gluconate used for pre-operative preparation of facial skin.[1]


1. Tabor E, *et al.* Corneal damage due to eye contact with chlorhexidine gluconate. *JAMA* 1989; **261:** 557–8.


**Effects on the nose.** Temporary hyposmia (reduced sense of smell) in some patients after transsphenoidal pituitary adenoma operation was assumed to be caused by pre-operative disinfection of the nasal cavity with chlorhexidine gluconate solution.[1]


1. Yamagishi M, *et al.* Impairment of olfactory epithelium treated with chlorhexidine digluconate (Hibitane). *Pract Otol* 1985; **78:** 399–409.


**Hypersensitivity.** Severe hypersensitivity reactions including anaphylactic shock have been reported following topical applications of chlorhexidine,[1-4] and from the use of chlorhexidine-containing lubricants for urinary catheterisation or cystoscopy.[5] There has been concern that similar reactions may occur with chlorhexidine-impregnated medical devices including intravenous catheters and implanted surgical mesh.[6] Occupational asthma has been attributed to an alcoholic chlorhexidine spray.[7]


1. Cheung J, O'Leary JJ. Allergic reaction to chlorhexidine in an anaesthetised patient. *Anaesth Intensive Care* 1985; **13:** 429–39.
2. Okano M, *et al.* Anaphylactic symptoms due to chlorhexidine gluconate. *Arch Dermatol* 1989; **125:** 50–2.
3. Evans RJ. Acute anaphylaxis due to topical chlorhexidine acetate. *BMJ* 1992; **304:** 686.
4. Chisholm DG, *et al.* Intranasal chlorhexidine resulting in an anaphylactic circulatory arrest. *BMJ* 1997; **315:** 785.
5. Visser LE, *et al.* Anafylaxie door chloorhexidine na cystoscopie of urethrale catheterisatie. *Ned Tijdschr Geneeskd* 1994; **138:** 778–80.

6. Anonymous. Hypersensitivity to chlorhexidine-impregnated medical devices. *JAMA* 1998; **279:** 1684.
7. Waclawski ER, *et al.* Occupational asthma in nurses caused by chlorhexidine and alcohol aerosols. *BMJ* 1989; **298:** 929–30.

**Poisoning.** Reports of adverse effects after ingestion of chlorhexidine salts include a neonate who developed multiple episodes of cyanosis and bradycardia;[1] the infant's mother had sprayed chlorhexidine onto her breasts to prevent mastitis. In contrast an 89-year-old woman only experienced mild giddiness, unusual laughter, and an increased appetite after mistakenly drinking 30 mL of a solution containing chlorhexidine gluconate 4% and isopropyl alcohol 4%.[2] There has also been a report of a patient who developed gastritis after ingesting a pre-operative skin preparation containing chlorhexidine gluconate 4% after using it as a mouthwash.[3] Another subject experienced much more serious effects in a suicide attempt after drinking about 150 mL of chlorhexidine gluconate solution, corresponding to about 30 g of the pure substance.[4] Besides pharyngeal oedema and necrotic oesophageal lesions, the patient had aminotransferase concentrations that rose to 30 times normal 5 days after ingestion and were still 8 times normal one week later. After one month the serum aspartate aminotransferase was returning to normal while the serum alanine aminotransferase was still 3 times normal. Six months after ingestion the aminotransferase levels were normal. A liver biopsy performed soon after the peak in aminotransferase levels showed diffuse fatty degeneration and lobular hepatitis suggesting that chlorhexidine was absorbed from the gastrointestinal tract in a concentration high enough to produce liver necrosis.

1. Quinn MW, Bini RM. Bradycardia associated with chlorhexidine spray. *Arch Dis Child* 1989; **64:** 892–3.
2. Emerson D, Pierce C. A case of a single ingestion of 4% Hibiclens. *Vet Hum Toxicol* 1988; **30:** 583.
3. Roche S, *et al.* Chlorhexidine-induced gastritis. *Postgrad Med J* 1991; **67:** 210–11.
4. Massano G, *et al.* Striking aminotransferase rise after chlorhexidine self-poisoning. *Lancet* 1982; **i:** 289.

## Precautions

Since chlorhexidine is irritant it is recommended that it should not be used on the brain, meninges, middle ear, or other sensitive tissues. Contact with the eye should be avoided except for dilute solutions expressly for use in the eyes. Chlorhexidine may be adsorbed by some soft contact lenses and cause eye irritation, although it may be suitable for use with others (see Contact Lens Care, p.1164). Syringes and needles that have been immersed in chlorhexidine solutions should be thoroughly rinsed with sterile water or saline before use.

Aqueous solutions of chlorhexidine salts may be susceptible to contamination with micro-organisms. To reduce this risk, a sterilised preparation should be used or, where necessary, solutions must be freshly prepared at the recommended concentration and appropriate measures should be taken to prevent contamination during storage or dilution.

Aqueous solutions of chlorhexidine used for instrument storage should contain sodium nitrite 0.1% to inhibit metal corrosion, and should be changed every 7 days. Commercial 5% concentrate contains a nonionic surfactant to prevent precipitation on dilution with hard water and is not suitable for use in body cavities or for disinfection of instruments containing cemented glass components; dilutions of the 20% concentrate should be used for this purpose.

**Contamination.** *Ralstonia pickettii* (*Burkholderia pickettii*; *Pseudomonas pickettii*) septicaemia developed in 6 patients after the use of aqueous chlorhexidine 0.05%, prepared with contaminated twice-distilled water, for skin disinfection before venepuncture and it was considered that unsterilised 0.05% solutions should not be used for such skin preparation.[1] Positive blood cultures of *Burkholderia cepacia* (*Pseudomonas cepacia*) were found in 2 patients after inappropriate use of a chlorhexidine handwash for the same purpose.[2] Further studies showed that the handwash supported pseudomonal growth only when diluted.[3]

1. Kahan A, *et al.* Is chlorhexidine an essential drug? *Lancet* 1984; **ii:** 759–60.
2. Gosden PE, Norman P. Pseudobacteraemia associated with contaminated skin cleansing agent. *Lancet* 1985; **ii** 671–2.
3. Norman P, *et al.* Pseudobacteraemia associated with contaminated skin cleansing agent. *Lancet* 1986; **i:** 209.

**Neonates.** Haemorrhagic skin necrosis associated with umbilical artery catheterisation in a premature infant was attributed to damage by the alcohol from the use of chlorhexidine 0.5% in spirit 70% as a disinfectant.[1]

For reference to the percutaneous absorption of chlorhexidine following topical use in neonates and infants, see Pharmacokinetics, below.

1. Harpin V, Rutter N. Percutaneous alcohol absorption and skin necrosis in a preterm infant. *Arch Dis Child* 1982; **57:** 477–9.

**Oral hygiene.** As toothpastes may contain anionic surfactants such as sodium laurilsulfate, which are incompatible with chlorhexidine, it has been recommended that at least 30 minutes should be allowed to elapse between the use of toothpaste and oral chlorhexidine preparations.[1]

1. Barkvoll P, *et al.* Interaction between chlorhexidine digluconate and sodium lauryl sulfate in vivo. *J Clin Periodontol* 1989; **16:** 593–5.

**Washing precautions.** Fabrics that have been in contact with chlorhexidine solution may develop a brown stain if bleached with a hypochlorite. A peroxide bleach may be used instead.

## Pharmacokinetics

Chlorhexidine is poorly absorbed from the gastrointestinal tract and skin.

**Neonates.** Occasional reports of the percutaneous absorption of chlorhexidine in neonates and infants include a study in which chlorhexidine was detected in low concentrations in the venous blood of 5 of 24 infants after washing them with a preparation containing chlorhexidine gluconate 4% (Hibiscrub); no adverse effects were observed.[1] Low concentrations have been found[2] in the venous blood of neonates following the topical use of a powder containing chlorhexidine 1%. Percutaneous absorption of chlorhexidine was reported in preterm neonates (but not full-term infants) treated with chlorhexidine 1% in alcohol for neonatal cord care; no such absorption occurred when a dusting powder containing chlorhexidine 1% and zinc oxide 3% was used.[3]

1. Cowen J, *et al.* Absorption of chlorhexidine from the intact skin of newborn infants. *Arch Dis Child* 1979; **54:** 379–83.
2. Alder VG, *et al.* Comparison of hexachlorophane and chlorhexidine powders in prevention of neonatal infection. *Arch Dis Child* 1980; **55:** 277–80.
3. Aggett PJ, *et al.* Percutaneous absorption of chlorhexidine in neonatal cord care. *Arch Dis Child* 1981; **56:** 878–91.

## Uses and Administration

Chlorhexidine is a bisbiguanide antiseptic and disinfectant that is bactericidal or bacteriostatic against a wide range of Gram-positive and Gram-negative bacteria. It is more effective against Gram-positive than Gram-negative bacteria, and some species of *Pseudomonas* and *Proteus* have low susceptibility. It is relatively ineffective against mycobacteria. Chlorhexidine inhibits some viruses and is active against some fungi. It is inactive against bacterial spores at room temperature. Chlorhexidine is most active at a neutral or slightly acid pH. Combinations of chlorhexidine with cetrimide (p.1172) or in alcoholic solution are used to enhance efficacy.

Chlorhexidine is formulated as lotions, washes, and creams for disinfection and cleansing of skin and wounds (p.1139), and as oral gels, sprays, and mouthwashes for mouth infections including candidiasis and to reduce dental plaque accumulation. It has also been used with neomycin to eliminate nasal carriage of staphylococci (p.147) and for disinfection of some contact lenses (but see Precautions, above). It has been suggested for use with propamidine isetionate for the treatment of Acanthamoeba keratitis and in spermicides to prevent transmission of HIV infection (p.623).

For pre-operative skin disinfection and hand-washing, chlorhexidine is used as a 0.5% solution of the acetate or gluconate in alcohol (70%) or as a 2 or 4% detergent solution of the gluconate. For disinfection of wounds, burns, or other skin damage or disorders chlorhexidine is used as a 0.05% aqueous solution of the acetate or gluconate, as a tulle dressing impregnated with chlorhexidine acetate 0.5%, or as a cream or powder containing chlorhexidine acetate or gluconate 1%. Preparations containing chlorhexidine acetate or gluconate 0.015% and cetrimide 0.15% are also used for cleansing and disinfection of skin and wounds. In obstetrics, chlorhexidine gluconate is used as a 0.05% aqueous solution or a 1% cream. The cream is also used as a barrier against bacterial hand infection.

Chlorhexidine gluconate is used in a 1% dental gel, 0.2% oral spray, and 0.1 to 0.2% mouthwash for the prevention of plaque and the prevention and treatment of gingivitis and in the treatment of oral candidiasis. A slow-release formulation for insertion into periodontal pockets is also available.

A 0.02% solution may be used as a bladder irrigation in some urinary-tract infections. A gel containing 0.25% chlorhexidine gluconate solution and lidocaine hydrochloride has been used in catheterisation and cystoscopy.

For the emergency disinfection of clean instruments, a 2-minute immersion in chlorhexidine acetate or gluconate 0.5% in alcohol (70%) is used; for the storage and disinfection of clean instruments a 30-minute immersion in a 0.05% aqueous solution containing 0.1% sodium nitrite to inhibit metal corrosion is used.

As an antimicrobial preservative, chlorhexidine is used at a concentration of 0.01% of the acetate or gluconate in eye drops. Solutions containing 0.002 to 0.006% of chlorhexidine gluconate have also been used for disinfection of hydrophilic contact lenses.

**Acanthamoeba infections.** As discussed on p.595, the optimal antiamoebic therapy for *Acanthamoeba* keratitis has yet to be determined. Propamidine isetionate is commonly used, usually in combinations including a biguanide. Chlorhexidine gluconate 0.02% with propamidine isetionate 0.1% has been suggested.[1] However, concern has been expressed over the possible toxicity of chlorhexidine at this concentration on the cornea.[2]

Chlorhexidine is also an effective disinfectant against *Acanthamoeba* cysts and most bacteria found in contact lens storage cases.[1]

Chlorhexidine has also been used to treat skin lesions associated with disseminated *Acanthamoeba* infection[3] as an adjunct to systemic therapy (see p.595).

1. Seal DV. Acanthamoeba keratitis. *BMJ* 1994; **308:** 1116–17.
2. Elder MJ, Dart JKG. Chemotherapy for acanthamoeba keratitis. *Lancet* 1995; **345:** 791–2.
3. Slater CA, *et al.* Brief report: successful treatment of disseminated Acanthamoeba infection in an immunocompromised patient. *N Engl J Med* 1994; **331:** 85–7.

**Contraception.** Bisbiguanides of the chlorhexidine type are reported to have the ability to diffuse into cervical mucus and render it impenetrable to sperm at concentrations as low as 1 mg/mL.[1] Higher concentrations of chlorhexidine structurally modify the mucus, producing a barrier to both the entry of sperm and chlorhexidine. The potency[1] of chlorhexidine in inhibiting sperm motility *in vitro* is identical to that of nonoxinol 9, but unlike spermicides containing nonoxinol 9, which tend to trickle out, the clearance of chlorhexidine from the vagina is delayed.[2] Chlorhexidine also has potential for reducing transmission of HIV infection as it does not disrupt the vaginal epithelium and has activity *in vitro* against the HIV virus in low concentrations.[2]

For a review of contraception, including the view that spermicides are not a particularly effective method unless used with other means of contraception, see p.1535.

1. Pearson RM. Update on vaginal spermicides. *Pharm J* 1985; **234:** 686–7.
2. Anonymous. Multipurpose spermicides. *Lancet* 1992; **340:** 211–13.

**Disinfection.** Viable bacterial counts on the hands were reduced by a mean of 97.9% by the application of chlorhexidine gluconate 0.5% in alcohol 95%.[1] The reduction was not so substantial with a 0.5% chlorhexidine aqueous solution (65.1% reduction in bacterial count) or a 4% detergent solution (86.7%). Hand disinfection with chlorhexidine gluconate 4% appeared to be more effective than the use of isopropyl alcohol 60% and soap in preventing nosocomial infections in a study conducted in intensive care units but this may have been partly due to better compliance with hand-washing instructions when using chlorhexidine.[2] In another study,[3] pre-operative total body bathing with a 4% detergent did not decrease the risk of wound infection in patients compared with bathing in detergent alone.

Chlorhexidine 1% nasal cream failed to control an epidemic of meticillin-resistant *Staphylococcus aureus* in a neurosurgical ward[4] and handwashing with chlorhexidine soap failed to control an outbreak of infection with *Staph. aureus* resistant to meticillin and gentamicin in a neonatal intensive care unit.[5] The organisms were subsequently eradicated by the use of nasal mupirocin and hexachlorophene handwashing, respectively.

1. Lowbury EJL, *et al.* Preoperative disinfection of surgeons' hands: use of alcoholic solutions and effects of gloves on skin flora. *BMJ* 1974; **4:** 369–72.
2. Doebbeling BN, *et al.* Comparative efficacy of alternative hand-washing agents in reducing nosocomial infections in intensive care units. *N Engl J Med* 1992; **327:** 88–93.
3. The European Working Party on Control of Hospital Infections. A comparison of the effects of preoperative whole-body bathing with detergent alone and with detergent containing chlorhexidine gluconate on the frequency of wound infections after clean surgery. *J Hosp Infect* 1988; **11:** 310–20.
4. Duckworth G. New method for typing Staphylococcus aureus resistant to methicillin. *BMJ* 1986; **293:** 885.
5. Reboli AC, *et al.* Epidemic methicillin-gentamicin-resistant Staphylococcus aureus in a neonatal intensive care unit. *Am J Dis Child* 1989; **143:** 34–9.

INJECTION SITE AND CATHETER CARE. See p.1165.

**Endocarditis.** Antiseptics applied immediately before dental procedures may reduce postextraction bacteraemia. Chlorhexidine mouthwash or gel may be used as an adjunct to antibacterial prophylaxis in dental patients at risk of bacterial endocarditis.[1,2] The protective cover required for such patients is discussed in detail on p.125.

1. Dajani AS, *et al.* Prevention of bacterial endocarditis: recommendations by the American Heart Association. *JAMA* 1997; **277:** 1794–1801.
2. Simmons NA, *et al.* Antibiotic prophylaxis and infective endocarditis. *Lancet* 1992; **339:** 1292–3.

**Mouth disorders.** Chlorhexidine mouthwashes, sprays, and gels are used to prevent accumulation of dental plaque (see Mouth Infections, p.136). Studies have generally shown chlorhexidine mouthwash 0.1 to 0.2% used 2 or 3 times daily to be effective in reducing plaque accumulation and gingivitis,[1-4] and to be superior to other disinfectant mouthwashes.[5] Its effect against subgingival plaque bacteria is enhanced by phenoxyethanol.[6] However, a 1% gel used nightly as a toothpaste was not more effective than placebo in reducing gingivitis in children.[7] Other studies have shown that chlorhexidine reduces gingivitis by 60 to 90% but its use is limited by its unpleasant taste and staining properties; special circumstances in which chlorhexidine is helpful include management of acute gingivitis, control of periodontal involvement in immunocompromised patients, and promotion of healing after periodontal treatment.[8]

Chlorhexidine gluconate may be useful in controlling secondary bacterial infections of aphthous ulcers (see Mouth Ulceration, p.1245). Local application of chlorhexidine has been reported to reduce the incidence[9] and duration and severity[10] of recurrent ulcers, although one study showed no benefit compared with placebo.[11]

Chlorhexidine may be a useful adjunct to antifungal treatment of oral candidiasis[12] (p.386).

For the need for a delay when using chlorhexidine with other oral hygiene preparations, see under Precautions, above.


1. Flötra L, *et al.* A 4-month study on the effect of chlorhexidine mouth washes on 50 soldiers. *Scand J Dent Res* 1972; **80:** 10–17.
2. O'Neil TCA, Figures KH. The effects of chlorhexidine and mechanical methods of plaque control on the recurrence of gingival hyperplasia in young patients taking phenytoin. *Br Dent J* 1982; **152:** 130–3.
3. de la Rosa M, *et al.* The use of chlorhexidine in the management of gingivitis in children. *J Periodontol* 1988; **59:** 387–9.
4. O'Neil TCA. The use of chlorhexidine mouthwash in the control of gingival inflammation. *Br Dent J* 1976; **141:** 276–80.
5. Brecx M, *et al.* Efficacy of Listerine, Meridol and chlorhexidine mouthrinses on plaque, gingivitis and plaque bacteria vitality. *J Clin Periodontol* 1990; **17:** 292–7.
6. Wilson M, *et al.* Effect of phenoxyethanol, chlorhexidine and their combination on subgingival plaque bacteria. *J Antimicrob Chemother* 1990; **25:** 921–9.
7. Hoyos DF, *et al.* The effect of chlorhexidine gel on plaque and gingivitis in children. *Br Dent J* 1977; **142:** 366–9.
8. Greene JC, *et al.* Preventive dentistry II: periodontal diseases, malocclusion, trauma, and oral cancer. *JAMA* 1990; **263:** 421–5.
9. Hunter L, Addy M. Chlorhexidine gluconate mouthwash in the management of minor aphthous ulceration. *Br Dent J* 1987; **162:** 106–10.
10. Addy M, *et al.* Management of recurrent aphthous ulceration: a trial of chlorhexidine gluconate gel. *Br Dent J* 1976; **141:** 118–20.
11. Matthews RW, *et al.* Clinical evaluation of benzydamine, chlorhexidine, and placebo mouthwashes in the management of recurrent aphthous stomatitis. *Oral Surg Oral Med Oral Pathol* 1987; **63:** 189–91.
12. WHO. *WHO model prescribing information: drugs used in skin diseases.* Geneva: WHO, 1997.


**Obstetric use.** Cleansing of the birth canal with chlorhexidine gluconate 0.25% has not been shown to reduce perinatal transmission of HIV except when membranes were ruptured for more than 4 hours before delivery,[1] although it has been reported to reduce neonatal morbidity and mortality from other neonatal infections in Africa.[2] In Swedish hospitals, flushing the vagina every 6 hours during labour with chlorhexidine acetate 0.2% reduced the incidence of transmission of group B streptococci but a reduction in neonatal morbidity was not demonstrated.[3,4] Comparable results have been reported with the use of chlorhexidine gluconate 1% obstetric cream at each examination during labour.[5]


1. Biggar RJ, *et al.* Perinatal intervention trial in Africa: effect of a birth canal cleansing intervention to prevent HIV transmission. *Lancet* 1996; **347:** 1647–50.
2. Taha TE, *et al.* Effect of cleansing the birth canal with antiseptic solution on maternal and newborn morbidity and mortality in Malawi: clinical trial. *BMJ* 1997; **315:** 216–20.
3. Burman LG, *et al.* Prevention of excess neonatal morbidity associated with group B streptococci by vaginal chlorhexidine disinfection during labour. *Lancet* 1992; **340:** 65–9.
4. Burman LG, Tullus K. Vaginal chlorhexidine disinfection during labour. *Lancet* 1992; **340:** 791–2.
5. Lindemann R, *et al.* Vaginal chlorhexidine disinfection during labour. *Lancet* 1992; **340:** 792.


**Urinary-tract infection.** Chlorhexidine solutions have been used in the management of catheter-related bladder infections and for urinary catheter maintenance. Twice-daily bladder irrigation with chlorhexidine acetate 0.02% did not produce a reduction in urinary bacterial counts in geriatric patients with indwelling catheters, and there was a tendency for overgrowth of *Proteus* spp. in patients given chlorhexidine.[1] In patients undergoing prostatectomy, intermittent pre-operative bladder irrigation with chlorhexidine gluconate 0.05% reduced the incidence of bacteraemia and severe wound infection, although urinary infections were eradicated in only 3 of the 13 patients treated.[2]

Addition of chlorhexidine to catheter drainage bags was not shown to reduce the frequency of urinary infections,[3] but infection rates were reduced by combining this technique with the use of a catheter lubricant containing chlorhexidine, disinfection of the urethral meatus, and aseptic nursing procedures.[4] The use of lubricating gel containing chlorhexidine did not reduce the risk of urinary-tract infections associated with short-term catheterisation.[5]

The treatment of urinary-tract infections is discussed on p.153.


1. Davies AJ, *et al.* Does instillation of chlorhexidine into the bladder of catheterized geriatric patients help reduce bacteriuria? *J Hosp Infect* 1987; **9:** 72–5.
2. Adesanya AA, *et al.* The use of intermittent chlorhexidine bladder irrigation in the prevention of post-prostatectomy infective complications. *Int Urol Nephrol* 1993; **25:** 359–67.
3. Gillespie WA, *et al.* Does the addition of disinfectant to urine drainage bags prevent infection in catheterised patients? *Lancet* 1983; **i:** 1037–9.
4. Southampton Infection Control Team. Evaluation of aseptic techniques and chlorhexidine on the rate of catheter-associated urinary-tract infection. *Lancet* 1982; **i:** 89–91.
5. Schiøtz HA. Antiseptic catheter gel and urinary tract infection after short-term postoperative catheterization in women. *Arch Gynecol Obstet* 1996; **258:** 97–100.


## Preparations

***BP 2003:*** Chlorhexidine Irrigation Solution; Chlorhexidine Mouthwash; Lidocaine and Chlorhexidine Gel;
***USP 27:*** Chlorhexidine Gluconate Oral Rinse.

**Proprietary Preparations** (details are given in Part 3)
***Arg.:*** Antiminth; Elgydium; Finaplac; Hexidin; Hexil; Hiboquad; Laclorhex; Plac Out; Strictus; ***Austral.:*** Anti-Plaque Chewing Gum†; Bactigras; Bush Formula†; Catheter Preparation; Chlorohex†; Clorhexitulle; Hexol; Hibiclens†; Hibitane†; Microshield 2, 4 and 5; Periogard Chlorohex†; Plaqacide†; Savacol Mouth and Throat Rinse†; ***Austria:*** Blend-a-Med Periochip; Chlorhexamed; Hexidin; Hibident; Kleenocid; Plak Out; Vitawund; ***Belg.:*** Astrexine; Baxil; Corsodyl; Golaseptine; Hibident†; Hibidil†; Hibiguard†; Hibiscrub†; Hibitane; Medisepta; Mefren Incolore; Mefren Pastilles; Pixidin†; Sterilon; Uro-Tainer; ***Braz.:*** Glucohex; Hibitane†; Marclorhex; Noplak; Periochip†; ***Canad.:*** Bactigras; Baxedin; Chlorhexseptic†; Hibidil; Hibitane; Oro-Clense†; Peridex; Rouhex-G†; Spectro Gram; Stanhexidine; ***Chile:*** AB; Agermin; Bucoseptil; Freshmel; Garonsept; Graneodin; Hibicrick; Hibiscrub; Oralgene; Ortoxine; Perident; Perio-Aid; Perioxidin; ***Denm.:*** Hibitane; Periochip; ***Fin.:*** Corsodyl; Hibiscrub†; Klorhexol; Travahex; ***Fr.:*** Biorgasept; Bucasept†; Collunovar; Corsodyl; D-Seb†; Diaseptyl; Dosiseptine; Elgydium; Elugel; Exoseptoplix; Hibidil; Hibiscrub; Hibisprint; Hibitane; Lysofon†; Merfene; Paroex; Plurexid; Prexidine; Septeal; ***Ger.:*** Bactigras; Cathejell S; Chlorhexamed; CHX Dental Gel; Cidegol C; Corsodyl†; Frubilurgyl; Gurgellosung Chauvin; Hansamed Spray; Lemocin CX; Mentopin Gurgellosung†; Nur 1 Tropfen Chlorhexidin; Periogard Chlorohex; Trachisan N; ***Hong Kong:*** Bactigras; Corsodyl; Hexol; Hibiscrub; Hibitane; Hydrex; ***Irl.:*** Corsodyl; Hibiscrub; Hibitane; Hydrex†; Rotersept†; ***Israel:*** Alcoxidine; Bactoscrub; Bactosept; Corsodyl; Medident; Medipe†; Periochip; Periodentix†; Pharma-Dentix; Septadine Scrub; Septal; Septalone; Septol; Tarodent; Uniscrub; Unisept; ***Ital.:*** Benodent CLX; Broxodin; Clorexident†; Clorosan; Contact†; Corsodyl; D-Seb†; Dempol; Dentosan Clorexidina; Dentosan Parodontale; Eburos; Effetre†; Ekuba; Esoform Mani; Golasan; Golasol†; Hibiscrub†; Lenil; Lenixil†; Lyasin†; Master-Aid; N32 Collutorio†; Neo Perginol; Neo-Destomygen; Neomercurocromo; Neoxene; Neoxinal; Odontoxina†; Oralsan†; Parodontax; Periogard Chlorohex; Plak; Plak Out; Sanoral†; Triseptil; Vaxidina†; ***Malaysia:*** Antibex; Antisol; Hibiscrub; Hibisol; Hibitane; Oradex; Sepsol; ***Mex.:*** Hibiscrub; Perioxidin; ***Neth.:*** Corsodyl; Hibiscrub†; Hibitane; Sterilon; Urogliss-S; ***Norw.:*** Corsodyl; Hexidin†; Hibiscrub; Hibitane; ***NZ:*** DP Hand Rub; Hibiclens†; Hibitane; Riotane; ***Port.:*** Bexident; Chlorohex†; Corsodyl†; Dialens; Hibiscrub†; Hibitane†; Periogard Chlorohex†; Plak Out; ***S.Afr.:*** Bactigras; Hibidil; Hibiscrub; Hibitane†; Orosept; ***Singapore:*** Chlorohex; Elugel; Hibiscrub†; Hibitane†; ***Spain:*** Antisept†; Clorxil; Cristalcrom; Cristalmina; Curafil; Cuvefilm; Deratin; Hibimax; Hibiscrub; Menalmina; Odol Med Dental†; Septisan; Sterilon†; ***Swed.:*** Cervitec; Corsodyl; Descutan; Hexident; Hibiscrub; Hibitane; Periochip; ***Switz.:*** Chlorhexamed; Chlorohex; Collunovar†; Corsodyl; Dentohexine; Hibidil; Hibiscrub; Hibitane; Lifo-Scrub; ***Thai.:*** Bacard Antiseptic; Bactigras; C-20; Chlorhex; Desmanol G; Hexene; Hexide; Hexol; Hibiscrub; Hibitane; Hidine; Hydrex; ***UAE:*** Zordyl; ***UK:*** Acriflex; Bactigras; Cepton; Chlorasept†; Chlorohex; Corsodyl; CX Powder; Elgydium; Hibiscrub; Hibitane; Hydrex; Periochip†; pHiso-MED†; Savlon Antiseptic Wound Wash; Serotulle; Spotoway; Sterets Unisept†; Sterexidine†; Steripod Chlorhexidine Gluconate; Uniscrub†; Uriflex C; ***USA:*** Betasept; Dyna-Hex; Exidine; Hibiclens; Hibistat; Peridex; Periochip; Periogard.

**Multi-ingredient:** ***Arg.:*** Antisepthic Hexil; Consil; Dexatopic; Drill; Elgyfluor; Eludril; Fluorexidina; Instillagel; Parodium; Periobacter; Periodent; Restaurene; ***Austral.:*** Curacleanse; Difflam-C; Egomycol†; Hamilton Body Lotion; Hamilton Cleansing Lotion; Hemocane; Hibicet†; Hibicol†; Hibitane†; Medi Creme†; Medi Pulv†; Microshield Antiseptic; Microshield Handrub; Microshield Tincture; Mycil Healthy Feet; Nasalate; Oralife Peppermint†; Paraderm Plus; Pro-PS†; Savlon Antiseptic; Seda-Gel; Silvazine; Soov Cream; Xylocaine Jelly with Chlorhexidine; ***Austria:*** Bepanthen Plus; Cathejell; Cathejell mit Lidocain; Dermaspray; Endosgel; Instillagel; Luuf-Halspastillen; Luuf-Halspastillen fur Kinder; Salbei-Halspastillen; Skinsept mucosa; Uromont; Vitawund; ***Belg.:*** Angiocine; Cetavlex; Dermaspray; HAC†; Hacdil-S†; Hibitane; Instillagel; Medica; Neo-Cutigenol; Neo-Golaseptine; Nestosyl†; Sedasept†; Vita-Mefren; ***Braz.:*** Effaclar; Flex-Care†; ***Canad.:*** Clearasil Sensitive Skin Cleanser†; Flamazine C; Ic-Gel†; Savlodil; Savlon†; Spectro Tar; ***Chile:*** AB Antitusivo; Endogel Esteril; Freshmel Tos; Graneodin N; Graneodin-Tos; Halita; Medisept; Oralgene; Perio-Aid c Cloruro de Cetilpiridinio; ***Denm.:*** Hexokain; Instillagel; Xylocain Klorhexidin†; ***Fin.:*** Citanest†; Dexatopic†; Duocort; Sibicort; Toncils; ***Fr.:*** Amygdol†; Antalyre; Aphtoral; Biseptine; Cantalene; Chlorispray; Collupressine†; Collustan†; Cyteal; Dacryne; Dermaspraid Antiseptique; Dermobacter; Desocort†; Dontopivalone†; Drill; Elgyfluor; Eludril; Instillagel; Isodril†; Lysofon†; Mercryl; Nostril; Parodium; Parogencyl anti-age gencives; Parogencyl sensibilite gencives; Paroplak; Posine; Sophtal; Spitaderm; Thiovalone; Visiodose†; ***Ger.:*** Cathejell mit Lidocain; Cathejell†; Desmanol; Endosgel; Hermalind; Hexoraletten N; Instillagel; Nystalocal; Skinman Intensiv†; Skinsept F; Skinsept mucosa; Trachisan; Uro-Stilloson; ***Hong Kong:*** Difflam-C; Hibicet Hospital Concentrate; Hibisol; Instillagel; Medicreme; Medipulv; Mycil; Norgotin†; Oragesic; Trachisan; ***India:*** Iteol-3; Silverex; ***Irl.:*** Alltracel S; Germolene First Aid†; Hibicet; Hibisol; Instillagel; Mycil; Naseptin; Nystaform; Nystaform-HC; Savlon; ***Israel:*** Bepanthen Plus; Cathejell; Cetrin; Dermaor†; Hexidin†; Instillagel; Merphen; Savior; Septacare; Septadine; Sterets H; Tisept; Travasept; Vita-Merfen NF; ***Ital.:*** Anadermin†; Baxidin; Benodent; Benodent Gel Gengivale; Cetrexidin; Cetrisan; Citromed; Citromed 80 and 85; Citromed Chirurgico; Citromedics Pronto; Citrosteril Pronto; Clorexan; Clorexan Ferri; Clorexident Ortodontico†; Clotramid; Cuprosodio Plus; Dentaton Antisettico†; Dentosan Azione Intensiva; Dentosan Mese; Dentosan Placca & Carie; Eso Ferri Plus; Eso S 80; Esoform Maniferri†; Esosan Pronto; Farvicett; Germozero Hospital†; Handexin; Hibicet†; Hibizene; Jalovis†; Larilon†; Levaknel†; Medical Pic†; Neo-Stomygen; Panseptil; PR 100-Cloressidina†; Rexichlor; Simp; Simpottantacinque; Spitaderm; Steridol; Videorelax; ***Malaysia:*** Difflam-C; Elan-Forte; Hibicet; Horf; Oral-Aid; Trachisan; ***Mex.:*** Instillagel; Perioxidin; ***Mon.:*** Akila mains et peau†; ***Neth.:*** Dexatopic†; Hibicet concentraat†; Hibicet verdunning†; Hibisol†; Urogliss; ***Norw.:*** Bacimycin; Citanest†; ***NZ:*** Acnederm Foaming Wash; Acnederm Wash; Conditioning Solution; Difflam-C; Egomycol; Hibicet†; Medicreme; Medipulv; Oralife Peppermint; Paraderm Plus; Savlon; Silvazine; Soov Cream; Xylocaine with Chlorhexidine; ***Port.:*** Alkagin; Alphacedre; Bepanthene; Bepanthene Plus; Biofluor; Cyteal; Drill; Eludril; Hibitane; Hibitane Menta; Lactigriet; Savlon†; ***S.Afr.:*** Andolex-C; Burnocaine†; Hibicet; Naseptin†; Orochlor; Savlon†; ***Singapore:*** Cyteal; Difflam-C; Eludril; Hibicet Hospital Concentrate†; Hibisol†; Oral-Aid; Savlon; Silvazine; Soov Cream; Trachisan; ***Spain:*** Angileptol; Bucodrin; Bucometasana; Bucospray; Cloraseptic†; Drill; Eludril; Faringesic; Gargaril; Garydol†; Hibitane; Mastiol; Menalcol; Mercryl Plus; Salvesept†; ***Swed.:*** Instillagel; ***Switz.:*** Adro-derm†; Antebor N; Bepanthene Plus; Cathejell N†; Collu-Blache; Collunosol-N; Eludril; Endosgel†; Eubucal; Galamila; Gleitmittel; Hibital; Hibitane Teinture; Instillagel†; Kamillosan†; Lidohex; Merfen; Nystacortone; Nystalocal; Rhinipan†; Secalan†; Trachisan†; Vita-Hexin; Vita-Merfen; ***Thai.:*** Bacard; Cathejell with Lidocaine; Chlorhex-C; Dekka; Frebac; Hibicet; Inhibac; Sepdine; Septone; ***UK:*** Cathejell with Lidocaine; Clearasil Pore Cleansing Lotion; Covonia Throat Spray; Dermol; Eludril; Germolene; Germoloids; Hibicet; Hibisol; Instillagel; Medi-Swab H; Medi-Wipe; Mycil; Naseptin; Nystaform; Nystaform-HC; Primahex†; Quinoderm Antibacterial Face Wash; Savlon Antiseptic Cream; Savlon Antiseptic Liquid; Sterets H; Steripod Chlorhexidine Gluconate with Cetrimide; Tisept; Torbetol; Travasept; Xylocaine Antiseptic†; ***USA:*** BactoShield.

---

## Chlorinated Lime

Bleaching Powder; Cal clorada; Calcaria Chlorata; Calcii Hypochloris; Calcium Hypochlorite; Calcium Hypochlorosum; Calx Chlorata; Calx Chlorinata; Chloride of Lime; Chlorkalk; Chlorure de Chaux; Cloruro de Cal.

*CAS — 7778-54-3.*

**Pharmacopoeias.** In *Br., Jpn,* and *Swiss.*

**BP 2003** (Chlorinated Lime). A dull white powder with a characteristic odour, containing not less than 30.0% w/w of 'available chlorine'. It becomes moist and gradually decomposes on exposure to air, carbon dioxide being absorbed and chlorine evolved. Partly soluble in water and in alcohol.

### Adverse Effects, Treatment, and Precautions

As for Sodium Hypochlorite, p.1192.

### Uses and Administration

Chlorinated lime is a disinfectant and antiseptic with the general properties of chlorine (p.1175).

Its action is rapid but brief, the 'available chlorine' soon being exhausted by combination with organic material. It is used to disinfect faeces, urine, and other organic material, and as a cleansing agent for lavatories, drains, and effluents.

Chlorinated lime is used in the preparation of Surgical Chlorinated Soda Solution (BPC 1973) (Dakin's Solution) which has been employed as a wound disinfectant, and Chlorinated Lime and Boric Acid Solution (BP 1993), (Eusol), which has been used as a disinfectant lotion and wet dressing, sometimes with equal parts of liquid paraffin. However, such solutions are irritant when applied undiluted, and are no longer recommended for use in this way. In addition, there is some evidence that such chlorine-releasing solutions may delay wound healing (see Disinfection, Wounds under Uses and Administration of Chlorine, p.1176).

### Preparations

***BPC 1973:*** Surgical Chlorinated Soda Solution.

---

# Chlorine

925; Cloro.

$Cl_2$ = 70.906.

*CAS — 7782-50-5.*

**Description.** Chlorine is a greenish-yellow gas with a suffocating odour; commonly available as a pressurised liquid.

## Adverse Effects and Treatment

Chlorine gas is irritant and corrosive producing inflammation, burns, and necrosis. Inhalation may result in coughing, choking, headache, dyspnoea, dizziness, expectoration of frothy white sputum (which may be blood stained), a burning chest pain, and nausea. Bronchospasm, laryngeal oedema, acute pulmonary oedema with cyanosis, and hypoxia may occur. There may be vomiting and development of acidosis. Death may result from hypoxia.

Some of the toxicity of chlorine may be due to its dissolution in tissue water to produce hydrochloric acid and hypochlorite. After exposure to chlorine, conjunctivitis may require a topical anaesthetic and frequent irrigations of water or saline. Respiratory distress should be treated with inhalations of humidified oxygen and bronchodilators; mechanical ventilation may be required. Corticosteroids have been given in an attempt to minimise pulmonary damage. Acidosis may require the intravenous use of sodium bicarbonate or other suitable alkalising agent.

◊ Experience gained from 186 cases of acute chlorine exposure indicated that medical support was required for only a short time even when exposure was repeated;[1] late sequelae were not observed, even in patients with abnormal respiratory function tests or blood gases on admission. Another report on 76 children with chlorine poisoning revealed that the longest period of hospitalisation was 12 hours.[2] There have been reports of deliberate inhalation of chlorine,[3,4] in one instance for pleasure,[3] leading to severe adverse effects. Some individuals may be unduly insensitive to chlorine-induced irritation and workers should be warned that concentrations of chlorine which can be tolerated for short periods without undue discomfort can still cause serious injury which may not be immediately apparent.[4]

1. Barret L, Faure J. Chlorine poisoning. *Lancet* 1984; **i:** 561–2.
2. Fleta J, *et al.* Intoxication of 76 children by chlorine gas. *Hum Toxicol* 1986; **5:** 99–100.
3. Rafferty P. Voluntary chlorine inhalation: a new form of self-abuse? *BMJ* 1980; **281:** 1178–9.
4. Dewhurst F. Voluntary chlorine inhalation. *BMJ* 1981; **282:** 565–6.

**Effects on the eyes.** Eye examinations performed on 50 subjects immediately before and after swimming in a chlorinated pool (chlorine range 1.0 to 1.5 ppm) showed that 68% had symptoms of corneal oedema and 94% had corneal epithelial erosions. No subject experienced a measurable decrease in visual acuity.[1]

1. Haag JR, Gieser RG. Effects of swimming pool water on the cornea. *JAMA* 1983; **249:** 2507–8.

## Precautions

The antimicrobial activity of chlorine disinfectants is reduced by the presence of organic material and by increasing pH. Hypochlorite solutions may delay wound healing (see Disinfection: Wounds under Uses and Administration, below).

## Uses and Administration

Chlorine is a disinfectant with a rapid potent brief bactericidal action. It is capable of killing most bacteria, and some fungi, yeasts, algae, viruses, and protozoa. It is slowly active against spores.

It is used as liquid chlorine for the treatment of water (p.1165), but for most other purposes it is used in the form of hypochlorites, organic and inorganic chloramines, chlorinated hydantoins, chlorinated isocyanurates, and similar oxidising compounds capable of releasing chlorine. In the presence of water these compounds produce hypochlorous acid (HOCl) and hypochlorite ion ($OCl^-$) and it is generally considered that the lethal action on micro-organisms is due to chlorination of cell protein or enzyme systems by non-ionised hypochlorous acid, although the hypochlorite ion may also contribute.

The activity of most of the compounds decreases with increase of pH, the activity of solutions of pH 4 to 7 being greater than those of higher pH values. However, stability is usually greater at an alkaline pH.

The potency of chlorine disinfectants is expressed in terms of **available chlorine**. This is based on the concept of chlorine gas ($Cl_2$) as the reference substance. Two atoms of chlorine (2 × Cl) yield in water only one molecule of hypochlorous acid (on which activity is based), while hypochlorites and chloramines yield one molecule of hypochlorous acid for each atom of chlorine as shown in the following equations:

$$Cl_2 + H_2O \leftrightarrow HOCl + H^+ + Cl^-$$

$$NaOCl + H_2O \leftrightarrow HOCl + NaOH$$

Thus the assayed chlorine in such compounds has to be multiplied by 2 to produce 'available chlorine'. The term 'active chlorine' has been used confusingly for either 'available chlorine' ($Cl_2$) or 'combined chlorine' (Cl).

Because they have relatively low residual toxicity, chlorine compounds are useful for the disinfection of relatively clean impervious surfaces, such as babies' feeding bottles, baths, and food and dairy equipment. A concentration of 100 to 300 ppm of 'available chlorine' is used; a detergent may be added to ensure wetting of the surface. Solutions containing 1000 ppm 'available chlorine' are recommended for minor surface contamination and as part of general good hygiene practice. Solutions containing 10 000 ppm 'available chlorine' are used to disinfect surfaces contaminated with spilled blood or body fluids; this strength is effective against viruses including human immunodeficiency virus (HIV) and hepatitis B virus (p.1165). A concentration providing 20 000 ppm 'available chlorine' is used for material from patients with Creutzfeldt-Jakob disease (p.1164).

On a large scale, chlorine gas is used to disinfect public water supplies. On a smaller scale, the use of chlorine compounds is more convenient and sodium hypochlorite, tosylchloramide sodium, chlorinated lime, chlorine dioxide, or halazone are used. After satisfying the chlorine demand (the amount of chlorine needed to react with organic matter and other substances), a free-residual content of 0.2 to 0.4 ppm 'available chlorine' should be maintained, though more is required for alkaline waters with a pH of 9 or more. For the disinfection of potentially contaminated water a concentration of 1 ppm is recommended. Excessive residual chlorine may be removed by adding a little citric acid or sodium thiosulfate.

For use in small swimming pools, sodium or calcium hypochlorite may be added daily to maintain a free-residual 'available chlorine' concentration of 1 to 3 ppm. Tosylchloramide sodium, chlorinated lime, and the isocyanurates (see Sodium Dichloroisocyanurate, p.1191) may also be used. To minimise irritation of the eyes, maintain disinfectant activity, prevent precipitation of salts, and prevent metal corrosion, a pH of 7.2 to 7.8 should be maintained.

Solutions of chlorine-releasing compounds are also used in wound desloughing and disinfection (but see below).

**Disinfection.** INSTRUMENTS. Needles and syringes should not usually be sterilised chemically. However, use of full-strength domestic bleach (about 5% sodium hypochlorite, about 2% of 'available chlorine') was reported to be effective for the cleaning by intravenous drug users of needles and syringes as a last resort in the absence of sterile equipment; a 30-second contact time was required.[1,2] A 1 in 10 dilution of bleach was not effective after 5 minutes' exposure.[2]

1. Donoghoe MC, Power R. Household bleach as disinfectant for use by injecting drug users. *Lancet* 1993; **341:** 1658.
2. Watters JK, *et al.* Household bleach as disinfectant for use by injecting drug users. *Lancet* 1993; **342:** 742–3.

WORMS. Sodium hypochlorite in aqueous solution at a concentration of 3.75% (or greater) is an effective ovicide for *Echinococcus* and may be used on hard surfaces, glassware, and sinks.[1]

1. Craig PS, Macpherson CNL. Sodium hypochlorite as an ovicide for Echinococcus. *Ann Trop Med Parasitol* 1988; **82:** 211–13.

WOUNDS. Hypochlorite solutions are now generally considered to be too irritant for use in the management of wounds (p.1139). Studies suggest that they may delay wound healing if repeatedly applied to open wounds.[1,2] It has been suggested that they may be of use in debriding burns (p.1134) or necrotic chronic wounds,[3] but also that any benefit that might be seen from the desloughing of necrotic tissue might be produced by damage of the superficial cell layer leading to separation[4] or from tissue hydration produced by wet dressing packs.[5] However, some burns units have found that hypochlorite as Dakin's solution (see Chlorinated Lime, above) produces better healing than other antibacterials.[6]

See also p.1165.

1. Thomas S, Hay NP. Wound healing. *Pharm J* 1985; **235:** 206.
2. Lineweaver W, *et al.* Topical antimicrobial toxicity. *Arch Surg* 1985; **120:** 267–70.
3. Leaper DJ. Eusol. *BMJ* 1992; **304:** 930–1.
4. Anonymous. Local applications to wounds—I: cleansers, antibacterials, debriders. *Drug Ther Bull* 1991; **29:** 93–5.
5. Thomas S. Milton and the treatment of burns. *Pharm J* 1986; **236:** 128–9.
6. Murphy KD, *et al.* Current pharmacotherapy for the treatment of severe burns. *Expert Opin Pharmacother* 2003; **4:** 369–84.

# Chlorine Dioxide

926.

$ClO_2$ = 67.45.
*CAS — 10049-04-4.*

## Profile

Chlorine dioxide is a strong oxidising agent with the general properties of chlorine (p.1175). It is rapidly active against vegetative bacteria, including mycobacteria, and viruses and is also sporicidal. It is used for disinfection of medical equipment either in gaseous form or in a solution that requires activation before use and yields 700 to 1100 ppm 'available chlorine' (see p.1176) . Chlorine dioxide is irritant to the skin, eyes, and respiratory tract and should be stored in sealed containers. It is potentially corrosive to many materials and solutions may contain corrosion inhibitors.

Chlorine dioxide is also used for treatment and disinfection of water supplies.

**Disinfection of endoscopes.** Chlorine dioxide solutions are used as an alternative to glutaral for the disinfection of endoscopes (p.1164).

**Halitosis.** Chlorine dioxide has been used in mouthrinses for the control of halitosis.[1]

1. Frascella J, *et al.* Odor reduction potential of a chlorine dioxide mouthrinse. *J Clin Dent* 1998; **9:** 39–42.

## Preparations

**Proprietary Preparations** (details are given in Part 3)
***UK:*** Retardent†; Retardex.

# Chloroacetamide

Chloracetamide; Cloroacetamida. 2-Chloroacetamide.
$C_2H_4ClNO$ = 93.51.
*CAS — 79-07-2.*

## Profile

Chloroacetamide is a preservative that has been used in topical pharmaceutical preparations and cosmetics.

# N-(3-Chloroallyl)hexaminium Chloride

N-(3-Cloroalil)hexaminio, cloruro de; Quaternium-15. 1-(3-Chloroallyl)-3,5,7-triaza-1-azoniaadamantane chloride.
$C_9H_{16}Cl_2N_4$ = 251.2.
*CAS — 4080-31-3.*

## Profile

*N*-(3-Chloroallyl)hexaminium chloride is an antimicrobial preservative used in pharmaceutical preparations and cosmetics. Skin reactions have been reported.

# Chlorobutanol *(BAN, rINN)*

Acetone-Chloroforme; Alcohol Trichlorisobutylicus; Chlorbutanol; Chlorbutanolum; Chlorbutol; Chloretone; Chlorobutanolum; Clorobutanol; Trichlorbutanolum. 1,1,1-Trichloro-2-methylpropan-2-ol.
$C_4H_7Cl_3O$ = 177.5.
*CAS — 57-15-8 (anhydrous chlorobutanol); 6001-64-5 (chlorobutanol hemihydrate).*
*ATC — A04AD04.*

**Pharmacopoeias.** *Eur.* (see p.vi), *Int.*, and *USNF* allow either the anhydrous form or the hemihydrate; *Eur.* includes them as separate monographs. *Chin.* specifies the hemihydrate. *Jpn* permits up to 6% of water.

**Ph. Eur. 5.0** (Chlorobutanol Hemihydrate; Chlorobutanol BP 2003). A white crystalline powder or colourless crystals. It sublimes readily. M.p. about 78°. Slightly soluble in water; very soluble in alcohol; soluble in glycerol (85%). Store in airtight containers.

**Ph. Eur. 5.0** (Chlorobutanol, Anhydrous). A white crystalline powder or colourless crystals. It sublimes readily. M.p. about 95°. Slightly soluble in water; very soluble in alcohol; soluble in glycerol (85%). Store in airtight containers.

**USNF 22** (Chlorobutanol). It is anhydrous or contains not more than one-half molecule of water of hydration. Colourless or white crystals with a characteristic, somewhat camphoraceous odour. M.p. about 76° for the hemihydrate and about 95° for the anhydrous form. Soluble 1 in 125 of water, 1 in 1 of alcohol, and 1 in 10 of glycerol; freely soluble in chloroform, in ether, and in volatile oils. Store in airtight containers.

**Incompatibility and stability.** The activity of chlorobutanol can be adversely affected by the presence of other compounds as well as by the packaging material. There may be sorption onto substances like magnesium trisilicate, bentonite, carmellose,[1] polyethylene,[2,3] or polyhydroxy-ethylmethacrylate that has been used in soft contact lenses.[4] Increasing heat[2,3] or pH[5,6] can reduce stability and activity.

1. Yousef RT, *et al.* Effect of some pharmaceutical materials on the bactericidal activities of preservatives. *Can J Pharm Sci* 1973; **8:** 54–6.
2. Friesen WT, Plein EM. The antibacterial stability of chlorobutanol stored in polyethylene bottles. *Am J Hosp Pharm* 1971; **28:** 507–12.
3. Holdsworth DG, *et al.* Fate of chlorbutol during storage in polyethylene dropper containers and simulated patient use. *J Clin Hosp Pharm* 1984; **9:** 29–39.
4. Richardson NE, *et al.* The interaction of preservatives with polyhydroxy-ethylmethacrylate (polyHEMA). *J Pharm Pharmacol* 1978; **30:** 469–75.
5. Nair AD, Lach JL. The kinetics of degradation of chlorobutanol. *J Am Pharm Assoc (Sci)* 1959; **48:** 390–5.
6. Patwa NV, Huyck CL. Stability of chlorobutanol. *J Am Pharm Assoc* 1966; **NS6:** 372–3.

## Adverse Effects

Acute poisoning with chlorobutanol may produce CNS depression with weakness, loss of consciousness, and depressed respiration. Delayed (type IV) hypersensitivity reactions have been reported rarely.

**Effects on the cardiovascular system.** Rapid falls in arterial blood pressure were observed following injections of heparin containing chlorobutanol in patients undergoing coronary bypass.[1] No fall in blood pressure was seen in patients who received preservative-free heparin injection.

1. Bowler GMR, *et al.* Sharp fall in blood pressure after injection of heparin containing chlorbutol. *Lancet* 1986; **i:** 848–9.

**Effects on mental function.** The sedative effects of chlorobutanol have been reported to be a problem in a patient dependent on large doses (0.9 to 1.5 g daily with salicylamide 1.8 to 3.0 g daily)[1] and in another patient given high doses of morphine in an infusion preserved with chlorobutanol.[2]

1. Borody T, *et al.* Chlorbutol toxicity and dependence. *Med J Aust* 1979; **i:** 288.
2. DeChristoforo R, *et al.* High-dose morphine infusion complicated by chlorobutanol-induced somnolence. *Ann Intern Med* 1983; **98:** 335–6.

**Hypersensitivity.** A delayed, cellular type of hypersensitivity reaction to chlorobutanol used to preserve heparin injection following subcutaneous injection has been reported.[1] Pruritus from intranasal desmopressin has been reported as being due to the chlorobutanol preservative.[2]

1. Dux S, *et al.* Hypersensitivity reaction to chlorbutanol-preserved heparin. *Lancet* 1981; **i:** 149.
2. Itabashi A, *et al.* Hypersensitivity to chlorobutanol in DDAVP solution. *Lancet* 1982; **i:** 108.

### Uses and Administration

Chlorobutanol has antibacterial and antifungal properties and it is used at a concentration of 0.5% as a preservative in injections and in eye drops as well as cosmetics.

Chlorobutanol has been used as a mild sedative and local analgesic but other compounds are preferred. It has been used in preparations for inflammatory and painful conditions of the ear and oropharynx.

### Preparations

**Proprietary Preparations** (details are given in Part 3)
***Port.:*** Vizoptal.

**Multi-ingredient:** ***Arg.:*** Eludril; Otocalmia; ***Austral.:*** Cerumol; ***Austria:*** Aleot; ***Belg.:*** Givalex; ***Braz.:*** Auritricin; Colirio Helios†; Lavolho†; Providex†; Visogenol†; ***Canad.:*** Aurisan†; Balminil Nasal Ointment; Cerumol; Gouttes pour Mal d'Oreilles†; Oralgar†; Outgro†; ***Fr.:*** Alodont; Angispray†; Balsamorhinol†; Eludril; Givalex; ***Ger.:*** Givalex; ***Hong Kong:*** Cerumol†; Fungifax; ***India:*** Andre; Waxolve; ***Irl.:*** Cerumol†; Karvol; ***Israel:*** Cepadont; Cerumol; Dentin; Karvol; Pitrisan; ***Ital.:*** Fialetta Odontalgica Dr Knapp; Odontalgiche (Dentali); ***Malaysia:*** Cerumol; ***NZ:*** Frador; ***Port.:*** Eludril; Otoceril; ***S.Afr.:*** Cerumol; Karvol; ***Singapore:*** Cerumol; Eludril; Karvol; ***Spain:*** Cloraseptic†; Eludril; Otocerum; ***Switz.:*** Alodont; Cerumenol; Demo baume†; Dental-Phenjoca†; Eludril; Spirogel†; ***Thai.:*** Opplin; Optal; ***UK:*** Aezodent†; Cerumol; Cetanorm; DDD; Dermidex; Eludril; Frador; Karvol; Monphytol; ***USA:*** Outgro.

## Chlorocresol *(USAN, rINN)*

Chlorkresolum; Chlorocresolum; Clorocresol; Parachlorometacresol; PCMC. *p*-Chloro-*m*-cresol; 4-Chloro-3-methylphenol.

$C_7H_7ClO$ = 142.6.
*CAS — 59-50-7.*

**Pharmacopoeias.** In *Eur.* (see p.vi) and *Int.* Also in *USNF.*

**Ph. Eur. 5.0** (Chlorocresol). A white or almost white, crystalline powder or compacted crystalline masses supplied as pellets or colourless or white crystals. M.p. 64° to 67°. Slightly soluble in water; very soluble in alcohol; freely soluble in fatty oils. It dissolves in solutions of alkali hydroxides. Protect from light.

**USNF 22** (Chlorocresol). Colourless or practically colourless crystals or crystalline powder with a characteristic nontarry odour; it is volatile in steam. M.p. 63° to 66°. Soluble 1 in 260 of water; more soluble in hot water; soluble 1 in 0.4 of alcohol; soluble in ether, in terpenes, in fixed oils, and in solutions of alkali hydroxides. Store in airtight containers. Protect from light.

**Incompatibility.** Chlorocresol has long been recognised to be incompatible with a range of compounds including: codeine phosphate, diamorphine hydrochloride, papaveretum, quinine hydrochloride,[1] methylcellulose,[2] and nonionic surfactants such as cetomacrogol 1000[3] and polysorbate 80.[4]

1. McEwan JS, Macmorran GH. The compatibility of some bactericides. *Pharm J* 1947; **158:** 260–2.
2. Harris WA. The inactivation of cationic antiseptics by bentonite suspensions. *Australas J Pharm* 1961; **42:** 583–8.
3. *PSGB Lab Report P/70/15* 1970.
4. Yousef RT, *et al.* Effect of some pharmaceutical materials on the bactericidal activities of preservatives. *Can J Pharm Sci* 1973; **8:** 54–6.

### Adverse Effects, Treatment, and Precautions

As for Phenol, p.1188. The antimicrobial activity of chlorocresol may be diminished through incompatibility (see above), through adsorption, through increasing pH, or through combination with organic matter (including oils and fats) or nonionic surfactants.

Chlorocresol is less toxic than phenol. Sensitisation reactions may follow application to the skin and hypersensitivity has occurred following systemic administration of injections containing chlorocresol as a preservative.

### Uses and Administration

Chlorocresol is a potent chlorinated phenolic disinfectant and antiseptic. It has bactericidal activity against Gram-positive and Gram-negative bacteria and is effective against fungi but has little activity against bacterial spores except at high temperatures. It is more active in acid than in alkaline solution.

Chlorocresol is used in various preparations for disinfection of the skin and wounds. It is also used as a preservative in cosmetics and in creams and other preparations for external use which contain water.

Chlorocresol is used as a preservative in aqueous injections issued in multidose containers. It may also be added to aqueous preparations that cannot be sterilised in their final containers and have to be prepared using aseptic precautions. Concentrations of 0.1% have generally been used. Injections prepared with chlorocresol should not be injected into the CSF, the eye, or the heart. Also such injections should generally not be administered in volumes greater than 15 mL. Sterilisation by heating with a bactericide such as chlorocresol in no longer a recommended practice.

### Preparations

***BPC 1973:*** Proflavine Cream.

**Proprietary Preparations** (details are given in Part 3)
***UK:*** Wright's Vaporizing Fluid†.

**Multi-ingredient:** ***Arg.:*** Perfungol; ***Austria:*** Ulcurilen; ***Chile:*** Perfungol; ***Fr.:*** Cicatryl; Cyteal; ***Ger.:*** Bacillotox†; Bomix; Grotanat†; Helipur; Ulcurilen N; ***Irl.:*** Anbesol; Valderma; ***Ital.:*** Helipur; Hygienist; ***Port.:*** Cyteal; ***Singapore:*** Cyteal; ***UK:*** Anbesol; Cymex; Valderma.

## Chlorothymol

Clorotimol; Monochlorothymol. 6-Chlorothymol; 4-Chloro-2-isopropyl-5-methylphenol.

$C_{10}H_{13}ClO$ = 184.7.
*CAS — 89-68-9.*

### Profile

Chlorothymol is a chlorinated phenolic antiseptic used as an ingredient of preparations for hand and skin disinfection and topical treatment of fungal infections. It has also been used in preparations for anorectal disorders, cold symptoms, and mouth disorders.

### Preparations

**Proprietary Preparations** (details are given in Part 3)
***Ital.:*** Pioral Pasta.

**Multi-ingredient:** ***Arg.:*** Solvex Liquido Fungicida; ***India:*** Karvol Plus; Sinarest Vapocaps; ***Ital.:*** Labocaina; Traumicid; Vagisil; ***Neth.:*** Rhinocaps†.

## Chloroxylenol *(BAN, USAN, rINN)*

Cloroxilenol; Parachlorometaxylenol; PCMX. 4-Chloro-3,5-xylenol; 4-Chloro-3,5-dimethylphenol.

$C_8H_9ClO$ = 156.6.
*CAS — 88-04-0.*
*ATC — D08AE05.*

**Pharmacopoeias.** In *Br.* and *US.*

**BP 2003** (Chloroxylenol). White or cream crystals or crystalline powder with a characteristic odour; volatile in steam. Very slightly soluble in water; freely soluble in alcohol; soluble in ether, in terpenes, in fixed oils, and in solutions of alkali hydroxides.

**USP 27** (Chloroxylenol). White crystals or crystalline powder with a characteristic odour; volatile in steam. Very slightly soluble in water; freely soluble in alcohol, in ether, in terpenes, in fixed oils, and in solutions of alkali hydroxides.

**Incompatibility.** Chloroxylenol has been reported to be incompatible with nonionic surfactants and methylcellulose.

### Adverse Effects and Precautions

Chloroxylenol in the recommended dilutions is generally non-irritant but skin sensitivity has occurred. There have been isolated reports of poisoning.

The antimicrobial activity of chloroxylenol may be diminished through combination with organic matter. Aqueous solutions of chloroxylenol may be susceptible to contamination with microorganisms. To reduce this risk, solutions must be freshly prepared at the recommended concentration and appropriate measures should be taken to prevent contamination during storage or dilution.

**Poisoning.** Reports of fatal[1] or severe[2,3] self-poisoning with chloroxylenol solution.

1. Meek D, *et al.* Fatal self-poisoning with Dettol. *Postgrad Med J* 1977; **53:** 229–31.
2. Joubert P, *et al.* Severe Dettol (chloroxylenol and terpineol) poisoning. *BMJ* 1978; **1:** 890.
3. Chan TYK, *et al.* Chemical gastro-oesophagitis, upper gastrointestinal haemorrhage and gastroscopic findings following Dettol poisoning. *Hum Exp Toxicol* 1995; **14:** 18–19.

### Uses and Administration

Chloroxylenol is a chlorinated phenolic antiseptic which is bactericidal against most Gram-positive bacteria but less active against staphylococci and Gram-negative bacteria, and is often inactive against *Pseudomonas* spp. Its activity against *Ps. aeruginosa* appears to be increased by the addition of edetic acid. It is inactive against bacterial spores.

Chloroxylenol Solution (BP 2003) is used for skin and wound disinfection, and chloroxylenol is used as a preservative in a variety of other topical formulations.

### Preparations

***BP 2003:*** Chloroxylenol Solution.

**Proprietary Preparations** (details are given in Part 3)
***Arg.:*** Espadol; Previnfec; Talowin; ***Austral.:*** Dettol Classic; ***Belg.:*** Dettol†; ***Canad.:*** Antiseptic Ointment; ***Hong Kong:*** Dettol; ***Irl.:*** Dettol; ***Ital.:*** Neomercurocromo; ***Malaysia:*** Dettol; ***NZ:*** Dettol; ***S.Afr.:*** Dettol†; ***Singapore:*** Dettol†; ***Thai.:*** Dettol; ***UK:*** Dettol; Prinsyl†.

**Multi-ingredient:** ***Arg.:*** Jabonacid; Kytinon; ZeaSorb; ***Austral.:*** Dettol Cream; Solyptol; ZeaSorb; ***Canad.:*** Acne-Aid†; Iba-Cide†; ZeaSorb; ***Chile:*** Acnaid; Dermac Crema; ZeaSorb; ***Ger.:*** Bacillotox†; Gehwol Fungizid; ZeaSorb†; ***Hong Kong:*** Acne-Aid; Dettol; ***India:*** Dettol Obstetric; Dettolin; ***Irl.:*** Dettol; ZeaSorb; ***Israel:*** Gargol; Hemo; Rexitol; ***Ital.:*** Foille Scottature; Foille Sole; Vironox†; ***Malaysia:*** Acne-Aid; Dettol; ZeaSorb; ***NZ:*** Dettol; ***S.Afr.:*** Dettol†; Respisniffers†; Woodwards Inhalant; ***Singapore:*** Acne-Aid; Dettol†; ZeaSorb; ***Thai.:*** Dettol; Johnson's Baby Prickly Heat Powder; ZeaSorb; ***UK:*** Dettol; Rinstead; Skintex; TCP; Waxwane; ZeaSorb; ***USA:*** Calamycin; Comfortine†; Cortane-B; Cortic; Cyotic; Dermacoat; Foille; Fungi-Nail; Gordochom; Lobana Peri-Garde; Otomar-HC; Pedi-Pro; PramOtic; Tri-Otic; Unguentine Plus; Zoto-HC.

## Cicliomenol *(rINN)*

2-Cyclohexyl-4-iodo-3,5-xylenol.

$C_{14}H_{19}IO$ = 330.2.
*CAS — 10572-34-6.*

### Profile

Cicliomenol is an antiseptic included in preparations intended for the topical treatment of mouth and throat infections.

### Preparations

**Proprietary Preparations** (details are given in Part 3)
***Ital.:*** Golamed.

**Multi-ingredient:** ***Fr.:*** Valda Septol†; ***Ital.:*** Golamed Due; Pastiglie Valda; Valda F3†.

## Cinnamic Acid

Cinámico, ácido; Cinnamylic Acid. *trans*-3-Phenylpropenoic acid.

$C_6H_5.CH:CH.CO_2H$ = 148.2.
*CAS — 621-82-9.*

**Pharmacopoeias.** In *Br.*

**BP 2003** (Cinnamic Acid). Colourless crystals with a faint balsamic odour. Very slightly soluble in water; freely soluble in alcohol; soluble in chloroform and in ether.

### Profile

Cinnamic acid has preservative properties. It is used with benzoic acid and other substances to simulate the flavour of tolu.

### Preparations

***BP 2003:*** Tolu-flavour Solution.

**Proprietary Preparations** (details are given in Part 3)

**Multi-ingredient:** ***Switz.:*** Spirogel†; ***UK:*** Hemocane; Potters Gees Linctus; Sanderson's Throat Specific.

## Cloponone *(BAN, rINN)*

(*RS*)-2,2-Dichloro-*N*-[4-chloro-α-(chloromethyl)phenacyl]acetamide.

$C_{11}H_9Cl_4NO_2$ = 329.0.
*CAS — 15301-50-5.*

### Profile

Cloponone is an antiseptic included in multi-ingredient preparations intended for the topical treatment of vaginal infections.

### Preparations

**Proprietary Preparations** (details are given in Part 3)

**Multi-ingredient:** ***Hong Kong:*** Ginetris.

## Clorophene *(USAN)*

Clorofene *(pINN)*; Clorfene; Clorofeno; NSC-59989; Septiphene. 2-Benzyl-4-chlorophenol.

$C_{13}H_{11}ClO$ = 218.7.
*CAS — 120-32-1.*

### Profile

Clorophene is a chlorinated phenolic antiseptic stated to be active against a wide range of bacteria, fungi, protozoa, and viruses. It is used as a skin disinfectant and for surface and instrument disinfection. Clorophene sodium has also been used.

### Preparations

**Proprietary Preparations** (details are given in Part 3)

**Multi-ingredient:** ***Belg.:*** Neo-Sabenyl; ***Canad.:*** Aseptone 1†; Aseptone 2†; Aseptone 5†; ***Fr.:*** Frekaderm†; ***Ger.:*** Bacillotox†; Bomix; Freka-Derm; Freka-Sept 80; Grotanat†; Helipur; ***Ital.:*** Helipur; Hygienist; ***Switz.:*** Frekaderm; ***UAE:*** Radol.

## Cresol

Cresylic Acid; Kresolum Venale; Tricresol; Trikresolum. Methylphenol.

$C_7H_8O$ = 108.1.
*CAS — 1319-77-3; 95-48-7 (o-cresol); 108-39-4 (m-cresol); 106-44-5 (p-cresol).*

NOTE. Some grades of mixed cresols may be equivalent to Tar Acids (p.1193).

**Pharmacopoeias.** In *Chin., Eur.* (see p.vi), and *Jpn.* Also in *USNF.*

*Eur.* also includes metacresol.

**Ph. Eur. 5.0** (Cresol, Crude; Cresolum Crudum). A mixture of *o*-, *m*-, and *p*-methylphenol. A colourless or pale brown liquid. Relative density 1.029 to 1.044. Sparingly soluble in water; miscible with alcohol and with dichloromethane. Protect from light.

**Ph. Eur. 5.0** (Metacresol; Metacresolum). A colourless or yellowish liquid. Relative density about 1.03. M.p. about 11°. Sparingly soluble in water; miscible with alcohol and with dichloromethane. Store in airtight containers. Protect from light.

**USNF 22** (Cresol). A mixture of cresol isomers obtained from coal tar or petroleum. A colourless, yellowish to brownish-yellow, or pinkish, highly refractive liquid, becoming darker with age or on exposure to light, with a phenol-like, sometimes empyreumatic odour. Specific gravity 1.030 to 1.038. Sparingly soluble in water, usually forming a cloudy solution; miscible with alcohol, with ether, and with glycerol; dissolves in solutions of fixed alkali hydroxides. A saturated solution in water is neutral or slightly acid to litmus. Store in airtight containers. Protect from light.

### Profile

Cresol is a disinfectant with a similar action to phenol (p.1188); suitable precautions should be taken to prevent absorption through the skin.

It has been used as Cresol and Soap Solution (BP 1968) (Lysol) as a general disinfectant but it has been largely superseded by other, less irritant, phenolic disinfectants. Cresol has been used in dentistry, alone or with formaldehyde, but is caustic to the skin and unsuitable for skin and wound disinfection. The cresols have been widely used in disinfectants for domestic and hospital use. Cresol is also used as an antimicrobial preservative in parenteral pharmaceutical preparations and in some topical formulations.

**Poisoning.** References to poisoning with cresol solutions.

1. Côté M-A, *et al.* Acute Heinz-body anaemia due to severe cresol poisoning: successful treatment with erythrocytapheresis. *Can Med Assoc J* 1984; **130:** 1319–22.
2. Wu ML, *et al.* Concentrated cresol intoxication. *Vet Hum Toxicol* 1998; **40:** 341–3.

### Preparations

**Proprietary Preparations** (details are given in Part 3)
***Ital.:*** Creolina.

**Multi-ingredient:** ***Arg.:*** Sulfanoral T; ***Austral.:*** Formo-Cresol Mitis†; ***Canad.:*** Gernel; ***Fr.:*** Eau Precieuse; ***Spain:*** Empapol†; Neodesfila†; Tifell; ***USA:*** Cresylate.

---

## Dehydroacetic Acid

Deshidroacético, ácido; Methylacetopyronone. 3-Acetyl-6-methyl-2*H*-pyran-2,4(3*H*)-dione (keto form); 3-Acetyl-4-hydroxy-6-methyl-2*H*-pyran-2-one (enol form).

$C_8H_8O_4$ = 168.1.

*CAS — 520-45-6 (keto form); 771-03-9 (enol form).*

## Sodium Dehydroacetate

Deshidroacetato sódico. The sodium salt of 3-acetyl-6-methyl-2*H*-pyran-2,4(3*H*)-dione.

$C_8H_7NaO_4$ = 190.1.

*CAS — 4418-26-2.*

**Pharmacopoeias.** In *USNF.*

**USNF 22** (Sodium Dehydroacetate). A white or practically white, odourless powder. Freely soluble in water, in glycerol, and in propylene glycol.

**Incompatibility.** The activity of sodium dehydroacetate may be reduced by alkaline pH or interaction with nonionic surfactants.

### Profile

Dehydroacetic acid and sodium dehydroacetate have some antifungal activity and have been used in the preservation of cosmetics.

---

## Dequalinium Chloride *(BAN, rINN)*

BAQD-10; Cloruro de decualinio; Decalinium Chloride; Decaminum; Dequalinii Chloridum. *N,N*-Decamethylenebis(4-amino-2-methylquinolinium chloride).

$C_{30}H_{40}Cl_2N_4$ = 527.6.

*CAS — 6707-58-0 (dequalinium); 522-51-0 (dequalinium chloride); 4028-98-2 (dequalinium acetate); 16022-70-1 (dequalinium salicylate).*

*ATC — D08AH01; G01AC05; R02AA02.*

**Pharmacopoeias.** In *Eur.* (see p.vi).

**Ph. Eur. 5.0** (Dequalinium Chloride). A white or yellowish-white, hygroscopic powder. Slightly soluble in water and in alcohol. Store in airtight containers.

**Incompatibility.** Dequalinium chloride is incompatible with soaps and other anionic surfactants, with phenol, and with chlorocresol.

### Profile

Dequalinium chloride is a bisquaternary quinolinium antiseptic, bactericidal against many Gram-positive and Gram-negative bacteria, and effective against fungi. It is mainly used in the form of lozenges in the treatment of minor infections of the mouth and throat. It has been applied topically in the treatment of skin and vaginal infections.

Dequalinium salicylate and undecenoate have also been used.

### Preparations

**Proprietary Preparations** (details are given in Part 3)
***Austria:*** Dequadin†; Dequavagyn; Evazol; Sorot; Tonsillol; ***Belg.:*** Anginol; Laryngarsol; ***Canad.:*** Dequadin; ***Chile:*** Larylin; ***Ger.:*** Efisol S†; Evazol; Fluomycin N; Gurgellosung-ratiopharm; Maltyl; Soor-Gel†; Sorot; ***Hong Kong:*** Delin; Dequadin; Roxine; ***Irl.:*** Dequadin; Labosept†; ***Ital.:*** Dequadin; Dequosangola; Faringina; Goladin†; Osangin; Pumilsan; ***Malaysia:*** Delin; Denium; DQM; SP Troches; Synti; Uphadeq; ***Mex.:*** Decatylen†; ***Neth.:*** Gargilon; ***NZ:*** Dequadin†; ***S.Afr.:*** Dequadin; ***Singapore:*** Dequadin; SP Troches; ***Spain:*** Dequadin; ***Switz.:*** Decatylene; Pastilles pour la gorge no 535; ***Thai.:*** Decho; Deo; Dequa/Delin†; Dequadin; V Day Lozenges; ***UK:*** Dequadin; Labosept; Mac Sugar Free†.

**Multi-ingredient:** ***Austria:*** Dequafungan; Dequalinetten; Dequonal; Eucillin; Fluorex Plus; Tetesept; ***Belg.:*** Anginol-Lidocaine; Bucco-Spray†; Buccosan; Dequalid; Dequalinium†; Ororhinathiol; Tricidine Dequalinium; ***Braz.:*** Dequadin C; ***Fin.:*** Septison; ***Fr.:*** Humex Mal de Gorge sans sucre; Oroseptol Lysozyme†; ***Ger.:*** Bakteriostat "Herbrand"†; Corti-Dynexan; De-menthasin†; Dequonal; Ephepect-Blocker-Pastillen N; Inspirol Halsschmerztabletten; Jasimenth CN; Mycatox; Neo-Pyodron; Otolitan N farblos; stas Halsschmerz-Tabletten†; Wick Sulagil; ***Hong Kong:*** Decatylen; Deq; Quadezyme; ***Irl.:*** Dequacaine; ***Israel:*** Dequasept; ***Ital.:*** Lisomucil Gola; Rinospray†; Transpulmina Gola; Tririnol†; ***Malaysia:*** Decatylen; Deq; Upha Lozenges; ***Norw.:*** Apolar med dekvalon; ***Port.:*** Anginova; Medifon; ***S.Afr.:*** Dequadin Mouth Paint; Dequamed†; ***Singapore:*** Decatylen; Deq; ***Spain:*** Anginovag; Dequadin Complex†; Roberfarin; Sedofarin; ***Switz.:*** Anginova; Arbid-top; Decasept N; Decatylene Neo; Dequonal; Gramipan; Neo-Bucosin†; Rhinipan†; Tyroqualine; ***Thai.:*** Deq; Detoch; Sentril; ***UK:*** Dequacaine.

---

## Diacetylaminoazotoluene

Diacetazotol; Pellidol. 4-Diacetylamino-2′,3-dimethylazobenzene.

$C_{18}H_{19}N_3O_2$ = 309.4.

*CAS — 83-63-6.*

### Profile

Diacetylaminoazotoluene is an antiseptic that has been used topically to promote wound healing.

### Preparations

**Proprietary Preparations** (details are given in Part 3)

**Multi-ingredient:** ***Austria:*** Dermowund.

---

## Dibrompropamidine Isetionate *(BANM, rINNM)*

Dibromopropamidine Isethionate; Isetionato de dibrompropamidina. 3,3′-Dibromo-4,4′-trimethylenedioxydibenzamidine bis(2-hydroxyethanesulphonate).

$C_{17}H_{18}Br_2N_4O_2,2C_2H_6O_4S$ = 722.4.

*CAS — 496-00-4 (dibrompropamidine); 614-87-9 (dibrompropamidine isetionate).*

*ATC — D08AC01; S01AX14.*

**Pharmacopoeias.** In *Br.*

**BP 2003** (Dibrompropamidine Isetionate). A white or almost white, odourless or almost odourless, crystalline powder. Freely soluble in water; sparingly soluble in alcohol; practically insoluble in chloroform, in ether, in fixed oils, and in liquid paraffin; soluble in glycerol. A 5% solution has a pH of 5.0 to 7.0.

### Profile

Dibrompropamidine isetionate is an aromatic diamidine antiseptic similar to propamidine (p.1191). It is bactericidal against Gram-positive bacteria but is less active against Gram-negative bacteria and spore-forming organisms. It also has antifungal properties. It is available as topical preparations for the local treatment of minor eye and skin infections.

### Preparations

**Proprietary Preparations** (details are given in Part 3)
***Austral.:*** Brolene; Brulidine†; ***Hong Kong:*** Brulidine†; ***Irl.:*** Brolene; Brulidine†; ***Norw.:*** Brulidine; ***NZ:*** Brolene; Brulidine†; ***UK:*** Brolene; Brulidine; Golden Eye Ointment; Pickles Antiseptic Cream.

**Multi-ingredient:** ***UK:*** Healthy Feet; No-Sor Nose Balm; RBC; Soleze†; Swarm.

---

## Dichlordimethylhydantoin

Diclorodimetilhidantoína. 1,3-Dichloro-5,5-dimethylhydantoin; 1,3-Dichloro-5,5-dimethylimidazolidine-2,4-dione.

$C_5H_6Cl_2N_2O_2$ = 197.0.

*CAS — 118-52-5.*

### Profile

Dichlordimethylhydantoin is a disinfectant used as a source of chlorine, for sterilising food and dairy equipment and as a bleach. It contains about 72% w/w of 'available chlorine' (see p.1176).

Bromochlorodimethylhydantoin ($C_5H_6N_2O_2BrCl$ = 241.5) is a closely related bromine-releasing compound used for the disinfection of swimming-pool water.

---

## Dichlorobenzyl Alcohol

Alcohol diclorobencílico; Dichlorophenylcarbinol. 2,4-Dichlorobenzyl alcohol.

$C_7H_6Cl_2O$ = 177.0.

*CAS — 1777-82-8.*

*ATC — R02AA03.*

### Profile

Dichlorobenzyl alcohol is an antiseptic used chiefly as an ingredient of lozenges in the treatment of minor infections of the mouth and throat.

### Preparations

**Proprietary Preparations** (details are given in Part 3)
***Ital.:*** Neo Borocillina Collutorio; Neo Borocillina Spray.

**Multi-ingredient:** ***Austral.:*** Ayrton's Antiseptic†; Logicin Rapid Relief; Sore Throat Chewing Gum†; Strepsils; Strepsils Plus; ***Austria:*** Coldangin; Neo-Angin; Sulgan 99; ***Belg.:*** Neofenox; Strepsils; Strepsils + Lidocaine; Strepsils Menthol; Strepsils Vit C; ***Canad.:*** Strepsils; ***Chile:*** Cornina; Hansaplast Antimicotico; ***Denm.:*** Strepsils; ***Fin.:*** Bafucin; Strepsils; Strepsils Menthol; ***Fr.:*** Strepsils; Strepsils Lidocaine; Strepsils Miel-Citron; Strepsils Vitamine C; Strepsilspray Lidocaine; ***Ger.:*** Neo-Angin N; ***Hong Kong:*** Logicin Rapid Relief; Strepsils; Strepsils Dual Action; ***Irl.:*** Strepsils; Strepsils Dual Action; Strepsils Vitamin C; ***Israel:*** Strepsils; Strepsils Plus; Strepsils with Vitamin C; ***Ital.:*** Arscolloid; Benagol; Benagol Mentolo-Eucaliptolo; Benagol Vitamina C; Bio-Arscolloid; Corti-Arscolloid; Farmagola; Neo Borocillina; Neo Borocillina Balsamica; Neo Borocillina C; Neo Borocillina Tosse Compresse; Oraseptic Gola†; ***Malaysia:*** Strepsils; Strepsils Dual Action; ***Neth.:*** Strepsils; Strepsils Menthol en Eucalyptus; Strepsils Sinaasappel en Vitamine C; ***NZ:*** Strepsils; Strepsils Plus Anaesthetic; Strepsils with Vitamin C; ***Port.:*** Dropcina; ***S.Afr.:*** Strepsils; Strepsils Eucalyptus Menthol; Strepsils Orange-C; Strepsils Plus; Strepsils Soothing Honey & Lemon†; ***Singapore:*** Floxil†; Strepsils; Strepsils Dual Action; ***Spain:*** Strepsils; Strepsils con Anestesico; Strepsils con Vitamina C; ***Swed.:*** Bafucin; Strepsils†; ***Switz.:*** Anginazol; Hextriletten; Lidazon; Neo-Angin au miel et citron; Neo-Angin avec vitamin C exempt de sucre; Neo-Angin exempt de sucre; Sulgan N; ***Thai.:*** Strepsils Plus Anaesthetic; Strepsils Plus Vit C; Strepsils Sugar Free; ***UK:*** Strepsils; Strepsils Pain Relief Plus†; Strepsils with Vitamin C.

---

## Dichloroxylenol *(BAN, rINN)*

DCMX; Dichlorometaxylenol. 2,4-Dichloro-3,5-xylenol; 2,4-Dichloro-3,5-dimethylphenol.

$C_8H_8Cl_2O$ = 191.1.

*CAS — 133-53-9.*

### Profile

Dichloroxylenol is a chlorinated phenolic antiseptic.

### Preparations

**Proprietary Preparations** (details are given in Part 3)

**Multi-ingredient:** ***India:*** Fairgenol; ***UAE:*** Radol.

---

## Didecyldimethylammonium Chloride

Didecildimetilamonio, cloruro de. *N*-Decyl-*N,N*-demethyl-l-decanaminium chloride.

$C_{22}H_{48}ClN$ = 362.1.

*ATC — D08AJ06.*

### Profile

Didecyldimethylammonium chloride is a quaternary ammonium disinfectant used in preparations for disinfection of the skin and mucous membranes. It is also used to disinfect instruments and surfaces.

### Preparations

**Proprietary Preparations** (details are given in Part 3)
***Ital.:*** Alfa; ***Thai.:*** Deconex 50FF.

**Multi-ingredient:** ***Fr.:*** Amphosept BV†; Aniospray; Bacterianos D; Chlorispray; Hexanios G+R; Sanytol; Ultrasept†; ***Ger.:*** Almyrol; Baccalin; Bacillocid rasant; Desoform; Freka-Nol; Fugisept; Gercid forte; Gigasept AF†; Gigasept Med; Hexaquart L; Hexaquart plus; Hexaquart S; Inova; Kohrsolin FF; Korsolex Extra; Korsolex FF; Korsolex Plus; Lysetol V†; Lysoformin 3000; Lysoformin spezial; Meliseptol Rapid; Melsept SF; Melsitt; Quatohex; Teta Extra; ***Ital.:*** Cedril Strumenti†; Cedril†; Melsept SF; ***Thai.:*** Deconex 53IN.

---

## Dodeclonium Bromide *(rINN)*

GR-412. [2-(*p*-Chlorophenoxy)ethyl]dodecyldimethylammonium bromide.

$C_{22}H_{39}BrClNO$ = 448.9.

*CAS — 15687-13-5.*

### Profile

Dodeclonium bromide is an antiseptic that has been included in multi-ingredient preparations intended for the treatment of skin and anorectal disorders.

### Preparations

**Proprietary Preparations** (details are given in Part 3)

**Multi-ingredient:** ***Fr.:*** Dermeol†; Phlebocreme†; Phlebosup†; Sedaplaie†; Sedorrhoide†.

## Domiphen Bromide (BAN, USAN, rINN)

Bromuro de domifeno; NSC-39415; PDDB; Phenododecinium Bromide. Dodecyldimethyl-2-phenoxyethylammonium bromide.

$C_{22}H_{40}BrNO = 414.5.$

*CAS — 13900-14-6 (domiphen); 538-71-6 (domiphen bromide).*

*ATC — A01AB06.*

**Pharmacopoeias.** In *Br. Chin.* includes the monohydrate.

**BP 2003** (Domiphen Bromide). Colourless or faintly yellow, crystalline flakes. Freely soluble in water and in alcohol; soluble in acetone.

**Incompatibility.** Domiphen bromide is incompatible with soaps and other anionic surfactants.

### Profile

Domiphen bromide is a quaternary ammonium antiseptic with actions and uses similar to those of other cationic surfactants (see Cetrimide, p.1172). Preparations containing domiphen bromide are used in the treatment of minor infections of the mouth and throat.

### Preparations

**Proprietary Preparations** (details are given in Part 3)

***Canad.:*** Antiseptique Pastilles; Bronchodex Pastilles; Oraseptic†; ***Ital.:*** Bradoral; ***Port.:*** Neobradoral.

**Multi-ingredient:** ***Austria:*** Bepanthen; Bradosol; ***Canad.:*** Mouthwash & Gargle†; Mouthwash Mint/Peppermint†; Nupercainal; Scope†; ***Fr.:*** Fluoselgine; ***Ital.:*** Golamed Oral†; Inalar; Nasalemed†; ***UK:*** Bradosol Plus†.

## Ethoxyquin

Etoxiquina. 6-Ethoxy-1,2-dihydro-2,2,4-trimethylquinoline.

$C_{14}H_{19}NO = 217.3.$

*CAS — 91-53-2.*

### Profile

Ethoxyquin has been used as an antoxidant for the prevention of common scald of apples and pears during storage and as an additive to animal feeds. Concern has been expressed over the toxicity of ethoxyquin and its residues on foodstuffs and its use is limited or restricted in some countries.

# Ethylene Oxide

Óxido de etileno; Oxirane.

$C_2H_4O = 44.05.$

*CAS — 75-21-8.*

**Description.** Ethylene oxide is a colourless flammable gas at room temperature and atmospheric pressure.

**Stability.** Mixtures of ethylene oxide with oxygen or air are explosive but the risk can be reduced by the addition of carbon dioxide or fluorocarbons.

## Adverse Effects and Precautions

Ethylene oxide irritates the eyes and respiratory tract and may also cause nausea and vomiting, diarrhoea, headache, vertigo, CNS depression, dyspnoea, and pulmonary oedema. Liver and kidney damage and haemolysis may occur. Fatalities have occurred. Excessive exposure of the skin to liquid or solution causes burns, blistering, irritation, and dermatitis; percutaneous absorption may lead to systemic effects.

Many materials including plastics and rubber adsorb ethylene oxide. If such materials are being sterilised with ethylene oxide all traces of the gas must be removed before the materials can be used; removal may be by ventilation or more active means. Hypersensitivity reactions, including anaphylaxis, have been associated with ethylene oxide-contaminated materials. Ethylene oxide may also react with materials being sterilised to produce substances such as ethylene chlorohydrin (with chloride) or ethylene glycol (with water); these may contribute to any toxicity.

Pharmaceutical manufacturers within the European Union have been advised to use ethylene oxide only when there is no alternative. Ethylene oxide has been shown to have carcinogenic and mutagenic properties and there is evidence of increased risk of neoplasms following occupational exposure.

◊ Reviews.

1. Ethylene oxide. *Environmental Health Criteria 55.* Geneva: WHO, 1985. Available at: http://www.inchem.org/documents/ehc/ehc/ehc55.htm (accessed 10/06/04)
2. Ethylene oxide health and safety guide. *IPCS Health and Safety Guide 16.* Geneva: WHO, 1988. Available at: http://www.inchem.org/documents/hsg/hsg/hsg016.htm (accessed 10/06/04)

**Carcinogenicity.** Exposure of workers to ethylene oxide has been associated with the development of lymphatic and haematopoietic cancer. However, epidemiological studies have not consistently shown an excess of cases among workers exposed to ethylene oxide, and excesses that have been seen have been small[1-4] although a trend towards increased risk related to cumulative exposure has been reported.[2,4]

1. Hogstedt C, *et al.* Epidemiologic support for ethylene oxide as a cancer-causing agent. *JAMA* 1986; **255:** 1575–8.
2. Steenland K, *et al.* Mortality among workers exposed to ethylene oxide. *N Engl J Med* 1991; **324:** 1402–7.
3. Hagmar L, *et al.* An epidemiological study of cancer risk among workers exposed to ethylene oxide using hemoglobin adducts to validate environmental exposure assessments. *Int Arch Occup Environ Health* 1991; **63:** 271–7.
4. Stayner L, *et al.* Exposure-response analysis of cancer mortality in a cohort of workers exposed to ethylene oxide. *Am J Epidemiol* 1993; **138:** 787–98.

**Effects on the nervous system.** Four men exposed to ethylene oxide at a concentration of greater than 700 ppm developed neurological disorders. One experienced headaches, nausea, vomiting, and lethargy followed by major motor seizures. The others experienced headaches, limb numbness and weakness, increased fatigue, trouble with memory and thought processes, and slurred speech. Three also developed cataracts, and one required bilateral cataract extractions.[1]

1. Jay WM, *et al.* Possible relationship of ethylene oxide exposure to cataract formation. *Am J Ophthalmol* 1982; **93:** 727–32.

**Hypersensitivity.** Anaphylactoid reactions in dialysis patients have resulted from the use of dialysis equipment sterilised with ethylene oxide.[1-3] There have also been reports of hypersensitivity[4] and anaphylactoid[5] reactions in plateletpheresis donors caused by residues of ethylene oxide in components of apheresis kits. The most common adverse reactions reported have been dyspnoea, wheezing, urticaria, flushing, headache, and hypotension, but acute severe bronchospasm, circulatory collapse, cardiac arrest, and death have also occurred. It was noted[6] that where severe, sometimes fatal, anaphylactoid reactions have occurred at the beginning of dialysis, ethylene oxide has almost universally been implicated, although exposure to cuprammonium cellulose (cuprophane) dialysis membranes may also have been involved.

It has been reported that there may be an increased risk of ethylene oxide-induced anaphylactic shock in children undergoing surgery for spina bifida.[7] Such children might be at increased risk of sensitisation and anaphylaxis, and came into frequent contact with ethylene oxide through multiple operations and catheterisations.

Occupational asthma and contact dermatitis have been attributed to residual ethylene oxide in surgical gloves.[8]

1. Bommer J, *et al.* Anaphylactoid reactions in dialysis patients: role of ethylene-oxide. *Lancet* 1985; **ii:** 1382–5.
2. Rumpf KW, *et al.* Association of ethylene-oxide-induced IgE antibodies with symptoms in dialysis patients. *Lancet* 1985; **ii:** 1385–7.
3. Röckel A, *et al.* Ethylene oxide hypersensitivity in dialysis patients. *Lancet* 1986; **i:** 382–3.
4. Leitman SF, *et al.* Allergic reactions in healthy plateletpheresis donors caused by sensitization to ethylene oxide gas. *N Engl J Med* 1986; **315:** 1192–6.
5. Muylle L, *et al.* Anaphylactoid reaction in platelet-pheresis donor with IgE antibodies to ethylene oxide. *Lancet* 1986; **ii:** 1225.
6. Nicholls A. Ethylene oxide and anaphylaxis during haemodialysis. *BMJ* 1986; **292:** 1221–2.
7. Moneret-Vautrin DA, *et al.* High risk of anaphylactic shock during surgery for spina bifida. *Lancet* 1990; **335:** 865–6.
8. Verraes S, Michel O. Occupational asthma induced by ethylene oxide. *Lancet* 1995; **346:** 1434–5.

**Pregnancy.** A study[1] of female hospital sterilising staff in all general hospitals in Finland showed that the incidence of spontaneous abortion (analysed according to employment at the time of conception and corrected for maternal age, parity, decade of pregnancy, smoking, and consumption of alcohol and coffee) was significantly increased in those exposed to ethylene oxide during pregnancy compared with those not so exposed. This study provoked criticism,[2,3] and the authors conceded that the study was not large enough to compare abortion rates and known ethylene oxide concentrations.[4]

1. Hemminki K, *et al.* Spontaneous abortions in hospital staff engaged in sterilising instruments with chemical agents. *BMJ* 1982; **285:** 1461–3.
2. Gordon JE, Meinhardt TJ. Spontaneous abortions in hospital sterilising staff. *BMJ* 1983; **286:** 1976.
3. Austin SG. Spontaneous abortions in hospital sterilising staff. *BMJ* 1983; **286:** 1976.
4. Hemminki K, *et al.* Spontaneous abortions in hospital sterilising staff. *BMJ* 1983; **286:** 1976–7.

## Pharmacokinetics

Ethylene oxide gas is rapidly absorbed through the lungs and distributed throughout the body. Percutaneous absorption can occur from aqueous solutions. It is rapidly metabolised by hydrolysis or conjugation with glutathione.

## Uses

Ethylene oxide is a bactericidal and fungicidal gaseous disinfectant which is effective against most micro-organisms, including viruses. It is also sporicidal. It is used for the gaseous sterilisation of heat-labile pharmaceutical and surgical materials that cannot be sterilised by other means.

Ethylene oxide forms explosive mixtures with air; this may be overcome by using mixtures containing 10% ethylene oxide in carbon dioxide, or by removing at least 95% of the air from the apparatus before admitting either ethylene oxide or a mixture of 90% ethylene oxide in carbon dioxide. Alternatively, non-flammable mixtures of dichlorodifluoromethane and trichlorofluoromethane with 9 to 12% w/w of ethylene oxide have been employed, but restrictions on the release of fluorocarbons or CFCs limit their use.

Effective sterilisation by ethylene oxide depends on exposure time, temperature, humidity, the amount and type of microbial contamination, and the partial pressure of the ethylene oxide in the exposure chamber. The material being sterilised must be permeable to ethylene oxide if occluded micro-organisms are present. The bactericidal action is accelerated by increase of temperature; a temperature of about 55° can be used for most heat-labile materials.

Moisture is essential for sterilisation by ethylene oxide. In practice, dry micro-organisms need to be rehydrated before ethylene oxide can be effective; humidification is normally carried out under vacuum prior to introduction of ethylene oxide. Relative humidities of 40 to 60% are used. Control of physical factors does not assure sterility, and the process should be monitored usually by employing standardised suspensions of aerobic spores such as those of *Bacillus subtilis* var. *niger.*

# Formaldehyde

$CH_2O = 30.03.$

*CAS — 50-00-0.*

### Formaldehyde Solution

Formaldehído, solución; Formaldehydi Solutio.

NOTE. The names formalin and formol have been used for formaldehyde solution but in some countries Formalin is a trade mark.

**Pharmacopoeias.** In *Chin., Eur.* (see p.vi), *Jpn, US,* and *Viet.*

**Ph. Eur. 5.0** (Formaldehyde Solution (35 per cent); Formaldehyde Solution BP 2003). It contains 34.5 to 38.0% w/w of formaldehyde with methyl alcohol as a stabiliser. It is a clear, colourless, liquid. Miscible with water and with alcohol. It may be cloudy after storage. Store at a temperature between 15° and 25°. Protect from light.

**USP 27** (Formaldehyde Solution). It contains not less than 36.5 or 37.0% w/w (depending on the packaging) of formaldehyde with methyl alcohol added to prevent polymerisation. It is a clear, colourless, or practically colourless liquid with a pungent, irritating odour. Miscible with water and with alcohol. Store at a temperature above 15° in airtight containers. It may become cloudy on standing due to the separation of paraformaldehyde, especially if the solution is kept in a cold place; the cloudiness disappears on warming.

**Strength of solutions.** Formaldehyde solution is sometimes known simply as formaldehyde and this has led to confusion in interpreting the strength and the form in which formaldehyde is being used. In practice formaldehyde is available as formaldehyde solution which is diluted before use, the percentage strength being expressed in terms of formaldehyde solution rather than formaldehyde. For example, in the UK, formaldehyde solution 3% consists of 3 volumes of Formaldehyde Solution (35 Per Cent) (Ph. Eur. 5.0) diluted to 100 volumes with water and thus contains 1.04 to 1.14% w/w of formaldehyde; it is *not* prepared by diluting Formaldehyde Solution (35 Per Cent) (Ph. Eur. 5.0) to arrive at a solution containing 3% w/w of formaldehyde.

**Incompatibility.** Formaldehyde reacts with protein and this may diminish its antimicrobial activity.

## Adverse Effects and Precautions

Concentrated formaldehyde solutions applied to the skin cause whitening and hardening. Contact dermatitis and sensitivity reactions have occurred after the use of conventional concentrations and after contact with residual formaldehyde in resins.

Ingestion of formaldehyde solution causes intense pain, with inflammation, ulceration, and necrosis of mucous membranes. There may be vomiting, haematemesis, blood-stained diarrhoea, haematuria, and anuria; metabolic acidosis, vertigo, convulsions, loss of consciousness, and circulatory failure may occur. Death has occurred after the ingestion of the equivalent of about 30 mL of formaldehyde solution. If the patient survives 48 hours, recovery is probable. Formaldehyde vapour is irritant to the eyes, nose, and upper respiratory tract, and may cause coughing, dysphagia, spasm and oedema of the larynx, bronchitis, pneumonia, and rarely, pulmonary oedema. Asthma has been reported after repeated exposure.

◊ General references.


1. Health and Safety Executive. Formaldehyde. *Toxicity Review 2.* London: HMSO, 1981.
2. Formaldehyde. *Environmental Health Criteria 89.* Geneva: WHO, 1989. Available at: http://www.inchem.org/documents/ehc/ehc/ehc89.htm (accessed 10/06/04)
3. Formaldehyde health and safety guide. *IPCS Health and Safety Guide 57.* Geneva: WHO, 1991. Available at: http://www.inchem.org/documents/hsg/hsg/hsg057.htm (accessed 10/06/04)


**Carcinogenicity.** There is controversy as to the risk formaldehyde presents as a carcinogen. Studies on the occupational exposure of medical personnel[1] and industrial workers[2-4] to formaldehyde have generally concluded that although the risk is small or non-existent, the possibility that formaldehyde is a human carcinogen cannot be excluded. Reanalyses of some studies have led to different interpretations of the results, with some workers concluding that the risk of cancer from formaldehyde is greater than originally thought.[5] In the USA, regulatory authorities consider formaldehyde to be a probable human carcinogen.[6]


1. Kreiger N. Formaldehyde and nasal cancer mortality. *Can Med Assoc J* 1983; **128:** 248–9.
2. Gérin M, *et al.* Cancer risks due to occupational exposure to formaldehyde: results of a multi-site case-control study in Montreal. *Int J Cancer* 1989; **44:** 53–8.
3. Blair A, *et al.* Mortality from lung cancer among workers employed in formaldehyde industries. *Am J Ind Med* 1990; **17:** 683–99.
4. Coggon D, *et al.* Extended follow-up of a cohort of British chemical workers exposed to formaldehyde. *J Natl Cancer Inst* 2003; **95:** 1608–15.
5. Sterling TD, Weinkam JJ. Mortality from respiratory cancers (including lung cancer) among workers employed in formaldehyde industries. *Am J Ind Med* 1994; **25:** 593–602.
6. Council on Scientific Affairs of the American Medical Association. Formaldehyde. *JAMA* 1989; **261:** 1183–7.


**Effects on the blood.** Haemolysis during chronic haemodialysis was due to formaldehyde eluted from filters.[1]


1. Orringer EP, Mattern WD. Formaldehyde-induced hemolysis during chronic hemodialysis. *N Engl J Med* 1976; **294:** 1416–20.


**Effects on the urinary tract.** Adverse effects of intravesical instillation of formaldehyde solutions in the treatment of haemorrhagic cystitis have included dysuria, suprapubic pain, ureteric and bladder fibrosis, hydronephrosis, vesicoureteral reflux, and fatal acute renal failure.[1] Intraperitoneal spillage through a fistula, leading to adverse systemic effects, has also occurred.[2] See also Haemorrhagic Cystitis under Uses, below.

There has also been a report[3] of 4 patients exposed to high levels of atmospheric formaldehyde who developed membranous nephropathy, suggesting that there may be genetic susceptibility for this effect.


1. Melekos M, Lalos J. Intravesical instillation of formalin and its complications. *Urology* 1983; **21:** 331–2.
2. Capen CV, *et al.* Intraperitoneal spillage of formalin after intravesical instillation. *Urology* 1982; **19:** 599–601.
3. Breysse P, *et al.* Membranous nephropathy and formaldehyde exposure. *Ann Intern Med* 1994; **120:** 396–7.


**Hypersensitivity.** Hypersensitivity to formaldehyde has had several manifestations. Effects on the skin have included acute exacerbation of eczema after injection of hepatitis B vaccine containing up to 20 micrograms of formaldehyde per mL.[1] In another case, formaldehyde sensitivity was characterised by pruritus, burning, and redness within minutes of exposure to sunlight.[2] Painful, enlarged, and haemorrhagic gingival margins have occurred following the use of a toothpaste containing a solution of formaldehyde.[3] There is conflicting evidence of the respiratory effects of formaldehyde: although a low concentration has been reported not to trigger an asthma attack in patients with severe bronchial hyperresponsiveness,[4] occupational asthma has been documented.[5] More severe manifestations of hypersensitivity include 7 cases of shock of possible toxic or anaphylactic aetiology, which occurred after the use of formaldehyde solutions during surgical removal of hydatid cysts.[6]

For mention of an allergic response to root canal paste containing paraformaldehyde, see p.1187.


1. Ring J. Exacerbation of eczema by formalin-containing hepatitis B vaccine in formaldehyde-allergic patients. *Lancet* 1986; **ii:** 522–3.
2. Shelley WB. Immediate sunburn-like reaction in a patient with formaldehyde photosensitivity. *Arch Dermatol* 1982; **118:** 117–18.
3. Laws IM. Toothpaste formulations. *Br Dent J* 1984; **156:** 240.
4. Harving H, *et al.* Low concentrations of formaldehyde in bronchial asthma: a study of exposure under controlled conditions. *BMJ* 1986; **293:** 310.
5. Heard BE. Low concentrations of formaldehyde in bronchial asthma. *BMJ* 1986; **293:** 821.
6. Galland MC, *et al.* Risques thérapeutiques de l'utilisation des solutions de formol dans le traitement chirurgical des kystes hydatiques du foie. *Therapie* 1980; **35:** 443–6.


## Treatment of Adverse Effects

Contaminated skin should be washed with soap and water. After ingestion water, milk, charcoal, and/or demulcents should be given; gastric lavage and emesis should be avoided. Assisted ventilation may be required and shock should be alleviated appropriately. Convulsions should be controlled with diazepam. Acidosis, resulting from metabolism of formaldehyde to formic acid, may require the intravenous administration of sodium bicarbonate or sodium lactate. The use of haemodialysis has been suggested.

## Uses and Administration

Formaldehyde solution is a bactericidal disinfectant also effective against fungi and many viruses. It is slowly effective against bacterial spores but its sporicidal effect is greatly increased by increase in temperature.

*Formaldehyde solution is usually used diluted and it is important to note that the strength of preparations is given in terms of the content of formaldehyde solution and not in terms of the final concentration of formaldehyde* (see under Strength of Solutions, above).

Formaldehyde solution is used in the disinfection of blankets and bedding and in the disinfection of the membranes in dialysis equipment. It is important to ensure that there are no traces of formaldehyde on any equipment before it is used. Formaldehyde solution is also used with succinic dialdehyde for instrument disinfection.

When applied to the unbroken skin, formaldehyde solution hardens the epidermis, renders it tough and whitish, and produces a local anaesthetic effect. Formaldehyde solution 3% v/v has been used for the treatment of warts on the palms of the hands and soles of the feet. It is used similarly as a water-miscible gel containing formaldehyde 0.75%. Sweating of the feet may be treated by the application of formaldehyde solution in glycerol or alcohol but such applications are liable to produce sensitisation reactions and other treatments are regarded as more effective (see Hyperhidrosis, p.1136).

After surgical removal of hydatid cysts, diluted formaldehyde solution has been used for irrigating the cavities to destroy scolices but other larvicides are preferred (see Echinococcosis, p.98). It is generally too irritant for use on mucous membranes but it has been used in mouthwashes and pastes as an antiseptic and hardening agent for the gums. In dentistry it has been used in endodontic treatment.

Formaldehyde solution in concentrations of up to 10% v/v in saline is used as a preservative for pathological specimens. It is not suitable for preserving urine for subsequent examination. Formaldehyde solution has been used for the inactivation of viruses in vaccine production.

Formaldehyde gas has little penetrating power and readily polymerises and condenses on surfaces and its effectiveness depends on it dissolving in a film of moisture before acting on micro-organisms; in practice a relative humidity of 80 to 90% is necessary. Formaldehyde gas is used for the disinfection of rooms and cabinets. The gas may be produced from 500 mL of undiluted formaldehyde solution by boiling with 1 litre of water or by addition of potassium permanganate or by heating a formaldehyde-containing solid such as paraformaldehyde (p.1187). Formaldehyde gas is used with low-temperature steam for the sterilisation of heat-sensitive items.

Other compounds which are thought to act by releasing formaldehyde include noxytiolin (p.1187) and methenamine (p.230).

**Haemorrhagic cystitis.** Formaldehyde has been used for local therapy of haemorrhagic cystitis, although there has been debate about the most appropriate regimen. The Fair regimen[1] for the intravesical administration of formaldehyde solution in haemorrhagic cystitis involves passive irrigation of the bladder with 500 to 1000 mL of formaldehyde solution 1% v/v for a total of 10 minutes, the bladder subsequently being emptied and washed out with 1 litre of distilled water. Stronger concentrations of formaldehyde solution and other methods can be used if bleeding does not stop.[2] In a review of 118 patients treated with solutions of formaldehyde for intractable haematuria, the authors felt that this was probably the most effective treatment, but also probably the most dangerous.[3] More concentrated instillations, containing formaldehyde solution 5 to 10% seem to be generally viewed as unnecessary, and associated with an increased risk of complications which precludes their use.[4-7] Instillation of intravesical alum (p.1652) has successfully controlled bleeding without complications and has been reported[7] to be a safe and effective treatment for intractable bladder bleeding; the authors considered that it should replace formaldehyde solution, no matter how dilute. Instillation of prostaglandins such as alprostadil (p.1513) or carboprost trometamol (p.1514) has also been used.


1. Fair WR. Formalin in the treatment of massive bladder hemorrhage: techniques, results, and complications. *Urology* 1974; **3:** 573–6.
2. Anonymous. Haemorrhagic cystitis after radiotherapy. *Lancet* 1987; **i:** 304–6.
3. Godec CJ, Gleich P. Intractable hematuria and formalin. *J Urol (Baltimore)* 1983; **130:** 688–91.
4. Bullock N, Whitaker RH. Massive bladder haemorrhage. *BMJ* 1985; **291:** 1522–3.
5. Donahue LA, Frank IN. Intravesical formalin for haemorrhagic cystitis: analysis of therapy. *J Urol (Baltimore)* 1989; **141:** 809–12.
6. Murray JA, *et al.* Massive bladder haemorrhage. *BMJ* 1986; **292:** 57.
7. Smith PJB, *et al.* Massive bladder haemorrhage. *BMJ* 1986; **292:** 412.


### Preparations

**Proprietary Preparations** (details are given in Part 3)
***Fr.:*** Emoform†; ***Ger.:*** Lysoform; ***Irl.:*** Veracur†; ***Spain:*** Diformil; ***UK:*** Veracur; ***USA:*** Formadon; Formalyde; Lazerformaldehyde.

**Multi-ingredient:** ***Arg.:*** Parodium; ***Austral.:*** Formo-Cresol Mitis†; ***Canad.:*** British Army Foot Powder; Duoplant; Sporex†; ***Fr.:*** Aniospray; Bacterianos D; Chlorispray; Ephydrol; Incidine; Parodium; Pipiol†; Veybirol-Tyrothyricine; ***Ger.:*** Aseptisol; Buraton 10 F†; Desoform; Gigasept FF†; Gigasept†; Incidin perfekt; Incidin Spezial; Indulfan plus†; Lysetol V†; Lysoformin; Melsept; Melsitt; Minutil; Prontocid N; Sekusept forte; Sekusept forte S; Sporcid; Ultrasol-F; Ultrasol-S†; ***Ital.:*** Melsept; ***Spain:*** Diformiltricina; Sudosin†; Tifell; Viberol Tirotricina.

## Glucoprotamine

Reaction product of L-glutamic acid and cocopropylene-1,3-diamine.

### Profile

Glucoprotamine is used as a disinfectant for surfaces and medical equipment.

◊ References.


1. Disch K. Glucoprotamine—a new antimicrobial substance. *Zentralbl Hyg Umweltmed* 1994; **195:** 357–65.
2. Meyer B, Kluin C. Efficacy of glucoprotamin containing disinfectants against different species of atypical mycobacteria. *J Hosp Infect* 1999; **42:** 151–4.
3. Widmer AE, Frei R. Antimicrobial activity of glucoprotamin: a clinical study of a new disinfectant for instruments. *Infect Control Hosp Epidemiol* 2003; **24:** 762–4.


### Preparations

**Proprietary Preparations** (details are given in Part 3)
***Ger.:*** Incidin Plus; Sekusept Plus.

**Multi-ingredient:** ***Ger.:*** Incidin extra N; Sekumatic FDR.

## Glutaral *(USAN, rINN)*

Glutaraldehyde; Glutaric Dialdehyde; Pentanedial. Pentane-1,5-dial.

$C_5H_8O_2$ = 100.1.
*CAS — 111-30-8.*
*ATC — D08AX09.*

**Pharmacopoeias.** Solutions of glutaral are included in *Br.*, *Chin.*, and *US.* A solution is also in *USNF.*

**BP 2003:** (Strong Glutaraldehyde Solution). It contains 47 to 53% w/w of glutaral. Store at a temperature not exceeding 15°.

**USP 27** (Glutaral Concentrate). It contains 50 to 52% w/w of glutaral and has a pH between 3.7 and 4.5. Store at a temperature not exceeding 40° in airtight containers. Protect from light.

**USNF 22** (Glutaral Disinfectant Solution). It has a pH between 2.7 and 3.7. Store at a temperature not exceeding 40° in airtight containers. Protect from light.

## Adverse Effects

As for Formaldehyde Solution, p.1179.

◊ In a brief review[1] of the occupational hazards of glutaral it was noted that several studies showed adverse effects, including nausea, headache, airway obstruction, asthma, rhinitis, eye irritation, and dermatitis, occurring among medical personnel exposed to glutaral, generally at concentrations below the recommended limits. Skin reactions were due to hypersensitivity or a direct irritant effect. It was concluded that, when using glutaral, workers should take suitable precautions to protect the skin and should avoid inhaling the vapour.

The risk of occupational exposure to glutaral vapour may be higher in warm climates.[2]

There has also been a report of accidental ocular contact with glutaral due to leakage of glutaral solution retained in an anaesthesia mask; moderate chemical conjunctivitis ensued.[3]

1. Burge PS. Occupational risks of glutaraldehyde. *BMJ* 1989; **299:** 342.
2. Mwaniki DL, Guthua SW. Occupational exposure to glutaraldehyde in tropical climates. *Lancet* 1992; **340:** 1476–7.
3. Murray WJ, Ruddy MP. Toxic eye injury during induction of anaesthesia. *South Med J* 1985; **78:** 1012–13.

**Effects on the gastrointestinal tract.** Insufficient rinsing of a glutaral 2% solution from flexible sigmoidoscopes after disinfection appeared to be responsible for an outbreak of fever and gastrointestinal symptoms including abdominal cramps, bloody diarrhoea, and nausea and vomiting in patients undergoing sigmoidoscopy.[1]

1. Durante L, *et al.* Investigation of an outbreak of bloody diarrhea: association with endoscopic cleaning solution and demonstration of lesions in an animal model. *Am J Med* 1992; **92:** 476–80.

## Uses and Administration

Glutaral is a bactericidal disinfectant that is rapidly effective against Gram-positive and Gram-negative bacteria. It is also effective against *Mycobacterium tuberculosis*, some fungi, and viruses, including hepatitis B virus and HIV, and is slowly effective against bacterial spores. Aqueous solutions show optimum activity between pH 7.5 and 8.5; such solutions are chemically stable for about 14 days. Solutions at lower pH values are more stable.

A 2% aqueous solution buffered to a pH of about 8 (activated glutaral; alkaline glutaral) is used for the sterilisation of endoscopic and dental instruments, rubber or plastic equipment, and for other equipment which cannot be sterilised by heat. Glutaral is non-corrosive towards most materials. Complete immersion in the solution for 10 to 20 minutes is sufficient for rapid disinfection of thoroughly cleansed instruments but exposure for up to 10 hours may be necessary for sterilisation. For further details, see Disinfection of Endoscopes, p.1164, and Disinfection in Hepatitis and HIV Infection, p.1165.

A 10% solution is applied twice daily for the treatment of warts (p.1139); a 5% solution and a 10% gel have also been used. Glutaral should not be used for facial or anogenital warts. Glutaral has also been used topically for treating hyperhidrosis of the palms and soles, although other agents are generally preferred (see p.1136).

### Preparations

***BP 2003:*** Glutaraldehyde Solution; Strong Glutaraldehyde Solution;
***USNF 22:*** Glutaral Disinfectant Solution;
***USP 27:*** Glutaral Concentrate.

**Proprietary Preparations** (details are given in Part 3)
***Arg.:*** Asepto-Glutaral; ***Austral.:*** Diswart; ***Braz.:*** Braudeide†; ***Canad.:*** Sonacide†; ***Fr.:*** Cidex; Endosporine†; Sekucid; Steranios; Verutal†; ***Ger.:*** Cidex; Korsolex-Endo-Disinfectant; Sekumatic FD; ***Irl.:*** Glutarol; Verucasep†; ***Ital.:*** Asporin 2†; Cidex†; Citrosteril Sterilferri; Diba; Eso Cem; Eso H1, HP, and HP1; Esoxid; Ferriseptil; H1†; SaniSteril Sterilferri; Sporacid; Sporex; Sporicidin; T5; ***NZ:*** Zenicide†; ***Switz.:*** Glutarol†; ***Thai.:*** Deconex 50FF; Glutarin†; Mycidal†; Pose-Dex†; Totacide†; ***UK:*** ASEP; Cidex†; Glutarol; ***USA:*** Cetylcide-G; Cidex.

**Multi-ingredient:** ***Fr.:*** Aniospray; Bacterianos D; Chlorispray; Incidine; Ultrasep†; ***Ger.:*** Aerodesin; Aseptisol; Bacillocid rasant; Bacillocid Spezial†; Bacillol plus; Baktobod†; Buraton 10 F†; Desoform; Helipur H plus N; Helipur H plus†; Incidin perfekt; Incidin Spezial; Incidur; Incidur Spray; Indulfan plus†; Kohrsolin; Kohrsolin FF; Kohrsolin iD†; Korsolex basic; Korsolex Extra; Korsolex FF; Lysetol FF; Lysetol V†; Lysoformin; Lysoformin 3000; Melsept; Melsept SF; Melsitt; Minutil; Prontocid N; Sekucid konz; Sekusept Extra N; Sekusept forte; Sekusept forte S; Sporcid; Ultrasol-F; Ultrasol-S†; ***Ital.:*** Asporin 0.5†; Bergon; Citrosteril Impronte; Diaril; Eso Din; Esoform 92; Iketoncid†; Incidin Spezial; Melsept; Melsept SF; Sekucid; Sekugerm†; Sekumatic; Sekusept Extra N; ***Mon.:*** Akila spray†.

---

## Glyoxal

Ethanedial; Glioxal; Oxalaldehyde. 1,2-Ethanedione.
$C_2H_2O_2$ = 58.04.
*CAS — 107-22-2.*

### Profile

Glyoxal is an aldehyde used for the disinfection of surfaces and of medical and surgical instruments.

### Preparations

**Proprietary Preparations** (details are given in Part 3)
***Thai.:*** Deconex 50FF.

**Multi-ingredient:** ***Fr.:*** Aniospray; Bacterianos D; Incidine; ***Ger.:*** Antifect†; Baktobod N†; Baktobod†; Buraton 10 F†; Desoform; Freka-Nol; Fugisept; Helipur H plus†; Incidin perfekt; Incidin Spezial; Incidur; Indulfan plus†; Lysoformin 3000; Meliseptol; Melsept; Melsept SF; Minutil; Pursept A†; Sekusept forte; Ultrasol-F; Ultrasol-S†; ***Ital.:*** Incidin Spezial; Indulfan; Melsept; Melsept SF; Melsept Spray; Sekugerm†.

---

The symbol † denotes a preparation no longer actively marketed

## Halazone *(rINN)*

Halazona; Pantocide. 4-(Dichlorosulphamoyl)benzoic acid.
$C_7H_5Cl_2NO_4S$ = 270.1.
*CAS — 80-13-7.*

**Pharmacopoeias.** In *US.*

**USP 27** (Halazone). A white crystalline powder with a characteristic odour of chlorine. Soluble 1 in more than 1000 of water and of chloroform, 1 in 140 of alcohol, and 1 in more than 2000 of ether; soluble in glacial acetic acid. It dissolves in solutions of alkali hydroxides and carbonates with the formation of a salt. Store in airtight containers. Protect from light.

### Profile

Halazone is a disinfectant with the general properties of chlorine (p.1175) in aqueous solution and is used for the disinfection of drinking water (p.1165). It contains about 52% of 'available chlorine' (see p.1176). One tablet containing 4 mg of halazone, stabilised with sodium carbonate and sodium chloride, may be sufficient to treat about 1 litre of water in about 30 minutes to 1 hour. The taste of residual chlorine may be removed by adding sodium thiosulfate.

### Preparations

***USP 27:*** Halazone Tablets for Solution.

**Proprietary Preparations** (details are given in Part 3)
***Ital.:*** Clordispenser†; Steridrolo a rapida idrolisi; ***Port.:*** Speton.

**Multi-ingredient:** ***Spain:*** Cloritines†.

---

## Hexachlorophene *(BAN, rINN)*

G-11; Hexachlorophane; Hexaclorofeno. 2,2′-Methylenebis(3,4,6-trichlorophenol).
$C_{13}H_6Cl_6O_2$ = 406.9.
*CAS — 70-30-4.*
*ATC — D08AE01.*

**Pharmacopoeias.** In *Br.* and *US.*

**BP 2003** (Hexachlorophene). A white or pale buff, odourless or almost odourless, crystalline powder. Practically insoluble in water; freely soluble in alcohol; very soluble in acetone and in ether. It dissolves in dilute solutions of alkali hydroxides. Protect from light.

**USP 27** (Hexachlorophene). A white or light tan, crystalline powder which is odourless or has a slight phenolic odour. Insoluble in water; freely soluble in alcohol, in acetone, and in ether; soluble in chloroform and in dilute solutions of fixed alkali hydroxides. Store in airtight containers. Protect from light.

**Incompatibility.** The activity of hexachlorophene may be reduced in the presence of blood or other organic material. It retains some activity in the presence of soap.

The activity has been reported[1] to be reduced by alkaline media and by nonionic surfactants such as polysorbate 80. It is extremely sensitive to iron, and to avoid discoloration due to traces of this metal in hexachlorophene detergent solutions, it is advisable to incorporate a sequestrant such as disodium edetate.[2]

1. Walter G, Gump W. Effect of pH on hexachlorophene. *Soap Chem Spec* 1963; **39:** 55–6.
2. Bell M. Hexachlorophene-based skin cleansers. *Specialities* 1965; **1:** 16–18.

### Adverse Effects and Treatment

Following ingestion, anorexia, nausea, vomiting, diarrhoea, abdominal cramps, dehydration, shock, and confusion may occur. Convulsions and death may follow. CNS stimulation, convulsions, and death have also occurred after absorption of hexachlorophene from burns and damaged skin. There have been reports showing that hexachlorophene can be absorbed through the skin of infants in amounts sufficient to produce spongy lesions of the brain, sometimes fatal.

Photosensitivity and skin sensitisation have occasionally occurred after repeated use of hexachlorophene.

Treatment of adverse effects is as for Phenol, p.1188.

**Effects on the respiratory system.** Asthma developed in a 43-year-old nurse after long-term exposure to hexachlorophene powder.[1]

1. Nagy L, Orosz M. Occupational asthma due to hexachlorophene. *Thorax* 1984; **39:** 630–1.

### Precautions

Hexachlorophene should not be applied to mucous membranes, large areas of skin, or to burnt, damaged, or denuded skin and should not be used vaginally, applied under occlusive dressings, or applied to areas affected by dermatoses. It should be used with caution on infants, especially premature and low birth-weight neonates. Its use is advised against in pregnancy.

Preparations of hexachlorophene are liable to contamination, especially with Gram-negative bacteria.

**Breast feeding.** The American Academy of Pediatrics[1] considers that, while no effects on the infant have been reported, there is a possibility of contamination of breast milk with hexachlorophene used by breast-feeding mothers for nipple wasting.

1. American Academy of Pediatrics. The transfer of drugs and other chemicals into human milk. *Pediatrics* 2001; **108:** 776–89. Correction. *ibid.*; 1029. Also available at: http://aappolicy.aappublications.org/cgi/content/full/pediatrics%3b108/3/776 (accessed 10/06/04)

**Neonates.** Spongiform encephalopathy has occurred in neonates who were treated topically with hexachlorophene.[1] Neonates with a birth-weight of 1.4 kg or less appeared to be most susceptible, whereas those weighing over 2 kg were not considered to be at risk.[1,2] Also most of the reports involved hexachlorophene applied in a concentration of 3%.

1. Anonymous. Hexachlorophene today. *Lancet* 1982; **i:** 87–8.
2. Plueckhahn VD, Collins RB. Hexachlorophene emulsions and antiseptic skin care of newborn infants. *Med J Aust* 1976; **1:** 815–19.

**Pregnancy.** Hexachlorophene is absorbed from the skin and crosses the placenta, but whether it has produced teratogenic effects is subject to debate.[1,2] However, it is considered best to avoid its use during pregnancy.

1. Halling H. Suspected link between exposure to hexachlorophene and malformed infants. *Ann N Y Acad Sci* 1979; **320:** 426–35.
2. Baltzar B, *et al.* Pregnancy outcome among women working in Swedish hospitals. *N Engl J Med* 1979; **300:** 627–8.

### Pharmacokinetics

Hexachlorophene is absorbed from the gastrointestinal tract after accidental ingestion, and through intact and denuded skin. Percutaneous absorption may be significant in premature infants and through damaged skin. Hexachlorophene crosses the placenta.

### Uses and Administration

Hexachlorophene is a chlorinated bisphenol antiseptic with a bacteriostatic action against Gram-positive organisms, but much less effective against Gram-negative organisms. It is most active at pH 5 to 6.

Hexachlorophene is mainly used in soaps and creams in a concentration of 0.23 to 3% and is an ingredient of various preparations used for skin disorders. After repeated use of these preparations for several days there is a marked diminution of the bacterial flora due to accumulation of hexachlorophene in the skin. This residual effect is rapidly lost after washing with unmedicated soap or alcohol.

A preparation containing 3% is used for the disinfection of the hands of surgeons and other health-care personnel. Thorough rinsing is recommended before drying. Hexachlorophene has been applied as a 0.33% dusting powder to the umbilical cord stump for the control of staphylococcal infection in the newborn. However, care is necessary when using hexachlorophene in neonates (see above).

Hexachlorophene sodium has also been used.

**Disinfection.** Eradication of an outbreak of infection with meticillin-resistant *Staphylococcus aureus* in a neonatal intensive care unit was achieved by use of hexachlorophene soap for hand washing. Previous infection-control measures including the use of chlorhexidine had failed.[1] For a discussion of staphylococcal infections and their treatment, see p.147.

1. Reboli AC, *et al.* Epidemic methicillin-gentamicin-resistant Staphylococcus aureus in a neonatal intensive care unit. *Am J Dis Child* 1989; **143:** 34–9.

### Preparations

***BP 2003:*** Hexachlorophene Dusting Powder;
***USP 27:*** Hexachlorophene Cleansing Emulsion; Hexachlorophene Liquid Soap.

**Proprietary Preparations** (details are given in Part 3)
***Canad.:*** Hexaphenyl†; Sapoderm†; ***Ger.:*** Aknefug simplex; ***Spain:*** Jabon Antiseptico Asens†; ***UK:*** Ster-Zac; ***USA:*** Septisol.

**Multi-ingredient:** ***Braz.:*** Lindanoxil†; Micosan†; ***Canad.:*** pHisoHex; ***Ger.:*** Aknefug-Emulsion; ***Irl.:*** Torbetol; ***Israel:*** Acnex; ***Port.:*** Anacal; ***Spain:*** Cresophene; Neo Visage†; Solarcaine†; ***Switz.:*** Acerbine; Acne-Med Wolff Simplex; ***Thai.:*** Cibis; ***USA:*** pHisoHex.

---

## Hexamidine Isetionate *(BANM, rINNM)*

Hexamidine Diisetionate; Hexamidine Isethionate; Hexamidini Diisetionas; Isetionato de hexamidina. 4,4′-(Hexamethylenedioxy)dibenzamidine bis(2-hydroxyethanesulphonate).
$C_{20}H_{26}N_4O_2,2C_2H_6O_4S$ = 606.7.
*CAS — 3811-75-4 (hexamidine); 659-40-5 (hexamidine isetionate).*
*ATC — D08AC04; R01AX07; R02AA18; S01AX08; S03AA05.*

NOTE. The name Hexamidinum has also been used for primidone.

**Pharmacopoeias.** In *Eur.* (see p.vi).
**Ph. Eur. 5.0** (Hexamidine Diisetionate; Hexamidine Isetionate BP 2003). A white or slightly yellow hygroscopic powder. Sparingly soluble in water; slightly soluble in alcohol; practically insoluble in dichloromethane. Store in airtight containers.

### Profile

Hexamidine isetionate has antibacterial and antifungal properties and is available in a variety of preparations for the local treatment of minor infections.

**Acanthamoeba keratitis.** Hexamidine was suggested[1] as a possible alternative to propamidine for the treatment of *Acanthamoeba* keratitis (p.595).

1. Perrine D, *et al.* Amoebicidal efficiencies of various diamidines against two strains of Acanthamoeba polyphaga. *Antimicrob Agents Chemother* 1995; **39:** 339–42.

### Preparations

**Proprietary Preparations** (details are given in Part 3)
***Arg.:*** Desomedine; ***Belg.:*** Hexomedine; Ophtamedine†; ***Fr.:*** Desomedine; Hexaseptine; Hexomedine; ***Ger.:*** Hexomedin N; Laryngomedin N; ***Hong Kong:*** Desomedine†; ***Neth.:*** Hexomedine†; ***Singapore:*** Desomedine; ***Spain:*** Hexomedin; ***Switz.:*** Desomedine; Hexomedine†.

**Multi-ingredient:** ***Austral.:*** Medi Creme†; Medi Pulv†; ***Belg.:*** Colludol; Pulvo 47†; ***Braz.:*** Hexomedine; ***Fr.:*** Amygdospray†; Aurigoutte; Colludol; Cyteal; Hexo-Imotryl†; Hexomedine; Oromedine; Otomide; Pulvo 47; Solutricine Maux de Gorge; ***Ger.:*** Imazol; Imazol comp; Pulvo; ***Hong Kong:*** Medicreme; Medipulv; ***NZ:*** Medicreme; Medipulv; ***Port.:*** Cyteal; ***Singapore:*** Cyteal; ***Spain:*** Tantum; ***Switz.:*** Imacort; Imazol; ***Thai.:*** Pulvo 47.

## Hexetidine *(BAN, rINN)*

Hexetidina; Hexetidinum. 5-Amino-1,3-bis(2-ethylhexyl)hexahydro-5-methylpyrimidine.
$C_{21}H_{45}N_3$ = 339.6.
*CAS — 141-94-6.*
*ATC — A01AB12.*

**Pharmacopoeias.** In *Eur.* (see p.vi).
**Ph. Eur. 5.0** (Hexetidine). An oily, colourless or slightly yellow liquid. Very slightly soluble in water; very soluble in alcohol, in acetone, and in dichloromethane. It dissolves in dilute mineral acids. Protect from light.

### Adverse Effects

Allergic contact dermatitis and alterations in taste and smell have occasionally been reported.

### Uses and Administration

Hexetidine is a bactericidal and fungicidal antiseptic. It is used for minor infections of mucous membranes, and in particular as a 0.1% mouthwash for local infections and oral hygiene.

**Mouth ulceration.** A mouthwash containing 0.1% hexetidine was no more effective than placebo in the management of patients with aphthous ulceration (p.1245) and provided no additional benefits to oral hygiene or gingival health.[1] However, such a mouthwash does appear to be of benefit in reducing supragingival plaque and gingival inflammation.[2]

1. Chadwick B, *et al.* Hexetidine mouthrinse in the management of minor aphthous ulceration and as an adjunct to oral hygiene. *Br Dent J* 1991; **171:** 83–7.
2. Sharma NC, *et al.* Antiplaque and antigingivitis effectiveness of a hexetidine mouthwash. *J Clin Periodontol* 2003; **30:** 590–4.

### Preparations

**Proprietary Preparations** (details are given in Part 3)
***Arg.:*** Duranil; ***Austria:*** Gurfix; Hexoral; Isozid-H; Kleenosept; ***Belg.:*** Hextril; ***Canad.:*** Steri/Sol; ***Chile:*** Muramyl; ***Fr.:*** Collu-Hextril; Hextril; ***Ger.:*** Doreperol N; Hexoral; Stas Gurgellosung†; Vagi-Hex; ***Gr.:*** Hexalen; ***Hong Kong:*** Bactidol; ***Irl.:*** Oraldene; ***Ital.:*** Oraseptic; ***Malaysia:*** Bactidol; ***Neth.:*** Hextril; ***NZ:*** Sterisol†; ***Port.:*** Collu-Hextril; Hexifluor†; Hextril; ***S.Afr.:*** Oraldine; ***Singapore:*** Bactidol; ***Spain:*** Hextril; Oraldine†; Oralspray†; ***Switz.:*** Drossadin; Hextril; Vagi-Hex; ***UK:*** Oraldene.

**Multi-ingredient:** ***Arg.:*** Buchex; Mantus; Pentadent; ***Austria:*** Neo-Angin; ***Belg.:*** Givalex; ***Fr.:*** Angispray†; Givalex; Nifluril†; ***Ger.:*** Anginasin N†; De-menthasin†; Givalex; Neo-Angin†; ***Hong Kong:*** Anso; ***Port.:*** Nifluril†; ***Spain:*** Abrasone Rectal; Anso; Mentamida.

## Hexylresorcinol *(BAN)*

Esilresorcina; Hexilresorcinol; Hexylresorc; Hexylresorcinolum. 4-Hexylbenzene-1,3-diol.
$C_{12}H_{18}O_2$ = 194.3.
*CAS — 136-77-6.*
*ATC — R02AA12.*

**Pharmacopoeias.** In *Eur.* (see p.vi) and *US.*
**Ph. Eur. 5.0** (Hexylresorcinol). A colourless, yellowish or reddish crystalline powder or needles, turning brownish-pink on exposure to light or air. It exhibits polymorphism. M.p. 66° to 68°; melting may occur at about 60° followed by solidification and a second melting at 66° to 68°. Very slightly soluble in water; freely soluble in alcohol and in dichloromethane. Store in airtight containers. Protect from light.
**USP 27** (Hexylresorcinol). M.p. 62° to 67°. Store in airtight containers. Protect from light.

**Incompatibility.** Hexylresorcinol is incompatible with alkalis and oxidising agents.

### Profile

Hexylresorcinol is a phenolic antiseptic that is used topically for the treatment of minor infections of the skin and mucous membranes, and in the form of lozenges for the treatment of sore throat. It has also been used in vaginal spermicidal preparations. High concentrations of hexylresorcinol are irritant and corrosive to skin and mucous membranes. Alcoholic solutions are vesicant.

It was formerly used as an anthelmintic.

### Preparations

***USP 27:*** Hexylresorcinol Lozenges.

**Proprietary Preparations** (details are given in Part 3)
***Austral.:*** Nyal Medithroat Anaesthetic Lozenges†; Strepsils Extra; ***Canad.:*** Antiseptic Throat Lozenges; Bradosol; Bronchodex Pastilles Antiseptiques; Soothe Aid; Sucrets Extra Strength; Throat Lozenges†; ***Israel:*** Sucrets; ***UK:*** Benylin Sore Throat Lozenge; Lemsip Sore Throat; Mac Dual Action†; Strepsils Extra; TCP; ***USA:*** ST 37; Sucrets Sore Throat.

**Multi-ingredient:** ***Arg.:*** Apracur Bucofaringeo; Bagociletas sin Anestesia; Balsamin; Caramelos Antibioticos; Caramelos Antibioticos Bucoangin; Caramelos Oriental; Fanaletas; Fungicida; Ixana; No-Tos Adultos; Pastillas Medex; Refenax Caramelos Expectorantes; Suavisan; Suavisan N; ***Braz.:*** Andriodermol; Micoz; ***Chile:*** Fittig; Lady Fittig; ***Fr.:*** Genola†; ***Ger.:*** Hexamon; Mycatox; ***India:*** Tytin; ***Ital.:*** Golamed Due; ***UK:*** Beechams Max Strength Sore Throat Relief; Beechams Throat-Plus.

## Hydrargaphen *(BAN, rINN)*

Hydraphen; Hygraphen; Phenylmercuric Dinaphthylmethanedisulfonate. μ-(2,2′-Binaphthalene-3-sulphonyloxy)bis(phenylmercury).
$C_{33}H_{24}Hg_2O_6S_2$ = 981.9.
*CAS — 14235-86-0.*

### Profile

Hydrargaphen is a mercurial antiseptic with antibacterial and antifungal properties. It has been used in the treatment of vaginitis, wounds, burns, and infections of the skin.

### Preparations

**Proprietary Preparations** (details are given in Part 3)
**Multi-ingredient:** ***Hong Kong:*** Penotran.

# Hydrogen Peroxide

Hydrogenii Peroxidum; Peróxido de hidrógeno.
$H_2O_2$ = 34.01.
*CAS — 7722-84-1.*
*ATC — A01AB02; D08AX01; S02AA06.*

NOTE. The BP 2003 directs that when Hydrogen Peroxide is prescribed or demanded, Hydrogen Peroxide Solution (6 per cent) shall be dispensed or supplied.

**Incompatibility.** Hydrogen peroxide solutions are incompatible with reducing agents, including organic matter and oxidisable substances, and with some metals, metallic salts, alkalis, iodides, permanganates, and other stronger oxidising agents.

**Stability.** Aqueous solutions of hydrogen peroxide gradually decompose on standing and if allowed to become alkaline. Decomposition is increased by light, agitation, and heat. Incompatibility may also produce decomposition. Solutions are comparatively stable in the presence of a slight excess of acid. Strong solutions are considered to be more stable than weak solutions.

**Storage.** Solutions of hydrogen peroxide should be stored in airtight containers at 15° to 30° (but see Hydrogen Peroxide Solution (30 per cent), below). Solutions should not be stored for long periods. Those not containing a stabiliser should be stored at a temperature not exceeding 15°. Protect from light.

## Hydrogen Peroxide Solution (3 per cent)

Dilute Hydrogen Peroxide Solution; Hydrogen Peroxide Solution (10-volume); Hydrogen Peroxide Topical Solution; Oxydol; Peróxido de hidrógeno, solución al 3%.
*ATC — A01AB02; D08AX01; S02AA06.*

**Pharmacopoeias.** In *Chin., Eur.* (see p.vi), *Jpn, Pol., US,* and *Viet.*
**Ph. Eur. 5.0** (Hydrogen Peroxide Solution (3 per cent)). A clear colourless liquid containing 2.5 to 3.5% w/w of $H_2O_2$ corresponding to about 10 times its volume of oxygen. It decomposes in contact with oxidisable organic matter and with certain metals and if allowed to become alkali. It may contain a suitable stabilising agent. Solutions not containing a stabilising agent should be stored at a temperature below 15°. Protect from light.
The BP 2003 directs that when Hydrogen Peroxide is prescribed or demanded, Hydrogen Peroxide Solution (6 per cent) shall be dispensed or supplied.
**USP 27** (Hydrogen Peroxide Topical Solution). It contains 2.5 to 3.5% w/v of $H_2O_2$. It may contain up to 0.05% of a suitable preservative or preservatives. Store in airtight containers at a temperature between 15° and 30°. Protect from light.

## Hydrogen Peroxide Solution (6 per cent)

Hydrog. Perox. Soln; Hydrogen Dioxide Solution; Hydrogen Peroxide Solution; Hydrogen Peroxide Solution (20-volume); Liq. Hydrog. Perox.; Liquor Hydrogenii Peroxidi; Peróxido de hidrógeno, solución al 6%; Solución de Bióxido de Hidrogeno; Soluté Officinal d'Eau Oxygénée; Wasserstoffsuperoxydlösung.
*ATC — A01AB02; D08AX01; S02AA06.*

**Pharmacopoeias.** In *Br.*
**BP 2003** (Hydrogen Peroxide Solution (6 per cent)). A clear colourless aqueous liquid containing 5.0 to 7.0% w/v of $H_2O_2$ corresponding to about 20 times its volume of available oxygen. It decomposes in contact with oxidisable organic matter and with certain metals and if allowed to become alkali. It may contain a suitable stabilising agent. It should not be stored for long periods. Solutions not containing a stabilising agent should be stored at a temperature below 15°. Protect from light.
The BP directs that when Hydrogen Peroxide is prescribed or demanded, Hydrogen Peroxide Solution (6 per cent) shall be dispensed or supplied.

## Hydrogen Peroxide Solution (27 per cent)

Hydrogenii Peroxidum; Perossido D'Idrogeno Soluzione; Peróxido de hidrógeno, solución al 27%; Solutio Hydrogenii Peroxydati; Strong Hydrog. Perox. Soln; Strong Hydrogen Peroxide Solution.
*ATC — A01AB02; D08AX01; S02AA06.*

**Description.** Hydrogen peroxide solution (27 per cent) is a clear, colourless aqueous solution containing 26 to 28% w/w of $H_2O_2$, corresponding to about 100 times its volume of available oxygen. It may contain a suitable stabilising agent.
The BP 2003 directs that when Hydrogen Peroxide is prescribed or demanded, Hydrogen Peroxide Solution (6 per cent) shall be dispensed or supplied.

## Hydrogen Peroxide Solution (30 per cent)

Hydrogen Peroxide Concentrate; Hydrogen Peroxide Solution (100-volume); Peróxido de hidrógeno, solución al 30%.
*ATC — A01AB02; D08AX01; S02AA06.*

**Pharmacopoeias.** In *Eur.* (see p.vi) and *Pol.*
*Chin.* specifies 26 to 28%.
*US* and *Viet.* specify 29 to 32%.
**Ph. Eur. 5.0** (Hydrogen Peroxide Solution (30 per cent)). A clear colourless liquid containing 29.0 to 31.0% w/w of $H_2O_2$ corresponding to about 110 times its volume of available oxygen. It decomposes in contact with oxidisable organic matter and with certain metals and if allowed to become alkali. It may contain a suitable stabilising agent. Solutions not containing a stabilising agent should be stored at a temperature below 15°. Protect from light.
The BP 2003 directs that when Hydrogen Peroxide is prescribed or demanded, Hydrogen Peroxide Solution (6 per cent) shall be dispensed or supplied.
**USP 27** (Hydrogen Peroxide Concentrate). A clear, colourless liquid containing 29 to 32% w/w of $H_2O_2$. It may contain up to 0.05% of a suitable preservative or preservatives. It is acid to litmus. It slowly decomposes and is affected by light. Store in partially-filled containers having a small vent in the closure, at a temperature of 8° to 15°.

## Adverse Effects and Precautions

Strong solutions of hydrogen peroxide produce irritating 'burns' on the skin and mucous membranes with a white eschar, but the pain disappears in about an hour. Continued use of hydrogen peroxide as a mouthwash may cause reversible hypertrophy of the papillae of the tongue.

It is dangerous to inject or instil hydrogen peroxide into closed body cavities from which the released oxygen has no free exit. Colonic lavage with solutions of hydrogen peroxide has been followed by gas embolism, rupture of the colon, proctitis, ulcerative colitis, and gangrene of the intestine.

**Closed body cavities.** Liberation of oxygen during the use of hydrogen peroxide in surgical procedures has resulted in oxygen embolism and local emphysema.[1-3] Gas embolism has also been reported after accidental ingestion of hydrogen peroxide solution.[4] Local damage to the colonic and rectal mucosa has followed the use of hydrogen peroxide 3% as an enema[5] and from residual hydrogen peroxide following disinfection of endoscopes.[6]

1. Sleigh JW, Linter SPK. Hazards of hydrogen peroxide. *BMJ* 1985; **291:** 1706.
2. Saïssy JM, *et al.* Risques de l'irrigation au peroxyde d'hydrogène en chirurgie de guerre. *Ann Fr Anesth Reanim* 1994; **13:** 749–53.
3. Konrad C, *et al.* Pulmonary embolism and hydrogen peroxide. *Can J Anaesth* 1997; **44:** 338–9.
4. Rackoff WR, Merton DF. Gas embolism after ingestion of hydrogen peroxide. *Pediatrics* 1990; **85:** 593–4.
5. Auroux J, *et al.* Rectocolite aiguë iatrogène après lavement à l'eau oxygénée. *Rev Geriatr* 1997; **22:** 21–4.
6. Ryan CK, Potter GD. Disinfectant colitis: rinse as well as you wash. *J Clin Gastroenterol* 1995; **21:** 6–9.

**Effects on the mouth.** Use of hydrogen peroxide 3% as a mouthwash has been reported to cause mouth ulceration.[1]

1. Rees TD, Orth CF. Oral ulcerations with use of hydrogen peroxide. *J Periodontol* 1986; **57:** 689–92.

**Intravascular administration.** Intravenous administration of hydrogen peroxide solutions as unconventional therapy for AIDS or cancer has resulted in severe acute haemolysis.[1,2]

Haemolysis was also reported following contamination of haemodialysis fluid with hydrogen peroxide.[3]


1. Jordan KS, *et al.* A 39-year-old man with acute hemolytic crisis secondary to intravenous injection of hydrogen peroxide. *J Emerg Nurs* 1991; **17:** 8–10.
2. Hirschtick RE, *et al.* Death from an unconventional therapy for AIDS. *Ann Intern Med* 1994; **120:** 694.
3. Gordon SM, *et al.* Hemolysis associated with hydrogen peroxide at a pediatric dialysis center. *Am J Nephrol* 1990; **10:** 123–7.


## Uses and Administration

Hydrogen peroxide is an oxidising agent used as an antiseptic, disinfectant, and deodorant. It has weak antibacterial activity and is also effective against viruses, including HIV. It also has a mild haemostatic action. It owes its antiseptic action to its ready release of oxygen when applied to tissues, but the effect lasts only as long as the oxygen is being released and is of short duration; in addition the antimicrobial effect of the liberated oxygen is reduced in the presence of organic matter. The mechanical effect of effervescence is probably more useful for wound cleansing than the antimicrobial action (but see p.1165).

Hydrogen peroxide solutions are used to cleanse wounds and ulcers in concentrations of up to 6%; creams containing 1 or 1.5% stabilised hydrogen peroxide are also used. Although hydrogen peroxide alone is not considered effective on intact skin, it is used with other antiseptics for the disinfection of hands, skin, and mucous membranes. Injection into closed body cavities is dangerous (see above). Adhering and blood-soaked dressings may be released by the application of a solution of hydrogen peroxide.

A 1.5% solution of hydrogen peroxide has been used as a mouthwash in the treatment of acute stomatitis and as a deodorant gargle. A suitable solution can be prepared by diluting 15 mL of hydrogen peroxide 6% in half a tumblerful of warm water. An oral gel has also been used.

Hydrogen peroxide ear drops have been used for the removal of wax. Such ear drops were prepared by diluting a 6% solution of hydrogen peroxide with 3 parts of water preferably just before use.

Hydrogen peroxide 3% is used for disinfecting soft contact lenses.

Immersion for 30 minutes in hydrogen peroxide 6% has been suggested for disinfecting cleaned equipment.

For bleaching hair and delicate fabrics hydrogen peroxide 6% should be diluted with an equal volume of water.

Strong solutions (27 per cent and 30 per cent) of hydrogen peroxide are used for the preparation of weaker solutions and should not be applied to tissues undiluted.

Hydrogen peroxide and other peroxides have many industrial uses as bleaching and oxidising agents.

**Disinfection.** CONTACT LENSES. Hydrogen peroxide 3% is particularly useful for disinfecting soft contact lenses (p.1164) and lens storage cases since it is effective against *Acanthamoeba* spp. However, it is irritant to the cornea and requires inactivating with sodium pyruvate, catalase, or sodium thiosulfate before the lenses are used.

DIALYSIS EQUIPMENT. A disinfectant containing hydrogen peroxide and peracetic acid (Renalin) was not completely effective in killing *Mycobacterium chelonae* in high-flux dialysers. This possibly led to infection of 5 dialysis patients.[1] For a report of haemolysis following inadvertent contamination of dialysis fluid with hydrogen peroxide, see Intravascular Administration under Adverse Effects and Precautions, above.


1. Lowry PW, *et al.* Mycobacterium chelonae infection among patients receiving high-flux dialysis in a hemodialysis clinic in California. *J Infect Dis* 1990; **161:** 85–90.


ENDOSCOPES. Peroxygen compounds have been suggested for disinfection of endoscopes as an alternative to glutaral (p.1164). Hydrogen peroxide solution 3% is fully effective against oocysts of *Cryptosporidium* and immersion for 30 minutes at room temperature has been recommended.[1] However, it has been pointed out that hydrogen peroxide damages external surfaces, particularly rubbers and plastics of the insertion tubes, and thus is not ideal for such purposes.[2] Other peroxygen-containing compounds have been assessed for disinfecting endoscopes but their activity against enteroviruses and mycobacteria may be inadequate.[3,4] Residual hydrogen peroxide solution can cause mucosal damage (see Closed Body Cavities, under Adverse Effects, above) and endoscopes should be thoroughly rinsed before use.


1. Casemore DP, *et al.* Cleaning and disinfection of equipment for gastrointestinal flexible endoscopy: interim recommendations of a working party of the British Society of Gastroenterology. *Gut* 1989; **30:** 1156.
2. Weller IVD, *et al.* Reply. *Gut* 1989; **30:** 1156–7.
3. Tyler R, *et al.* Virucidal activity of disinfectants: studies with the poliovirus. *J Hosp Infect* 1990; **15:** 339–45.
4. Broadley SJ, *et al.* Antimycobacterial activity of 'Virkon'. *J Hosp Infect* 1993; **23:** 189–97.


**Mouth ulceration and infection.** The use of antiseptic mouthwashes may be helpful in the management of mouth ulcers (p.1245), although the use of hydrogen peroxide 3% is not advisable. However, application of a 1.5% solution to individual ulcers with a topical corticosteroid may be useful. For oral candidal infections, specific antifungals are recommended (see p.386), and a hydrogen peroxide denture cleaner was not effective in either preventing re-infection or in reducing mucosal inflammation in a study of 49 patients.[1] See also Adverse Effects on the Mouth, above.


1. Walker DM, *et al.* The treatment of denture-induced stomatitis: evaluation of two agents. *Br Dent J* 1981; **151:** 416–19.


### Preparations

***BP 2003:*** Hydrogen Peroxide Mouthwash;
***USP 27:*** Hydrogen Peroxide Topical Solution.

**Proprietary Preparations** (details are given in Part 3)
***Austral.:*** Aosept†; Focus Care One Step†; Peroxyl; ***Austria:*** Aosept†; Austrosept†; Hioxyl†; Lensan A†; Lensept†; Les Yeux I†; Titmus Losung I†; ***Belg.:*** Crystacide; ***Braz.:*** Aosept; Oxysept; Peroxyl†; ***Canad.:*** Aosept; Consept Step I†; ***Denm.:*** Brintoverilte; Microcid; ***Fr.:*** Dentex; Dosoxygenee; ***Ger.:*** Crystacide; ***Hong Kong:*** Crystacide; ***Irl.:*** Crystacide; Hioxyl; ***Israel:*** Crystacide; ***Ital.:*** Crystacide; Oragard; ***NZ:*** Aosept; Crystacide; Focus Care One Step; ***Spain:*** Ahecan†; Crystacide; ***Swed.:*** Microcid; ***UK:*** Crystacide; Hioxyl; Peroxyl; ***USA:*** Oxysept; Peroxyl.

**Multi-ingredient:** ***Arg.:*** One Step; Plus & White; ***Austral.:*** Omnicare I Step†; Oxysept†; ***Austria:*** Oxy-Care; Septicon†; Skinsept mucosa; Soft Mate Consept I†; ***Canad.:*** UltraCare; ***Fr.:*** Spitaderm; ***Ger.:*** Oxysept Comfort†; Oxysept†; Peresal; Skinsept F; Skinsept mucosa; ***Israel:*** Omnicare†; Oxysept†; ***Ital.:*** Eso 70; Esoform 7 mc; Esoform 70 mc; Peresal; Spitaderm; ***Mon.:*** Akila mains et peau†; ***NZ:*** Omnicare I Step; Oxysept†; ***Spain:*** Oximen; ***USA:*** Aosept; MiraSept; Soft Mate Consept; UltraCare.

# Hydroxybenzoates

Parabenos; Parabens.

## Benzyl Hydroxybenzoate

Benzyl Parahydroxybenzoate; Benzylparaben; Parahidroxibenzoato de bencilo. Benzyl 4-hydroxybenzoate.

$C_{14}H_{12}O_3$ = 228.2.
*CAS — 94-18-8.*

**Pharmacopoeias.** In *Br.* and *Int.*

**BP 2003** (Benzyl Hydroxybenzoate). A white to creamy-white, odourless or almost odourless, crystalline powder. Practically insoluble in water; freely soluble in alcohol and in ether. It dissolves in solutions of alkali hydroxides. M.p. about 112°.

**Incompatibility.** The incompatibilities of hydroxybenzoates are described under Sodium Propyl Hydroxybenzoate, below.

## Butyl Hydroxybenzoate

Butilparabeno; Butyl Parahydroxybenzoate; Butylis Parahydroxybenzoas; Butylis Paraoxybenzoas; Butylparaben. Butyl 4-hydroxybenzoate.

$C_{11}H_{14}O_3$ = 194.2.
*CAS — 94-26-8.*

**Pharmacopoeias.** In *Eur.* (see p.vi) and *Jpn.* Also in *USNF.*

**Ph. Eur. 5.0** (Butyl Parahydroxybenzoate; Butyl Hydroxybenzoate BP 2003). Colourless crystals or a white or almost white crystalline powder. Very slightly soluble in water; freely soluble in alcohol and in methyl alcohol. M.p. 68° to 71°.

**USNF 22** (Butylparaben). Small colourless crystals or a white powder. Very slightly soluble in water and in glycerol; freely soluble in alcohol, in acetone, in ether, and in propylene glycol. M.p. 68° to 72°.

**Incompatibility.** The incompatibilities of hydroxybenzoates are described under Sodium Propyl Hydroxybenzoate, below.

## Ethyl Hydroxybenzoate

Aethylum Hydroxybenzoicum; E214; Ethyl Parahydroxybenzoate; Ethylis Parahydroxybenzoas; Ethylis Paraoxybenzoas; Ethylparaben; Etilparabeno. Ethyl 4-hydroxybenzoate.

$C_9H_{10}O_3$ = 166.2.
*CAS — 120-47-8.*
*ATC — D01AE10.*

**Pharmacopoeias.** In *Chin., Eur.* (p.vi), *Int., Jpn.,* and *Pol.* Also in *USNF.*

**Ph. Eur. 5.0** (Ethyl Parahydroxybenzoate; Ethyl Hydroxybenzoate BP 2003). Colourless crystals or a white or almost white crystalline powder. Very slightly soluble in water; freely soluble in alcohol and in methyl alcohol.

**USNF 22** (Ethylparaben). Small colourless crystals or a white powder. Slightly soluble in water and in glycerol; freely soluble in alcohol, in acetone, in ether, and in propylene glycol.

**Incompatibility.** The incompatibilities of hydroxybenzoates are described under Sodium Propyl Hydroxybenzoate, below.

## Methyl Hydroxybenzoate

E218; Metagin; Methyl Parahydroxybenzoate; Methylis Oxybenzoas; Methylis Parahydroxybenzoas; Methylis Paraoxibenzoas; Methylparaben *(USAN)*; Metilparabeno. Methyl 4-hydroxybenzoate.

$C_8H_8O_3$ = 152.1.
*CAS — 99-76-3.*

**Pharmacopoeias.** In *Eur.* (see p.vi), *Int., Jpn,* and *Pol.* Also in *USNF.*

**Ph. Eur. 5.0** (Methyl Parahydroxybenzoate; Methyl Hydroxybenzoate BP 2003). Colourless crystals or a white crystalline powder. Very slightly soluble in water; freely soluble in alcohol and in methyl alcohol. M.p. 125° to 128°.

**USNF 22** (Methylparaben). Colourless crystals or a white crystalline powder. Soluble 1 in 400 of water, 1 in 50 of water at 80°, 1 in 3 of alcohol, and 1 in 10 of ether; freely soluble in methyl alcohol. M.p. 125° to 128°.

**Incompatibility.** The incompatibilities of hydroxybenzoates are described under Sodium Propyl Hydroxybenzoate, below.

## Propyl Hydroxybenzoate

E216; Propagin; Propilparabeno; Propyl Parahydroxybenzoate; Propylis Oxybenzoas; Propylis Parahydroxybenzoas; Propylis Paraoxibenzoas; Propylparaben *(USAN)*. Propyl 4-hydroxybenzoate.

$C_{10}H_{12}O_3$ = 180.2.
*CAS — 94-13-3.*

**Pharmacopoeias.** In *Eur.* (see p.vi), *Int., Jpn,* and *Pol.* Also in *USNF.*

**Ph. Eur. 5.0** (Propyl Parahydroxybenzoate; Propyl Hydroxybenzoate BP 2003). A white crystalline powder. Very slightly soluble in water; freely soluble in alcohol and in methyl alcohol. M.p. 96° to 99°.

**USNF 22** (Propylparaben). Small colourless crystals or a white powder. Soluble 1 in 2500 of water, 1 in 400 of boiling water, 1 in 1.5 of alcohol, and 1 in 3 of ether. M.p. 95° to 98°.

**Incompatibility.** The incompatibilities of hydroxybenzoates are described under Sodium Propyl Hydroxybenzoate, below.

## Sodium Butyl Hydroxybenzoate

Butilparabeno sódico; Sodium Butyl Parahydroxybenzoate; Sodium Butylparaben.

$C_{11}H_{13}NaO_3$ = 216.2.
*CAS — 36457-20-2.*

**Pharmacopoeias.** In *Br.*

**BP 2003** (Sodium Butyl Hydroxybenzoate). A white, odourless or almost odourless, hygroscopic powder. Freely soluble in water and in alcohol. A 0.1% solution in water has a pH of 9.5 to 10.5.

**Incompatibility.** The incompatibilities of hydroxybenzoates are described under Sodium Propyl Hydroxybenzoate, below.

## Sodium Ethyl Hydroxybenzoate

E215.

$C_9H_9NaO_3$ = 188.2.
*CAS — 35285-68-8.*

**Pharmacopoeias.** In *Fr.* and *Ger.*

## Sodium Methyl Hydroxybenzoate

E219; Methylis Parahydroxybenzoas Natricum; Methylparaben Sodium *(USAN)*; Metilparabeno sódico; Sodium Methyl Parahydroxybenzoate; Sodium Methylparaben; Soluble Methyl Hydroxybenzoate.

$C_8H_7NaO_3$ = 174.1.
*CAS — 5026-62-0.*

**Pharmacopoeias.** In *Eur.* (see p.vi). Also in *USNF.*

**Ph. Eur. 5.0** (Sodium Methyl Parahydroxybenzoate; Sodium Methyl Hydroxybenzoate BP 2003). A white crystalline powder. Freely soluble in water; sparingly soluble in alcohol; practically insoluble in dichloromethane. A 0.1% solution in water has a pH of 9.5 to 10.5.

**USNF 22** (Methylparaben Sodium). A white, hygroscopic, powder. Freely soluble in water; sparingly soluble in alcohol; insoluble in fixed oils. A 0.1% solution in water has a pH of 9.5 to 10.5. Store in airtight containers.

**Incompatibility.** The incompatibilities of hydroxybenzoates are described under Sodium Propyl Hydroxybenzoate, below.

## Sodium Propyl Hydroxybenzoate

E217; Propilparabeno sódico; Propylis Parahydroxybenzoas Natricum; Propylparaben Sodium *(USAN)*; Sodium Propyl Parahydroxybenzoate; Sodium Propylparaben; Soluble Propyl Hydroxybenzoate.

$C_{10}H_{11}NaO_3$ = 202.2.
*CAS — 35285-69-9.*

**Pharmacopoeias.** In *Eur.* (see p.vi). Also in *USNF.*

**Ph. Eur. 5.0** (Sodium Propyl Parahydroxybenzoate; Sodium Propyl Hydroxybenzoate BP 2003). A white crystalline powder. Freely soluble in water; sparingly soluble in alcohol; practically insoluble in dichloromethane. A 0.1% solution in water has a pH of 9.5 to 10.5.

**USNF 22** (Propylparaben Sodium ). A white, hygroscopic, odourless powder. Freely soluble in water; sparingly soluble in alcohol; insoluble in fixed oils. A 0.1% solution in water has a pH of 9.5 to 10.5. Store in airtight containers.

**Incompatibility and stability.** The activity of hydroxybenzoates can be adversely affected by the presence of other excipients or active ingredients. There may be adsorption onto substances like magnesium trisilicate, aluminium magnesium silicate, talc, polysorbate 80,[1,2] carmellose sodium,[3] or plastics.[4] Nonionic surfactants can reduce hydroxybenzoate activity,[5] as may essential oils.[6] Other incompatibilities that have been reported include atropine,[7] iron,[4] sorbitol,[8] weak alkalis,[4] and strong acids.[4] Syrup preserved with hydroxybenzoates is incompatible with a range of compounds.[9,10] Methyl hydroxybenzoate 0.1% was reported[11] to be a poor preservative in insulin preparations, especially soluble insulin preparations. Increasing heat or pH can reduce stability and activity;[12] freeze-drying may also lead to a loss of activity.[13]

1. Yousef RT, *et al.* Effect of some pharmaceutical materials on the bactericidal activities of preservatives. *Can J Pharm Sci* 1973; **8:** 54–6.
2. Allwood MC. The adsorption of esters of p-hydroxybenzoic acid by magnesium trisilicate. *Int J Pharmaceutics* 1982; **11:** 101–7.
3. Fawcett JP, *et al.* Binding of parabens to sodium carboxymethylcellulose in oral liquid formulations. *Aust J Hosp Pharm* 1996; **26:** 552–4.
4. Rieger MM. Methylparaben. In: Rowe RC, *et al.* eds. *Handbook of pharmaceutical excipients.* 4th ed. London and Chicago: The Pharmaceutical Press and the American Pharmaceutical Association, 2003: 390–4.
5. Yamaguchi M, *et al.* Antimicrobial activity of butylparaben in relation to its solubilization behavior by nonionic surfactants. *J Soc Cosmet Chem* 1982; **33:** 297–307.
6. Chemburkar PB, Joslin RS. Effect of flavoring oils on preservative concentrations in oral liquid dosage forms. *J Pharm Sci* 1975; **64:** 414–17.
7. Deeks T. Oral atropine sulphate mixtures. *Pharm J* 1983; **230:** 481.
8. Runesson B, Gustavii K. Stability of parabens in the presence of polyols. *Acta Pharm Suec* 1986; **23:** 151–62.
9. *PSGB Lab Report P/79/2* 1979.
10. *PSGB Lab Report P/80/1* 1980.
11. Allwood MC. The effectiveness of preservatives in insulin injections. *Pharm J* 1982; **229:** 340.
12. Sunderland VB, Watts DW. Kinetics of the degradation of methyl, ethyl and n-propyl 4-hydroxybenzoate esters in aqueous solution. *Int J Pharmaceutics* 1984; **19:** 1–15.
13. Flora KP, *et al.* The loss of paraben preservatives during freeze drying. *J Pharm Pharmacol* 1980; **32:** 577–80.

## Adverse Effects and Precautions

Hypersensitivity reactions occur with the hydroxybenzoates. Generally these are of the delayed type, appearing as contact dermatitis. Immediate reactions with urticaria and bronchospasm have occurred rarely.

**Hypersensitivity.** Immediate hypersensitivity reactions have been reported following the injection of preparations containing hydroxybenzoates.[1,2] Delayed contact dermatitis occurs more frequently, usually after topical application but has also occurred after use of an ester or of *p*-hydroxybenzoic acid in oral preparations.[3-5] The North American Contact Dermatitis Group[6] provided an incidence of 3%, while another review[7] of a large number of patients gave an incidence of 2.2%. However, subjects with healthy skin exposed to hydroxybenzoates, for example in cosmetics, are considered to have a much lower incidence of reactions.[8] Unusually, patients who have reacted to a hydroxybenzoate with a contact dermatitis appear to be able to apply that preservative to another unaffected site and yet not suffer a reaction; this has been termed the 'paraben paradox'.[9]

Hypersensitivity reactions have occurred in patients given local anaesthetics containing hydroxybenzoates[1,10] and cross-sensitivity between the two groups of drugs has been proposed.[1]

1. Aldrete JA, Johnson DA. Allergy to local anaesthetics. *JAMA* 1969; **207:** 356–7.
2. Nagel JE, *et al.* Paraben allergy. *JAMA* 1977; **237:** 1594–5.
3. Michäelsson G, Juhlin L. Urticaria induced by preservatives and dye additives in food and drugs. *Br J Dermatol* 1973; **88:** 525–32.
4. Warin RP, Smith RJ. Challenge test battery in chronic urticaria. *Br J Dermatol* 1976; **94:** 401–6.
5. Kaminer Y, *et al.* Delayed hypersensitivity reaction to orally administered methylparaben. *Clin Pharm* 1982; **1:** 469–70.
6. North American Contact Dermatitis Group. Epidemiology of contact dermatitis in North America 1972. *Arch Dermatol* 1973; **108:** 537–40.
7. Moore J. Final report on the safety assessment of methylparaben, ethylparaben, propylparaben, and butylparaben. *J Am Coll Toxicol* 1984; **3:** 147–209.
8. Fisher AA. Cosmetic dermatitis. Part II; reactions to some commonly used preservatives. *Cutis* 1980; **26:** 136–7, 141–2, 147–8.
9. Fisher AA. Cortaid cream dermatitis and the "paraben paradox". *J Am Acad Dermatol* 1982; **6:** 116–7.
10. Lederman DA, *et al.* An unusual skin reaction following local anesthetic injection: review of the literature and report of four cases. *Oral Surg* 1980; **49:** 28–33.

**Neonates.** An *in-vitro* study on serum from neonates with hyperbilirubinaemia indicated that methyl hydroxybenzoate at a concentration of 200 micrograms/mL of serum increased the concentration of free unconjugated bilirubin and interfered with the binding of bilirubin to serum proteins. Methyl hydroxybenzoate was present in an injection of gentamicin sulfate at a concentration of 1.3 to 1.8 mg/mL. Neither gentamicin nor propyl hydroxybenzoate had a significant effect on bilirubin.[1]

1. Loria CJ, *et al.* Effect of antibiotic formulations in serum protein: bilirubin interaction of newborn infants. *J Pediatr* 1976; **89:** 479–82.

## Pharmacokinetics

**Neonates.** After intramuscular injection, methyl hydroxybenzoate present in a gentamicin preparation was excreted in the urine of preterm infants to a variable extent and mainly in the conjugated form.[1] *p*-Hydroxybenzoic acid was detected as a metabolite. The injection contained methyl hydroxybenzoate 3.6 mg, propyl hydroxybenzoate 400 micrograms, and gentamicin 80 mg. Propyl hydroxybenzoate was also detected in the urine samples.

1. Hindmarsh KW, *et al.* Urinary excretion of methylparaben and its metabolites in preterm infants. *J Pharm Sci* 1983; **72:** 1039–41.

## Uses

The hydroxybenzoate preservatives are alkyl esters of *p*-hydroxybenzoic acid with antibacterial and antifungal properties. They are active over a broad pH range (4 to 8), though are generally more active in acidic solutions. Activity increases with increasing alkyl chain length but aqueous solubility decreases, although this may be overcome by employing the more soluble sodium salts as long as the pH of the preparation is not increased. Activity may also be increased by combining two hydroxybenzoates with short alkyl chains. Another way of increasing activity is to use a hydroxybenzoate with propylene glycol.

Hydroxybenzoates are used as preservatives in pharmaceutical preparations in usual concentrations of up to 0.25%. Methyl hydroxybenzoate and propyl hydroxybenzoate are used together in some preparations. There have been reports of the hydroxybenzoates not being satisfactory preservatives for ophthalmic preparations because of their relative lack of efficacy against some Gram-negative bacteria, particularly *Pseudomonas aeruginosa.* The hydroxybenzoate preservatives are widely used in cosmetics and are also used for food preservation.

Hydroxybenzoates are also used for treating skin infections.

## Preparations

**Proprietary Preparations** (details are given in Part 3)
***Fr.:*** Nisapulvol; Nisaseptol; Nisasol; ***Malaysia:*** Nisapulvol.

**Multi-ingredient:** ***Austral.:*** Mycoderm; ***Braz.:*** Pelmic†; ***Ger.:*** Trachitol†; ***Hong Kong:*** Mycoderm; ***Malaysia:*** Mycoderm; ***UK:*** Brushtox†.

---

# Imidurea

*N,N''*-Methylenebis{*N'*-[3-(hydroxymethyl)-2,5-dioxo-4-imidazolidinyl]urea}.

$C_{11}H_{16}N_8O_8$ = 388.3.
*CAS — 39236-46-9.*

**Pharmacopoeias.** In *USNF.*

**USNF 22** (Imidurea). A white odourless powder. Soluble in water and in glycerol; sparingly soluble in propylene glycol; insoluble in most organic solvents. A 1% solution in water has a pH of 6.0 to 7.5. Store in airtight containers.

## Profile

Imidurea is used as an antimicrobial preservative in topical pharmaceutical and cosmetic preparations.

---

# Iodoform

Iodoformo. Tri-iodomethane.

$CHI_3$ = 393.7.
*CAS — 75-47-8.*

**Pharmacopoeias.** In *Jpn* and *US.*

**USP 27** (Iodoform). A lustrous greenish-yellow powder or lustrous crystals. It is slightly volatile at ordinary temperatures and distils slowly with steam. It decomposes at high temperatures emitting vapours of iodine. Practically insoluble in water; sparingly soluble in alcohol, in glycerol, and in olive oil; soluble in boiling alcohol; freely soluble in chloroform and in ether. Store in airtight containers at a temperature not exceeding 40°. Protect from light.

## Profile

Iodoform slowly releases iodine (p.1598) when applied to the tissues and is used for its mild antiseptic action. Bismuth Subnitrate and Iodoform Paste (BPC 1954) (BIPP) has been applied to wounds and abscesses. Sterile gauze impregnated with the paste has also been used for packing cavities after oral and otorhinological surgery.

**Adverse effects on the nervous system.** Encephalopathy has been associated with the use of bismuth subnitrate and iodoform paste for the packing of wound cavities after surgery to the head and neck,[1] although there is some debate as to whether the bismuth or the iodoform component is responsible.[1,2] However, encephalopathy has been reported after application of iodoform gauze without bismuth.[3,4]

1. Wilson APR. The dangers of BIPP. *Lancet* 1994; **344:** 1313–14.
2. Farrell RWR. Dangers of bismuth iodoform paraffin paste. *Lancet* 1994; **344:** 1637–8.
3. Roy P-M, *et al.* Dangers of bismuth iodoform paraffin paste. *Lancet* 1994; **344:** 1708.
4. Yamasaki K, *et al.* Delirium and a subclavian abscess. *Lancet* 1997; **350:** 1294.

## Preparations

***BPC 1954:*** Bismuth Subnitrate and Iodoform Paste; Compound Iodoform Paint.

**Proprietary Preparations** (details are given in Part 3)
***Ger.:*** Jodoform.

**Multi-ingredient:** ***Arg.:*** Aseptobron; ***Spain:*** Alvogil; ***Switz.:*** Alvogyl; Pate Iodoforme du Prof Dr Walkhoff†; ***UK:*** OxBipp.

---

# Isopropyl Alcohol

Alcohol isopropílico; Alcohol Isopropylicus; Dimethyl Carbinol; Isopropanol; 2-Propanol; Secondary Propyl Alcohol. Propan-2-ol.

$(CH_3)_2CHOH$ = 60.10.
*CAS — 67-63-0.*
*ATC — D08AX05.*

**Pharmacopoeias.** In *Eur.* (see p.vi), *Int., Jpn, Pol.,* and *US.*

**Ph. Eur. 5.0** (Isopropyl Alcohol). A clear colourless liquid. Miscible with water and with alcohol. Protect from light.

**USP 27** (Isopropyl Alcohol). A transparent, colourless, mobile, volatile, flammable liquid with a characteristic odour. Miscible with water, with alcohol, with chloroform, and with ether. Store in airtight containers remote from heat.

## Adverse Effects, Treatment, and Precautions

Isopropyl alcohol is considered to be more toxic than ethyl alcohol (p.1166), and the symptoms of intoxication appear to be similar, except that isopropyl alcohol has no initial euphoric action and gastritis, haemorrhage, pain, nausea, and vomiting are more prominent. The lethal dose by mouth is reported to be about 120 to 240 mL; however, toxic symptoms may be produced by as little as 20 mL. Ketoacidosis and ketonuria commonly occur due to the presence of the major metabolite, acetone, in the circulation. Inhalation of isopropyl alcohol vapour has been reported to produce coma.

Application of isopropyl alcohol to the skin may cause dryness and irritation; suitable precautions should be taken to prevent absorption through the skin.

Treatment of adverse effects is as for Alcohol, p.1166.

◊ General references.

1. 2-Propanol. *Environmental Health Criteria 103.* Geneva: WHO, 1990. Available at: http://www.inchem.org/documents/ehc/ehc/ehc103.htm (accessed 11/06/04)

**Children.** Reports of chemical skin burns caused by the topical application of isopropyl alcohol in premature infants.[1,2]

Haemorrhagic gastritis in a 2-year-old febrile child was attributed to topical absorption of isopropyl alcohol that had been used for sponge bathing and followed by wrapping the child tightly in a blanket.[3]

1. Schick JB, Milstein JM. Burn hazard of isopropyl alcohol in the neonate. *Pediatrics* 1981; **68:** 587–8.
2. Weintraub Z, Iancu TC. Isopropyl alcohol burns. *Pediatrics* 1982; **69:** 506.
3. Dyer S, *et al.* Hemorrhagic gastritis from topical isopropanol exposure. *Ann Pharmacother* 2002; **36:** 1733–5.

**Rectal absorption.** A report of intoxication and raised serum-creatinine concentrations due to absorption of isopropyl alcohol following its use as a rectal douche.[1]

1. Barnett JM, *et al.* Intoxication after an isopropyl alcohol enema. *Ann Intern Med* 1990; **113:** 638–9.

## Pharmacokinetics

Isopropyl alcohol is readily absorbed from the gastrointestinal tract but there appears to be little absorption through intact skin. The vapour may be absorbed through the lungs. Isopropyl alcohol is metabolised more slowly than ethyl alcohol and about 15% of an ingested dose is metabolised to acetone.

◊ For a report of rectal absorption of isopropyl alcohol, see above.

### Uses and Administration

Isopropyl alcohol is an antiseptic with bactericidal properties similar to those of alcohol (p.1167). It is used for pre-operative skin cleansing in concentrations of about 60 to 70%, and is an ingredient of preparations used for disinfection of hands and surfaces. Its marked degreasing properties may limit its usefulness in preparations used repeatedly. It is also used as a solvent, especially in cosmetics, perfumes and pharmaceutical preparations, and as a vehicle for other disinfectant compounds.

Propyl alcohol (p.1191) is also used as an antiseptic.

### Preparations

***USP 27:*** Azeotropic Isopropyl Alcohol; Isopropyl Rubbing Alcohol.

**Proprietary Preparations** (details are given in Part 3)
***Canad.:*** Alcojel; Alko Isol†; Auro-Dri; Duonalc; Friction Rub†; ***Ger.:*** Aktivin; ***Switz.:*** Avitracid; Mundisept†; ***UK:*** Alcowipe; Medi-Swab; Sterets; Steriwipe; ***USA:*** Auro-Dri.

**Multi-ingredient:** ***Austral.:*** Aquaear†; Ear Clear for Swimmer's Ear†; Hibicol†; Hibitane†; Unisolve; ***Austria:*** Braunoderm; Cleanomed; Cutasept; Dodesept; Dodesept Gefarbt; Dodesept N; Marcocid; Mycopol; Skinsept; Sterillium; ***Belg.:*** Braunoderm†; ***Canad.:*** Acnomel†; Diodine†; Duonalc-E; Iba-Cide†; Ic-Gel†; Snap Skin Cleanser Normal†; Swim-Ear; ***Chile:*** Solarcaine Spray Aerosol; ***Fr.:*** Clinogel; Manugel; Novospray†; Pulvispray†; Spitaderm; Sterillium; ***Ger.:*** Bacillol; Bacillol AF; Bacillol plus; Betaseptic; Braunoderm; Cutasept; Desmanol; Dibromol; Freka-Steril; Gercid forte; Helipur H plus N; Incidin; Incidin M Spray Extra; Kodan Tinktur Forte; Mucasept-A; Neo Kodan; Primasept Med; Promanum N; Rutisept extra; Sagrosept; Sanato-Rhev†; Sekucid konz; Skinman Soft; Skinsept F; Skinsept G; Softasept N; Spitacid; St-Tissues; Sterillium; ***Hong Kong:*** Hibisol; ***Irl.:*** Braunoderm†; Hibisol; ***Israel:*** Sterets H; ***Ital.:*** Bergon; Braunoderm; Citromed; Clorexan; Eso Ferri Alcolico Plus; Eso Ferri Plus; Esocetic; Esoform Maniferri†; Panseptil; SaniSteril Strumenti Alcolico; Sekucid; Spitaderm; ***Neth.:*** Hibisol†; ***NZ:*** Aqua Ear; ***Singapore:*** Hibisol†; ***Switz.:*** Aseptoman†; Betaseptic; Braunoderm; Cutasept; Desamon; Dolo-Arthrosenex sine Heparino; Dolorex†; Ederphyt; Hibital; Hibitane Teinture; Orosept†; Promanum N; Secalan†; Softasept N; ***UK:*** Hibisol; Manusept; Medi-Swab H; Sterets H; Sunspot†; Swim-Ear; ***USA:*** BactoShield; Cresylate; Dri/Ear; Ear-Dry; Fungi-Nail; Swim-Ear; Tinver.

## Isothiazolinones

Isotiazolinonas.

### Methylchloroisothiazolinone

Metilcloroisotiazolinona. 5-Chloro-2-methyl-3(2*H*)-isothiazolone; 5-Chloro-2-methyl-4-isothiazolin-3-one.
*CAS — 26172-55-4.*

### Methylisothiazolinone

Metilisotiazolinona. 2-Methyl-3(2*H*)-isothiazolone; 2-Methyl-4-isothiazolin-3-one.
*CAS — 2682-20-4.*

### Profile

A mixture of isothiazolinones consisting of methylchloroisothiazolinone and methylisothiazolinone in a ratio of approximately 3:1 is used as a preservative in industry and in cosmetic products. The mixture is often referred to as Kathon CG, one of its proprietary names.

Isothiazolinones may cause contact dermatitis and local irritation.

**Hypersensitivity.** There have been several reports of allergic contact dermatitis arising from the use of isothiazolinones in cosmetics.[1-4] One review[4] lists incidences ranging from 0.4 to 8.4% and considers that the risks are reduced when these preservatives are used in 'rinse-off' preparations such as shampoos at low concentrations. Irritant reactions can also occur,[1,3] and occupational asthma has been reported.[5]

1. Björkner B, *et al.* Contact allergy to the preservative Kathon CG. *Contact Dermatitis* 1986; **14:** 85–90.
2. De Groot AC, Bos JD. Preservatives in the European standard series for epicutaneous testing. *Br J Dermatol* 1987; **116:** 289–92.
3. Fransway AF. Sensitivity to Kathon CG: findings in 365 consecutive patients. *Contact Dermatitis* 1988; **19:** 342–7.
4. De Groot AC, Herxheimer A. Isothiazolinone preservative: cause of a continuing epidemic of cosmetic dermatitis. *Lancet* 1989; **i:** 314–16.
5. Bourke SJ, *et al.* Occupational asthma in an isothiazolinone manufacturing plant. *Thorax* 1997; **52:** 746–8.

### Preparations

**Proprietary Preparations** (details are given in Part 3)
**Multi-ingredient:** ***Switz.:*** Saltrates.

## Magenta

Aniline Red; Basic Fuchsin; Basic Magenta; CI Basic Violet 14; Colour Index No. 42510; Fuchsine; Fucsina.
*CAS — 569-61-9 (pararosaniline hydrochloride); 632-99-5 (rosaniline hydrochloride).*

**Description.** Magenta is a mixture of the hydrochlorides of pararosaniline {4-[(4-aminophenyl)(4-iminocyclohexa-2,5-dien-1-ylidene)-methyl]aniline} and rosaniline {4-[(4-aminophenyl)(4-iminocyclohexa-2,5-dien-1-ylidene)methyl]-2-methylaniline}.

**Pharmacopoeias.** In *US.*

**USP 27** (Basic Fuchsin). A mixture of rosaniline and pararosaniline hydrochlorides. It contains the equivalent of not less than 88% of rosaniline hydrochloride ($C_{20}H_{20}ClN_3$), calculated on the dried basis. A dark green powder or greenish glistening crystalline fragments with a bronze-like lustre and not more than a faint odour. Soluble in water, in alcohol, and in amyl alcohol; insoluble in ether.

### Profile

Magenta is a triphenylmethane antiseptic dye effective against Gram-positive bacteria and some fungi. Magenta Paint (BPC 1973) (Castellani's Paint) was formerly used in the treatment of superficial dermatophytoses.

Decolorised magenta solution (Schiff reagent) is used as a test for the presence of aldehydes.

Concerns about possible carcinogenicity have restricted the use of magenta.

**Carcinogenicity.** The handling of magenta was not thought to induce carcinogenesis but its actual manufacture may produce tumours.[1] Magenta was also considered to be unsafe for use in food.[2]

1. Glashan RW. Changes in compensation for occupationally induced bladder cancer. *BMJ* 1984; **288:** 1181–2.
2. FAO/WHO. Specifications for the identity and purity of food additives and their toxicological evaluation: food colours and some antimicrobials and antoxidants: eighth report of the joint FAO/WHO expert committee on food additives. *WHO Tech Rep Ser 309* 1965.

### Preparations

***BPC 1973:*** Magenta Paint;
***USP 27:*** Carbol-Fuchsin Topical Solution.

**Proprietary Preparations** (details are given in Part 3)
**Multi-ingredient:** ***Braz.:*** Antimic†; Fungol†; ***Ital.:*** Fucsina Fenica.

## Magnesium Peroxide

Magnesii Peroxidum; Magnesium Perhydrolum; Peróxido de magnesio.
*CAS — 1335-26-8; 14452-57-4.*
*ATC — A02AA03; A06AD03.*

**Pharmacopoeias.** In *Eur.* (see p.vi).

**Ph. Eur. 5.0** (Magnesium Peroxide). A mixture of magnesium peroxide and magnesium oxide. It contains not less than 22% and not more than 28% of $MgO_2$. A white or slightly yellow, amorphous, light powder. Practically insoluble in water and in alcohol; dissolves in mineral acids. Protect from light.

### Profile

Magnesium peroxide is used as an antiseptic. It is also an ingredient of preparations for gastrointestinal disorders.

### Preparations

**Proprietary Preparations** (details are given in Part 3)
***Austria:*** Ozovit†; ***Ger.:*** Ozovit.

**Multi-ingredient:** ***Fr.:*** Ektogan†; ***Israel:*** Digestif-Ara; ***Ital.:*** Carbonesia; Ektogan; ***Switz.:*** Magenpulver Hafter.

## Malachite Green

Aniline Green; China Green; CI Basic Green 4; Colour Index No. 42000; Diamond Green B; Verde de malaquita; Viride Malachitum. [4-(4-Dimethylaminobenzhydrylidene)cyclohexa-2,5-dienylidene]dimethylammonium chloride.
*CAS — 569-64-2.*

### Profile

Malachite green is a triphenylmethane antiseptic dye with actions similar to those of brilliant green (p.1171). It has been used for skin disinfection.

## Mecetronium Etilsulfate *(BAN, rINN)*

Etilsulfato de mecetronio; Mecetronium Ethylsulfate *(USAN)*; Mecetronium Ethylsulphate. Ethylhexadecyldimethylammonium ethyl sulphate.
$C_{22}H_{49}NO_4S = 423.7.$
*CAS — 3006-10-8.*

### Profile

Mecetronium etilsulfate is a quaternary ammonium antiseptic with actions and uses similar to those of other cationic surfactants (see Cetrimide, p.1172). It is active against bacteria, including mycobacteria, fungi, and viruses, including hepatitis B virus. It is used in alcoholic solution for disinfection of the skin and hard surfaces.

### Preparations

**Proprietary Preparations** (details are given in Part 3)
**Multi-ingredient:** ***Austria:*** Sterillium; ***Fr.:*** Sterillium; ***Ger.:*** Bacillol; St-Tissues; Sterillium.

## Merbromin *(rINN)*

Disodium 2,7-dibromo-4-hydroxymercurifluorescein; Merbromina; Mercurescéine Sodique; Mercurochrome; Mercurodibromofluorescein. The disodium salt of [2,7-dibromo-9-(2-carboxyphenyl)-6-hydroxy-3-oxo-3*H*-xanthen-5-yl]hydroxymercury.
$C_{20}H_8Br_2HgNa_2O_6 = 750.7.$
*CAS — 129-16-8.*
*ATC — D08AK04.*

NOTE. The use of the name Merbromin is limited; in some countries it is a trade-mark.

**Pharmacopoeias.** In *Fr., It., Jpn,* and *Viet.*

**Incompatibility.** Merbromin is incompatible with acids, most alkaloidal salts, many local anaesthetics, metals, and sulfides. Activity may be reduced in the presence of organic material.

### Adverse Effects and Treatment

As for Mercury, p.1713.

◊ Reports of merbromin toxicity have included contact dermatitis[1] and epidermal cell toxicity.[2] A fatality has occurred after transcutaneous absorption of merbromin during treatment of infected omphalocele (umbilical hernia)[3,4] and death due to shock, with aplastic anaemia, has followed application to surgical wounds and decubitus areas.[5] Anaphylaxis has also occurred.[6] Extensive absorption after ingestion has also been reported.[7]

1. Camarasa G. Contact dermatitis from mercurochrome. *Contact Dermatitis* 1976; **2:** 120.
2. Anonymous. Topical antiseptics and antibiotics. *Med Lett Drugs Ther* 1977; **19:** 83–4.
3. Yeh T-F, *et al.* Mercury poisoning from mercurochrome therapy of infected omphalocele. *Lancet* 1978; **i:** 210.
4. Yeh TF, *et al.* Mercury poisoning from mercurochrome therapy of an infected omphalocele. *Clin Toxicol* 1978; **13:** 463–7.
5. Slee PHTJ, *et al.* A case of Merbromin (mercurochrome) intoxication possibly resulting in aplastic anemia. *Acta Med Scand* 1979; **205:** 463–6.
6. Galindo PA, *et al.* Mercurochrome allergy: immediate and delayed hypersensitivity. *Allergy* 1997; **52:** 1138–41.
7. Magarey JA. Absorption of mercurochrome. *Lancet* 1993; **342:** 1424.

### Uses and Administration

Merbromin is a mercurial antiseptic that has been used for disinfection of skin and wounds.

### Preparations

**Proprietary Preparations** (details are given in Part 3)
***Belg.:*** Medichrom; ***Braz.:*** Mercurio Cromo†; ***Fr.:*** Pharmadose mercuresceine; Soluchrom; ***Ger.:*** Mercuchrom; ***Ital.:*** Cromocur; ***Mex.:*** Erthiol†; ***S.Afr.:*** Spraychrome†; ***Spain:*** Cinfacromin; Cromer Orto; Logacron†; Mercromina; Mercurin; Mercurobromo; Mercutina Brota; Pintacrom†; Super Cromer Orto.

**Multi-ingredient:** ***Braz.:*** Pomada Martel†; ***S.Afr.:*** Achromide; AMS†; Daromide; Ung Vernleigh; ***Spain:*** Argentocromo; Mercrotona.

## Mercurobutol *(rINN)*

L-542. 4-*tert*-Butyl-2-chloro-mercuriphenol.
$C_{10}H_{13}ClHgO = 385.3.$
*CAS — 498-73-7.*

**Pharmacopoeias.** In *Fr.*

### Profile

Mercurobutol is an organic mercurial antiseptic with antifungal properties. It has been used in the treatment of infections of the skin and mucous membranes.

### Preparations

**Proprietary Preparations** (details are given in Part 3)
***Spain:*** Mercryl Laurylet†.

## Metalkonium Chloride *(rINN)*

Dodecarbonium Chloride. Benzyl(dodecylcarbamoylmethyl)dimethylammonium chloride.
$C_{23}H_{41}ClN_2O = 397.0.$
*CAS — 100-95-8.*

### Profile

Metalkonium chloride is an antiseptic used for skin disinfection.

### Preparations

**Proprietary Preparations** (details are given in Part 3)
***Ital.:*** Theotex.

# Methylated Spirits

Alcoholes desnaturalizados.
*CAS — 8013-52-3 (ethyl alcohol-methyl alcohol mixture; industrial methylated spirit).*

**Description.** Three classes of methylated spirits are listed under the Methylated Spirits Regulations, 1987 (SI 1987: No. 2009): industrial methylated spirits, mineralised methylated spirits, and denatured ethanol (denatured alcohol).

Industrial Methylated Spirits is defined as 95 parts by volume of spirits mixed with wood naphtha (mostly methyl alcohol—p.1475) 5 parts by volume. Mineralised methylated spirits is spirits mixed with wood naphtha 9.5 parts by volume and crude pyridine 0.5 parts by volume, and to every 2000 litres of this mixture is added 7.5 litres of mineral naphtha (petroleum oil) and 3 g of synthetic organic dyestuff (methyl violet). This is the only variety that may be sold in Great Britain for general use. Denatured ethanol is 999 parts by volume of spirits (of a strength not less than 85%) mixed with 1 part by volume of tertiary butyl alcohol, and to this mixture is added Bitrex (denatonium benzoate) 10 mg/litre.

As Industrial Methylated Spirit may contain small amounts of acetone it should not be used for the preparation of iodine solutions, since an irritating compound is formed by reaction between iodine and acetone; for such preparations Industrial Methylated Spirit (Ketone-free) should be used.

**Pharmacopoeias.** *Br.* includes Industrial Methylated Spirit and Industrial Methylated Spirit (Ketone-free).

**BP 2003** (Industrial Methylated Spirit). A mixture of 19 volumes of ethyl alcohol of an appropriate strength with 1 volume of approved wood naphtha. Two strengths are available containing 99% and 95% v/v alcohol (also known as 74 OP and 66 OP respectively). It is a colourless, clear, mobile, volatile liquid with an odour which is spirituous and of wood naphtha. B.p. is about 78°. The BP 2003 gives Industrial Methylated Spirits and IMS as approved synonyms.

**BP 2003** (Industrial Methylated Spirit (Ketone-free)). A mixture of the same strength as Industrial Methylated Spirit, but it is substantially free from ketones, containing not more than the equivalent of 500 ppm of acetone.

## Adverse Effects

As for Alcohol, p.1166, and Methyl Alcohol, p.1475. Adverse effects are due chiefly to consumption of methylated spirits rather than its topical use as a disinfectant.

## Uses and Administration

Industrial methylated spirit, in a concentration of about 70%, is the usual form in which alcohol (p.1166) is used for disinfection. It is applied externally for its astringent action, but mucous membranes and excoriated skin surfaces must be protected. It may be used for skin preparation before injection.

Methylated spirits may be used in the form of Surgical Spirit (BP 2003), a mixture of methyl salicylate (0.5% v/v), diethyl phthalate (2% v/v), and castor oil (2.5% v/v) in industrial methylated spirit.

### Preparations

**BP 2003:** Surgical Spirit.

## Methylbenzethonium Chloride *(BAN, rINN)*

Cloruro de metilbencetonio. Benzyldimethyl-2-{2-[4-(1,1,3,3-tetramethylbutyl)-o-tolyloxy]ethoxy}ethylammonium chloride monohydrate.

$C_{28}H_{44}ClNO_2,H_2O$ = 480.1.

*CAS — 25155-18-4 (anhydrous methylbenzethonium chloride); 1320-44-1 (methylbenzethonium chloride monohydrate).*

**Pharmacopoeias.** In *US.*

**USP 27** (Methylbenzethonium Chloride). White hygroscopic crystals with a mild odour. Soluble 1 in 0.8 of water, 1 in 0.9 of alcohol, 1 in more than 10 000 of chloroform, and 1 in 0.7 of ether. Solutions are neutral or slightly alkaline to litmus. Store in airtight containers.

### Profile

Methylbenzethonium chloride is a quaternary ammonium disinfectant and antiseptic with actions and uses similar to those of other cationic surfactants (see Cetrimide, p.1172). It is used topically for minor infections or irritation of the skin.

**Leishmaniasis.** Topical treatment of cutaneous leishmaniasis (p.597) with methylbenzethonium chloride 5 or 12% and paromomycin sulfate has proved beneficial.

### Preparations

**USP 27:** Methylbenzethonium Chloride Lotion; Methylbenzethonium Chloride Ointment; Methylbenzethonium Chloride Topical Powder.

**Proprietary Preparations** (details are given in Part 3)

**Multi-ingredient:** ***Arg.:*** Lorophyn; ***Braz.:*** Leshcutan†; ***Israel:*** Leshcutan; ***Ital.:*** Traumicid; ***USA:*** Acnotex; Dermasept Antifungal; Drytex; Finac; Orasept.

## Methylrosanilinium Chloride *(rINN)*

CI Basic Violet 3; Cloruro de metilrosanilina; Colour Index No. 42555; Crystal Violet; Gentian Violet; Hexamethylpararosaniline Chloride; Kristallviolett; Methylrosaniline Chloride; Methylrosanilinii Chloridum; Pyoctaninum Caeruleum; Viola Crystallina. 4-[4,4′Bis(dimethylamino)benzhydrylidene]cyclohexa-2,5-dien-1-ylidenedimethylammonium chloride.

$C_{25}H_{30}ClN_3$ = 408.0.

*CAS — 548-62-9.*

*ATC — D01AE02; G01AX09.*

NOTE. The name methyl violet—CI Basic Violet 1; Colour Index No. 42535—has been used as a synonym for methylrosanilinium chloride, but is applied to a mixture of the hydrochlorides of the higher methylated pararosanilines consisting principally of the tetramethyl-, pentamethyl-, and hexamethyl- compounds.

**Pharmacopoeias.** In *Chin., Fr., Int.,* and *US.*

*Jpn* includes a mixture of hexamethylpararosaniline hydrochloride with the tetramethyl- and pentamethyl- compounds.

**USP 27** (Gentian Violet). A dark green powder or greenish, glistening pieces with a metallic lustre, and with not more than a faint odour. Sparingly soluble in water; soluble 1 in 10 of alcohol and 1 in 15 of glycerol; soluble in chloroform; insoluble in ether.

**Incompatibility.** The antimicrobial activity of methylrosanilinium chloride may be diminished through incompatibilities, decreasing pH, or through combination with organic matter.

The antibacterial activity of methylrosanilinium chloride was inhibited in suspensions of bentonite with which it formed a stable complex.[1]

1. Harris WA. The inactivation of cationic antiseptics by bentonite suspensions. *Australas J Pharm* 1961; **42:** 583–8.

### Adverse Effects and Precautions

Topical application of methylrosanilinium chloride can produce irritation and ulceration of mucous membranes. Ingestion of methylrosanilinium chloride during prolonged or frequent treatment for oral candidiasis has resulted in oesophagitis, laryngitis, and tracheitis; ingestion may also cause nausea, vomiting, diarrhoea, and abdominal pain. In the UK it is recommended that methylrosanilinium chloride should not be applied to mucous membranes or open wounds. Contact with the eyes or broken skin should be avoided. Methylrosanilinium chloride may stain skin and clothing.

*Animal* carcinogenicity has restricted its use.

**Carcinogenicity.** Methylrosanilinium chloride has been shown *in vitro* to be capable of interacting with DNA of living cells,[1] and has demonstrable carcinogenicity in *mice.*[2]

1. Rosenkranz HS, Carr HS. Possible hazard in use of gentian violet. *BMJ* 1971; **3:** 702–3.
2. MAFF Food Advisory Committee. Final report on the review of the Colouring Matter in Food Regulations 1973: FdAC/REP/4. London: HMSO, 1987.

**Effects on the skin and mucous membranes.** Necrotic skin reactions have been reported after the use of topical 1% aqueous solutions of methylrosanilinium chloride;[1] areas affected include the submammary folds, gluteal fold, genitalia, and toe-webs. Similar reactions were observed in 2 patients after use of 1% methylrosanilinium chloride or brilliant green on stripped skin.[1] Oral ulceration developed in all of 6 neonates treated with aqueous methylrosanilinium chloride 0.5 or 1% for oral candidiasis.[2]

In the UK it is recommended that methylrosanilinium chloride should not be applied to mucous membranes or open wounds.

1. Björnberg A, Mobacken H. Necrotic skin reactions caused by 1% gentian violet and brilliant green. *Acta Derm Venereol (Stockh)* 1972; **52:** 55–60.
2. Horsfield P, *et al.* Oral irritation with gentian violet. *BMJ* 1976; **2:** 529.

**Effects on the urinary tract.** Severe haemorrhagic cystitis rapidly occurred in a 32-year-old woman after accidental injection through the urethra of a solution of methylrosanilinium chloride 1% and alcohol 2%.[1] Severe cystitis was also reported after instillation into the bladder of a solution containing methylrosanilinium chloride and brilliant green 1:1 (Bonney's blue).[2]

1. Walsh C, Walsh A. Haemorrhagic cystitis due to gentian violet. *BMJ* 1986; **293:** 732.
2. Christmas TJ, *et al.* Bonney's blue. *Lancet* 1988; **ii:** 459–60.

**Porphyria.** Methylrosanilinium chloride has been associated with acute attacks of porphyria and is considered unsafe in porphyric patients.

### Uses and Administration

Methylrosanilinium chloride is a triphenylmethane antiseptic dye effective against some Gram-positive bacteria, particularly *Staphylococcus* spp., and some pathogenic fungi such as *Candida* spp. It is much less active against Gram-negative bacteria and ineffective against acid-fast bacteria and bacterial spores. Its activity increases as pH increases.

Methylrosanilinium chloride has been applied topically as a 0.25 to 2.0% aqueous solution or as a cream for the treatment of bacterial and fungal infections, but in the UK its use is now restricted to application to unbroken skin because of concern over *animal* carcinogenicity. However, it has been used as a 0.5% solution with brilliant green 0.5% (Bonney's blue) for skin marking before surgery.

In the UK, methylrosanilinium chloride is no longer permitted for use in foods.

### Preparations

**USP 27:** Gentian Violet Cream; Gentian Violet Topical Solution.

**Proprietary Preparations** (details are given in Part 3)

***Spain:*** Vigencial.

**Multi-ingredient:** ***Braz.:*** Vulgix†; ***Chile:*** Calmante De Aftas; Faxet; ***Fr.:*** Antiseptique-Calmante†; ***Ital.:*** Violgen†.

## Miripirium Chloride *(rINN)*

Cloruro de miripirio; Myristyl-gamma-picolinium Chloride. 4-Methyl-1-tetradecylpyridinium chloride.

$C_{20}H_{36}ClN$ = 326.0.

*CAS — 7631-49-4 (miripirium); 2748-88-1 (miripirium chloride).*

### Profile

Miripirium chloride is used as an antimicrobial preservative in some pharmaceutical products.

**Hypersensitivity.** Two patients displayed delayed hypersensitivity reactions to retrobulbar injection of methylprednisolone acetate suspension (Depo-Medrol).[1] Intradermal testing confirmed sensitivity to methylprednisolone and to miripirium chloride, included as a preservative in the formulation.

1. Mathias CGT, Robertson DB. Delayed hypersensitivity to a corticosteroid suspension containing methylprednisolone. *Arch Dermatol* 1985; **121:** 258–61.

## Miristalkonium Chloride *(BAN, rINN)*

Cloruro de miristalconio; Myristylbenzalkonium Chloride. Benzyldimethyltetradecylammonium chloride.

$C_{23}H_{42}ClN$ = 368.0.

*CAS — 139-08-2.*

### Profile

Miristalkonium chloride is a quaternary ammonium antiseptic with actions and uses similar to those of other cationic surfactants (see Cetrimide, p.1172). It has been used in creams and lotions for disinfection of the skin and has been an ingredient of sprays used for the treatment of minor infections of the mouth and throat. It is also used as a vaginal spermicide.

### Preparations

**Proprietary Preparations** (details are given in Part 3)

***Fr.:*** Alpagelle.

**Multi-ingredient:** ***Fr.:*** Sterlane; ***Ital.:*** Eburdent F.

## Monothioglycerol

α-Monothioglycerol; Monotioglicerol; Thioglycerol. 3-Mercaptopropane-1,2-diol.

$C_3H_8O_2S$ = 108.2.

*CAS — 96-27-5.*

**Pharmacopoeias.** In *USNF.*

**USNF 22** (Monothioglycerol). A colourless or pale yellow, viscous, hygroscopic liquid with a slight odour of sulfide. Freely soluble in water; miscible with alcohol; insoluble in ether. A 10% solution in water has a pH of 3.5 to 7.0. Store in airtight containers.

### Profile

Monothioglycerol is used as an antoxidant preservative in pharmaceutical preparations. It has some antimicrobial activity.

## Myralact *(BAN, pINN)*

(2-Hydroxyethyl)tetradecylammonium lactate.

$C_{19}H_{41}NO_4$ = 347.5.

*CAS — 15518-87-3.*

### Profile

Myralact is an antiseptic included in multi-ingredient preparations intended for the topical treatment of vaginal infections.

### Preparations

**Proprietary Preparations** (details are given in Part 3)

**Multi-ingredient:** ***Hong Kong:*** Ginetris.

## Nitromersol

5-Methyl-2-nitro-7-oxa-8-mercurabicyclo[4.2.0]octa-1,3,5-triene.

$C_7H_5HgNO_3$ = 351.7.

*CAS — 133-58-4.*

**Pharmacopoeias.** In *US.*

**USP 27** (Nitromersol). A brownish-yellow to yellow odourless powder or granules. Very slightly soluble in water, in alcohol, in acetone, and in ether; soluble in solutions of alkalis and of ammonia with the formation of salts. Store in airtight containers. Protect from light.

**Incompatibility.** Nitromersol is incompatible with metals and sulfides. Its antimicrobial activity may be diminished in the presence of organic material.

### Adverse Effects and Treatment

As for Mercury, p.1713.

Nitromersol occasionally gives rise to hypersensitivity reactions.

### Uses and Administration

Nitromersol is a mercurial antiseptic effective against some bacteria. It is not effective against spores or acid-fast bacteria. It has been used for superficial skin infections and for disinfection of the skin prior to surgical treatment.

### Preparations

***USP 27:*** Nitromersol Topical Solution.

**Proprietary Preparations** (details are given in Part 3)

**Multi-ingredient: *Austral.:*** Butesin Picrate; Cold Sore Balm†; ***NZ:*** Cold Sore Balm†.

## Nordihydroguaiaretic Acid

NDGA; Nordihidroguayarético, ácido. 4,4′-(2,3-Dimethyltetramethylene)bis(benzene-1,2-diol).

$C_{18}H_{22}O_4$ = 302.4.

*CAS — 500-38-9.*

### Profile

Nordihydroguaiaretic acid has been used as an antoxidant preservative. Allergic contact dermatitis has been reported.

## Noxytiolin *(BAN, rINN)*

Noxitiolina; Noxythiolin. 1-Hydroxymethyl-3-methyl-2-thiourea.

$C_3H_8N_2OS$ = 120.2.

*CAS — 15599-39-0.*

*ATC — B05CA07.*

### Adverse Effects

When noxytiolin is given initially by irrigation for the treatment of the purulent infected bladder there may be an intense reaction with a burning sensation and the passage of large fibrin clumps. Administration of a local anaesthetic such as tetracaine hydrochloride with noxytiolin may control the pain.

**Breath odour.** A pervasive sweet breath odour characteristic of decaying vegetables has been noted in patients treated with peritoneal dialysis fluid containing noxytiolin.[1] The odour was attributed to unidentified sulfur metabolites.

1. Stewart WK, Fleming LW. Use your nose. *Lancet* 1983; **i:** 426.

### Uses and Administration

Noxytiolin is an antiseptic with wide antibacterial and antifungal actions. It may act by slowly releasing formaldehyde in solution.

For instillation into, or irrigation of, the peritoneal cavity or other body cavities, a 1 to 2.5% solution is used. Solutions of noxytiolin should be warmed to 37° prior to instillation or irrigation. Treatment is usually for 3 to 7 days, modified or repeated thereafter as required. The normal total daily amount used in adults should not exceed 5 g for instillation or 10 g for continuous irrigation.

**Action.** Although noxytiolin has generally been thought to act, at least in part, by slowly releasing formaldehyde into solution, it has been reported[1] that much smaller amounts are released than have previously been thought and that the antimicrobial effects of noxytiolin solutions cannot be attributed solely to the presence of formaldehyde. There is evidence *in vitro* that noxytiolin might reduce the adherence of micro-organisms to epithelial surfaces.[2]

1. Gorman SP, *et al.* Formaldehyde release from noxythiolin solutions. *Pharm J* 1984; **234:** 62–3.
2. Anderson L, *et al.* Clinical implications of the microbial antiadherence properties of noxythiolin. *J Pharm Pharmacol* 1985; **37** (suppl): 64P.

**Infections of the pleural cavity.** Three patients with pleural empyema or pneumonectomy space infection were treated by irrigation of the cavity with noxytiolin 1% in normal saline for 3 hours, followed by drainage for 1 hour, the cycle being repeated 4-hourly. Infection was eradicated within 21 days in all 3 patients.[1]

1. Rosenfeldt FL, *et al.* Comparison between irrigation and conventional treatment for empyema and pneumonectomy space infection. *Thorax* 1981; **36:** 272–7.

### Preparations

**Proprietary Preparations** (details are given in Part 3)

***Fr.:*** Noxyflex; ***Irl.:*** Noxyflex S; ***UK:*** Noxyflex S.

## Octafonium Chloride *(BAN, rINN)*

Cloruro de octafonio; Octaphonium Chloride; Phenoctide. Benzyldiethyl-2-[4-(1,1,3,3-tetramethylbutyl)phenoxy]ethylammonium chloride monohydrate.

$C_{27}H_{42}ClNO,H_2O$ = 450.1.

*CAS — 15687-40-8 (anhydrous octafonium chloride); 78-05-7 (anhydrous octafonium chloride).*

### Profile

Octafonium chloride is a quaternary ammonium antiseptic with actions and uses similar to those of other cationic surfactants (see Cetrimide, p.1172). It is used in topical preparations for skin disinfection.

### Preparations

**Proprietary Preparations** (details are given in Part 3)

**Multi-ingredient: *Irl.:*** Germolene†; ***UK:*** Germolene.

## Octenidine Hydrochloride *(BANM, USAN, rINNM)*

Hidrocloruro de octenidina; Win-41464 (octenidine); Win-41464-2 (octenidine hydrochloride); Win-41464-6 (octenidine saccharin). 1,1′,4,4′-Tetrahydro-*N*,*N*′-dioctyl-1,1′-decamethylenedi-(4-pyridylideneamine) dihydrochloride.

$C_{36}H_{62}N_4,2HCl$ = 623.8.

*CAS — 71251-02-0 (octenidine); 70775-75-6 (octenidine hydrochloride).*

### Profile

Octenidine hydrochloride is a bispyridine bactericidal antiseptic with some antiviral and antifungal activity. It has been used for skin and mucous membrane disinfection.

### Preparations

**Proprietary Preparations** (details are given in Part 3)

***Fr.:*** Phisomain.

**Multi-ingredient: *Austria:*** Octenisept; ***Ger.:*** Neo Kodan; Octenisept; ***Switz.:*** Octenisept.

## Orthophenylphenol

2-Biphenylol; E231; E232 (sodium-o-phenylphenol); 2-Hydroxybiphenyl; *o*-Hydroxydiphenyl; Ortofenilfenol.

$C_{12}H_{10}O$ = 170.2.

*CAS — 90-43-7.*

*ATC — D08AE06.*

### Profile

Orthophenylphenol is a phenolic disinfectant with antimicrobial properties similar to those of chloroxylenol (p.1177). It is used for disinfection of skin, hands, instruments, and hard surfaces. It also has many industrial uses as a preservative for a wide range of materials, particularly against moulds and rots. Sodium-*o*-phenylphenol has been used similarly.

### Preparations

**Proprietary Preparations** (details are given in Part 3)

***Ger.:*** Amocid; Manusept†; ***Ital.:*** Citromedics Disinfettante; Citrosteril Aspiratori; Crescom; Esofenol 60; Helix I; Higesan; Neo Esoformolo; Vcanalare; ***Switz.:*** Manusept.

**Multi-ingredient: *Austria:*** Dodesept; Dodesept Gefarbt; ***Canad.:*** Aseptone 1†; Aseptone 2†; Aseptone 5†; ***Fr.:*** Frekaderm†; ***Ger.:*** Bacillotox†; Bomix; Desderman N; Freka-Derm; Freka-Sept 80; Grotanat†; Helipur; Incidin Extra; Kodan Tinktur Forte; Primasept Med; ***Ital.:*** Bergon; Diaril; Esofenol Ferri; Germozero Dermo; Germozero Plus; Helipur; Hygienist; Norica; Sangen Casa; Sterosan; ***Switz.:*** Frekaderm; Stellisept†.

## Oxychlorosene *(USAN)*

Monoxychlorosene; Oxicloroseno.

$C_{20}H_{34}O_3S,HOCl$ = 407.0.

*CAS — 8031-14-9.*

## Oxychlorosene Sodium *(USAN)*

Sodium Oxychlorosene.

*CAS — 52906-84-0.*

### Profile

Oxychlorosene is the hypochlorous acid complex of a mixture of the phenyl sulfonate derivatives of aliphatic hydrocarbons. It is a chlorine-releasing antiseptic with the general properties of chlorine, p.1175.

A 0.4% solution of oxychlorosene sodium has been used for cleansing wounds (although chlorine-releasing antiseptics are generally regarded as too irritant for this purpose—see Disinfection, Wounds, under Uses and Administration of Chlorine, p.1176) and for pre-operative skin preparation; a 0.1 or 0.2% solution has been used in urological and ophthalmological disinfection.

### Preparations

**Proprietary Preparations** (details are given in Part 3)

***Canad.:*** Clorpactin†; ***USA:*** Clorpactin WCS-90.

## Oxymethurea

Carbamol; Dihydroxymethyl Carbamide. *N,N*′-Bis(hydroxymethyl)urea.

$C_3H_8N_2O_3$ = 120.1.

*CAS — 140-95-4.*

### Profile

Oxymethurea is an antiseptic included in multi-ingredient preparations intended for the topical treatment of ear infections.

### Preparations

**Proprietary Preparations** (details are given in Part 3)

**Multi-ingredient: *Austria:*** Ciloprin cum Anaesthetico; ***Denm.:*** Ciloprin†; ***Fin.:*** Ciloprin cum Anaesthetico; ***Swed.:*** Ciloprin†; ***Switz.:*** Ciloprine ca.

## Parachlorophenol

Paraclorofenol. 4-Chlorophenol.

$C_6H_5ClO$ = 128.6.

*CAS — 106-48-9.*

**Pharmacopoeias.** In *Swiss* and *US.*

*US* also includes camphorated parachlorophenol.

**USP 27** (Parachlorophenol). It consists of white or pink crystals with a characteristic phenolic odour. M.p. about 42°; congealing temperature between 42° and 44°. Sparingly soluble in water and in liquid paraffin; very soluble in alcohol, in chloroform, in ether, in glycerol, and in fixed and volatile oils; soluble in soft paraffin. A 1% solution in water is acid to litmus. Store in airtight containers. Protect from light.

**USP 27** (Camphorated Parachlorophenol). It contains not less than 33% and not more than 37% of parachlorophenol and not less than 63% and not more than 67% of camphor, with the sum of the percentages of parachlorophenol and camphor not less than 97% and not more than 103%. Store in airtight containers. Protect from light.

### Profile

Parachlorophenol is a chlorinated phenolic disinfectant and antiseptic with similar properties to phenol (p.1188). Camphorated parachlorophenol has been used in dentistry in the treatment of infected root canals.

### Preparations

**Proprietary Preparations** (details are given in Part 3)

**Multi-ingredient: *Ital.:*** Esofenol Ferri; ***Spain:*** Cresophene; ***Switz.:*** Cresophene; Pate Iodoforme du Prof Dr Walkhoff†; Solution ChKM du Prof Dr Walkhoff†.

## Paraformaldehyde

Paraform; Paraformaldehído; Paraformic Aldehyde; Polymerised Formaldehyde; Polyoxymethylene; Trioxyméthylène.

$(CH_2O)_n$.

*CAS — 30525-89-4.*

**Pharmacopoeias.** In *Jpn* and *Swiss.*

### Adverse Effects, Treatment, and Precautions

As for Formaldehyde Solution, p.1179. There have been reports of allergic reactions and nerve damage associated with the dental use of paraformaldehyde as a root canal sealant; it should not extrude beyond the apex.

### Uses and Administration

Paraformaldehyde is a disinfectant and antiseptic with the properties and uses of formaldehyde (p.1180) and is used as a source of formaldehyde. To disinfect rooms it has been vapourised by heating. Tablets prepared for this purpose should be coloured by the addition of a suitable blue dye.

Paraformaldehyde has been used in lozenges for the treatment of minor throat infections. In dentistry, it has been used as an obtundent for sensitive dentine and as an antiseptic in mummifying pastes and for root canals.

### Preparations

**Proprietary Preparations** (details are given in Part 3)

**Multi-ingredient: *Austral.:*** Gartech†; ***Fr.:*** Gynescal†; ***Ital.:*** Eso 70; Esoform 7 mc; Esoform 70 mc; Pasta Devitalizzante; ***Switz.:*** Asphaline; Caustinerf forte; Rocanal Permanent Gangrene†; Rocanal Permanent Vital†.

## Peracetic Acid

Acetyl Hydroperoxide; Peracético, ácido; Peroxyacetic Acid.

$C_2H_4O_3$ = 76.05.

*CAS — 79-21-0.*

### Profile

Peracetic acid is a strong oxidising disinfectant which is corrosive to the skin. It is active against many micro-organisms including bacteria, spores, fungi, and viruses. It is used for disinfecting medical equipment including dialysers and endoscopes. It is used in the food industry and for disinfecting sewage sludge, and has been used as a spray for sterilisation of laboratories.

**Disinfection of dialysis equipment.** For use of peracetic acid with hydrogen peroxide in the disinfection of dialysis equipment, see under Hydrogen Peroxide, p.1183.

**Disinfection of endoscopes.** Peracetic acid has been used to disinfect endoscopes;[1,2] it is a possible alternative to glutaral (see p.1164).

1. Bradley CR, *et al.* Evaluation of the Steris system 1 peracetic acid endoscope processor. *J Hosp Infect* 1995; **29:** 143–51.
2. Middleton AM, *et al.* Disinfection of bronchoscopes, contaminated in vitro with Mycobacterium tuberculosis, Mycobacterium avium-intracellulare and Mycobacterium chelonae in sputum, using stabilized, buffered peracetic acid solution ('Nu-Cidex'). *J Hosp Infect* 1997; **37:** 137–43.

### Preparations

**Proprietary Preparations** (details are given in Part 3)

***Fr.:*** Dynacide; Nu-Cidex; ***Ger.:*** Sekusept; ***Ital.:*** Esodrox; Ferrister; SaniDrox; Sekusept N; Sporidox Plus.

**Multi-ingredient: *Ger.:*** Peresal; ***Ital.:*** Adaspor; Esocetic; Peresal.

## Phenethyl Alcohol *(BAN)*

Alcohol feniletílico; Benzyl Carbinol; Phenethanolum; Phenylethyl alcohol. 2-Phenylethanol.

$C_6H_5.CH_2.CH_2OH$ = 122.2.

*CAS — 60-12-8.*

**Pharmacopoeias.** In *Pol.* and *US.*

**USP 27** (Phenylethyl Alcohol). A colourless liquid with a rose-like odour. Soluble 1 in 60 of water, 1 in less than 1 of alcohol, of chloroform, of ether, of benzyl benzoate, and of diethyl phthalate, and 1 in 2 of alcohol 50%; very soluble in glycerol, in propylene glycol, and in fixed oils; slightly soluble in liquid paraffin. Store in airtight containers in a cool, dry place. Protect from light.

**Incompatibility.** Phenethyl alcohol is incompatible with oxidising agents and proteins. Activity may be reduced by nonionic surfactants or by adsorption onto low density polyethylene containers.

### Profile

Phenethyl alcohol is more active against Gram-negative than Gram-positive bacteria. It is used as a preservative in ophthalmic and parenteral solutions at a concentration of 0.25 to 0.5%, with another bactericide, and up to 1% in topical preparations. It is also used as an antiseptic in topical products in concentrations of up to 7.5%. It is also used as a component of flavouring essences and perfumes.

Phenethyl alcohol may cause eye irritation.

**Antimicrobial action.** Antimicrobial activity may be enhanced by the addition of phenethyl alcohol to solutions preserved with benzalkonium chloride, chlorhexidine acetate, phenylmercuric nitrate, chlorocresol, or chlorobutanol.[1]

1. Richards RME, McBride RJ. The preservation of ophthalmic solutions with antibacterial combinations. *J Pharm Pharmacol* 1972; **24:** 145–8.

### Preparations

**Proprietary Preparations** (details are given in Part 3)

***Multi-ingredient: Austral.:*** Sebirinse†; ***Canad.:*** Sclerodex; ***Ger.:*** Imazol; ***Irl.:*** Ceanel; ***NZ:*** Sebirinse; ***S.Afr.:*** Ceanel†; ***UK:*** Ceanel.

## Phenol

Carbolic Acid; Fenol; Phenic Acid; Phenolum; Phenyl Hydrate; Phenylic Acid. Hydroxybenzene.

$C_6H_5.OH$ = 94.11.

*CAS — 108-95-2.*

*ATC — C05BB05; D08AE03; N01BX03; R02AA19.*

**Pharmacopoeias.** In *Chin., Eur.* (see p.vi), *Jpn, Pol., US,* and *Viet.*

*Br., Swiss,* and *US* also include a monograph for Liquefied Phenol.

**Ph. Eur. 5.0** (Phenol). Colourless or faintly pink or faintly yellow deliquescent crystals or crystalline masses. F.p. not less than 39.5°. Soluble in water; very soluble in alcohol, in dichloromethane, and in glycerol. Store in airtight containers. Protect from light.

**BP 2003** (Liquified Phenol). An aqueous mixture containing phenol 77.0 to 81.5% w/w in purified water. A colourless to faintly coloured, caustic liquid with a characteristic and not tarry odour. Soluble in water; miscible with alcohol, with ether, and with glycerol. Protect from light. It may congeal or deposit crystals if stored at a temperature below 4°. It should be completely melted before use.

When phenol is to be mixed with collodion, fixed oils, or paraffins, melted phenol should be used, and not Liquefied Phenol.

**USP 27** (Phenol). Colourless to light pink, interlaced or separate, needle-shaped crystals, or a white to light pink crystalline mass, with a characteristic odour. It gradually darkens on exposure to light and air. Soluble 1 in 15 of water; very soluble in alcohol, in chloroform, in ether, in glycerol, and in fixed and volatile oils; soluble 1 in 70 of liquid paraffin. A solution of 1 g in 15 mL water is clear and is neutral or acid to litmus. Store in airtight containers. Protect from light.

**USP 27** (Liquefied Phenol). Phenol maintained in a liquid condition by the presence of about 10% of water; it contains not less than 89% by weight of phenol. It may contain a suitable stabiliser. A colourless to pink liquid which may develop a red tint upon exposure to air or light, and with a characteristic, somewhat aromatic odour. Miscible with alcohol, with ether, and with glycerol. Store in airtight glass containers. Protect from light.

When phenol is to be mixed with a fixed oil, liquid paraffin, or white soft paraffin, crystalline Phenol and not Liquefied Phenol should be used.

◊ NOTE. Phenol should not be used to preserve preparations that are to be freeze-dried.

**Incompatibility.** Phenol is incompatible with alkaline salts and nonionic surfactants. The antimicrobial activity of phenol may be diminished through increasing pH or through combination with blood and other organic matter.

### Adverse Effects

When ingested, phenol causes extensive local corrosion, with pain, nausea, vomiting, sweating, and diarrhoea. Excitation may occur initially but it is quickly followed by unconsciousness. There is depression of the CNS, with cardiac arrhythmias, and circulatory and respiratory failure, which may lead to death. Acidosis may develop and occasionally there is haemolysis and methaemoglobinaemia with cyanosis. The urine may become dark brown or green. Pulmonary oedema and myocardial damage may develop, and damage to the liver and kidneys may lead to organ failure.

Severe or fatal poisoning may occur from the absorption of phenol from unbroken skin or wounds and suitable precautions should be taken to prevent absorption. Applied to skin, phenol causes blanching and corrosion, sometimes with little pain. Aqueous solutions as dilute as 10% may be corrosive.

Toxic symptoms may also arise through absorption of phenol vapour by the skin or lungs. Phenol throat spray may cause local oedema.

Cresols and other phenolic substances have similar effects.

**Effects on the heart.** A 10-year-old boy developed life-threatening premature ventricular complexes during the application of a solution of phenol 40% and croton oil 0.8% in hexachlorophene soap and water for chemical peeling of a giant hairy naevus.[1] Cardiac arrhythmias have been reported after the use of phenol for chemical face peeling.[2] They were also seen in 3 of 16 children who received phenol 5% as a neurolytic.[3]

1. Warner MA, Harper JV. Cardiac dysrhythmias associated with chemical peeling with phenol. *Anesthesiology* 1985; **62:** 366–7.
2. Botta SA, *et al.* Cardiac arrhythmias in phenol face peeling: a suggested protocol for prevention. *Aesthetic Plast Surg* 1988; **12:** 115–17.
3. Morrison JE, *et al.* Phenol motor point blocks in children: plasma concentrations and cardiac dysrhythmias. *Anesthesiology* 1991; **75:** 359–62.

**Effects on the kidneys.** A 41-year-old man developed acute renal failure due to cutaneous absorption of phenol after falling into a shallow vat of industrial solvent containing 40% phenol in dichloromethane. No ingestion occurred. Other symptoms included 50% body-surface burns, cold extremities, nausea, vomiting, and respiratory distress. The patient required haemodialysis for 3 weeks; some abnormalities of renal function remained one year later.[1]

1. Foxall PJD, *et al.* Acute renal failure following accidental cutaneous absorption of phenol: application of NMR urinalysis to monitor the disease process. *Hum Toxicol* 1989; **9:** 491–6.

**Effects on sexual function.** Three patients developed urinary symptoms and impotence which lasted up to one year after each receiving phenol 5% in arachis oil sclerotherapy for haemorrhoids.[1]

1. Bullock N. Impotence after sclerotherapy of haemorrhoids: case reports. *BMJ* 1997; **314:** 419.

**Effects on the throat.** Acute life-threatening epiglottitis occurred in a 49-year-old woman after the use of a throat spray containing the equivalent of 1.4% phenol. The reaction may have been anaphylactic or due to a direct toxic effect of the spray.[1] The UK Committee on Safety of Medicines[2] reported in 1990 that it had received 4 reports of oedema of the epiglottis and/or larynx leading to respiratory difficulties. While the incidence was rare, the effects were severe; 1 patient died and 2 survived only after emergency hospital treatment.

1. Ho S-L, Hollinrake K. Acute epiglottitis and Chloraseptic. *BMJ* 1989; **298:** 1584.
2. Committee on Safety of Medicines. Chloraseptic throat spray and oedema of the epiglottis and larynx. *Current Problems 28* 1990.

### Treatment of Adverse Effects

If phenol has been swallowed, activated charcoal may be useful. Some sources suggest the cautious use of gastric lavage although this is generally inappropriate following ingestion of corrosive substances.

If phenol has been spilled on the skin removal of contaminated clothing and excess phenol should be followed by washing of the skin with glycerol or, alternatively, with copious amounts of water. Macrogol 300 and vegetable oils have also been used.

Contamination of the eyes should be treated by flooding with water or sodium chloride 0.9% only for at least 10 to 15 minutes.

The patient should be kept warm and given supportive treatment. Intravenous sodium bicarbonate should be given where there is metabolic acidosis.

### Precautions

Solutions containing phenol should not be applied to large areas of skin or large wounds since sufficient phenol may be absorbed to give rise to toxic symptoms.

Phenol should not be used as a throat spray in patients with epiglottitis, or in children aged under 6 years.

### Pharmacokinetics

Phenol is absorbed from the gastrointestinal tract and through skin and mucous membranes. It is metabolised to phenylglucuronide and phenyl sulfate, and small amounts are oxidised to catechol and quinol which are mainly conjugated. The metabolites are excreted in the urine; on oxidation to quinones they may tint the urine dark brown or green.

### Uses and Administration

Phenol is an antiseptic and disinfectant effective against vegetative Gram-positive and Gram-negative bacteria, mycobacteria, and some fungi, but only very slowly effective against spores. It is also active against certain viruses. Phenol is more active in acid solution.

Aqueous solutions up to 1% are bacteriostatic while stronger solutions are bactericidal.

A 0.5 to 1% solution has been used for its local anaesthetic effect to relieve itching.

A 1.4% solution is used for pain or irritation of the mouth and throat. Weak concentrations have also been used topically for disinfection. A 5% solution has been used as a disinfectant for excreta.

Oily Phenol Injection (BP 2003), up to 10 mL, has been injected into the tissues around internal haemorrhoids as an analgesic sclerosing agent, but alternative procedures may be preferred. Aqueous phenol has also used been as a sclerosant in the treatment of hydroceles.

Solutions of phenol in glycerol have been administered intrathecally for the alleviation of spasticity (p.1386) or injected intrathecally or into soft-tissue structures for the treatment of chronic low back pain. Other types of severe intractable pain may be relieved by injecting aqueous phenol close to motor nerves. Aqueous phenol has been used for chemical sympathectomy in peripheral vascular disorders and for the treatment of urinary incontinence.

Liquefied phenol has been used in the treatment of ingrowing toenails.

**Haemorrhoids.** Sclerotherapy with oily phenol injection has been used[1] to treat haemorrhoids (p.1243). The technique for preventing mucosal prolapse is to inject small volumes (about 2 or 3 mL) of a 5% solution of phenol in arachis oil into the submucous space above each of the 3 principal haemorrhoids. Rather than causing the haemorrhoidal veins to thrombose, the injection works by producing submucosal fibrosis, fixing the mucosa to the underlying muscle. Other techniques for mucosal fixation such as rubber band ligation or perhaps infra-red coagulation are more effective and associated with fewer complications.[2-5]

1. Alexander-Williams J. The management of piles. *BMJ* 1982; **285:** 1137–9.
2. Gartell PC, *et al.* A randomised clinical trial to compare rubber band ligation with phenol injection in the treatment of haemorrhoids. *Gut* 1984; **25:** A563.
3. Ambrose NS, *et al.* Prospective randomised trial of injection therapy against photocoagulation therapy in first and second degree haemorrhoids. *Gut* 1984; **25:** A563–4.
4. Johanson JF, Rimm A. Optimal nonsurgical treatment of hemorrhoids: a comparative analysis of infrared coagulation, rubber band ligation, and injection sclerotherapy. *Am J Gastroenterol* 1992; **87:** 1601–6.
5. MacRae HM, McLeod RS. Comparison of hemorrhoidal treatment modalities: a meta-analysis. *Dis Colon Rectum* 1995; **38:** 687–94.

**Ingrowing toenails.** Liquefied phenol ablation has been performed as an alternative to surgical avulsion in the treatment of ingrowing toenails.[1-5] Cauterisation with phenol 88% has also been successfully used to treat ingrowing toenails and onychogryposis.[6]

1. Shepherdson A. Nail matrix phenolization: a preferred alternative to surgical excision. *Practitioner* 1977; **219:** 725–8.
2. Cameron PF. Ingrowing toenails: an evaluation of two treatments. *BMJ* 1981; **283:** 821–2.
3. Morkane AJ, *et al.* Segmental phenolization of ingrowing toenails: a randomized controlled study. *Br J Surg* 1984; **71:** 526–7.
4. Sykes PA, Kerr R. Treatment of ingrowing toenails by surgeons and chiropodists. *BMJ* 1988; **297:** 335–6.
5. Leahy AL, *et al.* Ingrowing toenails: improving treatment. *Surgery* 1990; **107:** 566–7.
6. Andrew T, Wallace WA. Nail bed ablation—excise or cauterise? A controlled study. *BMJ* 1979; **1:** 1539.

**Pain.** The neurolytic use of phenol to produce destructive nerve block (p.1369) has produced variable results, and some consider the risk of complications outweighs the benefits.

**Spasmodic torticollis.** Intramuscular phenol was reported[1] to have produced improvement in 2 adult patients with moderately severe spasmodic torticollis (p.1391) who had not responded adequately to intramuscular injections of botulinum A toxin. Response was maintained by re-injection every 6 months.


1. Massey JM. Treatment of spasmodic torticollis with intramuscular phenol injection. *J Neurol Neurosurg Psychiatry* 1995; **58:** 258–9.


**Urinary incontinence.** Although injection of phenol into the pelvic plexus to produce partial denervation has been used in the management of severe intractable urge incontinence, its use has been largely abandoned. Some patients, especially those with detrusor hyperreflexia, have derived benefit[1,2] but overall efficacy can be poor and benefits short-lived.[3]


1. Ewing R, *et al.* Subtrigonal phenol injection therapy for incontinence in female patients with multiple sclerosis. *Lancet* 1983; **i:** 1304–5.
2. Blackford HN, *et al.* Results of transvesical infiltration of the pelvic plexuses with phenol in 116 patients. *Br J Urol* 1984; **56:** 647–9.
3. Rosenbaum TP, *et al.* Trans-trigonal phenol failed the test of time. *Br J Urol* 1990; **66:** 164–9.


### Preparations

***BP 2003:*** Aqueous Phenol Injection; Liquefied Phenol; Oily Phenol Injection; Phenol and Glycerol Injection;
***BPC 1973:*** Magenta Paint;
***USP 27:*** Camphorated Phenol Topical Gel; Carbol-Fuchsin Topical Solution; Liquefied Phenol; Phenolated Calamine Lotion.

**Proprietary Preparations** (details are given in Part 3)
***Austral.:*** Summers Eve Disposable†; ***Canad.:*** Chloraseptic Sore Throat Spray; P & S; ***Chile:*** Metapio; ***Irl.:*** Vicks Chloraseptic†; ***S.Afr.:*** Medi-Keel A; Septosol; ***UK:*** Ultra Chloraseptic; ***USA:*** Cheracol Sore Throat; P & S; Phenaseptic; Ulcerease; Vicks Children's Chloraseptic; Vicks Chloraseptic.

**Multi-ingredient:** ***Arg.:*** Aceite Esmeralda Moone; Callicida; Manzan; Piracalamina; Prurisedan; ***Austral.:*** Ayrton's Chilblain†; Calamine Lotion†; Egopsoryl TA; Nyal Toothache Drops; Sarna; ***Austria:*** Herposicc; Labisan; ***Belg.:*** Eucalyptine Pholcodine Le Brun; ***Braz.:*** Algidente; Axol†; Cloraseptic; Dordente†; Eucalyptine†; Nahora†; Osmogenol†; Otoloide; Otonax†; Pradente†; Timpanol; UM Instante†; Um Minuto†; Um Segundo†; Usedent†; ***Canad.:*** Anbesol; Blistex DCT Lip Balm; Blistex Lip Medex; Blistex Lip Ointment; Blistex Medicated Lip Conditioner Jar; Boil Ease; Bunion Salve†; Cepastat; Chapstick Medicated Lip Balm; Ictholin†; Lip Medex; Mecca; Ozonol; Phenoris; ***Chile:*** Blistex; Chapstick Medicated; ***Fr.:*** Brulex; Buccawalter†; Eau Precieuse; Otylol†; ***Hong Kong:*** Blistex Lip Ointment; Cepastat; Doans; Egopsoryl TA; ***Irl.:*** Germolene First Aid†; Germolene†; ***Ital.:*** Creosoto Composto; Diaril; Eso Din; Fucsina Fenica; Lavanda Sofar; Ondroly-A; Pinselina Knapp; ***Malaysia:*** Egopsoryl TA; Sarna; ***Mex.:*** Forcremol; ***Neth.:*** Agre-Gola; ***NZ:*** Egopsoryl TA; Toothache Drops; ***Port.:*** Tannosynt†; ***S.Afr.:*** Biohist; Burn-A-Sept†; Calasthetic; Cuticura; Lacto Calamine; ***Singapore:*** Cepastat; Egopsoryl TA; Sarna; ***Spain:*** Argentofenol; Carbocaina; Dermomycose Liquido; Odontocromil c Sulfamida; Otocerum; Otogen Calmante; Sabanotropico; ***Switz.:*** Caustinerf forte; Dental-Phenjoca†; Spirogel†; ***Thai.:*** Lanol; Sarna; ***UK:*** Blistex Relief Cream; Chymol; Colsor; Dermacreme; Germolene; Lacto Calamine; TCP; Vicks Chloraseptic†; ***USA:*** Anbesol; Blistex; Blistex Lip Balm; Boil Ease; Campho-Phenique; Castaderm; Cepastat; Cepastat Cherry; Chapstick Medicated Lip Balm; Columbia Antiseptic Powder; Debacterol; Heal Aid Plus; Lip Medex; Lipmagik; Massengill; Mycinette; Nasal Jelly; Orabase Lip; Orasol; Phylorinol; Skeeter Stik; Sting-Eze; Unguentine; Unguentine Plus.

## Phenoxyethanol

Ethyleneglycol Monophenylether; Fenoxietanol; Phenoxyaethanol; Phenoxyethanolum; β-Phenoxyethyl Alcohol. 2-Phenoxyethanol.

$C_8H_{10}O_2$ = 138.2.
*CAS — 122-99-6.*

**Pharmacopoeias.** In *Eur.* (see p.vi).

**Ph. Eur. 5.0** (Phenoxyethanol). A colourless slightly viscous liquid. Slightly soluble in water, in arachis oil and in olive oil; miscible with alcohol, with acetone, and with glycerol.

**Incompatibility.** The activity of phenoxyethanol may be reduced by interaction with nonionic surfactants and possibly by adsorption onto PVC.

### Profile

Phenoxyethanol is effective against strains of *Pseudomonas aeruginosa* but less so against other Gram-negative and Gram-positive bacteria. It has been used as a preservative in cosmetics and topical pharmaceuticals at a concentration of 0.5 to 1%. It is often used with other preservatives, commonly hydroxybenzoates, to obtain a wider spectrum of antimicrobial activity.

Phenoxyethanol is used in concentrations of about 2% as an antiseptic for minor infections of skin, wounds, and mucous membranes. Aqueous solutions may be prepared by shaking the phenoxyethanol with hot water until dissolved, then adjusting to final volume when cool. Preparation of the solution can be aided by propylene glycol.

Phenoxypropanol and chlorophenoxyethanol are related compounds used in topical preparations.

### Preparations

**Proprietary Preparations** (details are given in Part 3)
***Canad.:*** Lanohex†; ***Hong Kong:*** Lanohex†; ***Irl.:*** Biactol Antibacterial Facewash†; ***UK:*** Biactol Liquid; Clearasil Medicated Face Wash†.

**Multi-ingredient:** ***Arg.:*** Cicatul; Polviderm NF; ***Austral.:*** Dermocaine†; ***Austria:*** Octenisept; ***Belg.:*** Solubeol†; ***Chile:*** Eucerin; ***Fr.:*** Manugel; ***Ger.:*** Gigasept AF†; Gigasept Med; Lysetol Med; Octenisept; Terralin†; ***Ital.:*** Fitostimoline; Florigien†; ***Mex.:*** Fitoestimulina; Italdermol; ***NZ:*** Acnederm; Acnederm Foaming Wash; Dermocaine†; ***S.Afr.:*** Tantol Skin Cleanser†; ***Switz.:*** Ederphyt; Octenisept.



## Phenoxyisopropanol

Fenoxiisopropanol; Phenoxyisopropyl Alcohol. 1-phenoxypropan-2-ol.

$C_9H_{12}O_2$ = 152.2.
*CAS — 770-35-4.*

### Profile

Phenoxyisopropanol is used as a preservative and as an antiseptic in preparations for the treatment of acne, insect bites, and minor abrasions to the skin.

### Preparations

**Proprietary Preparations** (details are given in Part 3)
***Austral.:*** Clearasil Daily Face Wash.

# Phenylmercuric Salts

Fenilmercurio, sales.

## Phenylmercuric Acetate

Fenilmercurio, acetato de; Phenylhydrargyri Acetas; PMA. (Acetato)phenylmercury.

$C_8H_8HgO_2$ = 336.7.
*CAS — 62-38-4.*

**Pharmacopoeias.** In *Eur.* (see p.vi) and *Pol.* Also in *USNF.*

**Ph. Eur. 5.0** (Phenylmercuric Acetate). A white or yellowish crystalline powder or small, colourless crystals. Slightly soluble in water; soluble in alcohol and in acetone. Protect from light.

**USNF 22** (Phenylmercuric Acetate). A white to creamy-white, odourless, crystalline powder or small white prisms or leaflets. Soluble 1 in 180 of water, 1 in 225 of alcohol, 1 in 6.8 of chloroform, and 1 in 200 of ether; soluble in acetone. Store in airtight containers. Protect from light.

**Incompatibility.** The incompatibilities of phenylmercuric salts are described under Phenylmercuric Nitrate, below.

## Phenylmercuric Borate *(rINN)*

Borato de fenilmercurio; Hydrargyrum Phenyloboricum; Phenomerborum; Phenylhydrargyri Boras.

$C_6H_5HgOH, C_6H_5HgOB(OH)_2$ = 633.2 or $C_6H_5HgOH, C_6H_5HgBO_2$ = 615.2.
*CAS — 8017-88-7 ($C_{12}H_{13}BHg_2O_4$); 6273-99-0 ($C_{12}H_{11}BHg_2O_3$); 102-98-7 ($C_6H_7BHgO_3$).*
*ATC — D08AK02.*

**Pharmacopoeias.** In *Eur.* (see p.vi) and *Pol.*

**Ph. Eur. 5.0** (Phenylmercuric Borate). A compound consisting of equimolecular proportions of phenylmercuric orthoborate and phenylmercuric hydroxide ($C_{12}H_{13}BHg_2O_4$) or of the dehydrated form (metaborate, $C_{12}H_{11}BHg_2O_3$) or a mixture of the two compounds. Colourless shiny crystals or a white or slightly yellowish crystalline powder. Slightly soluble in water and in alcohol. Protect from light.

**Incompatibility.** The incompatibilities of phenylmercuric salts are described under Phenylmercuric Nitrate, below.

## Phenylmercuric Nitrate

Basic Phenylmercury Nitrate; Fenilmercurio, nitrato de; Phenylhydrargyri Nitras; PMN. Nitratophenylmercury.

$C_6H_5HgOH,C_6H_5HgNO_3$ = 634.4.
*CAS — 8003-05-2 ($C_6H_5HgOH,C_6H_5HgNO_3$); 55-68-5 ($C_6H_5HgNO_3$).*
*ATC — D09AA04.*

**Pharmacopoeias.** In *Eur.* (see p.vi), *Int.*, and *Pol.* Also in *USNF.*

**Ph. Eur. 5.0** (Phenylmercuric Nitrate). A mixture of phenylmercuric nitrate and phenylmercuric hydroxide. A white or pale yellow powder. Very slightly soluble in water and in alcohol; slightly soluble in hot water; dissolves in glycerol and in fatty oils. Protect from light.

**USNF 22** (Phenylmercuric Nitrate). A mixture of phenylmercuric nitrate and phenylmercuric hydroxide. A white crystalline powder. Soluble 1 in 600 of water; slightly soluble in alcohol and in glycerol; more soluble in the presence of nitric acid or alkali hydroxides. A saturated solution in water is acid to litmus. Store in airtight containers. Protect from light.

**Incompatibility.** The activity of phenylmercuric salts may be reduced by interaction with compounds such as kaolin, magnesium trisilicate, starch, and talc.[1,2] Disodium edetate and sodium thiosulfate can also produce inactivation.[3] Sodium metabisulfite can lead to precipitation,[3] or chemical destruction,[4] but it can also produce increased activity.[3] Other incompatibilities include bromides, iodides (chlorides to a lesser extent), metals, and ammonia and its salts.[5] There can be adsorption onto rubber and some plastics[5,6] although sorption by low density polyethylene can be inhibited by phosphate ions.[7] Some filters, though not membrane filters, used for sterilisation removed considerable amounts of phenylmercuric nitrate from solution.[8] The pH may also affect activity.[9]


1. Yousef RT, *et al.* Effect of some pharmaceutical materials on the bactericidal activities of preservatives. *Can J Pharm Sci* 1973; **8:** 54–6.
2. Horn NR, *et al.* Interactions between powder suspensions and selected quaternary ammonium and organomercurial preservatives. *Cosmet Toilet* 1980; **95:** 69–73.
3. Richards RME, Reary JME. Changes in antibacterial activity of thiomersal and PMN on autoclaving with certain adjuvants. *J Pharm Pharmacol* 1972; **24** (suppl): 84P–89P.
4. Collins AJ, *et al.* Incompatibility of phenylmercuric acetate with sodium metabisulphite in eye drop formulations. *J Pharm Pharmacol* 1985; **37** (suppl): 123P.
5. Owen SC. Phenylmercuric nitrate. In: Rowe RC, *et al.* eds. *Handbook of pharmaceutical excipients.* 4th ed. London and Chicago: The Pharmaceutical Press and the American Pharmaceutical Association, 2003: 438–41.
6. Aspinall JA, *et al.* The effect of low density polyethylene containers on some hospital-manufactured eyedrop formulations. *J Clin Hosp Pharm* 1980; **5:** 21–9.
7. Aspinall JE, *et al.* The effect of low density polyethylene containers on some hospital-manufactured eyedrop formulations II. Inhibition of the sorption of phenylmercuric acetate. *J Clin Hosp Pharm* 1983; **8:** 233–40.
8. Naido NT, *et al.* Preservative loss from ophthalmic solutions during filtration sterilisation. *Aust J Pharm Sci* 1972; **NS1:** 16–18.
9. Wessels JMC, Adema DMM. Some data on the relationship between fungicidal protection and pH. In: Walters AH, Elphick JJ, eds. *Biodeterioration of materials.* Amsterdam: Elsevier, 1968: 517–23.


### Adverse Effects and Precautions

While the adverse effects of inorganic mercury (p.1713) should be taken into account when considering the adverse effects of phenylmercuric compounds, there is little evidence of systemic toxicity arising from their use. They are irritant to the skin and may give rise to erythema and blistering. Hypersensitivity reactions have been reported. Topical application to eyes has been associated with mercurialentis and atypical band keratopathy; prolonged use of eye drops containing phenylmercuric preservatives is not recommended.

**Effects on the eyes.** References to primary atypical band keratopathy and pigmentation of the anterior capsule of the lens (mercurialentis) associated with the prolonged use of eye drops containing phenylmercuric preservative.


1. Kennedy RE, *et al.* Further observations on atypical band keratopathy in glaucoma patients. *Trans Am Ophthalmol Soc* 1974; **72:** 107–22.
2. Garron LK, *et al.* A clinical pathologic study of mercurialentis medicamentosus. *Trans Am Ophthalmol Soc* 1976; **74:** 295–320.
3. Brazier DJ, Hitchings RA. Atypical band keratopathy following long-term pilocarpine treatment. *Br J Ophthalmol* 1989; **73:** 294–6.


### Uses

Phenylmercuric salts have antibacterial and antifungal properties. They are primarily bacteriostatic compounds although they also have a slow bactericidal action. Their activity has been reported to be pH dependent.

Phenylmercuric compounds are used as preservatives in cosmetic, ophthalmic, or pharmaceutical preparations and as antiseptics. They have also been used as spermicides.

When employed as a preservative in eye drops, a concentration of 0.002% is usually used; in injection solutions, the concentration is usually 0.001%.

### Preparations

**Proprietary Preparations** (details are given in Part 3)
***Ger.:*** Soklinal†; ***Israel:*** Clean-N-Soak†.

**Multi-ingredient:** ***Austria:*** Panto Liquid; ***USA:*** Hem-Prep.

## o-Phthaldialdehyde

o-Phthalaldehyde. 1,2-Benzenedicarboxaldehyde.

$C_8H_6O_2$ = 134.1.
*CAS — 643-79-8.*

### Adverse Effects and Precautions

As for Formaldehyde Solution, p.1179.

The manufacturer warns that *o*-phthaldialdehyde should not be used to process equipment used to treat patients with a history of bladder cancer as there have been associated rare reports of anaphylactoid reactions in such patients.

### Uses and Administration

*o*-Phthaldialdehyde is a bactericidal disinfectant with similar actions to those of glutaral (p.1181) but it is reported to be more active against mycobacteria and to be stable at a wider pH range of 3 to 9. Unlike glutaral it requires no activation before use.

A 0.55% aqueous solution of *o*-phthaldialdehyde is used for high-level disinfection of medical equipment that cannot be sterilised by heat. It is non-corrosive towards most materials. Complete immersion in the solution for a minimum of 12 minutes at 20° or 5 minutes at 25° or higher is recommended. For further details, see Disinfection of Endoscopes, p.1164.

◊ References.


1. Cooke RPD, *et al.* An evaluation of Cidex OPA (0.55% orthophthalaldehyde) as an alternative to 2% glutaraldehyde for high-level disinfection of endoscopes. *J Hosp Infect* 2003; **54:** 226–31.

### Preparations

**Proprietary Preparations** (details are given in Part 3)
***Fr.:*** Cidex OPA; ***USA:*** Cidex OPA.

## Picloxydine Dihydrochloride *(BANM, rINNM)*

1,1′-[Piperazine-1,4-diylbis(formimidoyl)]bis[3-(4-chlorophenyl)guanidine] dihydrochloride.

$C_{20}H_{24}Cl_2N_{10},2HCl = 548.3$.

*CAS — 5636-92-0 (picloxydine); 19803-62-4 (picloxydine dihydrochloride).*

### Profile

Picloxydine is a biguanide disinfectant with properties similar to those of chlorhexidine (p.1173). It has been used in eye drops as the dihydrochloride for the treatment of superficial infections of the eye. It has also been used as a surface disinfectant with quaternary ammonium compounds.

### Preparations

**Proprietary Preparations** (details are given in Part 3)
***Fr.:*** Vitabact; ***Switz.:*** Vitabact.

## Policresulen *(rINN)*

α-(4-Hydroxy-2-methyl-5-sulfobenzyl)-ω-(4-hydroxy-5-sulfo-o-tolyl)poly[(4-hydroxy-2-methyl-5-sulfo-*m*-phenylene)methylene]; 2-hydroxy-*p*-toluenesulfonic acid, polymer with formaldehyde.

$(C_8H_9O_4S)(C_8H_8O_4S)_n(C_7H_7O_4S)$.

*CAS — 101418-00-2.*

*ATC — D08AE02; G01AX03.*

### Profile

Policresulen is an antiseptic used in infections of mucous membranes.

### Preparations

**Proprietary Preparations** (details are given in Part 3)
***Arg.:*** Albocresil; ***Braz.:*** Albocresil; ***Chile:*** Albocresil; ***Ital.:*** Emaftol.

**Multi-ingredient:** ***Arg.:*** Proctyl; ***Braz.:*** Proctil†; Proctyl; ***Fin.:*** Faktu; ***Ger.:*** Faktu; ***Hong Kong:*** Faktu; ***Mex.:*** Proctoacid; ***Port.:*** Faktu; ***Singapore:*** Faktu; ***Switz.:*** Faktu; ***Thai.:*** Faktu†.

## Polihexanide *(BAN, rINN)*

ICI-9073; Polihexanida; Polyhexamethylene Biguanide Hydrochloride; Polyhexanide. Poly(1-hexamethylenebiguanide hydrochloride).

$(C_8H_{17}N_5,HCl)_n$.

*CAS — 32289-58-0.*

*ATC — D08AC05.*

### Profile

Polihexanide has antibacterial and antiamoebic activity. It is used as a surface disinfectant and for disinfecting soft contact lenses (p.1164). It has been tried in the treatment of *Acanthamoeba* keratitis (p.595).

### Preparations

**Proprietary Preparations** (details are given in Part 3)
***Switz.:*** Lavasept.

**Multi-ingredient:** ***Fr.:*** Ampholysine Plus†; Hexanios G+R; Instruzyme†; Novospray†; ***Ger.:*** Complete†; Teta Extra; Teta-S; ***Israel:*** Complete All-In-One†.

## Polynoxylin *(BAN, rINN)*

Polinoxilina. Poly{[bis(hydroxymethyl)ureylene]methylene}.

$(C_4H_8N_2O_3)_n$.

*CAS — 9011-05-6.*

*ATC — A01AB05; D01AE05.*

### Profile

Polynoxylin is a condensation product of formaldehyde and urea. It is an antiseptic with antibacterial and antifungal actions and, like noxytiolin (p.1187), may act by the release of formaldehyde. It is used topically for the local treatment of minor infections, usually at a concentration of 10%.

### Preparations

**Proprietary Preparations** (details are given in Part 3)
***NZ:*** Ponoxylan; ***Singapore:*** Anaflex; ***UK:*** Anaflex.

## Potassium Nitrate

E252; Kalii Nitras; Kalium Nitricum; Nitrato potásico; Nitre; Saltpetre.

$KNO_3 = 101.1$.

*CAS — 7757-79-1.*

**Pharmacopoeias.** In *Eur.* (see p.vi), *Pol.*, and *US.*

**Ph. Eur. 5.0** (Potassium Nitrate). Colourless crystals or a white crystalline powder. Freely soluble in water; very soluble in boiling water; practically insoluble in alcohol.

**USP 27** (Potassium Nitrate). Colourless crystals or a white crystalline powder. Freely soluble in water; very soluble in boiling water; practically insoluble in alcohol; soluble in glycerol. Store in airtight containers.

**Nomenclature.** The name saltpetre has been used as a generic term for a number of potassium- and sodium-based preservatives used in food manufacture. For a report of poisoning when a mixture of sodium nitrate and sodium nitrite was supplied for saltpetre, see p.1192.

### Adverse Effects and Precautions

After ingestion potassium nitrate may be reduced to nitrite in the gastrointestinal tract by the action of bacteria and ingestion of large amounts can therefore cause methaemoglobinaemia. Gastrointestinal disturbances, vertigo, headache, flushing of the skin, hypotension, irregular pulse, cyanosis, convulsions, and collapse may occur. The toxic dose varies greatly; 15 g may prove fatal but much larger doses have been taken without serious effects. Poisoning has frequently been reported in infants given water from wells contaminated with nitrates.

Nitrites are precursors of nitrosamines, which are *animal* carcinogens, but a relationship with human cancer has not been established.

Concern has been expressed regarding the concentrations of nitrates and nitrites in the public drinking water supply. National limits are often set for permissible concentrations in drinking water.

**Handling.** Potassium nitrate has been used for the illicit preparation of explosives or fireworks; care is required with its supply.

### Uses and Administration

Potassium nitrate is used as a preservative in foods. It is also included in dentrifices to reduce the pain of hypersensitive teeth. When taken by mouth in dilute solution, it acts as a diuretic and was formerly used for this purpose.

### Preparations

***USP 27:*** Potassium Nitrate Solution.

**Proprietary Preparations** (details are given in Part 3)
***Chile:*** Crowne; ***USA:*** Denquel.

**Multi-ingredient:** ***Arg.:*** Oral-B Dientes Sensibles con Fluor; Sens-Out; Sensigel; ***Austral.:*** Mackenzies Menthoids†; Oral-B Sensitive†; Thermodent†; ***Braz.:*** Pilulas De Witt's; Sensodyne Antitartaro; Sensodyne C/Bicarbonato de Sodio; Sensodyne Fresh Mint; Sensodyne Protecao Total; ***Canad.:*** Sensodyne-F; ***Chile:*** Sensaid con Fluor; Sensilacer; ***Fr.:*** Emoform Gencives; Emoform Sensibles; Fluocaril dents sensibles; Sensigel; ***Ital.:*** Actisens; Benodent Gel Gengivale; Dentosan Sensibile; Fluocaril; ***Mex.:*** Dentsiblen; ***Port.:*** Biofluor Sensitive; ***Singapore:*** Sensigel; ***Switz.:*** Grafco batonnets de bois†; ***UK:*** Avoca; ***USA:*** Original Sensodyne; Sensitivity Protection Crest; Sensodyne-F.

## Potassium Permanganate

Kalii Permanganas; Kalium Hypermanganicum; Kalium Permanganicum; Permanganato potásico; Pot. Permang.

$KMnO_4 = 158.0$.

*CAS — 7722-64-7.*

*ATC — D08AX06; V03AB18.*

**Pharmacopoeias.** In *Chin., Eur.* (see p.vi), *Jpn, Pol., US,* and *Viet.*

**Ph. Eur. 5.0** (Potassium Permanganate). Dark purple or almost black crystals or a dark purple or brownish-black granular powder, usually with a metallic lustre. It decomposes in contact with certain organic substances. Soluble in cold water and freely soluble in boiling water.

**USP 27** (Potassium Permanganate). Dark purple crystals, almost opaque by transmitted light and with a blue metallic lustre by reflected light; its colour is sometimes modified by a dark bronze-like appearance. Soluble 1 in 15 of water and 1 in 3.5 of boiling water.

**Incompatibility.** Potassium permanganate is incompatible with iodides, reducing agents, and most organic substances.

### Adverse Effects, Treatment, and Precautions

The crystals and concentrated solutions of potassium permanganate are caustic and even fairly dilute solutions are irritant to tissues and stain skin brown.

Symptoms of poisoning following ingestion of potassium permanganate should be treated symptomatically; they include nausea, vomiting of a brownish-coloured material, corrosion, oedema, and brown coloration of the buccal mucosa, gastrointestinal haemorrhage, liver and kidney damage, and cardiovascular depression. The fatal dose is probably about 5 to 10 g and death may occur up to 1 month from the time of poisoning.

The insertion into the vagina of potassium permanganate for its supposed abortifacient action causes corrosive burns, severe vaginal haemorrhage, and perforation of the vaginal wall, leading to peritonitis. Vascular collapse may occur.

◊ Case reports of adverse effects following ingestion of potassium permanganate.

1. Mahomedy MC, *et al.* Methaemoglobinaemia following treatment dispensed by witch doctors: two cases of potassium permanganate poisoning. *Anaesthesia* 1975; **30:** 190–3.
2. Kochhar R, *et al.* Potassium permanganate induced oesophageal stricture. *Hum Toxicol* 1986; **5:** 393–4.
3. Southwood T, *et al.* Ingestion of potassium permanganate crystals by a three-year-old boy. *Med J Aust* 1987; **146:** 639–40.
4. Middleton SJ, *et al.* Haemorrhagic pancreatitis—a cause of death in severe potassium permanganate poisoning. *Postgrad Med J* 1990; **66:** 657–8.
5. Young RJ, *et al.* Fatal acute hepatorenal failure following potassium permanganate ingestion. *Hum Exp Toxicol* 1996; **15:** 259–61.
6. Ong KL, *et al.* Potassium permanganate poisoning—a rare cause of fatal self poisoning. *J Accid Emerg Med* 1997; **14:** 43–5.
7. Lifshitz M, *et al.* Fatal potassium permanganate intoxication in an infant. *J Toxicol Clin Toxicol* 1999; **37:** 801–2.

**Handling and storage.** Potassium permanganate may be explosive if it is brought into contact with organic or other readily oxidisable substances. It has been used for the illicit preparation of fireworks; care is required with its supply.

### Uses and Administration

Potassium permanganate possesses oxidising properties which in turn confer disinfectant and deodorising properties. It is also astringent. Though bactericidal *in vitro* its clinical value as a bactericide is minimised by its rapid reduction in the presence of body fluids.

Solutions are used as cleansing applications to wounds, ulcers, or abscesses and as wet dressings and in baths in eczematous conditions and acute dermatoses especially where there is secondary infection. It is often prepared as a concentrated 0.1% solution in water to be diluted 1 in 10 before use to provide a 0.01% (1 in 10 000) solution. Solutions have also been used in bromhidrosis, in mycotic infections such as athlete's foot, and in poison ivy dermatitis.

Potassium permanganate is added to formaldehyde solution to produce formaldehyde vapour for the disinfection of rooms and cabinets (see p.1180).

### Preparations

**Proprietary Preparations** (details are given in Part 3)
***UK:*** Permitabs.

## Povidone-Iodine *(BAN)*

Iodinated Povidone; Polyvidone-Iodine; Polyvinylpyrrolidone-Iodine Complex; Povidona yodada; Povidonum Iodinatum; PVP-Iodine.

*CAS — 25655-41-8.*

*ATC — D08AG02; D09AA09; D11AC06; G01AX11; R02AA15; S01AX18.*

**Pharmacopoeias.** In *Chin., Eur.* (see p.vi), *Jpn, Pol.,* and *US.*

**Ph. Eur. 5.0** (Povidone, Iodinated). A complex of iodine with povidone containing 9 to 12% of available iodine calculated with reference to the dried substance. Yellowish-brown or reddish-brown amorphous powder. It loses not more than 8% of its weight on drying. Soluble in water and in alcohol; practically insoluble in acetone. A 10% solution in water has a pH of 1.5 to 5.0. Protect from light.

**USP 27** (Povidone-Iodine). A complex of iodine with povidone containing 9 to 12% of available iodine calculated on the dried basis. A yellowish-brown to reddish-brown amorphous powder with a slight characteristic odour. It loses not more than 8% of its weight on drying. Soluble in water and in alcohol; practically insoluble in acetone, in carbon tetrachloride, in chloroform, in ether, and in petroleum spirit. Its solutions are acid to litmus. Store in airtight containers.

**Incompatibility.** Antimicrobial activity may be reduced at high pH.

Dermatological reactions, described as second- and third-degree burns, were observed in 4 patients in whom wounds were covered with a povidone-iodine soaked bandage secured to the skin by compound benzoin tincture. It was suggested that an interaction had occurred resulting in a more acidic pH.[1]

A mixture of povidone-iodine solution and hydrogen peroxide [brown bubbly] has caused explosions.[2]

1. Schillaci LJ, *et al.* Reduced pH associated with mixture of povidone-iodine and compound tincture of benzoin. *Am J Hosp Pharm* 1983; **40:** 1694–5.
2. Dannenberg E, Peebles J. Betadine-hydrogen peroxide irrigation solution incompatibility. *Am J Hosp Pharm* 1978; **35:** 525.

### Adverse Effects and Precautions

Povidone-iodine can cause hypersensitivity reactions and irritation of the skin and mucous membranes, although severe reactions are rare and povidone-iodine is considered to be less irritant than iodine.

The application of povidone-iodine to severe burns or to large areas otherwise denuded of skin may produce the systemic adverse effects associated with iodine (p.1598) and metabolic acidosis, hypernatraemia, and renal impairment. Hyperthyroidism or hypothyroidism may occur following ingestion of large quantities. Hypothyroidism has occurred in neonates both as a result of absorption of iodine from povidone-iodine applied to the neonate and also to the mother during pregnancy or breast feeding.

Regular or prolonged use should be avoided in patients with thyroid disorders or those receiving lithium therapy.

**Acidosis.** There have been a number of reports of acidosis in patients whose burns were treated topically with povidone-iodine.[1,2] Fatal metabolic acidosis[3] and seizures[4] have been reported following mediastinal irrigation with povidone-iodine.

1. Pietsch J, Meakins JL. Complications of povidone-iodine absorption in topically treated burn patients. *Lancet* 1976; **i:** 280–2.
2. Scoggin C, *et al.* Hypernatraemia and acidosis in association with topical treatment of burns. *Lancet* 1977; **i:** 959.
3. Glick PL, *et al.* Iodine toxicity in a patient treated by continuous povidone-iodine mediastinal irrigation. *Ann Thorac Surg* 1985; **39:** 478–80.
4. Zec N, *et al.* Seizures in a patient treated with continuous povidone-iodine mediastinal irrigation. *N Engl J Med* 1992; **326:** 1784.

**Breast feeding.** Use of povidone-iodine in a vaginal gel by a breast-feeding woman resulted in elevated iodine concentrations in the breast milk and an odour of iodine on the infant's skin.[1] Despite this report, the American Academy of Pediatrics considers however that the use of povidone-iodine is usually compatible with breast feeding.[2]

1. Pastellon DC, Aranow R. Iodine in mother's milk. *JAMA* 1982; **247:** 463.
2. American Academy of Pediatrics. The transfer of drugs and other chemicals into human milk. *Pediatrics* 2001; **108:** 776–89. Correction. *ibid.*; 1029. Also available at: http://aappolicy.aappublications.org/cgi/content/full/pediatrics%3b108/3/776 (accessed 11/06/04)

**Hypersensitivity.** Anaphylaxis was associated with vaginal application of povidone-iodine solution.[1]

1. Waran KD, Munsick RA. Anaphylaxis from povidone-iodine. *Lancet* 1995; **345:** 1506.

**Neonates.** Hypothyroidism has been reported in premature and very low birth-weight infants following the use of povidone-iodine for routine antisepsis,[1,2] and hyperthyroidism in a full-term infant following mediastinal lavage.[3]

Perinatal vaginal use of povidone-iodine may also cause neonatal thyroid dysfunction.[4]

1. Parravicini E, *et al.* Iodine, thyroid function, and very low birth weight infants. *Pediatrics* 1996; **98:** 730–4.
2. Linder N, *et al.* Topical iodine-containing antiseptics and subclinical hypothyroidism in preterm infants. *J Pediatr* 1997; **131:** 434–9.
3. Bryant WP, Zimmerman D. Iodine-induced hyperthyroidism in a newborn. *Pediatrics* 1995; **95:** 434–6. Correction. *ibid.*; **96:** 779.
4. l'Allemand D, *et al.* Iodine-induced alterations of thyroid function in newborn infants after prenatal and perinatal exposure to povidone iodine. *J Pediatr* 1983; **102:** 935–8.

## Uses and Administration

Povidone-iodine is an iodophore which is used as a disinfectant and antiseptic mainly for the treatment of contaminated wounds and pre-operative preparation of the skin and mucous membranes as well as for the disinfection of equipment.

Iodophores are loose complexes of iodine and carrier polymers. Solutions of povidone-iodine gradually release iodine to exert an effect against bacteria, fungi, viruses, protozoa, cysts, and spores; povidone-iodine is thus less potent than preparations containing free iodine but it is less toxic.

A wide variety of topical formulations is available, the majority containing about 4 to 10% of povidone-iodine; a 1% mouthwash has been used for oral infections including candidiasis and topical powders containing 0.5 to 5% povidone-iodine have been tried in the treatment and prevention of wound infection. For vaginal application povidone-iodine has also been used as pessaries containing 200 mg.

## Preparations

***BP 2003:*** Povidone-Iodine Mouthwash; Povidone-Iodine Solution;
***USP 27:*** Povidone-Iodine Cleansing Solution; Povidone-Iodine Ointment; Povidone-Iodine Topical Aerosol; Povidone-Iodine Topical Solution.

**Proprietary Preparations** (details are given in Part 3)
***Arg.:*** Clivasol; DG-6 Iodopovidona; Iodoasept; Iodomax; Pervinox; Povi Complex; Povibac; Povicler; Salguer; Tycoytycoy; ***Austral.:*** Betadine; EDP-Evans Dermal Powder†; Isodine; Logicin Sore Throat; Microshield PVP; Microshield PVP-S; Minidine; Nyal Medithroat Gargle†; Pl Antiseptic Ointment; Savlon Antiseptic†; Viodine; ***Austria:*** Betadona; Betaisodona; Betasan; Betaseptic; Braunol; Braunovidon; Wundesin; ***Belg.:*** Braunol; Iodex; Iso-Betadine; ***Braz.:*** Antisseptico†; Asteriodine; Braunoderm†; Braunol†; Marcodine; Povid-Derme†; Prepcare†; PVPI; Sabofen; Silvedine†; ***Canad.:*** Betadine; Massengill Medicated†; Metadyne†; Proviodine; ***Chile:*** Difexon; Neoyod; ***Fin.:*** Betadine; ***Fr.:*** Betadine; Poliodine; ***Ger.:*** Betaisodona; Braunol; Braunovidon; Freka-cid; Inadine; Jodobac; Polydona; Polysept; Sepso J; SP Betaisodona†; Traumasept; ***Gr.:*** Betadine; Drapix; Oxisept; ***Hong Kong:*** Betadine; Freka-cid; Pevidine†; Proviodine; Videne; ***India:*** Alphadine; Betadine; Betadine-AD; Povidine; Wokadine; ***Irl.:*** Betadine; Braunol†; Braunosan†; Braunovidon†; Inadine; ***Israel:*** Betadine†; Idovit; Iodiflor; Iodo-Vit; Massengill Medicated; Polydine; Polysept; Yodon; ***Ital.:*** Betadine; Betaseptic; Braunol; Citro Jod; Destrobac; Eso-Jod; Esoform Jod 35 and 75; Evadermin†; Gammadin; Garze Disinfettanti alla Pomata Betadine†; Golasept; Inadine; Iodocid†; Iodosteril; Iodoten; Jodocur; Jodogard; Oftasteril; Paniodal; Paniodine; Poviderm; ***Malaysia:*** Betadine; Freka-cid; Septi-Aid; Summers Eve Medicated; ***Mex.:*** Isodine; Solvin; Yodacua; Yodine; ***Neth.:*** Betadine; ***NZ:*** Betadine; Biocil; Riodine; Viodine; ***Port.:*** Betadine; Cromoseptil Plus†; Dinasepte; Isodine; Septil; ***S.Afr.:*** Betadine; Dermadine; Podine; Septadine; Septisooth; Steridine; ***Singapore:*** Betadine; Summers Eve Medicated†; ***Spain:*** Acydona; Betadine; Betatul; Braunoderm†; Braunol†; Curadona; Iodina; Kaput†; Orto Dermo P; Sanoyodo; Solucionic†; Topionic; ***Switz.:*** Betadine; Braunol; Braunosan; Braunosan H Plus; Braunovidon; Destrobac; Intersept; Jodoplex; Rocanal Intermediat†; ***Thai.:*** Annadine; Bactedene; Bernadine; Betadine; Cavodine; Eprodine; Isodine; Movidone; P-Vidine; Povadine; Sepfadine; Septidine; Videne; ***UK:*** Betadine; Brush Off†; Inadine; Savlon Dry; Videne; ***USA:*** ACU-dyne; Aerodine†; Betadine; Biodine; Efodine; Iodex; Massengill Medicated; Minidyne; Operand; Polydine; Summers Eve Medicated.

**Multi-ingredient:** ***Arg.:*** Pervinox D; ***Austral.:*** Microshield PVP Plus†; ***Austria:*** Braunoderm; ***Belg.:*** Braunoderm†; ***Braz.:*** Iodocaine†; ***Ger.:*** Betaseptic; Braunoderm; ***India:*** Eczo-Wokadine; ***Irl.:*** Braunoderm†; ***Ital.:*** Braunoderm; Jodieci; ***Jpn:*** U-Pasta; ***Switz.:*** Betaseptic; Braunoderm; Jodobac†; ***UK:*** Codella†; ***USA:*** Anbesol; Orasol; ProTech.

## Propamidine Isetionate *(BANM, rINNM)*

Isetionato de propamidina; M&B-782; Propamidine Isethionate. 4,4′-Trimethylenedioxydibenzamidine bis(2-hydroxyethanesulphonate).

$C_{17}H_{20}N_4O_2,2C_2H_6O_4S = 564.6.$
*CAS — 104-32-5 (propamidine); 140-63-6 (propamidine isetionate).*
*ATC — D08AC03; S01AX15.*

### Profile

Propamidine isetionate is an aromatic diamidine antiseptic which is active against Gram-positive bacteria, but less active against Gram-negative bacteria and spore-forming organisms. It also has antifungal properties and is active against *Acanthamoeba*. Ophthalmic solutions containing 0.1% of propamidine isetionate are used for the treatment of conjunctivitis and blepharitis.

**Acanthamoeba keratitis.** The optimal regimen for the treatment of *Acanthamoeba* keratitis (p.595) has yet to be determined. Propamidine isetionate 0.1% is commonly used, usually with neomycin[1,2] or a neomycin-polymyxin-gramicidin combination,[3] plus chlorhexidine gluconate,[4] or polihexanide.[5] However, reported resistance of some strains of *Acanthamoeba* to propamidine has prompted the suggestion that it should be replaced by another diamidine such as hexamidine.[6]

1. Wright P, *et al.* Acanthamoeba keratitis successfully treated medically. *Br J Ophthalmol* 1985; **69:** 778–82.
2. Varga JH, *et al.* Combined treatment of Acanthamoeba keratitis with propamidine, neomycin, and polyhexamethylene biguanide. *Am J Ophthalmol* 1993; **115:** 466–70.
3. Moore MB, McCulley JP. Acanthamoeba keratitis associated with contact lenses: six consecutive cases of successful management. *Br J Ophthalmol* 1989; **73:** 271–5.
4. Seal DV. Chlorhexidine or polyhexamethylene biguanide for acanthamoeba keratitis. *Lancet* 1995; **345:** 136.
5. Kilvington S. Chemotherapy for acanthamoeba keratitis. *Lancet* 1995; **345:** 792.
6. Perrine D, *et al.* Amoebicidal efficiencies of various diamidines against two strains of Acanthamoeba polyphaga. *Antimicrob Agents Chemother* 1995; **39:** 339–42.

### Preparations

**Proprietary Preparations** (details are given in Part 3)
***Austral.:*** Brolene; ***Irl.:*** Brolene; ***NZ:*** Brolene; ***S.Afr.:*** Brolene; ***UK:*** Brolene; Golden Eye Drops.

## Propiolactone *(BAN, USAN, rINN)*

BPL; NSC-21626; 2-Oxetanone; Propanolide; Propiolactona; β-Propiolactone. Propiono-3-lactone.

$C_3H_4O_2 = 72.06.$
*CAS — 57-57-8.*

### Profile

Propiolactone vapour is an irritant, mutagenic, possibly carcinogenic, disinfectant which is very active against most micro-organisms including viruses. It is rather less effective against bacterial spores.

Propiolactone vapour has been used for the gaseous sterilisation of pharmaceutical and surgical materials and for disinfecting large enclosed areas. It has low penetrating power. Propiolactone liquid has also been used.

## Propyl Alcohol

Alcohol propílico; Normal Propyl Alcohol; Primary Propyl Alcohol; Propanol; Propanolum. Propan-1-ol.

$CH_3.CH_2.CH_2OH = 60.10.$
*CAS — 71-23-8.*
*ATC — D08AX03.*

**Pharmacopoeias.** In *Eur.* (see p.vi).

**Ph. Eur. 5.0** (Propanol). A clear colourless liquid. Miscible with water and with dehydrated alcohol. Protect from light.

### Adverse Effects and Treatment

As for Alcohol, p.1166; propyl alcohol is considered more toxic.

◊ References.

1. 1-Propanol. *Environmental Health Criteria 102.* Geneva: WHO, 1990. Available at: http://www.inchem.org/documents/ehc/ehc/ehc102.htm (accessed 11/06/04)

### Uses and Administration

Propyl alcohol, an antiseptic with properties similar to those of alcohol (p.1167), is used in preparations for disinfection of the hands, skin, surfaces, and instruments.

Isopropyl alcohol (p.1185) is also used as an antiseptic.

### Preparations

**Proprietary Preparations** (details are given in Part 3)
**Multi-ingredient:** ***Austria:*** Dodesept; Marcocid; Sterillium; ***Fr.:*** Sterillium; ***Ger.:*** Aerodesin; Antifect†; Bacillol; Bacillol AF; Bacillol plus; Desmanol; Freka-Steril; Hospisept; Incidin; Incidur Spray; Kodan Tinktur Forte; Meliseptol; Meliseptol Rapid; Mikrozid†; Neo Kodan; Primasept Med; Sagrosept; Softa Man; St-Tissues; Sterillium; ***Ital.:*** Softa Man; ***Mon.:*** Akila mains et peau†; Akila spray†; ***Switz.:*** Adro-derm†; Jodobac†; Orosept†.

## Ritiometan *(rINN)*

Ritiometán. (Methylidynetrithio)triacetic acid.

$C_7H_{10}O_6S_3 = 286.3.$
*CAS — 34914-39-1.*
*ATC — R01AX05.*

### Profile

Ritiometan is used as the magnesium salt in an aerosol preparation for the treatment of infections of the nose and throat.

### Preparations

**Proprietary Preparations** (details are given in Part 3)
***Fr.:*** Necyrane.

## Scarlet Red

Biebrich Scarlet R Medicinal; CI Solvent Red 24; Colour Index No. 26105; Fat Ponceau R; Rojo escarlata; Rubrum Scarlatinum; Scharlachrot; Sudan IV. 1-[4-(o-Tolylazo)-o-tolylazo]naphth-2-ol.

$C_{24}H_{20}N_4O = 380.4.$
*CAS — 85-83-6.*

### Profile

Scarlet red is an antiseptic dye that has been used topically. It can be irritant.

## Sodium Azide

Azida sódica.

$N_3Na = 65.01.$
*CAS — 26628-22-8.*

### Adverse Effects and Precautions

Acute poisoning with sodium azide may cause nausea and vomiting, diarrhoea, life-threatening hypotension, tachycardia, convulsions, and severe headache. Fatalities have been reported. Solutions containing sodium azide must not be disposed of into drain pipelines containing copper, lead, or brass since highly explosive heavy metal azides may be produced.

◊ References to acute poisoning with sodium azide.

1. Edmonds OP, Bourne MS. Sodium azide poisoning in five laboratory technicians. *Br J Ind Med* 1982; **39:** 308–9.
2. Klein-Schwartz W, *et al.* Three fatal sodium azide poisonings. *Med Toxicol Adverse Drug Exp* 1989; **4:** 219–27.
3. Anonymous. Sodium azide contamination of hemodialysis water supplies. *JAMA* 1989; **261:** 2603.

### Uses

Sodium azide has been used as an antimicrobial preservative in laboratory reagents, serum samples, and dialysis equipment.

## Sodium Diacetate

Diacetato de sodio; E262. Sodium hydrogen diacetate.

$CH_3COONa,CH_3COOH(+xH_2O).$
*CAS — 126-96-5 (anhydrous sodium diacetate).*

### Profile

Sodium diacetate is used as a preservative in foods, particularly as an inhibitor of moulds and rope-forming micro-organisms in bread.

## Sodium Dichloroisocyanurate

Dicloroisocianurato sódico; Sodium Dichloro-s-triazinetrione; Sodium Troclosene. 1,3-Dichloro-1,3,5-triazine-2,4,6(1*H*,3*H*,5*H*)-trione sodium.

$C_3Cl_2N_3NaO_3 = 219.9.$
*CAS — 2893-78-9.*

### Profile

Sodium dichloroisocyanurate is a disinfectant with the general properties of chlorine (p.1175) and sodium hypochlorite (p.1192) but it remains active as pH increases from 6 to 10 and is reported to be less susceptible to inactivation by organic material. It contains about 65% of 'available chlorine' (see p.1176).

Sodium dichloroisocyanurate is used for disinfecting hard surfaces (see Disinfection in Hepatitis and HIV Infection, p.1165), babies' feeding bottles, and food and dairy equipment, for treating water (p.1165), for soft contact lens care (p.1164), and in various commercial bleach detergents and scouring powders as a relatively stable source of chlorine.

Dichloroisocyanuric acid ($C_3HCl_2N_3O_3 = 198.0$), potassium dichloroisocyanurate (potassium troclosene; troclosene potassium, $C_3Cl_2KN_3O_3 = 236.1$), and trichloroisocyanuric acid (symclosene, $C_3Cl_3N_3O_3 = 232.4$) are similarly used.

### Preparations

**Proprietary Preparations** (details are given in Part 3)
***Austral.:*** Milton Anti-Bacterial†; Puritabs†; ***Austria:*** Polyrinse Desinfektionssystem†; ***Fr.:*** Aquatabs; Milton†; Polycare†; Solusteril†; ***Hong Kong:*** Actichlor; ***Irl.:*** Aquatabs†; Klorsept†; Milton†; Sterinova†; ***Israel:*** Klor-De; Klorsept; Taharmayim; Taharsept; Tahartaf; ***Ital.:*** Dialster; Presept†; ***Mex.:*** Aquatabs†; ***NZ:*** Puritabs; Softab†; ***UK:*** Milton; Presept.
**Multi-ingredient:** ***Irl.:*** Klor-Kleen†.

## Sodium Formaldehyde Sulfoxylate

Formaldehído sulfoxilato sódico; Sodium Formaldehyde Sulphoxylate. Sodium hydroxymethanesulphinate dihydrate.
$CH_3NaO_3S,2H_2O$ = 154.1.
*CAS — 149-44-0 (anhydrous sodium formaldehyde sulfoxylate); 6035-47-8 (sodium formaldehyde sulfoxylate, dihydrate).*

**Pharmacopoeias.** In *Pol.* Also in *USNF.*
**USNF 22** (Sodium formaldehyde Sulfoxylate). White crystals or hard white masses with the characteristic odour of garlic. Soluble 1 in 3.4 of water, 1 in 510 of alcohol, 1 in 175 of chloroform, and 1 in 180 of ether; slightly soluble in benzene. A 2% solution in water has a pH of 9.5 to 10.5. Store at 15° to 30°. Protect from light.

### Profile

Sodium formaldehyde sulfoxylate is an antoxidant used as a preservative in pharmaceuticals. It has been used in the treatment of acute mercury poisoning (p.1713).

# Sodium Hypochlorite

Hipoclorito sódico.
$NaOCl,5H_2O$ = 164.5.
*CAS — 7681-52-9.*
*ATC — D08AX07.*

**Pharmacopoeias.** *Br., Fr., Jpn,* and *US* include sodium hypochlorite solutions.
**BP 2003** (Dilute Sodium Hypochlorite Solution). It contains 1% of available chlorine. Store away from acids at a temperature not exceeding 20°. Protect from light.
**BP 2003** (Strong Sodium Hypochlorite Solution). It contains not less than 8% of available chlorine. It should be diluted before use. Store away from acids at a temperature not exceeding 20°. Protect from light.
**USP 27** (Sodium Hypochlorite Solution). It contains not less than 4% and not more than 6% w/w of anhydrous sodium hypochlorite. It is not suitable for application to wounds. Store in airtight containers. Protect from light.
**USP 27** (Sodium Hypochlorite Topical Solution). It contains 0.025% sodium hypochlorite. Store in airtight containers. Protect from light.

**Incompatibility.** The antimicrobial activity of hypochlorites is rapidly reduced in the presence of organic material; it is also pH dependent being greater in acid pH although hypochlorites are more stable at alkaline pH.

Sodium hypochlorite solutions should not be mixed with solutions of strong acids or ammonia; the subsequent reactions release chlorine gas and tosylchloramide sodium gas, respectively.

**Stability.** The stability of sodium hypochlorite solutions increases with pH, solutions of pH 10 or more being most stable.[1] Stability studies have shown that solutions providing 0.04 to 0.12% 'available chlorine' stored in amber glass bottles at room temperature could carry a 23-month expiry date.[2]

1. Bloomfield SF, Sizer TJ. Eusol BPC and other hypochlorite formulations used in hospitals. *Pharm J* 1985; **235:** 153–5 and 157.
2. Fabian TM, Walker SE. Stability of sodium hypochlorite solutions. *Am J Hosp Pharm* 1982; **39:** 1016–17.

### Adverse Effects

Hypochlorite solutions release hypochlorous acid upon contact with gastric juice and acids, and ingestion causes irritation and corrosion of mucous membranes with pain and vomiting, oedema of the pharynx and larynx, and, rarely, perforation of the oesophagus and stomach. A fall in blood pressure, delirium, and coma may occur. Inhalation of hypochlorous fumes causes coughing and choking and may cause severe respiratory tract irritation and pulmonary oedema. Hypochlorite solutions may be irritating to the skin.

**Effects on wound healing.** For comment on the adverse effects of hypochlorite solutions on wound healing, see Disinfection: Wounds under Uses and Administration of Chlorine, p.1176.

**Effects on the blood.** An acute haemolytic crisis was reported in a child who had swum for about 4 hours in an indoor pool containing very high concentrations of sodium hypochlorite.[1] The child was subsequently found to have G6PD deficiency.

1. Ong SJ, Kearney B. Local swimming pool and G-6-PD deficiency. *Med J Aust* 1994; **161:** 226–7.

### Treatment of Adverse Effects

If sodium hypochlorite solution is ingested, water, milk, or other demulcents should be given; opinion over the use of antacids is divided. Sodium thiosulfate 1 to 2.5% solution has been used but is of little or no value. If spilled on skin, washing with copious amounts of water is recommended.

**Poisoning.** A patient who accidentally received an intravenous infusion of 150 mL of a 1% solution of sodium hypochlorite experienced a slow heart rate, mild hypotension, and increased respiratory rate. The slow heart rate persisted for 3 days but other parameters returned to normal after symptomatic treatment.[1]

1. Marroni M, Menichetti F. Accidental intravenous infusion of sodium hypochlorite. *DICP Ann Pharmacother* 1991; **25:** 1008–9.

### Precautions

Topically applied hypochlorites may dissolve blood clots and cause bleeding.

### Uses and Administration

Sodium hypochlorite is a disinfectant and antiseptic with the brief and rapid actions of chlorine (see p.1176). Sodium hypochlorite pentahydrate contains about 43% of 'available chlorine' (see p.1176); anhydrous sodium hypochlorite contains about 95%. Powders and solutions are commonly used for the rapid disinfection of hard surfaces (see Disinfection in Creutzfeldt-Jakob Disease, p.1164 and in Hepatitis and HIV Infection, p.1165), food and dairy equipment, babies' feeding bottles, excreta, and water (p.1165). Solutions for use as domestic bleaches contain about 5% of hypochlorite. Only diluted solutions containing up to 0.5% of 'available chlorine' are suitable for use on the skin and in wounds (but see Wound Disinfection, p.1165).

Solutions of hypochlorites used as disinfectants have included Labarraque's Solution containing sodium hypochlorite with an alkali, and Eau de Javel, containing sodium or potassium hypochlorite.

### Preparations

***BP 2003:*** Dilute Sodium Hypochlorite Solution; Strong Sodium Hypochlorite Solution;
***USP 27:*** Sodium Hypochlorite Solution; Sodium Hypochlorite Topical Solution.

**Proprietary Preparations** (details are given in Part 3)
***Arg.:*** Antibacter; ***Austral.:*** Milton Anti-Bacterial†; ***Belg.:*** Dakincooper; ***Braz.:*** Colix†; Liquido de Dakin; Milton†; ***Canad.:*** Hygeol; ***Fr.:*** Dakin; Milton†; ***Ger.:*** Maranon H; ***Irl.:*** Hypercidin†; Milton†; ***Israel:*** Chlorasol; ***Ital.:*** Amukine Med; Milton; Naclon†; ***UK:*** Chlorasol; Milton.
**Multi-ingredient:** ***Fr.:*** Amukine; ***Mex.:*** Amuchina.

## Sodium Nitrate

E251; Natrii Nitras; Natrium Nitricum; Nitrato sódico.
$NaNO_3$ = 84.99.
*CAS — 7631-99-4.*

NOTE. Crude sodium nitrate is known as Chile Saltpetre.

### Profile

Sodium nitrate has similar actions to potassium nitrate (p.1190) and is used as a preservative in foods, particularly in meat products.

Crude sodium nitrate is used as a fertiliser.

**Handling.** Sodium nitrate has been used for the illicit preparation of explosives or fireworks; care is required with its supply.

**Poisoning.** Cyanosis and methaemoglobinaemia has been reported[1] in 3 patients after eating sausages which had been preserved mistakenly with a mixture of sodium nitrate and sodium nitrite rather than with potassium nitrate (saltpetre). The name saltpetre is used as a generic term for a number of potassium- or sodium-based preservatives used in food manufacture.

1. Kennedy N, *et al.* Faulty sausage production causing methaemoglobinaemia. *Arch Dis Child* 1997; **76:** 367–8.

## Sodium Perborate

Natrii Perboras; Perborato sódico; Sod. Perbor.
$NaBO_2,H_2O_2,3H_2O$ = 153.9.
*CAS — 7632-04-4 (anhydrous sodium perborate); 10042-94-1 (sodium perborate hydrate).*
*ATC — A01AB19.*

NOTE. Sodium Perborate Monohydrate is *USAN.*

**Pharmacopoeias.** In *Eur.* (see p.vi).
**Ph. Eur. 5.0** (Sodium Perborate, Hydrated; Sodium Perborate BP 2003). Colourless prismatic crystals or a white powder, stable in crystalline form. Sparingly soluble in water, with slow decomposition. It dissolves in dilute mineral acids. Store in airtight containers.

### Adverse Effects

Frequent use of toothpowders containing sodium perborate may cause blistering and oedema. Hypertrophy of the papillae of the tongue has also been reported. The effects of swallowed sodium perborate are similar to those of boric acid (p.1662).

### Uses and Administration

Sodium perborate is a mild disinfectant and deodorant. It readily releases oxygen in contact with oxidisable matter and has been used in aqueous solutions for purposes similar to weak solutions of hydrogen peroxide.

Sodium perborate has also been used, with calcium carbonate, as a toothpowder. A freshly prepared solution is used as a mouthwash.

The less soluble $NaBO_2,H_2O_2$ known as sodium perborate monohydrate is used similarly.

### Preparations

**Proprietary Preparations** (details are given in Part 3)
***Arg.:*** Hifamonil; ***Canad.:*** Amosan; ***India:*** Steradent; ***Irl.:*** Bocasan†; ***Ital.:*** Kavosan; ***UK:*** Bocasan†; ***USA:*** Amosan.
**Multi-ingredient:** ***Arg.:*** Oral-B Enjuague Bucal Amosan; ***Austral.:*** Amosan; ***Belg.:*** Sulfaryl†; ***Braz.:*** Angino Tricin; Oticerim; ***Fr.:*** Bactident; Hydralin; ***Hong Kong:*** Hydralin; ***Ital.:*** Borossigeno Plus Stomatologico†; ***Port.:*** Dentolamina†; ***Spain:*** Lema C; ***Switz.:*** Saltrates Rodell; ***USA:*** Trichotine.

## Sodium Percarbonate

Sodium Carbonate Peroxide.
$Na_2CO_3,1\frac{1}{2}H_2O_2$ = 157.0.
*CAS — 15630-89-4.*

### Profile

Sodium percarbonate has similar uses to sodium perborate (p.1192).

### Preparations

**Proprietary Preparations** (details are given in Part 3)
**Multi-ingredient:** ***Arg.:*** Ascoxal; ***Austral.:*** Ascoxal†; ***Fin.:*** Ascoxal; ***Mex.:*** Ascoxal; ***Norw.:*** Ascoxal; ***Swed.:*** Ascoxal.

## Sorbates

Sorbatos.

## Sorbic Acid

Acidum Sorbicum; E200; Sórbico, ácido. (*E,E*)-Hexa-2,4-dienoic acid.
$C_6H_8O_2$ = 112.1.
*CAS — 22500-92-1.*

**Pharmacopoeias.** In *Chin., Eur.* (see p.vi), and *Pol.* Also in *USNF.*
**Ph. Eur. 5.0** (Sorbic Acid). A white or almost white, crystalline powder. Slightly soluble in water; freely soluble in alcohol. Protect from light.
**USNF 22** (Sorbic Acid). A free-flowing white crystalline powder with a characteristic odour. Soluble 1 in 1000 of water, 1 in 10 of alcohol, 1 in 8 of dehydrated alcohol, 1 in 15 of chloroform, 1 in 30 of ether, 1 in 8 of methyl alcohol, and 1 in 19 of propylene glycol. Store in airtight containers at a temperature not exceeding 40°. Protect from light.

**Incompatibility.** The incompatibility of sorbates is discussed under Potassium Sorbate, below.

## Potassium Sorbate

E202; Kalii Sorbas; Sorbato potásico. Potassium (*E,E*)-hexa-2,4-dienoate.
$C_6H_7KO_2$ = 150.2.
*CAS — 590-00-1; 24634-61-5;.*

**Pharmacopoeias.** In *Eur.* (see p.vi). Also in *USNF.*
**Ph. Eur. 5.0** (Potassium Sorbate). White or almost white granules or powder. Very soluble in water; slightly soluble in alcohol. Protect from light.
**USNF 22** (Potassium Sorbate). White crystals or powder with a characteristic odour. Soluble 1 in 4.5 of water, 1 in 35 of alcohol, and 1 in more than 1000 of chloroform and of ether. Store in airtight containers at a temperature not exceeding 40°. Protect from light.

**Incompatibility.** Sorbic acid can be inactivated by oxidation and to some extent by nonionic surfactants and plastics. Activity of the sorbates may be reduced by increases in pH.[1]

1. Beasley MW. Sorbic acid. In: Rowe RC, *et al.*, eds. *Handbook of pharmaceutical excipients.* 4th ed. London and Chicago: The Pharmaceutical Press and the American Pharmaceutical Association, 2003: 588–90.

### Adverse Effects and Precautions

The sorbates can be irritant and have caused contact dermatitis.

**Hypersensitivity.** References to allergic-type skin reactions[1] and non-allergic irritant-type reactions[2,3] with potassium sorbate or sorbic acid.

1. Saihan EM, Harman RRM. Contact sensitivity to sorbic acid in 'Unguentum Merck'. *Br J Dermatol* 1978; **99:** 583–4.

2. Soschin D, Leyden JJ. Sorbic acid-induced erythema and edema. *J Am Acad Dermatol* 1986; **14:** 234–41.
3. Fisher AA. Erythema limited to the face due to sorbic acid. *Cutis* 1987; **40:** 395–7.

### Uses

Potassium sorbate and sorbic acid possess antifungal, and to a lesser extent antibacterial, activity. They are relatively ineffective above a pH of about 6. They are used as preservatives in pharmaceutical preparations in concentrations of up to 0.2%, in enteral formulas, foods, and in cosmetic preparations.

### Preparations

**Proprietary Preparations** (details are given in Part 3)

**Multi-ingredient:** ***Austral.:*** Caprilate†; ***Austria:*** Onycho Phytex†; Phytex†; ***Ger.:*** Klysma Sorbit; ***Ital.:*** Bo-Gum†; Evasen Dischetti; Evasen Liquido; ***Mex.:*** Adapettes; ***UK:*** Relaxit; ***USA:*** Feminique.

## Sulfites and Sulfur Dioxide

Sulfitos y dióxido de azufre.

### Potassium Bisulfite

Bisulfito potásico; E228; Potassium Bisulphite; Potassium Hydrogen Sulphite.

$KHSO_3$ = 120.2.

*CAS — 7773-03-7.*

### Potassium Metabisulfite

Dipotassium Pyrosulphite; E224; Kalii Metabisulfis; Metabisulfito potásico; Potassium Metabisulphite; Potassium Pyrosulphite.

$K_2S_2O_5$ = 222.3.

*CAS — 16731-55-8.*

**Pharmacopoeias.** In *Eur.* (see p.vi). Also in *USNF.*

**Ph. Eur. 5.0** (Potassium Metabisulphite). A white powder or colourless crystals. Freely soluble in water; slightly soluble in alcohol. A 5% solution in water has a pH of 3.0 to 4.5. Store in airtight containers. Protect from light.

**USNF 22** (Potassium Metabisulfite). White or colourless, free-flowing crystals, crystalline powder, or granules, usually with an odour of sulfur dioxide. Gradually oxidises in air to the sulfate. Soluble in water; insoluble in alcohol. Its solutions are acid to litmus. Store in well-filled airtight containers at a temperature not exceeding 40°.

**Incompatibility.** The incompatibility of sulfites is discussed under Sulfur Dioxide, below.

### Sodium Bisulfite

Bisulfito sódico; E222; Sodium Bisulphite; Sodium Hydrogen Sulphite.

$NaHSO_3$ = 104.1.

*CAS — 7631-90-5.*

**Pharmacopoeias.** In *Chin.* and *Jpn,* described in both as consisting of a mixture of sodium bisulfite and sodium metabisulfite.

### Sodium Metabisulfite

Disodium Pyrosulphite; E223; Metabisulfito sódico; Natrii Disulfis; Natrii Metabisulfis; Sodium Disulphite; Sodium Metabisulphite; Sodium Pyrosulphite.

$Na_2S_2O_5$ = 190.1.

*CAS — 7681-57-4.*

**Pharmacopoeias.** In *Chin., Eur.* (see p.vi), *Jpn,* and *Pol.* Also in *USNF.*

**Ph. Eur. 5.0** (Sodium Metabisulphite). Colourless crystals or a white or almost white crystalline powder. Freely soluble in water; slightly soluble in alcohol. A 5% solution in water has a pH of 3.5 to 5.0. Protect from light.

**USNF 22** (Sodium Metabisulfite). White crystals or a white to yellowish crystalline powder with an odour of sulfur dioxide. Freely soluble in water and in glycerol; slightly soluble in alcohol. Store in well-filled airtight containers at a temperature not exceeding 40°.

**Incompatibility.** The incompatibility of sulfites is discussed under Sulfur Dioxide, below.

### Sodium Sulfite

Anhydrous Sodium Sulphite; E221; Exsiccated Sodium Sulphite; Natrii Sulfis Anhydricus; Natrii Sulfis Siccatus; Natrii Sulphis; Sodium Sulphite; Sulfito sódico.

$Na_2SO_3$ = 126.0.

*CAS — 7757-83-7.*

**Pharmacopoeias.** In *Chin., Eur.* (see p.vi), *Jpn,* and *Pol.*

*Eur.* and *Pol.* also include the heptahydrate.

**Ph. Eur. 5.0** (Sodium Sulphite, Anhydrous; Natri Sulfis Anhydricus). A white powder. Freely soluble in water; very slightly soluble in alcohol. Store in airtight containers.

**Ph. Eur. 5.0** (Sodium Sulphite Heptahydrate; Natrii Sulfis Heptahydricus). Colourless crystals. Freely soluble in water; very slightly soluble in alcohol.

**Incompatibility.** The incompatibility of sulfites is discussed under Sulfur Dioxide, below.

### Sulfur Dioxide

Dióxido de azufre; E220; Sulphur Dioxide.

$SO_2$ = 64.06.

*CAS — 7446-09-5.*

**Pharmacopoeias.** In *USNF.*

**USNF 22** (Sulfur Dioxide). A colourless non-flammable gas with a strong suffocating odour characteristic of burning sulfur. It condenses readily under pressure to a colourless liquid that boils at −10° and has a wt per mL of about 1.5 g. Soluble 36 in 1 of water and 114 in 1 of alcohol by vol. at 20° and standard pressure. Soluble in chloroform and in ether. Store in cylinders. It is usually packaged under pressure in liquid form.

**Incompatibility and stability.** Sulfite antoxidants can react with sympathomimetics such as adrenaline leading to their inactivation.[1] Measures need to be taken to prevent such a reaction if sulfites have to be used. Cisplatin is another compound that can be inactivated.[2] Phenylmercuric nitrate may be inactivated or its activity enhanced.[3,4] Sulfites are reported to react with chloramphenicol.[1] Hydrogen peroxide generation has been reported on exposure to light of amino acid solutions containing sulfites.[5] When used in foods there can be a noticeable taste and a reduction in thiamine content.[6] Stability is affected by air and moisture,[7] and there is decomposition at very low pH.[7] There can be adsorption on to rubber closures.[8]

1. Higuchi T, Schroeter LC. Reactivity of bisulfite with a number of pharmaceuticals. *J Am Pharm Assoc (Sci)* 1959; **48:** 535–40.
2. Garren KW, Repta AJ. Incompatibility of cisplatin and Reglan Injectable. *Int J Pharmaceutics* 1985; **24:** 91–9.
3. Richards RME, Reary JME. Changes in antibacterial activity of thiomersal and PMN on autoclaving with certain adjuvants. *J Pharm Pharmacol* 1972; **24** (suppl): 84P–89P.
4. Collins AJ, *et al.* Incompatibility of phenylmercuric acetate with sodium metabisulphite in eye drop formulations. *J Pharm Pharmacol* 1985; **37** (suppl): 123P.
5. Brawley V, *et al.* Effect of sodium metabisulfite on hydrogen peroxide production in light-exposed pediatric parenteral amino acid solutions. *Am J Health-Syst Pharm* 1998; **55:** 1288–92.
6. FAO/WHO. Evaluation of the toxicity of a number of antimicrobials and antioxidants: sixth report of the joint FAO/WHO expert committee on food additives. *WHO Tech Rep Ser 228* 1962.
7. Stewart JT. Sodium metabisulfite. In: Rowe RC, *et al.* eds. *Handbook of pharmaceutical excipients.* 4th ed. London and Chicago: The Pharmaceutical Press, and the American Pharmaceutical Association 2003: 571–3.
8. Schroeter LC. Sulfurous acid salts as pharmaceutical antioxidants. *J Pharm Sci* 1961; **50:** 891–901.

### Adverse Effects and Precautions

Gastric irritation due to liberation of sulfurous acid can follow ingestion of sodium metabisulfite and other sulfites. Large doses of sulfites may cause gastrointestinal upsets, respiratory or circulatory failure, and CNS disturbances.

Concentrated solutions of salts of sulfurous acid are irritant to skin and mucous membranes.

Sulfur dioxide is highly irritant to the eyes, skin, and mucous membranes. Inhalation results in irritation of the respiratory tract which may lead to bronchoconstriction and pulmonary oedema; very high concentrations may cause respiratory arrest and asphyxia. Contact with liquid sulfur dioxide results in acid burns.

Allergic reactions including anaphylaxis and deaths have been reported.

**Hypersensitivity.** Hypersensitivity reactions including bronchospasm, anaphylaxis, and some deaths have occurred in subjects, especially those with a history of asthma or atopic allergy, exposed to sulfites used as preservatives in foods.[1] These reactions have led to restrictions by the FDA on such use.[2] There have been case reports of reactions to sulfites in drugs;[3-7] such reports are considered to be few in number and the FDA has not extended the restriction on sulfites in foods to apply to their use in drugs since it was felt that in certain medications there was no suitable alternative to a sulfite.[2] It was even accepted that adrenaline recommended for use in treating allergic reactions could itself contain sulfite but that its presence should not preclude use of the adrenaline preparation even in sulfite-sensitive patients.[2]

1. Anonymous. Sulfites in drugs and food. *Med Lett Drugs Ther* 1986; **28:** 74–5.
2. Anonymous. Warning for prescription drugs containing sulfites. *FDA Drug Bull* 1987; **17:** 2–3.
3. Baker GJ, *et al.* Bronchospasm induced by metabisulphite-containing foods and drugs. *Med J Aust* 1981; **ii:** 614–17.
4. Twarog FJ, Leung DYM. Anaphylaxis to a component of isoetharine (sodium bisulfite). *JAMA* 1982; **248:** 2030–1.
5. Koepke JW, *et al.* Dose-dependent bronchospasm from sulfites in isoetharine. *JAMA* 1984; **251:** 2982–3.
6. Mikolich DJ, McCloskey WW. Suspected gentamicin allergy could be sulfite sensitivity. *Clin Pharm* 1988; **7:** 269.
7. Deziel-Evans LM, Hussey WC. Possible sulfite sensitivity with gentamicin infusion. *DICP Ann Pharmacother* 1989; **23:** 1032–3.

### Pharmacokinetics

Sulfites and metabisulfites are oxidised in the body to sulfate and excreted in the urine. Any sulfurous acid or sulfur dioxide is also converted to sulfate.

### Uses

Sulfur dioxide and the sulfites that produce sulfur dioxide and sulfurous acid are strong reducing agents and are used as antoxidants. Concentrations of the sulfites in pharmaceutical preparations have ranged from 0.01 to 1.0%. At higher concentrations and preferably at an acid pH sulfur dioxide and the sulfites exhibit antimicrobial activity.

Sulfur dioxide and the sulfites are used in the food industry as antoxidants, antimicrobial preservatives, and anti-browning agents. They are used in wine making where tabletted sodium metabisulfite is commonly known as Campden Tablets. Concentrations of sulfites above 500 ppm impart a noticeable unpleasant taste to preparations. There is concern over the risk of severe allergic reactions arising from the use of sulfites in foods (see Hypersensitivity, above).

### Preparations

**Proprietary Preparations** (details are given in Part 3)

**Multi-ingredient:** ***Switz.:*** Schwefelbad Dr Klopfer†.

## Tar Acids

Ácidos de alquitrán.

**Description.** Tar acids are phenolic substances derived from the distillation of coal tar or petroleum fractions. The lowest boiling fraction of coal tar, distilling at 188° to 205°, consists of mixed cresol isomers. The middle fraction, known as 'cresylic acids', distils at 205° to 230° and consists of cresols and xylenols. The 'high-boiling tar acids', distilling at 230° to 290°, consist mainly of alkyl homologues of phenol, with naphthalenes and other hydrocarbons. Cresol is described on p.1177.

- **Black Fluids** are homogeneous solutions of coal-tar acids, or similar acids derived from petroleum, or any mixture of these, with or without hydrocarbons and with a suitable emulsifying agent.
- **White Fluids** are finely dispersed emulsions of coal-tar acids, or similar acids derived from petroleum, or any mixture of these, with or without hydrocarbons.
- **Modified Black Fluids** and **Modified White Fluids** may contain, as an addition, any other active ingredients, but if these are used, the type and amount must be disclosed, if required.

### Adverse Effects and Treatment

As for Phenol, p.1188.

Tar acids are generally very irritant and corrosive to the skin, even when diluted to concentrations used for disinfection.

**Poisoning.** A report of fatal self-poisoning in a 59-year-old man following the ingestion of approximately 250 mL of a xylenol-containing disinfectant (Stericol Hospital Disinfectant).[1]

1. Watson ID, *et al.* Fatal xylenol self-poisoning. *Postgrad Med J* 1986; **62:** 411–12.

### Uses

Tar acids are phenolic disinfectants used in the preparation of a range of fluids of varied activity used for household and general disinfection purposes.

Hydrocarbons are often used to enhance the activity of the tar acids in disinfectant fluids; they also help to reduce crystallisation of phenols.

### Preparations

**Proprietary Preparations** (details are given in Part 3)

***UK:*** Clearsol†; Cresolox†; Printol†; Sterilite†; Sudol†.

## Tertiary Butylhydroquinone

Butilhidroquinona terciaria; TBHQ. 2-*tert*-butylhydroquinone.

$C_{10}H_{14}O_2$ = 166.2.

*CAS — 1948-33-0.*

### Profile

Tertiary butylhydroquinone is an antoxidant preservative used in foods. It has some antimicrobial activity.

## Tetrabromocresol

3,4,5,6-Tetrabromo-*o*-cresol.

$C_7H_4Br_4O$ = 423.7.

### Profile

Tetrabromocresol is a brominated phenolic antiseptic. It has been used for hand disinfection and is applied topically for the treatment of fungal infections of the skin.

### Preparations

**Proprietary Preparations** (details are given in Part 3)

**Multi-ingredient:** ***Austral.:*** Pedoz; ***Ger.:*** Gehwol Fungizid.

## Tetraglycine Hydroperiodide

Hidroperioduro de tetraglicina.

$C_{16}H_{42}I_7N_8O_{16}$ = 1490.9.

*CAS — 7097-60-1.*

### Profile

Tetraglycine hydroperiodide is an iodine-based disinfectant that is used in the emergency treatment of drinking water (p.1165).

### Preparations

**Proprietary Preparations** (details are given in Part 3)
***UK:*** Potable Aqua; ***USA:*** Potable Aqua.

## Thiomersal *(BAN, rINN)*

Mercurothiolate; Mercurothiolate Sodique; Sodium Ethyl Mercurithiosalicylate; Thimerosal; Thiomersalate; Thiomersalum; Tiomersal. Sodium (2-carboxyphenylthio)ethylmercury.

$C_9H_9HgNaO_2S$ = 404.8.

*CAS — 54-64-8.*

*ATC — D08AK06.*

**Pharmacopoeias.** In *Eur.* (see p.vi), *Pol.*, and *US.*

**Ph. Eur. 5.0** (Thiomersal). A white or almost white crystalline powder. Freely soluble in water; sparingly soluble or soluble in alcohol; practically insoluble in dichloromethane. A 0.8% solution in water has a pH of 6.0 to 8.0. Protect from light.

**USP 27** (Thimerosal). A light cream-coloured crystalline powder with a slight characteristic odour. Soluble 1 in 1 of water and 1 in 12 of alcohol; practically insoluble in ether. A 1% solution in water has a pH of about 6.7. Store in airtight containers. Protect from light.

**Incompatibility.** Thiomersal is incompatible with acids, metal ions, and iodine. It forms precipitates with many alkaloids. The rate of oxidation of thiomersal in solution is greatly increased by traces of copper ions. In slightly acid solution thiomersal may be precipitated as the corresponding acid which undergoes slow decomposition with the formation of insoluble products. The activity of thiomersal may also be reduced by boric acid, edetic acid, or sodium thiosulfate or by the presence of blood or organic matter. Thiomersal may be adsorbed by plastic or rubber packaging materials.

References.

1. Richards RME, Reary JME. Changes in antibacterial activity of thiomersal and PMN on autoclaving with certain adjuvants. *J Pharm Pharmacol* 1972; **24** (suppl): 84P–89P.
2. Reader MJ. Influence of isotonic agents on the stability of thimerosal in ophthalmic formulations. *J Pharm Sci* 1984; **73:** 840–1.
3. Morton DJ. EDTA reduces antimicrobial efficacy of thiomersal. *Int J Pharmaceutics* 1985; **23:** 357–8.

### Adverse Effects, Treatment, and Precautions

As for Mercury, p.1713.

Hypersensitivity reactions occasionally occur. Allergic conjunctivitis has been reported.

Appropriate measures should be taken to prevent contamination of thiomersal preparations during storage or dilution.

◊ The safety of thiomersal as a preservative for vaccines, eye and nose drops, and contact lens solutions has been questioned.[1] There have been reports of severe reactions to vaccines preserved with thiomersal,[2,3] and the regulatory authorities in both Europe[4] and the USA[5] issued statements recommending that the use of thiomersal in vaccines be phased out. More recently, however, studies have indicated a lack of association between thiomersal-containing vaccines and autism[6,7] or neurodevelopmental disorder and the European regulatory authority has issued a further statement[8] in which it confirmed that thiomersal could be used as a preservative when no alternative was available, subject to certain labelling requirements regarding hypersensitivity. The UK Committee on Safety of Medicines has similarly concluded[9] that there is no evidence of neurological adverse effects caused by the small amounts of thiomersal present in some vaccines; despite this, it endorsed the view that the use of vaccines without thiomersal would be a prudent precautionary measure.

Delayed hypersensitivity reactions have been associated with the use of thiomersal in contact lens solutions.[10] In one clinic, 7 of 116 patients with chronic blepharitis, who had never worn contact lenses, were found to be already sensitised to thiomersal.[1] Furthermore there has been an isolated report of acute laryngeal obstruction in a patient previously sensitised to thiomersal who used a throat spray preserved with thiomersal.[11] False positive reactions to old tuberculin have also been attributed to the presence of thiomersal.[12]

1. Seal D, *et al.* The case against thiomersal. *Lancet* 1991; **338:** 316–16.
2. Cox NH, Morley WN. Vaccination reactions and thiomersal. *BMJ* 1987; **294:** 250.
3. Noel I, *et al.* Hypersensitivity to thiomersal in hepatitis B vaccine. *Lancet* 1991; **338:** 705.
4. European Agency for the Evaluation of Medicinal Products (EMEA). EMEA public statement on thiomersal containing medicinal products. EMEA publication no. 20962/99. Full version: http://www.emea.eu.int/pdfs/human/press/pus/2096299EN.pdf (accessed 11/06/04)
5. American Academy of Pediatrics, United States Public Health Service. Thimerosal in vaccines: a joint statement of the American Academy of Pediatrics and the Public Health Service. *MMWR* 1999; **48:** 563–5.
6. Hviid A, *et al.* Association between thimerosal-containing vaccine and autism. *JAMA* 2003; **290:** 1763–6.
7. Madsen KM, *et al.* Thimerosal and the occurrence of autism: negative ecological evidence from Danish population-based data. *Pediatrics* 2003; **112:** 604–6.
8. European Agency for the Evaluation of Medicinal Products (EMEA). EMEA public statement on thiomersal in vaccines for human use—recent evidence supports safety of thiomersal-containing vaccines. EMEA publication no. 1194/04. Full version: http://www.emea.eu.int/pdfs/human/press/pus/119404en.pdf (accessed 05/07/04)
9. Committee on Safety of Medicines/Medicines and Healthcare Products Regulatory Agency. Safety of thiomersal-containing vaccines. *Current Problems* 2003; **29:** 9. Also available at: http://www.mca.gov.uk/ourwork/monitorsafequalmed/currentproblems/cpsept2003.pdf (accessed 11/06/04)
10. Wilson LA, *et al.* Delayed hypersensitivity to thiomersal in soft contact lens wearers. *Ophthalmology* 1981; **88:** 804–9.
11. Maibach H. Acute laryngeal obstruction presumed secondary to thiomersal (merthiolate) delayed hypersensitivity. *Contact Dermatitis* 1975; **1:** 221–2.
12. Hansson H, Möller H. Intracutaneous test reactions to tuberculin containing merthiolate as a preservative. *Scand J Infect Dis* 1971; **3:** 169–72.

**Poisoning.** Serious adverse effects have followed parenteral and topical use of thiomersal. Six poisonings (5 fatal) resulted from the use of 1000 times the normal concentration of thiomersal in a preparation of chloramphenicol for intramuscular injection.[1] Thiomersal used in topical antiseptic preparations was found to be toxic to epidermal cells.[2] After the death of 10 of 13 children as a result of treatment of omphaloceles (umbilical hernia) with a tincture of thiomersal, it was recommended that organic mercurial disinfectants be heavily restricted or withdrawn from hospital use as absorption occurred readily through intact membranes.[3]

1. Axton JHM. Six cases of poisoning after a parenteral organic mercurial compound (Merthiolate). *Postgrad Med J* 1972; **48:** 417–21.
2. Anonymous. Topical antiseptics and antibiotics: organic mercurials. *Med Lett Drugs Ther* 1977; **19:** 83.
3. Fagan DG, *et al.* Organ mercury levels in infants with omphaloceles treated with organic mercurial antiseptic. *Arch Dis Child* 1977; **52:** 962–4.

### Interactions

**Tetracyclines.** Nine patients using a contact lens solution containing 0.004% thiomersal developed varying degrees of ocular irritation after taking oral *tetracyclines* concurrently. Exposure to either the tetracyclines or thiomersal alone did not cause the response.[1]

1. Crook TG, Freeman JJ. Reactions induced by the concurrent use of thimerosal and tetracycline. *Am J Optom Physiol Opt* 1983; **60:** 759–61.

### Uses and Administration

Thiomersal is a bacteriostatic and fungistatic mercurial antiseptic that has been applied topically usually in a concentration of 0.1%.

Thiomersal, 0.001 to 0.01%, is used as a preservative in biological and pharmaceutical products. It has also been used to preserve solutions used in the care of contact lenses (p.1164).

### Preparations

***USP 27:*** Thimerosal Tincture; Thimerosal Topical Aerosol; Thimerosal Topical Solution.

**Proprietary Preparations** (details are given in Part 3)
***Arg.:*** Merthiolate; ***Braz.:*** Curativ†; Mercurio Cromo†; ***Fr.:*** Vitaseptol; ***Israel:*** LC-65†; ***Mex.:*** Mercural†; Septicol†; ***S.Afr.:*** Merthiolate; ***Thai.:*** Merthiolate; ***USA:*** Aeroaid; Mersol.

**Multi-ingredient:** ***Braz.:*** Flex-Care†; Nazotiran†; Rinocron†; ***Fr.:*** Collyrex†; Dermachrome; ***Israel:*** Cleaner No 4†; Hexidin†; ***Spain:*** Deltacina†; Proskin; Tintu. Mertiolato Asens†.

## Thymol

Acido Timico; Isopropylmetacresol; Thymolum; Timol. 2-Isopropyl-5-methylphenol.

$C_{10}H_{14}O$ = 150.2.

*CAS — 89-83-8.*

**Pharmacopoeias.** In *Eur.* (see p.vi), *Jpn*, and *Pol.* Also in *USNF.*

**Ph. Eur. 5.0** (Thymol). Colourless crystals. The melting range is 48° to 52°. Very slightly soluble in water; very soluble in alcohol; freely soluble in volatile and in fixed oils; sparingly soluble in glycerol; dissolves in dilute solutions of alkali hydroxides. Protect from light.

**USNF 22** (Thymol). Colourless, often large, crystals or a white crystalline powder with an aromatic thyme-like odour. The melting range is 48° to 51°; when melted it remains liquid at a considerably lower temperature. Soluble 1 in 1000 of water, 1 in 1 of alcohol and of chloroform, 1 in 1.5 of ether, and 1 in 2 of olive oil; soluble in glacial acetic acid and in fixed and volatile oils. Store in airtight containers. Protect from light.

**Incompatibility.** The antimicrobial activity of thymol is reduced by combination with protein.

### Adverse Effects, Treatment, and Precautions

As for Phenol, p.1188.

When ingested, thymol is less toxic than phenol. It is irritant to the gastric mucosa. Fats and alcohol increase absorption and aggravate the toxic symptoms.

Appropriate measures should be taken to avoid contamination of thymol preparations during storage or dilution.

**Hypersensitivity.** Contact allergy to a heparinoid cream was due to an allergen formed by the reaction between thymol and the degradation products of a triazine derivative, both present as preservatives.[1]

1. Smeenk G, *et al.* Contact allergy to a reaction product in Hirudoid cream: an example of compound allergy. *Br J Dermatol* 1987; **116:** 223–31.

### Uses and Administration

Thymol is a phenolic antiseptic with antibacterial and antifungal activity. It is more powerful than phenol but its use is limited by its low solubility in water, irritancy, and susceptibility to protein.

Thymol is used chiefly as a deodorant in mouthwashes and gargles such as Compound Thymol Glycerin (BP 1988), an aqueous mixture of thymol 0.05% and glycerol 10% with colouring and flavouring, which may be used undiluted or, alternatively, diluted with about 3 times its volume of warm water before use. Thymol has been used topically in the treatment of skin disorders and is also inhaled, with other volatile substances, for colds, coughs, and associated respiratory disorders.

Thymol 0.01% is added as an antoxidant to halothane, trichloroethylene, and tetrachloroethylene.

Thymol iodide is used in preparations for dental hygiene.

### Preparations

**Proprietary Preparations** (details are given in Part 3)
***Braz.:*** Balseptol†; ***Ger.:*** Medophyll; ***Switz.:*** Intrasol†.

**Multi-ingredient:** ***Arg.:*** Fungicida; Listerine Clasico; Listerine Cool Mint; Listerine Fresh Burst; Manzan; Novobroncol; Vagicural; ***Austral.:*** BFI†; Gartech†; SM-33; Thymol Mouthwash Red†; ***Austria:*** Alpicort; Criniton; DDD; Gingivan; Kinder Luuf; Linobion-Globuli†; Linobion-Salbenstift†; Luuf Balsam; Pe-Ce; Resol†; Spasmo Claim; Thrombocid; Wick Vaporub; ***Belg.:*** Balsoclase†; Borostyrol†; Dentophar; Perubore; Vicks Vaporub; ***Braz.:*** Anestesiol; Angi-a-Mid†; Angino-Rub; Axol†; Boralina†; Clorasep-tic; Cutisanol; Emplastro Salonpas†; Fluomint; Friccex†; Frixodont†; Gargotan†; Gyrol†; Higienex†; Lenidor; Listerine†; Mentolatum†; Passaja†; Pomalgex†; Relampago†; Salonpas†; Tabletes Valda†; Valda†; Vick Vaporub; ***Canad.:*** Antiseptic Mouthwash; Boil Ease; Buckley's White Rub; Carboseptol; Lipsorex; Listerine; Listerine Antiseptic Tartar Control; Mouthwash Antiseptic & Gargle; Nasal Jelly; Pastilles Valda†; Thermo-Gel; Valda; Vap Air; Vaporisateur Medicamente; Vaporizing Ointment; ***Chile:*** Balsamo Leon; Galutec; Hansaplast Descongestionante; Listerine; Listermint Con Fluor; Polisep; ***Fin.:*** Vicks Vaporub; ***Fr.:*** Borostyrol; Pastilles Medicinales Vicks; Perubore; Valda; Vicks Vaporub; ***Ger.:*** Alferm; Criniton; Customed†; DDD†; Denosol†; Em-eukal; Nasentropfen-ratiopharm; Oestrugol N; Parodontal F5 med†; Pulmotin; Pumilen-N†; Retterspitz Ausserlich†; Retterspitz Gelee†; Retterspitz Heilsalbe†; Retterspitz Quick†; Salviathymol N; Sedotussin Expectorans†; Thrombocid; ***Hong Kong:*** Burn Cream; Kamistad; Salomethyl; Valda; ***India:*** Anaebell; ***Irl.:*** Karvol; Listerine†; Valda; ***Israel:*** Gargol; Garonsept; Karvol; Pronaestin; Rectozorin; ***Ital.:*** Eucalipto Composto; Eugenol-Guaiacolo Composto; Florigien†; Pinselina Knapp; Resina Carbolica Dentilin†; Rinos†; Rinostil; Salonpas; ***Malaysia:*** Burnol Plus; Salonpas; ***Mon.:*** Glyco-Thymoline; ***Neth.:*** Vicks Vaporub; ***NZ:*** Listerine; Listerine Tartar Control; Solucol†; Thymol Mouthwash Red; Vicks Vaporub; ***Port.:*** Edoltar; Freimax; Listerine; Thrombocid; Valda; ***S.Afr.:*** Karvol; ***Singapore:*** Burnol Plus; Kamistad; Karvol; ***Spain:*** Balsamo Kneipp; Cloroboral†; Co Bucal; Contusin; Kneipp Balsamo†; Mentobox; Pastillas Antisep Garg M; Piorlis; Pomada Balsamica†; Sudosin†; Vicks Vaporub; ***Swed.:*** Vicks Vaporub; ***Switz.:*** Adrectal†; Asphaline; Borostyrol N; Butaparin; Cresophene; Dental-Phenjoca†; Ederphyt; Endomethasone†; Furodermal; Huile analgesique "Temple of Heaven" contre les maux de tete; Perubare; Rapura; Roliwol†; Sedasept; Sedotussin; Spirogel†; Thrombocid; Tumarol†; Vicks Vaporub N; ***Thai.:*** Burnol Plus; Flavinol; Kamistad; Stopain; ***UK:*** Antiseptic Mouthwash; Boots Vapour Rub†; DDD; Dragon Balm; Eftab†; Karvol; Listerine Antiseptic Mouthwash; No-Sor Vapour Rub; Potter's Catarrh Pastilles; ***USA:*** BFI; Boil Ease; Cool-Mint Listerine; FreshBurst Listerine; Listerine; Massengill; Vicks Menthol Cough Drops; Zonite.

## Toloconium Metilsulfate *(rINN)*

Metilsulfato de toloconio; Toloconium Methylsulphate. Trimethyl[1-(*p*-tolyl)dodecyl]ammonium methylsulphate.

$C_{23}H_{43}NO_4S$ = 429.7.

*CAS — 552-92-1.*

### Profile

Toloconium metilsulfate is a quaternary ammonium antiseptic that has been used for disinfection of skin, mucous membranes, and surgical instruments.

### Preparations

**Proprietary Preparations** (details are given in Part 3)
***Ital.:*** Desogen†.

## Tosylchloramide Sodium *(BAN, rINN)*

Chloramidum; Chloramine; Chloramine T; Chloraminum; Cloramina; Mianin; Natrium Sulfaminochloratum; Tosilcloramida sódica; Tosylchloramidum Natricum. Sodium *N*-chlorotoluene-*p*-sulphonimidate trihydrate.

$C_7H_7ClNNaO_2S,3H_2O$ = 281.7.

*CAS — 127-65-1 (anhydrous).*

*ATC — D08AX04.*

NOTE. The name Chloramin has been used for a preparation of chlorphenamine maleate.

**Pharmacopoeias.** In *Eur.* (see p.vi) and *Viet. Pol.* includes tosylchloramide sodium B.

**Ph. Eur. 5.0** (Tosylchloramide Sodium). A white or slightly yellow, crystalline powder. Freely soluble in water; soluble in alcohol. A 5% solution in water has a pH of 8.0 to 10.0. Store in airtight containers at a temperature of 8° to 15°. Protect from light.

### Adverse Effects and Treatment

Vomiting, cyanosis, circulatory collapse, frothing at the mouth, and respiratory failure can occur within a few minutes of tosylchloramide sodium ingestion. Fatalities have occurred. Tosylchloramide sodium in tap water has caused methaemoglobinaemia and haemolysis in patients undergoing dialysis. Bronchospasm has occurred after inhalation.

Treatment of adverse effects is similar to that for Sodium Hypochlorite, p.1192.

**Effects on the lungs.** Shortness of breath progressing to pneumonitis requiring emergency tracheostomy occurred in a previously healthy 53-year-old woman who used a mixture of household ammonia and bleach for cleaning purposes.[1] It was considered that inhalation of tosylchloramide sodium gas produced by reaction of the two cleaning products had caused the lung damage.

1. Tanen DA, *et al.* Severe lung injury after exposure to chloramine gas from household cleaners. *N Engl J Med* 1999; **341:** 848–9.

### Uses and Administration

Tosylchloramide sodium is an organic chlorine-releasing compound with the general properties of chlorine (p.1175). It contains about 25% w/w of 'available chlorine' (see p.1176). It is stable at an alkaline pH although it is much more active in acid media. It is more slowly active than hypochlorite solutions.

Tosylchloramide sodium is used for the treatment of minor wound infections and as a skin and hard surface disinfectant. It is also used for the treatment of drinking water (p.1165). It was formerly used as a spermicide.

Tosylchloramide sodium B (chlorogenium; sodium *N*-chlorobenzenesulphonimidate sesquihydrate) has been used similarly to tosylchloramide sodium.

### Preparations

**Proprietary Preparations** (details are given in Part 3)

***Belg.:*** Chloraseptine; Chlorazol; Chloronguent; Dercusan†; ***Fr.:*** Hydroclonazone; ***Ger.:*** Clorina; Trichlorol; ***Ital.:*** Citromed Chlor; Cloromi-T†; Dermedal; Disinclor†; Euclorina; Germozero; Minachlor; Ottoclor; Steridrolo; ***Spain:*** Clorina.

## Triclocarban *(USAN, rINN)*

NSC-72005; TCC; 3,4,4′-Trichlorocarbanilide; Triclocarbán. 1-(4-Chlorophenyl)-3-(3,4-dichlorophenyl)urea.

$C_{13}H_9Cl_3N_2O = 315.6.$
*CAS — 101-20-2.*

### Adverse Effects and Precautions

When subjected to prolonged high temperatures triclocarban can decompose to form toxic chloroanilines, which can be absorbed through the skin and cause methaemoglobinaemia. Mild photosensitivity has been seen in patch testing.

### Uses and Administration

Triclocarban is an anilide antiseptic. It is bacteriostatic against Gram-positive organisms in high dilutions but is less effective against Gram-negative organisms and some fungi. It is used in antiperspirants and soaps for disinfection of skin and mucous membranes.

### Preparations

**Proprietary Preparations** (details are given in Part 3)

***Arg.:*** Jabobip; Sodorant; Ungel; ***Braz.:*** Derso TCC; Stiefderm†; ***Fr.:*** Cutisan; Nobacter; Solubacter; ***Irl.:*** Valderma†; ***Ital.:*** Citrosil Sapone; Sangen Sapone Disinfettante; ***Mex.:*** Nutegen A; ***Port.:*** Solubacter†; ***UK:*** Valderma; ***USA:*** Cuticura.

**Multi-ingredient:** ***Arg.:*** Bacteroskin; LB Jabon con Purcelin; Sodorant; ***Fr.:*** Septivon; Septosan; ***Ger.:*** Ansudor; ***Mex.:*** Septosan; ***Spain:*** Cusiter†; ***Switz.:*** Septivon N.

## Triclosan *(BAN, USAN, rINN)*

CH-3565; Cloxifenol; Triclosán. 5-Chloro-2-(2,4-dichlorophenoxy)phenol; 2,4,4′-Trichloro-2′-hydroxydiphenyl ether.

$C_{12}H_7Cl_3O_2 = 289.5.$
*CAS — 3380-34-5.*
*ATC — D08AE04; D09AA06.*

**Pharmacopoeias.** In *US.*

**USP 27** (Triclosan). A fine whitish crystalline powder. M.p. about 57°. Practically insoluble in water; soluble in alcohol, in acetone, and in methyl alcohol; slightly soluble in petroleum spirit. Store in airtight containers. Protect from light.

### Profile

Triclosan is a chlorinated bisphenol antiseptic, effective against Gram-positive and most Gram-negative bacteria but with variable or poor activity against *Pseudomonas* spp. It is also active against fungi. It is used in soaps, creams, and solutions in concentrations of up to 2% for disinfection of the hands and wounds and for disinfection of the skin prior to surgery, injections, or venepuncture. It is also used in oral hygiene products and in preparations for acne. There have been isolated reports of contact dermatitis.

**MRSA control.** Reports of control of meticillin-resistant *Staphylococcus aureus* (MRSA) infection in surgical units involving handwashing and bathing with triclosan.[1-3] Triclosan resistance has been reported.[4,5]

1. Bartzokas CA, *et al.* Control and eradication of methicillin-resistant Staphylococcus aureus on a surgical unit. *N Engl J Med* 1984; **311:** 1422–5.
2. Bartzokas CA. Eradication of resistant Staphylococcus aureus on a surgical unit. *N Engl J Med* 1985; **312:** 858–9.
3. Brady LM, *et al.* Successful control of endemic MRSA in a cardiothoracic surgical unit. *Med J Aust* 1990; **152:** 240–5.
4. Cookson BD, *et al.* Transferable resistance to triclosan in MRSA. *Lancet* 1991; **337:** 1548–9.
5. Sasatsu M, *et al.* Triclosan-resistant Staphylococcus aureus. *Lancet* 1993; **341:** 756. Correction. *ibid.*; **342:** 248.

### Preparations

**Proprietary Preparations** (details are given in Part 3)

***Arg.:*** Daewo; ***Austral.:*** Bioband†; Dettol Liquid Wash; Gamophen†; Johnsons Clean & Clear Facial Cleansing Bar†; Johnsons Clean & Clear Foaming Facial Wash†; Liquid Soap Pre-Op; Microshield T; Neutrogena Acne Skin Cleanser†; Oxy Skin Wash; pHisoHex Face Wash; Sapoderm; Softwash†; Solyptol; ***Belg.:*** Dettol Liquid Wash†; ***Braz.:*** Babix†; Clean & Clear Sabonete Liquido Facial; Fisohex; Neutrogerm†; Proderm; Soapex; Theracne†; ***Canad.:*** Adasept; Clean & Clear Foaming Cleanser; Clearasil Face Wash; Clearskin Antibacterial; Clearskin Medicated Cleanser; Oxy Daily Facial Cleanser Regular; Oxy Gentle†; Oxy Medicated Soap; Promani†; Skin So Soft Antibacterial; Tersaseptic; Trisan; ***Chile:*** Antiseptin; Sanigermin; ***Hong Kong:*** Oxy Daily Wash; pHisoHex Reformulated; Prewash†; ***Israel:*** Dermax; ***Ital.:*** Cetriderm con Triclosan; Dermo-Steril†; Geroderm; Ippi Verde; Irgaman; Lactacyd Antibatterico; Oilatum AD; Till; ***Malaysia:*** pHisoHex; ***Mex.:*** Clearasil Jabon†; Clearasil Wash Antiseptico†; Septosan; ***NZ:*** Dalacin T Prewash; Liquid Soap Pre-Op; Oxy Daily Skin Wash; ***S.Afr.:*** Acneclear; ***Switz.:*** Cliniderm; Lipo Sol; Procoutol; Shampooing extra-doux; ***UK:*** Aquasept; Clearasil Medicated Moisturiser†; Clearasil Soap†; Gamophen; Oxy Facial Wash; Ster-Zac; ***USA:*** Ambi 10; Clearasil Daily Face Wash; Oxy Medicated Soap; Septi-Soft; Septisol; Stri-Dex Antibacterial Cleansing; Stri-Dex Face Wash.

**Multi-ingredient:** ***Arg.:*** Dettonjab; Esmedent con Fluor; Heduline; Hekabetol; Hydragenic; Neoceuticals Gel de Limpieza Facial; Odol Med Antiplaca; Odol Tratamiento de Encias; Prurigel; Tersoderm Cabellos Grasos; Ublosid; ***Austral.:*** Burnaid First Aid Burn Gel†; Clearasil Acne Treatment Cream; Dettol Cream; Microshield PVP Plus†; Oilatum Plus; ***Braz.:*** Babyglos†; Clearasil†; Cravo-Espin†; Efederm†; Nixoderm†; Traderm†; ***Canad.:*** Adasept; Oral Plan; PanOxyl Clear Acne; Solarcaine; Tersac†; ***Chile:*** Ac-Sal; Cariamyl; Cornina; Gingilacer; Hansaplast Antimicotico; Hansaplast Footcare; Kariax; Solarcaine Spray Aerosol; ***Fin.:*** Wicne; Wicnecarb; Wicnelact; Wicnevit; ***Fr.:*** Clinogel; Oilatum AD; Sanytol; Septosan; ***Ger.:*** Rutisept extra; Sicorten Plus; ***Hong Kong:*** Dettol; Oilatum Plus; Sicorten Plus; Solarcaine†; ***Irl.:*** Dettol; Oilatum Junior Flare-Up†; Oilatum Plus; ***Israel:*** Pedisol; Sicorten Plus; ***Ital.:*** Aknicare; Angstrom Viso; AZ Protezione Completa†; AZ Protezione Gengive; Dopo Pik; Geroderm Zolfo; Levaknel†; Plax; Steril Zeta; ***Malaysia:*** Dettol; Oilatum Plus Antibacterial; ***Mex.:*** Crema Axel; Dermobras; Periodentyl; Sebryl Plus; Septosan; ***NZ:*** Clearasil; Dettol; Oilatum Plus; Solarcaine; ***Port.:*** Aknicare; Alkagin; Antiacneicos Ac-Sal; Bexident; Disoderme†; Lambda; Sicorten Plus; ***S.Afr.:*** Dettol†; Oilatum Plus; Tantol Skin Cleanser†; ***Singapore:*** Burnaid; Dettol†; Oilatum Plus; pHisoHex Reformulated; QV Flare Up; Tinasolve; ***Spain:*** Anti-Acne†; Doctodermis; Poliglicol Anti Acne†; Sicorten Plus; Vaselatum; ***Switz.:*** Acne Creme; Acne Gel; Acne Lotion; Antebor N; Keroderm; Locacorten Triclosan†; Pixor Stick Anti-acne N; Saltrates; Sebo Creme; Sebo Shampooing; Sicorten Plus; Sulgan N; Teerol-H†; Tretinoine†; Turexan Emulsion; ***Thai.:*** Dettol; Oilatum Plus; ***UK:*** Actibrush†; Clearasil Active Treatment Cream; Dentyl pH; Dettol; Germolene; Manusept; Oilatum Junior Flare-Up; Oilatum Plus; Oxy Clean Facial Scrub; Oxy Cleanser; Oxy Dots; Oxy Duo Pads; Sensodyne-F; Solarcaine; TCP; ***USA:*** Clearasil Antibacterial; Solarcaine.

## Undebenzophene

Parahydroxybenzoate Phenoxyethanol. 2-Phenoxyethyl *p*-hydroxybenzoate.

$C_{15}H_{14}O_4 = 258.3.$
*CAS — 55468-88-7.*

### Profile

Undebenzophene is an antiseptic that has been included in multi-ingredient preparations intended for wound and burn disinfection.

### Preparations

**Proprietary Preparations** (details are given in Part 3)

**Multi-ingredient:** ***Ital.:*** Medical Pic†.

## Urea Hydrogen Peroxide

Carbamide Peroxide; Hydroperite; Peróxido de hidrógeno y urea; Urea Peroxide.

$NH_2.CO.NH_2,H_2O_2 = 94.07.$
*CAS — 124-43-6.*

**Pharmacopoeias.** In *US.*

**USP 27** (Carbamide Peroxide). Store in airtight containers at a temperature not exceeding 40°. Protect from light.

### Profile

Urea hydrogen peroxide consists of hydrogen peroxide and urea in equimolecular proportions. It is used for the extemporaneous preparation of hydrogen peroxide. It has been employed for infections of the ear, mouth, skin, and mucous membranes and for softening ear wax.

### Preparations

***USP 27:*** Carbamide Peroxide Topical Solution.

**Proprietary Preparations** (details are given in Part 3)

***Austral.:*** Ear Clear†; ***Braz.:*** Aceratun; ***Canad.:*** Murine; ***Ger.:*** Elawox; ***Irl.:*** Exterol; ***Israel:*** Exterol; ***Ital.:*** Debrox; Dermoxyl; Ginoxil; ***Mex.:*** Amosan†; ***NZ:*** Earclear; ***UK:*** Exterol; Otex; ***USA:*** Auraphene-B; Auro; Debrox; ERO; Gly-Oxide; Mollifene; Murine; Orajel Perioseptic; Proxigel†.

**Multi-ingredient:** ***Arg.:*** Hexiben Plus.

## Zinc Peroxide

Peróxido de zinc.
*CAS — 1314-22-3.*

### Profile

The action of zinc peroxide is similar to that of hydrogen peroxide (p.1182). Applied locally it has been used for disinfecting and deodorising burns, wounds, and various ulcers and lesions.

### Preparations

**Proprietary Preparations** (details are given in Part 3)

***Canad.:*** Neoderm†.

**Multi-ingredient:** ***Braz.:*** Anaseptil; ***Fr.:*** Bioxyol; Ektogan†; ***Ital.:*** Ektogan.

# Dopaminergics

Dopamine is a key neurotransmitter in the CNS; in particular, striatal dopamine depletion is associated with the clinical condition of parkinsonism. Dopamine also inhibits prolactin release from the pituitary and is believed to be the prolactin-release inhibiting factor (PRIF or PIF); dopamine deficiency in the pituitary is associated with conditions characterised by hyperprolactinaemia.

Accordingly, drugs that replenish central dopamine or that can act as stimulants of dopamine receptors (dopamine agonists), may alleviate the symptoms of parkinsonism (see below), hyperprolactinaemia (p.1315), and related disorders.

At least 5 subtypes of dopamine receptor are thought to exist: $D_1$ receptors appear to stimulate adenylate cyclase activity; $D_2$ receptors activate various systems and inhibit adenylate cyclase activity. $D_3$, $D_4$, and $D_5$ receptors have been less well studied but $D_3$ and $D_4$ are similar to $D_2$, forming the $D_2$-like group, whereas $D_1$ and $D_5$ form the $D_1$-like group. $D_2$ receptors have been implicated in the pathophysiology of parkinsonism and schizophrenia.

Dopaminergics, or drugs that enhance their actions, described in this chapter include:

- levodopa, which is converted by decarboxylation into dopamine in the body, and which, unlike dopamine itself, can penetrate the blood-brain barrier and supply a source of dopamine to the brain
- the peripheral dopa-decarboxylase inhibitors, benserazide and carbidopa, which have no dopaminergic action of their own but increase the availability of levodopa
- apomorphine, which is structurally related to dopamine and acts as a dopamine agonist
- the adamantanamines, amantadine and memantine, which may augment dopaminergic activity
- the ergot derivatives, bromocriptine, cabergoline, lisuride, and pergolide, which act as dopamine agonists
- various other non-ergot dopamine agonists, such as piribedil, pramipexole, quinagolide, and ropinirole
- the specific monoamine oxidase type B inhibitor, selegiline, which enhances the action of dopamine and levodopa
- the catechol-*O*-methyltransferase inhibitors (COMT-inhibitors), entacapone and tolcapone, which enhance the action of levodopa.

## Parkinsonism

The syndrome of parkinsonism is characterised by tremor, rigidity, akinesia or bradykinesia, and loss of postural reflexes, associated with reduced dopamine activity in the brain. It may be **classified** as follows:

- primary (idiopathic) parkinsonism, usually referred to as Parkinson's disease (formerly paralysis agitans)
- secondary (acquired) parkinsonism, including postencephalitic parkinsonism, drug-induced parkinsonism, and symptoms associated with manganese poisoning
- 'parkinsonism-plus' syndromes where parkinsonism is a feature of other degenerative diseases of the CNS, such as progressive supranuclear palsy and multiple system atrophy

'Arteriosclerotic parkinsonism' has been used to describe parkinsonism associated with cerebrovascular disease although this may be confusing since vascular brain damage is not a cause of Parkinson's disease.

The term parkinsonism is often used for the idiopathic form, that is, Parkinson's disease. Parkinson's disease and postencephalitic parkinsonism have been attributed primarily to depletion of striatal dopamine in the basal ganglia as a result of the loss of neurones in the substantia nigra. Striatal dopamine deficiency results in loss of the normal functional balance between dopaminergic and cholinergic activity and the aim of treatment is to increase the former and/or decrease the latter.

The **cause** of Parkinson's disease is not established, although environmental and genetic factors are probably superimposed on a background of neuronal loss related to ageing. MPTP (1-methyl-4-phenyl-1,2,3,6-tetrahydropyridine), a contaminant of an illicitly produced pethidine analogue MPPP (1-methyl-4-phenyl-4-propionoxypiperidine), causes irreversible parkinsonism similar to Parkinson's disease. This effect appears to follow conversion by monoamine oxidase B to the neurotoxic methylphenylpyridinium ion which is selectively concentrated in dopaminergic neurones in the substantia nigra. It has been proposed that free radicals produced during normal metabolism of dopamine in the brain by monoamine oxidase B might be similarly neurotoxic to dopaminergic neurones in the substantia nigra (the oxidant stress hypothesis). This has led to concern that administration of levodopa, by increasing the supply of dopamine, might therefore exacerbate neurodegeneration and hasten the progression of Parkinson's disease but compelling evidence of such an effect is lacking.

Drug-induced parkinsonism (see Extrapyramidal Disorders, p.677) can arise from depletion of presynaptic dopamine, as with reserpine and tetrabenazine, or from blockade of postsynaptic dopamine receptors in the striatum, as by antipsychotics and some antiemetics such as metoclopramide. It is generally reversible on drug withdrawal or dose reduction and may sometimes disappear gradually despite continuous drug therapy. Although the use of levodopa to overcome antipsychotic-induced blockade of dopamine receptors might appear rational, it has generally been reported to be ineffective or to increase psychiatric symptoms.

There is no cure for Parkinson's disease. Although the possibility of using drug therapy to slow neurodegeneration is being investigated, no drug so far has a proven neuroprotective effect. **Treatment** is palliative and symptomatic and consists mainly of drug therapy supplemented when necessary with physical treatment such as physiotherapy and speech therapy. Surgery is occasionally used and there is growing interest in the use of transplantation and in electrical devices for the control of tremor.

**Drugs used in Parkinson's disease.** Drug therapy consists largely of the use of dopaminergics or antimuscarinics in an attempt to restore the normal balance between dopaminergic and cholinergic activity. Dopaminergics may act by direct replacement of dopamine, by delaying the metabolism of endogenous dopamine, by stimulation of dopamine receptors directly, or by enhancement of release of endogenous dopamine. Drugs with differing actions are often used together to achieve optimum control of symptoms.

- *Levodopa* is the most effective symptomatic treatment. It is converted by decarboxylation into dopamine and, unlike dopamine, can penetrate the blood-brain barrier hence supplying a source of dopamine to the brain. Levodopa is usually given with a peripheral dopa-decarboxylase inhibitor such as *benserazide* or *carbidopa.* These drugs are unable to penetrate the blood-brain barrier and therefore prevent only extracerebral conversion of levodopa to dopamine. This allows effective concentrations of dopamine to be achieved in the brain with lower doses of levodopa and also reduces unwanted effects such as nausea and vomiting and cardiovascular effects associated with peripheral formation of dopamine.

  The majority of patients respond initially to levodopa and its use has improved the quality and duration of life. However, after 2 years or more, benefit is reduced as the disease progresses and late complications emerge. Apart from dyskinesias and psychiatric effects, a major problem with long-term levodopa treatment is the appearance of fluctuations in mobility, the two predominant forms being 'end-of-dose' deterioration ('wearing-off' effect) and the 'on-off' phenomenon (see Complications of Treatment, below). Thus, views differ as to the best time to start treatment and the dosage to employ in order to limit the long-term complications.

  Catechol-*O*-methyltransferase (COMT) inhibitors, such as *entacapone* and *tolcapone*, are selective and reversible inhibitors of catechol-*O*-methyltransferase (COMT), with mainly peripheral actions. They are given as adjunctive therapy to patients experiencing fluctuations in disability related to levodopa and dopa-decarboxylase inhibitor combinations; because of the risk of serious hepatotoxicity, tolcapone should be restricted to when other adjunctive therapy is ineffective or contra-indicated. When levodopa is used with a peripheral dopa-decarboxylase inhibitor, *O*-methylation becomes the predominant form of metabolism of levodopa; co-administration of a peripheral COMT inhibitor can thus extend the duration and effect of levodopa in the brain, and allow a reduction in the dose and frequency of administration of levodopa. They therefore can help to stabilise patients, especially those experiencing 'end-of-dose' deterioration.
- *Selegiline* is a selective inhibitor of monoamine oxidase type B, an enzyme involved in the metabolism of dopamine in the brain. When used with levodopa in severe parkinsonism it has a dose-sparing effect and is of use in patients experiencing fluctuations in mobility. Although early treatment with selegiline may delay the need for levodopa there is no evidence that it has a favourable effect on the long-term course of the disease. Whether any benefit obtained is due to a symptomatic or neuroprotective effect is unclear. Used alone, selegiline produces few side-effects but when used with levodopa it can provoke or worsen dyskinesias or psychiatric symptoms and doubts have been expressed on the safety of long-term use.
- Dopamine agonists such as *bromocriptine, cabergoline, lisuride, pergolide, pramipexole*, and *ropinirole* act by direct stimulation of remaining postsynaptic dopamine receptors. Dopamine agonists are increasingly used in the early treatment of younger patients with parkinsonism in an attempt to delay therapy with levodopa (younger patients are at an increased risk of motor complications with levodopa). However, their efficacy often decreases after a few years. In older patients they may be reserved for adjunctive use when levodopa is no longer effective alone or cannot be tolerated. They are sometimes useful in reducing 'off' periods with levodopa and in ameliorating fluctuations in mobility in the later stages of the disease. *Apomorphine* is a potent dopamine agonist, but must be given parenterally and with an antiemetic. Although this restricts its use, it has a role in stabilising patients who suffer unpredictable 'on-off' effects. It is also used in the differential diagnosis of parkinsonism.
- *Antimuscarinics* are considered to have a weak antiparkinsonian effect compared with levodopa. They may reduce tremor but have little effect on bradykinesia. They may be of use alone or with other drugs in the initial treatment of patients with mild symptoms, especially when tremor is pronounced, or later as an adjunct to levodopa such as in patients with refractory tremor or dystonias. Antimuscarinic side-effects occur frequently and can limit their use. However, some side-effects can ameliorate complications associated with Parkinson's disease; dry mouth may be an advantage in patients with sialorrhoea. There appear to be no important differences in the efficacy of antimuscarinics for Parkinson's disease but some patients may tolerate one drug better than another. Those commonly used for Parkinson's disease include *benzatropine, orphenadrine, procyclidine,* and *trihexyphenidyl.*
- *Amantadine* is a weak dopamine agonist with some antimuscarinic activity although its activity as an antagonist of *N*-methyl-D-aspartate may also have a beneficial effect in Parkinson's disease. It has mild antiparkinsonian effects compared with levodopa but is relatively free from side-effects. It can improve bradykinesia as well as tremor and rigidity but only a small proportion of patients derive much benefit. It is used similarly to antimuscarinics in early disease when symptoms are mild, but tolerance to its effects can occur rapidly.

**Choice and implementation of drug treatment.** If symptoms are mild, drug therapy may not be required in the early stages of the disease. When symptoms become troublesome but are still relatively mild *amantadine* or an *antimuscarinic* may be started; antimuscarinics are useful when tremor predominates but are generally more suitable for younger patients and in drug-induced rather than idiopathic parkinsonism. Some have initiated treatment with *selegiline* immediately, but there have been doubts over whether it has a neuroprotective effect, as postulated, and also over long-term safety. There is no consensus on when to initiate dopaminergic treatment or whether to begin with *levodopa* or a *dopamine agonist.* For most patients treatment with levodopa eventually becomes necessary, but many neurologists delay initial treatment with levodopa because of the increased risk of motor complications. New patients, especially younger patients, therefore often begin treatment with a dopamine agonist, with levodopa reserved for the elderly, the frail, or those with intercurrent illness or more severe symptoms.

When levodopa does become necessary, the usual practice is to start with small doses, together with a peripheral dopa-decarboxylase inhibitor, and increase slowly to a dose which reduces disability to an acceptable level. Variations in response and diminishing effectiveness over the years necessitate careful adjustment of the size and form of the dose and the schedule of administration.

**Complications of treatment**. Fluctuations in mobility have been reported in more than half of patients on levodopa after 5 years of therapy. They generally proceed through predictable **'end-of-dose'** deterioration to the **'on-off'** phenomenon with marked very sudden swings from mobility to immobility. The cause of the fluctuations is not known, but multiple factors including desensitisation of dopamine receptors, interference with the response to dopamine by other levodopa metabolites such as 3-*O*-methyldopa, fluctuating plasma concentrations, and erratic transport of levodopa from blood to the brain have been suggested. It appears that as the disease progresses the capacity of the nigrostriatal dopaminergic system to synthesise and store dopamine, and to act as a buffer in maintaining dopamine brain concentrations, declines. Dopamine concentrations therefore become more dependent on levodopa administration and the pattern of response will come to reflect more closely the rise and fall in levodopa concentrations. Eventually the effect of various factors that produce even small changes in plasma concentrations of levodopa will progressively become more pronounced.

Approaches to the management of 'end-of-dose' fluctuations include more frequent but smaller doses and the use of modified-release preparations. Addition of selegiline or partial replacement of levodopa by a dopamine agonist with a more prolonged action may also be tried.

Various attempts have been made to overcome the 'on-off' phenomenon. Those speculating that long-term treatment results in altered dopamine receptor sensitivity have used controlled withdrawal of levodopa for short periods ('drug holidays') but it is a dangerous procedure of doubtful value and no longer recommended.

Others have linked the 'on-off' phenomenon to variable plasma concentrations although, since transfer of levodopa into the brain involves active transport mechanisms, concentrations in plasma may not necessarily reflect those in the brain. Continuous intravenous infusion of levodopa has been shown to reduce fluctuations in mobility, which suggests that dopamine receptors are still sensitive, but this is not practical for day-to-day management. However, there is evidence that some patients may benefit from modified-release formulations of levodopa with a peripheral dopa-decarboxylase inhibitor. As levodopa competes with amino acids for uptake into the brain, attempts to lessen fluctuations in dopamine brain concentrations have included taking levodopa on an empty stomach and also delaying most of a day's protein consumption until the evening. Addition of selegiline or a dopamine agonist may also help to reduce 'on-off' phenomena. If fluctuations remain a problem subcutaneous apomorphine is often effective.

Other complications of treatment with levodopa can include **dyskinesia**, which may respond to dosage adjustment or partial replacement of levodopa with a dopamine agonist. Some patients with Parkinson's disease may experience **severe pain** and **dystonia** and it has been considered that measures to increase 'on' periods will reduce or eliminate pain in most patients.

Patients with Parkinson's disease can suffer from a range of **psychiatric effects** due to the adverse effects of drug therapy and to disease progression. It has been recommended that if patients develop psychotic reactions, an attempt to adjust their antiparkinsonian drugs should be tried before resorting to the use of antipsychotics. Although classical antipsychotics are usually contra-indicated because they can exacerbate parkinsonism, the atypical antipsychotic clozapine can be used in treatment-resistant psychosis—see Disturbed Behaviour, p.665. **Nausea and vomiting** induced by dopaminergics may be minimised by introducing the drug gradually and administering the dose with food, but if this is ineffective or apomorphine is being used these effects can be controlled by the antiemetic domperidone. Domperidone does not readily cross the blood-brain barrier and therefore acts mainly as a peripheral dopamine antagonist. Tolerance to the nausea usually develops after a few weeks and domperidone may then be withdrawn.

References.


1. Mizuno Y, *et al.* Potential of neuroprotective therapy in Parkinson's disease. *CNS Drugs* 1994; **1:** 45–56.
2. Quinn N. Drug treatment of Parkinson's disease. *BMJ* 1995; **310:** 575–9.
3. Harder S, *et al.* Concentration-effect relationship of levodopa in patients with Parkinson's disease. *Clin Pharmacokinet* 1995; **29:** 243–56.
4. Giron LT, Koller WC. Methods of managing levodopa-induced dyskinesias. *Drug Safety* 1996; **14:** 365–74.
5. Ahlskog JE. Treatment of early Parkinson's disease: are complicated strategies justified? *Mayo Clin Proc* 1996; **71:** 659–70.
6. Mendis T, *et al.* Drug-induced psychosis in Parkinson's disease: a review of management. *CNS Drugs* 1996; **5:** 166–74.
7. Hughes AJ. Drug treatment of Parkinson's disease in the 1990s. *Drugs* 1997; **53:** 195–205.
8. Gottwald MD, *et al.* New pharmacotherapy for Parkinson's disease. *Ann Pharmacother* 1997; **31:** 1205–17.
9. Lang AE, Lozano AM. Parkinson's disease. *N Engl J Med* 1998; **339:** 1044–53 and 1130–43.
10. Bhatia K, *et al.* Guidelines for the management of Parkinson's disease. *Hosp Med* 1998; **59:** 469–80.
11. Ahlskog JE. Medical treatment of later-stage motor problems of Parkinson disease. *Mayo Clin Proc* 1999; **74:** 1239–54.
12. Anonymous. Developments in the treatment of Parkinson's disease. *Drug Ther Bull* 1999; **37:** 36–40.
13. Olanow CW, *et al.* An algorithm (decision tree) for the management of Parkinson's disease (2001): treatment guidelines. *Neurology* 2001; **56** (suppl 5): S1–S88.
14. Miyasaki JM, *et al.* Practice parameter: initiation of treatment for Parkinson's disease: an evidence-based review: *Neurology* 2002; **58:** 11–17.
15. Clarke CE, Guttman M. Dopamine agonist monotherapy in Parkinson's disease. *Lancet* 2002; **360:** 1767–9.
16. Deleu D, *et al.* Clinical pharmacokinetic and pharmacodynamic properties of drugs used in the treatment of Parkinson's disease. *Clin Pharmacokinet* 2002; **41:** 261–309.
17. Korczyn AD, Nussbaum M. Emerging therapies in the pharmacological treatment of Parkinson's disease. *Drugs* 2002; **62:** 775–86.


## Amantadine Hydrochloride

*(BANM, USAN, pINNM)*

1-Adamantanamine Hydrochloride; Amantadini Hydrochloridum; EXP-105-1; Hidrocloruro de amantadina; NSC-83653. Tricyclo[3.3.1.1$^{3,7}$]dec-1-ylamine hydrochloride.

$C_{10}H_{17}N,HCl = 187.7.$

*CAS — 768-94-5 (amantadine); 665-66-7 (amantadine hydrochloride).*

*ATC — N04BB01.*

**Pharmacopoeias.** In *Chin., Eur.* (see p.vi), *Jpn,* and *US.*

**Ph. Eur. 5.0** (Amantadine Hydrochloride). A white or almost white crystalline powder. It sublimes on heating. Freely soluble in water and in alcohol.

**USP 27** (Amantadine Hydrochloride). A white or practically white crystalline powder. Soluble 1 in 2.5 of water, 1 in 5.1 of alcohol, 1 in 18 of chloroform, and 1 in 70 of macrogol 400. pH of a 20% solution in water is between 3.0 and 5.5.

### Amantadine Sulfate

Amantadina, sulfato de; Amantadine Sulphate.

$(C_{10}H_{17}N)_2,SO_4 = 398.6.$

*CAS — 31377-23-8.*

*ATC — N04BB01.*

### Adverse Effects

Most adverse effects associated with amantadine therapy appear to be dose-related and relatively mild; some resemble those of antimuscarinic drugs. They may be reversed by withdrawing therapy but many resolve despite continuation.

Livedo reticularis, sometimes associated with ankle oedema, is quite common in patients given amantadine long-term. CNS effects such as nervousness, inability to concentrate, dizziness, insomnia, nightmares, headache, and changes in mood may occur. Psychotic reactions, hallucinations, and confusion have been reported, especially in the elderly, patients with renal impairment, and those also receiving antimuscarinics.

Other adverse effects reported have included orthostatic hypotension, urinary retention, slurred speech, ataxia, lethargy, nausea, anorexia, vomiting, dry mouth, constipation, skin rash, diaphoresis, photosensitisation, and blurred vision. There have been isolated reports of congestive heart failure, palpitations, leucopenia, neutropenia, facial dyskinesias, oculogyric episodes, and convulsions.

**Effects on the cardiovascular system.** Congestive heart failure has been reported with amantadine;[1] the patient had been receiving combined treatment with amantadine, levodopa, and orphenadrine for 4 years. Others have considered that while amantadine sometimes causes ankle oedema, an association between amantadine and heart failure is not proven.[2] Livedo reticularis, a mottled blue discoloration of the skin due to prominence of the normal pattern of venous drainage, has been reported[2] to occur in about 50% of all elderly patients given amantadine 100 to 300 mg daily for 2 to 6 weeks and was associated with oedema in 5 to 10%. Both livedo and oedema have usually been confined to the legs and may result from the catecholamine-releasing action of amantadine in certain vascular beds; the oedema was unlikely to be due to heart failure. Angina, dyspnoea, pulmonary congestion, or distension of neck veins has also been reported[2] in 4 of 89 parkinsonian patients treated with amantadine; only 2 of these 4 had had ankle oedema before heart failure developed. No patient had been observed in whom heart failure seemed due directly to amantadine.

See also under Overdosage, below.


1. Vale JA, Maclean KS. Amantadine-induced heart-failure. *Lancet* 1977; **i:** 548.
2. Parkes JD, *et al.* Amantadine-induced heart-failure. *Lancet* 1977; **i:** 904.


**Effects on electrolytes.** For a report of a patient who developed hyponatraemia when given amantadine or levodopa, see under Effects on Kidney Function in Levodopa, p.1206.

**Effects on the eyes.** Superficial punctate keratitis and corneal abrasion with loss of visual acuity was observed in both eyes of a 64-year-old man about 3 weeks after starting treatment with amantadine 100 mg daily.[1] Symptoms resolved on discontinuation of amantadine but recurred when re-treatment with amantadine was attempted.


1. Nogaki H, Morimatsu M. Superficial punctate keratitis and corneal abrasion due to amantadine hydrochloride. *J Neurol* 1993; **240:** 388–9.


**Effects on mental function.** It has been suggested[1] that the ability of amantadine and memantine to cause psychotic disturbances in patients with Parkinson's disease might be related to their action as *N*-methyl-D-aspartate antagonists.


1. Riederer P, *et al.* Pharmacotoxic psychosis after memantine in Parkinson's disease. *Lancet* 1991; **338:** 1022–3.


**Effects on the nervous system.** Peripheral sensory motor neuropathy secondary to long-term (8 years) use of amantadine has been reported[1] in a 48-year-old woman with parkinsonism. Trophic skin ulcers, paraesthesias, and distal weakness resolved on discontinuation of amantadine.


1. Shulman LM, *et al.* Amantadine-induced peripheral neuropathy. *Neurology* 1999; **53:** 1862–5.


**Overdosage.** A patient with postencephalitic parkinsonism who had taken an estimated 2.8 g of amantadine hydrochloride in a suicide attempt suffered an acute toxic psychosis with disorientation, visual hallucinations, and aggressive behaviour.[1] Convulsions did not occur, possibly because he had been receiving phenytoin, which was continued. The patient was treated with hydration and chlorpromazine and recovered in 4 days.

A 2-year-old child who had ingested 600 mg of amantadine hydrochloride developed symptoms of acute toxicity, including agitation and dystonic posturing, despite emesis with 'syrup of ipecac'.[2] She responded immediately to a trial of physostigmine 500 micrograms intravenously, repeated after 10 minutes. Her pupils remained moderately dilated until about 20 hours after the ingestion; thereafter she made a full recovery.

Cardiac arrest developed 4 hours after a 37-year-old woman ingested 2.5 g of amantadine hydrochloride and was treated successfully.[3] However, ventricular arrhythmias, including torsade de pointes, continued over the ensuing 48 hours and may have been exacerbated by administration of isoprenaline and dopamine. The patient was subsequently stabilised with lidocaine by intravenous infusion, but died of respiratory failure 10 days after admission.


1. Fahn S, *et al.* Acute toxic psychosis from suicidal overdosage of amantadine. *Arch Neurol*, 1971; **25:** 45–8.
2. Berkowitz CD. Treatment of acute amantadine toxicity with physostigmine. *J Pediatr* 1979; **95:** 144–5.
3. Sartori M, *et al.* Torsade de pointe: malignant cardiac arrhythmia induced by amantadine poisoning. *Am J Med* 1984; **77:** 388–91.


### Precautions

Amantadine is usually contra-indicated in severe renal disease and in patients with a history of epilepsy or other seizure disorders or gastric ulceration. It should be used with caution in patients with cardiovascular or liver disease, renal impairment, recurrent eczema, or psychosis. Care should be taken in all elderly patients, who may be more sensitive to antimuscarinic effects, and in whom renal clearance is likely to be reduced.

In common with other drugs having antimuscarinic properties amantadine may cause blurred vision or impair alertness; patients so affected should not drive or operate machinery.

Treatment with amantadine should not be stopped abruptly in parkinsonian patients since they may experience a sudden marked clinical deterioration. There have been isolated reports of neuroleptic malignant syndrome associated with abrupt withdrawal of amantadine, especially in patients receiving concomitant treatment with antipsychotics.

**Antiviral resistance.** See under Influenza in Uses and Administration, below.

**Breast feeding.** Amantadine is distributed into breast milk and the manufacturer has reported that adverse effects have occurred in infants being breast fed by mothers taking amantadine.

**Pregnancy.** Amantadine should not be used during pregnancy; embryotoxicity and teratogenicity have been reported in *rats* given high doses.[1]

A complex cardiovascular lesion occurred in an infant whose mother had taken amantadine hydrochloride 100 mg daily during the first 3 months of pregnancy.[1]

1. Nora JJ, *et al.* Cardiovascular maldevelopment associated with maternal exposure to amantadine. *Lancet* 1975; **ii:** 607.

**Renal impairment.** Evidence of extremely limited excretion of amantadine was found in 12 patients who were either anephric or had negligible renal function following a single dose of 100 mg of amantadine hydrochloride.[1] Only small amounts were removed by dialysis. It was suggested that amantadine should be given with caution to patients requiring maintenance haemodialysis. It should be remembered that a single dose may provide adequate plasma concentrations for many days.[1]

Dosage regimens based on creatinine clearance[2] or fixed doses at extended intervals[3] have been published. However both regimens have been criticised, and a conservative approach to amantadine dosage in these patients recommended[4] (for the regimens recommended by the manufacturers see Administration in Renal Impairment, below). The need for caution in using amantadine in patients with renal impairment is highlighted by a report of a patient with end-stage renal disease who progressed from delirium to coma after receiving amantadine 100 mg twice daily for 3 days.[5]

1. Soung L-S, *et al.* Amantadine hydrochloride pharmacokinetics in hemodialysis patients. *Ann Intern Med* 1980; **93:** 46–9.
2. Horadam VW, *et al.* Pharmacokinetics of amantadine hydrochloride in subjects with normal and impaired renal function. *Ann Intern Med* 1981; **94:** 454–8.
3. Wu MJ, *et al.* Amantadine hydrochloride pharmacokinetics in patients with impaired renal function. *Clin Nephrol* 1982; **17:** 19–23.
4. Aoki FY, Sitar DS. Clinical pharmacokinetics of amantadine hydrochloride. *Clin Pharmacokinet* 1988; **14:** 35–51.
5. Macchio GJ, *et al.* Amantadine-induced coma. *Arch Phys Med Rehabil* 1993; **74:** 1119–20.

**Withdrawal.** Neuroleptic malignant syndrome occurred in a patient being treated for heat stroke when all his medication, including antipsychotics and amantadine, was withdrawn.[1] It is suggested that dopamine agonists should not be discontinued in patients with hyperpyrexia at risk from this syndrome.

1. Simpson DM, Davis GC. Case report of neuroleptic malignant syndrome associated with withdrawal from amantadine. *Am J Psychiatry* 1984; **141:** 796–7.

## Interactions

Amantadine may enhance the adverse effects of antimuscarinics and the dose of these drugs should be reduced when used with amantadine; adverse effects of levodopa may also be exacerbated.

The US manufacturer recommends that amantadine should be used with caution in patients receiving drugs with CNS stimulant properties. The rate of excretion of amantadine may be reduced by drugs that raise urinary pH.

**Antiarrhythmics.** Quinine and quinidine have been reported to reduce the renal clearance of amantadine in healthy male, but not female, subjects.[1] Patients taking these drugs concomitantly should be observed for signs of amantadine toxicity.

1. Gaudry SE, *et al.* Gender and age as factors in the inhibition of renal clearance of amantadine by quinine and quinidine. *Clin Pharmacol Ther* 1993; **54:** 23–7.

**Antimalarials.** See under Antiarrhythmics, above.

**Diuretics.** A patient with Parkinson's disease, previously stabilised on amantadine hydrochloride 300 mg daily, developed symptoms of amantadine toxicity, including ataxia, myoclonus, and confusion, 7 days after starting treatment with a preparation containing triamterene and hydrochlorothiazide (Dyazide).[1] It was postulated that the effect was due to reduction of the tubular secretion of amantadine.

1. Wilson TW, Rajput AH. Amantadine-Dyazide interaction. *Can Med Assoc J* 1983; **129:** 974–5.

**MAOIs.** Hypertension occurred about 48 hours after starting treatment with phenelzine sulfate in a patient already receiving amantadine.[1]

1. Jack RA, Daniel DG. Possible interaction between phenelzine and amantadine. *Arch Gen Psychiatry* 1984; **41:** 726.

## Pharmacokinetics

Amantadine hydrochloride is readily absorbed from the gastrointestinal tract; peak concentrations in the plasma appear within about 4 hours. It is mainly excreted unchanged in the urine by glomerular filtration and tubular secretion although small amounts of an acetylated metabolite have also been detected in urine; the plasma elimination half-life is reported to be about 11 to 15 hours in patients with normal renal function but is significantly prolonged in the elderly and in patients with renal impairment. The rate of elimination may be increased by acidification of the urine. Amantadine crosses the placenta and the blood-brain barrier. It is also distributed into breast milk. Plasma protein binding is reported to be about 67%.

◊ References.

1. Aoki FY, Sitar DS. Clinical pharmacokinetics of amantadine hydrochloride. *Clin Pharmacokinet* 1988; **14:** 35–51.

## Uses and Administration

Amantadine is a weak dopamine agonist with some antimuscarinic activity; it is also an antagonist at *N*-methyl-D-aspartate receptors. Amantadine has mild antiparkinsonian activity and is used in the management of parkinsonism, mainly in early disease when symptoms are mild. It may improve bradykinesia, rigidity, and tremor but tolerance can develop.

Amantadine is also an antiviral that inhibits replication of influenza type A virus. Variable activity has been reported *in vitro* against other viruses. It is used prophylactically against infection with influenza type A virus and to ameliorate symptoms when given during the early stages of infection.

Amantadine has also been used in the management of herpes zoster.

Amantadine is usually given by mouth as the hydrochloride and the doses below are expressed in terms of the hydrochloride.

In **parkinsonism**, treatment is usually started with 100 mg daily, increasing to 100 mg twice daily after a week or more. Doses of up to 400 mg daily have occasionally been used, but this dose should not be exceeded. The lowest effective dose should be used in patients over 65 years of age because of the potential for reduced renal clearance in this age group. Withdrawal of amantadine treatment for parkinsonism should be gradual to avoid exacerbating the condition; the manufacturers suggest decreasing the dose by half at weekly intervals.

The dose of amantadine in the UK for the treatment of **influenza A** is 100 mg, usually given daily for about 5 days. For the prophylaxis of influenza A the same dose is given for as long as protection from infection is required, which may be for about 6 weeks. If amantadine is being given with influenza vaccination then it is usually only given for up to 3 weeks after vaccination. Children aged 10 to 15 years may also be given 100 mg daily for the recommended period. A daily dose of less than 100 mg or 100 mg given at intervals greater than one day has been recommended for patients over 65 years of age. Doses in the USA are higher than those in the UK: for the treatment of influenza A the daily dose is 200 mg daily as a single dose or in two divided doses, continued for 24 to 48 hours after the disappearance of symptoms. The same dose is given for the prophylaxis of influenza A for at least 10 days following exposure. If given with vaccination then amantadine should be taken for the next 2 to 4 weeks. The dose of amantadine should be reduced to 100 mg daily in patients aged 65 years and over and in those who show intolerance to the higher dose. Children aged 1 to 9 years may be given 4.4 to 8.8 mg/kg daily to a maximum of 150 mg daily; older children may be given 100 mg twice daily.

In **herpes zoster**, treatment with 100 mg twice daily may be given for 14 days; if pain persists treatment may be continued for a further 14 days.

The dosage of amantadine should be reduced in patients with renal impairment (see below).

Amantadine sulfate has been used similarly to the hydrochloride; it has been given by mouth or by intravenous infusion.

**Administration.** Amantadine sulfate has been used successfully in doses of up to 600 mg daily by intravenous infusion in the management of akinetic crisis in patients with Parkinson's disease.[1]

1. Gadoth N, *et al.* I.V. amantadine sulfate for extrapyramidal crisis. *Clin Pharm* 1985; **4:** 146.

**Administration in renal impairment.** The dose of amantadine should be reduced in patients with renal impairment by either reducing the total daily dose or by increasing the dosage interval in accordance with the creatinine clearance (CC).

In the UK the following doses are recommended:

- CC over 35 mL/min: 100 mg daily
- CC 15 to 35 mL/min: 100 mg every 2 to 3 days
- CC less than 15 mL/min: not recommended.

In the USA the following doses are recommended:

- CC 30 to 50 mL/min: 200 mg on the first day followed by 100 mg daily thereafter
- CC 15 to 29 mL/min: 200 mg on the first day followed by 100 mg on alternate days
- CC less than 15 mL/min or those on haemodialysis: 200 mg every 7 days.

See also under Precautions, above.

**Extrapyramidal disorders.** Amantadine has been used as an alternative to antimuscarinics[1] in the short-term management of drug-induced extrapyramidal symptoms (p.677). However the development of tolerance has limited its usefulness. See also Parkinsonism, below.

1. König P, *et al.* Amantadine versus biperiden: a double-blind study of treatment efficacy in neuroleptic extrapyramidal movement disorders. *Neuropsychobiology* 1996; **33:** 80–4.

**Hiccup.** Amantadine[1] has been reported to have produced beneficial results in patients with intractable hiccups (p.682).

1. Askenasy JJM, *et al.* Persistent hiccup cured by amantadine. *N Engl J Med* 1988; **318:** 711.

**Influenza.** Amantadine has been used similarly to rimantadine (p.653) in the prophylaxis and symptomatic treatment of influenza A (p.624); the two are equally effective, but amantadine is associated with more adverse effects.[1] It reduced the duration of influenza A symptoms when given in a dose of 200 mg daily within 48 hours of the onset of symptoms.[2] Vaccination is usually the method of choice for prophylaxis of influenza but amantadine has been used in addition to vaccination in certain individuals or when vaccination is contra-indicated. Although amantadine is licensed in the UK for the prophylaxis and treatment of influenza A (in a dose of 100 mg daily), its use for such purposes is not recommended by the National Institute for Clinical Excellence.[3,4] This is not necessarily the advice of advisory bodies in other countries such as the USA[5] where higher doses of amantadine are used.

Treatment and prophylaxis failures may be due to the rapid emergence of drug-resistant viruses.[6] Some authorities recommend that to reduce the risk of resistance emerging, amantadine should not be used for both prophylaxis and treatment of influenza A in the same household.

1. Jefferson TO, *et al.* Amantadine and rimantadine for preventing and treating influenza A in adults. Available in The Cochrane Library; Issue 1. Chichester: John Wiley; 2004.
2. Nicholson KG, Wiselka MJ. Amantadine for influenza A. *BMJ* 1991; **302:** 425–6.
3. National Institute for Clinical Excellence. Guidance on the use of zanamivir, oseltamivir and amantadine for the treatment of influenza (issued February 2003). Available at: http://www.nice.org.uk/pdf/58_Flu_fullguidance.pdf (accessed 24/05/04)
4. National Institute for Clinical Excellence. Guidance on the use of oseltamivir and amantadine for the prophylaxis of influenza (issued September 2003). Available at: http://www.nice.org.uk/pdf/67_Flu_prophylaxis_guidance.pdf (accessed 24/05/04)
5. Centers for Disease Control. Prevention and control of influenza: recommendations of the Advisory Committee on Immunization Practices (ACIP). *MMWR* 2003; **52** (RR-8): 1–34. Correction. *ibid.*; 526. Also available at: http://www.cdc.gov/mmwr/PDF/rr/rr5208.pdf (accessed 24/05/04)
6. Belshe RB, *et al.* Resistance of influenza A virus to amantadine and rimantadine: results of one decade of surveillance. *J Infect Dis* 1989; **159:** 430–5.

**Multiple sclerosis.** Amantadine may help to alleviate fatigue[1,2] associated with multiple sclerosis (p.646).

1. Kemp BA, Gora ML. Amantadine and fatigue of multiple sclerosis. *Ann Pharmacother* 1993; **27:** 893–5.
2. Krupp LB, *et al.* Fatigue therapy in multiple sclerosis: results of a double-blind, randomized, parallel trial of amantadine, pemoline and placebo. *Neurology* 1995; **45:** 1956–61.

**Neuroleptic malignant syndrome.** Amantadine has been tried[1-3] in the treatment of the neuroleptic malignant syndrome (p.677).

1. McCarron MM, *et al.* A case of neuroleptic malignant syndrome successfully treated with amantadine. *J Clin Psychiatry* 1982; **43:** 381–2.
2. Amdurski S, *et al.* A therapeutic trial of amantadine in haloperidol-induced malignant neuroleptic syndrome. *Curr Ther Res* 1983; **33:** 225–9.
3. Woo J, *et al.* Neuroleptic malignant syndrome successfully treated with amantadine. *Postgrad Med J* 1986; **62:** 809–10.

**Parkinsonism.** Amantadine's mechanism of action in parkinsonism (p.1196) is unclear but may be due to its antimuscarinic activity and alterations in dopamine release and reuptake. It has also been suggested that amantadine's action as a non-competitive antagonist of *N*-methyl-D-aspartate may have a beneficial effect.[1,2] It has mild antiparkinsonian activity compared with levodopa but is relatively free from side-effects. It can improve bradykinesia as well as tremor and rigidity and is used in a similar manner to antimuscarinics mainly in the treatment of patients with early Parkinson's disease when symptoms are mild. It may also be useful for dyskinesias in more advanced disease.[3] However few patients obtain much benefit and tolerance to its effects can occur. The manufacturers suggest that the effectiveness of amantadine may be prolonged by withdrawing it for 3 to 4 weeks, continuing with existing antiparkinsonian therapy or initiating low dose levodopa treatment if clinically necessary in the meantime.

1. Laing P. Stroke treatment. *Lancet* 1991; **337:** 1601.
2. Greenamyre JT, O'Brien CF. N-Methyl-D-aspartate antagonists in the treatment of Parkinson's disease. *Arch Neurol* 1991; **48:** 977–81.
3. Thomas A, *et al.* Duration of amantadine benefit on dyskinesia of severe Parkinson's disease. *J Neurol Neurosurg Psychiatry* 2004; **75:** 141–3.

**Withdrawal syndromes.** COCAINE. Despite some early promising results a systematic review[1] considered that there was no evidence to support the use of dopamine agonists, including amantadine, in the treatment of cocaine dependence (p.1375).

1. Soares BGO, *et al.* Dopamine agonists for cocaine dependence. Available in The Cochrane Library; Issue 1. Chichester: John Wiley; 2004.

### Preparations

***BP 2003:*** Amantadine Capsules; Amantadine Oral Solution;
***USP 27:*** Amantadine Hydrochloride Capsules; Amantadine Hydrochloride Syrup.

**Proprietary Preparations** (details are given in Part 3)
***Arg.:*** Virosol; ***Austral.:*** Symmetrel; ***Austria:*** Hofcomant; Noctal; PK-Merz; Virucid; ***Belg.:*** Amantan; Mantadix†; ***Braz.:*** Mantidan; ***Canad.:*** Endantadine; Symmetrel; ***Chile:*** PK-Merz; Prayanol; ***Denm.:*** Virofral†; ***Fin.:*** Atarin; ***Fr.:*** Mantadix; ***Ger.:*** Adekin; Aman; Amanta; Amantagamma; Amixx; AMT; Cerebramed†; Grippin-Merz†; InfectoFlu; Infex; PK-Merz; tregor; Viregyt†; ***Gr.:*** Symmetrel; ***Hong Kong:*** PK-Merz; Symmetrel; ***India:*** Amantrel; ***Irl.:*** Symmetrel; ***Israel:*** A-Parkin; Influ-A; Paritrel; PK-Merz; Symmetrel†; ***Ital.:*** Mantadan; ***Malaysia:*** PK-Merz; ***Mex.:*** Padiken†; ***Neth.:*** Symmetrel; ***NZ:*** Symmetrel; ***Port.:*** Parkadina; Profil; ***S.Afr.:*** Antadine; Symmetrel; ***Singapore:*** Symmetrel; ***Swed.:*** Virofral†; ***Switz.:*** PK-Merz; Symmetrel; ***UK:*** Lysovir; Symmetrel; ***USA:*** Symmetrel.

**Multi-ingredient:** ***Mex.:*** Antiflu-Des.

## Apomorphine Hydrochloride *(BANM)*

Apomorfina, hidrocloruro de; Apomorphini Hydrochloridum.
6aβ-Aporphine-10,11-diol hydrochloride hemihydrate; (R)-10,11-Dihydroxy-6a-aporphine hydrochloride hemihydrate; (6aR)-5,6,6a,7-Tetrahydro-6-methyl-4H-dibenzo[de,g]quinoline-10,11-diol hydrochloride hemihydrate.

$C_{17}H_{17}NO_2,HCl,\frac{1}{2}H_2O = 312.8.$

*CAS — 58-00-4 (apomorphine); 314-19-2 (anhydrous apomorphine hydrochloride); 41372-20-7 (apomorphine hydrochloride, hemihydrate).*

*ATC — G04BE07; N04BC07.*

**Pharmacopoeias.** In *Chin., Eur.* (see p.vi), *Pol.,* and *US.*

**Ph. Eur. 5.0** (Apomorphine Hydrochloride). White or faintly yellow to green-tinged greyish crystals or crystalline powder, the green tinge becoming more pronounced on exposure to air and light. Sparingly soluble in water and in alcohol. A 1% solution in water has a pH of 4.0 to 5.0. Store in airtight containers. Protect from light.

**USP 27** (Apomorphine Hydrochloride). Odourless, minute white or greyish-white, glistening crystals or white powder. It gradually acquires a green colour on exposure to light and air. Soluble 1 in 50 of water and 1 in 20 of water at 80°; soluble 1 in 50 of alcohol; very slightly soluble in ether and in chloroform. Its solutions are neutral to litmus. Store in small, airtight containers. Containers from which it is to be taken for immediate use in compounding prescriptions contain no more than 350 mg. Protect from light.

**Stability.** Aqueous solutions of apomorphine hydrochloride decompose on storage and should not be used if they turn green or brown or contain a precipitate.

### Adverse Effects

*Treatment of parkinsonism.* Apomorphine usually produces nausea and vomiting when given in therapeutic doses but these effects can be controlled by treatment with domperidone. Apomorphine may induce dyskinesias during 'on' periods in patients with parkinsonism and these may be severe enough to require discontinuation of therapy; postural instability and falls may also be a problem. Transient sedation can be common during the first few weeks of treatment. Transient postural hypotension may also occur infrequently. Apomorphine can produce neuropsychiatric disturbances including increasing cognitive impairment, personality changes, confusion, and visual hallucinations. Signs of CNS stimulation including euphoria, lightheadedness, restlessness, tremor, tachycardia, and tachypnoea occur less frequently. Increased salivation and perspiration have also been reported. Eosinophilia has occurred rarely. The use of apomorphine with levodopa may cause haemolytic anaemia and treatment may need to be discontinued if this cannot be satisfactorily controlled through dosage adjustment. Induration, nodule formation, and panniculitis, sometimes leading to ulceration often develops at the site of subcutaneous injection.

*Management of erectile dysfunction.* The most common adverse effects have been nausea, headache, and dizziness. Other effects reported include yawning, rhinitis, pharyngitis, somnolence, infection, pain, increased cough, flushing, taste disturbances, and sweating. Fainting and syncope (vasovagal syndrome) have also occurred.

*Overdosage* with apomorphine can produce persistent vomiting, respiratory depression, bradycardia, hypotension, and coma; death may occur.

**Akinesia.** A 60-year-old man who was being investigated for parkinsonian symptoms became totally immobile and mute 15 minutes after receiving apomorphine 4 mg subcutaneously.[1] He remained conscious but was drowsy and sweating. Similar profound akinesia occurred on rechallenge with 2- and 6-mg doses. A diagnosis of probable nigrostriatal degeneration was made as the patient had previously shown no improvement after administration of levodopa but the mechanism of the idiosyncratic reaction to apomorphine was unclear.

1. Jenkins JR, Pearce JMS. Paradoxical akinetic response to apomorphine in parkinsonism. *J Neurol Neurosurg Psychiatry* 1992; **55:** 414–15.

**Effects on the heart.** A 67-year-old man developed palpitations with cold perspiration and chest pain, in addition to asthenia, salivation, nausea and vomiting, 5 minutes after receiving 3 mg apomorphine subcutaneously. An ECG demonstrated atrial fibrillation with a ventricular frequency of 140 beats/minute.[1]

1. Stocchi F, *et al.* Transient atrial fibrillation after subcutaneous apomorphine bolus. *Mov Disord* 1996; **11:** 584–5.

**Effects on mental function.** Severe confusion, hallucinations, and acute psychosis were reported in 4 of 6 parkinsonian patients given subcutaneous apomorphine.[1] Three of the 4 had previously experienced mental disturbances while receiving lisuride. However, other studies failed to note effects on mental function in parkinsonian patients given apomorphine[2,3] and it has been suggested that the risk of psychosis in patients with no history of confusion or hallucinations is low.[3] The UK manufacturer notes that apomorphine has been reported to exacerbate neuropsychiatric disturbances in patients with parkinsonism.

1. Ruggieri S, *et al.* Side-effects of subcutaneous apomorphine in Parkinson's disease. *Lancet* 1989; **i:** 566.
2. Stibe CMH, *et al.* Subcutaneous apomorphine in parkinsonian on-off oscillations. *Lancet* 1988; **i:** 403–6.
3. Poewe W, *et al.* Side-effects of subcutaneous apomorphine in Parkinson's disease. *Lancet* 1989; **i:** 1084–5.

**Hypersensitivity.** Allergic reactions including contact dermatitis, severe rhinitis, and respiratory distress have been reported in 2 workers who came into contact with apomorphine powder.[1] Contact allergy has also been reported in a patient who developed a swollen nose and lips after intranasal use of apomorphine.[2] Skin testing in all these cases[1,2] gave a positive reaction to apomorphine. Biopsy of subcutaneous nodules, which develop at the site of injection in most patients using apomorphine subcutaneously, has not been able to clarify what type of reaction was responsible for the development of panniculitis.[3] Although the nodules may slowly resolve the sites are often unsuitable for reuse as absorption from them is unpredictable; concern has been expressed that this may limit long-term use of apomorphine.[3]

1. Dahlquist I. Allergic reactions to apomorphine. *Contact Dermatitis* 1977; **3:** 349–50.
2. van Laar T, *et al.* Nasolabiale allergische reactie op intranasale toediening van apomorfine bij de ziekte van Parkinson. *Ned Tijdschr Geneeskd* 1992; **136** (suppl 47): 26–7.
3. Acland KM, *et al.* Panniculitis in association with apomorphine infusion. *Br J Dermatol* 1998; **138:** 480–2.

**Oedema.** A report of severe reversible oedema of the lower limbs in a patient receiving subcutaneous apomorphine.[1] Oedema recurred when apomorphine was reintroduced, but to a lesser extent.

1. Vermersch P. Severe oedema after subcutaneous apomorphine in Parkinson's disease. *Lancet* 1989; **ii:** 802.

**Stomatitis.** Stomatitis, severe enough to warrant discontinuation of treatment, occurred in 4 of 8 patients after 2 to 6 months of therapy with sublingual apomorphine.[1]

1. Montastruc JL, *et al.* Sublingual apomorphine in Parkinson's disease: a clinical and pharmacokinetic study. *Clin Neuropharmacol* 1991; **14:** 432–7.

### Treatment of Adverse Effects

Domperidone is usually given to control nausea and vomiting when apomorphine is used in the management of Parkinson's disease; pretreatment with domperidone for at least 2 days is advised before starting treatment with apomorphine. Usually domperidone can be withdrawn gradually over several weeks or longer although some patients may need to continue treatment indefinitely.

In overdosage an opioid antagonist such as naloxone has been given to treat excessive vomiting and CNS and respiratory depression.

◊ References.

1. Bonuccelli U, *et al.* Naloxone partly counteracts apomorphine side effects. *Clin Neuropharmacol* 1991; **14:** 442–9.

### Precautions

Apomorphine should not be given to patients with respiratory or CNS depression, hypersensitivity to opioids, neuropsychiatric problems, or dementia. It is not suitable for use in parkinsonian patients who have an 'on' response to levodopa marred by severe dyskinesia, hypotonia, or psychiatric effects; it should also not be used in parkinsonian patients with hepatic impairment.

The UK manufacturer warns that drugs for erectile dysfunction should be used with caution in patients with anatomical penile deformity.

It should be used with caution in patients prone to nausea and vomiting or when vomiting is likely to pose a risk. Apomorphine should also be used with care in patients with pulmonary, cardiovascular, or endocrine disease or with renal or hepatic impairment. Extra care is needed during initiation of treatment in elderly or debilitated patients and in those with a history of postural hypotension. In the management of parkinsonism periodic monitoring of hepatic, renal, haematopoietic, and cardiovascular function has been advised and the *British National Formulary* recommends that patients receiving apomorphine and levodopa together should be screened for haemolytic anaemia before starting treatment and then every 6 months.

Patients who develop anaemia, or those who have continuing confusion, or hallucinations during treatment with apomorphine require observation and dosage adjustment under specialist supervision; treatment may need to be discontinued.

Patients who experience dizziness, lightheadedness, or syncope should not drive or operate hazardous machinery. Excessive daytime sleepiness and sudden onset of sleep may also occur with apomorphine and caution is advised when driving or operating machinery; patients who suffer such effects should not drive or operate machinery until the effects have stopped recurring.

Local subcutaneous reactions can sometimes be reduced by using sodium chloride 0.9% to dilute injection solutions, by rotating injection sites, and possibly by use of ultrasound in areas of nodularity and induration.

### Interactions

Apomorphine should be used with caution in patients receiving antihypertensives or organic nitrates as it may potentiate their hypotensive effects. Enhanced hypotensive effects may also occur when alcohol is given with apomorphine. The therapeutic effects of apomorphine may be antagonised by antipsychotics and other drugs that act as CNS dopamine inhibitors. The effect of apomorphine is possibly enhanced by entacapone and memantine.

### Pharmacokinetics

Apomorphine is well absorbed following subcutaneous administration but undergoes extensive first-pass hepatic metabolism when given by mouth and oral bioavailability is low. However, it is readily absorbed following sublingual administration and peak plasma concentrations are achieved in about 40 to 60 minutes; bioavailability is reported to be about 17 to 18% compared with subcutaneous administration. Apomorphine is about 90% bound to plasma proteins.

Apomorphine is extensively metabolised in the liver, primarily by conjugation with glucuronic acid or sulfate; the major metabolite is apomorphine sulfate. It is also demethylated to produce norapomorphine. Most of a dose is excreted in urine, mainly as metabolites.

◊ References.

1. Neef C, van Laar T. Pharmacokinetic-pharmacodynamic relationships of apomorphine in patients with Parkinson's disease. *Clin Pharmacokinet* 1999; **37:** 257–71.

### Uses and Administration

Apomorphine is a morphine derivative with structural similarities to dopamine. It is a potent dopamine $D_1$- and $D_2$-receptor agonist used in the diagnosis and management of parkinsonism, especially in the control of the 'on-off' effect. It is also used in the management of erectile dysfunction. Apomorphine is given as the hydrochloride and doses are expressed in terms of this salt. The regimen for parkinsonism given below applies to the UK preparation; a similar preparation is available in the USA although the licensed maximum single and daily doses are less than those in the UK.

The optimal dose of apomorphine in the management of 'off' periods in **parkinsonism** should be established individually under specialist care. At least 2 days of pretreatment with the antiemetic domperidone is advised before starting apomorphine. After withholding antiparkinsonian therapy overnight to provoke an 'off' period, a test dose of 1 mg is given initially, followed by a second dose of 2 mg after 30 minutes, if necessary. Subsequent incremental increases should then be given at intervals of at least 40 minutes, as necessary, to determine the lowest dose producing a satisfactory response. Once the patient's normal antiparkinsonian therapy is re-established, the effective dose of apomorphine hydrochloride is given at the first signs of an 'off' period.

The dose and frequency of administration is further adjusted according to response; patients typically require 3 to 30 mg daily in divided doses but individual injections should not be greater than 10 mg. Patients who require more than 10 injections daily or those whose overall control of symptoms remains unsatisfactory with intermittent injections may benefit from continuous subcutaneous infusion. The infusion is started at a rate of 1 mg/hour and this may be increased in steps up to 0.5 mg/hour at intervals of not less than 4 hours up to a maximum rate of 4 mg/hour. It is advised that infusions should only be given during waking hours and that the infusion site should be changed every 12 hours; 24-hour infusions are not advised unless there are severe night-time symptoms. Patients usually need to supplement the infusion with intermittent bolus injections but the recommended maximum total daily dose given by infusion and/or injection is 100 mg.

In the management of **erectile dysfunction** the usual initial dose is 2 mg taken sublingually about 20 minutes before sexual activity. A dose of 3 mg may be used on subsequent occasions if necessary but a minimum of 8 hours should be allowed between doses.

Apomorphine stimulates the chemoreceptor trigger zone in the brain and can produce emesis within a few minutes of administration. However, the use of apomorphine for the induction of emesis in poisoning is considered dangerous owing to the risk of inducing protracted vomiting and shock, and is not recommended.

**Administration in renal impairment.** In the management of erectile dysfunction, the maximum dose of apomorphine hydrochloride should be limited to 2 mg sublingually in patients with severe renal impairment.

**Erectile dysfunction.** Apomorphine is among a wide range of drugs that has been used in the management of erectile dysfunction (p.1745) with some beneficial results. It is usually given by sublingual administration[1,2] although it has also been given subcutaneously.[3]

1. Heaton JPW, *et al.* Recovery of erectile function by the oral administration of apomorphine. *Urology* 1995; **45:** 200–6.
2. Dula E, *et al.* Efficacy and safety of fixed-dose and dose-optimization regimens of sublingual apomorphine versus placebo in men with erectile dysfunction. *Urology* 2000; **56:** 130–5.
3. Segraves RT, *et al.* Effect of apomorphine on penile tumescence in men with psychogenic impotence. *J Urol (Baltimore)* 1991; **145:** 1174–5.

**Parkinsonism.** Although apomorphine has produced benefit in Parkinson's disease (p.1196) when given orally, the high doses required to overcome extensive first-pass hepatic metabolism (up to 1.4 g daily in one study[1]), were associated with uraemia. The use of apomorphine in Parkinson's disease has therefore been limited by the need for parenteral administration. The current main use of apomorphine in Parkinson's disease is for the stabilisation of patients with 'on-off' fluctuations unresponsive to other dopamine agonists. It is usually given subcutaneously either by injection or infusion but a recent review[2] of the use of apomorphine in Parkinson's disease also discussed studies of rectal, sublingual, and intranasal administration.

1. Cotzias GC, *et al.* Treatment of Parkinson's disease with apomorphines. *N Engl J Med* 1976; **294:** 567–72.
2. Koller W, Stacy M. Other formulations and future considerations for apomorphine for subcutaneous injection therapy. *Neurology* 2004; **62**(suppl 4): S22–S26. 282–8.

DIAGNOSIS. Test doses of subcutaneous apomorphine have been used in the differential diagnosis of parkinsonian syndromes,[1-4] to distinguish forms responsive to dopaminergics from other parkinsonian syndromes such as Wilson's disease, corticobasal degeneration, and diffuse Lewy body dementia. Oral challenge with levodopa is still the best test of dopaminergic responsiveness[5,6] but apomorphine has proved of value in reassessing patients who have become less responsive to levodopa.[1,4]

1. Barker R, *et al.* Subcutaneous apomorphine as a diagnostic test for dopaminergic responsiveness in parkinsonian syndromes. *Lancet* 1989; **i:** 675.
2. Oertel WH, *et al.* Apomorphine test for dopaminergic responsiveness. *Lancet* 1989; **i:** 1262–3.
3. Frankel JP, *et al.* Use of apomorphine to test for dopamine responsiveness in Wilson's disease. *Lancet* 1989; **ii:** 801–2.
4. Hughes AJ, *et al.* Apomorphine test to predict dopaminergic responsiveness in parkinsonian syndromes. *Lancet* 1990; **336:** 32–4.
5. Steiger MJ, Quinn NP. Levodopa challenge test in Parkinson's disease. *Lancet* 1992; **339:** 751–2.
6. Müller T, *et al.* Repeated rating improves value of diagnostic dopaminergic challenge tests in Parkinson's disease. *J Neural Transm* 2003; **110:** 603–9.

### Preparations

***USP 27:*** Apomorphine Hydrochloride Tablets.

**Proprietary Preparations** (details are given in Part 3)
***Arg.:*** Apokinon; Uprima; ***Austral.:*** Apomine; ***Austria:*** Ixense; ***Belg.:*** Uprima; ***Braz.:*** Uprima; ***Chile:*** Noc; Uprima; ***Denm.:*** Uprima; ***Fin.:*** Uprima; ***Fr.:*** Apokinon; Ixense; Uprima; ***Ger.:*** Ixense; Uprima; ***Gr.:*** Uprima; ***Hong Kong:*** Uprima; ***Irl.:*** Uprima; ***Ital.:*** Apofin; Ixense; Taluvian; Uprima; ***Neth.:*** Britaject†; ***Norw.:*** Uprima; ***NZ:*** Apomine; Uprima; ***Port.:*** Uprima; ***S.Afr.:*** Uprima; ***Spain:*** APO-go Pen; Taluvian; Uprima; ***Swed.:*** Uprima; ***UK:*** APO-go; Britaject†; Uprima; ***USA:*** Apokyn.

## Benserazide *(BAN, USAN, rINN)*

Ro-4-4602. DL-Serine 2-(2,3,4-trihydroxybenzyl)hydrazide; 2-Amino-3-hydroxy-2′-(2,3,4-trihydroxybenzyl)propionohydrazide.

$C_{10}H_{15}N_3O_5$ = 257.2.
*CAS — 322-35-0.*

## Benserazide Hydrochloride *(BANM, rINNM)*

Benserazidi Hydrochloridum; Hidrocloruro de benserazida; Serazide Hydrochloride.

$C_{10}H_{15}N_3O_5,HCl$ = 293.7.
*CAS — 14919-77-8; 14046-64-1.*

NOTE. Compounded preparations of benserazide hydrochloride may be represented by the following names:

- Co-beneldopa *(BAN)*—benserazide 1 part and levodopa 4 parts (w/w).

**Pharmacopoeias.** In *Chin., Eur.* (see p.vi), and *Jpn.*
**Ph. Eur. 5.0** (Benserazide Hydrochloride). A white or yellowish-white or orange-white crystalline powder. It shows polymorphism. Freely soluble in water; very slightly soluble in dehydrated alcohol; practically insoluble in acetone. A 1% solution in water has a pH of 4.0 to 5.0. Protect from light.

**Solubility.** Benserazide is unstable in a neutral, alkaline, or strongly acidic medium.[1]

1. Schwartz DE, Brandt R. Pharmacokinetic and metabolic studies of the decarboxylase inhibitor benserazide in animals and man. *Arzneimittelforschung* 1978; **28:** 302–7.

### Adverse Effects and Precautions

◊ Early reports[1] noted developmental abnormalities of the *rat* skeleton, but others found no evidence of any disorder involving bone metabolism in man.[2] Nevertheless the manufacturers have recommended that benserazide should not be given to patients under 25 years of age or to pregnant women.

1. Theiss E, Schärer K. Toxicity of L-dopa and a decarboxylase inhibitor in animal experiments. In: de Ajuriaguerra J, Gauthier G, eds. *Monoamines Noyaux Gris Centraux et Syndrome de Parkinson.* Geneva: Georg, 1971: 497–504.
2. Ziegler WH, *et al.* Toxicity of L-dopa and a dopa decarboxylase inhibitor in humans. In: de Ajuriaguerra J, Gauthier G, eds. *Monoamines Noyaux Gris Centraux et Syndrome de Parkinson.* Geneva: Georg, 1971: 505–16.

### Pharmacokinetics

◊ Pharmacokinetic and metabolic studies of benserazide in *animals* and man.[1,2] Following oral administration to parkinsonian patients benserazide was rapidly absorbed to the extent of about 58%, simultaneous administration of levodopa tending to increase this slightly. It was rapidly excreted in the urine in the form of metabolites, mostly within the first 6 hours; 85% of urinary excretion had occurred within 12 hours. Benserazide is predominantly metabolised in the gut and appears to protect levodopa against decarboxylation primarily in the gut, but also in the rest of the organism, mainly by way of its metabolite trihydroxybenzylhydrazine. Benserazide did not cross the blood-brain barrier in *rats*.

1. Schwartz DE, *et al.* Pharmacokinetics of the decarboxylase benserazide in man: its tissue distribution in the rat. *Eur J Clin Pharmacol* 1974; **7:** 39–45.
2. Schwartz DE, Brandt R. Pharmacokinetic and metabolic studies of the decarboxylase inhibitor benserazide in animals and man. *Arzneimittelforschung* 1978; **28:** 302–7.

### Uses and Administration

Benserazide hydrochloride is a peripheral dopa-decarboxylase inhibitor with actions similar to those of carbidopa (p.1204) and is used similarly as an adjunct to levodopa in the treatment of parkinsonism (p.1196). For details of administration and dosage, see Levodopa, p.1209.

◊ References.

1. Dingemanse J, *et al.* Pharmacodynamics of benserazide assessed by its effects on endogenous and exogenous levodopa pharmacokinetics. *Br J Clin Pharmacol* 1997; **44:** 41–8.

### Preparations

***BP 2003:*** Co-beneldopa Capsules; Dispersible Co-beneldopa Tablets.

**Proprietary Preparations** (details are given in Part 3)
***Ger.:*** Restex.

**Multi-ingredient:** ***Arg.:*** Madopar; ***Austral.:*** Madopar; ***Austria:*** Dopamed; Levobens; Madopar; ***Belg.:*** Prolopa; ***Braz.:*** Prolopa; ***Canad.:*** Prolopa; ***Chile:*** Melitase; Prolopa; ***Denm.:*** Madopar; ***Fin.:*** Aktipar†; Madopar; ***Fr.:*** Modopar; ***Ger.:*** Levodopa comp B; Levopar; Madopar; PK-Levo; ***Gr.:*** Madopar; ***Hong Kong:*** Madopar; ***Irl.:*** Madopar; ***Israel:*** Levopar Plus; ***Ital.:*** Madopar; ***Mex.:*** Madopar; ***Neth.:*** Madopar; ***Norw.:*** Madopar; ***NZ:*** Madopar; ***Port.:*** Madopar; ***S.Afr.:*** Madopar; ***Singapore:*** Madopar; ***Spain:*** Madopar; ***Swed.:*** Madopark; ***Switz.:*** Madopar; ***Thai.:*** Madopar; Vopar; ***UK:*** Madopar.

## Bromocriptine Mesilate *(BANM, rINNM)*

Bromocriptine Mesylate *(USAN)*; Bromocriptine Methanesulphonate; Bromocriptini Mesilas; Bromocryptine Mesylate; 2-Bromo-α-ergocryptine Mesylate; 2-Bromoergocryptine Monomethanesulfonate; CB-154 (bromocriptine); Mesilato de bromocriptina. (5′S)-2-Bromo-12′-hydroxy-2′-(1-methylethyl)-5′-(2-methylpropyl)-ergotaman-3′,6′,18-trione methanesulphonate.

$C_{32}H_{40}BrN_5O_5,CH_4O_3S$ = 750.7.
*CAS — 25614-03-3 (bromocriptine); 22260-51-1 (bromocriptine mesilate).*
*ATC — G02CB01; N04BC01.*

**Pharmacopoeias.** In *Eur.* (see p.vi), *Jpn*, and *US.*
**Ph. Eur. 5.0** (Bromocriptine Mesilate). A white or slightly coloured fine crystalline powder. Practically insoluble in water; soluble in alcohol; sparingly soluble in dichloromethane; freely soluble in methyl alcohol. A 1% solution in a mixture of 2 parts methyl alcohol to 8 of water has a pH of 3.1 to 3.8. Store in airtight containers at a temperature not exceeding −15°. Protect from light.
**USP 27** (Bromocriptine Mesylate). A white or slightly coloured fine crystalline powder; odourless or having a weak characteristic odour. Store in airtight containers at a temperature not exceeding 8°. Protect from light.

### Adverse Effects

Nausea is the most common side-effect at the beginning of treatment with bromocriptine, but vomiting, dizziness, and orthostatic hypotension may also occur. Syncope has followed initial doses.

Side-effects are generally dose-related and may therefore be more frequent with the higher doses that have been used in the treatment of parkinsonism and acromegaly. Reduction of the dosage, followed in a few days by a more gradual increase, may alleviate many side-effects. Nausea may be reduced by taking bromocriptine with food.

Bromocriptine is a vasoconstrictor; digital vasospasm, induced by cold, and leg cramps have been reported. Other cardiovascular effects have included erythromelalgia, prolonged severe hypotension, arrhythmias, and exacerbation of angina. Very rarely hypertension, myocardial infarction, seizures or stroke (both sometimes preceded by severe headache or visual disturbances), and mental disorders have been reported in postpartum women given bromocriptine.

The use of ergot derivatives such as bromocriptine has been associated with retroperitoneal fibrosis, pleural thickening and effusions, and pericarditis and pericardial effusions.

Other side-effects reported include headache, nasal congestion, drowsiness, dry mouth, constipation, diarrhoea, and altered liver-function tests. Dyskinesias and psychomotor excitation have occurred in patients suffering from parkinsonism. Gastrointestinal bleeding has been reported in acromegalic patients. Psychosis, with hallucinations, delusions, and confusion, occurs particularly when high doses are used to treat parkinsonism, but has also been reported with low doses.

**Incidence of adverse effects.** In 27 published studies of bromocriptine in the treatment of Parkinson's disease, 217 of the 790 patients given bromocriptine had adverse effects.[1] Mental changes were noted in 90 patients, dyskinesia in 20, orthostatic hypotension in 40, and gastrointestinal effects in 40. The fewest adverse effects (9%) occurred with low-dose bromocriptine, more occurred with high-dose bromocriptine (27%) or with low-dose bromocriptine with levodopa (26%), and the most occurred with high-dose bromocriptine and levodopa (32%). However, those on high doses had more advanced disease and might be more susceptible to mental changes and dyskinesias.

An analysis by the manufacturer of published reports on patients treated with bromocriptine for 1 to 10 years concluded that in general, side-effects noted were no different from those associated with short-term treatment.[2]

1. Lieberman AN, Goldstein M. Bromocriptine in Parkinson disease. *Pharmacol Rev* 1985; **37:** 217–27.
2. Weil C. The safety of bromocriptine in long-term use: a review of the literature. *Curr Med Res Opin* 1986; **10:** 25–51.

**Effects on the blood.** Severe leucopenia and mild thrombocytopenia developed in a 23-year-old woman after treatment with bromocriptine 7.5 to 10 mg daily for about 3 months.[1]

1. Giampietro O, *et al.* Severe leukopenia and mild thrombocytopenia after chronic bromocriptine (CB-154) administration. *Am J Med Sci* 1981; **281:** 169–72.

**Effects on the cardiovascular system.** An early reviewer noted that asymptomatic **hypotension** occurred in many subjects given bromocriptine.[1] However, faintness and dizziness, sometimes accompanied by *nausea* and *vomiting*, were common at the start of treatment with bromocriptine and these symptoms rather than an anaphylactic type of reaction were likely to account for the collapse that occurred in a few sensitive patients. Two of 53 patients with Parkinson's disease fainted after an initial dose of 1.25 or 2.5 mg, but the exact incidence of shock-like syndromes was difficult to assess; the manufacturers had stated that 22 of over 10 000 subjects given bromocriptine had had hypotension and collapse, mainly at the start of treatment.

- All patients starting treatment should be warned of the possibility of fainting. The initial dose should not exceed 1.25 to 2.5 mg and should be taken with food and in bed.

If fainting does occur recovery is usually rapid and spontaneous. Tolerance to side-effects such as hypotension and nausea may develop rapidly.

*Hypertension, seizures, stroke*, and *myocardial infarction* have been associated with bromocriptine therapy, notably in postpartum women.[2-4] A study involving 1813 women suggested that the risk of **postpartum hypertension** was increased in women who experienced pregnancy-induced hypertension and that this risk was further increased in those who took bromocriptine for suppression of lactation.[5] A case-controlled study[6] involving 43 of the women who had had postpartum seizures while taking bromocriptine found that while the initial risk of seizures appeared to be lower in patients taking bromocriptine there was a small positive association with seizures occurring more than 72 hours after delivery.

- Although a causal relationship between the use of bromocriptine and these adverse effects in postpartum women has not been established the manufacturer recommends that bromocriptine should not be used postpartum or in the puerperium in women with high blood pressure, coronary artery disease, or symptoms or history of serious mental disorders.
- It is also recommended that when bromocriptine is used in postpartum women blood pressure should be carefully monitored, especially during the first few days and if hypertension, unremitting headache, or signs of CNS toxicity develop treatment should be discontinued immediately.

Fibrotic reactions (see also Effects on the Respiratory Tract, below) resulting in constrictive **pericarditis**[7] or **valvular heart disease**[8] have been reported.

1. Parkes D. Side effects of bromocriptine. *N Engl J Med* 1980; **302:** 749–50.
2. Anonymous. Postpartum hypertension, seizures, strokes reported with bromocriptine. *FDA Drug Bull* 1984; **14:** 3.
3. Ruch A, Duhring JL. Postpartum myocardial infarction in a patient receiving bromocriptine. *Obstet Gynecol* 1989; **74:** 448–51.
4. Larrazet F, *et al.* Possible bromocriptine-induced myocardial infarction. *Ann Intern Med* 1993; **118:** 199–200.
5. Watson DL, *et al.* Bromocriptine mesylate for lactation suppression: a risk for postpartum hypertension? *Obstet Gynecol* 1989; **74:** 573–6.
6. Rothman KJ, *et al.* Bromocriptine and puerperal seizures. *Epidemiology* 1990; **1:** 232–8.
7. Champagne S, *et al.* Chronic constrictive pericarditis induced by long-term bromocriptine therapy: report of two cases. *Ann Pharmacother* 1999; **33:** 1050–4.
8. Serratrice J, *et al.* Fibrotic valvular heart disease subsequent to bromocriptine treatment. *Cardiol Rev* 2002; **10:** 334–6.

**Effects on the ears.** Audiometric evidence of bilateral sensorineural hearing loss was reported in 3 patients receiving bromocriptine 15 or 20 mg daily for chronic hepatic encephalopathy.[1] Hearing improved when the dose was reduced to 10 mg daily.

1. Lanthier PL, *et al.* Bromocriptine-associated ototoxicity. *J Laryngol Otol* 1984; **98:** 399–404.

**Effects on electrolytes.** There have been isolated reports of severe hyponatraemia associated with the use of bromocriptine.[1,2]

1. Marshall AW, *et al.* Bromocriptine-associated hyponatraemia in cirrhosis. *BMJ* 1982; **285:** 1534–5.
2. Damase-Michel C, *et al.* Hyponatraemia in a patient treated with bromocriptine. *Drug Invest* 1993; **5:** 285–7.

**Effects on the eyes.** Blurred vision and diplopia has been reported in several patients receiving bromocriptine.[1] Reversible myopia also developed in a patient with hyperprolactinaemia given bromocriptine.[2]

In a patient with progressive visual loss due to compression of the optic chiasm by a large pituitary tumour, administration of bromocriptine caused total visual loss within hours.[3] Vision slowly returned to normal when the patient was placed in the supine position; the most likely cause of the visual loss was thought to be orthostatic hypotension with resultant decrease in perfusion pressure to the visual system.

Bromocriptine has been reported to cause visual cortical disturbances.[4] In some cases blurred vision and transient cortical blindness have preceded seizures and strokes.

1. Calne DB, *et al.* Long-term treatment of parkinsonism with bromocriptine. *Lancet* 1978; **i:** 735–7.
2. Manor RS, *et al.* Myopia during bromocriptine treatment. *Lancet* 1981; **i:** 102.
3. Couldwell WT, Weiss MH. Visual loss associated with bromocriptine. *Lancet* 1992; **340:** 1410–11.
4. Lane RJM, Routledge PA. Drug-induced neurological disorders. *Drugs* 1983; **26:** 124–47.

**Effects on mental function.** High doses of bromocriptine are well known to cause **psychotic reactions** in patients with parkinsonism.[1] However, mania has also been associated with the use of bromocriptine post partum[2,3] and it has been stated that psychological symptoms may occur with doses of only 2.5 to 5 mg daily.[4] It was also noted that, unlike the relatively mild and transient symptoms associated with levodopa, bromocriptine produces a severe psychosis in which the patient is violent and aggressive, suffering from intense delusions which are often hostile and violent; complete withdrawal of bromocriptine may still leave a residue of severe psychotic illness persisting for 1 to 3 weeks. Psychosis associated with low doses of bromocriptine has often occurred in patients with a history of psychotic illness or disturbances in behaviour and mood prior to treatment.[5-7] Drug-related psychotic reactions have also been reported in patients with no psychiatric history;[8,9] of 600 patients given bromocriptine or lisuride for the treatment of acromegaly or prolactinoma, 8 developed symptoms including anxiety, depression, auditory hallucinations, delusions, hyperactivity, disinhibition, euphoria, and insomnia and 4 had received doses only previously associated with psychosis in susceptible patients.[9]

For reference to **pathological gambling** reported in patients with Parkinson's disease receiving dopamine agonists, see under Levodopa, p.1206.

For reports of **daytime somnolence** occurring in patients receiving dopamine agonists including bromocriptine, see under Levodopa, p.1206.

1. Calne DB, *et al.* Long-term treatment of parkinsonism with bromocriptine. *Lancet* 1978; **i:** 735–7.
2. Vlissides DN, *et al.* Bromocriptine-induced mania? *BMJ* 1978; **1:** 510.
3. Brook NM, Cookson IB. Bromocriptine-induced mania? *BMJ* 1978; **1:** 790.
4. Pearce I, Pearce JMS. Bromocriptine in parkinsonism. *BMJ* 1978; **1:** 1402–4.
5. Pearson KC. Mental disorders from low-dose bromocriptine. *N Engl J Med* 1981; **305:** 173.
6. Le Feuvre CM, *et al.* Bromocriptine-induced psychosis in acromegaly. *BMJ* 1982; **285:** 1315.
7. Procter AW, *et al.* Bromocriptine induced psychosis in acromegaly. *BMJ* 1983; **286:** 50. Correction. *ibid.*; 311.
8. Einarson TR, Turchet EN. Psychotic reaction to low-dose bromocriptine. *Clin Pharm* 1983; **2:** 273–4.
9. Turner TH, *et al.* Psychotic reactions during treatment of pituitary tumours with dopamine agonists. *BMJ* 1984; **289:** 1101–3.

**Effects on the nervous system.** A report of 2 cases of cerebrospinal-fluid rhinorrhoea associated with the use of bromocriptine after partial surgical resection of prolactinoma.[1]

For reference to seizures associated with the use of bromocriptine in postpartum women, see under Effects on the Cardiovascular System, above.

1. Baskin DS, Wilson CB. CSF rhinorrhea after bromocriptine for prolactinoma. *N Engl J Med* 1982; **306:** 178.

**Effects on the respiratory tract.** Interstitial lung disease, with dyspnoea, chest pain, cough, and pulmonary fibrosis was reported in a patient after use of relatively high doses of bromocriptine (62 mg daily) for Parkinson's disease.[1] Respiratory symptoms largely resolved on withdrawal of the drug, although functional respiratory changes and moderate dyspnoea persisted after 6 months. A review of the literature revealed several other reports of pleuro-pulmonary fibrosis associated with relatively high doses of bromocriptine. Although the incidence of this effect did not seem to be high, similar cases continue to be reported.[2-4]

In April 2002 the UK Committee on Safety of Medicines calculated crude reporting rates of fibrotic reactions associated with the ergot derivative dopamine agonists (bromocriptine, cabergoline, lisuride, and pergolide), based on data submitted to its Yellow Card scheme and estimated drug exposure.[5] Pergolide was found to be associated with a higher reporting rate of fibrotic reactions compared with the other ergot derivatives; however, this result needed further investigation to see if it reflected a true increase in risk or was due to factors such as reporting biases.

1. Vergeret J, *et al.* Fibrose pleuro-pulmonaire et bromocriptine. *Sem Hop Paris* 1984; **60:** 741–4.
2. Kinnunen E, Viljanen A. Pleuropulmonary involvement during bromocriptine treatment. *Chest* 1988; **94:** 1034–6.
3. Macak IA, *et al.* Bromocriptine-induced pulmonary disease. *Can J Hosp Pharm* 1991; **44:** 37–8, xxiv.
4. Debove P, *et al.* Pleuropneumopathie à la bromocriptine chez un parkinsonien: revue de la littérature à propos d'une nouvelle observation. *Ann Med Interne (Paris)* 1998; **149:** 167–71.
5. Committee on Safety of Medicines/Medicines Control Agency. Fibrotic reactions with pergolide and other ergot-derived receptor agonists. *Current Problems* 2002; **28:** 3. Also available at: http://www.mca.gov.uk/ourwork/monitorsafequalmed/currentproblems/cpapril2002.pdf (accessed 13/04/04)

**Effects on sexual function.** Severe hypersexuality has been reported in a middle-aged man receiving bromocriptine and levodopa for Parkinson's disease.[1] About 3 years after the onset of hypersexuality he developed paranoid-hallucinatory psychoses that subsided on the reduction of dosage. It was apparent that addictive abuse of dopaminergic drugs had occurred. Clitoral tumescence and increased libido has been noted in a woman receiving bromocriptine to suppress lactation[2] but there has been a report of sexual dissatisfaction and decreased libido in 3 women receiving bromocriptine for hyperprolactinaemia.[3]

1. Vogel HP, Schiffter R. Hypersexuality—a complication of dopaminergic therapy in Parkinson's disease. *Pharmacopsychiatry* 1983; **16:** 107–10.
2. Blin O, *et al.* Painful clitoral tumescence during bromocriptine therapy. *Lancet* 1991; **337:** 1231–2.
3. Saleh AK, Moussa MAA. Sexual dysfunction in women due to bromocriptine. *BMJ* 1984; **289:** 228.

**Effects on the urinary tract.** Constant dribbling urinary incontinence developed in a woman receiving bromocriptine 2.5 mg daily for a recurrent pituitary growth; symptoms resolved on discontinuing the drug and recurred on rechallenge.[1] Bromocriptine has been shown to have two effects, one on the bladder outflow tract and one on the detrusor muscle, that could predispose to urinary incontinence.[2]

1. Sandyk R, Gillman MA. Urinary incontinence in patient on long-term bromocriptine. *Lancet* 1983; **ii:** 1260–1.
2. Caine M. Bromocriptine and urinary incontinence. *Lancet* 1984; **i:** 228.

**Hypersensitivity.** An allergic reaction developed in a 26-year-old woman being treated with bromocriptine for a prolactin-secreting microadenoma.[1] The patient reacted similarly to lisuride and treatment was continued with quinagolide.

1. Merola B, *et al.* Allergy to ergot-derived dopamine agonists. *Lancet* 1992; **339:** 620.

**Oedema.** Oedema poorly responsive to diuretics has been reported[1] in a patient given bromocriptine as part of treatment for prolactinoma. The oedema improved on substitution of pergolide but worsened with higher doses. Oedema resolved when treatment was changed to quinagolide. The reaction was considered to be idiosyncratic since enquiries by the author of the report had revealed only one similar case.

1. Blackard WG. Edema—an infrequently recognized complication of bromocriptine and other ergot dopaminergic drugs. *Am J Med* 1993; **94:** 445.

**Overdosage.** The most striking symptom in two children aged 2 and 2½ years who accidentally ingested an estimated 25 and 7.5 mg of bromocriptine, respectively, was lethargy with altered mental status.[1] The first child vomited and became sleepy. On admission he was markedly lethargic, but combative when disturbed, and also had hypotension, shallow breathing, dilated pupils, and hyperreflexic lower extremities. Nasogastric lavage was promptly performed and activated charcoal and then magnesium citrate administered. Blood pressure and ECG were monitored and glucose and sodium chloride solution infused. The other child vomited, became lethargic, and had dilated pupils. Ipecacuanha was administered and activated charcoal followed by magnesium citrate given by nasogastric tube. Both children recovered completely.

1. Vermund SH, *et al.* Accidental bromocriptine ingestion in childhood. *J Pediatr* 1984; **105:** 838–40.

**Withdrawal syndromes.** Transient galactorrhoea and hyperprolactinaemia occurred in a young woman after withdrawal of bromocriptine therapy for Parkinson's disease.[1] It was suggested the effects were due to a rebound phenomenon. For discussion of a syndrome resembling neuroleptic malignant syndrome that has developed on withdrawal of bromocriptine and other anti-parkinsonism drugs, see under Levodopa, p.1207.

1. Pentland B, Sawers JSA. Galactorrhoea after withdrawal of bromocriptine. *BMJ* 1980; **281:** 716.

## Precautions

Patients with hyperprolactinaemia should be investigated for the possibility of a pituitary tumour before treatment with bromocriptine. Annual gynaecological examinations (or every 6 months for postmenopausal women) are recommended. Treatment of women with hyperprolactinaemic amenorrhoea results in ovulation; such patients should be advised to use contraceptive measures other than an oral contraceptive. Acromegalic patients should be checked for symptoms of peptic ulceration before therapy and should immediately report symptoms of gastrointestinal discomfort during therapy.

Bromocriptine should be given with caution to patients with cardiovascular disease, Raynaud's syndrome, or a history of psychotic disorders. It is contra-indicated in patients with hypersensitivity to bromocriptine or other ergot alkaloids.

Bromocriptine is contra-indicated in the toxaemia of pregnancy. It should also not be used postpartum or in the puerperium in women with hypertension, coronary artery disease, or symptoms or a history of serious mental disorders. When used, blood pressure should be monitored carefully, especially during the first few days in postpartum women. Particular caution is necessary in patients who are receiving or who have recently received drugs that can alter blood pressure; use with ergot alkaloids during the puerperium is not recommended. Treatment in postpartum women should be discontinued immediately if hypertension, unremitting headache, or signs of CNS toxicity develop.

Hypotensive reactions may be disturbing in some patients during the first few days of treatment and those who drive or operate machinery should be warned of the possibility of dizziness and fainting during this period. Excessive daytime sleepiness and sudden onset of sleep may also occur with bromocriptine and caution is advised when driving or operating machinery; patients who suffer such effects should not drive or operate machinery until the effects have stopped recurring.

Patients on long-term, high-dose therapy should be monitored for signs of retroperitoneal fibrosis and bromocriptine withdrawn if fibrotic changes are diagnosed or suspected.

**Breast feeding.** The American Academy of Pediatrics[1] considers that bromocriptine should be given with caution to breast-feeding mothers, since it suppresses lactation and may be hazardous to the mother.

1. American Academy of Pediatrics. The transfer of drugs and other chemicals into human milk. *Pediatrics* 2001; **108:** 776–89. Correction. *ibid.*; 1029. Also available at: http://aappolicy.aappublications.org/cgi/content/full/pediatrics%3b108/3/776 (accessed 24/05/04)

**Porphyria.** Bromocriptine is considered to be unsafe in patients with porphyria because it has been shown to be porphyrinogenic in *in-vitro* systems.

**Pregnancy.** Details of various surveys of the effect of the use of bromocriptine during pregnancy have been published by the manufacturer.[1,2] The first survey was based on spontaneous reporting of all pregnancies between 1973 and 1980 in women who had taken bromocriptine after conception.[1] Information was obtained on 1410 pregnancies in 1335 women, the majority of whom had been treated for hyperprolactinaemic conditions, while in 256 pregnancies pituitary tumours and acromegaly were the primary diagnosis. Bromocriptine was generally taken at some time in the first 8 weeks after conception, the mean duration of treatment being 21 days. In 4 patients bromocriptine was not prescribed until late in pregnancy and in 9 with acromegaly and pituitary microadenoma it was taken continuously throughout gestation. There were 157 (11.1%) spontaneous abortions, 12 (0.9%) extrauterine pregnancies, 2 patients with 3 hydatidiform moles (0.2%), and an incidence of twin pregnancies of 1.8%. Major congenital abnormalities were detected in 12 (1%) infants at birth and minor abnormalities in 31 (2.5%). A second survey,[2] which consisted of formal monitoring of the use of bromocriptine at 33 clinics between 1979 and 1980, collected data on a further 743 pregnancies in 668 women and had similar findings. The incidence rates reported in these surveys were comparable with those quoted for normal populations and the data indicate that the use of bromocriptine in the treatment of women with infertility is not associated with an increased risk of abortion, multiple pregnancy, or congenital abnormalities. Furthermore, follow-up, for up to 9 years, of 546 children exposed to bromocriptine *in utero* found no evidence that bromocriptine had any adverse effect on postnatal development.[2] Nevertheless, since the risk of abortion is not increased by interruption of treatment, it is still recommended that bromocriptine therapy be stopped as soon as pregnancy is confirmed unless there is a definite indication for its continuation.

See also Pregnancy under Hyperprolactinaemia and Prolactinomas, below.

1. Turkalj I, *et al.* Surveillance of bromocriptine in pregnancy. *JAMA* 1982; **247:** 1589–91.
2. Krupp P, Monka C. Bromocriptine in pregnancy: safety aspects. *Klin Wochenschr* 1987; **65:** 823–7.

## Interactions

Dopamine antagonists such as the phenothiazines, butyrophenones, thioxanthenes, and metoclopramide (but see below) might be expected to reduce the prolactin-lowering and the antiparkinsonian effect of bromocriptine and domperidone might reduce its prolactin-lowering effect. Memantine may enhance the effects of bromocriptine. Concomitant administration of octreotide and bromocriptine increases the bioavailability of bromocriptine.

**Alcohol.** Alcohol intolerance was noted in 5 of 73 patients receiving bromocriptine 10 to 60 mg daily for the treatment of acromegaly.[1] Two patients who had gastrointestinal side-effects while taking low doses of bromocriptine had a marked reduction in their symptoms and were able to tolerate higher doses when they refrained completely from alcohol.[2]

1. Wass JAH, *et al.* Long-term treatment of acromegaly with bromocriptine. *BMJ* 1977; **1:** 875–8.
2. Ayres J, Maisey MN. Alcohol increases bromocriptine's side effects. *N Engl J Med* 1980; **302:** 806.

**Antibacterials.** Drowsiness, dystonia, choreoathetoid dyskinesias, and visual hallucinations occurred when *josamycin* was given to a patient receiving bromocriptine.[1]

The systemic bioavailability of a single oral dose of bromocriptine 5 mg was markedly increased in 5 healthy subjects following treatment with *erythromycin estolate* 250 mg four times daily for 4 days;[2] clearance of bromocriptine decreased by 70.6% and peak plasma concentrations of bromocriptine were more than 4 times higher than following the same dose before erythromycin administration.

1. Montastruc JL, Rascol A. Traitement de la maladie de Parkinson par doses élevées de bromocriptine: interaction possible avec la josamycine. *Presse Med* 1984; **13:** 2267–8.
2. Nelson MV, *et al.* Pharmacokinetic evaluation of erythromycin and caffeine administered with bromocriptine in normal subjects. *Clin Pharmacol Ther* 1990; **47:** 166.

**Antifungals.** The response to bromocriptine was blocked in a patient who was also receiving *griseofulvin*.[1]

1. Schwinn G, *et al.* Metabolic and clinical studies on patients with acromegaly treated with bromocriptine over 22 months. *Eur J Clin Invest* 1977; **7:** 101–7.

**Antipsychotics.** Serum concentrations of prolactin rose and visual fields deteriorated following administration of *thioridazine* to a 40-year-old man receiving bromocriptine therapy for a large prolactinoma.[1]

For a discussion of the effect of bromocriptine on patients receiving antipsychotics, see under Antiparkinsonian Drugs in Chlorpromazine on p.680.

1. Robbins RJ, *et al.* Interactions between thioridazine and bromocriptine in a patient with a prolactin-secreting pituitary adenoma. *Am J Med* 1984; **76:** 921–3.

**Metoclopramide.** As noted in Interactions, above, there are theoretical reasons to suppose that dopamine antagonists such as metoclopramide might reduce the effects of bromocriptine. However, an early study[1] in 10 patients with Parkinson's disease given single doses of bromocriptine 12.5 to 100 mg found that pretreatment with metoclopramide 60 mg had no consistent effect upon plasma concentrations of bromocriptine or growth hormone and no consistent effect upon clinical response.

1. Price P, *et al.* Plasma bromocriptine levels, clinical and growth hormone responses in parkinsonism. *Br J Clin Pharmacol* 1978; **6:** 303–9.

**Sympathomimetics.** There have been isolated reports[1,2] of severe hypertension, with headache and life-threatening complications, in patients taking bromocriptine with *isometheptene mucate* or *phenylpropanolamine*.

1. Kulig K, *et al.* Bromocriptine-associated headache: possible life-threatening sympathomimetic interaction. *Obstet Gynecol* 1991; **78:** 941–3.
2. Chan JCN, *et al.* Postpartum hypertension, bromocriptine and phenylpropanolamine. *Drug Invest* 1994; **8:** 254–6.

## Pharmacokinetics

Only about 30% of an oral dose of bromocriptine is absorbed from the gastrointestinal tract and, owing to extensive first-pass metabolism, the bioavailability is only about 6%. It is metabolised in the liver, mainly by hydrolysis to lysergic acid and peptides, and excreted chiefly in faeces via the bile, with small amounts in urine. It has been reported to be 90 to 96% bound to serum albumin *in vitro*.

◊ In a study involving 10 patients with Parkinson's disease, single doses of bromocriptine 12.5, 25, 50, and 100 mg resulted in very variable peak plasma concentrations ranging from 1.3 to 5.3, 1.4 to 3.5, 2.6 to 19.7, and 6.5 to 24.6 nanograms/mL, respectively, 30 to 210 minutes (mean 102 minutes) after dosage.[1] After 4 hours plasma concentrations were about 75% of the peak values. Clinical improvement was evident within 30 to 90 minutes of a dose with peak effect at about 130 minutes and in most patients improvement persisted throughout the 4-hour study period. Peak clinical response, peak fall in blood pressure, and peak rise in plasma concentrations of growth hormone occurred about 30, 60, and 70 minutes, respectively after peak plasma-bromocriptine concentrations but there was no significant relationship between them. However, there was a significant relationship between plasma concentrations and concurrent changes in clinical response compared with pretreatment scores. Dyskinesias occurred within 90 to 180 minutes of dosage in 5 of 10 patients.

Bromocriptine is well absorbed from standard oral tablets placed in the vagina and plasma concentrations sufficient to lower plasma prolactin concentrations have been achieved using this route.[2,3]

1. Price P, *et al.* Plasma bromocriptine levels, clinical and growth hormone responses in parkinsonism. *Br J Clin Pharmacol* 1978; **6:** 303–9.
2. Vermesh M, *et al.* Vaginal bromocriptine: pharmacology and effect on serum prolactin in normal women. *Obstet Gynecol* 1988; **72:** 693–8.
3. Katz E, *et al.* Successful treatment of a prolactin-producing pituitary macroadenoma with intravaginal bromocriptine mesylate: a novel approach to intolerance of oral therapy. *Obstet Gynecol* 1989; **73:** 517–20.

## Uses and Administration

Bromocriptine, an ergot derivative (p.1685), is a dopamine $D_2$-agonist. It inhibits the secretion of prolactin (p.1337) from the anterior pituitary and is used in the treatment of prolactinoma and in endocrinological disorders associated with hyperprolactinaemia, including amenorrhoea, galactorrhoea, hypogonadism, and infertility in both men and women. Bromocriptine is also used to suppress puerperal lactation for medical reasons; it is not recommended for the routine suppression of physiological lactation or for the treatment of postpartum breast pain and engorgement that may be adequately relieved with simple analgesics and breast support. Growth-hormone secretion may be suppressed by bromocriptine in some patients with acromegaly. Because of its dopaminergic activity bromocriptine is also used in the management of Parkinson's disease.

Bromocriptine is usually administered by mouth as the mesilate; doses are expressed in terms of the base. Bromocriptine mesilate 2.87 mg is approximately equivalent to 2.5 mg of bromocriptine. Oral doses should be taken with food. Bromocriptine mesilate has also been given intramuscularly as a depot injection for disorders associated with hyperprolactinaemia.

For the **prevention of puerperal lactation** bromocriptine 2.5 mg is given on the day of delivery followed by 2.5 mg twice daily for 14 days. The risk of hypotension and, more rarely, hypertension must be borne in mind and it has been recommended that bromocriptine should not be given until at least 4 hours after delivery. For the **suppression of established lactation** it is given in a dose of 2.5 mg daily for 2 to 3 days subsequently increased to 2.5 mg twice daily for 14 days.

For the treatment of other conditions (see below) the dose of bromocriptine is usually increased gradually. In the UK, typically, an initial dose of 1 to 1.25 mg at night is given, increased to 2 to 2.5 mg at night after 2 to 3 days, and subsequently increased by 1 to 2.5 mg at intervals of 2 to 3 days to a dose of 2.5 mg twice daily, or more if necessary. In the USA, increments of 2.5 mg are used, usually at intervals of 3 to 7 days.

In the **treatment of hypogonadism and galactorrhoea syndromes and infertility** bromocriptine is introduced gradually as described above. Most patients with hyperprolactinaemia respond to 7.5 mg daily but up to 30 mg daily may be required. Infertile patients without raised serum concentrations of prolactin are usually given 2.5 mg twice daily. In patients known to have **prolactinomas** the dose is increased gradually up to 5 mg every 6 hours but occasionally patients may require up to 30 mg daily.

In **cyclical benign breast and menstrual disorders** bromocriptine is introduced gradually up to a usual dosage of 2.5 mg twice daily.

Bromocriptine may be used as an adjunct to surgery and radiotherapy to reduce growth-hormone concentrations in plasma in **acromegalic patients**. It is introduced gradually up to a dose of 2.5 mg twice daily and may then be increased further by 2.5 mg every 2 to 3 days if necessary up to 5 mg every 6 hours, according to response.

In **Parkinson's disease** bromocriptine has been used alone, although it is usually given as an adjunct to levodopa treatment. It should be introduced even more gradually than the regimen above, and during this period patients already receiving levodopa can have their levodopa dosage decreased gradually until an optimal response is achieved. A suggested initial dose is the equivalent of 1 to 1.25 mg of bromocriptine at night during week 1, increased to 2 to 2.5 mg at night for week 2, 2.5 mg twice daily for week 3, and for week 4, 2.5 mg three times daily; the dose may be increased thereafter by 2.5 mg every 3 to 14 days depending on response. Most patients require doses within the range of 10 to 40 mg daily.

**Acromegaly.** Dopaminergics can produce a paradoxical reduction in growth hormone secretion and bromocriptine has been used in acromegaly (p.1312) as adjunctive therapy to surgery, radiotherapy, or somatostatin analogues to reduce circulating growth hormone levels. While it is less effective than octreotide, it can be given orally and is therefore more convenient to administer.

**Cushing's syndrome.** There have been occasional reports of benefit with the use of bromocriptine in the treatment of Cushing's syndrome (p.1313). Remission of ACTH-dependent Cushing's syndrome was maintained for 6 years by bromocriptine 2.5 mg twice daily in a patient who had initially received pituitary irradiation.[1] However, the same group subsequently reported that they had found that bromocriptine did not effectively reduce ACTH secretion following bilateral adrenalectomy.[2]


1. Atkinson AB, *et al.* Six year remission of ACTH-dependent Cushing's syndrome using bromocriptine. *Postgrad Med J* 1985; **61:** 239–42.
2. Atkinson AB. The treatment of Cushing's syndrome. *Clin Endocrinol (Oxf)* 1991; **34:** 507–13.


**Hyperprolactinaemia and prolactinomas.** Prolactinomas (prolactin-secreting pituitary adenomas) are among the commonest causes of hyperprolactinaemia. Raised serum-prolactin concentrations may result in reduced gonadotrophin production, which in turn may suppress gonadal function. Consequences may include oligomenorrhoea or amenorrhoea, and infertility in either sex. Galactorrhoea may also result from high prolactin levels and can occur in men as well as women.

Dopamine is the major inhibitory factor in the hypothalamus and directly inhibits the secretion of prolactin. Bromocriptine, a dopamine agonist, has been the first choice of treatment in many centres for the treatment of hyperprolactinaemia secondary to a prolactinoma although cabergoline is now preferred by some. Bromocriptine is extremely effective in controlling elevated circulating prolactin concentrations and restoring gonadal function; although it is rarely curative, it may produce considerable shrinkage of the adenoma.[1-5]

The sensitivity of hyperprolactinaemia to bromocriptine therapy can vary considerably between patients and this is reflected in the wide range of oral doses required to reduce prolactin concentrations to normal levels. Although methods such as initiating therapy with gradually increasing doses can minimise adverse effects it has been reported that about 5 to 10% of patients are unable to tolerate oral bromocriptine;[6] various other routes of administration have therefore been investigated. Bromocriptine is well absorbed from standard oral tablets placed in the vagina and appears to be both effective in lowering prolactin concentrations and well tolerated when given by this route.[7] However, limitations are considered to be the relatively short duration of action and the relatively low dose that can be administered.[6] Of the various injectable depot formulations that have been tried, one preparation given intramuscularly in a dose of 50 to 250 mg monthly has been found to be effective and well tolerated in long-term studies;[8,9] it is reported to be used in some centres to initiate treatment for macroprolactinomas.[6]

For discussions of the management of hyperprolactinaemia and associated disorders see p.1315 (hyperprolactinaemia), p.1313 (amenorrhoea), p.1316 (hypogonadism), p.1745 (erectile dysfunction), and p.1316 (infertility).


1. Prescott RWG, *et al.* Hyperprolactinaemia in men—response to bromocriptine therapy. *Lancet* 1982; **i:** 245–8.
2. Hancock KW, *et al.* Long term suppression of prolactin concentrations after bromocriptine induced regression of pituitary prolactinomas. *BMJ* 1985; **290:** 117–8.
3. Grossman A, Besser GM. Prolactinomas. *BMJ* 1985; **290:** 182–4.
4. Liuzzi A, *et al.* Low doses of dopamine agonists in the long-term treatment of macroprolactinomas. *N Engl J Med* 1985; **313:** 656–9.
5. Ho KY, Thorner MO. Therapeutic applications of bromocriptine in endocrine and neurological diseases. *Drugs* 1988; **36:** 67–82.
6. Ciccarelli E, Camanni F. Diagnosis and drug therapy of prolactinoma. *Drugs* 1996; **51:** 954–65.
7. Ginsburg J, *et al.* Vaginal bromocriptine. *Lancet* 1991; **338:** 1205–6.
8. Ciccarelli E, *et al.* Long term therapy of patients with macroprolactinoma using repeatable injectable bromocriptine. *J Clin Endocrinol Metab* 1993; **76:** 484–8.
9. Ciccarelli E, *et al.* Double blind randomized study using oral or injectable bromocriptine in patients with hyperprolactinaemia. *Clin Endocrinol (Oxf)* 1994; **40:** 193–8.


PREGNANCY. References to the management of prolactinoma during pregnancy.[1-3] Bromocriptine has been successfully used for management in pregnant women, particularly if there is symptomatic enlargement of the tumour, although there continues to be debate on the appropriateness of continuous therapy in less high-risk individuals.


1. Randeva HS, *et al.* Prolactinoma and pregnancy *Br J Obstet Gynaecol* 2000; **107:** 1064–8.
2. Bronstein MD, *et al.* Medical management of pituitary adenomas: the special case of management of the pregnant woman. *Pituitary* 2002; **5:** 99–107.
3. Chiodini I, Liuzzi A. PRL-secreting pituitary adenomas in pregnancy. *J Endocrinol Invest* 2003; **26:** 96–9.


**Lactation inhibition.** Because of its effects on prolactin, bromocriptine is a potent suppressor of lactation and has been widely used for the prevention of lactation in women who choose not to breast feed postpartum. However, bromocriptine has been associated with severe adverse effects in some women, and its use to suppress a physiological state has been criticised (see p.1317). Consequently, the manufacturers in a number of countries recommend that bromocriptine should only be used to suppress puerperal lactation for medical reasons; it is also not recommended for the treatment of postpartum breast pain and engorgement that may be adequately relieved with simple analgesics and breast support.

**Mastalgia.** Since mastalgia (p.1546) can improve spontaneously, treatment should rarely be considered unless pain has been present for about 6 months. Bromocriptine is one of the drugs that may be used to treat mastalgia.[1,2] It may improve symptoms in up to about 50% of patients with cyclical mastalgia, but is less effective in the non-cyclical form.[3,4] Adverse effects can be severe in some patients.


1. Gateley CA, Mansel RE. Management of the painful and nodular breast. *Br Med Bull* 1991; **47:** 284–94.
2. Anonymous. Cyclical breast pain—what works and what doesn't. *Drug Ther Bull* 1992; **30:** 1–3.
3. Pye JK, *et al.* Clinical experience of drug treatments for mastalgia. *Lancet* 1985; **ii:** 373–7.
4. Mansel RE, Dogliotti L. European multicentre trial of bromocriptine in cyclical mastalgia. *Lancet* 1990; **335:** 190–3.


**Neuroleptic malignant syndrome.** Bromocriptine has been used in doses of up to 30 mg daily,[1-6] usually alone or with dantrolene, in the treatment of neuroleptic malignant syndrome (p.677) although some workers have not found it to be of use.[7]


1. Mueller PS, *et al.* Neuroleptic malignant syndrome: successful treatment with bromocriptine. *JAMA* 1983; **249:** 386–8.
2. Dhib-Jalbut S, *et al.* Treatment of the neuroleptic malignant syndrome with bromocriptine. *JAMA* 1983; **250:** 484–5.
3. Clarke CE, *et al.* Clinical spectrum of neuroleptic malignant syndrome. *Lancet* 1988; **ii:** 969–70.
4. Guerrero RM, Shifrar KA. Diagnosis and treatment of neuroleptic malignant syndrome. *Clin Pharm* 1988; **7:** 697–701.
5. Lo TCM, *et al.* Neuroleptic malignant syndrome: another medical cause of acute abdomen. *Postgrad Med J* 1989; **65:** 653–5.
6. Chandran GJ, *et al.* Neuroleptic malignant syndrome: case report and discussion. *Can Med Assoc J* 2003; **169:** 439–42.
7. Rosebush PI, *et al.* The treatment of neuroleptic malignant syndrome: are dantrolene and bromocriptine useful adjuncts to supportive care? *Br J Psychiatry* 1991; **159:** 709–12.


**Parkinsonism.** Dopamine agonists such as bromocriptine are often used to begin treatment of parkinsonism (p.1196), particularly in younger patients, in an attempt to delay therapy with levodopa. They also have an adjunctive use when levodopa is no longer effective alone or cannot be tolerated and may sometimes be useful in reducing 'off' periods with levodopa and in ameliorating other fluctuations of mobility in the later stage of the disease.

References.


1. Temlett JA, *et al.* Adjunctive therapy with bromocriptine in Parkinson's disease. *S Afr Med J* 1990; **78:** 680–5.
2. Hely MA, *et al.* The Sydney Multicentre Study of Parkinson's disease: a randomised, prospective five year study comparing low dose bromocriptine with low dose levodopa-carbidopa. *J Neurol Neurosurg Psychiatry* 1994; **57:** 903–10.
3. Montastruc JL, *et al.* A randomised controlled study comparing bromocriptine to which levodopa was later added, with levodopa alone in previously untreated patients with Parkinson's disease: a five year follow up. *J Neurol Neurosurg Psychiatry* 1994; **57:** 1034–8.
4. Giménez-Roldán S, *et al.* Early combination of bromocriptine and levodopa in Parkinson's disease: a prospective randomized study of two parallel groups over a total follow-up period of 44 months including an initial 8-month double-blind stage. *Clin Neuropharmacol* 1997; **20:** 67–76.
5. Ogawa N, *et al.* Nationwide multicenter prospective study on the long-term effects of bromocriptine for Parkinson's disease: final report of a ten-year follow-up. *Eur Neurol* 1997; **38** (suppl 2): 37–49.
6. Lees AJ, *et al.* Ten-year follow-up of three different initial treatments in de-novo PD: a randomized trial. *Neurology* 2001; **57:** 1687–94.
7. Ramaker C, van Hilten JJ. Bromocriptine versus levodopa in early Parkinson's disease. Available in The Cochrane Library; Issue 1. Chichester: John Wiley; 2004.


**Polycystic ovary syndrome.** Bromocriptine has been tried in women with the polycystic ovary syndrome (p.1317) who have mild basal hyperprolactinaemia without evidence of a pituitary tumour.

**Restless legs syndrome.** The aetiology of restless legs syndrome (see Parasomnias, p.667) is obscure and treatment has largely been empirical but dopaminergic therapy has emerged as a common first line choice. Bromocriptine showed some benefit in a small study.[1]


1. Walters AS, *et al.* A double-blind randomized crossover trial of bromocriptine and placebo in restless legs syndrome. *Ann Neurol* 1988; **24:** 455–8.


**Withdrawal syndromes.** ALCOHOL. Studies of the efficacy of bromocriptine as an aid in the maintenance of abstinence from alcohol (p.1166) have yielded conflicting results.[1-4] However, it has been suggested[3] that response to bromocriptine might be linked to a specific genotype of the $D_2$ dopamine receptor.


1. Dongier M, *et al.* Bromocriptine in the treatment of alcohol dependence. *Alcohol Clin Exp Res* 1991; **15:** 970–7.
2. Naranjo CA, *et al.* Long-acting bromocriptine (B) does not reduce relapse in alcoholics. *Clin Pharmacol Ther* 1995; **57:** 161.
3. Lawford BR, *et al.* Bromocriptine in the treatment of alcoholics with the $D_2$ dopamine receptor A1 allele. *Nat Med* 1995; **1:** 337–41.
4. Powell BJ, *et al.* A double-blind, placebo-controlled study of nortriptyline and bromocriptine in male alcoholics subtyped by comorbid psychiatric disorders. *Alcohol Clin Exp Res* 1995; **19:** 462–8.


## Preparations

***BP 2003:*** Bromocriptine Capsules; Bromocriptine Tablets;
***USP 27:*** Bromocriptine Mesylate Capsules; Bromocriptine Mesylate Tablets.

**Proprietary Preparations** (details are given in Part 3)
***Arg.:*** Parlodel; Serocryptin; ***Austral.:*** Bromohexal; Bromolactin; Kripton; Parlodel; ***Austria:*** Broman†; Bromed; Cehapark; Parlodel; Umprel; ***Belg.:*** Parlodel; ***Braz.:*** Bagren; Parlodel; ***Canad.:*** Parlodel; ***Chile:*** Criten; Grifocriptina; Kriptonal; Parlodel; Prigost; ***Denm.:*** Bromergon; Bromopar†; Parlodel; ***Fin.:*** Parlodel; ***Fr.:*** Bromo-Kin; Parlodel; ***Ger.:*** Bromocrel; kirim; kirim gyn; Pravidel; ***Gr.:*** Parlodel; ***Hong Kong:*** Bromtine; Medocriptine; Parlodel; Serocryptin; Zolac†; ***India:*** Sicriptin; ***Irl.:*** Parlodel; ***Israel:*** Parilac; Parlodel; ***Ital.:*** Parlodel; ***Malaysia:*** Butin; Criptamine; Medocriptine; Parlodel; Zolac; ***Mex.:*** Broptin; Crilem; Cryocriptina; Inovapar†; Kriptiser; Lactess†; Mesiken†; Parlodel; Serocryptin; ***Neth.:*** Parlodel; ***Norw.:*** Parlodel; ***NZ:*** Parlodel†; ***Port.:*** Parlodel; ***S.Afr.:*** Parlodel; ***Singapore:*** Butin; Parlodel; Serocryptin†; Suplac; ***Spain:*** Parlodel; ***Swed.:*** Pravidel; ***Switz.:*** Parlodel; Serocryptin†; ***Thai.:*** Bromergon; Parlodel; Serocryptin†; Suplac; ***UAE:*** Antiprotin; ***UK:*** Parlodel; ***USA:*** Parlodel.

---

## Budipine *(rINN)*

Budipino. 1-*tert*-Butyl-4,4-diphenylpiperidine.
*$C_{21}H_{27}N$ = 293.4.*
*CAS — 57982-78-2.*
*ATC — N04BX03.*

### Profile

Budipine is a phenylpiperidine derivative used as adjunctive therapy in the treatment of parkinsonism. It is given by mouth as the hydrochloride in daily doses up to 60 mg.

◊ References.


1. Spieker S, *et al.* Tremorlytic activity of budipine: a quantitative study with long-term tremor recordings. *Clin Neuropharmacol* 1995; **18:** 266–72.
2. Groen H, *et al.* A study to investigate the pharmacokinetics and metabolism of budipine after administration of a single oral dose of [$^{14}$C]-B757-01 to six healthy volunteers. *Br J Clin Pharmacol* 1999; **48:** 771P–772P.
3. Malsch U, *et al.* Monotherapie der Parkinsonschen Erkrankung mit Budipin: ein randomisierter Doppelblindvergleich mit Amantadin. *Fortschr Neurol Psychiatr* 2001; **69:** 86–9.
4. Przuntek H, *et al.* Budipine provides additional benefit in patients with Parkinson disease receiving a stable optimum dopaminergic drug regimen. *Arch Neurol* 2002; **59:** 803–6.


## Preparations

**Proprietary Preparations** (details are given in Part 3)
***Ger.:*** Parkinsan.

---

# Cabergoline *(BAN, USAN, rINN)*

Cabergolina; FCE-21336. 1-[(6-Allylergolin-8β-yl)carbonyl]-1-[3-(dimethylamino)propyl]-3-ethylurea; (8*R*)-6-Allyl-*N*-[3-(dimethylamino)propyl]-*N*-(ethylcarbamoyl)ergoline-8-carboxamide.
*$C_{26}H_{37}N_5O_2$ = 451.6.*
*CAS — 81409-90-7.*
*ATC — G02CB03; N04BC06.*

## Adverse Effects and Precautions

As for Bromocriptine, p.1200, although patients unable to tolerate bromocriptine may tolerate cabergoline (and *vice versa*).

The manufacturer recommends that conception should be avoided for at least one month after treatment.

**Effects on mental function.** For reports of daytime somnolence occurring in patients receiving dopamine agonists including cabergoline, see Effects on Mental Function, under Adverse Effects of Levodopa, p.1206.

**Effects on the respiratory system.** A patient developed pleuropulmonary disease 16 months after starting treatment with cabergoline.[1] The patient had previously received bromocriptine for 10 years and had had a normal chest X-ray at the time of transer to cabergoline treatment. In another report, 2 cases of pleural effusion/pulmonary fibrosis, occurring after 10 to 11 months of treatment, were described.[2] One patient had modest pre-treatment lung alterations attributed to previous bromocriptine therapy. Withdrawal was associated with improvement in both cases. Congestive heart failure secondary to constrictive pericarditis, and severe pleuropulmonary fibrosis that resulted in persistent dyspnoea have also been reported in a patient receiving cabergoline.[3]


1. Bhatt MH, *et al.* Pleuropulmonary disease associated with dopamine agonist therapy. *Ann Neurol* 1991; **30:** 613–16.

2. Geminiani G, *et al.* Cabergoline in Parkinson's disease complicated by motor fluctuations. *Mov Disord* 1996; **11:** 495–500.
3. Ling LH, *et al.* Constrictive pericarditis and pleuropulmonary disease linked to ergot dopamine agonist therapy (cabergoline) for Parkinson's disease. *Mayo Clin Proc* 1999; **74:** 371–5.

**Oedema.** Three cases of lower limb oedema following chronic treatment with cabergoline have been reported.[1] In one case the oedema was severe enough to necessitate withdrawal of therapy.

1. Geminiani G, *et al.* Cabergoline in Parkinson's disease complicated by motor fluctuations. *Mov Disord* 1996; **11:** 495–500.

## Interactions

As for Bromocriptine, p.1202.

## Pharmacokinetics

Cabergoline is absorbed from the gastrointestinal tract and extensively metabolised to several metabolites that do not appear to contribute to its pharmacological activity. Plasma protein binding has been estimated to be about 40%. Cabergoline is mainly eliminated via the faeces; a small proportion is excreted in the urine.

◊ Pharmacokinetic studies of cabergoline have been hampered by lack of an assay method sensitive enough to detect plasma concentrations of cabergoline following therapeutic doses. However, the plasma elimination half-life of cabergoline has been estimated indirectly to be 63 to 68 hours in healthy subjects and 79 to 115 hours in patients with hyperprolactinaemia.[1]

1. Rains CP, *et al.* Cabergoline: a review of its pharmacological properties and therapeutic potential in the treatment of hyperprolactinaemia and inhibition of lactation. *Drugs* 1995; **49:** 255–79.

## Uses and Administration

Cabergoline, an ergot derivative, is a dopamine $D_2$-agonist with actions and uses similar to those of bromocriptine (p.1202). It is a potent and long-lasting inhibitor of prolactin secretion used in the management of disorders associated with hyperprolactinaemia. It is also used to suppress puerperal lactation for medical reasons; it is not recommended for the routine suppression of physiological lactation or for the treatment of postpartum breast pain and engorgement that may be adequately relieved with simple analgesics and breast support. Cabergoline is also used in the management of Parkinson's disease.

Cabergoline is administered by mouth and should be taken with food.

To **inhibit physiological lactation**, cabergoline is given as a single 1-mg dose on the first day postpartum. For **suppression of established lactation**, the dose is 250 micrograms every 12 hours for 2 days.

In the treatment of **disorders associated with hyperprolactinaemia**, the initial dose of cabergoline is 500 micrograms weekly. The dose is then increased at monthly intervals in increments of 500 micrograms weekly according to response. The weekly dose may be administered on a single occasion or divided into 2 doses on separate days; doses over 1 mg should be given as divided doses. The usual dose is 1 mg weekly but up to 4.5 mg has been used.

In **Parkinson's disease**, cabergoline is used as an adjunct in patients experiencing 'on-off' fluctuations in control with levodopa treatment. It should be introduced gradually and during this period the dose of levodopa may be reduced gradually until an optimal response is achieved. A suggested initial dose of cabergoline is 1 mg as a single daily dose. The dose may be increased in increments of 0.5 or 1 mg at intervals of 7 or 14 days. The recommended therapeutic dose range is 2 to 6 mg daily.

◊ General references.

1. Rains CP, *et al.* Cabergoline: a review of its pharmacological properties and therapeutic potential in the treatment of hyperprolactinaemia and inhibition of lactation. *Drugs* 1995; **49:** 255–79.

**Acromegaly.** Dopamine agonists have been used in acromegaly (p.1312) as adjuvants to surgery, radiotherapy, or somatostatin analogues to reduce circulating growth hormone concentrations, although they are less effective than the somatostatin analogue octreotide. However, a small study comparing cabergoline with depot bromocriptine and quinagolide failed to find evidence of its effectiveness (see p.1213).

**Hyperprolactinaemia and prolactinomas.** Dopamine agonists are widely used for the treatment of hyperprolactinaemia secondary to a prolactinoma (see p.1315). Although bromocriptine has been the first choice for this indication, some now prefer cabergoline,[1] which appears to be more effective and better tolerated.[2,3]

Further references.[4-8]

1. Webster J. A comparative review of the tolerability profiles of dopamine agonists in the treatment of hyperprolactinaemia and inhibition of lactation. *Drug Safety* 1996; **14:** 228–38. Correction. *ibid.*, 342.
2. Pascal-Vigneron V, *et al.* Amenorrhée hyperprolactinémique: traitement par cabergoline versus bromocriptine. *Presse Med* 1995; **24:** 753–7.
3. di Sarno A, *et al.* Resistance to cabergoline as compared with bromocriptine in hyperprolactinemia: prevalence, clinical definition, and therapeutic strategy. *J Clin Endocrinol Metab* 2001; **86:** 5256–61.
4. Webster J, *et al.* The efficacy and tolerability of long-term cabergoline therapy in hyperprolactinaemic disorders: an open, uncontrolled, multicentre study. *Clin Endocrinol (Oxf)* 1993; **39:** 323–9.
5. Webster J, *et al.* A comparison of cabergoline and bromocriptine in the treatment of hyperprolactinemic amenorrhea. *N Engl J Med* 1994; **331:** 904–9.
6. Verhelst J, *et al.* Cabergoline in the treatment of hyperprolactinaemia: a study in 455 patients. *J Clin Endocrinol Metab* 1999; **84:** 2518–22.
7. Colao A, *et al.* Macroprolactinoma shrinkage during cabergoline treatment is greater in naive patients than in patients pretreated with other dopamine agonists: a prospective study in 110 patients. *J Clin Endocrinol Metab* 2000; **85:** 2247–52.
8. Colao A, *et al.* Withdrawal of long-term cabergoline therapy for tumoral and nontumoral hyperprolactinemia. *N Engl J Med* 2003; **349:** 2023–33.

**Lactation inhibition.** A single 1-mg dose of cabergoline was found to be as effective as bromocriptine 2.5 mg given twice daily for 14 days for preventing puerperal lactation in a double-blind multicentre study involving 272 women.[1] It has been suggested that cabergoline would be a better choice than bromocriptine for lactation inhibition.[2] However, as discussed on p.1317, the routine use of dopaminergics such as bromocriptine or cabergoline is not recommended for the suppression of physiological lactation.

1. European Multicentre Study Group for Cabergoline in Lactation Inhibition. Single dose cabergoline versus bromocriptine in inhibition of puerperal lactation: randomised, double blind, multicentre study. *BMJ* 1991; **302:** 1367–71.
2. Webster J. A comparative review of the tolerability profiles of dopamine agonists in the treatment of hyperprolactinaemia and inhibition of lactation. *Drug Safety* 1996; **14:** 228–38. Correction. *ibid.*; 342.

**Parasomnias.** The aetiology of *restless legs syndrome* is obscure and treatment has been largely empirical (p.667) but dopaminergic therapy has emerged as a common first-line choice. Long acting drugs such as cabergoline may be preferred in order to avoid the complications associated with levodopa therapy. Results from a 12-week open label pilot study[1] in 9 patients with idiopathic restless legs syndrome given cabergoline following insufficient response to levodopa therapy were promising; doses of cabergoline ranged from 1 to 4 mg.

1. Stiasny K, *et al.* Treatment of idiopathic restless legs syndrome (RLS) with the D2-agonist cabergoline—an open clinical trial. *Sleep* 2000; **23:** 349–54.

**Parkinsonism.** Cabergoline is used as a long-acting dopamine agonist in Parkinson's disease (p.1196). Dopamine agonists are often used to begin treatment in an attempt to delay therapy with levodopa, particularly in younger patients. They also have an adjunctive use when levodopa is no longer effective alone or cannot be tolerated, and may sometimes be useful in reducing 'off' periods with levodopa and in ameliorating other fluctuations of mobility in the later stages of the disease.

References.

1. Inzelberg R, *et al.* Double-blind comparison of cabergoline and bromocriptine in Parkinson's disease patients with motor fluctuations. *Neurology* 1996; **47:** 785–8.
2. Geminiani G, *et al.* Cabergoline in Parkinson's disease complicated by motor fluctuations. *Mov Disord* 1996; **11:** 495–500.
3. Hutton JT, *et al.* Multicenter, placebo-controlled trial of cabergoline taken once daily in the treatment of Parkinson's disease. *Neurology* 1996; **46:** 1062–5.
4. Marsden CD. Clinical experience with cabergoline in patients with advanced Parkinson's disease treated with levodopa. *Drugs* 1998; **55** (suppl 1): 17–22.
5. Rinne UK, *et al.* Early treatment of Parkinson's disease with cabergoline delays the onset of motor complications: results of a double-blind levodopa controlled trial. *Drugs* 1998; **55** (suppl 1): 23–30.
6. Clarke CE, Deane KH. Cabergoline for levodopa-induced complications in Parkinson's disease. Available in The Cochrane Library; Issue 1. Chichester: John Wiley; 2004.
7. Clarke CE, Deane KD. Cabergoline versus bromocriptine for levodopa-induced complications in Parkinson's disease. Available in The Cochrane Library; Issue 1. Chichester: John Wiley; 2004.

## Preparations

**Proprietary Preparations** (details are given in Part 3)

***Arg.:*** Cabaser; Dostinex; Lactamax; Triaspar; ***Austral.:*** Cabaser; Dostinex; ***Austria:*** Cabaseril; Dostinex; ***Belg.:*** Dostinex; Sostilar; ***Braz.:*** Dostinex; ***Chile:*** Dostinex; ***Denm.:*** Cabaser; Dostinex; ***Fin.:*** Cabaser; Dostinex; ***Fr.:*** Dostinex; ***Ger.:*** Cabaseril; Dostinex; ***Gr.:*** Dostinex; ***Hong Kong:*** Dostinex; ***Irl.:*** Cabaser; Dostinex; ***Israel:*** Cabaser; Dostinex; ***Ital.:*** Actualene; Cabaser; Dostinex; ***Malaysia:*** Dostinex; ***Mex.:*** Dostinex; ***Neth.:*** Dostinex; ***Norw.:*** Cabaser; Dostinex; ***NZ:*** Dostinex; ***Port.:*** Dostinex; ***S.Afr.:*** Dostinex; ***Singapore:*** Dostinex; ***Spain:*** Dostinex; Sogilen; ***Swed.:*** Cabaser; Dostinex; ***Switz.:*** Cabaser; Dostinex; ***UK:*** Cabaser; Dostinex; ***USA:*** Dostinex.

# Carbidopa *(BAN, USAN, rINN)*

Carbidopum; α-Methyldopa Hydrazine; MK-486. (+)-2-(3,4-Dihydroxybenzyl)-2-hydrazinopropionic acid monohydrate; (−)-L-α-Hydrazino-3,4-dihydroxy-α-methylhydrocinnamic acid monohydrate.

$C_{10}H_{14}N_2O_4,H_2O = 244.2.$

*CAS — 28860-95-9 (anhydrous); 38821-49-7 (monohydrate).*

NOTE. The synonym MK-485 has been used for the racemic mixture.

Compounded preparations of carbidopa and levodopa may be represented by the following names:

- Co-careldopa *x/y* (*BAN*)—where *x* and *y* are the strengths in milligrams of carbidopa and levodopa respectively
- Co-careldopa (*PEN*)—carbidopa and levodopa.

**Pharmacopoeias.** In *Chin., Eur.* (see p.vi), *Int., Jpn,* and *US.*

**Ph. Eur. 5.0** (Carbidopa). A white or yellowish-white powder. Slightly soluble in water; very slightly soluble in alcohol; practically insoluble in dichloromethane; dissolves in dilute solutions of mineral acids. Protect from light.

**USP 27** (Carbidopa). A white to creamy-white, odourless or practically odourless powder. Slightly soluble in water and in methyl alcohol; practically insoluble in alcohol, in acetone, in chloroform, and in ether; freely soluble in 3N hydrochloric acid. Protect from light.

## Adverse Effects

**Hypersensitivity.** Henoch-Schönlein purpura which developed in a 68-year-old patient being treated for Parkinson's disease appeared to be due to either carbidopa or an excipient of the preparation containing the carbidopa (Sinemet).[1]

1. Niedermaier G, Briner V. Henoch-Schönlein syndrome induced by carbidopa/levodopa. *Lancet* 1997; **349:** 1071–2.

## Pharmacokinetics

Carbidopa is rapidly but incompletely absorbed from the gastrointestinal tract. It is rapidly excreted in the urine both unchanged and in the form of metabolites. It does not cross the blood-brain barrier. In *rats*, carbidopa has been reported to cross the placenta and to be distributed into breast milk.

## Uses and Administration

Carbidopa is a peripheral dopa-decarboxylase inhibitor with little or no pharmacological activity when given alone in usual doses. It inhibits the peripheral decarboxylation of levodopa to dopamine and as, unlike levodopa, it does not cross the blood-brain barrier, effective brain concentrations of dopamine are produced with lower doses of levodopa. At the same time reduced peripheral formation of dopamine reduces peripheral side-effects, notably nausea and vomiting, and cardiac arrhythmias, although the dyskinesias and adverse mental effects associated with levodopa therapy tend to develop earlier. Contrary to its effect in patients on levodopa alone, pyridoxine does not inhibit the response to levodopa in patients also receiving a peripheral dopa-decarboxylase inhibitor.

In the treatment of parkinsonism carbidopa is given with levodopa to enable a lower dosage of the latter to be used and a more rapid response to be obtained, and to decrease side-effects. For details of administration and dosage, see Levodopa, p.1209.

Carbidopa also inhibits the peripheral decarboxylation of the serotonin precursor oxitriptan (p.311).

◊ General references.

1. Pinder RM, *et al.* Levodopa and decarboxylase inhibitors: a review of their clinical pharmacology and use in the treatment of parkinsonism. *Drugs* 1976; **11:** 329–77.
2. Boshes B. Sinemet and the treatment of parkinsonism. *Ann Intern Med* 1981; **94:** 364–70.

## Preparations

***BP 2003:*** Co-careldopa Tablets;
***USP 27:*** Carbidopa and Levodopa Tablets.

**Proprietary Preparations** (details are given in Part 3)
***USA:*** Lodosyn.

**Multi-ingredient:** ***Arg.:*** Lebocar; Lecarge; Nervocur; Sinemet; ***Austral.:*** Kinson; Sinacarb†; Sinemet; ***Austria:*** Sinemet; ***Belg.:*** Sinemet; ***Braz.:*** Carbidol; Cronomet; Levocarb; Sinemet; ***Canad.:*** Apo-Levocarb; Nu-Levocarb; Sinemet; ***Chile:*** Grifoparkin; Levofamil; Saniter Compuesto; Sinemet; ***Denm.:*** Sinemet; ***Fin.:*** Kardopal; Sinemet; ***Fr.:*** Sinemet; ***Ger.:*** Dopadura C; Isicom; Levo-C; Levobeta C; Levocarb; Levocomp; Levodop; Levodopa Comp; Levodopa comp C; Levodopa-Carbi; Nacom†; Striaton; Tremopar; ***Gr.:*** Sinemet; Zimox; ***Hong Kong:*** Apo-Levocarb; Levomed; Levomet; Sinedopa; Sinemet; ***India:*** Levopa-C; Syndopa; ***Irl.:*** Half Sinemet; Sinemet; ***Israel:*** Dopicar; Sinemet; ***Ital.:*** Sinemet; ***Malaysia:*** Apo-Levocarb; Levomed; Sinemet; ***Mex.:*** Cloisone; Lemdopa; Racovel; Sinemet; ***Neth.:*** Sinemet; ***Norw.:*** Sinemet; ***NZ:*** Apo-Levocarb†; Sindopa; Sinemet; ***Port.:*** Sinemet; ***S.Afr.:*** Carbilev; Sinemet; ***Singapore:*** Cardopar; Levomet; Sinemet; ***Spain:*** Sinemet; ***Swed.:*** Sinemet; ***Switz.:*** Sinemet; ***Thai.:*** Levomed; Sinemet; Syndopa; ***UK:*** Half Sinemet; Sinemet; Stalevo; ***USA:*** Atamet; Sinemet.

# Droxidopa *(rINN)*

L-*threo*-3,4-Dihydroxyphenylserine. (−)-*threo*-3-(3,4-Dihydroxyphenyl)-L-serine.

$C_9H_{11}NO_5 = 213.2.$

*CAS — 23651-95-8.*

## Profile

Droxidopa is a precursor of noradrenaline that is used in the treatment of parkinsonism and some forms of orthostatic hypotension. The usual maintenance dose is 600 mg daily for the treatment of parkinsonism and 300 to 600 mg daily in orthostatic hypotension; daily doses should be divided.

The racemic form (DL-*threo*-3,4-dihydroxyphenylserine) has been studied for similar uses.

◊ References.


1. Iida N, *et al.* Treatment of dialysis-induced hypotension with L-threo-3, 4-dihydroxyphenylserine. *Nephrol Dial Transplant* 1994; **9:** 1130–5.
2. Freeman R, *et al.* The treatment of neurogenic orthostatic hypotension with 3,4-DL-threo-dihydroxyphenylserine: a randomized, placebo-controlled, crossover trial. *Neurology* 1999; **10:** 2151–7.
3. Akizawa T, *et al.* Clinical effects of L-threo-3,4-dihydroxyphenylserine on orthostatic hypotension in hemodialysis patients. *Nephron* 2002; **90:** 384–90.


### Preparations

**Proprietary Preparations** (details are given in Part 3)
***Jpn:*** Dops.

## Entacapone *(BAN, USAN, rINN)*

Entacapona; OR-611. (*E*)-α-Cyano-*N*,*N*-diethyl-3,4-dihydroxy-5-nitrocinnamamide; (*E*)-2-Cyano-3-(3,4-dihydroxy-5-nitrophenyl)-*N*,*N*-diethylacrylamide.

$C_{14}H_{15}N_3O_5$ = 305.3.
*CAS — 130929-57-6.*
*ATC — N04BX02.*

### Adverse Effects

The most frequent adverse effects produced by entacapone relate to increased dopaminergic activity and occur most commonly at the start of treatment; reduction of the levodopa dosage may reduce the severity and frequency of such effects. Adverse effects may include nausea, vomiting, abdominal pain, constipation, diarrhoea, dry mouth, and dyskinesias. Increases in liver enzyme values have been reported rarely; there have also been isolated cases of cholestatic hepatitis. Entacapone may produce a harmless reddish-brown discoloration of the urine.

### Precautions

Entacapone is contra-indicated in patients with phaeochromocytoma and in patients with a history of neuroleptic malignant syndrome or nontraumatic rhabdomyolysis. It should be avoided in patients with hepatic impairment, and given with caution to patients with biliary obstruction. Use with levodopa may cause dizziness and orthostatic hypotension; if affected patients should not drive or operate machinery. Excessive daytime sleepiness and sudden onset of sleep may also occur with combination use (see Effects on Mental Function, in Levodopa, p.1206) and caution is advised when driving or operating machinery; patients who suffer such effects should not drive or operate machinery until the effects have stopped recurring.

Treatment with entacapone should not be stopped abruptly; when necessary withdrawal should be made gradually, increasing the dose of levodopa as required.

### Interactions

Use of entacapone with a non-selective MAOI is contra-indicated. Entacapone should be used with caution in patients receiving drugs metabolised by catechol-*O*-methyltransferase (COMT) including adrenaline, apomorphine, dobutamine, dopamine, isoprenaline, methyldopa, noradrenaline, and rimiterol.

Entacapone may aggravate levodopa-induced orthostatic hypotension and should be used cautiously in patients who are taking other drugs which may cause orthostatic hypotension.

Entacapone may form chelates with iron preparations in the gastrointestinal tract; the two drugs should be taken at least 2 to 3 hours apart.

### Pharmacokinetics

There are large intra- and interindividual variations in the absorption of entacapone. Peak plasma concentrations are achieved about one hour after oral administration. Entacapone undergoes extensive first-pass metabolism and oral bioavailability is about 35%. Absorption is not affected significantly by food. Entacapone is about 98% bound to plasma proteins. It is eliminated mainly in the faeces with about 10 to 20% being excreted in the urine, mainly as glucuronide conjugates.

◊ Entacapone is rapidly absorbed from the gastrointestinal tract and bioavailability following oral administration has been reported to range from 29 to 46%. It does not cross the blood-brain barrier. Over half of a dose appears in the faeces with smaller amounts being excreted in the urine as glucuronides of entacapone and its (*Z*)-isomer. Elimination half-lives of about 1.6 to 3.4 hours have been reported for entacapone.

References.


1. Wikberg T, *et al.* Identification of major metabolites of the catechol-O-methyltransferase inhibitor entacapone in rats and humans. *Drug Metab Dispos* 1993; **21:** 81–92.
2. Keränen T, *et al.* Inhibition of soluble catechol-O-methyltransferase and single-dose pharmacokinetics after oral and intravenous administration of entacapone. *Eur J Clin Pharmacol* 1994; **46:** 151–7.


### Uses and Administration

Entacapone is a selective, reversible, peripheral inhibitor of catechol-*O*-methyltransferase (COMT), an enzyme involved in the metabolism of dopamine and levodopa. It is used as an adjunct to combination preparations of levodopa and dopa-decarboxylase inhibitors, in patients with Parkinson's disease and 'end-of-dose' motor fluctuations who cannot be stabilised on levodopa combinations alone. Entacapone is given by mouth in a dosage of 200 mg at the same time as each dose of levodopa with dopa-decarboxylase inhibitor, up to a maximum of 200 mg ten times daily. It is often necessary to gradually reduce the dosage of levodopa by about 10 to 30% within the first few weeks after starting treatment with entacapone.

Entacapone may also be given as a combination preparation with carbidopa and levodopa; for dosage details, see Levodopa, p.1209.

**Parkinsonism.** Entacapone is a selective and reversible inhibitor of catechol-*O*-methyltransferase (COMT), with mainly peripheral actions. It is given as adjunctive therapy to patients with Parkinson's disease (p.1196) experiencing fluctuations in disability related to levodopa and dopa-decarboxylase inhibitor combinations. When levodopa is given with a peripheral dopa-decarboxylase inhibitor, *O*-methylation then becomes the predominant form of metabolism of levodopa; therefore co-administration of a peripheral COMT inhibitor such as entacapone potentially extends the duration and effect of levodopa in the brain, and consequently allows a reduction in the dose and frequency of administration of levodopa.

References.


1. Holm KJ, Spencer CM. Entacapone: a review of its use in Parkinson's disease. *Drugs* 1999; **58:** 159–177.
2. Anonymous. Entacapone for Parkinson's disease. *Med Lett Drugs Ther* 2000; **42:** 7–8.
3. Chong BS, Mersfelder TL. Entacapone. *Ann Pharmacother* 2000; **34:** 1056–65.
4. Myllyla VV, *et al.* Twelve-month safety of entacapone in patients with Parkinson's disease. *Eur J Neurol* 2001; **8:** 53–60.
5. Poewe WH, *et al.* Efficacy and safety of entacapone in Parkinson's disease patients with suboptimal levodopa response: a 6-month randomized placebo-controlled double-blind study in Germany and Austria (Celomen study). *Acta Neurol Scand* 2002; **105:** 245–55.
6. Brooks DJ, *et al.* Entacapone is beneficial in both fluctuating and non-fluctuating patients with Parkinson's disease: a randomised, placebo controlled, double blind, six month study. *J Neurol Neurosurg Psychiatry* 2003; **74:** 1071–9.
7. Fenelon G, *et al.* Efficacy and tolerability of entacapone in patients with Parkinson's disease treated with levodopa plus a dopamine agonist and experiencing wearing-off motor fluctuations: a randomized, double-blind, multicentre study. *J Neural Transm* 2003; **110:** 239–51.
8. Olanow CW, Stocchi F. COMT inhibitors in Parkinson's disease: can they prevent and/or reverse levodopa-induced motor complications? *Neurology* 2004; **62** (suppl 1): S72–S81.


### Preparations

**Proprietary Preparations** (details are given in Part 3)
***Arg.:*** Comtan; ***Austral.:*** Comtan; ***Austria:*** Comtan; ***Belg.:*** Comtan; ***Braz.:*** Comtan; ***Canad.:*** Comtan; ***Denm.:*** Comtess; ***Fin.:*** Comtess; ***Fr.:*** Comtan; ***Ger.:*** Comtess; ***Gr.:*** Comtan; ***Hong Kong:*** Comtan; ***Irl.:*** Comtess; ***Israel:*** Comtan; ***Ital.:*** Comtan; ***Malaysia:*** Comtan; ***Mex.:*** Comtan; ***Neth.:*** Comtan; ***Norw.:*** Comtess; ***NZ:*** Comtan; ***Port.:*** Comtan; ***S.Afr.:*** Comtan; ***Singapore:*** Comtan; ***Spain:*** Comtan; ***Swed.:*** Comtess; ***Switz.:*** Comtan; ***Thai.:*** Comtan; ***UK:*** Comtess; ***USA:*** Comtan.

**Multi-ingredient:** ***UK:*** Stalevo.

## Lazabemide *(BAN, USAN, rINN)*

Lazabemida; Ro-19-6327; Ro-19-6327/000. *N*-(2-Aminoethyl)-5-chloropicolinamide.

$C_8H_{10}ClN_3O$ = 199.6.
*CAS — 103878-84-8 (lazabemide); 103878-83-7 (lazabemide hydrochloride).*

### Profile

Lazabemide is a reversible inhibitor of monoamine oxidase type B that was investigated in the management of parkinsonism, but development was discontinued when clinical trials highlighted a risk of severe hepatotoxicity.

## Levodopa *(BAN, USAN, rINN)*

Dihydroxyphenylalanine; L-Dopa; 3-Hydroxy-L-tyrosine; Laevodopa; Levodopum. (−)-3-(3,4-Dihydroxyphenyl)-L-alanine.

$C_9H_{11}NO_4$ = 197.2.
*CAS — 59-92-7.*
*ATC — N04BA01.*

NOTE. Compounded preparations of levodopa may be represented by the following names:

- Co-beneldopa (*BAN*)—benserazide 1 part and levodopa 4 parts (w/w)
- Co-careldopa *x/y* (*BAN*)—where *x* and *y* are the strengths in milligrams of carbidopa and levodopa respectively
- Co-careldopa (*PEN*)—carbidopa and levodopa.

**Pharmacopoeias.** In *Chin., Eur.* (see p.vi), *Int., Jpn,* and *US.*

**Ph. Eur. 5.0** (Levodopa). A white or slightly cream-coloured, crystalline powder. Slightly soluble in water; freely soluble in 1M hydrochloric acid but sparingly soluble in 0.1M hydrochloric acid; practically insoluble in alcohol. A 1% suspension in water has a pH of 4.5 to 7.0. Protect from light.

**USP 27** (Levodopa). A white to off-white, odourless, crystalline powder. In the presence of moisture, it is rapidly oxidised by atmospheric oxygen and darkens. Slightly soluble in water; freely soluble in 3N hydrochloric acid; insoluble in alcohol. Store in a dry place in airtight containers at a temperature not exceeding 40°. Protect from light.

**Stability.** Extemporaneously prepared oral liquid dosage forms may be unstable and manufacturers' formulations should be used where possible.[1] An extemporary formula is available for levodopa syrup. Water dispersible formulations of levodopa with benserazide are available in some countries but a method that can be used by patients to prepare daily solutions of levodopa with carbidopa has been suggested:[2] one litre of a solution in potable water may be prepared with ten crushed standard tablets of levodopa 100 mg with carbidopa 25 mg and 2 g of ascorbic acid added to stabilise the levodopa.


1. Walls TJ, *et al.* Problems with inactivation of drugs used in Parkinson's disease. *BMJ* 1985; **290:** 444–5.
2. Giron LT, Koller WC. Methods of managing levodopa-induced dyskinesias. *Drug Safety* 1996; **14:** 365–74.


### Adverse Effects

Gastrointestinal effects, notably nausea, vomiting, and anorexia are common early in treatment with levodopa, particularly if the dosage is increased too rapidly. Gastrointestinal bleeding has been reported in patients with a history of peptic ulcer disease.

The commonest cardiovascular effect is orthostatic hypotension, which is usually asymptomatic, but may be associated with faintness and dizziness. Cardiac arrhythmias have been reported and hypertension has occasionally occurred.

Psychiatric symptoms occur in a high proportion of patients, especially the elderly, and include agitation, anxiety, euphoria, nightmares, and insomnia, or sometimes drowsiness and depression. More serious effects, usually requiring a reduction in dosage or withdrawal of levodopa, include aggression, paranoid delusions, hallucinations, delirium, severe depression, with or without suicidal behaviour, and unmasking of psychoses. Psychotic reactions are more likely in patients with postencephalitic parkinsonism or a history of mental disorders.

Abnormal involuntary movements or dyskinesias are the most serious dose-limiting adverse effects of levodopa and are very common at the optimum dose required to control parkinsonism; their frequency increases with duration of treatment. Involuntary movements of the face, tongue, lips, and jaw often appear first and those of the trunk and extremities later. Severe generalised choreoathetoid and dystonic movements may occur after prolonged administration. Muscle twitching and blepharospasm may be early signs of excessive dosage. Exaggerated respiratory movements and exacerbated oculogyric crises have been reported in patients with postencephalitic parkinsonism. Re-emergence of bradykinesia and akinesia, in the form of 'end-of-dose' deterioration and the 'on-off' phenomenon, in patients with parkinsonism is a complication of long-term treatment, but may be due to progression of the disease rather than to levodopa (see also under Parkinsonism, p.1196).

A positive response to the direct Coombs' test may occur, usually without evidence of haemolysis although auto-immune haemolytic anaemia has occasionally been reported. Transient leucopenia has occurred rarely. The effects of levodopa on liver and kidney function are generally slight. Levodopa may cause discoloration of the urine; reddish at first then darkening on standing. Other body fluids may also be discoloured.

Some of the adverse effects reported may not be attributable directly to levodopa, but rather to the concomitant use of antimuscarinics, to increased mobility, or to the unmasking of underlying conditions as parkinsonism improves. Use with a peripheral dopa-decarboxylase inhibitor may reduce the severity of peripheral symptoms such as gastrointestinal and cardiovascular effects, but central effects such as dyskinesias and mental disturbances may occur earlier in treatment.

**Incidence of adverse effects.** The major adverse effects of levodopa are dyskinesia in 75% of patients and psychiatric disturbances in 25%.[1] Nausea and vomiting in 40 to 50% gradually regress and hypotension in 25 to 30% is generally asymptomatic. Less common adverse effects include cardiac arrhythmias, particularly atrial and ventricular ectopic beats and less commonly atrial flutter and fibrillation; palpitations and flushing often accompanied by excessive sweating; hypertension; polyuria, incontinence, and urinary retention, although antimuscarinic drugs often contribute to problems with micturition; and dark coloration of the urine and saliva. Rare adverse effects include abdominal pain, constipation, and diarrhoea; mydriasis, blurred vision, diplopia, and precipitation of glaucoma; headache; stridor; tachypnoea; and paraesthesias.


1. Calne DB, Reid JL. Antiparkinsonian drugs: pharmacological and therapeutic aspects. *Drugs* 1972; **4:** 49–74.


**Abnormal coloration.** Black pigmentation of rib cartilage has been noted at necropsy in patients treated with levodopa.[1,2] Abnormal pigmentation is generally not seen at other sites[2] but there have been isolated reports[2,3] of patients who also had pigmentation of the intervertebral discs. Although the pigmentation appears to be irreversible it was considered to be probably harmless.[2] It has been suggested that the pigmentation was due to deposition of dihydroxyphenylalanine (DOPA) in the cartilage.[1] It is known that DOPA will readily auto-oxidise *in vitro* in the presence of oxygen to a black pigment and this can also happen *in vivo* since black urine is a well known side-effect of levodopa. Dark sweat and pigmentation of the skin and teeth are also side-effects known to the manufacturers of levodopa.

See also Effects on the Skin and Hair, below.


1. Connolly CE, *et al.* Black cartilage associated with levodopa. *Lancet* 1986; **i:** 690.
2. Rausing A, Rosén U. Black cartilage after therapy with levodopa and methyldopa. *Arch Pathol Lab Med* 1994; **118:** 531–5.
3. Keen CE. *BMJ* 1998; **316:** 240.


**Dysgeusia.** A change in taste sensation was reported[1] in 23 of 514 patients treated with levodopa and a peripheral dopa-decarboxylase inhibitor; 2 of the 23 had total loss of taste initially. The altered taste was often described as insipid, metallic, or plastic, was first observed 3 to 32 weeks after beginning treatment, and lasted for 2 to 40 weeks. In an earlier report 22 of 100 patients receiving levodopa alone had experienced changes in taste.[2]


1. Siegfried J, Zumstein H. Changes in taste under L-DOPA therapy. *Z Neurol* 1971; **200:** 345–8.
2. Barbeau A. L-DOPA therapy: past, present and future. *Ariz Med* 1970; **27:** 1–4.


**Effects on the blood.** Reports of effects of levodopa on the blood are mostly confined to individual case reports. A study in 365 patients, receiving levodopa in a mean daily dosage of 4.04 g, found that 32 developed a positive direct Coombs' test, the majority after between 3 and 12 months of therapy, but none developed haemolytic anaemia.[1] However, occasional cases of auto-immune haemolytic anaemia have been reported;[2-4] in one case dosage reduction and addition of a peripheral dopa-decarboxylase inhibitor largely abolished haemolysis,[3] but in another, haemolysis recurred on re-institution of levodopa with carbidopa and required corticosteroid treatment.[4] A case of severe acute non-haemolytic anaemia related to levodopa therapy has also been reported.[5]

Although levodopa is widely stated to produce leucopenia in some patients, there are few published reports. However transient minor decreases in total leucocyte counts were reported in 3 of a group of 80 patients receiving levodopa.[6]

Severe thrombocytopenia occurred in a patient who had received levodopa for 3 years;[7] the condition was apparently an auto-immune response and responded to prednisone therapy.


1. Joseph C. Occurrence of positive Coombs test in patients treated with levodopa. *N Engl J Med* 1972; **286:** 1401–2.
2. Territo MC, *et al.* Autoimmune hemolytic anemia due to levodopa therapy. *JAMA* 1973; **226:** 1347–8.
3. Lindström FD, *et al.* Dose-related levodopa-induced haemolytic anaemia. *Ann Intern Med* 1977; **86:** 298–300.
4. Bernstein RM. Reversible haemolytic anaemia after levodopa-carbidopa. *BMJ* 1979; **1:** 1461–2.
5. Alkalay I, Zipoli T. Levodopa-induced acute non-hemolytic anemia. *Ann Allergy* 1977; **39:** 191.
6. Barbeau A. L-Dopa therapy in Parkinson's disease: a critical review of nine years' experience. *Can Med Assoc J* 1969; **101:** 791–800.
7. Wanamaker WM, *et al.* Thrombocytopenia associated with long-term levodopa therapy. *JAMA* 1976; **235:** 2217–19.


**Effects on the cardiovascular system.** There have been conflicting reports on the effects of peripheral dopa-decarboxylase inhibitors on orthostatic hypotension attributed to levodopa therapy. In a study[1] supine and erect systolic blood pressure was found to be significantly higher in parkinsonian patients given levodopa with carbidopa than in those receiving levodopa alone suggesting that the peripheral actions of dopamine contribute to levodopa-induced hypotension. However, another study[2] found no change in the incidence and degree of orthostatic hypotension after levodopa in association with carbidopa and, similarly, no difference in the frequency of ventricular arrhythmias.

See also Effects on Kidney Function, below and Cardiovascular Disorders, under Precautions, below.


1. Calne DB, *et al.* Action of L-α-methyldopahydrazine on the blood pressure of patients receiving levodopa. *Br J Pharmacol* 1972; **44:** 162–4.
2. Leibowitz M, Lieberman A. Comparison of dopa decarboxylase inhibitor (carbidopa) combined with levodopa and levodopa alone on the cardiovascular system of patients with Parkinson's disease. *Neurology* 1975; **25:** 917–21.


**Effects on electrolytes.** See under Effects on Kidney Function, below.

**Effects on the endocrine system.** Single doses of levodopa cause an increase in plasma concentrations of glucose, insulin, and glucagon, as well as of growth hormone, when given to healthy subjects[1] and there has been concern over the potential endocrine effects of levodopa therapy in patients with Parkinson's disease.[2] A study of carbohydrate metabolism in 24 patients with Parkinson's disease indicated that these patients had abnormally low rates of glucose utilisation when untreated, apparently due to impaired insulin release, and this was not altered when levodopa therapy was given.[3] However, a similar study completed by 19 patients[2] noted increased impairment of glucose utilisation following levodopa therapy for 1 year with a delayed hypersecretion of insulin in response to a glucose load similar to the metabolic changes of acromegaly. It was considered that patients receiving levodopa for parkinsonism should be monitored for evidence of diabetes mellitus or frank acromegaly.[2]

Postmenopausal bleeding occurred in varying degrees in 12 of 47 women treated with levodopa.[4] In one case bleeding was severe enough to warrant interrupting treatment and subsequent dosage reduction.


1. Rayfield EJ, *et al.* L-Dopa stimulation of glucagon secretion in man. *N Engl J Med* 1975; **293:** 589–91.
2. Sirtori CR, *et al.* Metabolic responses to acute and chronic L-dopa administration in patients with parkinsonism. *N Engl J Med* 1972; **287:** 729–33.
3. Van Woert MH, Mueller PS. Glucose, insulin, and free fatty acid metabolism in Parkinson's disease treated with levodopa. *Clin Pharmacol Ther* 1971; **12:** 360–7.
4. Wajsbort J. Post-menopausal bleeding after L-dopa. *N Engl J Med* 1972; **286:** 784.


**Effects on the eyes.** Both miosis[1] and mydriasis[2] have been reported with levodopa.

For a report of the exacerbation of oculogyric crises by levodopa, see under Extrapyramidal Effects, below.


1. Spiers ASD, *et al.* Miosis during L-dopa therapy. *BMJ* 1970; **2:** 639–40.
2. Weintraub MI, *et al.* Pupillary effects of levodopa therapy: development of anisocoria in latent Horner's syndrome. *N Engl J Med* 1970; **283:** 120–3.


**Effects on the gastrointestinal tract.** Although gastrointestinal bleeding has more commonly been reported in patients with a history of peptic ulceration there is a rare report[1] of acute melaena and non-specific gastritis associated with levodopa therapy in a 56-year-old man without any previous evidence of a gastric disorder.

See also Dysgeusia, above.


1. Riddoch D. Gastritis and L-dopa. *BMJ* 1972; **1:** 53–4.


**Effects on kidney function.** Administration of levodopa 1 to 2 g to 7 patients with idiopathic or postencephalitic Parkinson's disease produced significant increments in renal plasma flow, glomerular filtration rate, and sodium and potassium excretion.[1] It was considered that the natriuretic effects could contribute to the orthostatic hypotension commonly noted in patients receiving levodopa. There is a report of a patient who developed hyponatraemia when treated with levodopa with carbidopa.[2] The patient had previously had a similar reaction when given amantadine. On each occasion symptoms disappeared when dopaminergic medication was withdrawn and recurred on rechallenge. Inappropriate secretion of antidiuretic hormone was suggested as a possible mechanism.

Levodopa has also been reported to have a kaliuretic effect, resulting in hypokalaemia, in some parkinsonian patients;[3] the effect could be prevented by concomitant administration of a peripheral dopa-decarboxylase inhibitor.


1. Finlay GD, *et al.* Augmentation of sodium and potassium excretion, glomerular filtration rate and renal plasma flow by levodopa. *N Engl J Med* 1971; **284:** 865–70.
2. Lammers GJ, Roos RAC. Hyponatraemia due to amantadine hydrochloride and L-dopa/carbidopa. *Lancet* 1993; **342:** 439.
3. Granérus A-K, *et al.* Kaliuretic effect of L-dopa treatment in parkinsonian patients. *Acta Med Scand* 1977; **201:** 291–7.


**Effects on mental function. Psychiatric complications** were the single commonest reason for stopping levodopa treatment in a follow-up study of 178 patients with idiopathic Parkinson's disease, 81 of whom were still taking levodopa after 6 years.[1] Within 2 years levodopa was withdrawn because of toxic confusional states (21 patients), paranoid psychosis (6), unipolar depression (2), and mania (1). The incidence of visual hallucinations increased as treatment continued but, as with toxic confusional states, patients generally improved when levodopa was withdrawn. Before treatment 40 patients had suffered severe depression and levodopa produced sustained improvement in only 2. After 6 years, 20 of the 81 patients remaining were moderately or severely depressed and were rarely improved by withdrawal or reduction in dosage of levodopa. Increasing dementia affected 26 of the 81 patients after 6 years; withdrawal of levodopa in 5 failed to improve cognitive disabilities, but increased parkinsonism.

Another study[2] reported that 141 of 400 patients being treated for Parkinson's disease developed mental disorders. In this study certain acute states, particularly anxiety, on-off hallucinations, and fits of delirium were linked to treatment with levodopa, whereas dementia and depression were not.

A 12-month study of 1281 patients in the USA treated with dopamine agonists for Parkinson's disease found that 9 were suffering from **excessive gambling**.[3] All patients had received levodopa, 8 pramipexole, and the remaining patient pergolide. The rate of pathological gambling was 1.5% in the 529 patients taking pramipexole. The authors considered that this was not unexpected given the general availability of casinos in the local area and an incidence in the general US population of 0.3 to 1.3%. Similar behaviour described as being markedly increased in "on" periods has been reported in other patients treated with levodopa.[4] Pathological gambling has also been associated with misuse of dopaminergics.[5]

**Sleep-related complaints** have occurred and were reported by 74 of 100 patients with Parkinson's disease.[6] All 74 were on levodopa and the prevalence of symptoms increased with the duration of treatment. Symptoms included insomnia, excessive daytime somnolence, altered dream phenomena, nocturnal vocalisation, involuntary myoclonic movements, and rarely, sleep walking. Sleep fragmentation, which includes insomnia and somnolence, was the most common symptom overall. It has been suggested[7] that in patients with mild to moderate disease levodopa and dopamine agonists could cause sleep disruption. However, these drugs produce beneficial effects on nocturnal disabilities in patients with more severe disease. Reports[8-13] of daytime somnolence or sudden onset of sleep with various other dopamine agonists, including apomorphine, bromocriptine, cabergoline, lisuride, pergolide, piribedil, pramipexole, quinagolide, and ropinirole, suggest that this is a class effect of dopaminergic antiparkinsonian therapy, and patients should be warned of the possible risks (see Precautions, below). The risk of somnolence may be increased in those patients taking combinations of dopaminergics.[12,14]


1. Shaw KM, *et al.* The impact of treatment with levodopa on Parkinson's disease. *Q J Med* 1980; **49:** 283–93.
2. Rondot P, *et al.* Mental disorders in Parkinson's disease after treatment with L-dopa. *Adv Neurol* 1984; **40:** 259–69.
3. Driver-Dunckley E, *et al.* Pathological gambling associated with dopamine agonist therapy in Parkinson's disease. *Neurology* 2003; **61:** 422–3.
4. Molina JA, *et al.* Pathologic gambling in Parkinson's disease: a behavioral manifestation of pharmacologic treatment? *Mov Disord* 2000; **15:** 869–72.
5. Gschwandtner U, *et al.* Pathologic gambling in patients with Parkinson's disease. *Clin Neuropharmacol* 2001; **24:** 170–2.
6. Nausieda PA, *et al.* Psychiatric complications of levodopa therapy of Parkinson's disease. *Adv Neurol* 1984; **40:** 271–7.
7. van Hilten B, *et al.* Sleep disruption in Parkinson's disease: assessment by continuous activity monitoring. *Arch Neurol* 1994; **51:** 922–8.
8. Frucht S, *et al.* Falling asleep at the wheel: motor vehicle mishaps in persons taking pramipexole and ropinirole. *Neurology* 1999; **52:** 1908–10.
9. Schapira AHV. Sleep attacks (sleep episodes) with pergolide. *Lancet* 2000; **355:** 1332–3.
10. Ferreira JJ, *et al.* Sleep attacks and Parkinson's disease treatment. *Lancet* 2000; **355:** 1333–4.
11. Pirker W, Happe S. Sleep attacks in Parkinson's disease. *Lancet* 2000; **356:** 597–8.
12. Committee on Safety of Medicines/Medicines Control Agency. Dopaminergic drugs and sudden onset of sleep. *Current Problems* 2003; **29:** 9. Also available at: http://www.mca.gov.uk/ourwork/monitorsafequalmed/currentproblems/cpsept2003.pdf (accessed 24/05/04)
13. Houmann CN. *et al.* Sleep attacks in patients taking dopamine agonists: review. *BMJ* 2002; **324:** 1483–7.
14. Etminan M, *et al.* Increased risk of somnolence with the new dopamine agonists in patients with Parkinson's disease: a meta-analysis of randomised controlled trials. *Drug Safety* 2001; **24:** 863–8.


**Effects on respiration.** Respiratory crises, including attacks of gasping, panting, sniffing, puffing, and breath-holding, occurred in 12 of 25 patients with postencephalitic parkinsonism during treatment with levodopa.[1] A further 8 developed respiratory and phonatory tics, including sudden deep breaths, yawns, coughs, giggles, sighing, grunting, and moaning. All 20 patients also suffered tachypnoea, bradypnoea, and asymmetrical movement of both sides of the chest, paradoxical diaphragmatic movements, and reversal of inspiratory and expiratory phases. The induction of respiratory crises may be prompt or greatly delayed; 3 patients only developed crises after more than 9 months of treatment with levodopa. Crises were readily precipitated by psychophysiological arousals such as rage and exertion. Most of the patients who developed marked respiratory disorders had shown slight irregularities of respiratory rhythm, rate, and force before receiving levodopa.

In another report a distressing dose-related irregularity in the rate and depth of breathing occurred when a patient with Parkinson's disease was given levodopa with benserazide.[2] The respiratory abnormality was completely suppressed by use of tiapride, with no reduction in the efficacy of levodopa.


1. Sacks OW, *et al.* Side-effects of L-dopa in postencephalitic parkinsonism. *Lancet* 1970; **i:** 1006.
2. De Keyser J, Vincken W. L-Dopa-induced respiratory disturbance in Parkinson's disease suppressed by tiapride. *Neurology* 1985; **35:** 235–7.


**Effects on sexual function.** An increase in libido, over and above the effects of improved mobility and well-being, has been reported in parkinsonian patients receiving levodopa. One report noted increased libido but no improvement in sexual performance in 4 of 80 patients[1] while another reported a moderate increase in sexual interest in 4 of 7 male patients.[2] Reports of extreme hypersexuality are rare and include a patient receiving levodopa and bromocriptine who may have been abusing the drugs.[3] Hypersexual behaviour and hypergenitalism has also been reported in a pre-pubertal boy given levodopa for behaviour disturbances.[4]


1. Barbeau A. L-Dopa therapy in Parkinson's disease: a critical review of nine years' experience. *Can Med Assoc J* 1969; **101:** 791–9.
2. Brown E, *et al.* Sexual function and affect in parkinsonian men treated with L-dopa. *Am J Psychiatry* 1978; **135:** 1552–5.

3. Vogel HP, Schiffter R. Hypersexuality—a complication of dopaminergic therapy in Parkinson's disease. *Pharmacopsychiatry* 1983; **16:** 107–10.
4. Korten JJ, *et al.* Undesirable prepubertal effects of levodopa. *JAMA* 1973; **226:** 355.

**Effects on the skin and hair.** Two women who were given levodopa, up to 3 g daily, developed diffuse alopecia in addition to other adverse effects.[1] Repigmentation of hair has occurred in a white-bearded man after being treated with levodopa 1.5 g daily for 8 months.[2] Vitiligo has been reported[3] in a patient with Parkinson's disease following addition of tolcapone to his levodopa/carbidopa regimen. The development of vitiligo was attributed to the increase in plasma-levodopa concentrations brought about by concomitant use of tolcapone.

See also Melanoma, under Precautions, below.

1. Marshall A, Williams MJ. Alopecia and levodopa. *BMJ* 1971; **2:** 47.
2. Grainger KM. Pigmentation in Parkinson's disease treated with levodopa. *Lancet* 1973; **i:** 97–8.
3. Sabaté M, *et al.* Vitiligo associated with tolcapone and levodopa in a patient with Parkinson's disease. *Ann Pharmacother* 1999; **33:** 1228–9.

**Extrapyramidal effects.** Choreiform movements were the major dose-limiting complication of long-term treatment with levodopa in a follow-up study of 178 patients with idiopathic Parkinson's disease, 81 of whom were still taking levodopa after 6 years.[1] Dyskinesias usually appeared in the first year and became more severe and generalised with time. Certain distinctive patterns of involuntary movements occurred as follows:

- peak-dose movements affected 65 of the 81 patients and were dose-related. Movements were usually choreic, affecting the face and limbs, but dystonic and ballistic movements were also seen; characteristically they began 20 to 90 minutes after an oral dose and lasted from 10 minutes to 4 hours with a tendency to be more severe mid-way through the interdose period
- biphasic movements presenting as 2 distinct episodes of chorea or dystonia within each interdose period occurred in only 3 patients
- early morning and 'end-of-dose' dystonia was present in 15 patients after 6 years of treatment with levodopa, but rarely developed during the first 3 years
- nocturnal myoclonus occurred in 12 patients.

The frequency, intensity, and complexity of spontaneous fluctuations in performance were greatly enhanced by long-term levodopa therapy. Two clinically distinct types of fluctuation, 'end-of-dose' deterioration and the 'on-off' phenomenon, were related to treatment. 'End-of-dose' deterioration or the 'wearing-off' effect affected 52 patients after 6 years of treatment and was characterised by progressive reduction in the duration of benefit from each dose with a gradual return of nocturnal and early morning disability in some patients. The 'on-off' phenomenon affected 14 patients who experienced completely unpredictable swings from relative mobility, usually accompanied by involuntary movements, to periods of profound bradykinesia and hypotonia. In addition, 'freezing episodes' and abrupt falls became increasingly common and affected 50 patients after 6 years compared with 33 before therapy.

1. Shaw KM, *et al.* The impact of treatment with levodopa on Parkinson's disease. *Q J Med* 1980; **49:** 283–93.

OCULOGYRIC CRISIS. After initial remission, oculogyric crises in 5 of 25 patients with postencephalitic parkinsonism recurred and were subsequently severely exacerbated during treatment with levodopa.[1] One patient, who previously had not had oculogyric crises, developed severe crises in the fourth month of therapy with levodopa. During these crises forced gaze deviation was always accompanied by severe neurological and mental symptoms, some of which were scarcely tolerable.

1. Sacks OW, Kohl M. L-Dopa and oculogyric crises. *Lancet* 1970; **ii:** 215–16.

**Gout.** There have been reports of elevated serum uric acid concentrations in patients receiving levodopa, but some of these are of doubtful significance since levodopa has been shown to give falsely-elevated uric acid concentrations by colorimetric methods.[1] However, hyperuricaemia as measured by more specific methods,[2,3] with a few cases of overt gout,[2,3] has also been reported.

1. Cawein MJ, Hewins J. False rise in serum uric acid after L-dopa. *N Engl J Med* 1969; **281:** 1489–90.
2. Honda H, Gindin RA. Gout while receiving levodopa for parkinsonism. *JAMA* 1972; **219:** 55–7.
3. Calne DB, Fermaglich J. Gout induced by L-dopa and decarboxylase inhibitors. *Postgrad Med J* 1976; **52:** 232–3.

**Hypersensitivity.** Reports of hypersensitivity reactions to levodopa have included a vasculitis characterised by neuromyopathy, periarteriolitis with eosinophilia,[1] and a lupus-like autoimmune syndrome.[2]

1. Wolf S, *et al.* Neuromyopathy and periarteriolitis in a patient receiving levodopa. *Arch Intern Med* 1976; **136:** 1055–7.
2. Massarotti G, *et al.* Lupus-like autoimmune syndrome after levodopa and benserazide. *BMJ* 1979; **2:** 553.

**Overdosage.** Adverse effects following ingestion of 80 to 100 g of levodopa over a 12-hour period by a parkinsonian patient included hypertension initially, followed by hypotension of a few hours' duration, sinus tachycardia, and symptomatic orthostatic hypotension for more than a week.[1] Marked confusion, agitation, insomnia, and restlessness were the most prominent clinical symptoms and did not disappear completely for over a week; severe anorexia and insomnia persisted for 2 to 3 weeks. After the overdose the patient had virtually no signs of parkinsonism and received no levodopa or antimuscarinic medication for 6 days; rigidity and akinesia began to recur on the fourth day.

1. Hoehn MM, Rutledge CO. Acute overdose with levodopa: clinical and biochemical consequences. *Neurology* 1975; **25:** 792–4.

**Withdrawal syndromes.** Withdrawal of anti-parkinsonian drugs, particularly levodopa, has been implicated in the development of a syndrome resembling the neuroleptic malignant syndrome,[1-6] characterised by fever, muscle rigidity, profuse sweating, tachycardia, tachypnoea, and elevated muscle enzyme values.[1] Several fatalities have occurred.[1,2] It has been suggested that the neuroleptic malignant syndrome is associated with blockade of dopamine receptors in the striatum, leading to increased rigidity and heat production, and in the hypothalamus, resulting in impaired thermoregulation[7] and it seems reasonable that withdrawal of levodopa might have a similar effect in patients with depleted central dopamine concentrations. Thus, the use of a 'drug holiday' to manage fluctuations in response to levodopa (see under Parkinsonism, p.1196) is no longer recommended.

Fever, extrapyramidal symptoms and raised creatine kinase concentrations, resembling a very mild form of the neuroleptic malignant syndrome, have also been reported in parkinsonian patients exposed to stress such as dehydration or infection but without any change in medication.[8]

1. Friedman JH, *et al.* A neuroleptic malignantlike syndrome due to levodopa therapy withdrawal. *JAMA* 1985; **254:** 2792–5.
2. Sechi GP, *et al.* Fatal hyperpyrexia after withdrawal of levodopa. *Neurology* 1984; **34:** 249–51.
3. Figà-Talamanca L, *et al.* Hyperthermia after discontinuance of levodopa and bromocriptine therapy: impaired dopamine receptors a possible cause. *Neurology* 1985; **35:** 258–61.
4. Gibb WRG, Griffith DNW. Levodopa withdrawal syndrome identical to neuroleptic malignant syndrome. *Postgrad Med J* 1986; **62:** 59–60.
5. Serrano-Dueñas M. Neuroleptic malignant syndrome-like, or—dopaminergic malignant syndrome—due to levodopa therapy withdrawal: clinical features in 11 patients. *Parkinsonism Relat Disord* 2003; **9:** 175–8.
6. Mizuno Y, *et al.* Malignant syndrome in Parkinson's disease: concept and review of the literature. *Parkinsonism Relat Disord* 2003; **9** (suppl 1): S3–S9.
7. Henderson VW, Wooten GF. Neuroleptic malignant syndrome: a pathogenetic role for dopamine receptor blockade? *Neurology* 1981; **31:** 132–7.
8. Mezaki T, *et al.* Benign type of malignant syndrome. *Lancet* 1989; **i:** 49–50.

## Treatment of Adverse Effects

Reduction in dosage reverses most of the side-effects of levodopa. Nausea and vomiting may be diminished by increasing the dose of levodopa gradually, and/or by taking with or after meals, although taking levodopa on a full stomach may lead to lower plasma concentrations. Gastrointestinal effects may also be reduced by giving an antiemetic such as cyclizine or domperidone but not a phenothiazine (see Antipsychotics, under Interactions, below). Use with a peripheral dopa-decarboxylase inhibitor reduces peripheral but not central side-effects. Orthostatic hypotension may respond to the use of elastic stockings.

In acute overdosage gastric lavage and activated charcoal should be considered in patients who have taken more than 4 g or more than the total daily dose, whichever is greater, and who present within 1 hour; supportive measures should also be instituted. Pyridoxine may reverse some effects of levodopa (see Nutritional Agents, under Interactions, below) but its value in overdosage has not been established; it does not reverse the effects of levodopa given with a peripheral dopa-decarboxylase inhibitor.

**Nausea and vomiting.** For reference to the use of domperidone in the management of nausea and vomiting associated with levodopa in patients with Parkinson's disease, see under Uses and Administration of Domperidone, p.1264.

**Psychosis.** Atypical antipsychotics such as clozapine (p.689) have been tried in the management of psychosis occurring as a complication of parkinsonism and of drugs such as levodopa used in its treatment.

## Precautions

Levodopa is contra-indicated in patients with angle-closure glaucoma and should be used with caution in open-angle glaucoma. Caution is also required in patients with cardiovascular disease, pulmonary disease, endocrine disorders, psychiatric disturbances, osteomalacia, or a history of peptic ulceration. Periodic evaluations of hepatic, psychiatric, haematological, renal, and cardiovascular functions have been advised.

Since an association between levodopa and activation of malignant melanoma has been suspected (although not confirmed), it is generally recommended that levodopa should not be given to patients with (or with a history of) the disease or with skin disorders suggestive of it.

Parkinsonian patients who benefit from levodopa therapy should be warned to resume normal activities gradually to avoid the risk of injury. Treatment with levodopa should not be stopped abruptly.

Excessive daytime sleepiness and sudden onset of sleep may occur with levodopa and caution is advised when driving or operating machinery; patients who suffer such effects should not drive or operate machinery until the effects have stopped recurring.

Levodopa inhibits prolactin secretion and may therefore interfere with lactation.

Food interferes with the absorption of levodopa, though levodopa is usually given with or immediately after meals to reduce nausea and vomiting. However, patients experiencing the 'on-off' phenomenon may benefit from administration on an empty stomach (see under Parkinsonism, p.1196).

**Abuse.** Abuse of levodopa in patients with Parkinson's disease has been reported.[1-5] Patients had progressively increased the dosage of levodopa to obtain psychotropic effects such as euphoria despite accompanying dystonia and other extrapyramidal adverse effects. Discontinuation often led to craving, drug-seeking behaviour, and mood disturbances such as depression, features resembling a psychological dependence syndrome. Abuse in patients without parkinsonism has also occurred.[6]

1. Nausieda PA. Sinemet "abusers". *Clin Neuropharmacol* 1985; **8:** 318–27.
2. Soyka M, Huppert D. L-dopa abuse in a patient with former alcoholism. *Br J Addict* 1992; **87:** 117–18.
3. Spigset O, von Schéele C. Levodopa dependence and abuse in Parkinson's disease. *Pharmacotherapy* 1997; **17:** 1027–30.
4. Merims D, *et al.* Is there addiction to levodopa in patients with Parkinson's disease? *Mov Disord* 2000; **15:** 1014–16.
5. Müller U, *et al.* Levodopa-Abhängigkeit bei Parkinsonkrankheit: Fallbericht und Literaturübersicht. *Nervenarzt* 2002; **73:** 887–91.
6. Steiner I, Wirguin I. Levodopa addiction in non-parkinsonian patients. *Neurology* 2003; **61:** 1451.

**Cardiovascular disorders.** A high incidence of cardiovascular side-effects was reported in early studies of levodopa, but both Parkinson's disease and heart disease are common in the elderly and adverse cardiac effects of levodopa may be less prevalent than was first thought. A study in 40 patients[1] concluded that, apart from those with severe orthostatic hypotension or unstable coronary disease, levodopa may be used safely in parkinsonian patients with heart disease. Others[2] noted that levodopa and bromocriptine cause cardiac arrhythmias in less than 1% of all patients, the incidence for levodopa with a peripheral dopa-decarboxylase inhibitor being lower still. Nevertheless, caution is advised in patients with cardiovascular disease.

1. Jenkins RB, *et al.* Levodopa therapy of patients with parkinsonism and heart disease. *BMJ* 1972; **3:** 512–14.
2. Parkes JD, *et al.* Amantadine-induced heart failure. *Lancet* 1977; **i:** 904.

**Diabetes mellitus.** For reference to concern over the potential of levodopa to impair glucose utilisation, see Effects on the Endocrine System under Adverse Effects, above.

**Melanoma.** There has been concern over the effects of levodopa on melanoma in view of the ability of malignant melanoma cells to convert levodopa to melanin and isolated reports of melanoma developing or being exacerbated during levodopa therapy continue to appear. However, in a survey of 1099 patients with primary cutaneous malignant melanoma only one had taken levodopa.[1] It was concluded that levodopa therapy is not an important factor in the induction of malignant melanoma. Furthermore, use of levodopa in daily doses of up to 4 g with carbidopa to 17 patients with metastatic melanoma failed to provide any evidence that levodopa accelerated the progression of the disease.[2] Reviews[3,4] of these and later reports concluded that the purported link between levodopa and malignant melanoma was tenuous.

For a report of antineoplastic chemotherapy used for the treatment of melanoma reducing the efficacy of levodopa, see under Interactions, below.

1. Sober AJ, Wick MM. Levodopa therapy and malignant melanoma. *JAMA* 1978; **240:** 554–5.
2. Gurney H, *et al.* The use of L-dopa and carbidopa in metastatic malignant melanoma. *J Invest Dermatol* 1991; **96:** 85–7.
3. Siple JF, *et al.* Levodopa therapy and the risk of malignant melanoma. *Ann Pharmacother* 2000; **34:** 382–5.
4. Fiala KH, *et al.* Malignant melanoma and levodopa in Parkinson's disease: causality or coincidence? *Parkinsonism Relat Disord* 2003; **9:** 321–7.

**Pregnancy.** Levodopa alone and with carbidopa has been associated with fetal abnormalities in *animals* given high doses; no teratogenic effect has been noted with carbidopa alone. However, 2 women with parkinsonism who received levodopa with carbidopa or levodopa alone throughout their pregnancies gave birth to normal infants.[1]

1. Cook DG, Klawans HL. Levodopa during pregnancy. *Clin Neuropharmacol* 1985; **8:** 93–5.

**Withdrawal.** For adverse effects associated with withdrawal of levodopa, see under Adverse Effects, above.

## Interactions

The therapeutic or adverse effects of levodopa may be affected by interactions with a variety of drugs. Mechanisms may include effects on catecholamine metabolising enzymes, neurotransmitters, or receptor sites, effects on the endocrine system, and effects on gastrointestinal absorption. Drugs that modify gastric emptying may affect the absorption of levodopa.

**Antibacterials.** A study[1] in 7 healthy subjects showed that use of *spiramycin* with levodopa and carbidopa resulted in reduced plasma-levodopa concentrations and an increase in its peripheral metabolism.

A hypertensive reaction and severe tremor occurred when *isoniazid* was given to a patient receiving levodopa;[2] it was not certain whether isoniazid was acting as an MAOI.

1. Brion N, *et al.* Effect of a macrolide (spiramycin) on the pharmacokinetics of L-dopa and carbidopa in healthy volunteers. *Clin Neuropharmacol* 1992; **15:** 229–35.
2. Morgan JP. Isoniazid and levodopa. *Ann Intern Med* 1980; **92:** 434.

**Antidepressants.** BUPROPION. Caution has been advised with bupropion because of reports of a higher incidence of adverse effects during concomitant use with levodopa.

MAOIS. Administration of levodopa with non-specific MAOIs such as *phenelzine*, *pargyline*, *nialamide*, or *tranylcypromine* may cause dangerous hypertension;[1-4] it is recommended that levodopa should not be given within at least 14 days of stopping an MAOI. Hypertensive reactions to levodopa with *tranylcypromine* were inhibited by carbidopa,[5] but the manufacturers of preparations containing levodopa with carbidopa or benserazide still contra-indicate their use with MAOIs. The incidence of adverse effects may be increased if levodopa is used with *moclobemide*, a monoamine oxidase type A inhibitor (see p.308). *Selegiline*, a monoamine oxidase type B inhibitor, is used to enhance the antiparkinsonian effect of levodopa, see p.1214.

1. Hunter KR, *et al.* Monoamine oxidase inhibitors and L-dopa. *BMJ* 1970; **3:** 388.
2. Hodge JV. Use of monoamine oxidase inhibitors. *Lancet* 1965; **i:** 764–5.
3. Friend DG, *et al.* The action of L-dihydroxyphenylalanine in patients receiving nialamide. *Clin Pharmacol Ther* 1965; **6:** 362–6.
4. Sharpe J, *et al.* Idiopathic orthostatic hypotension treated with levodopa and MAO inhibitor: a preliminary report. *Can Med Assoc J* 1972; **107:** 296–300.
5. Teychenne PF, *et al.* Interactions of levodopa with inhibitors of monoamine oxidase and L-aromatic amino acid decarboxylase. *Clin Pharmacol Ther* 1975; **18:** 273–7.

SSRIS. There was some evidence from a prescribing study that SSRIs might exacerbate parkinsonism and necessitate increased doses of levodopa or addition of adjunctive drugs.[1]

1. van de Vijver DAMC, *et al.* Start of a selective serotonin reuptake inhibitor (SSRI) and increase of antiparkinsonian drug treatment in patients on levodopa. *Br J Clin Pharmacol* 2002; **54:** 168–70.

TRICYCLIC ANTIDEPRESSANTS. Although tricyclic antidepressants have been used safely with levodopa[1] hypertensive crises have occurred in patients receiving *amitriptyline* or *imipramine* and levodopa with carbidopa.[2,3] Imipramine has been reported to impair the rate of levodopa absorption,[4] presumably due to its antimuscarinic properties (for the effect of antimuscarinics on the absorption of levodopa, see below).

1. Hunter KR, *et al.* Use of levodopa with other drugs. *Lancet* 1970; **ii:** 1283–5.
2. Rampton DS. Hypertensive crisis in a patient given Sinemet, metoclopramide, and amitriptyline. *BMJ* 1977; **2:** 607–8.
3. Edwards M. Adverse interaction of levodopa with tricyclic antidepressants. *Practitioner* 1982; **226:** 1447–8.
4. Morgan JP, *et al.* Imipramine-mediated interference with levodopa absorption from the gastrointestinal tract in man. *Neurology* 1975; **25:** 1029–34.

TRYPTOPHAN. See Amino Acids under Nutritional Agents, below.

**Antiepileptics.** *Phenytoin* has been shown to diminish the therapeutic effect of levodopa in patients with parkinsonism or chronic manganese poisoning.[1] The mechanism of the interaction was considered uncertain.

1. Mendez JS. Diphenylhydantoin: blocking of levodopa effects. *Arch Neurol* 1975; **32:** 44–6.

**Antihypertensives.** Use of levodopa with *guanethidine* may cause increased hypotension.[1] *Clonidine* has been reported to inhibit the therapeutic effect of levodopa, possibly by stimulating central alpha-adrenoceptors.[2] *Methyldopa* and levodopa may enhance each other's therapeutic or adverse effects, although there has been mention of the inhibitory effect of methyldopa on the therapeutic response to levodopa.[3,4]

1. Hunter KR, *et al.* Use of levodopa with other drugs. *Lancet* 1970; **ii:** 1283–5.
2. Shoulson I, Chase TN. Clonidine and the anti-parkinsonian response to L-dopa or piribedil. *Neuropharmacology* 1976; **15:** 25–7.
3. Cotzias GC, *et al.* L-Dopa in Parkinson's syndrome. *N Engl J Med* 1969; **281:** 272.
4. Kofman O. Treatment of Parkinson's disease with L-dopa: a current appraisal. *Can Med Assoc J* 1971; **104:** 483–7.

**Antimuscarinics.** Antimuscarinic antiparkinsonian drugs may enhance the therapeutic effects of levodopa but by delaying gastric emptying they may reduce its absorption.[1]

1. Algeri S, *et al.* Effect of anticholinergic drugs on gastro-intestinal absorption of L-dopa in rats and in man. *Eur J Pharmacol* 1976; **35:** 293–9.

**Antineoplastics.** A patient with Parkinson's disease noted[1] that the efficacy of levodopa was reduced each time he received *dacarbazine* for the treatment of melanoma. As serum-dopamine concentrations were unchanged it was suggested[1] that dacarbazine might compete with levodopa at the blood-brain barrier.

1. Merello M, *et al.* Impaired levodopa response in Parkinson's disease during melanoma therapy. *Clin Neuropharmacol* 1992; **15:** 69–74.

**Antipsychotics.** The therapeutic effects of levodopa may be diminished by CNS dopamine inhibitors including phenothiazine derivatives[1] such as *prochlorperazine*.[2] Butyrophenones such as *haloperidol* and thioxanthenes such as *flupentixol* might be expected to have a similar effect due to their antidopaminergic properties.

1. Yahr MD, Duvoisin RC. Drug therapy of parkinsonism. *N Engl J Med* 1972; **287:** 20–4.
2. Duvoisin RC. Diphenidol for levodopa induced nausea and vomiting. *JAMA* 1972; **221:** 1408.

**Anxiolytics.** Reversible deterioration of parkinsonism has been reported in patients receiving levodopa who were given *benzodiazepines* such as *diazepam*,[1,2] *nitrazepam*[1] (although the evidence was equivocal), or *chlordiazepoxide*.[3] In one case parkinsonian symptoms resolved without alteration in the medication.[1]

1. Hunter KR, *et al.* Use of levodopa with other drugs. *Lancet* 1970; **ii:** 1283–5.
2. Wodak J, *et al.* Review of 12 months' treatment with L-dopa in Parkinson's disease, with remarks on unusual side effects. *Med J Aust* 1972; **2:** 1277–82.
3. Yosselson-Superstine S, Lipman AG. Chlordiazepoxide interaction with levodopa. *Ann Intern Med* 1982; **96:** 259–60.

**Baclofen.** Adverse effects including hallucinations, confusion, headache, and nausea and worsening of symptoms have been reported[1,2] in patients with Parkinson's disease taking levodopa when given baclofen.

1. Skausig OB, Korsgaard S. Hallucinations and baclofen. *Lancet* 1977; **i:** 1258.
2. Lees AJ, *et al.* Baclofen in Parkinson's disease. *J Neurol Neurosurg Psychiatry* 1978; **41:** 707–8.

**Gastrointestinal drugs.** ANTACIDS. Some studies have suggested that taking an antacid before a dose of levodopa enhances the absorption of levodopa, apparently by enhancing gastric emptying and reducing metabolism of levodopa in the stomach.[1,2] This was particularly marked in a case report in a patient with prolonged gastric emptying time.[1] However, another study in 8 patients with presumably normal gastric motility, only 3 of whom had Parkinson's disease, found no significant increase in overall absorption of levodopa when given with an antacid although there was some evidence of increased absorption in some of the patients.[3]

1. Rivera-Calimlim L, *et al.* L-Dopa treatment failure: explanation and correction. *BMJ* 1970; **4:** 93–4.
2. Pocelinko R, *et al.* The effect of an antacid on the absorption and metabolism of levodopa. *Clin Pharmacol Ther* 1972; **13:** 149.
3. Leon AS, Spiegel HE. The effect of antacid administration on the absorption and metabolism of levodopa. *J Clin Pharmacol* 1972; **12:** 263–7.

ANTIEMETICS. *Metoclopramide* accelerates gastric emptying and has been reported to increase the rate of levodopa absorption.[1] The importance of timing has been noted[2] since levodopa delayed gastric emptying and metoclopramide antagonised this effect. *Domperidone* has been reported to increase the bioavailability of levodopa slightly.[3]

1. Morris JGL, *et al.* Plasma dopa concentrations after different preparations of levodopa in normal subjects. *Br J Clin Pharmacol* 1976; **3:** 983–90.
2. Berkowitz DM, McCallum RW. Interaction of levodopa and metoclopramide on gastric emptying. *Clin Pharmacol Ther* 1980; **27:** 414–20.
3. Shindler JS, *et al.* Domperidone and levodopa in Parkinson's disease. *Br J Clin Pharmacol* 1984; **18:** 959–62.

PROKINETICS. Maximum plasma concentrations of levodopa are increased by concomitant administration of *cisapride*.[1]

See also Metoclopramide and Domperidone, under Antiemetics, above.

1. Neira WD, *et al.* The effects of cisapride on plasma L-dopa levels and the clinical response in Parkinson's disease. *Mov Disord* 1995; **10:** 66–70.

**General anaesthetics.** The general anaesthetics *cyclopropane* and *halothane* lower the threshold for ventricular arrhythmias to sympathomimetic amines, including dopamine, and should probably not be used within 6 to 8 hours of the administration of levodopa.[1,2] Although other general anaesthetics are now usually preferred, it was suggested that, in any case, levodopa could safely be taken before surgery when given with a peripheral dopa-decarboxylase inhibitor.[3]

1. Goldberg LI, Whitsett TL. Cardiovascular effects of levodopa. *Clin Pharmacol Ther* 1971; **12:** 376–82.
2. Bianchine JR, Sunyapridakul L. Interactions between levodopa and other drugs: significance in the treatment of Parkinson's disease. *Drugs* 1973; **6:** 364–88.
3. Anonymous. Surgery and long-term medication. *Drug Ther Bull* 1984; **22:** 73–6.

**Nutritional agents.** AMINO ACIDS. The transport of levodopa into the brain is subject to competition from chemically related L-amino acids, especially the other aromatic amino acids *phenylalanine*, *tyrosine*, *tryptophan*, and *histidine*.[1] A high-protein diet or the large neutral amino acids phenylalanine, *leucine*, or *isoleucine* have been shown to reduce the therapeutic effect of levodopa given by intravenous infusion to parkinsonian patients; such alterations in the absorption and transport of levodopa may contribute to the fluctuating responses seen in Parkinson's disease, the so-called 'on-off' phenomenon[2] (see also under Parkinsonism, p.1196). Other reported interactions with amino acids include *methionine*-antagonism of the therapeutic effect of levodopa in parkinsonism[3] and *tryptophan*-reduced blood concentrations of levodopa.[4]

1. Daniel PM, *et al.* Do changes in blood levels of other aromatic aminoacids influence levodopa therapy? *Lancet* 1976; **i:** 95.
2. Nutt JG, *et al.* The "on-off" phenomenon in Parkinson's disease: relation to levodopa absorption and transport. *N Engl J Med* 1984; **310:** 483–8.
3. Pearce LA, Waterbury LD. L-methionine: a possible levodopa antagonist. *Neurology* 1974; **24:** 640–1.
4. Weitbrecht W-U, Weigel K. Der Einfluß von L-Tryptophan auf die L-Dopa-Resorption. *Dtsch Med Wochenschr* 1976; **101:** 20–2.

IRON SALTS. Levodopa forms complexes with iron salts and administration with ferrous sulfate has reduced bioavailability of levodopa by about 50% in healthy subjects.[1] Administration of ferrous sulfate to 9 patients with Parkinson's disease receiving levodopa with carbidopa reduced the area under the curve by 30% and greater than 75% for levodopa and carbidopa, respectively. Although this was associated with deterioration in some patients' disability the average reduction in efficacy of therapy did not achieve statistical significance.[2]

1. Campbell NRC, Hasinoff BB. Iron supplements: a common cause of drug interactions. *Br J Clin Pharmacol* 1991; **31:** 251–5.
2. Campbell NRC, *et al.* Sinemet-ferrous sulphate interaction in patients with Parkinson's disease. *Br J Clin Pharmacol* 1990; **30:** 599–605.

PYRIDOXINE. The enzyme responsible for the decarboxylation of levodopa, L-amino acid decarboxylase, is dependent on pyridoxine and pyridoxine supplements have been reported to enhance the peripheral metabolism of levodopa to dopamine leaving less available to cross the blood-brain barrier for central conversion to dopamine;[1-4] pyridoxine therefore inhibits the action of levodopa but this can be stopped by use of a peripheral dopa-decarboxylase inhibitor.[3,4]

1. Carter AB. Pyridoxine and parkinsonism. *BMJ* 1973; **4:** 236.
2. Leon AS, *et al.* Pyridoxine antagonism of levodopa in parkinsonism. *JAMA* 1971; **218:** 1924–7.
3. Cotzias GC, Papavasiliou PS. Blocking the negative effects of pyridoxine on patients receiving levodopa. *JAMA* 1971; **215:** 1504–5.
4. Yahr MD, Duvoisin RC. Pyridoxine, levodopa, and L-α-methyldopa hydrazine regimen in parkinsonism. *JAMA* 1971; **216:** 2141.

**Papaverine.** Antagonism of the beneficial effects of levodopa in parkinsonism has been reported when patients were also given papaverine,[1,2] and it was recommended that the combination should be avoided.

1. Duvoisin RC. Antagonism of levodopa by papaverine. *JAMA* 1975; **231:** 845.
2. Posner DM. Antagonism of levodopa by papaverine. *JAMA* 1975; **233:** 768.

**Penicillamine.** Isolated case reports suggest that penicillamine increases plasma-levodopa concentrations.[1]

1. Mizuta E, *et al.* Effect of D-penicillamine on pharmacokinetics of levodopa in Parkinson's disease. *Clin Neuropharmacol* 1993; **16:** 448–50.

**Sympathomimetics.** It has been suggested that sympathomimetics such as *adrenaline* or *isoprenaline* may enhance the cardiac side-effects of levodopa.[1]

1. Goldberg LI, Whitsett TL. Cardiovascular effects of levodopa. *Clin Pharmacol Ther* 1971; **12:** 376–82.

## Pharmacokinetics

Levodopa is rapidly absorbed from the gastrointestinal tract by an active transport system. Most absorption takes place in the small intestine; absorption is very limited from the stomach, and since decarboxylation may take place in the stomach wall, delays in gastric emptying may reduce the amount of levodopa available for absorption.

Levodopa is rapidly decarboxylated by the enzyme aromatic L-amino acid decarboxylase, mostly in the gut, liver, and kidney, to dopamine, which is metabolised in turn, principally to dihydroxyphenylacetic acid (DOPAC) and homovanillic acid (HVA). Other routes of metabolism include *O*-methylation, transamination, and oxidation, producing a variety of minor metabolites including noradrenaline and 3-*O*-methyldopa; the latter may accumulate in the CNS due to its relatively long half-life. The plasma half-life of levodopa itself is reported to be about 1 to 3 hours.

Unlike dopamine, levodopa is actively transported across the blood-brain barrier, but because of the extent of peripheral decarboxylation very little is available to enter the CNS unless it is given with a peripheral dopa-decarboxylase inhibitor. In the presence of a peripheral dopa-decarboxylase inhibitor the major route of metabolism of levodopa becomes the formation of 3-*O*-methyldopa by the enzyme catechol-*O*-methyltransferase.

About 80% of an oral dose of levodopa is excreted in the urine within 24 hours, mostly as dihydroxyphenylacetic and homovanillic acids. Only small amounts of levodopa are excreted unchanged in the faeces.

Levodopa is reported to be distributed into breast milk.

◊ General references.


1. Nutt JG, Fellman JH. Pharmacokinetics of levodopa. *Clin Neuropharmacol* 1984; **7:** 35–49.
2. Cedarbaum JM. Clinical pharmacokinetics of anti-parkinsonian drugs. *Clin Pharmacokinet* 1987; **13:** 141–78.
3. Robertson DRC, *et al.* The effect of age on the pharmacokinetics of levodopa administered alone and in the presence of carbidopa. *Br J Clin Pharmacol* 1989; **28:** 61–9.
4. Robertson DRC, *et al.* The influence of levodopa on gastric emptying in man. *Br J Clin Pharmacol* 1990; **29:** 47–53.


## Uses and Administration

Levodopa, a naturally occurring amino acid, is the immediate precursor of the neurotransmitter dopamine. The actions of levodopa are mainly those of dopamine (p.907).

Unlike dopamine, levodopa can readily enter the CNS and is used in the treatment of conditions, such as Parkinson's disease, that are associated with depletion of dopamine in the brain. Levodopa is rapidly decarboxylated by peripheral enzymes so that very little unchanged drug is available to cross the blood-brain barrier for central conversion into dopamine. Consequently, levodopa is usually given with a peripheral dopa-decarboxylase inhibitor such as benserazide (p.1200) or carbidopa (p.1204) to increase the proportion of levodopa that can enter the brain. This enables the dosage of levodopa to be reduced and may diminish peripheral side-effects, such as nausea and vomiting and cardiac arrhythmias, by blocking the peripheral production of dopamine. It may also provide a more rapid response at the start of therapy.

The majority of patients with Parkinson's disease benefit from levodopa therapy, but after 2 years or more improvement in disability is gradually lost as the disease progresses and fluctuations in mobility emerge. Postencephalitic parkinsonism responds to levodopa, but a higher incidence of side-effects has been reported than in the idiopathic form so smaller doses are generally used. Levodopa has also been used to control the neurological symptoms of chronic manganese poisoning, which resemble those of parkinsonism. It should not be used in antipsychotic-induced parkinsonism.

Levodopa has an effect on pituitary function as a result of its conversion to dopamine. It may enhance growth-hormone secretion and has been used diagnostically as a provocative test for growth-hormone deficiency. Levodopa also inhibits prolactin secretion.

Response to levodopa varies considerably between patients. **Treatment of parkinsonism** should commence with small doses increased gradually, ideally to a dose which improves mobility without incurring side-effects. Levodopa should be taken with or after meals, although in later disease, it may be preferable to administer on an empty stomach (see Precautions, above). Once established, maintenance doses may need to be reduced as the patient ages. When given **without a peripheral dopa-decarboxylase inhibitor** (which is rare) a suggested initial dose is 125 mg twice daily by mouth increased gradually every 3 to 7 days, according to response, to up to 8 g daily in divided doses. The intervals between doses should be adjusted to meet individual needs; many patients find 4 or 5 divided doses daily to be satisfactory although some may require smaller, more frequent doses in order to control fluctuations in mobility. Maximum improvement may take up to 6 months or longer to occur.

When given **with a peripheral dopa-decarboxylase inhibitor** lower doses of levodopa are used. As high central dopamine concentrations can be achieved more quickly, both beneficial and adverse effects tend to occur more rapidly than with levodopa alone and patients should be monitored carefully. In those already receiving levodopa the drug should be discontinued and benserazide or carbidopa with levodopa started on the following day or after 24 hours if the patient was receiving a modified-release preparation of levodopa.

**Benserazide** is given as the hydrochloride but doses are expressed in terms of the base. Benserazide hydrochloride 28.5 mg is approximately equivalent to 25 mg of benserazide. Benserazide is usually given with levodopa in the ratio of 1 part of benserazide base to 4 parts of levodopa (co-beneldopa) and the doses for co-beneldopa that follow are expressed in terms of the levodopa component.

- An initial dose for *patients not previously treated with levodopa* is levodopa 50 mg three or four times daily by mouth increased gradually in increments of levodopa 100 mg once or twice weekly, according to response. If the disease is at an advanced stage, the initial starting dose may be increased to levodopa 100 mg three times daily. For some elderly patients, an initial dose of levodopa 50 mg once or twice daily, increased by 50 mg every third or fourth day, may be suitable. Maintenance doses usually lie within the range of levodopa 400 to 800 mg daily in divided doses, although most patients require no more than 600 mg daily. If optimal improvement has not been achieved after several weeks at the average dose, further increases may be made with caution; it is rarely necessary to give more than 1 g of levodopa daily.
- The initial dose of levodopa given with benserazide in *patients previously treated with levodopa alone* should be about 10 to 15% of the dose previously being taken, thus levodopa 300 mg would be appropriate for a patient previously taking levodopa 2 g daily. For *patients previously treated with other levodopa/dopa-decarboxylase inhibitor combinations* an initial dose is levodopa 50 mg given three or four times daily. In either situation, the dose may then be adjusted in a similar manner as described for previously untreated patients.
- Modified-release capsules containing the equivalent of benserazide 25 mg with levodopa 100 mg are available to reduce fluctuations in response to conventional preparations. For *patients not already receiving levodopa* the initial dose is one capsule three times daily adjusted every 2 to 3 days according to response; it is recommended that initial dosages should not exceed 600 mg of levodopa daily. For *patients already receiving a conventional preparation* of levodopa with benserazide, initially one capsule should be substituted for every 100 mg of levodopa and should be given at the same dosage frequency as before; increases in dosage can then be made every 2 to 3 days according to response. An average of 50% more levodopa may be required compared with previous therapy and titration may take up to 4 weeks. *Supplementary doses* of a conventional preparation of benserazide with levodopa may also be required with the first morning dose.

**Carbidopa** is usually given with levodopa (co-careldopa) as tablets in the ratio of 1 to 4 or 1 to 10, which allows dosage adjustments of either drug for individual patients. Carbidopa is given as the hydrous base although doses are expressed in terms of the anhydrous base; hydrous carbidopa 10.8 mg is approximately equivalent to 10 mg anhydrous carbidopa. Full inhibition of peripheral dopa-decarboxylase is reported to be achieved by 70 to 100 mg of carbidopa daily.

- A suggested initial dose for *patients not previously treated with levodopa* is carbidopa 25 mg with levodopa 100 mg three times daily by mouth, increased gradually, in increments of carbidopa 12.5 mg with levodopa 50 mg or carbidopa 25 mg with levodopa 100 mg every day or on alternate days, as necessary. The usual maintenance dosage range is carbidopa 75 to 200 mg with levodopa 750 mg to 2 g daily in divided doses. Carbidopa doses greater than 200 mg daily are not generally exceeded.
- The initial dose of levodopa with carbidopa in *patients previously treated with levodopa* should be about 20 to 25% of the dose previously being taken, thus for patients taking less than 1.5 g of levodopa daily a suggested initial dose is carbidopa 25 mg with levodopa 100 mg given three or four times daily; a suggested initial dose for patients taking more than 1.5 g of levodopa daily is carbidopa 25 mg with levodopa 250 mg given three or four times daily.
- Modified-release tablets containing carbidopa with levodopa in the ratio of 1 to 4 are available to reduce fluctuations in response to conventional preparations. For *patients not already receiving levodopa* therapy, or for *those currently receiving levodopa alone*, the initial dose is carbidopa 50 mg with levodopa 200 mg twice daily adjusted according to response at intervals of not less than 3 days. It is recommended that for patients who are not already receiving levodopa initial dosages should not exceed 600 mg of levodopa daily. For *patients already receiving a conventional preparation* of carbidopa with levodopa, the initial dose of the modified-release preparation should provide a similar daily amount of levodopa, but the dosing intervals should be prolonged and are normally between 4 to 12 hours. The initial substitution dose of the modified-release preparation should provide not more than 10% more levodopa than was previously given for doses of levodopa greater than 900 mg daily. Doses and intervals may then be altered according to clinical response, allowing at least 3 days between adjustments. Up to 30% more levodopa may be required in the modified-release preparation than was previously administered in the conventional preparation. Average maintenance doses of modified-release preparations lie within the range of carbidopa 100 mg with levodopa 400 mg to carbidopa 400 mg with levodopa 1.6 g. *Supplementary doses* of a conventional preparation of carbidopa with levodopa may be required in some patients.

Combination preparations of levodopa with carbidopa and the catechol-*O*-methyltransferase (COMT) inhibitor **entacapone** are also available; each tablet contains levodopa and carbidopa in a ratio of 4:1 with entacapone 200 mg. Such preparations are indicated for patients with end-of-dose motor fluctuations not stabilised on levodopa/peripheral dopa-decarboxylase inhibitor treatment. Patients should only take one combination tablet for each dose.

- *patients previously treated with standard-release levodopa with a peripheral dopa-decarboxylase and separate entacapone* should be transferred to the combination preparation at a dose that provides similar or slightly higher amounts of levodopa.
- for *patients not currently taking entacapone*, the dose of the combination preparation should normally provide a similar or slightly lower dose of levodopa to that previously taken. However, patients with *dyskinesia* or taking *levodopa doses above 800 mg daily* should start entacapone as a separate medication before being transferred to the combination preparation, as a 10 to 30% reduction in their levodopa dose may be needed when starting combination therapy.

In some countries a gel formulation of levodopa 20 mg/mL with carbidopa 5 mg/mL is available for infusion by an ambulatory pump into the duodenum.

**Drug-induced extrapyramidal disorders.** The management of drug-induced extrapyramidal disorders is discussed under the Adverse Effects of Chlorpromazine on p.677. Although the use of dopamine agonists, especially levodopa, to overcome antipsychotic-induced blockade of dopamine receptors might appear rational, levodopa has generally been reported to be ineffective or to increase psychiatric symptoms.

**Dysphagia.** Results of a small study[1] have suggested that levodopa may improve the impaired swallowing reflex in patients with basal ganglia infarctions and thereby help to prevent aspiration pneumonia.


1. Kobayashi H, *et al.* Levodopa and swallowing reflex. *Lancet* 1996; **348:** 1320–1.


**Dystonias.** A dystonia is a syndrome of sustained muscle contractions, frequently causing twisting and repetitive movements or abnormal postures; it may also have additional myoclonic or tremulous components. Typically it starts as a focal dystonia localised in one part of the body and to begin with may appear only during a specific motor act (action dystonia). If the syndrome is progressive the dystonias may become apparent at rest and spread first to more than one part of the body (segmental dystonia) and may eventually affect most or all of the body (generalised dystonia). Progression of the dystonia appears to be related to age of onset. Dystonia beginning in childhood usually starts in the legs and progresses to become segmental or generalised, whereas in adults the dystonia usually starts in other parts of the body and rarely becomes generalised. Examples of focal dystonias are blepharospasm (affecting the eye and surrounding facial muscles), writer's cramp (hand and arm), spasmodic torticollis (neck), spasmodic dysphonia, or dystonic dysphagia (larynx or pharynx), and leg dystonias. Some dystonias may be associated with metabolic disorders such as Wilson's disease or Lesch-Nyhan syndrome; with neurological disorders such as Huntington's disease; or with other causes including head trauma, manganese or carbon disulfide toxicity, or the side-effects of antipsychotics or antiparkinsonian drugs. However, in the majority of cases the disease is idiopathic.

There are no cures for most types of dystonia, but with appropriate **management** symptomatic relief is possible in many patients.[1-3]

- It has been suggested that all children and adolescents presenting with dystonia, particularly starting in the legs, should first be given a trial with *levodopa*.[2] A suggested regimen is to gradually build up to a dose of levodopa 200 mg with carbidopa 50 mg given three times daily and to maintain this dose for 3 months; if there is no useful response in this period the drug is withdrawn. Where there is benefit it is usually dramatic and is sustained as long as the drug is taken, which may be more than 10 years in some cases, in general without the long-term problems associated with levodopa for parkinsonism (see p.1196).
- In children and adolescents who fail to respond to levodopa an *antimuscarinic* such as trihexyphenidyl is second choice. Side-effects are minimised by starting with a low dose which is then gradually increased. General experience indicates that about half of all children and adolescents benefit from antimuscarinics; adults tolerate the drug less well and only about a fifth of adult patients with focal dystonia benefit.
- In patients who do not respond to levodopa or high-dose antimuscarinics other drugs may be used. Many benefit from *benzodiazepines* such as diazepam; a few have responded to *baclofen* or *carbamazepine*. *Antipsychotics* are sometimes useful but carry the risk of inducing tardive dyskinesia. *Tetrabenazine* carries less risk of tardive dyskinesia but may induce depression. In very severe dystonia combination therapy may be required: tetrabenazine with pimozide and trihexyphenidyl is sometimes effective.
- The response in patients with adult onset focal dystonia is usually poor. However, the use of *botulinum A toxin* can produce relief in blepharospasm, spasmodic torticollis, and spasmodic dysphonia, and is under investigation for writer's cramp and other occupational dystonias. Local injections into the affected muscles produce weakness over the next week or so, thereby reducing or abolishing dystonic spasms. The effect lasts some 2 to 4 months.

Further details of the management of blepharospasm and spasmodic torticollis can be found under Botulinum Toxins on p.1390. For a discussion of the management of antipsychotic-induced dystonic reactions, see under Extrapyramidal Disorders in the Adverse Effects of Chlorpromazine, p.677.

1. Anonymous. Dystonia: underdiagnosed and undertreated? *Drug Ther Bull* 1988; **26:** 33–6.
2. Marsden CD, Quinn NP. The dystonias. *BMJ* 1990; **300:** 139–44.
3. Williams A. Consensus statement for the management of focal dystonias. *Br J Hosp Med* 1993; **50:** 655–9.

**Neuroleptic malignant syndrome.** There have been isolated reports[1-4] that levodopa used alone or with bromocriptine has been successful in the treatment of patients with neuroleptic malignant syndrome (p.677). However, bromocriptine is usually preferred when a dopaminergic is required for the treatment of this condition.

1. Knezevic W, *et al.* Neuroleptic malignant syndrome. *Med J Aust* 1984; **140:** 28–30.
2. Clarke CE, *et al.* Clinical spectrum of neuroleptic malignant syndrome. *Lancet* 1988; **ii:** 969–70.
3. Lo TCN, *et al.* Neuroleptic malignant syndrome: another medical cause of acute abdomen. *Postgrad Med J* 1989; **65:** 653–5.
4. Shoop SA, Cernek PK. Carbidopa/levodopa in the treatment of neuroleptic malignant syndrome. *Ann Pharmacother* 1997; **31:** 119.

**Parasomnias.** The aetiology of *restless legs syndrome* and *periodic limb movements in sleep* is obscure and treatment has been largely empirical (p.667). Few of the treatments tried in these often co-existent disorders have been studied in a controlled manner but small controlled studies[1-6] have reported beneficial effects such as improved sleep quality and reduced leg movements from levodopa used with a peripheral dopa-decarboxylase inhibitor. Most patients received a bedtime dose of 50 to 200 mg of levodopa with possible additional doses during the night.

Levodopa has also been reported to have been of benefit in a study of 10 patients with *sleep bruxism*.[7]

1. von Scheele C. Levodopa in restless legs. *Lancet* 1986; **ii:** 426–7.
2. Brodeur C, *et al.* Treatment of restless legs syndrome and periodic movements during sleep with L-dopa: a double-blind controlled study. *Neurology* 1988; **38:** 1845–8.
3. Kaplan PW, *et al.* A double-blind, placebo-controlled study of the treatment of periodic limb movements in sleep using carbidopa/levodopa and propoxyphene. *Sleep* 1993; **16:** 717–23.
4. Trenkwalder C, *et al.* L-dopa therapy of uremic and idiopathic restless legs syndrome: a double-blind crossover trial. *Sleep* 1995; **18:** 681–8.
5. Beneš H, *et al.* Rapid onset of action of levodopa in restless legs syndrome: a double-blind, randomized, multicenter, crossover trial. *Sleep* 1999; **22:** 1073–81.
6. Janzen L, *et al.* An overview of levodopa in the management of restless legs syndrome in a dialysis population: pharmacokinetics, clinical trials, and complications of therapy. *Ann Pharmacother* 1999; **33:** 86–92.
7. Lobbezoo F, *et al.* The effect of the catecholamine precursor L-dopa on sleep bruxism: a controlled clinical trial. *Mov Disord* 1997; **12:** 73–8.

**Parkinsonism.** Levodopa is the mainstay in the treatment of Parkinson's disease (p.1196) but opinion varies on when it should be used in the course of the disease. Most patients respond to levodopa initially but after a few years benefit may be reduced. There may be problems with dyskinesias and psychiatric effects and fluctuations in mobility necessitating careful dosage adjustment or the use of adjunctive drugs. For most patients treatment with levodopa eventually becomes necessary, but many neurologists delay initial treatment with levodopa because of the increased risk of motor complications. New patients, especially younger patients, therefore often begin treatment with a dopamine agonist, with levodopa reserved for the elderly, the frail, or those with intercurrent illness or more severe symptoms. Levodopa should be given with a peripheral dopa-decarboxylase inhibitor; a peripheral catechol-*O*-methyltransferase (COMT) inhibitor may also be necessary for patients experiencing fluctuations in disability related to levodopa and dopa-decarboxylase inhibitor combinations. The various methods used for the pharmacokinetic optimisation of levodopa therapy as Parkinson's disease progresses include timing of administration, the use of modified-release formulations, oral solutions (but see Stability, p.1205) and dispersible formulations for immediate absorption, the timing of food intake, and the use of other drugs to increase the absorption of levodopa. In some countries a gel formulation of levodopa with carbidopa is available for intraduodenal infusion.

References.

1. Giron LT, Koller WC. Methods of managing levodopa-induced dyskinesias. *Drug Safety* 1996; **14:** 365–74.
2. Contin M, *et al.* Pharmacokinetic optimisation in the treatment of Parkinson's disease. *Clin Pharmacokinet* 1996; **30:** 463–81.
3. Murer MG, *et al.* Levodopa in Parkinson's disease: neurotoxicity issue laid to rest? *Drug Safety* 1999; **21:** 339–52.
4. Furlanut M, *et al.* Monitoring of L-dopa concentrations in Parkinson's disease. *Pharmacol Res* 2001; **43:** 423–7. Correction. *ibid.*; **44:** 149.
5. Carlsson A. Treatment of Parkinson's with L-DOPA: the early discovery phase, and a comment on current problems. *J Neural Transm* 2002; **109:** 777–87.
6. Katzenschlager R, Lees AJ. Treatment of Parkinson's disease: levodopa as the first choice. *J Neurol* 2002; **249** (suppl 2): II19–II24.
7. van Laar T. Levodopa-induced response fluctuations in patients with Parkinson's disease: strategies for management. *CNS Drugs* 2003; **17:** 475–89.
8. LeWitt PA, Nyholm D. New developments in levodopa therapy. *Neurology* 2004; **62** (suppl 1): S9–S16.
9. Stocchi F, Olanow CW. Continuous dopaminergic stimulation in early and advanced Parkinson's disease. *Neurology* 2004; **62** (suppl 1): S56–S63.

**Pituitary and hypothalamic disorders.** DIAGNOSIS AND TESTING. Diminished growth-hormone reserve is one of the earliest functional abnormalities in anterior pituitary failure and, since dopamine is believed to stimulate growth-hormone secretion, levodopa has been used as a provocative test for the diagnosis of growth-hormone deficiency.[1,2] Levodopa 500 mg has been given by mouth after an overnight fast and serum concentrations of growth hormone measured hourly at 0 to 3 hours; children may be given 10 mg/kg to a maximum of 500 mg. Transient nausea, vomiting, vertigo, and hypotension may occur and the patient should be kept recumbent during the test. A normal response is an increase in serum concentration of growth hormone of more than 5 nanograms/mL or to a level of more than 10 nanograms/mL, although 10 to 15% of normal subjects may not respond. However, there is some dispute as to whether stimulated growth hormone secretion tests are superior to measurements of circulating somatomedins in detecting growth hormone deficiency.[3-5] For a discussion of the management of growth retardation, including the problems of accurate diagnosis, see p.1314.

1. Abboud CF. Laboratory diagnosis of hypopituitarism. *Mayo Clin Proc* 1986; **61:** 35–48.
2. Müller EE, *et al.* Involvement of brain catecholamines and acetylcholine in growth hormone deficiency states: pathophysiological, diagnostic and therapeutic implications. *Drugs* 1991; **41:** 161–77.
3. Hoffmann DM, *et al.* Diagnosis of growth-hormone deficiency in adults. *Lancet* 1994; **343:** 1064–8. Correction. *ibid.*, **344:** 206.
4. de Boer H, *et al.* Diagnosis of growth hormone deficiency in adults. *Lancet* 1994; **343:** 1645–6.
5. Rosenfeld RG, *et al.* Diagnostic controversy: the diagnosis of childhood growth hormone deficiency revisited. *J Clin Endocrinol Metab* 1995; **80:** 1532–40.

**Strabismus.** Experimental studies have shown that centrally-acting drugs such as levodopa may improve vision in patients with amblyopia (see Strabismus, p.1487). However, their role in clinical practice remains to be established.[1]

1. Chatzistefanou KI, Mills MD. The role of drug treatment in children with strabismus and amblyopia. *Paediatr Drugs* 2000; **2:** 91–100.

**Tourette's syndrome.** Levodopa has been studied in the management of Tourette's syndrome (see Tics, p.664). A small pilot study[1] has produced encouraging results.

1. Black KJ, *et al.* Response to levodopa challenge in Tourette syndrome. *Mov Disord* 2000; **15:** 1194–8.

## Preparations

***BP 2003:*** Co-beneldopa Capsules; Co-careldopa Tablets; Dispersible Co-beneldopa Tablets; Levodopa Capsules; Levodopa Tablets;
***USP 27:*** Carbidopa and Levodopa Tablets; Levodopa Capsules; Levodopa Tablets.

**Proprietary Preparations** (details are given in Part 3)
***Ger.:*** Dopaflex; Restex; ***India:*** Levopa; ***Ital.:*** Levomet; ***USA:*** Dopar; Larodopa.

**Multi-ingredient:** ***Arg.:*** Lebocar; Lecarge; Madopar; Nervocur; Sinemet; ***Austral.:*** Kinson; Madopar; Sinacarb†; Sinemet; ***Austria:*** Dopamed; Levobens; Madopar; Sinemet; ***Belg.:*** Prolopa; Sinemet; ***Braz.:*** Carbidol; Cronomet; Levocarb; Prolopa; Sinemet; ***Canad.:*** Apo-Levocarb; Nu-Levocarb; Prolopa; Sinemet; ***Chile:*** Grifoparkin; Levofamil; Melitase; Prolopa; Saniter Compuesto; Sinemet; ***Denm.:*** Madopar; Sinemet; ***Fin.:*** Aktipar†; Kardopal; Madopar; Sinemet; ***Fr.:*** Modopar; Sinemet; ***Ger.:*** Dopadura C; Isicom; Levo-C; Levobeta C; Levocarb; Levocomp; Levodop; Levodopa Comp; Levodopa comp B; Levodopa comp C; Levodopa-Carbi; Levopar; Madopar; Nacom†; NeyDop N (Revitorgan-Dilutionen N Nr 97); PK-Levo; Striaton; Tremopar; ***Gr.:*** Madopar; Sinemet; Zimox; ***Hong Kong:*** Apo-Levocarb; Levomed; Levomet; Madopar; Sinedopa; Sinemet; ***India:*** Levopa-C; Syndopa; ***Irl.:*** Half Sinemet; Madopar; Sinemet; ***Israel:*** Dopicar; Levopar Plus; Sinemet; ***Ital.:*** Madopar; Sinemet; ***Malaysia:*** Apo-Levocarb; Levomed; Sinemet; ***Mex.:*** Cloisone; Lemdopa; Madopar; Racovel; Sinemet; ***Neth.:*** Madopar; Sinemet; ***Norw.:*** Madopar; Sinemet; ***NZ:*** Apo-Levocarb†; Madopar; Sindopa; Sinemet; ***Port.:*** Madopar; Sinemet; ***S.Afr.:*** Carbilev; Madopar; Sinemet; ***Singapore:*** Cardopar; Levomet; Madopar; Sinemet; ***Spain:*** Madopar; Sinemet; ***Swed.:*** Madopark; Sinemet; ***Switz.:*** Madopar; Sinemet; ***Thai.:*** Levomed; Madopar; Sinemet; Syndopa; Vopar; ***UK:*** Half Sinemet; Madopar; Sinemet; Stalevo; ***USA:*** Atamet; Sinemet.

# Lisuride Maleate *(BANM, rINNM)*

Lysuride Maleate; Maleato de lisurida; Methylergol Carbamide Maleate. 3-(9,10-Didehydro-6-methylergolin-8α-yl)-1,1-diethylurea hydrogen maleate; 8-Decarboxamido-8-(3,3-diethylureido)-D-lysergamide maleate.

$C_{20}H_{26}N_4O,C_4H_4O_4 = 454.5.$

*CAS — 18016-80-3 (lisuride); 19875-60-6 (lisuride maleate).*

*ATC — G02CB02; N02CA07.*

## Adverse Effects and Precautions

As for Bromocriptine, p.1200. Infusion of lisuride in parkinsonian patients has been associated with severe psychiatric adverse effects.

**Effects on mental function.** For reports of daytime somnolence occurring in patients receiving dopamine agonists including lisuride, see Effects on Mental Function, under Adverse Effects of Levodopa, p.1206.

**Effects on the respiratory tract.** A woman with Parkinson's disease developed bilateral pleural effusions after taking lisuride 4 mg daily for about 17 months.[1] Her condition improved on discontinuation of lisuride.

1. Bhatt MH, *et al.* Pleuropulmonary disease associated with dopamine agonist therapy. *Ann Neurol* 1991; **30:** 613–16.

**Porphyria.** Lisuride maleate is considered to be unsafe in patients with porphyria because it has been shown to be porphyrinogenic in *animals*.

## Interactions

As for Bromocriptine, p.1202.

## Pharmacokinetics

◊ Plasma concentrations varied widely following a single oral dose of lisuride maleate 300 micrograms in 11 patients with Parkinson's disease.[1] Absorption was rapid and the mean plasma elimination half-life was 2.2 hours. Only a mean of 0.05% of the dose was excreted unchanged in the urine in 24 hours. The mean oral bioavailability of lisuride maleate has been reported[2] to be 10% after a 100-microgram dose and 22% after a 300-microgram dose.

A single dose of lisuride 25 micrograms given by intravenous, intramuscular, or subcutaneous injection reduced plasma-prolactin concentrations by up to 60% in 11 of 12 healthy subjects, the effect lasting for about 10 hours.[3] Plasma concentrations after intravenous administration fell in 2 phases with half-lives of 14 minutes and 1.5 hours respectively. Peak plasma concentrations following subcutaneous and intramuscular injection were obtained after 12 and 15 minutes respectively.

1. Burns RS, *et al.* Disposition of oral lisuride in Parkinson's disease. *Clin Pharmacol Ther* 1984; **35:** 548–56.

2. Hümpel M, *et al.* Radioimmunoassay of plasma lisuride in man following intravenous and oral administration of lisuride hydrogen maleate; effect on plasma prolactin level. *Eur J Clin Pharmacol* 1981; **20:** 47–51.
3. Krause W, *et al.* The pharmacokinetics and pharmacodynamics of lisuride in healthy volunteers after intravenous, intramuscular, and subcutaneous injection. *Eur J Clin Pharmacol* 1991; **40:** 399–403.

## Uses and Administration

Lisuride maleate, an ergot derivative, is a dopamine $D_2$-agonist with actions and uses similar to those of bromocriptine (p.1200). It is also reported to have serotonergic activity. It is used similarly in the management of Parkinson's disease and has been used in disorders associated with hyperprolactinaemia. It is also used to suppress puerperal lactation for medical reasons; it is not recommended for the routine suppression of physiological lactation or for the treatment of postpartum breast pain and engorgement that may be adequately relieved with simple analgesics and breast support. Lisuride has been used in some countries for the treatment of acromegaly, and for the prophylaxis of migraine.

In the management of **Parkinson's disease** lisuride maleate has been given alone or added to treatment in patients experiencing 'on-off' fluctuations in control with levodopa. It is normally given by mouth; doses should be taken with food. Initially 200 micrograms is taken at bedtime and additional doses of 200 micrograms may be added, at intervals of one week, first at midday and then in the morning; further increases are made, until an optimum response is obtained, by adding 200 micrograms each week using the same sequence of increases, starting with the bedtime dose; dosage should not normally exceed 5 mg daily in divided doses.

**Acromegaly.** Dopaminergics can produce a paradoxical reduction in growth hormone secretion and may be used in the treatment of acromegaly as adjunctive therapy to surgery, radiotherapy, or somatostatin analogues to reduce circulating growth hormone levels, although they are less effective than octreotide (p.1312). While bromocriptine has been the main dopamine agonist used, lisuride has been used in some countries, typically in a dose of 100 micrograms three times daily.

**Hyperprolactinaemia and prolactinomas.** Dopamine agonists have been widely used for the treatment of hyperprolactinaemia secondary to a prolactinoma (p.1315). Lisuride has been used as an alternative to bromocriptine. There is a report of plasma-prolactin concentrations being reduced to normal in 4 female patients with macroprolactinomas given lisuride 400 to 800 micrograms daily for 2 years.[1] Subsequent dosage reduction in 3 was followed by a rise in prolactin values. In the fourth patient prolactin remained in the normal range when the dose was progressively reduced from 400 to 50 micrograms daily, although complete withdrawal was followed by an increase in prolactin concentration within 3 months.

Vaginal administration of lisuride has been studied in an attempt to avoid adverse effects associated with oral therapy. In a study[2] involving 40 women with hyperprolactinaemia a 200-microgram standard oral tablet placed in the vagina at night produced a similar reduction in prolactin concentrations to that obtained with 400 micrograms taken orally and was better tolerated.

1. Liuzzi A, *et al.* Low doses of dopamine agonists in the long-term treatment of macroprolactinomas. *N Engl J Med* 1985; **313:** 656–9.
2. Tasdemir M, *et al.* Vaginal lisuride for hyperprolactinaemia. *Lancet* 1995; **346:** 1362.

**Lactation inhibition.** Lisuride is used in some countries for the prevention of puerperal lactation (p.1317). However, the routine use of dopaminergics is not recommended for the suppression of physiological lactation.

References.

1. Venturini PL, *et al.* Effects of lisuride and bromocriptine on inhibition of lactation and on serum prolactin levels: comparative double-blind study. *Eur J Obstet Gynecol Reprod Biol* 1981; **11:** 395–400.

**Mastalgia.** In a small placebo-controlled trial,[1] lisuride 200 micrograms daily was effective in the treatment of cyclical mastalgia. However, since mastalgia (p.1546) can improve spontaneously, treatment should rarely be considered unless pain has been present for about 6 months.

1. Kaleli S, *et al.* Symptomatic treatment of premenstrual mastalgia in premenopausal women with lisuride maleate: a double-blind placebo-controlled randomized study. *Fertil Steril* 2001; **75:** 718–23.

**Migraine.** Although lisuride has been used in some countries for the prophylaxis of migraine (p.464), typically in doses up to 25 micrograms three times daily, it is not usually considered to be the drug of choice or even one of the main alternatives.

**Parkinsonism.** While some neurologists use dopamine agonists such as lisuride early in the treatment of parkinsonism (p.1196) in an attempt to delay therapy with levodopa others reserve them for adjunctive use when levodopa is no longer effective alone or cannot be tolerated. They are sometimes useful in reducing 'off' periods with levodopa and in ameliorating other fluctuations in mobility in the later stages of the disease.

References.

1. Rinne UK. Lisuride, a dopamine agonist in the treatment of early Parkinson's disease. *Neurology* 1989; **39:** 336–9.
2. Clarke CE, Speller JM. Lisuride for levodopa-induced complications in Parkinson's disease. Available in The Cochrane Library; Issue 1. Chichester: John Wiley; 2004.
3. Clarke CE, Speller JM. Lisuride versus bromocriptine for levodopa-induced complications in Parkinson's disease. Available in The Cochrane Library; Issue 1. Chichester: John Wiley; 2004.

ADMINISTRATION. Lisuride has been of benefit when administered by continuous intravenous or subcutaneous infusion in patients experiencing fluctuations in mobility with levodopa therapy[1-3] but severe psychiatric effects have been associated with the use of these routes.[3]

1. Obeso JA, *et al.* Intravenous lisuride corrects oscillations of motor performance in Parkinson's disease. *Ann Neurol* 1986; **19:** 31–5.
2. Obeso JA, *et al.* Lisuride infusion pump: a device for the treatment of motor fluctuations in Parkinson's disease. *Lancet* 1986; **i:** 467–70.
3. Critchley P, *et al.* Psychosis and the lisuride pump. *Lancet* 1986; **i:** 349.

## Preparations

**Proprietary Preparations** (details are given in Part 3)
***Arg.:*** Dopagon; ***Austria:*** Dopergin; Prolacam; ***Braz.:*** Dopergin†; ***Fr.:*** Arolac; Dopergine; ***Ger.:*** Cuvalit; Dopergin; ***Gr.:*** Dipergon; ***Israel:*** Dopergin; ***Ital.:*** Dopergin; ***Mex.:*** Dopergin; ***Neth.:*** Dopergin; ***NZ:*** Dopergin; ***Spain:*** Dopergin; ***Switz.:*** Dopergin; ***Thai.:*** Dopergin; ***UK:*** Revanil†.

---

# Metergoline *(BAN, rINN)*

FI-6337; MCE; Metergolina; Methergoline. Benzyl (8S,10S)-(1,6-dimethylergolin-8-ylmethyl)carbamate.

$C_{25}H_{29}N_3O_2$ = 403.5.
*CAS — 17692-51-2.*
*ATC — G02CB05.*

## Profile

Metergoline, an ergot derivative, is a dopamine agonist with actions and uses similar to those of bromocriptine (p.1200). It is also a serotonin antagonist. Metergoline has been used similarly to bromocriptine in disorders associated with hyperprolactinaemia and to inhibit lactation. In some countries it has also been used in the prophylaxis of migraine and other vascular headaches.

**Hyperprolactinaemia and prolactinomas.** Dopamine agonists have been widely used for the treatment of hyperprolactinaemia secondary to a prolactinoma (p.1315). There is a report of metergoline being tried in patients intolerant of bromocriptine.[1] In this report metergoline lowered plasma-prolactin concentrations, although not to normal, in 3 men and 8 women with hyperprolactinaemia. Galactorrhoea was abolished and/or a regular menstrual cycle established in 5 of the women. Prolactin concentrations and symptoms were unchanged in 3 further women with normoprolactinaemic galactorrhoea. Initial doses of 2 mg daily were increased over 2 weeks to 4 mg three times daily and at monthly re-assessment the dose was increased up to 24 mg daily in divided doses, according to response.

1. Casson IF, *et al.* Intolerance of bromocriptine: is metergoline a satisfactory alternative? *BMJ* 1985; **290:** 1783–4.

**Lactation inhibition.** Metergoline has been tried for the prevention of puerperal lactation (p.1317) in doses of 8 to 12 mg daily for 5 days.[1,2] However the routine use of dopaminergics is not recommended for the suppression of physiological lactation.

1. Delitala G, *et al.* Metergoline in the inhibition of puerperal lactation. *BMJ* 1977; **1:** 744–6.
2. Crosignani PG, *et al.* Suppression of puerperal lactation by metergoline. *Obstet Gynecol* 1978; **51:** 113–15.

**Migraine.** Although metergoline has been used in some countries for the prophylaxis of migraine (p.464) it is not usually considered to be the drug of choice or even one of the main alternatives.

## Preparations

**Proprietary Preparations** (details are given in Part 3)
***Ger.:*** Liserdol; ***Hong Kong:*** Liserdol; ***Ital.:*** Liserdol; ***S.Afr.:*** Liserdol†; ***Singapore:*** Liserdol; ***Switz.:*** Liserdol.

---

# Pergolide Mesilate *(BANM, rINNM)*

LY-127809; Mesilato de pergolida; Pergolide Mesylate *(USAN)*; Pergolidi Mesilas. 8β-Methylthiomethyl-6-propylergoline methanesulphonate; Methyl (8R,10R)-6-propylergolin-8-ylmethyl sulphide methanesulphonate.

$C_{19}H_{26}N_2S,CH_4O_3S$ = 410.6.
*CAS — 66104-22-1 (pergolide); 66104-23-2 (pergolide mesilate).*
*ATC — N04BC02.*

**Pharmacopoeias.** In *Eur.* (see p.vi) and *US.*

**Ph. Eur. 5.0** (Pergolide Mesilate). A white or almost white crystalline powder. Slightly soluble in water, in alcohol, and in dichloromethane; very slightly soluble in acetone; sparingly soluble in methyl alcohol. Protect from light.

**USP 27** (Pergolide Mesylate). A white to off-white powder. Slightly soluble in water, in dehydrated alcohol, and in chloroform; very slightly soluble in acetone; practically insoluble in ether; sparingly soluble in methyl alcohol. Store in airtight containers. Protect from light.

## Adverse Effects and Precautions

As for Bromocriptine, p.1200.

An increased incidence of uterine neoplasms has been reported in *rodents* given high doses of pergolide mesilate.

**Effects on the cardiovascular system.** The UK Committee on Safety of Medicines (CSM) has reported that pergolide has been associated with a small number of cases of cardiac valvulopathy;[1] since 1989, valvulopathy has been reported in fewer than 5 in 100 000 patients. The CSM also referred to a published case series[2] which reported on 3 patients with severe tricuspid regurgitation following long-term pergolide treatment. The authors of this case series and the CSM both considered that, based on the available evidence, there is a potential association between pergolide and cardiac valvulopathy.

Subsequently, the FDA stated that, up to the end of 2002, it was aware of 15 cases of valvular heart disease with pergolide treatment;[3] this figure included the 3 cases reported in the above series and 4 cases from the UK.

A recent study[4] that examined 78 patients taking pergolide for Parkinson's disease found evidence of restrictive valvular heart disease in 15 of 52 (29%) patients taking doses less than 5 mg daily and in 11 of 26 (42%) receiving doses of 5 mg or more daily.

1. Committee on Safety of Medicines/Medicines and Healthcare products Regulatory Agency. Pergolide (Celance) and cardiac valvulopathy. *Current Problems* 2003; **29:** 7. Also available at: http://medicines.mhra.gov.uk/ourwork/monitorsafequalmed/currentproblems/cpsept2003.pdf (accessed 24/05/04)
2. Pritchett AM, *et al.* Valvular heart disease in patients taking pergolide. *Mayo Clin Proc* 2002; **77:** 1280–6.
3. Flowers CM, *et al.* The US Food and Drug Administration's registry of patients with pergolide-associated valvular heart disease. *Mayo Clin Proc* 2003; **78:** 730–1.
4. Van Camp G, *et al.* Treatment of Parkinson's disease with pergolide and relation to restrictive valvular heart disease. *Lancet* 2004; **363:** 1179–83.

**Effects on mental function.** For reports of daytime somnolence occurring in patients receiving dopamine agonists including pergolide, see Effects on Mental Function, under Adverse Effects of Levodopa, p.1206.

## Interactions

As for Bromocriptine, p.1202.

## Pharmacokinetics

Pergolide mesilate is absorbed from the gastrointestinal tract. It is reported to be about 90% bound to plasma proteins. It is excreted mainly in the urine in the form of metabolites.

## Uses and Administration

Pergolide mesilate, an ergot derivative, is a dopamine $D_2$-agonist with actions and uses similar to those of bromocriptine (p.1202), but in contrast to bromocriptine (a dopamine $D_2$-agonist) it also has agonist properties at $D_1$ and $D_3$ receptors. Pergolide is used in the management of Parkinson's disease as monotherapy, or as an adjunct to levodopa therapy to reduce 'end-of-dose' or 'on-off' fluctuations in response. Pergolide is administered by mouth as the mesilate with doses expressed as the base. Pergolide mesilate 65.3 mg is approximately equivalent to 50 mg pergolide base.

For administration as *monotherapy* an initial dose equivalent to 50 micrograms of pergolide is given on the first evening of therapy. The dose is thereafter gradually increased: 50 micrograms twice daily is taken on days 2 to 4, then increased by 100 to 250 micrograms every 3 or 4 days, given in 3 divided doses, up to a daily dose of 1.5 mg at day 28. After day 30, the dose should be increased further by a maximum of 250 micrograms twice a week until an optimum response is achieved. Usual maintenance doses are 2.1 to 2.5 mg daily. The daily dose is usually given in 3 divided doses.

For administration as *adjunctive therapy* with levodopa, pergolide should be introduced gradually and during this period patients can have their levodopa dosage decreased gradually until an optimum response is achieved. The initial dose of pergolide is the equivalent of 50 micrograms daily for the first 2 days, increased gradually by 100 or 150 micrograms every third day over the next 12 days of therapy. Further increases of

250 micrograms may then be made every third day until an optimum response is achieved. A usual maintenance dose is 3 mg daily. The daily dose is usually given in 3 divided doses.

**Acromegaly.** Dopaminergics can produce a paradoxical reduction in growth hormone secretion and may be used in the treatment of acromegaly as adjunctive therapy to surgery, radiotherapy, or somatostatin analogues to reduce circulating growth hormone levels, although they are less effective than octreotide (p.1312). While bromocriptine has been the main dopamine agonist used pergolide has also been tried.[1]

1. Kleinberg DL, *et al.* Pergolide for the treatment of pituitary tumors secreting prolactin or growth hormone. *N Engl J Med* 1983; **309:** 704–9.

**Hyperprolactinaemia and prolactinomas.** Dopamine agonists are widely used for the treatment of hyperprolactinaemia secondary to a prolactinoma (p.1315). Pergolide has been suggested as an alternative to bromocriptine in this condition.

Studies[1-3] of pergolide mesilate in patients with hyperprolactinaemia indicate that single doses reduce serum-prolactin concentrations for more than 24 hours. In most patients, the effective dose was between 50 and 150 micrograms daily. Adverse effects were similar to those seen with bromocriptine, although some patients who could not take bromocriptine were able to tolerate pergolide (and *vice versa*). Pergolide reportedly lost favour for this indication following reports of an increased incidence of uterine neoplasms in *rodents* receiving high doses. However, the manufacturers point out that no cases of uterine malignancies have to date been reported in humans receiving pergolide. The long-term outcome of treatment of macroprolactinomas with pergolide has been examined in 23 patients,[4] and efficacy and relative safety of pergolide was demonstrated after an average of 27 months (range: 9 to 64 months) treatment.

1. Franks S, *et al.* Treatment of hyperprolactinaemia with pergolide mesylate: acute effects and preliminary evaluation of long-term treatment. *Lancet* 1981; **ii:** 659–61.
2. Franks S, *et al.* Effectiveness of pergolide mesylate in long-term treatment of hyperprolactinaemia. *BMJ* 1983; **286:** 1177–9.
3. Kleinberg DL, *et al.* Pergolide for the treatment of pituitary tumors secreting prolactin or growth hormone. *N Engl J Med* 1983; **309:** 704–9.
4. Freda PU, *et al.* Long-term treatment of prolactin-secreting macroadenomas with pergolide. *J Clin Endocrinol Metab* 2000; **85:** 8–13.

**Parkinsonism.** Dopamine agonists such as pergolide are often used to begin the treatment of parkinsonism (p.1196) in an attempt to delay therapy with levodopa, particularly in younger patients. They also have an adjunctive use when levodopa is no longer effective alone or cannot be tolerated, and may sometimes be useful in reducing 'off' periods with levodopa and in ameliorating other fluctuations in mobility in the later stages of the disease. Pergolide has a relatively long duration of action compared with other dopamine agonists commonly used. Although the duration of the clinical antiparkinsonian effect of pergolide remains to be determined, studies suggest it is of the order of 5 to 8 hours. Depending on the dose used the response to other dopamine agonists in late parkinsonism is 1 to 4 hours for levodopa, 2 to 4 hours for lisuride, and 4 to 6 hours for bromocriptine.

References.

1. Anonymous. Pergolide (Celance)—a third dopamine agonist. *Drug Ther Bull* 1991; **29:** 79.
2. Markham A, Benfield P. Pergolide: a review of its pharmacology and therapeutic use in Parkinson's disease. *CNS Drugs* 1997; **7:** 328–40.
3. Barone P, *et al.* Pergolide monotherapy in the treatment of early PD: a randomized, controlled study. *Neurology* 1999; **53:** 573–9.
4. Clarke CE, Speller JM. Pergolide for levodopa-induced complications in Parkinson's disease. Available in The Cochrane Library, Issue 1. Chichester: John Wiley; 2004.
5. Clarke CE, Speller JM. Pergolide versus bromocriptine for levodopa-induced complications in Parkinson's disease. Available in The Cochrane Library; Issue 1. Chichester: John Wiley; 2004.

**Restless legs syndrome.** The aetiology of restless legs syndrome (see Parasomnias, p.667) is obscure and treatment has largely been empirical although dopaminergic therapy has emerged as a common first-line choice. Pergolide has produced some benefit in small studies.[1-5]

1. Silber MH, *et al.* Pergolide in the management of restless legs syndrome: an extended study. *Sleep* 1997; **20:** 878–82.
2. Winkelmann J, *et al.* Treatment of restless legs syndrome with pergolide—an open clinical trial. *Mov Disord* 1998; **13:** 566–9.
3. Earley CJ, *et al.* Randomized, double-blind, placebo-controlled trial of pergolide in restless legs syndrome. *Neurology* 1998; **51:** 1599–1602.
4. Wetter TC, *et al.*. A randomized controlled study of pergolide in patients with restless legs syndrome. *Neurology* 1999; **52:** 944–50.
5. Stiasny K, *et al.* Long-term effects of pergolide in the treatment of restless legs syndrome. *Neurology* 2001; **56:** 1399–1402.

**Tourette's syndrome.** Pergolide has been studied in the management of Tourette's syndrome (see Tics, p.664). A preliminary study[1] has produced encouraging results, subsequently confirmed by placebo-controlled trials in children and adolescents.[2,3]

1. Lipinski JF, *et al.* Dopamine agonist treatment of Tourette disorder in children: results of an open-label trial of pergolide. *Mov Disord* 1997; **12:** 402–7.
2. Gilbert DL, *et al.* Tourette's syndrome improvement with pergolide in a randomized, double-blind, crossover trial. *Neurology* 2000; **54:** 1310–15.
3. Gilbert DL, *et al.* Tic reduction with pergolide in a randomized controlled trial in children. *Neurology* 2003; **60:** 606–11.

### Preparations

*USP 27:* Pergolide Tablets.

**Proprietary Preparations** (details are given in Part 3)
***Arg.:*** Aroltex; Celance; Geranil; Parlide; ***Austral.:*** Permax; ***Austria:*** Permax; ***Belg.:*** Permax; ***Braz.:*** Celance; ***Canad.:*** Permax; ***Chile:*** Celance; ***Denm.:*** Permax; ***Fin.:*** Permax; ***Fr.:*** Celance; ***Ger.:*** Parkotil; ***Gr.:*** Celance; ***Hong Kong:*** Celance; ***Irl.:*** Celance; ***Ital.:*** Nopar; ***Mex.:*** Permax; ***Neth.:*** Permax; ***NZ:*** Permax; ***Port.:*** Permax; ***S.Afr.:*** Permax; ***Singapore:*** Celance†; ***Spain:*** Pharken; ***Switz.:*** Permax; ***Thai.:*** Celance; ***UK:*** Celance; ***USA:*** Permax.

## Piribedil (*rINN*)

ET-495; EU-4200. 2-(4-Piperonylpiperazin-1-yl)pyrimidine.

$C_{16}H_{18}N_4O_2$ = 298.3.
*CAS — 3605-01-4.*
*ATC — C04AX13.*

### Profile

Piribedil is a non-ergot dopamine agonist that has been given by mouth in the treatment of parkinsonism (p.1196) and in circulatory disorders. Piribedil mesilate has been given by injection for circulatory disorders.

Adverse effects reported include nausea and vomiting, dizziness, hallucinations, confusion, drowsiness, hypothermia, dyskinesias, and occasional changes in liver function.

When used as monotherapy in Parkinson's disease a usual daily dose of piribedil is 150 to 250 mg given by mouth in divided doses; a daily dose of 80 to 140 mg may be suitable when used as an adjunct to levodopa.

**Effects on mental function.** For reports of daytime somnolence occurring in patients receiving dopamine agonists including piribedil, see Effects on Mental Function, under Adverse Effects of Levodopa, p.1206.

**Parkinsonism.** Piribedil is a dopamine $D_2$-agonist while its metabolite is reported to act on $D_1$ receptors. It has been mainly used as an adjunct to levodopa therapy.

References.

1. Montastruc JL, *et al.* Current status of dopamine agonists in Parkinson's disease management. *Drugs* 1993; **46:** 384–93.
2. Montastruc JL, *et al.* A randomized, double-blind study of a skin patch of a dopaminergic agonist, piribedil, in Parkinson's disease. *Mov Disord* 1999; **14:** 336–41.
3. Ziegler M, Rondot P. Activité du piribédil dans la maladie de Parkinson: étude multicentrique. *Presse Med* 1999; **28:** 1414–18.
4. Ziegler M, *et al.* Efficacy of piribedil as early combination to levodopa in patients with stable Parkinson's disease: a 6-month, randomized, placebo-controlled study. *Mov Disord* 2003; **18:** 418–25.

### Preparations

**Proprietary Preparations** (details are given in Part 3)
***Arg.:*** Trivastal; ***Braz.:*** Trivastal; ***Fr.:*** Trivastal; ***Ger.:*** Trivastal; ***India:*** Trivastal; ***Ital.:*** Trivastan; ***Malaysia:*** Trivastal; ***Port.:*** Trivastal; ***Singapore:*** Trivastal; ***Thai.:*** Trivastal.

## Pramipexole Hydrochloride

*(BANM, rINNM)*

Hidrocloruro de pramipexol; PNU-98528-E; Pramipexole Dihydrochloride *(USAN)*; SND-919-CL-2Y (pramipexole hydrochloride); SUD-919Y (pramipexole). (*S*)-2-Amino-4,5,6,7-tetrahydro-6-(propylamino)benzothiazole dihydrochloride monohydrate.

$C_{10}H_{17}N_3S,2HCl, H_2O$ = 302.3.
*CAS — 104632-26-0 (pramipexole); 104632-25-9 (anhydrous pramipexole hydrochloride); 191217-81-9 (pramipexole hydrochloride monohydrate).*
*ATC — N04BC05.*

### Adverse Effects and Precautions

As for Bromocriptine, p.1200.

Sudden onset of sleep, with or without any prior feeling of drowsiness, has been rarely reported and can occur at any time during treatment (see below). Patients affected should not drive or undertake other potentially hazardous activities such as operating machinery. A reduction in dosage or withdrawal of pramipexole will, in most cases, alleviate the problem.

Pramipexole should be used with caution in patients with renal impairment and reduced doses are recommended.

Ophthalmological monitoring is recommended at regular intervals or if vision abnormalities occur.

**Incidence of adverse effects.** References.

1. Etminan M, *et al.* Comparison of the risk of adverse events with pramipexole and ropinirole in patients with Parkinson's disease: a meta-analysis. *Drug Safety* 2003; **26:** 439–44.

**Effects on mental function.** Pramipexole has been associated with attacks of sudden onset of sleep. The UK manufacturer has reported that the incidence of daytime **somnolence** is increased at daily doses of pramipexole hydrochloride higher than 1.5 mg. A retrospective analysis[1] of data to evaluate the incidence and nature of somnolence experienced by patients receiving pramipexole in clinical trials showed that for patients with moderate or severe somnolence, the onset of worst-reported somnolence occurred at a mean dose of around 4 mg (range: 0.75 to 4.5 mg).

For further reports of daytime somnolence occurring in patients receiving dopamine agonists including pramipexole, see Effects on Mental Function, under Adverse Effects of Levodopa, p.1206.

For reference to **pathological gambling** reported in patients with Parkinson's disease receiving dopamine agonists, including pramipexole, see under Levodopa, p.1206.

1. Hauser RA, *et al.* Pramipexole-induced somnolence and episodes of daytime sleep. *Mov Disord* 2000; **15:** 658–63.

### Interactions

As for Bromocriptine, p.1202. Cimetidine is reported to reduce the renal clearance of pramipexole.

Caution is advised when other sedating drugs or alcohol are used with pramipexole because of possible additive effects and the risk of precipitating sudden onset of sleep (see above).

◊ References.

1. Wright CE, *et al.* Influence of probenecid and cimetidine on pramipexole pharmacokinetics. *Clin Pharmacol Ther* 1996; **59:** 183.

### Pharmacokinetics

Pramipexole is readily absorbed from the gastrointestinal tract and peak plasma concentrations have been reached within about 2 hours in fasting patients and in about 3 hours when given with food. Oral bioavailability is reported to be about 90%. Pramipexole is widely distributed throughout the body and its protein binding is less than 20%. Metabolism is minimal and more than 90% of a dose is excreted via renal tubular secretion unchanged into the urine. Elimination half-lives of 8 to 12 hours have been reported.

◊ References.

1. Wright CE, *et al.* Steady-state pharmacokinetic properties of pramipexole in healthy volunteers. *J Clin Pharmacol* 1997; **37:** 520–5.

### Uses and Administration

Pramipexole is a non-ergot dopamine agonist with actions similar to those of bromocriptine (p.1202). It is used similarly in the management of Parkinson's disease (p.1196) either alone or as an adjunct to levodopa therapy to reduce 'end-of-dose' or 'on-off' fluctuations in response. Pramipexole is given orally as the hydrochloride; doses have been described in terms of the hydrochloride (as below) or of the base. In terms of equivalency:

- Pramipexole hydrochloride 125 micrograms is approximately equivalent to pramipexole base 88 micrograms
- Pramipexole hydrochloride 250 micrograms is approximately equivalent to pramipexole base 180 micrograms
- Pramipexole hydrochloride 500 micrograms is approximately equivalent to pramipexole base 350 micrograms

The dose of pramipexole should be increased gradually and the dose of levodopa gradually reduced during the dose-titration and maintenance phases until an optimum response is achieved.

The initial dose of pramipexole *hydrochloride* is 125 micrograms given three times daily increased to 250 micrograms three times daily in the second week and then to 500 micrograms three times daily in the third week according to response. Thereafter the daily dose may be increased if necessary by 750 micrograms at weekly intervals to a maximum of 4.5 mg daily. The dosage should be reduced in patients with renal impairment (see below).

If it is necessary to discontinue pramipexole therapy, it should be withdrawn gradually. The UK manufacturer suggests tapering off the dose of pramipexole hydrochloride at a rate of 750 micrograms daily until a daily dose of 750 micrograms has been reached; thereafter, the dose should be reduced by 375 micrograms daily.

**Administration in renal impairment.** The elimination of pramipexole is dependent on renal function and the dosage of pramipexole hydrochloride should therefore be reduced in patients with renal impairment. The following dosage schedule has been suggested by the UK manufacturers for initiation of therapy according to the patient's creatinine clearance (CC):

- CC 20 to 50 mL/minute: 125 micrograms given twice daily
- CC less than 20 mL/minute: 125 micrograms once daily

If renal function declines during maintenance therapy it is recommended that the daily dose of pramipexole should be reduced by the same percentage as the decline in CC.

**Parasomnias.** The aetiology of *restless legs syndrome* (p.667) is obscure and treatment has largely been empirical although dopaminergic therapy has emerged as a common first-line choice. Pramipexole has produced some benefit in small studies.[1-3]

1. Lin S-C, *et al.* Effect of pramipexole in treatment of resistant restless legs syndrome. *Mayo Clin Proc* 1998; **73:** 497–500.
2. Montplaisir J, *et al.* Restless legs syndrome improved by pramipexole: a double-blind randomized trial. *Neurology* 1999; **52:** 938–43.
3. Montplaisir J, *et al.* Pramipexole in the treatment of restless legs syndrome: a follow-up study. *Eur J Neurol* 2000; **7** (suppl 1): 27–31.

**Parkinsonism.** Pramipexole is a dopamine agonist used in the treatment of Parkinson's disease (p.1196) as an adjunct to levodopa therapy to reduce 'off' periods with levodopa and ameliorate other fluctuations of mobility in the later stages of the disease. It is also used as monotherapy early in the course of the disease in an attempt to delay therapy with levodopa.

References.

1. Parkinson Study Group. Safety and efficacy of pramipexole in early Parkinson disease: a randomized dose-ranging study. *JAMA* 1997; **278:** 125–30.
2. Lieberman A, *et al.* Clinical evaluation of pramipexole in advanced Parkinson's disease: results of a double-blind, placebo-controlled, parallel-group study. *Neurology* 1997; **49:** 162–8.
3. Shannon KM, *et al.* Efficacy of pramipexole, a novel dopamine agonist, as monotherapy in mild to moderate Parkinson's disease. *Neurology* 1997; **49:** 724–8.
4. Guttman M. International Pramipexole-Bromocriptine Study Group. Double-blind comparison of pramipexole and bromocriptine treatment with placebo in advanced Parkinson's disease. *Neurology* 1997; **49:** 1060–5.
5. Parkinson Study Group. Pramipexole vs levodopa as initial treatment for Parkinson disease: a randomized controlled trial. *JAMA* 2000; **284:** 1931–8.
6. Clarke CE, *et al.* Pramipexole for levodopa-induced complications in Parkinson's disease. Available in The Cochrane Library; Issue 1. Chichester: John Wiley; 2004.
7. Clarke CE, *et al.* Pramipexole versus bromocriptine for levodopa-induced complications in Parkinson's disease. Available in The Cochrane Library; Issue 1. Chichester: John Wiley; 2004.

## Preparations

**Proprietary Preparations** (details are given in Part 3)

***Arg.:*** Mirapex; Sifrol; ***Belg.:*** Mirapexin; ***Braz.:*** Mirapex; Sifrol; ***Canad.:*** Mirapex; ***Chile:*** Sifrol; ***Denm.:*** Sifrol; ***Fin.:*** Sifrol; ***Ger.:*** Sifrol; ***Gr.:*** Mirapexin; ***Irl.:*** Mirapexin; ***Ital.:*** Mirapexin; ***Neth.:*** Sifrol; ***Norw.:*** Sifrol; ***S.Afr.:*** Pexola; ***Spain:*** Mirapexin; ***Swed.:*** Sifrol; ***Switz.:*** Sifrol; ***UK:*** Mirapexin; ***USA:*** Mirapex.

# Quinagolide Hydrochloride

*(BANM, rINNM)*

CV-205-502 (quinagolide); Hidrocloruro de quinagolida; SD2-CV-205-502 (quinagolide). (±)-*N*,*N*-Diethyl-*N*′-[(3*R**,4a*R**,10a*S**)-1,2,3,4,4a,5,10,10a-octahydro-6-hydroxy-1-propylbenzo[*g*]quinolin-3-yl]sulfamide hydrochloride.

$C_{20}H_{33}N_3O_3S,HCl = 432.0.$

*CAS — 87056-78-8 (quinagolide); 94424-50-7 (quinagolide hydrochloride).*

*ATC — G02CB04.*

## Adverse Effects and Precautions

As for Bromocriptine, p.1200, although it is not an ergot derivative and does not seem to be associated with fibrotic reactions or vasoconstriction. The manufacturers contra-indicate the use of quinagolide in patients with hepatic or renal impairment; however, this is based on a lack of data in such patients.

**Effects on mental function.** For reports of daytime somnolence occurring in patients receiving dopamine agonists including quinagolide, see Effects on Mental Function, under Adverse Effects of Levodopa, p.1206.

## Interactions

As for Bromocriptine, p.1202.

## Pharmacokinetics

Quinagolide is rapidly absorbed from the gastrointestinal tract and undergoes extensive first-pass metabolism to the *N*-desethyl analogue which is biologically active and the *N*,*N*-didesethyl analogue. Approximately equal amounts of a dose appear in the urine and the faeces; it is excreted in the urine as sulfate or glucuronide conjugates of quinagolide and its metabolites and in the faeces as the unconjugated forms. Protein binding has been reported to be about 90%. The elimination half-life of quinagolide at steady state is about 17 hours.

## Uses and Administration

Quinagolide is a non-ergot dopamine $D_2$-agonist that has actions and uses similar to those of bromocriptine (p.1202). It is used in the treatment of disorders associated with hyperprolactinaemia.

Quinagolide hydrochloride is given in single daily doses with food at bedtime; doses are expressed in terms of the base. Quinagolide hydrochloride 27.3 micrograms is approximately equivalent to quinagolide 25 micrograms. The initial dose is 25 micrograms daily for 3 days increasing thereafter at 3-day intervals in steps of 25 micrograms until the optimal response is achieved, which is usually within the range of 75 to 150 micrograms daily. If doses greater than 300 micrograms daily are required, increases may be made in steps of 75 to 150 micrograms daily at intervals of not less than 4 weeks.

Quinagolide has also been investigated in the treatment of acromegaly and lactation inhibition.

**Acromegaly.** Dopaminergics can produce a paradoxical reduction in growth hormone secretion and may be used in the treatment of acromegaly as adjunctive therapy to surgery, radiotherapy, or somatostatin analogues to reduce circulating growth hormone levels, although they are less effective than octreotide (p.1312). Bromocriptine has been the main dopamine agonist used, but quinagolide has been tried and results of an open study[1] in which quinagolide was administered to 17 patients with acromegaly suggest that quinagolide has a more prolonged effect on suppression of growth hormone secretion than bromocriptine. However, it was ineffective in bromocriptine-resistant patients. In another study involving 34 patients, quinagolide was more effective than either cabergoline or a depot preparation of bromocriptine in normalising circulating growth hormone and insulin-like growth factor.[2]

1. Chiodini PG, *et al.* CV 205-502 in acromegaly. *Acta Endocrinol (Copenh)* 1993; **128:** 389–93.
2. Colao A, *et al.* Effect of different dopaminergic agents in the treatment of acromegaly. *J Clin Endocrinol Metab* 1997; **82:** 518–23.

**Hyperprolactinaemia and prolactinomas.** Dopamine agonists such as quinagolide are widely used for the treatment of hyperprolactinaemia secondary to a prolactinoma (see p.1315).

References.

1. Vance ML, *et al.* Treatment of prolactin-secreting pituitary macroadenomas with the long-acting non-ergot dopamine agonist CV 205-502. *Ann Intern Med* 1990; **112:** 668–73.
2. Shoham Z, *et al.* CV 205-502—effectiveness, tolerability, and safety over 24-month study. *Fertil Steril* 1991; **55:** 501–6.
3. Rasmussen C, *et al.* Clinical response and prolactin concentration in hyperprolactinemic women during and after treatment for 24 months with the new dopamine agonist, CV 205-502. *Acta Endocrinol (Copenh)* 1991; **125:** 170–6.
4. Verhelst JA, *et al.* Acute and long-term effects of once-daily oral bromocriptine and a new long-acting non-ergot dopamine agonist, quinagolide, in the treatment of hyperprolactinemia: a double-blind study. *Acta Endocrinol (Copenh)* 1991; **125:** 385–91.
5. van der Heijden PFM, *et al.* CV205-502, a new dopamine agonist, versus bromocriptine in the treatment of hyperprolactinaemia. *Eur J Obstet Gynecol Reprod Biol* 1991; **40:** 111–18.
6. Vilar L, Burke CW. Quinagolide efficacy and tolerability in hyperprolactinaemic patients who are resistant to or intolerant of bromocriptine. *Clin Endocrinol (Oxf)* 1994; **41:** 821–6.
7. Rohmer V, *et al.* Efficacy of quinagolide in resistance to dopamine agonists: results of a multicenter study. *Ann Endocrinol (Paris)* 2000; **61:** 411–17.
8. Schultz PN, *et al.* Quinagolide in the management of prolactinoma. *Pituitary* 2000; **3:** 239–49.

**Lactation inhibition.** A small preliminary study[1] has suggested that quinagolide is of similar efficacy to bromocriptine for prevention of puerperal lactation. However, the routine use of dopaminergics is not recommended for the suppression of physiological lactation (see p.1317).

1. van der Heijden PFM, *et al.* Lactation inhibition by the dopamine agonist CV 205-502. *Br J Obstet Gynaecol* 1991; **98:** 270–6.

## Preparations

**Proprietary Preparations** (details are given in Part 3)

***Austria:*** Norprolac; ***Fin.:*** Norprolac; ***Fr.:*** Norprolac; ***Ger.:*** Norprolac; ***Gr.:*** Norprolac; ***Hong Kong:*** Norprolac; ***Israel:*** Norprolac; ***Mex.:*** Norprolac; ***Neth.:*** Norprolac; ***Norw.:*** Norprolac; ***S.Afr.:*** Norprolac; ***Spain:*** Norprolac; ***Swed.:*** Norprolac; ***Switz.:*** Norprolac; ***UK:*** Norprolac.

# Ropinirole Hydrochloride

*(BANM, USAN, pINNM)*

Hidrocloruro de ropinirol; SKF-101468 (ropinirole); SKF-0101468-A (ropinirole hydrochloride). 4-[2-(Dipropylamino)ethyl]-2-indolinone hydrochloride.

$C_{16}H_{24}N_2O,HCl = 296.8.$

*CAS — 91374-21-9 (ropinirole); 91374-20-8 (ropinirole hydrochloride).*

*ATC — N04BC04.*

## Adverse Effects and Precautions

As for Bromocriptine, p.1200. The manufacturers recommend that ropinirole should not be used in patients with hepatic or severe renal impairment; however, this is based on a lack of evidence in such patients.

Sudden onset of sleep, with or without any prior feeling of drowsiness, has been rarely reported and can occur at any time during treatment. Patients affected should not drive or undertake other potentially hazardous activities such as operating machinery. A reduction in dosage or withdrawal of ropinirole will, in most cases, alleviate the problem.

As with other dopaminergic agonists, ropinirole therapy should not be discontinued abruptly.

**Incidence of adverse effects.** References.

1. Etminan M, *et al.* Comparison of the risk of adverse events with pramipexole and ropinirole in patients with Parkinson's disease: a meta-analysis. *Drug Safety* 2003; **26:** 439–44.

**Effects on mental function.** For reports of daytime somnolence occurring in patients receiving dopamine agonists including ropinirole, see Effects on Mental Function, under Adverse Effects of Levodopa, p.1206.

## Interactions

Since it is a dopamine agonist, ropinirole may share some of the pharmacological interactions of bromocriptine, p.1202. In addition, high doses of oestrogens can increase plasma concentrations of ropinirole and dosage adjustments may be necessary if oestrogen therapy is started or withdrawn during treatment with ropinirole. Ropinirole is metabolised by the cytochrome P450 isoenzyme CYP1A2 and there is therefore the potential for interactions between ropinirole and other drugs that are metabolised similarly or are enzyme inducers or inhibitors.

Caution is advised when other sedating drugs or alcohol are used with ropinirole because of possible additive effects and the risk of precipitating sudden onset of sleep (see above).

## Pharmacokinetics

Ropinirole is rapidly absorbed from the gastrointestinal tract and mean peak plasma concentrations have been achieved 1.5 hours after oral administration; the rate of absorption, but not the extent, may be reduced if taken with food. Bioavailability is reported to be about 50%. Plasma protein binding of ropinirole is low (10 to 40%).

Ropinirole is metabolised primarily by the cytochrome P450 isoenzyme CYP1A2 and excreted in the urine as metabolites. A mean elimination half-life of about 6 hours has been reported for ropinirole.

◊ References.

1. Brefel C, *et al.* Effect of food on the pharmacokinetics of ropinirole in parkinsonian patients. *Br J Clin Pharmacol* 1998; **45:** 412–15.
2. Hubble J, *et al.* Linear pharmacokinetic behavior of ropinirole during multiple dosing in patients with Parkinson's disease. *J Clin Pharmacol* 2000; **40:** 641–6.
3. Kaye CM, Nicholls B. Clinical pharmacokinetics of ropinirole. *Clin Pharmacokinet* 2000; **39:** 243–54.

## Uses and Administration

Ropinirole is a non-ergot dopamine $D_2$-agonist with similar actions to those of bromocriptine (p.1202). It is given by mouth as the hydrochloride in the management of Parkinson's disease, either alone or as an adjunct to levodopa; doses are expressed in terms of the base. Ropinirole hydrochloride 1.14 mg is approximately equivalent to ropinirole 1 mg. It should be introduced gradually and during this period patients already receiving levodopa can have their levodopa dosage decreased gradually until an optimal response is achieved. The concurrent dose of levodopa may be reduced by about 20%. The daily dosage of ropinirole should be given in three divided doses, preferably with food. The initial daily dose of ropinirole is 750 micrograms increased at weekly intervals in steps of 750 micrograms until the optimal response is achieved, which is usually within the range of 3 to 9 mg daily; higher doses may be required if used with levodopa. If doses greater than 3 mg daily are required the weekly increments may be made in steps of up to 3 mg. The daily dosage should not exceed 24 mg.

If it is necessary to discontinue ropinirole therapy, it should be withdrawn gradually by reducing the number of daily doses over the period of one week.

◊ Reviews.

1. Tulloch IF. Pharmacologic profile of ropinirole: a nonergoline dopamine agonist. *Neurology* 1997; **49** (suppl 1): S58–S62.

**Parkinsonism.** Dopamine agonists such as ropinirole may be used to begin treatment of parkinsonism (p.1196) in an attempt to delay therapy with levodopa, particularly in younger patients. They also have an adjunctive use when levodopa is no longer effective alone or cannot be tolerated, and may be useful in reducing 'off' periods with levodopa and in ameliorating other fluctuations of mobility in the later stage of the disease.

References.

1. Rascol O, *et al.* A placebo-controlled study of ropinirole a new $D_2$ agonist, in the treatment of motor fluctuations of L-DOPA-treated parkinsonian patients. *Adv Neurol* 1996; **69:** 531–4.
2. Adler CH, *et al.* The Ropinirole Study Group. Ropinirole for the treatment of early Parkinson's disease. *Neurology* 1997; **49:** 393–9.
3. Rascol O, *et al.* Ropinirole in the treatment of early Parkinson's disease: a 6-month interim report of a 5-year levodopa-controlled study. *Mov Disord* 1998; **13:** 39–45.
4. Korczyn AD, *et al.* A 3-year randomized trial of ropinirole and bromocriptine in early Parkinson's disease. *Neurology* 1999; **53:** 364–70.
5. Matheson AJ, Spencer CM. Ropinirole: a review of its use in the management of Parkinson's disease. *Drugs* 2000; **60:** 115–37.
6. Whone AL, *et al.* Slower progression of Parkinson's disease with ropinirole versus levodopa: the REAL-PET study. *Ann Neurol* 2003; **54:** 93–101.
7. Clarke CE, Deane KHO. Ropinirole for levodopa-induced complications in Parkinson's disease. Available in The Cochrane Library; Issue 1. Chichester: John Wiley; 2004.
8. Clarke CE, Deane KHO. Ropinirole versus bromocriptine for levodopa-induced complications in Parkinson's disease. Available in The Cochrane Library: Issue 1. Chichester: John Wiley; 2004.

**Restless legs syndrome.** The aetiology of restless legs syndrome (see Parasomnias, p.667) is obscure and treatment has largely been empirical although dopaminergic therapy has emerged as a common first-line choice. In a study[1] in 284 patients, ropinirole, in a mean dose of 1.9 mg daily, was more effective than placebo in reducing the symptoms of restless legs syndrome and improving sleep.

1. Trenkwalder C, *et al.* Ropinirole in the treatment of restless legs syndrome: results from the TREAT RLS 1 study, a 12 week, randomised, placebo controlled study in 10 European countries. *J Neurol Neurosurg Psychiatry* 2004; **75:** 92–7.

## Preparations

**Proprietary Preparations** (details are given in Part 3)
***Arg.:*** Requip; ***Austria:*** Requip; ***Belg.:*** Requip; ***Canad.:*** Requip; ***Chile:*** Requip; ***Denm.:*** Requip; ***Fr.:*** Requip; ***Ger.:*** Requip; ***Gr.:*** Requip; ***Hong Kong:*** Requip; ***Irl.:*** Requip; ***Israel:*** Requip; ***Ital.:*** Requip; ***Neth.:*** Requip; ***Norw.:*** Requip; ***Port.:*** Requip; ***S.Afr.:*** Requip; ***Singapore:*** Requip; ***Spain:*** Requip; ***Swed.:*** Requip; ***Switz.:*** Requip; ***UK:*** Requip; ***USA:*** Requip.

# Selegiline Hydrochloride

*(BANM, USAN, rINNM)*

Deprenyl; L-Deprenyl; Hidrocloruro de selegilina; Selegilini Hydrochloridum. (−)-(R)-N,α-Dimethyl-N-(prop-2-ynyl)phenethylamine hydrochloride; (R)-Methyl(α-methylphenethyl)prop-2-ynylamine hydrochloride.

$C_{13}H_{17}N,HCl = 223.7.$

*CAS — 14611-51-9 (selegiline); 2079-54-1 (selegiline hydrochloride); 14611-52-0 (selegiline hydrochloride).*

*ATC — N04BD01.*

**Pharmacopoeias.** In *Eur.* (see p.vi) and *US.*

**Ph. Eur. 5.0** (Selegiline Hydrochloride). A white or almost white, crystalline powder. Freely soluble in water and in methyl alcohol; slightly soluble in acetone. A 2% solution in water has a pH of 3.5 to 4.5. Protect from light.

**USP 27** (Selegiline Hydrochloride). A white, odourless crystalline powder. Freely soluble in water, in chloroform, and in methyl alcohol. Store in airtight containers. Protect from light.

## Adverse Effects

Selegiline is often given as an adjunct to levodopa therapy and many of the adverse effects reported may be attributed to enhanced levodopa activity; dosage of levodopa may have to be reduced. However, most reported adverse effects, with the possible exception of increased dyskinesias and cardiac arrhythmias, have also been seen with selegiline monotherapy. Adverse effects have included hypotension, chest pain, nausea, vomiting, constipation, diarrhoea, confusion, headache, tremor, vertigo, dizziness, psychosis, depression, hallucinations, agitation, dry mouth, sore throat, difficulty in micturition, skin reactions, back pain, muscle cramps, joint pain, myopathy, and increased dyskinesias. The amfetamine metabolites of selegiline may cause insomnia and abnormal dreams; evening doses should be avoided. Transient increases in liver enzymes have been reported. Mouth ulcers and stomatitis may occur with the oral lyophilisate (Zelapar, UK).

Since the selectivity of selegiline is lost at higher doses, signs and symptoms of overdosage may resemble those of non-selective MAOIs such as phenelzine (see p.312).

**Effects on carbohydrate metabolism.** Profound hypoglycaemia developed in a 70-year-old man after selegiline was added to his existing medication for Parkinson's disease.[1] Hypoglycaemia was accompanied by hyperinsulinaemia and resolved 1 week after discontinuation of selegiline.

1. Rowland MJ, *et al.* Hypoglycemia caused by selegiline, an antiparkinsonian drug: can such side effects be predicted? *J Clin Pharmacol* 1994; **34:** 80–5.

**Effects on mortality.** For reference to a study which observed an increased mortality rate in patients with Parkinson's disease taking selegiline and levodopa compared with those taking levodopa alone, see under Parkinsonism in Uses and Administration, below.

## Precautions

Selegiline should be used with caution in patients with a history of peptic ulceration and avoided in those with active ulceration. It should also be used with caution in uncontrolled hypertension, arrhythmias, angina, or psychosis.

**Cardiovascular disorders.** An investigation[1] of the autonomic effects of selegiline as a potential cause of the unexpected mortality observed in one study[2] in patients with Parkinson's disease receiving selegiline and levodopa (see Parkinsonism, below) suggested that the risk of orthostatic hypotension with this combination may have been underestimated. It was considered prudent to withdraw selegiline from those with symptomatic orthostatic hypotension or concomitant cardiovascular or cerebrovascular disease. For those without symptomatic morbidity, but a greater than 20 mmHg fall in blood pressure on standing for 2 minutes, gradual withdrawal of selegiline with a concomitant retitration of levodopa dosage should be considered.

1. Churchyard A, *et al.* Autonomic effects of selegiline: possible cardiovascular toxicity in Parkinson's disease. *J Neurol Neurosurg Psychiatry* 1997; **63:** 228–34.
2. Parkinson's Disease Research Group of the United Kingdom. Comparison of therapeutic effects and mortality data of levodopa and levodopa combined with selegiline in patients with early, mild Parkinson's disease. *BMJ* 1995; **311:** 1602–7.

## Interactions

Selegiline is less likely than non-selective MAOIs, such as phenelzine, to interact with tyramine in food; such hypertensive reactions have been reported rarely at usual doses but the manufacturer has warned that its selectivity is lost at higher doses and it must be assumed that selegiline can usually only be used safely without dietary restrictions at doses of up to 10 mg daily. For dietary restrictions applicable to patients taking MAOIs, see p.314.

Even when given in therapeutic doses life-threatening interactions can occur between selegiline and pethidine. Serious reactions, sometimes fatal, have also been reported when selegiline has been used with tricyclic antidepressants or serotonin reuptake inhibitors including the SSRIs and venlafaxine. The manufacturer recommends that 14 days should elapse between discontinuation of selegiline and starting treatment with tricyclic or serotonergic antidepressants. Conversely, selegiline should not be given to patients who have recently received these antidepressants; at least 5 weeks should elapse between discontinuing fluoxetine and starting treatment with selegiline.

Selegiline is contra-indicated in patients receiving serotonin agonists such as sumatriptan.

**Antidepressants.** Although there have been studies in which patients with parkinsonism have received selegiline with *SSRIs* such as fluoxetine[1] or paroxetine[2] (apparently without any problems) there have been reports of reactions[3-5] such as shivering and sweating, hypertension, hyperactivity, and ataxia occurring when selegiline and fluoxetine have been used together. The FDA noted[6] that reactions similar to those between SSRIs and non-selective MAOIs had also been reported in patients taking selegiline with paroxetine or sertraline.

Severe reactions, sometimes fatal, have also occurred in patients taking selegiline and *tricyclic antidepressants*.[6] For a report of serotonin syndrome developing when *venlafaxine* was given after selegiline (despite a drug-free period) see p.322.

There has been a report[7] of a patient receiving the non-selective MAOI *iproniazid* who experienced severe orthostatic hypotension when given selegiline. Selegiline given with the reversible MAOI *moclobemide* to healthy subjects markedly increased the pressor response to tyramine compared with the effects of each drug used alone.[8] The authors concluded that dietary restriction of tyramine-containing foods would be necessary if these drugs were to be used together.

1. Waters CH. Fluoxetine and selegiline—lack of significant interaction. *Can J Neurol Sci* 1994; **21:** 259–61.
2. Toyama SC, Iacono RP. Is it safe to combine a selective serotonin reuptake inhibitor with selegiline? *Ann Pharmacother* 1994; **28:** 405–6.
3. Suchowersky O, de Vries JD. Interaction of fluoxetine and selegiline. *Can J Psychiatry* 1990; **35:** 571–2.
4. Jermain DM, *et al.* Potential fluoxetine-selegiline interaction. *Ann Pharmacother* 1992; **26:** 1300.
5. Montastruc JL, *et al.* Pseudophaeochromocytoma in parkinsonian patient treated with fluoxetine plus selegiline. *Lancet* 1993; **341:** 555.
6. Anonymous. Eldepryl and antidepressant interaction. *FDA Med Bull* 1995; **25** (Feb.): 6.
7. Pare CMB, *et al.* Attempts to attenuate the 'cheese effect': combined drug therapy in depressive illness. *J Affect Disord* 1985; **9:** 137–41.
8. Korn A, *et al.* Tyramine pressor sensitivity in healthy subjects during combined treatment with moclobemide and selegiline. *Eur J Clin Pharmacol* 1996; **49:** 273–8.

**Opioid analgesics.** Selegiline can produce life-threatening reactions when given with *pethidine*.[1]

1. Zornberg GL, *et al.* Severe adverse interaction between pethidine and selegiline. *Lancet* 1991; **337:** 246. Correction. *ibid.*; 440.

**Oral contraceptives.** The total area under the curve for selegiline given in single doses of 5 to 40 mg was raised 10- to 20-fold in 4 women who were using oral hormonal contraceptives when compared with 4 women receiving no concomitant medication.[1] It was suggested that use of selegiline and oral hormonal contraceptives should be avoided or the dosage of selegiline reduced.

1. Laine K, *et al.* Dose linearity study of selegiline pharmacokinetics after oral administration: evidence for strong drug interaction with female sex steroids. *Br J Clin Pharmacol* 1999; **47:** 249–54.

**Sympathomimetics.** The US manufacturers (Somerset, USA) have stated that there has been a report of hypertensive crisis in a patient taking recommended doses of selegiline and *ephedrine*. A hypertensive reaction following low-dose *dopamine* infusion has been reported[1] in a 75-year-old patient receiving selegiline 10 mg daily for Parkinson's disease. The authors suggest that this may indicate a non-specific action of selegiline at usual doses on peripheral monoamine oxidase inhibitor type-A.

1. Rose LM, *et al.* A hypertensive reaction induced by concurrent use of selegiline and dopamine. *Ann Pharmacother* 2000; **34:** 1020–4.

## Pharmacokinetics

Selegiline is readily absorbed from the gastrointestinal tract from conventional preparations and crosses the blood-brain barrier. It undergoes extensive first-pass metabolism in the liver to produce at least 5 metabolites, including *l*-(−)-desmethylselegiline (norselegiline), *l*-(−)-*N*-methylamfetamine, and *l*-(−)-amfetamine. Concentrations of selegiline metabolites are greatly reduced after administration of the oral lyophilisate preparation, the majority of which undergoes absorption through the buccal mucosa. Selegiline is excreted as metabolites mainly in the urine and about 15% appears in the faeces.

◊ References.

1. Heinonen EH, *et al.* Pharmacokinetic aspects of l-deprenyl (selegiline) and its metabolites. *Clin Pharmacol Ther* 1994; **56:** 742–9.
2. Mahmood I, *et al.* Clinical pharmacokinetics and pharmacodynamics of selegiline: an update. *Clin Pharmacokinet* 1997; **33:** 91–102.

## Uses and Administration

Selegiline is an irreversible selective inhibitor of monoamine oxidase type B, an enzyme involved in the metabolic degradation of dopamine in the brain. It enhances the effects of levodopa and is used in Parkinson's disease as an adjunct to levodopa therapy, usually when fluctuations in mobility have become a problem, but see Parkinsonism, below. Addition of selegiline to levodopa therapy may enable the dosage of levodopa to be reduced by about 10 to 50%. Selegiline may also be given alone in early Parkinson's disease in an attempt to delay the need for levodopa therapy.

Selegiline hydrochloride is given by mouth as conventional preparations such as tablets or oral liquid, or as oral lyophilisate tablets (Zelapar, UK). The dose of the conventional preparations is 10 mg daily, either as a single dose in the morning or in 2 divided doses of 5 mg at breakfast and lunchtime. The initial dose of the oral lyophilisate tablets is 1.25 mg daily at least 5 minutes before breakfast; patients already receiving 10 mg of conventional preparations can be transferred to 1.25 mg of the oral lyophilisate.

To avoid initial confusion and agitation, particularly in the elderly, it may be appropriate when using conventional preparations to start treatment with a dose of 2.5 mg daily.

Other conditions in which selegiline has been tried include dementia and depression.

◊ Some references to the actions of selegiline.


1. Youdim MBH, Finberg JPM. Pharmacological actions of l-deprenyl (selegiline) and other selective monoamine oxidase B inhibitors. *Clin Pharmacol Ther* 1994; **56:** 725–33.
2. Lange KW, *et al.* Biochemical actions of l-deprenyl (selegiline). *Clin Pharmacol Ther* 1994; **56:** 734–41.


**Dementia.** The hypothesis that neurodegeneration in Alzheimer's disease (p.1484) might be due to free radical formation has led to drugs such as selegiline being tried as antioxidant therapy.

Early double-blind studies[1,2] indicated that selegiline 10 mg daily might produce beneficial effects in patients with Alzheimer's disease but it was suggested that improvements in mood and cognitive function may have been due to a reduction in tension and depression.[3] A 15-month study in Alzheimers's patients with mild cognitive impairment showed selegiline 10 mg daily to have little effect,[4] although the authors pointed out that those with more severe dementia have shown more response in other studies. The conclusion of a later study[5] that selegiline 10 mg daily slowed progression in patients with moderate disease has been criticised[6] on the grounds that any effect was only evident after statistical adjustment to the original analysis. In addition a recent systematic review[7] that examined the effects of selegiline concluded that there was no meaningful evidence of a beneficial effect of selegiline on patients with Alzheimer's disease. They also considered that there was no longer any justification for its use in patients with Alzheimer's disease.


1. Piccinin GL, *et al.* Neuropsychological effects of L-deprenyl in Alzheimer's type dementia. *Clin Neuropharmacol* 1990; **13:** 147–63.
2. Mangoni A, *et al.* Effects of a MAO-B inhibitor in the treatment of Alzheimer disease. *Eur Neurol* 1991; **31:** 100–107.
3. Anonymous. Drugs for Alzheimer's disease. *Drug Ther Bull* 1990; **28:** 42–4.
4. Burke WJ, *et al.* L-Deprenyl in the treatment of mild dementia of the Alzheimer type: results of a 15-month trial. *J Am Geriatr Soc* 1993; **41:** 1219–25.
5. Sano M, *et al.* A controlled trial of selegiline, alpha-tocopherol, or both as treatment for Alzheimer's disease. *N Engl J Med* 1997; **336:** 1216–22.
6. Pincus MM. Alpha-tocopherol and Alzheimer's disease. *N Engl J Med* 1997; **337:** 572.
7. Birks J, Flicker L. Selegiline for Alzheimer's disease. Available in The Cochrane Library; Issue 1. Chichester: John Wiley; 2004.


**Depression.** Selegiline is a selective inhibitor of monoamine oxidase type B and there are reports of it producing improvement in depression.[1-3] However at the dosage level usually required to produce an antidepressant effect the specificity of oral selegiline is reported to be lost and it has been suggested that the efficacy of selegiline as an antidepressant might depend on inhibition of monoamine oxidase A rather than inhibition of monoamine oxidase B alone. Such a loss of specificity would mean that patients taking selegiline for depression would need to observe the dietary restrictions applicable to non-selective MAOIs.

To overcome the problems associated with the oral route, transdermal selegiline has also been tried and may be more effective than placebo in the treatment of depression.[4,5] The use of the transdermal route allows sustained blood levels of selegiline to be delivered without extensive inhibition of peripheral monoamine oxidase A.


1. Mendlewicz J, Youdim MBH. L-Deprenil, a selective monoamine oxidase type B inhibitor, in the treatment of depression: a double-blind evaluation. *Br J Psychiatry* 1983; **142:** 508–11.
2. Mann JJ, *et al.* A controlled study of the antidepressant efficacy and side-effects of (−)-deprenyl. *Arch Gen Psychiatry* 1989; **46:** 45–50.
3. Sunderland T, *et al.* High-dose selegiline in treatment-resistant older depressive patients. *Arch Gen Psychiatry* 1994; **51:** 607–15.
4. Bodkin JA, Amsterdam JD. Transdermal selegiline in major depression: a double-blind, placebo-controlled, parallel-group study in outpatients. *Am J Psychiatry* 2002; **159:** 1869–75.
5. Amsterdam JD. A double-blind, placebo-controlled trial of the safety and efficacy of selegiline transdermal system without dietary restrictions in patients with major depressive disorder. *J Clin Psychiatry* 2003; **64:** 208–14.


**Narcoleptic syndrome.** Small controlled studies[1,2] have suggested that selegiline 20 to 40 mg daily has a beneficial effect on symptoms of narcolepsy and cataplexy (p.1583); at such a dosage a low-tyramine diet is considered necessary.


1. Hublin C, *et al.* Selegiline in the treatment of narcolepsy. *Neurology* 1994; **44:** 2095–2101.
2. Mayer G, *et al.* Selegeline [sic] hydrochloride treatment in narcolepsy: a double-blind, placebo-controlled study. *Clin Neuropharmacol* 1995; **18:** 306–19.


**Parkinsonism.** As a selective monoamine oxidase type B inhibitor, selegiline reduces the metabolism of dopamine and thereby enhances its actions. It reduces levodopa's 'end-of-dose' effect and has a dose-sparing effect. Some have used it as **monotherapy** in an attempt to delay the need for levodopa. It has been postulated that progression of Parkinson's disease (p.1196) might be due to free radicals, generated during the metabolism of dopamine, having a cytotoxic effect on dopaminergic neurones in the substantia nigra. It has been suggested that selegiline might therefore slow disease progression by reducing the formation of free radicals generated by oxidation of dopamine by monoamine oxidase type B. In a large early study,[1] the DATATOP study, selegiline monotherapy delayed the need to start levodopa in patients with early Parkinson's disease. These findings were corroborated by other smaller studies.[2,3] There has been much debate over whether the benefit was due to a neuroprotective or symptomatic effect. Re-analysis of the DATATOP data by independent workers[4,5] and findings of other studies[6] support a symptomatic effect. Subsequent studies involving DATATOP patients have also been consistent with a symptomatic effect; any benefit produced by selegiline appeared to be less pronounced as the duration of treatment increased[7] and was lost completely long-term.[8,9] A later study[10] designed to minimise any symptomatic effect has cast doubt on whether the delay in progression of the signs and symptoms of Parkinson's disease obtained with selegiline is entirely due to a symptomatic effect.

Studies of the use of selegiline as an **adjunct** to levodopa therapy[6,11,12] indicate that selegiline permits a modest reduction in the dosage requirements of levodopa. An interim analysis of a study of the early addition of selegiline to levodopa has also suggested that selegiline might stabilise the long-term daily levodopa dosage.[13]

However, the use of selegiline in Parkinson's disease has been questioned after one UK study[11] found an unexpected increase in mortality in patients taking levodopa with selegiline compared with those taking levodopa alone. No difference in mortality had been detected at the 3-year follow-up[14] but after an average follow-up of 5.6 years[11] mortality was 60% higher in the group receiving selegiline. The study has been criticised on many grounds including the fact that mortality was very high in both arms of the study[15] and has been the subject of much debate.[16,17] The authors of the study[11] had stated that they would advise the study patients to withdraw selegiline therapy. Analysis of follow-up data[18] until the selegiline arm of the study was terminated (average 6.8 years) found an excess mortality of about 35%, a figure calculated[19] to be no longer significant. However, because of the premature termination of the study such results were considered[20] to be biased. Whether any excess in mortality is causally related to selegiline is still unclear. Some consider that changes in prescribing practice based on this study are not warranted.[16] Others[20] have made a cautious recommendation not to start combination treatment in patients with newly diagnosed Parkinson's disease but consider that there is little evidence to advise patients who have been using selegiline with levodopa for years without problem to change their treatment. An evaluation of mortality among patients taking antiparkinsonian drugs (using the UK General Practice Research Database) provided evidence against there being substantial excess mortality associated with the use of selegiline.[21] These results are supported by a meta-analysis[22] of 5 randomised, double-blind trials which found no increase in mortality associated with selegiline treatment regardless of concurrent levodopa. Furthermore, increased mortality was not observed in patients in the original DATATOP trial[1] after an average follow-up time of 8.2 years. However, it was noted that the delay of disability observed in the early phase of selegiline therapy[1,7] was not associated with longer life during follow-up.[23]


1. The Parkinson Study Group. Effect of deprenyl on the progression of disability in early Parkinson's disease. *N Engl J Med* 1989; **321:** 1364–71.
2. Tetrud JW, Langston JW. The effect of deprenyl (selegiline) on the natural history of Parkinson's disease. *Science* 1989; **245:** 519–22.
3. Allain H, *et al.* Selegiline in de novo parkinsonian patients: the French selegiline multicenter trial (FSMT). *Acta Neurol Scand* 1991; **84** (suppl 136): 73–8.
4. Schulzer M, *et al.* The antiparkinson efficacy of deprenyl derives from transient improvement that is likely to be symptomatic. *Ann Neurol* 1992; **32:** 795–8.
5. Ward CD. Does selegiline delay progression of Parkinson's disease? A critical re-evaluation of the DATATOP study. *J Neurol Neurosurg Psychiatry* 1994; **57:** 217–20.
6. Brannan T, Yahr MD. Comparative study of selegiline plus L-dopa–carbidopa versus L-dopa–carbidopa alone in the treatment of Parkinson's disease. *Ann Neurol* 1995; **37:** 95–8.
7. The Parkinson Study Group. Effects of tocopherol and deprenyl on the progression of disability in early Parkinson's disease. *N Engl J Med* 1993; **328:** 176–83.
8. Parkinson Study Group. Impact of deprenyl and tocopherol treatment on Parkinson's disease in DATATOP subjects not requiring levodopa. *Ann Neurol* 1996; **39:** 29–36.
9. Parkinson Study Group. Impact of deprenyl and tocopherol treatment on Parkinson's disease in DATATOP patients requiring levodopa. *Ann Neurol* 1996; **39:** 37–45.
10. Olanow CW, *et al.* The effect of deprenyl and levodopa on the progression of Parkinson's disease. *Ann Neurol* 1996; **38:** 771–7.
11. Parkinson's Disease Research Group of the United Kingdom. Comparison of therapeutic effects and mortality data of levodopa and levodopa combined with selegiline in patients with early, mild Parkinson's disease. *BMJ* 1995; **311:** 1602–7.
12. Myllylä VV, *et al.* Early selegiline therapy reduces levodopa dose requirement in Parkinson's disease. *Acta Neurol Scand* 1995; **91:** 177–82.
13. Larsen JP, Boas J. Norwegian-Danish Study Group. The effects of early selegiline therapy on long-term treatment and parkinsonian disability: an interim analysis of a Norwegian-Danish 5-year study. *Mov Disord* 1997; **12:** 175–82.
14. Parkinson's Disease Research Group in the United Kingdom. Comparisons of the therapeutic effects of levodopa, levodopa and selegiline, and bromocriptine in patients with early, mild Parkinson's disease: three year interim report. *BMJ* 1993; **307:** 467–72.
15. Olanow CW, *et al.* Patients taking selegiline may have received more levodopa than necessary. *BMJ* 1996; **312:** 702–3.
16. Ahlskog JE. Treatment of early Parkinson's disease: are complicated strategies justified? *Mayo Clin Proc* 1996; **71:** 659–70.
17. Mizuno Y, Kondo T. Mortality associated with selegiline in Parkinson's disease: what do the available data mean? *Drug Safety* 1997; **16:** 289–94.
18. Ben-Shlomo Y, *et al.* Investigation by Parkinson's Disease Research Group of United Kingdom into excess mortality seen with combined levodopa and selegiline treatment in patients with early, mild Parkinson's disease: further results of randomised trial and confidential inquiry. *BMJ* 1998; **316:** 1191–6.
19. Abrams KR. Monitoring randomised controlled trials. *BMJ* 1998; **316:** 1183–4.
20. Breteler MMB. Selegiline, or the problem of early termination of clinical trials. *BMJ* 1998; **316:** 1182–3.
21. Thorogood M, *et al.* Mortality in people taking selegiline: observational study. *BMJ* 1998; **317:** 252–4.
22. Olanow CW, *et al.* Effect of selegiline on mortality in patients with Parkinson's disease: a meta-analysis. *Neurology* 1998; **51:** 825–30.
23. The Parkinson Study Group. Mortality in DATATOP: A multicenter trial in early Parkinson's disease. *Ann Neurol* 1998; **43:** 318–25.


**Smoking cessation.** Selegiline has been investigated as an aid to smoking cessation (p.1721).

References.


1. George TP, *et al.* A preliminary placebo-controlled trial of selegiline hydrochloride for smoking cessation. *Biol Psychiatry* 2003; **53:** 136–43.
2. Biberman R, *et al.* A randomized controlled trial of oral selegiline plus nicotine skin patch compared with placebo plus nicotine skin patch for smoking cessation. *Addiction* 2003; **98:** 1403–7.


## Preparations

***BP 2003:*** Selegiline Oral Solution; Selegiline Tablets;
***USP 27:*** Selegiline Hydrochloride Tablets.

**Proprietary Preparations** (details are given in Part 3)

***Arg.:*** Brintenal; Jumex; Kinabide; ***Austral.:*** Eldepryl; Selgene; ***Austria:*** Amboneural; Cognitiv; Jumex; Regepar; ***Belg.:*** Eldepryl; ***Braz.:*** Deprilan; Elepril; Jumexil; Niar; Parkexin; ***Canad.:*** Eldepryl; ***Chile:*** Selgina; ***Denm.:*** Eldepryl; Tremorex†; ***Fin.:*** Eldepryl; ***Fr.:*** Deprenyl; Otrasel; ***Ger.:*** Amindan; Antiparkin; Deprenyl†; MAOtil; Movergan; Selegam; Selemerck; Selepark; Selgimed; Xilopar; ***Gr.:*** Cosmopril; Procythol; Resostyl; ***Hong Kong:*** Julab; Jumex; Sefmex; Selegos; ***India:*** Selgin; ***Irl.:*** Clondepryl†; Eldepryl; ***Israel:*** Apomex†; Jumex; ***Ital.:*** Egibren; Jumex; Selecom; Seledat; Selpar†; Xilopar; ***Malaysia:*** Ginex; Jumex; Selegos; ***Mex.:*** Niar; ***Neth.:*** Eldepryl; ***Norw.:*** Eldepryl; ***NZ:*** Eldepryl; Selgene; ***Port.:*** Jumex; Xilopar; ***S.Afr.:*** Eldepryl; ***Singapore:*** Elegelin†; Jumex; Selegos; ***Spain:*** Plurimen; ***Swed.:*** Eldepryl; ***Switz.:*** Jumexal; Regepar†; Selecim; ***Thai.:*** Elegelin; Julab; Jumex; Kinline; Sefmex; Selgene†; Seline; ***UK:*** Eldepryl; Vivapryl†; Zelapar; ***USA:*** Atapryl; Carbex; Eldepryl.

## Talipexole Hydrochloride *(rINNM)*

Alefexole Hydrochloride; B-HT-920; Hidrocloruro de talipexol.
6-Allyl-2-amino-5,6,7,8-tetrahydro-4*H*-thiazolo[4,5-*d*]azepine dihydrochloride.

$C_{10}H_{15}N_3S,2HCl = 282.2.$

*CAS — 101626-70-4 (talipexole); 36085-73-1 (talipexole hydrochloride).*

### Profile

Talipexole hydrochloride is a dopamine $D_2$-agonist that is used in the management of parkinsonism in usual doses of 1.2 to 3.6 mg daily, in divided doses by mouth. It has also been investigated in the treatment of schizophrenia.

◊ References.


1. Mizuno Y, *et al.* Preliminary study of B-HT 920, a novel dopamine agonist, for the treatment of Parkinson's disease. *Drug Invest* 1993; **5:** 186–92.
2. Ohmori T, *et al.* B-HT 920, a dopamine D2 agonist, in the treatment of negative symptoms of chronic schizophrenia. *Biol Psychiatry* 1993; **33:** 687–93.


### Preparations

**Proprietary Preparations** (details are given in Part 3)

***Jpn:*** Domin.

## Terguride *(rINN)*

Tergurida. 1,1-Diethyl-3-(6-methylergolin-8α-yl) urea.

$C_{20}H_{28}N_4O$ = 340.5.

*CAS — 37686-84-3.*

### Profile

Terguride, an ergot derivative, is a partial dopamine agonist with general properties similar to those of bromocriptine (p.1200). It is used in the treatment of disorders related to hyperprolactinaemia in a usual dose of 500 micrograms twice daily. It is also being investigated in the management of parkinsonism.

◊ References.

1. Krause W, *et al.* Pharmacokinetics and endocrine effects of terguride in healthy subjects. *Eur J Clin Pharmacol* 1990; **38:** 609–15.
2. Baronti F, *et al.* Partial dopamine agonist therapy of levodopa-induced dyskinesias. *Neurology* 1992; **42:** 1241–3.

### Preparations

**Proprietary Preparations** (details are given in Part 3)
***Jpn:*** Teluron.

## Tolcapone *(BAN, USAN, rINN)*

Ro-40-7592; Tolcapona. 3,4-Dihydroxy-4′-methyl-5-nitrobenzophenone; 3,4-Dihydroxy-5-nitrophenyl(4-methylphenyl)methanone.

$C_{14}H_{11}NO_5$ = 273.2.

*CAS — 134308-13-7.*

*ATC — N04BX01.*

### Adverse Effects

The most common adverse effects associated with tolcapone are diarrhoea, nausea, vomiting, constipation, abdominal pain, dry mouth, anorexia, dyskinesia, orthostatic hypotension, hallucinations, somnolence, headache, increased sweating, and sleep disorders. Diarrhoea may be severe enough to warrant discontinuation. Increases in liver enzyme values have occurred and hepatitis and hepatic failure, sometimes fatal, have been reported. Tolcapone and its metabolites can produce a yellow intensification in the colour of urine.

**Effects on the liver.** The UK Committee on Safety of Medicines had noted[1] that, following a report[2] in September 1998 of fatal acute hepatic failure associated with tolcapone, the European Committee for Proprietary Medicinal Products (CPMP) had reviewed all reports of hepatic injury with tolcapone. There had been 10 reports of serious hepatic adverse reactions since tolcapone was marketed in October 1997, which included 7 reports of hepatitis, 3 of which had a fatal outcome. Serious hepatic reactions occurred unpredictably and their development was not always predicted by liver function monitoring. Consequently, in the European Union, the marketing authorisation for tolcapone was suspended in November 1998. (This suspension was lifted in April 2004 by the CPMP following further review.)

In some countries such as the USA, tolcapone remained available albeit with restricted indications and strict monitoring requirements (see Precautions, below). There have been no further reports of fatal hepatic failure following the introduction of these measures although the number of patients eligible to receive the drug has been reduced.[3]

1. Committee on Safety of Medicines/Medicines Control Agency. Withdrawal of tolcapone (Tasmar). *Current Problems* 1999; **25:** 2. Also available at: http://www.mca.gov.uk/ourwork/monitorsafequalmed/currentproblems/volume25feb.htm (accessed 24/05/04)
2. Assal F, *et al.* Tolcapone and fulminant hepatitis. *Lancet* 1998; **352:** 958.
3. Borges N. Tolcapone-related liver dysfunction: implications for use in Parkinson's disease therapy. *Drug Safety* 2003; **26:** 743–7.

**Effects on the skin.** For reference to the development of vitiligo in a patient following addition of tolcapone to levodopa/carbidopa treatment, see under Levodopa, p.1207.

### Precautions

Tolcapone should not be given to patients with hepatic impairment or raised liver enzyme values. Liver enzymes should be monitored when starting treatment with tolcapone and then every 2 weeks for the first year of therapy, every 4 weeks for the next 6 months, and then every 8 weeks thereafter. If the dose is to be increased to 200 mg three times daily, liver enzyme monitoring should take place before increasing the dose and then re-initiated at the frequency above. Tolcapone should be discontinued if liver enzyme levels exceed the upper limit of normal or if signs or symptoms suggestive of the onset of hepatic failure occur. Tolcapone should not be reintroduced to patients who have developed evidence of hepatic injury while receiving tolcapone. Tolcapone should be used with caution in patients with severe renal impairment.

Tolcapone is contra-indicated in patients with a history of non-traumatic rhabdomyolysis or symptoms of hyperpyrexia and confusion possibly related to the neuroleptic malignant syndrome. Use with levodopa may cause dizziness and orthostatic hypotension; if affected patients should not drive or operate machinery.

Abrupt withdrawal or dose reduction of tolcapone should be monitored carefully because of the risk of developing symptoms resembling the neuroleptic malignant syndrome.

**Elderly.** Confusion occurred in 3 elderly patients with severe Parkinson's disease following the addition of tolcapone to their antiparkinsonian therapy.[1] It was suggested that a starting dose of tolcapone 100 mg daily might be more suitable in frail patients with severe disease. It was noted[2] that a reduction in levodopa dosage is generally recommended when tolcapone is given to patients such as these, who were receiving 500 to 600 mg of levodopa daily.

1. Henry C, Wilson JA. Catechol-O-methyltransferase inhibitors in Parkinson's disease. *Lancet* 1998; **351:** 1965–6.
2. Harper J, Vieira B. Catechol-O-methyltransferase inhibitors in Parkinson's disease. *Lancet* 1998; **352:** 578.

### Interactions

Tolcapone may influence the pharmacokinetics of drugs metabolised by catechol-*O*-methyltransferase; a dose reduction of such drugs should be considered when given with tolcapone. Increased concentrations of benserazide and its active metabolite have been reported during administration with tolcapone. The manufacturer advises that non-selective MAOIs should not be used with tolcapone.

### Pharmacokinetics

Tolcapone is rapidly absorbed from the gastrointestinal tract and maximum plasma concentrations have been obtained within 2 hours of a dose by mouth; food delays and decreases the absorption. Absolute bioavailability is reported to be about 65%. Tolcapone is more than 99% bound to plasma proteins and is not widely distributed into body tissues. It is extensively metabolised, mainly by conjugation to the inactive glucuronide, but methylation by catechol-*O*-methyltransferase to 3-*O*-methyltolcapone and metabolism by cytochrome P450 isoenzymes also occurs. About 60% of a dose is excreted in the urine with the remainder appearing in the faeces. The elimination half-life has been reported to be about 2 to 3 hours. The clearance of unbound tolcapone may be reduced by 50% in patients with moderate cirrhotic liver disorders.

◊ References.

1. Dingemanse J, *et al.* Integrated pharmacokinetics and pharmacodynamics of the novel catechol-O-methyltransferase inhibitor tolcapone during first administration to humans. *Clin Pharmacol Ther* 1995; **57:** 508–17.
2. Jorga KM, *et al.* Effect of liver impairment on the pharmacokinetics of tolcapone and its metabolites. *Clin Pharmacol Ther* 1998; **63:** 646–54.
3. Jorga K, *et al.* Metabolism and excretion of tolcapone, a novel inhibitor of catechol-O-methyltransferase. *Br J Clin Pharmacol* 1999; **48:** 513–20.
4. Jorga K, *et al.* Population pharmacokinetics of tolcapone in parkinsonian patients in dose finding studies. *Br J Clin Pharmacol* 2000; **49:** 39–48.

### Uses and Administration

Tolcapone is a peripheral inhibitor of catechol-*O*-methyltransferase (COMT), an enzyme involved in the metabolism of dopamine and levodopa. It has been used as an adjunct to levodopa and dopa-decarboxylase inhibitor combinations in the management of Parkinson's disease for patients who cannot be stabilised on these levodopa combinations or for those who experience 'end-of-dose' deterioration. Because of the risk of serious hepatotoxicity the FDA in the USA restricted its use to when other adjunctive therapy was ineffective or contra-indicated. In the European Union, tolcapone was withdrawn from the market in November 1998.

The usual recommended dosage of tolcapone is 100 mg given three times daily; up to a maximum of 200 mg three times daily may be considered if the clinical benefit justifies the increased risk of hepatotoxicity. The first dose of the day should be taken at the same time as the combined levodopa preparation. Most patients already taking more than 600 mg of levodopa daily will require a reduction in their dosage of levodopa; patients on lower levodopa doses may also require a dose reduction.

Tolcapone should be withdrawn if a substantial clinical benefit is not obtained within the first 3 weeks of treatment.

**Parkinsonism.** Tolcapone is a reversible peripheral inhibitor of catechol-*O*-methyltransferase (COMT), an enzyme involved in the metabolism of levodopa and dopamine.[1] It appears to differ from entacapone (p.1205) by being a more potent COMT inhibitor in the periphery and by penetrating into the brain (although the significance of any central effects of COMT inhibition are not known).[1] When given to patients with Parkinson's disease (p.1196) and levodopa-related fluctuations in disability or 'end-of-dose' effects, it has prolonged the clinical benefit obtained with levodopa and allowed the total daily dosage of levodopa to be reduced.[2,3] Benefit has also been reported[4] when added to levodopa therapy in patients with stable Parkinson's disease.

1. Nutt JG. Catechol-O-methyltransferase inhibitors for treatment of Parkinson's disease. *Lancet* 1998; **351:** 1221–2.
2. Kurth MC, *et al.* Tolcapone improves motor function and reduces levodopa requirement in patients with Parkinson's disease experiencing motor fluctuations: a multicenter, double-blind, randomized, placebo-controlled trial. *Neurology* 1997; **48:** 81–7.
3. Rajput AH, *et al.* Tolcapone improves motor function in parkinsonian patients with the "wearing-off" phenomenon: a double-blind placebo-controlled, multicenter trial. *Neurology* 1997; **49:** 1066–71.
4. Waters CH, *et al.* Tolcapone Stable Study Group. Tolcapone in stable Parkinson's disease: efficacy and safety of long-term treatment. *Neurology* 1997; **49:** 665–71.

### Preparations

**Proprietary Preparations** (details are given in Part 3)
***Arg.:*** Tasmar; ***Austria:*** Tasmar; ***Braz.:*** Tasmar; ***Chile:*** Tasmar; ***Hong Kong:*** Tasmar; ***Mex.:*** Tasmar†; ***Norw.:*** Tasmar†; ***NZ:*** Tasmar; ***S.Afr.:*** Tasmar; ***Singapore:*** Tasmar†; ***Switz.:*** Tasmar; ***Thai.:*** Tasmar†; ***USA:*** Tasmar.

# Electrolytes


Acid-base Balance, p.1217
Metabolic acidosis, p.1217
Metabolic alkalosis, p.1217
Calcium Homoeostasis, p.1217
Hypercalcaemia, p.1218
Hypercalcaemia of malignancy, p.1218
Hyperparathyroidism, p.1218
Vitamin D-mediated hypercalcaemia, p.1218
Hypocalcaemia, p.1218
Magnesium Homoeostasis, p.1218
Hypermagnesaemia, p.1218
Hypomagnesaemia, p.1219
Phosphate Homoeostasis, p.1219
Hyperphosphataemia, p.1219
Hypophosphataemia, p.1219
Potassium Homoeostasis, p.1219
Hyperkalaemia, p.1219
Hyperkalaemic periodic paralysis, p.1219
Hypokalaemia, p.1219
Bartter's syndrome, p.1220
Diuretic-induced hypokalaemia, p.1220
Hypokalaemic periodic paralysis, p.1220
Sodium Homoeostasis, p.1220
Hypernatraemia, p.1220
Hyponatraemia, p.1220


Electrolytes are used to correct disturbances in fluid and electrolyte homoeostasis or acid-base balance and to re-establish osmotic equilibrium of specific ions. The osmotic effects of solutions may be expressed in terms of osmolality, which is defined as the 'molal' concentration in moles (or osmoles) per kg of solvent, or in terms of osmolarity, which is the 'molar' concentration in moles (or osmoles) per litre of solution. In clinical practice, solute concentrations are measured per litre of solution and are expressed as millimoles (mmol) per litre or sometimes as milliequivalents (mEq) per litre. Milliequivalents are converted to millimoles by dividing by the valency of the ion. Positively charged ions are known as *cations* and include calcium, magnesium, potassium, and sodium ions. Negatively charged ions are known as *anions* and include bicarbonate, chloride, and phosphate ions. The ions principally involved in fluid and electrolyte homoeostasis and acid-base balance are sodium, chloride, bicarbonate, and potassium. Calcium, phosphate, and magnesium have a central role in the formation of bone mineral.

## Acid-base Balance

Within the body, acid is mostly produced during cellular respiration in the form of carbon dioxide. Small amounts of various non-volatile acids are generated via metabolism, including lactic acid, uric acid, keto acids, and some inorganic acids such as sulfuric and phosphoric acids. For normal tissue function, the pH of the body needs to be held within a narrow range. The pH of arterial blood is normally maintained between about 7.38 and 7.42 by means of compensatory respiratory, renal, and buffering mechanisms.

The most important buffer system in the extracellular fluid is the bicarbonate-carbonic acid system. Bicarbonate and hydrogen ions are in equilibrium with carbonic acid which is in turn in equilibrium with carbon dioxide in the body fluid, as expressed by:

$$H^+ + HCO_3^- \leftrightarrow H_2CO_3 \leftrightarrow CO_2 + H_2O$$

A normal plasma-bicarbonate concentration in adults is in the range of 20 to 30 mmol/litre and arterial partial pressure of carbon dioxide ($P_aCO_2$) is normally 4.7 to 5.7 kPa (35 to 43 mmHg).

Ultimately, excess acid must be removed from the body and base regenerated. $P_aCO_2$ is under respiratory control with carbon dioxide being excreted by the lungs. Plasma-bicarbonate concentrations are regulated by the kidneys, where bicarbonate is actively regenerated or reabsorbed. Organic acids such as lactic acid may be eliminated by metabolism; and other non-volatile acids, such as the inorganic acids of phosphate and sulfate, are excreted via the kidneys with simultaneous regeneration of bicarbonate.

The relationship between plasma pH, $P_aCO_2$, and bicarbonate is defined by the Henderson-Hasselbalch equation which is used to assess acid-base balance. For clinical purposes, this equation becomes

$$pH = pK_{CO_2} + \log\left(\frac{C_{HCO_3}}{\alpha \times P_aCO_2}\right)$$

where pH is the plasma pH, $pK_{CO_2}$ is the carbonic acid dissociation constant (6.1), $C_{HCO_3}$ is the plasma-bicarbonate concentration, $\alpha$ is a value representing carbon dioxide solubility, and $P_aCO_2$ is the arterial partial pressure of carbon dioxide. Disorders of acid-base balance may be due to a change in plasma-bicarbonate concentrations (metabolic) or to a change in $P_aCO_2$ (respiratory), although mixed disorders do occur.

The 4 major acid-base disturbances are:

- metabolic acidosis—a decrease in the plasma-bicarbonate concentration
- metabolic alkalosis—an increase in the plasma-bicarbonate concentration
- respiratory acidosis—hypoventilation and a raised $P_aCO_2$
- respiratory alkalosis—hyperventilation and a reduced $P_aCO_2$

A further measure that may provide useful information in the assessment of metabolic acidosis is the plasma anion gap. This is the difference in ionic charge between the principal plasma cation (sodium) and anions (chloride and bicarbonate), and provides an estimation of unmeasured serum anions, which include inorganic and organic acids.


◊ References.

1. Gluck SL. Acid-base. *Lancet* 1998; **352:** 474–9.
2. Hood VL, Tannen RL. Protection of acid-base balance by pH regulation of acid production. *N Engl J Med* 1998; **339:** 819–26.
3. Kraut JA, Madias NE. Approach to patients with acid-base disorders. *Respir Care* 2001; **46:** 392–403.
4. Epstein SK, Singh N. Respiratory acidosis. *Respir Care* 2001; **46:** 366–83.
5. Foster GT, *et al.* Respiratory alkalosis. *Respir Care* 2001; **46:** 384–91.
6. Madias NE, Adrogué HJ. Cross-talk between two organs: how the kidney responds to disruption of acid-base balance by the lung. *Nephron Physiol* 2003; **93:** 61–6.


**Metabolic acidosis.** Metabolic acidosis, characterised by a low plasma-bicarbonate concentration and a tendency towards a fall in arterial pH, is the most frequent acid-base abnormality.

Metabolic acidosis with a *normal anion gap* is usually caused by excessive losses of bicarbonate from the gastro-intestinal tract (as in severe diarrhoeas) or failure of the kidneys to reabsorb or regenerate adequate bicarbonate (as in the renal tubular acidoses). Ingestion of acidifying salts such as ammonium chloride, which generate hydrochloric acid, can also result in this type of acidosis. Metabolic acidosis characterised by an *increased anion gap* is often due to a reduction in the renal excretion of inorganic acids such as phosphates and sulfates as in renal failure (uraemic acidosis), or to the net accumulation of organic acids as, for example, in lactic acidosis or diabetic ketoacidosis.

Metabolic acidosis is diagnosed and monitored by measurement of serum electrolytes, arterial pH, and $P_aCO_2$. There is often hyperventilation with reduced cardiac function, constriction of peripheral veins, inhibition of the hepatic metabolism of lactate, and impairment of consciousness.

The main aim of **treatment** is to manage any underlying disorder,[1,2] and in some cases this will be sufficient to enable the body's homoeostatic mechanisms to correct the acid-base imbalance. The advantages of more active treatment of the acidosis must be balanced against the risks, including over-alkalinisation, and in consequence such therapy tends to be reserved for more persistent or severe cases.

The usual alkalinising agent is sodium bicarbonate. It may be given orally to replace bicarbonate losses in various chronic metabolic acidoses such as uraemic acidosis or renal tubular acidosis. Potassium bicarbonate may be preferred if the acidosis is associated with potassium deficiency. Potassium citrate and sodium citrate have also been used. More severe and acute cases (particularly where arterial pH is below 7.1) may require intravenous sodium bicarbonate therapy. Intravenous sodium bicarbonate has a role in acute metabolic acidoses attributable to severe renal failure, severe secretory diarrhoeas, and renal tubular acidosis. Although hypertonic solutions have been used, for example, in patients with circulatory overload, roughly isotonic bicarbonate solutions are otherwise preferred; arterial pH and plasma bicarbonate should be raised a little at a time and the patient's response monitored.

Although the role of bicarbonate is accepted in the forms of metabolic acidosis mentioned, its use in the treatment of metabolic acidosis with concomitant tissue hypoxia, particularly lactic acidosis, is controversial.[1-4] The administration of bicarbonate generates carbon dioxide which, if not appropriately eliminated, due to poor tissue perfusion or impaired ventilation or both, diffuses rapidly into the cells exacerbating intracellular acidosis. In addition, in metabolic acidosis associated with organic acids such as lactic acid, there is a risk of over-alkalinisation due to the metabolism of the acid after correction of the arterial pH.

For similar reasons, the use of sodium bicarbonate in advanced cardiac life support (p.812) is no longer routine, although current guidelines permit consideration of its use to correct acidosis if the resuscitation effort is prolonged.

The role of bicarbonate in the management of diabetic ketoacidosis is also limited, although it may be appropriate in certain situations—see Diabetic Emergencies, p.328.

Because of concerns about the effects of bicarbonate, other agents have been investigated for the treatment of metabolic acidosis, including trometamol (THAM) and sodium dichloroacetate.[1-4] Alkalinising agents that have to be metabolised to bicarbonate before they have an effect, such as sodium lactate, are not generally used as many patients with acute acidosis have impaired metabolic activity, particularly of lactate.

Peritoneal dialysis, haemodialysis, or haemofiltration is required for refractory metabolic acidosis associated with acute renal failure (p.1221).


1. Swenson ER. Metabolic acidosis. *Respir Care* 2001; **46:** 342–53.
2. Levraut J, Grimaud D. Treatment of metabolic acidosis. *Curr Opin Crit Care* 2003; **9:** 260–5.
3. Arieff AI. Indications for use of bicarbonate in patients with metabolic acidosis. *Br J Anaesth* 1991; **67:** 165–77.
4. Adrogué HJ, Madias NE. Management of life-threatening acid-base disorders. *N Engl J Med* 1998; **338:** 26–34. Correction. *ibid.* 1999; **340:** 247.


**Metabolic alkalosis.** Metabolic alkalosis with an increased plasma-bicarbonate concentration and a sustained elevation in arterial pH results from excessive renal reabsorption and/or regeneration of bicarbonate. It is commonly seen with volume contraction (chloride depletion), potassium depletion, or mineralocorticoid excess, and may occur with excessive alkali intake as in the milk-alkali syndrome. If the metabolic alkalosis is severe, cardiac arrhythmias and hypoventilation may develop and there can be symptoms of concomitant hypokalaemia such as muscle weakness.

**Treatment** is generally aimed at the underlying disturbances.[1-3] Correcting volume depletion by giving a chloride salt often obviates the need for other treatment; sodium chloride is normally used. However, potassium chloride may also be required if there is potassium depletion, particularly if this is severe. Rarely, direct acidification with ammonium chloride, dilute hydrochloric acid, or acidifying salts such as lysine hydrochloride or arginine hydrochloride may be required if the alkalosis is severe.


1. Adrogué HJ, Madias NE. Management of life-threatening acid-base disorders. *N Engl J Med* 1998; **338:** 107–11.
2. Galla JH. Metabolic alkalosis. *J Am Soc Nephrol* 2000; **11:** 369–75.
3. Khanna A, Kurtzman NA. Metabolic alkalosis. *Respir Care* 2001; **46:** 354–65.


## Calcium Homoeostasis

The adult body contains about 1.2 kg of calcium, of which about 99% is incorporated into the skeleton where its primary role is structural. The remaining 1% is found in body tissues and fluids and is essential for normal nerve conduction, muscle activity, and blood coagulation.

The concentration of calcium in plasma is normally kept within a narrow range (total calcium about 2.15 to 2.60 mmol/litre) by homoeostatic mechanisms involving parathyroid hormone, calcitonin, and vitamin D. Normally about 50% of calcium in plasma is in the ionised physiologically active form (giving a usual range of about 1.1 to 1.3 mmol/litre), about 10% is complexed with anions such as phosphate or citrate, and the remainder is bound to proteins, principally albumin. If the plasma-albumin concentration is raised (as in dehydration) or reduced (as is common in malignancy) it will affect the proportion of ionised calcium. Thus, the total plasma-calcium concentration is commonly adjusted for plasma albumin.

**Hypercalcaemia.** Hypercalcaemia, an increase in plasma-calcium concentration above the normal range, is most commonly due to primary hyperparathyroidism or malignant disease.[1,2] Less common causes of hypercalcaemia include vitamin D intoxication, granulomatous diseases such as sarcoidosis, familial benign hypercalcaemia, renal failure, thyrotoxicosis, and excess calcium carbonate ingestion (milk-alkali syndrome).[1,2]

Mild asymptomatic hypercalcaemia is often associated with a plasma-concentration elevated above the normal but below 3.00 mmol/litre. Severe symptomatic hypercalcaemia is broadly correlated with a plasma-calcium concentration of more than 3.50 mmol/litre.

Symptoms of hypercalcaemia include thirst, polyuria, anorexia, constipation, muscle weakness, fatigue, and confusion. In severe cases, there may be nausea and vomiting; cardiac arrhythmias may develop but are rare. Extreme hypercalcaemia may result in coma and death. Chronic hypercalcaemia can lead to interstitial nephritis and calcium renal calculi.

Mild asymptomatic hypercalcaemia is best corrected by increasing oral fluid intake and treating any identified underlying disease. Patients with more severe hypercalcaemia, and/or significant symptoms, need prompt **treatment** to reduce plasma-calcium concentrations independent of the cause.[2,3]

The first step is rehydration with intravenous sodium chloride 0.9% to restore the intravascular volume and to promote renal excretion of calcium. Furosemide or other loop diuretics may help the latter, but only in the presence of adequate volume expansion and control of other electrolyte losses. Large doses, for example 80 to 100 mg of furosemide given intravenously every 1 to 2 hours, may be required. Thiazide diuretics should be avoided as they increase the renal tubular reabsorption of calcium. Peritoneal dialysis or haemodialysis with calcium-free dialysate should be considered in patients with renal failure for whom urinary excretion of calcium is inadequate.

In life-threatening hypercalcaemia, more specific immediate therapy is generally required in addition to saline.[2,3] Most experience has been gained in the treatment of hypercalcaemia of malignancy (see below) using drugs that inhibit bone resorption such as bisphosphonates. Calcitonins are useful as they have a rapid onset of action. However, their effect is moderate and generally short-lived, and drugs with a more sustained effect may also be required. Corticosteroids have been used to prolong the efficacy of calcitonin. Intravenous phosphates have been used to rapidly lower plasma-calcium concentrations but can cause soft tissue calcification resulting in serious adverse effects such as irreversible renal damage and hypotension, and are best avoided. Another drug that has been used for the emergency treatment of hypercalcaemia is trisodium edetate.

Choice of subsequent therapy is likely to depend on the specific cause.

1. Heath D. Hypercalcaemia. *Prescribers' J* 1999; **39:** 234–41.
2. Bushinsky DA, Monk RD. Calcium. *Lancet* 1998; **352:** 306–11.
3. Bilezikian JP. Management of acute hypercalcemia. *N Engl J Med* 1992; **326:** 1196–1203.

• HYPERCALCAEMIA OF MALIGNANCY. About 10% of patients with cancer develop hypercalcaemia of malignancy, which is typically severe and progressive.[1,2] The condition is generally thought to be due to either the production of parathyroid hormone-related protein by a tumour (humoral hypercalcaemia of malignancy) or to the release of bone-resorbing factors (osteoclast-activating factors), which include cytokines such as tumour necrosis factor, growth factors, and interleukin-1, from the site of bone metastases (local osteolytic hypercalcaemia of malignancy). Humoral hypercalcaemia is frequently associated with squamous cell carcinomas of the lung and head and neck whereas local osteolytic hypercalcaemia tends to occur with breast cancer or myeloma.[3]

Bisphosphonates are the preferred drugs for **treating** hypercalcaemia once the patient has been adequately rehydrated (see Hypercalcaemia, above). Pamidronate has been widely used and is considered by many to be the drug of choice.[1-4] However, zoledronic acid has now been shown to have a faster onset, higher response rate, and longer duration of action than pamidronate.[5] It also has a shorter infusion time than pamidronate.[6] Clodronate has also been given, first by intravenous infusion and then orally. Etidronate, administered by intravenous infusion on 3 successive days, has been found to reduce hypercalcaemia but has been reported to be less effective than pamidronate[4,6] and to have a shorter duration of action. Subsequent oral therapy with daily doses of etidronate can prolong the period of normocalcaemia but may cause osteomalacia. There is some evidence that the bisphosphonates may be less effective for humoral than for osteolytic hypercalcaemia.[7]

Calcitonin has a rapid onset of action, and is particularly useful in life-threatening hypercalcaemia.[1,4] This effect, however, is short-lived, and calcitonin is generally used as adjunctive therapy.

Plicamycin, a cytotoxic antibiotic with particular activity against osteoclasts, has been used to obtain a rapid (within 24 hours) and sustained reduction in plasma-calcium concentrations in severe hypercalcaemia. However, it is highly toxic and safer drugs such as the bisphosphonates and calcitonins are generally preferred. Gallium nitrate also inhibits bone resorption; initial studies in patients with hypercalcaemia associated with malignancy have indicated beneficial effects but clinical experience is limited; again, the bisphosphonates are likely to be preferred.[1,2]

Corticosteroids are useful in hypercalcaemia associated with corticosteroid-sensitive haematological malignancies such as lymphoma or myeloma.[2] In addition they may be useful to overcome renal tubular resistance to calcitonin[8] but otherwise are not usually effective.[9] There have been individual reports of beneficial results using somatostatin analogues such as octreotide for the treatment of hypercalcaemia of malignancy.

1. Chisholm MA, *et al.* Acute management of cancer-related hypercalcemia. *Ann Pharmacother* 1996; **30:** 507–13.
2. Watters J, *et al.* The management of malignant hypercalcaemia. *Drugs* 1996; **52:** 837–48.
3. Mundy GR, Guise TA. Hypercalcemia of malignancy. *Am J Med* 1997; **103:** 134–45.
4. Davidson TG. Conventional treatment of hypercalcemia of malignancy. *Am J Health-Syst Pharm* 2001; **58** (suppl 3): S8–S15.
5. Major P, *et al.* Zoledronic acid is superior to pamidronate in the treatment of hypercalcemia of malignancy: a pooled analysis of two randomized, controlled clinical trials. *J Clin Oncol* 2001; **19:** 558–67.
6. Berenson JR. Treatment of hypercalcemia of malignancy with bisphosphonates. *Semin Oncol* 2002; **29** (suppl 21): 12–18.
7. Gurney H, *et al.* Parathyroid hormone-related protein and response to pamidronate in tumour-induced hypercalcaemia. *Lancet* 1993; **341:** 1611–13.
8. Hosking DJ, *et al.* Potentiation of calcitonin by corticosteroids during the treatment of the hypercalcaemia of malignancy. *Eur J Clin Pharmacol* 1990; **38:** 37–41.
9. Percival RC, *et al.* Role of glucocorticoids in management of malignant hypercalcaemia. *BMJ* 1984; **389:** 287.

• HYPERPARATHYROIDISM. Excess secretion of parathyroid hormone in primary hyperparathyroidism is characterised by hypercalcaemia, which is most frequently asymptomatic, and by hypophosphataemia. Oral phosphates and bisphosphonates have been used to control hypercalcaemia. However, in the long term, hypercalcaemia associated with primary hyperparathyroidism appears to be best managed by parathyroidectomy (p.765). Symptomatic hypocalcaemia may occur after surgery, requiring short-term treatment with calcium supplements and vitamin D.

• VITAMIN D-MEDIATED HYPERCALCAEMIA. Hypercalcaemia can occur because of increased gastrointestinal absorption of calcium mediated by the active metabolite of vitamin D, 1,25-dihydroxycholecalciferol (calcitriol). This may be a feature of diseases associated with increased vitamin D sensitivity or increased vitamin D production, or may occur due to overdose of vitamin D. For example, granulomatous diseases such as sarcoidosis (p.1087) are associated with unregulated production of 1,25-dihydroxycholecalciferol. Hypercalcaemia due to vitamin D is most commonly seen in patients with renal failure receiving vitamin D analogues such as ergocalciferol.

**Treatment** of severe hypercalcaemia requires prompt rehydration regardless of the cause (see Hypercalcaemia, above). Where hypercalcaemia is due to excessive doses of a vitamin D analogue, it should be discontinued until normocalcaemia is achieved. Corticosteroids effectively reduce gastrointestinal absorption of calcium, and these may be used intravenously as adjuncts to rehydration in severe hypercalcaemia, and orally for milder hypercalcaemia or longer term therapy. Oral sodium cellulose phosphate, which binds calcium in the gastrointestinal tract, and a low-calcium diet may also be considered. Oral chloroquine or hydroxychloroquine have been used in hypercalcaemia associated with sarcoidosis. Ketoconazole may be useful as an alternative to corticosteroids.

References.

1. Adams JS. Vitamin D metabolite-mediated hypercalcemia. *Endocrinol Metab Clin North Am* 1989; **18:** 765–78.
2. Sharma OP. Vitamin D, calcium, and sarcoidosis. *Chest* 1996; **109:** 535–9.

**Hypocalcaemia.** Hypocalcaemia, a decrease in plasma-calcium concentration below the normal range, may be due to impaired or reduced absorption of calcium from the gastrointestinal tract, as with vitamin D deficiency disorders (see Osteomalacia, p.762) and chronic renal failure (see Renal Osteodystrophy, p.764). Alternatively, it may be due to deficient parathyroid hormone secretion and/or action as in hypoparathyroidism (p.765) and hypomagnesaemia (see below). Excessive phosphate administration is also a cause of hypocalcaemia (see Hyperphosphataemia, below). Rarely, hypocalcaemia may follow repeated infusions of citrate ions, for example, during transfusions utilising citrated blood, as the citrate complexes with the calcium ion. Respiratory alkalosis due to hyperventilation can also lead to depression of ionised plasma-calcium concentrations.

Where symptoms of hypocalcaemia occur, they are typically associated with increased neuromuscular excitability; paraesthesias can occur and in more severe cases, carpopedal spasm, muscle cramps, tetany, and convulsions may develop.[1-3] Other symptoms include ECG changes and mental disturbances such as irritability and depression. Prolonged hypocalcaemia can lead to dental defects, cataract formation, and in children can result in mental retardation.

In patients with hypocalcaemia due to an underlying disease, long-term management should be aimed at **treating** this disease. Vitamin D supplements are widely used to enhance calcium absorption and correct vitamin D deficiency disorders and hypoparathyroidism. Oral supplements of calcium salts are often also given. Acute hypocalcaemia or hypocalcaemic tetany require emergency treatment with intravenous calcium salts.

1. Lebowitz MR, Moses AM. Hypocalcemia. *Semin Nephrol* 1992; **12:** 146–58.
2. Reber PM, Heath H. Hypocalcemic emergencies. *Med Clin North Am* 1995; **79:** 93–106.
3. Bushinsky DA, Monk RD. Calcium. *Lancet* 1998; **352:** 306–11.

## Magnesium Homoeostasis

Magnesium is an essential body cation that is involved in numerous enzymatic reactions and physiological processes including energy transfer and storage, skeletal development, nerve conduction, and muscle contraction. Over half of the magnesium in the body is found in bone, about 40% is present in muscle and soft tissue, and only about 1% is present in the extracellular fluid. A normal concentration for magnesium in plasma is from about 0.7 to 1.0 mmol/litre.

Magnesium homoeostasis appears to be primarily regulated by the kidney where magnesium is extensively reabsorbed. Bone may act as a magnesium reservoir to reduce plasma-magnesium fluctuations. Magnesium is actively absorbed from the gastrointestinal tract and this is enhanced to some extent by 1,25-dihydroxycholecalciferol (calcitriol).

**Hypermagnesaemia.** Hypermagnesaemia is an increase in the plasma concentration of magnesium above the normal range, as may follow excessive parenteral doses of salts such as magnesium sulfate. Hypermagnesaemia due to oral intake is uncommon as the kidneys are able to excrete a relatively large magnesium load. However, it may occur in patients with impaired renal function taking large amounts of magnesium, for example, in antacids or laxatives.

Symptoms of hypermagnesaemia include nausea, vomiting, CNS and respiratory depression, hyporeflexia, muscle weakness, and cardiovascular effects including peripheral vasodilatation, hypotension, bradycardia, and cardiac arrest.

**Treatment** of mild hypermagnesaemia is usually limited to restricting magnesium intake. In severe hypermagnesaemia, ventilatory and circulatory support may be required. Slow intravenous administration of 10 to 20 mL of calcium gluconate 10% is recommended to reverse the effects on cardiovascular and respiratory systems. If renal function is normal, adequate fluids should be given to promote renal magnesium clearance. This may be increased by the use of furosemide. Haemodialysis using a magnesium-free dialysis solution effectively removes magnesium, and this may be necessary in patients with renal impairment, or for whom other methods prove ineffective.

**Hypomagnesaemia.** Hypomagnesaemia, a plasma-magnesium concentration below the normal range, may result from a reduced magnesium intake as in dietary deficiency or malabsorption syndromes. Alternatively, it may be due to excessive magnesium loss either via the kidney because of inadequate reabsorption or more often from the gut, for example, during chronic diarrhoea. Drugs that may cause renal magnesium wasting include aminoglycosides, cisplatin (see Effects on Electrolytes, p.538), and diuretics.

Hypomagnesaemia is closely associated with other electrolyte disturbances, especially hypocalcaemia (see above) and hypokalaemia (see below), and rarely occurs alone. Specific symptoms are therefore difficult to determine but may include anorexia, nausea, weakness, neuromuscular dysfunction such as tetany, tremor, and muscle fasciculations, and rarely seizures. Cardiac arrhythmias may occur, but the relative contribution of hypomagnesaemia and hypokalaemia to these is uncertain.

Magnesium salts can be given by mouth for the **treatment** of chronic or asymptomatic magnesium deficiency.[1,2] Parenteral therapy may be preferred in patients with poor gastrointestinal absorption of magnesium or who are unable to tolerate oral supplements (usually because they cause diarrhoea); magnesium sulfate can be given by intravenous or intramuscular injection. In acute symptomatic hypomagnesaemia, rapid replacement therapy with intravenous magnesium salts may be necessary. Renal function and plasma-magnesium concentrations should be monitored.

1. Whang R, *et al.* Magnesium homeostasis and clinical disorders of magnesium deficiency. *Ann Pharmacother* 1994; **28:** 220–6.
2. Weisinger JR, Bellorín-Font E. Magnesium and phosphorus. *Lancet* 1998; **352:** 391–6.

## Phosphate Homoeostasis

Phosphate is an essential bone mineral; about 80% of phosphorus in an adult body is incorporated into the skeleton as a calcium salt where it is required to give rigidity. The remainder is present in the soft tissues and is involved in several metabolic and enzymatic reactions including energy storage and transfer.

Phosphate exists in body fluids mainly as the divalent $HPO_4^{2-}$ ion (about 80%) or monovalent $H_2PO_4^-$ ion (about 20%). Phosphate measurements are usually expressed as inorganic phosphorus to avoid confusion with the anion content. A normal range for phosphorus in plasma in adults is about 0.85 to 1.45 mmol/litre, but as only a small proportion of body phosphate is found in the extracellular fluid, plasma-phosphorus levels may not always reflect total body stores or predict replacement needs.

Phosphate concentrations in plasma are primarily regulated by renal excretion; parathyroid hormone reduces the renal tubular reabsorption of phosphate. Intestinal absorption of phosphate is enhanced by the vitamin D metabolite, 1,25-dihydroxycholecalciferol.

**Hyperphosphataemia.** Hyperphosphataemia, an abnormally raised plasma-phosphorus concentration, is usually associated with renal failure and may lead to renal osteodystrophy (p.764). Hyperphosphataemia may also be a consequence of release of phosphate from cells; this can occur in conditions of cell breakdown such as haemolysis or rhabdomyolysis, during chemotherapy (when it may be part of the tumour lysis syndrome), or as a result of acidoses. Hypoparathyroidism may also lead to hyperphosphataemia due to decreased levels of parathyroid hormone (see Hypoparathyroidism, p.765). Other causes include excessive phosphate doses during treatment of hypophosphataemia, overuse of phosphate enemas or oral phosphate bowel preparations, and excessive vitamin D intake.

Hyperphosphataemic symptoms include those of associated hypocalcaemia (see above). Complexation with calcium may lead to metastatic calcification.

The **treatment** of hyperphosphataemia[1] usually involves control of the relevant underlying condition, and the use of low-phosphate diets, and if necessary oral phosphate-binding agents, such as calcium acetate or carbonate or aluminium hydroxide. Sevelamer, a polymer capable of binding phosphate, may also be given.[2] Lanthanum carbonate is under investigation.[2,3] Haemodialysis has been used to correct hyperphosphataemia in renal failure.[3]

1. Weisinger JR, Bellorín-Font E. Magnesium and phosphorus. *Lancet* 1998; **352:** 391–6.
2. Bleyer AJ. Phosphate binder usage in kidney failure patients. *Expert Opin Pharmacother* 2003; **4:** 941–7.
3. Albaaj F, Hutchison AJ. Hyperphosphataemia in renal failure: causes, consequences and current management. *Drugs* 2003; **63:** 577–96.

**Hypophosphataemia.** Hypophosphataemia, a reduction in plasma-phosphorus concentrations below the normal range, may be due to insufficient absorption of phosphate or increased renal clearance as in primary hyperparathyroidism, vitamin D deficiency, or X-linked familial hypophosphataemia. An increased cell uptake of phosphate can also result in hypophosphataemia, as for example, in chronic respiratory alkalosis and related disorders including alcoholism, hepatic failure, and septicaemia. As phosphate is widely available in most foods, dietary deficiency is rare though it may occur in infants of low birth-weight fed exclusively on human breast milk (see Rickets of Prematurity, p.1232). The absorption of phosphate from the gastrointestinal tract can be reduced if phosphate-binding antacids are taken in large amounts.

Hypophosphataemia is usually asymptomatic but clinical symptoms become apparent when plasma-phosphorus concentrations fall below 0.3 mmol/litre.[1-3] Symptoms include neuromuscular dysfunction such as muscle weakness and paraesthesias, convulsions, cardiomyopathy, respiratory failure, and haematological abnormalities. Prolonged hypophosphataemia can result in rickets or osteomalacia (p.762).

**Treatment** of hypophosphataemia primarily involves correction of any underlying disease. Milk or oral phosphate supplements may be appropriate if a phosphate deficiency is identified or in certain disorders such as X-linked hypophosphataemic rickets. Intravenous phosphate may be required for severe hypophosphataemia (see p.1231), but this should be used cautiously to avoid hypocalcaemia and metastatic calcification.[2,3] Consideration should be given to correcting concomitant electrolyte disturbances such as hypomagnesaemia.

1. Larner AJ. Clinical applicability of inorganic phosphate measurements. *Br J Hosp Med* 1992; **48:** 748–53.
2. Lloyd CW, Johnson CE. Management of hypophosphatemia. *Clin Pharm* 1988; **7:** 123–8.
3. Weisinger JR, Bellorín-Font E. Magnesium and phosphorus. *Lancet* 1998; **352:** 391–6.

## Potassium Homoeostasis

Potassium is mainly an intracellular cation, primarily found in muscle; only about 2% is present in the extracellular fluid. It is essential for numerous metabolic and physiological processes including nerve conduction, muscle contraction, and acid-base regulation. A normal concentration of potassium in plasma is about 3.5 to 5.0 mmol/litre, but factors influencing transfer between intracellular and extracellular fluids such as acid-base disturbances can distort the relationship between plasma concentrations and total body stores. The body content of potassium is primarily regulated by renal glomerular filtration and tubular secretion. Aldosterone enhances the renal secretion of potassium and several other factors such as sodium excretion, dietary potassium intake, and plasma pH can modulate the excretion of potassium by the kidney. Insulin, $beta_2$ agonists, and aldosterone, and increases in plasma pH, can promote the cellular uptake of potassium. The passage of potassium into the cells and retention against the concentration gradient requires active transport via the $Na^+/K^+$ ATPase enzyme.

**Hyperkalaemia.** Hyperkalaemia, an abnormally raised plasma-potassium concentration, can occur if the potassium intake is increased, if the renal excretion decreases (as in renal failure or adrenocortical insufficiency), or if there is a sudden efflux of potassium from intracellular stores, (as in acidosis, or cell destruction due to tissue trauma, burns, haemolysis, or rhabdomyolysis). Renal failure is the commonest cause of severe hyperkalaemia.[1] Hyperkalaemia may also be induced by drugs such as the potassium-sparing diuretics, ciclosporin, tacrolimus, NSAIDs, or ACE inhibitors.[2,3] Usually the renal mechanisms for potassium excretion adapt readily to an increased potassium load, and hyperkalaemia due to increased dietary intake is rare unless renal function is also impaired.

Hyperkalaemia mainly affects the heart, but skeletal muscle function may also be affected. Symptoms include ECG abnormalities, ventricular arrhythmias, cardiac arrest, and also neuromuscular dysfunction such as muscle weakness and paralysis.[3,4]

**Treatment** involves giving calcium to counteract the negative effects of hyperkalaemia on cardiac excitability, drugs such as insulin or sodium bicarbonate to promote the transfer of potassium from the extracellular to the intracellar fluid compartment, and enhancing potassium excretion with exchange resins or dialysis.[3,4] The methods used depend largely on the severity of the hyperkalaemia and critically, any associated ECG changes. Hyperkalaemia associated with a plasma concentration of potassium above 6.0 to 7.0 mmol/litre or with ECG changes is usually considered a medical emergency.

If effects on the heart are present, then first-line therapy should be with a calcium salt given intravenously; typically 10 to 20 mL of calcium gluconate 10% is given by slow intravenous injection, the dosage being titrated and adjusted based on ECG improvement.

Calcium will not, however, reduce the plasma-potassium concentration. In moderate to severe hyperkalaemia, insulin, together with glucose to prevent hypoglycaemia, is given intravenously in order to reduce the potassium concentration by stimulating the uptake of potassium by cells.[1] Insulin is given as a rapid-acting soluble insulin and typical doses are 5 to 10 units with 50 mL of glucose 50% given slowly over 5 to 15 minutes. Doses may need to be repeated as necessary. Alternatively or additionally, intravenous sodium bicarbonate may be used to correct acidosis and promote cellular uptake of potassium (but see Metabolic Acidosis above). Opinions vary on its value and on the appropriate dose and concentration, but it may be indicated where there is severe associated acidosis (pH less than 7.2).[1]

The $beta_2$ agonist, salbutamol, given intravenously or by a nebuliser, has also been found to enhance the cellular uptake of potassium and reduce plasma-potassium concentrations.[3-5] However, its effect may be inconsistent,[5] and some clinicians prefer to avoid $beta_2$ agonists because of fears that large doses may induce cardiac arrhythmias.[6] Some consider that it should only ever be used in conjunction with insulin, as up to 40% of patients may not respond.[1]

After the plasma-potassium concentration has been reduced in the immediate term by enhancing cellular potassium uptake, treatments are often required that will remove excess potassium from the body over the longer term. Cation exchange resins such as calcium or sodium polystyrene sulfonate can be given orally or rectally and, after about 1 to 2 hours, will begin to remove potassium from the body. Haemodialysis removes potassium from the body very effectively and is particularly useful in patients with acute renal failure, hypervolaemia, hypernatraemia, or severe hyperkalaemia. Peritoneal dialysis is effective in some patients.

1. Ahee P, Crowe AV. The management of hyperkalaemia in the emergency department. *J Accid Emerg Med* 2000; **17:** 188–91.
2. Perazella MA. Drug-induced hyperkalemia: old culprits and new offenders. *Am J Med* 2000; **109:** 307–14.
3. Gennari FJ. Disorders of potassium homeostasis: hypokalemia and hyperkalemia. *Crit Care Clin* 2002; **18:** 273–88.
4. Rastergar A, Soleimani M. Hypokalaemia and hyperkalaemia. *Postgrad Med J* 2001; **77:** 759–64. Correction. *ibid.* 2002; **78:** 126.
5. Wong S-L, Maltz HC. Albuterol for the treatment of hyperkalemia. *Ann Pharmacother* 1999; **33:** 103–6.
6. Halperin ML, Kamel KS. Potassium. *Lancet* 1998; **352:** 135–40.

• HYPERKALAEMIC PERIODIC PARALYSIS. Hyperkalaemic periodic paralysis is an inherited disorder in which sudden increases in plasma-potassium concentrations cause muscle paralysis, sometimes followed by myotonia. An acute attack may require intravenous calcium gluconate and insulin with glucose (see above). Inhalation of a $beta_2$ agonist such as salbutamol has been used to treat or abort attacks.[1,2] Diuretics such as acetazolamide or the thiazides are used prophylactically to reduce the frequency of attacks.[2,3]

1. Hanna MG, *et al.* Salbutamol treatment in a patient with hyperkalaemic periodic paralysis due to a mutation in the skeletal muscle sodium channel gene (SCN4A). *J Neurol Neurosurg Psychiatry* 1998; **65:** 248–50.
2. Bond EF. Channelopathies: potassium-related periodic paralyses and similar disorders. *AACN Clin Issues* 2000; **11:** 261–70.
3. Meola G, Sansone V. Therapy in myotonic disorders and in muscle channelopathies. *Neurol Sci* 2000; **21** (suppl): S953–61.

**Hypokalaemia.** Chronic hypokalaemia, a prolonged reduction of the plasma concentration of potassium, usually indicates a reduction in total body potassium. It may result from an inadequate intake, or gastrointestinal losses, for example in patients with secretory diarrhoeas, or from excessive renal losses as in hyperaldosteronism, Cushing's syndrome, or chronic metabolic alkalosis. Thiazides or loop diuretics increase urinary-potassium losses. Other drugs, notably corticosteroids and some antibacterials such as gentamicin, also have this effect. Hypokalaemia can also be caused by an increased cellular uptake of potassium rather than excess body losses. This may occur with drugs such as beta$_2$ agonists or xanthines, during insulin therapy, acute alkalosis, or possibly be induced by catecholamines after myocardial infarction. Hypokalaemia secondary to hypomagnesaemia (see above) can occur.

Hypokalaemia results in neuromuscular disturbances ranging from muscle weakness to paralysis and respiratory insufficiency and can also cause rhabdomyolysis, ECG abnormalities, and ileus. Chronic hypokalaemia may lead to renal tubular damage (hypokalaemic nephropathy). Hypokalaemia increases the risk of digoxin toxicity.

**Treatment** involves correcting any underlying disorder and replacement therapy with potassium salts. Oral potassium supplements are generally preferred but in severe hypokalaemia associated with cardiac arrhythmias, paralysis or diabetic ketoacidosis, parenteral therapy may be necessary. Potassium salts, usually potassium chloride, may be given by intravenous infusion but must be administered slowly to avoid causing hyperkalaemia and associated cardiac toxicity; plasma-potassium concentrations should be closely monitored and ECG monitoring may be required. The choice of salt for oral potassium replacement depends on co-existing acid-base and electrolyte disturbances. Potassium chloride is generally the drug of choice for the treatment of hypokalaemia in patients with metabolic alkalosis with hypochloraemia, whereas a salt such as the bicarbonate may be preferred in patients with hyperchloraemic acidosis as in some renal tubular acidoses. Hypokalaemia secondary to hypomagnesaemia requires magnesium replacement therapy.

References.


1. Halperin ML, Kamel KS. Potassium. *Lancet* 1998; **352:** 135–40.
2. Gennari FJ. Hypokalemia. *N Engl J Med* 1998; **339:** 451–8.
3. Cohn JN, *et al.* New guidelines for potassium replacement in clinical practice: a contemporary review by the National Council on Potassium in Clinical Practice. *Arch Intern Med* 2000; **160:** 2429–36.


• BARTTER'S SYNDROME. Bartter's syndrome is a set of closely related disorders thought to result from inherited defects in ion transport in various sections of the renal tubule.[1,2] Patients exhibit hyperplasia of the juxtaglomerular cells, hypokalaemia and metabolic alkalosis, and excess aldosterone, prostaglandin, and renin production. Symptoms are primarily those of the hypokalaemia, including muscle weakness; polyuria and enuresis, and growth retardation in children, can occur. In contrast to other hyperreninaemic states, patients do not have hypertension or oedema.

**Treatment** rarely completely corrects hypokalaemia. Potassium supplementation may be given, while a cyclo-oxygenase inhibitor such as indometacin, or an ACE inhibitor such as captopril, can produce benefit.[2] There are reports[3,4] of benefit with rofecoxib. Spironolactone and propranolol have also been tried and magnesium salts may be given if there is hypomagnesaemia.[2]


1. Guay-Woodford LM. Bartter syndrome: unraveling the pathophysiologic enigma. *Am J Med* 1998; **105:** 151–61.
2. Amirlak I, Dawson KP. Bartter syndrome: an overview. *Q J Med* 2000; **93:** 207–15.
3. Kleta R, *et al.* New treatment options for Bartter's syndrome. *N Engl J Med* 2000; **343:** 661–2.
4. Haas NA, *et al.* Successful management of an extreme example of neonatal hyperprostaglandin-E syndrome (Bartter's syndrome) with the new cyclooxygenase-2 inhibitor rofecoxib. *Pediatr Crit Care Med* 2003; **4:** 249–51.


• DIURETIC-INDUCED HYPOKALAEMIA. Reduced potassium concentrations may result from the use of potassium-losing diuretics, particularly thiazides and loop diuretics. Clinically significant hypokalaemia is unlikely at the doses used in hypertension and the routine use of potassium supplements is no longer recommended. However, the concomitant use of a potassium-sparing diuretic such as amiloride or, less usually, a potassium supplement, may be necessary in patients at risk of hypokalaemia (see also Hydrochlorothiazide, Effects on Electrolyte Balance, p.933).

• HYPOKALAEMIC PERIODIC PARALYSIS. Hypokalaemic periodic paralysis is an inherited disorder in which episodes of hypokalaemia with muscle weakness or paralysis appear to be associated with a shift in potassium from the extracellular to the intracellular fluid. Acute attacks are treated with potassium, given orally or intravenously. Prophylaxis with acetazolamide has been found to reduce the frequency and severity of attacks.[1,2]


1. Ahlawat SK, Sachdev A. Hypokalaemic paralysis. *Postgrad Med J* 1999; **75:** 193–7.
2. Bond EF. Channelopathies: potassium-related periodic paralyses and similar disorders. *AACN Clin Issues* 2000; **11:** 261–70.


## Sodium Homoeostasis

Sodium is the principal cation in the extracellular fluid and is responsible for the maintenance of the extracellular fluid volume and osmolality. In addition, sodium is also involved in nerve conduction, muscle contraction, acid-base balance, and cell nutrient uptake. A usual plasma concentration of sodium would be expected to be within 135 to 145 mmol/litre.

Sodium homoeostasis is complex and closely associated with fluid balance. The osmolality and volume of the extracellular fluid are tightly regulated. Small changes in osmolality (plasma-sodium concentrations) are corrected by alteration of extracellular volume. This balance of plasma osmolality is achieved by the secretion or suppression of antidiuretic hormone (ADH; vasopressin), which primarily controls water excretion by the kidney. A tendency towards hyponatraemia suppresses ADH secretion and promotes renal loss of water; an increase in ADH secretion increases water reabsorption by the renal distal tubules. Changes in extracellular volume will also affect ADH release independently of osmolality. In addition, changes in extracellular volume result in modulation of the renal excretion of sodium.

Total body sodium content is regulated by renal sodium excretion, which can vary widely depending on dietary intake. Various mechanisms are involved in controlling renal sodium excretion including the renin-angiotensin system, glomerular filtration rate, and natriuretic factors. A reduction in extracellular fluid volume leads to the production of angiotensin II which stimulates the secretion of aldosterone. Aldosterone promotes the reabsorption of sodium ions by the distal tubules. There may be significant effects on sodium homoeostasis if adrenal insufficiency or mineralocorticoid excess disturb this mechanism.

**Hypernatraemia.** Hypernatraemia is an abnormal rise in the plasma-sodium concentration with a simultaneous rise in plasma osmolality. It is generally associated with volume depletion when water intake is less than water losses through renal or extrarenal routes. The causes include impaired thirst, as in coma or essential hypernatraemia, osmotic diuresis (solute diuresis), as in diabetic ketoacidosis (see Diabetic Emergencies, p.328) or after mannitol administration, and excessive water losses, either from the kidney, as in diabetes insipidus (p.1314), or extrarenally, for example, because of excessive sweating or diarrhoea.

Hypernatraemia can also occur following excessive oral sodium intake (but this is uncommon) and after inappropriate use of intravenous sodium chloride.

The clinical manifestations of hypernatraemia are caused by the effect of increased plasma osmolality on the brain and include somnolence, confusion, respiratory paralysis, and coma. CNS symptoms are more severe when hypernatraemia develops rapidly. In the presence of volume depletion, other symptoms such as hypotension, tachycardia, and various symptoms of circulatory insufficiency may occur concomitantly. A high volume of dilute urine is seen in patients with abnormal renal water conservation, whereas a low volume of concentrated urine is expected in patients with impaired thirst or excessive extrarenal water loss.

**Treatment** of hypernatraemia usually requires water replacement, and drinking water may be sufficient for some patients. In more severe conditions, glucose 5% may be given by slow intravenous infusion. Alternatively, some recommend the use of sodium chloride 0.9% if volume depletion is severe. Care is required as too rapid correction can induce cerebral oedema, particularly in chronic conditions.

If the total body sodium is too high, loop diuretics may be used to increase sodium excretion with fluid losses being replaced by an infusion of glucose 5% and potassium chloride. It has also been suggested that dialysis may be necessary if there is significant renal impairment, if the patient is moribund, or if the serum-sodium concentration is greater than 200 mmol/litre.

References.


1. Adrogué HJ, Madias NE. Hypernatremia. *N Engl J Med* 2000; **342:** 1493–9.
2. Kang SK, *et al.* Pathogenesis and treatment of hypernatremia. *Nephron* 2002; **92** (suppl): 14–17.


**Hyponatraemia.** Hyponatraemia, an abnormal fall in the plasma-sodium concentration, usually with a simultaneous fall in the plasma osmolality, is not uncommon, and may occur in diseases as diverse as heart failure, cirrhosis, adrenocortical insufficiency, hyperglycaemia, and AIDS.

The kidney is able to conserve sodium and sodium depletion due to low salt intake is rare. Sodium depletion may occur if there are abnormal losses, either from the gut as a consequence of repeated diarrhoea and/or vomiting or from the kidney, for example, due to various renal disorders or the overuse of diuretics (see under Hydrochlorothiazide, Effects on Electrolyte Balance, p.934).

The most common cause of hyponatraemia is dilution. This may result from excessive fluid intake, for example the ingestion of large volumes of water in patients with primary polydipsia (psychogenic polydipsia). More often, however, it is a result of reduced water excretion, as in renal impairment or the syndrome of inappropriate secretion of antidiuretic hormone (SIADH—p.1318). Postoperative hyponatraemia is a frequent complication which can be exacerbated by the inappropriate intravenous administration of hypotonic,[1] or even isotonic,[2] fluids.

Hyponatraemia due to sodium depletion in the presence of volume contraction may cause orthostatic hypotension and circulatory insufficiency. Dilutional hyponatraemia may be asymptomatic but headache, confusion, nausea, vomiting, somnolence, and weakness can occur. If severe, cerebral oedema is present, and respiratory arrest, convulsions, and coma may ensue. CNS symptoms are more common when the condition is acute.

**Therapy** is guided by the rate of development and degree of hyponatraemia, accompanying symptoms, and the state of water balance, and should also take into account the underlying cause. Mild asymptomatic hyponatraemia does not usually require specific therapy. Chronic mild to moderate sodium depletion, such as occurs in salt-losing bowel or renal disease, may be treated with oral sodium chloride supplements while ensuring adequate fluid intake.

When there is substantial volume depletion, volume replacement is necessary and intravenous sodium chloride 0.9% is often used.

Chronic dilutional hyponatraemia, which is often asymptomatic, can generally be managed by correcting the underlying disease; water restriction may also be necessary and drugs that interfere with the action of ADH such as demeclocycline or lithium carbonate may be useful in SIADH.[3,4] Furosemide plus oral sodium chloride supplements have also been used.

Acute symptomatic hyponatraemia (water intoxication) is generally associated with plasma-sodium concentrations below 120 mmol/litre and requires more aggressive therapy. This involves giving hypertonic or isotonic sodium chloride intravenously, often with a loop diuretic such as furosemide, especially if fluid overload is likely to be a problem.[3,4] The aim is to render the patient asymptomatic, with a plasma-sodium concentration of 120 to 130 mmol/litre; the plasma-sodium concentration should not be corrected to normal values nor should hypernatraemia be allowed to develop.[3,4] Plasma-sodium concentrations and the total body-water volume should be monitored throughout.

A rare neurological syndrome known as central pontine myelinolysis (osmotic demyelination) has been associated with the over-rapid correction of symptomatic hyponatraemia, particularly if the condition is well established, and it has been recommended that the plasma-sodium concentration should be increased at a rate not exceeding 0.5 mmol/litre per hour,[5,6] though the best correction rate is debatable.[4,7] Some have suggested an initial prompt increase in plasma sodium of about 10% or 10 mmol/litre, followed by correction at a rate not exceeding 1.0 to 1.5 mmol/litre per hour or 15 mmol/litre per 24 hours,[8] while others recommend an initial rate of correction of 1 to 2 mmol/litre per hour for several hours, to a maximum of 8 mmol/litre per 24 hours.[9] However, the association of hyponatraemia with central pontine myelinolysis is controversial and some authorities do not consider the rate of correction to be a factor in hyponatraemic brain injury.[4]


1. Moritz ML, Ayus JC. Prevention of hospital-acquired hyponatremia: a case for using isotonic saline. *Pediatrics* 2003; **111:** 227–30.
2. Steele A, *et al.* Postoperative hyponatremia despite near-isotonic saline infusion: a phenomenon of desalination. *Ann Intern Med* 1997; **126:** 20–5.
3. Swales JD. Management of hyponatraemia. *Br J Anaesth* 1991; **67:** 146–53.
4. Arieff AI. Management of hyponatraemia. *BMJ* 1993; **307:** 305–8.
5. Cluitmans FHM, Meinders AE. Management of severe hyponatremia: rapid or slow correction? *Am J Med* 1990; **88:** 161–6.

6. Laureno R, Karp BI. Myelinolysis after correction of hyponatremia. *Ann Intern Med* 1997; **126:** 57–62.
7. Sterns RH. The treatment of hyponatremia: first, do no harm. *Am J Med* 1990; **88:** 557–60.
8. Kumar S, Berl T. Sodium. *Lancet* 1998; **352:** 220–8.
9. Adrogué HJ, Madias NE. Hyponatremia. *N Engl J Med* 2000; **342:** 1581–9.

# Dialysis Solutions

Soluciones para diálisis.

**Pharmacopoeias.** In *Eur.* (see p.vi), which includes separate monographs for solutions for haemodialysis, haemofiltration and haemodiafiltration, and peritoneal dialysis.

## Dialysis and Haemofiltration

Dialysis and filtration solutions are solutions of electrolytes formulated in concentrations similar to those of extracellular fluid or plasma. They always contain sodium and chloride and bicarbonate or a bicarbonate precursor. In addition, they often contain calcium and magnesium, and rarely potassium. Glucose may be added as an osmotic agent. These solutions allow the removal of water and metabolites and the replacement of electrolytes.

In *haemodialysis*, the exchange of ions between the solution and the patient's blood is made across a semipermeable membrane, primarily by diffusion. Excess fluid is removed by ultrafiltration achieved by a pressure gradient. Membranes are either derived from cellulose (e.g. cuprophane) or are synthetic. Bicarbonate rather than a bicarbonate precursor is increasingly preferred as the bicarbonate source in haemodialysis since the problems of precipitation of calcium and magnesium have been overcome by changes in dialysis technique. Acetate is still used in some dialysers, but is thought to have vasodilator and cardiodepressant actions, and may not be converted to bicarbonate fast enough for high-flux haemodialysis or in patients with liver disease. Haemodialysis solutions are provided in a sterile concentrated form for dilution with water before use; this water need not be sterile.

In *peritoneal dialysis*, the exchange is made across the membranes of the peritoneal cavity primarily by diffusion. Excess fluid is removed by ultrafiltration achieved by the use of osmotic agents such as glucose. The problems of calcium bicarbonate precipitation have not yet been overcome, and lactate is generally used as the bicarbonate precursor. Peritoneal dialysis solutions must be sterile and apyrogenic.

In *haemofiltration*, blood is filtered rather than dialysed. Metabolites are removed by convective transport, and excess water by hydrostatic ultrafiltration. Fluid and electrolytes are replaced by direct intravenous infusion. Most haemofiltration solutions use acetate or lactate as the bicarbonate source. Haemofiltration solutions must be sterile and apyrogenic.

## Adverse Effects

Adverse effects occurring during *haemodialysis* include nausea, vomiting, hypotension, muscle cramps, and air embolus. Effects related to vascular access include infection, thrombosis, and haemorrhage. Adverse effects occurring during *haemofiltration* are similar to those for haemodialysis.

The most common adverse effects associated with *peritoneal dialysis* include peritonitis, hernias, hyperglycaemia, protein malnutrition, and catheter complications.

Long-term complications in dialysed patients, some of which may relate to renal failure itself, include haemodialysis-related amyloidosis, acquired cystic kidney disease, and accelerated atherosclerosis. Dialysis dementia is a special hazard of aluminium overload. Long-term peritoneal dialysis results in progressive structural changes to the peritoneal membrane ultimately resulting in dialysis failure.

**Aluminium overload.** Accumulation of aluminium in patients on dialysis may result in dialysis dementia, anaemia, and aluminium-related bone disease (see also p.1652). Sources of aluminium include the water used for preparation of dialysis fluids and aluminium-containing phosphate binders used in treating renal osteodystrophy (p.764). It is therefore important that water used for the preparation of dialysis fluids has a low aluminium concentration; Ph. Eur. 5.0 specifies a limit for aluminium of 10 micrograms/litre. Non-aluminium-containing phosphate binders such as calcium acetate or calcium carbonate may be preferred for long-term therapy. Aluminium overload in patients on dialysis has been treated with desferrioxamine (p.1035).

**Copper toxicity.** Liver and haematological toxicity has occurred as a result of absorption of copper from dialysis fluids (p.1426).

**Haemodialysis-induced cramp.** Muscle cramps commonly occur during haemodialysis procedures, and are often associated with hypotension as a result of inappropriate volume removal. In addition, they may be exacerbated by cellulose-derived membranes or the use of acetate as a bicarbonate precursor. Sodium chloride tablets (p.1234), intravenous sodium chloride 0.9%, intravenous hypertonic glucose (p.1433), and quinine (p.463) have been used in the prevention or treatment of haemodialysis-induced cramp.

**Hypersensitivity.** For anaphylactic reactions associated with the use of ethylene oxide for the disinfection of dialysis equipment, see p.1179.

**Infections.** Patients undergoing haemodialysis are at risk of infections from microbial contamination of dialysis fluid, and from inadequate care of vascular access sites. Maximum microbial counts and limits for endotoxins have been specified for water used in dialysis fluids. Bicarbonate-based dialysis solutions are more susceptible to microbial growth than acetate-based solutions.

Peritonitis is common in patients receiving peritoneal dialysis. The risk of infection may be minimised by using disconnect systems, good aseptic technique, and by good care of catheters. Treatment of bacterial peritonitis requires intraperitoneal administration of antibacterials, which are usually added to the dialysis fluid (see p.140).

Dialysis equipment should be regularly disinfected with agents such as formaldehyde (p.1180) or ethylene oxide (p.1179), but for mention of ethylene oxide anaphylactoid reactions, see p.1179.

**Metabolic complications.** The high concentrations of glucose in peritoneal dialysis solutions required to form an osmotic gradient can lead to weight gain, hyperglycaemia, hyperlipidaemia, and increased protein loss. Alternative osmotic agents such as icodextrin (p.1427) can be used, and amino acid-based solutions are also available.

## Precautions

Peritoneal dialysis is not appropriate for patients with abdominal sepsis, previous abdominal surgery, or severe inflammatory bowel disease.

Haemodialysis should be used with caution in patients with unstable cardiovascular disease or active bleeding. During haemodialysis and haemofiltration, heparin (see Extracorporeal Circulation, p.930) or epoprostenol (Uses, p.1517) are required to prevent clotting of the blood in the extracorporeal circuit.

Dialysis solutions should be warmed to body temperature with dry heat because wet heat carries a risk of microbial contamination.

## Interactions

The effects of dialysis and filtration procedures on drug concentrations in the body can be complex. More drug may be removed by one dialysis technique than another. In general, drugs of low molecular weight, high water solubility, low volume of distribution, low protein binding, and high renal clearance are most extensively removed by dialysis. For example, aminoglycosides are extensively removed by dialysis procedures, and extra doses may be needed to replace losses. Specific drug dosage adjustments for dialysis procedures may be used where these are known. For drugs where the effect of dialysis is unknown, it is usual to give maintenance doses after dialysis. Dialysis has been used to remove some drugs in the treatment of overdosage (see below).

Dialysis-induced changes in fluids and electrolytes have the potential to alter the effects of some drugs. For example, hypokalaemia predisposes to digoxin toxicity.

In patients undergoing peritoneal dialysis, drugs such as insulin and antibacterials may be added to the dialysis fluid. Consideration should be given to the possibility of adsorption of drugs onto the PVC bags.

◊ References.

1. Aronson JK. The principles of prescribing in renal failure. *Prescribers' J* 1992; **32:** 220–31.
2. Cotterill S. Antimicrobial prescribing in patients on haemofiltration. *J Antimicrob Chemother* 1995; **36:** 773–80.
3. Aronoff GR, *et al. Drug prescribing in renal failure: dosing guidelines for adults.* 4th ed. Philadelphia: American College of Physicians, 1999.

## Uses and Administration

Dialysis and filtration procedures are used in renal failure to correct electrolyte imbalance, correct fluid overload, and remove metabolites. They also have a limited role in the treatment of overdosage and poisoning. The two main techniques are haemodialysis and peritoneal dialysis; haemofiltration is used less frequently. The choice of technique will depend on the condition to be treated, the clinical state of the patient, patient preference, and availability.

Haemodialysis is more efficient than peritoneal dialysis at clearing small molecules such as urea, whereas peritoneal dialysis may be better at clearing larger molecules. Haemodialysis is considered to be less physiological as it alternates periods of high clearance with periods of no clearance.

**Haemodialysis** is usually performed intermittently (often 3 times a week); a typical session takes 3 to 5 hours. More recently high-flux dialysers have been developed which have reduced the time required for dialysis sessions.

**Peritoneal dialysis** may be performed continuously or intermittently. Continuous ambulatory peritoneal dialysis (CAPD) is the most commonly used technique. Patients remain mobile, except during exchanges, and can carry out the procedure themselves. There is always dialysis solution in the peritoneal cavity, and this is drained and replaced 3 to 5 times daily. Continuous cycle peritoneal dialysis (CCPD) is similar, except that exchanges are carried out automatically overnight, and patients do not have to carry out any exchanges during the day. Intermittent peritoneal dialysis (IPD) requires the patient to be connected to a dialysis machine for 12 to 24 hours 2 to 4 times a week. During this time, dialysis solution is pumped into and out of the peritoneal cavity, with a dwell time of about 10 to 20 minutes.

**Haemofiltration** is usually performed as a continuous technique and, as it is not portable, its principal use is in intensive care units. It may also be used intermittently as an adjunct to haemodialysis in patients with excess fluid weight gain. Continuous arteriovenous or venovenous haemodiafiltration (CAVHD or CVVHD) combines dialysis and filtration.

Assessing serum concentrations of urea or creatinine before the next dialysis session is not a good measure of the adequacy of the dialysis, so various other measures have been developed including the urea reduction ratio and urea kinetic modelling. The use of such measures is more established for haemodialysis than for peritoneal dialysis.

◊ References.

1. Zucchelli P, Santoro A. How to achieve optimal correction of acidosis in end-stage renal failure patients. *Blood Purif* 1995; **13:** 375–84.
2. Carlsen DB, Wild ST. Grams to milliequivalents: a concise guide to adjusting hemodialysate composition. *Adv Ren Replace Ther* 1996; **3:** 261–5.
3. Passlick-Deetjen J, Kirchgessner J. Bicarbonate: the alternative buffer for peritoneal dialysis. *Perit Dial Int* 1996; **16** (suppl 1): S109–S113.
4. Pastan S, Bailey J. Dialysis therapy. *N Engl J Med* 1998; **338:** 1428–37.
5. Ifudu O. Care of patients undergoing hemodialysis. *N Engl J Med* 1998; **339:** 1054–62.
6. Mallick NP, Gokal R. Haemodialysis. *Lancet* 1999; **353:** 737–42.
7. Gokal R, Mallick NP. Peritoneal dialysis. *Lancet* 1999; **353:** 823–8.

**Acute renal failure.** Acute renal failure is characterised by a rapid decline in kidney function, and has a variety of causes.[1-6] It is often classified by origin as *prerenal* (e.g. due to hypovolaemia such as that associated with shock, burns, or dehydration; congestive heart failure; or renal artery obstruction), *renal* (such as acute tubular necrosis or interstitial nephritis of various causes, including nephrotoxic drugs and infections), or *postrenal* (acute urinary tract obstruction). The prognosis depends on the underlying disease, which should be identified and treated if possible, but the mortality may still be as high as 60%, particularly after surgery or trauma and in patients who become oliguric. Management is essentially supportive in the hope that renal function will recover. Complications of acute renal failure include extracellular volume overload and hyponatraemia, hyperkalaemia, metabolic acidosis, hyperphosphataemia and hypocalcaemia. Those complications requiring urgent treatment, often including the use of dialysis, are severe hyperkalaemia (p.1219), pulmonary oedema, pericarditis, and severe metabolic acidosis (p.1217). The use of dialysis before clinical signs of uraemia is a matter of debate since it does not appear to hasten recovery *per se*,[1] but all save the shortest episodes of acute renal failure will require some form of renal replacement therapy with dialysis or filtration. Intermittent haemodialysis and peritoneal dialysis are both used, but the newer haemofiltration techniques have theoretical advantages in terms of volume control and cardiovascular stability, and are increasingly preferred.[2,7,8]

Numerous drugs have been tried in attempts to attenuate renal injury or hasten recovery in patients with acute tubular necrosis due to ischaemia or nephrotoxins.[1,5,9,10] These include drugs to increase renal blood flow (e.g. low-dose dopamine, atrial natriuretic peptide, or prostaglandins), drugs to increase urine flow and protect the epithelial cells (mannitol and loop diuretics, calcium-channel blockers), or the use of chelating agents or antidotes against specific nephrotoxins. Consistent clinical benefit has not, however, been demonstrated.

Acute renal failure is reversible in about 95% of patients who survive the complications. A few patients who survive acute renal failure will require long-term dialysis or kidney transplantation (p.1346).


1. Brady HR, Singer GG. Acute renal failure. *Lancet* 1995; **346:** 1533–40.
2. Morgan AG. The management of acute renal failure. *Br J Hosp Med* 1996; **55:** 167–70.
3. Evans JHC. Acute renal failure in children. *Br J Hosp Med* 1994; **52:** 159–61.
4. Klahr S, Miller SB. Acute oliguria. *N Engl J Med* 1998; **338:** 671–5.
5. Dishart MK, Kellum JA. An evaluation of pharmacological strategies for the prevention and treatment of acute renal failure. *Drugs* 2000; **59:** 79–91.
6. Ashley C, Holt S. Acute renal failure. *Pharm J* 2001; **266:** 625–8.
7. McCarthy JT. Renal replacement therapy in acute renal failure. *Curr Opin Nephrol Hypertens* 1996; **5:** 480–4.
8. Joy MS, *et al*. A primer on continuous renal replacement therapy for critically ill patients. *Ann Pharmacother* 1998; **32:** 362–75.
9. Albright RC. Acute renal failure: a practical update. *Mayo Clin Proc* 2001; **76:** 67–74.
10. Pruchnicki MC, Dasta JF. Acute renal failure in hospitalized patients: part II. *Ann Pharmacother* 2002; **36:** 1430–42.


**Chronic renal failure.** Chronic renal failure is the irreversible, usually progressive, loss of renal function that eventually results in end-stage renal disease (ESRD) and the need for renal replacement therapy (dialysis or renal transplantation). The rate of decline in renal function is generally constant for each patient and is usually monitored by measuring serum-creatinine concentrations as an indirect index of the glomerular filtration rate (GFR). In its early stages when the patient is asymptomatic, progressive loss of renal function is described as diminished renal reserve or chronic renal insufficiency. When the limits of renal reserve have been exceeded and symptoms become apparent, it is termed chronic renal failure or overt renal failure. When renal function is diminished to such an extent that life is no longer sustainable (GFR less than 5 mL/minute), the condition is termed ESRD or uraemia. Many diseases can lead to ESRD, the most common being diabetes (p.326), glomerulonephritis (p.1080), and hypertension (p.825).

The management of patients with chronic renal failure prior to ESRD involves measures to conserve renal function and compensate for renal insufficiency. Methods to slow the progression of renal failure include the treatment of hypertension, reduction of proteinuria with dietary protein restriction (p.1418) or in some cases ACE inhibitors (p.847), or both, and the reduction of hyperlipidaemia (p.823). Anaemia (p.749), hyperphosphataemia (p.1219), and renal osteodystrophy (p.764) often require active treatment. Nephrotoxic drugs, including NSAIDs, should be avoided.

The choice between haemodialysis, peritoneal dialysis, and organ transplantation is considered, and the patient prepared, before it is actually required. In patients for whom transplantation is the preferred option, dialysis may still be required while waiting for a kidney. Kidney transplantation is discussed on p.1346. There are differences between countries in the choice of dialysis technique for patients with ESRD. For example, in-centre haemodialysis is used in about 80% of patients in the USA, whereas CAPD is used in over 50% of patients in the UK. Overall survival appears to be similar between the 2 techniques, but more patients on CAPD will eventually require a change to another dialysis method because of treatment failure.

Unlike renal transplant patients, dialysis patients still require replacement therapy with hormones that are usually produced by the kidney. Thus, recombinant erythropoietin and hydroxylated vitamin D analogues are commonly given.

References.


1. NIH. Morbidity and mortality of dialysis. *NIH Consens Statement* 1993; **11:** 1–33.
2. Friedman AL. Etiology, pathophysiology, diagnosis, and management of chronic renal failure in children. *Curr Opin Pediatr* 1996; **8:** 148–51.
3. Steinman TI. Kidney protection: how to prevent or delay chronic renal failure. *Geriatrics* 1996; **51:** 28–35.
4. Walker R. General management of end stage renal disease. *BMJ* 1997; **315:** 1429–32.
5. McCarthy JT. A practical approach to the management of patients with chronic renal failure. *Mayo Clin Proc* 1999; **74:** 269–73. Correction. *ibid.*; 538.
6. Morlidge C, Richards T. Managing chronic renal disease. *Pharm J* 2001; **266:** 655–7.
7. Currie A, O'Brien P. Renal replacement therapies. *Pharm J* 2001; **266:** 679–83.
8. Ruggenenti P, *et al*. Progression, remission, regression of chronic renal diseases. *Lancet* 2001; **357:** 1601–8.
9. Renal Association. *Treatment of adults and children with renal failure: standards and audit measures*. 3rd ed. London: Royal College of Physicians of London and the Renal Association, 2002. Also available at: http://www.renal.org/Standards/RenalStandards_2002b.pdf (accessed 18/05/04)


**Electrolyte disturbances.** Haemodialysis with magnesium-free dialysis solution has been used to remove magnesium from the body in severe hypermagnesaemia (p.1218). Similarly, haemodialysis, and sometimes peritoneal dialysis, has been used in treating hypercalcaemia (p.1218), hyperkalaemia (p.1219), hypernatraemia (p.1220), and hyperphosphataemia (p.1219).

**Overdosage and poisoning.** Haemodialysis, or less often peritoneal dialysis, can be used to remove some substances from the body after overdosage or poisoning. Substances most readily removed have a low molecular weight, low volume of distribution, low protein binding, high water solubility, and high renal clearance. Examples of agents for which haemodialysis may have a role in the treatment of severe overdosage include alcohol (p.1166), ethylene glycol (p.1685), methyl alcohol (p.1475), lithium (p.302), and salicylates such as aspirin (p.15). Dialysis may be particularly important when poisoning with these agents is complicated by renal failure.

## Preparations

***Ph. Eur.:*** Solutions for Haemodialysis; Solutions for Haemofiltration and for Haemodiafiltration; Solutions for Peritoneal Dialysis.

**Proprietary Preparations** (details are given in Part 3)

***Austral.:*** Dianeal; Extraneal; ***Austria:*** Acetat-Haemodialyse†; Dianeal; Extraneal; HAMFL; Hamofiltrasol†; Monosol; Nutrineal PD4; Peritofundin†; Physioneal; ***Braz.:*** Extraneal†; HD†; HF†; Nutrineal†; Peritofundin†; Solurin; ***Canad.:*** Nutrineal PD4†; ***Chile:*** Concentrado Acido; ***Denm.:*** Bicbag†; CAPD/DPCA; Dianeal; Extraneal; Gambrosol; Hemosol Bicar; Lockolys†; Nutrineal PD4; Physioneal; ***Fin.:*** Dianeal; Extraneal; Gambrosol; Lockolys†; Physioneal; ***Fr.:*** Dialysol Acide†; Dialysol Bicarbonate†; Dialytan H; DPCA 2†; ***Ger.:*** Extraneal; Nutrineal PD4; Physioneal; ***Israel:*** CAPD; D-204; D-248; D-300; D-326; Dialine; Dianeal; G-204; G-248; Nutrineal PD4; ***Ital.:*** Extraneal; Icodial; Nutrineal PD2 and PD4; Physioneal; ***Mex.:*** Bipodial; Solucion DP; ***Port.:*** Dianeal†; Nutrineal†; Peritofundinas†; Renofundina†; ***Spain:*** Bicaflac; CAPD; CAPD/DPCA; Dialisis Perit; Dialisol†; Dianeal; Extraneal; Gambrosol; Hemofiltracion E2 and E3; Hemofiltracion E4 and E5; Hemofiltracion HF 01; Hemofiltracion HF 02; Hemofiltracion HF 11 and HF 23; Icodial; Nutrineal PD4; Peritoflex†; Physioneal Glucosa; ***Swed.:*** Altracart II†; BiCart†; Bicbag†; Biorenal†; Biosol A†; Biosol B†; CAPD/DPCA; Dianeal; Dicalys 11; Dicalys 17; Duolys A†; Duolys B†; Extraneal; Gambrolys†; Gambrosol; Haemovex 4; Haemovex 8; Hemofiltrasol; Hemofiltrationslosning 401; Hemoset A glucos†; Hemoset A†; Hemosol B0; HF-BIC35+HF-EL010; HF-BIC35+HF-EL210; Nutrineal PD4; Physioneal; Schiwalys Hemofiltration; ***Switz.:*** Clear-Flex Formula 13, 15, 55, 62, 91, AA, AB, AC†; Dianeal; DPCA; Extraneal; Gambrosol†; HF; Nutrineal PD4; Physioneal; SK-F, BIC-F†; ***Thai.:*** Dialyte; ***UK:*** Dianeal†; Nutrineal PD4; Physioneal; ***USA:*** Dialyte; Extraneal.

# Oral Rehydration Solutions

Soluciones de rehidratación oral.

Oral rehydration solutions have 4 main constituents:

- electrolytes—typically sodium chloride and potassium chloride
- a bicarbonate source to correct or prevent metabolic acidosis, such as sodium bicarbonate or sodium citrate
- water to replace fluid losses
- a carbohydrate source to maximise absorption of fluid and electrolytes—typically glucose, although cereal-based formulations may also be used.

They are most commonly available as oral powders (oral rehydration salts) that are reconstituted with water before use, but effervescent tablets and ready-to-use oral solutions are also available.

## Adverse Effects

Vomiting can occur after administration of oral rehydration solution, and may be an indication that it was given too quickly. If vomiting occurs, administration should be halted for 10 minutes then resumed in smaller, more frequent, amounts.

The risk of hypernatraemia or overhydration after administration of oral rehydration solutions is low in patients with normal renal function. Overdosage of oral rehydration solutions in patients with renal impairment may lead to hypernatraemia and hyperkalaemia.

## Precautions

Oral rehydration salts or effervescent tablets should be reconstituted only with water and at the volume stated. Fresh drinking water is generally appropriate, but freshly boiled and cooled water is preferred when the solution is for infants or when drinking water is not available. The solution should not be boiled after it is prepared. Other ingredients such as sugar should not be added. Unused solution should be stored in a refrigerator and discarded within 24 hours of preparation.

Oral rehydration solutions are not appropriate for patients with gastrointestinal obstruction, oliguric or anuric renal failure, or when parenteral rehydration therapy is indicated as in severe dehydration or intractable vomiting.

## Uses and Administration

Oral rehydration solutions are used for oral replacement of electrolytes and fluids in patients with dehydration, particularly that associated with acute diarrhoea of various aetiologies (p.1241).

The dosage of oral rehydration solutions should be tailored to the individual based on body-weight and the stage and severity of the condition. The initial aim of treatment is to rehydrate the patient, and, subsequently, to maintain hydration by replacing any further losses due to continuing diarrhoea and vomiting and normal losses from respiration, sweating, and urination. Initial rehydration should be rapid, over 3 to 4 hours, unless the patient is hypernatraemic, in which case rehydration over 12 hours is appropriate.

For adults, a usual dose of 200 to 400 mL of oral rehydration solution for every loose motion has been suggested. The dosage for children is 200 mL for every loose motion, and for infants is 1 to 1.5 times their usual feed volume. Normal feeding can continue after the initial fluid deficit has been corrected. Breast feeding should continue between administrations of oral rehydration solution.

**Sodium content and osmolarity.** The original standard WHO oral rehydration solution contains 90 mmol/litre of sodium and 111 mmol/litre of glucose.[1-3] While it has been used safely and effectively,[4] it does not reduce the volume or duration of diarrhoea,[3] and solutions with reduced sodium content and osmolarity have been suggested to be more effective.[1,2] WHO and UNICEF now recommend a solution containing 75 mmol/litre of sodium and 75 mmol/litre of glucose, with a reduced osmolarity.[4] However, there are concerns that the reduced sodium content of this formulation may increase the risk of hyponatraemia in patients with cholera.[3,5,6] Solutions containing less sodium have been recommended in more developed countries: 60 mmol/litre in Europe,[7] and 45 to 90 mmol/litre in the USA.[8]

For discussion of modified formulations of oral rehydration solutions in the treatment of diarrhoea, including the use of cereal-based and low osmolarity preparations, see oral rehydration therapy under Diarrhoea, p.1241.


1. Hahn S, *et al*. Reduced osmolarity oral rehydration solution for treating dehydration caused by acute diarrhoea in children. Available in The Cochrane Library; Issue 2. Chichester: John Wiley; 2004.
2. CHOICE Study Group. Multicenter, randomized, double-blind clinical trial to evaluate the efficacy and safety of a reduced osmolarity oral rehydration salts solution in children with acute watery diarrhea. *Pediatrics* 2001; **107:** 613–18.
3. Fuchs GJ. A better oral rehydration solution? An important step, but not a leap forward. *BMJ* 2001; **323:** 59–60.
4. Anonymous. New formula oral rehydration salts. *WHO Drug Inf* 2002; **16:** 121–2.
5. Hirschhorn N, *et al*. Formulation of oral rehydration solution. *Lancet* 2002; **360:** 340–1.
6. Cash R, *et al*. Oral rehydration and hyponatraemia. *Lancet* 1999; **354:** 1733–4.
7. Booth I, *et al*. Recommendations for composition of oral rehydration solutions for the children of Europe: report of an ESPGAN working group. *J Pediatr Gastroenterol Nutr* 1992; **14:** 113–15.
8. American Academy of Pediatrics. Practice parameter: the management of acute gastroenteritis in young children. *Pediatrics* 1996; **97:** 424–35. Also available at: http://aappolicy.aappublications.org/cgi/reprint/pediatrics;97/3/424.pdf (accessed 02/06/04)


## Preparations

***BP 2003:*** Oral Rehydration Salts;
***USP 27:*** Oral Rehydration Salts;
***WHO/UNICEF:*** Oral Rehydration Salts.

**Proprietary Preparations** (details are given in Part 3)

***Arg.:*** Dixidrol; Pedialyte; SRO; ***Austral.:*** E-Lyte; Gastrolyte; Gastrolyte-R; Gold Cross Gluco-lyte; Hydralyte; Pedialyte†; Repalyte; ***Austria:*** Eloverlan; Milupa GES; Normhydral; Normolyt; Oralpadon; ***Braz.:*** Baby-Drax; Dietasal; Emidrat; Golac†; H-Sal†; Hidra Plus; Hidra-Ped†; Hidrabene; Hidrafix; Hidrafix 90; Hidrolyte†; Hidroral; Hydrax; Hydroplus†; Isolyte†; Pedia-Trict†; Pedialyte; Phosphocalcina Iodada; Reafix; Rehidrat; Reidramax; Sindrat†; Turgoral†; Wassertrat†; ***Canad.:*** Enfalac Enfalyte; Enfalac Lytren†; Gastrolyte; Lytren; Lytren RHS†; Pedialyte; Pediatric Electrolyte; Rehydralyte; ***Chile:*** Pedialyte; Rehsal; ***Denm.:*** Revolyt; ***Fin.:*** Osmosal; ***Fr.:*** Adiaril; Alhydrate; Caril; Carogil; Fanolyte; GES 45; Hydrigoz; Lytren; Picolite; Viatol; ***Ger.:*** D-Iso†; Elotrans; InfectoDyspept†; Isolyt†; Isotonic; Oralpadon; Saltadol; Santalyt; ***Gr.:*** Almora; ***Hong Kong:*** Gastrolyte-R†; GES 45†; Pedialyte; ***India:*** Coslyte; Dextrolyte; Electral; Electrobion; Emlyte; Emlyte-S; Leclyte; Peditral; Ricelyt; Walyte; ***Irl.:*** Dioralyte; Electrolade; Rapolyte; Rehidrat; ***Israel:*** Electrorice; Hydran; Orset; Rehidrat†; ***Ital.:*** Alhydrate; Dicodral; Floridral; Milupa GES; Pedialyte; Reidrax†; Sodioral con Inulina; ***Malaysia:*** ORS Bicarbonate; Servidrat Low Sodium; Uphalyte; ***Mex.:*** Cobirolyte; Electrolit; Electrolit Pediatrico; Hidraplus; Hydrasor; ***Neth.:*** Dioralyte; Dioralyte Rice; ***Norw.:*** Gem; ***NZ:*** E-Lyte; Gastrolyte; Pedialyte; ***Port.:*** Dioralyte; Redrate; ***S.Afr.:*** Darrow-Liq; Darrowped†; Electrona†; Electropak; Enterolyte; Hydrol; Kaostatex; Pectrolyte; Rehidrat; Resalt; Scriptolyte; ***Singapore:*** GES 45†; Hydralyte; Pedialyte; Repalyte; Servidrat; ***Spain:*** Bebesales; Citorsal; Didrica; Oral Rehidr Sal Farmasur; Oralesper; Reemplazante Intesti†; Sueroral; ***Switz.:*** Elotrans; GES 45; Normolytoral; Oralpadon; ***Thai.:*** Infanolyte; Oreda; Oris; Osaline; Osra; Pedialyte; Rehydralyte; Servidrat†; ***UK:*** Diocalm Replenish†; Dioralyte; Dioralyte Effervescent; Dioralyte Relief; Electrolade; Entrocalm Replace; Rapolyte; Rehidrat†; Replavite†; ***USA:*** Infalyte; Naturalyte; Pedialyte; Rehydralyte; Resol.

# Bicarbonate

Bicarbonato.

**Description.** Bicarbonate is an alkalinising agent given as bicarbonate-containing salts (sodium or potassium bicarbonate) or bicarbonate-producing salts (acetate, citrate, or lactate salts). Allowance should be made for the effect of the cation.

**Incompatibility.** Bicarbonate-producing or bicarbonate-containing solutions have been reported to be incompatible with a wide range of drugs. In many cases this incompatibility is a function of the alkaline nature of the bicarbonate solution. Precipitation of insoluble carbonates may occur, as may production of gaseous carbon dioxide when the bicarbonate ion is reduced by acidic solutions.

## Potassium Bicarbonate

Bicarbonato de potasio; E501; Kalii Hydrogenocarbonas; Monopotassium Carbonate; Potassium Hydrogen Carbonate.

$KHCO_3$ = 100.1.
*CAS — 298-14-6.*

**Pharmacopoeias.** In *Eur.* (see p.vi), *Pol.*, and *US.*

**Ph. Eur. 5.0** (Potassium Hydrogen Carbonate; Potassium Bicarbonate BP 2003). A white, crystalline powder or colourless crystals. Freely soluble in water; practically insoluble in alcohol. When heated in the dry state or in solution, it is gradually converted to potassium carbonate. A freshly prepared 5% solution in water has a pH of not more than 8.6.

**USP 27** (Potassium Bicarbonate). Colourless, odourless, transparent monoclinic prisms or white granular powder. Freely soluble in water; practically insoluble in alcohol. Its solutions are neutral or alkaline to phenolphthalein.

**Equivalence.** Each g of potassium bicarbonate represents approximately 10 mmol of potassium and of bicarbonate. Potassium bicarbonate 2.56 g is approximately equivalent to 1 g of potassium.

## Potassium Citrate

Citrato de potasio; E332; Kalii Citras; Tripotassium Citrate. Tripotassium 2-hydroxypropane-1,2,3-tricarboxylate monohydrate.

$C_6H_5K_3O_7,H_2O$ = 324.4.
*CAS — 866-84-2 (anhydrous potassium citrate); 6100-05-6 (potassium citrate monohydrate).*
*ATC — A12BA02.*

**Pharmacopoeias.** In *Chin., Eur.* (see p.vi), *Int.*, and *US.*

**Ph. Eur. 5.0** (Potassium Citrate). Transparent, hygroscopic crystals or a white granular powder. Very soluble in water; practically insoluble in alcohol. Store in airtight containers.

**USP 27** (Potassium Citrate). Transparent crystals or a white granular powder. It is odourless and is deliquescent in moist air. Soluble 1 in 1 of water and 1 in 2.5 of glycerol; almost insoluble in alcohol. Store in airtight containers.

**Equivalence.** Each g of potassium citrate (anhydrous) represents approximately 9.8 mmol of potassium and 3.26 mmol of citrate. Each g of potassium citrate (monohydrate) represents approximately 9.3 mmol of potassium and 3.08 mmol of citrate. Potassium citrate (monohydrate) 2.77 g is approximately equivalent to 1 g of potassium.

## Sodium Acetate

Acetato de sodio; E262; Natrii Acetas Trihydricus; Natrium Aceticum.

$CH_3.CO_2Na,3H_2O$ = 136.1.
*CAS — 127-09-3 (anhydrous sodium acetate); 6131-90-4 (sodium acetate trihydrate).*
*ATC — B05XA08.*

**Pharmacopoeias.** In *Eur.* (see p.vi), *Jpn, Pol.*, and *US.*

*US* also allows the anhydrous form.

**Ph. Eur. 5.0** (Sodium Acetate Trihydrate). Colourless crystals. Very soluble in water; soluble in alcohol. A 5% solution in water has a pH of 7.5 to 9.0. Store in airtight containers.

**USP 27** (Sodium Acetate). It contains three molecules of water of hydration or is anhydrous. Colourless, transparent crystals, or a white, granular crystalline powder, or white flakes. It is odourless or has a faint acetous odour. It is efflorescent in warm dry air. Soluble 1 in 0.8 of water, 1 in 0.6 of boiling water, and 1 in 19 of alcohol. pH of a solution in water containing the equivalent of 3% of anhydrous sodium acetate is between 7.5 and 9.2. Store in airtight containers.

**Equivalence.** Each g of sodium acetate (anhydrous) represents approximately 12.2 mmol of sodium and of acetate. Each g of sodium acetate (trihydrate) represents approximately 7.3 mmol of sodium and of acetate. Sodium acetate (anhydrous) 3.57 g is approximately equivalent to 1 g of sodium. Sodium acetate (trihydrate) 5.92 g is approximately equivalent to 1 g of sodium.

## Sodium Acid Citrate

Citrato ácido de sodio; Disodium Hydrogen Citrate; E331; Natrium Citricum Acidum.

$C_6H_6Na_2O_7,1\frac{1}{2}H_2O$ = 263.1.
*CAS — 144-33-2.*

**Pharmacopoeias.** In *Br.*

**BP 2003** (Sodium Acid Citrate). A white, odourless or almost odourless, powder. Freely soluble in water; practically insoluble in alcohol. A 3% solution in water has a pH of 4.9 to 5.2.

The BP gives Disodium Hydrogen Citrate as an approved synonym.

**Equivalence.** Each g of sodium acid citrate (sesquihydrate) represents approximately 7.6 mmol of sodium and 3.8 mmol of citrate. Sodium acid citrate (sesquihydrate) 5.72 g is approximately equivalent to 1 g of sodium.

## Sodium Bicarbonate

Baking Soda; Bicarbonato de sodio; E500; Monosodium Carbonate; Natrii Bicarbonas; Natrii Hydrogenocarbonas; Sal de Vichy; Sodium Acid Carbonate; Sodium Hydrogen Carbonate.

$NaHCO_3$ = 84.01.
*CAS — 144-55-8.*
*ATC — B05CB04; B05XA02.*

**Pharmacopoeias.** In *Chin., Eur.* (see p.vi), *Int., Jpn, Pol., US,* and *Viet.*

**Ph. Eur. 5.0** (Sodium Hydrogen Carbonate; Sodium Bicarbonate BP 2003). A white, crystalline powder. Soluble in water; practically insoluble in alcohol. The pH of a freshly prepared 5% solution in water is not more than 8.6. When heated in the dry state or in solution, it gradually changes into sodium carbonate.

**USP 27** (Sodium Bicarbonate). A white crystalline powder that slowly decomposes in moist air. Soluble 1 in 12 of water; insoluble in alcohol. Its solutions, when freshly prepared with cold water, without shaking, are alkaline to litmus; alkalinity increases on standing, agitation, or heating.

**Equivalence.** Each g of sodium bicarbonate (anhydrous) represents approximately 11.9 mmol of sodium and of bicarbonate. Sodium bicarbonate 3.65 g is approximately equivalent to 1 g of sodium.

## Sodium Citrate

Citrato de sodio; E331; Natrii Citras; Trisodium Citrate. Trisodium 2-hydroxypropane-1,2,3-tricarboxylate dihydrate.

$C_6H_5Na_3O_7,2H_2O$ = 294.1.
*CAS — 68-04-2 (anhydrous sodium citrate); 6132-04-3 (sodium citrate dihydrate).*
*ATC — B05CB02.*

**Pharmacopoeias.** In *Chin., Eur.* (see p.vi), *Int., Jpn, Pol.*, and *Viet.*

*Int.* and *US* specify anhydrous or dihydrate.

**Ph. Eur. 5.0** (Sodium Citrate). A white, crystalline powder or white, granular crystals; slightly deliquescent in moist air. Freely soluble in water; practically insoluble in alcohol. Store in airtight containers.

**USP 27** (Sodium Citrate). It is anhydrous or contains two molecules of water of hydration. Colourless crystals, or a white crystalline powder. The hydrous form is soluble 1 in 1.5 of water and 1 in 0.6 of boiling water; insoluble in alcohol. Store in airtight containers.

**Equivalence.** Each g of sodium citrate (anhydrous) represents approximately 11.6 mmol of sodium and 3.9 mmol of citrate. Each g of sodium citrate (dihydrate) represents approximately 10.2 mmol of sodium and 3.4 mmol of citrate. Sodium citrate (anhydrous) 3.74 g is approximately equivalent to 1 g of sodium. Sodium citrate (dihydrate) 4.26 g is approximately equivalent to 1 g of sodium.

**Storage.** Sterilised solutions when stored may cause separation of particles from glass containers and solutions containing such particles must not be used.

## Sodium Lactate

E325; Lactato de sodio. Sodium 2-hydroxypropionate.

$C_3H_5NaO_3$ = 112.1.
*CAS — 72-17-3.*

**Pharmacopoeias.** *Chin., Eur.* (see p.vi), and *US* include preparations of sodium lactate.

**Ph. Eur. 5.0** (Sodium Lactate Solution). It contains a minimum of 50% w/w of sodium lactate and is a mixture of the two enantiomers in approximately equal proportions. Sodium (*S*)-Lactate Solution contains a minimum of 50% w/w of sodium lactate, not less than 95% of which is the (*S*)-enantiomer. The solutions are clear, colourless, slightly syrupy liquids. Miscible with water and with alcohol. pH 6.5 to 9.0.

**USP 27** (Sodium Lactate Solution). It is an aqueous solution containing at least 50% sodium lactate. A clear, colourless or practically colourless, slightly viscous liquid, odourless or having a slight, not unpleasant, odour. Miscible with water. pH between 5.0 and 9.0. Store in airtight containers.

**Equivalence.** Each g of sodium lactate (anhydrous) represents approximately 8.9 mmol of sodium and of lactate. Sodium lactate (anhydrous) 4.88 g is approximately equivalent to 1 g of sodium.

## Adverse Effects and Treatment

Excessive administration of bicarbonate or bicarbonate-forming compounds may lead to hypokalaemia and metabolic alkalosis, especially in patients with impaired renal function. Symptoms include mood changes, tiredness, slow breathing, muscle weakness, and irregular heartbeat. Muscle hypertonicity, twitching, and tetany may develop, especially in hypocalcaemic patients. Treatment of metabolic alkalosis associated with bicarbonate overdose consists mainly of appropriate correction of fluid and electrolyte balance. Replacement of calcium, chloride, and potassium ions may be of particular importance.

Excessive doses of *sodium salts* may also lead to sodium overloading and hyperosmolality (see Adverse Effects of Sodium, p.1233). Sodium bicarbonate given orally can cause stomach cramps, belching, and flatulence. Extravasation of irritant hypertonic sodium bicarbonate solutions resulting in local tissue necrosis has been reported after intravenous administration.

Excessive doses of *potassium salts* may lead to hyperkalaemia (see Adverse Effects of Potassium, p.1232). Oral administration of potassium salts can cause gastrointestinal adverse effects, and tablet formulations may cause contact irritation due to high local concentrations of potassium.

Excessive oral administration of *citrate salts* may have a laxative effect.

**Effects on the gastrointestinal tract.** In addition to minor gastrointestinal effects (see above), spontaneous rupture of the stomach, although an exceedingly rare event, has been reported on several occasions following ingestion of sodium bicarbonate. The bicarbonate was believed to have resulted in the rapid production of enough carbon dioxide to rupture a stomach already distended with food, liquid, or air.[1,2]


1. Mastrangelo MR, Moore EW. Spontaneous rupture of the stomach in a healthy adult man after sodium bicarbonate ingestion. *Ann Intern Med* 1984; **101:** 649.
2. Lazebnik N, *et al.* Spontaneous rupture of the normal stomach after sodium bicarbonate ingestion. *J Clin Gastroenterol* 1986; **8:** 454–6.


**Effects on mental state.** Sodium lactate infusions have been reported to induce panic attacks, especially in patients with anxiety states, and have been used as a pharmacological model in the evaluation of mechanisms involved in panic disorder.[1] However, the mechanism that underlies panic attacks induced by lactate remains unknown,[1] and it has been suggested[2] that rapid administration of the large sodium load may be involved. There has also been a report[3] of a patient receiving oral lactate (as calcium lactate) who was suffering from panic disorder associated with agoraphobia; when lactate was discontinued, the patient reported a reduction in panic intensity without a decrease in the frequency of attacks.


1. Bourin M, *et al.* Provocative agents in panic disorder. *Therapie* 1995; **50:** 301–6.
2. Peskind ER, *et al.* Sodium lactate and hypertonic sodium chloride induce equivalent panic incidence, panic symptoms, and hypernatremia in panic disorder. *Biol Psychiatry* 1998; **44:** 1007–16.
3. Robinson D, *et al.* Possible oral lactate exacerbation of panic disorder. *Ann Pharmacother* 1995; **29:** 539–40.


**Epileptogenic effect.** Alkalosis may precipitate seizures; however, absence seizures have also been reported to be associated with sodium bicarbonate administration in a child in whom the serum pH was normal.[1]


1. Reif S, *et al.* Absence seizures associated with bicarbonate therapy and normal serum pH. *JAMA* 1989; **262:** 1328–9.


## Precautions

It is generally recommended that bicarbonate or bicarbonate-forming compounds should not be given to patients with metabolic or respiratory alkalosis, hypocalcaemia, or hypochlorhydria. During treatment of acidosis, frequent monitoring of serum-electrolyte concentrations and acid-base status is essential.

*Sodium-containing salts* should be administered extremely cautiously to patients with heart failure, oedema, renal impairment, hypertension, eclampsia, or aldosteronism (see Sodium, p.1234).

*Potassium-containing salts* should be administered with considerable care to patients with renal or adrenocortical insufficiency, cardiac disease, or other conditions that may predispose to hyperkalaemia (see Potassium, p.1232).

**Abuse.** High doses of bicarbonate have been taken by athletes to enhance performance in endurance sports by buffering hydrogen ions produced in conjunction with lactic acid.[1] Bicarbonates have also been used to alkalinise the urine and prolong the half-life of basic drugs, notably sympathomimetics and stimulants, thereby avoiding detection; however, such a practice may enhance toxicity.

1. Kennedy M. Drugs and athletes—an update. *Adverse Drug React Bull* 1994; (Dec): 639–42.

## Interactions

The effect of oral bicarbonate or bicarbonate-forming compounds in raising intra-gastric pH may reduce or increase the rate and/or extent of absorption of a number of drugs (see also Antacids, p.1239). Alkalinisation of the urine leads to increased renal clearance of acidic drugs such as salicylates, tetracyclines, and barbiturates. Conversely, it prolongs the half-life of basic drugs and may result in toxicity (see also under Abuse, above).

*Sodium bicarbonate* enhances lithium excretion. The use of *potassium-containing salts* with drugs that increase serum-potassium concentrations such as ACE inhibitors and potassium-sparing diuretics should generally be avoided (p.1232). *Citrate salts* taken orally can enhance the absorption of aluminium from the gastrointestinal tract (see p.1249 under Adverse Effects of Aluminium Hydroxide). Patients with impaired renal function are particularly susceptible to aluminium accumulation and citrate-containing oral preparations, including many effervescent or dispersible tablets, are best avoided by patients with renal failure taking aluminium-containing compounds.

## Pharmacokinetics

Oral bicarbonate, such as sodium bicarbonate, neutralises gastric acid with the production of carbon dioxide. Bicarbonate not involved in that reaction is absorbed and in the absence of a deficit of bicarbonate in the plasma, bicarbonate ions are excreted in the urine, which is rendered alkaline, and there is an accompanying diuresis.

Acetates such as potassium acetate and sodium acetate, citrates such as potassium citrate, sodium acid citrate, and sodium citrate, and lactates such as sodium lactate are metabolised, after absorption, to bicarbonate.

## Uses and Administration

Bicarbonate-providing salts are alkalinising agents used for a variety of purposes including the correction of metabolic acidosis, alkalinisation of the urine, and as antacids.

When an alkalinising agent is indicated for treating acute or chronic **metabolic acidosis** (p.1217), sodium bicarbonate is usually used. In conditions when acute metabolic acidosis is associated with tissue hypoxia, such as *cardiac arrest* and *lactic acidosis*, the role of such alkalinising agents is controversial (see p.1217, and for guidelines on advanced cardiac life support, p.812). Sodium lactate has been given as an alternative to sodium bicarbonate in acute metabolic acidosis, but is no longer recommended because of the risk of precipitating lactic acidosis. In *chronic hyperchloraemic acidosis* associated with potassium deficiency, potassium bicarbonate may be preferred to sodium bicarbonate. The citrate salts of potassium or sodium have also been used as alternatives to sodium bicarbonate in treating chronic metabolic acidosis resulting from *renal disorders*. Sodium bicarbonate, lactate and acetate, and potassium acetate are used as bicarbonate sources in *dialysis fluids* (p.1221).

The dose of bicarbonate required for the treatment of acidotic states must be calculated on an individual basis, and is dependent on the acid-base balance and electrolyte status of the patient. In the treatment of chronic acidosis bicarbonate has been given by mouth and doses providing 57 mmol (4.8 g sodium bicarbonate) or more daily may be required. In severe acidosis, sodium bicarbonate has been given intravenously by continuous infusion usually as a 1.26% (150 mmol/litre) solution or by slow intravenous injection of a stronger (hypertonic) solution of up to 8.4% (1000 mmol/litre) sodium bicarbonate (but see the discussion on metabolic acidosis, p.1217). For the correction of acidosis during advanced cardiac life support procedures, doses of 50 mmol of sodium bicarbonate (50 mL of an 8.4% solution) may be given intravenously to adults. Frequent monitoring of serum-electrolyte concentrations and acid-base status is essential during treatment of acidosis.

Sodium bicarbonate may be used in the management of **hyperkalaemia** (p.1219) to promote the intracellular uptake of potassium and correct associated acidosis, although there is some debate as to its value. Some sources suggest that 50 to 100 mL of an 8.4% solution may be given in severe hyperkalaemia accompanied by acidosis, although more dilute solutions have been used, and care is required, particularly if there is accompanying renal impairment.

Sodium bicarbonate, sodium citrate, and potassium citrate cause **alkalinisation of the urine**. They may therefore be given to relieve discomfort in mild *urinary-tract infections* (p.153) and to prevent the development of uric-acid renal calculi in the initial stages of *uricosuric* therapy for hyperuricaemia in chronic gout (for example, see Probenecid, p.416). In both cases, they are administered with a liberal fluid intake, usually by mouth, in divided doses of up to about 10 g daily. Sodium bicarbonate has also been used with a diuretic in the treatment of *acute poisoning* from weakly acidic drugs to enhance their excretion, but this process, which is known as 'forced alkaline diuresis', is generally no longer recommended.

When given by mouth, sodium bicarbonate and potassium bicarbonate neutralise acid secretions in the gastrointestinal tract and sodium bicarbonate in particular is therefore frequently included in **antacid** preparations (p.1239). To relieve *dyspepsia* doses of about 1 to 5 g of sodium bicarbonate in water have been taken when required. Sodium citrate has been widely used as a 'clear' (non-particulate) antacid, usually with an $H_2$-antagonist, for the *prophylaxis of acid aspiration* associated with anaesthesia (p.1240). Sodium bicarbonate is also used in various preparations for *double-contrast radiography* where production of gas (carbon dioxide) in the gastrointestinal tract is necessary. Similarly, solutions containing sodium bicarbonate or citrate have been used to treat acute *oesophageal impaction*.

Sodium bicarbonate and sodium or potassium citrate are used as buffering or alkalinising agents in *pharmaceutical formulation*. Sodium or potassium bicarbonate and anhydrous sodium citrate are used in effervescent tablet formulations.

Individual salts also have **other specific uses**. A 5% solution of sodium bicarbonate can be administered as ear drops to soften and remove *ear wax* (p.1262). Sodium bicarbonate injection has been used to treat *extravasation of anthracycline antineoplastics* (p.496) although as mentioned in Adverse Effects, above, hypertonic solutions may themselves cause necrosis.

Sodium citrate has anti-clotting properties and is used, as sodium acid citrate, with other agents in solutions for the anticoagulation and preservation of blood for *transfusion* purposes. Similarly, sodium citrate 3% irrigation may be useful for the dissolution of *blood clots in the bladder* as an alternative to sodium chloride 0.9%. Enemas containing sodium citrate are given rectally as *osmotic laxatives*. Sodium citrate is also a common ingredient in *cough* mixtures.

**Eye disorders.** Sodium citrate eye drops have been employed in the management of certain ocular injuries. It has been suggested that corneal epithelial defects due to chemical weapon injuries, and lasting for more than one week or accompanied by limbal ischaemia, require intensive topical therapy with eye drops of sodium citrate 10% and of potassium ascorbate 10%. Such therapy is said to prevent late corneal melting and to permit the continuation of local corticosteroid therapy as necessary.[1] The two types of eye drops are given in alternate doses and are believed to act by mopping up free oxygen radicals after chemical burns.[2]

Sodium bicarbonate is also used in the management of blepharitis, an inflammation of the margin of the eyelids with various causes. It may be allergic in nature or associated with seborrhoea of the scalp. Infection of the eyelids can produce ulcerative blepharitis, a condition characterised by the formation of yellow crusts which may glue the eyelashes together. Parasites occasionally cause blepharitis. The condition is first treated by cleaning the eyes and eyelids with sodium bicarbonate solution or a suitable bland eye lotion; simple eye ointment or diluted baby shampoo can also be used to soften crusts to aid removal. If an infection is present, antibacterials may be required (p.127). Long-term management consists of daily cleansing of the lid margins with a bland eye lotion.

1. Wright P. Injuries due to chemical weapons. *BMJ* 1991; **302:** 239.
2. Anonymous. Citrate/ascorbate eye-drops for chemical weapons injuries. *Pharm J* 1991; **246:** 145.

**Osteoporosis.** Potassium bicarbonate 1 to 2 mmol/kg daily by mouth improved mineral balance and bone metabolism in a short-term study.[1] However, the authors cautioned against the use of bicarbonate to treat or prevent osteoporosis (p.763) without further study.[2]

1. Sebastian A, *et al.* Improved mineral balance and skeletal metabolism in postmenopausal women treated with potassium bicarbonate. *N Engl J Med* 1994, **330:** 1776–81.
2. Sebastian A, Morris RC. Improved mineral balance and skeletal metabolism in postmenopausal women treated with potassium bicarbonate. *N Engl J Med* 1994; **331:** 279.

**Renal calculi.** Citrate forms soluble complexes with calcium, thereby reducing urinary saturation of stone-forming calcium salts. Potassium citrate has a hypocalciuric effect when given by mouth, probably due to enhanced renal calcium absorption. Urinary calcium excretion is unaffected by sodium citrate, since the alkali-mediated hypocalciuric effect is offset by a sodium-linked calciuresis.[1] Potassium citrate may be beneficial in reducing the rate of stone formation in patients with hypocitraturia[2,3] or hypercalciuria.[4] As mentioned in Uses above, sodium bicarbonate or sodium or potassium citrate may also be used for their alkalinising action, as an adjunct to a liberal fluid intake, to prevent development of uric-acid renal calculi during uricosuric therapy.

Other causes of renal calculi and their treatment are discussed on p.936.

Urinary alkalinisation with sodium bicarbonate, sodium citrate, or potassium citrate may be useful in the management of cystine stone formation in patients with cystinuria (see under Penicillamine, p.1049).

1. Anonymous. Citrate for calcium nephrolithiasis. *Lancet* 1986; **i:** 955.
2. Pak CYC, Fuller C. Idiopathic hypocitraturic calcium-oxalate nephrolithiasis successfully treated with potassium citrate. *Ann Intern Med* 1986; **104:** 33–7.
3. Tekin A, *et al.* Oral potassium citrate treatment for idiopathic hypocitruria in children with calcium urolithiasis. *J Urol (Baltimore)* 2002; **168:** 2572–4.
4. Pak CYC, *et al.* Prevention of stone formation and bone loss in absorptive hypercalciuria by combined dietary and pharmacological interventions. *J Urol (Baltimore)* 2003; **169:** 465–9.

## Preparations

***BP 2003:*** Alkaline Gentian Mixture; Aromatic Magnesium Carbonate Mixture; Compound Magnesium Trisilicate Oral Powder; Compound Sodium Bicarbonate Tablets; Compound Sodium Chloride Mouthwash; Kaolin and Morphine Mixture; Kaolin Mixture; Magnesium Trisilicate Mixture; Potassium Citrate Mixture; Sodium Bicarbonate Ear Drops; Sodium Bicarbonate Eye Lotion; Sodium Bicarbonate Intravenous Infusion; Sodium Citrate Eye Drops; Sodium Citrate Irrigation Solution; Sodium Lactate Intravenous Infusion;
***BPC 1968:*** Effervescent Potassium Tablets;
***Ph. Eur.:*** Anticoagulant Acid-Citrate-Glucose Solutions (ACD); Anticoagulant Citrate-Phosphate-Glucose Solution (CPD);
***USP 27:*** Anticoagulant Citrate Dextrose Solution; Anticoagulant Citrate Phosphate Dextrose Adenine Solution; Anticoagulant Citrate Phosphate Dextrose Solution; Anticoagulant Sodium Citrate Solution; Half-strength Lactated Ringer's and Dextrose Injection; Lactated Ringer's and Dextrose Injection; Lactated Ringer's Injection; Magnesium Carbonate and Sodium Bicarbonate for Oral Suspension; Potassium and Sodium Bicarbonates and Citric Acid Effervescent Tablets for Oral Solution; Potassium Bicarbonate and Potassium Chloride Effervescent Tablets for Oral Solution; Potassium Bicarbonate and Potassium Chloride for Effervescent Oral Solution; Potassium Bicarbonate Effervescent Tablets for Oral Solution; Potassium Chloride in Lactated Ringer's and Dextrose Injection; Potassium Chloride, Potassium Bicarbonate, and Potassium Citrate Effervescent Tablets for Oral Solution; Potassium Citrate And Citric Acid Oral Solution; Potassium Citrate Extended-release Tablets; Potassium Gluconate and Potassium Citrate Oral Solution; Potassium Gluconate, Potassium Citrate, and Ammonium Chloride Oral Solution; Sodium Acetate Injection; Sodium Acetate Solution; Sodium Bicarbonate Injection; Sodium Bicarbonate Oral Powder; Sodium Bicarbonate Tablets; Sodium Citrate and Citric Acid Oral Solution; Sodium Lactate Injection; Sodium Lactate Solution; Tricitrates Oral Solution; Trikates Oral Solution.

**Proprietary Preparations** (details are given in Part 3)
***Arg.:*** Urokit; ***Austral.:*** Chlorvescent; Sodibic; Urocit-K; ***Austria:*** Bullrich Salz; Oxalyt; Uralyt-U; ***Belg.:*** Uralyt-U; ***Braz.:*** Acalka; Citrosodine; Litocit; ***Canad.:*** Brioschi; Bromo Seltzer; Eno; K-Lyte; Polycitra-K; ***Chile:*** Acalka; Eucerin; Sal De Yasta; ***Fr.:*** Elgydium Bicarbonate; Soludial†; ***Ger.:*** Alkala T; Blanel; Kalitrans; Kalium; Kohlensaurebad Bastian; Nephrotrans; Uralyt-U; ***Hong Kong:*** Urocit-K; ***India:*** Alkasol; Citralka; Oricitral; ***Irl.:*** Cystopurin; ***Israel:*** Babic; Uralyt-U; ***Ital.:*** Citrosodina; Kation†; Uralyt-U; ***Jpn:*** Meylon; ***Malaysia:*** Urocit-K; ***Mex.:*** Betsol Z; Bicarnat; Debonal; ***Norw.:*** Kajos; ***NZ:*** Citravescent; ***Port.:*** Acalka; Uralyt-U; ***S.Afr.:*** Crystacit; Nitrocit†; Uralyt-U; ***Singapore:*** Gripe Water; Urocit-K†; ***Spain:*** Acalka; Apir Bicarbonato Sod†; Plurisalina; ***Swed.:*** Kajos; ***Switz.:*** Nephrotrans; Uralyt-U; ***Thai.:*** Uralyt-U; ***UK:*** Boots Gripe Mixture 1 Month Plus; Canesten Oasis; Cystemme; Cystitis Relief; Cystocalm; Cystofem†; Cystoleve†; Cystopurin; ***USA:*** Citra pH; K + Care; K-Lyte; Neut; Urocit-K.

**Multi-ingredient:** numerous preparations are listed in Part 3.

# Calcium

Calcio.

Ca = 40.078.

**Description.** Calcium is a cation given as various calcium-containing salts.

**Incompatibility.** Calcium salts have been reported to be incompatible with a wide range of drugs. Complexes may form resulting in the formation of a precipitate.

## Calcium Acetate

Calcio, acetato de; E263.

$C_4H_6CaO_4$ = 158.2.

*CAS — 62-54-4.*

*ATC — A12AA12.*

**Pharmacopoeias.** In *Br.* and *US.*

**BP 2003** (Calcium Acetate). A white, hygroscopic, odourless or almost odourless, powder. Freely soluble in water; slightly soluble in alcohol. A 5% solution in water has a pH of 7.2 to 8.2.

**USP 27** (Calcium Acetate). A white, odourless or almost odourless, hygroscopic, crystalline powder. It decomposes to calcium carbonate and acetone when heated to above 160°. Freely soluble in water; slightly soluble in methyl alcohol; practically insoluble in dehydrated alcohol, in acetone, and in benzene. A 5% solution in water has a pH of 6.3 to 9.6. Store in airtight containers.

**Equivalence.** Each g of calcium acetate (anhydrous) represents approximately 6.3 mmol of calcium. Calcium acetate (anhydrous) 3.95 g is approximately equivalent to 1 g of calcium.

## Calcium Chloride

Calcii Chloridum; Calcio, cloruro de; Calcium Chloratum; Cloreto de Cálcio; Cloruro de Calcio; E509.

$CaCl_2,xH_2O$ = 110.0 (anhydrous); 147.0 (dihydrate).

*CAS — 10043-52-4 (anhydrous calcium chloride); 7774-34-7 (calcium chloride hexahydrate); 10035-04-8 (calcium chloride dihydrate).*

*ATC — A12AA07; B05XA07; G04BA03.*

**Pharmacopoeias.** *Chin., Eur.* (see p.vi), *Jpn, US,* and *Viet.* include the dihydrate.

*Eur.* also specifies the hexahydrate. *Pol.* only specifies the hexahydrate.

**Ph. Eur. 5.0** (Calcium Chloride Dihydrate; Calcii Chloridum Dihydricum). A white, hygroscopic, crystalline powder. Freely soluble in water; soluble in alcohol. Store in airtight containers.

**Ph. Eur. 5.0** (Calcium Chloride Hexahydrate; Calcii Chloridum Hexahydricum). A white, crystalline mass or colourless crystals. Very soluble in water; freely soluble in alcohol. F.p. about 29°.

**USP 27** (Calcium Chloride). White, hard, odourless fragments or granules. Is deliquescent. Soluble 1 in 0.7 of water, 1 in 0.2 of boiling water, 1 in 4 of alcohol, and 1 in 2 of boiling alcohol. pH of a 5% solution in water is between 4.5 and 9.2. Store in airtight containers.

**Equivalence.** Each g of calcium chloride (dihydrate) represents approximately 6.8 mmol of calcium and 13.6 mmol of chloride. Calcium chloride (dihydrate) 3.67 g is approximately equivalent to 1 g of calcium.

Each g of calcium chloride (hexahydrate) represents approximately 4.56 mmol of calcium and 9.13 mmol of chloride. Calcium chloride (hexahydrate) 5.47 g is approximately equivalent to 1 g of calcium.

## Calcium Citrate

Calcio, citrato de; Tricalcium Citrate. Tricalcium 2-hydroxypropane-1,2,3-tricarboxylate tetrahydrate.

$C_{12}H_{10}Ca_3O_{14},4H_2O$ = 570.5.

*CAS — 5785-44-4.*

**Pharmacopoeias.** In *US.*

**USP 27** (Calcium Citrate). A white, odourless, crystalline powder. Slightly soluble in water; insoluble in alcohol; freely soluble in diluted 3N hydrochloric acid and in diluted 2N nitric acid.

**Equivalence.** Each g of calcium citrate (tetrahydrate) represents approximately 5.3 mmol of calcium and 3.5 mmol of citrate. Calcium citrate (tetrahydrate) 4.74 g is approximately equivalent to 1 g of calcium.

## Calcium Glubionate *(USAN, rINN)*

Calcium Gluconate Lactobionate Monohydrate; Calcium Gluconogalactogluconate Monohydrate; Glubionato de calcio. Calcium D-gluconate lactobionate monohydrate.

$(C_{12}H_{21}O_{12},C_6H_{11}O_7)Ca,H_2O$ = 610.5.

*CAS — 31959-85-0 (anhydrous calcium glubionate); 12569-38-9 (calcium glubionate monohydrate).*

*ATC — A12AA02.*

**Pharmacopoeias.** *US* includes Calcium Glubionate Syrup.

**Equivalence.** Each g of calcium glubionate (monohydrate) represents approximately 1.6 mmol of calcium. Calcium glubionate (monohydrate) 15.2 g is approximately equivalent to 1 g of calcium.

## Calcium Gluceptate

Calcium Glucoheptonate *(pINN)*; Calcii Glucoheptonas; Glucoheptonato de calcio.

$C_{14}H_{26}CaO_{16}$ = 490.4.

*CAS — 17140-60-2 (anhydrous calcium gluceptate); 29039-00-7 (anhydrous calcium gluceptate).*

*ATC — A12AA10.*

**Pharmacopoeias.** In *Eur.* (see p.vi). *US* allows anhydrous or with varying amounts of water of hydration.

**Ph. Eur. 5.0** (Calcium Glucoheptonate). A mixture in variable proportions of calcium di(D-*glycero*-D-*gulo*-heptonate) and calcium di(D-*glycero*-D-*ido*-heptonate). A white or very slightly yellow, hygroscopic, amorphous powder. Very soluble in water; practically insoluble in alcohol and in acetone. A 10% solution in water has a pH of 6.0 to 8.0. Store in airtight containers.

**USP 27** (Calcium Gluceptate). It is anhydrous or contains varying amounts of water of hydration. It consists of the calcium salt of the alpha-epimer of glucoheptonic acid or of a mixture of the alpha and beta epimers of glucoheptonic acid. A white to faintly yellow amorphous powder. It is stable in air, but the hydrous forms may lose part of their water of hydration on standing. Freely soluble in water; insoluble in alcohol and in many other organic solvents. pH of a 10% solution in water is between 6.0 and 8.0.

**Equivalence.** Each g of calcium gluceptate (anhydrous) represents approximately 2 mmol of calcium. Calcium gluceptate (anhydrous) 12.2 g is approximately equivalent to 1 g of calcium.

## Calcium Gluconate

Calcii Gluconas; Calcio, gluconato de; Calcium Glyconate; E578. Calcium D-gluconate monohydrate.

$C_{12}H_{22}CaO_{14},H_2O$ = 448.4.

*CAS — 299-28-5 (anhydrous calcium gluconate); 18016-24-5 (calcium gluconate monohydrate).*

*ATC — A12AA03; D11AX03.*

**Pharmacopoeias.** In *Chin., Eur.* (see p.vi), *Int., Jpn, Pol.,* and *Viet.* Also in *US* as the anhydrous or the monohydrate form.

Calcium borogluconate is included as an injection in *BP(Vet).*

**Ph. Eur. 5.0** (Calcium Gluconate). A white, crystalline or granular, powder. Sparingly soluble in water; freely soluble in boiling water.

**USP 27** (Calcium Gluconate). It is anhydrous or contains one molecule of water of hydration. White, odourless, crystalline granules or powder. Slowly soluble 1 in 30 of water; soluble 1 in 5 of boiling water; insoluble in alcohol. Its solutions are neutral to litmus.

**Equivalence.** Each g of calcium gluconate (monohydrate) represents approximately 2.2 mmol of calcium. Calcium gluconate (monohydrate) 11.2 g is approximately equivalent to 1 g of calcium.

## Calcium Glycerophosphate

Calcii Glycerophosphas; Calcio, glicerofosfato de; Calcium Glycerinophosphate; Calcium Glycerylphosphate.

$C_3H_7CaO_6P(+xH_2O)$ = 210.1 (anhydrous).

*CAS — 27214-00-2 (anhydrous calcium glycerophosphate).*

*ATC — A12AA08.*

**Pharmacopoeias.** In *Eur.* (see p.vi) and *Viet.*

**Ph. Eur. 5.0** (Calcium Glycerophosphate). A mixture in variable proportions of calcium (*RS*)-2,3-dihydroxypropyl phosphate and of calcium 2-hydroxy-1-(hydroxymethyl)ethyl phosphate, which may be hydrated. It contains not less than 18.6% and not more than 19.4% of calcium, calculated with reference to the dried substance. A white hygroscopic powder. Sparingly soluble in water; practically insoluble in alcohol. It loses not more than 12% of its weight on drying.

**Equivalence.** Each g of calcium glycerophosphate (anhydrous) represents approximately 4.8 mmol of calcium. Calcium glycerophosphate (anhydrous) 5.24 g is approximately equivalent to 1 g of calcium.

## Calcium Hydrogen Phosphate

Calcii et Hydrogenii Phosphas; Calcii Hydrogenophosphas; Calcio, hidrogenofosfato de; Calcium Hydrophosphoricum; Calcium Monohydrogen Phosphate; Dicalcium Orthophosphate; Dicalcium Phosphate; E341. Calcium hydrogen orthophosphate.

$CaHPO_4$ = 136.1 (anhydrous); 172.1 (dihydrate).

*CAS — 7757-93-9 (anhydrous calcium hydrogen phosphate); 7789-77-7 (calcium hydrogen phosphate dihydrate).*

**Pharmacopoeias.** In *Chin., Eur.* (see p.vi), *Jpn, Pol.,* and *US,* which include specifications for the anhydrous substance, the dihydrate form, or both.

**Ph. Eur. 5.0** (Calcium Hydrogen Phosphate, Anhydrous; Calcii Hydrogenophosphas Anhydricus). A white crystalline powder or colourless crystals. Practically insoluble in water and in alcohol; dissolves in dilute hydrochloric acid and in dilute nitric acid.

**Ph. Eur. 5.0** (Calcium Hydrogen Phosphate Dihydrate; Calcii Hydrogenophosphas Dihydricus; Calcium Hydrogen Phosphate BP 2003). A white, crystalline powder. Practically insoluble in cold water and in alcohol; dissolves in dilute hydrochloric acid and in dilute nitric acid.

The BP 2003 gives Dibasic Calcium Phosphate as an approved synonym.

**USP 27** (Dibasic Calcium Phosphate). It is anhydrous or contains two molecules of water of hydration. A white, odourless, powder. Practically insoluble in water; insoluble in alcohol; soluble in 3N hydrochloric acid and in 2N nitric acid.

**Equivalence.** Each g of calcium hydrogen phosphate (dihydrate) represents approximately 5.8 mmol of calcium and of phosphate. Calcium hydrogen phosphate (dihydrate) 4.29 g is approximately equivalent to 1 g of calcium.

## Calcium Lactate

Calcii Lactas; Calcio, lactato de; E327. Calcium 2-hydroxypropionate.

$C_6H_{10}CaO_6,xH_2O$ = 218.2 (anhydrous); 308.3 (pentahydrate); 272.3 (trihydrate).

*CAS — 814-80-2 (anhydrous calcium lactate); 41372-22-9 (hydrated calcium lactate); 5743-47-5 (calcium lactate pentahydrate); 63690-56-2 (calcium lactate pentahydrate).*

*ATC — A12AA05.*

**Pharmacopoeias.** In *Chin., Eur.* (see p.vi), *Jpn, Pol.,* and *US.* *Eur.* and *Viet.* have separate monographs for the pentahydrate and the trihydrate. *US* allows anhydrous or hydrous forms.

**Ph. Eur. 5.0** (Calcium Lactate Trihydrate; Calcii Lactas Trihydricus). A white or almost white, crystalline or granular powder. Soluble in water; freely soluble in boiling water; very slightly soluble in alcohol.

**Ph. Eur. 5.0** (Calcium Lactate Pentahydrate; Calcii Lactas Pentahydricus). A white or almost white, slightly efflorescent, crystalline or granular powder. Soluble in water; freely soluble in boiling water; very slightly soluble in alcohol.

The BP 2003 gives Calcium Lactate as an approved synonym.

**USP 27** (Calcium Lactate). White, practically odourless, granules or powder. The pentahydrate is somewhat efflorescent and at 120° becomes anhydrous. The pentahydrate is soluble 1 in 20 of water and practically insoluble in alcohol. Store in airtight containers.

**Equivalence.** Each g of calcium lactate (trihydrate) represents approximately 3.7 mmol of calcium. Each g of calcium lactate (pentahydrate) represents approximately 3.2 mmol of calcium. Calcium lactate (pentahydrate) 7.7 g and calcium lactate (trihydrate) 6.8 g are approximately equivalent to 1 g of calcium.

## Calcium Lactate Gluconate

Calcio, gluconato lactato de.

$Ca_5(C_3H_5O_3)_6,(C_6H_{11}O_7)_4,2H_2O$ = 1551.4.

*ATC — A12AA06.*

**Equivalence.** Each g of calcium lactate gluconate (dihydrate) represents approximately 3.2 mmol of calcium. Calcium lactate gluconate (dihydrate) 7.74 g is approximately equivalent to 1 g of calcium.

## Calcium Lactobionate

Calcio, lactobionato de; Calcium Lactobionate Dihydrate. Calcium 4-*O*-β-D-galactopyranosyl-D-gluconate dihydrate.

$C_{24}H_{42}CaO_{24},2H_2O$ = 790.7.

*CAS — 110638-68-1.*

**Pharmacopoeias.** In *US.*

**USP 27** (Calcium Lactobionate). pH of a 5% solution in water is between 5.4 and 7.4.

**Equivalence.** Each g of calcium lactobionate (dihydrate) represents approximately 1.3 mmol of calcium. Calcium lactobionate (dihydrate) 19.7 g is approximately equivalent to 1 g of calcium.

## Calcium Levulinate *(BAN)*

Calcii Levulinas Dihydricum; Calcio, levulinato de; Calcium Laevulate; Calcium Laevulinate; Lévulinate Calcique. Calcium 4-oxovalerate dihydrate.

$C_{10}H_{14}CaO_6,2H_2O$ = 306.3.

*CAS — 591-64-0 (anhydrous calcium levulinate); 5743-49-7 (calcium levulinate dihydrate).*

*ATC — A12AA30.*

**Pharmacopoeias.** In *Eur.* (see p.vi) and *US.*

**Ph. Eur. 5.0** (Calcium Levulinate Dihydrate). A white or almost white, crystalline powder. Freely soluble in water; very slightly soluble in alcohol; practically insoluble in dichloromethane. A 10% solution in water has a pH of 6.8 to 7.8. Protect from light.

**USP 27** (Calcium Levulinate). A white crystalline or amorphous powder, having a faint odour suggestive of burnt sugar. Freely soluble in water; slightly soluble in alcohol; insoluble in chloroform and in ether. pH of a 10% solution in water is between 7.0 and 8.5.

**Equivalence.** Each g of calcium levulinate (dihydrate) represents approximately 3.3 mmol of calcium. Calcium levulinate (dihydrate) 7.64 g is approximately equivalent to 1 g of calcium.

## Calcium Phosphate

Calcio, fosfato de; Calcium Orthophosphate; E341; Fosfato Tricalcico; Phosphate Tertiaire de Calcium; Precipitated Calcium Phosphate; Tricalcii Phosphas; Tricalcium Phosphate.

*CAS — 7758-87-4 (tricalcium diorthophosphate); 12167-74-7 (calcium hydroxide phosphate).*

*ATC — A12AA01.*

**Description.** Calcium phosphate is not a clearly defined chemical entity but is a mixture of calcium phosphates that has been most frequently described as either tricalcium diorthophosphate, $Ca_3(PO_4)_2$ = 310.2, or calcium hydroxide phosphate, $Ca_5(OH)(PO_4)_3$ = 502.3.

**Pharmacopoeias.** In *Eur.* (see p.vi), *Pol.*, and *Viet.* Also in *USNF.*

**Ph. Eur. 5.0** (Calcium Phosphate). It consists of a mixture of calcium phosphates and contains 35 to 40% of Ca. A white or almost white powder. Practically insoluble in water; dissolves in dilute hydrochloric acid and in dilute nitric acid.

The BP 2003 gives Tribasic Calcium Phosphate as an approved synonym.

**USNF 22** (Tribasic Calcium Phosphate). It consists of a variable mixture of calcium phosphates having the approximate composition $10CaO.3P_2O_5.H_2O$. It contains not less than 34% and not more than 40% of calcium. A white, odourless, powder. Practically insoluble in water; insoluble in alcohol; readily soluble in 3N hydrochloric acid and in 2N nitric acid.

## Calcium Pidolate *(pINNM)*

Calcium Pyroglutamate; Pidolato de calcio. Calcium 5-oxopyrrolidine-2-carboxylate.

$Ca(C_5H_6NO_3)_2$ = 296.3.

*CAS — 31377-05-6.*

**Equivalence.** Each g of calcium pidolate (anhydrous) represents approximately 3.4 mmol of calcium. Calcium pidolate (anhydrous) 7.39 g is approximately equivalent to 1 g of calcium.

## Calcium Silicate

Calcio, silicato de; E552.

*CAS — 1344-95-2; 10101-39-0 (calcium metasilicate); 10034-77-2 (calcium diorthosilicate); 12168-85-3 (calcium trisilicate).*

*ATC — A02AC02.*

**Description.** A naturally occurring mineral, the most common forms being calcium metasilicate ($CaSiO_3$ = 116.2), calcium diorthosilicate ($Ca_2SiO_4$ = 172.2), and calcium trisilicate ($Ca_3SiO_5$ = 228.3). It is usually found in hydrated forms containing various amounts of water of crystallisation. Commercial calcium silicate is prepared synthetically.

**Pharmacopoeias.** In *USNF.*

**USNF 22** (Calcium Silicate). A compound of calcium oxide and silicon dioxide containing not less than 4% of CaO and not less than 45% of $SiO_2$. A white to off-white free-flowing powder. Insoluble in water; with mineral acids it forms a gel. A 5% aqueous suspension has a pH of 8.4 to 10.2.

## Calcium Sodium Lactate

Calcio, lactato sódico de.

$2C_3H_5NaO_3,(C_3H_5O_3)_2Ca,4H_2O$ = 514.4.

**Equivalence.** Each g of calcium sodium lactate (tetrahydrate) represents approximately 1.9 mmol of calcium and 3.9 mmol of sodium and of lactate. Calcium sodium lactate (tetrahydrate) 12.8 g is approximately equivalent to 1 g of calcium.

### Adverse Effects and Treatment

Oral calcium salts can cause gastrointestinal irritation; calcium chloride is generally considered to be the most irritant of the commonly used calcium salts.

Injection of calcium salts can also produce irritation, and intramuscular or subcutaneous injection in particular can cause local reactions including sloughing or necrosis of the skin; solutions of calcium chloride are extremely irritant and should not be injected intramuscularly or subcutaneously. Soft-tissue calcification has followed the use of calcium salts parenterally.

Excessive amounts of calcium salts may lead to hypercalcaemia. This complication is usually associated with parenteral administration, but can occur after oral dosage, usually in patients with renal failure or who are also taking vitamin D. Symptoms of hypercalcaemia include anorexia, nausea, vomiting, constipation, abdominal pain, muscle weakness, mental disturbances, polydipsia, polyuria, nephrocalcinosis, renal calculi, and, in severe cases, cardiac arrhythmias and coma. Too rapid intravenous injection of calcium salts may also lead to symptoms of hypercalcaemia, as well as a chalky taste, hot flushes, and peripheral vasodilatation. Mild asymptomatic hypercalcaemia will usually resolve if calcium and other contributory drugs such as vitamin D are stopped (see also Vitamin D-mediated Hypercalcaemia, p.1218). If hypercalcaemia is severe, urgent treatment is required as outlined on p.1218.

### Precautions

Solutions of calcium salts, particularly calcium chloride, are irritant, and care should be taken to prevent extravasation during intravenous injection. Calcium salts should be given cautiously to patients with renal impairment, or diseases associated with hypercalcaemia such as sarcoidosis and some malignancies. In addition, they should generally be avoided in patients with calcium renal calculi, or a history of renal calculi. Calcium chloride, because of its acidifying nature, is unsuitable for the treatment of hypocalcaemia caused by renal insufficiency or in patients with respiratory acidosis or failure.

Plasma-calcium concentrations should be monitored closely in patients with renal impairment and during parenteral administration and if large doses of vitamin D are used concurrently.

### Interactions

Hypercalcaemia has occurred when calcium salts are given with thiazide diuretics or vitamin D. Vitamin D increases the gastrointestinal absorption of calcium and thiazide diuretics decrease its urinary excretion. Plasma-calcium concentrations should be monitored in patients receiving the drugs together.

Bran decreases the gastrointestinal absorption of calcium, and may therefore decrease the efficacy of calcium supplements. Corticosteroids also reduce calcium absorption.

Calcium enhances the effects of digitalis glycosides on the heart and may precipitate digitalis intoxication; parenteral calcium therapy is best avoided in patients receiving cardiac glycosides. Citrate salts increase the absorption of aluminium from the gastrointestinal tract (see under Adverse Effects of Aluminium Hydroxide, p.1249), therefore patients with renal failure taking aluminium compounds should avoid taking calcium citrate. Calcium salts reduce the absorption of a number of other drugs such as bisphosphonates, fluoride, some fluoroquinolones, and tetracyclines; administration should be separated by at least 3 hours.

### Pharmacokinetics

Calcium is absorbed mainly from the small intestine by active transport and passive diffusion. About one-third of ingested calcium is absorbed although this can vary depending upon dietary factors and the state of the small intestine; also absorption is increased in calcium deficiency and during periods of high physiological requirement such as during childhood or pregnancy and lactation. 1,25-Dihydroxycholecalciferol (calcitriol), a metabolite of vitamin D, enhances the active phase of absorption.

Excess calcium is predominantly excreted renally. Unabsorbed calcium is eliminated in the faeces, together with that secreted in the bile and pancreatic juice. Minor amounts are lost in the sweat, skin, hair, and nails. Calcium crosses the placenta and is distributed into breast milk.

### Human Requirements

Calcium is the most abundant mineral in the body and is an essential body electrolyte. However, defining individual calcium requirements has proved difficult and guidelines vary widely by country and culture. Some authorities have adopted a factorial approach. For example, in the UK the dietary reference value (DRV) represents the apparent calcium requirements of healthy people under the prevailing dietary circumstances. The amount of calcium absorbed varies according to several factors including the requirements of the body, but is normally only about 30 to 40% of the dietary intake.

The richest dietary sources of calcium are milk and milk products. Significant amounts can also be consumed in green leafy vegetables, fortified flour, the soft bones of fish, and hard water.

**UK and US recommended dietary intake.** In the UK dietary reference values (DRV—see p.1419) have been published for calcium.[1] In the USA recommended dietary allowances (RDA) had been set,[2] but have been replaced by dietary reference intakes (see p.1419).[3] In the UK the estimated average requirement (EAR) for adults is 525 mg (13.1 mmol) daily and the reference nutrient intake (RNI) for adults is 700 mg (17.5 mmol) daily; these figures are based on a mean absorption of calcium of 30% from mixed diets. In the USA the traditional RDA was 800 mg daily for adults aged over 25 years; this figure was based on an absorption rate of 40%. Under the new dietary reference intakes, adequate intakes (AI) for calcium have been set, which are higher in some age groups than the previous RDAs.[3] For adults aged up to 50 years the AI is 1 g daily, and for those 51 years or older, it is 1.2 g daily.[3] The tolerable upper intake is considered to be 2.5 g daily.[3]


1. DoH. Dietary reference values for food energy and nutrients for the United Kingdom: report of the panel on dietary reference values of the committee on medical aspects of food policy. *Report on health and social subjects 41.* London: HMSO, 1991.
2. Subcommittee on the tenth edition of the RDAs, Food and Nutrition Board, Commission on Life Sciences, National Research Council. *Recommended dietary allowances.* 10th ed. Washington, DC: National Academy Press, 1989. Also available at: http://www.nap.edu/catalog/1349.html (accessed 03/06/04)
3. Standing Committee on the Scientific Evaluation of Dietary Reference Intakes of the Food and Nutrition Board. *Dietary Reference Intakes for calcium, phosphorus, magnesium, vitamin D, and fluoride.* Washington, DC: National Academy Press, 1999. Also available at: http://www.nap.edu/catalog/5776.html (accessed 03/06/04)


### Uses and Administration

Calcium salts are used in the management of **hypocalcaemia** (p.1218) and **calcium deficiency states** resulting from dietary deficiency or ageing (see also Osteoporosis, p.763). Doses may be expressed in terms of mmol or mEq of calcium, mass (mg) of calcium, or mass of calcium salt (for comparative purposes, see Table 1, below).

In simple deficiency states calcium salts may be given by mouth, usually in doses of 10 to 50 mmol (400 mg to 2 g) of calcium daily adjusted to the individual patient's requirements.

In severe acute hypocalcaemia or hypocalcaemic tetany parenteral administration is necessary, generally by slow intravenous injection or continuous infusion of calcium chloride or calcium gluconate (see also Administration, below). A typical dose is 2.25 to 4.5 mmol of calcium by slow intravenous injection, either repeated as required, or followed by continuous intravenous infusion of about 9 mmol daily. 2.25 mmol of calcium is provided by 10 mL of calcium gluconate 10%. Calcium gluceptate and calcium glycerophosphate with calcium lactate have been given by the intramuscular route; the chloride and gluconate are unsuitable for this route because of their irritancy. The intravenous route is used in children.

Intravenous calcium salts are also used to reverse the toxic cardiac effects of potassium in the emergency

**Table 1.** Some calcium salts and their calcium content.

| | Calcium content per g | | |
|---|---|---|---|
| Calcium salt | mg | mmol | mEq |
| Calcium acetate (anhydrous) | 253 | 6.3 | 12.6 |
| Calcium carbonate | 400 | 10.0 | 20.0 |
| Calcium chloride (dihydrate) | 273 | 6.8 | 13.6 |
| Calcium chloride (hexahydrate) | 183 | 4.6 | 9.1 |
| Calcium citrate (tetrahydrate) | 211 | 5.3 | 10.5 |
| Calcium glubionate (monohydrate) | 66 | 1.6 | 3.3 |
| Calcium glucoheptonate (anhydrous) | 82 | 2.0 | 4.1 |
| Calcium gluconate (monohydrate) | 89 | 2.2 | 4.5 |
| Calcium glycerophosphate (anhydrous) | 191 | 4.8 | 9.5 |
| Calcium lactate (anhydrous) | 184 | 4.6 | 9.2 |
| Calcium lactate (trihydrate) | 147 | 3.7 | 7.3 |
| Calcium lactate (pentahydrate) | 130 | 3.2 | 6.5 |
| Calcium lactate gluconate (dihydrate) | 129 | 3.2 | 6.4 |
| Calcium lactobionate (dihydrate) | 51 | 1.3 | 2.5 |
| Calcium levulinate (dihydrate) | 131 | 3.3 | 6.5 |
| Calcium hydrogen phosphate (dihydrate) | 233 | 5.8 | 11.6 |
| Calcium phosphate [$10CaO.3P_2O_5.H_2O$] | 399 | 10.0 | 19.9 |
| Calcium pidolate (anhydrous) | 135 | 3.4 | 6.7 |
| Calcium silicate [$CaSiO_3$] | 345 | 8.6 | 17.2 |
| Calcium sodium lactate (tetrahydrate) | 78 | 1.9 | 3.9 |

treatment of severe **hyperkalaemia** (p.1219), and as an antidote to magnesium in severe **hypermagnesaemia** (p.1218). For these indications, 2.25 to 4.5 mmol of calcium (10 to 20 mL of calcium gluconate 10%) is commonly used.

Individual calcium salts have specific uses. Calcium carbonate (p.1254) or acetate are effective phosphate binders and are given by mouth to reduce phosphate absorption from the gut in patients with **hyperphosphataemia**; this is particularly relevant to patients with chronic renal failure in order to prevent the development of renal osteodystrophy (p.764). The initial dose of calcium carbonate is 2.5 g daily titrated to a maximum of 17 g daily. A typical initial dose of calcium acetate is 3 or 4 g daily; most patients require 6 to 12 g daily.

Calcium carbonate and calcium silicate, given orally, are used for their **antacid** properties (p.1239).

Some of the calcium salts discussed here also have *pharmaceutical uses* as diluents in capsules and tablets, buffers and dissolution aids in dispersible tablets, disintegrant and anticaking agents, and as a basis or abrasive in dental preparations.

Calcium phosphate (Calcarea Phosphorica; Calc. Phos.) is used in homoeopathic medicine.

**Administration.** Some prefer calcium chloride to calcium gluconate for parenteral preparations,[1,2] because retention of the chloride is greater and more predictable than of the gluconate, and results in a more predictable increase in extracellular ionised calcium concentration. However, calcium chloride is considered to be the most irritant of the calcium salts in general use (see Adverse Effects, above).

Calcium gluconate has been given by the intraperitoneal route[3] for the treatment of chronic hypocalcaemia after parathyroidectomy in a patient undergoing continuous ambulatory peritoneal dialysis, resulting in improved systemic bioavailability compared with oral and intravenous administration.


1. Worthley LIG, Phillips PJ. Intravenous calcium salts. *Lancet* 1980; **ii:** 149.
2. Broner CW, *et al.* A prospective, randomized, double-blind comparison of calcium chloride and calcium gluconate therapies for hypocalcemia in critically ill children. *J Pediatr* 1990; **117:** 986–9.
3. Stamatakis MK, Seth SK. Treatment of chronic hypocalcemia with intraperitoneal calcium. *Am J Health-Syst Pharm* 1995; **52:** 201–3.


**Bites and stings.** Calcium gluconate 10% solution has been given intravenously as an alternative to the use of conventional muscle relaxants for the management of pain and muscle spasm associated with neurotoxic spider envenomation (p.1640). Mention has been made of such use of calcium in the management of *Latrodectus mactans* (black widow spider) envenomation.[1,2] Although the precise mechanism of action of calcium in the alleviation of neuromuscular symptoms is unknown it is believed to be due to the replenishment of calcium stores in the sarcoplasmic reticulum of muscle depleted by stimulation.


1. Binder LS. Acute arthropod envenomation: incidence, clinical features and management. *Med Toxicol Adverse Drug Exp* 1989; **4:** 163–73.
2. Woestman R, *et al.* The black widow: is she deadly to children? *Pediatr Emerg Care* 1996; **12:** 360–4.


**Bone disease.** Calcium is essential for the development and maintenance of normal bone, and calcium salts may be indicated in the treatment of some bone disorders associated with calcium deficiency, such as certain types of osteomalacia and rickets (p.762). Doses of 1 to 3 g of calcium daily are used in osteomalacia.

Oral calcium supplements can also be used as an adjunct in the management of osteoporosis (p.763) and corticosteroid-induced osteoporosis (see Effects on Bones and Joints, under Corticosteroids, p.1069).

**Cramps.** Calcium salts are one of a number of interventions that have been tried in the management of cramps (see Muscle Spasm, p.1386). However, evidence for these interventions is mostly lacking and a small systematic review concluded that oral calcium was not of benefit for leg cramps during pregnancy.[1]


1. Young GL, Jewell D. Interventions for leg cramps in pregnancy. Available in The Cochrane Library; Issue 2. Chichester: John Wiley; 2004.


**Diagnosis of insulinoma.** Calcium stimulates the release of insulin from insulinomas. Intra-arterial calcium gluconate, followed by hepatic venous sampling, has been found to be accurate and sensitive in the diagnosis and localisation of insulinomas,[1-3] even when other investigations have been negative.[4,5]


1. Doppman JL, *et al.* Localization of insulinomas to regions of the pancreas by intra-arterial stimulation with calcium. *Ann Intern Med* 1995; **123:** 269–73.
2. Lo CY, *et al.* Value of intra-arterial calcium stimulated venous sampling for regionalization of pancreatic insulinomas. *Surgery* 2000; **128:** 903–9.
3. Brändle M, *et al.* Assessment of selective arterial calcium stimulation and hepatic venous sampling to localize insulin-secreting tumours. *Clin Endocrinol (Oxf)* 2001; **55:** 357–62.
4. O'Shea D, *et al.* Localization of insulinomas by selective intraarterial calcium injection. *J Clin Endocrinol Metab* 1996; **81:** 1623–7.
5. Pereira PL, *et al.* Insulinoma and islet cell hyperplasia: value of the calcium intraarterial stimulation test when findings of other preoperative studies are negative. *Radiology* 1998; **206:** 703–9.


**Fluoride toxicity.** Inorganic fluoride is corrosive to skin and mucous membranes and acute intoxication disrupts many physiological systems; severe burns and profound hypocalcaemia may ensue. Absorption of the fluoride can be prevented by conversion to an insoluble form such as calcium fluoride and thus irrigation of skin (or gastric lavage as appropriate) with lime water, milk, or a 1% solution of calcium gluconate is recommended. Immediate treatment should also consist of 10 mL of calcium gluconate 10% intravenously, repeated after one hour; 30 mL should be given if tetany is present. In the short term affected skin and tissue should be injected with a 10% solution of calcium gluconate at a dose of 0.5 mL/cm$^2$ and burnt skin treated with a calcium gluconate 2.5% gel.[1]

See also under Hydrofluoric Acid, p.1699.


1. McIvor ME. Acute fluoride toxicity: pathophysiology and management. *Drug Safety* 1990; **5:** 79–85.


**Hypertension.** Meta-analysis suggests that calcium supplementation results in a small reduction in systolic and diastolic blood pressure.[1] Although the effect was too small to support the use of calcium supplementation for preventing or treating hypertension (p.825), it is possible that calcium supplementation might have beneficial effects on blood pressure in those with an inadequate intake. In a controlled trial, calcium with vitamin D supplementation reduced systolic blood pressure more effectively than calcium alone.[2]


1. Griffith LE, *et al.* The influence of dietary and nondietary calcium supplementation on blood pressure: an updated metaanalysis of randomized controlled trials. *Am J Hypertens* 1999; **12:** 84–92.
2. Pfeifer M, *et al.* Effects of a short-term vitamin $D_3$ and calcium supplementation on blood pressure and parathyroid hormone levels in elderly women. *J Clin Endocrinol Metab* 2001; **86:** 1633–7.


PREGNANCY. Despite an earlier meta-analysis[1] which concluded that calcium supplementation during pregnancy reduced systolic and diastolic blood pressure and the incidence of pre-eclampsia and hypertension, results from a double-blind, placebo-controlled trial in a total of 4589 women indicated that calcium supplementation during normal pregnancy did not prevent pre-eclampsia, pregnancy-associated hypertension without pre-eclampsia, and a number of other related disorders.[2] The inclusion criteria for the meta-analysis have been criticised.[3,4] However, subsequent systematic reviews also concluded that calcium supplementation reduced hypertension and pre-eclampsia in pregnant women, although the benefit was most pronounced in women at high risk of hypertension or in communities with low dietary calcium intake.[5,6]

For discussions of hypertension in pregnancy and eclampsia and pre-eclampsia, see p.825 and p.352, respectively.


1. Bucher HC, *et al.* Effect of calcium supplementation on pregnancy-induced hypertension and preeclampsia: a meta-analysis of randomized controlled trials. *JAMA* 1996; **275:** 1113–17. Correction. *ibid.*; **276:** 1388.
2. Levine RJ, *et al.* Trial of calcium to prevent preeclampsia. *N Engl J Med* 1997; **337:** 69–76.
3. Roberts JM, D'Abarno J. Effects of calcium supplementation on pregnancy-induced hypertension. *JAMA* 1996; **276:** 1386–7.
4. Levine R, DerSimonian R. Effects of calcium supplementation on pregnancy-induced hypertension. *JAMA* 1996; **276:** 1387.
5. DerSimonian R, Levine RJ. Resolving discrepancies between a meta-analysis and a subsequent large controlled trial. *JAMA* 1999; **282:** 664–70.
6. Atallah AN, *et al.* Calcium supplementation during pregnancy for preventing hypertensive disorders and related problems. Available in The Cochrane Library; Issue 2. Chichester: John Wiley; 2004.


**Malignant neoplasms.** There is some evidence that calcium supplementation may modestly reduce the risk[1,2] of colorectal cancer and its recurrence.[3-5]


1. Wu K, *et al.* Calcium intake and risk of colon cancer in women and men. *J Natl Cancer Inst* 2002; **94:** 437–46.
2. McCullough ML, *et al.* Calcium, vitamin D, dairy products, and risk of colorectal cancer in the Cancer Prevention Study II Nutrition Cohort (United States). *Cancer Causes Control* 2003; **14:** 1–12.
3. Baron JA, *et al.* Calcium supplements for the prevention of colorectal adenomas. *N Engl J Med* 1999; **340:** 101–7.
4. Bonithon-Kopp C, *et al.* Calcium and fibre supplementation in prevention of colorectal adenoma recurrence: a randomised intervention trial. *Lancet* 2000; **356:** 1300–6.
5. Martínez ME, *et al.* Calcium, vitamin D, and risk of adenoma recurrence (United States). *Cancer Causes Control* 2002; **13:** 213–20.


**Premenstrual syndrome.** Calcium supplementation was effective in relieving the luteal phase symptoms of premenstrual syndrome (p.1551) in 1 study.[1] A review of this and other studies suggested that calcium supplementation at a dose of 1.2 to 1.6 g daily should be considered in patients with premenstrual syndrome.[2]


1. Thys-Jacobs S, *et al.* Calcium carbonate and the premenstrual syndrome: effects on premenstrual and menstrual symptoms. *Am J Obstet Gynecol* 1998; **179:** 444–52.
2. Ward MW, Holimon TD. Calcium treatment for premenstrual syndrome. *Ann Pharmacother* 1999; **33:** 1356–8.


## Preparations

***BP 2003:*** Calcium and Ergocalciferol Tablets; Calcium Chloride Injection; Calcium Gluconate Injection; Calcium Gluconate Tablets; Calcium Lactate Tablets; Effervescent Calcium Gluconate Tablets;
***BPC 1973:*** Calcium with Vitamin D Tablets;
***USP 27:*** Aluminum Sulfate and Calcium Acetate Tablets for Topical Solution; Calcium Acetate Tablets; Calcium Chloride Injection; Calcium Glubionate Syrup; Calcium Gluceptate Injection; Calcium Gluconate Injection; Calcium Gluconate Tablets; Calcium Lactate Tablets; Calcium Levulinate Injection; Calcium with Vitamin D Tablets; Dibasic Calcium Phosphate Tablets; Half-strength Lactated Ringer's and Dextrose Injection; Lactated Ringer's and Dextrose Injection; Lactated Ringer's Injection; Potassium Chloride in Lactated Ringer's and Dextrose Injection.

**Proprietary Preparations** (details are given in Part 3)
***Arg.:*** Calcimax; Calcio Cit Simple; Calcium-Sandoz; Citramar; Ostram; Raffo-Ca; Regucal; Royen; ***Austral.:*** Celloids CP 57†; Citracal; Nephrex†; Sandocal†; ***Austria:*** Calcilin†; Calcium Fresenius; Calcium Novartis; Calcium-Sandoz; ***Belg.:*** Sandoz Calcium; ***Braz.:*** Bromocal†; Calcium-Sandoz; Calcium-Sandoz F; Miocalven; Osteocalcic; Ostram†; Phosfonema†; Solucalcine†; ***Canad.:*** Cal Gel†; Calais†; Calciject; Calcimax†; Calcium-Rougier; Calcium-Sandoz; ***Chile:*** Elcal I; Ostram; Phoslo; ***Denm.:*** Calcium-Sandoz; ***Fin.:*** Calcium-Sandoz; Phos-Ex; ***Fr.:*** CAL Ocean; Calcium Corbiere†; Calcium-Sandoz; Glucalcium†; Kalcikidz; Ostram; Sandocal†; ***Ger.:*** Calcipot†; Calciretard; Calcitrat; Calcium Eifelfango; Calcium Fresenius; Calcium-Sandoz; Cerasorb; Endobon; Eubiolac; Phos-Ex; RMS; ***Gr.:*** Neocalcit; Osteus; ***Hong Kong:*** Calcium Unison; Calcium-Sandoz; Citracal; Gluco-Calcium; Mega-Cal; Nephrex†; ***India:*** Calcium-Sandoz; Phosforid; ***Irl.:*** Calcium-Sandoz; Sandocal; ***Israel:*** Calcium-Sandoz; ***Ital.:*** Calcetat; Calcium-Sandoz; Rubrocalcium†; ***Malaysia:*** Ca Lac; Citracal; Trocium; ***Mex.:*** Bon-Ker; Calcium-Sandoz; Calcival; Ostram; Rical†; ***Neth.:*** Calcium-Sandoz; ***Norw.:*** Calcium-Sandoz; Phos-Ex; ***NZ:*** Calcium-Sandoz; ***Port.:*** Calcium-Sandoz; Sandocal; ***S.Afr.:*** Calcium-Sandoz; Kalci-300†; ***Singapore:*** Calcium-Sandoz; Citracal†; Hydrofluoric Acid Antidote; Os-Cal; ***Spain:*** Calbion†; Calcio 20 Emulsion; Calcium-Sandoz; Calcium-Sandoz Forte; Ibercal; Ostram; Royen; Tepox Cal; ***Swed.:*** Calcium-Sandoz; Ostram†; Phos-Ex; ***Switz.:*** Calcium-Sandoz; ***Thai.:*** Calcibon; Calcium Unison; Calcium-Sandoz; Calsorp; Caltrate; Lo-P-Caps; ***UK:*** Calcium-Sandoz; Ostram†; Phos-Ex; Sandocal; ***USA:*** Cal-Citrate; Cal-Lac; Calphron†; Citracal; Neo-Calglucon†; Oyster Calcium; PhosLo; Posture.

**Multi-ingredient:** numerous preparations are listed in Part 3.

# Magnesium

Magnesio.
Mg = 24.305.

**Description.** Magnesium is a cation given as various magnesium-containing salts.

**Incompatibility.** Magnesium salts have been reported to be incompatible with a wide range of drugs.

## Magnesium Acetate

Magnesii Acetas Tetrahydricus; Magnesio, acetato de.
$C_4H_6MgO_4,4H_2O$ = 214.5.
*CAS — 142-72-3 (anhydrous magnesium acetate); 16674-78-5 (magnesium acetate tetrahydrate).*

**Pharmacopoeias.** In *Eur.* (see p.vi).

**Ph. Eur. 5.0** (Magnesium Acetate Tetrahydrate). Colourless crystals or a white crystalline powder. Freely soluble in water and in alcohol. A 5% solution in water has a pH of 7.5 to 8.5.

**Equivalence.** Each g of magnesium acetate (tetrahydrate) represents approximately 4.7 mmol of magnesium and the equivalent of bicarbonate. Magnesium acetate (tetrahydrate) 8.83 g is approximately equivalent to 1 g of magnesium.

## Magnesium Ascorbate

Magnesio, ascorbato de.
$(C_6H_7O_6)_2Mg$ = 374.5.
*CAS — 15431-40-0.*

**Equivalence.** Each g of magnesium ascorbate (anhydrous) represents approximately 2.7 mmol of magnesium. Magnesium ascorbate (anhydrous) 15.4 g is approximately equivalent to 1 g of magnesium.

## Magnesium Aspartate

Magnesii Aspartas Dihydricus; Magnesio, aspartato de; Magnesium Aspartate Dihydrate. Magnesium aminosuccinate dihydrate; Magnesium di[(*S*)-2-aminohydrogenobutane-1,4-dioate].
$C_8H_{12}MgN_2O_8,2H_2O$ = 324.5.
*CAS — 18962-61-3 (anhydrous magnesium aspartate); 2068-80-6 (anhydrous magnesium aspartate or magnesium aspartate dihydrate); 7018-07-7 (magnesium aspartate tetrahydrate);.*
*ATC — A12CC05.*

**Pharmacopoeias.** *Eur.* (see p.vi) includes the dihydrate form of the (*S*)-aspartate. *Ger.* includes the tetrahydrate form of the racemic aspartate.

**Ph. Eur. 5.0** (Magnesium Aspartate Dihydrate; Magnesium Aspartate BP 2003). A white, crystalline powder or colourless crystals. Freely soluble in water. A 2.5% solution in water has a pH of 6.0 to 8.0.

**Equivalence.** Each g of magnesium aspartate (dihydrate) represents approximately 3.1 mmol of magnesium. Magnesium aspartate (dihydrate) 13.4 g is approximately equivalent to 1 g of magnesium.

Each g of magnesium aspartate (tetrahydrate) represents approximately 2.8 mmol of magnesium. Magnesium aspartate (tetrahydrate) 14.8 g is approximately equivalent to 1 g of magnesium.

## Magnesium Chloride

Chlorure de Magnésium Cristallisé; Cloreto de Magnésio; E511; Magnesio, cloruro de; Magnesium Chloratum.

$MgCl_2,xH_2O$ = 95.21 (anhydrous); 203.3 (hexahydrate).

*CAS — 7786-30-3 (anhydrous magnesium chloride); 7791-18-6 (magnesium chloride hexahydrate).*

*ATC — A12CC01; B05XA11.*

**Pharmacopoeias.** *Eur.* (see p.vi), *Pol., US,* and *Viet.* include the hexahydrate.

*Eur.* also includes magnesium chloride 4.5-hydrate.

**Ph. Eur. 5.0** (Magnesium Chloride Hexahydrate; Magnesii Chloridum Hexahydricum). Colourless, hygroscopic crystals. Very soluble in water; freely soluble in alcohol. Store in airtight containers.

**Ph. Eur. 5.0** (Magnesium Chloride 4.5-Hydrate; Magnesii Chloridum 4.5-Hydricum; Partially Hydrated Magnesium Chloride BP 2003). A white or almost white, hygroscopic, granular powder. Very soluble in water; freely soluble in alcohol. Store in airtight containers.

**USP 27** (Magnesium Chloride). Colourless, odourless, deliquescent flakes or crystals, which lose water when heated to 100° and lose hydrochloric acid when heated to 110°. Very soluble in water; freely soluble in alcohol. pH of a 5% solution in water is between 4.5 and 7.0. Store in airtight containers.

**Equivalence.** Each g of magnesium chloride (hexahydrate) represents approximately 4.9 mmol of magnesium and 9.8 mmol of chloride. Magnesium chloride (hexahydrate) 8.36 g is approximately equivalent to 1 g of magnesium.

## Magnesium Gluceptate

Magnesio, glucoheptonato de; Magnesium Glucoheptonate.

$C_{14}H_{26}MgO_{16}$ = 474.7.

**Equivalence.** Each g of magnesium gluceptate (anhydrous) represents approximately 2.1 mmol of magnesium. Magnesium gluceptate (anhydrous) 19.5 g is approximately equivalent to 1 g of magnesium.

## Magnesium Gluconate

Magnesio, gluconato de. Magnesium D-gluconate hydrate.

$C_{12}H_{22}MgO_{14}(+xH_2O)$ = 414.6 (anhydrous).

*CAS — 3632-91-5 (anhydrous magnesium gluconate); 59625-89-7 (magnesium gluconate dihydrate).*

*ATC — A12CC03.*

**Pharmacopoeias.** In *US* which allows either anhydrous or the dihydrate.

**USP 27** (Magnesium Gluconate). Colourless crystals or a white powder or granules. Is odourless. Freely soluble in water; very slightly soluble in alcohol; insoluble in ether. pH of a 5% solution in water is between 6.0 and 7.8.

**Equivalence.** Each g of magnesium gluconate (anhydrous) represents approximately 2.4 mmol of magnesium. Magnesium gluconate (anhydrous) 17.1 g is approximately equivalent to 1 g of magnesium.

## Magnesium Glycerophosphate

Magnesii Glycerophosphas; Magnesio, glicerofosfato de; Magnesium Glycerinophosphate.

$C_3H_7MgO_6P(+xH_2O)$ = 194.4 (anhydrous).

*CAS — 927-20-8 (anhydrous magnesium glycerophosphate).*

**Pharmacopoeias.** In *Eur.* (see p.vi).

**Ph. Eur. 5.0** (Magnesium Glycerophosphate). A mixture, in variable proportions, of magnesium *(R,S)*-2,3-dihydroxypropyl phosphate and magnesium 2-hydroxy-1-(hydroxymethyl)ethyl phosphate. It may be hydrated. A white, hygroscopic powder. Practically insoluble in alcohol; dissolves in dilute solutions of acids. Store in airtight containers.

**Equivalence.** Each g of magnesium glycerophosphate (anhydrous) represents approximately 5.1 mmol of magnesium. Magnesium glycerophosphate (anhydrous) 8 g is approximately equivalent to 1 g of magnesium.

## Magnesium Lactate

Magnesio, lactato de. Magnesium 2-hydroxypropionate.

$C_6H_{10}MgO_6$ = 202.4.

*CAS — 18917-93-6.*

*ATC — A12CC06.*

**Equivalence.** Each g of magnesium lactate (anhydrous) represents approximately 4.9 mmol of magnesium. Magnesium lactate (anhydrous) 8.33 g is approximately equivalent to 1 g of magnesium.

## Magnesium Phosphate

Magnesio, fosfato de; Tribasic Magnesium Phosphate; Trimagnesium Phosphate.

$Mg_3(PO_4)_2,5H_2O$ = 352.9.

*CAS — 7757-87-1 (anhydrous magnesium phosphate); 10233-87-1 (magnesium phosphate pentahydrate).*

*ATC — B05XA10.*

**Pharmacopoeias.** In *US.*

*Ger.* includes Dibasic Magnesium Phosphate Trihydrate (Magnesium Hydrogen Phosphate Trihydrate).

**USP 27** (Magnesium Phosphate). A white, odourless, powder. Almost insoluble in water; readily soluble in dilute mineral acids.

**Equivalence.** Each g of magnesium phosphate (pentahydrate) represents approximately 8.5 mmol of magnesium and 5.7 mmol of phosphate. Magnesium phosphate (pentahydrate) 4.84 g is approximately equivalent to 1 g of magnesium.

## Magnesium Pidolate *(pINNM)*

Magnesii Pidolas; Magnesium Pyroglutamate; Pidolato de magnesio. Magnesium 5-oxopyrrolidine-2-carboxylate.

$(C_5H_6NO_3)_2Mg$ = 280.5.

*CAS — 62003-27-4.*

*ATC — A12CC08.*

**Pharmacopoeias.** In *Eur.* (see p.vi).

**Ph. Eur. 5.0** (Magnesium Pidolate). An amorphous, white or almost white, hygroscopic powder. Very soluble in water; practically insoluble in dichloromethane; soluble in methyl alcohol. A 10% solution in water has a pH of 5.5 to 7.0. Store in airtight containers.

**Equivalence.** Each g of magnesium pidolate (anhydrous) represents approximately 3.6 mmol of magnesium. Magnesium pidolate (anhydrous) 11.5 g is approximately equivalent to 1 g of magnesium.

## Magnesium Sulfate

518; Epsom Salts; Magnesio, sulfato de; Magnesium Sulphate; Sal Amarum; Sel Anglais; Sel de Sedlitz.

$MgSO_4,xH_2O$ = 120.4 (anhydrous); 246.5 (heptahydrate).

*CAS — 7487-88-9 (anhydrous magnesium sulfate); 10034-99-8 (magnesium sulfate heptahydrate).*

*ATC — A06AD04; A12CC02; B05XA05; D11AX05; V04CC02.*

**Pharmacopoeias.** *Chin., Eur.* (see p.vi), *Jpn, Pol.,* and *Viet.* include the heptahydrate.

*US* allows the dried form, the monohydrate, or the heptahydrate form.

The dried form is included in *Br.* and *Pol.*

**Ph. Eur. 5.0** (Magnesium Sulphate Heptahydrate; Magnesii Sulfas Heptahydricus). A white, crystalline powder or brilliant, colourless crystals. Freely soluble in water; very soluble in boiling water; practically insoluble in alcohol.

The BP 2003 gives Epsom Salts as an approved synonym.

**BP 2003** (Dried Magnesium Sulphate). A white odourless or almost odourless powder, prepared by drying magnesium sulfate (heptahydrate) at 100° until it has lost about 25% of its weight; it contains 62 to 70% of $MgSO_4$. Freely soluble in water; more rapidly soluble in hot water.

The BP gives Dried Epsom Salts as an approved synonym.

**USP 27** (Magnesium Sulfate). It is the dried form, monohydrate, or the heptahydrate. Small, colourless crystals, usually needle-like. It effloresces in warm dry air. Soluble 1 in 0.8 of water and 1 in 0.5 of boiling water; freely but slowly soluble 1 in 1 of glycerol; sparingly soluble in alcohol. pH of a 5% solution in water is between 5.0 and 9.2.

**Equivalence.** Each g of magnesium sulfate (heptahydrate) represents approximately 4.1 mmol of magnesium. Magnesium sulfate (heptahydrate) 10.1 g is approximately equivalent to 1 g of magnesium.

### Adverse Effects

Excessive parenteral doses of magnesium salts lead to the development of hypermagnesaemia, important signs of which are loss of deep tendon reflexes and respiratory depression, both due to neuromuscular blockade. Other symptoms of hypermagnesaemia may include nausea, vomiting, flushing of the skin, thirst, hypotension due to peripheral vasodilatation, drowsiness, confusion, slurred speech, double vision, muscle weakness, bradycardia, coma, and cardiac arrest.

Hypermagnesaemia is uncommon after oral magnesium salts except in the presence of renal impairment. Ingestion of magnesium salts may cause gastrointestinal irritation and watery diarrhoea.

**Effects on the gastrointestinal tract.** There are isolated reports of paralytic ileus in patients receiving magnesium salts.[1,2] See also Pregnancy, under Precautions, below.


1. Hill WC, *et al.* Maternal paralytic ileus as a complication of magnesium sulfate tocolysis. *Am J Perinatol* 1985; **2:** 47–8.
2. Golzarian J, *et al.* Hypermagnesemia-induced paralytic ileus. *Dig Dis Sci* 1994; **39:** 1138–42.


**Hypersensitivity.** Hypersensitivity reactions characterised by urticaria were described in 2 women after receiving magnesium sulfate intravenously.[1]


1. Thorp JM, *et al.* Hypersensitivity to magnesium sulfate. *Am J Obstet Gynecol* 1989; **161:** 889–90.


### Treatment of Adverse Effects

The management of hypermagnesaemia is reviewed on p.1218.

**Hypermagnesaemia.** A patient with hypermagnesaemia of a degree that is normally fatal was successfully treated using assisted ventilation, calcium chloride administered intravenously, and forced diuresis with mannitol infusions.[1]


1. Bohman VR, Cotton DB. Supralethal magnesemia with patient survival. *Obstet Gynecol* 1990; **76:** 984–6.


### Precautions

Parenteral magnesium salts should generally be avoided in patients with heart block or severe renal impairment. They should be used with caution in less severe degrees of renal impairment and in patients with myasthenia gravis. Patients should be monitored for clinical signs of excess magnesium (see Adverse Effects, above), particularly when being treated for conditions not associated with hypomagnesaemia such as eclampsia. An intravenous preparation of a calcium salt should be available in case of toxicity. When used for hypomagnesaemia, serum-magnesium concentrations should be monitored.

Magnesium crosses the placenta. When used in pregnant women, fetal heart rate should be monitored and use within 2 hours of delivery should be avoided (see also Pregnancy, below).

Oral magnesium salts should be used cautiously in patients with renal impairment. Taking with food may decrease the incidence of diarrhoea. Chronic diarrhoea from long-term use may result in electrolyte imbalance.

**Breast feeding.** In breast milk samples from 10 pre-eclamptic women given magnesium sulfate, mean magnesium concentrations 24 hours after delivery were about 6.4 mg per 100 mL, and significantly higher than those in control subjects. However, by 48 and 72 hours after delivery, values were not significantly different. In both treated and control subjects, milk-magnesium concentrations were about twice those of maternal plasma concentrations. Although total doses of magnesium given to mothers may differ, the authors considered any increased magnesium load to a breast-fed infant to be quite small, about 1.5 mg of additional magnesium daily, and unlikely to significantly alter magnesium clearance from the neonate.[1] Based on this, the American Academy of Pediatrics considers that use of magnesium sulfate is therefore usually compatible with breast feeding.[2]


1. Cruikshank DP, *et al.* Breast milk magnesium and calcium concentrations following magnesium sulfate treatment. *Am J Obstet Gynecol* 1982; **143:** 685–8.
2. American Academy of Pediatrics. The transfer of drugs and other chemicals into human milk. *Pediatrics* 2001; **108:** 776–89. Correction. *ibid.*; 1029. Also available at: http://aappolicy.aappublications.org/cgi/content/full/pediatrics%3b108/3/776 (accessed 18/05/04)


**Hepatic disorders.** Severe hypermagnesaemia and hypercalcaemia developed in 2 patients with hepatic encephalopathy following the use of magnesium sulfate enemas; both patients died, one during and one after asystole. It was recommended that patients with liver disease who might develop renal impairment, or in whom renal failure is established, should not be prescribed enemas containing magnesium for treatment of hepatic encephalopathy as serious magnesium toxicity can occur, which may contribute to death.[1]


1. Collinson PO, Burroughs AK. Severe hypermagnesaemia due to magnesium sulphate enemas in patients with hepatic coma. *BMJ* 1986; **293:** 1013–14. Correction. *ibid.*; 1222.


**Pregnancy.** The meconium-plug syndrome (abdominal distention and failure to pass meconium) has been described in 2 neonates who were hypermagnesaemic after their mothers had received magnesium sulfate for eclampsia.[1] It was believed that the hypermagnesaemia may have depressed the function of intestinal smooth muscle. See also Effects on the Gastrointestinal Tract, above. In 36 hypermagnesaemic infants born to pre-eclamptic mothers treated with magnesium sulfate, significant neurobehavioural impairment persisted for over 24 hours after birth. Impairment was manifest by prolonged weakness in activities such as head lag, ventral suspension, suck reflex, and cry response; improvement corresponded to the decrease in plasma-magnesium concentrations.[2]

In studies in women with[3] and without[4] pre-eclampsia there were decreases in short-term fetal heart rate variability when women were given intravenous magnesium sulfate; however, although variability is considered a sign of fetal well-being the decrease was considered clinically insignificant.


1. Sokal MM, *et al.* Neonatal hypermagnesemia and the meconium-plug syndrome. *N Engl J Med* 1972; **286:** 823–5.
2. Rasch DK, *et al.* Neurobehavioral effects of neonatal hypermagnesemia. *J Pediatr* 1982; **100:** 272–6.
3. Atkinson MW, *et al.* The relation between magnesium sulfate therapy and fetal heart rate variability. *Obstet Gynecol* 1994; **83:** 967–70.
4. Hallak M, *et al.* The effect of magnesium sulfate on fetal heart rate parameters: a randomized, placebo-controlled trial. *Am J Obstet Gynecol* 1999; **181:** 1122–7.

## Interactions

Parenteral administration of magnesium sulfate potentiates the effects of competitive and depolarising neuromuscular blockers (p.1401). The neuromuscular blocking effects of parenteral magnesium and aminoglycoside antibacterials may be additive. Similarly, parenteral magnesium sulfate and nifedipine have been reported to have additive effects (p.969).

Oral magnesium salts decrease the absorption of tetracyclines and bisphosphonates, and administration should be separated by a number of hours.

## Pharmacokinetics

About one-third of magnesium is absorbed from the small intestine after oral doses and even soluble magnesium salts are generally very slowly absorbed. The fraction of magnesium absorbed increases if magnesium intake decreases. In plasma, about 25 to 30% of magnesium is protein bound. Parenterally administered magnesium salts are excreted mainly in the urine, and orally administered magnesium salts are eliminated in the urine (absorbed fraction) and the faeces (unabsorbed fraction). Small amounts are distributed into breast milk. Magnesium crosses the placenta.

## Human Requirements

Magnesium is the second most abundant cation in intracellular fluid and is an essential body electrolyte which is a cofactor in numerous enzyme systems.

The body is very efficient at maintaining magnesium concentrations by regulating absorption and renal excretion, and symptoms of deficiency are rare. It is therefore difficult to establish a daily requirement.

Foods rich in magnesium include nuts, unmilled grains, and green vegetables.

**UK and US recommended dietary intake.** In the United Kingdom dietary reference values (DRV—see p.1419)[1] and in the United States recommended daily allowances (RDA)[2] have been published for magnesium. In the UK the estimated average requirement (EAR) is 200 mg (or 8.2 mmol) daily for adult females and 250 mg (or 10.3 mmol) daily for adult males; the reference nutrient intake (RNI) is 270 mg (or 10.9 mmol) daily for adult females and 300 mg (or 12.3 mmol) daily for adult males; no increment is recommended during pregnancy but an increment of 50 mg (or 2.1 mmol) daily in the RNI is advised during lactation. In the USA under the new dietary reference intakes an EAR of 330 to 350 mg daily has been set in adult males and 255 to 265 mg daily in adult females; the corresponding RDAs are 400 to 420 mg and 310 to 320 mg daily.[2] An increase in RDA to 350 to 360 mg is recommended during pregnancy but the standard RDA is considered adequate during lactation. A tolerable upper intake level of 350 mg daily has been set for adults.[2]

1. DoH. Dietary reference values for food energy and nutrients for the United Kingdom: report of the panel on dietary reference values of the committee on medical aspects of food policy. *Report on health and social subjects 41*. London: HMSO, 1991.
2. Standing Committee on the Scientific Evaluation of Dietary Reference Intakes of the Food and Nutrition Board. *Dietary Reference Intakes for calcium, phosphorus, magnesium, vitamin D, and fluoride*. Washington, DC: National Academy Press, 1999. Also available at: http://www.nap.edu/catalog/5776.html (accessed 03/06/04)

## Uses and Administration

Magnesium salts have a variety of actions and uses. Many are given as a source of magnesium ions in the treatment of **magnesium deficiency and hypomagnesaemia** (p.1219). Doses may be expressed in terms of mmol or mEq of magnesium, mass (mg) of magnesium, or mass of magnesium salt (for comparative purposes, see Table 2, opposite).

In simple deficiency states magnesium salts may be given by mouth in doses of up to 50 mmol of magnesium daily adjusted according to individual requirements. Salts that are, or have been, used include magnesium aspartate, magnesium chloride, magnesium gluceptate, magnesium gluconate, magnesium glycerophosphate, magnesium lactate, magnesium levulinate, magnesium orotate, and magnesium pidolate. In acute or severe hypomagnesaemia, magnesium may be given parenterally, usually as the chloride or sulfate. A suggested regimen is 35 to 75 mmol of magnesium given by slow intravenous infusion (in glucose 5%) on the first day followed by 25 mmol daily until the hypomagnesaemia is corrected; up to a total of 160 mmol may be required. Alternatively, magnesium sulfate has been given by intramuscular or slow intravenous injection. Careful monitoring of plasma-magnesium and other electrolyte concentrations is essential. Doses should be reduced in renal impairment. Other salts which are, or have been, used parenterally include magnesium acetate, magnesium ascorbate, magnesium aspartate hydrochloride, magnesium levulinate, and magnesium pidolate.

Several magnesium salts such as the carbonate, hydroxide, oxide, and trisilicate are widely used for their **antacid** properties (p.1239). Magnesium salts also act as **osmotic laxatives** (see Constipation, p.1240); the salts generally used for this purpose are magnesium sulfate (an oral dose of 5 to 10 g in 250 mL of water being administered for rapid bowel evacuation) and magnesium hydroxide (p.1272).

Parenterally administered magnesium sulfate has some specific uses. It is used for the emergency treatment of some **arrhythmias** such as torsade de pointes (p.816) and those associated with hypokalaemia (p.1219). The usual dose is 2 g of magnesium sulfate (8 mmol of magnesium) given intravenously over 10 to 15 minutes and repeated once if necessary.

Parenteral magnesium sulfate is also used for the prevention of recurrent seizures in pregnant women with **eclampsia** (see below). A variety of dosage regimens have been used and debate continues as to which is most appropriate. Typically an intravenous loading dose of 4 g of magnesium sulfate (16 mmol of magnesium) is administered over 5 to 15 minutes. This is then followed by either an infusion of 1 g (4 mmol magnesium) per hour or deep intramuscular administration of 5 g (20 mmol magnesium) into each buttock then 5 g intramuscularly every 4 hours for at least 24 hours after the last seizure. Should seizures recur under either regimen, then an additional intravenous dose of 2 to 4 g can be given. It is essential to monitor for signs of hypermagnesaemia, and to stop magnesium administration should this occur. Doses should be reduced in renal impairment.

The use of magnesium sulfate in **acute myocardial infarction** and **premature labour** is discussed below.

Dried magnesium sulfate has been used in the form of Magnesium Sulphate Paste (BP 2003) as an application to inflammatory skin conditions such as boils and carbuncles, but prolonged or repeated use may damage the surrounding skin.

◊ General references.

1. McLean RM. Magnesium and its therapeutic uses: a review. *Am J Med* 1994; **96:** 63–76.
2. Fawcett WJ, *et al.* Magnesium: physiology and pharmacology. *Br J Anaesth* 1999; **83:** 302–20.
3. Fox C, *et al.* Magnesium: its proven and potential clinical significance. *South Med J* 2001; **94:** 1195–1201.

**Anaesthesia.** Magnesium sulfate has been used to prevent the undesirable haemodynamic response sometimes associated with intubation (p.1397). It has also been tried in the treatment of postanaesthetic shivering (p.1295).

**Table 2.** Some magnesium salts and their magnesium content.

| Magnesium salt | Magnesium content per g | | |
|---|---|---|---|
| | mg | mmol | mEq |
| Magnesium acetate (tetrahydrate) | 113 | 4.7 | 9.3 |
| Magnesium ascorbate (anhydrous) | 65 | 2.7 | 5.3 |
| Magnesium aspartate (dihydrate) | 75 | 3.1 | 6.2 |
| Magnesium aspartate (tetrahydrate) | 67 | 2.8 | 5.5 |
| Magnesium chloride (hexahydrate) | 120 | 4.9 | 9.8 |
| Magnesium gluceptate (anhydrous) | 51 | 2.1 | 4.2 |
| Magnesium gluconate (anhydrous) | 59 | 2.4 | 4.8 |
| Magnesium glycerophosphate (anhydrous) | 125 | 5.1 | 10.3 |
| Magnesium lactate (anhydrous) | 120 | 4.9 | 9.9 |
| Magnesium phosphate (pentahydrate) | 207 | 8.5 | 17.0 |
| Magnesium pidolate (anhydrous) | 87 | 3.6 | 7.1 |
| Magnesium sulfate (heptahydrate) | 99 | 4.1 | 8.1 |

**Eclampsia and pre-eclampsia.** Magnesium sulfate has become the preferred treatment for seizures associated with **eclampsia** (p.352). Studies and systematic reviews have shown it to be more effective than phenytoin,[1,2] diazepam,[1,3] or lytic cocktail,[4] as well as causing fewer adverse effects. Its advantages included a rapid effect and lack of sedation in the mother or the infant.[5] It was also considered to have a wide safety margin with the added security of calcium gluconate being an easily available antidote should overdose occur. Subsequent meta-analysis[6] and systematic review[2-4] reinforced this favourable view.

Magnesium sulfate may also be used to prevent eclampsia in **pre-eclamptic** patients; trials have shown it to be more effective than phenytoin,[7] or nimodipine.[8] A randomised placebo-controlled trial[9] involving over 10 000 women in 33 countries found that treatment with magnesium sulfate approximately halved the risk of developing eclampsia; the number of maternal deaths was also less in the treatment group although the differences in risk between this group and the placebo group were not significant.

Despite some concerns about the effects of *early* use of magnesium sulfate on the fetus (see Premature Labour, below), many,[10,11] including WHO, consider magnesium sulfate the drug of choice for both treatment and prevention of eclampsia.

1. The Eclampsia Trial Collaborative Group. Which anticonvulsant for women with eclampsia: evidence from the Collaborative Eclampsia Trial. *Lancet* 1995; **345:** 1455–63. Correction. *ibid.*; **346:** 258.
2. Duley L, Henderson-Smart D. Magnesium sulphate versus phenytoin for eclampsia. Available in The Cochrane Library; Issue 2. Chichester: John Wiley; 2004.
3. Duley L, Henderson-Smart D. Magnesium sulphate versus diazepam for eclampsia. Available in The Cochrane Library; Issue 2. Chichester: John Wiley; 2004.
4. Duley L, Gulmezoglu AM. Magnesium sulphate versus lytic cocktail for eclampsia. Available in The Cochrane Library; Issue 2. Chichester: John Wiley; 2004.
5. Saunders N, Hammersley B. Magnesium for eclampsia. *Lancet* 1995; **346:** 788–9.
6. Chien PFW, *et al.* Magnesium sulphate in the treatment of eclampsia and pre-eclampsia: an overview of the evidence from randomised trials. *Br J Obstet Gynaecol* 1996; **103:** 1085–91.
7. Lucas MJ, *et al.* A comparison of magnesium sulfate with phenytoin for the prevention of eclampsia. *N Engl J Med* 1995; **333:** 201–5.
8. Belfort MA, *et al.* A comparison of magnesium sulfate and nimodipine for the prevention of eclampsia. *N Engl J Med* 2003; **348:** 304–11.
9. The Magpie Trial Collaborative Group. Do women with pre-eclampsia, and their babies, benefit from magnesium sulphate? The Magpie Trial: a randomised placebo-controlled trial. *Lancet* 2002; **359:** 1877–90.
10. Roberts JM, *et al.* Preventing and treating eclamptic seizures. *BMJ* 2002; **325:** 609–10.
11. WHO. Managing complications in pregnancy and childbirth: a guide for midwives and doctors: headache, blurred vision, convulsions or loss of consciousness, elevated blood pressure. Available at: http://www.who.int/reproductive-health/impac/Symptoms/Headache_blood_pressure_S35_S56.html (accessed 18/05/04)

**Hypokalaemia.** Potassium and magnesium homoeostasis are linked, and hypokalaemia with increased urine potassium excretion may occur in patients with hypomagnesaemia. In this situation, correction of potassium deficit usually requires concomitant magnesium administration. Administration of magnesium sulfate at doses greater than those required to correct hypomagnesaemia has been associated with greater improvements in potassium balance than doses just sufficient to correct hypomagnesaemia.[1]

1. Hamill-Ruth RJ, McGory R. Magnesium repletion and its effect on potassium homeostasis in critically ill adults: results of a double-blind, randomized, controlled trial. *Crit Care Med* 1996; **24:** 38–45.

**Migraine.** Low magnesium concentrations are thought to be important in the pathogenesis of migraine (p.464), but the precise role of magnesium supplementation in the disorder remains to be determined.[1] In a double-blind study,[2] 24 mmol magnesium daily (in the form of magnesium citrate) reduced the incidence of migraine headache by 42% compared with a reduction of 16% with placebo. However, in another similar study,[3] 20 mmol magnesium daily (in the form of magnesium aspartate hydrochloride) was no more effective than placebo in producing a 50% reduction in migraine frequency or intensity. Intravenous magnesium sulfate has shown benefit in the treatment of migraine attacks,[4] especially in those with aura,[5,6] or in patients with low serum-magnesium levels.[7]

1. Mauskop A, Altura BM. Role of magnesium in the pathogenesis and treatment of migraines. *Clin Neurosci* 1998; **5:** 24–7.
2. Peikert A, *et al.* Prophylaxis of migraine with oral magnesium: results from a prospective, multi-center, placebo-controlled and double-blind randomized study. *Cephalalgia* 1996; **16:** 257–63.
3. Pfaffenrath V, *et al.* Magnesium in the prophylaxis of migraine: a double-blind placebo-controlled study. *Cephalalgia* 1996; **16:** 436–40.
4. Demirkaya Ş, *et al.* Efficacy of intravenous magnesium sulfate in the treatment of acute migraine attacks. *Headache* 2001; **41:** 171–7.
5. Bigal ME, *et al.* Intravenous magnesium sulphate in the acute treatment of migraine without aura and migraine with aura: a randomized, double-blind, placebo-controlled study. *Cephalalgia* 2002; **22:** 345–53.
6. Bigal ME, *et al.* Eficácia de três drogas sobre a aura migranosa: um estudo randomizado placebo controlado. *Arq Neuropsiquiatr* 2002; **60:** 406–9.
7. Mauskop A, *et al.* Intravenous magnesium sulphate relieves migraine attacks in patients with low serum ionized magnesium levels: a pilot study. *Clin Sci* 1995; **89:** 633–6.

**Myocardial infarction.** Magnesium has an important physiological role in maintaining the ion balance in muscle including the myocardium. Magnesium might have an antiarrhythmic effect and might protect the myocardium against reperfusion injury including myocardial stunning (delayed recovery of myocardial contractility function). Intravenous magnesium salts have been used for cardiac arrhythmias and in an overview of studies in patients with suspected myocardial infarction their administration, generally within 12 hours of the onset of chest pain, had reduced mortality.[1] The beneficial effect on mortality appeared to be confirmed by the LIMIT-2 study[2] in which 8 mmol of magnesium was given by intravenous injection before thrombolysis and followed by a maintenance infusion of 65 mmol over the next 24 hours. Benefit was confirmed at follow-up an average of 2.7 years later;[3] however, there was no evidence of an antiarrhythmic effect. These beneficial effects were not borne out by the larger ISIS-4 study,[4] although there were slight differences in the magnesium regimen and its timing which might have played a part in these contradictory results. In an attempt to resolve the controversy, the MAGIC trial[5] was designed to test the hypothesis that early administration of magnesium in a similar dose to that used in the LIMIT-2 study would reduce short-term mortality in patients with ST elevation myocardial infarction. No benefit or harm of magnesium was observed, and at present the routine use of magnesium in myocardial infarction (p.828) cannot be recommended.

Patients with acute myocardial infarction may have magnesium deficiency and long-term treatment with oral magnesium has been tried, but in one study was associated with an increased risk of adverse cardiac events and could not be recommended for secondary prevention.[6]


1. Teo KK, *et al.* Effects of intravenous magnesium in suspected acute myocardial infarction: overview of randomised trials. *BMJ* 1991; **303:** 1499–1503.
2. Woods KL, *et al.* Intravenous magnesium sulphate in suspected acute myocardial infarction: results of the second Leicester Intravenous Magnesium Intervention Trial (LIMIT-2). *Lancet* 1992; **339:** 1553–8.
3. Woods KL, Fletcher S. Long-term outcome after intravenous magnesium sulphate in suspected acute myocardial infarction: the second Leicester Intravenous Magnesium Intervention Trial (LIMIT-2). *Lancet* 1994; **343:** 816–19.
4. Fourth International Study of Infarct Survival Collaborative Group. ISIS–4: a randomised factorial trial assessing early oral captopril, oral mononitrate, and intravenous magnesium sulphate in 58 050 patients with suspected acute myocardial infarction. *Lancet* 1995; **345:** 669–85.
5. The Magnesium in Coronaries (MAGIC) Trial Investigators. Early administration of intravenous magnesium to high-risk patients with acute myocardial infarction in the Magnesium in Coronaries (MAGIC) trial: a randomised controlled trial. *Lancet* 2002; **360:** 1189–96.
6. Galløe AM, *et al.* Influence of oral magnesium supplementation on cardiac events among survivors of an acute myocardial infarction. *BMJ* 1993; **307:** 585–7.


**Porphyria.** Magnesium sulfate is one of the drugs that has been used for seizure prophylaxis in patients with porphyria (p.353) who continue to experience convulsions while in remission.

**Premature labour.** Magnesium sulfate has been given intravenously to suppress initial uterine contractions in the management of premature labour[1-3] (p.794). Although it has been found to possess similar efficacy to beta$_2$ agonists,[4,5] and is widely used in the USA in particular, a systematic review[6] has concluded it is ineffective at delaying birth or preventing preterm birth. Other magnesium salts have also sometimes been given by mouth.[7,8] Retrospective observational studies found a lower incidence of cerebral palsy in children with birth-weights of less than 1500 g when mothers were treated with magnesium sulfate for pre-eclampsia, eclampsia or premature labour.[9,10] However, increased total paediatric mortality was noted in an interim analysis of a trial of antenatal magnesium sulfate in preterm labour,[11] and the trial was subsequently discontinued. Although they considered the safety of magnesium sulfate well established in gestation at term, the authors cautioned against the use of magnesium sulfate in very preterm labour. Subsequent studies found that magnesium sulfate was associated with increased perinatal mortality in low birth-weight offspring, particularly when doses of more than 48 g were used,[12] and that neonates with intraventricular haemorrhage (p.740) had mothers with higher serum-magnesium concentrations at delivery.[13] Some studies have commented[14,15] on other results, including trials of magnesium for treatment and prevention of eclampsia (see above), and have concluded, along with a systematic review[6] that its use as a tocolytic increases the risk of infant mortality.


1. Amon E, *et al.* Tocolysis with advanced cervical dilatation. *Obstet Gynecol* 2000; **95:** 358–62.
2. Terrone DA, *et al.* A prospective, randomized, controlled trial of high and low maintenance doses of magnesium sulfate for acute tocolysis. *Am J Obstet Gynecol* 2000; **182:** 1477–82.
3. Katz VL, Farmer RM. Controversies in tocolytic therapy. *Clin Obstet Gynecol* 1999; **42:** 802–19.
4. Wilkins IA, *et al.* Efficacy and side effects of magnesium sulfate and ritodrine as tocolytic agents. *Am J Obstet Gynecol* 1988; **159:** 685–9.
5. Chau AC, *et al.* A prospective comparison of terbutaline and magnesium for tocolysis. *Obstet Gynecol* 1992; **80:** 847–51.
6. Crowther CA, *et al.* Magnesium sulphate for preventing preterm birth in threatened preterm labour. Available in The Cochrane Library; Issue 2. Chichester: John Wiley; 2004.
7. Martin RW, *et al.* Comparison of oral ritodrine and magnesium gluconate for ambulatory tocolysis. *Am J Obstet Gynecol* 1988; **158:** 1440–3.
8. Ridgway LE, *et al.* A prospective randomized comparison of oral terbutaline and magnesium oxide for the maintenance of tocolysis. *Am J Obstet Gynecol* 1990; **163:** 879–82.
9. Nelson KB, Grether JK. Can magnesium sulfate reduce the risk of cerebral palsy in very low birthweight infants? *Pediatrics* 1995; **95:** 263–9.
10. Schendel DE, *et al.* Prenatal magnesium sulfate exposure and the risk for cerebral palsy or mental retardation among very low-birth-weight children aged 3 to 5 years. *JAMA* 1996; **276:** 1805–10.
11. Mittendorf R, *et al.* Is tocolytic magnesium sulphate associated with increased total paediatric mortality? *Lancet* 1997; **350:** 1517–18.
12. Scudiero R, *et al.* Perinatal death and tocolytic magnesium sulfate. *Obstet Gynecol* 2000; **96:** 178–82.
13. Mittendorf R, *et al.* Association between maternal serum ionized magnesium levels at delivery and neonatal intraventricular hemorrhage. *J Pediatr* 2002; **140:** 540–6.
14. Mittendorf R, *et al.* If tocolytic magnesium sulfate is associated with excess total pediatric mortality, what is its impact? *Obstet Gynecol* 1998; **92:** 308–11.
15. Mittendorf R, *et al.* The Magpie trial. *Lancet* 2002; **360:** 1330–1.


**Pulmonary hypertension of the newborn.** Preliminary studies have suggested that intravenous magnesium sulfate may be effective in treating persistent pulmonary hypertension of the newborn, as mentioned on p.832.

**Respiratory disorders.** Magnesium sulfate, given intravenously over 20 minutes in doses of 1.2 g to patients with acute exacerbations of chronic obstructive pulmonary disease (p.779) who had received inhaled salbutamol, appeared to have moderate efficacy.[1]

Infusion of magnesium has been reported to be of benefit in some patients with acute asthma (p.777), but results have been conflicting;[2-5] meta-analyses of these and other studies concluded that its routine use was not justified, but that it may benefit some patients with severe exacerbations.[6,7] Inhalation of magnesium has also been investigated, with promising results, either alone[8] or with salbutamol.[9,10]


1. Skorodin MS, *et al.* Magnesium sulfate in exacerbations of chronic obstructive pulmonary disease. *Arch Intern Med* 1995; **155:** 496–500.
2. Skobeloff EM, *et al.* Intravenous magnesium sulfate for the treatment of acute asthma in the emergency department. *JAMA* 1989; **262:** 1210–13.
3. Green SM, Rothrack SG. Intravenous magnesium for acute asthma: failure to decrease emergency treatment duration or need for hospitalization. *Ann Emerg Med* 1992; **21:** 260–5.
4. Ciarallo L, *et al.* Intravenous magnesium therapy for moderate to severe pediatric asthma: results of a randomized, placebo-controlled trial. *J Pediatr* 1996; **129:** 809–14.
5. Silverman RA, *et al.* IV magnesium sulfate in the treatment of acute severe asthma: a multicenter randomized controlled trial. *Chest* 2002; **122:** 489–97.
6. Rowe BH, *et al.* Magnesium sulfate for treating exacerbations of acute asthma in the emergency department. Available in The Cochrane Library; Issue 2. Chichester: John Wiley; 2004.
7. Alter HJ, *et al.* Intravenous magnesium as an adjuvant in acute bronchospasm: a meta-analysis. *Ann Emerg Med* 2000; **36:** 191–7.
8. Mangat HS, *et al.* Nebulized magnesium sulphate versus nebulized salbutamol in acute bronchial asthma: a clinical trial. *Eur Respir J* 1998; **12:** 341–4.
9. Nannini LJ, *et al.* Magnesium sulfate as a vehicle for nebulized salbutamol in acute asthma. *Am J Med* 2000; **108:** 193–7.
10. Hughes R, *et al.* Use of isotonic nebulised magnesium sulphate as an adjuvant to salbutamol in treatment of severe asthma in adults: randomised placebo-controlled trial. *Lancet* 2003; **361:** 2114–17.


**Tetanus.** Magnesium sulfate has been found to minimise autonomic disturbance in ventilated patients and control spasms in non-ventilated patients when used in the treatment of tetanus (p.1398).

References.


1. Attygalle D, Rodrigo N. Magnesium as first line therapy in the management of tetanus: a prospective study of 40 patients. *Anaesthesia* 2002; **57:** 811–17.
2. William S. Use of magnesium to treat tetanus. *Br J Anaesth* 2002; **88:** 152–3.


## Preparations

***BP 2003:*** Magnesium Chloride Injection; Magnesium Sulphate Injection; Magnesium Sulphate Mixture; Magnesium Sulphate Paste;
***USP 27:*** Magnesium Gluconate Tablets; Magnesium Sulfate in Dextrose Injection; Magnesium Sulfate Injection.

**Proprietary Preparations** (details are given in Part 3)
***Arg.:*** Biomag; Holomagnesio; Magnebe; Magnesoide; ***Austral.:*** Celloids MP 65†; Mag 50†; Magmin†; ***Austria:*** Cormagnesin; Emgecard; FX Passage; Magium; Magnesium Diasporal; Magvital; Mg 5-Longoral; Solumag; Ultra-Mag; ***Belg.:*** Magnespasmyl; Ultra-Mg; ***Braz.:*** Magnolat; Magnoston; Pidomag; ***Canad.:*** Mag 2†; Maglucate; Magnolex; Magnorol; Proflavanol C; Slow-Mag; ***Chile:*** Mag-Tab; ***Fr.:*** Efimag; Ionimag; Mag 2; Magnespasmyl; Magnogene; Megamag; Solumag; Spasmag; Top-Mag; Vivamag; ***Ger.:*** Basti-Mag; Cormagnesin; FX Passage; Magium; Magnaspart; Magnerot; Magnerot A; magnerot Classic; Magnesiocard; Magnesium Diasporal; Magnesium Tonil†; Magnesium Verla; Magnesorot; Magnorbin†; metamagnesol; Mg 5-Granulat; Mg 5-Longoral; Mg 5-Sulfat; Mg-nor; Nourymag; Power Orot; ***Gr.:*** Mag 2; ***Ital.:*** Actimag; Mag 2; MG 50; Olimag; Solumag; ***Mex.:*** Conducat; Ifupeptol Magnesiado; Magnefusin; ***Mon.:*** Oromag; ***Port.:*** Magnesiocard; Magnesona; Magnespasmil; Magnoral; ***S.Afr.:*** Be-Lax; Magnesit; Slow-Mag; ***Spain:*** Actimag; Mag 2†; Magnesioboi; Sulmetin; ***Switz.:*** Mag 2; Mag-Min; Magnesiocard; Magnesium Biomed; Magnesium Vital; Magnespasmyl; Magnogene; Magvital†; Mg 5-Granoral; Mg 5-Longoral; Mg 5-Oraleff; Mg 5-Sulfat; Solmag; ***UK:*** Kest; ***USA:*** Almora; Mag-G; Mag-SR; Mag-Tab SR; Magtrate; Slow-Mag.

**Multi-ingredient:** numerous preparations are listed in Part 3.

---

# Phosphate

Fosfato.

**Description.** Phosphate is an anion given as various potassium or sodium salts.

**Incompatibility.** Phosphates are incompatible with calcium salts; the mixing of calcium and phosphate salts can lead to the formation of insoluble calcium-phosphate precipitates. Incompatibility has also been reported with magnesium salts.

## Monobasic Potassium Phosphate

E340; Fosfato de potasio, dihidrógeno; Kalii Dihydrogenophosphas; Monopotassium Phosphate; Potassium Acid Phosphate; Potassium Biphosphate; Potassium Dihydrogen Phosphate. Potassium dihydrogen orthophosphate.

$KH_2PO_4$ = 136.1.
*CAS — 7778-77-0.*

**Pharmacopoeias.** In *Eur.* (see p.vi). Also in *USNF.*

**Ph. Eur. 5.0** (Potassium Dihydrogen Phosphate). A white, crystalline powder or colourless crystals. Freely soluble in water; practically insoluble in alcohol. A 5% solution in water has a pH of 4.2 to 4.5.

**USNF 22** (Monobasic Potassium Phosphate). Colourless crystals or a white granular or crystalline powder. Is odourless. Freely soluble in water; practically insoluble in alcohol. pH of a 1% solution in water is about 4.5. Store in airtight containers.

**Equivalence.** Each g of monobasic potassium phosphate represents approximately 7.3 mmol of potassium and of phosphate.

## Dibasic Potassium Phosphate

Dikalii Phosphas; Dipotassium Hydrogen Phosphate; Dipotassium Phosphate; E340; Fosfato de potasio, hidrógeno; Potassium Phosphate. Dipotassium hydrogen orthophosphate.

$K_2HPO_4$ = 174.2.
*CAS — 7758-11-4.*

**Pharmacopoeias.** In *Eur.* (see p.vi) and *US.*

**Ph. Eur. 5.0** (Dipotassium Phosphate; Dipotassium Hydrogen Phosphate BP 2003). A very hygroscopic, white powder or colourless crystals. Very soluble in water; very slightly soluble in alcohol. Store in airtight containers.

**USP 27** (Dibasic Potassium Phosphate). Colourless or white, somewhat hygroscopic, granular powder. Freely soluble in water; very slightly soluble in alcohol. pH of a 5% solution in water is between 8.5 and 9.6.

**Equivalence.** Each g of dibasic potassium phosphate represents approximately 11.5 mmol of potassium and 5.7 mmol of phosphate.

## Monobasic Sodium Phosphate

E339; Fosfato de sodio, dihidrógeno; Natrii Dihydrogenophosphas; Natrium Phosphoricum Monobasicum; Sodium Acid Phosphate; Sodium Biphosphate; Sodium Dihydrogen Phosphate. Sodium dihydrogen orthophosphate.

$NaH_2PO_4,xH_2O$.
*CAS — 7558-80-7 (anhydrous monobasic sodium phosphate); 10049-21-5 (monobasic sodium phosphate monohydrate); 13472-35-0 (monobasic sodium phosphate dihydrate); 10028-24-7 (monobasic sodium phosphate dihydrate).*
*ATC — A06AD17; A06AG01.*

**Pharmacopoeias.** In *Eur.* (see p.vi) and *Pol.* (with $2H_2O$); in *Chin.* (with $1H_2O$). *Br.* also includes monographs for the anhydrous and monohydrate forms. *US* permits the anhydrous, monohydrate, and dihydrate forms.

**Ph. Eur. 5.0** (Sodium Dihydrogen Phosphate Dihydrate; Natrii Dihydrogenophosphas Dihydricus). A white powder or colourless crystals. Very soluble in water; very slightly soluble in alcohol. A 5% solution in water has a pH of 4.2 to 4.5.

The BP 2003 gives Sodium Acid Phosphate as an approved synonym.

**BP 2003** (Anhydrous Sodium Dihydrogen Phosphate). A white, slightly deliquescent, crystals or granules. Very soluble in water; very slightly soluble in alcohol. A 5% solution in water has a pH of 4.2 to 4.5.

**BP 2003** (Sodium Dihydrogen Phosphate Monohydrate). A white powder or colourless crystals. Very soluble in water; very slightly soluble in alcohol. A 5% solution in water has a pH of 4.2 to 4.5.

**USP 27** (Monobasic Sodium Phosphate). It contains one or two molecules of water of hydration, or is anhydrous. Colourless crystals or white crystalline powder. Is odourless and is slightly deliquescent. Freely soluble in water; practically insoluble in alcohol. Its solutions are acid to litmus and effervesce with sodium carbonate. pH of a 5% solution in water of the monohydrate form is between 4.1 and 4.5.

**Equivalence.** Each g of monobasic sodium phosphate (anhydrous) represents approximately 8.3 mmol of sodium and of phosphate. Each g of monobasic sodium phosphate (monohydrate) represents approximately 7.2 mmol of sodium and of phosphate. Each g of monobasic sodium phosphate (dihydrate) represents approximately 6.4 mmol of sodium and of phosphate.

### Dibasic Sodium Phosphate

Dinatrii Phosphas; Disodium Hydrogen Phosphate; Disodium Phosphate; E339; Fosfato de sodio, hidrógeno; Natrii Phosphas; Sodium Phosphate. Disodium hydrogen orthophosphate.

$Na_2HPO_4,xH_2O$.

*CAS — 7558-79-4 (anhydrous dibasic sodium phosphate); 10028-24-7 (dibasic sodium phosphate dihydrate); 7782-85-6 (dibasic sodium phosphate heptahydrate); 10039-32-4 (dibasic sodium phosphate dodecahydrate).*

*ATC — A06AD17; A06AG01; B05XA09; V10XX01 ($^{32}P$).*

**Pharmacopoeias.** In *Eur.* (see p.vi), *Jpn, Pol.,* and *US.* The pharmacopoeias may specify one or more states of hydration; monographs and specifications can be found for:
the anhydrous form ($Na_2HPO_4$ = 142.0),
the dihydrate ($Na_2HPO_4,2H_2O$ = 178.0),
the heptahydrate ($Na_2HPO_4,7H_2O$ = 268.1),
and the dodecahydrate ($Na_2HPO_4,12H_2O$ = 358.1), although not necessarily all will be found in any one pharmacopoeia.

**Ph. Eur. 5.0** (Disodium Phosphate, Anhydrous; Dinatrii Phosphas Anhydricus; Anhydrous Disodium Hydrogen Phosphate BP 2003). A white, hygroscopic powder. Soluble in water; practically insoluble in alcohol. Store in airtight containers.

**Ph. Eur. 5.0** (Disodium Phosphate Dihydrate; Dinatrii Phosphas Dihydricus; Disodium Hydrogen Phosphate Dihydrate BP 2003). A white or almost white powder or colourless crystals. Soluble in water; practically insoluble in alcohol.

The BP 2003 gives Sodium Phosphate Dihydrate as an approved synonym.

**Ph. Eur. 5.0** (Disodium Phosphate Dodecahydrate; Dinatrii Phosphas Dodecahydricus; Disodium Hydrogen Phosphate Dodecahydrate BP 2003). Colourless, transparent, very efflorescent crystals. Very soluble in water; practically insoluble in alcohol.

**USP 27** (Dibasic Sodium Phosphate). It is dried, or contains one, two, seven, or twelve molecules of water of hydration.

The dried substance is a white powder that readily absorbs moisture. It is soluble 1 in 8 of water; insoluble in alcohol.

The heptahydrate is a colourless or white, granular or caked salt that effloresces in warm, dry air. It is freely soluble in water; very slightly soluble in alcohol. Its solutions are alkaline to phenolphthalein, a 0.1M solution having a pH of about 9.

Store all forms in airtight containers.

**Equivalence.** Each g of dibasic sodium phosphate (anhydrous) represents approximately 14.1 mmol of sodium and 7.0 mmol of phosphate. Each g of dibasic sodium phosphate (dihydrate) represents approximately 11.2 mmol of sodium and 5.6 mmol of phosphate. Each g of dibasic sodium phosphate (heptahydrate) represents approximately 7.5 mmol of sodium and 3.7 mmol of phosphate. Each g of dibasic sodium phosphate (dodecahydrate) represents approximately 5.6 mmol of sodium and 2.8 mmol of phosphate.

### Tribasic Sodium Phosphate

E339; Fosfato de sodio; Trisodium Orthophosphate; Trisodium Phosphate.

$Na_3PO_4$ = 163.9.

*CAS — 7601-54-9.*

*ATC — A06AD17; A06AG01.*

**Pharmacopoeias.** In *USNF.*

**USNF 22** (Tribasic Sodium Phosphate). It is anhydrous or contains 1 to 12 molecules of water of hydration. White, odourless crystals or granules, or a crystalline powder. Freely soluble in water; insoluble in alcohol. pH of a 1% solution in water is between 11.5 and 12.0. Store in airtight containers at a temperature not exceeding 40°. Do not allow to freeze.

**Equivalence.** Each g of tribasic sodium phosphate (anhydrous) represents approximately 18.3 mmol of sodium and 6.1 mmol of phosphate.

## Adverse Effects and Treatment

Excessive doses of intravenous phosphate cause hyperphosphataemia, particularly in patients with renal failure. Hyperphosphataemia leads in turn to hypocalcaemia, which may be severe, and to ectopic calcification, particularly in patients with initial hypercalcaemia. Tissue calcification may cause hypotension and organ damage and result in acute renal failure. Hyperphosphataemia, hypocalcaemia, and tissue calcification are rare after oral or rectal phosphate administration (but see also Effects on Electrolytes, below).

Adverse effects of oral phosphates may include nausea, vomiting, diarrhoea, and abdominal pain. When they are being used for indications other than their laxative effects, diarrhoea may necessitate a reduction in dosage. Sodium phosphates given rectally for bowel evacuation may cause local irritation.

Phosphates are given as the potassium or sodium salts or both, and may thus be associated with hyperkalaemia, and hypernatraemia and dehydration. Sodium phosphate may cause hypokalaemia.

Treatment of adverse effects involves withdrawal of phosphate, general supportive measures, and correction of serum-electrolyte concentrations, especially calcium. Measures to remove excess phosphate such as oral phosphate binders and haemodialysis may be required (see also Hyperphosphataemia, p.1219).

**Effects on electrolytes.** Although less common than after intravenous therapy, hyperphosphataemia, accompanied by hypocalcaemia or other severe electrolyte disturbances and resulting in tetany[1,2] and even death,[2] has been reported on a number of occasions following the use of phosphate enemas. Similar effects have also been reported with the use of oral phosphate laxatives,[3-5] and in the USA, the FDA has issued warnings of the risk of electrolyte disturbances following the use of high oral doses of sodium phosphate, particularly in vulnerable patients.[6] Infants or children,[2,7,8] the elderly,[4,9] and those with renal impairment,[1,4,9] or congestive heart failure[4] have often been the subjects of these adverse effects. Soft tissue calcification appears to occur rarely with oral phosphate, but nephrocalcinosis has been reported in children with hypophosphataemic rickets treated with calcitriol and phosphate supplements, and was found to be associated with the phosphate dose.[10]


1. Haskell LP. Hypocalcaemic tetany induced by hypertonic-phosphate enema. *Lancet* 1985; **ii:** 1433.
2. Martin RR, *et al.* Fatal poisoning from sodium phosphate enema: case report and experimental study. *JAMA* 1987; **257:** 2190–2.
3. Peixoto Filho AJ, Lassman MN. Severe hyperphosphatemia induced by a phosphate-containing oral laxative. *Ann Pharmacother* 1996; **30:** 141–3.
4. Adverse Drug Reactions Advisory Committee. Electrolyte disturbances with oral phosphate bowel preparations. *Aust Adverse Drug React Bull* 1997; **16:** 2. Also available at: http://www.tga.health.gov.au/docs/html/aadrbltn/aadr9702.htm (accessed 18/05/04)
5. Ullah N, *et al.* Fatal hyperphosphatemia from a phosphosoda bowel preparation. *J Clin Gastroenterol* 2002; **34:** 457–8.
6. Food and Drug Administration. Safety of Sodium Phosphates Oral Solution. Available at: http://www.fda.gov/cder/drug/safety/sodiumphospate.htm (accessed 18/05/04)
7. McCabe M, *et al.* Phosphate enemas in childhood: cause for concern. *BMJ* 1991; **302:** 1074.
8. Harrington L, Schuh S. Complications of Fleet® enema administration and suggested guidelines for use in the pediatric emergency department. *Pediatr Emerg Care* 1997; **13:** 225–6.
9. Boivin MA, Kahn SR. Symptomatic hypocalcemia from oral sodium phosphate: a report of two cases. *Am J Gastroenterol* 1998; **93:** 2577–9.
10. Verge CF, *et al.* Effects of therapy in X-linked hypophosphatemic rickets. *N Engl J Med* 1991; **325:** 1843–8.


**Local toxicity.** Rectal gangrene has been associated with the use of phosphate enemas in elderly patients and was believed to be due to a direct necrotising effect of the phosphate on the rectum.[1]


1. Sweeney JL, *et al.* Rectal gangrene: a complication of phosphate enema. *Med J Aust* 1986; **144:** 374–5.


## Precautions

Phosphates should not generally be given to patients with severe renal impairment. They should be avoided in patients who may have low serum-calcium concentrations, as these may decrease further, and in patients with infected phosphate renal calculi. Potassium phosphates should be avoided in patients with hyperkalaemia and sodium phosphates should generally be avoided in patients with congestive heart failure, hypertension, and oedema. Serum electrolytes and renal function should be monitored during therapy, particularly if phosphates are given parenterally.

Oral or rectal sodium phosphate preparations for bowel evacuation should not be used in patients with gastrointestinal obstruction, inflammatory bowel disease, and conditions where there is likely to be increased colonic absorption. They should be used cautiously in elderly and debilitated patients, and in those with pre-existing electrolyte disturbances (see Effects on Electrolytes, above).

## Interactions

Oral phosphate supplements should not be used with aluminium, calcium, or magnesium salts as these will bind phosphate and reduce its absorption. Vitamin D increases the gastrointestinal absorption of phosphates and therefore increases the potential for hyperphosphataemia.

Hyperphosphataemia, hypocalcaemia, and hypernatraemia are more likely to occur with phosphate enemas or oral laxatives if these are given to patients receiving diuretics or other drugs that may affect serum electrolytes. The risk of ectopic calcification may be increased by concurrent use of calcium supplements or calcium-containing antacids.

The risk of hyperkalaemia is increased if potassium phosphates are given with drugs that can increase serum-potassium concentrations.

## Pharmacokinetics

About two-thirds of ingested phosphate is absorbed from the gastrointestinal tract. Excess phosphate is mainly excreted in the urine, the remainder being excreted in the faeces.

◊ References.


1. Larson JE, *et al.* Laxative phosphate poisoning: pharmacokinetics of serum phosphorus. *Hum Toxicol* 1986; **5:** 45–9.


## Human Requirements

Phosphorus requirements are usually regarded as equal to those of calcium.

Most foods contain adequate amounts of phosphate, particularly meat and dairy products, hence deficiency is virtually unknown except in certain disease states, in patients receiving total parenteral nutrition, or in those who have received phosphate-binding drugs for prolonged periods; for further details see under Hypophosphataemia, p.1219.

**UK and US recommended dietary intake.** In the UK dietary reference values (DRV—see p.1419)[1] and in the USA dietary reference intakes including recommended dietary allowances (RDA)[2] have been published for phosphorus. In the UK the reference nutrient intake (RNI) for adults is approximately 550 mg (17.5 mmol) daily; no additional amount is recommended for pregnancy although an additional amount of about 440 mg (14.3 mmol) daily is advised during lactation. In the USA the RDA is 1250 mg daily for those aged 9 to 18 years and 700 mg daily in adults; no increase in RDA is recommended during pregnancy and lactation. A tolerable upper intake level of 4 g daily has been set in adults aged up to 70 years; in those older than 70 a maximum of 3 g daily is recommended.[2]


1. DoH. Dietary reference values for food energy and nutrients for the United Kingdom: report of the panel on dietary reference values of the committee on medical aspects of food policy. *Report on health and social subjects 41.* London: HMSO, 1991.
2. Standing Committee on the Scientific Evaluation of Dietary Reference Intakes of the Food and Nutrition Board. *Dietary Reference Intakes for calcium, phosphorus, magnesium, vitamin D, and fluoride.* Washington, DC: National Academy Press, 1999. Also available at: http://www.nap.edu/catalog/5776.html (accessed 03/06/04)


## Uses and Administration

Phosphates are used in the management of **hypophosphataemia** caused by phosphate deficiency or hypophosphataemic states (p.1219). Doses of up to 100 mmol of phosphate daily may be given orally. The intravenous route is seldom necessary, but a dose of up to 9 mmol of phosphate as monobasic potassium phosphate may be given over 12 hours and repeated every 12 hours as necessary for severe hypophosphataemia (see also below). Plasma-electrolyte concentrations, especially phosphate and calcium, and renal function should be carefully monitored. Reduced doses may be necessary in patients with renal impairment. Phosphate supplements are used in total parenteral nutrition regimens; typical daily requirements are 20 to 30 mmol of phosphate.

Phosphates act as mild osmotic **laxatives** (p.1239) when given orally as dilute solutions or by the rectal route. Phosphate enemas or concentrated oral solutions are used for bowel cleansing before surgery or endoscopy procedures. Preparations typically combine monobasic and dibasic sodium phosphates but the composition and dosage do vary slightly. Phosphate enemas act within 2 to 5 minutes, whereas the oral solutions act within 30 minutes to 6 hours.

Phosphates also have **other uses**. They lower the pH of urine and have been given as adjuncts to urinary antibacterials that depend on an acid urine for their activity. Phosphates have also been used for the prophylaxis of calcium renal calculi; the phosphates reduce urinary excretion of calcium thus preventing calcium deposition. A suggested dose for both uses is 7.4 mmol of phosphate four times daily by mouth.

Butafosfan (1-butylamino-1-methylethylphosphinic acid) and the sodium salt of toldimfos (4-dimethylamino-*O*-tolylphosphinic acid) are used as phosphorus sources in veterinary medicine.

**Hypercalcaemia.** Intravenous phosphates have been used to lower plasma-calcium concentrations in hypercalcaemic emergencies (p.1218), but because of their potential to cause serious adverse effects other drugs are now preferred. Oral phosphates may be used to prevent gastrointestinal absorption of calcium in the treatment of hypercalcaemia. The dose in adults is up to 100 mmol phosphate daily adjusted according to response.

**Hypophosphataemia.** Phosphate salts are given in the management of hypophosphataemia when a phosphate deficiency is identified, as discussed in Uses and Administration, above. Intravenous phosphates are associated with serious adverse effects if hypophosphataemia is over-corrected, and the rise in serum-phosphorus concentration cannot be predicted from a given dose. Consequently, it has been recommended[1-4] that intravenous phosphate be used cautiously in the treatment of severe hypophosphataemia (for the standard rate and dose see Uses and Administration, above). However, some advocate a more aggressive fixed-dose regimen in critically ill patients.[5-7]

1. Vannatta JB, *et al.* Efficacy of intravenous phosphorus therapy in the severely hypophosphataemic patient. *Arch Intern Med* 1981; **141:** 885–7.
2. Anonymous. Treatment of severe hypophosphatemia. *Lancet* 1981; **ii:** 734.
3. Lloyd CW, Johnson CE. Management of hypophosphatemia. *Clin Pharm* 1988; **7:** 123–8.
4. Coyle S, *et al.* Treatment of hypophosphataemia. *Lancet* 1992; **340:** 977.
5. Perreault MM, *et al.* Efficacy and safety of intravenous phosphate replacement in critically ill patients. *Ann Pharmacother* 1997; **31:** 683–8.
6. Miller DW, Slovis CM. Hypophosphatemia in the emergency department therapeutics. *Am J Emerg Med* 2000; **18:** 457–61.
7. Charron T, *et al.* Intravenous phosphate in the intensive care unit: more aggressive repletion regimens for moderate and severe hypophosphatemia. *Intensive Care Med* 2003; **29:** 1273–8.

**Osteomalacia.** Vitamin D deficiency, or its abnormal metabolism, is the most usual cause of osteomalacia and rickets (p.762); however, phosphate depletion may also contribute, and phosphate supplementation may be given as appropriate. A suggested dose for vitamin-D-resistant hypophosphataemic osteomalacia in adults is 65 to 100 mmol phosphate daily, and for vitamin D-resistant rickets in children is 32 to 48 mmol phosphate daily.

RICKETS OF PREMATURITY. Dietary deficiency of phosphorus is unusual, but can occur in small premature infants fed exclusively on human breast milk. The phosphate intake in these infants appears to be inadequate to meet the needs of bone mineralisation, and hypophosphataemic rickets can develop. It has been proposed that this condition, variably called metabolic bone disease of prematurity, or rickets of prematurity, could be prevented by giving phosphorus supplements to very low-birth-weight babies (less than about 1000 g) fed on breast milk alone.[1] A suggested regimen is to add 10 to 15 mg of phosphorus per 100 mL of feed (as buffered sodium phosphate) until the infant reached 2000 g. Concomitant calcium and vitamin D supplementation are also recommended.[1] A placebo-controlled study[2] in infants weighing less than 1250 g at birth confirmed that phosphate supplements (50 mg daily) could prevent the development of the bone defects of rickets of prematurity.

1. Brooke OG, Lucas A. Metabolic bone disease in preterm infants. *Arch Dis Child* 1985; **60:** 682–5.
2. Holland PC, *et al.* Prenatal deficiency of phosphate, phosphate supplementation, and rickets in very-low-birthweight infants. *Lancet* 1990; **335:** 697–701. Correction. *ibid.*; 1408–9.

## Preparations

***BP 2003:*** Dipotassium Hydrogen Phosphate Injection; Phosphates Enema; Sterile Potassium Dihydrogen Phosphate Concentrate;
***Ph. Eur.:*** Anticoagulant Citrate-Phosphate-Glucose Solution (CPD);
***USP 27:*** Anticoagulant Citrate Phosphate Dextrose Adenine Solution; Anticoagulant Citrate Phosphate Dextrose Solution; Potassium Phosphates Injection; Sodium Phosphates Injection; Sodium Phosphates Oral Solution; Sodium Phosphates Rectal Solution.

**Proprietary Preparations** (details are given in Part 3)
***Arg.:*** Dicofan; Enemol; Fleet Enema; Fosfo-Dom; Fosfoadital; Silaxa; Tekfema; ***Austral.:*** Celloids PP 85†; Celloids SP 96†; Kwikprep†; Phosphate-Sandoz; Phosphoprep; ***Austria:*** Fleet Phospho-Soda; Relaxyl; ***Belg.:*** Fleet Phospho-Soda; ***Canad.:*** Fleet Phospho-Soda; ***Chile:*** Fabulaxol; Fleet Enema; Fleet Fosfosoda; ***Fin.:*** K-Fosfosteril; ***Fr.:*** Fleet Phospho-Soda; ***Ger.:*** Fleet Phospho-Soda; ***Hong Kong:*** Fleet Phospho-Soda; Uni-Ma; ***India:*** Exit; ***Mex.:*** Deplecat; ***NZ:*** Fleet Phosphate Enema; Fleet Phospho-Soda; ***Singapore:*** Fleet Phospho-Soda; ***Spain:*** Clisma Bieffe Medital†; Fosfoevac; Fosfosoda; ***Swed.:*** Phosphoral; ***UK:*** Fleet Phospho-Soda; New Era Calm & Clear†; ***USA:*** Fleet Phospho-Soda; K-Phos Original; Visicol.
**Multi-ingredient:** numerous preparations are listed in Part 3.

# Potassium

Potasio.
K = 39.0983.

**Description.** Potassium salts covered in this section are those principally given as a source of potassium ions, but consideration should also be given to the effect of the anion. Phosphate salts of potassium are covered under Phosphate, p.1230, and the bicarbonate and citrate salts under Bicarbonate, p.1223.

## Potassium Acetate

E261; Kalii Acetas; Potasio, acetato de.
$CH_3.CO_2K$ = 98.14.
*CAS — 127-08-2.*

**Pharmacopoeias.** In *Eur.* (see p.vi), *Pol.*, and *US.*
**Ph. Eur. 5.0** (Potassium Acetate). Deliquescent white, crystalline powder or colourless crystals. Very soluble in water; freely soluble in alcohol. A 5% solution in water has a pH of 7.5 to 9.0. Protect from moisture.
**USP 27** (Potassium Acetate). Colourless, monoclinic crystals, or a white crystalline powder. It is odourless or has a faint acetous odour. Deliquesces on exposure to moist air. Soluble 1 in 0.5 of water, 1 in 0.2 of boiling water, and 1 in 3 of alcohol. pH of a 5% solution in water is between 7.5 and 8.5. Store in airtight containers.

**Equivalence.** Each g of potassium acetate (anhydrous) represents approximately 10.2 mmol of potassium. Potassium acetate (anhydrous) 2.51 g is approximately equivalent to 1 g of potassium.

## Potassium Chloride

Cloreto de Potássio; E508; Kalii Chloridum; Kalium Chloratum; Potasio, cloruro de.
KCl = 74.55.
*CAS — 7447-40-7.*
*ATC — A12BA01; B05XA01.*

**Pharmacopoeias.** In *Chin., Eur.* (see p.vi), *Int., Jpn, Pol., US,* and *Viet.*
**Ph. Eur. 5.0** (Potassium Chloride). A white, crystalline powder or colourless crystals. Freely soluble in water; practically insoluble in dehydrated alcohol.
**USP 27** (Potassium Chloride). Colourless, elongated, prismatic, or cubical crystals, or a white, granular powder. Is odourless. Soluble 1 in 2.8 of water, and 1 in 2 of boiling water; insoluble in alcohol. Its solutions are neutral to litmus.

**Equivalence.** Each g of potassium chloride represents approximately 13.4 mmol of potassium. Potassium chloride 1.91 g is approximately equivalent to 1 g of potassium.

## Potassium Gluconate

E577; Potasio, gluconato de. Potassium D-gluconate.
$CH_2OH.[CH(OH)]_4.CO_2K$ = 234.2.
*CAS — 299-27-4 (anhydrous potassium gluconate); 35398-15-3 (potassium gluconate monohydrate).*
*ATC — A12BA05.*

**Pharmacopoeias.** In *Fr.*
*US* permits anhydrous or the monohydrate.
**USP 27** (Potassium Gluconate). It is anhydrous or contains one molecule of water of hydration. A white or yellowish-white, odourless, crystalline powder or granules. Soluble 1 in 3 of water; practically insoluble in dehydrated alcohol, in chloroform, in ether, and in benzene. Its solutions are slightly alkaline to litmus. Store in airtight containers.

**Equivalence.** Each g of potassium gluconate (anhydrous) represents approximately 4.3 mmol of potassium. Each g of potassium gluconate (monohydrate) represents approximately 4 mmol of potassium. Potassium gluconate (anhydrous) 5.99 g and potassium gluconate (monohydrate) 6.45 g are each approximately equivalent to 1 g of potassium.

## Potassium Sulfate

E515; Kalii Sulfas; Kalium Sulfuricum; Potasio, sulfato de; Potassii Sulphas; Potassium Sulphate; Tartarus Vitriolatus.
$K_2SO_4$ = 174.3.
*CAS — 7778-80-5.*

**Pharmacopoeias.** In *Eur.* (see p.vi) and *Jpn.*
**Ph. Eur. 5.0** (Potassium Sulphate; Potassium Sulphate for Homoeopathic Use BP 2003). A white crystalline powder or colourless crystals. Soluble in water; practically insoluble in dehydrated alcohol.

**Equivalence.** Each g of potassium sulfate represents approximately 11.5 mmol of potassium. Potassium sulfate 2.23 g is approximately equivalent to 1 g of potassium.

## Potassium Tartrate

E336; Potasio, tartrato de.
$C_4H_4K_2O_6,\frac{1}{2}H_2O$ = 235.3.
*CAS — 921-53-9 (anhydrous potassium tartrate).*

**Equivalence.** Each g of potassium tartrate (hemihydrate) represents approximately 8.5 mmol of potassium. Potassium tartrate (hemihydrate) 3.00 g is approximately equivalent to 1 g of potassium.

## Adverse Effects

Excessive doses of potassium may lead to the development of hyperkalaemia (p.1219), especially in patients with renal impairment. Symptoms include paraesthesia of the extremities, muscle weakness, paralysis, cardiac arrhythmias, heart block, cardiac arrest, and confusion. Cardiac toxicity is of particular concern after intravenous administration.

Pain or phlebitis may occur during intravenous administration via the peripheral route, particularly at higher concentrations.

Nausea, vomiting, diarrhoea, and abdominal cramps may occur following oral administration of potassium salts. There have been numerous reports of gastrointestinal ulceration, sometimes with haemorrhage and perforation or with the late formation of strictures, after the use of enteric-coated tablets of potassium chloride. Ulceration has also occurred after the use of sustained-release tablets.

## Treatment of Adverse Effects

The treatment of hyperkalaemia discussed on p.1219 also applies when hyperkalaemia occurs during potassium therapy. However, in mild hyperkalaemia that has developed on long-term treatment, discontinuation of the potassium supplement and other drugs that may increase plasma-potassium concentrations, and avoidance of foods with a high potassium content may be sufficient to correct the hyperkalaemia.

In cases of acute oral overdosage of potassium supplements, the stomach should be emptied by gastric lavage in addition to the measures described on p.1219.

## Precautions

Potassium salts should be given with considerable care to patients with cardiac disease or conditions predisposing to hyperkalaemia such as renal or adrenocortical insufficiency, acute dehydration, or extensive tissue destruction as occurs with severe burns. Excessive use of potassium-containing salt substitutes or potassium supplements may lead to accumulation of potassium especially in patients with renal insufficiency. Regular monitoring of clinical status, serum electrolytes, and the ECG is advisable in patients receiving potassium therapy, particularly those with cardiac or renal impairment.

Liquid or effervescent preparations are preferred to solid dosage forms for oral administration; use of the former, with or after food, may reduce gastric irritation. Solid oral dosage forms of potassium salts should not be given to patients with gastrointestinal ulceration or obstruction. They should be given with care to patients in whom passage through the gastrointestinal tract may be delayed, as in pregnant patients. Treatment should be discontinued if severe nausea, vomiting, or abdominal distress develops.

Potassium chloride should not be used in patients with hyperchloraemia.

Direct injection of potassium chloride concentrates without appropriate dilution may cause instant death. For the view that glucose-containing solutions should not be used for the initial intravenous administration of potassium in hypokalaemia see Administration, below.

## Interactions

Potassium supplements should be used with caution, if at all, in patients receiving drugs that increase serum-potassium concentrations. These include potassium-sparing diuretics, ACE inhibitors, ciclosporin, and drugs that contain potassium such as the potassium salts of penicillin. Similarly, the concomitant use of potassium-containing salt substitutes for flavouring food should be avoided. Antimuscarinics delay gastric emptying and consequently may increase the risk of gastrointestinal adverse effects in patients receiving solid oral dosage forms of potassium.

## Pharmacokinetics

Potassium salts other than the phosphate, sulfate, and tartrate are generally readily absorbed from the gastrointestinal tract. Potassium is excreted mainly by the kidneys; it is secreted in the distal tubules in exchange for sodium or hydrogen ions. Some potassium is excreted in the faeces and small amounts may also be excreted in sweat.

## Human Requirements

Potassium is an essential body electrolyte. However, requirements are difficult to determine and have been estimated from the amount accumulated during growth and reported urinary and faecal excretion.

Over 90% of dietary potassium is absorbed from the gastrointestinal tract. Potassium is particularly abundant in vegetables, potatoes, and fruit.

**UK and US recommended dietary intake.** In the UK dietary reference values (DRV—see p.1419)[1] have been estimated for potassium. The reference nutrient intake (RNI) for adults is 3.5 g (90 mmol) daily. In the USA, no recommended dietary allowance (RDA) has been established for potassium. However a daily intake of 1.6 to 2 g (40 to 50 mmol) is considered adequate for adults.

1. DoH. Dietary reference values for food energy and nutrients for the United Kingdom: report of the panel on dietary reference values of the committee on medical aspects of food policy. *Report on health and social subjects 41.* London: HMSO, 1991.

## Uses and Administration

Potassium salts in this section are used for the prevention and treatment of potassium depletion and/or **hypokalaemia** (p.1219) and have been used in the prevention of **diuretic-induced hypokalaemia** (see Hydrochlorothiazide, Effects on Electrolyte Balance, p.933). Doses may be expressed in terms of mmol or mEq of potassium, mass (mg) of potassium, or mass of potassium salt (for comparative purposes see Table 3, below). Treatment should be monitored by plasma-potassium estimations because of the risk of inducing hyperkalaemia, especially where there is renal impairment.

**Table 3.** Some potassium salts and their potassium content.

| | Potassium content per g | | |
|---|---|---|---|
| Potassium salt | mg | mmol | mEq |
| Potassium acetate (anhydrous) | 398 | 10.2 | 10.2 |
| Potassium bicarbonate | 391 | 10.0 | 10.0 |
| Potassium chloride | 524 | 13.4 | 13.4 |
| Potassium citrate (anhydrous) | 383 | 9.8 | 9.8 |
| Potassium citrate (monohydrate) | 361 | 9.3 | 9.3 |
| Potassium gluconate (anhydrous) | 167 | 4.3 | 4.3 |
| Potassium gluconate (monohydrate) | 155 | 4.0 | 4.0 |
| Potassium sulfate (anhydrous) | 449 | 11.5 | 11.5 |
| Potassium tartrate (hemihydrate) | 332 | 8.5 | 8.5 |

Potassium chloride is probably the most commonly used potassium salt; this is because hypochloraemic alkalosis, which is often associated with hypokalaemia, can be corrected by the chloride ions. An alkalinising salt such as potassium acetate, potassium bicarbonate, or potassium citrate may be preferable if a metabolic acidosis, such as occurs in renal tubular acidosis, accompanies the hypokalaemia (see p.1217). Other salts that are or have been used in the management of potassium deficiency include potassium ascorbate, potassium aspartate, potassium benzoate, potassium gluceptate, potassium gluconate, potassium phosphate, and potassium tartrate. Typical doses for the prevention of hypokalaemia may be up to 50 mmol daily and similar doses may be adequate in mild potassium deficiency. However, higher doses may be needed in more severe deficiency. Patients with renal impairment should receive correspondingly lower doses. Oral treatment is used for prophylaxis and is also suitable for treating most cases of hypokalaemia. Oral potassium salts are more irritating than the corresponding sodium salts; they should be taken with or after meals with plenty of fluid; liquid preparations are preferable.

Intravenous administration of a potassium salt may be required in severe acute hypokalaemia. This is normally carried out by infusing a solution containing 20 mmol of potassium in 500 mL over 2 to 3 hours under ECG control. A recommended maximum dose is 2 to 3 mmol/kg of potassium in 24 hours. Higher concentrations have been given when an infusion pump has been used (see Administration below). Adequate urine flow must be ensured and careful monitoring of plasma-potassium and other electrolyte concentrations is essential. Potassium chloride is the salt most commonly used and solutions intended for intravenous use that are in a concentrated form (such as 1.5 or 2 mmol/mL) *must* be diluted to the appropriate concentration before administration. There should be careful and thorough mixing when adding concentrated potassium chloride solutions to infusion fluids. Potassium chloride is also available as premixed infusions with sodium chloride and/or glucose containing 10 to 40 mmol/litre of potassium (but see also Administration, below). Potassium acetate is also given intravenously.

Amongst **other uses**, the sulfate, and tartrate salts of potassium have been given orally as osmotic laxatives (p.1239).

Some potassium salts are used as sodium-free condiments when sodium intake must be restricted.

Potassium chloride is sometimes used as an excipient in pharmaceutical formulations.

**Administration.** The standard concentration and rate of administration of potassium chloride for infusion is discussed in Uses and Administration, above. However, higher concentrations (200 or 300 mmol/litre) and faster infusion rates have been used, via an infusion pump, for cases of severe symptomatic hypokalaemia, especially with fluid overload.[1,2]

There has been controversy regarding the preferred route of administration of these higher concentrations of potassium chloride.[1] The central route avoids the problems of pain and phlebitis when potassium is given peripherally. However, it has been suggested that high concentrations of potassium given centrally may carry a greater risk of cardiac toxicity if the infusion is carried directly to the heart. Use of lidocaine has improved tolerability of peripheral administration of potassium chloride.[2]

Intravenous potassium is usually given in sodium chloride and/or glucose infusion. However, it has been pointed out that glucose can reduce serum-potassium concentrations, and that glucose-free solutions should be used for the initial intravenous administration of potassium in hypokalaemia.[3]

1. Kruse JA, Carlson RW. Rapid correction of hypokalemia using concentrated intravenous potassium chloride infusions. *Arch Intern Med* 1990; **150:** 613–17.
2. Pucino F, *et al.* Patient tolerance to intravenous potassium chloride with and without lidocaine. *Drug Intell Clin Pharm* 1988; **22:** 676–9.
3. Agarwal A, Wingo CS. Treatment of hypokalaemia. *N Engl J Med* 1999; **340:** 154–5.

**Diabetic ketoacidosis.** As discussed under Diabetic Emergencies on p.328, potassium replacement is given in diabetic ketoacidosis to restore total body stores of potassium and thereby prevent the hypokalaemia induced by the administration of insulin.

**Hypertension.** A meta-analysis[1] has reported that potassium supplementation results in reductions of both systolic and diastolic blood pressure. The size of the effect in hypertensive patients was sufficiently great to suggest a possible role in the treatment of hypertension (p.825); effects in normotensive subjects were less marked but consistent with a role for potassium supplementation in preventing hypertension.

1. Whelton PK, *et al.* Effects of oral potassium on blood pressure: meta-analysis of randomized controlled clinical trials. *JAMA* 1997; **277:** 1624–32.

**Myocardial infarction.** There is some evidence to suggest that a glucose, insulin, and potassium infusion may be beneficial in acute myocardial infarction (see p.342).

**Termination of pregnancy.** Solutions of potassium chloride are used to reduce fetal numbers in multifetal pregnancies[1-3] or for severe fetal malformation by abolishing the fetal cardiac activity. The solution is injected into the thorax of the fetus without affecting the others which are allowed to continue to term. Alternatively, potassium chloride may be injected into the umbilical vein when access to the fetal heart is difficult. A retrospective comparison[4] found both techniques to be effective. Significantly smaller doses were required for the umbilical route, possibly because a sustained dose is delivered directly to the fetal heart and myocardium, compared with intraventricular injection.

1. Wapner RJ, *et al.* Selective reduction of multifetal pregnancies. *Lancet* 1990; **335:** 90–3.
2. Berkowitz RL, *et al.* The current status of multifetal pregnancy reduction. *Am J Obstet Gynecol* 1996; **174:** 1265–72.
3. De Catte L, Foulon W. Obstetric outcome after fetal reduction to singleton pregnancies. *Prenat Diagn* 2002; **22:** 206–10.
4. Bhide A, *et al.* Comparison of feticide carried out by cordocentesis versus cardiac puncture. *Ultrasound Obstet Gynecol* 2002; **20:** 230–2.

## Preparations

***BP 2003:*** Bumetanide and Slow Potassium Tablets; Effervescent Potassium Chloride Tablets; Potassium Chloride and Glucose Intravenous Infusion; Potassium Chloride and Sodium Chloride Intravenous Infusion; Potassium Chloride, Sodium Chloride and Glucose Intravenous Infusion; Slow Potassium Chloride Tablets; Sterile Potassium Chloride Concentrate;
***USP 27:*** Half-strength Lactated Ringer's and Dextrose Injection; Lactated Ringer's and Dextrose Injection; Lactated Ringer's Injection; Potassium Acetate Injection; Potassium Bicarbonate and Potassium Chloride Effervescent Tablets for Oral Solution; Potassium Bicarbonate and Potassium Chloride for Effervescent Oral Solution; Potassium Chloride Extended-release Capsules; Potassium Chloride Extended-release Tablets; Potassium Chloride for Injection Concentrate; Potassium Chloride for Oral Solution; Potassium Chloride in Dextrose and Sodium Chloride Injection; Potassium Chloride in Dextrose Injection; Potassium Chloride in Lactated Ringer's and Dextrose Injection; Potassium Chloride in Sodium Chloride Injection; Potassium Chloride Oral Solution; Potassium Chloride, Potassium Bicarbonate, and Potassium Citrate Effervescent Tablets for Oral Solution; Potassium Gluconate and Potassium Chloride for Oral Solution; Potassium Gluconate and Potassium Chloride Oral Solution; Potassium Gluconate and Potassium Citrate Oral Solution; Potassium Gluconate Elixir; Potassium Gluconate Tablets; Potassium Gluconate, Potassium Citrate, and Ammonium Chloride Oral Solution; Trikates Oral Solution.

**Proprietary Preparations** (details are given in Part 3)
***Arg.:*** Co-Salt; Control K; Kaon; Orakit; ***Austral.:*** Celloids PC 73†; Celloids PS 29†; Chlorvescent; Duro-K; KSR; Slow-K; Span-K; ***Austria:*** KCl-retard; Micro-Kalium; Rekawan†; ***Belg.:*** Chloropotassuril; Kali-Sterop; Kalium Durettes; Steropotassium; Ultra-K; ***Braz.:*** Clotassio; Kloren†; Slow-K†; ***Canad.:*** Apo-K; K-10; K-Dur; K-Lor; K-Lyte/Cl; Kalium Durules†; Kaochlor†; Kaon; Micro-K; Potassium-Rougier; Proflavanol C; Roychlor; Slow-K; ***Chile:*** Kaion Retard; Sal Dietetica; Slow K; Yonka; ***Denm.:*** Kaleorid; Kalinorm†; ***Fin.:*** Durekal; Kalinorm; Kalisol; Kalisteril; Kalium Duretter†; ***Fr.:*** Diffu-K; Kaleorid; Nati-K†; ***Ger.:*** Kalinor-retard P; Kalitrans retard†; Kalium; Kalium-Duriles; KCl-retard; Rekawan; ***Gr.:*** Sopa-K; ***Hong Kong:*** Addi-K; Apo-K; Kalium; KSR; Slow-K; Span-K; ***India:*** Diucontin-K; Keylyte; Potklor; ***Irl.:*** Kay-Cee-L; Slow-K; ***Israel:*** Slow-K; ***Ital.:*** K-Flebo; Kadalex; Lento-Kalium; ***Malaysia:*** Apo-K; Beacon K; KSR; Slow-K; ***Mex.:*** Ceposil; Clor-K-Zaf; K-Dur; Kaliolite; Kasele; Kelefusin; Potasoral; ***Neth.:*** Kalium Durettes; Slow-K; ***Norw.:*** Kaleorid; Kalinorm†; ***NZ:*** Chlorvescent; K-SR; Slow-K; Span-K†; ***S.Afr.:*** Plenish-K; Slow-K; Swiss-Kal SR; ***Singapore:*** Addi-K; Kalium Durules†; KSR; ***Spain:*** AP Inyec Cloruro Potasic; Boi K; Boi K Aspartico; Potasion; Potasion Solucion; ***Swed.:*** Kaleorid; Kalitabs; Kalium Duretter; Kalium Retard; ***Switz.:*** Kaliglutol; Plus Kalium retard; ***Thai.:*** Addi-K; Enpott; Kaliject; Potassride; ***UK:*** Kay-Cee-L; Slow-K; ***USA:*** Cena-K; Gen-K; K + 10; K + 8; K-Dur; K-G Elixir; K-Lease; K-Lor; K-Lyte/Cl; K-Norm; K-Tab; Kaochlor†; Kaon; Kaon-Cl; Kay Ciel; Klor-Con; Klorvess; Klotrix; Micro-K; Potasalan; Rum-K; Slow-K; Ten-K.

**Multi-ingredient:** numerous preparations are listed in Part 3.

# Sodium

Sodio.
Na = 22.98977.

**Description.** Sodium chloride is the principal sodium salt used as a source of sodium ions. Sodium salts used chiefly as sources of bicarbonate ions, such as the acetate, bicarbonate, citrate, and lactate, are covered under Bicarbonate, p.1223. Phosphate salts of sodium are covered under Phosphate, p.1230.

## Sodium Chloride

Chlorure de Sodium; Cloreto de Sódio; Natrii Chloridum; Salt; Sodio, cloruro de.
NaCl = 58.44.
*CAS — 7647-14-5.*
*ATC — A12CA01; B05CB01; B05XA03.*

NOTE. An aqueous solution of sodium chloride 0.9% is often known as physiological saline.
SALINE is a code approved by the BP 2003 for use on single unit doses of eye drops containing sodium chloride 0.9% where the individual container may be too small to bear all the appropriate labelling information. HECL is a similar code approved for hyetellose and sodium chloride eye drops.

**Pharmacopoeias.** In *Chin., Eur.* (see p.vi), *Int., Jpn, Pol., US,* and *Viet.*

**Ph. Eur. 5.0** (Sodium Chloride). A white, crystalline powder or colourless crystals or white pearls. Freely soluble in water; practically insoluble in dehydrated alcohol.

**USP 27** (Sodium Chloride). Colourless cubic crystals or white crystalline powder. Soluble 1 in 2.8 of water, 1 in 2.7 of boiling water, and 1 in 10 of glycerol; slightly soluble in alcohol.

**Equivalence.** Each g of sodium chloride represents approximately 17.1 mmol of sodium and of chloride. Sodium chloride 2.54 g is approximately equivalent to 1 g of sodium.

**Storage.** Solutions of some sodium salts, including sodium chloride, when stored, may cause separation of solid particles from glass containers and solutions containing such particles must not be used.

## Adverse Effects

Adverse effects of sodium salts are attributable to electrolyte imbalances from excess sodium; there may also be effects due to the specific anion.

Retention of excess sodium in the body usually occurs when there is defective renal sodium excretion. This leads to the accumulation of extracellular fluid to maintain normal plasma osmolality, which may result in pulmonary and peripheral oedema and their consequent effects.

Hypernatraemia (a rise in plasma osmolality) is usually associated with inadequate water intake, or excessive water losses (see p.1220). It rarely occurs after therapeutic doses of sodium chloride, but has occurred with the use of hypertonic saline for induction of emesis or for gastric lavage and after errors in the formulation of infant feeds. Hypernatraemia may also occur after inappropriate intravenous administration of hypertonic saline.

The most serious effect of hypernatraemia is dehydration of the brain which causes somnolence and confusion progressing to convulsions, coma, respiratory failure, and death. Other symptoms include thirst, reduced salivation and lachrymation, fever, sweating, tachycardia, hypertension or hypotension, headache, dizziness, restlessness, irritability, weakness, and muscular twitching and rigidity.

Gastrointestinal effects associated with acute oral ingestion of hypertonic solutions or excessive amounts of sodium chloride include nausea, vomiting, diarrhoea, and abdominal cramps.

Excessive use of chloride salts may cause a loss of bicarbonate with an acidifying effect.

Intra-amniotic injection of hypertonic solutions of sodium chloride, which has been used for termination of pregnancy, has been associated with serious adverse effects including disseminated intravascular coagulation, renal necrosis, cervical and uterine lesions, haemorrhage, pulmonary embolism, pneumonia, and death.

◊ General references.


1. Moder KG, Hurley DL. Fatal hypernatremia from exogenous salt intake: report of a case and review of the literature. *Mayo Clin Proc* 1990; **65:** 1587–94. Correction. *ibid.* 1991; **66:** 439.
2. Martos Sánchez I, *et al.* Hipernatremia grave por administración accidental de sal común. *An Esp Pediatr* 2000; **53:** 495–8.
3. Adeleye O, *et al.* Hypernatremia in the elderly. *J Natl Med Assoc* 2002; **94:** 701–5.
4. Coulthard MG, Haycock GB. Distinguishing between salt poisoning and hypernatraemic dehydration in children. *BMJ* 2003; **326:** 157–60. Correction. *ibid.*; 497.


## Treatment of Adverse Effects

In patients with mild sodium excess, oral administration of water and restriction of sodium intake is sufficient. However, in the event of recent acute oral overdose of sodium chloride, gastric lavage should be carried out along with general symptomatic and supportive treatment. Serum-sodium concentrations should be measured, and if severe hypernatraemia is present this should be treated (see p.1220).

## Precautions

Sodium salts should be used with caution in patients with hypertension, heart failure, peripheral or pulmonary oedema, renal impairment, pre-eclampsia, or other conditions associated with sodium retention.

When sodium supplements are given orally, adequate water intake should be maintained. Sustained-release tablets should not be given to patients with gastrointestinal disorders associated with strictures or diverticula because of the risk of obstruction.

Sodium chloride solutions should *not* be used to induce emesis; this practice is dangerous and deaths from resulting hypernatraemia have been reported.

## Pharmacokinetics

Sodium chloride is well absorbed from the gastrointestinal tract. Excess sodium is mainly excreted by the kidney, and small amounts are lost in the faeces and sweat.

## Human Requirements

The body contains about 4 mol (92 g) of sodium of which about one-third is found in the skeleton and about half is present in the extracellular fluid.

The body can adapt to a wide range of intakes by adjustment of renal excretion through physical and hormonal factors. Loss through the skin is significant only if excessive sweating occurs. Sodium requirements may be increased with exercise or exposure to high ambient temperatures in the short term, until the body adjusts.

Sodium is widely available in foods and is also added as salt during processing, cooking, and at the table. Dietary deficiency of sodium is therefore extremely rare and more concern has been expressed that current intakes are excessive. Restriction of sodium intake, by limiting the amount of culinary salt consumed, may be a useful aid in the management of some patients with hypertension (p.825).

**UK and US recommended dietary intake.** In the UK dietary reference values (DRV—see p.1419)[1] have been published for sodium. The reference nutrient intake (RNI) for adults is 1.6 g of sodium (70 mmol) daily, which is about 4 g of sodium chloride. In the USA, it has been recommended that daily intakes of sodium be limited to 2.4 g (6 g of sodium chloride) or less.[2] Dietary intake is often in excess of these recommendations, and may be a factor in essential hypertension,[3] and osteoporosis.[4]


1. DoH. Dietary reference values for food energy and nutrients for the United Kingdom: report of the panel on dietary reference values of the committee on medical aspects of food policy. *Report on health and social subjects 41.* London: HMSO, 1991.
2. Subcommittee on the tenth edition of the RDAs, Food and Nutrition Board, Commission on Life Sciences, National Research Council. *Recommended dietary allowances.* 10th ed. Washington, DC: National Academy Press, 1989. Also available at: http://www.nap.edu/catalog/1349.html (accessed 03/06/04)
3. Midgley JP, *et al.* Effect of reduced dietary sodium on blood pressure: a meta-analysis of randomized controlled trials. *JAMA* 1996; **275:** 1590–7.
4. Devine A, *et al.* A longitudinal study of the effect of sodium and calcium intakes on regional bone density in postmenopausal women. *Am J Clin Nutr* 1995; **62:** 740–5.


## Uses and Administration

Sodium chloride is used in the management of deficiencies of sodium and chloride ions in salt-losing conditions (see Hyponatraemia, p.1220). Sodium chloride solutions are used as a source of sodium chloride and water for hydration.

A 0.9% solution in water is iso-osmotic, and thus in most cases isotonic with serum and lachrymal secretions. Doses may be expressed in terms of mEq or mmol of sodium, mass (mg) of sodium, or mass of sodium salt. For comparative purposes, see Table 4, below.

**Table 4.** Some sodium salts and their sodium content.

| Sodium salt | Sodium content per g | | |
|---|---|---|---|
| | mg | mmol | mEq |
| Sodium acetate (anhydrous) | 280 | 12.2 | 12.2 |
| Sodium acetate (trihydrate) | 169 | 7.3 | 7.3 |
| Sodium acid citrate | 175 | 7.6 | 7.6 |
| Sodium bicarbonate | 274 | 11.9 | 11.9 |
| Sodium chloride | 394 | 17.1 | 17.1 |
| Sodium citrate (anhydrous) | 267 | 11.6 | 11.6 |
| Sodium citrate (dihydrate) | 235 | 10.2 | 10.2 |
| Sodium lactate | 205 | 8.9 | 8.9 |

A typical oral replacement dose of sodium chloride in **chronic salt-losing conditions** is about 2.4 to 4.8 g (about 40 to 80 mmol of sodium) daily as a modified-release preparation, accompanied by a suitable fluid intake; doses of up to 12 g daily may be necessary in severe cases. Oral supplements are also used for the prevention of muscle cramps during routine haemodialysis; a suggested dose is about 6 to 10 g of a modified-release preparation per dialysis session.

Glucose facilitates the absorption of sodium from the gastrointestinal tract, and solutions containing sodium chloride and glucose usually with additional electrolytes (see p.1222) are used for oral rehydration in acute diarrhoea (p.1241).

The concentration and dosage of sodium chloride solutions for intravenous use is determined by several factors including the age, weight, and clinical condition of the patient and in particular the patients' hydration state. Serum-electrolyte concentrations should be carefully monitored. In severe sodium depletion, 2 to 3 litres of sodium chloride 0.9% may be given over 2 to 3 hours and thereafter at a slower rate. If there is combined water and sodium depletion a 1 to 1 mixture of sodium chloride 0.9% and glucose 5% may be appropriate. Although hypertonic sodium chloride solutions may be used in certain patients with severe acute dilutional hyponatraemia, over-rapid correction may have severe neurological adverse effects (see p.1220). Solutions containing 1.8 to 5% are available.

In **hypernatraemia** with volume depletion (p.1220), sodium chloride 0.9% may be used to maintain plasma-sodium concentrations with expanding fluid volume. Sodium chloride 0.9% (or rarely, in marked hypernatraemia, 0.45%) is used for fluid replacement in diabetic ketoacidosis (see Diabetic Emergencies, p.328).

Among its **other uses**, sodium chloride solution 0.9%, being isotonic, is a useful fluid for sterile irrigations, for example, of the eye or bladder, and general skin or wound cleansing. The 0.9% concentration is also widely used as a vehicle or diluent for the parenteral administration of other drugs. Nasal drops of sodium chloride 0.9% are used to relieve nasal congestion. A mouthwash containing sodium chloride is also available for oral hygiene.

Sodium chloride solutions should *not* be used to induce emesis; this practice is dangerous and deaths from resulting hypernatraemia have been reported.

Sodium chloride (Natrium muriaticum; Nat. Mur.) is used in homoeopathic medicine. It is also sometimes used as an excipient in capsules and tablets.

**Catheters and cannulas.** For reference to sodium chloride 0.9% being used to maintain the patency of catheters and cannulas, and to its equivalent efficacy to heparin, see Catheters and Cannulas under Uses and Administration of Heparin, p.930.

**Termination of pregnancy.** Trans-abdominal intra-amniotic instillation of sodium chloride 20% (maximum volume 200 to 250 mL) has been used for the termination of second-trimester pregnancy. However, serious adverse effects have occurred (see above), and other methods are generally preferred (p.1512).

## Preparations

***BP 2003:*** Compound Sodium Chloride Mouthwash; Potassium Chloride and Sodium Chloride Intravenous Infusion; Potassium Chloride, Sodium Chloride and Glucose Intravenous Infusion; Sodium Chloride and Glucose Intravenous Infusion; Sodium Chloride Eye Drops; Sodium Chloride Eye Lotion; Sodium Chloride Intravenous Infusion; Sodium Chloride Irrigation Solution; Sodium Chloride Solution; Sodium Chloride Tablets;
***USP 27:*** Bacteriostatic Sodium Chloride Injection; Dextrose and Sodium Chloride Injection; Fructose and Sodium Chloride Injection; Half-strength Lactated Ringer's and Dextrose Injection; Inulin in Sodium Chloride Injection; Lactated Ringer's and Dextrose Injection; Lactated Ringer's Injection; Mannitol in Sodium Chloride Injection; Potassium Chloride in Dextrose and Sodium Chloride Injection; Potassium Chloride in Lactated Ringer's and Dextrose Injection; Potassium Chloride in Sodium Chloride Injection; Sodium Chloride and Dextrose Tablets; Sodium Chloride Inhalation Solution; Sodium Chloride Injection; Sodium Chloride Irrigation; Sodium Chloride Ophthalmic Ointment; Sodium Chloride Ophthalmic Solution; Sodium Chloride Tablets; Sodium Chloride Tablets for Solution.

**Proprietary Preparations** (details are given in Part 3)
***Arg.:*** Hypersol; Muro 128; Nasomicina Salina; ***Austral.:*** Bausch & Lomb Saline Plus†; Bausch & Lomb Sensitive Eyes Saline†; Fess; Hypergel; Lens Plus†; Mucolyt; Narium†; Slow-Sodium; Softwear†; ***Austria:*** Ery-Set; Otrisal; Polyrinse-Aufnahmelosung†; Uro-Pract; ***Belg.:*** Naaprep; Natriclo; Physiologica; Physiorhine; ***Braz.:*** Afrin Natural; Fisiologico†; Fluimucil Solucao Nasal†; Lens Plus†; Narisoro; Nasoflux†; Nasolac; Nazosoro; Nefrosol†; Nesoro†; Novo Rino-S; Rino-Ped; Rinoben; Rinoflux; Rinox Pediatrico†; Sinustrat Solucao Natural; Snif; Soroliv; Soroneo; ***Canad.:*** Certified Nasal; EFA Steri†; Lens Plus Buffered Saline Solution; Muro 128; Physium†; Rhinaris Saline; Safeway Nasal; Salinex; Softwear; Thalaris†; ***Chile:*** Fisiolimp; Fludrop; Larmabak; Printan; Rinodan; Suero Fisiologico; ***Denm.:*** Viskose ojendraber; ***Fin.:*** Natrosteril; ***Fr.:*** Aequalyre†; Aquarhine†; Erjean; Hypergel; Irriclens; Larmabak; Larmes Artificielles; Normlgel; Physiologica; Physiomer; Physiosoin; Polyrinse; Proceane Isotonique; Selgine; Serophy†; Unilarm; Uro 3000†; Versol; Vesirig; ***Ger.:*** Adsorbonac; Freka-Drainjet; Isogutt akut; Isotone Kochsalz; Olynth salin; Otrisal; Rhinomer; Rhinospray Atlantik; Rhinoton plus; Tetrisal; Uro-Pract N†; ***Gr.:*** Clinofar; Otrisalin; Phy-O; Selva N; ***Hong Kong:*** Adsorbonac†; Atomic Enema; Larmabak; Unison Enema; ***Irl.:*** Slow-Sodium†; ***Israel:*** Baby AF; Clean-AF; Drossanose; Normasol; Otrivini; Tinok AF; Tipotaf; Uro-Tainer; ***Ital.:*** Adsorbonac; Hydrabak; Libenar; Naribel; Physiodose; Physiomer; Rinowash; Sterimar; ***Mex.:*** Alcacat; Corni Limp†; Hiperton; ***NZ:*** Hydrocare Preserved Saline†; Narium; ***Port.:*** Libenar; Lyomer; Rhinomer; Sterimar; Tonimer; ***Singapore:*** Adsorbonac†; Larmabak; ***Spain:*** Antiedema; Apir Clorurado; Apiroflex Clorurado†; Estericlean†; Fisiologica; Fisiologico; Fisiologico Bieffe M; Fisiologico Braun†; Fisiologico Farmacelsia; Fisiologico Isoton; Fisiologico Mein; Fisiologico Vitulia; Flebobag Fisio; Fleboplast Fisio; Freeflex Cloruro Sodico; Irrigacion CLNA; Lavaflac†; Libenar†; Liberanas†; Meinvenil Fisiologico; Plast Apyr Fisio Irrigac†; Plast Apyr Fisiologico; Respitol†; Solucion Fisio; Suero Fisiologico; Suero Fisiologico Vitulia; ***Swed.:*** Tresal†; ***Switz.:*** Amuchina Med; Drossa-Nose; Fluimare; Naaprep; Nasben Soft†; nasmer; Nose Fresh; Physiologic; Physiosoin; Rhinomer; Serophy; Sterimar; Triomer; ***UAE:*** Normaline; ***UK:*** Askina; Irriclens; Normasol; Rhinomer†; Slow-Sodium; Steracf; Stericlens; Steripod; Tubilux; Uriflex S; Uro-Tainer M; ***USA:*** Adsorbonac; Afrin Moisturizing Saline Mist; Ak-NaCl; Ayr Saline; Breathe Free; Broncho Saline; Dristan Saline Spray; HuMist Nasal Mist; Marlin Salt System; Muro 128; Muroptic; NaSal; Nasal Moist; Normaline; Ocean; Pretz; Salinex; SeaMist; Your Choice.

**Multi-ingredient:** numerous preparations are listed in Part 3.

# Gases

This chapter includes monographs on gases with medical or pharmaceutical uses and applications (such as oxygen, carbon dioxide, helium, and nitrogen) as well as those where the medical interest lies primarily in management of their toxicity or adverse effects (such as carbon monoxide or hydrogen sulfide). Also included are some compressed and liquefied gases used as refrigerants and aerosol propellants. Nitric oxide gas is used in bronchopulmonary disorders and is discussed in Cardiovascular Drugs (p.973). Other gases with medical uses can be found in Disinfectants and Preservatives (p.1164) and General Anaesthetics (p.1295).

## Refrigerants and Aerosol Propellants

A number of compressed and liquefied gases are used as refrigerants and as aerosol propellants; these include nitrogen, nitrous oxide, carbon dioxide, propane, and the butanes. Chlorofluorocarbons (CFCs) were widely used but because of environmental hazards their general use has been severely restricted and they are being phased out in medicine and pharmacy. Hydrogenated chlorofluorocarbons (hydrochlorofluorocarbons) and nonchlorinated fluorocarbons (hydrofluorocarbons) are being developed as alternatives, although neither are devoid of environmental effects.

The evaporation of halogenated hydrocarbon propellants produces an intense cold that numbs the tissues, and they have been used as topical analgesics (p.4).

Refrigerants and aerosol propellants have been subject to deliberate abuse. Inhalation of high concentrations of halogenated hydrocarbons for their euphoriant effect may result in CNS depression, cardiac arrhythmias, respiratory depression, and death. Propane and butane can act as simple asphyxiants. Heat can cause the decomposition of halogenated hydrocarbons into irritant and toxic gases such as hydrogen chloride and phosgene.

**Toxicity.** Reviews have covered the toxicity and adverse effects that may occur as a consequence of the deliberate abuse of aerosol propellants[1-3] as well as the hazards associated with occupational exposure.[4] Further references relevant to the toxicity of individual agents are given in the monographs.


1. Volatile substance abuse—an overview. *Hum Toxicol* 1989; **8:** 255–344.
2. Ashton CH. Solvent abuse. *BMJ* 1990; **300:** 1356–6.
3. Anderson HR. Increase in deaths from deliberate inhalation of fuel gases and pressurised aerosols. *BMJ* 1990; **301:** 41.
4. Matthews G. Toxic gases. *Postgrad Med J* 1989; **65:** 224–32.


## Bromochlorodifluoromethane

Bromoclorodifluorometano.

$CBrClF_2$ = 165.4.

### Profile

Bromochlorodifluoromethane has been employed as a fire-extinguishing agent.

◊ Reports of toxicity following the misuse or abuse of fire extinguishers containing bromochlorodifluoromethane.[1,2]


1. Steadman C, *et al.* Abuse of fire-extinguishing agent and sudden death in adolescents. *Med J Aust* 1984; **141:** 115–17.
2. Lerman Y, *et al.* Fatal accidental inhalation of bromochlorodifluoromethane (Halon 1211). *Hum Exp Toxicol* 1991; **10:** 125–8.


## Butane

*n*-Butane; Butano; E943a.

$C_4H_{10}$ = 58.12.
*CAS — 106-97-8.*

**Pharmacopoeias.** In *USNF.*

**USNF 22** (Butane). A colourless gas. It is highly flammable and explosive. Store in airtight cylinders at a temperature not exceeding 40°.

### Profile

Butane is used as an aerosol propellant (above). It is widely used as a fuel.

**Abuse.** Reports of toxicity associated with the abuse of butane.[1-3]


1. Gunn J, *et al.* Butane sniffing causing ventricular fibrillation. *Lancet* 1989; **i:** 617.
2. Siegel E, Wason S. Sudden death caused by inhalation of butane and propane. *N Engl J Med* 1990; **323:** 1638.
3. Roberts MJD, *et al.* Asystole following butane gas inhalation. *Br J Hosp Med* 1990; **44:** 294.


### Preparations

**Proprietary Preparations** (details are given in Part 3)
**Multi-ingredient:** ***Arg.:*** Batistol; Frionex.

## Carbon Dioxide

Carbonei Dioxidum; Carbonei Dioxydum; Carbonic Acid Gas; Carbonic Anhydride; Dióxido de carbono; E290.

$CO_2$ = 44.01.
*CAS — 124-38-9.*
*ATC — V03AN02.*

NOTE. Carbon dioxide is about 1½ times as heavy as air.

**Pharmacopoeias.** In *Chin., Eur.* (see p.vi), *Jpn,* and *US.*

**Ph. Eur. 5.0** (Carbon Dioxide). A colourless gas. Soluble 1 in about 1 of water by volume at 20° and at a pressure of 101 kpA. Store liquefied under pressure in suitable containers.

The BP 2003 directs that carbon dioxide should be kept in approved metal cylinders which are painted grey and carry a label stating 'Carbon Dioxide'. In addition, 'Carbon Dioxide' or the symbol '$CO_2$' should be stencilled in paint on the shoulder of the cylinder.

**USP 27** (Carbon Dioxide). A colourless, odourless gas. Its solutions are acid to litmus. One volume dissolves in about 1 volume of water. Store in cylinders.

### Adverse Effects

Above a concentration of 6%, carbon dioxide causes headache, dizziness, confusion, palpitations, hypertension, dyspnoea, increased depth and rate of respiration, and CNS depression. Concentrations of about 20% and higher produce convulsions and loss of consciousness; inhalation of 50% carbon dioxide is reported to produce central effects similar to anaesthetics. The inhalation of high concentrations may produce respiratory acidosis.

Abrupt withdrawal of carbon dioxide after prolonged inhalation commonly produces pallor, hypotension, dizziness, severe headache, and nausea or vomiting.

Skin contact with solid carbon dioxide may cause frostbite.

### Uses and Administration

Carbon dioxide has been added to the oxygen in certain types of pump oxygenators to maintain the carbon dioxide content of the blood.

Although carbon dioxide stimulates respiration, it is seldom used for this purpose. Treatment of carbon monoxide poisoning with carbon dioxide/oxygen mixtures is discouraged due to the risk of respiratory acidosis.

Inhalation of carbon dioxide has been tried for relief of intractable hiccup (p.682). Carbonated vehicles are useful for masking the unpleasant taste of some medicinal preparations.

Solid carbon dioxide, or 'dry ice' has a temperature of −80° and has been used to treat warts (p.1139) and naevi by cryotherapy.

Carbon dioxide may be used as the insufflating gas for laparoscopy and as a contrast agent in radiography (p.1059).

### Preparations

**Proprietary Preparations** (details are given in Part 3)
**Multi-ingredient:** ***Ger.:*** Ensinger Schiller-Quelle Heilwasser.

## Carbon Monoxide

Monóxido de carbono.

CO = 28.01.
*CAS — 630-08-0.*

**Description.** Carbon monoxide is a colourless, odourless, tasteless, highly flammable gas.

### Adverse Effects

Carbon monoxide is produced by incomplete combustion of organic materials and is highly toxic when inhaled; infants, small children, and elderly people are particularly susceptible. Although the number of cases of poisoning in countries such as the UK has fallen as the availability of coal gas has declined and as changes have been made to motor vehicles to improve their exhaust fumes, carbon monoxide is still a major cause of poisoning. Common sources of carbon monoxide include poorly maintained and ventilated heating systems and improperly burnt fuel in domestic fires.

When inhaled, carbon monoxide combines with haemoglobin in the blood to form carboxyhaemoglobin, which is unable to transport oxygen; the symptoms of carbon monoxide poisoning are largely due to anoxia. The skin and tissues may turn a classic cherry red in patients poisoned with carbon monoxide although this is seen most often after death.

The symptoms of carbon monoxide poisoning are varied and depend on the degree and duration of exposure. Unconsciousness may occur suddenly but is commonly preceded by headache, dizziness, weakness, nausea, and vomiting, which may be misdiagnosed as a viral illness or food poisoning. Other symptoms may include skin lesions, excessive sweating, pyrexia, increased respiration, mental dullness and confusion, visual disturbances, convulsions, hypotension, tachycardia or other cardiac arrhythmias, myocardial ischaemia, and possibly myocardial infarction. Death may result from respiratory failure, pulmonary oedema, cardiovascular failure, or cerebral damage. The lethal concentration of carboxyhaemoglobin in the blood is about 50% or more. Concentrations over 1000 ppm of carbon monoxide in inspired air may be fatal in 1 hour. Neurological and psychiatric sequelae may develop some weeks later in the survivors of severe poisoning and therefore a prolonged follow-up of such patients is advised; symptoms include memory impairment, apathy, mutism, irritability, personality change, gait disturbance, and urinary and faecal incontinence. Chronic carbon monoxide exposure may present as a non-specific illness with headache, nausea, and flu-like symptoms.

◊ General references.


1. Meredith T, Vale A. Carbon monoxide poisoning. *BMJ* 1988; **296:** 77–9.
2. Crawford R, *et al.* Carbon monoxide poisoning in the home: recognition and treatment. *BMJ* 1990; **301:** 977–9.
3. Ernst A, Zibrak JD. Carbon monoxide poisoning. *N Engl J Med* 1998; **339:** 1603–8.
4. Carbon Monoxide. *Environmental Health Criteria 213.* Geneva: WHO, 1999. Available at: http://www.inchem.org/documents/ehc/ehc/ehc213.htm (accessed 05/07/04)


### Treatment of Adverse Effects

The patient should be removed from the contaminated atmosphere and an effective airway established. Oxygen (100%) should be given until the blood carboxyhaemoglobin concentration has fallen below dangerous levels (usually 5%). Management is then usually symptomatic and supportive with attention being given to the possible need to treat or correct any cardiovascular disorders, metabolic acidosis, or cerebral oedema. Hyperbaric oxygen therapy may be considered in pregnant patients or in severe poisoning (if the patient is, or has been, unconscious; if the carboxyhaemoglobin concentration exceeds 20%; or if there are neurological symptoms or cardiac complications) but is of unproven benefit (see below) and its use is controversial.

◊ References.


1. Anonymous. Treatment of carbon monoxide poisoning. *Drug Ther Bull* 1988; **26:** 77–9.
2. Ely EW, *et al.* Warehouse workers' headache: emergency evaluation and management of 30 patients with carbon monoxide poisoning. *Am J Med* 1995; **98:** 145–55.


**Hyperbaric oxygen therapy.** The use of hyperbaric oxygen therapy in the management of carbon monoxide poisoning is controversial. It is of theoretical benefit since it increases the rate at which carboxyhaemoglobin dissociates, and beneficial results have been reported in patients with carbon monoxide poisoning.[1,2] Its use has therefore been widely recommended, particularly in patients with severe poisoning. However, the availability of hyperbaric oxygen is limited, and it remains unclear which patients should receive therapy. A controlled trial[3] comparing hyperbaric oxygen with normobaric oxygen (at higher levels than commonly used) in patients with severe poisoning found no benefit from hyperbaric oxygen, but a later study[4] using a different regimen did find a reduction in cognitive sequelae. Hyperbaric oxygen has been successfully used in pregnant patients with carbon monoxide poisoning[5] and its use should possibly be considered earlier in pregnant patients due to the risks to the fetus from hypoxia.


1. Gorman DF. Problems and pitfalls in the use of hyperbaric oxygen for the treatment of poisoned patients. *Med Toxicol Adverse Drug Exp* 1989; **4:** 393–9.
2. Hawkins M, *et al.* Severe carbon monoxide poisoning: outcome after hyperbaric oxygen therapy. *Br J Anaesth* 2000; **84:** 584–6.
3. Scheinkestel CD, *et al.* Hyperbaric or normobaric oxygen for acute carbon monoxide poisoning: a randomised controlled clinical trial. *Med J Aust* 1999; **170:** 203–10.
4. Weaver LK, *et al.* Hyperbaric oxygen for acute carbon monoxide poisoning. *N Engl J Med* 2002; **347:** 1057–67.
5. Van Hoesen KB, *et al.* Should hyperbaric oxygen be used to treat the pregnant patient for acute carbon monoxide poisoning: a case report and literature review. *JAMA* 1989; **261:** 1039–43. Correction. *ibid.* 1990; **263:** 2750.


### Uses

Carbon monoxide has been used in low concentrations as a tracer gas in measurements of lung function. Carbon monoxide labelled with carbon-11 may also be used to assess the blood volume.

## Chlorofluorocarbons

CFCs; Clorofluorocarbonos.

## Cryofluorane *(rINN)*

CFC-114; Criofluorano; Dichlorotetrafluoroethane; Propellant 114; Refrigerant 114; Tetrafluorodichloroethane. 1,2-Dichloro-1,1,2,2-tetrafluoroethane.

$C_2Cl_2F_4$ = 170.9.
*CAS — 76-14-2.*

**Pharmacopoeias.** In *USNF.*

**USNF 22** (Dichlorotetrafluoroethane). A clear, colourless gas having a faint ethereal odour. Store in airtight cylinders at a temperature not exceeding 40°.

## Dichlorodifluoromethane

CFC-12; Diclorodifluorometano; Difluorodichloromethane; Propellant 12; Refrigerant 12.

$CCl_2F_2$ = 120.9.
*CAS — 75-71-8.*

**Pharmacopoeias.** In *USNF.*

**USNF 22** (Dichlorodifluoromethane). A clear, colourless gas having a faint ethereal odour. Store in airtight cylinders at a temperature not exceeding 40°.

## Trichlorofluoromethane

CFC-11; Fluorotrichloromethane; Propellant 11; Refrigerant 11; Trichloromonofluoromethane; Triclorofluorometano.

$CCl_3F$ = 137.4.
*CAS — 75-69-4.*

NOTE. Trichlorofluoromethane is a gas above 24°.

**Pharmacopoeias.** In *USNF.*

**USNF 22** (Trichloromonofluoromethane). A clear, colourless gas having a faint ethereal odour. Store in airtight cylinders at a temperature not exceeding 40°.

### Profile

Chlorofluorocarbons are used as refrigerants and as aerosol propellants (p.1235). They may also be used as a spray for topical anaesthesia, the intense cold produced by the rapid evaporation of the spray making the tissues insensitive.

### Preparations

**Proprietary Preparations** (details are given in Part 3)
***Arg.:*** Algispray; ***Austria:*** Pharmaethyl†; ***Ger.:*** Provotest†.
**Multi-ingredient: *Austral.:*** Derm-Freeze†; ***Fr.:*** Dynacold†; ***USA:*** Aerofreeze; Fluori-Methane; Fluro-Ethyl.

## Dimethyl Ether

Dimethyl Oxide; Éter dimetílico; Methoxymethane; Oxybismethane.

$C_2H_6O$ = 46.07.
*CAS — 115-10-6.*

### Profile

Dimethyl ether is used as a refrigerant, aerosol propellant (p.1235), and topical anaesthetic.

### Preparations

**Proprietary Preparations** (details are given in Part 3)
**Multi-ingredient: *Austral.:*** Histofreezer; ***Fr.:*** Histofreezer; ***Irl.:*** Wartner; ***NZ:*** Wartner; ***UK:*** PR Freeze Spray; Ralgex Freeze Spray; Wartner.

## Helium

E939; Helio.

He = 4.002602.
*CAS — 7440-59-7.*
*ATC — V03AN03.*

**Pharmacopoeias.** In *US.*

**USP 27** (Helium). A colourless, odourless, tasteless gas which is not combustible and does not support combustion. Very slightly soluble in water. Store in cylinders.

### Profile

As helium is less dense than nitrogen, breathing a mixture of 80% helium and 20% oxygen requires less effort than breathing air. Thus mixtures containing various concentrations of oxygen ('Heliox') have been used in patients with respiratory disorders. Due to the low solubility of helium, mixtures of helium and oxygen are used by divers or others working under high pressure to prevent the development of decompression sickness (caisson disease); they are preferred to compressed air as they do not cause nitrogen narcosis. Helium has been used in pulmonary function testing.

Breathing helium increases vocal pitch and causes voice distortion. Cerebral artery gas embolism has been reported after inhalation of helium from a pressurised container.

◊ Reviews.

1. Rodrigo GJ, *et al.* Use of helium-oxygen mixtures in the treatment of acute asthma: a systematic review. *Chest* 2003; **123:** 891–6.

## Hydrochlorofluorocarbons

HCFCs; Hidroclorofluorocarbonos.

## Chlorodifluoroethane

Clorodifluoroetano; Propellant 142b; Refrigerant 142b. 1-Chloro-1,1-difluoroethane.

$C_2H_3ClF_2$ = 100.5.
*CAS — 75-68-3.*

## Chlorodifluoromethane

Clorodifluorometano; Propellant 22; Refrigerant 22.

$CHClF_2$ = 86.47.
*CAS — 75-45-6.*

### Profile

Hydrochlorofluorocarbons are used as refrigerants and as aerosol propellants (p.1235).

## Hydrofluorocarbons

HFAs; HFCs; Hidrofluorocarbonos; Hydrofluroalkanes.

## Apaflurane *(BAN, rINN)*

Heptafluoropropane; HFA-227; HFC-227. 1,1,1,2,3,3,3-Heptafluoropropane.

$C_3HF_7$ = 170.0.
*CAS — 431-89-0.*

## Difluoroethane

Difluoroetano; Ethylene Fluoride; HFC-152a; Propellant 152a; Refrigerant 152a. 1,1-Difluoroethane.

$C_2H_4F_2$ = 66.05.
*CAS — 75-37-6.*

## Norflurane *(BAN, USAN, rINN)*

Fluorocarbon 134a; GR-106642X; HFA-134a; HFC-134a; Norflurano; Propellant 134a; Refrigerant 134a. 1,1,1,2-Tetrafluoroethane.

$C_2H_2F_4$ = 102.0.
*CAS — 811-97-2.*

### Profile

Hydrofluorocarbons are used as refrigerants and as aerosol propellants (p.1235). They are nonchlorinated and cause less ozone depletion than chlorinated fluorocarbons, which may lead to less detrimental effects on the environment. They are gradually replacing chlorinated fluorocarbons as propellants in medicinal inhalers.

◊ References.

1. Denyer LH, *et al.* GR106642X, a non-chlorinated propellant for use in metered-dose inhalers: safety, tolerability and pharmacokinetics in healthy volunteers. *Br J Clin Pharmacol* 1994; **38:** 509P.
2. Taggart SCO, *et al.* GR106642X: a new, non-ozone depleting propellant for inhalers. *BMJ* 1995; **310:** 1639–40.

## Hydrogen Sulfide

Hydrogen Sulphide; Sulfuro de hidrógeno; Sulphuretted Hydrogen.

$H_2S$ = 34.08.
*CAS — 7783-06-4.*

**Description.** Hydrogen sulfide is a colourless flammable gas with a characteristic odour.

### Adverse Effects

Hydrogen sulfide is a common industrial hazard and is encountered in such places as chemical works, mines, sewage works, and stores of decomposing protein. Concentrations of 0.1 to 0.2% in the atmosphere may be fatal in a few minutes. At concentrations of about 0.005% and above hydrogen sulfide causes anosmia and its unpleasant odour is no longer detectable. Pulmonary irritation, oedema, and respiratory failure usually occur after acute poisoning; prolonged exposure to low concentrations may cause severe conjunctivitis with photophobia and corneal opacity, irritation of the respiratory tract, cough, nausea, vomiting and diarrhoea, pharyngitis, headache, dizziness, and lassitude. There are some similarities to poisoning with cyanides.

◊ General references.

1. Hydrogen Sulfide. *Environmental Health Criteria 19.* Geneva: WHO, 1981. Available at: http://www.inchem.org/documents/ehc/ehc/ehc019.htm (accessed 05/07/04)

### Treatment of Adverse Effects

In poisoning with hydrogen sulfide the patient should be removed from the contaminated atmosphere and an effective airway established. Inhalation of amyl nitrite or parenteral therapy with sodium nitrite have been suggested; this produces methaemoglobin, which may bind sulfide. Oxygen should be given; hyperbaric oxygen therapy has also been suggested. The conjunctival sacs should be carefully washed out if eye irritation is severe. Management is then usually symptomatic and supportive.

◊ References.

1. Gorman DF. Problems and pitfalls in the use of hyperbaric oxygen for the treatment of poisoned patients. *Med Toxicol Adverse Drug Exp* 1989; **4:** 393–9.

### Uses

Hydrogen sulfide is widely employed in many industrial processes.

## Isobutane

E943b; Isobutano; 2-Methylpropane.

$C_4H_{10}$ = 58.12.

**Pharmacopoeias.** In *USNF.*

**USNF 22** (Isobutane). A colourless gas. It is highly flammable and explosive. Store in airtight cylinders at a temperature not exceeding 40°.

### Profile

Isobutane is used as an aerosol propellant (p.1235).

### Preparations

**Proprietary Preparations** (details are given in Part 3)
**Multi-ingredient: *Austral.:*** Histofreezer.

## Nitrogen

Azote; E941; Nitrogenium; Nitrógeno.

$N_2$ = 28.0134.
*CAS — 7727-37-9.*
*ATC — V03AN04.*

**Pharmacopoeias.** In *Eur.* (see p.vi) and *Jpn.* Also in *USNF.*

**Ph. Eur. 5.0** (Nitrogen). The monograph applies to nitrogen for medicinal use. A colourless, odourless gas. Soluble 1 in about 62 of water and 1 in about 10 of alcohol by volume at 20° and at a pressure of 101 kpA. Store as a compressed gas or a liquid in appropriate containers.

The BP 2003 directs that nitrogen should be kept in approved metal cylinders, the shoulders of which are painted black and the remainder grey. The cylinder should carry a label stating 'Nitrogen'.

**Ph. Eur. 5.0** (Nitrogen, Low-oxygen). The monograph applies to nitrogen used in the production of an inert atmosphere for finished medicinal products that are particularly sensitive to degradation by oxygen. A colourless, odourless gas. Soluble 1 in about 62 of water and 1 in about 10 of alcohol by volume at 20° and at a pressure of 101 kpA. Store as a compressed gas or a liquid in appropriate containers.

**USNF 22** (Nitrogen). A colourless, odourless, tasteless gas. It is non-flammable and does not support combustion. Soluble 1 in about 65 of water v/v and 1 in about 9 of alcohol v/v at 20° and at a pressure of 760 mmHg. Store in cylinders.

**USNF 22** (Nitrogen 97 Percent). It contains not less than 97% v/v of nitrogen. Store in cylinders or in a low-pressure collecting tank.

### Adverse Effects

Nitrogen narcosis has been reported after use of nitrogen at high pressure as in deep-water diving. Under high pressure, nitrogen dissolves in blood and lipid. If decompression is too rapid, nitrogen effervesces from body stores producing gas emboli and leads to the syndrome of decompression sickness. Skin contact with liquid nitrogen causes frostbite or burns.

◊ References.

1. Roblin P, *et al.* Liquid nitrogen injury: a case report. *Burns* 1997; **23:** 638–40.
2. Kernbach-Wighton G, *et al.* Clinical and morphological aspects of death due to liquid nitrogen. *Int J Legal Med* 1998; **111:** 191–5.
3. Koplewitz BZ, *et al.* Gastric perforation attributable to liquid nitrogen ingestion. *Pediatrics* 2000; **105:** 121–3.

### Uses and Administration

Nitrogen is used as a diluent for pure oxygen or other active gases and as an inert gas to replace air in containers holding oxidisable substances. Liquid nitrogen is used as a cryotherapeutic agent for the removal of warts (p.1139) and for preservation of tissues and organisms.

## Oxygen

E948; Ossigeno; Oxígeno; Oxygenium; Sauerstoff.

$O_2$ = 31.9988.
*CAS — 7782-44-7.*
*ATC — V03AN01.*

**Pharmacopoeias.** In *Chin., Eur.* (see p.vi), *Int., Jpn, US,* and *Viet.*

**Ph. Eur. 5.0** (Oxygen). A colourless, odourless gas. Soluble 1 in about 32 of water by volume at 20° and at a pressure of 101 kPa. Store as a compressed gas or liquid in appropriate containers.

The BP 2003 directs that oxygen should be kept in approved metal cylinders, the shoulders of which are painted white and the remainder black. The cylinder should carry a label stating 'Oxygen'. In addition, 'Oxygen' or the symbol '$O_2$' should be stencilled in paint on the shoulder of the cylinder.

**Ph. Eur. 5.0** (Air, Medicinal; Aer Medicinalis). It is compressed ambient air containing not less than 20.4% and not more than 21.4% of oxygen. A colourless, odourless gas. Soluble 1 in about 50 of water by volume at 20° and at a pressure of 101 kPa. Store as a gas in suitable containers.

**Ph. Eur. 5.0** (Air, Synthetic Medicinal; Aer Medicinalis Artificiosus; Synthetic Air BP 2003). It is a mixture of nitrogen and oxygen containing between 21.0% and 22.5% of oxygen. A colourless, odourless gas. Soluble 1 in about 50 of water by volume at 20° and at a pressure of 101 kPa. Store as a compressed gas in suitable containers.

**USP 27** (Oxygen). A colourless, odourless, tasteless gas that supports combustion more energetically than does air. Soluble 1 in about 32 of water v/v and 1 in about 7 of alcohol v/v at 20° and at a pressure of 760 mmHg. Store in cylinders or in a pressurised storage tank.

**USP 27** (Medical Air). A natural or synthetic mixture of gases consisting largely of nitrogen and oxygen. It contains not less than 19.5% and not more than 23.5% of oxygen. Store in cylinders or in a low pressure collecting tank.

**USP 27** (Oxygen 93 Percent). It contains not less than 90% v/v and not more than 96% v/v of oxygen, the remainder consisting mostly of argon and nitrogen. Store in cylinders or in a low-pressure collecting tank.

## Adverse Effects

Oxygen toxicity depends upon both the inspired pressure (a function of concentration and barometric pressure) and the duration of exposure, the safe duration decreasing as the pressure increases. At lower pressures of up to 2 atmospheres absolute, pulmonary toxicity occurs before CNS toxicity; at higher pressures, the reverse applies. Symptoms of pulmonary toxicity include a decrease in vital capacity, cough, and substernal distress. Symptoms of CNS toxicity include nausea, mood changes, vertigo, twitching, convulsions, and loss of consciousness.

**Hyperbaric oxygen therapy.** In a review of hyperbaric oxygen therapy[1] the following were mentioned as potential complications: barotrauma (ear or sinus trauma, tympanic membrane rupture, or rarely pneumothorax or air embolism); oxygen toxicity (CNS toxicity or pulmonary toxicity); and reversible visual changes.

1. Grim PS, *et al.* Hyperbaric oxygen therapy. *JAMA* 1990; **263:** 2216–20.

**Retinopathy of prematurity.** In the 1940s and 1950s an epidemic of retinopathy of prematurity, affecting perhaps 10 000 babies, was attributed to excessive use of oxygen in neonates. This resulted in the use of oxygen being reduced or curtailed and the incidence of the condition fell dramatically. However, in the 1970s and later an unexpected resurgence of retinopathy of prematurity occurred (probably *not* due to excessive oxygen use). It was suggested[1,2] that oxygen plays only a minor part and that retinopathy of prematurity is a multifactorial condition that affects the most immature and sick children; the increased incidence may reflect the improved survival of these very premature neonates. A study[3] of supplemental oxygen in infants with prethreshold retinopathy of prematurity suggested that therapy was safe, but a beneficial effect could not be confirmed. However, a retrospective study[4] in premature neonates given supplemental oxygen found that retinopathy of prematurity was more common in those maintained at higher oxygen saturations.

1. Anonymous. Retinopathy of prematurity. *Lancet* 1991; **337:** 83–4.
2. Holmström G. Retinopathy of prematurity. *BMJ* 1993; **307:** 694–5.
3. The STOP-ROP Multicenter Study Group. Supplemental therapeutic oxygen for prethreshold retinopathy of prematurity (STOP-ROP), a randomized, controlled trial. I: Primary outcomes. *Pediatrics* 2000; **105:** 295–310.
4. Tin W, *et al.* Pulse oximetry, severe retinopathy, and outcome at one year in babies of less than 28 weeks gestation. *Arch Dis Child Fetal Neonatal Ed* 2001; **84:** F106–F110.

## Precautions

Any fire or spark is highly dangerous in the presence of increased oxygen concentrations especially when oxygen is used under pressure.

Metal cylinders containing oxygen should be fitted with a reducing valve by which the rate of flow can be controlled. It is important that the reducing valve should be free from all traces of oil or grease, as otherwise a violent explosion may occur. Combustible material soaked in liquid oxygen is potentially explosive and the low temperature of liquid oxygen may cause unsuitable equipment to become brittle and crack. Liquid oxygen should not be allowed to come into contact with the skin as it produces severe 'cold burns'.

Oxygen intended for aviation or mountain rescue must have a sufficiently low moisture content to avoid blocking of valves by ice on freezing.

High concentrations of oxygen should be avoided in patients whose respiration is dependent upon hypoxic drive, otherwise carbon dioxide retention and respiratory depression may ensue.

**Neonates.** The use of supplemental oxygen in neonates is controversial. Although current resuscitation guidelines[1] recommend the use of 100% oxygen for the resuscitation of asphyxiated term neonates, a number of studies[2,3] have suggested that use of room air (21% oxygen) is equally effective and possibly safer than 100% oxygen. Use of supplemental oxygen in preterm neonates has been associated with an increased risk of retinopathy of prematurity, although other factors are probably also involved (see under Adverse Effects, above). However, another study[4] has reported that supplemental oxygen has beneficial effects on sleep patterns in premature neonates.

1. The American Heart Association in collaboration with the International Liaison Committee on Resuscitation (ILCOR). International guidelines 2000 for cardiopulmonary resuscitation and emergency cardiovascular care: part 11: neonatal resuscitation. *Circulation* 2000; **102** (suppl I): 1343–1357. Also published in *Resuscitation* 2000; **46:** 401–16.
2. Saugstad OD, *et al.* Resuscitation of newborn infants with 21% or 100% oxygen: follow-up at 18 to 24 months. *Pediatrics* 2003; **112:** 296–300.
3. Vento M, *et al.* Oxidative stress in asphyxiated term infants resuscitated with 100% oxygen. *J Pediatr* 2003; **142:** 240–6. Correction. *ibid.*; 616.
4. Simakajornboon N, *et al.* Effect of supplemental oxygen on sleep architecture and cardiorespiratory events in preterm infants. *Pediatrics* 2002; **110:** 884–8.

## Uses and Administration

Oxygen is given by inhalation to correct hypoxaemia in conditions causing respiratory failure (below) and in conditions where the oxygen content of the air breathed is inadequate such as in high-altitude disorders (p.822). Oxygen is of value in the treatment of poisoning with a number of substances, including carbon monoxide (p.1235), cyanides (p.1506), and dichloromethane (p.1473). It provides enhanced oxygenation in inhalation injury. Oxygen is also given by inhalation to subjects working in pressurised spaces and to divers to reduce the concentration of nitrogen inhaled. It is used as a diluent of volatile and gaseous anaesthetics.

Oxygen is usually administered by means of nasal prongs or via a face mask; these can usually deliver concentrations of up to 60%. Tight-fitting anaesthetic-type masks, or delivery via an endotracheal tube or oxygen tent, can provide higher concentrations of up to 100%. Face masks are commonly employed for domiciliary oxygen therapy when flow rates are 2 or 4 litres/minute. Oxygen is commonly supplied compressed in metal cylinders although oxygen concentrators, which produce oxygen-enriched air, are useful for domiciliary therapy, especially in patients using large quantities of oxygen. Oxygen may also be supplied at low temperature in insulated containers as liquid oxygen.

In respiratory failure in conditions not usually associated with retention of carbon dioxide, such as pneumonia, pulmonary oedema, or fibrosing alveolitis, oxygen should be given in high concentrations (usually 40 to 100%). Concentrations of 40 to 60% should be used in acute severe asthma even though carbon dioxide retention may have increased as the patient's condition deteriorated. High concentrations of oxygen should always be reduced as soon as possible to the lowest concentration needed to correct hypoxaemia in order to prevent development of any associated oxygen toxicity, including increased carbon dioxide retention. High concentrations of oxygen should be used in carbon monoxide poisoning and, in selected patients, treatment with hyperbaric oxygen considered.

In respiratory failure associated with chronic obstructive pulmonary disease (conditions such as chronic bronchitis and emphysema) oxygen is usually administered to initially give an inspired concentration of up to 28%. High concentrations are to be avoided as they may enhance carbon dioxide retention and narcosis.

Oxygen at a pressure greater than 1 atmosphere absolute, i.e. hyperbaric oxygen therapy (below), is administered by enclosing the patient in a special high-pressure chamber. It may be used in carbon monoxide poisoning, as an adjunct in the treatment of severe anaerobic infections, especially gas gangrene, and for the treatment of decompression sickness and gas emboli.

◊ General references.

1. Naylor-Shepherd MF, *et al.* Oxygen homeostasis: theory, measurement, and therapeutic implications. *DICP Ann Pharmacother* 1990; **24:** 1195–1203.
2. Gribbin HR. Management of respiratory failure. *Br J Hosp Med* 1993; **49:** 461–77.
3. Tarpy SP, Celli BR. Long-term oxygen therapy. *N Engl J Med* 1995; **333:** 710–14.
4. Bateman NT, Leach RM. ABC of oxygen: acute oxygen therapy. *BMJ* 1998; **317:** 798–801.
5. Rees PJ, Dudley F. ABC of oxygen: oxygen therapy in chronic lung disease. *BMJ* 1998; **317:** 871–4.
6. Rees PJ, Dudley F. ABC of oxygen: provision of oxygen at home. *BMJ* 1998; **317:** 935–8.
7. Treacher DF, Leach RM. ABC of oxygen: oxygen transport: basic principles. *BMJ* 1998; **317:** 1302–6.
8. Leach RM, Treacher DF. ABC of oxygen: oxygen transport: tissue hypoxia. *BMJ* 1998; **317:** 1370–3.

**Cluster headache.** Inhalation of 100% oxygen can provide rapid and effective treatment of cluster headache attacks (p.464) but practical difficulties associated with its use result in other drugs being preferred.

References.

1. Fogan L. Treatment of cluster headache: a double-blind comparison of oxygen v air inhalation. *Arch Neurol* 1985; **42:** 362–3.

**Hyperbaric oxygen therapy.** The use of hyperbaric oxygen therapy, which involves the intermittent inhalation of 100% oxygen under a pressure of greater than 1 atmosphere in a specialised chamber, has been the subject of reviews.[1-3] In the 1960s hyperbaric therapy was used for disorders such as *myocardial infarction, stroke, senility,* and *cancer* but clinical studies and experience have shown little benefit and enthusiasm has since waned. Hyperbaric oxygen therapy has also been tried in *multiple sclerosis* but there is little evidence of benefit. There are, however, other disorders for which the evidence supporting the efficacy of hyperbaric oxygen is much stronger.

Hyperbaric oxygen is a safe and effective primary therapy for *decompression sickness* and *air or gas embolism*. The effect is achieved through the mechanical reduction in bubble size in the blood brought about by an increase in ambient pressure; the increased oxygenation of blood due to the additional pressure employed for these conditions (often 6 rather than 2 or 3 atmospheres) is also beneficial.

The role of hyperbaric oxygen therapy in *carbon monoxide poisoning* is unclear but it should be considered in selected patients (see p.1235). Its mechanism of action is not fully understood; it increases the rate at which carboxyhaemoglobin concentrations decline, increases intracellular delivery of oxygen, and may also reduce lipid peroxidation and thus spare neuronal cell membranes.

Hyperbaric oxygen is used as adjunctive therapy in *clostridial infections (gas gangrene)* (p.127). Early treatment appears to reduce systemic toxic reactions (probably by inhibiting the production of alpha toxin by the anaerobic bacteria, *Clostridium*) thus enabling patients to tolerate surgery more readily; additionally there is a clearer demarcation of viable and nonviable tissue. *Necrotising fasciitis* (p.136) is another infection in which hyperbaric oxygen therapy may be useful.

There is some evidence that hyperbaric oxygen may be useful in other types of *wounds*. In an *acute crush injury* therapy may reduce oedema via vasoconstriction and reverse ischaemia by increased oxygen delivery. In *problem wounds*, including venous ulcers, therapy may increase the tissue oxygen tension and stimulate angioneogenesis but it is emphasised that it is adjunctive therapy and not a replacement for meticulous local care. Other wounds in which therapy may be beneficial include thermal burns and compromised skin grafts and flaps. The management of burns and wounds is described on p.1134 and p.1139, respectively.

*Radiation therapy* can damage normal adjacent tissue resulting in tissue hypoxia and eventual cell death. Hyperbaric oxygen therapy appears to aid in salvaging such tissue by stimulating angioneogenesis in marginally viable tissue and has been demonstrated to be beneficial in osteoradionecrosis, radiation-induced cystitis,[4] and other radiation-damaged soft tissue.

There has been interest in the use of hyperbaric oxygen in children with *cerebral palsy*, although a randomised study[5] found that it was no better than pressurised air.

1. Grim PS, *et al.* Hyperbaric oxygen therapy. *JAMA* 1990; **263:** 2216–20.
2. Tibbles PM, Edelsberg JS. Hyperbaric-oxygen therapy. *N Engl J Med* 1996; **334:** 1642–8.
3. Leach RM, *et al.* ABC of oxygen: hyperbaric oxygen therapy. *BMJ* 1998; **317:** 1140–3.
4. Bevers RFM, *et al.* Hyperbaric oxygen treatment for haemorrhagic radiation cystitis. *Lancet* 1995; **346:** 803–5.
5. Collet J-P, *et al.* Hyperbaric oxygen for children with cerebral palsy: a randomised multicentre trial. *Lancet* 2001; **357:** 582–6.

**Respiratory failure.** Respiratory failure occurs when the arterial plasma partial pressure of oxygen ($P_aO_2$) and of carbon dioxide ($P_aCO_2$) cannot be maintained within normal physiological limits.[1] Respiratory failure can be classified into 2 types, both of which are characterised by a low $P_aO_2$ (hypoxaemia). However, in type I the $P_aCO_2$ is normal or low whereas in type II, referred to as ventilatory failure, $P_aCO_2$ is raised (hypercapnia). Some conditions, for example asthma, can produce either type of respiratory failure.

Management of respiratory failure primarily involves administration of oxygen to reverse hypoxaemia, and specific therapy for any underlying condition. Respiratory stimulants may be considered in some situations.

In type I respiratory failure oxygen is administered in high concentrations. Nasal prongs and certain face masks can provide concentrations of up to 60% but if concentrations higher than this are needed then tight-fitting anaesthetic-type masks or methods of delivery such as by endotracheal intubation have to be used.

In type II respiratory failure both high and low concentrations are used according to need.

Patients with *acute severe asthma* (p.777) should usually be given oxygen at high concentrations of 40 to 60%. Low controlled concentrations of oxygen (beginning with about 24 to 28%) are used in the management of respiratory failure in patients with chronic respiratory disorders such as *chronic obstructive pulmonary disease* (p.779) the aim being to improve hypoxaemia without increasing hypercapnia and respiratory acidosis. Patients with exacerbations of chronic ventilatory failure already have an increased central drive to the respiratory muscles and therefore respiratory stimulants such as doxapram have a limited role but may be indicated for short-term use if hypercapnia worsens as a result of the administration of oxygen. For most patients with chronic obstructive pulmonary disease, non-invasive ventilation is probably preferred.[2] Respiratory stimulants may be considered in the management of *postanaesthetic hypoventilation*. Although naloxone can reverse respiratory depression caused by opioid analgesics careful dosage adjustment is required as it can also abolish analgesia. Specific antagonists such as naloxone and flumazenil are also used to treat hypoventilation associated with opioid and benzodiazepine overdosage, respectively. If oxygen therapy fails to raise $P_aO_2$ in respiratory failure and there is worsening hypercapnia and respiratory acidosis the use of artificial ventilation should be considered.

Severe respiratory failure in *neonates* may result from various disorders. Administration of surfactant or inhaled nitric oxide may be of benefit in some cases but extracorporeal membrane oxygenation (ECMO), where blood is removed from the neonate, oxygenated, and re-injected in a continuous circuit that also removes carbon dioxide, may be required.[3] ECMO has also been used in older children and in adults,[4] but is less well established.

1. Gribbin HR. Management of respiratory failure. *Br J Hosp Med* 1993; **49:** 461–77.
2. Plant PK, Elliott MW. Chronic obstructive pulmonary disease 9: management of ventilatory failure in COPD. *Thorax* 2003; **58:** 537–42.

3. Barrington KJ, Finer NN. Care of near term infants with respiratory failure. *BMJ* 1997; **315:** 1215–18.
4. Peek GJ, *et al.* Extracorporeal membrane oxygenation: potential for adults and children? *Hosp Med* 1998; **59:** 304–8.

**Wounds.** Hyperbaric oxygen therapy may have a role in the management of infected and problem wounds (see above). Supplemental normobaric oxygen has been tried in the prevention of postoperative wound infections, but results of controlled studies[1,2] have been contradictory and its role is not established.

1. Greif R, *et al.* Supplemental perioperative oxygen to reduce the incidence of surgical-wound infection. *N Engl J Med* 2000; **342:** 161–7.
2. Pryor KO, *et al.* Surgical site infection and the routine use of perioperative hyperoxia in a general surgical population: a randomized controlled trial. *JAMA* 2004; **291:** 79–87.

## Preparations

**Proprietary Preparations** (details are given in Part 3)
**Multi-ingredient:** ***S.Afr.:*** Entonox; ***UK:*** Entonox; Equanox.

# Propane

Dimethylmethane; E944; Propano; Propyl Hydride.
$C_3H_8$ = 44.10.
*CAS — 74-98-6.*

**Pharmacopoeias.** In *USNF.*

**USNF 22** (Propane). A colourless gas. It is highly flammable and explosive. Store in airtight cylinders at a temperature not exceeding 40°.

## Profile

Propane is used as a refrigerant and as an aerosol propellant (p.1235). It is also widely used as a fuel.

◊ Reports of toxicity associated with the abuse or misuse of propane.[1,2]

1. James NK, Moss ALH. Cold injury from liquid propane. *BMJ* 1989; **299:** 950–1.
2. Siegel E, Wason S. Sudden death caused by inhalation of butane and propane. *N Engl J Med* 1990; **323:** 1638.

## Preparations

**Proprietary Preparations** (details are given in Part 3)
**Multi-ingredient:** ***Austral.:*** Histofreezer; ***Fr.:*** Histofreezer; ***Irl.:*** Wartner; ***NZ:*** Wartner; ***UK:*** Wartner.

# Gastrointestinal Drugs

Gastrointestinal Drug Groups, p.1239
- Antacids, p.1239
- Antidiarrhoeals, p.1239
- Antiemetics, p.1239
- Antisecretory drugs, p.1239
- Laxatives, p.1239
- Mucosal protectants, p.1240
- Prokinetic drugs, p.1240

Management of Gastrointestinal Disorders, p.1240
- Aspiration syndromes, p.1240
- Collagenous colitis, p.1240
- Constipation, p.1240
- Decreased gastrointestinal motility, p.1241
- Diarrhoea, p.1241
- Diverticular disease, p.1241
- Dumping syndrome, p.1242
- Dyspepsia, p.1242
- Gastrointestinal spasm, p.1242
- Gastro-oesophageal reflux disease, p.1242
- Haemorrhoids, p.1243
- Hepatic encephalopathy, p.1243
- Inflammatory bowel disease, p.1243
- Irritable bowel syndrome, p.1244
- Mouth ulceration, p.1245
- Nausea and vomiting, p.1245
- Oesophageal motility disorders, p.1246
- Peptic ulcer disease, p.1246
- Zollinger-Ellison syndrome, p.1247

This chapter describes the principal drugs used in the treatment of gastrointestinal disorders, and the choice of treatment for some of the main disorders.

## Gastrointestinal Drug Groups

### Antacids

Antacids are basic compounds that neutralise hydrochloric acid in the gastric secretions. They are used in the symptomatic management of gastrointestinal disorders associated with gastric hyperacidity such as dyspepsia, gastro-oesophageal reflux disease, and peptic ulcer disease (see below).

Antacids do not reduce the volume of hydrochloric acid secreted and elevation of the gastric pH may actually promote an increase in acid and pepsin secretion. However, this is usually minor and short-lived except after large doses of calcium carbonate. Antacids are normally given between meals and at bedtime when symptoms of gastric hyperacidity usually occur; the presence of food in the stomach can prolong the neutralising activity. Some calculate doses as mEq or mmol of acid-neutralising capacity, but the relationship between neutralising capacity and beneficial effect is not straightforward. Other factors, including formulation (liquid preparations are more effective than solids) and duration of action (relatively insoluble antacids are longer acting) are also important.

Aluminium salts tend to produce constipation and to delay gastric emptying, while magnesium salts have the reverse effect; a combination of the two may reduce adverse gastrointestinal effects. Another advantage of combined antacid formulations is that a slow-acting antacid such as aluminium hydroxide may be combined with a more rapidly acting drug such as magnesium hydroxide to improve the onset and duration of effect. Alternatively, complexes containing both aluminium and magnesium may be used, such as almasilate, hydrotalcite, and magaldrate. Other drugs that may be combined with antacid formulations include simeticone, which acts as a defoaming agent to reduce excess gas in the stomach, and alginates, which form a gel or foam on the surface of the stomach contents thereby impeding reflux and protecting the oesophageal mucosa from acid attack.

Calcium carbonate and sodium bicarbonate are both rapidly acting but have disadvantages: calcium carbonate is usually reserved for short-term treatment because of the risks of rebound acid secretion and metabolic alkalosis, while sodium bicarbonate is absorbed and is contra-indicated in patients who must control sodium intake (e.g. in heart failure, hypertension, renal failure, cirrhosis, or pregnancy).

Antacids may interact with numerous other drugs, affecting the rate and extent of their absorption, and in some cases their renal elimination. Changes in gastric pH affect the dissolution of other drugs, and together with altered gastric emptying can markedly influence absorption. Aluminium compounds in particular are noted for their propensity to adsorb other drugs and to form insoluble complexes that are not absorbed. Antacids that alter urinary pH will affect renal clearance of drugs that are weak acids or bases. Several mechanisms may play a part in any particular interaction. Interactions can be minimised by giving antacids and other medication 2 to 3 hours apart.

Antacids in this chapter include aluminium salts, magnesium salts, and calcium carbonate. For sodium bicarbonate, see p.1223.

Described in this chapter are
- Aceglutamide Aluminium, p.1248
- Alexitol Sodium, p.1248
- Almagate, p.1248
- Almasilate, p.1248
- Aloglutamol, p.1248
- Aluminium Glycinate, p.1249
- Aluminium Hydroxide, p.1249
- Aluminium Hydroxide-Magnesium Carbonate Co-dried Gel, p.1250
- Aluminium Phosphate, p.1250
- Aluminium Sodium Silicate, p.1250
- Basic Aluminium Carbonate, p.1249
- Bismuth Compounds, p.1252
- Calcium Carbonate, p.1254
- Dihydroxyaluminum Sodium Carbonate, p.1261
- Hydrotalcite, p.1267
- Magaldrate, p.1271
- Magnesium Carbonate, p.1272
- Magnesium Hydroxide, p.1272
- Magnesium Oxide, p.1272
- Magnesium Trisilicate, p.1272

### Antidiarrhoeals

Antidiarrhoeals are used as adjuncts in the symptomatic treatment of diarrhoea (see below), although the main aim in the management of *acute* diarrhoea is the correction of fluid and electrolyte depletion with rehydration therapy; this is especially important in infants and young children and antidiarrhoeals are not generally recommended for this age group. Their use is also limited in *chronic* diarrhoea since treatment aimed at the underlying disorder will often alleviate the diarrhoea.

Described in this chapter are drugs that reduce intestinal motility such as the opioid analogues diphenoxylate and loperamide, and adsorbents such as attapulgite and kaolin. Bulking agents (which include bran and ispaghula) have also been used for diarrhoea and for adjusting faecal consistency in patients with colostomies.

Described in this chapter are
- Albumin Tannate, p.1248
- Attapulgite, p.1251
- Bismuth Compounds, p.1252
- Bran, p.1253
- Chalk, p.1255
- Difenoxin, p.1261
- Diphenoxylate, p.1261
- Ispaghula, p.1268
- Kaolin, p.1268
- Lidamidine, p.1270
- Loperamide, p.1271
- Racecadotril, p.1285
- Zaldaride, p.1294

### Antiemetics

Antiemetics are a diverse group of drugs used to treat or prevent nausea and vomiting, including that associated with cancer therapy, anaesthesia, and motion sickness (see below).

The choice of drug depends partly on the cause of nausea and vomiting. For example, hyoscine or an antihistamine are used in motion sickness whereas dopamine antagonists (such as metoclopramide and domperidone) and serotonin 5-$HT_3$-receptor antagonists (5-$HT_3$ antagonists), such as ondansetron, are ineffective. Conversely, nausea and vomiting associated with cancer chemotherapy is often hard to control and special regimens have been devised including the use of the 5-$HT_3$ antagonists, dexamethasone, and, more recently, the neurokinin-1 receptor antagonist aprepitant.

Described in this chapter are
- Alizapride, p.1248
- Aprepitant, p.1250
- Azasetron, p.1251
- Bromopride, p.1254
- Cerium Oxalate, p.1255
- Clebopride, p.1260
- Difenidol, p.1261
- Dolasetron, p.1262
- Domperidone, p.1263
- Dronabinol, p.1264
- Ginger, p.1267
- Granisetron, p.1267
- Itopride, p.1268
- Metoclopramide, p.1274
- Metopimazine, p.1276
- Nabilone, p.1277
- Ondansetron, p.1281
- Palonosetron, p.1282
- Ramosetron, p.1285
- Tropisetron, p.1293

### Antisecretory drugs

Antisecretory drugs are used in the treatment and prophylaxis of peptic ulcer disease (below); some are also employed in other disorders associated with gastric hyperacidity such as gastro-oesophageal reflux disease and dyspepsia (below). They may be divided into:

- *Histamine $H_2$-receptor antagonists* ($H_2$-antagonists), which act by blocking histamine $H_2$-receptors on gastric parietal cells, thereby antagonising the normal stimulatory effect of endogenous histamine on gastric acid production. Those described in this chapter include cimetidine, famotidine, nizatidine, and ranitidine.
- *Proton pump inhibitors*, which act by blocking the enzyme system responsible for active transport of protons into the gastrointestinal lumen, namely the hydrogen/potassium adenosine triphosphatase ($H^+/K^+$ ATPase) of the gastric parietal cell, also known as the 'proton pump'. Those described in this chapter include lansoprazole, omeprazole, pantoprazole, and rabeprazole.
- *Selective antimuscarinics*, which block cholinergic stimulation of gastric acid production with fewer adverse effects than standard antimuscarinics (p.475), but have largely been superseded. Pirenzepine (p.488) is an example.
- *Prostaglandin analogues*, which inhibit gastric acid secretion by a direct action on the parietal cell and may also inhibit gastrin release and possess cytoprotective properties. Misoprostol (p.1519) is an example.

Described in this chapter are
- Cimetidine, p.1255
- Ebrotidine, p.1264
- Esomeprazole, p.1265
- Famotidine, p.1265
- Lafutidine, p.1269
- Lansoprazole, p.1269
- Niperotidine, p.1277
- Nizatidine, p.1277
- Omeprazole, p.1278
- Pantoprazole, p.1283
- Rabeprazole, p.1285
- Ranitidine, p.1285
- Roxatidine, p.1288
- Urogastrone, p.1294

### Laxatives

Laxatives (purgatives or cathartics) promote defaecation and are used in the treatment of constipation (see below) and for bowel evacuation before investigational procedures, such as endoscopy or radiological examination, or before surgery.

Laxatives are frequently employed for self-medication. Abuse of laxatives is a well-known phenomenon that may occasionally lead to toxicity.

Laxatives may be classified according to their mode of action. There is, however, a degree of overlap between the various groups and in some cases the precise mechanisms of action are not fully understood. Many traditionally used laxatives have fallen from use owing to the violence of their action or their adverse effect profile.

- *Bulk laxatives* (bulk-forming laxatives or bulking agents) cause retention of fluid and an increase in faecal mass resulting in stimulation of peristalsis. Owing to their hydrophilic nature, bulk laxatives may also be used to control diarrhoea and to regulate the consistency of effluent in colostomy patients. Those described in this chapter include bran, ispaghula, and sterculia.
- *Stimulant laxatives* (contact laxatives) act by directly stimulating nerve endings in the colonic mucosa, thereby increasing intestinal motility. It is this group of laxatives which is most commonly associated with abuse. Those described in this chapter include bisacodyl, cascara, phenolphthalein, senna, and sodium picosulfate.
- *Osmotic laxatives* act by increasing intestinal osmotic pressure thereby promoting retention of fluid within the bowel. Those described in this chapter include saline laxatives such as magnesium citrate, magnesium hydroxide, and sodium sulfate (for magnesium sulfate and sodium phosphate see p.1228 and p.1230 respectively). Lactulose may also be classified as an osmotic laxative because its breakdown products exert a similar effect. Also included in this group are the hyperosmotic laxatives such as glycerol (p.1694) and sorbitol (p.1446), and the macrogols (p.1708).
- *Faecal softeners* (emollient laxatives) are claimed to act by decreasing surface tension and increasing penetration of intestinal fluid into the faecal mass. Those described in this chapter include docusate (which is also believed to have a stimulant action).

For the lubricant laxative liquid paraffin see p.1479.

Described in this chapter are
- Aloes, p.1248
- Aloin, p.1248
- Bisacodyl, p.1251
- Bisoxatin, p.1253
- Bran, p.1253
- Liquorice, p.1270
- Magnesium Citrate, p.1272
- Magnesium Hydroxide, p.1272
- Magnesium Oxide, p.1272
- Manna, p.1273

Buckthorn, p.1254
Casanthranol, p.1255
Cascara, p.1255
Cassia Pulp, p.1255
Colocynth, p.1260
Croton Oil, p.28
Dantron, p.1261
Docusates, p.1262
Euonymus, p.1265
Fig, p.1266
Frangula, p.1266
Ipomoea, p.1267
Ispaghula, p.1268
Jalap, p.1268
Lactitol, p.1269
Lactulose, p.1269
Oxyphenisatine, p.1282
Pentaerythritol, p.1283
Phenolphthalein, p.1284
Polycarbophil, p.1284
Potassium Acid Tartrate, p.1284
Potassium Sodium Tartrate, p.1284
Prune, p.1285
Psyllium Seed, p.1268
Rhubarb, p.1287
Senna, p.1288
Sodium Picosulfate, p.1289
Sodium Sulfate, p.1290
Sodium Tartrate, p.1290
Sterculia, p.1290
Tamarind, p.1293

### Mucosal protectants

Cytoprotective drugs (mucosal protectants) play a role in the management of peptic ulcer disease (below). They may be divided into:

- *Chelates or complexes*, which coat the gastric mucosa preferentially at sites of ulceration by forming an adherent complex with proteins. Those described in this chapter include sucralfate and tripotassium dicitratobismuthate (which also has an antibacterial role in regimens aimed at eradicating *Helicobacter pylori*)
- *Miscellaneous drugs* include liquorice and its derivatives, such as carbenoxolone, which may act by stimulating the synthesis of protective mucus

Described in this chapter are

Benexate, p.1251
Carbenoxolone, p.1254
Cetraxate, p.1255
Ebrotidine, p.1264
Ecabet, p.1264
Enoxolone Aluminium, p.1264
Gefarnate, p.1267
Irsogladine, p.1267
Liquorice, p.1270
Plaunotol, p.1284
Polaprezinc, p.1284
Rebamipide, p.1287
Sucralfate, p.1290
Sulglicotide, p.1293
Teprenone, p.1293
Tripotassium Dicitratobismuthate, p.1252
Troxipide, p.1294

### Prokinetic drugs

Prokinetic drugs stimulate the motility of the gastrointestinal tract. Gastrointestinal smooth muscle exhibits intrinsic motor activity which is modified by autonomic innervation, local reflexes, and gastrointestinal hormones. This activity produces peristaltic waves, which move the gut contents from stomach to anus, and segmentations, which encourage digestion. Prokinetic drugs may act at various points within this complex system to enhance gastrointestinal movement. Those described in this chapter include metoclopramide, cisapride, and domperidone. Other drugs with prokinetic properties include parasympathomimetics such as bethanechol (p.1487) or neostigmine (p.1492), and the macrolide antibacterial erythromycin (p.208).

Described in this chapter are

Bromopride, p.1254
Cinitapride, p.1259
Cisapride, p.1259
Clebopride, p.1260
Domperidone, p.1263
Itopride, p.1268
Metoclopramide, p.1274
Mosapride, p.1276
Renzapride, p.1287
Tegaserod, p.1293

## Management of Gastrointestinal Disorders

The management of some gastrointestinal disorders is discussed below.

### Aspiration syndromes

Regurgitation and aspiration of gastric contents (Mendelson's syndrome) is an important cause of morbidity and mortality associated with anaesthesia, especially in obstetrics and in emergency surgery. Chemical pneumonitis and respiratory distress result from the acid aspiration, the risk of which is increased by the drugs given as adjuncts to anaesthesia such as opioid analgesics and atropine.

Apart from good anaesthetic technique, including a prohibition on oral intake before elective procedures, efforts to **prevent** or reduce the problem have focussed mainly on increasing the pH of gastric contents to above 2.5, and in reducing gastric volume. However, there is little evidence to show that reduced gastric acidity or volume is associated with decreased morbidity or mortality in patients who have aspirated gastric contents,[1] and some do not recommend the routine pre-operative use of pharmacological prophylaxis in patients undergoing elective surgery with no apparent increased risk for pulmonary aspiration.[1]

The *$H_2$-antagonists* decrease gastric acid secretion and may decrease gastric fluid volume. However, they do not affect the pH of fluid already in the stomach; they must therefore be given some time before anaesthesia, which limits their value in emergency procedures. Cimetidine is considered effective in most patients, although where more prolonged reduction of acidity is required $H_2$-antagonists with a longer duration of action such as ranitidine or famotidine may be preferred. Nizatidine has the advantage of a relatively rapid onset of action.[2] The *proton pump inhibitors*, have also been tried, but results have been variable. Combination with a prokinetic drug may produce better results.[3]

Because of the lack of effect of antisecretory drugs on the pH of existing gastric fluid $H_2$-antagonists may be combined with *antacids* to neutralise gastric acidity. Although magnesium trisilicate has been extensively used[4] without apparent problems particulate antacids are potentially toxic to the lung, which is why soluble antacids such as sodium citrate have been widely used. An effervescent formulation of sodium citrate with cimetidine has been reported to raise gastric pH above 2.5 in more than 98% of patients undergoing caesarean section.[5]

A third component of prophylactic regimens for acid aspiration may be use of a *prokinetic drug* such as metoclopramide. These increase gastric emptying and thereby decrease the volume of stomach contents, and also increase pressure at the lower oesophageal sphincter. The ability of metoclopramide to reverse the effects of opioids on gastric emptying appears to depend on the route of administration: 10 mg given intravenously after opioid analgesia is reported to be effective in promoting gastric emptying, whereas the same dose intramuscularly is not.[6]

If aspiration occurs, pulmonary damage may result within seconds; **treatment** has included removal of any particulate matter, and measures to maintain the airway and ensure adequate oxygenation. Corticosteroids have been used but are no longer considered helpful.[7]


1. American Society of Anesthesiologists Task Force on Preoperative Fasting. Practice guidelines for preoperative fasting and the use of pharmacologic agents to reduce the risk of pulmonary aspiration: application to healthy patients undergoing elective procedures. *Anesthesiology* 1999; **90:** 896–905.
2. Popat MT, *et al.* Comparison of the effects of oral nizatidine and ranitidine on gastric volume and pH in patients undergoing gynaecological laparoscopy. *Anaesthesia* 1991; **46:** 816–19.
3. Orr DA, *et al.* Effects of omeprazole, with and without metoclopramide, in elective obstetric anaesthesia. *Anaesthesia* 1993; **48:** 114–19.
4. Sweeney BL, Wright I. The use of antacids as a prophylaxis against Mendelson's syndrome in the United Kingdom: a survey. *Anaesthesia* 1986; **41:** 419–22.
5. Ormezzano X, *et al.* Aspiration pneumonitis prophylaxis in obstetric anaesthesia: comparison of effervescent cimetidine–sodium citrate mixture and sodium citrate. *Br J Anaesth* 1990; **64:** 503–6.
6. McNeill MJ, *et al.* Effect of iv metoclopramide on gastric emptying after opioid premedication. *Br J Anaesth* 1990; **64:** 450–2.
7. Ryan DW. Pulmonary aspiration: high dose steroids should be abandoned. *BMJ* 1984; **289:** 51.


### Collagenous colitis

Collagenous colitis is a rare condition that presents as persistent watery diarrhoea and is associated with a thickened band of collagen immediately below the surface epithelium of the colonic mucosa. Treatment is largely symptomatic.[1-3] A suggested approach from analysis of data from 163 patients was to try antidiarrhoeal therapy with loperamide initially, and then sulfasalazine if this was ineffective.[2] In unresponsive patients colestyramine, prednisolone, antibacterials such as metronidazole, or mepacrine, or an immunosuppressant such as methotrexate, might all be tried. Mesalazine and olsalazine seemed to be less effective than sulfasalazine,[2] although they may be useful where sulfasalazine is not tolerated.[2,4]

More recently, budesonide has been shown to improve symptoms and histology in patients with collagenous colitis (see p.1095) and this beneficial effect has been supported by a systematic review.[5] However, the usefulness of such treatment in induction or maintenance of remission has not been studied.


1. Rams H, *et al.* Collagenous colitis. *Ann Intern Med* 1987; **106:** 108–13.
2. Bohr J, *et al.* Collagenous colitis: a retrospective study of clinical presentation and treatment in 163 patients. *Gut* 1996; **39:** 846–51.
3. Weldon M. A useful collagenous colitis registry. *Lancet* 1997; **349:** 1410–11.
4. O'Mahony S, *et al.* Coeliac disease and collagenous colitis. *Postgrad Med J* 1990; **66:** 238–41.
5. Chande N, *et al.* Interventions for treating collagenous colitis. Available in The Cochrane Library; Issue 1. Chichester: John Wiley; 2004.


### Constipation

The pattern of normal defaecation is extremely variable. Constipation may be considered to occur if there is a change in that pattern with 2 or more of the following features: a reduced frequency of defaecation, a hardening of the stool, straining on defaecation, or a feeling of incomplete evacuation or anorectal blockage.[1] It is of serious clinical concern when faecal impaction is likely. Constipation can be a symptom of a range of disorders or of drug toxicity[2] and the necessary attention to these underlying causes can resolve it. Constipation can also reflect a change in lifestyle.

An increase in fibre intake, preferably through a high-fibre diet, will help to relieve constipation in the majority of patients[3] without the need for laxatives. Laxatives are often taken unnecessarily and their regular use can lead to problems of abuse, but when dietary modification is difficult or unacceptable a *bulk laxative* may be appropriate.[3,4] The choice of bulk laxative includes bran, ispaghula, methylcellulose and related compounds, psyllium, or sterculia. Bulk laxatives generally have an effect after 1 to 3 days and are of particular value in those with small hard stools; a gradual increase in dose is advisable to avoid flatulence and distension.[1] They may not be the first choice for elderly patients who are frail or immobile since the resulting soft faeces may result in faecal incontinence.[5]

If constipation fails to respond to an increase in fibre intake or use of a bulk laxative, other laxatives should be considered, the choice depending on the clinical condition.[6] For short-term treatment a *stimulant laxative* may be given. Many traditional stimulant laxatives have fallen from use due to adverse effects, and their prolonged use or abuse may irreversibly damage colonic nerves and muscles.[4,6] Provided appropriate stimulant laxatives are used infrequently and at the minimal effective dose, however, they are unlikely to cause significant harm.[4] Commonly used stimulant laxatives include anthraquinone-containing drugs such as senna, and diphenylmethane derivatives such as bisacodyl or sodium picosulfate. Stimulant laxatives have a more rapid onset of action than bulk laxatives, usually proving effective within 6 to 12 hours.[6] Combined preparations are also available, and a combination of senna and fibre has been found to be more effective than the osmotic laxative lactulose in elderly patients with chronic constipation.[7]

*Osmotic laxatives* such as magnesium hydroxide and magnesium sulfate have a very rapid action and are also useful for short-term treatment, but the resultant watery stool, urgency, and occasional incontinence may limit their value.[4] Lactulose and sorbitol have a similar, but slower, action, and may be useful for chronic constipation when a bulk-forming agent is unsuitable.[6] Macrogol 3350 or 4000 is also used as an osmotic laxative.

*Other laxatives* include surfactants such as docusates, which are relatively ineffective alone but are often combined with a stimulant laxative,[6] and may be of value for patients with haemorrhoids or anal fissures, or those in whom straining is potentially hazardous (such as the elderly or those with existing cardiovascular disease). Liquid paraffin should be used with caution owing to its adverse effects, which include anal seepage and the risks of granulomatous disease of the gastrointestinal tract or of lipoid pneumonia on aspiration. Although it has been recommended in some countries for constipation in children,[8,9] the UK Committee on Safety of Medicines considers it should not be used in those under 3 years of age.

*Rectal administration* of laxatives using enemas or suppositories is appropriate in patients requiring rapid relief from constipation. Enemas, which usually combine osmotic and stimulant laxatives, are generally easier for patients to retain than suppositories.[6] Phosphate enemas should be used with caution in patients with renal impairment because of the risks of absorption of significant amounts of phosphate.[6] Glycerol may be administered rectally as suppositories to promote faecal evacuation, and usually acts within 15 to 30 minutes; its action is probably due to an osmotic effect although it may have additional stimulant, lubricating, or faecal-softening properties. Bisacodyl suppositories also have a rapid stimulant effect on the bowel.[6]

**Faecal impaction** is the inability to pass a hard collection of stool, and may result in overflow diarrhoea. Faecal impaction should be treated with a laxative enema and/or manual disimpaction.[2,5,6] Oral laxatives should not be used because of the risk of colonic perforation.[5] When all stool has been cleared, it is important to institute measures, often including regular laxatives, to prevent constipation and recurrent impaction.[5]


1. Lembo A, Camilleri M. Chronic constipation. *N Engl J Med* 2003; **349:** 1360–8.
2. Moriarty KJ, Irving MH. Constipation. *BMJ* 1992; **304:** 1237–40.
3. Taylor R. Management of constipation 1: high fibre diets work. *BMJ* 1990; **300:** 1063–4.
4. Spiller R. Management of constipation 2: when fibre fails. *BMJ* 1990; **300:** 1064–5.

5. Romero Y, *et al.* Constipation and fecal incontinence in the elderly population. *Mayo Clin Proc* 1996; **71:** 81–92.
6. Bateman DN. Management of constipation. *Prescribers' J* 1991; **31:** 7–15.
7. Passmore AP, *et al.* Chronic constipation in long stay elderly patients: a comparison of lactulose and a senna-fibre combination. *BMJ* 1993; **307:** 769–71.
8. Baker SS, *et al.* Constipation in infants and children: evaluation and treatment: a medical position statement of the North American Society for Pediatric Gastroenterology and Nutrition. *J Pediatr Gastroenterol Nutr* 1999; **29:** 612–26. Correction. *ibid.* 2000; **30:** 109. Also available at: http://www.naspghan.org/PDF/constipation.pdf (accessed 06/05/04)
9. Sharif F, *et al.* Liquid paraffin: a reappraisal of its role in the treatment of constipation. *Arch Dis Child* 2001; **85:** 121–4.

## Decreased gastrointestinal motility

Decreased gastrointestinal motility may occur in any part of the gastrointestinal tract, with symptoms depending on the site. It is of varying aetiology and often secondary to some other disorder, such as infection, metabolic or electrolyte disturbance (for example in gastroparesis due to diabetic neuropathy—see also p.326), or insult to the gastrointestinal tract (for example, paralytic or adynamic ileus is frequently a consequence of abdominal surgery and is a serious adverse effect of some drugs).

Acute loss of gastrointestinal motility is often self-limiting once the underlying cause has been treated. Provided the ability of gastrointestinal smooth muscle to contract has not been lost, however, prokinetic drugs such as metoclopramide or domperidone, or erythromycin, or drugs capable of stimulating functional contraction including parasympathomimetics such as neostigmine or bethanechol, may be employed.

Drugs are less successful in chronic conditions such as chronic intestinal pseudo-obstruction where neuromuscular function of the gastrointestinal tract has some intrinsic abnormality.

References.

1. Malagelada J-R, Distrutti E. Management of gastrointestinal motility disorders: a practical guide to drug selection and appropriate ancillary measures. *Drugs* 1996; **52:** 494–506.
2. Luckas M, Buckett W. Acute colonic pseudo-obstruction in the obstetric patient. *Br J Hosp Med* 1997; **57:** 378–81.
3. Mann SD, *et al.* Clinical characteristics of chronic idiopathic intestinal pseudo-obstruction in adults. *Gut* 1997; **41:** 675–81.
4. Laine L. Management of acute colonic pseudo-obstruction. *N Engl J Med* 1999; **341:** 192–3.
5. Rabine JC, Barnett JL. Management of the patient with gastroparesis. *J Clin Gastroenterol* 2001; **32:** 11–18.
6. Holte K, Kehlet H. Postoperative ileus: progress towards effective management. *Drugs* 2002; **62:** 2603–15.

## Diarrhoea

Diarrhoea is characterised by liquid stools and increased stool weight and frequency of defaecation. Although diarrhoea is commonly associated with infection (see Gastro-enteritis, p.127), it may also result from the accumulation of nonabsorbed osmotically active solutes in the gastrointestinal lumen, such as in lactase deficiency, or from the gastrointestinal effects of secretory stimuli, other than the enterotoxins from an infection. It may also occur when intestinal motility or morphology is altered.

**Acute diarrhoea** may lead to excessive water and electrolyte loss and dehydration, and is potentially life-threatening in infants; frail and elderly patients are also at risk. Severe dehydration associated with acute diarrhoea (greater than 10% loss of body-weight), requires *intravenous rehydration therapy* preferably with Ringer's lactate solution.[1,2] Intravenous therapy is also needed for patients who are unable to drink. Otherwise, *oral rehydration therapy* to correct fluid and electrolyte depletion forms the basis of treatment for acute diarrhoea[1-6] and an oral rehydration solution containing essential electrolytes (sodium, potassium, chloride, and bicarbonate or citrate) and glucose is indicated regardless of the age of the patient or the cause of the diarrhoea. A rehydration phase, which involves the replenishment of fluid and electrolytes lost through the diarrhoea, is followed by a maintenance phase to replace continuing losses. Oral rehydration therapy does not stop diarrhoea, which usually continues for a limited period, although it can reduce stool output and vomiting. Oral rehydration therapy may need to be modified if the diarrhoea is associated with malnutrition.[7] (Malnourished children may also benefit from zinc supplementation in acute diarrhoea—see p.1470; vitamin A supplementation may also be important in reducing mortality—see p.1453.) The rationale[4] for the composition of oral rehydration solutions is that glucose promotes the active transport of electrolytes, the absorption of which theoretically increases in efficiency as the ratio of carbohydrate to sodium approaches 1:1.

WHO originally recommended a solution containing 90 mmol/litre of sodium and 111 mmol/litre of glucose; this type of preparation has been used effectively in developing countries where diarrhoeas are commonly bacterial in origin. However, there is now evidence from studies and meta-analyses to suggest that solutions of reduced sodium content and osmolarity are safe and effective and may be preferable to the original standard WHO solution, even in developing countries,[8-11] and WHO and UNICEF now recommend a solution containing 75 mmol/litre of sodium and 75 mmol/litre of glucose, with a reduced total osmolarity of 245 mmol/litre.[12] However, there are concerns regarding the possible increased risk of hyponatraemia with the use of the reduced osmolarity solutions in patients with cholera.[12-14]

In developed countries viral diarrhoeas, which are associated with less electrolyte loss, are more common. Commercial preparations available in the UK therefore usually provide 50 to 60 mmol/litre of sodium and 90 to 111 mmol/litre of glucose; the total osmolarity is slightly hypotonic (about 250 mmol/litre) to prevent possible induction of osmotic diarrhoea.[15]

Areas of debate include the necessity for inclusion of citrate or bicarbonate,[15] and whether cereal-based rather than glucose-based rehydration solutions would be preferable.[16-19] There is considerable evidence that cereal-based solutions tend to produce more rapid resolution of diarrhoea, although one study has suggested that the reduction in stool output is temporary,[20] and another found that a glucose-based solution was equally effective when combined with early re-introduction of feeding.[17] In 1994, a review of clinical trials concluded that a rice-based rehydration solution should be recommended for patients with cholera, but that there was no reason to change from WHO's glucose-based formulation for children with non-cholera diarrhoea,[21] a view confirmed by a recent systematic review.[22] A study in 48 patients with cholera compared the use of standard glucose-based oral rehydration therapy, standard therapy plus rice flour, and standard therapy plus amylase-resistant starch.[23] The addition of amylase-resistant starch to standard oral rehydration solution was shown to reduce stool output and to reduce the duration of diarrhoea,[23] although the methodology of this study was questioned[24] and further investigation of such solutions is required.

Home remedies[1,2] that have been used for oral rehydration include coconut water, rice water, soups, weak tea, and solutions of various salts and sugars; these may be of value when more conventional oral rehydration solutions are unavailable. The use of cordials and soft drinks with low pH and high osmolality, however, may exacerbate diarrhoea and infant deaths have been associated with their use for rehydration.[25]

Oral rehydration therapy should be combined with *dietary measures*, particularly in children, to avoid malnutrition owing to low food intake during the illness, and as mentioned above, may need to be modified if the diarrhoea is associated with malnutrition. Breast feeding should be continued throughout rehydration therapy.[15,25,26] In the case of cows' milk formula feeds dilution has been advocated because of the possibility of lactose intolerance[27] but is usually not necessary.[28,29] Withholding food during diarrhoea in both adults and children is not recommended:[1,10] feeding may decrease stool output and shorten the duration of diarrhoea.[6]

Oral rehydration therapy prevents dehydration, but does not necessarily shorten the duration of the diarrhoea, and patients therefore frequently desire the symptomatic relief provided by *drug therapy*. Use of such therapy should be balanced against the risk that it may distract from the need for oral rehydration therapy and may have undesirable side-effects. WHO considers that antidiarrhoeal drug therapy is of limited value for acute infectious diarrhoea, does not reduce fluid and electrolyte loss, may delay the expulsion of causative micro-organisms, and should never be used in children.[30] Nevertheless, short courses of antidiarrhoeals are occasionally used if symptoms are causing considerable discomfort.[31]

The main groups of antidiarrhoeal drugs are adsorbents such as attapulgite, kaolin, and pectin, and drugs that reduce intestinal motility such as diphenoxylate, loperamide, and codeine. Bulk laxatives such as methylcellulose have also been used for symptomatic treatment because of their absorptive capacity. Bismuth salicylate is another compound used in diarrhoea and is favoured in the USA when antidiarrhoeal therapy is deemed desirable.[31] Racecadotril is an enkephalinase inhibitor used in the treatment of acute diarrhoea; the calmodulin inhibitor zaldaride has also been investigated.

Antibacterial and antiprotozoal drugs have been used for infective diarrhoeas, including the prophylaxis and treatment of travellers' diarrhoea (see Gastro-enteritis, p.127 and p.596), but their overuse encourages the development of resistance and prophylaxis is not recommended. Vaccines are being developed for the prevention of rotaviral diarrhoeas (p.1637).

**Chronic diarrhoea** may be associated with underlying disease and therefore symptomatic relief is less appropriate than treatment of the disease itself. For example, colestyramine will reduce the diarrhoea associated with bile acid malabsorption. Where the disease process responsible for chronic diarrhoea cannot be satisfactorily suppressed, however, symptomatic relief may be appropriate, for example in diabetic diarrhoea (see under Diabetic Complications, p.326).

1. WHO. *The management and prevention of diarrhoea: practical guidelines*. 3rd ed. Geneva: WHO, 1993.
2. Sack DA. Use of oral rehydration therapy in acute watery diarrhoea: a practical guide. *Drugs* 1991; **41:** 566–73.
3. WHO Diarrhoeal Diseases Control Programme/Fédération Internationale Pharmaceutique. *The treatment of acute diarrhoea: information for pharmacists*. Geneva: (WHO/CDD/SER/87.11).
4. Avery ME, Snyder JD. Oral therapy for acute diarrhea: the underused simple solution. *N Engl J Med* 1990; **323:** 891–4.
5. Balistreri WF. Oral rehydration in acute infantile diarrhoea. *Am J Med* 1990; **88** (suppl 6A): 30S–33S.
6. American Academy of Pediatrics. Practice parameter: the management of acute gastroenteritis in young children. *Pediatrics* 1996; **97:** 424–35. Also available at: http://aappolicy.aappublications.org/cgi/reprint/pediatrics;97/3/424.pdf (accessed 07/05/04)
7. Golden MHN, Briend A. Treatment of malnutrition in refugee camps. *Lancet* 1993; **342:** 360.
8. International Study Group on Reduced-osmolarity ORS Solutions. Multicentre evaluation of reduced-osmolarity oral rehydration salts solution. *Lancet* 1995; **345:** 282–5.
9. Santosham M, *et al.* A double-blind clinical trial comparing World Health Organization oral rehydration solution with a reduced osmolarity solution containing equal amounts of sodium and glucose. *J Pediatr* 1996; **128:** 45–51.
10. Alam NH, *et al.* Efficacy and safety of oral rehydration solution with reduced osmolarity in adults with cholera: a randomised double-blind clinical trial. *Lancet* 1999; **354:** 296–9.
11. Hahn S, *et al.* Reduced osmolarity oral rehydration solution for treating dehydration caused by acute diarrhoea in children. Available in The Cochrane Library; Issue 1. Chichester: John Wiley; 2004.
12. Anonymous. New formula oral rehydration salts. *WHO Drug Inf* 2002; **16:** 121–2.
13. Fuchs GJ. A better oral rehydration solution? An important step, but not a leap forward. *BMJ* 2001; **323:** 59–60.
14. Hirschhorn N, *et al.* Formulation of oral rehydration solution. *Lancet* 2002; **360:** 340–1.
15. Murphy MS. Guidelines for managing acute gastroenteritis based on a systematic review of published research. *Arch Dis Child* 1998; **79:** 279–84.
16. Gore SM, *et al.* Impact of rice-based oral rehydration solution on stool output and duration of diarrhoea: metaanalysis of 13 clinical trials. *BMJ* 1992; **304:** 287–91.
17. Fayad IM, *et al.* Comparative efficacy of rice-based and glucose-based oral rehydration salts plus early reintroduction of food. *Lancet* 1993; **342:** 772–5.
18. Bang A. Towards better oral rehydration. *Lancet* 1993; **342:** 755–6.
19. Islam A, *et al.* Is rice-based oral rehydration therapy effective in young infants? *Arch Dis Child* 1994; **71:** 19–23.
20. Molina S, *et al.* Clinical trial of glucose-oral rehydration solution (ORS), rice dextrin-ORS, and rice flour-ORS for the management of children with acute diarrhea and mild or moderate dehydration. *Pediatrics* 1995; **95:** 191–7.
21. Bhan MK, *et al.* Clinical trials of improved oral rehydration salt formulations: a review. *Bull WHO* 1994; **72:** 945–55.
22. Fontaine O, *et al.* Rice-based oral rehydration solution for treating diarrhoea. Available in The Cochrane Library; Issue 1. Chichester: John Wiley; 2004.
23. Ramakrishna BS, *et al.* Amylase-resistant starch plus oral rehydration solution for cholera. *N Engl J Med* 2000; **342:** 308–13.
24. Pierce NF, *et al.* Amylase-resistant starch plus oral rehydration solution for cholera. *N Engl J Med* 2000; **342:** 1995–6.
25. Elliott EJ. Viral diarrhoeas in childhood. *BMJ* 1992; **305:** 1111–12.
26. Jelliffe DB, Jelliffe EFP. *Dietary management of young children with acute diarrhoea*. 2nd ed. Geneva: WHO, 1991.
27. Kleinman RE. We have the solution: now what's the problem? *Pediatrics* 1992; **90:** 113–15.
28. Chew F, *et al.* Is dilution of cows' milk formula necessary for dietary management of acute diarrhoea in infants aged less than 6 months? *Lancet* 1993; **341:** 194–7.
29. Duggan C, Nurko S. 'Feeding the gut': the scientific basis for continued enteral nutrition during acute diarrhea. *J Pediatr* 1997; **131:** 801–8.
30. WHO. *The rational use of drugs in the management of acute diarrhoea in children*. Geneva: WHO, 1990.
31. Aranda-Michel J, Giannella RA. Acute diarrhoea: a practical review. *Am J Med* 1999; **106:** 670–6.

## Diverticular disease

Diverticula are small hernias or pouches of mucosa that develop through the muscular wall of the gut (especially the colon) or other hollow organs; they increase in prevalence with increasing age. Diverticular disease (the presence of colonic diverticula) is usually asymptomatic, but may be associated with symptoms of abdominal pain and altered bowel habit (diverticulosis). Occasionally there may be severe life-threatening complications such as inflammation and necrosis of diverticula (diverticulitis), perforation, fistula formation, obstruction, or haemorrhage.

In uncomplicated diverticular disease, treatment is with a high-fibre diet, gradually supplemented if necessary with a bulk laxative such as bran or ispaghula, to ease constipation, but such supplements may not relieve the other symptoms of diverticular disease. Antispasmodics such as antimuscarinics or mebeverine may be useful in relieving pain due to muscle spasm.

Diverticulitis requires treatment with broad-spectrum antibacterials and fluid support; analgesia may be needed for severe pain. If peritonitis or abscess develops, surgical intervention may be necessary. Surgical resection is usually considered when fistula, perforation, or obstruction are present.

References.


1. Ferzoco LB, *et al*. Acute diverticulitis. *N Engl J Med* 1998; **338:** 1521–6.
2. Stollman N, Raskin JB. Diverticular disease of the colon. *Lancet* 2004; **363:** 631–9.


## Dumping syndrome

The word dumping in this context is used to describe the unnaturally rapid transport of gastric contents to the small intestine. The dumping syndrome is an important cause of morbidity following gastrointestinal surgery, and is thought to be due to the destruction of normal regulatory mechanisms in the upper gastrointestinal tract.[1,2] Early dumping begins within 10 to 30 minutes of the ingestion of a meal (typically, symptoms are precipitated by hyperosmolar, carbohydrate-rich food) and comprises gastrointestinal symptoms (fullness, abdominal pain, nausea and vomiting, explosive diarrhoea) and vasomotor symptoms (sweating, weakness, dizziness, flushing, and palpitations). The effects are thought to be due to fluid shifts from the intravascular space to the bowel lumen. Some patients experience late dumping, 1 to 4 hours after a meal, which comprises only the vasomotor symptoms and appears to be due to reactive hypoglycaemia following high carbohydrate concentrations in the small intestine.

The mainstays of therapy are dietary modifications, taking small frequent meals low in carbohydrate, followed by liquids 30 minutes later. Attempts to slow or reduce carbohydrate absorption have involved the use of dietary fibre (guar gum or pectin) or α-glucosidase inhibitors such as acarbose; acarbose and pectin have also been tried in combination.[3] However, such agents may themselves cause gastrointestinal disturbances and they do not seem to be helpful in most patients.[2] More recently, beneficial results with somatostatin have led to the use of its longer-acting analogue, octreotide.[2,4] Octreotide substantially reduces the symptoms of both early and late dumping, probably by slowing gastric emptying and by inhibiting the release of gastrointestinal mediators (peptide hormones such as neurotensin), and prevents hyperinsulinaemia and subsequent reactive hypoglycaemia. It may be given up to 2 hours before a meal.

In the minority of patients who do not respond to medical therapy surgery may be required.[1,2]


1. Eagon JC, *et al*. Postgastrectomy syndromes. *Surg Clin North Am* 1992; **72:** 445–65.
2. Carvajal SH, Mulvihill SJ. Postgastrectomy syndromes: dumping and diarrhea. *Gastroenterol Clin North Am* 1994; **23:** 261–79.
3. Speth PAJ, *et al*. Effect of acarbose, pectin, a combination of acarbose with pectin, and placebo on postprandial reactive hypoglycaemia after gastric surgery. *Gut* 1983; **24:** 799–802.
4. Li-Ling J, Irving M. Therapeutic value of octreotide for patients with severe dumping syndrome—a review of randomised controlled trials. *Postgrad Med J* 2001; **77:** 441–2.


## Dyspepsia

Dyspepsia, also commonly known as indigestion, is a frequent but ill-defined disorder primarily associated with epigastric discomfort or pain. It may be a symptom of specific diseases such as peptic ulcer disease, gastro-oesophageal reflux disease, gastric carcinoma, chronic pancreatitis, or gallstones. However, in many patients there is no identifiable systemic disease, in which case it is known as non-ulcer dyspepsia or functional dyspepsia.

A number of reviews and recommendations have addressed the subject of dyspepsia,[1-6] and, in the UK, guidelines have been issued by the Scottish Intercollegiate Guidelines Network[7] and the British Society of Gastroenterology.[8] The initial management of non-ulcer dyspepsia usually includes advice to avoid alcohol, caffeine, smoking, and aggravating foods, and to eat small regular meals to aid digestion. Results of studies of drugs for non-ulcer dyspepsia have been variable and difficult to evaluate since the condition tends to be self-limiting, and there is often a large placebo response.

Drugs to suppress gastric acid such as antacids or antisecretory drugs are commonly used. Antacids may give some symptomatic relief, and are widely used for self-medication. Similarly, $H_2$-antagonists are often tried, especially for symptoms of reflux, although studies in non-ulcer dyspepsia have been largely disappointing. Proton pump inhibitors are also widely used, although again the evidence suggests that their value in non-ulcer dyspepsia is limited, and in the UK the National Institute for Clinical Excellence does not recommend such use.[9] However, they may be of value in patients with uninvestigated dyspepsia, many of whom have peptic ulcer disease or gastro-oesophageal reflux disease. Most authorities consider that a short course of drug therapy may be given to younger patients (under 40 to 45 years of age) lacking obvious symptoms of organic disease before any investigation needs to be performed. However, the use of antisecretory drugs can mask the symptoms of gastric carcinoma, and in older patients who are at greater risk, early investigation may be desirable.

Alternatively, prokinetic drugs such as metoclopramide may be given, particularly if an underlying gastrointestinal motility disorder is suspected. Meta-analysis has suggested that prokinetic therapy may be more effective than an $H_2$-antagonist in non-ulcer dyspepsia.[10] Other approaches to drug therapy include the use of an insoluble bismuth salt, and the use of antimuscarinics to relieve spasm. It is not clear whether *Helicobacter pylori* plays any role in the pathology of non-ulcer dyspepsia, but eradication in *H. pylori*-positive patients has been suggested on the grounds that it will benefit patients with undiagnosed peptic ulcer disease and reduce the need for endoscopy.[2] An analysis of five *H. pylori*-eradication trials suggested a modest improvement in symptoms in patients with non-ulcer dyspepsia.[11] Although a subsequent study found no evidence of benefit from *H. pylori* eradication,[12] others have suggested that response to omeprazole may be greater in *H. pylori*-positive patients.[13] Meta-analyses have come to opposite conclusions regarding the benefits of eradication.[14,15]


1. Whitaker MJ, *et al*. Controversy and consensus in the management of upper gastrointestinal disease in primary care. *Int J Clin Pract* 1997; **51:** 239–43.
2. Agréus L, Talley N. Challenges in managing dyspepsia in general practice. *BMJ* 1997; **315:** 1284–8.
3. Fisher RS, Parkman HP. Management of nonulcer dyspepsia. *N Engl J Med* 1998; **339:** 1376–81.
4. Locke GR. Nonulcer dyspepsia: what it is and what it is not. *Mayo Clin Proc* 1999; **74:** 1011–15.
5. Delaney B, *et al*. The management of dyspepsia: a systematic review. *Health Technol Assess* 2000; **4:** (39). Also available at: http://www.ncchta.org/ProjectData/3_project_record_published.asp?PjtId=1017 (accessed 07/05/04)
6. Stanghellini V, *et al*. New developments in the treatment of functional dyspepsia. *Drugs* 2003; **63:** 869–92.
7. Scottish Intercollegiate Guidelines Network. Dyspepsia: a national clinical guideline (March 2003). Available at: http://www.sign.ac.uk/pdf/sign68.pdf (accessed 06/05/04)
8. British Society of Gastroenterology. Dyspepsia management guidelines (revised April 2002). Available at: http://www.bsg.org.uk/clinical_prac/guidelines/dyspepsia.htm (accessed 06/05/04)
9. National Institute for Clinical Excellence. Guidance on the use of proton pump inhibitors in the treatment of dyspepsia (issued July 2000). Available at: http://www.nice.org.uk/pdf/proton.pdf (accessed 06/05/04)
10. Finney JS, *et al*. Meta-analysis of antisecretory and gastrokinetic compounds in functional dyspepsia. *J Clin Gastroenterol* 1998; **26:** 312–20.
11. Jaakkimainen RL, *et al*. Is *Helicobacter pylori* associated with non-ulcer dyspepsia and will eradication improve symptoms? A meta-analysis. *BMJ* 1999; **319:** 1040–4.
12. Talley NJ, *et al*. Absence of benefit of eradicating Helicobacter pylori in patients with nonulcer dyspepsia. *N Engl J Med* 1999; **341:** 1106–11.
13. Blum AL, *et al*. Short course acid suppressive treatment for patients with functional dyspepsia: results depend on Helicobacter pylori status. *Gut* 2000; **47:** 473–80.
14. Moayyedi P, *et al*. Eradication of Helicobacter pylori for non-ulcer dyspepsia. Available in The Cochrane Library; Issue 1. Chichester: John Wiley; 2004.
15. Laine L, *et al*. Therapy for Helicobacter pylori in patients with nonulcer dyspepsia: a meta-analysis of randomized, controlled trials. *Ann Intern Med* 2001; **134:** 361–9.


## Gastrointestinal spasm

Pain or discomfort of the gastrointestinal tract may be associated with spasm of the smooth muscle of the gut; such pain and spasm may be associated with the irritable bowel syndrome (see below), dyspepsia (see above), or diverticular disease (see above). Antispasmodic drugs have traditionally been used in patients thought to have gastrointestinal spasm, and have mainly been of two types: antimuscarinics such as dicycloverine, and direct smooth muscle relaxants such as mebeverine; use of antimuscarinics, in particular, has tended to be limited by concern about their adverse effects.

Colic is a general term used to describe spasmodic or griping pain, usually of the viscera, and when not otherwise qualified is often understood to refer to pain in the gastrointestinal tract. Infant colic is common in the first few months of childhood,[1] and tends to be managed by nonpharmacological measures and assessment of the feeding technique. Elimination of cows' milk protein appears to be of benefit, but use of a low-lactose formula is not.[1] Tilactase has been added to feeds to aid lactose digestion but the extent of any benefit is unclear. Traditional remedies such as gripe water, which contains essential oils of dill or fennel and is mildly carminative, are of dubious efficacy. Antimuscarinic antispasmodics, although effective[1] may be associated with adverse effects, and are no longer considered appropriate.[2] Simeticone suspension, given before feeds, is commonly used but has been found to be no better than placebo.[2,3] It has been reported that sucrose, given as a 12% solution, improves infant colic.[4]


1. Lucassen PLBJ, *et al*. Effectiveness of treatments for infantile colic: systematic review. *BMJ* 1998; **316:** 1563–9.
2. Garrison MM, Christakis DA. A systematic review of treatments for infant colic. *Pediatrics* 2000; **106** (suppl): 184–90.
3. Metcalf TJ, *et al*. Simethicone in the treatment of infant colic: a randomized, placebo-controlled, multicenter trial. *Pediatrics* 1994; **94:** 29–34.
4. Markestad T. Use of sucrose as a treatment for infant colic. *Arch Dis Child* 1997; **76:** 356–8.


## Gastro-oesophageal reflux disease

Gastro-oesophageal reflux disease results from the reflux of gastric or duodenal contents into the oesophagus. Symptoms include heartburn, acid regurgitation, and dysphagia (difficulty in swallowing); oesophageal inflammation and ulceration (reflux oesophagitis), and stricture formation may occur. Protracted reflux over several years can lead to the development of Barrett's oesophagus (columnar epithelial metaplasia), which is a risk factor for malignancy.

Lifestyle measures for **management** of the disease include avoidance of alcohol and aggravating foods such as chocolate and coffee.[1-6] Raising the head of the bed for patients with nocturnal symptoms,[4] and avoiding lying down within 2 to 3 hours of a meal may be useful.[1,3] Cessation of smoking does not appear to alter reflux symptoms.[4,6] Withdrawing drugs that reduce gastro-oesophageal sphincter tone and hence exacerbate reflux may be considered:[3] such drugs include theophylline and antimuscarinics.

- *Antacids* are used for mild disease and as adjuncts to other therapies. Alginate-containing antacids are said to form an alkaline 'raft' that floats on the surface of the stomach contents to impede reflux and protect the oesophageal mucosa; they are more effective than simple antacids for symptomatic relief.[3]
- Should more vigorous therapy be needed suppression of gastric acid secretion is a likely next step. In the first instance, particularly in patients with mild oesophagitis, this may be with a *histamine $H_2$-antagonist* such as cimetidine or ranitidine.[1,2] Although $H_2$-antagonists have been found to relieve symptoms and reduce antacid consumption, rates of oesophageal healing depend on the severity of the disease and duration of therapy. There do not appear to be useful gains in efficacy from doubling the standard dose of $H_2$-antagonists,[4] but use of divided doses may possibly be of additional benefit.[4,5]
- Alternatively, a *prokinetic drug* such as metoclopramide may improve gastro-oesophageal sphincter function and accelerate gastric emptying. These appear to be as effective as $H_2$-antagonists. The combination of an $H_2$-antagonist and cisapride may be more effective than either drug alone.[4] However, concern over the risk of cardiotoxicity and potential for serious interactions with cisapride has led to severe restrictions on its use.
- A better alternative for resistant disease, or for initial therapy in patients with moderate or severe disease, may be treatment with a *proton pump inhibitor* such as omeprazole or lansoprazole. Proton pump inhibitors are more effective than $H_2$-antagonists in terms of both rate and extent of reduction in symptoms and healing of oesophagitis.[7,8] Consequently, some advocate the use of proton pump inhibitors as first-line drugs even in mild disease, using a step-down approach after successful therapy.[4,6]

In patients with mild disease, a trial of withdrawal of drug therapy is appropriate after successful initial drug therapy.[4,6] Short courses of therapy as and when symptoms demand (intermittent treatment) may be effective in uncomplicated disease.[9] However, in patients with severe oesophagitis, long-term **maintenance** therapy is likely to be required.[4] Maintenance with $H_2$-antagonists has generally been disappointing although some patients respond. A proton pump inhibitor is more effective.[8] Another approach is to use a combination for maintenance and in one study omeprazole with cisapride provided more effective maintenance than ranitidine or cisapride alone or in combination.[10] Again, however, cisapride is now unlikely to be used in practice because of the risks.

**Eradication** of *Helicobacter pylori* infection does not heal or prevent relapse of gastro-oesophageal reflux disease.[4] However, eradication of *H. pylori* has been suggested on the basis that treatment with proton pump inhibitors is associated with worsening of gastritis in *H. pylori*-infected patients. Conversely, epidemiological evidence suggests that *H. pylori* infection protects against gastro-oesophageal reflux disease.[11]

In patients who have a poor response to drug therapy, or in those with complications such as oesophageal stricture or ulceration, **surgery** to re-establish gastro-oesophageal competence may be considered.[4] Elimination of acid reflux by surgery or proton pump inhibitors has at best modest effects on metaplasia in Barrett's oesophagus,[12] although proton pump inhibitors remain the mainstay of therapy.[13] Combining acid suppression with thermal ablation or photodynamic therapy (5-aminolevulinic acid or porfimer) has been investigated.[12]

In **infants**, gastro-oesophageal reflux is common but usually resolves spontaneously with increasing age and requires no treatment. Occasionally, it may be associated with complications such as failure to thrive, oesophagitis, and pulmonary symptoms of acid regurgitation, but can be managed by upright positioning and the use of thickened foods; drug therapy is controversial. It has been suggested that where drug therapy is needed, an alginate-antacid combination may be appropriate initially;[14] cisapride, alone[14] or with an antisecretory drug,[15] has been given but the risk of cardiotoxicity makes the use of cisapride in infants extremely problematic (see p.1259).

Gastro-oesophageal reflux is commonly encountered during normal **pregnancy**, and is generally managed by lifestyle and dietary modifications.[16] If drug therapy is required, nonsystemically absorbed antacids or sucralfate should be tried first. If these are ineffective, ranitidine may be tried.[16] Proton pump inhibitors are not licensed for use during pregnancy although the relative risk associated with exposure seems to be quite low (see under Precautions of Omeprazole, p.1279).


1. Klinkenberg-Knol EC, *et al.* Pharmacological management of gastro-oesophageal reflux disease. *Drugs* 1995; **49:** 695–710.
2. Anonymous. The medical management of gastro-oesophageal reflux. *Drug Ther Bull* 1996; **34:** 1–4.
3. Galmiche JP, *et al.* Treatment of gastro-oesophageal reflux disease in adults. *BMJ* 1998; **316:** 1720–3.
4. Dent J, *et al.* An evidence-based appraisal of reflux disease management—the Genval Workshop Report. *Gut* 1999; **44** (suppl 2): S1–S16.
5. De Vault KR, *et al.* Updated guidelines for the diagnosis and treatment of gastroesophageal reflux disease. *Am J Gastroenterol* 1999; **94:** 1434–42.
6. Dent J, *et al.* Management of gastro-oesophageal reflux disease in general practice. *BMJ* 2001; **322:** 344–7.
7. Chiba N, *et al.* Speed of healing and symptom relief in grade II to IV gastroesophageal reflux disease: a meta-analysis. *Gastroenterology* 1997; **112:** 1798–810.
8. Dekel R, *et al.* The role of proton pump inhibitors in gastro-oesophageal reflux disease. *Drugs* 2004; **64:** 277–95.
9. Bardhan KD, *et al.* Symptomatic gastro-oesophageal reflux disease: double blind controlled study of intermittent treatment with omeprazole or ranitidine. *BMJ* 1999; **318:** 502–7.
10. Vigneri S, *et al.* A comparison of five maintenance therapies for reflux esophagitis. *N Engl J Med* 1995; **333:** 1106–10.
11. Labenz J, Malfertheiner P. Helicobacter pylori in gastro-oesophageal reflux disease: causal agent, independent or protective factor? *Gut* 1997; **41:** 277–80.
12. Cameron AJ. Management of Barrett's esophagus. *Mayo Clin Proc* 1998; **73:** 457–61.
13. Fass R, Sampliner RE. Barrett's oesophagus: optimal strategies for prevention and treatment. *Drugs* 2003; **63:** 555–64.
14. Anonymous. Managing childhood gastro-oesophageal reflux. *Drug Ther Bull* 1997; **35:** 77–80.
15. Faubion WA, Zein NN. Gastroesophageal reflux in infants and children. *Mayo Clin Proc* 1998; **73:** 166–73.
16. Broussard CN, Richter JE. Treating gastro-oesophageal reflux disease during pregnancy and lactation: what are the safest therapy options? *Drug Safety* 1998; **19:** 325–37.


## Haemorrhoids

Haemorrhoids ('piles') are venous swellings of the tissues around the anus: those above the dentate line (the point where the modified skin of the outer anal canal becomes gut epithelium), which usually protrude into the anal canal, are termed internal haemorrhoids, while those below this point are called external haemorrhoids. Due to internal pressure, internal haemorrhoids tend to congest, bleed, and eventually prolapse; with external haemorrhoids painful thrombosis may develop.

Initial treatment of internal haemorrhoids involves a high-fibre diet and avoidance of straining at stool, so bulk laxatives and faecal softeners may be indicated. Small bleeding haemorrhoids may be injected with a sclerosing agent such as oily phenol injection, but rubber band ligation, or perhaps a technique such as infra-red coagulation, is more effective and associated with fewer complications.[1,2] More severe and prolonged prolapse generally requires surgery.[3] Surgical excision to remove the clot is used for thrombosed external haemorrhoids.

An enormous range of mainly topical drug treatments is available for symptomatic relief, but in many cases their value is at best unproven.

Topical preparations are usually made up in a lubricating or emollient base. Local anaesthetics may be included to relieve pain, and corticosteroids may be used where infection is not present: preparations containing either group of drugs are intended only for short-term use. Inclusion of antibacterials is thought to be of little value and may encourage the development of resistant organisms. Some preparations include heparinoids. Other agents frequently included for their soothing properties include various bismuth salts, zinc oxide, hamamelis, resorcinol, and peru balsam.

Bioflavonoids and various derivatives of aesculus may also be included in topical preparations; they have also been given systemically in some countries as have some other compounds such as calcium dobesilate and tribenoside, presumably for their supposed action on venous capillary walls. Oral micronised bioflavonoid preparations may reduce symptoms as an adjunct to surgery.[3,4]

Other agents that have been used in the treatment of haemorrhoids include pilewort (ficaria) and combinations of yeast extract with shark-liver oil.


1. Johanson JF, Rimm A. Optimal nonsurgical treatment of hemorrhoids: a comparative analysis of infrared coagulation, rubber band ligation, and injection sclerotherapy. *Am J Gastroenterol* 1992; **87:** 1601–6.
2. MacRae HM, McLeod RS. Comparison of hemorrhoidal treatment modalities: a meta-analysis. *Dis Colon Rectum* 1995; **38:** 687–94.
3. Nisar PJ, Scholefield JH. Managing haemorrhoids. *BMJ* 2003; **327:** 847–51.
4. Lyseng-Williamson KA, Perry CM. Micronised purified flavonoid fraction: a review of its use in chronic venous insufficiency, venous ulcers and haemorrhoids. *Drugs* 2003; **63:** 71–100.


## Hepatic encephalopathy

Hepatic encephalopathy (portal systemic encephalopathy) is a metabolically related dysfunction of the brain associated with abnormalities of liver function. It may be acute, as in patients with fulminant hepatic failure, or chronic, with acute episodes precipitated by some triggering factor, as in patients with cirrhosis or other chronic liver disease.

Treatment is aimed at identifying and correcting any precipitating factor, decreasing the production and absorption of ammonia in the gut, and increasing metabolism of ammonia in the tissues. Precipitating factors include infection, increased protein load due to gastrointestinal haemorrhage or high protein intake, alcohol abuse, electrolyte imbalance, and certain drugs (notably anxiolytics, hypnotics, and diuretics).

Restriction of dietary protein intake is a mainstay of short-term treatment, but in the long-term, care must be taken to provide adequate protein to avoid malnutrition. A daily protein intake of 0.5 to 1.5 g/kg body-weight has been recommended.[1] There is some evidence that vegetable protein is better tolerated than animal protein.[2,3] The administration of branched-chain amino acids (valine, isoleucine, and leucine) by infusion or as dietary supplements may facilitate adequate protein intake in some patients.[1-3] Supplementation with ornithine aspartate has been used to increase metabolic conversion of ammonia to urea and glutamine.[2,3] Sodium benzoate has also been tried.[2,3]

Active drug treatment may be initiated with bowel cleansing by means of a magnesium sulfate enema, especially if the patient is constipated. Lactulose is subsequently the treatment of choice in many cases, particularly in the elderly, the constipated, and those with renal impairment. It is usually given by mouth although it may be used rectally when oral use is not feasible.[3] It reduces colonic pH and absorption of ammonia and aromatic amino acids. The lactulose analogue lactitol is also used.[4] However, a recent meta-analysis[5] was unable to find sufficient evidence to support or refute the use of nonabsorbable disaccharides, such as lactulose and lactitol, for hepatic encephalopathy. Another approach that has been investigated is the use of the disaccharidase inhibitor voglibose to reduce intestinal uptake of disaccharides and promote fermentation, with effects similar to lactulose.[3]

Alternatively, locally active antibacterials have been given to reduce the urease-producing bacteria. Neomycin is the traditional drug but adverse effects such as ototoxicity and nephrotoxicity may be a problem, particularly if used long-term. Metronidazole is also used,[2] and rifaximin has been tried. A combination of lactulose and neomycin[2] or metronidazole has been tried in patients who fail to respond to single-drug therapy.

Another approach that has been tried in low grade chronic recurrent encephalopathy is the oral ingestion of *Lactobacillus acidophilus* or *Enterococcus faecium* SF68, in an attempt to produce a more favourable bowel flora. Results have been inconsistent.[3,6] *Helicobacter pylori* is a urease-producing organism, but the relevance of *H. pylori* infection to hepatic encephalopathy is unclear.[7]

Investigational therapy has also attempted to affect cerebral function directly. Flumazenil, a benzodiazepine antagonist, has been tried, on the basis of the suspected role of endogenous benzodiazepine-like agonists.[8] A meta-analysis[9] concluded that flumazenil did produce short-term improvement of hepatic encephalopathy but had no effect on recovery or survival; it might be considered for patients with chronic liver disease and hepatic encephalopathy but routine clinical use was not recommended.

Liver transplantation (p.1346) is the ultimate therapy for end-stage cirrhosis, acute liver failure, or patients with severe refractory hepatic encephalopathy.[2]


1. Plauth M, *et al.* ESPEN guidelines for nutrition in liver disease and transplantation. *Clin Nutr* 1997; **16:** 43–55.
2. Riordan SM, Williams R. Treatment of hepatic encephalopathy. *N Engl J Med* 1997; **337:** 473–9.
3. Gerber T, Schomerus H. Hepatic encephalopathy in liver cirrhosis: pathogenesis, diagnosis and management. *Drugs* 2000; **60:** 1353–70.
4. Cammà C, *et al.* Lactitol in treatment of chronic hepatic encephalopathy: a meta-analysis. *Dig Dis Sci* 1993; **38:** 916–22.
5. Als-Nielsen B, *et al.* Nonabsorbable disaccharides for hepatic encephalopathy. Available in The Cochrane Library; Issue 2. Chichester: John Wiley; 2004.
6. Loguercio C, *et al.* Long-term effects of Enterococcus faecium SF68 versus lactulose in the treatment of patients with cirrhosis and grade 1-2 hepatic encephalopathy. *J Hepatol* 1995; **23:** 39–46.
7. Taylor-Robinson SD, *et al.* Helicobacter pylori, ammonia and the brain. *Gut* 1997; **40:** 805–6.
8. Basile AS, *et al.* The pathogenesis and treatment of hepatic encephalopathy: evidence for the involvement of benzodiazepine receptor ligands. *Pharmacol Rev* 1991; **43:** 27–71.
9. Als-Nielsen B, *et al.* Benzodiazepine receptor antagonists for hepatic encephalopathy. Available in The Cochrane Library; Issue 2. Chichester: John Wiley; 2004.


## Inflammatory bowel disease

Inflammatory bowel disease covers chronic non-specific inflammatory conditions of the gastrointestinal tract, of which the two major forms are **Crohn's disease** and **ulcerative colitis.**

Crohn's disease is characterised by thickened areas of the gastrointestinal wall, with inflammation extending through all layers, deep ulceration and fissuring of the mucosa, and the presence of granulomas; affected areas may occur in any part of the gastrointestinal tract, interspersed with areas of relatively normal tissue; the terminal ileum is frequently involved. Symptoms depend on the site of disease but may include abdominal pain, diarrhoea, fever, weight loss, and rectal bleeding. Extra-intestinal manifestations may include joint inflammation, skin lesions, mouth ulcers, and liver disorders.

In ulcerative colitis, disease is confined to the colon and rectum, inflammation is superficial but continuous over the affected area, and granulomas are rare. In mild disease, the rectum alone may be affected (proctitis); in severe disease, ulceration is extensive and much of the mucosa may be lost, with an increased risk of toxic dilatation of the colon, a potentially life-threatening complication. Symptoms include diarrhoea and rectal bleeding. The extra-intestinal manifestations are similar to those of Crohn's disease.

Although there are important differences between Crohn's disease and ulcerative colitis which affect their management, the broad principles of treatment, and the drugs used, are similar.[1-6] The aminosalicylate derivatives are generally the first choice in mild to moderate active disease, and are of particular value for maintenance treatment of ulcerative colitis; the role of maintenance treatment in Crohn's disease is less well established. Corticosteroids are also used in the initial treatment of active disease, dosage and route varying with disease site and severity. Immunosuppressant therapy may be helpful in chronic active disease. For Crohn's disease an elemental diet (see p.1417) may have some value in active disease, but diet plays a lesser role in ulcerative colitis.

**Active disease.**

The major group of drugs used to induce remission in moderate to severe *active ulcerative colitis* and *Crohn's disease* (including ileal disease) is the **corticosteroids**. Oral prednisolone or prednisone is often used; in the most severe cases hydrocortisone or methylprednisolone may be given intravenously. Dosage is high initially, and is reduced gradually as symptoms improve, but adverse effects remain a problem, hence the interest in poorly absorbed or rapidly metabolised corticosteroids such as beclometasone, budesonide, or tixocortol. Oral budesonide is effective in inducing remission in Crohn's disease,[7-10] and is probably comparable in effect to conventional corticosteroids;[10] although some suggest that it may be slightly less effective,[9] adverse effects are reduced. It appears to be more effective than the 5-aminosalicylate mesalazine in inducing remission of Crohn's disease affecting the ileum and/or colon.[11]

In patients with disease confined to the *distal colon* or *rectum*, local topical therapy may be appropriate. Suppositories of prednisolone or mesalazine may be suitable in *mild proctitis*. However, *proctocolitis* involving more of the distal colon is usually treated with enemas of corticosteroids or of mesalazine. Meta-analysis has suggested that rectal mesalazine is more effective than rectal corticosteroids in the management of distal ulcerative colitis.[12] Combined oral and rectal mesalazine may be more effective for ulcerative colitis than either alone.[13,14] Systemic corticosteroids are reserved for patients who fail to respond to topical therapy.

Oral sulfasalazine, a **5-aminosalicylate** derivative (5-aminosalicylic acid linked to sulfapyridine), is of value in producing remission of mild ulcerative colitis and in Crohn's disease affecting the colon, but has produced equivocal results in Crohn's ileitis.[15-17]

The discovery that 5-aminosalicylate was the active component of sulfasalazine led to the development of numerous derivatives, including mesalazine (5-aminosalicylic acid itself in slow-release or enteric-coated form), olsalazine (2 molecules of 5-aminosalicylic acid joined by an azo bond), and a variety of forms, such as balsalazide, in which the active moiety was joined to inert carriers. All the above have been shown to be effective in *active ulcerative colitis*, and may be better tolerated than sulfasalazine, since many of the latter's adverse effects are due to its sulfonamide portion. However, in patients who can tolerate sulfasalazine, the newer drugs have no clinical advantage for remission induction.[17] Nevertheless, the risk of adverse effects on starting sulfasalazine therapy has led to increasing use of the newer derivatives.

Other drugs used in active inflammatory bowel disease include **immunosuppressants**. The majority of studies have been with azathioprine, or its metabolite mercaptopurine. Because they have a slow onset of action (months) their use in acute disease is limited, but they are of benefit in remission induction in patients with chronically active disease, particularly corticosteroid-resistant or corticosteroid-dependent disease. Low-dose methotrexate also appears to be useful in active Crohn's disease, and probably in ulcerative colitis. Conversely, ciclosporin has not generally proved useful in chronically active inflammatory bowel disease but may have some value in the short-term treatment of acute severe ulcerative colitis. Other immunosuppressants that have been used with some success include tacrolimus and mycophenolate mofetil, although further studies are needed to evaluate the role of these drugs. Infliximab, a monoclonal antibody to tumour necrosis factor, is effective in active Crohn's disease refractory to other treatments, especially in fistulising Crohn's disease. Thalidomide, a tumour necrosis factor inhibitor, has also been tried in Crohn's disease with some benefit,[18] but another such inhibitor, pentoxifylline, was ineffective.[19]

**Metronidazole** is useful in *perineal Crohn's disease* and may be used in colonic Crohn's disease. It is usually given for 3 months. Ciprofloxacin is an alternative, and has also been given with metronidazole,[20] although the combination is not very well tolerated. Antibacterials do not have a role in ulcerative colitis, except for infection prophylaxis in severe attacks.

A wide variety of **other drugs** are or have been tried in inflammatory bowel disease, including immunoglobulins, some interleukins, interferons, ICAM-antisense oligonucleotides, short-chain fatty acids, heparin, factor XIII, omega-3 triglycerides (fish oils), and aminosalicylic acid (4-aminosalicylic acid as opposed to 5-aminosalicylic acid). Nicotine has been tried, based on the observation that ulcerative colitis is rare in smokers. Studies have suggested that nicotine, supplied via transdermal patch, may have benefit in active disease, although it is ineffective for maintenance.[21] Rectal and oral formulations of nicotine are under investigation. There has also been some interest in manipulation of the bowel flora through administration of lactobacilli and other probiotic bacteria.

Correction of nutritional deficiencies may be necessary in severe disease. In Crohn's disease, enteral feeding, often with an elemental diet is effective in inducing remission (p.1417), but corticosteroids are more effective.[22] Elemental diets are useful in children and those unable to tolerate corticosteroids.

**Maintenance of remission.**

Treatment in patients who achieve remission depends on disease type. The 5-aminosalicylates are of value in the maintenance of remission in *ulcerative colitis* and are widely used for this purpose; sulfasalazine may be more effective than other aminosalicylates.[23] One study found that treatment with non-pathogenic *Escherichia coli* was equivalent to mesalazine in maintaining remission in ulcerative colitis.[24] Maintenance therapy for *Crohn's disease* is less well established.[25,26] Aminosalicylate maintenance is less effective in Crohn's disease than ulcerative colitis, but may still be considered, particularly to reduce postsurgical recurrence;[27] most studies have used mesalazine. Metronidazole may also reduce postsurgical recurrence. It is generally agreed that conventional corticosteroids have no role in the maintenance of remission of either ulcerative colitis or Crohn's disease,[28] although there is limited evidence that budesonide may modestly prolong the time to relapse in patients with Crohn's disease.[29,30] Azathioprine and mercaptopurine are used for maintenance treatment in Crohn's disease. Once the disease has been in remission for 4 years it may be possible to withdraw therapy.[31] Infliximab is also used in maintenance and is effective in patients with fistulising Crohn's disease.[32] Ciclosporin has not proved effective in maintaining remission of Crohn's disease. There has been interest in the possible role of *Mycobacterium paratuberculosis* in Crohn's disease, but there is currently insufficient evidence to support the use of antituberculous therapy for maintenance therapy.[33] A controlled diet, excluding foods that precipitated symptoms, has been reported to maintain remission in patients with Crohn's disease brought to remission by an elemental diet.[34] Unlike patients with ulcerative colitis (see above) those with Crohn's disease may have an increased risk of relapse if they smoke and should be particularly encouraged to stop.

**Surgery.**

In patients with ulcerative colitis in whom medical therapy is inadequate surgical colectomy is curative, and may avoid the risks of long-term corticosteroid therapy and the increased risk of bowel cancer to which patients with inflammatory bowel disease are subject. Formation of an ileoanal pouch, which acts as a reservoir for the ileal contents, avoids the necessity for a standard ileostomy and maintains a degree of continence in suitable patients. Curative surgery is not possible in Crohn's disease, since recurrence elsewhere in the gut is almost inevitable, but resection of the affected area becomes necessary in many patients during the course of their illness.


1. Kornbluth A, Sachar DB. Ulcerative colitis practice guidelines in adults. *Am J Gastroenterol* 1997; **92:** 204–11.
2. Stein RB, Hanauer SB. Medical therapy for inflammatory bowel disease. *Gastroenterol Clin North Am* 1999; **28:** 297–321.
3. Rampton DS. Management of Crohn's disease. *BMJ* 1999; **319:** 1480–85.
4. Farrell RJ, Peppercorn MA. Ulcerative colitis. *Lancet* 2002; **359:** 331–40.
5. Podolsky DK. Inflammatory bowel disease. *N Engl J Med* 2002; **347:** 417–29.
6. Shanahan F. Crohn's disease. *Lancet* 2002; **359:** 62–9.
7. Greenberg GR, *et al.* Oral budesonide for active Crohn's disease. *N Engl J Med* 1994; **331:** 836–41.
8. Rutgeerts P, *et al.* A comparison of budesonide with prednisolone for active Crohn's disease. *N Engl J Med* 1994; **331:** 842–5.
9. Anonymous. Controlled-release budesonide in Crohn's disease. *Drug Ther Bull* 1997; **35:** 30–1.
10. Campieri M, *et al.* Oral budesonide is as effective as oral prednisolone in active Crohn's disease. *Gut* 1997; **41:** 209–14.
11. Thomsen OØ, *et al.* A comparison of budesonide and mesalamine for active Crohn's disease. *N Engl J Med* 1998; **339:** 370–4.
12. Marshall JK, Irvine EJ. Rectal corticosteroids versus alternative treatments in ulcerative colitis: a meta-analysis. *Gut* 1997; **40:** 775–81.
13. d'Albasio G, *et al.* Combined therapy with 5-aminosalicylic acid tablets and enemas for maintaining remission in ulcerative colitis: a randomized double-blind study. *Am J Gastroenterol* 1997; **92:** 1143–7.
14. Safdi M, *et al.* A double-blind comparison of oral versus rectal mesalamine versus combination therapy in the treatment of distal ulcerative colitis. *Am J Gastroenterol* 1997; **92:** 1867–71.
15. Summers RW, *et al.* National cooperative Crohn's disease study: results of drug treatment. *Gastroenterology* 1979; **77:** 847–69.
16. Malchow H, *et al.* European cooperative Crohn's disease study (ECCDS): results of drug treatment. *Gastroenterology* 1984; **86:** 249–66.
17. Sutherland LR, MacDonald JK. Oral 5-aminosalicylic acid for induction of remission in ulcerative colitis. Available in The Cochrane Library; Issue 1. Chichester: John Wiley; 2004.
18. Sands BE, Podolsky DK. New life in a sleeper: thalidomide and Crohn's disease. *Gastroenterology* 1999; **117:** 1485–98.
19. Bauditz J, *et al.* Treatment with tumour necrosis factor inhibitor oxpentifylline does not improve corticosteroid dependent chronic active Crohn's disease. *Gut* 1997; **40:** 470–4.
20. Prantera C, *et al.* An antibiotic regimen for the treatment of active Crohn's disease: a randomized, controlled clinical trial of metronidazole plus ciprofloxacin. *Am J Gastroenterol* 1996; **91:** 328–32.
21. Guslandi M. Nicotine treatment for ulcerative colitis. *Br J Clin Pharmacol* 1999; **48:** 481–4.
22. Zachos M, *et al.* Enteral nutritional therapy for induction of remission in Crohn's disease. Available in The Cochrane Library; Issue 1. Chichester: John Wiley; 2004.
23. Sutherland L, *et al.* Oral 5-aminosalicylic acid for maintenance of remission in ulcerative colitis. Available in The Cochrane Library; Issue 1. Chichester: John Wiley; 2004.
24. Rembacken BJ, *et al.* Non-pathogenic Escherichia coli versus mesalazine for the treatment of ulcerative colitis: a randomised trial. *Lancet* 1999; **354:** 635–9.
25. Stark ME, Tremaine WJ. Maintenance of symptomatic remission in patients with Crohn's disease. *Mayo Clin Proc* 1993; **68:** 1183–90.
26. Greenberger NJ, Miner PB. Is maintenance therapy effective in Crohn's disease? *Lancet* 1994; **344:** 900–1.
27. Cammà C, *et al.* Mesalamine in the maintenance treatment of Crohn's disease: a meta-analysis adjusted for confounding variables. *Gastroenterology* 1997; **113:** 1465–73.
28. Steinhart AH, *et al.* Corticosteroids for maintenance of remission in Crohn's disease. Available in The Cochrane Library; Issue 1. Chichester: John Wiley; 2004.
29. Löfberg R, *et al.* Budesonide prolongs time to relapse in ileal and ileocaecal Crohn's disease: a placebo controlled one year study. *Gut* 1996; **39:** 82–6.
30. Greenberg GR, *et al.* Oral budesonide as maintenance treatment for Crohn's disease: a placebo-controlled, dose-ranging study. *Gastroenterology* 1996; **110:** 45–51.
31. Bouhnik Y, *et al.* Long-term follow-up of patients with Crohn's disease treated with azathioprine or 6-mercaptopurine. *Lancet* 1996; **347:** 215–19.
32. Sands BE, *et al.* Infliximab maintenance therapy for fistulizing Crohn's disease. *N Engl J Med* 2004; **350:** 876–85.
33. Borgaonkar M, *et al.* Anti-tuberculous therapy for maintenance of remission in Crohn's disease. Available in The Cochrane Library; Issue 1. Chichester: John Wiley; 2004.
34. Riordan AM, *et al.* Treatment of active Crohn's disease by exclusion diet: East Anglian Multicentre Controlled Trial. *Lancet* 1993; **342:** 1131–4.


## Irritable bowel syndrome

Irritable bowel syndrome is a functional gastrointestinal disorder of abdominal pain and altered bowel habit; pain is characteristically relieved by defaecation and may be associated with increase or decrease in stool frequency. There may be abdominal bloating. Women are more frequently affected than men. The value of drug therapy is difficult to prove, given the heterogeneity of symptoms and the high rate of response to placebo.[1,2] Primary treatment comprises counselling and when necessary dietary modification; short-term drug therapy may bring some benefit if directed at individual symptoms,[1-7] as follows:

- in patients in whom *diarrhoea* is predominant, loperamide may be considered; it is preferred to other opioid antidiarrhoeal drugs because it does not pass the blood-brain barrier. Alternatively, colestyramine may be of benefit. The 5-$HT_3$ antagonist alosetron is also available in some countries for use in women with severe symptoms unresponsive to conventional therapy; it was previously withdrawn due to gastrointestinal toxicity
- in *constipation-predominant* forms of the syndrome bran or ispaghula should be tried to increase dietary fibre. Fibre supplementation should be gradual to avoid bloating. Nevertheless, a proportion of patients are intolerant of bran, which will exacerbate symptoms such as abdominal distension and pain. An osmotic laxative or stool softener may be added in patients who fail to respond to fibre, but stimulant laxatives should be avoided. Tegaserod, a partial agonist at 5-$HT_4$ receptors, is also effective in this group of patients
- in patients with *abdominal pain*, 'as-needed' antispasmodics or antimuscarinics may be tried. These should be taken before meals if abdominal pain occurs principally after eating. Examples include alverine, dicycloverine, hyoscine, mebeverine, and peppermint oil. Antidepressants are also effective. Analgesic use should be minimised
- patients whose symptoms are associated with mild or masked *depression* may obtain benefit from antidepressant therapy; a depressed patient with increased bowel frequency and abdominal pain may benefit from a tricyclic antidepressant, which slows intestinal transit. It has been suggested that patients with constipation may be better treated with an SSRI.

Many other drugs have been tried in the irritable bowel syndrome, including cromoglicate, leuprorelin, and naloxone, with variable results.[8] Newer approaches being investigated are cholecystokinin antagonists (loxiglumide), kappa opioid agonists (fedotozine), antibacterials (such as neomycin), and somatostatin analogues (octreotide).[1,2,8,9]


1. Talley NJ. Evaluation of drug treatment in irritable bowel syndrome. *Br J Clin Pharmacol* 2003; **56:** 362–9.
2. Mertz HR. Irritable bowel syndrome. *N Engl J Med* 2003; **349:** 2136–46.

3. Malcolm A, Kellow JE. Irritable bowel syndrome. *Med J Aust* 1998; **169:** 274–9.
4. Camilleri M. Review article: clinical evidence to support current therapies of irritable bowel syndrome. *Aliment Pharmacol Ther* 1999; **13** (suppl. 2): 48–53.
5. Jones J, *et al.* British Society of Gastroenterology guidelines for the management of the irritable bowel syndrome. *Gut* 2000; **47** (suppl 2): ii1–ii19. Also available at: http://www.bsg.org.uk/pdf_word_docs/man_ibd.pdf (accessed 07/05/04)
6. American Gastroenterological Association. American Gastroenterological Association medical position statement: irritable bowel syndrome. *Gastroenterology* 2002; **123:** 2105–7.
7. Talley NJ, Spiller R. Irritable bowel syndrome: a little understood organic bowel disease? *Lancet* 2002; **360:** 555–64.
8. Farthing MJG. New drugs in the management of the irritable bowel syndrome. *Drugs* 1998; **56:** 11–21.
9. Horwitz BJ, Fisher RS. The irritable bowel syndrome. *N Engl J Med* 2001; **344:** 1846–50.


## Mouth ulceration

Recurrent ulceration of the oral mucosa is usually idiopathic and self-limiting and is known as recurrent aphthous stomatitis or recurrent aphthous ulceration. However, oral ulcers (canker sores) may also be caused by mechanical trauma, nutritional deficiencies (particularly iron, folic acid, or vitamin $B_{12}$), drug reactions, or underlying disease such as Behçet's syndrome (p.1076).

Management includes identifying any underlying disease or nutritional deficiency and treating these as appropriate. Usually no underlying cause can be found, and treatment is purely symptomatic including topical anti-inflammatories, local anaesthetics, antiseptics, astringents, or antihistamines. The value of many of these drugs in reducing symptoms remains anecdotal, and no treatments have yet been proven to reduce the incidence of recurrences.

Where ulceration is due to minor trauma frequent use of a warm saline or compound thymol glycerin mouthwash may be all that is required to relieve discomfort and swelling. Alternatively, pain relief may be obtained with local anaesthetics or analgesics, but their effectiveness in oral ulceration is limited by their relatively short duration of action when applied topically. Salicylates are widely used, mainly as choline salicylate gel, although they themselves have the potential for local irritation and ulceration. Benzydamine spray or mouthwash may also be helpful. Lidocaine, as a gel or lozenges, may be of value in pain that has not responded to other measures. Topical corticosteroids are probably the most effective symptomatic treatment for recurrent aphthous stomatitis. Pellets or lozenges of hydrocortisone are allowed to dissolve next to an ulcer, or triamcinolone in an oral paste formulation may be used, although the paste may sometimes be difficult to apply. Mouthwashes have been employed particularly when ulceration is widespread in the mouth and a dexamethasone mouthwash has been used effectively. The healing properties of carbenoxolone have also been employed as a gel or mouthwash, and the mast-cell stabilising agent amlexanox is also used as an oral paste.

Mechanical protection may be provided by a paste or powder of carmellose sodium, although application may be difficult.

Use of an antiseptic mouthwash such as chlorhexidine or povidone-iodine may be helpful, since secondary bacterial infection can delay healing. Chlorhexidine is also available as a gel. Tetracyclines, used as mouthwashes, reportedly reduce ulcer pain and duration, but their potential for adverse effects if swallowed must be borne in mind. Use of hydrogen peroxide 3% is inadvisable, as it can cause ulceration, but application of a 1.5% solution to individual ulcers in combination with a topical corticosteroid may be helpful in producing resolution.

A wide variety of other drugs have been tried in aphthous ulceration. Sucralfate may be of benefit. Drugs such as levamisole and thalidomide, although possibly beneficial, are unlikely to be suitable in most cases because of their adverse effects, although thalidomide is used, for example, for aphthous stomatitis in patients with AIDS. Pentoxifylline, which, like thalidomide, inhibits tumour necrosis factor production, has been used in patients with minor recurrent aphthous ulceration. Systemic corticosteroids are generally reserved for cases with severe underlying disease.

References.


1. Burgess JA, *et al.* Pharmacological management of recurrent oral mucosal ulceration. *Drugs* 1990; **39:** 54–65.
2. Fischman SL. Oral ulcerations. *Semin Dermatol* 1994; **13:** 74–7.
3. Woo SB, Sonis ST. Recurrent aphthous ulcers: a review of diagnosis and treatment. *J Am Dent Assoc* 1996; **127:** 1202–13.
4. Porter SR, *et al.* Recurrent aphthous stomatitis. *Crit Rev Oral Biol Med* 1998; **9:** 306–21.


## Nausea and vomiting

Vomiting follows stimulation of the vomiting centre in the medulla of the brain. This may be via the chemoreceptor trigger zone, which is sensitive to many drugs and to certain metabolic disturbances, or following actions on other areas such as the vestibular apparatus of the ear (in motion sickness), the cerebral cortex (in psychogenic vomiting), and multiple peripheral receptors. In adults vomiting is almost invariably preceded by a sensation of nausea.

In situations where it can be anticipated, such as motion sickness, surgery, and cancer therapy, antiemetic drugs are given prophylactically, but if this fails they may need to be given therapeutically. Vomiting of unknown origin should ideally not be treated until the underlying cause has been found. If vomiting is prolonged, dehydration, hypokalaemia, and alkalosis may occur and replacement of fluid and electrolytes may be necessary, especially in young children and the elderly.

**Cancer chemotherapy**. Nausea and vomiting are common adverse effects of cancer chemotherapy and for many patients represent a major drawback to treatment. Once experienced, anticipatory vomiting may occur at the sight of medical staff or a needle and this problem may be severe enough in some cases to hinder or prevent further treatment.

Antineoplastic or cytotoxic drugs may induce vomiting by both a central action on the chemoreceptor trigger zone and a peripheral action on the gastrointestinal tract. The cerebral cortex is probably responsible for anticipatory vomiting. Mechanisms involving $5\text{-HT}_3$-receptors are important in the pathogenesis of *acute cisplatin-associated vomiting*, whereas different mechanisms are probably involved in *delayed emesis*.

The emetic potential of antineoplastics varies in terms of severity and incidence. Vomiting may be

- *very severe* with cisplatin, dacarbazine, dactinomycin, chlormethine, high-dose cyclophosphamide, and streptozocin, and occurs in most patients
- *moderate* with the taxanes, doxorubicin, more modest doses of cyclophosphamide, and high-dose methotrexate
- *milder* and less common with vinca alkaloids, fluorouracil, lower doses of methotrexate, chlorambucil, bleomycin, and etoposide.

Emetogenicity may depend to some extent on the dose, route, and schedule of administration. Some combination therapy has resulted in a higher incidence of vomiting than would be expected from the constituents.

The *onset and duration* of vomiting also varies from drug to drug. For cisplatin the onset may be between 4 and 8 hours after a dose, while the duration may be up to 48 hours or occasionally even longer; a persistent feeling of nausea, and sometimes vomiting, lasting for several days may also occur. After chlormethine, vomiting may begin within a half to 2 hours, whereas after cyclophosphamide there may be a latent interval of 9 to 18 hours, but in both cases vomiting is generally less prolonged than with cisplatin. *Acute emesis* (that occurring within 24 hours of chemotherapy) has generally been easier to control than *delayed emesis* (that occurring more than 24 hours after chemotherapy) or *anticipatory emesis*.

MANAGEMENT. Guidelines for the management of nausea and vomiting associated with chemotherapy have been produced.[1-3] It is important that effective antiemetic prophylaxis is given from the first course of chemotherapy, to avoid subsequent problems with anticipatory vomiting. With the antiemetic drugs now available it should be possible to control *acute emesis*; *delayed emesis* is more resistant. A variety of drugs has been used in antiemetic regimens including:

- dopamine antagonists such as metoclopramide, domperidone, and some phenothiazines such as prochlorperazine
- corticosteroids such as dexamethasone
- $5\text{-HT}_3$ antagonists such as ondansetron
- cannabinoids such as nabilone
- benzodiazepines such as lorazepam
- antihistamines such as diphenhydramine.

The choice depends on the emetogenicity of the cancer chemotherapy regimen, as well as factors such as the age of the patient.

- For prophylaxis of *acute emesis* associated with *highly emetogenic chemotherapy*, $5\text{-HT}_3$ antagonists are used, often with dexamethasone. At equipotent doses, granisetron, ondansetron, dolasetron, and tropisetron are effective and equally safe.[1-3] High-dose metoclopramide was formerly used, but frequently caused extrapyramidal adverse effects, particularly in patients under 30 years of age; diphenhydramine was used to reduce these effects
- For prophylaxis of *acute emesis* associated with *moderately emetogenic chemotherapy*, dexamethasone alone is preferred
- No routine prophylactic antiemetic needs to be given for chemotherapy of low emetic risk; however, as-needed or prophylactic use of prochlorperazine, domperidone, or metoclopramide is common
- Lorazepam may be used for its amnestic, sedative, and anxiolytic effects as an adjunct to antiemetics when *anticipatory emesis* is a problem
- Good control of acute emesis is important in preventing delayed emesis. In addition, for prophylaxis of *delayed emesis*, dexamethasone alone or combined with oral metoclopramide or perhaps a $5\text{-HT}_3$ antagonist or prochlorperazine, is used. More recently, the neurokinin-1 ($NK_1$) receptor antagonists such as aprepitant have shown promise in the prevention of acute and delayed nausea and vomiting due to highly emetogenic chemotherapy;[4,5] aprepitant is used in combination with a $5\text{-HT}_3$ antagonist and dexamethasone.

Cannabinoids such as dronabinol and nabilone have been used for chemotherapy-induced nausea and vomiting, usually as second-line drugs.

**Motion sickness** has been described as a normal reaction to stimuli that occur during passive transportation and to which the individual is not adapted. The term embraces all forms of travel sickness including sea sickness, car sickness, train sickness, and air sickness. It is a type of vertigo in which autonomic symptoms predominate, therefore signs and symptoms include pallor, sweating, increased salivation, yawning, malaise, and hyperventilation.

MANAGEMENT. The aim is to *prevent* motion sickness and antiemetics are more effective if given prophylactically before nausea and vomiting has developed. The principal drugs used are the antimuscarinic hyoscine and some of the centrally acting antihistamines.[6] Antiemetic drugs *not* effective against motion sickness include metoclopramide, domperidone, chlorpromazine, and $5\text{-HT}_3$ antagonists. Ginger has been tried.

For short-term protection against motion sickness hyoscine hydrobromide by mouth is often the drug of choice. It is taken about 30 minutes before a journey followed by further doses every 6 hours if necessary. Transdermal administration of hyoscine markedly prolongs the duration of action, but the patches need to be applied to the skin several hours before travelling.

Antihistamines may be slightly less effective than hyoscine against motion sickness, but are often better tolerated. They are usually given by mouth and include cinnarizine, cyclizine, dimenhydrinate, meclozine, and promethazine; all have similar efficacy, but differ in onset and duration of action and in the extent of side-effects such as drowsiness. Their antimuscarinic properties may contribute to their effects. Non-sedating antihistamines (e.g. astemizole and terfenadine) penetrate poorly into the CNS and do not appear to be effective against motion sickness.

Once motion sickness has developed, gastric motility is inhibited and it may be preferable to administer antiemetics intramuscularly rather than by mouth. In one study promethazine was preferred to hyoscine for intramuscular use because of its longer duration of action.[7]

**Palliative care.** Nausea and vomiting are common in terminal illness, and may be prolonged. There are various causes, and more than one cause may occur in the same patient. They include unpalatable or excess food, gastric irritation or delayed emptying, constipation or intestinal obstruction, renal failure, increased intracranial pressure, hypercalcaemia, infection, and treatments such as chemotherapy (see above), radiotherapy (see below), opioid analgesics, NSAIDs, or corticosteroids.[8,9]

MANAGEMENT. Nausea and vomiting can often be *reduced* by treatment of associated symptoms such as pain, anxiety, and cough. Non-drug measures include appropriate diet and avoidance of unpleasant odours, adequate fluid intake, and regular mouth care. Drugs used for *prevention and treatment* are selected depending on the cause of nausea and vomiting. These include haloperidol, some phenothiazines such as prochlorperazine and promethazine, antihistamines such as cyclizine and hydroxyzine, the antimuscarinic hyoscine, prokinetics such as metoclopramide and domperidone, $5\text{-HT}_3$ antagonists such as ondansetron and granisetron, corticosteroids such as dexamethasone, benzodiazepines, and cannabinoids. Although antiemetic treatments are given orally, patients with severe vomiting will require drug administration by other routes such as subcutaneous infusion.[8,9] Octreotide may be helpful to reduce intestinal secretions and vomiting.

**Postoperative nausea and vomiting** is a common and distressing side-effect of anaesthesia and surgery; it may sometimes be more of a problem than pain, especially in day-case surgery.[10-12] The incidence depends on many factors, including the type of anaesthetic, the type and duration of operation, and the sex of the patient (women are more at risk than men). Patients with a history of postoperative vomiting or of motion sickness may be more susceptible.

MANAGEMENT. The aim is prevention and most studies have been directed at this rather than treatment. Routine antiemetic prophylaxis is not necessary in all surgical patients.[2,10,12,13] Widely used drugs for the *prevention and treatment* of postoperative nausea and vomiting include dopamine antagonists such as metoclopramide, droperidol, and some phenothiazines such as prochlorperazine; 5-$HT_3$ antagonists such as ondansetron; and antihistamines (including phenothiazine antihistamines such as promethazine). In a meta-analysis[14] of studies comparing ondansetron, droperidol, and metoclopramide for *prophylaxis*, ondansetron and droperidol were more effective than metoclopramide for preventing vomiting, and droperidol was more effective than metoclopramide for preventing nausea. An analysis[15] of studies comparing metoclopramide with placebo concluded that metoclopramide was not an effective antiemetic in the doses currently used in anaesthesia, and that doses are likely to be too low. When intravenous ondansetron was compared with phenothiazines for prevention of nausea and vomiting after surgery, it was equivalent to intravenous perphenazine in one study,[16] and less effective than intramuscular prochlorperazine in another.[17] In high-risk patients combination antiemetic regimens should be considered.[12,13,18] Ondansetron or granisetron used with dexamethasone are reportedly more effective than the 5-$HT_3$ antagonist alone.[19] Ondansetron has also been given with droperidol for the prophylaxis of postoperative emesis although opinions vary as to the additional benefit.[18,20]

In the *treatment* of established nausea and vomiting, ondansetron was no different to droperidol[21] and at least as effective as metoclopramide,[21,22] with an overall efficacy of only about 25% greater than placebo.[21]

Other drugs that have been tried include transdermal hyoscine, clonidine,[23] ginger,[24,25] and ephedrine.[26,27] The use of propofol for maintenance anaesthesia may be associated with a reduction in risk of postoperative nausea and vomiting (see p.1307). Some nonpharmacological techniques to prevent postoperative nausea and vomiting may be effective in adults.[12,28]

**Pregnancy**. Nausea and vomiting or 'morning sickness' is common in the first trimester of pregnancy, but is generally mild and does not require drug therapy. Dietary modification such as eating small frequent carbohydrate meals often helps. There is also some evidence that pyridoxine can reduce nausea in pregnancy.[29] On rare occasions short-term therapy with an antihistamine such as promethazine may be required if vomiting is severe. For reference to the controversy that has surrounded the risk to the fetus of antiemetic therapy during pregnancy, see under the Precautions of Antihistamines, p.420. Persistent vomiting and severe nausea may progress to *hyperemesis gravidarum* if adequate hydration cannot be maintained; the condition occurs in up to 1% of pregnancies.[30] Management of hyperemesis includes hospitalisation for intravenous fluid and electrolyte replacement, and this is usually sufficient. Routine thiamine supplementation, by mouth if tolerated otherwise parenterally, has been recommended to reduce the risk of Wernicke's encephalopathy[30,31] (p.1455), although there is some dissent from this view.[32] If hyperemesis fails to respond to rehydration, antiemetics should be used; options include domperidone, phenothiazines, and antihistamines.[30] There is some evidence that hyperemesis unresponsive to conventional therapy may respond to oral prednisolone or intravenous hydrocortisone.[30] There have also been anecdotal reports of ondansetron being used successfully in life-threatening hyperemesis gravidarum unresponsive to conventional treatment,[33] although a double-blind pilot study found it to be no more effective than promethazine.[34]

**Radiotherapy**. The risk of emesis with radiotherapy varies with the treatment given, particularly the area of the body irradiated. However, emetic risk, and recommendations for use of antiemetics, are less clearly defined than in the situation of chemotherapy-induced nausea and vomiting.[2,3] Total body irradiation is considered to have high emetogenic potential, but is not a common treatment. It has been suggested[2] that a prophylactic 5-$HT_3$ antagonist should be given before each fraction, perhaps combined with a corticosteroid. For radiotherapy of intermediate emetogenic risk, such as that to the abdomen, prophylactic antiemetics may also be considered; options are dopamine antagonists (metoclopramide, domperidone) or 5-$HT_3$ antagonists. Dexamethasone has also been effective.[35] For radiotherapy of low emetogenic potential, treatment on an as-needed only basis has been suggested.[3]


1. Fauser AA, *et al.* Guidelines for anti-emetic therapy: acute emesis. *Eur J Cancer* 1999; **35:** 361–70.
2. American Society of Health-System Pharmacists. ASHP therapeutic guidelines on the pharmacologic management of nausea and vomiting in adult and pediatric patients receiving chemotherapy or radiation therapy or undergoing surgery. *Am J Health-Syst Pharm* 1999; **56:** 729–64. Also available at: http://www.ashp.org/bestpractices/tg/Therapeutic%20Guideline%20Pharmacologic%20Management%20of%20Nausea%20and%20Vomiting%20in%20Adult%20and%20Pediatric.pdf (accessed 07/05/04)
3. Gralla RJ, *et al.* Recommendations for the use of antiemetics: evidence-based, clinical practice guidelines. *J Clin Oncol* 1999; **17:** 2971–94. Correction. *ibid.* 2000; **18:** 3064.
4. Navari RM, *et al.* Reduction of cisplatin-induced emesis by a selective neurokinin-1-receptor antagonist. *N Engl J Med* 1999; **340:** 190–5.
5. Diemunsch P, Grélot L. Potential of substance P antagonists as antiemetics. *Drugs* 2000; **60:** 533–46.
6. Gahlinger PM. Motion sickness: how to help your patients avoid travel travail. *Postgrad Med* 1999; **106:** 177–84.
7. Wood CD, *et al.* Effectiveness and duration of intramuscular antimotion sickness medications. *J Clin Pharmacol* 1992; **32:** 1008–12.
8. WHO. Nausea and vomiting. In: *Symptom relief in terminal illness.* Geneva: WHO, 1998.
9. Baines MJ. ABC of palliative care: nausea, vomiting, and intestinal obstruction. *BMJ* 1997; **315:** 1148–50.
10. Watcha MF, White PF. Postoperative nausea and vomiting: its etiology, treatment, and prevention. *Anesthesiology* 1992; **77:** 162–84.
11. Sung Y-F. Risks and benefits of drugs used in the management of postoperative nausea and vomiting. *Drug Safety* 1996; **14:** 181–97.
12. Kovac AL. Prevention and treatment of postoperative nausea and vomiting. *Drugs* 2000; **59:** 213–43.
13. Rose JB, Watcha MF. Postoperative nausea and vomiting in paediatric patients. *Br J Anaesth* 1999; **83:** 104–17.
14. Domino KB, *et al.* Comparative efficacy and safety of ondansetron, droperidol, and metoclopramide for preventing postoperative nausea and vomiting: a meta-analysis. *Anesth Analg* 1999; **88:** 1370–9.
15. Henzi I, *et al.* Metoclopramide in the prevention of postoperative nausea and vomiting: a quantitative systematic review of randomized, placebo-controlled studies. *Br J Anaesth* 1999; **83:** 761–71.
16. Desilva PHDP, *et al.* The efficacy of prophylactic ondansetron, droperidol, perphenazine, and metoclopramide in the prevention of nausea and vomiting after major gynecologic surgery. *Anesth Analg* 1995; **81:** 139–43.
17. Chen JJ, *et al.* Efficacy of ondansetron and prochlorperazine for the prevention of postoperative nausea and vomiting after total hip replacement or total knee replacement procedures: a randomized, double-blind, comparative trial. *Arch Intern Med* 1998; **158:** 2124–8.
18. Habib AS, Gan TJ. Pharmacotherapy of postoperative nausea and vomiting. *Expert Opin Pharmacother* 2003; **4:** 457–73.
19. Henzi I, *et al.* Dexamethasone for the prevention of postoperative nausea and vomiting: a quantitative systematic review. *Anesth Analg* 2000; **90:** 186–94.
20. Eberhart LH, *et al.* Droperidol and 5-$HT_3$-receptor antagonists, alone or in combination, for prophylaxis of postoperative nausea and vomiting: a meta-analysis of randomised controlled trials. *Acta Anaesthesiol Scand* 2000; **44:** 1252–7.
21. Tramèr MR, *et al.* A quantitative systematic review of ondansetron in treatment of established postoperative nausea and vomiting. *BMJ* 1997; **314:** 1088–92.
22. Diemunsch P, *et al.* Ondansetron compared with metoclopramide in the treatment of established postoperative nausea and vomiting. *Br J Anaesth* 1997; **79:** 322–6.
23. Mikawa K, *et al.* Oral clonidine premedication reduces vomiting in children after strabismus surgery. *Can J Anaesth* 1995; **42:** 977–81.
24. Phillips S, *et al.* Zingiber officinale (ginger)—an antiemetic for day case surgery. *Anaesthesia* 1993; **48:** 715–17.
25. Arfeen Z, *et al.* A double-blind randomized controlled trial of ginger for the prevention of postoperative nausea and vomiting. *Anaesth Intensive Care* 1995; **23:** 449–52.
26. Rothenberg DM, *et al.* Efficacy of ephedrine in the prevention of postoperative nausea and vomiting. *Anesth Analg* 1991; **72:** 58–61.
27. Liu Y-C, *et al.* Comparison of antiemetic effect among ephedrine, droperidol and metoclopramide in pediatric inguinal hernioplasty. *Acta Anaesthesiol Sin* 1992; **32:** 37–42.
28. Lee A, *et al.* The use of nonpharmacologic techniques to prevent postoperative nausea and vomiting: a meta-analysis. *Anesth Analg* 1999; **88:** 1362–9.
29. Vutyavanich T, *et al.* Pyridoxine for nausea and vomiting of pregnancy: a randomized, double-blind, placebo-controlled trial. *Am J Obstet Gynecol* 1995; **173:** 881–4.
30. Nelson-Piercy C. Treatment of nausea and vomiting in pregnancy: when should it be treated and what can be safely taken? *Drug Safety* 1998; **19:** 155–64.
31. Child TJ. Management of hyperemesis in pregnant women. *Lancet* 1999; **353:** 325.
32. Dickson MJ. Management of hyperemesis in pregnant women. *Lancet* 1999; **353:** 325.
33. World MJ. Ondansetron and hyperemesis gravidarum. *Lancet* 1993; **341:** 185.
34. Sullivan CA, *et al.* A pilot study of intravenous ondansetron for hyperemesis gravidarum. *Am J Obstet Gynecol* 1996; **174:** 1565–8.
35. Kirkbride P, *et al.* Dexamethasone for the prophylaxis of radiation-induced emesis: a National Cancer Institute of Canada Clinical Trials Group phase III study. *J Clin Oncol* 2000; **18:** 1960–6.


## Oesophageal motility disorders

Oesophageal disorders, many due to disturbances in oesophageal motility, may produce non-cardiac chest pain, similar to that of angina pectoris, from which they must be differentiated.

**Achalasia** is obstruction caused by failure of the lower oesophageal sphincter to relax and permit passage of food into the stomach. It is accompanied by dilatation and abnormal peristalsis in the oesophagus, which becomes a reservoir for the unassimilated matter; symptoms include dysphagia and sometimes pain. The treatment of choice is mechanical dilatation of the sphincter or, if necessary, surgery. Laparoscopic techniques have reduced the risks associated with surgery, and this may become the preferred treatment. Taking isosorbide dinitrate or nifedipine before eating results in some improvement in achalasia, but these drugs have a role only as a temporary measure, or when other options are not suitable. More recently, injection of botulinum toxin into the lower oesophageal sphincter has been found to be effective, but remission in the long-term is better with mechanical dilatation than botulinum toxin. Therefore, it has been recommended that botulinum toxin be reserved for patients thought to be at risk from mechanical dilatation or surgery.

**Oesophageal spasm**, although frequently asymptomatic, can produce dysphagia and pain. Drug treatment of diffuse oesophageal spasm, or its variant 'nutcracker oesophagus' which is characterised by high amplitude peristalsis in the oesophagus, is often ineffective. Antimuscarinics, nitrates, and calcium-channel blockers have been tried in an attempt to relax the smooth muscle, but results are often disappointing; experience with nifedipine in patients with nutcracker oesophagus suggests that decrease in oesophageal pressure may not correlate with reduction in pain. As with achalasia, minimally invasive surgery is effective for these conditions, and is likely to be preferred.

Reviews.


1. Patti MG, Way LW. Evaluation and treatment of primary esophageal motility disorders. *West J Med* 1997; **166:** 263–9.
2. Vaezi MF, Richter JE. Current therapies for achalasia: comparison and efficacy. *J Clin Gastroenterol* 1998; **27:** 21–35.
3. Spiess AE, Kahrilas PJ. Treating achalasia: from whalebone to laparoscope. *JAMA* 1998; **280:** 638–42.
4. Storr M, *et al.* Current concepts on pathophysiology, diagnosis and treatment of diffuse oesophageal spasm. *Drugs* 2001; **61:** 579–91.
5. Richter JE. Oesophageal motility disorders. *Lancet* 2001; **358:** 823–8.


## Peptic ulcer disease

Peptic ulceration is a common condition consisting of a distinct break in the gastrointestinal mucosa, usually of the stomach or duodenum. Duodenal ulcers are rarely malignant but gastric ulcers are more commonly associated with malignancy.

The aetiology of peptic ulcer disease is probably multifactorial but the bacterium *Helicobacter pylori* plays an important role. Abnormalities of normal mucosal defence mechanisms, and, in the case of gastric ulcer, reflux of duodenal contents into the stomach or delayed gastric emptying may also be involved. Other factors include emotional stress, smoking, alcohol, and drugs such as NSAIDs or corticosteroids.

Peptic ulcer disease usually presents as dyspeptic pain, sometimes associated with nausea, vomiting, anorexia, heartburn, or bloating. Patients may develop complications such as bleeding, obstruction, or perforation.

Certain simple measures such as bed rest, dietary modification, and cessation of smoking, may accelerate ulcer healing, but these play an adjuvant role, and the basis of treatment is pharmacological. Treatment is aimed at eradicating *H. pylori* with antibacterials and neutralising or inhibiting acid activity with antisecretory drugs, and a number of guidelines are available.[1-4] Surgical treatment is used in patients with acute complications such as perforation, haemorrhage, obstruction, or pyloric stenosis, or in patients with recurrent or intractable ulcer disease, or where there is suspicion of malignancy.

**Anti-Helicobacter therapy**. The presence of *H. pylori* should usually be confirmed before therapy to eradicate the infection is started. The urea breath test is the most widely used method to test for *H. pylori*, but may produce false-negatives if used soon after treatment with proton pump inhibitors (see under Omeprazole, p.1279) or antibacterials. The best eradication regimen has not yet been established, and the number of regimens being tried is large.[5-7] The most widely used regimens comprise so-called **'triple therapy'** with a proton pump inhibitor and two antibacterials. The initial choice of antibacterial is normally between clarithromycin, a nitroimidazole (metronidazole or tinidazole), and amoxicillin, and depends on the likelihood of metronidazole or clarithromycin resistance. In the UK, the *British National Formulary* recommends a regimen containing amoxicillin and clarithromycin for initial therapy, and one with amoxicillin and metronidazole if this fails. Ranitidine bismuth citrate may replace the proton pump inhibitor. Other regimens, including those combining clarithromycin and metronidazole, are considered best used in specialist settings. Therapy is usually given for 7 to 14 days with the drugs given twice daily. Two-week triple therapy regimens are associated with high eradication rates, but adverse effects are common and compliance is a problem, so consensus favours the shorter 7-day course. Such regimens can produce eradication of *H. pylori* in over 80 to 90% of patients. Two-week triple therapy with a bismuth compound and 2 antibacterials (metronidazole and tetracycline) was formerly used, but is not as effective as proton pump inhibitor-based regimens.[5] Two-week **dual therapy** of omeprazole with amoxicillin or clarithromycin has also been used, but although less complex than triple therapy, it is also less effective. Two-week **quadruple therapy** in which omeprazole is added to a conventional bismuth-based triple therapy regimen may have a role in refractory *H. pylori* infection.[8] Although continuation of acid suppressive therapy for 4 to 8 weeks after eradication of *H. pylori* is often recommended to promote healing, some consider this unwarranted except for large or complicated lesions.[9] The recurrence rate of duodenal or gastric ulcers after successful eradication of *H. pylori* has generally been reported to be low (about 4 to 8%),[10] but in one analysis a 6-month recurrence rate of 20% was reported.[11]

Before the advent of *H. pylori* eradication therapy, drug treatment of gastric and duodenal ulcers relied mainly on antisecretory therapy. Four to 8 weeks of $H_2$-antagonist or proton pump inhibitor therapy was required for ulcer healing. Because of the high incidence of relapse, these drugs were then often given as maintenance therapy. Numerous other drugs were formerly used in peptic ulcer disease before the development of $H_2$-antagonists and proton pump inhibitors, including antacids, antimuscarinics such as pirenzepine, and mucosal protectants such as sucralfate.

**NSAID-induced ulceration**. The ulcerogenic effects of NSAIDs have been attributed to inhibition of prostaglandin synthesis and mucosal cell proliferation, and the ulcers they cause may differ from non-iatrogenic ulcers in their pathology and prognosis.[12,13] In particular, they are not directly related to *H. pylori* infection.[14] If peptic ulceration develops during treatment with an NSAID the drug should be withdrawn if possible. If this can be done, the ulcer may be treated with an antisecretory drug such as an $H_2$-antagonist or proton pump inhibitor given for 4 to 8 weeks. If NSAIDS have to be continued, *treatment* is with antisecretory drugs or the prostaglandin analogue misoprostol.[12,13] Ulcers tend to heal more slowly with $H_2$-antagonists if NSAIDs are continued, whereas the rate of ulcer healing with proton pump inhibitors appears not to be affected. There is also some evidence that omeprazole is more effective at healing NSAID-associated ulceration than misoprostol.[15] Patients at high risk of NSAID-associated gastrointestinal complications, including those with a history of these events, should receive *prophylactic therapy*.[12,13] A systematic review[16] concluded that misoprostol, proton pump inhibitors, and double-dose $H_2$ antagonists are effective at preventing chronic NSAID-associated gastric and duodenal ulcers. Standard doses of $H_2$-antagonists prevent NSAID-associated duodenal ulceration, but appear to be less effective in preventing gastric ulceration. After healing of NSAID-associated ulceration, omeprazole prophylaxis was more effective than ranitidine,[17] and was more effective and better tolerated than misoprostol.[15] It is not clear whether eradication of *H. pylori* infection reduces the occurrence of NSAID-induced ulcer,[18,19] and despite a European guideline indicating that eradication should be considered in planned NSAID therapy[2] some doubt the benefits of such a policy.[20] Treatment to eradicate infection only in patients with a history of peptic ulcer has been suggested.[12]

**Stress ulceration** may occur in the stomach or the duodenum following major physical trauma such as burns or surgery, or after severe sepsis or illness. $H_2$-antagonists and sucralfate are widely used for the prevention of stress ulceration in high-risk patients in intensive care units.[21,22] Pirenzepine is used in a few countries, and some[21] prefer it in neurosurgical patients and those with head trauma. $H_2$-antagonists may be given by mouth, nasogastric tube, or by intermittent or continuous intravenous administration. It has been suggested that the rise in gastric pH which results from such use may predispose patients to nosocomial pneumonia due to bacterial overgrowth in the stomach and retrograde colonisation of the pharynx. Sucralfate does not increase gastric pH, and meta-analysis has indicated that it may be as effective as an $H_2$-antagonist in reducing bleeding, and is associated with lower rates of pneumonia and mortality.[23] The findings of a subsequent large randomised study[24] by the same authors were at odds with those of this meta-analysis, suggesting that intravenous ranitidine was more effective than sucralfate given orally or via nasogastric tube in reducing clinically significant gastrointestinal bleeding. Moreover, there was no difference in rate of ventilator-associated mortality between ranitidine and sucralfate recipients. A further meta-analysis[25] has in turn raised doubts about the efficacy of ranitidine; no significant benefit was found for ranitidine, compared with placebo, in the prevention of bleeding. One clinical guideline suggests that, given the conflicting evidence, the choice between antacids, $H_2$-antagonists, and sucralfate be made on an institutional basis.[22]

**Bleeding ulcer**. Peptic ulceration is responsible for about 50% of all cases of upper gastrointestinal bleeding. Although many patients cease to bleed without a specific intervention, the condition is potentially life-threatening and in severe cases prompt resuscitation with intravenous fluids and blood may be required. Endoscopic therapy has substantially improved management of patients with severe bleeding or at high risk of rebleeding.[26,27] Endoscopic treatments include local injection therapy with adrenaline, sclerosants such as alcohol, and thermal therapy with lasers or electrocoagulation. Adrenaline injection will achieve haemostasis in up to 95% of patients although bleeding will recur in up to 20% of these; there is little evidence that addition of sclerosants reduces the rate of rebleeding, and their use may lead to life-threatening necrosis of the injected area.[28] Combining injection and thermal therapies has not been conclusively proven to be better than single therapies.[28] Investigational injection therapies include a fibrin glue,[29] and thrombin.[30] If endoscopic treatments fail to stop bleeding, or rebleeding occurs, further endoscopic therapy may be considered, but otherwise patients require surgery.

There is little evidence that treatment with $H_2$-antagonists[31] is useful in the acute management of bleeding, although some consider that there is evidence of benefit for omeprazole;[32] evidence of value for tranexamic acid or somatostatin is ambiguous.[27] However, once haemorrhage has been controlled, long-term treatment with an antisecretory drug to promote healing and reduce the risk of rebleeding is often given, particularly in frail and elderly patients. Eradication of *H. pylori* is generally recommended, using an appropriate regimen.[26]


1. Soll AH. Medical treatment of peptic ulcer disease: practice guidelines. *JAMA* 1996; **275:** 622–9.
2. Peura D. The report of the Digestive Health Initiative International Update Conference on Helicobacter pylori. *Gastroenterology* 1997; **113:** S4–S8.
3. Hunt RH, *et al.* Canadian Helicobacter pylori Consensus Conference update: infections in adults. *Can J Gastroenterol* 1999; **13:** 213–17.
4. Malfertheiner P, *et al.* Current concepts in the management of Helicobacter pylori infection—the Maastricht 2-2000 Consensus Report. *Aliment Pharmacol Ther* 2002; **16:** 167–80.
5. Unge P, Berstad A. Pooled analysis of anti-Helicobacter pylori treatment regimens. *Scand J Gastroenterol* 1996; **31** (suppl 220): 27–40.
6. Penston JG, McColl KEL. Eradication of Helicobacter pylori: an objective assessment of current therapies. *Br J Clin Pharmacol* 1997; **43:** 223–43.
7. Huang J-Q, Hunt RH. The importance of clarithromycin dose in the management of Helicobacter pylori infection: a meta-analysis of triple therapies with a proton pump inhibitor, clarithromycin and amoxycillin or metronidazole. *Aliment Pharmacol Ther* 1999; **13:** 719–29.
8. Peitz U, *et al.* A practical approach to patients with refractory Helicobacter pylori infection, or who are re-infected after standard therapy. *Drugs* 1999; **57:** 905–20.
9. Treiber G, Lambert JR. The impact of Helicobacter pylori eradication on peptic ulcer healing. *Am J Gastroenterol* 1998; **93:** 1080–4.
10. Hopkins RJ, *et al.* Relationship between Helicobacter pylori eradication and reduced duodenal and gastric ulcer recurrence: a review. *Gastroenterology* 1996; **110:** 1244–52.
11. Laine L, *et al.* Has the impact of Helicobacter pylori therapy on ulcer recurrence in the United States been overstated? A meta-analysis of rigorously designed trials. *Am J Gastroenterol* 1998; **93:** 1409–15.
12. Wolfe MM, *et al.* Gastrointestinal toxicity of nonsteroidal antiinflammatory drugs. *N Engl J Med* 1999; **340:** 1888–99.
13. La Corte R, *et al.* Prophylaxis and treatment of NSAID-induced gastroduodenal disorders. *Drug Safety* 1999; **20:** 527–43.
14. Barkin J. The relationship between Helicobacter pylori and nonsteroidal anti-inflammatory drugs. *Am J Med* 1998; **105** (suppl 5A): 22S–27S.
15. Hawkey CJ, *et al.* Omeprazole compared with misoprostol for ulcers associated with nonsteroidal antiinflammatory drugs. *N Engl J Med* 1998; **338:** 727–34.
16. Rostom A, *et al.* Prevention of NSAID-induced gastroduodenal ulcers. Available in The Cochrane Library; Issue 1. Chichester: John Wiley; 2004.
17. Yeomans ND, *et al.* A comparison of omeprazole with ranitidine for ulcers associated with nonsteroidal antiinflammatory drugs. *N Engl J Med* 1998; **338:** 719–26.
18. Chan FKL, *et al.* Randomised trial of eradication of Helicobacter pylori before non-steroidal anti-inflammatory drug therapy to prevent peptic ulcers. *Lancet* 1997; **350:** 975–9.
19. Hawkey CJ, *et al.* Randomised controlled trial of Helicobacter pylori eradication in patients on non-steroidal anti-inflammatory drugs: HELP NSAIDs study. *Lancet* 1998; **352:** 1016–21. Correction. *ibid.*; 1634.
20. Hawkey CJ, *et al.* Helicobacter pylori, NSAIDs, and peptic ulcers. *Lancet* 1998; **351:** 61.
21. Tryba M, Cook D. Current guidelines on stress ulcer prophylaxis. *Drugs* 1997; **54:** 581–96.
22. ASHP Commission on Therapeutics. ASHP therapeutic guidelines on stress ulcer prophylaxis. *Am J Health-Syst Pharm* 1999; **56:** 347–79. Also available at: http://www.ashp.org/bestpractices/tg/Therapeutic%20Guideline%20Stress%20Ulcer%20Prophylaxis.pdf (accessed 07/05/04)
23. Cook DJ, *et al.* Stress ulcer prophylaxis in critically ill patients: resolving discordant meta-analyses. *JAMA* 1996; **275:** 308–14.
24. Cook D, *et al.* A comparison of sucralfate and ranitidine for the prevention of upper gastrointestinal bleeding in patients requiring mechanical ventilation. *N Engl J Med* 1998; **338:** 791–7.
25. Messori A, *et al.* Bleeding and pneumonia in intensive care patients given ranitidine and sucralfate for prevention of stress ulcer: meta-analysis of randomised controlled trials. *BMJ* 2000; **321:** 1103–6.
26. Laine L, Peterson WL. Bleeding peptic ulcer. *N Engl J Med* 1994; **331:** 717–27.
27. Villanueva C, Balanzó J. A practical guide to the management of bleeding ulcers. *Drugs* 1997; **53:** 389–403.
28. British Society of Gastroenterology Endoscopy Committee. Non-variceal upper gastrointestinal haemorrhage: guidelines. *Gut* 2002; **51:** (suppl IV): iv1–iv6. Also available at: http://www.bsg.org.uk/pdf_word_docs/nonvar3.pdf (accessed 07/05/04)
29. Rutgeerts P, *et al.* Randomised trial of single and repeated fibrin glue compared with injection of polidocanol in treatment of bleeding peptic ulcer. *Lancet* 1997; **350:** 692–6.
30. Kubba AK, *et al.* Endoscopic injection for bleeding peptic ulcer: a comparison of adrenaline alone with adrenaline plus human thrombin. *Gastroenterology* 1996; **111:** 623–8.
31. Peterson WL, Cook DJ. Antisecretory therapy for bleeding peptic ulcer. *JAMA* 1998; **280:** 877–8.
32. Erstad BL. Proton-pump inhibitors for acute peptic ulcer bleeding. *Ann Pharmacother* 2001; **35:** 730–40.


## Zollinger-Ellison syndrome

Zollinger-Ellison syndrome is a rare disorder characterised by the presence of a gastrin-producing tumour (gastrinoma), which leads to hypersecretion of gastric acid and consequent peptic ulcer disease (often with complications such as perforation or bleeding), diarrhoea, or malabsorption. Gastrinomas usually occur in the non-beta islet cells of the pancreas or in the duodenal wall. Up to two-thirds are malignant. About 20 to 25% of cases are seen in patients with multiple endocrine neoplasia type 1 (MEN-1) syndrome.

Initial treatment is aimed at controlling the hypersecretion of gastric acid with an antisecretory drug. Giving enough medication just to control symptoms is not considered adequate, and it is important that acid secretion is reduced below 10 mmol/hour. Intravenous $H_2$-antagonists or proton pump inhibitors may be required initially. Once the symptoms have been controlled the tumour can be investigated for surgical removal. When complete removal is not possible then antisecretory therapy is continued indefinitely. A proton pump inhibitor is the drug of choice; it profoundly reduces acid secretion with once- or twice-daily use, although relatively high doses are required compared with those used in other conditions. An $H_2$-antagonist such as cimetidine or ranitidine may be used as an alternative to omeprazole, and, as with omeprazole, daily doses are higher than those used for other conditions; they are given in 3 or 4 divided doses. The somatostatin analogue octreotide can be used to reduce serum gastrin, but has to be given subcutaneously, and is not well tolerated.

Parietal cell vagotomy may be performed to reduce acid secretion if the tumour is not found, to allow lower doses of antisecretory drugs to be used.

References.


1. Maton PN. Zollinger-Ellison syndrome: recognition and management of acid hypersecretion. *Drugs* 1996; **52:** 33–44.
2. Qureshi W, Rashid S. Zollinger-Ellison syndrome: improved treatment options for this complex disorder. *Postgrad Med* 1998; **104:** 155–164.

## Aceglutamide Aluminium (USAN, rINNM)

Aceglutamida de aluminio; KW-110. Pentakis ($N^2$-acetyl-L-glutaminato)tetrahydroxytrialuminium.

$C_{35}H_{59}Al_3N_{10}O_{24}$ = 1084.8.

*CAS — 12607-92-0.*

**Pharmacopoeias.** In *Jpn.*

### Profile

Aceglutamide aluminium, a complex of aceglutamide with aluminium hydroxide, is an antacid with general properties similar to those of aluminium hydroxide (p.1249). It is given by mouth in a usual dose of 700 mg three times daily.

### Preparations

**Proprietary Preparations** (details are given in Part 3)
***Jpn:*** Glumal; ***Spain:*** Glumal†.

## Albumin Tannate

Albúmina, tanato de; Albutannin; Tannin Albuminate.

*CAS — 9006-52-4.*
*ATC — A07XA01.*

**Pharmacopoeias.** In *Jpn.*

### Profile

Albumin tannate, a compound of tannin with albumin, is given by mouth for its astringent properties in the treatment of diarrhoea (p.1241). It is stated to liberate tannic acid (p.1751) in the gastrointestinal tract.

### Preparations

**Proprietary Preparations** (details are given in Part 3)
***Austria:*** Tannalbin; ***Ger.:*** Tannalbin; ***Neth.:*** Entosorbine-N; Tannalbin; ***Port.:*** Tanalbina†; ***Spain:*** Cunticina†.

**Multi-ingredient:** ***Austria:*** Neoplex; ***Belg.:*** Tanalone; ***Fin.:*** Tannopon; ***Ger.:*** Tannacomp; ***Spain:*** Demusin; Salitanol Estreptomicina.

## Alexitol Sodium (BAN, rINN)

Alexitol sódico. Sodium poly(hydroxyaluminium) carbonate-hexitol complex.

*CAS — 66813-51-2.*

### Profile

Alexitol sodium is an antacid with general properties similar to those of aluminium hydroxide (p.1249). It is given in doses of 360 to 720 mg by mouth when required, up to a maximum of sixteen 360-mg tablets in 24 hours.

### Preparations

**Proprietary Preparations** (details are given in Part 3)
***Hong Kong:*** Actal; ***Malaysia:*** Actal; ***S.Afr.:*** Actan†; ***Singapore:*** Actal; ***Thai.:*** Actal; ***UK:*** Actal.

**Multi-ingredient:** ***Malaysia:*** Actal Plus.

## Alizapride Hydrochloride (rINNM)

Hidrocloruro de alizaprida. N-(1-Allyl-2-pyrrolidinylmethyl)-6-methoxy-1H-benzotriazole-5-carboxamide hydrochloride.

$C_{16}H_{21}N_5O_2,HCl$ = 351.8.

*CAS — 59338-93-1 (alizapride); 59338-87-3 (alizapride hydrochloride).*
*ATC — A03FA05.*

### Adverse Effects and Precautions

As for Metoclopramide, (see p.1274).

### Pharmacokinetics

Alizapride is well absorbed from the gastrointestinal tract. It is mainly excreted unchanged in the urine and has an elimination half-life of about 3 hours.

### Uses and Administration

Alizapride is a substituted benzamide similar to metoclopramide (p.1276), which is used to control nausea and vomiting (p.1245) associated with a variety of disorders. It is given as the hydrochloride but doses are expressed in terms of the base. Alizapride 50 mg is approximately equivalent to alizapride hydrochloride 55.8 mg.

Alizapride hydrochloride is given by mouth in usual doses equivalent to 100 to 300 mg of alizapride daily in divided doses; children have been given 5 mg/kg daily. It is also given by intravenous or intramuscular injection in doses equivalent to 50 to 200 mg of alizapride daily.

For patients receiving cancer chemotherapy usual daily doses equivalent to alizapride 2 to 5 mg/kg have been given intravenously or intramuscularly in 2 divided doses, one 30 minutes before and one 4 to 8 hours after cytotoxic drug administration. For highly emetic cytotoxic regimens requiring doses above 5 mg/kg it may be given by intravenous infusion over 15 minutes every 2 hours for 5 doses, starting 30 minutes before cytotoxic administration. It has been recommended that the total dose given with a course of chemotherapy does not exceed 4.5 g.

### Preparations

**Proprietary Preparations** (details are given in Part 3)
***Arg.:*** Gastriveran; ***Belg.:*** Litican; ***Braz.:*** Superan; ***Fr.:*** Plitican; ***Ger.:*** Vergentan; ***Hong Kong:*** Plitican†; ***Ital.:*** Limican; Nausilen†; ***Neth.:*** Litican†; ***Port.:*** Plitican; ***Switz.:*** Plitican†.

## Almagate (BAN, USAN, rINN)

Almagato; Almagatum; LAS-3876. Aluminium trimagnesium carbonate heptahydroxide dihydrate.

$AlMg_3(CO_3)(OH)_7,2H_2O$ = 315.0.

*CAS — 66827-12-1 (almagate); 72526-11-5 (anhydrous almagate).*
*ATC — A02AD03.*

**Pharmacopoeias.** In *Eur.* (see p.vi).

**Ph. Eur. 5.0** (Almagate). A white or almost white, fine crystalline powder. It contains 15.0 to 17.0% aluminium calculated as aluminium oxide, 36.0 to 40.0% magnesium calculated as magnesium oxide, and 12.5 to 14.5% carbonic acid calculated as carbon dioxide. Practically insoluble in water, in alcohol, and in dichloromethane. It dissolves with effervescence and heating in dilute mineral acids. The filtrate of a 4% suspension in water has a pH of 9.1 to 9.7. Store in airtight containers.

### Profile

Almagate is a hydrated aluminium-magnesium hydroxycarbonate. It is an antacid with general properties similar to those of aluminium hydroxide (p.1249) and magnesium carbonate (p.1272). It is given in doses of 1 to 1.5 g by mouth.

### Preparations

**Proprietary Preparations** (details are given in Part 3)
***Spain:*** Almax; Deprece; Obetine.

## Almasilate (BAN, rINN)

Almasilato; Aluminium Magnesium Silicate Hydrate; Magnesium Aluminosilicate Hydrate; Magnesium Aluminum Silicate Hydrate.

$Al_2O_3.MgO.2SiO_2,xH_2O$ = 262.4 (anhydrous).

*CAS — 71205-22-6; 50958-44-6.*
*ATC — A02AD05.*

### Profile

Almasilate is an artificial form of aluminium magnesium silicate hydrate. It is an antacid (p.1239) that is given in doses of up to about 1 g by mouth.

A hydrated native aluminium magnesium silicate (p.1577) is used as a suspending, thickening, and stabilising agent in pharmaceutical preparations. Attapulgite (p.1251) is another native form.

### Preparations

**Proprietary Preparations** (details are given in Part 3)
***Austria:*** Gelusil; ***Ger.:*** Gelusil; Lac 4 n†; Megalac; Simagel; ***Spain:*** Alubifar; Sinegastrin†; ***Switz.:*** Gelusil†.

**Multi-ingredient:** ***Austria:*** Gastripan; ***Ger.:*** Gelusil-Lac; Neo-Pyodron; Ultilac N; ***Spain:*** Dolcopin; ***Switz.:*** Gelusil-Lac.

## Aloes

Acibar; Áloe.

*CAS — 8001-97-6; 67479-27-0 (aloe gum).*

NOTE. Do not confuse with Aloe vera (p.1141).

**Pharmacopoeias.** In *Chin., Eur.* (see p.vi), *Jpn, Pol.,* and *US.*

**Ph. Eur. 5.0** (Aloes, Barbados; Aloe barbadensis). The concentrated and dried juice of the leaves of *Aloe barbadensis.* It contains not less than 28% of hydroxyanthracene derivatives expressed as barbaloin and calculated with reference to the dried drug. Dark brown masses, slightly shiny or opaque with a conchoidal fracture, or a brown powder. Partly soluble in boiling water; soluble in hot alcohol. Store in airtight containers. Protect from light.

The BP 2003 lists Curaçao Aloes as an approved synonym.

**Ph. Eur. 5.0** (Aloes, Cape; Aloe capensis). The concentrated and dried juice of the leaves of various species of *Aloe,* mainly *Aloe ferox* and its hybrids. It contains not less than 18% of hydroxyanthracene derivatives expressed as barbaloin and calculated with reference to the dried drug. Dark brown masses tinged with green and having a shiny conchoidal fracture, or a greenish-brown powder. Partly soluble in boiling water; soluble in hot alcohol; practically insoluble in ether. Store in airtight containers. Protect from light.

**USP 27** (Aloe). The dried latex of the leaves of *Aloe barbadensis (A. vera)* known in commerce as Curaçao Aloe, or of *A. ferox* and its hybrids, known in commerce as Cape Aloe (Liliaceae). It yields not less than 50% of water-soluble extractive. It has a characteristic, somewhat sour and disagreeable, odour. Curaçao Aloe is brownish-black, opaque masses with a fractured, uneven, waxy, and somewhat resinous surface. Cape Aloe is dusty to dark brown irregular masses, the surfaces of which are often covered with a yellowish powder. Its fracture is smooth and glassy.

### Adverse Effects and Precautions

As for Senna, p.1288, although aloes has a more drastic and irritant action.

### Uses and Administration

Aloes is an anthraquinone stimulant laxative (p.1239) but other less toxic drugs are generally preferred.

It has also been used in homoeopathic medicine.

### Preparations

***BP 2003:*** Compound Benzoin Tincture;
***Ph. Eur.:*** Aloes Dry Extract, Standardised;
***USP 27:*** Compound Benzoin Tincture.

**Proprietary Preparations** (details are given in Part 3)
***Fr.:*** Contre-Coups de l'Abbe Perdrigeon; Vulcase; ***Ger.:*** Aristo L†; Dr Janssens Teebohnen; Krauterlax A; Rheogen; ***Switz.:*** Elixir Rebleuten†.

**Multi-ingredient:** ***Arg.:*** Genolaxante; ***Austral.:*** Herbal Cleanse†; Lexat†; Peritone†; ***Austria:*** Abfuhrdragees; Abfuhrdragees mild; Aristochol†; Artin; Dragees Neunzehn; Pserhofer's; ***Belg.:*** Grains de Vals; ***Braz.:*** Camomila†; ***Canad.:*** Extra Strong Formula 12; Laxative; ***Chile:*** Aloelax; Bulgarolax; ***Fr.:*** Ideolaxyl; Opobyl; Petites Pilules Carters; Tonilax†; ***Ger.:*** Aristochol; Befelka-Tinktur†; Chol-Kugeletten Neu; Cholhepan N; Pascoletten N; Redaxa Lax†; Reducelle†; Schwedentrunk mit Ginseng†; Schwedentrunk†; ***Hong Kong:*** Rheogen†; ***Israel:*** Laxative Comp; ***Ital.:*** Cura†; Frerichs Maldifassi; Grani di Vals; Lassativi Vetegali; Neutrogena Anti-Acne†; Pillole Fattori†; ***Mon.:*** Akipic; ***Port.:*** Emopads†; ***Spain:*** Alofedina; Cinaro Bilina†; Crislaxo; Cynaro Bilina; Laxante Sanatorium; Nico Hepatocyn; Opobyl; Pildoras Zeninas; ***Switz.:*** Adistop Lax†; Ajaka†; Aloinophen†; Dragees laxatives no 510†; Kneipp Woerisettes†; Opobyl†; Padma-Lax; Physiolax†; Phytolax†; PhytoLaxin; Schweden-Mixtur H nouvelle formulation; Tavolax†; ***UK:*** Dual-Lax Normal Strength; Gerard House Gladlax†; Laxative Tablets; Natural Herb Tablets; Out-of-Sorts; Sure-Lax (Herbal); ***USA:*** Diaparene Corn Starch; Natures Remedy†; Vagisil.

## Aloglutamol

2-Amino-2-hydroxymethylpropane-1,3-diol gluconate dihydroxyaluminate.

$C_{10}H_{24}AlNO_{12}$ = 377.3.

*ATC — A02AB06.*

### Profile

Aloglutamol has been used as an antacid (p.1239).

### Preparations

**Proprietary Preparations** (details are given in Part 3)
***Mex.:*** Sabro.

## Aloin (BAN)

Alloin; Aloína.

*CAS — 5133-19-7; 8015-61-0; 1415-73-2 (barbaloin).*

### Profile

Aloin is a crystalline substance obtained from aloes (see above). It consists of *C*-glycosides such as barbaloin. Aloin is an anthraquinone stimulant laxative. Like aloes it is very irritant and other less toxic laxatives are generally preferred. Aloin is used as a flavouring agent.

### Preparations

**Proprietary Preparations** (details are given in Part 3)
***Chile:*** Felaxen; ***UK:*** Calsalettes.

**Multi-ingredient:** ***Austral.:*** Ford Pills†; ***Belg.:*** Sanicolax†; ***Braz.:*** Pilulas Ross; ***Canad.:*** Aid-Lax†; Alsiline†; Bicholate; Laxa†; Thunas Bilettes†; Triolax†; ***Irl.:*** Alophen†; ***Israel:*** Laxative; Laxative Comp; ***Ital.:*** Boldina He; Cuscutine; Grani di Vals; ***Mex.:*** Redotex NF; ***Spain:*** Laxante Bescansa Aloico; ***Switz.:*** Ajaka†; Carter Petites Pilules†; ***UK:*** Alophen†; Dual-Lax Extra Strong; Modern Herbals Laxative.

## Alosetron Hydrochloride (BANM, USAN, rINNM)

GR-68755C. 2,3,4,5-Tetrahydro-5-methyl-2-[(5-methyl-imidazol-4-yl)methyl]-1H-pyrido[4,3-b]indol-1-one hydrochloride.

$C_{17}H_{18}N_4O,HCl$ = 330.8.

*CAS — 122852-42-0 (alosetron); 122852-69-1 (alosetron hydrochloride).*
*ATC — A03AE01.*

### Adverse Effects

Serious gastrointestinal adverse effects including severe constipation and ischaemic colitis have occurred following the use of alosetron, and as a result, alosetron was withdrawn from the market in the USA and subsequently re-introduced with more restricted indications. Complications of severe constipation such as obstruction, perforation, impaction, toxic megacolon, and colonic ischaemia have been observed. Fatalities have been reported.

Other gastrointestinal effects reported include abdominal distension and pain, nausea, reflux, and haemorrhoids. Adverse effects reported rarely include cardiac arrhythmias, cholecystitis, altered bilirubin levels, and CNS effects such as confusion, depression, and sedation.

### Precautions

Alosetron should be discontinued immediately in patients who develop constipation or symptoms of ischaemic colitis such as new or worsening abdominal pain or blood in the stool. Treatment with alosetron should not be resumed in patients who develop ischaemic colitis.

Alosetron should not be used in patients with a history of severe or chronic constipation, intestinal obstruction or stricture, toxic megacolon, or gastrointestinal perforation or adhesions. It is also contra-indicated in patients with a history of ischaemic colitis, impaired intestinal circulation, thrombophlebitis, or hypercoagulable state, and those with current or previous inflammatory bowel disease or diverticulitis.

Alosetron should be used with caution in patients with hepatic impairment.

### Pharmacokinetics

Alosetron is rapidly absorbed from the gastrointestinal tract; peak plasma concentrations are reached about 1 hour after an oral dose. Bioavailability is about 60%; the extent and rate of absorption are slightly reduced by food. Plasma protein binding is about 82%. Alosetron is extensively metabolised to numerous metabolites which are subsequently excreted in the urine and faeces; only 6% of a dose is recovered unchanged from the urine. The terminal elimination half-life of alosetron is reported to be about 1.5 hours.

### Uses and Administration

Alosetron is a 5-$HT_3$ antagonist used in the treatment of severe diarrhoea-predominant irritable bowel syndrome (p.1244) in women who have not responded to conventional therapy; effectiveness in men has not been established. It is given as the hydrochloride but doses are expressed in terms of the base; alosetron hydrochloride 1.12 mg is approximately equivalent to 1 mg alosetron.

The initial dose is the equivalent of alosetron 1 mg daily for 4 weeks; if tolerated, the dose may then be increased to 1 mg twice daily. If symptoms are not adequately controlled after 4 weeks' treatment with the higher dose, alosetron should be discontinued.

Alosetron has also been investigated for schizophrenia and other mental disorders.

◊ References.

1. Lembo A, *et al.* Alosetron in irritable bowel syndrome: strategies for its use in a common gastrointestinal disorder. *Drugs* 2003; **63:** 1895–905.
2. Mayer EA, Bradesi S. Alosetron and irritable bowel syndrome. *Expert Opin Pharmacother* 2003; **4:** 2089–98.
3. Cremonini F, *et al.* Efficacy of alosetron in irritable bowel syndrome: a meta-analysis of randomized controlled trials. *Neurogastroenterol Motil* 2003; **15:** 79–86.
4. Andresen V, Hollerbach S. Reassessing the benefits and risks of alosetron: what is its place in the treatment of irritable bowel syndrome? *Drug Safety* 2004; **27:** 283–92.

### Preparations

**Proprietary Preparations** (details are given in Part 3)
***Arg.:*** Lotronex; ***Mex.:*** Liminos; ***USA:*** Lotronex.

## Basic Aluminium Carbonate *(USAN)*

Aluminium Hydroxycarbonate; Carbonato básico de aluminio.

### Profile

Basic aluminium carbonate is a combination of aluminium hydroxide and aluminium carbonate. It is an antacid with general properties similar to those of aluminium hydroxide (below). Doses are given in terms of the equivalent amount of aluminium hydroxide; a dose equivalent to about 1 g of aluminium hydroxide is usually taken.

Basic aluminium carbonate may also be given by mouth as a phosphate binder in the treatment of hyperphosphataemia. For a discussion of the choice of phosphate binders, see Renal Osteodystrophy, p.764.

### Preparations

**Proprietary Preparations** (details are given in Part 3)
***Fr.:*** Lithiagel†; ***USA:*** Basaljel†.
**Multi-ingredient:** ***Fr.:*** Dextomat†.

## Aluminium Glycinate

Aluminio, glicinato de; Basic Aluminium Aminoacetate; Dihydroxyaluminum Aminoacetate. (Glycinato-*N*,*O*)dihydroxyaluminium hydrate.

$C_2H_6AlNO_4(+xH_2O)$ = 135.1 (anhydrous).
*CAS — 13682-92-3 (anhydrous aluminium glycinate); 41354-48-7 (aluminium glycinate hydrate).*
*ATC — A02AB07.*

**Pharmacopoeias.** In *Br.* and *US.*

**BP 2003** (Aluminium Glycinate). A white or almost white, odourless or almost odourless, powder. It contains 34.5 to 38.5% of $Al_2O_3$ calculated on the dried substance, and not more than 12% loss of weight on drying. Practically insoluble in water and in organic solvents; it dissolves in dilute mineral acids and in aqueous solutions of alkali hydroxides. A 4% suspension in water has a pH of 6.5 to 7.5.

**USP 27** (Dihydroxyaluminum Aminoacetate). A white, odourless, powder. It may contain small amounts of aluminium oxide and aminoacetic acid. It loses not more than 14.5% of its weight on drying. Insoluble in water and in organic solvents; soluble in dilute mineral acids and in solutions of fixed alkalis. A 4% suspension in water has a pH of 6.5 to 7.5.

### Profile

Aluminium glycinate is an antacid with general properties similar to those of aluminium hydroxide (below). It has been given in doses of up to 1 g by mouth.

### Preparations

***USP 27:*** Dihydroxyaluminum Aminoacetate Magma.
**Proprietary Preparations** (details are given in Part 3)
**Multi-ingredient:** ***Arg.:*** Dafne; ***Austria:*** Acidrine†; Gastripan; ***Belg.:*** Acidrine†; Alucid; Normacidine†; ***Braz.:*** Betazon†; ***Chile:*** Sinacid; ***Denm.:*** Alminox; ***Fr.:*** Acidrine; Gastralgine†; ***Ger.:*** Acidrine; ***Gr.:*** Novalox; ***Ital.:*** Acidrine; Gastrostop†; ***Spain:*** Digestinas Super†; Gastroglutal; Jorkil†; Meteoril; Natrocitral; Secrepat.

*Used as an adjunct in:* ***Austria:*** Ambene N; Indobene; ***Braz.:*** Reumix†; Somalgin; ***Canad.:*** Bufferin; ***Chile:*** Flexono; ***Ger.:*** Indomet-ratiopharm m; ***Hong Kong:*** Trabit†; ***Ital.:*** Aspirina 03 and 05; ***Switz.:*** Bonidon; ***USA:*** Buffex.

## Aluminium Hydroxide

Aluminium Oxidum Hydricum; Aluminum Hydroxide; Hidróxido de aluminio; Wasserhaltiges Aluminiumoxid.
*CAS — 21645-51-2 [$Al(OH)_3$].*
*ATC — A02AB01.*

NOTE. Algeldrate (*USAN, pINN*) is defined as a hydrated aluminium hydroxide with the general formula of $Al(OH)_3,xH_2O$.

Compounded preparations of aluminium hydroxide may be represented by the following names:

- Co-magaldrox *x/y* (*BAN*)—where *x* and *y* are the strengths in milligrams of magnesium hydroxide and aluminium hydroxide respectively.

**Pharmacopoeias.** In *Chin., Eur.* (see p.vi), *Int., Jpn, Pol., US,* and *Viet.*

**Ph. Eur. 5.0** (Aluminium Oxide, Hydrated; Dried Aluminium Hydroxide BP 2003). It contains the equivalent of 47 to 60% $Al_2O_3$. It is a white amorphous powder. Practically insoluble in water; it dissolves in dilute mineral acids and in solutions of alkali hydroxides. Store in airtight containers at a temperature not exceeding 30°.

**Ph. Eur. 5.0** (Aluminium Hydroxide, Hydrated, for Adsorption; Aluminii Hydroxidum Hydricum ad Adsorptionem). A white or almost white, translucent, viscous, colloidal gel. A supernatant may be formed upon standing. A clear or almost clear solution is obtained with alkali hydroxide solutions and with mineral acids. pH 5.5 to 8.5. Store at a temperature not exceeding 30°. Do not allow to freeze.

**USP 27** (Aluminum Hydroxide Gel). A suspension of amorphous aluminium hydroxide in which there is a partial substitution of carbonate for hydroxide. It is a white viscous suspension from which small amounts of clear liquid may separate on standing. It has a pH of between 5.5 and 8.0. Store in airtight containers. Avoid freezing.

**USP 27** (Dried Aluminum Hydroxide Gel). An amorphous form of aluminium hydroxide in which there is a partial substitution of carbonate for hydroxide. It contains the equivalent of not less than 76.5% of $Al(OH)_3$ and may contain varying quantities of basic aluminium carbonate and bicarbonate. The labelling requirements states that 1 g of dried aluminium hydroxide gel is equivalent to 765 mg of $Al(OH)_3$. It is a white, odourless, tasteless, amorphous powder. Insoluble in water and in alcohol; soluble in dilute mineral acids and in solutions of fixed alkali hydroxides. A 4% aqueous dispersion has a pH of not more than 10.0. Store in airtight containers.

### Adverse Effects and Precautions

Aluminium hydroxide, like other aluminium compounds, is astringent and may cause constipation; large doses can cause intestinal obstruction.

Excessive doses, or even normal doses in patients with low-phosphate diets, may lead to phosphate depletion accompanied by increased bone resorption and hypercalciuria with the risk of osteomalacia.

Aluminium salts are not, in general, well absorbed from the gastrointestinal tract, and systemic effects are therefore rare in patients with normal renal function. However, care is necessary in patients with chronic renal impairment: osteomalacia or adynamic bone disease, encephalopathy, dementia, and microcytic anaemia have been associated with aluminium accumulation in such patients given large doses of aluminium hydroxide as a phosphate-binding agent. Similar adverse effects have also been associated with the aluminium content of dialysis fluids.

Aluminium hydroxide used as an adjuvant in adsorbed vaccines has been associated with the formation of granulomas.

**Porphyria.** Aluminium hydroxide is considered to be unsafe in patients with porphyria because it has been shown to be porphyrinogenic in *animals*.

**Toxicity.** References to aluminium toxicity in dialysis patients and the possible association between aluminium ingestion and Alzheimer's disease are included under Aluminium (see p.1652).

Aluminium accumulation does not generally appear to be significant in patients with normal renal function taking therapeutic doses of aluminium-containing antacids, and there is little evidence that such antacids are a risk factor for Alzheimer's disease.[1] Elevated plasma-aluminium concentrations have been reported in infants with normal renal function given aluminium-containing antacids but there were no obvious signs of toxicity.[2] However, aluminium accumulation resulting in osteomalacia or encephalopathy with seizures and dementia has been reported in children with renal failure treated with aluminium-containing phosphate binders.[3-7] Aluminium-containing antacids should therefore be used with caution in patients with chronic renal failure, especially in children. Hypophosphataemia and metabolic bone disease have been reported in an infant given an excess of an antacid containing aluminium hydroxide and magnesium hydroxide.[8]

Oral citrate salts increase the absorption of aluminium from the gastrointestinal tract[9] and patients with renal failure taking aluminium compounds should avoid citrate-containing preparations, which include many effervescent or dispersible tablets.[10,11] Ascorbic acid has also been reported to enhance aluminium absorption.[12]

1. Flaten TP, *et al.* Mortality from dementia among gastroduodenal ulcer patients. *J Epidemiol Community Health* 1991; **45:** 203–6.
2. Tsou VM, *et al.* Elevated plasma aluminum levels in normal infants receiving antacids containing aluminum. *Pediatrics* 1991; **87:** 148–51.
3. Pedersen S, Nathan E. Water treatment and dialysis dementia. *Lancet* 1982; **ii:** 1107.
4. Griswold WR, *et al.* Accumulation of aluminum in a nondialyzed uremic child receiving aluminum hydroxide. *Pediatrics* 1983; **71:** 56–8.
5. Randall ME. Aluminium toxicity in an infant not on dialysis. *Lancet* 1983; **i:** 1327–8.
6. Sedman AB, *et al.* Encephalopathy in childhood secondary to aluminum toxicity. *J Pediatr* 1984; **105:** 836–8.
7. Andreoli SP, *et al.* Aluminum intoxication from aluminum-containing phosphate binders in children with azotemia not undergoing dialysis. *N Engl J Med* 1984; **310:** 1079–84.
8. Robinson RF, *et al.* Metabolic bone disease after chronic antacid administration in an infant. *Ann Pharmacother* 2004 **38:** 265–8.
9. Walker JA, *et al.* The effect of oral bases on enteral aluminum absorption. *Arch Intern Med* 1990; **150:** 2037–9.
10. Mees EJD, Başçi A. Citric acid in calcium effervescent tablets may favour aluminium intoxication. *Nephron* 1991; **59:** 322.
11. Main J, Ward MK. Potentiation of aluminium absorption by effervescent analgesic tablets in a haemodialysis patient. *BMJ* 1992; **304:** 1686.
12. Domingo JL, *et al.* Effect of ascorbic acid on gastrointestinal aluminium absorption. *Lancet* 1992; **338:** 1467.

### Interactions

As outlined on p.1239, aluminium compounds used as antacids interact with many other drugs, both by alterations in gastric pH and emptying, and by direct adsorption and formation of complexes that are not absorbed. Interactions can be minimised by giving the aluminium compound and any other medication 2 to 3 hours apart. The absorption of aluminium from the gastrointestinal tract may be enhanced if aluminium compounds are taken with citrates or ascorbic acid (see above).

### Pharmacokinetics

Aluminium hydroxide, given by mouth, slowly reacts with the hydrochloric acid in the stomach to form soluble aluminium chloride, some of which is absorbed. The presence of food or other factors that decrease gastric emptying prolongs the availability of aluminium hydroxide to react and may increase the amount of aluminium chloride formed. About 100 to 500 micrograms of the cation is reported to be absorbed from standard daily doses of an aluminium-containing antacid, leading to about a doubling of usual aluminium concentrations in the plasma of patients with normal renal function.

Absorbed aluminium is eliminated in the urine, and patients with renal failure are therefore at particular risk of accumulation (especially in bone and the CNS), and aluminium toxicity (see above).

The aluminium compounds remaining in the gastrointestinal tract, which account for most of a dose, form insoluble, poorly absorbed aluminium salts in the intestines including hydroxides, carbonates, phosphates and fatty acid derivatives, which are excreted in the faeces.

### Uses and Administration

Aluminium hydroxide is used as an antacid (p.1239). It is given in doses of up to about 1 g by mouth. In order to reduce the constipating effects, aluminium hydroxide is often given with a magnesium-containing antacid, such as magnesium oxide or magnesium hydroxide.

Aluminium hydroxide binds phosphate in the gastrointestinal tract to form insoluble complexes and reduces phosphate absorption. It is thus used to treat hyperphosphataemia in patients with chronic renal failure (see Renal Osteodystrophy, p.764). With this use the dose must be adjusted to the individual patient's requirement but up to about 10 g daily by mouth may be given in divided doses.

Aluminium hydroxide is also used as an adjuvant in adsorbed vaccines.

**Polymyositis and dermatomyositis.** Corticosteroids form the basis of the management of polymyositis (p.1086) but the calcinosis that may occur in dermatomyositis does not always respond well. Aluminium hydroxide 1.68 to 2.24 g daily produced clinical improvement with complete clearing of most calcified nodules after 1 year in a patient with calcinosis cutis complicating juvenile dermatomyositis.[1] The calcified masses are made up of hydroxyapatite and amorphous calcium phosphate and reduction in phosphate absorption by aluminium hydroxide probably helped to reverse their formation. Subsequent cases[2,3] have also reported benefit from aluminium hydroxide treatment in the management of calcinosis.

1. Wang W-J, *et al.* Calcinosis cutis in juvenile dermatomyositis: remarkable response to aluminium hydroxide therapy. *Arch Dermatol* 1988; **124:** 1721–2.
2. Nakagawa T, Takaiwa T. Calcinosis cutis in juvenile dermatomyositis responsive to aluminium hydroxide treatment. *J Dermatol* 1993; **20:** 558–60.
3. Wananukul S, *et al.* Calcinosis cutis presenting years before other clinical manifestations of juvenile dermatomyositis: report of two cases. *Australas J Dermatol* 1997; **38:** 202–5.

### Preparations

***BP 2003:*** Aluminium Hydroxide Oral Suspension; Aluminium Hydroxide Tablets; Co-magaldrox Oral Suspension; Co-magaldrox Tablets; Compound Magnesium Trisilicate Tablets;
***USP 27:*** Alumina and Magnesia Oral Suspension; Alumina and Magnesia Tablets; Alumina and Magnesium Carbonate Oral Suspension; Alumina and Magnesium Carbonate Tablets; Alumina and Magnesium Trisilicate Oral Suspension; Alumina and Magnesium Trisilicate Tablets; Alumina, Magnesia, and Calcium Carbonate Oral Suspension; Alumina, Magnesia, and Calcium Carbonate Tablets; Alumina, Magnesia, and Simethicone Oral Suspension; Alumina, Magnesia, and Simethicone Tablets; Alumina, Magnesia, Calcium Carbonate, and Simethicone Tablets; Alumina, Magnesium Carbonate, and Magnesium Oxide Tablets; Aluminum Hydroxide Gel; Aspirin, Alumina, and Magnesia Tablets; Aspirin, Alumina, and Magnesium Oxide Tablets; Dried Aluminum Hydroxide Gel; Dried Aluminum Hydroxide Gel Capsules; Dried Aluminum Hydroxide Gel Tablets.

**Proprietary Preparations** (details are given in Part 3)
***Arg.:*** Pepsamar; ***Austral.:*** Alu-Tab; Amphojel†; ***Austria:*** Anti-Phosphat; ***Braz.:*** Aldrox†; Aludroxil; Anacidron-H†; Aziram; Ductogel; Fluagel; Gelpan†; Kaogel; Mylanta Plus; Natusgel†; No-Acid†; Pepsamar; Peptgel; ***Canad.:*** Alu-Tab; Alugel; Amphojel; Basaljel; ***Chile:*** Risthal; ***Ger.:*** Aludrox; Antacidum OPT†; Anti-Phosphat; Gastracops A†; ***Gr.:*** Alu-cap; Pepsamar; ***Hong Kong:*** Alu-Tab; ***India:*** Aludrox; Tricaine-MPS; ***Irl.:*** Aludrox; ***Israel:*** Alu-Cap; ***Ital.:*** Polisilon; ***Malaysia:*** Alu-Tab; ***Mex.:*** Galcdexan†; Magnalum†; ***NZ:*** Alu-Tab; Amphojel; ***Port.:*** Almigastrico†; Gelumina; Pepsamar; ***S.Afr.:*** Acidex†; Alukon†; Amphojel†; ***Singapore:*** Alu-Tab; ***Spain:*** Alugel; Dialume†; Pepsamar; ***Switz.:*** Anti-Phosphate; Gastracol; ***UK:*** Alu-Cap†; Aludrox; ***USA:*** ALternaGEL; Alu-Cap; Alu-Tab; Amphojel; Dialume; Nephrox.

**Multi-ingredient:** numerous preparations are listed in Part 3.

## Aluminium Hydroxide-Magnesium Carbonate Co-dried Gel

F-MA 11; Hidróxido de aluminio y carbonato de magnesio desecado, gel de.

### Profile

Aluminium hydroxide-magnesium carbonate co-dried gel is a co-precipitate of aluminium hydroxide and magnesium carbonate dried to contain a proportion of water for antacid activity. It is an antacid with general properties similar to those of aluminium hydroxide (above) and magnesium carbonate (p.1272). It is given in doses of about 400 to 800 mg by mouth.

### Preparations

**Proprietary Preparations** (details are given in Part 3)
***Denm.:*** Link; ***Fin.:*** Link; PeeHoo; ***Gr.:*** ReglaPh; ***Mex.:*** Gelasim; ***Norw.:*** Link; ***Swed.:*** Link; ***UK:*** Dijex†.

**Multi-ingredient:** ***Austral.:*** Algicon†; ***Belg.:*** Barexal; Gastropulgite†; Nozid; Regla pH Forte; Syngel; ***Braz.:*** Acidex†; Algicote†; Andursil; ***Canad.:*** Amphojel Plus†; Diovol; Diovol Plus; Gastrinol†; Gastrocalm; Thunas Hyperacidity Tablets; ***Chile:*** Algicote; Ditopax; ***Fin.:*** PH maxi†; ***Fr.:*** Gastropulgite; ***Ger.:*** Colina Spezial; Duoventrinetten N; Gastropulgit†; ***Gr.:*** Simeco; ***Hong Kong:*** Diovol Plus; Simeco; Veragel; ***Irl.:*** Algicon; ***Israel:*** Silain; ***Mex.:*** Algicon; Ditopax; Ditopax-F; ***Neth.:*** Algicon; Regla pH; Rigoletten; ***Norw.:*** Algicon†; ***Port.:*** Di-Gel; Di-Gel Forte; ***S.Afr.:*** Tacid-4†; ***Singapore:*** Meclosil; Simeco†; Tocid†; Veragel DMS; ***Spain:*** Acylene; ***Switz.:*** Anacidol; Andursil; Combacid; Gastropulgite; Refluxine; ***Thai.:*** Defomil; Diovol; Kremil; Kremil-S; Machto; Simeco; Veragel; ***UK:*** Algicon; Aludrox†; Simeco; ***USA:*** Maalox Heartburn Relief†.

## Aluminium Phosphate

Aluminii Phosphas; Aluminum Phosphate; Fosfato de aluminio.
*CAS — 7784-30-7 ($AlPO_4$).*
*ATC — A02AB03.*

**Pharmacopoeias.** In *Pol.* and *Viet.*
*Eur.* (see p.vi) includes hydrated aluminium phosphate. *US* includes as a gel.

**Ph. Eur. 5.0** (Aluminium Phosphate, Hydrated; Aluminii Phosphas Hydricus; Dried Aluminium Phosphate BP 2003). A white or almost white powder. Very slightly soluble in water; practically insoluble in alcohol. It dissolves in dilute solutions of alkali hydroxides and mineral acids. A 4% suspension in water has a pH of 5.5 to 7.2. Store in airtight containers.

**USP 27** (Aluminum Phosphate Gel). A 4 to 5% suspension of aluminium phosphate ($AlPO_4$) in water and has a pH of 6.0 to 7.2. It is a white viscous suspension from which small amounts of water separate on standing. Store in airtight containers.

### Profile

Aluminium phosphate is an antacid with general properties similar to those of aluminium hydroxide (p.1249), but it does not produce phosphate depletion.

Aluminium phosphate is also used as an adjuvant in adsorbed vaccines.

### Preparations

***USP 27:*** Aluminum Phosphate Gel.

**Proprietary Preparations** (details are given in Part 3)
***Austria:*** Phosphalugel; ***Belg.:*** Phosphalugel; ***Fr.:*** Phosphalugel; ***Ger.:*** Phosphalugel; ***Ital.:*** Fosfalugel; ***Port.:*** Phosphalugel; ***Spain:*** Fosfalumina†; ***Switz.:*** Phosphalugel.

**Multi-ingredient:** ***Austria:*** Phoscortil; ***Fr.:*** Isudrine†; Moxydar.

## Aluminium Sodium Silicate

E554; Silicato de sodio y de aluminio; Sodium Aluminium Silicate; Sodium Aluminosilicate; Sodium Silicoaluminate.
*CAS — 1344-00-9.*

### Profile

Aluminium sodium silicate is an antacid with general properties similar to those of aluminium hydroxide (p.1249). Aluminium silicate has been used similarly. They are also used as food additives.

### Preparations

**Proprietary Preparations** (details are given in Part 3)
***Fr.:*** Sulfuryl; ***Port.:*** Acnoil Free.

**Multi-ingredient:** ***Austria:*** Diphlogen; ***Belg.:*** Mucal†; ***Braz.:*** Diteutrin†; ***Fr.:*** Anti-H; Cerat Inalterable; Sulfuryl; ***Ger.:*** Enelbin-Paste N; Mucal†; Sulfredox; ***Port.:*** Gastroplex†; Mucal; ***Spain:*** Doctogaster†; ***Switz.:*** TRI-OM†; ***Thai.:*** Ulgastrin.

## Alverine Citrate *(BANM, USAN, rINNM)*

Citrato de alverina; Dipropyline Citrate; Phenpropamine Citrate.
*N*-Ethyl-3,3′-diphenyldipropylamine citrate.
$C_{20}H_{27}N,C_6H_8O_7 = 473.6.$
*CAS — 150-59-4 (alverine); 5560-59-8 (alverine citrate).*
*ATC — A03AX08.*

### Adverse Effects and Precautions

Nausea, headache, pruritus, rash, and dizziness have been reported. Allergic reactions, including anaphylaxis, have also occurred. Alverine is contra-indicated in patients with intestinal obstruction or paralytic ileus.

### Pharmacokinetics

Alverine is absorbed from the gastrointestinal tract following oral administration and is rapidly metabolised to an active metabolite, peak plasma concentrations of which occur 1 to 1.5 hours after an oral dose. Further metabolism to inactive metabolites occurs; metabolites are excreted in the urine by active renal secretion.

### Uses and Administration

Alverine is an antispasmodic that acts directly on intestinal and uterine smooth muscle. It is used for the relief of smooth muscle spasm in the treatment of gastrointestinal disorders such as irritable bowel syndrome (p.1244). It is also used in the treatment of dysmenorrhoea (p.6).

Alverine is given by mouth as the citrate in doses of 60 to 120 mg one to three times daily. It has also been given by suppository as the base in doses of 80 mg two or three times daily. Alverine citrate 67.3 mg is approximately equivalent to 40 mg of alverine.

### Preparations

**Proprietary Preparations** (details are given in Part 3)
***Belg.:*** Spasmine; ***Fr.:*** Spasmaverine†; ***Hong Kong:*** Profenil; Spasmonal; ***Irl.:*** Spasmonal; ***Malaysia:*** Spasmonal; ***Singapore:*** Spasmonal; ***Thai.:*** Spasmonal; ***UK:*** Relaxyl; Spasmonal.

**Multi-ingredient:** ***Austral.:*** Alvercol; ***Belg.:*** Normacol Antispasmodique; ***Fr.:*** Hepatoum; Meteospasmyl; Schoum; Spasmaverine†; ***Hong Kong:*** Alvercol†; Meteospasmyl†; ***Irl.:*** Alvercol†; ***Malaysia:*** Meteospasmyl; ***S.Afr.:*** Alvercol; ***Singapore:*** Meteospasmyl; ***Thai.:*** Meteospasmyl; ***UK:*** Spasmonal Fibre†.

## Alvimopan *(rINN)*

ADL-8-2698; LY-246736. [((2*S*)-2-{[(3*R*,4*R*)-4-(3-Hydroxyphenyl)-3,4-dimethylpiperidin-1-yl]methyl}-3-phenylpropanoyl)amino]acetic acid.
$C_{25}H_{32}N_2O_4 = 424.5.$
*CAS — 156053-89-3 (alvimopan); 170098-38-1 (alvimopan dihydrate).*

NOTE. Alvimopan (USAN) is the dihydrate.

### Profile

Alvimopan is a peripherally acting selective antagonist of opioid μ-receptors that is under investigation for postoperative ileus and constipation.

◊ References.

1. Taguchi A, *et al.* Selective postoperative inhibition of gastrointestinal opioid receptors. *N Engl J Med* 2001; **345:** 935–40.

## Aprepitant *(USAN, rINN)*

MK-0869. 3-[((2*R*,3*S*)-3-(*p*-Fluorophenyl)-2-{[(αR)-α-methyl-3,5-bis(trifluoromethyl)benzyl]oxy}morpholino)methyl]-$\Delta^2$-1,2,4-triazolin-5-one.
$C_{23}H_{21}F_7N_4O_3 = 534.4.$
*CAS — 170729-80-3.*

### Adverse Effects and Precautions

The most common adverse effects associated with aprepitant are headache, constipation, dyspepsia, anorexia, fatigue, hiccups, and an increase in alanine aminotransferase (ALT) concentrations. Other reported effects have included abdominal pain, dizziness, tinnitus, and flushing. Stevens-Johnson syndrome and angioedema with urticaria have been reported.

The manufacturers recommend caution in patients with severe hepatic impairment as clinical data is lacking in this patient group.

### Interactions

Aprepitant is both a moderate inhibitor and, within 2 weeks of therapy, an inducer of cytochrome P450 isoenzyme CYP3A4. Caution is therefore required when using it with drugs that are primarily metabolised by this isoenzyme. As aprepitant is also a substrate for CYP3A4, drugs that inhibit or induce this isoenzyme may increase or decrease plasma concentrations of aprepitant. Aprepitant is also an inducer of CYP2C9 and may lower plasma concentrations of drugs metabolised by this isoenzyme, such as warfarin, phenytoin, or tolbutamide.

Aprepitant may increase systemic exposure to corticosteroids; when given together the manufacturers recommend that the usual dose of oral dexamethasone be reduced by 50%, and the dose of methylprednisolone by about 25% when given intravenously, and by 50% when given orally. It should be noted that the dose of dexamethasone in the regimen recommended by the manufacturers of aprepitant already accounts for this interaction (see below).

Aprepitant may reduce the efficacy of oral contraceptives.

### Pharmacokinetics

Aprepitant is absorbed from the gastrointestinal tract with peak plasma concentrations achieved after approximately 4 hours. Bioavailability is about 60% at usual doses. It crosses the blood-brain barrier; plasma protein binding is reported to be more than 95%. Aprepitant is extensively metabolised in the liver, mainly via oxidation by cytochrome P450 isoenzyme CYP3A4 and with minor metabolism by CYP1A2 and CYP2C19. The resultant metabolites have only weak activity and they are excreted in the urine and in the faeces. Aprepitant is not excreted unchanged in the urine. The terminal half-life is about 9 to 13 hours.

### Uses and Administration

Aprepitant is a neurokinin-1 ($NK_1$) receptor antagonist, given by mouth in doses up to 125 mg in combination with a corticosteroid and a 5-$HT_3$ antagonist, in the prevention of acute and delayed nausea and vomiting associated with highly emetogenic cancer chemotherapy (for details, see Administration, below).

◊ References.

1. Campos D, *et al.* Prevention of cisplatin-induced emesis by the oral neurokinin-1 antagonist, MK-869, in combination with granisetron and dexamethasone or with dexamethasone alone. *J Clin Oncol* 2001; **19:** 1759–67.
2. Poli-Bigelli S, *et al.* Addition of the neurokinin 1 receptor antagonist aprepitant to standard antiemetic therapy improves control of chemotherapy-induced nausea and vomiting: results from a randomized, double-blind, placebo-controlled trial in Latin America. *Cancer* 2003; **97:** 3090–8.

3. de Wit R, *et al.* Addition of the oral $NK_1$ antagonist aprepitant to standard antiemetics provides protection against nausea and vomiting during multiple cycles of cisplatin-based chemotherapy. *J Clin Oncol* 2003; **21:** 4105–11.
4. Hesketh PJ, *et al.* The oral neurokinin-1 antagonist aprepitant for the prevention of chemotherapy-induced nausea and vomiting: a multinational, randomized, double-blind, placebo-controlled trial in patients receiving high-dose cisplatin—the Aprepitant Protocol 052 Study Group. *J Clin Oncol* 2003; **21:** 4112–19.

**Administration.** The manufacturers of aprepitant suggest the following 4-day regimen for the prevention of acute and delayed nausea and vomiting associated with highly emetogenic cancer chemotherapy:

- day 1: aprepitant 125 mg (given 1 hour before chemotherapy) with oral dexamethasone 12 mg and intravenous ondansetron 32 mg (both 30 minutes before chemotherapy)
- days 2 and 3: aprepitant 80 mg with oral dexamethasone 8 mg in the morning
- day 4: oral dexamethasone 8 mg in the morning.

### Preparations

**Proprietary Preparations** (details are given in Part 3)
***UK:*** Emend; ***USA:*** Emend.

## Attapulgite

Atapulgita.
*CAS — 1337-76-4; 12174-11-7.*
*ATC — A07BC04.*

**Pharmacopoeias.** In *Br.*
Activated attapulgite is included in *Br., It.,* and *US.* Colloidal activated attapulgite is included in *US.*
**BP 2003** (Attapulgite). A purified native hydrated aluminium magnesium silicate essentially consisting of the clay mineral palygorskite. A light, cream or buff, very fine powder, free or almost free from gritty particles. A 5% suspension in water has a pH of 7.0 to 9.5.
**BP 2003** (Activated Attapulgite). Attapulgite that has been carefully heated to increase its adsorptive capacity.
**USP 27** (Activated Attapulgite). Processed native aluminium magnesium silicate which has been carefully heated. It is a cream-coloured, micronised, nonswelling powder, free from gritty particles. Insoluble in water.
**USP 27** (Colloidal Activated Attapulgite). A native aluminium magnesium silicate which has been purified. It is a cream-coloured, micronised, nonswelling powder, free from gritty particles. Insoluble in water. A 10% suspension in water has a pH of 7.0 to 9.5.

◊ NOTE. Another native aluminium magnesium silicate is described on p.1577.

### Profile

Attapulgite is highly adsorbent and is used in a wide range of products including fertilisers, pesticides, and pharmaceuticals. Activated attapulgite is an adsorbent antidiarrhoeal used as an adjunct in the management of diarrhoea (p.1241) in a daily dose of up to 9 g by mouth in divided doses.

### Preparations

**Proprietary Preparations** (details are given in Part 3)
***Belg.:*** Actapulgite; ***Canad.:*** Fowlers; Kaopectate; ***Fr.:*** Actapulgite; Norgagil†; ***Hong Kong:*** Diatabs; ***Malaysia:*** Entox-P; ***Switz.:*** Actapulgite; ***Thai.:*** Attat; Entox-P; ***UAE:*** Kaptin II; ***USA:*** Diasorb; Donnagel†; K-Pek; Kaopectate Advanced Formula; Kaopectate Maximum Strength; Rheaban Maximum Strength.

**Multi-ingredient:** ***Arg.:*** Enterobacticel; ***Austral.:*** Diareze; ***Belg.:*** Gastropulgite†; Mucipulgite†; ***Braz.:*** Atacolyt; Diapoolt†; Diazol; Dispeptrin†; Ductrin Enterico†; Entercal†; Enterocler†; Enteropen†; Enterovit†; Fluocal com Pectina†; Linadin†; Magnostase†; ***Canad.:*** Diban†; Donnagel-PG†; ***Chile:*** Diaren; Diarfin; Entero Micinovo; Enterol; Nifurat; ***Fr.:*** Gastropulgite; Mucipulgite; ***Ger.:*** Gastropulgit†; ***Ital.:*** Streptomagma; ***S.Afr.:*** Kantrexil; ***Spain:*** Terpalate†; ***Switz.:*** Gastropulgite; Mucipulgite; ***Thai.:*** Attafur†; ***UK:*** Diocalm Dual Action; Entrotabs†.

## Azasetron Hydrochloride *(rINNM)*

Hidrocloruro de azasetrón; Nazasetron Hydrochloride; Y-25130. (±)-6-Chloro-3,4-dihydro-4-methyl-3-oxo-*N*-3-quinuclidinyl-2*H*-1,4-benzoxazine-8-carboxamide hydrochloride.
$C_{17}H_{20}ClN_3O_3,HCl$ = 386.3.
*CAS — 123040-69-7 (azasetron); 141922-90-9 (azasetron hydrochloride).*

### Profile

Azasetron is a 5-$HT_3$ antagonist with general properties similar to those of ondansetron (p.1281). It is used as an antiemetic in the management of nausea and vomiting induced by cytotoxic therapy. It is given as the hydrochloride in a usual dose of 10 mg once daily by mouth or intravenously.

### Preparations

**Proprietary Preparations** (details are given in Part 3)
***Arg.:*** Serotone; ***Jpn:*** Serotone.

## Balsalazide Sodium *(BANM, rINNM)*

Balsalazida sódica; Balsalazide Disodium *(USAN)*; Balsalazine Disodium; BX-661A. 5-[4-(2-Carboxyethylcarbamoyl)phenylazo]salicylic acid, disodium salt, dihydrate.
$C_{17}H_{13}N_3Na_2O_6,2H_2O$ = 437.3.
*CAS — 80573-04-2 (balsalazide); 150399-21-6 (balsalazide disodium dihydrate).*
*ATC — A07EC04.*

### Adverse Effects and Precautions

As for Mesalazine, p.1273. If a blood dyscrasia is suspected treatment should be stopped immediately and a blood count performed. Patients or their carers should be told how to recognise signs of haematotoxicity and should be advised to seek immediate medical attention if symptoms such as fever, sore throat, mouth ulcers, bruising, or bleeding develop. Balsalazide should not be used in patients with severe hepatic impairment or moderate or severe renal impairment; care is required in those with lesser degrees of hepatic or renal impairment, and in asthma, bleeding disorders, or active peptic ulcer disease.

**Hypersensitivity.** A case of acute pericarditis, cholestasis, and vasculitis resulting from hypersensitivity to balsalazide has been reported.[1] The authors noted similarities to mesalazine-associated pericarditis and lupus-like syndrome (see Effects on the Cardiovascular System, p.1273).

1. Adhiyaman V, *et al.* Hypersensitivity reaction to balsalazide. *BMJ* 2000; **320:** 613.

### Pharmacokinetics

The absorption of intact balsalazide from the gastrointestinal tract is negligible. It is split by bacteria in the colon to 5-aminosalicylic acid (mesalazine), which is active, and 4-aminobenzoylalanine, which is considered to be an inert carrier. About 25% of the released mesalazine is absorbed and acetylated, as described under mesalazine (p.1274). A small proportion of 4-aminobenzoylalanine is absorbed and acetylated on first pass through the liver. The acetylated metabolites are excreted in the urine.

### Uses and Administration

Balsalazide consists of mesalazine linked to 4-aminobenzoylalanine via an azo bond. This bond is broken by colonic bacteria releasing the active mesalazine (p.1274). Balsalazide sodium is given by mouth in the treatment of mild to moderate active ulcerative colitis (p.1243), in a dose of 2.25 g three times daily until remission or for up to 12 weeks. For maintenance of remission of ulcerative colitis a dose of 1.5 g twice daily is recommended, adjusted as necessary up to 6 g daily.

◊ Reviews.

1. Muijsers RBR, Goa KL. Balsalazide: a review of its therapeutic use in mild-to-moderate ulcerative colitis. *Drugs* 2002; **62:** 1689–705.

### Preparations

**Proprietary Preparations** (details are given in Part 3)
***Denm.:*** Premid; ***Ital.:*** Balzide; ***Norw.:*** Colazid; ***UK:*** Colazide; ***USA:*** Colazal.
**Multi-ingredient:** ***Swed.:*** Colazid.

## Benexate Hydrochloride *(rINNM)*

Hidrocloruro de benexato. Benzyl salicylate *trans*-4-(guanidinomethyl)cyclohexanecarboxylate hydrochloride.
$C_{23}H_{27}N_3O_4,HCl$ = 445.9.
*CAS — 78718-52-2 (benexate); 78718-25-9 (benexate hydrochloride); 91574-91-3 (benexate hydrochloride betadex).*

### Profile

Benexate hydrochloride has been used in the management of peptic ulcer disease. It has been given by mouth as the clathrate with β-cyclodextrin, benexate hydrochloride betadex, in a dose of 400 mg twice daily.

### Preparations

**Proprietary Preparations** (details are given in Part 3)
***Jpn:*** Ulgut.

## Bisacodyl *(BAN, rINN)*

Bisacodilo; Bisacodylum. 4,4′-(2-Pyridylmethylene)di(phenyl acetate).
$C_{22}H_{19}NO_4$ = 361.4.
*CAS — 603-50-9 (bisacodyl); 1336-29-4 (bisacodyl tannex).*
*ATC — A06AB02; A06AG02.*

NOTE. Bisacodyl Tannex is *USAN.*

**Pharmacopoeias.** In *Chin., Eur.* (see p.vi), *Jpn, Pol.,* and *US.*
**Ph. Eur. 5.0** (Bisacodyl). A white or almost white crystalline powder. Practically insoluble in water; sparingly soluble in alcohol; soluble in acetone. It dissolves in dilute mineral acids. Protect from light.
**USP 27** (Bisacodyl). A white to off-white crystalline powder. Practically insoluble in water; soluble in benzene; soluble 1 in 210 of alcohol, 1 in 2.5 of chloroform, and 1 in 275 of ether; sparingly soluble in methyl alcohol.

### Adverse Effects

Bisacodyl and other stimulant laxatives may cause abdominal discomfort such as colic or cramps. Prolonged use or overdosage can result in diarrhoea with excessive loss of water and electrolytes, particularly potassium; there is also the possibility of developing an atonic non-functioning colon. Hypersensitivity reactions, including angioedema and anaphylactoid reactions, have been reported rarely. When given rectally, bisacodyl sometimes causes irritation and repeated use may cause proctitis or sloughing of the epithelium. To avoid gastric irritation bisacodyl tablets are enteric-coated.

### Precautions

As with other laxatives, prolonged use should be avoided. Bisacodyl should not be given to patients with intestinal obstruction or acute abdominal conditions such as appendicitis; care should also be taken in patients with inflammatory bowel disease. It should not be used in patients with severe dehydration. The suppositories should preferably be avoided in patients with anal fissures, proctitis, or ulcerated haemorrhoids.

**Handling.** Inhalation of bisacodyl powder and contact with eyes, skin, and mucous membranes should be avoided.

### Pharmacokinetics

Following oral or rectal administration bisacodyl is converted to the active desacetyl metabolite bis(*p*-hydroxyphenyl)pyridyl-2-methane by intestinal and bacterial enzymes. Absorption from the gastrointestinal tract is minimal with enteric-coated tablets or suppositories; the small amount absorbed is excreted in the urine as the glucuronide. Bisacodyl is mainly excreted in the faeces.

### Uses and Administration

Bisacodyl is a diphenylmethane stimulant laxative (p.1239) used for the treatment of constipation (p.1240) and for bowel evacuation before investigational procedures or surgery. Its action is mainly in the large intestine and it is usually effective within 6 to 12 hours after oral administration, within 15 to 60 minutes after rectal administration by suppository, and within 5 to 20 minutes of administration by enema. Bisacodyl tablets should be swallowed whole and should not be taken within 1 hour of milk or antacids.

For constipation, bisacodyl is given in usual doses of 5 to 10 mg daily as enteric-coated tablets administered at night or 10 mg as a suppository or enema administered in the morning. Doses of 10 to 20 mg are given by mouth for complete bowel evacuation, followed by 10 mg as a suppository the next morning.

Children under 10 years of age may be given 5 mg rectally in the morning for constipation; those over 4 years may alternatively be given 5 mg by mouth at night. For bowel evacuation the dose is 5 mg by mouth the night before and 5 mg rectally the morning of the procedure. Children over 10 years of age may be given doses similar to those for adults.

A complex of bisacodyl with tannic acid (bisacodyl tannex) has been given with a barium sulfate enema before radiographic examination of the colon.

### Preparations

***BP 2003:*** Bisacodyl Suppositories; Bisacodyl Tablets;
***USP 27:*** Bisacodyl Delayed-release Tablets; Bisacodyl Rectal Suspension; Bisacodyl Suppositories.

**Proprietary Preparations** (details are given in Part 3)
***Arg.:*** Dulcolax; Laxamin; Modaton; ***Austral.:*** Bisalax; Durolax; Fleet Laxative; ***Austria:*** Dulcolax; Laxbene; ***Belg.:*** Carters; Dulcolax; Mucinum†; Purgo-Pil; ***Braz.:*** Dislax†; Dulcolax; ***Canad.:*** Alophen; Bisacolax; Carters Little Pills; Correctol; Dulcolax; Feen-A-Mint; Laxcodyl; Soflax EX; ***Chile:*** Alsylax; ***Denm.:*** Dulcolax; Perilax; Toilax; ***Fin.:*** Metalax; Toilax; ***Fr.:*** Contalax; Dulcolax; ***Ger.:*** Agaroletten; Bekunis Bisacodyl; Bisco-Zitron; Darmol Bisacodyl†; Drix Bisacodyl; Dulcolax; Florisan N; Laxagetten; Laxanin N; Laxans-ratiopharm; Laxbene; Laxoberal Bisa; Laxysat Burger; Mandrolax†; Marienbader Pillen N; Mediolax; Pyrilax; Rhabarex B†; Stadalax; Tempolax; Tirgon; Vinco Forte†; Vinco-Abfuhr-Perlen; ***Gr.:*** Dulcolax; ***Hong Kong:*** Correctol†; Dulcolax; ***India:*** Dulcolax; JuLax; JuLax-M; ***Irl.:*** Dulcolax; Toilax; ***Israel:*** Contalax; Laxadin; ***Ital.:*** Alaxa; Confetto CM; Dulcolax; Normalene; Verecolene CM; ***Malaysia:*** Beacolux; Dulcolax; ***Mex.:*** Dulcolan; ***Neth.:*** Dulcolax; Nourilax†; Zwitsalax/N†; ***Norw.:*** Dulcolax; Toilax; ***NZ:*** Dulcolax; Fleet Laxative; ***Port.:*** Dulcolax; Moderlax; ***S.Afr.:*** Dulcolax; Megalax; ***Singapore:*** Dulcolax; ***Spain:*** Dulco Laxo; Medesup†; ***Swed.:*** Dulcolax; Toilax; ***Switz.:*** Bekunis Dragees; Demolaxin; Dulcolax; Ercolax†; Muxol; Prontolax; Tavolax nouvelle formule; ***Thai.:*** Dulcolax; Emulax; Gencolax; Kadolax; Laxcodyl; Laxitab; Vacolax; ***UAE:*** Laxocodyl; ***UK:*** Biolax; Dulcolax; Entrolax; ***USA:*** Alophen; Bisa-Lax; Correctol; Doxidan; Dulcolax; Evac-Q-Kwik Suppository†; Evac-Q-Tabs; Feen-A-Mint; Fleet Bisacodyl; Fleet Laxative; Gentlax; Modane.

**Multi-ingredient:** ***Arg.:*** En-Ga-Lax; Laxicona; Nigalax; ***Austral.:*** Coloxyl; Durolax X-Pack; Go Kit; Go Kit Plus; ***Austria:*** Laxbene; Prepacol; Purgazen; Purigoa; ***Belg.:*** Prepacol; Softene; ***Braz.:*** Cronoplex; Humectol†; ***Canad.:*** Bicholate; Evac-Q-Kwik†; Extra Strong Formula 12; Fruitatives; Royvac Kit; ***Chile:*** Laxogeno; ***Fr.:*** Prepacol; ***Ger.:*** Potsilo N; Prepacol; ***Gr.:*** Florisan; ***NZ:*** Coloxyl; ***Port.:*** Bekunis†; ***Spain:*** Bekunis Complex; Boldolaxin; ***Switz.:*** Aloinophen†; Drix†; Tavolax†; ***Thai.:*** Bisolax; ***USA:*** Fleet Prep Kit No. 1; Fleet Prep Kit No. 2; Fleet Prep Kit No. 3; X-Prep Bowel Evacuant Kit-1; X-Prep Bowel Evacuant Kit-2†.

## Bismuth Compounds

Bismuto, compuestos de.

Bismuth compounds have been used for their astringent and antidiarrhoeal properties in a variety of gastrointestinal disorders, and have been applied topically in skin disorders and anorectal disorders such as haemorrhoids. Certain salts are active against *Helicobacter pylori* and are used in the treatment of peptic ulcer disease.

### Bismuth Aluminate *(USAN)*

Aluminato de bismuto; Aluminum Bismuth Oxide.
$Bi_2(Al_2O_4)_3,10H_2O$ = 952.0.
*CAS — 12284-76-3 (anhydrous bismuth aluminate).*

**Pharmacopoeias.** In *Chin.* and *Fr.*

### Bismuth Citrate

Citrato de bismuto.
*CAS — 813-93-4.*

**Pharmacopoeias.** In *US.*

**USP 27** (Bismuth Citrate). A white, amorphous or crystalline powder. Insoluble in water and in alcohol; soluble in dilute ammonia solution and in solutions of alkali citrates. Store in airtight containers. Protect from light. Prevent exposure to temperatures above 40°.

### Bismuth Oxide

Bismuth Trioxide; Óxido de bismuto.
$Bi_2O_3$ = 466.0.
*CAS — 1304-76-3.*

### Bismuth Salicylate

Basic Bismuth Salicylate; Bismuth Oxysalicylate; Bismuth Subsalicylate *(USAN)*; Bismuthi Subsalicylas; Salicilato de bismuto.
$C_7H_5BiO_4$ = 362.1.
*CAS — 14882-18-9.*

**Pharmacopoeias.** In *Eur.* (see p.vi) and *US.*

**Ph. Eur. 5.0** (Bismuth Subsalicylate). A complex of bismuth and salicylic acid. It contains not less than 56% and not more than 59.4% of Bi, calculated with reference to the dried substance. A white powder. Practically insoluble in water and in alcohol; dissolves in mineral acids with decomposition. Protect from light.

**USP 27** (Bismuth Subsalicylate). A basic salt corresponding to $C_7H_5BiO_4$ = 362.1 and containing not less than 56.0% and not more than 59.4% of Bi and not less than 36.5% and not more than 39.3% of total salicylates. It is a fine, odourless, white to off-white microcrystalline powder. Practically insoluble in water, in alcohol, and in ether. It reacts with alkalis and mineral acids. Store in airtight containers. Protect from light.

### Bismuth Subcarbonate *(USAN)*

Basic Bismuth Carbonate; Basisches Wismutkarbonat; Bism. Carb.; Bismuth Carbonate; Bismuth Oxycarbonate; Bismuthi Subcarbonas; Bismutylum Carbonicum; Carbonato de Bismutila; Subcarbonato de bismuto.
*CAS — 5892-10-4 (anhydrous bismuth subcarbonate); 5798-45-8 (bismuth subcarbonate hemihydrate).*

**Pharmacopoeias.** In *Chin., Eur.* (see p.vi), and *US.*

**Ph. Eur. 5.0** (Bismuth Subcarbonate). A white or almost white powder. Practically insoluble in water and in alcohol. It dissolves in mineral acids with effervescence. Protect from light.

**USP 27** (Bismuth Subcarbonate). A white or almost white powder. Practically insoluble in water, in alcohol, and in ether; dissolves in dilute acids with effervescence. Protect from light.

### Bismuth Subgallate *(USAN)*

Basic Bismuth Gallate; Basisches Wismutgallat; Bism. Subgall.; Bismuth Oxygallate; Bismuthi Subgallas; Subgalato de bismuto.
$C_7H_5BiO_6$ = 394.1.
*CAS — 99-26-3.*

**Pharmacopoeias.** In *Eur.* (see p.vi), *Jpn, Pol.,* and *US.*

**Ph. Eur. 5.0** (Bismuth Subgallate). A complex of bismuth and gallic acid. It contains not less than 48% and not more than 51% of Bi, calculated with reference to the dried substance. A yellow powder. Practically insoluble in water and in alcohol; dissolves in mineral acids with decomposition and in alkali hydroxides, producing a reddish-brown liquid. Protect from light.

**USP 27** (Bismuth Subgallate). A basic salt containing 52 to 57% of $Bi_2O_3$ when dried at 105° for 3 hours. It is an odourless amorphous bright yellow powder. Practically insoluble in water, in alcohol, in chloroform, and in ether; insoluble in very dilute mineral acids; dissolves readily with decomposition in warm, moderately dilute hydrochloric, nitric, or sulfuric acids; readily dissolves in solutions of alkali hydroxides to form a clear yellow liquid which rapidly becomes deep red. Store in airtight containers. Protect from light.

### Bismuth Subnitrate

Basic Bismuth Nitrate; Basisches Wismutnitrat; Bism. Subnit.; Bismuth Hydroxide Nitrate Oxide; Bismuth Nitrate, Heavy; Bismuth Oxynitrate; Bismuth (Sous-Nitrate de) Lourd; Bismuthi Subnitras; Bismuthyl Nitrate; Magistery of Bismuth; Nitrato de Bismutilo; Subazotato de Bismuto; Subnitrato de bismuto; White Bismuth.
$Bi_5O(OH)_9(NO_3)_4$ = 1462.0.
*CAS — 1304-85-4.*
*ATC — A02BX12.*

**Pharmacopoeias.** In *Eur.* (see p.vi), *Jpn, Pol.,* and *US.*
*Fr.* also includes Bismuth (Sous-Nitrate de) Léger (Bismuthi Subnitras Levis) which is described as a variable mixture of bismuth hydroxide, carbonate, and subnitrate.

**Ph. Eur. 5.0** (Bismuth Subnitrate, Heavy). It contains not less than 71% and not more than 74% of Bi, calculated with reference to the dried substance. A white powder. Practically insoluble in water and in alcohol; dissolves in mineral acids with decomposition.

**USP 27** (Bismuth Subnitrate). A basic salt containing not less than 79% of $Bi_2O_3$ calculated on the dried basis. It is a white, slightly hygroscopic powder. Practically insoluble in water and in alcohol; readily dissolves in nitric and hydrochloric acids.

### Tripotassium Dicitratobismuthate

Colloidal Bismuth Subcitrate; Dicitratobismutato tripotásico.
*CAS — 57644-54-9.*
*ATC — A02BX05.*

## Adverse Effects, Treatment, and Precautions

The bismuth compounds listed above are insoluble or very poorly soluble, and bismuth toxicity does not appear to be common with them if they are used for limited periods. However, excessive or prolonged dosage may produce symptoms of bismuth poisoning, and for this reason long-term systemic therapy is not recommended. Reversible encephalopathy (see below) was once a problem in some countries, notably France and Australia; bone and joint toxicity had also occurred, sometimes associated with the encephalopathy. This led to restrictions on the use of bismuth salts and a virtual disappearance of these toxic effects.

Nausea and vomiting have been reported. Darkening or blackening of the faeces and tongue may occur due to conversion to bismuth sulfide in the gastrointestinal tract.

The effects of *acute bismuth intoxication* include gastrointestinal disturbances, skin reactions, stomatitis, and discoloration of mucous membranes; a characteristic blue line may appear on the gums. There may be renal failure and liver damage.

Other adverse effects may not be related to the bismuth content. With bismuth subnitrate given orally there is a risk of the nitrate being reduced in the intestines to nitrite and the development of methaemoglobinaemia. Absorption of salicylate occurs after oral administration of bismuth salicylate and therefore the adverse effects, treatment of adverse effects, and precautions of aspirin (p.15) should be considered.

Gastric lavage should be considered following overdosage; activated charcoal by mouth and the use of a chelating agent such as dimercaprol, succimer, or unithiol have been recommended (see also Overdosage, below). Renal function should be monitored for 10 days following acute overdosage.

Bismuth compounds should not be given to patients with moderate to severe renal impairment.

**Encephalopathy.** Reviews[1,2] and reports[3-10] of bismuth encephalopathy. Many of the original reports implicated bismuth subgallate or subnitrate, in most but not all cases at high doses or for prolonged periods; toxicity has also occurred with other salts.[6-9] Patients receiving the subcitrate (480 mg daily) or the subnitrate (1.8 g daily) for 8 weeks in the treatment of *Helicobacter pylori* infection, showed no evidence of neurological changes compared with a control group.[11]


1. Winship KA. Toxicity of bismuth salts. *Adverse Drug React Acute Poisoning Rev* 1983; **2:** 103–21.
2. Slikkerveer A, de Wolff FA. Pharmacokinetics and toxicity of bismuth compounds. *Med Toxicol Adverse Drug Exp* 1989; **4:** 303–23.
3. Morrow AW. Request for reports: adverse reactions with bismuth subgallate. *Med J Aust* 1973; **1:** 912.
4. Martin-Bouyer G. Intoxications par les sels de bismuth administrés par voie orale: enquête épidémiologique. *Therapie* 1976; **31:** 683–702.
5. Stahl JP, *et al.* Encéphalites au sel insoluble de bismuth: toujours d'actualité. *Nouv Presse Med* 1982; **11:** 3856.
6. Hasking GJ, Duggan JM. Encephalopathy from bismuth subsalicylate. *Med J Aust* 1982; **2:** 167.
7. Weller MPI. Neuropsychiatric symptoms following bismuth intoxication. *Postgrad Med J* 1988; **64:** 308–10.
8. Mendelowitz PC, *et al.* Bismuth absorption and myoclonic encephalopathy during bismuth subsalicylate therapy. *Ann Intern Med* 1990; **112:** 140–1.
9. Playford RJ, *et al.* Bismuth induced encephalopathy caused by tri potassium dicitrato bismuthate in a patient with chronic renal failure. *Gut* 1990; **31:** 359–60.
10. Von Bose MJ, Zaudig M. Encephalopathy resembling Creutzfeldt-Jakob disease following oral, prescribed doses of bismuth nitrate. *Br J Psychiatry* 1991; **158:** 278–80.
11. Noach LA, *et al.* Bismuth salts and neurotoxicity: a randomised, single-blind and controlled study. *Hum Exp Toxicol* 1995; **14:** 349–55.


FOLLOWING TOPICAL APPLICATION. Encephalopathy has been associated with the use of bismuth iodoform paraffin paste (BIPP) for the packing of wound cavities after surgery to the head and neck, although there is some debate as to whether the bismuth or the iodoform component is responsible—see p.1184.

**Overdosage.** Bismuth salicylate or tripotassium dicitratobismuthate in recommended doses are rarely associated with serious adverse effects but there are reports of renal failure,[1-4] encephalopathy,[5-7] and neurotoxicity[1] following acute[1-4,6] or chronic[5,7] overdose. Bismuth has been detected in the blood, urine, stools, and kidneys of these patients; a blood concentration of 1.6 micrograms/mL was found[2] 4 hours after a dose of 9.6 g.

The optimal treatment of bismuth overdosage is unknown. Gastric lavage, purgation, and hydration should be considered, even if the patient presents late, as bismuth may be absorbed from the colon.[1,2] Chelating agents may be effective; unithiol has been reported to increase the renal clearance of bismuth with a reduction in the blood concentration.[5] Haemodialysis may be necessary[1-3] but whether this hastens tissue clearance is uncertain.

Prolonged ingestion of bismuth salicylate in excessive doses by an elderly diabetic was associated with hearing disturbances, vertigo, acid-base abnormalities and mild clotting disturbances.[8] The toxicity was thought to be due to the salicylate component of the drug.


1. Hudson M, Mowat NAG. Reversible toxicity in poisoning with colloidal bismuth subcitrate. *BMJ* 1989; **299:** 159.
2. Taylor EG, Klenerman P. Acute renal failure after colloidal bismuth subcitrate overdose. *Lancet* 1990; **335:** 670–1.
3. Huwez F, *et al.* Acute renal failure after overdose of colloidal bismuth subcitrate. *Lancet* 1992; **340:** 1298.
4. Akpolat I, *et al.* Acute renal failure due to overdose of colloidal bismuth. *Nephrol Dial Transplant* 1996; **11:** 1890–8.
5. Playford RJ, *et al.* Bismuth induced encephalopathy caused by tri potassium dicitrato bismuthate in a patient with chronic renal failure. *Gut* 1990; **31:** 359–60.
6. Hasking GJ, Duggan JM. Encephalopathy from bismuth subsalicylate. *Med J Aust* 1982; **2:** 167.
7. Mendelowitz PC, *et al.* Bismuth absorption and myoclonic encephalopathy during bismuth subsalicylate therapy. *Ann Intern Med* 1990; **112:** 140–1.
8. Vernace MA, *et al.* Chronic salicylate toxicity due to consumption of over-the-counter bismuth subsalicylate. *Am J Med* 1994; **97:** 308–9.


## Interactions

Bismuth salts given by mouth reduce the absorption of tetracyclines, possibly by chelation or by reducing tetracycline solubility as a result of increasing the gastric pH. This interaction can be minimised by separating doses of the two drugs by a couple of hours. The clinical significance of this interaction to the use of bismuth salts for peptic ulcer disease is unclear; tripotassium dicitratobismuthate or bismuth salicylate have been given at the same time as tetracycline as part of triple therapy for the eradication of *Helicobacter pylori*.

**Antisecretory drugs.** Pretreatment with *omeprazole* resulted in about a threefold increase in absorption of bismuth from tripotassium dicitratobismuthate in 6 healthy subjects.[1] The mean peak plasma concentration of bismuth following a single dose of 240 mg of tripotassium dicitratobismuthate was increased from 36.7 to 86.7 nanograms/mL after omeprazole suggesting an increased risk of toxicity from combined therapy. The mechanism was thought to be the increase in gastric pH produced by the antisecretory drug as similar results had been reported with *ranitidine*.[2] However, the clinical significance of these interactions to the use of antisecretory drugs with bismuth compounds for eradication of *Helicobacter pylori* is unclear; bismuth compounds have been combined with proton pump inhibitors or $H_2$ antagonists in short-term regimens as part of triple or quadruple therapy.


1. Treiber G, *et al.* Omeprazole-induced increase in the absorption of bismuth from tripotassium dicitrato bismuthate. *Clin Pharmacol Ther* 1994; **55:** 486–91.
2. Nwokolo CU, *et al.* The effect of histamine $H_2$-receptor blockade on bismuth absorption from three ulcer-healing compounds. *Gastroenterology* 1991; **101:** 889–94.


## Pharmacokinetics

Poorly soluble bismuth compounds are largely converted to insoluble bismuth oxide, hydroxide, and oxychloride in the acidic environment of the stomach. Most of the bismuth compounds included in this monograph are thus only slightly absorbed. Increased gastric pH may increase bismuth absorption—see Antisecretory Drugs, above. Unabsorbed bismuth is excreted in the faeces. Absorbed bismuth is distributed throughout body tissues, including bone, and is slowly excreted in the urine and bile. It has a plasma half-life of about 5 days and continues to be excreted for about 12 weeks after stopping therapy.

◊ References.


1. Nwokolo CU, *et al.* The absorption of bismuth from oral doses of tripotassium dicitrato bismuthate. *Aliment Pharmacol Ther* 1989; **3:** 29–39.
2. Froomes PRA, *et al.* Absorption and elimination of bismuth from oral doses of tripotassium dicitrato bismuthate. *Eur J Clin Pharmacol* 1989; **37:** 533–6.
3. Lacey LF, *et al.* Comparative pharmacokinetics of bismuth from ranitidine bismuth citrate (GR122311X), a novel anti-ulcerant and tripotassium dicitrato bismuthate (TDB). *Eur J Clin Pharmacol* 1994; **47:** 177–80.


## Uses and Administration

Some insoluble salts of bismuth are given by mouth for their supposed antacid action and for their mildly astringent action in various gastrointestinal disorders, including diarrhoea (p.1241) and dyspepsia (p.1242). Such salts include the aluminate, salicylate, subcarbonate, and subnitrate. Bismuth salicylate, which is given as an antidiarrhoeal and weak antacid in doses up to about 4 g daily in divided doses, possesses in addition the properties of the salicylates.

Tripotassium dicitratobismuthate is used as a mucosal protectant for the treatment of peptic ulcer disease (p.1246). It is active against *Helicobacter pylori* and has been used as triple therapy (with metronidazole and either tetracycline or amoxicillin) to eradicate this organism and thereby prevent relapse of duodenal ulcer. Bismuth salicylate is also active against *H. pylori* and has been used similarly.

The usual dose of tripotassium dicitratobismuthate in benign gastric and duodenal ulceration is 240 mg twice daily, or 120 mg four times daily by mouth before food. Treatment is for a period of 4 weeks, extended to 8 weeks if necessary. Maintenance therapy with tripotassium dicitratobismuthate is not recommended although treatment may be repeated after a drug-free interval of one month. When used as part of triple therapy the usual dose of tripotassium dicitratobismuthate has been 120 mg four times daily for 2 weeks. The usual dose of bismuth salicylate as part of triple therapy is 525 mg four times daily for 2 weeks. Appropriate antisecretory treatment with a histamine $H_2$-antagonist or a proton pump inhibitor is usually added to these regimens.

A complex of bismuth citrate with ranitidine, ranitidine bismuth citrate (p.1287), is also used in the treatment of peptic ulcer disease.

Some insoluble salts of bismuth have been used topically in the treatment of skin disorders, wounds, and burns. Some have been used as ingredients of ointments or suppositories (sometimes containing more than one bismuth salt) in the treatment of haemorrhoids and other anorectal disorders (p.1243). Bismuth compounds that have been used topically and/or rectally include the oxide, subgallate, and subnitrate; bismuth resorcinol compounds have also been used. For the use of bismuth subnitrate and iodoform paste as a wound dressing, see Iodoform, p.1184.

Numerous other salts and compounds of bismuth have been promoted for various therapeutic purposes. Glycobiarsol was formerly used by mouth as an amoebicide.

Bismuth (Bismuthum) is used in homoeopathic medicine.

### Preparations

***BPC 1954:*** Bismuth Subnitrate and Iodoform Paste;
***USP 27:*** Bismuth Subsalicylate Magma; Compound Resorcinol Ointment; Milk of Bismuth.

**Proprietary Preparations** (details are given in Part 3)
***Arg.:*** Re-Dux; ***Austral.:*** De-Nol†; ***Belg.:*** De-Nol†; ***Braz.:*** Pepto-Bismol; Peptulan; Senophile; Ulcerosol†; ***Canad.:*** Bismed; Bismylate†; Neo-Laryngobis; Pepto-Bismol; Personnel; Pink Bismuth Rose†; ***Fr.:*** Amygdorectol; ***Ger.:*** Angass S; Dermatol; Haemo-Exhirud Bufexamac; Jatrox†; Katulcin-R; Noemin N†; Telen; Ulcolind Wismut†; Ulgastrin Bis†; Ulkowis; ***Gr.:*** De-Nol; ***Hong Kong:*** De-Nol; ***India:*** Trymo; ***Irl.:*** De-Nol†; De-Noltab; ***Israel:*** De-Nol†; Kalbeten; ***Ital.:*** De-Nol; ***Mex.:*** Biselic; Bismofarma; Bismopepsin†; Bisval; Pepto-Bismol; Sucrato; ***Neth.:*** De-Nol; ***Norw.:*** De-Nol†; ***NZ:*** De-Nol; ***Port.:*** De-Nol; ***S.Afr.:*** De-Nol; Ulcerone†; ***Spain:*** Gastrodenol; Rectamigdol; ***Switz.:*** Amygdorectol; Bismuth Tulasne†; De-Nol†; ***Thai.:*** De-Nol†; ***UK:*** De-Noltab; Pepto-Bismol; ***USA:*** Bismatrol; Children's Kaopectate; Devrom; Kaopectate; Peptic Relief; Pepto-Bismol.

**Multi-ingredient: *Arg.:*** Anusol; Anusol Duo S; Colistop; Colistoral; Cutidermin; Gastop; Histidanol; Mabis; ***Austral.:*** BFI†; Helidac†; ***Belg.:*** Amazyl†; Baseler Haussalbe†; Gastrofilm; Procto-Synalar; Rectovasol; ***Braz.:*** Anusol-HC; Bisuisan; Claudemor; Cutisanol; Magnesia Bisurada; Neoseptil†; Neutracido†; Salicilato de Bismuto Composto; Senophile; ***Canad.:*** Bismed†; Bismutal; Eczema Ointment†; Onrectal; Pepto-Bismol; Thunas Pile; ***Denm.:*** Xylocain Comp†; ***Fin.:*** Tannopon; ***Fr.:*** Anoreine; Anusol; Bi-Qui-Nol†; Bismurectol†; Cutiphile; Paps; Pholcones Bismuth; ***Ger.:*** Angass; Anisan; Anusept†; Bismofalk†; Bismolan; Bismolan H Corti; Bismolan N; Bufeproct†; Combustin Heilsalbe; Duoventrin; Eulatin N; Eulatin NN; Faktu akut; Friosmin N; Haemomac†; Hamo-ratiopharm N; Hamoagil plus; Karaya Bismuth†; Katulcin-Rupha†; Mastu S; Nervogastrol N; Pascomag; Proctoparf†; Sagittaproct S†; Sagittaproct†; Siozwo N†; Spasmo-Nervogastrol; Tamposit N; Varitan N†; Ventricon N; Vit-u-pept; Wismut comp; ***Hong Kong:*** Anusol; Anusol-HC†; Anuzinc†; Biscasil†; Bismofalk†; Mastu S; Rowatanal; ***Irl.:*** Anugesic-HC; Anusol; Anusol-HC; Rowatanal; ***Israel:*** Anusol; Contra Combustiones†; Hemo; Rectozorin; Rekiv; ***Ital.:*** Antiemorroidali; Anusol; ***Malaysia:*** Rowatanal; ***Mex.:*** Ercal†; Heliton; ***Neth.:*** Anusol; Theranal; Zwitsanal†; ***Norw.:*** Biserirte Magnesia†; ***Port.:*** Claudemor; Gastroplex†; Servetinal; Synalar Rectal; ***S.Afr.:*** Anugesic; Anusol; Anusol-HC†; Arola Rosebalm; Biskapect; Bisma Rex; Chloropect; Collodyne†; Dyrosol†; Enterodyne; Kantrexil; ***Singapore:*** Anusol; Rowatanal; ***Spain:*** Grietalgen; Grietalgen Hidrocort; Hemodren Compuesto; Metagliz Bismutico†; Nasopomada; Pomada Infantil Vera; Roter Complex†; Sabanotropico; Stomosan†; Sualyn†; Synalar Rectal; Talco Antihistam Calber†; Talkosona†; Talquissar†; ***Switz.:*** Bismorectal; Cicafissan; Euproctol N; Fissan; Furodermal; Furodermil†; Haemocortin; Haemolan; Magenpulver Hafter; Magentabletten Hafter; Rectoseptal-Neo bismuthe; ***Thai.:*** Anusol; Biodan; Mastu S; Roter†; Ulgastrin; ***UK:*** Anugesic-HC; Anusol; Anusol-HC, Plus HC; Bisma-Rex; Hemocane; Moorland; OxBipp; Stomach Mixture; ***USA:*** Anumed; Anumed HC; BFI; Calmol; Helidac; Hem-Prep; Hemril; K-C; Kao-Paverin; Kaodene Non-Narcotic; Mammol; Rectagene Medicated Rectal Balm.

---

## Bisoxatin Acetate *(BANM, USAN, rINNM)*

Acetato de bisoxatina; Bisoxatin Diacetate; Wy-8138. 2,2-Bis(4-hydroxyphenyl)-1,4-benzoxazin-3(2*H*,4*H*)-one diacetate.
$C_{24}H_{19}NO_6$ = 417.4.
*CAS — 17692-24-9 (bisoxatin); 14008-48-1 (bisoxatin acetate).*
*ATC — A06AB09.*

### Profile

Bisoxatin acetate is a stimulant laxative that has been used in the treatment of constipation (p.1240).

### Preparations

**Proprietary Preparations** (details are given in Part 3)
***Belg.:*** Wylaxine†.

---

# Bran

Crusca; Farelo; Kleie; Salvado; Son.

**Description.** Bran consists of the fibrous outer layers of cereal grains. It contains celluloses, polysaccharides or hemicelluloses, protein, fat, minerals, and moisture and may contain part of the germ or embryo. Bran provides water-insoluble fibre and, depending on the source, may also provide water-soluble fibre (see also Dietary Role, below). It comprises about 12% of the weight of the grain and is a byproduct of flour milling. It is available in various grades.

**Pharmacopoeias.** *US* includes wheat bran.

**USP 27** (Wheat Bran). The outer fraction of the cereal grain (comprising the pericarp, seed coat (testa), nucellar tissue, and aleurone layer) derived from *Triticum aestivum*, *T. compactum*, *T. durum*, or other common einkorn and emmer wheat cultivars. It is obtained by milling and processing the whole wheat grain, and is available in a variety of particle sizes depending on the degree of milling. It contains not less than 36% of dietary fibre. It is a light tan powder having a characteristic aroma. Practically insoluble in cold water and in alcohol.

## Adverse Effects

Large quantities of bran may temporarily increase flatulence and abdominal distension, and intestinal obstruction may occur rarely.

**Diarrhoea.** A report of diarrhoea induced by a dramatic increase in fibre intake. Reduction of dietary fibre led to a return to normal bowel habit in 2 to 3 days.[1]


1. Saibil F. Diarrhea due to fiber overload. *N Engl J Med* 1989; **320:** 599.


**Intestinal obstruction.** Intestinal obstruction associated with excessive bran intake has been reported.[1-3]


1. Allen-Mersh T, De Jode LR. Is bran useful in diverticular disease? *BMJ* 1982; **284:** 740.
2. Cooper SG, Tracey EJ. Small-bowel obstruction caused by oat-bran bezoar. *N Engl J Med* 1989; **320:** 1148–9.
3. Miller DL, *et al.* Small-bowel obstruction from bran cereal. *JAMA* 1990; **263:** 813–14.


## Precautions

Bran is contra-indicated in patients with intestinal obstruction or with undiagnosed abdominal symptoms. There is a particular risk of intestinal or oesophageal obstruction if bulk laxatives are swallowed dry; they should be taken with sufficient fluid and should not be taken immediately before going to bed. Wheat bran should be avoided in gluten enteropathies and coeliac disease.

## Interactions

Bran may reduce the absorption of some drugs when given concomitantly by mouth. Interference with iron, zinc, and calcium absorption has been reported; calcium phosphate may be added to bran to neutralise fytic acid, which can contribute to such interference.

## Uses and Administration

The main use of bran is as a bulk laxative and source of dietary fibre in the management of disorders of the gastrointestinal tract such as constipation (p.1240), especially in diverticular disease (p.1241) and the irritable bowel syndrome (p.1244). It should always be taken with plenty of fluid.

Bran is used as the basis for some breakfast cereals.

**Dietary role.** There is no precise definition for the complex mixture of substances known as dietary fibre. It has been defined as plant polysaccharides and lignin resistant to hydrolysis by the digestive enzymes of humans but this covers many substances other than cell-wall and related polysaccharides. Non-starch polysaccharides are the major component of the plant cell wall and are used as an index of dietary fibre. They comprise water-soluble fibres such as pectins, gums, and mucilages and water-insoluble fibres such as cellulose. Wheat, maize, and rice contain mainly insoluble non-starch polysaccharides whereas oats, barley, and rye have a significant proportion of soluble fibres.

In the UK, dietary reference values (DRV) have been published for non-starch polysaccharides.[1] It has been proposed[1] that adult diets should contain an average for the population of 18 g daily (individual range 12 to 24 g daily) non-starch polysaccharide from a variety of foods whose constituents contain it as a naturally integrated component. Children should receive proportionately less non-starch polysaccharide according to body size. No evidence exists for benefit of intakes of non-starch polysaccharide in excess of 32 g daily, and therefore there is no advantage in exceeding this amount.

In the USA, an adult dietary fibre intake of 20 to 35 g daily has been suggested; children should consume an amount equivalent to their age plus 5 g daily.[2]


1. DOH. Dietary reference values for food energy and nutrients for the United Kingdom: report of the panel on dietary reference values of the committee on medical aspects of food policy. *Report on health and social subjects 41.* London: HMSO, 1991.
2. Marlett JA, *et al.* Position of the American Dietetic Association: health implications of dietary fiber. *J Am Diet Assoc* 2002; **102:** 993–1000. Also available at: http://www.eatright.org/images/journal/0702/adar2.pdf (accessed 07/05/04)


**Disease prevention.** Diseases such as colorectal cancer, ischaemic heart disease, diabetes mellitus, and obesity are common in affluent developed countries but occur rarely in rural Africa. This difference in disease patterns has been linked to the low fibre intake in developed countries compared with rural Africans. However, there are many other differences in diet and lifestyle, such as a lower intake of fat, protein, and sugar in rural Africans and less exposure to toxins and pollutants, any of which could contribute to the difference. The excessive consumption of energy-rich foods may be more to blame for diseases of affluence than is deficiency of dietary fibre.[1] Furthermore, there is some concern that the use of fibre supplements is not entirely without harmful effects: it has been pointed out that fermentable fibre substrates can stimulate cell proliferation in the colon.[2] However, the role of cell proliferation as a marker for the development of colonic **cancer** is questioned by some authors.[3] Results from the Nurses' Health Study, a large prospective cohort study, failed to support any *reduction in risk* of colon cancer associated with a high intake of dietary fibre.[4] In contrast, subsequent multicentre studies in the USA[5] and in Europe[6] have shown an association between an increased intake of dietary fibre and a decreased risk of colonic adenoma and of colorectal cancer, respectively.

Controlled trials of the effect of dietary intervention, over 3 to 4 years, on the *recurrence rate* of colorectal adenomas have also been reported. Neither a high fibre diet based on wheat bran cereal supplements,[7] nor a diet of low fat, high fibre foods, fruit and vegetables,[8] were found to reduce the recurrence of colorectal adenomas. However, although adenomas are precursors of colorectal cancer, most adenomas do not develop into cancer, and so the relevance of these study results for the prevention of colorectal cancer is unclear.[9]

A small randomised crossover study[10] in patients with type 2 **diabetes mellitus** suggested that an increased intake of dietary fibre was associated with improved glycaemic control, decreased hyperinsulinaemia, and lower plasma lipid concentrations.


1. Anonymous. The bran wagon. *Lancet* 1987; **i:** 782–3.
2. Wasan HS, Goodlad RA. Fibre-supplemented foods may damage your health. *Lancet* 1996; **348:** 319–20.
3. Hill MJ, Leeds AR. Fibre and colorectal cancer. *Lancet* 1996; **348:** 957.
4. Fuchs CS, *et al.* Dietary fibre and the risk of colorectal cancer and adenoma in women. *N Engl J Med* 1999; **340:** 169–76.
5. Peters U, *et al.* Dietary fibre and colorectal adenoma in a colorectal cancer early detection programme. *Lancet* 2003; **361:** 1491–5.
6. Bingham SA, *et al.* Dietary fibre in food and protection against colorectal cancer in the European Prospective Investigation into Cancer and Nutrition (EPIC): an observational study. *Lancet* 2003; **361:** 1496–1501. Correction. *ibid.*; **362:** 1000.
7. Alberts DS, *et al.* Lack of effect of a high-fiber cereal supplement on the recurrence of colorectal adenomas. *N Engl J Med* 2000; **342:** 1156–62.
8. Schatzkin A, *et al.* Lack of effect of a low-fat, high-fiber diet on the recurrence of colorectal adenomas. *N Engl J Med* 2000; **342:** 1149–55.
9. Byers T. Diet, colorectal adenomas, and colorectal cancer. *N Engl J Med* 2000; **342:** 1206–7.
10. Chandalia M, *et al.* Beneficial effects of high dietary fiber intake in patients with type 2 diabetes mellitus. *N Engl J Med* 2000; **342:** 1392–8.


### Preparations

**Proprietary Preparations** (details are given in Part 3)
***Braz.:*** Dietoman†; Fibrocol†; Trifibra Mix†; ***Canad.:*** Fibyrax†; ***Fr.:*** Celluson†; Doses-O-Son; Infibran†; ***Irl.:*** Trifyba; ***Ital.:*** Crusken; Dialibra†; ***Port.:*** Infibran; ***Switz.:*** Fibion; ***UK:*** Trifyba†.

**Multi-ingredient:** ***Arg.:*** Centella Queen Reductora; Gurfi Fibras; Salutaris; ***Austral.:*** Fibyrax†; Neo-Trim Fibre†; Procholt†; Proslender†; ***Austria:*** Herbelax; ***Ital.:*** Crusken†; Ecofibra; Fibrovit†; Levoplus; Melaprugna†; Plurilac; Resource Benefiber; Sedastip; ***Mex.:*** Psilumax; ***Port.:*** Stimulance.

## Bromopride *(rINN)*

Bromoprida; CM-8252; VAL-13081. 4-Amino-5-bromo-*N*-(2-diethylaminoethyl)-o-anisamide.
$C_{14}H_{22}BrN_3O_2$ = 344.2.
*CAS — 4093-35-0.*
*ATC — A03FA04.*

### Profile

Bromopride is a substituted benzamide similar to metoclopramide (p.1274), used in a variety of gastrointestinal disorders including nausea and vomiting (p.1245) and motility disorders. It is given in a usual dose of 20 to 60 mg daily by mouth in divided doses, or 20 mg daily by intramuscular or intravenous injection. The hydrochloride is also used.

### Preparations

**Proprietary Preparations** (details are given in Part 3)
***Braz.:*** Bilenzima†; Bromoprid; Digecap†; Digerex; Digesan; Digesprid; Digestil†; Digestina; Digeston; Eme-Ped†; Pangest; Plamet; Pridecil; ***Ger.:*** Cascapride†; ***Ital.:*** Opridan†; Procirex; Valopride.

**Multi-ingredient:** ***Braz.:*** Digecap-Zimatico; Enziprid†; Normopride Enzimatico†; Primeral; ***Port.:*** Modulanzime.

## Buckthorn

Bacca Spinae Cervinae; Espino Cerval; Espino cerval; Kreuzdorn; Nerprun.

NOTE. Distinguish from Sea Buckthorn (p.1742).

**Pharmacopoeias.** In *Ger.*

### Profile

Buckthorn is the dried ripe fruit of *Rhamnus cathartica* (Rhamnaceae); the bark is also occasionally used. Buckthorn is an anthraquinone stimulant laxative.

### Preparations

**Proprietary Preparations** (details are given in Part 3)
***Ger.:*** Laxysat mono†.

**Multi-ingredient:** ***Austral.:*** Neo-Cleanse†; ***Canad.:*** Floralaxative†; ***Ger.:*** Salus Abfuhr-Tee Nr. 2†; ***UK:*** Cleansing Herbs; Lion Cleansing Herbs.

## Calcium Carbonate

Calcii Carbonas; Carbonato de calcio; Creta Preparada; E170; Precipitated Calcium Carbonate; Precipitated Chalk.
$CaCO_3$ = 100.1.
*CAS — 471-34-1.*
*ATC — A02AC01; A12AA04.*

**Pharmacopoeias.** In *Chin., Eur.* (see p.vi), *Int., Jpn, Pol., US,* and *Viet.*

**Ph. Eur. 5.0** (Calcium Carbonate). A white powder. Practically insoluble in water.

**USP 27** (Calcium Carbonate). A fine, white, odourless, microcrystalline powder. Practically insoluble in water; its solubility in water is increased by the presence of carbon dioxide or ammonium salts although the presence of any alkali hydroxide reduces its solubility; insoluble in alcohol; dissolves with effervescence in acetic acid, in hydrochloric acid, and in nitric acid.

### Adverse Effects, Treatment, and Precautions

Calcium carbonate may occasionally cause constipation. Flatulence from released carbon dioxide may occur in some patients. High doses or prolonged use may lead to gastric hypersecretion and acid rebound. Like other calcium salts (see p.1226), calcium carbonate can cause hypercalcaemia, particularly in patients with renal impairment or after high doses. Alkalosis (p.1217) may also occur as a result of the carbonate anion. There have been rare reports of the milk-alkali syndrome, see below, and tissue calcification.

For precautions to be observed with the use of calcium carbonate, see Calcium, p.1226.

**Milk-alkali syndrome.** The milk-alkali syndrome of hypercalcaemia, alkalosis and renal impairment was first identified in the 1920s and may still occur in patients who ingest large amounts of calcium and absorbable alkali.[1] However, the milk-alkali syndrome has also been reported in a patient taking recommended doses of antacids containing calcium carbonate for chronic epigastric discomfort.[2] Metastatic calcification can develop.[3]

For reference to thiazide diuretics increasing the risk of the milk-alkali syndrome in patients taking moderately large doses of calcium carbonate, see p.935.


1. Orwoll ES. The milk-alkali syndrome: current concepts. *Ann Intern Med* 1982; **97:** 242–8.
2. Camidge R, Peaston R. Recommended dose antacids and severe hypercalcaemia. *Br J Clin Pharmacol* 2001; **52:** 341–2.
3. Duthie JS, *et al.* Milk-alkali syndrome with metastatic calcification. *Am J Med* 1995; **99:** 102–3.


### Interactions

As for other calcium salts, p.1226.

As outlined on p.1239, antacids, including calcium salts, interact with many other drugs both by alterations in gastric pH and emptying, and by formation of complexes that are not absorbed. Interactions can be minimised by giving calcium carbonate and any other medication 2 to 3 hours apart.

### Pharmacokinetics

Calcium carbonate is converted to calcium chloride by gastric acid. Some of the calcium is absorbed from the intestines and the unabsorbed portion is excreted in the faeces, as described for other calcium salts, p.1226.

### Uses and Administration

Calcium carbonate is used as an antacid (p.1239), usually in doses of up to about 1.5 g by mouth. It is often given with other antacids, especially magnesium-containing antacids.

Calcium carbonate is also used as a calcium supplement in deficiency states and as an adjunct in the management of osteoporosis, as described under Calcium, p.1226.

Calcium carbonate binds phosphate in the gastrointestinal tract to form insoluble complexes and reduces phosphate absorption. It is used to treat hyperphosphataemia in patients with chronic renal failure (see Renal Osteodystrophy, p.764). For this purpose, initial doses of 2.5 g daily by mouth in divided doses have been given, increased to up to 17 g daily in divided doses.

A preparation of a native calcium carbonate (Calcarea Carbonica; Calc. Carb.) is used in homoeopathic medicine.

Calcium carbonate is also used as a food additive.

### Preparations

***BP 2003:*** Calcium and Colecalciferol Tablets; Chewable Calcium Carbonate Tablets;
***USP 27:*** Alumina, Magnesia, and Calcium Carbonate Oral Suspension; Alumina, Magnesia, and Calcium Carbonate Tablets; Alumina, Magnesia, Calcium Carbonate, and Simethicone Tablets; Aluminum Subacetate Topical Solution; Calcium and Magnesium Carbonates Oral Suspension; Calcium and Magnesium Carbonates Tablets; Calcium Carbonate and Magnesia Tablets; Calcium Carbonate Lozenges; Calcium Carbonate Oral Suspension; Calcium Carbonate Tablets; Calcium Carbonate, Magnesia, and Simethicone Tablets.

**Proprietary Preparations** (details are given in Part 3)
***Arg.:*** Bica; Calcional; Calcium-Sandoz; Cavirox Junior; Mylanta Pocket; Pluscal; Renacalcio; Titralac; Tums; Ultracalcium; ***Austral.:*** Andrews Tums Antacid; Cal-Sup; Caltrate; Sandocal†; Titralac; ***Austria:*** Calcihexal; Calcium Novartis; Calcium-Sandoz; Dreisacarb; Kalzonorm†; Tetesept Calcium; ***Belg.:*** Cacit; Calci-Chew†; Sandoz Calcium; Steocar; ***Braz.:*** Calcium-Sandoz F; Calciumvit; Calsan; Natecal; Nutricalcio; Os-Cal; Osporin; Tums†; ***Canad.:*** Apo-Cal; Cal-500; Calcite; Calcium Oyster Shell; Calcium-Sandoz; Calsan; Caltrate; Hi Potency Cal; Maalox Quick Dissolve; Neo Cal; Nu-Cal; Os-Cal; Prevencal†; Titralac†; Tums; ***Chile:*** Aplical; Calcefor; Calcefor Cap; Calcium Factor; Calcium-Sandoz; Calcivorin; Caprimida; Elcal; Levucal; Natecal; ***Denm.:*** Calcium-Sandoz; ***Fin.:*** Calcichew; Calcium-Sandoz; Kalcidon; Kalcipos; Maxi-Calsorf†; ***Fr.:*** Cacit; Calcidia; Calcidose; Calciprat; Calcium-Sandoz; Calperos; Calprimum; Caltrate; Densical; Eucalcic; Fixical; Osteocal; Perical; Sandocal†; ***Ger.:*** Basti-Cal; Biolectra Calcium; Calcedon†; Calci-Gry; Calcigamma; Calcilos†; Calcimagon; Calcimed; Calcitridin; Calcium AL; Calcium beta; Calcium Dago; Calcium Heumann; Calcium Hexal; Calcium Stada; Calcium Verla; Calcium von CT; Calcium-dura; Calcium-Sandoz; CC-Nefro; Dreisacarb; Frubiase Calcium†; Loscalcon; Ospur Ca; Vivural; ***Gr.:*** Alcamex; Calcioral; Tums; ***Hong Kong:*** Apo-Cal; Calcichew; Calcium-Sandoz; Caltrate; Os-Cal; Titralac; ***India:*** Calcium-Sandoz; Sandocal; ***Irl.:*** Cacit; Calcichew; Remegel†; Rennie Rap-Eze; Rowarolan; Sandocal; Setlers Tums†; Tums; ***Israel:*** Cal-ci-Rav; Calcimore; Calcium-Sandoz; Caltrate; Tums; ***Ital.:*** Adiecal; Biocalcium; Cacit; Cal-Car; Calbisan; Calciodie; Calciopiu; Calcium-Sandoz; Calma; Carbo; Carbosint; Carbotop; Citracal; Effercal†; Fervical; Lubical; Metocal; Recal; Remegel†; Salicalcium; Savecal; Top Calcium; Unical; ***Malaysia:*** Apo-Cal; Cal-Sup; Caltrate; ***Mex.:*** Calcifar; Calcium-Sandoz; Calsan; Caltrate; Ciocar; Grisical; Osteomin; ***Mon.:*** Orocal; ***Neth.:*** Cacit; Calci-Chew; Calcium-Sandoz; ***Norw.:*** Calcium-Sandoz; Titralac; ***NZ:*** Cal-Sup†; Calcium-Sandoz; Caltrate; Oscal†; Osteo; Titralac; ***Port.:*** Calcior; Calcioral; Calcitab; Calcium-Sandoz; Sandocal; Tums; ***S.Afr.:*** Calcium-Sandoz; Caltrate; Titralac; ***Singapore:*** Cal-Sup; Calcium-Sandoz; Caltrate; ***Spain:*** Calcio 20; Calcium-Sandoz Forte; Caosina; Carbocal†; Cimascal; Densical; Fortical; Mastical; Natecal; ***Swed.:*** Calcitugg; Calcium-Sandoz; Kalcidon; Kalcipos; Kalcitena; ***Switz.:*** Calcium-Sandoz; Calperos; Calsan†; Fixateur phospho-calcique; Maxi-calc; ***Thai.:*** Bo-Ne-Ca; Calcanate; Calcium-Sandoz; Calsum Forte; Caltab; Prima-Cal; Sorcal; ***UK:*** Adcal; Cacit; Calcette†; Calcichew; Calcidrink†; Rap-eze; Remegel; Rennie Gold†; Rennie Soft Chews; Sandocal; Sea-Cal; Setlers; Titralac†; Tums; ***USA:*** Alka-Mints; Alkets; Amitone; Antacid; Cal-Plus†; Calci-Chew; Calci-Mix; Calciday†; Caltrate; Caltrate Jr†; Chooz; Equilet; Gencalc†; Maalox Antacid/Calcium; Maalox Quick Dissolve; Mallamint; Mylanta; Nephro-Calci; Os-Cal; Oysco; Oyst-Cal; Oyster Shell Calcium†; Oystercal†; Surpass; Titralac Extra Strength; Trial Antacid; Tums.

**Multi-ingredient:** numerous preparations are listed in Part 3.

## Carbenoxolone Sodium *(BANM, USAN, rINNM)*

Carbenoxolona sódica; Disodium Enoxolone Succinate. 3β-(3-Carboxypropionyloxy)-11-oxo-olean-12-en-30-oic acid, Disodium Salt.
$C_{34}H_{48}Na_2O_7$ = 614.7.
*CAS — 5697-56-3 (carbenoxolone); 7421-40-1 (carbenoxolone disodium).*
*ATC — A02BX01.*

**Pharmacopoeias.** In *Br.*

**BP 2003** (Carbenoxolone Sodium). A white or pale cream-coloured, hygroscopic powder. Freely soluble in water; sparingly soluble in alcohol; practically insoluble in chloroform and in ether. A 10% solution in water has a pH of 8.0 to 9.2.

### Adverse Effects

Carbenoxolone sodium has mineralocorticoid-like effects and ingestion may produce sodium and water retention and hypokalaemia. This may cause or exacerbate hypertension, heart failure, oedema, alkalosis, and muscle weakness and damage. If hypokalaemia is prolonged, renal impairment can occur.

◊ Muscle weakness,[1-5] muscle necrosis,[4] myopathy,[1] hypertension,[2] headache,[2] cardiac failure,[2] mental confusion,[4] areflexia,[3] renal tubular dysfunction,[5] and acute tubular necrosis[4] have all been associated with carbenoxolone-induced hypokalaemia. Carbenoxolone-induced hypertension may have precipitated the onset of fatal polyarteritis in a patient predisposed to this condition.[6]


1. Fyfe T, *et al.* Myopathy and hypokalaemia in carbenoxolone therapy. *BMJ* 1969; **3:** 476.
2. Davies GJ, *et al.* Complications of carbenoxolone therapy. *BMJ* 1974; **3:** 400–2.
3. Royston A, Prout BJ. Carbenoxolone-induced hypokalaemia simulating Guillain-Barré syndrome. *BMJ* 1976; **2:** 150–1.
4. Descamps C, *et al.* Rhabdomyolysis and acute tubular necrosis associated with carbenoxolone and diuretic treatment. *BMJ* 1977; **1:** 272.

5. Dickinson RJ, Swaminathan R. Total body potassium depletion and renal tubular dysfunction following carbenoxolone therapy. *Postgrad Med J* 1978; **54:** 836–7.
6. Sloan J, Weaver JA. A case of polyarteritis developing after carbenoxolone therapy. *Ir Med J* 1968; **1:** 505–7.

### Precautions

Systemic use of carbenoxolone sodium is contra-indicated in patients with hypokalaemia, in pregnancy, in the elderly, and in children. It should be used with caution, if at all, in patients with cardiac disease, hypertension, or hepatic or renal impairment.

**Handling.** Carbenoxolone sodium powder is irritant to nasal membranes.

### Interactions

Because of the risk of toxicity, carbenoxolone should not be taken with digitalis glycosides unless serum-electrolyte concentrations are measured at weekly intervals and measures are taken to avoid hypokalaemia.

Although amiloride or spironolactone relieve sodium and water retention, they antagonise the efficacy of systemic carbenoxolone and should not be used concomitantly. The hypokalaemia associated with diuretics may be exacerbated by carbenoxolone.

### Pharmacokinetics

Carbenoxolone sodium is absorbed from the gastrointestinal tract, mainly from the stomach. It is highly bound to plasma proteins. Carbenoxolone is chiefly excreted in the faeces via the bile. It appears to undergo enterohepatic circulation.

### Uses and Administration

Carbenoxolone sodium is a synthetic derivative of glycyrrhizinic acid (see Liquorice, p.1270) that was formerly used as a mucosal protectant in peptic ulcer disease and may be given in gastro-oesophageal reflux disease (p.1242). The suggested dosage of carbenoxolone sodium in gastro-oesophageal reflux disease is 20 mg three times daily by mouth and 40 mg at night for 6 to 12 weeks, as a preparation also containing antacids and alginic acid.

Carbenoxolone sodium is one of many topical treatments for the symptomatic management of mouth ulceration (p.1245). It is used as a 2% gel or as a 1% mouthwash.

### Preparations

**Proprietary Preparations** (details are given in Part 3)
***Austral.:*** Bioral; ***Austria:*** Rowadermat; ***Hong Kong:*** Herpesan; ***Irl.:*** Carbosan; ***Malaysia:*** Herpesan; ***Singapore:*** Herpesan; ***Spain:*** Sanodin; ***UK:*** Bioplex; Bioral.

**Multi-ingredient:** ***Irl.:*** Pyrogastrone; ***UK:*** Pyrogastrone.

---

## Casanthranol *(USAN)*

Casantranol.
*CAS — 8024-48-4.*

**Pharmacopoeias.** In *US.*

**USP 27** (Casanthranol). It is obtained from cascara. It contains not less than 20% of total hydroxyanthracene derivatives calculated on the dried basis, of which not less than 80% consists of cascarosides, both calculated as cascaroside A.

It is a light tan to brown, amorphous, hygroscopic powder. Freely soluble in water with some residue; partially soluble in methyl alcohol and in hot isopropyl alcohol; practically insoluble in acetone. Store in airtight containers at a temperature not exceeding 30°. Protect from light.

### Profile

Casanthranol is an anthraquinone stimulant laxative with general properties similar to those of senna (p.1288). It is given in usual doses of 30 to 60 mg daily by mouth, together with a faecal softener. In severe cases a dose of 90 mg daily, or 60 mg twice daily, may be given.

### Preparations

**Proprietary Preparations** (details are given in Part 3)
***Belg.:*** Cascalax.

**Multi-ingredient:** ***Arg.:*** Bil 13; En-Ga-Lax; ***Canad.:*** Peri-Colace; ***Hong Kong:*** Softon Plus†; ***Spain:*** Laxvital; ***USA:*** Black-Draught†; Docusoft Plus; Genasoft Plus Softgels†; Laxative & Stool Softener; Peri-Colace†; Peri-Dos Softgels†; Silace-C†.

---

## Cascara

Cáscara sagrada; Cascararinde; Chittem Bark; Rhamni Purshianae Cortex; Rhamni Purshiani Cortex; Sacred Bark.
*CAS — 8047-27-6; 8015-89-2 (cascara sagrada extract).*
*ATC — A06AB07.*

**Pharmacopoeias.** In *Eur.* (see p.vi) and *US.*

**Ph. Eur. 5.0** (Cascara). The dried, whole or fragmented bark of *Rhamnus purshianus* (=*Frangula purshiana*). It contains not less than 8.0% of hydroxyanthracene glycosides of which not less than 60% consists of cascarosides, both expressed as cascaroside A ($C_{27}H_{32}O_{14}$ = 580.5). and calculated with reference to the dried drug. Protect from light.

**USP 27** (Cascara Sagrada). The dried bark of *Rhamnus purshianus* (Rhamnaceae). It contains not less than 7% of total hydroxyanthracene derivatives calculated on the dried basis, of which not less than 60% consists of cascarosides, both calculated as cascaroside A. It has a distinct odour.

### Profile

Cascara is an anthraquinone stimulant laxative with general properties similar to those of senna (p.1288). It has been used in the treatment of constipation in doses equivalent to up to about 20 to 70 mg of total hydroxyanthracene derivatives daily by mouth.

**Breast feeding.** No adverse effects have been observed in breast-fed infants whose mothers were receiving cascara, and the American Academy of Pediatrics considers[1] that it is therefore usually compatible with breast feeding. For a contrary view see p.1288.

1. American Academy of Pediatrics. The transfer of drugs and other chemicals into human milk. *Pediatrics* 2001; **108:** 776–89. Correction. *ibid.*; 1029. Also available at: http://aappolicy.aappublications.org/cgi/content/full/pediatrics%3b108/3/776 (accessed 07/05/04)

### Preparations

***BP 2003:*** Cascara Dry Extract; Cascara Tablets;
***USP 27:*** Aromatic Cascara Fluidextract; Cascara Sagrada Extract; Cascara Sagrada Fluidextract; Cascara Tablets.

**Proprietary Preparations** (details are given in Part 3)
***Arg.:*** Natulax; ***Canad.:*** Le 500 D†; ***Fr.:*** Peristaltine; ***Ger.:*** Legapas; ***Ital.:*** Bonlax†; Colamin†; Sagrada-Lax†; ***Port.:*** Laxolen; Mucinum; ***Switz.:*** Legapas†.

**Multi-ingredient:** ***Arg.:*** Bilidren; Calculina; Cascara Sagrada Puler; Cascara Sagrada Sanaplex; Veracolate; Yuyo; ***Austral.:*** Peritone†; ***Austria:*** Cascara-Salax; Dragees Neunzehn; Silberne; ***Belg.:*** Grains de Vals; Vethoine; ***Braz.:*** Bilifel†; Boldobeba†; Boldopeptan; Chofranina; Composto Emagrecedor; Dioctosal†; Emagrevit; Enterotonus†; Epagogo†; Eparema; Epatovis†; Fideine†; Figadosan†; Gotas Hepaticas†; Hepato-Flux†; Hepatophil†; Hepavirmo†; Jurubileno†; Licor de Cacau†; Metionina Composta†; Pilulas De Witt's; Prisoventril; Purgoleite†; Solvobil; Ventre Livre; ***Canad.:*** Aid-Lax†; Alsilax†; Alsiline†; Bicholate; Caroid†; Cholasyn; Cholasyn II; Control; Doulax; Extra Strong Formula 12; Herbal Laxative; Herbalax; Herbalax Forte†; Herbolax†; Herborex; Lapidar†; Laxa†; Laxaco; Laxative; Le 100 B†; Mucinum; Phytolax†; Thunas Bilettes†; Thunas Laxative; Triolax†; Vesilax†; ***Chile:*** Bulgarolax; ***Denm.:*** Cosylan†; ***Fr.:*** Aromabyl†; Dragees Fuca; Dragees Vegetales Rex; Grains de Vals; Imegul; Mucinum a l'Extrait de Cascara; Spevin†; ***Ger.:*** Cascara-Salax†; Legapas comp†; Reducelle†; ***Hong Kong:*** Mucinum Cascara; ***Ital.:*** Amaro Medicinale; Amaro Padil†; Bitteridina†; Certobil†; Coladren; Confetti Lassativi CM; Critichol; Depurativo†; Digelax; Dis-Cinil Complex; Eparema; Eparema-Levul; Eupatol; Fave di Fuca; Grani di Vals; Hepasil Composto†; Hepatos; Hepatos B12; Lassatina; Magisbile; Mepalax; Neo-Heparbil†; Pillole Fattori†; Raboldo†; Schias-Amaro Medicinale; Sintobil†; Solvobil; Stimolfit; Vadolax; Vegebyl†; ***Norw.:*** Cosylan; ***Port.:*** Caroid; ***S.Afr.:*** Veracolate; ***Spain:*** Crislaxo; Laxante Derly†; Laxo Vian†; Lipograsil; Menabil Complex; Nico Hepatocyn; Pildoras Zeninas; ***Swed.:*** Cosylan†; Emulax; ***Switz.:*** Cascara-Salax†; Fuca†; Grains de Vals†; Laxativum Nouvelle Formule†; Padma-Lax; Tavolax†; ***Thai.:*** Flatulence Gastulence; Hemolax; Veracolate; ***UK:*** Dual-Lax Extra Strong; Dual-Lax Normal Strength; Jacksons Herbal Laxative; Laxative Tablets; Modern Herbals Laxative; Modern Herbals Pile; Natural Herb Tablets; Out-of-Sorts; Pileabs; Piletabs; Pilewort Compound†; Rhuaka†; Skin Eruptions Mixture; ***USA:*** Concentrated Milk of Magnesia-Cascara; Natures Remedy†; Veracolate†.

---

## Cassia Pulp

Pulpa de caña fístula.

### Profile

Cassia pulp is the evaporated aqueous extract of crushed ripe cassia fruits (cassia pods), *Cassia fistula* (Leguminosae). It is a mild anthraquinone stimulant laxative with general properties similar to those of senna (p.1288).

### Preparations

**Proprietary Preparations** (details are given in Part 3)

**Multi-ingredient:** ***Braz.:*** Fitolax; Florlax; Fontolax; Forlax; Frutalax; Frutarine†; Laxan†; Laxarine; Laxtam; Novolax†; Sene Composta†; Tamaril; Tamarine; Tamarix; ***Ital.:*** Tamarine; ***Mex.:*** Naturetti; ***Spain:*** Pruina; ***Switz.:*** Tamarine†.

---

## Cerium Oxalate

Oxalato de cerio.
*CAS — 139-42-4 (anhydrous cerous oxalate).*
*ATC — A04AD02.*

NOTE. The chemically defined substance $Ce_2(C_2O_4)_3$ is cerous oxalate.

### Profile

Cerium oxalate is used as an antiemetic.

### Preparations

**Proprietary Preparations** (details are given in Part 3)

**Multi-ingredient:** ***Spain:*** Novonausin.

---

## Cetraxate Hydrochloride *(USAN, rINNM)*

DV-1006; Hidrocloruro de cetraxato. 4-(2-Carboxyethyl)phenyl tranexamate hydrochloride; 4-(2-Carboxyethyl)phenyl *trans*-4-aminomethylcyclohexanecarboxylate hydrochloride.
$C_{17}H_{23}NO_4$,HCl = 341.8.
*CAS — 34675-84-8 (cetraxate); 27724-96-5 (cetraxate hydrochloride).*

**Pharmacopoeias.** In *Jpn.*

### Profile

Cetraxate hydrochloride is stated to be a mucosal protectant with actions on gastric microcirculation as well as prostaglandin synthesis and kallikrein. It is used in the treatment of gastritis and peptic ulcer disease (p.1246) in doses of 600 to 800 mg daily in divided doses.

### Preparations

**Proprietary Preparations** (details are given in Part 3)
***Hong Kong:*** Neuer†; ***Jpn:*** Neuer.

---

## Chalk

Creta; Prepared Chalk.
$CaCO_3$ = 100.1.
*CAS — 13397-25-6.*

**Pharmacopoeias.** In *Br.*

**BP 2003** (Chalk). A native form of calcium carbonate freed from most of its impurities by elutriation and dried. It consists of the calcareous shells and detritus of various foraminifera and contains not less than 97.0% and not more than 100.5% of $CaCO_3$, calculated with reference to the dried substance.

White or greyish-white, odourless or almost odourless, amorphous, earthy, small friable masses, usually conical in form, or in powder. Practically insoluble in water; slightly soluble in water containing carbon dioxide; it absorbs water readily.

### Profile

Chalk has been used as an adsorbent antidiarrhoeal. Calcium carbonate (precipitated chalk) is used as an antacid, calcium supplement, and phosphate binder, see p.1254.

### Preparations

***BP 2003:*** Compound Magnesium Trisilicate Oral Powder.

---

## Cilansetron *(rINN)*

KC-9946; KC-9946. (−)-(*R*)-5,6,9,10-Tetrahydro-10-[(2-methylimidazol-1-yl)methyl]-4*H*-pyrido[3,2,1-*jk*]carbazol-11(8*H*)-one.
$C_{20}H_{21}N_3O$ = 319.4.
*CAS — 120635-74-7.*

### Profile

Cilansetron is a 5-$HT_3$ antagonist under investigation for the treatment of diarrhoea-predominant irritable bowel syndrome.

---

## Cimetidine *(BAN, USAN, rINN)*

Cimetidina; Cimetidinum; SKF-92334. 2-Cyano-1-methyl-3-[2-(5-methylimidazol-4-ylmethylthio)ethyl]guanidine.
$C_{10}H_{16}N_6S$ = 252.3.
*CAS — 51481-61-9.*
*ATC — A02BA01.*

**Pharmacopoeias.** In *Chin., Eur.* (see p.vi), *Int., Jpn, Pol., US,* and *Viet.*

**Ph. Eur. 5.0** (Cimetidine). A white or almost white, polymorphic powder. Slightly soluble in water; soluble in alcohol; practically insoluble in dichloromethane. It dissolves in dilute mineral acids. Store in airtight containers. Protect from light.

**USP 27** (Cimetidine). A white to off-white crystalline powder, odourless or with a slight mercaptan odour. Slightly soluble in water and in chloroform; soluble in alcohol and in macrogol 400; practically insoluble in ether; sparingly soluble in isopropyl alcohol; freely soluble in methyl alcohol. Store in airtight containers. Protect from light.

## Cimetidine Hydrochloride *(BANM, USAN, rINNM)*

Cimetidini Hydrochloridum.
$C_{10}H_{16}N_6S$,HCl = 288.8.
*CAS — 70059-30-2.*
*ATC — A02BA01.*

**Pharmacopoeias.** In *Eur.* (see p.vi) and *US.*

**Ph. Eur. 5.0** (Cimetidine Hydrochloride). A white or almost white, crystalline powder. Freely soluble in water; sparingly soluble in dehydrated alcohol. A 1% solution in water has a pH of 4.0 to 5.0. Store in airtight containers. Protect from light.

**USP 27** (Cimetidine Hydrochloride). Store in airtight containers. Protect from light.

### Adverse Effects

Adverse reactions to cimetidine and other histamine $H_2$-antagonists are generally infrequent. The commonest side-effects reported have been diarrhoea and other gastrointestinal disturbances, dizziness, tiredness, headache, and rashes.

Altered liver function tests have occurred and there have been rare reports of hepatotoxicity. Reversible confusional states, especially in the elderly or in seriously ill patients such as those with renal failure, have occasionally occurred. Other adverse effects that have been reported rarely are hypersensitivity reactions and fever, arthralgia and myalgia, blood disorders including agranulocytosis and thrombocytopenia, acute pancreatitis, hallucinations and depression, and cardiovascular disorders including bradycardia and heart block.

Cimetidine has a weak anti-androgenic effect and gynaecomastia and impotence have also occasionally occurred in men receiving relatively high doses for conditions such as the Zollinger-Ellison syndrome.

**Incidence of adverse effects.** In a meta-analysis of 24 double-blind placebo-controlled studies,[1] the incidence of adverse effects with cimetidine was not significantly different from placebo. The most common adverse effects reported by patients taking cimetidine who were followed up for at least one year[2,3] were diarrhoea, headache, fatigue, skin rash or pruritus, and gynaecomastia. The incidence of adverse effects was dose-related and decreased with length of treatment.[3] No fatal adverse effect of cimetidine could be found in a mortality survey involving 9928 patients taking cimetidine and 9351 controls;[4] although the mortality rate was higher in the cimetidine patients, this was explained by the presence of underlying disease (known or unknown) before starting cimetidine treatment and the use of cimetidine to counter adverse gastric effects of other drugs. Follow-up of 9377 of these cimetidine-treated patients for a further 3 years[5] still revealed no fatal disorder attributable to cimetidine treatment and a steady fall in the excess death rate in cimetidine users was observed with increasing length of follow-up; by the fourth year there was little difference between the observed and expected death rate. Cimetidine still appeared to be safe after 10 years of follow-up.[6]

1. Richter JM, *et al.* Cimetidine and adverse reactions: a meta-analysis of randomized clinical trials of short-term therapy. *Am J Med* 1989; **87:** 278–84.
2. Colin Jones DG, *et al.* Post-marketing surveillance of the safety of cimetidine: twelve-month morbidity report. *Q J Med* 1985; **54:** 253–68.
3. Bardhan KD, *et al.* Safety of longterm cimetidine (CIM) treatment: the view from one centre. *Gut* 1990; **31:** A599.
4. Colin-Jones DG, *et al.* Postmarketing surveillance of the safety of cimetidine: 12 month mortality report. *BMJ* 1983; **286:** 1713–16.
5. Colin-Jones DG, *et al.* Postmarketing surveillance of the safety of cimetidine: mortality during second, third, and fourth years of follow up. *BMJ* 1985; **291:** 1084–8.
6. Colin-Jones DG, *et al.* Postmarketing surveillance of the safety of cimetidine: 10 year mortality report. *Gut* 1992; **33:** 1280–4.

**Carcinogenicity.** An association between $H_2$-antagonists and gastric cancer was proposed following individual case reports, the finding of tumours in long-term high-dose *animal* studies, and the possibility that nitrites and nitroso compounds may be produced, but seemed of little clinical relevance.[1,2] The excess risk of gastric cancer reported in patients taking cimetidine[3-6] or ranitidine[6] decreases with time and there is no evidence for any long-term persistence of the effect.[6] The increased risk may be explained by misdiagnosis and inappropriate cimetidine treatment of existing malignancy.[3-5] An apparently protective effect has been observed for $H_2$-antagonist use starting 10 or more years before diagnosis of gastric cancer.[6]

The observed excess risk for cancers of the respiratory system is probably related to smoking, since this is causally related to both peptic ulcer and lung cancer and the excess risk does not decline with time.[3-5]

1. Penston J, Wormsley KG. $H_2$-receptor antagonists and gastric cancer. *Med Toxicol* 1986; **1:** 163–8.
2. Møller H, *et al.* Use of cimetidine and other peptic ulcer drugs in Denmark 1977–1990 with analysis of the risk of gastric cancer among cimetidine users. *Gut* 1992; **33:** 1166–9.
3. Colin-Jones DG, *et al.* Postmarketing surveillance of the safety of cimetidine: 12 month mortality report. *BMJ* 1983; **286:** 1713–16.
4. Colin-Jones DG, *et al.* Postmarketing surveillance of the safety of cimetidine: mortality during second, third, and fourth years of follow up. *BMJ* 1985; **291:** 1084–8.
5. Møller H, *et al.* Cancer occurrence in a cohort of patients treated with cimetidine. *Gut* 1989; **30:** 1558–62.
6. La Vecchia C, *et al.* Histamine-2-receptor antagonists and gastric cancer risk. *Lancet* 1990; **336:** 355–7.

**Effects on the blood.** A review[1] in 1988 noted that leucopenia, thrombocytopenia, and pancytopenia have all been reported with cimetidine and ranitidine, with neutropenia and agranulocytosis occurring most often. There were also isolated reports of haemolytic anaemia and leucocytosis associated with cimetidine therapy. The overall incidence of cimetidine-associated blood cytopenia was estimated as 2.3 per 100 000 treated patients; the incidence for ranitidine was less and although there were reports with famotidine the incidence had not been determined. A subsequent case-control study,[2] concluded that the risk of hospitalisation due to neutropenia in patients receiving a 6-week course of cimetidine was no more than 1 in 116 000, while agranulocytosis did not occur in more than 1 in 573 000 patients.

A review[3] of the safety profile of famotidine noted that as of May 1992 there had been 60 reports of serious blood dyscrasias in patients receiving famotidine, of which 22 were considered possibly related to drug therapy (6 cases of pancytopenia or bone marrow depression, 5 of thrombocytopenia, 4 of leucopenia, 3 of combined leucopenia and thrombocytopenia, and 3 of agranulocytosis).

1. Aymard J-P, *et al.* Haematological adverse effects of histamine $H_2$-receptor antagonists. *Med Toxicol* 1988; **3:** 430–48.
2. Strom BL, *et al.* Is cimetidine associated with neutropenia? *Am J Med* 1995; **99:** 282–90.
3. Howden CW, Tytgat GNJ. The tolerability and safety profile of famotidine. *Clin Ther* 1996; **18:** 36–54.

**Effects on the cardiovascular system.** Bradycardia,[1-4] atrioventricular block,[5,6] tachycardia,[7] and hypotension[4,8] have been reported during cimetidine treatment given by mouth and by intravenous injection or infusion. Although there are studies in patients[9] and healthy subjects[10,11] that have found no significant cardiovascular effects associated with cimetidine treatment, it is likely that a small proportion of patients are more susceptible to the cardiovascular effects of cimetidine. Caution is recommended if the drug is given intravenously to patients with cardiovascular disease (see Precautions, below).

See also under Overdosage, below.

1. Jefferys DB, Vale JA. Cimetidine and bradycardia. *Lancet* 1978; **i:** 828.
2. Ligumsky M, *et al.* Cimetidine and arrhythmia suppression. *Ann Intern Med* 1978; **89:** 1008–9.
3. Tanner LA, Arrowsmith JB. Bradycardia and $H_2$ antagonists. *Ann Intern Med* 1988; **109:** 434–5.
4. Drea EJ, *et al.* Cimetidine-associated adverse reaction. *DICP Ann Pharmacother* 1990; **24:** 581–3.
5. Tordjman T, *et al.* Complete atrioventricular block and long-term cimetidine therapy. *Arch Intern Med* 1984; **144:** 861.
6. Ishizaki M, *et al.* First-degree atrioventricular block induced by oral cimetidine. *Lancet* 1987; **i:** 225–6.
7. Dickey W, Symington M. Broad-complex tachycardia after intravenous cimetidine. *Lancet* 1987; **i:** 99–100.
8. Mahon WA, Kolton M. Hypotension after intravenous cimetidine. *Lancet* 1978; **i:** 828.
9. Jackson G, Upward JW. Cimetidine, ranitidine, and heart rate. *Lancet* 1982; **ii:** 265.
10. Hughes DG, *et al.* Cardiovascular effects of $H_2$-receptor antagonists. *J Clin Pharmacol* 1989; **29:** 472–7.
11. Hilleman DE, *et al.* Impact of chronic oral $H_2$-antagonist therapy on left ventricular systolic function and exercise capacity. *J Clin Pharmacol* 1992; **32:** 1033–7.

**Effects on the endocrine system.** Cimetidine has dose-related mild anti-androgenic properties and reduced sperm counts and raised serum-prolactin concentrations have been reported in men during cimetidine treatment[1] as have gynaecomastia, breast tenderness, and impotence.[2] Those symptoms resolved following withdrawal of cimetidine,[1,2] reduction of the dose,[2] or transfer to ranitidine.[2]

A study by the Boston Collaborative Drug Surveillance Program, using data from 81 535 men in the UK, found that cimetidine was associated with an incidence of 3.29 cases of gynaecomastia per 1000 person years, representing a relative risk 7.2 times greater than that of non-users.[3] The period at highest risk seemed to be between the seventh and twelfth month after starting treatment, and the occurrence was related to dose, with most of the risk associated with doses over 1 g daily. This large study found no significant risk of gynaecomastia with ranitidine or omeprazole. However, there have been isolated reports of gynaecomastia or impotence with ranitidine (p.1285), nizatidine (p.1277), and famotidine (p.1265).

1. Wang C, *et al.* Effect of cimetidine on gonadal function in man. *Br J Clin Pharmacol* 1982; **13:** 791–4.
2. Jensen RT, *et al.* Cimetidine-induced impotence and breast changes in patients with gastric hypersecretory states. *N Engl J Med* 1983; **308:** 883–7.
3. García Rodríguez LA, Jick H. Risk of gynaecomastia associated with cimetidine, omeprazole, and other antiulcer drugs. *BMJ* 1994; **308:** 503–6. Correction. *ibid.*; 819.

**Effects on the eyes.** Ocular pain, blurred vision, and a rise in intra-ocular pressure occurred in a patient with chronic glaucoma during treatment with cimetidine; ocular symptoms associated with raised intra-ocular pressure subsequently developed during ranitidine treatment.[1] However, a study suggested that cimetidine had no effect on intra-ocular pressure.[2] A cohort study involving 140 128 patients receiving anti-ulcer therapy, 68 504 of whom received cimetidine, found no evidence that any of the drugs were associated with a major increased risk of vascular or inflammatory disorders of the eye.[3]

1. Dobrilla G, *et al.* Exacerbation of glaucoma associated with both cimetidine and ranitidine. *Lancet* 1982; **i:** 1078.
2. Feldman F, Cohen MM. Intraocular pressure and $H_2$ receptor antagonists. *Lancet* 1982; **i:** 1359.
3. García Rodríguez LA, *et al.* A cohort study of the ocular safety of anti-ulcer drugs. *Br J Clin Pharmacol* 1996; **42:** 213–16.

**Effects on the kidneys.** A review[1] of the nephrotoxicity and hepatotoxicity of $H_2$-antagonists noted that mild elevation of serum-creatinine was relatively common following use of cimetidine but appeared to have no clinical significance. However, the authors found 25 published reports of acute interstitial nephritis associated with this class of drug (20 with cimetidine, 4 with ranitidine, and 1 with famotidine) and 16 cases reported to the Australian Drug Reaction Advisory Committee (ADRAC) between 1972 and 1999 (11 with cimetidine, 4 with ranitidine, and 1 with famotidine). Symptoms were mostly nonspecific, and did not seem to be associated with the rash, arthralgia, and flank pain that may be seen in nephritis induced by other drugs. Nephritis invariably resolved when the drug was withdrawn; in 6 cases, rechallenge resulted in prompt return of clinical features, although there was some evidence that patients who developed nephrotoxicity with one $H_2$-antagonist might be able to tolerate substitution with another. The effect was rare (an earlier analysis estimated an incidence of around 1 in 100 000 treated patients[2]) but with the increasing availability of over-the-counter $H_2$-antagonist formulations it was important to be aware of the risk.

1. Fisher AA, Le Couteur DG. Nephrotoxicity and hepatotoxicity of histamine $H_2$ receptor antagonists. *Drug Safety* 2001; **24:** 39–57.
2. Rowley-Jones D, Flind AC. Cimetidine-induced renal failure. *BMJ* 1982; **285:** 1422–3.

**Effects on the liver.** A cohort study[1] involving 108 891 patients who had received cimetidine, ranitidine, famotidine, or omeprazole between 1990 and 1993, found 33 cases meeting the authors' definition of clinically serious liver injury (cholestatic in 8 cases, hepatocellular in 15 and mixed in 10), most of whom presented with jaundice. Of these cases of liver injury, 12 were among current users of cimetidine, compared with 5 among users of ranitidine and 1 omeprazole user. It was estimated that the incidence of hepatotoxicity among patients using cimetidine was 2.3 cases per 10 000 users, and the adjusted relative risk was 5.5 times that of non-users. The relative risk for use of ranitidine or omeprazole was calculated at 1.7 and 2.1 respectively. The risk with cimetidine was greatest at high doses (800 mg daily or above) and at the beginning of therapy. For reports of liver damage with famotidine, see p.1265.

1. García Rodríguez LA, *et al.* The risk of acute liver injury associated with cimetidine and other acid-suppressing anti-ulcer drugs. *Br J Clin Pharmacol* 1997; **43:** 183–8.

**Effects on the nervous system.** Cimetidine has been associated with a number of adverse neurological effects including confusion,[1-8] bizarre behaviour,[9] reversible brain stem syndrome (with ataxia, dysarthria, visual impairment, deafness, and paraesthesia),[10] coma,[8,11] convulsions,[7] encephalopathy,[12] visual hallucinations,[9,13,14] paranoia,[5] chorea,[15,16] myopathy,[17] and neuropathy.[18,19] These reactions occur mainly in patients who are elderly, critically ill, or with impaired renal or hepatic function, in whom there may be increased penetration of the blood-brain barrier by cimetidine. Single-dose studies in young healthy subjects[20] have found no adverse changes in performance, central nervous function, or subjective assessment of mood after administration of cimetidine 200 or 400 mg by mouth.

There is no clear evidence that cimetidine is a more frequent cause of CNS reactions than ranitidine, famotidine, or nizatidine.[21]

1. Robinson TJ, Mulligan TO. Cimetidine and mental confusion. *Lancet* 1977; **ii:** 719.
2. Spears JB. Cimetidine and mental confusion. *Am J Hosp Pharm* 1978; **35:** 1035.
3. Wood CA, *et al.* Cimetidine and mental confusion. *JAMA* 1978; **239:** 2550–1.
4. McMillen MA, *et al.* Cimetidine and mental confusion. *N Engl J Med* 1978; **298:** 284–5.
5. Kinnell HG, Webb A. Confusion associated with cimetidine. *BMJ* 1979; **ii:** 1438.
6. Mogelnicki SR, *et al.* Physostigmine reversal of cimetidine-induced mental confusion. *JAMA* 1979; **241:** 826–7.
7. Edmonds ME, *et al.* Cimetidine: does neurotoxicity occur? Report of three cases. *J R Soc Med* 1979; **72:** 172–5.
8. Sonnenblick M, *et al.* Neurological and psychiatric side effects of cimetidine—report of 3 cases with review of the literature. *Postgrad Med J* 1982; **58:** 415–18.
9. Papp KA, Curtis RM. Cimetidine-induced psychosis in a 14-year-old girl. *Can Med Assoc J* 1984; **131:** 1081–4.
10. Cumming WJK, Foster JB. Cimetidine-induced brainstem dysfunction. *Lancet* 1978; **i:** 1096.
11. Levine ML. Cimetidine-induced coma in cirrhosis of the liver. *JAMA* 1978; **240:** 1238.
12. Niv Y, *et al.* Cimetidine and encephalopathy. *Ann Intern Med* 1986; **105:** 977.
13. Agarwal SK. Cimetidine and visual hallucinations. *JAMA* 1978; **240:** 214.
14. Rushton AR. Pseudohypoparathyroidism, cimetidine, and neurologic toxicity. *Ann Intern Med* 1983; **98:** 677.
15. Kushner MJ. Chorea and cimetidine. *Ann Intern Med* 1982; **96:** 126.
16. Lehmann AB. Reversible chorea due to ranitidine and cimetidine. *Lancet* 1988; **ii:** 158.
17. Feest TG, Read DJ. Myopathy associated with cimetidine? *BMJ* 1980; **281:** 1284–5.
18. Walls TJ, *et al.* Motor neuropathy associated with cimetidine. *BMJ* 1980; **281:** 974–5.
19. Atkinson AB, *et al.* Neurological dysfunction in two patients receiving captopril and cimetidine. *Lancet* 1980; **ii:** 36–7.
20. Nicholson AN, Stone BM. The $H_2$-antagonists, cimetidine and ranitidine: studies on performance. *Eur J Clin Pharmacol* 1984; **26:** 579–82.
21. Cantú TG, Korek JS. Central nervous system reactions to histamine-2 receptor blockers. *Ann Intern Med* 1991; **114:** 1027–34.

**Effects on the skin.** Widespread erythrosis-like lesions in a 36-year-old man were probably induced by cimetidine.[1] There has been a report[2] of a skin eruption clinically consistent with erythema annulare centrifugum developing in a patient after 6 months of treatment with cimetidine; the eruption resolved after withdrawal of cimetidine and reappeared on rechallenge. The condition had not recurred during therapy with ranitidine. Erythema multiforme eruptions occurred after both cimetidine and famotidine administration in one patient (see p.1265). There have been reports of the Stevens-Johnson syndrome during cimetidine treatment in patients with a history of hypersensitivity to penicillin[3] or sulfonamides,[4] and a report of toxic epidermal necrolysis.[5]

Urticarial vasculitis[6] and alopecia[7] have also been associated with cimetidine treatment.

1. Angelini G, *et al.* Cimetidine and erythrosis-like lesions. *BMJ* 1979; **i:** 1147–8.
2. Merrett AC, *et al.* Cimetidine-induced erythema annulare centrifugum: no cross-sensitivity with ranitidine. *BMJ* 1981; **283:** 698.
3. Ahmed AH, *et al.* Stevens-Johnson syndrome during treatment with cimetidine. *Lancet* 1978; **ii:** 433.
4. Guan R, Yeo PPB. Stevens-Johnson syndrome: was it cimetidine? *Aust N Z J Med* 1983; **13:** 182.
5. Tidwell BH, *et al.* Cimetidine-induced toxic epidermal necrolysis. *Am J Health-Syst Pharm* 1998; **55:** 163–4.
6. Mitchell GG, *et al.* Cimetidine-induced cutaneous vasculitis. *Am J Med* 1983; **75:** 875–6.
7. Khalsa JH, *et al.* Cimetidine-associated alopecia. *Int J Dermatol* 1983; **22:** 202–4.

**Fever.** Reports of febrile reactions associated with cimetidine. Fever has also been reported with famotidine (p.1265) and ranitidine (p.1286).


1. Ramboer C. Drug fever with cimetidine. *Lancet* 1978; **i:** 330–1.
2. McLoughlin JC, *et al.* Cimetidine fever. *Lancet* 1978; **ii:** 499–500.
3. Corbett CL, Holdsworth CD. Fever, abdominal pain, and leucopenia during treatment with cimetidine. *BMJ* 1978; **i:** 753–4.
4. Landolfo K, *et al.* Cimetidine-induced fever. *Can Med Assoc J* 1984; **130:** 1580.


**Hypersensitivity.** Facial oedema,[1] laryngospasm,[1] pruritus,[2,3] rash,[2,3] angioedema[3] and anaphylaxis[4] have been reported in patients receiving cimetidine by mouth or intravenously.

See also under Effects on the Skin, above.


1. Delaunois L. Hypersensitivity to cimetidine. *N Engl J Med* 1979; **300:** 1216.
2. Hadfield WA. Cimetidine and giant urticaria. *Ann Intern Med* 1979; **91:** 128–9.
3. Sandhu BS, Requena R. Hypersensitivity to cimetidine. *Ann Intern Med* 1982; **97:** 138.
4. Knapp AB, *et al.* Cimetidine-induced anaphylaxis. *Ann Intern Med* 1982; **97:** 374–5.


**Infection.** Treatment with $H_2$-antagonists may predispose patients to salmonella infection, probably because the decrease in gastric acidity reduces the gastric killing of ingested organisms.[1] The greatest increase in risk was seen in patients over 65 years of age. There are conflicting data on whether the use of $H_2$-antagonists for prophylaxis of stress ulcers in critically ill patients increases the risk for pneumonia (see under Peptic Ulcer Disease, p.1246).


1. Neal KR, *et al.* Recent treatment with $H_2$ antagonists and antibiotics and gastric surgery as risk factors for salmonella infection. *BMJ* 1994; **308:** 176.


**Overdosage.** No serious toxic effects were noted in reports[1-3] of overdosage in patients who took cimetidine 5.2 to 20 g (including one patient who took about 12 g daily for 5 days[1]). Resultant plasma concentrations had been up to 57 micrograms/mL compared with a usual peak plasma concentration of 1 microgram/mL after a 200-mg dose. However, an overdose of about 12 g produced high pulse rate, dilated pupils, speech disturbances, agitation and disorientation in one patient[4] and respiratory depression in another patient who had chronic schizophrenia and was also taking trifluoperazine and hydroxyzine.[5] Also, fatal bradycardia has been reported after overdosage with an unknown amount of cimetidine and diazepam.[6] In a review of 881 cases of cimetidine overdose, excluding cases where several drugs were taken, it was concluded that the toxicity of cimetidine after acute overdose was very low.[7] No symptoms were observed in 79% of cases, which included ingestions of up to 15 g of cimetidine, and only 3 patients had moderate clinical manifestations (dizziness and bradycardia; CNS depression; vomiting). No patients had major medical outcomes and there were no fatalities. Gastric emptying was performed in 34% of cases.

Emptying the stomach, for example by gastric lavage, has been used in overdosage, provided that not more than 4 hours have elapsed since ingestion of the drug, but supportive measures and symptomatic treatment alone may be adequate. Forced diuresis does not appear to enhance the excretion of cimetidine from the body, and is not recommended.[3]


1. Gill GV. Cimetidine overdose. *Lancet* 1978; **i:** 99.
2. Illingworth RN, Jarvie DR. Absence of toxicity in cimetidine overdosage. *BMJ* 1979; **i:** 453–4.
3. Meredith TJ, Volans GN. Management of cimetidine overdose. *Lancet* 1979; **ii:** 1367.
4. Nelson PG. Cimetidine and mental confusion. *Lancet* 1977; **ii:** 928.
5. Wilson JB. Cimetidine overdosage. *BMJ* 1979; **i:** 955.
6. Hiss J, *et al.* Fatal bradycardia after intentional overdose of cimetidine and diazepam. *Lancet* 1982; **ii:** 982.
7. Krenzelok EP, *et al.* Cimetidine toxicity: an assessment of 881 cases. *Ann Emerg Med* 1987; **1:** 1217–21.


## Precautions

Before giving cimetidine or other histamine $H_2$-antagonists to patients with gastric ulcers the possibility of malignancy should be considered since these drugs may mask symptoms and delay diagnosis. They should be given in reduced dosage to patients with renal impairment.

Intravenous injections of cimetidine should be given slowly and intravenous infusion is preferred, particularly for high doses and in patients with cardiovascular impairment.

**Breast feeding.** In the UK, manufacturers advise that mothers receiving cimetidine avoid breast feeding. Cimetidine is reported to be actively transported into breast milk, resulting in a milk:serum ratio 5.5 times higher than that expected with passive diffusion.[1] In one case, where cimetidine was detected in the milk of a nursing mother in concentrations higher than in her plasma, it was calculated[2] that the maximum amount of cimetidine that an infant could ingest assuming an intake of about 1 litre of milk daily and fed at the time of peak concentrations would be about 6 mg. However, the Committee on Drugs of the American Academy of Pediatrics has pointed out that there was no evidence of signs or symptoms attributable to the drug in the infant in this case,[3] despite 6 months of breast feeding, and cimetidine has been classified by that body as usually compatible with breast feeding.[4]


1. Oo CY, *et al.* Active transport of cimetidine into human milk. *Clin Pharmacol Ther* 1995; **58:** 548–55.
2. Somogyi A, Gugler R. Cimetidine excretion into breast milk. *Br J Clin Pharmacol* 1979; **7:** 627–9.
3. Berlin CM. Cimetidine and breast-feeding. *Pediatrics* 1991; **88:** 1294.
4. American Academy of Pediatrics. The transfer of drugs and other chemicals into human milk. *Pediatrics* 2001; **108:** 776–89. Correction. *ibid.*; 1029. Also available at: http://aappolicy.aappublications.org/cgi/content/full/pediatrics%3b108/3/776 (accessed 07/05/04)


**Burns.** The clearance of cimetidine has been reported to be increased in burn patients, with the increase correlating to the size of the burn.[1] Despite another study that reported a decreased renal clearance (but an increased non-renal clearance) early in the evolution of burn injury,[2] it has been recommended that the dosage of cimetidine be increased in patients with burns, depending on the extent of injury. A requirement for increased dosage has also been noted in paediatric burns patients.[3]


1. Martyn JAJ, *et al.* Increased cimetidine clearance in burn patients. *JAMA* 1985; **253:** 1288–91.
2. Ziemniak JA, *et al.* Cimetidine kinetics during resuscitation from burn shock. *Clin Pharmacol Ther* 1984; **36:** 228–33.
3. Martyn JAJ, *et al.* Alteration by burn injury of the pharmacokinetics and pharmacodynamics of cimetidine in children. *Eur J Clin Pharmacol* 1989; **36:** 361–7.


**Helicobacter pylori testing.** In one study,[1] 2 of 11 patients with *Helicobacter pylori* infection had false-negative urea breath tests while receiving high dose ranitidine (600 mg daily). The breath test became positive again within 5 days of stopping therapy. The manufacturers of the breath test recommend it should not be performed for at least 2 weeks after stopping antisecretory drug therapy.


1. Chey WD, *et al.* Lansoprazole and ranitidine affect the accuracy of the $^{14}$C-urea breath test by a pH-dependent mechanism. *Am J Gastroenterol* 1997; **92:** 446–50.


**Hepatic impairment.** An increased resistance to $H_2$-receptor antagonists has been reported in patients with cirrhosis, see Ranitidine, p.1286. For a suggestion that dosage reduction of cimetidine may be required in patients with portal systemic encephalopathy, see Administration in Hepatic Impairment, below.

**Porphyria.** Cimetidine is considered to be unsafe in patients with porphyria although there is conflicting experimental evidence of porphyrinogenicity.

For reference to clinical and biochemical improvement in porphyric patients receiving cimetidine, see below.

**Renal impairment.** The clearance of cimetidine is reduced in renal impairment and dosage reduction is recommended (see under Administration in Renal Impairment, below).

## Interactions

Cimetidine and other $H_2$-antagonists can reduce the absorption of drugs such as ketoconazole, and possibly itraconazole, whose absorption is dependent on an acid gastric pH.

Cimetidine may inhibit the hepatic metabolism of many drugs by binding to cytochrome P450 isoenzymes, notably CYP1A2, CYP2C9, CYP2D6, and CYP3A4. Although many such interactions may occur, only a few are considered clinically significant, notably those with phenytoin, theophylline, lidocaine, and oral anticoagulants. Avoidance of the combination, or a reduction in the dosage of these drugs may be required.

◊ Cimetidine can affect a wide range of drugs[1-4] but these interactions are of clinical significance for only a few, particularly those that have a narrow therapeutic index where the risk of toxicity may necessitate adjustment of dosage. The majority of interactions are due to binding of cimetidine to cytochrome P450 isoenzymes in the liver with subsequent inhibition of microsomal oxidative metabolism and increased bioavailability or plasma concentrations of drugs metabolised by these enzymes. A few interactions are due to competition for renal tubular secretion. Other mechanisms of interaction such as changes in hepatic blood flow play only a minor role.

Significant or potentially significant interactions have occurred with

- antiepileptics such as phenytoin (p.374) and carbamazepine (p.356)
- biguanide antidiabetics (p.330)
- ciclosporin (p.1356)
- lidocaine (p.1378)
- nifedipine (p.969)
- pethidine (p.73)
- procainamide (p.988)
- theophylline (p.803)
- tricyclic antidepressants such as amitriptyline (p.285)
- warfarin and other oral anticoagulants (p.1026)
- zalcitabine (p.657)
- zolmitriptan (p.473)

Combinations of these drugs and cimetidine should be avoided or used with caution, with monitoring of effects or plasma-drug concentrations and reductions in dosage as appropriate.

Famotidine, nizatidine, and ranitidine do not inhibit cytochrome P450, and the potential for drug interactions is therefore reduced.


1. Penston J, Wormsley KG. Adverse reactions and interactions with $H_2$-receptor antagonists. *Med Toxicol* 1986; **i:** 192–216.
2. Somogyi A, Muirhead M. Pharmacokinetic interactions of cimetidine 1987. *Clin Pharmacokinet* 1987; **12:** 321–66.
3. Smith SR, Kendall MJ. Ranitidine versus cimetidine: a comparison of their potential to cause clinically important drug interactions. *Clin Pharmacokinet* 1988; **15:** 44–56.
4. Shinn AF. Clinical relevance of cimetidine drug interactions. *Drug Safety* 1992; **7:** 245–67.


**Alcohol.** Any interaction between $H_2$-antagonists and alcohol is generally thought unlikely to be clinically significant (see p.1167).

**Antacids.** Single-dose studies of the interaction between cimetidine and antacids[1] have shown reduced bioavailability of cimetidine as well as no interaction. The neutralising capacity of the antacid appears to be a factor in determining whether an interaction occurs and a dose with less than 50 mmol neutralising capacity will have little, if any, effect on cimetidine absorption. There is no evidence that the therapeutic efficacy of cimetidine is reduced and with long-term use of the combination the bioavailability of cimetidine is unlikely to be reduced.


1. Gugler R, Allgayer H. Effects of antacids on the clinical pharmacokinetics of drugs: an update. *Clin Pharmacokinet* 1990; **18:** 210–19.


**Antimuscarinics.** The antimuscarinic *propantheline* delays gastric emptying and reduces intestinal motility and has been reported to reduce the bioavailability of cimetidine.[1]


1. Kanto J, *et al.* The effect of metoclopramide and propantheline on the gastrointestinal absorption of cimetidine. *Br J Clin Pharmacol* 1981; **11:** 629–31.


**Prokinetic drugs.** *Metoclopramide* may reduce the bioavailability of cimetidine possibly due to reduction of gastrointestinal transit time.[1-3] A similar interaction has been reported between cimetidine and the prokinetic drug *cisapride*.[4] The clinical significance of this interaction is questionable since such combinations may be clinically effective, although the use of cisapride is now restricted in many countries.


1. Gugler R, *et al.* Impaired cimetidine absorption due to antacids and metoclopramide. *Eur J Clin Pharmacol* 1981; **20:** 225–8.
2. Kanto J, *et al.* The effect of metoclopramide and propantheline on the gastrointestinal absorption of cimetidine. *Br J Clin Pharmacol* 1981; **11:** 629–31.
3. Barzaghi N, *et al.* Effects on cimetidine bioavailability of metoclopramide and antacids given two hours apart. *Eur J Clin Pharmacol* 1989; **37:** 409–10.
4. Kirch W, *et al.* Cisapride-cimetidine interactions; enhanced cisapride bioavailability and accelerated cimetidine absorption. *Ther Drug Monit* 1989; **11:** 411–14.


**Sucralfate.** The manufacturers of the mucosal protectant sucralfate state that it has been shown to reduce the bioavailability of cimetidine and other $H_2$ antagonists, presumably due to binding in the gastrointestinal tract. The effect can be avoided by separating doses of the two drugs by 2 hours, but it is not clear whether the interaction has a clinical significance.

## Pharmacokinetics

Cimetidine is readily absorbed from the gastrointestinal tract and peak plasma concentrations are obtained about an hour after administration on an empty stomach; a second peak may be seen after about 3 hours. Food delays the rate and may slightly decrease the extent of absorption, with the peak plasma concentration occurring after about 2 hours.

The bioavailability of cimetidine after oral administration is about 60 to 70%. Cimetidine is widely distributed and has a volume of distribution of about 1 litre/kg and is weakly bound, about 20%, to plasma proteins. The elimination half-life from plasma is about 2 hours and is increased in renal impairment. Cimetidine is partially metabolised in the liver to the sulfoxide and to hydroxymethylcimetidine. About 50% of an oral dose, and 75% of an intravenous dose, is excreted unchanged in the urine in 24 hours. Cimetidine crosses the placental barrier and is distributed into breast milk.

◊ Reviews.


1. Somogyi A, Gugler R. Clinical pharmacokinetics of cimetidine. *Clin Pharmacokinet* 1983; **8:** 463–95.
2. Lin JH. Pharmacokinetic and pharmacodynamic properties of histamine $H_2$-receptor antagonists: relationship between intrinsic potency and effective plasma concentrations. *Clin Pharmacokinet* 1991; **20:** 218–36.
3. Gladziwa U, Klotz U. Pharmacokinetics and pharmacodynamics of $H_2$-receptor antagonists in patients with renal insufficiency. *Clin Pharmacokinet* 1993; **24:** 319–32.


**Children.** Renal function is limited in the first few months of life and half-lives of 1.1 to 3.7 hours have been reported for cimetidine in neonates.[1-3] A dosage regimen for neonates based on renal function has been suggested[1] with 15 to 20 mg/kg daily for full-term neonates, but with lower doses for premature neonates and those with renal dysfunction. However, single doses of 5 to

7 mg/kg may be sufficient to suppress gastric acid secretion in neonates.[3]

In older infants and children maturation of renal function is complete and the clearance of cimetidine is increased compared with that in adults while younger children show higher clearance values than older children. A typical dosage regimen for children is 30 mg/kg daily, in 3 or 4 divided doses.[4] However, even this dose might not produce optimal control of gastric acid.[5]

1. Ziemniak JA, *et al.* The pharmacokinetics and metabolism of cimetidine in neonates. *Dev Pharmacol Ther* 1984; **7:** 30–8.
2. Lloyd CW, *et al.* The pharmacokinetics of cimetidine and metabolites in a neonate. *Drug Intell Clin Pharm* 1985; **19:** 203–5.
3. Stile IL, *et al.* Pharmacokinetic evaluation of cimetidine in newborn infants. *Clin Ther* 1985; **7:** 361–4.
4. Somogyi A, *et al.* Cimetidine pharmacokinetics and dosage requirements in children. *Eur J Pediatr* 1985; **144:** 72–6.
5. Lambert J, *et al.* Efficacy of cimetidine for gastric acid suppression in pediatric patients. *J Pediatr* 1992; **120:** 474–8.

## Uses and Administration

Cimetidine is a histamine $H_2$-antagonist and inhibits actions of histamine mediated by $H_2$-receptors such as gastric acid secretion and pepsin output. It is used where inhibition of gastric acid secretion may be beneficial, as in peptic ulcer disease, including stress ulceration (p.1246), gastro-oesophageal reflux disease (p.1242), selected cases of persistent dyspepsia (p.1242), pathological hypersecretory states such as the Zollinger-Ellison syndrome (p.1247), and in patients at risk of acid aspiration (p.1240) during general anaesthesia or child birth. Cimetidine may also be used to reduce malabsorption and fluid loss in patients with the short bowel syndrome and to reduce the degradation of enzyme supplements given to patients with pancreatic insufficiency.

Cimetidine may be given by mouth, by the nasogastric route, or parenterally by the intravenous or intramuscular routes; the total daily dose by any route should not normally exceed 2.4 g. Although some formulations are prepared as the hydrochloride, strengths and doses are expressed in terms of the base. Cimetidine 100 mg is approximately equivalent to cimetidine hydrochloride 114.4 mg. Doses should be reduced in renal impairment and may also need to be reduced in hepatic impairment (see below).

SPECIFIC DISEASE DOSES.

In the management of benign **gastric** and **duodenal ulceration** a single daily dose of 800 mg by mouth at bedtime is recommended, which should be given initially for at least 4 weeks in the case of duodenal, and for at least 6 weeks in the case of gastric, ulcers. Where appropriate a maintenance dose of 400 mg may then be given once daily at bedtime, or twice daily in the morning and at bedtime. Other regimens have also been used for treatment and maintenance.

In **gastro-oesophageal reflux disease** the recommended dose is 400 mg by mouth four times daily (with meals and at bedtime), or 800 mg twice daily, for 4 to 8 weeks. In pathological hypersecretory conditions, such as the **Zollinger-Ellison syndrome**, a dose of 300 or 400 mg by mouth four times daily is normally used, although sometimes higher doses may be necessary.

Doses of 200 to 400 mg by mouth, by nasogastric administration, or parenterally (200 mg only for direct intravenous injection) every 4 to 6 hours are recommended for the management of patients at risk from **stress ulceration** of the upper gastrointestinal tract. In patients at risk of developing the **acid aspiration syndrome**, a dose of 400 mg by mouth may be given 90 to 120 minutes before the induction of anaesthesia, or at the start of labour (in obstetric practice), and doses of up to 400 mg (by the parenteral route if appropriate, see below) may be repeated at intervals of 4 hours if required.

Doses of up to 200 mg four times daily have been taken for non-ulcer **dyspepsia**; 100 mg at night has been used in the prophylaxis of nocturnal heartburn.

To reduce the degradation of pancreatic enzyme supplements, patients with **pancreatic insufficiency**, as in cystic fibrosis (p.123), may be given cimetidine 800 to 1600 mg daily by mouth in 4 divided doses, 60 to 90 minutes before meals.

PARENTERAL ADMINISTRATION.

In the UK, the usual dose of cimetidine by intravenous injection is 200 mg, which should be given slowly over at least 5 minutes and may be repeated every 4 to 6 hours. If a larger dose is required, or if the patient has cardiovascular impairment, intravenous infusion is recommended. For an intermittent intravenous infusion the recommended dose is 200 to 400 mg every 4 to 6 hours if necessary. For a continuous intravenous infusion the recommended rate is 50 to 100 mg/hour. The usual intramuscular dose is 200 mg which may be repeated at intervals of 4 to 6 hours. In the USA, dosage recommendations for parenteral administration are 300 mg every 6 to 8 hours by intramuscular injection or by slow intravenous injection over at least 5 minutes. The same dosage may be given by intermittent intravenous infusion over 15 to 20 minutes; for continuous intravenous infusion the recommended rate is 37.5 mg/hour, which may be preceded by 150 mg as an intravenous loading dose. However, a rate of 50 mg/hour is recommended for prevention of stress ulceration.

CHILDREN'S DOSES.

For **children** over one year of age 25 to 30 mg/kg daily may be given in divided doses, by mouth or parenterally. Under 1 year of age, 20 mg/kg daily in divided doses has been used (see also under Pharmacokinetics, above).

**Administration in hepatic impairment.** The bioavailability of cimetidine may be increased in patients with cirrhosis[1,2] and a dosage reduction of up to 40% has been suggested in patients with portal systemic encephalopathy.[3] However, UK and US licensed drug information does not include recommendations for dosage adjustment in hepatic impairment.

1. Gugler R, *et al.* Altered disposition and availability of cimetidine in liver cirrhotic patients. *Br J Clin Pharmacol* 1982; **14:** 421–30.
2. Cello JP, Øie S. Cimetidine disposition in patients with Laennec's cirrhosis during multiple dosing therapy. *Eur J Clin Pharmacol* 1983; **25:** 223–9.
3. Ziemniak JA, *et al.* Hepatic encephalopathy and altered cimetidine kinetics. *Clin Pharmacol Ther* 1983; **34:** 375–82.

**Administration in renal impairment.** The dosage of cimetidine should be reduced in patients with renal impairment; suggested doses according to creatinine clearance (CC) are:

- CC over 50 mL/minute: normal dosage
- CC 30 to 50 mL/minute: 200 mg four times daily
- CC 15 to 30 mL/minute: 200 mg three times daily
- CC 0 to 15 mL/minute: 200 mg twice daily

Cimetidine is removed by haemodialysis, but not significantly removed by peritoneal dialysis.

**Dapsone toxicity.** Cimetidine might reduce the haemolysis and methaemoglobinaemia associated with dapsone. For references supporting this suggestion, see Effects on the Blood, under Dapsone, p.202.

**Diagnostic use.** Cimetidine blocks renal tubular secretion of creatinine and has been used experimentally to improve the accuracy of estimations of glomerular filtration rate from creatinine clearance in patients with renal disease.[1] Best results were achieved with a bolus dose of 1.2 g and the use of such a high dose was questioned.[2]

1. van Acker BAC, *et al.* Creatinine clearance during cimetidine administration for measurement of glomerular filtration rate. *Lancet* 1992; **340:** 1326–9.
2. Agarwal R. Creatinine clearance with cimetidine for measurement of GFR. *Lancet* 1993; **341:** 188.

**Echinococcosis.** Cimetidine has been given with albendazole to increase its effect (by inhibiting its metabolism) in the treatment of echinococcosis (p.98).

**Immunomodulation.** Studies in *mice* and humans have shown that $H_2$-antagonists have an immunoregulatory effect.[1] T-lymphocyte suppressor cells have histamine $H_2$ receptors and cimetidine has been reported to reduce activity of these cells, thus enhancing immune response.[1,2] There is also some evidence that it enhances cellular immunity, notably natural killer cell activity.[3] This discovery has led to the investigation of cimetidine in a number of disorders associated with alteration of the immune response including eosinophilic fasciitis, herpesvirus infections, mucocutaneous candidiasis,[4] hypogammaglobulinaemia,[5] and various malignancies.[1]

1. Kumar A. Cimetidine: an immunomodulator. *DICP Ann Pharmacother* 1990; **24:** 289–95.
2. Snyman JR, *et al.* Cimetidine as modulator of the cell-mediated immune response in vivo using the tuberculin skin test as parameter. *Br J Clin Pharmacol* 1990; **29:** 257–60.
3. Katoh J, *et al.* Cimetidine and immunoreactivity. *Lancet* 1996; **348:** 404–5.
4. Polizzi B, *et al.* Successful treatment with cimetidine and zinc sulphate in chronic mucocutaneous candidiasis. *Am J Med Sci* 1996; **311:** 189–90.
5. White WB, Ballow M. Modulation of suppressor-cell activity by cimetidine in patients with common variable hypogammaglobulinemia. *N Engl J Med* 1985; **312:** 198–202.

EOSINOPHILIC FASCIITIS. Eosinophilic fasciitis is a scleroderma-like syndrome of inflammation of the muscle fascia and associated eosinophilia and hypergammaglobulinaemia. Although it responds well to corticosteroid therapy in most cases, cimetidine has also been tried. The effect of cimetidine on eosinophilic fasciitis is unpredictable with both remission[1-4] and lack of response[5,6] having been reported in a few patients.

1. Solomon G, *et al.* Eosinophilic fasciitis responsive to cimetidine. *Ann Intern Med* 1982; **97:** 547–9.
2. Laso FJ, *et al.* Cimetidine and eosinophilic fasciitis. *Ann Intern Med* 1983; **98:** 1026.
3. Garcia-Morteo O, *et al.* Cimetidine and eosinophilic fasciitis. *Ann Intern Med* 1984; **100:** 318–19.
4. Farrell AM, *et al.* Eosinophilic fasciitis associated with autoimmune thyroid disease and myelodysplasia treated with pulsed methylprednisolone and antihistamines. *Br J Dermatol* 1999; **140:** 1185–7.
5. Loftin EB. Cimetidine and eosinophilic fasciitis. *Ann Intern Med* 1983; **98:** 111–12.
6. Herson S, *et al.* Cimetidine in eosinophilic fasciitis. *Ann Intern Med* 1990; **113:** 412–13.

HERPESVIRUS AND PAPILLOMAVIRUS INFECTIONS. Although there have been numerous isolated and anecdotal reports of a beneficial response to cimetidine in patients with infections due to various *herpesviruses* (p.619), including genital herpes simplex,[1] infectious mononucleosis,[2,3] and herpes zoster[4-7] some of these reports have been criticised[8,9] mainly on the grounds that the majority of cases of herpes zoster will resolve within 2 to 3 weeks whether any treatment is given or not. Also, a double-blind placebo-controlled study involving 63 patients with herpes zoster[10] found no evidence that cimetidine relieved the pain or accelerated the rate of healing of lesions.

There are reports[11] of benefit from the use of cimetidine in patients with *viral warts* (p.1139), but controlled studies have failed to show significant benefit.[12,13]

1. Wakefield D. Cimetidine in recurrent genital herpes simplex infection. *Ann Intern Med* 1984; **101:** 882.
2. Goldstein JA. Cimetidine and mononucleosis. *Ann Intern Med* 1983; **99:** 410–11.
3. Goldstein JA. Cimetidine, ranitidine, and Epstein-Barr virus infection. *Ann Intern Med* 1986; **105:** 139.
4. Hayne ST, Mercer JB. Herpes zoster: treatment with cimetidine. *Can Med Assoc J* 1983; **129:** 1284–5.
5. Shandera R. Treatment of herpes zoster with cimetidine. *Can Med Assoc J* 1984; **131:** 279.
6. Mavligit GM, Talpaz M. Cimetidine for herpes zoster. *N Engl J Med* 1984; **310:** 318–19.
7. Arnot RS. Herpes zoster and cimetidine. *Med J Aust* 1984; **141:** 903.
8. Tyrrell DL. Course of herpes zoster. *Can Med Assoc J* 1984; **130:** 1109.
9. Giles KE. Herpes zoster and cimetidine. *Med J Aust* 1985; **142:** 283.
10. Levy DW, *et al.* Cimetidine in the treatment of herpes zoster. *J R Coll Physicians Lond* 1985; **19:** 96–8.
11. Glass AT, *et al.* Cimetidine therapy for recalcitrant warts in adults. *Arch Dermatol* 1996; **132:** 680–2.
12. Karabulut AA, *et al.* Is cimetidine effective for nongenital warts: a double-blind, placebo-controlled study. *Arch Dermatol* 1997; **133:** 533–4.
13. Rogers CJ, *et al.* Cimetidine therapy for recalcitrant warts in adults: is it any better than placebo? *J Am Acad Dermatol* 1999; **41:** 123–7.

MALIGNANT NEOPLASMS. Because of its immunomodulatory effects cimetidine has been tried, with some reported benefit,[1-3] as an adjuvant in the management of a variety of malignant neoplasms such as those of the gastrointestinal tract (see p.516). However, a large randomised study[4] failed to show any benefit for cimetidine compared with placebo in gastric cancer. A similar study with ranitidine also failed to show any significant benefit.[5]

1. Tønnesen H, *et al.* Effect of cimetidine on survival after gastric cancer. *Lancet* 1988; **ii:** 990–2.
2. Adams WJ, Morris DL. Short-course cimetidine and survival with colorectal cancer. *Lancet* 1994; **344:** 1768–9.
3. Matsumoto S. Cimetidine and survival with colorectal cancer. *Lancet* 1995; **346:** 115.
4. Langman MJS, *et al.* Prospective, double-blind, placebo-controlled randomized trial of cimetidine in gastric cancer. *Br J Cancer* 1999; **81:** 1356–62.
5. Primrose JN, *et al.* A prospective randomised controlled study of the use of ranitidine in patients with gastric cancer. *Gut* 1998; **42:** 17–19.

**Mastocytosis.** Cimetidine, alone or in combination with an antihistamine (histamine $H_1$-antagonist), has been reported to relieve gastrointestinal symptoms,[1,2] pruritus, and urticaria[3,4] in patients with mastocytosis (p.797).

1. Hirschowitz BI, Groarke JF. Effect of cimetidine on gastric hypersecretion and diarrhea in systemic mastocytosis. *Ann Intern Med* 1979; **90:** 769–71.
2. Linde R, *et al.* Combination H1 and H2 receptor antagonist therapy in mastocytosis. *Ann Intern Med* 1980; **92:** 716.
3. Simon RA. Treatment of systemic mastocytosis. *N Engl J Med* 1980; **302:** 231.
4. Frieri M, *et al.* Comparison of the therapeutic efficacy of cromolyn sodium with that of combined chlorpheniramine and cimetidine in systemic mastocytosis: results of a double-blind clinical trial. *Am J Med* 1985; **78:** 9–14.

**Paracetamol toxicity.** It has been suggested that cimetidine might be of use in the treatment of paracetamol poisoning (see p.76) because of its inhibition of the cytochrome P450 system. However, there is no current evidence to support the claims of benefit made in some anecdotal reports.[1]

1. Kaufenberg AJ, Shepherd MF. Role of cimetidine in the treatment of acetaminophen poisoning. *Am J Health-Syst Pharm* 1998; **55:** 1516–19.

**Porphyria.** There are reports[1,2] of patients with acute intermittent porphyria (p.1040) showing clinical and biochemical improvement during treatment with cimetidine. Cimetidine is, however, considered to be unsafe in patients with porphyria (see above).

1. Baccino E, *et al.* Cimetidine in the treatment of acute intermittent porphyria. *JAMA* 1989; **262:** 3000.
2. Horie Y, *et al.* Clinical usefulness of cimetidine treatment for acute relapse in intermittent porphyria. *Clin Chim Acta* 1995; **234:** 171–5.

**Skin disorders.** Cimetidine has been used alone[1-8] or with an antihistamine ($H_1$-antagonist)[5,8,9] in various skin disorders. $H_2$-antagonists such as cimetidine and ranitidine have produced improvement in certain types of *urticaria* (p.1138), especially those associated with cold or angioedema. Their routine use in urticaria is controversial, but in practice their addition to conventional treatment can be tried in resistant cases.[10-12] Little additional benefit has been found with combination therapy in dermographic urticaria.[13] Although they may act by antagonism of $H_2$-receptors on cutaneous blood vessels, other mechanisms of action may be involved.[8] Patients with *pruritus* (p.1137) of various causes may also respond to $H_2$-antagonists,[1,2,6,7,9] but studies in larger groups of patients have demonstrated no benefit.[3-5,14]

1. Easton P, Galbraith PR. Cimetidine treatment of pruritus in polycythemia vera. *N Engl J Med* 1978; **299:** 1134.
2. Hess CE. Cimetidine for the treatment of pruritus. *N Engl J Med* 1979; **300:** 370.
3. Harrison AR, *et al.* Pruritus, cimetidine and polycythemia. *N Engl J Med* 1979; **300:** 433–4.
4. Scott GL, Horton RJ. Pruritus, cimetidine and polycythemia. *N Engl J Med* 1979; **300:** 434. Correction. *ibid.*; 936.
5. Zappacosta AR, Hauss D. Cimetidine doesn't help pruritus of uremia. *N Engl J Med* 1979; **300:** 1280.
6. Schapira DV, Bennett JM. Cimetidine for pruritus. *Lancet* 1979; **i:** 726–7.
7. Aymard JP, *et al.* Cimetidine for pruritus in Hodgkin's disease. *BMJ* 1980; **280:** 151–2.
8. Theoharides TC. Histamine$_2$ ($H_2$)-receptor antagonists in the treatment of urticaria. *Drugs* 1989; **37:** 345–55.
9. Deutsch PH. Dermatographism treated with hydroxyzine and cimetidine and ranitidine. *Ann Intern Med* 1984; **101:** 569.
10. Advenier C, Queille-Roussel C. Rational use of antihistamines in allergic dermatological conditions. *Drugs* 1989; **38:** 634–44.
11. Ormerod AD. Urticaria: recognition, causes, and treatment. *Drugs* 1994; **48:** 717–30.
12. Greaves MW. Chronic urticaria. *N Engl J Med* 1995; **332:** 1767–72.
13. Sharpe GR, Shuster S. In dermographic urticaria $H_2$ receptor antagonists have a small but therapeutically irrelevant additional effect compared with $H_1$ antagonists alone. *Br J Dermatol* 1993; **129:** 575–9.
14. Raisch DW, *et al.* Evaluation of a non-food and drug administration-approved use of cimetidine: treatment of pruritus resulting from epidural morphine analgesia. *DICP Ann Pharmacother* 1991; **25:** 716–8.

## Preparations

***BP 2003:*** Cimetidine Injection; Cimetidine Oral Solution; Cimetidine Oral Suspension; Cimetidine Tablets;
***USP 27:*** Cimetidine in Sodium Chloride Injection; Cimetidine Injection; Cimetidine Tablets.

**Proprietary Preparations** (details are given in Part 3)
***Arg.:*** Tagamet; Ulcerfen; ***Austral.:*** Cimehexal; Cimetimax†; Magicul; Sigmetadine; Tagamet; ***Austria:*** Cimetag; Neutromed; Neutronorm; Sodexx; Ulcometin; Ulcostad; ***Belg.:*** Nuardin; Tagamet; ***Braz.:*** Cimetidan; Cimetil†; Cimetin; Cimetina; Cimetinax; Cimetival; Cimext†; Cinton; Climatidine; Duomet; Gastidin†; Gastrodine†; Laveran†; Prometidine; Stomakon; Stomet†; Tagaliv; Tagamet; Tranimet; Ulcedine; Ulcedor†; Ulcenon; Ulcerac; Ulceracid; Ulcerase†; Ulcimet; Ulcinax; Ulcitag; Ulcitrat; Ulgastrin†; Up Mep†; Zagastrol†; ***Canad.:*** Gaviscon Prevent; Novo-Cimetine; Nu-Cimet; Peptol†; Tagamet; ***Denm.:*** Aciloc; Acinil; Cimecodan; Hocimin; Metinet†; Novamet; Tagamet†; ***Fin.:*** Cimex†; ***Fr.:*** Stomedine; Tagamet; ***Ger.:*** Altramet†; Azucimet; Cime; Cimebeta; Cimehexal; Cimemerck†; Cimephil†; Cimet; CimLich; Ciuk†; Contracid†; duraH2; Gastroprotect; H 2 Blocker; Jenametidin†; Sigacimet; Tagagel†; Tagamet; Ulcolind H$_2$†; Ulcubloc†; ***Gr.:*** Besidin; Gastrolene; Tagamet; Tamper; ***Hong Kong:*** Altramet†; Cementin; Cimedine; Cimeta; Cimulcer; Citidine; Gastab; Gastidine; Megadin†; Neutronorm†; Pallia†; Simaglen; Syncomet; Tagadine; Tagamet; Ulcomet; Ultec†; ***Irl.:*** Cedine; Cimagen; Cimeldine; Dyspamet; Galenamet; Geramet; Pinamet; Tagamet; ***Israel:*** Cemidin; Cimetag; Cimi; Tagamet; ***Ital.:*** Biomag; Brumetidina; Citimid†; Dina; Eureceptor†; Gastromet†; Neo Gastrausil†; Notul; Stomet; Tagamet; Tametin†; Temic; Ulcedin; Ulcestop†; Ulcodina; Ulcomedina; Ulis; Vagolisal†; ***Malaysia:*** Cimulcer; Shintamet; Tagamet; Ulcidine; Xepamet; ***Mex.:*** Alcatex; Antil†; Asaurex†; Beamat†; Blocan†; Cimebec; Cimedul; Cimetase; Colimet; Columina†; Dimetigal†; Gastrodina; Gastrolem†; Inesfay†; Novamet†; Procimeti; Sercim; Sinegastrin; Tagamet; Ulcerim†; Ulogen†; Ulserral; Zimerol†; Zymerol†; ***Neth.:*** Tagamet; ***Norw.:*** Acinil†; Cimal; Cimetid†; Gastrobitan†; Tagamet; ***NZ:*** Cytine; Duomet†; Tagamet†; ***Port.:*** Cim; Evicer; Tagamet; Ulceridine; ***S.Afr.:*** Aci-Med; Acidown†; Cimlok; Cinadine; Duomet†; Hexamet; Lenamet; Secadine; Tagamet; Ulcim†; ***Singapore:*** Cementin; Cimulcer; Citidine; Erlmetin; Gastromet; Shintamet; Tagamet; Xepamet; ***Spain:*** Ali Veg; Fremet; Gastro H2†; Mansal; Tagamet; ***Swed.:*** Aciloc†; Acinil; Tagamet; ***Switz.:*** Malimed; Tagamet; ***Thai.:*** Aidar; Alserine; Cencamet; Cidine; Cigamet; Cimag†; Cimet-P; Cimetine; Cimidine; Cimulcer; Citidine; Clinimet; CMD; Duotric; Gastrodin; Histodil†; Iwamet; Manomet; Med-Gastramet; Milamet; Peptica; Pondarmett; Pose-CM†; Rinadine; Servicimet†; Siamidine; Simaglen; Simex; Tagamet; Ulcedine; Ulcemet; Ulcimet; ***UAE:*** Cimetag; ***UK:*** Acid-Eze†; Acitak; Dyspamet; Galenamet; Peptimax; Tagamet; Ultec; Zita; ***USA:*** Tagamet.
**Multi-ingredient:** ***Irl.:*** Algitec†; ***Neth.:*** Aciflux.

## Cinitapride (rINN)

Cinitaprida. 4-Amino-N-[1-(3-cyclohexen-1-ylmethyl)-4-piperidyl]-2-ethoxy-5-nitrobenzamide.
$C_{21}H_{30}N_4O_4$ = 402.5.
*CAS — 66564-14-5.*

### Profile

Cinitapride is a substituted benzamide used for its prokinetic properties. It is given by mouth as the acid tartrate in doses of 1 mg three times daily before meals in the management of gastroparesis and gastro-oesophageal reflux disease (p.1242).

### Preparations

**Proprietary Preparations** (details are given in Part 3)
***Arg.:*** Paxapride; Rogastril; ***Spain:*** Blaston; Cidine.

## Cisapride (BAN, USAN, rINN)

Cisaprida; Cisapridum; R-51619. *cis*-4-Amino-5-chloro-N-{1-[3-(4-fluorophenoxy)propyl]-3-methoxy-4-piperidyl}-2-methoxybenzamide monohydrate.
$C_{23}H_{29}ClFN_3O_4,H_2O$ = 484.0.
*CAS — 81098-60-4 (anhydrous cisapride).*
*ATC — A03FA02.*

**Pharmacopoeias.** In *Eur.* (see p.vi) and *Pol.*

**Ph. Eur. 5.0** (Cisapride Monohydrate; Cisapride BP 2003). A white or almost white powder; it exhibits polymorphism. Practically insoluble in water; soluble in dichloromethane; freely soluble in dimethylformamide; sparingly soluble in methyl alcohol. Protect from light.

## Cisapride Tartrate (BANM, rINNM)

Cisapridi Tartras.
$C_{27}H_{35}ClFN_3O_{10}$ = 616.0.

**Pharmacopoeias.** In *Eur.* (see p.vi).

**Ph. Eur. 5.0** (Cisapride Tartrate). A white or almost white powder. It exhibits polymorphism. Slightly soluble in water and in methyl alcohol; very slightly soluble in alcohol; freely soluble in dimethylformamide. Protect from light.

### Adverse Effects

The most commonly reported side-effects with cisapride are gastrointestinal disturbances including abdominal cramps, borborygmi, and diarrhoea. Headache and lightheadedness may also occur. Hypersensitivity (including rash, pruritus, and bronchospasm), convulsions, extrapyramidal effects, and increased urinary frequency, have occasionally been reported. Cases of arrhythmia, including ventricular tachycardia, ventricular fibrillation, torsade de pointes, and QT interval prolongation have occurred rarely; fatalities have resulted, and have led to severe restrictions on its use (see Effects on the Heart, below). There have been a few cases of disturbances in liver function among patients receiving cisapride.

**Incidence of adverse effects.** A comparison of data from prescription-event monitoring in over 13 000 recipients of cisapride and from a further 9726 recipients involved in a controlled study showed that diarrhoea, in about 2 to 4% of patients, was the commonest adverse effect reported.[1] Other relatively common adverse effects were headache, abdominal pain, nausea and vomiting, and constipation, all in around 1 to 1.5% of patients. There were 46 reports in the prescription-event monitoring data of increased urinary frequency (plus a further 20 among the controlled study patients), and 5 reports of arrhythmias.

1. Wager E, *et al.* A comparison of two cohort studies evaluating the safety of cisapride: prescription-event monitoring and a large phase IV study. *Eur J Clin Pharmacol* 1997; **52:** 87–94.

**Effects on the heart.** Seven reports[1] of cardiac effects associated with cisapride were submitted to the WHO Programme for International Drug Monitoring between 1989 and 1991. They included palpitations in 4, tachycardia and hypertension in 1, and extrasystole in 2. Subsequent reports implicated cisapride in the development of prolonged QT interval and torsade de pointes or ventricular fibrillation or both.[2,3] By December 1999 the FDA had received 341 reports of heart rhythm abnormalities associated with cisapride use, including 80 reports of deaths. Most patients were either receiving other drugs known to impair cisapride metabolism (see Interactions, below) or had other factors predisposing to arrhythmias. In the light of earlier reports of cardiac effects and of evidence for a direct effect of cisapride on the heart at therapeutic concentrations, in 1998 the UK Committee on Safety of Medicines (CSM) **contra-indicated**[2] the use of cisapride in patients receiving drugs that could inhibit cisapride metabolism or that prolong the QT interval, as well as in patients with a history of QT interval prolongation, ventricular arrhythmia, or torsade de pointes, or other risk factors for arrhythmia (see Precautions, below). Neonates[4] (especially of low gestational age[5]) are vulnerable to cisapride-induced QT interval prolongation, and the CSM also specifically contra-indicated use in premature neonates[2] and noted that there were insufficient data to support use in children up to the age of 12. Other studies have also noted a prolongation of QT interval in children.[6,7] However, some commentators have questioned the general contra-indication in prematurity,[8] and one retrospective analysis estimated the rate of serious adverse events such as arrhythmia in premature newborns to be less than 1 in 11 000, excluding those cases related to concurrent treatment with a contra-indicated drug or to overdose.[9] Conversely, others emphasise the lack of objective evidence for benefit for cisapride in most paediatric indications.[10] The European Society of Paediatric Gastroenterology, Hepatology and Nutrition has published recommendations on the use of cisapride in paediatric gastro-oesophageal reflux disease,[11] including that the total daily dose of cisapride should rarely exceed 800 micrograms/kg, and that ECG monitoring should be performed before and after 3 days of treatment in certain groups such as premature infants.

The use of cisapride has also been the subject of warnings and restrictions in other countries. In the USA, prescribing information was amended in January 2000 to recommend that all patients should receive an ECG before beginning cisapride therapy and extending the contra-indications to use; the drug was subsequently **withdrawn** from general supply, remaining available only in severely restricted cases. In July 2000 cisapride was also withdrawn completely from the UK market.[12]

1. Olsson S, Edwards IR. Tachycardia during cisapride treatment. *BMJ* 1992; **305:** 748–9.
2. Committee on Safety of Medicines/Medicines Control Agency. Cisapride (Prepulsid): risk of arrhythmias. *Current Problems* 1998; **24:** 11. Also available at: http://www.mca.gov.uk/ourwork/monitorsafequalmed/currentproblems/volume24aug.htm (accessed 07/05/04)
3. Wysowski DK, Bacsanyi J. Cisapride and fatal arrhythmia. *N Engl J Med* 1996; **335:** 290–1.
4. Bernardini S, *et al.* Effect of cisapride on QTc interval in neonates. *Arch Dis Child Fetal Neonatal Ed* 1997; **77:** F241–3.
5. Dubin A, *et al.* Cisapride associated with QTc prolongation in very low birth weight preterm infants. *Pediatrics* 2001; **107:** 1313–16.
6. Hill SL, *et al.* Proarrhythmia associated with cisapride in children. *Pediatrics* 1998; **101:** 1053–6.
7. Khongphatthanayothin A, *et al.* Effects of cisapride on QT interval in children. *J Pediatr* 1998; **133:** 51–6.
8. Lander A, Desai A. The risks and benefits of cisapride in premature neonates, infants, and children. *Arch Dis Child* 1998; **79:** 469–71.
9. Ward RM, *et al.* Cisapride: a survey of the frequency of use and adverse events in premature newborns. *Pediatrics* 1999; **103:** 469–72.
10. Cairns P. The risks and benefits of cisapride. *Arch Dis Child* 1999; **80:** 493.
11. Vandenplas Y, *et al.* The role of cisapride in the treatment of pediatric gastroesophageal reflux: the European Society of Paediatric Gastroenterology, Hepatology and Nutrition. *J Pediatr Gastroenterol Nutr* 1999; **28:** 518–28.
12. Committee on Safety of Medicines/Medicines Control Agency. Cisapride (Prepulsid) withdrawn. *Current Problems* 2000; **26:** 9–10. Also available at: http://www.mca.gov.uk/ourwork/monitorsafequalmed/currentproblems/cpsept2000.pdf (accessed 07/05/04)

**Effects on the respiratory system.** Chest tightness, wheezing, and a fall in peak flow rate occurred in a patient with severe brittle asthma after taking cisapride 10 mg.[1] Four other cases of bronchospasm associated with cisapride use have been discussed in a subsequent report;[2] in 2 of these cases symptoms resolved on withdrawal and recurred on rechallenge.

1. Nolan P, *et al.* Cisapride and brittle asthma. *Lancet* 1990; **336:** 1443.
2. Pillans P. Bronchospasm associated with cisapride. *BMJ* 1995; **311:** 1472.

**Effects on the urinary tract.** There had been 12 cases of urinary disturbances associated with use of cisapride[1] reported to the Australian Adverse Drug Reactions Advisory Committee between March 1991 and July 1993. Five reports were of urinary incontinence, 8 involved frequency, and individual reports involved cystitis, hesitancy, and urinary retention. The majority of the cases involved women, and most patients were elderly.

1. Boyd IW, Rohan AP. Urinary disorders associated with cisapride. *Med J Aust* 1994; **160:** 579–80.

### Precautions

Cisapride should not be used when stimulation of muscular contractions might adversely affect gastrointestinal conditions as in gastrointestinal haemorrhage, obstruction, perforation, or immediately after surgery.

Cisapride is **contra-indicated** in the following patients:

- those receiving potent inhibitors of the cytochrome P450 isoenzyme CYP3A4 such as macrolide antibacterials, azole antifungals, HIV-protease inhibitors, or nefazodone (see also under Interactions, below)
- those taking other drugs that predispose to electrolyte disturbances or that prolong the QT interval
- those with a personal or family history of QT interval prolongation
- those with a previous history of ventricular arrhythmia or torsade de pointes

Furthermore, it should not be given to those with other risk factors for arrhythmia including:

- clinically significant heart disease
- uncorrected electrolyte disturbances (particularly hypokalaemia and hypomagnesaemia)
- renal failure
- respiratory failure

Use is also contra-indicated in premature infants for up to 3 months after birth.

Cisapride should be used with caution and in reduced doses in patients with hepatic or renal impairment. All patients should have their ECG, serum electrolytes, and renal function monitored before and during treatment.

Care should be taken not to exceed the recommended dose.

**Breast feeding.** No adverse effects have been observed in breast-fed infants whose mothers were receiving cisapride, and the American Academy of Pediatrics considers[1] that it is therefore usually compatible with breast feeding.

1. American Academy of Pediatrics. The transfer of drugs and other chemicals into human milk. *Pediatrics* 2001; **108:** 776–89. Correction. *ibid.*; 1029. Also available at: http://aappolicy.aappublications.org/cgi/content/full/pediatrics%3b108/3/776 (accessed 07/05/04)

## Interactions

Cisapride is metabolised by the cytochrome P450 isoenzyme CYP3A4. Use with drugs that significantly inhibit this enzyme is contra-indicated as it may result in increased plasma concentrations of cisapride and hence a greater risk of QT interval prolongation and ventricular arrhythmias. Examples of such drugs include the azole antifungals ketoconazole, fluconazole, itraconazole, and miconazole; the macrolide antibacterials troleandomycin, erythromycin, and clarithromycin; the non-nucleoside reverse transcriptase inhibitors delavirdine and efavirenz; and the HIV-protease inhibitors indinavir and ritonavir. Nefazodone may interact similarly. Cisapride should not be used in patients receiving other medication known to prolong the QT interval, including quinine or halofantrine, terfenadine, astemizole, certain antiarrhythmics such as amiodarone or quinidine, some antidepressants such as amitriptyline, phenothiazine antipsychotics, and sertindole. Cimetidine may enhance cisapride bioavailability. Grapefruit juice also increases the bioavailability of cisapride and concomitant use should be avoided. In addition, drugs such as potassium-sparing diuretics, or insulin in acute settings, can result in altered electrolyte balance, and use with cisapride may also increase the risk of arrhythmias.

Antimuscarinics and possibly opioid analgesics may antagonise the gastrointestinal effects of cisapride. Because cisapride increases intestinal motility it may affect the absorption of other drugs, either diminishing absorption from the stomach or enhancing absorption from the small intestine. Prothrombin times may be increased in some patients receiving oral anticoagulants, and the effects of alcohol and some other CNS depressants may be enhanced.

◊ Reviews.

1. Bedford TA, Rowbotham DJ. Cisapride: drug interactions of clinical significance. *Drug Safety* 1996; **15:** 167–75.
2. Michalets EL, Williams CR. Drug interactions with cisapride: clinical implications. *Clin Pharmacokinet* 2000; **39:** 49–75.

**Antidepressants.** It has been pointed out[1] that a number of antidepressants, including *fluoxetine, fluvoxamine, nefazodone,* and *sertraline* all appear to markedly inhibit cytochrome P450 isoenzyme CYP3A4, and therefore might interact with cisapride. See also above.

1. Caley CF. Cisapride interaction with antidepressants. *Ann Pharmacother* 1996; **30:** 684.

**Antimicrobials.** Of 57 cases of prolonged QT interval or torsade de pointes reported to the US FDA as of April 1996 in patients receiving cisapride, 32 (56%) were also receiving azole antifungals (*fluconazole, itraconazole, ketoconazole,* or *miconazole*) or macrolide antibacterials (*erythromycin* or *clarithromycin*).[1] Subsequently, use of cisapride with clarithromycin has been shown to prolong the QT interval in healthy subjects,[2] and further cases of torsade de pointes[3,4] and QT prolongation with syncope[5] have been reported in patients receiving the combination. A case of torsade de pointes in a patient receiving erythromycin and cisapride has also been reported.[6] There is a theoretical possibility of a serious interaction with *quinupristin/dalfopristin.* Similar interactions could also be anticipated with *non-nucleoside reverse transcriptase inhibitor antiretrovirals* and *HIV-protease inhibitors.*

1. Wysowski DK, Bacsanyi J. Cisapride and fatal arrhythmia. *N Engl J Med* 1996; **335:** 290–1.
2. van Haarst AD, *et al.* The influence of cisapride and clarithromycin on QT intervals in healthy volunteers. *Clin Pharmacol Ther* 1998; **64:** 542–6.
3. Mekkarie MA. Torsade de pointes in two chronic renal failure patients treated with cisapride and clarithromycin. *Am J Kidney Dis* 1997; **30:** 437–9.
4. Piquette RK. Torsade de pointes induced by cisapride/clarithromycin interaction. *Ann Pharmacother* 1999; **33:** 22–6.
5. Seals Gray V. Syncopal episodes associated with cisapride and concurrent drugs. *Ann Pharmacother* 1998; **32:** 648–51.
6. Tierney MG, *et al.* Potential cisapride-erythromycin interaction. *Can J Clin Pharmacol* 1997; **4:** 82–4.

**Cardiovascular drugs.** Near syncope and a prolonged QT interval occurred in a patient taking cisapride and *diltiazem.*[1] Diltiazem may have inhibited the metabolism of cisapride. For mention of cisapride possibly reducing the absorption of *digoxin,* see p.898.

1. Thomas AR, *et al.* Prolongation of the QT interval related to cisapride-diltiazem interaction. *Pharmacotherapy* 1998; **18:** 381–5.

**Grapefruit juice.** Grapefruit juice increased the oral bioavailability of cisapride, with large interindividual variation, in healthy volunteers.[1,2] The manufacturer advises that the combination be avoided.

1. Gross AS, *et al.* Influence of grapefruit juice on cisapride pharmacokinetics. *Clin Pharmacol Ther* 1999; **65:** 395–401.
2. Kivistö KT, *et al.* Repeated consumption of grapefruit juice considerably increases plasma concentrations of cisapride. *Clin Pharmacol Ther* 1999; **66:** 448–53.

**$H_2$-antagonists.** *Cimetidine*[1] but not *ranitidine*[2] has been reported to enhance the bioavailability of oral cisapride, possibly by inhibition of cisapride metabolism (cimetidine is an inhibitor of the cytochrome P450 isoenzyme CYP3A4). Cisapride conversely increases the rate of absorption and decreases the oral bioavailability of both cimetidine[1] and ranitidine (see p.1286).

1. Kirch W, *et al.* Cisapride-cimetidine interaction: enhanced cisapride bioavailability and accelerated cimetidine absorption. *Ther Drug Monit* 1989; **11:** 411–14.
2. Rowbotham DJ, *et al.* Effect of single doses of cisapride and ranitidine administered simultaneously on plasma concentrations of cisapride and ranitidine. *Br J Anaesth* 1991; **67:** 302–305.

## Pharmacokinetics

Cisapride is readily absorbed from the gastrointestinal tract, with peak plasma concentrations achieved 1 to 2 hours after a dose by mouth. It undergoes extensive first-pass metabolism in the liver and gut wall, resulting in an absolute bioavailability of 35 to 40%. The main metabolic pathways are oxidative *N*-dealkylation by the cytochrome P450 isoenzyme CYP3A4, producing the major metabolite norcisapride, and aromatic hydroxylation. More than 90% of a dose is excreted as metabolites in the urine and faeces in about equal amounts. A small amount is distributed into breast milk. The elimination half-life is about 10 hours. Cisapride is about 98% bound to plasma proteins.

## Uses and Administration

Cisapride is a substituted benzamide used for its prokinetic properties. It stimulates gastrointestinal motility, probably by increasing the release of acetylcholine in the gut wall at the level of the myenteric plexus, increases the resting tone of the lower oesophageal sphincter, and increases the amplitude of lower oesophageal contractions. Gastric emptying is accelerated and the mouth-to-caecum transit time is reduced. Colonic peristalsis is also increased which decreases colonic transit time. Cisapride apparently lacks antidopaminergic effects (unlike metoclopramide, p.1274, to which it is chemically related) or direct parasympathomimetic activity and it does not affect prolactin release or gastric secretion. It is reported to be an agonist at serotonin-4 ($5\text{-}HT_4$) receptors.

Cisapride has been used mainly in the treatment of gastro-oesophageal reflux disease (p.1242), in disorders associated with decreased gastric motility (below), and in non-ulcer dyspepsia. However, as mentioned under Effects on the Heart, above, its use is severely restricted by its propensity to cause cardiac arrhythmias, and it has been withdrawn completely in the UK.

Cisapride is given as the monohydrate, but doses are calculated in terms of the anhydrous substance. Cisapride monohydrate 10.39 mg is approximately equivalent to 10 mg of anhydrous cisapride. It is taken by mouth 15 to 30 minutes before a meal and at bedtime, if necessary. Where still licensed, a usual oral dose is 5 to 10 mg three to four times daily up to a maximum daily dose of 40 mg. Neonates, infants, and children have been given 0.2 mg/kg three to four times daily up to a maximum daily dose of 0.8 mg/kg (but see below for further discussion on the use of cisapride in children). A dose of 10 mg twice daily or 20 mg at night has been given for maintenance treatment in adults; the maintenance dose might be increased to 20 mg twice daily in severe cases.

Doses of cisapride should be reduced in patients with hepatic or renal impairment (see below).

◊ Reviews.

1. Barone JA, *et al.* Cisapride: a gastrointestinal prokinetic drug. *Ann Pharmacother* 1994; **28:** 488–500.
2. Wiseman LR, Faulds D. Cisapride: an updated review of its pharmacology and therapeutic efficacy as a prokinetic agent in gastrointestinal motility disorders. *Drugs* 1999; **47:** 116–52.

**Administration in children.** There are safety concerns over the use of cisapride in children because of the risk of cardiac arrhythmias (see Effects on the Heart, above). Particular care is needed in neonates and cisapride is contra-indicated in premature neonates for 3 months after birth due to the increased risk of QT interval prolongation in this patient group.

Its efficacy has also been questioned and a systematic review[1] of the use of cisapride in children found no clear evidence that cisapride had a statistically significant effect in reducing symptoms of gastro-oesophageal reflux disease compared with placebo.

1. Augood C, *et al.* Cisapride treatment for gastro-oesophageal reflux in children. Available in The Cochrane Library; Issue 1. Chichester: John Wiley; 2004.

**Administration in hepatic or renal impairment.** In patients with hepatic impairment the dose of cisapride should be half the usual dose, followed by adjustment depending on clinical response. In cases where renal impairment is not considered to contra-indicate the use of cisapride, a similar reduction in dose has been recommended.

**Decreased gastrointestinal motility.** Some benefit has been reported from the use of cisapride in patients with chronic intestinal pseudo-obstruction[1-3] and also in the acute form.[4,5] For a general discussion of decreased gastrointestinal motility and its treatment, see p.1241. Cisapride has also been used in diabetic gastroparesis (below).

1. Camilleri M, *et al.* Impaired transit of chyme in chronic intestinal pseudoobstruction: correction by cisapride. *Gastroenterology* 1986; **91:** 619–26.
2. Puntis JWL, *et al.* Cisapride in neonatal short gut. *Lancet* 1986; **ii:** 108–9.
3. Coombs RC, Booth IW. Small intestinal motor activity response to cisapride in children with dysmotility syndromes. *Gut* 1989; **30:** A1473.
4. Vantrappen G. Acute colonic pseudo-obstruction. *Lancet* 1993; **341:** 152–3.
5. Lander A, *et al.* Cisapride reduces neonatal postoperative ileus: randomised placebo controlled trial. *Arch Dis Child Fetal Neonatal Ed* 1997; **77:** F119–22.

**Diabetes mellitus.** Cisapride has been used as an alternative to metoclopramide in the management of diabetic gastroparesis. For a discussion of diabetic complications, and their management, see p.326.

References.

1. Chang CS, *et al.* Effect of cisapride on gastric dysrhythmia and emptying of indigestible solids in type-II diabetic patients. *Scand J Gastroenterol* 1998; **33:** 600–4.
2. Stacher G, *et al.* Cisapride versus placebo for 8 weeks on glycemic control and gastric emptying in insulin-dependent diabetes: a double blind cross-over trial. *J Clin Endocrinol Metab* 1999; **84:** 2357–62.

## Preparations

**Proprietary Preparations** (details are given in Part 3)

***Arg.:*** Cisap; Cispride; Digenormotil; Etacril; Fabrapride; Kinetizine; Prepulsid; Pulsar; Regalisa; ***Austral.:*** Prepulsid; ***Austria:*** Prepulsid; Pulsitil†; ***Belg.:*** Cyprid†; Prepulsid; ***Braz.:*** Cinetic†; Cisapan†; Cisatec†; Cispride†; Enteropride†; Prepulsid; ***Canad.:*** Prepulsid†; ***Chile:*** Gastrokin; Gastromet; Marovil; Ondax; Prepulsid; Tono-Cis; ***Denm.:*** Prepulsid; ***Fin.:*** Prepulsid; ***Fr.:*** Prepulsid; ***Ger.:*** Alimix†; Propulsin†; ***Gr.:*** Bozaktral; ***Hong Kong:*** Prepulsid; ***India:*** Alipride; Cisalone; ***Irl.:*** Prepulsid; ***Israel:*** Prepulsid; ***Ital.:*** Alimix†; Cipril†; Prepulsid†; ***Mex.:*** Enteropride; Eriken; Kinestase; Prepulsid; Presistin; Sapriken; Unamol; ***Neth.:*** Prepulsid; ***Norw.:*** Prepulsid; ***NZ:*** Prepulsid; ***Port.:*** Prepulsid; ***S.Afr.:*** Prepulsid; ***Singapore:*** Prepulsid†; ***Spain:*** Arcasin; Fisiogastrol; Kelosal; Kinet†; Prepulsid; Trautil†; ***Swed.:*** Prepulsid; ***Switz.:*** Prepulsid; ***Thai.:*** Cipasid; Cipride; Cisapin; Esorid; Metison; Palcid; Prepulsid; Pri-De-Sid†; ***UAE:*** Prokinate†; ***UK:*** Prepulsid†; ***USA:*** Propulsid†.

**Multi-ingredient: *Arg.:*** Digenormotil Plus; Gastrimet; Gastrimet Enzimatico; Pulsar Enzimatico; Pulsar Plus.

---

## Clebopride *(BAN, USAN, rINN)*

LAS-9273. 4-Amino-*N*-(1-benzyl-4-piperidyl)-5-chloro-*o*-anisamide.

$C_{20}H_{24}ClN_3O_2$ = 373.9.
*CAS — 55905-53-8.*
*ATC — A03FA06.*

## Clebopride Malate *(BANM, rINNM)*

Clebopridi Malas; Malato de cleboprida.

$C_{20}H_{24}ClN_3O_2,C_4H_6O_5$ = 508.0.
*CAS — 57645-91-7.*
*ATC — A03FA06.*

**Pharmacopoeias.** In *Eur.* (see p.vi).

**Ph. Eur. 5.0** (Clebopride Malate). A white or almost white, crystalline powder. Sparingly soluble in water and in methyl alcohol; slightly soluble in dehydrated alcohol; practically insoluble in dichloromethane. The pH of a 1% solution in water is 3.8 to 4.2. Protect from light.

## Profile

Clebopride is a substituted benzamide similar to metoclopramide (p.1274), that is used for its antiemetic and prokinetic actions in nausea and vomiting (p.1245) and various other gastrointestinal disorders. It is given as the malate but doses are expressed in terms of the base. Clebopride malate 679 micrograms is approximately equivalent to clebopride 500 micrograms.

Clebopride malate is given in a usual dose equivalent to clebopride 0.5 mg by mouth three times daily before meals or 0.5 to 1 mg by intramuscular or intravenous injection for acute symptoms. Adolescents aged 12 to 20 years may be given 0.25 mg by mouth three times daily; an oral dose of 15 to 20 micrograms/kg daily in 3 divided doses has been recommended for children.

## Preparations

**Proprietary Preparations** (details are given in Part 3)

***Arg.:*** Gastridin; ***Ital.:*** Motilex; ***Port.:*** Clebofex; Clebutec; ***Spain:*** Clanzol†; Cleboril; Maduraset†.

**Multi-ingredient: *Arg.:*** Eudon; Gastridin-E; ***Spain:*** Clanzoflat; Flatoril.

---

## Colocynth

Bitter Apple; Bitter Cucumber; Colocinto; Colocynth Pulp; Colocynthis; Coloquinte; Coloquintidas; Koloquinthen.

NOTE. The synonym Bitter Apple has also been applied to the fruits of *Solanum incanum*.

## Profile

Colocynth is the dried pulp of the fruit of *Citrullus colocynthis* (Cucurbitaceae). It has a drastic purgative and irritant action and has been superseded by less toxic laxatives. Colocynth is used in homoeopathic medicine.

---

## Dantron *(BAN, rINN)*

Antrapurol; Chrysazin; Danthron; Dantrón; Dianthon; Dioxyanthrachinonum. 1,8-Dihydroxyanthraquinone.

$C_{14}H_8O_4$ = 240.2.

*CAS — 117-10-2.*

*ATC — A06AB03.*

NOTE. Compounded preparations of dantron may be represented by the following names:

- Co-danthramer *x/y* (*BAN*)—where *x* and *y* are the strengths in milligrams of dantron and poloxamer respectively
- Co-danthrusate (*BAN*)—dantron 5 parts and docusate sodium 6 parts (w/w).

**Pharmacopoeias.** In *Br.*

**BP 2003** (Dantron). An orange, odourless or almost odourless, crystalline powder. Practically insoluble in water; very slightly soluble in alcohol; soluble in chloroform; slightly soluble in ether; dissolves in solutions of alkali hydroxides.

### Adverse Effects and Precautions

As for Senna, p.1288. Dantron may colour the urine pink or red. Discoloration and superficial sloughing of perianal skin can occur after prolonged contact, therefore dantron should not be used in infants wearing nappies (diapers) and should be used with caution in incontinent patients. The mucosa of the large intestine may be discoloured with prolonged use or high dosage.

In *rodents*, dantron has been associated with the development of intestinal and liver tumours. Consequently, its use has been restricted, see below.

◊ References to adverse effects occurring with dantron-containing laxatives include individual cases of leucopenia with liver damage,[1] greyish-blue skin discoloration,[2] and orange vaginal discharge.[3] There has also been a report of intestinal sarcoma in an 18-year-old girl with a history of prolonged use of a dantron-containing laxative.[4] In May 2000 the UK Committee on Safety of Medicines restricted the use of dantron to terminally ill patients on the grounds that pre-clinical evidence had increased and dantron was now established as a potential human carcinogen.[5]


1. Tolman KG, *et al.* Possible hepatotoxicity of Doxidan. *Ann Intern Med* 1976; **84:** 290–2.
2. Darke CS, Cooper RG. Unusual case of skin discoloration. *BMJ* 1978; **1:** 1188–9.
3. Greer IA. Orange periods. *BMJ* 1984; **289:** 323.
4. Patel PM, *et al.* Anthraquinone laxatives and human cancer: an association in one case. *Postgrad Med J* 1989; **65:** 216–17.
5. Committee on Safety of Medicines/Medicine Control Agency. Danthron restricted to constipation in the terminally ill. *Current Problems* 2000; **26:** 4. Also available at: http://www.mca.gov.uk/ourwork/monitorsafequalmed/currentproblems/cpmay2000.pdf (accessed 07/05/04)


**Breast feeding.** The American Academy of Pediatrics[1] state that, although usually compatible with breast feeding, use of dantron by breast-feeding mothers has been reported to cause increased bowel activity in the infant.


1. American Academy of Pediatrics. The transfer of drugs and other chemicals into human milk. *Pediatrics* 2001; **108:** 776–89. Correction. *ibid.*; 1029. Also available at: http://aappolicy.aappublications.org/cgi/content/full/pediatrics%3b108/3/776 (accessed 07/05/04)


### Pharmacokinetics

Dantron is metabolised by bacteria in the colon. Dantron or its metabolites are absorbed from the gastrointestinal tract, as indicated by discoloration of urine in some patients. Dantron or its metabolites are excreted in the faeces and the urine, and also in other secretions including breast milk.

### Uses and Administration

Dantron is an anthraquinone stimulant laxative, but unlike senna (p.1288), it is not a glycoside. It is given by mouth to treat constipation (p.1240) and is effective within 6 to 12 hours. However, because of concern over *rodent* carcinogenicity it has been withdrawn in some countries, and its use restricted in others. In the UK, it may be used only in terminally ill patients.

Dantron is given in doses of 25 to 75 mg when given with poloxamer 188 (p.1414) as co-danthramer, and in doses of 50 to 150 mg when given with docusate sodium (p.1262) as co-danthrusate. Doses are usually given at bedtime. Children have been given dantron 12.5 to 25 mg as co-danthramer or, in those aged 6 to 12 years, 50 mg as co-danthrusate.

### Preparations

***BP 2003:*** Co-danthrusate Capsules.

**Proprietary Preparations** (details are given in Part 3)

**Multi-ingredient:** ***Braz.:*** Fenogar†; Perlax†; ***Canad.:*** Doss†; Regulex-D†; ***Chile:*** Modane; ***Irl.:*** Ailax; Codalax; Cotron; ***Mex.:*** Modaton; ***NZ:*** Codalax; Conthram; ***UK:*** Ailax†; Capsuvac; Codalax; Danlax; Normax.

---

## Difenidol Hydrochloride *(BANM, rINNM)*

Diphenidol Hydrochloride *(USAN)*; Hidrocloruro de difenidol; SKF-478 (difenidol); SKF-478-A; SKF-478-J (difenidol embonate). 1,1-Diphenyl-4-piperidinobutan-1-ol hydrochloride.

$C_{21}H_{27}NO,HCl$ = 345.9.

*CAS — 972-02-1 (difenidol); 3254-89-5 (difenidol hydrochloride); 26363-46-2 (difenidol embonate).*

**Pharmacopoeias.** In *Chin.* and *Jpn.*

### Profile

Difenidol hydrochloride is an antiemetic that probably acts through the chemoreceptor trigger zone. It is claimed to control vertigo by means of a specific effect on the vestibular apparatus. Difenidol also has a weak peripheral antimuscarinic action.

It has been used in the treatment of some forms of nausea and vomiting (p.1245) such as those associated with surgery, radiotherapy, and cancer chemotherapy. It has also been used for the symptomatic treatment of vertigo (p.423), nausea and vomiting due to Ménière's disease (p.422), and other labyrinthine disturbances.

It has been given in doses equivalent to 25 to 50 mg of difenidol by mouth every 4 hours as required. Difenidol hydrochloride has also been given parenterally.

### Preparations

**Proprietary Preparations** (details are given in Part 3)

***Braz.:*** Vontrol; ***Chile:*** Vontrol; ***Hong Kong:*** Cephadol; ***Jpn:*** Cephadol; ***Malaysia:*** Cephadol; ***Mex.:*** Biomitin; Dicavin†; Hemetiken†; Laudefen†; Nautrol†; Normavom; Normitrol†; Serratol; Vernausin†; Vontrol; ***Singapore:*** Cephadol; ***Thai.:*** Cephadol.

---

## Difenoxin *(BAN, USAN)*

Difenoxilic Acid; Diphenoxylic Acid; McN-JR-15403-11. 1-(3-Cyano-3,3-diphenylpropyl)-4-phenylpiperidine-4-carboxylic acid.

$C_{28}H_{28}N_2O_2$ = 424.5.

*CAS — 28782-42-5.*

*ATC — A07DA04.*

## Difenoxin Hydrochloride *(BANM, rINNM)*

Difenoxylic Acid Hydrochloride; Diphenoxylic Acid Hydrochloride; Hidrocloruro de difenoxina; R-15403.

$C_{28}H_{28}N_2O_2,HCl$ = 461.0.

*CAS — 35607-36-4.*

*ATC — A07DA04.*

### Profile

Difenoxin is the principal active metabolite of diphenoxylate (p.1261) and has similar actions and uses. It is given by mouth as the hydrochloride, but doses are in terms of the base; difenoxin hydrochloride 1.1 mg is approximately equivalent to 1 mg of difenoxin.

In the treatment of diarrhoea (p.1241), the usual dose in adults is the equivalent of difenoxin 2 mg initially, followed by 1 mg after each loose stool or every 3 to 4 hours as required, up to a maximum of 8 mg daily.

Preparations of difenoxin usually contain subclinical amounts of atropine sulfate in an attempt to discourage abuse.

### Preparations

**Proprietary Preparations** (details are given in Part 3)

***USA:*** Motofen.

---

## Dihydroxyaluminum Sodium Carbonate

Aluminium Sodium Carbonate Hydroxide; Carbaldrate; Carbonato sódico de dihidroxialuminio; Dihydroxyaluminium Sodium Carbonate. Sodium (carbonato)dihydroxyaluminate(1-).

$CH_2AlNaO_5$ = 144.0.

*CAS — 12011-77-7; 16482-55-6.*

**Pharmacopoeias.** In *US.*

**USP 27** (Dihydroxyaluminum Sodium Carbonate). A fine white odourless powder. It loses not more than 14.5% of its weight on drying. Practically insoluble in water and in organic solvents; soluble in dilute mineral acids with the evolution of carbon dioxide. A 4% suspension in water has a pH of 9.9 to 10.2. Store in airtight containers.

### Profile

Dihydroxyaluminum sodium carbonate is an antacid with general properties similar to aluminium hydroxide (p.1249) that is given in doses of about 300 to 600 mg by mouth.

### Preparations

***USP 27:*** Dihydroxyaluminum Sodium Carbonate Tablets.

**Proprietary Preparations** (details are given in Part 3)

***Austria:*** Antacidum; ***Denm.:*** Noacid; ***Ger.:*** Kompensan; ***Port.:*** Kompensan; ***Switz.:*** Kompensan.

**Multi-ingredient:** ***Ger.:*** Kompensan-S; ***Port.:*** Kompensan-S.

---

## Diisopromine Hydrochloride *(rINNM)*

Di-isopromine Hydrochloride; Hidrocloruro de diisopromina. *NN*-Di-isopropyl-3,3-diphenylpropylamine hydrochloride.

$C_{21}H_{29}N,HCl$ = 331.9.

*CAS — 5966-41-6 (diisopromine); 24358-65-4 (diisopromine hydrochloride).*

*ATC — A03AX02.*

### Profile

Diisopromine hydrochloride is an antispasmodic used with sorbitol in various gastrointestinal disorders.

### Preparations

**Proprietary Preparations** (details are given in Part 3)

**Multi-ingredient:** ***Belg.:*** Bilagol†; ***Braz.:*** Biliflux; ***Fr.:*** Megabyl†; ***S.Afr.:*** Agofell.

---

## Diphenoxylate Hydrochloride

*(BANM, rINNM)*

Diphenoxylati Hydrochloridum; Hidrocloruro de difenoxilato; R-1132. Ethyl 1-(3-cyano-3,3-diphenylpropyl)-4-phenylpiperidine-4-carboxylate hydrochloride.

$C_{30}H_{32}N_2O_2,HCl$ = 489.0.

*CAS — 915-30-0 (diphenoxylate); 3810-80-8 (diphenoxylate hydrochloride).*

*ATC — A07DA01.*

NOTE. Compounded preparations of diphenoxylate hydrochloride may be represented by the following names:

- Co-phenotrope (*BAN*)—diphenoxylate hydrochloride 100 parts and atropine sulfate 1 part (w/w).

**Pharmacopoeias.** In *Chin., Eur.* (see p.vi), *Int.*, and *US.*

**Ph. Eur. 5.0** (Diphenoxylate Hydrochloride). A white or almost white, crystalline powder. Very slightly soluble in water; sparingly soluble in alcohol; freely soluble in dichloromethane. Protect from light.

**USP 27** (Diphenoxylate Hydrochloride). A white odourless crystalline powder. Slightly soluble in water and in isopropyl alcohol; sparingly soluble in alcohol and in acetone; freely soluble in chloroform; practically insoluble in ether and in petroleum spirit; soluble in methyl alcohol. A saturated solution in water has a pH of about 3.3.

### Dependence and Withdrawal

Preparations of diphenoxylate usually contain subclinical amounts of atropine sulfate in an attempt to discourage abuse. Short-term administration of diphenoxylate with atropine in the recommended dosage carries a negligible risk of dependence, although prolonged use or use of high doses may produce dependence of the morphine type (see p.71).

### Adverse Effects and Treatment

Diphenoxylate is related to the opioid analgesics (p.72), and its adverse effects and their treatment are similar, particularly in overdosage. Reported side-effects include: gastrointestinal effects such as anorexia, nausea and vomiting, abdominal distension or discomfort, paralytic ileus, toxic megacolon, and pancreatitis; nervous system effects such as headache, drowsiness, dizziness, restlessness, euphoria, depression, numbness of the extremities; and hypersensitivity reactions including angioedema, urticaria, pruritus, and swelling of the gums. Signs of overdosage may be delayed and patients should be observed for at least 48 hours. Young children are particularly susceptible to the effects of overdosage.

The presence of subclinical doses of atropine sulfate in preparations containing diphenoxylate may give rise to the side-effects of atropine in susceptible individuals or in overdosage—see Atropine Sulfate, p.477.

### Precautions

Diphenoxylate hydrochloride should be avoided in patients with jaundice, intestinal obstruction, antibiotic-associated colitis, or diarrhoea associated with enterotoxin-producing bacteria, and should be used with caution in patients with hepatic impairment. It should also be used with caution in young children because of a greater variability of response in this age group, and is not generally recommended for use in infants. Patients with inflammatory bowel disease receiving diphenoxylate should be carefully observed for signs of toxic megacolon and diphenoxylate discontinued promptly should abdominal distention occur.

### Interactions

Because of the structural relationship of diphenoxylate to pethidine there is a theoretical risk of hypertensive crisis if diphenoxylate is used with MAOIs. Diphenoxylate may potentiate the effects of other CNS depressants such as alcohol, barbiturates, and some anxiolytics.

### Pharmacokinetics

Diphenoxylate hydrochloride is well absorbed from the gastrointestinal tract. It is rapidly and extensively metabolised in the liver principally to diphenoxylic acid (difenoxin, p.1261), which has antidiarrhoeal activity; other metabolites include hydroxydiphenoxylic acid. It is excreted mainly as metabolites and their conjugates in the faeces; lesser amounts are excreted in urine. It may be distributed into breast milk.

### Uses and Administration

Diphenoxylate hydrochloride is a synthetic derivative of pethidine with little or no analgesic activity; it reduces intestinal motility and is used in the symptomatic treatment of acute and chronic diarrhoea (p.1241). It may also be used to reduce the frequency and fluidity of the stools in patients with colostomies or ileostomies.

In acute diarrhoea the usual initial dose for adults is 10 mg by mouth followed by 5 mg every six hours, later reduced as the diarrhoea is controlled. In the UK, diphenoxylate hydrochloride is not recommended for children under 4 years of age. Suggested initial doses for children are: 4 to 8 years, 2.5 mg three times daily; 9 to 12 years, 2.5 mg four times daily; over 12 years, 5 mg three times daily. In the USA, diphenoxylate is not recommended for children under the age of 2 years and an initial dose of 0.3 to 0.4 mg/kg (up to an effective maximum of 10 mg) daily in 4 divided doses is suggested for children aged 2 to 12 years. (For the view that antidiarrhoeal drugs should not be used at all in children, see p.1241.)

Similar initial doses are used for chronic diarrhoea, and subsequently reduced as necessary. If clinical improvement is not observed after 10 days' treatment with the maximum daily dose of 20 mg (in adults) further administration is unlikely to result in any benefit.

Preparations of diphenoxylate usually contain subclinical amounts of atropine sulfate in an attempt to discourage abuse.

**Substance dependence.** Diphenoxylate may be useful[1] in the symptomatic management of diarrhoea associated with opioid withdrawal syndromes (p.71).

1. DOH. *Drug misuse and dependence: guidelines on clinical management*. London: HMSO, 1999. Also available at: http://www.dh.gov.uk/assetRoot/04/07/81/98/04078198.pdf (accessed 07/05/04)

### Preparations

**USP 27:** Diphenoxylate Hydrochloride and Atropine Sulfate Oral Solution; Diphenoxylate Hydrochloride and Atropine Sulfate Tablets.

**Proprietary Preparations** (details are given in Part 3)

***Austral.:*** Lofenoxal; Lomotil; ***Belg.:*** Reasec†; ***Braz.:*** Lomotil; ***Canad.:*** Lomotil; ***Denm.:*** Retardin†; ***Fr.:*** Diarsed; ***Ger.:*** Reasec†; ***Hong Kong:*** Dhamotil; Lomotil; ***India:*** Lomotil; ***Irl.:*** Lomotil; ***Ital.:*** Reasec†; ***Malaysia:*** Atrotil; Beamotil; Dhamotil; Lomotil; Setmotil; ***NZ:*** Diastop; Lomotil; ***Port.:*** Lomotil; ***S.Afr.:*** Eldox†; Lomotil; ***Singapore:*** Dhamotil; Erlotyl†; Lomotil; Remodil; ***Switz.:*** Reasec†; ***Thai.:*** Dilomil; Ditropine†; Lomotil; ***UAE:*** Intard; ***UK:*** Dymotil; Lomotil; Lotharin†; Tropergen†; ***USA:*** Logen; Lomotil; Lonox.

**Multi-ingredient:** ***Braz.:*** Colestase; Magnostase†; ***India:*** Lomofen.

# Docusates

Docusatos.

## Docusate Calcium *(USAN)*

Dioctyl Calcium Sulfosuccinate; Dioctyl Calcium Sulphosuccinate; Docusato cálcico. Calcium 1,4-bis(2-ethylhexyl) sulphosuccinate.

$C_{40}H_{74}CaO_{14}S_2$ = 883.2.

*CAS — 128-49-4.*

**Pharmacopoeias.** In *US.*

**USP 27** (Docusate Calcium). A white amorphous solid with the characteristic odour of octil alcohol. Soluble 1 in 3300 of water; very soluble in alcohol, in macrogol 400, and in maize oil.

## Docusate Potassium *(USAN)*

Dioctyl Potassium Sulfosuccinate; Dioctyl Potassium Sulphosuccinate; Docusato potásico. Potassium 1,4-bis(2-ethylhexyl) sulphosuccinate.

$C_{20}H_{37}KO_7S$ = 460.7.

*CAS — 7491-09-0.*

**Pharmacopoeias.** In *US.*

**USP 27** (Docusate Potassium). A white amorphous solid with a characteristic odour suggestive of octil alcohol. Sparingly soluble in water; soluble in alcohol and in glycerol; very soluble in petroleum spirit.

## Docusate Sodium *(BAN, USAN, rINN)*

Dioctyl Sodium Sulfosuccinate; Dioctyl Sodium Sulphosuccinate; Docusato sódico; Docusatum Natricum; DSS; Natrii Docusas; Sodium Dioctyl Sulphosuccinate. Sodium 1,4-bis(2-ethylhexyl) sulphosuccinate.

$C_{20}H_{37}NaO_7S$ = 444.6.

*CAS — 577-11-7.*

*ATC — A06AA02.*

NOTE. Compounded preparations of docusate sodium may be represented by the following names:

- Co-danthrusate (*BAN*)—docusate sodium 6 parts and dantron 5 parts.

**Pharmacopoeias.** In *Eur.* (see p.vi) and *US.*

**Ph. Eur. 5.0** (Docusate Sodium). White or almost white, hygroscopic, waxy masses or flakes. Sparingly soluble in water; freely soluble in alcohol and in dichloromethane. Store in airtight containers.

**USP 27** (Docusate Sodium). A white wax-like plastic solid with a characteristic odour suggestive of octil alcohol. Slowly soluble 1 in 70 of water; freely soluble in alcohol and in glycerol; very soluble in petroleum spirit.

### Adverse Effects and Precautions

Adverse effects occur rarely with docusates; diarrhoea, nausea, abdominal cramps, and skin rash have been reported. Anorectal pain or bleeding have occasionally occurred following rectal administration.

Like all laxatives, docusates should not be used when intestinal obstruction or undiagnosed abdominal symptoms are present; prolonged use should be avoided. Docusate sodium should not be given rectally to patients with haemorrhoids or anal fissures.

Docusate sodium should not be used to soften ear wax when the ear is inflamed or the ear drum perforated.

**Pregnancy.** Hypomagnesaemia, manifested by jitteriness, in a neonate was considered to be secondary to maternal hypomagnesaemia caused by the use of docusate sodium by the mother during pregnancy.[1]

1. Schindler AM. Isolated neonatal hypomagnesaemia associated with maternal overuse of stool softener. *Lancet* 1984; **ii:** 822.

### Interactions

Docusates may enhance the gastrointestinal uptake of other drugs, such as liquid paraffin (which should not be given concomitantly). Dosage of anthraquinone laxatives may need to be reduced if used with docusates. It has also been suggested that concomitant administration of docusates and aspirin increases the incidence of adverse effects on the gastrointestinal mucosa.

### Pharmacokinetics

Docusate salts are absorbed from the gastrointestinal tract and excreted in bile. Docusate sodium is also distributed into breast milk.

### Uses and Administration

Docusates are administered as the calcium or sodium salt and are used as laxatives in the management of constipation (p.1240). They are also used as adjuncts for bowel evacuation before abdominal radiological procedures. Docusate potassium has also been used.

Docusates are anionic surfactants which have been considered to act primarily by increasing the penetration of fluid into the faeces, but may also have other effects on intestinal fluid secretion, and probably act both as stimulants and as faecal softening agents.

The usual daily dose by mouth of docusate calcium is 240 mg. Docusate sodium is given in usual doses of 50 to 300 mg daily in divided doses by mouth, although doses of up to 500 mg daily may be used. Suggested doses for children have been up to 120 mg daily. The effect is usually seen within 12 to 72 hours. When used as an adjunct to abdominal radiological procedures, a dose of 400 mg by mouth is given with the barium meal. It is also given rectally as an enema in doses of 50 to 120 mg; the effect is usually seen in 5 to 20 minutes. Docusate sodium is also used in combination with anthraquinone stimulant laxatives such as casanthranol (p.1255), dantron (p.1261), and senna (p.1288).

Docusate sodium is used for softening wax in the ear as ear drops containing 0.5 or 5%.

Docusate sodium and other docusate salts are widely used as anionic surfactants in pharmaceutical formulations.

**Ear wax removal.** Cerumen or ear wax is a normal secretion of the ceruminous glands present in the lining of the external auditory canal. Excessive accumulation or impaction of ear wax may decrease hearing acuity, and may also produce tinnitus and otalgia.

Syringing of the external auditory canal with warm water is the favoured method for removing wax from the ear; a suitable dispersing agent may be given as ear drops for 7 days beforehand.[1] Such agents may also be used alone for self-medication. Traditionally, a fixed oil such as olive oil or almond oil has been favoured;[1] other dispersing agents that have been reported as effective include docusates,[2] peroxides such as hydrogen peroxide or urea hydrogen peroxide,[3] choline salicylate,[4] and an oily solution of paradichlorobenzene and chlorobutanol.[4] Glycerol and sodium bicarbonate solution have also been used. However, a comparative study *in vitro* of the efficacy of various wax dispersing agents found the most effective to be water, which had originally been included as a control,[5] and a systematic review[6] concluded that saline or water ear drops seemed to be as good as proprietary agents for the removal of ear wax, although there was a lack of good quality trials on which to base recommendations.

1. Sharp JF, *et al.* Ear wax removal: a survey of current practice. *BMJ* 1990; **301:** 1251–3.
2. Chen DA, Caparosa RJ. A nonprescription cerumenolytic. *Am J Otol* 1991; **12:** 475–6.
3. Fahmey S, Whitefield M. Multicentre clinical trial of Exterol as a cerumenolytic. *Br J Clin Pract* 1982; **36:** 197–204.
4. Drummer DS, *et al.* A single-blind, randomized study to compare the efficacy of two ear drop preparations ('Audax' and 'Cerumol') in the softening of ear wax. *Curr Med Res Opin* 1992; **13:** 26–30.
5. Andaz C, Whittet HB. An in vitro study to determine efficacy of different wax-dispersing agents. *ORL J Otorhinolaryngol Relat Spec* 1993; **55:** 97–9.
6. Burton MJ, Dorée CJ. Ear drops for the removal of ear wax. Available in The Cochrane Library; Issue 1. Chichester: John Wiley; 2004.

### Preparations

***BP 2003:*** Co-danthrusate Capsules; Compound Docusate Enema; Docusate Capsules; Docusate Oral Solution; Paediatric Docusate Oral Solution;

***USP 27:*** Docusate Calcium Capsules; Docusate Potassium Capsules; Docusate Sodium Capsules; Docusate Sodium Solution; Docusate Sodium Syrup; Docusate Sodium Tablets; Ferrous Fumarate and Docusate Sodium Extended-release Tablets.

**Proprietary Preparations** (details are given in Part 3)

***Arg.:*** Cerumex; Otoclean Solucion de Limpieza; ***Austral.:*** Coloxyl; Rectalad; Waxsol; ***Belg.:*** Norgalax; ***Canad.:*** Calax; Colace; Colax-C†; Colax-S†; Correctol Stool Softener; Dioctyl†; Doxate-C†; Doxate-S†; Ex-Lax Stool Softener; Laxagel†; Regulex; Selax; Silace; Soflax; Surfak; ***Chile:*** Regal; ***Fr.:*** Jamylene; Norgalax; ***Ger.:*** Norgalax†; Otitex; Otowaxol; ***Hong Kong:*** Hisof†; Norgalax; Softon†; Waxsol; ***India:*** Desol; Laxicon; ***Irl.:*** Fletchers Enemette†; Norgalax; Waxsol; ***Israel:*** Docusoft†; ***Malaysia:*** Waxsol; ***Mex.:*** Correctol; ***Neth.:*** Norgalax; ***NZ:*** Coloxyl; Waxsol; ***S.Afr.:*** Waxsol NF; ***Singapore:*** Norgalax; Waxsol; ***Spain:*** Dama-Lax†; Tirolaxo†; ***Switz.:*** Norgalax; ***Thai.:*** Cusate; Dewax; Pedoc†; Waxsol; ***UK:*** Clear Ear; Dioctyl; Docusol; Fletchers Enemette; Molcer; Norgalax; Waxsol; ***USA:*** Colace; D-S-S; DC Softgels; Dioeze†; Docusoft; DOK; DOS Softgel; Ex-Lax Stool Softener; Modane Soft†; Pro-Cal-Soft†; Regulax SS; Silace; Surfak.

**Multi-ingredient:** ***Arg.:*** Nigalax; ***Austral.:*** Chemists Own Natural Laxative with Softener; Coloxyl; Coloxyl with Senna; Sennesoft; ***Austria:*** Purigoa; Yal; ***Belg.:*** Laxavit; Softene; ***Braz.:*** Dioctosal†; Humectol†; Ventre Livre; ***Canad.:*** Calcium Docuphen†; Doss†; Doxidan†; Ex-Lax Gentle Strength; Ex-Lax Light†; Fruitatives; Peri-Colace; Phillips Gelcaps†; Regulex-D†; Senokot-S; ***Denm.:*** Analka; Glyoktyl; Klyx; ***Fin.:*** Klyx; ***Fr.:*** Neo-Boldolaxine†; ***Ger.:*** Norgalax Miniklistier; Yal; ***Gr.:*** Florisan; ***Hong Kong:*** Softon Plus†; ***India:*** Hepasules; Pursennid-In; ***Israel:*** Migraleve; ***Ital.:*** Macrolax; Sorbiclis; ***Mex.:*** Clyss-Go; ***Norw.:*** Klyx; ***NZ:*** Coloxyl; Coloxyl with Senna; Laxsol; ***Port.:*** Clyss-Go; ***Spain:*** Boldolaxin; Laxvital; Migraleve; ***Swed.:*** Emulax; Klyx; ***Switz.:*** Elle-care†; Klyx Magnum; Tavolax†; Yal; ***Thai.:*** Bisolax; Hemorhin; ***UK:*** Capsuvac; Normax; ***USA:*** Docusoft Plus; Doxidan†; Ex-Lax Extra Gentle Pills†; Ex-Lax Gentle Strength; Genasoft Plus Softgels†; Laxative & Stool Softener; Peri-Colace†; Peri-Dos Softgels†; Senokot-S; Silace-C†; Therevac Plus; Therevac SB; X-Prep Bowel Evacuant Kit-1.

*Used as an adjunct in:* ***Hong Kong:*** Ferosoft†; ***Spain:*** Glutaferro; ***USA:*** Anemagen OB; Ferro-Dok; Hem Fe; Hemaspan; Natal Extra; Nephron FA; Obstetrix; Prenatal; TriHEMIC; Vinate GT.

# Dolasetron Mesilate *(BANM, rINNM)*

Dolasetron Mesylate *(USAN)*; MDL-73147EF (dolasetron or dolasetron mesilate); Mesilato de dolasetrón. (6R,8r,9aS)-3-Oxoperhydro-2*H*-2,6-methanoquinolizin-8-yl indole-3-carboxylate methanesulphonate.

$C_{19}H_{20}N_2O_3,CH_4O_3S$ = 420.5.

*CAS — 115956-12-2 (dolasetron); 115956-13-3 (dolasetron mesilate).*

*ATC — A04AA04.*

**Pharmacopoeias.** In *US.*

**USP 27** (Dolasetron Mesylate). A white to off-white powder. Freely soluble in water and in propylene glycol; slightly soluble in alcohol and in sodium chloride 0.9%. Protect from light.

### Adverse Effects and Precautions

As for Ondansetron, p.1281. Diarrhoea and abdominal pain may also occur. Various ECG changes have been noted with dolasetron. Dolasetron should be used with caution in patients who have or may develop prolongation of the QT interval, or other alterations in cardiac conduction intervals. No dosage reduction is considered necessary in renal or hepatic impairment, despite possible reductions in clearance.

**Effects on the cardiovascular system.** References.


1. Benedict CR, *et al.* Single-blind study of the effects of intravenous dolasetron mesylate versus ondansetron on electrocardiographic parameters in normal volunteers. *J Cardiovasc Pharmacol* 1996; **28:** 53–9.


## Interactions

Plasma concentrations of hydrodolasetron, the active metabolite of dolasetron, are increased by cimetidine and atenolol and decreased by rifampicin. Dolasetron should be used with caution in patients taking drugs that prolong the QT interval.

## Pharmacokinetics

Dolasetron given by mouth and intravenously is rapidly converted to the active metabolite hydrodolasetron by carbonyl reductase, a ubiquitous enzyme. Peak plasma concentrations of hydrodolasetron occur 1 hour after oral, and 0.6 hours after intravenous, dolasetron administration. The apparent oral bioavailability of dolasetron determined as hydrodolasetron is about 75%. It has a mean elimination half-life of about 7 to 8 hours.

Some hydrodolasetron is metabolised by cytochrome P450 isoenzymes CYP2D6 and CYP3A, while about 50 to 60% is eliminated unchanged in the urine. Two thirds of a dose of dolasetron is recovered in the urine and one third in the faeces.

Clearance of hydrodolasetron is increased in children, but is not altered in the elderly. Clearance is reduced in severe hepatic and severe renal impairment.

◊ References.


1. Lerman J, *et al.* Pharmacokinetics of the active metabolite (MDL 74,156) of dolasetron mesylate after oral or intravenous administration to anesthetized children. *Clin Pharmacol Ther* 1996; **60:** 485–92.
2. Dempsey E, *et al.* Pharmacokinetics of single intravenous and oral doses of dolasetron mesylate in healthy elderly volunteers. *J Clin Pharmacol* 1996; **36:** 903–10.
3. Stubbs K, *et al.* Pharmacokinetics of dolasetron after oral and intravenous administration of dolasetron mesylate in healthy volunteers and patients with hepatic dysfunction. *J Clin Pharmacol* 1997; **37:** 926–36.
4. Dimmitt DC, *et al.* Pharmacokinetics of oral and intravenous dolasetron mesylate in patients with renal impairment. *J Clin Pharmacol* 1998; **38:** 798–806.
5. Dimmitt DC, *et al.* Effect of infusion rate on the pharmacokinetics and tolerance of intravenous dolasetron mesylate. *Ann Pharmacother* 1998; **32:** 39–44.


## Uses and Administration

Dolasetron is a 5-$HT_3$ antagonist with antiemetic actions similar to those of ondansetron (see p.1281). It is used as the mesilate in the prevention of nausea and vomiting (p.1245) associated with chemotherapy, and in the prevention and treatment of postoperative nausea and vomiting.

For *prevention* of acute **nausea and vomiting** associated with **chemotherapy** dolasetron mesilate may be given by mouth in a dose of 100 mg (in the USA) or 200 mg (in most other countries including the UK) within 1 hour before treatment. Alternatively, it may be given in a dose of 1.8 mg/kg, or 100 mg, by intravenous injection at a rate of up to 100 mg over 30 seconds about 30 minutes before chemotherapy; the same dose may be diluted to 50 mL with a suitable infusion solution and given intravenously over up to 15 minutes. To protect against delayed emesis, a further dose of dolasetron mesilate 200 mg orally once daily may be given; in Europe and the UK dolasetron may not normally be given for more than 4 consecutive days per chemotherapy cycle although some countries permit use for up to 7 days.

When given for the *prevention* of **postoperative** nausea and vomiting the recommended dose is usually 50 mg of dolasetron mesilate by mouth before induction of anaesthesia or 12.5 mg intravenously at the end of anaesthesia. In the USA, it is given in a dose of 100 mg of dolasetron mesilate by mouth within 2 hours before surgery, or 12.5 mg intravenously approximately 15 minutes before the end of anaesthesia. The same intravenous dose may be given for the *treatment* of postoperative nausea and vomiting.

**Children** over 2 years of age may be given dolasetron mesilate 1.8 mg/kg orally (within 1 hour before chemotherapy) or intravenously (about 30 minutes before chemotherapy), up to a maximum dose of 100 mg, to prevent acute chemotherapy-induced nausea and vomiting. For prevention of postoperative nausea and vomiting, 1.2 mg/kg by mouth, up to a maximum of 100 mg, may be given within 2 hours before surgery; or 350 micrograms/kg, up to a maximum of 12.5 mg, may be given intravenously 15 minutes before the end of anaesthesia. The same intravenous dose may be given to treat established postoperative nausea and vomiting.

◊ Reviews.


1. Balfour JA, Goa KL. Dolasetron: a review of its pharmacology and therapeutic potential in the management of nausea and vomiting induced by chemotherapy, radiotherapy or surgery. *Drugs* 1997; **54:** 273–98.
2. Anonymous. Dolasetron for prevention of nausea and vomiting due to cancer chemotherapy. *Med Lett Drug Ther* 1998; **40:** 53–4.


## Preparations

***USP 27:*** Dolasetron Mesylate Injection; Dolasetron Mesylate Tablets.

**Proprietary Preparations** (details are given in Part 3)
***Arg.:*** Anzemet; ***Austral.:*** Anzemet; ***Austria:*** Anzemet; ***Braz.:*** Anzemet; ***Canad.:*** Anzemet; ***Fin.:*** Anzemet; ***Fr.:*** Anzemet; ***Ger.:*** Anemet; ***Gr.:*** Anzemet; ***Ital.:*** Anzemet; ***Mex.:*** Anzemet; ***S.Afr.:*** Zamanon; ***Switz.:*** Anzemet; ***UK:*** Anzemet; ***USA:*** Anzemet.

---

# Domperidone *(BAN, USAN, rINN)*

Domperidona; Domperidonum; R-33812. 5-Chloro-1-{1-[3-(2-oxobenzimidazolin-1-yl)propyl]-4-piperidyl}benzimidazolin-2-one.

$C_{22}H_{24}ClN_5O_2$ = 425.9.
*CAS — 57808-66-9.*
*ATC — A03FA03.*

**Pharmacopoeias.** In *Eur.* (see p.vi).

**Ph. Eur. 5.0** (Domperidone). A white or almost white powder. Practically insoluble in water; slightly soluble in alcohol and in methyl alcohol; soluble in dimethylformamide. Protect from light.

## Domperidone Maleate *(BANM, rINNM)*

Domperidoni Maleas; Maleato de domperidona.

$C_{22}H_{24}ClN_5O_2,C_4H_4O_4$ = 542.0.
*CAS — 99497-03-7.*
*ATC — A03FA03.*

**Pharmacopoeias.** In *Eur.* (see p.vi).

**Ph. Eur. 5.0** (Domperidone Maleate). A white or almost white powder; it exhibits polymorphism. Very slightly soluble in water and in alcohol; sparingly soluble in dimethylformamide; slightly soluble in methyl alcohol. Protect from light.

## Adverse Effects

Plasma-prolactin concentrations may be increased, which may lead to galactorrhoea or gynaecomastia. There have been reports of reduced libido, and rashes and other allergic reactions. Domperidone does not readily cross the blood-brain barrier and the incidence of central effects such as extrapyramidal reactions or drowsiness may be lower than with metoclopramide (p.1274); however, there have been reports of dystonic reactions.

Domperidone by injection has been associated with convulsions, arrhythmias, and cardiac arrest. Fatalities have restricted administration by this route.

**Effects on the cardiovascular system.** Sudden death has occurred in cancer patients given domperidone intravenously in high doses.[1-3] Four cancer patients experienced cardiac arrest after high intravenous doses[4] and 2 of 4 similar patients had ventricular arrhythmias.[5] After such reports the manufacturers withdrew the injection from general use in the UK.


1. Joss RA, *et al.* Sudden death in cancer patient on high-dose domperidone. *Lancet* 1982; **i:** 1019.
2. Giaccone G, *et al.* Two sudden deaths during prophylactic antiemetic treatment with high doses of domperidone and methylprednisolone. *Lancet* 1984; **ii:** 1336–7.
3. Weaving A, *et al.* Seizures after antiemetic treatment with high dose domperidone: report of four cases. *BMJ* 1984; **288:** 1728.
4. Roussak JB, *et al.* Cardiac arrest after treatment with intravenous domperidone. *BMJ* 1984; **289:** 1579.
5. Osborne RJ, *et al.* Cardiotoxicity of intravenous domperidone. *Lancet* 1985; **ii:** 385.


**Effects on the endocrine system.** Reports of galactorrhoea with gynaecomastia[1] or mastalgia[2,3] generally associated with raised serum-prolactin concentrations. Gynaecomastia without galactorrhoea has also been reported.[4]


1. Van der Steen M, *et al.* Gynaecomastia in a male infant given domperidone. *Lancet* 1982; **ii:** 884–5.
2. Cann PA, *et al.* Galactorrhoea as side effect of domperidone. *BMJ* 1983; **286:** 1395–6.
3. Cann PA, *et al.* Oral domperidone: double blind comparison with placebo in irritable bowel syndrome. *Gut* 1983; **24:** 1135–40.
4. Keating JP, Rees M. Gynaecomastia after long-term administration of domperidone. *Postgrad Med J* 1991; **67:** 401–2.


**Extrapyramidal effects.** Reports of extrapyramidal symptoms, including acute dystonic reactions, in individual patients given domperidone.


1. Sol P, *et al.* Extrapyramidal reactions due to domperidone. *Lancet* 1980; **ii:** 802.
2. Debontridder O. Extrapyramidal reactions due to domperidone. *Lancet* 1980; **ii:** 802. Correction, *ibid.*; 1259.
3. Casteels-Van Daele M, *et al.* Refusal of further cancer chemotherapy due to antiemetic drug. *Lancet* 1984; **i:** 57.


## Precautions

Domperidone is not recommended for chronic use or for the routine prophylaxis of postoperative nausea and vomiting. Domperidone should be used with great caution if given intravenously, because of the risk of arrhythmias, especially in patients predisposed to cardiac arrhythmias or hypokalaemia.

**Breast feeding.** No adverse effects have been observed in breast-fed infants whose mothers were receiving domperidone, and the American Academy of Pediatrics considers[1] that it is therefore usually compatible with breast feeding. However, the FDA in the USA has issued a warning against the use of domperidone to increase milk production because of the possibility of serious adverse effects.[2]


1. American Academy of Pediatrics. The transfer of drugs and other chemicals into human milk. *Pediatrics* 2001; **108:** 776–89. Correction. *ibid.*; 1029. Also available at: http://aappolicy.aappublications.org/cgi/content/full/pediatrics%3b108/3/776 (accessed 07/05/04)
2. FDA. FDA warns against women using unapproved drug, domperidone, to increase milk production (June 7, 2004). Available at: http://www.fda.gov/bbs/topics/ANSWERS/2004/ANS01292.html (accessed 30/06/04)


## Interactions

As with other dopamine antagonists (see Metoclopramide, p.1275), there is a theoretical potential that domperidone may antagonise the hypoprolactinaemic effect of drugs such as bromocriptine. In addition, the prokinetic effects of domperidone may alter the absorption of some drugs. Opioid analgesics and antimuscarinics may antagonise the prokinetic effects of domperidone.

## Pharmacokinetics

The systemic bioavailability of domperidone is only about 15% in fasting subjects given a dose by mouth, although this is increased when domperidone is given after food. The low bioavailability is thought to be due to first-pass hepatic and intestinal metabolism. The bioavailability of rectal domperidone is similar to that following oral administration, although peak plasma concentrations are only achieved after about an hour, compared with 30 minutes after a dose by mouth.

Domperidone is more than 90% bound to plasma proteins, and has a terminal elimination half-life of about 7.5 hours. It is chiefly cleared from the blood by extensive metabolism. About 30% of an oral dose is excreted in urine within 24 hours, almost entirely as metabolites; the remainder of a dose is excreted in faeces over several days, about 10% as unchanged drug. It does not readily cross the blood-brain barrier.

Small amounts of domperidone are distributed into breast milk, reaching concentrations about one-quarter of those in maternal serum.

## Uses and Administration

Domperidone is a dopamine antagonist with actions and uses similar to those of metoclopramide (p.1276). It is used as an antiemetic for the short-term treatment of nausea and vomiting of various aetiologies (p.1245). It is not considered suitable for chronic nausea and vomiting, nor for the routine prophylaxis of postoperative vomiting.

Domperidone is also used for its prokinetic actions in dyspepsia (p.1242) and has been tried in diabetic gastroparesis (see Diabetic Complications, p.326). It is given with paracetamol in the symptomatic treatment of migraine (p.464).

Domperidone is used as the maleate in tablet preparations and as the base in suppositories and the oral suspension; doses are expressed in terms of the base. Domperidone maleate 12.73 mg is approximately equivalent to 10 mg domperidone. Domperidone has been given parenterally, but this route has been associated with severe adverse effects (see above).

For the treatment of **nausea and vomiting** domperidone may be given by mouth in doses of 10 to 20 mg three or four times daily up to a maximum daily dose of 80 mg or it may be given rectally in a dose of 60 mg twice daily. In children, doses of 250 to 500 micrograms/kg may be given by mouth three to four times daily, up to a maximum daily dose of 2.4 mg/kg and should not exceed a total of 80 mg daily. Alternatively, children weighing more than 15 kg may be given a rectal dose of 30 mg twice daily.

For the symptomatic treatment of non-ulcer **dyspepsia**, adults may be given 10 mg by mouth 3 times daily before meals and at night. Depending on clinical response the dose may be increased to 20 mg if necessary. A course of treatment should not normally exceed 2 weeks. In **migraine**, a dose of 20 mg by mouth may be taken up to every 4 hours, in combination with paracetamol, as required, up to a maximum of 4 doses in 24 hours.

◊ Reviews.


1. Prakash A, Wagstaff AJ. Domperidone: a review of its use in diabetic gastropathy. *Drugs* 1998; **56:** 429–45.
2. Barone JA. Domperidone: a peripherally acting dopamine$_2$-receptor antagonist. *Ann Pharmacother* 1999; **33:** 429–40.


**Parkinsonism.** Domperidone is used to control gastrointestinal effects of dopaminergic drugs given in the management of parkinsonism (p.1196). It may be of use in those patients who experience peripheral effects with levodopa despite the use of peripheral dopa-decarboxylase inhibitors and for patients using dopamine agonists such as bromocriptine or apomorphine since peripheral dopa-decarboxylase inhibitors are ineffective for preventing the peripheral effects of these drugs. Although domperidone does not readily cross the blood-brain barrier there have been isolated reports of extrapyramidal effects associated with its use (see above). Consequently there has been concern over its potential to produce central effects and some consider that domperidone should only be used in patients with parkinsonism when safer antiemetic measures have failed.[1,2] However, this view has been contested both by the manufacturers and other workers.[3,4] In a subsequent review of the use of domperidone in Parkinson's disease it was considered[5] that domperidone might produce central blockade of the therapeutic effects of levodopa if given at a high oral dosage such as 120 mg daily for prolonged periods but also noted that such high doses were rarely required to control levodopa-induced vomiting.


1. Leeser J, Bateman DN. Domperidone. *BMJ* 1985; **290:** 241.
2. Bateman DN. Domperidone. *BMJ* 1985; **290:** 1079.
3. Lake-Bakaar G, Cameron HA. Domperidone. *BMJ* 1985; **290:** 241–2.
4. Critchley P, *et al.* Domperidone. *BMJ* 1985; **290:** 788.
5. Parkes JD. Domperidone and Parkinson's disease. *Clin Neuropharmacol* 1986; **9:** 517–32.


### Preparations

**BP 2003:** Domperidone Tablets.

**Proprietary Preparations** (details are given in Part 3)
***Arg.:*** Ecuamon; Euciton; Moperidona; Motilium; ***Austral.:*** Motilium; ***Austria:*** Motilium; ***Belg.:*** Motilium; Zilium; ***Braz.:*** Domperol†; Motilium; Peridal†; Pleiadon†; ***Canad.:*** Motilidone†; Motilium; ***Chile:*** Donegal; Dosin; Idon; Restol; ***Denm.:*** Motilium; ***Fr.:*** Motilium; Motilyo; Peridys; ***Ger.:*** Motilium; ***Gr.:*** Cilroton; ***Hong Kong:*** Costi; Dompeon; Motilium; Rabugen; ***India:*** Domstal; Nautigo; ***Irl.:*** Motilium; ***Israel:*** Motilium; ***Ital.:*** Digestivo Giuliani; Fobidon; Gastronorm; Mod†; Motilium; Peridon; ***Malaysia:*** Domper; Motilium; ***Mex.:*** Biolix; Emiken†; Motilium; Seronex; ***Neth.:*** Gastrocure; Motilium; ***NZ:*** Motilium; ***Port.:*** Cinet; Mogasinte; Motilium; Nordonil; Remotil; ***S.Afr.:*** Motilium; Vomidon; ***Singapore:*** Dompel; Dompenyl; Domper; Doridone; Mirax; Motilium; ***Spain:*** Motilium; Nauzelin†; ***Switz.:*** Motilium; ***Thai.:*** Costi†; Dany; Dolium; Domerdon; Domidone; Domilium†; Domper-M; Domperdone; Donum; Mirax; Mocydone; Modomed; Molax; Moticon; Motidom; Motilium; Movelium; Ninlium; Peptomet; Pondperdone; Poselium†; ***UK:*** Motilium; Vivadone.

**Multi-ingredient:** ***Arg.:*** Alplax Net; Bigetric; Bilagol; Dom-Polienzim; Euciton Complex; Faradil Novo; Megalex; Moperidona AF; Moperidona Enzimatica; Praxis; Tetralgin Novo; Vegestabil Digest; ***Belg.:*** Touristil; ***UK:*** Domperamol.

## Dosmalfate *(rINN)*

F-3616; F-3616. {$\mu_7$-[(Diosmin heptasulfato)(7-)]}tetracontahydroxytetradecaaluminium.

$C_{28}H_{60}Al_{14}O_{71}S_7$ = 2134.9.
*CAS — 122312-55-4.*

### Profile

Dosmalfate is a cytoprotective drug derived from diosmin (p.1688), that is used for the prevention and treatment of NSAID-associated peptic ulcer disease (p.1246) in a dose of 1.5 g twice daily.

### Preparations

**Proprietary Preparations** (details are given in Part 3)
***Spain:*** Diotul.

## Dronabinol *(USAN, rINN)*

NSC-134454; Δ⁹-Tetrahydrocannabinol; Δ⁹-THC. (6aR,10aR)-6a,7,8,10a-Tetrahydro-6,6,9-trimethyl-3-pentyl-6*H*-dibenzo[*b*,*d*]pyran-1-ol.

$C_{21}H_{30}O_2$ = 314.5.
*CAS — 1972-08-3.*
*ATC — A04AD10.*

**Pharmacopoeias.** In *US.*

**USP 27** (Dronabinol). Store at a temperature between 8° and 15° in airtight glass containers in an inert atmosphere. Protect from light.

### Adverse Effects and Precautions

As for Nabilone, p.1277. The most frequent adverse effects of dronabinol include abdominal pain, nausea and vomiting, dizziness, euphoria, paranoid reactions, and somnolence.

**Abuse.** The abuse liability of dronabinol was rated as being substantially lower than that of cannabis.[1]


1. WHO. WHO expert committee on drug dependence: twenty-seventh report. *WHO Tech Rep Ser 808* 1991.


**Breast feeding.** The US manufacturer states that dronabinol is concentrated in breast milk and recommends that it should not be used in breast-feeding mothers.

### Pharmacokinetics

Following oral administration dronabinol is slowly and erratically absorbed from the gastrointestinal tract; the bioavailability of an oral dose is about 10 to 20%, due to extensive first-pass metabolism. Peak plasma concentrations of dronabinol and its 11-hydroxy metabolite are achieved about 2 to 3 hours after a dose by mouth. It is widely distributed and is extensively protein bound, with a volume of distribution of approximately 10 litres/kg.

Dronabinol is extensively metabolised; the primary metabolite, 11-hydroxydronabinol is also active, and has an elimination half-life of 15 to 18 hours. The 11-hydroxy metabolite is converted to other, more polar and acidic compounds which are excreted in faeces via the bile, and in the urine. About 50% of an oral dose is recovered in faeces within 72 hours and 10 to 15% in urine. Many of the metabolites have relatively prolonged half-lives of 25 to 36 hours, and accumulation may occur with repeated administration.

Dronabinol is distributed into breast milk.

### Uses and Administration

Dronabinol, the major psychoactive constituent of cannabis (p.1666), has antiemetic properties and is used for the control of nausea and vomiting associated with cancer chemotherapy (p.1245) in patients who have failed to respond adequately to conventional antiemetics.

The usual initial dose of dronabinol by mouth is 5 mg/m² body-surface given 1 to 3 hours before the first dose of the antineoplastic drug with subsequent doses being given every 2 to 4 hours after chemotherapy to a maximum of 4 to 6 doses daily. If necessary, the dose may be increased by increments of 2.5 mg/m² to a maximum dose of 15 mg/m², if adverse effects permit.

Dronabinol also has appetite-stimulant effects and is used in the treatment of anorexia associated with weight loss in patients with AIDS. For this purpose 2.5 mg may be taken twice daily by mouth, before lunch and supper, reduced to a single 2.5-mg dose in the evening in patients who tolerate the drug poorly. If necessary, and if adverse effects permit, doses may also be increased up to 20 mg daily in divided doses.

◊ General references.


1. Voth EA, Schwartz RH. Medicinal applications of delta-9-tetrahydrocannabinol and marijuana. *Ann Intern Med* 1997; **126:** 791–8.
2. Williamson EM, Evans FJ. Cannabinoids in clinical practice. *Drugs* 2000; **60:** 1303–14.
3. Tramer MR, *et al.* Cannabinoids for control of chemotherapy induced nausea and vomiting: quantitative systematic review. *BMJ* 2001; **323:** 16–21.


**Anorexia.** Dronabinol is used for the management of anorexia in patients with HIV-associated wasting and diarrhoea (p.623). However, although dronabinol may stimulate appetite and prevent weight loss,[1] it does not appear to produce significant weight gain, and may produce less benefit than megestrol acetate.[2] Benefits were also less than those of megestrol in patients with anorexia associated with malignant disease.[3]


1. Beal JE, *et al.* Dronabinol as a treatment for anorexia associated with weight loss in patients with AIDS. *J Pain Symptom Manage* 1995; **10:** 89–97.
2. Timpone JG, *et al.* The safety and pharmacokinetics of single-agent and combination therapy with megestrol acetate and dronabinol for the treatment of HIV wasting syndrome. *AIDS Res Hum Retroviruses* 1997; **13:** 305–15.
3. Jatoi A, *et al.* Dronabinol versus megestrol acetate versus combination therapy for cancer-associated anorexia: a North Central Cancer Treatment Group study. *J Clin Oncol* 2002; **20:** 567–73.


### Preparations

***USP 27:*** Dronabinol Capsules.

**Proprietary Preparations** (details are given in Part 3)
***Canad.:*** Marinol; ***Israel:*** Ronabin; ***S.Afr.:*** Elevat†; ***USA:*** Marinol.

## Ebrotidine *(rINN)*

Ebrotidina. *p*-Bromo-*N*-[(*E*)-({2-[({2-[(diaminomethylene)amino]-4-thiazolyl}methyl)thio]ethyl}amino)methylene]benzenesulfonamide.

$C_{14}H_{17}BrN_6O_2S_3$ = 477.4.
*CAS — 100981-43-9.*

### Profile

Ebrotidine is a histamine $H_2$-antagonist with general properties similar to those of cimetidine (p.1255), but which also has cytoprotective actions. It has been used in peptic ulcer disease. Serious liver damage has been reported.

◊ References.


1. Patel SS, Wilde MI. Ebrotidine. *Drugs* 1996; **51:** 974–80.
2. Various. Ebrotidine: a new generation $H_2$-receptor antagonist and gastroprotective agent. *Arzneimittelforschung* 1997; **47:** 427–590.
3. Andrade RJ, *et al.* Acute liver injury associated with the use of ebrotidine, a new $H_2$-receptor antagonist. *J Hepatol* 1999; **31:** 641–6.


## Ecabet Sodium *(rINNM)*

Ecabet sódico; 12-Sulphodehydroabietic Acid, Monosodium Salt; TA-2711. 13-Isopropyl-12-sulphopodocarpa-8,11,13-trien-15-oic acid pentahydrate, sodium salt.

$C_{20}H_{27}NaO_5S,5H_2O$ = 492.6.
*CAS — 33159-27-2 (ecabet); 86408-72-2 (ecabet sodium).*

### Profile

Ecabet sodium is a cytoprotective drug used in the treatment of peptic ulcer disease (p.1246). The suggested dose is 1 g of ecabet sodium by mouth twice daily.

◊ References.


1. Shibata K, *et al.* Bactericidal activity of a new antiulcer agent, ecabet sodium, against Helicobacter pylori under acidic conditions. *Antimicrob Agents Chemother* 1995; **39:** 1295–9.
2. Ohkusa T, *et al.* Prospective evaluation of a new anti-ulcer agent, ecabet sodium, for the treatment of Helicobacter pylori infection. *Aliment Pharmacol Ther* 1998; **12:** 457–61.


### Preparations

**Proprietary Preparations** (details are given in Part 3)
***Jpn:*** Gastrom.

## Enoxolone Aluminium *(BANM, rINNM)*

Aluminium Glycyrrhetate; Aluminium Glycyrrhetinate; Enoxolona de aluminio; Enoxolone Aluminum. 3β-Hydroxy-11-oxo-olean-12-en-30-oic acid, aluminium salt.

$(C_{30}H_{46}O_4)_3.Al$ = 1439.0.
*CAS — 4598-66-7.*

### Profile

Enoxolone aluminium is an analogue of carbenoxolone (p.1254) that has been used in preparations for the treatment of peptic ulcer disease and other gastrointestinal disorders. It has also been used in preparations for skin disorders and mouth and throat disorders.

### Preparations

**Proprietary Preparations** (details are given in Part 3)
**Multi-ingredient:** ***Spain:*** Gastroalgine; Terpalate†.

## Esomeprazole Magnesium

*(BANM, USAN, rINNM)*

Esomeprazol magnésico; H199/18 (esomeprazole); Perprazole (esomeprazole). 5-Methoxy-2-{(S)-[(4-methoxy-3,5-dimethyl-2-pyridyl)methyl]sulfinyl}benzimidazole magnesium (2:1) trihydrate.

$C_{34}H_{36}MgN_6O_6S_2,3H_2O$ = 767.2.

*CAS — 119141-88-7 (esomeprazole); 217087-09-7 (esomeprazole magnesium).*

*ATC — A02BC05.*

## Esomeprazole Sodium *(BANM, USAN, rINNM)*

$C_{17}H_{19}N_3NaO_3S$ = 368.4.

*CAS — 161796-78-7.*

*ATC — A02BC05.*

### Adverse Effects and Precautions

As for Omeprazole, p.1278.

### Interactions

As for Omeprazole, p.1279.

◊ References.

1. Andersson T, *et al.* Drug interaction studies with esomeprazole, the (S)-isomer of omeprazole. *Clin Pharmacokinet* 2001; **40:** 523–37.

### Pharmacokinetics

Esomeprazole is rapidly absorbed following oral administration, with peak plasma levels occurring after about 1 to 2 hours. It is acid labile and an enteric-coated formulation has been developed. Bioavailability of esomeprazole increases with both dose and repeated administration to about 68 and 89% for doses of 20 and 40 mg respectively. Food delays and decreases the absorption of esomeprazole, but this does not significantly change its effect on intragastric acidity. Esomeprazole is about 97% bound to plasma proteins. It is extensively metabolised in the liver by the cytochrome P450 isoenzyme CYP2C19 to hydroxy and desmethyl metabolites, which have no effect on gastric acid secretion. The remainder is metabolised by the cytochrome P450 isoenzyme CYP3A4 to esomeprazole sulfone. With repeated administration, there is a decrease in first-pass metabolism and systemic clearance, probably caused by an inhibition of the CYP2C19 isoenzyme. However, there is no accumulation during once daily administration. The plasma elimination half-life is about 1.3 hours. Almost 80% of an oral dose is eliminated as metabolites in the urine, the remainder in the faeces.

◊ References.

1. Andersson T, *et al.* Pharmacokinetic studies with esomeprazole, the (S)-isomer of omeprazole. *Clin Pharmacokinet* 2001; **40:** 411–26.

### Uses and Administration

Esomeprazole is the *S*-isomer of the proton pump inhibitor omeprazole (p.1278) and is used similarly in the treatment of peptic ulcer disease (p.1246) and gastro-oesophageal reflux disease (p.1242). It is given as the magnesium or sodium salt but doses are calculated in terms of esomeprazole. Esomeprazole magnesium 22.2 mg and esomeprazole sodium 21.3 mg are each approximately equivalent to 20 mg of esomeprazole.

Usual doses for **peptic ulcer disease**, as a component of a triple therapy regimen with amoxicillin and clarithromycin, are the equivalent of 20 mg esomeprazole by mouth twice daily for 7 days, or 40 mg once daily for 10 days. In the UK, the dose for treatment of severe (erosive) **gastro-oesophageal reflux disease** is 40 mg once daily for 4 weeks, extended for a further 4 weeks if necessary; in the USA, where doses of 20 or 40 mg daily are permitted for initial treatment, a further 4 to 8 weeks of treatment may be considered for patients who do not heal after 4 to 8 weeks. For maintenance, or for symptomatic disease without erosive oesophagitis, doses equivalent to 20 mg of esomeprazole daily may be used in both countries.

Similar doses may be given as the sodium salt by slow intravenous injection or by intravenous infusion over 10 to 30 minutes.

Doses of esomeprazole may need to be reduced in patients with hepatic impairment (see below).

◊ General references.

1. Maton PN, *et al.* Safety and efficacy of long term esomeprazole therapy in patients with healed erosive oesophagitis. *Drug Safety* 2001; **24:** 625–35.
2. Scott LJ, *et al.* Esomeprazole: a review of its use in the management of acid-related disorders. *Drugs* 2002; **62:** 1503–38.

**Administration in hepatic impairment.** For patients with severe hepatic impairment the maximum daily dose of esomeprazole is 20 mg.

### Preparations

**Proprietary Preparations** (details are given in Part 3)
***Arg.:*** Nexium; ***Austral.:*** Nexium; ***Austria:*** Nexium; ***Belg.:*** Nexiam; ***Braz.:*** Nexium; ***Canad.:*** Nexium; ***Chile:*** Nexium; ***Denm.:*** Nexium; ***Fin.:*** Nexium; ***Fr.:*** Inexium; ***Ger.:*** Nexium; ***Hong Kong:*** Nexium; ***India:*** Sompraz; ***Irl.:*** Nexium; ***Israel:*** Nexium; ***Ital.:*** Axagon; Esopral; Lucen; Nexium; ***Malaysia:*** Nexium; ***Neth.:*** Nexium; ***Norw.:*** Nexium; ***Port.:*** Nexium; ***S.Afr.:*** Nexiam; ***Singapore:*** Nexium; ***Spain:*** Axiago; Nexium; ***Swed.:*** Nexium; ***Switz.:*** Nexium; ***Thai.:*** Nexium; ***UK:*** Nexium; ***USA:*** Nexium.

**Multi-ingredient:** ***Swed.:*** Nexium Hp.

---

## Euonymus

Evónimo; Fusain Noir Pourpré; Spindle Tree Bark; Wahoo Bark.

### Profile

Euonymus is the dried root-bark of *Euonymus atropurpureus* (=*Evonymus atropurpurea*) (Celastraceae). It is reported to have laxative, choleretic, and diuretic activity.

### Preparations

**Proprietary Preparations** (details are given in Part 3)
**Multi-ingredient:** ***Fr.:*** Jecopeptol; ***Port.:*** Solucao Stago†; ***UK:*** Acidosis; GB Tablets; Indigestion Mixture.

---

## Famotidine *(BAN, USAN, rINN)*

Famotidina; Famotidinum; L-643341; MK-208; YM-11170. 3-[2-(Diaminomethyleneamino)thiazol-4-ylmethylthio]-*N*-sulphamoylpropionamidine.

$C_8H_{15}N_7O_2S_3$ = 337.4.

*CAS — 76824-35-6.*

*ATC — A02BA03.*

**Pharmacopoeias.** In *Chin., Eur.* (see p.vi), *Jpn*, and *US.*

**Ph. Eur. 5.0** (Famotidine). A white or yellowish-white, crystalline powder or crystals. It exhibits polymorphism. Very slightly soluble in water and in dehydrated alcohol; freely soluble in glacial acetic acid; practically insoluble in ethyl acetate. It dissolves in dilute mineral acids. Protect from light.

**USP 27** (Famotidine). A white to pale yellowish-white crystalline powder. Very slightly soluble in water; practically insoluble in alcohol, in acetone, in chloroform, in ether, and in ethyl acetate; freely soluble in dimethylformamide and in glacial acetic acid; slightly soluble in methyl alcohol. Protect from light.

**Stability.** References.

1. Quercia RA, *et al.* Stability of famotidine in an extemporaneously prepared oral liquid. *Am J Hosp Pharm* 1993; **50:** 691–3.
2. Dentinger PJ, *et al.* Stability of famotidine in an extemporaneously compounded oral liquid. *Am J Health-Syst Pharm* 2000; 1340–2.

### Adverse Effects

As for Cimetidine, p.1255. Unlike cimetidine, famotidine is reported to have little or no anti-androgenic effect, although there are isolated reports of gynaecomastia and impotence.

◊ General references.

1. Howden CW, Tytgat GNJ. The tolerability and safety profile of famotidine. *Clin Ther* 1996; **18:** 36–54.

**Effects on the blood.** For reports of blood dyscrasias, some serious, occurring with famotidine, see under Cimetidine p.1256.

**Effects on the cardiovascular system.** Famotidine 40 mg daily by mouth reduced cardiac output and stroke volume, compared with placebo, cimetidine, or ranitidine in healthy subjects.[1] Similar effects observed in another study[2] were delayed by pretreatment with ranitidine. However, other workers have found that oral famotidine had no effect on exercise capacity or left ventricular systolic function in healthy subjects,[3] and that famotidine 20 mg intravenously had no effect on any of the haemodynamic parameters measured in 11 critically ill patients.[4] As with other $H_2$-antagonists (p.1256), bradycardia and atrioventricular block has been reported with famotidine,[5] as has a case of QT prolongation.[6]

1. Hinrichsen H, *et al.* Hemodynamic effects of different $H_2$-receptor antagonists. *Clin Pharmacol Ther* 1990; **48:** 302–8.
2. Mescheder A, *et al.* Changes in the effects of nizatidine and famotidine on cardiac performance after pretreatment with ranitidine. *Eur J Clin Pharmacol* 1993; **45:** 151–6.
3. Hillermann DE, *et al.* Impact of chronic oral $H_2$-antagonist therapy of left ventricular systolic function and exercise capacity. *J Clin Pharmacol* 1992; **32:** 1033–7.
4. Heiselman DE, *et al.* Hemodynamic status during famotidine infusion. *DICP Ann Pharmacother* 1990; **24:** 1163–5.
5. Schoenwald PK, *et al.* Complete atrioventricular block and cardiac arrest following intravenous famotidine administration. *Anesthesiology* 1999; **90:** 623–6.
6. Endo T, *et al.* Famotidine and acquired long QT syndrome. *Am J Med* 2000; **108:** 438–9.

**Effects on the endocrine system.** Hyperprolactinaemia and breast engorgement occurred in a woman during the fourth month of treatment with famotidine 80 mg daily;[1] she had mistakenly been given twice the usual maximum dose. Recovery occurred when famotidine was withdrawn. Transient hyperprolactinaemia and galactorrhoea have also been reported in a woman after standard doses (40 mg daily) of famotidine.[2] There have been a few instances of impotence.[3]

1. Delpre G, *et al.* Hyperprolactinaemia during famotidine therapy. *Lancet* 1993; **342:** 868.
2. Güven K. Hyperprolactinemia and galactorrhea with standard-dose famotidine therapy. *Ann Pharmacother* 1995; **29:** 788.
3. Kassianos GC. Impotence and nizatidine. *Lancet* 1989; **i:** 963.

**Effects on the kidney.** For mention of acute interstitial nephritis associated with $H_2$-antagonists, including famotidine, see under Cimetidine, p.1256.

**Effects on the liver.** Mixed hepatocellular jaundice[1] and acute hepatitis[2] have been associated with famotidine administration; in the latter case the patient subsequently experienced a recurrence when given cimetidine.

1. Ament PW, *et al.* Famotidine-induced mixed hepatocellular jaundice. *Ann Pharmacother* 1994; **28:** 40–2.
2. Hashimoto F, *et al.* Hepatitis following treatments with famotidine and then cimetidine. *Ann Pharmacother* 1994; **28:** 37–9.

**Effects on the nervous system.** Similarly to other $H_2$-antagonists (p.1256), CNS reactions have occurred with famotidine, particularly in the elderly and those with renal failure.[1-3] In one report,[1] convulsions and mental deterioration in 2 elderly patients with renal failure were associated with grossly elevated plasma and CSF concentrations of the drug; symptoms resolved within 3 days of withdrawing famotidine. In another elderly patient with renal impairment, delirium was associated with use of famotidine but did not occur with cimetidine.[4]

1. Yoshimoto K, *et al.* Famotidine-associated central nervous system reactions and plasma and cerebrospinal drug concentrations in neurosurgical patients with renal failure. *Clin Pharmacol Ther* 1994; **55:** 693–700.
2. Catalano G, *et al.* Famotidine-associated delirium: a series of six cases. *Psychosomatics* 1996; **37:** 349–55.
3. Odeh M, Oliven A. Central nervous system reactions associated with famotidine: report of five cases. *J Clin Gastroenterol* 1998; **27:** 253–4.
4. Yuan R-Y, *et al.* Delirium following a switch from cimetidine to famotidine. *Ann Pharmacother* 2001; **35:** 1045–8.

**Effects on the skin.** Toxic epidermal necrolysis or erythema multiforme have been reported after use of famotidine;[1,2] the second patient had a recurrence with cimetidine.

1. Brunner M, *et al.* Toxic epidermal necrolysis (Lyell syndrome) following famotidine administration. *Br J Dermatol* 1995; **133:** 814–15.
2. Horiuchi Y, Ikezawa K. Famotidine-induced erythema multiforme: cross-sensitivity with cimetidine. *Ann Intern Med* 1999; **131:** 795.

**Fever.** Famotidine 20 mg intravenously every 12 hours was associated with hyperpyrexia in a patient with facial and cranial trauma.[1] Rectal temperature in the 24 hours after starting famotidine was 40.5° and remained elevated for the 5 days of famotidine treatment, despite use of antipyretics. Withdrawal of famotidine resulted in a return to normal temperature within 24 hours.

1. Norwood J, *et al.* Famotidine and hyperpyrexia. *Ann Intern Med* 1990; **112:** 632.

### Precautions

As for Cimetidine, p.1257.

**Hepatic impairment.** For a report of increased resistance to $H_2$-antagonists in patients with liver cirrhosis, see Ranitidine, p.1286.

**Renal impairment.** In patients with renal impairment, famotidine clearance is reduced and the elimination half-life increased, resulting in increased serum-drug concentrations and in some cases clinical sequelae (see Effects on the Nervous System, above). The half-life of famotidine in healthy subjects is about 3 hours, but in patients with a creatinine clearance less than 38 mL/minute[1] or those with end-stage renal disease[2] it has been reported to be 19.3 hours and 27.2 hours respectively. A 50% reduction in the dose of famotidine in patients with renal impairment has therefore been recommended. However, it may not be sufficient to adjust the dose only on the basis of creatinine clearance since famotidine is partly eliminated by tubular secretion, which may also be diminished.[1]

Haemodialysis does not effectively remove famotidine from the systemic circulation. The proportion removed depends on the type of membrane used; with a high flux polysulfone membrane about 16% is reported to be removed, but only 6% with a cuprophan membrane.[2] Continuous ambulatory peritoneal dialysis is reported to remove about 5% of a dose.[2] Continuous haemofiltration may remove about 16% of a dose;[2] intermittent haemofiltration is reported to remove about 4%[3] or 8%.[2] Dosage supplements of famotidine are not required during or after dialysis or filtration procedures.

1. Inotsume N, *et al.* Pharmacokinetics of famotidine in elderly patients with and without renal insufficiency and in healthy young volunteers. *Eur J Clin Pharmacol* 1989; **36:** 517–20.

2. Gladziwa U, *et al.* Pharmacokinetics and dynamics of famotidine in patients with renal failure. *Br J Clin Pharmacol* 1988; **26:** 315–21.
3. Saima S, *et al.* Hemofiltrability of $H_2$-receptor antagonist, famotidine, in renal failure patients. *J Clin Pharmacol* 1990; **30:** 159–62.

## Interactions

Unlike cimetidine (see p.1257) famotidine does not inhibit cytochrome P450, and therefore is considered to have little effect on the metabolism of other drugs. However, like other $H_2$-antagonists its effects on gastric pH may affect the absorption of some other drugs.

**Antacids.** Giving famotidine 40 mg with a 10-mL dose of antacid containing 800 mg *aluminium hydroxide* with 800 mg *magnesium hydroxide*,[1] resulted in a decrease in the bioavailability of famotidine that was considered clinically insignificant. Giving famotidine with a 30-mL dose of the same antacid resulted in a greater reduction in the absorption of famotidine from the gastrointestinal tract, but the interaction could be minimised by separating ingestion by 2 hours.[2]

1. Lin JH, *et al.* Effects of antacids and food on absorption of famotidine. *Br J Clin Pharmacol* 1987; **24:** 551–3.
2. Barzaghi N, *et al.* Impaired bioavailability of famotidine given concurrently with a potent antacid. *J Clin Pharmacol* 1989; **29:** 670–2.

**Probenecid.** Probenecid in a total dose of 1500 mg had a significant effect on the pharmacokinetics of famotidine 20 mg in 8 healthy subjects.[1] The maximum serum concentration of famotidine and the area under the concentration/time curve were significantly increased and renal clearance significantly reduced. These effects were explained by inhibition of the renal tubular secretion of famotidine by probenecid.

1. Inotsume N, *et al.* The inhibitory effect of probenecid on renal excretion of famotidine in young, healthy volunteers. *J Clin Pharmacol* 1990; **30:** 50–6.

**Theophylline.** Although famotidine is considered not to interfere with the metabolism of other drugs there is a report of a clinically significant interaction with theophylline—see p.803.

## Pharmacokinetics

Famotidine is readily but incompletely absorbed from the gastrointestinal tract with peak concentrations in plasma occurring 1 to 3 hours after administration by mouth. The bioavailability of famotidine following oral administration is about 40 to 45% and is not significantly affected by the presence of food.

The elimination half-life from plasma is reported to be about 3 hours and is prolonged in renal impairment. Famotidine is weakly bound, about 15 to 20%, to plasma proteins. A small proportion of famotidine is metabolised in the liver to famotidine *S*-oxide. About 25 to 30% of an oral dose, and 65 to 70% of an intravenous dose, is excreted unchanged in the urine in 24 hours, primarily by active tubular secretion. Famotidine is also found in breast milk.

◊ Reviews.

1. Echizen H, Ishizaki T. Clinical pharmacokinetics of famotidine. *Clin Pharmacokinet* 1991; **21:** 178–94.

**Children.** Famotidine 300 micrograms/kg intravenously was given to 10 children aged 2 to 7 years, after cardiac surgery and before extubation, to prevent aspiration.[1] This dose (equivalent to about 20 mg in adults) induced a rise in the intragastric pH within 1 hour of administration and the pH remained above 3.5 for about 9 hours. The mean elimination half-life was 3.3 hours, similar to the value in healthy adults and it was considered that doses in children need therefore only be adjusted according to body-weight and renal function. This conclusion was supported by a review of 8 studies in children over 1 year of age.[2] Conversely, in infants aged 5 to 19 days, the mean elimination half-life was prolonged (10.5 hours) secondary to reduced renal clearance.[3]

1. Kraus G, *et al.* Famotidine: pharmacokinetic properties and suppression of acid secretion in paediatric patients following cardiac surgery. *Clin Pharmacokinet* 1990; **18:** 77–81.
2. James LP, Kearns GL. Pharmacokinetics and pharmacodynamics of famotidine in paediatric patients. *Clin Pharmacokinet* 1996; **31:** 103–10.
3. James LP, *et al.* Pharmacokinetics and pharmacodynamics of famotidine in infants. *J Clin Pharmacol* 1998; **38:** 1089–95. Correction. *ibid.* 2000; **40:** 1298.

**Distribution into breast milk.** The peak concentration of famotidine in breast milk which occurred in 8 lactating women 6 hours after an oral dose of 40 mg was similar to the peak plasma concentration which occurred 2 hours after the dose.[1]

1. Courtney TP, *et al.* Excretion of famotidine in breast milk. *Br J Clin Pharmacol* 1988; **26:** 639P.

**Enterohepatic recirculation.** Some individuals exhibit a second peak in the plasma concentration of famotidine, which could be due to enterohepatic recirculation. However, a maximum of 0.43% of a dose of famotidine was excreted in the bile of 2 patients following single doses of 20 mg intravenously or 40 mg by mouth indicating that significant recirculation had not occurred.[1]

1. Klotz U, Walker S. Biliary excretion of $H_2$-receptor antagonists. *Eur J Clin Pharmacol* 1990; **39:** 91–2.

## Uses and Administration

Famotidine is a histamine $H_2$-antagonist with actions and uses similar to those of cimetidine (see p.1258).

Famotidine may be given by mouth or parenterally by the intravenous route.

In the management of benign **gastric** and **duodenal ulceration** (p.1246) the dose is 40 mg daily by mouth at bedtime, for 4 to 8 weeks. A dose of 20 mg twice daily has also been given. A maintenance dose of 20 mg at bedtime may be given to prevent recurrence of duodenal ulceration. In **gastro-oesophageal reflux disease** (p.1242) the recommended dose is 20 mg by mouth twice daily for 6 to 12 weeks, or up to 40 mg twice daily if there is oesophageal ulceration. A maintenance dose of 20 mg twice daily may be given to prevent recurrence. For the short-term symptomatic relief of heartburn or non-ulcer **dyspepsia** (p.1242) a dose of 10 mg up to twice daily is suggested. In the **Zollinger-Ellison syndrome** (p.1247) the initial dose by mouth is 20 mg every 6 hours, increased as necessary; doses up to 800 mg daily have been used.

The usual dose of famotidine by the intravenous route is 20 mg and may be given by injection over at least 2 minutes or as an infusion over 15 to 30 minutes; the dose may be repeated every 12 hours.

Doses of famotidine should be reduced in patients with renal impairment (see below).

**Administration.** Although famotidine is most usually given as a film-coated tablet, an alternative wafer formulation, designed to dissolve on the tongue without the need for water, has also been developed.[1]

Parenteral formulations of famotidine are also available in some countries. Although the manufacturers recommend that intravenous injections be given over at least 2 minutes, a study that compared rapid intravenous injection (over up to 1 minute) with slow intravenous infusion found both to be safe.[2] Continuous infusion has however been reported by others[3] to be more effective in the prevention of stress ulceration than bolus injection.

1. Schwartz JI, *et al.* Novel oral medication delivery system for famotidine. *J Clin Pharmacol* 1995; **35:** 362–7.
2. Fish DN. Safety and cost of rapid iv injection of famotidine in critically ill patients. *Am J Health-Syst Pharm* 1995; **52:** 1889–94.
3. Baghaie AA, *et al.* Comparison of the effect of intermittent administration and continuous infusion of famotidine on gastric pH in critically ill patients: results of a prospective, randomized, crossover study. *Crit Care Med* 1995; **23:** 687–91.

**Administration in renal impairment.** The dosage of famotidine should be reduced in patients with renal impairment. In the UK, a 50% reduction is suggested for patients whose creatinine clearance is less than 10 mL/minute; in the USA this reduction is recommended in all those with creatinine clearance less than 50 mL/minute. Alternatively, the dosage interval may be prolonged to 36 to 48 hours.

**Schizophrenia.** There are reports of improvement in schizophrenic symptoms (p.665) in patients given famotidine.[1-4]

1. Kaminsky R, *et al.* Effect of famotidine on deficit symptoms of schizophrenia. *Lancet* 1990; **335:** 1351–2.
2. Rosse RB, *et al.* Famotidine adjunctive pharmacotherapy of schizophrenia: a case report. *Clin Neuropharmacol* 1995; **18:** 369–74.
3. Rosse RB, *et al.* An open-label study of the therapeutic efficacy of high-dose famotidine adjuvant pharmacotherapy in schizophrenia: preliminary evidence for treatment efficacy. *Clin Neuropharmacol* 1996; **19:** 341–8.
4. Martinez MC. Famotidine in the management of schizophrenia. *Ann Pharmacother* 1999; **33:** 742–7.

## Preparations

***BP 2003:*** Famotidine Tablets;
***USP 27:*** Famotidine Tablets.

**Proprietary Preparations** (details are given in Part 3)
***Arg.:*** Ulcelac; ***Austral.:*** Amfamox; Pepcid; Pepcidine; ***Austria:*** Eradix; Pepcid; Pepcidine; Tetacid; Ulcusan; ***Belg.:*** Pepcidine; ***Braz.:*** Famodine; Famoset; Famotid; Famotil; Famox; Famoxil; ***Canad.:*** Acid Control; Acid Halt; Maalox $H_2$ Acid Controller; Pepcid; Peptic Guard; Ulcidine; ***Chile:*** Anulbet; Fibonel; Gastrium; ***Denm.:*** Pepcidin; ***Fin.:*** Pepcid; Pepcidin; ***Fr.:*** Pepcidac; Pepdine; ***Ger.:*** Fadul; Famo; Famobeta; Famonerton; Ganor†; Pepcid; Pepdul; ***Gr.:*** Ansilan; Banatin; Cepal; Esseldon; Gasterogen; Imposergon; Mostrelan; Panalba; Peptan; Rosagenus; Sedanium-R; Vexurat; ***Hong Kong:*** Actidine†; Fadine; Famine; Famodine; Famolta; Famopsin; Famox; Gastrodomina; Motidine; Pepcid†; Pepcidine; Pepzan†; Quamatel; Servipep; Ulceran; Vida Famodine; ***India:*** Blocacid; Famowal; Famtac; Fudone; ***Irl.:*** Pepcid; ***Israel:*** Apogastine; Famo; Gastro; Rogasti; Zarex; ***Ital.:*** Famodil; Gastridin; Motiax; ***Jpn:*** Gaster; ***Malaysia:*** Acidine; Fadine; Famopsin; Pepcidine; Pepzan; Ulceran; Voker; ***Mex.:*** Amofat†; Durater; Fabutin; Fagatrim; Famoxal; Farmotex†; Fatoril; Fawodin†; Pepcidine; Sertidine; Sigafam; Ultidin†; ***Neth.:*** Pepcid; Pepcidin; ***Norw.:*** Famotal; Pepcid; Pepcidin; ***NZ:*** Famox; Pepcid; Pepcidine; Pepzan; ***Port.:*** Dinul; Dipsin; Fatidin; Gastopride; Gastrifam; Lasa; Mensoma; Nulceran; Pepcidina; ***S.Afr.:*** Pepcid†; ***Singapore:*** Blocacid; Famoc; Famocid†; Famopril; Famopsin; Famotin; Famox; Motidine; Pepcidine; Pepzan; Servipep†; Ulceran†; ***Spain:*** Brolin; Confobos; Cronol; Digervin; Dispromil; Eviantrina; Fagastril; Famokey; Famulcer; Fanosin; Fanox; Gastrion; Gastrodomina; Gastropen; Ingastri; Invigan; Muclox†; Nos; Nulcerin; Pepcid; Rubacina; Tairal; Tameran†; Tamin; Tipodex; Ulcetrax; Ulgarine; Vagostal; ***Swed.:*** Pepcid; Pepcidin; ***Switz.:*** Pepcid; Pepcidine; ***Thai.:*** Agufam; Fadine; Famoc; Famocid; Famonox; Famopsin; Famotab; Famotin; Fasidine; Motidine; Pepcidine; Pepcine; Pepdenal; Pepfamin; Peptoci; Pepzan; Pharmotidine; Servipep†; Ulceran; Ulcofam; Ulfamet; ***UAE:*** Famotec; ***UK:*** Pepcid; Ultra Heartburn Relief; ***USA:*** Mylanta AR Acid Reducer; Pepcid.

**Multi-ingredient:** ***Canad.:*** Pepcid Complete; ***Fin.:*** Pepcid Duo; ***Fr.:*** Pepcidduo; ***Ger.:*** Pepciddual; ***Ital.:*** Pepciddual; ***Norw.:*** Pepcidduo; ***Spain:*** Pepdual; ***Swed.:*** Pepcid Duo; ***UK:*** Pepcidtwo; ***USA:*** Pepcid Complete.

## Fedotozine *(rINN)*

Fedotozina. (+)-(*R*)-α-Ethyl-*N*,*N*-dimethyl-α-{[(3,4,5-trimethoxybenzyl)oxy]methyl}benzylamine.

$C_{22}H_{31}NO_4$ = 373.5.

*CAS — 123618-00-8.*

### Profile

Fedotozine is a peripherally acting selective agonist of opioid κ-receptors that is under investigation in dyspepsia and the irritable bowel syndrome.

◊ References.

1. Fraitag B, *et al.* Double-blind dose-response multicenter comparison of fedotozine and placebo in treatment of nonulcer dyspepsia. *Dig Dis Sci* 1994; **39:** 1072–7.
2. Read NW, *et al.* Efficacy and safety of the peripheral kappa agonist fedotozine versus placebo in the treatment of functional dyspepsia. *Gut* 1997; **41:** 664–8.
3. Delvaux M, *et al.* The kappa agonist fedotozine relieves hypersensitivity to colonic distention in patients with irritable bowel syndrome. *Gastroenterology* 1999; **116:** 38–45.
4. Delvaux M. Pharmacology and clinical experience with fedotozine. *Expert Opin Invest Drugs* 2001; **10:** 97–110.

## Fig

Carica; Ficus; Higo.

**Pharmacopoeias.** In *Br.* and *Swiss.*

**BP 2003** (Fig). The sun-dried succulent fruit of *Ficus carica* containing not less than 60.0% of water-soluble extractive. Store in a dry place.

### Profile

Fig is a mild laxative and demulcent usually used with other laxatives.

### Preparations

**Proprietary Preparations** (details are given in Part 3)

**Multi-ingredient:** ***Austria:*** Carilax; Frugelletten; Herbelax; Naturaform Fruchtewurfel mit Manna; Neda Fruchtewurfel; Sinolax-Milder; ***Braz.:*** Bilifel†; Limao Bravo†; ***Denm.:*** Figen; ***Ger.:*** florabio Mann-Feigen-Sirup mit Senna; ***Switz.:*** Agarol Soft; Dragees aux figues avec du sene; Fruttasan; Pursana; Valverde Dragees laxatives; Valverde Sirop laxatif; ***UK:*** Califig.

## Frangula Bark

Alder Buckthorn Bark; Amieiro Negro; Bourdaine; Corteza de frángula; Faulbaumrinde; Frangulae Cortex; Rhamni Frangulae Cortex.

*CAS — 8057-57-6 (frangula extract).*

**Pharmacopoeias.** In *Eur.* (see p.vi) and *Pol.*

**Ph. Eur. 5.0** (Frangula Bark). The dried, whole or fragmented bark of the stems and branches of *Rhamnus frangula (=Frangula alnus)*. It contains not less than 7.0% of glucofrangulins, expressed as glucofrangulin A ($C_{27}H_{30}O_{14}$ = 578.5) and calculated with reference to the dried drug. Protect from light.

### Profile

Frangula bark is an anthraquinone stimulant laxative with actions and uses similar to those of senna (p.1288).

It is also used in homoeopathic medicine.

### Preparations

***Ph. Eur.:*** Frangula Bark Dry Extract, Standardised.

**Proprietary Preparations** (details are given in Part 3)
***Fr.:*** Depuratif des Alpes; ***Switz.:*** Arkocaps; Emodella†; ***UK:*** Heath & Heather Inner Fresh Tablets†.

**Multi-ingredient:** ***Austral.:*** Granocol; Herb-a-Lax†; Normacol Plus; ***Austria:*** Abfuhrdragees mild; Abfuhrtee; Artin; Dr Ernst Richter's Abfuhrtee-tassenfertig†; Dr Ernst Richter's Abfuhrtee†; Dr. Ernst Richter's Abfuhrtee-Filterbeutel†; Dragees Neunzehn; Gallesyn; Laxalpin; Laxolind†; Mag Kottas May-Cur-Tee; Planta Lax; Pserhofer's; St Bonifatius-Tee; ***Belg.:*** Grains de Vals; Normacol Plus; Tisane Antibiliaire et Stomachique†; Tisane Contre la Tension†; Tisane Depurative "les 12 Plantes"†; Tisane Purgative†; ***Canad.:*** Constipation; Extra Strong Formula 12; Herbalax; Lapidar†; ***Denm.:*** Ferroplex-frangula; ***Fr.:*** Boldoflorine†; Bronpax†; Dragees Fuca; Dragees Vegetales Rex; Mediflor Tisane Antirhumatismale No 2; Mediflor Tisane Circulation du Sang No 12; Mucinum†; Normacol a la Bourdaine; Santane $C_6$†; Sirop Pectoral enfant†; Tisane des Familles†; Tisane Grande Chartreuse†; Tisane Mexicaine†; Tisane Touraine†; Tisanes de l'Abbe Hamon no 17†; Tisanes de l'Abbe Hamon no 3†; Tonilax†; ***Ger.:*** Floradix Maskam†; Heumann Abfuhrtee Solubilax N; Hevertolax duo; ***Hong Kong:*** Hepatofalk; Normacol Plus; ***India:*** Kanormal; ***Irl.:*** Normacol Plus; ***Israel:*** Encypalmed; Rekiv; ***Ital.:*** Fave di Fuca; Fitodorf Alghe Marine†; Frangulina; Ginolax†; Hepasil Composto†; Lactolas; Neo-Heparbil†; Sintobil†; Tisana Arnaldi†; ***Mex.:*** Normacol†; ***Neth.:*** Normacol Plus; ***NZ:*** Granocol; Normacol Plus; ***Port.:*** Normacol Plus; ***S.Afr.:*** Normacol Plus; ***Singapore:*** Normacol Plus; ***Spain:*** Caved-S†; Doctogaster†; Jarabe Manzanas Siken†; Normacol Forte; Rabro†; Roter Complex†; ***Switz.:*** Adistop Lax†; Boldoflorine†; Caved-S†; Colosan plus;

Drix†; Fuca†; Lapidar 10; Linoforce; Normacol (avec bourdaine); Optilax†; Padma-Lax; Phyto-Laxia; Phytolax†; PhytoLaxin; The laxatif Solubilax†; ***Thai.:*** Roter†; ***UK:*** Herbulax; Lustys Herbalene; Normacol Plus.

## Gefarnate *(BAN, rINN)*

DA-688; Gefarnato; Geranyl Farnesylacetate. A mixture of stereoisomers of 3,7-dimethylocta-2,6-dienyl 5,9,13-trimethyltetradeca-4,8,12-trienoate.

$C_{27}H_{44}O_2$ = 400.6.
*CAS — 51-77-4.*
*ATC — A02BX07.*

### Profile

Gefarnate is a cytoprotective agent that has been used in the treatment of peptic ulcer disease and gastritis.

## Ginger

Gengibre; Gingembre; Ingwer; Jengibre; Zingib.; Zingiber; Zingiberis Rhizoma.

**Pharmacopoeias.** In *Chin., Eur.* (see p.vi), and *Jpn.* Also in *USNF.*

**Ph. Eur. 5.0** (Ginger). The dried, whole or cut rhizome of *Zingiber officinale*, with the cork removed, either completely or from the wide flat surfaces only. Whole or cut, it contains not less than 1.5% of essential oil, calculated with reference to the anhydrous drug. It has a characteristic aromatic odour. Protect from light.

The BP 2003 states that ginger may be known in commerce as unbleached ginger.

**USNF 22** (Ginger). The scraped or unscraped rhizome of *Zingiber officinale* (Zingiberaceae), known in commerce as unbleached ginger. It contains not less than 4.5% of alcohol-soluble extractive and not less than 10% of water-soluble extractive. Protect from light and moisture.

### Profile

Ginger has carminative properties. It is used as a flavouring agent and has been tried for the prophylaxis of motion sickness and postoperative nausea and vomiting (p.1245).

It is also used in homoeopathic medicine.

**Nausea and vomiting.** References.


1. Grøntved A, Hentzer E. Vertigo-reducing effect of ginger root: a controlled clinical study. *ORL J Otorhinolaryngol Relat Spec* 1986; **48:** 282–6.
2. Bone ME, *et al.* Ginger root—a new antiemetic: the effect of ginger root on postoperative nausea and vomiting after major gynaecological surgery. *Anaesthesia* 1990; **45:** 669–71.
3. Stewart JJ, *et al.* Effects of ginger on motion sickness susceptibility and gastric function. *Pharmacology* 1991; **42:** 111–20.
4. Phillips S, *et al.* Zingiber officinale (ginger)—an antiemetic for day case surgery. *Anaesthesia* 1993; **48:** 715–17.
5. Arfeen Z, *et al.* A double-blind randomized controlled trial of ginger for the prevention of postoperative nausea and vomiting. *Anaesth Intensive Care* 1995; **23:** 449–52.
6. Ernst E, Pittler MH. Efficacy of ginger for nausea and vomiting: a systematic review of randomized clinical trials. *Br J Anaesth* 2000; **84:** 367–71.
7. Vutyavanich T, *et al.* Ginger for nausea and vomiting in pregnancy: randomized, double-masked, placebo-controlled trial. *Obstet Gynecol* 2001; **97:** 577–82.


### Preparations

***BP 2003:*** Aromatic Cardamom Tincture; Strong Ginger Tincture; Weak Ginger Tincture;
***USNF 22:*** Ginger Tincture.

**Proprietary Preparations** (details are given in Part 3)
***Austral.:*** Travacalm Natural†; ***Austria:*** Zintona; ***Ger.:*** Zintona; ***Hong Kong:*** Zinaxin†; ***Singapore:*** Zinaxin†; ***Switz.:*** Zintona; ***Thai.:*** Zinaxin; ***UK:*** Travel Sickness; Travellers†; Zinaxin.

**Multi-ingredient:** ***Austral.:*** Bioglan Ginger-Vite Forte†; Bioglan Psylli-Mucil Plus†; Cal Alkyline†; Digestive Aid†; Extralife Arthri-Care†; Feminine Herbal Complex†; Ginkgo Plus Herbal Plus Formula 10†; Herbal Cleanse†; Herbal Digestive Formula†; Lifesystem Herbal Plus Formula 11 Ginkgo†; PC Regulax†; Peritone†; PMS Support†; PMT Complex†; Travelaide†; ***Austria:*** Mariazeller; Sanvita Magen; Synpharma Aromatische Tinktur; ***Braz.:*** Broncol; Catuaba†; Catuama†; Geripan†; Pulmoiodo†; Tussifen; ***Canad.:*** Cayenne Plus; Chase Kolik Gripe Water; ***Fr.:*** Evacrine; ***Ger.:*** Fovysat; Gallexier; Gastricard; Gastrosecur; Imbak†; JuViton; Majocarmin forte; Presselin Dyspeptikum; Unex Amarum; ***Hong Kong:*** Gl†; Magesto; ***India:*** Carmicide; ***Ital.:*** Cura†; Donalg; Lozione Same Urto; ***Malaysia:*** Zinaxin Plus; ***Singapore:*** Artrex; ***Switz.:*** Padma-Lax; ***Thai.:*** Carmicide; Flatulence Gastulence; Magesto; Mesto-Of; Papytazyme; ***UK:*** Digestive; HRI Golden Seal Digestive; Indian Brandee; Indigestion Relief; Neo Gripe Mixture; Super Mega B+C; Travel-Caps†; Traveleeze; Wind & Dyspepsia Relief.

## Granisetron Hydrochloride

*(BANM, USAN, rINNM)*

BRL-43694A; Hidrocloruro de granisetrón. 1-Methyl-*N*-(9-methyl-9-azabicyclo[3.3.1]non-3-yl)-1*H*-indazole-3-carboxamide hydrochloride.

$C_{18}H_{24}N_4O,HCl$ = 348.9.
*CAS — 109889-09-0 (granisetron); 107007-99-8 (granisetron hydrochloride).*
*ATC — A04AA02.*

### Adverse Effects and Precautions

As for Ondansetron, p.1281.

◊ The manufacturer has reported an increased incidence of hepatic neoplasms in *rodents* given very high doses of granisetron for prolonged periods, but the relevance of these results to the clinical situation is unknown. Although mutagenicity and genotoxicity have not been seen in some tests, others have reported an increased incidence of polyploidy or unscheduled DNA synthesis in exposed cells.

### Pharmacokinetics

Granisetron is absorbed after oral administration, with peak plasma concentrations occurring about 2 hours after a dose. Oral bioavailability is about 60% as a result of first-pass hepatic metabolism. It has a large volume of distribution of around 3 litres/kg; plasma protein binding is about 65%. The pharmacokinetics of granisetron exhibit considerable interindividual variation, and the elimination half-life is reported to be around 3 to 4 hours in healthy subjects but about 9 to 12 hours in cancer patients. It is metabolised in the liver, primarily by 7-hydroxylation, with less than 20% of a dose recovered unchanged in urine, the remainder being excreted in faeces and urine as metabolites. Granisetron clearance is not affected by renal impairment, but is lower in the elderly and in patients with hepatic impairment.

### Uses and Administration

Granisetron is a 5-$HT_3$ antagonist with an antiemetic action similar to that of ondansetron (p.1281). It is used in the management of nausea and vomiting induced by cytotoxic chemotherapy and radiotherapy and for the prevention and treatment of postoperative nausea and vomiting (p.1245). Granisetron is administered as the hydrochloride, but doses are expressed in terms of the base. Granisetron hydrochloride 1.1 mg is approximately equivalent to 1 mg of granisetron base.

For acute **nausea and vomiting** associated with **chemotherapy** granisetron is used in *prevention* and *treatment* in similar doses.

- In the UK, a dose equivalent to 3 mg of granisetron is diluted to a volume of 20 to 50 mL with a suitable infusion solution and given intravenously over 5 minutes before the start of chemotherapy; alternatively this dose may be administered in 15 mL of infusion solution and given as a bolus over not less than 30 seconds. The dose may be repeated up to twice in 24 hours; doses should be given at least 10 minutes apart and a total daily dose of 9 mg should not be exceeded. The efficacy of granisetron may be enhanced by the use of dexamethasone. The recommended dose by mouth is 1 to 2 mg within one hour before therapy begins, then 2 mg daily as a single dose or in 2 divided doses.
- In children, an intravenous infusion of 40 micrograms/kg, up to a maximum total dose of 3 mg, has been recommended, dissolved in 10 to 30 mL of infusion fluid and given over 5 minutes. This dose may be repeated once within 24 hours, but at least 10 minutes after the original infusion. Alternatively, children may be given 20 micrograms/kg (up to 1 mg) twice daily by mouth for up to 5 days during therapy; the first dose should be administered within 1 hour of the start of chemotherapy.
- In the USA, lower intravenous doses of the equivalent of 10 micrograms of granisetron per kg are recommended in both adults and children over 2 years of age, beginning within 30 minutes before chemotherapy. Doses by mouth are the same as those described above.

For the *prevention* of nausea and vomiting associated with **radiotherapy** the recommended adult dosage is 2 mg daily by mouth taken within 1 hour of irradiation. It has also been given intravenously.

For the *prevention* of **postoperative** nausea and vomiting 1 mg is diluted to 5 mL and given by intravenous injection over 30 seconds. Administration should be completed before induction of anaesthesia. The same dose may be given up to twice daily for the *treatment* of established postoperative nausea and vomiting.

◊ References.


1. Anonymous. Granisetron to prevent vomiting after cancer chemotherapy. *Med Lett Drugs Ther* 1994; **36:** 61–2.
2. Yarker YE, McTavish D. Granisetron: an update of its therapeutic use in nausea and vomiting induced by antineoplastic therapy. *Drugs* 1994; **48:** 761–93.
3. Adams VR, Valley AW. Granisetron: the second serotonin-receptor antagonist. *Ann Pharmacother* 1995; **29:** 1240–51. Correction. *ibid.* 1996; **30:** 1043.
4. Wilson AJ, *et al.* Single-dose i.v. granisetron in the prevention of postoperative nausea and vomiting. *Br J Anaesth* 1996; **76:** 515–18.
5. Taylor AM, *et al.* A double-blind, parallel-group, placebo-controlled, dose-ranging, multicenter study of intravenous granisetron in the treatment of postoperative nausea and vomiting in patients undergoing surgery with general anesthesia. *J Clin Anesth* 1997; **9:** 658–63.


**Pain.** For reference to the use of granisetron in various painful syndromes see under Uses and Administration of Ondansetron, p.1282

### Preparations

**Proprietary Preparations** (details are given in Part 3)
***Arg.:*** Aludal; Eumetic; Granitron; Kytril; Rigmoz; ***Austral.:*** Kytril; ***Austria:*** Kytril; ***Belg.:*** Kytril; ***Braz.:*** Kytril; ***Canad.:*** Kytril; ***Chile:*** Kytril; ***Denm.:*** Kytril; ***Fin.:*** Kytril; ***Fr.:*** Kytril; ***Ger.:*** Kevatril; ***Gr.:*** Kytril; ***Hong Kong:*** Kytril; ***India:*** Granicip; ***Irl.:*** Kytril; ***Israel:*** Kytril; Setron; ***Ital.:*** Kytril; ***Mex.:*** Kytril; ***Neth.:*** Kytril; ***Norw.:*** Kytril; ***Port.:*** Kytril; ***S.Afr.:*** Kytril; ***Singapore:*** Kytril; ***Spain:*** Kytril; ***Swed.:*** Kytril; ***Switz.:*** Kytril; ***Thai.:*** Kytril; ***UK:*** Kytril; ***USA:*** Kytril.

## Hydrotalcite *(BAN, rINN)*

Hidrotalcita. Aluminium magnesium carbonate hydroxide hydrate.

$Mg_6Al_2(OH)_{16}CO_3,4H_2O$ = 604.0.
*CAS — 12304-65-3.*
*ATC — A02AD04.*

NOTE. Compounded preparations of hydrotalcite may be represented by the following names:

- Co-simalcite *x/y* (*BAN*)—where *x* and *y* are the strengths in milligrams of simeticone and hydrotalcite respectively.

**Pharmacopoeias.** In *Br.*

**BP 2003** ( Hydrotalcite). A hydrated form of an aluminium magnesium basic carbonate corresponding to the formula $Al_2Mg_6(OH)_{16}CO_3,4H_2O$. It contains not less than 15.3% and not more than 18.7% of $Al_2O_3$ and not less than 36.0% and not more than 44.0% of MgO. The ratio of $Al_2O_3$ to MgO is not less than 0.40 and not more than 0.45. A white or almost white, free-flowing, granular powder. Practically insoluble in water; it dissolves in dilute mineral acids with slight effervescence. A 4% suspension in water has a pH of 8.0 to 10.0.

### Profile

Hydrotalcite is an antacid (see p.1239) that is given in doses of up to about 1 g by mouth.

### Preparations

***BP 2003:*** Hydrotalcite Tablets.

**Proprietary Preparations** (details are given in Part 3)
***Austria:*** Talcid; Talidat; ***Fr.:*** Ultacite†; ***Ger.:*** Ancid; Megalac; Talcid; Talidat; ***Gr.:*** Talcid; ***Israel:*** Talcid; ***Malaysia:*** Swecon; ***Mex.:*** Talcid; ***Neth.:*** Ultacit; ***S.Afr.:*** Altacite†; ***Spain:*** Hidralma†; Talcid; Talidat†; ***UK:*** Actal†; Altacite†.

**Multi-ingredient:** ***Hong Kong:*** Gl†; ***Irl.:*** Altacite Plus†; ***UK:*** Altacite Plus.

## Ipomoea

Ipomoea Root; Mexican Scammony Root; Orizaba Jalap Root; Scammony Root.

## Ipomoea Resin

Mexican Scammony Resin; Resina de ipomoea; Scammony Resin.
*CAS — 9000-34-4.*

### Profile

Ipomoea is the dried root of *Ipomoea orizabensis* (Convolvulaceae). Ipomoea resin is a mixture of glycosidal resins obtained from ipomoea and it has a drastic purgative and irritant action. It has been superseded by less toxic laxatives.

### Preparations

**Proprietary Preparations** (details are given in Part 3)
**Multi-ingredient:** ***Fr.:*** Mucinum†.

## Irsogladine Maleate *(rINNM)*

Maleato de irsogladina; MN-1695. 2,4-Diamino-6-(2,5-dichlorophenyl)-*S*-triazine maleate.

$C_9H_7Cl_2N_5.C_4H_4O_4$ = 372.2.
*CAS — 57381-26-7 (irsogladine); 84504-69-8 (irsogladine maleate).*

### Profile

Irsogladine maleate is a cytoprotective drug that is used in the treatment of peptic ulcer disease (p.1246) in a usual dose of 4 mg daily by mouth.

### Preparations

**Proprietary Preparations** (details are given in Part 3)
***Jpn:*** Gaslon N.

## Ispaghula

Ispágula.

**Pharmacopoeias.** Monographs for the husk and seed are included in *Eur.* (see p.vi), *Pol.*, and *US*.

**Ph. Eur. 5.0** (Ispaghula Husk; Plantaginis Ovatae Seminis Tegumentum). The episperm and collapsed adjacent layers removed from the seeds of *Plantago ovata* (*P. ispaghula*). The powdered drug loses not more than 12.0% of its weight on drying. Protect from light.

**Ph. Eur. 5.0** (Ispaghula Seed; Plantaginis Ovatae Semen). The dried ripe seeds of *Plantago ovata* (*P. ispaghula*). The powdered drug loses not more than 10.0% of its weight on drying. Protect from light.

**USP 27** (Psyllium Husk). The cleaned, dried seed coat (epidermis), in whole or in powdered form, separated by winnowing and threshing from the seeds of *Plantago ovata* (known in commerce as Blond Psyllium, Indian Psyllium, Indian Plantago, or Ispaghula), or from *Plantago psyllium*, or from *Plantago indica* (*P. arenaria*) known in commerce as Spanish or French Psyllium.

**USP 27** (Plantago Seed). The cleaned, dried, ripe seed of *Plantago ovata*, or of *Plantago psyllium*, or of *Plantago indica* (*P. arenaria*).

### Psyllium Seed

Flea Seed; Psyllii Semen; Semilla de psilio.

**Pharmacopoeias.** In *Eur.* (see p.vi) and *Pol.* Also in *US* under the title of Plantago Seed.

**Ph. Eur. 5.0** (Psyllium Seed). The ripe, whole, dry seeds of *Plantago afra* (*P. psyllium*) or *Plantago indica* (*P. arenaria*). It loses not more than 14.0% of its weight on drying. Protect from light and moisture.

**USP 27** (Plantago Seed). The cleaned, dried, ripe seed of *Plantago ovata*, or of *Plantago psyllium*, or of *Plantago indica* (*P. arenaria*) (see also Ispaghula, above).

### Adverse Effects and Precautions

Large quantities of ispaghula and other bulk laxatives may temporarily increase flatulence and abdominal distension; hypersensitivity reactions have been reported. There is a risk of intestinal or oesophageal obstruction and faecal impaction, especially if such compounds are swallowed dry. Therefore, they should always be taken with sufficient fluid and should not be taken immediately before going to bed. They should be avoided by patients who have difficulty swallowing.

Bulk laxatives should not be given to patients with pre-existing faecal impaction, intestinal obstruction, or colonic atony.

**Hypersensitivity.** Hypersensitivity reactions associated with the ingestion or inhalation of ispaghula or psyllium have been reported;[1-6] symptoms have included rhinitis, urticaria, bronchospasm, and anaphylactic shock. In most patients, sensitisation was thought to have occurred during occupational exposure.

1. Busse WW, Schoenwetter WF. Asthma from psyllium in laxative manufacture. *Ann Intern Med* 1975; **83:** 361–2.
2. Gross R. Acute bronchospasm associated with inhalation of psyllium hydrophilic mucilloid. *JAMA* 1979; **241:** 1573–4.
3. Suhonen R, *et al.* Anaphylactic shock due to ingestion of psyllium laxative. *Allergy* 1983; **38:** 363–5.
4. Zaloga GP, *et al.* Anaphylaxis following psyllium ingestion. *J Allergy Clin Immunol* 1984; **74:** 79–80.
5. Kaplan MJ. Anaphylactic reaction to "Heartwise". *N Engl J Med* 1990; **323:** 1072–3.
6. Lantner RR, *et al.* Anaphylaxis following ingestion of a psyllium-containing cereal. *JAMA* 1990; **264:** 2534–6.

### Interactions

There is a possibility that ispaghula may reduce or delay gastrointestinal absorption of other drugs.

**Lithium.** For reference to ispaghula possibly reducing the absorption of lithium, see Gastrointestinal Drugs, p.304.

### Uses and Administration

Ispaghula seed, ispaghula husk, and psyllium seed are bulk laxatives (p.1239). They absorb water in the gastrointestinal tract to form a mucilaginous mass which increases the volume of faeces and hence promotes peristalsis. They are used in the treatment of constipation (p.1240), especially in diverticular disease (p.1241) and irritable bowel syndrome (p.1244), and when excessive straining at stool must be avoided, for example following anorectal surgery or in the management of haemorrhoids. The ability to absorb water and increase faecal mass means that they may also be used in the management of diarrhoea (p.1241) and for adjusting faecal consistency in patients with colostomies.

The usual dose is about 3.5 g one to three times daily by mouth, although higher doses have been given. It should be taken immediately after mixing in at least 150 mL water or fruit juice. The full effect may not be achieved for up to 3 days.

Ispaghula is also given for mild to moderate hypercholesterolaemia as an adjunct to a lipid-lowering diet. The recommended dose is about 3.5 g in at least 150 mL water twice daily by mouth. A higher dose of 5.25 g twice daily may be given for the initial 2 or 3 months of treatment if necessary.

**Hyperlipidaemias.** Preparations of ispaghula have been reported[1-4] to lower serum-cholesterol concentrations in patients with mild to moderate hypercholesterolaemia. They have also been given with reduced doses of a bile-acid binding resin in the treatment of hyperlipidaemia,[5] which is reported to be effective and better tolerated than full doses of the resin alone. However, ispaghula or psyllium should be regarded as adjuncts to dietary modification rather than substitutes for it. For a discussion of the hyperlipidaemias and their management, see p.823.

1. Anderson JW, *et al.* Cholesterol-lowering effect of psyllium hydrophilic mucilloid for hypercholesterolemic men. *Arch Intern Med* 1988; **148:** 292–6.
2. Bell LP, *et al.* Cholesterol-lowering effects of psyllium hydrophilic mucilloid: adjunct therapy to a prudent diet for patients with mild to moderate hypercholesterolemia. *JAMA* 1989; **261:** 3419–23.
3. Anderson JW, *et al.* Cholesterol-lowering effects of psyllium intake adjunctive to diet therapy in men and women with hypercholesterolemia: meta-analysis of 8 controlled trials. *Am J Clin Nutr* 2000; **71:** 472–9.
4. Anderson JW, *et al.* Long-term cholesterol-lowering effects of psyllium as an adjunct to diet therapy in the treatment of hypercholesterolemia. *Am J Clin Nutr* 2000; **71:** 1433–8.
5. Spence JD, *et al.* Combination therapy with colestipol and psyllium mucilloid in patients with hyperlipidemia. *Ann Intern Med* 1995; **123:** 493–9.

### Preparations

***BP 2003:*** Ispaghula Husk Effervescent Granules; Ispaghula Husk Granules; Ispaghula Husk Oral Powder;
***USP 27:*** Psyllium Hydrophilic Mucilloid for Oral Suspension.

**Proprietary Preparations** (details are given in Part 3)
***Arg.:*** Agarol Fibras Naturales; Herbaccion Laxante; Konsyl; Metamucil; Motional; Mucofalk; Plantaben; ***Austral.:*** Agiofibe; Ford Fibre†; Fybogel; Metamucil†; Mucilax; Natural Fibre†; ***Austria:*** Agiocur; Agiolind; Effersyllium†; Laxans; Metamucil; Pascomucil†; Plantocur; ***Belg.:*** Colofiber; Fybogel; Metamucil†; Mucivital†; ***Braz.:*** Agiofibra; Loraga†; Metamucil; Plantaben; ***Canad.:*** Fibrepur†; Floralax†; Karacil†; Laxagel†; Laxucil; Metamucil; Mucilloid†; Natural Source Laxative; Naturcil†; Novo-Mucilax; Prodiem Plain; ***Chile:*** Euromucil; Fibrasol; Metamucil; Plantaben; ***Denm.:*** Vi-Siblin; ***Fin.:*** Agiocur; Laxamucil; Vi-Siblin; ***Fr.:*** Mucivital; Phytofibre†; Spagulax; Spagulax Mucilage; Transilane; ***Ger.:*** Agiocur; Agiolax Ballast†; Bekunis Leicht†; Flosa; Flosine; Kneipp Abfuhr Herbagran†; Laxiplant Soft; Metamucil; Mucofalk; Pascomucil; Plantocur†; ***Hong Kong:*** Agiocur; Fybogel; Metamucil; Mucofalk; Vitalax†; ***India:*** Isogel; ***Irl.:*** Fybogel; Regulan; ***Israel:*** Agiocur; Konsyl; Metamucil†; Mucivital; Planten; ***Ital.:*** Fibrolax; Mucivital†; Planten; ***Malaysia:*** Fybogel; Mucofalk; ***Mex.:*** Agiofibra; Fibromucil; Fybogel; Hormolax; Konsyl; Laxen†; Metabyn†; Metamucil; Novagon; Pygosal†; Tagozzard†; ***Mon.:*** Psylia; ***Neth.:*** Metamucil; Volcolon; ***Norw.:*** Lunelax; Vi-Siblin; ***NZ:*** Isogel; Konsyl†; Metamucil; Mucilax; ***Port.:*** Agiocur; Bekunis Fibra†; Metamucil†; Mucofalk; ***S.Afr.:*** Agiobulk; Fybogel; Metamucil; ***Singapore:*** Fybogel; Isogel†; Metamucil†; Mucilin; Mucofalk; ***Spain:*** Biolid; Biopasal Fibra†; Cenat; Fibramucil†; Fybogel†; Laxisoft; Metamucil; Plantaben; ***Swed.:*** Lunelax; Vi-Siblin; ***Switz.:*** Agiolax mite; Bekunis Plantago Granule†; Colosoft; Dulconatur†; Konsyl†; Laxiplant Soft; Metamucil; Mucilar; Valverde regulateur du transit intestinal granules; ***Thai.:*** Agiocur; Fybogel; Metamucil; Mucilin; Mucofalk; ***UK:*** Fybogel; Fybozest†; Isogel; Ispagel; Konsyl; Regulan; ***USA:*** Alramucil Instant Mix†; Alramucil†; Fiberall; Hydrocil Instant; Konsyl; Konsyl-D; Maalox Daily Fiber†; Metamucil; Modane Bulk†; Mylanta Natural Fiber; Perdiem Fiber†; Reguloid; Restore†; Serutan; Syllact.

**Multi-ingredient:** ***Arg.:*** Agiolax; Cholesterol Reducing Plan; Medilaxan; Prompt; Rapilax Fibras; Salutaris; ***Austral.:*** Agiolax; Bioglan Psylli-Mucil Plus†; Enterocare†; Herb-a-Lax†; Herbal Cleanse†; Nucolox; PC Regulax†; ***Austria:*** Abbiofort; Agiolax; ***Belg.:*** Agiolax; ***Braz.:*** Agiolax; Plantax; Prompt†; ***Canad.:*** Prodiem Plus; ***Chile:*** Bilaxil; ***Fin.:*** Agiolax; ***Fr.:*** Agiolax; Filigel; Imegul; Parapsyllium; Spagulax au Citrate de Potassium; Spagulax au Sorbitol; ***Ger.:*** Agiolax; Kneipplax N†; ***Hong Kong:*** Agiolax; Fybogel Mebeverine; ***Irl.:*** Fybogel Mebeverine; ***Israel:*** Agiolax; ***Ital.:*** Agiolax; Duolaxan; Fibrolax Complex; Ginolax†; ***Mex.:*** Agiolax; Psilumax; ***Neth.:*** Agiolax; ***NZ:*** Nucolox; ***Port.:*** Agiolax; ***S.Afr.:*** Agiolax; ***Singapore:*** Fybogel Mebeverine†; ***Spain:*** Agiolax; Laxiplant†; ***Swed.:*** Lunelax comp†; Vi-Siblin S; ***Switz.:*** Agiolax; Bronchalin†; Laxiplant cum Senna†; Mucilar Avena; ***Thai.:*** Agiolax; ***UK:*** Cleansing Herbs; Fibre Dophilus; Fibre Plus; Fybogel Mebeverine; Lion Cleansing Herbs; Lipolest†; Manevac; ***USA:*** Perdiem; Syllamalt†.

## Itopride Hydrochloride *(rINNM)*

HC-803; Hidrocloruro de itoprida; HSR-803. *N*-{*p*-[2-(Dimethylamino)ethoxy]benzyl}veratramide hydrochloride.

$C_{20}H_{26}N_2O_4,HCl = 394.9$.

*CAS — 122898-67-3 (itopride).*

### Profile

Itopride hydrochloride is a substituted benzamide with general properties similar to those of metoclopramide (p.1274) that has been used for its prokinetic and antiemetic actions in doses of 50 mg by mouth three times daily before meals.

### Preparations

**Proprietary Preparations** (details are given in Part 3)
***Jpn:*** Ganaton.

## Jalap

Jalap Root; Jalap Tuber; Jalapa; Jalapenwurzel; Vera Cruz Jalap.

## Jalap Resin

Jalapenharz; Resina de jalapa.

*CAS — 9000-35-5.*

### Profile

Jalap is the dried tubercles of *Ipomoea purga* (*=Exogonium purga*) (Convolvulaceae). Jalap resin is a mixture of glycosidal resins obtained by extraction of jalap with alcohol and it has a drastic purgative and irritant action. It has been superseded by less toxic laxatives.

### Preparations

**Proprietary Preparations** (details are given in Part 3)
**Multi-ingredient:** ***Braz.:*** Jalapa Composta.

## Kaolin

Bolus Alba; Caolin; E559; Weisser Ton.

*CAS — 1332-58-7.*

*ATC — A07BC02.*

**Pharmacopoeias.** In *Chin.*, *Eur.* (see p.vi), *Int.*, *Jpn*, *US*, and *Viet.* Some pharmacopoeias do not differentiate between the heavy and light varieties.

**Ph. Eur. 5.0** (Kaolin, Heavy). A purified, natural, hydrated aluminium silicate of variable composition. It is a fine, white or greyish-white, unctuous powder. Practically insoluble in water and in organic solvents.

**BP 2003** (Light Kaolin). A native hydrated aluminium silicate, freed from most of its impurities by elutriation, and dried. It contains a suitable dispersing agent. It is a light, white, odourless or almost odourless, unctuous powder free from gritty particles. Practically insoluble in water and in mineral acids.

The BP 2003 directs that when Kaolin or Light Kaolin is prescribed or demanded, Light Kaolin shall be dispensed or supplied, unless it is ascertained that Light Kaolin (Natural) is required.

**BP 2003** (Light Kaolin (Natural)). It is Light Kaolin which does not contain a dispersing agent. It is a light, white, odourless or almost odourless, unctuous powder free from gritty particles. Practically insoluble in water and in mineral acids.

The BP 2003 directs that when Kaolin or Light Kaolin is prescribed or demanded, Light Kaolin shall be dispensed or supplied, unless it is ascertained that Light Kaolin (Natural) is required.

**USP 27** (Kaolin). A native hydrated aluminium silicate, powdered and freed from gritty particles by elutriation. It is a soft, white or yellowish-white powder or lumps with an earthy or clay-like taste and when moistened with water assumes a darker colour and develops a marked clay-like odour. Insoluble in water, in cold dilute acids, and in solutions of alkali hydroxides.

### Profile

Light kaolin and light kaolin (natural) are adsorbent antidiarrhoeal agents that have been used as adjuncts to rehydration therapy in the management of diarrhoea (p.1241). Up to about 24 g daily may be taken by mouth in divided doses. Kaolin is often given in combination with other antidiarrhoeals, especially pectin.

Kaolin can form insoluble complexes with a number of other drugs in the gastrointestinal tract and reduce their absorption; concomitant oral administration should be avoided.

Externally, light kaolin is used as a dusting powder. Kaolin is liable to be heavily contaminated with bacteria, and when used in dusting powders, it should be sterilised.

Heavy kaolin is used in the preparation of kaolin poultice, which is applied topically with the intention of reducing inflammation and alleviating pain (see Rubefacients and Topical Analgesia, p.4).

Light kaolin is also used as a food additive.

### Preparations

***BP 2003:*** Kaolin and Morphine Mixture; Kaolin Mixture; Kaolin Poultice.

**Proprietary Preparations** (details are given in Part 3)
***Braz.:*** Kaogel; ***Ital.:*** Kao-Pront†; ***UK:*** Childrens Diarrhoea Mixture; Entrocalm.

**Multi-ingredient:** ***Arg.:*** Anusol-A; Endomicina; Gastranil; Opocarbon; Opocler; ***Austral.:*** Bis-Pectin; Chemists Own Diarrhoea Mixture; De Witt's Antacid†; Diarcalm†; Donnagel; Kaomagma with Pectin†; Kaomagma†; Kaopectate†; ***Belg.:*** Alopate; Kaopectate†; Neutroses†; ***Braz.:*** Atalin; Digastril†; Eviprostat†; Gastrobene; Kal Sept†; Kaomagma; Kaopectate†; Kaopectin†; Kaostase Suspension†; Kaostase†; Neutracido†; Pectalin†; Pectimax†; Plexo Enterin†; ***Canad.:*** Bebia†; Diarex†; Donnagel-PG†; ***Chile:*** Furazolidona; ***Fr.:*** Anti-H; Antiphlogistine; Argeal; Gastropax; Gelogastrine†; Kaobrol; Kaologeais; Kaomuth; Karayal; Keracnyl; Neutroses; ***Ger.:*** Kaoprompt-H; rohasal; ***Gr.:*** Kaopectate; ***Hong Kong:*** Calamine-D; Uni-Kaotin; ***Irl.:*** Kaopectate; ***Israel:*** Digestif-Ara; Kaopectin; Kapectin Forte; Zincod; ***Ital.:*** Carbotiol†; Katoxyn; Magnesia Bisurata†; Neo Zeta-Foot†; Neutrose S Pellegrino; Streptomagma; ***Malaysia:*** Beakopectin; Kaopectate; ***Mex.:*** Caopecfar; Colfur; Contefur; Coralzul; Dibapec Compuesto; Facetin-D; Farpectol; Fuzotyl; Hidromagma; Isocar; Kaomycin; Kaopectate; Lactopectin; Neo-Kap; Neoxil; Olam; Optazol;

Quimefuran; Tapzol con Neomicina; Tapzol†; Treda; Trilor; Yodozona; ***S.Afr.:*** Betapect; Bipectinol; Biskapect; Chloropect; Collodyne†; Enterolyte; Gastropect; Kao; Kaopectin; Kaostatex; Pectin-K; Pectrolyte; ***Singapore:*** Kaopectate; ***Switz.:*** Argent; Cicafissan; Fissan; Gyrosan; Kaopectate†; Neo-Decongestine; Neutroses; Padma-Lax; ***Thai.:*** Alkamine; Alupep; Antacil; Coccila; Di-Su-Frone; Difuran; Diolin†; Disento; Disento PF; Droximag; Furasian; Furopectin; Kaopectal; Kaopectal-N†; Kaopectate†; Med-Kafuzone; ***UAE:*** Kaptin; ***UK:*** Codella†; Collis Browne's; De Witt's Antacid; Enterosan†; Junior Kao-C; Kaodene; KLN; Moorland; Opazimes; ***USA:*** K-C; Kao-Paverin; Kao-Spen; Kaodene Non-Narcotic; Mexsana.

## Lactitol *(BAN, rINN)*

E966; β-Galactosido-sorbitol; Lactit; Lactitolum; Lactobiosit; Lactositol. 4-*O*-(β-D-Galactopyranosyl)-D-glucitol.

$C_{12}H_{24}O_{11}$ = 344.3.

*CAS — 585-86-4.*

*ATC — A06AD12.*

**Pharmacopoeias.** In *USNF. Eur.* (see p.vi) includes the monohydrate.

**Ph. Eur. 5.0** (Lactitol Monohydrate). A white crystalline powder. Very soluble in water; slightly soluble in alcohol; practically insoluble in dichloromethane.

**USNF 22** (Lactitol). It may be the anhydrous form, the monohydrate, or the dihydrate.

### Profile

Lactitol is a disaccharide analogue of lactulose (below) and has similar actions and uses.

Lactitol monohydrate is used as an oral powder in the management of hepatic encephalopathy (p.1243) and in constipation (p.1240). Lactitol monohydrate 1.05 g is approximately equivalent to 1 g of anhydrous lactitol.

In the treatment of hepatic encephalopathy, lactitol monohydrate is given in usual doses of 500 to 700 mg/kg daily by mouth in 3 divided doses at meal times. The dose is subsequently adjusted to produce 2 soft stools daily.

In the treatment of constipation, lactitol monohydrate is given in an initial dose of 20 g daily by mouth as a single dose with the morning or evening meal, subsequently adjusted to produce one stool daily. A dose of 10 g daily may be sufficient for many patients.

Doses should be mixed with food or liquid, and 1 to 2 glasses of liquid should be drunk with the meal.

Lactitol is a permitted sweetener in foods.

### Preparations

**Proprietary Preparations** (details are given in Part 3)

***Austria:*** Importal; Portolac; Pselac; ***Belg.:*** Importal; Normolaxil; Portolac; ***Denm.:*** Importal; ***Fin.:*** Importal†; Lalax; ***Fr.:*** Importal; ***Ger.:*** Importal; Neda Lactiv Importal†; ***Gr.:*** Importal; ***Israel:*** Importal; Novolax; ***Ital.:*** Portolac; ***Jpn:*** Portolac; ***Neth.:*** Importal; ***Norw.:*** Importal; ***NZ:*** Importal; ***Port.:*** Importal; ***S.Afr.:*** Importal†; ***Spain:*** Emportal; Oponaf; ***Swed.:*** Importal; ***Switz.:*** Importal; ***Thai.:*** Importal.

**Multi-ingredient:** ***Fr.:*** Fucafibres†; ***Ital.:*** Levoplus.

## Lactulose *(BAN, USAN, rINN)*

Lactulosa; Lactulosum. 4-*O*-β-D-Galactopyranosyl-D-fructose.

$C_{12}H_{22}O_{11}$ = 342.3.

*CAS — 4618-18-2.*

*ATC — A06AD11.*

**Pharmacopoeias.** In *Eur.* (see p.vi) and *Jpn. Chin.* only contains specifications for a solution. *US* only contains specifications for a solution and a concentrated liquid.

**Ph. Eur. 5.0** (Lactulose). A white or almost white, crystalline powder. Freely soluble in water; sparingly soluble in methyl alcohol; practically insoluble in toluene.

**Ph. Eur. 5.0** (Lactulose, Liquid; Lactulose Solution BP 2003). An aqueous solution of lactulose. It contains not less than 62.0% w/v of lactulose; it may contain lesser amounts of other sugars including lactose, epilactose, galactose, tagatose, and fructose. It may contain a suitable antimicrobial preservative. It is a clear, colourless or pale brownish-yellow, viscous liquid. Miscible with water. It may be a supersaturated solution or may contain crystals that disappear on heating.

**USP 27** (Lactulose Concentrate). A colourless to amber syrupy liquid that may exhibit some precipitation and darkening on standing. Miscible with water. Store in airtight containers preferably at a temperature between 2° and 30°.

### Adverse Effects

Lactulose may cause abdominal discomfort associated with flatulence or cramps. Nausea and vomiting have occasionally been reported after high doses. Some consider the taste to be unpleasant. Prolonged use or excessive dosage may result in diarrhoea with excessive loss of water and electrolytes, particularly potassium. Hypernatraemia has been reported.

**Lactic acidosis.** Severe lactic acidosis developed in a patient with adynamic ileus who was being given lactulose for hepatic encephalopathy.[1]


1. Mann NS, *et al.* Lactulose and severe lactic acidosis. *Ann Intern Med* 1985; **103:** 637.


### Precautions

Lactulose should not be given to patients with galactosaemia or intestinal obstruction. It should not be used in patients on a low galactose diet and care should be taken in patients with lactose intolerance or in diabetic patients because of the presence of some free galactose and lactose.

### Pharmacokinetics

Following administration by mouth, lactulose passes essentially unchanged into the large intestine where it is metabolised by saccharolytic bacteria with the formation of simple organic acids, mainly lactic acid and small amounts of acetic and formic acids. The small amount of absorbed lactulose is subsequently excreted unchanged in the urine.

### Uses and Administration

Lactulose is a synthetic disaccharide osmotic laxative (p.1239) used in the treatment of constipation (p.1240) and in hepatic encephalopathy (p.1243). Lactulose is broken down by colonic bacteria mainly into lactic acid. This exerts a local osmotic effect in the colon resulting in increased faecal bulk and stimulation of peristalsis. It may take up to 48 hours before an effect is obtained. When larger doses are given for hepatic encephalopathy the pH in the colon is reduced significantly and the absorption of ammonium ions and other toxic nitrogenous compounds is decreased, leading to a fall in blood-ammonia concentration and an improvement in mental function.

Lactulose is usually given as a solution containing approximately 3.35 g of lactulose per 5 mL together with other sugars such as galactose and lactose; an oral powder formulation is also available in some countries. In the treatment of **constipation**, the usual initial dose is 10 to 20 g (15 to 30 mL) given daily by mouth in a single dose or in 2 divided doses; doses up to 40 g (60 mL) daily have been given. The dose is gradually adjusted according to the patient's needs. Children aged 5 to 10 years may be given initial doses of 10 mL twice daily; 1 to 5 years, 5 mL twice daily; under 1 year, 2.5 mL twice daily.

In **hepatic encephalopathy**, 60 to 100 g (90 to 150 mL) is given daily by mouth in 3 divided doses. The dose is subsequently adjusted to produce 2 or 3 soft stools each day. Lactulose solution 300 mL mixed with 700 mL of water or sodium chloride 0.9% has been used as a retention enema; the enema is retained for 30 to 60 minutes, repeated every 4 to 6 hours until the patient is able to take oral medication.

◊ References.


1. Clausen MR, Mortensen PB. Lactulose, disaccharides and colonic flora: clinical consequences. *Drugs* 1997; **53:** 930–42.


**Diagnosis and testing.** THE SUGAR ABSORPTION TEST. In healthy individuals lactulose is largely unabsorbed from the gastrointestinal tract, but in, for example, coeliac disease (p.1417) there is increased permeability to disaccharides such as lactulose and a paradoxical decrease in the absorption of monosaccharides. This led to the development of the differential sugar absorption test in which 2 sugars are given simultaneously by mouth and the urinary recovery of each is determined; mannitol is commonly used as the monosaccharide component and lactulose as the disaccharide. Alternatives include mannitol plus cellobiose and rhamnose plus lactulose. This absorption test is useful in the investigation of intestinal disease.[1]

THE LACTOSE BREATH TEST (hydrogen breath test). Lactulose is converted by bacteria in the large bowel to short chain fatty acids with the production of small quantities of hydrogen gas. The hydrogen is rapidly absorbed and is exhaled in the breath and measurement of its production is used to measure orocaecal transit time and carbohydrate malabsorption. However, even small doses of lactulose shortens transit time, which may limit the value of this test.[2]


1. Uil JJ, *et al.* Clinical implications of the sugar absorption test: intestinal permeability test to assess mucosal barrier function. *Scand J Gastroenterol* 1997; **223** (suppl): 70–8.
2. Miller MA, *et al.* Comparison of scintigraphy and lactulose breath hydrogen test for assessment of orocecal transit: lactulose accelerates small bowel transit. *Dig Dis Sci* 1997; **42:** 10–18.


### Preparations

***BP 2003:*** Lactulose Oral Powder;
***Ph. Eur.:*** Liquid Lactulose;
***USP 27:*** Lactulose Solution.

**Proprietary Preparations** (details are given in Part 3)

***Arg.:*** Genocolan; Lactulon; Tenualax; ***Austral.:*** Actilax; Duphalac; Genlac; Lac-Dol; ***Austria:*** Bifiteral; Darmol Lactulose; Duphalac; Floralac; Laevolac; Lose.Lax; Medilet; ***Belg.:*** Bifiteral; Certalac; Duphalac; ***Braz.:*** Farlac; Lactulona; ***Canad.:*** Acilac; Cephulac†; Chronulac†; Comalose-R†; Duphalac†; Gen-Lac; Lactulax†; Laxilose; ***Chile:*** Disman Sobres; Duphalac; Rencef; ***Denm.:*** Danilax; Medilax; ***Fin.:*** Duphalac; Levolac; Loraga; ***Fr.:*** Duphalac; Fitaxal†; Laxaron; ***Ger.:*** Bifinorma; Bifiteral; Eugalac; Hepa-Merz Lact; Hepaticum-Lac-Medice; Kattwilact; Lactocur; Lactofalk†; Lactuflor; Lactuverlan; Laevilac S; Laxomundin†; Mandrolax Lactu†; Medilet; Natulax†; Tulotract; ***Gr.:*** Duphalac; ***Hong Kong:*** Danilax; Duphalac; ***India:*** Livo Luk; ***Irl.:*** Dulax; Duphalac; Gerelax; Laxose; ***Israel:*** Avilac; Gerelax; Lactulax; Sirolax†; ***Ital.:*** Biolac; Dia-Colon; Duphalac; Epalat EPS; Epalfen; Idrolac†; Lactoger; Lactyl†; Laevolac; Lassifar; Lattubio; Lattulac; Lis; Normase; Osmolac; Sintolatt; Verelait; ***Jpn:*** Monilac; ***Malaysia:*** Duphalac; Lactul; Lactumed; ***Mex.:*** Lactulax; Regulact; ***Neth.:*** Duphalac; Legendal; ***Norw.:*** Duphalac; Levolac; ***NZ:*** Duphalac†; Laevolac; ***Port.:*** Colsanac; Duphalac; Laevolac; ***S.Afr.:*** Adco-Liquilax; Duphalac; Lacson; Laevolac†; Laxette; ***Singapore:*** Dhactulose; Duphalac; ***Spain:*** Belmalax; Duolax†; Duphalac; Gatinar†; ***Swed.:*** Betulac†; Duphalac; Laktipex; Loraga; ***Switz.:*** Duphalac; Gatinar; Laevolac†; Legendal; Rudolac; ***Thai.:*** Duphalac; Hepalac; ***UAE:*** Soflax; ***UK:*** Duphalac; Lactugal; Lemlax; Regulose; ***USA:*** Cephulac; Cholac; Chronulac; Constilac; Constulose; Duphalac; Enulose; Evalose†; Heptalac†; Kristalose.

**Multi-ingredient:** ***Arg.:*** Bifidosa; ***Fr.:*** Melaxose; Transulose; ***Ger.:*** Eugalan Topfer forte; ***Ital.:*** Dimalosio†; Lactolas; Lactomannan; Levoplus; Naturalass.

## Lafutidine *(rINN)*

FRG-8813. (±)-2-(Furfurylsulfinyl)-*N*-[(*Z*)-4-{[4-(piperidinomethyl)-2-pyridyl]oxy}-2-butenyl]acetamide.

$C_{22}H_{29}N_3O_4S$ = 431.5.

*CAS — 118288-08-7.*

*ATC — A02BA08.*

### Profile

Lafutidine, like cimetidine (p.1255), is a histamine $H_2$-antagonist. It is used in the management of peptic ulcer disease.

◊ References.


1. Uesugi T, *et al.* The efficacy of lafutidine in improving preoperative gastric fluid property: a comparison with ranitidine and rabeprazole. *Anesth Analg* 2002; **95:** 144–7.
2. Mikawa K, *et al.* Lafutidine vs cimetidine to decrease gastric fluid acidity and volume in children. *Can J Anaesth* 2003; **50:** 425–6.
3. Isomoto H, *et al.* Lafutidine, a novel histamine H2-receptor antagonist, vs lansoprazole in combination with amoxicillin and clarithromycin for eradication of Helicobacter pylori. *Helicobacter* 2003; **8:** 111–19.


### Preparations

**Proprietary Preparations** (details are given in Part 3)
***Jpn:*** Stogar.

## Lansoprazole *(BAN, USAN, rINN)*

A-65006; AG-1749; Lansoprazol. 2-({3-Methyl-4-(2,2,2-trifluoroethoxy)-2-pyridyl)methyl} sulphinylbenzimidazole.

$C_{16}H_{14}F_3N_3O_2S$ = 369.4.

*CAS — 103577-45-3.*

*ATC — A02BC03.*

**Pharmacopoeias.** In *US.*

**USP 27** (Lansoprazole). Protect from light.

### Adverse Effects and Precautions

As for Omeprazole, p.1278.

◊ Reviews.


1. Freston JW, *et al.* Safety profile of lansoprazole: the US clinical trial experience. *Drug Safety* 1999; **20:** 195–205.


**Effects on the gastrointestinal tract.** Glossitis (associated in some cases with black tongue or stomatitis) has been reported in a few patients taking lansoprazole as part of a triple therapy regimen for *Helicobacter pylori* elimination in peptic ulcer disease.[1] Discoloured tongue has been reported in a patient taking lansoprazole alone.[2]

An increase in gastritis was observed in patients infected with *Helicobacter pylori* when treated with long term lansoprazole therapy.[3] For further discussion of the link between *H. pylori*, gastritis, and proton pump inhibitor use, see Gastrointestinal Tumours, p.1279.


1. Greco S, *et al.* Glossitis, stomatitis, and black tongue with lansoprazole plus clarithromycin and other antibiotics. *Ann Pharmacother* 1997; **31:** 1548.
2. Scully C. Discoloured tongue: a new cause? *Br J Dermatol* 2001; **144:** 1293–4.
3. Berstad AE, *et al.* Helicobacter pylori gastritis and epithelial cell proliferation in patients with reflux oesophagitis after treatment with lansoprazole. *Gut* 1997; **41:** 740–7.


**Effects on the skin.** For mention of skin reactions to lansoprazole, see p.1279.

**Musculoskeletal effects.** For reference to a case of eosinophilia and myalgia related to lansoprazole therapy, see p.1279.

### Interactions

As for Omeprazole, p.1279. Antacids and sucralfate may reduce the bioavailability of lansoprazole, and should not be taken within 1 hour of a dose of lansoprazole.

◊ For reference to a lack of effect of lansoprazole on diazepam, see Gastrointestinal Drugs, p.694, and for a clinically insignificant effect on theophylline clearance, see p.803. For reference to glossitis occurring when lansoprazole was used with some antibacterials, see Effects on the Gastrointestinal Tract, above.

## Pharmacokinetics

Lansoprazole is rapidly absorbed after oral administration, with peak plasma concentrations achieved about 1.5 hours after a dose by mouth. Bioavailability is reported to be 80% or more even with the first dose, although the drug must be given in an enteric-coated form since lansoprazole is unstable at acid pH. It is extensively metabolised in the liver primarily by cytochrome P450 isoenzyme CYP2C19 to form 5-hydroxyl-lansoprazole and by CYP3A to form lansoprazole sulfone. Metabolites are excreted primarily in faeces via the bile; only about 15 to 30% of a dose is excreted in urine. The plasma elimination half-life is around 1 to 2 hours but the duration of action is much longer. Lansoprazole is about 97% bound to plasma protein. Clearance is decreased in elderly patients, and in liver disease.

◊ References.


1. Hussein Z, *et al.* Age-related differences in the pharmacokinetics and pharmacodynamics of lansoprazole. *Br J Clin Pharmacol* 1993; **36:** 391–8.
2. Flouvat B, *et al.* Single and multiple dose pharmacokinetics of lansoprazole in elderly subjects. *Br J Clin Pharmacol* 1993; **36:** 467–9.
3. Delhotal-Landes B, *et al.* Pharmacokinetics of lansoprazole in patients with renal or liver disease of varying severity. *Eur J Clin Pharmacol* 1993; **45:** 367–71.
4. Delhotal Landes B, *et al.* Clinical pharmacokinetics of lansoprazole. *Clin Pharmacokinet* 1995; **28:** 458–70.
5. Karol MD, *et al.* Lansoprazole pharmacokinetics in subjects with various degrees of kidney function. *Clin Pharmacol Ther* 1997; **61:** 450–8.
6. Tran A, *et al.* Pharmacokinetic-pharmacodynamic study of oral lansoprazole in children. *Clin Pharmacol Ther* 2002; **71:** 359–67.


**Metabolism.** As for omeprazole (p.1280), the cytochrome P450 isoenzyme CYP2C19 (*S*-mephenytoin hydroxylase) is involved in the hydroxylation of lansoprazole, and individuals who are deficient in this enzyme are poor metabolisers of lansoprazole.

References.


1. Pearce RE, *et al.* Identification of the human P450 enzymes involved in lansoprazole metabolism. *J Pharmacol Exp Ther* 1996; **277:** 805–16.
2. Sohn DR, *et al.* Metabolic disposition of lansoprazole in relation to the S-mephenytoin 4′-hydroxylation phenotype status. *Clin Pharmacol Ther* 1997; **61:** 574–82.


## Uses and Administration

Lansoprazole is a proton pump inhibitor with actions and uses similar to those of omeprazole (p.1280). It is used in the treatment of peptic ulcer disease and in other conditions where inhibition of gastric acid secretion may be beneficial.

Lansoprazole is usually given by mouth as capsules, dispersible tablets, or suspension containing enteric-coated granules. Once daily regimens are taken before food in the morning. An intravenous formulation is also available.

For the relief of acid-related **dyspepsia** (p.1242) intermittent courses of lansoprazole may be given in doses of 15 or 30 mg once daily, for 2 to 4 weeks.

In the treatment of **gastro-oesophageal reflux disease** (p.1242) the dose is 30 mg once daily for 4 to 8 weeks; thereafter maintenance therapy can be continued with 15 or 30 mg once daily according to response. In patients unable to take oral therapy, lansoprazole may be given by intravenous infusion for the treatment of erosive oesophagitis for up to 7 days; a dose of 30 mg over 30 minutes daily is recommended.

Lansoprazole is given for the treatment of **peptic ulcer disease** (p.1246) in doses of 30 mg once daily. Treatment is continued for 4 weeks for duodenal and 8 weeks for gastric ulcer. In the USA, a dose of 15 mg daily for 4 weeks is recommended for duodenal ulcer. When appropriate, 15 mg daily may be used as maintenance therapy for the prevention of relapse of duodenal ulcer. Lansoprazole may be combined with antibacterials in one-week **triple therapy** regimens for the eradication of *Helicobacter pylori*. Effective regimens include lansoprazole 30 mg twice daily combined with clarithromycin 500 mg twice daily and either amoxicillin 1 g twice daily or metronidazole 400 mg twice daily; lansoprazole with amoxicillin and metronidazole has also been used. In patients with **NSAID-associated ulceration** a dose of 15 or 30 mg daily for 4 to 8 weeks is recommended; the same dose may be used as prophylaxis for patients who require continued NSAID treatment.

In the treatment of pathological hypersecretory states such as the **Zollinger-Ellison syndrome** (p.1247) the initial dose is 60 mg daily, adjusted as required. Doses of up to 90 mg twice daily have been used. Daily doses greater than 120 mg should be given in divided doses.

In the USA, **children** over the age of 1 year may be given lansoprazole for the short-term treatment of erosive oesophagitis and symptomatic gastro-oesophageal reflux disease. Children weighing less than 30 kg should be given 15 mg daily, and those weighing more than 30 kg are given 30 mg daily. Doses of up to 30 mg twice daily have been used.

Doses of lansoprazole may need to be reduced in patients with hepatic impairment (see below).

◊ General references. For general reviews of proton pump inhibitors, see Omeprazole, p.1280.


1. Anonymous. Lansoprazole—another proton pump inhibitor. *Drug Ther Bull* 1995; **33:** 36–7.
2. Anonymous. Lansoprazole. *Med Lett Drugs Ther* 1995; **37:** 63–4.
3. Blum RA. Lansoprazole and omeprazole in the treatment of acid peptic disorders. *Am J Health-Syst Pharm* 1996; **53:** 1401–15.
4. Garnett WR. Lansoprazole: a proton pump inhibitor. *Ann Pharmacother* 1996; **30:** 1425–36.
5. Langtry HD, Wilde MI. Lansoprazole: an update of its pharmacological properties and clinical efficacy in the management of acid-related disorders. *Drugs* 1997; **54:** 473–500.
6. Matheson AJ, Jarvis B. Lansoprazole: an update of its place in the management of acid-related disorders. *Drugs* 2001; **61:** 1801–33.


**Administration.** Lansoprazole capsules should be swallowed whole and not crushed or chewed. Lansoprazole dispersible tablets should be placed on the tongue and allowed to disintegrate and the resultant granules swallowed; alternatively, the tablets may be swallowed whole with a glass of water. The tablets should not be crushed or chewed. Lansoprazole granules for oral suspension should be reconstituted in a little water and swallowed immediately. Where the suspension formulation is not available, the contents of the capsules (enteric-coated granules) can be sprinkled on apple sauce or mixed with a little fruit juice and swallowed.

**Administration in hepatic impairment.** Care is required in patients with severe hepatic impairment, and doses of lansoprazole should not exceed 30 mg daily.

## Preparations

***USP 27:*** Lansoprazole Delayed-Release Capsules.

**Proprietary Preparations** (details are given in Part 3)
***Arg.:*** Ilsatec; Lanzopral; Mesactol; Ogasto; ***Austral.:*** Zoton; ***Austria:*** Agopton; ***Belg.:*** Dakar; ***Braz.:*** Diprox†; Ilsatec†; Lanogastro; Lanz; Lanzol; Ogastro; Prazol; ***Canad.:*** Prevacid; ***Chile:*** Fudermex; Gastride; Lanzopral; Ogasto; Unival; ***Denm.:*** Lanzo; ***Fin.:*** Lanzo; ***Fr.:*** Lanzor; Ogast; ***Ger.:*** Agopton; Lanzor; ***Gr.:*** Laprazol; ***Hong Kong:*** Takepron; ***India:*** Lanzol; ***Irl.:*** Zoton; ***Israel:*** Zoton; ***Ital.:*** Lansox; Limpidex; Zoton; ***Jpn:*** Takepron; ***Malaysia:*** Prevacid; ***Mex.:*** Ilsatec; Keval; Ogastro; Uldapril; Ulpax; ***Neth.:*** Prezal; ***Norw.:*** Lanzo; ***NZ:*** Zoton; ***Port.:*** Alexin; Gastrex; Gastroliber; Lansox; Lanzogastro; Lizul; Monolitum; Ogasto; Pampe; Pepzol; Ulcertec; ***S.Afr.:*** Lanzor; ***Singapore:*** Prevacid; ***Spain:*** Bamalite; Estomil; Monolitum; Opiren; Pro Ulco; ***Swed.:*** Lanzo; ***Switz.:*** Agopton; ***Thai.:*** Prevacid; ***UAE:*** Lanfast; ***UK:*** Zoton; ***USA:*** Prevacid.

**Multi-ingredient:** ***Arg.:*** Heliklar; ***Braz.:*** Anzopac; Helicopac; Heliklar; Pyloripac; ***Canad.:*** Hp-Pac; ***Fin.:*** Helipak A; Helipak K; Helipak T; ***UK:*** Heliclear; HeliMet; ***USA:*** Prevpac.

*Used as an adjunct in:* ***USA:*** Prevacid NapraPAC.

## Lidamidine Hydrochloride *(USAN, rINNM)*

Hidrocloruro de lidamidina; WHR-1142A. *N*-(2,6-Dimethylphenyl)-*N*′-[imino(methylamino)methyl]urea hydrochloride.

$C_{11}H_{16}N_4O,HCl = 256.7.$

*CAS — 66871-56-5 (lidamidine); 65009-35-0 (lidamidine hydrochloride).*

### Profile

Lidamidine is an alpha$_2$-adrenergic receptor stimulant used as the hydrochloride for the management of diarrhoea.

### Preparations

**Proprietary Preparations** (details are given in Part 3)
***Mex.:*** Idealid; Supra.

## Liquorice

Alcaçuz; Glycyrrhiza; Licorice; Liquiritiae Radix; Liquorice Root; Orozuz; Raiz de Regaliz; Regaliz; Süssholzwurzel.

**Description.** Liquorice is the dried rhizome and roots of *Glycyrrhiza glabra.* Those of *G. glabra* var. *typica* are known in commerce as Spanish Liquorice, those of *G. glabra* var. *glandulifera* as Russian Liquorice, and those of *G. glabra* var. *β-violacea* as Persian Liquorice.

**Pharmacopoeias.** In *Chin., Eur.* (see p.vi), and *Jpn.* Also in *USNF,* which also includes Powdered Licorice and Powdered Licorice Extract. *Eur.* also includes Ammonium Glycyrrhizate ($C_{42}H_{65}NO_{16}$ = 840.0).

**Ph. Eur. 5.0** (Liquorice Root; Liquorice BP 2003). The dried unpeeled or peeled, whole or cut root and stolons of *Glycyrrhiza glabra* containing not less than 4% of glycyrrhizinic acid. Protect from light.

**USNF 22** (Licorice). The roots, rhizomes, and stolons of *Glycyrrhiza glabra* or *G. uralensis*. It contains not less than 2.5% of glycyrrhizinic acid, calculated on the dried basis. Store in a cool, dry place.

### Adverse Effects and Precautions

Liquorice has mineralocorticoid-like actions manifesting as sodium and water retention and hypokalaemia (see below).

Deglycyrrhizinised liquorice is not usually associated with such adverse effects.

**Effects on fluid and electrolyte homoeostasis.** Mineralocorticoid effects have been reported following excessive ingestion of liquorice. The liquorice may be ingested in confectionery (including liquorice-flavoured chewing gum), soft drinks, medicines, or by chewing tobacco. Adverse effects reported include hypokalaemia,[1-15] hypertension,[1,2,6,9,14] congestive heart failure,[1] arrhythmias,[13,16] fatal cardiac arrest,[10] headache,[1] muscle weakness,[1,6,9,13] myopathy,[3,7,8] myoglobinuria,[5] paralysis,[5,11,15] hyperprolactinaemia,[4] and amenorrhoea.[4] The effects are thought to be due to inhibition of 11-β-hydroxysteroid dehydrogenase (cortisol oxidase) by glycyrrhetinic acid, (a metabolite produced by the hydrolysis of glycyrrhizinic acid), resulting in increased concentrations of cortisol in the body.[12,17-19]


1. Chamberlain TJ. Licorice poisoning, pseudoaldosteronism, and heart failure. *JAMA* 1970; **213:** 1343.
2. Wash LK, Bernard JD. Licorice-induced pseudoaldosteronism. *Am J Hosp Pharm* 1975; **32:** 73–4.
3. Bannister B, *et al.* Cardiac arrest due to liquorice-induced hypokalaemia. *BMJ* 1977; **2:** 738–9.
4. Werner S, *et al.* Hyperprolactinaemia and liquorice. *Lancet* 1979; **i:** 319.
5. Cumming AMM, *et al.* Severe hypokalaemia with paralysis induced by small doses of liquorice. *Postgrad Med J* 1980; **56:** 526–9.
6. Blachley JD, Knochel JP. Tobacco chewer's hypokalemia: licorice revisited. *N Engl J Med* 1980; **302:** 784–5.
7. Lai F, *et al.* Licorice, snuff, and hypokalemia. *N Engl J Med* 1980; **303:** 463.
8. Nightingale S, *et al.* Anorexia nervosa, liquorice and hypokalaemic myopathy. *Postgrad Med J* 1981; **57:** 577–9.
9. Cereda JM, *et al.* Liquorice intoxication caused by alcohol-free pastis. *Lancet* 1983; **i:** 1442.
10. Haberer JP, *et al.* Severe hypokalaemia secondary to overindulgence in alcohol-free "pastis". *Lancet* 1984; **i:** 575–6.
11. Nielsen I, Pedersen RS. Life-threatening hypokalaemia caused by liquorice ingestion. *Lancet* 1984; **i:** 1305.
12. Farese RV, *et al.* Licorice-induced hypermineralocorticoidism. *N Engl J Med* 1991; **325:** 1223–7.
13. Bauchart J-J, *et al.* Alcohol-free pastis and hypokalaemia. *Lancet* 1995; **346:** 1701.
14. de Klerk GJ, *et al.* Hypokalaemia and hypertension associated with use of liquorice flavoured chewing gum. *BMJ* 1997; **314:** 731–2.
15. Elinav E, Chajek-Shaul T. Licorice consumption causing severe hypokalemic paralysis. *Mayo Clin Proc* 2003; **78:** 767–8.
16. Eriksson JW, *et al.* Life-threatening ventricular tachycardia due to liquorice-induced hypokalaemia. *J Intern Med* 1999; **245:** 307–10.
17. Edwards CRW. Lessons from licorice. *N Engl J Med* 1991; **325:** 1242–3.
18. Teelucksingh S, *et al.* Liquorice. *Lancet* 1991; **337:** 1549.
19. Walker BR, Edwards CR. Licorice-induced hypertension and syndromes of apparent mineralocorticoid excess. *Endocrinol Metab Clin North Am* 1994; **23:** 359–77.


**Pregnancy.** Studies in Finnish women indicated that heavy consumption of liquorice (equivalent to ≥ 500 mg/week of glycyrrhizinic acid) during pregnancy was associated with an increased risk of preterm delivery.[1,2] Consumption of large amounts of liquorice was a social habit noted to occur in some northern European countries.


1. Strandberg TE, *et al.* Birth outcome in relation to licorice consumption during pregnancy. *Am J Epidemiol* 2001; **153:** 1085–8.
2. Strandberg TE, *et al.* Preterm birth and licorice consumption during pregnancy. *Am J Epidemiol* 2002; **156:** 803–5.


### Uses and Administration

Liquorice is used as a flavouring and sweetening agent. It has demulcent and expectorant properties and has been used in cough preparations. It has ulcer-healing properties that may result from stimulation of mucus synthesis. It also has mild anti-inflammatory and mineralocorticoid properties associated with the presence of glycyrrhizinic acid and its metabolite glycyrrhetinic acid, which is an inhibitor of cortisol metabolism. Liquorice may also possess some antispasmodic and laxative properties.

Deglycyrrhizinised liquorice has a reduced mineralocorticoid activity and has been used, usually with antacids, for the treatment of peptic ulcer disease (p.1246).

### Preparations

***Ph. Eur.:*** Liquorice Ethanolic Liquid Extract, Standardised;
***USNF 22:*** Licorice Fluidextract.

**Proprietary Preparations** (details are given in Part 3)
***Braz.:*** Brefus; ***Fr.:*** Depiderm; Trio D; ***Ger.:*** Fichtensirup N; Lakriment Neu; Suczulen mono; Ulgastrin Neu†.

**Multi-ingredient:** numerous preparations are listed in Part3

## Loperamide Hydrochloride

*(BANM, USAN, rINNM)*

Hidrocloruro de loperamida; Loperamidi Hydrochloridum; R-18553. 4-(4-*p*-Chlorophenyl-4-hydroxypiperidino)-*NN*-dimethyl-2,2-diphenylbutyramide hydrochloride.

$C_{29}H_{33}ClN_2O_2,HCl$ = 513.5.

*CAS — 53179-11-6 (loperamide); 34552-83-5 (loperamide hydrochloride).*

*ATC — A07DA03.*

**Pharmacopoeias.** In *Chin.*, *Eur.* (see p.vi), *Int.*, and *US.*

**Ph. Eur. 5.0** (Loperamide Hydrochloride). A white or almost white powder. It exhibits polymorphism. Slightly soluble in water; freely soluble in alcohol and in methyl alcohol. Protect from light.

**USP 27** (Loperamide Hydrochloride). A white to slightly yellow powder. Slightly soluble in water and in dilute acids; freely soluble in chloroform, in isopropyl alcohol, and in methyl alcohol.

### Loperamide Oxide *(BAN, rINN)*

R-58425.

$C_{29}H_{33}ClN_2O_3$ = 493.0.

*CAS — 106900-12-3.*

*ATC — A07DA05.*

**Pharmacopoeias.** *Eur.* (see p.vi) includes the monohydrate.

**Ph. Eur. 5.0** (Loperamide Oxide Monohydrate; Loperamidi Oxidum Monohydricum). A white or almost white, slightly hygroscopic, powder. Practically insoluble in water; freely soluble in alcohol and in dichloromethane. Store in airtight containers. Protect from light.

### Adverse Effects and Treatment

Abdominal pain or bloating, nausea, constipation, dry mouth, dizziness, fatigue, and hypersensitivity reactions including skin rashes have been reported. Loperamide has been associated with paralytic ileus, particularly in infants and young children, and deaths have been reported. Depression of the CNS, to which children may be more sensitive, may be seen in overdosage, and naloxone hydrochloride (see p.1045) has been recommended for its treatment.

◊ Some references to loperamide toxicity covering toxic megacolon[1,2] and severe effects in young children including coma,[3] paralytic ileus with death,[4] and delirium.[5]


1. Brown JW. Toxic megacolon associated with loperamide therapy. *JAMA* 1979; **241:** 501–2.
2. Walley T, Milson D. Loperamide related toxic megacolon in Clostridium difficile colitis. *Postgrad Med J* 1990; **66:** 582.
3. Minton NA, Smith PGD. Loperamide toxicity in a child after a single dose. *BMJ* 1987; **294:** 1383.
4. Bhutta TI, Tahir KI. Loperamide poisoning in children. *Lancet* 1990; **335:** 363.
5. Schwartz RH, Rodriguez WJ. Toxic delirium possibly caused by loperamide. *J Pediatr* 1991; **118:** 656–7.


### Precautions

Loperamide should not be used when inhibition of peristalsis is to be avoided, in particular where ileus or constipation occur, and should be avoided in patients with abdominal distension, acute inflammatory bowel disease, or antibiotic-associated colitis. Loperamide should not be used alone in patients with dysentery.

Loperamide should be used with caution in patients with hepatic impairment because of its considerable first-pass metabolism in the liver. It should also be used with caution in young children because of a greater variability of response in this age group; it is not recommended for use in infants (see Uses and Administration, below).

**Breast feeding.** The American Academy of Pediatrics[1] states that there have been no reports of any clinical effect on the infant associated with the use of loperamide by breast-feeding mothers, and that therefore it may be considered to be usually compatible with breast feeding.


1. American Academy of Pediatrics. The transfer of drugs and other chemicals into human milk. *Pediatrics* 2001; **108:** 776–89. Correction. *ibid.*; 1029. Also available at: http://aappolicy.aappublications.org/cgi/content/full/pediatrics%3b108/3/776 (accessed 07/05/04)


### Interactions

**Co-trimoxazole.** Concomitant administration with co-trimoxazole increases the bioavailability of loperamide,[1] apparently by inhibiting its first-pass metabolism.


1. Kamali F, Huang ML. Increased systemic availability of loperamide after oral administration of loperamide and loperamide oxide with cotrimoxazole. *Br J Clin Pharmacol* 1996; **41:** 125–8.


### Pharmacokinetics

About 40% of a dose of loperamide is reported to be absorbed from the gastrointestinal tract to undergo first-pass metabolism in the liver and excretion in the faeces via the bile as inactive conjugate; there is slight urinary excretion. Little intact drug reaches the systemic circulation. The elimination half-life is reported to be about 10 hours.

### Uses and Administration

Loperamide is a synthetic opioid analogue which inhibits gut motility and may also reduce gastrointestinal secretions. It is given by mouth as an antidiarrhoeal drug as an adjunct in the management of acute and chronic diarrhoeas and may also be used in the management of colostomies or ileostomies to reduce the volume of discharge.

In acute diarrhoea the usual initial dose for adults is loperamide hydrochloride 4 mg followed by 2 mg after each loose stool to a maximum of 16 mg daily; the usual daily dose is 6 to 8 mg. In the UK, it is not recommended for children under 4 years of age. Suggested doses for older children are: 4 to 8 years, 1 mg three or four times daily for up to 3 days; 9 to 12 years, 2 mg four times daily for up to 5 days. In the USA, loperamide is not recommended for children under the age of 2 years and an initial dose of 1 mg three times daily is suggested for children aged 2 to 5 years. (For restrictions on the use of loperamide in children and the view that antidiarrhoeal drugs should not be used at all in children, see Diarrhoea, below.)

In chronic diarrhoea the usual initial dose for adults is 4 to 8 mg daily in divided doses subsequently adjusted as necessary; doses of 16 mg daily should not be exceeded. If no improvement has been observed after treatment with 16 mg daily for at least 10 days, further administration is unlikely to be of benefit.

Loperamide is also given as the prodrug, loperamide oxide, which is converted to loperamide in the gastrointestinal tract. It has been given for acute diarrhoea in doses of 2 to 4 mg initially followed by 1 mg after each loose stool, to a maximum of 8 mg daily.

**Diarrhoea.** The mainstay of treatment for acute diarrhoea (p.1241) is rehydration therapy. Antidiarrhoeals like loperamide have a limited role for symptomatic relief in adults with acute diarrhoea, but WHO does not recommend the use of *any* antidiarrhoeal drug in children with diarrhoea. There have been problems regarding the use of antidiarrhoeals such as loperamide in young children in developing countries. Manufacturers have considered that a lower age limit is acceptable in those countries than is recommended in the UK or USA; even that lower limit is not always observed in practice and there have been reports of serious toxicity in very young children.[1] In response to such reports the manufacturers withdrew concentrated drops of loperamide worldwide and the syrup from countries where the WHO had a programme for control of diarrhoeal diseases,[2] but tablets and capsules remain available. In some countries the use of antidiarrhoeals is now restricted by law.


1. Bhutta TI, Tahir KI. Loperamide poisoning in children. *Lancet* 1990; **335:** 363.
2. Gussin RZ. Withdrawal of loperamide drops. *Lancet* 1990; **335:** 1603–4.


◊ References to the use of *loperamide oxide* in diarrhoea.


1. Van Den Eynden B, *et al.* New approaches to the treatment of patients with acute, nonspecific diarrhea: a comparison of the effects of loperamide and loperamide oxide. *Curr Ther Res* 1995; **56:** 1132–41.
2. Hughes IW, *et al.* First-line treatment in acute non-dysenteric diarrhoea: clinical comparison of loperamide oxide, loperamide and placebo. *Br J Clin Pract* 1995; **49:** 181–5.
3. van Outryve M, Toussaint J. Loperamide oxide for the treatment of chronic diarrhoea in Crohn's disease. *J Int Med Res* 1995; **23:** 335–41.


### Preparations

***BP 2003:*** Loperamide Capsules;
***USP 27:*** Loperamide Hydrochloride Capsules; Loperamide Hydrochloride Oral Solution; Loperamide Hydrochloride Tablets.

**Proprietary Preparations** (details are given in Part 3)
***Arg.:*** Colifilm; Contem; Custey; Dotalsec; Elcoman; Ionet; Lanseka; Plorinoc; Regulane; Salvaxil; Suprasec; Viltar; ***Austral.:*** Chemists Own Diarrhoea Relief; Gastro-Stop; Harmonise; Imodium; ***Austria:*** Arestal†; Enterobene; Imodium; ***Belg.:*** Ercestopyl†; Imodium; Toriac†; ***Braz.:*** Closecs†; Diafuran; Diarresec; Diasec; Enteronorm†; Imosec; Obstar†; ***Canad.:*** Anti-Diarrheal; Diahalt; Diarr-Eze; Diarrhea Relief; Imodium; Loperacap; ***Chile:*** Capent; Coliper; Lopediar; ***Denm.:*** Imodium; Propiden; Travello; ***Fin.:*** Imocur; Imodium; Lopex; ***Fr.:*** Altocel; Antidiar†; Arestal; Celkalm†; Diaretyl; Dyspagon; Ercestop; Imodium; Imossel; Indiaral; Lodiarid†; Lopelin†; Nabutil; Nimaz†; Peracel†; ***Ger.:*** Aperamid†; Azuperamid; Boxolip; D-Stop†; duralopid; Endiaron; Imodium; Lop-Dia; Lopalind; Lopedium; Lopepham; Loperamerck†; Loperhoe; Lopetrans†; Mandros Diarstop†; Metifex-L†; Sanifug†; ***Gr.:*** Imodium; Neo-enteroseptol; ***Hong Kong:*** Colodium; Imodium; Loperax; Loperium; Lopermide; Reximide; Vacontil; Vidaperamide; ***India:*** Diarlop; Lopamide; ***Irl.:*** Arret; Diarrest RF; Imodium; ***Israel:*** Imodium; Kamidex†; Loperid; Loperium; Rekamide; Stopit; ***Ital.:*** Diarstop; Diarzero; Dissenten; Imodium; Lodis†; Lopemid; Loperyl†; Ramidox; Tebloc; ***Malaysia:*** Beamodium; Imocap; Imodium; Imotab; Loperium; Lopermide; Loramide; Miraton; Vacontil; ***Mex.:*** Acanol; Acqta; Biolid; Cryoperacid; Dialacid; Dilostop; F9; Imodium; Lomotil; Pramidal; Raxamida†; Raxedin†; Rediarin; Top-Dal; Valfam; ***Neth.:*** Arestal; Diacure; Imodium; ***Norw.:*** Imodium; Travello; ***NZ:*** Dicap; Imodium; ***Port.:*** Imodium; Loride; ***S.Afr.:*** Betaperamide; Gastron; Imodium; Lenide-T; Lopedium; Loperastat; Norimode; Prodium; ***Singapore:*** Colodium; IMD; Imodium; Loperamil; Lopermide; Loramide; Lorpa; Vacontil†; ***Spain:*** Elissan; Fortasec; Imodium; Imosec; Loperan; Loperkey; Orulop†; Protector; Salvacolina NF; Taguinol; ***Swed.:*** Dimor; Imodium; Primodium; Travello; ***Switz.:*** Binaldan; Imodium; Lopimed; ***Thai.:*** Diarent; Diarodil; Entermid; Imodium; Impelium; Imporе†; Lomide; Lomy; Lopamine; Lopela; Lopercin; Loperdium; Loperia; Lopermide; Operium; Perasian; SBOB; Vacontil†; ***UK:*** Arret; Diah-Limit; Diaquitte; Diareze; Diasorb†; Diocalm Ultra; Diocaps; Entrocalm; Imodium; LoperaGen†; Norimode; Normaloe; ***USA:*** Imodium; K-Pek II; Kao-Paverin; Kaopectate II; Maalox Anti-Diarrheal†; Neo-Diaral; Pepto Diarrhea Control.

**Multi-ingredient:** ***Arg.:*** Neo Kef; Neomas L; Regulane AF; ***Austral.:*** Imodium Advanced; ***Austria:*** Imodium Plus; ***Braz.:*** Imodium Plus; ***Canad.:*** Imodium Advanced; ***Denm.:*** Imodium med Simethicon; ***Fr.:*** Imosselduo; ***Ger.:*** Imodium Plus; ***Mex.:*** Imodium Plus; ***Neth.:*** Diacure Plus; ***NZ:*** Imodium Advanced; ***S.Afr.:*** Imodium Plus; ***Spain:*** Imodium Plus; ***Switz.:*** Imodium Plus; ***UK:*** Imodium Plus; ***USA:*** Imodium Advanced.

## Loxiglumide *(rINN)*

CR-1505; Loxiglumida. (±)-4-(3,4-Dichlorobenzamido)-*N*-(3-methoxypropyl)-*N*-pentylglutaramic acid.

$C_{21}H_{30}Cl_2N_2O_5$ = 461.4.

*CAS — 107097-80-3.*

### Profile

Loxiglumide is a specific cholecystokinin antagonist related to proglumide (see p.1284), and has been investigated in biliary and gastrointestinal dyskinesias, constipation and irritable bowel syndrome, and pancreatitis.

The *R*-isomer of loxiglumide, dexloxiglumide is also under investigation for constipation-predominant irritable bowel syndrome.

◊ References.


1. Setnikar I, *et al.* Pharmacokinetics and tolerance of repeated oral doses of loxiglumide. *Arzneimittelforschung* 1989; **39:** 1454–9.
2. Meier R, *et al.* Therapeutic effects of loxiglumide, a cholecystokinin antagonist, on chronic constipation in elderly patients: a prospective, randomized, double-blind, controlled trial. *J Gastrointest Mot* 1993; **5:** 129–35.
3. Lieverse RJ, *et al.* Effects of somatostatin and loxiglumide on gallbladder motility. *Eur J Clin Pharmacol* 1995; **47:** 489–92.
4. Shiratori K, *et al.* Clinical evaluation of oral administration of a cholecystokinin-A receptor antagonist (loxiglumide) to patients with acute, painful attacks of chronic pancreatitis: a multicenter dose-response study in Japan. *Pancreas* 2002; **25:** e1–e5.


## Magaldrate *(BAN, USAN, rINN)*

Aluminum Magnesium Hydroxide Sulfate; AY-5710; Magaldrato; Magaldratum.

$Al_5Mg_{10}(OH)_{31}(SO_4)_2,xH_2O$ = 1097.3 (anhydrous).

*CAS — 74978-16-8.*

*ATC — A02AD02.*

NOTE. Magaldrate was formerly described as Aluminium Magnesium Hydroxide ($AlMg_2(OH)_7$ monohydrate, *CAS—1317-26-6*).

**Pharmacopoeias.** In *Eur.* (see p.vi) and *US.*

**Ph. Eur. 5.0** (Magaldrate). A combination of aluminium and magnesium hydroxides (see p.1249 and p.1272 respectively) and sulfates. It contains the equivalent of 90 to 105% of $Al_5Mg_{10}(OH)_{31}(SO_4)_2$, calculated with reference to the dried substance. A white or almost white crystalline powder. Practically insoluble in water and in alcohol; soluble in dilute mineral acids. It loses between 10 and 20% of its weight on drying at 200° for 4 hours.

**USP 27** (Magaldrate). A combination of aluminium and magnesium hydroxides and sulfates. It contains the equivalent of 90 to 105% of $Al_5Mg_{10}(OH)_{31}(SO_4)_2$, calculated on the dried basis. A white odourless crystalline powder. Insoluble in water and in alcohol; soluble in dilute solutions of mineral acids. It loses between 10 and 20% of its weight on drying at 200° for 4 hours.

### Profile

Magaldrate is an antacid (see p.1239) that is given in doses of up to about 2 g by mouth.

### Preparations

***BP 2003:*** Magaldrate Oral Suspension;
***USP 27:*** Magaldrate and Simethicone Oral Suspension; Magaldrate and Simethicone Tablets; Magaldrate Oral Suspension; Magaldrate Tablets.

**Proprietary Preparations** (details are given in Part 3)
***Arg.:*** Riopan; ***Austria:*** Riopan; ***Belg.:*** Gastricalm; Riopan; ***Braz.:*** Riopan; Selanac†; ***Canad.:*** Riopan; ***Fr.:*** Riopan; ***Ger.:*** Gastrimagal†; Gastripan; Gastrostad†; Glysan; Hevert-Mag; Magalphil†; Magasan†; Magastron; Magmed†; Marax; ProWohl†; Riopan; Simaphil; ***Gr.:*** Felfar; Riopan; ***Ital.:*** Gadral; Magralibi; Riopan; ***Neth.:*** Riopan; ***Port.:*** Riopan; ***S.Afr.:*** Gastrobon†; Riopone†; ***Spain:*** Bemolan; Gastromol; Magion; Minoton; ***Switz.:*** Riopan; ***UK:*** Dyneset†; ***USA:*** Iosopan; Riopan.

**Multi-ingredient:** ***Arg.:*** Aci Tip; Carbogasol Antiacido; ***Austral.:*** Mylanta Heartburn Relief; ***Braz.:*** Riopan Plus; ***Canad.:*** Riopan Plus; ***Chile:*** Aci-Tip; Antiax; ***Hong Kong:*** Nilcid-MPS; ***India:*** pH4; Rolac Plus; Ulgel; ***Mex.:*** Nilcid; Riopan; ***Spain:*** Compagel; ***UK:*** Bisodol Heartburn Relief; ***USA:*** Iosopan Plus; Lowsium Plus; Riopan Plus.

## Magnesium Carbonate

E504; Magnesii Subcarbonas; Magnesio, carbonato de.

*CAS — 546-93-0 (anhydrous magnesium carbonate); 23389-33-5 (hydrated normal magnesium carbonate); 39409-82-0 (hydrated basic magnesium carbonate).*

*ATC — A02AA01; A06AD01.*

**Pharmacopoeias.** In *Chin., Eur.* (see p.vi), *Jpn, Pol., US,* and *Viet.* Some pharmacopoeias include a single monograph that permits both the light and heavy varieties while some have 2 separate monographs for the 2 varieties.

**Ph. Eur. 5.0** (Magnesium Carbonate, Heavy; Magnesii Subcarbonas Ponderosus). A hydrated basic magnesium carbonate containing the equivalent of 40 to 45% of MgO. 15 g has an apparent volume before settling of about 30 mL. Practically insoluble in water; dissolves in dilute acids with strong effervescence.

**Ph. Eur. 5.0** (Magnesium Carbonate, Light; Magnesii Subcarbonas Levis). A hydrated basic magnesium carbonate containing the equivalent of 40 to 45% of MgO. 15 g has an apparent volume before settling of about 180 mL. Practically insoluble in water; dissolves in dilute acids with strong effervescence.

**USP 27** (Magnesium Carbonate). A basic hydrated magnesium carbonate or a normal hydrated magnesium carbonate containing the equivalent of 40.0 to 43.5% of MgO. It is an odourless, bulky white powder or light, white, friable masses. Practically insoluble in water; insoluble in alcohol; dissolves in dilute acids with effervescence.

### Profile

Magnesium carbonate is an antacid with general properties similar to those of magnesium hydroxide (below) that is given in doses of up to about 500 mg by mouth. When administered by mouth, it reacts with gastric acid to form soluble magnesium chloride and carbon dioxide in the stomach; the carbon dioxide may cause flatulence and eructation. Magnesium carbonate is often given with aluminium-containing antacids such as aluminium hydroxide, which counteract its laxative effect.

Magnesium carbonate may be used as a magnesium supplement. It is also used as a food additive.

### Preparations

***BP 2003:*** Aromatic Magnesium Carbonate Mixture; Compound Magnesium Trisilicate Oral Powder; Kaolin Mixture; Magnesium Sulphate Mixture; Magnesium Trisilicate Mixture;

***USP 27:*** Alumina and Magnesium Carbonate Oral Suspension; Alumina and Magnesium Carbonate Tablets; Alumina, Magnesium Carbonate, and Magnesium Oxide Tablets; Calcium and Magnesium Carbonates Oral Suspension; Calcium and Magnesium Carbonates Tablets; Magnesium Carbonate and Citric Acid for Oral Solution; Magnesium Carbonate and Sodium Bicarbonate for Oral Suspension; Magnesium Citrate Oral Solution.

**Proprietary Preparations** (details are given in Part 3)

***Arg.:*** Polvo Roge; ***Austria:*** Magnofit; Tetesept Magnesium; ***Belg.:*** Magnezyme†; ***Canad.:*** Cepasium†; ***Fr.:*** Mag 2; Magnosol; ***Ger.:*** Palmicol; ***Ital.:*** Magnofit; ***S.Afr.:*** Be-Lax; ***USA:*** Mag-Carb.

**Multi-ingredient:** numerous preparations are listed in Part 3.

## Magnesium Citrate

Magnesio, citrato de.

$C_{12}H_{10}Mg_3O_{14}$ = 451.1.

*CAS — 3344-18-1.*

*ATC — A06AD19; A12CC04; B05CB03.*

**Pharmacopoeias.** In *Fr.* and *US.*

**USP 27** (Magnesium Citrate). A 5% suspension in water has a pH of 5.0 to 9.0. Store in airtight containers.

### Profile

Magnesium citrate is an osmotic laxative (p.1239) used as a bowel evacuant prior to investigational procedures or surgery of the colon. In the UK, an aqueous solution containing 17.7 g of magnesium citrate is prepared from a sachet (*Citramag*) containing magnesium carbonate and anhydrous citric acid by mixing with 200 mL of hot water. After the solution has cooled, one dose is taken by mouth at 8 a.m. the day before the procedure, and a second dose between 2 and 4 p.m. Dosages with other preparations have ranged from about 11 to 25 g of magnesium citrate. A high fluid intake and low residue diet are needed with such bowel preparations. It is also used in combination with sodium picosulfate, p.1289.

Magnesium citrate is also used as a magnesium supplement in doses of up to about 1.9 g daily by mouth.

For the general properties of magnesium salts, see p.1227.

**Migraine.** For mention of the use of magnesium supplementation, including magnesium citrate, for the prophylaxis of migraine, see p.1229.

### Preparations

***USP 27:*** Magnesium Citrate for Oral Solution.

**Proprietary Preparations** (details are given in Part 3)

***Arg.:*** Holomagnesio; ***Austral.:*** Mag Cit Prep; ***Austria:*** Magnesium Diasporal; Magnofit; ***Belg.:*** Magnetop; ***Canad.:*** Citro-Mag; ***Ger.:*** Magnesium Diasporal; Magnesium Tonil N†; Magnesium Verla; Magnorell†; Presselin Heilozon P; ***Hong Kong:*** Citro-Mag; ***Mon.:*** Oromag; ***Switz.:*** Magnesium Biomed; Magnesium Diasporal; ***UK:*** Citramag; ***USA:*** Evac-Q-Mag.

**Multi-ingredient:** ***Arg.:*** Magnebe; ***Austral.:*** Go Kit; Go Kit Plus; ***Austria:*** Biovital Weissdorn; ***Belg.:*** Carbobel; ***Canad.:*** Evac-Q-Kwik†; Royvac Kit; ***Chile:*** Laxogeno; ***Fr.:*** Citrocholine†; ***Ger.:*** Acidovert; Lithurex S; Magnerot N; ***Irl.:*** Picolax; ***Spain:*** Salmagne; ***UK:*** Picolax; Porosis D†.

# Magnesium Hydroxide

E528; Magnesii Hydroxidum; Magnesio, hidróxido de; Magnesium Hydrate.

$Mg(OH)_2$ = 58.32.

*CAS — 1309-42-8.*

*ATC — A02AA04; G04BX01.*

NOTE. Compounded preparations of magnesium hydroxide may be represented by the following names:

- Co-magaldrox *x/y* (*BAN*)—where *x* and *y* are the strengths in milligrams of magnesium hydroxide and aluminium hydroxide respectively.

**Pharmacopoeias.** In *Eur.* (see p.vi), *Int., US,* and *Viet.*

**Ph. Eur. 5.0** (Magnesium Hydroxide). A fine white amorphous powder. Practically insoluble in water; dissolves in dilute acids. A solution in water is alkaline to phenolphthalein.

**USP 27** (Magnesium Hydroxide). A bulky white powder. Practically insoluble in water, in alcohol, in chloroform, and in ether; soluble in dilute acids. Store in airtight containers.

## Adverse Effects, Treatment, and Precautions

As for magnesium salts in general, see p.1228. Magnesium hydroxide may cause diarrhoea, an effect that is dose-dependent. Hypermagnesaemia may occur, usually in patients with renal impairment.

**Hypermagnesaemia.** Reports of hypermagnesaemia in infants given magnesium-containing antacids,[1,2] and in a patient with normal renal function but bowel obstruction.[3]

1. Brand JM, Greer FR. Hypermagnesemia and intestinal perforation following antacid administration in a premature infant. *Pediatrics* 1990; **85:** 121–4.
2. Alison LH, Bulugahapitiya D. Laxative induced magnesium poisoning in a 6 week old infant. *BMJ* 1990; **300:** 125.
3. Laughlin SA, McKinney PE. Antacid-induced hypermagnesemia in a patient with normal renal function and bowel obstruction. *Ann Pharmacother* 1998; **32:** 312–15.

## Interactions

As outlined on p.1239, antacids, including magnesium salts, interact with many other drugs both by alterations in gastric pH and emptying, and by formation of complexes that are not absorbed. Interactions can be minimised by giving the antacid and any other medications 2 to 3 hours apart.

## Pharmacokinetics

Magnesium hydroxide, given by mouth, reacts relatively rapidly with hydrochloric acid in the stomach to form magnesium chloride and water. About 30% of the magnesium ions are absorbed from the small intestine, as described for Magnesium Salts, p.1229.

## Uses and Administration

Magnesium hydroxide is an antacid (see p.1239) that is given in doses of up to about 1 g by mouth. It is often given with aluminium-containing antacids such as aluminium hydroxide which counteract its laxative effect.

Magnesium hydroxide is also given as an osmotic laxative (p.1239) in doses of about 2 to 5 g by mouth.

Magnesium hydroxide has also been used as a food additive and as a magnesium supplement in deficiency states.

## Preparations

***BP 2003:*** Co-magaldrox Oral Suspension; Co-magaldrox Tablets; Liquid Paraffin and Magnesium Hydroxide Oral Emulsion; Magnesium Hydroxide Mixture;

***USP 27:*** Alumina and Magnesia Oral Suspension; Alumina and Magnesia Tablets; Alumina, Magnesia, and Calcium Carbonate Oral Suspension; Alumina, Magnesia, and Calcium Carbonate Tablets; Alumina, Magnesia, and Simethicone Oral Suspension; Alumina, Magnesia, and Simethicone Tablets; Alumina, Magnesia, Calcium Carbonate, and Simethicone Tablets; Aspirin, Alumina, and Magnesia Tablets; Calcium Carbonate and Magnesia Tablets; Calcium Carbonate, Magnesia, and Simethicone Tablets; Magnesia Tablets; Magnesium Hydroxide Paste; Milk of Magnesia.

**Proprietary Preparations** (details are given in Part 3)

***Arg.:*** Leche de Magnesia Phillips; Magnesia San Pellegrino; ***Braz.:*** Leite de Magnesia de Phillips; Leite de Magnesia†; Magnesia Fluida†; Magnesiol; Mylanta Plus; ***Canad.:*** Phillips' Milk of Magnesia; ***Chile:*** Leche de Magnesia Phillips; Magnesia Pasteur; Tabletas Antiacidas; ***Denm.:*** Magnesia; ***Fin.:*** Emgesan; Magnesiamaito; ***Fr.:*** Carbonex; Magnesie S Pellegrino; ***Gr.:*** Milk of Magnesia; ***India:*** Tricaine-MPS; ***Irl.:*** Milk of Magnesia; ***Israel:*** Magnesia S Pellegrino†; ***Ital.:*** Citrato Espresso S. Pellegrino; Magnesia S Pellegrino; Magnesia Volta; ***Mon.:*** Chlorumagene; ***Port.:*** Leite de Magnesia; ***S.Afr.:*** Deopens; ***Spain:*** Crema de Magnesia†; Magnesia; Magnesia San Pellegrino; ***Swed.:*** Emgesan; ***Switz.:*** Chlorumagene†; Magnesia S Pellegrino; ***UK:*** Milk of Magnesia; ***USA:*** Milk of Magnesia; Phillips' Chewable; Phillips' Milk of Magnesia.

**Multi-ingredient:** numerous preparations are listed in Part 3.

## Magnesium Oxide

E530; Magnesii Oxidum; Magnesio, óxido de.

MgO = 40.30.

*CAS — 1309-48-4.*

*ATC — A02AA02; A06AD02; A12CC10.*

**Pharmacopoeias.** In *Chin., Eur.* (see p.vi), *Int., Jpn, Pol., US,* and *Viet.* Some pharmacopoeias include a single monograph that permits both the light and heavy varieties while some have 2 separate monographs for the 2 varieties.

**Ph. Eur. 5.0** (Magnesium Oxide, Heavy; Magnesii Oxidum Ponderosum). A fine, white powder. 15 g has an apparent volume before settling of about 30 mL. Practically insoluble in water; dissolves in dilute acids with at most slight effervescence.

**Ph. Eur. 5.0** (Magnesium Oxide, Light; Magnesii Oxidum Leve). A fine, white, amorphous powder. 15 g has an apparent volume before settling of about 150 mL. Practically insoluble in water; dissolves in dilute acids with at most slight effervescence.

**USP 27** (Magnesium Oxide). It is either the heavy or light variety. Heavy magnesium oxide is a relatively dense white powder with 5 g occupying a volume of about 10 to 20 mL. Light magnesium oxide is a very bulky white powder with 5 g occupying a volume of about 40 to 50 mL. Both varieties are practically insoluble in water; insoluble in alcohol; soluble in dilute acids. Store in airtight containers.

### Profile

Magnesium oxide is an antacid with general properties similar to those of magnesium hydroxide (above). It is given in usual doses of about 400 mg by mouth. It is often given with aluminium-containing antacids such as aluminium hydroxide, which counteract its laxative effect.

Magnesium oxide has been used for its osmotic laxative properties in bowel preparation; doses of 3.5 g by mouth are given for this purpose, combined with bisacodyl or sodium picosulfate.

Magnesium oxide is also used as a magnesium supplement in deficiency states in doses of up to 800 mg (20 mmol) daily by mouth. It is also used as a food additive.

### Preparations

***USP 27:*** Alumina, Magnesium Carbonate, and Magnesium Oxide Tablets; Aromatic Cascara Fluidextract; Aspirin, Alumina, and Magnesium Oxide Tablets; Citric Acid, Magnesium Oxide, and Sodium Carbonate Irrigation; Magnesium Oxide Capsules; Magnesium Oxide Tablets.

**Proprietary Preparations** (details are given in Part 3)

***Arg.:*** Magneforte; Polvo Roge; ***Austria:*** Magnihexal; Magnofit; Magnonorm; Magnotab; ***Denm.:*** Salilax; ***Fr.:*** Magnosol; Magocean; ***Ger.:*** Biolectra Magnesium; Magium; Magnesium Diasporal; Magnetrans forte; Magno Sanol; ***NZ:*** Mylanta Effervescent; ***S.Afr.:*** Solumag; ***Swed.:*** Salilax; ***Thai.:*** Magoral; ***USA:*** Mag-200; Mag-Ox; Maox; Uro-Mag.

**Multi-ingredient:** numerous preparations are listed in Part 3.

## Magnesium Trisilicate

E553(a); Magnesii Trisilicas; Magnesio, trisilicato de.

*CAS — 14987-04-3 (anhydrous magnesium trisilicate); 39365-87-2 (magnesium trisilicate hydrate).*

**Description.** Magnesium trisilicate is a hydrated magnesium silicate. The code E553(a) has been applied to both magnesium silicate and to magnesium trisilicate.

**Pharmacopoeias.** In *Chin., Eur.* (see p.vi), *Jpn, US,* and *Viet.*

**Ph. Eur. 5.0** (Magnesium Trisilicate). It has a variable composition corresponding approximately to the formula $Mg_2Si_3O_8.xH_2O$ containing not less than 29% of magnesium oxide and not less than the equivalent of 65% of silicon dioxide, both calculated with reference to the ignited substance. A white powder. Practically insoluble in water and in alcohol.

**USP 27** (Magnesium Trisilicate). A compound of magnesium oxide and silicon dioxide with varying proportions of water. It contains not less than 20% of magnesium oxide and not less than 45% of silicon dioxide. A fine, white, odourless, powder, free from grittiness. Insoluble in water and in alcohol. It is readily decomposed by mineral acids.

### Profile

Magnesium trisilicate is a hydrated magnesium silicate. It is an antacid with general properties similar to those of magnesium hydroxide (p.1272). It has been given in doses of up to about 2 g by mouth. When given orally it reacts more slowly with hydrochloric acid in the stomach than magnesium hydroxide. Magnesium trisilicate is often given with aluminium-containing antacids such as aluminium hydroxide, which counteract its laxative effect.

Magnesium trisilicate is also used as a food additive and as a pharmaceutical excipient.

**Effects on the kidneys.** A 68-year-old man with a history of renal calculus passed a 300-mg stone which was found to consist chiefly of silica.[1] He had been taking the equivalent of 2 g of magnesium trisilicate daily for many years.

1. Joekes AM, *et al.* Multiple renal silica calculi. *BMJ* 1973; **1:** 146–7.

### Preparations

***BP 2003:*** Compound Magnesium Trisilicate Oral Powder; Compound Magnesium Trisilicate Tablets; Magnesium Trisilicate Mixture;

***USP 27:*** Alumina and Magnesium Trisilicate Oral Suspension; Alumina and Magnesium Trisilicate Tablets; Magnesium Trisilicate Tablets.

**Proprietary Preparations** (details are given in Part 3)
***Ger.:*** Solitab†; ***Spain:*** Mabosil†; Silimag†.

**Multi-ingredient:** numerous preparations are listed in Part 3.

## Manna

Maná; Manne en Larmes.

### Profile

Manna is the dried exudation from the bark of the European flowering ash, *Fraxinus ornus* (Oleaceae), containing about 40 to 60% of mannitol (p.950). It has been used as an osmotic laxative.

### Preparations

**Proprietary Preparations** (details are given in Part 3)

**Multi-ingredient:** ***Austria:*** Krauterdoktor Entschlackungs-Elixier; Naturaform Fruchtewurfel mit Manna; Sinolax-Milder; St Radegunder Entschlackungs-Elixier; ***Ger.:*** florabio Mann-Feigen-Sirup mit Senna; Infitract; Schwedentrunk mit Ginseng†; Schwedentrunk†; ***Ital.:*** Certobil†.

## Mebeverine Hydrochloride *(BANM, USAN, rINNM)*

CSAG-144; Hidrocloruro de mebeverina. 4-[Ethyl(4-methoxy-α-methylphenethyl)amino]butyl veratrate hydrochloride.

$C_{25}H_{35}NO_5,HCl$ = 466.0.

*CAS — 3625-06-7 (mebeverine); 2753-45-9 (mebeverine hydrochloride).*

*ATC — A03AA04.*

**Pharmacopoeias.** In *Br.*

**BP 2003** (Mebeverine Hydrochloride). A white or almost white crystalline powder. Very soluble in water; freely soluble in alcohol; practically insoluble in ether. A 2% solution in water has a pH of 4.5 to 6.5. Store in airtight containers at a temperature not exceeding 30°. Protect from light.

### Adverse Effects and Precautions

Although adverse effects appear rare, gastrointestinal disturbances, dizziness, headache, insomnia, anorexia, and decreased heart rate have been reported in patients receiving mebeverine. Mebeverine should be avoided in patients with paralytic ileus. Based on theoretical concerns, it should be used with care in patients with marked hepatic or renal impairment, and those with cardiac disorders such as heart block.

◊ A 24-year-old man with cystic fibrosis, prescribed mebeverine hydrochloride for lower abdominal pain and constipation, was found to have a perforated stercoral ulcer with generalised peritonitis.[1] It was suggested that mebeverine produced colonic stasis, which predisposed the patient to ulceration,[1] but the manufacturers[2] considered that the concomitant development of constipation and distal intestinal syndrome (meconium ileus equivalent) in this patient precipitated the development of stercoral ulceration. It was recommended[1] that antispasmodics such as mebeverine should not be used for the symptomatic treatment of distal intestinal syndrome in cystic fibrosis.


1. Hassan W, Keaney N. Mebeverine-induced perforated colon in distal intestinal syndrome of cystic fibrosis. *Lancet* 1990; **335:** 1225.
2. Whitehead AM. Perforation of colon in distal intestinal syndrome of cystic fibrosis. *Lancet* 1990; **336:** 446.


**Porphyria.** Mebeverine hydrochloride is considered to be unsafe in patients with porphyria because it has been shown to be porphyrinogenic in *in-vitro* systems.

### Pharmacokinetics

Mebeverine is rapidly absorbed after oral administration with peak plasma concentrations occurring in 1 to 3 hours. It is 75% bound to albumin in plasma. Mebeverine is completely metabolised by hydrolysis to veratric acid and mebeverine alcohol, the latter of which may then be conjugated. The metabolites are excreted in the urine.

### Uses and Administration

Mebeverine hydrochloride is an antispasmodic with a direct action on the smooth muscle of the gastrointestinal tract. It is used in conditions such as irritable bowel syndrome (p.1244) in a usual dose of 135 mg three times daily by mouth before meals; 100 mg three times daily may also be used. A modified-release preparation is also available, taken as 200 mg twice daily. The embonate is also used in a dose equivalent to 150 mg of the hydrochloride three times daily.

### Preparations

***BP 2003:*** Mebeverine Tablets.

**Proprietary Preparations** (details are given in Part 3)
***Arg.:*** Duspatalin; ***Austral.:*** Colese; Colofac; ***Austria:*** Colofac; ***Belg.:*** Duspatalin; Spasmonal; ***Braz.:*** Duspatalin; ***Chile:*** Doloverina; Duspatal; Evadol; Meditoina; ***Denm.:*** Duspatalin; ***Fr.:*** Colopriv; Duspatalin; Spasmopriv; ***Ger.:*** Duspatal; Mebemerck; ***Gr.:*** Duspatalin; ***Hong Kong:*** Duspatalin; ***India:*** Colospa; ***Irl.:*** Colofac; ***Israel:*** Colotal; ***Ital.:*** Duspatal; ***Malaysia:*** Duspatalin; ***Neth.:*** Duspatal; ***NZ:*** Colofac; ***Port.:*** Duspatal; ***S.Afr.:*** Bevispas; Colofac; ***Singapore:*** Duspatalin; Mebetin; ***Spain:*** Duspatalin; ***Switz.:*** Duspatalin; ***Thai.:*** Colofac; Duspatin; Menosor; ***UK:*** Colofac; Equilon; IBS Relief.

**Multi-ingredient:** ***Hong Kong:*** Fybogel Mebeverine; ***Irl.:*** Fybogel Mebeverine; ***Singapore:*** Fybogel Mebeverine†; ***UK:*** Fybogel Mebeverine.

## Mesalazine *(BAN, rINN)*

5-Aminosalicylic Acid; 5-ASA; Fisalamine; Mesalamine *(USAN)*; Mesalazina; Mesalazinum. 5-Amino-2-salicylic acid.

$C_7H_7NO_3$ = 153.1.

*CAS — 89-57-6.*

*ATC — A07EC02.*

NOTE. Distinguish from 4-aminosalicylic acid (Aminosalicylic Acid, p.154) which is used in the treatment of tuberculosis.

**Pharmacopoeias.** In *Eur.* (see p.vi) and *US.*

**Ph. Eur. 5.0** (Mesalazine). An almost white or light grey or light pink powder or crystals. Very slightly soluble in water; practically insoluble in alcohol. It dissolves in dilute solutions of alkali hydroxides and in dilute hydrochloric acid. Store in airtight containers. Protect from light.

**USP 27** (Mesalamine). Light tan to pink needle-shaped crystals, odourless or with a slight characteristic odour. The colour may darken on exposure to air. Slightly soluble in water; very slightly soluble in dehydrated alcohol, in acetone, and in methyl alcohol; practically insoluble in butyl alcohol, in chloroform, in dichloromethane, in ether, in ethyl acetate, in *n*-hexane, and in propyl alcohol; soluble in dilute hydrochloric acid and in dilute alkali hydroxides. A 2.5% suspension in water has a pH of 3.5 to 4.5. Store in airtight containers. Protect from light.

### Adverse Effects and Precautions

Mesalazine may cause headache and gastrointestinal disturbances, such as nausea, diarrhoea, and abdominal pain. Hypersensitivity reactions may occasionally occur. Some patients may experience exacerbation of symptoms of colitis. There are some reports of myocarditis, pericarditis, pancreatitis, interstitial nephritis, nephrotic syndrome, allergic lung reaction, increased liver enzyme values, hepatitis, lupus-like syndrome, skin reactions, alopecia, myalgia, and arthralgia. There have been rare reports of blood disorders including aplastic anaemia, agranulocytosis, leucopenia, neutropenia, thrombocytopenia, and methaemoglobinaemia.

Mesalazine should not be given to patients with severe renal or hepatic impairment, or salicylate hypersensitivity. It should be used with caution in the elderly, and in mild to moderate renal or hepatic impairment, active peptic ulceration, or sulfasalazine allergy.

If a blood dyscrasia is suspected treatment should be stopped immediately and a blood count performed. Patients or their carers should be told how to recognise signs of blood toxicity and should be advised to seek immediate medical attention if symptoms such as fever, sore throat, mouth ulcers, bruising, or bleeding develop. It is recommended that renal function is monitored before and during therapy, (see Effects on the Kidneys, below).

◊ Many of the adverse effects associated with sulfasalazine therapy have been attributed to the sulfapyridine moiety and most patients unable to tolerate sulfasalazine because of hypersensitivity or adverse reactions can be transferred to mesalazine without adverse effects occurring.[1-4] However, a small number of patients also experience adverse effects while taking mesalazine and these are often very similar to those seen with sulfasalazine.[1-4] They may include nausea, abdominal discomfort or pain, exacerbation of diarrhoea, headache, fever, and rashes. Mesalazine is not associated with sulfasalazine's adverse effects on sperm. An analysis of adverse reactions reported to the UK Committee on Safety of Medicines between 1991 and 1998 found no evidence of a significant difference in the frequency of serious adverse effects for mesalazine and sulfasalazine in the treatment of inflammatory bowel disease.[5] Reports of pancreatitis and interstitial nephritis (see Effects on the Kidneys, below), were more common with mesalazine. However, it has been pointed out that 80% of patients intolerant to sulfasalazine will tolerate mesalazine without problems.[6]

Mesalazine therapy should be initiated cautiously in patients with a history of sulfasalazine **hypersensitivity** and it should be withdrawn if signs of sensitivity develop or if there is diarrhoea or rectal bleeding. It has been suggested[2] that patients with a history of sulfasalazine hypersensitivity should be given test doses of mesalazine before starting a full course.


1. Dew MJ, *et al.* Treatment of ulcerative colitis with oral 5-aminosalicylic acid in patients unable to take sulphasalazine. *Lancet* 1983; **ii:** 801.
2. Campieri M, *et al.* 5-Aminosalicylic acid as rectal enema in ulcerative colitis patients unable to take sulphasalazine. *Lancet* 1984; **i:** 403.
3. Donald IP, Wilkinson SP. The value of 5-aminosalicylic acid in inflammatory bowel disease for patients intolerant or allergic to sulphasalazine. *Postgrad Med J* 1985; **61:** 1047–8.
4. Rao SS, *et al.* Clinical experience of the tolerance of mesalazine and olsalazine in patients intolerant of sulphasalazine. *Scand J Gastroenterol* 1987; **22:** 332–6.
5. Ransford RAJ, Langman MJS. Sulphasalazine and mesalazine: serious adverse reactions re-evaluated on the basis of suspected adverse reaction reports to the Committee on Safety of Medicines. *Gut* 2002; **51:** 536–9.
6. D'Haens G, van Bodegraven AA. Mesalazine is safe for the treatment of IBD. *Gut* 2004; **53:** 155.


**Breast feeding.** The concentrations of mesalazine in maternal plasma and breast milk in a lactating woman taking 500 mg three times daily, were 410 and 110 nanograms/mL respectively.[1] Although it was considered that the amount of mesalazine distributed into breast milk was small and that it was safe during breast feeding,[2,3] maternal use of mesalazine 500 mg suppositories twice daily has been associated with watery diarrhoea in a breast-fed infant[2] and for this reason the American Academy of Pediatrics considers that mesalazine should be given with caution to breast-feeding mothers.[4]


1. Jenss H, *et al.* 5-Aminosalicylic acid and its metabolite in breast milk during lactation. *Am J Gastroenterol* 1990; **85:** 331.
2. Nelis GF. Diarrhoea due to 5-aminosalicylic acid in breast milk. *Lancet* 1989; **i:** 383.
3. Klotz U, Harings-Kaim A. Negligible excretion of 5-aminosalicylic acid in breast milk. *Lancet* 1993; **342:** 618–19.
4. American Academy of Pediatrics. The transfer of drugs and other chemicals into human milk. *Pediatrics* 2001; **108:** 776–89. Correction. *ibid.*; 1029. Also available at: http://aappolicy.aappublications.org/cgi/content/full/pediatrics%3b108/3/776 (accessed 07/05/04)


**Effects on the blood.** Although uncommon, mesalazine-associated adverse effects on the blood have been reported, including thrombocytopenia,[1] neutropenia,[2] fatal aplastic anaemia,[3] and pancytopenia.[4] In July 1995 the UK Committee on Safety of Medicines stated that it had been notified of 49 haematological reactions suspected of being associated with mesalazine,[5] including 5 reports of aplastic anaemia, 1 of agranulocytosis, 11 of leucopenia, and 17 of thrombocytopenia. There had been 3 fatalities. They recommended a blood count and immediate withdrawal of the drug if a dyscrasia was suspected. Antilymphocyte immunoglobulin has been used in the management of mesalazine-associated aplastic anaemia.[6]


1. Daneshmend TK. Mesalazine-associated thrombocytopenia. *Lancet* 1991; **337:** 1297–8.
2. Wyatt S, *et al.* Filgrastim for mesalazine-associated neutropenia. *Lancet* 1993; **341:** 1476.
3. Abboudi ZH, *et al.* Fatal aplastic anaemia after mesalazine. *Lancet* 1994; **343:** 542.
4. Kotanagi H, *et al.* Pancytopenia associated with 5-aminosalicylic acid use in a patient with Crohn's disease. *J Gastroenterol* 1998; **33:** 571–4.
5. Committee on Safety of Medicines/Medicines Control Agency. Blood dyscrasias and mesalazine. *Current Problems* 1995; **21:** 5–6.
6. Laidlaw ST, Reilly JT. Antilymphocyte globulin for mesalazine-associated aplastic anaemia. *Lancet* 1994; **343:** 981–2.


**Effects on the cardiovascular system.** Myocarditis associated with chest pain and ECG abnormalities has been reported[1,2] in 2 patients taking mesalazine; 1 patient died in cardiogenic shock.[2] It was suggested that mesalazine or sulfasalazine should be replaced by glucocorticoids if cardiac symptoms arise during treatment.[2] Pericarditis[3,4] together with fever, rash, dyspnoea, pleural and pericardial effusions, and arthritis, has also been described, and is considered to constitute a drug-induced lupus-like syndrome.


1. Agnholt J, *et al.* Cardiac hypersensitivity to 5-aminosalicylic acid. *Lancet* 1989; **i:** 1135.
2. Kristensen KS, *et al.* Fatal myocarditis associated with mesalazine. *Lancet* 1990; **335:** 605.
3. Dent MT, *et al.* Mesalazine induced lupus-like syndrome. *BMJ* 1992; **305:** 159.
4. Lim AG, Hine KR. Fever, vasculitic rash, arthritis, pericarditis, and pericardial effusion after mesalazine. *BMJ* 1994; **308:** 113.


**Effects on the hair.** For a report of accelerated hair loss from the scalp in 2 patients receiving mesalazine enemas, see under Sulfasalazine, p.1292.

**Effects on the kidneys.** The risk of nephrotoxicity may be low for mesalazine and the related compounds sulfasalazine and olsalazine.[1] Even so, adverse effects on the kidneys have occurred and between February 1988 and December 1990 the UK Committee on Safety of Medicines[2] received 9 reports of serious nephrotoxic reactions associated with the use of Asacol, a modified-release mesalazine preparation. The reactions included 4 cases of interstitial nephritis, 3 of severe renal failure, and 2 cases of nephrotic syndrome. A subsequent case report[3] indicated that by September 1998 the number of such reports for mesalazine totalled 104, including 35 cases of interstitial nephritis. The authors considered that monitoring of renal function was required in patients receiving mesalazine. A protocol for such monitoring was subsequently suggested,[4] and a similar protocol has been adopted in UK licensing information for mesalazine, with serum creatinine estimated:

- before treatment
- every 3 months for the first year
- every 6 months for the next 4 years
- annually thereafter

The nephrotic syndrome[5] and interstitial nephritis[6] have also been reported with sulfasalazine, and interstitial nephritis with olsalazine (see p.1278).


1. Anonymous. Choosing an oral 5-aminosalicylic acid preparation for ulcerative colitis. *Drug Ther Bull* 1992; **30:** 50–2.
2. Committee on Safety of Medicines. Nephrotoxicity associated with mesalazine (Asacol). *Current Problems 30* 1990.
3. Popoola J, *et al.* Late onset interstitial nephritis associated with mesalazine treatment. *BMJ* 1998; **317:** 795–7.

4. Corrigan G, Stevens PE. Review article: interstitial nephritis associated with the use of mesalazine in inflammatory bowel disease. *Aliment Pharmacol Ther* 2000; **14:** 1–6.
5. Barbour VM, Williams PF. Nephrotic syndrome associated with sulphasalazine. *BMJ* 1990; **301:** 818.
6. Dwarakanath AD, *et al.* Sulphasalazine induced renal failure. *Gut* 1992; **33:** 1006–1007.

**Effects on the liver.** A case of chronic hepatitis and liver fibrosis has been reported after prolonged mesalazine administration.[1] The authors considered that mesalazine should be discontinued when liver dysfunction occurred.

1. Deltenre P, *et al.* Mesalazine (5-aminosalicylic acid) induced chronic hepatitis. *Gut* 1999; **44:** 886–8.

**Effects on the nervous system.** Peripheral neuropathy,[1] mainly affecting the legs, has occurred during mesalazine treatment. The symptoms resolved on discontinuing the drug. Mononeuritis multiplex was part of the presentation of an eosinophilic reaction attributed to mesalazine in an asthmatic patient;[2] Churg-Strauss syndrome developed after withdrawal of mesalazine, but the patient subsequently recovered without sequelae.

1. Woodward DK. Peripheral neuropathy and mesalazine. *BMJ* 1989; **299:** 1224.
2. Morice AH, *et al.* Mesalazine activation of eosinophil. *Lancet* 1997; **350:** 1105.

**Effects on the pancreas.** Reports of pancreatitis, with abdominal pain and raised serum amylase activity, in 2 patients taking mesalazine.[1,2] The reaction was confirmed by rechallenge in both patients and symptoms resolved on withdrawal of mesalazine. The UK Committee on Safety of Medicines had received 15 reports[3] of pancreatitis associated with mesalazine therapy at February 1994.

1. Sachedina B, *et al.* Acute pancreatitis due to 5-aminosalicylate. *Ann Intern Med* 1989; **110:** 490–2.
2. Deprez P, *et al.* Pancreatitis induced by 5-aminosalicylic acid. *Lancet* 1989; **ii:** 445–6.
3. Committee on Safety of Medicines. Drug-induced pancreatitis. *Current Problems* 1994; **20:** 2–3.

**Effects on the respiratory system.** Pulmonary complications occur rarely with sulfasalazine (see p.1292). It is not known which component of sulfasalazine is responsible although, following a report of alveolitis in a patient with ulcerative colitis given mesalazine,[1] it was concluded that both sulfasalazine and 5-aminosalicylate (mesalazine) could induce hypersensitivity lung disease. Similar cases have since been reported,[2-4] and pulmonary symptoms may also manifest as part of a broader lupus-like syndrome (see Effects on the Cardiovascular System, above).

1. Welte T, *et al.* Mesalazine alveolitis. *Lancet* 1991; **338:** 1273. Correction. *ibid.* 1992; **339:** 70.
2. Honeybourne D. Mesalazine toxicity. *BMJ* 1994; **308:** 533–4.
3. Pascual-Lledó JF, *et al.* Interstitial pneumonitis due to mesalamine. *Ann Pharmacother* 1997; **31:** 499.
4. Sesin GP, *et al.* Mesalamine-associated pleural effusion with pulmonary infiltration. *Am J Health-Syst Pharm* 1998; **55:** 2304–5.

**Lupus.** For reports of lupus-like syndrome occurring with mesalazine, see Effects on the Cardiovascular System, above.

**Pregnancy.** Renal insufficiency in a neonate whose mother received mesalazine 2 to 4 g daily by mouth during the second trimester of pregnancy was suggested to be due to the drug,[1] although the proposed mechanism, inhibition of prostaglandin synthesis in the neonatal kidney, has been questioned.[2] A subsequent case-control study[3] found that use of oral mesalazine in 165 pregnant women with inflammatory bowel disease was not associated with a greater incidence of malformations. However, women treated with mesalazine were more likely to have preterm deliveries and newborns with decreased birth-weights, although the disease may have been a factor in this finding. A commentator on this study,[4] considered that active inflammatory bowel disease was a greater risk to pregnancy than drug treatment. In a further cohort of 123 pregnancies,[5] oral mesalazine at doses of 3 g daily or less did not increase the risk of fetal malformations or affect pregnancy outcome. The researchers concluded that further information was required on doses higher than 3 g daily. In another study,[6] all of 19 pregnancies in women receiving rectal mesalazine were full-term with no fetal abnormalities. For a discussion of sulfasalazine in pregnancy, see p.1292.

1. Colombel J-F, *et al.* Renal insufficiency in infant: side-effect of prenatal exposure to mesalazine? *Lancet* 1994; **344:** 620–1.
2. Marteau P, Devaux CB. Mesalazine during pregnancy. *Lancet* 1994; **344:** 1708–9.
3. Diav-Citrin O, *et al.* The safety of mesalamine in human pregnancy: a prospective controlled cohort study. *Gastroenterology* 1998; **114:** 23–8.
4. Sachar D. Exposure to mesalamine during pregnancy increased preterm deliveries (but not birth defects) and decreased birth weight. *Gut* 1998; **43:** 316.
5. Marteau P, *et al.* Foetal outcome in women with inflammatory bowel disease treated during pregnancy with oral mesalazine microgranules. *Aliment Pharmacol Ther* 1998; **12:** 1101–8.
6. Bell CM, Habal FM. Safety of topical 5-aminosalicylic acid in pregnancy. *Am J Gastroenterol* 1997; **92:** 2201–2.

## Interactions

Preparations formulated to release mesalazine in the colon should not be given with drugs such as lactulose that lower colonic pH as they may prevent the release of mesalazine (but see Gastrointestinal Drugs below).

**Anticoagulants.** For reference to a case of mesalazine reducing the effect of *warfarin*, see Gastrointestinal Drugs, p.1026.

**Antineoplastics.** For mention of 5-aminosalicylates such as mesalazine inhibiting the metabolism of thiopurine antineoplastics, and increasing their toxicity, see Mercaptopurine, p.567.

**Gastrointestinal drugs.** Although it has been suggested that *lactulose* could delay the intestinal release of mesalazine from modified release preparation, a study found no evidence that lactulose co-administration influenced the release or disposition of mesalazine.[1] Similarly, *omeprazole* did not appear to increase the likelihood of premature mesalazine release.

1. Hussain FN, *et al.* Mesalazine release from a pH dependent formulation: effects of omeprazole and lactulose co-administration. *Br J Clin Pharmacol* 1998; **46:** 173–5.

## Pharmacokinetics

Following oral administration of conventional formulations, mesalazine would be extensively absorbed from the upper gastrointestinal tract, with little of the drug reaching the colon. Oral preparations are therefore generally formulated to release the drug in the terminal ileum and colon, where it is thought to exert a mainly local action. The specific release characteristics differ somewhat between formulations and this, together with interindividual variation, makes comparison of pharmacokinetic data between studies difficult. Some 20 to 50% of an oral dose is thought to be lost to absorption in healthy subjects, but absorption is lower in patients with active inflammatory bowel disease. Absorption from rectal dosage forms has also varied widely, with factors such as the dose, the formulation, and the pH also playing a role, but mean absorption of around 10 to 20% of a rectal dose has been reported in several studies.

The absorbed portion of mesalazine is almost completely acetylated in the gut wall and in the liver to acetyl-5-aminosalicylic acid. The rate of acetylation, and hence the concentration of parent drug and metabolite in the systemic circulation, is independent of the acetylator status. The acetylated metabolite is excreted mainly in urine by tubular secretion, together with traces of the parent compound; a clearance of about 3 to 4 mL/minute per kg has been reported for the former.

The elimination half-life of mesalazine is reported to be about 1 hour and it is 40 to 50% bound to plasma proteins; the acetylated metabolite has a half-life of up to 10 hours and is about 80% bound to plasma proteins.

Only negligible quantities of mesalazine cross the placenta. Amounts distributed into breast milk are very small.

◊ Reviews.

1. Klotz U. Clinical pharmacokinetics of sulphasalazine, its metabolites and other prodrugs of 5-aminosalicylic acid. *Clin Pharmacokinet* 1985; **10:** 285–302.
2. De Vos M. Clinical pharmacokinetics of slow release mesalazine. *Clin Pharmacokinet* 2000; **39:** 85–97.

## Uses and Administration

Mesalazine is an anti-inflammatory drug structurally related to the salicylates and active in inflammatory bowel disease (p.1243); it is considered to be the active moiety of sulfasalazine (p.1291). Its mode of action is uncertain, but may be due, at least in part, to its ability to inhibit local prostaglandin and leukotriene synthesis in the gastrointestinal mucosa.

Mesalazine is given by mouth or rectally in the treatment of *acute attacks* of mild to moderate ulcerative colitis or the *maintenance of remission* of ulcerative colitis or Crohn's disease. An oral dose of 400 mg of mesalazine is theoretically equivalent to 1 g of sulfasalazine.

There are several differently formulated oral preparations of mesalazine available, and dosage recommendations vary. Recommended doses for some UK preparations are as follows:

- *Asacol* tablets (Procter and Gamble, UK), *Ipocol* tablets (Sandoz, UK), *Mesren* tablets (IVAX, UK): acute attack, initially 2.4 g daily in divided doses; maintenance of remission, 1.2 to 2.4 g daily in divided doses
- *Pentasa Slow Release* tablets (Ferring, UK): acute attack, initially up to 4 g daily in 2 or 3 divided doses; maintenance of remission, adjusted individually from an initial dose of 1.5 g daily in 2 or 3 divided doses
- *Pentasa Slow Release* granules (Ferring, UK): acute attack, initially, up to 4 g daily in 2 to 4 divided doses; maintenance of remission, 2 g daily in 2 divided doses
- *Salofalk* tablets (Provalis, UK): acute attack, initially 1.5 g daily in 3 divided doses; maintenance of remission, 0.75 to 1.5 g daily in divided doses
- *Salofalk* granules (Provalis, UK): acute attack, initially 1.5 to 3 g daily in 3 divided doses; maintenance of remission, 1.5 g daily in 3 divided doses.

When given rectally, the suggested dose is 0.5 to 3 g daily as suppositories. In the UK, 1 or 2 g has been given daily as an enema, but in the USA an enema containing 4 g of mesalazine has been given.

◊ Reviews.

1. Clemett D, Markham A. Prolonged-release mesalazine: a review of its therapeutic potential in ulcerative colitis and Crohn's disease. *Drugs* 2000; **59:** 929–56.
2. Sutherland L, *et al.* Oral 5-aminosalicylic acid for maintenance of remission in ulcerative colitis. Available in The Cochrane Library; Issue 1. Chichester: John Wiley; 2004.

**Administration.** Because the release characteristics of different formulations of mesalazine vary, they should not be regarded as interchangeable.[1] This applies even to those formulations where the dosage is apparently similar.[2]

1. Forbes A, Chadwick C. Mesalazine preparations. *Lancet* 1997; **350:** 1329.
2. Benbow AG, Gould I. Mesalazine preparations. *Lancet* 1998; **351:** 68.

## Preparations

***USP 27:*** Mesalamine Delayed-Release Tablets; Mesalamine Extended-Release Capsules; Mesalamine Rectal Suspension.

**Proprietary Preparations** (details are given in Part 3)
***Arg.:*** Bufexan; Pentasa; ***Austral.:*** Mesasal; Salofalk; ***Austria:*** Claversal; Pentasa; Salofalk; ***Belg.:*** Asacol; Claversal; Colitofalk; Pentasa; ***Braz.:*** Asalit; Pentasa†; ***Canad.:*** Asacol; Mesasal; Pentasa; Quintasa†; Salofalk; ***Chile:*** Pentasa; Salofalk; ***Denm.:*** Asacol; Mesasal; Pentasa; ***Fin.:*** Asacol; Pentasa; ***Fr.:*** Fivasa; Pentasa; Rowasa; ***Ger.:*** Asacolitin; Claversal; Pentasa; Salofalk; ***Gr.:*** Asacol; Asalazin; Laboxantryl; Mesagin; Pentasa; Salofalk; ***Hong Kong:*** Asacol; Pentasa; Salofalk; ***India:*** Mesacol; ***Irl.:*** Asacolon; Pentasa; Salofalk; ***Israel:*** Asacol; Pentasa; Rafassal; ***Ital.:*** Asacol; Asalex; Asamax; Claversal; Enterasin; Lextrasa; Mesaflor; Pentacol; Pentasa; Salofalk; Xalazin; ***Jpn:*** Pentasa; ***Malaysia:*** Pentasa; Salofalk; ***Mex.:*** Asacol; Kenzomyl; Pentasa; Salofalk; ***Neth.:*** Asacol; Pentasa; Salofalk; ***Norw.:*** Asacol; Mesasal; Pentasa; ***NZ:*** Asacol; Pentasa; ***Port.:*** Asacol; Claversal; Pentasa; Salofalk; ***S.Afr.:*** Asacol; Pentasa; ***Singapore:*** Asacol; Mesacol†; Pentasa; Salofalk; ***Spain:*** Claversal; Lixacol; Pentasa; Quintasa†; ***Swed.:*** Asacol; Mesasal; Pentasa; ***Switz.:*** Asacol; Asazine; Pentasa; Salofalk; ***Thai.:*** Asacol; Mesacol; Salofalk; ***UK:*** Asacol; Ipocol; Mesren; Pentasa; Salofalk; ***USA:*** Asacol; Canasa; Pentasa; Rowasa.

---

# Metoclopramide *(BAN, rINN)*

Metoclopramidum. 4-Amino-5-chloro-*N*-(2-diethylaminoethyl)-2-methoxybenzamide.

$C_{14}H_{22}ClN_3O_2$ = 299.8.

*CAS — 364-62-5.*

*ATC — A03FA01.*

**Pharmacopoeias.** In *Chin.*, *Eur.* (see p.vi), and *Jpn.*

**Ph. Eur. 5.0** (Metoclopramide ). A white or almost white, fine powder. It exhibits polymorphism. Practically insoluble in water; sparingly soluble in alcohol; sparingly soluble in dichloromethane.

## Metoclopramide Hydrochloride *(BANM, USAN, rINNM)*

AHR-3070-C; DEL-1267; Hidrocloruro de metoclopramida; Metoclopramidi Hydrochloridum; MK-745.

$C_{14}H_{22}ClN_3O_2,HCl,H_2O$ = 354.3.

*CAS — 7232-21-5 (anhydrous metoclopramide hydrochloride); 54143-57-6 (metoclopramide hydrochloride monohydrate); 2576-84-3 (anhydrous metoclopramide dihydrochloride).*

*ATC — A03FA01.*

**Pharmacopoeias.** In *Eur.* (see p.vi), *Int.*, *Pol.*, and *US.*

**Ph. Eur. 5.0** (Metoclopramide Hydrochloride). A white or almost white, crystalline powder or crystals. Very soluble in water; freely soluble in alcohol; sparingly soluble in dichloromethane. A 10% solution in water has a pH of 4.5 to 6.0. Protect from light.

**USP 27** (Metoclopramide Hydrochloride). A white or practically white, odourless or practically odourless, crystalline powder. Very soluble in water; freely soluble in alcohol; sparingly soluble in chloroform; practically insoluble in ether. Store in airtight containers. Protect from light.

**Incompatibility.** Proprietary preparations of metoclopramide hydrochloride are stated to be incompatible with cephalothin sodium, chloramphenicol sodium, and sodium bicarbonate. Cisplatin, cyclophosphamide, and doxorubicin hydrochloride are stated to be compatible with metoclopramide hydrochloride but compatibility is dependent upon factors such as the particular formulation, drug concentration, and temperature.

## Adverse Effects

Metoclopramide is a dopamine antagonist and may cause extrapyramidal symptoms (usually acute dystonic reactions); these are more common in children and young adults, especially if female, and at daily doses above 500 micrograms/kg. Parkinsonism and tardive dyskinesia have occasionally occurred, usually during prolonged treatment in elderly patients.

Other adverse effects include restlessness, drowsiness, and diarrhoea. Hypotension, hypertension, dizziness, headache, and depression may occur and there are isolated reports of blood disorders, hypersensitivity reactions (rash, bronchospasm), and neuroleptic malignant syndrome. Disorders of cardiac conduction have been reported with intravenous metoclopramide.

Metoclopramide stimulates prolactin secretion and may cause galactorrhoea or related disorders. Transient increases in plasma-aldosterone concentrations have been reported.

**Effects on the blood.** A report[1] of agranulocytosis associated with use of metoclopramide on 2 separate occasions. Both episodes resolved within 2 to 3 weeks of withdrawing metoclopramide. Methaemoglobinaemia[2] has also been reported.

1. Harvey RL, Luzar MJ. Metoclopramide-induced agranulocytosis. *Ann Intern Med* 1988; **108:** 214–15.
2. Grant SCD, *et al.* Methaemoglobinaemia produced by metoclopramide in an adult. *Eur J Clin Pharmacol* 1994; **47:** 89.

**Effects on the cardiovascular system.** Reports of hypotension,[1] hypertension,[2,3] and supraventricular tachycardia[4] associated with metoclopramide. Bradycardia followed by total heart block,[5] and sinus arrest,[6] have also been reported.

1. Park GR. Hypotension following metoclopramide administration during hypotensive anaesthesia for intracranial aneurysm. *Br J Anaesth* 1978; **50:** 1268–9.
2. Sheridan C, *et al.* Transient hypertension after high doses of metoclopramide. *N Engl J Med* 1982; **307:** 1346.
3. Filibeck DJ, *et al.* Metoclopramide-induced hypertensive crisis. *Clin Pharm* 1984; **3:** 548–9.
4. Bevacqua BK. Supraventricular tachycardia associated with postpartum metoclopramide administration. *Anesthesiology* 1988; **68:** 124–5.
5. Midttun M, Øberg B. Total heart block after intravenous metoclopramide. *Lancet* 1994; **343:** 182–3.
6. Malkoff MD, *et al.* Sinus arrest after administration of intravenous metoclopramide. *Ann Pharmacother* 1995; **29:** 381–3.

**Effects on the endocrine system.** ALDOSTERONISM. Metoclopramide has been reported to increase plasma-aldosterone concentrations in healthy individuals[1] and in patients with liver cirrhosis and ascites associated with secondary hyperaldosteronism.[2] Increased plasma aldosterone after metoclopramide administration has also been associated with the development of oedema in a patient with congestive heart failure.[3] The metoclopramide-induced aldosterone response was blunted by prior administration of neostigmine.[1]

1. Sommers DK, *et al.* Effect of neostigmine on metoclopramide-induced aldosterone secretion in man. *Eur J Clin Pharmacol* 1989; **36:** 411–13.
2. Mazzacca G, *et al.* Metoclopramide and secondary hyperaldosteronism. *Ann Intern Med* 1983; **98:** 1024–5.
3. Zumoff B. Metoclopramide and edema. *Ann Intern Med* 1983; **98:** 557.

HYPERPROLACTINAEMIA. Hyperprolactinaemia, galactorrhoea, and pituitary adenoma occurred in a 49-year-old woman with reflux oesophagitis who had received metoclopramide for 3 months.[1] Her plasma-prolactin concentrations fell to normal and her symptoms resolved over 4 months following withdrawal of metoclopramide. The pituitary tumour was considered to be incidental to, and not caused by, metoclopramide therapy.

1. Cooper BT, *et al.* Galactorrhoea, hyperprolactinaemia, and pituitary adenoma presenting during metoclopramide therapy. *Postgrad Med J* 1982; **58:** 314–15.

**Effects on mental state.** There are isolated reports of dose-related delirium, depression, and uncontrollable crying in patients treated with metoclopramide in doses of 40 to 80 mg daily.[1-3] Symptoms resolved on reducing the dose or withdrawing metoclopramide and tolerance could be achieved by gradually increasing the dose.

Insomnia, with or without daytime drowsiness, has also been reported in patients taking metoclopramide 40 mg daily.[4]

1. Bottner RK, Tullio CJ. Metoclopramide and depression. *Ann Intern Med* 1985; **103:** 482.
2. Adams CD. Metoclopramide and depression. *Ann Intern Med* 1985; **103:** 960.
3. Fishbain DA, Rogers A. Delirium secondary to metoclopramide hydrochloride. *J Clin Psychopharmacol* 1987; **7:** 281–2.
4. Saxe TG. Metoclopramide side effects. *Ann Intern Med* 1983; **98:** 674.

**Extrapyramidal effects.** The Adverse Reactions Register of the UK Committee on Safety of Medicines for the years 1967-82 contained 479 reports of extrapyramidal reactions in which metoclopramide was the suspected drug: 455 were for dystonic-dyskinetic reactions, 20 for parkinsonism, and 4 for tardive dyskinesia.[1]

Acute **dystonic-dyskinetic** reactions occur most commonly in children and young adults[1-3] and about 70% of reactions are in females;[1,3] a substantial proportion of reactions are associated with doses in excess of those recommended by the manufacturers.[1,3,4] Symptoms reported include oculogyric crisis,[4,5] opisthotonus,[6] torticollis,[5,7] trismus,[5,7] a tetanus-like reaction,[8] and blue coloration of the tongue;[6] akathisia following the use of metoclopramide alone,[9] or with droperidol[10] or haloperidol[9] has been reported. The effects usually occur within 72 hours of starting treatment[1] but have been reported within 30 minutes of receiving metoclopramide.[4] They may occur in patients who have previously received metoclopramide without complications[5,8,10] and may be precipitated by other drugs. Although generally self-limiting, deaths have occurred.[1,5] The reactions are readily reversed by an antihistamine such as diphenhydramine,[7] or an antimuscarinic such as benzatropine;[4,6] prophylactic use of diphenhydramine has been suggested for patients with a history of extrapyramidal reactions and in those less than 30 years of age.[7,8]

Metoclopramide-associated **parkinsonism** is thought to occur less commonly than the acute dystonias and is seen predominantly in older patients. Symptoms usually appear several months after starting metoclopramide, but may occur within days or not for several years. Withdrawal of metoclopramide usually results in resolution of symptoms, although it may take several months.[1] A study has suggested that metoclopramide-induced parkinsonism (misdiagnosed as idiopathic Parkinson's disease) may be more common in the elderly than generally realised.[11]

**Tardive dyskinesia** may rarely be associated with metoclopramide administration. The reaction is usually confined to elderly patients following prolonged oral use,[12,13] but it has been reported after short-term high-dose parenteral use as an antiemetic in cancer chemotherapy,[14] and a case has been reported in an 8-year-old child treated with metoclopramide for gastro-oesophageal reflux disease in usual doses.[15] The average duration of treatment before the onset of symptoms was 14 months (range 4 to 44 months) in a report of 11 cases[13] and 26 months (range 8 to 60 months) in a report of 12 cases;[16] some patients did not experience symptoms until after withdrawal of metoclopramide. Tardive dyskinesia is potentially irreversible and its management is difficult.[16] Some patients improve after withdrawal of metoclopramide but symptoms persisting during follow-up periods of up to 3 years have been reported[12,13] The emphasis must be on prevention hence the recommendation that metoclopramide should not be prescribed for the long-term treatment of minor symptoms, especially in elderly patients.[16]

1. Bateman DN, *et al.* Extrapyramidal reactions with metoclopramide. *BMJ* 1985; **291:** 930–2.
2. Anonymous. Measuring therapeutic risk. *Lancet* 1989; **ii:** 139–40.
3. Adverse Drug Reactions Advisory Committee. Metoclopramide—choose the dose carefully. *Aust Adverse Drug React Bull* 1990; Feb.
4. Tait P, *et al.* Metoclopramide side effects in children. *Med J Aust* 1990; **152:** 387.
5. Pollera CF, *et al.* Sudden death after acute dystonic reaction to high-dose metoclopramide. *Lancet* 1984; **ii:** 460–1.
6. Alroe C, Bowen P. Metoclopramide and prochlorperazine: "the blue-tongue sign". *Med J Aust* 1989; **150:** 724–5.
7. Kris MG, *et al.* Extrapyramidal reactions with high-dose metoclopramide. *N Engl J Med* 1983; **309:** 433–4.
8. Della Valle R, *et al.* Metoclopramide-induced tetanus-like dystonic reaction. *Clin Pharm* 1985; **4:** 102–3.
9. Akagi H, Kumar TM. Akathisia: overlooked at a cost. *BMJ* 2002; **324:** 1506–7.
10. Barnes TRE, *et al.* Acute akathisia after oral droperidol and metoclopramide preoperative medication. *Lancet* 1982; **ii:** 48–9.
11. Avorn J, *et al.* Increased incidence of levodopa therapy following metoclopramide use. *JAMA* 1995; **274:** 1780–2.
12. Grimes JD, *et al.* Long-term follow-up of tardive dyskinesia due to metoclopramide. *Lancet* 1982; **ii:** 563.
13. Wiholm B-E, *et al.* Tardive dyskinesia associated with metoclopramide. *BMJ* 1984; **288:** 545–7.
14. Breitbart W. Tardive dyskinesia associated with high-dose intravenous metoclopramide. *N Engl J Med* 1986; **315:** 518.
15. Putnam PE, *et al.* Tardive dyskinesia associated with use of metoclopramide in a child. *J Pediatr* 1992; **121:** 983–5.
16. Orme ML'E, Tallis RC. Metoclopramide and tardive dyskinesia in the elderly. *BMJ* 1984; **289:** 397–8.

**Neuroleptic malignant syndrome.** Neuroleptic malignant syndrome has occurred very rarely with metoclopramide. In a report of a case with a fatal outcome, it was noted that 17 additional cases had been published in the years 1978 to 1998, three of which resulted in death.[1] Metoclopramide should be stopped immediately if the syndrome occurs, and the patient treated urgently with bromocriptine.

1. Nonino F, Campomori A. Neuroleptic malignant syndrome associated with metoclopramide. *Ann Pharmacother* 1999; **33:** 644–5.

## Precautions

Metoclopramide should not be used when stimulation of muscular contractions might adversely affect gastrointestinal conditions, as in gastrointestinal haemorrhage, obstruction, perforation, or immediately after surgery. There have been reports of hypertensive crises in patients with phaeochromocytoma given metoclopramide, thus its use is not recommended in such patients.

Children, young patients, and the elderly should be treated with care as they are at increased risk of extrapyramidal reactions; in the UK, use of metoclopramide is restricted in patients under 20 years (see Uses and Administration, below). Patients on prolonged therapy should be reviewed regularly. Care should also be taken when metoclopramide is administered to patients with renal impairment, epilepsy, Parkinson's disease, or a history of depression.

Metoclopramide may cause drowsiness or impaired reactions; patients so affected should not drive or operate machinery.

**Breast feeding.** The American Academy of Pediatrics[1] considers that the use of metoclopramide by mothers during breast feeding may be of concern, owing to its dopamine-receptor blocking activity.

1. American Academy of Pediatrics. The transfer of drugs and other chemicals into human milk. *Pediatrics* 2001; **108:** 776–89. Correction. *ibid.*; 1029. Also available at: http://aappolicy.aappublications.org/cgi/content/full/pediatrics%3b108/3/776 (accessed 07/05/04)

**Hepatic impairment.** The UK manufacturers recommend that the dose of metoclopramide should be reduced in patients with clinically significant hepatic impairment, although the US manufacturers note that it has been used safely in some patients with advanced liver disease and make no such recommendation. Decreases in clearance and increases in half-life and area under the plasma concentration-time curve have been reported in patients with cirrhosis given metoclopramide.[1,2]

1. Hellstern A, *et al.* Absolute bioavailability of metoclopramide given orally or by enema in patients with normal liver function or with cirrhosis of the liver. *Arzneimittelforschung* 1987; **37:** 733–6.
2. Magueur E, *et al.* Pharmacokinetics of metoclopramide in patients with liver cirrhosis. *Br J Clin Pharmacol* 1991; **31:** 185–7.

**Porphyria.** Metoclopramide has been associated with acute attacks of porphyria and is considered to be unsafe in porphyric patients, although there is conflicting evidence of porphyrinogenicity, and indeed some have used it successfully in the management of acute attacks.[1]

1. Elder GH, *et al.* Metoclopramide and acute porphyria. *Lancet* 1997; **350:** 1104.

**Renal impairment.** Total clearance of metoclopramide is significantly reduced in patients with renal impairment[1-3] and the elimination half-life is prolonged to up to 19 hours.[2] This may be due to impaired metabolism[1,2] or to an alteration in enterohepatic circulation of metoclopramide.[1] Accumulation of metoclopramide could therefore occur in renal impairment with a possible increased risk of side-effects. Dosage reductions of at least 50% have therefore been recommended in patients with moderate to severe renal impairment.[1,2]

Patients undergoing haemodialysis do not require dosage supplements since relatively little metoclopramide is cleared by this process.[2,3]

1. Bateman DN, *et al.* The pharmacokinetics of single doses of metoclopramide in renal failure. *Eur J Clin Pharmacol* 1981; **19:** 437–41.
2. Lehmann CR, *et al.* Metoclopramide kinetics in patients with impaired renal function and clearance by haemodialysis. *Clin Pharmacol Ther* 1985; **37:** 284–9.
3. Wright MR, *et al.* Effect of haemodialysis on metoclopramide kinetics in patients with severe renal failure. *Br J Clin Pharmacol* 1988; **26:** 474–7.

## Interactions

Caution should be observed when using metoclopramide in patients taking other drugs that can also cause extrapyramidal reactions, such as the phenothiazines. Increased toxicity may occur if metoclopramide is used in patients receiving lithium, and caution is advisable with other centrally active drugs such as antiepileptics. Antimuscarinics and opioid analgesics antagonise the gastrointestinal effects of metoclopramide.

The absorption of other drugs may be affected by metoclopramide; it may either diminish absorption from the stomach (as with digoxin) or enhance absorption from the small intestine (for example, with ciclosporin, aspirin, or paracetamol). It inhibits serum cholinesterase and may prolong neuromuscular blockade produced by suxamethonium (see p.1408) and mivacurium (p.1404). Metoclopramide may also increase prolactin blood concentrations and therefore interfere with drugs which have a hypoprolactinaemic effect such as bromocriptine (but see p.1202). It has been suggested that it should not be given to patients receiving MAOIs.

**Carbamazepine.** For a report of neurotoxicity associated with the use of metoclopramide with carbamazepine, see p.356.

**Hydroxyzine.** Acute anxiety, rigidity, generalised tremor, opisthotonus, and hypertension developed in a 20-year-old man after administration of metoclopramide 10 mg intravenously and hydroxyzine 100 mg intramuscularly.[1] The side-effects occurred 30 minutes after giving hydroxyzine and it was suggested that hydroxyzine potentiated the onset of the reaction.

1. Fouilladieu JL, *et al.* Possible potentiation by hydroxyzine of metoclopramide's undesirable side effects. *Anesth Analg* 1985; **64:** 1227–8.

## Pharmacokinetics

Metoclopramide is rapidly and almost completely absorbed from the gastrointestinal tract following a dose by mouth, although conditions such as vomiting or impaired gastric motility may reduce absorption. However, it undergoes hepatic first-pass metabolism, which varies considerably between subjects, and hence absolute bioavailability and plasma concentrations are subject to wide interindividual variation. On average, the bioavailability of oral metoclopramide is about 75%, but it varies between about 30 and 100%. Peak plasma concentrations of metoclopramide occur about 1 to 2 hours after an oral dose. Bioavailability is equally variable following rectal or intranasal administration, although it may be somewhat better if the drug is given intramuscularly.

Metoclopramide is widely distributed in the body, with an apparent volume of distribution of about 3.5 litres/kg. It readily crosses the blood-brain barrier into the CNS. It also freely crosses the placenta, and has been reported to attain concentrations in fetal plasma about 60 to 70% of those in maternal plasma. Concentrations higher than those in maternal plasma may be reached in the breast milk of lactating mothers, particularly in the early puerperium, although concentrations decrease somewhat in the late puerperium.

Elimination of metoclopramide is biphasic, with a terminal elimination half-life of about 4 to 6 hours, although this may be prolonged in renal impairment, with consequent elevation of plasma concentrations. It is excreted in the urine, about 85% of a dose being eliminated in 72 hours, 20 to 30% as unchanged metoclopramide and the remainder as sulfate or glucuronide conjugates, or as metabolites. About 5% of a dose is excreted in faeces via the bile.

## Uses and Administration

Metoclopramide hydrochloride is a substituted benzamide used for its prokinetic and antiemetic properties. It stimulates the motility of the upper gastrointestinal tract without affecting gastric, biliary, or pancreatic secretion and increases gastric peristalsis, leading to accelerated gastric emptying. Duodenal peristalsis is also increased which decreases intestinal transit time. The resting tone of the gastro-oesophageal sphincter is increased and the pyloric sphincter is relaxed. Metoclopramide possesses parasympathomimetic activity as well as being a dopamine-receptor antagonist with a direct effect on the chemoreceptor trigger zone. It may have serotonin-receptor ($5\text{-}HT_3$) antagonist properties.

Metoclopramide is used in disorders of decreased gastrointestinal motility (p.1241) such as gastroparesis or ileus; in gastro-oesophageal reflux disease (p.1242) and dyspepsia (p.1242); and in nausea and vomiting (p.1245) associated with various gastrointestinal disorders, with migraine, following surgery, and with cancer therapy. Metoclopramide is of no value in the prevention or treatment of motion sickness. It may be used to stimulate gastric emptying during radiographic examinations, to facilitate intubation of the small bowel, and in the management of aspiration syndromes (p.1240).

It is usually given as the hydrochloride monohydrate with doses expressed as the anhydrous hydrochloride. In the USA, the strength of preparations of the hydrochloride monohydrate is usually expressed in terms of the base. Metoclopramide hydrochloride 10.5 mg is approximately equivalent to 10.0 mg of the anhydrous substance, which is approximately equivalent to 8.9 mg of the anhydrous base.

For most purposes the total daily dose should not exceed 500 micrograms/kg; dosage reduction is recommended in renal and perhaps hepatic impairment (see Precautions, above).

- In the UK, the recommended dose by mouth, intramuscularly, or by slow intravenous injection, is 10 mg (expressed as anhydrous metoclopramide hydrochloride) three times daily.
- In the USA, the recommended dose is 10 to 15 mg (expressed as the base) up to four times daily.
- Single doses of 10 to 20 mg (expressed as anhydrous base or anhydrous hydrochloride) should be considered where appropriate.

In the UK, the use of metoclopramide is restricted in patients under 20 years of age to severe intractable vomiting of known cause, chemotherapy- or radiotherapy-induced vomiting, as an aid to gastrointestinal intubation, and in premedication. Suggested doses are:

- for those aged 15 to 19 years and weighing 60 kg and over: 10 mg three times daily
- 15 to 19 years (30 to 59 kg): 5 mg three times daily
- 9 to 14 years (30 kg and over): 5 mg three times daily
- 5 to 9 years (20 to 29 kg): 2.5 mg three times daily
- 3 to 5 years (15 to 19 kg): 2 mg two or three times daily
- 1 to 3 years (10 to 14 kg): 1 mg two or three times daily
- under 1 year (up to 10 kg): 1 mg twice daily

Where body-weight is below that specified for a given age group, the dose should reflect the weight rather than the age, so that a lower dose is chosen.

An intranasal formulation of metoclopramide is available in some countries.

The base, the dihydrochloride, and the glycyrrhizinate have also been used.

**High-dose therapy.** High doses of metoclopramide have been used in the treatment of the nausea and vomiting associated with cancer chemotherapy often in combination with other agents such as dexamethasone. The loading dose of metoclopramide given before cancer therapy is 2 to 4 mg/kg administered as a continuous intravenous infusion over 15 to 20 minutes and is followed by a maintenance dose of 3 to 5 mg/kg, again as a continuous intravenous infusion, administered over 8 to 12 hours. Alternatively, initial doses of up to 2 mg/kg by intravenous infusion over at least 15 minutes may be given before cancer therapy and repeated every 2 or 3 hours. The total dosage by either continuous or intermittent infusion should not normally exceed 10 mg/kg in 24 hours.

**Administration.** INTRANASAL. References.

1. Ormrod D, Goa KL. Intranasal metoclopramide. *Drugs* 1999; **58:** 315–22. Commentaries. *ibid.*; 323–4.

**Administration in hepatic or renal impairment.** For discussion of dosage in hepatic or renal impairment see under Precautions, above.

**Hiccup.** Metoclopramide has been used with chlorpromazine in protocols for the management of intractable hiccup. For a discussion of hiccup and its management see p.682.

**Lactation induction.** Metoclopramide has been used for its dopamine antagonist properties to stimulate lactation in women who wish to breast feed and in whom mechanical stimulation of the nipple alone is inadequate. Doses of 10 mg three times daily have been used for this purpose, but should be viewed as adjunctive to mechanical methods and the duration of therapy should probably be limited to 7 to 14 days.[1] Young women are at increased risk of extrapyramidal effects from metoclopramide—see under Adverse Effects, above. There has also been concern about the presence of the drug in breast milk. For a discussion of lactation inhibition and induction, see p.1317.

1. Anderson PO, Valdés V. Increasing breast milk supply. *Clin Pharm* 1993; **12:** 479–80.

**Migraine.** Metoclopramide is used in the treatment of migraine (p.464) to alleviate nausea and vomiting and gastric stasis, which commonly develop as a migraine attack progresses and can lead to poor absorption of oral antimigraine preparations. It may also be given to counteract nausea and vomiting from the use of ergotamine. Metoclopramide is included in some combination analgesic preparations for the treatment of acute attacks of migraine. In a study lysine aspirin with metoclopramide was as effective as sumatriptan in the treatment of migraine.[1]

Metoclopramide given intravenously can relieve the pain of migraine attacks;[2,3] this effect may be related to its action as a dopamine antagonist and may be worth trying in patients who require parenteral treatment and do not respond to sumatriptan or dihydroergotamine.

1. Tfelt-Hansen P, *et al.* The effectiveness of combined oral lysine acetylsalicylate and metoclopramide compared with oral sumatriptan for migraine. *Lancet* 1995; **346:** 923–6.
2. Tek DS, *et al.* A prospective, double-blind study of metoclopramide hydrochloride for the control of migraine in the emergency department. *Ann Emerg Med* 1990; **19:** 1083–7.
3. Ellis GL, *et al.* The efficacy of metoclopramide in the treatment of migraine. *Ann Emerg Med* 1993; **22:** 191–5.

**Orthostatic hypotension.** Metoclopramide has been tried in the management of some patients with orthostatic hypotension, as mentioned on p.1100.

**Variceal haemorrhage.** Metoclopramide 20 mg intravenously controlled bleeding from oesophageal varices within 15 minutes in 10 of 11 patients compared with 4 of 11 patients given placebo; all patients were treated by sclerotherapy.[1] Lower oesophageal sphincter pressure is increased by metoclopramide, thus reducing blood flow to varices and achieving haemostasis; another study[2] found a combination of metoclopramide and intravenous glyceryl trinitrate to be more effective than glyceryl trinitrate alone in reducing intravariceal pressure.

For a discussion of variceal haemorrhage and its management, see p.1716.

1. Hosking SW, *et al.* Pharmacological constriction of the lower oesophageal sphincter: a simple method of arresting variceal haemorrhage. *Gut* 1988; **29:** 1098–1102.
2. Sarin SK, Saraya A. Effects of intravenous nitroglycerin and nitroglycerin and metoclopramide on intravariceal pressure: a double blind, randomized study. *Am J Gastroenterol* 1995; **90:** 48–53.

### Preparations

***BP 2003:*** Metoclopramide Injection; Metoclopramide Oral Solution; Metoclopramide Tablets;
***USP 27:*** Metoclopramide Injection; Metoclopramide Oral Solution; Metoclopramide Tablets.

**Proprietary Preparations** (details are given in Part 3)
***Arg.:*** Celit; Fonderyl; Lizarona; Metoc; Midatenk; Novomit; Primavera-N; Primperil; Reliveran; Rilaquin; Sintegran; ***Austral.:*** Maxolon; Pramin; ***Austria:*** Gastro-Timelets; Gastronerton; Gastrosil; Metogastron; Nausigon†; Paspertin; ***Belg.:*** Dibertil; Movistal; Primperan; ***Braz.:*** Aristopramida; Citroplus; Clopra†; Dart†; Emetic†; Estomaplus†; Eucil; Metoclosan; Metosix†; Metovit†; Nausil†; Neolasil; No-Vomit; Plagex; Plamidasil; Plamin†; Plamivon; Plasil; Vomix†; Vonil†; Vopax; ***Canad.:*** Apo-Metoclop; Maxeran†; Reglan†; ***Chile:*** Hemibe; Itan; ***Denm.:*** Emperal; Gastro-Timelets; Primperan; ***Fin.:*** Metopram; Primperan; ***Fr.:*** Anausin; Primperan; ***Ger.:*** Cerucal; duraMCP†; Gastro-Timelets†; Gastronerton; Gastrosil; Gastrotranquil; Hyrin; MCP; MCPham; Paspertin; ***Gr.:*** Primeran; ***Hong Kong:*** Apo-Metoclop†; Maxolon; Metocyl; Metram; Primperan; ***India:*** Maxeron; Metocontin; Perinorm; Reglan; Tomid; ***Irl.:*** Antimet; Gastrobid Continus; Maxolon; Metocyl; ***Israel:*** Pramin; ***Ital.:*** Citroplus; Clopan; Plasil; Pramidin; Randum; ***Jpn:*** Primperan; ***Malaysia:*** Maril; Maxolon; Metocyl; Primperan; Pulin; ***Mex.:*** Biopram; Carnotprim; Cirulan; Clorimet-Z; Meclomid; Midetol; Mipramid; Plasil; Pramilem; Pramotil; Primperan; Propace†; Vonifin†; ***Mon.:*** Prokinyl; ***Neth.:*** Primperan†; ***Norw.:*** Afipran; Primperan; ***NZ:*** Maxolon; Metamide; ***Port.:*** Metoclan; Primperan; Reglan; ***S.Afr.:*** Acumet†; Ametic†; Betaclopramide; Clopamon; Contromet; Maxolon; Metalon; Metcon†; Perinorm; Setin; ***Singapore:*** Maril; Maxolon; Metocyl; Metolon; Primperan; Pulin; ***Spain:*** Metagliz; Primperan; ***Swed.:*** Primperan; ***Switz.:*** Gastro-Timelets†; Gastrosil; Paspertin; Primperan; ***Thai.:*** Elitan†; Emetal; Gensil; H-Peran; Hawkperan; Maril; Meramide; Met-Sil; Metoclor; Metono†; Nausil; Plasil; Vasil†; ***UAE:*** Premosan; ***UK:*** Gastrobid Continus; Gastroflux; Gastromax†; Maxolon; Mygdalon†; Parmid†; Primperan; ***USA:*** Clopra; Maxolon; Octamide; Reclomide; Reglan.

**Multi-ingredient:** ***Arg.:*** Bil 13 Enzimatico; Bitecain AA; Digesplen; Facilgest; Factorine; Faradil; Faradil Enzimatico; Migral Compositum; Pakinase; Pankreon Total; Tetralgin; Vacuobil Plus; ***Austria:*** Ceolat Compositum; Paspertase; ***Belg.:*** Migpriv; ***Braz.:*** Cefalium; Diagrin†; Digeplus; Digest†; Emetrol; Essen; Estac; Plagon†; Plasil Enzimatico; Plasonil†; Sintozima; Vominil; Vomistop†; Vonil Enzimatico†; ***Chile:*** Aero Itan; Aeroflat; Aerogastrol; Digespar; Garceptol; Gaseofin; No-Ref; Pangastren; ***Denm.:*** Migpriv; ***Fin.:*** Migpriv; ***Fr.:*** Cephalgan; Migpriv; Primperoxane†; ***Ger.:*** Migraeflux MCP; Migrane-Neuridal; Migranerton; Paspertase; ***India:*** Paramet; ***Irl.:*** Paramax; ***Ital.:*** Ede†; Geffer; Migpriv; Migraprim; ***Mex.:*** Digenor Plus; Espaven MD; Plasil Enzimatico; Pramigel; Primpesasy; ***Neth.:*** Migrafin; ***Norw.:*** Migpriv; ***NZ:*** Paramax; ***Spain:*** Aero Plus; Aeroflat; Anti Anorex Triple; Edym Sedante†; Gastro Gobens†; Jorkil†; Liberbil†; Metagliz Bismutico†; Novo Aerofil Sedante; Paidozim; Primperan Complex†; Salcemetic; Starlep†; Sualyn†; Surifarm†; Suxidina; ***Swed.:*** Migpriv; ***Switz.:*** Migpriv; ***UK:*** Migramax; Migravess†; Paramax.

---

## Metopimazine *(BAN, USAN, rINN)*

EXP-999; Metopimazina; RP-9965. 1-[3-(2-Methylsulphonylphenothiazin-10-yl)propyl]piperidine-4-carboxamide.

$C_{22}H_{27}N_3O_3S_2$ = 445.6.
*CAS — 14008-44-7.*
*ATC — A04AD05.*

**Pharmacopoeias.** In *Fr.*

### Profile

Metopimazine, a phenothiazine dopamine antagonist, is an antiemetic with general properties similar to those of chlorpromazine (p.675). It is used in the management of nausea and vomiting, including that associated with cancer chemotherapy (p.1245). It is given in usual doses of 15 to 30 mg daily by mouth, in 2 to 4 divided doses; similar doses have been given by rectum. It has also been given by injection in a dose of 10 to 20 mg daily, usually intramuscularly but occasionally by the intravenous route. Higher doses of 30 to 50 mg daily by intramuscular injection or intravenous infusion have been given for chemotherapy-induced nausea and vomiting.

### Preparations

**Proprietary Preparations** (details are given in Part 3)
***Belg.:*** Vogalene†; ***Denm.:*** Vogalene; ***Fr.:*** Vogalene; Vogalib; ***Israel:*** Vogalene†.

---

## Mosapride Citrate *(rINNM)*

AS-4370; Citrato de mosaprida; Rimopride Citrate. (±)-4-Amino-5-chloro-2-ethoxy-*N*-{[4-(*p*-fluorobenzyl)-2-morpholinyl]-methyl}benzamide citrate dihydrate.

$C_{21}H_{25}ClFN_3O_3,C_6H_8O_7,2H_2O$ = 650.0.
*CAS — 112885-41-3 (mosapride); 112885-42-4 (mosapride citrate).*

### Profile

Mosapride is a substituted benzamide used for its prokinetic properties. It is reported to be an agonist at 5-$HT_4$ receptors, increasing acetylcholine release and stimulating gastrointestinal motility (see also Cisapride, p.1260), as well as having 5-$HT_3$ antagonist properties. It is given by mouth as the citrate dihydrate, but doses are expressed as the anhydrous citrate, and are 5 mg three times daily before or after meals.

◊ References.

1. Sakashita M, *et al.* Pharmacokinetics of the gastrokinetic agent mosapride citrate after single and multiple oral administrations in healthy subjects. *Arzneimittelforschung* 1993; **43:** 867–72.
2. Ruth M, *et al.* The effect of mosapride, a novel prokinetic, on acid reflux variables in patients with gastro-oesophageal reflux disease. *Aliment Pharmacol Ther* 1998; **12:** 35–40.

### Preparations

**Proprietary Preparations** (details are given in Part 3)
***Arg.:*** Galopran; Intesul; Mosar; ***Jpn:*** Gasmotin.

## Nabilone *(BAN, USAN, rINN)*

Compound 109514; Lilly-109514; Nabilona. (±)-(6a*R*,10a*R*)-3-(1,1-Dimethylheptyl)-6a,7,8,9,10,10a-hexahydro-1-hydroxy-6,6-dimethyl-6*H*-benzo[*c*]chromen-9-one.
$C_{24}H_{36}O_3$ = 372.5.
*CAS — 51022-71-0.*
*ATC — A04AD11.*

### Adverse Effects

Nabilone may produce adverse effects similar to those of cannabis (see p.1666). The most common side-effect is reported to be drowsiness; other neurological side-effects have included confusion, disorientation, dizziness, euphoria, dysphoria, hallucinations, psychosis, depression, headache, decreased concentration, blurred vision, sleep disturbances, decreased coordination, and tremors. Adverse cardiovascular reactions including postural hypotension and tachycardia have occurred. Dry mouth, decreased appetite, and abdominal cramp have also been reported.

### Precautions

Nabilone is extensively metabolised and largely excreted in bile, and therefore is not recommended in patients with severe hepatic impairment. It should be used with caution in patients with a history of psychosis or depression, or those with hypertension or heart disease.

Because of the possibility of CNS depression patients should be warned not to drive or operate machinery.

The possibility of dependence similar to that of cannabis should be borne in mind.

### Interactions

Nabilone has been shown to have an additive CNS depressant effect when given with alcohol, diazepam, or other CNS depressants.

### Pharmacokinetics

Nabilone is well absorbed from the gastrointestinal tract and is rapidly and extensively metabolised; one or more of the metabolites may be active. The major excretory pathway is the biliary system; about 65% of a dose is excreted in the faeces and about 20% in the urine. The elimination half-life of nabilone is about 2 hours, but the half-life of its combined metabolites is about 35 hours after a dose by mouth.

◊ References.

1. Rubin A, *et al.* Physiologic disposition of nabilone, a cannabinol derivative, in man. *Clin Pharmacol Ther* 1977; **22:** 85–91.

### Uses and Administration

Nabilone, a synthetic cannabinoid with antiemetic and anxiolytic properties, is used for the control of nausea and vomiting associated with cancer chemotherapy in patients who have failed to respond adequately to conventional antiemetics (p.1245).

The usual initial dose for adults is 1 mg twice daily by mouth, increased to 2 mg twice daily if necessary. The first dose should be given the evening before initiation of chemotherapy with the second dose of nabilone being given 1 to 3 hours before the first dose of the antineoplastic. Nabilone may be given throughout each cycle of chemotherapy and for 48 hours after the last dose of chemotherapy, if required. The dose of nabilone should not exceed 6 mg daily in 3 divided doses.

◊ Reviews.

1. Tramer MR, *et al.* Cannabinoids for control of chemotherapy induced nausea and vomiting: quantitative systematic review. *BMJ* 2001; **323:** 16–21.

**Multiple sclerosis.** There is a report of reduction in spasticity and nocturia, and improvement in mood and well-being, in a patient with multiple sclerosis (p.646) who received nabilone 1 mg every second day.[1] Given that there are also anecdotal reports of improvement in symptoms in patients with multiple sclerosis who took cannabis, it was suggested that synthetic cannabinoids might be worthy of study in the treatment of spasticity.

1. Martyn CN, *et al.* Nabilone in the treatment of multiple sclerosis. *Lancet* 1995; **345:** 579.

### Preparations

**Proprietary Preparations** (details are given in Part 3)
***Canad.:*** Cesamet; ***Irl.:*** Cesamet; ***UK:*** Cesamet†.

## Niperotidine Hydrochloride *(rINNM)*

Hidrocloruro de niperotidina; Piperonyl Ranitidine Hydrochloride. *N*-[2-({5-[(Dimethylamino)methyl]furfuryl}thio)ethyl]-2-nitro-*N'*-piperonyl-1,1-ethenediamine hydrochloride.
$C_{20}H_{26}N_4O_5S,HCl$ = 471.0.
*CAS — 84845-75-0 (niperotidine).*
*ATC — A02BA05.*

### Profile

Niperotidine hydrochloride is a histamine $H_2$-receptor antagonist with general properties similar to those of cimetidine (p.1255). Severe hepatic disorders have occurred in patients receiving niperotidine.

◊ References.

1. Gasbarrini G, *et al.* Acute liver injury related to the use of niperotidine. *J Hepatol* 1997; **27:** 583–6.

## Nizatidine *(BAN, USAN, rINN)*

LY-139037; Nizatidina; Nizatidinum; ZL-101. 4-[2-(1-Methylamino-2-nitrovinylamino)ethylthiomethyl]thiazol-2-ylmethyl(dimethyl)amine; *N*-[2-(2-Dimethylaminomethylthiazol-4-ylmethylthio)ethyl]-*N'*-methyl-2-nitrovinylidenediamine.
$C_{12}H_{21}N_5O_2S_2$ = 331.5.
*CAS — 76963-41-2.*
*ATC — A02BA04.*

**Pharmacopoeias.** In *Eur.* (see p.vi) and *US.*

**Ph. Eur. 5.0** (Nizatidine). An almost white or slightly brownish, crystalline powder. Sparingly soluble in water; soluble in methyl alcohol. A 1% solution in water has a pH of 8.5 to 10.0.

**USP 27** (Nizatidine). An off-white to buff crystalline solid. Sparingly soluble in water; freely soluble in chloroform; soluble in methyl alcohol. Store in airtight containers. Protect from light.

### Adverse Effects

As for Cimetidine, p.1255. Some patients taking nizatidine may experience excessive sweating and urticaria; anaemia may also occur.

Nizatidine is considered to have little or no anti-androgenic activity although there are isolated reports of gynaecomastia and impotence.

**Effects on the cardiovascular system.** Nizatidine has been reported to reduce heart rate in healthy subjects,[1,2] an effect that was not seen when they were pretreated with ranitidine[1] or also given the antimuscarinic pirenzepine.[2] As with other $H_2$-antagonists (see Cimetidine, p.1256), tachycardia, bradycardia, postural hypotension and syncope have been reported rarely with rapid intravenous injection of nizatidine.

1. Mescheder A, *et al.* Changes in the effects of nizatidine and famotidine on cardiac performance after pretreatment with ranitidine. *Eur J Clin Pharmacol* 1993; **45:** 151–6.
2. Hinrichsen H, *et al.* Dose-dependent heart rate reducing effect of nizatidine, a histamine $H_2$-receptor antagonist. *Br J Clin Pharmacol* 1993; **35:** 461–6.

**Effects on the endocrine system.** A report of reversible impotence in a patient taking nizatidine 300 mg at night.[1]

1. Kassianos GC. Impotence and nizatidine. *Lancet* 1989; **i:** 963.

**Effects on the skin.** Similarly to cimetidine (p.1256), vasculitis has been reported with nizatidine.[1] Exfoliative dermatitis has also occurred.

1. Suh J-G, *et al.* Leukocytoclastic vasculitis associated with nizatidine therapy. *Am J Med* 1997; **102:** 216–17.

### Precautions

As for Cimetidine, p.1257.

### Interactions

Unlike cimetidine (p.1257) nizatidine does not inhibit cytochrome P450, and therefore is considered to have little effect on the metabolism of other drugs. However, like other $H_2$-antagonists its effects on gastric pH may affect the absorption of some other drugs.

### Pharmacokinetics

Nizatidine is readily and almost completely absorbed from the gastrointestinal tract. The bioavailability of nizatidine after oral administration exceeds 70% and may be slightly increased by the presence of food. It is widely distributed and is about 35% bound to plasma proteins.

The elimination half-life of nizatidine is 1 to 2 hours and is prolonged in renal impairment. Nizatidine is partly metabolised in the liver: nizatidine *N*-2-oxide, nizatidine *S*-oxide, and *N*-2-monodesmethylnizatidine have been identified, the latter having about 60% of the activity of nizatidine.

More than 90% of a dose of nizatidine is excreted in the urine, in part by active tubular secretion, within 12 hours, about 60% as unchanged drug. Less than 6% is excreted in the faeces. Nizatidine is distributed into breast milk.

◊ Reviews.

1. Callaghan JT, *et al.* A pharmacokinetic profile of nizatidine in man. *Scand J Gastroenterol* 1987; **22** (suppl 136): 9–17.

**Distribution into breast milk.** About 0.1% of an oral dose of nizatidine was secreted in breast milk in a study in lactating women.[1] The milk to serum ratio varied (from 1:1 to 4.9:1) with the time of samples.

1. Obermeyer BD, *et al.* Secretion of nizatidine into human breast milk after single and multiple doses. *Clin Pharmacol Ther* 1990; **47:** 724–30.

### Uses and Administration

Nizatidine is a histamine $H_2$-antagonist with actions and uses similar to those of cimetidine (see p.1258). It is given by mouth and by intravenous infusion.

In the management of benign **gastric** and **duodenal ulceration** (p.1246) a single daily dose of nizatidine 300 mg by mouth at night is recommended, which should be given initially for 4 weeks and may be extended to 8 weeks if necessary; alternatively 150 mg may be given twice daily in the morning and evening. Where appropriate a maintenance dose of 150 mg daily may be given at night. In patients who are unsuited to receive oral therapy nizatidine may be given on a short-term basis by continuous intravenous infusion of 10 mg/hour; alternatively 100 mg may be diluted in 50 mL of infusion fluid and be given over 15 minutes, three times daily. The total intravenous dose should not exceed 480 mg daily.

In **gastro-oesophageal reflux disease** (p.1242) a dose of 150 to 300 mg twice daily by mouth is recommended for up to 12 weeks.

For the short-term symptomatic relief of **dyspepsia** a dose of 75 mg, repeated if necessary up to a maximum of 150 mg daily may be taken by mouth for up to 14 days.

Doses of nizatidine should be reduced in patients with renal impairment (see below).

**Administration in renal impairment.** The dosage of nizatidine should be reduced in patients with renal impairment according to creatinine clearance (CC):

- CC 20 to 50 mL/minute: doses should be reduced by 50%, or where the standard dose would be 150 mg, given on alternate days
- CC less than 20 mL/minute: doses are reduced by 75%, or where the standard dose would be 150 mg, given every third day

### Preparations

***USP 27:*** Nizatidine Capsules.

**Proprietary Preparations** (details are given in Part 3)
***Austral.:*** Tazac; ***Austria:*** Ulxit; ***Belg.:*** Panaxid; ***Braz.:*** Axid; Nizax†; ***Canad.:*** Axid; ***Chile:*** Nizaxid; ***Denm.:*** Izatax; Nizax; ***Fin.:*** Nizax; ***Fr.:*** Nizaxid; ***Ger.:*** Gastrax; Nizax; ***Gr.:*** Axid; Flexidon; ***Hong Kong:*** Axid; ***Irl.:*** Axid; ***Ital.:*** Cronizat; Nizax; Zanizal; ***Malaysia:*** Axid; ***Mex.:*** Axid; Uldadin; ***Neth.:*** Axid; Naxidine†; ***Port.:*** Nizaxid; ***S.Afr.:*** Antizid; Axid†; ***Spain:*** Distaxid; Ulcosal†; ***Swed.:*** Nizax; ***Switz.:*** Calmaxid; ***Thai.:*** Axid; ***UK:*** Axid; Zinga†; ***USA:*** Axid.

## Olsalazine Sodium (BANM, USAN, rINNM)

Azodisal Sodium; CI Mordant Yellow 5; Colour Index No. 14130; CJ-91B; Olsalazina sódica; Olsalazinum Natricum; Sodium Azodisalicylate. Disodium 5,5′-azodisalicylate.

$C_{14}H_8N_2Na_2O_6$ = 346.2.

*CAS — 6054-98-4.*

*ATC — A07EC03.*

**Pharmacopoeias.** In *Eur.* (see p.vi).

**Ph. Eur. 5.0** (Olsalazine Sodium). A yellow, fine, crystalline powder; it exhibits polymorphism. Sparingly soluble in water; soluble in dimethyl sulfoxide; very slightly soluble in methyl alcohol.

### Adverse Effects and Precautions

As for Mesalazine, p.1273. The most common adverse effects associated with olsalazine sodium are diarrhoea, arthralgia, and skin rashes. Diarrhoea may be watery in some patients; it may resolve with dosage reduction but can be severe enough to require withdrawal of treatment. Diarrhoea is less likely if the drug is taken after meals. There have been a few reports of blood dyscrasias. If a blood dyscrasia is suspected treatment should be stopped immediately and a blood count performed. Patients or their carers should be told how to recognise signs of haematotoxicity and should be advised to seek immediate medical attention if symptoms such as fever, sore throat, mouth ulcers, bruising, or bleeding develop.

**Incidence of adverse effects.** In an open study[1] of olsalazine 1 g daily by mouth involving 160 patients with active ulcerative colitis and a history of sulfasalazine intolerance, 103 (64.4%) patients experienced no side-effects; 29 patients reported only minor side-effects: gastrointestinal disturbances in 22 patients, transient skin rash in 3, and headache, increased salivation, cough, and irritability each in one patient. The most common side-effect was frequent loose stools which affected 25 patients, 20 of whom had to discontinue treatment. This side-effect occurred early in treatment, within 10 hours of the first dose in 13 patients. Severe diarrhoea was more frequent in patients with widespread disease, but the incidence of diarrhoea did not correlate with disease severity.

A subsequent study[2] in healthy subjects has shown that olsalazine has a significant inhibitory effect on water and electrolyte absorption in the small intestine, which may account, at least in part, for the induction of diarrhoea. Patients with extensive colitis have reduced colonic absorptive function and may be less able to assimilate the increased colonic inflow volumes.

1. Sandberg-Gertzén H, *et al.* Azodisal sodium in the treatment of ulcerative colitis: a study of tolerance and relapse-prevention properties. *Gastroenterology* 1986; **90:** 1024–30.
2. Raimundo AH, *et al.* Effects of olsalazine and sulphasalazine on jejunal and ileal water and electrolyte absorption in normal human subjects. *Gut* 1991; **32:** 270–4.

**Effects on the blood.** As of July 1995, the UK Committee on Safety of Medicines had received 4 reports of blood dyscrasias associated with olsalazine, none of them fatal.[1] It was recommended that a blood count be performed and the drug stopped immediately if there was suspicion of a dyscrasia. See also under Mesalazine, p.1273.

1. Committee on Safety of Medicines/Medicines Control Agency. Blood dyscrasias and mesalazine. *Current Problems* 1995; **21:** 5–6.

**Effects on the kidneys.** A report of nephrotoxicity, characterised by interstitial nephritis, was associated with the use of olsalazine.[1] Symptoms resolved on discontinuation of the drug. See also under Mesalazine, p.1273.

1. Wilcox GM, *et al.* Nephrotoxicity associated with olsalazine. *Am J Med* 1996; **100:** 238–40.

### Interactions

**Antineoplastics.** For mention of 5-aminosalicylates such as olsalazine inhibiting the metabolism of thiopurine antineoplastics, and increasing their toxicity, see Mercaptopurine, p.567.

### Pharmacokinetics

Very little of an oral dose of olsalazine is absorbed via the upper gastrointestinal tract, and almost the entire dose reaches its site of action in the colon intact. It is broken down by the colonic bacterial flora into 2 molecules of 5-aminosalicylic acid (mesalazine). Some mesalazine is absorbed and acetylated (see p.1274) but systemic concentrations of mesalazine and its metabolite are lower than after comparable doses of mesalazine by mouth, perhaps because there is less release of mesalazine in the small intestine, where absorption is better. Mesalazine concentrations in the colon following a dose of olsalazine are stated to be about 1000 times greater than systemic concentrations.

The small amounts (1 to 2% of the dose or less) of intact olsalazine which are absorbed are excreted mainly in urine; the elimination half-life after an intravenous dose has been calculated at about 1 hour. Some olsalazine is metabolised by sulfate conjugation in the liver: the elimination half-life of the metabolite is reported to be about 7 days.

◊ References.

1. Ryde EM. Pharmacokinetic aspects of drugs targeted for the colon, with special reference to olsalazine. *Acta Pharm Suec* 1988; **25:** 327–8.
2. Laursen LS, *et al.* Disposition of 5-aminosalicylic acid by olsalazine and three mesalazine preparations in patients with ulcerative colitis: comparison of intraluminal colonic concentrations, serum values, and urinary excretion. *Gut* 1990; **31:** 1271–6.

### Uses and Administration

Olsalazine consists of two molecules of mesalazine (p.1273) linked with an azo bond. It is activated in the colon where the active mesalazine is released. It is used as the sodium salt in the management of acute mild ulcerative colitis and for the maintenance of remission (see Inflammatory Bowel Disease, p.1243). The usual initial dose of olsalazine sodium is 1 g by mouth daily in divided doses and this is gradually increased, if necessary, over one week, to a maximum dose of 3 g daily. The usual dose for the maintenance of remission is 500 mg twice daily. Doses should be taken after meals and a single dose should not exceed 1 g.

### Preparations

**Proprietary Preparations** (details are given in Part 3)
***Arg.:*** Dipentum; ***Austral.:*** Dipentum; ***Austria:*** Dipentum; ***Canad.:*** Dipentum; ***Chile:*** Dipentum; ***Denm.:*** Dipentum; ***Fin.:*** Dipentum; ***Fr.:*** Dipentum; ***Ger.:*** Dipentum; ***Gr.:*** Dipentum; ***Hong Kong:*** Dipentum; ***Irl.:*** Dipentum; ***Israel:*** Dipentum; ***Ital.:*** Dipentum; ***Neth.:*** Dipentum; ***Norw.:*** Dipentum; ***NZ:*** Dipentum; ***S.Afr.:*** Dipentum; ***Spain:*** Rasal; ***Swed.:*** Dipentum; ***Switz.:*** Dipentum; ***UK:*** Dipentum; ***USA:*** Dipentum.

## Omeprazole (BAN, USAN, rINN)

H-168/68; Omeprazol; Omeprazolum. (*RS*)-5-Methoxy-2-(4-methoxy-3,5-dimethyl-2-pyridylmethylsulphinyl)benzimidazole.

$C_{17}H_{19}N_3O_3S$ = 345.4.

*CAS — 73590-58-6.*

*ATC — A02BC01.*

**Pharmacopoeias.** In *Eur.* (see p.vi) and *US.*

**Ph. Eur. 5.0** (Omeprazole). A white or almost white powder. It exhibits polymorphism. Very slightly soluble in water; sparingly soluble in alcohol and in methyl alcohol; soluble in dichloromethane. It dissolves in dilute solutions of alkali hydroxides. Store in airtight containers at a temperature between 2° and 8°. Protect from light.

**USP 27** (Omeprazole). A white to off-white powder. Very slightly soluble in water; sparingly soluble in alcohol and in methyl alcohol; soluble in dichloromethane. Store in airtight containers at a temperature not exceeding 8°. Protect from moisture.

## Omeprazole Magnesium (BANM, USAN, rINNM)

Omeprazol magnésico.

$C_{34}H_{36}MgN_6O_6S_2$ = 713.1.

*CAS — 95382-33-5.*

*ATC — A02BC01.*

## Omeprazole Sodium (BANM, USAN, rINNM)

Omeprazol sódico; Omeprazolum Natricum.

$C_{17}H_{18}N_3NaO_3S$ = 367.4.

*CAS — 95510-70-6.*

*ATC — A02BC01.*

**Pharmacopoeias.** In *Eur.* (see p.vi).

**Ph. Eur. 5.0** (Omeprazole Sodium). A white or almost white, hygroscopic powder. Freely soluble in water and in alcohol; very slightly soluble in dichloromethane; soluble in propylene glycol. The pH of a 2% solution in water is 10.3 to 11.3. Store in airtight containers. Protect from light.

### Adverse Effects

Adverse effects reported most frequently with omeprazole and other proton pump inhibitors have been headache, diarrhoea, and skin rashes; they have sometimes been severe enough to require discontinuation of treatment. Other effects include pruritus, dizziness, fatigue, constipation, nausea and vomiting, flatulence, abdominal pain, arthralgia and myalgia, urticaria, and dry mouth. Isolated cases of photosensitivity, bullous eruption, erythema multiforme, angioedema, and anaphylaxis have been reported. Effects on the CNS include occasional insomnia, somnolence, and vertigo; reversible confusional states, agitation, depression, and hallucinations have occurred in severely ill patients. Raised liver enzymes, and isolated cases of hepatitis, jaundice, and hepatic encephalopathy, have been reported. Other adverse effects reported rarely or in isolated cases include paraesthesia, blurred vision, alopecia, stomatitis, sweating, taste disturbances, peripheral oedema, malaise, hyponatraemia, blood disorders (including agranulocytosis, leucopenia, and thrombocytopenia), and interstitial nephritis.

Proton pump inhibitors may increase the risk of gastrointestinal infections because of their acid suppressive effects.

Early toxicological studies identified carcinoid-like tumours of the gastric mucosa in *rats* given very high doses of omeprazole over long periods; this is reviewed in more detail under Gastrointestinal Tumours, below.

**Incidence of adverse effects.** General references.

1. Martin RM, *et al.* The rates of common adverse events reported during treatment with proton pump inhibitors used in general practice in England: cohort studies. *Br J Clin Pharmacol* 2000; **50:** 366–72.

**Effects on the blood.** There have been rare cases of leucopenia, agranulocytosis, thrombocytopenia, and pancytopenia, with omeprazole and other proton pump inhibitors.

References.

1. Holt TL, *et al.* Neutropenia associated with omeprazole. *Med J Aust* 1999; **170:** 141–2.
2. Zlabek JA, Anderson CG. Lansoprazole-induced thrombocytopenia. *Ann Pharmacother* 2002; **36:** 809–11.

**Effects on the endocrine system.** Up to December 1991, WHO had received 30 reports of impotence or gynaecomastia which might have been due to omeprazole;[1] of these reports 15 were of impotence, 13 of gynaecomastia in men, and 2 of breast enlargement in women. For reference to a case-control study showing no statistical link between gynaecomastia and omeprazole, see under Cimetidine, p.1256.

1. Lindquist M, Edwards IR. Endocrine adverse effects of omeprazole. *BMJ* 1992; **305:** 451–2.

**Effects on the eyes.** Visual disturbances associated with the use of omeprazole have included 6 cases of irreversible blindness or visual impairment in severely ill patients given the drug intravenously, and 13 cases of visual disturbances associated with oral use.[1] As a result of concern about these effects the availability of intravenous omeprazole was restricted in Germany; however, the consensus appears to be that a causal link has not been established between omeprazole and these ocular effects. Suggestions that visual (and also auditory[2]) impairment could follow drug-induced vasculitis[2-4] appear to be contentious.[1,5-7] A cohort study involving 140 128 patients receiving antisecretory therapy, 33 988 of whom received omeprazole, found no evidence that any of the drugs used was associated with a major increase in risk of vascular or inflammatory disorders of the eye;[8] however, the statistical power of this study was not high.[9]

1. Creutzfeldt WC, Blum AL. Safety of omeprazole. *Lancet* 1994; **343:** 1098.
2. Schönhöfer PS. Intravenous omeprazole and blindness. *Lancet* 1994; **343:** 665.
3. Schönhöfer PS. Safety of omeprazole and lansoprazole. *Lancet* 1994; **343:** 1369–70.
4. Schönhöfer PS, *et al.* Ocular damage associated with proton pump inhibitors. *BMJ* 1997; **314:** 1805.
5. Colin-Jones D. Safety of omeprazole and lansoprazole. *Lancet* 1994; **343:** 1369.
6. Lessell S. Omeprazole and ocular damage. *BMJ* 1998; **316:** 67.
7. Sachs G. Omeprazole and ocular damage. *BMJ* 1998; **316:** 67–8.
8. García Rodríguez LA, *et al.* A cohort study of the ocular safety of anti-ulcer drugs. *Br J Clin Pharmacol* 1996; **42:** 213–16.
9. Merlo J, Ranstam J. Ocular safety of anti-ulcer drugs. *Br J Clin Pharmacol* 1997; **43:** 449.

**Effects on the kidneys.** Acute interstitial nephritis developed in 2 elderly patients receiving omeprazole for the treatment of gastro-oesophageal reflux disease.[1,2] Following discontinuation, renal function improved rapidly in 1, but recurred upon rechallenge,[1] while in the other renal function remained severely affected for several months.[2] It was postulated that this adverse effect might have an allergic mechanism.[2] In these cases interstitial nephritis was associated with rash and eosinophilia; however, a further 2 cases of acute interstitial nephritis associated with omeprazole therapy in elderly patients[3,4] did not exhibit these symptoms. In another report, associated rash without eosinophiluria was seen.[5]

The Australian Adverse Drug Reactions Advisory Committee (ADRAC)[6] stated in April 2003 that it had received 18 biopsy-confirmed reports of interstitial nephritis associated with the use of omeprazole. These patients had presented with symptoms including weight loss, malaise, fever, and nausea; polyuria and polydipsia occurred in one case. Most patients had raised plasma-urea and/or plasma-creatinine concentrations. ADRAC had also received 2 reports of interstitial nephritis associated with rabeprazole.[6] Acute interstitial nephritis has also been associated with the use of pantoprazole in an elderly woman for the treatment of gastro-oesophageal reflux disease.[7]

1. Ruffenach SJ, *et al.* Acute interstitial nephritis due to omeprazole. *Am J Med* 1992; **93:** 472–3.
2. Christensen PB, *et al.* Renal failure after omeprazole. *Lancet* 1993; **341:** 55.

3. Assouad M, *et al.* Recurrent acute interstitial nephritis on rechallenge with omeprazole. *Lancet* 1994; **344:** 549.
4. Jones B, *et al.* Acute interstitial nephritis due to omeprazole. *Lancet* 1994; **344:** 1017–18.
5. Kuiper JJ. Omeprazole-induced acute interstitial nephritis. *Am J Med* 1993; **95:** 248.
6. Adverse Drug Reactions Advisory Committee. Interstitial nephritis with the proton pump inhibitors. *Aust Adverse Drug React Bull* 2003; **22:** 3. Also available at: http://www.tga.health.gov.au/adr/aadrb/aadr0304.htm (accessed 07/05/04)
7. Ra A, Tobe SW. Acute interstitial nephritis due to pantoprazole. *Ann Pharmacother* 2004; **38:** 41–5.

**Effects on the liver.** Raised liver enzymes have occurred with omeprazole and other proton pump inhibitors, and there have been isolated cases of hepatotoxicity. For a study suggesting a relatively low incidence of acute liver injury in patients receiving omeprazole see Cimetidine, p.1256.

References.

1. Jochem V, *et al.* Fulminant hepatic failure related to omeprazole. *Am J Gastroenterol* 1992; **87:** 523–5.
2. Kourg SI, *et al.* Omeprazole and the development of acute hepatitis. *Eur J Emerg Med* 1998; **5:** 467–9.

**Effects on the nervous system.** A report of ataxia in a patient receiving omeprazole;[1] symptoms resolved on discontinuing the drug.

1. Varona L, *et al.* Gait ataxia during omeprazole therapy. *Ann Pharmacother* 1996; **30:** 192.

**Effects on the skin.** An extensive blistering erythematous skin rash in an elderly woman given omeprazole[1] was characteristic of acute disseminated epidermal necrosis. The UK Committee on Safety of Medicines (CSM) had received 223 reports of cutaneous reactions to omeprazole up to August 1992, including 6 of erythema multiforme, but none of this severity. Other severe reactions that have subsequently been reported include a toxic bullous skin reaction,[2] exfoliative dermatitis,[3,4] erythema multiforme,[4] and toxic erythema.[4] One patient developed exfoliative dermatitis with both omeprazole and lansoprazole.[4] The authors of this report noted that by January 1998 a total of 1296 skin reactions to omeprazole, 500 to lansoprazole, and 44 to pantoprazole, had been reported to the CSM. Most were non-specific rashes, pruritus, urticaria, erythematous rashes, and photosensitive eruptions. A lichenoid reaction that occurred in a patient during omeprazole treatment cleared after ceasing the drug, but recurred during treatment with both lansoprazole and pantoprazole.[5]

For a report of urticaria and angioedema possibly associated with the formulation of omeprazole see Hypersensitivity, below. For the association of rash with interstitial nephritis, see Effects on the Kidneys, above.

1. Cox NH. Acute disseminated epidermal necrosis due to omeprazole. *Lancet* 1992; **340:** 857.
2. Stenier C, *et al.* Bullous skin reaction induced by omeprazole. *Br J Dermatol* 1995; **133:** 343–4.
3. Epelde Gonzalo FD, *et al.* Exfoliative dermatitis related to omeprazole. *Ann Pharmacother* 1995; **29:** 82–3.
4. Cockayne SE, *et al.* Severe erythrodermic reactions to the proton pump inhibitors omeprazole and lansoprazole. *Br J Dermatol* 1999; **141:** 173–5.
5. Bong JL, *et al.* Lichenoid drug eruption with proton pump inhibitors. *BMJ* 2000; **320:** 283.

**Gastrointestinal tumours.** Early toxicological studies in *rats* given high doses of omeprazole over 2 years identified carcinoid tumours of the gastric mucosa associated with complete block of gastric acid secretion leading to *hypergastrinaemia and hyperplasia of enterochromaffin-like cells.*[1] This has been the main issue concerning the safety of omeprazole and other proton pump inhibitors and initially led to restrictions in use and duration of treatment. A drug manufacturer, Glaxo, developed a new test to detect genotoxicity of antisecretory drugs which indicated that a genotoxic effect of omeprazole could not be discounted.[2] This study was heavily criticised; more established genotoxicity tests have been reported to be negative for omeprazole,[3-5] and other groups have not been able to replicate the findings with the new test.[6] The lowest doses at which Glaxo found a genotoxic effect of omeprazole were 10 to 20 mg/kg body-weight[2] and the clinical significance of their results was questioned.[3] Long-term studies of omeprazole in patients with Zollinger-Ellison syndrome have found no increase in fasting serum-gastrin concentrations and no evidence of gastric carcinoid tumours.[7,8] For mention of the risk of proton pump inhibitors delaying the diagnosis of gastric carcinoma, see under Precautions, below. Hypergastrinaemia can occur with both short- and long-term omeprazole therapy,[9] and may be higher in patients with *Helicobacter pylori* infection.[10] Patients who had *H. pylori* eradicated before long-term omeprazole treatment had lower gastrin concentrations than those who did not, since *H. pylori* eradication reduced the pretreatment gastrin concentrations.[11]

*H. pylori* is also a cause of *atrophic gastritis*, another risk factor for stomach cancer, and one study found that omeprazole increased the risk of atrophic gastritis in *H. pylori*-positive patients with gastro-oesophageal reflux disease.[12] However, the results of this study require confirmation since it was nonrandomised and retrospective. Nevertheless, some have suggested that it may be appropriate to eradicate *H. pylori* before long-term treatment with a proton pump inhibitor.[11,12] Conversely, there is some evidence that *H. pylori* may be protective in gastro-oesophageal reflux disease.[13]

There has been a report of *gastric polyps* developing in 3 of 8 patients after receiving omeprazole 20 or 40 mg daily for one year.[14] In a subsequent report it was noted that these omeprazole-induced fundic gland polyps had remained asymptomatic and non-malignant for up to five years after their onset.[15]

Further long-term studies of omeprazole may be needed before a realistic risk assessment can be made.

1. Ekman L, *et al.* Toxicological studies on omeprazole. *Scand J Gastroenterol* 1985; **20** (suppl 108): 53–69.
2. Burlinson B, *et al.* Genotoxicity studies of gastric acid inhibiting drugs. *Lancet* 1990; **335:** 419.
3. Ekman L, *et al.* Genotoxicity studies of gastric acid inhibiting drugs. *Lancet* 1990; **335:** 419–20.
4. Wright NA, Goodlad RA. Omeprazole and genotoxicity. *Lancet* 1990; **335:** 909–10.
5. Helander HF, *et al.* Omeprazole and genotoxicity. *Lancet* 1990; **335:** 910–11.
6. Goodlad RA. Acid suppression and claims of genotoxicity: what have we learned? *Drug Safety* 1994; **10:** 413–19.
7. Lloyd-Davies KA, *et al.* Omeprazole in the treatment of Zollinger-Ellison syndrome: a 4-year international study. *Aliment Pharmacol Ther* 1988; **2:** 13–32.
8. Maton PN, *et al.* Long-term efficacy and safety of omeprazole in patients with Zollinger-Ellison syndrome: a prospective study. *Gastroenterology* 1989; **97:** 827–36.
9. Koop H, *et al.* Serum gastrin levels during long-term omeprazole treatment. *Aliment Pharmacol Ther* 1990; **4:** 131–8.
10. Sanduleanu S, *et al.* Serum gastrin and chromogranin A during medium- and long-term acid suppressive therapy: a case-control study. *Aliment Pharmacol Ther* 1999; **13:** 145–53.
11. El-Nujumi A, *et al.* Eradicating Helicobacter pylori reduces hypergastrinaemia during long term omeprazole treatment. *Gut* 1998; **42:** 159–65.
12. Kuipers EJ, *et al.* Atrophic gastritis and Helicobacter pylori infection in patients with reflux esophagitis treated with omeprazole or fundoplication. *N Engl J Med* 1996; **334:** 1018–22.
13. Labenz J, Malfertheiner P. Helicobacter pylori in gastro-oesophageal reflux disease: causal agent, independent or protective factor? *Gut* 1997; **41:** 277–80.
14. Graham JR. Gastric polyposis: onset during long-term therapy with omeprazole. *Med J Aust* 1992; **157:** 287–8.
15. Graham JR. Gastric acne: omeprazole-induced fundic gland polyposis. *Med J Aust* 1998; **168:** 93.

**Hypersensitivity.** Cases of anaphylactic reactions following treatment with omeprazole, lansoprazole, and pantoprazole, have been reported in the literature and to WHO.[1]

Urticaria, facial angioedema, and bronchospasm in a patient given omeprazole capsules did not recur when the patient was given omeprazole granules and the reaction might have been precipitated by the ingredients of the capsule shell.[2]

See also under Effects on the Kidney, above, and Musculoskeletal Effects, below.

1. Natsch S, *et al.* Anaphylactic reactions to proton-pump inhibitors. *Ann Pharmacother* 2000; **34:** 474–6.
2. Haeney MR. Angio-oedema and urticaria associated with omeprazole. *BMJ* 1992; **305:** 870.

**Infection.** Oesophageal candidiasis occurred in 2 elderly patients receiving omeprazole but was successfully treated with antifungal therapy. It was postulated that gastric acid secretion and a degree of physiological reflux of acid into the oesophagus might normally play a protective role in preventing candidal infection.[1] The profound reduction in acid secretion produced by omeprazole may also predispose to gastrointestinal infection; there is some evidence for an increased risk of campylobacter infection,[2] as well as a report of recurrent salmonellal infection.[3]

1. Larner AJ, Lendrum R. Oesophageal candidiasis after omeprazole therapy. *Gut* 1992; **33:** 860–1.
2. Neal KR, *et al.* Omeprazole as a risk factor for campylobacter gastroenteritis: case-control study. *BMJ* 1996; **312:** 414–15.
3. Wingate DL. Acid reduction and recurrent enteritis. *Lancet* 1990; **335:** 222.

**Lupus syndrome.** For a report of drug-induced lupus syndrome associated with omeprazole therapy, see Musculoskeletal Effects, below.

**Malabsorption.** Omeprazole has been reported to result in a substantial reduction in cyanocobalamin (vitamin $B_{12}$) absorption,[1] probably related to the increase in gastric pH, and indicating a potential risk of vitamin deficiency with long-term therapy.[2] Fat malabsorption, secondary to increased deconjugation of bile acids caused by bacterial overgrowth in the jejunum, has also been reported with omeprazole treatment.[3]

1. Marcuard SP, *et al.* Omeprazole therapy causes malabsorption of cyanocobalamin (vitamin $B_{12}$). *Ann Intern Med* 1994; **120:** 211–15.
2. Termanini B, *et al.* Effect of long-term gastric acid suppressive therapy on serum vitamin $B_{12}$ levels in patients with Zollinger-Ellison syndrome. *Am J Med* 1998; **104:** 422–30.
3. Shindo K, *et al.* Omeprazole induces altered bile acid metabolism. *Gut* 1998; **42:** 266–71.

**Musculoskeletal effects.** Progressive muscular weakness suggestive of *myopathy* developed in a 78-year-old patient given omeprazole.[1] After 4 weeks of treatment the patient required assistance in walking and rising from squatting. Weakness resolved on withdrawal of the drug, but returned on rechallenge.

A report of 5 cases of *arthralgia*, sometimes associated with swelling of the affected joints, in patients receiving omeprazole,[2] also noted that some reported cases of omeprazole-associated headache were accompanied by arthralgia or *myalgia*. In another case[3] arthralgia in a patient with a hereditary myopathy receiving omeprazole appeared to represent one aspect of a drug-induced *lupus* syndrome, being accompanied by malaise, fever, Raynaud's phenomenon, raised antinuclear antibody titres, and anticardiolipin and antihistone antibodies. Symptoms resolved on withdrawal of the drug.

A case of eosinophilia and myalgia related to lansoprazole treatment has been reported.[4]

There has also been a report of 2 cases of acute *gout* associated with omeprazole;[5] in one patient symptoms, which resolved on withdrawal, recurred on rechallenge. However, case control studies have failed to show an increased risk of polyarthralgia[6] or gout[7] associated with omeprazole use.

1. Garrote FJ, *et al.* Subacute myopathy during omeprazole therapy. *Lancet* 1992; **340:** 672.
2. Beutler M, *et al.* Arthralgias and omeprazole. *BMJ* 1994; **309:** 1620.
3. Sivakumar K, Dalakas MC. Autoimmune syndrome induced by omeprazole. *Lancet* 1994; **344:** 619–20.
4. Smith JD, *et al.* Possible lansoprazole-induced eosinophilic syndrome. *Ann Pharmacother* 1998; **32:** 196–200.
5. Kraus A, Flores-Suárez LF. Acute gout associated with omeprazole. *Lancet* 1995; **345:** 461–2.
6. Meier CR, Jick H. Omeprazole, $H_2$ blockers, and polyarthralgia: case-control study. *BMJ* 1997; **315:** 1283.
7. Meier CR, Jick H. Omeprazole, other antiulcer drugs and newly diagnosed gout. *Br J Clin Pharmacol* 1997; **44:** 175–8.

**Overdosage.** A report of 2 cases of overdosage with omeprazole.[1] The major clinical features were drowsiness, headache (possibly due to a metabolite), and tachycardia. Both patients recovered uneventfully without specific treatment.

1. Ferner RE, Allison TR. Omeprazole overdose. *Hum Exp Toxicol* 1993; **12:** 541–2.

## Precautions

Before giving omeprazole or other proton pump inhibitors to patients with gastric ulcers the possibility of malignancy should be considered since these drugs may mask symptoms and delay diagnosis. Omeprazole and other proton pump inhibitors should be used with caution in hepatic impairment.

**Gastric carcinoma.** Proton pump inhibitors relieve dyspeptic symptoms associated with gastric carcinoma and can therefore delay its diagnosis. In addition, there is some evidence that they may also endoscopically 'heal' early gastric carcinoma so that the diagnosis is missed.[1] Consequently, some commentators recommend that proton pump inhibitors should not be prescribed for symptom control prior to endoscopy in patients at risk for gastric carcinoma.[2]

1. Wayman J, *et al.* The response of early gastric cancer to proton-pump inhibitors. *N Engl J Med* 1998; **338:** 1924–5.
2. Griffin SM, Raimes SA. Proton pump inhibitors may mask early gastric cancer: dyspeptic patients over 45 should undergo endoscopy before these drugs are started. *BMJ* 1998; **317:** 1606–7.

**Helicobacter infection.** Treatment with proton pump inhibitors may cause false-negative results in the urea breath test for *Helicobacter pylori* infection. In one study in patients with *H. pylori* infection, 4 weeks treatment with lansoprazole 30 mg daily caused 33% of patients to have negative urea breath tests.[1] The breath test became positive again in all patients within 2 weeks of stopping lansoprazole therapy. In a similar study, 52% of patients had negative urea breath tests for *H. pylori* while receiving omeprazole 20 mg daily, and the breath test became positive again in all patients within 2 to 6 days of stopping treatment.[2] The manufacturers of the urea breath test for *H. pylori* recommend that it should not be performed for at least 2 weeks after stopping treatment with an antisecretory drug.

For a discussion of the link between proton pump inhibitors, *H. pylori*, and gastritis, see under Gastrointestinal Tumours above.

1. Laine L, *et al.* Effect of proton-pump inhibitor therapy on diagnostic testing for Helicobacter pylori. *Ann Intern Med* 1998; **129:** 547–50.
2. Connor SJ, *et al.* The effect of dosing with omeprazole on the accuracy of the $^{13}$C-urea breath test in Helicobacter pylori-infected subjects. *Aliment Pharmacol Ther* 1999; **13:** 1287–93.

**Hepatic impairment.** In patients with cirrhosis an increase in omeprazole bioavailability, and elimination half-life has been reported.[1] For dosage adjustment in hepatic impairment see under Uses and Administration, below.

1. Andersson T, *et al.* Pharmacokinetics of [$^{14}$C]omeprazole in patients with liver cirrhosis. *Clin Pharmacokinet* 1993; **24:** 71–8.

**Pregnancy.** Proton pump inhibitors are not generally licensed for use during pregnancy, but a meta-analysis[1] of 5 studies of exposure to proton pump inhibitors during the first trimester, involving 593 exposed infants, found the relative risk of major abnormalities associated with such exposure to be only 1.18, with a 95% confidence interval ranging from 0.72 to 1.94. Meta-analysis of exposures to omeprazole (from 4 studies only) gave a relative risk of 1.05 (95% confidence interval 0.59 to 1.85). It was concluded that exposure to proton pump inhibitors, and omeprazole in particular, did not pose an important teratogenic risk. A retrospective epidemiological study of data from the Swedish Medical Birth Registry, which identified 955 exposed infants, also found no evidence of significant risk following exposure to omeprazole during pregnancy.[2]

1. Nikfar S, *et al.* Use of proton pump inhibitors during pregnancy and rates of major malformations: a meta-analysis. *Dig Dis Sci* 2002; **47:** 1526–9.
2. Källén BAJ. Use of omeprazole during pregnancy–no hazard demonstrated in 955 infants exposed during pregnancy. *Eur J Obstet Gynecol Reprod Biol* 2001; **96:** 63–8.

## Interactions

Omeprazole and other proton pump inhibitors are metabolised by the cytochrome P450 system, primarily by isoenzyme CYP2C19, and may alter the metabolism of some drugs metabolised by these enzymes. Omeprazole may prolong the elimination of diazepam, phenytoin, and warfarin (but see below). Omeprazole and other proton pump inhibitors can reduce the absorption of drugs such as ketoconazole, and possibly itraconazole, whose absorption is dependent on an acid gastric pH. With voriconazole, the plasma concentration of both drugs may be increased and a reduced dose of omeprazole is recommended.

◊ Omeprazole is metabolised primarily by the cytochrome P450 isoenzyme CYP2C19 (see Metabolism, below) and therefore may interact with diazepam (see under Gastrointestinal Drugs, p.694). Some metabolism of phenytoin (see p.374), tolbutamide, and the *R*-enantiomer of warfarin (see p.1026) also takes place by CYP2C19, but the effects seen have been minor.[1] Although some induction of CYP1A2, which metabolises caffeine and theophylline (p.803), has been reported this does not appear to be clinically significant.[2] Omeprazole does not appear to have a significant effect on CYP3A4, which is an important cytochrome for drug metabolism.[1,3] (For a study *in vitro* suggesting that omeprazole affected CYP3A4 metabolism of tacrolimus, see under Interactions of Tacrolimus, p.1364.)

For reference to the possibility of enhanced digoxin absorption with omeprazole, see p.898. For a study suggesting that omeprazole reduces the absorption of cyanocobalamin, see Malabsorption, above. For reference to possible interactions between methotrexate and omeprazole, see p.571.

1. Andersson T. Pharmacokinetics, metabolism and interactions of acid pump inhibitors: focus on omeprazole, lansoprazole and pantoprazole. *Clin Pharmacokinet* 1996; **31:** 9–28.
2. Rizzo N, *et al.* Omeprazole and lansoprazole are not inducers of cytochrome P4501A2 under conventional therapeutic conditions. *Eur J Clin Pharmacol* 1996; **49:** 491–5.
3. Tateishi T, *et al.* Omeprazole does not affect measured CYP3A4 activity using the erythromycin breath test. *Br J Clin Pharmacol* 1995; **40:** 411–12.

**Clarithromycin.** Studies in healthy subjects have indicated that use of omeprazole with clarithromycin results in an approximate 30% increase in peak plasma concentrations of omeprazole, and an increase in its mean half-life from 1.2 to 1.6 hours.[1] At the same time, plasma concentrations of clarithromycin were also modestly increased, as were local concentrations in gastric tissue and mucus.[1] Clarithromycin inhibits[2] the metabolism of omeprazole mediated by the cytochrome P450 isoenzyme CYP3A4. The interaction may contribute to the benefits of combined therapy for *Helicobacter pylori* infection.

1. Gustavson LE, *et al.* Effect of omeprazole on concentrations of clarithromycin in plasma and gastric tissue at steady state. *Antimicrob Agents Chemother* 1995; **39:** 2078–83.
2. Furuta T, *et al.* Effects of clarithromycin on the metabolism of omeprazole in relation to CYP2C19 genotype status in humans. *Clin Pharmacol Ther* 1999; **66:** 265–74.

## Pharmacokinetics

Omeprazole is rapidly but variably absorbed after oral administration. Absorption is not affected by food. Omeprazole is acid-labile and pharmacokinetics may vary between the various formulations developed to improve oral bioavailability. The absorption of omeprazole also appears to be dose-dependent; increasing the dosage above 40 mg has been reported to increase the plasma concentrations in a non-linear fashion because of saturable first-pass hepatic metabolism. In addition, absorption is higher after long-term use.

Bioavailability of omeprazole may be increased in elderly patients, in some ethnic groups such as Chinese, and in patients with hepatic impairment, but is not markedly affected in patients with renal impairment.

Following absorption, omeprazole is almost completely metabolised in the liver, primarily by the cytochrome P450 isoenzyme CYP2C19 to form hydroxyomeprazole, and to a small extent by CYP3A to form omeprazole sulfone. The metabolites are inactive, and are excreted mostly in the urine and to a lesser extent in bile. The elimination half-life from plasma is reported to be about 0.5 to 3 hours. Omeprazole is about 95% bound to plasma proteins.

◊ References.

1. Andersson T, *et al.* Pharmacokinetics of various single intravenous and oral doses of omeprazole. *Eur J Clin Pharmacol* 1990; **39:** 195–7.
2. Andersson T, Regårdh C-G. Pharmacokinetics of omeprazole and metabolites following single intravenous and oral doses of 40 and 80 mg. *Drug Invest* 1990; **2:** 255–63.
3. Ching MS, *et al.* Oral bioavailability of omeprazole before and after chronic therapy in patients with duodenal ulcer. *Br J Clin Pharmacol* 1991; **31:** 166–70.
4. Landahl S, *et al.* Pharmacokinetic study of omeprazole in elderly healthy volunteers. *Clin Pharmacokinet* 1992; **23:** 469–76.
5. Andersson T, *et al.* Pharmacokinetics of [$^{14}$C]omeprazole in patients with liver cirrhosis. *Clin Pharmacokinet* 1993; **24:** 71–8.
6. Jacqz-Aigrain E, *et al.* Pharmacokinetics of intravenous omeprazole in children. *Eur J Clin Pharmacol* 1994; **47:** 181–5.

**Metabolism.** The major enzyme involved in omeprazole metabolism is cytochrome P450 isoenzyme CYP2C19. This enzyme is polymorphically expressed, and individuals who are deficient in the enzyme are poor metabolisers of omeprazole. This occurs in about 3% of Caucasians and 15% of Chinese, Japanese, and Koreans. These individuals have markedly higher plasma concentrations of omeprazole, and they may require dosage adjustment. Some omeprazole is metabolised by CYP3A to form omeprazole sulfone and hydroxy-omeprazole, and some by CYP2D6 to form desmethylomeprazole.

References.

1. Andersson T, *et al.* Identification of human liver cytochrome P450 isoforms mediating omeprazole metabolism. *Br J Clin Pharmacol* 1993; **36:** 521–30.
2. Caraco Y, *et al.* Ethnic and genetic determinants of omeprazole disposition and effect. *Clin Pharmacol Ther* 1996; **60:** 157–67.
3. Karam WG, *et al.* Human CYP2C19 is a major omeprazole 5-hydroxylase, as demonstrated with recombinant cytochrome P450 enzymes. *Drug Metab Dispos* 1996; **24:** 1081–7.

## Uses and Administration

Omeprazole is a proton pump inhibitor. It inhibits secretion of gastric acid by irreversibly blocking the enzyme system of hydrogen/potassium adenosine triphosphatase ($H^+/K^+$ ATPase), the 'proton pump' of the gastric parietal cell. It is used in conditions where inhibition of gastric acid secretion may be beneficial, including aspiration syndromes (p.1240), dyspepsia (p.1242), gastro-oesophageal reflux disease (p.1242), peptic ulcer disease (p.1246), and the Zollinger-Ellison syndrome (p.1247).

Esomeprazole (p.1265), an isomer of omeprazole, is also used.

Omeprazole may be given by mouth as the base or magnesium salt, or intravenously as the sodium salt. Doses are expressed in terms of the base. Omeprazole magnesium 10.32 mg and omeprazole sodium 10.64 mg are each approximately equivalent to 10 mg of omeprazole.

For the relief of acid-related **dyspepsia** omeprazole is given in usual doses of 10 or 20 mg daily by mouth for 2 to 4 weeks.

The usual dose for the treatment of **gastro-oesophageal reflux disease** is 20 mg by mouth once daily for 4 weeks, followed by a further 4 to 8 weeks if not fully healed. In refractory oesophagitis, a dose of 40 mg daily may be used. Maintenance therapy after healing of oesophagitis is 20 mg once daily, and for acid reflux is 10 mg daily. In children over 2 years, doses in the range 0.7 to 1.4 mg/kg daily, up to a maximum daily dose of 40 mg, have been given for 4 to 12 weeks.

In the management of **peptic ulcer disease** a single daily dose of 20 mg by mouth, or 40 mg in severe cases, is given. Treatment is continued for 4 weeks for duodenal ulcer and 8 weeks for gastric ulcer. Where appropriate, a dose of 10 to 20 mg once daily may be given for maintenance.

For the eradication of *Helicobacter pylori* in peptic ulceration omeprazole may be combined with antibacterials in dual or triple therapy. Effective **triple therapy** regimens include omeprazole 20 mg twice daily combined with: amoxicillin 500 mg and metronidazole 400 mg, both three times daily; clarithromycin 500 mg and metronidazole 400 mg (or tinidazole 500 mg) both twice daily; or with amoxicillin 1 g and clarithromycin 500 mg both twice daily. These regimens are given for 1 week. **Dual therapy** regimens such as omeprazole 40 mg daily with either amoxicillin 750 mg to 1 g twice daily or clarithromycin 500 mg three times daily, are less effective and must be given for 2 weeks. Omeprazole alone may be continued for a further 2 to 8 weeks.

Doses of 20 mg daily are used in the treatment of **NSAID-associated ulceration**; a dose of 20 mg daily may also be used for prophylaxis in patients with a previous history of gastroduodenal lesions who require continued NSAID treatment.

The initial recommended dosage for patients with the **Zollinger-Ellison syndrome** is 60 mg by mouth once daily, adjusted as required. The majority of patients are effectively controlled by doses in the range 20 to 120 mg daily, but doses up to 120 mg three times daily have been used. Daily doses above 80 mg should be administered in divided doses (usually 2).

Omeprazole is also used for the prophylaxis of **acid aspiration** during general anaesthesia, in a dose of 40 mg the evening before surgery and a further 40 mg two to six hours before the procedure.

The dose of omeprazole may need to be reduced in patients with hepatic impairment (see below).

PARENTERAL DOSAGE.

In patients who are unsuited to receive oral therapy omeprazole sodium may be given on a short-term basis by intravenous infusion, in a usual dose equivalent to 40 mg of the base over a period of 20 to 30 minutes in 100 mL of sodium chloride 0.9% or glucose 5%. It may also be given by slow intravenous injection. Higher intravenous doses have been given to patients with Zollinger-Ellison syndrome.

◊ General reviews.

1. Richardson P, *et al.* Proton pump inhibitors: pharmacology and rationale for use in gastrointestinal disorders. *Drugs* 1998; **56:** 307–35.
2. Langtry HD, Wilde MI. Omeprazole: a review of its use in Helicobacter pylori infection, gastro-oesophageal reflux disease and peptic ulcers induced by nonsteroidal anti-inflammatory drugs. *Drugs* 1998; **56:** 447–86.
3. Berardi RR, Welage LS. Proton-pump inhibitors in acid-related diseases. *Am J Health-Syst Pharm* 1998; **55:** 2289–98.
4. Brown GJE, Yeomans ND. Prevention of the gastrointestinal adverse effects of nonsteroidal anti-inflammatory drugs: the role of proton pump inhibitors. *Drug Safety* 1999; **21:** 503–12.
5. Erstad BL. Proton-pump inhibitors for acute peptic ulcer bleeding. *Ann Pharmacother* 2001; **35:** 730–40.

**Administration.** Omeprazole is given by mouth as tablets or capsules containing enteric-coated pellets or granules which should be swallowed whole and not crushed or chewed. In patients with swallowing difficulties the manufacturers generally recommend that the tablet be dispersed in water, fruit juice, or yogurt before swallowing. Similarly the contents of the capsules can be mixed with a little fruit juice or yogurt and swallowed.

**Administration in hepatic impairment.** Consideration should be given to reducing the dose of omeprazole in patients with hepatic impairment. In the UK, a maximum daily dose of 20 mg is recommended for such patients. In the USA, it is merely recommended that dose adjustment should be considered, particularly where maintenance treatment is required.

**Asthma.** Gastro-oesophageal reflux has been suggested as a potential exacerbating factor for asthma (p.777), and acid suppressive therapy with omeprazole has been reported to reduce asthma symptoms in some[1] but not other[2] studies. A meta-analysis of acid suppressive therapy concluded it was not effective in improving asthma symptoms in patients with gastro-oesophageal reflux,[3] and the link between reflux and asthma symptoms has been disputed.[4]

1. Harding SM, *et al.* Asthma and gastroesophageal reflux: acid suppressive therapy improves asthma outcome. *Am J Med* 1996; **100:** 395–405.
2. Ford GA, *et al.* Omeprazole in the treatment of asthmatics with nocturnal symptoms and gastro-oesophageal reflux: a placebo-controlled cross-over study. *Postgrad Med J* 1994; **70:** 350–4.
3. Coughlan JL, *et al.* Medical treatment for reflux oesophagitis does not consistently improve asthma control: a systematic review. *Thorax* 2001; **56:** 198–204.
4. Field SK. A critical review of the studies of the effects of simulated or real gastroesophageal reflux on pulmonary function in asthmatic adults. *Chest* 1999; **115:** 848–56.

**Dyspepsia.** UK guidelines[1] on the use of proton pump inhibitors in patients with dyspepsia (p.1242) consider that although they are valuable in patients with peptic ulcer disease, NSAID-associated ulcer, or gastro-oesophageal reflux disease, proton pump inhibitors should not be routinely used in patients with non-ulcer dyspepsia. Nonetheless, they are often effective in patients with dyspepsia of undiagnosed cause, since some patients will have reflux or peptic ulcer disease, but the evidence suggests they are only marginally more effective than placebo in patients with true non-ulcer dyspepsia. However, they have no serious contraindications for the vast majority of users.

1. National Institute for Clinical Excellence. Guidance on the use of proton pump inhibitors in the treatment of dyspepsia (issued July 2000). Available at: http://www.nice.org.uk/pdf/proton.pdf (accessed 07/05/04)

**Inflammatory bowel disease.** There are a few reports[1-3] of responses to omeprazole in patients with inflammatory bowel disease (p.1243). Combination of omeprazole with mesalazine has also been tried.[2]

1. Heinzow U, Schlegelberger T. Omeprazole in ulcerative colitis. *Lancet* 1994; **343:** 477.
2. Dickinson JB. Is omeprazole helpful in inflammatory bowel disease? *J Clin Gastroenterol* 1994; **18:** 317–19.
3. Guslandi M, Tittobello A. Symptomatic response to omeprazole in inflammatory bowel disease. *J Clin Gastroenterol* 1996; **22:** 159–60.

**Scleroderma.** Gastro-oesophageal reflux is one of the gastrointestinal manifestations of systemic sclerosis, and proton pump inhibitors such as omeprazole play a major role in the management of such gastrointestinal disease.[1] For a discussion of the broader management of the condition see p.1348.

1. Williamson DJ. Update on scleroderma. *Med J Aust* 1995; **162:** 599–601.

## Preparations

**Proprietary Preparations** (details are given in Part 3)

***Arg.:*** Acimed; Danlox; Fabrazol; Fendiprazol; Gastec; Gastrotem; Klomeprax; Losec; Omeprasec; Pepticus; Procelac; Regulacid; Timezol; Ulcozol; Zoltenk; ***Austral.:*** Acimax; Losec; Maxor; Probitor; ***Austria:*** Antra; Helicostad; Losec; Probitor; Semiglen; ***Belg.:*** Logastric; Losec; ***Braz.:*** Estomepe; Eupept†; Fegran; Gasec; Gaspiren; Gastrib†; Gastrium; Gastrozol; Klispel; Lomepral; Loprazol; Losaprol; Losar; Losec; Lozap; Meprazan; Mesopran; Neoprazol; Omep; Omeprasec†; Omeprazin; Omeprotec; Oprazon; Peprazol; Pepsicaps†; Prazonil; Ulcefor; Ulconar†; Ulcozol; Uniprazol; Victrix; Zolpramex†; ***Canad.:*** Losec; ***Chile:*** Lomex; Losec; Micromex; Omeprax; Pepticum; Prazolo; Ulc-Out; Ulcelac; Ulcrux; Zatrol; Zomepral; ***Denm.:*** Losec; ***Fin.:*** Losec; ***Fr.:*** Mopral; Zoltum; ***Ger.:*** Antra; Gastroloc†; Ome-nerton; Ome-Puren; Omebeta; Omelind; Omep; ***Gr.:*** Belifax; Elkostop; Elkotheran; Eselan; Ezipol; Gertalgin; Glaveral; Kerlofin; Lanex; Lenar; Loproc; Losec; Lozaprin; Malortil; Odamesol; Odasol; Ofnimarex; Omeprol; Penrazol; Pipacid; Probitor; Rythmogastryl; Sieral; Ufonitren; Veralox; ***Hong Kong:*** Losec; ***India:*** Biocid; Lomac; Ocid; Omezol; Ulzol; ***Irl.:*** Losamel; Losec; ***Israel:*** Losec; Omepradex; ***Ital.:*** Antra; Losec; Mepral; Omeprazen; ***Jpn:*** Omepral; ***Malaysia:*** Gasec; Losec; Omesec; Omezole; Romesec; Zenpro; ***Mex.:*** Alboz; Aleprozil; Azoran; Danovag; Domer; Hopram; Inhibitron; Losec; Medral; Mopral; Olexin; Osiren; Ozoken; Plazolit†; Prazidec; Prazolit; Suifac; Ulsen; Vulcasid; ***Neth.:*** Losec; ***Norw.:*** Losec; ***NZ:*** Losec; ***Port.:*** Belmazol; Gasec; Losec; Mepraz; Nuclosina; Omepra; Omerol; Ometon; Omezolan; Prazentol; Prazolene; Proclor; Proton; ***S.Afr.:*** Losec; Ulzec; ***Singapore:*** Losec; Omesec; Penrazole; Proceptin; Romesec; Zimor; ***Spain:*** Audazol; Aulcer; Belmazol; Ceprandal; Elgam; Emeproton; Gastrimut; Indurgan; Losec; Miol; Mopral; Norpramin; Nuclosina; Omapren; Ompranyt; Parizac; Pepticum; Prysma; Sanamidol; Secrepina†; Ulceral; Ulcesep; Ulcometion; Zimor; ***Swed.:*** Losec; ***Switz.:*** Antra; Antramups; ***Thai.:*** Airomet; Desec; Dosate; Duogas; Eucid; Gomec; Lomac; Losec; Madiprazole; Meiceral; Metsec; Miracid; Nocid; O-Sid; Omez; OMP†; Oprazole; Peptizole†; Probitor; Severon; Stomec; Ulprazole; Zefxon; ***UAE:*** Risek; ***UK:*** Losec; Zanprol; ***USA:*** Prilosec.

**Multi-ingredient:** ***Austral.:*** Klacid HP 7; Losec Helicopak†; Losec Hp 7; ***Braz.:*** Erradic; ***Canad.:*** Losec 1-2-3 A; Losec 1-2-3 M; ***Fin.:*** Losec Helira; ***NZ:*** Helicosec†; Klacid HP 7; Losec Hp 7; ***S.Afr.:*** Losec 20 Triple.

# Ondansetron *(BAN, rINN)*

GR-38032; Ondansetrón. (±)-1,2,3,9-Tetrahydro-9-methyl-3-(2-methylimidazol-1-ylmethyl)-carbazol-4(9*H*)-one.

$C_{18}H_{19}N_3O$ = 293.4.

*CAS — 99614-02-5; 116002-70-1.*

*ATC — A04AA01.*

## Ondansetron Hydrochloride *(BANM, USAN, rINNM)*

GR-38032F; Hidrocloruro de ondansetrón; Ondansetroni Hydrochloridum; SN-307.

$C_{18}H_{19}N_3O,HCl,2H_2O$ = 365.9.

*CAS — 103639-04-9.*

*ATC — A04AA01.*

**Pharmacopoeias.** In *Eur.* (see p.vi) and *US*.

**Ph. Eur. 5.0** (Ondansetron Hydrochloride Dihydrate). A white or almost white powder. Sparingly soluble in water and in alcohol; slightly soluble in dichloromethane; soluble in methyl alcohol. Protect from light.

**USP 27** (Ondansetron Hydrochloride). A white to off-white powder. Sparingly soluble in water and in alcohol; very slightly soluble in acetone, in chloroform, and in ethyl acetate; slightly soluble in dichloromethane and in isopropyl alcohol; soluble in methyl alcohol. Store in airtight containers at a temperature of 25°, excursions permitted between 15° and 30°. Protect from light.

**Incompatibility.** Ondansetron hydrochloride and dexamethasone sodium phosphate were not compatible when high concentrations were combined in polypropylene syringes.[1] Lower concentrations (up to 640 micrograms/mL of ondansetron and 400 micrograms/mL of dexamethasone phosphate) were stable in 50 mL containers of infusion fluid for 30 days under refrigeration. Compatibility has been reported for 24 hours in plastic syringes at 4° or 23° with a variety of other drugs,[2] and with several antineoplastics (cytarabine, dacarbazine, doxorubicin, etoposide, or methotrexate) in PVC infusion bags for 48 hours at room temperature.[3]

1. Hagan RL, *et al.* Stability of ondansetron hydrochloride and dexamethasone sodium phosphate in infusion bags and syringes for 32 days. *Am J Health-Syst Pharm* 1996; **53:** 1431–5.
2. Stewart JT, *et al.* Stability of ondansetron hydrochloride and 12 medications in plastic syringes. *Am J Health-Syst Pharm* 1998; **55:** 2630–4.
3. Stewart JT, *et al.* Stability of ondansetron hydrochloride and five antineoplastic medications. *Am J Health-Syst Pharm* 1996; **53:** 1297–1300.

## Adverse Effects and Precautions

Ondansetron and other 5-$HT_3$ antagonists may cause headache, a sensation of flushing or warmth, and constipation. A transient rise in liver enzymes has occasionally occurred. There have been rare reports of immediate hypersensitivity reactions, including anaphylaxis. Chest pain, hypotension, tachycardia, and bradycardia have been reported rarely. Dizziness and transient visual disturbances such as blurred vision have been reported during rapid intravenous administration.

5-$HT_3$ antagonists should generally not be used in patients who have had a hypersensitivity reaction to a member of this drug class. They should be used with care in patients with signs of subacute intestinal obstruction or ileus. Ondansetron should be given in reduced doses to patients with moderate to severe hepatic impairment.

**Effects on the cardiovascular system.** Chest pain and/or cardiac arrhythmias that might have been associated with ondansetron were reported[1] in 4 patients, 2 of whom died. In 3 subsequent patients who developed severe chest or anginal pain, treatment with ondansetron was discontinued.

The manufacturers (Glaxo) had at that time no evidence of a causal relationship between ondansetron and episodes of chest pain and cardiac abnormalities.[2] Administration of ondansetron 32 mg intravenously over 15 minutes produced no clinically important cardiovascular changes in a study in 12 healthy subjects.[3] A review[4] of the electrocardiographic and cardiovascular effects of the 5-$HT_3$ antagonists concluded that although this class of drugs may cause small, transient ECG changes, the clinical benefits of the drugs outweighed the small theoretical risk of any clinically significant cardiovascular events.

1. Ballard HS, *et al.* Ondansetron and chest pain. *Lancet* 1992; **340:** 1107.
2. Palmer JBD, Greenstreet YL. Ondansetron and chest pain. *Lancet* 1992; **340:** 1410.
3. Boike SC, *et al.* Cardiovascular effects of i.v. granisetron at two administration rates and of ondansetron in healthy adults. *Am J Health-Syst Pharm* 1997; **54:** 1172–6.
4. Navari RM, Koeller JM. Electrocardiographic and cardiovascular effects of the 5-hydroxytryptamine$_3$ receptor antagonists. *Ann Pharmacother* 2003; **37:** 1276–86.

**Effects on the liver.** Although disturbances in liver enzyme values have been reported in patients receiving ondansetron, more severe symptoms of liver disorder appear to be very rare; however, there is a report of severe jaundice associated with ondansetron as an antiemetic for chemotherapy.[1] Symptoms did not recur when the patient was given granisetron.

1. Verrill M, Judson I. Jaundice with ondansetron. *Lancet* 1994; **344:** 190–1.

**Effects on the nervous system.** Tonic-clonic movements and frothing at the mouth occurred in a patient 90 minutes after an infusion of ondansetron;[1] the patient responded to diazepam intravenously. The manufacturers had observed 10 patients who developed *seizures* during initial clinical studies, but considered that, unlike this case, all these patients had predisposing factors. Seizures have also been reported occasionally in patients receiving other 5-$HT_3$ antagonists. *Extrapyramidal reactions* in patients receiving ondansetron as part of a chemotherapy regimen[2,3] and for post-operative nausea and vomiting[4] have also been reported.

1. Sargent AI, *et al.* Seizure associated with ondansetron. *Clin Pharm* 1993; **12:** 613–15.
2. Krstenansky PM, *et al.* Extrapyramidal reaction caused by ondansetron. *Ann Pharmacother* 1994; **28:** 280.
3. Mathews HG, Tancil CG. Extrapyramidal reaction caused by ondansetron. *Ann Pharmacother* 1996; **30:** 196.
4. Stonell C. An extrapyramidal reaction to ondansetron. *Br J Anaesth* 1998; **81:** 658.

**Hypersensitivity.** Anaphylactoid reactions have been reported in patients receiving ondansetron injection. The FDA stated in October 1993 that it had received 24 reports of such reactions,[1] mostly occurring after the first ondansetron dose of the second or third chemotherapy cycle, and characterised by urticaria, angioedema, hypotension, bronchospasm, and dyspnoea.

In a subsequent report, 2 patients who had had a mild hypersensitivity reaction to a 5-$HT_3$ antagonist developed a more severe reaction after exposure to another drug of the same class.[2] In the first case severe acute asthma, cyanosis, and loss of consciousness developed after ondansetron in a patient who had previously experienced an asthmatic reaction after tropisetron. The second patient had developed pruritus after a tropisetron injection and urticaria after ondansetron, and subsequently developed anaphylactic shock 5 minutes after a further dose of tropisetron. It was recommended that another 5-$HT_3$ antagonist should not be given as a replacement to patients who developed a hypersensitivity reaction to a drug of this class.

1. Chen M, *et al.* Anaphylactoid-anaphylactic reactions associated with ondansetron. *Ann Intern Med* 1993; **119:** 862.
2. Kataja V, de Bruijn KM. Hypersensitivity reactions associated with 5-hydroxytryptamine$_3$-receptor antagonists: a class effect? *Lancet* 1996; **347:** 584–5.

## Interactions

**Antibacterials.** *Rifampicin* pretreatment reduced the area under the plasma concentration-time curve of oral ondansetron by 65% and of intravenous ondansetron by 48% in healthy subjects.[1] Use of rifampicin, or other potent inducers of cytochrome P450 isoenzyme CYP3A4, with ondansetron may reduce antiemetic efficacy.

1. Villikka K, *et al.* The effect of rifampin on the pharmacokinetics of oral and intravenous ondansetron. *Clin Pharmacol Ther* 1999; **65:** 377–81.

**Antineoplastics.** For mention of retrospective studies suggesting a change of pharmacokinetic parameters of high-dose cyclophosphamide and cisplatin when given with an ondansetron-containing antiemetic regimen, see Gastrointestinal Drugs, p.541.

## Pharmacokinetics

Following oral administration, ondansetron is rapidly absorbed with peak plasma concentrations being reported about 1.5 to 2 hours after an oral dose of 8 mg. The absolute bioavailability is about 60%, due mainly to hepatic first-pass metabolism. It is extensively distributed in the body; results *in vitro* suggest that about 70 to 75% of the drug in plasma is protein bound. It is cleared from the systemic circulation predominantly by hepatic metabolism through multiple enzymatic pathways, with less than 5% of a dose being excreted in urine unchanged: clearances of around 6 mL/minute per kg have been reported in young, healthy subjects. In elderly subjects, bioavailability may be somewhat higher (65%) and clearance lower (4 to 5 mL/minute per kg), presumably due to reduced hepatic metabolism. The terminal elimination half-life is about 3 hours in younger subjects, prolonged to about 5 hours in the elderly and in those with renal impairment. These differences are not considered sufficient to warrant dosage adjustment; however, in patients with severe hepatic impairment, in whom bioavailability may approach 100% and clearance is markedly slowed, with elimination half-lives of 15 to 32 hours, dosage restriction is advisable (see Administration in Hepatic Impairment, below). Children also have reduced clearance, which is age-related; use of weight-based doses compensates for this change.

◊ References.

1. Roila F, Del Favero A. Ondansetron clinical pharmacokinetics. *Clin Pharmacokinet* 1995; **29:** 95–109.
2. Figg WD, *et al.* Pharmacokinetics of ondansetron in patients with hepatic insufficiency. *J Clin Pharmacol* 1996; **36:** 206–15.
3. Van Den Berg CM, *et al.* Pharmacokinetics of three formulations of ondansetron hydrochloride in healthy volunteers: 24-mg oral tablet, rectal suppository, and iv infusion. *Am J Health-Syst Pharm* 2000; **57:** 1046–50.

## Uses and Administration

Ondansetron is a 5-$HT_3$ antagonist (5-$HT_3$-receptor antagonist) with antiemetic activity. It is used in the management of **nausea and vomiting** induced by cytotoxic chemotherapy and radiotherapy. It is also used for the prevention and treatment of postoperative nausea and vomiting. For the management of nausea and vomiting, and the important role of 5-$HT_3$ antagonists, see p.1245.

Ondansetron is given by intramuscular or slow intravenous injection as the hydrochloride, by mouth as the hydrochloride or base, or rectally as the base. Doses are expressed in terms of the base. Ondansetron hydrochloride 4.99 mg is approximately equivalent to 4 mg of ondansetron base.

For *highly emetogenic chemotherapy* the following dose schedules appear to be equally effective in preventing acute emesis:

- a single dose of 8 mg by slow intravenous or intramuscular injection immediately before treatment

*or*

- 8 mg by slow intravenous or intramuscular injection immediately before treatment, either followed by a continuous intravenous infusion of 1 mg/hour for up to 24 hours, or by a further two doses of 8 mg two to four hours apart

*or*

- a single dose of 32 mg given by intravenous infusion over at least 15 minutes immediately before treatment

*or*

- a 16-mg suppository rectally, given 1 to 2 hours before treatment

The efficacy of ondansetron in highly emetogenic chemotherapy may be enhanced by intravenous administration of dexamethasone sodium phosphate 20 mg before chemotherapy.

For preventing acute emesis with *less emetogenic chemotherapy* and *radiotherapy*:

- 8 mg may be given as a slow intravenous or intramuscular injection immediately before treatment

*or*

- 16 mg rectally can be given 1 to 2 hours before treatment

*or*

- 8 mg can be given by mouth 1 to 2 hours before treatment followed by 8 mg 12 hours later

To protect against delayed emesis these regimens are followed by ondansetron 8 mg by mouth twice daily, or 16 mg rectally once daily, for up to 5 days after the end of a course of chemotherapy.

For children a recommended dose is 5 mg/m$^2$ body-surface intravenously immediately before chemotherapy, followed by 4 mg orally 12 hours later. A dose of 4 mg orally twice daily may be continued for up to 5 days after the end of chemotherapy.

To *prevent postoperative nausea and vomiting* adults may be given:

- 16 mg by mouth an hour before anaesthesia

*or*

- 8 mg by mouth an hour before anaesthesia followed by 2 further doses of 8 mg at 8-hour intervals

*or*

- a single dose of 4 mg by intramuscular or slow intravenous injection at induction of anaesthesia

For the *treatment of postoperative nausea and vomiting* a single 4-mg dose by intramuscular or slow intravenous injection is recommended.

Children aged 2 years and over may be given 100 micrograms/kg by slow intravenous injection, up to a maximum dose of 4 mg, both for the prevention and treatment of postoperative nausea and vomiting.

In patients with moderate or severe *hepatic impairment* the manufacturers have recommended that the total daily dose of ondansetron should not exceed 8 mg (see below).

◊ Reviews.


1. Markham A, Sorkin EM. Ondansetron: an update of its therapeutic use in chemotherapy-induced and postoperative nausea and vomiting. *Drugs* 1993; **45:** 931–52.
2. Wilde MI, Markham A. Ondansetron: a review of its pharmacology and preliminary clinical findings in novel applications. *Drugs* 1996; **52:** 773–94.
3. Perez EA. A risk-benefit assessment of serotonin 5-HT$_3$ receptor antagonists in antineoplastic therapy-induced emesis. *Drug Safety* 1998; **18:** 43–56.
4. Gregory RE, Ettinger DS. 5-HT$_3$ receptor antagonists for the prevention of chemotherapy-induced nausea and vomiting: a comparison of their pharmacology and clinical efficacy. *Drugs* 1998; **55:** 173–89.
5. Lindley C, Blower P. Oral serotonin type 3-receptor antagonists for prevention of chemotherapy-induced emesis. *Am J Health-Syst Pharm* 2000; **57:** 1685–97.
6. Culy CR, *et al.* Ondansetron: a review of its use as an antiemetic in children. *Paediatr Drugs* 2001; **3:** 441–79.
7. Gridelli C. 5-HT$_3$-receptor antagonists in the control of delayed-onset emesis. *Anticancer Res* 2003; 23: 2773–82.


**Administration.** A report[1] of the successful use of ondansetron by continuous subcutaneous infusion to control intractable nausea and vomiting. Despite concern about the low pH of ondansetron injection there was no problem with the skin at the infusion site.


1. Mulvenna PM, Regnard CFB. Subcutaneous ondansetron. *Lancet* 1992; **339:** 1059.


**Administration in hepatic impairment.** The manufacturers recommend that the dose of ondansetron should not exceed 8 mg daily in patients with moderate or severe hepatic impairment. When this dose was given intravenously to patients with various degrees of impairment it was found that in those who were severely impaired there was an increase in the area under the plasma concentration/time curve and in the terminal plasma half-life, and a decrease in plasma clearance.[1] The authors of this study, some of whom worked for the manufacturers, considered that ondansetron should be restricted to once daily dosage in severe hepatic impairment.


1. Blake JC, *et al.* The pharmacokinetics of intravenous ondansetron in patients with hepatic impairment. *Br J Clin Pharmacol* 1993; **35:** 441–3.


**Bulimia nervosa.** A combination of counselling, support, psychotherapy, and antidepressants is the usual treatment of bulimia nervosa. Preliminary reports have indicated that ondansetron may be of benefit in the treatment of this disorder.[1,2]


1. Faris PL, *et al.* Effect of decreasing afferent vagal activity with ondansetron on symptoms of bulimia nervosa: a randomised, double-blind trial. *Lancet* 2000; **355:** 792–7.
2. Fung SM, Ferrill MJ. Treatment of bulimia nervosa with ondansetron. *Ann Pharmacother* 2001; **35:** 1270–3.


**Pain.** Preliminary results from a small crossover study[1] indicated that ondansetron was more effective than paracetamol in relieving the pain of fibromyalgia, a chronic disorder that responds poorly to conventional analgesics. Other 5-HT$_3$ antagonists such as granisetron[2-4] and tropisetron[5,6] have also been investigated in various painful syndromes.


1. Hrycaj P, *et al.* Pathogenetic aspects of responsiveness to ondansetron (5-hydroxytryptamine type 3 receptor antagonist) in patients with primary fibromyalgia syndrome—a preliminary study. *J Rheumatol* 1996; **23:** 1418–23.
2. Voog O, *et al.* Immediate effects of the serotonin antagonist granisetron on temporomandibular joint pain in patients with systemic inflammatory disorders. *Life Sci* 2000; **68:** 591–602.
3. Dubey PK, Prasad SS. Pain on injection of propofol: the effect of granisetron pretreatment. *Clin J Pain* 2003; **19:** 121–4.
4. Ernberg M, *et al.* Effects on muscle pain by intramuscular injection of granisetron in patients with fibromyalgia. *Pain* 2003; **101:** 275–82.
5. Farber L, *et al.* Short-term treatment of primary fibromyalgia with the 5-HT3-receptor antagonist tropisetron: results of a randomized, double-blind, placebo-controlled multicenter trial in 418 patients. *Int J Clin Pharmacol Res* 2001; **21:** 1–13.
6. Stratz T, *et al.* Local treatment of tendinopathies: a comparison between tropisetron and depot corticosteroids combined with local anesthetics. *Scand J Rheumatol* 2002; **31:** 366–70.


**Pruritus.** There are several case reports of cholestatic pruritus (p.1137) responding to intravenous or oral ondansetron,[1,2] but its value has been questioned, although one study suggested a modest effect from 8 mg by mouth 3 times daily.[3] It is similarly unclear if ondansetron is of benefit in pruritus due to renal failure[4,6] but a controlled study reported excellent results from intravenous use for opioid-induced pruritus.[5]


1. Schwörer H, Ramadori G. Improvement of cholestatic pruritus by ondansetron. *Lancet* 1993; **341:** 1277.
2. Raderer M, *et al.* Ondansetron for pruritus due to cholestasis. *N Engl J Med* 1994; **330:** 1540.
3. Müller C, *et al.* Treatment of pruritus in chronic liver disease with the 5-hydroxytryptamine receptor type 3 antagonist ondansetron: a randomized, placebo-controlled, double-blind cross-over trial. *Eur J Gastroenterol Hepatol* 1998; **10:** 865–70.
4. Balaskas EV, *et al.* Histamine and serotonin in uremic pruritus: effect of ondansetron in CAPD-pruritic patients. *Nephron* 1998; **78:** 395–402.
5. Borget A, Stirnemann HR. Ondansetron is effective to treat spinal or epidural morphine-induced pruritus. *Anesthesiology* 1999; **90:** 432–6.
6. Murphy M, *et al.* A randomized, placebo-controlled, double-blind trial of ondansetron in renal itch. *Br J Dermatol* 2003; **148:** 314–7.


**Psychiatric disorders.** Ondansetron has been tried experimentally in a number of psychiatric disorders including schizophrenia[1] and psychosis in patients with parkinsonism,[2] and may be of value in moderating tardive dyskinesia.[3] It is also reported to be under investigation in the management of panic attacks (p.663). For the more conventional management of schizophrenia and parkinsonism see p.665 and p.1196, respectively.


1. White A, *et al.* Ondansetron in the treatment of schizophrenia. *Lancet* 1991; **337:** 1173.
2. Zoldan J, *et al.* Psychosis in advanced Parkinson's disease: treatment with ondansetron, a 5-HT$_3$ receptor antagonist. *Neurology* 1995; **45:** 1305–8.
3. Sirota P, *et al.* Use of the selective serotonin 3 receptor antagonist ondansetron in the treatment of neuroleptic-induced tardive dyskinesia. *Am J Psychiatry* 2000; **157:** 287–9.


**Substance dependence.** Ondansetron is being studied in the management of alcohol dependence (p.1166). However, in one study[1] a significant reduction in alcohol consumption was found only in lighter drinkers after subgroup analysis. Another study[2] found a reduction in alcohol consumption by patients with early-onset alcoholism (onset before age 25) who took ondansetron compared with placebo. No such effect was seen, however, in patients with late-onset alcoholism.


1. Sellers EM, *et al.* Clinical efficacy of the 5-HT$_3$ antagonist ondansetron in alcohol abuse and dependence. *Alcohol Clin Exp Res* 1994; **18:** 879–85.
2. Johnson BA, *et al.* Ondansetron for reduction of drinking among biologically predisposed alcoholic patients. *JAMA* 2000; **284:** 963–71.


## Preparations

***USP 27:*** Ondansetron Injection.

**Proprietary Preparations** (details are given in Part 3)

***Arg.:*** Cetron; Dantenk; Dismolan; Emivox; Espasevit; Finaber; Finoxi; Tiosalis; Zofran; ***Austral.:*** Zofran; ***Austria:*** Zofran; ***Belg.:*** Zofran; ***Braz.:*** Ansentron; Modificial; Nausedron; Ontrax; Zofran; ***Canad.:*** Zofran; ***Chile:*** Amilene; Gardoton; Izofran; Odanex; Trorix; ***Denm.:*** Zofran; ***Fin.:*** Zofran; ***Fr.:*** Zophren; ***Ger.:*** Zofran; ***Gr.:*** Zofron; ***Hong Kong:*** Zofran; ***India:*** Emeset; ***Irl.:*** Zofran; ***Israel:*** Zofran; ***Ital.:*** Zofran; ***Malaysia:*** Zofran; ***Mex.:*** Zofran; ***Neth.:*** Zofran; ***Norw.:*** Zofran; ***NZ:*** Zofran; ***Port.:*** Zofran; ***S.Afr.:*** Zofran; ***Singapore:*** Zofran; ***Spain:*** Fixca†; Helmine†; Yatrox; Zofran; ***Swed.:*** Zofran; ***Switz.:*** Zofran; ***Thai.:*** Emeset; Onsia; Vomitron; Zetron; Zofran; ***UK:*** Zofran; ***USA:*** Zofran.

## Oxyphenisatine *(BAN, rINN)*

Dihydroxyphenylisatin; Oxifenisatina; Oxyphenisatin. 3,3-Bis(4-hydroxyphenyl)indolin-2-one.

$C_{20}H_{15}NO_3$ = 317.3.

*CAS — 125-13-3.*

## Oxyphenisatine Acetate *(rINNM)*

Acetato de oxifenisatina; Acetphenolisatin; Bisatin; Diacetoxydiphenylisatin; Diacetyldiphenolisatin; Diasatin; Diphesatin; Isaphenin; NSC-59687; Oxyphenisatin Acetate *(USAN)*; Oxyphenisatin Diacetate; Oxyphenisatine Diacetate *(BANM)*; Phenlaxine.

$C_{24}H_{19}NO_5$ = 401.4.

*CAS — 115-33-3.*

*ATC — A06AB01.*

### Profile

Oxyphenisatine is a stimulant laxative that has been used by mouth and as an enema. Liver damage has occurred, usually after prolonged use by mouth, and has led to it being withdrawn in some countries.

◊ References.


1. Reynolds TB, *et al.* Chronic active and lupoid hepatitis caused by a laxative, oxyphenisatin. *N Engl J Med* 1971; **285:** 813–20.
2. Gjone E, Stave R. Liver disease associated with a "non-constipating" iron preparation. *Lancet* 1973; **i:** 421–2.
3. Kotha P, *et al.* Liver damage induced by oxyphenisatin. *BMJ* 1980; **281:** 1530.


# Palonosetron Hydrochloride

*(USAN, rINNM)*

RS-25259-197. (3a*S*)-2,3,3a,4,5,6-Hexahydro-2-[(3*S*)-3-quinuclidinyl]-1*H*-benz[*de*]isoquinolin-1-one hydrochloride.

$C_{19}H_{24}N_2O,HCl$ = 332.9.

*CAS — 135729-56-5 (palonosetron); 135729-55-4 (palonosetron hydrochloride); 135729-62-3 (palonosetron hydrochloride).*

## Adverse Effects and Precautions

As for Ondansetron, p.1281, although no dosage reduction is considered necessary in hepatic impairment. Diarrhoea, fatigue, and abdominal pain may also occur. Palonosetron should be used with caution in patients who have or may develop prolongation of the QT interval.

## Pharmacokinetics

Palonosetron has a volume of distribution of around 8 litres/kg; plasma protein binding is about 62%. About 50% of a dose is metabolised in the liver by cytochrome P450 isoenzymes and about 80% of a dose is recovered in the urine within 144 hours, as palonosetron and its metabolites. The mean elimination half-life is reported to be about 40 hours.

## Uses and Administration

Palonosetron is a 5-HT$_3$ antagonist used in the prevention of acute and delayed nausea and vomiting associated with initial and repeat courses of moderately and highly emetogenic cancer chemotherapy. Palonosetron is given as the hydrochloride but doses are expressed in terms of the base; 280.8 micrograms of palonosetron hydrochloride is approximately equivalent to 250 micrograms of palonosetron base. A dose of 250 micrograms is given intravenously over 30 seconds about 30 minutes before chemotherapy. Repeated dosing within 7 days is not recommended.

◊ References.


1. Eisenberg P, *et al.* Improved prevention of moderately emetogenic chemotherapy-induced nausea and vomiting with palonosetron, a pharmacologically novel 5-HT3 receptor antagonist: results of a phase III, single-dose trial versus dolasetron. *Cancer* 2003; **98:** 2473–82.
2. Gralla R, *et al.* Palonosetron improves prevention of chemotherapy-induced nausea and vomiting following moderately emetogenic chemotherapy: results of a double-blind randomized phase III trial comparing single doses of palonosetron with ondansetron. *Ann Oncol* 2003; **14:** 1570–7.


## Preparations

**Proprietary Preparations** (details are given in Part 3)

***USA:*** Aloxi.

## Pantoprazole (BAN, USAN, rINN)

BY-1023; Pantoprazol; SKF-96022. 5-Difluoromethoxybenzimidazol-2-yl 3,4-dimethoxy-2-pyridylmethyl sulphoxide.
$C_{16}H_{15}F_2N_3O_4S$ = 383.4.
*CAS — 102625-70-7.*
*ATC — A02BC02.*

## Pantoprazole Sodium (BANM, USAN, rINNM)

Pantoprazole sodium sesquihydrate.
$C_{16}H_{14}F_2N_3NaO_4S,1\frac{1}{2}H_2O$ = 432.4.
*CAS — 138786-67-1 (pantoprazole sodium); 164579-32-2 (pantoprazole sodium sesquihydrate).*
*ATC — A02BC02.*

### Adverse Effects and Precautions

As for Omeprazole, p.1278. Dosage may need to be reduced in severe hepatic impairment; liver function should be monitored regularly.

### Interactions

As for Omeprazole, p.1279.

◊ For reference to a lack of effect of pantoprazole on diazepam, see Gastrointestinal Drugs, p.694, for a lack of effect on theophylline, see p.803, and for a lack of effect on warfarin, see p.1026. For a report of severe generalised myalgia and bone pain attributed to the concomitant use of methotrexate and pantoprazole, see Gastrointestinal Drugs, p.571.

### Pharmacokinetics

Peak plasma-pantoprazole concentrations are achieved about 2 to 2.5 hours after a dose by mouth. The oral bioavailability is about 77% with the enteric-coated tablet formulation, and does not vary after single or multiple doses. Pantoprazole is 98% bound to plasma proteins. It is extensively metabolised in the liver, primarily by the cytochrome P450 isoenzyme CYP2C19, to desmethylpantoprazole; small amounts are also metabolised by CYP3A4, CYP2D6, and CYP2C9. Metabolites are excreted principally (about 80%) in the urine, with the remainder being excreted in bile. The terminal elimination half-life is about 1 hour, and is prolonged in hepatic impairment; the half-life in patients with cirrhosis was 3 to 6 hours.

◊ References.

1. Pue MA, *et al.* Pharmacokinetics of pantoprazole following single intravenous and oral administration to healthy male subjects. *Eur J Clin Pharmacol* 1993; **44:** 575–8.

### Uses and Administration

Pantoprazole is a proton pump inhibitor with actions and uses similar to those of omeprazole (p.1280). It is given as the sodium salt but doses are expressed in terms of the base. Pantoprazole sodium 11.28 mg is approximately equivalent to 10 mg pantoprazole. Once-daily doses should be taken in the morning.

In the treatment of **gastro-oesophageal reflux disease** (p.1242), the usual dose by mouth is 20 to 40 mg once daily for 4 weeks, increased to 8 weeks if necessary; in the USA, up to 16 weeks' therapy is permitted for healing of erosive oesophagitis. For maintenance therapy, treatment can be continued with 20 to 40 mg daily.

The usual dose for the treatment of **peptic ulcer disease** (p.1246) is 40 mg once daily. Treatment is usually given for 2 to 4 weeks for duodenal ulceration, or 4 to 8 weeks for benign gastric ulceration. For the eradication of *Helicobacter pylori* pantoprazole may be combined with two antibacterials in a 1-week **triple therapy** regimen. Effective regimens include pantoprazole 40 mg twice daily combined with clarithromycin 500 mg twice daily and either amoxicillin 1 g twice daily or metronidazole 400 mg twice daily.

Patients who require prophylaxis for **NSAID-associated ulceration** may take 20 mg daily.

In the treatment of pathological hypersecretory states such as the **Zollinger-Ellison syndrome** (p.1247), the initial dose is 80 mg daily, adjusted as required. Doses of up to 240 mg daily have been used. Daily doses greater than 80 mg should be given in 2 divided doses.

Pantoprazole may also be given intravenously, as the sodium salt, in recommended doses of 40 mg daily given over 2 to 15 minutes. A dose of 80 mg daily may be used for Zollinger-Ellison syndrome or up to 240 mg daily in divided doses if rapid control is required.

Doses of pantoprazole may need to be reduced in patients with hepatic impairment (see below).

◊ Reviews.

1. Anonymous. Pantoprazole—a third proton pump inhibitor. *Drug Ther Bull* 1997; **35:** 93–4.
2. Poole P. Pantoprazole. *Am J Health-Syst Pharm* 2001; **58:** 999–1008.
3. Cheer SM, *et al.* Pantoprazole: an update of its pharmacological properties and therapeutic use in the management of acid-related disorders. *Drugs* 2003; **63:** 101–32.

**Administration in hepatic impairment.** Dosage of pantoprazole may need to be reduced in severe hepatic impairment, or doses given only on alternate days. A maximum dose of 20 mg daily, or 40 mg on alternate days, has been suggested.

**Administration in renal impairment.** Most studies have not found the pharmacokinetics of pantoprazole to be altered in patients with renal impairment[1] and licensed drug information in the UK and US generally does not recommend dosage adjustment in this group; however some UK sources, including the *British National Formulary*, suggest that a maximum dose of 40 mg daily should be observed.

1. Cheer SM, *et al.* Pantoprazole: an update of its pharmacological properties and therapeutic use in the management of acid-related disorders. *Drugs* 2003; **63:** 101–132.

### Preparations

**Proprietary Preparations** (details are given in Part 3)
***Arg.:*** Gastromax; Pangest; Pantop; Pantus; Peptazol; Supracam; Ulserch; Zurcal; ***Austral.:*** Somac; ***Austria:*** Pantoloc; Zurcal; ***Belg.:*** Pantozol; Zurcale; ***Braz.:*** Noprop; Pantocal; Pantopaz; Pantozol; Ziprol; Zurcal; ***Canad.:*** Panto; Pantoloc; ***Chile:*** Singastril; Ulcemex; Zurcal; ***Denm.:*** Pantoloc; ***Fin.:*** Somac; ***Fr.:*** Eupantol; Inipomp; ***Ger.:*** Pantozol; Pantozol-Rifun; Rifun; ***Gr.:*** Controloc; Zurcazol; ***Hong Kong:*** Pantoloc; ***India:*** Pantodac; ***Irl.:*** Protium; ***Israel:*** Controloc; ***Ital.:*** Pantecta; Pantopan; Pantorc; Peptazol; ***Malaysia:*** Controloc; ***Mex.:*** Pantozol; Zurcal; ***Neth.:*** Pantozol; ***Norw.:*** Somac; ***NZ:*** Somac; ***Port.:*** Apton; Pantoc; Zurcal; ***S.Afr.:*** Controloc; Pantoloc; ***Singapore:*** Controloc; ***Spain:*** Anagastra; Pantecta; Pantocarm; Ulcotenal; ***Swed.:*** Pantoloc; ***Switz.:*** Pantozol; Zurcal; ***Thai.:*** Controloc; ***UK:*** Protium; ***USA:*** Protonix.

**Multi-ingredient:** ***Austral.:*** Somac-MA†; ***Ger.:*** ZacPac; ***Malaysia:*** Klacid HP 7; ***Neth.:*** PantoPAC.

## Pentaerythritol

Pentaeritritol; Tetramethylolmethane. 2,2-Bis(hydroxymethyl)propane-1,3-diol.
$C_5H_{12}O_4$ = 136.1.
*CAS — 115-77-5.*

### Profile

Pentaerythritol is an osmotic laxative used in the treatment of constipation (p.1240) in doses of 5 to 15 g daily.

### Preparations

**Proprietary Preparations** (details are given in Part 3)
***Fr.:*** Auxitrans; Hydrafuca.

## Peppermint Leaf

Black Mint; Hoja de Menta; Hortelã-Pimenta; Menta piperita, hoja de; Menth. Pip.; Mentha Piperita; Menthae Piperitae Folium; Menthe Poivrée; Peppermint; Pfefferminzblätter; White Mint.

**Pharmacopoeias.** In *Eur.* (see p.vi) and *Pol.*

**Ph. Eur. 5.0** (Peppermint Leaf). The whole or cut dried leaves of *Mentha × piperita*, containing not less than 1.2% v/w of essential oil if whole, or not less than 0.9% v/w if cut. It has a characteristic and penetrating odour and a characteristic aromatic taste. Protect from light.

**USNF 22** (Peppermint). The dried leaf and flowering top of *Mentha piperita* (Labiatae). It has an aromatic, characteristic odour and a pungent taste, and produces a cooling sensation in the mouth.

## Peppermint Oil

Essence de Menthe Poivrée; Essência de Hortelã-Pimenta; Menta piperita, aceite esencial de; Menthae Piperitae Aetheroleum; Ol. Menth. Pip.; Oleum Menthae Piperitae; Pfefferminzöl.
*CAS — 8006-90-4.*

**Pharmacopoeias.** In *Eur.* (see p.vi) and *Pol.* Also in *USNF.*

**Ph. Eur. 5.0** (Peppermint Oil). It is obtained by steam distillation from the fresh overground parts of the flowering plant of *Mentha × piperita*. It contains 30.0 to 55.0% menthol, 14.0 to 32.0% menthone, and 2.8 to 10.0% menthyl acetate, 3.5 to 14.0% cineole, 1.5 to 10.0% isomenthone, 1.0 to 9.0% menthofuran, 1.0 to 5.0% limonene, not more than 4.0% pulegone, and not more than 1.0% carvone; the ratio of eucalyptol content to limonene content is greater than two.

It is a colourless, pale yellow, or pale greenish-yellow liquid with a characteristic odour and taste followed by a sensation of cold. Miscible with alcohol and with dichloromethane. Store in well-filled, airtight containers. Protect from light and heat.

**USNF 22** (Peppermint Oil). The volatile oil distilled with steam from the fresh overground parts of the flowering plant *Mentha piperita* (Labiatae), rectified by distillation, and neither partially nor wholly dementholised. It yields not less than 5% of esters calculated as menthyl acetate and not less than 50% of total menthol, free and as esters.

It is a colourless or pale yellow liquid with a strong, penetrating, characteristic odour and a pungent taste, followed by a sensation of cold when air is drawn into the mouth. Soluble 1 in 3 of alcohol (70%) with not more than slight opalescence. Store in airtight containers at a temperature not exceeding 40°.

**Storage.** The Pharmaceutical Society of Great Britain's Department of Pharmaceutical Sciences found that PVC bottles softened and distorted fairly rapidly in the presence of peppermint oil, which should not be stored or dispensed in such bottles.[1]

1. Department of Pharmaceutical Sciences of the Pharmaceutical Society of Great Britain. Plastic medicine bottles of rigid PVC. *Pharm J* 1973; **210:** 100.

### Adverse Effects and Precautions

Peppermint oil can be irritant and may rarely cause hypersensitivity reactions. Reported reactions include erythematous skin rash, headache, bradycardia, muscle tremor, and ataxia. Heartburn has also been reported.

**Effects on the cardiovascular system.** Idiopathic atrial fibrillation occurred in 2 patients addicted to 'peppermints'. Normal rhythm was restored when peppermint-sucking ceased.[1]

1. Thomas JG. Peppermint fibrillation. *Lancet* 1962; **i:** 222.

**Hypersensitivity.** Exacerbation of asthma, with wheezing and dyspnoea, associated with the use of paste-based toothpastes containing peppermint or wintergreen as a flavouring.[1]

1. Spurlock BW, Dailey TM. Shortness of (fresh) breath—toothpaste-induced bronchospasm. *N Engl J Med* 1990; **323:** 1845–6.

### Interactions

Adverse effects may be more likely if peppermint oil is taken with alcohol. Enteric-coated capsules containing peppermint oil should not be taken immediately after food or with antacids. There is some evidence that peppermint oil can inhibit the cytochrome P450 isoenzyme CYP3A4, and may affect the clearance of drugs whose metabolism is mediated by this enzyme.

◊ References.

1. Dresser GK, *et al.* Evaluation of peppermint oil and ascorbyl palmitate as inhibitors of cytochrome P4503A4 activity in vitro and in vivo. *Clin Pharmacol Ther* 2002; **72:** 247–55.

### Uses and Administration

Peppermint oil is an aromatic carminative that relaxes gastrointestinal smooth muscle and relieves flatulence and colic. Enteric-coated capsules containing peppermint oil are used for the relief of symptoms of the irritable bowel syndrome or gastrointestinal spasm secondary to other disorders. Usual doses are 0.2 mL three times daily by mouth, (increased to 0.4 mL three times daily if necessary) for up to 2 to 3 months. The capsules should be taken half to one hour before food and swallowed whole, not chewed.

Peppermint oil is also used as a flavour and with other volatile agents in preparations for respiratory-tract disorders.

Peppermint leaf, the source of the oil, has also been used for its carminative and flavouring properties.

**Gastrointestinal disorders.** Menthol, the major constituent of peppermint oil, has properties similar to those of calcium-channel blockers on smooth muscle such as that in the human gut.[1-3] A review[4] of randomised studies of peppermint oil in irritable bowel syndrome (p.1244) concluded that there was some evidence of its benefit but that further studies were required.

The relaxant effect of peppermint oil on the gastrointestinal tract has been used to reduce colonic spasm during endoscopy by injecting the oil or a diluted suspension of the oil along the biopsy channel of the colonoscope.[5] Addition of peppermint oil to barium enema has also been tried and appears to reduce spasm and reduce the need for intravenous antispasmodics.[6]

1. Taylor BA, *et al.* Inhibitory effect of peppermint oil on gastrointestinal smooth muscle. *Gut* 1983; **24:** A992.
2. Taylor BA, *et al.* Inhibitory effect of peppermint oil and menthol on human isolated coli. *Gut* 1984; **25:** A1168–9.
3. Taylor BA, *et al.* Calcium antagonist activity of menthol on gastrointestinal smooth muscle. *Br J Clin Pharmacol* 1985; **20:** 293P–4P.
4. Pittler MH, Ernst E. Peppermint oil for irritable bowel syndrome: a critical review and metaanalysis. *Am J Gastroenterol* 1998; **93:** 1131–5.
5. Leicester RJ, Hunt RH. Peppermint oil to reduce colonic spasm during endoscopy. *Lancet* 1982; **ii:** 989.
6. Sparks MJW, *et al.* Does peppermint oil relieve spasm during barium enema? *Br J Radiol* 1995; **68:** 841–3.

### Preparations

***BP 2003:*** Concentrated Peppermint Emulsion; Gastro-resistant Peppermint Oil Capsules; Peppermint Spirit;
***USNF 22:*** Peppermint Water;
***USP 27:*** Peppermint Spirit.

**Proprietary Preparations** (details are given in Part 3)
***Austral.:*** Mintec†; ***Austria:*** Aponatura Herz; China-Ol; Colpermin; Japomin; ***Canad.:*** Colpermin†; ***Ger.:*** Carminetum†; Chiana; China-Oel; Cholaktol†; Euminz; Inspirol Heilpflanzenol; Leukona-Mintol†; Mentacur; Ni-No-Fluid N†; spasmo gallo sanol mint; SX Mentha†; ***Hong Kong:*** Colpermin; ***Irl.:*** Colpermin; ***Ital.:*** Carmint; ***Mex.:*** Colpermin; ***NZ:*** Colpermin†; Mintec; ***Port.:*** Colominte; ***Switz.:*** Colpermin; ***Thai.:*** Colpermin; ***UK:*** Colpermin; Equilon Herbal; Kiminto†; Mintec; Obbekjaers.

**Multi-ingredient:** numerous preparations are listed in Part3.

## Phenolphthalein (BAN, rINN)

Dihydroxyphthalophenone; Fenolftaleína; Phenolphtaleinum; Phenolphthaleinum. 3,3-Bis(4-hydroxyphenyl)phthalide.

$C_{20}H_{14}O_4$ = 318.3.

*CAS — 77-09-8.*

*ATC — A06AB04.*

**Pharmacopoeias.** In *Chin.* and *Eur.* (see p.vi).

**Ph. Eur. 5.0** (Phenolphthalein). A white or almost white powder. Practically insoluble in water; soluble in alcohol. Protect from light.

### Adverse Effects and Precautions

As for Bisacodyl, p.1251. Hypersensitivity reactions, usually as skin rashes or eruptions, have occurred with phenolphthalein. Phenolphthalein may cause pink discoloration of alkaline urine.

Tumours have occurred in *rats* and *mice* given very high doses of phenolphthalein; there does not appear to be evidence of carcinogenicity in humans, but phenolphthalein-containing products have been withdrawn in many countries because of concerns about long-term safety.

**Effects on the skin.** Reports of skin reactions associated with phenolphthalein include fixed drug eruptions,[1,2] erythema multiforme reactions,[1,3] and toxic epidermal necrolysis.[4,5]


1. Baer RL, Harris H. Types of cutaneous reactions to drugs. *JAMA* 1967; **202:** 710–13.
2. Savin JA. Current causes of fixed drug eruptions. *Br J Dermatol* 1970; **83:** 546–9.
3. Shelley WB, *et al.* Demonstration of intercellular immunofluorescence and epidermal hysteresis in bullous fixed drug eruption due to phenolphthalein. *Br J Dermatol* 1972; **86:** 118–25.
4. Kar PK, *et al.* Toxic epidermal necrolysis in a patient induced by phenolphthalein. *J Indian Med Assoc* 1986; **84:** 189–93.
5. Artymowicz RJ, *et al.* Phenolphthalein-induced toxic epidermal necrolysis. *Ann Pharmacother* 1997; **31:** 1157–9.


**Overdosage.** The most likely consequence of phenolphthalein overdosage is excessive purgation, which may require fluid and electrolyte replacement. However, a possible association with acute pancreatitis occurred in a 34-year-old man who inadvertently ingested phenolphthalein 2 g. There was complete recovery with no sequelae from the pancreatitis.[1] Widespread organ failure with disseminated intravascular coagulation, massive liver damage, pulmonary oedema, renal failure, and myocardial damage in a second patient[2] were attributed to self-poisoning with an unknown quantity of phenolphthalein-containing laxative, although the diagnosis was problematic. The patient died despite intensive support.


1. Lambrianides AL, Rosin RD. Acute pancreatitis complicating excessive intake of phenolphthalein. *Postgrad Med J* 1984; **60:** 491–2.
2. Sidhu PS, *et al.* Fatal phenolphthalein poisoning with fulminant hepatic failure and disseminated intravascular coagulation. *Hum Toxicol* 1989; **8:** 381–4.


### Pharmacokinetics

Up to 15% of phenolphthalein given by mouth is subsequently excreted in the urine. Enterohepatic circulation occurs and the glucuronide is excreted in the bile. Elimination may take several days.

### Uses and Administration

Phenolphthalein is a diphenylmethane stimulant laxative that has been used for the treatment of constipation (p.1240) and for bowel evacuation before investigational procedures or surgery. It has been withdrawn in many countries because of concern over its carcinogenic potential following reports of tumours in *rodents*.

It has been given in pills or tablets, and as an emulsion with liquid paraffin. Yellow phenolphthalein, an impure form, has been used similarly.

### Preparations

**Proprietary Preparations** (details are given in Part 3)

***Arg.:*** Fructines; ***Austral.:*** Laxettes†; ***Belg.:*** Caolax†; ***Braz.:*** Teutolax†; ***Canad.:*** Espotabs†; Neo-Prunex†; ***Chile:*** Felaxen; ***Fr.:*** Purganol†; ***Hong Kong:*** Regulim†; ***Israel:*** Easylax; ***S.Afr.:*** Laxicaps P; ***Singapore:*** Regulim; ***Spain:*** Laxen Busto†; Purgante†; Sure-Lax†; ***Switz.:*** Euchessina†; Regulets; ***Thai.:*** Purmolax; Regulim; ***UK:*** Bonomint†; Brooklax†; Sure-Lax†.

**Multi-ingredient:** ***Arg.:*** Cascara Sagrada Puler; Cascara Sagrada Sanaplex; Genolaxante; Veracolate; ***Austral.:*** Ford Pills†; Mackenzies Menthoids†; ***Austria:*** Abfuhrdragees; ***Belg.:*** Grains de Vals; Sanicolax†; ***Braz.:*** Agarol; Dioctosal†; Emagrex†; Esbelt†; Esbeltrat†; Fenogar†; Fideine†; Lacto-Purga†; Laxantil†; Macroten†; Magroton†; Manolio†; Manon†; Normagrin†; Obesidex; Obesifran; Prisoventril; Purgoleite†; ***Canad.:*** Agarol†; Aid-Lax†; Alsiline†; Calcium Docuphen†; Caroid†; Doulax†; Doxidan†; Evac-Q-Kwik†; Ex-Lax Light†; Herbalax Forte†; Laxa†; Laxarol†; Le 100 B†; Phillips Gelcaps†; Phytolax†; Thunas Bilettes†; Triolax†; Vesilax†; ***Chile:*** Bulgarolax; Fenokomp 39; Fenolftaleina Compuesta; Oblax A-1-1; ***Fr.:*** Mucinum†; ***Ger.:*** Vencipon N; ***India:*** Agarol; Jetomisol-P; ***Irl.:*** Agarol†; Alophen†; Petrolagar No. 2†; Petrolagar with Phenolphthalein†; ***Israel:*** Laxative; Laxative Comp; ***Port.:*** Byl; Caroid; ***S.Afr.:*** Agarol†; Redupon; Veracolate; ***Spain:*** Agarol†; Laxante Bescansa Aloico; Laxante Bescansa†; Laxo Vian†; Mahiou; ***Switz.:*** Agarol†; Carter Petites Pilules†; Paragar; ***Thai.:*** Agarol; Emulax; Veracolate; Zenda; ***UK:*** Agarol†; Alophen†; Fam-Lax; Juno Junipah†; ***USA:*** Agoral; Doxidan†; Ex-Lax Extra Gentle Pills†; Veracolate†.

---

## Plaunotol (rINN)

CS-684. (2Z,6E)-2-[(3E)-4,8-Dimethyl-3,7-nonadienyl]-6-methyl-2,6-octadiene-1,8-diol.

$C_{20}H_{34}O_2$ = 306.5.

*CAS — 64218-02-6.*

### Profile

Plaunotol is a complex aliphatic alcohol extracted from the Thai medicinal plant plau-noi (*Croton sublyratus* (Euphorbiaceae)). It is reported to possess cytoprotective properties and has been used in the treatment of gastritis and peptic ulcer disease in a dose of 80 mg three times daily by mouth.

### Preparations

**Proprietary Preparations** (details are given in Part 3)

***Jpn:*** Kelnac; ***Thai.:*** Kelnac.

---

## Polaprezinc (rINN)

Z-103. *catena*-Poly{zinc-μ-[β-alanyl-L-histidinato(2-)-*N*,*N*^N^,*O*:*N*^τ^]}.

$(C_9H_{12}N_4O_3Zn)_n$.

*CAS — 107667-60-7.*

### Profile

Polaprezinc is a cytoprotective agent used in the treatment of peptic ulcer disease.

◊ References.


1. Kashimura H, *et al.* Polaprezinc, a mucosal protective agent, in combination with lansoprazole, amoxycillin and clarithromycin increases the cure rate of Helicobacter pylori infection. *Aliment Pharmacol Ther* 1999; **13:** 483–7.


---

## Polycarbophil (BAN, rINN)

Policarbofilo.

*CAS — 9003-97-8.*

**Pharmacopoeias.** In *US.*

**USP 27** (Polycarbophil). It is polyacrylic acid cross-linked with divinyl glycol. White to creamy-white granules, with a characteristic, ester-like odour. Swells in water to a range of volumes, depending primarily on the pH. Insoluble in water, in common organic solvents, and in dilute acids and alkalis. A 1% mixture in water has a pH of not more than 4.0. Store in airtight containers.

## Polycarbophil Calcium (BANM, rINNM)

AHR-3260B; Calcium Polycarbophil (USAN); Policarbofilo cálcico; Polycarbophilum Calcii; WI-140.

*CAS — 126040-58-2.*

*ATC — A06AC08.*

**Pharmacopoeias.** In *US.*

**USP 27** (Calcium Polycarbophil). A white to creamy-white powder. Insoluble in water, in common organic solvents, and in dilute acids and alkalis. It loses not more than 10% of its weight on drying and contains not less than 18% and not more than 22% of calcium, calculated on the dried basis. Store in airtight containers.

### Adverse Effects and Precautions

As for Ispaghula, p.1268. Polycarbophil calcium releases calcium ions in the gastrointestinal tract and should be avoided by patients who must restrict their calcium intake.

There is a risk of intestinal or oesophageal obstruction and faecal impaction, especially if such bulk laxatives are swallowed dry. Therefore, they should always be taken with sufficient fluid and should not be taken immediately before going to bed. They should be avoided by patients who have difficulty swallowing.

### Interactions

The calcium component of polycarbophil calcium may produce interactions typical of calcium salts (p.1226), such as reducing the absorption of tetracyclines from the gastrointestinal tract; it should be taken at least 1 hour before or 2 hours after the antibacterial.

### Uses and Administration

Polycarbophil calcium has similar properties to ispaghula (p.1268) and is used as a bulk laxative and for adjusting faecal consistency. Following ingestion calcium ions are replaced by hydrogen ions from gastric acid and the resultant polycarbophil exerts a hydrophilic effect in the intestines.

It is given by mouth in a usual dose equivalent to 1 g of polycarbophil up to four times daily, as necessary. Doses should be taken with at least 250 mL of water.

Polycarbophil is used topically as a vaginal moisturiser and as an ocular lubricant.

◊ Reviews.


1. Danhof IE. Pharmacology, toxicology, clinical efficacy, and adverse effects of calcium polycarbophil, an enteral hydrosorptive agent. *Pharmacotherapy* 1982; **2:** 18–28.


### Preparations

**Proprietary Preparations** (details are given in Part 3)

***Arg.:*** Fibercon; ***Austral.:*** Replens; ***Austria:*** Fibercon; ***Belg.:*** Replens; ***Canad.:*** Replens; ***Israel:*** Fibercon; ***Ital.:*** Modula; Pursennid Fibra†; Replens; ***Mex.:*** Fibercon; ***Port.:*** Replens†; ***Spain:*** Replens; ***Swed.:*** Replens; ***Thai.:*** Fibercon; ***USA:*** Equalactin; Fiber-Lax; Fiberall†; Fibercon; FiberNorm; Mitrolan†; Replens.

**Multi-ingredient:** ***Ital.:*** Ormobyl CM; Pursennid Complex†; ***USA:*** Aquasite.

---

## Potassium Acid Tartrate

E336; Kalii Hydrogenotartras; Kalium Hydrotartaricum; Potassium Bitartrate (USAN); Potassium Hydrogen Tartrate; Purified Cream of Tartar; Tartarus Depuratus; Tartrato ácido de potasio; Weinstein.

$C_4H_5KO_6$ = 188.2.

*CAS — 868-14-4.*

*ATC — A12BA03.*

**Pharmacopoeias.** In *Eur.* (see p.vi) and *US.*

**Ph. Eur. 5.0** (Potassium Hydrogen Tartrate). A white crystalline powder or colourless crystals. Slightly soluble in water; practically insoluble in alcohol. It dissolves in dilute solutions of mineral acids and alkali hydroxides.

**USP 27** (Potassium Bitartrate). Colourless or slightly opaque crystals or a white, crystalline powder. Slightly soluble in water; soluble in boiling water; very slightly soluble in alcohol. A saturated solution is acid to litmus. Store in airtight containers.

### Profile

Potassium acid tartrate is given with sodium bicarbonate as a suppository for the treatment of constipation (p.1240) and for bowel evacuation before investigational procedures or surgery. Carbon dioxide gas is produced in the rectum, which stimulates defaecation within 5 to 30 minutes.

Potassium acid tartrate is used as a food additive and pharmaceutical aid.

Potassium acid tartrate has been used as an ingredient of preparations for potassium supplementation, although other potassium salts are usually preferred. For the general properties of potassium salts, see p.1232.

### Preparations

***BPC 1968:*** Effervescent Potassium Tablets.

**Proprietary Preparations** (details are given in Part 3)

**Multi-ingredient:** ***Austria:*** Lecicarbon; ***Braz.:*** Circanetten†; Varicell; ***Ital.:*** Potassion; ***Mon.:*** Eductyl; ***Swed.:*** Relaxit; ***Thai.:*** Circanetten; ***USA:*** Ceo-Two.

---

## Potassium Sodium Tartrate

E337; Kalii Natrii Tartras; Kalium Natrium Tartaricum; Rochelle Salt; Seignette Salt; Sodii et Potassii Tartras; Sodium Potassium Tartrate; Tartarus Natronatus; Tartrato de potasio y de sodio.

$C_4H_4KNaO_6,4H_2O$ = 282.2.

*CAS — 304-59-6 (anhydrous sodium potassium tartrate); 6381-59-5 (sodium potassium tartrate tetrahydrate); 6100-16-9 (sodium potassium tartrate tetrahydrate).*

**Pharmacopoeias.** In *Eur.* (see p.vi) and *US.*

**Ph. Eur. 5.0** (Potassium Sodium Tartrate Tetrahydrate). A white crystalline powder or colourless transparent crystals. Very soluble in water; practically insoluble in alcohol.

**USP 27** (Potassium Sodium Tartrate). Colourless crystals or a white, crystalline powder, with a cooling, saline taste. It effloresces slightly in warm dry air, the crystals often being coated with a white powder. Soluble 1 in 1 of water; practically insoluble in alcohol. Store in airtight containers.

### Profile

Potassium sodium tartrate has been used as an osmotic laxative (p.1239). It is also used as a food additive.

For the general properties of potassium salts, see p.1232, and of sodium salts, see p.1233.

### Preparations

***BPC 1973:*** Compound Effervescent Powder.

**Proprietary Preparations** (details are given in Part 3)

**Multi-ingredient:** ***Austria:*** Laxalpin; ***Fr.:*** Romarene; ***UK:*** Jaaps Health Salt.

---

## Proglumide (BAN, USAN, rINN)

CR-242; Proglumida; W-5219; Xylamide. (±)-4-Benzamido-*N*,*N*-dipropylglutaramic acid.

$C_{18}H_{26}N_2O_4$ = 334.4.

*CAS — 6620-60-6.*

*ATC — A02BX06.*

**Pharmacopoeias.** In *Chin.* and *Jpn.*

### Profile

Proglumide is a cholecystokinin antagonist with an inhibitory effect on gastric secretion. It is used in the treatment of peptic ulcer disease (p.1246) and other gastrointestinal disorders in usual doses of 400 mg two to three times daily by mouth before meals. It may also be given by intramuscular or intravenous injection in a dose of 400 to 800 mg daily.

### Preparations

**Proprietary Preparations** (details are given in Part 3)

***Austria:*** Milid; ***Ger.:*** Milid†; ***Hong Kong:*** Milid†; ***Ital.:*** Milid; ***Port.:*** Milid; ***Thai.:*** Milid†.

### Prune

Ameixa; Ciruela; Prunus.

#### Profile

Prune is the dried ripe fruits of *Prunus domestica* and some other species of *Prunus* (Rosaceae). It has laxative and demulcent properties.

#### Preparations

**Proprietary Preparations** (details are given in Part 3)

**Multi-ingredient: Arg.:** Cirulaxia; **Austral.:** Neo-Cleanse†; Prolax†; **Braz.:** Lumbriquil†; **Canad.:** Fruitatives; **Chile:** Tamarine; **Spain:** Jarabe Manzanas Siken†.

## Rabeprazole Sodium *(BANM, USAN, rINNM)*

E-3810; LY-307640; Rabeprazol sódico; Sodium Pariprazole. 2-({[4-(3-Methoxypropoxy)-3-methyl-2-pyridyl]methyl}sulfinyl)-1*H*-benzimidazole sodium.

$C_{18}H_{20}N_3NaO_3S$ = 381.4.

*CAS — 117976-89-3 (rabeprazole); 117976-90-6 (rabeprazole sodium).*

*ATC — A02BC04.*

#### Adverse Effects and Precautions

As for Omeprazole, p.1278.

#### Interactions

As for Omeprazole, p.1279. In healthy subjects, clinically significant interactions with diazepam, phenytoin, theophylline, or warfarin have not been demonstrated.

#### Pharmacokinetics

Peak plasma-rabeprazole concentrations are reached about 3.5 hours after a dose by mouth. The oral bioavailability is about 52% with the enteric-coated tablet formulation, because of first-pass metabolism, and does not appear to vary after single or repeated doses. Rabeprazole is 97% bound to plasma proteins. It is extensively metabolised in the liver by cytochrome P450 isoenzymes CYP2C19 and CYP3A4 to the thioether, thioether carboxylic acid, sulfone, and desmethylthioether. Metabolites are excreted principally in the urine (about 90%) with the remainder in the faeces. The plasma half-life is about 1 hour, increased two to threefold in hepatic impairment, 1.6 times in CYP2C19 slow metabolisers (see also Metabolism under Omeprazole, p.1280), and by 30% in the elderly.

◊ References.


1. Yasuda S, *et al.* Comparison of the kinetic disposition and metabolism of E3810, a new proton pump inhibitor, and omeprazole in relation to S-mephenytoin 4-hydroxylation status. *Clin Pharmacol Ther* 1995; **58:** 143–54.
2. Keane WF, *et al.* Rabeprazole: pharmacokinetics and tolerability in patients with stable, end-stage renal failure. *J Clin Pharmacol* 1999; **39:** 927–33.


#### Uses and Administration

Rabeprazole is a proton pump inhibitor with actions and uses similar to those of omeprazole (p.1280). It is given by mouth as rabeprazole sodium in the form of enteric-coated tablets. It is normally taken in the morning.

In the treatment of severe (erosive or ulcerative) **gastro-oesophageal reflux disease** (p.1242), the usual dose of rabeprazole sodium is 20 mg once daily for 4 to 8 weeks; in the USA, a further 8-week course is permitted for healing of erosive oesophagitis. Thereafter, maintenance therapy can be continued with 10 or 20 mg daily depending on the response. For symptomatic disease without erosive or ulcerative oesophagitis a dose of 10 mg may be given once daily for 4 weeks; once symptoms have resolved, a dose of 10 mg once daily may be given as necessary.

For the treatment of active **peptic ulcer disease** (p.1246), 20 mg daily is given for 4 to 8 weeks for duodenal ulcer and 6 to 12 weeks for gastric ulcer. For the eradication of *Helicobacter pylori* rabeprazole sodium may be combined with two antibacterials in a 1-week **triple therapy** regimen. Effective regimens include 20 mg twice daily combined with clarithromycin 500 mg twice daily and either amoxicillin 1 g twice daily or metronidazole 400 mg twice daily.

For **Zollinger-Ellison syndrome** (p.1247), the starting dose is 60 mg daily, adjusted according to response. Doses of up to 60 mg twice daily have been used.

◊ Reviews.


1. Prakash A, Faulds D. Rabeprazole. *Drugs* 1998; **55:** 261–7.
2. Anonymous. Rabeprazole. *Med Lett Drug Ther* 1999; **41:** 110–12.
3. Carswell CI, Goa KL. Rabeprazole: an update of its use in acid-related disorders. *Drugs* 2001; **61:** 2327–2356.


#### Preparations

**Proprietary Preparations** (details are given in Part 3)

**Arg.:** Pariet; Rabec; **Austral.:** Pariet; **Austria:** Pariet; **Belg.:** Pariet; **Braz.:** Pariet; **Chile:** Gastrodine; **Denm.:** Pariet; **Fin.:** Pariet; **Fr.:** Pariet; **Ger.:** Pariet; **Gr.:** Pariet; **Hong Kong:** Pariet; **India:** Rabeloc; **Irl.:** Pariet; **Ital.:** Pariet; **Jpn:** Pariet; **Malaysia:** Pariet; **Mex.:** Pariet; **Neth.:** Pariet; **Port.:** Pariet; **S.Afr.:** Pariet; **Singapore:** Pariet; **Spain:** Pariet; **Swed.:** Pariet; **Switz.:** Pariet; **Thai.:** Pariet; **UK:** Pariet; **USA:** Aciphex.

### Racecadotril *(rINN)*

Acetorphan; Racecadotrilo. (±)-*N*-{2-[(Acetylthio)methyl]-1-oxo-3-phenylpropyl}glycine phenylmethyl ester; *N*-[(*R*,*S*)-3-acetylthio-2-benzylpropanoyl]glycine benzyl ester; (±)-*N*-[α-(Mercaptomethyl)hydrocinnamoyl]glycine benzyl ester acetate.

$C_{21}H_{23}NO_4S$ = 385.5.

*CAS — 81110-73-8.*

*ATC — A07XA04.*

#### Profile

Racecadotril is an enkephalinase inhibitor that inhibits the breakdown of endogenous opioids thus reducing intestinal secretions. It is given by mouth in doses of 100 mg three times daily before meals for up to 7 days for the symptomatic management of acute diarrhoea (p.1241).

The *S*-form of racecadotril (sinorphan, ecadotril—see Natriuretic Peptides, p.964) has been investigated for hypertension and heart failure.

◊ References.


1. Baumer P, *et al.* Effects of acetorphan, an enkephalinase inhibitor, on experimental and acute diarrhoea. *Gut* 1992; **33:** 753–8.
2. Roge J, *et al.* The enkephalinase inhibitor, acetorphan, in acute diarrhoea: a double-blind, controlled clinical trial versus Loperamide. *Scand J Gastroenterol* 1993; **28:** 352–4.
3. Beaugerie L, *et al.* Treatment of refractory diarrhoea in AIDS with acetorphan and octreotide: a randomized crossover study. *Eur J Gastroenterol Hepatol* 1996; **8:** 485–9.
4. Salazar-Lindo E, *et al.* Racecadotril in the treatment of acute watery diarrhea in children. *N Engl J Med* 2000; **343:** 463–7.
5. Matheson AJ, Noble S. Racecadotril. *Drugs* 2000; **59:** 829–35.


#### Preparations

**Proprietary Preparations** (details are given in Part 3)

**Braz.:** Tiorfan; **Fr.:** Tiorfan; **Spain:** Tiorfan; **Thai.:** Hidrasec.

### Ramosetron Hydrochloride *(rINNM)*

Hidrocloruro de ramosetrón; YM-060. (−)-(*R*)-1-Methylindol-3-yl 4,5,6,7-tetrahydro-5-benzimidazolyl ketone hydrochloride.

$C_{17}H_{17}N_3O,HCl$ = 315.8.

*CAS — 132036-88-5 (ramosetron); 132907-72-3 (ramosetron hydrochloride).*

#### Profile

Ramosetron is a 5-$HT_3$ antagonist with general properties similar to those of ondansetron (p.1281). It is given as the hydrochloride for its antiemetic properties in the management of nausea and vomiting induced by cancer chemotherapy in usual doses of 300 micrograms once daily intravenously, or 100 micrograms once daily by mouth.

#### Preparations

**Proprietary Preparations** (details are given in Part 3)

**Jpn:** Nasea; **Thai.:** Nasea.

## Ranitidine *(BAN, USAN, rINN)*

AH-19065. *NN*-Dimethyl-5-[2-(1-methylamino-2-nitrovinylamino)ethylthiomethyl]furfurylamine.

$C_{13}H_{22}N_4O_3S$ = 314.4.

*CAS — 66357-35-5.*

*ATC — A02BA02.*

### Ranitidine Hydrochloride *(BANM, rINNM)*

AH-19065; Hidrocloruro de ranitidina; Ranitidini Hydrochloridum.

$C_{13}H_{22}N_4O_3S,HCl$ = 350.9.

*CAS — 66357-59-3.*

*ATC — A02BA02.*

**Pharmacopoeias.** In *Chin., Eur.* (see p.vi), *Jpn*, and *US.*

**Ph. Eur. 5.0** (Ranitidine Hydrochloride). A white or pale yellow, crystalline powder. It exhibits polymorphism. Freely soluble in water and in methyl alcohol; sparingly soluble in dehydrated alcohol; very slightly soluble in dichloromethane. A 1% solution in water has a pH of 4.5 to 6.0. Store in airtight containers. Protect from light.

**USP 27** (Ranitidine Hydrochloride). A white to pale yellow, practically odourless, crystalline powder. It is sensitive to light and to moisture. Very soluble in water; sparingly soluble in alcohol. A 1% solution in water has a pH of 4.5 to 6.0. Store in airtight containers. Protect from light.

**Stability and incompatibility.** References.


1. Chilvers MR, Lysne JM. Visual compatibility of ranitidine hydrochloride with commonly used critical-care medications. *Am J Hosp Pharm* 1989; **46:** 2057–8.
2. Wohlford JG, *et al.* More information on the visual compatibility of hetastarch with injectable critical-care drugs. *Am J Hosp Pharm* 1990; **47:** 297–8.
3. Williams MF, *et al.* In vitro evaluation of the stability of ranitidine hydrochloride in total parenteral nutrition mixtures. *Am J Hosp Pharm* 1990; **47:** 1574–9.
4. Galante LJ, *et al.* Stability of ranitidine hydrochloride at dilute concentration in intravenous infusion fluids at room temperature. *Am J Hosp Pharm* 1990; **47:** 1580–4.
5. Galante LJ, *et al.* Stability of ranitidine hydrochloride with eight medications in intravenous admixtures. *Am J Hosp Pharm* 1990; **47:** 1606–10.
6. Stewart JT, *et al.* Stability of ranitidine in intravenous admixtures stored frozen, refrigerated, and at room temperature. *Am J Hosp Pharm* 1990; **47:** 2043–6.
7. Montoro JB, Pou L. Comment on stability of ranitidine hydrochloride in total nutrient admixtures. *Am J Hosp Pharm* 1991; **48:** 2384.
8. Stewart JT, *et al.* Stability of ranitidine hydrochloride and seven medications. *Am J Hosp Pharm* 1994; **51:** 1802–7.
9. Crowther RS, *et al.* In vitro stability of ranitidine hydrochloride in enteral nutrient formulas. *Ann Pharmacother* 1995; **29:** 859–62.


#### Adverse Effects

As for Cimetidine, p.1255. Unlike cimetidine, ranitidine has little or no anti-androgenic effect, despite isolated reports of gynaecomastia and impotence.

◊ General references.


1. Wormsley KG. Safety profile of ranitidine: a review. *Drugs* 1993; **46:** 976–85.


**Carcinogenicity.** For a discussion of the possible association between histamine $H_2$-antagonists and cancer, including mention of a study with ranitidine, see Cimetidine, p.1256.

**Effects on the blood.** For a discussion of the adverse haematological effects of $H_2$-antagonists, see Cimetidine, p.1256.

**Effects on the cardiovascular system.** Similarly to cimetidine (p.1256), bradycardia,[1,2] atrioventricular block,[2] and cardiac arrest[3] have been reported rarely during ranitidine therapy. A positive inotropic effect, without significant changes in heart rate or blood pressure, has also been reported in healthy subjects[4] and pretreatment with ranitidine has blocked the cardiac depressant effects seen in some subjects given famotidine or nizatidine.[5] Although studies in critically ill patients[6] and healthy subjects[7,8] have found no adverse haemodynamic effects associated with ranitidine, it is likely that a small proportion of patients are more susceptible to the cardiovascular effects of ranitidine. Caution is recommended when ranitidine is given intravenously, particularly in patients with cardiovascular disease.


1. Johnson WS, Miller DR. Ranitidine and bradycardia. *Ann Intern Med* 1988; **108:** 493.
2. Tanner LA, Arrowsmith JB. Bradycardia and $H_2$ antagonists. *Ann Intern Med* 1988; **109:** 434–5.
3. Hart AM. Cardiac arrest associated with ranitidine. *BMJ* 1989; **299:** 519.
4. Meyer EC, *et al.* Inotropic effects of ranitidine. *Eur J Clin Pharmacol* 1990; **39:** 301–3.
5. Mescheder A, *et al.* Changes in the effects of nizatidine and famotidine on cardiac performance after pretreatment with ranitidine. *Eur J Clin Pharmacol* 1993; **45:** 151–6.
6. Vohra SB, *et al.* The haemodynamic effects of ranitidine injected centrally in optimally resuscitated patients. *Br J Hosp Med* 1989; **42:** 149.
7. Hughes DG, *et al.* Cardiovascular effects of $H_2$-receptor antagonists. *J Clin Pharmacol* 1989; **29:** 472–7.
8. Hilleman DE, *et al.* Impact of chronic oral $H_2$-antagonist therapy on left ventricular systolic function and exercise capacity. *J Clin Pharmacol* 1992; **32:** 1033–7.


**Effects on the endocrine system.** Unlike cimetidine (p.1256), ranitidine does not bind to androgen receptors and has little, if any, anti-androgenic effect. Studies in males taking ranitidine for the management of duodenal ulcer[1,2] reported no significant changes in the plasma concentrations of testosterone, luteinising hormone, follicle-stimulating hormone, or prolactin after up to 2 years of treatment; no significant changes in sperm concentration, motility, or morphology were noted.[1] There have been isolated reports of gynaecomastia,[3] loss of libido,[4] and impotence[5] associated with ranitidine, but in 9 patients with cimetidine-induced breast changes and impotence, transfer to ranitidine resulted in resolution of these symptoms.[6]


1. Wang C, *et al.* Ranitidine does not affect gonadal function in man. *Br J Clin Pharmacol* 1983; **16:** 430–2.
2. Knigge U, *et al.* Plasma concentrations of pituitary and peripheral hormones during ranitidine treatment for two years in men with duodenal ulcer. *Eur J Clin Pharmacol* 1989; **37:** 305–7.
3. Tosi S, Cagnoli M. Painful gynaecomastia with ranitidine. *Lancet* 1982; **i:** 160.
4. Smith RN, Elsdon-Dew RW. Alleged impotence with ranitidine. *Lancet* 1983; **ii:** 798.
5. Kassianos GC. Impotence and nizatidine. *Lancet* 1989; **i:** 963.
6. Jensen RT, *et al.* Cimetidine-induced impotence and breast changes in patients with gastric hypersecretory states. *N Engl J Med* 1983; **308:** 883–7.

**Effects on the eyes.** For a report of an increase in intra-ocular pressure associated with ranitidine, see under Cimetidine, p.1256. A cohort study involving 140 128 patients receiving anti-ulcer therapy, 70 389 of whom received ranitidine, found no evidence that any of the drugs studied were associated with a major increased risk of vascular or inflammatory disorders of the eye.[1]

For reference to loss of colour vision in a child receiving ranitidine see under Effects on the Nervous System, below.

1. García Rodríguez LA, *et al.* A cohort study of the ocular safety of anti-ulcer drugs. *Br J Clin Pharmacol* 1996; **42:** 213–16.

**Effects on the kidneys.** For reference to interstitial nephritis associated with $H_2$-antagonists including ranitidine, see under Cimetidine, p.1256.

**Effects on the liver.** There have been some case reports of ranitidine hepatotoxicity.[1] The increase in relative risk seen in a large cohort study involving 108 891 patients receiving antisecretory therapy was less for ranitidine (1.7:1) than for cimetidine (see p.1256).

1. Souza Lima MA. Ranitidine and hepatic injury. *Ann Intern Med* 1986; **105:** 140.

**Effects on the nervous system.** Ranitidine has been associated with adverse neurological effects including confusion,[1-8] loss of colour vision,[4] aggressiveness,[2,4,6] lethargy,[8] somnolence,[8] disorientation,[8] depression,[8] hallucinations,[1,7-9] and severe headache.[10] As with cimetidine (p.1256) these reactions occur mainly in the elderly, the severely ill, or patients with renal or hepatic impairment. Single-dose studies in young healthy subjects have found no adverse changes in performance, CNS function, or subjective assessment of mood after administration of ranitidine 150 or 300 mg by mouth.[11]

1. Hughes JD, *et al.* Mental confusion associated with ranitidine. *Med J Aust* 1983; **2:** 12–13.
2. Silverstone PH. Ranitidine and confusion. *Lancet* 1984; **i:** 1071.
3. Epstein CM. Ranitidine and confusion. *Lancet* 1984; **i:** 1071.
4. De Giacomo C, *et al.* Ranitidine and loss of colour vision in a child. *Lancet* 1984; **ii:** 47.
5. Mani RB, *et al.* $H_2$-receptor blockers and mental confusion. *Lancet* 1984; **ii:** 98.
6. Mandal SK. Psychiatric side effects of ranitidine. *Br J Clin Pract* 1986; **40:** 260.
7. MacDermott AJ, *et al.* Acute confusional episodes during treatment with ranitidine. *BMJ* 1987; **294:** 1616.
8. Slugg PH, *et al.* Ranitidine pharmacokinetics and adverse central nervous system reactions. *Arch Intern Med* 1992; **152:** 2325–9.
9. Price W, *et al.* Ranitidine-associated hallucinations. *Eur J Clin Pharmacol* 1985; **29:** 375–6.
10. Epstein CM. Ranitidine. *N Engl J Med* 1984; **310:** 1602.
11. Nicholson AN, Stone BM. The $H_2$-antagonists, cimetidine and ranitidine: studies on performance. *Eur J Clin Pharmacol* 1984; **26:** 579–82.

**Effects on the skin.** A report of vasculitic rash occurring in 3 patients undergoing ranitidine therapy.[1] In each case the rash cleared following withdrawal of the drug.

See also under Hypersensitivity, below, and also Cimetidine, p.1256.

1. Haboubi N, Asquith P. Rash mediated by immune complexes associated with ranitidine treatment. *BMJ* 1988; **296:** 897.

**Fever.** A report[1] of pyrexia associated with ranitidine. Apart from raised temperature the patient was otherwise well; fever resolved on discontinuation and recurred on rechallenge with ranitidine.

1. Kavanagh GM, *et al.* Ranitidine fever. *Lancet* 1993; **341:** 1422.

**Hypersensitivity.** Respiratory stridor and an urticarial rash occurred in a patient shortly after taking the first dose of ranitidine;[1] the symptoms responded to adrenaline subcutaneously.

1. Brayko CM. Ranitidine. *N Engl J Med* 1984; **310:** 1601–2.

**Meningitis.** A 30-year-old man developed aseptic meningitis on 3 occasions after use of ranitidine.[1] In each case symptoms resolved rapidly on withdrawal of the drug.

1. Durand JM, *et al.* Ranitidine and aseptic meningitis. *BMJ* 1996; **312:** 886. Correction. *ibid.*; 1392.

## Precautions

As for Cimetidine, p.1257.

**Helicobacter pylori testing.** For reference to the effect of ranitidine on the urea breath test for *Helicobacter pylori*, see p.1257.

**Hepatic impairment.** Sixteen of 27 patients with cirrhosis of the liver and indications for treatment with an $H_2$-antagonist (peptic ulcer, gastritis, or reflux oesophagitis) failed to respond to ranitidine 300 mg compared with 6 failures from 32 patients without cirrhosis. Famotidine 40 mg was given to 10 of the cirrhotic nonresponders and 8 still exhibited no response; 7 of these patients were given cimetidine 800 mg and only 1 responded. In the control group, all 3 patients given famotidine did not respond and only 1 responded when given cimetidine. It was concluded that the incidence of non-response to $H_2$-antagonists is increased in patients with liver cirrhosis but no explanation could be given for this effect.[1] Interestingly there is an earlier report of patients with cirrhosis demonstrating increased bioavailability and decreased clearance of ranitidine.[2]

1. Walker S, *et al.* Frequent non-response to histamine $H_2$-receptor antagonists in cirrhotics. *Gut* 1989; **30:** 1105–9.
2. Young CJ, *et al.* Effects of cirrhosis and ageing on the elimination and bioavailability of ranitidine. *Gut* 1982; **23:** 819–23.

**Porphyria.** Ranitidine is considered to be unsafe in patients with porphyria although there is conflicting experimental evidence of porphyrinogenicity.

**Renal impairment.** For evidence of reduced clearance of ranitidine in patients with renal impairment see Administration in Renal Impairment, below.

## Interactions

Unlike cimetidine (p.1257), ranitidine does not seem to affect cytochrome P450 to any great extent, and therefore is considered to have little effect on the metabolism of other drugs. However, as with other $H_2$-antagonists, its effects on gastric pH may alter the absorption of some other drugs.

◊ A review comparing the drug interactions of ranitidine with those of cimetidine.[1]

1. Smith SR, Kendall MJ. Ranitidine versus cimetidine: a comparison of their potential to cause clinically important drug interactions. *Clin Pharmacokinet* 1988; **15:** 44–56.

**Cisapride.** Peak plasma concentrations of ranitidine were achieved more rapidly in 12 healthy subjects who also took cisapride.[1] The clinical significance is questionable and such combinations have been used clinically, although the use of cisapride is now restricted in most countries.

1. Rowbotham DJ, *et al.* Effect of single doses of cisapride and ranitidine administered simultaneously on plasma concentrations of cisapride and ranitidine. *Br J Anaesth* 1991; **67:** 302–305.

## Pharmacokinetics

Ranitidine is readily absorbed from the gastrointestinal tract with peak concentrations in plasma occurring about 2 to 3 hours after administration by mouth. Food does not significantly impair absorption. The bioavailability of ranitidine following oral administration is about 50%. Ranitidine is rapidly absorbed following intramuscular injection, with peak plasma concentrations occurring in about 15 minutes. It is weakly bound, about 15%, to plasma proteins.

The elimination half-life is about 2 to 3 hours and is increased in renal impairment. A small proportion of ranitidine is metabolised in the liver to the *N*-oxide, the *S*-oxide, and desmethylranitidine; the *N*-oxide is the major metabolite but accounts for only about 4 to 6% of a dose. Approximately 30% of an oral dose and 70% of an intravenous dose is excreted unchanged in the urine in 24 hours, primarily by active tubular secretion; there is some excretion in the faeces. Ranitidine crosses the placental barrier and is distributed into breast milk.

**Distribution into breast milk.** A study in a mother given multiple doses of ranitidine showed higher concentrations in breast milk than in serum; the minimum milk concentration occurred between 1 and 2 hours after administration and the highest concentration was towards the end of the 12-hour dosing interval.[1] The amount that would be ingested by the infant could not be reliably estimated because of the variable milk to serum ratio.

1. Kearns GL, *et al.* Appearance of ranitidine in breast milk following multiple dosing. *Clin Pharm* 1985; **4:** 322–4.

**Enterohepatic recycling.** Some individuals exhibit a second peak in the plasma concentration of ranitidine, which could be due to enterohepatic recirculation. However, only 0.7 to 2.6% and 0.3 to 1.0% of a dose of ranitidine was excreted into the bile of 3 patients in 24 hours following 50 mg given intravenously or 300 mg by mouth, indicating that significant recirculation did not occur.[1]

1. Klotz U, Walker S. Biliary excretion of $H_2$-receptor antagonists. *Eur J Clin Pharmacol* 1990; **39:** 91–2.

**Neonates.** Renal function is limited in the first month of life, and reduced clearance of ranitidine would be expected. Blood samples taken from 27 full-term neonates given a single intravenous dose of ranitidine 2.4 mg/kg revealed the following pharmacokinetic data: elimination half-life, 3.45 hours; total volume of distribution, 1.52 litres/kg; total plasma clearance, 5.02 mL/kg per minute.[1] None of the infants had renal or hepatic impairment. In another study,[2] an elimination half-life of 6.61 hours was found in 13 full-term neonates administered ranitidine 2 mg/kg. See also Administration in Children, below.

1. Fontana M, *et al.* Ranitidine pharmacokinetics in newborn infants. *Arch Dis Child* 1993; **68:** 602–3.
2. Wells TG, *et al.* Pharmacokinetics and pharmacodynamics of ranitidine in neonates treated with extracorporeal membrane oxygenation. *J Clin Pharmacol* 1998; **38:** 402–7.

## Uses and Administration

Ranitidine is a histamine $H_2$-antagonist with actions and uses similar to those of cimetidine (p.1258).

Ranitidine may be given by mouth or parenterally by the intravenous or intramuscular routes. Although most preparations contain ranitidine hydrochloride, strengths and doses are expressed in terms of the base. Ranitidine hydrochloride 111.6 mg is approximately equivalent to 100 mg of ranitidine.

In the management of benign **gastric** and **duodenal ulceration** (p.1246) a single daily dose of 300 mg by mouth at bedtime or 150 mg twice daily (in the morning and at bedtime) is given initially for at least 4 weeks. A dose of 300 mg twice daily may also be used in duodenal ulcer. Where appropriate a maintenance dose of 150 mg daily may be given at bedtime. Ranitidine 150 mg twice daily may be given during therapy with NSAIDs for prophylaxis against duodenal ulceration. A suggested dose for the treatment of peptic ulcer in children is 2 to 4 mg/kg twice daily to a maximum of 300 mg in 24 hours.

For duodenal ulcer associated with *Helicobacter pylori* infection ranitidine in a usual dose of 300 mg once daily or 150 mg twice daily by mouth may be given as part of triple therapy in combination with amoxicillin 750 mg and metronidazole 500 mg, both three times daily, for 2 weeks. Therapy with ranitidine should then be continued for a further 2 weeks.

In **gastro-oesophageal reflux disease** (p.1242) the dose is 150 mg twice daily by mouth or 300 mg at bedtime for up to 8 weeks or, if required, 12 weeks. This may be increased to 150 mg four times daily for up to 12 weeks in severe cases. In pathological hypersecretory conditions, such as the **Zollinger-Ellison syndrome,** (p.1247) the initial oral dose is usually 150 mg twice or three times daily and may be increased if necessary; doses of up to 6 g daily have been used. Alternatively, an intravenous infusion may be given, initially at a rate of 1 mg/kg per hour; the rate may be increased by increments of 500 micrograms/kg per hour, beginning after 4 hours, if required.

For the management of patients at risk from **stress ulceration** of the upper gastrointestinal tract, parenteral therapy may be given as a slow intravenous injection of a 50-mg priming dose followed by a continuous intravenous infusion of 125 to 250 micrograms/kg per hour. Doses of 150 mg twice daily by mouth may be given once oral feeding is resumed.

In patients at risk of developing the **acid aspiration syndrome** (p.1240) during general anaesthesia, a dose of 150 mg by mouth may be given 2 hours before the induction of anaesthesia and preferably also 150 mg the previous evening. Alternatively, a dose of 50 mg may be given by intramuscular or slow intravenous injection 45 to 60 minutes before the induction of anaesthesia. In obstetric patients, at the start of labour a dose of 150 mg by mouth may be given and may be repeated at intervals of 6 hours if required.

In patients with chronic episodic **dyspepsia** (p.1242), a dose of 150 mg twice daily by mouth for up to 6 weeks may be given. For the short-term symptomatic relief of dyspepsia a dose of 75 mg, repeated if necessary up to a maximum of 4 doses daily, may be taken. Treatment should be restricted to a maximum of 2 weeks' continuous use at one time.

PARENTERAL DOSAGE.

The usual dose of ranitidine by intramuscular or intravenous injection is 50 mg, which may be repeated every 6 to 8 hours; the intravenous injection should be given slowly over not less than 2 minutes and should be diluted to contain 50 mg in 20 mL. For an intermittent intravenous infusion the recommended dose in the UK is 25 mg/hour given for 2 hours which may be repeated every 6 to 8 hours. A rate of 6.25 mg/hour has been suggested for continuous intravenous infusion although higher rates may be employed for conditions such as Zollinger-Ellison syndrome or in patients at risk from stress ulceration (see above).

DOSAGE IN RENAL IMPAIRMENT.

For dosage in renal impairment, see below.

**Administration in children.** The disposition of ranitidine in children is not significantly different from that in young adults and a dose of 2 mg/kg (approximately equal to an adult dose of 150 mg) by mouth has been used for the prevention of acid aspiration in children undergoing surgery.[1] A study in premature infants being treated with dexamethasone for bronchopulmonary dysplasia found that infusion of ranitidine 62.5 micrograms/kg per hour was sufficient to raise and maintain gastric pH above 4 to help protect against gastrointestinal bleeding and perforation.[2] Another study found 500 micrograms/kg twice daily to be sufficient for preterm infants, but that 1.5 mg/kg three times daily was needed for full-term infants.[3] A minimum dosage of 3 mg/kg daily was suggested for stress ulcer prophylaxis in older infants and children.[4]


1. Christensen S, *et al.* Effects of ranitidine and metoclopramide on gastric fluid pH and volume in children. *Br J Anaesth* 1990; **65:** 456–60.
2. Kelly EJ, *et al.* The effect of intravenous ranitidine on the intragastric pH of preterm infants receiving dexamethasone. *Arch Dis Child* 1993; **69:** 37–9.
3. Kuusela A-L. Long term gastric pH monitoring for determining optimal dose of ranitidine for critically ill preterm and term neonates. *Arch Dis Child Fetal Neonatal Ed* 1998; **78:** F151–F153.
4. Harrison AM, *et al.* Gastric pH control in critically ill children receiving intravenous ranitidine. *Crit Care Med* 1998; **26:** 1433–6.


**Administration in renal impairment.** A study in patients with varying degrees of renal impairment[1] found that the mean terminal half-life of ranitidine was increased from 2.09 hours in subjects with normal renal function to between 4.23 and 8.45 hours in patients with renal impairment, the degree of prolongation being proportional to the degree of impairment as measured by glomerular filtration rate. As a result of these findings it was recommended that the dose of ranitidine should be halved in patients with a glomerular filtration rate of 20 mL/minute or less. Licensed drug information therefore recommends that dosage of ranitidine be reduced in patients with severe renal impairment; in the UK the suggested doses for those with severe renal impairment are 150 mg daily by mouth or 25 mg for parenteral administration.

Ranitidine 150 mg daily provided adequate serum concentrations without excessive accumulation in 20 patients undergoing regular haemodialysis.[2] The serum-ranitidine concentrations fell by about 50% during a 4-hour haemodialysis session but less than 3% of the administered dose was removed and supplemental doses after dialysis were considered unnecessary.


1. Dixon JS, *et al.* The effect of renal function on the pharmacokinetics of ranitidine. *Eur J Clin Pharmacol* 1994; **46:** 167–71.
2. Comstock TJ, *et al.* Ranitidine accumulation in patients undergoing chronic hemodialysis. *J Clin Pharmacol* 1988; **28:** 1081–5.


**Cystic fibrosis.** A comparative study involving 29 patients with cystic fibrosis (p.123) found that ranitidine was more effective than cisapride in improving dyspeptic symptoms and gastric emptying and distension.[1] Antisecretory drugs are also used in this condition to decrease the inactivation of orally administered pancreatic enzymes.


1. Cucchiara S, *et al.* Ultrasound measurement of gastric emptying time in patients with cystic fibrosis and effect of ranitidine on delayed gastric emptying. *J Pediatr* 1996; **128:** 485–8.


**Immunomodulation.** Like cimetidine (see p.1258), ranitidine has been proposed to have immunoregulatory effects. However, ranitidine 300 mg twice daily had no effect on absolute CD4 cell counts or plasma HIV RNA in patients with HIV infection in a placebo-controlled trial.[1] Similarly, ranitidine had no significant benefit in patients with gastric cancer (see Malignant Neoplasms, p.1258).


1. Bartlett JA, *et al.* A placebo-controlled trial of ranitidine in patients with early human immunodeficiency virus infection. *J Infect Dis* 1998; **177:** 231–4.


**Skin disorders.** As with cimetidine (p.1259), ranitidine has been tried in various skin disorders. Ranitidine 300 mg twice daily by mouth has been reported to be of benefit as an adjuvant to local treatment with corticosteroids and a moisturising ointment in patients with *atopic dermatitis*.[1] There are reports of improvements in *psoriasis* (p.1137) following use of ranitidine,[2-4] although this is a field that is notoriously difficult to evaluate because of the chronic relapsing and remitting nature of the disease, and others have failed to show benefit.[5]


1. Veien NK, *et al.* Ranitidine treatment of hand eczema in patients with atopic dermatitis: a double-blind placebo-controlled trial. *J Am Acad Dermatol* 1995; **32:** 1056–7.
2. Witkamp L, *et al.* An open prospective clinical trial with systemic ranitidine in the treatment of psoriasis. *J Am Acad Dermatol* 1993; **28:** 778–81.
3. Smith KC. Ranitidine useful in the management of psoriasis in a patient with acquired immunodeficiency syndrome. *Int J Dermatol* 1994; **33:** 220–1.
4. Kristensen JK, *et al.* Systemic high-dose ranitidine in the treatment of psoriasis: an open prospective clinical trial. *Br J Dermatol* 1995; **133:** 905–8.
5. Çetin L, *et al.* High-dose ranitidine is ineffective in the treatment of psoriasis. *Br J Dermatol* 1997; **137:** 1021–2.


## Preparations

***BP 2003:*** Ranitidine Injection; Ranitidine Oral Solution; Ranitidine Tablets; ***USP 27:*** Ranitidine in Sodium Chloride Injection; Ranitidine Injection; Ranitidine Oral Solution; Ranitidine Tablets.

**Proprietary Preparations** (details are given in Part 3)
***Arg.:*** Acidex; Aludrox AC; Dualid; Fendibina; Gastrial; Gastrolets; Gastrosedol; Gastrozac; Insuflen; Luvier; Notrab; Ranitic; Ranitidi GNO; Ranitral; Ranitul; Raticina; Sustac; Taural; Telus; Teogrand; Tomag; Ulcotenk; Urgis; Vingional; Vizerul; Zantac; ***Austral.:*** Ausran; Rani 2; Ranihexal; Ranitic; Ranoxyl; Zantac; ***Austria:*** Digestosan†; Ranic; Ranityrol; Ulsal; Zantac; Zantarac; ***Belg.:*** Ranic†; Zantac; ***Braz.:*** Antagon; Antak; Antanidina†; Antidin; Aziliv; Gastrat†; Label; Logat; Neosac; Radan; Ranidin; Ranidina; Raniflex; Ranitak; Ranitil; Ranitinol; Ranition; Ranitrat; Regalil†; Tazepin; Ulcerit; Ulcerocin; Ulcoren; Zadine; Zilak†; Zylium; ***Canad.:*** Acid Reducer; Novo-Ranidine; Nu-Ranit; Peptic Relief†; Zantac; ***Chile:*** Aciflux; Ranicel; Ranitax; Tipac; Zantac; ***Denm.:*** Aducin; Kuracid; Ranicodan; Ranikur; Zantac; ***Fin.:*** Esofex; Ranicur; Ranil; Ranimex; Ranixal; Zantac; ***Fr.:*** Azantac; Raniplex; Ulcirex†; Zidac†; ***Ger.:*** Azuranit; Phamoranit; Ran Lich; Rani; Rani-nerton; Raniberl; Ranibeta; Ranibloc; Ranicux; Ranidura T; Ranimerck; Raniprotect; Ranitic; Ranitidoc; Sostril; Ulcolind Rani†; Zantic; ***Gr.:*** Alphadine; Aova; B-Alcerin; Baroxal; Bindazac; Blumol; Brixoral; Ceftrinal; Epadoren; Ezopta; Galebiron; Gaproxen; Gertocalm; Lomadryl; Lumaren; Narigen; Nipodur; Nitised; Odanet; Ptinolin; Raniclon; Restopon; Rothonal; Semuele; Smaril; Soredine; Specinor; Synthomanet; Tupast; Verlost; Zantac; Zoliden; Zurfix; ***Hong Kong:*** Gastril; Hyzan; Novo-Ranidine; Radin; Ranolta; Simetac; Synitidine; Zantac; ***India:*** Aciloc; Consec; Histac; R-Loc; Rantac; Zinetac; ***Irl.:*** Gertac; Ranitic; Ranopine; Xanomel; Zandine; Zantac; ***Israel:*** Apozan†; Zanidex; Zantab; Zantac; ***Ital.:*** Dolilux; Duoran; Raniben; Ranibloc; Ranidil; Sensigard; Ulcex; Zantac; ***Malaysia:*** Histac; Hyzan; Rintac; Vesyca; X'tac; Zantac; ***Mex.:*** Acloral; Agpisen; Alter-$H_2$†; Alvidina; Anistal; Apoprin†; Avintac; Azantac; Cauteridol†; Credaxol; Danitin†; Dinaxin; Galidrin; Gastrec; Gasyran; Iqfadina; Katalem; Microdit†; Microtid†; Neugal; Offentina; Radyn†; Ranepal; Ranifarma†; Ranifur; Ranisen; Ranulin; Ranzil†; Raudil; Redacid; Serranit; Serviradine; Sinhcloran†; Sirani†; Suronit†; Terodul; Ulcedin; Ulkodin; Ulsaven; Ultran; Zerandin†; ***Neth.:*** Zantac; ***Norw.:*** Noktone†; Ranacid†; Zantac; ***NZ:*** Zanidin†; Zantac; ***Port.:*** Gastridina; Gastrolav; Gastrulcer; Pep-Rani; Peptab; Peptifar; Quardin; Ran; Ranitine; Stacer; Ulcecur; Ulcerol; Zantac; ***S.Afr.:*** Histak; Ranihexal; Ranteen; Ulcaid; Ultak; Zantac; ***Singapore:*** Gastran; Histac; Hyzan; Lumaren; Neoceptin-R; Rani; Ranidine; Xanidine; Zantac; Zendhin; Zoran; ***Spain:*** Alquen; Arcid; Ardoral; Coralen; Denulcer; Fagus; Lake; Meticel; Quantor; Ran H2; Ranidin; Ranilonga†; Ranivel†; Ranix; Ranuber; Rubiulcer; Tanidina; Terposen; Toriol; Zantac; ***Swed.:*** Artonil; Inside; Rani-Q; Zantac; ***Switz.:*** Ranimed; Ranisifar; Ulcidine; Zantic; ***Thai.:*** Aciloc; Histac; Radine; Ranicid; Ranidine; Ratic; Ratica; Xanidine; Zanamet; Zantac; Zantidon; ***UAE:*** Rantag; ***UK:*** Gavilast; Indigestion Relief†; Ranitic; Rantec; Ranzac; Vivatak; Zaedoc; Zantac; ***USA:*** Zantac.

**Multi-ingredient:** ***Arg.:*** Duo Vizerul; Megalex.

# Ranitidine Bismuth Citrate *(BAN, USAN)*

A complex of ranitidine and bismuth citrate; Citrato de bismuto y ranitidina; GR-122311X; Ranitidine Bismutrex. *N*-[2-({5-[(Dimethylamino)methyl]furfuryl}thio)-ethyl]-*N'*-methyl-2-nitro-1,1-ethenediamine, compound with bismuth(3+) citrate (1:1).

$C_{13}H_{22}N_4O_3S,C_6H_5BiO_7$ = 712.5.

*CAS — 128345-62-0.*

*ATC — A02BA07.*

## Adverse Effects and Precautions

Ranitidine bismuth citrate would be expected to combine the adverse effects of both bismuth compounds (p.1252) and ranitidine (p.1285). Blackening of the tongue and faeces is common, and gastrointestinal disturbances, headache, mild anaemia, and altered liver enzyme values have been reported. Rarely, hypersensitivity reactions (including anaphylaxis), have occurred.

Ranitidine bismuth citrate should not be given to patients with moderate to severe renal impairment. It is not suitable for long-term or maintenance therapy because of the risk of bismuth accumulation. As with other antisecretory drugs, the possibility of malignancy should be considered when giving ranitidine bismuth citrate to patients with gastric ulcers since the drug may mask symptoms and delay diagnosis.

## Interactions

Ranitidine bismuth citrate would be expected to have the interactions of bismuth compounds (p.1252), and ranitidine (p.1286).

## Pharmacokinetics

Following oral administration, ranitidine bismuth citrate dissociates into its ranitidine and bismuth components in the stomach. For the pharmacokinetics of ranitidine, see p.1286, and for those of bismuth, see p.1253.

◊ References.


1. Lacey LF, *et al.* Comparative pharmacokinetics of bismuth from ranitidine bismuth citrate (GR122311X), a novel anti-ulcerant and tripotassium dicitrato bismuthate (TDB). *Eur J Clin Pharmacol* 1994; **47:** 177–80.
2. Koch KM, *et al.* Pharmacokinetics of bismuth and ranitidine following single doses of ranitidine bismuth citrate. *Br J Clin Pharmacol* 1996; **42:** 201–5.
3. Koch KM, *et al.* Pharmacokinetics of bismuth and ranitidine following multiple doses of ranitidine bismuth citrate. *Br J Clin Pharmacol* 1996; **42:** 207–11.


## Uses and Administration

Ranitidine bismuth citrate is a complex of ranitidine with bismuth and citrate, which releases ranitidine and bismuth in the gastrointestinal tract and therefore possesses both the actions of the bismuth compounds (p.1253) and of ranitidine (p.1286). It is used in the management of peptic ulcer disease (p.1246), and may be given in combination with antibacterials for the eradication of *Helicobacter pylori* infection and the prevention of relapse of peptic ulcer disease.

Doses are 400 mg twice daily by mouth; treatment is usually given for 4 to 8 weeks for duodenal ulceration and for 8 weeks for benign gastric ulceration. Ranitidine bismuth citrate should not be used for maintenance therapy, and a maximum of 16 weeks of treatment (two 8-week courses or four 4-week courses) may be given in a 12-month period. For duodenal ulceration where *H. pylori* infection is present, ranitidine bismuth citrate may be given as part of a 7-day triple therapy regimen, typically combined with any two of clarithromycin 500 mg twice daily, amoxicillin 1 g twice daily, or metronidazole 400 mg twice daily. Alternatively, a 14-day dual therapy regimen of ranitidine bismuth citrate combined with clarithromycin 500 mg two or three times daily may be given. In both regimens ranitidine bismuth citrate alone may be continued to a total of 28 days.

◊ References.


1. Bardhan KD, *et al.* GR122311X (ranitidine bismuth citrate), a new drug for the treatment of duodenal ulcer. *Aliment Pharmacol Ther* 1995; **9:** 497–506.
2. Peterson WL, *et al.* Ranitidine bismuth citrate plus clarithromycin is effective for healing duodenal ulcers, eradicating H.pylori and reducing ulcer recurrence. *Aliment Pharmacol Ther* 1996; **10:** 251–61.
3. Anonymous. Pylorid, H. pylori and peptic ulcer. *Drug Ther Bull* 1996; **34:** 69–70.
4. van der Wouden EJ, *et al.* One-week triple therapy with ranitidine bismuth citrate, clarithromycin and metronidazole versus two-week dual therapy with ranitidine bismuth citrate and clarithromycin for Helicobacter pylori infection: a randomized, clinical trial. *Am J Gastroenterol* 1998; **93:** 1228–31.


## Preparations

**Proprietary Preparations** (details are given in Part 3)
***Arg.:*** Pylorid; ***Austria:*** Helirad; Pylorisin; ***Belg.:*** Pylorid; ***Braz.:*** Pylorid; ***Canad.:*** Pylorid†; ***Denm.:*** Pylorid; ***Fin.:*** Pylorid; ***Gr.:*** Pylorid; ***Hong Kong:*** Pylorid; ***Irl.:*** Pylorid; ***Ital.:*** Elicodil; Pylorid; ***Mex.:*** Azanplus; ***Neth.:*** Pylorid; ***Norw.:*** Pylorid; ***Port.:*** Gastrimut†; Pylorid; ***Singapore:*** Pylorid†; ***Spain:*** Pylorid; ***Switz.:*** Pylorid; ***Thai.:*** Pylorid; ***UK:*** Pylorid; ***USA:*** Tritec†.

**Multi-ingredient:** ***Austral.:*** Pylorid-KA.

# Rebamipide *(rINN)*

Rebamipida. (±)-α-(*p*-Chlorobenzamido)-1,2-dihydro-2-oxo-4-quinolinepropionic acid.

$C_{19}H_{15}ClN_2O_4$ = 370.8.

*CAS — 90098-04-7; 111911-87-6.*

## Profile

Rebamipide is stated to possess cytoprotective properties and is used in the treatment of peptic ulcer disease (p.1246) and gastritis in usual doses of 100 mg by mouth three times daily.

## Preparations

**Proprietary Preparations** (details are given in Part 3)
***Jpn:*** Mucosta.

# Renzapride *(BAN, rINN)*

ATL-1251; BRL-24924A; Renzaprida. (±)-*endo*-4-Amino-*N*-(1-azabicyclo[3.3.1]non-4-yl)-5-chloro-*o*-anisamide.

$C_{16}H_{22}ClN_3O_2$ = 323.8.

*CAS — 88721-77-1; 112727-80-7.*

## Profile

Renzapride is a substituted benzamide with prokinetic actions on gastrointestinal motility. It also has 5-$HT_4$ agonist and 5-$HT_3$ antagonist activity. It is under investigation for the management of gastrointestinal disorders including irritable bowel syndrome.

◊ References.


1. Robertson CS, *et al.* A double-blind dose ranging study of BRL 24924 and metoclopramide on lower oesophageal sphincter pressure in healthy volunteers. *Br J Clin Pharmacol* 1989; **28:** 323–7.
2. Mackie A, *et al.* BRL 24924, a novel prokinetic agent, potentially valuable in diabetic gastroparesis. *Gut* 1989; **30:** A1489.
3. Staniforth DH, Pennick M. Human pharmacology of renzapride: a new gastrokinetic benzamide without dopamine antagonist properties. *Eur J Clin Pharmacol* 1990; **38:** 161–4.
4. Mackie ADR, *et al.* The effects of renzapride, a novel prokinetic agent, in diabetic gastroparesis. *Aliment Pharmacol Ther* 1991; **5:** 135–42.


# Rhubarb

Chinese Rhubarb; Rabarbaro; Rhabarber; Rhei Radix; Rhei Rhizoma; Rheum; Rhubarb Rhizome; Ruibarbo.

**Description.** Indian rhubarb (Himalayan rhubarb) consists of the dried rhizome and roots of *Rheum emodi*, *R. webbianum*, or some other related species of *Rheum*.

Rhapontic rhubarb (Chinese rhapontica) consists of the dried rhizomes of *R. rhaponticum*. It may occur as an adulterant of rhubarb, and pharmacopoeias specify a test to confirm its absence.

Garden rhubarb, of which the leaf-stalks are used as food, is derived from *R. rhaponticum*.

**Pharmacopoeias.** In *Chin., Eur.* (see p.vi), *Jpn*, and *Pol. Chin.* and *Jpn* also permit *Rheum tanguticum*, and *Jpn* also permits *R. coreanum*.

**Ph. Eur. 5.0** (Rhubarb). The whole or cut, dried underground parts of *Rheum palmatum* or of *R. officinale* or of hybrids of these two species or of a mixture. The underground parts are often divided; the stem and most of the bark with the rootlets are removed. It contains not less than 2.2% of hydroxyanthracene derivatives, expressed as rhein ($C_{15}H_8O_6$ = 284.2), calculated with reference to the dried drug. Protect from light.

### Adverse Effects and Precautions

As for Senna, p.1288.

### Uses and Administration

Rhubarb is an anthraquinone stimulant laxative used similarly to senna (p.1288). It also exerts an astringent action due to the presence of gallic acid derivatives and tannins.

It is used in homoeopathic medicine when it is known as Rheum.

### Preparations

***BP 2003:*** Compound Rhubarb Tincture.

**Proprietary Preparations** (details are given in Part 3)
***Ger.:*** Phytoestrol N.

**Multi-ingredient:** ***Arg.:*** Calculina; Oralsone Topic; Parodium; ***Austral.:*** Betaine Digestive Aid†; Hamamelis Complex†; Neo-Cleanse†; Pyralvex; SM-33 Adult Formula; ***Austria:*** Abfuhrtee; Eucarbon; Novocholin; Pyralvex; Sabatif; Silberne; St Bonifatius-Tee; ***Belg.:*** Eucarbon†; Pyralvex; ***Braz.:*** Bilifel†; Bisuisan; Boldopeptan; Camomila†; Epagogo†; Eparema; Epatovis†; Fargestium†; Fideine†; Figadosan†; Funchicorea†; Gotas Hepaticas†; Gotas Preciosas†; Hepatophil†; Puersan†; Regulador Xavier n-2†; Steitonit†; ***Canad.:*** Extra Strong Formula 12; Gasmol†; Herbal Laxative; Herbalax; Herbolax†; ***Fr.:*** Depuratum; Parodium; Pyralvex; Tisanes de l'Abbe Hamon no 17†; ***Ger.:*** Floradix Maskam†; Pyralvex; Redaxa Lax†; ***Hong Kong:*** Hepatofalk; Rheogen†; ***Irl.:*** Pyralvex; ***Israel:*** Davilla; Encypalmed; Eucarbon; Novicarbon; ***Ital.:*** Amaro Medicinale; Caramelle alle Erbe Digestive; Carbondifer†; Certobil†; Colax; Critichol; Depurativo†; Digelax; Dis-Cinil Complex; Eparema; Eparema-Levul; Eucarbon; Eupatol; Fitodorf Alghe Marine†; Fitodorf Rabarbaro†; Frerichs Maldifassi; Hepasil Composto†; Lactolas; Lassatina; Lassativi Vetegali; Magisbile; Mepalax; Neo-Heparbil†; Pillole Fattori†; Pyralvex; Rabarbaroni†; Raboldo†; Schias-Amaro Medicinale; Stimolfit; Tisana Arnaldi†; Tisana Cisbey†; Vegebyl†; ***Malaysia:*** Eucarbon; ***Neth.:*** Pyralvex; ***Port.:*** Pyralvex; ***S.Afr.:*** Pyralvex; Rubilax; ***Singapore:*** Pyralvex; ***Spain:*** Crislaxo; Laxante Bescansa Aloico; Menabil Complex; Pildoras Ferrug Sanatori†; Pyralvex; Solucion Schoum; ***Switz.:*** Dragees laxatives no 510†; Eucarbon†; Optilax†; Padma-Lax; Pyralvex; Schweden-Mixtur H nouvelle formulation; ***UK:*** Acidosis; Digestive; Fam-Lax; Fam-Lax Senna; HRI Golden Seal Digestive; Indian Brandee; Jacksons Herbal Laxative; Liminate†; Pegina; Pyralvex; Rhuaka†; Stomach Mixture; Wind & Dyspepsia Relief; ***USA:*** Black-Draught†.

---

## Roxatidine Acetate Hydrochloride

*(BANM, USAN, rINNM)*

Hidrocloruro de acetato de roxatidina; Hoe-062 (roxatidine); Hoe-760; Pifatidine Hydrochloride; TZU-0460. *N*-{3-[(α-Piperidino-*m*-tolyl)oxy]propyl}glycolamide acetate monohydrochloride.

$C_{17}H_{26}N_2O_3,C_2H_2O,HCl$ = 384.9.

*CAS — 78273-80-0 (roxatidine); 97900-88-4 (roxatidine hydrochloride); 78628-28-1 (roxatidine acetate); 93793-83-0 (roxatidine acetate hydrochloride).*

*ATC — A02BA06.*

### Adverse Effects and Precautions

As for Cimetidine, p.1255.

### Interactions

Unlike cimetidine (p.1257) roxatidine does not appear to affect cytochrome P450, and therefore is considered to have little effect on the metabolism of other drugs. However, like other $H_2$-antagonists its effects on gastric pH may alter the absorption of some other drugs.

### Pharmacokinetics

Roxatidine acetate hydrochloride is rapidly and almost completely absorbed from the gastrointestinal tract with peak concentrations in plasma occurring about 1 to 3 hours after administration by mouth. It is rapidly hydrolysed to the active desacetyl metabolite, roxatidine, by esterases in the liver, small intestine, and serum.

Over 90% of a dose is excreted in the urine as roxatidine and other metabolites. The elimination half-life of roxatidine is about 6 hours and is prolonged in renal impairment.

Small amounts of roxatidine have been reported to be distributed into breast milk.

### Uses and Administration

Roxatidine acetate hydrochloride is an $H_2$-antagonist with actions and uses similar to those of cimetidine (p.1258).

In the management of peptic ulcer disease the dose is 150 mg by mouth at bedtime or 75 mg twice daily for 4 to 8 weeks. Where appropriate a maintenance dose of 75 mg at bedtime may be given to prevent the recurrence of duodenal ulcers. In gastro-oesophageal reflux disease the recommended dose is 75 mg twice daily.

Roxatidine acetate hydrochloride may also be given intravenously for the treatment of upper gastrointestinal tract haemorrhage in a dose of 75 mg twice daily by slow intravenous injection or by intravenous infusion.

For dosage in renal impairment, see below.

◊ Reviews.

1. Murdoch D. Roxatidine acetate: a review of its pharmacodynamic and pharmacokinetic properties, and its therapeutic potential in peptic ulcer disease and related disorders. *Drugs* 1991; **42:** 240–60.

**Administration in renal impairment.** The dosage of roxatidine acetate hydrochloride should be reduced in patients with renal impairment. Suggested oral doses, based on creatinine clearance (CC), for patients on acute therapy are:

- CC 20 to 50 mL/minute: 75 mg at bedtime
- CC less than 20 mL/minute: 75 mg every 2 days

However, results in 6 patients with chronic renal failure and CC less than 20 mL/minute indicated that administration of the recommended dose of roxatidine acetate hydrochloride, 75 mg every other day, was inadequate to maintain gastric pH above 4 for more than 6 hours. Subsequent study in 8 patients showed that a dose of 75 mg daily was well tolerated and effective.[1]

1. Gladziwa U, *et al.* Pharmacokinetics and pharmacodynamics of roxatidine in patients with renal insufficiency. *Br J Clin Pharmacol* 1995; **39:** 161–7.

### Preparations

**Proprietary Preparations** (details are given in Part 3)
***Austria:*** Roxane†; ***Ger.:*** Roxit; ***Gr.:*** Roxane; ***India:*** Rotane; ***Ital.:*** Gastralgin; Neo H2; Roxit; ***Jpn:*** Altat; ***Neth.:*** Roxit; ***S.Afr.:*** Roxit†; ***Singapore:*** Roxane†; ***Spain:*** Roxiwas; Sarilen†; Zarocs.

---

## Senna

Sen.

*CAS — 8013-11-4.*

*ATC — A06AB06.*

**Description.** Senna obtained commercially from *Cassia senna* (*C. acutifolia*) (Leguminosae) is known as Alexandrian senna or Khartoum senna and that from *Cassia angustifolia* (Leguminosae) as Tinnevelly senna.

**Pharmacopoeias.** Senna fruit, from Alexandrian and Tinnevelly senna is included in *Eur.* (see p.vi) and *Int.* Senna leaf, from Alexandrian or Tinnevelly senna or both, is included in *Chin., Eur., Int., Jpn, Pol.*, and *US.*

**Ph. Eur. 5.0** (Senna Pods, Alexandrian; Sennae Fructus Acutifoliae; Alexandrian Senna Fruit BP 2003). The dried fruit of *Cassia senna* (*Cassia acutifolia*) containing not less than 3.4% of hydroxyanthracene glycosides, calculated as sennoside B ($C_{42}H_{38}O_{20}$ = 862.7) with reference to the dried drug. Protect from light and moisture.

**Ph. Eur. 5.0** (Senna Pods, Tinnevelly; Sennae Fructus Angustifoliae; Tinnevelly Senna Fruit BP 2003). The dried fruit of *Cassia angustifolia* containing not less than 2.2% of hydroxyanthracene glycosides, calculated as sennoside B ($C_{42}H_{38}O_{20}$ = 862.7) with reference to the dried drug. Protect from light and moisture.

**Ph. Eur. 5.0** (Senna Leaf; Sennae Folium). The dried leaflets of *Cassia senna* (=*Cassia acutifolia*), known as Alexandrian or Khartoum senna, or *Cassia angustifolia*, known as Tinnevelly senna, or a mixture of the two species. It contains not less than 2.5% of hydroxyanthracene glycosides, calculated as sennoside B ($C_{42}H_{38}O_{20}$ = 862.7) with reference to the dried drug. Protect from light and moisture.

**USP 27** (Senna). The dried leaflet of *Cassia acutifolia*, known in commerce as Alexandria senna, or *Cassia angustifolia*, known in commerce as Tinnevelly senna (Leguminosae).

### Sennosides

*CAS — 81-27-6 (sennoside A); 128-57-4 (sennoside B); 52730-36-6 (sennoside A, calcium salt); 52730-37-7 (sennoside B, calcium salt).*

**Pharmacopoeias.** In *US.*

**USP 27** (Sennosides). A partially purified natural complex of anthraquinone glucosides found in senna, isolated from *Cassia acutifolia* or *Cassia angustifolia* as calcium salts. It is a brownish powder. Soluble 1 in 35 of water, 1 in 2100 of alcohol, 1 in 3700 of chloroform, and 1 in 6100 of ether. A 10% solution in water has a pH of 6.3 to 7.3.

### Adverse Effects

Senna may cause mild abdominal discomfort such as colic or cramps. Prolonged use or overdosage can result in diarrhoea with excessive loss of water and electrolytes, particularly potassium; there is also the possibility of developing an atonic non-functioning colon. Anthraquinone derivatives may colour the urine yellowish-brown at acid pH, and red at alkaline pH. Reversible melanosis coli has been reported following chronic use.

**Abuse.** Prolonged use or abuse of senna laxatives has been associated with reversible finger clubbing,[1-4] hypokalaemia[3] and tetany,[1] hypertrophic osteoarthropathy,[4] intermittent urinary excretion of aspartylglucosamine,[2] hypogammaglobulinaemia,[3] reversible cachexia,[3] and hepatitis.[5]

1. Prior J, White I. Tetany and clubbing in patient who ingested large quantities of senna. *Lancet* 1978; **ii:** 947.
2. Malmquist J, *et al.* Finger clubbing and aspartylglucosamine excretion in a laxative-abusing patient. *Postgrad Med J* 1980; **56:** 862–4.
3. Levine D, *et al.* Purgative abuse associated with reversible cachexia, hypogammaglobulinaemia, and finger clubbing. *Lancet* 1981; **i:** 919–20.
4. Armstrong RD, *et al.* Hypertrophic osteoarthropathy and purgative abuse. *BMJ* 1981; **282:** 1836.
5. Beuers U, *et al.* Hepatitis after chronic abuse of senna. *Lancet* 1991; **337:** 372–3.

**Hypersensitivity.** Hypersensitivity reactions manifesting as asthma and rhinoconjunctivitis have been reported in those manufacturing[1] or dispensing[2] senna products. However, a study of 125 workers involved in the manufacture of laxatives found only 4 cases of occupational asthma, although sensitisation to senna or ispaghula dust was present in 18 and 9 of the workers respectively, and other airway, eye, and skin symptoms were relatively frequent.[3]

1. Helin T, Mäkinen-Kiljunen S. Occupational asthma and rhinoconjunctivitis caused by senna. *Allergy* 1996; **51:** 181–4.
2. Baggaley P. A shared allergy. *Pharm J* 1997; **259:** 724.
3. Marks GB, *et al.* Asthma and allergy associated with occupational exposure to ispaghula and senna products in a pharmaceutical work force. *Am Rev Respir Dis* 1991; **144:** 1065–9.

### Precautions

Senna should not be given to patients with undiagnosed abdominal pain or intestinal obstruction; care should also be taken in patients with inflammatory bowel disease. Prolonged use should generally be avoided.

Although anthraquinone derivatives may be distributed into breast milk the concentration achieved after usual maternal dosage is thought to be insufficient to affect the nursing infant (see also below).

**Breast feeding.** No adverse effects have been observed in breast-fed infants whose mothers were receiving senna, and the American Academy of Pediatrics considers[1] that it is therefore usually compatible with breast feeding. However, the *British National Formulary* states that anthraquinones (and particularly cascara and dantron) should be avoided in women who are breast feeding.

1. American Academy of Pediatrics. The transfer of drugs and other chemicals into human milk. *Pediatrics* 2001; **108:** 776–89. Correction. *ibid.*; 1029. Also available at: http://aappolicy.aappublications.org/cgi/content/full/pediatrics%3b108/3/776 (accessed 07/05/04)

**Colonic perforation.** There were early reports of colonic perforation with faecal peritonitis,[1,2] in one case fatal,[1] following the use of a senna preparation containing total sennosides 142 mg for bowel preparation prior to barium enema. In 1985, the strength of the UK preparation was halved to contain 72 mg of total sennosides; it was subsequently discontinued, although a similar preparation, at the higher strength, remains available in some countries. To reduce the risk of colonic perforation, patients with suspected stricture, inflammatory bowel disease, or impending obstruction should not receive a bowel stimulant.[2]

1. Galloway D, *et al.* Faecal peritonitis after laxative preparation for barium enema. *BMJ* 1982; **284:** 472.
2. Cave-Bigley D. Faecal peritonitis after laxative preparation for barium enema. *BMJ* 1982; **284:** 740.

### Pharmacokinetics

There is some absorption of anthraquinone laxatives after oral administration. Absorbed anthraquinones are metabolised in the liver. Unabsorbed senna is hydrolysed in the colon by bacteria to release the active free anthraquinones. Anthraquinones are excreted in urine and faeces and distributed into breast milk.

### Uses and Administration

Senna is an anthraquinone stimulant laxative (p.1239) that is used to treat constipation (p.1240) and for bowel evacuation before investigational procedures or surgery. The active anthraquinones are liberated into the colon from the sennoside glycosides by colonic bacteria and an effect usually occurs within 6 to 12 hours of administration by mouth.

For constipation, senna is usually given as tablets, granules, or syrup. It has also been given rectally as suppositories. In the UK, doses of senna preparations are usually expressed in terms of total sennosides calculated as sennoside B. The usual adult dose is 15 to 30 mg given by mouth as a single dose at bedtime. Children over 6 years of age have been given one-half the adult dose, and those aged 2 to 6 years one-quarter the adult dose. In the USA, the usual adult dose is 15 to 30 mg once or twice daily, expressed in terms of total sennosides.

For bowel evacuation before investigational procedures, a dose of 130 mg of sennosides may be given as a liquid preparation by mouth on the day before the procedure. A dose of 72 mg was formerly given in the UK, see Colonic Perforation under Precautions, above.

The purified sennosides (sennosides A and B), and their calcium salts (calcium sennoside A and calcium sennoside B) are used similarly to senna.

Senna is used in homoeopathic medicine.

### Preparations

***BP 2003:*** Senna Liquid Extract; Senna Tablets; Standardised Senna Granules;
***Ph. Eur.:*** Senna Leaf Dry Extract, Standardised;
***USP 27:*** Senna Fluidextract; Senna Syrup; Sennosides Tablets.

**Proprietary Preparations** (details are given in Part 3)

***Austral.:*** Bekunis Herbal Tea†; Bekunis Instant†; Laxettes; SennaPlus; Sennetabs†; Senokot; ***Austria:*** Bekunis; Colonorm; Darmol; Dragees Neunzehn Senna; Tara Abfuhrsirup†; X-Prep; ***Belg.:*** Darlin; Midro; Prunasine; Senokot†; Transix; ***Canad.:*** Agarol Extra; Agarol with Sennosides; Castoria†; Ex-Lax; Glysennid; GNC Herbal Laxative; Herbal Laxative; Laxative Pills; Natures Remedy; Senokot; Senolax†; X-Prep; ***Chile:*** Cholax; Naturlax; ***Denm.:*** Pursennid; ***Fin.:*** Exprep; Pursennid; Sennapur; ***Fr.:*** Herbesan Instantane; Senokot; X-Prep; ***Ger.:*** Abfuhrtee N; Bekunis Instant; Bekunis-Krautertee N; Depuran; Drix Abfuhr-Dragees†; Hermes Drix Abfuhr-Tee†; Hevertolax Phyto†; JuLax S†; Kneipp Abfuhr Tee N†; Kneipp Worisetten S†; Krauterlax-S†; Liquidepur; Maskam Krauter-Tee†; Midro Abfuhr; Midro Tee; Neda Fruchtewurfel; Ramend; Regulax N; X-Prep; ***Gr.:*** Bekunis; Pursennid; X-Prep; ***Hong Kong:*** Senokot; ***Irl.:*** Bekunis†; Senokot; ***Israel:*** Bekunis; Florilax; Jungborn; Laxikal Forte; X-Prep†; ***Ital.:*** Falquilax; Tisana Kelemata; X-Prep; ***Malaysia:*** Senokot; ***Mex.:*** Lagenbach; Sekalax; Senokot; ***Neth.:*** Sennocol; X-Praep; ***Norw.:*** Senokot; X-Prep; ***NZ:*** Senokot; ***Port.:*** Bekunis†; Pursennide; Senolax; X-Prep; ***S.Afr.:*** Black Forest Herbal Tea; Depuran; Senokot; Silaxon†; Soflax; X-Prep; ***Singapore:*** Senokot; ***Spain:*** Depuran†; Diolaxil; Justelax†; Laxante Bescansa Normal; Laxante Olan; Laxante Salud; Takata; X-Prep; ***Swed.:*** Pursennid; ***Switz.:*** Bekunis; Darmol; Demodon Neo; Fuca N; Grains de Vals Nouvelle formule; Midro; Tisane laxative H nouvelle formulation; Woerisetten S; X-Prep; ***Thai.:*** Senokot; ***UAE:*** Laxal; ***UK:*** Ex-Lax; Nylax with Senna; Senlax†; Senokot; Sure-Lax; ***USA:*** Black-Draught; Dosaflex; Dosalax†; Ex-Lax; Ex-Lax Gentle Nature†; Fletchers Castoria; Lax Pills; Maximum Relief Ex-Lax; Senexon; Senna-Gen; Senokot; Senokotxtra; X-Prep.

**Multi-ingredient:** ***Arg.:*** Agiolax; Calculina; Cirulaxia; Medilaxan; Prompt; Rapilax Fibras; ***Austral.:*** Agiolax; Chemists Own Natural Laxative with Softener; Coloxyl with Senna; Herb-a-Lax†; Neo-Cleanse†; Peritone†; Prolax†; Sennesoft; ***Austria:*** Abfuhrtee; Abfuhrtee EF-EM-ES; Agiolax; Carilax; Dr Ernst Richter's Abfuhrtee-tassenfertig†; Dr Ernst Richter's Abfuhrtee†; Dr. Ernst Richter's Abfuhrtee-Filterbeutel†; Entschlackender Abfuhrtee EF-EM-ES; Eucarbon; Frugelletten; Herbelax; Illings Bozner Maycur-Tee; Laxalpin; Laxolind†; Mag Kottas May-Cur-Tee; Midro Tee; Neda Fruchtewurfel; Planta Lax; Pursennid; Sabatif; St Bonifatius-Tee; The Chambard-Tee; ***Belg.:*** Agiolax; Eucarbon†; Manceau†; Solucamphre†; Tamarine†; Tisane Antibiliaire et Stomachique†; Tisane Depurative "les 12 Plantes"†; Tisane pour le Foie†; Tisane Purgative†; Tux; ***Braz.:*** Agiolax; Circanetten†; Estomafitino†; Fitolax; Florlax; Fontolax; Frutalax; Frutarine†; Laxan†; Laxarine; Laxtam; Novolax†; Plantax; Prompt†; Sene Composta†; Steitonit†; Tamaril; Tamarine; Tamarix; Varicell; ***Canad.:*** Cennlacs†; Cholasyn; Cholasyn II; Constipation; Control; Doulax; Ex-Lax Gentle Strength; Extra Strong Formula 12; Floralaxative†; Herbal Laxative; Herbalax; Herbolax†; Lapidar†; Laxaco; Mucinum; Prodiem Plus; Senokot-S; Thunas Laxative; ***Chile:*** Bilaxil; Naturlax; Tamarine; ***Denm.:*** Figen; ***Fin.:*** Agiolax; ***Fr.:*** Actisane Constipation Occasionnelle†; Agiolax; Boldoflorine†; Grains de Vals; Herbesan; Ideolaxyl; Laxasan†; Mediflor Tisane Contre la Constipation Passagere No 7; Mediflor Tisane Hepatique No 5; Modane; Mucinum a l'Extrait de Cascara; Mucinum†; Neo-Boldolaxine†; Pursennide; Santane $C_6$†; Tamarine; Tisane Clairo†; Tisane des Familles†; Tisane Grande Chartreuse†; Tisane Mexicaine†; Tisane Touraine†; Vegelax; ***Ger.:*** Agiolax; Alasenn; Dralinsa†; Floradix Maskam†; Heumann Abfuhrtee Solubilax N; Hevertolax duo; Kneipplax N†; Presselin Stoffwechsel-Tee Hapeka 225 N; Ramend Krauter; Salus Abfuhr-Tee Nr. 2†; Schwedentrunk mit Ginseng†; Schwedentrunk†; Sirmia Abfuhrkapseln†; ***Hong Kong:*** Agiolax; Mucinum Cascara; ***India:*** Pursennid-In; ***Irl.:*** Pripsen; ***Israel:*** Agiolax; Eucarbon; Jungborn; Lido Tea; Midro-Tea; Novicarbon; Pursennid†; ***Ital.:*** Agiolax; Carbondifer†; Colax; Confetti Lassativi CM; Cura†; Cuscutine; Depurativo†; Eucarbon; Fibrolax Complex; Fitolinea†; Florerbe Lassativa†; Lactolas; Lassatina; Midro; Ormobyl CM; Ortisan; Pursennid; Pursennid Complex†; Senna-Specie Composta; Stimolfit; Tamarine; Tisana Arnaldi†; Tisana Kelemata; ***Malaysia:*** Eucarbon; ***Mex.:*** Agiolax; Naturetti; ***Neth.:*** Agiolax; ***Norw.:*** Pursennid; ***NZ:*** Coloxyl with Senna; Laxsol; ***Port.:*** Agiolax; Bekunis†; Midro; Xarope de Macas Rainetas; ***S.Afr.:*** Agiolax; Rubilax; ***Spain:*** Agiolax; Bekunis Complex; Crislaxo; Jarabe Manceau; Jarabe Manzanas Siken†; Laxante Derly†; Laxante Sanatorium; Laxiplant†; Laxomax; Modane; Natusor Malvasen; Pruina; Puntual; Puntualex; Pursenid; Senalsor; Vegetalin†; ***Swed.:*** Lunelax comp†; ***Switz.:*** Adistop Lax†; Agiolax; Boldoflorine†; Capsules laxatives Nattermann Nr. 13†; Dragees aux figues avec du sene; Drix†; Eucarbon†; Fruttasan; Grains de Vals†; Lapidar 10; Laxativum Nouvelle Formule†; Laxiplant cum Senna†; Laxomild†; Linoforce; Optilax†; Phyto-Laxia; PhytoLaxin; Pursennide; Schweden-Mixtur H nouvelle formulation; Tamarine†; Tavolax†; The Brioni†; The Franklin†; The laxatif Solubilax†; Tisane laxative; Tisane laxative Natterman no 13 instant†; Tisane laxative Natterman no 13†; Tisane Provencale No1; Valverde Dragees laxatives; Valverde Sirop laxatif; ***Thai.:*** Agiolax; Circanetten; ***UK:*** Athera; Califig; Clairo Tea†; Cleansing Herbs; Dual-Lax Extra Strong; Dual-Lax Normal Strength; Fam-Lax Senna; Fibre Plus; Jacksons Herbal Laxative; Kas-Bah; Laxative Tablets; Liminate†; Lion Cleansing Herbs; Lustys Herbalene; Manevac; Modern Herbals Laxative; Modern Herbals Menopause; Natural Herb Tablets; Out-of-Sorts; Pilewort Compound†; Pripsen; Rhuaka†; Skin Cleansing; Tabritis; ***USA:*** Black-Draught†; Ex-Lax Gentle Strength; Perdiem; Senokot-S; X-Prep Bowel Evacuant Kit-1; X-Prep Bowel Evacuant Kit-2†.

## Simeticone *(BAN, rINN)*

Activated Dimethicone; Activated Dimethylpolysiloxane; Antifoam A; Antifoam AF; Simethicone *(USAN)*; Simeticona; Simeticonum.

*CAS — 8050-81-5.*

NOTE. Compounded preparations of simeticone may be represented by the following names:

- Co-simalcite *x/y (BAN)*—where *x* and *y* are the strengths in milligrams of simeticone and hydrotalcite respectively.

**Pharmacopoeias.** In *Eur.* (see p.vi) and *US.*

**Ph. Eur. 5.0** (Simeticone). It is prepared by incorporation of 4 to 7% silica into poly(dimethylsiloxane) with a degree of polymerisation between 20 and 400. It contains 90.5 to 99.0% of poly(dimethylsiloxane). It is a greyish-white, opalescent, viscous liquid. Practically insoluble in water and in methyl alcohol; very slightly soluble to practically insoluble in dehydrated alcohol; partly miscible with dichloromethane, with ethyl acetate, with methyl ethyl ketone, and with toluene.

**USP 27** (Simeticone). A mixture of fully methylated linear siloxane polymers containing repeating units of the formula $[-(CH_3)_2SiO-]_n$, stabilised with trimethylsiloxy end-blocking units of the formula $[(CH_3)_3SiO-]$, and silicon dioxide. It contains not less than 90.5% and not more than 99% of polydimethylsiloxane and not less than 4% and not more than 7% of silicon dioxide. A translucent, grey, viscous fluid. Insoluble in water, in alcohol, and in dehydrated alcohol; the liquid phase is soluble 1 in 10 of chloroform, of ether, and of benzene, leaving a residue of silicon dioxide. Store in airtight containers.

### Profile

Simeticone is a mixture of liquid dimeticones containing finely divided silicon dioxide to enhance the defoaming properties of the silicone. It lowers surface tension and when administered by mouth causes bubbles of gas in the gastrointestinal tract to coalesce, thus aiding their dispersion.

Simeticone is used for the relief of flatulence and abdominal discomfort due to excess gastrointestinal gas in disorders such as dyspepsia (p.1242) and gastro-oesophageal reflux disease (p.1242). Doses of 100 to 250 mg three or four times daily have been given. For many gastrointestinal disorders, it is given with an antacid.

Doses of 20 to 40 mg of simeticone have been given with feeds to relieve colic in infants (see Gastrointestinal Spasm, p.1242).

Simeticone is also used as a defoaming agent in radiography or endoscopy of the gastrointestinal tract.

◊ A brief review of the use of simeticone for gastrointestinal symptoms concluded that although it was commonly prescribed in combination with an antacid, there was no good evidence that it provided additional benefit. When used alone it probably helped to relieve minor postoperative and postprandial symptoms and it was a useful aid in upper gastrointestinal endoscopy.[1] However, some considered there was no convincing evidence that it was effective for the treatment of eructation, flatulence, or other signs or symptoms of excess gastrointestinal gas.[2]


1. Anonymous. Dimethicone for gastrointestinal symptoms? *Drug Ther Bull* 1986; **24:** 21–2.
2. Anonymous. Simethicone for gastrointestinal gas. *Med Lett Drugs Ther* 1996; **38:** 57–8.


### Preparations

***BP 2003:*** Simeticone for Oral Use; Simeticone Suspension for Infants;
***USP 27:*** Alumina, Magnesia, and Simethicone Oral Suspension; Alumina, Magnesia, and Simethicone Tablets; Alumina, Magnesia, Calcium Carbonate, and Simethicone Tablets; Calcium Carbonate, Magnesia, and Simethicone Tablets; Magaldrate and Simethicone Oral Suspension; Magaldrate and Simethicone Tablets; Simethicone Capsules; Simethicone Emulsion; Simethicone Oral Suspension; Simethicone Tablets.

**Proprietary Preparations** (details are given in Part 3)

***Arg.:*** Aesim; Aflat; Carbogasol; Carbogasol Forte; Factor AG; Mylanta Gas; Simecon; ***Austral.:*** Degas; Degas Infant Drops; Infacol; Medefoam; ***Austria:*** Disflatyl; Lefaxin; SAB Simplex; Setlers; ***Belg.:*** Polysilon†; Sili-Met-San; ***Braz.:*** Anflat; Dimezin; Finigas; Flagass; Flatex; Flatol; For Gas; Gastroflat; Gazyme†; Luftal; Mylanta Plus; Sanagas; Silidron; ***Canad.:*** Babys Own Infant Drops†; Gas-X; Maalox GRF†; Ovol; Phazyme; Silgas; ***Chile:*** Flapex; Gasorbol; Pepsidol; ***Denm.:*** Aeropax; Ceolat†; Minifom†; Mylicon; ***Fin.:*** Ceolat†; Cuplaton; Disflatyl; Minifom; ***Fr.:*** Siligaz; ***Ger.:*** Absorber HFV; Aegrosan; Busala†; Ceolat; Elugan; Endo-Paractol; Espumisan; Ilio-Funkton; Kompensan Dimeticon; Lefax; Meteosan; SAB Simplex; ***Gr.:*** Ceolat; ***Hong Kong:*** Dentinox Colic Drops; Disflatyl; Gasteel; Infacol; Ovol; ***India:*** Dimol; Tricaine-MPS; ***Irl.:*** Infacol; ***Israel:*** Simicol; ***Ital.:*** Meteosim; Mylicon; Polisilon; ***Malaysia:*** Cuplaton; Dentinox Colic Drops; Disflatyl; Gascoal; Gastyl; ***Mex.:*** Espaven Pediatrico; Liberan; ***Neth.:*** Ceolat; ***Norw.:*** Ceolat; Minifom; Siloxan; ***NZ:*** De-Gas; Infacol; Medefoam; ***Port.:*** Aero-Om; ***S.Afr.:*** Telament; ***Singapore:*** Cuplaton; Gascoal; Infacol; ***Spain:*** Aero Red; Disflatyl†; Enterosilicona; Pergastric†; Phazyme†; ***Swed.:*** Ceolat†; Minifom; ***Switz.:*** Aeropax†; Disflatyl; Flatulex; Lefax; Polysilane; Sili-Met-San†; Simet-AF; ***Thai.:*** Air-X; Babcon; Disflatyl; Gas-MM; Gas-X; Gassi; Gastyl; Logastin; Mylom; Ovol; Semeth; Sigas; Simcone; Simecon; Simetyl; ***UAE:*** Salinal; ***UK:*** Asilone Windcheaters; Dentinox Colic Drops; Infacol; Wind-Eze; Woodwards Colic Drops†; ***USA:*** Colicon; Degas; Extra Strength Mintox Plus; Flatulex; Gas Relief; Gas-X; Maalox Anti-Gas; Maalox Extra Strength Anti-Gas; Major-Con; Mylanta Gas; Mylicon; Phazyme; SonoRx.

**Multi-ingredient:** numerous preparations are listed in Part 3.

## Sodium Picosulfate *(BAN, rINN)*

DA-1773; LA-391; Natrii Picosulfas; Picosulfato de sodio; Picosulphol; Sodium Picosulphate. Disodium 4,4′-(2-pyridylmethylene)di(phenyl sulphate).

$C_{18}H_{13}NNa_2O_8S_2,H_2O = 499.4.$

*CAS — 10040-45-6.*

*ATC — A06AB08.*

**Pharmacopoeias.** In *Eur.* (see p.vi) and *Jpn.*

**Ph. Eur. 5.0** (Sodium Picosulfate). A white or almost white, crystalline powder. Freely soluble in water; slightly soluble in alcohol.

### Adverse Effects and Precautions

As for Bisacodyl, p.1251.

**Bowel evacuation.** Sodium picosulfate with magnesium citrate was considered a safe and effective bowel cleansing agent in adults[1] and children[2] with inflammatory bowel disease. They tolerated the preparation as well as patients with other colonic disorders with no adverse effect on their disease symptoms. Patients should be kept well hydrated (it may be appropriate to carry out bowel preparation in hospital in frail or elderly patients to avoid the risks of over- or underhydration[3,4]), and this procedure should not be used in suspected toxic dilatation of the colon.

In Australia, the Adverse Drug Reactions Advisory Committee has warned that low volume sodium picosulfate solutions may cause marked dehydration, hyponatraemia, other electrolyte abnormalities, and associated complications. Patients at particular risk include infants, the elderly, the frail, and those with congestive heart failure or with renal impairment.[5]


1. McDonagh AJG, *et al.* Safety of Picolax (sodium picosulphate-magnesium citrate) in inflammatory bowel disease. *BMJ* 1989; **299:** 776–7.
2. Evans M, *et al.* Safety of Picolax in inflammatory bowel disease. *BMJ* 1989; **299:** 1101–2.
3. Lewis M, *et al.* Bowel preparation at home in elderly people. *BMJ* 1997; **314:** 74.
4. Hanning CD. Bowel preparation at home in elderly people. *BMJ* 1997; **314:** 74.
5. Adverse Drug Reactions Advisory Committee. Electrolyte disturbances with sodium picosulphate bowel cleansing products. *Aust Adverse Drug React Bull* 2002; **21:** 2. Also available at: http://www.tga.health.gov.au/docs/html/aadrbltn/aadr0202.htm (accessed 07/05/04)


### Pharmacokinetics

Like bisacodyl (p.1251), sodium picosulfate is metabolised by colonic bacteria to the active compound bis(*p*-hydroxyphenyl)pyridyl-2-methane.

### Uses and Administration

Sodium picosulfate is a stimulant laxative related to bisacodyl (p.1251) used for the treatment of constipation (p.1240) and for evacuation of the colon before investigational procedures or surgery. When taken by mouth it stimulates bowel movements following metabolism by colonic bacteria. It is usually effective within 6 to 12 hours although when used with magnesium citrate for bowel evacuation an effect may be seen within 3 hours.

For constipation it is given by mouth as a single dose of 5 to 10 mg, usually at bedtime. Doses of 2.5 to 5 mg at night have been given to children aged 4 to 10 years; children aged less than 4 years have received 250 micrograms/kg.

For bowel evacuation, a dose of sodium picosulfate 10 mg with magnesium citrate (p.1272) is given in the morning and again in the afternoon of the day before examination. Doses are reduced in children.

### Preparations

***BP 2003:*** Sodium Picosulfate Oral Powder.

**Proprietary Preparations** (details are given in Part 3)

***Arg.:*** Agarol; Cirulaxia; Dagol; Dulcolax; Feen-A-Mint; Gotalax; Granulax; Kritel; Laxamin; Modaton; Modernel; Opalino; Rapilax; Rogelina; Trali; Verilax; Yodolin; ***Austral.:*** Durolax SP; ***Austria:*** Agaffin; Agiopic; Guttalax; ***Belg.:*** Dulcolax Picosulphate; Fructines†; Guttalax; Laxoberon; Obstilax†; Picolaxine†; ***Braz.:*** Diltin; Dulcolax Liquid†; Guttalax; Picolax†; Rapilax†; ***Chile:*** Aguala; Cronolax; Guttalax; Laxantil; Laxoberal; ***Denm.:*** Laxoberal; Picolon; ***Fin.:*** Laxoberon; ***Fr.:*** Fructines; ***Ger.:*** Abführtropfen†; Agiolax Pico; AgioPico Plus†; Darmol; Darmol Pico; Dulcolax NP; Laxans-ratiopharm Pico; Laxoberal; Mandrolax Pico†; Midro Pico; Regulax Picosulfat; ***Gr.:*** Guttalax; Laxatol; ***Hong Kong:*** Sur-Lax; ***India:*** Cremalax; ***Irl.:*** Laxoberal; ***Ital.:*** Euchessina CM; Falquigut; Gocce Antonetto†; Gocce Lassative Aicardi; Guttalax; ***Jpn:*** Laxoberon; ***Mex.:*** Anara; Laxoberon; ***Neth.:*** Dulcodruppels; ***Norw.:*** Laxoberal; ***Port.:*** Guttalax; Laxodal; ***Singapore:*** Sur-Lax†; ***Spain:*** Contumax; Elimin†; Evacuol; Gutalax; Laxonol†; Lubrilax; Skilax; **Swed.:** Cilaxoral; Laxoberal; **Switz.:** Fructines; Guttalax†; Laxoberon; **UK:** Dulcolax; Laxoberal.

**Multi-ingredient:** **Arg.:** Agarol; **Austral.:** Colonprep; Picolax; Picoprep; Prep Kit-C; **Belg.:** Pilules de Vichy†; **Braz.:** Cronoplex; Forlax; **Irl.:** Picolax; **Israel:** Pico-Salax†; **Malaysia:** Picroprep; **Norw.:** Pico-Salax†; **NZ:** Picoprep; **Spain:** Emuliquen Laxante; **Swed.:** Pico-Salax†; **Switz.:** Laxasan; Pico-Salax†; **UK:** Picolax.

## Anhydrous Sodium Sulfate

Anhydrous Sodium Sulphate; Dried Sodium Sulphate; Exsiccated Sodium Sulphate; Natrii Sulfas Anhydricus; Natrium Sulfuricum Siccatum; Sulfato sódico anhidro.

$Na_2SO_4$ = 142.0.
*CAS — 7757-82-6.*
*ATC — A06AD13; A12CA02.*

**Pharmacopoeias.** In *Chin., Eur.* (see p.vi), *Int., Pol.,* and *Viet. US* includes a single monograph for both the anhydrous form and the decahydrate.

**Ph. Eur. 5.0** (Sodium Sulphate, Anhydrous). A white, hygroscopic powder. Freely soluble in water. Store in airtight containers.

**USP 27** (Sodium Sulfate). It contains 10 molecules of water of hydration or is anhydrous. The decahydrate loses between 51 and 57% of its weight on drying and the anhydrous form loses not more than 0.5% of its weight. Large, colourless, odourless, transparent crystals or a granular powder. It effloresces rapidly in air, liquefies in its water of hydration at about 33°, and loses all of its water of hydration at about 100°. Freely soluble in water; insoluble in alcohol; soluble in glycerol. Store in airtight containers, preferably at a temperature not exceeding 30°.

## Sodium Sulfate

E514; Glauber's Salt; Natrii Sulfas Decahydricus; Natrii Sulphas; Natrium Sulfuricum Crystallisatum; Sodium Sulphate; Sodium Sulphate Decahydrate; Sulfato sódico.

$Na_2SO_4,10H_2O$ = 322.2.
*CAS — 7727-73-3 (sodium sulfate decahydrate).*
*ATC — A06AD13; A12CA02.*

**Pharmacopoeias.** In *Chin., Eur.* (see p.vi), *Int., Pol.,* and *Viet. US* includes a single monograph for both the anhydrous form and the decahydrate.

**Ph. Eur. 5.0** (Sodium Sulphate Decahydrate; Sodium Sulphate BP 2003). A white, crystalline powder or colourless, transparent crystals. Freely soluble in water; practically insoluble in alcohol. It partly dissolves in its own water of crystallisation at about 33°. It loses between 52.0 and 57.0% of its weight on drying.

**USP 27** (Sodium Sulfate). It contains 10 molecules of water of hydration or is anhydrous. The decahydrate loses between 51 and 57% of its weight on drying and the anhydrous form loses not more than 0.5% of its weight. Large, colourless, odourless, transparent crystals or a granular powder. It effloresces rapidly in air, liquefies in its water of hydration at about 33°, and loses all of its water of hydration at about 100°. Freely soluble in water; insoluble in alcohol; soluble in glycerol. Store in airtight containers, preferably at a temperature not exceeding 30°.

### Profile

Sodium sulfate is an osmotic laxative (p.1239). It has been given by mouth in a usual dose of 5 to 10 g daily. It is also given in dilute solution with a high molecular weight macrogol for prompt bowel evacuation before investigational procedures or surgery (see Macrogols, p.1709).

Sodium sulfate is also used as a diluent for colours in foods.

For the general properties of sodium salts, see p.1233.

### Preparations

***USP 27:*** Sodium Sulfate Injection.

**Proprietary Preparations** (details are given in Part 3)
**Austral.:** Celloids SS 69†; **UK:** Fynnon Salt†.

**Multi-ingredient:** **Arg.:** Magnesia Phosphorica I Oligoplex; **Austral.:** Duo Celloids SPSS†; Duo Celloids SSMP†; Duo Celloids SSPC†; Duo Celloids SSS†; Iron Compound†; Liv-Detox†; Silybum Complex†; **Belg.:** Kruschels†; Normogastryl†; **Canad.:** Normo Gastryl; **Fr.:** Actisoufre; Azym†; Digedryl; Hepargitol; Jecobiase†; Normogastryl; Oxyboldine; Prefagyl; **Ital.:** Argirofedrina; Carbotiol†; **Spain:** Boldosal†; Darmen Salt; Digestovital; Leberetic; Lebersal; Normogastryl†; Salcedol; **Switz.:** Drix†; Normogastryl†; Padma-Lax; Thiorubrol†; **Thai.:** Ulgastrin; **UK:** Juno Junipah†; New Era Zief†; **USA:** Triv.

## Sodium Tartrate

E335 (sodium tartrate or monosodium tartrate); Tartrato sódico.

$C_2H_4O_2(CO_2Na)_2,2H_2O$ = 230.1.
*CAS — 868-18-8 (anhydrous sodium tartrate); 6106-24-7 (sodium tartrate dihydrate).*
*ATC — A06AD21.*

### Profile

Sodium tartrate has been used as an osmotic laxative. It is used as a food additive.

For the general properties of sodium salts, see p.1233.

### Preparations

**Proprietary Preparations** (details are given in Part 3)

**Multi-ingredient:** **Arg.:** Oral-B Enjuague Bucal Amosan; **Port.:** Dentolamina†; Sais Zitos†.

## Sterculia

E416; Goma Esterculia; Indian Tragacanth; Karaya; Karaya Gum; Sterculia Gum.

*CAS — 9000-36-6.*
*ATC — A06AC03.*

**Pharmacopoeias.** In *Br.* and *Fr.*

**BP 2003** (Sterculia). The gum obtained from *Sterculia urens* and other species of *Sterculia*. Irregular or vermiform pieces, greyish-white with a brown or pink tinge, with an odour resembling that of acetic acid. It contains not less than 14.0% of volatile acid (or not less than 10.0% if supplied in powdered form), calculated as acetic acid. Sparingly soluble in water, but swells into a homogeneous, adhesive, gelatinous mass; practically insoluble in alcohol. Store at a temperature not exceeding 25°.

### Adverse Effects and Precautions

As for Ispaghula, p.1268. There is a risk of intestinal or oesophageal obstruction and faecal impaction, especially if such compounds are swallowed dry. Therefore they should always be taken with sufficient fluid and should not be taken immediately before going to bed. They should be avoided by patients who have difficulty swallowing.

### Uses and Administration

Sterculia is used similarly to ispaghula (p.1268) as a bulk laxative and for adjusting faecal consistency. It has also been used as an aid to appetite control in the management of obesity (p.1583) but there is little evidence of efficacy. It is usually taken in the form of granules by mouth once or twice daily after meals. The granules are washed down without chewing with plenty of water. They may also be taken sprinkled onto soft foods such as yogurt.

Sterculia is used topically, as a paste or powder, for skin protection and sealing in the fitting of ileostomy and colostomy appliances. It has also been used in dental fixative powders, and as an emulsifier and stabiliser in foods.

### Preparations

***BP 2003:*** Sterculia Granules.

**Proprietary Preparations** (details are given in Part 3)
**Austral.:** Normafibe; **Belg.:** Calox†; Normacol; **Braz.:** Corega; **Canad.:** Normacol; **Fr.:** Enteromucilage†; Inolaxine; Norgagil†; Normacol; Prefinet†; **Ger.:** Decorpa; Granamon; **Hong Kong:** Inolaxine†; Normacol; **Irl.:** Normacol; **Ital.:** Normacol; **Malaysia:** Normacol; **Neth.:** Normacol; **NZ:** Normacol; **S.Afr.:** Normacol; **Singapore:** Normacol; **Swed.:** Inolaxol; **Switz.:** Colosan mite; Inolaxine; Normacol; **Thai.:** Normacol; **UK:** Normacol.

**Multi-ingredient:** **Austral.:** Alvercol; Enterocare†; Granocol; Normacol Plus; **Belg.:** Normacol Antispasmodique; Normacol Plus; **Braz.:** Formitonicum†; **Fr.:** Kaologeais; Karayal; Normacol a la Bourdaine; Poly-Karaya; **Ger.:** Karaya Bismuth†; **Hong Kong:** Alvercol†; Normacol Plus; **India:** Kanormal; **Irl.:** Alvercol†; Normacol Plus; **Neth.:** Normacol Plus; **NZ:** Granocol; Normacol Plus; **Port.:** Normacol Plus; **S.Afr.:** Alvercol; Normacol Plus; **Singapore:** Normacol Plus; **Spain:** Normacol Forte; **Switz.:** Colosan plus; Normacol (avec bourdaine); Poly-Karaya†; **UK:** Normacol Plus; Spasmonal Fibre†.

## Sucralfate *(BAN, USAN, rINN)*

Sucralfato. Sucrose hydrogen sulphate basic aluminium salt; Sucrose octakis(hydrogen sulphate) aluminium complex; β-D-Fructofuranosyl-α-D-glucopyranoside octakis (hydrogen sulphate) aluminium complex.

$C_{12}H_mAl_{16}O_nS_8$.
*CAS — 54182-58-0.*
*ATC — A02BX02.*

**Pharmacopoeias.** In *Chin., Jpn,* and *US.*

**USP 27** (Sucralfate). The hydrous basic aluminium salt of sucrose octasulfate. Store in airtight containers.

### Adverse Effects and Precautions

Constipation is the most frequently reported adverse effect of sucralfate although diarrhoea, nausea, or gastric discomfort may also occur. Dry mouth, dizziness, drowsiness, headache, vertigo, back pain, skin rashes, and hypersensitivity reactions such as pruritus have been reported.

Great caution is needed in patients with renal impairment (below) as absorption and accumulation of aluminium may cause adverse effects.

**Bezoar formation.** As of March 1999, the UK Committee on Safety of Medicines was aware of 7 reports worldwide of bezoar formation associated with sucralfate use in intensive care patients.[1] It advised caution in the use of sucralfate in seriously ill patients because of the risks of bezoar formation and intestinal obstruction.[1] Patients with delayed gastric emptying or receiving concomitant enteral feeds may be at increased risk.

1. Committee on Safety of Medicines/Medicines Control Agency. Bezoar formation with sulcralfate [sic] (Antepsin). *Current Problems* 1999; **25:** 6. Also available at: http://www.mca.gov.uk/ourwork/monitorsafequalmed/currentproblems/volume25mar.htm (accessed 07/05/04)

**Renal impairment.** Sucralfate under acid conditions can release aluminium ions that may be absorbed systemically. Significant increases in the urinary excretion of aluminium have been observed in healthy subjects given sucralfate 4 g daily,[1,2] reflecting gastrointestinal absorption of aluminium; aluminium concentrations in serum and urine were significantly higher in patients with chronic renal insufficiency than in subjects with normal renal function.[3] Aluminium toxicity in patients with normal renal function receiving sucralfate would not be expected, but seizures, muscle weakness, bone pain,[1] and severe aluminium encephalopathy[4] have been reported in patients with end-stage renal disease requiring dialysis. Sucralfate should be used with caution in patients with renal impairment, especially if other aluminium-containing agents are also taken, and such patients should be monitored for signs of aluminium toxicity.[5]

1. Robertson JA, *et al.* Sucralfate, intestinal aluminium absorption, and aluminium toxicity in a patient on dialysis. *Ann Intern Med* 1989; **111:** 179–81.
2. Allain P, *et al.* Plasma and urine aluminium concentrations in healthy subjects after administration of sucralfate. *Br J Clin Pharmacol* 1990; **29:** 391–5.
3. Burgess E, *et al.* Aluminum absorption and excretion following sucralfate therapy in chronic renal insufficiency. *Am J Med* 1992; **92:** 471–5.
4. Withers DJ, *et al.* Encephalopathy in patient taking aluminium-containing agents, including sucralfate. *Lancet* 1989; **ii:** 674.
5. Hemstreet BA. Use of sucralfate in renal failure. *Ann Pharmacother* 2001; **35:** 360–4.

### Interactions

Sucralfate may interfere with the absorption of other drugs and it has been suggested that there should be an interval of 2 hours between the administration of sucralfate and other concurrent non-antacid medication. Some of the drugs reported to be affected by sucralfate include cimetidine, ranitidine, digoxin, ketoconazole, phenytoin, fluoroquinolone antibacterials, tetracycline, quinidine, theophylline, levothyroxine, and possibly warfarin. The recommended interval between sucralfate and antacids is 30 minutes. An interval of 1 hour should elapse between sucralfate administration and enteral feeding.

### Pharmacokinetics

Sucralfate is only slightly absorbed from the gastrointestinal tract following oral administration. However, there can be some release of aluminium ions and of sucrose sulfate and small quantities of sucrose sulfate may be absorbed and excreted, primarily in the urine; some absorption of aluminium may also occur (see Renal Impairment, above).

### Uses and Administration

Sucralfate is a cytoprotective drug that, under acid gastrointestinal conditions, forms an adherent complex with proteins which coats the gastric mucosa and is reported to have a special affinity for ulcer sites. It also inhibits the action of pepsin and adsorbs bile salts.

Sucralfate is used in the treatment of peptic ulcer disease (p.1246) and chronic gastritis. It is given by mouth and should be taken on an empty stomach before meals and at bedtime. The usual dose is 1 g four times daily or 2 g twice daily for 4 to 8 weeks; if necessary the dose may be increased to a maximum of 8 g daily. If longer-term therapy is required sucralfate may be given for up to 12 weeks. Where appropriate a maintenance dose of 1 g twice daily may be given to prevent the recurrence of duodenal ulcers.

For prophylaxis of stress ulceration the usual dose of sucralfate is 1 g six times daily; a dose of 8 g daily should not be exceeded.

**Gastrointestinal bleeding.** Sucralfate is an effective drug for the prophylaxis and management of stress-induced gastrointestinal bleeding in severely ill patients, and may reduce the risk of late-onset pneumonia compared with an $H_2$-antagonist.[1] For further discussion of stress ulceration and bleeding, including the use of sucralfate, see under Peptic Ulcer Disease, p.1246. There is also some evidence from another study[2] that sucralfate reduces gastrointestinal bleeding associated with NSAID use, although it does not prevent drug-induced gastric erosion.


1. Prod'hom G, *et al.* Nosocomial pneumonia in mechanically ventilated patients receiving antacid, ranitidine, or sucralfate as prophylaxis for stress ulcer: a randomized controlled trial. *Ann Intern Med* 1994; **120:** 653–62.
2. Hudson N, *et al.* Effect of sucralfate on aspirin induced mucosal injury and impaired haemostasis in humans. *Gut* 1997; **41:** 19–23.


**Gastro-oesophageal reflux disease.** Although sucralfate has been tried for gastro-oesophageal reflux disease (p.1242) the results of studies have been inconsistent.[1-3]


1. Orlando RC. Sucralfate therapy and reflux esophagitis: an overview. *Am J Med* 1991; **91** (suppl 2A): 123S–124S.
2. Klinkenberg-Knol EC, *et al.* Pharmacological management of gastro-oesophageal reflux disease. *Drugs* 1995; **49:** 695–710.
3. Simon B, *et al.* Sucralfate gel versus placebo in patients with non-erosive gastro-oesophageal reflux disease. *Aliment Pharmacol Ther* 1996; **10:** 441–6.


**Mouth ulceration.** Sucralfate has been investigated as a mouth rinse in the treatment and prophylaxis of stomatitis induced by cancer chemotherapy[1-3] although evidence of benefit for any drug is ambiguous (see Mucositis, p.497). One study[2] in 40 patients found a significant reduction in symptoms among 23 evaluable patients given sucralfate prophylactically. Seven patients withdrew due to aggravation of chemotherapy-induced nausea. It was suggested that to overcome this problem, the suspension should have a neutral taste, should not be swallowed after rinsing, and that rinsing should not be commenced until nausea had ceased. However, another study[4] involving 80 patients treated with fluorouracil for colorectal cancer found no significant difference in self-reported mucositis symptoms between patients given sucralfate suspension and those given placebo.

Sucralfate has also been reported to be of benefit in patients with recurrent aphthous stomatitis (mouth ulceration—p.1245). A study involving 21 such patients over 2 years found that topical application of sucralfate suspension 4 times daily was superior to treatment with an antacid (aluminium hydroxide with magnesium hydroxide) or placebo.[5]


1. Pfeiffer P, *et al.* A prospective pilot study on the effect of sucralfate mouth-swishing in reducing stomatitis during radiotherapy of the oral cavity. *Acta Oncol* 1990; **29:** 471–3.
2. Pfeiffer P, *et al.* Effect of prophylactic sucralfate suspension on stomatitis induced by cancer chemotherapy: a randomized, double-blind cross-over study. *Acta Oncol* 1990; **29:** 171–3.
3. Allison RR, *et al.* Symptomatic acute mucositis can be minimized or prophylaxed [sic] by the combination of sucralfate and fluconazole. *Cancer Invest* 1995; **13:** 16–22.
4. Nottage M, *et al.* Sucralfate mouthwash for prevention and treatment of 5-fluorouracil-induced mucositis: a randomized, placebo-controlled trial. *Support Care Cancer* 2003; **11:** 41–7.
5. Rattan J, *et al.* Sucralfate suspension as a treatment of recurrent aphthous stomatitis. *J Intern Med* 1994; **236:** 341–3.


**Skin ulceration.** Sucralfate has reportedly been applied topically with some success to treat bleeding skin ulcers (p.1139) associated with malignancy,[1] and to promote the healing of venous stasis ulcers.[2] It has been suggested that sucralfate promotes angiogenesis by binding to, and preventing degradation of, basic fibroblast growth factor (bFGF).[2]


1. Regnard CFB. Control of bleeding in advanced cancer. *Lancet* 1991; **337:** 974.
2. Tsakayannis D, *et al.* Sucralfate and chronic venous stasis ulcers. *Lancet* 1994; **343:** 424–5.


## Preparations

**USP 27:** Sucralfate Tablets.

**Proprietary Preparations** (details are given in Part 3)

**Arg.:** Antepsin; Netunal; Sucralmax; **Austral.:** Carafate; Ulcyte; **Austria:** Citogel; Sucralan; Sucralbene; Sucralstad; Sucramed; Sucratyrol; Ulceral; Ulcogant; **Belg.:** Ulcogant; **Braz.:** Antepsin†; Sucrafilm; **Canad.:** Novo-Sucralate; Sulcrate; **Chile:** Gastrocol; Mulcatel; Sulcran; **Denm.:** Antepsin; Hexagastron; **Fin.:** Alsucral; Antepsin; **Fr.:** Keal; Ulcar; **Ger.:** Sucrabest; Sucraphil; Ulcogant; **Gr.:** Peptonorm; **Hong Kong:** Sucari; Ulsanic; **India:** Ulcekon; **Irl.:** Antepsin; **Israel:** Ulsanic; **Ital.:** Antepsin; Citogel; Crafilm; Escudo; Gastrogel; Ipagastril; Sucrager; Sucral; Sucralfin; Sucramal; Sucrate; Sucroril; Sugar; Sugast; Suril; Ulcrast; Zenodian; **Jpn:** Ulcerlmin; **Malaysia:** Alsucral; Ulcertec; **Mex.:** Unival; **Neth.:** Ulcogant; **Norw.:** Antepsin; **NZ:** Carafate; **Port.:** Calfate; Sucralum; Ulcermin; **S.Afr.:** Cralsanic†; Ulcefate†; Ulsanic; **Singapore:** Alsucral; Ulcertec; **Spain:** Gastral†; Ulcufato†; Urbal; **Swed.:** Andapsin; Succosa†; **Switz.:** Gastrogel†; Ulcogant; **Thai.:** Sucrafen; Sucral; Sucrate; Ulcefate; Ulcrafate; Ulsanic; **UAE:** Sucralose; **UK:** Antepsin; **USA:** Carafate.

**Multi-ingredient: Fr.:** Cicalfate.

*Used as an adjunct in:* **Ital.:** Ketodol.

# Sulfasalazine *(BAN, USAN, rINN)*

Salazosulfapyridine; Salicylazosulfapyridine; SI-88; Sulfasalazina; Sulfasalazinum; Sulphasalazine. 4-Hydroxy-4′-(2-pyridylsulphamoyl)azobenzene-3-carboxylic acid.

$C_{18}H_{14}N_4O_5S$ = 398.4.

*CAS — 599-79-1.*

*ATC — A07EC01.*

**Pharmacopoeias.** In *Chin., Eur.* (see p.vi), *Int., Jpn, Pol.,* and *US.*

**Ph. Eur. 5.0** (Sulfasalazine). A bright yellow or brownish-yellow, fine powder. Practically insoluble in water and in dichloromethane; very slightly soluble in alcohol; dissolves in dilute solutions of alkali hydroxides. Protect from light.

**USP 27** (Sulfasalazine). A fine odourless bright yellow or brownish-yellow powder. Practically insoluble in water, in chloroform, in ether, and in benzene; soluble 1 in 2900 of alcohol, and 1 in 1500 of methyl alcohol; soluble in aqueous solutions of alkali hydroxides. Store in airtight containers. Protect from light.

## Adverse Effects and Precautions

Since sulfasalazine is metabolised to sulfapyridine and 5-aminosalicylic acid (mesalazine), its adverse effects and precautions are similar to those of sulfonamides (see Sulfamethoxazole, p.261) and of mesalazine (p.1273). Many adverse effects have been attributed to the sulfapyridine moiety and appear to be more common if serum-sulfapyridine concentrations are greater than 50 micrograms/mL, if the daily dose of sulfasalazine is 4 g or more, or in slow acetylators of sulfapyridine.

The most commonly reported adverse effects include nausea and vomiting, abdominal discomfort, headache, fever, and skin rash.

Adverse effects can be broadly divided into 2 groups:

- dose-related effects are dependent on acetylator phenotype, and largely predictable; this group includes nausea and vomiting, headache, haemolytic anaemia, and methaemoglobinaemia
- hypersensitivity reactions are essentially unpredictable and usually occur at the start of treatment; this group includes skin rash, aplastic anaemia, hepatic and pulmonary dysfunction, and auto-immune haemolysis

Oligospermia, reversible on withdrawal of sulfasalazine, has also been reported. Administration of sulfasalazine may result in yellow-orange discoloration of skin, urine, and other body fluids. Some soft contact lenses may be stained.

Sulfasalazine should not be given to patients with a history of sensitivity to sulfonamides or salicylates. Use in children under 2 years of age is contra-indicated because of the risk of kernicterus.

Blood counts should be performed at the start of therapy and at least once a month for a minimum of the first 3 months of treatment. If a blood dyscrasia is suspected treatment should be stopped immediately and a blood count performed. Patients or their carers should be told how to recognise signs of blood toxicity and should be advised to seek immediate medical attention if symptoms such as fever, sore throat, mouth ulcers, bruising or bleeding develop. Care is advisable in patients with G6PD deficiency because of the risk of haemolytic anaemia.

Sulfasalazine should be used with caution in hepatic or renal impairment. Liver function tests should be carried out at monthly intervals for the first 3 months of treatment. Periodic monitoring of kidney function has also been recommended.

◊ Reviews of the adverse effects associated with the administration of sulfasalazine in patients with inflammatory bowel disease[1] or rheumatoid arthritis.[2,3] The type and incidence of adverse effects appear to be similar in both groups of patients.[2] Although most reactions are minor and patients may continue therapy at the same or reduced dosage, some patients discontinue treatment because of adverse effects and in these cases a hyposensitisation regimen may be considered.[1,4,5] Hyposensitisation should not be attempted in patients with a history of a serious adverse effect such as agranulocytosis, toxic epidermal necrolysis, erythema multiforme, frank haemolysis, or a severe hypersensitivity reaction.[1,4,5] An alternative to hyposensitisation in patients with inflammatory bowel disease who cannot tolerate sulfasalazine is to try a drug that supplies the active 5-aminosalicylic acid component without sulfapyridine, as the latter is thought to be responsible for many of the adverse effects. Examples include mesalazine and olsalazine; however, some patients still experience hypersensitivity, see under Mesalazine, p.1273.


1. Taffet SL, Das KM. Sulfasalazine: adverse effects and desensitization. *Dig Dis Sci* 1983; **28:** 833–42.
2. Amos RS, *et al.* Sulphasalazine for rheumatoid arthritis: toxicity in 774 patients monitored for one to 11 years. *BMJ* 1986; **293:** 420–3.
3. Farr M, *et al.* Side effect profile of 200 patients with inflammatory arthritides treated with sulphasalazine. *Drugs* 1986; **32** (suppl 1): 49–53.
4. Purdy BH, *et al.* Desensitization for sulfasalazine skin rash. *Ann Intern Med* 1984; **100:** 512–14.
5. Bax DE, Amos RS. Sulphasalazine in rheumatoid arthritis: desensitising the patient with a skin rash. *Ann Rheum Dis* 1986; **45:** 139–40.


**Breast feeding.** Small amounts of sulfasalazine and its sulfapyridine metabolites are excreted in breast milk; the concentrations of sulfasalazine and total sulfapyridine may be up to 30% and 50% of maternal serum concentrations.[1] Bloody diarrhoea in a breast-fed infant whose mother was taking sulfasalazine 3 g daily has been reported.[2] The mother was a slow acetylator with a relatively high blood concentration of sulfapyridine which contributed to the appearance of the drug in the infant's blood. Based on this report, the American Academy of Pediatrics[3] considers that sulfasalazine should be given with caution to breast-feeding mothers. However, others consider that continued treatment with sulfasalazine can generally be recommended to breast-feeding mothers of healthy infants.[4]


1. Khan AKA, Truelove SC. Placental and mammary transfer of sulphasalazine. *BMJ* 1979; **2:** 1553.
2. Branski D, *et al.* Bloody diarrhea—a possible complication of sulfasalazine transferred through human breast milk. *J Pediatr Gastroenterol Nutr* 1986; **5:** 316–17.
3. American Academy of Pediatrics. The transfer of drugs and other chemicals into human milk. *Pediatrics* 2001; **108:** 776–89. Correction. *ibid.*; 1029. Also available at: http://aappolicy.aappublications.org/cgi/content/full/pediatrics%3b108/3/776 (accessed 07/05/04)
4. Peppercorn MA. Sulfasalazine and related new drugs. *J Clin Pharmacol* 1987; **27:** 260–5.


**Effects on the blood.** Blood disorders constitute 19% of all reactions reported with sulfasalazine.[1] As of June 1993 the UK Committee on Safety of Medicines was aware of 191 reports of neutropenia, leucopenia, or agranulocytosis (22 fatal), 44 reports of bone marrow depression or aplastic anaemia (13 fatal) and 30 reports of thrombocytopenia (1 fatal).[1]

Although blood dyscrasias were initially thought to be caused by the sulfapyridine moiety, subsequent experience has shown that the aminosalicylates can also cause haematological reactions (see Mesalazine, p.1273). The risk of blood dyscrasias with sulfasalazine has been estimated at 0.6 per 1000 in those given the drug for inflammatory bowel disease, but approximately 10 times greater in patients receiving sulfasalazine for rheumatoid arthritis.[2]

Sulfasalazine inhibits folic acid absorption, interferes with its metabolism, and can increase folic acid requirements through haemolysis of red blood cells.[3,4] These effects are not usually significant in patients with inflammatory bowel disease unless there are additional factors causing folate deficiency such as intercurrent illness or an exacerbation of bowel disease.[3,4] However, clinical folate deficiency with macrocytosis, megaloblastic anaemia, or pancytopenia has been reported rarely.[3,4] Macrocytic anaemia associated with sulfasalazine may occur more commonly in patients with rheumatoid arthritis; it was found in 7 of 50 patients within 3 to 4 months of starting treatment with sulfasalazine.[5] The effects of sulfasalazine on folic acid metabolism appear to be dose-related and respond to withdrawal or dosage reduction, and folic acid supplements;[3-5] intravenous folinic acid may sometimes be needed.[4] Although the effects may be potentially serious, they are not a contra-indication to continuing sulfasalazine treatment.[4,5]

Patients with a history of leucopenia associated with administration of gold for rheumatoid arthritis should not be given sulfasalazine since a similar reaction may occur.[6]


1. Committee on Safety of Medicines/Medicines Control Agency. Sulphasalazine and fatal blood dyscrasias. *Current Problems* 1993; **19:** 6.
2. Committee on Safety of Medicines/Medicines Control Agency. Blood dyscrasias and mesalazine. *Current Problems* 1995; **21:** 5–6.
3. Swinson CM, *et al.* Role of sulphasalazine in the aetiology of folate deficiency in ulcerative colitis. *Gut* 1981; **22:** 456–61.
4. Logan ECM, *et al.* Sulphasalazine associated pancytopenia may be caused by acute folate deficiency. *Gut* 1986; **27:** 868–72.
5. Prouse PJ, *et al.* Macrocytic anaemia in patients treated with sulphasalazine for rheumatoid arthritis. *BMJ* 1986; **293:** 1407.
6. Bliddal H, *et al.* Gold-induced leucopenia may predict a similar adverse reaction to sulphasalazine. *Lancet* 1987; **i:** 390.


**Effects on the cardiovascular system.** Reports include Raynaud's syndrome with sulfasalazine[1] and myocarditis with sulfasalazine and with mesalazine.[2] Myocarditis leading to fatal cardiogenic shock has been reported in a patient receiving mesalazine and it has been recommended that sulfasalazine or mesalazine should be replaced by glucocorticoids if cardiac symptoms arise.[3]


1. Reid J, *et al.* Raynaud's phenomenon induced by sulphasalazine. *Postgrad Med J* 1980; **56:** 106–7.
2. Agnholt J, *et al.* Cardiac hypersensitivity to 5-aminosalicylic acid. *Lancet* 1989; **i:** 1135.
3. Kristensen KS, *et al.* Fatal myocarditis associated with mesalazine. *Lancet* 1990; **335:** 605.


**Effects on fertility.** Although successful pregnancies have been reported in the partners of men taking sulfasalazine,[1,2] male infertility is a well recognised complication of sulfasalazine treatment. Untreated inflammatory bowel disease is not associated with abnormal seminal quality or infertility, but oligospermia, reduced sperm motility, and an increase in morphological abnormalities are seen after treatment with sulfasalazine which may lead to infertility.[1-4] Oligospermia has been reported in 86% of men with inflammatory bowel disease treated with sulfasalazine.[1] Seminal characteristics and fertility return to normal within 2 to 3 months of withdrawing sulfasalazine and successful pregnancies have been reported following withdrawal.[1-3] The mechanism involved is thought to be a direct toxic effect on immature and developing spermatozoa, possibly due to the sulfapyridine moiety.[2-4] Improvement in seminal characteristics and successful pregnancies have been reported following substitution of mesalazine[4,5] or balsalazide[6] for sulfasalazine in patients with ulcerative colitis.

1. Birnie GG, *et al.* Incidence of sulphasalazine-induced male infertility. *Gut* 1981; **22:** 452–5.
2. Riley SA, *et al.* Sulphasalazine induced seminal abnormalities in ulcerative colitis: results of mesalazine substitution. *Gut* 1987; **28:** 1008–12.
3. Toovey S, *et al.* Sulphasalazine and male infertility: reversibility and possible mechanism. *Gut* 1981; **22:** 445–51.
4. Ó'Moráin C, *et al.* Reversible male infertility due to sulphasalazine: studies in man and rat. *Gut* 1984; **25:** 1078–84.
5. Cann PA, Holdsworth CD. Reversal of male infertility on changing treatment from sulphasalazine to 5-aminosalicylic acid. *Lancet* 1984; **i:** 1119.
6. McIntyre PB, Lennard-Jones JE. Reversal with balsalazide of infertility caused by sulphasalazine. *BMJ* 1984; **288:** 1652–3.

**Effects on the gastrointestinal tract.** Sulfasalazine-induced exacerbations of ulcerative colitis have been reported[1,2] and are probably caused by the salicylate moiety rather than sulfapyridine.[3] Other reported effects include a dose-related metallic taste[4] and intestinal villous atrophy.[5]

1. Schwartz AG, *et al.* Sulfasalazine-induced exacerbation of ulcerative colitis. *N Engl J Med* 1982; **306:** 409–12.
2. Ring FA, *et al.* Sulfasalazine-induced colitis complicating idiopathic ulcerative colitis. *Can Med Assoc J* 1984; **131:** 43–5.
3. Shanahan F, Targan S. Sulfasalazine and salicylate-induced exacerbation of ulcerative colitis. *N Engl J Med* 1987; **317:** 455.
4. Ogburn RM. Sulfamethazine-related dysgeusia. *JAMA* 1979; **241:** 837.
5. Smith MA, *et al.* Angioimmunoblastic lymphadenopathy, sulphasalazine exposure and villous atrophy. *Postgrad Med J* 1985; **61:** 337–8.

**Effects on the hair.** Alopecia occurred on 2 occasions[1] after starting sulfasalazine 2 or 3 g daily in a patient with ulcerative colitis. On both occasions normal hair growth returned after treatment was stopped, and the patient was later successfully desensitised. However, alopecia that developed in another patient during sulfasalazine treatment did not recur on rechallenge.[2] In this case postpartum alopecia was considered to be the cause and these authors doubted whether sulfasalazine causes alopecia at all. Hair loss has been reported in 2 patients receiving mesalazine enemas.[3] However, remission of alopecia universalis has been reported during sulfasalazine treatment of rheumatoid arthritis.[4]

1. Breen EG, Donnelly S. Alopecia associated with sulphasalazine (Salazopyrin). *BMJ* 1986; **292:** 802.
2. Fich A, Eliakim R. Does sulfasalazine induce alopecia? *J Clin Gastroenterol* 1988; **10:** 466.
3. Kutty PK, *et al.* Hair loss and 5-aminosalicylic acid enemas. *Ann Intern Med* 1982; **97:** 785–6.
4. Jawad ASM, Scott DGI. Remission of alopecia universalis during sulphasalazine treatment for rheumatoid arthritis. *BMJ* 1989; **298:** 675.

**Effects on the kidneys.** For reports of nephrotic syndrome and of interstitial nephritis associated with sulfasalazine treatment, see under Adverse Effects of Mesalazine, p.1273.

**Effects on the pancreas.** The UK Committee on Safety of Medicines had received 6 reports of pancreatitis associated with sulfasalazine as of February 1994.[1] There had been further reports associated with mesalazine (see p.1274).

1. Committee on Safety of Medicines/Medicines Control Agency. Drug-induced pancreatitis. *Current Problems* 1994; **20:** 2–3.

**Effects on the respiratory system.** Sulfasalazine-induced pulmonary complications are reported rarely. Most reports include dyspnoea, cough, pulmonary infiltrates, fever, and eosinophilia, usually developing in the first few months of treatment although they may occur after several years.[1,2] Symptoms are generally readily reversible on withdrawal of sulfasalazine, although death due to fibrosing alveolitis has been reported.[1] These effects have also occurred with mesalazine, p.1274; they have been reported in patients with a history of sensitivity to salicylates, sulfonamides, or with no known sensitivity to these drugs.[1,2]

1. Wang KK, *et al.* Pulmonary infiltrates and eosinophilia associated with sulfasalazine. *Mayo Clin Proc* 1984; **59:** 343–6.
2. Jordan A, Cowan RE. Reversible pulmonary disease and eosinophilia associated with sulphasalazine. *J R Soc Med* 1988; **81:** 233–5.

**Lupus.** A study in 11 patients with sulfasalazine-induced lupus found that induction of disease was more likely in patients who were slow acetylators of sulfapyridine, and who had HLA haplotypes associated with idiopathic systemic lupus erythematosus (SLE).[1] Furthermore, the risk of developing persistent SLE and lupus nephritis increased with duration of treatment and cumulative dose of sulfasalazine. Lupus-like syndrome has also occurred with mesalazine, see Effects on the Cardiovascular System, p.1273.

1. Gunnarsson I, *et al.* Predisposing factors in sulphasalazine-induced systemic lupus erythematosus. *Br J Rheumatol* 1997; **36:** 1089–94.

**Porphyria.** Sulfasalazine has been associated with acute attacks of porphyria and is considered unsafe in porphyric patients.

**Pregnancy.** Sulfasalazine and its sulfapyridine metabolites readily cross the placenta resulting in similar concentrations in the cord serum and maternal serum at delivery.[1,2] The concentration of the 5-aminosalicylic acid component of sulfasalazine in both cord serum and maternal serum is negligible.[1] There have been isolated reports of congenital abnormalities associated with use of sulfasalazine during pregnancy including coarctation of the aorta with a ventricular septal defect,[3,4] and genito-urinary disorders.[4] There is also a theoretical risk of kernicterus in the neonate if sulfasalazine is given close to delivery (see p.261). However, given the concentrations of sulfasalazine and its metabolites found in cord blood, the risk of kernicterus from maternal use is considered minimal.[2] There have been many successful and uncomplicated pregnancies during sulfasalazine therapy and the general consensus favours continuing sulfasalazine throughout pregnancy when indicated.[1,3-6] (See also Mesalazine, p.1274.) The minimum effective dose should be used and since sulfasalazine may precipitate folate deficiency (see Effects on the Blood, above), folic acid supplements are recommended.[7]

1. Khan AKA, Truelove SC. Placental and mammary transfer of sulphasalazine. *BMJ* 1979; **2:** 1553.
2. Järnerot G, *et al.* Placental transfer of sulphasalazine and sulphapyridine and some of its metabolites. *Scand J Gastroenterol* 1981; **16:** 693–7.
3. Hoo JJ, *et al.* Possible teratogenicity of sulfasalazine. *N Engl J Med* 1988; **318:** 1128.
4. Newman NM, Correy JF. Possible teratogenicity of sulphasalazine. *Med J Aust* 1983; **1:** 528–9.
5. Peppercorn MA. Sulfasalazine and related new drugs. *J Clin Pharmacol* 1987; **27:** 260–5.
6. Korelitz BI. Commentary: observations on sulfasalazine in Crohn's disease and ulcerative colitis. *J Clin Pharmacol* 1987; **27:** 265–6.
7. Byron MA. Treatment of rheumatic diseases. *BMJ* 1987; **294:** 236–8.

## Interactions

Administration of sulfasalazine with antibacterial therapy may reduce conversion of sulfasalazine to its active metabolite (see below).

Sulfasalazine has been reported to interfere with the absorption of digoxin (p.898) or folic acid (see Effects on the Blood, above) from the gastrointestinal tract.

**Antibacterials.** Since the effects of sulfasalazine depend on release of 5-aminosalicylic acid by bacterial metabolism in the gut, any drug that reduces the intestinal microflora may reduce the production of active metabolite. Evidence for this has been seen in patients given *rifampicin* and *ethambutol*,[1] or subjects given *ampicillin*,[2] concurrently with sulfasalazine. However, a decrease in clinical effect does not seem to have been demonstrated.

1. Shaffer JL, Houston JB. The effect of rifampicin on sulphapyridine plasma concentrations following sulphasalazine administration. *Br J Clin Pharmacol* 1985; **19:** 526–8.
2. Houston JB, *et al.* Azo reduction of sulphasalazine in healthy volunteers. *Br J Clin Pharmacol* 1982; **14:** 395–8.

**Antineoplastics.** For mention of 5-aminosalicylates such as sulfasalazine inhibiting the metabolism of thiopurine antineoplastics, and increasing their toxicity, see Mercaptopurine, p.567.

## Pharmacokinetics

Following oral administration up to about 15% of a dose of sulfasalazine is absorbed from the small intestine, although some of this is subsequently returned to the intestine in bile via enterohepatic circulation. The great majority of the dose reaches the colon where the azo bond is cleaved by the action of the intestinal flora, producing sulfapyridine and 5-aminosalicylic acid (mesalazine). Results in patients who have undergone colectomy suggest that between 60 and 90% of the total dose is metabolised in this way, but the degree of metabolism depends both on the activity of the intestinal flora and the speed of intestinal transit; colonic metabolism is reduced in patients with diarrhoea (for example, in active inflammatory bowel disease).

The small amount of intact sulfasalazine that is absorbed is extensively protein bound and subsequently excreted unchanged in urine. It crosses the placenta and is found in breast milk.

Following cleavage of the sulfasalazine molecule about 60 to 80% of available sulfapyridine is absorbed and undergoes extensive metabolism by acetylation, hydroxylation, and glucuronidation. Peak steady-state concentrations of sulfapyridine are higher in slow acetylators than fast acetylators after similar doses and the former are 2 to 3 times more likely to experience adverse effects. Some 60% of the original dose of sulfasalazine is excreted in urine as sulfapyridine and its metabolites. As with sulfasalazine, absorbed sulfapyridine crosses the placenta and is found in breast milk.

The 5-aminosalicylic acid (5-ASA) moiety is much less well absorbed. About one-third of liberated 5-ASA is absorbed and almost all of this is acetylated and excreted in urine. For further details of the pharmacokinetics of 5-aminosalicylic acid see under Mesalazine, p.1274.

◊ Reviews.

1. Klotz U. Clinical pharmacokinetics of sulphasalazine, its metabolites and other prodrugs of 5-aminosalicylic acid. *Clin Pharmacokinet* 1985; **10:** 285–302.

## Uses and Administration

Sulfasalazine is a compound of a sulfonamide, sulfapyridine, with 5-aminosalicylic acid (mesalazine). Its activity is generally considered to lie in the 5-aminosalicylic acid moiety, which is released in the colon by bacterial metabolism, although intact sulfasalazine has some anti-inflammatory properties in its own right.

In inflammatory bowel disease (p.1243) it is used alone or as an adjunct to corticosteroids in the treatment of active ulcerative colitis and is effective in maintaining remission. Sulfasalazine may also be effective in the treatment of active Crohn's disease, particularly of the colon, but it does not appear to be of value in maintaining remissions. Sulfasalazine is also used as a disease modifying drug in the treatment of severe or progressive rheumatoid arthritis (below).

In **inflammatory bowel disease** the usual initial adult dose of sulfasalazine is 1 to 2 g by mouth 4 times daily in the UK, although doses over 4 g daily are associated with an increased risk of toxicity. In the USA, therefore, the usual dose is 1 g given 3 or 4 times daily, and an initial dose of 500 mg every 6 to 12 hours may be recommended to lessen gastrointestinal adverse effects. Enteric-coated tablets are also claimed to reduce the incidence of adverse gastrointestinal effects. The overnight interval between doses should not exceed 8 hours. On remission the dose in patients with ulcerative colitis is gradually reduced to 2 g daily and then generally continued indefinitely. For children 2 years of age or older doses should be proportional to body-weight; initially 40 to 60 mg/kg may be given daily in divided doses reduced to 20 to 30 mg/kg daily for the maintenance of remission.

Sulfasalazine is also given rectally, as suppositories, in an adult dose of 0.5 to 1 g night and morning, either alone or as an adjunct to treatment by mouth; it may also be given by enema in a dose of 3 g at bedtime.

In adult **rheumatoid arthritis** treatment is usually commenced with a dose of 500 mg daily by mouth, as enteric-coated tablets, for the first week; dosage is then increased by 500 mg each week to a maximum of 3 g daily given in 2 to 4 divided doses. Sulfasalazine can also be used for polyarticular juvenile rheumatoid arthritis in children aged 6 years and older who have not responded adequately to salicylates or other NSAIDs. A dose of 30 to 50 mg/kg daily is given in two divided doses, to a maximum dose of 2 g daily. To reduce adverse gastrointestinal effects, an enteric-coated tablet is used and the initial dose should be a quarter to a third of the planned maintenance; it is then increased weekly to reach the maintenance dose after one month.

**Psoriasis.** In a double-blind placebo-controlled study involving 50 patients with moderate to severe plaque-type psoriasis (p.1137), sulfasalazine 3 to 4 g daily produced a significantly greater clinical improvement than placebo after 4 weeks of treatment with a further improvement at 8 weeks.[1]

See also Psoriatic Arthritis, below.

1. Gupta AK, *et al.* Sulfasalazine improves psoriasis: a double-blind analysis. *Arch Dermatol* 1990; **126:** 487–93.

**Pyoderma gangrenosum.** Sulfasalazine is licensed in some countries for the treatment of pyoderma gangrenosum (p.1138), a condition that may be associated with inflammatory bowel disease, although published evidence of benefit is scanty.

References.

1. Shenefelt PD. Pyoderma gangrenosum associated with cystic acne and hidradenitis suppurativa controlled by adding minocycline and sulfasalazine to the treatment regimen. *Cutis* 1996; **57:** 315–9.

**Rheumatoid arthritis.** Sulfasalazine is considered to be a useful disease-modifying antirheumatic drug (DMARD) in the treatment of rheumatoid arthritis (p.9). Meta-analyses[1,2] of generally short-term comparative studies suggest that sulfasalazine is roughly comparable in efficacy to methotrexate, intramuscular gold (sodium aurothiomalate), and penicillamine, and some rheumatologists use it as one of the DMARDs of first choice.[3] In an open study[4] of 200 patients with rheumatoid arthritis who were randomly allocated to treatment with sulfasalazine or auranofin, 31% of the sulfasalazine recipients were still taking the drug after 5 years compared with 15% of auranofin recipients. Improvement over baseline was still significant at 5 years for those patients receiving sulfasalazine but not in those treated with auranofin. Although one study[5] failed to find convincing evidence that using sulfasalazine with methotrexate was more effective than either drug alone, other studies have shown that combination treatment with sulfasalazine plus methotrexate and hydroxychloroquine was more effective than methotrexate alone or with sulfasalazine or hydroxychloroquine or the combination of sulfasalazine with hydroxychloroquine.[6,7]

1. Felson DT, *et al.* The comparative efficacy and toxicity of second-line drugs in rheumatoid arthritis. *Arthritis Rheum* 1990; **33:** 1449–61.
2. Capell HA, *et al.* Second line (disease modifying) treatment in rheumatoid arthritis: which drug for which patient? *Ann Rheum Dis* 1993; **52:** 423–8.
3. Rains CP, *et al.* Sulfasalazine: a review of its pharmacological properties and therapeutic efficacy in the treatment of rheumatoid arthritis. *Drugs* 1995; **50:** 137–56.
4. McEntegart A, *et al.* Sulfasalazine has a better efficacy/toxicity profile than auranofin—evidence from a 5 year prospective, randomized trial. *J Rheumatol* 1996; **23:** 1887–90.
5. Dougados M, *et al.* Combination therapy in early rheumatoid arthritis: a randomised, controlled, double blind 52 week clinical trial of sulphasalazine and methotrexate compared with the single components. *Ann Rheum Dis* 1999; **58:** 220–5.
6. O'Dell JR, *et al.* Treatment of rheumatoid arthritis with methotrexate alone, sulfasalazine and hydroxychloroquine, or a combination of all three medications. *N Engl J Med* 1996; **334:** 1287–91.
7. O'Dell JR, *et al.* Treatment of rheumatoid arthritis with methotrexate and hydroxychloroquine, methotrexate and sulfasalazine, or a combination of the three medications: results of a two-year, randomized, double-blind, placebo-controlled trial. *Arthritis Rheum* 2002; **46:** 1164–70.

JUVENILE IDIOPATHIC ARTHRITIS. Juvenile idiopathic arthritis (p.9) is generally managed similarly to rheumatoid arthritis, but there is limited experience with the use of some antirheumatic drugs in children. Sulfasalazine has produced significant improvement in open studies of patients with juvenile chronic arthritis.[1] Beneficial results were also reported in a controlled study of 69 patients with juvenile chronic arthritis of articular onset who received either sulfasalazine or placebo for 24 weeks.[2] The dose of sulfasalazine used was 50 mg/kg daily, starting with one-quarter of the total dose and increased weekly by increments of one-quarter of the total dose. Improvements in some, but not all, disease severity scores and laboratory tests were greater for sulfasalazine than placebo. Adverse effects were also more frequent in the sulfasalazine group, and included gastrointestinal disturbances, skin rashes, headache, elevated liver enzyme concentrations, leucopenia, and hypoimmunoglobulinaemia.

1. Imundo LF, Jacobs JC. Sulfasalazine therapy for juvenile rheumatoid arthritis. *J Rheumatol* 1996; **23:** 360–6.
2. van Rossum MAJ, *et al.* Sulfasalazine in the treatment of juvenile chronic arthritis: a randomized, double-blind, placebo-controlled, multicenter study. *Arthritis Rheum* 1998; **41:** 808–16.

**Spondyloarthropathies.** ANKYLOSING SPONDYLITIS. Sulfasalazine has been found to be effective[1] in the treatment of active ankylosing spondylitis (p.11), but there is evidence that it is more useful in the treatment of peripheral articular manifestations than in the management of chronic long-standing disease.[2,3] The active moiety appears to be sulfapyridine rather than mesalazine.[4]

1. Ferraz MB, *et al.* Meta-analysis of sulfasalazine in ankylosing spondylitis. *J Rheumatol* 1990; **17:** 1482–6.
2. Clegg DO, *et al.* Comparison of sulfasalazine and placebo in the treatment of ankylosing spondylitis: a Department of Veterans Affairs Cooperative study. *Arthritis Rheum* 1996; **39:** 2004–12.
3. Clegg DO, *et al.* Comparison of sulfasalazine and placebo for the treatment of axial and peripheral articular manifestations of the seronegative spondyloarthropathies: a Department of Veterans Affairs cooperative study. *Arthritis Rheum* 1999; **42:** 2325–9.
4. Taggart A, *et al.* Which is the active moiety of sulfasalazine in ankylosing spondylitis? A randomized, controlled study. *Arthritis Rheum* 1996; **39:** 1400–5.

PSORIATIC ARTHRITIS. A systematic review[1] of interventions for psoriatic arthritis (see p.11) concluded that sulfasalazine was one of only two drugs with well demonstrated published efficacy in psoriatic arthritis (the other being high-dose parenteral methotrexate).

See also under Psoriasis, above.

1. Jones G, *et al.* Interventions for treating psoriatic arthritis. Available in The Cochrane Library, Issue 1. Chichester: John Wiley; 2004.

## Preparations

***BP 2003:*** Sulfasalazine Tablets;
***USP 27:*** Sulfasalazine Delayed-release Tablets; Sulfasalazine Tablets.

**Proprietary Preparations** (details are given in Part 3)
***Arg.:*** Azulfidine; ***Austral.:*** Pyralin; Salazopyrin; ***Austria:*** Colo-Pleon; Salazopyrin; ***Belg.:*** Salazopyrine; ***Braz.:*** Aculfin†; Azulfin; Salazoprin; ***Canad.:*** Salazopyrin; SAS; ***Chile:*** Azulfidine; ***Denm.:*** Salazopyrin; ***Fin.:*** Salazopyrin; ***Fr.:*** Salazopyrine; ***Ger.:*** Azulfidine; Colo-Pleon; Pleon RA; ***Gr.:*** Salopyrine; ***Hong Kong:*** Salazopyrin; ***India:*** Sazo; ***Irl.:*** Salazopyrin; ***Israel:*** Salazine†; Salazopyrin; ***Ital.:*** Salazopyrin; ***Malaysia:*** Salazopyrin; ***Neth.:*** Salazopyrine; ***Norw.:*** Salazopyrin; ***NZ:*** Salazopyrin; ***Port.:*** Salazopirina; ***S.Afr.:*** Salazopyrin; ***Singapore:*** Salazopyrin; ***Spain:*** Salazopyrina; ***Swed.:*** Salazopyrin; ***Switz.:*** Salazopyrin; ***Thai.:*** Salazopyrin; Saridine; ***UK:*** Salazopyrin; Sulazine; Ucine†; ***USA:*** Azulfidine.

## Sulglicotide *(BAN, rINN)*

Sulglicotida; Sulglycotide.
*CAS — 54182-59-1.*
*ATC — A02BX08.*

### Profile

Sulglicotide is a sulfated glycopeptide with cytoprotective properties extracted from pig duodenum. It is used in the treatment of peptic ulcer disease (p.1246) and other gastrointestinal disorders in a usual dose of 200 mg three times daily by mouth.

◊ References.

1. Luminari M, *et al.* Effectiveness of sulglycotide treatment for active chronic superficial gastritis. *Acta Ther* 1988; **14:** 45–54.
2. Psilogenis M, *et al.* A multicenter double-blind study of sulglycotide versus sucralfate in nonulcer dyspepsia. *Int J Clin Pharmacol Ther Toxicol* 1990; **28:** 369–74.
3. Bianchi Porro G, *et al.* Sulglycotide in the prevention of nonsteroidal anti-inflammatory drug-induced gastroduodenal mucosal injury: a controlled double-blind, double-dummy, randomized endoscopic study versus placebo in rheumatic patients. *Scand J Gastroenterol* 1993; **28:** 875–8.
4. De Conca V, *et al.* Effect of sulglycotide in the prevention of duodenal ulcer relapse. *Eur J Gastroenterol Hepatol* 1995; **7:** 25–8.

### Preparations

**Proprietary Preparations** (details are given in Part 3)
***Ital.:*** Gliptide.

## Tamarind

Tamarindo; West Indian Tamarind.
**Pharmacopoeias.** In *Fr.*

### Profile

Tamarind is the fruits of *Tamarindus indica* (Leguminosae) freed from the brittle outer part of the pericarp and preserved with sugar or syrup. It contains tartaric, citric, and malic acid and their salts. Tamarind is used as a laxative in combination with senna.

### Preparations

**Proprietary Preparations** (details are given in Part 3)
***Fr.:*** Delabarre.

**Multi-ingredient:** ***Arg.:*** Tamarine; ***Austria:*** Frugelletten; Naturaform Fruchtewurfel mit Manna; Neda Fruchtewurfel; ***Belg.:*** Tamarine†; ***Braz.:*** Fitolax; Florlax; Fontolax; Frutalax; Frutarine†; Laxan†; Laxarine; Laxtam; Novolax†; Tamaril; Tamarine; Tamarix; ***Chile:*** Tamarine; ***Fr.:*** Actisane Constipation Occasionnelle†; Laxasan†; Tamarine; ***Ital.:*** Ortisan; Tamarine; ***Mex.:*** Naturetti; ***Spain:*** Dentomicin; Pruina; ***Switz.:*** Tamarine†.

## Tegaserod Maleate *(BANM, USAN, rINNM)*

HTF-919; Maleato de tegaserod; SDZ-HTF-919. 1-{[(5-Methoxyindol-3-yl)methylene]amino}-3-pentylguanidine maleate.
$C_{16}H_{23}N_5O,C_4H_4O_4$ = 417.5.
*CAS — 145158-71-0 (tegaserod); 189188-57-6 (tegaserod maleate).*
*ATC — A03AE02.*

### Adverse Effects

The most common adverse effects of tegaserod are gastrointestinal disturbances including abdominal pain, diarrhoea, nausea, and flatulence. Diarrhoea generally occurs within the first week of treatment and is usually transient but may be severe. Ischaemic colitis has been reported. Headache, dizziness, migraine, leg or back pain, and arthropathy have also been commonly reported. Other adverse effects include cardiovascular effects such as hypotension and arrhythmias, effects on the nervous system such as depression, and other gastrointestinal effects including bilirubinaemia, cholecystitis, and elevated liver transaminases.

**Effects on the gastrointestinal tract.** Severe diarrhoea, leading to hypovolaemia, hypotension, and syncope has been seen occasionally in patients receiving tegaserod. Some patients required hospitalisation for rehydration, and patients should be advised to stop taking the drug and seek medical attention if severe diarrhoea or associated dizziness or lightheadedness develop. In addition, ischaemic colitis has been reported rarely, and the drug should be discontinued immediately in patients who develop symptoms such as rectal bleeding, bloody diarrhoea, or new and worsening abdominal pain.[1]

1. Novartis, Canada. Important safety update: diarrhea and ischemic colitis in patients using Zelnorm (tegaserod hydrogen maleate) (issued 28/04/04). Available at: http://www.hc-sc.gc.ca/hpfb-dgpsa/tpd-dpt/zelnorm_hpc_e.html (accessed 10/05/04)

### Precautions

Tegaserod is contra-indicated in patients with a history of bowel obstruction, symptomatic gallbladder disease, suspected sphincter of Oddi dysfunction, or abdominal adhesions. Tegaserod should also not be given to patients who have diarrhoea or who frequently experience diarrhoea. It should be discontinued in patients with new or sudden worsening of abdominal symptoms, hypertension, or syncope. Tegaserod should not be used in patients with severe renal impairment or moderate to severe hepatic impairment.

### Pharmacokinetics

Tegaserod is rapidly absorbed from the gastrointestinal tract with peak plasma levels occurring after about 1 hour. The absolute bioavailability of an oral dose is 10%; this is reduced by the presence of food. Tegaserod is widely distributed into the tissues and is about 98% bound to plasma proteins. Presystemic acid-catalysed hydrolysis in the stomach, followed by oxidation and glucuronidation, produces the main metabolite, which is inactive; direct systemic glucuronidation also occurs. Two-thirds of an oral dose is excreted unchanged in the faeces and one-third excreted in the urine primarily as the main metabolite. The terminal half-life of tegaserod is about 11 hours.

◊ Reviews.

1. Appel-Dingemanse S. Clinical pharmacokinetics of tegaserod, a serotonin 5-$HT_4$ receptor partial agonist with promotile activity. *Clin Pharmacokinet* 2002; **41:** 1021–42.

### Uses and Administration

Tegaserod is a partial agonist at 5-$HT_4$ receptors and has prokinetic properties. It is used in women for the short-term treatment of irritable bowel syndrome, particularly the constipation-predominant form. It is also under investigation for the treatment of chronic constipation.

Tegaserod is given orally as the maleate but doses are expressed in terms of the base. 1.39 mg of tegaserod maleate is approximately equivalent to 1 mg of tegaserod. It is given in a dose of 6 mg twice daily before food for 4 to 6 weeks; a further 4 to 6 weeks of treatment may be given if a beneficial response is seen.

◊ References.

1. Scott LJ, Perry CM. Tegaserod. *Drugs* 1999; **58:** 491–8.
2. Wagstaff AJ, *et al.* Tegaserod: a review of its use in the management of irritable bowel syndrome with constipation in women. *Drugs* 2003; **63:** 1101–20.
3. Lea R, Whorwell PJ. Benefit-risk assessment of tegaserod in irritable bowel syndrome. *Drug Safety* 2004; **27:** 229–42.

### Preparations

**Proprietary Preparations** (details are given in Part 3)
***Austral.:*** Zelmac; ***Braz.:*** Zelmac; ***Singapore:*** Zelmac; ***Switz.:*** Zelmac; ***Thai.:*** Zelmac; ***USA:*** Zelnorm.

## Teprenone *(rINN)*

E-671; Geranylgeranylacetone (5*E*, 9*E*,13*E* isomer); Teprenona. 6,10,14,18-Tetramethyl-5,9,13,17-nonadecatetraen-2-one, mixture of (5*E*,9*E*,13*E*) and (5*Z*,9*E*,13*E*) isomers.
$C_{23}H_{38}O$ = 330.5.
*CAS — 6809-52-5 (teprenone); 3796-63-2 (5E,9E,13E isomer); 3796-64-3 (5Z,9E,13E isomer).*

### Profile

Teprenone is a cytoprotective drug that is used in the treatment of gastritis and peptic ulcer disease (p.1246) in a usual dose of 50 mg three times daily by mouth.

### Preparations

**Proprietary Preparations** (details are given in Part 3)
***Jpn:*** Selbex; ***Thai.:*** Selbex.

## Tropisetron *(BAN, rINN)*

Tropisetrón. 1α*H*,5α*H*-Tropan-3α-yl indole-3-carboxylate.
$C_{17}H_{20}N_2O_2$ = 284.4.
*CAS — 89565-68-4.*
*ATC — A04AA03.*

## Tropisetron Hydrochloride *(BANM, rINNM)*

Hidrocloruro de tropisetrón; ICS-205-930.
$C_{17}H_{20}N_2O_2,HCl$ = 320.8.
*CAS — 105826-92-4.*
*ATC — A04AA03.*

### Adverse Effects and Precautions

As for Ondansetron, p.1281. Fatigue, abdominal pain, and diarrhoea may also occur. Visual hallucinations, and an increase in blood pressure in patients with pre-existing hypertension, have been noted at high repeated doses. ECG changes such as prolongation of QT interval have been noted with high-dose intravenous tropisetron. The drug should therefore be used with caution in patients with cardiac rhythm or conduction disturbances. The manufacturers have warned that care should be taken when driving or operating machinery.

◊ Adverse effects reported with tropisetron include headache and mild sedation.[1] There have been reports of fever requiring drug withdrawal;[2,3] one patient[3] also experienced mild hypotension, macular rash, joint aches, and cervical lymphadenopathy.

The manufacturer has reported an increased incidence of hepatic neoplasms in male *mice* given high doses of tropisetron but it is suggested that these effects are both species and sex specific.

1. Leibundgut U, Lancranjan I. First results with ICS 205-930 (5-$HT_3$ receptor antagonist) in prevention of chemotherapy-induced emesis. *Lancet* 1987; **i:** 1198.
2. Anderson JV, *et al.* Remission of symptoms in carcinoid syndrome with a new 5-hydroxytryptamine M receptor antagonist. *BMJ* 1987; **294:** 1129.
3. Coupe M. Adverse reaction to 5-$HT_3$ antagonist ICS 205930. *Lancet* 1987; **i:** 1494.

### Interactions

Drugs that induce or inhibit hepatic enzymes may affect plasma concentrations of tropisetron. The manufacturer considers that any changes are usually unlikely to be clinically relevant with the recommended doses.

Tropisetron should be used with caution with antiarrhythmics, beta blockers, or drugs likely to prolong the QT interval.

## Pharmacokinetics

Tropisetron is well absorbed following oral administration. Peak plasma concentrations are achieved within 3 hours. Absolute bioavailability depends on the dose since first-pass metabolism is saturable. It is 71% bound to plasma proteins. Tropisetron is metabolised by hydroxylation and conjugation, and metabolites are excreted mainly in the urine with a small amount in the faeces. The cytochrome P450 isoenzyme CYP2D6 is involved in tropisetron metabolism, and shows genetic polymorphism. The elimination half-life is about 8 hours in extensive metabolisers and up to 45 hours in poor metabolisers. Clearance is also reduced in patients with renal impairment.

## Uses and Administration

Tropisetron is a 5-$HT_3$ antagonist with an antiemetic action similar to that of ondansetron (p.1281). It is used in the prevention of nausea and vomiting induced by cytotoxic therapy and in the treatment and prevention of postoperative nausea and vomiting (p.1245).

Tropisetron is given by slow intravenous injection or infusion, as the hydrochloride or by mouth as the base; doses are calculated in terms of tropisetron base. 5.64 mg of tropisetron hydrochloride is approximately equivalent to 5 mg of tropisetron base.

For the *prophylaxis* of acute **nausea and vomiting** associated with cytotoxic **chemotherapy** a single dose of 5 mg may be given by slow intravenous injection or infusion on the day of treatment, shortly before chemotherapy. Subsequent doses of 5 mg daily are given by mouth, at least one hour before food, for a further 5 days. Children over 2 years of age may be given 200 micrograms/kg (maximum dose 5 mg) by intravenous injection over at least 1 minute, or by infusion, before chemotherapy. In children weighing less than 25 kg the same dose may be given intravenously once daily for up to a further 4 days as required. In those weighing more than 25 kg, a dose of 5 mg may be given orally once daily for up to a further 5 days; if oral administration is not possible the same dose may be given intravenously.

For the *treatment* of **postoperative** nausea and vomiting in adults 2 mg may be given by slow intravenous injection, or by infusion, within 2 hours of the end of anaesthesia. For *prophylaxis*, the same dose may be given shortly before induction of anaesthesia.

◊ References.


1. Lee CR, *et al.* Tropisetron: a review of its pharmacodynamic and pharmacokinetic properties, and therapeutic potential as an antiemetic. *Drugs* 1993; **46:** 925–43.
2. Simpson K, *et al.* Tropisetron: an update of its use in the prevention of chemotherapy-induced nausea and vomiting. *Drugs* 2000; **59:** 1297–1315.


**Anxiety disorders.** A dose-dependent anxiolytic effect was reported for tropisetron when studied in patients with generalised anxiety,[1] but clinical evidence for the benefit of 5-$HT_3$ antagonists in anxiety disorders is lacking.[2]


1. Lecrubier Y, *et al.* A randomized double-blind placebo-controlled study of tropisetron in the treatment of outpatients with generalized anxiety disorder. *Psychopharmacology (Berl)* 1993; **112:** 129–33.
2. Greenshaw AJ, Silverstone PH. The non-antiemetic uses of serotonin 5-$HT_3$ receptor antagonists: clinical pharmacology and therapeutic applications. *Drugs* 1997; **53:** 20–39.


**Pain.** For reference to the use of tropisetron in various painful syndromes, see under Uses and Administration of Ondansetron, p.1282.

### Preparations

**Proprietary Preparations** (details are given in Part 3)
***Arg.:*** Navoban; ***Austral.:*** Navoban; ***Austria:*** Navoban; ***Belg.:*** Novaban; ***Braz.:*** Navoban; ***Chile:*** Navoban; ***Denm.:*** Navoban; ***Fin.:*** Navoban; ***Fr.:*** Navoban; ***Ger.:*** Navoban; ***Gr.:*** Navoban; ***Hong Kong:*** Navoban; ***Irl.:*** Navoban†; ***Israel:*** Navoban; ***Ital.:*** Navoban; ***Jpn:*** Navoban; ***Malaysia:*** Navoban; ***Mex.:*** Navoban; ***Neth.:*** Novaban; ***Norw.:*** Navoban; ***NZ:*** Navoban; ***Port.:*** Navoban; ***S.Afr.:*** Navoban; ***Spain:*** Navoban; ***Swed.:*** Navoban; ***Switz.:*** Navoban; ***Thai.:*** Navoban; ***UK:*** Navoban.

## Troxipide *(rINN)*

Troxipida. (±)-3,4,5-Trimethoxy-*N*-3-piperidylbenzamide.
$C_{15}H_{22}N_2O_4$ = 294.3.
*CAS — 30751-05-4.*
*ATC — A02BX11.*

### Profile

Troxipide is used for its cytoprotective properties in the treatment of gastritis and peptic ulcer disease (p.1246) in a usual dose of 100 mg three times daily by mouth.

### Preparations

**Proprietary Preparations** (details are given in Part 3)
***Jpn:*** Aplace.

## Urogastrone

Anthelone; EGF-URO; Epidermal Growth Factor; Murodermina; Uroanthelone; Uroenterone.
*CAS — 9010-53-1.*

### Uses

Urogastrone is a polypeptide first isolated from human urine. Two forms have been identified, β and γ urogastrone. The β form consists of 53 amino acids and is distinguishable from the γ form by an additional terminal arginine residue. The β form is reported to be identical to human epidermal growth factor and this term is widely used in the literature.

Urogastrone inhibits gastric acid secretion and has been tried in the treatment of peptic ulcer disease and other gastrointestinal disorders but its rapid destruction in the stomach has limited its clinical use.

It is a potent stimulator of cellular proliferation and has also been used as an aid to wound healing.

◊ Reviews[1,2] of epidermal growth factor (EGF) and transforming growth factor (TGF).


1. Burgess AW. Epidermal growth factor and transforming growth factor α. *Br Med Bull* 1989; **45:** 401–24.
2. Miyazawa K. Role of epidermal growth factor in obstetrics and gynecology. *Obstet Gynecol* 1992; **79:** 1032–40.


**Gastrointestinal disorders.** Intravenous infusion of urogastrone 250 nanograms/kg over 1 hour has been reported[1,2] to reduce the secretion of gastric acid in patients with duodenal ulcer (p.1246) or the Zollinger-Ellison syndrome (p.1247). Ulcer pain was relieved 30 to 60 minutes after the start of the infusion.[2] A dose of 100 nanograms/kg per hour by intravenous infusion has been used with partial success in an infant with microvillous atrophy[3] and was apparently beneficial in an infant with necrotising enteritis.[4]

Human epidermal growth factor has also shown some promise in the treatment of active ulcerative colitis. In a small study,[5] patients received daily enemas containing either recombinant human epidermal growth factor (5 micrograms in 100 mL) or placebo; all patients also received oral mesalazine. Ten of the 12 patients in the urogastrone group were in remission after 2 weeks treatment compared with 1 of the 12 patients in the placebo group, and this benefit was maintained for up to 12 weeks.


1. Koffman CG, *et al.* Effect of urogastrone on gastric secretion and serum gastrin concentration in patients with duodenal ulceration. *Gut* 1982; **23:** 951–6.
2. Elder JB, *et al.* Effect of urogastrone in the Zollinger-Ellison syndrome. *Lancet* 1975; **ii:** 424–7.
3. Walker-Smith JA, *et al.* Intravenous epidermal growth factor/urogastrone increases small-intestinal cell proliferation in congenital microvillous atrophy. *Lancet* 1985; **ii:** 1239–40.
4. Sullivan PB, *et al.* Epidermal growth factor in necrotising enteritis. *Lancet* 1991; **338:** 53–4.
5. Sinha A, *et al.* Epidermal growth factor enemas with oral mesalamine for mild-to-moderate left-sided ulcerative colitis or proctitis. *N Engl J Med* 2003; **349:** 350–7.


**Wound healing.** In a randomised double-blind study in 61 patients with diabetic foot ulcers, adding human epidermal growth factor 0.04% to an ulcer cream containing protein-free bovine blood extract was shown to significantly enhance wound healing and reduce healing time compared with either the cream alone or the cream plus human epidermal growth factor 0.02%.[1]

The effect on the rate of wound healing (p.1139) of a cream containing sulfadiazine silver plus recombinant human epidermal growth factor (10 micrograms/mL) was compared with sulfadiazine silver alone in 12 patients each requiring skin grafts at 2 donor sites.[2] The cream containing epidermal growth factor accelerated the rate of epidermal regeneration in all patients and reduced the average time to 100% healing by about 1.5 days. Patients were followed up for a maximum of 1 year after cessation of therapy and no complications or clinical evidence of neoplasia at the healed donor sites occurred.

In contrast, recombinant human epidermal growth factor as an ophthalmic solution containing 30 or 100 micrograms/mL was investigated in patients who had undergone keratoplasty, but the weaker solution had no effect on the rate of re-epithelialisation, and the more concentrated one was actually associated with slower healing.[3]


1. Tsang MW, *et al.* Human epidermal growth factor enhances healing of diabetic foot ulcers. *Diabetes Care* 2003; **26:** 1856–61.
2. Brown GL, *et al.* Enhancement of wound healing by topical treatment with epidermal growth factor. *N Engl J Med* 1989; **321:** 76–9.
3. Dellaert MMMJ, *et al.* Influence of topical human epidermal growth factor on postkeratoplasty re-epithelialisation. *Br J Ophthalmol* 1997; **81:** 391–5.


### Preparations

**Proprietary Preparations** (details are given in Part 3)
**Multi-ingredient:** ***Chile:*** Hebermin.

## Zaldaride *(rINN)*

CGS-9343B (zaldaride maleate); Zaldarida. (±)-1-{1-[(4-Methyl-4*H*,6*H*-pyrrolo[1,2-*a*][4,1]benzoxazepin-4-yl)methyl]-4-piperidyl}-2-benzimidazolinone.
$C_{26}H_{28}N_4O_2$ = 428.5.
*CAS — 109826-26-8 (zaldaride); 109826-27-9 (zaldaride maleate).*

### Profile

Zaldaride is a calmodulin antagonist that has been investigated as the maleate for the treatment of diarrhoea.

**Diarrhoea.** Studies in patients with travellers' diarrhoea have indicated that zaldaride in doses of 20 mg by mouth as the maleate four times daily is an effective antidiarrhoeal.[1,2] It was somewhat less effective then loperamide when given without a loading dose,[2] but a regimen of 40 mg initially, followed by 20 mg approximately every 6 hours was as effective as loperamide 4 mg initially followed by 2 mg after each unformed stool.[3] Although antidiarrhoeal drugs may be given for symptom control in adults, the mainstay of therapy for acute diarrhoea (p.1241) should still be fluid and electrolyte replacement.


1. DuPont HL, *et al.* Zaldaride maleate, an intestinal calmodulin inhibitor, in the therapy of travelers' diarrhea. *Gastroenterology* 1993; **104:** 709–15.
2. Okhuysen PC, *et al.* Zaldaride maleate (a new calmodulin antagonist) versus loperamide in the treatment of traveler's diarrhea: randomized, placebo-controlled trial. *Clin Infect Dis* 1995; **21:** 341–4.
3. Silberschmidt G, *et al.* Treatment of travellers' diarrhoea: zaldaride compared with loperamide and placebo. *Eur J Gastroenterol Hepatol* 1995; **7:** 871–5.

# General Anaesthetics

This chapter includes drugs used for the induction and maintenance of general anaesthesia. General anaesthetics are given either by inhalation or by intravenous or occasionally intramuscular injection (see below).

| Injectable | Inhalational |
|---|---|
| *Barbiturate* | *Halogenated* |
| Methohexital | Chloroform |
| Thiamylal | Desflurane |
| Thiopental | Enflurane |
| | Halothane |
| *Miscellaneous* | Isoflurane |
| Alfadolone | Methoxyflurane |
| Alfaxolone | Sevoflurane |
| Etomidate | Trichloroethylene |
| Ketamine | *Miscellaneous* |
| Propanidid | Cyclopropane |
| Propofol | Anaesthetic Ether |
| Sodium Oxybate | Nitrous Oxide |
| Tiletamine | Xenon |

## Adverse Effects of General Anaesthetics

The complex regimens used in general anaesthesia may produce complications both during and after the procedure. Adverse effects that may occur with general anaesthesia include involuntary muscle movements, hiccup, coughing, bronchospasm, laryngospasm, respiratory depression, hypotension, cardiac arrhythmias, and mild hypothermia.

Following general anaesthesia many patients will experience drowsiness and impaired mental performance for at least 24 hours. Postoperative nausea with or without vomiting is common in the absence of antiemetic prophylaxis; nausea may last for 2 days but vomiting seldom persists beyond the first day. Other relatively common postanaesthetic effects include anorexia, malaise, fatigue, dizziness, and headache. Delirium has been noted in at least 10% of elderly general surgical patients and in up to 50% of elderly patients undergoing hip fracture repair.

Sore throat is frequent in patients who have been intubated or have had a throat pack inserted. Dry mouth as a result of premedication can add to the patient's discomfort. Manipulations for the maintenance of a clear airway may result in postoperative jaw pain.

Muscle pain, typically involving the neck, shoulders, and upper abdomen, may occur if the neuromuscular blocker suxamethonium has been given. It is usually worse on the second postoperative day and may last up to 6 days. Shoulder ache after laparoscopy resolves after 24 hours; it is due to accumulation of carbon dioxide under the diaphragm. Backache may occur after epidural or spinal anaesthesia. Urinary retention may follow regional block, cystoscopic or gynaecological surgery, or when there is prostatism.

Malignant hyperthermia (malignant hyperpyrexia—see under Dantrolene, p.1394) is a rare but potentially fatal complication of general anaesthesia that may be induced by inhalational anaesthetics (mainly halogenated hydrocarbons).

Sensitisation of the myocardium to beta-adrenergic stimulation occurs with some anaesthetics.

There has been concern over the possible danger to anaesthetists, dentists, and other personnel from exposure to volatile anaesthetics.

◊ References.


1. Anonymous. Following up day case anaesthesia in general practice. *Drug Ther Bull* 1990; **28:** 81–2.
2. Rowbotham DJ, Smith G, eds. Postoperative nausea and vomiting. *Br J Anaesth* 1992; **69** (suppl 1): 1S–68S.
3. O'Keeffe ST, NíChonchubhair A. Postoperative delirium in the elderly. *Br J Anaesth* 1994; **73:** 673–87.
4. Marcantonio ER, *et al.* A clinical prediction rule for delirium after elective noncardiac surgery. *JAMA* 1994; **271:** 134–9.
5. Davies CJ, *et al.* Delayed adverse reactions to drugs used in anaesthesia. *Adverse Drug React Bull* 1995 (Apr.); 647–50.
6. Klafta JM, *et al.* Neurological and psychiatric adverse effects of anaesthetics: epidemiology and treatment. *Drug Safety* 1995; **13:** 281–95.
7. Fee JPH, Thompson GH. Comparative tolerability profiles of the inhaled anaesthetics. *Drug Safety* 1997; **16:** 157–70.


**Hypersensitivity.** Type I hypersensitivity reactions have occurred with general anaesthetics.[1] In most patients the release of histamine and other mediators such as prostaglandins and leukotrienes is of no clinical importance but in a few susceptible individuals anaphylaxis may result. Numerous factors to identify those at risk have been proposed over the years along with suggested modifications for anaesthetic management. Of the drugs used in anaesthesia, neuromuscular blockers are associated with the highest incidence of anaphylaxis; the most commonly implicated is reported to be suxamethonium, followed by alcuronium[2] (see under the Adverse Effects of Suxamethonium, p.1407). It has been suggested[3] that routine prophylaxis with histamine $H_1$- and histamine $H_2$-antagonists should be considered as part of anaesthetic management but others[2] thought it better to avoid the use of combinations such as thiopental, suxamethonium, and alcuronium that are well known to cause histamine release.


1. McKinnon RP, Wildsmith JAW. Histaminoid reactions in anaesthesia. *Br J Anaesth* 1995; **74:** 217–28.
2. O'Connor B, Edwards ND. Reactions to gelatin plasma expanders. *Lancet* 1994; **344:** 328.
3. Lorenz W, *et al.* Incidence and clinical importance of perioperative histamine release: randomised study of volume loading and antihistamines after induction of anaesthesia. *Lancet* 1994; **343:** 933–40.


**Nausea and vomiting.** For a discussion on postoperative nausea and vomiting and its management, see p.1245.

**Shivering and its treatment.** Postoperative shivering, also referred to as spontaneous postanaesthetic tremor, can occur in up to 65% of patients recovering from general anaesthesia;[1,2] its aetiology and relationship to thermoregulation is unclear.[1,3,4] Postoperative shivering may be part of a more generalised neurological disturbance associated with anaesthesia.[1] It also occurs following regional anaesthesia, especially when given epidurally, but this is probably produced by different mechanisms.[3] Muscular activity during shivering greatly increases metabolic rate, oxygen consumption, and cardiac output and may cause complications in patients with cardiac or respiratory disorders. It can also strain surgical sutures, raise intra-ocular pressure, and impede haemodynamic monitoring.

Although the relationship between postoperative shivering, body temperature, and heat loss is unclear, patients may respond to warming their environment and the use of blankets.[1,3] Postoperative shivering may sometimes be an appropriate thermoregulatory response to a low body temperature,[3] and it is important before starting therapy to check the patient's temperature and take suitable steps to avoid hypothermia.[1]

Numerous drugs have been tried for the management of postoperative shivering including the central and respiratory stimulant doxapram, the $\alpha_2$-agonist clonidine, and the opioid analgesic pethidine.[2,4] Reviews have discussed[1-4] a number of other opioids that have been tried including morphine, alfentanil, butorphanol, fentanyl, and sufentanil but studies suggest that not all opioids are effective or that some may only be effective when given epidurally. However, this may be due to the use of insufficient doses rather than a true difference between opioids.[5] Tramadol and nefopam have also been tried.[2] Neuromuscular blockers have been used after cardiac surgery in order to reduce cardiovascular stress.[6] Vecuronium might be preferable to pancuronium as it does not increase myocardial work and may be associated with fewer complications.[7] However, as profound neuromuscular block is required to inhibit shivering, repeated or higher doses of vecuronium might be required to prevent recurrence. Other drugs that have been investigated include ketanserin,[2] ketamine,[8] and magnesium sulfate.[2]


1. Crossley AWA. Postoperative shivering. *Br J Hosp Med* 1993; **49:** 204–8.
2. Alfonsi P. Postanaesthetic shivering: epidemiology, pathophysiology, and approaches to prevention and management. *Drugs* 2001; **61:** 2193–2205.
3. Anonymous. Perioperative shivering. *Lancet* 1991; **338:** 547–8.
4. Kranke P, *et al.* Pharmacological treatment of postoperative shivering: a quantitative systematic review of randomized controlled trials. *Anesth Analg* 2002; **94:** 453–60.
5. Alfonsi P, *et al.* Fentanyl, as pethidine, inhibits post anaesthesia shivering. *Br J Anaesth* 1993; **70** (suppl 1): 38.
6. Cruise C, *et al.* Comparison of meperidine and pancuronium for the treatment of shivering after cardiac surgery. *Can J Anaesth* 1992; **39:** 563–8.
7. Dupuis J-Y, *et al.* Pancuronium or vecuronium for treatment of shivering after cardiac surgery. *Anesth Analg* 1994; **79:** 472–81.
8. Sharma DR, Thakur JR. Ketamine and shivering. *Anaesthesia* 1990; **45:** 252–3.


## Precautions for General Anaesthetics

Patients with impaired function of the adrenal cortex, for example, those who are being treated, or have recently been treated, with corticosteroids, may experience hypotension with the stress of anaesthesia. Treatment with corticosteroids, pre-operatively and postoperatively, may be necessary. Patients taking other long-term medication such as aspirin, oral anticoagulants, oestrogens, MAOIs, or lithium, may require a change in dosage or cessation of therapy before major elective surgery.

Patients with chronic diseases such as diabetes or hypertension may require adjustment to their therapy prior to anaesthesia. Anaesthetics should be used with caution in patients with cardiac, respiratory, renal, or hepatic impairment and care may be needed in elderly or obese patients.

Patients should not undertake hazardous tasks such as driving for at least 24 hours after a general anaesthetic; alcohol should also be avoided.

**Intraoperative awareness.** The use of neuromuscular blockers has enabled anaesthetic doses to be reduced. However, lack of a reliable method for detecting conscious awareness in patients with complete neuromuscular block has resulted in paralysed patients who have received inadequate anaesthesia being aware during surgery.[1,2] Recommendations to control this problem include premedication with sedative or amnesic drugs, induction with sufficient doses of intravenous anaesthetic, the use of effective analgesic techniques during surgery, and, in particular, adequate concentrations of inspired anaesthetic gas. However, even patients given lorazepam or opioids may have some recall and there is no certain way to avoid awareness in paralysed patients. One commentator[3] considered that the routine use of neuromuscular blockers during surgery should be re-assessed since modern anaesthetics and analgesics could provide good operating conditions without paralysis for most major surgical procedures.


1. Brighouse DI, Norman J. To wake in fright. *BMJ* 1992; **304:** 1327–8.
2. Jones JG. Memory of intraoperative events. *BMJ* 1994; **309:** 967–8.
3. Ponte J. Neuromuscular blockers during general anaesthesia. *BMJ* 1995; **310:** 1218–19.


## Interactions of General Anaesthetics

Sensitisation of the myocardium to beta-adrenergic stimulation occurs with some anaesthetics and ventricular fibrillation may occur if *sympathomimetics* such as adrenaline and isoprenaline are used concomitantly. Enhanced hypotensive effects may result when anaesthetics are given with *ACE inhibitors, tricyclic antidepressants* (which may also increase the risk of arrhythmias), *MAOIs* (see also Anaesthesia, under Precautions for Phenelzine, p.313), *antihypertensives, antipsychotics*, or *beta blockers*. The effects of *competitive neuromuscular blockers* may be increased by inhalational anaesthetics. The use of anaesthetics with other *CNS depressant drugs* such as those used for premedication may produce synergistic effects on the CNS and, in some cases, a smaller dose of general anaesthetic should be given.

◊ Reviews.


1. Wood M. Pharmacokinetic drug interactions in anaesthetic practice. *Clin Pharmacokinet* 1991; **21:** 285–307.
2. Ransom ES, Mueller RA. Safety considerations in the use of drug combinations during general anaesthesia. *Drug Safety* 1997; **16:** 88–103.


## Uses of General Anaesthetics

General anaesthetics depress the CNS and cause loss of consciousness associated with an inability to perceive pain. An ideal anaesthetic would produce unconsciousness, analgesia, and muscle relaxation suitable for all surgical procedures and would be metabolically inert and rapidly eliminated. No anaesthetic fulfils all these requirements in safe concentrations and it is customary to use a number of drugs to achieve the required conditions while minimising the risk of toxicity.

The activity of any anaesthetic is dependent on its ability to reach the brain. With inhalational anaesthetics there has to be a transfer from the alveolar space to the blood, then to the brain; recovery is a function of the removal of the anaesthetic from the brain. With injectable anaesthetics their activity is similarly dependent on their ability to penetrate the blood/brain barrier and recovery in turn is governed by their redistribution and excretion. The potency of inhalational anaesthetics is often expressed in terms of *minimum alveolar concentrations*, known as MAC values. The MAC of an anaesthetic is the concentration at 1 atmosphere that will produce immobility in 50% of subjects exposed to a noxious stimulus. Values given under the individual monographs are based on use without nitrous oxide as the latter can reduce the MAC. Other factors including age, body temperature, and concurrent medication such as opioid analgesics can also affect MAC values.

◊ General references.

1. Royston D, Cox F. Anaesthesia: the patient's point of view. *Lancet* 2003; **362:** 1648–58.
2. García-Miguel FJ, *et al.* Preoperative assessment. *Lancet* 2003; **362:** 1749–57.
3. Buhre W, Rossaint R. Perioperative management and monitoring in anaesthesia. *Lancet* 2003; **362:** 1839–46.
4. Kehlet H, Dahl JB. Anaesthesia, surgery, and challenges in post-operative recovery. *Lancet* 2003; **362:** 1921–8.

**Anaesthesia.** Many drugs are involved in achieving and maintaining conditions suitable for surgery. Conventional general anaesthesia may be divided into a number of stages including:

- premedication
- induction
- muscle relaxation and intubation
- maintenance
- analgesia
- reversal

A brief outline of the drugs typically used in each stage follows.

For **premedication**, benzodiazepines and some phenothiazines such as promethazine or alimemazine may be given to sedate and relieve *anxiety* in apprehensive patients. Butyrophenones such as droperidol have also been used. The benzodiazepines have useful amnesic and muscle-relaxant properties and short-acting oral analogues are common in current regimens. The phenothiazines and butyrophenones are rarely used now although their antiemetic actions may be useful to control *postoperative nausea and vomiting* (see p.1245). Cloral hydrate is still used in some countries for pre-operative sedation. The use of barbiturates has largely ceased. For sedation of children the oral route is often preferred to injections, or the rectal route may be used in exceptional circumstances.

Antimuscarinics such as atropine, glycopyrronium, and hyoscine may be given to inhibit excessive *bronchial* and *salivary secretions* induced by intubation and some anaesthetics, although such use is less common nowadays. Antimuscarinics are also given as premedicants to reduce the intra-operative bradycardia and hypotension induced by drugs such as suxamethonium, halothane, or propofol or following vagal stimulation. Hyoscine also provides some degree of amnesia.

Opioids, including morphine and its derivatives, papaveretum and pethidine, have been widely used before surgery to reduce anxiety, smooth induction of anaesthesia, reduce overall anaesthetic requirements, and provide pain relief during and after surgery. The routine use of opioids as premedicants is now rare and generally restricted to patients already in pain. However, they continue to find a role at induction (below).

Patients may also be given drugs that reduce the danger from regurgitation and *aspiration* of gastric contents (see under Aspiration Syndromes, p.1240), such as the histamine $H_2$-antagonists, cimetidine and ranitidine, and the proton pump inhibitor, omeprazole. Cardiovascular drugs may be required during surgery to control *blood pressure* and counteract *arrhythmias*.

The aim of **induction** is to produce anaesthesia rapidly and smoothly. Induction may be achieved with intravenous or inhalational anaesthetics but intravenous induction may be more pleasant for the patient. Intravenous drugs used include the barbiturate thiopental, the benzodiazepine midazolam, and other anaesthetics such as etomidate, propofol, or ketamine. Small doses of short-acting opioids, for example alfentanil, fentanyl, or remifentanil, given before or at induction allow the use of smaller induction doses of some drugs used for anaesthesia, and this technique is particularly suitable for poor-risk patients.

Following induction, **muscle relaxation** with a rapidly acting depolarising neuromuscular blocker such as suxamethonium facilitates **intubation** of the patient. Longer acting, competitive neuromuscular blockers may then be given to allow procedures such as abdominal surgery to be carried out under lighter anaesthesia. For more detail, see Anaesthesia, p.1397.

**Maintenance of anaesthesia** may be achieved with an inhalational anaesthetic, an intravenous anaesthetic, or an intravenous opioid, either alone or in combination.

Opioid analgesics may also be given for **analgesia** as supplements during general anaesthesia (see also Balanced Anaesthesia, under Anaesthetic Techniques, below). Long-acting opioids such as morphine or papaveretum may cause postoperative respiratory depression. The short-acting opioid fentanyl, and its congeners alfentanil and sufentanil, appear to produce fewer circulatory changes and may be preferred to other opioids, especially in cardiovascular surgery; remifentanil may be valuable for its very short duration of action. Various combinations of analgesic techniques, including the use of pre-emptive analgesia, are used or are being investigated for the management of surgical pain (see Postoperative Analgesia, p.4).

At the end of surgery drugs are sometimes given to accelerate recovery by **reversal** of the effects of the various agents used during anaesthesia. The *neuromuscular block* produced by competitive neuromuscular blockers may be reversed with anticholinesterases such as neostigmine and edrophonium but concomitant use of atropine or glycopyrronium is required to prevent bradycardia and other muscarinic actions developing. The opioid antagonist naloxone has been given to reverse opioid-induced *respiratory depression*. However, it may antagonise the analgesic effects of the opioids in the control of postoperative pain and the increasing use of short-acting intravenous opioid analgesics should reduce the need for its use. Flumazenil is a benzodiazepine antagonist that is used to reverse the *central sedative effects* of benzodiazepines in anaesthetic procedures.

ANAESTHETIC TECHNIQUES. A balanced combination of drugs with different actions is often used to provide the various components of general anaesthesia including unconsciousness, muscle relaxation, and analgesia. This technique, termed **balanced anaesthesia**, has been reported to minimise intra-operative cardiovascular depression, to facilitate a rapid return of consciousness, and to have a low incidence of postoperative adverse effects such as nausea and vomiting, and excitation. Typically an opioid is given before or with induction and anaesthesia is induced using nitrous oxide and an intravenous barbiturate such as thiopental. The opioid is then given in small incremental doses to achieve and maintain adequate analgesia during surgery. Opioid analgesics commonly used in this technique include morphine, fentanyl, sufentanil, and alfentanil; buprenorphine and nalbuphine have also been used.

In **total intravenous anaesthesia** (TIVA), induction and maintenance of anaesthesia is achieved with one or more anaesthetics given intravenously. This allows a high inspired oxygen concentrations in situations where hypoxaemia may otherwise occur, and is advantageous in surgery where delivery of inhaled anaesthetic may be difficult (for example in bronchoscopy). Combinations used in TIVA include propofol with alfentanil or fentanyl, and midazolam with alfentanil. Neuromuscular blockers are given to produce muscle relaxation but there can be difficulty in assessing the depth of anaesthesia in patients who are paralysed for mechanical ventilation, and there have been reports of awareness during procedures under total intravenous anaesthesia (see also under Intraoperative Awareness in Precautions, above).

Although now largely obsolete, use of a neuroleptic with an opioid analgesic produces an altered state of consciousness known as **neuroleptanalgesia** in which the patient is calm and indifferent to the surroundings yet is responsive to commands. The technique was used for diagnostic or therapeutic procedures such as minor surgery, endoscopy, and changing dressings. Neuroleptanalgesia can be converted to **neuroleptanaesthesia** by the concurrent administration of nitrous oxide in oxygen; a muscle relaxant may also be included. Neuroleptanaesthesia is particularly useful if the patient's cooperation is required, as consciousness soon returns once the nitrous oxide is discontinued. The neuroleptic most commonly employed was droperidol and it was usually used with fentanyl although other opioids have also been employed. These procedures have since evolved into **conscious sedation** techniques employing newer drugs.

Ketamine used alone can produce a state of **dissociative anaesthesia** similar to that of neuroleptanalgesia in which the patient may appear to be awake but is unconscious. Marked analgesia and amnesia are produced, but there may be an increase in muscle tone and emergence reactions. Dissociative anaesthesia is considered suitable for use in various diagnostic procedures, dressing changes, and in minor surgery not requiring muscle relaxation.

Techniques using **local anaesthetics** are discussed on p.1370.

## Alfadolone Acetate *(BANM, rINNM)*

Acetato de alfadolona; Alphadolone Acetate; GR-2/1574. 3α,21-Dihydroxy-5α-pregnane-11,20-dione 21-acetate.

$C_{23}H_{34}O_5$ = 390.5.

*CAS — 14107-37-0 (alfadolone); 23930-37-2 (alfadolone acetate).*

**Pharmacopoeias.** In *BP(Vet).*

**BP(Vet) 2003** (Alfadolone Acetate). A white to creamy white powder. Practically insoluble in water and in petroleum spirit; soluble in alcohol; freely soluble in chloroform.

### Profile

Alfadolone acetate has been used to enhance the solubility of alfaxalone (below). It possesses some anaesthetic properties and is considered to be about half as potent as alfaxalone.

## Alfaxalone *(BAN, rINN)*

Alfaxalona; Alphaxalone; GR-2/234. 3α-Hydroxy-5α-pregnane-11,20-dione.

$C_{21}H_{32}O_3$ = 332.5.

*CAS — 23930-19-0.*

*ATC — N01AX05.*

**Pharmacopoeias.** In *BP(Vet).*

**BP(Vet) 2003** (Alfaxalone). A white to creamy white powder. Practically insoluble in water and in petroleum spirit; soluble in alcohol; freely soluble in chloroform.

### Profile

Alfaxalone was formerly used with alfadolone acetate (above) ['Althesin'], as an intravenous anaesthetic for induction and maintenance of general anaesthesia.

Adverse reactions associated with polyethoxylated castor oil (present as a vehicle) led to the general withdrawal of alfaxalone with alfadolone acetate from human use. It is still used in veterinary medicine.

**Porphyria.** Alfaxalone:alfadolone has been associated with acute attacks of porphyria and is considered unsafe in porphyric patients.

## Chloroform

Chloroformium Anesthesicum; Chloroformum; Chloroformum pro Narcosi; Cloroformo. Trichloromethane.

$CHCl_3$ = 119.4.

*CAS — 67-66-3.*

*ATC — N01AB02.*

**Pharmacopoeias.** In *Br., Chin.,* and *Viet.*

**BP 2003** (Chloroform). A colourless volatile liquid with a characteristic odour. Not more than 5.0% v/v distils below 60° and the remainder distils at 60° to 62°. It contains 1.0 to 2.0% v/v of ethyl alcohol; amylene 50 micrograms/mL is permitted as an alternative to ethyl alcohol.

Slightly soluble in water; miscible with dehydrated alcohol, with ether, with fixed and volatile oils, and with most other organic solvents. Store in containers with glass stoppers or other suitable closures. Protect from light. The label should state whether it contains ethyl alcohol or amylene.

**Stability.** The addition of the small percentage of alcohol greatly retards the gradual oxidation which occurs when chloroform is exposed to air and light, and which results in its becoming contaminated with the very poisonous carbonyl chloride (phosgene) and with chlorine; the alcohol also serves to decompose any carbonyl chloride that may have been formed.

From a study[1] of chloroform losses from chloroform water and from 6 typical BPC mixtures under various conditions of storage the following shelf-lives were recommended: chloroform solutions and non-sedimented mixtures could be stored in well-closed well-filled containers for 2 months at ambient temperatures; when stored in partially-filled containers periodically opened the shelf-life should not exceed 2 weeks; sedimented mixtures could be stored for 2 months in well-closed well-filled containers, but because loss of chloroform could be expected in containers periodically opened such mixtures should be prepared as required or packed in their final containers; for chloroform-containing mixtures in the home a shelf-life of 2 weeks was suggested.

1. Lynch M, *et al.* Chloroform as a preservative in aqueous systems: losses under "in-use" conditions and antimicrobial effectiveness. *Pharm J* 1977; **219:** 507–10.

**Storage.** It has been recommended[1] that PVC bottles should not be used for storing or dispensing Chloroform and Morphine Tincture, aqueous mixtures containing more than 5% thereof, mixtures or dispersions in which chloroform was present in excess of its aqueous solubility, aqueous mixtures containing chloroform and high concentrations of electrolytes, or Chloroform Water (BP) or mixtures containing it if the period of use would exceed 6 weeks.

1. Anonymous. Plastics medicine bottles of rigid PVC. *Pharm J* 1973; **210:** 100.

### Adverse Effects and Precautions

Chloroform depresses respiration and produces hypotension. Cardiac output is reduced and arrhythmias may develop. Poisoning may therefore lead to respiratory depression and cardiac arrest. Delayed hepatotoxic and nephrotoxic reactions may occur 6 to 24 hours after a dose; symptoms may include abdominal pain, vomiting, and, at a later stage, jaundice.

Liquid chloroform is irritant to the skin and mucous membranes and may cause burns if spilt on them. Suitable precautions should be taken to avoid skin contact with chloroform as it can penetrate skin and produce systemic toxicity. Chloroform is not flammable. Care should be taken not to vaporise chloroform in the presence of a flame because of the production of toxic gases.

In the UK medicinal products are limited to a chloroform content of not more than 0.5% (w/w or v/v as appropriate) of chloroform. Exceptions include supply by a doctor or dentist, or in accordance with his prescription, to a particular patient, and supply for anaesthetic purposes.

In the USA the FDA has banned the use of chloroform in medicines and cosmetics, because of reported carcinogenicity in *animals*. It has also been withdrawn from systemic use in other countries.

The sale within or import into England and Wales and Scotland of food containing any added chloroform is prohibited.

See also Adverse Effects and Precautions for General Anaesthetics, p.1295.

**Breast feeding.** No adverse effects have been observed in breast-fed infants whose mothers were receiving chloroform, and the American Academy of Pediatrics[1] considers that it is therefore usually compatible with breast feeding.

1. American Academy of Pediatrics. The transfer of drugs and other chemicals into human milk. *Pediatrics* 2001; **108:** 776–89. Correction. *ibid.*; 1029. Also available at: http://aappolicy.aappublications.org/cgi/content/full/pediatrics%3b108/3/776 (accessed 25/05/04)

**Porphyria.** Chloroform has been associated with acute attacks of porphyria and is considered unsafe in porphyric patients.

### Uses and Administration

Chloroform is a volatile halogenated anaesthetic that was administered by inhalation but safer drugs are now preferred in general anaesthesia.

Chloroform is used as a carminative and as a flavouring agent and preservative. For these purposes it is usually employed as Chloroform Spirit (BP 2003) or Chloroform Water (BP 2003) but doubts have been cast on the safety of the long-term use of chloroform in mixtures.

Externally, chloroform has a rubefacient action.

Chloroform is also used as a solvent.

◊ An historical review of the use of chloroform in clinical anaesthesia.[1]

1. Payne JP. Chloroform in clinical anaesthesia. *Br J Anaesth* 1981; **53:** 11S–15S.

### Preparations

***BP 2003:*** Chloroform and Morphine Tincture; Chloroform Spirit; Chloroform Water; Double-strength Chloroform Water.

**Proprietary Preparations** (details are given in Part 3)

**Multi-ingredient: *Belg.:*** Baume Dalet†; Dentophar; Dolpyc†; ***Fr.:*** Baume Dalet†; Dolpyc†; Lao-Dal†.

---

## Cyclopropane *(rINN)*

Ciclopropano; Trimethylene.

$C_3H_6$ = 42.08.

*CAS — 75-19-4.*

**Pharmacopoeias.** In *US.*

**USP 27** (Cyclopropane). A colourless highly flammable gas with a characteristic odour and pungent taste. Freely soluble in alcohol; soluble in fixed oils. One volume dissolves in about 2.7 volumes of water at 15°.

**Stability.** CAUTION. Mixtures of cyclopropane with oxygen or air at certain concentrations are explosive. Cyclopropane should not be used in the presence of an open flame or of any electrical apparatus liable to produce a spark. Precautions should be taken against the production of static electrical discharge.

**Storage and supply.** Cyclopropane is supplied compressed in metal cylinders. National standards are usually in operation for the labelling and marking of such cylinders.

### Adverse Effects and Precautions

Cyclopropane depresses respiration to a greater extent than many other anaesthetics. Laryngospasm, cardiac arrhythmias, or hepatic injury may occur. Cyclopropane increases the sensitivity of the heart to sympathomimetic amines. Malignant hyperthermia has also been reported. Postoperative nausea, vomiting, and headache are frequent.

Cyclopropane should be used with caution in patients with bronchial asthma and cardiovascular disorders. Premedication with atropine may be advisable to reduce vagal tone.

See also Adverse Effects and Precautions for General Anaesthetics, p.1295.

**Abuse.** Two of 4 deaths from abuse of volatile anaesthetics in operating rooms were attributed to cyclopropane.[1]

1. Bass M. Abuse of inhalation anesthetics. *JAMA* 1984; **251:** 604.

**Malignant hyperthermia.** Malignant hyperthermia was associated with cyclopropane.[1]

1. Lips FJ, *et al.* Malignant hyperthermia triggered by cyclopropane during cesarean section. *Anesthesiology* 1982; **56:** 144–6.

### Interactions

Care is advised if adrenaline or other sympathomimetics are given during cyclopropane anaesthesia. Potentiation of competitive neuromuscular blockers occurs after cyclopropane administration.

See also Interactions for General Anaesthetics, p.1295.

### Uses and Administration

Cyclopropane is an anaesthetic that has been administered by inhalation for analgesia and induction and maintenance of general anaesthesia. It produces skeletal muscle relaxation, is non-irritant, and induction and recovery are rapid, but it is difficult to use and handle and other anaesthetics are generally preferred. Because of the risk of explosion, the usual method of administration has been by means of a closed circuit. It has a minimum alveolar concentration (MAC) value (see Uses of General Anaesthetics, p.1295) of 9.2%.

---

## Desflurane *(USAN, rINN)*

Desflurano; I-653. (±)-2-Difluoromethyl 1,2,2,2-tetrafluoroethyl ether.

$C_3H_2F_6O$ = 168.0.

*CAS — 57041-67-5.*

*ATC — N01AB07.*

**Pharmacopoeias.** In *US.*

**USP 27** (Desflurane). Store in airtight containers. Protect from light.

### Adverse Effects and Precautions

As with other halogenated anaesthetics, respiratory depression, hypotension, and arrhythmias may occur. Desflurane may rarely precipitate malignant hyperthermia in susceptible individuals. It appears to sensitise the myocardium to sympathomimetics to a lesser extent than halothane or enflurane. Nausea and vomiting have been reported in the postoperative period.

Desflurane is irritant to the airways and may provoke breath holding, apnoea, coughing, increased salivation, and laryngospasm. It is therefore not recommended for induction of anaesthesia in paediatric patients.

As with other halogenated anaesthetics, patients with known or suspected susceptibility to malignant hyperthermia should not be anaesthetised with desflurane. Desflurane may increase CSF pressure and should therefore be used with caution in patients with, or at risk from, raised intracranial pressure.

In order to minimise the risk of developing elevated carboxyhaemoglobin levels carbon dioxide absorbents in anaesthetic apparatus should not be allowed to dry out when delivering volatile anaesthetics such as desflurane (see below).

See also Adverse Effects and Precautions of General Anaesthetics, p.1295.

**Carbon dioxide absorbents.** Significant carboxyhaemoglobinaemia may develop rarely during anaesthesia with volatile anaesthetics given by circle breathing systems containing carbon dioxide absorbents.[1] The effect is only seen when the absorbent has become excessively dried out. The use of barium hydroxide lime (which is not available in the UK) as an absorbent produces more carbon monoxide than soda lime, particularly at low water content. No cases of this complication had been reported to date in the UK.

1. Committee on Safety of Medicines/Medicines Control Agency. Safety issues in anaesthesia: volatile anaesthetic agents and carboxyhaemoglobinaemia. *Current Problems* 1997; **23:** 7. Also available at: http://www.mca.gov.uk/ourwork/monitorsafequalmed/currentproblems/volume24.htm (accessed 25/05/04)

**Effects on the cardiovascular system.** A review[1] of *animal* and human studies concluded that the cardiorespiratory effects of desflurane were similar to those of isoflurane but that there might be better control of arterial pressure with desflurane during stressful stimuli. A study[2] in patients undergoing coronary artery bypass surgery demonstrated that a state of haemodynamic stability suitable for patients at risk of myocardial ischaemia could be maintained when desflurane was supplemented with the opioid analgesic fentanyl.

1. Warltier DC, Pagel PS. Cardiovascular and respiratory actions of desflurane: is desflurane different from isoflurane? *Anesth Analg* 1992; **75:** S17–S31.
2. Parsons RS, *et al.* Comparison of desflurane and fentanyl-based anaesthetic techniques for coronary artery bypass surgery. *Br J Anaesth* 1994; **72:** 430–8.

**Effects on the liver.** Although considered to be less hepatotoxic than some other halogenated anaesthetics (see under Adverse Effects of Halothane, p.1300), delayed hepatotoxicity has occurred in a 65-year-old woman following maintenance anaesthesia involving desflurane.[1] She had received halothane on two previous occasions which may have caused sensitisation. Investigation of hepatocellular integrity (by measuring glutathione transferase alpha) in 30 women who had received desflurane indicated a mild subclinical disturbance.[2]

1. Martin JL, *et al.* Hepatotoxicity after desflurane anesthesia. *Anesthesiology* 1995; **83:** 1125–9.
2. Tiainen P, *et al.* Changes in hepatocellular integrity during and after desflurane or isoflurane anaesthesia in patients undergoing breast surgery. *Br J Anaesth* 1998; **80:** 87–9.

**Effects on the respiratory tract.** The irritant effect of desflurane on the lungs limits its role in the induction of anaesthesia, especially in children. Pre-operative use of nebulised lidocaine 4% failed to alleviate the response[1] although pretreatment with intravenous opioids may reduce the irritation.[2]

1. Bunting HE, *et al.* Effect of nebulized lignocaine on airway irritation and haemodynamic changes during induction of anaesthesia with desflurane. *Br J Anaesth* 1995; **75:** 631–3.
2. Kong CF, *et al.* Intravenous opioids reduce airway irritation during induction of anaesthesia with desflurane in adults. *Br J Anaesth* 2000; **85:** 364–7.

### Interactions

The effects of competitive neuromuscular blockers such as atracurium are enhanced by desflurane (see p.1401). Lower doses of desflurane are required in those receiving opioids, benzodiazepines or other sedatives. Care is advised if adrenaline or other sympathomimetics are given to patients during desflurane anaesthesia.

See also Interactions of General Anaesthetics, p.1295.

◊ References.

1. Dale O. Drug interactions in anaesthesia: focus on desflurane and sevoflurane. *Baillieres Clin Anaesthesiol* 1995; **9:** 105–17.

### Pharmacokinetics

Desflurane has a low blood/gas partition coefficient and following inhalation its absorption, distribution, and elimination are reported to be more rapid than for other halogenated anaesthetics such as isoflurane or halothane. It is excreted mainly unchanged through the lungs. A small amount diffuses through the skin. About 0.02% of administered desflurane is metabolised in the liver and trichloroacetic acid has been detected in the serum and urine of patients given desflurane.

◊ References.

1. Caldwell JE. Desflurane clinical pharmacokinetics and pharmacodynamics. *Clin Pharmacokinet* 1994; **27:** 6–18.
2. Eger EI. Physicochemical properties and pharmacodynamics of desflurane. *Anaesthesia* 1995; **50** (suppl): 3–8.
3. Wissing H, *et al.* Pharmacokinetics of inhaled anaesthetics in a clinical setting: comparison of desflurane, isoflurane and sevoflurane. *Br J Anaesth* 2000; **84:** 443–9.
4. Lu CC, *et al.* Pharmacokinetics of desflurane uptake into the brain and body. *Anaesthesia* 2004; **59:** 216–21.

### Uses and Administration

Desflurane is a volatile halogenated anaesthetic administered by inhalation. It is structurally similar to isoflurane and has anaesthetic actions similar to those of halothane (p.1300). The minimum alveolar concentration (MAC) value (see Uses of General Anaesthetics, p.1295) ranges from about 6% in the elderly to about 11% in infants. It is non-flammable and non-explosive in clinical concentrations but, because of its low boiling-point, it must be delivered by a special vaporiser, preferably within a closed circuit system.

Desflurane is used for induction and maintenance of general anaesthesia (p.1296), but because of its pungency is not recommended for induction in children. Concentrations of 4 to 11% v/v have been used for induction and usually produce surgical anaesthesia in 2 to 4 minutes. Concentrations of 2 to 6% v/v with nitrous oxide or 2.5 to 8.5% v/v in oxygen or oxygen-enriched air may be used to maintain anaesthesia. Higher concentrations of desflurane have been used but it is important to ensure adequate oxygenation; concentrations in excess of 17% v/v are not recommended.

As with other volatile halogenated anaesthetics supplemental neuromuscular blockers may be required. Recovery from anaesthesia is reported to be more rapid than with other halogenated anaesthetics.

**Administration in hepatic or renal impairment.** Desflurane concentrations of 1 to 4% v/v in oxygen and nitrous oxide have been used in patients with chronic renal or hepatic impairment and during renal transplantation surgery.

**Anaesthesia.** The characteristics of desflurane have been discussed in a number of reviews.[1-5] Its advantages are considered to include rapid induction and emergence from anaesthesia, and minimal metabolism makes end-organ toxicity unlikely. Emergence from anaesthesia and recovery of psychomotor and cognitive skills with desflurane is more rapid than after anaesthesia with other halogenated volatile anaesthetics such as isoflurane and possibly than after the intravenous anaesthetic propofol. This is considered to be of particular advantage for outpatient treatment, but studies so far have found no difference in time to discharge with desflurane or other general anaesthetics. Furthermore, the incidence of nausea and vomiting with desflurane is significantly greater than after the use of propofol. Desflurane's pungency may also limit its use for induction especially in children, although it is suitable for maintenance in this group and may be particularly suitable for neonates.[4]

1. Caldwell JE. Desflurane clinical pharmacokinetics and pharmacodynamics. *Clin Pharmacokinet* 1994; **27:** 6–18.
2. Patel SS, Goa KL. Desflurane: a review of its pharmacodynamic and pharmacokinetic properties and its efficacy in general anaesthesia. *Drugs* 1995; **50:** 742–67.
3. Young CJ, Apfelbaum JL. Inhalational anesthetics: desflurane and sevoflurane. *J Clin Anesth* 1995; **7:** 564–77.
4. Hatch DJ. New inhalation agents in paediatric anaesthesia. *Br J Anaesth* 1999; **83:** 42–9.
5. Umbrain V, *et al.* Desflurane: a reappraisal. *Acta Anaesthesiol Belg* 2002; **53:** 187–91.

## Preparations

**Proprietary Preparations** (details are given in Part 3)
***Arg.:*** Suprane; ***Austral.:*** Suprane†; ***Austria:*** Suprane; ***Belg.:*** Suprane†; ***Braz.:*** Suprane†; ***Canad.:*** Suprane; ***Denm.:*** Suprane; ***Fin.:*** Suprane; ***Ger.:*** Suprane; ***Gr.:*** Suprane; ***Irl.:*** Suprane†; ***Israel:*** Suprane; ***Ital.:*** Suprane; ***Mex.:*** Suprane†; ***Neth.:*** Suprane; ***Norw.:*** Suprane†; ***NZ:*** Suprane; ***S.Afr.:*** Suprane; ***Singapore:*** Suprane†; ***Spain:*** Suprane; ***Swed.:*** Suprane; ***Switz.:*** Suprane; ***UK:*** Suprane; ***USA:*** Suprane.

# Enflurane *(BAN, USAN, rINN)*

Anaesthetic Compound No. 347; Compound 347; Enflurano; Methylflurether; NSC-115944. 2-Chloro-1,1,2-trifluoroethyl difluoromethyl ether; 2-Chloro-1-(difluoromethoxy)-1,1,2-trifluoroethane.

$C_3H_2ClF_5O$ = 184.5.

*CAS — 13838-16-9.*

*ATC — N01AB04.*

**Pharmacopoeias.** In *Jpn* and *US.*

**USP 27** (Enflurane). A clear colourless volatile liquid having a mild sweet odour. Non-flammable. Distilling range 55.5° to 57.5°. Slightly soluble in water; miscible with organic solvents, with fats, and with oils. Store in airtight containers at a temperature not exceeding 40°. Protect from light.

## Adverse Effects

As with other halogenated anaesthetics, respiratory depression, hypotension, and arrhythmias have been reported although the incidence of arrhythmias is lower with enflurane than with halothane. It sensitises the myocardium to sympathomimetics to a lesser extent than halothane. Compared with halothane, enflurane has a stimulant effect on the CNS and convulsions may occur when concentrations of enflurane are high or hypocapnia is present. Malignant hyperthermia has also been reported. Asthma and bronchospasm may occur. There have been reports of elevated serum-fluoride concentrations although resulting renal damage appears to be rare. There have been changes in measurements of hepatic enzymes and a number of reports of liver damage. Shivering, nausea, and vomiting have been reported in the postoperative period.

See also Adverse Effects of General Anaesthetics, p.1295.

**Effects on the blood.** The development of carboxyhaemoglobinaemia in patients anaesthetised with volatile anaesthetics is discussed under Precautions, below.

**Effects on the kidneys.** The nephrotoxicity of volatile anaesthetics has been reviewed.[1] Although enflurane released inorganic fluoride it appeared to be safe in patients with normal renal function. It had also been given to patients with mild to moderate renal impairment without any further deterioration. There was an increase in serum-fluoride concentrations when enflurane was given to a group of patients who had been receiving isoniazid, but there was no change in kidney function. Pretreatment of patients with a single dose of disulfiram before anaesthesia was found to produce a consistent and almost complete inhibition of enflurane metabolism as shown by substantial reductions in plasma-fluoride concentrations and urinary excretion of fluoride.[2]

1. Mazze RI. Nephrotoxicity of fluorinated anaesthetic agents. *Clin Anaesthesiol* 1983; **1:** 469–83.
2. Kharasch ED, *et al.* Clinical enflurane metabolism by cytochrome P450 2E1. *Clin Pharmacol Ther* 1994; **55:** 434–40.

**Effects on the liver.** A review[1] of 58 cases of suspected enflurane hepatitis considered enflurane to be the likely cause of the liver damage in 24. There was biochemical evidence of liver damage in 23 of these cases. Histology reports were available for 15 patients and all showed some degree of hepatocellular necrosis and degeneration.

While the incidence of liver damage from enflurane seemed to be lower than from halothane, the character of the injury was similar.

Another review[2] of the same cases plus an additional 30 (88 in all) came to different conclusions; the main author was a consultant to the manufacturer of enflurane. Of the 88 patients with suspected enflurane hepatitis, 30 were rejected because of insufficient evidence and 43 were considered to have other factors known to produce liver injury. This left 15 possible cases of enflurane hepatitis compared with the 24 identified by the first review. While agreeing that in the rare patient unexplained liver damage follows enflurane anaesthesia, it was considered that the incidence was too small to suggest an association. No consistent histological pattern was identified in this study.

See also under Adverse Effects in Halothane, p.1300.

1. Lewis JH, *et al.* Enflurane hepatotoxicity: a clinicopathologic study of 24 cases. *Ann Intern Med* 1983; **98:** 984–92.
2. Eger EI, *et al.* Is enflurane hepatotoxic? *Anesth Analg* 1986; **65:** 21–30.

**Effects on respiration.** Overall, enflurane is considered to produce more respiratory depression than halothane or isoflurane.[1,2]

1. Quail AW. Modern inhalation anaesthetic agents: a review of halothane, isoflurane and enflurane. *Med J Aust* 1989; **150:** 95–102.
2. Merrett KL, Jones RM. Inhalational anaesthetic agents. *Br J Hosp Med* 1994; **52:** 260–3.

## Precautions

Enflurane should be used with caution in patients with convulsive disorders. High concentrations of enflurane may cause uterine relaxation. In order to minimise the risk of developing elevated carboxyhaemoglobin levels, carbon dioxide absorbents in anaesthetic apparatus should not be allowed to dry out when delivering volatile anaesthetics such as enflurane.

As with other halogenated anaesthetics, patients with known or suspected susceptibility to malignant hyperthermia should not be anaesthetised with enflurane.

See also Precautions for General Anaesthetics, p.1295.

**Abuse.** Report[1] of a fatality in a 29-year-old student nurse anaesthetist who had applied enflurane to the herpes simplex lesions of her lower lip. She was found with an empty 250 mL bottle of enflurane.

1. Lingenfelter RW. Fatal misuse of enflurane. *Anesthesiology* 1981; **55:** 603.

**Carbon dioxide absorbents.** Significant carboxyhaemoglobinaemia may develop rarely during anaesthesia with volatile anaesthetics given by circle breathing systems containing carbon dioxide absorbents.[1] The effect is only seen when the absorbent has become excessively dried out. The use of barium hydroxide lime (which is not available in the UK) as an absorbent produces more carbon monoxide than soda lime, particularly at low water content. No cases of this complication had been reported to date in the UK.

1. Committee on Safety of Medicines/Medicines Control Agency. Safety issues in anaesthesia: volatile anaesthetic agents and carboxyhaemoglobinaemia. *Current Problems* 1997; **23:** 7. Also available at: http://www.mca.gov.uk/ourwork/monitorsafequalmed/currentproblems/volume24.htm (accessed 25/02/04)

**Porphyria.** Enflurane is considered to be unsafe in patients with porphyria because it has been shown to be porphyrinogenic in *animals.*

## Interactions

Care is advised if adrenaline or other sympathomimetics are given to patients during enflurane anaesthesia. The effects of competitive neuromuscular blockers such as atracurium are enhanced by enflurane (see p.1401).

See also Interactions of General Anaesthetics, p.1295.

**Antibacterials.** For the effects of *isoniazid* on enflurane defluorination, see Effects on the Kidneys under Adverse Effects, above.

**Antidepressants.** It appeared likely that the enflurane-induced seizure activity observed in 2 patients could have been enhanced by *amitriptyline.*[1] It may be advisable to avoid the use of enflurane in patients requiring tricyclic antidepressants, especially when the patient has a history of seizures or when hyperventilation or high enflurane concentrations are a desired part of the anaesthetic technique.

1. Sprague DH, Wolf S. Enflurane seizures in patients taking amitriptyline. *Anesth Analg* 1982; **61:** 67–8.

**Disulfiram.** For the effect of disulfiram on the metabolism of enflurane, see Effects on the Kidneys under Adverse Effects, above.

## Pharmacokinetics

Enflurane is absorbed on inhalation. The blood/gas partition coefficient is low. It is mostly excreted unchanged through the lungs. Up to 10% of administered enflurane is metabolised in the liver, mainly to inorganic fluoride.

◊ References.

1. Bengtson JP, *et al.* Uptake of enflurane and isoflurane during spontaneous and controlled ventilation. *Anaesth Intensive Care* 1992; **20:** 191–5.
2. Devchand D, *et al.* The uptake of enflurane during anaesthesia. *Anaesthesia* 1995; **50:** 491–5.

## Uses and Administration

Enflurane is a volatile halogenated anaesthetic administered by inhalation. It is an isomer of isoflurane. It has anaesthetic actions similar to those of halothane (p.1300). Enflurane has a minimum alveolar concentration (MAC) value (see Uses of General Anaesthetics, p.1295) ranging from 1.7% in middle age to 2.5% in children. Enflurane is administered using a calibrated vaporiser for induction and maintenance of general anaesthesia (p.1296); it is also used in subanaesthetic doses to provide analgesia in obstetrics and other painful procedures.

To avoid CNS excitement a short-acting barbiturate or other intravenous induction agent is recommended before the inhalation of enflurane. Anaesthesia is induced starting at an enflurane concentration of 0.4% v/v in air, oxygen, or nitrous oxide-oxygen mixtures and increasing by increments of 0.5% v/v every few breaths to a maximum of 4.5%. Anaesthesia may be maintained with a concentration of 0.5 to 3% v/v of enflurane in nitrous oxide-oxygen; a concentration of 3% v/v should not be exceeded during spontaneous respiration. Although enflurane is reported to possess muscle relaxant properties, neuromuscular blockers may nevertheless be required. Postoperative analgesia may be necessary.

**Pain.** Enflurane is used in subanaesthetic doses to provide analgesia in obstetrics and other painful procedures although a study[1] was unable to confirm that it had an analgesic effect at subanaesthetic concentrations.

1. Tomi K, *et al.* Alterations in pain threshold and psychomotor response associated with subanaesthetic concentrations of inhalation anaesthetics in humans. *Br J Anaesth* 1993; **70:** 684–6.

## Preparations

**Proprietary Preparations** (details are given in Part 3)
***Arg.:*** Enforan; Inhelthran; ***Austral.:*** Alyrane†; Ethrane; ***Austria:*** Ethrane; ***Belg.:*** Alyrane†; Ethrane†; ***Braz.:*** Enfluthane; Etrane; ***Canad.:*** Ethrane†; ***Denm.:*** Alyrane†; Efrane; ***Fin.:*** Efrane; ***Ger.:*** Ethrane; ***Hong Kong:*** Ethrane†; ***Irl.:*** Ethrane; ***Israel:*** Alyrane; Ethrane; ***Mex.:*** Enfran; Enlirane†; Ethrane; ***Neth.:*** Alyrane†; Ethrane; ***Norw.:*** Efrane†; ***S.Afr.:*** Alyrane†; Ethrane; ***Swed.:*** Alyrane†; Efrane; ***Switz.:*** Ethrane; ***UK:*** Alyrane†; ***USA:*** Ethrane.

# Anaesthetic Ether

Aether ad Narcosin; Aether Anaesthesticus; Aether pro Narcosi; Aether Purissimus; Diethyl Ether; Éter anestésico; Éter Puríssimo; Ether; Ether Anesthesicus; Ethyl Ether.

$(C_2H_5)_2O$ = 74.12.

*CAS — 60-29-7.*

*ATC — N01AA01.*

**Pharmacopoeias.** In *Chin., Eur.* (see p.vi), *Int., Jpn, Pol., US,* and *Viet.*

**Ph. Eur. 5.0** (Ether, Anaesthetic). Diethyl ether to which an appropriate quantity of a non-volatile antoxidant may have been added. It contains not more than 2 g/litre of water. A clear, colourless, volatile, highly flammable, and very mobile liquid. Distillation range 34° to 35°.

Soluble 1 in 15 of water; miscible with alcohol and with fatty oils. Store at a temperature of 8° to 15° in airtight containers. Protect from light. Ether remaining in a partly used container may deteriorate rapidly. The label should state the name and concentration of any added non-volatile antoxidant.

**USP 27** (Ether). It consists of 96 to 98% of $C_4H_{10}O$, the remainder consisting of alcohol and water. Ether for anaesthetic use contains not more than 0.2% of water. It is a colourless, mobile, highly flammable, highly volatile liquid, having a characteristic sweet, pungent odour. It is slowly oxidised by the action of air and light, with the formation of peroxides. Its vapour, when mixed with air and ignited, may explode. B.p. about 35°.

Soluble 1 in 12 of water; miscible with alcohol, with chloroform, with dichloromethane, with petroleum spirit, with benzene, and with fixed and volatile oils; soluble in hydrochloric acid. Store in partly-filled, airtight containers, remote from fire and at a temperature not exceeding 40°. Protect from light. Ether to be used for anaesthesia must be preserved in airtight containers of not more than 3 kg capacity and is not to be used for anaesthesia if it has been removed from the original container longer than 24 hours.

**Labelling.** The label should state that it is suitable for use as an anaesthetic.

**Stability.** Ether is very volatile and flammable and mixtures of its vapour with oxygen, nitrous oxide, or air at certain concentrations are explosive. It should not be used in the presence of an open flame or any electrical apparatus liable to produce a spark. Precautions should be taken against the production of static electrical discharge.

**Storage.** The Pharmaceutical Society of Great Britain's Department of Pharmaceutical Sciences found that free ether, even in low concentrations, caused softening of PVC bottles and was associated with loss by permeation.[1]

1. Anonymous. Plastics medicine bottles of rigid PVC. *Pharm J* 1973; **210:** 100.

### Adverse Effects

Ether has an irritant action on the mucous membrane of the respiratory tract; it stimulates salivation and increases bronchial secretion. Laryngeal spasm may occur. Ether causes vasodilatation which may lead to a severe fall in blood pressure and it reduces blood flow to the kidneys; it also increases capillary bleeding. The bleeding time is unchanged but the prothrombin time may be prolonged. Ether may cause malignant hyperthermia in certain individuals. Alterations in kidney and liver function have been reported. Convulsions occasionally occur. Hyperglycaemia due to gluconeogenesis has been noted.

Recovery is slow from prolonged ether anaesthesia and postoperative vomiting commonly occurs. Acute overdosage of ether is characterised by respiratory failure and cardiac arrest.

Dependence on ether or ether vapour has been reported. Prolonged contact with ether spilt on any tissue produces necrosis.

See also Adverse Effects of General Anaesthetics, p.1295.

### Precautions

Ether anaesthesia is contra-indicated in patients with diabetes mellitus, impaired kidney function, raised CSF pressure, and severe liver disease. Its use is not advisable in hot and humid conditions in patients with fever as convulsions are liable to occur, particularly in children and in patients who have been given atropine.

See also Precautions for General Anaesthetics, p.1295.

### Interactions

Ether enhances the action of competitive neuromuscular blockers to a greater degree than most other anaesthetics. Potentiation of the arrhythmogenic effect of sympathomimetics, including adrenaline, by ether is less than that seen with other inhalational anaesthetics.

See also Interactions of General Anaesthetics, p.1295.

### Uses and Administration

Ether is an anaesthetic administered by inhalation. It has a minimum alveolar concentration (MAC) value (see Uses of General Anaesthetics, p.1295) of 1.92%. Ether is still used in some countries for the induction and maintenance of general anaesthesia although it has been replaced in many other countries by the halogenated anaesthetics. It possesses a respiratory stimulant effect in all but the deepest planes of anaesthesia. Ether also possesses analgesic and muscle relaxant properties. Premedication with an antimuscarinic such as atropine is necessary to reduce salivary and bronchial secretions.

Solvent ether is described on p.1474.

---

## Etomidate *(BAN, USAN, rINN)*

Etomidato; Etomidatum; R-16659; R-26490 (etomidate sulfate).
R-(+)-Ethyl 1-(α-methylbenzyl)imidazole-5-carboxylate.
$C_{14}H_{16}N_2O_2$ = 244.3.
*CAS — 33125-97-2.*
*ATC — N01AX07.*

**Pharmacopoeias.** In *Chin.* and *Eur.* (see p.vi).

**Ph. Eur. 5.0** (Etomidate). A white or almost white powder. M.p. about 68°. Very slightly soluble in water; freely soluble in alcohol and in dichloromethane. Protect from light.

### Adverse Effects and Precautions

Excitatory phenomena (especially involuntary myoclonic muscle movements, which are sometimes severe) are common following injection of etomidate, but may be reduced by the prior administration of an opioid analgesic or a short-acting benzodiazepine. Pain on injection may be reduced by giving it into a large vein in the arm rather than into the hand, or, again, by premedication with an opioid analgesic. Convulsions may occur rarely as may laryngospasm and cardiac arrhythmias. Hypersensitivity reactions including anaphylaxis have been reported. Etomidate is associated with less hypotension than other drugs commonly used for induction.

Because etomidate inhibits adrenocortical function during maintenance anaesthesia (see below) its use is limited to induction of anaesthesia. In addition it should not be used in patients whose adrenocortical function is already reduced or at risk of being reduced. Etomidate should be used with care in the elderly, who may be more prone to cardiac depression; lower doses may be required. The dose of etomidate should also be reduced in patients with hepatic cirrhosis. Caution may be appropriate in patients with pre-existing epilepsy.

See also Adverse Effects and Precautions for General Anaesthetics, p.1295.

**Effects on the endocrine system.** Etomidate used for sedation in an intensive care unit was implicated in an increase in mortality.[1] The UK Committee on Safety of Medicines agreed that etomidate could cause a significant fall in circulating plasma-cortisol concentrations, unresponsive to corticotropin stimulation.[2] As a result of this effect, use of etomidate is restricted to induction of anaesthesia. The manufacturers advise that the postoperative rise in serum-cortisol concentration, which has been observed after thiopental induction, is delayed for about 3 to 6 hours when etomidate is used for induction.

A study comparing the effects of etomidate with those of methohexital on the adrenocortical function of neonates borne by mothers who received these agents for induction of anaesthesia before caesarean section indicated that there was no evidence to preclude the use of etomidate in such patients. However, regardless of which anaesthetic agent was used, early feeding was recommended to avoid neonatal hypoglycaemia.[3]

1. Ledingham IM, Watt I. Influence of sedation on mortality in critically ill multiple trauma patients. *Lancet* 1983; **i:** 1270.
2. Goldberg A. Etomidate. *Lancet* 1983; **ii:** 60.
3. Crozier TA, *et al.* Effects of etomidate on the adrenocortical and metabolic adaptation of the neonate. *Br J Anaesth* 1993; **70:** 47–53.

**Hypersensitivity.** Reactions involving immediate widespread cutaneous flushing or urticaria attributed to etomidate have been described.[1] There have also been reports[2,3] of anaphylactic reactions following injection of etomidate.

1. Watkins J. Etomidate: an 'immunologically safe' anaesthetic agent. *Anaesthesia* 1983; **38** (suppl): 34–8.
2. Sold M, Rothhammer A. Lebensbedrohliche anaphylaktoide reaktion nach etomidat. *Anaesthesist* 1985; **34:** 208–10.
3. Krumholz W, *et al.* Ein fall von anaphylaktoider reaktion nach gabe von etomidat. *Anaesthesist* 1984; **33:** 161–2.

**Porphyria.** Etomidate is considered to be unsafe in patients with porphyria because it has been shown to be porphyrinogenic in *animals*.

### Interactions

A reduced dose of etomidate may be necessary in patients who have received antipsychotics, sedatives, or opioids. The hypnotic effect of etomidate has been potentiated by other sedative drugs.

See also Interactions of General Anaesthetics, p.1295.

**Calcium-channel blockers.** Prolonged anaesthesia and Cheyne-Stokes respiration following etomidate injection has been reported in 2 patients given concomitant treatment with *verapamil*.[1]

1. Moore CA, *et al.* Potentiation of etomidate anesthesia by verapamil: a report of two cases. *Hosp Pharm* 1989; **24:** 24–5.

**General anaesthetics.** For a report of synergy between *propofol* and etomidate, see p.1306.

### Pharmacokinetics

After injection, etomidate is rapidly redistributed from the CNS to other body tissues, and undergoes rapid metabolism in the liver and plasma. Pharmacokinetics are complex and have been described by both 2- and 3-compartment models. Etomidate is about 76% bound to plasma protein. It is mainly excreted in the urine, but some is excreted in the bile. It may cross the placenta and is distributed into breast milk.

◊ References.

1. Levron JC, Assoune P. Pharmacocinétique de l'étomidate. *Ann Fr Anesth Reanim* 1990; **9:** 123–6.
2. Sfez M, *et al.* Comparaison de la pharmacocinétique de l'étomidate chez l'enfant et chez l'adulte. *Ann Fr Anesth Reanim* 1990; **9:** 127–31.
3. Esener Z, *et al.* Thiopentone and etomidate concentrations in maternal and umbilical plasma, and in colostrum. *Br J Anaesth* 1992; **69:** 586–8.

### Uses and Administration

Etomidate is an intravenous anaesthetic administered for the induction of general anaesthesia (p.1296). Anaesthesia is rapidly induced and may last for 6 to 10 minutes with a single usual dose. Recovery is usually rapid without hangover effect. Etomidate has no analgesic activity.

For the induction of anaesthesia, the usual dose is 300 micrograms/kg of etomidate given slowly, preferably into a large vein in the arm. An initial dose of 150 to 200 micrograms/kg is recommended in the elderly, subsequently adjusted according to effects. Dosage should also be reduced in hepatic cirrhosis. Children may require up to 30% more than the standard adult dose. Opioid analgesics or benzodiazepines as premedication reduce myoclonic muscle movements; opioids also reduce injection site pain. A neuromuscular blocker is necessary if intubation is required.

**Administration in the elderly.** A study[1] in elderly patients has demonstrated that although reducing the rate of intravenous administration of etomidate reduces the speed of induction, the dosage required is also reduced. Administration of etomidate 0.2% solution at a rate of 10 mg/minute induced anaesthesia in a mean of 89.6 seconds and required a mean dose of 0.11 mg/kg. Corresponding values for an administration rate of 40 mg/minute were 47.7 seconds and 0.26 mg/kg, respectively.

1. Berthoud MC, *et al.* Comparison of infusion rates of three i.v. anaesthetic agents for induction in elderly patients. *Br J Anaesth* 1993; **70:** 423–7.

**Anaesthesia.** Etomidate might be useful for induction if rapid tracheal intubation is required with a competitive neuromuscular blocker as it has been shown to reduce the time to onset of block with vecuronium.[1,2]

1. Gill RS, Scott RPF. Etomidate shortens the onset time of neuromuscular block. *Br J Anaesth* 1992; **69:** 444–6.
2. Bergen JM, Smith DC. A review of etomidate for rapid sequence intubation in the emergency department. *J Emerg Med* 1997; **15:** 221–30.

**Status epilepticus.** Anaesthesia in conjunction with assisted ventilation may be instituted to control refractory tonic-clonic status epilepticus (p.352). A short-acting barbiturate such as thiopental is usually used, but other anaesthetics including etomidate have also been tried[1] for intractable convulsive status epilepticus. However, like a number of other anaesthetics there have been reports of seizures associated with its use in anaesthesia,[2] especially in patients with epilepsy.

1. Yeoman P, *et al.* Etomidate infusions for the control of refractory status epilepticus. *Intensive Care Med* 1989; **15:** 255–9.
2. Nicoll K, Callender J. Etomidate-induced convulsion prior to electroconvulsive therapy. *Br J Psychiatry* 2000; **177:** 373.

### Preparations

**Proprietary Preparations** (details are given in Part 3)
***Austria:*** Hypnomidate; ***Belg.:*** Hypnomidate; ***Braz.:*** Hypnomidate; ***Chile:*** Hypnomidate; ***Fr.:*** Hypnomidate; ***Ger.:*** Hypnomidate; Radenarcon†; ***Gr.:*** Hypnomidate; ***Mex.:*** Hypnomidate; ***Neth.:*** Hypnomidate; ***S.Afr.:*** Hypnomidate; ***Spain:*** Hypnomidate; ***UK:*** Hypnomidate; ***USA:*** Amidate.

---

## Halothane *(BAN, rINN)*

Alotano; Halotano; Halothanum; Phthorothanum. (*RS*)-2-Bromo-2-chloro-1,1,1-trifluoroethane.
$CHBrCl.CF_3$ = 197.4.
*CAS — 151-67-7.*
*ATC — N01AB01.*

**Pharmacopoeias.** In *Chin.*, *Eur.* (see p.vi), *Int.*, *Jpn*, *Pol.*, and *US.*

**Ph. Eur. 5.0** (Halothane). A clear, colourless, mobile, dense, non-flammable liquid. Distillation range 49° to 51°. Slightly soluble in water; miscible with dehydrated alcohol and with trichloroethylene. Halothane contains 0.01% w/w of thymol. Store at a temperature not greater than 25° in airtight containers. Protect from light.

**USP 27** (Halothane). A colourless, mobile, non-flammable, heavy liquid having a characteristic odour resembling that of chloroform. It contains not less than 0.008% and not more than 0.012% of thymol, by weight, as a stabiliser. It should contain not more than 0.03% of water. Distillation range 49° to 51°. Slightly soluble in water; miscible with alcohol, with chloroform, with ether, and with fixed oils. Store in airtight containers at a temperature not greater than 40°. Protect from light. Dispense only in the original container.

**Incompatibility.** In the presence of moisture, halothane reacts with many metals. Rubber and some plastics deteriorate when in contact with halothane vapour or liquid.

**Stability.** Halothane contains 0.01% w/w of thymol as a stabiliser; some commercial preparations may also contain up to 0.00025% w/w of ammonia. Thymol does not volatilise with halothane and therefore accumulates in the vaporiser. It may give a yellow colour to any remaining liquid; halothane that has discoloured should be discarded.

### Adverse Effects

As with other halogenated anaesthetics, halothane has a depressant action on the cardiovascular system and reduces blood pressure; signs of overdosage are bradycardia and profound hypotension. It is also a respiratory depressant and can cause cardiac arrhythmias; there have been instances of cardiac arrest. The sensitivity of the heart to sympathomimetic amines is increased.

Adverse effects on the liver have limited its use in recent years (see below); these effects range from liver dysfunction to fatal hepatitis and necrosis and are more frequent following repeated use.

Halothane can produce nausea, vomiting, and shivering. Malignant hyperthermia has been reported.

See also Adverse Effects of General Anaesthetics, p.1295.

**Effects on the cardiovascular system.** The incidence of cardiac arrhythmias is higher with halothane than with enflurane or isoflurane; also the arrhythmogenic threshold with injected adrenaline is lower with halothane than isoflurane or enflurane.

Arrhythmias are considered to be very common in children anaesthetised with halothane and in the UK it is recommended that it should not be used for dental procedures outside hospital in those under 18 years old.

**Effects on the kidneys.** Renal failure has been reported following halothane anaesthesia,[1,2] sometimes with concurrent liver failure.[2]

1. Cotton JR, *et al.* Acute renal failure following halothane anesthesia. *Arch Pathol Lab Med* 1976; **100:** 628–9.
2. Gelman ML, Lichtenstein NS. Halothane-induced nephrotoxicity. *Urology* 1981; **17:** 323–7.

**Effects on the liver.** Liver damage has been recognised as an adverse effect of halothane for many years.[1-3] It may be severe, and associated with a high mortality.

Two types of hepatotoxicity are recognised; in **type I** there is a minor disturbance in liver function shown by increases in liver enzyme values; this may occur in up to 30% of patients given halothane,[4] or more if activity is measured by glutathione S-transferase rather than serum aminotransferase.[5] Subsequent re-exposure to halothane is not necessarily associated with liver damage.[2,6]

**Type II** hepatotoxicity, which is rarer, involves massive liver cell necrosis; reported incidences[2] range from 1 in 2500 to 1 in 36 000. Type II liver toxicity is characterised by several clinical features: non-specific gastrointestinal upset, delayed pyrexia, jaundice, eosinophilia, serum autoantibodies, rash, and arthralgia.[1,3] Biochemical tests of liver function show changes typical of hepatocellular damage; histological features are typified by centrilobular necrosis.[1] Several **risk factors** for development of serious toxicity have become apparent;[1-3] they include repeated exposure, previous adverse reactions to halothane (jaundice, pyrexia), female gender, obesity, middle age, genetic predisposition, enzyme induction, and a history of drug allergy.

The **causes** of halothane hepatotoxicity have been debated. Type I reactions may result from toxic products of halothane metabolism, possibly influenced by genetic factors or from an imbalance between hepatic oxygen supply and demand. Changes in cellular calcium homoeostasis may also be involved. Type II reactions are most likely immune-mediated.[1,2] It has been suggested[4] that metabolism of halothane produces a reactive metabolite which binds covalently to proteins in the endoplasmic reticulum of hepatocytes. In susceptible patients it is believed that these metabolite-modified proteins provoke an immune response which is responsible for the liver damage. Recent findings[7,8] have implicated the cytochrome P450 isoenzyme CYP2E1 as having a major role in the metabolism of halothane and patients with high levels of this isoenzyme may be predisposed to developing immune-medicated liver damage following halothane exposure.

The UK Committee on Safety of Medicines,[9] after receiving 84 further reports of hepatotoxicity between 1978 and 1985, issued the following **guidelines** on **precautions** to be taken before using halothane:

- a careful anaesthetic history should be taken to determine previous exposure and previous reactions to halothane
- repeated exposure to halothane within a period of at least 3 months should be avoided unless there are overriding clinical circumstances. An opinion has been expressed that the 3-month interval between exposures would be unlikely to prevent hepatotoxicity[2]
- a history of unexplained jaundice or pyrexia in a patient following exposure to halothane is an absolute contra-indication to its future use in that patient.

These guidelines were reiterated in 1997 after the CSM were notified of a further 15 cases of acute liver failure all requiring transplantation.[10]

The problem of patients sensitised to halothane who require **subsequent anaesthesia** with a volatile anaesthetic has been discussed.[4] Although the incidence of hepatotoxicity produced by *enflurane* appears to be less than with halothane it is of a similar nature and there have been reports of several patients who apparently had cross-sensitivity to both. Hepatotoxicity with *isoflurane* appears to be rare and it was suggested that for the majority of patients sensitised to halothane, isoflurane would be likely to be free from hepatotoxic effects. However, there has been a report[11] of a patient who had had two previous exposures to isoflurane and subsequently developed liver function abnormalities after receiving halothane. Hepatotoxicity with *desflurane* (see p.1297) might also be associated with sensitisation to halothane.

1. Ray DC, Drummond GB. Halothane hepatitis. *Br J Anaesth* 1991; **67:** 84–99.
2. Neuberger JM. Halothane and hepatitis: incidence, predisposing factors and exposure guidelines. *Drug Safety* 1990; **5:** 28–38.
3. Rosenak D, *et al.* Halothane and liver damage. *Postgrad Med J* 1989; **65:** 129–35.
4. Kenna JG, Neuberger JM. Immunopathogenesis and treatment of halothane hepatitis. *Clin Immunother* 1995; **3:** 108–24.
5. Allan LG, *et al.* Hepatic glutathione S-transferase release after halothane anaesthesia: open randomised comparison with isoflurane. *Lancet* 1987; **i:** 771–4.
6. Neuberger J, Williams R. Halothane anaesthesia and liver damage. *BMJ* 1984; **289:** 1136–9.
7. Kharasch ED, *et al.* Identification of the enzyme responsible for oxidative halothane metabolism: implications for prevention of halothane hepatitis. *Lancet* 1996; **347:** 1367–71.
8. Kenna JC, *et al.* Formation of the C[F]$_3$CO-protein antigens implicated in the pathogenesis of halothane hepatitis is catalyzed in human liver microsomes in vitro by CYP 2E1. *Br J Clin Pharmacol* 1997; **43:** 209.
9. Committee on Safety of Medicines. Halothane hepatotoxicity. *Current Problems 18* 1986.
10. Committee on Safety of Medicines/Medicines Control Agency. Safety issues in anaesthesia: reminder: hepatotoxicity with halothane. *Current Problems* 1997; **23:** 7. Also available at: http://www.mca.gov.uk/ourwork/monitorsafequalmed/currentproblems/volume24.htm (accessed 25/05/04)
11. Slayter KL, *et al.* Halothane hepatitis in a renal transplant patient previously exposed to isoflurane. *Ann Pharmacother* 1993; **27:** 101.

## Precautions

The risk of halothane hepatitis led the UK Committee on Safety of Medicines to issue guidelines on its use (see Effects on the Liver, under Adverse Effects, above). It is also recommended that patients be informed of any reactions and that this be done in addition to the updating of the patients' medical records.

It is recommended in the UK that halothane should not be used for dental procedures outside hospital in patients under 18 years old.

Halothane reduces uterine muscle tone during pregnancy and generally its use is not recommended in obstetrics because of the increased risk of postpartum haemorrhage.

Premedication with atropine has been recommended to reduce vagal tone and to prevent bradycardia and severe hypotension.

Allowance may need to be made for any increase in CSF pressure or in cerebral blood flow. Halothane should be used with caution in patients with phaeochromocytoma.

As with other halogenated anaesthetics, patients with known or suspected susceptibility to malignant hyperthermia should not be anaesthetised with halothane.

See also Precautions for General Anaesthetics, p.1295.

**Abuse.** A brief review[1] of abuse of volatile anaesthetics found that of 14 patients who had ingested or sniffed halothane 10 had died. Another patient who had injected halothane intravenously also died. There has also been another report[2] of fatalities resulting from acute pulmonary oedema after intravenous injection of halothane.

1. Yamashita M, *et al.* Illicit use of modern volatile anaesthetics. *Can Anaesth Soc J* 1984; **31:** 76–9.
2. Berman P, Tattersal M. Self-poisoning with intravenous halothane. *Lancet* 1982; **i:** 340.

**Breast feeding.** No adverse effects have been observed in breast-fed infants whose mothers were receiving halothane, and the American Academy of Pediatrics[1] considers that it is therefore usually compatible with breast feeding.

Trace amounts of halothane have been detected in the breast milk of a lactating anaesthetist exposed to environmental halothane in the operating theatre.[2]

1. American Academy of Pediatrics. The transfer of drugs and other chemicals into human milk. *Pediatrics* 2001; **108:** 776–89. Correction. *ibid.*; 1029. Also available at: http://aappolicy.aappublications.org/cgi/content/full/pediatrics%3b108/3/776 (accessed 25/05/04)
2. Coté CJ, *et al.* Trace concentrations of halothane in human breast milk. *Br J Anaesth* 1976; **48:** 541–3.

**Porphyria.** Halothane has been associated with acute attacks of porphyria and is considered unsafe in porphyric patients.

## Interactions

Adrenaline and most other sympathomimetics, and theophylline should be avoided during halothane anaesthesia since they can produce cardiac arrhythmias; the risk of arrhythmias is also increased if halothane is used in patients receiving dopaminergics. The effects of competitive neuromuscular blockers such as atracurium, and of ganglion blockers such as trimetaphan are enhanced by halothane and if required they should be given in reduced dosage. Morphine increases the depressant effects of halothane on respiration. Chlorpromazine also enhances the respiratory depressant effect of halothane. The effects of both ergometrine and oxytocin on the parturient uterus are diminished by halothane.

See also Interactions of General Anaesthetics, p.1295.

**Antiepileptics.** For a case of *phenytoin* intoxication associated with halothane anaesthesia, see p.372.

**Benzodiazepines.** *Midazolam* has been reported to potentiate the anaesthetic action of halothane.[1]

1. Inagaki Y, *et al.* Anesthetic interaction between midazolam and halothane in humans. *Anesth Analg* 1993; **76:** 613–17.

**General anaesthetics.** For a report that halothane increases serum concentrations of *propofol*, see p.1306

**Neuromuscular blockers.** For the potentiation of the neuromuscular blockade of neuromuscular blockers such as *atracurium* by halothane, see p.1401. For increased toxicity during halothane anaesthesia, see *suxamethonium* p.1408.

**Trichloroethane.** A report[1] of 2 patients showing evidence of chronic cardiac toxicity following repeated exposure to trichloroethane. In both cases there was circumstantial evidence of a deterioration after routine anaesthetic use of halothane.

1. McLeod AA, *et al.* Chronic cardiac toxicity after inhalation of 1,1,1-trichloroethane. *BMJ* 1987; **294:** 727–9.

**Xanthines.** For references to increased cardiotoxicity when patients taking *theophylline* were anaesthetised with halothane, see p.803.

## Pharmacokinetics

Halothane is absorbed on inhalation. It has a relatively low solubility in blood and is more soluble in the neutral fats of adipose tissue than in the phospholipids of brain cells. Up to 80% of administered halothane is excreted unchanged through the lungs. Up to 20% is metabolised by the liver by oxidative and, under hypoxic conditions, reductive pathways. Urinary metabolites include trifluoroacetic acid and bromide and chloride salts (oxidative pathway) and fluoride salts (reductive pathway). Halothane diffuses across the placenta and has been detected in breast milk.

## Uses and Administration

Halothane is a volatile halogenated anaesthetic administered by inhalation. It has a minimum alveolar concentration (MAC) value (see Uses of General Anaesthetics, p.1295) ranging from 0.64% in the elderly to 1.08% in infants. It is non-flammable and is not explosive when mixed with oxygen at normal atmospheric pressure. It is not irritant to the skin and mucous membranes and does not produce necrosis when spilt on tissues. It suppresses salivary, bronchial, and gastric secretions and dilates the bronchioles. However, its use has diminished due to the risk of hepatotoxicity.

Halothane is used for the induction and maintenance of general anaesthesia (p.1296) and is given using a calibrated vaporiser to provide close control over the concentration of inhaled vapour.

Anaesthesia may be induced with 2 to 4% v/v of halothane in oxygen or mixtures of nitrous oxide and oxygen; induction may also be started at a concentration of 0.5% v/v and increased gradually to the required level. For induction in children a concentration of 1.5 to 2% v/v has been used. It takes up to about 5 minutes to attain surgical anaesthesia and halothane produces little or no excitement in the induction period. The more usual practice is to induce anaesthesia with an intravenous agent. Anaesthesia is maintained with concentrations of 0.5 to 2% v/v depending on the flow rate used; the lower concentration is usually suitable for the elderly.

Adequate muscle relaxation is only achieved with deep anaesthesia so a neuromuscular blocker is given to increase muscular relaxation if necessary.

◊ Reviews.

1. Quail AW. Modern inhalational anaesthetic agents: a review of halothane, isoflurane and enflurane. *Med J Aust* 1989; **150:** 95–102.

## Preparations

**Proprietary Preparations** (details are given in Part 3)

***Arg.:*** Ineltano; ***Austral.:*** Fluothane; ***Austria:*** Fluothane; ***Belg.:*** Fluothane†; ***Braz.:*** Fluothane; ***Chile:*** Fluothane; ***Fr.:*** Fluothane; ***Ger.:*** Fluothane; ***Gr.:*** Fluothane; ***Hong Kong:*** Fluothane†; ***India:*** Fluothane; ***Irl.:*** Fluothane†; ***Israel:*** Fluothane; ***Ital.:*** Fluothane†; ***Malaysia:*** Fluothane; ***Mex.:***

Fluothane†; **Neth.:** Fluothane†; **Norw.:** Fluothane†; **NZ:** Fluothane; **Port.:** Fluothane†; **S.Afr.:** Fluothane; **Spain:** Fluothane; **Swed.:** Fluothane; **Switz.:** Fluothane†; **Thai.:** Fluothane†; **UK:** Fluothane†; **USA:** Fluothane.

## Isoflurane *(BAN, USAN, rINN)*

Compound 469; Isoflurano; Isofluranum. 1-Chloro-2,2,2-trifluoroethyl difluoromethyl ether; 2-Chloro-2-(difluoromethoxy)-1,1,1-trifluoroethane.

$C_3H_2ClF_5O$ = 184.5.

*CAS — 26675-46-7.*

*ATC — N01AB06.*

**Pharmacopoeias.** In *Eur.* (see p.vi) and *US.*

**Ph. Eur. 5.0** (Isoflurane). A clear, colourless, mobile, heavy liquid. B.p. about 48°. It is non-flammable. Practically insoluble in water; miscible with dehydrated alcohol and with trichloroethylene. Store in airtight containers. Protect from light.

**USP 27** (Isoflurane). A clear, colourless, volatile liquid having a slight odour. B.p. about 49°. Insoluble in water; miscible with common organic solvents and with fats and oils. Store in airtight containers at a temperature of 25°, excursions permitted between 15° and 30°.

### Adverse Effects and Precautions

As with other halogenated anaesthetics, respiratory depression, hypotension, arrhythmias, and malignant hyperthermia have been reported; patients with known or suspected susceptibility to malignant hyperthermia should not be anaesthetised with isoflurane. Isoflurane differs from halothane and enflurane in that it produces less cardiac depression than either drug and heart rate may be increased. Also isoflurane sensitises the myocardium to sympathomimetics to a lesser extent than halothane and enflurane. The incidence of cardiac arrhythmias is lower with isoflurane than with halothane. Shivering, nausea, and vomiting have been reported in the postoperative period.

Induction with isoflurane is not as smooth as with halothane and this may be connected with its pungency; breath holding, coughing, and laryngospasm may occur. It has been reported to increase the cerebrospinal pressure and should be used with caution in patients with raised intracranial pressure. Isoflurane relaxes the uterine muscle; increased blood loss may occur after curettage or termination of pregnancy.

In order to minimise the risk of developing elevated carboxyhaemoglobin levels, carbon dioxide absorbents in anaesthetic apparatus should not be allowed to dry out when delivering volatile anaesthetics such as isoflurane (see below).

See also Adverse Effects and Precautions of General Anaesthetics, p.1295.

◊ A comparison[1] of isoflurane and halothane for outpatient dental anaesthesia in children considered that isoflurane would produce fewer arrhythmias than halothane, but that the ease of induction and the quality of anaesthesia was inferior to that with halothane. Others[2] also found a higher incidence of coughing, salivation, and laryngospasm with isoflurane than halothane, but felt that it could be used as an alternative.

Further information on the adverse effects profile of isoflurane can be obtained from the report of and commentaries on an extensive multicentre study of patients undergoing anaesthesia with this agent.[3,4]


1. Cattermole RW, *et al.* Isoflurane and halothane for outpatient dental anaesthesia in children. *Br J Anaesth* 1986; **58:** 385–9.
2. McAteer PM, *et al.* Comparison of isoflurane and halothane in outpatient paediatric dental anaesthesia. *Br J Anaesth* 1986; **58:** 390–3.
3. Forrest JB, *et al.* A multi-centre clinical evaluation of isoflurane. *Can Anaesth Soc J* 1982; **29** (suppl): S1–S69.
4. Levy WJ. Clinical anaesthesia with isoflurane: a review of the multicentre study. *Br J Anaesth* 1984; **56:** 101S–112S.


**Carbon dioxide absorbents.** Significant carboxyhaemoglobinaemia may develop rarely during anaesthesia with volatile anaesthetics given by circle breathing systems containing carbon dioxide absorbents.[1] The effect is only seen when the absorbent has become excessively dried out. The use of barium hydroxide lime (which is not available in the UK) as an absorbent produces more carbon monoxide than soda lime, particularly at low water content. No cases of this complication had been reported to date in the UK.


1. Committee on Safety of Medicines/Medicines Control Agency. Safety issues in anaesthesia: volatile anesthetic agents and carboxyhaemoglobinaemia. *Current Problems* 1997; **23:** 7. Also available at: http://www.mca.gov.uk/ourwork/monitorsafequalmed/currentproblems/volume24.htm (accessed 25/05/04)


**Effects on the cardiovascular system.** Isoflurane is considered to produce less cardiovascular depression than halothane. However, the results of a study[1] suggest that while this may be true for young patients, in elderly patients isoflurane appears to have a cardiac depressant effect similar to that of halothane.


1. McKinney MS, *et al.* Cardiovascular effects of isoflurane and halothane in young and elderly adult patients. *Br J Anaesth* 1993; **71:** 696–701.


CEREBRAL BLOOD FLOW. Autoregulation of cerebral blood flow appears to be impaired at higher concentrations of isoflurane. A study[1] in healthy subjects found that increasing isoflurane anaesthesia from a concentration of 1 to 2 MAC increased cerebral blood flow and reduced cerebral oxygen metabolism.


1. Olsen KS, *et al.* Effect of 1 or 2 MAC isoflurane with or without ketanserin on cerebral blood flow autoregulation in man. *Br J Anaesth* 1994; **72:** 66–71.


CORONARY CIRCULATION. Halothane, enflurane, and isoflurane decrease coronary perfusion pressure, coronary blood flow, ventricular function, and myocardial oxygen demand. Halothane and enflurane have a variable effect on coronary vascular resistance, but isoflurane dilates coronary vessels.[1] There has been concern over the potential of isoflurane to produce coronary steal and whether this effect is detrimental in patients with ischaemic heart disease.[2] However, despite conflicting results of individual studies[3-6] an early review[7] concluded that isoflurane could be used safely even in high-risk patients with coronary artery disease provided that blood pressure and heart rate were maintained close to baseline concentrations. A subsequent review[8] considered that more recent evidence supported the use of isoflurane as the anaesthetic agent of choice in patients with coronary heart disease.


1. Quail AW. Modern inhalational anaesthetic agents: a review of halothane, isoflurane and enflurane. *Med J Aust* 1989; **150:** 95–102.
2. Stoelting RK. Anesthesiology. *JAMA* 1991; **265:** 3103–5.
3. Buffington CW, *et al.* The prevalence of steal-prone coronary anatomy in patients with coronary artery disease: an analysis of the coronary artery surgery study registry. *Anesthesiology* 1988; **69:** 721–7.
4. Inoue K, *et al.* Does isoflurane lead to a higher incidence of myocardial infarction and perioperative death than enflurane in coronary artery surgery? A clinical study of 1178 patients. *Anesth Analg* 1990; **71:** 469–74.
5. Slogoff S, *et al.* Steal-prone coronary anatomy and myocardial ischemia associated with four primary anesthetic agents in humans. *Anesth Analg* 1991; **72:** 22–7.
6. Stühmeier KD, *et al.* Isoflurane does not increase the incidence of intraoperative myocardial ischaemia compared with halothane during vascular surgery. *Br J Anaesth* 1992; **69:** 602–6.
7. Hogue CW, *et al.* Anesthetic-induced myocardial ischemia: the isoflurane-coronary steal controversy. *Coron Artery Dis* 1993; **4:** 413–19.
8. Agnew NM, *et al.* Isoflurane and coronary heart disease. *Anaesthesia* 2002; **57:** 338–47.


**Effects on the kidneys.** See under Metabolism in Pharmacokinetics, below.

**Effects on the liver.** Of 45 cases of isoflurane-associated hepatotoxicity reported to the FDA between 1981 and 1984 there was some other cause for the liver damage in 29. While isoflurane might have been one of the causes of the damage in the other 16 cases, there was not a reasonable likelihood of an association between isoflurane and postoperative liver impairment.[1] Subsequent rare cases of hepatotoxicity,[2-6] sometimes fatal,[2,5] have suggested that isoflurane may induce hepatitis, though much less frequently than halothane, and that there may be cross-sensitisation with other halogenated anaesthetics.

See also under the Adverse Effects of Halothane, p.1300.


1. Stoelting RK, *et al.* Hepatic dysfunction after isoflurane anesthesia. *Anesth Analg* 1987; **66:** 147–53.
2. Carrigan TW, Straughen WJ. A report of hepatic necrosis and death following isoflurane anesthesia. *Anesthesiology* 1987; **67:** 581–3.
3. Sinha A, *et al.* Isoflurane hepatotoxicity: a case report and review of the literature. *Am J Gastroenterol* 1996; **91:** 2406–9.
4. Hasan F. Isoflurane hepatotoxicity in a patient with a previous history of halothane-induced hepatitis. *Hepatogastroenterology* 1998; **45:** 518–22.
5. Turner GB, *et al.* Fatal hepatotoxicity after re-exposure to isoflurane: a case report and review of the literature. *Eur J Gastroenterol Hepatol* 2000; **12:** 955–9.
6. Malnick SDH, *et al.* Acute cholestatic hepatitis after exposure to isoflurane. *Ann Pharmacother* 2002; **36:** 261–3.


**Effects on the nervous system.** Seizures associated with induction of anaesthesia with isoflurane have been reported in patients without known neurological abnormalities and not undergoing neurosurgery.[1,2] However, data from a retrospective analysis of patients undergoing intracranial surgery indicated that when convulsions occurred postoperatively in these conditions, it was the neurosurgical procedures rather than the anaesthetics that were responsible.[3]

See also under Status Epilepticus in Uses, below.


1. Poulton TJ, Ellingson RJ. Seizure associated with induction of anesthesia with isoflurane. *Anesthesiology* 1984; **61:** 471–6.
2. Hymes JA. Seizure activity during isoflurane anesthesia. *Anesth Analg* 1985; **64:** 367–8.
3. Christys AR, *et al.* Retrospective study of early postoperative convulsions after intracranial surgery with isoflurane or enflurane anaesthesia. *Br J Anaesth* 1989; **62:** 624–7.


**Effects on the respiratory tract.** A study[1] conducted mainly in adults found that humidification of anaesthetic mixtures containing isoflurane could reduce respiratory complications such as coughing, laryngospasm, and breath-holding that were usually associated with the use of isoflurane for induction. However, a similar study[2] in children failed to confirm these findings.


1. van Heerden PV, *et al.* Effect of humidification on inhalation induction with isoflurane. *Br J Anaesth* 1990; **64:** 235–7.
2. McAuliffe GL, *et al.* Effect of humidification on inhalation induction with isoflurane in children. *Br J Anaesth* 1994; **73:** 587–9.


**Effects on the skin.** There have been rare reports of contact dermatitis to isoflurane in anaesthetists.[1,2]


1. Caraffini S, *et al.* Isoflurane: an uncommon cause of occupational airborne contact dermatitis. *Contact Dermatitis* 1998; **38:** 286.
2. Muncaster A, *et al.* Allergic contact dermatitis to isoflurane. *Br J Dermatol* 1999; **141:** (suppl 55): 96–7.


**Porphyria.** Isoflurane is considered to be unsafe in patients with porphyria because it has been shown to be porphyrinogenic in *animals*.

### Interactions

The effects of competitive neuromuscular blockers such as atracurium are enhanced by isoflurane (see p.1401). Care is advised if adrenaline and other sympathomimetics are given during isoflurane anaesthesia. See also Interactions of General Anaesthetics, p.1295.

**General anaesthetics.** For a report that isoflurane increases serum concentrations of *propofol*, see p.1306.

### Pharmacokinetics

Isoflurane is absorbed on inhalation. The blood/gas partition coefficient is lower than that of enflurane or halothane. It is mostly excreted unchanged through the lungs. About 0.2% of administered isoflurane is metabolised mainly to inorganic fluoride.

**Metabolism.** In 26 patients sedated with isoflurane for 24 hours, plasma fluoride ion concentration increased from a mean of 4.03 nanomol/mL to 13.57 nanomol/mL in 12 hours after stopping sedation.[1] These fluoride concentrations were considered to be too low to cause clinical renal dysfunction. In 30 patients sedated with isoflurane for up to 127 hours (mean duration was 36 hours), mean plasma fluoride ion concentration increased[2] to 20.01 nanomol/mL during sedation and continued rising for 16 hours after discontinuing isoflurane to a maximum mean concentration of 25.34 nanomol/mL; thereafter, levels gradually declined to normal values by the fifth day. Despite the increased plasma fluoride ion concentrations, no biochemical or clinical evidence of deterioration in renal function was found. Administration of isoflurane for 34 days to a patient with tetanus who required sedation to facilitate mechanical ventilation resulted[3] in sustained fluoride ion concentrations of 50 nanomol/mL and a peak concentration of 87 nanomol/mL. Although such concentrations are considered to be potentially nephrotoxic no clinical effect on renal function was found.


1. Kong KL, *et al.* Isoflurane sedation for patients undergoing mechanical ventilation: metabolism to inorganic fluoride and renal effects. *Br J Anaesth* 1990; **64:** 159–62.
2. Spencer EM, *et al.* Plasma inorganic fluoride concentrations during and after prolonged (>24h) isoflurane sedation: effect on renal function. *Anesth Analg* 1991; **73:** 731–7.
3. Stevens JJWM, *et al.* Prolonged use of isoflurane in a patient with tetanus. *Br J Anaesth* 1993; **70:** 107–109.


### Uses and Administration

Isoflurane is a volatile halogenated anaesthetic administered by inhalation. It is an isomer of enflurane and has anaesthetic actions similar to those of halothane (p.1300). Isoflurane has a minimum alveolar concentration (MAC) value (see Uses of General Anaesthetics, p.1295) ranging from 1.05% in the elderly to 1.87% in infants. It is employed in the induction and maintenance of general anaesthesia (p.1296) although induction is more often carried out using an intravenous anaesthetic. Isoflurane is also used in subanaesthetic doses to provide analgesia in obstetrics and other painful procedures.

Isoflurane is administered using a calibrated vaporiser. If it is used for induction then it is given with oxygen or oxygen and nitrous oxide mixtures and induction should start with an isoflurane concentration of 0.5% v/v increased to 1.5 to 3% v/v which generally produces surgical anaesthesia within 10 minutes. Its pungency may limit the rate of induction. Anaesthesia may be maintained with a concentration of 1 to 2.5% v/v with oxygen and nitrous oxide mixtures; 1.5 to 3.5% v/v may be required if used only with oxygen. Isoflurane 0.5 to 0.75% v/v with oxygen and nitrous oxide mixtures is suitable to maintain anaesthesia for caesarean section. Although isoflurane is reported to possess muscle relaxant properties, neuromuscular blockers may nevertheless be required. Recovery is rapid.

**Anaesthesia.** CAESAREAN SECTION. Isoflurane 0.8% v/v has been found to be a suitable supplement to nitrous oxide-oxygen anaesthesia for patients undergoing caesarean section.[1] It has been suggested[2] that an overpressure technique might be of use to further reduce awareness in such patients. Administration of isoflurane at a concentration of 2% v/v for 5 minutes followed by concentrations of 1.5% v/v for the next 5 minutes and 0.8% v/v thereafter produced higher arterial concentrations of isoflurane in patients undergoing caesarean section than when it was given at a concentration of 1% v/v throughout.[2]

1. Dwyer R, *et al.* Uptake of halothane and isoflurane by mother and baby during Caesarean section. *Br J Anaesth* 1995; **74:** 379–83.
2. McCrirrick A, *et al.* Overpressure isoflurane at Caesarean section: a study of arterial isoflurane concentrations. *Br J Anaesth* 1994; **72:** 122–4.

**Pain.** Isoflurane is used in subanaesthetic doses to provide analgesia in obstetrics and other painful procedures but studies[1,2] have been unable to confirm that it had an analgesic effect at subanaesthetic concentrations. The use of isoflurane 0.2 or 0.25% v/v in a mixture of nitrous oxide 50% v/v and oxygen 50% v/v has been studied.[3,4]

1. Tomi K, *et al.* Alterations in pain threshold and psychomotor response associated with subanaesthetic concentrations of inhalation anaesthetics in humans. *Br J Anaesth* 1993; **70:** 684–6.
2. Roth D, *et al.* Analgesic effect in humans of subanaesthetic isoflurane concentrations evaluated by evoked potentials. *Br J Anaesth* 1996; **76:** 38–42.
3. Wee MYK, *et al.* Isoflurane in labour. *Anaesthesia* 1993; **48:** 369–72.
4. Bryden FM, *et al.* Isoflurane for removal of chest drains after cardiac surgery. *Br J Anaesth* 1994; **73:** 712P–713P.

**Sedation.** INTENSIVE CARE. The various drugs used to provide sedation in intensive care are discussed on p.666. Isoflurane is not usually considered for such a purpose but in a comparative 24-hour study[1] in 60 patients requiring mechanical ventilation, isoflurane 0.1 to 0.6% v/v in an air-oxygen mixture produced satisfactory sedation for a greater proportion of time than did the continuous infusion of midazolam 10 to 200 micrograms/kg per hour. Patients given isoflurane also recovered more rapidly. Isoflurane has also been used successfully for sedation over 5 days in a 3-year-old infant who required ventilation for pneumonia, a complication of the child's myasthenia gravis.[2] However, there has been some concern over high plasma fluoride concentrations following prolonged use of isoflurane (see under Metabolism in Pharmacokinetics, above).

1. Kong KL, *et al.* Isoflurane compared with midazolam for sedation in the intensive care unit. *BMJ* 1989; **298:** 1277–80.
2. McBeth C, Watkins TGL. Isoflurane for sedation in a case of congenital myasthenia gravis. *Br J Anaesth* 1996; **77:** 672–4.

**Status epilepticus.** Anaesthesia in conjunction with assisted ventilation may be instituted to control refractory tonic-clonic status epilepticus (p.352). A short-acting barbiturate such as thiopental is usually used. Despite rare reports of seizures associated with the use of isoflurane in anaesthetic procedures (see under Adverse Effects, above) concentrations of 0.5 to 1% v/v have been used successfully in isolated patients[1,2] to control refractory convulsive status epilepticus. Although some[3] consider that isoflurane-induced coma may be more easy to control than barbiturate-induced coma, the use of isoflurane may be limited by the need for special anaesthetic equipment and continuous EEG monitoring.

1. Meeke RI, *et al.* Isoflurane for the management of status epilepticus. *DICP Ann Pharmacother* 1989; **23:** 579–81.
2. Hilz MJ, *et al.* Isoflurane anaesthesia in the treatment of convulsive status epilepticus. *J Neurol* 1992; **239:** 135–7.
3. Bauer J, Elger CE. Management of status epilepticus in adults. *CNS Drugs* 1994; **1:** 26–44.

### Preparations

**Proprietary Preparations** (details are given in Part 3)
***Arg.:*** Forane; Zuflax; ***Austral.:*** AErrane; Forthane; ***Austria:*** Forane; ***Belg.:*** AErrane†; Forene; ***Braz.:*** Forane; Isoforine; Isothane; ***Canad.:*** Forane; ***Denm.:*** Forene; ***Fin.:*** Forene; ***Ger.:*** Forene; ***Gr.:*** Forenium; ***Hong Kong:*** Forane; ***Irl.:*** AErrane†; Forane; ***Israel:*** AErrane; Forane; ***Ital.:*** AErrane; Forane; ***Malaysia:*** Forane; ***Mex.:*** Forane; Lisorane†; Sofloran; ***Neth.:*** AErrane; Forene; ***Norw.:*** Forene; ***NZ:*** AErrane; Forane; ***S.Afr.:*** AErrane; Forane; ***Singapore:*** Forane; ***Spain:*** AErrane; Forane; ***Swed.:*** Forene; ***Switz.:*** Forene; ***Thai.:*** AErrane†; Forane; ***UK:*** AErrane; Isoflurane; ***USA:*** Forane.

## Ketamine Hydrochloride

*(BANM, USAN, rINNM)*

CI-581; CL-369; CN-52372-2; Hidrocloruro de ketamina; Ketamini Hydrochloridum. (±)-2-(2-Chlorophenyl)-2-methylaminocyclohexanone hydrochloride.

$C_{13}H_{16}ClNO,HCl = 274.2.$

*CAS — 6740-88-1 (ketamine); 1867-66-9 (ketamine hydrochloride).*

*ATC — N01AX03.*

**Pharmacopoeias.** In *Chin., Eur.* (see p.vi), *Int., Jpn,* and *US.*

**Ph. Eur. 5.0** (Ketamine Hydrochloride). A white crystalline powder. Freely soluble in water and in methyl alcohol; soluble in alcohol. A 10% solution in water has a pH of 3.5 to 4.1. Protect from light.

**USP 27** (Ketamine Hydrochloride). A white crystalline powder having a slight characteristic odour. Soluble 1 in 4 of water, 1 in 14 of alcohol, 1 in 60 of dehydrated alcohol and of chloroform, and 1 in 6 of methyl alcohol; practically insoluble in ether. pH of a 10% solution in water is between 3.5 and 4.1. Store at a temperature of 25°, excursions permitted between 15° and 30°.

**Incompatibility.** Ketamine hydrochloride is incompatible with soluble barbiturates. The US manufacturer has recommended that when concomitant use of diazepam and ketamine is required they should be given separately and not mixed in the same giving equipment.

## Esketamine Hydrochloride *(BANM, rINNM)*

Esketamini Hydrochloridum; S-Ketamine Hydrochloride.

*CAS — 33643-46-8 (esketamine).*

*ATC — N01AX14.*

**Pharmacopoeias.** In *Eur.* (see p.vi).

**Ph. Eur. 5.0** (Esketamine Hydrochloride). A white crystalline powder. Freely soluble in water and in methyl alcohol; soluble in alcohol. A 10% solution in water has a pH of 3.5 to 4.5. Protect from light.

### Adverse Effects

Emergence reactions are common during recovery from ketamine anaesthesia and include vivid often unpleasant dreams, confusion, hallucinations, and irrational behaviour. Children and elderly patients appear to be less sensitive. Patients may also experience increased muscle tone, sometimes resembling seizures. Blood pressure and heart rate may be temporarily increased by ketamine; hypotension, arrhythmias, and bradycardia have occurred rarely.

Respiration may be depressed following rapid intravenous injection or with high doses. Apnoea and laryngospasm have occurred. Diplopia and nystagmus may occur. Nausea and vomiting, lachrymation, hypersalivation, and raised intra-ocular and CSF pressure have also been reported. Transient skin rashes and pain at the site of injection may occur.

See also Adverse Effects of General Anaesthetics, p.1295.

**Effects on the cardiovascular system.** Ketamine has been advocated by some for maintaining or increasing cardiovascular performance in selected patients during induction of anaesthesia as it may increase blood pressure and heart rate.[1] However, there have been reports of reduced cardiac and pulmonary performance in severely ill patients[1] and of arrhythmias.[2]

Some of the cardiovascular effects of ketamine may be attenuated by premedication with diazepam[2] or clonidine.[3]

1. Waxman K, *et al.* Cardiovascular effects of anesthetic induction with ketamine. *Anesth Analg* 1980; **59:** 355–8.
2. Cabbabe EB, Behbahani PM. Cardiovascular reactions associated with the use of ketamine and epinephrine in plastic surgery. *Ann Plast Surg* 1985; **15:** 50–2.
3. Tanaka M, Nishikawa T. Oral clonidine premedication attenuates the hypertensive response to ketamine. *Br J Anaesth* 1994; **73:** 758–62.

**Effects on the liver.** Changes in serum-enzyme levels have occurred following ketamine in an initial dose of 1 mg/kg followed by continuous infusion as a 0.1% solution.[1]

1. Dundee JW, *et al.* Changes in serum enzyme levels following ketamine infusions. *Anaesthesia* 1980; **35:** 12–16.

**Effects on mental state.** Mental disturbances following ketamine anaesthesia may vary in incidence from less than 5% to greater than 30%.[1] See also Abuse, below.

1. White PF, *et al.* Ketamine—its pharmacology and therapeutic uses. *Anesthesiology* 1982; **56:** 119–36.

**Effects on the skin.** Harlequin-like colour skin changes were reported[1] in a 9-month-old boy during anaesthesia with ketamine 15 mg.

1. Wagner DL, Sewell AD. Harlequin color change in an infant during anesthesia. *Anesthesiology* 1985; **62:** 695.

**Malignant hyperthermia.** Malignant hyperthermia has been reported in a patient given ketamine.[1]

1. Rasore-Quartino A, *et al.* Forma atipica di ipertermia maligna: osservazione di un caso da ketamina. *Pathologica* 1985; **77:** 609–17.

### Precautions

Ketamine is contra-indicated in patients in whom elevation of blood pressure would be a serious hazard including those with hypertension or a history of cerebrovascular accident. Cardiac function should be monitored in patients found to have hypertension or cardiac decompensation. Ketamine should be used with caution in patients with elevated CSF pressure. It can raise intra-ocular pressure and should not be used in the presence of eye injury or increased intra-ocular pressure.

Ketamine does not reliably suppress pharyngeal and laryngeal reflexes and mechanical stimulation of the pharynx should be avoided unless a muscle relaxant is used.

The use of ketamine should be avoided in patients prone to hallucinations or psychotic disorders. Verbal, tactile, and visual stimuli should be kept to a minimum during recovery in an attempt to reduce the risk of emergence reactions.

See also Precautions for General Anaesthetics, p.1295.

**Abuse.** Health care workers in the USA were alerted to the dangers associated with the abuse of ketamine as long ago as 1979.[1] Similar concern had also been voiced in the UK[2] over the abuse of ketamine at social gatherings where it has been taken intranasally or orally under the names of 'vitamin K', 'super K', or 'special K'. Street names in the USA have also included 'K', 'keets', 'kit-kat', 'jet', and 'super acid'.[3]

Ketamine produces a state of psychological dissociation resulting in hallucinations and out of body or near death experiences. It can induce a state of helplessness in which the user loses awareness of the environment and this together with severe loss of coordination and pronounced analgesia can put the user at great risk. Furthermore, some users experience a state in which they are unconcerned about whether they live or die. Ketamine has the potential for compulsive repeated use and there have been reports of users self-injecting ketamine several times a day for prolonged periods. Dependency may develop[3,4] and withdrawal symptoms requiring detoxification can occur.[3] Frequent use may produce long-lasting memory impairment.[5] Other adverse effects include a report[6] of an acute dystonic reaction in a 20-year old man following self-administration of ketamine intravenously.

In one case series[7] of 20 patients presenting to hospital after ketamine abuse the most common symptoms included anxiety, chest pain, and palpitations. Frequent complications included agitation and rhabdomyolysis. Symptoms were generally short lived with most patients discharged within 5 hours.

Some[2] suggest that patients seeking medical attention are best placed in a quiet darkened room to recover with diazepam being given for unresponsive panic attacks while others advocate that such patients should be admitted to an intensive care unit for close monitoring.[8] The use of intravenous fluids to prevent rhabdomyolysis has also been recommended.[7]

Ketamine is tasteless, odourless, and colourless and has been misused to incapacitate the victim and produce amnesia in sexual assaults and drug-facilitated rape ('date rape').[3]

1. Anonymous. Ketamine abuse. *FDA Drug Bull* 1979; **9:** 24.
2. Jansen KLR. Non-medical use of ketamine. *BMJ* 1993; **306:** 601–2.
3. Smith KM, *et al.* Club drugs: methylenedioxymethamphetamine, flunitrazepam, ketamine hydrochloride, and γ-hydroxybutyrate. *Am J Health-Syst Pharm* 2002; **59:** 1067–76.
4. Jansen KLR, Darracot-Cankovic R. The nonmedical use of ketamine, part two: A review of problem use and dependence. *J Psychoactive Drugs* 2001; **33:** 151–8.
5. Curran HV, Monaghan L. In and out of the K-hole: a comparison of the acute and residual effects of ketamine in frequent and infrequent ketamine users. *Addiction* 2001; **96:** 749–60.
6. Felser JM, Orban DJ. Dystonic reaction after ketamine abuse. *Ann Emerg Med* 1982; **11:** 673–5.
7. Weiner AL, *et al.* Ketamine abusers presenting to the emergency department: a case series. *J Emerg Med* 2000; **18:** 447–51.
8. Gill PA. Non-medical use of ketamine. *BMJ* 1993; **306:** 1340.

### Interactions

Inhalational anaesthetics, such as ether and halothane, and other cerebral depressants may prolong the effect of ketamine and delay recovery. Prolonged recovery has also occurred when barbiturates and/or opioids have been given concomitantly with ketamine. It has been recommended that ketamine should not be used with ergometrine.

See also Interactions of General Anaesthetics, p.1295.

**Neuromuscular blockers.** For the enhancement of the effect of *tubocurarine* or *atracurium* by ketamine, see p.1401.

**Thyroid drugs.** For a reference to increased cardiovascular adverse effects with *thyroid drugs*, see p.1601.

**Xanthines.** For a reference to seizures and tachycardia attributed to an interaction between ketamine and *theophylline*, see p.803.

### Pharmacokinetics

After intravenous bolus administration, ketamine shows a bi- or triexponential pattern of elimination. The alpha phase lasts about 45 minutes with a half-life of 10 to 15 minutes. This first phase, which represents ketamine's anaesthetic action, is terminated by redistribution from the CNS to peripheral tissues and hepatic biotransformation to an active metabolite norketamine. Other metabolic pathways include hydroxylation of the cyclohexone ring and conjugation with glucuronic acid. The beta phase half-life is about 2.5 hours. Ketamine is excreted mainly in the urine as metabolites. It crosses the placenta.

◊ References.


1. Clements JA, Nimmo WS. Pharmacokinetics and analgesic effect of ketamine in man. *Br J Anaesth* 1981; **53:** 27–30.
2. Grant IS, *et al.* Pharmacokinetics and analgesic effects of IM and oral ketamine. *Br J Anaesth* 1981; **53:** 805–9.
3. Grant IS, *et al.* Ketamine disposition in children and adults. *Br J Anaesth* 1983; **55:** 1107–11. **14:** 144P.
4. Geisslinger G, *et al.* Pharmacokinetics and pharmacodynamics of ketamine enantiomers in surgical patients using a stereoselective analytical method. *Br J Anaesth* 1993; **70:** 666–71.
5. Malinovsky J-M, *et al.* Ketamine and norketamine plasma concentrations after iv, nasal and rectal administration in children. *Br J Anaesth* 1996; **77:** 203–7.


## Uses and Administration

Ketamine is an anaesthetic administered by intravenous injection, intravenous infusion, or intramuscular injection. It produces dissociative anaesthesia characterised by a trance-like state, amnesia, and marked analgesia which may persist into the recovery period. There is often an increase in muscle tone and the patient's eyes may remain open for all or part of the period of anaesthesia. Ketamine is used in general anaesthesia for diagnostic or short surgical operations that do not require skeletal muscle relaxation, for the induction of anaesthesia to be maintained with other drugs, and as a supplementary anaesthetic (see p.1296). It also has good analgesic properties in subanaesthetic doses. It is considered to be of particular value in children requiring frequent repeated anaesthesia. Recovery is relatively slow.

Ketamine is administered as the hydrochloride but doses are expressed in terms of the equivalent amount of base; ketamine hydrochloride 1.15 mg is approximately equivalent to 1 mg of ketamine base.

- For induction the dose given by *intravenous injection* may range from the equivalent of 1 to 4.5 mg/kg of ketamine; a dose of 2 mg/kg given intravenously over 60 seconds usually produces surgical anaesthesia within 30 seconds of the end of the injection and lasting for 5 to 10 minutes.
- The initial *intramuscular* dose may range from 6.5 to 13 mg/kg; an intramuscular dose of 10 mg/kg usually produces surgical anaesthesia within 3 to 4 minutes lasting for 12 to 25 minutes. For diagnostic or other procedures not involving intense pain an initial intramuscular dose of 4 mg/kg has been used. Additional doses may be given for maintenance.
- For induction by *intravenous infusion* a total dose of 0.5 to 2 mg/kg is usually given at an appropriate infusion rate. Maintenance is achieved with 10 to 45 micrograms/kg per minute, the infusion rate being adjusted according to response.

Administration should be preceded by atropine or another suitable antimuscarinic. Diazepam or another benzodiazepine may be given before surgery or as an adjunct to ketamine to reduce the incidence of emergence reactions.

The *S*-isomer, esketamine, is also being investigated for similar uses in anaesthesia.

◊ Reviews.


1. Hirota K, Lambert DG. Ketamine: its mechanism(s) of action and unusual clinical uses. *Br J Anaesth* 1996; **77:** 441–4.


**Administration.** Although ketamine hydrochloride is usually given intravenously or intramuscularly, oral[1,2] and rectal[3] administration has been used successfully in children. Intranasal administration of ketamine with midazolam in a neonate requiring anaesthesia has also been reported.[4] Unfortunately the onset of sedation with these three routes is too slow for emergency procedures and therefore a jet-injector of ketamine was developed[5] to provide non-traumatic, painless, and rapid anaesthesia in children. Intranasal and transdermal administration may be useful in the management of pain (see below); oral, rectal, and subcutaneous administration has also been tried.[6]


1. Tobias JD, *et al.* Oral ketamine premedication to alleviate the distress of invasive procedures in pediatric oncology patients. *Pediatrics* 1992; **90:** 537–41.
2. Gutstein HB, *et al.* Oral ketamine preanesthetic medication in children. *Anesthesiology* 1992; **76:** 28–33.
3. Lökken P, *et al.* Conscious sedation by rectal administration of midazolam or midazolam plus ketamine as alternatives to general anesthesia for dental treatment of uncooperative children. *Scand J Dent Res* 1994; **102:** 274–80.
4. Louon A, *et al.* Sedation with nasal ketamine and midazolam for cryotherapy in retinopathy of prematurity. *Br J Ophthalmol* 1993; **77:** 529–30.
5. Zsigmond EK, *et al.* A new route, jet-injection for anesthetic induction in children–ketamine dose-range finding studies. *Int J Clin Pharmacol Ther* 1996; **34:** 84–8.
6. Kronenberg RH. Ketamine as an analgesic: parenteral, oral, rectal, subcutaneous, transdermal and intranasal administration. *J Pain Palliat Care Pharmacother* 2002; **16:** 27–35.


**Nonketotic hyperglycinaemia.** Ketamine was tried with strychnine in a newborn infant with severe nonketotic hyperglycinaemia (p.1750) and resulted in neurological improvement, although motor development remained unsatisfactory.[1] It was thought that ketamine might act by blocking N-methyl-D-aspartate (NMDA) receptors, which are activated in the CNS by glycine.


1. Tegtmeyer-Metadorf H, *et al.* Ketamine and strychnine treatment of an infant with nonketotic hyperglycinaemia. *Eur J Pediatr* 1995; **154:** 649–53.


**Pain.** For a discussion of pain and its management, see p.2. Ketamine is used for its analgesic action in neuropathic or other pain unresponsive to conventional analgesics. (For mention of its use for outpatient procedures in children, see p.3.) Systematic reviews[1,2] have found the evidence for such use to be limited, but it has been suggested[1] that ketamine is a reasonable third-line option where standard analgesics have failed. Subcutaneous, intramuscular, intravenous, epidural, intrathecal, intranasal, transdermal, rectal, and oral administration have all been tried.[1,3]


1. Hocking G, Cousins MJ. Ketamine in chronic pain management: an evidence-based review. *Anesth Analg* 2003; **97:** 1730–9.
2. Bell R, *et al.* Ketamine as an adjuvant to opioids for cancer pain. Available in The Cochrane Library; Issue 1. Chichester: John Wiley; 2004.
3. Kronenberg RH. Ketamine as an analgesic: parenteral, oral, rectal, subcutaneous, transdermal and intranasal administration. *J Pain Palliat Care Pharmacother* 2002; **16:** 27–35.


### Preparations

***BP 2003:*** Ketamine Injection;
***USP 27:*** Ketamine Hydrochloride Injection.

**Proprietary Preparations** (details are given in Part 3)
***Arg.:*** Cost; Inducmina; Ketalar; Ketanest; ***Austral.:*** Ketalar; ***Austria:*** Ketalar†; Ketanest; ***Belg.:*** Ketalar; ***Braz.:*** Ketalar; ***Canad.:*** Ketalar; ***Denm.:*** Ketalar; ***Fin.:*** Ketalar; Ketanest; ***Fr.:*** Ketalar†; ***Ger.:*** Keta; Ketanest; Velonarcon†; ***Hong Kong:*** Ketalar; ***India:*** Ketalar; Ketmin; ***Irl.:*** Ketalar; ***Israel:*** Ketalar; ***Ital.:*** Ketalar†; ***Malaysia:*** Calypsol; Ketava; ***Mex.:*** Ketalin; Ketina†; ***Neth.:*** Ketalar; Ketanest; ***Norw.:*** Ketalar; ***NZ:*** Ketalar; ***S.Afr.:*** Brevinaze†; ***Spain:*** Ketolar; ***Swed.:*** Ketalar; ***Switz.:*** Ketalar; ***Thai.:*** Calypsol; Keta-Hameln; Ketalar; ***UK:*** Ketalar; ***USA:*** Ketalar.

## Methohexital *(BAN, rINN)*

Methohexitone; Metohexital. (±)-5-Allyl-1-methyl-5-(1-methylpent-2-ynyl)barbituric acid; 1-Methyl-5-(1-methyl-2-pentynyl)-5-(2-propenyl)-2,4,6(1*H*,3*H*,5*H*)-pyrimidinetrione.

$C_{14}H_{18}N_2O_3$ = 262.3.

*CAS — 151-83-7; 18652-93-2.*

*ATC — N01AF01; N05CA15.*

**Pharmacopoeias.** In *US.*

**USP 27** (Methohexital). A white to faintly yellowish-white crystalline odourless powder. M.p. 92° to 96° but the range between beginning and end of melting does not exceed 3°. Very slightly soluble in water; slightly soluble in alcohol, in chloroform, and in dilute alkalis.

### Methohexital Sodium *(BANM, rINNM)*

Compound 25398; Enallynymalnatrium; Methohexitone Sodium; Metohexital sódico.

$C_{14}H_{17}N_2NaO_3$ = 284.3.

*CAS — 309-36-4; 22151-68-4; 60634-69-7.*

*ATC — N01AF01; N05CA15.*

**Pharmacopoeias.** *US* includes Methohexital Sodium for Injection.

**USP 27** (Methohexital Sodium for Injection). A freeze-dried sterile mixture of methohexital sodium and anhydrous sodium carbonate as a buffer, prepared from an aqueous solution of methohexital, sodium hydroxide, and sodium carbonate. It is a white to off-white, essentially odourless, hygroscopic powder. pH of a 5% solution in water is between 10.6 to 11.6.

**Incompatibility.** Solutions of methohexital sodium are incompatible with acidic substances including a number of antibacterials, antipsychotics, neuromuscular blockers, antimuscarinics, and analgesics. Compounds commonly listed as incompatible include atropine sulfate, pethidine hydrochloride, metocurine iodide, fentanyl citrate, morphine sulfate, pentazocine lactate, silicones, suxamethonium chloride, tubocurarine chloride, and compound sodium lactate injection. Only preservative-free diluents should be used to reconstitute methohexital sodium; precipitation may occur if a diluent containing a bacteriostatic agent is used.

**Stability.** Solutions of methohexital sodium in Water for Injections are stable for at least 6 weeks at room temperature; however reconstituted solutions should be stored no longer than 24 hours as they contain no bacteriostatic agent. Solutions in glucose or sodium chloride injections are stable only for about 24 hours.

## Adverse Effects and Precautions

As for Thiopental Sodium, p.1309.

Excitatory phenomena are more common and induction less smooth with methohexital than with thiopental. Methohexital should be used with caution, if at all, in patients with a history of epilepsy.

See also Adverse Effects and Precautions for General Anaesthetics, p.1295.

◊ In a study of 4379 administrations of methohexital to 2722 dental patients the total dose ranged from 20 mg to 560 mg (with a mean of 151 mg), and the duration of treatment was 8 to 32 minutes.[1] Complications included: restlessness not controlled by diazepam (292 cases), respiratory complications (214), uncontrollable crying during recovery (73), pain along vein (45) with thrombophlebitis (5), jactitations (22), and allergic reactions (10).


1. McDonald D. Methohexitone in dentistry. *Aust Dent J* 1980; **25:** 335–42.


**Breast feeding.** No adverse effects have been observed in breast-feeding infants whose mothers were receiving methohexital, and the American Academy of Pediatrics[1] considers that it is therefore usually compatible with breast feeding.

In a study[2] of 9 breast-feeding women undergoing general anaesthesia, it was estimated that the exposure of a breast-fed infant to methohexital would be less than 1% of the maternal dose following induction with methohexital. Breast feeding was not interrupted during the study and none of the infants appeared drowsy or sedated.


1. American Academy of Pediatrics. The transfer of drugs and other chemicals into human milk. *Pediatrics* 2001; **108:** 776–89. Correction. *ibid.*; 1029. Also available at: http://aappolicy.aappublications.org/cgi/content/full/pediatrics%3b108/3/776 (accessed 26/05/04)
2. Borgatta L, *et al.* Clinical significance of methohexital, meperidine, and diazepam in breast milk. *J Clin Pharmacol* 1997; **37:** 186–92.


**Effects on the nervous system.** Two case reports of seizures induced by methohexital in children with seizure disorders.[1] Seizures are considered a rare adverse effect of methohexital. In 48 000 patients given methohexital, only 3 developed clonic-type seizures.[2]

A case of a tonic-clonic seizure possibly due to an interaction between paroxetine and methohexital is discussed below.


1. Rockoff MA, Goudsouzian NG. Seizures induced by methohexital. *Anesthesiology* 1981; **54:** 333–5.
2. Metriyakool K. Seizures induced by methohexital. *Anesthesiology* 1981; **55:** 718.


**Pain on injection.** Methohexital is associated with severe pain particularly if veins on the back of the hands are used. The incidence of pain on injection may be reduced by using a forearm vein or by pre-injection with lidocaine.

**Porphyria.** Methohexital is considered to be unsafe in patients with porphyria because it has been shown to be porphyrinogenic in *animals.*

**Rebound anaesthesia.** Rebound of anaesthesia with abolition of reflexes and depression of respiration occurred in a 6-year-old boy[1] 100 minutes after anorectal induction with 27.6 mg/kg methohexital.


1. Kaiser H, Al-Rafai S. Wie sicher ist die rektale Narkoseeinleitung mit Methohexital in der Kinderanaesthesie? *Anaesthesist* 1985; **34:** 359–60.


## Interactions

As for Thiopental Sodium, p.1309.

**Antidepressants.** A 42-year-old woman[1] suffered a generalised tonic-clonic seizure immediately after being anaesthetised with methohexital for the last in a series of 6 electroconvulsive therapies. She had been receiving *paroxetine* throughout the series. A previous course, without concurrent paroxetine, had been uneventful.


1. Folkerts H. Spontaneous seizure after concurrent use of methohexital anesthesia for electroconvulsive therapy and paroxetine: a case report. *J Nerv Ment Dis* 1995; **183:** 115–16.


## Pharmacokinetics

Methohexital is less lipid soluble than thiopental but concentrations sufficient to produce anaesthesia are attained in the brain within 30 seconds of an intravenous dose. Methohexital is also absorbed when given rectally, producing an effect within about 5 to 11 minutes. Recovery from anaesthesia occurs quickly as a result of rapid metabolism and redistribution into other body tissues. Methohexital does not appear to concentrate in fatty tissues to the same extent as other barbiturate anaesthetics. Protein binding has been reported to be about 73%. Methohexital is rapidly metabolised in the liver through demethylation and oxidation. The terminal half-life ranges from 1.5 to 6 hours. Methohexital diffuses across the placenta and has been detected in breast milk.

◊ References.


1. Swerdlow BN, Holley FO. Intravenous anaesthetic agents: pharmacokinetic-pharmacodynamic relationships. *Clin Pharmacokinet* 1987; **12:** 79–110.

2. Le Normand Y, *et al.* Pharmacokinetics and haemodynamic effects of prolonged methohexitone infusion. *Br J Clin Pharmacol* 1988; **26:** 589–94.
3. Redke F, *et al.* Pharmacokinetics and clinical experience of 20-h infusions of methohexitone in intensive care patients with postoperative pyrexia. *Br J Anaesth* 1991; **66:** 53–9.
4. van Hoogdalem EJ, *et al.* Pharmacokinetics of rectal drug administration, part I: general considerations and clinical applications of centrally acting drugs. *Clin Pharmacokinet* 1991; **21:** 11–26.

## Uses and Administration

Methohexital is a short-acting barbiturate anaesthetic that has actions similar to those of thiopental (p.1310) but it is about 2 to 3 times more potent. It is administered as the sodium salt and has similar uses to thiopental in anaesthesia. Induction of anaesthesia is less smooth than with thiopental and there may be excitatory phenomena. It has a shorter duration of action than thiopental and recovery after an induction dose occurs within 5 to 7 minutes although drowsiness may persist for some time.

As with other barbiturate anaesthetics the dose of methohexital required varies greatly according to the state of the patient and the nature of other drugs also being used (see under Precautions of Thiopental, p.1309, and Interactions of Thiopental, p.1309, for further details). Methohexital sodium is usually given intravenously as a 1% solution. Higher concentrations may markedly increase the incidence of adverse effects. A typical dose for induction of anaesthesia is 50 to 120 mg given at a rate of about 10 mg (1 mL of a 1% solution) every 5 seconds. For the maintenance of general anaesthesia methohexital sodium may be given by intravenous injection in doses of 20 to 40 mg every 4 to 7 minutes as required or it may be given as a 0.2% solution by continuous intravenous infusion at a rate of 3 mL/minute.

For dosage in children, see below.

**Administration in children.** Although intravenous administration is considered preferable in adults, in the USA methohexital sodium is licensed for use in children only by the intramuscular and rectal routes: usual doses for the induction of anaesthesia are 6.6 to 10 mg/kg intramuscularly, as a 5% solution, or 25 mg/kg rectally, as a 1% solution. In some countries methohexital sodium has also been given intravenously to children: doses in the range of 1 to 2 mg/kg have been used.

**Administration in the elderly.** It is usually recommended that the dosage of barbiturate anaesthetics is reduced in the elderly. A study[1] in elderly patients has demonstrated that although reducing the rate of intravenous administration reduces the speed of induction, the dosage required is also reduced. Administration of methohexital sodium 0.5% at a rate of 25 mg/minute induced anaesthesia in a mean of 83.8 seconds and required a mean dose of 0.56 mg/kg. Corresponding values for an administration rate of 100 mg/minute were 43.6 seconds and 1 mg/kg, respectively.

1. Berthoud MC, *et al.* Comparison of infusion rates of three i.v. anaesthetic agents for induction in elderly patients. *Br J Anaesth* 1993; **70:** 423–7.

**Dental sedation.** Some anaesthetics are used as sedatives in dental procedures (see p.666). Methohexital has been tried for patient-controlled sedation in oral surgery under local anaesthesia.[1] In a group of 42 patients, results with 2.5 mg of methohexital compared favourably with those obtained in patients receiving 5 mg of propofol on demand, although patients in the methohexital group experienced a greater degree of postoperative drowsiness.

1. Hamid SK, *et al.* Comparison of patient-controlled sedation with either methohexitone or propofol. *Br J Anaesth* 1996; **77:** 727–30.

### Preparations

***USP 27:*** Methohexital Sodium for Injection.

**Proprietary Preparations** (details are given in Part 3)
***Austral.:*** Brietal; ***Austria:*** Brietal; ***Canad.:*** Brietal†; ***Denm.:*** Brietal†; ***Ger.:*** Brevimytal; ***Irl.:*** Brietal†; ***Israel:*** Brietal; ***Neth.:*** Brietal; ***Norw.:*** Brietal†; ***NZ:*** Brietal†; ***S.Afr.:*** Brietal†; ***Singapore:*** Brietal†; ***Swed.:*** Brietal†; ***Switz.:*** Brietal†; ***USA:*** Brevital.

## Methoxyflurane *(BAN, USAN, rINN)*

Metoxiflurano; NSC-110432. 2,2-Dichloro-1,1-difluoro-1-methoxyethane; 2,2-Dichloro-1,1-difluoroethyl methyl ether.

$C_3H_4Cl_2F_2O$ = 165.0.
*CAS — 76-38-0.*
*ATC — N01AB03.*

**Pharmacopoeias.** In *US.*

**USP 27** (Methoxyflurane). A clear, practically colourless, mobile liquid having a characteristic odour. It may contain a suitable stabiliser. B.p. about 105°. Soluble 1 in 500 of water; miscible with alcohol, with acetone, with chloroform, with ether, and with fixed oils. Store in airtight containers at a temperature not exceeding 40°. Protect from light.

### Adverse Effects

As with other halogenated anaesthetics respiratory depression, hypotension, and malignant hyperthermia have been reported. Methoxyflurane sensitises the myocardium to sympathomimetics to a lesser extent than halothane; arrhythmias appear to be rare.

Methoxyflurane impairs renal function in a dose-related manner due to the effect of the released fluoride on the distal tubule and may cause polyuric or oliguric renal failure, oxaluria being a prominent feature. Nephrotoxicity is greater with methoxyflurane than with other halogenated anaesthetics because of slower metabolism over several days resulting in prolonged production of fluoride ions, and metabolism to other potentially nephrotoxic substances.

There have also been occasional reports of hepatic dysfunction, jaundice, and fatal hepatic necrosis. Headache has been reported by some patients. Cardiac arrest, gastrointestinal side-effects, delirium, and prolonged postoperative somnolence have been observed.

See also Adverse Effects of General Anaesthetics, p.1295.

### Precautions

The use of methoxyflurane is limited because of its potential to cause renal toxicity. It should not be used to achieve deep anaesthesia or for surgical procedures expected to last longer than 4 hours. Methoxyflurane is contra-indicated in the presence of renal impairment. Renal function and urine output should be monitored during anaesthesia. As with other halogenated anaesthetics it is advisable not to administer methoxyflurane to patients who have shown signs of liver damage or fever after previous anaesthesia involving halogenated anaesthetics. Patients with known, or suspected, susceptibility to malignant hyperthermia should not be anaesthetised with methoxyflurane. Allowance may need to be made for any increase in CSF pressure or in cerebral blood flow.

There is significant absorption of methoxyflurane by the rubber and soda lime in anaesthetic circuits. PVC plastics are partially soluble in methoxyflurane.

See also Precautions for General Anaesthetics, p.1295.

**Abuse.** A 27-year-old nurse suffered from progressive renal disease and painful diffuse and multifocal periostitis, which had developed as a probable consequence of intermittent self-exposure to methoxyflurane possibly over a 9-year period.[1] There has also been a report[2] of hepatitis in a 39-year-old physician who repeatedly self-administered subanaesthetic concentrations of methoxyflurane for insomnia. Inhalation of about 2 mL of methoxyflurane had occurred once or twice almost every day for 6 weeks. A 125-mL bottle of methoxyflurane had been consumed in about 1 month.

1. Klemmer PJ, Hadler NM. Subacute fluorosis: a consequence of abuse of an organofluoride anesthetic. *Ann Intern Med* 1978; **89:** 607–11.
2. Okuno T, *et al.* Hepatitis due to repeated inhalation of methoxyflurane in subanaesthetic concentrations. *Can Anaesth Soc J* 1985; **32:** 53–5.

**Porphyria.** Methoxyflurane is considered to be unsafe in patients with porphyria because it has been shown to be porphyrinogenic in *animals* or *in-vitro* systems.

### Interactions

Care is advised if adrenaline or other sympathomimetics are given to patients during methoxyflurane anaesthesia. The effects of competitive neuromuscular blockers are enhanced by methoxyflurane. The chronic use of hepatic enzyme-inducing drugs may enhance the metabolism of methoxyflurane thereby increasing the risk of nephrotoxicity. Use of nephrotoxic drugs with methoxyflurane should be avoided.

See also Interactions of General Anaesthetics, p.1295.

### Pharmacokinetics

Methoxyflurane is absorbed on inhalation. The blood/gas partition coefficient is high. Methoxyflurane is metabolised to a greater extent than other inhalational anaesthetics. About 50 to 70% of absorbed methoxyflurane undergoes metabolism in the liver to free fluoride, oxalic acid, difluoromethoxyacetic acid, and dichloroacetic acid. Methoxyflurane is very soluble in adipose tissue and excretion may be slow. Peak plasma concentrations of fluoride occur 2 to 4 days after administration. Methoxyflurane crosses the placenta.

### Uses and Administration

Methoxyflurane is a volatile halogenated anaesthetic administered by inhalation. It has a minimum alveolar concentration (MAC) value (see Uses of General Anaesthetics, p.1295) of 0.16%, but because of its low vapour pressure, induction of general anaesthesia with methoxyflurane is slow. In recommended concentrations it is non-flammable and not explosive when mixed with oxygen. Methoxyflurane possesses good analgesic properties. It does not produce appreciable skeletal muscle relaxation at the concentrations used. Methoxyflurane does not relax the uterus and has little effect on uterine contractions during labour. It is used in subanaesthetic doses to provide analgesia for painful procedures. In anaesthetic doses, it has been used mainly for maintenance of general anaesthesia (p.1296), but safer anaesthetics are preferred because of its nephrotoxicity.

Concentrations of 0.3 to 0.8% v/v are used to provide analgesia in a variety of situations. The recommended maximum dose for self-administration for analgesia is 6 mL of liquid per day or 15 mL/week.

For maintenance of general anaesthesia, a concentration of up to 2% v/v methoxyflurane in at least 50% v/v nitrous oxide and oxygen has been given for not more than 5 minutes and then progressively reduced to the lowest concentration that would maintain adequate anaesthesia. The production of deep anaesthesia with methoxyflurane is not recommended, and a maximum of 4 hours exposure to a concentration of 0.25% v/v or the equivalent total dosage is suggested. Recovery may be prolonged.

### Preparations

**Proprietary Preparations** (details are given in Part 3)
***Austral.:*** Penthrox.

## Nitrous Oxide

Azoto Protossido; Dinitrogen Oxide; Dinitrogenii Oxidum; Distickstoffmonoxid; E942; Laughing Gas; Nitrogen Monoxide; Nitrogen Oxide; Nitrogenii Monoxidum; Nitrogenii Oxidum; Nitrogenium Oxydulatum; Óxido nitroso; Oxyde Nitreux; Oxydum Nitrosum; Protoxyde d'Azote; Stickoxydul.

$N_2O$ = 44.01.
*CAS — 10024-97-2.*
*ATC — N01AX13.*

**Pharmacopoeias.** In *Chin., Eur.* (see p.vi), *Int., Jpn,* and *US.*

**Ph. Eur. 5.0** (Nitrous Oxide). A colourless gas. One vol. measured at a pressure of 101 kPa dissolves, at 20°, in about 1.5 vol. of water. Store liquefied under pressure in suitable containers complying with the legal regulations.

The BP 2003 directs that Nitrous Oxide should be kept in approved metal cylinders which are painted blue and carry a label stating 'Nitrous Oxide'. In addition, 'Nitrous Oxide' or the symbol '$N_2O$' should be stencilled in paint on the shoulder of the cylinder.

**USP 27** (Nitrous Oxide). A colourless gas, without appreciable odour or taste. One litre at 0° and at a pressure of 760 mmHg weighs about 1.97 g. One volume dissolves in about 1.4 volumes of water at 20° and at a pressure of 760 mmHg; freely soluble in alcohol; soluble in ether and in oils.

**Flammability.** Nitrous oxide supports combustion.

**Storage and supply.** Nitrous oxide is supplied compressed in metal cylinders. National standards are usually in operation for the labelling and marking of such cylinders.

Cylinders containing 50% nitrous oxide and 50% oxygen should be protected from the cold to prevent separation of the gases. Cylinders exposed to temperatures lower than −7° should be rolled at room temperature to ensure mixing or alternatively stored horizontally for 24 hours at a temperature of not less than 10°.

### Adverse Effects

The main complications following the use of nitrous oxide are those due to varying degrees of hypoxia. Prolonged administration has been followed by megaloblastic anaemia and peripheral neuropathy. Depression of white cell formation may also occur. There is a risk of increased pressure and volume from the diffusion of nitrous oxide into air-containing cavities. Malignant hyperthermia has been reported rarely.

See also Adverse Effects of General Anaesthetics, p.1295.

◊ Reviews.

1. Louis-Ferdinand RT. Myelotoxic, neurotoxic and reproductive adverse effects of nitrous oxide. *Adverse Drug React Toxicol Rev* 1994; **13:** 193–206.
2. Donaldson D, Meechan JG. The hazards of chronic exposure to nitrous oxide: an update. *Br Dent J* 1995; **178:** 95–100.
3. Weimann J. Toxicity of nitrous oxide. *Best Pract Res Clin Anaesthesiol* 2003; **17:** 47–61.

**Effects on the blood.** Nitrous oxide interacts with vitamin $B_{12}$. This blocks the transmethylation reaction for which vitamin $B_{12}$ is a coenzyme and results in depletion of methionine and tetrahydrofolate. Metabolic consequences have been attributed to depletion of either or both. Interference by nitrous oxide with DNA synthesis prevents production of both leucocytes and red blood cells by the bone marrow. Megaloblastic changes in bone marrow and impaired granulocyte production are found in patients exposed to anaesthetic concentrations of nitrous oxide for 24 hours. In patients with normal bone marrow, stores of mature granulocytes will normally be adequate to prevent leucopenia during exposure for up to 3 days; in patients exposed to nitrous oxide for longer periods of time, leucopenia will develop and exposure for 4 days or longer can result in agranulocytosis. In general, healthy surgical patients can be given nitrous oxide for up to 24 hours without harm. In situations where nitrous oxide is used for more than 24 hours, folinic acid 30 mg twice daily has been given to protect the haematopoietic system. Repeat exposure to nitrous oxide at intervals of less than 3 days will have a cumulative effect on DNA synthesis and megaloblastic marrow changes have been reported following multiple short-term exposure.[1] Depletion of methionine has been implicated in the neurological deficit (see below) seen mainly after chronic use of nitrous oxide. It may also account for the fetotoxicity observed in *rats*, see below.

1. Nunn JF. Clinical aspects of the interaction between nitrous oxide and vitamin $B_{12}$. *Br J Anaesth* 1987; **59:** 3–13.

**Effects on the nervous system.** Neurological disorders (mainly myeloneuropathies and neuropathies) have occurred in chronic abusers of nitrous oxide.[1] Similar effects have been noted after repeated administration of nitrous oxide in hospitalised patients. These neurological effects are considered to be due to nitrous oxide-induced methionine deficiency (see Effects on the Blood, above).

In patients with undiagnosed subclinical deficiency of vitamin $B_{12}$ (a coenzyme involved in methionine synthesis) neurological manifestations, including those consistent with subacute combined degeneration of the spinal cord, have occurred following a single exposure to nitrous oxide for anaesthesia.[2,3]

1. Miller MA, *et al.* Nitrous oxide "whippit" abuse presenting as clinical B12 deficiency and ataxia. *Am J Emerg Med* 2004; **22:** 124.
2. Schilling RF. Is nitrous oxide a dangerous anesthetic for vitamin $B_{12}$-deficient subjects? *JAMA* 1986; **255:** 1605–6.
3. Nestor PJ, Stark RJ. Vitamin $B_{12}$ myeloneuropathy precipitated by nitrous oxide anaesthesia. *Med J Aust* 1996; **165:** 174.

**Malignant hyperthermia.** An 11-year-old girl whose father had died from malignant hyperthermia after anaesthesia developed hyperthermia after anaesthesia with nitrous oxide and oxygen.[1]

1. Ellis FR, *et al.* Malignant hyperpyrexia induced by nitrous oxide and treated with dexamethasone. *BMJ* 1974; **4:** 270–1.

## Precautions

Hypoxic anaesthesia is dangerous and nitrous oxide should always be given with at least 20 to 30% oxygen. Nitrous oxide diffuses into gas-filled body cavities and care is essential when using it in patients at risk from such diffusion such as those with abdominal distension, occlusion of the middle ear, pneumothorax, or similar cavities in the pericardium or peritoneum. Care is also required in patients during or after air encephalography. Oxygen should be given during emergence from prolonged anaesthesia with nitrous oxide to prevent diffusion hypoxia where the alveolar oxygen concentration is diminished. See also Precautions for General Anaesthetics, p.1295. In addition to the above precautions, mixtures of equal parts of nitrous oxide and oxygen should not be used for analgesia in patients with head injuries with impairment of consciousness, maxillofacial injuries, decompression sickness, or those heavily sedated.

Nitrous oxide has been subject to abuse.

**Driving.** A slight but quantified impairment in driving ability was found up to 30 minutes after 15 minutes' inhalation of nitrous oxide/oxygen mixtures.[1]

1. Moyes DG, *et al.* Driving after anaesthetics. *BMJ* 1979; **1:** 1425.

**Epidural anaesthesia.** Nitrous oxide diffuses into gas-filled body cavities and can increase the size of any air bubbles injected into the epidural space to determine placement of the needle in epidural anaesthesia.[1] This could result in uneven spread of the local anaesthetic and produce inadequate analgesia. The volume of air injected should be limited or another technique used to determine placement of the needle if nitrous oxide is to be given subsequently.

1. Stevens R, *et al.* Fate of extradural air bubbles during inhalation of nitrous oxide. *Br J Anaesth* 1994; **72:** 482P–483P.

**Hazard to user.** A scavenging system and effective ventilation may be necessary to control the nitrous oxide pollution that can occur when this gas is used for analgesia or anaesthesia. Risk areas include, in addition to operating theatres, delivery rooms and dental surgeries.[1-3] Occupational exposure can lead to serious toxicity with bone-marrow and neurological impairment.[2,3] Reduced fertility has been reported in female dental workers exposed to high concentrations of nitrous oxide;[4] such women also appear to have a higher rate of spontaneous abortion.[5] It has been suggested that nitrous oxide can also affect male fertility;[6] in one study a dose-related increase in the incidence of spontaneous abortion was found in the wives of men with occupational exposure to nitrous oxide.[7]

1. Munley AJ, *et al.* Exposure of midwives to nitrous oxide in four hospitals. *BMJ* 1986; **293:** 1063–4. Correction. *ibid.*; 1280.
2. Sweeney B, *et al.* Toxicity of bone marrow in dentists exposed to nitrous oxide. *BMJ* 1985; **291:** 567–9.
3. Brodsky JB, *et al.* Exposure to nitrous oxide and neurologic disease among dental professionals. *Anesth Analg* 1981; **60:** 297–301.
4. Rowland AS, *et al.* Reduced fertility among women employed as dental assistants exposed to high levels of nitrous oxide. *N Engl J Med* 1992; **327:** 993–7.
5. Rowland AS, *et al.* Nitrous oxide and fertility. *N Engl J Med* 1993; **328:** 284.
6. Brodsky JB. Nitrous oxide and fertility. *N Engl J Med* 1993; **328:** 284–5.
7. Cohen EN, *et al.* Occupational disease in dentistry and chronic exposure to trace anesthetic gases. *J Am Dent Assoc* 1980; **101:** 21–31.

**Pregnancy.** Nitrous oxide is fetotoxic in *rats*.[1] However, retrospective reviews,[2] and individual case reports[3] have not shown nitrous oxide anaesthesia to be fetotoxic in humans. See also under Hazard to User, above.

1. Lane GA, *et al.* Anesthetics as teratogens: nitrous oxide is fetotoxic, xenon is not. *Science* 1980; **210:** 899–901.
2. Aldridge LM, Tunstall ME. Nitrous oxide and the fetus: a review and the results of a retrospective study of 175 cases of anaesthesia for insertion of Shirodkar suture. *Br J Anaesth* 1986; **58:** 1348–56.
3. Park GR, *et al.* Normal pregnancy following nitrous oxide exposure in the first trimester. *Br J Anaesth* 1986; **58:** 576–7.

**Vitamin $B_{12}$ deficiency.** For reports of neurological dysfunction associated with the use of nitrous oxide in patients with undiagnosed subclinical vitamin $B_{12}$ deficiency, see Effects on the Nervous System, above.

## Interactions

Use of nitrous oxide with an inhalational anaesthetic accelerates the uptake of the latter from the lungs. This phenomenon is known as the *second gas effect.* It is due to the disproportionate absorption of nitrous oxide into the blood resulting in an increased alveolar concentration of the second gas.

The use of high doses of opioids such as fentanyl with nitrous oxide may result in a drop in heart rate and cardiac output.

See also Interactions for General Anaesthetics, p.1295.

**Methotrexate.** Combined use of nitrous oxide and methotrexate may increase the side-effects of methotrexate therapy, see p.571.

## Pharmacokinetics

Nitrous oxide is rapidly absorbed on inhalation. The blood/gas partition coefficient is low and most of the inhaled nitrous oxide is rapidly eliminated unchanged through the lungs though small amounts diffuse through the skin.

## Uses and Administration

Nitrous oxide is an anaesthetic administered by inhalation. It is a weak anaesthetic with a minimum alveolar concentration (MAC) value (see Uses of General Anaesthetics, p.1295) of 110%. It has strong analgesic properties, but produces little muscle relaxation. Nitrous oxide must be administered with oxygen, otherwise hypoxia will occur.

Nitrous oxide with oxygen may be used in the induction and maintenance of general anaesthesia (p.1296). However, it is now mainly employed as an adjuvant to other inhalational or intravenous anaesthetics, permitting them to be used at significantly lower concentrations. It is also used, with oxygen, in subanaesthetic concentrations for analgesia and sedation in emergency care and obstetric and other painful procedures, including dental procedures (see p.666).

Induction of anaesthesia may be carried out using a mixture containing about 70% nitrous oxide with 30% v/v of oxygen; similar or more dilute mixtures may be used for maintenance. Recovery is usually rapid from nitrous oxide anaesthesia.

Nitrous oxide 25 to 50% v/v with oxygen is used for analgesia; cylinders containing premixed nitrous oxide 50% v/v and oxygen 50% v/v are available in some countries.

**Alcohol withdrawal syndrome.** The symptoms of acute alcohol withdrawal (p.1166) are usually managed with benzodiazepines but nitrous oxide has been reported[1] to reduce symptoms when tried in alcohol withdrawal. In mild to moderate cases a single administration of up to 20 minutes' duration of a nitrous oxide-oxygen mixture in analgesic doses has been used. However, a more recent controlled trial[2] did not find that treatment with nitrous oxide relieved the symptoms of alcohol withdrawal or reduce cravings.

1. Gillman MA, Lichtigfeld FJ. Analgesic nitrous oxide for alcohol withdrawal: a critical appraisal after 10 years' use. *Postgrad Med J* 1990; **66:** 543–6.
2. Alho H, *et al.* Long-term effects of and physiological responses to nitrous oxide gas treatment during alcohol withdrawal: a double-blind, placebo-controlled trial. *Alcohol Clin Exp Res* 2002; **26:** 1816–22.

**Pain.** A mixture of nitrous oxide 50% v/v and oxygen 50% v/v can provide good relief of pain (see Choice of Analgesic, p.2) without loss of consciousness and is suitable for self-administration. It has been widely used for analgesia and sedation during dental procedures. It is also used for short procedures such as dressing changes,[1,2] for pain relief during childbirth,[3] in the management of postoperative pain,[1] as an aid to postoperative physiotherapy, and for acute pain in emergency situations such as in ambulances. Continuous inhalation of nitrous oxide-oxygen has been tried for periods longer than 24 hours in the management of pain in terminal cancer.[4] However, such a practice is not usually otherwise recommended[1] as it may result in megaloblastic bone-marrow changes.

1. Hull CJ. Control of pain in the perioperative period. *Br Med Bull* 1988; **44:** 341–56.
2. Gaukroger PB. Pediatric analgesia: which drug, which dose? *Drugs* 1991; **41:** 52–9.
3. Brownridge P. Treatment options for the relief of pain during childbirth. *Drugs* 1991; **41:** 69–80.
4. Fosburg MT, Crone RK. Nitrous oxide analgesia for refractory pain in the terminally ill. *JAMA* 1983; **250:** 511–13.

## Preparations

**Proprietary Preparations** (details are given in Part 3)
**Multi-ingredient:** ***S.Afr.:*** Entonox; ***UK:*** Entonox; Equanox.

---

## Propanidid *(BAN, USAN, rINN)*

Bayer-1420; FBA-1420; TH-2180; WH-5668. Propyl 4-diethylcarbamoylmethoxy-3-methoxyphenylacetate.

$C_{18}H_{27}NO_5$ = 337.4.
*CAS — 1421-14-3.*
*ATC — N01AX04.*

### Profile

Propanidid has been used as an intravenous anaesthetic for rapid induction and for maintenance of general anaesthesia of short duration.

Commercial preparations of propanidid were provided as a liquid in polyethoxylated castor oil. Anaphylactoid reactions associated with the vehicle led to the general withdrawal of propanidid from use.

**Porphyria.** Propanidid is considered to be unsafe in patients with porphyria although there is conflicting experimental evidence of porphyrinogenicity.

### Preparations

**Proprietary Preparations** (details are given in Part 3)
***Arg.:*** Progray; ***Mex.:*** Inductol†; Panitol.

---

# Propofol *(BAN, USAN, rINN)*

Disoprofol; ICI-35868; Propofolum. 2,6-Di-isopropylphenol; 2,6-Bis(1-methylethyl)phenol.

$C_{12}H_{18}O$ = 178.3.
*CAS — 2078-54-8.*
*ATC — N01AX10.*

**Pharmacopoeias.** In *Eur.* (see p.vi) and *US.*

**Ph. Eur. 5.0** (Propofol). A colourless or very light yellow, clear liquid. Very slightly soluble in water; miscible with hexane and with methyl alcohol. Store under an inert gas. Protect from light.

**USP 27** (Propofol). A clear, colourless to slightly yellowish liquid. Very slightly soluble in water; very soluble in dehydrated alcohol and in methyl alcohol; slightly soluble in cyclohexane and in isopropyl alcohol. Store under an inert gas in airtight containers at a temperature of 25°, excursions permitted between 15° and 30°. Protect from light.

## Adverse Effects

Early studies with propofol employed a preparation formulated with polyethoxylated castor oil. Because of anaphylactoid reactions the preparation was reformulated with a vehicle of soya oil and purified egg phosphatide. Adverse effects with this preparation include pain on injection especially if the injection is into a small vein. Local pain may be reduced by injection into a large vein or by injection of intravenous lidocaine. Apnoea may be frequent; apnoea lasting longer than 60 seconds has been reported to occur in 12% of patients. There are isolated reports of pulmonary oedema. Cardiovascular effects include a reduction in blood pressure and bradycardia. There have been reports of convulsions (sometimes delayed in onset) and involuntary movements. Fever has occurred. Discoloration of urine has been reported following prolonged use. Anaphylactic-like reactions have been reported. Nausea, vomiting, and headache may occur during recovery.

Children who have received propofol for prolonged sedation have suffered severe reactions and there have been fatalities, see below.

See also Adverse Effects of General Anaesthetics, p.1295.

◊ In May 1989 the UK Committee on Safety of Medicines commented on the 268 reports of adverse reactions to propofol that it had received since propofol was introduced to the UK market, during which period about 2 million patients had been anaesthetised with the drug.[1] These included reports of:

- seizures (37 cases, 13 in known epileptics)
- involuntary movements (16 cases)
- opisthotonus (10 cases)
- anaphylactic reactions (32 cases)
- cardiac arrest (13 cases)
- delayed recovery (8 cases)

In 1992 the CSM pointed to the risk of **delayed convulsions** with propofol and its particular importance for day-case surgery.[2] While the incidence of convulsions was low (170 reports), 31% of the reports described the convulsions as delayed.

In June 1992 the CSM commented on the dangers of propofol for the **sedation of children** in intensive care,[3] a use for which it is contra-indicated in the UK. (This prohibition does not apply to its use for the sedation of ventilated adults—but see below—or to propofol's use as an anaesthetic in children. Sedation in children undergoing surgical and diagnostic procedures is not contra-indicated but is an unlicensed use, and is not recommended.[4])

The CSM reported that there had been 66 reports worldwide of serious adverse effects in children sedated with propofol and some fatalities had ensued. The children had suffered neurological, cardiac, and renal effects, hyperlipidaemia, hepatomegaly, and metabolic acidosis. Five deaths had been reported to the CSM. These 5 children[5] were aged 4 weeks to 6 years and doses of propofol ranged from 4 to 10.7 mg/kg per hour. They developed metabolic acidosis, bradyarrhythmia, and progressive myocardial failure resistant to treatment. The latter has been reported by others to be significantly associated with the use of long-term, **high-dose** propofol infusions.[6]

Similar adverse effects resulting in fatalities have also been reported in **adult** patients with head injuries who received high doses of propofol infusion (greater than 5 mg/kg per hour) for long-term sedation.[7] The CSM subsequently reminded prescribers that the recommended dose range for sedation (up to 4 mg/kg per hour) should not be exceeded.[8]


1. Committee on Safety of Medicines. Propofol—convulsions, anaphylaxis and delayed recovery from anaesthesia. *Current Problems 26* 1989.
2. Committee on Safety of Medicines. Propofol and delayed convulsions. *Current Problems 35* 1992.
3. Committee on Safety of Medicines. Serious adverse effects and fatalities in children associated with the use of propofol (Diprivan) for sedation. *Current Problems 34* 1992.
4. Committee on Safety of Medicines/Medicines Control Agency. Clarification: propofol (Diprivan) infusion contraindication. *Current Problems* 2002; **28:** 6. Also available at: http://www.mca.gov.uk/ourwork/monitorsafequalmed/currentproblems/cpapril2002.pdf (accessed 26/05/04)
5. Parke TJ, *et al.* Metabolic acidosis and fatal myocardial failure after propofol infusion in children: five case reports. *BMJ* 1992; **305:** 613–16.
6. Bray RJ. Propofol infusion syndrome in children. *Paediatr Anaesth* 1998; **8:** 491–9.
7. Cremer OL, *et al.* Long-term propofol infusion and cardiac failure in adult head-injured patients. *Lancet* 2001; **357:** 117–18.
8. Committee on Safety of Medicines/Medicines Control Agency. Long term, high dose propofol (Diprivan) infusion. *Current Problems* 2001; **27:** 6. Also available at: http://www.mca.gov.uk/ourwork/monitorsafequalmed/currentproblems/cpfeb2001.pdf (accessed 26/05/04)


**Effects on the cardiovascular system.** The main effect of propofol on the cardiovascular system is a fall in both systolic and diastolic blood pressure of 20 to 30%. The compensatory tachycardia seen after a fall in arterial pressure with other intravenous anaesthetics is not usually seen with propofol. Propofol can also decrease systemic vascular resistance, cardiac output, myocardial blood flow, and myocardial oxygen consumption. Bradycardia can occur even in those premedicated with antimuscarinics and can occasionally be profound with asystole developing.[1] Despite these cardiodepressant effects propofol in doses of 1.5 to 2.5 mg/kg does not generally cause unacceptable haemodynamic changes in patients with a healthy cardiovascular system although concern has been expressed regarding its safety in cardiac surgical patients.[2]

Patients (especially children) who have received propofol for continuous sedation in intensive care units have suffered adverse cardiac reactions with bradyarrhythmia, progressive myocardial failure, and death—see above.


1. Tramèr MR, *et al.* Propofol and bradycardia: causation, frequency and severity. *Br J Anaesth* 1997; **78:** 642–51.
2. Ginsberg R, Lippmann M. Haemodynamic effects of propofol. *Br J Anaesth* 1994; **72:** 370–1.


**Effects on lipids.** Prolonged administration of propofol may be associated with increases in serum triglycerides. In one patient this was believed to have been the cause of necrotising pancreatitis.[1]


1. Metkus AP, *et al.* A firefighter with pancreatitis. *Lancet* 1996; **348:** 1702.


**Effects on mental function.** There have been anecdotal reports[1] of disinhibited behaviour or sexually orientated hallucinations associated with the use of propofol, but a study using subanaesthetic doses found no evidence that propofol produced euphoria or other mood changes.[2]


1. Canaday BR. Amorous, disinhibited behaviour associated with propofol. *Clin Pharm* 1993; **12:** 449–51.
2. Whitehead C, *et al.* The subjective effects of low-dose propofol. *Br J Anaesth* 1994; **72** (suppl 1): 89.


**Effects on the nervous system.** See under Precautions, below.

**Effects on respiration.** See under Precautions, below.

**Hypersensitivity.** Anaphylactic reactions associated with polyethoxylated castor oil used in propofol preparations had prompted a change to the use of soya oil and egg phosphatide in the formulation. A group of workers have reported a patient who experienced anaphylactic shock when given the reformulated emulsion.[1] A possible case of anaphylaxis to this formulation has also been reported in a child with allergies to egg and peanut oil.[2]


1. Laxenaire MC, *et al.* Anaphylactic shock due to propofol. *Lancet* 1988; **ii:** 739–40.
2. Hofer KN, *et al.* Possible anaphylaxis after propofol in a child with food allergy. *Ann Pharmacother* 2003; **37:** 398–401.


**Infection.** Between June 1990 and February 1993 62 cases of postsurgical infections identified in 7 hospitals in the USA were attributed to improper handling of propofol.[1] The infusion was not prepared aseptically and the syringes used in the infusion pumps were reused for several patients. Propofol is formulated as a soybean fat emulsion and the injection contains no antimicrobial preservative although, in the USA, the formulation now contains the microbial-retarding agent, disodium edetate (see under Administration, below). However, either formulation still has the potential to support microbial growth. The UK and USA manufacturers now warn of the importance of aseptic technique in the preparation and administration of propofol. Microbial multiplication did not appear to be clinically significant when propofol infusions were prepared and administered using conventional aseptic techniques.[2]


1. Bennett SN, *et al.* Postoperative infections traced to contamination of an intravenous anesthetic, propofol. *N Engl J Med* 1995; **333:** 147–54.
2. Farrington M, *et al.* Do infusions of midazolam and propofol pose an infection risk to critically ill patients? *Br J Anaesth* 1994; **72:** 415–17.


**Malignant hyperthermia.** From an *in-vitro* study it was concluded that propofol does not trigger malignant hyperthermia.[1] There is a report of the safe use of propofol in 19 patients considered susceptible to malignant hyperthermia.[2]


1. Denborough M, Hopkinson KC. Propofol and malignant hyperpyrexia. *Lancet* 1988; **i:** 191.
2. Harrison GG. Propofol in malignant hyperthermia. *Lancet* 1991; **337:** 503.


**Pain on injection.** The manufacturers have suggested the use of lidocaine to reduce the pain associated with injection of propofol; alternatively, the larger veins in the forearm and antecubital fossa can be used. Studies indicate that alfentanil[1] and metoclopramide[2] might also be effective. It has been suggested[3] that the analgesic action of lidocaine and possibly metoclopramide is due to a pH-lowering effect, rather than to a local anaesthetic action, permitting more propofol to exist in the oily phase of the emulsion. Propofol concentrated in the aqueous phase is believed to be responsible for the pain on injection. However, iontophoretically applied lidocaine has also been found to be effective.[4]


1. Fletcher JE, *et al.* Pretreatment with alfentanil reduces pain caused by propofol. *Br J Anaesth* 1994; **72:** 342–4.
2. Ganta R, Fee JPH. Pain on injection of propofol: comparison of lignocaine with metoclopramide. *Br J Anaesth* 1992; **69:** 316–17.
3. Eriksson M, *et al.* Effect of lignocaine and pH on propofol-induced pain. *Br J Anaesth* 1997; **78:** 502–6.
4. Sadler PJ, *et al.* Iontophoretically applied lidocaine reduces pain on propofol injection. *Br J Anaesth* 1999; **82:** 432–4.


**Urine discoloration.** A case report of dark green urine in a 16-year-old during a prolonged infusion of propofol.[1]


1. Bodenham A, *et al.* Propofol infusion and green urine. *Lancet* 1987; **ii:** 740.


## Precautions

Propofol should not be given to patients known to be allergic to it. Propofol should be administered with caution to patients with hypovolaemia, epilepsy, or lipid metabolism disorders, and to the elderly. Since there have been reports of delayed convulsions associated with the use of propofol it is recommended that special care should be taken when propofol is used for day-case surgery. When used in patients with increased intracranial pressure it should be administered slowly to avoid a substantial decrease in mean arterial pressure and a resultant decrease in cerebral perfusion pressure. It is also recommended that propofol should not be used with ECT. Premedication with an antimuscarinic may be advisable since propofol does not cause vagal inhibition.

Propofol is used to provide continuous sedation for ventilated adult patients under intensive care. Account should be taken of increasing the patient's lipid load. If the duration of sedation is in excess of 3 days, lipid concentrations should be monitored. Children aged 16 years or less should not be sedated in this manner with propofol (see under Adverse Effects, above). Propofol is not recommended for use in obstetrics including caesarean section. See also Precautions for General Anaesthetics, p.1295.

For the need for aseptic handling of propofol see Administration, below.

**CNS effects.** Epileptic activity was seen[1] on the EEGs of 3 patients given propofol and it was suggested that it might be useful in ECT, but others[2,3] found that the duration of seizures was less with propofol anaesthesia than with methohexital anaesthesia. It has been suggested that propofol should not be used with ECT[4] and this is the advice of the manufacturer.

Some consider that abnormal movements induced by propofol are not associated with cortical seizure activity.[5,6] These appear to be more frequent with low doses of propofol[6] and can be abolished in children by increasing the induction dose of propofol from 3 to 5 mg/kg.


1. Hodkinson BP, *et al.* Propofol and the electroencephalogram. *Lancet* 1987; **ii:** 1518.
2. Simpson KH, *et al.* Seizure duration after methohexitone or propofol for induction of anaesthesia for electroconvulsive therapy (ECT). *Br J Anaesth* 1987; **59:** 1323P–1324P.
3. Rampton AJ, *et al.* Propofol and electroconvulsive therapy. *Lancet* 1988; **i:** 296–7.
4. Anonymous. Addendum: propofol better avoided with ECT at present. *Drug Ther Bull* 1990; **28:** 72.
5. Borgeat A, *et al.* Spontaneous excitatory movements during recovery from propofol anaesthesia in an infant: EEG evaluation. *Br J Anaesth* 1993; **70:** 459–61.
6. Borgeat A, *et al.* Propofol and epilepsy: time to clarify. *Anesth Analg* 1994; **78:** 198–9.


**Impaired respiration.** The manufacturer has stated[1] that some patients who have received propofol for sedation in regional anaesthesia have experienced bradypnoea or hypoxaemia, or both. A reduction in oxygen saturation has also been noted in other patients sedated for endoscopy.[2] The manufacturer therefore recommends that oxygen saturation should be monitored and that oxygen supplementation should be readily available.


1. Arnold BDC. Sedation with propofol during regional anaesthesia. *Br J Anaesth* 1993; **70:** 112.
2. Patterson KW, *et al.* Propofol sedation for outpatient upper gastrointestinal endoscopy: comparison with midazolam. *Br J Anaesth* 1991; **67:** 108–11.


## Interactions

The use of propofol with other CNS depressants including those used in premedication may increase the sedative, anaesthetic, and cardiorespiratory depressant effects of propofol. It is recommended that propofol is given after opioids so that the dose of propofol can be carefully titrated against the response. The dosage of propofol should be reduced if used with nitrous oxide or halogenated anaesthetics. Although propofol does not potentiate the effects of neuromuscular blockers, bradycardia and asystole have occurred after use of propofol with atracurium or suxamethonium (but see under Adverse Effects, above for the effects of propofol itself on the cardiovascular system).

See also Interactions of General Anaesthetics, p.1295.

**Benzodiazepines.** Propofol and *midazolam* have been reported to act synergistically.[1-3]


1. Short TG, Chui PT. Propofol and midazolam act synergistically in combination. *Br J Anaesth* 1991; **67:** 539–45.
2. McClune S, *et al.* Synergistic interaction between midazolam and propofol. *Br J Anaesth* 1992; **69:** 240–5.
3. Teh J, *et al.* Pharmacokinetic interactions between midazolam and propofol: an infusion study. *Br J Anaesth* 1994; **72:** 62–5.


**Clonidine.** Premedication with clonidine has been reported[1] to reduce intraoperative requirements of propofol.


1. Guglielminotti J, *et al.* Effects of premedication on dose requirements for propofol: comparison of clonidine and hydroxyzine. *Br J Anaesth* 1998; **80:** 733–6.


**Gastrointestinal drugs.** The dose of propofol required for induction is reduced in patients given *metoclopramide*.[1]


1. Page VJ, Chhipa JH. Metoclopramide reduces the induction dose of propofol. *Acta Anaesthesiol Scand* 1997; **41:** 256–9.


**General anaesthetics.** Concomitant administration of *halothane* or *isoflurane* has been reported to increase serum concentrations of propofol.[1] Synergy has been reported between propofol and *etomidate*.[2]


1. Grundmann U, *et al.* Propofol and volatile anaesthetics. *Br J Anaesth* 1994; **72** (suppl 1): 88.
2. Drummond GB, Cairns DT. Do propofol and etomidate interact kinetically during induction of anaesthesia? *Br J Anaesth* 1994; **73:** 272P.


**Local anaesthetics.** A reduction in the amount of propofol required to provide adequate hypnosis[1] or sedation[2] has been reported after the administration of *bupivacaine*[1] or *lidocaine*.[1,2]


1. Ben-Shlomo I, *et al.* Hypnotic effect of iv propofol is enhanced by im administration of either lignocaine or bupivacaine. *Br J Anaesth* 1997; **78:** 375–7.
2. Mallick A, *et al.* Local anaesthesia to the airway reduces sedation requirements in patients undergoing artificial ventilation. *Br J Anaesth* 1996; **77:** 731–4.


**Opioids.** In a study mean blood concentrations of propofol were higher in patients pretreated with *fentanyl* compared with patients maintained only on nitrous oxide.[1] However, others[2] were unable to confirm this interaction.

1. Cockshott ID, *et al.* Pharmacokinetics of propofol in female patients. *Br J Anaesth* 1987; **59:** 1103–10.
2. Dixon J, *et al.* Study of the possible interaction between fentanyl and propofol using a computer-controlled infusion of propofol. *Br J Anaesth* 1990; **64:** 142–7.

## Pharmacokinetics

The pharmacokinetics of propofol are best described by a 3-compartment model. After a single bolus dose, two distribution phases are seen. The first phase has a half-life of 2 to 4 minutes. This is followed by a slow distribution phase with a half-life of 30 to 60 minutes. Significant metabolism of propofol occurs during the second phase. The termination of anaesthetic effect after a single intravenous bolus or maintenance infusion is due to extensive redistribution from the brain to other tissues and to metabolic clearance. Propofol is over 95% bound to plasma proteins. It undergoes extensive hepatic metabolism to conjugates which are eliminated in the urine. The terminal half-life ranges from 3 to 12 hours; with prolonged use, the terminal half-life may be longer. The pharmacokinetics of propofol do not appear to be altered by gender, chronic hepatic cirrhosis, or chronic renal impairment. Propofol crosses the placental barrier and is distributed into breast milk.

◊ References.

1. Saint-Maurice C, *et al.* Pharmacokinetics of propofol in young children after a single dose. *Br J Anaesth* 1989; **63:** 667–70.
2. Kanto J, Gepts E. Pharmacokinetic implications for the clinical use of propofol. *Clin Pharmacokinet* 1989; **17:** 308–26.
3. Gin T, *et al.* Pharmacokinetics of propofol in women undergoing elective caesarean section. *Br J Anaesth* 1990; **64:** 148–53.
4. Servin F, *et al.* Pharmacokinetics of propofol infusions in patients with cirrhosis. *Br J Anaesth* 1990; **65:** 177–83.
5. Jones RDM, *et al.* Pharmacokinetics of propofol in children. *Br J Anaesth* 1990; **65:** 661–7.
6. Morgan DJ, *et al.* Pharmacokinetics of propofol when given by intravenous infusion. *Br J Clin Pharmacol* 1990; **30:** 144–8.
7. Gin T, *et al.* Disposition of propofol at caesarean section and in the postpartum period. *Br J Anaesth* 1991; **67:** 49–53.
8. Bailie GR, *et al.* Pharmacokinetics of propofol during and after long term continuous infusion for maintenance of sedation in ICU patients. *Br J Anaesth* 1992; **68:** 486–91.
9. Altmayer P, *et al.* Propofol binding in human blood. *Br J Anaesth* 1994; **72** (suppl 1): 86.
10. Oei-Lim VLB, *et al.* Pharmacokinetics of propofol during conscious sedation using target-controlled infusion in anxious patients undergoing dental treatment. *Br J Anaesth* 1998; **80:** 324–31.

## Uses and Administration

Propofol is a short-acting anaesthetic given intravenously for the induction and maintenance of general anaesthesia (p.1296). It is also used for sedation (p.666) in adult patients undergoing diagnostic procedures, in those undergoing surgery in conjunction with local or regional anaesthesia, and in ventilated adult patients under intensive care. When used for anaesthesia, induction is rapid, as is recovery. Propofol has no analgesic activity and supplementary analgesia may be required.

Propofol is available as a 1 or 2% emulsion. The 1% emulsion may be given by intravenous injection or infusion, but the 2% emulsion is for infusion only. Infusions and injections should be prepared using aseptic techniques, see under Administration, below.

Induction of **anaesthesia** is generally carried out by giving propofol by injection or infusion at a rate of 40 mg every 10 seconds; a rate of 20 mg every 10 seconds may be used in high-risk patients including elderly, neurosurgical, and debilitated patients. Most *adults* under 55 years of age can be anaesthetised by a dose of 1.5 to 2.5 mg/kg; high-risk patients usually require a dose of 1 to 1.5 mg/kg.

When used for maintenance propofol is infused at a rate of between 4 to 12 mg/kg per hour (or 3 to 6 mg/kg per hour for elderly and debilitated patients); alternatively intermittent bolus injections of 20 to 50 mg may be given; rapid administration of bolus doses should be avoided in high-risk patients.

A novel delivery system is also available for the induction and maintenance of anaesthesia in adults. The Diprifusor target-controlled infusion system allows the speed of induction and depth of anaesthesia to be controlled by specifying target blood concentrations of propofol. Initial target concentrations for induction range from 4 to 8 micrograms/mL for patients under 55 years of age; lower initial target concentrations should be used in older and debilitated patients and should be increased gradually thereafter in steps of 0.5 to 1 microgram/mL at intervals of 1 minute to achieve a gradual induction of anaesthesia. Target concentrations for maintenance are 3 to 6 micrograms/mL.

In the UK, *children* aged 1 month and over may be given propofol for the induction and maintenance of anaesthesia. The dose should be adjusted for weight and age and administered slowly until the onset of anaesthesia. Most children over 8 years require an induction dose of 2.5 mg/kg; younger children may require a higher dose within the range of 2.5 to 4 mg/kg. Doses of 9 to 15 mg/kg per hour by intravenous infusion or intermittent bolus injections are suitable for maintenance. The 2% emulsion formulation of propofol should only be used in children over 3 years. In the USA, children aged 3 years and over may be given propofol for the induction of anaesthesia; those aged 2 months and over may also receive propofol for maintenance of anaesthesia. Doses are similar to those used in the UK.

For **sedation** in diagnostic and surgical procedures in *adults* an initial infusion of 6 to 9 mg/kg per hour may be given for 3 to 5 minutes; alternatively 0.5 to 1 mg/kg may be injected slowly over 1 to 5 minutes. An infusion of 1.5 to 4.5 mg/kg per hour may be used for maintenance of sedation. High-risk patients usually require a 20% reduction in the maintenance dose.

For the sedation of ventilated adults propofol can be given by intravenous infusion in a dose of 0.3 to 4 mg/kg per hour. If the duration of sedation is in excess of 3 days, lipid concentrations should be monitored.

Propofol is contra-indicated for sedation in *children* aged 16 years or less.

◊ Reviews.

1. Langley MS, Heel RC. Propofol: a review of its pharmacodynamic and pharmacokinetic properties and use as an intravenous anaesthetic. *Drugs* 1988; **35:** 334–72.
2. Larijani GE, *et al.* Clinical pharmacology of propofol: an intravenous anesthetic agent. *DICP Ann Pharmacother* 1989; **23:** 743–9.
3. Bryson HM, *et al.* Propofol: an update of its use in anaesthesia and conscious sedation. *Drugs* 1995; **50:** 513–59.
4. Fulton B, Sorkin EM. Propofol: an overview of its pharmacology and a review of its clinical efficacy in intensive care sedation. *Drugs* 1995; **50:** 636–57.

**Administration.** Propofol is formulated as an oil in water emulsion for injection. Strict aseptic techniques must be maintained when handling propofol as, in some countries including the UK, the parenteral product contains no antimicrobial preservatives and the vehicle can support rapid growth of microorganisms. Aseptic techniques must also be applied to formulations, such as those available in the USA, that contain the microbial-retarding agent disodium edetate as microbial growth is still possible. An emulsion containing 1% of propofol may be diluted with glucose 5% immediately before administration but it should not be diluted to a concentration of less than 2 mg/mL. An emulsion containing 2 % of propofol should not be diluted. The use of a 5-micron filter needle to withdraw propofol emulsion from an ampoule does not cause significant loss of drug.[1] A reduction in concentration of propofol can occur when the diluted emulsion is run through polyvinyl chloride intravenous tubing.[1] Propofol 1 or 2% may be administered into a running intravenous infusion through a Y-site close to the injection site and under these circumstances it is compatible with glucose 5%, sodium chloride 0.9%, and glucose with sodium chloride intravenous solutions.

1. Bailey LC, *et al.* Effect of syringe filter and I.V. administration set on delivery of propofol emulsion. *Am J Hosp Pharm* 1991; **48:** 2627–30.

**Nausea and vomiting.** It is commonly believed that propofol is associated with less postoperative nausea and vomiting than some other anaesthetics.[1,2] However, a review[3] concluded that any reduction in nausea and vomiting when using propofol anaesthesia may be short term and clinically relevant only for maintenance anaesthesia in procedures with an inherent risk of nausea and vomiting.

There are also reports[4-8] indicating that propofol may have some intrinsic antiemetic action when used in sub-hypnotic doses although a study[9] of the effect of sedative and non-sedative (sub-hypnotic) doses against apomorphine-induced vomiting has suggested that any antiemetic effect is probably due to sedation.

1. McCollum JSC, *et al.* The antiemetic action of propofol. *Anaesthesia* 1988; **43:** 239–40.
2. Woodward WM, *et al.* Comparison of post-operative nausea and vomiting after thiopentone/isoflurane or propofol infusion for 'bat-ear' correction in children. *Br J Anaesth* 1994; **72** (suppl 1): 92.
3. Tramèr M, *et al.* Propofol anaesthesia and postoperative nausea and vomiting: quantitative systematic review of randomized controlled studies. *Br J Anaesth* 1997: **78:** 247–55.
4. Borgeat A, *et al.* Adjuvant propofol for refractory cisplatin-associated nausea and vomiting. *Lancet* 1992; **340:** 679–80.
5. Törn K, *et al.* Effects of sub-hypnotic doses of propofol on the side effects of intrathecal morphine. *Br J Anaesth* 1994; **73:** 411–12.
6. Borgeat A, *et al.* Adjuvant propofol enables better control of nausea and emesis secondary to chemotherapy for breast cancer. *Can J Anaesth* 1994; **41:** 1117–19.
7. Ewalenko P, *et al.* Antiemetic effect of subhypnotic doses of propofol after thyroidectomy. *Br J Anaesth* 1996; **77:** 463–7.
8. Gan TJ, *et al.* Determination of plasma concentrations of propofol associated with 50% reduction in postoperative nausea. *Anesthesiology* 1997; **87:**779–84.
9. Thörn S-E, *et al.* Propofol effects upon apomorphine induced vomiting. *Br J Anaesth* 1994; **72** (suppl 1): 90.

**Pruritus.** Propofol is one of many drugs that have been tried in the management of pruritus (p.1137). Sub-hypnotic doses of propofol appear to have an antipruritic action. It has produced conflicting results in the treatment and prophylaxis of pruritus associated with epidural and intrathecal morphine[1-4] although it appears to be able to relieve cholestasis-associated pruritus.[5] It has been suggested that propofol might act by suppression of the spinal transmission of pruritic signals.

1. Borgeat A, *et al.* Subhypnotic doses of propofol relieve pruritus induced by epidural and intrathecal morphine. *Anesthesiology* 1992; **76:** 510–12.
2. Törn K, *et al.* Effects of sub-hypnotic doses of propofol on the side effects of intrathecal morphine. *Br J Anaesth* 1994; **73:** 411–12.
3. Warwick JP, *et al.* The effect of subhypnotic doses of propofol on the incidence of pruritus after intrathecal morphine for caesarean section. *Anaesthesia* 1997; **52:** 270–5.
4. Beilin Y, *et al.* Subhypnotic doses of propofol do not relieve pruritus induced by intrathecal morphine after cesarean section. *Anesth Analg* 1998; **86:** 310–3.
5. Borgeat A, *et al.* Subhypnotic doses of propofol relieve pruritus associated with liver disease. *Gastroenterology* 1993; **104:** 244–7.

**Status epilepticus.** Anaesthesia in conjunction with assisted ventilation may be instituted to control refractory tonic-clonic status epilepticus (p.352). A short-acting barbiturate such as thiopental is usually used. Propofol is also used[1,2] although good controlled studies of its effectiveness are lacking, and it has caused seizures when used in anaesthesia (see under Precautions, above) and should be given with caution to patients with epilepsy. It has a rapid onset of action and its effects are maintained while the infusion is maintained; recovery is rapid on discontinuation. However, the risks of respiratory and cerebral depression, as well as of lipid overload with prolonged therapy, should be borne in mind. It may induce involuntary movements and care is required to distinguish these from seizures. A suggested regimen for management[2] is an initial intravenous bolus of 1 to 2 mg/kg followed by an infusion of 2 to 10 mg/kg per hour guided by EEG monitoring. The dose should be gradually reduced and the infusion tapered 12 hours after seizure activity is halted. Lower doses should be used in the elderly. A study[3] comparing propofol with high-dose barbiturates in patients with refractory status epilepticus concluded that recurrent seizures were common when propofol infusions were suddenly discontinued but not when the infusions were gradually tapered.

1. Brown LA, Levin GM. Role of propofol in refractory status epilepticus. *Ann Pharmacother* 1998; **32:** 1053–9.
2. Lowenstein DH, Alldredge BK. Status epilepticus. *N Engl J Med* 1998; **338:** 970–6.
3. Stecker MM, *et al.* Treatment of refractory status epilepticus with propofol: clinical and pharmacokinetic findings. *Epilepsia* 1998; **39:** 18–26.

**Tetanus.** Sedation with propofol has been used in the treatment of tetanus (p.1398) to control spasms and rigidity.

## Preparations

**Proprietary Preparations** (details are given in Part 3)
***Arg.:*** Diprivan; Oleo-Lax; Recofol; ***Austral.:*** Diprivan; Recofol; ***Austria:*** Diprivan; ***Belg.:*** Diprivan; ***Braz.:*** Bioprofol; Diprivan; Profolen; Pronest; Propoabbott; Propovan; Provive; ***Canad.:*** Diprivan; ***Chile:*** Diprivan; ***Denm.:*** Diprivan; Recofol†; ***Fin.:*** Diprivan; Recofol; ***Fr.:*** Diprivan; ***Ger.:*** Disoprivan; Klimofol†; ***Gr.:*** Diprivan; ***Hong Kong:*** Diprivan; ***Irl.:*** Diprivan; ***Israel:*** Diprivan; Diprofol; Recofol; ***Ital.:*** Diprivan; ***Malaysia:*** Diprivan; ***Mex.:*** Cryotol; Diprivan; Fresofol; Propocam; Recofol; ***Neth.:*** Diprivan; ***Norw.:*** Diprivan; Recofol; ***NZ:*** Diprivan; Recofol; ***Port.:*** Diprivan; Recofol; ***S.Afr.:*** Diprivan; ***Singapore:*** Diprivan; Pofol; Recofol; ***Spain:*** Diprivan; Ivofol; Recofol; ***Swed.:*** Diprivan; Recofol; ***Switz.:*** Ansiven; Disoprivan; Recofol; ***Thai.:*** Diprivan; Pofol; Recofol; ***UK:*** Diprivan; ***USA:*** Diprivan.

# Sevoflurane *(BAN, USAN, rINN)*

BAX-3084; MR-654; Sevoflurano. Fluoromethyl 2,2,2-trifluoro-1-(trifluoromethyl)ethyl ether; 1,1,1,3,3,3-Hexafluoro-2-(fluoromethoxy)-propane.

$C_4H_3F_7O$ = 200.1.

*CAS — 28523-86-6.*

*ATC — N01AB08.*

## Adverse Effects

As with other halogenated anaesthetics sevoflurane may cause cardiorespiratory depression, hypotension, and malignant hyperthermia. However, the effects of sevoflurane on heart rate have only been seen at higher concentrations and it appears to have little effect on heart rhythm in comparison to other halogenated anaesthetics. Sevoflurane appears to sensitise the myocardium to sympathomimetics to a lesser extent than halothane or enflurane. Other effects seen with sevoflurane include agitation, especially in children, laryngospasm, and increased cough and salivation. Acute renal failure has also been noted. Shivering, nausea, and vomiting have been reported in the postoperative period.

See also Adverse Effects of General Anaesthetics, p.1295.

**Effects on the cardiovascular system.** The cardiovascular effects of sevoflurane are similar to those of isoflurane (see p.1301) but it does not produce coronary steal. Also sevoflurane produces less tachycardia than isoflurane suggesting that it may be preferable in those predisposed to myocardial ischaemia.

**Effects on the kidneys.** Investigations[1] of the nephrotoxic potential of sevoflurane have found no evidence of renal function impairment despite peak plasma-fluoride ion concentrations greater than 50 nanomol/mL (a level considered to be nephrotoxic) being recorded in some patients at the end of sevoflurane anaesthesia,[2] and clinical experience would tend to support this.[3] The lack of renal toxicity with sevoflurane may be due to low concentrations of intrarenally generated fluoride ions;[4] in comparison, methoxyflurane defluorination in the kidney is much greater and may contribute to its known nephrotoxicity.

Compound A, formed by the breakdown of sevoflurane by carbon dioxide absorbents (see under Precautions, below), is nephrotoxic in *rats*.[1] However, studies in humans undergoing sevoflurane anaesthesia have detected no renal impairment postoperatively even when compound A was detected in the anaesthetic circuits.


1. Malan TP. Sevoflurane and renal function. *Anesth Analg* 1995; **81:** S39–S45.
2. Kobayashi Y, *et al.* Serum and urinary inorganic fluoride concentrations after prolonged inhalation of sevoflurane in humans. *Anesth Analg* 1992; **74:** 753–7.
3. Gentz BA, Malan TP. Renal toxicity with sevoflurane: a storm in a teacup? *Drugs* 2001; **61:** 2155–62.
4. Kharasch ED, *et al.* Human kidney methoxyflurane and sevoflurane metabolism: intrarenal fluoride production as a possible mechanism of methoxyflurane nephrotoxicity. *Anesthesiology* 1995; **82:** 689–99.


**Effects on the liver.** There have been signs of hepatotoxicity in *animal* studies but in studies in humans, markers for hepatocellular dysfunction were no greater following sevoflurane anaesthesia than those after isoflurane.[1] Also the metabolism of sevoflurane differs from other halogenated anaesthetics in such a way that metabolites implicated in liver toxicity are not formed (see Pharmacokinetics, below).


1. Darling JR, *et al.* Comparison of the effects of sevoflurane with those of isoflurane on hepatic glutathione-S-transferase concentrations after body surface surgery. *Br J Anaesth* 1994; **73:** 268P.


**Effects on the nervous system.** Clonic and tonic seizure-like movements of the extremities have been reported[1] in a child during induction of anaesthesia using sevoflurane. It was considered that this might have been a result of seizure activity in the CNS or due to myoclonus of the extremities.


1. Adachi M, *et al.* Seizure-like movements during induction of anaesthesia with sevoflurane. *Br J Anaesth* 1992; **68:** 214–15.


## Precautions

As with other halogenated anaesthetics, patients with known or suspected susceptibility to malignant hyperthermia should not be anaesthetised with sevoflurane. Although the effects of sevoflurane on cerebral pressure is minimal in normal patients, safety in those with raised intracranial pressure has not been established and therefore sevoflurane should be used with caution. As emergence and recovery are particularly rapid with sevoflurane patients may require early postoperative pain relief.

See also Precautions for General Anaesthetics, p.1295.

**Carbon dioxide absorbents.** The breakdown of sevoflurane by carbon dioxide absorbents (such as soda lime) results in the formation of pentafluoroisopropenyl fluoromethyl ether (PIFE; compound A), and trace amounts of pentafluoromethoxy isopropyl fluoromethyl ether (PMFE; Compound B). Compound A has been shown to be nephrotoxic in *rats* (see under Effects on the Kidneys, above). Even during short exposure times, as required for induction of anaesthesia, use of moist soda lime is important to minimise sevoflurane degradation, which is aggravated by a high potassium hydroxide content of the soda lime.[1]

The manufacturers state that increased amounts of compound A may be formed if barium hydroxide lime is used as a carbon dioxide absorbent rather than soda lime.

The use of desiccated carbon dioxide absorbents with sevoflurane has also been associated with rare cases of extreme heat and smoke or fire developing in the anaesthetic apparatus.[2]


1. Funk W, *et al.* Dry soda lime markedly degrades sevoflurane during simulated inhalation induction. *Br J Anaesth* 1999; **82:** 193–8.
2. Abbott Laboratories, Canada. Important safety information regarding the use of Sevorane AF (sevoflurane) in conjunction with anesthesia machines. Available at: http://www.hc-sc.gc.ca/hpfb-dgpsa/tpd-dpt/sevorane_hpc_e.pdf (accessed 26/05/04)


## Interactions

Care is advised if adrenaline or other sympathomimetics are given during sevoflurane anaesthesia. The effects of competitive neuromuscular blockers such as atracurium are enhanced by sevoflurane (see p.1401). The metabolism, and hence toxicity, of sevoflurane may be increased by drugs or compounds that induce cytochrome P450 isoenzyme CYP2E1 including isoniazid and alcohol.

See also Interactions of General Anaesthetics, p.1295.

◊ References.


1. Dale O. Drug interactions in anaesthesia: focus on desflurane and sevoflurane. *Baillieres Clin Anaesthesiol* 1995; **9:** 105–17.


## Pharmacokinetics

Sevoflurane is absorbed on inhalation. The blood/gas partition coefficient is low. Up to 5% of the absorbed dose of sevoflurane is metabolised in the liver by the cytochrome P450 isoenzyme CYP2E1 and defluorinated to its major metabolites hexafluoroisopropanol (HFIP), inorganic fluoride, and carbon dioxide. HFIP is rapidly conjugated with glucuronic acid and eliminated in the urine. Sevoflurane crosses the placenta.

◊ References.


1. Behne M, *et al.* Clinical pharmacokinetics of sevoflurane. *Clin Pharmacokinet* 1999; **36:** 13–26.


## Uses and Administration

Sevoflurane is a volatile halogenated anaesthetic administered by inhalation. It has a minimum alveolar concentration (MAC) value (see Uses of General Anaesthetics, p.1295) ranging from 1.4% in the elderly to 3.3% in neonates. It is employed for the induction and maintenance of general anaesthesia (p.1296). It is non-flammable. Sevoflurane has a nonpungent odour and does not cause respiratory irritation. It also has muscle relaxant properties which may be sufficient for some surgical procedures to be performed without a neuromuscular blocker. However, it possesses no analgesic properties.

Sevoflurane is administered using a calibrated vaporiser. For induction, sevoflurane is given in concentrations of up to 5% v/v in adults, with oxygen or a mixture of oxygen and nitrous oxide. Concentrations of up to 7% v/v may be used in children. A short-acting barbiturate or other intravenous induction agent may be given before inhaling sevoflurane. Induction with sevoflurane is rapid (surgical anaesthesia in less than 2 minutes) and smooth because of its nonpungent odour. Maintenance of anaesthesia is achieved with a concentration of 0.5 to 3% v/v with or without nitrous oxide.

◊ Reviews.


1. Patel SS, Goa KL. Sevoflurane: a review of its pharmacodynamic and pharmacokinetic properties and its clinical use in general anaesthesia. *Drugs* 1996; **51:** 658–700.
2. Smith I, *et al.* Sevoflurane—a long-awaited volatile anaesthetic. *Br J Anaesth* 1996; **76:** 435–45.
3. Grounds RM, Newman PJ. Sevoflurane. *Br J Hosp Med* 1997; **57:** 43–6.
4. Goa KL, *et al.* Sevoflurane in paediatric anaesthesia: a review. *Paediatr Drugs* 1999; **1:** 127–53.
5. Ghatge S, *et al.* Sevoflurane: an ideal agent for adult day-case anesthesia? *Acta Anaesthesiol Scand* 2003; **47:** 917–31.


## Preparations

**Proprietary Preparations** (details are given in Part 3)

***Arg.:*** Sevorane; ***Austral.:*** Sevorane; ***Austria:*** Sevorane; ***Belg.:*** Sevorane; ***Braz.:*** Sevocris; Sevorane; ***Canad.:*** Sevorane; ***Denm.:*** Sevorane; ***Fin.:*** Sevorane; ***Fr.:*** Sevorane; ***Ger.:*** Sevorane; ***Gr.:*** Sevorane; ***Hong Kong:*** Sevorane; ***Irl.:*** Sevorane; ***Israel:*** Sevorane; ***Ital.:*** Sevorane; ***Malaysia:*** Sevorane; ***Mex.:*** Sevorane; ***Neth.:*** Sevorane; ***Norw.:*** Sevorane; ***NZ:*** Sevorane; ***S.Afr.:*** Ultane; ***Singapore:*** Sevorane; ***Spain:*** Sevorane; ***Swed.:*** Sevorane; ***Switz.:*** Sevorane; ***Thai.:*** Sevorane; ***USA:*** Ultane.

## Sodium Oxybate *(USAN)*

NSC-84223; Oxibato sódico; Sodium Gamma-hydroxybutyrate; Wy-3478. Sodium 4-hydroxybutyrate.

$C_4H_7NaO_3$ = 126.1.

*CAS — 502-85-2.*

**Pharmacopoeias.** In *Chin.*

## Adverse Effects

When used in general anaesthesia side-effects with sodium oxybate include abnormal muscle movements during the induction period and nausea and vomiting. Occasional emergence delirium has been reported. Bradycardia frequently occurs. Respiration may be slowed and hypokalaemia has been reported.

Patients receiving sodium oxybate orally for the management of narcolepsy may experience dizziness, lightheadedness, and confusion; gastrointestinal effects and enuresis occur occasionally.

See also Adverse Effects of General Anaesthetics, p.1295.

**Effects on electrolyte balance.** A report of severe metabolic disorders occurring during therapy with sodium oxybate and tetracosactide in 4 patients with severe head injuries.[1] The disorders consisted of hypernatraemia, hypokalaemia, and metabolic acidosis.


1. Béal JL, *et al.* Troubles métaboliques induits par l'association gamma-hydroxy butyrate de sodium et tétracosactide chez le traumatisé crânien. *Therapie* 1983; **38:** 569–71.


## Precautions

Sodium oxybate should not be given to patients with severe hypertension, bradycardia, conditions associated with defects of cardiac conduction, epilepsy, eclampsia, renal impairment, or alcohol abuse.

See also Precautions for General Anaesthetics, p.1295.

**Abuse.** Reports[1] of acute poisoning with sodium oxybate following illicit use led the FDA in the USA to issue warnings[2] about its potential for abuse. It is usually supplied illicitly as the sodium salt under a variety of names including GHB or GBH, gamma-hydroxybutyrate, liquid ecstasy, liquid X, sodium oxybutyrate, and somatomax PM and has been promoted for body building, weight loss, as a psychedelic substance, and as a sleep aid. Adverse effects include vomiting, drowsiness, amnesia, hypotonia, vertigo, respiratory depression, and involuntary movements. Seizure-like activity, bradycardia, hypotension, and respiratory arrest have also been reported. Resolution of symptoms occurs spontaneously over 2 to 96 hours. However, some patients have required hospitalisation and respiratory support and deaths have been reported in both the UK[3] and USA.[4] Severity of symptoms depends on the dose of sodium oxybate and the presence of other drugs such as alcohol, benzodiazepines, cannabis, or amfetamines. Prolonged use of large doses may lead to a withdrawal syndrome on discontinuation.[5,6]

There is also a report of CNS depression following ingestion of a chemical derivative, gamma-butyrolactone (GBL).[7] Another derivative, 1,4-butanediol is abused similarly.[6]


1. Centers for Disease Control. Multistate outbreak of poisonings associated with illicit use of gamma hydroxy butyrate. *JAMA* 1991; **265:** 447–8.
2. Food and Drug Administration. Warning about GHB. *JAMA* 1991; **265:** 1802.
3. Anonymous. GBH death indicates increasing problem. *Pharm J* 1996; **256:** 441.
4. Centers for Disease Control. Gamma hydroxy butyrate use—New York and Texas, 1995–1996. *JAMA* 1997; **277:** 1511.
5. Galloway GP, *et al.* Physical dependence on sodium oxybate. *Lancet* 1994; **343:** 57.
6. Rodgers J, *et al.* Liquid ecstasy: a new kid on the dance floor. *Br J Psychiatry* 2004; **184:** 104–6.
7. LoVecchio F, *et al.* Butyrolactone-induced central nervous system depression after ingestion of RenewTrient, a "dietary supplement" *N Engl J Med* 1998; **339:** 847–8.


**Porphyria.** Sodium oxybate is considered to be unsafe in patients with porphyria because it has been shown to be porphyrinogenic in *animals* or *in-vitro* systems.

## Interactions

Sodium oxybate enhances the effects of opioid analgesics and competitive neuromuscular blockers. The action of sodium oxybate may be potentiated by benzodiazepines or antipsychotics.

See also Interactions of General Anaesthetics, p.1295.

## Pharmacokinetics

Following oral administration sodium oxybate is absorbed from the gastrointestinal tract and rapidly metabolised in the liver to carbon dioxide and water. In one study the mean values for the terminal half-life ranged from 20 to 23 minutes. It crosses the blood-brain barrier and the placental barrier.

◊ References.


1. Palatini P, *et al.* Dose-dependent absorption and elimination of gamma-hydroxybutyric acid in healthy volunteers. *Eur J Clin Pharmacol* 1993; **45:** 353–6.
2. Scharf MB, *et al.* Pharmacokinetics of gammahydroxybutyrate (GHB) in narcoleptic patients. *Sleep* 1998; **21:** 507–14.


## Uses and Administration

Sodium oxybate has hypnotic properties and, in its endogenous form, gamma-hydroxybutyrate (a catabolite of gamma-aminobutyric acid), increases dopamine concentrations in the brain. It is given intravenously usually with an opioid analgesic and a neuroleptic to produce general anaesthesia (p.1296). Skeletal muscle relaxants may also be necessary. Sodium oxybate given orally is used in the treatment of cataplexy in patients with narcolepsy.

In general anaesthesia a solution of sodium oxybate equivalent to 20% of the acid is administered slowly by intravenous injection, usually in a dose of 60 mg/kg; further smaller doses may be required in long procedures. In children up to 100 mg/kg may be necessary.

For the treatment of cataplexy, sodium oxybate is given by mouth in initial doses of 4.5 g daily, as two equally-divided doses. The first dose should be taken at bedtime while in bed; the second dose should be taken 2.5 to 4 hours later also while sitting in bed. Both doses should be prepared before going to bed: each dose should be diluted with 60 mL of water. The initial dose may be increased in increments of 1.5 g daily (0.75 g per dose) every 2 weeks to a maximum dose of 9 g daily. Reduced doses are recommended in patients with hepatic impairment (see below).

**Administration in hepatic impairment.** The recommended initial oral dose of sodium oxybate (see above) should be halved in patients with hepatic impairment. Subsequent increases should be monitored against effect.

**Alcohol withdrawal syndrome.** Gamma-hydroxybutyric acid has been reported[1] to be effective in reducing symptoms of alcohol withdrawal (p.1166) and to be of use as an aid in the maintenance of abstinence.[2,3] However, following reports of CNS toxicity associated with abuse of gamma-hydroxybutyric acid its role in the treatment of substance abuse disorders appears questionable.[4]

1. Gallimberti L, *et al.* Gamma-hydroxybutyric acid for treatment of alcohol withdrawal syndrome. *Lancet* 1989; **ii:** 787–9.
2. Gallimberti L, *et al.* Gamma-hydroxybutyric acid in the treatment of alcohol dependence: a double blind study. *Alcohol Clin Exp Res* 1992; **16:** 673–6.
3. Addolorato G, *et al.* Maintaining abstinence from alcohol with γ-hydroxybutyric acid. *Lancet* 1998; **351:** 38.
4. Quinn DI, *et al.* Pharmacokinetic and pharmacodynamic principles of illicit drug use and treatment of illicit drug users. *Clin Pharmacokinet* 1997; **33:** 344–400.

**Narcoleptic syndrome.** Sodium oxybate[1-5] given at night is used to improve cataplexy in patients with narcoleptic syndrome (p.1583).

For a reference to the pharmacokinetics of sodium oxybate in narcoleptic patients, see above.

1. Scharf MB, *et al.* The effects and effectiveness of γ-hydroxybutyrate in patients with narcolepsy. *J Clin Psychiatry* 1985; **46:** 222–5.
2. Mamelak M, *et al.* Treatment of narcolepsy with γ-hydroxybutyrate: a review of clinical and sleep laboratory findings. *Sleep* 1986; **9:** 285–9.
3. Scrima L, *et al.* Efficacy of gamma-hydroxybutyrate versus placebo in treating narcolepsy-cataplexy: double-blind subjective measures. *Biol Psychiatry* 1989; **26:** 331–43.
4. US Xyrem Multicenter Study Group. A randomized, double blind, placebo-controlled multicenter trial comparing the effects of three doses of orally administered sodium oxybate with placebo for the treatment of narcolepsy. *Sleep* 2002; **25:** 42–9.
5. US Xyrem Multicenter Study Group. A 12-month, open-label, multicenter extension trial of orally administered sodium oxybate for the treatment of narcolepsy. *Sleep* 2003; **26:** 31–5.

### Preparations

**Proprietary Preparations** (details are given in Part 3)
***Austria:*** Alcover; ***Fr.:*** Gamma-OH; ***Ger.:*** Somsanit; ***Ital.:*** Alcover.
**Multi-ingredient:** ***USA:*** Xyrem.

## Thiamylal Sodium

Tiamilal sódico. Sodium 5-allyl-5-(1-methylbutyl)-2-thiobarbiturate.

$C_{12}H_{17}N_2NaO_2S$ = 276.3.
*CAS — 77-27-0 (thiamylal); 337-47-3 (thiamylal sodium).*

**Pharmacopoeias.** In *Jpn.*

### Profile

Thiamylal sodium is a short-acting intravenous barbiturate anaesthetic. It is possibly slightly more potent than thiopental sodium (p.1310) and has similar actions and uses. It has been used for the production of complete anaesthesia of short duration, for the induction of general anaesthesia, or for inducing a hypnotic state.

# Thiopental Sodium *(BANM, rINN)*

Natrium Isopentylaethylthiobarbituricum (cum Natrio Carbonico); Penthiobarbital Sodique; Soluble Thiopentone; Thiomebumalnatrium cum Natrii Carbonate; Thiopental Sodium and Sodium Carbonate; Thiopentalum Natricum; Thiopentalum Natricum et Natrii Carbonas; Thiopentobarbitalum Solubile; Thiopentone Sodium; Tiopental sódico. Sodium 5-ethyl-5-(1-methylbutyl)-2-thiobarbiturate.

$C_{11}H_{17}N_2NaO_2S$ = 264.3.
*CAS — 76-75-5 (thiopental); 71-73-8 (thiopental sodium).*
*ATC — N01AF03; N05CA19.*

NOTE. The name thiobarbital has been applied to thiopental and has also been used to describe a barbiturate of different composition.

**Pharmacopoeias.** In *Chin., Eur.* (see p.vi), *Int., Jpn, US,* and *Viet.* Some include thiopental sodium with, some without, anhydrous sodium carbonate; some only include a sterile mixture for injection.

**Ph. Eur. 5.0** (Thiopental Sodium and Sodium Carbonate; Thiopental Sodium BP 2003). A yellowish-white hygroscopic powder. It contains 84 to 87% thiopental and 10.2 to 11.2% sodium. Freely soluble in water; partly soluble in dehydrated alcohol. Store in airtight containers. Protect from light.

**USP 27** (Thiopental Sodium). A white to off-white crystalline powder, or yellowish-white to pale greenish-yellow hygroscopic powder. May have a disagreeable odour. Its solutions are alkaline to litmus, decompose on standing, and on boiling, precipitation occurs. Soluble in water and in alcohol; insoluble in ether, in petroleum spirit, and in benzene. Store in airtight containers.

**Incompatibility.** Solutions of thiopental sodium are incompatible with acidic and oxidising substances including some antibacterials, neuromuscular blockers and analgesics. Compounds commonly listed as incompatible include amikacin sulfate, benzylpenicillin salts, cefapirin sodium, codeine phosphate, ephedrine sulfate, fentanyl citrate, glycopyrronium bromide, morphine sulfate, pentazocine lactate, prochlorperazine edisilate, suxamethonium salts, and tubocurarine chloride. Solutions decompose on standing and precipitation occurs on boiling.

Loss of thiopental in PVC and cellulose propionate delivery systems has been reported,[1,2] but in another study,[3] no loss of potency was noted.

1. Kowaluk EA, *et al.* Interactions between drugs and polyvinyl chloride infusion bags. *Am J Hosp Pharm* 1981; **38:** 1308–14.
2. Kowaluk EA, *et al.* Interactions between drugs and intravenous delivery systems. *Am J Hosp Pharm* 1982; **39:** 460–7.
3. Martens HJ, *et al.* Sorption of various drugs in polyvinyl chloride, glass, and polyethylene-lined infusion containers. *Am J Hosp Pharm* 1990; **47:** 369–73.

## Adverse Effects and Treatment

As for Phenobarbital, p.368.

Excitatory phenomena such as coughing, hiccuping, sneezing, and muscle twitching or jerking may occur with any of the barbiturate anaesthetics, particularly during induction, but they occur more frequently with methohexital than with thiopental. Cough, sneezing, and laryngeal spasm or bronchospasm may also occur during induction. The intravenous injection of concentrated solutions of thiopental sodium such as 5% may result in thrombophlebitis. Extravasation of barbiturate anaesthetics may cause tissue necrosis. Intra-arterial injection causes severe arterial spasm with burning pain and may cause prolonged blanching of the forearm and hand and gangrene of digits. Hypersensitivity reactions have been reported. Barbiturate anaesthetics can cause respiratory depression. They depress cardiac output and often cause an initial fall in blood pressure, and overdosage may result in circulatory failure. Arrhythmias may occur. Postoperative vomiting is infrequent but shivering may occur and there may be persistent drowsiness, confusion, and amnesia. Headache has also been reported.

See also under Adverse Effects of General Anaesthetics, p.1295.

**Hypersensitivity.** Anaphylactic reactions to thiopental have been reported[1,2] although such reactions are rare. There has also been a report of haemolytic anaemia and renal failure in association with the development of an anti-thiopental antibody in a patient who had undergone general anaesthesia induced by thiopental.[3]

1. Westacott P, *et al.* Anaphylactic reaction to thiopentone: a case report. *Can Anaesth Soc J* 1984; **31:** 434–8.
2. Moneret-Vautrin DA, *et al.* Simultaneous anaphylaxis to thiopentone and a neuromuscular blocker: a study of two cases. *Br J Anaesth* 1990; **64:** 743–5.
3. Habibi B, *et al.* Thiopental-related immune hemolytic anemia and renal failure: specific involvement of red-cell antigen I. *N Engl J Med* 1985; **312:** 353–5. Correction. *ibid.*; 1136.

**Intra-arterial injection.** Accidental intra-arterial injection of thiopental sodium produces severe arterial spasm with intense burning pain. Anaesthesia, paresis, paralysis, and gangrene may occur. Therapy has concentrated on dilution of injected thiopental, prevention and treatment of arterial spasm, prophylaxis of thrombosis, thrombectomy and other measures to sustain good blood flow. There has been a report[1] of the successful use of urokinase intra-arterially in the management of one patient accidentally given thiopental intra-arterially.

1. Vangerven M, *et al.* A new therapeutic approach to accidental intra-arterial injection of thiopentone. *Br J Anaesth* 1989; **62:** 98–100.

## Precautions

Barbiturate anaesthetics are contra-indicated when there is dyspnoea or respiratory obstruction such as in acute severe asthma or when maintenance of an airway cannot be guaranteed.

Barbiturate anaesthetics should be used with caution in shock and dehydration, hypovolaemia, severe anaemia, hyperkalaemia, toxaemia, myasthenia gravis, myxoedema and other metabolic disorders, or in severe renal disease. Caution is also required in patients with cardiovascular disease, muscular dystrophies, adrenocortical insufficiency, or with increased intracranial pressure. Reduced doses are required in the elderly and in severe hepatic disease.

See also Precautions for General Anaesthetics, p.1295.

**Breast feeding.** No adverse effects have been observed in breast-fed infants whose mothers received thiopental, and the American Academy of Pediatrics[1] considers that it is therefore usually compatible with breast feeding.

In two groups of 8 women undergoing induction with thiopental, the milk-to-plasma ratio was less than 1 in both groups and it was considered that the effects of thiopental on breast-fed infants would be negligible.[2]

1. American Academy of Pediatrics. The transfer of drugs and other chemicals into human milk. *Pediatrics* 2001; **108:** 776–89. Correction. *ibid.*; 1029. Also available at: http://aappolicy.aappublications.org/cgi/content/full/pediatrics%3b108/3/776 (accessed 26/05/04)
2. Andersen LW, *et al.* Concentrations of thiopentone in mature breast milk and colostrum following an induction dose. *Acta Anaesthesiol Scand* 1987; **31:** 30–2.

**Porphyria.** Barbiturates including thiopental sodium have been associated with acute attacks of porphyria and are considered unsafe in porphyric patients.

## Interactions

Difficulty may be experienced in producing anaesthesia with the usual dose of barbiturate anaesthetics in patients accustomed to taking alcohol or other CNS depressants; additional anaesthetics may be necessary. Care is required when anaesthetising patients being treated with phenothiazine antipsychotics since there may be increased hypotension. Some phenothiazines, especially promethazine, may increase the incidence of excitatory phenomena produced by barbiturate anaesthetics; cyclizine may possibly have a similar effect. Opioid analgesics can potentiate the respiratory depressant effect of barbiturate anaesthetics and the dose of the anaesthetic may need to be reduced. Use with nitrous oxide greatly reduces the dose of barbiturate anaesthetics required for anaesthesia. Reduced doses of thiopental may be required in patients receiving sulfafurazole.

See also Interactions of General Anaesthetics, p.1295.

**Antidepressants.** Potentiation of barbiturate anaesthesia may be expected in patients receiving *tricyclic antidepressants* or *MAOIs* (see under Anaesthesia in Precautions for Amitriptyline, p.283 and for Phenelzine, p.313, respectively).

**Antipsychotics.** For mention of the effect of *droperidol* on thiopental see under Gastrointestinal Drugs, below.

**Aspirin.** Pretreatment with aspirin, a highly protein-bound drug, has been shown to potentiate thiopental anaesthesia.[1]

1. Dundee JW, *et al.* Aspirin and probenecid pretreatment influences the potency of thiopentone and the onset of action of midazolam. *Eur J Anaesthesiol* 1986; **3:** 247–51.

**Gastrointestinal drugs.** *Metoclopramide* profoundly reduced the dose of thiopental required to produce hypnosis in female patients; *droperidol* had a similar effect.[1]

1. Mehta D, *et al.* Metoclopramide decreases thiopental hypnotic requirement. *Anesth Analg* 1993; **77:** 784–7.

**Probenecid.** Pretreatment with probenecid, a highly protein-bound drug, has been shown to potentiate thiopental anaesthesia.[1]

1. Dundee JW, *et al.* Aspirin and probenecid pretreatment influences the potency of thiopentone and the onset of action of midazolam. *Eur J Anaesthesiol* 1986; **3:** 247–51.

## Pharmacokinetics

Thiopental is highly lipid soluble and when it is administered intravenously as the sodium salt, concentrations sufficient to produce unconsciousness are achieved in the brain within 30 seconds. Onset of action occurs within 8 to 10 minutes when thiopental sodium is given rectally but absorption may be unpredictable if a suspension rather than a solution is used. Recovery from anaesthesia is also rapid due to redistribution to other tissues, particularly fat. About 80% of thiopental may be bound to plasma proteins, although reports show a wide range of figures. Thiopental is metabolised almost entirely in the liver, but as it is only released slowly from lipid stores this occurs at a very slow rate.

It is mostly metabolised to inactive metabolites but a small amount is desulfurated to pentobarbital. Repeated or continuous administration can lead to accumulation of thiopental in fatty tissue and this can result in prolonged anaesthesia and respiratory and cardiovascular depression. Elimination of thiopental following bolus injection can be described by a triexponential curve. The terminal elimination half-life has been reported to be 10 to 12 hours in adults and about 6 hours in children. However, values of 26 to 28 hours have been reported in obese patients and pregnant patients at term. Thiopental readily diffuses across the placenta and is distributed into breast milk.

◊ References.


1. Gaspari F, *et al.* Elimination kinetics of thiopentone in mothers and their newborn infants. *Eur J Clin Pharmacol* 1985; **28:** 321–5.
2. Swerdlow BN, Holley FO. Intravenous anaesthetic agents: pharmacokinetic-pharmacodynamic relationships. *Clin Pharmacokinet* 1987; **12:** 79–110.
3. Esener Z, *et al.* Thiopentone and etomidate concentrations in maternal and umbilical plasma, and in colostrum. *Br J Anaesth* 1992; **69:** 586–8.
4. Gedney JA, Ghosh S. Pharmacokinetics of analgesics, sedatives and anaesthetic agents during cardiopulmonary bypass. *Br J Anaesth* 1995; **75:** 344–51.


## Uses and Administration

Thiopental is a short-acting barbiturate anaesthetic. It is given intravenously, usually for the induction of general anaesthesia (p.1296), but may be used as the sole anaesthetic to maintain anaesthesia for short procedures with minimal painful stimuli. It is also used in anaesthesia as a supplement to other anaesthetics, as a hypnotic in balanced anaesthesia, and, when given rectally, for basal anaesthesia or basal narcosis. Thiopental sodium may also be used intravenously in the control of refractory tonic-clonic status epilepticus and in neurosurgical patients to reduce increased intracranial pressure.

Thiopental does not usually produce excitation and induction of anaesthesia is usually smooth. It has poor muscle relaxant properties and a muscle relaxant must be administered before intubation is attempted. Thiopental also has poor analgesic properties and small doses may even lower the pain threshold. Recovery from moderate doses usually occurs within 10 to 30 minutes, but the patient may remain sleepy or confused for several hours. Large doses, repeated smaller doses, or continuous administration may markedly delay recovery.

In **anaesthesia**, the dosage of thiopental varies greatly according to the state of the patient and the nature of other drugs being used concurrently (see under Precautions above and Interactions above for further details). Thiopental is usually administered intravenously as the sodium salt as a 2.5% solution but a 5% solution is occasionally used. A typical dose for inducing anaesthesia is 100 to 150 mg injected over 10 to 15 seconds, repeated after 30 to 60 seconds according to response. Some prefer to initiate induction with a test dose of 25 to 75 mg. The UK manufacturer recommends that the total dosage used in pregnant patients should not exceed 250 mg. Children's doses range from 2 to 7 mg/kg. When thiopental is used as the sole anaesthetic, anaesthesia can be maintained by repeat doses as needed or by continuous intravenous infusion of a 0.2 or 0.4% solution.

To **reduce elevations of intracranial pressure** in neurological patients, thiopental sodium is licensed for use as intermittent bolus injections of 1.5 to 3 mg/kg if adequate ventilation is provided (but see also Cerebrovascular Disorders, below). Higher doses have been tried.

A suggested dose in refractory tonic-clonic **status epilepticus** is 75 to 125 mg intravenously (see also under Status Epilepticus, below).

◊ References.


1. Russo H, Bressolle F. Pharmacodynamics and pharmacokinetics of thiopental. *Clin Pharmacokinet* 1998; **35:** 95–134.


**Administration in the elderly.** It is usually recommended that the dosage of barbiturate anaesthetics is reduced in the elderly. A study[1] in elderly patients demonstrated that although reducing the rate of intravenous administration reduced the speed of induction, the dosage required was also reduced. Administration of thiopental sodium 2.5% solution at a rate of 125 mg/minute induced anaesthesia in a mean of 90.8 seconds and required a mean dose of 2.8 mg/kg. Corresponding values for an administration rate of 500 mg/minute were 40.8 seconds and 5 mg/kg, respectively.


1. Berthoud MC, *et al.* Comparison of infusion rates of three i.v. anaesthetic agents for induction in elderly patients. *Br J Anaesth* 1993; **70:** 423–7.


**Anaesthesia.** Some of the adverse effects of the neuromuscular blocker suxamethonium may be reduced when thiopental is used as part of the anaesthetic regimen. For a suggestion that thiopental may help to counteract the rise in intra-ocular pressure associated with the use of suxamethonium for intubation, see under Anaesthesia, p.1397.

**Cerebrovascular disorders.** Barbiturates are considered to be suitable anaesthetics for use in patients with or at risk of raised intracranial pressure. Barbiturate-induced coma (commonly with pentobarbital or thiopental) has been used, both therapeutically and prophylactically, to protect the brain from ischaemia resulting from neurological insults including head injury, stroke, Reye's syndrome, and hepatic encephalopathy.[1-3] Rationale includes the ability of barbiturates to reduce intracranial pressure and to reduce metabolic demands of cerebral tissues. Although thiopental protected patients against the neuropsychiatric complications of cardiopulmonary bypass,[4] the Brain Resuscitation Clinical Trial I Study Group[5] found no cerebral benefit from thiopental in comatose survivors of cardiac arrest. Nor did others[6] observe any benefit from thiopental-induced coma in infants with severe birth asphyxia. A review in 1989 considered that there was no convincing evidence of improvement in neurological outcome to justify the risks of the procedure in conditions causing global ischaemia, although administration of barbiturates without necessarily inducing coma might have a limited role in reduction of raised intracranial pressure refractory to other therapy. Use of barbiturates in the setting of regional cerebral ischaemia, including use during cardiopulmonary bypass to prevent focal neurological complications, remained controversial.[1] A recent systematic review[7] came to similar conclusions, pointing out that although the barbiturates may reduce intracranial pressure their hypotensive effects are likely to offset any beneficial action on cerebral perfusion, perhaps accounting for the lack of evidence for any clinical benefit.

For a discussion of the treatment of raised intracranial pressure, including a mention of the use of barbiturates, see p.833.


1. Rogers MC, Kirsch JR. Current concepts in brain resuscitation. *JAMA* 1989; **261:** 3143–7.
2. Lyons MK, Meyer FB. Cerebrospinal fluid physiology and the management of increased intracranial pressure. *Mayo Clin Proc* 1990; **65:** 684–707.
3. Woster PS, LeBlanc KL. Management of elevated intracranial pressure. *Clin Pharm* 1990; **9:** 762–72.
4. Nussmeier NA, *et al.* Neuropsychiatric complications after cardiopulmonary bypass: cerebral protection by a barbiturate. *Anesthesiology* 1986; **64:** 165–70.
5. Abramson NS, *et al.* Randomized clinical study of thiopental loading in comatose survivors of cardiac arrest. *N Engl J Med* 1986; **314:** 397–403.
6. Eyre JA, Wilkinson AR. Thiopentone induced coma after severe birth asphyxia. *Arch Dis Child* 1986; **61:** 1084–9.
7. Roberts I. Barbiturates for acute traumatic brain injury. Available in The Cochrane Library; Issue 1. Chichester: John Wiley; 2004.


**Status epilepticus.** Anaesthesia in conjunction with assisted ventilation may be instituted to control refractory tonic-clonic status epilepticus (p.352). A short-acting barbiturate such as thiopental is usually used. A loading dose of 5 mg/kg given intravenously has been suggested.[1] This may be followed after 30 minutes by an infusion given at a rate of 1 to 3 mg/kg per hour adjusted to maintain a maximum blood concentration of 60 to 100 micrograms/mL.[1] It has been recommended that administration should be continued for at least 12 hours after seizure activity has ceased and then slowly discontinued.[2] Recovery may be prolonged.[3]


1. O'Brien MD. Management of major status epilepticus in adults. *BMJ* 1990; **301:** 918.
2. Bauer J, Elger CE. Management of status epilepticus in adults. *CNS Drugs* 1994; **1:** 26–44.
3. Parviainen I, *et al.* High-dose thiopental in the treatment of refractory status epilepticus in intensive care unit. *Neurology* 2002; **59:** 1249–51.


## Preparations

***BP 2003:*** Thiopental Injection;
***USP 27:*** Thiopental Sodium for Injection.

**Proprietary Preparations** (details are given in Part 3)
***Arg.:*** Bensulf; Hipnopento; Pentothal; ***Austral.:*** Pentothal; ***Belg.:*** Nesdonal†; Pentothal; ***Braz.:*** Thionembutal; Thiopentax; ***Canad.:*** Pentothal; ***Chile:*** Penthotal; ***Denm.:*** Pentothal; ***Fin.:*** Pentothal; ***Ger.:*** Trapanal; ***Hong Kong:*** Intraval Sodium†; Pentothal; ***India:*** Anesthal; ***Irl.:*** Intraval Sodium; ***Israel:*** Pentothal; ***Ital.:*** Farmotal; Pentothal; ***Mex.:*** Inductal†; Pensodital†; Pentothal; Sodipental; ***Neth.:*** Nesdonal†; ***Norw.:*** Pentothal; ***NZ:*** Intraval; Pentothal†; ***S.Afr.:*** Intraval Sodium†; ***Singapore:*** Pentothal; ***Spain:*** Pentothal; Tiobarbital; ***Swed.:*** Pentothal; ***Switz.:*** Pentothal; ***Thai.:*** Intraval Sodium†; Pentothal; ***UK:*** Intraval Sodium†; ***USA:*** Pentothal.

---

## Tiletamine Hydrochloride *(BANM, USAN, rINNM)*

CI-634; CL-399; CN-54521-2; Hidrocloruro de tiletamina. 2-Ethylamino-2-(2-thienyl)cyclohexanone hydrochloride.
$C_{12}H_{17}NOS,HCl$ = 259.8.
*CAS — 14176-49-9 (tiletamine); 14176-50-2 (tiletamine hydrochloride).*

**Pharmacopoeias.** In *US* for veterinary use only.

**USP 27** (Tiletamine Hydrochloride). A white to off-white crystalline powder. Freely soluble in water; slightly soluble in chloroform; practically insoluble in ether; soluble in methyl alcohol; freely soluble in 0.1N hydrochloric acid. pH of a 10% solution in water is between 3.0 and 5.0. Store in airtight containers.

### Profile

Tiletamine has similar properties to ketamine (p.1302). It is used as the hydrochloride with zolazepam (p.728) for general anaesthesia in veterinary medicine.

---

## Trichloroethylene *(rINN)*

Trichlorethylene; Trichlorethylenum; Trichloroethene; Trichloroethylenum; Tricloroetileno.
$CHCl:CCl_2$ = 131.4.
*CAS — 79-01-6.*
*ATC — N01AB05.*

**Stability.** NOTE. Trichloroethylene used for anaesthetic purposes contains thymol 0.01% w/v as a stabiliser and is coloured blue for identification. It is non-flammable.

### Adverse Effects and Precautions

Trichloroethylene increases the rate and decreases the depth of respiration and may be followed by apnoea. The sensitivity of the heart to beta-adrenergic activity may increase, possibly with ventricular arrhythmias.

Acute exposure to trichloroethylene may be followed by dizziness, lightheadedness, lethargy, nausea, and vomiting; hepatic and renal dysfunction may follow. Fatalities have occurred, although temporary unconsciousness is a more common manifestation.

Chronic poisoning may result in visual disturbances, intolerance to alcohol as manifested by transient redness of the face and neck (degreasers' or trichloroethylene flush), impairment of performance, hearing defects, neuralgia, and mild liver dysfunction. Prolonged contact with trichloroethylene can cause dermatitis, eczema, burns, and conjunctivitis.

Dependence has been reported in medical personnel and factory workers who regularly inhale trichloroethylene vapour.

If trichloroethylene is used as an anaesthetic it should not be used in closed-circuit apparatus since there is a reaction with soda lime to produce a toxic end product that may cause cranial nerve paralysis and possibly death.

See also Adverse Effects and Precautions for General Anaesthetics, p.1295.

◊ Reviews of the toxicity of trichloroethylene.


1. Health and Safety Executive. Trichloroethylene. *Toxicity Review 6.* London: HMSO, 1982.
2. Trichloroethylene. *Environmental Health Criteria 50.* Geneva: WHO, 1985. Available at: http://www.inchem.org/documents/ehc/ehc/ehc50.htm (accessed 26/05/04)
3. Davidson IWF, Beliles RP. Consideration of the target organ toxicity of trichloroethylene in terms of metabolite toxicity and pharmacokinetics. *Drug Metab Rev* 1991; **23:** 493–599.


**Abuse.** Toxicity associated with inhalation of volatile substances including trichloroethylene has been reviewed.[1,2] Trichloroethylene can damage the kidney, liver, heart, and lung. However, in young healthy subjects, organ toxicity becomes apparent only with intensive and protracted abuse of volatile substances.


1. Marjot R, McLeod AA. Chronic non-neurological toxicity from volatile substance abuse. *Hum Toxicol* 1989; **8:** 301–6.
2. Anonymous. Solvent abuse: little progress after 20 years. *BMJ* 1990; **300:** 135–6.


**Carcinogenicity.** The use of trichloroethylene in foods, drugs, and cosmetics was banned by the FDA following studies demonstrating that hepatocellular carcinomas could be induced in *mice* by chronic exposure to very high doses. However, similar effects have not been found in *rats* and larger species and several epidemiologic studies have failed to demonstrate an increased incidence of liver tumours, total mortality or mortality due to cancer in workers exposed to trichloroethylene. Suggestions that the carcinogenicity of trichloroethylene is due to one of its intermediate metabolites, cloral hydrate, have raised concern over the continuing use of cloral hydrate as a medicine. For further details, see p.684.

**Effects on the liver.** References[1,2] to hepatotoxicity following occupational exposure to trichloroethylene. See also under Carcinogenicity, above.


1. McCunney RJ. Diverse manifestations of trichloroethylene. *Br J Ind Med* 1988; **45:** 122–6.
2. Schattner A, Malnick SDH. Anicteric hepatitis and uveitis in a worker exposed to trichloroethylene. *Postgrad Med J* 1990; **66:** 730–1.


**Effects on the skin.** A report[1] of scleroderma in 3 patients occupationally exposed to trichloroethylene and, in 2 cases, also to trichloroethane.


1. Flindt-Hansen H, Isager H. Scleroderma after occupational exposure to trichlorethylene and trichlorethane. *Acta Derm Venereol (Stockh)* 1987; **67:** 263–4.


### Interactions

The arrhythmogenic effects of trichloroethylene may be potentiated by sympathomimetics such as adrenaline. Alcohol consumption after chronic exposure to trichloroethylene may result in a reddening of the skin (see under Adverse Effects and Precautions, above).

See also Interactions of General Anaesthetics, p.1295.

### Pharmacokinetics

Trichloroethylene is rapidly absorbed by inhalation and ingestion. Percutaneous absorption can occur. Some of the inhaled trichloroethylene is slowly eliminated through the lungs; trichloroethylene is metabolised primarily in the liver, cloral hydrate (see p.684) being the first stable major metabolite formed; most is then metabolised to trichloroethanol and trichloroacetic acid which are excreted in the urine. The latter may be used as an indicator of industrial exposure. Trichloroethylene diffuses across the placenta.

### Uses and Administration

Trichloroethylene is a volatile halogenated anaesthetic administered by inhalation. It has been used in some countries for the maintenance of light anaesthesia (p.1296) but it has weak anaesthetic properties compared to other halogenated anaesthetics and poor muscle relaxant activity, and safer anaesthetics are generally preferred. It has also been used to supplement anaesthesia with nitrous oxide-oxygen or halothane. Trichloroethylene is a potent analgesic and has been used in subanaesthetic concentrations to provide analgesia for obstetrics, emergency management of trauma, and other acutely painful procedures.

Trichloroethylene is used in industry as a solvent for oils and fats, for degreasing metals, and for dry cleaning. It has also been used in typewriter correction fluids but is no longer included in most brands.

## Xenon

Xenón.

Xe = 131.293.

### Profile

Xenon is a non-explosive gas. Mixtures of 60 or 70% v/v xenon with oxygen have been tried as a general anaesthetic.

◊ References.


1. Lachmann B, *et al.* Safety and efficacy of xenon in routine use as an inhalational anaesthetic. *Lancet* 1990; **335:** 1413–15.
2. Yagi M, *et al.* Analgesic and hypnotic effects of subanaesthetic concentrations of xenon in human volunteers: comparison with nitrous oxide. *Br J Anaesth* 1995; **74:** 670–3.
3. Goto T, *et al.* Emergence times from xenon anaesthesia are independent of the duration of anaesthesia. *Br J Anaesth* 1997; **79:** 595–9.
4. Rossaint R, *et al.* Multicenter randomized comparison of the efficacy and safety of xenon and isoflurane in patients undergoing elective surgery. *Anesthesiology* 2003; **98:** 6–13.
5. Sanders RD, *et al.* Xenon: no stranger to anaesthesia. *Br J Anaesth* 2003; **91:** 709–17.
6. Bedi A, *et al.* Use of xenon as a sedative for patients receiving critical care. *Crit Care Med* 2003; **31:** 2470–7.
7. Preckel B, Schlack W. Xenon—cardiovascularly inert? *Br J Anaesth* 2004; **92:** 786–9.

# Hypothalamic and Pituitary Hormones


Acromegaly and gigantism, p.1312
Amenorrhoea, p.1313
Cryptorchidism, p.1313
Cushing's syndrome, p.1313
Delayed puberty, p.1314
Diabetes insipidus, p.1314
Endometriosis, p.1314
Growth retardation, p.1314
Hyperprolactinaemia, p.1315
Hypogonadism, p.1316
Infertility, p.1316
Lactation inhibition and induction, p.1317
Ovarian dysfunction, p.1317
Polycystic ovary syndrome, p.1317
Turner's syndrome, p.1317
Precocious puberty, p.1318
Premenstrual syndrome, p.1318
Syndrome of inappropriate ADH secretion, p.1318


The pituitary gland or hypophysis in humans is composed of the adenohypophysis, which is the anterior lobe, and the neurohypophysis, which comprises the posterior lobe and the neural stalk, above which lies the hypothalamus. The anterior lobe is linked to the hypothalamus by a portal vascular system but there is no vascular link between the posterior lobe and the hypothalamus.

The hormones secreted by the anterior lobe of the **pituitary**, each by its own specialised cells, are: adrenocorticotrophic hormone (ACTH; corticotropin); the gonadotrophic hormones (gonadotrophins), follicle-stimulating hormone and luteinising hormone; growth hormone (somatropin); lactogenic hormone (prolactin); and thyroid-stimulating hormone (thyrotrophin). In some mammals, but apparently not in humans, the pituitary also secretes melanocyte-stimulating hormone.

Oxytocin and antidiuretic hormone (ADH; vasopressin) are synthesised in the **hypothalamus**. They become associated with carrier proteins, neurophysins, and are then transported down nerve fibres to the posterior pituitary where they are stored until required. The release of oxytocin and vasopressin appears to be controlled mainly by nervous reflex responses.

The secretion of anterior pituitary hormones, in which the hypothalamus plays a major part, is regulated by a complex interaction between stimulatory and inhibitory neural and hormonal influences. A stylised representation of the hypothalamic-pituitary-endocrine axis is depicted in Figure 1, below. The hypothalamus produces transmitter substances that regulate pituitary secretion. These substances are secreted by hypothalamic neurones called neuroendocrine transducers, and stored in the median eminence of the hypothalamus. On receipt of an appropriate stimulus they are released into the blood of the hypophyseal portal system which carries them to the anterior pituitary. Conventionally these substances are known as factors until their structure and function is reasonably well established, when they may be referred to as hormones.

Hypothalamic releasing factors or hormones stimulate release of anterior pituitary hormones into the systemic circulation. Growth hormone is under a system of double regulation, since the hypothalamus secretes a release-inhibiting hormone (somatostatin) as well as growth hormone-releasing hormone (somatorelin). For others, secretion of the releasing factor is controlled by feedback mechanisms involving target organ hormones, pituitary hormones, and perhaps the hypothalamic hormones themselves as well as by excitatory and inhibitory impulses from different parts of the brain.

The major groups of hypothalamic and pituitary hormones and their analogues described in this chapter are summarised in Table 1, p.1313.

**Figure 1.** A stylised representation of the hypothalamic-pituitary-endocrine axis.

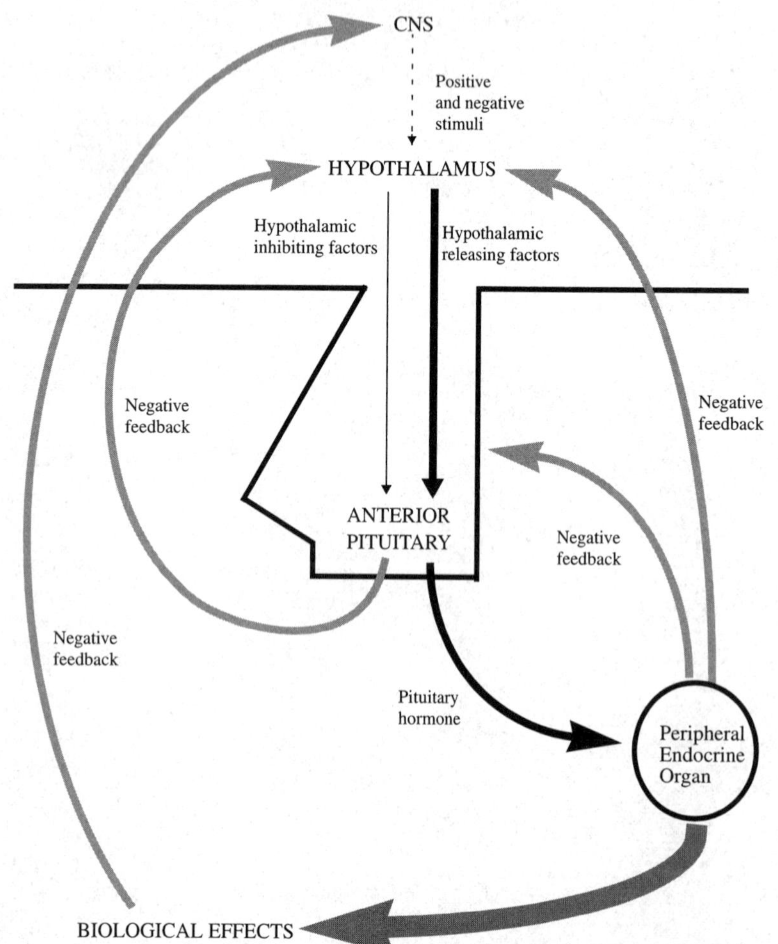


## Use of Hypothalamic and Pituitary Hormones

A number of disorders associated with hypothalamic or pituitary dysfunction are discussed below. Some other endocrine disorders that may be due to dysfunction of the hypothalamic-pituitary-endocrine axes include adrenocortical insufficiency (p.1075), and hyperthyroidism (p.1594) or hypothyroidism (p.1595), as well as some of the disorders discussed in the chapter on Sex Hormones (p.1527).

### Acromegaly and gigantism

Acromegaly and gigantism are syndromes of excess growth hormone secretion, usually associated with a secretory pituitary adenoma (somatropinoma).

Excessive growth hormone secretion in childhood, while the epiphyses of the long bones are open, results in **gigantism**, with a proportional growth spurt and skeletal enlargement. Subsequently skeletal deformities develop, including kyphosis and deformity of the chest wall, as a consequence of osteoporosis. Puberty, with the increase in sex hormone secretion that leads to epiphyseal fusion, may be delayed by concomitant hypogonadism, leading to attainment of an even greater ultimate height. If growth hormone excess persists into adulthood, features of acromegaly may be superimposed on gigantism.

When excess growth hormone secretion develops first in adulthood the condition is known as **acromegaly**. Signs and symptoms tend to develop slowly and may be missed, sometimes for years. Growth hormone concentrations, and hence those of insulin-like growth factor I (IGF-I), which is produced in the liver in response to growth hormone, are elevated, sometimes markedly. The facial features become coarser, the jaw enlarges (prognathism), and hands and feet become enlarged. Peripheral neuropathy and carpal tunnel syndrome due to nerve entrapment, arthropathy, osteoarthritis, and muscle weakness, abnormal glucose tolerance, hypertension and left ventricular hypertrophy are all common, as is nodular goitre. Daytime somnolence may occur due to sleep apnoea. Acromegalics have an increased mortality if left untreated, largely due to cardiovascular disease.

**Treatment**. The biochemical goal of treatment is to normalise growth hormone and IGF-I concentrations. Although mean 24-hour growth hormone concentrations of less than 2.5 micrograms/litre have been used to define diagnosis and cure,[1] more sensitive assays have changed the criteria. In patients with acromegaly, growth hormone concentrations are not suppressed during oral glucose tolerance testing, and this measurement of growth hormone is used both diagnostically and to assess treatment efficacy; a concentration of less than 2 micrograms/litre has been used to define successful therapy,[1] and more recently concentrations below 1 microgram/litre have been suggested.[2,3] Random IGF-I concentrations should be reduced to normal for age and sex.[2,3] It is not yet clear, however, whether any form of treatment to reduce growth hormone concentrations reduces mortality from cardiorespiratory or neoplastic disease in patients with acromegaly.[1]

As for most pituitary tumours, **surgery** is the mainstay of treatment. The success rate depends on surgical expertise and the size and extension of the mass, with success rates higher for microadenomas (about 70 to 80%) than macroadenomas (less than 50%) depending on criteria.[1,2] In elderly patients with macroadenomas, where surgery may carry considerable risks, drug therapy with octreotide may be a better option.[1]

**Drug therapy** for acromegaly is indicated for patients who refuse surgery, are at increased risk from surgery, have active disease after surgery, or are awaiting the effects of radiotherapy (see below). The somatostatin analogues, octreotide and lanreotide, reduce growth hormone secretion in most patients, but not all will have persistent suppression and normalisation of growth hormone levels.[4]

Reported response rates vary, but effective growth hormone suppression occurs in about 50 to 55% of patients, and IGF-I is normalised in about 50 to 65%. Somatostatin analogues also produce tumour shrinkage, reducing tumour size by 20 to 50% in about 30% of patients, and improve signs and symptoms of acromegaly, including improvements in cardiac structure and function. Octreotide and lanreotide are given as sustained-release intramuscular injections.[4] Octreotide may be more effective than lanreotide, but data from comparative trials are limited. Octreotide can also be given by subcutaneous injection, but must be given three times daily, making it less attractive for long-term therapy. There have been some promising reports of the use of somatostatin analogues for primary therapy, but when there is visual or neurological compromise then surgery is preferred because drug therapy may not provide enough tumour shrinkage to relieve pressure on the optic chiasm.[4] There is some data to suggest that pre-operative use of somatostatin analogues could improve cardiovascular, respiratory, and metabolic functions and hence reduce morbidity associated with surgery, and improve remission rates, but further study is needed.[4,5] Dopaminergics, particularly bromocriptine, can produce a paradoxical reduction in growth hormone secretion in some patients with acromegaly, providing symptomatic relief. However, they produce acceptable suppression of growth hormone secretion in only about 10 to 20% of patients, and they are generally added to somatostatin analogue therapy.[3,4] Another dopaminergic, quinagolide, has been reported to produce better results than a depot preparation of bromocriptine, or cabergoline.[6] Pegvisomant is a growth hormone-receptor antagonist that may be used when other therapies have failed or are inappropriate. It is reported[7,8] to lower IGF-I concentrations, improve signs and symptoms of acromegaly, and be well tolerated.

Tumour regression induced by **radiotherapy** is a possible alternative when surgery cannot be performed, there is residual pituitary disease following surgery, or medical therapy has failed.[3] Although it reduces growth hormone concentrations in about 90% of patients[2] and tumour recurrence is rare[3] its effects are slow and it often produces hypopituitarism. Some consider these to be disadvantages and prefer to use drug treatment for management of tumours that persist after surgery.[3] Since it may take several years for growth hormone concentrations to fall, drug therapy is also given until the effects of radiation therapy are satisfactory.[1,3]


1. Colao A, Lombardi G. Growth-hormone and prolactin excess. *Lancet* 1998; **352:** 1455–61.
2. Giustina A, *et al.* Criteria for cure of acromegaly: a consensus statement. *J Clin Endocrinol Metab* 2000; **85:** 526–9.
3. Melmed S, *et al.* Guidelines for acromegaly management. *J Clin Endocrinol Metab* 2002; **87:** 4054–8.
4. Freda PU. Somatostatin analogs in acromegaly. *J Clin Endocrinol Metab* 2002; **87:** 3013–18.
5. Ben-Shlomo A, Melmed S. The role of pharmacotherapy in perioperative management of patients with acromegaly. *J Clin Endocrinol Metab* 2003; **88:** 963–8.
6. Colao A, *et al.* Effect of different dopaminergic agents in the treatment of acromegaly. *J Clin Endocrinol Metab* 1997; **82:** 518–23.
7. Trainer PJ, *et al.* Treatment of acromegaly with the growth hormone-receptor antagonist pegvisomant. *N Engl J Med* 2000; **342:** 1171–7.
8. van der Lely AJ, *et al.* Long-term treatment of acromegaly with pegvisomant, a growth hormone receptor antagonist. *Lancet* 2001; **358:** 1754–9.


**Table 1.** Hypothalamic and pituitary hormones.

| | |
|---|---|
| *Antidiuretic hormones*<br>Argipressin<br>Lypressin<br>Desmopressin<br>Felypressin<br>Ornipressin<br>Terlipressin<br>Powdered Pituitary, Posterior Lobe<br>Vasopressin | *Oxytocic hormones*<br>Carbetocin<br>Demoxytocin<br>Oxytocin<br>Powdered Pituitary, Posterior Lobe<br>*Oxytocin antagonists*<br>Atosiban |
| *Corticotrophic hormones*<br>Corticotropin<br>Tetracosactide<br>*Corticotrophic releasing hormone*<br>Corticorelin | *Somatotrophic hormones*<br>Mecasermin<br>Somatrem<br>Somatropin<br>*Somatotrophic hormone receptor antagonists*<br>Pegvisomant<br>*Somatotrophic releasing hormones*<br>Sermorelin<br>Somatorelin<br>*Somatotrophic release inhibitors*<br>Lanreotide<br>Octreotide<br>Somatostatin<br>Vapreotide |
| *Gonadotrophic hormones*<br>Choriogonadotropin Alfa<br>Chorionic Gonadotrophin<br>Follicle-stimulating Hormone<br>Follitropin Alfa<br>Follitropin Beta<br>Luteinising Hormone<br>Lutropin Alfa<br>Menotrophin<br>Urofollitropin<br>*Gonadotrophic releasing hormones*<br>Buserelin<br>Deslorelin<br>Gonadorelin<br>Goserelin<br>Histrelin<br>Leuprorelin<br>Nafarelin<br>Triptorelin<br>*Gonadotrophic releasing hormone antagonists*<br>Abarelix<br>Cetrorelix<br>Ganirelix | *Thyrotrophic hormones*<br>Thyrotrophin<br>Thyrotropin Alfa<br>*Thyrotrophic releasing hormones*<br>Posatirelin<br>Protirelin<br>Taltirelin |
| *Lactotrophic hormones*<br>Prolactin | |

## Amenorrhoea

Amenorrhoea is the absence of menstruation: a break in menstruation of 6 months or more is considered pathological in an adult woman who is not pregnant, lactating, or menopausal. Amenorrhoea occurring from the time of puberty is known as primary, while amenorrhoea developing later in life is referred to as secondary. Pathological amenorrhoea is usually associated with infertility (see also below). Hirsutism (p.1545) may also be present.

The causes of amenorrhoea (or oligomenorrhoea—infrequent and erratic periods) are most often ovarian or hypothalamic/pituitary in origin. Ovarian causes include failure of normal gonadal development, as in Turner's syndrome (below); premature ovarian failure including that due to trauma, drugs, radiotherapy, or autoimmunity; and conditions such as the polycystic ovary syndrome (below). Hypothalamic or pituitary causes include reduced production of gonadotrophins due to inadequate nutrition, excessive exercise, or pituitary trauma (see also Hypogonadism, below); or excess prolactin production (see Hyperprolactinaemia, below). Other causes, including adrenal disorders, thyroid disorders, abnormalities of the vagina or uterus, or testicular feminisation, may be found rarely.

The management of amenorrhoea essentially involves the identification of any underlying disorder and its correction, if possible. When the cause cannot be corrected, oestrogen replacement therapy, usually in the form of an oral contraceptive, is appropriate to minimise the consequences of long-term oestrogen deficiency.

References.


1. Crosignani PG, Vegetti W. A practical guide to the diagnosis and management of amenorrhoea. *Drugs* 1996; **52:** 671–81.
2. McIver B, *et al.* Evaluation and management of amenorrhea. *Mayo Clin Proc* 1997; **72:** 1161–9.
3. Baird DT. Amenorrhoea. *Lancet* 1997; **350:** 275–9.


## Cryptorchidism

The testes are formed within the abdomen and subsequently descend the inguinal canal to the scrotum. Failure of the testes to descend (cryptorchidism) occurs in about 3 to 6% of newborn males but in many the testes descend during the first year of life decreasing the prevalence to about 1%. In children with cryptorchidism, pathological testicular damage has been noted by the age of 2 years, which may result in subsequent infertility;[1,2] cryptorchidism also significantly increases the risk of testicular cancer. Abnormalities of the testes and anatomical abnormalities such as inguinal hernia may contribute to maldescent, and both primary testicular disease and gonadotrophin deficiency may be associated with cryptorchidism. For discussions of Hypogonadism and Infertility, see below. Cryptorchidism should be distinguished from retractile testes in which the testes develop normally and for which treatment is usually not required.[1]

If sterility is to be avoided, treatment should be carried out preferably before 18 months of age.[2] Surgery remains the treatment with the best success rate but in most clinics boys are referred for surgery only after the failure of hormonal therapy.[3] Meta-analysis[4] suggests that gonadorelin, and probably chorionic gonadotrophin, are more effective than placebo with a success rate of about 20% overall, although this may be considerably lower when care is taken to exclude retractile testes. The lower the position of the undescended testis, the more likely benefit from hormonal therapy appears to be.[4-6] Results may perhaps be improved by combined therapy with gonadorelin and chorionic gonadotrophin.[5] Chorionic gonadotrophin may also be useful as an adjuvant before surgery, in order to cause a non-palpable testis to become palpable;[7] however, changes suggestive of inflammation in the testis have been reported following such treatment.[6]


1. Palmer JM. The undescended testicle. *Endocrinol Metab Clin North Am* 1991; **20:** 231–40.
2. Cilento BG, *et al.* Cryptorchidism and testicular torsion. *Pediatr Clin North Am* 1993; **40:** 1133–49.
3. Müller J, Skakkebaek NE. Cryptorchidism. *Curr Ther Endocrinol Metab* 1997; **6:** 363–6.
4. Pyörälä S, *et al.* A review and meta-analysis of hormonal treatment of cryptorchidism. *J Clin Endocrinol Metab* 1995; **80:** 2795–9.
5. Nane I, *et al.* Primary gonadotropin releasing hormone and adjunctive human chorionic gonadotropin treatment in cryptorchidism: a clinical trial. *Urology* 1997; **49:** 108–11.
6. Kaleva M, *et al.* Treatment with human chorionic gonadotrophin for cryptorchidism: clinical and histological effects. *Int J Androl* 1996; **19:** 293–8.
7. Polascik TJ, *et al.* Reappraisal of the role of human chorionic gonadotropin in the diagnosis and treatment of the nonpalpable testis: a 10 year-old experience. *J Urol (Baltimore)* 1996; **156:** 804–6.


## Cushing's syndrome

Cushing's syndrome is the result of a chronic excess of glucocorticoids. It is commonly divided into those forms independent of adrenocorticotrophic hormone (ACTH; corticotropin) secretion (either due to an adrenal tumour secreting cortisol, or to administration of exogenous corticosteroids) and those which are ACTH-dependent (caused by excessive ACTH secretion from a pituitary adenoma—Cushing's disease proper, pituitary hyperplasia, or an ectopic ACTH-secreting tumour elsewhere—usually bronchus or lung cancer). About two-thirds of all cases are due to Cushing's disease, which is 8 times more common in women than men.

Symptoms may develop insidiously over several years and include obesity, particularly of the trunk, rounding of the face, atrophy of the skin leading to striae, poor wound healing, muscle weakness, osteoporosis, hypertension, diabetes mellitus, and depression and other psychological disturbances. Hypokalaemia is rare in Cushing's disease but common in other forms of the syndrome. Women may experience hirsutism due to adrenal androgen secretion, and both sexes may develop hypogonadism and loss of libido.

**Diagnosis** of Cushing's syndrome may be problematic because no test is wholly reliable.[1,2] Where there is suspicion, options for initial screening include measurement of urinary cortisol, late-night salivary cortisol, midnight plasma-cortisol, and overnight low-dose dexamethasone suppression testing. A dexamethasone-corticorelin test may be used to identify pseudo-Cushing's conditions such as depression or alcoholism. Once a diagnosis of Cushing's syndrome has been made, plasma-ACTH measurements are used to distinguish between ACTH-dependent and ACTH-independent forms. High-dose dexamethasone suppression testing and corticorelin stimulation testing have been used to differentiate between pituitary and ectopic ACTH-dependent Cushing's syndrome, but they both have disadvantages and their usefulness has been debated. For further discussion of dexamethasone suppression testing, see p.1098, and for corticorelin stimulation testing, see p.1321. Imaging techniques and sampling of central (petrosal) venous blood are additional procedures that may be used for localising tumours.

Appropriate **treatment** depends on accurate identification of the cause of the syndrome.[1] The usual treatment in Cushing's disease is transsphenoidal resection of the tumour, which when carried out by an experienced surgeon produces a successful response in the great majority of patients. Pituitary radiotherapy is slower than surgery to take effect, produces a lower remission rate, and is more likely to produce hypopituitarism. It is therefore usually used as second-line therapy when initial surgery has not been curative and a second operation is considered unsuitable. If pituitary surgery or radiotherapy fails, bilateral adrenalectomy may be considered (although this has some risks including that of Nelson's syndrome due to hyperactivity of residual pituitary tumour). Patients who undergo such surgery require glucocorticoid and mineralocorticoid replacement therapy for life. Surgery is also the treatment of choice for a resectable adrenal tumour or ectopic ACTH-secreting tumour; even where there is metastasis it may be useful in moderating symptoms.

A number of drugs have been used in patients with Cushing's disease, but their role appears to be mainly adjuvant.[1,3] Drugs acting at the hypothalamic-pituitary level, aimed at reducing ACTH secretion, do not seem to be of much value; there have been occasional reports of benefit with bromocriptine, cyproheptadine, and sodium valproate. Drugs that inhibit steroid synthesis in the adrenal gland are more effective, and include mitotane, metyrapone, aminoglutethimide, and ketoconazole. These may be used to control severe complications quickly, prepare patients for surgery, or provide cover while radiotherapy takes effect. Mifepristone acts as a glucocorticoid receptor antagonist, and has been used successfully in a few patients with Cushing's syndrome.

In patients with the ectopic ACTH syndrome in whom surgery is unsuitable or ineffective, chemotherapy aimed at the primary tumour is the treatment of choice but is likely to be only palliative. Inhibitors of steroid synthesis can be used to control symptoms, and somatostatin analogues such as octreotide may decrease ACTH secretion by ectopic tumours that have somatostatin receptors.[1]

Surgery is the preferred treatment for an adrenal tumour but, although this is usually curative for adrenal adenoma, it is less successful for adrenal carcinoma and in these patients mitotane, alone or with chemotherapy, is generally used.[1]

In patients who are successfully treated for Cushing's syndrome adrenocortical replacement therapy (see p.1075) is usually required until the hypothalamic-pituitary-adrenal axis recovers normal function, a process which may take many months.

1. Boscaro M, *et al.* Cushing's syndrome. *Lancet* 2001; **357:** 783–91.
2. Raff H, Findling JW. A physiologic approach to diagnosis of the Cushing syndrome. *Ann Intern Med* 2003; **138:** 980–91.
3. Nieman LK. Medical therapy of Cushing's disease. *Pituitary* 2002; **5:** 77–82.

## Delayed puberty

Puberty in boys usually begins between the ages of 9 and 14 years; in girls pubertal development starts about 2 years earlier than in boys and 95% of normal girls in the UK experience menstruation by 15 years of age. Delay beyond these norms should lead to investigation to try and eliminate the possibility of an underlying organic disorder. In addition to the various causes of hypogonadism (see below), some of which may be difficult to diagnose, severe systemic illness such as asthma or diabetes, or hypothyroidism, may cause delay in sexual maturation. Where no apparent cause can be found a family history of delayed maturation may suggest constitutional delayed puberty, in which normal pubertal development can eventually be expected.

Where pubertal delay is secondary to some other condition appropriate management of the precipitating cause is required. In constitutional delayed puberty small doses of oestrogens in girls, or androgens (such as oxandrolone or a testosterone ester) in boys, may be given to promote growth and sexual development if psychological problems are apparent. Care is required as overly aggressive therapy with sex hormones may lead to premature closure of the epiphyses and compromise final adult height. Treatment should be interrupted periodically to see if spontaneous pubertal development has begun. The use of chorionic gonadotrophin or a gonadorelin analogue has no advantage in such patients, although they have a role in hypogonadotrophic hypogonadism, which may be difficult to distinguish from constitutional delay.

## Diabetes insipidus

Diabetes insipidus deprives the kidney of its capacity to produce a concentrated urine, resulting in the passage of large volumes of dilute urine (polyuria) and excessive thirst (polydipsia). Patients generally have moderately raised serum-sodium concentrations but are prone to more severe hypernatraemia (p.1220) when fluid is restricted.

The syndrome of diabetes insipidus is caused either by a deficiency in secretion of antidiuretic hormone (ADH; vasopressin) from the posterior pituitary gland (cranial, pituitary, or neurogenic diabetes insipidus), or by a failure in activity of secreted ADH on renal tubules (nephrogenic diabetes insipidus). Cranial diabetes insipidus is most commonly idiopathic (although it is now increasingly suspected to have an auto-immune basis) or occurs following surgery or trauma when it may be temporary. More rarely, it results from neoplasms, infections, or infiltrations of the CNS, or forms part of the familial DIDMOAD syndrome (diabetes insipidus, diabetes mellitus, optic atrophy, and deafness). Nephrogenic diabetes insipidus may occur as a familial X-linked recessive disorder in male infants, but is more often secondary to hypercalcaemia, hypokalaemia, or drug therapy (including lithium salts, foscarnet, and demeclocycline).

The mainstay of diagnosis of diabetes insipidus is measurement of serum and urine osmolality, urine specific gravity, and serum-sodium concentration. If these are found to be normal a formal water deprivation test may be performed, with careful monitoring of urine volume, osmolality, and body-weight. The test should be discontinued if more than 3 litres of urine is passed or 3% of total body-weight is lost, although this is in any case virtually diagnostic of diabetes insipidus. A dose of ADH in the form of desmopressin is then given to test renal responsiveness—prompt urine concentration is indicative of cranial diabetes insipidus, while failure indicates the nephrogenic form.

Cranial diabetes insipidus is usually treated by replacement therapy with ADH in the form of intranasal desmopressin, although tablets are now also available and may be preferred in children; desmopressin has greater antidiuretic efficacy and considerably less vasoconstrictor activity than lypressin or vasopressin itself.

Nephrogenic diabetes insipidus is by definition unresponsive to ADH therapy and water replacement tends to be the mainstay of treatment. Thiazide diuretics, notably hydrochlorothiazide, are given with some restriction of sodium intake to patients with nephrogenic diabetes insipidus; the resultant mild sodium depletion enhances proximal renal tubular sodium and water resorption. The co-administration of amiloride has been reported to have an additive effect while also preventing hypokalaemia.

Other drugs have also been tried in the management of diabetes insipidus. Chlorpropamide stimulates ADH secretion and augments the activity of residual ADH in patients with partial cranial disease and as in nephrogenic disease the thiazides may be useful. Clofibrate and carbamazepine have also been found to promote ADH secretion in these patients. Indometacin and other prostaglandin synthetase inhibitors decrease urine volume in all types of the condition. Combination of indometacin with a thiazide and desmopressin has been investigated.

References.

1. Seckl JR, Dunger DB. Diabetes insipidus: current treatment recommendations. *Drugs* 1992; **44:** 216–24.
2. Knoers N, Monnens LAH. Nephrogenic diabetes insipidus: clinical symptoms, pathogenesis, genetics and treatment. *Pediatr Nephrol* 1992; **6:** 476–82.
3. Singer I, *et al.* The management of diabetes insipidus in adults. *Arch Intern Med* 1997; **157:** 1293–1301.
4. Baylis PH, Cheetham T. Diabetes insipidus. *Arch Dis Child* 1998; **79:** 84–9.
5. Bendz H, Aurell M. Drug-induced diabetes insipidus. *Drug Safety* 1999; **21:** 449–56.

## Endometriosis

Gonadorelin analogues are used in the management of endometriosis (see p.1546) but the need for long-term therapy to prevent recurrence limits their value because of the risk of osteoporosis; 'add-back' therapy, with concomitant hormone replacement, can be used to prevent this.

## Growth retardation

Stature follows a normal (bell-shaped) distribution within the population and there may be some difficulty in deciding at what point short stature becomes abnormal; to some extent this is determined by cultural as well as physiological norms. However, certain disorders are associated with well-defined deficiencies of growth which may be severe enough to warrant the description dwarfism. Some forms are associated with disorders of bone or cartilage growth (skeletal dysplasias), and many of these result additionally in disproportionate growth, as in the short-limbs and large head characteristic of achondroplasia. Other important causes of dwarfism include inadequate production of growth hormone (idiopathic growth hormone deficiency), either alone (isolated growth hormone deficiency) or combined with other pituitary hormone deficiencies as part of hypopituitarism; resistance to circulating growth hormone, as in Laron-type dwarfism, where there is a mutation of the growth hormone receptor; or defects in somatomedin synthesis. Some other endocrine causes of short stature include hypothyroidism, Cushing's syndrome, and Turner's syndrome. Severe chronic disease in childhood such as asthma, chronic renal failure, or liver disorders can result in some growth retardation as can inadequate nutrition due to malabsorption syndromes such as coeliac disease.

Endocrine causes of growth retardation are significant because they may generally be treatable by appropriate replacement therapy. Isolated growth hormone deficiency, or growth hormone and gonadotrophin deficiencies, are the commonest congenital forms of hypopituitarism. The deficiency is rarely complete, and since most children with short stature will not have growth hormone deficiency care is required in its diagnosis. Although provocative growth hormone tests, which use non-physiological means to stimulate growth hormone secretion, have long been considered the gold standard for diagnosis of growth hormone deficiency they have a number of limitations and some consider measurement of circulating somatomedins (insulin-like growth factors; IGFs) or their binding proteins to be more useful.[1] Different assays may give different results, and it has been advised that therapeutic decisions should be based on a combination of comprehensive clinical and height assessments, biochemical tests, and radiological evaluation.[2]

In children with confirmed growth hormone deficiency replacement therapy is appropriate, and is given by subcutaneous injections of synthetic human growth hormone (somatropin) or its methionyl analogue (somatrem). Treatment improves bone density and growth velocity.[3-6] The greatest increase in the latter occurs in the first year of treatment, and subsequently declines,[3] perhaps due to downregulation of the growth hormone receptor; intermittent[7] or pulsatile[8] administration do not appear to have any advantage in this regard.

The extent of the benefit in terms of increase in final height is unclear. A cohort study of French children registered to receive growth hormone between 1973 and 1993 suggested that the eventual outcome was not as good as expected, and treated individuals remained short.[9] However, others are of the opinion that many growth-hormone deficient children achieve their genetic height potential with replacement therapy, and that most attain adult heights significantly greater than untreated children.[10] A further cohort study[11] from the same register for 1987 to 1996 found that adult heights were similar whether patients completed treatment or stopped before reaching adult height, and that patients with severe growth hormone deficiency may respond better than those with less severe deficiency.

Increasing the dose or the frequency of administration may improve outcome[12] but the most important prognostic factor is age. For optimum results, treatment should be started as early as possible.[3,9,12,13] In patients with multiple pituitary hormone deficiencies, genetic defects in growth hormone synthesis, or severe organic growth hormone deficiency, growth hormone therapy should be continued into adulthood. In other patients, growth hormone deficiency may or may not persist into adult life, and retesting should be done after the patient reaches adult height and after 1 to 3 months without therapy.[2,14] In those patients who need continued treatment, the dose of growth hormone should be gradually reduced in order to maintain IGF-I concentrations within the normal range.[14]

Somatorelin (growth hormone-releasing hormone) or its analogue sermorelin have also been tried to boost growth hormone secretion in patients with growth hormone deficiency,[15-17] and improved growth rates have been reported in some children. Another peptide analogue, pralmorelin is also under investigation.[18,19] There is a report that the effects of releasing hormone can be enhanced by concomitant use of a beta blocker.[20]

In patients with Laron dwarfism, conventional growth hormone therapy is ineffective because of defects in the growth hormone receptors. However, replacement therapy with mecasermin, the recombinant form of insulin-like growth factor-I, may be of substantial benefit in the treatment of this disorder.[21]

The use of growth hormone in short stature other than that due to indisputable growth hormone deficiency is controversial. Benefit has been reported from growth hormone therapy in children with chronic renal failure,[22,23] in girls with Turner's syndrome (but see below), and in young children (6 months to 3 years of age) with Down's syndrome,[24,25] all of which are associated with marked growth retardation. However, many commentators see such interventions as essentially cosmetic. The treatment of short stature for which no underlying disorder can be identified, in particular, poses problems as the risks and also the benefits in terms of final height are uncertain.[26] Children who are born small for gestational age usually experience catch-up growth by 2 years of age. In those who do not achieve this, growth hormone therapy can induce catch-up growth and improve childhood height scores; data on adult height are limited, however.[27] Guidelines suggest that therapy is justifiable in renal insufficiency and in Turner's syndrome,[10,28] but that evidence of benefit is lacking for other growth disorders including non-growth hormone deficient short stature and growth retardation associated with Down's syndrome.[10] It was considered that growth hormone should not be given to children with constitutional delay of growth.

Although sex hormones have effects on growth they may also cause premature closure of the epiphyses when given to prepubertal or pubertal children, and this has limited their use. Nonetheless, anabolic drugs such as testosterone,[29] oxandrolone[30] and fluoxymesterone[31] have been used in boys with constitutional delay of growth associated with delayed puberty (see also above) and oestrogens such as ethinylestradiol have been reported to increase growth rate in some girls, for example those with Turner's syndrome.[32]

A number of other drugs have been investigated in growth retardation. Clonidine, which can promote growth hormone-releasing hormone release, has been given to children with growth hormone deficiency as well as to short children without proven deficiency, but results have been contradictory and largely unsatisfactory.[33-35] A possible association of growth with zinc or vitamin A has led to preliminary studies of the benefits of supplementation with these agents.[36,37] Gonadorelin analogues have also been given with growth hormone to short girls without growth hormone deficiency, in an attempt to slow bone maturation and delay puberty, thereby improving adult height.[38] However, a decrease in bone mineral density may outweigh any modest increase in height.[39]


1. Rosenfeld RG, *et al.* Diagnostic controversy: the diagnosis of childhood growth hormone deficiency revisited. *J Clin Endocrinol Metab* 1995; **80:** 1532–40.
2. GH Research Society. Consensus guidelines for the diagnosis and treatment of growth hormone (GH) deficiency in childhood and adolescence: summary statement of the GH Research Society. *J Clin Endocrinol Metab* 2000; **85:** 3990–3.
3. Milner RDG, *et al.* Experience with human growth hormone in Great Britain: the report of the MRC working party. *Clin Endocrinol (Oxf)* 1979; **11:** 15–38.
4. Clayton PE, *et al.* Growth hormone state after completion of treatment with growth hormone. *Arch Dis Child* 1987; **62:** 222–6.
5. Leiper AD, *et al.* Growth in children treated for acute lymphoblastic leukaemia. *Lancet* 1988; **i:** 943.
6. Saggese G, *et al.* Effects of long-term treatment with growth hormone on bone and mineral metabolism in children with growth hormone deficiency. *J Pediatr* 1993; **122:** 37–45.
7. Hakeem V, *et al.* Intermittent versus continuous administration of growth hormone treatment. *Arch Dis Child* 1993; **68:** 783–4.
8. Smith PJ, *et al.* Single dose and pulsatile treatment with human growth hormone in growth hormone deficiency. *Arch Dis Child* 1987; **62:** 849–51.
9. Coste J, *et al.* Long term results of growth hormone treatment in France in children of short stature: population, register based study. *BMJ* 1997; **315:** 708–13.
10. Drug and Therapeutics Committee, Lawson Wilkins Pediatric Endocrine Society. Guidelines for the use of growth hormone in children with short stature. *J Pediatr* 1995; **127:** 857–67.
11. Carel J-C, *et al.* Adult height after long term treatment with recombinant growth hormone for idiopathic isolated growth hormone deficiency: observational follow up study of the French population based registry. *BMJ* 2002; **325:** 70–3.
12. Blethen SL, *et al.* Factors predicting the response to growth hormone (GH) therapy in prepubertal children with GH deficiency. *J Clin Endocrinol Metab* 1993; **76:** 574–9.
13. Smith PJ, *et al.* Contribution of dose and frequency of administration to the therapeutic effect of growth hormone. *Arch Dis Child* 1988; **63:** 491–4.
14. Wilson TA, *et al.* Update of guidelines for the use of growth hormone in children: the Lawson Wilkins Pediatric Endocrinology Society Drug and Therapeutics Committee. *J Pediatr* 2003; **143:** 415–21.
15. Wit JM, *et al.* Short-term effect on growth of two doses of GRF 1-44 in children with growth hormone deficiency: comparison with growth induced by methionyl-GH administration. *Horm Res* 1987; **27:** 181–9.
16. Ross RJM, *et al.* Treatment of growth hormone deficiency with growth-hormone-releasing hormone. *Lancet* 1987; **i:** 5–8.
17. Smith PJ, Brook CGD. Growth hormone releasing hormone or growth hormone treatment in growth hormone insufficiency? *Arch Dis Child* 1988; **63:** 629–34.
18. Mericq V, *et al.* Effects of eight months treatment with graded doses of a growth hormone (GH)-releasing peptide in GH-deficient children. *J Clin Endocrinol Metab* 1998; **83:** 2355–60.
19. Gondo RG, *et al.* Growth hormone-releasing peptide-2 stimulates GH secretion in GH-deficient patients with mutated GH-releasing hormone receptor. *J Clin Endocrinol Metab* 2001; **86:** 3279–83.
20. Cassorla F, *et al.* The effects of β-1-adrenergic blockade on the growth response to growth hormone (GH)-releasing hormone therapy in GH-deficient children. *J Clin Endocrinol Metab* 1995; **80:** 2997–3001.
21. Laron Z. Somatomedin-1 (insulin-like growth factor-I) in clinical use: facts and potential. *Drugs* 1993; **45:** 1–8.
22. Haffner D, *et al.* Effect of growth hormone treatment on the adult height of children with chronic renal failure. *N Engl J Med* 2000; **343:** 923–30.
23. Vimalachandra D, *et al.* Growth hormone for children with chronic renal failure. Available in The Cochrane Library; Issue 1. Chichester: John Wiley; 2004.
24. Annerén G, *et al.* Normalized growth velocity in children with Down's syndrome during growth hormone therapy. *J Intellect Disabil Res* 1993; **37:** 381–7.
25. Annerén G, *et al.* Growth hormone treatment in young children with Down's syndrome: effects on growth and psychomotor development. *Arch Dis Child* 1999; **80:** 334–8.
26. Bryant J, *et al.* Recombinant growth hormone for idiopathic short stature in children and adolescents. Available in The Cochrane Library; Issue 1. Chichester: John Wiley; 2004.
27. Lee PA, *et al.* International Small for Gestational Age Advisory Board consensus development conference statement: management of short children born small for gestational age, April 24–October 1, 2001. *Pediatrics* 2003; **111:** 1253–61.
28. National Institute for Clinical Excellence. Guidance on the use of human growth hormone (somatropin) in children with growth failure (May 2002). Available at: http://www.nice.org.uk/pdf/HGHinChild-42-ALS.pdf (accessed 01/04/04)
29. Brown DC, *et al.* A double blind, placebo controlled study of the effects of low dose testosterone undecanoate on the growth of small for age, prepubertal boys. *Arch Dis Child* 1995; **73:** 131–5.
30. Stanhope R, *et al.* Double blind placebo controlled trial of low dose oxandrolone in the treatment of boys with constitutional delay of growth and puberty. *Arch Dis Child* 1988; **63:** 501–5.
31. Strickland AL. Long-term results of treatment with low-dose fluoxymesterone in constitutional delay of growth and puberty and in genetic short stature. *Pediatrics* 1993; **91:** 716–20.
32. Ross JL, *et al.* A preliminary study of the effect of estrogen dose on growth in Turner's syndrome. *N Engl J Med* 1983; **309:** 1104–6.
33. Pintor C, *et al.* Clonidine treatment for short stature. *Lancet* 1987; **i:** 1226–30.
34. Pescovitz OH, Tan E. Lack of benefit of clonidine treatment for short stature in a double-blind, placebo-controlled trial. *Lancet* 1988; **ii:** 874–7.
35. Allen DB. Effects of nightly clonidine administration on growth velocity in short children without growth hormone deficiency: a double-blind, placebo-controlled study. *J Pediatr* 1993; **122:** 32–6.
36. Nakamura T, *et al.* Mild to moderate zinc deficiency in short children: effect of zinc supplementation on linear growth velocity. *J Pediatr* 1993; **123:** 65–9.
37. Evain-Brion D, *et al.* Vitamin A deficiency and nocturnal growth hormone secretion in short children. *Lancet* 1994; **343:** 87–8.
38. Saggese G, *et al.* Combination treatment with growth hormone and gonadotropin-releasing hormone analogs in short normal girls. *J Pediatr* 1995; **126:** 468–73.
39. Yanovski JA, *et al.* Treatment with a luteinizing hormone-releasing hormone agonist in adolescents with short stature. *N Engl J Med* 2003; **348:** 908–17.


### Hyperprolactinaemia

Hyperprolactinaemia is a condition of elevated circulating prolactin concentrations. It occurs for physiological reasons in pregnancy or following mechanical stimulation of the nipple, as in suckling. However, hyperprolactinaemia may also be induced pharmacologically as an adverse effect of drugs that inhibit dopaminergic function such as antipsychotics and metoclopramide; other drugs causing hyperprolactinaemia include opioid analgesics, methyldopa, reserpine, oestrogens, SSRIs, and verapamil. Furthermore, pathological hyperprolactinaemia may be associated with prolactin-secreting pituitary adenomas (prolactinomas), damage to the pituitary stalk or hypothalamus (including that caused by non-secreting tumours), or trauma to the chest wall; it may also be associated with disorders such as Cushing's syndrome or hypothyroidism. Prolactinomas are amongst the commonest pathological causes, and so-called idiopathic hyperprolactinaemia, in which no apparent cause is found, may in fact represent undetected microadenoma.

The consequences of hyperprolactinaemia include suppression of ovarian function in women, leading to erratic cycles or amenorrhoea, and infertility (see also above and below); in men, in whom the condition is less common, reduced gonadotrophin production leads to testosterone deficiency, diminished libido, and impotence. Both sexes may develop unwanted milk flow (galactorrhoea), although this depends on the concomitant presence of oestrogens; men may rarely develop gynaecomastia (p.1546) due to the change in oestrogen/androgen balance.

Management of hyperprolactinaemia depends on its cause. Pathological hyperprolactinaemia must be distinguished from physiological, and where it is secondary to another disease this should be managed appropriately; any drug thought likely to be causative should be withdrawn if possible. Some patients are asymptomatic, or are untroubled by their symptoms; whether such patients should be treated has been a matter of some controversy, although the risk of osteoporosis in women with prolonged suppression of ovarian function has been cited as a reason for such treatment.[1]

In many cases hyperprolactinaemia will be secondary to a prolactinoma. These are generally classified as microadenomas (less than 10 mm in size) or macroadenomas (over 10 mm in size); macroadenomas are often associated with prolactin concentrations more than 10 times the normal upper limit and their rapid expansion may result in visual defects and headache. Initially a course of treatment with a dopamine agonist such as bromocriptine, while rarely curative, is extremely effective in controlling hyperprolactinaemia and restoring gonadal function.[2-6] Surgical removal is now rarely indicated, although transsphenoidal decompression may be necessary for macroadenomas despite bromocriptine therapy, and ultimately radiotherapy may also be required.

The most extensively used dopamine agonist has been bromocriptine; it decreases prolactin secretion and reduces tumour size in the majority of patients.[5] There are reports of maintained normoprolactinaemia and reduced tumour size when bromocriptine has been withdrawn after about 2 to 4 years of treatment.[7] However, this occurs in only a minority of patients, and macroadenomas in particular can re-expand, sometimes rapidly, when treatment is stopped.[5] It has been suggested[6] that when the prolactin level has been normal for 2 years and the tumour has decreased by at least 50%, the dose of bromocriptine can be gradually reduced, with close follow-up to detect tumour enlargement. The short half-life and the adverse effects of bromocriptine may pose problems, although depot formulations can minimise these. Combination of oral prednisolone with intramuscular depot injection of bromocriptine has been reported to produce a reduced incidence of adverse effects.[8]

Treatment of hyperprolactinaemia restores ovulation in the majority of female patients. In those who become pregnant it is generally advised that fetal exposure to the dopamine agonist should be as short as possible, and therefore stopped when pregnancy is confirmed. Bromocriptine is the drug of choice for patients who are planning pregnancy, because most experience exists with its use compared with other dopamine agonists. The hyperoestrogenic state of pregnancy itself can stimulate prolactinoma growth and patients must be carefully monitored throughout gestation. If symptomatic tumour growth occurs, bromocriptine may be restarted, which is probably less harmful to the mother and fetus than surgery. Surgical debulking prior to pregnancy has been advocated by some, but may not prevent symptomatic tumour enlargement during pregnancy.[5,9]

More recently a number of alternative dopaminergic drugs have become available, including cabergoline, lisuride, metergoline, quinagolide, and terguride. All of these can suppress prolactin secretion, but it is not clear whether most of them offer much advantage over bromocriptine. Quinagolide appears to be of similar efficacy,[10,11] but may possibly be useful in patients intolerant of or unresponsive to other drugs.[12] However, cabergoline appears to be both more effective than bromocriptine[13-15] (and probably quinagolide[16]), and better tolerated, and as a result some centres now reportedly use it as first-line treatment in many hyperprolactinaemic patients,[17] although bromocriptine may still be favoured in women who wish to become pregnant. Pergolide has also been tried, with similar efficacy to bromocriptine, but it is not licensed for such use.[5]


1. Klibanski A, Greenspan SL. Increase in bone mass after treatment of hyperprolactinemic amenorrhea. *N Engl J Med* 1986; **315:** 542–6.
2. Ciccarelli E, Camanni F. Diagnosis and drug therapy of prolactinoma. *Drugs* 1996; **51:** 954–65.
3. Andrews DW. Pituitary adenomas. *Curr Opin Oncol* 1997; **9:** 55–60.
4. Molitch ME, *et al.* Therapeutic controversy: management of prolactinomas. *J Clin Endocrinol Metab* 1997; **82:** 996–1000.
5. Molitch ME. Medical management of prolactin-secreting pituitary adenomas. *Pituitary* 2002; **5:** 55–65.
6. Schlechte JA. Prolactinoma. *N Engl J Med* 2003; **349:** 2035–41.
7. Passos VQ, *et al.* Long-term follow-up of prolactinomas: normoprolactinemia after bromocriptine withdrawal. *J Clin Endocrinol Metab* 2002; **87:** 3578–82.
8. Jenkins PJ, *et al.* Oral prednisolone supplement abolishes the acute adverse effects following initiation of depot bromocriptine therapy. *Clin Endocrinol (Oxf)* 1996; **45:** 447–51.
9. Randeva HS, *et al.* Prolactinoma and pregnancy. *Br J Obstet Gynaecol* 2000; **107:** 1064–8.
10. Verhelst JA, *et al.* Acute and long-term effects of once-daily oral bromocriptine and a new long-acting non-ergot dopamine agonist, quinagolide, in the treatment of hyperprolactinemia: a double-blind study. *Acta Endocrinol (Copenh)* 1991; **125:** 385–91.
11. van der Heijden PFM, *et al.* CV205-502, a new dopamine agonist, versus bromocriptine in the treatment of hyperprolactinaemia. *Eur J Obstet Gynecol Reprod Biol* 1991; **40:** 111–18.
12. Vilar L, Burke CW. Quinagolide efficacy and tolerability in hyperprolactinaemic patients who are resistant to or intolerant of bromocriptine. *Clin Endocrinol (Oxf)* 1994; **41:** 821–6.
13. Webster J, *et al.* A comparison of cabergoline and bromocriptine in the treatment of hyperprolactinemic amenorrhea. *N Engl J Med* 1994; **331:** 904–9.
14. Pascal-Vigneron V, *et al.* Aménorrhée hyperprolactinémique: traitement par cabergoline versus bromocriptine. *Presse Med* 1995; **24:** 753–7.

15. Di Sarno A, *et al.* Resistance to cabergoline as compared with bromocriptine in hyperprolactinemia: prevalence, clinical definition, and therapeutic strategy. *J Clin Endocrinol Metab* 2001; **86:** 5256–61.
16. Giusti M, *et al.* A cross-over study with the two novel dopaminergic drugs cabergoline and quinagolide in hyperprolactinemic patients. *J Endocrinol Invest* 1994; **17:** 51–7.
17. Webster J. A comparative review of the tolerability profiles of dopamine agonists in the treatment of hyperprolactinaemia and inhibition of lactation. *Drug Safety* 1996; **14:** 228–38. Correction. *ibid.*; 342.

## Hypogonadism

Hypogonadism (decreased or absent gonadal function) may occur in both men and women, and may be either primary, due to some dysfunction of the gonads themselves, or secondary, due to hypopituitarism or some other cause of decreased gonadotrophic stimulation.

Causes of ovarian dysfunction are discussed under Ovarian Dysfunction, below. Primary testicular dysfunction may be due to congenital disorders such as Klinefelter's syndrome (associated with an XXY chromosome constitution); the effects of chemotherapy, radiotherapy, infections (particularly mumps), or trauma; and a few other conditions such as testicular degeneration.

Secondary hypogonadism may be due to general hypopituitarism, or to a specific deficiency of gonadotrophin production, or gonadorelin production. Kallmann's syndrome is a congenital disorder of hypogonadotrophic hypogonadism due to gonadorelin deficiency associated with anosmia or hyposmia. The causes of pituitary or hypothalamic failure include neoplasms, trauma, or infiltrative granulomatous diseases such as tuberculosis. Gonadotrophin production may also be suppressed by various drugs (notably exogenous sex steroids and continuous, rather than pulsatile, administration of gonadorelin analogues), by weight loss or inadequate nutrition, by excessive exercise, by severe systemic illness, and by hyperprolactinaemia (see above).

The fundamental treatment for primary hypogonadism is replacement therapy with sex hormones to produce appropriate sexual development and activity and counteract effects such as osteoporosis, but fertility cannot usually be restored. In prepubertal children, the induction of secondary sexual characteristics must be balanced against a possible reduction in final height due to stimulation of premature closure of the bone epiphyses. Women may be given an oestrogen with a progestogen (for a discussion on the management of ovarian dysfunction, see below) and men are treated with androgens, often in the form of a long-acting testosterone ester such as the cipionate or enantate given intramuscularly. The transdermal administration of testosterone is also effective.

The cause of secondary hypogonadism should be determined and managed appropriately if possible. In some cases this may be adequate to restore gonadal function but in other cases sex hormone replacement therapy as in primary hypogonadism will be required. Where there is no fundamental defect in gonadal function the possibility of using a gonadotrophic hormone or stimulating the release of gonadotrophins also exists. In general, however, such therapy is often reserved for patients desiring restoration of fertility, since it is inconvenient and expensive. For a discussion on the management of infertility including the use of agents such as clomifene, gonadotrophins, and the pulsatile administration of gonadorelin and its analogues in men and women with hypogonadism, see under Infertility, below.

## Infertility

Although about one couple in 6 may experience sufficient difficulty in conceiving children to seek medical help, most are subfertile rather than infertile, and may eventually conceive, with or without treatment. A number of possible treatments are available, but which is used depends upon the cause of the problem. Reduced fertility may have its origins in the male or the female partner or may be due to a combination of factors from both.[1-7]

The most obvious cause of infertility is a failure of either ovulation in the female or spermatogenesis in the male. Such failures may be due to damage or abnormal formation of the gonads, a failure of hypothalamic/pituitary stimulation, abnormal feedback as in the polycystic ovary syndrome, or suppression of gonadal function as in hyperprolactinaemia. These conditions and their management are briefly discussed under Hypogonadism (above), Ovarian Dysfunction (below), Polycystic Ovary Syndrome (below), and Hyperprolactinaemia (above).

The primary problem in about 25 to 30% of infertile couples is anovulation.[1] *Clomifene* has been reported to produce ovulation in up to 70% of anovulatory women,[1,2] or to increase the odds of ovulation more than 6 times in those with oligomenorrhoea,[8] although amenorrhoeic women are claimed to respond less well.[2] Because of concerns about a possibly increased risk of ovarian cancer opinion on the maximum number of cycles that clomifene should be used for varies (see p.1542). It has been suggested that no more than 6 cycles of clomifene therapy should be given: some consider that as few as 3 cycles of treatment at increasing doses are enough to tell if the patient will ovulate.[1,2] Combination of clomifene with a mid-cycle injection of *chorionic gonadotrophin* has also been tried,[2] with variable results.[9,10] *Tamoxifen* is an alternative in those who cannot tolerate clomifene,[11,12] and may be useful where abnormalities of cervical mucus contribute to infertility.

Direct administration of *gonadotrophins with follicle-stimulating activity*, such as human menopausal gonadotrophins or recombinant human follicle-stimulating hormone,[13,14] may be appropriate in hypogonadotrophic women with low oestrogen levels, and can be effective even in others.

The risks of ovarian hyperstimulation and multiple pregnancies are considerable however, and close monitoring is mandatory, using ovarian ultrasound to assess follicle development.[1,2] Once one to three follicles are sufficiently mature, chorionic gonadotrophin is given to induce ovulation, and thereafter for luteal support. Aggregate pregnancy rates of about 10 to 25% per cycle have been reported with such treatment.[1] Combination of gonadotrophin treatment with intra-uterine insemination may be more effective than either method alone.[15] Women with polycystic ovary syndrome (see below) respond less well to gonadotrophins than hypogonadotrophic patients,[1,2] and are at greater risk of the ovarian hyperstimulation syndrome.[2,16]

Another method used for anovulation is pulsatile administration of *gonadorelin*[16] (gonadotrophin-releasing hormone) or its analogues. It is primarily indicated in women with hypothalamic causes of anovulation, in whom pregnancy rates approaching 30% per cycle have been stated to occur,[1,2] and again is less effective in women with polycystic ovary syndrome than in hypogonadotrophic patients. However, the risks of ovarian hyperstimulation and multiple pregnancy are lower than with direct administration of gonadotrophins.

Where anovulation is secondary to hyperprolactinaemia treatment with dopamine agonists such as bromocriptine can restore fertility (see Hyperprolactinaemia, above). The use of bromocriptine in infertility of unknown cause does not seem to be justified.[1]

Current UK guidelines[16] recommend that ovulation disorders characterised by hypothalamic amenorrhoea or hypogonadotrophic hypogonadism should be offered gonadotrophins with luteinising hormone activity or pulsatile administration of gonadorelin. For those with ovulation disorders characterised by hypothalamic dysfunction, such as polycystic ovary syndrome, the treatment of choice is considered to be clomifene or tamoxifen. Women who ovulate with clomifene treatment but do not become pregnant within 6 months should be offered intra-uterine insemination in addition to clomifene. Patients who fail to ovulate with clomifene and have a body-mass of more than 25, may be given combined treatment with clomifene and metformin. Alternatively these patients may be treated with ovarian drilling (laparoscopic diathermy of follicles) or gonadotrophins; human menopausal gonadotrophin, urofollitropin, and recombinant follicle-stimulating hormone are considered to be equally effective.

Producing a response in men with impaired sperm production can be difficult.[3-6,17] In men with hypogonadotrophic hypogonadism, replacement therapy with a substance with luteinising hormone activity, such as chorionic gonadotrophin, is given to stimulate spermatogenesis and is followed if necessary by the addition of an agent such as menopausal gonadotrophins with follicle-stimulating and luteinising activity.[5,18,19] Treatment must often be continued for 12 months or more to permit development and maturation of spermatozoa, but 70% of these men have shown some degree of spermatogenesis with this therapy.[4] Once initiated, spermatogenesis may be maintained with chorionic gonadotrophin therapy alone. Pulsatile administration of gonadorelin may restore gonadotrophin secretion and correct infertility in men with hypogonadotrophic hypogonadism in whom the pituitary-gonadal axis is intact, such as those with Kallmann's syndrome.[19-21] Again, 12 months' therapy or more may be required.[4]

In idiopathic oligospermia, results of drug therapy have been disappointing, including trials with gonadorelin, and with testolactone and mesterolone; testosterone rebound therapy (in which high doses are given to suppress endogenous pituitary function, and then abruptly stopped, in the hope of provoking a rebound) is not recommended.[5] The anti-oestrogens, clomifene and tamoxifen have both been used in sub-fertile men,[5,6] but with little convincing evidence of benefit. Autoantibodies to spermatozoa in some men may interfere with sperm motility; immunosuppression with corticosteroids (prednisolone[22] or methylprednisolone[23]) has been associated with successful pregnancy in such cases, but the usual risks of corticosteroid therapy apply and must be balanced against the equivocal evidence of benefit;[4,6] such treatment is not recommended in UK guidelines.[16]

Where infertility is due to obstruction or inflammation of the fallopian tubes in the woman or the ductal system in the man treatment may be difficult, and the return of normal fertility unlikely. Microsurgical techniques may offer hope for a return of patency, but many patients will require *in-vitro* fertilisation in order to conceive. Where infection is the cause, appropriate anti-infective agents may be useful.[3,4,19] (See also under Pelvic Inflammatory Disease, p.139.)

Endometriosis (p.1546) is another important cause of infertility in women, although the reason for the association is not fully understood. Medical treatment of endometriosis does not enhance fertility, although conservative surgery may do so.[7,16]

In the absence of the above disorders and when infertility is otherwise unexplained the UK guidelines[16] indicate that treatment with clomifene should be offered.

Various other drugs have been used, on a more or less empirical basis, in the management of infertility. Such drugs include NSAIDs, guaifenesin to improve cervical mucus quality, kallidinogenase because of its supposed role in male genital-tract function, and pentoxifylline to increase sperm count and motility. Growth hormone or one of its analogues has been used as an adjunct to ovarian stimulation with gonadotrophins but is not considered to improve pregnancy rates.[16]

Where other methods fail, assisted reproduction may be considered, including *in-vitro* fertilisation or gamete or zygote intrafallopian transfer.[1,2,4,6] In particular, intracytoplasmic sperm injection has reportedly revolutionised the treatment of male factor infertility.[17,19] Gonadotrophins with or without clomifene, together with a gonadorelin analogue to desensitise the pituitary, are used to stimulate follicular maturation and ovulation so that the ova can be collected. So called 'long protocols' in which gonadorelin agonists are started in the midluteal phase of the menstrual cycle or earlier and are maintained until chorionic gonadotrophin is given, appear to give better results than short ('flare-up') or ultrashort regimens, in which gonadorelin agonists are given for less time.[24-26] One study has suggested that results may be better if nafarelin is used rather than leuprorelin.[27] Although individual studies[28] may suggest a difference in efficacy for recombinant follicle-stimulating hormone, urofollitropin, and human menopausal gonadotrophins a meta-analysis indicated that they were equally effective.[16] Gonadorelin (gonadotrophin-releasing hormone) antagonists such as cetrorelix have been used as an alternative to gonadorelin analogues for pituitary desensitisation[29] but may be associated with reduced pregnancy rates.[16] Progesterone is the preferred drug for luteal support for *in-vitro* fertilisation procedures because of the increased likelihood of ovarian hyperstimulation syndrome with chorionic gonadotrophin.[16]

1. Collins JA, Hughes EG. Pharmacological interventions for the induction of ovulation. *Drugs* 1995; **50:** 480–94.
2. Hamilton M. Treatment of infertility: anovulatory infertility in women. *Prescribers' J* 1996; **36:** 46–54.
3. Skakkebaek NE, *et al.* Pathogenesis and management of male infertility. *Lancet* 1994; **343:** 1473–9.
4. Wu FC-W. Treatment of infertility: infertility in men. *Prescribers' J* 1996; **36:** 55–61.
5. Howards SS. Treatment of male infertility. *N Engl J Med* 1995; **332:** 312–17.
6. Wardle PG. Treatment of male infertility. *Prescribers' J* 1990; **30:** 124–30.
7. Templeton A. Infertility and the establishment of pregnancy—overview. *Br Med Bull* 2000; **56:** 577–87.
8. Hughes E, *et al.* Clomiphene citrate for ovulation induction in women with oligo-amenorrhoea. Available in The Cochrane Library; Issue 1. Chichester: John Wiley; 2004.
9. Nash LD. The treatment of luteal phase dysfunction with clomiphene citrate and human chorionic gonadotrophin (HCG). *Infertility* 1982; **5:** 87–104.
10. Fisch P, *et al.* Unexplained infertility: evaluation of treatment with clomiphene citrate and human chorionic gonadotropin. *Fertil Steril* 1989; **51:** 828–33.
11. Messinis IE, Nillius SJ. Comparison between tamoxifen and clomiphene for induction of ovulation. *Acta Obstet Gynecol Scand* 1982; **61:** 377–9.

12. Roumen FJME, *et al.* Treatment of infertile women with a deficient postcoital test with two antiestrogens: clomiphene and tamoxifen. *Fertil Steril* 1984; **41:** 237–43.
13. Chuong CJ, *et al.* Successful pregnancy after treatment with recombinant human follicle stimulating hormone. *Lancet* 1993; **341:** 1101.
14. Hornnes P, *et al.* Recombinant human follicle-stimulating hormone treatment leads to normal follicular growth, estradiol secretion, and pregnancy in a World Health Organization group II anovulatory woman. *Fertil Steril* 1993; **60:** 724–6.
15. Guzick DS, *et al.* Efficacy of superovulation and intrauterine insemination in the treatment of infertility. *N Engl J Med* 1999; **340:** 177–83.
16. National Collaborating Centre for Women's and Children's Health. Fertility: assessment and treatment for people with fertility problems. February 2004. Available at: http://www.rcog.org.uk/resources/Public/Fertility_full.pdf (accessed 21/04/04)
17. Lewis-Jones DI, Gazvani MR. Male infertility: modern management and prognosis. *Br J Hosp Med* 1997; **58:** 271–6.
18. Finkel DM, *et al.* Stimulation of spermatogenesis by gonadotropins in men with hypogonadotropic hypogonadism. *N Engl J Med* 1985; **313:** 651–5.
19. Haidl G. Management strategies for male factor infertility. *Drugs* 2002; **62:** 1741–53.
20. Shargil AA. Treatment of idiopathic hypogonadotropic hypogonadism in men with luteinizing hormone-releasing hormone: a comparison of treatment with daily injections and with the pulsatile infusion pump. *Fertil Steril* 1987; **47:** 492–501.
21. Crowley WF, Whitcomb RW. Gonadotropin-releasing hormone deficiency in men: diagnosis and treatment with exogenous gonadotropin-releasing hormone. *Am J Obstet Gynecol* 1990; **163:** 1752–8.
22. Hendry WF, *et al.* Comparison of prednisolone and placebo in subfertile men with antibodies to spermatozoa. *Lancet* 1990; **335:** 85–8.
23. Shulman JF, Shulman S. Methylprednisolone treatment of immunologic infertility in the male. *Fertil Steril* 1982; **38:** 591–9.
24. Tan S-L, *et al.* Cumulative conception and live-birth rates after in vitro fertilization with and without the use of long, short, and ultrashort regimens of the gonadotropin-releasing hormone agonist buserelin. *Am J Obstet Gynecol* 1994; **171:** 513–20.
25. Filicori M, *et al.* Different gonadotropin and leuprorelin ovulation induction regimens markedly affect follicular fluid hormone levels and folliculogenesis. *Fertil Steril* 1996; **65:** 387–93.
26. Urbancsek J, Witthaus E. Midluteal buserelin is superior to early follicular phase buserelin in combined gonadotropin-releasing hormone analog and gonadotropin stimulation in in vitro fertilization. *Fertil Steril* 1996; **65:** 966–71.
27. Martin MC, *et al.* The choice of a gonadotropin-releasing hormone analog influences outcome of in vitro fertilization treatment. *Am J Obstet Gynecol* 1994; **170:** 1629–34.
28. Out HJ, *et al.* Recombinant follicle stimulating hormone (follitropin beta, Puregon) yields higher pregnancy rates in in vitro fertilization than urinary gonadotropins. *Fertil Steril* 1997; **68:** 138–42.
29. Olivennes F, *et al.* The use of a GnRH antagonist (Cetrorelix) in a single dose protocol in IVF-embryo transfer: a dose finding study of 3 versus 2 mg. *Hum Reprod* 1998; **13:** 2411–14.


### Lactation inhibition and induction

Lactation is the physiological secretion of milk post partum. Milk production by the breast is induced by prolactin while oxytocin promotes milk ejection into the milk ducts; both prolactin and oxytocin secretion are stimulated by suckling.

**Lactation inhibition.** The breast engorgement with consequent discomfort and galactorrhoea triggered by prolactin secretion post partum can be problematic in women who choose not to breast feed or are unable to do so. Nonsteroidal or synthetic oestrogens were historically used to suppress lactation in such women, but this use is now considered inappropriate because of an increased risk of thromboembolism. Bromocriptine is a potent inhibitor of prolactin secretion: it has been given post partum in short treatment courses (about 14 days) to suppress lactation[1,2] and is more effective than an oestrogen for this purpose.[2] However, bromocriptine is a potent drug which has also been associated with severe adverse effects in some women receiving it, and its use for lactation suppression is no longer advocated in a number of countries. Other dopaminergics with similar actions such as cabergoline, lisuride, metergoline, and quinagolide have also been used to suppress lactation. Although one commentator has suggested that cabergoline, which is generally better tolerated than bromocriptine, may be a better choice for lactation inhibition,[3] the same general objections as for bromocriptine apply to all these drugs. Non-pharmacological methods, such as the avoidance of nipple stimulation, and if necessary the use of mild analgesics, are generally to be preferred.

**Lactation induction.** Drug therapy has sometimes been used to help stimulate lactation, although mechanical stimulation of the nipple remains the primary method.[4] Dopamine antagonists, of which metoclopramide has been the most widely used, can produce modest increases in breast milk production but carry a risk of adverse effects including dystonias. If used, such therapy should be limited to 1 or 2 weeks; there has also been some concern about the presence of these drugs in breast milk.[4,5] Domperidone has also been reported to increase milk production,[6] and may cause fewer adverse central effects than metoclopramide. Nevertheless, the FDA has warned against the use of domperidone because of the potential risks of adverse effects in both mother and infant.[7] Protirelin has been given intranasally to stimulate lactation by increasing serum prolactin concentrations, but is expensive, and a suitable commercial preparation is unavailable.[4] The use of oxytocin nasal spray to promote milk ejection is not recommended, as mothers may become dependent upon its action.[4]


1. Duchesne C, Leke R. Bromocriptine mesylate for prevention of postpartum lactation. *Obstet Gynecol* 1981; **57:** 464–7.
2. Walker S, *et al.* Controlled trial of bromocriptine, quinoestrol, and placebo in suppression of puerperal lactation. *Lancet* 1975; **ii:** 842–5.
3. Webster J. A comparative review of the tolerability profiles of dopamine agonists in the treatment of hyperprolactinaemia and inhibition of lactation. *Drug Safety* 1996; **14:** 228–38. Correction. *ibid.*; 342.
4. Anderson PO, Valdés V. Increasing breast milk supply. *Clin Pharm* 1993; **12:** 479–80.
5. Kauppila A, *et al.* Metoclopramide and breast feeding: transfer into milk and the newborn. *Eur J Clin Pharmacol* 1983; **25:** 819–23.
6. da Silva OP, *et al.* Effect of domperidone on milk production in mothers of premature newborns: a randomized, double-blind, placebo-controlled trial. *Can Med Assoc J* 2001; **164:** 17–21.
7. FDA. FDA warns against women using unapproved drug, domperidone, to increase milk production (June 7, 2004). Available at: http://www.fda.gov/bbs/topics/ANSWERS/2004/ANS01292.html (accessed 30/06/04)


### Ovarian dysfunction

Primary ovarian dysfunction may be due to failure of the ovaries to form normally, as in Turner's syndrome (see below), or their degeneration before puberty; there may be premature failure, effectively an early menopause, due to low initial follicle numbers or to destruction of follicles by autoantibodies, chemotherapy, radiotherapy, infection, or trauma; or there may be some other condition such as the polycystic ovary syndrome (see below). Alternatively, ovarian dysfunction can be secondary to decreased gonadotrophic stimulation, which may occur with weight loss or due to a defect in the hypothalamic/pituitary axis (see also under Hypogonadism, above).

Primary dysfunction is often associated with high concentrations of circulating gonadotrophins, whereas in hypothalamic or pituitary dysfunction the gonadotrophin concentrations are of course low.

Women with primary ovarian dysfunction generally require HRT. Conception is rarely possible in such women. In women with chronic anovulation secondary to gonadotrophin deficiency due to hypothalamic or pituitary dysfunction, ovulation may be induced with clomifene, gonadotrophins, or the pulsatile administration of gonadorelin (see under Infertility, above).

**Polycystic ovary syndrome.** The polycystic ovary syndrome comprises enlargement of the ovaries with multiple follicular cysts and a thickened, whitish, capsule; there is persistent elevation of serum luteinising hormone concentrations, with a tendency to increased androgen and oestrogen concentrations. Women typically present with erratic menstruation, hirsutism, and obesity, although not all these features may be present; fertility is also often impaired. There is often associated hyperinsulinaemia with insulin resistance, and increased risk of developing hyperlipidaemia, hypertension, and ischaemic heart disease.[1]

Management is essentially symptomatic. Patients should be encouraged to lose weight if obese; weight loss alone may be sufficient to improve menstrual regularity, hirsutism, and fertility. Symptoms of hyperandrogenism can be treated with an anti-androgen, such as cyproterone acetate or spironolactone, with an oestrogen or a combined contraceptive pill;[2-5] flutamide has also been used as an anti-androgen in these patients (see also the discussion of the management of hirsutism, p.1545). In women who do not desire pregnancy, a low-dose oral contraceptive is also the recommended means of treating amenorrhoea or oligomenorrhoea.[3,4] Alternatively a progestogen that lacks androgenic properties may be given cyclically, in order to induce withdrawal bleeding (anovular women who do not receive hormonal treatment may be at increased risk of endometrial cancer).[3-5]

In patients who wish to conceive, clomifene citrate is the initial treatment of choice to induce ovulation, but although ovulation may be induced in up to 80% of cases, pregnancy rates are only about half this figure.[4] Tamoxifen may be used as an alternative. In patients who do not respond, a human menopausal gonadotrophin with follicle-stimulating activity may be tried (see also Infertility, above). Human gonadotrophins such as urofollitropin or recombinant follicle-stimulating hormone, which both lack luteinising hormone activity, may be preferable[6] as patients with polycystic ovary syndrome already have raised luteinising hormone concentrations. The use of pulsatile gonadorelin and its analogues in patients with polycystic ovary syndrome appears to be less effective than in hypogonadotrophic hypogonadism (see Infertility, above) and is held to be contra-indicated by some manufacturers. However, pretreatment with a gonadorelin analogue given continuously for 8 weeks, to suppress gonadotrophin production, before the pulsatile administration of gonadorelin, has produced improved ovulation and pregnancy rates.[7] Patients must be monitored carefully during any therapy to induce ovulation, as women with polycystic ovaries are more prone to multiple follicle development and ovarian hyperstimulation;[2] a low-dose regimen of follicle stimulating hormone has been reported to reduce this risk.[6,8]

Insulin resistance is a feature of polycystic ovary syndrome, particularly in obese women. Small non-randomised studies of metformin have reported improvements in insulin metabolism, a reduction in circulating androgen concentrations, small reductions in body-mass index or waist/hip ratio, and improvements in menstrual cycles.[9] Controlled studies have found that metformin alone can improve ovulation rates and menstrual cycles, and that rates can be improved further by the addition of clomifene citrate.[9,10] Metformin may also improve responses to ovulation induction using follicle-stimulating hormone.[9] Long-term effects of metformin in polycystic ovary syndrome have not been studied, however, and any reduction in cardiovascular risks is yet to be established. There has also been some interest in the use of thiazolidinediones, such as rosiglitazone, but these drugs can increase body-mass, which is undesirable in women who are already overweight.[9]

Occasional reports have suggested some benefit from octreotide[11] and bromocriptine[12] in normalising the hormonal environment; the latter is most likely to be useful in women with associated hyperprolactinaemia—see above.

An alternative to drug therapy is the use of laparoscopic ovarian diathermy, which appears to be as effective as gonadotrophin therapy in inducing ovulation in women resistant to clomifene, with reduced rates of multiple pregnancy.[13]


1. Lobo RA, Carmina E. The importance of diagnosing the polycystic ovary syndrome. *Ann Intern Med* 2000; **132:** 989–93.
2. White MC, Turner EI. Polycystic ovary syndrome 2: diagnosis and management. *Br J Hosp Med* 1994; **51:** 349–52. Correction. *ibid.*; **52:** 122.
3. Franks S. Polycystic ovary syndrome. *N Engl J Med* 1995; **333:** 853–61. Correction. *ibid.*; 1435.
4. Harrington DJ, Balen AH. Polycystic ovary syndrome: aetiology and management. *Br J Hosp Med* 1996; **56:** 17–20.
5. Anonymous. Tackling polycystic ovary syndrome. *Drug Ther Bull* 2001; **39:** 1–5.
6. Shoham Z, *et al.* Polycystic ovarian syndrome: safety and effectiveness of stepwise and low-dose administration of purified follicle-stimulating hormone. *Fertil Steril* 1991; **55:** 1051–6.
7. Filicori M, *et al.* Polycystic ovary syndrome: abnormalities and management with pulsatile gonadotropin-releasing hormone and gonadotropin-releasing hormone analogs. *Am J Obstet Gynecol* 1990; **163:** 1737–42.
8. White DM, *et al.* Induction of ovulation with low-dose gonadotropins in polycystic ovary syndrome: an analysis of 109 pregnancies in 225 women. *J Clin Endocrinol Metab* 1996; **81:** 3821–4.
9. Harborne L, *et al.* Descriptive review of the evidence for the use of metformin in polycystic ovary syndrome. *Lancet* 2003; **361:** 1894–1901.
10. Lord JM, *et al.* Insulin-sensitising drugs (metformin, troglitazone, rosiglitazone, pioglitazone, D-chiro-inositol) for polycystic ovary syndrome. Available in The Cochrane Library; Issue 1. Chichester: John Wiley; 2004.
11. Prelević GM, *et al.* Inhibitory effect of Sandostatin on secretion of luteinising hormone and ovarian steroids in polycystic ovary syndrome. *Lancet* 1990; **336:** 900–3.
12. Pehrson JJ, *et al.* Bromocriptine, sex steroid metabolism, and menstrual patterns in the polycystic ovary syndrome. *Ann Intern Med* 1986; **105:** 129–30.
13. Farquhar C, *et al.* Laparoscopic "drilling" by diathermy or laser for ovulation induction in anovulatory polycystic ovary syndrome. Available in The Cochrane Library; Issue 1. Chichester: John Wiley; 2004.


**Turner's syndrome.** Turner's syndrome is a congenital disorder associated with the absence of an X or Y chromosome, resulting in an individual with only a single X chromosome who is female in phenotype but in whom the ovaries do not develop. In addition to this gonadal dysgenesis, which results in infertility and primary amenorrhoea, various physical abnormalities may be present including short stature, a short webbed neck and characteristic facial appearance, shield-like chest, multiple naevi, and certain renal and cardiovascular abnormalities. Hypothyroidism and glucose intolerance may occur.

As with other forms of ovarian failure, HRT with oestrogen and intermittent progestogen is indicated in women with Turner's syndrome, in order to produce sexual maturation and the development of secondary sexual characteristics as well as to avoid complications such as osteoporosis. Clinical opinion has generally been that therapy should begin with low doses of oestrogen in girls of prepubertal age, gradually increasing the dose to promote slow development of secondary sexual characteristics and eventual breakthrough bleeding, at which point a cyclic progestogen should be added to oestrogen maintenance.[1-3] In the UK ethinylestradiol has been widely used in girls with Turner's syndrome, but commentators in both the UK and the USA suggest that this is inappropriate,[1,2] and that replacement should be with a natural oestrogen such as estradiol, in suitably modest doses. (Good comparative studies of these options are lacking.[4]) Application of a transdermal estradiol patch may be a convenient way to achieve oestrogen replacement in these women, although during adolescence oestrogen requirements are greater than those in normal menopausal women, for whom most transdermal formulations have been developed.[2] Oral contraceptives have been used for maintenance in adult women with Turner's syndrome (again often containing ethinylestradiol)[1] but it has been suggested that these supply too high a dose of oestrogen.[2]

A minority of patients with Turner's syndrome have some residual ovarian function, and there are a few reports of pregnancy in such patients.[2] In women without ovaries it may be possible to maintain pregnancy by appropriate endocrine replacement following implantation of a fertilised donor egg.

Short stature is the most common clinical manifestation of Turner's syndrome. Growth hormone therapy has been widely used and may be considered from as early as 2 years of age,[5] but there is considerable debate about the extent of the benefit in terms of final height. Results from 622 girls enrolled in the National Cooperative Growth Study[6] suggested a mean height gain of 6.4 ± 4.9 cm, and another cohort database[7] of 485 girls found that when treatment was started before puberty a mean increase in final height of 5 cm or more would be expected. A systematic review[8] of 4 controlled trials found that growth hormone increased short-term growth, but that there was limited controlled data on final height. It has been suggested[3] that a final height of 150 cm is an achievable goal for most patients. Growth hormone therapy during childhood and adolescence may also be important in maximising bone mass and reducing the risk of osteoporosis.[9] Although it is generally recommended that oestrogen replacement be delayed where growth promotion is a priority,[3,5] optimal oestrogen replacement therapy may also be important in maximising final height.[10] In a comparison[11] of the introduction of conjugated oestrogen therapy at 12 or 15 years of age, the combination of growth hormone and oestrogen initially stimulated growth velocity and bone maturation more than growth hormone alone, but subsequently declined after about 2 years. Patients who received growth hormone for a longer period before the initiation of oestrogen therapy attained greater adult height, a finding also noted in another study;[12] it was suggested that early use of growth hormone could allow oestrogen therapy to be begun at a more appropriate, younger age without compromising final height. Combination of growth hormone with a non-aromatisable anabolic steroid such as oxandrolone is recommended as an option in girls aged 8 to 12 years if therapy is begun late,[3] or if response to growth hormone is inadequate.[5]

Adult women with Turner's syndrome require multidisciplinary management including cardiovascular monitoring, psychological support, and a programme of prevention for diabetes, osteoporosis, and hypertension.[3,5]

1. Masters KW. Treatment of Turner's syndrome—a concern. *Lancet* 1996; **348:** 681–2.
2. Saenger P. Turner's syndrome. *N Engl J Med* 1996; **335:** 1749–54.
3. Saenger P, *et al.* Recommendations for the diagnosis and management of Turner syndrome. *J Clin Endocrinol Metab* 2001; **86:** 3061–9.
4. Conway GS, *et al.* Treatment of Turner's syndrome. *Lancet* 1996; **348:** 1590–1.
5. Frías JL, *et al.* Health supervision for children with Turner syndrome. *Pediatrics* 2003; **111:** 692–702.
6. Plotnick L, *et al.* Growth hormone treatment of girls with Turner syndrome: the National Cooperative Growth Study experience. *Pediatrics* 1998; **102:** 479–81.
7. Betts PR, *et al.* A decade of growth hormone treatment in girls with Turner syndrome in the UK. *Arch Dis Child* 1999; **80:** 221–5.
8. Cave CB, *et al.* Recombinant growth hormone in children and adolescents with Turner syndrome. Available in The Cochrane Library; Issue 1. Chichester: John Wiley; 2004.
9. Rubin K. Turner syndrome and osteoporosis: mechanisms and prognosis. *Pediatrics* 1998; **102** (suppl): 481–5.
10. Rosenfield RL, *et al.* Optimizing estrogen replacement treatment in Turner syndrome. *Pediatrics* 1998; **102** (suppl): 486–8.
11. Chernausek SD, *et al.* Growth hormone therapy of Turner syndrome: the impact of age of estrogen replacement on final height. *J Clin Endocrinol Metab* 2000; **85:** 2439–45.
12. Reiter EO, *et al.* Early initiation of growth hormone treatment allows age-appropriate estrogen use in Turner's syndrome. *J Clin Endocrinol Metab* 2001; **86:** 1936–41.

### Precocious puberty

Precocious puberty is commonly understood to mean the development of secondary sexual characteristics before the age of 8 years in girls or 9 years in boys; it is four to five times more common in girls. However, the age limit used to define precocious puberty in girls has been questioned.[1] Recent data from the United States suggests that puberty is occurring earlier in girls, at age 7 years for white girls, and 6 years for African-American girls. Precocious puberty is either central, due to premature activation of the hypothalamic-pituitary-gonadal axis, or peripheral, due to secretion of extrapituitary gonadotrophins or gonadal steroids independent of gonadorelin secretion from the hypothalamus or pituitary gonadotrophins. In many cases the cause is not apparent, and they are classified as idiopathic. A small proportion of cases are due to tumours. Central precocious puberty may be caused by CNS lesions secondary to diseases such as encephalitis, meningitis, or granuloma, or due to head trauma. Peripheral precocious puberty can be associated with congenital or familial syndromes such as McCune-Albright syndrome or familial testotoxicosis (familial male precocious puberty). Congenital adrenal hyperplasia (see p.1078) can also produce premature sexual development in boys and virilisation in girls.

Apart from early sexual maturation and the associated emotional distress, the chief clinical consequence of precocious puberty is short stature as an adult, due to premature closure of the epiphyses under the influence of sex steroids.[2-4]

Gonadorelin analogues have replaced drugs such as medroxyprogesterone acetate (which suppressed secondary sexual characteristics but were often ineffective in preventing epiphyseal fusion) as the treatment of choice in central precocious puberty.[3,4] The continuous rather than pulsatile administration of gonadorelin can paradoxically suppress gonadotrophin secretion by desensitisation and down regulation of pituitary receptors. Although originally given daily, by subcutaneous injection or nasal insufflation, intramuscular depot preparations[5,6] are more convenient, and are now more widely used.[4] Treatment with gonadorelin analogues suppresses sexual development and also skeletal maturation and most studies have reported an improvement in final height.[3,7,8] Cyproterone acetate has been given at the beginning of treatment to prevent the initial stimulatory effect of the gonadorelin analogue.[4] However, the treatment of girls with borderline early puberty (between 6 and 8 years of age) has been questioned, as studies suggest that most will reach adult height within the normal range without treatment.[1] Such girls with idiopathic slowly progressing puberty, and no evidence of advanced bone age, may not require gonadorelin therapy, but should be monitored for an onset of rapid pubertal development.[1,9] Children with concomitant growth hormone deficiency (for example after cranial irradiation) may need additional therapy with somatropin or its analogues for maximum benefit.[10] Discontinuation of treatment should be individualised on the basis of final height potential and the patient and family's wishes.[4]

In the peripheral forms of precocious puberty the gonadorelin analogues are ineffective.[3] Any underlying condition such as a gonadal or adrenal neoplasm should be sought and treated appropriately. Otherwise, therapy is aimed at suppressing premature sexual maturation. Medroxyprogesterone acetate retains some usefulness in these conditions.[3] In girls with precocious puberty associated with the McCune-Albright syndrome, the aromatase inhibitor testolactone has been used with some success to block oestrogen biosynthesis,[11,12] and tamoxifen has been reported to be beneficial.[13] Although ineffective when given alone, testolactone was reported to be of benefit when used with the anti-androgen, spironolactone, in boys with testotoxicosis;[14] a reduction in the rate of bone maturation was reported. Response diminished with long-term treatment, but could be restored by the addition of a gonadorelin analogue, deslorelin, to therapy.[15] This regimen has also been reported[16] to improve predicted adult height. Other drugs with anti-androgenic properties such as ketoconazole[4] have also been tried in boys with precocious puberty.

1. Kaplowitz PB, *et al.* Reexamination of the age limit for defining when puberty is precocious in girls in the United States: implications for evaluation and treatment. *Pediatrics* 1999; **104:** 936–41.
2. Anonymous. Precocious puberty. *Lancet* 1991; **337:** 1194–5.
3. Wheeler MD, Styne DM. Drug treatment in precocious puberty. *Drugs* 1991; **41:** 717–28.
4. Merke DP, Cutler GB. Evaluation and management of precocious puberty. *Arch Dis Child* 1996; **75:** 269–71.
5. Neely EK, *et al.* Two-year results of treatment with depot leuprolide acetate for central precocious puberty. *J Pediatr* 1992; **121:** 634–40.
6. Paterson WF, *et al.* Efficacy of Zoladex LA (goserelin) in the treatment of girls with central precocious or early puberty. *Arch Dis Child* 1998; **79:** 323–7.
7. Paul D, *et al.* Long term effect of gonadotropin-releasing hormone agonist therapy on final and near-final height in 26 children with true precocious puberty treated at a median age of less than 5 years. *J Clin Endocrinol Metab* 1995; **80:** 546–51.
8. Klein KO, *et al.* Increased final height in precocious puberty after long-term treatment with LHRH agonists: the National Institutes of Health experience. *J Clin Endocrinol Metab* 2001; **86:** 4711–16.
9. Léger J, *et al.* Do all girls with apparent idiopathic precocious puberty require gonadotropin-releasing hormone agonist treatment? *J Pediatr* 2000; **137:** 819–25.
10. Cara JF, *et al.* Height prognosis of children with true precocious puberty and growth hormone deficiency: effect of combination therapy with gonadotropin releasing hormone agonist and growth hormone. *J Pediatr* 1992; **120:** 709–15.
11. Feuillan PP, *et al.* Treatment of precocious puberty in the McCune-Albright syndrome with the aromatase inhibitor testolactone. *N Engl J Med* 1986; **315:** 1115–19.
12. Feuillan PP, *et al.* Long term testolactone therapy for precocious puberty in girls with the McCune-Albright syndrome. *J Clin Endocrinol Metab* 1993; **77:** 647–51.
13. Eugster EA, *et al.* Tamoxifen treatment for precocious puberty in McCune-Albright syndrome: a multicenter trial. *J Pediatr* 2003; **143:** 60–6.
14. Laue L, *et al.* Treatment of familial male precocious puberty with spironolactone and testolactone. *N Engl J Med* 1989; **320:** 496–502.
15. Laue L, *et al.* Treatment of familial male precocious puberty with spironolactone, testolactone, and deslorelin. *J Clin Endocrinol Metab* 1993; **76:** 151–5.
16. Leschek EW, *et al.* Six-year results of spironolactone and testolactone treatment of familial male-limited precocious puberty with addition of deslorelin after central puberty onset. *J Clin Endocrinol Metab* 1999; **84:** 175–8.

### Premenstrual syndrome

Gonadorelin analogues have been used to treat patients with severe symptoms attributable to the premenstrual syndrome (p.1551), with 'add-back' therapy with oestrogen plus progestogen to prevent the symptoms of oestrogen deficiency.

### Syndrome of inappropriate ADH secretion

In some patients secretion of antidiuretic hormone (ADH; vasopressin) occurs despite hypotonicity of the extracellular fluid and normal or raised fluid volume, and such patients are said to have the syndrome of inappropriate ADH secretion (SIADH). With severe water excess, the resultant hyponatraemia may result in symptoms ranging from lassitude or headache to profound neurological symptoms such as confusion, convulsions, or coma. Some patients may experience inappropriate thirst as well as ADH secretion, thus exacerbating their condition. For a discussion of sodium homoeostasis and dilutional hyponatraemia, see p.1220.

Conditions which may precipitate SIADH include CNS disorders, infections such as encephalitis and meningitis, head trauma, porphyria, or pulmonary diseases such as tuberculosis and pneumonia. ADH may also be secreted ectopically from a variety of malignancies, most commonly from small-cell bronchial carcinoma. Alternatively, SIADH may be drug-induced; drugs associated with the condition include carbamazepine, chlorpropamide, cytotoxic drugs such as cyclophosphamide and the vinca alkaloids, oxytocin, some antipsychotics, tricyclic antidepressants, and SSRIs.

Diagnosis of SIADH is initially prompted by the presence of hyponatraemia and corresponding plasma hypo-osmolality with or without neurological symptoms. Hypervolaemia, persistent excess sodium excretion, lack of oedema, and normality of both renal and adrenal function are confirmatory.

Mild degrees of water excess are frequently asymptomatic and may not require specific therapy, but patients with SIADH often have a more severe disorder and initially treatment is best aimed at the underlying cause. If such treatment is not possible or if symptoms persist, water restriction may be considered. However, fluid restriction is an unpleasant form of treatment, particularly for patients who retain inappropriate thirst, and may not be tolerable. In these patients demeclocycline may be given to antagonise the effect of ADH on the renal tubules. Lithium has been given as an alternative but has a high frequency of adverse effects, and phenytoin has been used occasionally to inhibit pituitary ADH secretion. Diuretics such as furosemide (used with oral sodium chloride) have also been tried in an attempt to optimise diuresis while retaining sodium. In patients with life-threatening severe acute water intoxication (see Hyponatraemia, p.1220), treatment initially involves cautious improvement of the profound hyponatraemia with intravenous infusion of hypertonic (usually 3%) or isotonic sodium chloride often with concurrent furosemide or other loop diuretic to avoid volume expansion. A group of drugs that act directly in the renal tubules as vasopressin $V_2$ receptor antagonists is under investigation.

References.


1. Kinzie BJ. Management of the syndrome of inappropriate secretion of antidiuretic hormone. *Clin Pharm* 1987; **6:** 625–33.
2. Kovacs L, Robertson GL. Syndrome of inappropriate antidiuresis. *Endocrinol Metab Clin North Am* 1992; **21:** 859–75.
3. Miller M. Syndromes of excess antidiuretic hormone release. *Crit Care Clin* 2001; **17:** 11–23.


## Abarelix *(USAN, rINN)*

PPI-149; R-3827. N-Acetyl-3-(2-naphthyl)-D-alanyl-4-chloro-D-phenylalanyl-3-(3-pyridyl)-D-alanyl-L-seryl-N-methyl-L-tyrosyl-D-asparaginyl-L-leucyl-$N^6$-isopropyl-L-lysyl-L-prolyl-D-alaninamide.

$C_{72}H_{95}ClN_{14}O_{14}$ = 1416.1.

*CAS — 183552-38-7.*

### Adverse Effects and Precautions

Immediate hypersensitivity reactions, including urticaria, pruritus, hypotension, and syncope, can occur with abarelix, and the cumulative risk of such a reaction increases with repeated doses. Patients should be monitored for at least 30 minutes after each injection. Hot flushes, sleep disturbance, breast enlargement and tenderness may result from testosterone reduction. Prolongation of the QT interval has occurred in patients receiving abarelix.

Elevations in transaminase concentrations have occurred, and liver function should be monitored before starting treatment, and periodically during treatment. The effectiveness of abarelix in the management of prostate cancer decreases with duration of therapy, and may be further reduced in patients weighing more than about 100 kg (225 pounds).

### Uses and Administration

Like cetrorelix (p.1320), abarelix is a gonadorelin (gonadotrophin-releasing hormone) antagonist. It is used to reduce testosterone concentrations in the palliative hormonal therapy of prostate cancer (p.521). A dose of abarelix 100 mg is given intramuscularly on days 1, 15, and 29, and then every 4 weeks thereafter.

Abarelix is under investigation for the treatment of endometriosis.

◊ References.


1. Tomera K, *et al.* The gonadotropin-releasing hormone antagonist abarelix depot versus luteinizing hormone releasing hormone agonists leuprolide or goserelin: initial results of endocrinological and biochemical efficacies in patients with prostate cancer. *J Urol (Baltimore)* 2001; **165:** 1585–9.


### Preparations

**Proprietary Preparations** (details are given in Part 3)
**USA:** Plenaxis.

## Atosiban *(BAN, USAN, rINN)*

ORF-22164; RWJ-22164. 1-(3-Mercaptopropionic acid)-2-[3-(p-ethoxyphenyl)-D-alanine]-4-L-threonine-8-L-ornithineoxytocin; [1-(3-Sulfanylpropanoyl),2-(4-O-ethyltyrosine),4-L-threonine-8-L-ornithine]oxytocin.

$C_{43}H_{67}N_{11}O_{12}S_2$ = 994.2.

*CAS — 90779-69-4.*

*ATC — G02CX01.*

### Adverse Effects and Precautions

Adverse effects reported in women receiving atosiban for premature labour include nausea and vomiting, headache, dizziness, flushes, tachycardia, hypotension, hyperglycaemia, and injection site reactions. Atosiban should not be used where continuation of pregnancy is hazardous to mother or fetus, including where gestational age is below 24 or over 33 weeks, in eclampsia or severe pre-eclampsia, intra-uterine growth retardation and abnormal fetal heart rate, suspected intra-uterine infection, placenta praevia, or abruptio placentae. Monitoring of uterine contractions and fetal heart rate is recommended during use, and blood loss should be monitored after delivery.

Although there has been some concern about fetal exposure, the manufacturers report that no specific adverse effects on the newborn have been reported.

### Pharmacokinetics

In women in premature labour, atosiban reaches steady-state plasma concentrations within one hour of the start of infusion, and has a terminal half-life of 1.7 hours after ceasing infusion. Atosiban is 46 to 48% bound to plasma proteins, and crosses the placenta. It is metabolised to an active metabolite, which is excreted in the urine; both atosiban and this metabolite are distributed into breast milk.

### Uses and Administration

Atosiban is a peptide analogue of oxytocin (p.1336) but with oxytocin antagonist properties. It is used as a tocolytic in the management of premature labour. Atosiban is given intravenously as the acetate, but doses are expressed in terms of the base. An initial bolus dose equivalent to atosiban 6.75 mg is given by intravenous injection (as a solution containing 7.5 mg/mL) over one minute. This is immediately followed by a continuous infusion of 300 micrograms/minute for 3 hours, then 100 micrograms/minute for up to 45 hours, as a solution containing 750 micrograms/mL. The total duration of treatment should not exceed 48 hours, and the total dose should not exceed 330 mg.

◊ References.


1. Valenzuela GJ, *et al.* Placental passage of the oxytocin antagonist atosiban. *Am J Obstet Gynecol* 1995; **172:** 1304–6.
2. Goodwin TM, *et al.* Dose ranging study of the oxytocin antagonist atosiban in the treatment of preterm labor. *Obstet Gynecol* 1996; **88:** 331–6.
3. Romero R, *et al.* An oxytocin receptor antagonist (atosiban) in the treatment of preterm labor: a randomized, double-blind, placebo-controlled trial with tocolytic rescue. *Am J Obstet Gynecol* 2000; **182:** 1173–83.
4. Valenzuela GJ, *et al.* Maintenance treatment of preterm labor with the oxytocin antagonist atosiban: the Atosiban PTL-098 Study Group. *Am J Obstet Gynecol* 2000; **182:** 1184–90.
5. Moutquin JM, *et al.* Double-blind, randomized, controlled trial of atosiban and ritodrine in the treatment of preterm labor: a multicenter effectiveness and safety study. *Am J Obstet Gynecol* 2000; **182:** 1191–9.
6. The Worldwide Atosiban versus Beta-agonists Study Group. Effectiveness and safety of the oxytocin antagonist atosiban versus beta-adrenergic agonists in the treatment of preterm labour. *Br J Obstet Gynaecol* 2001; **108:** 133–42.
7. The European Atosiban Study Group. The oxytocin antagonist atosiban versus the beta-agonist terbutaline in the treatment of preterm labor: a randomized, double-blind, controlled study. *Acta Obstet Gynecol Scand* 2001; **80:** 413–22.


### Preparations

**Proprietary Preparations** (details are given in Part 3)
**Arg.:** Tractocile; **Belg.:** Tractocile; **Denm.:** Tractocile; **Fin.:** Tractocile; **Fr.:** Tractocile; **Ger.:** Tractocile; **Hong Kong:** Tractocile; **Irl.:** Tractocile; **Ital.:** Tractocile; **Neth.:** Tractocile; **Norw.:** Tractocile; **NZ:** Tractocile; **Port.:** Tractocile; **Spain:** Tractocile; **Swed.:** Tractocile; **UK:** Tractocile.

# Buserelin *(BAN, rINN)*

Buserelinum; S74-6766. (6-O-tert-Butyl-D-serine)-des-10-glycinamidegonadorelin ethylamide; 5-Oxo-L-prolyl-L-histidyl-L-tryptophyl-L-seryl-L-tyrosyl-O-tert-butyl-D-seryl-L-leucyl-L-arginyl-N-ethyl-L-prolinamide.

$C_{60}H_{86}N_{16}O_{13}$ = 1239.4.

*CAS — 57982-77-1.*

*ATC — L02AE01.*

**Pharmacopoeias.** In *Eur.* (see p.vi).

**Ph. Eur. 5.0** (Buserelin). A white or slightly yellowish hygroscopic powder. Sparingly soluble in water and in dilute acids. Store at 2° to 8°. Protect from light and moisture.

## Buserelin Acetate *(BANM, USAN, rINNM)*

Acetato de buserelina; Hoe-766; D-Ser $(Bu^t)^6$ $Pro^9$ NEt LHRH acetate.

$C_{60}H_{86}N_{16}O_{13},C_2H_4O_2$ = 1299.5.

*CAS — 68630-75-1.*

*ATC — L02AE01.*

### Adverse Effects and Precautions

As for Gonadorelin, p.1325.

**Effects on the bones.** In a study[1] involving 46 patients with symptomatic locally advanced or metastatic prostate cancer, buserelin or triptorelin in various doses produced objective improvement in 26 of 35 given buserelin and 8 of 11 given triptorelin. However 17 of 32 patients who had bone pain at the start of treatment had an increase in bone pain which resolved after the first week; one patient who had no initial bone pain developed such pain on receiving the gonadorelin analogue. Additional symptoms included lymphoedema in 4, increased serum-creatinine concentration in 1, and one patient who developed signs of compression of the spinal cord with complete sphincter dysfunction and weakness in the legs.

To prevent adverse effects arising from the initial increase in circulating testosterone, cyproterone acetate has been given for 3 days before and for 1 week after initiation of gonadorelin analogue therapy.[2] Another anti-androgen, nilutamide, has been given with buserelin for a similar purpose.[3]

Bone loss has been reported in premenopausal women given buserelin for endometriosis.[4,5]


1. Waxman J, *et al.* Importance of early tumour exacerbation in patients treated with long acting analogues of gonadotrophin releasing hormone for advanced prostatic cancer. *BMJ* 1985; **291:** 1387–8.
2. Waxman J. Early tumour exacerbation in patients treated with long acting analogues of gonadotrophin releasing hormones. *BMJ* 1986; **292:** 58.
3. Kuhn J-M, *et al.* Prevention of the transient adverse effects of a gonadotropin-releasing hormone analogue (buserelin) in metastatic prostatic carcinoma by administration of an antiandrogen (nilutamide). *N Engl J Med* 1989; **321:** 413–18.
4. Matta WH, *et al.* Hypogonadism induced by luteinising hormone releasing hormone agonist analogues: effects on bone density in premenopausal women. *BMJ* 1987; **294:** 1523–4.
5. Devogelaer J-P, *et al.* LHRH analogues and bone loss. *Lancet* 1987; **i:** 1498.


**Effects on the cardiovascular system.** Hypertension in one patient associated with buserelin acetate.[1]


1. Barrett JFR, Dalton ME. Hypertension in association with buserelin. *BMJ* 1987; **294:** 1101.


### Interactions

As for Gonadorelin, p.1325.

### Pharmacokinetics

Buserelin is completely absorbed following subcutaneous injection, with peak plasma concentrations occurring about 1 hour after a dose. It accumulates in liver and kidneys as well as in the anterior pituitary. It is metabolised by tissue peptidases and is excreted in urine and bile as unchanged drug and metabolites. The half-life after injection is stated to be about 80 minutes.

### Uses and Administration

Buserelin is an analogue of gonadorelin (p.1325) with similar properties. It is used for the suppression of testosterone in the treatment of malignant neoplasms of the prostate; it is also used in the treatment of endometriosis and as an adjunct to ovulation induction with gonadotrophins in the treatment of infertility. It has also been used in precocious puberty and has been tried in the treatment of uterine fibroids (see below). Buserelin is usually given as the acetate but doses are expressed in terms of the base; 105 micrograms of buserelin acetate is approximately equivalent to 100 micrograms of buserelin.

In advanced prostatic carcinoma treatment is started with doses of 500 micrograms being injected subcutaneously every 8 hours for 7 days. On the eighth day treatment is changed to the nasal route with 100 micrograms sprayed into each nostril 6 times daily (usually before and after meals). An acceptable response should be achieved within 4 to 6 weeks. Since there is an initial increase in circulating testosterone, an anti-androgen such as cyproterone acetate may be given for at least 3 days before beginning buserelin therapy, and continued for at least 3 weeks, to avoid the risk of a disease flare. Long-acting subcutaneous depot preparations that release buserelin over a 2- or 3-month period are also available.

In endometriosis a dose of 150 micrograms is sprayed into each nostril three times daily. The usual duration of therapy is 6 months which should not be exceeded.

In infertility, pituitary desensitisation before ovulation induction with gonadotrophins is achieved by giving 150 micrograms intranasally four times daily, beginning either in the early follicular phase (day 1) or midluteal phase (day 21) of the menstrual cycle. Alternatively, 200 to 500 micrograms may be given daily as a subcutaneous injection. Therapy should be continued until pituitary downregulation occurs, which normally takes 1 to 3 weeks; if necessary 300 micrograms four times daily intranasally, or 500 micrograms twice daily subcutaneously may be given. Gonadotrophin treatment is then added to buserelin therapy until an appropriate stage of follicular development, when both are withdrawn and chorionic gonadotrophin is given to induce ovulation.

◊ General reviews of buserelin.


1. Brogden RN, *et al.* Buserelin: a review of its pharmacodynamic and pharmacokinetic properties, and clinical profile. *Drugs* 1990; **39:** 399–437.


**Endometriosis.** Gonadorelin analogues such as buserelin have a role in the management of endometriosis (p.1546), but the need for long-term therapy limits their value because of the risk of osteoporosis; 'add-back' therapy with concomitant hormone replacement can be used to prevent this.

References.


1. Lemay A, *et al.* Efficacy of intranasal or subcutaneous luteinizing hormone-releasing hormone agonist inhibition of ovarian function in the treatment of endometriosis. *Am J Obstet Gynecol* 1988; **158:** 233–6.
2. Donnez J, *et al.* Administration of nasal buserelin as compared with subcutaneous buserelin implant for endometriosis. *Fertil Steril* 1989; **52:** 27–30.
3. Nieto A, *et al.* Long term follow-up of endometriosis after two different therapies (gestrinone and buserelin). *Clin Exp Obstet Gynecol* 1996; **23:** 198–204.
4. Regidor P-A, *et al.* Long-term follow-up on the treatment of endometriosis with the GnRH-agonist buserelin acetate. *Eur J Obstet Gynecol Reprod Biol* 1997; **73:** 153–60.
5. Takeuchi H, *et al.* A prospective randomized study comparing endocrinological and clinical effects of two types of GnRH agonists in cases of uterine leiomyomas or endometriosis. *J Obstet Gynaecol Res* 2000; **26:** 325–31.

**Fibroids.** Like other gonadorelin analogues (see also p.1326) buserelin has been used to reduce the volume of uterine fibroids.

References.


1. Maheux R, *et al.* Use of intranasal luteinizing hormone-releasing hormone agonist in uterine leiomyomas. *Fertil Steril* 1987; **47:** 229–33.
2. Matta WHM, *et al.* Long-term follow-up of patients with uterine fibroids after treatment with the LHRH agonist buserelin. *Br J Obstet Gynaecol* 1989; **96:** 200–6.
3. Fedele L, *et al.* Intranasal buserelin versus surgery in the treatment of uterine leiomyomata: long-term follow-up. *Eur J Obstet Gynecol Reprod Biol* 1991; **38:** 53–7.
4. Ueki M, *et al.* Endocrinological and histological changes after treatment of uterine leiomyomas with danazol or buserelin. *J Obstet Gynaecol* 1995; **21:** 1–7.


**Infertility.** Buserelin is given with gonadotrophic hormone therapy for induction of ovulation and as an aid to improving *in-vitro* fertilisation procedures. Buserelin with gonadotrophic hormones has been found to result in pregnancies in women previously unresponsive to clomifene citrate,[1,2] although there may be a greater risk of multiple births.[3]

The regimens used in *in-vitro* fertilisation may be characterised as long, in which the gonadorelin analogue is given for 2 weeks or more; short, in which it is given for about 8 to 10 days of the menstrual cycle; and ultrashort, where it is given for 3 days only. A comparative study of such regimens found that the best results in all age groups were consistently associated with the long buserelin protocol.[4] The timing of buserelin administration may also be important. Starting buserelin in the midluteal phase of the cycle has been reported to produce more rapid pituitary down regulation and higher pregnancy rates from *in-vitro* fertilisation than when buserelin was begun in the early follicular phase.[5]

For a general discussion of the management of infertility, see p.1316.


1. Armitage M, *et al.* Successful treatment of infertility due to polycystic ovary disease using a combination of luteinising hormone releasing hormone agonist and low dosage menotrophin. *BMJ* 1987; **295:** 96.
2. Owen EJ, *et al.* The use of a short regimen of buserelin, a gonadotrophin-releasing hormone agonist, and human menopausal gonadotrophin in assisted conception cycles. *Hum Reprod* 1989; **4:** 749–53.
3. Rutherford AJ, *et al.* Improvement of in vitro fertilisation after treatment with buserelin, an agonist of luteinising hormone releasing hormone. *BMJ* 1988; **296:** 1765–8.
4. Tan S-L, *et al.* Cumulative conception and live-birth rates after in vitro fertilization with and without the use of long, short, and ultrashort regimens of the gonadotrophin-releasing hormone agonist buserelin. *Am J Obstet Gynecol* 1994; **171:** 513–20.
5. Urbancsek J, Witthaus E. Midluteal buserelin is superior to early follicular phase buserelin in combined gonadotropin-releasing hormone analog and gonadotropin stimulation in in vitro fertilization. *Fertil Steril* 1996; **65:** 966–71.


**Malignant neoplasms.** The long-term use of buserelin in men decreases the testicular concentration of testosterone. For this reason it is used in the treatment of prostatic cancer (p.521), which is androgen-dependent.[1-6] Gonadorelin analogues are an effective alternative to orchidectomy, sometimes combined with an anti-androgen for enhanced effect, and play a major role in the management of advanced, incurable disease.

Other reports of malignant neoplasms treated with buserelin include its use in metastatic breast cancer[7,8] (p.514).


1. Waxman JH, *et al.* Treatment with gonadotrophin releasing hormone analogue in advanced prostatic cancer. *BMJ* 1983; **286:** 1309–12.
2. Lock MTWT, *et al.* Long-term effects of buserelin on plasma testosterone and luteinizing hormone concentrations. *Lancet* 1985; **ii:** 1236–7.
3. Volmer MC, *et al.* Lung metastases of prostate carcinoma cleared by intranasal GRH analogue. *Lancet* 1985; **i:** 1507.
4. Klign JGM, *et al.* Combined treatment with buserelin and cyproterone acetate in metastatic prostatic carcinoma. *Lancet* 1985; **ii:** 493.
5. Labrie F, *et al.* Combined treatment with flutamide and surgical or medical (LHRH agonist) castration in metastatic prostatic cancer. *Lancet* 1986; **i:** 48–9.
6. Waxman J, *et al.* A pharmacological evaluation of a new 3-month depot preparation of buserelin for prostatic cancer. *Cancer Chemother Pharmacol* 1989; **25:** 219–20.
7. Klijn JGM, de Jong FH. Treatment with a luteinising-hormone-releasing-hormone analogue (buserelin) in premenopausal patients with metastatic breast cancer. *Lancet* 1982; **i:** 1213–16.
8. Falkson G, Falkson HC. CAF and nasal buserelin in the treatment of premenopausal women with metastatic breast cancer. *Eur J Cancer Clin Oncol* 1989; **25:** 737–41.


**Porphyria.** Buserelin given with medroxyprogesterone acetate suppressed cyclic and premenstrual exacerbations of porphyria (p.1040) in 2 patients. Doses used were 300 micrograms buserelin intranasally in the evenings of days 1 to 21 of the menstrual cycle and 10 mg medroxyprogesterone acetate daily by mouth from day 12 to 21. Both patients were free from porphyric attacks during the reported 11 months of treatment.[1] Intranasal buserelin has also been used in 1 patient to prevent premenstrual exacerbation of coproporphyria.[2] The initial dose of 900 micrograms daily could be tapered to 150 micrograms daily, with only 1 minor attack in 5 years of treatment. The authors of this report also noted a number of case reports of buserelin used in acute intermittent porphyria.


1. Bargetzi MJ, *et al.* Premenstrual exacerbations in hepatic porphyria: prevention by intermittent administration of an LH-RH agonist in combination with a gestagen. *JAMA* 1989; **261:** 864.
2. Yamamori I, *et al.* Prevention of premenstrual exacerbation of hereditary coproporphyria by gonadotropin-releasing hormone analogue. *Intern Med* 1999; **38:** 365–8.


**Precocious puberty.** The gonadorelin analogues have largely replaced other treatments in the management of central precocious puberty (p.1318). For some references to the use of buserelin in precocious puberty, see below.


1. Drop SLS, *et al.* The effect of treatment with an LH-RH agonist (buserelin) on gonadal activity growth and bone maturation in children with central precocious puberty. *Eur J Pediatr* 1987; **146:** 272–8.
2. Cacciari E, *et al.* Long-term follow-up and final height in girls with central precocious puberty treated with luteinizing hormone-releasing hormone analogue nasal spray. *Arch Pediatr Adolesc Med* 1994; **148:** 1194–9.
3. Juul A, *et al.* Serum insulin-like growth factor I (IGF-I) and IGF-binding protein 3 levels are increased in central precocious puberty: effects of two different treatment regimens with gonadotropin-releasing hormone agonists, without or in combination with an antiandrogen (cyproterone acetate). *J Clin Endocrinol Metab* 1995; **80:** 3059–67.
4. Bertelloni S, *et al.* Effect of central precocious puberty and gonadotropin-releasing hormone analogue treatment on peak bone mass and final height in females. *Eur J Pediatr* 1998; **157:** 363–7.


**Premenstrual syndrome.** For reference to the use of buserelin or other gonadorelin analogues with HRT to prevent menopausal symptoms in women unresponsive to other drug treatment, see under Gonadorelin, p.1326.

## Preparations

**Proprietary Preparations** (details are given in Part 3)
***Arg.:*** Suprefact; ***Austria:*** Suprecur; Suprefact; ***Belg.:*** Suprefact; ***Braz.:*** Suprefact; ***Canad.:*** Suprefact; ***Denm.:*** Suprecur; Suprefact; ***Fin.:*** Suprecur; Suprefact; ***Fr.:*** Bigonist; Suprefact; ***Ger.:*** Profact; Suprecur; ***Gr.:*** Suprefact; ***Hong Kong:*** Suprecur; Suprefact†; ***Irl.:*** Suprecur; Suprefact; ***Israel:*** Suprefact; ***Ital.:*** Suprefact; ***Malaysia:*** Suprefact; ***Mex.:*** Suprefact; ***Neth.:*** Suprecur; Suprefact; ***Norw.:*** Suprecur; Suprefact; ***NZ:*** Suprefact; ***Port.:*** Suprefact; ***S.Afr.:*** Suprefact; ***Singapore:*** Suprecur†; Suprefact; ***Spain:*** Suprefact; ***Swed.:*** Suprecur; Suprefact; ***Switz.:*** Suprefact; ***Thai.:*** Suprefact; ***UK:*** Suprecur; Suprefact.

# Carbetocin *(BAN, rINN)*

Carbetocina. 2,1-Desamino-4,1-desthio-$O^{4,2}$-methyl[1-homocysteine]oxytocin; 1-Butyric acid-2-[3-(*p*-methoxyphenyl)-L-alanine]oxytocin.

$C_{45}H_{69}N_{11}O_{12}S$ = 988.2.
*CAS — 37025-55-1.*
*ATC — H01BB03.*

## Profile

Carbetocin is a synthetic analogue of oxytocin (p.1336) reported to have a longer duration of action. For the prevention of uterine atony and excessive bleeding following caesarean section a single dose of 100 micrograms may be given by intravenous injection after delivery. It should not be given before delivery.

◊ References.


1. Sweeney G, *et al.* Pharmacokinetics of carbetocin, a long-acting oxytocin analogue, in nonpregnant women. *Curr Ther Res* 1990; **47:** 528–40.
2. Hunter DJS, *et al.* Effect of carbetocin, a long-acting oxytocin analog on the postpartum uterus. *Clin Pharmacol Ther* 1992; **52:** 60–7.
3. Dansereau J, *et al.* Double-blind comparison of carbetocin versus oxytocin in prevention of uterine atony after cesarean section. *Am J Obstet Gynecol* 1999; **180:** 670–6.


**Breast feeding.** In 5 lactating women who were 7 to 14 weeks postpartum, carbetocin was measured in the breast milk within 90 minutes of a single 70-microgram intramuscular dose.[1] The ratio of milk to plasma concentrations was low, suggesting that very little carbetocin was distributed into breast milk. The American Academy of Pediatrics considers that the use of carbetocin is usually compatible with breast feeding.[2]


1. Silcox J, *et al.* Transfer of carbetocin into human breast milk. *Obstet Gynecol* 1993; **82:** 456–9.
2. American Academy of Pediatrics. The transfer of drugs and other chemicals into human milk. *Pediatrics* 2001; **108:** 776–89. Correction. *ibid.*; 1029. Also available at: http://aappolicy.aappublications.org/cgi/content/full/pediatrics%3b108/3/776 (accessed 01/04/04)


## Preparations

**Proprietary Preparations** (details are given in Part 3)
***Arg.:*** Duratocin; ***Canad.:*** Duratocin; ***UK:*** Lonactene†.

# Cetrorelix Acetate *(BANM, USAN, rINNM)*

D-20761; NS-75A; SB-75 (cetrorelix); SB-075 (cetrorelix). *N*-Acetyl-3-(2-naphthyl)-D-alanyl-*p*-chloro-D-phenylalanyl-3-(3-pyridyl)-D-alanyl-L-seryl-L-tyrosyl-$N^5$-carbamoyl-D-ornithyl-L-leucyl-L-arginyl-L-prolyl-D-alaninamide acetate.

$C_{70}H_{92}ClN_{17}O_{14},xC_2H_4O_2$ = 1431.0 (cetrorelix).
*CAS — 120287-85-6 (cetrorelix); 145672-81-7 (cetrorelix acetate).*
*ATC — H01CC02.*

## Adverse Effects and Precautions

Transient reactions at the injection site, including erythema, pruritus, and swelling, may occur. Nausea and headache have been reported occasionally. Systemic hypersensitivity reactions have been reported rarely.

Cetrorelix should not be used in patients with moderate to severe renal or hepatic impairment.

## Pharmacokinetics

The bioavailability of cetrorelix after subcutaneous injection is about 85%. The mean terminal half-life after a subcutaneous injection of 3 mg is about 60 hours.

◊ References.


1. Pechstein B, *et al.* Pharmacokinetic-pharmacodynamic modeling of testosterone and luteinizing hormone suppression by cetrorelix in healthy volunteers. *J Clin Pharmacol* 2000; **40:** 266–74.
2. Nagaraja NV, *et al.* Pharmacokinetic and pharmacodynamic modeling of cetrorelix, an LH-RH antagonist, after subcutaneous administration in healthy premenopausal women. *Clin Pharmacol Ther* 2000; **68:** 617–25.


## Uses and Administration

Cetrorelix is a gonadorelin (gonadotrophin-releasing hormone) antagonist used as a component of ovarian stimulation regimens for assisted reproduction in infertility (p.1316). It has also been tried in benign prostatic hyperplasia and malignant neoplasms of the prostate, and for uterine fibroids. Cetrorelix is given by subcutaneous injection as the acetate; an intramuscular depot formulation containing cetrorelix embonate is reported to be under development. For assisted reproduction, doses of cetrorelix acetate equivalent to cetrorelix 250 micrograms daily may be given either in the morning beginning on day 5 or 6 of ovarian stimulation or in the evening beginning on day 5, and continued until ovulation induction. Alternatively a single dose equivalent to 3 mg of cetrorelix may be given on day 7; if follicle growth does not allow ovulation induction within 4 days, additional doses of cetrorelix 250 micrograms once daily may be given until the day of ovulation induction.

◊ References.


1. Albano C, *et al.* Comparison of different doses of gonadotropin-releasing hormone antagonist cetrorelix during controlled ovarian hyperstimulation. *Fertil Steril* 1997; **67:** 917–22.
2. Gonzalez-Barcena D, *et al.* Treatment of uterine leiomyomas with luteinizing hormone-releasing hormone antagonist cetrorelix. *Hum Reprod* 1997; **12:** 2028–35.
3. Comaru-Schally AM, *et al.* Efficacy and safety of luteinizing hormone-releasing hormone antagonist cetrorelix in the treatment of symptomatic benign prostatic hyperplasia. *J Clin Endocrinol Metab* 1998; **83:** 3826–31.
4. Felberbaum RE, *et al.* Treatment of uterine fibroids with a slow-release formulation of the gonadotrophin releasing hormone antagonist cetrorelix. *Hum Reprod* 1998; **13:** 1660–8.
5. Duijkers IJ, *et al.* Single and multiple dose pharmacokinetics of the gonadotrophin-releasing hormone antagonist cetrorelix in healthy female volunteers. *Hum Reprod* 1998; **13:** 2392–8.
6. Olivennes F, *et al.* The use of a GnRH antagonist (cetrorelix) in a single dose protocol in IVF-embryo transfer: a dose finding study of 3 versus 2 mg. *Hum Reprod* 1998; **13:** 2411–14.
7. Huirne JAF, Lambalk CB. Gonadotropin-releasing-hormone-receptor antagonists. *Lancet* 2001; **358:** 1793–1803.


## Preparations

**Proprietary Preparations** (details are given in Part 3)
***Arg.:*** Cetrotide; ***Austral.:*** Cetrotide; ***Austria:*** Cetrotide; ***Belg.:*** Cetrotide†; ***Denm.:*** Cetrotide; ***Fin.:*** Cetrotide; ***Fr.:*** Cetrotide; ***Ger.:*** Cetrotide; ***Gr.:*** Cetrotide; ***Hong Kong:*** Cetrotide; ***Israel:*** Cetrotide; ***Ital.:*** Cetrotide; ***Neth.:*** Cetrotide; ***Norw.:*** Cetrotide; ***NZ:*** Cetrotide; ***Port.:*** Cetrotide; ***Singapore:*** Cetrotide; ***Spain:*** Cetrotide; ***Swed.:*** Cetrotide; ***Thai.:*** Cetrotide; ***UK:*** Cetrotide; ***USA:*** Cetrotide.

# Chorionic Gonadotrophin *(BAN, rINN)*

CG; Choriogonadotrophin; Chorionic Gonadotropin; Gonadotrofina coriónica; Gonadotrophinum Chorionicum; Gonadotropinum Chorionicum; HCG; hCG; Human Chorionic Gonadotrophin; Pregnancy-urine Hormone; PU.

*CAS — 9002-61-3.*
*ATC — G03GA01.*

**Pharmacopoeias.** In *Chin., Eur.* (see p.vi), *Jpn,* and *US.*

**Ph. Eur. 5.0** (Gonadotrophin, Chorionic). A dry preparation of placental glycoproteins extracted from the urine of pregnant women. The potency is not less than 2500 units/mg. A white to yellowish-white, amorphous powder. Soluble in water. Store at 2° to 8° in airtight containers. Protect from light.

**USP 27** (Chorionic Gonadotropin). A gonad-stimulating polypeptide hormone obtained from the urine of pregnant women. It has a potency of not less than 1500 USP units/mg. A white or practically white, amorphous powder. Freely soluble in water. Store in airtight containers at 2° to 8°.

# Choriogonadotropin Alfa *(BAN, USAN, rINN)*

Coriogonadotropina alfa.

*CAS — 177073-44-8 (choriogonadotropin alfa); 56832-30-5 (α subunit); 56832-34-9 (β subunit).*
*ATC — G03GA08.*

## Adverse Effects and Precautions

Side-effects that have been reported with chorionic gonadotrophin include headache, tiredness, changes in mood, depression, restlessness, oedema (especially in males), and pain on injection. Treatment for cryptorchidism may produce premature epiphyseal closure or precocious puberty. Gynaecomastia has been reported. Ovarian hyperstimulation may occur, with marked ovarian enlargement or cyst formation, acute abdominal pain, ascites, pleural effusion, hypovolaemia, shock, and thromboembolic disorders in severe cases.

Chorionic gonadotrophin should be given with care to patients in whom androgen-induced fluid retention might be a hazard as in asthma, epilepsy, migraine, or cardiovascular disorders, including hypertension, or renal disorders. Hypersensitivity reactions may occur and it is recommended that patients suspected to be susceptible should be given skin tests before treatment. It should not be given to patients with disorders that might be exacerbated by androgen release such as carcinoma of the prostate or precocious puberty. Use should also be avoided in the presence of breast, uterine, ovarian, and testicular tumours, as well as tumours of the hypothalamus, pituitary, thyroid, and adrenal glands.

## Pharmacokinetics

Following intramuscular administration peak concentrations of chorionic gonadotrophin occur about 6 hours after a dose. It is distributed primarily to the gonads. Blood concentrations decline in a biphasic manner, with half-lives of about 6 to 11 hours and 23 to 38 hours, respectively. About 10 to 12% of an intramuscular dose is excreted in urine within 24 hours.

Following subcutaneous administration, choriogonadotropin alfa has a bioavailability of about 40%. It is metabolised and excreted similarly to chorionic gonadotrophin.

## Uses and Administration

Chorionic gonadotrophin is a hormone produced by the placenta and obtained from the urine of pregnant women. Its effects are predominantly those of the gonadotrophin, luteinising hormone (p.1332), which is responsible for triggering ovulation and formation of the corpus luteum in women, and stimulates the production of testosterone by the testes in men. Choriogonadotropin alfa is a recombinant form of chorionic gonadotrophin.

Chorionic gonadotrophin is given to women with anovulatory infertility due to absent or low concentrations of gonadotrophins, to induce ovulation after follicular development has been stimulated with follicle-stimulating hormone or human menopausal gonadotrophins. A single dose of 5000 to 10 000 units of chorionic gonadotrophin is given by intramuscular injection to mimic the midcycle peak of luteinising hormone which normally stimulates ovulation. Up to 3 repeat injections of up to 5000 units each may be given within the following 9 days to prevent insufficiency of the corpus luteum. Chorionic gonadotrophin is also given with menotrophin and sometimes also clomifene citrate as an adjunct to *in-vitro* fertilisation procedures and other assisted conception techniques involving superovulation and oocyte collection.

Choriogonadotropin alfa is used similarly to induce ovulation in the treatment of anovulatory infertility, or as an adjunct to *in-vitro* fertilisation procedures and other assisted conception techniques. A single dose of 250 micrograms is given, by subcutaneous injection, when optimal stimulation of follicular growth is achieved.

In males, chorionic gonadotrophin has been used in the treatment of prepubertal cryptorchidism. Regimens vary widely, but doses usually range from 500 to 4000 units three times weekly by intramuscular injection.

Chorionic gonadotrophin is also given for male infertility associated with hypogonadotrophic hypogonadism. Again, there is considerable variation in the dosage regimen, and doses have varied from 500 to 4000 units two to three times weekly by intramuscular injection. A drug with follicle-stimulating activity such as menotrophin is often added to enable normal spermatogenesis.

In the treatment of delayed puberty associated with hypogonadism in males, an initial dose of chorionic gonadotrophin 500 to 1500 units is given twice weekly by intramuscular injection; the dose should be titrated against plasma-testosterone concentration.

Chorionic gonadotrophin has also been administered by subcutaneous injection.

**Cryptorchidism.** Although surgery remains the treatment with the best success rate in cryptorchidism it is often reserved for boys who do not respond to a trial of hormonal therapy (see p.1313). Gonadorelin or chorionic gonadotrophin appear to be of some benefit, although only a minority of cases will respond;[1] they may be given in combination.[2] Chorionic gonadotrophin is also used as an adjuvant to surgery, to render the testes palpable.[3]

1. Pyörälä S, *et al.* A review and meta-analysis of hormonal treatment of cryptorchidism. *J Clin Endocrinol Metab* 1995; **80:** 2795–9.
2. Nane I, *et al.* Primary gonadotropin releasing hormone and adjunctive human chorionic gonadotropin treatment in cryptorchidism: a clinical trial. *Urology* 1997; **49:** 108–11.
3. Polascik TJ, *et al.* Reappraisal of the role of human chorionic gonadotropin in the diagnosis and treatment of the nonpalpable testis: a 10-year experience. *J Urol (Baltimore)* 1996; **156:** 804–6.

**Delayed puberty.** Use of chorionic gonadotrophin may be appropriate in boys with delayed puberty due to hypogonadotrophic hypogonadism (p.1314).

**Infertility.** In women with anovulatory infertility chorionic gonadotrophin and choriogonadotropin alfa can be used to provoke ovulation and provide luteal support once maturation of a suitable number of follicles has been stimulated by other means. They are used similarly in the various protocols for assisted reproduction. However, use is not recommended in patients at risk of ovarian hyperstimulation, such as those with polycystic ovary syndrome. In men with hypogonadotrophic hypogonadism chorionic gonadotrophin is used to stimulate and maintain spermatogenesis. The management of male and female infertility, including the role of chorionic gonadotrophin, is discussed on p.1316.

**Malignant neoplasms.** Control of Kaposi's sarcoma (p.524) has been reported in a few patients given high-dose intramuscular chorionic gonadotrophin, but regrowth occurred when dosage was reduced or withdrawn.[1] Another study, using lower doses, was discontinued due to toxicity and lack of benefit,[2] but others have confirmed benefit following intralesional injection.[3] There is some suggestion that preparations vary in their activity against the tumour, and that it is not chorionic gonadotrophin itself, but some impurity, (perhaps a ribonuclease[4] or the degradation product of the β-subunit[5]) which is the active principle.[3,6,7] Some contaminants may have a stimulant effect on the neoplasm, which might also contribute to the variable results.[5]

Chorionic gonadotrophin has also been investigated[8] in the treatment of acute myeloid leukaemias (p.506).

1. Harris PJ. Treatment of Kaposi's sarcoma and other manifestations of AIDS with human chorionic gonadotropin. *Lancet* 1995; **346:** 118–19.
2. Bower M, *et al.* Human chorionic gonadotropin for AIDS-related Kaposi's sarcoma. *Lancet* 1995; **346:** 642.
3. Gill PS, *et al.* The effects of preparations of human chorionic gonadotropin on AIDS-related Kaposi's sarcoma. *N Engl J Med* 1996; **335:** 1261–9. Correction. *ibid.* 1997; **336:** 1115.
4. Griffiths SJ, *et al.* Ribonuclease inhibits Kaposi's sarcoma. *Nature* 1997; **390:** 568.
5. Simonart T, *et al.* Treatment of Kaposi's sarcoma with human chorionic gonadotropin. *Dermatology* 2002; **204:** 330–3.
6. Gill PS, *et al.* Intralesional human chorionic gonadotropin for Kaposi's sarcoma. *N Engl J Med* 1997; **336:** 1188.
7. von Overbeck J, *et al.* Human chorionic gonadotropin for AIDS-related Kaposi's sarcoma. *Lancet* 1995; **346:** 642–3.
8. Feldman EJ, *et al.* In vitro effects and clinical evaluation of a human chorionic gonadotrophin preparation in acute leukemia. *Leukemia* 1998; **12:** 1749–55.

**Obesity.** A meta-analysis[1] involving 24 trials concluded that there was no evidence that chorionic gonadotrophin was effective in the treatment of obesity (p.1583).

1. Lijesen GKS, *et al.* The effect of human chorionic gonadotropin (HCG) in the treatment of obesity by means of the Simeons therapy: a criteria-based meta-analysis. *Br J Clin Pharmacol* 1995; **40:** 237–43.

## Preparations

***BP 2003:*** Chorionic Gonadotrophin Injection;
***USP 27:*** Chorionic Gonadotropin for Injection.

**Proprietary Preparations** (details are given in Part 3)
***Arg.:*** Endocorion; Gonacor; Ovidrel; Pregnyl; Profasi; ***Austral.:*** APL†; Pregnyl; Profasi; ***Austria:*** Pregnyl; Profasi; ***Belg.:*** Pregnyl; ***Braz.:*** Choragon†; Pregnyl; Profasi HP; ***Canad.:*** APL†; Pregnyl; Profasi HP; ***Chile:*** APL; Pregnyl; Profasi; ***Denm.:*** Ovitrelle; Pregnyl; Profasi; ***Fin.:*** Ovitrelle; Pregnyl; Profasi; ***Ger.:*** Choragon; Ovitrelle; Predalon; Pregnesin; Primogonyl; ***Gr.:*** Pregnyl; Profasi; ***Hong Kong:*** Choriomon; Ovidrel; Pregnyl; Profasi; ***India:*** Corion; Profasi; Pubergen; ***Irl.:*** Choragon†; Gonadotraphon LH†; Pregnyl; Profasi; ***Israel:*** Chorigon; Pregnyl; ***Ital.:*** Gonasi HP; Pregnyl; Profasi HP; ***Malaysia:*** Pregnyl; Profasi; ***Mex.:*** Gonadotropyl C; Gonaplex†; Gonasone†; Pregnyl; Profasi; ***Neth.:*** Ovitrelle; Pregnyl; Profasi; ***Norw.:*** Ovitrelle; Pregnyl; Profasi; ***NZ:*** Pregnyl†; Profasi; ***Port.:*** Ovitrelle; Pregnyl; Profasi HP; ***S.Afr.:*** APL†; Pregnyl; Profasi; ***Singapore:*** Pregnyl; Profasi; ***Spain:*** Ovidrelle; Physex†; Pregnyl†; Profasi HP; ***Swed.:*** Ovitrelle; Pregnyl; Profasi; ***Switz.:*** Choriomon; Pregnyl; Profasi; ***Thai.:*** Pregnyl; Profasi; ***UK:*** Choragon; Ovitrelle; Pregnyl; Profasi†; ***USA:*** APL†; Chorex; Choron; Gonic; Novarel; Ovidrel; Pregnyl; Profasi.

**Multi-ingredient:** ***Ger.:*** AntiFocal N; NeyNormin N (Revitorgan-Dilutionen N Nr 65); ***Mex.:*** Gonakor.

## Corticorelin *(rINN)*

Corticoliberin; Corticorelina; Corticotrophin-releasing Hormone; Corticotropin-releasing Factor; CRF; CRH.

$C_{208}H_{344}N_{60}O_{63}S_2$ = 4757.5 (human);
$C_{205}H_{339}N_{59}O_{63}S$ = 4670.3 (ovine).
*CAS — 86784-80-7 (corticorelin (human)); 79804-71-0 (corticorelin (ovine)).*
*ATC — V04CD04.*

## Corticorelin Triflutate *(rINNM)*

Corticorelin Trifluoroacetate.

$C_{205}H_{339}N_{59}O_{63}S,xC_2HF_3O_2$ (ovine).
*CAS — 121249-14-7 (corticorelin ovine triflutate).*
*ATC — V04CD04.*

NOTE. Corticorelin Ovine Triflutate is *USAN.*

## Adverse Effects

Flushing of the face, neck, and upper chest, and mild dyspnoea may follow intravenous injection of corticorelin, and last for about 3 to 5 minutes. Prolonged flushing, tachycardia, hypotension, and chest tightness have been reported following large doses.

**Effects on the cardiovascular system.** Loss of consciousness, lasting for 10 seconds to 5 minutes, occurred in 3 patients, two of whom had Cushing's disease and one who had secondary adrenal insufficiency, following intravenous injection of corticorelin 200 micrograms.[1] The 2 patients with Cushing's disease had a slight accompanying fall in blood pressure. In a fourth patient, receiving corticosteroid and thyroid hormone replacement therapy, injection of corticorelin was associated with a sharp fall in systolic blood pressure and subsequent asystole. These serious side-effects were not noted by others[2,3] and were variously attributed to impurities,[2] high dosage,[2] vasovagal syncope,[3] or to the fact that the corticorelin used in the study was of ovine rather than human origin.[3] The authors of the original study[1] have since stated[4] that lowering of the dose from 200 micrograms given intravenously over 10 seconds to 100 micrograms over 60 seconds has stopped serious adverse effects but that ovine corticorelin was still preferred because of its longer duration of action and lower incidence of hypotensive adverse effects. There has, however, been a further report of chest pain accompanied by a fall in blood pressure in a patient receiving corticorelin at a dose of 100 micrograms.[5]

1. Hermus A, *et al.* Serious reactions to corticotropin-releasing factor. *Lancet* 1983; **i:** 776.
2. Schulte HM, *et al.* Safety of corticotropin-releasing factor. *Lancet* 1983; **i:** 1222.
3. Oppermann D. Safety of human and ovine corticotropin-releasing hormone. *Lancet* 1986; **ii:** 1031–2.
4. Hermus ARMM, *et al.* Safety of human and ovine corticotropin-releasing hormone. *Lancet* 1986; **ii:** 1032–3.
5. Paloma VC, *et al.* Chest pain after intravenous corticotropin-releasing hormone. *Lancet* 1989; **i:** 222.

## Uses and Administration

Corticorelin is a polypeptide hypothalamic releasing hormone that stimulates the release of corticotropin (p.1322) from the anterior pituitary. It is used in the differential diagnosis of Cushing's syndrome (p.1313) and other adrenal disorders. Corticorelin is usually given as the triflutate, but doses are expressed in terms of corticorelin (human or ovine). Doses of 100 micrograms, or of 1 microgram/kg, are given by intravenous injection over 30 seconds. Higher doses and more rapid administration have been used but may be associated with an increased risk of adverse effects (see above).

It is also under investigation in other disorders including asthma and cerebral oedema.

**Administration.** Corticorelin was well absorbed following subcutaneous injection and bioavailability was calculated to be about 60 to 70%; absorption was slower with high doses, suggesting that it may be a saturable process. Given the preservation of bioactivity, the subcutaneous route was considered an attractive alternative to intravenous administration.[1]

1. Angst MS, *et al.* Pharmacokinetics, cortisol release, and hemodynamics after intravenous and subcutaneous injection of human corticotropin-releasing factor in humans. *Clin Pharmacol Ther* 1998; **64:** 499–510.

**Diagnosis and testing.** Corticorelin may be used in the diagnosis of adrenal disorders including Cushing's syndrome (p.1313). In the initial diagnosis of Cushing's syndrome, a dexamethasone-corticorelin test may be used to identify pseudo-Cushing's conditions such as depression or alcoholism in patients with mild hypercortisolism and equivocal results on other diagnostic tests. This combination is reportedly more accurate than either alone,[1] but it is cumbersome and difficult to carry out on an ambulatory basis.[2]

When a diagnosis of ACTH-dependent Cushing's syndrome has been established, corticorelin may be used for differential diagnosis of the subtype. Patients with pituitary Cushing's syndrome have an exaggerated increase in plasma-corticotropin and plasma-cortisol concentrations in response to corticorelin, whereas those with adrenal or ectopic syndrome have no response.[3,4] The corticorelin stimulation test is of comparable diagnostic efficacy to the dexamethasone suppression test,[5,6] although false results have been obtained with both tests.[2,5] The corticorelin stimulation test is also considered somewhat unreliable if the disease is due to low-grade ectopic secretion of corticotropin by small tumours.[7] Again, a combination of the dexamethasone and corticorelin tests is reportedly more accurate than either alone.[6] The most reliable test to distinguish between pituitary and nonpituitary forms of Cushing's syndrome is to measure the difference between central and peripheral concentrations of ACTH following the administration of corticorelin.[2] However, this requires sampling of central (petrosal) venous blood, an invasive procedure needing considerable expertise.


1. Yanovski JA, *et al.* Corticotropin-releasing hormone stimulation following low-dose dexamethasone administration: a new test to distinguish Cushing's syndrome from pseudo-Cushing's states. *JAMA* 1993; **269:** 2232–8.
2. Raff H, Findling JW. A physiologic approach to diagnosis of the Cushing syndrome. *Ann Intern Med* 2003; **138:** 980–91.
3. Chrousos GP, *et al.* The corticotropin-releasing factor stimulation test: an aid in the evaluation of patients with Cushing's syndrome. *N Engl J Med* 1984; **310:** 622–6.
4. Newell-Price J, *et al.* Optimal response criteria for the human CRH test in the differential diagnosis of ACTH-dependent Cushing's syndrome. *J Clin Endocrinol Metab* 2002; **87:** 1640–5.
5. Hermus AR, *et al.* The corticotropin-releasing-hormone test versus the high-dose dexamethasone test in the differential diagnosis of Cushing's syndrome. *Lancet* 1986; **ii:** 540–4.
6. Nieman LK, *et al.* The ovine corticotropin-releasing hormone stimulation test and the dexamethasone suppression test in the differential diagnosis of Cushing's syndrome. *Ann Intern Med* 1986; **105:** 862–7.
7. McCarthy MI, *et al.* CRH test. *Lancet* 1991; **337:** 233–4.


### Preparations

**Proprietary Preparations** (details are given in Part 3)
***Austria:*** CRH; ***Fr.:*** Stimu-ACTH; ***Ger.:*** Corticrel; CRH; ***Neth.:*** CRH; ***USA:*** Acthrel.

## Corticotropin *(BAN, rINN)*

ACTH; Adrenocorticotrophic Hormone; Adrenocorticotrophin; Corticotrophin; Corticotropina; Corticotropinum.
*CAS — 9002-60-2 (corticotropin); 9050-75-3 (corticotropin zinc hydroxide); 8049-55-6 (corticotropin zinc hydroxide).*
*ATC — H01AA01.*

**Pharmacopoeias.** In *US* as preparations for injection.

### Units

5 units of porcine corticotropin for bioassay are contained in approximately 50 micrograms (with lactose 5 mg) in one ampoule of the third International Standard (1962).

### Adverse Effects

Corticotropin stimulates the adrenals to produce cortisol (hydrocortisone) and mineralocorticoids; it therefore has the potential to produce similar adverse glucocorticoid and mineralocorticoid effects to those of the corticosteroids (see p.1068). In particular, its mineralocorticoid properties may produce marked sodium and water retention; considerable potassium loss may also occur.

Corticotropin can induce sensitisation, and severe hypersensitivity reactions, including anaphylaxis, may occur. This is generally considered to be due to the porcine component of the peptide.

Whereas corticosteroids replace endogenous cortisol (hydrocortisone) and thereby induce adrenal atrophy, corticotropin's stimulant effect induces hypertrophy. Nevertheless, the ability of the hypothalamic-pituitary-adrenal axis to respond to stress is still reduced, and abrupt withdrawal of corticotropin may result in symptoms of adrenal insufficiency (see Withdrawal, below).

◊ Reports of the adverse effects observed in children given corticotropin for infantile spasms.


1. Riikonen R, Donner M. ACTH therapy in infantile spasms: side effects. *Arch Dis Child* 1980; **55:** 664–72.
2. Hanefeld F, *et al.* Renal and pancreatic calcification during treatment of infantile spasms with ACTH. *Lancet* 1984; **i:** 901.
3. Riikonen R, *et al.* Disturbed calcium and phosphate homeostasis during treatment with ACTH of infantile spasms. *Arch Dis Child* 1986; **61:** 671–6.
4. Perheentupa J, *et al.* Adrenocortical hyporesponsiveness after treatment with ACTH of infantile spasms. *Arch Dis Child* 1986; **61:** 750–3.


### Withdrawal

Corticotropin administration may depress the hypothalamic-pituitary-adrenal axis. Abrupt withdrawal of corticotropin may therefore produce adrenocortical and pituitary unresponsiveness, and therapy should be stopped gradually. An increase in corticosteroid requirements associated with the stress of infection, or accidental or surgical trauma, may also precipitate acute adrenocortical insufficiency. See also Withdrawal under Corticosteroids, p.1070.

### Precautions

As for Corticosteroids, p.1071.

**Phaeochromocytoma.** A hypertensive crisis following intravenous administration of tetracosactide resulted in the discovery of an adrenaline-secreting phaeochromocytoma in a patient.[1] It was suggested that caution should be observed when using corticotropin in patients with orthostatic hypotension in whom the diagnosis of phaeochromocytoma has not been excluded.


1. Jan T, *et al.* Epinephrine-producing pheochromocytoma with hypertensive crisis after corticotropin injection. *Am J Med* 1990; **89:** 824–5.


### Interactions

Interactions seen with corticotropin are liable to be similar to those with corticosteroids (p.1072).

### Uses and Administration

Corticotropin is a naturally occurring hormone of the anterior lobe of the pituitary gland. It stimulates the adrenal glands to secrete adrenocortical hormones, especially cortisol (hydrocortisone), some mineralocorticoids, such as corticosterone, and, to a lesser extent, androgens. It has little effect on aldosterone secretion, which proceeds independently.

Secretion of corticotropin by the functioning pituitary gland is controlled by the release of corticorelin from the hypothalamus and is also regulated by a negative feedback mechanism involving concentrations of circulating glucocorticoids. Conditions of stress may also stimulate secretion.

Corticotropin may be used diagnostically to investigate adrenocortical insufficiency. It has also been used therapeutically in most of the conditions (with the exception of the adrenal deficiency states and adrenocortical overactivity) for which systemic corticosteroid therapy is indicated (p.1073). Such use is now fairly limited. However, corticotropin may be used in certain neurological disorders such as infantile spasms and multiple sclerosis. The synthetic polypeptide tetracosactide (p.1340), which has the same amino-acid sequence as the first 24 residues of human corticotropin, may be used as an alternative. Tosactide is another polypeptide analogue of corticotropin; it has the same sequence as the first 28 residues.

Corticotropin has been available for injection in two forms. One form is a plain injection that may be administered by the subcutaneous, intramuscular, or intravenous routes. The other form includes the long-acting depot preparations in which the viscosity is increased by the addition of gelatin or in which corticotropin is combined with zinc hydroxide. The gelatin-containing depot preparation is administered subcutaneously or intramuscularly, the zinc hydroxide-containing depot preparation is administered intramuscularly; neither should be given intravenously. Individual responses to therapeutic corticotropin vary considerably and doses must be adjusted accordingly.

For diagnostic purposes the corticotropin test is based on the measurement of plasma-cortisol concentrations before and after injection. The plain preparation is used in doses of 10 to 25 units in 500 mL of glucose 5% infused intravenously over 8 hours.

For therapeutic purposes typical initial doses for the plain type of injection have been up to 20 units four times daily by the subcutaneous or intramuscular routes, and for the depot preparations about 20 to 80 units every 24 to 72 hours by the subcutaneous route (for the gelatin-containing preparation) or the intramuscular route (for both types of depot preparation). As soon as possible the dosage should be reduced gradually to the minimum necessary to control symptoms.

**Epilepsy.** The use of corticotropin in the management of infantile spasms is referred to under Corticosteroids, p.1080.
References.


1. Hrachovy RA, *et al.* High-dose, long-duration versus low-dose, short-duration corticotropin therapy for infantile spasms. *J Pediatr* 1994; **124:** 803–6.
2. Baram TZ, *et al.* High-dose corticotropin (ACTH) versus prednisone for infantile spasms: a prospective, randomized, blinded study. *Pediatrics* 1996; **97:** 375–9.


**Multiple sclerosis.** Short-term courses of corticotropin have been used to speed recovery from acute exacerbations of multiple sclerosis (p.646) but corticosteroids, usually methylprednisolone, are now preferred.

**Post-dural puncture headache.** There are anecdotal reports of the relief of post-dural puncture headache by corticotropin (or tetracosactide),[1,2] although, as discussed on p.1368, in many cases patients respond to conservative measures.


1. Collier BB. Treatment for postdural puncture headache. *Br J Anaesth* 1994; **72:** 366–7.
2. Foster P. ACTH treatment for post-lumbar puncture headache. *Br J Anaesth* 1994; **73:** 429.


### Preparations

***USP 27:*** Corticotropin for Injection; Corticotropin Injection; Corticotropin Zinc Hydroxide Injectable Suspension; Repository Corticotropin Injection.

**Proprietary Preparations** (details are given in Part 3)
***Arg.:*** Acthelea; ***Irl.:*** Acthar; ***S.Afr.:*** Acthar†; ***UK:*** Acthar†; ***USA:*** Acthar.

## Demoxytocin *(rINN)*

Deamino-oxytocin; Demoxitocina; Desamino-oxytocin; ODA-914. 1-(3-Mercaptopropionic acid)-oxytocin.
$C_{43}H_{65}N_{11}O_{12}S_2$ = 992.2.
*CAS — 113-78-0.*
*ATC — H01BB01.*

### Profile

Demoxytocin is a synthetic analogue of oxytocin (p.1336) and has similar properties. It has been given as buccal tablets for the induction and augmentation of labour. It has also been given before nursing to stimulate milk ejection, although it is generally recommended that oxytocics should not be used for this purpose (see p.1317).

### Preparations

**Proprietary Preparations** (details are given in Part 3)
***Ital.:*** Demopart†; Sandopart†.

## Deslorelin *(BAN, USAN, rINN)*

Deslorelina; D-Trp LHRH-PEA. 5-Oxo-L-prolyl-L-histidyl-L-tryptophyl-L-seryl-L-tyrosyl-D-tryptophyl-L-leucyl-L-arginyl-*N*-ethyl-L-prolinamide.
$C_{64}H_{83}N_{17}O_{12}$ = 1282.5.
*CAS — 57773-65-6.*

### Profile

Deslorelin is an analogue of gonadorelin (p.1325) investigated in the treatment of precocious puberty and for prostate cancer; it has also been tried in endometriosis.

◊ References.


1. Anonymous. Deslorelin: D-Trp-LHRH-PEA, LHRH agonist analogue, Somagard. *Drugs R D* 1999; **2:** 420–2.
2. Klein KO, *et al.* Increased final height in precocious puberty after long-term treatment with LHRH agonists: the National Institutes of Health experience. *J Clin Endocrinol Metab* 2001; **86:** 4711–16.


## Desmopressin *(BAN, rINN)*

DDAVP; Desmopresina; Desmopressinum. 1-(3-Mercaptopropionic acid)-8-D-arginine-vasopressin; [1-Deamino,8-D-arginine]vasopressin.
$C_{46}H_{64}N_{14}O_{12}S_2$ = 1069.2.
*CAS — 16679-58-6.*
*ATC — H01BA02.*

**Pharmacopoeias.** In *Eur.* (see p.vi).
**Ph. Eur. 5.0** (Desmopressin). A white fluffy powder. Soluble in water, in alcohol, and in glacial acetic acid. Store at 2° to 8°. Protect from light and moisture.

### Desmopressin Acetate *(BANM, USAN, rINNM)*

Acetato de desmopresina.
$C_{46}H_{64}N_{14}O_{12}S_2,C_2H_4O_2,3H_2O$ = 1183.3.
*CAS — 62288-83-9 (anhydrous desmopressin acetate); 62357-86-2 (desmopressin acetate trihydrate).*
*ATC — H01BA02.*

### Units

27 units of desmopressin are contained in approximately 27 micrograms of desmopressin (with 5 mg of human albumin and citric acid) in one ampoule of the first International Standard (1980).

### Adverse Effects and Precautions

Adverse effects with desmopressin include headache, nausea, and mild abdominal cramps; there may be pain and swelling at the site of injection. With large intravenous doses hypotension, with tachycardia and facial flushing, may occur; some patients may experience an increase in blood pressure. Occasionally there may be cerebral or coronary thrombosis. Hypersensitivity reactions have also occurred. The antidiuretic action of desmopressin may produce water intoxication and hyponatraemia, occasionally leading to convulsions. Nasal administration may cause local irritation, congestion, and epistaxis.

Precautions to be observed during the use of desmopressin are similar to those for vasopressin (see p.1343). It should not be given to patients with type IIB von Willebrand's disease, in whom the release of clotting factors may lead to platelet aggregation and thrombocytopenia. When desmopressin is used diagnostically, or for the treatment of enuresis, the fluid intake should be limited to a minimum and only to satisfy thirst from 1 hour before to 8 hours after administration (see also Effects on Electrolytes, below).

**Effects on the cardiovascular system.** Facial flushing and warmth following intravenous desmopressin reflect a vasodilator action[1] or may be due to an opioid mechanism in the CNS.[2] A drop in diastolic blood pressure of about 14 mmHg and an increase in heart rate of 20 beats/minute are the rule during intravenous infusion of desmopressin in doses of 400 nanograms/kg or more.[1] The hypotensive effects of desmopressin were responsible for a serious reaction, involving cyanosis and dyspnoea, in a 21-month-old child with cyanotic heart disease.[3] Thrombosis (including myocardial infarction)[4-6] and cerebral infarction[7] have been associated rarely with the use of intravenous desmopressin.

Manufacturers also warn of the possibility of an increase in blood pressure.

1. Brommer EJP, *et al.* Desmopressin and hypotension. *Ann Intern Med* 1985; **103:** 962.
2. Pigache RM. Facial flushing induced by vasopressin-like peptides lacking pressor activity. *J Clin Pharmacol* 1984; **17:** 369–71.
3. Israels SJ, Kobrinsky NL. Serious reaction to desmopressin in a child with cyanotic heart disease. *N Engl J Med* 1989; **320:** 1563–4.
4. Anonymous. Desmopressin and arterial thrombosis. *Lancet* 1989; **i:** 938–9.
5. Mannucci PM, Lusher JM. Desmopressin and thrombosis. *Lancet* 1989; **ii:** 675–6.
6. Hartmann S, Reinhart W. Fatal complication of desmopressin. *Lancet* 1995; **345:** 1302–3. Correction. *ibid.;* 1648.
7. Grunwald Z, Sather SDC. Intraoperative cerebral infarction after desmopressin administration in infant with end-stage renal disease. *Lancet* 1995; **345:** 1364–5.

**Effects on electrolytes.** There have been a number of reports of seizures due to hyponatraemia and water intoxication following intranasal[1-7] or intravenous[8] desmopressin. The UK Committee on Safety of Medicines noted in March 1996 that it had received reports of hyponatraemic convulsions in 21 children and 3 adults receiving desmopressin (which it somewhat inaccurately described as vasopressin).[9] It was recommended that when this drug was used to treat primary nocturnal enuresis the risks of concomitant hyponatraemia should be minimised by

- avoiding concomitant use of drugs, such as *tricyclic antidepressants*, that increase endogenous ADH secretion
- keeping to the recommended starting dose
- avoiding excessive fluid intake, including during swimming
- stopping treatment temporarily if vomiting or diarrhoea occurred, to allow recovery of normal fluid and electrolyte balance.

Some have suggested that serum sodium concentrations be measured 24 to 48 hours, 1 week, and 1 month after starting treatment with desmopressin.[7]

1. Simmonds EJ, *et al.* Convulsions and coma after intranasal desmopressin in cystic fibrosis. *BMJ* 1988; **297:** 1614.
2. Salvatoni A, *et al.* Hyponatremia and seizures during desmopressin acetate treatment in hypothyroidism. *J Pediatr* 1990; **116:** 835–6.
3. Davis RC, *et al.* Nocturnal enuresis. *Lancet* 1992; **340:** 1550.
4. Hamed M, *et al.* Hyponatraemic convulsion associated with desmopressin and imipramine treatment. *BMJ* 1993; **306:** 1169.
5. Hourihane J, Salisbury AJ. Use caution in prescribing desmopressin for nocturnal enuresis. *BMJ* 1993; **306:** 1545.
6. Robson WLM, Leung AKC. Hyponatraemia following desmopressin. *BMJ* 1993; **307:** 64–5.
7. Odeh M, Oliven A. Coma and seizures due to severe hyponatremia and water intoxication in an adult with intranasal desmopressin therapy for nocturnal enuresis. *J Clin Pharmacol* 2001; **41:** 582–4.
8. Shepherd LL, *et al.* Hyponatremia and seizures after intravenous administration of desmopressin acetate for surgical hemostasis. *J Pediatr* 1989; **114:** 470–2.
9. Committee on Safety of Medicines/Medicines Control Agency. Hyponatraemic convulsions in patients with enuresis treated with vasopressin. *Current Problems* 1996; **22:** 4.

**Effects on the eyes.** Pseudotumor cerebri associated with desmopressin treatment has been reported in one patient.[1]

1. Neely DE, *et al.* Desmopressin (DDAVP)-induced pseudotumor cerebri. *J Pediatr* 2003; **143:** 808.

**Effects on mental function.** Paranoid psychosis occurred after desmopressin therapy in a patient with Alzheimer's dementia.[1]

1. Collins GB, *et al.* Paranoid psychosis after DDAVP therapy for Alzheimer's dementia. *Lancet* 1981; **ii:** 808.

**Tolerance.** In 3 uraemic patients desmopressin infusion produced an initial shortening of the bleeding time but following repeated infusions this response was reduced and there was even some increase in baseline bleeding times.[1] Two infusions of desmopressin 300 nanograms/kg in one day appear to induce a near maximum response; different treatment is required subsequently.

1. Canavese C, *et al.* Reduced response of uraemic bleeding time to repeated doses of desmopressin. *Lancet* 1985; **i:** 867–8.

## Interactions

As for Vasopressin, p.1343. See also under Effects on Electrolytes, above. NSAIDs, such as ibuprofen (see Effects on Electrolytes under Ibuprofen, p.46) and indometacin, may enhance the antidiuretic effect of desmopressin.

## Pharmacokinetics

Desmopressin is absorbed from the nasal mucosa with a bioavailability of 10 to 20%. Following oral administration it is largely destroyed in the gastrointestinal tract but sufficient is absorbed following high doses to produce therapeutic effects. When given intravenously desmopressin exhibits biphasic pharmacokinetics, with half-lives of about 8 minutes and 75 minutes for the 2 phases respectively.

◊ References.

1. Fjellestad-Paulsen A, *et al.* Pharmacokinetics of 1-deamino-8-D-arginine vasopressin after various routes of administration in healthy volunteers. *Clin Endocrinol (Oxf)* 1993; **38:** 177–82.
2. Lam KSL, *et al.* Pharmacokinetics, pharmacodynamics, long-term efficacy and safety of oral 1-deamino-8-D-arginine vasopressin in adult patients with central diabetes insipidus. *Br J Clin Pharmacol* 1996; **42:** 379–85.

## Uses and Administration

Desmopressin is a synthetic analogue of vasopressin (p.1342). It has greater antidiuretic activity and a more prolonged action than vasopressin or lypressin. It also stimulates factor VIII and plasminogen activator activity in the blood, but has little pressor activity.

Desmopressin is used in the diagnosis and treatment of cranial diabetes insipidus, in the treatment of nocturnal enuresis, and in tests of renal function. It is also used in the management of mild or moderate haemophilia and type I von Willebrand's disease, and in tests of fibrinolytic response.

It is given as the acetate, by mouth, as a solution intranasally, and by injection. The intranasal dose is approximately ten times that required intravenously and the oral dose about ten times greater than the intranasal dose.

In the control of **cranial diabetes insipidus**, desmopressin acetate is given by mouth to adults and children in usual initial doses of 100 micrograms three times daily. Doses may be adjusted according to response, with maintenance doses usually between 100 and 200 micrograms three times daily though total doses of between 100 micrograms and 1200 micrograms daily have been used. It may also be used intranasally in usual doses of 10 to 40 micrograms of desmopressin acetate daily as a single dose or in divided doses; children aged 3 months to 12 years may be given 5 to 30 micrograms intranasally daily. It may also be given subcutaneously, intramuscularly, or intravenously in a dose of 1 to 4 micrograms daily; a dose from 400 nanograms may be used for children and infants.

A single intranasal dose of 20 micrograms or 2 micrograms subcutaneously or intramuscularly has been given to adults and children in the diagnosis of diabetes insipidus.

In the **testing of renal function**, it has been given intranasally in single doses of 40 micrograms for adults, 20 micrograms for children aged 1 to 15 years, and 10 micrograms for infants. It has also been given subcutaneously or intramuscularly in doses of 2 micrograms for adults and children, and 400 nanograms for infants.

In the management of **primary nocturnal enuresis**, children aged 5 years and older (the *British National Formulary* suggests preferably over 7 years) and adults are given desmopressin acetate in usual doses of 200 to 400 micrograms by mouth or 10 to 40 micrograms intranasally at bedtime. The need for continued treatment should be reassessed after 3 months by withdrawing desmopressin for at least 1 week. For the control of **nocturia** in adults with multiple sclerosis 10 to 20 micrograms intranasally at bedtime is recommended (but see Urinary Incontinence, below).

Desmopressin acetate is given by intravenous infusion to boost concentrations of factor VIII before surgical procedures in patients with mild to moderate **haemophilia** or **type I von Willebrand's disease**. The usual dose for adults and children is 300 or 400 nanograms/kg by slow intravenous infusion over 15 to 30 minutes just before surgery. It may be used similarly to treat spontaneous or trauma-induced bleeding episodes in these patients. It is also given intranasally in doses of 150 micrograms (in patients weighing less than 50 kg) or 300 micrograms; it should be given 2 hours before surgery.

For **testing of fibrinolytic response** desmopressin acetate may be given to adults and children by intravenous infusion in doses of 400 nanograms/kg over 20 minutes; a sample of venous blood is taken 20 minutes after completing the infusion and tested for fibrinolytic activity on fibrin plates.

**Diabetes insipidus.** Desmopressin is the usual treatment for cranial diabetes insipidus (p.1314).

**Haemorrhagic disorders.** Desmopressin is used in the management of patients with mild haemophilia A, carriers of haemophilia with low factor VIII concentrations, and patients with von Willebrand's disease, as discussed on p.737. The use of desmopressin results in a two- to sixfold increase in plasma concentrations of factor VIII and von Willebrand factor,[1] and patients must have measurable baseline concentrations of these factors in order to respond to desmopressin.[1,2] In general, a baseline factor VIII concentration of 0.1 to 0.15 units/mL is needed to achieve post-injection concentrations of about 0.3 to 0.5 units/mL, which are generally sufficient for minor bleeding or lesser procedures. Concentrations of at least 0.7 to 1 unit/mL must be achieved for major surgery.[1] Desmopressin can be given subcutaneously, but the peak levels of factor VIII are reached later than after intravenous administration. Intranasal use is also effective and can be used by patients to treat bleeding episodes themselves, without delay, outside hospital.[1] The use of desmopressin as an alternative to blood products has been recommended whenever possible in the treatment of these disorders, as a precaution against blood-borne infection.[1]

Bleeding due to liver disease has been controlled by desmopressin,[3,4] as has that associated with uraemia[5-8] (but for a report of tolerance to the effects of repeated doses of desmopressin in uraemic patients, see under Adverse Effects and Precautions, above), and there are reports of bleeding being controlled in other disorders such as telangiectasia,[9] and platelet storage deficiency,[10] and in patients with acquired antibodies to factor VIII.[11] See also Variceal Haemorrhage, in Vasopressin (p.1343) and Terlipressin (p.1340).

Desmopressin has been tried in surgical procedures with conflicting results.[12-15] A meta-analysis, which mainly included trials in cardiac surgery, found no evidence that desmopressin reduces perioperative blood transfusion in patients who do not have congenital bleeding disorders.[16] It has been suggested that desmopressin may only be useful in patients with inadequate haemostatic mechanisms undergoing cardiac surgery[17] and that its usefulness in non-cardiac surgery needs further study.[18] A possible role for desmopressin has been proposed in the control of surgical bleeding in patients whose religious beliefs preclude the use of blood products.[19] It has been reported to be effective in postoperative aspirin-related bleeding that was previously unresponsive to administration of clotting factors,[20] and may be helpful for the prevention of excessive blood loss in patients who have received aspirin within 7 days of cardiac bypass surgery.[21]

1. Lethagen S. Desmopressin in mild hemophilia A: indications, limitations, efficacy, and safety. *Semin Thromb Hemost* 2003; **29:** 101–5.
2. Mannucci PM. Desmopressin (DDAVP) in the treatment of bleeding disorders: the first 20 years. *Blood* 1997; **90:** 2515–21.
3. Burroughs AK, *et al.* Desmopressin and bleeding time in patients with cirrhosis. *BMJ* 1985; **291:** 1377–81.
4. Rak K, *et al.* Desmopressin and bleeding time in patients with cirrhosis. *BMJ* 1986; **292:** 138.
5. Mannucci PM, *et al.* Deamino-8-D-arginine vasopressin shortens the bleeding time in uremia. *N Engl J Med* 1983; **308:** 8–12.
6. Shapiro MD, Kelleher SP. Intranasal deamino-8-D-arginine vasopressin shortens the bleeding time in uremia. *Am J Nephrol* 1984; **4:** 260–1.
7. Viganò GL, *et al.* Subcutaneous desmopressin (DDAVP) shortens the bleeding time in uremia. *Am J Hematol* 1989; **31:** 32–5.
8. Jacquot C, *et al.* Addition of desmopressin to recombinant human erythropoietin in treatment of haemostatic defect of uraemia. *Lancet* 1988; **i:** 420.
9. Quitt M, *et al.* The effect of desmopressin on massive gastrointestinal bleeding in hereditary telangiectasia unresponsive to treatment with cryoprecipitate. *Arch Intern Med* 1990; **150:** 1744–6.
10. Nieuwenhuis HK, Sixma JJ. 1-Desamino-8-D-arginine vasopressin (desmopressin) shortens the bleeding time in storage pool deficiency. *Ann Intern Med* 1988; **108:** 65–7.
11. Naorose-Abidi SM, *et al.* Desmopressin therapy in patients with acquired factor VIII inhibitors. *Lancet* 1988; **i:** 366.
12. Salzman EW, *et al.* Treatment with desmopressin acetate to reduce blood loss after cardiac surgery: a double-blind randomized trial. *N Engl J Med* 1986; **314:** 1402–6.

13. Kobrinsky NL, *et al.* 1-Desamino-8-D-arginine vasopressin (desmopressin) decreases operative blood loss in patients having Harrington rod spinal fusion surgery: a randomized, double-blinded, controlled trial. *Ann Intern Med* 1987; **107:** 446–50. Correction. *ibid.* 1988; **108:** 496.
14. Hackmann T, *et al.* A trial of desmopressin (1-desamino-8-D-arginine vasopressin) to reduce blood loss in uncomplicated cardiac surgery. *N Engl J Med* 1989; **321:** 1437–43.
15. Cattaneo M, Mannucci PM. Desmopressin and blood loss after cardiac surgery. *Lancet* 1993; **342:** 812.
16. Carless PA, *et al.* Desmopressin for minimising perioperative allogeneic blood transfusion. Available in The Cochrane Library; Issue 1. Chichester: John Wiley; 2004.
17. Salzman EW. Desmopressin and surgical hemostasis. *N Engl J Med* 1990; **322:** 1085.
18. Anonymous. Can drugs reduce surgical blood loss? *Lancet* 1988; **i:** 155–6.
19. Martens PR. Desmopressin and Jehovah's witness. *Lancet* 1989; **i:** 1322.
20. Chard RB, *et al.* Use of desmopressin in the management of aspirin-related and intractable haemorrhage after cardiopulmonary bypass. *Aust N Z J Surg* 1990; **60:** 125–8.
21. Sheridan DP, *et al.* Use of desmopressin acetate to reduce blood transfusion requirements during cardiac surgery in patients with acetylsalicylic-acid-induced platelet dysfunction. *Can J Surg* 1994; **37:** 33–6.

**Nocturnal enuresis.** Desmopressin is one of the main drugs used as an alternative or adjunct to nonpharmacological methods for the treatment of nocturnal enuresis in children (p.475). Secretion of vasopressin during the night in normal individuals reduces urine output and it has been suggested that nocturnal enuresis in some children might be due to impaired nocturnal secretion of vasopressin. However, one study[1] found no difference in nocturnal vasopressin levels or urine production in enuretic and non-enuretic children, but did find that children with nocturnal enuresis required a greater output of vasopressin to regulate plasma osmolality; other evidence has suggested that developmental delay in 2 separate areas of the CNS is involved.[2] Furthermore, there have been cases[3,4] of patients with both nocturnal enuresis and nephrogenic diabetes insipidus (which is resistant to desmopressin) in which desmopressin did not reduce urine output but did decrease the frequency of bed wetting; this suggested that the effects of desmopressin in nocturnal enuresis may not be due to increased renal concentrating capacity, but to some other mechanism. Nonetheless, it has been shown that use of the synthetic vasopressin analogue, desmopressin, at night can be effective in the short-term control of nocturnal enuresis[5] and many now consider it to be the drug of choice in terms of safety. However, a meta-analysis suggested that benefit might not be sustained once the drug was discontinued.[6] It should not be given when enuresis is due to polydipsia as desmopressin may provoke water intoxication and convulsions due to hyponatraemia. For precautions to be observed when desmopressin is used to treat enuresis see under Effects on Electrolytes, above.

1. Eggert P, Kühn B. Antidiuretic hormone regulation in patients with primary nocturnal enuresis. *Arch Dis Child* 1995; **73:** 508–11.
2. Koff SA. Cure of nocturnal enuresis: why isn't desmopressin very effective? *Pediatr Nephrol* 1996; **10:** 667–70.
3. Jonat S, *et al.* Effect of DDAVP on nocturnal enuresis in a patient with nephrogenic diabetes insipidus. *Arch Dis Child* 1999; **81:** 57–9.
4. Müller D, *et al.* Desmopressin for nocturnal enuresis in nephrogenic diabetes insipidus. *Lancet* 2002; **359:** 495–7.
5. Moffat MEK, *et al.* Desmopressin acetate and nocturnal enuresis: how much do we know? *Pediatrics* 1993; **92:** 420–5.
6. Glazener CMA, Evans JHC. Desmopressin for nocturnal enuresis in children. Available in The Cochrane Library; Issue 1. Chichester: John Wiley; 2004.

**Orthostatic hypotension.** The first drug tried in patients with orthostatic hypotension (p.1100) who cannot be managed by nonpharmacological methods is usually fludrocortisone, but desmopressin is sometimes useful in patients with central neurological abnormalities.[1]

1. Mathias CJ, *et al.* The effect of desmopressin on nocturnal polyuria, overnight weight loss, and morning postural hypotension in patients with autonomic failure. *BMJ* 1986; **293:** 353–4.

**Post-dural puncture headache.** Desmopressin acetate has been given to adults in a dose of 4 micrograms subcutaneously or intramuscularly for the treatment or prophylaxis of headache due to lumbar puncture, repeated if necessary after 24 hours. However, results have generally been disappointing and as mentioned on p.1368 many patients respond to conservative treatment.

References.

1. Durward WF, Harrington H. Headache after lumbar puncture. *Lancet* 1976; **ii:** 1403–4.
2. Widerlöv E, Lindström L. DDAVP and headache after lumbar puncture. *Lancet* 1979; **i:** 548.
3. Hansen PE, Hansen JH. DDAVP, a synthetic analogue of vasopressin, in prevention of headache after lumbar puncture and lumbar pneumoencephalography. *Acta Neurol Scand* 1979; **60:** 183–8.
4. Cowan JMA, *et al.* DDAVP in the prevention of headache after lumbar puncture. *BMJ* 1980; **280:** 224.

**Renal colic.** Intranasal desmopressin is being studied[1] in the management of the pain of acute renal colic (p.4).

1. Zabihi N, Teichman JMH. Dealing with the pain of renal colic. *Lancet* 2001; **358:** 437–8.

**Urinary incontinence.** Desmopressin given intranasally appeared to be effective in reducing voiding frequency/incontinence when studied in 26 patients with multiple sclerosis whose bladder dysfunction had previously been unresponsive to antimuscarinic therapy.[1] However, a review of studies using desmopressin to treat nocturia in patients with multiple sclerosis cast doubt on the clinical relevance of the limited reductions achieved in voiding frequency.[2] Oral desmopressin has been reported to have a favourable effect on measures such as the number of nocturnal voids and duration of sleep until the first nocturnal void in women[3] and men[4] with nocturia.

For the usual treatment of incontinence, see Urinary Incontinence and Retention, p.476.

1. Fredrikson S. Nasal spray desmopressin treatment of bladder dysfunction in patients with multiple sclerosis. *Acta Neurol Scand* 1996; **94:** 31–4.
2. Ferreira E, Letwin SR. Desmopressin for nocturia and enuresis associated with multiple sclerosis. *Ann Pharmacother* 1998; **32:** 114–16.
3. Lose G, *et al.* Efficacy of desmopressin (Minirin) in the treatment of nocturia: a double-blind placebo-controlled study in women. *Am J Obstet Gynecol* 2003; **189:** 1106–13.
4. Mattiasson A, *et al.* Efficacy of desmopressin in the treatment of nocturia: a double-blind placebo-controlled study in men. *BJU Int* 2002; **89:** 855–62.

## Preparations

***BP 2003:*** Desmopressin Injection; Desmopressin Intranasal Solution.

**Proprietary Preparations** (details are given in Part 3)
***Arg.:*** Emosint; Octostim; ***Austral.:*** Minirin; Octostim; ***Austria:*** Minirin; Nocutil; Octostim; ***Belg.:*** Minirin; ***Braz.:*** DDAVP†; Octostim†; ***Canad.:*** DDAVP; Octostim; ***Chile:*** DDAVP; Octostim; ***Denm.:*** Minirin; Octostim; ***Fin.:*** Minirin; Octostim; ***Fr.:*** Minirin; Octim; ***Ger.:*** DDAVP†; Desmogalen; Minirin; Nocutil; Octostim; ***Gr.:*** DDAVP; Defirin; Minirin; ***Hong Kong:*** Minirin; Octostim; ***India:*** D-Void; ***Irl.:*** DDAVP; Desmospray; Desmotabs; ***Israel:*** Minirin; Octostim; ***Ital.:*** Emosint; Minirin/DDAVP; ***Malaysia:*** Minirin; ***Mex.:*** DDAVP; Minirin; ***Neth.:*** Minirin; Octostim; ***Norw.:*** Minirin; Octostim; ***NZ:*** Minirin; Octostim; ***Port.:*** DDAVP; Desmospray; Minirin; ***S.Afr.:*** DDAVP; ***Singapore:*** Minirin; Octostim; ***Spain:*** Minurin; ***Swed.:*** Minirin; Octostim; ***Switz.:*** Minirin; Nocutil; Octostim; ***Thai.:*** Minirin; ***UK:*** DDAVP; Desmospray; Desmotabs; Nocutil; Presinex; ***USA:*** DDAVP; Minirin; Stimate.

---

## Felypressin *(BAN, USAN, rINN)*

Felipresina; Phelypressine; PLV2. [2-Phenylalanine,8-lysine]vasopressin; Cys-Phe-Phe-Gln-Asn-Cys-Pro-Lys-Gly-$NH_2$.

$C_{46}H_{65}N_{13}O_{11}S_2$ = 1040.2.
*CAS — 56-59-7.*

### Profile

Felypressin is a synthetic analogue of vasopressin (p.1342) with similar actions. Its antidiuretic effects are less than those of vasopressin. It is used as a vasoconstrictor in local anaesthetic injections for dental use when sympathomimetics should be avoided. It is also an ingredient of preparations that have been used in the treatment of pain and inflammation of the mouth.

### Preparations

**Proprietary Preparations** (details are given in Part 3)
**Multi-ingredient:** ***Fr.:*** Collupressine†.

*Used as an adjunct in:* ***Austral.:*** Citanest Dental; ***Braz.:*** Citanest; Citocaina; ***Denm.:*** Citanest Octapressin; ***Fin.:*** Citanest Octapressin; ***Ger.:*** Xylonest; ***Irl.:*** Citanest with Octapressin†; ***Ital.:*** Citanest con Octapressin; ***Mex.:*** Citanest Octapresin; ***Neth.:*** Citanest Octapressine†; ***Norw.:*** Citanest Octapressin; ***NZ:*** Citanest with Octapressin; ***Port.:*** Citanest Octapressin†; ***Spain:*** Citanest Octapressin; ***Swed.:*** Citanest Octapressin; ***Switz.:*** Xylonest-Octapressin†; ***UK:*** Citanest with Octapressin.

---

# Follicle-stimulating Hormone

Folitropina; FSH.

## Follitropin Alfa *(BAN, rINN)*

Folitropina alfa.

$C_{437}H_{682}N_{122}O_{134}S_{13}$ = 10 206 (α-subunit);
$C_{538}H_{833}N_{145}O_{171}S_{13}$ = 12 485 (β-subunit).
*CAS — 9002-68-0 (follitropin alfa); 56832-30-5 (α-subunit); 110909-60-9 (β-subunit); 146479-72-3 (follitropin alfa).*
*ATC — G03GA05.*

## Follitropin Beta *(BAN, rINN)*

Folitropina beta; Org-32489.

$C_{437}H_{682}N_{122}O_{134}S_{13}$ = 10 206 (α-subunit);
$C_{538}H_{833}N_{145}O_{171}S_{13}$ = 12 485 (β-subunit).
*CAS — 169108-34-3 (follitropin beta); 150490-84-9 (follitropin beta); 56832-30-5 (α-subunit); 110909-60-9 (β-subunit).*
*ATC — G03GA06.*

## Units

80 units of human pituitary follicle-stimulating hormone are contained in approximately 4.17 micrograms (with 5 mg of mannitol and 1 mg human serum albumin) in one ampoule of the first International Standard (1986).

138 units of recombinant human follicle-stimulating hormone for bioassay are contained in one ampoule of the first International Standard (1995).

## Adverse Effects and Precautions

As for Human Menopausal Gonadotrophins, p.1330.

**Spongiform encephalopathies.** In a few countries, gonadotrophins derived from cadaver pituitary glands have been used in the treatment of infertility, and a small number of patients are reported to have acquired Creutzfeldt-Jakob disease from such preparations.[1] However, most countries have preferred to use gonadotrophins derived from urine,[1] and these in their turn are being replaced with recombinant products;[2] such preparations do not carry the risk of transmitting the disease.

1. Healy DL, Evans J. Creutzfeldt-Jakob disease after pituitary gonadotrophins. *BMJ* 1993; **307:** 517–18.
2. Eshkol A, Page ML. Human gonadotrophin preparations. *BMJ* 1994; **308:** 789.

## Pharmacokinetics

Follitropins alfa and beta are slowly absorbed following subcutaneous or intramuscular injection, with an absolute bioavailability of about 70 to 80%. Peak plasma concentrations of follitropin beta have been stated to occur about 12 hours after subcutaneous or intramuscular injection. Accumulation occurs with repeated doses, reaching a steady state within 3 to 4 days. Follitropins are slowly eliminated from the body, with a terminal half-life ranging from 12 to 70 hours. About one-eighth of a dose of follitropin alfa is reported to be excreted in the urine.

◊ References.

1. Karlsson MO, *et al.* The population pharmacokinetics of recombinant- and urinary-human follicle stimulating hormone in women. *Br J Clin Pharmacol* 1998; **45:** 13–20.

## Uses and Administration

Follicle-stimulating hormone is secreted by the anterior lobe of the pituitary gland, with another gonadotrophin, luteinising hormone (p.1332).

These gonadotrophins stimulate the normal functioning of the gonads and the secretion of sex hormones in both men and women. In women, follicle-stimulating hormone stimulates the development and maturation of the follicles and ova; in men it has a role in spermatogenesis.

Recombinant human follicle-stimulating hormones (follitropins alfa or beta) are used in the treatment of female infertility due to anovulation, in women who have not responded to treatment with clomifene. Follitropins are also used for the stimulation of spermatogenesis in the management of male infertility caused by hypogonadotrophic hypogonadism (see Infertility, p.1316).

The dosage and schedule of treatment for female infertility must be determined according to the needs of each patient; it is usual to monitor response by studying the patient's urinary oestrogen excretion or by ultrasonic visualisation of follicles or both. Treatment is usually begun with 75 to 150 units daily by subcutaneous or intramuscular injection for 7 or 14 days; if there is no response, dosage is increased at 7- or 14-day intervals until an adequate but not excessive response is achieved. Treatment is then stopped and followed after 1 or 2 days by a single dose of chorionic gonadotrophin 5000 to 10 000 units to induce ovulation. In menstruating patients treatment should be started within the first 7 days of the menstrual cycle. It has been suggested by the UK manufacturers of follitropin alfa that a daily dose of 225 units is the usual maximum, and that if a patient fails to respond adequately after 4 weeks of treatment that cycle should be abandoned and the patient should subsequently begin the next cycle at a higher starting dose.

Follitropins are also used as part of *in-vitro* fertilisation or other assisted reproductive technologies. For this purpose doses of 150 to 225 units daily are generally given, for at least 4 days, commencing on the second or third day of the menstrual cycle. Thereafter the dose may be adjusted individually based on ovarian response to a usual maximum of about 450 units; adequate follicular development generally occurs within about 5 to 10 days of treatment. Pituitary downregulation with a gonadorelin analogue may be used with follitropin therapy, in which case the gonadorelin analogue is generally begun about 2 weeks before follitropin, and the 2 are then continued concomitantly until follicular development is adequate. A single dose of up to 10 000 units of chorionic gonadotrophin is then given to induce final follicular maturation and oocyte retrieval performed about 35 hours later.

Follitropins are used for the stimulation of spermatogenesis in the management of male infertility caused by hypogonadotrophic hypogonadism. Before starting follitropin therapy, chorionic gonadotrophin is given to raise serum testosterone concentrations to the normal range, which may take 3 to 6 months. A dose of 150 units subcutaneously three times weekly is then used, with continued chorionic gonadotrophin; doses of follitropin alfa up to 300 units three times weekly may be required. Treatment is continued for at least 4 months, and more than 18 months' treatment may be needed. A dose of follitropin beta 75 units daily or two or three times weekly has been used similarly.

Other substances with follicle-stimulating activity are used similarly: these include human menopausal gonadotrophins (p.1330), which have both luteinising and follicle-stimulating activity, and urofollitropin (p.1342).

## Preparations

**Proprietary Preparations** (details are given in Part 3)

***Arg.:*** Gonal-F; Puregon; ***Austral.:*** Gonal-F; Puregon; ***Austria:*** Gonal-F; Puregon; ***Belg.:*** Puregon; ***Braz.:*** Gonal-F; Puregon; ***Canad.:*** Gonal-F; Puregon; ***Chile:*** Puregon; ***Denm.:*** Gonal-F; Puregon; ***Fin.:*** Gonal-F; Puregon; ***Fr.:*** Gonal-F; Puregon; ***Ger.:*** Gonal-F; Puregon; ***Gr.:*** Gonal-F; Puregon; ***Hong Kong:*** Gonal-F; Puregon; ***India:*** Gonal-F; ***Irl.:*** Gonal-F; Puregon; ***Israel:*** Gonal-F; Puregon; ***Ital.:*** Gonal-F; Puregon; ***Malaysia:*** Gonal-F; Puregon; ***Mex.:*** Gonal-F; Puregon; ***Neth.:*** Gonal-F; Puregon; ***Norw.:*** Gonal-F; Puregon; ***NZ:*** Gonal-F; Puregon; ***Port.:*** Gonal-F; Puregon; ***S.Afr.:*** Gonal-F; Puregon; ***Singapore:*** Gonal-F; Puregon; ***Spain:*** Gonal-F; Puregon; ***Swed.:*** Gonal-F; Puregon; ***Switz.:*** Gonal-F; Puregon; ***Thai.:*** Gonal-F; Puregon; ***UK:*** Gonal-F; Puregon; ***USA:*** Follistim; Gonal-F.

---

## Ganirelix Acetate *(BANM, USAN, rINNM)*

Acetato de ganirelix; Org-37462; RS-26306. *N*-Acetyl-3-(2-naphthyl)-D-alanyl-*p*-chloro-D-phenylalanyl-3-(3-pyridyl)-D-alanyl-L-seryl-L-tyrosyl-$N^6$-(*N*,*N*′-diethylamidino)-D-lysyl-L-leucyl-$N^6$-(*N*,*N*′-diethylamidino)-L-lysyl-L-prolyl-D-alaninamide acetate.

$C_{80}H_{113}ClN_{18}O_{13},2C_2H_4O_2$ = 1690.4.

*CAS — 124904-93-4 (ganirelix); 129311-55-3 (ganirelix acetate).*

*ATC — H01CC01.*

### Adverse Effects and Precautions

As for Cetrorelix, p.1320.

### Uses and Administration

Like cetrorelix (p.1320), ganirelix is a gonadorelin (gonadotrophin-releasing hormone) antagonist. It is used as the acetate as a component of ovarian stimulation regimens for assisted reproduction in infertility (p.1316). Ganirelix acetate is given by subcutaneous injection for the prevention of premature luteinising hormone surges in women undergoing controlled ovarian hyperstimulation for assisted reproduction techniques. Doses are expressed in terms of the acetate or the equivalent amount of base. Ganirelix acetate 108 mg is approximately equivalent to ganirelix 100 mg. In the UK a dose equivalent to ganirelix 250 micrograms is given once daily, starting on day 6 of ovarian stimulation and continued until ovulation induction. In the USA a dose of ganirelix acetate 250 micrograms is used similarly.

◊ References.


1. The Ganirelix Dose-finding Study Group. A double-blind, randomized, dose-finding study to assess the efficacy of the gonadotrophin-releasing hormone antagonist ganirelix (Org 37462) to prevent premature luteinizing hormone surges in women undergoing ovarian stimulation with recombinant follicle stimulating hormone (Puregon). *Hum Reprod* 1998; **13:** 3023–31.
2. Gillies PS, *et al.* Ganirelix. *Drugs* 2000; **59:** 107–11.


### Preparations

**Proprietary Preparations** (details are given in Part 3)

***Arg.:*** Orgalutran; ***Austral.:*** Orgalutran; ***Braz.:*** Orgalutran; ***Denm.:*** Orgalutran; ***Fin.:*** Orgalutran; ***Fr.:*** Orgalutran; ***Ger.:*** Orgalutran; ***Gr.:*** Orgalutran; ***Irl.:*** Orgalutran; ***Ital.:*** Orgalutran; ***Norw.:*** Orgalutran; ***Spain:*** Orgalutran; ***Swed.:*** Orgalutran; ***Switz.:*** Orgalutran; ***UK:*** Orgalutran; ***USA:*** Antagon.

---

# Gonadorelin *(BAN, rINN)*

Follicle Stimulating Hormone-releasing Factor; GnRH; Gonadoliberin; Gonadorelina; Gonadorelinum; Gonadotrophin-releasing Hormone; Hoe-471; LH/FSH-RF; LH/FSH-RH; LH-RF; LH-RH; Luliberin; Luteinising Hormone-releasing Factor. 5-Oxo-L-prolyl-L-histidyl-L-tryptophyl-L-seryl-L-tyrosylglycyl-L-leucyl-L-arginyl-L-prolylglycinamide.

$C_{55}H_{75}N_{17}O_{13}$ = 1182.3.

*CAS — 33515-09-2.*

*ATC — H01CA01; V04CM01.*



## Gonadorelin Acetate *(BANM, USAN, rINNM)*

Abbott-41070; Acetato de gonadorelina.

$C_{55}H_{75}N_{17}O_{13},xC_2H_4O_2,yH_2O$.

*CAS — 34973-08-5 (anhydrous gonadorelin diacetate); 52699-48-6 (gonadorelin diacetate tetrahydrate).*

*ATC — H01CA01; V04CM01.*

**Pharmacopoeias.** In *Eur.* (see p.vi).

**Ph. Eur. 5.0** (Gonadorelin Acetate). The acetate form of a hypothalamic peptide that stimulates the release of follicle-stimulating hormone and luteinising hormone from the pituitary gland. It is obtained by chemical synthesis. A white or slightly yellowish powder; soluble in water and in 1% v/v glacial acetic acid; sparingly soluble in methyl alcohol. Store in airtight containers at a temperature of 2° to 8°. Protect from light.

## Gonadorelin Hydrochloride *(BANM, USAN, rINNM)*

AY-24031; Hidrocloruro de gonadorelina.

$C_{55}H_{75}N_{17}O_{13},2HCl$ = 1255.2.

*CAS — 51952-41-1.*

*ATC — H01CA01; V04CM01.*

**Pharmacopoeias.** In *Br.* and *US.*

**BP 2003** (Gonadorelin Hydrochloride). The chloride form of a hypothalamic peptide that stimulates the release of follicle-stimulating hormone and luteinising hormone from the pituitary gland. It is obtained by synthesis. A white or slightly yellowish-white powder; soluble in water and in 1% v/v glacial acetic acid; sparingly soluble in methyl alcohol. Store at a temperature of 2° to 8°. Protect from light and moisture.

**USP 27** (Gonadorelin Hydrochloride). A synthetic polypeptide hormone having the property of stimulating the release of the luteinising hormone from the hypothalamus. It is extremely hygroscopic. Protect from exposure to moisture and store in airtight well-sealed containers, in a desiccator.

## Adverse Effects

Gonadorelin and its analogues are generally well tolerated but may cause gastrointestinal adverse effects, usually nausea and abdominal pain or discomfort. There may be headache or lightheadedness, and an increase in menstrual bleeding. Continued therapy with gonadorelin analogues results in paradoxical suppression of the pituitary gonadal axis; in premenopausal women this may produce menopausal symptoms, including vaginal dryness, hot flushes, and loss of libido. If sufficiently prolonged the suppression of circulating oestrogens may lead to osteoporosis. In men, hot flushes and sexual dysfunction have occurred. Breast swelling and tenderness in men have been reported infrequently with gonadorelin analogues. Other adverse effects reportedly associated with gonadorelin analogue therapy, and presumably related to changes in the hormonal milieu, include mood changes, nervousness, palpitations, acne and dry skin, alterations in liver function tests and blood lipids, decreased glucose tolerance, and changes in scalp and body hair. Ovarian hyperstimulation (as seen with chorionic gonadotrophin, p.1320), although rare, has occurred in women given gonadorelin.

Reactions or pain may occur at the site of injection with rash (local or generalised), thrombophlebitis, swelling, or pruritus. Hypersensitivity reactions, including bronchospasm and anaphylaxis, have been reported.

Other effects may be a consequence of the particular use of gonadorelin or its analogues. Tumour flare, due to an initial surge in testosterone concentrations, has been reported in the initial stages of treatment for cancer of the prostate and concomitant anti-androgen therapy may be given prophylactically. Flare may manifest as an increase in bone pain; occasionally there has been spinal cord compression, or a worsening of urinary-tract symptoms with haematuria and urinary obstruction. Acute degeneration of submucous fibroids with severe bleeding has been reported following use of leuprorelin. An initial increase in signs and symptoms has also been reported in women with breast cancer receiving gonadorelin analogues; hypercalcaemia has occurred in those with metastatic disease.

**Hypersensitivity.** Acquired hypersensitivity led to an anaphylactic reaction following intravenous administration of gonadorelin to a man who had been receiving pulsatile subcutaneous gonadorelin therapy for 10 weeks.[1]


1. Potashnik G, *et al.* Anaphylactic reaction to gonadotropin-releasing hormone. *N Engl J Med* 1993; **328:** 815.


**Osteoporosis.** Long-term use of a gonadorelin analogue results in oestrogen deficiency-associated osteoporosis. Various drugs have been investigated for their ability to reduce this effect including parathyroid hormone,[1,2] or 'add-back' therapy with tibolone[3] or oestrogen plus progestogen.


1. Finkelstein JS, *et al.* Parathyroid hormone for the prevention of bone loss induced by estrogen deficiency. *N Engl J Med* 1994; **331:** 1618–23.
2. Finkelstein JS, *et al.* Prevention of estrogen deficiency-related bone loss with human parathyroid hormone-(1-34): a randomized controlled trial. *JAMA* 1998; **280:** 1067–73.
3. Lindsay PC, *et al.* The effect of add-back treatment with tibolone (Livial) on patients treated with the gonadotropin-releasing hormone agonist triptorelin (Decapeptyl). *Fertil Steril* 1996; **65:** 342–8.


## Precautions

Gonadorelin or its analogues should not generally be used in patients with pituitary adenoma as haemorrhagic infarction (pituitary apoplexy) has sometimes occurred. It has also been recommended that patients with weight-related amenorrhoea should not receive these drugs until their weight is corrected. While it has been recommended by at least one manufacturer that gonadorelin should not be used in women with polycystic ovary disease or with endometriotic cysts, gonadorelin and its analogues have produced improvement in polycystic disease and in uterine fibroids, and gonadorelin analogues have been used with benefit in endometriosis. Gonadorelin or its analogues should be discontinued if the patient becomes pregnant. Contraceptive measures should be taken to protect against unwanted ovulation. Men at risk from tumour flare should be carefully monitored in the first month of therapy.

## Interactions

Drugs affecting pituitary secretion of gonadotrophins may alter the response to gonadorelin or its analogues; other hormonal therapy and corticosteroids can affect the response. Spironolactone and levodopa can stimulate gonadotrophins while phenothiazines, dopamine antagonists, digoxin, and sex hormones can inhibit gonadotrophin secretion.

## Pharmacokinetics

Gonadorelin is poorly absorbed from the gastrointestinal tract. It has a terminal plasma half-life of only 10 to 40 minutes after intravenous injection. It is hydrolysed in the plasma and excreted in the urine as inactive metabolites.

Gonadorelin analogues are absorbed following oral, intramuscular, intranasal, or rectal administration and have a longer half-life.

## Uses and Administration

Gonadorelin is a synthetic form of hypothalamic gonadotrophin-releasing hormone. It stimulates the synthesis and release of follicle-stimulating hormone and, in particular, luteinising hormone in the anterior lobe of the pituitary. The secretion of endogenous gonadotrophin-releasing hormone is pulsatile and is controlled by several factors including circulating sex hormones. Gonadotrophic hormones (gonadotrophins), released from the pituitary gland in response to gonadorelin, stimulate secretion of sex hormones from the gonads. A single dose of gonadorelin or one of its analogues has the effect of increasing circulating sex hormones; continued administration leads to down-regulation of gonadorelin-receptor synthesis in the pituitary and results in a paradoxical reduction in sex-hormone secretion.

Gonadorelin is used in the diagnosis of hypothalamic-pituitary-gonadal dysfunction. Assessment is usually based on the response to a dose of gonadorelin of 100 micrograms by intravenous or subcutaneous injection. In females, where possible, it should be given early in the follicular stage of the menstrual cycle.

Gonadorelin is also used in the treatment of amenorrhoea and infertility associated with hypogonadotrophic hypogonadism and multifollicular ovaries. Weight-related amenorrhoea should have been corrected by diet. Treatment in such conditions is based on an intermittent pulse pump providing 5 to 20 micrograms over one minute every 90 minutes for up to 6 months or until conception.

Gonadorelin, or more usually its analogues such as buserelin, goserelin, leuprorelin, nafarelin, and triptorelin (which are more potent and have a longer duration of action) are used in cryptorchidism, malignant neoplasms (especially of the prostate), and in delayed and precocious puberty.

Gonadorelin is sometimes used as the hydrochloride or acetate.

**Benign prostatic hyperplasia.** The gonadorelin analogues have been tried in the management of benign prostatic hyperplasia (p.1555) but are considered unsatisfactory for indefinite use. See also under Leuprorelin Acetate, p.1331, and Nafarelin Acetate, p.1332.

**Cryptorchidism.** Whether gonadorelin or its analogues have a role in the management of cryptorchidism is a matter of debate; surgery remains the treatment with the best success rate, but hormonal therapy, with gonadorelin or chorionic gonadotrophin or both, is widely employed (see p.1313). Meta-analysis has suggested a success rate of about 20% overall, although this may be reduced when care is taken to exclude retractile testes.[1]

1. Pyörälä S, *et al.* A review and meta-analysis of hormonal treatment of cryptorchidism. *J Clin Endocrinol Metab* 1995; **80:** 2795–9.

**Delayed and precocious puberty.** For mention of the use of gonadorelin or its analogues in delayed and precocious puberty, see p.1314 and p.1318 respectively. Benefit in delayed puberty is most likely in those cases where it is secondary to hypogonadism (see p.1316).

**Diagnosis of hypothalamic and pituitary dysfunction.** References to gonadorelin in the diagnosis of hypothalamic-pituitary-gonadal dysfunction[1-6] including one[5] suggesting its abandonment on the grounds that it offered no help in classifying patients with amenorrhoea or determining the therapeutic potential of treatment with gonadorelin.

1. Mortimer CH, *et al.* Luteinizing hormone and follicle stimulating hormone-releasing hormone test in patients with hypothalamic-pituitary-gonadal dysfunction. *BMJ* 1973; **4:** 73–7.
2. Yoshimoto Y, *et al.* Restoration of normal pituitary gonadotropin reserve by administration of luteinizing-hormone-releasing hormone in patients with hypogonadotropic hypogonadism. *N Engl J Med* 1975; **292:** 242–5.
3. Sagel J, *et al.* The role of luteinizing hormone-releasing hormone in the diagnosis of constitutional delayed puberty. *Postgrad Med J* 1975; **51:** 611–14.
4. Ginsburg J, *et al.* Use of clomiphene and luteinizing hormone/follicle stimulating hormone-releasing hormone in investigation of ovulatory failure. *BMJ* 1975; **3:** 130–3.
5. Adulwahid NA, *et al.* Diagnostic tests with luteinising hormone releasing hormone should be abandoned. *BMJ* 1985; **291:** 1471–2.
6. Eckert KL, *et al.* A single-sample, subcutaneous gonadotropin-releasing hormone test for central precocious puberty. *Pediatrics* 1996; **97:** 517–19.

**Disturbed behaviour.** For mention of the use of triptorelin in men with paraphilias, see p.1341.

**Endometriosis.** Gonadorelin analogues are effective in the management of endometriosis (p.1546), but the need for long-term therapy to prevent recurrence limits their value, because of the risk of osteoporosis. 'Add-back' therapy with concomitant hormone replacement may be given in an attempt to reduce bone mineral density loss and vasomotor symptoms.

Some references to gonadorelin analogues in endometriosis are listed below. For further references, see Buserelin Acetate, p.1319, Goserelin Acetate, p.1327, Leuprorelin Acetate, p.1331, and Nafarelin Acetate, p.1333.

1. Gargiulo AR, Hornstein MD. The role of GnRH agonists plus add-back therapy in the treatment of endometriosis. *Semin Reprod Endocrinol* 1997; **15:** 273–84.
2. Hemmings R. Combined treatment of endometriosis: GnRH agonists and laparoscopic surgery. *J Reprod Med* 1998; **43** (suppl 3): 316–20.
3. Pickersgill A. GnRH agonists and add-back therapy: is there a perfect combination? *Br J Obstet Gynaecol* 1998; **105:** 475–85.
4. Surrey ES. Add-back therapy and gonadotropin-releasing hormone agonists in the treatment of patients with endometriosis: can a consensus be reached? *Fertil Steril* 1999; **71:** 420–4.
5. Prentice A, *et al.* Gonadotrophin-releasing hormone analogues for pain associated with endometriosis. Available in The Cochrane Library; Issue 1. Chichester: John Wiley; 2004.

**Fibroids.** Uterine fibroids (leiomyomas) are benign tumours of uterine smooth muscle.[1,2] They are found in about 25% of women, most of whom are aged in their 30s or 40s when the condition becomes symptomatic. Fibroids may give rise to menstrual problems, particularly menorrhagia, pelvic discomfort, infertility, and miscarriage. Although small fibroids may not require treatment, the management of symptomatic fibroids has traditionally been surgical. However, because fibroids are oestrogen responsive, gonadorelin analogues have also been tried as medical treatment for their ability to induce a hypogonadotrophic hypogonadal state. These drugs produce a significant reduction in uterine and fibroid volume, and amenorrhoea, but when treatment stops uterine and fibroid volume tend to return to pretreatment values. The hypoestrogenism produced during treatment also causes menopausal symptoms such as hot flushes and vaginal dryness, and bone loss may occur. The administration of oestrogens or progestogens, once the uterine fibroid size has significantly reduced, has been tried as 'add-back' therapy to counteract these side-effects.[3] Tibolone has also been reported to reduce bone loss and vasomotor symptoms.[2] Subcutaneous injection of long-acting depot preparations of gonadorelin or its analogues appear to be the preferred method of administration and it is considered that this treatment is a valuable pre-operative adjunct to surgery, simplifying the procedure by reducing uterine and fibroid volume and intra-operative blood loss, as well as correcting pre-operative iron-deficiency anaemia.[4] However, concern has been expressed that the use of gonadorelin analogues for treating fibroids may complicate the differentiation of benign and malignant growths.[5]

For further references to gonadorelin analogues being used in the treatment of fibroids, see Buserelin Acetate, p.1320, Goserelin Acetate, p.1327, Leuprorelin Acetate, p.1331, Nafarelin Acetate, p.1333, and Triptorelin, p.1341.

Other drugs that are under investigation for fibroids include gonadorelin antagonists such as cetrorelix and ganirelix, and mifepristone. Danazol and gestrinone have also been tried in a small number of patients.[2]

1. Stewart EA. Uterine fibroids. *Lancet* 2001; **357:** 293–8.
2. De Leo V, *et al.* A benefit-risk assessment of medical treatment for uterine leiomyomas. *Drug Safety* 2002; **25:** 759–79.
3. Friedman AJ, *et al.* Efficacy and safety considerations in women with uterine leiomyomas treated with gonadotropin-releasing hormone agonists: the estrogen threshold hypothesis. *Am J Obstet Gynecol* 1990; **163:** 1114–19.
4. Lethaby A, *et al.* Pre-operative GnRH analogue therapy before hysterectomy or myomectomy for uterine fibroids. Available in The Cochrane Library; Issue 1. Chichester: John Wiley; 2004.
5. Meyer WR, *et al.* Unsuspected leiomyosarcoma: treatment with a gonadotropin-releasing hormone analogue. *Obstet Gynecol* 1990; **75** (suppl): 529–32.

**Growth retardation.** The use of a gonadorelin analogue to delay precocious puberty may improve the final height of children with the disorder. However, the use of a gonadorelin analogue with growth hormone in short but otherwise normal children is controversial—see under Triptorelin, p.1341.

**Hirsutism.** For reference to the use of gonadorelin analogues such as leuprorelin in the treatment of hirsutism, see p.1331.

**Infertility.** Gonadorelin and its analogues are used in the management of infertility related to hypogonadotrophic hypogonadism in both women and men (p.1316). Some further references are given below. See also under Buserelin Acetate, p.1320, Leuprorelin Acetate, p.1331, and Nafarelin Acetate, p.1333.

1. Lingle L, Hart LL. Gonadotropin-releasing hormone in infertility. *DICP Ann Pharmacother* 1989; **23:** 246–8.
2. Thomas AK, *et al.* Induction of ovulation with subcutaneous pulsatile gonadotropin-releasing hormone: correlation with body weight and other parameters. *Fertil Steril* 1989; **51:** 786–90.
3. Homburg R, *et al.* One hundred pregnancies after treatment with pulsatile luteinising hormone releasing hormone to induce ovulation. *BMJ* 1989; **298:** 809–12.
4. Kovacs GT, *et al.* Induction of ovulation with gonadotrophin-releasing hormone—life-table analysis of 50 courses of treatment. *Med J Aust* 1989; **151:** 21–6.
5. Santoro N. Efficacy and safety of intravenous pulsatile gonadotropin-releasing hormone: Lutrepulse for injection. *Am J Obstet Gynecol* 1990; **163:** 1759–64.
6. Nachtigall LB, *et al.* Adult-onset idiopathic hypogonadotropic hypogonadism–a treatable form of male infertility. *N Engl J Med* 1997; **336:** 410–15.

**Malignant neoplasms.** Gonadorelin analogues are used in the treatment of prostatic cancer (p.521) where they provide an alternative to orchidectomy in the management of advanced disease. They may also be used for ovarian ablation in premenopausal women with breast cancer (p.514). Gonadorelin analogues have been tried in neoplasms of the endometrium (p.516) and ovary, but their use is much less well established.

Analogues used include buserelin (p.1320), goserelin (p.1327), leuprorelin (p.1332), and triptorelin (p.1342).

**Mastalgia.** Gonadorelin analogues such as goserelin may be effective in severe refractory mastalgia (p.1546).

**Polycystic ovary syndrome.** Gonadorelin and its analogues have been tried in polycystic ovary syndrome (p.1317) even though they are contra-indicated in this condition by some manufacturers. Pulsatile gonadorelin achieves a higher ovulatory rate in women with multifollicular ovaries than in those with large polycystic ovaries and the incidences of early miscarriage and abortion are higher in those with polycystic ovaries. Nonetheless there is a suggestion that addition of gonadorelin analogues to gonadotrophin stimulation results in better pregnancy rates in women with polycystic ovaries than do gonadotrophins alone.[1] Ovulation rate can be improved by pretreatment with a gonadorelin analogue for 8 weeks before using gonadorelin; 38% of patients achieved pregnancy in one study using this technique.[2] The rate of spontaneous abortion was also decreased from 50 to 38% after administration.

1. Nugent D, *et al.* Gonadotrophin therapy for ovulation induction in subfertility associated with polycystic ovary syndrome. Available in The Cochrane Library; Issue 1. Chichester: John Wiley; 2004.
2. Filicori M, *et al.* Polycystic ovary syndrome: abnormalities and management with pulsatile gonadotropin-releasing hormone and gonadotropin-releasing hormone analogs. *Am J Obstet Gynecol* 1990; **163:** 1737–42.

**Porphyria.** For mention of the use of gonadorelin analogues to suppress cyclic premenstrual exacerbations of acute porphyria, see Buserelin, p.1320, Nafarelin, p.1333, and Triptorelin, p.1342.

**Premenstrual syndrome.** In women in whom other drug treatments for premenstrual syndrome (p.1551) are ineffective, use of a gonadorelin analogue, usually with HRT to prevent menopausal symptoms, may be considered. Short-term therapy (3 months) has been used to confirm the diagnosis of premenstrual syndrome, or to predict the response to bilateral oophorectomy when this is being considered. Some references to the use of gonadorelin analogues in premenstrual syndrome are given below.[1-4]

1. Mortola JF, *et al.* Successful treatment of severe premenstrual syndrome by combined use of gonadotropin-releasing hormone agonist and estrogen/progestin. *J Clin Endocrinol Metab* 1991; **72:** 252A–F.
2. Hussain SY, *et al.* Buserelin in premenstrual syndrome. *Gynecol Endocrinol* 1992; **6:** 57–64.
3. Mortola JF. Applications of gonadotropin-releasing hormone analogues in the treatment of premenstrual syndrome. *Clin Obstet Gynecol* 1993; **36:** 753–63.
4. Mezrow G, *et al.* Depot leuprolide acetate with estrogen and progestin add-back for long-term treatment of premenstrual syndrome. *Fertil Steril* 1994; **62:** 932–7.

## Preparations

***BP 2003:*** Gonadorelin Injection;
***USP 27:*** Gonadorelin for Injection.

**Proprietary Preparations** (details are given in Part 3)
***Arg.:*** Luteoliberina; ***Austral.:*** HRF†; ***Austria:*** Kryptocur; Lutrelef; Relefact LH-RH; ***Belg.:*** HRF†; Kryptocur†; ***Braz.:*** HRF†; Parlib; Relisorm L†; ***Canad.:*** Factrel†; Lutrepulse; Relisorm†; ***Fr.:*** Lutrelef; Stimu-LH; ***Ger.:*** Kryptocur; Lutrelef; Relefact LH-RH; ***Gr.:*** Relefact LH-RH; ***Hong Kong:*** Relisorm L; ***Irl.:*** HRF; ***Israel:*** Lutrelef; Relefact LH-RH; ***Ital.:*** Kryptocur; Lutrelef; ***Mex.:*** Relisorm L†; ***Neth.:*** Cryptocur; HRF; Lutrelef; Relefact LH-RH; ***NZ:*** HRF; ***S.Afr.:*** HRF†; ***Spain:*** Luforan; ***Swed.:*** Lutrelef; ***Switz.:*** Kryptocur; Lutrelef; Relisorm L; ***UK:*** HRF; ***USA:*** Factrel; Lutrepulse†.

# Goserelin *(BAN, USAN, rINN)*

Goserelinum; ICI-118630. 3-[5-Oxo-L-prolyl-L-histidyl-L-tryptophyl-L-seryl-L-tyrosyl-(3-*O*-*tert*-butyl)-D-seryl-L-leucyl-L-arginyl-L-prolyl]carbazamide.

$C_{59}H_{84}N_{18}O_{14}$ = 1269.4.
*CAS — 65807-02-5.*
*ATC — L02AE03.*

**Pharmacopoeias.** In *Eur.* (see p.vi).

**Ph. Eur. 5.0** (Goserelin). A nonapeptide analogue of the hypothalamic decapeptide, gonadorelin. It is obtained by chemical synthesis and is available as an acetate. A white or almost white powder. Soluble in water; freely soluble in glacial acetic acid. It dissolves in dilute solutions of mineral acids and alkali hydroxides. Store at 2° to 8° in airtight containers. Protect from light.

## Goserelin Acetate *(BANM, rINNM)*

Acetato de goserelina; D-Ser (Bu$^t$)$^6$ Azgly$^{10}$-LHRH Acetate.
$C_{59}H_{84}N_{18}O_{14},C_2H_4O_2$ = 1329.5.
*CAS — 145781-92-6.*
*ATC — L02AE03.*

## Adverse Effects and Precautions

As for Gonadorelin, p.1325. Some women may experience vaginal bleeding during initial therapy, which normally resolves spontaneously. Arthralgia and paraesthesias have been reported.

**Pituitary apoplexy.** A report of pituitary apoplexy (a clinical syndrome caused by haemorrhage and infarction of a pituitary adenoma) in an elderly patient with a symptomless pituitary adenoma who was given goserelin for advanced prostate cancer.[1] The patient developed headache, vomiting, visual disturbances, gradual impairment of consciousness, intermittent fever, and progressive hyponatraemia. Symptoms responded to prednisolone replacement therapy.

1. Ando S, *et al.* Pituitary apoplexy after goserelin. *Lancet* 1995; **345:** 458.

## Pharmacokinetics

Goserelin is almost completely absorbed following subcutaneous injection, and has a serum elimination half-life of 2 to 4 hours, which may be increased in patients with impaired renal function. More than 90% of a dose is excreted in urine, as unchanged drug and metabolites.

◊ Reviews.

1. Cockshott ID. Clinical pharmacokinetics of goserelin. *Clin Pharmacokinet* 2000; **39:** 27–48.

## Uses and Administration

Goserelin is an analogue of gonadorelin (p.1325) with similar properties. It is used for the suppression of gonadal sex hormone production in the treatment of malignant neoplasms of the prostate, in breast cancer in pre- and peri-menopausal women, and in the management of endometriosis and uterine fibroids. It is also given before surgery for endometrial reduction and as an adjunct to ovulation induction with gonadotrophins in the treatment of infertility. Goserelin is usually given as the acetate but doses are expressed in terms of the base; 10.5 mg of goserelin acetate is approximately equivalent to 10 mg of goserelin.

Goserelin acetate is available as depot preparations; with one such preparation a dose equivalent to 3.6 mg of goserelin injected subcutaneously into the anterior abdominal wall provides effective suppression of oestradiol or testosterone for 28 days. A full response should be achieved by the end of this period and treatment is continued with repeated doses at 28-day intervals; in endometriosis, therapy is given for up to 6 months while in women with anaemia as a result of uterine fibroids it is continued, with concomitant iron supplementation, for up to 3 months before surgery. In men with prostate cancer preparations supplying the equivalent of 10.8 mg of goserelin, given every 12 weeks, may also be employed.

In the treatment of prostatic cancer an anti-androgen such as cyproterone acetate may be given for several days before beginning goserelin therapy and continued for at least 3 weeks, to avoid the risk of a disease flare.

Regimens for oocyte collection for *in-vitro* fertilisation employ gonadorelin analogues for pituitary desensitisation before ovulation induction with gonadotrophins. The equivalent of 3.6 mg of goserelin is given as a subcutaneous depot injection and serum-oestradiol concentrations monitored until they decline to levels similar to those in the early follicular phase, a process which usually takes 7 to 21 days. Once downregulation occurs gonadotrophin (follicle stimulating) therapy is begun until an appropriate stage of follicular development, when it is withdrawn and chorionic gonadotrophin is given to induce ovulation.

Goserelin has also been given in other sex-hormone-related conditions.

◊ Reviews of goserelin.


1. Chrisp P, Goa KL. Goserelin: a review of its pharmacodynamic and pharmacokinetic properties, and clinical use in sex hormone-related conditions. *Drugs* 1991; **41:** 254–88.
2. Perry CM, Brogden RN. Goserelin: a review of its pharmacodynamic and pharmacokinetic properties, and therapeutic use in benign gynaecological disorders. *Drugs* 1996; **51:** 319–46.


**Endometriosis.** Gonadorelin analogues such as goserelin are effective in the management of endometriosis (p.1546), but the need for long-term therapy to prevent recurrence limits their value because of the risk of osteoporosis. 'Add-back' therapy, with concomitant hormone replacement, may be given in an attempt to reduce bone mineral density loss and vasomotor symptoms in women receiving goserelin.

References.


1. Shaw RW, *et al.* An open randomized comparative study of the effect of goserelin depot and danazol in the treatment of endometriosis. *Fertil Steril* 1992; **58:** 265–72.
2. Schlaff WD. Extending the treatment boundaries: Zoladex and add-back. *Int J Gynaecol Obstet* 1999; **64** (suppl 1): S25–S31.
3. Franke HR, *et al.* Gonadotropin-releasing hormone agonist plus "add-back" hormone replacement therapy for treatment of endometriosis: a prospective, randomized, placebo-controlled, double-blind trial. *Fertil Steril* 2000; **74:** 534–9.
4. Pierce SJ, *et al.* Long-term use of gonadotropin-releasing hormone analogs and hormone replacement therapy in the management of endometriosis: a randomized trial with a 6-year follow-up. *Fertil Steril* 2000; **74:** 964–8.


**Fibroids.** Gonadorelin analogues such as goserelin have been tried as an adjunct or an alternative to surgery in the treatment of uterine fibroids (p.1326) although there has been some concern that this might complicate the diagnosis of malignancy. Some further references are listed below.


1. Lumsden MA, *et al.* Goserelin therapy before surgery for uterine fibroids. *Lancet* 1987; **i:** 36–7.
2. Lumsden MA, *et al.* Treatment with the gonadotrophin releasing hormone-agonist goserelin before hysterectomy for uterine fibroids. *Br J Obstet Gynaecol* 1994; **101:** 438–42.
3. Benagiano G, *et al.* Zoladex (goserelin acetate) and the anemic patient: results of a multicenter fibroid study. *Fertil Steril* 1996; **66:** 223–9.


**Malignant neoplasms.** Goserelin is effective in the treatment of prostate cancer (p.521). It has produced a response similar to that of orchidectomy (surgical removal of the testes) in patients with metastatic prostate cancer.[1] Goserelin has been combined with an anti-androgen such as flutamide to provide maximum androgen blockade, but this appears to produce modest additional benefits at most. There is some evidence that adjuvant therapy with goserelin may improve survival in patients with locally advanced prostate cancer when combined with radiotherapy.[2]

Goserelin may also be used as hormonal therapy in premenopausal women with advanced breast cancer (p.514), either alone[3,4] or combined with tamoxifen,[5] and is said to be as effective as oophorectomy.[4] It is also used as an alternative to chemotherapy in pre- or peri-menopausal women with oestrogen-receptor positive early breast cancer.[6,7]


1. Seidenfeld J, *et al.* Single-therapy androgen suppression in men with advanced prostate cancer: a systematic review and meta-analysis. *Ann Intern Med* 2000; **132:** 566–77.
2. Bolla M, *et al.* Improved survival in patients with locally advanced prostrate cancer treated with radiotherapy and goserelin. *N Engl J Med* 1997; **337:** 295–300.
3. Dixon AR, *et al.* Goserelin (Zoladex) in premenopausal advanced breast cancer: duration of response and survival. *Br J Cancer* 1990; **62:** 868–70.
4. Bajetta E, *et al.* Goserelin in premenopausal advanced breast cancer: clinical and endocrine evaluation of responsive patients. *Oncology* 1994; **51:** 262–9.
5. Jonat W, *et al.* A randomised study to compare the effect of the luteinising hormone releasing hormone (LHRH) analogue goserelin with or without tamoxifen in pre- and perimenopausal patients with advanced breast cancer. *Eur J Cancer* 1995; **31A:** 137–42.
6. Jakesz R, *et al.* Randomized adjuvant trial of tamoxifen and goserelin versus cyclophosphamide, methotrexate, and fluorouracil: evidence for the superiority of treatment with endocrine blockade in premenopausal patients with hormone-responsive breast cancer—Austrian Breast and Colorectal Cancer Study Group Trial 5. *J Clin Oncol* 2002; **20:** 4621–7.
7. Jonat W, *et al.* Goserelin versus cyclophosphamide, methotrexate, and fluorouracil as adjuvant therapy in premenopausal patients with node-positive breast cancer: the Zoladex Early Breast Cancer Research Association Study. *J Clin Oncol* 2002; **20:** 4628–35.


**Mastalgia.** For reference to the use of goserelin in mastalgia, see under Danazol, p.1546.

## Preparations

**Proprietary Preparations** (details are given in Part 3)
***Arg.:*** Larmadex; Zoladex; ***Austral.:*** Zoladex; ***Austria:*** Zoladex; ***Belg.:*** Zoladex; ***Braz.:*** Zoladex; ***Canad.:*** Zoladex; ***Chile:*** Vacromil; Zoladex; ***Denm.:*** Zoladex; ***Fin.:*** Zoladex; ***Fr.:*** Zoladex; ***Ger.:*** Zoladex; ***Gr.:*** Zoladex; ***Hong Kong:*** Zoladex; ***Irl.:*** Zoladex; ***Israel:*** Zoladex; ***Ital.:*** Zoladex; ***Malaysia:*** Zoladex; ***Mex.:*** Zoladex; ***Neth.:*** Zoladex; ***Norw.:*** Zoladex; ***NZ:*** Zoladex; ***Port.:*** Zoladex; ***S.Afr.:*** Zoladex; ***Singapore:*** Zoladex; ***Spain:*** Zoladex; ***Swed.:*** Zoladex; ***Switz.:*** Zoladex; ***Thai.:*** Zoladex; ***UK:*** Zoladex; ***USA:*** Zoladex.

---

# Growth Hormone *(BAN)*

GH; Phyone; Somatotrophin; Somatotropin; Somatotropina; STH.
*CAS — 9002-72-6.*

## Somatrem *(BAN, USAN, pINN)*

Met-HGH; Methionyl Human Growth Hormone.
$C_{995}H_{1537}N_{263}O_{301}S_8$ = 22 256.
*CAS — 82030-87-3.*
*ATC — H01AC02.*

**Description.** Somatrem is an analogue of somatropin containing an additional (methionyl) amino-acid residue. It may be produced in bacteria from recombinant DNA.
Sometribove (*BAN*) is methionyl bovine growth hormone.
Sometripor (*BAN*) is methionyl porcine growth hormone.

## Somatropin *(BAN, USAN, rINN)*

CB-311; HGH; Human Growth Hormone; LY-137998; Somatropina; Somatropinum.
$C_{990}H_{1528}N_{262}O_{300}S_7$ = 22 125.
*CAS — 12629-01-5.*
*ATC — H01AC01.*

**Description.** Somatropin is synthetic human growth hormone having the normal structure of the major (22K) component of natural human pituitary growth hormone. It consists of a single polypeptide chain of 191 amino acids with disulfide linkages between positions 53 and 165 and between 182 and 189. For labelling purposes, the name may carry in parentheses an approved code in lower case letters indicative of the method of production: (epr) indicates production by enzymatic conversion of a precursor produced by a bacterium genetically modified by recombinant DNA technology; (rbe) indicates production from bacteria genetically modified by recombinant DNA technology; (rmc) indicates production from genetically engineered and transformed mammalian (mouse) cells.
Somidobove (*BAN*) is synthetic bovine growth hormone.

**Pharmacopoeias.** In *Chin.* and *Eur.* (see p.vi).
**Ph. Eur. 5.0** (Somatropin). A protein having the structure (191 amino acid residues) of the major component of growth hormone produced by the human pituitary. A white or almost white powder, containing not less than 2.5 units/mg. Store at 2° to 8° in airtight containers.
**Ph. Eur. 5.0** (Somatropin Bulk Solution). A clear or slightly turbid, colourless solution. It may contain buffer salts and other auxiliary substances. Store at –20° in airtight containers. Avoid repeated freezing and thawing.

## Units

4.4 units of human growth hormone (somatropin) are contained in 1.75 mg of freeze-dried purified human growth hormone, with 20 mg of glycine, 2 mg of mannitol, 2 mg of lactose, and 2 mg of sodium bicarbonate, in one ampoule of the first International Standard (1987).

The first International Standard for Somatropin (1994) has a defined content of 2 mg of protein per ampoule, with a specific activity of 3 units/mg of protein. Commercial preparations vary somewhat in the number of units/mg.

◊ References.


1. WHO. WHO Expert Committee on biological standardization: forty-fourth report. *WHO Tech Rep Ser 848* 1994.
2. WHO. WHO Expert Committee on biological standardization: forty-fifth report *WHO Tech Rep Ser 858* 1995.


## Adverse Effects and Precautions

Antibodies to growth hormone have been formed in some patients but these rarely seem to affect growth. There may be redness, itching, lumps, or lipoatrophy at the site of injection. Transient dose-related fluid retention with peripheral oedema and carpal tunnel syndrome has occurred; headache, muscle and joint pain, and cases of benign intracranial hypertension have been reported. Although growth hormone has diabetogenic effects, high acute dosage has been associated with hypoglycaemia followed by hyperglycaemia.

Growth hormone therapy is contra-indicated in patients with active neoplasms or intracranial lesions and should be discontinued if evidence of tumour growth develops. Growth hormones should not be used for growth promotion in patients with closed epiphyses. Because of the diabetogenic effect of growth hormone it should be given with care to patients with diabetes mellitus; adjustment of antidiabetic therapy may be necessary. Hypothyroidism may develop during treatment, and may result in suboptimal response. For the suggestion that growth hormone should not be used to treat acute catabolic states, as in patients with severe burns or who are otherwise critically ill, see Burns, under Uses and Administration, below.

**Benign intracranial hypertension.** Benign intracranial hypertension (pseudotumor cerebri) had occurred[1] in 22 children and 1 adult given growth hormone treatment between 1986 and 1993. Eight further cases were identified in a subsequent report[2] in 1995. Three patients treated with mecasermin also developed benign intracranial hypertension. Symptoms such as headache and papilloedema resolved when treatment was stopped. In an analysis[3] of a postmarketing surveillance database (1985 to 2000) of almost 40 000 children and adolescents who had been treated with growth hormone for various conditions, there was an increased prevalence of benign intracranial hypertension compared with the general paediatric population. The incidence in new patients starting growth hormone therapy was estimated to be about 30 in 100 000, and had occurred more frequently in patients with renal failure or Turner's syndrome. Headache and papilloedema were the most common symptom and sign, but these did not occur in all patients, and most cases had an onset of a few months. The condition was effectively managed with discontinuation of growth hormone. A small number of patients were rechallenged after the benign intracranial hypertension had resolved, and most could be treated with doses that were 25 to 50% of the original dose. In a report of another case[4] it was pointed out that diagnosis may be complicated by the not infrequent occurrence of headache in patients receiving growth hormone; these normally resolved spontaneously.


1. Malozowski S, *et al.* Growth hormone, insulin-like growth factor I, and benign intracranial hypertension. *N Engl J Med* 1993; **329:** 665–6.
2. Malozowski S, *et al.* Benign intracranial hypertension in children with growth hormone deficiency treated with growth hormone. *J Pediatr* 1995; **126:** 996–9.
3. Reeves GD, Doyle DA. Growth hormone treatment and pseudotumor cerebri: coincidence or close relationship? *J Pediatr Endocrinol Metab* 2002; **15** (suppl 2): 723–30.
4. Price DA, *et al.* Benign intracranial hypertension induced by growth hormone treatment. *Lancet* 1995; **345:** 458–9.


**Carcinogenicity.** Despite fears to the contrary, studies in children given growth hormone after cranial irradiation for brain tumours or CNS leukaemia have found no evidence that therapy with growth hormone increased the relapse rate.[1-3]

Cases of acute leukaemia have been reported among patients treated with growth hormones. An international workshop convened in 1988 to review known leukaemia cases in patients treated with growth hormones in Europe, North America, Japan, and Australia since 1959 found the observed incidence of leukaemia in growth hormone-treated patients to represent a twofold increase over the expected rate.[4] After a careful review of the data it was concluded that there may be a small increase in leukaemia incidence associated with growth hormone treatment of growth hormone-deficient patients, but that it was not clear that this was actually attributable to growth hormone. A later study involving 6284 patients treated with growth hormone between 1963 and 1985 in the USA confirmed an increase of about 2.5-fold in the incidence of leukaemia in this population, but noted that many of the patients had other risk factors for leukaemia.[5] It has been suggested that growth hormone deficiency is itself a risk factor for leukaemia and that perhaps this, rather than growth hormone treatment, is related to the increased incidence of leukaemia in these patients.[6] If there is any risk it is relatively small, and in view of the essential nature of growth hormone therapy in growth hormone-deficient children it was considered inappropriate and unwise to withhold it.[4] Further large cohort studies of survivors of childhood cancers[3] or patients treated for idiopathic growth hormone deficiency[7] have found that the use of growth hormone was not associated with an increased risk of leukaemia.

There is some evidence to suggest that growth hormone may increase the risk of solid tumours. The risk of secondary solid tumours was increased in a cohort of childhood cancer survivors, but the authors considered that the risk was probably quite small compared with the benefits of growth hormone therapy in these patients.[3] Another cohort of patients who had been treated for idiopathic growth hormone deficiency showed increased risks in the incidence and mortality of colorectal cancer.[7]

Further reports of malignancies associated with growth hormone therapy include two children with Bloom's syndrome (a rare chromosomal disorder affecting DNA replication), one of whom developed B-cell non-Hodgkin's lymphoma and the other stem-cell leukaemia.[8]

1. Packer RJ, *et al.* Growth hormone replacement therapy in children with medulloblastoma: use and effect on tumor control. *J Clin Oncol* 2001; **19:** 480–7.
2. Swerdlow AJ, *et al.* Growth hormone treatment of children with brain tumors and risk of tumor recurrence. *J Clin Endocrinol Metab* 2000; **85:** 4444–9.
3. Sklar CA, *et al.* Risk of disease recurrence and second neoplasms in survivors of childhood cancer treated with growth hormone: a report from the Childhood Cancer Survivor Study. *J Clin Endocrinol Metab* 2002; **87:** 3136–411.
4. Fisher DA, *et al.* Leukaemia in patients treated with growth hormone. *Lancet* 1988; **i:** 1159–60.
5. Fradkin JE, *et al.* Risk of leukemia after treatment with pituitary growth hormone. *JAMA* 1993; **270:** 2829–32.
6. Rapaport R, *et al.* Relationship of growth hormone deficiency and leukemia. *J Pediatr* 1995; **126:** 759–61.
7. Swerdlow AJ, *et al.* Risk of cancer in patients treated with human pituitary growth hormone in the UK, 1959–85: a cohort study. *Lancet* 2002; **360:** 273–7.
8. Brock PR, *et al.* Malignant disease in Bloom's syndrome children treated with growth hormone. *Lancet* 1991; **337:** 1345–6.

**Creutzfeldt-Jakob disease.** Reports in 1985 of a small number of deaths from Creutzfeldt-Jakob disease in patients under 40 years of age who had received growth hormone extracted from human pituitary glands resulted in the suspension of the distribution of pituitary-derived growth hormone by the licensing authorities in a number of countries, including Australia, Canada, the Netherlands, the UK, and the USA.[1-5] Preparations of non-pituitary-derived growth hormone are now available that are free from contamination with Creutzfeldt-Jakob agent. However, because of the long incubation period of the disease, cases are still being reported in patients who had received pituitary-derived growth hormone years previously.[6-10]

1. Brown P, *et al.* Potential epidemic of Creutzfeldt-Jakob disease from human growth hormone therapy. *N Engl J Med* 1985; **313:** 728–33. Correction. *ibid.*; 967.
2. Powell-Jackson J, *et al.* Creutzfeldt-Jakob disease after administration of human growth hormone. *Lancet* 1985; **ii:** 244–6.
3. Anonymous. Human growth hormone distribution discontinued. *FDA Drug Bull* 1985; **15:** 17–18.
4. Lazarus L. Suspension of the Australian human pituitary hormone programme. *Med J Aust* 1985; **143:** 57–9.
5. Bannister BA, McCormick A. Creutzfeldt-Jakob disease with reference to the safety of pituitary growth hormone. *J Infect* 1987; **14:** 7–12.
6. Fradkin JE, *et al.* Creutzfeldt-Jakob disease in pituitary growth hormone recipients in the United States. *JAMA* 1991; **265:** 880–4.
7. Buchanan CR, *et al.* Mortality, neoplasia, and Creutzfeldt-Jakob disease in patients treated with human pituitary growth hormone in the United Kingdom. *BMJ* 1991; **302:** 824–8.
8. Billette de Villemeur T, *et al.* Creutzfeldt-Jakob disease in children treated with growth hormone. *Lancet* 1991; **337:** 864–5.
9. Macario ME, *et al.* Pituitary growth hormone and Creutzfeldt-Jakob disease. *BMJ* 1991; **302:** 1149.
10. Croes EA, *et al.* Creutzfeldt-Jakob disease 38 years after diagnostic use of human growth hormone. *J Neurol Neurosurg Psychiatry* 2002; **72:** 792–3.

**Effects on carbohydrate metabolism.** A retrospective analysis[1] of data from a pharmacoepidemiological survey of children treated with growth hormone found a higher incidence of type 2 diabetes, compared with that found in untreated children. The researchers speculated that growth hormone treatment might precipitate the onset of type 2 diabetes in predisposed patients, and proposed that patients with risk factors for diabetes, including Turner's syndrome, Prader-Willi syndrome, or intrauterine growth retardation, be monitored. Studies of growth hormone have reported rises in serum concentrations of insulin, fasting and postprandial blood-glucose, and glycosylated haemoglobin, although these changes were generally small.[2] It has been noted that these effects appear to regress during treatment, but not always, and in some patients glucose intolerance and diabetes mellitus is not reversible after withdrawal of growth hormone.

Nonketotic hyperglycaemia developed within weeks of beginning growth hormone therapy in a 22-month-old child, leading to convulsions and metabolic acidosis; the patient died despite correction of the hyperglycaemia.[3]

1. Cutfield WS, *et al.* Incidence of diabetes mellitus and impaired glucose tolerance in children and adolescents receiving growth-hormone treatment. *Lancet* 2000; **355:** 610–13.
2. Jeffcoate W. Growth hormone therapy and its relationship to insulin resistance, glucose intolerance and diabetes mellitus: a review of recent evidence. *Drug Safety* 2002; **25:** 199–212.
3. Garg AK. Hyperglycemia during replacement growth hormone therapy. *J Pediatr* 1994; **125:** 329.

**Effects on immune function.** Growth hormone is generally considered to interact with the immune system although there is a lack of evidence that this is clinically significant.[1,2] There has been a report of acute renal transplant rejection in 2 children receiving treatment for growth retardation with somatropin.[3] In both children renal function of the transplant was stable for several years before somatropin was started, and growth hormone therapy had continued for some months before rejection occurred. It was suggested that during the first months of growth hormone therapy in transplant recipients, immunosuppressive therapy should be increased and transplant function carefully monitored.

1. Church JA, *et al.* Immune functions in children treated with biosynthetic growth hormone. *J Pediatr* 1989; **115:** 420–3.
2. Rapaport R, Oleske J. Immune function during growth hormone therapy. *J Pediatr* 1990; **116:** 669–70.
3. Tydén G, *et al.* Acute renal graft rejection after treatment with human growth hormone. *Lancet* 1990; **336:** 1455–6.

**Effects on skeletal muscle.** A report of mild inflammatory myositis, with myalgia and muscle weakness, in 2 patients receiving growth hormone therapy.[1] It was suggested that the effect might be due to *m*-cresol used as a preservative in the preparation.

1. Yordam N. Myositis associated with growth hormone therapy. *J Pediatr* 1994; **125:** 671.

**Gynaecomastia.** A report of 22 cases of prepubertal gynaecomastia diagnosed during growth hormone treatment.[1]

1. Malozowski S, Stadel BV. Prepubertal gynecomastia during growth hormone therapy. *J Pediatr* 1995; **126:** 659–61.

**Hypersensitivity.** Generalised urticaria in a patient given somatropin was overcome by a desensitisation regimen.[1] The patient was subsequently maintained uneventfully on daily injections of somatropin.

1. Walker SB, *et al.* Systemic reaction to human growth hormone treated with acute desensitization. *Pediatrics* 1992; **90:** 108–9.

**Iron deficiency.** The view has been expressed[1] that given the increased production of haemoglobin and the prevalence of iron deficiency in patients treated with growth hormone, supplementation with iron should be considered in patients receiving growth hormone treatment.

1. Vihervuori E, *et al.* Increases in hemoglobin concentration and iron needs in response to growth hormone treatment. *J Pediatr* 1994; **125:** 242–5.

**Pancreatitis.** A report of acute pancreatitis in a patient with pseudohypoparathyroidism and growth hormone deficiency following the institution of growth hormone treatment.[1] Ten further cases of acute pancreatitis associated with growth hormone treatment had been reported to the FDA at the time of writing.

1. Malozowski S, *et al.* Acute pancreatitis associated with growth hormone therapy for short stature. *N Engl J Med* 1995; **332:** 401–2.

**Prader-Willi syndrome.** One US manufacturer of somatropin has stated that as of April 2003 it was aware of 7 reports of death in children with Prader-Willi syndrome treated with growth hormone.[1] The patients shared one or more of the following risk factors: severe obesity, a history of respiratory impairment or sleep apnoea, or unidentified respiratory infection. It was recommended that patients with Prader-Willi syndrome should be evaluated for upper airway obstruction, before beginning treatment, and if signs of such obstruction, such as snoring, developed during treatment therapy should be suspended. Somatropin was considered contra-indicated in these patients if they were severely obese or had severe respiratory impairment; licensed drug information in the USA had been amended accordingly. Early diagnosis and aggressive treatment of respiratory infections was also recommended.

1. Pharmacia, USA. 2003 Safety alert: Genotropin (somatropin [rDNA origin] for injection). Available at: http://www.fda.gov/medwatch/SAFETY/2003/genotropin.htm (accessed 02/04/04)

## Interactions

High doses of corticosteroids may inhibit the growth promoting effects of growth hormone.

## Pharmacokinetics

Somatropin is well absorbed after subcutaneous or intramuscular injection with a bioavailability varying from about 60 to 80%; peak serum concentrations may not be achieved for several hours. After intravenous injection it has a half-life of about 20 to 30 minutes but after subcutaneous or intramuscular administration serum concentrations decline with a half-life of 3 to 5 hours, due to more prolonged release from the injection site. It is metabolised in the liver and kidneys and excreted in bile.

◊ Studies of the pharmacokinetics of somatropin following transdermal jet injection in healthy subjects suggested that absorption was more rapid and peak serum concentration higher than after conventional subcutaneous injection of the same dose.[1,2] However this did not seem to result in any difference in the total amount absorbed, nor in the biological effect.

1. Verhagen A, *et al.* Pharmacokinetics and pharmacodynamics of a single dose of recombinant human growth hormone after subcutaneous administration by jet-injection: comparison with conventional needle-injection. *Eur J Clin Pharmacol* 1995; **49:** 69–72.
2. Agersø H, *et al.* Pharmacokinetics and pharmacodynamics of a new formulation of recombinant human growth hormone administered by ZomaJet 2 Vision, a new needle-free device, compared to subcutaneous administration using a conventional syringe. *J Clin Pharmacol* 2002; **42:** 1262–8.

## Uses and Administration

Somatropin is synthetic human growth hormone and somatrem its methionyl analogue.

Growth hormone is an anabolic hormone secreted by the anterior lobe of the pituitary, varying in size and amino-acid sequence between animal species. It promotes growth of skeletal, muscular, and other tissues, stimulates protein anabolism, and affects fat and mineral metabolism. The hormone has a diabetogenic action on carbohydrate metabolism. Secretion is pulsatile and dependent on neural and hormonal influences including a hypothalamic release-inhibiting hormone (see Somatostatin, p.1339), and a hypothalamic releasing hormone (see Somatorelin, p.1339). Sleep, hypoglycaemia, and physical or emotional stress result in increased secretion of growth hormone. The effects of growth hormone on skeletal growth are mediated by the somatomedins (see p.1338).

Somatropin or somatrem is given to children with open epiphyses for the treatment of short stature due to growth hormone deficiency (pituitary dwarfism) following assessment of pituitary function. Somatropin is also used in children with some other forms of growth retardation, for example in Turner's syndrome, or that due to chronic renal insufficiency, or in short children born small for gestational age. In Prader-Willi syndrome, somatropin is given to improve growth and body composition (but see also under Adverse Effects and Precautions, above). In adults, somatropin is given for confirmed growth hormone deficiency. It is also used in the management of wasting or cachexia associated with AIDS.

Doses should be individualised for each patient. Manufacturers vary somewhat in their estimates of the number of units/mg for somatropin and although some countries specify labelling in mg, others require labelling in units or both. Somatrem may be given in doses similar to those of somatropin.

In children with growth hormone deficiency, the usual daily dose in the UK is 25 to 35 micrograms/kg by subcutaneous injection (0.07 to 0.1 units/kg), or 0.7 to 1 mg/m$^2$ (2 to 3 units/m$^2$). Similar doses are used in other countries, by subcutaneous or intramuscular injection, and the total weekly dose may be divided into 3, 6, or 7 doses. A suspension of somatropin for subcutaneous depot injection is also available, given in a dose of 1.5 mg/kg on the same day of each month. Alternatively, the dose can be given as 750 micrograms/kg twice monthly (for example, on days 1 and 15 of each month).

In Turner's syndrome (gonadal dysgenesis) higher doses are used, such as a subcutaneous daily dose of 45 to 50 micrograms/kg (0.14 units/kg), or 1.4 mg/m$^2$ (4.3 units/m$^2$). Similar doses may be employed in children with growth retardation due to chronic renal insufficiency.

In children with growth retardation who were born small for gestational age, the licensed daily dose in the UK is 35 micrograms/kg by subcutaneous injection (0.1 units/kg), or 1 mg/m$^2$ (3 units/m$^2$). In the USA, the licensed dose is somewhat higher, at 480 micrograms/kg weekly, divided into 6 or 7 doses.

In children with Prader-Willi syndrome, a daily dose of about 35 micrograms/kg, or 1 mg/m$^2$, is given subcutaneously; daily doses should not exceed 2.7 mg.

In adults with growth hormone deficiency lower doses are recommended. The initial dose is not more than 6 micrograms/kg (0.018 units/kg) subcutaneously daily. The dose can then be gradually increased according to patient response, to a usual maximum of

12.5 micrograms/kg daily, although doses up to 25 micrograms/kg daily have been used for patients younger than 35 years of age. Alternatively, an initial dose in the range of 150 to 300 micrograms daily (0.45 to 0.9 units) is increased gradually at monthly intervals, based on clinical response, to a maintenance dose of no more than 1 mg daily. Dosage requirements may decline with increasing age. In the UK, it has been recommended that treatment should be re-assessed 9 months after starting therapy.

In the treatment of HIV-associated wasting or cachexia somatropin is given in doses of 100 micrograms/kg daily by subcutaneous injection at bedtime.

Somatropin is also used in short bowel syndrome to increase intestinal absorption of water, electrolytes, and nutrients. It has been given subcutaneously in a dose of about 100 micrograms/kg daily (to a maximum of 8 mg daily) for 4 weeks.

**Administration in adults.** Growth hormone continues to be secreted in adult life, although secretion and activity gradually decline with increasing age, and it appears to play a role in maintaining skeletal and lean body-mass amongst other things. In adults with growth hormone deficiency (usually secondary to pituitary adenoma or its treatment) replacement therapy with growth hormone is reported to decrease body fat and abdominal adiposity, increase lean body-mass, and improve lipid profiles.[1-3] It may also increase bone density,[1,3] and improve strength, exercise capacity, and some other cardiovascular risk factors.[3] There are also reports of improvements in quality of life[3] but not all studies have found benefit.[4] Long-term data are not yet available to determine whether growth hormone therapy reduces the mortality rate in this group of patients. Guidelines on the use of growth hormone in adults with growth hormone deficiency have been issued in the UK.[5]

Less well established is the use of growth hormone in otherwise healthy elderly patients. Considerable controversy has attended suggestions that growth hormone therapy may retard or reverse some of the metabolic effects of ageing, and there is some concern that these patients may be at increased risk of adverse effects.[6] Studies[7,8] have shown that growth hormone can increase lean body-mass and decrease body fat, but functional ability does not necessarily improve and common adverse effects include peripheral oedema, carpal tunnel syndrome, and arthralgias.

Other uses for growth hormone in adult patients are discussed below.


1. Götherström G, *et al.* A prospective study of 5 years of GH replacement therapy in GH-deficient adults: sustained effects on body composition, bone mass, and metabolic indices. *J Clin Endocrinol Metab* 2001; **86:** 4657–65.
2. Attanasio AF, *et al.* Human growth hormone replacement in adult hypopituitary patients: long-term effects on body composition and lipid status—3-year results from the HypoCCS Database. *J Clin Endocrinol Metab* 2002; **87:** 1600–6.
3. Verhelst J, Abs R. Long-term growth hormone replacement therapy in hypopituitary adults. *Drugs* 2002; **62:** 2399–2412.
4. Baum HBA, *et al.* Effects of physiological growth hormone (GH) therapy on cognition and quality of life in patients with adult-onset GH deficiency. *J Clin Endocrinol Metab* 1998; **83:** 3184–9.
5. National Institute for Clinical Excellence. Human growth hormone (somatropin) in adults with growth hormone deficiency (issued August 2003). Available at: http://www.nice.org.uk/pdf/TA64_HGHadults_fullguidance.pdf (accessed 08/04/04)
6. Vance ML. Can growth hormone prevent aging? *N Engl J Med* 2003; **348:** 779–80.
7. Papadakis MA, *et al.* Growth hormone replacement in healthy older men improves body composition but not functional ability. *Ann Intern Med* 1996; **124:** 708–16.
8. Blackman MR, *et al.* Growth hormone and sex steroid administration in healthy aged women and men: a randomized controlled trial. *JAMA* 2002; **288:** 2282–92.


**Burns.** In children with severe burns requiring skin grafts, somatropin 200 micrograms/kg daily by intramuscular injection reduced donor-site healing times and hospitalisation times; subcutaneous somatropin 100 micrograms/kg daily was ineffective.[1] Treatment also subsequently ameliorates burn-induced growth delays in such children.[2] However, the manufacturers have recommended that somatropin should not be used to treat acute catabolic states in critically ill and burn patients, as there is some evidence in adults that mortality may be increased.[3] The management of burns is described on p.1134.


1. Herndon DN, *et al.* Effects of recombinant human growth hormone on donor-site healing in severely burned children. *Ann Surg* 1990; **212:** 424–9.
2. Low JFA, *et al.* Effect of growth hormone on growth delay in burned children: a 3-year follow-up study. *Lancet* 1999; **354:** 1789.
3. Takala J, *et al.* Increased mortality associated with growth hormone treatment in critically ill adults. *N Engl J Med* 1999; **341:** 785–92.


**Cachexia and lipodystrophy.** Treatment with subcutaneous growth hormone has been reported[1-3] to reverse weight loss and improve body wasting in subjects with HIV disease (p.623). Dosage may be important: most studies have used doses of around 100 micrograms/kg, but a study using lower doses, alone or combined with mecasermin, reported only modest improvement.[4] Mecasermin alone was of uncertain value.

Some benefit has been reported[5,6] with growth hormone therapy in HIV-associated lipodystrophy, but its use is currently investigational.

Growth hormone therapy has also been reported to improve metabolic indicators of malnutrition when given with parenteral nutrition to patients undergoing haemodialysis.[7]


1. Krentz AJ, *et al.* Anthropometric, metabolic, and immunological effects of recombinant human growth hormone in AIDS and AIDS-related complex. *J Acquir Immune Defic Syndr* 1993; **6:** 245–51.
2. Mulligan K, *et al.* Anabolic effects of recombinant human growth hormone in patients with wasting associated with human immunodeficiency virus infection. *J Clin Endocrinol Metab* 1993; **77:** 956–62.
3. Schambelan M, *et al.* Recombinant human growth hormone in patients with HIV-associated wasting: a randomized, placebo-controlled trial. *Ann Intern Med* 1996; **125:** 873–82.
4. Waters D, *et al.* Recombinant human growth hormone, insulin-like growth factor 1, and combination therapy in AIDS-associated wasting: a randomized, double-blind, placebo-controlled trial. *Ann Intern Med* 1996; **125:** 865–72.
5. Lo JC, *et al.* The effects of recombinant human growth hormone on body composition and glucose metabolism in HIV-infected patients with fat accumulation. *J Clin Endocrinol Metab* 2001; **86:** 3480–7.
6. Tai VW, *et al.* Effects of recombinant human growth hormone on fat distribution in patients with human immunodeficiency virus–associated wasting. *Clin Infect Dis* 2002; **35:** 1258–62.
7. Schulman G, *et al.* The effects of recombinant human growth hormone and intradialytic parenteral nutrition in malnourished haemodialysis patients. *Am J Kidney Dis* 1993; **21:** 527–34.


**Cardiovascular disorders.** A few small uncontrolled studies have reported improvements in heart failure (p.820) with the use of growth hormone.[1] However, in a controlled study, growth hormone given for 12 weeks to patients with heart failure secondary to dilated cardiomyopathy (p.818) produced an increase in left-ventricular mass but no improvement in clinical status.[2] A study[3] of 6 months' treatment in patients with ischaemic cardiac failure found no improvement in left-ventricular function or mass.


1. Volterrani M, *et al.* Role of growth hormone in chronic heart failure: therapeutic implications. *Drugs* 2000; **60:** 711–19.
2. Osterziel KJ, *et al.* Randomised, double-blind, placebo-controlled trial of human recombinant growth hormone in patients with chronic heart failure due to dilated cardiomyopathy. *Lancet* 1998; **351:** 1233–7.
3. Smit JWA, *et al.* Six months of recombinant human GH therapy in patients with ischemic cardiac failure does not influence left ventricular function and mass. *J Clin Endocrinol Metab* 2001; **86:** 4638–43.


**Fibromyalgia.** Symptomatic improvement was reported after several months in a study of daily subcutaneous growth hormone injection in women with fibromyalgia,[1] a painful form of soft-tissue rheumatism (p.11), and low levels of insulin-like growth factor I (IGF-I).


1. Bennett RM, *et al.* A randomized, double-blind, placebo-controlled study of growth hormone in the treatment of fibromyalgia. *Am J Med* 1998; **104:** 227–31.


**Growth retardation.** Growth hormone is a mainstay of the management of growth retardation (p.1314) and various guidelines[1-3] have been issued concerning its appropriate use.


1. Drug and Therapeutics Committee, Lawson Wilkins Pediatric Endocrine Society. Guidelines for the use of growth hormone in children with short stature. *J Pediatr* 1995; **127:** 857–67.
2. GH Research Society. Consensus guidelines for the diagnosis and treatment of growth hormone (GH) deficiency in childhood and adolescence: summary statement of the GH Research Society. *J Clin Endocrinol Metab* 2000; **85:** 3990–3. Also available at: http://jcem.endojournals.org/cgi/reprint/85/11/3990.pdf (accessed 02/04/04)
3. National Institute for Clinical Excellence. Guidance on the use of human growth hormone (somatropin) in children with growth failure (May 2002). Available at: http://www.nice.org.uk/pdf/HGHinChild-42-ALS.pdf (accessed 02/04/04)


**Infertility.** Studies[1,2] have found that somatropin sensitises the ovary to stimulation by gonadotrophins and it has been suggested that it may have a role in the management of female infertility in patients resistant to conventional ovarian stimulation, although not in those with no previous history of poor stimulation.[3] However, some have found it of little value[4] and current UK guidelines[5] for the treatment of infertility do not recommend its use. Growth hormone has also been tried similarly to enhance spermatogenesis in infertile men unresponsive to conventional therapy.[6,7]

For a discussion of infertility and the more usual drugs used in its management, see p.1316.


1. Homburg R, *et al.* Cotreatment with human growth hormone and gonadotropins for induction of ovulation: a controlled clinical trial. *Fertil Steril* 1990; **53:** 254–60.
2. Yoshimura Y, *et al.* Effects of growth hormone on follicle growth, oocyte maturation, and ovarian steroidogenesis. *Fertil Steril* 1993; **59:** 917–23.
3. Harper K, *et al.* Growth hormone for in vitro fertilization. Available in The Cochrane Library; Issue 1. Chichester: John Wiley; 2004.
4. Levron J, *et al.* No beneficial effects of human growth hormone therapy in normal ovulatory patients with a poor ovarian response to gonadotropins. *Gynecol Obstet Invest* 1993; **35:** 65–8.
5. National Collaborating Centre for Women's and Children's Health. Fertility: assessment and treatment for people with fertility problems. February 2004. Available at: http://www.rcog.org.uk/resources/Public/Fertility_full.pdf (accessed 21/04/04)
6. Shoham Z, *et al.* Cotreatment with growth hormone for induction of spermatogenesis in patients with hypogonadotropic hypogonadism. *Fertil Steril* 1992; **57:** 1044–51.
7. Ovesen PG. *et al.* Vaeksthormonbehandling af maend med nedsat saedkvalitet. *Ugeskr Laeger* 1998; **160:** 176–80.


**Osteogenesis imperfecta.** For reference to possible benefit from growth hormone therapy in patients with osteogenesis imperfecta, see p.762.

**Osteomalacia.** As mentioned on p.762, there has been some interest in the use of growth hormone in children with hypophosphataemic rickets.

**Prader-Willi syndrome.** Growth hormone treatment may be of benefit in the management of Prader-Willi syndrome (p.1584), but see also under Adverse Effects and Precautions, above.

References.


1. Lindgren AC, *et al.* Five years of growth hormone treatment in children with Prader-Willi syndrome. *Acta Paediatr Suppl* 1999; **433:** 109–11.
2. Myers SE, *et al.* Physical effects of growth hormone treatment in children with Prader-Willi syndrome. *Acta Paediatr Suppl* 1999; **433:** 112–14.
3. Carrel AL, *et al.* Growth hormone improves body composition, fat utilization, physical strength and agility, and growth in Prader-Willi syndrome: a controlled study. *J Pediatr* 1999; **134:** 215–21.
4. Myers SE, *et al.* Sustained benefit after 2 years of growth hormone on body composition, fat utilization, physical strength and agility, and growth in Prader-Willi syndrome. *J Pediatr* 2000; **137:** 42–9.
5. Carrel AL, *et al.* Benefits of long-term GH therapy in Prader-Willi syndrome: a 4-year study. *J Clin Endocrinol Metab* 2002; **87:** 1581–5.
6. Whitman BY, *et al.* The behavioral impact of growth hormone treatment for children and adolescents with Prader-Willi syndrome: a 2-year, controlled study. *Pediatrics* 2002; **109:** 308–9. Full version: http://pediatrics.aappublications.org/cgi/content/full/109/2/e35 (accessed 02/04/04)


**Veterinary and agricultural use.** Bovine growth hormone or bovine somatotrophin (bovine somatotropin; BST) can increase milk yield. Some references to the debate on the safety of this practice follow.


1. Daughaday WH, Barbano DM. Bovine somatotropin supplementation of dairy cows: is the milk safe? *JAMA* 1990; **264:** 1003–5. Correction. *ibid.* 1991; **265:** 1393.
2. Mepham TB. Bovine somatotrophin and public health. *BMJ* 1991; **302:** 483–4.
3. Kronfeld DS. Bovine somatotropin. *JAMA* 1991; **265:** 1389.
4. Daughaday WH, Barbano DM. Bovine somatotropin. *JAMA* 1991; **265:** 1389–90.
5. Morris K. Bovine somatotrophin—who's crying over spilt milk? *Lancet* 1999; **353:** 306.


## Preparations

***BP 2003:*** Somatropin Injection.

**Proprietary Preparations** (details are given in Part 3)

***Arg.:*** Biotropin; Genotropin; HHT; Hutrope; Norditropin; Saizen; Serostim; ***Austral.:*** Genotropin; Humatro-Pen; Humatrope; Norditropin; Saizen; Scitropin; ***Austria:*** Genotropin; Humatrope; Norditropin; Saizen; Zomacton; ***Belg.:*** Genotonorm; Humatrope; Norditropin; Zomacton; ***Braz.:*** Biotropin; Genotropin; Humatrope; Norditropin†; Saizen; Somatrop; Somatropil†; ***Canad.:*** Humatrope; Nutropin; Protropin; Saizen; Serostim; ***Chile:*** Genotonorm; Humatrope; Norditropin; ***Denm.:*** Genotropin; Humatrope; Norditropin; Zomacton; ***Fin.:*** Genotropin; Humatrope; Norditropin; Saizen; Zomacton; ***Fr.:*** Genotonorm; Maxomat; Norditropine; Saizen; Umatrope; Zomacton; ***Ger.:*** Genotropin; Humatrope; Norditropin; Saizen; Zomacton; ***Gr.:*** Genotropin; Humatrope; Norditropin; Saizen; Zomacton; ***Hong Kong:*** Genotropin; Humatrope; Norditropin; Saizen; Scitropin; Serostim; ***India:*** Saizen; ***Irl.:*** Genotropin; Norditropin; Saizen; Zomacton; ***Israel:*** Bio-Tropin; Genotropin; Norditropin; Saizen†; ***Ital.:*** Genotropin; Humatrope; Norditropin; Saizen; Zomacton; ***Jpn:*** Growject; Norditropin; ***Malaysia:*** Genotropin; Norditropin; Saizen; ***Mex.:*** Bio-Tropin†; Cryo-Tropin; Genotropin; Humatrope; Norditropin; Saizen; Serostim; ***Neth.:*** Genotropin; Humatrope; Norditropin; Zomacton; ***Norw.:*** Genotropin; Humatrope; Norditropin; Saizen; Zomacton; ***NZ:*** Genotropin; Norditropin; Saizen; ***Port.:*** Genotropin; Humatrope; Norditropin; Saizen; Zomacton; ***S.Afr.:*** Genotropin; Humatrope; Norditropin; Saizen; ***Singapore:*** Genotropin; Humatrope; Norditropin; Saizen; Scitropin; Serostim†; ***Spain:*** Genotonorm; Humatrope; Norditropin; Saizen; Zomacton; ***Swed.:*** Genotropin; Humatrope; Norditropin; Saizen; Zomacton; ***Switz.:*** Genotropin; Humatrope; Norditropine; Saizen; ***UK:*** Genotropin; Humatrope; Norditropin; Nutropin; Saizen; Zomacton; ***USA:*** Genotropin; Humatrope; Norditropin; Nutropin; Protropin; Saizen; Serostim; Tev-Tropin; Zorbtive.

## Histrelin *(USAN, rINN)*

ORF-17070; RWJ-17070. 5-Oxo-L-prolyl-L-histidyl-L-tryptophyl-L-seryl-L-tyrosyl-$N^{\tau}$-benzyl-D-histidyl-L-leucyl-L-argininyl-*N*-ethyl-L-prolinamide.

$C_{66}H_{86}N_{18}O_{12}$ = 1323.5.
*CAS — 76712-82-8.*
*ATC — H01CA03.*

## Histrelin Acetate *(rINNM)*

Acetato de histrelina.

$C_{66}H_{86}N_{18}O_{12},xC_2H_4O_2,yH_2O$.
*CAS — 220810-26-4.*
*ATC — H01CA03.*

### Adverse Effects and Precautions

As for Gonadorelin, p.1325.

### Uses and Administration

Histrelin is an analogue of gonadorelin (p.1325) with similar properties. It is used for the suppression of gonadal sex hormone production in children with central precocious puberty (p.1318). It is given by subcutaneous injection as the acetate, in usual doses equivalent to histrelin 10 micrograms/kg daily.

Histrelin is under investigation in the treatment of malignant neoplasms of the prostate (p.521). It has also been investigated in disorders related to the menstrual cycle, and in the treatment of acute intermittent porphyria.

◊ References.


1. Anderson KE, *et al.* A gonadotropin releasing hormone analogue prevents cyclical attacks of porphyria. *Arch Intern Med* 1990; **150:** 1469–74.
2. Mortola JF, *et al.* Successful treatment of severe premenstrual syndrome by combined use of gonadotropin-releasing hormone agonist and estrogen/progestin. *J Clin Endocrinol Metab* 1991; **72:** 252A–F.
3. Barradell LB, McTavish D. Histrelin: a review of its pharmacological properties and therapeutic role in central precocious puberty. *Drugs* 1993; **45:** 570–88.
4. Cheung AP, Chang RJ. Pituitary responsiveness to gonadotrophin-releasing hormone agonist stimulation: a dose-response comparison of luteinizing hormone/follicle-stimulating hormone secretion in women with polycystic ovary syndrome and normal women. *Hum Reprod* 1995; **10:** 1054–9.
5. Feuillan PP, *et al.* Reproductive axis after discontinuation of gonadotropin-releasing hormone analog treatment of girls with precocious puberty: long term follow-up comparing girls with hypothalamic hamartoma to those with idiopathic precocious puberty. *J Clin Endocrinol Metab* 1999; **84:** 44–9.
6. Chertin B, *et al.* An implant releasing the gonadotropin hormone-releasing hormone agonist histrelin maintains medical castration for up to 30 months in metastatic prostate cancer. *J Urol (Baltimore)* 2000; **163:** 838–44.
7. Klein KO, *et al.* Increased final height in precocious puberty after long-term treatment with LHRH agonists: the National Institutes of Health experience. *J Clin Endocrinol Metab* 2001; **86:** 4711–16.


### Preparations

**Proprietary Preparations** (details are given in Part 3)
***USA:*** Supprelin.

## Human Menopausal Gonadotrophins *(BAN)*

Gonadotropina menopáusica humana; HMG; Org-31338; Urogonadotrophin.

*ATC — G03GA02.*

**Description.** A purified extract of human postmenopausal urine containing follicle-stimulating hormone (FSH) and luteinising hormone (LH); the relative *in-vivo* activity is expressed as a ratio. Human menopausal gonadotrophins with a ratio of FSH:LH of 1:1 are known as menotrophin (see below).

### Menotrophin *(BAN)*

Menotropina; Menotropins *(USAN)*; Menotropinum.

*CAS — 9002-68-0.*

**Pharmacopoeias.** In *Br., Chin.,* and *US.*

**BP 2003** (Menotrophin). A dry preparation containing glycoprotein gonadotrophins possessing follicle-stimulating and luteinising activities. It contains not less than 40 units of follicle-stimulating hormone activity per mg. The ratio of units of luteinising hormone activity to units of follicle-stimulating hormone activity is approximately 1. The preparation is exclusively or predominantly of pituitary origin and obtained from the urine of postmenopausal women but, when necessary, chorionic gonadotrophin obtained from the urine of pregnant women may be added to achieve the above ratio. An almost white or slightly yellow powder. Soluble in water. Store in airtight containers. Protect from light.

**USP 27** (Menotropins). An extract of human postmenopausal urine containing both follicle-stimulating hormone and luteinising hormone. It has a potency of not less than 40 follicle-stimulating hormone units and not less than 40 luteinising hormone units per mg. The ratio of units is approximately 1. Chorionic Gonadotropin obtained from the urine of pregnant women may be added to achieve this ratio. Not more than 30% of the luteinising hormone activity is contributed by Chorionic Gonadotropin. Store in airtight containers at 2° to 8°.

### Adverse Effects

Human menopausal gonadotrophins may cause dose-related ovarian hyperstimulation varying from mild ovarian enlargement and abdominal discomfort to severe hyperstimulation with marked ovarian enlargement or cyst formation, acute abdominal pain, ascites, pleural effusion, hypovolaemia, shock and thromboembolic disorders. Rupture of ovarian cysts and intraperitoneal haemorrhage has occurred, usually after pelvic examination. Fatalities have been reported.

Hypersensitivity reactions and local reactions at the injection site may occur. Nausea and vomiting, joint pains and fever have been reported; gynaecomastia, acne, and weight gain have occurred in men.

**Carcinogenicity.** In a case-control study of 4575 women with primary invasive breast cancer, an evaluation of risk factors found that, overall, the use of infertility drugs was not associated with an increased risk of breast cancer.[1] However, subgroup analysis of individual drugs found that the use of human menopausal gonadotrophins for at least 6 months or 6 treatment cycles was associated with a risk of breast cancer that was 2 to 3 times greater than for women who had never received any fertility treatment. The authors of this study noted that these results were based on small numbers and that other studies had failed to show an association between fertility treatment and breast cancer.


1. Burkman RT, *et al.* Infertility drugs and the risk of breast cancer: findings from the National Institute of Child Health and Human Development Women's Contraceptive and Reproductive Experiences Study. *Fertil Steril* 2003; **79:** 844–51.


**Effects on the ovary.** Ovarian hyperstimulation syndrome occurring with human menopausal gonadotrophins treatment in 4 women progressed to acute adnexal torsion[1] and in another became severe and was accompanied by deep-vein thrombosis.[2]


1. Kemmann E, *et al.* Adnexal torsion in menotropin-induced pregnancies. *Obstet Gynecol* 1990; **76:** 403–6.
2. Kaaja R, *et al.* Severe ovarian hyperstimulation syndrome and deep venous thrombosis. *Lancet* 1989; **ii:** 1043.


### Precautions

Human menopausal gonadotrophins should not be given to pregnant patients. Use should be avoided in patients with abnormal genital bleeding, hormone sensitive malignancies such as those of the breast, uterus, prostate, ovaries or testes, or ovarian cysts or enlargement not caused by the polycystic ovary syndrome. Pituitary or hypothalamic lesions, adrenal or thyroid disorders, and hyperprolactinaemia should be treated appropriately to exclude them as causes of infertility before attempting therapy with human menopausal gonadotrophins. Patients who experience ovarian enlargement are at risk of rupture; pelvic examinations should be avoided or carried out with care and the recommendation has been made that sexual intercourse should be avoided while there is such a risk.

There is a risk of multiple births.

### Interactions

In women who show evidence of excessive ovarian stimulation while receiving human menopausal gonadotrophins the use of drugs with luteinising-hormone (LH) activity increases the risk of ovarian hyperstimulation syndrome.

### Uses and Administration

Human menopausal gonadotrophins possess both follicle-stimulating hormone (FSH) activity (see p.1324) and luteinising hormone (LH) activity (see p.1332).

Human menopausal gonadotrophins are used in the treatment of male and female infertility due to hypogonadism. In anovulatory infertility unresponsive to clomifene, human menopausal gonadotrophins are administered to induce follicular maturation and are followed by treatment with chorionic gonadotrophin to stimulate ovulation and corpus luteum formation, a topic discussed further on p.1316. In women with polycystic ovary syndrome a gonadorelin analogue may be given beforehand to suppress pituitary gonadotrophin production (see p.1317).

The dosage and schedule of treatment for female infertility must be determined according to the needs of each patient; it is usual to monitor response by studying the patient's urinary oestrogen excretion or by ultrasonic visualisation of follicles, or both. Human menopausal gonadotrophins may be given daily by intramuscular or subcutaneous injection to provide a dose of 75 to 150 units of FSH and gradually adjusted if necessary until an adequate response is achieved. Treatment is then stopped and followed after 1 or 2 days by single doses of chorionic gonadotrophin 5000 to 10 000 units (see p.1321). In menstruating patients treatment should be started within the first 7 days of the menstrual cycle. In the UK it has been suggested that the treatment course should be abandoned if no response is seen in 3 weeks although in the US the manufacturers recommend that an individual course should not exceed 12 days. This course may be repeated at least twice more if necessary.

An alternative schedule is to give three equal doses by intramuscular or subcutaneous injection, each providing 225 to 375 units of FSH on alternate days followed by chorionic gonadotrophin one week after the first dose.

In fertilisation procedures *in vitro*, or other assisted conception techniques, human menopausal gonadotrophins are used with chorionic gonadotrophin and sometimes also clomifene citrate or a gonadorelin analogue. Stimulation of follicular growth is produced by human menopausal gonadotrophins given by intramuscular or subcutaneous injection, in a dose providing 75 to 300 units of FSH daily, usually beginning on the 2nd or 3rd day of the menstrual cycle. An example of a combined regimen involves clomifene citrate 100 mg on days 2 to 6, with human menopausal gonadotrophins beginning on day 5 in a dose providing 150 to 225 units of FSH daily. Treatment is continued until an adequate response is obtained and the final injection of human menopausal gonadotrophins is followed 1 to 2 days later with up to 10 000 units of chorionic gonadotrophin. Oocyte retrieval is carried out about 32 to 36 hours later.

In men with infertility due to hypogonadotrophic hypogonadism (see Infertility, p.1316), spermatogenesis is stimulated with chorionic gonadotrophin and then human menopausal gonadotrophins are added in a dose of 75 or 150 units of FSH two or three times weekly by intramuscular or subcutaneous injection. Treatment should be continued for at least 3 or 4 months.

**Infertility.** Anecdotal reports suggest that human menopausal gonadotrophins may be more effective than urofollitropin in treating anovulatory infertility,[1] perhaps because the luteinising hormone content plays some role in follicular development. However, meta-analyses indicate that urinary derived gonadotrophins have no advantage over traditional human menopausal gonadotrophin preparations.[2,3] However, in contrast, others have found the use of a pure recombinant follicle-stimulating hormone to be associated with higher pregnancy rates than human menopausal gonadotrophins when employed in regimens for *in-vitro* fertilisation.[4]

For a discussion of infertility and its management, including the role of human menopausal gonadotrophins, see p.1316.


1. Vine S, *et al.* Human gonadotrophin preparations. *BMJ* 1994; **308:** 1509–10.
2. Nugent D, *et al.* Gonadotrophin therapy for ovulation induction in subfertility associated with polycystic ovary syndrome. Available in The Cochrane Library, Issue 1. Chichester: John Wiley; 2004.
3. National Collaborating Centre for Women's and Children's Health. Fertility: assessment and treatment for people with fertility problems. February 2004. Available at: http://www.rcog.org.uk/resources/Public/Fertility_full.pdf (accessed 21/04/04)
4. Out HJ, *et al.* Recombinant follicle-stimulating hormone (follitropin beta, Puregon) yields higher pregnancy rates in in vitro fertilization than urinary gonadotropins. *Fertil Steril* 1997; **68:** 138–42.


### Preparations

***BP 2003:*** Menotrophin Injection;
***USP 27:*** Menotropins for Injection.

**Proprietary Preparations** (details are given in Part 3)
***Arg.:*** HMG Massone; Pergonal; ***Austral.:*** Humegon; ***Austria:*** Humegon†; Menopur; ***Belg.:*** Humegon†; Menogon†; Menopur; ***Braz.:*** Humegon†; Menogon†; Merional-HMG; Pergonal; ***Canad.:*** Humegon; Pergonal; ***Chile:*** Pergonal; ***Denm.:*** Menogon; Menopur; ***Fin.:*** Menogon; ***Fr.:*** Menogon†; Menopur; Neo-Pergonal†; ***Ger.:*** Humegon; Menogon; Pergonal†; ***Gr.:*** Altermon; Menogon; Pergogreen; Pergonal; ***Hong Kong:*** Humegon†; Menogon; Merional; Pergonal; ***India:*** Pergonal; Pregnorm; ***Irl.:*** Humegon; Menogon; Menopur; Pergonal†; ***Israel:*** Humegon; Menogon; Menopur; Pergonal; ***Ital.:*** Humegon; Menogon; Pergogreen†; ***Mex.:*** HMG Massone†; Humegon†; Pergonal; ***Neth.:*** Humegon†; Menogon; Menopur; Pergonal†; ***Port.:*** Humegon; ***S.Afr.:*** Humegon; Pergonal; ***Singapore:*** Humegon†; Menogon; Pergonal†; ***Spain:*** HMG; Menogon†; Menopur; Pergonal; ***Switz.:*** Humegon†; Menogon; Merional; Pergogreen†; Pergonal; ***Thai.:*** Humegon†; Pergonal†; ***UK:*** Menogon; Menopur; Merional; ***USA:*** Humegon; Pergonal; Repronex.

## Lanreotide Acetate *(BANM, USAN, rINNM)*

Acetato de lanreotida; BIM-23014C; BN-52030 (lanreotide). 3-(2-Naphthyl)-D-alanyl-L-cysteinyl-L-tyrosyl-D-tryptophyl-L-lysyl-L-valyl-L-cysteinyl-L-threoninamide cyclic (2→7)-disulfide acetate.

$C_{54}H_{69}N_{11}O_{10}S_2,x(C_2H_4O_2)$.

*CAS — 108736-35-2 (lanreotide); 127984-74-1 (lanreotide acetate).*

*ATC — H01CB03.*

### Adverse Effects and Precautions

As for Octreotide Acetate, p.1333.

### Interactions

As for Octreotide Acetate, p.1333.

### Pharmacokinetics

Following intravenous injection lanreotide has a terminal half-life of about 2.5 hours. Lanreotide is available as sustained-release preparations, and following subcutaneous or intramuscular administration of these an initial rapid liberation of the drug is followed by more prolonged release with an apparent half-life of about 5 to 30 days. The absolute bioavailability is stated to range from about 50 to 80%, depending on the product.

### Uses and Administration

Lanreotide is a somatostatin analogue with similar properties to those of octreotide (p.1333). It is given, as a long-acting depot injection, in the treatment of acromegaly (p.1312) and thyrotrophic adenoma, as well as in the symptomatic management of carcinoid syndrome (p.504).

Lanreotide is given as the acetate, but doses are usually expressed in terms of the base. The usual starting dose is equivalent to lanreotide 30 mg by intramuscular depot injection every 14 days. In acromegaly and carcinoid syndrome, this may be increased if necessary to 30 mg every 7 to 10 days; in thyrotrophic adenoma it may be increased to 30 mg every 10 days. An alternative preparation, given by deep subcutaneous injection every 28 days, delivers doses equivalent to 60, 90, or 120 mg of lanreotide.

Lanreotide has been tried for the prevention of restenosis in coronary blood vessels following angioplasty (see Reperfusion and Revascularisation Procedures, p.834).

◊ References.

1. Emanuelsson H, *et al.* Long-term effects of angiopeptin treatment in coronary angioplasty: reduction in clinical events but not angiographic restenosis. *Circulation* 1995; **91:** 1689–96.
2. Eriksson B, *et al.* The use of new somatostatin analogues, lanreotide and octastatin, in neuroendocrine gastro-intestinal tumours. *Digestion* 1996; **57** (suppl 1): 77–80.
3. Caron P, *et al.* Three year follow-up of acromegalic patients treated with intramuscular slow-release lanreotide. *J Clin Endocrinol Metab* 1997; **82:** 18–22.
4. Wymenga ANM, *et al.* Efficacy and safety of prolonged-release lanreotide in patients with gastrointestinal neuroendocrine tumors and hormone-related symptoms. *J Clin Oncol* 1999; **17:** 1111–17.
5. Baldelli R, *et al.* Two-year follow-up of acromegalic patients treated with slow release lanreotide (30 mg). *J Clin Endocrinol Metab* 2000; **85:** 4099–4103.
6. Kuhn JM, *et al.* Evaluation of the treatment of thyrotropin-secreting pituitary adenomas with a slow release formulation of the somatostatin analog lanreotide. *J Clin Endocrinol Metab* 2000; **85:** 1487–91.
7. Caron P, *et al.* Efficacy of the new long-acting formulation of lanreotide (Lanreotide Autogel) in the management of acromegaly. *J Clin Endocrinol Metab* 2002; **87:** 99–104.
8. Ayuk J, *et al.* Long-term safety and efficacy of depot long-acting somatostatin analogs for the treatment of acromegaly. *J Clin Endocrinol Metab* 2002; **87:** 4142–6.
9. Attanasio R, *et al.* Lanreotide 60 mg, a new long-acting formulation: effectiveness in the chronic treatment of acromegaly. *J Clin Endocrinol Metab* 2003; **88:** 5258–65.

**Administration in renal impairment.** The clearance of lanreotide, given by intravenous bolus, was reduced in patients with severe chronic renal impairment requiring haemodialysis.[1] The authors of this study suggested that considering the wide therapeutic window of lanreotide, depot formulations may be given at the usual initial dose, with further doses adjusted according to response. The manufacturers of one depot formulation recommend that dose adjustment is not necessary.

1. Barbanoj M, *et al.* Pharmacokinetics of the somatostatin analog lanreotide in patients with severe chronic renal insufficiency. *Clin Pharmacol Ther* 1999; **66:** 485–91.

### Preparations

**Proprietary Preparations** (details are given in Part 3)
***Arg.:*** Somatuline; ***Austral.:*** Somatuline; ***Austria:*** Somatuline†; ***Belg.:*** Somatuline; ***Denm.:*** Ipstyl; ***Fin.:*** Somatuline; ***Fr.:*** Somatuline; ***Gr.:*** Somatuline; ***Hong Kong:*** Somatuline; ***Irl.:*** Somatuline; ***Israel:*** Somatuline; ***Ital.:*** Ipstyl; ***Norw.:*** Ipstyl; ***Port.:*** Somatulina; ***Singapore:*** Somatuline; ***Spain:*** Somatulina; ***Swed.:*** Somatuline; ***Switz.:*** Somatulin; ***UK:*** Somatuline.

---

## Leuprorelin *(BAN, rINN)*

Leuprolide; Leuprorelinum. 5-Oxo-L-prolyl-L-histidyl-L-tryptophyl-L-seryl-L-tyrosyl-D-leucyl-L-leucyl-L-arginyl-N-ethyl-L-prolinamide.

$C_{59}H_{84}N_{16}O_{12}$ = 1209.4.
*CAS — 53714-56-0.*
*ATC — L02AE02.*

**Pharmacopoeias.** In *Eur.* (see p.vi).

**Ph. Eur. 5.0** (Leuprorelin). A synthetic nonapeptide analogue of the hypothalamic peptide gonadorelin. It is obtained by chemical synthesis and is available as an acetate. A white or almost white, hygroscopic, powder. Store in airtight containers at a temperature not exceeding 30°. Protect from light.

### Leuprorelin Acetate *(BANM, rINNM)*

Abbott-43818; Acetato de leuprorelina; Leuprolide Acetate *(USAN)*; TAP-144.

$C_{59}H_{84}N_{16}O_{12},C_2H_4O_2$ = 1269.5.
*CAS — 74381-53-6.*
*ATC — L02AE02.*

### Adverse Effects and Precautions

As for Gonadorelin, p.1325. Thrombocytopenia and leucopenia have been reported rarely.

**Benign intracranial hypertension.** Increased intracranial pressure associated with leuprorelin treatment has been reported in one patient.[1]

1. Arber N, *et al.* Pseudotumor cerebri associated with leuprorelin acetate. *Lancet* 1990; **335:** 668.

**Effects on the eyes.** Leuprorelin may be associated with blurred vision, usually lasting 1 to 2 hours after injection, but in rare instances longer.[1] Haemorrhage or occlusion of intra-ocular blood vessels, ocular pain, and lid oedema have also been reported but the association is less well established.

1. Fraunfelder FT, Edwards R. Possible ocular adverse effects associated with leuprolide injections. *JAMA* 1995; **273:** 773–4.

**Hypersensitivity.** A report of recurrent anaphylaxis in a patient given a depot injection of leuprorelin acetate, requiring both acute and chronic management.[1]

1. Letterie GS, *et al.* Recurrent anaphylaxis to a depot form of GnRH analogue. *Obstet Gynecol* 1991; **78:** 943–6.

**Local reactions.** Local reactions, including erythema, pain, induration, and sterile abscess are particularly associated with depot injections of gonadorelin analogues such as leuprorelin and triptorelin;[1-4] they may also occur with subcutaneous daily injection.[1] It has been suggested that the depot vehicle, a lactic acid-glycolic acid copolymer, may be responsible for many, although not all, such reactions.[1-4] Reactions are claimed to be more prevalent in children than in adults:[4] an incidence of about 5% of patients has been suggested. Reactions are apparently idiosyncratic and may occur at any time during therapy, may be intermittent, or may never recur.[4]

1. Manasco PK, *et al.* Local reactions to depot leuprolide therapy for central precocious puberty. *J Pediatr* 1993; **123:** 334–5.
2. Neely EK, *et al.* Local reactions to depot leuprolide therapy for central precocious puberty. *J Pediatr* 1993; **123:** 335.
3. Tonini G, *et al.* Local reactions to luteinizing hormone releasing hormone analog therapy. *J Pediatr* 1995; **126:** 159.
4. Neely EK, *et al.* Local reactions to luteinizing hormone releasing hormone analog therapy. *J Pediatr* 1995; **126:** 159–60.

### Interactions

As for Gonadorelin, p.1325.

### Pharmacokinetics

Leuprorelin acetate is not active when given orally but is well absorbed following subcutaneous or intramuscular injection. Following parenteral administration it has an elimination half-life of about 3 hours.

◊ References.

1. Sennello LT, *et al.* Single-dose pharmacokinetics of leuprolide in humans following intravenous and subcutaneous administration. *J Pharm Sci* 1986; **75:** 158–60.
2. Periti P, *et al.* Clinical pharmacokinetics of depot leuprorelin. *Clin Pharmacokinet* 2002; **41:** 485–504.

### Uses and Administration

Leuprorelin is an analogue of gonadorelin (p.1325) with similar properties. Continuous administration is used for the suppression of gonadal sex hormone production in the treatment of malignant neoplasms of the prostate, in central precocious puberty, and in the management of endometriosis and uterine fibroids. It is also given before uterine surgery for endometrial reduction, and may be used in the treatment of breast cancer in premenopausal women. Leuprorelin is used as the acetate.

In the management of advanced prostate cancer, leuprorelin acetate may be given by subcutaneous injection in a usual single daily dose of 1 mg. It is also given subcutaneously or intramuscularly as depot preparations but the dosage and route of these may differ between countries. In the UK, 3.75 mg may be given once a month, by subcutaneous or intramuscular injection, or 11.25 mg may be given subcutaneously every 3 months. In the USA, however, the dose administered is 7.5 mg monthly, 22.5 mg every 3 months, or 30 mg every 4 months, and the preparation is given intramuscularly. A nonbiodegradable titanium alloy implant is also available, which is inserted subcutaneously into the inner part of the upper arm. It contains 72 mg of leuprorelin acetate and delivers the drug at a controlled rate of 120 micrograms daily. After 12 months it must be removed, but can be replaced by another implant to continue therapy. An anti-androgen such as cyproterone acetate may be given for several days before beginning leuprorelin therapy and continued for about 3 weeks, to avoid the risk of a disease flare.

For the management of endometriosis and uterine fibroids, leuprorelin acetate 3.75 mg monthly may be given as a single depot injection, intramuscularly or subcutaneously. Alternatively, 11.25 mg may be given as an intramuscular depot every 3 months. Treatment is initiated during the first 5 days of the menstrual cycle, and may be continued for up to 6 months for endometriosis, while in women with anaemia due to uterine fibroids it is continued, with concomitant iron supplementation, usually for up to 3 months. To prepare for uterine surgery a single 3.75 mg depot injection may be given 5 to 6 weeks before the procedure.

In the management of central precocious puberty leuprorelin acetate has been given by intramuscular depot injection in a dose of 300 micrograms/kg every 4 weeks, adjusted according to response. Doses of 50 micrograms/kg daily by subcutaneous injection, adjusted according to response, have also been used.

Leuprorelin acetate has also been given in other sex-hormone-related disorders and has been tried in some gastrointestinal disorders such as irritable bowel syndrome (p.1244).

◊ General references.

1. Plosker GL, Brogden RN. Leuprorelin: a review of its pharmacology and therapeutic use in prostatic cancer, endometriosis and other sex hormone-related disorders. *Drugs* 1994; **48:** 930–67.

**Benign prostatic hyperplasia.** For a discussion of the management of benign prostatic hyperplasia, including mention of the use of gonadorelin analogues and the view that they are unsatisfactory for indefinite therapy, see p.1555.

References to the use of leuprorelin.

1. Gabrilove JL, *et al.* Effect of long-acting gonadotropin-releasing hormone analog (leuprolide) therapy on prostatic size and symptoms in 15 men with benign prostatic hypertrophy. *J Clin Endocrinol Metab* 1989; **69:** 629–32.
2. Eri LM, Tveter KJ. A prospective, placebo-controlled study of the luteinizing hormone-releasing hormone agonist leuprolide as treatment for patients with benign prostatic hyperplasia. *J Urol (Baltimore)* 1993; **150:** 359–64.
3. Eri LM, Tveter KJ. Safety, side effects and patient acceptance of the luteinizing hormone releasing hormone agonist leuprolide in treatment of benign prostatic hyperplasia. *J Urol (Baltimore)* 1994; **152:** 448–52.
4. Eri LM, *et al.* Effects on the endocrine system of long-term treatment with the luteinizing hormone-releasing hormone agonist leuprolide in patients with benign prostatic hyperplasia. *Scand J Clin Lab Invest* 1996; **56:** 319–25.

**Endometriosis.** Gonadorelin analogues are effective in the management of endometriosis (p.1546) but the need for long-term therapy to prevent recurrence limits their value because of the risk of osteoporosis; 'add-back' therapy, with concomitant hormone replacement, can be used to prevent this.

References to the use of leuprorelin.

1. Hornstein MD, *et al.* Leuprolide acetate depot and hormonal add-back in endometriosis: a 12-month study. *Obstet Gynecol* 1998; **91:** 16–24.
2. Ling FW. Randomized controlled trial of depot leuprolide in patients with chronic pelvic pain and clinically suspected endometriosis. *Obstet Gynecol* 1999; **93:** 51–8.
3. Takeuchi H, *et al.* A prospective randomized study comparing endocrinological and clinical effects of two types of GnRH agonists in cases of uterine leiomyomas or endometriosis. *J Obstet Gynaecol Res* 2000; **26:** 325–31.

**Fibroids.** Gonadorelin analogues may be of some benefit as an adjunct or alternative to surgery in women with uterine fibroids (p.1326), although there has been some concern that this might complicate the diagnosis of malignancy.

References to the use of leuprorelin.

1. Friedman AJ, *et al.* Treatment of leiomyomata with intranasal or subcutaneous leuprolide, a gonadotropin-releasing hormone agonist. *Fertil Steril* 1987; **48:** 560–4.
2. Friedman AJ, *et al.* Treatment of leiomyomata uteri with leuprolide acetate depot: a double-blind, placebo-controlled, multicenter study. *Obstet Gynecol* 1991; **77:** 720–5.
3. Friedman AJ, *et al.* Long-term medical therapy for leiomyomata uteri: a prospective, randomized study of leuprolide acetate depot plus either oestrogen-progestin or progestin 'add-back' for 2 years. *Hum Reprod* 1994; **9:** 1618–25.
4. Zullo F, *et al.* A prospective randomized study to evaluate leuprolide acetate treatment before laparoscopic myomectomy: efficacy and ultrasonographic predictors. *Am J Obstet Gynecol* 1998; **178:** 108–112.
5. Scialli AR, Levi AJ. Intermittent leuprolide acetate for the nonsurgical management of women with leiomyomata uteri. *Fertil Steril* 2000; **74:** 540–6.

**Hirsutism.** The mainstay of drug treatment for hirsutism (p.1545) has been an anti-androgen, usually cyproterone acetate or spironolactone. Although gonadorelin analogues have been used, and are effective, they must be given parenterally or nasally and may produce menopausal effects, notably osteoporosis.

References to the use of leuprorelin.

1. Rittmaster RS, Thompson DL. Effect of leuprolide and dexamethasone on hair growth and hormone levels in hirsute women: the relative importance of the ovary and the adrenal in the pathogenesis of hirsutism. *J Clin Endocrinol Metab* 1990; **70:** 1096–1102.
2. Elkind-Hirsch KE, *et al.* Combination gonadotropin-releasing hormone agonist and oral contraceptive therapy improves treatment of hirsute women with ovarian hyperandrogenism. *Fertil Steril* 1995; **63:** 970–8.

**Infertility.** Gonadorelin analogues are used in the treatment of infertility—see p.1316. References to the use of leuprorelin.

1. Stone BA, *et al.* Gonadotrophin and estradiol levels during ovarian stimulation in women treated with leuprolide acetate. *Obstet Gynecol* 1989; **73:** 990–5.

2. Sathanandan M, *et al.* Adjuvant leuprolide in normal, abnormal, and poor responders to controlled ovarian hyperstimulation for in vitro fertilization/gamete intrafallopian transfer. *Fertil Steril* 1989; **51:** 998–1006.
3. Filicori M, *et al.* Different gonadotropin and leuprorelin ovulation induction regimens markedly affect follicular fluid hormone levels and folliculogenesis. *Fertil Steril* 1996; **65:** 387–93.

**Malignant neoplasms.** Gonadorelin analogues are used as an alternative to orchidectomy in the management of advanced malignant neoplasms of the prostate (p.521). Such therapy is as effective as orchidectomy in prolonging survival;[1] combination of leuprorelin or other gonadorelin analogues with nonsteroidal anti-androgens to produce maximal androgen blockade produces only modest additional benefit.[2] Leuprorelin is also used for ovarian ablation[3] in premenopausal women with breast cancer (p.514).

There are also isolated reports of endometrial cancer (p.516),[4] and ovarian cancer[5] responding to leuprorelin, but the role of the gonadorelin analogues in these conditions is much less well established.

1. Seidenfeld J, *et al.* Single-therapy androgen suppression in men with advanced prostate cancer: a systematic review and meta-analysis. *Ann Intern Med* 2000; **132:** 566–77.
2. Prostate Cancer Trialists' Collaborative Group. Maximum androgen blockade in advanced prostate cancer: an overview of the randomised trials. *Lancet* 2000; **355:** 1491–8.
3. Schmid P, *et al.* Cyclophosphamide, methotrexate and fluorouracil (CMF) versus hormonal ablation with leuprorelin acetate as adjuvant treatment of node-positive, premenopausal breast cancer patients: preliminary results of the TABLE-study (Takeda Adjuvant Breast cancer study with Leuprorelin Acetate). *Anticancer Res* 2002; **22:** 2325–32.
4. Noci I, *et al.* Longstanding survival without cancer progression in a patient affected by endometrial carcinoma treated primarily with leuprolide. *Br J Cancer* 2001; **85:** 333–6.
5. Paskeviciute L, *et al.* No rules without exception: long-term complete remission observed in a study using a LH-RH agonist in platinum-refractory ovarian cancer. *Gynecol Oncol* 2002; **86:** 297–301.

**Precocious puberty.** The gonadorelin analogues have replaced other agents as the drugs of choice for the treatment of central precocious puberty (p.1318).

References to the use of leuprorelin.

1. Lee PA, *et al.* Effects of leuprolide in the treatment of central precocious puberty. *J Pediatr* 1989; **114:** 321–4.
2. Clemons RD, *et al.* Long-term effectiveness of depot gonadotropin-releasing hormone analogue in the treatment of children with central precocious puberty. *Am J Dis Child* 1993; **147:** 653–7.
3. Carel JC, *et al.* Treatment of central precocious puberty with depot leuprorelin. *Eur J Endocrinol* 1995; **132:** 699–704.
4. Carel J-C, *et al.* Treatment of central precocious puberty by subcutaneous injections of leuprorelin 3-month depot (11.25 mg). *J Clin Endocrinol Metab* 2002; **87:** 4111–16.

**Premenstrual syndrome.** For reference to the use of leuprorelin or other gonadorelin analogues with HRT to prevent menopausal symptoms in women unresponsive to other drug therapy, see under Gonadorelin, p.1326.

### Preparations

**Proprietary Preparations** (details are given in Part 3)
***Arg.:*** Lectrum; Lupron; Reliser; ***Austral.:*** Eligard; Lucrin; ***Austria:*** Enantone; Trenantone; ***Belg.:*** Lucrin; ***Braz.:*** Lupron; Reliser; ***Canad.:*** Lupron; ***Chile:*** Lupron; ***Denm.:*** Enanton; Procren; ***Fin.:*** Enanton; Procren; ***Fr.:*** Enantone; Lucrin; ***Ger.:*** Carcinil†; Enantone; Enantone-Gyn; Trenantone; Uno-Enantone; ***Gr.:*** Daronda; Elityran; ***Hong Kong:*** Enantone; Lucrin; ***India:*** Lupride; ***Irl.:*** Prostap; ***Israel:*** Lucrin; ***Ital.:*** Enantone; ***Jpn:*** Leuplin; ***Malaysia:*** Lucrin; ***Mex.:*** Lucrin; Reliser; ***Neth.:*** Lucrin; ***Norw.:*** Enanton; Procren; ***NZ:*** Lucrin; ***Port.:*** Lucrin; ***S.Afr.:*** Lucrin; ***Singapore:*** Lucrin; ***Spain:*** Ginecrin; Procrin; ***Swed.:*** Enanton; Procren; ***Switz.:*** Lucrin; ***Thai.:*** Enantone; ***UK:*** Prostap; ***USA:*** Eligard; Lupron; Viadur.

## Luteinising Hormone

Human Interstitial-cell-stimulating Hormone; ICSH; LH; Lutropin; Lutropina.
*CAS — 9002-67-9; 39341-83-8 (human).*

## Lutropin Alfa *(BAN, USAN, rINN)*

Lutropina alfa.
*CAS — 152923-57-4 (lutropin alfa); 56832-30-5 (α subunit); 53664-53-2 (βsubunit).*
*ATC — G03GA07.*

### Units

35 units of human pituitary luteinising hormone are contained in approximately 5.8 micrograms (with 1 mg of human albumin, 5 mg of mannitol, and 1 mg of sodium chloride) in one ampoule of the second International Standard (1988).

10 units of the alpha subunit of human pituitary luteinising hormone are contained in approximately 10 micrograms (with 0.5 mg of human albumin, 2.5 mg of lactose, and 45 micrograms of sodium chloride) in one ampoule of the first International Standard (1984).

10 units of the beta subunit of human pituitary luteinising hormone are contained in 10 micrograms (with 0.5 mg of human albumin, 2.5 mg of lactose, and 45 micrograms of sodium chloride) in one ampoule of the first International Standard (1984).

### Adverse Effects and Precautions

As for Human Menopausal Gonadotrophins, p.1330.

### Pharmacokinetics

The absolute bioavailability of lutropin alfa after subcutaneous administration is about 60%, and the terminal half-life is at least 10 to 12 hours.

### Uses and Administration

Luteinising hormone (LH) is secreted with follicle-stimulating hormone (FSH) (p.1324), another gonadotrophin, by the anterior pituitary lobe.

These gonadotrophins stimulate the normal functioning of the gonads and the secretion of sex hormones in both men and women. In women, follicle-stimulating hormone stimulates the development and maturation of the follicles and ova. As the follicle develops it produces oestrogen in increasing amounts which at mid-cycle stimulates the release of LH. This causes rupture of the follicle with ovulation and converts the follicle into the corpus luteum which secretes progesterone. In men, luteinising hormone stimulates the interstitial cells of the testis to secrete testosterone, which in turn has a direct effect on the seminiferous tubules.

Gonadotrophic substances with luteinising or follicle-stimulating activity or both are used in the treatment of infertility (p.1316), chiefly in females but also in males. Such substances include chorionic gonadotrophin (p.1321) which possesses LH activity and human menopausal gonadotrophins (p.1330) which possess both LH and FSH activity.

Lutropin alfa is a recombinant human luteinising hormone (rechLH) used to induce ovulation in women with severe deficiency of luteinising and follicle-stimulating hormones. It is used at the same time as a preparation with follicle-stimulating activity, usually follitropin alfa. The dosage and schedule of treatment for female infertility must be determined according to the needs of each patient; it is usual to monitor response by studying the patient's urinary oestrogen excretion or by ultrasonic visualisation of follicles or both. Treatment is usually begun with 75 units of lutropin alfa daily by subcutaneous injection for 7 to 14 days, accompanied by FSH. If there is no response, the FSH dosage may be increased at 7- or 14-day intervals until an adequate but not excessive response is achieved. A treatment cycle of up to 5 weeks may be needed. Treatment is then stopped and followed after 1 or 2 days by a single dose of chorionic gonadotrophin 5000 to 10 000 units to induce ovulation. These patients are generally amenorrhoeic and treatment may be started at any time.

◊ References.

1. Hull M, *et al.* Recombinant human luteinising hormone: an effective new gonadotropin preparation. *Lancet* 1994; **344:** 334–5.
2. Imthurn B, *et al.* Recombinant human luteinising hormone to mimic mid-cycle LH surge. *Lancet* 1996; **348:** 332–3.
3. Agrawal R, *et al.* Pregnancy after treatment with three recombinant gonadotropins. *Lancet* 1997; **349:** 29–30.
4. The European Recombinant LH Study Group. Human recombinant luteinizing hormone is as effective as, but safer than, urinary human chorionic gonadotropin in inducing final follicular maturation and ovulation in in vitro fertilization procedures: results of a multicenter double-blind study. *J Clin Endocrinol Metab* 2001; **86:** 2607–18.

### Preparations

**Proprietary Preparations** (details are given in Part 3)
***Arg.:*** Luveris; ***Denm.:*** Luveris; ***Fin.:*** Luveris; ***Fr.:*** Luveris; ***Ger.:*** Luveris; ***Neth.:*** Luveris; ***Norw.:*** Luveris; ***Port.:*** Luveris; ***Spain:*** Luveris; ***Swed.:*** Luveris; ***UK:*** Luveris.

## Melanocyte-stimulating Hormone

B Hormone; Chromatophore Hormone; Intermedin; Intermedina; Melanotropin; MSH; Pigment Hormone.
*CAS — 9002-79-3.*

### Profile

Melanocyte-stimulating hormone is a polypeptide isolated from the pars intermedia of the pituitary of fish and amphibia which causes dispersal of melanin granules in the skin of fish and amphibia and allows adaptation to the environment.

In adult humans, the pituitary gland lacks a distinct intermediate lobe, and the pituitary is not thought to secrete melanocyte-stimulating hormone (MSH) directly. However, the precursor molecule, pro-opiomelanocortin, is cleaved in the pituitary into corticotropin (p.1322), the glycoprotein β-lipotrophin (β-LPH), and an amino-terminal peptide. Subsequent processing in other tissues, such as the brain and gastrointestinal tract, may yield three forms of MSH, α-MSH (via corticotropin cleavage), β-MSH, and γ-MSH. The presence and function of these melanocyte-stimulating hormones in man are uncertain. A receptor analogous to that in amphibians is apparently lacking in humans; effects on skin pigmentation emanating from the pituitary are primarily mediated by corticotropin.

Release of melanocyte-stimulating hormone is inhibited in animals by melanostatin; there is also evidence for a hypothalamic releasing factor (MRF).

Melanocyte-stimulating hormone is under investigation, as α-MSH, in the prevention and treatment of ischaemic intrinsic acute renal failure.

◊ Alpha melanocyte-stimulating hormone (α-MSH) has neurotrophic actions during development and has been investigated for its potential in promoting recovery of nerve function after injury.[1]

1. Choo V. Healing with recovery of function. *Lancet* 1993; **342:** 673.

## Melanostatin

Intermedin-inhibiting Factor; Melanocyte-stimulating-hormone-release-inhibiting Factor; Melanostatina; Melanotropin Release-inhibiting Factor; MIF. Pro-Leu-Gly-$NH_2$.
*CAS — 9083-38-9.*

### Profile

Melanostatin is a tripeptide, obtained from the hypothalamus, that inhibits the release of melanocyte-stimulating hormone (see above) in animals. However, there is little evidence of its activity in man. It has been tried in the treatment of depression and parkinsonism but with little benefit.

## Nafarelin Acetate *(BANM, USAN, rINNM)*

Acetato de nafarelina; D-Nal(2)[6]-LHRH acetate hydrate; RS-94991298. 5-Oxo-L-prolyl-L-histidyl-L-tryptophyl-L-seryl-L-tyrosyl-3-(2-naphthyl)-D-alanyl-L-leucyl-L-arginyl-L-prolylglycinamide acetate hydrate.
$C_{66}H_{83}N_{17}O_{13},xC_2H_4O_2,yH_2O$.
*CAS — 76932-56-4 (nafarelin); 86220-42-0 (nafarelin acetate).*
*ATC — H01CA02.*

### Adverse Effects and Precautions

As for Gonadorelin, p.1325.

**Effects on electrolytes.** A report of severe hyperkalaemia in a woman receiving nafarelin therapy for uterine fibroids.[1] Despite serum potassium greater than 10 mmol/litre she had no symptoms and the electrocardiogram was normal. Hyperkalaemia resolved without treatment following discontinuation of nafarelin.

1. Hata T, *et al.* Severe hyperkalaemia with nafarelin. *Lancet* 1996; **347:** 333.

### Interactions

As for Gonadorelin, p.1325.

### Pharmacokinetics

Nafarelin is rapidly absorbed following intranasal administration with peak plasma concentrations achieved within 20 minutes of a dose, although bioavailability is only about 3%. The plasma half-life is about 3 to 4 hours. Nafarelin is metabolised by peptidases in the body; following subcutaneous administration it is excreted in urine, as metabolites and a small amount of unchanged drug, and in the faeces.

### Uses and Administration

Nafarelin acetate is an analogue of gonadorelin (p.1325) with similar properties. It is used in the treatment of endometriosis and central precocious puberty, and as an adjunct to ovulation induction with gonadotrophins in the treatment of infertility.

For endometriosis it is given in usual doses equivalent to 200 micrograms of nafarelin twice daily intranasally, doubled after 2 months if amenorrhoea has not occurred. Treatment should begin on days 2 to 4 of the menstrual cycle, and may be continued for up to 6 months.

For central precocious puberty the usual dose is the equivalent of nafarelin 800 micrograms intranasally (400 micrograms in each nostril) twice daily. If adequate suppression is not achieved at this dose it may be increased to 600 micrograms three times daily in alternate nostrils (1800 micrograms daily).

Regimens for oocyte collection for *in-vitro* fertilisation employ gonadorelin analogues for pituitary desensitisation before ovulation induction with gonadotrophins; the equivalent of 400 micrograms of nafarelin is given intranasally twice daily, beginning either in the early follicular phase (day 2) or midluteal phase (day 21) of the menstrual cycle. Therapy should be continued until downregulation is achieved; if this does not occur within 12 weeks therapy should be withdrawn. Once downregulation occurs gonadotrophin treatment is added to nafarelin therapy until an appropriate stage of follicular development, when both are withdrawn and chorionic gonadotrophin is given to induce ovulation.

Nafarelin has also been given in other sex hormone-related conditions.

**Benign prostatic hyperplasia.** For a discussion of the management of benign prostatic hyperplasia, including mention of the use of gonadorelin analogues and the view that they are unsatisfactory for indefinite therapy, see p.1555.

Prostate size decreased by a mean of 24.2% in 9 men treated for benign prostatic hyperplasia for 6 months with nafarelin acetate 400 micrograms daily subcutaneously.[1] Six months after the end of treatment, prostate size approached that of pretreatment values.

1. Peters CA, Walsh PC. The effect of nafarelin acetate, a luteinizing-hormone-releasing hormone agonist, on benign prostatic hyperplasia. *N Engl J Med* 1987; **317:** 599–604.

**Endometriosis.** Gonadorelin analogues are effective in the management of endometriosis (p.1546), but the need for long-term therapy to prevent recurrence limits their value because of the risk of osteoporosis; 'add-back' therapy, with concomitant hormone replacement, can be used to prevent this.

References to the use of nafarelin.

1. Schriock E, *et al.* Treatment of endometriosis with a potent agonist of gonadotropin-releasing hormone (nafarelin). *Fertil Steril* 1985; **44:** 583–8.
2. Henzl MR, *et al.* Administration of nasal nafarelin as compared with oral danazol for endometriosis: a multicenter double-blind comparative clinical trial. *N Engl J Med* 1988; **318:** 485–9.
3. Burry KA. Nafarelin in the management of endometriosis: quality of life assessment. *Am J Obstet Gynecol* 1992; **166:** 735–9.
4. Hornstein MD, *et al.* Retreatment with nafarelin for recurrent endometriosis symptoms: efficacy, safety, and bone mineral density. *Fertil Steril* 1997; **67:** 1013–18.

**Fibroids.** Gonadorelin analogues have been tried as an adjunct or alternative to surgery in the treatment of uterine fibroids (see p.1326), although there has been some concern that this might complicate the diagnosis of malignancy.

References to the use of nafarelin.

1. Minaguchi H, *et al.* Clinical use of nafarelin in the treatment of leiomyomas: a review of the literature. *J Reprod Med* 2000; **45:** 481–9.

**Infertility.** Gonadorelin analogues are used in the treatment of infertility (p.1316). As well as being used directly they are employed in regimens to induce superovulation to enable ova collection and *in-vitro* fertilisation, and use of nafarelin has been reported to produce a higher rate of successful pregnancies than leuprorelin in one *in-vitro* fertilisation programme.[1]

1. Martin MC, *et al.* The choice of a gonadotropin-releasing hormone analog influences outcome of in vitro fertilization treatment. *Am J Obstet Gynecol* 1994; **170:** 1629–34.

**Porphyria.** Nafarelin nasal spray was used to prevent menstrual exacerbations of acute intermittent porphyria (p.1040) in 2 sisters.[1]

1. McNulty SJ, Hardy KJ. Two patients with acute intermittent porphyria treated with nafarelin to prevent menstrual exacerbations. *J R Soc Med* 2000; **93:** 429–30.

**Precocious puberty.** Nafarelin preserved adult height potential in girls with idiopathic precocious puberty (p.1318) having a poor initial height prognosis.[1] However, reviewers have noted that results from earlier studies into other features of precocious puberty have been equivocal.[2]

1. Kreiter M, *et al.* Preserving adult height potential in girls with idiopathic true precocious puberty. *J Pediatr* 1990; **117:** 364–70.
2. Chrisp P, Goa KL. Nafarelin: a review of its pharmacodynamic and pharmacokinetic properties, and clinical potential in sex hormone-related conditions. *Drugs* 1990; **39:** 523–51.

## Preparations

**Proprietary Preparations** (details are given in Part 3)
***Arg.:*** Synrelin; ***Austral.:*** Synarel; ***Belg.:*** Synarel†; ***Braz.:*** Synarel; ***Canad.:*** Synarel; ***Denm.:*** Synarela; ***Fin.:*** Synarela; ***Fr.:*** Synarel; ***Ger.:*** Synarela; ***Hong Kong:*** Synarel; ***India:*** Nasarel; ***Irl.:*** Synarel; ***Israel:*** Synarel; ***Mex.:*** Synarel; ***Neth.:*** Synarel; ***Norw.:*** Synarela; ***NZ:*** Synarel; ***S.Afr.:*** Synarel; ***Spain:*** Synarel; ***Swed.:*** Synarela; ***Switz.:*** Synrelina; ***UK:*** Synarel; ***USA:*** Synarel.

# Octreotide Acetate *(BANM, USAN, rINNM)*

Acetato de octreotida; SMS-201-995 (octreotide). 2-(D-Phenylalanyl-L-cystyl-L-phenylalanyl-D-tryptophyl-L-lysyl-L-threonyl-L-cystyl)-(2*R*,3*R*)-butane-1,3-diol acetate; D-Phenylalanyl-L-cysteinyl-L-phenylalanyl-D-tryptophyl-L-lysyl-L-threonyl-*N*-[(1*R*,2*R*)-2-hydroxy-1-(hydroxymethyl)propyl]-L-cysteinamide cyclic (2→7) disulphide acetate.

$C_{49}H_{66}N_{10}O_{10}S_2,xC_2H_4O_2$ = 1019.2 (octreotide).

*CAS — 83150-76-9 (octreotide); 79517-01-4 (octreotide acetate).*

*ATC — H01CB02.*

**Incompatibility.** Apparent loss of insulin has been reported from a total parenteral nutrient solution containing octreotide; there may be an incompatibility.[1] Also the manufacturers had suggested that octreotide might be adsorbed onto plastics. However, a solution containing octreotide 200 micrograms/mL as the acetate was reported to be stable at 5° or −20° for up to 60 days when stored in polypropylene syringes.[2]

1. Rosen GH. Potential incompatibility of insulin and octreotide in total parenteral nutrient solutions. *Am J Hosp Pharm* 1989; **46:** 1128.
2. Ripley RG, *et al.* Stability of octreotide acetate in polypropylene syringes at 5 and −20°C. *Am J Health-Syst Pharm* 1995; **52:** 1910–11.

## Adverse Effects and Precautions

There may be a transient local reaction at the site of injection of octreotide. Systemic side-effects are mainly gastrointestinal and may include anorexia, nausea, vomiting, diarrhoea and steatorrhoea, abdominal discomfort, and flatulence. Administration between meals or at bedtime may reduce these gastrointestinal effects.

Gallstones may develop on long-term therapy; there have been isolated reports of hepatic dysfunction and of biliary colic associated with drug withdrawal. Checks should be made for gallstones before prolonged therapy and at 6- to 12-month intervals during treatment. Hypoglycaemia may occur, especially in patients with insulinomas, but there is also a risk of hyperglycaemia or impaired glucose tolerance. Thyroid function should be monitored during octreotide therapy because of the possibility of hypothyroidism. Pituitary tumours that secrete growth hormone can expand during treatment, causing serious complications; patients should be monitored for signs of tumour expansion, such as visual field defects. Cardiac rhythm should be monitored during intravenous administration of octreotide. Doses may need to be adjusted in patients with end-stage renal failure, in whom the clearance of octreotide is reduced.

**Effects on the biliary tract.** Octreotide has an inhibitory effect on gallbladder motility accounting for the development of gallstones and biliary colic.[1-8]

1. McKnight JA, *et al.* Changes in glucose tolerance and development of gall stones during high dose treatment with octreotide for acromegaly. *BMJ* 1989; **299:** 604–5.
2. Ho KY, *et al.* Therapeutic efficacy of the somatostatin analog SMS 201-995 (octreotide) in acromegaly: effects of dose and frequency and long-term safety. *Ann Intern Med* 1990; **112:** 173–81.
3. Bigg-Wither GW, *et al.* Effects of long term octreotide on gall stone formation and gall bladder function. *BMJ* 1992; **304:** 1611–12.
4. Redfern JS, Fortuner WJ. Octreotide-associated biliary tract dysfunction and gallstone formation: pathophysiology and management. *Am J Gastroenterol* 1995; **90:** 1042–52.
5. Tauber JP, *et al.* The impact of continuous subcutaneous infusion of octreotide on gallstone formation in acromegalic patients. *J Clin Endocrinol Metab* 1995; **80:** 3262–6.
6. Hussaini SH, *et al.* Roles of gall bladder emptying and intestinal transit in the pathogenesis of octreotide induced gall bladder stones. *Gut* 1996; **38:** 775–83.
7. Trendle MC, *et al.* Incidence and morbidity of cholelithiasis in patients receiving chronic octreotide for metastatic carcinoid and malignant islet cell tumors. *Cancer* 1997; **79:** 830–4.
8. Moschetta A, *et al.* Severe impairment of postprandial cholecystokinin release and gall-bladder emptying and high risk of gallstone formation in acromegalic patients during Sandostatin LAR. *Aliment Pharmacol Ther* 2001; **15:** 181–5.

**Effects on carbohydrate metabolism.** Changes in glucose tolerance were observed over 12 months in patients treated with octreotide 600 to 1500 micrograms daily subcutaneously for acromegaly.[1] Of 3 patients with normal glucose tolerance initially, one remained normal, one developed impaired glucose tolerance, and one became diabetic. Of 4 with impaired glucose tolerance initially, 2 remained unchanged, one became diabetic, and the other returned to normal. There has been a report of deterioration in glucose tolerance leading to death from diabetic ketoacidosis occurring after cessation of octreotide treatment in a patient with acromegaly and insulin-resistant diabetes mellitus.[2]

See also Diabetes Mellitus and Hyperinsulinism under Uses and Administration, below.

1. McKnight JA, *et al.* Changes in glucose tolerance and development of gall stones during high dose treatment with octreotide for acromegaly. *BMJ* 1989; **299:** 604–5.
2. Abrahamson MJ. Death from diabetic ketoacidosis after cessation of octreotide in acromegaly. *Lancet* 1990; **336:** 318–19.

**Effects on the hair.** Diffuse loss of scalp hair has been reported in 4 of 7 women who received octreotide; after withdrawal of octreotide in 3 of the women there was a complete recovery of scalp hair.[1] Other similar cases have also been reported. In one case, diffuse alopecia in a male patient was completely reversed when octreotide was replaced with lanreotide.[2]

1. Jönsson A, Manhem P. Octreotide and loss of scalp hair. *Ann Intern Med* 1991; **115:** 913.
2. Lami M-C, *et al.* Hair loss in three patients with acromegaly treated with octreotide. *Br J Dermatol* 2003; **149:** 655–6.

**Effects on the liver.** Hepatitis occurred during treatment of an acromegalic patient with octreotide 300 micrograms daily subcutaneously.[1] Liver enzyme values returned to normal within 2 months of withdrawing octreotide.

1. Arosio M, *et al.* Acute hepatitis after treatment of acromegaly with octreotide. *Lancet* 1988; **ii:** 1498.

**Effects on the pancreas.** There have been reports of pancreatitis associated with octreotide.[1-3] It has been suggested that octreotide-induced pancreatitis may result from spasm of the sphincter of Oddi, resulting in retention of activated pancreatic enzymes due to outflow obstruction.[3]

1. Fredenrich A, *et al.* Acute pancreatitis after short-term octreotide. *Lancet* 1991; **338:** 52–3.
2. Sadoul J-L, *et al.* Acute pancreatitis following octreotide withdrawal. *Am J Med* 1991; **90:** 763–4.
3. Bodemar G, Hjortswang H. Octreotide-induced pancreatitis: an effect of increased contractility of Oddi sphincter. *Lancet* 1996; **348:** 1668–9.

**Pregnancy.** A report of a woman who received octreotide during pregnancy also reviewed 6 other cases in the literature. Most were receiving the drug for the treatment of acromegaly. No maternal complications or congenital anomalies were described.[1]

1. Mikhail N. Octreotide treatment of acromegaly during pregnancy. *Mayo Clin Proc* 2002; **77:** 297–8.

## Interactions

Octreotide has been associated with alterations in nutrient absorption and there is a theoretical possibility that it may affect the absorption of orally administered drugs. Patients receiving insulin or oral hypoglycaemics may require dose adjustments of these drugs if octreotide is given concomitantly. The bioavailability of bromocriptine is increased by administration with octreotide. It has been suggested that dosage of beta blockers, calcium-channel blockers, or drugs to control fluid and electrolyte balance may also need to be adjusted.

**Ciclosporin.** For a reference to octreotide reducing serum concentrations of ciclosporin, see p.1356.

## Pharmacokinetics

Octreotide is rapidly absorbed following subcutaneous injection, with peak plasma concentrations reached about 25 to 30 minutes after a dose, and is distributed to body tissues. It is said to exhibit non-linear pharmacokinetics, with reduced clearance at high doses. Octreotide is removed from the body with a plasma elimination half-life of about 1.5 hours; half-life is prolonged in elderly patients and in renal impairment. About a third of a dose is excreted unchanged in the urine. Octreotide diffuses across the placenta.

## Uses and Administration

Octreotide is an octapeptide analogue of somatostatin (p.1339) with similar properties but a longer duration of action.

It is used as the acetate in the symptomatic management of carcinoid tumours and other secretory neoplasms such as VIPomas and glucagonomas. Octreotide acetate is also used in the treatment of acromegaly and the prevention of complications following pancreatic surgery, and may be used in the treatment of other disorders including variceal haemorrhage and HIV-associated diarrhoea. It has also been investigated in a variety of other disorders including the dumping syndrome.

In the management of **secretory neoplasms** octreotide acetate is given subcutaneously in an initial dose equivalent to 50 micrograms of octreotide once or twice daily gradually increased, according to response, to up to 600 micrograms daily in 2 to 4 divided doses. Higher doses have been used.

Where a rapid response is required, the initial dose may be given by the intravenous route. In the UK the manufacturers state that it should be diluted not less than 1 in 1 or not more than 1 in 9 in sodium chloride 0.9%, but in the USA the manufacturers permit the use of the undiluted solution as an intravenous bolus in emergencies; alternatively the dose may be given by intermittent infusion over 15 to 30 minutes, diluted in 50 to 200 mL of sodium chloride 0.9% or glucose 5%.

Once control has been established maintenance therapy with a depot preparation may be possible; initially 20 mg by intramuscular injection every 4 weeks is suggested. Subcutaneous injection with a rapid-acting preparation should be continued for 2 weeks after the first depot injection to provide symptomatic cover, and may be added to therapy when necessary thereafter. Maintenance doses of the depot preparation may be adjusted after 2 or 3 months to between 10 and 30 mg every 4 weeks, as necessary.

In **acromegaly**, the usual dose is the equivalent of 100 to 200 micrograms of octreotide three times daily by subcutaneous injection. In the USA it is suggested that dosage begin with 50 micrograms three times daily in order to minimise gastrointestinal disturbance. Once control has been established maintenance therapy with a depot preparation is possible; an initial dose equivalent to 20 mg of octreotide given intramuscularly once a month has been recommended for patients with acromegaly, adjusted after 3 months to between 10 and 30 mg monthly.

For the prevention of complications following **pancreatic surgery** the equivalent of 100 micrograms of octreotide may be given three times daily by subcutaneous injection of a rapid-acting preparation; treatment is given for 7 consecutive days, beginning at least 1 hour before laparotomy on the day of operation.

◊ General reviews of octreotide.


1. Mosdell KW, Visconti JA. Emerging indications for octreotide therapy, part 1. *Am J Hosp Pharm* 1994; **51:** 1184–92.
2. Mosdell KW, Visconti JA. Emerging indications for octreotide therapy, part 2. *Am J Hosp Pharm* 1994; **51:** 1317–30.
3. Bloom SR, O'Shea D. Octreotide. *Prescribers' J* 1996; **36:** 120–4.
4. Lamberts SWJ, *et al.* Octreotide. *N Engl J Med* 1996; **334:** 246–54.


**Acromegaly.** Although surgery remains the most important method of treatment, octreotide has a useful role in the management of acromegaly (p.1312). It can reduce growth hormone concentrations, normalise IGF-I concentrations, reduce tumour size, and improve signs and symptoms.[1-4] There is also some evidence that it may improve cardiac function, which is usually compromised in these patients.[5-7] Octreotide can be given subcutaneously, and continuous subcutaneous infusion may be more effective than intermittent injection.[8] Intramuscular sustained-release octreotide is effective for maintenance therapy.[4,7,9] There is also increasing interest in the role of octreotide for primary therapy of acromegaly, instead of surgery.[9,10]


1. Vance ML, Harris AG. Long-term treatment of 189 acromegalic patients with the somatostatin analog octreotide: results of the International Multicenter Acromegaly Study Group. *Arch Intern Med* 1991; **151:** 1573–8.
2. Ezzat S, *et al.* Octreotide treatment of acromegaly: a randomized, multicenter study. *Ann Intern Med* 1992; **117:** 711–18.
3. van der Lely AJ, *et al.* A risk-benefit assessment of octreotide in the treatment of acromegaly. *Drug Safety* 1997; **17:** 317–24.
4. Freda PU. Somatostatin analogs in acromegaly. *J Clin Endocrinol Metab* 2002; **87:** 3013–18.
5. Colao A, *et al.* Cardiovascular effects of depot long-acting somatostatin analog Sandostatin LAR in acromegaly. *J Clin Endocrinol Metab* 2000; **85:** 3132–40.
6. Colao A, *et al.* Is the acromegalic cardiomyopathy reversible? Effect of 5-year normalization of growth hormone and insulin-like growth factor I levels on cardiac performance. *J Clin Endocrinol Metab* 2001; **86:** 1551–7.
7. McKeage K, *et al.* Octreotide long-acting release (LAR): a review of its use in the management of acromegaly. *Drugs* 2003; **63:** 2473–99.
8. Harris AG, *et al.* Continuous versus intermittent subcutaneous infusion of octreotide in the treatment of acromegaly. *J Clin Pharmacol* 1995; **35:** 59–71.
9. Ayuk J, *et al.* Long-term safety and efficacy of depot long-acting somatostatin analogs for the treatment of acromegaly. *J Clin Endocrinol Metab* 2002; **87:** 4142–6.
10. Bevan JS, *et al.* Primary medical therapy for acromegaly: an open, prospective, multicenter study of the effects of subcutaneous and intramuscular slow-release octreotide on growth hormone, insulin-like growth factor-I, and tumor size. *J Clin Endocrinol Metab* 2002; **87:** 4554–63.


**Carcinoid syndrome and other secretory neoplasms.** For a discussion of carcinoid tumours and other secretory neoplasms, including reference to the important role of octreotide, see p.504.

**Cardiovascular disorders.** There have been reports of benefit from octreotide in patients with postprandial hypotension and orthostatic hypotension (p.1100) associated with autonomic neuropathy.[1-4] Octreotide has also produced cardiac improvement in patients with acromegaly (see above). Promising results have been reported in patients with primary hypertrophic cardiomyopathy.[5,6]


1. Hoeldtke RD, *et al.* Treatment of autonomic neuropathy with a somatostatin analogue SMS-201-995. *Lancet* 1986; **ii:** 602–5.
2. Hoeldtke RD, Israel BC. Treatment of orthostatic hypotension with octreotide. *J Clin Endocrinol Metab* 1989; **68:** 1051–9.
3. Woo J, *et al.* Treatment of severe orthostatic hypotension with the somatostatin analogue octreotide. *Aust N Z J Med* 1990; **20:** 822–3.
4. Hoeldtke RD, *et al.* Treatment of orthostatic hypotension with midodrine and octreotide. *J Clin Endocrinol Metab* 1998; **83:** 339–43.
5. Günal AI, *et al.* Short term reduction of left ventricular mass in primary hypertrophic cardiomyopathy by octreotide injections. *Heart* 1996; **76:** 418–21.
6. Demirtas E, *et al.* Effects of octreotide in patients with hypertrophic obstructive cardiomyopathy. *Jpn Heart J* 1998; **39:** 173–81.


**Chylous effusion.** Chylous effusion results in accumulation of a milky lymphatic fluid containing raised concentrations of white blood cells, triglycerides, and cholesterol. Chylothorax, when the effusion affects the pleural cavity, is generally a complication of malignancy or chest surgery, or may be idiopathic. Treatment usually involves catheter drainage and dietary modification; surgery is used when these measures fail. Octreotide has been used successfully in a number of cases, given subcutaneously or by continuous infusion, to treat chylothorax.[1-5] There are also reports of octreotide being ineffective.[6] Octreotide has also been used in chyloperitoneum.[7]


1. Demos NJ, *et al.* Somatostatin in the treatment of chylothorax. *Chest* 2001; **119:** 964–6.
2. Cheung Y, *et al.* Octreotide for treatment of postoperative chylothorax. *J Pediatr* 2001; **139:** 157–9.
3. Ottinger JG. Octreotide for persistent chylothorax in a pediatric patient. *Ann Pharmacother* 2002; **36:** 1106–7.
4. Demos NJ. Octreotide in the treatment of chylothorax. *Chest* 2002; **121:** 2080–1.
5. Al-Zubairy SA, Al-Jazairi AS. Octreotide as a therapeutic option for management of chylothorax. *Ann Pharmacother* 2003; **37:** 679–82.
6. Mikroulis D, *et al.* Octreotide in the treatment of chylothorax. *Chest* 2002; **121:** 2079–80.
7. Bhatia C, *et al.* Octreotide therapy: a new horizon in treatment of iatrogenic chyloperitoneum. *Arch Dis Child* 2001; **85:** 234–5.


**Cushing's syndrome.** It has been suggested[1,2] that octreotide may be useful in the diagnosis, and possibly the treatment, of selected patients with Cushing's syndrome (p.1313).


1. Woodhouse NJY, *et al.* Acute and long-term effects of octreotide in patients with ACTH-dependent Cushing's syndrome. *Am J Med* 1993; **95:** 305–8.
2. de Herder WW, Lamberts SWJ. Is there a role for somatostatin and its analogs in Cushing's syndrome? *Metabolism* 1996; **45** (suppl): 83–5.


**Diabetes mellitus.** Although octreotide has been reported to impair glucose tolerance, and even precipitate frank diabetes (see Effects on Carbohydrate Metabolism, under Adverse Effects, above), its variable effects on blood glucose and insulin have led to investigations[1-3] of its possible benefits in diabetes mellitus (p.324). There is also some suggestion that it may be of benefit in the treatment or prevention of diabetic nephropathy[4] and retinopathy.[5] Benefit has been reported from the use of octreotide in patients with diabetic diarrhoea—see Gastrointestinal Disorders, below.


1. Rios MS, *et al.* Somatostatin analog SMS 201-995 and insulin needs in insulin-dependent diabetic patients studied by means of an artificial pancreas. *J Clin Endocrinol Metab* 1986; **63:** 1071–4.
2. Hadjidakis DJ, *et al.* The effects of the somatostatin analogue SMS 201-995 on carbohydrate homeostasis of insulin-dependent diabetics as assessed by the artificial endocrine pancreas. *Diabetes Res Clin Pract* 1988; **5:** 91–8.
3. Candrina R, Giustina G. Effect of a new long-acting somatostatin analogue (SMS 201-995) on glycemic and hormonal profiles in insulin-treated type II diabetic patients. *J Endocrinol Invest* 1988; **11:** 501–7.
4. Serri O, *et al.* Somatostatin analogue, octreotide, reduces increased glomerular filtration rate and kidney size in insulin-dependent diabetes. *JAMA* 1991; **265:** 888–92.
5. Grant MB, *et al.* The efficacy of octreotide in the therapy of severe nonproliferative and early proliferative diabetic retinopathy: a randomized controlled trial. *Diabetes Care* 2000; **23:** 504–9.


**Diagnosis and testing.** Radiolabelled octreotide or derivatives such as pentetreotide may be used successfully to visualise various malignant neoplasms which express somatostatin receptors.[1-6] Somatostatin receptor scintigraphy is the most sensitive method for imaging lesions in patients with Zollinger-Ellison syndrome.[6]

Octreotide may also have a role in the diagnosis of Cushing's syndrome, see above.


1. Krenning EP, *et al.* Localisation of endocrine-related tumours with radioiodinated analogue of somatostatin. *Lancet* 1989; **i:** 242–4.
2. Lamberts SWJ, *et al.* Somatostatin-receptor imaging in the localization of endocrine tumors. *N Engl J Med* 1990; **323:** 1246–9.
3. van Eijck CHJ, *et al.* Somatostatin-receptor scintigraphy in primary breast cancer. *Lancet* 1994; **343:** 640–3.
4. McCready VR, Hickish TF. Somatostatin imaging function. *Lancet* 1994; **343:** 617.
5. Dominioni L, *et al.* Localisation of carcinoid tumour with radiolabelled octreotide and intraoperative gamma detection. *Lancet* 1994; **344:** 1783.
6. Gibril F, *et al.* Somatostatin receptor scintigraphy: its sensitivity compared with that of other imaging methods in detecting primary and metastatic gastrinomas: a prospective study. *Ann Intern Med* 1996; **125:** 26–34.


**Eye disorders.** A report of response to octreotide in a patient with bilateral cystoid macular oedema, a refractory form of retinal oedema.[1] The problem recurred when octreotide was twice discontinued and each time responded to resumption of octreotide injections.


1. Kuijpers RWAM, *et al.* Treatment of cystoid macular edema with octreotide. *N Engl J Med* 1998; **338:** 624–6.


**Gastrointestinal disorders.** Somatostatin inhibits gastric and intestinal secretion and the production of various active substances in the gastrointestinal tract. It also reduces splanchnic arterial blood flow and portal and gastric mucosal blood flow. These properties are made use of, usually in the form of octreotide, in the management of a number of gastrointestinal disorders. Octreotide is used particularly in the treatment of carcinoid syndrome arising from **endocrine tumours** (see Carcinoid Tumours, p.504).

The antisecretory properties of octreotide have been of benefit in patients with **diarrhoea** associated with a variety of conditions including amyloidosis,[1,2] diabetes mellitus,[3-5] microvillous atrophy,[6] bone marrow transplantation,[7] and enterocolitis induced by gold therapy.[8] There have also been reports of benefit in refractory AIDS-associated diarrhoea,[9] but a double-blinded, controlled study found octreotide to be no more beneficial than placebo.[10] Octreotide may be useful in decreasing faecal mass or jejunal efflux in patients with the short-bowel syndrome and jejunostomies or ileostomies.[11,12] Octreotide has also been used in the management of postoperative small-bowel **fistulae**. There have been mixed reports, but some have found reduced fistula output,[13,14] with the time to spontaneous fistula closure either reduced[13] or unchanged.[14] Octreotide has also been reported to accelerate healing of pancreatic cutaneous fistulae.[15] A systematic review[16] of controlled trials commented on the variation in trial methods and conflicting results, but concluded that there is probably benefit in giving octreotide pre-operatively to prevent complications of pancreatic surgery, and that in established postoperative fistulae it may have a limited role in reducing fistula output and reducing the time to fistula closure.

There have been mixed results with octreotide in the treatment of **gastrointestinal bleeding**. Although a large multicentre study[17] showed that octreotide had no benefit compared with placebo in the management of bleeding upper gastrointestinal ulcers, a later meta-analysis suggested there might be some benefit.[18] Octreotide is used to control acute **variceal haemorrhage** (p.1716). It appears to be as effective as balloon tamponade,[19] and there is some evidence that it is as effective as sclerotherapy.[20] Two large controlled studies have suggested that combination of octreotide with endoscopic ligation[21] or sclerotherapy[22] reduces the risk of rebleeding. A subsequent meta-analysis[23] of trials comparing octreotide with other therapies for the control of acute variceal bleeding came to similar conclusions, and also found octreotide treatment to be more effective and associated with fewer major complications than vasopressin or terlipressin. However, there was no evidence of mortality benefit associated with octreotide use. Octreotide has also produced some benefit (combined with regular sclerotherapy), in the long-term management of patients with cirrhotic portal hypertension.[24]

Other gastrointestinal disorders in which octreotide might be useful include **dumping syndrome**[25,26] (further discussed on p.1242), reactive (or postprandial) **hypoglycaemia**,[27,28] **protein-losing enteropathy** associated with intestinal lymphangiectasia,[29] prevention of **NSAID-induced gastric injury**,[30] and **vomiting** secondary to bowel obstruction in patients terminally ill with cancer.[31,32] The *British National Formulary* states that in palliative care a dose of 300 to 600 micrograms may be given by subcutaneous infusion over 24 hours to reduce intestinal secretions and vomiting.


1. O'Connor CR, O'Dorisio TM. Amyloidosis, diarrhea, and a somatostatin analogue. *Ann Intern Med* 1989; **110:** 665–6.
2. Gilanders IA, *et al.* Octreotide therapy for diarrhoea. *Postgrad Med J* 1997; **73:** 62.
3. Tsai S-T, *et al.* Diabetic diarrhea and somatostatin. *Ann Intern Med* 1986; **104:** 894.
4. Michaels PE, Cameron RB. Octreotide is cost-effective therapy in diabetic diarrhea. *Arch Intern Med* 1991; **151:** 2469.
5. Mourad FH, *et al.* Effective treatment of diabetic diarrhoea with somatostatin analogue, octreotide. *Gut* 1992; **33:** 1578–80.
6. Couper RTL, *et al.* Clinical response to the long acting somatostatin analogue SMS 201-995 in a child with congenital microvillus atrophy. *Gut* 1989; **30:** 1020–4.
7. Crouch MA, *et al.* Octreotide acetate in refractory bone marrow transplant-associated diarrhea. *Ann Pharmacother* 1996; **30:** 331–6.
8. Dorta G, *et al.* Treatment of gold-induced enteritis with octreotide. *Lancet* 1993; **342:** 179.
9. Montaner JSG, *et al.* Octreotide therapy in AIDS-related, refractory diarrhea: results of a multicentre Canadian-European study. *AIDS* 1995: **9:** 209–10.
10. Simon DM, *et al.* Multicenter trial of octreotide in patients with refractory acquired immunodeficiency syndrome–associated diarrhea. *Gastroenterology* 1995; **108:** 1753–60. Correction. *ibid.*; **109:** 1024.
11. Ladefoged K, *et al.* Effect of a long acting somatostatin analogue SMS 201-995 on jejunostomy effluents in patients with severe short bowel syndrome. *Gut* 1989; **30:** 943–9.
12. Nightingale JMD, *et al.* Jejunal efflux in short bowel syndrome. *Lancet* 1990; **336:** 765–8.
13. Nubiola-Calonge P, *et al.* Blind evaluation of the effect of octreotide (SMS 201-995), a somatostatin analogue, on small-bowel fistula output. *Lancet* 1987; **ii:** 672–4.
14. Alivizatos V, *et al.* Evaluation of the effectiveness of octreotide in the conservative treatment of postoperative enterocutaneous fistulas. *Hepatogastroenterology* 2002; **49:** 1010–12.
15. Prinz RA, *et al.* Treatment of pancreatic cutaneous fistulas with a somatostatin analog. *Am J Surg* 1988; **155:** 36–42.
16. Li-Ling J, Irving M. Somatostatin and octreotide in the prevention of postoperative pancreatic complications and the treatment of enterocutaneous pancreatic fistulas: a systematic review of randomized controlled trials. *Br J Surg* 2001; **88:** 190–9.
17. Christiansen J, *et al.* Placebo-controlled trial with the somatostatin analogue SMS 201-995 in peptic ulcer bleeding. *Gastroenterology* 1989; **97:** 568–74.
18. Imperiale TF, Birgisson S. Somatostatin or octreotide compared with $H_2$ antagonists and placebo in the management of acute nonvariceal upper gastrointestinal hemorrhage: a meta-analysis. *Ann Intern Med* 1997; **127:** 1062–71. Correction. *ibid.* 1998; **128:** 245.
19. O'Donnell LJD, Farthing MJG. Octreotide and bleeding oesophageal varices. *Lancet* 1989; **ii:** 1276.
20. Jenkins SA, *et al.* A multicentre randomised trial comparing octreotide and injection sclerotherapy in the management and outcome of acute variceal haemorrhage. *Gut* 1997; **41:** 526–33.
21. Sung JJY, *et al.* Prospective randomised study of effect of octreotide on rebleeding from oesophageal varices after endoscopic ligation. *Lancet* 1995; **346:** 1666–9.
22. Besson I, *et al.* Sclerotherapy with or without octreotide for acute variceal bleeding. *N Engl J Med* 1995; **333:** 555–60.
23. Corley DA, *et al.* Octreotide for acute esophageal variceal bleeding: a meta-analysis. *Gastroenterology* 2001; **120:** 946–54.
24. Jenkins SA, *et al.* Randomised trial of octreotide for long term management of cirrhosis after variceal haemorrhage. *BMJ* 1997; **315:** 1338–41.
25. Hopman WPM, *et al.* Treatment of the dumping syndrome with the somatostatin analogue SMS 201-995. *Ann Surg* 1988; **207:** 155–9.
26. Farthing MJA. Octreotide in dumping and short bowel syndromes. *Digestion* 1993; **54** (suppl 1): 47–52.
27. D'Cruz DP, *et al.* Long-term symptomatic relief of postprandial hypoglycaemia following gastric surgery with a somatostatin analogue. *Postgrad Med J* 1989; **65:** 116–17.
28. Lehnert H, *et al.* Treatment of severe reactive hypoglycemia with a somatostatin analogue (SMS 201-995). *Arch Intern Med* 1990; **150:** 2401–2.

29. Bac DJ, *et al.* Octreotide for protein-losing enteropathy with intestinal lymphangiectasia. *Lancet* 1995; **345:** 1639.
30. Scheiman JM, *et al.* Reduction of non-steroidal anti-inflammatory drug induced gastric injury and leucocyte endothelial adhesion by octreotide. *Gut* 1997; **40:** 720–5.
31. Khoo D,*et al.* Control of emesis in bowel obstruction in terminally ill patients. *Lancet* 1992; **339:** 375–6.
32. Crawford R, Quigley C. Octreotide. *Prescribers' J* 1996; **36:** 231–2.

**Hypercalcaemia.** There have been individual reports of hypercalcaemia associated with raised plasma concentrations of parathyroid hormone-related protein (humoral hypercalcaemia of malignancy—p.1218) being successfully controlled with octreotide in patients with malignant pancreatic endocrine tumours[1,2] and adrenal phaeochromocytoma.[3] In two of these patients,[2,3] hypercalcaemia had previously been resistant to treatment with bisphosphonates. Octreotide also resolved hypercalcaemia occurring in a patient with VIPoma and vasoactive intestinal peptide concentrations declined.[4]

1. Wynick D, *et al.* Treatment of a malignant pancreatic endocrine tumour secreting parathyroid hormone related protein. *BMJ* 1990; **300:** 1314–15.
2. Dodwell D, *et al.* Treatment of a pancreatic tumour secreting parathyroid hormone related protein. *BMJ* 1990; **300:** 1653.
3. Harrison M, *et al.* Somatostatin analogue treatment for malignant hypercalcaemia. *BMJ* 1990; **300:** 1313–14. Correction. *ibid.*; **301:** 97 [dosage error].
4. Venkatesh S, *et al.* Somatostatin analogue: use in the treatment of vipoma with hypercalcaemia. *Am J Med* 1989; **87:** 356–7.

**Hyperinsulinism.** As well as reactive hypoglycaemia (see Gastrointestinal Disorders, above), octreotide has been used to control inappropriate insulin secretion, both in the short-term and long-term, in children with hypoglycaemia of infancy,[1-4] or nesidioblastosis.[5-7] It has also been used to treat a patient with hyperinsulinaemia induced by quinine.[8] For mention of investigations of octreotide for the reverse effect, see Diabetes Mellitus, above.

1. Kirk JMW, *et al.* Somatostatin analogue in short term management of hyperinsulinism. *Arch Dis Child* 1988; **63:** 1493–4.
2. DeClue TJ, *et al.* Linear growth during long-term treatment with somatostatin analog (SMS 201-995) for persistent hyperinsulinemic hypoglycemia of infancy. *J Pediatr* 1990; **116:** 747–50.
3. Thornton PS, *et al.* Short- and long-term use of octreotide in the treatment of congenital hyperinsulinism. *J Pediatr* 1993; **123:** 637–43.
4. Aynsley-Green A, *et al.* Practical management of hyperinsulinism in infancy. *Arch Dis Child Fetal Neonatal Ed* 2000; **82:** F98–F107.
5. Hindmarsh P, Brook CGD. Short-term management of nesidioblastosis using the somatostatin analogue SMS 201-995. *N Engl J Med* 1987; **316:** 221–2.
6. Delemarre-van de Waal HA, *et al.* Long-term treatment of an infant with nesidioblastosis using a somatostatin analogue. *N Engl J Med* 1987; **316:** 222–3.
7. Behrens R, *et al.* Unusual course of neonatal hyperinsulinaemic hypoglycaemia (nesidioblastosis). *Arch Dis Child* 1998; **78:** F156.
8. Phillips RE, *et al.* Effectiveness of SMS 201-995, a synthetic, long-acting somatostatin analogue, in treatment of quinine-induced hyperinsulinaemia. *Lancet* 1986; **i:** 713–16.

**Infertility.** Octreotide reduced circulating insulin and luteinising hormone concentrations and lowered androgen production in women with polycystic ovary syndrome.[1,2] This should assist in the development of ovulatory cycles. However, a small placebo-controlled study in women with infertility associated with polycystic ovary syndrome and clomifene resistance did not find octreotide to be of value in reversing the latter,[3] although some evidence suggested it might reduce the risk of ovarian hyperstimulation.

There has been a report of a pregnancy occurring in a previously infertile woman, resistant to clomifene, who was treated with octreotide for acromegaly.[4] The neonate had no malformations and developed normally. For a further reference to the use of octreotide during pregnancy, see Pregnancy, above.

1. Prelević GM, *et al.* Inhibitory effect of Sandostatin on secretion of luteinising hormone and ovarian steroids in polycystic ovary syndrome. *Lancet* 1990; **336:** 900–3.
2. Prelevic GM, *et al.* The effects of the somatostatin analogue octreotide on ovulatory performance in women with polycystic ovaries. *Hum Reprod* 1995; **10:** 28–32.
3. Morris RS, *et al.* Octreotide is not useful for clomiphene citrate resistance in patients with polycystic ovary syndrome but may reduce the likelihood of ovarian hyperstimulation syndrome. *Fertil Steril* 1999; **71:** 452–6.
4. Landolt AM, *et al.* Successful pregnancy in a previously infertile woman treated with SMS-201-995 for acromegaly. *N Engl J Med* 1989; **320:** 671–2.

**Malignant neoplasms.** See also Carcinoid Syndrome, above. For mention of the use of octreotide to treat vomiting associated with malignant gastrointestinal obstruction see Gastrointestinal Disorders, above. Octreotide has also proved of benefit in bone pain due to metastatic gastrinoma (see Pain, below). An unconventional regimen using octreotide or somatostatin with melatonin, bromocriptine, and a solution of retinoids (the Di Bella regimen) was investigated in patients with a variety of advanced malignancies and found to be ineffective.[1,2]

1. Italian Study Group for the Di Bella Multitherapy Trials. Evaluation of an unconventional cancer treatment (the Di Bella multitherapy): results of phase II trials in Italy. *BMJ* 1999; **318:** 224–8.
2. Buiatti E, *et al.* Results from a historical survey of the survival of cancer patients given Di Bella multitherapy. *Cancer* 1999; **86:** 2143–9.

HEPATOCELLULAR CARCINOMA. In a study in 58 patients with advanced hepatocellular carcinoma (p.518) treatment with octreotide was associated with prolongation of survival compared with no treatment.[1] However, another study of long-acting octreotide in patients with advanced hepatocellular carcinoma failed to demonstrate any benefit.[2]

1. Kouroumalis E, *et al.* Treatment of hepatocellular carcinoma with octreotide: a randomised controlled study. *Gut* 1998; **42:** 442–7.
2. Yuen M-F, *et al.* A randomized placebo-controlled study of long-acting octreotide for the treatment of advanced hepatocellular carcinoma. *Hepatology* 2002; **36:** 687–91.

MENINGIOMA. Octreotide has been reported to suppress headaches and visual disturbances associated with meningioma in a small number of patients.[1-3] Doses were generally started at 100 micrograms three times daily subcutaneously, but were increased to 500 micrograms three times daily in some cases because of tolerance. Although it was thought that octreotide may have had a beneficial effect on the meningioma size in one case,[1] others found no evidence of tumour shrinkage.[2,3]

1. Rünzi MW, *et al.* Successful treatment of meningioma with octreotide. *Lancet* 1989; **i:** 1074.
2. García-Luna PP, *et al.* Clinical use of octreotide in unresectable meningiomas: a report of three cases. *J Neurosurg Sci* 1993; **37:** 237–41.
3. Jaffrain-Rea M-L, *et al.* Visual improvement during octreotide therapy in a case of episellar meningioma. *Clin Neurol Neurosurg* 1998; **100:** 40–3.

THYMOMA. A patient with thymoma and pure red cell aplasia, in whom corticosteroids alone failed to control anaemia, experienced complete remission following treatment with octreotide and prednisone, and subsequently remained well on long-term maintenance therapy with octreotide 500 micrograms twice daily and prednisone 200 micrograms/kg daily.[1] In a study[2] that included 32 patients with thymoma and a positive octreotide scan, octreotide therapy alone (500 micrograms subcutaneously three times daily for up to 1 year) or with prednisone (600 micrograms/kg daily) had modest activity; there were 2 complete and 10 partial responses overall.

1. Palmieri G, *et al.* Successful treatment of a patient with a thymoma and pure red-cell aplasia with octreotide and prednisone. *N Engl J Med* 1997; **336:** 263–5.
2. Loehrer PJ, *et al.* Octreotide alone or with prednisone in patients with advanced thymoma and thymic carcinoma: an Eastern Cooperative Oncology Group phase II trial. *J Clin Oncol* 2004; **22:** 293–9.

**Nesidioblastosis.** For reference to the use of octreotide in nesidioblastosis, see Hyperinsulinism, above.

**Pain.** Octreotide 120 to 480 micrograms daily was administered by continuous intrathecal infusion to 5 patients with cancer pain that had been poorly controlled by opioid analgesics.[1] All patients obtained good pain relief, 3 reporting pain to be totally absent. Sustained decrease in incapacitating bone pain has also been reported in a patient with skeletal metastasis of a gastrinoma who was given subcutaneous octreotide 100 micrograms three times daily.[2] The pain of hypertrophic pulmonary osteoarthropathy (a paraneoplastic syndrome of periostitis, arthropathy, and gynaecomastia seen particularly with squamous cell lung cancer) has also been reported to respond to octreotide.[3] However, a controlled study of octreotide in cancer pain found that it was no better than placebo in most patients.[4] (General guidelines for the management of cancer pain are discussed on p.5.) Octreotide has also been reported to ease headache associated with meningioma (above), and pituitary adenoma (see below).

1. Penn RD, *et al.* Intrathecal octreotide for cancer pain. *Lancet* 1990; **335:** 738.
2. Burgess JR, *et al.* Effective control of bone pain by octreotide in a patient with metastatic gastrinoma. *Med J Aust* 1996; **164:** 725–7.
3. Johnson SA, *et al.* Treatment of resistant pain in hypertrophic pulmonary osteoarthropathy with subcutaneous octreotide. *Thorax* 1997; **52:** 298–9.
4. De Conno F, *et al.* Subcutaneous octreotide in the treatment of pain in advanced cancer patients. *J Pain Symptom Manage* 1994; **9:** 34–8.

**Pancreatic disorders.** Octreotide has been tried in the treatment of acute pancreatitis, but was found to be ineffective.[1] For reference to the use of octreotide in the management of pancreatic endocrine tumours, see under Carcinoid Tumours (p.504); for its use in pancreatic fistulae, see Gastrointestinal Disorders, above.

1. Uhl W, *et al.* A randomised, double blind, multicentre trial of octreotide in moderate to severe acute pancreatitis. *Gut* 1999; **45:** 97–104.

**Pituitary adenoma.** Pituitary adenomas, which may be responsible for conditions such as acromegaly (p.1312), or hyperprolactinaemia (p.1315), may respond to therapy with octreotide by shrinkage of the tumour and an improvement in symptoms such as headaches and visual disturbances or reduction in the secretion of active hormones, or both.

References.

1. Williams G, *et al.* Analgesic effect of somatostatin analogue (octreotide) in headache associated with pituitary tumours. *BMJ* 1987; **295:** 247–8.
2. Orme SM, *et al.* Shrinkage of thyrotrophin secreting pituitary adenoma treated with octreotide. *Postgrad Med J* 1991; **67:** 466–8.
3. Donckier J, *et al.* Shrinkage of inoperable adenomas in cavernous sinus with high-dose octreotide. *Lancet* 1993; **342:** 301.
4. Chanson P, *et al.* Octreotide therapy for thyroid-stimulating hormone-secreting pituitary adenomas: a follow-up of 52 patients. *Ann Intern Med* 1993; **119:** 236–40.
5. Thapar K, *et al.* Antiproliferative effect of the somatostatin analogue octreotide on growth hormone-producing pituitary tumors: results of a multicenter randomized trial. *Mayo Clin Proc* 1997; **72:** 893–900.

**Pretibial myxoedema.** Pretibial myxoedema (deposition of glycosaminoglycans in the subcutaneous tissue of the shins) is associated with Graves' disease (see Hyperthyroidism, p.1594). There are reports of apparent benefit from the use of octreotide for this condition. In one case,[1] octreotide given for 6 months following surgical removal of the myxoedematous tissue may have prevented its recurrence. In another,[2] octreotide injected intralesionally was reported to improve and control the condition.

1. Derrick EK, *et al.* Successful surgical treatment of severe pretibial myxoedema. *Br J Dermatol* 1995; **133:** 317–18.
2. Shinohara M, *et al.* Refractory pretibial myxoedema with response to intralesional insulin-like growth factor 1 antagonist (octreotide): downregulation of hyaluronic acid production by the lesional fibroblasts. *Br J Dermatol* 2000; **143:** 1083–6.

**Raised intracranial pressure.** For a reference to octreotide being tried in benign intracranial hypertension, see p.833.

**Sleep apnoea.** There have been reports of improvement in the severity of sleep apnoea in acromegalic patients treated with octreotide.[1,2]

1. Grunstein RR, *et al.* Effect of octreotide, a somatostatin analog, on sleep apnea in patients with acromegaly. *Ann Intern Med* 1994; **121:** 478–83.
2. Buyse B, *et al.* Relief of sleep apnoea after treatment of acromegaly: report of three cases and review of the literature. *Eur Respir J* 1997; **10:** 1401–4.

**Sulfonylurea overdose.** Octreotide has been used in the treatment of severe refractory cases of sulfonylurea-induced hypoglycaemia (see p.346).

## Preparations

**Proprietary Preparations** (details are given in Part 3)
***Arg.:*** Sandostatin; ***Austral.:*** Sandostatin; ***Austria:*** Sandostatin; ***Belg.:*** Sandostatine; ***Braz.:*** Sandostatin; ***Canad.:*** Sandostatin; ***Chile:*** Sandostatin; ***Denm.:*** Sandostatin; ***Fin.:*** Sandostatin; ***Fr.:*** Sandostatine; ***Ger.:*** Sandostatin; ***Gr.:*** Sandostatin; ***Hong Kong:*** Sandostatin; ***India:*** Sandostatin; ***Irl.:*** Sandostatin; ***Israel:*** Sandostatin; ***Ital.:*** Longastatina; Samilstin; Sandostatina; ***Malaysia:*** Sandostatin; ***Mex.:*** Sandostatina; ***Neth.:*** Sandostatine; ***Norw.:*** Sandostatin; ***NZ:*** Sandostatin; ***Port.:*** Sandostatina; ***S.Afr.:*** Sandostatin; ***Singapore:*** Sandostatin; ***Spain:*** Sandostatin; ***Swed.:*** Sandostatin; ***Switz.:*** Sandostatine; ***Thai.:*** Sandostatin; ***UK:*** Sandostatin; ***USA:*** Sandostatin.

# Ornipressin *(rINN)*

Ornipresina. [8-Ornithine]-vasopressin.
$C_{45}H_{63}N_{13}O_{12}S_2$ = 1042.2.
*CAS — 3397-23-7.*
*ATC — H01BA05.*

## Profile

Ornipressin is a synthetic derivative of vasopressin (p.1342) with similar actions. It is reported to be a strong vasoconstrictor with only weak antidiuretic properties and is used to reduce bleeding during surgery. A solution containing up to 5 units in 20 to 60 mL of sodium chloride 0.9% is infiltrated into the area involved. Ornipressin is also used for bleeding oesophageal varices (p.1716). For this purpose it has been given by intravenous infusion: a dose of 20 units over 20 minutes, diluted in 100 mL of sodium chloride 0.9% has been suggested. Continuous infusion over 24 or 48 hours has also been advocated.

◊ References.

1. Kam PC, Tay TM. The pharmacology of ornipressin (POR-8): a local vasoconstrictor used in surgery. *Eur J Anaesthesiol* 1998; **15:** 133–9.
2. De Kock M, *et al.* Ornipressin (Por 8): an efficient alternative to counteract hypotension during combined general/epidural anesthesia. *Anesth Analg* 2000; **90:** 1301–7.

**Adverse effects.** Acute pulmonary oedema occurred in a patient following infiltration of ornipressin (12 units in 40 mL isotonic saline) as a local vasoconstrictor during surgery.[1] It was suggested that no more than 0.1 unit/kg should be administered in this manner.

1. Borgeat A, *et al.* Acute pulmonary oedema following administration of ornithine-8-vasopressin. *Br J Anaesth* 1990; **65:** 548–51.

**Hepatorenal syndrome.** Ornipressin has been found to be of benefit[1-3] in the hepatorenal syndrome, a form of renal insufficiency associated with cirrhosis of the liver, and thought to be due to severe renal vasoconstriction secondary to systemic arterial vasodilatation. However, caution in its use has been urged[2] because of the risk of ischaemic complications.

1. Lenz K, *et al.* Ornipressin in the treatment of functional renal failure in decompensated liver cirrhosis: effects on renal hemodynamics and atrial natriuretic factor. *Gastroenterology* 1991; **101:** 1060–7.
2. Guevara M, *et al.* Reversibility of hepatorenal syndrome by prolonged administration of ornipressin and plasma volume expansion. *Hepatology* 1998; **27:** 35–41.
3. Gülberg V, *et al.* Long-term therapy and retreatment of hepatorenal syndrome type 1 with ornipressin and dopamine. *Hepatology* 1999; **30:** 870–5.

## Preparations

**Proprietary Preparations** (details are given in Part 3)
***Austral.:*** POR 8; ***Austria:*** POR 8; ***Ger.:*** POR 8†; ***NZ:*** POR 8†; ***S.Afr.:*** POR 8; ***Switz.:*** POR 8†.

## Oxytocin *(BAN, rINN)*

Alpha-hypophamine; Oxitocina; Oxytocinum. Cys-Tyr-Ile-Gln-Asn-Cys-Pro-Leu-Gly-$NH_2$ cyclic (1→6) disulphide; [2-Leucine,7-isoleucine]vasopressin.

$C_{43}H_{66}N_{12}O_{12}S_2$ = 1007.2.

*CAS — 50-56-6.*

*ATC — H01BB02.*

**Pharmacopoeias.** In *Chin., Eur.* (see p.vi), *Jpn,* and *US.*

**Ph. Eur. 5.0** (Oxytocin). A cyclic nonapeptide having the structure of the hormone produced by the posterior lobe of the pituitary that stimulates contraction of the uterus and milk ejection in receptive mammals. It is obtained by chemical synthesis and is available in the freeze-dried form as an acetate. A white or almost white, hygroscopic powder. Very soluble in water and in dilute solutions of dehydrated alcohol and of acetic acid. A 2% solution in water has a pH of 3.0 to 6.0. Store at 2° to 8° in airtight containers. Protect from light.

**Ph. Eur. 5.0** (Oxytocin Bulk Solution). A solution of oxytocin with a concentration of not less than 250 micrograms of oxytocin per mL. It may contain a suitable antimicrobial preservative. A clear colourless liquid with a pH of 3.0 to 5.0. Store at 2° to 8°. Protect from light.

**USP 27** (Oxytocin). A nonapeptide hormone having the property of causing the contraction of uterine smooth muscle and of the myoepithelial cells within the mammary glands. It is prepared by synthesis or obtained from the posterior lobe of the pituitary of healthy domestic animals used for food by man. Its oxytocic activity is not less than 400 units/mg. Store in airtight containers at 2° to 8°.

### Units

12.5 units of oxytocin for bioassay are contained in approximately 21.4 micrograms of synthetic peptide (with human albumin 5 mg and citric acid) in one ampoule of the fourth International Standard (1978).

### Adverse Effects

Administration of oxytocin in high doses or to those hypersensitive to it may cause violent uterine contractions leading to uterine rupture and extensive laceration of the soft tissues, fetal bradycardia, fetal arrhythmias, and fetal asphyxiation, and perhaps fetal or maternal death.

Maternal deaths from severe hypertension and subarachnoid haemorrhage have occurred. Postpartum haemorrhage and fatal afibrinogenaemia have been reported but may be due to obstetric complications. Water retention leading to hyponatraemia and intoxication, with pulmonary oedema, convulsions, coma, and even death may occur, especially when oxytocin is given intravenously over prolonged periods. Vasopressin-like activity (see p.1342) is more likely with oxytocin of natural origin but may occur even with the synthetic peptide.

Anaphylactic and other hypersensitivity reactions, cardiac arrhythmias, pelvic haematomas, and nausea and vomiting may occur. Rapid intravenous injection has produced acute transient hypotension with flushing and reflex tachycardia.

There are reports of neonatal jaundice and retinal haemorrhage associated with the use of oxytocin in the management of labour. Adverse effects following the intranasal administration of oxytocin have included nasal irritation, rhinorrhoea, lachrymation, uterine bleeding, and violent uterine contractions.

**Inappropriate use.** In a 1988 comment on the misuse of oxytocin in labour,[1] it was observed that statements on the management of labour were often misinterpreted as meaning that all labouring women who failed to make adequate progress in terms of cervical dilatation should be given oxytocin. This was only true if poor progress was due to poor uterine action, and would be dangerous where there was disproportion; the decision to use oxytocin required careful assessment by an experienced obstetrician. In the previous 2 years the authors had seen one case of fractured pelvis, 2 of ruptured uterus, and 7 of cerebral palsy from fetal hypoxia, all of which were thought to be due to the ill-advised use of oxytocin to augment labour.

For reference to haemorrhage and to neonatal hyperbilirubinaemia occurring after an oxytocin challenge test, see under Uses and Administration, below.

1. Taylor RW, Taylor M. Misuse of oxytocin in labour. *Lancet* 1988; **i:** 352.

**Neonatal jaundice.** Analysis of neonatal jaundice in 12 461 single births confirmed a higher incidence of jaundice in offspring of mothers given oxytocin, independent of gestational age at birth, sex, race, epidural analgesia, method of delivery, and birth-weight, each of which was also associated with jaundice.[1] In a total of 90 infants born to mothers after oxytocin-induced labour in 2 studies,[2,3] haematological disturbances were noted. These included erythrocyte fragility or reduction in erythrocyte deformability, hyponatraemia, hypo-osmolality, and an increase in serum-bilirubin concentration. Glucose injection, used as a vehicle for oxytocin may have further aggravated these changes.[3]

See also under Oxytocin Challenge Test in Uses and Administration, below.

1. Friedman L, *et al.* Factors influencing the incidence of neonatal jaundice. *BMJ* 1978; **1:** 1235–7.
2. Buchan PC. Pathogenesis of neonatal hyperbilirubinaemia after induction of labour with oxytocin. *BMJ* 1979; **2:** 1255–7.
3. Singhi S, Singh M. Pathogenesis of oxytocin-induced neonatal hyperbilirubinaemia. *Arch Dis Child* 1979; **54:** 400–2.

**Water intoxication.** Oxytocin-induced water intoxication is most likely to arise as a result of prolonged attempts to empty the uterus in missed abortion or mid-trimester termination of pregnancy, but it has also been described after oxytocin infusion in other conditions including induction of labour.[1] Irrespective of the oxytocin concentration, patients in virtually all the reported cases have received more than 3.5 litres of infused fluid. Convulsions and somnolence associated with hyponatraemia have also been reported in a patient who was drinking more than 5 litres of herbal tea daily while using intranasal oxytocin 8 times or more a day.[2]

Another factor contributing to hyponatraemia is the antidiuretic effect of the pethidine and morphine commonly used for analgesia with oxytocin infusions. Water intoxication usually presents with fits and loss of consciousness but in some cases there may be preceding signs such as raised venous pressure, bounding pulse, and tachycardia. Diagnosis is confirmed by profound hyponatraemia; the mechanism appears to be more complex than simply haemodilution by the infused water. Treatment consists of controlling convulsions and maintaining an airway; oxytocin infusion must be stopped and isotonic, or even hypertonic, saline may be infused. Diuresis may then be assisted with furosemide. The prime objective, however, should be prevention; no patient should receive more than 3 litres of fluid containing oxytocin, and a careful fluid balance record is essential.

1. Feeney JG. Water intoxication and oxytocin. *BMJ* 1982; **285:** 243.
2. Mayer-Hubner B. Pseudotumour cerebri from intranasal oxytocin and excessive fluid intake. *Lancet* 1996; **347:** 623.

### Precautions

Oxytocin should not be given where spontaneous labour or vaginal delivery are liable to harm either the mother or the fetus. This includes significant cephalopelvic disproportion or unfavourable presentation of the fetus, placenta praevia or vasa praevia, cord presentation or prolapse, mechanical obstruction to delivery, fetal distress or hypertonic uterine contractions. It should not be used where there is a predisposition to uterine rupture, as in multiple pregnancy or high parity, polyhydramnios, or the presence of a uterine scar from previous caesarean section. Oxytocin should not be employed for prolonged periods in resistant uterine inertia, severe pre-eclampsia, or severe cardiovascular disorders.

When given for induction or enhancement of labour particular care is needed in borderline cephalopelvic disproportion, less severe degrees of cardiovascular disease, and in patients over 35 years of age or with other risk factors. Careful monitoring of fetal heart rate and uterine motility is essential so that dosage of oxytocin can be adjusted to individual response; the drug should be given by intravenous infusion, preferably by means of a syringe pump. Infusion should be discontinued immediately if fetal distress or uterine hyperactivity occur.

Over-vigorous labour should be avoided in cases of fetal death *in utero,* or where there is meconium-stained amniotic fluid, because there is a risk of amniotic fluid embolism.

The risk of water intoxication should be borne in mind, particularly when high doses of oxytocin are given over a long time. Infusion volumes should be kept low, and in such circumstances an electrolyte-based infusion fluid should be used rather than glucose solution. Fluid intake by mouth should be restricted and a fluid balance chart maintained; serum electrolytes should be measured if electrolyte imbalance is suspected.

**Oxytocin challenge test.** For the suggestion that oxytocin challenge testing should be used with caution in women whose offspring might be at risk of hyperbilirubinaemia, see under Uses and Administration, below.

### Interactions

Oxytocin may enhance the vasopressor effects of sympathomimetics. Some inhalational anaesthetics, such as cyclopropane or halothane, may enhance the hypotensive effect of oxytocin and reduce its oxytocic effect; cardiac arrhythmias may occur. Prostaglandins and oxytocin may potentiate the effects of each other on the uterus.

### Pharmacokinetics

Oxytocin undergoes enzymatic destruction in the gastrointestinal tract but it is rapidly absorbed from the mucous membranes when administered buccally or intranasally. It is metabolised by the liver and kidneys with a plasma half-life of only a few minutes. Only small amounts are excreted unchanged in the urine.

◊ References.

1. Seitchik J, *et al.* Oxytocin augmentation of dysfunctional labor IV: oxytocin pharmacokinetics. *Am J Obstet Gynecol* 1984; **150:** 225–8.

### Uses and Administration

Oxytocin is a cyclic nonapeptide secreted by the hypothalamus and stored in the posterior lobe of the pituitary gland. It may be prepared from the gland of mammals or by synthesis.

Oxytocin causes contraction of the uterus, the effect increasing with the duration of pregnancy due to proliferation of oxytocin receptors. Small doses increase the tone and amplitude of the uterine contractions; large or repeated doses result in tetany. Oxytocin also stimulates the smooth muscle associated with the secretory epithelium of the lactating breast causing the ejection of milk but having no direct effect on milk secretion. It has a weak antidiuretic action.

Oxytocin is used for the induction and augmentation of labour, to control postpartum bleeding and uterine hypotonicity in the third stage of labour, and to promote lactation in cases of faulty milk ejection. It is also used in missed abortions, but other measures may be preferred.

For the **induction** or **augmentation of labour** oxytocin may be given by slow intravenous infusion preferably by means of an infusion pump. A solution containing 5 units in 500 mL of a physiological electrolyte solution such as sodium chloride 0.9% has been recommended but more concentrated solutions may be given via infusion pump, and current UK guidelines suggest 10 or 30 units in 500 mL of diluent. Infusion is begun at a recommended initial rate of 1 to 2 milliunits/minute and then gradually increased at intervals of at least 30 minutes, until a maximum of 3 or 4 contractions are occurring every 10 minutes. A rate of up to 6 milliunits/minute is reported to produce plasma oxytocin concentrations comparable to those in natural labour, and 12 milliunits/minute is usually the most that is needed but doses of up to 20 milliunits/minute or more may be required. UK guidelines suggest that 32 milliunits/minute should not be exceeded, and no more than a total of 5 units should be given in 1 day. Fetal heart rate and uterine contractions should be monitored continuously. Once labour is progressing, oxytocin infusion may be gradually withdrawn.

For the treatment and prevention of **postpartum haemorrhage** oxytocin may be given by slow intravenous injection in a dose of 5 units; this may be followed in severe cases by intravenous infusion of 5 to 20 units (the *British National Formulary* suggests up to 30 units) in 500 mL of a suitable non-hydrating diluent. An alternative for the prophylaxis of postpartum haemorrhage in the routine management of the third stage of labour is the intramuscular injection of oxytocin 5 units with ergometrine maleate 500 micrograms with or after delivery of the baby's shoulders. In the USA a dose of 10 units of oxytocin, by intravenous infusion at a rate of 20 to 40 milliunits/minute, or as an intramuscular injection, has been recommended for treatment of postpartum haemorrhage.

In **missed abortion** a suggested dose in the UK is 5 units by slow intravenous injection, followed if necessary by intravenous infusion at a rate of 20 to 40 milliunits/minute or higher.

Oxytocin nasal spray is used to facilitate **lactation**; a dose of one spray, delivering 4 units, into one nostril 5 minutes before suckling has been used. However, there is a danger that the mother may become dependent upon its action and such usage is not generally recommended (see p.1317).

Oxytocin citrate has been given in the form of a buccal tablet to induce labour; however, absorption is irregular following buccal administration and this route has been superseded by intravenous infusion.

An **oxytocin challenge test** has been used to evaluate fetal distress in pregnant patients at high-risk.

Synthetic derivatives of oxytocin such as demoxytocin (p.1322) have been used similarly.

**Labour induction and augmentation.** Oxytocin infusions have proved to be one of the most successful agents for induction and augmentation of labour, as discussed on p.1511. There have been numerous studies on the dosage of oxytocin required to induce or augment labour,[1-9] which increasingly favour low-dose regimens, starting at infusion rates of 1 milliunit/minute or less. UK guidelines favour a starting dose of 1 to 2 milliunits/minute, increased at intervals of 30 minutes, and titrated against contractions.[10] However, it has been pointed out that no one regimen has been clearly proved superior.[11]


1. Seitchik J, Castillo M. Oxytocin augmentation of dysfunctional labor I: clinical data. *Am J Obstet Gynecol* 1982; **144:** 899–905.
2. Seitchik J, Castillo M. Oxytocin augmentation of dysfunctional labor III: multiparous patients. *Am J Obstet Gynecol* 1983; **145:** 777–80.
3. Seitchik J, *et al.* Oxytocin augmentation of dysfunctional labor V: an alternative oxytocin regimen. *Am J Obstet Gynecol* 1985; **151:** 757–61.
4. Wein P. Efficacy of different starting doses of oxytocin for induction of labor. *Obstet Gynecol* 1989; **74:** 863–8.
5. Blakemore KJ, *et al.* A prospective comparison of hourly and quarter-hourly oxytocin dose increase intervals for the induction of labor at term. *Obstet Gynecol* 1990; **75:** 757–61.
6. Mercer B, *et al.* Labor induction with continuous low-dose oxytocin infusion: a randomized trial. *Obstet Gynecol* 1991; **77:** 659–63.
7. Akoury HA, *et al.* Oxytocin augmentation of labour and perinatal outcome in nulliparas. *Obstet Gynecol* 1991; **78:** 227–30.
8. Satin AJ, *et al.* High versus low-dose oxytocin for labor stimulation. *Obstet Gynecol* 1992; **80:** 111–16.
9. Merrill DC, Zlatnik FJ. Randomized, double-masked comparison of oxytocin dosage in induction and augmentation of labor. *Obstet Gynecol* 1999; **94:** 455–63.
10. Royal College of Obstetricians and Gynaecologists. Induction of labour: evidence-based clinical guideline number 9 (issued June 2001). Available at: http://www.nice.org.uk/pdf/inductionoflabourrcogrep.pdf (accessed 02/04/04)
11. Xenakis EM-J, Piper JM. Chemotherapeutic induction of labour: a rational approach. *Drugs* 1997; **54:** 61–8.


**Oxytocin challenge test.** The oxytocin challenge test (OCT) is designed to detect placental insufficiency, and identify fetuses at risk of still-birth or complications during labour. In a study, it was performed on 399 occasions in 305 women with pregnancies at risk and a gestational age of 36 weeks or more.[1] Oxytocin 1 milliunit/minute was given by infusion pump and increased every 5 to 10 minutes until a contraction rate of 3 per 10 minutes was achieved. Less than 10% of late or variable decelerations of fetal heart rate (FHR) was judged negative; 10 to 29% was judged equivocal; and 30% or more was judged positive. The finding of a positive or equivocal response to the OCT was considered a prediction of decelerations of the FHR during parturition, though the type of risk might vary. After 100 OCTs in 90 pregnant women considered at risk[2] it was concluded that a negative result is a reliable test of fetal well-being which should encourage obstetricians to await spontaneous onset of labour in preference to intervention. However, there have been reports of fetal death occurring despite a negative response to the OCT.[3-5] Adverse effects associated with the OCT have included haemorrhage occurring in a patient after the second of two tests (the patient was found to have a major placenta praevia)[6] and neonatal hyperbilirubinaemia.[7] The latter effect led to the suggestion that the OCT should be used with caution in women whose babies might be at risk from hyperbilirubinaemia.


1. Schulman H, *et al.* Quantitative analysis in the oxytocin challenge test. *Am J Obstet Gynecol* 1977; **129:** 239–44.
2. Sellappah S, Wagman H. Oxytocin challenge test as an out patient procedure. *Br J Clin Pract* 1984; **38:** 255–8.
3. Marcum RG. False negative oxytocin challenge test. *Am J Obstet Gynecol* 1977; **127:** 894.
4. Lorenz RP, Pagano JS. A case of intrauterine fetal death after a negative oxytocin challenge test. *Am J Obstet Gynecol* 1978; **130:** 232.
5. Dittman R, Belcher J. False-negative oxytocin challenge test. *N Engl J Med* 1978; **298:** 56.
6. Ng KH, Wong WP. Risk of haemorrhage in oxytocin stress test. *BMJ* 1976; **2:** 698–9.
7. Peleg D, Goldman JA. Oxytocin challenge test and neonatal hyperbilirubinaemia. *Lancet* 1976; **ii:** 1026.


**Postpartum haemorrhage.** Oxytocin is used for the prophylaxis and treatment of postpartum haemorrhage (p.1684). In the active management of the third stage of labour, the combination of oxytocin and ergometrine may be associated with a small reduction in the risk of postpartum haemorrhage compared with oxytocin alone, but a higher incidence of nausea, vomiting, and hypertension.

**Retained placenta.** Oxytocin injected into the vein of the umbilical cord has been used to assist the removal of retained placenta. A meta-analysis[1] of 12 studies found evidence that oxytocin reduced the incidence of manual removal of the retained placenta, although there was no apparent benefit in terms of other measures including blood loss, curettage, and infection. The removal of the placenta is important to allow contraction of the myometrium and prevention of excessive blood loss, and is one reason for the use of oxytocin in the active management of the third stage of labour, as discussed under Postpartum Haemorrhage—see above and on p.1684.


1. Carroli G, Bergel E. Umbilical vein injection for management of retained placenta. Available in The Cochrane Library; Issue 1. Chichester: John Wiley; 2004.


### Preparations

***BP 2003:*** Ergometrine and Oxytocin Injection; Oxytocin Injection;
***USP 27:*** Oxytocin Injection; Oxytocin Nasal Solution.

**Proprietary Preparations** (details are given in Part 3)
***Arg.:*** Hipofisina; Syntocinon; Veracuril; ***Austral.:*** Syntocinon; ***Austria:*** Syntocinon; ***Belg.:*** Syntocinon; ***Braz.:*** Naox; Orastina; Oxiton; Syntocinon; ***Chile:*** Syntocinon; ***Denm.:*** Syntocinon; ***Fin.:*** Syntocinon; ***Fr.:*** Syntocinon; ***Ger.:*** Orasthin; Syntocinon; ***Hong Kong:*** Syntocinon; ***India:*** Pitocin; Syntocinon; ***Irl.:*** Syntocinon; ***Israel:*** Partocon†; Syntocinon†; ***Ital.:*** Syntocinon; ***Malaysia:*** Syntocinon; ***Mex.:*** Oxitopisa; Syntocinon; Xitocin; ***Neth.:*** Syntocinon; ***Norw.:*** Pitocin†; Syntocinon; ***NZ:*** Syntocinon; ***Port.:*** Syntocinon; ***S.Afr.:*** Syntocinon; ***Singapore:*** Syntocinon; ***Spain:*** Syntocinon; ***Swed.:*** Partocon†; Syntocinon; ***Switz.:*** Syntocinon; ***Thai.:*** Syntocinon†; ***UK:*** Syntocinon; ***USA:*** Pitocin.

**Multi-ingredient:** ***Austral.:*** Syntometrine; ***Ger.:*** Syntometrin; ***Hong Kong:*** Syntometrine; ***Irl.:*** Syntometrine; ***Israel:*** Syntometrine†; ***Malaysia:*** Syntometrine; ***NZ:*** Syntometrine; ***S.Afr.:*** Syntometrine; ***UK:*** Syntometrine.

---

## Pegvisomant *(USAN, rINN)*

B2036-PEG.
*ATC — H01AX01.*

### Adverse Effects and Precautions

Adverse effects commonly reported with the use of pegvisomant include gastrointestinal disturbances, elevated liver function tests, flu-like symptoms, fatigue, injection site reactions, arthralgia, myalgia, headache, dizziness, somnolence, tremor, sweating, pruritus, rash, sleep disorders, hypercholesterolaemia, weight gain, hyperglycaemia, hunger, and hypertension.

Liver function tests should be measured before starting pegvisomant, then every 4 to 6 weeks for the first 6 months of therapy, and periodically thereafter.

### Interactions

Pegvisomant may increase insulin sensitivity. In patients with diabetes, doses of insulin or oral hypoglycaemics may need to be decreased because of the increased risk of hypoglycaemia.

### Uses and Administration

Pegvisomant is a growth hormone-receptor antagonist used for the treatment of acromegaly (p.1312). A loading dose of 40 or 80 mg is given subcutaneously, followed by 10 mg daily. Further dose adjustments, in increments of 5 mg, are made according to serum concentrations of IGF-I, which should be measured every 4 to 6 weeks. The maintenance dose should not exceed 30 mg daily.

◊ References.


1. Trainer PJ, *et al.* Treatment of acromegaly with the growth hormone-receptor antagonist pegvisomant. *N Engl J Med* 2000; **342:** 1171–7.
2. Herman-Bonert VS, *et al.* Growth hormone receptor antagonist therapy in acromegalic patients resistant to somatostatin analogs. *J Clin Endocrinol Metab* 2000; **85:** 2958–61.
3. van der Lely AJ, *et al.* Control of tumor size and disease activity during cotreatment with octreotide and the growth hormone receptor antagonist pegvisomant in an acromegalic patient. *J Clin Endocrinol Metab* 2001; **86:** 478–81.
4. van der Lely AJ, *et al.* Long-term treatment of acromegaly with pegvisomant, a growth hormone receptor antagonist. *Lancet* 2001; **358:** 1754–9.


### Preparations

**Proprietary Preparations** (details are given in Part 3)
***UK:*** Somavert; ***USA:*** Somavert.

---

## Posatirelin *(rINN)*

Posatirelina; RGH-2202. (2*S*)-*N*-[(1*S*)-1-[[(2*S*)-2-Carbamoyl-1-pyrrolidinyl]carbonyl]-3-methylbutyl]-6-oxopipecolamide.
$C_{17}H_{28}N_4O_4$ = 352.4.
*CAS — 78664-73-0.*

### Profile

Posatirelin is an analogue of protirelin (p.1337). It is claimed to have beneficial effects on CNS function, and has been investigated in the management of dementia of various causes.

◊ References.


1. Parnetti L, *et al.* Posatirelin for the treatment of late-onset Alzheimer's disease: a double-blind multicentre study vs citicoline and ascorbic acid. *Acta Neurol Scand* 1995; **92:** 135–40.
2. Parnetti L, *et al.* Posatirelin in the treatment of vascular dementia: a double-blind multicentre study vs placebo. *Acta Neurol Scand* 1996; **93:** 456–63.
3. Reboldi G, *et al.* Pharmacokinetic profile and endocrine effects of posatirelin treatment in healthy elderly subjects. *J Clin Pharmacol* 1996; **36:** 823–31.


---

## Powdered Pituitary (Posterior Lobe)

Hipófisis pulverizada (neurohipófisis); Hypophysis Cerebri Pars Posterior; Hypophysis Sicca; Ipofisi Posteriore; Pituitarium Posterius Pulveratum; Pituitary; Posterior Pituitary.

NOTE. Pituitary Extract (Posterior) is *BAN*.

**Pharmacopoeias.** In *Chin.*

### Adverse Effects, Treatment, and Precautions

Similar to those for oxytocin (p.1336) and for vasopressin (p.1342). Hypersensitivity reactions, including anaphylaxis, have occasionally been reported.

### Uses and Administration

Powdered pituitary (posterior lobe) is a preparation from the posterior lobes of mammalian pituitary bodies. It has oxytocic, pressor, antidiuretic, and hyperglycaemic actions and has generally been replaced by compounds or preparations with more specific actions such as oxytocin (p.1336) and desmopressin (p.1323).

It has been included as an ingredient of a number of preparations of combined tissue extracts promoted as tonics or for a variety of non-endocrine disorders.

---

## Prolactin

Galactin; Lactogen; Lactogenic Hormone; Lactotropin; LMTH; LTH; Luteomammotropic Hormone; Luteotrophic Hormone; Luteotropin; Mammotropin; Prolactina.
*CAS — 9002-62-4; 12585-34-1 (sheep); 56832-36-1 (ox); 9046-05-3 (pig).*

### Profile

Prolactin is a water-soluble protein from the anterior pituitary; it is structurally related to growth hormone (p.1327). In *animals*, prolactin has a wide variety of actions and is involved in reproduction, parental care, feeding of the young, electrolyte balance, and growth and development. In humans it has a definite role in inducing milk production; oxytocin (p.1336) stimulates milk ejection. Relatively high concentrations of prolactin have been found in amniotic fluid. Placental lactogen has been shown to have prolactin-like activity. Prolactin secretion is stimulated by suckling and, for a few months after delivery, it has an inhibitory effect on the ovaries, acting as a natural contraceptive.

The hypothalamus can both stimulate and inhibit prolactin secretion by the anterior pituitary; the inhibitory influence is predominant and is mediated through a dopaminergic system. Dopamine binds to the lactotrope $D_2$ receptor to inhibit prolactin synthesis and release. Noradrenaline and gamma-aminobutyric acid are also inhibitory as are dopaminergic drugs such as bromocriptine. Although protirelin (below) has prolactin-releasing activity, there is evidence for the existence of a separate hypothalamic releasing factor (PRF). Prolactin secretion may also be stimulated by methyldopa, metoclopramide, reserpine, opioid analgesics, and phenothiazine or butyrophenone antipsychotics.

Hyperprolactinaemia, which is associated with a variety of other endocrine disorders, is discussed on p.1315.

Prolactin has been given by intramuscular injection in the management of lactation disorders and some forms of menstrual disturbance.

---

## Protirelin *(BAN, USAN, rINN)*

Abbott-38579; Lopremone; Protirelina; Protirelinum; Synthetic TRH; Thyrotrophin-releasing Hormone; Thyrotropin-releasing Hormone; TRF; TRH. L-Pyroglutamyl-L-histidyl-L-prolinamide; 1-[*N*-(5-Oxo-L-prolyl)-L-histidyl]-L-prolinamide; Glu-His-Pro-$NH_2$.
$C_{16}H_{22}N_6O_4$ = 362.4.
*CAS — 24305-27-9.*
*ATC — V04CJ02.*

**Pharmacopoeias.** In *Eur.* (see p.vi) and *Jpn*, which also includes the tartrate.

**Ph. Eur. 5.0** (Protirelin). A synthetic tripeptide with the same sequence of amino acids as the natural hypothalamic neurohormone, that stimulates the release and synthesis of thyrotrophin. A white or yellowish-white hygroscopic powder. Very soluble in water; freely soluble in methyl alcohol. Store at a temperature of 2° to 8°. Protect from light and moisture.

### Adverse Effects

Protirelin given by intravenous injection may cause headache, nausea, a desire to micturate, flushing, dizziness, and a strange taste. These effects have been attributed to contraction of smooth muscles by the bolus injection. Hypertension and an increased pulse rate, or hypotension, have occasionally been reported as have a few cases of amaurosis and convulsions.

**Amaurosis.** Of 4 patients with pituitary tumours who developed severe headache after protirelin injection, one also developed amaurosis, apparently associated with pituitary apoplexy.[1] Visual acuity improved after surgery.


1. Drury PL, *et al.* Transient amaurosis and headache after thyrotropin releasing hormone. *Lancet* 1982; **i:** 218–19.

**Effects on the cardiovascular system.** Increased blood pressure has been reported in women given protirelin antenatally,[1,2] and the view has been expressed that although the magnitude of the change is unlikely to be clinically significant in normotensive women, a much greater rise seen in pre-eclamptic women was severe enough to increase the risk of cerebral haemorrhage.[2]

1. ACTOBAT Study Group. Australian collaborative trial of antenatal thyrotropin-releasing hormone (ACTOBAT) for prevention of neonatal respiratory disease. *Lancet* 1995; **345:** 877–82.
2. Peek MJ, *et al.* Hypertensive effect of antenatal thyrotropin-releasing hormone in pre-eclampsia. *Lancet* 1995; **345:** 793. Correction. *ibid.*; 1124.

**Effects on the CNS.** Adverse effects reported following injection of 400 micrograms of protirelin included unconsciousness, hypotension, and convulsions.[1] In another patient with a history of convulsions, a 500-microgram injection induced epileptic seizures.[2]

1. Dolva LØ, *et al.* Side effects of thyrotrophin releasing hormone. *BMJ* 1983; **287:** 532.
2. Maeda K, Tanimoto K. Epileptic seizures induced by thyrotropin releasing hormone. *Lancet* 1981; **i:** 1058–9.

**Effects on the respiratory system.** A report of bronchospasm in an asthmatic boy given protirelin intravenously.[1]

For the suggestion that protirelin may provoke bronchospasm in patients with motor neurone disease, see under Precautions, below.

1. McFadden RG, *et al.* TRH and bronchospasm. *Lancet* 1981; **ii:** 758–9.

**Effect on sexual function.** On questioning, 7 of 16 women reported a sensation of mild vaginal sexual arousal occurring 1 to 3 minutes after intravenous injection of protirelin.[1] Four women also experienced urinary sensations, and 3 described an urge to urinate with no sexual component.

1. Blum M, Pulini M. Vaginal sensations after injection of thyrotropin releasing hormone. *Lancet* 1980; **ii:** 43.

**Pituitary apoplexy.** Pituitary apoplexy has been reported following combined testing of anterior pituitary function in patients with a pituitary tumour.[1,2] Of the drugs given, protirelin was thought most likely to have an aetiological role. Pituitary apoplexy has also been reported following the use of protirelin alone.[3]

See also Amaurosis, above.

1. Chapman AJ, *et al.* Pituitary apoplexy after combined test of anterior pituitary function. *BMJ* 1985; **291:** 26.
2. Dökmetaş HS, *et al.* Pituitary apoplexy probably due to TRH and GnRH stimulation tests in a patient with acromegaly. *J Endocrinol Invest* 1999; **22:** 698–700.
3. Szabolcs I, *et al.* Apoplexy of a pituitary macroadenoma as a severe complication of preoperative thyrotropin-releasing hormone (TRH) testing. *Exp Clin Endocrinol Diabetes* 1997; **105:** 234–6.

## Precautions

Protirelin should be given with care to patients with ischaemic heart disease, obstructive airways disease, or severe hypopituitarism. Administration of protirelin while the patient is lying down may reduce the incidence of hypotension.

**Eclampsia.** For the suggestion that the hypertensive effects of protirelin increase the risk of cerebral haemorrhage in pre-eclamptic women, see Effects on the Cardiovascular System under Adverse Effects, above.

**Motor neurone disease.** In some patients with amyotrophic lateral sclerosis intravenous injection of protirelin resulted in acute bronchospasm.[1] Five of 25 patients experienced falls in $FEV_1$ of more than 20%; in 2, a 15% decrease in arterial-oxygen pressure occurred. Patients with sclerosis and weakened respiratory muscles should be warned of this potential side-effect.

1. Braun SR, *et al.* Pulmonary effects of thyrotropin-releasing hormone in amyotrophic lateral sclerosis. *Lancet* 1984; **ii** 529–30.

## Interactions

◊ Drugs influencing the response to protirelin have been reviewed.[1] The secretion of thyrotrophin appears to be modulated by dopaminergic and noradrenergic pathways at both the hypothalamic and pituitary level. Dopamine and bromocriptine have depressed the response to protirelin; levodopa is a powerful depressant. Partial depression has been reported after the administration of chlorpromazine, thioridazine, and phentolamine, all of which have alpha-receptor blocking properties. Beta-receptors do not appear to be involved in the thyrotrophin response to protirelin whereas the antiserotonin drug, cyproheptadine, has an inhibitory effect. Aspirin and corticosteroids with predominantly glucocorticoid activity have also depressed the response. An enhanced response to protirelin has been seen after the administration of theophylline. Oestrogens may also increase the response in men but not usually in women; when combined with a progestogen a slightly depressed response has been reported.

Other drugs reported to depress the response to protirelin include lithium[2] and ranitidine.[3]

1. Lamberg B-A, Gordin A. Abnormalities of thyrotrophin secretion and clinical implications of the thyrotrophin releasing hormone stimulation test. *Ann Clin Res* 1978; **10:** 171–83.
2. Lauridsen UB, *et al.* Lithium and the pituitary-thyroid axis in normal subjects. *J Clin Endocrinol Metab* 1974; **39:** 383–5.
3. Tarditi E, *et al.* Impaired TSH response to TRH after intravenous ranitidine in man. *Experientia* 1983; **39:** 109–10.

## Uses and Administration

Protirelin is a hypothalamic releasing hormone which stimulates the release of thyrotrophin (p.1341) from the anterior lobe of the pituitary. It also has prolactin-releasing activity. It may be obtained by synthesis.

Protirelin may be used in the assessment of the hypothalamic-pituitary-thyroid axis in the diagnosis of mild hyperthyroidism (p.1594) or hypothyroidism (p.1595), and ophthalmic Graves' disease, although in many cases immunoassays for thyroid-stimulating hormone are now preferred. The response to protirelin may be used for differentiating between primary and secondary hypothyroidism but care is required in interpreting the results of the test and it should not be used alone in establishing the diagnosis. Protirelin is given with gonadorelin (p.1325) in the assessment of anterior pituitary function.

Protirelin is given intravenously usually in doses of 200 to 400 micrograms. A suggested intravenous dose in children is 1 microgram/kg in the UK, but in other countries a dose of 7 micrograms/kg has been recommended.

Protirelin has been investigated in the treatment of neurological diseases, and in the prevention of neonatal respiratory distress syndrome, but results have been variable.

Protirelin tartrate has been given in the treatment of neurological disorders.

**Lactation induction.** Intranasal protirelin has been tried for stimulation of lactation (p.1317) but there is no suitable commercial preparation, and in any case mechanical stimulation is preferable to drug treatment.

**Neonatal respiratory distress syndrome.** The regulation of fetal lung development is under multihormonal control and thyroid hormones appear to stimulate pulmonary maturation. However, the thyroid hormones and thyrotrophin do not cross the placenta sufficiently for them to be employed for prenatal treatment in premature labour where neonatal respiratory distress syndrome (p.1084) may develop, and therefore therapy with protirelin has been investigated.[1] Protirelin has been given with corticosteroids to the mother and some beneficial effects have been noted.[1] One study using protirelin 400 micrograms every 8 hours for 4 doses indicated that antenatal protirelin reduced the incidence of chronic lung disease when given with corticosteroids but did not affect the incidence of respiratory distress syndrome.[2] However, 2 large multicentre studies had found that addition of protirelin to corticosteroid treatment had no beneficial effects on outcome compared with corticosteroids only;[3,4] in fact, in the earlier of these studies,[3] respiratory distress syndrome and the need for ventilation were greater in the offspring of mothers given protirelin. Subsequent follow-up appeared to confirm the disadvantages of protirelin in this cohort;[5] however the unexpected conclusions of this study aroused some controversy.[6-8] The second study noted no difference in outcome in the 2 groups of infants.[4] A meta-analysis concluded[9] that prenatal treatment with protirelin was not beneficial, and that it was associated with more adverse effects than the use of corticosteroids alone.

1. de Zegher F, *et al.* Prenatal treatment with thyrotrophin releasing hormone to prevent neonatal respiratory distress. *Arch Dis Child* 1992; **67:** 450–4.
2. Ballard RA, *et al.* Respiratory disease in very-low-birthweight infants after prenatal thyrotropin-releasing hormone and glucocorticoid. *Lancet* 1992; **339:** 510–5.
3. ACTOBAT Study Group. Australian collaborative trial of antenatal thyrotropin-releasing hormone (ACTOBAT) for prevention of neonatal respiratory disease. *Lancet* 1995; **345:** 877–82.
4. Ballard RA, *et al.* Antenatal thyrotropin-releasing hormone to prevent lung disease in preterm infants. *N Engl J Med* 1998; **338:** 493–8.
5. Crowther CA, *et al.* Australian collaborative trial of antenatal thyrotropin-releasing hormone: adverse effects at 12-month follow-up. *Pediatrics* 1997; **99:** 311–17.
6. Ballard RA, *et al.* Thyrotropin-releasing hormone for prevention of neonatal respiratory disease. *Lancet* 1995; **345:** 1572.
7. Moya FR, Maturana A. Thyrotropin-releasing hormone for prevention of neonatal respiratory disease. *Lancet* 1995; **345:** 1572–3.
8. McCormick MC. The credibility of the ACTOBAT follow-up study. *Pediatrics* 1997; **99:** 476–8.
9. Crowther CA, *et al.* Prenatal thyrotropin-releasing hormone for preterm birth. Available in the Cochrane Library; Issue 1. Chichester: John Wiley; 2004.

**Neurological disorders.** Reports of the use of protirelin in various neurological disorders.

1. Bonuccelli U, *et al.* Oral thyrotropin-releasing hormone treatment in inherited ataxias. *Clin Neuropharmacol* 1988; **11:** 520–8.
2. Filla A, *et al.* Sperimentazione cronica del TRH per via intramuscolare nelle degenerazioni spino-cerebellari: studio in doppio cieco cross-over su 30 soggetti. *Riv Neurol* 1989; **59:** 83–8.
3. Mellow AM, *et al.* A peptide enhancement strategy in Alzheimer's disease: pilot study with TRH-physostigmine infusions. *Biol Psychiatry* 1993; **34:** 271–3.
4. Tanaka C, *et al.* Successful treatment of progressive myoclonus epilepsy with TRH. *Pediatr Neurol* 1998; **18:** 442–4.
5. Chemaly R, *et al.* Myélinolyse extra-pontine: traitement par T.R.H. *Rev Neurol (Paris)* 1998; **154:** 163–5.

## Preparations

**Proprietary Preparations** (details are given in Part 3)
***Arg.:*** TRH; Trhelea; ***Austria:*** Antepan; Relefact TRH; Thyroliberin TRH; ***Belg.:*** TRH; ***Braz.:*** RTH†; TRH†; ***Canad.:*** Relefact TRH; ***Denm.:*** Thyrefact†; ***Fr.:*** Stimu-TSH; ***Ger.:*** Antepan; Relefact TRH; Thyroliberin; TRH; ***Gr.:*** Relefact; ***Israel:*** Relefact TRH; TRH; ***Ital.:*** Irtonin; Xantium; ***Jpn:*** Hirtonin; ***Neth.:*** Relefact TRH; ***Spain:*** TRH Prem; ***Swed.:*** Thyrefact†; ***Switz.:*** Relefact TRH; ***USA:*** Thypinone†; Thyrel-TRH†.

# Somatomedins

IGFs; Insulin-like Growth Factors; Somatomedinas; Sulphation Factors.

**Description.** Somatomedins are a group of polypeptide hormones related to insulin and usually known individually as insulin-like growth factors (IGFs), with molecular weights of about 7000 to 8000. They are synthesised in the liver, kidney, muscle, and other tissues.

### Mecasermin *(BAN, USAN, rINN)*

CEP-151; IGF-I; Insulin-like growth factor I (human); Mecasermina; rhIGF-1; Somatomedin C.

$C_{331}H_{512}N_{94}O_{101}S_7$ = 7648.6.
*CAS — 68562-41-4; 67763-96-6.*
*ATC — H01AC03.*

## Units

150 000 units of insulin-like growth factor I are contained in one ampoule of the first International Standard (1994). For practical purposes 1 international unit can be assumed to be equivalent to 1 microgram of insulin-like growth factor I.

## Adverse Effects

Since the somatomedins are considered to be responsible for many of the actions of growth hormone similar adverse effects (see p.1327) might be expected.

◊ Syncope in the absence of hypoglycaemia has been reported in patients given mecasermin by intravenous bolus, accompanied in some cases by convulsions, asystole, bradycardia, hypotension, or dizziness.[1] Reports appear to have ceased since recommendations that mecasermin should not be given intravenously at rates greater than 24 micrograms/kg per hour. In addition, mid- and long-term effects of treatment have resulted in adverse effects similar to those associated with growth hormone therapy, including benign intracranial hypertension, gynaecomastia, and acromegalic changes of the features.[1] Arthralgia, nerve palsies, and hypophosphataemia and dyspnoea have been associated with high-dose intravenous bolus therapy.[2]

For a reference to benign intracranial hypertension associated with mecasermin therapy, see under Growth Hormone, p.1327. For concerns about an increased risk of retinopathy in diabetic patients receiving mecasermin, see under Diabetes Mellitus, below.

1. Malozowski S, Stadel B. Risks and benefits of insulin-like growth factor. *Ann Intern Med* 1994; **121:** 549.
2. Usala A-L. Risks and benefits of insulin-like growth factor. *Ann Intern Med* 1994; **121:** 550.

## Uses and Administration

The somatomedins are a group of polypeptide hormones, some of which are involved in mediating the effects of growth hormone in the body. IGF-I (mecasermin) is believed to be responsible for many of the anabolic effects of growth hormone. It is secreted primarily by the liver, regulated principally by growth hormone and insulin secretion; IGF-I may also be secreted in other tissues, where it may exert local hormonal (paracrine) effects. In the circulation, IGF-I is almost completely protein bound; 6 binding proteins have been identified, production of some of which is also under the control of growth hormone. In addition to its anabolic effects IGF-I, which is structurally related to insulin, also has potent hypoglycaemic properties.

IGF-I is available as mecasermin, a product of recombinant DNA technology. It has been used in the treatment of children with Laron-type dwarfism, in whom an abnormality of the growth hormone receptor results in an inability to secrete endogenous IGF-I. Long-term administration (several months) with a dose of 150 micrograms/kg daily by subcutaneous injection has been reported to produce significant improvement in linear growth in children with this condition. It has also been given to children with growth-attenuating antibodies to growth hormone.

Mecasermin is also being investigated in the management of diabetes mellitus and insulin resistance and is being tried in various other disorders including motor neurone disease, osteoporosis, and cachexia.

A recombinant protein complex of IGF-I and its most abundant binding protein, insulin-like growth factor binding protein-3, (rhIGF-I/rhIGFBP-3) is under investigation for the treatment of Laron-type dwarfism, diabetes mellitus, osteoporosis, and severe burns.

IGF-II is thought to play an important role in fetal growth, although its function in adults is uncertain. It is closely related in structure to IGF-I, but is not under the control of growth hormone.

◊ General reviews.


1. Laron Z. Somatomedin-1 (insulin-like growth factor-I) in clinical use: facts and potential. *Drugs* 1993; **45:** 1–8.
2. Bondy CA, *et al.* Clinical uses of insulin-like growth factor I. *Ann Intern Med* 1994; **124:** 593–601.
3. Le Roith D. Insulin-like growth factors. *N Engl J Med* 1997; **336:** 633–40.


**Diabetes mellitus.** There has been considerable interest in the therapeutic potential of mecasermin in diabetes mellitus;[1,2] in particular, several reports and small studies have suggested it can improve insulin sensitivity in patients with insulin resistance.[3-7] Randomised studies[8,9] have found that mecasermin 40 micrograms/kg daily by subcutaneous injection improves metabolic control in the short term when added to insulin therapy in patients with type 1 diabetes. Although there was no evidence of an increase in diabetic complications in these studies, the known proliferative effects of mecasermin have raised concern about a possibly increased risk of diabetic retinopathy;[10] some studies have been halted because of this possibility.

For a general discussion of diabetes mellitus and its management, see p.324.


1. Kolaczynski JW, Caro JF. Insulin-like growth factor-1 therapy in diabetes: phyiologic basis, clinical benefits, and risks. *Ann Intern Med* 1994; **120:** 47–55.
2. Dunger DB. Insulin and insulin-like growth factors in diabetes mellitus. *Arch Dis Child* 1995; **72:** 469–71.
3. Usala A-L, *et al.* Brief report: treatment of insulin-resistant diabetic ketoacidosis with insulin-like growth factor I in an adolescent with insulin-dependent diabetes. *N Engl J Med* 1992; **327:** 853–7.
4. Hussain MA, Froesch ER. Treatment of type A insulin resistance with insulin-like growth factor-I. *Lancet* 1993; **341:** 1536–7.
5. Ishihama H, *et al.* Long term follow up in type A insulin resistant syndrome treated by insulin-like growth factor I. *Arch Dis Child* 1994; **71:** 144–6.
6. Moses AC, *et al.* Insulin-like growth factor I (rhIGF-I) as a therapeutic agent for hyperinsulinemic insulin-resistant diabetes mellitus. *Diabetes Res Clin Pract* 1995; **28** (suppl): 185–94.
7. Hirano T, Adachi M. Insulin-like growth factor 1 therapy for type B insulin resistance. *Ann Intern Med* 1997; **127:** 245–6.
8. Acerini CL, *et al.* Randomised placebo-controlled trial of human recombinant insulin-like growth factor I plus intensive insulin therapy in adolescents with insulin-dependent diabetes mellitus. *Lancet* 1997; **350:** 1199–1204.
9. Thrailkill KM, *et al.* Cotherapy with recombinant human insulin-like growth factor I and insulin improves glycemic control in type 1 diabetes. *Diabetes Care* 1999; **22:** 585–92.
10. Møller N, Ørskov H. Does IGF-I therapy in insulin-dependent diabetes mellitus limit complications? *Lancet* 1997; **350:** 1188–9.


**Growth retardation.** References[1,2] to the use of mecasermin in patients with Laron-type dwarfism (growth hormone resistance). For a discussion of growth retardation and its management see p.1314.


1. Laron Z, *et al.* Effect of acute administration of insulin-like growth factor I in patients with Laron-type dwarfism. *Lancet* 1988; **ii:** 1170–72.
2. Laron Z, *et al.* Effects of insulin-like growth factor on linear growth, head circumference, and body fat in patients with Laron-type dwarfism. *Lancet* 1992; **339:** 1258–61.


**Motor neurone disease.** Mecasermin is under investigation for the management of amyotrophic lateral sclerosis,[1] a form of motor neurone disease (p.1739).


1. Lai EC, *et al.* Effect of recombinant human insulin-like growth factor-1 on progression of ALS: a placebo-controlled study. *Neurology* 1997; **49:** 1621–30.


**Osteoporosis.** Mecasermin has been investigated as a stimulant of bone formation in osteoporosis (p.763).

References.


1. Ebeling PR, *et al.* Short-term effects of recombinant human insulin-like growth factor I on bone turnover in normal women. *J Clin Endocrinol Metab* 1993; **77:** 1384–7.
2. Rubin CG, *et al.* Treating a patient with the Werner syndrome and osteoporosis using recombinant human insulin-like growth factor. *Ann Intern Med* 1994; **121:** 655–8.
3. Boonen S, *et al.* The prevention or treatment of age-related osteoporosis in the elderly by systemic recombinant growth factor therapy (rhIGF-I or rhTGF beta): a perspective. *J Intern Med* 1997; **242:** 285–90.


## Somatorelin *(rINN)*

GHRF; GHRH; GRF; GRF-44; Growth Hormone-releasing Factor (Human); Growth Hormone-releasing Hormone; Somatoliberin; Somatorelina.

$C_{215}H_{358}N_{72}O_{66}S$ = 5039.7.

*CAS — 83930-13-6.*

*ATC — V04CD05.*

### Sermorelin Acetate *(BANM, USAN, rINNM)*

Acetato de sermorelina; GRF(1-29)$NH_2$; Growth Hormone-releasing Factor (Human)-(1-29)-peptide Amide. Tyr-Ala-Asp-Ala-Ile-Phe-Thr-Asn-Ser-Tyr-Arg-Lys-Val-Leu-Gly-Gln-Leu-Ser-Ala-Arg-Lys-Leu-Leu-Gln-Asp-Ile-Met-Ser-Arg-$NH_2$ acetate hydrate.

$C_{149}H_{246}N_{44}O_{42}S.xC_2H_4O_2.yH_2O$ = 3357.9 (sermorelin).

*CAS — 86168-78-7 (sermorelin); 114466-38-5 (sermorelin acetate).*

*ATC — H01AC04; V04CD03.*

### Adverse Effects and Precautions

Facial flushing and pain at the injection site may occur after injection of sermorelin acetate. Headache, nausea and vomiting, dysgeusia, and tightness in the chest have also been reported. Antibodies to somatorelin may develop on repeated administration.

Sermorelin should be used with care in patients with epilepsy. Uncontrolled hypothyroidism, obesity, hyperglycaemia, or elevated plasma fatty acids may impair response to sermorelin. Sermorelin should not be used to treat growth retardation in children whose growth hormone response to stimulation tests is inadequate. Treatment should cease once the epiphyses have closed.

### Uses and Administration

Somatorelin is a peptide, secreted by the hypothalamus, that promotes the release of growth hormone from the anterior pituitary. It exists as 44-, 40-, and 37-amino-acid peptides; the 44-amino acid form may possibly be converted to the smaller forms but all are reported to be active, the activity residing in the first 29 amino-acid residues. Sermorelin is a synthetic peptide corresponding to the 1–29 amino acid sequence of somatorelin.

Sermorelin acetate is used for the diagnosis of growth hormone deficiency. The usual dose is the equivalent of sermorelin 1 microgram/kg by intravenous injection in the morning following an overnight fast. A normal response to sermorelin indicates that the somatotrophs are functional, but does not exclude growth hormone deficiency due to hypothalamic dysfunction; to establish a diagnosis it must be used with other tests. Somatorelin acetate is used similarly.

Sermorelin has also been used for the treatment of growth hormone deficiency in children; doses equivalent to 30 micrograms/kg, as the acetate, may be given once daily at bedtime by subcutaneous injection.

Sermorelin has also been tried as an adjunct to gonadotrophin therapy in the induction of ovulation and has been investigated in the treatment of HIV-associated wasting.

◊ Somatorelin (in its 40- or 44-amino-acid forms) has been used in the assessment of growth hormone deficiency.[1-3] It has usually been given as a single intravenous injection in doses of 1 microgram/kg or total doses of up to 200 micrograms. Subsequent normal or exaggerated increases in serum-growth hormone concentrations have occurred in healthy subjects,[1,2] and in patients with hypothalamic tumours[3] or acromegaly,[2] but not in patients with hypopituitarism.[2] A synthetic 29-amino-acid sequence of somatorelin, sermorelin acetate is now available for the diagnosis of growth hormone deficiency. However, it has been suggested that the test is not useful for screening as it does not test the hypothalamic-pituitary axis, and that it should not be used in routine clinical practice.[4] The use of sermorelin with the synthetic hexapeptide growth-hormone-releasing peptide-6 has also been reported.[5]

The 44- and 40-amino-acid forms of somatorelin, known as GRF(1-44) and GRF(1-40) (hpGRF-40), as well as sermorelin, have been investigated for the treatment of growth hormone deficiency.[6-9] Generally an increase in growth hormone secretion occurred accompanied by an increase in growth rate. Various treatment regimens have been tried. Patients have received somatorelin or sermorelin subcutaneously. Somatorelin has been given in 3-hourly pulses day and night,[6] in 4 nocturnal pulses,[7] or once daily.[9] Sermorelin has been given twice daily.[7,8] For a discussion of growth retardation and its management, including mention of the use of growth hormone-releasing hormone as an alternative to growth hormone treatment, see p.1314.

Sermorelin has also been investigated for intranasal administration.[10]


1. Thorner MO, *et al.* Human pancreatic growth-hormone-releasing factor selectively stimulates growth-hormone secretion in man. *Lancet* 1983; **i:** 24–8. Correction. *ibid.*; 256.
2. Wood SM, *et al.* Abnormalities of growth hormone release in response to human pancreatic growth hormone releasing factor (GRF (1-44)) in acromegaly and hypopituitarism. *BMJ* 1983; **286:** 1687–91.
3. Grossman A, *et al.* Growth-hormone-releasing factor in growth hormone deficiency: demonstration of a hypothalamic defect in growth hormone release. *Lancet* 1983; **ii:** 137–8.
4. Hindmarsh PC, Swift PGF. An assessment of growth hormone provocation tests. *Arch Dis Child* 1995; **72:** 362–8.
5. Popovic V, *et al.* GH-releasing hormone and GH-releasing peptide-6 for diagnostic testing in GH-deficient adults. *Lancet* 2000; **356:** 1137–42.
6. Thorner MO, *et al.* Acceleration of growth in two children treated with human growth hormone-releasing factor. *N Engl J Med* 1985; **312:** 4–9.
7. Smith PJ, Brook CGD. Growth hormone releasing hormone or growth hormone treatment in growth hormone insufficiency? *Arch Dis Child* 1988; **63:** 629–34.
8. Ross RJM, *et al.* Treatment of growth-hormone deficiency with growth-hormone-releasing hormone. *Lancet* 1987; **i:** 5–8.
9. Wit JM, *et al.* Short-term effect on growth of two doses of GRF 1-44 in children with growth hormone deficiency: comparison with growth induced by methionyl-GH administration. *Horm Res* 1987; **27:** 181–9.
10. Vance ML, *et al.* The effect of intravenous, subcutaneous, and intranasal GH-RH analog, [$Nle^{27}$]GHRH(1-29)-$NH_2$, on growth hormone secretion in normal men: dose-response relationships. *Clin Pharmacol Ther* 1986; **40:** 627–33.


### Preparations

**Proprietary Preparations** (details are given in Part 3)

***Austria:*** Geref; ***Belg.:*** GHRH; ***Canad.:*** Geref†; ***Denm.:*** Somatrel; ***Fin.:*** Geref; ***Fr.:*** Stimu-GH; ***Ger.:*** GHRH; ***Hong Kong:*** Geref; ***Irl.:*** Geref; ***Israel:*** Geref†; ***Ital.:*** Geref; GHRH; ***Mex.:*** Geref†; ***Neth.:*** GHRH; ***Norw.:*** Geref; ***Port.:*** Geref; ***S.Afr.:*** Geref†; ***Spain:*** Geref; ***Swed.:*** Geref; ***Switz.:*** Geref; ***Thai.:*** Geref†; ***UK:*** Geref; GHRH; ***USA:*** Geref.

## Somatostatin *(BAN, rINN)*

GH-RIF; GHRIH; Growth-hormone-release-inhibiting Hormone; Somatostatina; Somatostatinum; Somatotrophin-release-inhibiting Factor. Ala-Gly-Cys-Lys-Asn-Phe-Phe-Trp-Lys-Thr-Phe-Thr-Ser-Cys cyclic (3→14) disulphide.

$C_{76}H_{104}N_{18}O_{19}S_2$ = 1637.9.

*CAS — 38916-34-6.*

*ATC — H01CB01.*

**Pharmacopoeias.** In *Eur.* (see p.vi).

**Ph. Eur. 5.0** (Somatostatin). A cyclic tetradecapeptide having the structure of the hypothalamic hormone that inhibits the release of human growth hormone. It is produced by chemical synthesis and contains not more than 15% w/w of acetic acid. A white amorphous powder. Freely soluble in water and in acetic acid; practically insoluble in dichloromethane. Store in airtight containers at a temperature of 2° to 8°. Protect from light and moisture.

### Adverse Effects and Precautions

Abdominal discomfort, flushing, nausea, and bradycardia have been associated with too rapid administration. Because of the short half-life of somatostatin adverse effects are generally transitory on stopping or reducing the infusion. Concomitant parenteral nutrition has been suggested because of the inhibitory effects of somatostatin on intestinal absorption; blood glucose should be monitored since somatostatin may interfere with the secretion of insulin and glucagon.

**Effects on the kidneys.** Somatostatin has been reported to have an inhibitory effect on renal function[1,2] and severe water retention and hyponatraemia have been reported.[3]


1. Walker BJ, *et al.* Somatostatin and water excretion. *Lancet* 1983; **i:** 1101–2.
2. Vora JP, *et al.* Effect of somatostatin on renal function. *BMJ* 1986; **292:** 1701–2.
3. Halma C, *et al.* Life-threatening water intoxication during somatostatin therapy. *Ann Intern Med* 1987; **107:** 518–20.


### Uses and Administration

Somatostatin is a polypeptide obtained from the hypothalamus or by synthesis. The naturally occurring form has a cyclic structure. Although somatostatin derived from the hypothalamus is a 14-amino-acid peptide, a longer, 28-amino-acid form also exists in some tissues. It inhibits the release of growth hormone (p.1327) from the anterior pituitary. Somatostatin also inhibits the release of thyrotrophin (p.1341) and corticotropin (p.1322) from the pituitary, glucagon and insulin from the pancreas, and appears to have a role in the regulation of duodenal and gastric secretions. In the CNS it appears to play a role in the perception of pain.

It has been tried in a variety of disorders such as upper gastrointestinal haemorrhage including variceal haemorrhage (p.1716), insulin resistance, and the management of hormone-secreting tumours and other hypersecretory disorders. However, it has a very short duration of action and several analogues of somatostatin have been produced in an attempt to prolong its activity as well as making its inhibitory effects more specific. Octreotide (p.1333) and lanreotide (p.1330) are such analogues.

Somatostatin is usually given as the acetate. In the treatment of gastrointestinal haemorrhage, such as acute bleeding from oesophageal varices, somatostatin acetate equivalent to somatostatin 250 micrograms has been given by intravenous bolus over 3 to 5 minutes, followed by a continuous infusion of 250 micrograms/hour (about 3.5 micrograms/kg per hour) until the bleeding has stopped, which is usually within 12 to 24 hours. The infusion may then be continued for a further 48 to 72 hours to prevent recurrent bleeding.

**Malignant neoplasms.** Somatostatin given with melatonin, bromocriptine, and a solution of retinoids (the Di Bella regimen) was ineffective in the treatment of advanced malignancies (see Malignant Neoplasms, under Uses and Administration of Octreotide, p.1335).

## Preparations

**Proprietary Preparations** (details are given in Part 3)
***Arg.:*** Stilamin; ***Austria:*** Curastatin; Somatin; Somatolan; Stilamin; ***Belg.:*** Modustatine; ***Braz.:*** Stilamin; ***Canad.:*** Stilamin; ***Fr.:*** Modustatine; ***Ger.:*** Aminopan; ***Gr.:*** Somabion; Somastin; Stilamin; ***Hong Kong:*** Stilamin; ***India:*** Stilamin; ***Ital.:*** Etaxene; Ikestatina; Modustatina; Nastoren; Resurmide; Stilamin; Zecnil; ***Mex.:*** Stilamin; ***Neth.:*** Somatofalk†; ***Port.:*** Stilamin; ***S.Afr.:*** Stilamin; ***Singapore:*** Stilamin†; ***Spain:*** Biostatine†; Somiaton; Somonal; ***Switz.:*** Stilamin; ***Thai.:*** Etaxene; Somatosan†; Stilamin.

## Taltirelin *(rINN)*

TA-0910; Taltirelina. (−)-*N*-{[(*S*)-Hexahydro-1-methyl-2,6-dioxo-4-pyrimidinyl]carbonyl}-L-histidyl-L-prolinamide.

$C_{17}H_{23}N_7O_5$ = 405.4.

*CAS — 103300-74-9.*

### Profile

Taltirelin is an analogue of protirelin (p.1337) and is claimed to have beneficial effects on CNS function. It is used in the treatment of spinocerebellar degeneration.

## Terlipressin *(BAN, rINN)*

Terlipresina; Triglycyl-lysine-vasopressin. *N*-[*N*-(*N*-Glycylglycyl)glycyl]lypressin; Gly-Gly-Gly-Cys-Tyr-Phe-Gln-Asn-Cys-Pro-Lys-Gly-$NH_2$ cyclic (4→9) disulphide.

$C_{52}H_{74}N_{16}O_{15}S_2$ = 1227.4.

*CAS — 14636-12-5.*

*ATC — H01BA04.*

## Terlipressin Acetate *(BANM, rINNM)*

Terlipressin Diacetate.

$C_{52}H_{74}N_{16}O_{15}S_2,2C_2H_4O_2,5H_2O$ = 1437.6.

*ATC — H01BA04.*

### Adverse Effects, Treatment, and Precautions

As for Vasopressin, p.1342.

The pressor and antidiuretic effects of terlipressin are reported to be less marked than those of vasopressin.

**Effects on electrolytes.** A report of hypokalaemia in a patient receiving terlipressin.[1]

1. Stéphan F, Paillard F. Terlipressin-exacerbated hypokalaemia. *Lancet* 1998; **351:** 1249–50.

### Uses and Administration

Terlipressin is an inactive prodrug which is slowly converted in the body to lypressin, and has the general physiological actions of vasopressin (p.1343).

Terlipressin acetate is used to control bleeding oesophageal varices and is given by intravenous injection in doses of 2 mg, followed by 1 or 2 mg every 4 to 6 hours if necessary, until bleeding is controlled, for up to 72 hours.

**Hepatorenal syndrome.** Terlipressin has been found to be of benefit in the hepatorenal syndrome, a form of renal insufficiency associated with cirrhosis of the liver. A retrospective study[1] found that it had been given in doses of about 3 mg/day for about 11 days, and that this appeared to improve renal function in 58 of 91 patients; it may also have improved survival. Further prospective studies have also reported beneficial effects on renal function; these used doses of terlipressin 1 mg every 4 hours for 7 to 15 days,[2] and 1 mg every 12 hours for up to 15 days.[3]

1. Moreau R, *et al.* Terlipressin in patients with cirrhosis and type 1 hepatorenal syndrome: a retrospective multicenter study. *Gastroenterology* 2002; **122:** 923–30.
2. Alessandria C, *et al.* Renal failure in cirrhotic patients: role of terlipressin in clinical approach to hepatorenal syndrome type 2. *Eur J Gastroenterol Hepatol* 2002; **14:** 1363–8.
3. Solanki P, *et al.* Beneficial effects of terlipressin in hepatorenal syndrome: a prospective, randomized placebo-controlled clinical trial. *J Gastroenterol Hepatol* 2003; **18:** 152–6.

**Shock.** Terlipressin has vasopressor effects and has been tried in the management of septic shock (p.835). In a group of 8 patients who could not be adequately managed with conventional vasopressor therapy, an intravenous bolus of terlipressin 1 to 2 mg produced a progressive increase in mean arterial pressure over 10 to 20 minutes that was sustained for at least 5 hours, allowing reduction or cessation of noradrenaline.[1]

1. O'Brien A, *et al.* Terlipressin for norepinephrine-resistant septic shock. *Lancet* 2002; **359:** 1209–10.

**Variceal haemorrhage.** Meta-analysis has indicated[1] that terlipressin is effective in the management of acute oesophageal variceal haemorrhage (p.1716), and reduces the relative risk of mortality by about one-third. Differences in effectiveness from other therapies could not be conclusively demonstrated. Comparison of a regimen of terlipressin given by intravenous bolus injection, plus glyceryl trinitrate given sublingually, with balloon tamponade in variceal bleeding has suggested similar efficacy.[2] However, tamponade was successful in all patients that were previously unresponsive to terlipressin plus glyceryl trinitrate whereas this drug combination failed in all patients previously unresponsive to tamponade. A comparison of terlipressin and endoscopic injection sclerotherapy found them to be equally effective for the control of acute variceal bleeding.[3]

1. Ioannou G, *et al.* Terlipressin for acute esophageal variceal hemorrhage. Available in The Cochrane Library; Issue 1. Chichester: John Wiley; 2004.
2. Fort E, *et al.* A randomized trial of terlipressin plus nitroglycerin vs balloon tamponade in the control of acute variceal hemorrhage. *Hepatology* 1990; **11:** 678–81.
3. Escorsell À, *et al.* Multicenter randomized controlled trial of terlipressin versus sclerotherapy in the treatment of acute variceal bleeding: the TEST study. *Hepatology* 2000; **32:** 471–6.

## Preparations

**Proprietary Preparations** (details are given in Part 3)
***Arg.:*** Glycylpressin; ***Austria:*** Glycylpressin; ***Belg.:*** Glypressin; ***Braz.:*** Glypressin†; ***Denm.:*** Glypressin; ***Fin.:*** Glypressin; ***Fr.:*** Glypressine; ***Ger.:*** Glycylpressin; Haemopressin; ***Hong Kong:*** Glypressin; ***Irl.:*** Glypressin; ***Ital.:*** Glipressina; ***Malaysia:*** Glypressin; ***Neth.:*** Glypressin; ***Singapore:*** Glypressin; ***Spain:*** Glypressin; ***Switz.:*** Glypressine; ***Thai.:*** Glypressin†; ***UK:*** Glypressin.

# Tetracosactide *(BAN, rINN)*

$\alpha^{1-24}$-Corticotrophin; $\beta^{1-24}$-Corticotrophin; Cosyntropin *(USAN)*; Tetracosactida; Tetracosactido; Tetracosactidum; Tetracosactrin. Corticotrophin-(1–24)-tetracosapeptide; Ser-Tyr-Ser-Met-Glu-His-Phe-Arg-Trp-Gly-Lys-Pro-Val-Gly-Lys-Lys-Arg-Arg-Pro-Val-Lys-Val-Tyr-Pro.

$C_{136}H_{210}N_{40}O_{31}S$ = 2933.4.

*CAS — 16960-16-0 (tetracosactide); 22633-88-1 (tetracosactide hexaacetate); 60189-34-6 (tetracosactide xacetate).*

*ATC — H01AA02.*

**Pharmacopoeias.** In *Eur.* (see p.vi).

**Ph. Eur. 5.0** (Tetracosactide). A synthetic tetracosapeptide in which the sequence of amino acids is the same as that of the first 24 residues of human corticotropin. It is available as an acetate and contains water. It increases the rate at which corticoid hormones are secreted by the adrenal gland. The potency is not less than 800 units/mg. A white or yellow, amorphous powder. Sparingly soluble in water. Store under nitrogen at a temperature of 2° to 8°. Protect from light.

### Adverse Effects, Withdrawal, and Precautions

As for Corticotropin, p.1322. Although hypersensitivity reactions, including anaphylaxis, may occur with the use of tetracosactide, it is reported to be less immunogenic than corticotropin; the US manufacturer suggests that patients with a history of hypersensitivity to corticotropin may tolerate tetracosactide. In the UK, however, previous hypersensitivity to corticotropin or tetracosactide is considered a contra-indication to tetracosactide use. Tetracosactide is also contra-indicated in patients with a history of allergic disorders such as asthma.

Since hypersensitivity reactions may occur up to 1 hour after injection, sufficient time should be allowed for recovery after administration at the hospital or surgery. Self-administration is not recommended.

### Interactions

As for Corticosteroids, p.1072.

### Pharmacokinetics

Following intravenous injection tetracosactide exhibits triphasic pharmacokinetics. It is rapidly eliminated from plasma, mostly by distribution to the adrenal glands and kidneys. It is metabolised by serum endopeptidases into inactive oligopeptides, and then by aminopeptidases into free amino acids. Most of a dose is excreted in urine within 24 hours. The terminal half-life of tetracosactide is about 3 hours.

### Uses and Administration

Tetracosactide is a synthetic polypeptide with general properties similar to those of corticotropin (p.1322). Tetracosactide is used diagnostically to investigate adrenocortical insufficiency (p.1075).

Although tetracosactide, like corticotropin, has also been used therapeutically for most of the conditions in which systemic corticosteroid therapy is indicated, it is now rarely used for such indications.

Tetracosactide is usually used in the form of the acetate although doses are often expressed in terms of tetracosactide itself.

For diagnostic purposes tetracosactide acetate is used intramuscularly or intravenously as a plain injection in the first instance then, if results are inconclusive, intramuscularly as a long-acting depot injection. The initial test using the plain injection is based on the measurement of plasma-cortisol concentrations immediately before and exactly 30 minutes after an intramuscular or intravenous injection equivalent to 250 micrograms of tetracosactide; adrenocortical function may be regarded as normal if there is a rise in the cortisol concentration of at least 200 nanomoles/litre (70 micrograms/litre). A suggested intravenous dose in children has been 250 micrograms per 1.73 $m^2$.

If the results of this test are equivocal the long-acting depot preparation may be used, the adult dose being 1 mg of tetracosactide acetate given intramuscularly with adrenocortical function being regarded as normal if plasma-cortisol concentrations have steadily increased to 1000 to 1800 nanomoles/litre 5 hours after the injection. A three day test, for example with 1 mg of the depot preparation given each morning, is also used to differentiate between primary and secondary adrenocortical insufficiency; this is preceded on the first day and followed on the fourth day by the test using the plain injection. A marked improvement in the second assessment suggests secondary adrenocortical insufficiency.

For therapeutic purposes tetracosactide acetate has been given by intramuscular injection as the long-acting depot preparation. The usual initial adult dose of tetracosactide acetate has been 1 mg daily (or 1 mg every 12 hours in acute cases), reduced after the acute symptoms have been controlled to 0.5 to 1 mg every 2 or 3 days or 1 mg weekly. For children aged 3 to 5 years, a dose of 250 to 500 micrograms intramuscularly has been given daily initially, and then every 2 to 8 days for maintenance. A dose of 0.25 to 1 mg has been used similarly in children aged 5 to 12 years.

◊ Reviews.

1. Dorin RI, *et al.* Diagnosis of adrenal insufficiency. *Ann Intern Med* 2003; **139:** 194–204.

## Preparations

***BP 2003:*** Tetracosactide Injection; Tetracosactide Zinc Injection.

**Proprietary Preparations** (details are given in Part 3)
***Austral.:*** Synacthen; ***Austria:*** Synacthen; ***Belg.:*** Synacthen; ***Braz.:*** Cortrosina†; ***Canad.:*** Cortrosyn; Synacthen Depot; ***Chile:*** Synacthen; ***Denm.:*** Synacthen; ***Fr.:*** Synacthene; ***Ger.:*** Synacthen; Synacthen Depot; ***Gr.:*** Cortrosyn; Synacthene; ***Hong Kong:*** Cortrosyn; ***Irl.:*** Synacthen; ***Israel:*** Cortrosyn; Synacthen; ***Ital.:*** Cortrosyn; Synacthen; ***Neth.:*** Synacthen; ***NZ:*** Synacthen; ***Port.:*** Synacthen; ***S.Afr.:*** Synacthen Depot; ***Spain:*** Nuvacthen Depot; ***Swed.:*** Synacthen; ***Switz.:*** Synacthen; Synacthen Retard; ***UK:*** Synacthen; Synacthen Depot; ***USA:*** Cortrosyn.

## Thyrotrophin *(BAN, rINN)*

Thyroid-stimulating Hormone; Thyrotrophic Hormone; Thyrotropin; Tirotrofina; TSH.

*CAS — 9002-71-5.*
*ATC — H01AB01; V04CJ01.*

**Description.** Thyrotrophin is a glycoprotein from the anterior pituitary with a molecular weight in man of about 30 000.

## Thyrotropin Alfa *(BAN, USAN, rINN)*

rhTSH; Tirotropina alfa.

*CAS — 194100-83-9.*
*ATC — V04CJ01.*

### Units

0.037 units of human pituitary thyrotrophin for immunoassay and bioassay are contained in approximately 7.5 micrograms of thyrotrophin, with albumin 1 mg and lactose 5 mg, in one ampoule of the second International Reference Preparation (1983).

### Adverse Effects

Infrequent side-effects of thyrotrophin include nausea, vomiting, headache, a desire to micturate, and flushing. High doses may produce excessive thyroid stimulation, with angina, tachycardia or arrhythmias, dyspnoea, sweating, nervousness and irritability. Hypersensitivity reactions, including skin rash and urticaria, erythema and swelling at the injection site, and anaphylaxis have occurred, particularly on repeated administration.

### Precautions

Thyrotrophin should not be given to patients with recent myocardial infarction or uncorrected adrenocortical insufficiency, including adrenocortical insufficiency secondary to hypopituitarism. Care is also required in patients with cardiovascular disease.

### Uses and Administration

Thyrotrophin is a glycoprotein secreted by the anterior lobe of the pituitary and with an alpha subunit essentially the same as that of the gonadotrophins. Its main actions are to increase iodine uptake by the thyroid and the formation and secretion of the thyroid hormones. It may produce hyperplasia of thyroid tissue. Thyrotrophin secretion is controlled by a hypothalamic releasing hormone (Protirelin, p.1337) and by circulating thyroid hormones; somatostatin (p.1339) may inhibit the release of thyrotrophin.

Thyrotrophin has been used with radio-iodine in the diagnosis of hypothyroidism (p.1595) and to differentiate between primary and secondary hypothyroidism, but direct radio-immunoassay of circulating endogenous thyroid-stimulating hormone may be preferred. Thyrotrophin increases the uptake of radio-iodine by the thyroid and has been used as a diagnostic tool and as an adjunct in the treatment of certain types of thyroid cancer.

The usual dose is 10 units daily by intramuscular or subcutaneous injection; depending upon the indication this dose may be given for between 1 and 8 days.

Thyrotropin alfa is a recombinant form of thyrotrophin used in the follow-up of patients with thyroid cancer. The usual dose is 900 micrograms intramuscularly, every 24 hours for two doses, or every 72 hours for three doses, given before serum-thyroglobulin testing with or without radio-iodine imaging.

**Malignant neoplasms of the thyroid.** Patients with well-differentiated thyroid carcinoma (p.523) undergo surgery, with or without iodine-131 treatment. They then receive thyroid hormone therapy to suppress thyrotrophin (TSH), because most differentiated thyroid cancers express TSH receptors and grow in response to thyrotrophin stimulation. Monitoring for tumour recurrence in subsequent years requires interruption of thyroid hormone treatment so that thyrotrophin levels rise, and stimulate the uptake of iodine-131 by any residual or recurrent tumour. However, this results in hypothyroidism, with associated symptoms that may be severe in some patients.[1] Studies[2,3] have compared administration of thyrotropin alfa with withdrawal of thyroid hormones as a prelude to radio-iodine scanning. They found that thyrotropin alfa did stimulate radio-iodine uptake, although the sensitivity of scanning may depend on the technique used, and that thyrotropin alfa might be considered an alternative to thyroid hormone withdrawal. In patients with CNS or spinal metastases, or who have substantial disease in the thyroid bed, the administration of thyrotropin alfa may cause tumour expansion with acute complications; it has been recommended[1] that prophylactic corticosteroid therapy should be considered in these cases.


1. Basaria M, *et al.* The use of recombinant thyrotropin in the follow-up of patients with differentiated thyroid cancer. *Am J Med* 2002; **112:** 721–5.
2. Ladenson PW, *et al.* Comparison of administration of recombinant human thyrotropin with withdrawal of thyroid hormone for radioactive iodine scanning in patients with thyroid carcinoma. *N Engl J Med* 1997; **337:** 888–96.
3. Haugen BR, *et al.* A comparison of recombinant human thyrotropin and thyroid hormone withdrawal for the detection of thyroid remnant or cancer. *J Clin Endocrinol Metab* 1999: **84:** 3877–85.


### Preparations

**Proprietary Preparations** (details are given in Part 3)
***Braz.:*** Thyrogen; ***Denm.:*** Thyrogen; ***Ger.:*** Thyrogen; ***Israel:*** Thyrogen; Thytropar; ***Ital.:*** Thyrogen; ***Norw.:*** Thyrogen; ***Spain:*** Thyrogen; ***Swed.:*** Thyrogen; ***UK:*** Thyrogen; ***USA:*** Thyrogen; Thytropar†.



## Triptorelin *(BAN, USAN, rINN)*

AY-25650; BIM-21003; BN-52014; CL-118532; Triptorelina; Triptoreline; D-Trp$^6$-LHRH; [6-D-Tryptophan] luteinising hormone-releasing factor. 5-Oxo-L-prolyl-L-histidyl-L-tryptophyl-L-seryl-L-tyrosyl-D-tryptophyl-L-leucyl-L-arginyl-L-prolylglycinamide.

$C_{64}H_{82}N_{18}O_{13}$ = 1311.4.
*CAS — 57773-63-4.*
*ATC — L02AE04.*

## Triptorelin Acetate *(BANM, rINNM)*

$C_{64}H_{82}N_{18}O_{13},C_2H_4O_2$ = 1371.5.
*CAS — 140194-24-7.*
*ATC — L02AE04.*

## Triptorelin Diacetate *(BANM, rINNM)*

$C_{64}H_{82}N_{18}O_{13},2C_2H_4O_2$ = 1431.6.
*CAS — 105581-02-0.*
*ATC — L02AE04.*

## Triptorelin Embonate *(BANM, rINNM)*

Triptorelin Pamoate *(USAN)*.

$C_{64}H_{82}N_{18}O_{13},C_{23}H_{16}O_6$ = 1699.8.
*CAS — 124508-66-3.*
*ATC — L02AE04.*

### Adverse Effects and Precautions

As for Gonadorelin, p.1325.

◊ For a report of disease flare in patients given triptorelin for prostatic cancer, see Effects on the Bones, under Adverse Effects of Buserelin Acetate, p.1319.

**Local reactions.** For reference to local reactions occurring following injection of gonadorelin analogues, including triptorelin, see Leuprorelin Acetate, p.1331.

**Sepsis.** A report of 2 patients in whom triptorelin therapy led to sepsis caused by expulsion of necrotic fibroids through the cervix.[1]


1. Ellenbogen A, *et al.* Complication of triptorelin treatment for uterine myomas. *Lancet* 1989; **ii:** 167–8.


### Interactions

As for Gonadorelin, p.1325.

### Pharmacokinetics

Triptorelin is rapidly absorbed following subcutaneous injection, with peak plasma concentrations achieved about 40 minutes after a dose. The biological half-life has been stated to be about 7.5 hours, although longer half-lives have been reported in patients with prostate cancer, and shorter half-lives in some groups of healthy subjects.

◊ References.


1. Müller FO, *et al.* Pharmacokinetics of triptorelin after intravenous bolus administration in healthy males and in males with renal or hepatic insufficiency. *Br J Clin Pharmacol* 1997; **44:** 335–41.


### Uses and Administration

Triptorelin is an analogue of gonadorelin (p.1325) with similar properties. It is used for the suppression of gonadal sex hormone production in the treatment of malignant neoplasms of the prostate, in precocious puberty, and in the management of endometriosis, female infertility, and uterine fibroids. Triptorelin may be used as the base, acetate, diacetate, or embonate, although for preparations containing the acetate or diacetate it is not always obvious which has been used. Doses are usually given in terms of the base, and the following are each approximately equivalent to 1 mg of triptorelin:

- triptorelin acetate, 1.05 mg
- triptorelin diacetate, 1.09 mg
- triptorelin embonate, 1.30 mg

It is given as a daily subcutaneous injection, or as an intramuscular depot preparation lasting a month or longer.

In the treatment of prostate cancer, a dose equivalent to triptorelin 3 or 3.75 mg is given intramuscularly as a depot preparation every 4 weeks; the first dose may be preceded by 100 micrograms daily for 7 days by subcutaneous injection. A longer-acting depot preparation that contains the equivalent of triptorelin 11.25 mg is given once every 12 to 13 weeks. An anti-androgen such as cyproterone acetate may be given for several days before beginning therapy with triptorelin and continued for about 3 weeks to avoid the risk of a disease flare.

Similar doses of the 3 or 3.75 mg depot preparations may be given for up to 6 months in the management of endometriosis or uterine fibroids, with treatment begun during the first 5 days of the menstrual cycle. In the management of female infertility doses of 100 micrograms subcutaneously daily, with gonadotrophins, have been recommended from the second day of the menstrual cycle for about 10 to 12 days.

In children with precocious puberty a dose equivalent to triptorelin 50 micrograms/kg from the 3-mg depot preparation may be given intramuscularly every 4 weeks. Alternatively, using the 3.75-mg preparation, doses of 1.875 mg for children weighing less than 20 kg, 2.5 mg for children of 20 to 30 kg, or 3.75 mg for children of more than 30 kg may be given; the first 3 doses should be given at 14-day intervals, with further doses given every 4 weeks.

**Delayed and precocious puberty.** Gonadorelin analogues such as triptorelin[1-4] are used in the management of central precocious puberty (p.1318). They may also be effective in delayed puberty (p.1314) although they are most likely to be helpful where this is due to hypogonadism. Triptorelin has been used to differentiate gonadotrophin deficiency from constitutional delayed puberty.[5]


1. Roger M, *et al.* Long term treatment of male and female precocious puberty by periodic administration of a long-acting preparation of D-trp$^6$-luteinizing hormone-releasing hormone microcapsules. *J Clin Endocrinol Metab* 1986; **62:** 670–7.
2. Oostdijk W, *et al.* Final height in central precocious puberty after long term treatment with a slow release GnRH agonist. *Arch Dis Child* 1996; **75:** 292–7.
3. Cassio A, *et al.* Randomised trial of LHRH analogue treatment on final height in girls with onset of puberty aged 7.5—8.5 years. *Arch Dis Child* 1999; **81:** 329–32.
4. Heger S, *et al.* Long-term outcome after depot gonadotropin-releasing hormone agonist treatment of central precocious puberty: final height, body proportions, body composition, bone mineral density, and reproductive function. *J Clin Endocrinol Metab* 1999; **84:** 4583–90.
5. Zamboni G, *et al.* Use of the gonadotropin-releasing hormone agonist triptorelin in the diagnosis of delayed puberty in boys. *J Pediatr* 1995; **126:** 756–8.


**Disturbed behaviour.** Combined therapy with triptorelin, which suppressed testosterone secretion by inhibiting the pituitary-gonadal axis, and supportive psychotherapy, has been tried in the treatment of men with paraphilias (see p.665): a reduction in abnormal sexual thoughts and behaviours has been reported, although the study was uncontrolled.[1]


1. Rösler A, Witztum E. Treatment of men with paraphilia with a long-acting analogue of gonadotropin-releasing hormone. *N Engl J Med* 1998; **338:** 416–22.


**Endometriosis.** Gonadorelin analogues are effective in the management of endometriosis (p.1546), but the need for long-term therapy to prevent recurrence limits their value because of the risk of osteoporosis; 'add-back' therapy, with concomitant hormone replacement, can be used to prevent this.

References.


1. Lindsay PC, *et al.* The effect of add-back treatment with tibolone (Livial) on patients treated with the gonadotropin-releasing hormone agonist triptorelin (Decapeptyl). *Fertil Steril* 1996; **65:** 342–8.


**Fibroids.** Gonadorelin analogues have been used as an alternative to surgery in the treatment of uterine fibroids (see p.1326), despite some concern that this may complicate the diagnosis of malignancy.

References to the use of triptorelin.


1. Schneider D, *et al.* GnRH analogue-induced uterine shrinkage enabling a vaginal hysterectomy and repair in large leiomyomatous uteri. *Obstet Gynecol* 1991; **78:** 540–1.
2. van Leusden HA. Symptom-free interval after triptorelin treatment of uterine fibroids: long-term results. *Gynecol Endocrinol* 1992; **6:** 189–98.
3. Golan A, *et al.* Pre-operative gonadotrophin-releasing hormone agonist treatment in surgery for uterine leiomyomata. *Hum Reprod* 1993; **8:** 450–2.
4. Broekmans FJ, *et al.* Two-step gonadotropin-releasing hormone agonist treatment of uterine leiomyomas: standard-dose therapy followed by reduced-dose therapy. *Am J Obstet Gynecol* 1996; **175:** 1208–16.
5. Vercellini P, *et al.* Treatment with a gonadotrophin releasing hormone agonist before hysterectomy for leiomyomas: results of a multicentre, randomised controlled trial. *Br J Obstet Gynaecol* 1998; **105:** 1148–54.


**Growth retardation.** As discussed on p.1314 gonadorelin analogues have been given with growth hormone to short girls without growth hormone deficiency, in an attempt to delay puberty and bone maturation and thus maximise the final height achieved. However, there is some doubt about the extent of benefit, and in any case the concept of such treatment in children who are not clinically deficient in growth hormone is controversial, and some authorities do not consider it appropriate.

References to the use of triptorelin.

1. Saggese G, *et al.* Combination treatment with growth hormone and gonadotropin-releasing hormone analogs in short normal girls. *J Pediatr* 1995; **126:** 468–73.
2. Kamp GA, *et al.* A randomized controlled trial of three years growth hormone and gonadotropin-releasing hormone agonist treatment in children with idiopathic short stature and intrauterine growth retardation. *J Clin Endocrinol Metab* 2001; **86:** 2969–75.

**Infertility.** Gonadorelin analogues are used in the management of infertility related to hypogonadotrophic hypogonadism in both men and women. For a discussion of infertility and its management, including the role of gonadorelin analogues, see p.1316.

**Malignant neoplasms.** Triptorelin, like other gonadorelin analogues, may be used in the production of androgen blockade in patients with prostate cancer (p.521).

References.

1. Klippel KF, *et al.* Wirksamkeit und Vertraglichkeit von 2 Applikationsformen (s.c. und i.m.) von Decapeptyl Depot bei Patienten mit fortgeschrittenem Prostatakarzinom. *Urologe* 1999; **38:** 270–5.
2. Heyns CF, *et al.* Comparative efficacy of triptorelin pamoate and leuprolide acetate in men with advanced prostate cancer. *BJU Int* 2003; **92:** 226–31.

**Porphyria.** Triptorelin has been used successfully to suppress premenstrual exacerbations of acute intermittent porphyria (p.1040), in doses of 3.75 mg by intramuscular depot injection given monthly.[1,2] To reduce the risk of osteoporosis, 'add-back' therapy with topical oestrogen and oral calcium was used in one case,[1] and tibolone in another.[2]

1. De Block CEM, *et al.* Premenstrual attacks of acute intermittent porphyria: hormonal and metabolic aspects – a case report. *Eur J Endocrinol* 1999; **141:** 50–4.
2. Castelo-Branco C, *et al.* Use of gonadotropin-releasing hormone analog with tibolone to prevent cyclic attacks of acute intermittent porphyria. *Metabolism* 2001; **50:** 995–6.

## Preparations

**Proprietary Preparations** (details are given in Part 3)

***Arg.:*** Decapeptyl; Gonapeptyl; ***Austria:*** Decapeptyl; ***Belg.:*** Decapeptyl; ***Braz.:*** Neo Decapeptyl; ***Chile:*** Decapeptyl; ***Denm.:*** Decapeptyl; ***Fin.:*** Decapeptyl; ***Fr.:*** Decapeptyl; ***Ger.:*** Decapeptyl; ***Gr.:*** Arvekap; ***Hong Kong:*** Decapeptyl; Diphereline; ***India:*** Decapeptyl; ***Irl.:*** Decapeptyl; ***Israel:*** Decapeptyl; Diphereline; ***Ital.:*** Decapeptyl; ***Malaysia:*** Decapeptyl; ***Neth.:*** Decapeptyl; ***NZ:*** Decapeptyl†; ***Port.:*** Decapeptyl; ***S.Afr.:*** Decapeptyl; ***Singapore:*** Decapeptyl; ***Spain:*** Decapeptyl; ***Swed.:*** Decapeptyl; ***Switz.:*** Decapeptyl; ***Thai.:*** Decapeptyl; Diphereline; ***UK:*** Decapeptyl; Gonapeptyl; ***USA:*** Trelstar.

---

## Urofollitropin *(BAN, USAN, rINN)*

Urofolitropina; Urofollitrophin; Urofollitropinum.

*CAS — 97048-13-0.*

*ATC — G03GA04.*

**Pharmacopoeias.** In *Eur.* (see p.vi).

**Ph. Eur. 5.0** (Urofollitropin). A dry preparation containing menopausal gonadotrophin obtained from the urine of postmenopausal women. It has follicle-stimulating activity and no or virtually no luteinising activity. The potency is not less than 90 units of follicle-stimulating hormone per mg; the ratio of units of luteinising hormone to units of follicle-stimulating hormone is not more than 1:60. An almost white or slightly yellow powder. Soluble in water. Store in airtight containers at a temperature of 2° to 8°. Protect from light.

### Adverse Effects and Precautions

As for Human Menopausal Gonadotrophins, p.1330.

### Pharmacokinetics

Following multiple intramuscular or subcutaneous dosing of urofollitropin, the maximum plasma concentration of follicle-stimulating hormone occurs about 10 hours after a dose, and has an elimination half-life of about 15 or 20 hours respectively.

### Uses and Administration

Urofollitropin is a gonadotrophin, obtained from the urine of postmenopausal women, possessing follicle-stimulating hormone (FSH) activity but virtually no luteinising activity. For details of the actions of FSH, see p.1324.

Urofollitropin is used similarly to human menopausal gonadotrophins (p.1330) in the treatment of female infertility with the exception that, being without luteinising hormone activity, it can be used in patients where any increase in luteinising hormone activity is not required, as in polycystic ovarian disease. Urofollitropin is given subcutaneously or intramuscularly in a dosage adjusted according to the patient's response. Usually a dose providing 75 to 150 units of FSH daily is given initially. When an adequate response is achieved, as determined by oestrogen monitoring or ultrasonic visualisation of follicles, treatment is stopped and after 1 or 2 days a single dose of chorionic gonadotrophin 5000 to 10 000 units is administered to induce ovulation. Treatment with urofollitropin should be discontinued if there is no response after 4 weeks although treatment may be attempted again in future cycles. US manufacturers have recommended that a maximum daily dose of 450 units should not be exceeded, and that courses of treatment should be no longer than 12 days.

Urofollitropin is also used with other drugs as part of *in-vitro* fertilisation procedures. It is typically given in a dose providing 150 to 225 units of FSH daily, usually beginning from day 2 or 3 of the menstrual cycle. Alternatively, therapy has been initiated with clomifene citrate and continued with urofollitropin, or urofollitropin may be given after suppression of gonadotrophin release with a gonadorelin analogue. Treatment is continued until an adequate response is obtained and the final injection of urofollitropin is followed 1 to 2 days later by 5000 to 10 000 units of chorionic gonadotrophin. Oocyte retrieval is performed 34 to 35 hours later.

Urofollitropin is also used with chorionic gonadotrophin to stimulate spermatogenesis in the treatment of male infertility, although a preparation with combined luteinising activity, such as human menopausal gonadotrophins, may be preferred. The usual dose of urofollitropin provides 150 units of FSH three times a week. Treatment with urofollitropin and chorionic gonadotrophin should be continued for at least 4 months. For a brief discussion of hypogonadism see p.1316.

**Infertility.** For reference to the use of preparations with follicle-stimulating hormone activity in infertility, see p.1316. The management of women with polycystic ovary syndrome is discussed in more detail on p.1317. Some further references are listed below.

1. Remorgida V, *et al.* Administration of pure follicle-stimulating hormone during gonadotropin-releasing hormone agonist therapy in patients with clomiphene-resistant polycystic ovarian disease: hormonal evaluations and clinical perspectives. *Am J Obstet Gynecol* 1989; **160:** 108–13.
2. Buvat J, *et al.* Purified follicle-stimulating hormone in polycystic ovary syndrome: slow administration is safer and more effective. *Fertil Steril* 1989; **52:** 553–9.
3. McFaul PB, *et al.* Treatment of clomiphene citrate-resistant polycystic ovarian syndrome with pure follicle-stimulating hormone or human menopausal gonadotropin. *Fertil Steril* 1990; **53:** 792–7.
4. European Metrodin HP Study Group. Efficacy and safety of highly purified urinary follicle-stimulating hormone with human chorionic gonadotropin for treating men with isolated hypogonadotropic hypogonadism. *Fertil Steril* 1998; **70:** 256–62.

## Preparations

***BP 2003:*** Urofollitropin Injection.

**Proprietary Preparations** (details are given in Part 3)

***Arg.:*** Follitrin; ***Austral.:*** Metrodin; ***Braz.:*** Metrodin; ***Canad.:*** Fertinorm; Metrodin†; ***Fr.:*** Fostimon; Metrodine†; ***Ger.:*** Fertinorm†; ***Gr.:*** Metrodin; ***Hong Kong:*** Follimon; Fostimon; Metrodin; ***India:*** Gonotrop F; Metrodin; ***Irl.:*** Metrodin; ***Israel:*** Metrodin; ***Ital.:*** Fostimon; Metrodin; ***Mex.:*** Follitrin†; ***Neth.:*** Follegon; Metrodin†; ***NZ:*** Metrodin†; ***Port.:*** Metrodin; ***S.Afr.:*** Metrodin; ***Singapore:*** Metrodin; ***Spain:*** Neo Fertinorm; ***Switz.:*** Fostimon; Metrodin; ***Thai.:*** Metrodin†; ***UK:*** Metrodin†; ***USA:*** Bravelle; Fertinex; Metrodin.

---

## Vapreotide *(BAN, USAN, rINN)*

BMY-41606; RC-160; Vapreotida. D-Phenylalanyl-L-cysteinyl-L-tyrosyl-D-tryptophyl-L-lysyl-L-valyl-L-cysteinyl-L-tryptophanamide cyclic (2→7)-disulfide.

$C_{57}H_{70}N_{12}O_9S_2$ = 1131.4.

*CAS — 103222-11-3.*

### Profile

Vapreotide is a somatostatin analogue similar to octreotide (p.1333). It is under investigation in the management of various disorders, including bleeding oesophageal varices, gastrointestinal and pancreatic fistulas, acromegaly, carcinoid tumours, hepatocellular carcinoma, and for the prevention of postoperative complications following pancreatic surgery.

◊ References.

1. Eriksson B, *et al.* The use of new somatostatin analogues, lanreotide and octastatin, in neuroendocrine gastro-intestinal tumours. *Digestion* 1996; **57** (suppl 1): 77–80.
2. Calès P, *et al.* Early administration of vapreotide for variceal bleeding in patients with cirrhosis. *N Engl J Med* 2001; **344:** 23–8.
3. Anonymous. Vapreotide: BMY 41606, RC 160, Sanvar. *Drugs R D* 2003; **4:** 326–30.

---

# Vasopressin

ADH; Antidiuretic Hormone; Beta-Hypophamine; Vasopresina.

*CAS — 11000-17-2 (vasopressin injection).*

*ATC — H01BA01.*

NOTE. Vasopressin Injection is *rINN*.

**Pharmacopoeias.** In *US*, which includes both argipressin and lypressin in this title.

An injection is included in *Jpn*.

**USP 27** (Vasopressin). A polypeptide hormone having the properties of causing the contraction of vascular and other smooth muscles, and of antidiuresis. It is prepared by synthesis or obtained from the posterior lobe of the pituitary of healthy, domestic animals used for food by humans. Its vasopressor activity is not less than 300 USP units/mg. Store in airtight containers at 2° to 8°.

## Argipressin *(BAN, rINN)*

[8-Arginine]vasopressin; Argipresina; AVP; CI-107 (argipressin tannate). Cys-Tyr-Phe-Gln-Asn-Cys-Pro-Arg-Gly-$NH_2$ cyclic (1→6) disulphide.

$C_{46}H_{65}N_{15}O_{12}S_2$ = 1084.2.

*CAS — 113-79-1.*

*ATC — H01BA06.*

NOTE. Argipressin Tannate is *USAN*.

**Description.** Argipressin is a form of vasopressin obtained from most mammals including man but excluding pig. It is usually prepared synthetically. Lypressin (see below) is vasopressin from pig.

### Units

8.2 units of argipressin for bioassay are contained in approximately 20 micrograms of synthetic peptide acetate (with human albumin 5 mg and citric acid) in one ampoule of the first International Standard (1978).

## Lypressin *(BAN, USAN, rINN)*

L-8; Lipresina; Lipressina; LVP. [8-Lysine]vasopressin; Cys-Tyr-Phe-Gln-Asn-Cys-Pro-Lys-Gly-$NH_2$ cyclic (1→6) disulphide.

$C_{46}H_{65}N_{13}O_{12}S_2$ = 1056.2.

*CAS — 50-57-7.*

*ATC — H01BA03.*

**Description.** Lypressin is the form of vasopressin present in the posterior pituitary of pigs.

**Pharmacopoeias.** *US* includes Lypressin Nasal Solution.

### Units

7.7 units of lypressin are contained in approximately 23.4 micrograms of synthetic peptide (with albumin 5 mg and citric acid) in one ampoule of the first International Standard (1978).

## Adverse Effects

Large parenteral doses of vasopressin may give rise to marked pallor, pounding headache, vertigo, sweating, tremor, nausea, vomiting, diarrhoea, eructation, cramp, and a desire to defaecate; some of these effects may also occur after large intranasal doses of lypressin. In women, vasopressin may cause uterine cramps of a menstrual character. Hyponatraemia with water retention and signs of water intoxication can occur.

Hypersensitivity reactions have occurred and include urticaria and bronchial constriction. Anaphylactic shock and cardiac arrest have been reported.

Vasopressin may constrict coronary arteries. Chest pain, myocardial ischaemia, and infarction have occurred following injection, and fatalities have been reported. Other cardiovascular effects include occasional reports of arrhythmias and bradycardia, as well as hypertension. Peripheral vasoconstriction has resulted in gangrene, and thrombosis as well as local irritation at the injection site may occur.

Nasal congestion, irritation, and ulceration have been reported occasionally after intranasal use, usually as lypressin; systemic effects at usual intranasal doses are mostly reported to be mild.

**Effects on the heart.** Arrhythmias, including ventricular tachycardia and fibrillation,[1] torsade de pointes,[2-4] and asystole[5] are among the adverse effects of vasopressin administration. Paradoxical bradycardia and hypotension has also been reported.[6]

1. Kelly KJ, *et al.* Vasopressin provocation of ventricular dysrhythmia. *Ann Intern Med* 1980; **92:** 205–6.
2. Eden E, *et al.* Ventricular arrhythmia induced by vasopressin: torsade de pointes related to vasopressin-induced bradycardia. *Mt Sinai J Med* 1983; **50:** 49–51.
3. Stein LB, *et al.* Fatal torsade de pointes occurring in a patient receiving intravenous vasopressin and nitroglycerin. *J Clin Gastroenterol* 1992; **15:** 171–4.
4. Faigel DO, *et al.* Torsade de pointes complicating the treatment of bleeding esophageal varices: association with neuroleptics, vasopressin, and electrolyte imbalance. *Am J Gastroenterol* 1995; **90:** 822–4.
5. Fitz JD. Vasopressin induction of ventricular ectopy. *Arch Intern Med* 1982; **142:** 644.
6. Kraft W, *et al.* Paradoxical hypotension and bradycardia after intravenous arginine vasopressin. *J Clin Pharmacol* 1998; **38:** 283–6.

**Ischaemia.** Reports of ischaemia and infarction associated with vasopressin.[1-8]

1. Greenwald RA, *et al.* Local gangrene: a complication of peripheral Pitressin therapy for bleeding esophageal varices. *Gastroenterology* 1978; **74:** 744–6.
2. Colombani P. Upper extremity gangrene secondary to superior mesenteric artery infusion of vasopressin. *Dig Dis Sci* 1982; **27:** 367–9.
3. Lambert M, *et al.* Reversible ischemic colitis after intravenous vasopressin therapy. *JAMA* 1982; **247:** 666–7.
4. Anderson JR, Johnston GW. Development of cutaneous gangrene during continuous peripheral infusion of vasopressin. *BMJ* 1983; **287:** 1657–8.

5. Reddy KR, *et al.* Bilateral nipple necrosis after intravenous vasopressin therapy. *Arch Intern Med* 1984; **144:** 835–6.
6. Brearly S, *et al.* A lethal complication of peripheral vein vasopressin infusion. *Hepatogastroenterology* 1985; **32:** 224–5.
7. Sweren BS, Bohlman ME. Gastric and splenic infarction: a complication of intraarterial vasopressin infusion. *Cardiovasc Intervent Radiol* 1989; **12:** 207–9.
8. Maceyko RF, *et al.* Vasopressin-associated cutaneous infarcts, alopecia, and neuropathy. *J Am Acad Dermatol* 1994; **31:** 111–13.


## Treatment of Adverse Effects

The antidiuretic effects on water retention and sodium imbalance may be treated by water restriction and a temporary withdrawal of vasopressin. Severe cases may require osmotic diuresis alone or with furosemide.

◊ A report of the localised intravenous and intra-arterial administration of guanethidine in the treatment of a patient with extravasation of vasopressin.[1] The intra-arterial administration of guanethidine was considered to have helped to avoid necrotic changes.


1. Crocker MC. Intravascular guanethidine in the treatment of extravasated vasopressin. *N Engl J Med* 1981; **304:** 1430.


## Precautions

Vasopressin should not be used in patients with chronic nephritis with nitrogen retention. It should be avoided or given only with extreme care, and in small doses, to patients with vascular disease, especially of the coronary arteries.

It should be given with care to patients with asthma, epilepsy, migraine, heart failure, or other conditions which might be aggravated by water retention. Fluid intake should be adjusted to avoid hyponatraemia and water intoxication. Care is also required in hypertension or other conditions that may be exacerbated by a rise in blood pressure. Nasal absorption of vasopressin may be impaired in patients with rhinitis.

**Abuse.** Vasopressin or its analogues have been abused as so-called 'smart drugs' for their supposed effect on memory recall and cognition.

**Resistance.** Antibodies to vasopressin were detected in 6 of 28 patients being treated for diabetes insipidus, all of whom experienced a decrease in antidiuretic effect with previously effective argipressin or lypressin therapy;[1] desmopressin and chlorpropamide remained effective in these patients. There have been reports of patients with diabetes insipidus of pregnancy unresponsive to argipressin but responsive to desmopressin.[2] This was probably due to excessive placental production of vasopressinase, an enzyme which degrades argipressin.


1. Vokes TJ, *et al.* Antibodies to vasopressin in patients with diabetes insipidus: implications for diagnosis and therapy. *Ann Intern Med* 1988; **108:** 190–5.
2. Shah SV, Thakur V. Vasopressinase and diabetes insipidus of pregnancy. *Ann Intern Med* 1988; **109:** 435–6.


## Interactions

The antidiuretic effects of vasopressins might be expected to be enhanced in some patients receiving chlorpropamide, clofibrate, carbamazepine, fludrocortisone, urea, or tricyclic antidepressants. Lithium, heparin, demeclocycline, noradrenaline, and alcohol may decrease the antidiuretic effect. Ganglion-blocking drugs may increase sensitivity to the pressor effects of vasopressins.

**Cimetidine.** A report of severe bradycardia and heart block leading to asystole in a patient given combined vasopressin and cimetidine therapy.[1]


1. Nikolic G, Singh JB. Cimetidine, vasopressin and chronotropic incompetence. *Med J Aust* 1982; **2:** 435–6.


## Uses and Administration

Vasopressin is secreted by the hypothalamus and stored in the posterior lobe of the pituitary gland. It may be prepared from the gland of mammals or by synthesis. Vasopressin has a direct antidiuretic action on the kidney, increasing tubular reabsorption of water. It also constricts peripheral blood vessels and causes contraction of the smooth muscle of the intestine, gallbladder, and urinary bladder. It has practically no oxytocic activity.

Vasopressin, which is usually administered parenterally or intranasally in the synthetic forms of argipressin or lypressin, is used in the treatment of cranial diabetes insipidus due to a deficiency in antidiuretic hormone. It is ineffective in nephrogenic diabetes insipidus. Argipressin has also been used in the prevention and treatment of postoperative abdominal distension, and was formerly given to remove gas in abdominal visualisation procedures. Argipressin or lypressin are used in the treatment of bleeding oesophageal varices. Argipressin may have a role in cardiopulmonary resuscitation and shock due to vasodilatation.

In the treatment of cranial diabetes insipidus to control polyuria, argipressin may be given subcutaneously or intramuscularly; the dose in the UK is 5 to 20 units every 4 hours. In the USA, 5 to 10 units given 2 or 3 times daily or more has been used. Alternatively, argipressin or lypressin has been given as a nasal spray; dosage should be individually adjusted as required. A long-acting oily suspension of vasopressin tannate was formerly used by intramuscular injection in diabetes insipidus.

In the initial control of variceal bleeding argipressin is given in an initial dose of 20 units in 100 mL of glucose 5% infused intravenously over 15 minutes. Lypressin has also been given for bleeding oesophageal varices.

Vasopressin has also been used as a vasoconstrictor in local anaesthetic injections.

**Administration.** Results[1] suggesting that although intravenous administration of argipressin produced much higher plasma concentrations than intranasal administration, the latter evoked a greater CNS response.


1. Pietrowsky R, *et al.* Brain potential changes after intranasal vs intravenous administration of vasopressin: evidence for a direct nose-brain pathway for peptide effects in humans. *Biol Psychiatry* 1996; **39:** 332–40.


**Administration in children.** Vasopressin given by continuous intravenous infusion in an average dose of 9 milliunits/kg per hour was safe and effective in 5 children who had diabetes insipidus as a manifestation of severe brain injury.[1] It has also been used safely in 2 children aged 3 years and under with postoperative diabetes insipidus; the dose used was 1.5 to 3 milliunits/kg per hour.[2] Similar initial doses of argipressin were used in 3 comatose children with cranial diabetes insipidus,[3] while a published algorithm for the management of acute cranial diabetes insipidus has recommended an initial dose of vasopressin of 0.25 to 1 milliunits/kg per hour, subsequently titrated to achieve an appropriate output and specific gravity of urine, and a serum sodium value of between 140 and 145 mmol/litre.[4]


1. Ralston C, Butt W. Continuous vasopressin replacement in diabetes insipidus. *Arch Dis Child* 1990; **65:** 896–7.
2. McDonald JA, *et al.* Treatment of the young child with postoperative central diabetes insipidus. *Am J Dis Child* 1989; **143:** 201–4.
3. Lee Y-J, *et al.* Continuous infusion of vasopressin in comatose children with neurogenic diabetes insipidus. *J Pediatr Endocrinol Metab* 1995; **8:** 257–62.
4. Lugo N, *et al.* Diagnosis and management algorithm of acute onset of central diabetes insipidus in critically ill children. *J Pediatr Endocrinol Metab* 1997; **10:** 633–9.


**Advanced cardiac life support.** Vasopressin (as argipressin) may be used as an alternative to adrenaline in cardiopulmonary resuscitation (see p.812). In a preliminary study argipressin 40 units by intravenous injection appeared to be of value in the treatment of cardiac arrest due to ventricular fibrillation.[1] Spontaneous circulation returned in 16 of 20 patients so treated; 14 were successfully resuscitated on arrival in hospital and 8 survived to be discharged. In comparison, of 20 patients treated with 1 mg of adrenaline intravenously only 7 were resuscitated and 3 survived till discharge. However, a larger study[2] found no difference between vasopressin and adrenaline in the rates of survival to hospital admission for patients with ventricular fibrillation or pulseless electrical activity, although vasopressin was associated with a higher rate of hospital admission and discharge among patients with asystole. It also found that two doses of vasopressin followed by a single dose of adrenaline resulted in a better survival rate than three doses of adrenaline. Another large study[3] of patients who experienced cardiac arrest while in hospital and were treated with either vasopressin 40 units or adrenaline 1 mg, found no difference in survival to discharge from hospital.


1. Lindner KH, *et al.* Randomised comparison of epinephrine and vasopressin in patients with out-of-hospital ventricular fibrillation. *Lancet* 1997; **349:** 535–7.
2. Wenzel V, *et al.* A comparison of vasopressin and epinephrine for out-of-hospital cardiopulmonary resuscitation. *N Engl J Med* 2004; **350:** 105–13.
3. Stiell IG, *et al.* Vasopressin versus epinephrine for inhospital cardiac arrest: a randomised controlled trial. *Lancet* 2001; **358:** 105–9.


**Diabetes insipidus.** For a discussion of diabetes insipidus and its management, including reference to the use of vasopressin analogues (particularly desmopressin), see p.1314.

**Nocturnal enuresis.** For references to the use of the vasopressin analogue, desmopressin, in nocturnal enuresis, see p.1324.

**Shock.** Argipressin has been reported to have beneficial vasopressor effects in the management of shock (p.835) due to vasodilatation. It has been given by continuous intravenous infusion at a dose of about 2 to 6 units/hour as supplemental therapy in patients who could not be adequately managed with conventional vasopressor therapy.[1]


1. Dünser MW, *et al.* Management of vasodilatory shock: defining the role of arginine vasopressin. *Drugs* 2003; **63:** 237–56.


**Variceal haemorrhage.** Vasopressin has been widely used to control bleeding from oesophageal varices, as discussed on p.1716. However, terlipressin, and more recently octreotide, have been found to have some advantages over vasopressin, including bolus administration and fewer side-effects, and octreotide is increasingly preferred for this purpose. Glyceryl trinitrate has been given with the aim of counteracting the adverse cardiac effects of vasopressin while potentiating its beneficial effects on portal pressure.[1-4]

References listed below also give information on the use of vasopressin in the management of some other haemorrhagic disorders, including massive haemorrhage in Crohn's disease, blood loss in abortion or caesarean section, and haemoptysis.[5-8]


1. Stump DL, Hardin TC. The use of vasopressin in the treatment of upper gastrointestinal haemorrhage. *Drugs* 1990; **39:** 38–53.
2. Williams SGJ, Westaby D. Management of variceal haemorrhage. *BMJ* 1994; **308:** 1213–17.
3. Sung JJY. Non-surgical treatment of variceal haemorrhage. *Br J Hosp Med* 1997; **57:** 162–6.
4. McCormack G, McCormack PA. A practical guide to the management of oesophageal varices. *Drugs* 1999; **57:** 327–35.
5. Mellor JA, *et al.* Massive gastrointestinal bleeding in Crohn's disease: successful control by intra-arterial vasopressin infusion. *Gut* 1982; **23:** 872–4.
6. Schulz KF, *et al.* Vasopressin reduces blood loss from second-trimester dilatation and evacuation abortion. *Lancet* 1985; **ii:** 353–6.
7. Noseworthy TW, Anderson BJ. Massive hemoptysis. *Can Med Assoc J* 1986; **135:** 1097–9.
8. Lurie S, *et al.* Subendometrial vasopressin to control intractable placental bleeding. *Lancet* 1997; **349:** 698.


## Preparations

***USP 27:*** Lypressin Nasal Solution; Vasopressin Injection.

**Proprietary Preparations** (details are given in Part 3)

***Austral.:*** Pitressin; ***Canad.:*** Pressyn; ***Fr.:*** Diapid†; ***Ger.:*** Pitressin; Vasopressin†; ***Irl.:*** Pitressin; Syntopressin†; ***NZ:*** Pitressin†; ***UK:*** Pitressin; ***USA:*** Diapid†; Pitressin.

*Used as an adjunct in:* ***Ger.:*** Neo-Lidocaton†; ***Thai.:*** Neo-Lidocaton.

# Immunosuppressants

Asthma, p.1344
Blood disorders, p.1344
Diabetes mellitus, p.1344
Gastrointestinal disorders, p.1344
Inflammatory bowel disease, p.1344
Liver disorders, p.1344
Lung disorders, p.1344
Diffuse parenchymal lung disease, p.1344
Neurological disorders, p.1344
Multiple sclerosis, p.1344
Myasthenia gravis, p.1344
Ocular disorders, p.1344
Organ and tissue transplantation, p.1344
Corneal transplantation, p.1344
Haematopoietic stem cell transplantation, p.1344
Heart transplantation, p.1345
Intestinal transplantation, p.1346
Kidney transplantation, p.1346
Liver transplantation, p.1346
Lung transplantation, p.1347
Pancreatic transplantation, p.1347
Renal disorders, p.1348
Rheumatoid arthritis, p.1348
Sarcoidosis, p.1348
Scleroderma, p.1348
Skin and connective tissue disorders, p.1348

The compounds described in this chapter are used in diseases considered to have an auto-immune component, and in organ and tissue transplantation. The choice of an immunosuppressant is discussed below.

### Asthma

Immunosuppressant drugs do not play a role in the regular management of asthma (p.777). In individual patients requiring oral corticosteroids for chronic severe asthma immunosuppressants have however been investigated for their anti-inflammatory and corticosteroid-sparing properties.

### Blood disorders

For the use of immunosuppressants in aplastic anaemia, see p.732.

### Diabetes mellitus

For a discussion of diabetes mellitus and its treatment, including the experimental use of immunosuppressants, see p.324. See also Pancreatic Transplantation, below.

### Gastrointestinal disorders

**Inflammatory bowel disease.** A number of immunosuppressants have been tried in inflammatory bowel disease (p.1243), with some success, but the mainstays of drug therapy remain the aminosalicylates and the corticosteroids. Immunosuppressants may be valuable in some circumstances for their corticosteroid-sparing effect and for chronic active disease refractory to other treatments.

### Liver disorders

For a discussion of the role of immunosuppressants, and particularly azathioprine, in the management of chronic active hepatitis, see p.1078. For the use of immunosuppressants in primary biliary cirrhosis see under Ursodeoxycholic Acid, p.1761.

### Lung disorders

**Diffuse parenchymal lung disease.** Corticosteroids are the mainstay of treatment for diffuse parenchymal lung disease (p.1079) such as cryptogenic fibrosing alveolitis, usually in combination with azathioprine (or occasionally cyclophosphamide).

### Neurological disorders

**Multiple sclerosis.** Immunosuppressants have been tried in the treatment of multiple sclerosis (p.646), although in some studies the benefit obtained may have been outweighed by toxicity.

**Myasthenia gravis.** Patients with myasthenia gravis (p.1486) who require immunosuppression are usually treated with corticosteroids. Azathioprine is used mainly in myasthenia gravis for its corticosteroid-sparing effect but may also be of use when corticosteroids are contra-indicated or when response to corticosteroids alone is insufficient. Ciclosporin and mycophenolate mofetil have been tried similarly.

### Ocular disorders

Immunosuppressants have been used with some success in a variety of ocular disorders with inflammatory or immunological components. In *scleritis* and *uveitis* (see p.1088 and p.1090) corticosteroids, given topically, intra-ocularly, or systemically are widely used when treatment is needed, but in unresponsive disease, or in patients with unacceptable adverse effects, immunosuppressants such as azathioprine, ciclosporin, or mycophenolate mofetil, may be given. Daclizumab, leflunomide, sirolimus, and tacrolimus have also been tried in uveitis. Immunosuppressants may be valuable in the management of the ocular lesions of *Behçet's disease, rheumatoid arthritis*, or *Wegener's granulomatosis*, (see p.1076, p.9, and p.1090, respectively). Ciclosporin or azathioprine have been used with corticosteroids in the management of both ocular and vascular symptoms of *Cogan's syndrome* (p.1078). Ciclosporin has also been used topically in corneal ulceration, see p.1358.

In *Graves' ophthalmopathy*, see under Hyperthyroidism, (p.1594), immunosuppressants, particularly ciclosporin, have been tried with equivocal results.

Reviews.

1. McCluskey PJ, *et al.* Management of chronic uveitis. *BMJ* 2000; **320:** 555–8.
2. Jabs DA, *et al.* Guidelines for the use of immunosuppressive drugs in patients with ocular inflammatory disorders: recommendations of an expert panel. *Am J Ophthalmol* 2000; **130:** 492–513.
3. Kulkarni P. Review: uveitis and immunosuppressive drugs. *J Ocul Pharmacol Ther* 2001; **17:** 181–7.

### Organ and tissue transplantation

Although surgical techniques suitable for the removal of organs and tissues from a donor, and their engraftment into a host, have existed for many years, such grafts would not normally survive for long. The host's CD4 T-cells recognise foreign antigens from donor cells. A CD4 cell is subsequently activated by antigen-presenting cells to secrete interleukin-2 and induce T-cell proliferation. Activated T-cells then mediate a rejection response, by increasing the activity and function of B-cells, cytotoxic CD8 T-cells, and macrophages, either directly, or by cytokine release. Only from the 1960s with the development of drugs capable of attenuating or suppressing this response, did transplantation start to become a feasible mode of treatment.

The drugs available vary in their mechanisms of action, and are often combined for optimum effect. The glucocorticoids act at several points in the immune cascade, including antigen recognition and production of lymphokines. Ciclosporin and polypeptide immunosuppressants such as tacrolimus prevent formation of cytotoxic T-cells by inhibiting calcineurin activation, an important step in the release of interleukin-2 from helper T-cells, while polyclonal or monoclonal antibodies such as antilymphocyte immunoglobulins and muromonab-CD3 bind to and deplete T-cell populations. Basiliximab and daclizumab function as interleukin-2 receptor antagonists. Anti-proliferative drugs such as azathioprine and mycophenolate mofetil act by preventing cell division of lymphocytes. Sirolimus is an anti-proliferative drug that inhibits the T-cell response to cytokines.

Immunosuppressant regimens may be divided into those aimed at

- prevention of rejection in the early period after transplantation
- long-term maintenance prophylaxis
- treatment of acute episodes of rejection.

In bone marrow transplantation, where an immunologically competent tissue is transplanted, it is the donor cells which attack host tissues (graft-versus-host disease), and immunosuppression is required for prophylaxis of this condition.

Because of the critical nature of the early stage, when the organ or tissue must recover normal function, and perhaps to permit better long-term tolerance, initial immunosuppressant regimens tend to use higher doses than maintenance therapy. Standard protocols are usually based around ciclosporin or tacrolimus, combined with corticosteroids and an anti-proliferative agent (triple therapy). Where appropriate, a course of antilymphocyte antibodies is added to the standard regimen for induction (quadruple therapy). This is usually only required in individuals at increased risk of acute rejection, such as children or patients with a previous transplant or pregnancy, multiple blood transfusions, or a poor HLA-matching. However, it also enables delayed introduction of ciclosporin or tacrolimus in patients at risk of nephrotoxicity, and the use of low-dose regimens, allowing for withdrawal of corticosteroids.

No one immunosuppressive regimen has been identified as being superior to others in pregnancy, and although there are known theoretical risks to mother and fetus, successful pregnancies are now common in transplant recipients. The incidence of structural malformation has not been noted to be increased compared with the general population, but newer regimens have yet to be evaluated.

Since immunosuppressant therapy must in most cases be given for the lifetime of the graft, in long-term maintenance the toxicity of the drugs used, and the risks of infection, neoplasia, post-transplant diabetes mellitus, hyperlipidaemia, and osteoporosis, must be considered. Doses and numbers of agents used tend to be reduced, and in particular there is a tendency to taper or even eliminate the doses of corticosteroids used in maintenance regimens because of the potential sequelae of prolonged corticosteroid use. Post-transplant cardiovascular disease is a leading cause of death and graft loss. The risk varies between types of transplant, and specific recommendations for prophylaxis may differ.

The use of less intensive maintenance regimens must be balanced against the risk of an acute rejection episode, and the likelihood of its responding to therapy. High-dose corticosteroids and polyclonal or monoclonal antilymphocyte antibodies often play a role in the rescue therapy of patients with acute rejection episodes, although much depends upon the severity of the reaction, and whether such episodes have occurred previously.

The management of immunosuppression for the transplantation of particular organs is discussed in more detail below. With the use of suitable immunosuppressant regimens long-term graft survival can be obtained following transplantation of heart, kidney or liver; the transplantation of other organs such as bowel, lung, or pancreas remains more experimental. Ultimately, however, the complications of chronic rejection are likely to lead to loss of the graft: the induction of specific tolerance to the donor organ remains the goal of much research. In allogeneic bone marrow transplantation, where the aim of immunosuppression is prevention of graft-versus-host disease rather than rejection, immunosuppressant therapy can often be tapered off and eventually withdrawn.

Much recent interest has been aroused by the possibility of organ transplants from *animals*, genetically modified to reduce complement-mediated hyperacute rejection. It is not clear whether such xenotransplantation will require modified immunosuppressive regimens.

◊ Reviews.

1. Denton MD, *et al.* Immunosuppressive strategies in transplantation. *Lancet* 1999; **353:** 1083–91.
2. Hong JC, Kahan BD. Immunosuppressive agents in organ transplantation: past, present, and future. *Semin Nephrol* 2000; **20:** 108–25.
3. Chapman LE, Bloom ET. Clinical xenotransplantation. *JAMA* 2001; **285:** 2304–6.
4. del Mar Fernández de Gatta M, *et al.* Immunosuppressive therapy for paediatric transplant patients: pharmacokinetic considerations. *Clin Pharmacokinet* 2002; **41:** 115–35.
5. Bostom AD, *et al.* Prevention of post-transplant cardiovascular disease - report and recommendations of an ad hoc group. *Am J Transplant* 2002; **2:** 491–500.

**Corneal transplantation.** For reference to the use of immunosuppressants to treat graft rejection after corneal transplant see Corneal Graft Rejection, under Uses of Corticosteroids, p.1079.

**Haematopoietic stem cell transplantation.** Haematopoietic stem cell transplantation is used in the treatment of a variety of malignancies, notably leukaemias and lymphomas; to permit the use of very high-dose chemotherapy in the management of some solid tumours (bone marrow rescue); and to treat some other serious disorders affecting the bone marrow, such as aplastic anaemia and the haemoglobinopathies.[1] Two types of haematopoietic stem cell transplant are in use: in autologous transplantation, the patient's own stem cells are harvested from bone marrow or peripheral blood, while in allogeneic transplantation stem cells are harvested from the bone marrow, peripheral blood or umbilical cord blood of a healthy donor matched for HLA type.[2] Peripheral blood stem cell use is convenient as collection does not require hospitalisation or general anaesthesia for the donor, and clinical trials have demonstrated more rapid engraftment of neutrophils and platelets compared with bone marrow transplants.[3] However, peripheral blood stem cell transplantation appears to increase the risk of both acute and chronic graft-versus-host disease[4] (see below). Umbilical cord blood is mainly used for transplants in children, since the total number of stem cells in a donation often falls short of the levels deemed necessary for engraftment in an adult. Use of umbilical cord blood is associated with slightly delayed engraftment, but a lower risk of graft-versus-host disease (see below).

With autologous transplants problems of compatibility do not arise, but if abnormal cell clones are present in the marrow (as in leukaemia) or stem cells they may be transferred back into the patient and cause disease relapse. Allogeneic bone marrow transplants require immunosuppression for about 6 months[5,6] to prevent graft-versus-host disease (see below) until a new immunological balance is achieved.

The patient is normally prepared by conditioning with total body irradiation, or myeloablative chemotherapy with drugs such as cyclophosphamide or busulfan, or more often both, in order to destroy host bone marrow cells. In autologous procedures, harvesting of bone marrow or peripheral blood must be carried out before conditioning. Bone marrow is aspirated from the donor, and infused into the recipient via an indwelling catheter or directly into a peripheral vein. Peripheral blood stem cells are collected by cell separation after mobilisation, which is best achieved by a combination of chemotherapy and granulocyte or granulocyte-macrophage colony-stimulating factor.[3] Infection is a major cause of morbidity and mortality after transplantation, so prophylactic cover with antimicrobials and normal immunoglobulins is recommended,[7] although the value of the latter has been questioned.[8]

In addition to such supportive care, patients who have received allogeneic transplants require immunosuppressive therapy aimed at the prevention of **graft-versus-host disease** (GVHD). GVHD is usually characterised as acute or chronic depending on the manifestations, and the time of presentation[9] (by convention acute disease occurs within a hundred days of transplantation, and chronic disease after this time, although in practice there is considerable overlap). The organ systems primarily affected are skin, liver, and gastrointestinal tract. Both forms are marked by maculopapular rashes, which in severe disease may progress to bullous lesions and epidermal necrolysis. Liver disease may include cholestatic jaundice (usually in the acute form) and hepatitis; symptoms may need to be distinguished from the veno-occlusive disease which sometimes complicates bone marrow transplantation and is due to the pre-transplant conditioning regimen (the latter may respond to treatment with antithrombin III[10] or defibrotide[11]). Ursodeoxycholic acid has been investigated for the prophylaxis of hepatic complications.[12] The primary symptom of gastrointestinal GVHD is diarrhoea, often severe and painful. In patients with chronic GVHD other manifestations may include arthritis, mucositis, lung disease, and scleroderma.

Most modern regimens for the prophylaxis of GVHD after allogeneic bone marrow transplantation are based on ciclosporin. Although GVHD still occurs in many ciclosporin-treated patients, morbidity is much reduced and survival improved. Combination regimens have been tried for prophylaxis, particularly ciclosporin or tacrolimus with methotrexate, but also combinations with other drugs including antilymphocyte immunoglobulins, corticosteroids, mycophenolate mofetil, and sirolimus.[5,6] Monoclonal antibodies have been used to produce T-cell depletion or reduce the effects of circulating cytokines.[5,13,14]

Acute GVHD is usually treated primarily by the addition of corticosteroids (usually methylprednisolone[5,6]) to the prophylactic regimen until symptoms are controlled, followed by gradual tapering of the dose. Mycophenolate mofetil, antilymphocyte immunoglobulins, and monoclonal antibodies such as daclizumab have also been tried.[5,6] Chronic GVHD requires long-term immunosuppression, and combination therapy results in increased disease-free survival,[5] although a small, further study did not confirm this.[15] Ciclosporin, with or without a corticosteroid is commonly used,[5,13,16] but thalidomide and azathioprine have also been tried.[5] Tacrolimus with mycophenolate mofetil, and pentostatin are under investigation.[6] PUVA therapy has been used in refractory cutaneous GVHD and extracorporeal photopheresis has been investigated.[5] Octreotide is recommended for the symptomatic treatment of diarrhoea.[17]

However, a degree of acute GVHD may be desirable in some stem cell transplants, since it can result in a 'graft-versus-malignancy' effect which reduces relapse. Indeed, many leukaemia patients who relapse following allogeneic transplant can be reinduced into remission by an additional infusion of donor lymphocytes.[18] Consequently, too effective an immunosuppressant regimen may not always be desirable, and leukaemic patients given bone marrow transplants purged of T-cells, which virtually abolishes GVHD, do not have a better survival rate than those given conventional prophylaxis (engraftment too is reduced in the absence of all T-cells). Specific donor marrow T-cell depletion has been investigated as the sole form of GVHD prophylaxis, with favourable outcomes.[19] The observation of graft-versus-malignancy effects has led to the development of low-dose non-myeloablative preparative regimens (with or without donor lymphocyte infusions) for elderly or more sensitive patients who might have been unable to receive the standard aggressive therapy.[2,18,20]

The combination of irradiation, chemotherapy, and immunosuppression can cause the development of secondary malignant neoplasms in long-term survivors of bone marrow transplantation.[21]


1. Goldman JM, *et al.* Allogeneic and autologous transplantation for haematological diseases, solid tumours and immune disorders: current practice in Europe in 1998. *Bone Marrow Transplant* 1998; **21:** 1–7.
2. Lennard AL, Jackson GH. Stem cell transplantation. *BMJ* 2000; **321:** 433–7.
3. Demirer T, *et al.* Peripheral blood stem cell mobilization for high-dose chemotherapy. *J Hematother* 1999; **8:** 103–13.
4. Cutler C, *et al.* Acute and chronic graft-versus-host disease after allogeneic peripheral-blood stem-cell and bone marrow transplantation: a meta-analysis. *J Clin Oncol* 2001; **19:** 3685–91.
5. Flowers MED, *et al.* Pathophysiology and treatment of graft-versus-host disease. *Hematol Oncol Clin North Am* 1999; **13:** 1091–1112.
6. Jacobsohn DA, Vogelsang GB. Novel pharmacotherapeutic approaches to prevention and treatment of GVHD. *Drugs* 2002; **62:** 879–89.
7. Centers for Disease Control and Prevention. Guidelines for preventing opportunistic infections among hematopoietic stem cell transplant recipients: recommendations of CDC, the Infectious Disease Society of America, and the American Society of Blood and Marrow Transplantation. *MMWR* 2000; **49** (RR-10): 1–128.
8. Cordonnier C, *et al.* Should immunoglobulin therapy be used in allogeneic stem-cell transplantation? A randomized, double-blind, dose effect, placebo-controlled, multicenter trial. *Ann Intern Med* 2003; **139:** 8–18.
9. Antin JH. Long-term care after hematopoietic-cell transplantation in adults. *N Engl J Med* 2002; **347:** 36–42.
10. Morris JD, *et al.* Antithrombin-III for the treatment of chemotherapy-induced organ dysfunction following bone marrow transplantation. *Bone Marrow Transplant* 1997; **20:** 871–8.
11. Chopra R, *et al.* Defibrotide for the treatment of hepatic veno-occlusive disease: results of the European compassionate-use study. *Br J Haematol* 2000; **111:** 1122–9.
12. Essell JH, *et al.* Ursodiol prophylaxis against hepatic complications of allogeneic bone marrow transplantation: a randomized, double-blind, placebo-controlled trial. *Ann Intern Med* 1998; **128:** 975–81.
13. Hiscott A, McLellan DS. Graft-versus-host disease in allogeneic bone marrow transplantation: the role of monoclonal antibodies in prevention and treatment. *Br J Biomed Sci* 2000; **57:** 163–9.
14. Ferrara JLM, *et al.* Monoclonal antibody and receptor antagonist therapy for GVHD. *Cancer Treat Res* 1999; **101:** 331–68.
15. Koc S, *et al.* Therapy for chronic graft-versus-host disease: a randomized trial comparing cyclosporine plus prednisone versus prednisone alone. *Blood* 2002; **100:** 48–51.
16. Bhushan V, Collins RH. Chronic graft-vs-host disease. *JAMA* 2003; **290:** 2599–2603.
17. Kornblau S, *et al.* Management of cancer treatment-related diarrhea: issues and therapeutic strategies. *J Pain Symptom Manage* 2000; **19:** 118–29.
18. Champlin R, *et al.* Reinventing bone marrow transplantation: reducing toxicity using nonmyeloablative, preparative regimens and induction of graft-versus-malignancy. *Curr Opin Oncol* 1999; **11:** 87–95.
19. Soiffer RJ, *et al.* CD6+ donor marrow T-cell depletion as the sole form of graft-versus-host disease prophylaxis in patients undergoing allogeneic bone marrow transplant from unrelated donors. *J Clin Oncol* 2001; **19:** 1152–9.
20. Appelbaum FR. Hematopoietic cell transplantation as a form of immunotherapy. *Int J Hematol* 2002; **75:** 222–7.
21. Kolb HJ, *et al.* Malignant neoplasms in long-term survivors of bone marrow transplantation. *Ann Intern Med* 1999; **131:** 738–44.


**Heart transplantation.** Marked improvements have been seen in outcome following heart transplantation since the introduction of ciclosporin, which has resulted in a reduced incidence and severity of rejection episodes. The 1-year survival rate is approximately 80%.[1]

A common **immunosuppressive regimen** consists of triple therapy with ciclosporin, azathioprine and corticosteroids.[2-4] Some centres use induction therapy with antilymphocyte immunoglobulins or muromonab-CD3,[2,4] which increases the risk of infection and lymphoproliferative disorders, but does delay the first rejection episode and allows transplantation in higher risk groups. It also enables ciclosporin use to be delayed in patients with initial poor renal function and corticosteroids to be stopped as maintenance therapy in some groups of patients.[2] It has been suggested that the high doses of corticosteroids used increase the risk of cardiac adverse events in the longer term, and protocols that wean patients from corticosteroids after 6 months postoperatively have been used,[5] without apparent increases in infection or rejection. Basiliximab and daclizumab are being evaluated for induction therapy.[3]

There does not seem to be any significant difference in efficacy between tacrolimus and ciclosporin in heart transplant patients,[2,6] although there is some evidence[7] of a higher incidence of acute rejection in black patients receiving ciclosporin microemulsion than in those given tacrolimus. It has been suggested that tacrolimus be substituted for ciclosporin in those patients suffering persistent rejection, or adverse effects associated with ciclosporin,[8] or with hyperlipidaemia or hypertension.[9] Ciclosporin microemulsion may be associated with less rejection than the oil-based formulation,[10] and a small, preliminary study[11] found that patients with lower levels of unbound ciclosporin were more prone to cardiac rejection. The use of mycophenolate mofetil instead of azathioprine in triple therapy has been shown to reduce mortality and rejection in the first year after heart transplantation,[12] and a retrospective review[13] concluded that the advent of mycophenolate mofetil has contributed to improved survival in cardiac transplant recipients. Although lower mycophenolic acid (MPA) concentrations may be associated with an increased allograft rejection,[14] there appears to be no benefit in monitoring MPA concentrations beyond the first year in heart transplant recipients,[15] and MPA levels may be affected by concomitant immunosuppression, see under Mycophenolate Mofetil, p.1361. Substituting cyclophosphamide for azathioprine for 6 weeks after transplantation is reported to reduce the development of anti-muromonab-CD3 antibodies from induction therapy.[16] Substitution of mycophenolate mofetil with intravenous pulse cyclophosphamide for 4 months post-transplantation appeared to decrease the risk of rejection in a small, non-randomised trial in sensitised allograft recipients.[17]

In the early post-transplant period, the most significant **causes of morbidity** are infection and rejection episodes.[2] Co-trimoxazole is used to protect against *Pneumocystis carinii* infection, and ganciclovir as prophylaxis against cytomegalovirus.[3] Rejection is usually treated with corticosteroids, but other drugs have been used for corticosteroid-resistant cases,[2] including antilymphocyte immunoglobulins and muromonab-CD3.[4] In repetitive rejection, tacrolimus may be substituted for ciclosporin, and mycophenolate mofetil for azathioprine.[4] Adjunctive methotrexate, total lymphoid irradiation and photopheresis have all been tried.[2,6] Newer drugs under investigation include sirolimus and basiliximab.[4,6]

In the late post-transplant period, malignancy and coronary artery disease are the most significant problems.[2,3] Coronary artery vasculopathy is a major cause of death and prevention of its progression is a major therapeutic goal.[3,18] It is thought to be mainly an immunological response, but can be accelerated by the classical risk factors of dyslipidaemia, obesity, glucose intolerance, and smoking, as well as by postoperative cytomegalovirus infection, and immunosuppression itself.[2,3] Calcium-channel blockers and HMG-CoA reductase inhibitors such as pravastatin and simvastatin have been used to decrease the incidence of coronary artery disease, but it has remained a difficult complication to treat.[19] Supplementation with antoxidant vitamins such as C or E may reduce the progression of arteriosclerosis after transplantation,[20] and a small trial[21] found that omega-3 triglycerides improved blood pressure control in hypertensive transplant recipients.

Improved surgical techniques and the use of ciclosporin have also made possible successful combined *heart-lung* transplants, although these may require enhanced or modified immunosuppression to prevent obliterative bronchiolitis, a possible manifestation of chronic rejection.[22] Early rejection after transplantation is the most important risk factor for the development of bronchiolitis obliterans syndrome although pathogenesis is unclear.[23] Lung infection,[22] or oxidative stress and lack of glutathione[23] may be factors in the aggravation or onset of bronchiolitis obliterans syndrome.


1. Hosenpud JD, *et al.* The registry of the International Society for Heart and Lung Transplantation: seventeenth official report—2000. *J Heart Lung Transplant* 2000; **19:** 909–31.
2. Hunt SA. Current status of cardiac transplantation. *JAMA* 1998; **280:** 1692–8.
3. Deng MC. Cardiac transplantation. *Heart* 2002; **87:** 177–84.
4. Baran DA, *et al.* Current practices: immunosuppression induction, maintenance, and rejection regimens in contemporary post-heart transplant patient treatment. *Curr Opin Cardiol* 2002; **17:** 165–70.

5. Oaks TE, *et al.* Steroid-free maintenance immunosuppression after heart transplantation. *Ann Thorac Surg* 2001; **72:** 102–6.
6. Kobashigawa JA. Advances in immunosuppression for heart transplantation. *Adv Card Surg* 1998; **10:** 155–74.
7. Mehra MR, *et al.* A randomized comparison of an immunosuppressive strategy using tacrolimus and cyclosporine in black heart transplant recipients. *Transplant Proc* 2001; **33:** 1606–7.
8. De Bonis M, *et al.* Tacrolimus as a rescue immunosuppressant after heart transplantation. *Eur J Cardiothorac Surg* 2001; **19:** 690–5.
9. Taylor DO, *et al.* Suggested guidelines for the use of tacrolimus in cardiac transplant recipients. *J Heart Lung Transplant* 2001; **20:** 734–8.
10. Eisen HJ, *et al.* Safety, tolerability, and efficacy of cyclosporine microemulsion in heart transplant recipients: a randomized, multicenter, double-blind comparison with the oil-based formulation of cyclosporine—results at 24 months after transplantation. *Transplantation* 2001; **71:** 70–8.
11. Akhlaghi F, *et al.* Unbound cyclosporine and allograft rejection after heart transplantation. *Transplantation* 1999; **67:** 54–9.
12. Kobashigawa J, *et al.* A randomized active-controlled trial of mycophenolate mofetil in heart transplant recipients. *Transplantation* 1998; **66:** 507–15.
13. John R, *et al.* Long-term outcomes after cardiac transplantation: an experience based on different eras of immunosuppressive therapy. *Ann Thorac Surg* 2001; **72:** 440–9.
14. DeNofrio D, *et al.* Mycophenolic acid concentrations are associated with cardiac allograft rejection. *J Heart Lung Transplant* 2000; **19:** 1071–6.
15. Cantin B, *et al.* Mycophenolic acid concentrations in long-term heart transplant patients: relationship with calcineurin antagonists and acute rejection. *Clin Transplant* 2002; **16:** 196–201.
16. Taylor DO, *et al.* A prospective, randomized comparison of cyclophosphamide and azathioprine for early rejection prophylaxis after cardiac transplantation: decreased sensitization to OKT3. *Transplantation* 1994; **58:** 645–9.
17. Itescu S, *et al.* Intravenous pulse administration of cyclophosphamide is an effective and safe treatment for sensitized cardiac allograft recipients. *Circulation* 2002; **105:** 1214–19.
18. John R, *et al.* Factors affecting long-term survival (>10 years) after cardiac transplantation in the cyclosporine era. *J Am Coll Cardiol* 2001; **37:** 189–94.
19. Cotts WG, Johnson MR. The challenge of rejection and cardiac allograft vasculopathy. *Heart Fail Rev* 2001; **6:** 227–40.
20. Fang JC, *et al.* Effect of vitamins C and E on progression of transplant-associated arteriosclerosis: a randomised trial. *Lancet* 2002; **359:** 1108–13.
21. Holm T, *et al.* Omega-3 fatty acids improve blood pressure control and preserve renal function in hypertensive heart transplant recipients. *Eur Heart J* 2001; **22:** 428–36.
22. Harringer W, Haverich A. Heart and heart-lung transplantation: standards and improvements. *World J Surg* 2002; **26:** 218–25.
23. Behr J, *et al.* Evidence for oxidative stress in bronchiolitis obliterans syndrome after lung and heart-lung transplantation. *Transplantation* 2000; **69:** 1856–60.

**Intestinal transplantation.** Transplantation of the *small bowel* is becoming more common, especially in children.[1] There are 3 types of intestinal allograft: the isolated intestine, combined liver and intestine, and the multivisceral graft, which can also include the pancreas, stomach, and kidneys.[2] Combined liver and small intestine transplants are used for patients with TPN dependence and irreversible intestinal and hepatic failure, while intestine-only transplants tend to be used for intestinal failure in patients with severe progressive complications of parenteral nutrition, such as recurring sepsis and impending loss of central venous access.[1,3,4] Transplantation of the *colon* is avoided because of poorer outcomes and increased risk of sepsis.[5] Overall patient and graft survival varies according to the type of intestinal allograft, and between transplant centres, but is increasing, and reported to be about 50% at 5 years post-transplant.[1]

Tacrolimus and tapered corticosteroid doses[1,2,5] are the basis of the standard immunosuppressive regimen; prostaglandins[5] may also be given. Induction therapy with interleukin-2 receptor antibodies such as daclizumab is also used to prevent rejection.[1,5,6] Sirolimus has also been tried.[1,5,6]

Substantial morbidity occurs and acute rejection, manifested by diarrhoea, fever, and ileus, is common.[1,2,5] Treatment includes increasing the dose of tacrolimus or corticosteroid, or the use of muromonab-CD3 or antilymphocyte immunoglobulins.[1,2,5] Azathioprine, sirolimus, and mycophenolate mofetil have also been used if tacrolimus toxicity occurs,[1] although the use of mycophenolate mofetil in intestinal transplantation has been questioned.[6,7] Chronic rejection, a common cause of late graft dysfunction, is more difficult to treat.[1,5,7] Bacterial, viral, and fungal infections are also common post-transplant,[1,2,5,7] and may be confused with rejection.[7] The high level of immunosuppression necessary in intestinal transplantation makes recipients particularly susceptible to post-transplant lymphoproliferative disease associated with Epstein-Barr virus infection.[1-3,7] Controlling rejection by more potent immunosuppression is difficult because of these complications, so the induction of immune tolerance through adjunctive bone marrow infusion is being investigated.[1,2,6] Graft-versus-host disease (see Haematopoietic Stem Cell Transplantation, p.1344) may occur and there may be a recurrence of the original disease.[2]

1. Park BK. Intestinal transplantation in pediatric patients. *Prog Transplant* 2002; **12:** 97–115.
2. Kato T, *et al.* Intestinal and multivisceral transplantation. *World J Surg* 2002; **26:** 226–37.
3. Kaufman SS, *et al.* Indications for pediatric intestinal transplantation: a position paper of the American Society of Transplantation. *Pediatr Transplant* 2001; **5:** 80–7.
4. Benedetti E, *et al.* Surgical approaches and intestinal transplantation. *Best Pract Res Clin Gastroenterol* 2003; **17:** 1017–40.
5. Ghanekar A, Grant D. Small bowel transplantation. *Curr Opin Crit Care* 2001; **7:** 133–7.
6. Pirenne J, *et al.* Recent advances and future prospects in intestinal and multi-visceral transplantation. *Pediatr Transplant* 2001; **5:** 452–6.
7. Kaufman SS. Small bowel transplantation: selection criteria, operative techniques, advances in specific immunosuppression, prognosis. *Curr Opin Pediatr* 2001; **13:** 425–8.

**Kidney transplantation.** The transplantation of kidneys is now established as the ultimate therapy for end-stage renal disease. There is no single generally accepted immunosuppressant regimen, and different centres have achieved good results with a variety of strategies.[1] Therapy should be tailored to the individual patient. A number of factors affect the intensity of immunotherapy required, including the donor source (living or cadaveric) and degree of HLA histocompatibility, and the age, race and panel reactive antibody titre of the recipient.[1] A widely used approach consists of **triple therapy** with ciclosporin or tacrolimus, azathioprine or mycophenolate mofetil, and prednisolone.[2,3] Triple therapy is popular because it allows the use of lower doses of nephrotoxic ciclosporin, and the eventual tapering or even elimination of corticosteroids in some patients.[1] Azathioprine has largely been replaced by mycophenolate mofetil which lowers the incidence of acute rejection and reduces the risk of chronic allograft failure.[4] Tacrolimus has been substituted for ciclosporin because it appears to be more effective in preventing acute rejection than either the older oil-based formulation,[4] or the newer microemulsion.[5,6] It may also have a superior cardiovascular risk profile,[5,7] but has been associated with an increase in the incidence of diabetes mellitus.[1,4,8] There is some evidence of synergism between sirolimus and ciclosporin[9] and addition of sirolimus to ciclosporin-based regimens may reduce the incidence of acute rejection.[4,10] However, there is some suggestion that sirolimus may augment the nephrotoxicity of ciclosporin.[2] Combining sirolimus with tacrolimus instead of ciclosporin may be even more effective.[4]

**Sequential quadruple therapy** is also used. Induction therapy with antilymphocyte immunoglobulins or muromonab-CD3 is given postoperatively, in addition to triple therapy.[2] The antibodies are stopped once good graft function is achieved.[1] The regimen may improve long-term graft survival in patients with delayed graft function.[11] However, such strongly immunosuppressive regimens can increase the risk of cytomegalovirus and other infections and some centres have reverted to the use of triple therapy.[12] There is some evidence that the incidence of complications is lower with antilymphocyte immunoglobulins than with muromonab-CD3.[13] The more specific interleukin-2 receptor antibodies basiliximab and daclizumab have also been added to initial therapy and appear to reduce the incidence of rejection episodes without increased toxicity.[4,11,14]

As immunosuppressant regimens have developed the role of **corticosteroids** has come to be questioned, mainly because of the adverse effects associated with their prolonged use.[4] Studies indicate that corticosteroid withdrawal is feasible in many patients initially receiving triple therapy,[1,8] although there is debate about the long-term consequences of this for graft survival.[4] Induction therapy with antilymphocyte immunoglobulin, combined with a calcineurin inhibitor and mycophenolate mofetil may allow the use of corticosteroid-free regimens.[4]

Where an **acute rejection** episode occurs treatment is likely to be with high-dose corticosteroids, or with drugs such as antilymphocyte immunoglobulins, or muromonab-CD3, which are potent and effective reversers of rejection.[1,2] European guidelines recommend that the antibody preparations be reserved for corticosteroid-resistant rejection or more severe episodes,[11] but approaches remain varied.[1] Tacrolimus,[4] mycophenolate mofetil,[4] sirolimus,[15] and gusperimus[3] have been effective in reversing acute rejection episodes. Ciclosporin and azathioprine are ineffective in treating established rejection. Interleukin-2 receptor antibodies have not been shown to reverse established rejection episodes.[3] There has also been evidence that asymptomatic cytomegalovirus infection may be associated with episodes of late acute rejection;[16] ganciclovir is reported to improve graft function in such circumstances. However, augmented or rescue immunosuppressive therapy predisposes the patient to infections such as cytomegalovirus, which may itself mimic late acute rejection, and contribute to chronic rejection.[17]

Severe, recurrent, late episodes of acute rejection are considered to be a major risk factor for the development of **chronic rejection**. Manifested clinically by declining renal function, hypertension, and low-grade proteinuria, the term chronic allograft nephropathy is used.[4] Long-term calcineurin inhibitor treatment and inadequate immunosuppression may contribute to this, but there is some suggestion that the addition of mycophenolate mofetil can delay this process.[4]

Although newer drugs have decreased the incidence of acute rejection, there is only limited evidence that this has improved longer-term **graft survival**.[18-20] The one-year cadaveric graft survival is about 88% and about 60% at 10 years.[21] Pentoxifylline[22] and gusperimus[23] may improve graft survival. Morbidity and mortality have improved following reductions in cardiac, vascular and infectious complications, but there has been no decrease in death from malignancy, and the risk of developing cancer has been estimated to be approximately 100% by 30 years post-transplant.[24] Recurrence of the original disease or *de novo* renal disease may also cause graft failure.[25]

Nonmyeloablative conditioning regimens allowing for the development of immunological tolerance specific to the donor remains the ultimate goal of renal transplantation.[4,26]

1. First MR. Clinical application of immunosuppressive agents in renal transplantation. *Surg Clin North Am* 1998; **78:** 61–76.
2. Fisher JS, *et al.* Kidney transplantation: graft monitoring and immunosuppression. *World J Surg* 2002; **26:** 185–93.
3. Luke PPW, Jordan ML. Contemporary immunosuppression in renal transplantation. *Urol Clin North Am* 2001; **28:** 733–50.
4. Pascual M, *et al.* Strategies to improve long-term outcomes after renal transplantation. *N Engl J Med* 2002; **346:** 580–90.
5. Margreiter R. Efficacy and safety of tacrolimus compared with ciclosporin microemulsion in renal transplantation: a randomised multicentre study. *Lancet* 2002; **359:** 741–6.
6. Tanabe K. Calcineurin inhibitors in renal transplantation: what is the best option? *Drugs* 2003; **63:** 1535–48. Correction. *ibid.*; 2234.
7. Gaston RS. Maintenance immunosuppression in the renal transplant recipient: an overview. *Am J Kidney Dis* 2001; **38** (suppl 6): S25–S35. Correction. *ibid.* 2002; **39:** 898.
8. Gonin JM. Maintenance immunosuppression: new agents and persistent dilemmas. *Adv Ren Replace Ther* 2000; **7:** 95–116.
9. Kahan BD, Kramer WG. Median effect analysis of efficacy versus adverse effects of immunosuppressants. *Clin Pharmacol Ther* 2001; **70:** 74–81.
10. MacDonald AS. A worldwide, phase III, randomized, controlled, safety and efficacy study of a sirolimus/cyclosporine regimen for prevention of acute rejection in recipients of primary mismatched renal allografts. *Transplantation* 2001; **71:** 271–80.
11. EBPG Expert Group on Renal Transplantation. European best practice guidelines for renal transplantation (part 1). *Nephrol Dial Transplant* 2000; **15** (suppl 7): 1–85.
12. Verran D, *et al.* Quadruple immunosuppression in renal allografts—the Auckland experience. *N Z Med J* 1991; **104:** 517–18.
13. Bock HA, *et al.* A randomized prospective trial of prophylactic immunosuppression with ATG-Fresenius versus OKT3 after renal transplantation. *Transplantation* 1995; **59:** 830–40.
14. Adu D, *et al.* Interleukin-2 receptor monoclonal antibodies in renal transplantation: meta-analysis of randomised trials. *BMJ* 2003; **326:** 789–91.
15. Hong JC, Kahan BD. Sirolimus rescue therapy for refractory rejection in renal transplantation. *Transplantation* 2001; **71:** 1579–84.
16. Reinke P, *et al.* Late-acute renal allograft rejection and symptomless cytomegalovirus infection. *Lancet* 1994; **344:** 1737–8.
17. Tanphaichitr NT, Brennan DC. Infectious complications in renal transplant recipients. *Adv Ren Replace Ther* 2000; **7:** 131–46.
18. Szczech LA, *et al.* The effect of antilymphocyte induction therapy on renal allograft survival: a meta-analysis of individual patient-level data. *Ann Intern Med* 1998; **128:** 817–26.
19. Ojo AO, *et al.* Mycophenolate mofetil reduces late renal allograft loss independent of acute rejection. *Transplantation* 2000; **69:** 2405–9.
20. Hariharan S, *et al.* Improved graft survival after renal transplantation in the United States, 1988 to 1996. *N Engl J Med* 2000; **342:** 605–12.
21. Andrews PA. Renal transplantation. *BMJ* 2002; **324:** 530–4.
22. Noel C, *et al.* Immunomodulatory effect of pentoxifylline during human allograft rejection: involvement of tumor necrosis factor-α and adhesion molecules. *Transplantation* 2000; **69:** 1102–7.
23. Amada N, *et al.* Prophylactic use of deoxyspergualin improves long-term graft survival in living related renal transplant recipients transfused with donor-specific blood. *Transplant Proc* 2001; **33:** 2256–7.
24. Mathew TH. Optimal long-term immunotherapy protocols. *Transplant Proc* 1999; **31:** 1102–3.
25. Ponticelli C. Renal transplantation strengths and shortcomings. *J Nephrol* 2001; **14** (suppl 4): S1–S6.
26. Cosimi AB, Sachs DH. Mixed chimerism and transplantation tolerance. *Transplantation* 2004; **77:** 943–6.

**Liver transplantation.** Marked improvements have occurred in the outcome and reliability of liver transplantation in recent years, and it is now seen as standard therapy for acute and chronic hepatic failure, regardless of aetiology,[1,2] and some metabolic disorders.[3] The 1-year patient and graft survival rates[2-4] are approximately 90%.

Current immunosuppressive regimens generally combine a calcineurin inhibitor (ciclosporin or tacrolimus) with a corticosteroid and azathioprine or mycophenolate mofetil (triple therapy), and with such regimens it is possible to avoid acute rejection episodes in the majority of cases.[5-7] Double therapy with ciclosporin or tacrolimus and corticosteroids is also used,[6,8] and monotherapy with a calcineurin inhibitor alone has been proposed, allowing for complete corticosteroid withdrawal or avoidance.[1,4,9,10] The liver induces some tolerance and liver transplant recipients usually require less immunosuppression than other solid organ transplant patients.[11] Up to 85% of patients can be withdrawn from corticosteroids within a few months of transplantation, and some centres have performed liver transplants without the use of corticosteroids.[8,11-13] Patients with underlying auto-immune hepatitis or inflammatory bowel disease may be relatively refractory to corticosteroid withdrawal.[8] It may be feasible to reduce or stop all immunosuppression in up to 40 to 50% of long-term stable liver transplant patients.[11]

Tacrolimus is increasingly used as the first-line calcineurin inhibitor in liver transplant recipients, as the incidence of rejection appears to be lower than that with ciclosporin-based regimens, although patient and graft survival does not appear to differ significantly between the two.[3,6,7] Studies of different formulations of ciclosporin found a reduced incidence of rejection with the microemulsion compared to the older oil-based formulation.[4]

Mycophenolate mofetil has been used in place of azathioprine, to reduce the dose of the calcineurin inhibitor or corticosteroid used, and possibly prevent rejection.[2,6] However, although substitution of calcineurin inhibitors with mycophenolate mofetil has been suggested, in an attempt to improve renal function, a small study has suggested that this monotherapy carries a high risk of rejection.[14] The role of sirolimus in liver transplantation has yet to be evaluated. Although there have been reports of efficacy when combined with a calcineurin inhibitor,[1,7] and as such may allow dose reduction[7] or discontinuation of therapy[4] in patients evidencing toxicity on tacrolimus or ciclosporin, excess mortality, graft loss, and hepatic artery thrombosis has been associated with such use.

Induction therapy with antilymphocyte immunoglobulins or muromonab-CD3 has declined due to the high incidence of infection and lymphoproliferative disease associated with their use, and they are generally reserved for the treatment of corticosteroid-resistant acute rejection.[2,3,6,7] The use of interleukin-2 receptor antibodies, such as basiliximab, daclizumab, and inolimomab, is still being evaluated, although initial studies suggest they decrease the number of rejection episodes.[6,7]

Most **acute rejection** episodes occur during the first 3 to 6 months of therapy.[8] Early acute rejection does not affect patient or graft survival[11,15] and, if mild, may be associated with increased survival.[1] Late acute rejection, occurring after 30 days post-transplant may be related to reduction or withdrawal of immunosuppressive therapy.[16] Corticosteroids are used in the first-line treatment of acute rejection. For corticosteroid-resistant rejection, muromonab-CD3 or antilymphocyte immunoglobulins are used, and increasing the dose of tacrolimus, or conversion from ciclosporin to tacrolimus, may also be effective.[2,3,7] Mycophenolate mofetil is used in patients not responding to conventional therapies, but there have been no controlled trials to determine its efficacy.[17] **Chronic rejection** is almost always preceded by one or more episodes of corticosteroid-resistant acute rejection,[16] and although its incidence has decreased[4,16] to less than 5%, it remains difficult to treat. Corticosteroids are generally ineffective, and tacrolimus is the most effective drug available.[17]

The main **complications** encountered with liver transplants are infection in the early post-transplant period, vascular and biliary complications, recurrent disease (particularly viral recurrence), and adverse effects due to immunosuppressants.[3,11,16]

Sepsis is an important cause of death in the early post-transplant period.[11] Patients at increased risk, including those with malnutrition, fulminant liver failure, or renal insufficiency, require particularly cautious immunosuppression and more aggressive antibacterial and antifungal prophylaxis regimens.

Recurrence of hepatitis B infection is common.[18] Although the introduction of hepatitis B immunoglobulins and lamivudine have improved the prospects for these patients, combination antiviral therapy and a modified immunosuppression protocol are usually needed.[5,11,15] Hepatitis C recurrence is almost universal in infected patients,[19] with a probable reduction in long-term graft survival.[5,15] The use of corticosteroids and muromonab-CD3 appears to be associated with more severe recurrence of hepatitis C. Treatment with a combination of interferon alfa and ribavirin appears promising.[18-20]

Nephrotoxicity from ciclosporin or tacrolimus can be a significant problem after long-term therapy. Long-term renal function is affected by the function in the early post-transplant period, so serum creatinine concentrations at 1 and 3 months are often used to predict toxicity.[5] Cardiovascular complications may follow metabolic abnormalities such as diabetes mellitus, hypertension, hyperlipidaemia, and obesity. Dose reduction or change of the calcineurin inhibitor used, corticosteroid withdrawal, or use of statins could minimise the cardiovascular risk post-transplantation.[21,22] Malignancy may occur following prolonged immunosuppression.[3,15] The induction of immune tolerance remains the ultimate goal in liver transplantation.[23,24]


1. Raimondo ML, Burroughs AK. Single-agent immunosuppression after liver transplantation: what is possible? *Drugs* 2002; **62:** 1587–97.
2. Keeffe EB. Liver transplantation: current status and novel approaches to liver replacement. *Gastroenterology* 2001; **120:** 749–62.
3. Bramhall SR, *et al.* Liver transplantation in the UK. *World J Gastroenterol* 2001; **7:** 602–11.
4. Levy GA. Long-term immunosuppression and drug interactions. *Liver Transpl* 2001; **7** (suppl 1): S53–9.
5. McMaster P, *et al.* Liver transplantation: changing goals in immunosuppression. *Transplant Proc* 1998; **30:** 1819–21.
6. Moser MAJ. Options for induction immunosuppression in liver transplant recipients. *Drugs* 2002; **62:** 995–1011.
7. Cohen SM. Current immunosuppression in liver transplantation. *Am J Ther* 2002; **9:** 119–25.
8. Everson GT, *et al.* Early steroid withdrawal in liver transplantation is safe and beneficial. *Liver Transpl Surg* 1999; **5** (suppl 1): S48–57.
9. Lerut JP, *et al.* Adult liver transplantation and steroid-azathioprine withdrawal in cyclosporine (Sandimmun)-based immunosuppression – 5 year results of a prospective study. *Transpl Int* 2001; **14:** 420–8.
10. Chau TN, *et al.* Histological patterns of rejection using oral microemulsified cyclosporine and tacrolimus (FK506) as monotherapy induction after orthotopic liver transplantation. *Liver* 2001; **21:** 329–34.
11. Pirenne J, Koshiba T. Present status and future prospects in liver transplantation. *Int Surg* 1999; **84:** 297–304.
12. Ringe B, *et al.* A novel management strategy of steroid-free immunosuppression after liver transplantation: efficacy and safety of tacrolimus and mycophenolate mofetil. *Transplantation* 2001; **71:** 508–15.
13. Reding R, *et al.* Steroid-free liver transplantation in children. *Lancet* 2003; **362:** 2068–70.
14. Schlitt HJ, *et al.* Replacement of calcineurin inhibitors with mycophenolate mofetil in liver-transplant patients with renal dysfunction: a randomised controlled study. *Lancet* 2001; **357:** 587–91.
15. Neuberger J. Liver transplantation. *J Hepatol* 2000; **32** (suppl 1): 198–207.
16. Wiesner RH, Menon KVN. Late hepatic allograft dysfunction *Liver Transpl* 2001; **7** (suppl 1): S60–73.
17. Millis JM. Treatment of liver allograft rejection. *Liver Transpl Surg* 1999; **5** (suppl 1): S98–106.
18. Rosen HR. Hepatitis B and C in the liver transplant recipient: current understanding and treatment. *Liver Transpl* 2001; **7** (suppl 1): S87–98.
19. Sponseller CA, Ramrakhiani S. Treatment of hepatitis B and C following liver transplantation. *Curr Gastroenterol Rep* 2002; **4:** 52–62.
20. Charlton M. Hepatitis C infection in liver transplantation. *Am J Transplant* 2001; **1:** 197–203.
21. Neal DAJ, Alexander GJM. Can the potential benefits of statins in general medical practice be extrapolated to liver transplantation? *Liver Transpl* 2001; **7:** 1009–14.
22. Reuben A. Long-term management of the liver transplant patient: diabetes, hyperlipidemia, and obesity. *Liver Transpl* 2001; **7** (suppl 1): S13–21.
23. Bishop GA, McCaughan GW. Immune activation is required for the induction of liver allograft tolerance: implications for immunosuppressive therapy. *Liver Transpl* 2001; **7:** 161–72.
24. Goddard S, Adams DH. New approaches to immunosuppression in liver transplantation. *J Gastroenterol Hepatol* 2002; **17:** 116–26.


**Lung transplantation.** Lung transplantation has become accepted therapy[1,2] for end-stage pulmonary disease such as pulmonary hypertension, cystic fibrosis, emphysema, and pulmonary fibrosis, with a 1-year survival of 70% or more.[1] The rate of death is highest in the first year following transplantation, with infection[3] and primary graft failure[1] the leading causes of early death.

Immunosuppressant therapy is usually with a triple therapy regimen of ciclosporin or tacrolimus, azathioprine or mycophenolate mofetil, and a corticosteroid.[1,4-6] Antilymphocyte immunoglobulins, daclizumab, or muromonab-CD3 may be added in the early post-transplant period as induction therapy to reduce the incidence of early acute rejection,[7] although some consider evidence for this to be lacking.[1] Acute rejection occurs more frequently with lung transplants than with other solid organ transplants; the prevalence has been estimated to range from 60 to 100%.[2] High doses of intravenous corticosteroids are generally used to control acute episodes of rejection.[1,5] Patients at risk from cytomegalovirus should be given ganciclovir.[5] Several other drugs have been tried for corticosteroid-resistant episodes, including tacrolimus, inhaled ciclosporin, antilymphocyte immunoglobulins and muromonab-CD3.[2] The main complication encountered in the long term is chronic rejection manifesting as bronchiolitis obliterans syndrome (obliterative bronchiolitis). This is characterised by progressive airway obstruction and may be present in up to 40% of patients at 2 years, and in 60 to 70% who survive for 5 years.[5] The frequency and severity of acute rejection episodes are the main risk factors for the development of bronchiolitis obliterans, but cytomegalovirus infection, airway ischaemia and HLA mismatching may also play a part.[1,4,5,8] The syndrome is often refractory to immunosuppressants[1,2] and the prognosis is poor, with 40% mortality within 3 years of diagnosis.[5]

Sirolimus, everolimus, and the induction of donor-specific tolerance are under investigation in human lung transplantation.[1,2,4] However, cases of fatal bronchial anastomotic dehiscence have been reported with the use of sirolimus in immunosuppressive regimens in lung transplant recipients.


1. Arcasoy SM, Kotloff RM. Lung transplantation. *N Engl J Med* 1999; **340:** 1081–91.
2. van den Berg JWK, *et al.* New immunosuppressive drugs and lung transplantation: last or least? *Thorax* 1999; **54:** 550–3.
3. Alexander BD, Tapson VF. Infectious complications of lung transplantation. *Transpl Infect Dis* 2001; **3:** 128–37.
4. Estenne M, Hertz MI. Bronchiolitis obliterans after human lung transplantation. *Am J Respir Crit Care Med* 2002; **166:** 440–4.
5. DeMeo DL, Ginns LC. Clinical status of lung transplantation. *Transplantation* 2001; **72:** 1713–24.
6. Knoop C, *et al.* Immunosuppressive therapy after human lung transplantation. *Eur Respir J* 2004; **23:** 159–71.
7. Brock MV, *et al.* Induction therapy in lung transplantation: a prospective, controlled clinical trial comparing OKT3, anti-thymocyte globulin, and daclizumab. *J Heart Lung Transplant* 2001; **20:** 1282–90.
8. Sharples LD, *et al.* Risk factors for bronchiolitis obliterans: a systematic review of recent publications. *J Heart Lung Transplant* 2002; **21:** 271–81.


**Pancreatic transplantation.** Transplantation of the pancreas may be considered in some diabetic patients. In the vast majority of cases, pancreatic grafts have been transplanted together with a kidney in patients with end-stage diabetic nephropathy, which has produced better graft survival than transplanting the pancreas alone.[1-3] However, pancreas transplants after renal allografting, or solitary pancreatic transplantation, are becoming more common,[3] and approaching comparable survival rates.[2,4] Advances in surgical and preservation techniques, together with new immunosuppressants, have helped to improve survival.[1,5] Overall patient survival in the USA has been estimated to be 92% at 1 year and 81% at 5 years, with graft survival of 76% and 61% at 1 and 5 years, respectively.[5]

The pancreas is a highly immunogenic organ, so extensive immunosuppression is required. Standard treatment often consists of quadruple therapy.[2] Antilymphocyte immunoglobulins, basiliximab, daclizumab, or muromonab-CD3 are used as induction therapy, followed by maintenance therapy with a calcineurin inhibitor (ciclosporin or tacrolimus), corticosteroids, and azathioprine or mycophenolate mofetil.[2] Tacrolimus is increasingly preferred to ciclosporin as it appears to allow for rapid tapering of corticosteroids and less rejection.[2-4] However, if the regimen also includes mycophenolate mofetil, which is now preferred to azathioprine,[2] there appears to be little difference in the incidence of rejection between tacrolimus and ciclosporin microemulsion.[2,5] Although the precise role of sirolimus in pancreatic transplantation has yet to be defined, it may be used as an adjunctive immunosuppressant to allow for lower doses of tacrolimus and improve renal function.[2] Episodes of rejection are treated with corticosteroids or antilymphocyte immunoglobulins.[2] Conversion to tacrolimus from ciclosporin is used, and for those patients on tacrolimus, sirolimus has been tried.[2]

Pancreatic transplantation facilitates normal carbohydrate metabolism and has the potential to improve patient survival and reduce the incidence of diabetic nephropathy. However, there has been concern over the long-term effects of immunosuppression,[5,6] and whether islet-cell autoantibodies might produce diabetes in the transplanted graft (although this is certainly not inevitable with adequate immunosuppression).[5] One possible alternative to complete pancreatic transplantation is an *islet-cell* graft. These have rarely been successful,[1] with insulin independence at 1 year[3] only in about 10% of cases. However, the use of carefully prepared islet cells from more than one donor and a modified immunosuppressant protocol[7] has produced greatly improved results. In this 'Edmonton Protocol', corticosteroids were completely avoided because of diabetogenic effects. Induction therapy with daclizumab was used, followed by maintenance with sirolimus and low-dose tacrolimus.[7] Multicentre trials of this protocol are being conducted.[8,9] See also under Diabetes Mellitus, p.324.

The induction of tolerance[3,6,8] and the possibility of neogenesis of beta cells from pancreatic stem or precursor cells[6,8,10] remain the ultimate challenge in islet transplantation.


1. Robertson RP, *et al.* Pancreas and islet transplantation for patients with diabetes. *Diabetes Care* 2000; **23:** 112–16.
2. Odorico JS, Sollinger HW. Technical and immunosuppressive advances in transplantation for insulin-dependent diabetes mellitus. *World J Surg* 2002; **26:** 194–211.
3. Bottino R, *et al.* Pancreas and islet cell transplantation. *Best Pract Res Clin Gastroenterol* 2002; **16:** 457–74.
4. Sutherland DER, *et al.* Lessons learned from more than 1,000 pancreas transplants at a single institution. *Ann Surg* 2001; **233:** 463–501.
5. Stratta RJ. Review of immunosuppressive usage in pancreas transplantation. *Clin Transplant* 1999; **13:** 1–12.
6. Pipeleers D, *et al.* A view on beta cell transplantation in diabetes. *Ann N Y Acad Sci* 2002; **958:** 69–76.
7. Shapiro AMJ, *et al.* Islet transplantation in seven patients with type 1 diabetes mellitus using a glucocorticoid-free immunosuppressive regimen. *N Engl J Med* 2000; **343:** 230–8.
8. Shapiro AMJ, *et al.* Pancreatic islet transplantation in the treatment of diabetes mellitus. *Best Pract Res Clin Endocrinol Metab* 2001; **15:** 241–64.
9. Robertson RP. Islet transplantation as a treatment for diabetes—a work in progress. *N Engl J Med* 2004; **350:** 694–705.
10. García-Ocaña A, *et al.* Using β-cell growth factors to enhance human pancreatic islet transplantation. *J Clin Endocrinol Metab* 2001; **86:** 984–8.


### Renal disorders

Corticosteroids and immunosuppressants are commonly used in the treatment of glomerular kidney disease (p.1080).

### Rheumatoid arthritis

Disease-modifying antirheumatic drugs (DMARDs) including immunosuppressants may be given to patients with rheumatoid arthritis (p.9) in an attempt to modify the course of the disease. The most widely used immunosuppressant is probably low-dose methotrexate which produces clear short-term clinical benefits. Ciclosporin also appears to be effective, but adverse effects have been a problem. The use of low-dose regimens may help to minimise nephrotoxicity. Use of ciclosporin with methotrexate has produced clinical improvement in patients who had only partial responses to methotrexate alone, but some investigators found that a combination of methotrexate, ciclosporin and intra-articular corticosteroids was no more effective than standard DMARD therapy.

The role of other immunosuppressants in rheumatoid arthritis is more debatable. Azathioprine has been used, with beneficial short-term effects, but is reported to be no more effective than other DMARDs and significantly more toxic; it may however be useful with prednisone in rheumatoid vasculitis. Mycophenolate mofetil and tacrolimus may be effective in rheumatoid arthritis, but further studies are needed.

References.


1. Drosos AA. Newer immunosuppressive drugs: their potential role in rheumatoid arthritis therapy. *Drugs* 2002; **62:** 891–907.


### Sarcoidosis

Where drug therapy is required for sarcoidosis (p.1087), corticosteroids are the usual treatment. In patients in whom these are ineffective or poorly tolerated, immunosuppressants have been given, with variable results.

### Scleroderma

The term scleroderma has been used for both systemic sclerosis, a multisystem disease characterised by collagen proliferation and fibrosis throughout the body, and for localised fibrotic changes of the skin (morphea) without involvement of other organs. Systemic sclerosis is an uncommon disease which has been linked to various environmental toxins as well as to genetic factors. Vascular involvement produces Raynaud's syndrome, which usually precedes any skin changes, and there may be ulceration or ischaemic changes of the digits. A long history of Raynaud's syndrome before skin changes occur suggests a more indolent course (limited cutaneous disease) as opposed to the more aggressive diffuse cutaneous form. Skin oedema is followed by thickening and tightening of the skin of hands and face, and sometimes limbs and trunk, before progressing to atrophy and contractures. There may be decreased gastrointestinal motility, dysphagia and gastro-oesophageal reflux, arthritis, muscle weakness, and cardiac involvement. Among the most serious potential symptoms, which may result in death, are pulmonary disease and renal failure with malignant hypertension.

There is a paucity of adequately controlled trials for scleroderma; no treatment has been clearly demonstrated to affect the progression of the disease, and much management is essentially symptomatic. Immunosuppressants are probably appropriate in the early oedematous stages of diffuse scleroderma.[1,2] Antilymphocyte immunoglobulins have been tried as an induction therapy in early stages of the disease.[1] Ciclosporin has been found to be beneficial, both for skin and visceral manifestations, but its use has been limited by nephrotoxicity and hypertension.[1-3] Tacrolimus has also been tried, though again adverse effects limit its benefit,[1,3] and mycophenolate mofetil is under investigation.[2] Other novel immunosuppressive strategies include bone marrow ablation followed by peripheral blood stem cell transplantation,[1,2] photopheresis with a psoralen, and the induction of oral tolerance with native bovine type I collagen.[1]

Penicillamine has been widely used as an antifibrotic drug, but with variable effects, and there appears to be no benefit in using high doses.[1,2] Interferons alfa and gamma showed promising results in early trials, but larger scale studies have failed to confirm any benefit.[1] Some other drugs are being investigated for their antifibrotic properties, including halofuginone, minocycline and relaxin.[1] There is some evidence that oxidative stress is involved in the pathogenesis of scleroderma, so antoxidants like probucol may also be useful.[1] Other drugs that have been investigated include potassium aminobenzoate, sulfasalazine, and thymopentin.

Many patients will require therapy for organ-specific symptoms. Skin flexibility may be maintained by emollients,[4] and systemic antihistamines can relieve itching, an early feature of diffuse cutaneous scleroderma.[1] Methotrexate has been used with some benefit.[1,2] Treatment of Raynaud's syndrome (p.833) may involve vasodilators such as the calcium-channel blockers, nifedipine and diltiazem.[2,4] Topical nitrates have been used in acute situations,[2] and intravenous prostacyclin analogues such as epoprostenol and iloprost are used in severe attacks.[1,2] Calcitonin gene-related peptide is being investigated as an alternative to iloprost.[2] Because elevated levels of serotonin have been found in patients with Raynaud's phenomenon, SSRIs and ketanserin have been used.[2] Dietary supplementation with antoxidant vitamins, fish oils, and evening primrose oil has been of anecdotal benefit.[1,2] ACE inhibitors have substantially improved the prognosis for patients with renal scleroderma, but over 30% of patients will still require renal replacement therapy.[1] Lung fibrosis is treated with cyclophosphamide, usually with prednisolone, while calcium-channel blockers, ACE inhibitors, and intravenous iloprost may be used for pulmonary hypertension.[1,2] Proton pump inhibitors such as omeprazole, sometimes with prokinetic drugs, are extremely effective for oesophageal involvement, and broad spectrum antibiotics are helpful for small bowel bacterial overgrowth.[1,2] Cardiac involvement may be underdiagnosed;[1] ACE inhibitors or digoxin may be used.[2]

NSAIDs and corticosteroids must be used with care in scleroderma because of the risk of exacerbating renal and other problems.[1,2]


1. Denton CP, Black CM. Scleroderma and related disorders: therapeutic aspects. *Baillieres Best Pract Res Clin Rheumatol* 2000; **14:** 17–35.
2. Leighton C. Drug treatment of scleroderma. *Drugs* 2001; **61:** 419–27.
3. Morton SJ, Powell RJ. Cyclosporin and tacrolimus: their use in a routine clinical setting for scleroderma. *Rheumatology (Oxford)* 2000; **39:** 865–9.
4. Sontheimer RD. Skin manifestations of systemic autoimmune connective tissue disease: diagnostics and therapeutics. *Best Pract Res Clin Rheumatol* 2004; **18:** 429–62.


### Skin and connective tissue disorders

Immunosuppressants are used in various skin and connective tissue disorders, including Behçet's syndrome (p.1076), eczema (p.1135), pemphigus and pemphigoid (p.1137), polymyositis (p.1086), psoriasis (p.1137), systemic lupus erythematosus (p.1088), and the various vasculitic syndromes (p.1090). See also Scleroderma, above.

---

## Abetimus Sodium *(USAN, rINNM)*

LJP-394.

*CAS — 169147-32-4.*

### Profile

Abetimus sodium is an immunomodulator that arrests the production of antibodies to double-stranded DNA and is under investigation for the treatment of lupus nephritis.

◊ References.


1. Furie RA, *et al.* Treatment of systemic lupus erythematosus with LJP 394. *J Rheumatol* 2001; **28:** 257–65.


---

## Antilymphocyte Immunoglobulins

Inmunoglobulinas antilinfocitarias.

**Description.** Antilymphocyte immunoglobulins are polyclonal antibodies to human lymphocytes produced by the purification of sera from appropriately immunised animals. The term antilymphocyte immunoglobulin (ALG; lymphocyte immune globulin) implies a product raised against all lymphocyte subsets. The term antithymocyte immunoglobulin (antithymocyte gammaglobulin; antithymocyte globulin; ATG) implies specificity for T-cells (thymus lymphocytes or thymocytes). However, in practice the nomenclature does not seem to be used consistently, and both terms tend to be used for antibodies raised against T-cells. Nomenclature normally includes an indication of the animal source of the immunoglobulin e.g. antithymocyte immunoglobulin (horse), or antithymocyte immunoglobulin (rabbit).

In addition to the purified immunoglobulins the native sera (antilymphocyte serum and antithymocyte serum, sometimes referred to as lymphocytic antiserum and thymitic antiserum) have also been used as immunosuppressants.

**Pharmacopoeias.** *Eur.* (see p.vi) includes an anti-T lymphocyte immunoglobulin.

**Ph. Eur. 5.0** (Anti-T Lymphocyte Immunoglobulin for Human Use, Animal; Immunoglobulinum Anti-T Lymphocytorum ex Animale ad Usum Humanum). A liquid or freeze-dried preparation containing immunoglobulins, obtained from serum or plasma of animals, mainly rabbits or horses, immunised with human lymphocytic antigens. It has the property of diminishing the number and function of immunocompetent cells, in particular T-lymphocytes. It contains principally immunoglobulin G, and may contain antibodies against other lymphocyte subpopulations and against other cells. It is intended for intravenous administration, after dilution with a suitable diluent where applicable. Protect from light.

### Adverse Effects and Precautions

Common adverse reactions to antilymphocyte immunoglobulins include fever, chills, and skin reactions including rash, pruritus, and urticaria, which may be manifestations of hypersensitivity. Dyspnoea, hypotension, chest, back or flank pain may indicate anaphylaxis, which can occur in up to 1% of patients. Rashes and arthralgia may represent serum sickness, especially in patients with aplastic anaemia. Use with other immunosuppressants may reduce the incidence or severity of hypersensitivity but increase the risk of acquired systemic infections, such as cytomegalovirus or herpes simplex. Enhanced immunosuppression may also increase the incidence of post-transplant lymphoproliferative disease or other malignancies.

Leucopenia and thrombocytopenia are also common. Although usually transient, dosage adjustment may be necessary if they become severe or prolonged, and if unremitting, they may warrant stopping therapy. Other adverse effects include headache, abdominal pain, gastrointestinal disturbances, hypertension, peripheral oedema, asthenia, hyperkalaemia, and tachycardia. Nephrotoxicity has been reported.

Intra-uterine contraceptive devices should be used with caution during immunosuppressive treatment as there is an increased risk of infection. Use of live vaccines should generally be avoided for the same reason. Thrombophlebitis may be avoided by infusion into a vein with a rapid blood flow. To identify those at risk of anaphylaxis, patients should be tested for skin sensitivity before infusion. Facilities for management of anaphylaxis (see p.855) should be available during treatment, and the patient should be observed continuously.

### Uses and Administration

Antilymphocyte immunoglobulins are antibodies, raised in *animals*, which act against lymphocytes, and in particular against T-cells, to produce suppression of cell-mediated immunity.

They may be added to existing immunosuppressant regimens to treat acute rejection episodes in patients who have undergone organ or tissue transplantation. Alternatively, they may be given prophylactically as part of a combination immunosuppressant regimen with several other agents. For discussion of the role of antilymphocyte immunoglobulins in transplantation, see p.1344 *et seq.*

Antilymphocyte immunoglobulins are also used in the treatment of aplastic anaemia (p.732) in patients unsuitable for bone marrow transplantation, and have been tried in other immunological disorders. They are under investigation for the treatment of myelodysplastic syndromes (p.508).

Different antilymphocyte preparations may vary in their activity, as may different lots of the same preparation. However, daily doses in transplantation have usually ranged from 10 to 30 mg/kg of **equine** immunoglobulin, or 1.5 mg/kg of **rabbit** immunoglobulin. Doses are given as a slow intravenous infusion diluted in sodium chloride 0.9%, or other suitable diluent. It has been recommended that the final dilution should contain no more than 1 mg/mL of immunoglobulin and be given over 4 hours or more, via an in-line filter.

**Organ and tissue transplantation.** Antithymocyte immunoglobulin derived from *rabbits* has been found to be more effective than the equine product in preventing renal graft rejection.[1] In bone marrow transplant recipients, those given rabbit antilymphocyte immunoglobulin prior to an unrelated donor (UD) transplant had comparable outcomes to those given matched related donor (MRD) transplants but no antilymphocyte immunoglobulin; the authors supposed that the use of antilymphocyte immunoglobulin caused UD recipients to behave clinically like MRD recipients.[2]


1. Gaber AO, *et al.* Results of the double-blind, randomized, multicenter, phase III clinical trial of Thymoglobulin versus Atgam in the treatment of acute graft rejection episodes after renal transplantation. *Transplantation* 1998; **66:** 29–37.
2. Duggan P, *et al.* Unrelated donor BMT recipients given pretransplant low-dose antithymocyte globulin have outcomes equivalent to matched sibling BMT: a matched pair analysis. *Bone Marrow Transplant* 2002; **30:** 681–6.


## Preparations

**Ph. Eur.:** Anti-T Lymphocyte Immunoglobulin for Human Use, Animal.

**Proprietary Preparations** (details are given in Part 3)

***Arg.:*** Apasmil; Linfoglobulina; Timoglobulina; ***Austral.:*** Atgam; ***Belg.:*** ATG†; Atgam†; Lymphoglobuline†; Thymoglobuline†; ***Braz.:*** Gat Globulina Antitimocitaria†; Lymphoglobuline; Thymoglobuline; ***Canad.:*** Atgam; ***Chile:*** Linfoglobulina; Timoglobulina; ***Denm.:*** Thymoglobuline; ***Fr.:*** Lymphoglobuline; Thymoglobuline; ***Ger.:*** Lymphoglobulin; Tecelac; Thymoglobulin; ***Gr.:*** Lymphoglobulin; Thymoglobulin; ***Hong Kong:*** ATG; Atgam; Lymphoglobuline†; Thymoglobuline†; ***Israel:*** ATG-S; Atgam†; Lymphoglobuline; Thymoglobuline; ***Ital.:*** Lymphoglobuline; Thymoglobuline; Uman-Gal E†; ***Malaysia:*** Atgam; ***Mex.:*** Atgam; ***Neth.:*** Lymphoglobuline; Thymoglobuline; ***NZ:*** Atgam; ***S.Afr.:*** Atgam; Lymphoglobuline; Thymoglobuline; ***Singapore:*** ATG; Atgam; Lymphoglobuline; Thymoglobuline; ***Spain:*** Atege; Atgam; Linfoglobulina; Timoglobulina; ***Switz.:*** ATG; Atgam; Lymphoglobuline; Thymoglobuline; ***Thai.:*** ATG; Lymphoglobuline; Thymoglobuline; ***USA:*** Atgam.

# Azathioprine *(BAN, USAN, rINN)*

Azathioprinum; Azatioprina; BW-57322; NSC-39084. 6-(1-Methyl-4-nitroimidazol-5-ylthio)purine.

$C_9H_7N_7O_2S$ = 277.3.

*CAS — 446-86-6.*

*ATC — L04AX01.*

NOTE. The abbreviation AZT, which has sometimes been used for azathioprine, has also been used to denote the antiviral zidovudine.

**Pharmacopoeias.** In *Chin., Eur.* (see p.vi), *Int., Jpn, Pol.,* and *US.*

**Ph. Eur. 5.0** (Azathioprine). A pale yellow powder. Practically insoluble in water and in alcohol; soluble in dilute solutions of alkali hydroxides; sparingly soluble in dilute mineral acids. Protect from light.

**USP 27** (Azathioprine). A pale yellow, odourless powder. Insoluble in water; very slightly soluble in alcohol and in chloroform; sparingly soluble in dilute mineral acids; soluble in dilute solutions of alkali hydroxides. Store in airtight containers. Protect from light.

## Adverse Effects

Dose-related bone-marrow depression may be manifested as leucopenia or, less often, thrombocytopenia or anaemia, and may occasionally be delayed. Macrocytic, including megaloblastic, anaemia has occurred. Azathioprine has also been associated with the development of liver damage; it has been suggested that cholestatic symptoms may be due to the mercaptopurine moiety. Rarely, delayed and potentially fatal veno-occlusive liver disease has occurred.

Other side-effects associated with azathioprine include gastrointestinal disturbances, reversible alopecia, and symptoms including rashes, muscle and joint pains, fever, rigors, pneumonitis, pancreatitis, tachycardia, renal dysfunction, and hypotension, some or all of which may represent hypersensitivity reactions.

Solutions for injection are irritant.

◊ References.


1. Lawson DH, *et al.* Adverse effects of azathioprine. *Adverse Drug React Acute Poisoning Rev* 1984; **3:** 161–71.


**Carcinogenicity.** Immunosuppression, including that with azathioprine, may be associated with an increased risk of certain neoplasms such as lymphomas and skin cancers in transplant recipients[1] and in patients with rheumatoid arthritis.[2,3] Rheumatic diseases may themselves be associated with an increased risk of malignancy that is independent of treatment, but one study[3] concluded that there is a further risk related to the duration of exposure to immunosuppressive drugs, including azathioprine. Conversely, a study in 755 patients given azathioprine for inflammatory bowel disease and followed for up to 29 years failed to show any increased risk of neoplasia.[4]

Skin cancer may be a particular risk in immunosuppressed patients with a history of high sun exposure.[5] A synergistic clastogenic effect has been noted with azathioprine and long-wave ultraviolet light.


1. Kinlen LJ, *et al.* Collaborative United Kingdom-Australasian study of cancer in patients treated with immunosuppressive drugs. *BMJ* 1979; **2:** 1461–6.
2. Silman AJ, *et al.* Lymphoproliferative cancer and other malignancy in patients with rheumatoid arthritis treated with azathioprine: a 20 year follow up study. *Ann Rheum Dis* 1988; **47:** 988–92.
3. Asten P, *et al.* Risk of developing certain malignancies is related to duration of immunosuppressive drug exposure in patients with rheumatic diseases. *J Rheumatol* 1999; **26:** 1705–14.
4. Connell WR, *et al.* Long-term neoplasia risk after azathioprine treatment in inflammatory bowel disease. *Lancet* 1994, **343:** 1249–52.
5. Boyle J, *et al.* Cancer, warts, and sunshine in renal transplant patients: a case-control study. *Lancet* 1984; **i:** 702–5.


**Effects on the blood.** Neutropenia in patients receiving mercaptopurine has been reported to correlate negatively with the concentration of the metabolite tioguanine nucleotide in erythrocytes,[1] and it has been suggested that measurement of metabolite concentrations in erythrocytes,[2] or activity of the enzyme thiopurine methyltransferase (TPMT),[3-6] permits prediction of those individuals likely to experience severe bone-marrow toxicity with mercaptopurine and the related drugs tioguanine and azathioprine. However, not all studies have found such correlations,[7] and effects on the bone marrow with this class of drugs are probably multifactorial;[8,9] low activity of other enzymes such as lymphocyte 5-nucleotidase,[10] and other factors, may contribute to toxicity. A review[9] of studies investigating TPMT activity in patients with Crohn's disease concluded that measurement of TPMT activity at initiation of azathioprine treatment has a role in identifying those at risk of severe myelosuppression. Lower TPMT activities correlate with low neutrophil counts in the initial 4 months of thiopurine therapy; identification of the heterozygote might allow for safer management (see Therapeutic Drug Monitoring, below). However, in those patients established on therapy, TPMT did not predict clinical response or toxicity.


1. Lennard L, *et al.* Childhood leukaemia: a relationship between intracellular 6-mercaptopurine metabolites and neutropenia. *Br J Clin Pharmacol* 1983; **16:** 359–63.
2. Maddocks JL, *et al.* Azathioprine and severe bone marrow depression. *Lancet* 1986; **i:** 156.
3. Schütz E, *et al.* Azathioprine-induced myelosuppression in thiopurine methyltransferase deficient heart transplant recipient. *Lancet* 1993; **341:** 436.
4. Lennard L, *et al.* Congenital thiopurine methyltransferase deficiency and 6-mercaptopurine toxicity during treatment for acute lymphoblastic leukaemia. *Arch Dis Child* 1993; **69:** 577–9.
5. Jackson AP, *et al.* Thiopurine methyltransferase levels should be measured before commencing patients on azathioprine. *Br J Dermatol* 1997; **136:** 133–4.
6. Black AJ, *et al.* Thiopurine methyltransferase genotype predicts therapy-limiting severe toxicity from azathioprine. *Ann Intern Med* 1998; **129:** 716–18.
7. Boulieu R, *et al.* Intracellular thiopurine nucleotides and azathioprine myelotoxicity in organ transplant patients. *Br J Clin Pharmacol* 1997; **43:** 116–18.
8. Soria-Royer C, *et al.* Thiopurine-methyl-transferase activity to assess azathioprine myelotoxicity in renal transplant recipients. *Lancet* 1993; **341:** 1593–4.
9. Lennard L. TPMT in the treatment of Crohn's disease with azathioprine. *Gut* 2002; **51:** 143–6.
10. Kerstens PJSM, *et al.* 5-Nucleotidase and azathioprine-related bone-marrow toxicity. *Lancet* 1993; **342:** 1245–6.


**Effects on the liver.** A review[1] of drug-related hepatotoxicity noted that azathioprine has been associated with hepatocanalicular cholestasis, in which the interference with bile flow is combined with hepatocyte damage, and with several hepatic vascular disorders, including focal sinusoidal dilatation, peliosis, and veno-occlusive disease. A later review[2] grouped reported cases into three syndromes: hypersensitivity, idiosyncratic cholestatic reaction, and presumed endothelial cell injury, with the imidazole and 6-mercaptopurine components of azathioprine playing different roles in pathogenesis.


1. Sherlock S. The spectrum of hepatotoxicity due to drugs. *Lancet* 1986; **ii:** 440–4.
2. Romagnuolo J, *et al.* Cholestatic hepatocellular injury with azathioprine: a case report and review of the mechanisms of hepatotoxicity. *Can J Gastroenterol* 1998; **12:** 479–83.


**Hypersensitivity.** In 2 of 5 renal transplant recipients with acute allergic reactions associated with azathioprine, the symptoms (interstitial nephritis) were initially mistaken for acute rejection episodes.[1] In another report,[2] shock, fever, and acute renal insufficiency in a patient led to an initial mistaken diagnosis of sepsis, and it was recommended that a hypersensitivity reaction be considered as a cause if any of these symptoms occurred within 4 weeks of azathioprine ingestion.


1. Parnham AP, *et al.* Acute allergic reactions associated with azathioprine. *Lancet* 1996; **348:** 542–3.
2. Fields CL, *et al.* Hypersensitivity reaction to azathioprine. *South Med J* 1998; **91:** 471–4.


## Precautions

Regular monitoring of blood counts is required. Patients with renal or hepatic impairment require more frequent monitoring of blood counts and reduced doses; liver function tests should be performed in hepatic impairment. Intra-uterine devices should be used with caution during immunosuppressive treatment as there is an increased risk of infection. Use of live vaccines should be avoided for the same reason. Azathioprine should generally be avoided in pregnancy (see below).

**Breast feeding.** Low concentrations of mercaptopurine have been found in human colostrum and breast milk of patients taking azathioprine.[1] Breast feeding by these patients has not been recommended because of the potential risk of immunosuppression in the infant.[1,2] However, there are reports[1,2] of 3 breast-fed infants, whose mothers had been taking doses of 75 or 100 mg of azathioprine daily, in whom no evidence of immunosuppression was found. All 3 had normal blood counts, no increase in infections, and above average growth rate. In one case, the levels of mercaptopurine were determined at 2 days and after 2 weeks of breast feeding,[1] and in the other 2 cases, no levels were determined.[2]


1. Coulam CB, *et al.* Breast-feeding after renal transplantation. *Transplant Proc* 1982; **14:** 605–9.
2. Grekas DM, *et al.* Immunosuppressive therapy and breast-feeding after renal transplantation. *Nephron* 1984; **37:** 68.


**Pregnancy.** Despite reports of chromosomal aberrations[1] or fetal growth retardation[2] in the offspring of mothers who received azathioprine during pregnancy, there seems to be little evidence that azathioprine is teratogenic in humans.[1,3-5] Given the nature of the severe chronic conditions for which azathioprine is generally used, discontinuing therapy in patients who become pregnant may not be necessary or desirable, but it seems prudent to avoid its use where possible during pregnancy. Leucopenia has been reported in neonates whose mothers received azathioprine during pregnancy.[6]


1. The Registration Committee of the European Dialysis and Transplant Association. Successful pregnancies in women treated by dialysis and kidney transplantation. *Br J Obstet Gynaecol* 1980; **87:** 839–45.
2. Pirson Y, *et al.* Retardation of fetal growth in patients receiving immunosuppressive therapy. *N Engl J Med* 1985; **313:** 328.
3. Hou S. Retardation of fetal growth in patients receiving immunosuppressive therapy. *N Engl J Med* 1985; **313:** 328.
4. Whittle MJ, Hanretty KP. Prescribing in pregnancy: identifying abnormalities. *BMJ* 1986; **293:** 1485–8.
5. Alstead EM, *et al.* Safety of azathioprine in pregnancy in inflammatory bowel disease. *Gastroenterology* 1990; **99:** 443–6.
6. Davison JM, *et al.* Maternal azathioprine therapy and depressed haemopoiesis in the babies of renal allograft patients. *Br J Obstet Gynaecol* 1985; **92:** 233–9.


## Interactions

The effects of azathioprine are enhanced by allopurinol and the dose of azathioprine should be reduced to one-third to one-quarter of the usual dose when allopurinol is given.

◊ In addition to being affected by allopurinol, azathioprine may itself affect other drugs including the following:

- competitive neuromuscular blockers (antagonism, see under Immunosuppressants on p.1401)
- vaccines (reduced response or generalised infection, see p.1606)
- warfarin (inhibition, see Immunosuppressants p.1027).

**Gastrointestinal drugs.** For mention of *5-aminosalicylates* inhibiting the metabolism of thiopurines such as azathioprine, and increasing their toxicity, see Mercaptopurine, p.567.

## Pharmacokinetics

Azathioprine is well absorbed from the gastrointestinal tract when given by mouth. After oral or intravenous doses it disappears rapidly from the circulation and is extensively metabolised to mercaptopurine (which is then further metabolised—see p.568). Both azathioprine and mercaptopurine are about 30% bound to plasma proteins. About 10% of a dose of azathioprine is reported to be split between the sulfur and the purine ring to give 1-methyl-4-nitro-5-thioimidazole. The proportion of different metabolites is reported to vary between patients. Metabolites and small amounts of unchanged azathioprine and mercaptopurine are eliminated in the urine. Azathioprine is distributed into breast milk in low concentrations.

**Therapeutic drug monitoring.** Although plasma concentrations of 6-thiouric acid (the inactive product of mercaptopurine, and hence of azathioprine) can be readily measured in patients who have been receiving azathioprine, they are of little value in therapeutic drug monitoring.[1] The active moieties are the tioguanine nucleotides (6-TGN) formed intracellularly, which appear to have extremely long half-lives,[2] and mean erythrocyte concentrations of which appear to vary considerably between individuals.[2] The formation of other inactive metabolites is catalysed by thiopurine methyltransferase (TPMT) and its activity is genetically determined, with a trimodal distribution in the general population; 0.3% have low activity of TPMT, 11% have intermediate activity, and 89% have normal or high activity. Patients with low or intermediate activity appear to shift metabolism toward production of 6-TGN. Because excess concentrations of 6-TGN have been associated with leucopenia, it has been suggested[3] that patients with normal or high TPMT activity receive standard doses of azathioprine or mercaptopurine, those with intermediate TPMT activity have reduced doses, and those with low activity not be treated with either drug (but see Effects on the Blood, above). Because low concentrations of erythrocyte 6-TGN have been associated with disease relapse in lymphomas and leukaemias, a small study[4] of patients with inflammatory bowel disease attempted to define a therapeutic window of drug efficacy. Without monitoring TPMT genotype, treatment efficacy was found to correlate with erythrocyte 6-TGN levels. It was concluded that patients who remain symptomatic despite apparently therapeutic 6-TGN concentrations should be treated with adjunctive or alternative immunosuppression or surgery. However, a large study[5] did not confirm disease correlation with 6-TGN concentrations, and concluded that therapeutic drug monitoring of 6-TGN may be premature. It was noted that methodological differences, such as assay technique, existed between their study and others. As the role of routine monitoring of 6-TGN remains controversial,[6,7] it has been suggested that selective monitoring, such as in those with low or intermediate TPMT activity, be considered.[3]


1. Chan GLC, *et al.* Pharmacokinetics of 6-thiouric acid and 6-mercaptopurine in renal allograft recipients after oral administration of azathioprine. *Eur J Clin Pharmacol* 1989; **36:** 265–71.
2. Chan GLC, *et al.* Azathioprine metabolism: pharmacokinetics of 6-mercaptopurine, 6-thiouric acid and 6-thioguanine nucleotides in renal transplant patients. *J Clin Pharmacol* 1990; **30:** 358–63.
3. Sandborn WJ. Rational dosing of azathioprine and 6-mercaptopurine. *Gut* 2001; **48:** 591–2.
4. Cuffari C, *et al.* Utilisation of erythrocyte 6-thioguanine metabolite levels to optimise azathioprine therapy in patients with inflammatory bowel disease. *Gut* 2001; **48:** 642–6.
5. Lowry PW, *et al.* Measurement of thiopurine methyltransferase activity and azathioprine metabolites in patients with inflammatory bowel disease. *Gut* 2001; **49:** 665–70.
6. Dubinsky MC. Monitoring of AZA/6-MP treatment in children with IBD is necessary. *Inflamm Bowel Dis* 2003; **9:** 386–8.
7. Griffiths AM. Monitoring of azathioprine/6-mercaptopurine treatment in children with IBD is not necessary. *Inflamm Bowel Dis* 2003; **9:** 389–91.


## Uses and Administration

Azathioprine is an immunosuppressive antimetabolite with similar actions to those of mercaptopurine (p.567), to which it is converted in the body. Its effects may not be seen for several weeks after a dose. It is given by mouth, but in patients in whom oral use is not feasible it may be given by slow intravenous injection or by infusion as azathioprine sodium.

Azathioprine is mainly used as an immunosuppressant for the prevention of rejection in **organ and tissue transplantation** (p.1344). The dose for this purpose varies from 1 to 5 mg/kg daily and depends partly on the regimen employed; the higher doses are used initially, adjusted according to clinical response and haematological tolerance.

Azathioprine is also used in **auto-immune diseases** or conditions that are considered to have an auto-immune component, see below. The usual dose of azathioprine in these conditions is in the range of 1 to 3 mg/kg daily by mouth.

Use of azathioprine with a corticosteroid (p.1073) may have a corticosteroid-sparing effect.

Blood counts should be carried out regularly during treatment and azathioprine withdrawn or the dosage reduced at the first indication of bone-marrow depression.

**Blood disorders.** Immunosuppressants such as azathioprine are occasionally tried in auto-immune haemolytic anaemia (p.733) refractory to other treatment and may permit reduction of corticosteroid dosage. Similarly in patients with idiopathic thrombocytopenic purpura (p.1082), immunosuppressants may be tried as a last resort.

**Cogan's syndrome.** Azathioprine has been used with corticosteroids for severe Cogan's syndrome with large-vessel vasculitis (see p.1078).

**Connective tissue and muscular disorders.** Azathioprine is one of many agents tried for disease control in Behçet's syndrome[1] (p.1076) and systemic lupus erythematosus[2] (p.1088). In polymyositis (p.1086), combined therapy with azathioprine and a corticosteroid has been found to be better than a corticosteroid alone for maintenance long-term.[3] However, there is also some evidence that methotrexate may be more effective in refractory polymyositis than azathioprine.[4]


1. Yazici H, *et al.* A controlled trial of azathioprine in Behçet's syndrome. *N Engl J Med* 1990; **322:** 281–5.
2. Abu-Shakra M, Shoenfeld Y. Azathioprine therapy for patients with systemic lupus erythematosus. *Lupus* 2001; **10:** 152–3.
3. Bunch TW. Prednisone and azathioprine for polymyositis: long-term followup. *Arthritis Rheum* 1981; **24:** 45–8.
4. Joffe MM, *et al.* Drug therapy of the idiopathic inflammatory myopathies; predictors of response to prednisone, azathioprine, and methotrexate and a comparison of their efficacy. *Am J Med* 1993; **94:** 379–87.


**Inflammatory bowel disease.** Azathioprine, or its metabolite mercaptopurine, is used to induce remission in chronically active inflammatory bowel disease (p.1243), and to maintain remission, particularly in Crohn's disease.[1-4] They have a useful corticosteroid-sparing effect. In patients who have been in remission for 4 years, it may be possible to stop treatment.[5] The onset of benefit from oral azathioprine may be delayed for several months. One study[6] reported that a more rapid response could be achieved with an intravenous loading dose but a later study failed to confirm this.[7]


1. Lamers CB, *et al.* Azathioprine: an update on clinical efficacy and safety in inflammatory bowel disease. *Scand J Gastroenterol* 1999; **230** (suppl): 111–15.
2. Sandborn W, *et al.* Azathioprine or 6-mercaptopurine for induction of remission in Crohn's disease. Available in The Cochrane Library; Issue 2. Chichester: John Wiley; 2004.
3. Pearson DC, *et al.* Azathioprine for maintenance of remission in Crohn's disease. Available in The Cochrane Library; Issue 2. Chichester: John Wiley; 2004.
4. Fraser AG, *et al.* The efficacy of azathioprine for the treatment of inflammatory bowel disease: a 30 year review. *Gut* 2002; **50:** 485–9.
5. Bouhnik Y, *et al.* Long-term follow-up of patients with Crohn's disease treated with azathioprine or 6-mercaptopurine. *Lancet* 1996; **347:** 215–19.
6. Sandborn WJ, *et al.* An intravenous loading dose of azathioprine decreases the time to response in patients with Crohn's disease. *Gastroenterology* 1995; **109:** 1808–17.
7. Sandborn WJ, *et al.* Lack of effect of intravenous administration on time to respond to azathioprine for steroid-treated Crohn's disease: North American Azathioprine Study Group. *Gastroenterology* 1999; **117:** 527–35.


**Liver disorders.** Azathioprine has been widely used with corticosteroids to produce and maintain remission of chronic active hepatitis,[1-5] as discussed on p.1078, and such combination therapy, which also permits a reduction in corticosteroid dosage, is generally thought to be more effective than azathioprine alone.[1,3] Patients successfully maintained in remission for at least a year on azathioprine with a corticosteroid can subsequently be maintained on azathioprine (at a dose of 2 mg/kg daily) alone.[6] Results in patients with primary biliary cirrhosis (p.1761) have been more equivocal, and initial studies did not indicate much benefit from azathioprine,[7,8] although a later study did seem to indicate improved survival and disease retardation.[9]


1. Giusti G, *et al.* Immunosuppressive therapy in chronic active hepatitis (CAH): a multicentric retrospective study on 867 patients. *Hepatogastroenterology* 1984; **31:** 24–9.
2. Vegnente A, *et al.* Duration of chronic active hepatitis and the development of cirrhosis. *Arch Dis Child* 1984; **59:** 330–5.
3. Stellon AJ, *et al.* Randomised controlled trial of azathioprine withdrawal in autoimmune chronic active hepatitis. *Lancet* 1985; **i:** 668–70.
4. Brunner G, Hopf U. Relapse after azathioprine withdrawal in autoimmune chronic active hepatitis. *Lancet* 1985; **i:** 1216.
5. Czaja AJ. Drug therapy in the management of type 1 autoimmune hepatitis. *Drugs* 1999; **57:** 49–68.
6. Johnson PJ, *et al.* Azathioprine for long-term maintenance of remission in autoimmune hepatitis. *N Engl J Med* 1995; **333:** 958–63.
7. Heathcote J, *et al.* A prospective controlled trial of azathioprine in primary biliary cirrhosis. *Gastroenterology* 1976; **70:** 656–60.
8. Crowe J, *et al.* Azathioprine in primary biliary cirrhosis: a preliminary report of an international trial. *Gastroenterology* 1980; **78:** 1005–10.
9. Christensen E, *et al.* Beneficial effect of azathioprine and prediction of prognosis in primary biliary cirrhosis: final results of an international trial. *Gastroenterology* 1985; **89:** 1084–91.


**Lung disorders.** Although corticosteroids remain the mainstay of treatment for the various forms of diffuse parenchymal lung disease (p.1079) including cryptogenic fibrosing alveolitis (CFA), there is some evidence that combined therapy with azathioprine improves survival in the latter condition,[1] and the British Thoracic Society now recommends that initial treatment of CFA should be with oral prednisolone plus azathioprine 2 to 3 mg/kg daily.[2]


1. Raghu G, *et al.* Azathioprine combined with prednisone in the treatment of idiopathic pulmonary fibrosis: a prospective double-blind, randomized, placebo-controlled clinical trial. *Am Rev Respir Dis* 1991; **144:** 291–6.
2. British Thoracic Society. The diagnosis, assessment and treatment of diffuse parenchymal lung disease in adults. *Thorax* 1999; **54** (suppl 1): S1–S30. Also available at: http://www.brit-thoracic.org.uk/docs/Parenchymaltext.pdf (accessed 17/05/04)


**Neuromuscular disorders.** Azathioprine may be used for its corticosteroid-sparing properties[1,2] in patients who require corticosteroid treatment for myasthenia gravis (p.1486). It may also be of use when corticosteroids are contra-indicated or when response to corticosteroids alone is insufficient.[3] Azathioprine is not usually used alone because it may be several months before any beneficial effect is seen. Studies have also indicated modest benefit from azathioprine[4,5] in patients with multiple sclerosis (p.646). It has been suggested that the benefits are too slight to justify the toxicity of the required doses,[6] but it has also been pointed out that in terms of relapse reduction azathioprine appears as effective as newer treatments such as interferon beta.[7]


1. Mantegazza R, *et al.* Azathioprine as a single drug or in combination with steroids in the treatment of myasthenia gravis. *J Neurol* 1988; **235:** 449–53.
2. Palace J, *et al.* A randomized double-blind trial of prednisolone alone or with azathioprine in myasthenia gravis. *Neurology* 1998; **50:** 1778–83.
3. Gajdos P, *et al.* Myasthenia Gravis Clinical Study Group. A randomised clinical trial comparing prednisone and azathioprine in myasthenia gravis: results of the second interim analysis. *J Neurol Neurosurg Psychiatry* 1993; **56:** 1157–63.
4. British and Dutch Multiple Sclerosis Azathioprine Trial Group. Double-masked trial of azathioprine in multiple sclerosis. *Lancet* 1988; **ii:** 179–83.
5. Ellison GW, *et al.* A placebo-controlled, randomized, double-masked, variable dosage, clinical trial of azathioprine with and without methylprednisolone in multiple sclerosis. *Neurology* 1989; **39:** 1018–26.
6. Yudkin PL, *et al.* Overview of azathioprine treatment in multiple sclerosis. *Lancet* 1991; **338:** 1051–5.
7. Palace J, Rothwell P. New treatments and azathioprine in multiple sclerosis. *Lancet* 1997; **350:** 261.


**Ocular disorders.** For mention of the use of azathioprine in various disorders characterised by ocular lesions such as scleritis or uveitis, see p.1344.

**Polymyalgia rheumatica.** Azathioprine may be used for its corticosteroid-sparing properties in patients who require corticosteroid treatment for polymyalgia rheumatica (p.1086) and in whom withdrawal is difficult.

**Psoriatic arthritis.** Azathioprine may be useful for severe or progressive cases of psoriatic arthritis (see under Spondyloarthropathies, p.11) when the arthritis is not controlled by physical therapy and NSAIDs.

**Rheumatoid arthritis.** Although azathioprine may be beneficial in rheumatoid arthritis (p.9) in the short-term, its toxicity is significantly more severe than other disease-modifying antirheumatic drugs (DMARDs).[1] It may, however, be useful in patients with severe disease unresponsive to other DMARDs especially in those with extra-articular manifestations such as vasculitis.[2]


1. Suarez-Almazor ME, *et al.* Azathioprine for treating rheumatoid arthritis. Available in The Cochrane Library; Issue 2. Chichester: John Wiley; 2004.
2. Heurkens AHM, *et al.* Prednisone plus azathioprine treatment in patients with rheumatoid arthritis complicated by vasculitis. *Arch Intern Med* 1991; **151:** 2249–54.


**Sarcoidosis.** Cytotoxic immunosuppressants such as azathioprine have been tried in patients with sarcoidosis (p.1087) who do not respond to or cannot tolerate corticosteroids.

**Skin disorders.** Like other immunosuppressants, azathioprine has been tried in various refractory skin disorders, notably in pemphigus (see below). Other conditions in which it has been tried include atopic eczema,[1-5] nodular prurigo,[6] chronic actinic dermatitis,[1,4] pyoderma gangrenosum,[2] erythema multiforme,[2,7] pompholyx, and plaque psoriasis,[4] as well as in the skin manifestations of systemic disorders such as dermatomyositis and lupus erythematosus.


1. Younger IR, *et al.* Azathioprine in dermatology. *J Am Acad Dermatol* 1991; **25:** 281–6.
2. Tan BB, *et al.* Azathioprine in dermatology: a survey of current practice in the UK. *Br J Dermatol* 1997; **136:** 351–5.
3. Lear JT, *et al.* A retrospective review of the use of azathioprine in severe atopic dermatitis. *Br J Dermatol* 1996; **135** (suppl 47): 38.
4. Scerri L. Azathioprine in dermatological practice: an overview with special emphasis on its use in non-bullous inflammatory dermatoses. *Adv Exp Med Biol* 1999; **455:** 343–8.
5. Murphy L-A, Atherton D. A retrospective evaluation of azathioprine in severe childhood atopic eczema, using thiopurine methyltransferase levels to exclude patients at high risk of myelosuppression. *Br J Dermatol* 2002; **147:** 308–15.
6. Lear JT, *et al.* Nodular prurigo responsive to azathioprine. *Br J Dermatol* 1996; **134:** 1151.
7. Schofield JK, *et al.* Recurrent erythema multiforme: clinical features and treatment in a large series of patients. *Br J Dermatol* 1993; **128:** 542–5.


PEMPHIGUS AND PEMPHIGOID. Corticosteroids are the main treatment for blistering in pemphigus and pemphigoid (p.1137). Immunosuppressive therapy, including azathioprine,[1] has been used with corticosteroids to permit a reduction in corticosteroid dosage. However, it has been suggested that evidence for the corticosteroid-sparing effect is lacking and that immunosuppressants should be reserved for patients who cannot tolerate corticosteroids or in whom they are contra-indicated.[2]


1. Aberer W, *et al.* Azathioprine in the treatment of pemphigus vulgaris: a long-term follow-up. *J Am Acad Dermatol* 1987; **16:** 527–33.
2. Bystryn J-C, Steinman NM. The adjuvant therapy of pemphigus: an update. *Arch Dermatol* 1996; **132:** 203–12.


**Vasculitic syndromes.** Azathioprine has been tried in a number of the vasculitic syndromes, including giant cell arteritis (p.1080), microscopic polyangiitis (p.1085), Churg-Strauss syndrome (p.1078), Takayasu's arteritis (p.1089), and Wegener's granulomatosis (p.1090). In general it is most useful in maintenance for its corticosteroid-sparing effect. Cyclophosphamide tends to be preferred where a more aggressive regimen is required, as in some combinations for induction of remission.

## Preparations

***BP 2003:*** Azathioprine Tablets;
***USP 27:*** Azathioprine Sodium for Injection; Azathioprine Tablets.

**Proprietary Preparations** (details are given in Part 3)
***Arg.:*** Imuran; ***Austral.:*** Azahexal; Azamun; Imuran; Thioprine; ***Austria:*** Imurek; ***Belg.:*** Imuran; ***Braz.:*** Imunen; Imuran; ***Canad.:*** Imuran; ***Chile:*** Azafalk; Imuran; ***Denm.:*** Imurel; ***Fin.:*** Azamun; Imuprin; Imurel; ***Fr.:*** Imurel; ***Ger.:*** Azafalk; Azamedac; Azathiodura; Colinsan; Imurek; Zytrim; ***Gr.:*** Imuran; ***Hong Kong:*** Azamun; Imuran; ***India:*** Azoran; Imuran; Transimune; ***Irl.:*** Azopine†; Imuger; Imuran; ***Israel:*** Azopi; Imuran; ***Malaysia:***

Imuran; **Mex.:** Aseroprim†; Azatrilem; Imuran; Satedon†; Tiosalprin†; **Neth.:** Imuran; **Norw.:** Imurel; **NZ:** Azamun; Imuran; Thioprine; **Port.:** Imuran; **S.Afr.:** Azapress; Imuran; **Singapore:** Imuran; **Spain:** Imurel; **Swed.:** Imurel; **Switz.:** Imurek; **Thai.:** Imuran; **UK:** Immunoprin; Imuran; Oprisine†; **USA:** Azasan; Imuran.

## Basiliximab *(BAN, USAN, rINN)*

SDZ-CHI-621.

*CAS — 179045-86-4.*

*ATC — L04AA09.*

### Adverse Effects and Precautions

As for Daclizumab, p.1359. Bolus administration of basiliximab may cause nausea, vomiting, and local reactions.

### Pharmacokinetics

Basiliximab has a terminal half-life of about 7 days in adults and about 9 days in children.

### Uses and Administration

Basiliximab is a chimeric murine/human monoclonal antibody similar to daclizumab (p.1359) that functions as an interleukin-2 receptor antagonist by binding to the alpha chain (CD25 antigen) of the interleukin-2 receptor on the surface of activated T-lymphocytes. It is used in the prevention of acute graft rejection episodes in patients undergoing renal transplantation as part of an immunosuppressive regimen that includes ciclosporin and corticosteroids; azathioprine or mycophenolate mofetil may also be added to the regimen. The recommended dose for adults and children over 35 kg is 20 mg, given within 2 hours before surgery and repeated once after 4 days. Children under 35 kg may receive 10 mg, repeated after 4 days. Doses are administered either as an intravenous bolus, or diluted to a usual concentration of 0.4 mg/mL in sodium chloride 0.9% or glucose 5%, for infusion over 20 to 30 minutes.

**Organ and tissue transplantation.** A course of basiliximab with dual therapy (ciclosporin and corticosteroids) reduced the incidence of acute rejection episodes in the first year after kidney transplantation (p.1346) compared with placebo, but there was no overall difference in graft survival.[1,2] In a pooled analysis of these 2 trials, superior graft survival was evident in diabetic patients treated with basiliximab.[3] A further study[4] showed that addition of basiliximab to triple therapy (ciclosporin, corticosteroids, and azathioprine) also reduced the incidence of acute allograft rejection without a concurrent increase in adverse events, infections, or malignancy. Similar results have been found in 2 small paediatric studies.[5,6] Two reviews[7,8] concluded that the use of basiliximab in renal transplantation was safe and effective, with reduced rates of acute rejection, but no long-term benefit in terms of graft survival; basiliximab appears to allow the safe withdrawal of corticosteroids or the use of corticosteroid-free immunosuppressive regimens.

In a randomised, controlled trial,[9] a course of basiliximab with dual therapy reduced the incidence of acute rejection episodes in the first year after liver transplantation (p.1346) compared with placebo, including patients positive for hepatitis C. In a small, retrospective, pilot study, basiliximab with dual therapy reduced the incidence of acute graft rejection in children.[10] A small retrospective comparison of paediatric liver transplant recipients found that a corticosteroid-free immunosuppressive regimen using basiliximab and tacrolimus was associated with significantly lower rejection rates at 1 year than a corticosteroid-based regimen.[11]

Basiliximab is under investigation in immunosuppressant regimens for heart (p.1345) and pancreatic (p.1347) transplantation.


1. Nashan B, *et al.* Randomised trial of basiliximab versus placebo for control of acute cellular rejection in renal allograft recipients. *Lancet* 1997; **350:** 1193–8. Correction. *ibid.*; 1484.
2. Kahan BD, *et al.* Reduction of the occurrence of acute cellular rejection among renal allograft recipients treated with basiliximab, a chimeric anti-interleukin-2-receptor monoclonal antibody. *Transplantation* 1999; **67:** 276–84.
3. Thistlethwaite JR, *et al.* Reduced acute rejection and superior 1-year renal allograft survival with basiliximab in patients with diabetes mellitus. *Transplantation* 2000; **70:** 784–90.
4. Ponticelli C, *et al.* A randomized, double-blind trial of basiliximab immunoprophylaxis plus triple therapy in kidney transplant recipients. *Transplantation* 2001; **72:** 1261–7.
5. Swiatecka-Urban A, *et al.* Basiliximab induction improves the outcome of renal transplants in children and adolescents. *Pediatr Nephrol* 2001; **16:** 693–6.
6. Pape L, *et al.* Single centre experience with basiliximab in paediatric renal transplantation. *Nephrol Dial Transplant* 2002; **17:** 276–80.
7. Chapman TM, Keating GM. Basiliximab: a review of its use as induction therapy in renal transplantation. *Drugs* 2003; **63:** 2803–35.
8. Boggi U, *et al.* A benefit-risk assessment of basiliximab in renal transplantation. *Drug Safety* 2004; **27:** 91–106.
9. Neuhaus P, *et al.* Improved treatment response with basiliximab immunoprophylaxis after liver transplantation: results from a double-blind randomized placebo-controlled trial. *Liver Transpl* 2002; **8:** 132–42.
10. Ganschow R, *et al.* First experience with basiliximab in pediatric liver graft recipients. *Pediatr Transplant* 2001; **5:** 353–8.
11. Reding R, *et al.* Steroid-free liver transplantation in children. *Lancet* 2003; **362:** 2068–70.


**Skin disorders.** There are a few case reports of successful treatment with basiliximab in psoriasis[1-4] (p.1137), chronic atopic dermatitis[5] (see Eczema, p.1135), and epidermolysis bullosa acquisita[6] (p.1135).


1. Salim A, *et al.* Successful treatment of severe generalized pustular psoriasis with basiliximab (interleukin-2 receptor blocker). *Br J Dermatol* 2000; **143:** 1121–2.
2. Mrowietz U, *et al.* Treatment of severe psoriasis with anti-CD25 monoclonal antibodies. *Arch Dermatol* 2000; **136:** 675–6.
3. Owen CM, Harrison PV. Successful treatment of severe psoriasis with basiliximab, an interleukin-2 receptor monoclonal antibody. *Clin Exp Dermatol* 2000; **25:** 195–7.
4. Bell HK, Parslew RAG. Use of basiliximab as a cyclosporin-sparing agent in palmoplantar pustular psoriasis with myalgia as an adverse effect. *Br J Dermatol* 2002; **147:** 606–7.
5. Kägi MK, Heyer G. Efficacy of basiliximab, a chimeric anti-interleukin-2 receptor monoclonal antibody, in a patient with severe chronic atopic dermatitis. *Br J Dermatol* 2001; **145:** 350–1.
6. Haufs MG, Haneke E. Epidermolysis bullosa acquisita treated with basiliximab, an interleukin-2 receptor antibody. *Acta Derm Venereol (Stockh)* 2001; **81:** 72.


### Preparations

**Proprietary Preparations** (details are given in Part 3)
**Arg.:** Simulect; **Austral.:** Simulect; **Belg.:** Simulect; **Braz.:** Simulect; **Canad.:** Simulect; **Chile:** Simulect; **Denm.:** Simulect; **Fin.:** Simulect; **Fr.:** Simulect; **Ger.:** Simulect; **Gr.:** Simulect; **Hong Kong:** Simulect; **Irl.:** Simulect; **Israel:** Simulect; **Ital.:** Simulect; **Malaysia:** Simulect; **Mex.:** Simulect; **Neth.:** Simulect; **Norw.:** Simulect; **NZ:** Simulect; **Port.:** Simulect; **S.Afr.:** Simulect; **Singapore:** Simulect†; **Spain:** Simulect; **Swed.:** Simulect; **Switz.:** Simulect; **Thai.:** Simulect; **UK:** Simulect; **USA:** Simulect.

## Brequinar Sodium *(USAN, rINNM)*

Brequinar sódico; DuP-785; NSC-368390. Sodium 6-fluoro-2-(2′-fluoro-4-biphenylyl)-3-methyl-4-quinolinecarboxylate.

$C_{23}H_{14}F_2NO_2Na = 397.3.$

*CAS — 96187-53-0 (brequinar); 96201-88-6 (brequinar sodium).*

### Profile

Brequinar sodium is an inhibitor of pyrimidine metabolism with potent immunosuppressant properties that has been investigated for the prevention and treatment of rejection episodes following organ and tissue transplantation and for treating various cancers.

◊ References.


1. Arteaga CL, *et al.* Phase I clinical and pharmacokinetic trial of brequinar sodium (DuP-785; NSC-368390). *Cancer Res* 1989; **49:** 4648–53.
2. Jaffee BD, *et al.* The unique immunosuppressive activity of brequinar sodium. *Transplant Proc* 1993; **25** (suppl 2): 19–22.
3. Cramer DV. Brequinar sodium. *Transplant Proc* 1996; **28:** 960–3.
4. Joshi AS, *et al.* Phase I safety and pharmacokinetic studies of brequinar sodium after single ascending oral doses in stable renal, hepatic, and cardiac allograft recipients. *J Clin Pharmacol* 1997; **37:** 1121–8.
5. Burris HA, *et al.* Pharmacokinetic and phase I studies of brequinar (DUP 785; NSC 368390) in combination with cisplatin in patients with advanced malignancies. *Invest New Drugs* 1998; **16:** 19–27.


## Ciclosporin *(BAN, rINN)*

27-400; Ciclosporina; Ciclosporinum; Cyclosporin; Cyclosporin A; Cyclosporine *(USAN)*; OL-27-400. Cyclo{-[4-(*E*)-but-2-enyl-*N*,4-dimethyl-L-threonyl]-L-homoalanyl-(*N*-methylglycyl)-(*N*-methyl-L-leucyl)-L-valyl-(*N*-methyl-L-leucyl)-L-alanyl-D-alanyl-(*N*-methyl-L-leucyl)-(*N*-methyl-L-leucyl)-(*N*-methyl-L-valyl)-}.

$C_{62}H_{111}N_{11}O_{12} = 1202.6.$

*CAS — 59865-13-3.*

*ATC — L04AA01.*

**Pharmacopoeias.** In *Chin., Eur.* (see p.vi), *Int., Jpn,* and *US.*

**Ph. Eur. 5.0** (Ciclosporin). A substance produced by *Beauveria nivea* (=*Tolypocladium inflatum* Gams) or obtained by any other means. A white or almost white powder; practically insoluble in water; freely soluble in dehydrated alcohol and in dichloromethane. Store in airtight containers. Protect from light.

**USP 27** (Cyclosporine). A white to almost white powder. Practically insoluble in water; soluble in alcohol, in acetone, in chloroform, in dichloromethane, in ether, and in methyl alcohol; slightly soluble in saturated hydrocarbons. Store in airtight containers. Protect from light.

**Incompatibility.** The plasticiser diethylhexyl phthalate, which is a possible carcinogen, was leached from PVC containers by ciclosporin preparations containing polyethoxylated castor oil.[1] Such preparations should not be given through PVC tubing nor stored in PVC containers. Polysorbate 80, which is an excipient in other ciclosporin preparations, also leached plasticiser from PVC,[1] and similar precautions would apply to preparations so formulated. UK manufacturers further recommend that containers and stoppers be free of silicone oil and fatty substances.


1. Pearson SD, Trissel LA. Leaching of diethylhexyl phthalate from polyvinyl chloride containers by selected drugs and formulation components. *Am J Hosp Pharm* 1993; **50:** 1405–9.


**Stability.** Ciclosporin was stable over 72 hours following dilution in glucose 5% or glucose/amino-acid solutions and storage at room temperature in the dark; similar stability was seen following dilution in lipid emulsion, but dilutions in sodium chloride 0.9% were considered to be stable only for 8 hours.[1] In all cases miscibility in the diluent was poor and vigorous shaking was required after addition to produce even distribution of ciclosporin. An extemporaneously compounded paste produced from ciclosporin oral solution (Sandimmun) in an oral gel base was found to be stable[2] for at least 31 days in aluminium-lined ointment tubes stored at 2° to 37°.


1. McLeod HL, *et al.* Stability of cyclosporin in dextrose 5%, NaCl 0.9%, dextrose/amino acid solution, and lipid emulsion. *Ann Pharmacother* 1992; **26:** 172–5.
2. Ghnassia LT, *et al.* Stability of cyclosporine in an extemporaneously compounded paste. *Am J Health-Syst Pharm* 1995; **52:** 2204–7.


### Adverse Effects and Treatment

Nephrotoxicity, manifesting as raised serum creatinine and urea, is the major adverse effect of ciclosporin and occurs in approximately one-third of all patients. It is related to drug-plasma concentrations and is usually reversible on reduction of the dose. In renal graft recipients episodes of nephrotoxicity may be difficult to distinguish from graft rejection. Interstitial fibrosis may develop during long-term therapy.

Other frequent adverse effects include hypertension, gastrointestinal disturbances, hepatotoxicity, hypertrichosis, gum hyperplasia, tremor, headaches, hyperlipidaemias, electrolyte disturbances (hyperkalaemia, hypomagnesaemia), paraesthesia, hyperuricaemia, and muscle cramps and myalgia. Less commonly, anaemia, rashes, weight increase, oedema, pancreatitis, myopathy, neuropathy, and convulsions have been reported. Optic disc oedema, including papilloedema secondary to benign intracranial hypertension, has occurred rarely.

Anaphylactoid reactions have occurred following intravenous administration; it has been suggested that these represent a reaction to the polyethoxylated castor oil vehicle of the intravenous preparation.

There is an increased incidence of certain malignancies and a predisposition to infection in patients receiving ciclosporin therapy.

**Alopecia.** Although ciclosporin is more often associated with reports of hypertrichosis, there have been cases of alopecia areata developing in patients receiving ciclosporin,[1] sometimes with complete hair loss (alopecia universalis).[2,3]


1. Davies MG, Bowers PW. Alopecia areata arising in patients receiving cyclosporin immunosuppression. *Br J Dermatol* 1995; **132:** 835–6.
2. Monti M, *et al.* Alopecia universalis in liver transplant patients treated with cyclosporin. *Br J Dermatol* 1995; **133:** 663–4.
3. Parodi A, *et al.* Alopecia universalis and cyclosporin A. *Br J Dermatol* 1996; **135:** 657.


**Carcinogenicity.** The use of ciclosporin in organ transplant recipients is associated with an increased incidence of malignancy, notably lymphoma,[1] and also skin cancer and Kaposi's sarcoma. The manufacturers have stated that of an estimated 5550 transplant patients who had been treated with ciclosporin by February 1984, lymphoproliferative disorders had been reported in 40; this represented an overall incidence of 0.7%, varying from 0.2 to 8% in different series.[2] In 1991, a report of 12 cases of lymphoproliferative disorders among 132 paediatric liver graft recipients estimated the incidence at about 2.8% per year for the first 6 years after transplantation, giving a cumulative risk of nearly 20% after 7 years.[3] There is evidence that the incidence of malignancy is related to dose,[2,4] and is greater when ciclosporin is used with other potent immunosuppressants.[2] In addition, the incidence of malignancy varies geographically, possibly reflecting environmental triggers and genetic susceptibility.[5]

It has been suggested that these lymphomas represent proliferation of B-cells under the influence of Epstein-Barr virus, a process normally prevented by the T-cells which are specifically inhibited by ciclosporin.[3] The resultant, usually polyclonal, lymphoproliferative tumours appear to regress on prompt excision of the affected tissue and reduction or discontinuation of the immunosuppressant regimen, in most cases without graft loss.[6] However, the need for vigilance and rapid response to these conditions has been stressed, since the responsive polyclonal disorder may evolve into a monoclonal, frankly malignant form; where the presentation is indistinguishable from a classic non-Hodgkins lymphoma the prognosis is much less good.[3] Interestingly, use of lower dose ciclosporin regimens appears to maintain normal elimination of Epstein-Barr virus-infected B-cells by specific T-cells,[7] and may lead to a reduced incidence of malignancy compared with earlier results.[4,7]

The risk of skin cancers in ciclosporin recipients is further increased by the exposure to sunlight.[8] Prophylactic retinoid therapy may prevent skin cancer in patients with renal transplants.[9]

There is no clear evidence that ciclosporin is associated with an increased incidence of malignancy compared with other immunosuppressants, although in one study dysplastic skin lesions were found in 14 of 64 transplant patients receiving ciclosporin compared with 3 of 33 previous similar patients who had received azathioprine.[10] However, such comparisons are difficult, not least because many transplant patients tend to have received multiple immunosuppressant agents.


1. Penn I. Cancers following cyclosporine therapy. *Transplantation* 1987; **43:** 32–5.
2. Beveridge T, *et al.* Lymphomas and lymphoproliferative lesions developing under cyclosporin therapy. *Lancet* 1984; **i:** 788.

3. Malatack JJ, *et al.* Orthotopic liver transplantation, Epstein-Barr virus, cyclosporine, and lymphoproliferative disease: a growing concern. *J Pediatr* 1991; **118:** 667–75.
4. Dantal J, *et al.* Effect of long-term immunosuppression in kidney-graft recipients on cancer incidence: randomised comparison of two cyclosporin regimens. *Lancet* 1998; **351:** 623–8.
5. Newstead CG. Assessment of risk of cancer after renal transplantation. *Lancet* 1998; **351:** 610–11.
6. Starzl TE, *et al.* Reversibility of lymphomas and lymphoproliferative lesions developing under cyclosporin-steroid therapy. *Lancet* 1984; **i:** 583–7.
7. Crawford DH, Edwards JMB. Immunity to Epstein-Barr virus in cyclosporin A-treated renal allograft recipients. *Lancet* 1982; **i:** 1469–70.
8. Stockfleth E, *et al.* Epithelial malignancies in organ transplant patients: clinical presentation and new methods of treatment. *Recent Results Cancer Res* 2002; **160:** 251–8.
9. Bavinck JN, *et al.* Prevention of skin cancer and reduction of keratotic skin lesions during acitretin therapy in renal transplant recipients: a double-blind, placebo-controlled study. *J Clin Oncol* 1995; **13:** 1933–8.
10. Shuttleworth D, *et al.* Epidermal dysplasia and cyclosporine therapy in renal transplant patients: a comparison with azathioprine. *Br J Dermatol* 1989; **120:** 551–4.


**Dysmorphic changes.** There was pronounced coarsening of facial features in 11 children who were treated with prednisone and ciclosporin for renal transplantation and followed up for more than 6 months.[1] The changes resembled those seen with phenytoin therapy. In a 13-year-old patient given ciclosporin as part of an immunosuppressive regimen following lung transplantation, facial dysmorphism, which developed along with follicular disturbances, later improved upon conversion to tacrolimus.[2]


1. Reznik VM, *et al.* Changes in facial appearance during cyclosporin treatment. *Lancet* 1987; **i:** 1405–7.
2. Chastain MA, Millikan LE. Pilomatrix dysplasia in an immunosuppressed patient. *J Am Acad Dermatol* 2000; **43:** 118–22.


**Effects on the blood.** Erythraemia[1,2] and thrombocytosis[3] have both been reported with ciclosporin treatment, both of which may contribute to **thromboembolic complications.** One retrospective study reported 17 thromboembolic events (pulmonary embolism, renal-vein or deep-vein thrombosis, or haemorrhoidal thrombosis) in 13 of 90 renal allograft recipients treated with ciclosporin and corticosteroids, compared with only 1 episode of superficial thrombophlebitis in 90 similar patients treated with an azathioprine-based regimen.[4] However, other authors dispute that the incidence of thromboembolic events is any greater after ciclosporin than azathioprine,[5-7] and one group found the reverse.[8]

**Other effects** that have been associated with ciclosporin therapy include cases of the haemolytic-uraemic syndrome,[9] and thrombocytopenia,[10] or leucopenia.[11] Post-transplant thrombotic microangiopathy has also been reported.[12] This syndrome can include haemolytic anaemia and thrombocytopenia, and must be distinguished from rejection in renal transplant recipients. In those patients with a history of thrombotic microangiopathy, the risk of recurrence is high, irrespective of ciclosporin treatment.


1. Tatman AJ, *et al.* Erythraemia in renal transplant recipients treated with cyclosporin. *Lancet* 1988; **i:** 1279.
2. Innes A, *et al.* Cyclosporin and erythraemia. *Lancet* 1988; **ii:** 285.
3. Itami N, *et al.* Thrombocytosis after cyclosporin therapy in child with nephrotic syndrome. *Lancet* 1988; **ii:** 1018.
4. Vanrenterghem Y, *et al.* Thromboembolic complications and haemostatic changes in cyclosporin-treated cadaveric kidney allograft recipients. *Lancet* 1985; **i:** 999–1002.
5. Bergentz S-E, *et al.* Venous thrombosis and cyclosporin. *Lancet* 1985; **ii:** 101–2.
6. Zazgornik J, *et al.* Venous thrombosis and cyclosporin. *Lancet* 1985; **ii:** 102.
7. Choudhury N, *et al.* Thromboembolic complications in cyclosporin-treated kidney allograft recipients. *Lancet* 1985; **ii:** 606.
8. Allen RD, *et al.* Venous thrombosis and cyclosporin. *Lancet* 1985; **ii:** 1004.
9. Bonser RS, *et al.* Cyclosporin-induced haemolytic uraemic syndrome in liver allograft recipient. *Lancet* 1984; **ii:** 1337.
10. Dejong DJ, Sayler DJ. Possible cyclosporine-associated thrombocytopenia. *DICP Ann Pharmacother* 1990; **24:** 1007.
11. Michel F, *et al.* Bone marrow toxicity of cyclosporin in a kidney transplant patient. *Lancet* 1986; **ii:** 394.
12. Pisoni R, *et al.* Drug-induced thrombotic microangiopathy: incidence, prevention and management. *Drug Safety* 2001; **24:** 491–501.


**Effects on the cardiovascular system.** The principal cardiovascular adverse effect of ciclosporin is **hypertension.** This may be severe,[1] appears to be dose-related,[1,2] and is particularly common in recipients of cardiac or heart-lung grafts.[3,4] There may be an association with low serum-magnesium concentrations.[5] A variety of mechanisms have been suggested to contribute to ciclosporin-induced hypertension, including impaired sodium excretion,[6] enhanced sympathetic nervous activity,[3,7] effects on renal prostaglandin metabolism,[2] and direct damage to endothelial cells[8] with release of the potent vasoconstrictor endothelin,[9] all of which may be due to calcineurin inhibition.[10] Thus hypertension may occur independently of nephrotoxicity,[2,7] and may be difficult to treat with conventional antihypertensive regimens.[6] Calcium-channel blockers are the preferred class of antihypertensives for hypertension that develops after transplantation.[1,11] It is important to choose one that does not interact with ciclosporin (see Cardiovascular Drugs under Interactions, below).[1] Beta blockers may also be used. Diuretics are usually avoided.[11] For mention of the ability of calcium-channel blockers to ameliorate the nephrotoxic effects of ciclosporin, see Effects on the Kidneys, below. Occasionally, hypertension may be irreversible.[2,12]

**Raynaud's syndrome** has been reported with ciclosporin.[13] For a discussion of possible thromboembolic complications, see Effects on the Blood, above.


1. Textor SC, *et al.* Cyclosporine-induced hypertension after transplantation. *Mayo Clin Proc* 1994; **69:** 1182–93.
2. Porter GA, *et al.* Cyclosporine-associated hypertension. *Arch Intern Med* 1990; **150:** 280–3.
3. Scherrer U, *et al.* Cyclosporine-induced sympathetic activation and hypertension after heart transplantation. *N Engl J Med* 1990; **323:** 693–9.
4. Weidle PJ, Vlasses PH. Systemic hypertension associated with cyclosporine: a review. *Drug Intell Clin Pharm* 1988; **22:** 443–51.
5. June CH, *et al.* Correlation of hypomagnesemia with the onset of cyclosporine-associated hypertension in marrow transplant patients. *Transplantation* 1986; **41:** 47–51.
6. Weinman EJ. Cyclosporine-associated hypertension. *Am J Med* 1989; **86:** 256–7.
7. Mark AL. Cyclosporine, sympathetic activity, and hypertension. *N Engl J Med* 1990; **323:** 748–50.
8. Zaal MJW, *et al.* Is cyclosporin toxic to endothelial cells? *Lancet* 1988; **ii:** 956–7.
9. Deray G, *et al.* Increased endothelin level after cyclosporine therapy. *Ann Intern Med* 1991; **114:** 809.
10. Koomans HA, Ligtenberg G. Mechanisms and consequences of arterial hypertension after renal transplantation. *Transplantation* 2001; **72:** S9–12.
11. Taler SJ, *et al.* Cyclosporin-induced hypertension: incidence, pathogenesis and management. *Drug Safety* 1999; **20:** 437–49.
12. Sennesael JJ, *et al.* Hypertension and cyclosporine. *Ann Intern Med* 1986; **104:** 729.
13. Deray G, *et al.* Cyclosporin and Raynaud phenomenon. *Lancet* 1986; **ii:** 1092–3.


**Effects on the gastrointestinal tract.** There have been reports[1,2] of severe non-specific colitis associated with both elevated[1] and therapeutic[2] blood or serum concentrations of ciclosporin.


1. Innes A, *et al.* Cyclosporin toxicity and colitis. *Lancet* 1988; **ii:** 957. Correction. *ibid.*; 1094.
2. Bowen JRC, Sahi S. Cyclosporin induced colitis. *BMJ* 1993; **307:** 484.


**Effects on glucose tolerance.** There is some evidence that ciclosporin, particularly in high doses, may be associated with reduced insulin production,[1] impaired glucose tolerance,[2] and occasional overt diabetes mellitus,[3,4] although ciclosporin has also been tried, with some apparent benefit, in the treatment of recent-onset diabetes mellitus (for mention of the use of immunosuppressants in diabetes mellitus, see p.324). The incidence of fasting hyperglycaemia has been estimated at about 8% in ciclosporin-treated renal transplant recipients, compared with about 5% in those given an azathioprine-based regimen.[4]


1. Scott JP, Higenbottam TW. Adverse reactions and interactions of cyclosporin. *Med Toxicol* 1983; **3:** 107–27.
2. Gunnarsson R, *et al.* Deterioration in glucose metabolism in pancreatic transplant recipients given cyclosporin. *Lancet* 1983; **ii:** 571–2.
3. Bending JJ, *et al.* Diabetogenic effect of cyclosporin. *BMJ* 1987; **294:** 401–2.
4. Yagisawa T, *et al.* Deterioration in glucose metabolism in cyclosporine-treated kidney transplant recipients and rats. *Transplant Proc* 1986; **18:** 1548–51.


**Effects on the kidneys.** The use of ciclosporin is associated with nephrotoxicity, characterised by fluid retention, increased serum creatinine and urea concentrations, a fall in glomerular filtration rate, and decreased sodium and potassium excretion.[1,2] In renal graft recipients it may be difficult to distinguish nephrotoxicity from graft rejection.[1] Symptoms are usually chronic, dose-related, and reversible,[1] and increase with the duration of exposure.[2]

- Extremely *high intravenous doses* (21 mg/kg per 24 hours for 60 hours) have been reported to be associated with fatal acute tubular necrosis;[3] in another patient prescribed 30 mg/kg per 24 hours, the error was detected after 18 hours, and the necrosis was deemed to be partially reversible[4]
- *Prolonged use* has been associated with progressive irreversible renal dysfunction in heart transplant patients,[5] despite plasma ciclosporin concentrations below 400 nanograms/mL, the value above which nephrotoxicity is more frequent.[1] However, impairment of renal function has been reported to be reversible, after stopping the drug, in psoriatic patients who had received low-dose ciclosporin for 5 years[6]
- One study[7] of paediatric heart transplant recipients found that decline in renal function correlated with *early exposure* to ciclosporin, and subsequently recommended a target trough level of 300 nanograms/mL or less during early, aggressive immunosuppression

It has been pointed out that with current regimens, which tend to use low doses of ciclosporin, the majority of transplant and other patients receiving ciclosporin long-term tolerate the drug without evidence of progressive nephrotoxicity.[6,8,9]

There is some evidence suggesting that the renal effects are due to a *toxic metabolite*,[10,11] thus, total ciclosporin and metabolite concentrations, as given by radio-immunoassay, may be more helpful in predicting toxicity than concentration of the parent drug alone.[10]

In addition to these chronic changes ciclosporin has also been associated with a syndrome of *acute renal failure*, occurring shortly after beginning treatment.[2,12] This may be due to arteriolar vasoconstriction secondary to inhibition of renal prostaglandin synthesis, with serious consequences in patients with clinical conditions in which prostaglandin-induced renal vasodilatation is necessary to maintain glomerular perfusion.[12] Such a mechanism would be in line with suggestions that inhibition of prostaglandin $E_2$ or prostacyclin synthesis can play a role in the development of chronic ciclosporin-induced nephrotoxicity.[13-15] However, endothelin has also been proposed as a causative agent,[16] and the relationship between the renal and vascular effects of ciclosporin has been a matter of some debate.[2]

Drugs tried to *ameliorate* the nephrotoxic effects of ciclosporin in patients who have undergone transplantation include calcium-channel blockers (see Transplantation, under Diltiazem, p.902, Nifedipine, p.972, and Verapamil, p.1022), clonidine, co-dergocrine,[17-19] omega-3 triglycerides,[20] and misoprostol and other prostaglandin analogues.[21,22] Although benefits have been reported with some of these, hydration, careful monitoring of ciclosporin concentrations, and the use where possible of low-dose or intermittent regimens of ciclosporin appear to remain the major means of minimising nephrotoxicity. Calcium-channel blockers are used if hypertension occurs (see Effects on the Cardiovascular System, above).


1. Bennett WM, Pulliam JP. Cyclosporine nephrotoxicity. *Ann Intern Med* 1983; **99:** 851–4.
2. Scott JP, Higenbottam TW. Adverse reactions and interactions of cyclosporin. *Med Toxicol* 1988; **3:** 107–27.
3. Shechter P. Acute tubular necrosis following high-dose cyclosporine A therapy. *Eur J Clin Pharmacol* 1996; **49:** 521–3.
4. Dussol B, *et al.* Acute tubular necrosis induced by high level of cyclosporine A in a lung transplant. *Transplantation* 2000; **70:** 1234–6.
5. Myers BD, *et al.* Cyclosporine-associated chronic nephropathy. *N Engl J Med* 1984; **311:** 699–705.
6. Powles AV, *et al.* Renal function after 10 years' treatment with cyclosporin for psoriasis. *Br J Dermatol* 1998; **138:** 443–9.
7. Hornung TS, *et al.* Renal function after pediatric cardiac transplantation: the effect of early cyclosporin dosage. *Pediatrics* 2001; **107:** 1346–50.
8. Burke JF, *et al.* Long-term efficacy and safety of cyclosporine in renal-transplant recipients. *N Engl J Med* 1994; **331:** 358–63.
9. Leaker B, Cairns HS. Clinical aspects of cyclosporin nephrotoxicity. *Br J Hosp Med* 1994; **52:** 529–34.
10. Leunissen KML, *et al.* Cyclosporin metabolites and nephrotoxicity. *Lancet* 1986; **ii:** 1398.
11. Lucey MR, *et al.* Cyclosporin toxicity at therapeutic blood levels and cytochrome P-450 IIIA. *Lancet* 1990; **335:** 11–15.
12. Praga M, *et al.* Cyclosporine-induced acute renal failure in the nephrotic syndrome. *Ann Intern Med* 1987; **107:** 786–7.
13. Duarte R. Cyclosporine: renal effects and prostacyclin. *Ann Intern Med* 1985; **102:** 420.
14. Adu D, *et al.* Cyclosporine and prostaglandins. *Ann Intern Med* 1985; **103:** 303.
15. Stahl RAK, *et al.* Cyclosporine and renal prostaglandin $E_2$ production. *Ann Intern Med* 1985; **103:** 474.
16. Cairns HS, *et al.* Endothelin and cyclosporin nephrotoxicity. *Lancet* 1988; **ii:** 1496–7.
17. Heinrichs DA, *et al.* The effects of co-dergocrine on cyclosporin A pharmacokinetics and pharmacodynamics. *Br J Clin Pharmacol* 1987; **24:** 117–18.
18. Nussenblatt RB, *et al.* Hydergine and cyclosporin nephrotoxicity. *Lancet* 1986; **i:** 1220–1.
19. Kho TL, *et al.* Hydergine and reversibility of cyclosporin nephrotoxicity. *Lancet* 1986; **ii:** 394–5.
20. Stoof TJ, *et al.* Does fish oil protect renal function in cyclosporin-treated psoriasis patients? *Br J Dermatol* 1990; **123:** 535.
21. Moran M, *et al.* Prevention of acute graft rejection by the prostaglandin $E_1$ analogue misoprostol in renal-transplant recipients treated with cyclosporine and prednisone. *N Engl J Med* 1990; **322:** 1183–8.
22. Di Palo FQ, *et al.* Role of a prostaglandin $E_1$ analogue in the prevention of acute graft rejection by cyclosporine. *N Engl J Med* 1990; **323:** 832.


**Effects on lipids.** Marked hyperlipidaemia has been associated with ciclosporin therapy, with notable increases reported in low-density lipoprotein cholesterol,[1,2] and triglycerides. An increase in lipoprotein (a) has been reported,[3] but this was disputed.[4-6] Ciclosporin has been reported to have greater effects on lipids than azathioprine[7] or tacrolimus[8] post-transplantation. The use of corticosteroids with ciclosporin appears to have an additive adverse effect on lipids.[9] Lipid regulating drugs are used to decrease hypercholesterolaemia in transplant patients.


1. Luke DR, *et al.* Longitudinal study of cyclosporine and lipids in patients undergoing bone marrow transplantation. *J Clin Pharmacol* 1990; **30:** 163–9.
2. Ballantyne CM, *et al.* Effects of cyclosporine therapy on plasma lipoprotein levels. *JAMA* 1989; **262:** 53–6.
3. Webb AT, *et al.* Does cyclosporin increase lipoprotein(a) concentrations in renal transplant recipients? *Lancet* 1993; **341:** 268–70.
4. Kronenberg F, *et al.* Cyclosporin and serum lipids in renal transplant recipients. *Lancet* 1993; **341:** 765.
5. Segarra A, *et al.* Cyclosporin and serum lipids in renal transplant recipients. *Lancet* 1993; **341:** 766.
6. Hunt BJ, *et al.* Does cyclosporin affect lipoprotein(a) concentrations? *Lancet* 1994; **343:** 119–20.
7. Van den Dorpel MA, *et al.* Conversion from cyclosporine A to azathioprine treatment improves LDL oxidation in kidney transplant recipients. *Kidney Int* 1997; **51:** 1608–12.
8. Taylor DO, *et al.* A randomized, multicenter comparison of tacrolimus and cyclosporine immunosuppressive regimens in cardiac transplantation: decreased hyperlipidemia and hypertension with tacrolimus. *J Heart Lung Transplant* 1999; **18:** 336–45.
9. Moore R, *et al.* Calcineurin inhibitors and post-transplant hyperlipidaemias. *Drug Safety* 2001; **24:** 755–66.


**Effects on the nervous system.** Adverse effects of ciclosporin on the CNS include tremor,[1-3] ataxia,[1-3] confusion[1,2] or agitation,[2] mental depression,[3] headache and sleep disturbances,[2] lethargy,[1,2,4] or coma[2,4] (in one case coma persisted for 44 days),[5] convulsions,[2,3,6-9] leukoencephalopathy,[2,5,6] cortical blindness,[2,6] diplopia,[10] and spasticity or paralysis of the limbs.[1,2] Convulsions have sometimes been associated with hypertension and fluid retention,[8] but this is by no means always the case.[6,7] Severe CNS toxicity has been stated to vary in incidence from 0.1% in renal transplant patients to about 1.6% in bone marrow transplant recipients.[9] There is some evidence for an association of serious neurological effects with low total serum-cholesterol concentrations,[2] and the use of the intravenous formulation.[2] Neurotoxicity may also be associated with the use of lipid solutions.[11] An association with hypomagnesaemia has also been proposed[3] but may just represent concomitant nephrotoxicity.[12] Convulsions may be more likely or more severe in patients with a familial history of epilepsy,[13] subclinical aluminium overload,[14] or in those also given high-dose corticosteroids.[15,16] The mechanism of toxicity is unknown but may be associated with disturbance of the blood-brain barrier;[7,9,17] it has been suggested that the metabolite M-17, or possibly other metabolites, are responsible for neurotoxicity.[4] Ciclosporin may be selectively toxic for glial cells, and alteration of sympathetic outflow by calcineurin inhibition may also mediate neurotoxicity.[18] Although neurotoxicity usually manifests within a month of beginning treatment, it may be delayed, and in one case occurred only after 3 years of ciclosporin therapy.[19]

1. Atkinson K, *et al.* Cyclosporine-associated central-nervous-system toxicity after allogeneic bone-marrow transplantation. *N Engl J Med* 1984; **310:** 527.
2. de Groen PC, *et al.* Central nervous system toxicity after liver transplantation: the role of cyclosporine and cholesterol. *N Engl J Med* 1987; **317:** 861–6.
3. Thompson CB, *et al.* Association between cyclosporin neurotoxicity and hypomagnesaemia. *Lancet* 1984; **ii:** 1116–20.
4. Kunzendorf U, *et al.* Cyclosporin metabolites and central-nervous-system toxicity. *Lancet* 1988; **i:** 1223.
5. Berden JHM, *et al.* Severe central-nervous-system toxicity associated with cyclosporin. *Lancet* 1985; **i:** 219–20.
6. Hughes RL. Cyclosporine-related central nervous system toxicity in cardiac transplantation. *N Engl J Med* 1990; **323:** 420–1.
7. Gottrand F, *et al.* Cyclosporine neurotoxicity. *N Engl J Med* 1991; **324:** 1744–5.
8. Joss DV, *et al.* Hypertension and convulsions in children receiving cyclosporin A. *Lancet* 1982; **i:** 906.
9. Krupp P, *et al.* Encephalopathy associated with fat embolism induced by solvent for cyclosporin. *Lancet* 1989; **i:** 168–9.
10. Openshaw H. Eye movement abnormality associated with cyclosporin. *J Neurol Neurosurg Psychiatry* 2001; **70:** 809.
11. De Klippel N. Cyclosporin leukoencephalopathy induced by intravenous lipid solution. *Lancet* 1992; **339:** 1114.
12. Allen RD, *et al.* Cyclosporin and magnesium. *Lancet* 1985; **i:** 1283–4.
13. Velu T, *et al.* Cyclosporin-associated fatal convulsions. *Lancet* 1985; **i:** 219.
14. Nordal KP, *et al.* Aluminium overload, a predisposing condition for epileptic seizures in renal-transplant patients treated with cyclosporin. *Lancet* 1985; **ii:** 153–4.
15. Durrant S, *et al.* Cyclosporin A, methylprednisolone, and convulsions. *Lancet* 1982; **ii:** 829–30.
16. Boogaerts MA, *et al.* Cyclosporin, methylprednisolone, and convulsions. *Lancet* 1982; **ii:** 1216–17.
17. Sloane JP, *et al.* Disturbance of blood-brain barrier after bone-marrow transplantation. *Lancet* 1985; **ii:** 280–1.
18. Bechstein WO. Neurotoxicity of calcineurin inhibitors: impact and clinical management. *Transpl Int* 2000; **13:** 313–26.
19. Welge-Lüssen UC, Gerhartz HH. Late onset of neurotoxicity with cyclosporin. *Lancet* 1994; **343:** 293.

**Effects on skeletal muscle.** Ciclosporin has been associated with a number of reports of myopathy.[1-4] The manufacturer noted that 29 cases had been reported by December 1990, which appeared to be divided into cases of toxic or non-specific myopathy or mild sensory motor neuropathy, which were generally dose-related; and rhabdomyolysis, often, but not always, associated with concomitant medication with lovastatin or colchicine.[5] Rhabdomyolysis has also been reported with concomitant use of other statins and ciclosporin, see Lipid Regulating Drugs, under Interactions, below.

1. Noppen M, *et al.* Cyclosporine and myopathy. *Ann Intern Med* 1987; **107:** 945–6.
2. Goy J-J. Myopathy as possible side-effect of cyclosporin. *Lancet* 1989; **i:** 1446–7.
3. Grezard O, *et al.* Cyclosporin-induced muscular toxicity. *Lancet* 1990; **335:** 177.
4. Fernandez-Sola J, *et al.* Reversible cyclosporin myopathy. *Lancet* 1990; **335:** 362–3.
5. Arellano F, Krupp P. Muscular disorders associated with cyclosporin. *Lancet* 1991; **337:** 915.

**Hyperplasia.** Ciclosporin is well known to be associated with the development of gingival hyperplasia or gingival overgrowth: one review[1] has estimated the incidence at about 30% in transplant patients, while noting that reported values in the literature range from about 7 to 70%. A large study[2] found dosage and serum concentration of ciclosporin to be the most significant risk factors in the development of gingival hyperplasia. The presence of dental plaque may exacerbate the response, and good oral hygiene is important in preventing or minimising of gingival overgrowth.[1] The concomitant use of nifedipine (which can itself produce hyperplasia) may exacerbate overgrowth;[3] a cohort study[4] of renal transplant recipients found that amlodipine was associated with a greater prevalence of overgrowth than nifedipine. Overgrowth is generally reversible following dosage reduction or withdrawal of ciclosporin; where this is not feasible, surgical excision is recommended.[1] However, improvement or resolution of the overgrowth may also be produced by a course of azithromycin.[5-7] Similar benefit has been reported for metronidazole in some[8,9] but not all patients.[10] There are reports[11,12] of marked improvement in hyperplasia after changing treatment from ciclosporin to tacrolimus, including a case apparently resistant to azithromycin.[13]

Enlargement of the papillae of the tongue[14] and sebaceous gland hyperplasia[15] have also occurred in association with ciclosporin.

1. Brunet L, *et al.* Gingival enlargement induced by drugs. *Drug Safety* 1996; **15:** 219–31.
2. Thomas DW, *et al.* Risk factors in the development of cyclosporine-induced gingival overgrowth. *Transplantation* 2000; **69:** 522–6.
3. Slavin J, Taylor J. Cyclosporin, nifedipine, and gingival hyperplasia. *Lancet* 1987; **ii:** 739.
4. James JA, *et al.* The calcium channel blocker used with cyclosporin has an effect on gingival overgrowth. *J Clin Periodontol* 2000; **27:** 109–15.
5. Jucglà A, *et al.* The use of azithromycin for cyclosporin-induced gingival overgrowth. *Br J Dermatol* 1998; **138:** 198–9.
6. Nash MM, Zaltzman JS. Efficacy of azithromycin in the treatment of cyclosporine-induced gingival hyperplasia in renal transplant recipients. *Transplantation* 1998; **65:** 1611–15.
7. Citterio F, *et al.* Azithromycin treatment of gingival hyperplasia in kidney transplant recipients is effective and safe. *Transplant Proc* 2001; **33:** 2134–5.
8. Wong W, *et al.* Resolution of cyclosporin-induced gingival hypertrophy with metronidazole. *Lancet* 1994; **343:** 986.
9. Cecchin E, *et al.* Treatment of cyclosporine-induced gingival hypertrophy. *Ann Intern Med* 1997; **126:** 409–10.
10. Aufricht C, *et al.* Oral metronidazole does not improve cyclosporine A-induced gingival hyperplasia. *Pediatr Nephrol* 1997; **11:** 552–5.
11. Thorp M, *et al.* The effect of conversion from cyclosporine to tacrolimus on gingival hyperplasia, hirsutism and cholesterol. *Transplantation* 2000; **69:** 1218–20.
12. James JA, *et al.* Reduction in gingival overgrowth associated with conversion from cyclosporin A to tacrolimus. *J Clin Periodontol* 2000; **27:** 144–8.
13. Vallejo C, *et al.* Resolution of cyclosporine-induced gingival hyperplasia resistant to azithromycin by switching to tacrolimus. *Haematologica* 2001; **86:** 110.
14. Silverberg NB, *et al.* Lingual fungiform papillae hypertrophy with cyclosporin A. *Lancet* 1996; **348:** 967.
15. Boschnakow A, *et al.* Ciclosporin A-induced sebaceous gland hyperplasia. *Br J Dermatol* 2003; **149:** 198–200.

**Hypersensitivity.** Anaphylactoid reactions in 5 of 21 patients given intravenous ciclosporin infusions were found to be associated with improper mixing of the ciclosporin concentrate, which has a polyethoxylated castor oil vehicle, with the infusion solution.[1] It was concluded that this had led to an initial bolus of polyethoxylated castor oil which had triggered the anaphylactic reactions. Subsequent study indicated that peak concentrations of up to 9 times the intended concentration of ciclosporin and polyethoxylated castor oil were present in the first 10 minutes of a poorly mixed infusion.[2] Anaphylactic shock after ingestion of ciclosporin capsules has been reported. The microemulsion base containing corn oil and polyoxyl 40 hydrogenated castor oil, which is related to the polyethoxylated castor oil vehicle used in the intravenous formulation, was considered to be the likely cause.[3]

1. Liau M, *et al.* High incidence of anaphylactoid reactions to iv cyclosporin A caused by improper dissolution of Cremophor EL. *Clin Pharmacol Ther* 1995; **57:** 209.
2. Liau-Chu M, *et al.* Mechanism of anaphylactoid reactions: improper preparation of high-dose intravenous cyclosporine leads to bolus infusion of Cremophor EL and cyclosporine. *Ann Pharmacother* 1997; **31:** 1287–91.
3. Kuiper RAJ, *et al.* Cyclosporine-induced anaphylaxis. *Ann Pharmacother* 2000; **34:** 858–61.

**Hyperuricaemia.** Ciclosporin therapy may be associated with marked hyperuricaemia,[1-3] which may lead (predominantly in male patients[1]) to episodes of severe gouty arthritis.[1-3] It has been suggested that ciclosporin specifically reduces urate clearance by the kidney independently of its effects on glomerular filtration,[4,5] but this has been disputed.[6] Treatment of ciclosporin-induced gout can be difficult since interactions with NSAIDs may lead to enhanced renal toxicity[5] and patients who are also receiving azathioprine may experience increased bone-marrow toxicity if given allopurinol.[7] Benzbromarone appears to be an alternative[8] for treating hyperuricaemia in renal transplant recipients with a creatinine clearance greater than 25 mL/minute.

1. Lin H-Y, *et al.* Cyclosporine-induced hyperuricemia and gout. *N Engl J Med* 1989; **321:** 287–92.
2. Kahl LE, *et al.* Gout in the heart transplant recipient: physiologic puzzle and therapeutic challenge. *Am J Med* 1989; **87:** 289–94.
3. Burack DA, *et al.* Hyperuricemia and gout among heart transplant recipients receiving cyclosporine. *Am J Med* 1992; **92:** 141–6.
4. Noordzij TC, *et al.* Cyclosporine-induced hyperuricemia and gout. *N Engl J Med* 1990; **322:** 335.
5. Farge D, *et al.* Hyperuricemia and gouty arthritis in heart transplant recipients. *Am J Med* 1990; **88:** 553.
6. Zürcher RM, *et al.* Hyperuricaemia in cyclosporin-treated patients: a GFR-related effect. *Nephrol Dial Transplant* 1996; **11:** 153–8.
7. Figg WD. Cyclosporine-induced hyperuricemia and gout. *N Engl J Med* 1990; **332:** 334–5.
8. Zürcher RM, *et al.* Excellent uricosuric efficacy of benzbromarone in cyclosporin-A-treated renal transplant patients: a prospective study. *Nephrol Dial Transplant* 1994; **9:** 548–51.

**Overdosage.** Anxiety, diarrhoea, vomiting, and perspiration, with weak and irregular pulse, occurred in a patient accidentally injected with 250 mg (estimated 6.25 mg/kg) of ciclosporin.[1] The patient subsequently developed atrial fibrillation, which was treated with digoxin, and in the following 36 hours showed signs of slight renal insufficiency. Two days later no adverse effects were apparent. Atrial fibrillation also developed in another patient accidentally administered 1 g of oral ciclosporin microemulsion.[2] No adverse renal, hepatic, or neurological effects were seen in a third patient[3] who took 25 g of ciclosporin over 8 days. There was a mild increase in blood pressure and other symptoms included burning sensations in the mouth and the extremities, dysgeusia, facial flushing, and gastrointestinal disturbances. Symptoms resolved within 2 weeks of stopping ciclosporin.

A patient accidentally given intravenous ciclosporin at 30 mg/hour for 13 hours, developed massive intracerebral oedema and brainstem compression and died despite stopping the infusion.[4]

For reference to tubular necrosis following ciclosporin overdose, see under Effects on the Kidneys, above.

1. Wallemacq PE, Lesne ML. Accidental massive IV administration of cyclosporine in man. *Drug Intell Clin Pharm* 1985; **19:** 29–30.
2. LoVecchio FA, Goltz HR. Atrial fibrillation following acute overdose with oral cyclosporine. *Ann Pharmacother* 2000; **34:** 405.
3. Baumhefner RW, *et al.* Huge cyclosporin overdose with favourable outcome. *Lancet* 1987; **ii:** 332.
4. de Perrot M, *et al.* Massive cerebral edema after i.v. cyclosporin overdose. *Transplantation* 2000; **70:** 1259–60.

## Precautions

Regular monitoring of renal and hepatic function, blood pressure, and serum electrolytes (chiefly potassium and magnesium) is required in patients receiving ciclosporin. Serum lipids should also be monitored. Monitoring of plasma ciclosporin concentrations is mandatory in transplant patients. Dosage adjustment may frequently be necessary in patients with renal impairment or other factors affecting plasma ciclosporin concentrations. Care is required in patients with hyperuricaemia, and intravenous formulations should be given cautiously to those who have previously received parenteral drugs formulated in polyethoxylated castor oil, or to those with a history of allergic reactions.

Ciclosporin should not be used to treat atopic dermatitis, psoriasis, or rheumatoid arthritis in patients with persistently raised creatinine, uncontrolled hypertension, uncontrolled infections, or malignancy. An exception is patients with treated malignant or pre-malignant lesions of the skin who may receive ciclosporin as a last resort for psoriasis. Psoriatic patients should not be given concomitant ultraviolet irradiation and should avoid excessive sun exposure. Ciclosporin may increase the risk of benign intracranial hypertension.

The commercially available oral formulations of ciclosporin differ in their bioavailability, and patients should not be transferred from one to another without appropriate monitoring. Intra-uterine contraceptive devices should be used with caution during immunosuppressive treatment as there is an increased risk of infection. Immunosuppressants may reduce the response to vaccines and use with live vaccines should generally be avoided as there is a possibility of generalised infection, see below.

**Oral formulation.** Following development of the oral microemulsion formulation of ciclosporin patients were switched from the old formulation on a 1:1 basis by weight initially, with monitoring of resultant ciclosporin concentrations and subsequent dosage adjustment. Despite some reports of nephrotoxicity or rejection in previously stable grafts,[1-4] most consider the new formulation superior. A meta-analysis[5] concluded that of *de novo* transplant recipients, those receiving the microemulsion formulation had significantly fewer instances of rejection, and, in liver transplant recipients, significantly fewer adverse events.

1. Bennett WM, *et al.* Which cyclosporin formulation? *Lancet* 1996; **348:** 205.
2. Olyaei AJ, *et al.* Switching between cyclosporin formulations: what are the risks? *Drug Safety* 1997; **16:** 366–73.
3. Filler G, Ehrich J. Which cyclosporin formulation? *Lancet* 1996; **348:** 1176–7.
4. Gennery A, *et al.* Which cyclosporin formulation? *Lancet* 1996; **348:** 1177.
5. Shah MB, *et al.* A meta-analysis to assess the safety and tolerability of two formulations of cyclosporine: Sandimmune and Neoral. *Transplant Proc* 1998; **30:** 4048–53.

**Breast feeding.** The American Academy of Pediatrics considers that ciclosporin may possibly suppress the immune system in a nursing infant.[1] However, a study[2] in the breast-fed infants of 7 women receiving ciclosporin found that the amounts ingested produced undetectable blood concentrations in the infants. In another case it was estimated that a breast-fed infant received less than 100 micrograms/kg of ciclosporin daily.[3]

1. American Academy of Pediatrics. The transfer of drugs and other chemicals into human milk. *Pediatrics* 2001; **108:** 776–89. Correction. *ibid.*; 1029. Also available at: http://aappolicy.aappublications.org/cgi/content/full/pediatrics%3b108/3/776 (accessed 22/06/04)
2. Nyberg G, *et al.* Breast feeding during treatment with cyclosporine. *Transplantation* 1998; **65:** 253–5.
3. Thiru Y, *et al.* Successful breast feeding while mother was taking cyclosporin. *BMJ* 1997; **315:** 463.

**Porphyria.** Ciclosporin is considered to be unsafe in patients with porphyria because it has been shown to be porphyrinogenic in *animals*. However, there has been a report of a patient with acute intermittent porphyria given ciclosporin for 5 days pretransplant with no exacerbation of symptoms.[1]

1. Barone GW, *et al.* The tolerability of newer immunosuppressive medications in a patient with acute intermittent porphyria. *J Clin Pharmacol* 2001; **41:** 113–15.

**Pregnancy.** Ciclosporin has been used successfully in pregnant women. However, in common with other immunosuppressants, fetal growth retardation may be a significant problem.[1-4] Patients with hypertension or graft dysfunction are more likely to have adverse outcomes, so patients should have stable graft function and be on maintenance therapy before considering pregnancy.[1,2] Serum ciclosporin concentrations may fall during pregnancy,[2,3,5] but although frequent monitoring is necessary, the suppressed auto-immune state of pregnancy may protect against rejection episodes.[5] Ciclosporin should be used at the lowest possible dose to maintain efficacy, and one review[3] has recommended that the daily dose should be kept below 5 mg/kg.

One case of osseous malformation, resulting in hypoplasia of the right leg has been reported in an infant born to a ciclosporin-treated mother.[6]

1. Armenti VT, *et al.* Variables affecting birthweight and graft survival in 197 pregnancies in cyclosporine-treated female kidney transplant recipients. *Transplantation* 1995; **59:** 476–9.
2. Armenti VT, *et al.* National Transplantation Pregnancy Registry (NTPR): cyclosporine dosing and pregnancy outcome in female renal transplant recipients. *Transplant Proc* 1996; **28:** 2111–12.
3. Huynh LA, Min DI. Outcomes of pregnancy and the management of immunosuppressive agents to minimize fetal risks in organ transplant patients. *Ann Pharmacother* 1994; **28:** 1355–6.
4. Lamarque V, *et al.* Analysis of 629 pregnancy outcomes in transplant recipients treated with Sandimmun. *Transplant Proc* 1997; **29:** 2480.
5. Thomas AG, *et al.* The effect of pregnancy on cyclosporine levels in renal allograft patients. *Obstet Gynecol* 1997; **90:** 916–19.
6. Pujals JM, *et al.* Osseous malformation in baby born to woman on cyclosporin. *Lancet* 1989; **i:** 667.

## Interactions

Ciclosporin is extensively metabolised in the liver and plasma-ciclosporin concentrations may be affected by inducers or competitive inhibitors of hepatic enzymes, particularly cytochrome P450 isoenzyme CYP3A4. For example, use of carbamazepine, phenytoin, phenobarbital, rifampicin, and other inducers of hepatic enzymes may lead to lower plasma concentrations of ciclosporin, and increased plasma concentrations have been reported with some antifungals, macrolide antibiotics, some calcium-channel blockers, sex hormones, corticosteroids and grapefruit juice. In transplant patients frequent measurement of plasma ciclosporin and, if necessary, ciclosporin dosage adjustment is required, particularly during the introduction or withdrawal of other drugs.

Concurrent use of statins may increase the risk of myopathy and rhabdomyolysis. Potassium-sparing diuretics should be avoided because of the risk of hyperkalaemia, and patients taking ciclosporin should avoid a high dietary intake of potassium. The risk of gingival hyperplasia may be increased by amlodipine or nifedipine.

During treatment with ciclosporin, vaccination may be less effective, and the use of live vaccines should generally be avoided.

Care should be taken when ciclosporin is given concomitantly with other nephrotoxic drugs.

◊ Reviews of the interactions of ciclosporin.

1. Yee GC, McGuire TR. Pharmacokinetic drug interactions with cyclosporin. *Clin Pharmacokinet* 1990; **19:** 319–32 and 400–15.
2. Lake KD, Canafax DM. Important interactions of drugs with immunosuppressive agents used in transplant recipients. *J Antimicrob Chemother* 1995; **36** (suppl B): 11–22.
3. Campana C, *et al.* Clinically significant drug interactions with cyclosporin: an update. *Clin Pharmacokinet* 1996; **30:** 141–79.
4. Chan L-N. Drug-nutrient interactions in transplant recipients. *J Parenter Enteral Nutr* 2001; **25:** 132–41.

**Allopurinol.** A patient who had been receiving maintenance doses of ciclosporin for some years, with consistent whole-blood trough concentrations of around 130 nanograms/mL at doses of 175 mg twice daily experienced a rise in ciclosporin concentrations to 410 nanograms/mL following 2 months of treatment with allopurinol 200 mg daily.[1] Ciclosporin concentrations returned to their previous levels over several weeks following discontinuation of allopurinol, and rose again on rechallenge. Dosage of ciclosporin was then reduced. For a report of a low dose of allopurinol being added to a ciclosporin-containing immunosuppressive regimen, see p.414.

1. Gorrie M, *et al.* Allopurinol interaction with cyclosporin. *BMJ* 1994; **308:** 113.

**Antibacterials.** AMINOGLYCOSIDES. Increased nephrotoxicity has been reported with the concomitant use of aminoglycosides with ciclosporin.[1,2] However, a retrospective analysis in 21 patients given ciclosporin for allogeneic bone marrow transplant, in whom aminoglycosides were used if fever and neutropenia developed, showed no greater incidence of nephrotoxicity than in 20 autologous bone marrow recipients who did not receive ciclosporin, suggesting that these drugs can be given together provided careful monitoring is maintained.[3]

1. Termeer A, *et al.* Severe nephrotoxicity cause by the combined use of gentamicin and cyclosporine in renal allograft recipients. *Transplantation* 1986; **42:** 220–1.
2. Morales JM, *et al.* Reversible acute renal toxicity by toxic sinergic effect between gentamicin and cyclosporine. *Clin Nephrol* 1988; **29:** 272.
3. Chandrasekar PH, Cronin SM. Nephrotoxicity in bone marrow transplant recipients receiving aminoglycoside plus cyclosporine or aminoglycoside alone. *J Antimicrob Chemother* 1991; **27:** 845–9.

CHLORAMPHENICOL. Two cases of marked rises in plasma-ciclosporin concentrations have been reported when chloramphenicol was given.[1,2]

1. Steinfort CL, McConachy KA. Cyclosporin-chloramphenicol drug interaction in a heart-lung transplant recipient. *Med J Aust* 1994; **161:** 455.
2. Bui LL, Huang DD. Possible interaction between cyclosporine and chloramphenicol. *Ann Pharmacother* 1999; **33:** 252–3.

MACROLIDES. Markedly raised blood concentrations of ciclosporin have been reported in patients also given *erythromycin*.[1-4] The mechanism involved appears to be a combination of decreased hepatic metabolism of ciclosporin and increased gastrointestinal absorption.[5] Similar elevations of ciclosporin concentrations have been noted following use with other macrolide antibiotics, including *clarithromycin*,[6-8] *josamycin*,[9,10] *midecamycin*,[11] *midecamycin acetate*,[12] and the structurally-related streptogramins, *pristinamycin*[13] and *quinupristin/dalfopristin*.[14] Small increases in ciclosporin concentrations have been seen with *roxithromycin*.[15] An increase in ciclosporin concentrations was attributed to *azithromycin* in 1 patient,[16] but a study in 6 patients found no effect.[17] *Spiramycin* does not appear to affect the pharmacokinetics of ciclosporin.[18,19]

1. Ptachcinski RJ, *et al.* Effect of erythromycin on cyclosporine levels. *N Engl J Med* 1985; **313:** 1416–17.
2. Martell R, *et al.* The effects of erythromycin in patients treated with cyclosporine. *Ann Intern Med* 1986; **104:** 660–1.
3. Wadhwa NK, *et al.* Interaction between erythromycin and cyclosporine in a kidney and pancreas allograft recipient. *Ther Drug Monit* 1987; **9:** 123–5.
4. Gupta SK, *et al.* Cyclosporin-erythromycin interaction in renal transplant patients. *Br J Clin Pharmacol* 1989; **27:** 475–81.
5. Ignoffo RJ, Kim LE. Erythromycin and cyclosporine drug interaction. *DICP Ann Pharmacother* 1991; **25:** 30–1.
6. Ferrari SL, *et al.* The interaction between clarithromycin and cyclosporine in kidney transplant recipients. *Transplantation* 1994; **58:** 725–7.
7. Treille S, *et al.* Kidney graft dysfunction after drug interaction between clarithromycin and cyclosporin. *Nephrol Dial Transplant* 1996; **11:** 1192–3.
8. Sádaba B, *et al.* Concurrent clarithromycin and cyclosporin A treatment. *J Antimicrob Chemother* 1998; **42:** 393–5.
9. Kreft-Jais C, *et al.* Effect of josamycin on plasma cyclosporine levels. *Eur J Clin Pharmacol* 1987; **32:** 327–8.
10. Azanza JR, *et al.* Possible interaction between cyclosporine and josamycin: a description of three cases. *Clin Pharmacol Ther* 1992; **51:** 572–5.
11. Alfonso I, *et al.* Interaction between cyclosporine A and midecamycin. *Eur J Clin Pharmacol* 1997; **52:** 79–80.
12. Couet W, *et al.* Effect of ponsinomycin on cyclosporin pharmacokinetics. *Eur J Clin Pharmacol* 1990; **39:** 165–7.
13. Garraffo R, *et al.* Pristinamycin increases cyclosporin blood levels. *Med Sci Res* 1987; **15:** 461.
14. Stamatakis MK, Richards JG. Interaction between quinupristin/dalfopristin and cyclosporine. *Ann Pharmacother* 1997; **31:** 576–8.
15. Billaud EM, *et al.* Interaction between roxithromycin and cyclosporin in heart transplant patients. *Clin Pharmacokinet* 1990; **19:** 499–502.
16. Ljutic D, Rumboldt Z. Possible interaction between azithromycin and cyclosporin: a case report. *Nephron* 1995; **70:** 130.
17. Gomez E, *et al.* Interaction between azithromycin and cyclosporin? *Nephron* 1996; **73:** 724.
18. Vernillet L, *et al.* Lack of effect of spiramycin on cyclosporin pharmacokinetics. *Br J Clin Pharmacol* 1989; **27:** 789–94.
19. Kessler M, *et al.* Lack of effect of spiramycin on cyclosporin pharmacokinetics. *Br J Clin Pharmacol* 1990; **29:** 370–1.

PENICILLINS. Decreased plasma-ciclosporin concentrations and effect were seen in a patient given *nafcillin*.[1] Conversely, another study reported increased nephrotoxicity with the concomitant use of ciclosporin and nafcillin without an apparent increase in ciclosporin concentrations.[2]

1. Veremis SA, *et al.* Subtherapeutic cyclosporine concentrations during nafcillin therapy. *Transplantation* 1987; **43:** 913–15.
2. Jahansouz F, *et al.* Potentiation of cyclosporine nephrotoxicity by nafcillin in lung transplant recipients. *Transplantation* 1993; **55:** 1045–8.

QUINOLONES. A number of reports have indicated that the quinolone *ciprofloxacin* has no effect on the pharmacokinetics of ciclosporin.[1-3] However, there is a report of enhanced nephrotoxicity without a change in ciclosporin concentrations in a patient given ciprofloxacin,[4] and another report showing both enhanced nephrotoxicity and increased ciclosporin concentrations.[5] Furthermore, a small case-control study suggested an increase in transplant rejection with ciprofloxacin.[6] *Norfloxacin* has been reported to decrease clearance and increase blood concentrations of ciclosporin in paediatric patients,[7] probably by inhibition of ciclosporin metabolism. *Levofloxacin* did not alter ciclosporin pharmacokinetics in healthy volunteers.[8]

1. Hooper TL, *et al.* Ciprofloxacin: a preferred treatment for legionella infections in patients receiving cyclosporin A. *J Antimicrob Chemother* 1988; **22:** 952–3.
2. Tan KKC, *et al.* Co-administration of ciprofloxacin and cyclosporin: lack of evidence for a pharmacokinetic interaction. *Br J Clin Pharmacol* 1989; **28:** 185–7.
3. Krüger HU, *et al.* Investigation of potential interaction of ciprofloxacin with cyclosporine in bone marrow transplant recipients. *Antimicrob Agents Chemother* 1990; **34:** 1048–52.
4. Elston RA, Taylor J. Possible interaction of ciprofloxacin with cyclosporin A. *J Antimicrob Chemother* 1988; **21:** 679–80.
5. Nasir M, *et al.* Interaction between ciclosporin and ciprofloxacin. *Nephron* 1991; **57:** 245–6.
6. Wrishko RE, *et al.* Investigation of a possible interaction between ciprofloxacin and cyclosporine in renal transplant patients. *Transplantation* 1997; **64:** 996–9.
7. McLellan RA, *et al.* Norfloxacin interferes with cyclosporine disposition in pediatric patients undergoing renal transplantation. *Clin Pharmacol Ther* 1995; **58:** 322–7.
8. Doose DR, *et al.* Levofloxacin does not alter cyclosporine disposition. *J Clin Pharmacol* 1998; **38:** 90–93.

RIFAMYCINS. Concomitant use of *rifampicin* has been associated with marked decreases in blood-ciclosporin concentrations,[1-3] and has resulted in graft rejection.[1,3] Although it has been assumed that this effect represents induction of the hepatic metabolism of ciclosporin by rifampicin, there is some suggestion that rifampicin may decrease the absorption of ciclosporin or induce intestinal metabolism, resulting in reduced bioavailability.[4] Topical application of *rifamycin* has also been associated with a decrease in blood-ciclosporin concentrations in another patient;[5] ciclosporin concentrations rose immediately after withdrawal of rifamycin, suggesting that the effect was not due to enzyme induction.

1. Langhoff E, Madsen S. Rapid metabolism of cyclosporin and prednisone in kidney transplant patient receiving tuberculostatic treatment. *Lancet* 1983; **ii:** 1031.
2. Daniels NJ, *et al.* Interaction between cyclosporin and rifampicin. *Lancet* 1984; **ii:** 639.
3. Allen RDM, *et al.* Cyclosporin and rifampicin in renal transplantation. *Lancet* 1985; **i:** 980.
4. Hebert MF, *et al.* Bioavailability of cyclosporine with concomitant rifampin administration is markedly less than predicted by hepatic enzyme induction. *Clin Pharmacol Ther* 1992; **52:** 453–7.
5. Renoult E, *et al.* Effect of topical rifamycin SV treatment on cyclosporin A blood levels in a renal transplant recipient. *Eur J Clin Pharmacol* 1991; **40:** 433–4.

STREPTOGRAMINS. Increased plasma concentrations of ciclosporin have occurred following therapy with *pristinamycin* and *quinupristin/dalfopristin* (see Macrolides, above).

SULFONAMIDES. Intravenous, but not oral, therapy with *sulfadimidine* and *trimethoprim* has been associated with falls in ciclosporin concentrations to subtherapeutic values.[1,2] Oral *sulfadiazine* has had a similar effect.[3] Conversely, *trimethoprim* and *co-trimoxazole* can cause rises in serum creatinine, and therefore may contribute to ciclosporin-induced nephrotoxicity.[4,5]

1. Wallwork J, *et al.* Cyclosporin and intravenous sulphadimidine and trimethoprim therapy. *Lancet* 1983; **i:** 366–7.
2. Jones DK, *et al.* Serious interaction between cyclosporin A and sulphadimidine. *BMJ* 1986; **292:** 728–9.
3. Spes CH, *et al.* Sulfadiazine therapy for toxoplasmosis in heart transplant recipients decreases cyclosporine concentration. *Clin Invest* 1992; **70:** 752–4.
4. Thompson JF, *et al.* Nephrotoxicity of trimethoprim and cotrimoxazole in renal allograft recipients treated with cyclosporine. *Transplantation* 1983; **36:** 204–6.
5. Ringden O, *et al.* Nephrotoxicity by co-trimoxazole and cyclosporin in transplanted patients. *Lancet* 1984; **i:** 1016.

**Antidepressants.** Giving *fluoxetine* to a patient receiving ciclosporin as part of an immunosuppressant regimen after cardiac transplantation was associated with a subsequent marked increase in ciclosporin trough blood concentrations to about twice their original value, necessitating a reduction in ciclosporin dosage.[1] Following subsequent withdrawal of fluoxetine, ciclosporin concentrations fell, and dosage had to be increased. However, a study in 13 other patients receiving ciclosporin with fluoxetine failed to find any evidence of altered ciclosporin concentrations.[2] A nearly tenfold increase in ciclosporin concentration was seen in a cardiac transplant patient after use of *nefazodone*,[3] and there are 2 case reports[4] of ciclosporin toxicity due to interactions with nefazodone and *fluvoxamine* in renal transplant recipients.

1. Horton RC, Bonser RS. Interaction between cyclosporin and fluoxetine. *BMJ* 1995; **311:** 422.
2. Strouse TB, *et al.* Fluoxetine and cyclosporine in organ transplantation: failure to detect significant drug interactions or adverse clinical events in depressed organ recipients. *Psychosomatics* 1996; **37:** 23–30.
3. Wright DH, *et al.* Nefazodone and cyclosporine drug-drug interaction. *J Heart Lung Transplant* 1999; **18:** 913–15.
4. Vella JP, Sayegh MH. Interactions between cyclosporine and newer antidepressant medications. *Am J Kidney Dis* 1998; **31:** 320–3.

HYPERICUM. Ciclosporin plasma levels are reduced by hypericum. This has lead to acute rejection episodes in transplant patients,[1-4] and the two drugs should not be used together.[5]

1. Ruschitzka F, *et al.* Acute heart transplant rejection due to Saint John's wort. *Lancet* 2000; **355:** 548–9.
2. Breidenbach T, *et al.* Drug interaction of St John's wort with ciclosporin. *Lancet* 2000; **355:** 1912.
3. Barone GW, *et al.* Drug interaction between St John's wort and cyclosporine. *Ann Pharmacother* 2000; **34:** 1013–16.
4. Karliova M, *et al.* Interaction of Hypericum perforatum (St. John's wort) with cyclosporin A metabolism in a patient after liver transplantation. *J Hepatol* 2000; **33:** 853–5.
5. Committee on Safety of Medicines/Medicines Control Agency. Reminder: St John's wort (Hypericum perforatum) interactions. *Current Problems* 2000; **26:** 6–7. Also available at: http://www.mca.gov.uk/ourwork/monitorsafequalmed/currentproblems/cpmay2000.pdf (accessed 21/06/04)

**Antiepileptics.** The antiepileptics *carbamazepine*,[1,2] *phenobarbital*,[3] and *phenytoin*,[4] which are all inducers of hepatic cytochrome P450, have been associated with a reduction in blood-ciclosporin concentrations when given concomitantly. *Valproate* has been successfully used in ciclosporin-treated patients without apparent interaction.[1,2]


1. Hillebrand G, *et al.* Valproate for epilepsy in renal transplant recipients receiving cyclosporine. *Transplantation* 1987; **43:** 915–16.
2. Schofield OMV, *et al.* Cyclosporin A in psoriasis: interaction with carbamazepine. *Br J Dermatol* 1990; **122:** 425–6.
3. Carstensen H, *et al.* Interaction between cyclosporin A and phenobarbitone. *Br J Clin Pharmacol* 1986; **21:** 550–1.
4. Freeman DJ, *et al.* Evaluation of cyclosporin-phenytoin interaction with observations on cyclosporin metabolites. *Br J Clin Pharmacol* 1984; **18:** 887–93.


**Antifungals.** The imidazole *ketoconazole* is a potent inhibitor of hepatic cytochrome P450 and markedly increased blood-ciclosporin concentrations have resulted when conventional formulations of the latter were given with the antifungal.[1-4] The interaction has been used, similarly to the calcium-channel blockers (see below), to permit therapeutic blood concentrations of ciclosporin to be achieved at lower doses;[5,6] however, this method may result in considerable variations in ciclosporin pharmacokinetics, and has been criticised on several grounds.[7] It was noted[8] that this improved bioavailability of ciclosporin was not seen when the microemulsion formulation (see Absorption under Pharmacokinetics, below) was given with ketoconazole, suggesting that bioavailability was already maximal. Increased ciclosporin concentrations also appear to occur with the related drugs *itraconazole*,[9] and *voriconazole*,[10] and there is a single report of such an interaction with *miconazole*.[11] However, although such an interaction has also been reported with *fluconazole*,[12,13] a small study has failed to note any significant interaction;[14,15] it has been suggested that an interaction may take place only at high doses of fluconazole,[16] or that sex and ethnicity may play a role.[13]

Increased nephrotoxicity may occur if ciclosporin is used with *amphotericin B*,[17] while liposomal amphotericin B has been reported possibly to exacerbate ciclosporin neurotoxicity.[18] There is a report of decreased ciclosporin concentrations in a patient following addition of *griseofulvin* to therapy.[19] Modest decreases have also been seen in ciclosporin concentrations when *terbinafine* was given.[20]


1. Ferguson RM, *et al.* Ketoconazole, cyclosporin metabolism, and renal transplantation. *Lancet* 1982; **ii:** 882–3.
2. Dieperink H, Møller J. Ketoconazole and cyclosporin. *Lancet* 1982; **ii:** 1217.
3. Shepard JH, *et al.* Cyclosporine-ketoconazole: a potentially dangerous drug-drug interaction. *Clin Pharm* 1986; **5:** 468.
4. Gomez DY, *et al.* The effects of ketoconazole on the intestinal metabolism and bioavailability of cyclosporine. *Clin Pharmacol Ther* 1995; **58:** 15–19.
5. First MR, *et al.* Concomitant administration of cyclosporin and ketoconazole in renal transplant recipients. *Lancet* 1989; **ii:** 1198–1201.
6. Keogh A, *et al.* Ketoconazole to reduce the need for cyclosporine after cardiac transplantation. *N Engl J Med* 1995; **333:** 628–33.
7. Frey FJ. Concomitant cyclosporin and ketoconazole. *Lancet* 1990; **335:** 109–10.
8. Akhlaghi F, *et al.* Pharmacokinetics of cyclosporine in heart transplant recipients receiving metabolic inhibitors. *J Heart Lung Transplant* 2001; **20:** 431–8.
9. Kramer MR, *et al.* Cyclosporine and itraconazole interaction in heart and lung transplant recipients. *Ann Intern Med* 1990; **113:** 327–9.
10. Romero AJ, *et al.* Effect of voriconazole on the pharmacokinetics of cyclosporine in renal transplant patients. *Clin Pharmacol Ther* 2002; **71:** 226–34.
11. Horton CM, *et al.* Cyclosporine interactions with miconazole and other azole-antimycotics: a case report and review of the literature. *J Heart Lung Transplant* 1992; **11:** 1127–32.
12. Collignon P, *et al.* Interaction of fluconazole with cyclosporin. *Lancet* 1989; **i:** 1262.
13. Mathis AS, *et al.* Sex and ethnicity may chiefly influence the interaction of fluconazole with calcineurin inhibitors. *Transplantation* 2001; **71:** 1069–75.
14. Krüger HU, *et al.* Absence of significant interaction of fluconazole with cyclosporin. *J Antimicrob Chemother* 1989; **24:** 781–6.
15. Ehninger G, *et al.* Interaction of fluconazole with cyclosporin. *Lancet* 1989; **ii:** 104–5.
16. López-Gil JA. Fluconazole-cyclosporine interaction: a dose-dependent effect? *Ann Pharmacother* 1993; **27:** 427–30.
17. Kennedy MS, *et al.* Acute renal toxicity with combined use of amphotericin B and cyclosporine after marrow transplantation. *Transplantation* 1983; **35:** 211–15.
18. Ellis ME, *et al.* Is cyclosporin neurotoxicity enhanced in the presence of liposomal amphotericin B? *J Infect* 1994; **29:** 106–7.
19. Abu-Romeh SH, *et al.* Ciclosporin A and griseofulvin: another drug interaction. *Nephron* 1991; **58:** 237.
20. Lo ACY, *et al.* The interaction of terbinafine and cyclosporine A in renal transplant patients. *Br J Clin Pharmacol* 1997; **43:** 340–1.


**Antimalarials.** A large rise in serum-ciclosporin concentration was seen on 2 occasions in a renal graft recipient when *chloroquine* was added to his medication for malaria prophylaxis.[1] *Quinine* has been reported to reduce ciclosporin concentrations.[2]


1. Finielz P, *et al.* Interaction between cyclosporin and chloroquine. *Nephron* 1993; **65:** 333.
2. Tan HW, Ch'ng SL. Drug interaction between cyclosporine A and quinine in a renal transplant patient with malaria. *Singapore Med J* 1991; **32:** 189–90.


**Antineoplastics.** Elevated plasma-ciclosporin concentrations and an increased incidence of nephrotoxic effects and hypertension have been reported in patients receiving ciclosporin for psoriasis who had been previously,[1] or concurrently,[2] treated with *methotrexate*. Conversely, methotrexate has been used effectively with reduced-dose ciclosporin in graft-versus-host disease.[3] Severe renal failure has been reported when standard oral doses of ciclosporin were given after high-dose intravenous *melphalan* (used as a bone marrow conditioning agent before allogeneic bone marrow transplantation).[4]

Ciclosporin increases plasma-*doxorubicin* concentrations and toxicity (see p.549), and has been used to increase oral absorption of *paclitaxel* (see p.578). For the effects of ciclosporin on the pharmacokinetics of *teniposide* and *etoposide*, see p.587 and p.552, respectively.

Ciclosporin and its analogues have been given with antineoplastics for their ability to inhibit the P-glycoprotein cellular pump responsible for multidrug resistance, thus resulting in raised intracellular concentrations of the other drug.


1. Powles AV, *et al.* Cyclosporin toxicity. *Lancet* 1990; **i:** 610.
2. Korstanje MJ, *et al.* Cyclosporine and methotrexate: a dangerous combination. *J Am Acad Dermatol* 1990; **23:** 320–1.
3. Stockschlaeder M, *et al.* A pilot study of low-dose cyclosporin for graft-versus-host prophylaxis in marrow transplantation. *Br J Haematol* 1992; **80:** 49–54.
4. Morgenstern GR, *et al.* Cyclosporin interaction with ketoconazole and melphalan. *Lancet* 1982; **ii:** 1342.


**Antivirals.** For a report of mutual elevations in the area under the plasma concentration-time curves for ciclosporin and the HIV-protease inhibitor *saquinavir*, see Indinavir, p.639.

**Cardiovascular drugs.** ACE INHIBITORS. There may be an increased risk of hyperkalaemia when ACE inhibitors are used with ciclosporin. Acute renal failure, associated with concomitant use of *enalapril*, has been reported in 2 patients receiving ciclosporin after renal transplantation.[1] Renal function recovered when the ACE inhibitor was withdrawn.


1. Murray BM, *et al.* Enalapril-associated acute renal failure in renal transplants: possible role of cyclosporine. *Am J Kidney Dis* 1990; **16:** 66–9.


ANTIARRHYTHMICS. Marked rises in serum-ciclosporin concentrations despite reductions in dose have been noted in recipients of heart or heart-lung transplants following treatment with *amiodarone*.[1,2] A rise in serum ciclosporin has similarly been seen in a patient given both ciclosporin and *propafenone*.[3]


1. Mamprin F, *et al.* Amiodarone-cyclosporine interaction in cardiac transplantation. *Am Heart J* 1992; **123:** 1725–6.
2. Egami J, *et al.* Increase in cyclosporine levels due to amiodarone therapy after heart and heart-lung transplantation. *J Am Coll Cardiol* 1993; **21:** 141A.
3. Spes CH, *et al.* Ciclosporin-propafenone interaction. *Klin Wochenschr* 1990; **68:** 872.


ANTICOAGULANTS. Treatment with *warfarin* for deep-vein thrombosis in a patient maintained on ciclosporin for pure red cell aplasia resulted in a relapse of the latter and a significant fall in ciclosporin blood concentrations.[1] Increase in the ciclosporin dose restored control of the aplasia but resulted in a marked increase in prothrombin activity requiring an increase in warfarin dosage. The results suggest that each drug interferes with the activity of the other. The influence of the patient's other medications (including phenobarbital and folic acid), if any, is unknown, although it has been suggested[2,3] that the phenobarbital had enhanced the metabolism of both drugs. In another report,[2] a patient on long-term warfarin for deep-vein thrombosis was started on ciclosporin for lymphoma relapse, and subsequently required larger doses of warfarin. During concomitant use of *acenocoumarol* and ciclosporin, the dose of ciclosporin had to be increased[3] in one patient and both drugs decreased[4] in another. It appears that the interaction between ciclosporin and anticoagulants is unpredictable[3] and dependent on the anticoagulant used.[2]


1. Snyder DS. Interaction between cyclosporine and warfarin. *Ann Intern Med* 1988; **108:** 311.
2. Turri D, *et al.* Oral anticoagulants and cyclosporin A. *Haematologica* 2000; **85:** 893–4.
3. Borrás-Blasco J, *et al.* Interaction between cyclosporine and acenocoumarol in a patient with nephrotic syndrome. *Clin Nephrol* 2001; **55:** 338–40.
4. Campistol JM, *et al.* Interaction between ciclosporin A and Sintrom. *Nephron* 1989; **53:** 291–2.


ANTIPLATELET DRUGS. *Ticlopidine* decreased serum ciclosporin concentrations in isolated cases,[1,2] but a study in 20 heart transplant patients failed to show any interaction between ciclosporin and low-dose ticlopidine.[3]


1. Birmelé B, *et al.* Interaction of cyclosporin and ticlopidine. *Nephrol Dial Transplant* 1991; **6:** 150–1.
2. Verdejo A, *et al.* Probable interaction between cyclosporin A and low dose ticlopidine. *BMJ* 2000; **320:** 1037.
3. Boissonnat P, *et al.* A drug interaction study between ticlopidine and cyclosporin in heart transplant recipients. *Eur J Clin Pharmacol* 1997; **53:** 39–45.


BETA BLOCKERS. Ciclosporin plasma concentrations increased when *carvedilol* was added to treatment regimens of 21 renal transplant patients.[1] Considerable interindividual variation was seen, so it is recommended that ciclosporin concentrations should be monitored carefully if the drugs are used together.


1. Kaijser M, *et al.* Elevation of cyclosporin A blood levels during carvedilol treatment in renal transplant patients. *Clin Transplant* 1997; **11:** 577–81.


BOSENTAN. There appears to be a complex interaction between ciclosporin and bosentan. In a pharmacokinetic study in healthy subjects,[1] ciclosporin increased the concentration of bosentan. However, doses of ciclosporin needed adjustment to achieve target ciclosporin trough levels; had the dose adjustment not been made, bosentan might have significantly reduced exposure to ciclosporin. The authors recommended that should the two drugs be used together, the dose of bosentan be reduced and the dose of ciclosporin increased. However, the manufacturer of bosentan contra-indicates use with ciclosporin.


1. Binet I, *et al.* Renal hemodynamics and pharmacokinetics of bosentan with and without cyclosporine A. *Kidney Int* 2000; **57:** 224–31.


CALCIUM-CHANNEL BLOCKERS. The calcium-channel blockers *diltiazem*,[1-3] *nicardipine*,[4,5] and *verapamil*[6,7] have all been associated with increases in ciclosporin blood concentrations. It has been suggested that such an interaction can be used to obtain effective ciclosporin concentrations with lower doses.[8] In addition, there is some evidence of mitigation of ciclosporin-induced nephrotoxicity when calcium-channel blockers are given concomitantly (see Effects on the Kidneys, above), and they are useful for ciclosporin-induced hypertension (see Effects on the Cardiovascular System, above). However, some caution is required: one report has pointed out that diltiazem does not increase ciclosporin concentrations in all cases,[9] while others have found that concomitant use alters the pattern of ciclosporin metabolites, and that pharmacokinetic changes are greater in female than in male patients.[10] Therefore, some prefer a calcium-channel blocker that does not alter ciclosporin pharmacokinetics for hypertension and renal protection. *Nifedipine* has not been shown to increase blood-ciclosporin concentrations.[6] For a report of increased nifedipine toxicity with ciclosporin see Immunosuppressants, p.969. Other calcium-channel blockers that do not appear to affect ciclosporin pharmacokinetics include *felodipine*[7,11] and *isradipine*.[7,12] Ciclosporin concentrations have been reported to increase[13] or to remain unchanged[14] with *amlodipine*. Use of amlodipine or nifedipine with ciclosporin may exacerbate the problem of gingival hyperplasia—see Hyperplasia under Adverse Effects, above.


1. Brockmöller J, *et al.* Pharmacokinetic interaction between cyclosporin and diltiazem. *Eur J Clin Pharmacol* 1990; **38:** 237–42.
2. Bourge RC, *et al.* Diltiazem-cyclosporine interaction in cardiac transplant recipients: impact on cyclosporine dose and medication costs. *Am J Med* 1991; **90:** 402–4.
3. Åsberg A, *et al.* Pharmacokinetic interactions between microemulsion formulated cyclosporine A and diltiazem in renal transplant recipients. *Eur J Clin Pharmacol* 1999; **55:** 383–7.
4. Todd P, *et al.* Nicardipine interacts with cyclosporin. *Br J Dermatol* 1989; **121:** 820.
5. Kessler M, *et al.* Influence of nicardipine on renal function and plasma cyclosporin in renal transplant patients. *Eur J Clin Pharmacol* 1989; **36:** 637–8.
6. Tortorice KL, *et al.* The effects of calcium channel blockers on cyclosporine and its metabolites in renal transplant patients. *Ther Drug Monit* 1990; **12:** 321–8.
7. Yildiz A, *et al.* Interaction between cyclosporine A and verapamil, felodipine, and isradipine. *Nephron* 1999; **81:** 117–18.
8. Sketris IS, *et al.* Effect of calcium-channel blockers on cyclosporine clearance and use in renal transplant patients. *Ann Pharmacother* 1994; **28:** 1227–31.
9. Jones TE, Morris RG. Diltiazem does not always increase blood cyclosporin concentration. *Br J Clin Pharmacol* 1996; **42:** 642–4.
10. Bleck JS, *et al.* Diltiazem increases blood concentrations of cyclized cyclosporine metabolites resulting in different cyclosporine metabolite patterns in stable male and female renal allograft recipients. *Br J Clin Pharmacol* 1996; **41:** 551–6.
11. Cohen DJ, *et al.* Influence of oral felodipine on serum cyclosporine concentrations. *Clin Transplant* 1994; **8:** 541–5.
12. Endresen L, *et al.* Lack of effect of the calcium antagonist isradipine on cyclosporine pharmacokinetics in renal transplant patients. *Ther Drug Monit* 1991; **13:** 490–5.
13. Pesavento TE, *et al.* Amlodipine increases cyclosporin levels in hypertensive renal transplant patients: results of a prospective study. *J Am Soc Nephrol* 1996; **7:** 831–5.
14. Toupance O, *et al.* Antihypertensive effect of amlodipine and lack of interference with cyclosporine metabolism in renal transplant recipients. *Hypertension* 1994; **24:** 297–300.


CARDIAC GLYCOSIDES. For reference to the effect of ciclosporin on serum-digoxin concentrations, see under Digoxin, p.898.

CLONIDINE. Addition of clonidine to the regimen of a 3-year-old child who had developed hypertension after a renal transplant resulted in a marked increase in whole blood ciclosporin concentrations, despite a reduction in ciclosporin dose.[1] Ciclosporin concentrations fell rapidly on withdrawal of clonidine.


1. Gilbert RD, *et al.* Interaction between clonidine and cyclosporine A. *Nephron* 1995; **71:** 105.


DIURETICS. Enhanced nephrotoxicity, without apparent change in ciclosporin blood concentrations, has been seen in individual patients following addition of *metolazone*[1] or *amiloride* with *chlorothiazide*[2] to their regimen. Severe nephrotoxicity, resulting in loss of graft function, has been seen in a renal transplant patient given *mannitol* with ciclosporin;[3] graft function recovered on withdrawal of the diuretic.


1. Christensen P, Leski M. Nephrotoxic drug interaction between metolazone and cyclosporin. *BMJ* 1987; **294:** 578.
2. Deray G, *et al.* Enhancement of cyclosporin nephrotoxicity by diuretic therapy. *Clin Nephrol* 1989; **32:** 47.
3. Brunner FP, *et al.* Mannitol potentiates cyclosporine nephrotoxicity. *Clin Nephrol* 1986; **25** (suppl 1): S130–6.


**Colchicine.** Use of ciclosporin with colchicine may result in myopathy or rhabdomyolysis—see Effects on Skeletal Muscle, under Adverse Effects, above. For reports of adverse effects and increased serum-ciclosporin concentrations following concurrent therapy with colchicine, see also p.415.

**Corticosteroids.** It has been suggested that use of ciclosporin with corticosteroids increases plasma concentrations of both drugs, but not all studies support this—see Immunosuppressants, p.1072.

**Gastrointestinal drugs.** Administration of *cisapride* to renal transplant recipients receiving ciclosporin has been reported to increase peak ciclosporin concentrations and increase the speed of absorption.[1] *Cimetidine*,[2,3] *ranitidine*,[2] or *famotidine*,[3] do not appear to affect ciclosporin pharmacokinetics. A literature review[4] noted that although there are reports of cimetidine influencing peak concentrations of ciclosporin, there is no support for a pharmacokinetic interaction. A pharmacodynamic interaction between ciclosporin and histamine $H_2$-receptor antagonists, resulting in a potentiation of nephrotoxicity, is also unlikely.

1. Finet L, *et al.* Effects of cisapride on the intestinal absorption of cyclosporine in renal transplant recipients. *Gastroenterology* 1991; **100:** A209.
2. Barri YM, *et al.* Cimetidine or ranitidine in renal transplant patients receiving cyclosporine. *Clin Transplant* 1996; **10:** 34–8.
3. Shaefer MS, *et al.* Evaluation of the pharmacokinetic interaction between cimetidine or famotidine and cyclosporine in healthy men. *Ann Pharmacother* 1995; **29:** 1088–91.
4. Lewis SM, McCloskey WW. Potentiation of nephrotoxicity by $H_2$-antagonists in patients receiving cyclosporine. *Ann Pharmacother* 1997; **31:** 363–5.

**Grapefruit juice.** Grapefruit juice increases the bioavailability of oral ciclosporin,[1-4] including the microemulsion formulation,[5] leading to marked increases in blood-ciclosporin concentrations; intravenous ciclosporin is unaffected. The effect appears to be due to inhibition of cytochrome P450 enzymes in the gut wall by substances present in grapefruit juice,[3] resulting in transiently reduced ciclosporin metabolism. Although it has been suggested that the effect might be used similarly to that of calcium-channel blockers or ketoconazole in reducing the required dose of ciclosporin,[2] others have pointed out that grapefruit juice is not standardised and its effects are variable.[6]

1. Proppe DG, *et al.* Influence of chronic ingestion of grapefruit juice on steady-state blood concentrations of cyclosporine A in renal transplant patients with stable graft function. *Br J Clin Pharmacol* 1995; **39:** 337–8.
2. Yee GC, *et al.* Effect of grapefruit juice on blood cyclosporin concentration. *Lancet* 1995; **345:** 955–6.
3. Hollander AAMJ, *et al.* The effect of grapefruit juice on cyclosporine and prednisone metabolism in transplant patients. *Clin Pharmacol Ther* 1995; **57:** 318–24.
4. Ducharme MP, *et al.* Disposition of intravenous and oral cyclosporine after administration with grapefruit juice. *Clin Pharmacol Ther* 1995; **57:** 485–91.
5. Ku Y-M, *et al.* Effect of grapefruit juice on the pharmacokinetics of microemulsion cyclosporine and its metabolite in healthy volunteers: does the formulation difference matter? *J Clin Pharmacol* 1998; **38:** 959–65.
6. Johnston A, Holt DW. Effect of grapefruit juice on blood cyclosporin concentration. *Lancet* 1995; **346:** 122–3.

**Hypoglycaemic drugs.** Use of *glibenclamide* with ciclosporin in 6 patients was associated with a mean 57% increase in the steady-state plasma concentration of ciclosporin, suggesting that dosage adjustment may be necessary when these drugs are given concomitantly.[1]

*Troglitazone* decreased ciclosporin-blood concentrations by 32%, necessitating an increase in ciclosporin dosage.[2]

1. Islam SI, *et al.* Possible interaction between cyclosporine and glibenclamide in posttransplant diabetic patients. *Ther Drug Monit* 1996; **18:** 624–6.
2. Burgess SJ, *et al.* Effect of troglitazone on cyclosporine whole blood levels. *Transplantation* 1998; **66:** 272–3.

**Immunosuppressants.** There has been a report of altered ciclosporin requirements in paediatric renal graft patients treated with *basiliximab*,[1] but others have failed to note such an effect,[2] and whether an interaction exists is unclear.

Treatment of acute rejection of kidney grafts in 10 patients using *muromonab-CD3* resulted in increases in mean trough ciclosporin concentrations, despite a reduction in ciclosporin dosage.[3] Once muromonab-CD3 was withdrawn the ciclosporin dosage had to be increased again to provide adequate concentrations. In a retrospective study[4] of renal transplant recipients given ciclosporin and either muromonab-CD3 or antilymphocyte immunoglobulin, ciclosporin trough concentrations were found to be raised on day 5 postoperatively in the patients receiving muromonab-CD3. Although no differences were found in trough concentrations on days 7 and 10, the doses of ciclosporin had by then been adjusted based on the levels obtained on day 5.

For the effects of ciclosporin on the pharmacokinetics of *everolimus, mycophenolate mofetil,* and *sirolimus*, see p.1360, p.1361, and p.1363 respectively.

*Tacrolimus* inhibits ciclosporin metabolism *in vitro*[5] but did not alter the pharmacokinetics of intravenous ciclosporin in 7 liver transplant patients.[6] However, there is a possibility of increased nephrotoxicity when the drugs are used together, so the manufacturers recommend avoiding such use.

1. Strehlau J, *et al.* Interleukin-2 receptor antibody-induced alterations of ciclosporin dose requirements in paediatric transplant recipients. *Lancet* 2000; **356:** 1327–8.
2. Vester U, *et al.* Basiliximab in paediatric liver-transplant recipients. *Lancet* 2001; **357:** 388–9.
3. Vrahnos D, *et al.* Cyclosporin levels during OKT3 treatment of acute renal allograft rejection. *Pharmacotherapy* 1991; **11:** 278.
4. Vasquez EM, Pollak R. OKT3 therapy increases cyclosporine blood levels. *Clin Transplant* 1997; **11:** 38–41.
5. Venkataramanan R, *et al.* Pharmacokinetics of FK 506 in transplant patients. *Transplant Proc* 1991; **23:** 2736–40.
6. Jain AB, *et al.* Pharmacokinetics of cyclosporine and nephrotoxicity in orthotopic liver transplant patients rescued with FK 506. *Transplant Proc* 1991; **23:** 2777–9.

**Lipid regulating drugs.** A study in 10 renal transplant recipients indicated that concomitant use of ciclosporin and *probucol* markedly reduced the whole blood and plasma concentrations of the former in 9 of them, compared with use of ciclosporin alone.[1] *Bezafibrate* has been reported to increase blood concentrations of ciclosporin, with resultant nephrotoxicity.[2]

In 1 study, *simvastatin* increased the unbound fraction of ciclosporin in the blood, resulting in a modest increase in apparent ciclosporin clearance.[3] In renal transplant recipients, *atorvastatin* increased ciclosporin blood concentrations in 4 out of 10 patients in one study[4] but was deemed to have minimal clinical effect in others.[5,6] Ciclosporin concentrations were unaffected by *cerivastatin*,[4,7] *fluvastatin*,[8] *lovastatin*,[9] and *pravastatin*.[9,10] A literature review concluded that the statins do not interact with ciclosporin to a clinically relevant degree; however, given the narrow therapeutic range of ciclosporin, and reports of rhabdomyolysis when used together, the authors advise that ciclosporin levels be monitored when starting statin therapy, and that lower doses of statins be used.[11] For the effects of ciclosporin on plasma levels of statins and reports of rhabdomyolysis, see Immunosuppressants, under Interactions of Simvastatin, p.999.

1. Gallego C, *et al.* Interaction between probucol and cyclosporine in renal transplant patients. *Ann Pharmacother* 1994; **28:** 940–3.
2. Hirai M, *et al.* Elevated blood concentrations of cyclosporine and kidney failure after bezafibrate in renal graft recipient. *Ann Pharmacother* 1996; **30:** 883–4.
3. Akhlaghi F, *et al.* Effect of simvastatin on cyclosporine unbound fraction and apparent blood clearance in heart transplant recipients. *Br J Clin Pharmacol* 1997; **44:** 537–42.
4. Renders L, *et al.* Efficacy and drug interactions of the new HMG-CoA reductase inhibitors cerivastatin and atorvastatin in CsA-treated renal transplant recipients. *Nephrol Dial Transplant* 2001; **16:** 141–6.
5. Åsberg A, *et al.* Bilateral pharmacokinetic interaction between cyclosporine A and atorvastatin in renal transplant recipients. *Am J Transplant* 2001; **1:** 382–6.
6. Taylor PJ, *et al.* Effect of atorvastatin on cyclosporine pharmacokinetics in liver transplant recipients. *Ann Pharmacother* 2004; **38:** 205–8.
7. Mück W, *et al.* Increase in cerivastatin systemic exposure after single and multiple dosing in cyclosporine-treated kidney transplant recipients. *Clin Pharmacol Ther* 1999; **65:** 251–61.
8. Goldberg R, Roth D. Evaluation of fluvastatin in the treatment of hypercholesterolemia in renal transplant recipients taking cyclosporine. *Transplantation* 1996; **62:** 1559–64.
9. Olbricht C, *et al.* Accumulation of lovastatin, but not pravastatin, in the blood of cyclosporine-treated kidney graft patients after multiple doses. *Clin Pharmacol Ther* 1997; **62:** 311–21.
10. Regazzi MB, *et al.* Altered disposition of pravastatin following concomitant drug therapy with cyclosporin A in transplant recipients. *Transplant Proc* 1993; **25:** 2732–4.
11. Åsberg A. Interactions between cyclosporin and lipid-lowering drugs: implications for organ transplant recipients. *Drugs* 2003; **63:** 367–78.

**NSAIDs.** Raised serum-ciclosporin trough concentrations, together with small increases in serum creatinine and BUN concentrations, followed the use of *sulindac* in a previously-stabilised renal graft recipient taking an immunosuppressive regimen including ciclosporin.[1] Increased renal impairment was seen when sulindac or *naproxen* were added to ciclosporin therapy in patients with rheumatoid arthritis.[2] Nephrotoxicity, in the absence of significantly raised blood-ciclosporin concentrations, has been reported in other patients given *diclofenac* with ciclosporin.[3] Ciclosporin may also increase plasma-diclofenac concentrations, see p.33. In general, because of the known potential of NSAIDs to adversely affect renal function, careful monitoring of renal function is advised if these drugs are added to ciclosporin therapy or their dosages altered.

1. Sesin GP, *et al.* Sulindac-induced elevation of serum cyclosporine concentration. *Clin Pharm* 1989; **8:** 445–6.
2. Altman RD, *et al.* Interaction of cyclosporine A and nonsteroidal anti-inflammatory drugs on renal function in patients with rheumatoid arthritis. *Am J Med* 1992; **93:** 396–402.
3. Branthwaite JP, Nicholls A. Cyclosporin and diclofenac interaction in rheumatoid arthritis. *Lancet* 1991; **337:** 252.

**Octreotide.** A marked reduction in ciclosporin serum concentrations was seen in 10 diabetic patients with pancreatic transplants when octreotide was given concomitantly;[1] it was suggested that if these 2 drugs are given together the oral dosage of ciclosporin needs to be increased on average by 50%.

1. Landgraf R, *et al.* Effect of somatostatin analogue (SMS 201-995) on cyclosporine levels. *Transplantation* 1987; **44:** 724–5.

**Orlistat.** A reduction in ciclosporin concentrations to subtherapeutic levels has been reported[1-3] in transplant recipients following concomitant use of orlistat. It was postulated[2] that the interaction was a result of reduced absorption of ciclosporin in the presence of orlistat and that at least 2 hours should elapse between doses of these two drugs. However, despite this dosing interval, there has been a further report[3] of subtherapeutic plasma levels of ciclosporin. The patient had experienced severe diarrhoea, and the subsequent decreased absorption of fats was thought to have decreased the absorption of ciclosporin.

1. Nägele H, *et al.* Effect of orlistat on blood cyclosporin concentration in an obese heart transplant patient. *Eur J Clin Pharmacol* 1999; **55:** 667–9.
2. Colman E, Fossler M. Reduction in blood cyclosporine concentrations by orlistat. *N Engl J Med* 2000; **342:** 1141–2.
3. Barbaro D, *et al.* Obesity in transplant patients: case report showing interference of orlistat with absorption of cyclosporine and review of literature. *Endocr Pract* 2002; **8:** 124–6.

**Retinoids.** Following a report of increased whole-blood ciclosporin concentrations and nephrotoxicity in a patient given *etretinate* with ciclosporin, *in-vitro* results indicated that etretinate inhibited hepatic microsomal metabolism of ciclosporin, as did *acitretin* and *isotretinoin*.[1] However, a study failed to find evidence of such an interaction *in vitro*.[2]

1. Shah IA, *et al.* The effects of retinoids and terbinafine on the human hepatic microsomal metabolism of cyclosporin. *Br J Dermatol* 1993; **129:** 395–8.
2. Webber IR, Back DJ. Effect of etretinate on cyclosporin metabolism in vitro. *Br J Dermatol* 1993; **128:** 42–4.

**Sex hormones.** Raised ciclosporin concentrations in blood have been seen when therapy with *danazol*,[1] *methyltestosterone*,[2] or *norethisterone*[1] was given with ciclosporin, and clinical evidence of both nephrotoxicity[1,2] and hepatotoxicity[2] has been seen. Severe hepatotoxicity and raised plasma-ciclosporin trough values also resulted when an oral contraceptive containing *levonorgestrel* and *ethinylestradiol* was taken by a woman receiving ciclosporin;[3] she had taken the same contraceptive before beginning ciclosporin without ill-effects.

1. Ross WB, *et al.* Cyclosporin interaction with danazol and norethisterone. *Lancet* 1986; **i:** 330.
2. Møller BB, Ekelund B. Toxicity of cyclosporine during treatment with androgens. *N Engl J Med* 1985; **313:** 1416.
3. Deray G, *et al.* Oral contraceptive interaction with cyclosporin. *Lancet* 1987; **i:** 158.

**Vaccines.** Efficacy of immunoprophylaxis may be expected to be diminished during ciclosporin therapy, and use of live virus vaccines, in particular, is contra-indicated in immunocompromised patients.[1] Further, there is some evidence that antigens given during ciclosporin therapy may induce tolerance, which might result in increased susceptibility to the diseases one wishes to protect against.

1. Grabenstein JD, Baker JR. Comment: cyclosporine and vaccination. *Drug Intell Clin Pharm* 1985; **19:** 679–80.

**Vitamins.** For reference to increased absorption of ciclosporin when given with a water-soluble macrogol derivative of *vitamin E*, see Absorption, under Pharmacokinetics, below.

## Pharmacokinetics

The pharmacokinetics of ciclosporin are variable and difficult to determine. Results vary depending on the assay used, and values obtained by different methods are not strictly comparable.

Absorption of conventional formulations of ciclosporin from the gastrointestinal tract is variable and incomplete. An oral microemulsion formulation with improved absorption characteristics is available and is more rapidly and completely absorbed, with peak concentrations achieved about 1.5 to 2 hours after a dose.

Ciclosporin is widely distributed throughout the body. Distribution in the blood is concentration-dependent, with between 41 and 58% in erythrocytes and 10 to 20% in leucocytes; the remainder is found in plasma, about 90% protein-bound, mostly to lipoprotein. Because of distribution into blood cells whole blood concentrations are higher than, and not comparable with, plasma concentrations; where peak plasma concentrations are reported to be approximately 1 nanogram/mL (by specific HPLC assay) for each mg of oral ciclosporin, whole blood concentrations for each mg range from about 1.4 to 2.7 nanograms/mL. Ciclosporin is reported to cross the placenta, and to be distributed into breast milk.

Clearance from the blood is biphasic. The terminal elimination half-life of an oral dose is reported to range from about 5 to 20 hours; clearance in children is more rapid.

Ciclosporin is extensively metabolised in the liver and primarily excreted in faeces via the bile. About 6% of a dose is reported to be excreted in urine, less than 0.1% unchanged.

**Absorption.** Ingestion of conventional formulations of ciclosporin with food may increase its bioavailability, although the effect only appears to be significant when the meal is high in fat;[1] ingestion with food and added bile acids may also increase absorption moderately.[2] A micelle-forming macrogol derivative of vitamin E (tocofersolan) has also been reported to markedly increase ciclosporin absorption.[3,4]

Because of the problems of variable oral absorption, an oral microemulsion has been developed which offers greatly improved and more predictable bioavailability,[5-8] particularly in liver transplant patients with impaired bile flow.[5] It should be noted that the formulation of this microemulsion in fact includes a vitamin E compound.

However, a study[9] has suggested that contrary to previous assumptions, conventional formulations of ciclosporin are quite well absorbed, and that the low bioavailability is due to extensive cytochrome-mediated metabolism in the gut wall (see also Metabolism, below). If this were the case, the improved bioavailability seen with the microemulsion formulation is presumably less to do with improved absorption than with protection from such metabolism.


1. Gupta SK, *et al.* Effect of food on the pharmacokinetics of cyclosporine in healthy subjects following oral and intravenous administration. *J Clin Pharmacol* 1990; **30:** 643–53.
2. Lindholm A, *et al.* The effect of food and bile acid administration on the relative bioavailability of cyclosporin. *Br J Clin Pharmacol* 1990; **29:** 541–8.
3. Sokol RJ, *et al.* Improvement of cyclosporin absorption in children after liver transplantation by means of water-soluble vitamin E. *Lancet* 1991; **338:** 212–15.
4. Chang T, *et al.* The effect of water-soluble vitamin E on cyclosporine pharmacokinetics in healthy volunteers. *Clin Pharmacol Ther* 1996; **59:** 297–303.
5. Trull AK, *et al.* Absorption of cyclosporin from conventional and new microemulsion oral formulations in liver transplant recipients with external biliary diversion. *Br J Clin Pharmacol* 1995; **39:** 627–31.
6. van den Borne BEEM, *et al.* Relative bioavailability of a new oral form of cyclosporin A in patients with rheumatoid arthritis. *Br J Clin Pharmacol* 1995; **39:** 172–5.
7. Friman S, Bäckman L. A new microemulsion formulation of cyclosporin: pharmacokinetic and clinical features. *Clin Pharmacokinet* 1996; **30:** 181–93.
8. Schädeli F, *et al.* Population pharmacokinetic model to predict steady-state exposure to once-daily cyclosporin microemulsion in renal transplant recipients. *Clin Pharmacokinet* 2002; **41:** 59–69.
9. Wu C-Y, *et al.* Differentiation of absorption and first-pass gut and hepatic metabolism in humans: studies with cyclosporine. *Clin Pharmacol Ther* 1995; **58:** 492–7.


**Ethnicity and sex.** Gender-dependent racial differences in the pharmacokinetics of ciclosporin have been suggested.[1] African American women showed larger clearances of intravenous and oral ciclosporin (microemulsion formulation) than African American men, and white women. There were no significant differences in clearance between men of different ethnic origin, or between white men and women. Overall bioavailability was also lower in African Americans compared with white subjects. However, other studies[2,3] found no differences in relative bioavailability between races.


1. Min DI, *et al.* Gender-dependent racial difference in disposition of cyclosporine among healthy African American and white volunteers. *Clin Pharmacol Ther* 2000; **68:** 478–86.
2. Stein CM, *et al.* Cyclosporine pharmacokinetics and pharmacodynamics in African American and white subjects. *Clin Pharmacol Ther* 2001; **69:** 317–23.
3. Pollak R, *et al.* Cyclosporine bioavailability of Neoral and Sandimmune in white and black de novo renal transplant recipients. *Ther Drug Monit* 1999; **21:** 661–3.


**Metabolism.** *In vitro*[1] and *in vivo*[2-4] evidence indicates that the low oral bioavailability of ciclosporin is due to first-pass metabolism in the gastrointestinal tract rather than the liver.


1. Tjia JF, *et al.* Cyclosporin metabolism by the gastrointestinal mucosa. *Br J Clin Pharmacol* 1991; **31:** 344–6.
2. Kolars JC, *et al.* First-pass metabolism of cyclosporin by the gut. *Lancet* 1991; **338:** 1488–90.
3. Hoppu K, *et al.* Evidence for pre-hepatic metabolism of oral cyclosporine in children. *Br J Clin Pharmacol* 1991; **32:** 477–81.
4. Wu C-Y, *et al.* Differentiation of absorption and first-pass gut and hepatic metabolism in humans: studies with cyclosporine. *Clin Pharmacol Ther* 1995; **58:** 492–7.


**Therapeutic drug monitoring.** Considerable debate has attended the necessity for therapeutic monitoring of ciclosporin concentrations and also on the questions of which assay methods to use and whether to measure drug concentrations in whole blood or plasma.

Before the introduction of specific monoclonal radio-immunoassay the HPLC assay for ciclosporin had the advantage of being specific for the parent compound, and some suggested it to be the method of choice.[1,2] However, it is a more complex procedure, is not universally available, and is slower to perform than radio-immunoassay.[1,3-5] Specific monoclonal radio-immunoassays are now widely available; a comparative study of specific and non-specific radio-immunoassays, HPLC, and polyclonal fluorescence polarisation immunoassay (FPIA) found that the specific assays, used on whole blood samples, gave the best correlation with clinical events.[6]

Because the distribution of ciclosporin between blood cells and plasma is temperature-dependent,[7] plasma concentrations may be twice as high at 37° as at 21°. The temperature at which samples are stored and processed may therefore considerably influence results. In consequence, measurement of drug concentrations in whole blood is to be preferred.[1,3,4,8] However, many, particularly early, clinical studies have given plasma or serum concentrations, which makes comparison of literature data difficult. This problem is compounded by a considerable degree of variation between laboratories,[9,10] even when the same technique is used,[10] and by circadian variations in ciclosporin metabolism which mean that samples should be taken at the same time of day.[11]

Because of the variability in results caused by difficulties in monitoring it has proved difficult to determine precisely the ciclosporin concentrations associated with therapeutic benefit and toxicity,[1,3-5] and it has been suggested that measurement of the therapeutic concentrations is unnecessary (provided the patient's clinical condition and renal function are monitored) when low-dose ciclosporin is being given (for example, in psoriasis).[12] However, others consider that it is always critical that ciclosporin blood trough concentrations are regularly measured,[13] in addition to other monitoring. It has been suggested[14] that trough ciclosporin concentrations, measured by a specific method in whole blood, should not be less than 150 nanograms/mL during the first month after renal transplantation, although lower concentrations are subsequently acceptable; trough concentrations of 250 to 300 nanograms/mL are recommended in the 3 months following liver transplantation.

Other methods of monitoring ciclosporin therapy include monitoring the area under the concentration-time curve, limited sampling strategies, and Bayesian forecasting.[13,15,16] However, these methods also have limitations, often requiring several samples at inconvenient times for the patient, and can involve complex calculations. A large study[17] in liver transplant recipients found that measuring peak ciclosporin concentration at 2 hours postdose was superior to trough concentration monitoring, resulting in a reduction of the incidence and severity of rejection. It has been pointed out that these results cannot necessarily be extrapolated to different transplant groups and that analysis when sampling high ciclosporin concentrations needs to be extremely accurate.[18] However, there is some suggestion that ciclosporin concentration at 2 hours postdose predicts rejection better than trough concentrations in renal transplant recipients also.[19]


1. Ptachcinski RJ, *et al.* Cyclosporine concentration determinations for monitoring and pharmacokinetic studies. *J Clin Pharmacol* 1986; **26:** 358–66.
2. Varghese Z, *et al.* How to measure cyclosporin. *Lancet* 1984; **i:** 1407–8.
3. Faynor SM, *et al.* Therapeutic drug monitoring of cyclosporine. *Mayo Clin Proc* 1984; **59:** 571–2.
4. Burkle WS. Cyclosporine pharmacokinetics and blood level monitoring. *Drug Intell Clin Pharm* 1985; **19:** 101–5.
5. Rodighiero V. Therapeutic drug monitoring of cyclosporin: practical applications and limitations. *Clin Pharmacokinet* 1989; **16:** 27–37.
6. Lindholm A, *et al.* A prospective study of cyclosporine concentration in relation to its therapeutic effect and toxicity after renal transplantation. *Br J Clin Pharmacol* 1990; **30:** 443–52.
7. Dieperink H. Temperature dependency of cyclosporin plasma levels. *Lancet* 1983; **i:** 416.
8. Bandini G, *et al.* Measuring cyclosporin in plasma. *Lancet* 1983; **i:** 762.
9. Moyer TP. Measurement of cyclosporine: a challenge to the professional laboratory organizations. *Ther Drug Monit* 1985; **7:** 123–4.
10. Johnston A, *et al.* The United Kingdom Cyclosporin Quality Assessment Scheme. *Ther Drug Monit* 1986; **8:** 200–204.
11. Venkataramanan R, *et al.* Diurnal variation in cyclosporine kinetics. *Ther Drug Monit* 1986; **8:** 380–1.
12. Heydendael VMR, *et al.* Cyclosporin trough levels: is monitoring necessary during short-term treatment in psoriasis? A systematic review and clinical data on trough levels. *Br J Dermatol* 2002; **147:** 122–9.
13. Dumont RJ, Ensom MHH. Methods for clinical monitoring of cyclosporin in transplant patients. *Clin Pharmacokinet* 2000; **38:** 427–47.
14. Lindholm A. Therapeutic monitoring of cyclosporin—an update. *Eur J Clin Pharmacol* 1991; **41:** 273–83.
15. David O, Johnston A. Limited sampling strategies. *Clin Pharmacokinet* 2000; **39:** 311–13.
16. Leger F, *et al.* Maximum A Posteriori Bayesian estimation of oral cyclosporin pharmacokinetics in patients with stable renal transplants. *Clin Pharmacokinet* 2002; **41:** 71–80.
17. Levy G, *et al.* Improved clinical outcomes for liver transplant recipients using cyclosporine monitoring based on 2-hr post-dose levels ($C_2$). *Transplantation* 2002; **73:** 953–9.
18. Holt DW. Cyclosporine monitoring based on $C_2$ sampling. *Transplantation* 2002; **73:** 840–1.
19. Pescovitz MD, *et al.* Two-hour post-dose cyclosporine level is a better predictor than trough level of acute rejection of renal allografts. *Clin Transplant* 2002; **16:** 378–82.


## Uses and Administration

Ciclosporin is a powerful immunosuppressant which appears to act specifically on lymphocytes, mainly helper T-cells. It inhibits the activation of calcineurin, an important step in the production of lymphokines including interleukin-2, resulting in a depression of cell-mediated immune response. Unlike cytotoxic immunosuppressants such as cyclophosphamide it has little effect on bone marrow.

Ciclosporin is used, usually with corticosteroids (and often with other immunosuppressants), in organ and tissue transplantation for the prophylaxis of graft rejection, or in the management of graft rejection in patients previously treated with other immunosuppressants. It is also used in severe forms of atopic dermatitis, psoriasis, or rheumatoid arthritis, usually when conventional therapy is ineffective or inappropriate, and is used in nephrotic syndrome.

Ciclosporin has been tried in various other diseases considered to have an auto-immune component as indicated by the cross-references given below; they include aplastic anaemia, asthma, Behçet's syndrome, chronic active hepatitis, multiple sclerosis, myasthenia gravis, sarcoidosis, scleritis or uveitis, scleroderma, and various skin disorders.

Ciclosporin is given by mouth as liquid-filled capsules or as an oily solution, which may be diluted with milk or fruit juice (not grapefruit) immediately before administration to improve palatability. Microemulsion formulations with improved bioavailability are available in a number of countries. When changing between preparations, the initial dose of the new formulation should be the same (mg for mg), and should subsequently be adjusted as necessary based on blood-ciclosporin concentrations, serum creatinine, and blood pressure monitoring. The daily dose of ciclosporin is taken in 2 divided doses, although the conventional formulation is sometimes given as a single daily dose.

In **organ transplantation** the usual initial dose of ciclosporin is 10 to 15 mg/kg daily, given by mouth, beginning 4 to 12 hours before transplantation, and continued for 1 to 2 weeks; lower initial doses may be given with other immunosuppressants (e.g. with corticosteroids or as part of 'triple' or 'quadruple' therapy). Dosage may subsequently be reduced gradually to a daily maintenance dose of 2 to 6 mg/kg.

Kidney function and blood pressure should be monitored regularly, as well as blood concentrations of ciclosporin (see Therapeutic Drug Monitoring, above), and dosage should be adjusted as necessary. Hepatic function should also be monitored.

Ciclosporin may also be given intravenously, at one-third of the oral dose, in patients in whom oral dosage is not feasible. It is given by slow intravenous infusion over 2 to 6 hours, the 5% concentrate being diluted 1:20 to 1:100 in sodium chloride 0.9% or glucose 5%, to give a 0.05 to 0.25% solution of ciclosporin. Because of the risk of anaphylactoid reactions, which have been attributed to the polyethoxylated castor oil vehicle, patients should be transferred to oral therapy as soon as possible.

For the prevention of graft rejection in **bone marrow transplantation**, and prevention and treatment of graft-versus-host disease, an initial dose of 3 to 5 mg/kg daily by the intravenous route is recommended, starting the day before transplantation and continuing for up to 2 weeks until maintenance by mouth, in doses of 12.5 mg/kg daily can be instituted. If oral treatment is used to initiate therapy the recommended dose is 12.5 to 15 mg/kg daily followed by 12.5 mg/kg daily for maintenance. The maintenance dose is continued for at least 3 to 6 months, then gradually reduced until ciclosporin is withdrawn altogether; this may take up to a year after transplantation.

In the treatment of **psoriasis**, ciclosporin may be given in usual initial doses of 2.5 mg/kg daily (a maximum of 5 mg/kg daily is recommended in the UK and 4 mg/kg daily in the USA), in 2 divided doses by mouth, reduced once remission is achieved to the lowest effective maintenance dose. Treatment should be stopped if there is insufficient response to the maximum dose within 6 weeks. A similar dosage range may be given for a maximum of 8 weeks in the treatment of severe **atopic dermatitis**.

In **rheumatoid arthritis** ciclosporin may be given by mouth in initial daily doses of 2.5 mg/kg, divided into two doses, for a period of 6 or 8 weeks. If the clinical effect is insufficient dosage may then be gradually increased to a maximum of 4 mg/kg daily; if there is no response after 3 to 4 months, treatment should be stopped.

For **nephrotic syndrome** secondary to glomerular kidney disease (minimal change nephropathy, focal glomerulosclerosis, or membranous nephropathy) dosage of ciclosporin depends on age and renal function. To induce remission in patients with normal renal function 5 mg/kg daily may be given to adults and 6 mg/kg daily to children, in 2 divided doses by mouth. In patients with renal impairment the initial dose should not exceed 2.5 mg/kg daily. Treatment may be stopped if there is no response after 3 months (or 6 months in patients with membranous nephropathy). In patients who do respond, maintenance doses should be gradually reduced to the minimum effective value.

Eye drops containing ciclosporin 0.05% are used in the management of **dry eye** associated with ocular inflammation.

Ciclosporin can inhibit the P-glycoprotein cellular pump responsible for multidrug resistance, and has been given with antineoplastics to raise their intracellular concentrations. Nonimmunosuppressive ciclosporin analogues such as valspodar (p.591) are also being investigated for their ability to reverse multidrug resistance.

**Administration.** It has been suggested that calculating doses in mg/kg may not be the best way to achieve the desired blood concentrations of ciclosporin.[1] (See also Therapeutic Drug Monitoring, above) Retrospective study of 1071 renal transplant recipients indicated that blood ciclosporin concentrations were not significantly correlated with patient weight, the best prediction of trough blood concentration being given by the formula:

$$\text{Blood concentration (nanograms/mL)} = \text{dose in mg/day} \times (1.34 + 0.00011 \times \text{days after transplant} - 0.0049 \times \text{height in cm})$$

This formula appeared useful in predicting blood concentrations in prospective studies; from the seventh day after transplantation target trough concentrations could be expected to be about 0.3 times the daily ciclosporin dose in mg.


1. Bock HA, *et al.* Weight-independent dosing of cyclosporine—an alternative to the mg/kg doctrine. *Transplantation* 1994; **57:** 1484–9.


INHALATION. Aerosolised ciclosporin given by inhalation has proved effective in the management of acute graft rejection in lung transplantation.[1,2] Doses were up to 300 mg daily via a nebuliser, in either propylene glycol or ethanol solvents.[3] Pulmonary delivery of ciclosporin has been reviewed.[3]


1. Keenan RJ, *et al.* Efficacy of inhaled cyclosporine in lung transplant recipients with refractory rejection: correlation of intragraft cytokine gene expression with pulmonary function and histologic characteristics. *Surgery* 1995; **118:** 385–91.
2. Iacono AT, *et al.* Dose-related reversal of acute lung rejection by aerosolized cyclosporine. *Am J Respir Crit Care Med* 1997; **155:** 1690–8.
3. Klyashchitsky BA, Owen AJ. Nebulizer-compatible liquid formulations for aerosol pulmonary delivery of hydrophobic drugs: glucocorticoids and cyclosporine. *J Drug Target* 1999; **7:** 79–99.


ORAL. The newer microemulsion formulation of ciclosporin has been reviewed.[1,2] For discussion of the potential problems involved in converting from conventional to microemulsion oral formulations see under Precautions, above.


1. Noble S, Markham A. Cyclosporin: a review of the pharmacokinetic properties, clinical efficacy and tolerability of a microemulsion-based formulation (Neoral). *Drugs* 1995; **50:** 924–41.
2. Dunn CJ, *et al.* Cyclosporin: an updated review of the pharmacokinetic properties, clinical efficacy and tolerability of a microemulsion-based formulation (Neoral®) in organ transplantation. *Drugs* 2001; **61:** 1957–2016.


**Aplastic anaemia.** Ciclosporin, usually combined with antilymphocyte immunoglobulin, is used in patients with aplastic anaemia when bone marrow transplantation is unsuitable (see p.732).

**Asthma.** Ciclosporin is being considered as a potential treatment for some cases of asthma (p.777). A controlled study[1] in patients with chronic severe asthma requiring long-standing oral corticosteroid treatment found that addition of ciclosporin in an initial dose of 5 mg/kg daily to their regimen resulted in significant improvement in lung function and a reduced frequency of disease exacerbation, compared with placebo. The results were interesting because of the improvement in what had been considered 'irreversible' airflow obstruction. A subsequent study[2] from the same centre involving 39 patients with severe corticosteroid-dependent asthma found that low-dose ciclosporin by mouth (an initial dose of 5 mg/kg daily) permitted a reduction in the daily dosage of prednisolone, from a median of 10 to 3.5 mg daily. However, a systematic review[3] considered that, given the adverse effects of ciclosporin, any clinical benefit was debatable.


1. Alexander AG, *et al.* Trial of cyclosporin in corticosteroid-dependent chronic severe asthma. *Lancet* 1992; **339:** 324–8.
2. Lock SH, *et al.* Double-blind, placebo-controlled study of cyclosporin A as a corticosteroid-sparing agent in corticosteroid-dependent asthma. *Am J Respir Crit Care Med* 1996; **153:** 509–14.
3. Evans DJ, *et al.* Cyclosporin as an oral corticosteroid sparing agent in stable asthma. Available in The Cochrane Library; Issue 2. Chichester: John Wiley; 2004.


**Behçet's syndrome.** Ciclosporin has been tried in Behçet's syndrome, see p.1076.

**Cogan's syndrome.** Ciclosporin has been used with corticosteroids for severe Cogan's syndrome with large-vessel vasculitis (see p.1078).

**Corneal ulcer.** Ciclosporin 1% eye drops, with lamellar keratoplasty, proved effective in treating Mooren's ulcer, a possibly auto-immune corneal disease that is difficult to manage and can lead to blindness.[1] Treatment with topical ciclosporin alone may also be useful[2] in patients with sterile corneal ulcers associated with rheumatoid disease.


1. Chen J, *et al.* Mooren's ulcer in China: a study of clinical characteristics and treatment. *Br J Ophthalmol* 2000; **84:** 1244–9.
2. Gottsch JD, Akpek EK. Topical cyclosporin stimulates neovascularization in resolving sterile rheumatoid central corneal ulcers. *Trans Am Ophthalmol Soc* 2000; **98:** 81–90.


**Diabetes mellitus.** Immunosuppressants have been used in attempts to prolong the so called 'honeymoon period' in recently diagnosed diabetics (p.324). Ciclosporin has apparently produced modest benefits in such a context,[1-3] but its overall value remains to be determined.


1. Bougneres PF, *et al.* Factors associated with early remission of type 1 diabetes in children treated with cyclosporine. *N Engl J Med* 1988; **318:** 663–70.
2. The Canadian-European Randomized Control Trial Group. Cyclosporin-induced remission of IDDM after early intervention: association of 1 yr of cyclosporin treatment with enhanced insulin secretion. *Diabetes* 1988; **37:** 1574–82.
3. Carel JC, *et al.* Cyclosporine delays but does not prevent clinical onset in glucose intolerant pre-type 1 diabetic children. *J Autoimmun* 1996; **9:** 739–45.


**Dry eye.** Topical ciclosporin has been found to be beneficial[1] for keratoconjunctivitis sicca (dry eye—see p.1576). Further studies[2,3] found ciclosporin 0.05% and 0.1% to be the most appropriate formulations since no additional benefit was found with higher concentrations[2] and both were significantly better than placebo.[3]


1. Laibovitz RA, *et al.* Pilot trial of cyclosporine 1% ophthalmic ointment in the treatment of keratoconjunctivitis sicca. *Cornea* 1993; **12:** 315–23.
2. Stevenson D, *et al.* Efficacy and safety of cyclosporin A ophthalmic emulsion in the treatment of moderate-to-severe dry eye disease: a dose-ranging, randomized trial. *Ophthalmology* 2000; **107:** 967–74.
3. Sall K, *et al.* Two multicenter, randomized studies of the efficacy and safety of cyclosporine ophthalmic emulsion in moderate to severe dry eye disease. *Ophthalmology* 2000; **107:** 631–9.


**Eczema.** Ciclosporin is effective in atopic eczema (atopic dermatitis),[1-3] where it is employed as adjunctive therapy (see p.1135). It is generally reserved for short-term treatment (up to 8 weeks) in patients with severe disease unresponsive to all conventional therapies, although reports have described long-term use in adult patients.[4] It has also been suggested[5] that long-term remission is possible, even in those treated with short courses. Ciclosporin has been used for both short courses[6,7] and continuous therapy in children.[8] In a small, open, crossover study,[9] the microemulsion was considered equivalent or superior in tolerability and efficacy when compared with the lipophilic formulation. Responses have also been reported in severe eczematisation associated with Darier's disease[10] (p.1134).


1. van Joost T, *et al.* Cyclosporin in atopic dermatitis: a multicentre placebo-controlled study. *Br J Dermatol* 1994; **130:** 634–40.
2. Munro CS, *et al.* Maintenance treatment with cyclosporin in atopic eczema. *Br J Dermatol* 1994; **130:** 376–80.
3. Granlund H, *et al.* Cyclosporin in atopic dermatitis: time to relapse and effect of intermittent therapy. *Br J Dermatol* 1995; **132:** 106–12.
4. Berth-Jones J, *et al.* Long-term efficacy and safety of cyclosporin in severe adult atopic dermatitis. *Br J Dermatol* 1997; **136:** 76–81.
5. Granlund H, *et al.* Long-term follow-up of eczema patients treated with cyclosporine. *Acta Derm Venereol (Stockh)* 1998; **78:** 40–3.
6. Zaki I, *et al.* Treatment of severe atopic dermatitis in childhood with cyclosporin. *Br J Dermatol* 1996; **135** (suppl 48): 21–4.
7. Berth-Jones J, *et al.* Cyclosporine in severe childhood atopic dermatitis: a multicenter study. *J Am Acad Dermatol* 1996; **34:** 1016–21.
8. Harper JI, *et al.* Cyclosporin for severe childhood atopic dermatitis: short course versus continuous therapy. *Br J Dermatol* 2000; **142:** 52–8.
9. Chawla M, *et al.* Comparison of the steady state pharmacokinetics of two formulations of cyclosporin in patients with atopic dermatitis. *Br J Dermatol* 1996; **135** (suppl 48): 9–14.
10. Shahidullah H, *et al.* Darier's disease: severe eczematization successfully treated with cyclosporin. *Br J Dermatol* 1994; **131:** 713–16.


**Glaucoma.** Topical ciclosporin has produced some encouraging results[1] when used as an adjunct to reduce formation of scar tissue and improve outcome of glaucoma filtering surgery (p.1485). It has been suggested[2] that topical ciclosporin 0.5% may be substituted for topical corticosteroids in the treatment of postkeratoplasty glaucoma.


1. Turaçli E, *et al.* A comparative clinical trial of mitomycin C and cyclosporin A in trabeculectomy. *Eur J Ophthalmol* 1996; **6:** 398–401.
2. Perry HD, *et al.* Topical cyclosporin A in the management of postkeratoplasty glaucoma. *Cornea* 1997; **16:** 284–8.


**Glomerular kidney disease.** Ciclosporin has been tried in a number of forms of glomerular kidney disease (p.1080) but use has been cautious because of fears about nephrotoxicity. Nonetheless, responses have been seen in patients with corticosteroid-resistant minimal change nephropathy,[1,2] focal glomerulosclerosis,[1-3] and membranous nephropathy.[4,5]


1. Nyrop M, Olgaard K. Cyclosporin A treatment of severe steroid resistant nephrotic syndrome in adults. *J Intern Med* 1990; **227:** 65–8.
2. Niaudet P, *et al.* Steroid-resistant idiopathic nephrotic syndrome and ciclosporin. *Nephron* 1991; **57:** 481.
3. Chishti AS, *et al.* Long-term treatment of focal segmental glomerulosclerosis in children with cyclosporine given as a single daily dose. *Am J Kidney Dis* 2001; **38:** 754–60.
4. Cattran DC, *et al.* A controlled trial of cyclosporine in patients with progressive membranous nephropathy. *Kidney Int* 1995; **47:** 1130–5.
5. Cattran DC, *et al.* Cyclosporine in patients with steroid-resistant membranous nephropathy: a randomized trial. *Kidney Int* 2001; **59:** 1484–90.


**Hepatitis.** In chronic active hepatitis (p.1078), some evidence suggests that ciclosporin may offer an alternative therapy in patients with severe auto-immune (non-viral) disease where corticosteroids alone or with azathioprine do not suffice.

References.


1. Mistilis SP, *et al.* Cyclosporin, a new treatment for autoimmune chronic active hepatitis. *Med J Aust* 1985; **143:** 463–5.
2. Sherman KE, *et al.* Cyclosporine in the management of corticosteroid-resistant type 1 autoimmune chronic active hepatitis. *J Hepatol* 1994; **21:** 1040–7.
3. Debray D, *et al.* Efficacy of cyclosporin A in children with type 2 autoimmune hepatitis. *J Pediatr* 1999; **135:** 111–14.


**Histiocytic syndromes.** As mentioned in the discussion on p.505 ciclosporin has been tried in patients with advanced Langerhans-cell histiocytosis.

**Inflammatory bowel disease.** Ciclosporin has been tried with variable success as a second-line drug in inflammatory bowel disease (p.1243). Intravenous high-dose ciclosporin has shown some efficacy in refractory ulcerative colitis,[1-3] and may also be useful if given by enema.[4] However, benefit in Crohn's disease is less clear. Although intravenous therapy is reportedly useful in healing refractory fistulae,[5] lower oral doses have produced disappointing results in adults and children with chronic active Crohn's disease,[6,7] and for maintenance of remission.[8] However, since these studies used the older lipophilic formulation, a small study[9] investigated the pharmacokinetics of the microemulsion in patients with inflammatory bowel disease. Absorption was greater in patients with ulcerative colitis than in those with Crohn's disease. Despite few differences in the pharmacokinetics of the microemulsion in patients with inflammatory bowel disease and healthy volunteers, the authors believe the newer formulation may offer increased absorption and bioavailability, and that studies are needed, specifically comparing the two oral formulations in patients with inflammatory bowel disease.


1. Lichtiger S, *et al.* Cyclosporine in severe ulcerative colitis refractory to steroid therapy. *N Engl J Med* 1994; **330:** 1841–5.
2. Hyde GM, *et al.* Intravenous cyclosporin as rescue therapy in severe ulcerative colitis: time for a reappraisal? *Eur J Gastroenterol Hepatol* 1998; **10:** 411–13.
3. Loftus CG, *et al.* Cyclosporin for refractory ulcerative colitis. *Gut* 2003; **52:** 172–3.
4. Sandborn WJ, *et al.* Cyclosporine enemas for treatment-resistant, mildly to moderately active, left-sided ulcerative colitis. *Am J Gastroenterol* 1993; **88:** 640–5.
5. Hanauer SB, Smith MB. Rapid closure of Crohn's disease fistulas with continuous intravenous cyclosporin A. *Am J Gastroenterol* 1993; **88:** 646–9.
6. Nicholls S, *et al.* Cyclosporin as initial treatment for Crohn's disease. *Arch Dis Child* 1994; **71:** 243–7.
7. Stange EF, *et al.* European trial of cyclosporine in chronic active Crohn's disease: a 12-month study. *Gastroenterology* 1995; **109:** 774–82.
8. Feagan BG, *et al.* Low-dose cyclosporine for the treatment of Crohn's disease. *N Engl J Med* 1994; **330:** 1846–51.
9. Latteri M, *et al.* Pharmacokinetics of cyclosporin microemulsion in patients with inflammatory bowel disease. *Clin Pharmacokinet* 2001; **40:** 473–83.


**Lichen planus.** Lichen planus is a skin disorder generally controlled with corticosteroids (see p.1136), although ciclosporin has also been used. Ciclosporin has been given successfully in relatively low doses (3 to 5 mg/kg by mouth) to produce remission of severe lichen planus,[1] but such therapy may be associated with the development of hypertension and impairment of renal function. Use of ciclosporin oral solution as a mouthwash for oral lichen planus has been tried, but results have been variable.[2-7] One such study failed to note any benefit long-term from either ciclosporin mouthwash or corticosteroid oral paste.[7]


1. Pigatto PD, *et al.* Cyclosporin A for treatment of severe lichen planus. *Br J Dermatol* 1990; **121:** 121–3.
2. Eisen D, *et al.* Cyclosporin wash for oral lichen planus. *Lancet* 1990; **335:** 535–6.
3. Eisen D, *et al.* Effect of topical cyclosporine rinse on oral lichen planus: a double-blind analysis. *N Engl J Med* 1990; **323:** 290–4.
4. Levell NJ, *et al.* Lack of effect of cyclosporin mouthwash in oral lichen planus. *Lancet* 1991; **337:** 796–7.
5. Ho VC, Conklin RJ. Effect of topical cyclosporine rinse on oral lichen planus. *N Engl J Med* 1991; **325:** 435.
6. Porter SR, *et al.* The efficacy of topical cyclosporin in the management of desquamative gingivitis due to lichen planus. *Br J Dermatol* 1993; **129:** 753–5.
7. Sieg P, *et al.* Topical cyclosporin in oral lichen planus: a controlled, randomized prospective trial. *Br J Dermatol* 1995; **132:** 790–4.


**Lupus nephritis.** As mentioned on p.1088, ciclosporin has been investigated for systemic lupus erythematosus, particularly lupus nephritis,[1-3] but controlled trials are needed.


1. Fu LW, *et al.* Clinical efficacy of cyclosporin A Neoral in the treatment of paediatric lupus nephritis with heavy proteinuria. *Br J Rheumatol* 1998; **37:** 217–21.
2. Tam LS, *et al.* Long-term treatment of lupus nephritis with cyclosporin A. *Q J Med* 1998; **91:** 573–80.
3. Hallegua D, *et al.* Cyclosporine for lupus membranous nephritis: experience with ten patients and review of the literature. *Lupus* 2000; **9:** 241–51.


**Multiple sclerosis.** As noted on p.646, immunosuppressants, including ciclosporin,[1,2] have produced modest benefit in patients with multiple sclerosis. However, it has been concluded that the scanty benefits of therapy are outweighed by the toxicity of the doses required.


1. Rudge P, *et al.* Randomised double blind controlled trial of cyclosporin in multiple sclerosis. *J Neurol Neurosurg Psychiatry* 1989; **52:** 559–65.
2. The Multiple Sclerosis Study Group. Efficacy and toxicity of cyclosporine in chronic progressive multiple sclerosis: a randomized, double-blinded, placebo-controlled clinical trial. *Ann Neurol* 1990; **27:** 591–605.


**Muscular dystrophies.** A study in 15 boys with Duchenne muscular dystrophy (p.1083) given ciclosporin 5 mg/kg daily by mouth in divided doses, adjusted according to trough serum concentrations of ciclosporin, found that muscular force generation was improved during treatment, but declined again once treatment ceased.[1] The clinical significance, if any, of this effect remains to be established.


1. Sharma KR, *et al.* Cyclosporine increases muscular force generation in Duchenne muscular dystrophy. *Neurology* 1993; **43:** 527–32.


**Myasthenia gravis.** Ciclosporin may be of use as an alternative to azathioprine in the management of myasthenia gravis (p.1486) for its corticosteroid-sparing effect[1] or when patients are intolerant of or unresponsive to corticosteroids and azathioprine.[2,3] It appears to be of similar efficacy to azathioprine[4] with a more rapid effect but serious adverse effects such as nephrotoxicity may limit its use.


1. Tindall RSA, *et al.* A clinical therapeutic trial of cyclosporine in myasthenia gravis. *Ann N Y Acad Sci* 1993; **681:** 539–51.
2. Bonifati DM, Angelini C. Long-term cyclosporine treatment in a group of severe myasthenia gravis patients. *J Neurol* 1997; **244:** 542–7.
3. Ciafaloni E, *et al.* Retrospective analysis of the use of cyclosporine in myasthenia gravis. *Neurology* 2000; **55:** 448–50.
4. Schalke BCG, *et al.* Ciclosporin A vs azathioprine in the treatment of myasthenia gravis: final results of a randomized, controlled double-blind clinical trial. *Neurology* 1988; **38** (suppl 1): 135.


**Organ and tissue transplantation.** Ciclosporin has greatly improved the prospects for successful organ and tissue transplantation, and is a mainstay of regimens used to prevent rejection of solid organ grafts as well as being used for the prevention of graft-versus-host disease in bone marrow transplantation. For more detailed discussion of organ and tissue transplantation and the role of ciclosporin, see p.1344. Ciclosporin has also occasionally been used for corneal graft rejection (p.1079) in high-risk patients, where corticosteroids alone are insufficient.

**Pemphigus.** Although pemphigus is usually treated with corticosteroids (see p.1137), ciclosporin has also been tried in a few patients with pemphigus vulgaris, with variable results.[1-3] A small, randomised trial[4] found that combination treatment with corticosteroids and ciclosporin had no advantage over corticosteroids alone.


1. Luisi AF, Stoukides CA. Cyclosporine for the treatment of pemphigus vulgaris. *Ann Pharmacother* 1994; **28:** 1183–5.
2. Vardy DA, Cohen AD. Cyclosporine therapy should be considered for maintenance of remission in patients with pemphigus. *Arch Dermatol* 2001; **137:** 505.
3. Gooptu C, Staughton RCD. Use of topical cyclosporin in oral pemphigus. *J Am Acad Dermatol* 1998; **38:** 860–1.
4. Ioannides D, *et al.* Ineffectiveness of cyclosporine as an adjuvant to corticosteroids in the treatment of pemphigus. *Arch Dermatol* 2000; **136:** 868–72.


**Polymyositis and dermatomyositis.** Ciclosporin may be of benefit[1-3] in refractory polymyositis and dermatomyositis (see p.1086).


1. Heckmatt J, *et al.* Cyclosporin in juvenile dermatomyositis. *Lancet* 1989; **i:** 1063–6.
2. Lueck CJ, *et al.* Cyclosporin in the management of polymyositis and dermatomyositis. *J Neurol Neurosurg Psychiatry* 1991; **54:** 1007–8.
3. Qushmaq KA, *et al.* Cyclosporin A in the treatment of refractory adult polymyositis/dermatomyositis: population based experience in 6 patients and literature review. *J Rheumatol* 2000; **27:** 2855–9.


**Primary biliary cirrhosis.** In primary biliary cirrhosis (p.1761) some benefit has been reported with ciclosporin,[1] but there are problems with toxicity.


1. Lombard M, *et al.* Cyclosporin A treatment in primary biliary cirrhosis: results of a long-term placebo controlled trial. *Gastroenterology* 1993; **104:** 519–26.


**Psoriasis.** Ciclosporin is used to induce remission or prevent relapse in severe refractory psoriasis (p.1137).

References.


1. Laburte C, *et al.* Efficacy and safety of oral cyclosporin A (CyA; Sandimmun) for long-term treatment of chronic severe plaque psoriasis. *Br J Dermatol* 1994; **130:** 366–75.
2. Berth-Jones J, *et al.* Treatment of psoriasis with intermittent short course cyclosporin (Neoral): a multicentre study. *Br J Dermatol* 1997; **136:** 527–30.
3. Ho VC, *et al.* Intermittent short courses of cyclosporin (Neoral) for psoriasis unresponsive to topical therapy: a 1-year multicentre, randomized study. *Br J Dermatol* 1999; **141:** 283–91.
4. Faerber L, *et al.* Cyclosporine in severe psoriasis: results of a meta-analysis in 579 patients. *Am J Clin Dermatol* 2001; **2:** 41–7.


**Psoriatic arthritis.** One study[1] has shown that low-dose ciclosporin effectively improves joint complaints in psoriatic arthritis (see under Spondyloarthropathies, p.11), and another[2] found ciclosporin to be more effective than sulfasalazine.


1. Mahrle G, *et al.* Anti-inflammatory efficacy of low-dose cyclosporin A in psoriatic arthritis: a prospective multicentre study. *Br J Dermatol* 1996; **135:** 752–7.
2. Salvarani C, *et al.* A comparison of cyclosporine, sulfasalazine, and symptomatic therapy in the treatment of psoriatic arthritis. *J Rheumatol* 2001; **28:** 2274–82.


**Pyoderma gangrenosum.** There have been reports[1-4] of responses to ciclosporin in patients with pyoderma gangrenosum (p.1138).


1. Schmitt EC, *et al.* Pyoderma gangrenosum treated with low-dose cyclosporin. *Br J Dermatol* 1993; **128:** 230–1.
2. Fearfield LA, *et al.* Pyoderma gangrenosum associated with Takayasu's arteritis responding to cyclosporin. *Br J Dermatol* 1999; **141:** 339–43.
3. Sassolas B, *et al.* Pyoderma gangrenosum with pathergic phenomenon in pregnancy. *Br J Dermatol* 2000; **142:** 827–8.
4. Vena GA, Cassano N. Can we still suggest the topical cyclosporin treatment in cutaneous disorders? *J Eur Acad Dermatol Venereol* 2001; **15:** 18–19.


**Rheumatoid arthritis.** Various disease-modifying antirheumatic drugs (DMARDs) are used in rheumatoid arthritis (p.9) in an attempt to modify the disease process. Ciclosporin has produced responses in active disease,[1-4] and there is some evidence that it can slow radiological progression of disease[4] as well as providing symptomatic relief; a systematic review[5] has concluded it has an important clinical benefit in the short-term (up to one year) treatment of progressive disease. There has been some concern about associated nephrotoxicity,[1] but the use of low-dose regimens may help to minimise this. Ciclosporin has also been combined with other DMARDs. A combination of ciclosporin with methotrexate has reportedly produced responses in patients unresponsive to methotrexate alone,[6] but some investigators found that a combination of methotrexate, ciclosporin and intra-articular corticosteroids was no more effective than standard DMARD therapy.[7]

International consensus recommendations exist for the use of ciclosporin in rheumatoid arthritis.[8] These suggest that the use of ciclosporin may be considered in patients who are candidates for DMARDs and who do not have risk factors such as malignancy, uncontrolled hypertension, renal dysfunction, cytopenias, or marked disorder of liver function. They recommend a starting dose of between 2.5 and 3 mg/kg daily, increased if necessary after 4 to 8 weeks, in increments of 0.5 or 1 mg/kg at 1 to 2 month intervals, up to a maximum of 5 mg/kg daily, particular care being taken at doses over 4 mg/kg daily. Once the patient's disease has been stable for at least 3 months the daily dose should be decreased monthly or bimonthly in decrements of 0.5 mg/kg to the lowest effective dose. If it is only partially effective after 3 months at the maximum tolerable dose another medication should be considered instead or in addition; if there is no response to the maximum tolerable dose after 3 months, ciclosporin should be discontinued. Patients should be carefully monitored before and during therapy.

Ciclosporin has been shown to have a corticosteroid-sparing effect and control the fever of juvenile idiopathic arthritis.[9]


1. Yocum DE, *et al.* Cyclosporin A in severe, treatment-refractory rheumatoid arthritis: a randomized study. *Ann Intern Med* 1988; **109:** 863–9.
2. Tugwell P, *et al.* Low-dose cyclosporin versus placebo in patients with rheumatoid arthritis. *Lancet* 1990; **335:** 1051–5.
3. Landewé RBM, *et al.* A randomized, double-blind, 24-week controlled study of low-dose cyclosporine versus chloroquine for early rheumatoid arthritis. *Arthritis Rheum* 1994; **37:** 637–43.
4. Førre Ø, *et al.* Radiologic evidence of disease modification in rheumatoid arthritis patients treated with cyclosporine: results of a 48-week multicenter study comparing low-dose cyclosporine with placebo. *Arthritis Rheum* 1994; **37:** 1506–12.
5. Wells G, *et al.* Cyclosporine for treating rheumatoid arthritis. Available in The Cochrane Library; Issue 2. Chichester: John Wiley; 2004.
6. Tugwell P, *et al.* Combination therapy with cyclosporine and methotrexate in severe rheumatoid arthritis. *N Engl J Med* 1995; **333:** 137–41.
7. Proudman SM, *et al.* Treatment of poor-prognosis early rheumatoid arthritis. *Arthritis Rheum* 2000; **43:** 1809–19.
8. Panayi GS, Tugwell P. The use of cyclosporin A microemulsion in rheumatoid arthritis: conclusions of an international review. *Br J Rheumatol* 1997; **36:** 808–11.
9. Gerloni V, *et al.* Efficacy and safety profile of cyclosporin A in the treatment of juvenile chronic (idiopathic) arthritis: results of a 10-year prospective study. *Rheumatology (Oxford)* 2001; **40:** 907–13.


**Sarcoidosis.** Corticosteroids are the usual therapy for symptomatic sarcoidosis (p.1087), and other agents are very much second-line; ciclosporin is one of a number of immunosuppressants that have been tried with variable results.

**Scleritis.** Ciclosporin is used alone or with corticosteroids in the treatment of scleritis (see p.1088).

**Scleroderma.** There are a few reports of responses to ciclosporin in patients with scleroderma (p.1348).

**Uveitis.** Ciclosporin is used in uveitis, see p.1090.

**Vasculitic syndromes.** For the use of ciclosporin in Takayasu's arteritis and Wegener's granulomatosis, see p.1089 and p.1090, respectively.

## Preparations

***USP 27:*** Cyclosporine Capsules; Cyclosporine Injection; Cyclosporine Oral Solution.

**Proprietary Preparations** (details are given in Part 3)

***Arg.:*** Cermox; Gengraf; Sandimmun; ***Austral.:*** Cysporin; Neoral; Sandimmun; ***Austria:*** Sandimmun; ***Belg.:*** Neoral-Sandimmun; Sandimmun; ***Braz.:*** Gengraf; Sandimmun; Sigmasporin†; ***Canad.:*** Neoral; Sandimmune; ***Chile:*** Sandimmun; ***Denm.:*** Sandimmun; ***Fin.:*** Sandimmun; ***Fr.:*** Neoral; Sandimmun; ***Ger.:*** Cicloral; Sandimmun; ***Gr.:*** Sandimmun; Sandimmun Neoral; ***Hong Kong:*** Gengraf; Sandimmun; ***India:*** Imusporin; Panimun Bioral; Sandimmun Neoral; ***Irl.:*** Neoral; Sandimmun; ***Israel:*** Deximune; Sandimmun; Sangcya; ***Ital.:*** Sandimmun; ***Malaysia:*** Sandimmun; ***Mex.:*** Colosina†; Immulem; Sandimmun; ***Neth.:*** Neoral; Sandimmune; ***Norw.:*** Sandimmun; ***NZ:*** Neoral; Sandimmun; ***Port.:*** Sandimmun; ***S.Afr.:*** Ciclohexal; Sandimmun; ***Singapore:*** Sandimmun Neoral†; ***Spain:*** Sandimmun; ***Swed.:*** Sandimmun; ***Switz.:*** Neoral; Sandimmun; ***Thai.:*** Consupren; Sandimmun; ***UAE:*** Sigmasporin; ***UK:*** Neoral; Sandimmun; Sangcya†; ***USA:*** Gengraf; Neoral; Restasis; Sandimmune.

## Daclizumab *(BAN, USAN, rINN)*

Dacliximab; Humanised Anti-Tac Antibody; Ro-24-7375.

*CAS — 152923-56-3.*
*ATC — L04AA08.*

### Adverse Effects and Precautions

Severe hypersensitivity reactions have occurred rarely; facilities for the treatment of such reactions should be available during use.

◊ Increased mortality was reported in cardiac transplant recipients who received an immunosuppressive regimen of daclizumab with ciclosporin, mycophenolate mofetil, and corticosteroids. Some deaths were associated with severe infection and concomitant use of antilymphocyte immunoglobulins.[1]


1. Roche, USA. 2003 safety alert: Zenapax (daclizumab). Available at: http://www.fda.gov/medwatch/SAFETY/2003/zenapax.htm (accessed 22/06/04)


### Pharmacokinetics

The recommended regimen of daclizumab (see below) should result in serum concentrations sufficient to saturate interleukin-2 receptors for more than 90 days. The terminal elimination half-life of daclizumab has ranged from 11 to 38 days.

### Uses and Administration

Daclizumab is a humanised monoclonal murine antibody that functions as an interleukin-2 receptor antagonist by binding to the alpha chain (CD25 antigen, Tac subunit) of the interleukin-2 receptor on the surface of activated T-lymphocytes. It is used in the prevention of acute graft rejection following kidney transplantation as part of an immunosuppressive regimen that includes ciclosporin and corticosteroids. It is given in a dose of 1 mg/kg intravenously over 15 minutes within 24 hours before surgery and repeated at intervals of 2 weeks for a total of 5 doses. The required dose is diluted in 50 mL of sodium chloride 0.9%, and may be infused either centrally or peripherally. Daclizumab is also under investigation for its immunosuppressant properties in other forms of transplantation (see below) and in various diseases with an auto-immune component.

◊ Reviews.


1. Wiseman LR, Faulds D. Daclizumab: a review of its use in the prevention of acute rejection in renal transplant recipients. *Drugs* 1999; **58:** 1029–42.
2. Carswell CI, *et al.* Daclizumab: a review of its use in the management of organ transplantation. *BioDrugs* 2001; **15:** 745–73.


**Organ and tissue transplantation.** Daclizumab reduced the incidence of acute rejection episodes in the first 6 months,[1,2] and the first 12 months[3] after kidney transplantation (p.1346) when compared with placebo, but did not affect the graft survival rate. Compared with placebo, daclizumab improved patient survival when added to double therapy (ciclosporin plus corticosteroids),[2] but this effect was not seen when daclizumab was added to triple therapy (ciclosporin, corticosteroids, plus azathioprine).[1] When added to another triple therapy regimen (tacrolimus, corticosteroids, plus mycophenolate mofetil) and retrospectively compared with muromonab-CD3, daclizumab reduced the incidence of acute rejection episodes in the first 6 months after renal transplantation, but again did not affect patient or graft survival.[4] In a small, retrospective analysis[5] of simultaneous kidney-pancreas transplant recipients (p.1347), patients receiving 1 to 3 doses of daclizumab in addition to triple therapy (tacrolimus, corticosteroids plus mycophenolate mofetil) experienced a significantly higher incidence of rejection than those receiving 4 to 5 doses. There was no difference in patient or graft survival.

Daclizumab has been investigated in the prevention of acute rejection following heart,[6] liver,[7] and lung[8] transplantation (see p.1345) but increased mortality has followed its use in patients receiving heart grafts (see under Adverse Effects and Precautions, above). It has also been tried in the management of acute graft-versus-host disease (see Haematopoietic Stem Cell Transplantation, p.1344).


1. Vincenti F, *et al.* Interleukin-2-receptor blockade with daclizumab to prevent acute rejection in renal transplantation. *N Engl J Med* 1998; **338:** 161–5.
2. Nashan B, *et al.* Reduction of acute renal allograft rejection by daclizumab. *Transplantation* 1999; **67:** 110–15.
3. Bumgardner GL, *et al.* Results of 3-year phase III clinical trials with daclizumab prophylaxis for prevention of acute rejection after renal transplantation. *Transplantation* 2001; **72:** 839–45.

4. Ciancio G, *et al.* Daclizumab induction, tacrolimus, mycophenolate mofetil and steroids as an immunosuppression regimen for primary kidney transplant recipients. *Transplantation* 2002; **73:** 1100–6.
5. Bruce DS, *et al.* Multicenter survey of daclizumab induction in simultaneous kidney-pancreas transplant recipients. *Transplantation* 2001; **72:** 1637–43.
6. Beniaminovitz A, *et al.* Prevention of rejection in cardiac transplantation by blockade of the interleukin-2 receptor with a monoclonal antibody. *N Engl J Med* 2000; **342:** 613–19.
7. Niemeyer G, *et al.* Long-term safety, tolerability and efficacy of daclizumab (Zenapax®) in a two-dose regimen in liver transplant recipients. *Am J Transplant* 2002; **2:** 454–60.
8. Garrity ER, *et al.* Low rate of acute lung allograft rejection after the use of daclizumab, an interleukin 2 receptor antibody. *Transplantation* 2001; **71:** 773–7.


**Psoriasis.** A report[1] of a response to daclizumab in a patient with severe intractable psoriasis.


1. Wohlrab J, *et al.* Treatment of recalcitrant psoriasis with daclizumab. *Br J Dermatol* 2001; **144:** 209–10.


## Preparations

**Proprietary Preparations** (details are given in Part 3)
***Arg.:*** Zenapax; ***Austral.:*** Zenapax; ***Austria:*** Zenapax; ***Belg.:*** Zenapax; ***Braz.:*** Zenapax; ***Canad.:*** Zenapax; ***Chile:*** Zenapax; ***Denm.:*** Zenapax; ***Fin.:*** Zenapax; ***Fr.:*** Zenapax; ***Ger.:*** Zenapax; ***Gr.:*** Zenapax; ***Hong Kong:*** Zenapax; ***Irl.:*** Zenapax; ***Israel:*** Zenapax; ***Ital.:*** Zenapax; ***Mex.:*** Zenapax; ***Neth.:*** Zenapax; ***NZ:*** Zenapax; ***Port.:*** Zenapax; ***S.Afr.:*** Zenapax; ***Singapore:*** Zenapax; ***Spain:*** Zenapax; ***Swed.:*** Zenapax; ***Switz.:*** Zenapax; ***Thai.:*** Zenapax; ***UK:*** Zenapax; ***USA:*** Zenapax.

# Everolimus *(USAN, rINN)*

Everolimús; RAD-001. (3*S*,6*R*,7*E*,9*R*,10*R*,12*R*,14*S*,15*E*,17*E*,19*E*,21*S*,23*S*,26*R*,27*R*,34a*S*)-9,10,12,13,14,21,22,23,24,25,26,27,32,33,34,34a-Hexadecahydro-9,27-dihydroxy-3-{(1*R*)-2-[(1*S*,3*R*,4*R*)-4-(2-hydroxyethoxy)-3-methoxycyclohexyl]-1-methylethyl}-10,21-dimethoxy-6,8,12,14,20,26-hexamethyl-23,27-epoxy-3*H*-pyrido[2,1-*c*][1,4]oxaazacyclohentriacontine-1,5,11,28,29(4*H*,6*H*,31*H*)-pentone.

$C_{53}H_{83}NO_{14}$ = 958.2.
*CAS — 159351-69-6.*
*ATC — L04AA18.*

## Adverse Effects

Leucopenia, thrombocytopenia, and anaemia occur commonly with everolimus. Haemolysis has been reported rarely. Other common adverse effects include hypercholesterolaemia, hyperlipidaemia, hypertriglyceridaemia, hypertension, lymphocele, venous thromboembolism, and gastrointestinal upsets. Pneumonia, pneumonitis, hepatitis, jaundice, renal tubular necrosis, and pyelonephritis may occur. Acne and oedema occur frequently; rashes and myalgia occur rarely.

## Interactions

Everolimus is metabolised in the liver and to some extent in the gastrointestinal wall; plasma concentrations may be affected by inducers or competitive inhibitors of P-glycoprotein, or hepatic enzymes, particularly cytochrome P450 isoenzyme CYP3A4. Use with live vaccines should be avoided.

**Ciclosporin.** The bioavailability of everolimus was significantly increased when given with ciclosporin,[1] and dose adjustment of everolimus may be necessary if the ciclosporin dose is altered (see Administration, below).


1. Kovarik JM, *et al.* Differential influence of two cyclosporine formulations on everolimus pharmacokinetics: a clinically relevant pharmacokinetic interaction. *J Clin Pharmacol* 2002; **42:** 95–9.


**Rifampicin.** In a pharmacokinetic study,[1] rifampicin increased the clearance of everolimus, decreasing exposure to everolimus by about 63%. The manufacturers recommend against the combined use of these drugs.


1. Kovarik JM, *et al.* Effect of rifampin on apparent clearance of everolimus. *Ann Pharmacother* 2002; **36:** 981–5.


## Pharmacokinetics

Peak plasma concentrations of everolimus occur about 1 to 2 hours after an oral dose. Plasma protein binding is about 74%. Everolimus is metabolised in the liver and to some extent in the gastrointestinal wall; the majority of metabolites are excreted in the faeces with a minor amount found in urine.

◊ References.


1. Kirchner GI, *et al.* Clinical pharmacokinetics of everolimus. *Clin Pharmacokinet* 2004; **43:** 83–95.


**Therapeutic drug monitoring.** The manufacturers recommend routine monitoring of whole blood everolimus concentrations. Patients with trough levels of 3 nanograms/mL or greater have been found to have a lower incidence of acute rejection in both renal and cardiac transplantation; an upper limit of 8 nanograms/mL is recommended. Monitoring is considered especially important in those with hepatic impairment (see under Uses, below) and if ciclosporin formulation or dosage is changed (see Administration, below).

## Uses and Administration

Everolimus is a derivative of sirolimus (p.1363). It is used in the prevention of graft rejection episodes in patients undergoing renal or cardiac transplantation as part of an immunosuppressive regimen that includes ciclosporin (microemulsion) and corticosteroids. The recommended adult dose is 750 micrograms twice daily by mouth, begun as soon as possible after transplantation, and given at the same time as ciclosporin microemulsion (see Administration, below). Doses of everolimus should be reduced in patients with hepatic impairment, see below.

◊ References.


1. Kovarik JM, *et al.* Exposure-response relationships for everolimus in de novo kidney transplantation: defining a therapeutic range. *Transplantation* 2002; **73:** 920–5.
2. Eisen HJ, *et al.* Everolimus for the prevention of allograft rejection and vasculopathy in cardiac-transplant recipients. *N Engl J Med* 2003; **349:** 847–58.
3. Chapman TM, Perry CM. Everolimus. *Drugs* 2004; **64:** 861–72.


**Administration.** Everolimus is given with ciclosporin and corticosteroids. Ciclosporin exposure reduction is recommended 1 month after transplantation. Because ciclosporin interacts with everolimus, and the dose adjustments of ciclosporin will affect exposure to everolimus, the manufacturer of everolimus recommends that levels of both drugs be monitored to minimise the risk of graft rejection. Before dose reduction of ciclosporin, everolimus whole blood concentrations should be at least 3 nanograms/mL (see Therapeutic Drug Monitoring, above, and under Ciclosporin, p.1357).

In renal transplantation, ciclosporin doses should be adjusted to the following target ciclosporin concentration ranges, as measured 2 hours after the dose of ciclosporin:

- weeks 0-4: 1000 to 1400 nanograms/mL
- weeks 5-8: 700 to 900 nanograms/mL
- weeks 9-12: 550 to 650 nanograms/mL
- weeks 13-52: 350 to 450 nanograms/mL

In cardiac transplantation, ciclosporin levels are adjusted according to ciclosporin blood trough levels.

**Administration in hepatic impairment.** The clearance of everolimus was significantly reduced in patients with moderate hepatic impairment.[1] The manufacturers state that the dose should be reduced by 50% in mild to moderate hepatic impairment with further titration of the dose based on therapeutic drug monitoring (see under Pharmacokinetics, above). Everolimus has not been studied in severe hepatic impairment.


1. Kovarik JM, *et al.* Influence of hepatic impairment on everolimus pharmacokinetics: implications for dose adjustment. *Clin Pharmacol Ther* 2001; **70:** 425–30.


# Gavilimomab *(rINN)*

*CAS — 244096-20-6.*

## Profile

Gavilimomab is an anti-CD147 monoclonal antibody of murine origin that has been used for the treatment of acute graft-versus-host disease.

◊ References.


1. Deeg HJ, *et al.* Treatment of steroid-refractory acute graft-versus-host disease with anti-CD147 monoclonal antibody ABX-CBL. *Blood* 2001; **98:** 2052–8.


# Gusperimus Hydrochloride *(rINNM)*

BMS-181173; BMY-42215-1; Deoxyspergualin Hydrochloride; 15-Deoxyspergualin Hydrochloride; Gusperimus Trihydrochloride *(USAN)*; Hidrocloruro de gusperimús; NKT-01; NSC-356894. (±)-*N*-[{[4-[(3-Aminopropyl)amino]butyl}carbamoyl)hydroxymethyl]-7-guanidinoheptanamide trihydrochloride.

$C_{17}H_{37}N_7O_3,3HCl$ = 496.9.
*CAS — 104317-84-2 (gusperimus); 89149-10-0 (gusperimus); 85468-01-5 (gusperimus hydrochloride).*
*ATC — L04AA19.*

## Profile

Gusperimus is a guanidine derivative that inhibits both cell-mediated and antibody-mediated immunity. It is used in the treatment of graft rejection, and has been investigated in the management of graft-versus-host disease and Wegener's granulomatosis. For mention of its role in reversing acute graft rejection in kidney transplantation, see p.1346.

Gusperimus is used as the hydrochloride. A dose of 3 to 5 mg/kg of gusperimus hydrochloride given daily for 7 days, by intravenous infusion over 3 hours, has been suggested in the treatment of acute renal graft rejection. Treatment may be continued for a further 3 days if required.

Adverse effects reported with gusperimus include bone-marrow depression, numbness of face and extremities, headache, gastrointestinal disturbances, alterations in liver enzyme values, and facial flushing. Rapid injection should be avoided as an acute increase in plasma concentration may produce respiratory depression.

◊ References.


1. Amemiya H, *et al.* A novel rescue drug, 15-deoxyspergualin: first clinical trials for recurrent graft rejection in renal recipients. *Transplantation* 1990; **49:** 337–43.
2. Gores PF. Deoxyspergualin: clinical experience. *Transplant Proc* 1996; **28:** 871–2.
3. Ramos EL, *et al.* Deoxyspergualin: mechanism of action and pharmacokinetics. *Transplant Proc* 1996; **28:** 873–5.
4. Tanabe K, *et al.* Effect of deoxyspergualin on the long-term outcome of renal transplantation. *Transplant Proc* 2000; **32:** 1745–6.
5. Amada N, *et al.* Prophylactic use of deoxyspergualin improves long-term graft survival in living related renal transplant recipients transfused with donor-specific blood. *Transplant Proc* 2001; **33:** 2256–7.


## Preparations

**Proprietary Preparations** (details are given in Part 3)
***Jpn:*** Spanidin.

# Inolimomab *(rINN)*

BT-563.
*CAS — 152981-31-2.*

## Profile

Inolimomab is a murine/human monoclonal antibody similar to daclizumab (p.1359) that acts as an interleukin-2 receptor antagonist at the alpha chain (CD25) of the interleukin-2 receptor on the surface of activated T-lymphocytes. It is under investigation for its immunosuppressant properties in the treatment and prevention of rejection episodes following organ transplantation (p.1344).

◊ References.


1. van Gelder T, *et al.* Intragraft monitoring of rejection after prophylactic treatment with monoclonal anti-interleukin-2 receptor antibody (BT563) in heart transplant recipients. *J Heart Lung Transplant* 1995; **14:** 346–50.
2. van Gelder T, *et al.* A double-blind, placebo-controlled study of monoclonal anti-interleukin-2 receptor antibody (BT563) administration to prevent acute rejection after kidney transplantation. *Transplantation* 1995; **60:** 248–52.
3. Cahn JY, *et al.* Treatment of acute graft-versus-host disease with methylprednisolone and cyclosporine with or without an anti-interleukin-2 receptor monoclonal antibody: a multicenter phase III study. *Transplantation* 1995; **60:** 939–42.
4. Langrehr JM, *et al.* A prospective randomized trial comparing interleukin-2 receptor antibody versus antithymocyte globulin as part of a quadruple immunosuppressive induction therapy following orthotopic liver transplantation. *Transplantation* 1997; **63:** 1772–81.
5. van Gelder T, *et al.* Blockade of the interleukin (IL)-2/IL-2 receptor pathway with a monoclonal anti-IL-2 receptor antibody (BT563) does not prevent the development of acute heart allograft rejection in humans. *Transplantation* 1998; **65:** 405–10.
6. Langrehr JM, *et al.* A randomized, placebo-controlled trial with anti-interleukin-2 receptor antibody for immunosuppressive induction therapy after liver transplantation. *Clin Transplant* 1998; **12:** 303–12.
7. Winkler M. Inolimomab (OPi). *Curr Opin Investig Drugs* 2002; **3:** 1464–7.


# Mizoribine *(rINN)*

HE-69; Mizoribina. 5-Hydroxy-1-β-D-ribofuranosylimidazole-4-carboxamide.

$C_9H_{13}N_3O_6$ = 259.2.
*CAS — 50924-49-7.*

## Profile

Mizoribine is an oral immunosuppressant that is used in the treatment of rheumatoid arthritis, and in organ and tissue transplantation.

◊ References.


1. Tanabe K, *et al.* Long-term results in mizoribine-treated renal transplant recipients: a prospective, randomized trial of mizoribine and azathioprine under cyclosporine-based immunosuppression. *Transplant Proc* 1999; **31:** 2877–9.
2. Yoshioka K, *et al.* A multicenter trial of mizoribine compared with placebo in children with frequently relapsing nephrotic syndrome. *Kidney Int* 2000; **58:** 317–24.
3. Yokota S. Mizoribine: mode of action and effects in clinical use. *Pediatr Int* 2002; **44:** 196–8.
4. Takei S. Mizoribine in the treatment of rheumatoid arthritis and juvenile idiopathic arthritis. *Pediatr Int* 2002; **44:** 205–9.
5. Honda M. Nephrotic syndrome and mizoribine in children. *Pediatr Int* 2002; **44:** 210–6.
6. Nagaoka R, *et al.* Mizoribine treatment for childhood IgA nephropathy. *Pediatr Int* 2002; **44:** 217–23.
7. Tsuzuki K. Role of mizoribine in renal transplantation. *Pediatr Int* 2002; **44:** 224–31.


# Muromonab-CD3 *(USAN, rINN)*

OKT3.
*ATC — L04AA02.*

**Description.** A murine monoclonal antibody comprising a purified $IgG_{2a}$ immunoglobulin with a heavy chain having a molecular weight of about 50 000 daltons and a light chain with a molecular weight of approximately 25 000 daltons.

## Adverse Effects, Treatment, and Precautions

An acute cytokine release syndrome ranging from fever, chills, gastrointestinal disturbances, myalgia, and tremor to dyspnoea, pulmonary oedema, collapse, and cardiac arrest has occurred, typically 30 to 60 minutes after the first few doses of muromonab-CD3 although risk persists for some 48 hours after a dose. Frequency and severity tend to decrease with successive doses, while prophylactic corticosteroids may reduce initial adverse reactions (see Uses and Administration, below). Reversible impairment of renal function may also be associated with the syndrome.

Other reported effects of muromonab-CD3 include encephalopathy, cerebral oedema, and a syndrome resembling aseptic meningitis, with headache, fever, stiff neck, and photophobia; seizures have also occurred. Hypersensitivity reactions, including anaphylaxis, have been reported and may be difficult to distinguish from the cytokine release syndrome.

As with other potent immunosuppressants, treatment with muromonab-CD3 may increase the risk of serious infections and the development of certain malignancies. Intra-uterine devices should be used with caution during immunosuppressive therapy as there is an increased risk of infection. Use of live vaccines should be avoided for the same reason.

Muromonab-CD3 should not be given to patients with pre-existing fever, or uncontrolled hypertension, or in patients hypersensitive to products of murine origin. It should be avoided in patients with a history of seizures. Because fluid overload is associated with an increased risk of pulmonary oedema due to the cytokine release syndrome, muromonab-CD3 is contra-indicated in patients who have undergone a more than 3% weight gain in the week preceding therapy, or who have radiographic evidence of fluid overloading. Repeated courses of muromonab-CD3 may be less effective because of the development of antibodies to the drug. Paediatric patients may be at increased risk of serious adverse effects following muromonab-CD3 therapy.

**Effects on the blood.** THROMBOEMBOLISM. Intragraft thromboses developed in 9 of 93 consecutive kidney transplant recipients given high-dose muromonab-CD3 (10 mg daily) as part of their immunosuppressive regimen.[1] In one patient the thrombosis was in the renal artery, and in 3 in the renal vein; the remainder had thromboses in the glomerular capillaries and thrombotic microangiopathy similar to that of haemolytic-uraemic syndrome. The authors suggested that muromonab-CD3 has procoagulant effects, perhaps mediated by released tumour necrosis factor; these effects had also been seen in 3 patients receiving muromonab-CD3 at conventional doses (5 mg daily). Another group[2] has also reported an apparently increased incidence of acute vascular thrombosis in patients given muromonab-CD3 at conventional doses, but in the experience of others,[3] despite evidence of activation of coagulation by the drug, treatment of acute rejection with 5 mg daily was not associated with thromboembolic complications.

1. Abramowicz D, *et al.* Induction of thromboses within renal grafts by high-dose prophylactic OKT3. *Lancet* 1992; **339:** 777–8.
2. Gomez E, *et al.* Main graft vessels thromboses due to conventional-dose OKT3 in renal transplantation. *Lancet* 1992; **339:** 1612–13.
3. Raasveld MHM, *et al.* Thromboembolic complications and dose of monoclonal OKT3 antibody. *Lancet* 1992; **339:** 1363–4.

**Effects on the ears.** Bilateral sensorineural hearing loss has occurred following muromonab-CD3 therapy. In one case series, 5 out of 7 patients were affected, showing a mean hearing loss of 18 decibels.[1] Tinnitus may also occur.[1,2] Although symptoms are generally reversible,[1,2] one patient still showed a deficit in hearing after 6 months.[3]

1. Hartnick CJ, *et al.* Reversible sensorineural hearing loss following administration of muromonab-CD3 (OKT3) for cadaveric renal transplant immunosuppression. *Ann Otol Rhinol Laryngol* 2000; **109:** 45–7.
2. Hartnick CJ, *et al.* Reversible sensorineural hearing loss after renal transplant immunosuppression with OKT3 (muromonab-CD3). *Ann Otol Rhinol Laryngol* 1997; **106:** 640–2.
3. Michals M, *et al.* Hearing loss associated with muromonab-CD3 therapy. *Clin Pharm* 1988; **7:** 867–8.

**Effects on the nervous system.** Generalised seizures were reported in 2 uraemic kidney-graft recipients following administration of muromonab-CD3.[1] Delayed graft function may result in the accumulation of uraemic toxins which combine with cytokines released by the immunosuppressant to produce the effects on the CNS. Seizures and encephalopathy were reported in siblings given muromonab-CD3 following renal transplantation, and appeared to predispose one of them to develop ciclosporin neurotoxicity.[2]

1. Seifeldin RA, *et al.* Generalized seizures associated with the use of muromonab-CD3 in two patients after kidney transplantation. *Ann Pharmacother* 1997; **31:** 586–9.
2. Thaisetthawatkul P, *et al.* Muromonab-CD3-induced neurotoxicity: report of two siblings, one of whom had subsequent cyclosporin-induced neurotoxicity. *J Child Neurol* 2001; **16:** 825–31.

## Uses and Administration

Muromonab-CD3 is a murine monoclonal antibody to the T3 (CD3) antigen of human T-lymphocytes, which is essential to antigen recognition and response; the antibody thus specifically blocks T-cell generation and function, to exert an immunosuppressant effect without affecting the bone marrow.

It is used in the treatment of acute allograft rejection in organ transplant recipients, in doses of 5 mg daily by intravenous injection for 10 to 14 days. An initial dose of 2.5 mg daily is recommended in children weighing 30 kg or less, subsequently adjusted if necessary in increments of 2.5 mg according to response. The dose of any other immunosuppressant therapy may need to be reduced. Patients should be monitored closely after the first few doses of muromonab-CD3 because of the risk of cytokine release syndrome and hypersensitivity reactions. The first dose may be preceded by intravenous methylprednisolone sodium succinate, in a dose of 8 mg/kg, 1 to 4 hours before muromonab-CD3. Paracetamol and antihistamines may also be given with muromonab-CD3 to reduce early reactions.

Muromonab-CD3 has also been given experimentally as part of regimens for the prophylaxis of graft rejection. For further details of the use of muromonab-CD3 in the treatment and prophylaxis of graft rejection see p.1344, *et seq.*

◊ References.

1. Wilde MI, Goa KL. Muromonab CD3: a reappraisal of its pharmacology and use as prophylaxis of solid organ transplant rejection. *Drugs* 1996; **51:** 865–94.
2. Burk ML, Matuszewski KA. Muromonab-CD3 and antithymocyte globulin in renal transplantation. *Ann Pharmacother* 1997; **31:** 1370–7.
3. ten Berge IJM, *et al.* Guidelines for optimal use of muromonab CD3 in transplantation. *BioDrugs* 1999; **11:** 277–84.
4. Flechner SM. A randomized prospective trial of low-dose OKT3 induction therapy to prevent rejection and minimize side effects in recipients of kidney transplants. *Transplantation* 2000; **69:** 2374–81.

### Preparations

**Proprietary Preparations** (details are given in Part 3)
***Austral.:*** Orthoclone OKT3; ***Belg.:*** Orthoclone OKT3; ***Braz.:*** Anti CD3†; Orthoclone OKT3; ***Canad.:*** Orthoclone OKT3; ***Chile:*** Ior T3; ***Fin.:*** Orthoclone OKT3; ***Fr.:*** Orthoclone OKT3; ***Ger.:*** Orthoclone OKT3; ***Hong Kong:*** Orthoclone OKT3; ***Israel:*** Orthoclone OKT3; ***Ital.:*** Orthoclone OKT3; ***Malaysia:*** Orthoclone OKT3; ***Mex.:*** Ior T3; Orthoclone OKT3; ***Neth.:*** Orthoclone OKT3; ***Norw.:*** Orthoclone OKT3; ***NZ:*** Orthoclone OKT3; ***Swed.:*** Orthoclone OKT3; ***Switz.:*** Orthoclone OKT3; ***Thai.:*** Orthoclone OKT3; ***USA:*** Orthoclone OKT3.

## Mycophenolate Mofetil *(BANM, USAN, rINNM)*

Micofenolato de mofetilo; Mycophenolate Morpholinoethyl; RS-61443; RS-61443-190 (mycophenolate mofetil hydrochloride).
2-Morpholinoethyl (*E*)-6-(4-hydroxy-6-methoxy-7-methyl-3-oxo-5-phthalanyl)-4-methyl-4-hexenoate.
$C_{23}H_{31}NO_7$ = 433.5.
*CAS — 24280-93-1 (mycophenolic acid); 115007-34-6 (mycophenolate mofetil); 116680-01-4 (mycophenolate mofetil hydrochloride); 37415-62-6 (mycophenolate sodium).*
*ATC — L04AA06.*

**Stability.** Solutions of mycophenolate mofetil 1, 5, or 10 mg/mL were stable for 7 days when stored at 4° or 25° in PVC infusion bags.[1] However, it was noted that a progressive discoloration occurred in bags unprotected from light and stored at 25°; further study was required to determine the source of the discoloration.

1. Certain E, *et al.* Stability of i.v. mycophenolate mofetil in 5% dextrose injection in polyvinyl chloride infusion bags. *Am J Health-Syst Pharm* 2002; **59** 2434–9.

### Adverse Effects, Treatment, and Precautions

Mycophenolate mofetil is associated with gastrointestinal disturbances, particularly diarrhoea and vomiting; gastrointestinal haemorrhage and perforation has occurred. Leucopenia may develop; as with other immunosuppressants there is an increased risk of infection and certain malignancies in patients receiving mycophenolate mofetil. Other reported adverse effects include asthenia, fever, pain, headache, anaemia, thrombocytopenia, renal tubular necrosis, haematuria, hypertension, hyperglycaemia, disturbances of electrolytes and blood lipids, peripheral oedema, dyspnoea, cough, acne, dizziness, insomnia, and tremor. Hypersensitivity reactions have occurred. Pancreatitis has been reported rarely. Mycophenolate is teratogenic in *animals*.

Mycophenolate mofetil should be given with care to patients with severe renal impairment or active disorders of the gastrointestinal tract. Intra-uterine devices should be used with caution during immunosuppressive treatment as there is an increased risk of infection. Concomitant use of live vaccines should be avoided for the same reason.

**Effects on the gastrointestinal tract.** The adverse effects of mycophenolate mofetil on the gastrointestinal tract appeared to be mostly of an irritative nature and included diarrhoea, abdominal pain, nausea and vomiting, anorexia, dyspepsia, and occasionally gastrointestinal haemorrhage or perforation.[1] Paediatric patients tended to have a higher incidence of adverse gastrointestinal events than adults. There was some evidence that adverse effects were related to peak plasma concentrations of the drug.

1. Behrend M. Adverse gastrointestinal effects of mycophenolate mofetil: aetiology, incidence and management. *Drug Safety* 2001; **24:** 645–63.

**Infection.** The use of mycophenolate mofetil was not found to increase the risk of cytomegalovirus (CMV) infection in 2 small studies.[1,2] However, its use did appear to be associated with an increased frequency[1] and severity[2] of CMV disease (defined as CMV infection plus evidence of viral syndrome). The number of organs affected in patients with CMV disease was also higher in those treated with mycophenolate mofetil.[2]

A retrospective study[3] found that the use of a protocol containing mycophenolate mofetil and tacrolimus was an independent risk factor for the development of CMV disease, but that the dose of mycophenolate mofetil was not. The authors interpreted this to mean that either the combination of mycophenolate mofetil and tacrolimus had an overall stronger immunosuppressive effect than other regimens, or that this protocol bore a specific risk for the development of CMV disease. The pharmacokinetics of mycophenolic acid (MPA), a metabolite of mycophenolate mofetil, and its interaction with tacrolimus, must be considered, with further studies taking MPA levels into account (see under Interactions, below).

In contrast to these findings, another retrospective study[4] found that, although no patient developed CMV disease, the use of mycophenolate mofetil was an independent risk factor for the development of CMV infection in those patients initially seropositive for the CMV antigen.

1. ter Meulen CG, *et al.* The influence of mycophenolate mofetil on the incidence and severity of primary cytomegalovirus infections and disease after renal transplantation. *Nephrol Dial Transplant* 2000; **15:** 711–14.
2. Sarmiento JM, *et al.* Mycophenolate mofetil increases cytomegalovirus invasive organ disease in renal transplant patients. *Clin Transplant* 2000; **14:** 136–8.
3. Kuypers DRJ, *et al.* Role of immunosuppressive drugs in the development of tissue-invasive cytomegalovirus infection in renal transplant recipients. *Transplant Proc* 2002; **34:** 1164–70.
4. Hambach L, *et al.* Increased risk of complicated CMV infection with the use of mycophenolate mofetil in allogeneic stem cell transplantation. *Bone Marrow Transplant* 2002; **29:** 903–6.

### Interactions

Mycophenolate mofetil may compete with other drugs that undergo active renal tubular secretion, resulting in increased concentrations of either drug. Antacids or colestyramine may result in reduced absorption of mycophenolate. See above for precautions about use with live vaccines.

**Antacids.** Although giving mycophenolate mofetil with an antacid mixture (aluminium and magnesium hydroxides) or food both resulted in reductions in peak plasma concentrations of mycophenolic acid, the differences were small compared with interindividual variation, and were considered unlikely to be clinically significant.[1]

1. Bullingham R, *et al.* Effects of food and antacid on the pharmacokinetics of single doses of mycophenolate mofetil in rheumatoid arthritis patients. *Br J Clin Pharmacol* 1996; **41:** 513–16.

**Immunosuppressants.** Stopping *ciclosporin* therapy was found to increase serum concentrations of mycophenolic acid (MPA),[1,2] leading to the hypothesis that ciclosporin inhibits the enterohepatic recirculation of MPA. In contrast,[3,4] *tacrolimus* therapy increased serum concentrations of MPA, apparently by inhibiting conversion to mycophenolic acid glucuronide. While the studies have been criticised,[5] it has been pointed out that an interaction cannot be excluded.[6] An increased incidence of cytomegalovirus disease has been reported in renal transplant recipients given a triple therapy regimen containing tacrolimus and mycophenolate mofetil.[7] Based on a study[8] in children it has been recommended that mycophenolate mofetil be given in initial doses of 600 mg/m² twice daily with ciclosporin but 300 mg/m² twice daily with tacrolimus; 500 mg/m² twice daily was suggested if no calcineurin inhibitor was given. It is also recommended that dose adjustments are made using therapeutic drug monitoring. However, a pharmacokinetic study[9] demonstrated that changes in MPA exposure with tacrolimus varied with the dose of mycophenolate mofetil used and that this effect was not adequately reflected by MPA trough concentrations (see Therapeutic Drug Monitoring, below). While not commenting on dose adjustment when used with tacrolimus, one manufacturer of mycophenolate mofetil recommends no dose adjustment when it is given with ciclosporin.

1. Smak Gregoor PJH, *et al.* Effect of cyclosporine on mycophenolic acid trough levels in kidney transplant recipients. *Transplantation* 1999; **68:** 1603–6.

2. Shipkova M, *et al.* Effect of cyclosporine withdrawal on mycophenolic acid pharmacokinetics in kidney transplant recipients with deteriorating renal function: preliminary report. *Ther Drug Monit* 2001; **23:** 717–21.
3. Zucker K, *et al.* Unexpected augmentation of mycophenolic acid pharmacokinetics in renal transplant patients receiving tacrolimus and mycophenolate mofetil in combination therapy, and analogous in vitro findings. *Transpl Immunol* 1997; **5:** 225–32.
4. Hübner GI, *et al.* Drug interaction between mycophenolate mofetil and tacrolimus detectable within therapeutic mycophenolic acid monitoring in renal transplant patients. *Ther Drug Monit* 1999; **21:** 536–9.
5. van Gelder T, *et al.* [Drug interaction between mycophenolate mofetil and tacrolimus detectable within therapeutic mycophenolic acid monitoring in renal transplant patients]. *Ther Drug Monit* 2000; **22:** 639.
6. Hübner GI, Sziegoleit W. [Drug interaction between mycophenolate mofetil and tacrolimus detectable within therapeutic mycophenolic acid monitoring in renal transplant patients.] *Ther Drug Monit* 2000; **22:** 498–9.
7. Kuypers DRJ, *et al.* Role of immunosuppressive drugs in the development of tissue-invasive cytomegalovirus infection in renal transplant recipients. *Transplant Proc* 2002; **34:** 1164–70.
8. Filler G, *et al.* Pharmacokinetics of mycophenolate mofetil are influenced by concomitant immunosuppression. *Pediatr Nephrol* 2000; **14:** 100–104.
9. Kuypers DRJ, *et al.* Long-term changes in mycophenolic acid exposure in combination with tacrolimus and corticosteroids are dose dependent and not reflected by trough plasma concentration: a prospective study in 100 de novo renal allograft recipients. *J Clin Pharmacol* 2003; **43:** 866–80.

**Iron.** Absorption of mycophenolate mofetil following oral administration was markedly reduced by iron preparations in a study in 7 healthy subjects:[1] mean peak serum concentrations of mycophenolic acid were reduced from 20.1 to 1.3 micrograms/mL.

1. Morii M, *et al.* Impairment of mycophenolate mofetil absorption by iron ion. *Clin Pharmacol Ther* 2000; **68:** 613–6.

## Pharmacokinetics

Mycophenolate mofetil is rapidly and extensively absorbed from the gastrointestinal tract, and undergoes presystemic metabolism to active mycophenolic acid (MPA). It undergoes enterohepatic recirculation. MPA is metabolised by glucuronidation and excreted primarily in the urine; about 6% of a dose is recovered in faeces. MPA is 97% bound to plasma albumin. The half-life of MPA after oral doses of mycophenolate has been variously stated to be about 12 or 18 hours depending on the preparation.

◊ References.

1. Bullingham RES, *et al.* Clinical pharmacokinetics of mycophenolate mofetil. *Clin Pharmacokinet* 1998; **34:** 429–55.
2. Gabardi S, *et al.* Enteric-coated mycophenolate sodium. *Ann Pharmacother* 2003; **37:** 1685–93.

**Metabolism.** Mycophenolate mofetil is rapidly de-esterified in the body to active mycophenolic acid (MPA) which is subsequently converted to inactive mycophenolic acid glucuronide (MPAG) in the gastrointestinal tract, liver and possibly kidney. This conversion to MPAG is considered to be the most important and rate limiting step.[1] MPA undergoes enterohepatic circulation, with MPAG formed in the liver being excreted into bile and converted back to MPA in the gastrointestinal tract. A further metabolite, the acyl glucuronide, has been shown to be active *in vitro*, inhibiting human inosine monophosphate dehydrogenase (IMPDH),[1,2] and may have implications in therapeutic drug monitoring (see below). MPA is extensively bound to albumin in patients with normal renal and hepatic function, but this binding may be affected in transplant patients by several factors such as hypoalbuminaemia, hyperbilirubinaemia, and uraemia. Accumulation of MPAG leads to an increase in unbound MPA, and a subsequent increase in MPA clearance.[2]

1. Shaw LM, *et al.* Pharmacokinetic, pharmacodynamic, and outcome investigations as the basis for mycophenolic acid therapeutic drug monitoring in renal and heart transplant patients. *Clin Biochem* 2001; **34:** 17–22.
2. Shaw LM, *et al.* Current issues in therapeutic drug monitoring of mycophenolic acid: report of a roundtable discussion. *Ther Drug Monit* 2001; **23:** 305–15.

**Therapeutic drug monitoring.** Mycophenolic acid (MPA) concentration appears to correlate with efficacy and toxicity and therapeutic drug monitoring of mycophenolate mofetil is considered necessary.[1] Patients with low MPA concentrations may be at increased risk of transplant rejection,[2,3] and there is some evidence that a high MPA concentration correlates with increased adverse effects.[4] Other immunosuppressants can affect MPA concentrations, see under Interactions, above. Assay procedures to measure MPA concentrations include high performance liquid chromatography (HPLC) and an enzyme-multiplied immunoassay technique (EMIT). However, the acyl glucuronide metabolite of MPA (see Metabolism, above) may cross-react with the latter method, leading to higher measured concentrations than with HPLC.[5] Another suggested approach is to measure inosine monophosphate dehydrogenase (IMPDH) activity directly, (see above) but this has produced variable results.[6]

A review[5] concluded that while some studies show a correlation between MPA trough concentration and acute allograft rejection, MPA area under the concentration-time curve (AUC) is predictive of the risk for rejection, and that both have limitations. An abbreviated AUC involving more practical blood sampling regimens may be more appropriate, and a trough concentration between 1 and 3.5 mg/litre has been proposed. Measurements of unbound MPA concentrations may be of benefit in patients with renal or hepatic impairment, as factors such as hypoalbuminaemia and renal dysfunction affect the binding of MPA.[5]

A study in 6 patients with psoriasis concluded that MPA trough concentrations (measured by EMIT) did not predict efficacy or toxicity, but instead were useful to evaluate compliance.[7]

For the view that MPA trough concentrations may not adequately reflect exposure in patients also receiving tacrolimus, see Interactions, Immunosuppressants, above.

1. Mourad M, *et al.* Therapeutic monitoring of mycophenolate mofetil in organ transplant recipients: is it necessary? *Clin Pharmacokinet* 2002; **41:** 319–27.
2. van Gelder T, *et al.* A randomized double-blind, multicenter plasma concentration controlled study of the safety and efficacy of oral mycophenolate mofetil for the prevention of acute rejection after kidney transplantation. *Transplantation* 1999; **68:** 261–6.
3. DeNofrio D, *et al.* Mycophenolic acid concentrations are associated with cardiac allograft rejection. *J Heart Lung Transplant* 2000; **19:** 1071–6.
4. Mourad M, *et al.* Correlation of mycophenolic acid pharmacokinetic parameters with side effects in kidney transplant patients treated with mycophenolate mofetil. *Clin Chem* 2001; **47:** 88–94.
5. Shaw LM, *et al.* Current issues in therapeutic drug monitoring of mycophenolic acid: report of a roundtable discussion. *Ther Drug Monit* 2001: **23:** 305–15.
6. Shaw LM, *et al.* Monitoring of mycophenolic acid in clinical transplantation. *Ther Drug Monit* 2002; **24:** 68–73.
7. Daudén E, *et al.* Plasma trough levels of mycophenolic acid do not correlate with efficacy and safety of mycophenolate mofetil in psoriasis. *Br J Dermatol* 2004; **150:** 132–5.

## Uses and Administration

Mycophenolic acid is an immunosuppressant derived from *Penicillium stoloniferum*. It is a reversible inhibitor of inosine monophosphate dehydrogenase and thus inhibits purine synthesis, with potent cytostatic effects on both T- and B-lymphocytes. It has been used mainly as the morpholinoethyl derivative, mycophenolate mofetil. It is given with other immunosuppressants, for the prevention of graft rejection, and has also been tried in various diseases with an auto-immune or immune-mediated inflammatory component.

An enteric-coated formulation of mycophenolate sodium (the sodium salt of mycophenolic acid) is available in some countries. Doses are expressed in terms of the acid; mycophenolate sodium 769 mg is approximately equivalent to 720 mg of mycophenolic acid.

In the prophylaxis of acute renal graft rejection, the conventional formulation of mycophenolate mofetil is given by mouth in doses of 1 g twice daily; 1.5 g twice daily is recommended in the prophylaxis of cardiac graft rejection. For prevention of renal graft rejection in children and adolescents aged 2 to 18 years a dose of 600 mg/m$^2$ may be given by mouth twice daily, up to a maximum of 1 g twice daily; patients with a body-surface of 1.25 to 1.5 m$^2$ may be given 750 mg twice daily.

The enteric-coated formulation is given for the prophylaxis of acute renal graft rejection to adults in a dose of 720 mg twice daily; the two formulations cannot be indiscriminately interchanged or substituted.

In patients to whom oral therapy cannot initially be given, mycophenolate mofetil may be given for up to 14 days by intravenous infusion. Infusions are given as the hydrochloride salt, dissolved in glucose 5%, over 2 hours. Doses are described in terms of the base and are equivalent to those by mouth. For use in hepatic transplantation, the equivalent of 1 g twice daily is given for the first 4 days following transplantation, with subsequent conversion to 1.5 g twice daily by mouth as soon as it can be tolerated. Therapy should begin as soon as possible after transplantation, together with ciclosporin and corticosteroids. Patients should undergo regular blood counts; if neutropenia develops consideration should be given to interrupting mycophenolate therapy or reducing the dose.

◊ Mycophenolate mofetil has been investigated in a number of conditions with an auto-immune component: these include IgA nephropathy (see Glomerular Kidney Disease, p.1080), myasthenia gravis (p.1486), and rheumatoid arthritis (p.9). It has also been reported to be of benefit in uveitis (p.1090), and chronic active hepatitis (p.1078), and is under investigation for the treatment of lupus nephritis (p.1088).

**Eczema.** Mycophenolate mofetil has been tried in severe eczema.[1]

1. Neuber K, *et al.* Treatment of atopic eczema with oral mycophenolate mofetil. *Br J Dermatol* 2000; **143:** 385–91.

**Inflammatory bowel disease.** Mycophenolate mofetil has been investigated as an alternative to azathioprine in Crohn's disease (see Inflammatory Bowel Disease, p.1243). A randomised trial in 70 patients compared therapy with corticosteroids plus mycophenolate mofetil or azathioprine in patients with moderate or severe Crohn's disease. The authors concluded that the mycophenolate regimen produced a clinical response earlier than the azathioprine regimen, and that mycophenolate should be considered in patients allergic or unresponsive to azathioprine or mercaptopurine.[1] However, it has been suggested[2] that the trial may have been too short to draw definite conclusions, due to the known delayed therapeutic effect of azathioprine. A beneficial effect for 5 out of 6 patients with severe Crohn's disease was reported[3] after 3 months of therapy with mycophenolate mofetil, but this effect was not sustained beyond 6 months.[4] Others have also noted relapse or lack of response to be relatively common;[5,6] while mycophenolate may have a role in those who cannot tolerate, or are refractory to, azathioprine, the latter remains the immunosuppressant of choice due to its greater ability to prevent flare-ups.[2]

1. Neurath MF, *et al.* Randomised trial of mycophenolate mofetil versus azathioprine for treatment of chronic active Crohn's disease. *Gut* 1999; **44:** 625–8.
2. Miehsler W, *et al.* Is mycophenolate mofetil an effective alternative in azathioprine-intolerant patients with chronic active Crohn's disease? *Am J Gastroenterol* 2001; **96:** 782–7.
3. Florin THJ, *et al.* Treatment of steroid refractory inflammatory bowel disease (IBD) with mycophenolate mofetil (MMF). *Aust N Z J Med* 1998; **28:** 344–5.
4. Radford-Smith GL, *et al.* Mycophenolate mofetil in IBD patients. *Lancet* 1999; **354:** 1386–7.
5. Ford AC, *et al.* Mycophenolate mofetil in refractory inflammatory bowel disease. *Aliment Pharmacol Ther* 2003; **17:** 1365–9.
6. Wenzl HH, *et al.* Mycophenolate mofetil for Crohn's disease: short-term efficacy and long-term outcome. *Aliment Pharmacol Ther* 2004; **19:** 427–34.

**Organ and tissue transplantation.** Mycophenolate mofetil is used for the prophylaxis of graft rejection in kidney (p.1346), heart (p.1345), and liver transplantation (p.1346), and has also been employed following transplantation of the lung (p.1347), pancreas (p.1347) and intestines (p.1346). It has been employed as an alternative to, or replacement for, azathioprine, and may result in fewer rejections. It has also been tried for the prophylaxis of graft-versus-host disease following bone marrow transplantation (see Haematopoietic Stem Cell Transplantation, p.1344).

A few selected references to the use of mycophenolate mofetil in transplantation are given below.

1. European Mycophenolate Mofetil Cooperative Study Group. Placebo-controlled study of mycophenolate mofetil combined with cyclosporin and corticosteroids for prevention of acute rejection. *Lancet* 1995; **345:** 1321–5.
2. Fulton B, Markham A. Mycophenolate mofetil: a review of its pharmacodynamic and pharmacokinetic properties and clinical efficacy in renal transplantation. *Drugs* 1996; **51:** 278–98.
3. Simmons WD, *et al.* Preliminary risk-benefit assessment of mycophenolate mofetil in transplant rejection. *Drug Safety* 1997; **17:** 75–92.
4. Halloran P, *et al.* Mycophenolate mofetil in renal allograft recipients: a pooled efficacy analysis of three randomized, double-blind, clinical studies in prevention of rejection. *Transplantation* 1997; **63:** 39–47. Correction. *ibid.*; 618.
5. Mathew TH. A blinded, long-term, randomized multicenter study of mycophenolate mofetil in cadaveric renal transplantation: results at three years. *Transplantation* 1998; **65:** 1450–4. Correction. *ibid.*; **66:** 817.
6. Gruessner RW, *et al.* Mycophenolate mofetil in pancreas transplantation. *Transplantation* 1998; **66:** 318–23.
7. Kobashigawa J, *et al.* A randomized active-controlled trial of mycophenolate mofetil in heart transplant recipients. *Transplantation* 1998; **66:** 507–15.
8. Jain AB, *et al.* A prospective randomized trial of tacrolimus and prednisone versus tacrolimus, prednisone, and mycophenolate mofetil in primary adult liver transplant recipients: an interim report. *Transplantation* 1998; **66:** 1395–8.
9. Shapiro R, *et al.* A prospective, randomized trial of tacrolimus/prednisone versus tacrolimus/prednisone/mycophenolate mofetil in renal transplant recipients. *Transplantation* 1999; **67:** 411–15.
10. Oh JM, *et al.* Comparison of azathioprine and mycophenolate mofetil for the prevention of acute rejection in recipients of pancreas transplantation. *J Clin Pharmacol* 2001; **41:** 861–9.

**Pemphigus and pemphigoid.** Mycophenolate mofetil has been used successfully in the treatment of pemphigus and pemphigoid (p.1137), both with prednisolone[1-5] and alone.[6] It may be of benefit in patients who cannot tolerate, or do not respond to, azathioprine.[7]

1. Böhm M, *et al.* Bullous pemphigoid treated with mycophenolate mofetil. *Lancet* 1997; **349:** 541.
2. Enk AH, Knop J. Treatment of pemphigus vulgaris with mycophenolate mofetil. *Lancet* 1997; **350:** 494.
3. Enk AH, Knop J. Mycophenolate is effective in the treatment of pemphigus vulgaris. *Arch Dermatol* 1999; **135:** 54–6.
4. Williams JV, *et al.* Use of mycophenolate mofetil in the treatment of paraneoplastic pemphigus. *Br J Dermatol* 2000; **142:** 506–8.
5. Powell AM, *et al.* An evaluation of the usefulness of mycophenolate mofetil in pemphigus. *Br J Dermatol* 2003; **149:** 138–45.
6. Bredlich R-O, *et al.* Mycophenolate mofetil monotherapy for pemphigus vulgaris. *Br J Dermatol* 1999; **141:** 934.
7. Stanley JR. Therapy of pemphigus vulgaris. *Arch Dermatol* 1999; **135:** 76–8.

**Psoriasis.** Mycophenolate mofetil has proved successful in some cases of psoriasis (p.1137) refractory to conventional therapies,[1,2] and topical application is being investigated.[3]

1. Grundmann-Kollmann M, *et al.* Treatment of chronic plaque-stage psoriasis and psoriatic arthritis with mycophenolate mofetil. *J Am Acad Dermatol* 2000; **42:** 835–7.

2. Geilen CC, *et al.* Mycophenolate mofetil as a systemic antipsoriatic agent: positive experience in 11 patients. *Br J Dermatol* 2001; **144:** 583–6.
3. Wohlrab J, *et al.* Topical application of mycophenolate mofetil in plaque-type psoriasis. *Br J Dermatol* 2001; **144:** 1263–4.

**Vasculitic syndromes.** Mycophenolate mofetil has been tried in a number of the vasculitic syndromes, including Churg-Strauss syndrome (p.1078), polyarteritis nodosa and microscopic polyangiitis (p.1085), Takayasu's arteritis (p.1089), and Wegener's granulomatosis (p.1090).

## Preparations

**Proprietary Preparations** (details are given in Part 3)
***Arg.:*** CellCept; ***Austral.:*** CellCept; ***Austria:*** CellCept; ***Belg.:*** CellCept; ***Braz.:*** CellCept; ***Canad.:*** CellCept; ***Chile:*** CellCept; ***Denm.:*** CellCept; ***Fin.:*** CellCept; ***Fr.:*** CellCept; ***Ger.:*** CellCept; ***Gr.:*** Cellcept; ***Hong Kong:*** CellCept; ***Irl.:*** CellCept; ***Israel:*** CellCept; ***Ital.:*** CellCept; ***Jpn:*** CellCept; ***Mex.:*** CellCept; ***Neth.:*** CellCept; ***Norw.:*** CellCept; ***NZ:*** CellCept; ***Port.:*** CellCept; ***S.Afr.:*** CellCept; ***Singapore:*** CellCept; ***Spain:*** CellCept; ***Swed.:*** CellCept; ***Switz.:*** CellCept; ***Thai.:*** CellCept; ***UK:*** CellCept; ***USA:*** CellCept.

## Repertaxin L-lysine

### Profile

Repertaxin L-lysine is an inhibitor of interleukin-8 that is under investigation for the prevention of delayed graft function in organ transplantation.

## Sirolimus *(BAN, USAN, rINN)*

AY-22989; AY-022989; NSC-226080; Rapamycin; Sirolimús; Wy-090217.
(3*S*,6*R*,7*E*,9*R*,10*R*,12*R*,14*S*,15*E*,17*E*,19*E*,21*S*,23*S*,26*R*,27*R*,34a*S*)-9,10,12,13,14,21,22,23,24,25,26,27,32,33,34,34a-Hexadecahydro-9,27-dihydroxy-3-{(1*R*)-2-[(1*S*,3*R*,4*R*)-4-hydroxy-3-methoxycyclohexyl]-1-methylethyl}-10,21-dimethoxy-6,8,12,14,20,26-hexamethyl-23,27-epoxy-3*H*-pyrido[2,1-*c*][1,4]oxaazacyclohentriacontine-1,5,11,28,29(4*H*,6*H*,31*H*)-pentone.
$C_{51}H_{79}NO_{13}$ = 914.2.
*CAS — 53123-88-9.*
*ATC — L04AA10.*

### Adverse Effects and Precautions

The most frequent adverse effects of sirolimus include peripheral oedema, lymphocele, hyperlipidaemia, hypercholesterolaemia, tachycardia, venous thromboembolism, gastrointestinal disturbances, stomatitis, epistaxis, acne, rash, and bone necrosis. Anaemia, thrombocytopenia, and leucopenia have occurred, especially at higher doses. Arthralgia, hypokalaemia, and pyelonephritis are frequent. Hypersensitivity, including anaphylactic reactions, and pancreatitis have been reported rarely. Infections, including cytomegalovirus and *Pneumocystis carinii* pneumonia, are also common, and antimicrobial prophylaxis for pneumonia is recommended for the first year following transplantation. Thrombotic thrombocytopenic purpura and the haemolytic-uraemic syndrome may occur. Renal impairment may also occur, and there are reports of hepatotoxicity, and rarely, fatal hepatic necrosis. Excess mortality, graft loss, and hepatic artery thrombosis has been associated with the use of sirolimus in immunosuppressive regimens in liver transplant recipients and therefore use in such patients is not recommended. Interstitial lung disease has been reported, including some fatalities, although other cases resolved upon discontinuation or dose reduction of sirolimus. Abnormal wound healing following transplant surgery has been reported with the use of sirolimus; bronchial anastomotic dehiscence, including some fatal cases, has occurred in lung transplant recipients and such use is not recommended.

Immunosuppressants may reduce the response to vaccines, and the use of live vaccines should be avoided. Intra-uterine devices should be used with caution during immunosuppressive therapy, as there is an increased risk of infection.

Hypersensitivity reactions and subacute thrombosis have occurred with use of the sirolimus-eluting stent; fatalities have been reported.

### Interactions

Inhibitors of the cytochrome P450 isoenzyme CYP3A4, such as ketoconazole and diltiazem may increase plasma concentrations of sirolimus. Conversely, inducers of this isoenzyme, such as rifampicin, may reduce plasma concentrations of sirolimus. Grapefruit juice should not be taken with sirolimus. Ciclosporin can affect the rate and extent of sirolimus absorption and it is recommended that these drugs be given 4 hours apart. See above for precautions about use with live vaccines.

**Ciclosporin.** Concentrations of sirolimus, and area under the concentration-time curve were significantly higher when sirolimus and ciclosporin were given together than when the 2 drugs were given 4 hours apart,[1,2] and a synergistic effect has been suggested.[3] This effect may allow for lower doses[4] or early withdrawal[5] of ciclosporin, resulting in improved renal function and less nephrotoxicity.

1. Kaplan B, *et al.* The effects of relative timing of sirolimus and cyclosporine microemulsion formulation coadministration on the pharmacokinetics of each agent. *Clin Pharmacol Ther* 1998; **63:** 48–53.
2. Zimmerman JJ, *et al.* Pharmacokinetic interactions between sirolimus and microemulsion cyclosporine when orally administered jointly and 4 hours apart in healthy volunteers. *J Clin Pharmacol* 2003; **43:** 1168–76.
3. Kahan BD, Kramer WG. Median effect analysis of efficacy versus adverse effects of immunosuppressants. *Clin Pharmacol Ther* 2001; **70:** 74–81.
4. Reitamo S, *et al.* Efficacy of sirolimus (rapamycin) administered concomitantly with a subtherapeutic dose of cyclosporin in the treatment of severe psoriasis: a randomized controlled trial. *Br J Dermatol* 2001; **145:** 438–45.
5. Johnson RWG, *et al.* Sirolimus allows early cyclosporine withdrawal in renal transplantation resulting in improved renal function and lower blood pressure. *Transplantation* 2001; **72:** 777–86.

### Pharmacokinetics

Sirolimus is rapidly absorbed after doses of the oral solution, with a time to peak concentration of about 2 hours. Absorption is variably affected by food, especially high-fat meals. Sirolimus is extensively bound to plasma proteins. It is metabolised by the cytochrome P450 isoenzyme CYP3A4. Metabolism occurs by demethylation or hydroxylation, and the majority of a dose is excreted via the faeces, with only about 2% excreted in the urine. In healthy subjects, the bioavailability of a single dose of the tablet formulation is about 27% higher than the oral solution, bioavailability of which is only about 14%. However, this difference is less marked in renal transplant recipients, and when switching between formulations, the manufacturers recommend giving the same dose, with trough concentrations verified 1 to 2 weeks later.

◊ References.

1. Mahalati K, Kahan BD. Clinical pharmacokinetics of sirolimus. *Clin Pharmacokinet* 2001; **40:** 573–85.

### Uses and Administration

Sirolimus is a macrolide compound obtained from *Streptomyces hygroscopicus* and has potent immunosuppressant properties. It is used for the prevention of graft rejection in kidney transplantation (p.1346), and is being investigated for induction of remission in some auto-immune diseases. Sirolimus-releasing stents have been developed to reduce restenosis after coronary artery stent placement.

For prevention of graft rejection, sirolimus is given with ciclosporin and corticosteroids as soon as possible after transplantation. A loading dose of 6 mg is given orally, followed by a maintenance dose of 2 mg daily, 4 hours after ciclosporin. In patients 13 years of age or more who weigh less than 40 kg a loading dose of 3 $mg/m^2$, followed by initial maintenance doses of 1 $mg/m^2$ daily, is recommended. In the UK, it is recommended that the dose of sirolimus should be adjusted to obtain whole blood trough concentrations of 4 to 12 nanograms/mL (by chromatographic assay), and the doses of ciclosporin and corticosteroids gradually reduced. After 2 to 3 months, ciclosporin should be gradually stopped over 4 to 8 weeks, and the dose of sirolimus adjusted to obtain trough concentrations of 12 to 20 nanograms/mL. In patients in whom ciclosporin withdrawal is unsuccessful or cannot be attempted, sirolimus should not be used for more than 3 months after transplantation.

Sirolimus has been shown to possess antifungal and antineoplastic properties. It is under investigation for gene regulation in gene therapy.

**Organ and tissue transplantation.** References.

1. Vasquez EM. Sirolimus: a new agent for prevention of renal allograft rejection. *Am J Health-Syst Pharm* 2000; **57:** 437–51.
2. Kahan BD. Efficacy of sirolimus compared with azathioprine for reduction of acute renal allograft rejection: a randomised multicentre study. *Lancet* 2000; **356:** 194–202.
3. Ingle GR, *et al.* Sirolimus: continuing the evolution of transplant immunosuppression. *Ann Pharmacother* 2000; **34:** 1044–55.
4. Ponticelli C, *et al.* Phase III trial of Rapamune versus placebo in primary renal allograft recipients. *Transplant Proc* 2001; **33:** 2271–2.
5. Kahan BD, Camardo JS. Rapamycin: clinical results and future opportunities. *Transplantation* 2001; **72:** 1181–93.
6. Trotter JF. Sirolimus in liver transplantation. *Transplant Proc* 2003; **35** (suppl): 193S–200S.
7. MacDonald AS. Rapamycin in combination with cyclosporine or tacrolimus in liver, pancreas, and kidney transplantation. *Transplant Proc* 2003; **35** (suppl): 201S–208S.
8. Neff GW, *et al.* Ten years of sirolimus therapy in orthotopic liver transplant recipients. *Transplant Proc* 2003; **35** (suppl): 209S–216S.
9. Fairbanks KD, *et al.* Renal function improves in liver transplant recipients when switched from a calcineurin inhibitor to sirolimus. *Liver Transpl* 2003; **9:** 1079–85.
10. Fisher A, *et al.* Effect of sirolimus on infection incidence in liver transplant recipients. *Liver Transpl* 2004; **10:** 193–8.
11. Lo A, *et al.* Comparison of sirolimus-based calcineurin inhibitor-sparing and calcineurin inhibitor-free regimens in cadaveric renal transplantation. *Transplantation* 2004; **77:** 1228–35.

**Psoriasis.** Sirolimus has been investigated both systemically[1,2] and topically[3] in the treatment of psoriasis.

1. Reitamo S, *et al.* A double-blind study in patients with severe psoriasis to assess the clinical activity and safety of rapamycin (sirolimus) alone or in association with a reduced dose of cyclosporine. *Br J Dermatol* 1999; **141:** 978–9.
2. Reitamo S, *et al.* Efficacy of sirolimus (rapamycin) administered concomitantly with a subtherapeutic dose of cyclosporin in the treatment of severe psoriasis: a randomized controlled trial. *Br J Dermatol* 2001; **145:** 438–45.
3. Ormerod AD, *et al.* Penetration, safety and efficacy of the topical immunosuppressive sirolimus in psoriasis. *Br J Dermatol* 1999; **141:** 975.

**Reperfusion and revascularisation procedures.** References.

1. Sousa JE, *et al.* Lack of neointimal proliferation after implantation of sirolimus-coated stents in human coronary arteries: a quantitative coronary angiography and three-dimensional intravascular ultrasound study. *Circulation* 2001; **103:** 192–5.
2. Sousa JE, *et al.* Sustained suppression of neointimal proliferation by sirolimus-eluting stents: one-year angiographic and intravascular ultrasound follow-up. *Circulation* 2001; **104:** 2007–11.
3. Morice M-C, *et al.* A randomized comparison of a sirolimus-eluting stent with a standard stent for coronary revascularization. *N Engl J Med* 2002; **346:** 1773–80.
4. Serruys PW, *et al.* Rapamycin eluting stent: the onset of a new era in interventional cardiology. *Heart* 2002; **87:** 305–7.
5. Moses JW, *et al.* Sirolimus-eluting stents versus standard stents in patients with stenosis in a native coronary artery. *N Engl J Med* 2003; **349:** 1315–23.
6. Lemos PA, *et al.* Early outcome after sirolimus-eluting stent implantation in patients with acute coronary syndromes: insights from the Rapamycin-Eluting Stent Evaluated At Rotterdam Cardiology Hospital (RESEARCH) registry. *J Am Coll Cardiol* 2003; **41:** 2093–9.
7. Brara PS, *et al.* Pilot trial of oral rapamycin for recalcitrant restenosis. *Circulation* 2003; **107:** 1722–4. Correction. *ibid.*; **108:** 2170.
8. Holmes DR, *et al.* Analysis of 1-year clinical outcomes in the SIRIUS trial: a randomized trial of a sirolimus-eluting stent versus a standard stent in patients at high risk for coronary restenosis. *Circulation* 2004; **109:** 634–40.

### Preparations

**Proprietary Preparations** (details are given in Part 3)
***Arg.:*** Rapamune; ***Austral.:*** Rapamune; ***Belg.:*** Rapamune; ***Braz.:*** Rapamune; ***Canad.:*** Rapamune; ***Chile:*** Rapamune; ***Denm.:*** Rapamune; ***Fin.:*** Rapamune; ***Fr.:*** Rapamune; ***Ger.:*** Rapamune; ***Gr.:*** Rapamune; ***Irl.:*** Rapamune; ***Israel:*** Rapamune; ***Ital.:*** Rapamune; ***Mex.:*** Rapamune; ***Norw.:*** Rapamune; ***NZ:*** Rapamune; ***Spain:*** Rapamune; ***Swed.:*** Rapamune; ***Switz.:*** Rapamune; ***UK:*** Rapamune; ***USA:*** Rapamune.

## Tacrolimus *(BAN, USAN, rINN)*

FK-506; FR-900506; Tacrolimús. (−)-(3*S*,4*R*,5*S*,8*R*,9*E*,12*S*,14*S*,15*R*,16*S*,18*R*,19*R*,26a*S*)-8-Allyl-5,6,8,11,12,13,14,15,16,17,18,19,24,25,26,26a-hexadecahydro-5,19-dihydroxy-3-{(*E*)-2-[(1*R*,3*R*,4*R*)-4-hydroxy-3-methoxycyclohexyl]-1-methylvinyl}-14,16,-dimethoxy-4,10,12,18-tetramethyl-15,19-epoxy-3*H*-pyrido[2,1-*c*][1,4]oxaazacyclotricosine-1,7,20,21(4*H*,23*H*)-tetrone monohydrate.
$C_{44}H_{69}NO_{12},H_2O$ = 822.0.
*CAS — 104987-11-3 (anhydrous tacrolimus); 109581-93-3 (tacrolimus monohydrate).*
*ATC — D11AX14; L04AA05.*

### Adverse Effects and Precautions

Systemic exposure to tacrolimus may produce nephrotoxicity and neurotoxicity. The most common adverse effects after **systemic** use include tremor, headache, paraesthesias, nausea and diarrhoea, hypertension, leucocytosis, and impaired renal function. Anaemia, leucopenia, and thrombocytopenia also occur commonly. Disturbances of serum electrolytes, notably hyperkalaemia occur frequently. Other adverse effects include mood changes, sleep disturbances, confusion, dizziness, tinnitus, visual disturbances, and convulsions; disturbances of carbohydrate metabolism or frank diabetes mellitus; ECG changes and tachycardia, as well as hypertrophic cardiomyopathy (particularly in children); constipation, dyspepsia, and gastrointestinal haemorrhage; dyspnoea, asthma, pleural effusions; alopecia, hirsutism, skin rash and pruritus; and arthralgia or myalgia, spasm, leg cramps, peripheral oedema, liver dysfunction, and coagulation disorders.

Tacrolimus injection is formulated with polyethoxylated castor oil: anaphylactoid reactions have occurred, and appropriate means for their management should be available in patients given the injection. Use of tacrolimus should be avoided in patients hypersensitive to macrolides. Dosage reduction may be necessary in patients with hepatic impairment. Care is also required in patients with pre-existing renal impairment, and dosage reduction may prove advisable in such patients. Monitoring of blood concentrations of tacrolimus is recommended in all patients. Renal and hepatic function, blood pressure, serum glucose and electrolytes, and haematological and cardiac function, as well as visual function should be monitored regularly. As with other immunosuppressants, patients receiving tacrolimus are at increased risk of infection and malignancy. Intra-uterine devices should be used with caution during immunosuppressive therapy as there is an increased risk of infection. Use of live vaccines should be avoided for the same reason. Tacrolimus may affect visual or neurological function, and patients so affected should not drive or operate dangerous machinery.

**Topical** tacrolimus has been associated with local irritation and skin disorders including an increased incidence of herpes simplex and zoster infections; headache and 'flu-like' symptoms have also been reported. Exposure of the skin to sunlight should be minimised and the use of artificial sources of ultraviolet light avoided.

**Breast feeding.** Tacrolimus concentrations were measured in milk from a liver transplant recipient on a dose of 0.1 mg/kg daily. The authors estimated that the infant would ingest only 0.06% (0.06 micrograms/kg daily) of the mother's weight-adjusted dose. No adverse effects were noted in the infant at 2.5 months of age.[1]

1. French AE, *et al.* Milk transfer and neonatal safety of tacrolimus. *Ann Pharmacother* 2003; **37:** 815–18.

**Effects on the blood.** Severe anaemia due to selective depression of erythropoiesis in a patient given tacrolimus resolved when tacrolimus was replaced with ciclosporin.[1] More generalised bone marrow suppression,[2] and post-transplant thrombotic microangiopathy[3] have also been reported.

1. Winkler M, *et al.* Anaemia associated with FK 506 immunosuppression. *Lancet* 1993; **341:** 1035–6.
2. de-la-Serna-Higuera C, *et al.* Tacrolimus-induced bone marrow suppression. *Lancet* 1997; **350:** 714–15.
3. Trimarchi HM, *et al.* FK506-associated thrombotic microangiopathy: report of two cases and review of the literature. *Transplantation* 1999; **67:** 539–44.

**Effects on carbohydrate metabolism.** The development of diabetes mellitus after solid organ transplantation is common.[1,2] Post-transplant diabetes mellitus has been attributed to the diabetogenic effects of immunosuppressive drugs, and incidence has appeared to be increased in both adult[3] and paediatric[4] renal transplant recipients given tacrolimus. However, a retrospective review found no significant difference in incidence between patients receiving tacrolimus or ciclosporin.[2] This review found instead a correlation between the absence of an antiproliferative agent and the development of diabetes. Since post-transplant diabetes is potentially reversible,[5] guidelines for management, including the monitoring of blood glucose and the tapering of corticosteroids, have been proposed.[2] A retrospective study of liver transplant recipients found that, although those given tacrolimus had a greater incidence of diabetes mellitus, hepatitis C infection was the only factor predictive of its development.[1]

1. AlDosary AA, *et al.* Post-liver transplantation diabetes mellitus: an association with hepatitis C. *Liver Transpl* 2002; **8:** 356–61.
2. First MR, *et al.* Posttransplant diabetes mellitus in kidney allograft recipients: incidence, risk factors, and management. *Transplantation* 2002; **73:** 379–86.
3. Pirsch JD, *et al.* A comparison of tacrolimus (FK506) and cyclosporine for immunosuppression after cadaveric renal transplantation. *Transplantation* 1997; **63:** 977–83.
4. Al-Uzri A, *et al.* Posttransplant diabetes mellitus in pediatric renal transplant recipients: a report of the North American Pediatric Renal Transplant Cooperative Study (NAPRTCS). *Transplantation* 2001; **72:** 1020–4.
5. Vincenti F, *et al.* A long-term comparison of tacrolimus (FK506) and cyclosporine in kidney transplantation: evidence for improved allograft survival at five years. *Transplantation* 2002; **73:** 775–82. Correction. *ibid.*; 1370.

**Effects on the cardiovascular system.** Hypertrophic cardiomyopathy, and in some cases heart failure, has been described in paediatric patients receiving tacrolimus after organ grafting (small bowel or liver).[1] Symptoms largely resolved on discontinuation or dosage reduction. A similar case had been found *post mortem* in an adult,[2] and the UK Committee on Safety of Medicines[3] was aware of 29 reported cases worldwide as of July 1995. Echocardiographic monitoring of patients receiving tacrolimus has been recommended, with dose reduction or withdrawal in those who developed hypertrophic changes.[3] However, echocardiographic abnormalities may be quite common after orthotopic liver transplantation in adults, with no obvious relationship to the use of tacrolimus,[4] and a retrospective analysis concluded that tacrolimus is not a risk factor for hypertrophic cardiomyopathy in adult transplant recipients.[5]

Severe hypertension was documented in 5 out of 10 paediatric patients who received intravenous tacrolimus following renal transplant surgery. All patients responded to intravenous labetalol. By contrast none of 11 children who received ciclosporin at the same institution developed hypertension.[6] However, a review[7] concluded that tacrolimus causes less hypertension than ciclosporin, resulting in a better cardiovascular risk profile in renal transplant recipients, and possibly ultimately prolonging graft survival.

1. Atkison P, *et al.* Hypertrophic cardiomyopathy associated with tacrolimus in paediatric transplant patients. *Lancet* 1995; **345:** 894–6.
2. Natazuka T, *et al.* Immunosuppressive drugs and hypertrophic cardiomyopathy. *Lancet* 1995; **345:** 1644.
3. Committee on Safety of Medicines/Medicines Control Agency. Tacrolimus (Prograf) and hypertrophic cardiomyopathy in transplant patients. *Current Problems* 1995; **21:** 6.
4. Dollinger MM, *et al.* Tacrolimus and cardiotoxicity in adult liver transplant recipients. *Lancet* 1995; **346:** 507.
5. Coley KC, *et al.* Lack of tacrolimus-induced cardiomyopathy. *Ann Pharmacother* 2001; **35:** 985–9.
6. Booth CJ, *et al.* Intravenous tacrolimus may induce severe hypertension in renal transplant recipients. *Arch Dis Child* 1999; **80** (suppl 1): A27.
7. Koomans HA, Ligtenberg G. Mechanisms and consequences of arterial hypertension after renal transplantation. *Transplantation* 2001; **72** (suppl): S9–12.

**Effects on the kidney.** A comparison in patients who had undergone liver transplantation suggested that nephrotoxicity was more of a problem in those receiving tacrolimus than in those given a ciclosporin-based regimen.[1] In particular intravenous tacrolimus during the first week after transplantation was associated with acute renal failure in 4 of 20 patients. Furthermore, on follow-up for 1 year, GFR was somewhat lower in the tacrolimus-treated group. A small study compared GFR and effective renal plasma flow (ERPF), at various stages after transplantation, in renal and liver transplant recipients given tacrolimus.[2] In renal transplant patients, the GFR, although lower than normal, was increased after transplant, and remained stable over 3 months. ERPF, however, was significantly lower at 3 months. In liver transplant recipients, despite being lower than normal, GFR and ERPF were unchanged at 1 year post-transplant.

1. Porayko MK, *et al.* Nephrotoxic effects of primary immunosuppression with FK-506 and cyclosporine regimens after liver transplantation. *Mayo Clin Proc* 1994; **69:** 105–11.
2. Agarwala S, *et al.* Evaluation of renal function in transplant patients on tacrolimus therapy. *J Clin Pharmacol* 2002; **42:** 798–805.

**Effects on the nervous system.** Severe peripheral neuropathy together with signs of cerebral dysfunction has been reported in 2 patients receiving tacrolimus.[1] Among other central effects, tacrolimus has also been associated with speech disorders, including severe dysarthria and mutism in 1 patient;[2] some degree of speech dysfunction, in the form of an apparent Norwegian accent, appeared to be permanent in this case. Although many of the symptoms of neurotoxicity induced by tacrolimus are similar to those of ciclosporin (p.1352), some symptoms such as headaches, tremor, and sleep disturbances, appear to be more prevalent with tacrolimus, and the incidence of tacrolimus-induced neurotoxicity appears to be higher in liver transplant recipients.[3]

1. Ayres RCS, *et al.* Peripheral neurotoxicity with tacrolimus. *Lancet* 1994; **343:** 862–3.
2. Boeve BF, *et al.* Dysarthria and apraxia of speech associated with FK-506 (tacrolimus). *Mayo Clin Proc* 1996; **71:** 969–72.
3. Bechstein WO. Neurotoxicity of calcineurin inhibitors: impact and clinical management. *Transpl Int* 2000; **13:** 313–26.

**Effects on skeletal muscle.** Severe acute rhabdomyolysis, leading to fatal acute renal failure, developed in an 18-month-old child given tacrolimus after bone marrow transplantation.[1]

1. Hibi S, *et al.* Severe rhabdomyolysis associated with tacrolimus. *Lancet* 1995; **346:** 702.

**Hepatitis.** For the suggestion that dosage requirements of tacrolimus may be reduced in children with hepatitis C see Administration, below.

**Infection.** For a report of an increased incidence of cytomegalovirus disease in renal transplant recipients given a regimen combining tacrolimus and mycophenolate mofetil see under Interactions, p.1361.

**Overdosage.** A report[1] of 12 cases of acute overdose with tacrolimus described overdoses of up to 30 times the prescribed dose. Three patients were asymptomatic, while 7 showed mild transient renal and hepatic impairment, nausea, and mild hand tremors. One patient suffered renal failure, histoplasmosis, and sepsis 48 hours after admission for the overdose. The outcome was unknown in one patient. All 8 symptomatic patients recovered when tacrolimus concentrations returned to normal. No specific treatment regimen has been recommended, but patients have been treated with gastric lavage, oral activated charcoal, and phenytoin. The latter is used both to prevent seizures and to enhance tacrolimus metabolism by stimulation of cytochrome P450. Patients should be closely monitored for known signs and symptoms of tacrolimus toxicity. In a further series of 5 cases,[2] acute ingestion of tacrolimus was reported to be well tolerated, and adequately managed with conservative treatment.

1. Curran CF, *et al.* Acute overdoses of tacrolimus. *Transplantation* 1996; **62:** 1376.
2. Mrvos R, *et al.* Tacrolimus (FK 506) overdose: a report of five cases. *J Toxicol Clin Toxicol* 1997; **35:** 395–9.

## Interactions

Increased nephrotoxicity may result if tacrolimus is given with other potentially nephrotoxic drugs: use with ciclosporin should be avoided for this reason. Potassium-sparing diuretics should also be avoided in patients receiving tacrolimus.

Tacrolimus is metabolised by the cytochrome P450 isoenzyme CYP3A4, and drugs which inhibit this enzyme system, such as azole antifungals, bromocriptine, calcium-channel blockers, cimetidine, some corticosteroids, ciclosporin, danazol, HIV-protease inhibitors, macrolide antibacterials, and metoclopramide, may produce increased blood concentrations of tacrolimus. The metabolism of tacrolimus may also be inhibited by grapefruit juice and concomitant use should be avoided. Equally, inducers of this enzyme system (such as carbamazepine, phenobarbital, phenytoin, and rifampicin) may reduce blood concentrations of tacrolimus. For a warning concerning the use of live vaccines in patients receiving immunosuppressants see Adverse Effects and Precautions, above.

Facial flushing or skin irritation may occur if alcohol is consumed by patients using topical tacrolimus.

◊ The cytochrome P450 isoenzyme subfamily CYP3A, and P-glycoprotein, are involved in the pharmacokinetic pathways of tacrolimus.[1] Drugs known to interact with these systems will probably affect tacrolimus concentrations, primarily by influencing oral bioavailability rather than clearance.[2] A study[3] *in vitro* found that metabolism of tacrolimus by CYP3A in human liver microsomes was inhibited by bromocriptine, corticosterone, dexamethasone, ergotamine, erythromycin, ethinylestradiol, josamycin, ketoconazole, miconazole, midazolam, nifedipine, omeprazole, tamoxifen, troleandomycin, and verapamil. No effect on tacrolimus metabolism was seen with aspirin, amphotericin B, captopril, cefotaxime, ciprofloxacin, diclofenac, diltiazem, doxycycline, furosemide, glibenclamide, imipramine, lidocaine, paracetamol, prednisolone, progesterone, ranitidine, sulfamethoxazole, trimethoprim, or vancomycin.

1. van Gelder T. Drug interactions with tacrolimus. *Drug Safety* 2002; **25:** 707–12.
2. Christians U, *et al.* Mechanisms of clinically relevant drug interactions associated with tacrolimus. *Clin Pharmacokinet* 2002; **41:** 813–51.
3. Christians U, *et al.* Identification of drugs inhibiting the in vitro metabolism of tacrolimus by human liver microsomes. *Br J Clin Pharmacol* 1996; **41:** 187–90.

**Antibacterials.** Increased concentrations of tacrolimus in plasma have been reported with *erythromycin*;[1] the interaction was accompanied by some evidence of nephrotoxicity. A similar interaction has been reported between tacrolimus and *clarithromycin*.[2,3] For reference to the effects of macrolides on tacrolimus metabolism *in vitro* see above.

Treatment with *rifampicin* has been found to substantially decrease tacrolimus concentrations.[4,5] A pharmacokinetic study found that rifampicin induces metabolism of tacrolimus in both the liver and intestine, probably by induction of the cytochrome P450 isoenzyme subfamily CYP3A and P-glycoprotein.[6] Both *metronidazole*[7] and *chloramphenicol*[8] increased the blood concentrations of tacrolimus. This is probably due to inhibition of metabolism, and dosage reduction of the immunosuppressant may be necessary when either drug is given with tacrolimus.

Plasma concentrations of tacrolimus are also increased by *quinupristin/dalfopristin*.

1. Jensen C, *et al.* Interaction between tacrolimus and erythromycin. *Lancet* 1994; **344:** 825.
2. Wolter K, *et al.* Interaction between FK 506 and clarithromycin in a renal transplant patient. *Eur J Clin Pharmacol* 1994; **47:** 207–8.
3. Ibrahim RB, *et al.* Tacrolimus-clarithromycin interaction in a patient receiving bone marrow transplantation. *Ann Pharmacother* 2002; **36:** 1971–2.
4. Furlan V, *et al.* Interactions between FK506 and rifampicin or erythromycin in pediatric liver recipients. *Transplantation* 1995; **59:** 1217–18.
5. Chenhsu R-Y, *et al.* Renal allograft dysfunction associated with rifampin-tacrolimus interaction. *Ann Pharmacother* 2000; **34:** 27–31.
6. Hebert MF, *et al.* Effects of rifampin on tacrolimus pharmacokinetics in healthy volunteers. *J Clin Pharmacol* 1999; **39:** 91–6.
7. Herzig K, Johnson DW. Marked elevation of blood cyclosporin and tacrolimus levels due to concurrent metronidazole therapy. *Nephrol Dial Transplant* 1999; **14:** 521–3.
8. Schulman SL, *et al.* Interaction between tacrolimus and chloramphenicol in a renal transplant recipient. *Transplantation* 1998; **65:** 1397–8.

**Antidepressants.** Tacrolimus trough concentrations reduced sharply in a patient who took *hypericum*, and returned to previous levels on stopping the hypericum.[1] Hypericum induces cytochrome P450 isoenzyme CYP3A4, enhancing the metabolism of tacrolimus. A pharmacokinetic study[2] confirmed this, finding an increase in tacrolimus clearance; the authors concluded that potential consequences of this interaction in transplant recipients are rejection and graft loss.

1. Bolley R, *et al.* Tacrolimus-induced nephrotoxicity unmasked by induction of the CYP3A4 system with St John's wort. *Transplantation* 2002; **73:** 1009.
2. Hebert MF, *et al.* Effects of St. John's wort (Hypericum perforatum) on tacrolimus pharmacokinetics in healthy volunteers. *J Clin Pharmacol* 2004; **44:** 89–94.

**Antiepileptics.** For the effect of tacrolimus on *phenytoin*, see Immunosuppressants in Phenytoin, p.374.

**Antifungals.** Elevated plasma-tacrolimus concentrations have been reported in patients given *clotrimazole*,[1] *fluconazole*,[2] or *voriconazole*[3]; a reduction in the dose of tacrolimus was likely to be necessary if it were given with an azole antifungal. A study involving tacrolimus and *ketoconazole* suggested that an increase in the oral bioavailability of tacrolimus from a mean of 14 to 30% when given with the azole was probably due to decreased cytochrome P450 isoenzyme CYP3A4 metabolism in the gut wall, or improved absorption due to inhibition of P-glycoprotein mediated efflux, rather than an effect on hepatic metabolism.[4] Similarly, a 50% reduction in tacrolimus dosage was found to be necessary when the drug was given with *itraconazole*.[5] It has been suggested that the interaction could be exploited to reduce the cost of immunosuppressant regimens.[6]

1. Mieles L, *et al.* Interaction between FK506 and clotrimazole in a liver transplant recipient. *Transplantation* 1991; **52:** 1086–7.

2. Mañez R, *et al.* Fluconazole therapy in transplant recipients receiving FK506. *Transplantation* 1994; **57:** 1521–3.
3. Venkataramanan R, *et al.* Voriconazole inhibition of the metabolism of tacrolimus in a liver transplant recipient and in human liver microsomes. *Antimicrob Agents Chemother* 2002; **46:** 3091–3.
4. Floren LC, *et al.* Tacrolimus oral bioavailability doubles with coadministration of ketoconazole. *Clin Pharmacol Ther* 1997; **62:** 41–9.
5. Capone D, *et al.* Effects of itraconazole on tacrolimus blood concentrations in a renal transplant recipient. *Ann Pharmacother* 1999; **33:** 1124–5.
6. Kramer MR, *et al.* Dose adjustment and cost of itraconazole prophylaxis in lung transplant recipients receiving cyclosporine and tacrolimus (FK506). *Transplant Proc* 1997; **29:** 2657–9.

**Antivirals.** In 6 HIV-positive liver transplant recipients receiving tacrolimus-based immunosuppressive therapy, antiretroviral therapy including a protease inhibitor was started postoperatively.[1] To maintain therapeutic tacrolimus trough concentrations, ten- to fiftyfold reductions in tacrolimus dosage were necessary. This effect was more pronounced with *nelfinavir* than *indinavir.* In contrast, 4 HIV-positive kidney transplant recipients received antiretroviral therapy without protease inhibitors, and required only conventional doses of tacrolimus. The authors caution that some protease inhibitors can act as both inducers and inhibitors of the cytochrome P450 isoenzyme CYP3A4. While the inhibitory effect appears to predominate when given with tacrolimus, if the protease inhibitor is withdrawn suddenly the CYP3A4 system may remain induced, and a sudden decrease in tacrolimus concentration may occur; this had occurred in one case. For this reason, they concluded that great caution and frequent tacrolimus monitoring are necessary when protease inhibitors are introduced or withdrawn in transplant recipients receiving tacrolimus.

1. Jain AKB, *et al.* The interaction between antiretroviral agents and tacrolimus in liver and kidney transplant patients. *Liver Transpl* 2002; **8:** 841–5.

**Calcium-channel blockers.** Dosage requirements for tacrolimus were substantially reduced in 22 liver graft recipients who also received *nifedipine*, compared with 28 patients who did not, in a 1-year retrospective study.[1]

1. Seifeldin RA, *et al.* Nifedipine interaction with tacrolimus in liver transplant recipients. *Ann Pharmacother* 1997; **31:** 571–5.

**Danazol.** Nephrotoxicity and tremors associated with elevated concentrations of tacrolimus developed in a patient given danazol with the immunosuppressant.[1] The effect might be due to inhibition of the metabolism of tacrolimus.

1. Shapiro R, *et al.* FK 506 interaction with danazol. *Lancet* 1993; **341:** 1344–5.

**Gastrointestinal drugs.** In a renal transplant recipient, tacrolimus trough concentrations increased markedly after introduction of *lansoprazole* and returned to normal after its discontinuation.[1] For a study *in vitro* suggesting that *omeprazole* affected CYP3A4 metabolism of tacrolimus, see above.

1. Takahashi K, *et al.* Lansoprazole-tacrolimus interaction in Japanese transplant recipient with CYP2C19 polymorphism. *Ann Pharmacother* 2004; **38:** 791–4.

**Immunosuppressants.** Tacrolimus may inhibit *ciclosporin* metabolism *in vitro*, with the possibility of increased nephrotoxicity (see under Ciclosporin, p.1356). Tacrolimus may also increase concentrations of mycophenolic acid, a metabolite of *mycophenolate mofetil* (see under Mycophenolate Mofetil, p.1361), and the risk of infection may be increased if used together.

## Pharmacokinetics

Absorption of tacrolimus after oral doses is reported to be erratic. Oral bioavailability varies very widely, although a bioavailability of about 15 to 20% seems common. There is little or no systemic exposure to tacrolimus following topical use (but see Absorption, below). Following intravenous administration it is widely distributed to the tissues; in the blood, about 80% is bound to erythrocytes, and variations in red cell binding account for much of the variability in pharmacokinetics. The portion in plasma is approximately 99% bound to plasma proteins. Tacrolimus is extensively metabolised in the liver, principally by cytochrome P450 isoenzyme CYP3A4, and excreted, primarily in bile, almost entirely as metabolites. Some metabolism may occur in the gastrointestinal tract. Whole-blood elimination half-life has been reported to average 43 hours in healthy volunteers, and to range from about 12 to 16 hours in transplant patients.

◊ References.

1. Gruber SA, *et al.* Pharmacokinetics of FK506 after intravenous and oral administration in patients awaiting renal transplantation. *J Clin Pharmacol* 1994; **34:** 859–64.
2. Jusko WJ, *et al.* Pharmacokinetics of tacrolimus in liver transplant patients. *Clin Pharmacol Ther* 1995; **57:** 281–90.
3. Venkataramanan R, *et al.* Clinical pharmacokinetics of tacrolimus. *Clin Pharmacokinet* 1995; **29:** 404–30.
4. Wallemacq PE, Verbeeck RK. Comparative clinical pharmacokinetics of tacrolimus in paediatric and adult patients. *Clin Pharmacokinet* 2001; **40:** 283–95.
5. Bekersky I, *et al.* Comparative tacrolimus pharmacokinetics: normal versus mildly hepatically impaired subjects. *J Clin Pharmacol* 2001; **41:** 628–35.
6. Reding R, *et al.* Efficacy and pharmacokinetics of tacrolimus oral suspension in pediatric liver transplant recipients. *Pediatr Transplant* 2002; **6:** 124–6.

**Absorption.** In an infant treated with topical tacrolimus for chronic dermatitis, a single application of 0.1% ointment resulted in high serum concentrations of the drug (24 nanograms/mL). Tacrolimus levels decreased over 7 days, after which another smaller, single application of 0.03% tacrolimus ointment again resulted in high serum concentrations. The authors cautioned against its use in young children and diseases with decreased skin barrier function.[1] In another report,[2] elevated blood tacrolimus concentrations were observed after application of 0.1% tacrolimus ointment to a large area of the body of a patient with erythroderma; again, caution in conditions where the skin barrier is disrupted was advised.

1. Kameda G, *et al.* Unexpected high serum levels of tacrolimus after a single topical application in an infant. *J Pediatr* 2003; **143:** 280. Correction. *ibid.*; 462.
2. Teshima D, *et al.* Increased topical tacrolimus absorption in generalized leukemic erythroderma. *Ann Pharmacother* 2003; **37:** 1444–7.

**Bioavailability.** Bioavailability of tacrolimus appears to be influenced by the type and timing of meals. Food, particularly high-fat meals, significantly reduced bioavailability, compared with the fasting state.[1] Ingestion of tacrolimus up to 1.5 hours after a meal also considerably reduced absorption.[2] The manufacturer therefore recommends that tacrolimus should be taken consistently with respect to meals. Gastrointestinal metabolism of tacrolimus is thought to be extensive, significantly affecting its bioavailability,[3] and differences in this metabolism may account for apparent differences in availability according to ethnic origin.[4]

1. Bekersky I, *et al.* Effect of low- and high-fat meals on tacrolimus absorption following 5 mg single oral doses to healthy human subjects. *J Clin Pharmacol* 2001; **41:** 176–82.
2. Bekersky I, *et al.* Effect of time of meal consumption on bioavailability of a single oral 5 mg tacrolimus dose. *J Clin Pharmacol* 2001; **41:** 289–97.
3. Tuteja S, *et al.* The effect of gut metabolism on tacrolimus bioavailability in renal transplant recipients. *Transplantation* 2001; **71:** 1301–7.
4. Mancinelli LM, *et al.* The pharmacokinetics and metabolic disposition of tacrolimus: a comparison across ethnic groups. *Clin Pharmacol Ther* 2001; **69:** 24–31.

**Therapeutic drug monitoring.** Microparticle enzyme immunoassay (MEIA) and enzyme-linked immunosorbent assay (ELISA) have both been used to measure tacrolimus whole blood concentrations. A study[1] of liver transplant recipients found that increasing trough tacrolimus concentrations, as measured by the ELISA, correlated with decreasing risk of acute rejection, but increasing risk of nephrotoxicity. The authors suggested a trough blood concentration of less than 15 nanograms/mL to minimise nephrotoxicity.

Bayesian forecasting has also been used.[2]

1. Venkataramanan R, *et al.* Clinical utility of monitoring tacrolimus blood concentrations in liver transplant patients. *J Clin Pharmacol* 2001; **41:** 542–51.
2. Fukudo M, *et al.* Forecasting of blood tacrolimus concentrations based on the Bayesian method in adult patients receiving living-donor liver transplantation. *Clin Pharmacokinet* 2003; **42:** 1161–78.

## Uses and Administration

Tacrolimus is a potent macrolide (macrolactam) immunosuppressant derived from *Streptomyces tsukubaensis*, and has actions similar to those of ciclosporin (see p.1357). It is used to prevent or reverse rejection in patients receiving organ transplants, as indicated by the cross-references given below, and has been tried in a few patients with refractory auto-immune or immune-mediated disorders. Tacrolimus is also applied topically in the management of moderate to severe atopic eczema.

The manufacturer recommends that oral tacrolimus should be taken consistently with respect to the timing of ingestion of food.

For **transplantation**, the initial dose recommended in the UK for liver graft recipients is 100 to 200 micrograms/kg daily by mouth, in 2 divided doses. The initial oral dose in kidney transplant patients is 150 to 300 micrograms/kg daily in 2 divided doses. Dosage should begin about 6 hours after completion of liver grafting and within 24 hours of a kidney transplant. If the patient's condition does not permit oral use, therapy may be commenced intravenously, by continuous 24-hour infusion: suggested initial doses are 10 to 50 micrograms/kg daily for liver transplants and 50 to 100 micrograms/kg daily for kidney transplants. In the USA, initial oral doses in patients with liver grafts are 100 to 150 micrograms/kg daily, in 2 divided doses, and in kidney grafts 200 micrograms/kg daily, in 2 divided doses. The recommended starting dose of intravenous tacrolimus is 30 to 50 micrograms/kg daily. Dosage should be adjusted according to whole-blood or plasma trough concentrations in individual patients: it is suggested that most patients can be satisfactorily maintained at whole-blood concentrations below 20 nanograms/mL. Children generally require doses 1.5 to 2 times greater than those recommended in adults to achieve the same blood concentrations.

For the treatment of **atopic eczema**, where conventional therapies are ineffective or unsuitable, tacrolimus may be applied twice daily as a 0.03 or 0.1% ointment. Treatment should be continued for 1 week after resolution of signs and symptoms of the disease.

◊ Reviews.

1. Hooks MA. Tacrolimus, a new immunosuppressant—a review of the literature. *Ann Pharmacother* 1994; **28:** 501–11.
2. Winkler M, Christians U. A risk-benefit assessment of tacrolimus in transplantation. *Drug Safety* 1995; **12:** 348–57.
3. Plosker GL, Foster RH. Tacrolimus: a further update of its pharmacology and therapeutic use in the management of organ transplantation. *Drugs* 2000; **59:** 323–89.
4. Skaehill PA. Tacrolimus in dermatologic disorders. *Ann Pharmacother* 2001; **35:** 582–8.

**Administration.** The mean dose of tacrolimus required to produce a standard trough concentration of 10 to 15 nanograms/mL was reported to be 96% higher in 7 black renal graft recipients than in 20 such patients of white or Asian descent.[1] (For mention of the effect of ethnicity on the bioavailability of tacrolimus see under Pharmacokinetics, above.)

There is limited evidence that children with hepatitis C required on average one-third of the dose of tacrolimus needed by children without the virus.[2]

1. Andrews PA, *et al.* Racial variation in dosage requirements of tacrolimus. *Lancet* 1996; **348:** 1446.
2. Moreno M, *et al.* Monitoring of tacrolimus as rescue therapy in pediatric liver transplantation. *Ther Drug Monit* 1998; **20:** 376–9.

**Eczema.** Topical tacrolimus has been found to be safe and effective[1-3] for short-term use in the treatment of moderate to severe atopic eczema (p.1135). In adult patients,[4] the efficacy of 0.1% tacrolimus ointment was similar to that of 0.1% hydrocortisone butyrate ointment, whereas in paediatric patients,[5,6] both 0.03 and 0.1% tacrolimus were significantly more effective than 1% hydrocortisone acetate ointment. In 18 of 19 patients with facial atopic eczema resistant to 0.03% tacrolimus ointment,[7] there was significant improvement upon application of a 0.03% lotion formulation, and 6 patients were positive to a patch test for white petrolatum, an ingredient of the commercial ointment.

1. Gianni LM, Sulli MM. Topical tacrolimus in the treatment of atopic dermatitis. *Ann Pharmacother* 2001; **35:** 943–6.
2. Allen BR. Tacrolimus ointment: its place in the therapy of atopic dermatitis. *J Allergy Clin Immunol* 2002; **109:** 401–3.
3. Anonymous. Topical tacrolimus—a role in atopic dermatitis? *Drug Ther Bull* 2002; **40:** 73–5.
4. Reitamo S, *et al.* Efficacy and safety of tacrolimus ointment compared with that of hydrocortisone butyrate ointment in adult patients with atopic dermatitis. *J Allergy Clin Immunol* 2002; **109:** 547–55.
5. Reitamo S, *et al.* Efficacy and safety of tacrolimus ointment compared with that of hydrocortisone acetate ointment in children with atopic dermatitis. *J Allergy Clin Immunol* 2002; **109:** 539–46.
6. Reitamo S, *et al.* 0.03% Tacrolimus ointment applied once or twice daily is more efficacious than 1% hydrocortisone acetate in children with moderate to severe atopic dermatitis: results of a randomized double-blind controlled trial. *Br J Dermatol* 2004; **150:** 554–62.
7. Sugiura H, *et al.* An open study of a lotion formulation to improve tolerance of tacrolimus in facial atopic dermatitis. *Br J Dermatol* 2001; **145:** 795–8.

**Glomerular kidney disease.** Tacrolimus used with corticosteroids induced a sustained remission in proteinuria in patients with idiopathic focal glomerulosclerosis (p.1080) refractory to standard therapy.[1]

1. Segarra A, *et al.* Combined therapy of tacrolimus and corticosteroids in cyclosporin-resistant or -dependent idiopathic focal glomerulosclerosis: a preliminary uncontrolled study with prospective follow-up. *Nephrol Dial Transplant* 2002; **17:** 655–62.

**Hepatitis.** In auto-immune chronic active hepatitis (p.1078), some evidence suggests that tacrolimus may offer an alternative therapy when corticosteroids alone or with azathioprine do not suffice.

References.

1. Van Thiel DH, *et al.* Tacrolimus: a potential new treatment for autoimmune chronic active hepatitis: results of an open-label preliminary trial. *Am J Gastroenterol* 1995; **90:** 771–6.
2. Heneghan MA, *et al.* Low dose tacrolimus as treatment of severe autoimmune hepatitis: potential role in remission induction. *Gut* 1999; **44** (suppl 1): A61.

**Ichthyosis.** For mention of the use of tacrolimus in ichthyosis see p.1136.

**Inflammatory bowel disease.** There are reports of response to tacrolimus in patients with inflammatory bowel disease (p.1243). Tacrolimus has been given orally,[1-3] intravenously,[1] or topically,[4] in the treatment of ulcerative colitis[1,3] and Crohn's disease,[1-4] refractory to standard therapy. However, further controlled trials are needed.

1. Fellermann K, *et al.* Tacrolimus: a new immunosuppressant for steroid refractory inflammatory bowel disease. *Transplant Proc* 2001; **33:** 2247–8.
2. Ierardi E, *et al.* Oral tacrolimus long-term therapy in patients with Crohn's disease and steroid resistance. *Aliment Pharmacol Ther* 2001; **15:** 371–7.
3. Bousvaros A, *et al.* Oral tacrolimus treatment of severe colitis in children. *J Pediatr* 2000; **137:** 794–9.
4. Casson DH, *et al.* Topical tacrolimus may be effective in the treatment of oral and perineal Crohn's disease. *Gut* 2000; **47:** 436–40.

**Myasthenia gravis.** Tacrolimus was effective in the management of myasthenia gravis (p.1486) in a patient in whom the use of standard therapy was contra-indicated.[1]

1. Evoli A, *et al.* Successful treatment of myasthenia gravis with tacrolimus. *Muscle Nerve* 2002; **25:** 111–14.

**Ocular disorders.** For mention of the use of tacrolimus in various disorders characterised by ocular lesions such as uveitis, see p.1344.

**Organ and tissue transplantation.** Tacrolimus has been used both for primary immunosuppression and for the control of graft rejection. Much of the initial experience with the drug was for liver grafts, (p.1346), but it is also employed in the transplantation of heart (p.1345), kidney (p.1346), lung (p.1347), pancreas (p.1347), and intestines (p.1346). It has also been tried for the prophylaxis of graft-versus-host disease following bone marrow transplantation (see Haematopoietic Stem Cell Transplantation, p.1344).

A few selected references to the use of tacrolimus in transplantation are given below.

1. European FK506 Multicentre Liver Study Group. Randomised trial comparing tacrolimus (FK506) and cyclosporin in prevention of liver allograft rejection. *Lancet* 1994; **344:** 423–8.
2. The US Multicenter FK506 Liver Study Group. A comparison of tacrolimus (FK506) and cyclosporine for immunosuppression in liver transplantation. *N Engl J Med* 1994; **331:** 1110–15.
3. Klein A. Tacrolimus rescue in liver transplant patients with refractory rejection or intolerance or malabsorption of cyclosporine. *Liver Transpl Surg* 1999; **5:** 502–8.
4. Gruessner RW. Tacrolimus in pancreas transplantation: a multicenter analysis. *Clin Transplant* 1997; **11:** 299–312.
5. Gruessner RWG, *et al.* Suggested guidelines for the use of tacrolimus in pancreas/kidney transplantation. *Clin Transplant* 1998; **12:** 260–2.
6. Reichart B, *et al.* European Multicenter Tacrolimus (FK506) Heart Pilot Study: one-year results. *J Heart Lung Transplant* 1998; **17:** 775–81.
7. Wiesner RH. A long-term comparison of tacrolimus (FK506) versus cyclosporine in liver transplantation: a report of the United States FK506 Study Group. *Transplantation* 1998; **66:** 493–9.
8. Taylor DO, *et al.* A randomized, multicenter comparison of tacrolimus and cyclosporine immunosuppressive regimens in cardiac transplantation: decreased hyperlipidemia and hypertension with tacrolimus. *J Heart Lung Transplant* 1999; **18:** 336–45.
9. Margreiter R. Efficacy and safety of tacrolimus compared with ciclosporin microemulsion in renal transplantation: a randomised multicentre study. *Lancet* 2002; **359:** 741–6.
10. O'Grady JG, *et al.* Tacrolimus versus microemulsified ciclosporin in liver transplantation: the TMC randomised controlled trial. *Lancet* 2002; **360:** 1119–25.
11. Scott LJ, *et al.* Tacrolimus: a further update of its use in the management of organ transplantation. *Drugs* 2003; **63:** 1247–97.

**Psoriasis.** Tacrolimus has been shown to be effective in the treatment of psoriasis (p.1137) when used orally[1] or topically.[2,3]

1. The European FK 506 Multicentre Psoriasis Study Group. Systemic tacrolimus (FK 506) is effective for the treatment of psoriasis in a double-blind, placebo-controlled study. *Arch Dermatol* 1996; **132:** 419–23.
2. Remitz A, *et al.* Tacrolimus ointment improves psoriasis in a microplaque assay. *Br J Dermatol* 1999; **141:** 103–7.
3. Clayton TH, *et al.* Topical tacrolimus for facial psoriasis. *Br J Dermatol* 2003; **149:** 419–20.

**Pyoderma gangrenosum.** There are reports of response to tacrolimus, given orally[1-4] or topically,[4-7] in patients with pyoderma gangrenosum (p.1138). A small study[8] found topical tacrolimus 0.3% in carmellose sodium paste to be more effective than clobetasol propionate 0.05% for peristomal pyoderma gangrenosum.

1. Abu-Elmagd K, *et al.* Resolution of severe pyoderma gangrenosum in a patient with streaking leukocyte factor disease after treatment with tacrolimus (FK 506). *Ann Intern Med* 1993; **119:** 595–8.
2. D'Incà R, *et al.* Tacrolimus to treat pyoderma gangrenosum resistant to cyclosporine. *Ann Intern Med* 1998; **128:** 783–4.
3. Lyon CC, *et al.* Recalcitrant pyoderma gangrenosum treated with systemic tacrolimus. *Br J Dermatol* 1999; **140:** 562–4.
4. Jolles S, *et al.* Combination oral and topical tacrolimus in therapy-resistant pyoderma gangrenosum. *Br J Dermatol* 1999; **140:** 564–5.
5. Schuppe H-C, *et al.* Topical tacrolimus for pyoderma gangrenosum. *Lancet* 1998; **351:** 832.
6. Reich K, *et al.* Topical tacrolimus for pyoderma gangrenosum. *Br J Dermatol* 1998; **139:** 755–7.
7. Vidal D, Alomar A. Successful treatment of periostomal pyoderma gangrenosum using topical tacrolimus. *Br J Dermatol* 2004; **150:** 387–8.
8. Lyon CC, *et al.* Topical tacrolimus in the management of peristomal pyoderma gangrenosum. *J Dermatol Treat* 2001; **12:** 13–17.

**Rheumatoid arthritis.** In a small, open-label study[1] of 12 patients with rheumatoid arthritis (p.9) refractory to other disease-modifying antirheumatic drugs including ciclosporin, 7 had significant response to tacrolimus after treatment for 6 months, with 4 of these patients maintaining this response after 2 years of therapy. In a larger controlled trial,[2] tacrolimus improved disease activity in patients with rheumatoid arthritis resistant to methotrexate.

1. Gremillion RB, *et al.* Tacrolimus (FK506) in the treatment of severe, refractory rheumatoid arthritis: initial experience in 12 patients. *J Rheumatol* 1999; **26:** 2332–6.
2. Furst DE, *et al.* Efficacy of tacrolimus in rheumatoid arthritis patients who have been treated unsuccessfully with methotrexate: a six-month, double-blind, randomized, dose-ranging study. *Arthritis Rheum* 2002; **46:** 2020–8.

**Scleroderma.** There are reports of response to tacrolimus in patients with scleroderma (p.1348).

## Preparations

**Proprietary Preparations** (details are given in Part 3)

***Arg.:*** Prograf; ***Austral.:*** Prograf; ***Austria:*** Prograf; ***Belg.:*** Prograft; ***Braz.:*** Prograf; ***Canad.:*** Prograf; ***Chile:*** Prograf; ***Denm.:*** Prograf; ***Fin.:*** Prograf; ***Fr.:*** Prograf; ***Ger.:*** Prograf; ***Gr.:*** Prograf; ***Hong Kong:*** Prograf; ***Irl.:*** Prograf; Protopic; ***Israel:*** Prograf; ***Ital.:*** Prograf; ***Jpn:*** Prograf; Protopic; ***Malaysia:*** Prograf; ***Mex.:*** Prograf; ***Norw.:*** Prograf; ***NZ:*** Prograf; ***Port.:*** Prograf; Protopic; ***S.Afr.:*** Prograf; ***Singapore:*** Prograf; ***Spain:*** Prograf; Protopic; ***Swed.:*** Prograf; ***Switz.:*** Prograf; ***Thai.:*** Prograf; ***UK:*** Prograf; Protopic; ***USA:*** Prograf; Protopic.

# Local Anaesthetics

Local anaesthetics produce reversible loss of function or sensation by preventing or diminishing the conduction of nerve impulses near to the site of their application or injection. Because their mode of action is to decrease permeability of the nerve cell membrane to sodium ions, they also have a membrane stabilising effect.

Most clinically useful local anaesthetics have the same general chemical configuration of an amine portion joined to an aromatic residue by an ester or amide link. The type of linkage is important in determining the properties of the drug.

For a classification of local anaesthetics, see Table 1, below.

**Table 1.** Classification of local anaesthetics.

| Amide type | Ester type |
|---|---|
| Articaine | *Esters of benzoic acid* |
| Bupivacaine | Amylocaine |
| Cinchocaine | Cocaine |
| Ethyl parapiperidino-acetylaminobenzoate | Propanocaine |
| Etidocaine | *Esters of meta-aminobenzoic acid* |
| Levobupivacaine | Proxymetacaine |
| Lidocaine | |
| Mepivacaine | *Esters of para-aminobenzoic acid* |
| Oxetacaine | Benzocaine |
| Prilocaine | Butacaine |
| Ropivacaine | Butoxycaine |
| Tolycaine | Butyl aminobenzoate |
| Trimecaine | Chloroprocaine |
| **Miscellaneous** | Oxybuprocaine |
| Diperodon | Parethoxycaine |
| Dyclonine | Procaine |
| Ethyl chloride | Propoxycaine |
| Ketocaine | Tetracaine |
| Myrtecaine | Tricaine |
| Octacaine | |
| Pramocaine | |
| Propipocaine | |
| Quinisocaine | |

## Adverse Effects

Adverse effects apparent after local anaesthesia may be caused by the anaesthetic or errors in technique, or may be the result of blockade of the sympathetic nervous system. Local anaesthetics may produce systemic adverse effects as a result of raised plasma concentrations that occur when the rate of uptake into the circulation exceeds the rate of breakdown, for example, following

- accidental intravascular injection
- excessive dosage or rate of administration
- absorption of large amounts through mucous membranes or damaged skin
- absorption of large amounts from inflamed or highly vascular areas.

The systemic toxicity of local anaesthetics mainly involves the CNS and the cardiovascular system. Excitation of the CNS may be manifested by restlessness, excitement, nervousness, paraesthesias, dizziness, tinnitus, blurred vision, nausea and vomiting, muscle twitching and tremors, and convulsions. Numbness of the tongue and perioral region, and lightheadedness followed by sedation may appear as early signs of systemic toxicity. Excitation when it occurs may be transient and followed by depression with drowsiness, respiratory failure, and coma. There may be effects on the cardiovascular system with myocardial depression and peripheral vasodilatation resulting in hypotension and bradycardia; arrhythmias and cardiac arrest may occur. Hypotension often accompanies spinal and epidural anaesthesia; inappropriate positioning of the patient may be a contributory factor for women in labour.

Hypersensitivity reactions are rare and generally limited to local anaesthetics of the ester type. There appears to be no cross-sensitivity between ester- and amide-type local anaesthetics. Idiosyncrasy to local anaesthetics has been reported. Hypersensitivity reactions to preservatives in local anaesthetic preparations have also occurred.

Some local anaesthetics cause methaemoglobinaemia.

Fetal intoxication has occurred after the use of local anaesthetics in labour, either as a result of transplacental diffusion or after accidental injection of the fetus.

Prolonged use of topical anaesthetics in the eye causes corneal damage.

Adverse effects may also be caused by concomitantly administered vasoconstrictors.

◊ Reviews.


1. McCaughey W. Adverse effects of local anaesthetics. *Drug Safety* 1992; **7:** 178–189.
2. Berde CB. Toxicity of local anesthetics in infants and children. *J Pediatr* 1993; **122** (suppl): S14–S20.
3. Naguib M, *et al.* Adverse effects and drug interactions associated with local and regional anaesthesia. *Drug Safety* 1998; **18:** 221–50.
4. Dalens BJ, Mazoit J-X. Adverse effects of regional anaesthesia in children. *Drug Safety* 1998; **19:** 251–68.
5. Cox B, *et al.* Toxicity of local anaesthetics. *Best Pract Res Clin Anaesthesiol* 2003; **17:** 111–36.


**Adverse effects of central block.** Central nerve block (see Local Anaesthetic Techniques, below), comprising spinal or epidural block, is very widely used and certain adverse effects are particularly associated with the technique. Systemic effects (see Adverse Effects, above) are more likely with epidural than with spinal block, because of the larger doses used.

Total spinal anaesthesia from extreme spread of a block or accidental penetration of the dura during an epidural block produces unconsciousness, hypotension, and respiratory arrest. Less extensive spread to the cervical region is usually associated with nausea, agitation, and hypotension.

Hypotension (associated with venodilatation and decreased cardiac output secondary to sympathetic block) is the **cardiovascular** effect most often associated with the technique, and may be especially problematic in pregnancy. Other cardiovascular complications may include bradycardia or heart block; cardiac arrest has also been reported unexpectedly after spinal anaesthesia.

Post-dural puncture headache (see Treatment of Adverse Effects, below) is probably the most common **neurological complication** related to these procedures and may be accompanied by tinnitus or photophobia. Headache following spinal block may rarely be caused by meningitis. Backache is a frequent postoperative complication following epidural, spinal, or general anaesthesia. Cranial nerve lesions and reversible loss of hearing in the low frequency range, usually affecting both ears, have been reported rarely following spinal block. Neurological complications associated with these blocks may also rarely include paraplegia caused by arachnoiditis, or trauma or compression of the spinal cord following development of a haematoma or abscess. Transient radicular irritation involving the lower back, buttocks, and thighs may develop within 24 hours of spinal block; recovery is usually within 1 week. Cauda equina syndrome, the symptoms of which include urinary retention, loss of perineal sensation, loss of sexual function, and faecal incontinence, is also a rare complication which can present many months after spinal block. There is some evidence that, although still rare, the incidence of neurotoxic complications after spinal anaesthesia is greater with lidocaine than with other commonly used local anaesthetics such as bupivacaine and tetracaine. The incidence of persistent lumbosacral neuropathy may be as high as 1 in 200 after continuous spinal anaesthesia with lidocaine.

Perioperative shivering has been associated with epidural block.

References.


1. Kalmanovitch DVA, Simmons P. Post-anaesthetic complications in the home. *Prescribers' J* 1988; **28:** 124–31.
2. Wildsmith JAW, Lee JA. Neurological sequelae of spinal anaesthesia. *Br J Anaesth* 1989; **63:** 505–7.
3. Parnass SM, Schmidt KJ. Adverse effects of spinal and epidural anaesthesia. *Drug Safety* 1990; **5:** 179–94.
4. Anonymous. Perioperative shivering. *Lancet* 1991; **338:** 547–8.
5. Broome IJ. Hearing loss and dural puncture. *Lancet* 1993: **341:** 667–8.
6. Russell R, *et al.* Assessing long term backache after childbirth. *BMJ* 1993; **306:** 1299–1303.
7. Harding SA, *et al.* Meningitis after combined spinal-extradural anaesthesia in obstetrics. *Br J Anaesth* 1994; **73:** 545–7.
8. Gielen M. Spinal anaesthesia: hearing loss, failure, transient radicular irritation. *Anaesthesia* 1998; **53** (suppl 2): 23–5.
9. Horlocker TT, Wedel DJ. Neurologic complications of spinal and epidural anesthesia. *Reg Anesth Pain Med* 2000; **25:** 88–98.
10. Johnson ME. Potential neurotoxicity of spinal anesthesia with lidocaine. *Mayo Clin Proc* 2000; **75:** 921–32.


**Effects on the ears.** Symptoms such as vertigo, nausea, and nystagmus, which have been reported after the use of local anaesthetics in the external[1] or middle ear,[2] may result from penetration of the local anaesthetic into the inner ear. For reference to hearing loss associated with spinal block, see under Adverse Effects of Central Block, above.


1. Raine NMN, Whittet HB. Emla cream and induced vertigo. *Br J Hosp Med* 1994; **51:** 614–15.
2. Blair Simmons F, *et al.* Lidocaine in the middle ear: a unique cause of vertigo. *Arch Otolaryngol* 1973; **98:** 42–3.


**Hypersensitivity.** Local anaesthetics may provoke types I and IV hypersensitivity reactions. Type I reactions (e.g. anaphylaxis) to local anaesthetics are generally rare. They occur more often with the ester-type than with the amide-type drugs, probably because of the metabolism of the former to para-aminobenzoic acid (PABA). Nevertheless, severe or fatal reactions have been associated not only with ester-type local anaesthetics such as tetracaine[1] and procaine[2] but also with the amide-type local anaesthetics lidocaine[3-7] and prilocaine.[3] Intolerance may also have been the cause of death in a patient who received mepivacaine for paracervical anaesthesia.[8] Hypotension during dental anaesthesia is usually a vasovagal response unrelated to the type of local anaesthetic used and may be prevented by the use of diazepam. Patients sensitised by topical application may then develop anaphylactic reactions when treated systemically.[9] The use of drugs such as benzocaine or tetracaine in lozenges or throat sprays may also sensitise patients.[10]

Some patients diagnosed as being hypersensitive to local anaesthetics may have reacted to preservatives in the preparations.[11] Cross-hypersensitivity reactions may also occur between some ester-type local anaesthetics and topical preparations, such as sunscreens, that contain PABA or related compounds.[12]

Skin testing may be of benefit in patients who will require future local anaesthesia and when a patient's history does not rule out a possible allergic reaction. However, testing itself can cause severe or anaphylactic reactions.[9,13]

Type IV reactions (i.e. delayed reactions) to local anaesthetics have also been reported, albeit rarely.[14-16]

For reports of the incidence of allergy to local anaesthetics determined by patch testing, see under individual monographs.


1. Moriwaki K, *et al.* A case report of anaphylactic shock induced by tetracaine used for spinal anesthesia. *Masui* 1986; **35:** 1279–84.
2. MacLachlan D, Forrest AL. Procaine and malignant hyperthermia. *Lancet* 1974; **i:** 355.
3. Fisher MM, Pennington JC. Allergy to local anaesthesia. *Br J Anaesth* 1982; **54:** 893–4.
4. Howard JJ, *et al.* Adult respiratory distress syndrome following administration of lidocaine. *Chest* 1982; **81:** 644–5.
5. Promisloff RA, DuPont DC. Death from ARDS and cardiovascular collapse following lidocaine administration. *Chest* 1983; **83:** 585.
6. Ruffles SP, Ayres JG. Fatal bronchospasm after topical lignocaine before bronchoscopy. *BMJ* 1987; **294:** 1658–9.
7. Ball IA. Allergic reactions to lignocaine. *Br Dent J* 1999; **186:** 224–6.
8. Grimes DA, Cates W. Deaths from paracervical anesthesia used for first-trimester abortion, 1972–1975. *N Engl J Med* 1976; **295:** 1397–9.
9. Mulvey PM. Allergy to local anaesthetics. *Med J Aust* 1980; **1:** 386.
10. Verbov J. Drug eruptions. *Practitioner* 1979; **222:** 400–9.
11. Wildsmith JAW, *et al.* Alleged allergy to local anaesthetic drugs. *Br Dent J* 1998; **184:** 507–10.
12. Parnass SM, Schmidt KJ. Adverse effects of spinal and epidural anesthesia. *Drug Safety* 1990; **5:** 179–94.
13. Brown DT, *et al.* Allergic reaction to an amide local anaesthetic. *Br J Anaesth* 1981; **53:** 435–7.
14. Klein CE, Gall H. Type IV allergy to amide-type local anesthetics. *Contact Dermatitis* 1991; **25:** 45–8.
15. Craft DV, Good RP. Delayed hypersensitivity reaction of the knee after injection of arthroscopy portals with bupivacaine (Marcaine). *Arthroscopy* 1994; **10:** 305–8.
16. Bircher AJ, *et al.* Delayed-type hypersensitivity to subcutaneous lidocaine with tolerance to articaine: confirmation by in vivo and in vitro tests. *Contact Dermatitis* 1996; **34:** 387–9.


**Methaemoglobinaemia.** Methaemoglobinaemia has been reported with several local anaesthetics including tetracaine,[1] benzocaine,[1-3] and lidocaine[1,4] but is more commonly associated with the use of prilocaine.[5-7] It may occur after local injection or topical administration. It has been suggested that the effect is due to the presence of an aniline group in the structure or, in the case of lidocaine and prilocaine, metabolism to an aniline-like structure. Methaemoglobinaemia may result from the use of usual doses as well as exposure to toxic concentrations of local anaesthetic;[1,7] with prilocaine doses of 8 mg/kg or more [above recommended maxima] usually produce symptoms.[8]

Methaemoglobinaemia has occurred after the topical application of a eutectic preparation of prilocaine and lidocaine.[6] Although increases in methaemoglobin concentrations are generally small following the use of this mixture in infants[9,10] and children,[11] some infants may be particularly susceptible to induced methaemoglobinaemia during the first 3 months of life probably due to their limited enzyme capacity.[9] The *British National Formulary* states that eutectic prilocaine/lidocaine cream may be used under specialist supervision in infants over 1 month of age, and in some other countries the cream is also licensed for limited use in neonates (see also Surface Anaesthesia under Lidocaine, p.1380). However, the UK manufacturers do not recommend its use in children under 1 year old.

Use with drugs such as sulfonamides[6] or antimalarials[8] may predispose to methaemoglobinaemia. Patients with haemoglobinopathies or G6PD deficiency may also be at greater risk.[1]


1. Olson ML, McEvoy GK. Methemoglobinemia induced by local anesthetics. *Am J Hosp Pharm* 1981; **38:** 89–93.
2. Rodriguez LF, *et al.* Benzocaine-induced methemoglobinemia: report of a severe reaction and review of the literature. *Ann Pharmacother* 1994; **28:** 643–9.
3. Tush GM, Kuhn RJ. Methemoglobinemia induced by an over-the-counter medication. *Ann Pharmacother* 1996; **30:** 1251–4.

4. Karim A, *et al.* Methemoglobinemia complicating topical lidocaine used during endoscopic procedures. *Am J Med* 2001; **111:** 150–3.
5. Mandel S. Methemoglobinemia following neonatal circumcision. *JAMA* 1989; **261:** 702.
6. Jakobson B, Nilsson A. Methemoglobinemia associated with a prilocaine-lidocaine cream and trimetoprim-sulphamethoxazole: a case report. *Acta Anaesthesiol Scand* 1985; **29:** 453–5.
7. Knobeloch L, *et al.* Prilocaine-induced methemoglobinemia—Wisconsin, 1993. *JAMA* 1994; **272:** 1403–4.
8. Reynolds F. Adverse effects of local anaesthetics. *Br J Anaesth* 1987; **59:** 78–95.
9. Nilsson A, *et al.* Inverse relationship between age-dependent erythrocyte activity of methaemoglobin reductase and prilocaine-induced methaemoglobinaemia during infancy. *Br J Anaesth* 1990; **64:** 72–6.
10. Brisman M, *et al.* Methaemoglobin formation after the use of EMLA cream in term neonates. *Acta Paediatr* 1998; **87:** 1191–4.
11. Frayling IM, *et al.* Methaemoglobinaemia in children treated with prilocaine-lignocaine cream. *BMJ* 1990; **301:** 153–4.

**Pregnancy.** As mentioned under Adverse Effects of Central Block, above, hypotension may be particularly problematic for patients receiving epidural or spinal block for analgesia during labour. In addition it has been suggested that patients receiving epidural analgesia during labour may have an increased risk of pyrexia, which can lead to fetal compromise.[1] See also under Labour Pain on p.6.

The use of paracervical block has fallen out of favour because of serious adverse effects on the fetus.

1. Fusi L, *et al.* Maternal pyrexia associated with the use of epidural analgesia in labour. *Lancet* 1989; **i:** 1250–2.

**Effects on wound healing.** A review of the literature[1] found evidence that local infiltration of local anaesthetics can have detrimental effects on the first two stages of wound healing. The size of the effect on mature wound strength remains to be determined.

1. Brower MC, Johnson ME. Adverse effects of local anesthetic infiltration on wound healing. *Reg Anesth Pain Med* 2003; **28:** 233–40.

## Treatment of Adverse Effects

At the first signs of local anaesthetic toxicity due to parenteral administration, the injection should be stopped; in some cases it may also be possible to apply a tourniquet to limit further systemic absorption. Subsequent management, regardless of the route of administration, is supportive. In the event of systemic reactions developing steps should be taken to maintain the circulation and respiration and to control convulsions. A patent airway must be established and oxygen given, together with assisted ventilation if necessary. The circulation should be maintained with infusions of intravenous fluids. Vasopressors have been suggested in the treatment of marked hypotension although their use is accompanied by a risk of CNS excitation. Ephedrine is preferred for the management of hypotension associated with spinal or epidural block, particularly in pregnancy. Vasopressors should not be given to patients receiving oxytocic drugs. Convulsions may be controlled with intravenous benzodiazepines such as diazepam although these drugs may also depress respiration and the circulation. Intravenous phenobarbital is used for persistent convulsions.

Methaemoglobinaemia may be treated by the intravenous administration of methylthioninium chloride.

**Post-dural puncture headache.** Headache following puncture of the dura mater during procedures such as lumbar puncture or central nerve blocks is thought to be caused by subsequent leakage of CSF. The incidence of such post-dural puncture headache is significantly reduced by the use of small, blunt needles which produce a smaller hole in the dura and separate its fibres rather than cutting them.

When treatment is necessary conservative therapy such as analgesics and hydration will relieve symptoms in the majority of patients with mild post-dural puncture headache within 1 to 2 days. Bed rest does not reduce the incidence but once headache develops the patient may feel some relief when recumbent. If the headache persists for a further 24 hours measures such as epidural saline or dextran or the use of intravenous caffeine and sodium benzoate may be effective; oral caffeine has also been shown to be of benefit. If such measures are unsuccessful then the epidural injection of autologous blood to form a blood patch over the dural puncture is extremely effective. There have been anecdotal reports of success using corticotropin or tetracosactide. Anecdotal reports of relief with sumatriptan were not confirmed by a controlled study.

References.

1. Choi A, *et al.* Pharmacologic management of postdural puncture headache. *Ann Pharmacother* 1996; **30:** 831–9.
2. Broadley SA, Fuller GN. Lumbar puncture needn't be a headache. *BMJ* 1997; **315:** 1324–5.
3. Serpell MG, *et al.* Prevention of headache after lumbar puncture: questionnaire survey of neurologists and neurosurgeons in United Kingdom. *BMJ* 1998; **316:** 1709–10.
4. Turnbull DK, Shepherd DB. Post-dural puncture headache: pathogenesis, prevention and treatment. *Br J Anaesth* 2003; **91:** 718–29.

## Precautions

As with any drug local anaesthetics are contra-indicated in patients with known hypersensitivity. However, it might be possible to avoid reactions by using a local anaesthetic of the alternative chemical type. Facilities for resuscitation should be available when local anaesthetics are administered parenterally.

Local anaesthetics should not be used in patients with complete heart block. They should be given cautiously to the elderly, to the debilitated, to children, and to patients with epilepsy, impaired cardiac conduction or respiratory function, shock, or hepatic impairment; patients with myasthenia gravis are particularly susceptible to the effects of local anaesthetics. Ester-type local anaesthetics are contra-indicated in patients with low plasma-cholinesterase concentrations. Techniques such as epidural or spinal block should not be employed in patients with cerebrospinal diseases, cardiogenic or hypovolaemic shock, or altered coagulation status. Because of the risk of transmitting infection into the CNS these techniques should not be employed where there is pyogenic infection of the skin at or adjacent to the injection site.

Because of the risk of systemic adverse effects when local anaesthetics are absorbed too rapidly, they should not be injected into or applied to inflamed or infected tissues or to damaged skin or mucosa. For similar reasons, the rate of injection should not be too rapid and great care must be taken to avoid inadvertent intravascular injection. The risk of adverse effects from the uptake of local anaesthetics into the circulation may be reduced by the inclusion of adrenaline to produce vasoconstriction, but the lowest effective concentration of adrenaline should be used. Solutions containing adrenaline should not, however, be used for producing anaesthesia in appendages such as digits, because the profound ischaemia that follows may lead to gangrene. Mepivacaine and prilocaine tend to produce less vasodilatation at low concentrations than other local anaesthetics and may be useful where the addition of vasoconstrictors is contra-indicated (but see also under Action, below).

When used in the mouth or throat, local anaesthetics may impair swallowing and increase the risk of aspiration. Patients who have received local anaesthetics for procedures such as laryngoscopy or tracheoscopy should be cautioned not to eat or drink for at least 3 to 4 hours after the anaesthetic.

The cornea may be damaged by prolonged topical application of local anaesthetics, particularly cocaine. Patients should be warned not to rub or touch the eye while anaesthesia persists and the anaesthetised eye should be protected from dust and bacterial contamination.

Local anaesthetics may be ototoxic and should not be instilled into the middle ear.

The application of local anaesthetics to the skin for prolonged periods or to extensive areas should be avoided.

**Precautions for central block.** Epidural or spinal block may rarely result in paraplegia caused by an induced haematoma or abscess, and have thus been considered unsuitable in patients with pre-existing neurological disease, infection at the puncture site, or blood disorders, or in those receiving aspirin or full-dose anticoagulant therapy. Such therapy may be discontinued at an appropriate time before surgery if central block is planned. It is necessary to balance the risk of withholding anticoagulation against the risk of bleeding in the individual patient. Epidural or spinal block in patients receiving low-dose anticoagulant therapy to prevent postoperative deep-vein thrombosis is still controversial. For further discussion and recommendations on concomitant use see Spinal Anaesthesia, p.929.

A study in the USA[1] involving 891 patients found that low-dose aspirin during pregnancy did not increase the risk of bleeding complications during epidural anaesthesia compared with placebo; it was considered that the recommendation to stop aspirin 7 to 10 days before delivery was unjustified.

1. Sibai BM, *et al.* Low-dose aspirin in correlation between bleeding time and maternal-neonatal bleeding complications. *Am J Obstet Gynecol* 1995; **172:** 1553–7.

**Pregnancy.** For discussions covering the precautions associated with the use of epidural or spinal blocks during labour, see under Labour Pain, p.6.

**Tachyphylaxis.** The effect of successive epidural injections of 2% solutions of lidocaine, mepivacaine, or prilocaine was reduced by 25 to 30% with each injection when the interval between the disappearance of analgesia and re-injection was more than 10 minutes but anaesthesia was augmented if this interval was less than 10 minutes.[1] Such tachyphylaxis, associated with the prolonged epidural administration of all local anaesthetics, has also been reviewed.[2]

1. Bromage PR, *et al.* Tachyphylaxis in epidural analgesia 1: augmentation and decay of local anesthesia. *J Clin Pharmacol* 1969; **9:** 30–8.
2. Mogensen T. Tachyphylaxis to epidural local anaesthetics. *Dan Med Bull* 1995; **42:** 141–6.

**Test dose.** A test dose is recommended in epidural block to check for accidental intravenous or intrathecal injection but negative results should be treated with caution.[1] Accidental intravenous placement of the needle is notoriously more difficult to detect than inadvertent subarachnoid placement. Adrenaline has been added to the test solution to aid detection of intravenous injection but is considered by some to be of little value.[2,3]

1. Scott DB. Test doses in extradural block. *Br J Anaesth* 1988; **61:** 129–30.
2. Thornburn J. Limitations of adrenaline test doses in obstetric patients undergoing extradural anaesthesia. *Br J Anaesth* 1989; **62:** 578–81.
3. Narchi P, *et al.* Heart rate response to an iv test dose of adrenaline and lignocaine with and without atropine pretreatment. *Br J Anaesth* 1991; **66:** 583–6.

## Interactions

The metabolism of ester-type local anaesthetics may be inhibited by anticholinesterases, increasing the risk of systemic toxicity.

Ester derivatives such as tetracaine, benzocaine, or procaine that are hydrolysed to para-aminobenzoic acid may antagonise the activity of aminosalicylic acid or sulfonamides. Ester-type local anaesthetics such as procaine and cocaine that are hydrolysed by plasma cholinesterase may competitively enhance the neuromuscular blocking activity of suxamethonium; the amide local anaesthetic, lidocaine may have a similar effect.

There is an increased risk of myocardial depression when amide-type local anaesthetics such as bupivacaine, levobupivacaine, lidocaine, or ropivacaine are administered with antiarrhythmics.

If local anaesthetics containing adrenaline are given for epidural or paracervical block during labour the use of an oxytocic drug post partum may lead to severe hypertension. Although there is no clinical evidence of dangerous interactions between adrenaline-containing local anaesthetics and MAOIs or tricyclic antidepressants, great care should nevertheless be taken to avoid inadvertent intravenous administration of the local anaesthetic preparation.

For further details of interactions between local anaesthetics and other drugs, see under individual monographs.

## Pharmacokinetics

Most local anaesthetics are readily absorbed through mucous membranes, and through damaged skin. Local anaesthetics are weak bases and at tissue pH can diffuse through connective tissue and cellular membranes to reach the nerve fibre where ionisation can occur.

Anaesthetics of the ester type are hydrolysed by esterases in the plasma and, to a lesser extent, in the liver. The effect of spinal anaesthetics lasts until the drug is taken up into the blood circulation since there is little esterase in the spinal fluid.

Amide-type anaesthetics are metabolised in the liver and, in some cases, the kidneys. While there is little protein binding with most ester-type anaesthetics, the amide types are considerably bound.

◊ References.

1. Tucker GT. Pharmacokinetics of local anaesthetics. *Br J Anaesth* 1986; **58:** 717–31.
2. Burm AGL. Clinical pharmacokinetics of epidural and spinal anaesthesia. *Clin Pharmacokinet* 1989; **16:** 283–311.

3. Smith C. Pharmacology of local anaesthetic agents. *Br J Hosp Med* 1994; **52:** 455–60.
4. Mazoit J-X, Dalens BJ. Pharmacokinetics of local anaesthetics in infants and children. *Clin Pharmacokinet* 2004; **43:** 17–32.

## Uses and Administration

Local anaesthetics act by preventing the generation and transmission of impulses along nerve fibres and at nerve endings; depolarisation and ion-exchange are inhibited. The effects are reversible. They are used for the local relief of painful conditions, and to prevent pain and discomfort of various medical and surgical procedure (see below). In general, loss of pain (analgesia) occurs before loss of sensory and autonomic function (anaesthesia) and loss of motor function (paralysis), but this may depend on the drug used and the site of administration.

Local anaesthetics vary in their potency and speed of onset and duration of action. The anaesthetic must penetrate the lipoprotein nerve sheath in its unionised form before it can act and therefore drugs with high lipid-solubility tend to have a greater potency and duration of action and a faster onset than drugs with low lipid-solubility. The most protein-bound drugs tend to have the longest duration of action.

The potency of local anaesthetics is traditionally compared against that of procaine, which is low; chloroprocaine, lidocaine, mepivacaine, and prilocaine are similar or somewhat more potent; etidocaine is of intermediate potency, bupivacaine and ropivacaine highly potent, and tetracaine extremely potent.

Speed of onset and duration of action also depend on the technique employed (see Local Anaesthetic Techniques, below), the type of block, and the site of administration.

The speed of onset and duration of action of local anaesthetics may be increased by the addition of a vasoconstrictor, which has the effect of reducing the uptake of the local anaesthetic into the circulation from the injection site. Solutions containing adrenaline 1 in 200 000 are generally advocated, although higher concentrations such as 1 in 80 000 may be used in dentistry where the total dose is small. The total amount of adrenaline injected should not exceed 500 micrograms although the amount of adrenaline absorbed varies considerably with the site of administration; some consider that the maximum dose should be 200 micrograms. Other vasoconstrictors including noradrenaline are also used, but the *Dental Practitioners' Formulary* in the UK considers that noradrenaline should not be used since it presents no advantages and when given at relatively high concentrations has occasionally been associated with severe hypertensive episodes. Vasoconstrictors should not be used when producing a nerve block in an appendage such as a digit, as gangrene may occur. Vasoconstrictors have been added to injections for spinal block, but their use is not recommended because of the danger of reducing the blood supply to the spinal cord.

Local anaesthetics are generally administered as acidic solutions of the water-soluble hydrochloride salts; alkalinisation of these solutions or formulation as a carbonated base may increase the speed of onset (see under Administration, below).

The dosage of individual local anaesthetics depends on the injection site and the procedure used. The smallest effective dose and the lowest effective concentration should be used. Smaller doses are usually needed in the elderly, in children, in debilitated patients, and in cardiac disease. Doses should also be reduced in the presence of hepatic disease. Meticulous attention to technique is essential particularly in nerve block and spinal procedures. Injections for central nerve blocks, such as epidural (including caudal block) and spinal block should not contain preservatives.

**Action.** The intrinsic vasoactivity of a local anaesthetic can influence its rate of removal from the site of action and therefore its duration of action. Ester-type local anaesthetics such as tetracaine and procaine are more likely to produce vasodilatation than amide-type local anaesthetics such as cinchocaine, lidocaine, mepivacaine, and prilocaine following intradermal administration.[1] However, cocaine differs from other ester-type local anaesthetics in that it produces vasoconstriction. The amide-type local anaesthetics can produce vasoconstriction but, apart from prilocaine, their vasoconstrictor activity has generally been found to decline with increasing concentration,[1,2] and, in a study, lidocaine and bupivacaine produced more vasodilatation than vasoconstriction at the higher concentrations tested.[2] Mepivacaine has produced greater and more consistent vasoconstriction than lidocaine, cinchocaine, or prilocaine following intradermal injection[1] but this greater vasoactivity is not always evident.[3]

1. Willatts DG, Reynolds F. Comparison of the vasoactivity of amide and ester local anaesthetics: an intradermal study. *Br J Anaesth* 1985; **57:** 1006–11.
2. Aps C, Reynolds F. The effect of concentration on vasoactivity of bupivacaine and lignocaine. *Br J Anaesth* 1976; **48:** 1171–4.
3. Goebel WM, *et al.* Comparative circulatory levels of 2 per cent mepivacaine and 2 per cent lignocaine. *Br Dent J* 1980; **148:** 261–4.

**Administration.** Systemic toxic effects of local anaesthetics are related to blood concentrations and, as absorption varies considerably according to the site of injection, it has been suggested[1,2] that recommendation of a single maximum dose without regard to the site of the procedure is meaningless. If a plasma-lidocaine concentration of 5 micrograms/mL were required for toxicity then this would be achieved by injection of 300 mg in the intercostal area, 500 mg epidurally, 600 mg in the region of the brachial plexus, or 1000 mg subcutaneously. The reduction of peak concentrations obtained by the addition of adrenaline was also dependent on the site of injection. Furthermore, most cases of severe toxicity did not result from overdosage but from inadvertent intravascular injection or too rapid injection.

1. Scott DB. "Maximum recommended doses" of local anaesthetic drugs. *Br J Anaesth* 1989; **63:** 373–4.
2. Scott DB. Safe use of lignocaine. *BMJ* 1989; **299:** 56.

CARBONATED SOLUTIONS. The use of carbonated solutions of local anaesthetics instead of the usual hydrochloride salts has been discussed in several reviews.[1-3] Although some early studies indicated that carbonated solutions of bupivacaine, lidocaine, or prilocaine produced earlier onset of anaesthesia and improved the quality of epidural or brachial plexus blocks not all subsequent studies have confirmed these results. A method for preparing carbonated solutions has been published[4] but proprietary preparations of such solutions of bupivacaine or lidocaine may be available in some countries.

1. Covino BG. Pharmacology of local anaesthetic agents. *Br J Anaesth* 1986; **58:** 701–16.
2. Burm AGL. Clinical pharmacokinetics of epidural and spinal anaesthesia. *Clin Pharmacokinet* 1989; **16:** 283–311.
3. Carrie LES. Extradural, spinal or combined block for obstetric surgical anaesthesia. *Br J Anaesth* 1990; **65:** 225–33.
4. Bromage PR. Improved conduction blockade in surgery and obstetrics: carbonated local anesthetics. *Can Med Assoc J* 1967; **97:** 1377–84.

PH OF SOLUTIONS. The pain associated with infiltration of local anaesthetics can be reduced by buffering the solution to physiological pH with sodium bicarbonate.[1,2] Although buffering itself does not appear to compromise the efficacy of anaesthesia,[2] alkalinisation of the solution may reduce the solubility of the local anaesthetic and cause precipitation.[2-4] To enhance stability local anaesthetic solutions are usually prepared to have an acidic pH and it is therefore recommended that if solutions are buffered they should be used immediately.[2] (Solutions containing adrenaline require an acidic pH.)

Similar pH adjustments of solutions for intravenous regional anaesthesia have been reported to reduce the amount of local venous irritation and thrombophlebitis[5] and to increase the speed of onset and the duration of the block.[6] However, it has been noted that at alkaline pH lidocaine can lower surface tension, thereby altering drop size and potentially resulting in a decreased dose if such solutions are infused via a drop counting device rather than a volume pump.[7] Alkalinisation of a solution used for epidural block for caesarean section has been reported to result in a more rapid onset of action and denser block.[8]

Alkalinisation has also been used to hasten the onset of peripheral nerve block[9] by increasing the proportion of the lipid-soluble nonionised free base but the effect in epidural block has been inconsistent.[10,11]

1. McKay W, *et al.* Sodium bicarbonate attenuates pain on skin infiltration with lidocaine, with or without epinephrine. *Anesth Analg* 1987; **66:** 572–4.
2. Cristoph RA, *et al.* Pain reduction in local anesthetic administration through pH buffering. *Ann Emerg Med* 1988; **17:** 117–20.
3. Bourget P, *et al.* Factors influencing precipitation of pH-adjusted bupivacaine solutions. *J Clin Pharm Ther* 1990; **15:** 197–204.
4. Nakano NI. Temperature-dependent aqueous solubilities of lidocaine, mepivacaine, and bupivacaine. *J Pharm Sci* 1979; **68:** 667–8.
5. Yudenfreund SM, *et al.* pH-Buffered 2-chloroprocaine for intravenous regional anesthesia. *DICP Ann Pharmacother* 1989; **23:** 614–15.
6. Armstrong P, *et al.* Effect of alkalinization of prilocaine on IV regional anaesthesia. *Br J Anaesth* 1989; **63:** 625P–626P.
7. Leor R, *et al.* The influence of pH on the intravenous delivery of lidocaine solutions. *Eur J Clin Pharmacol* 1990; **39:** 521–3.
8. Fernando R, Jones HM. Comparison of plain and alkalinized local anaesthetic mixtures of lignocaine and bupivacaine for elective extradural caesarean section. *Br J Anaesth* 1991; **67:** 699–703.
9. Coventry DM, Todd JG. Alkalinization of bupivacaine for sciatic nerve blockade. *Br J Anaesth* 1989; **62:** 227P.
10. Burm AGL. Clinical pharmacokinetics of epidural and spinal anaesthesia. *Clin Pharmacokinet* 1989; **16:** 283–311.
11. Carrie LES. Extradural, spinal or combined block for obstetric surgical anaesthesia. *Br J Anaesth* 1990; **65:** 225–33.

**Anorectal disorders.** See under Surface Anaesthesia, below.

**Cough.** Drugs such as lidocaine or bupivacaine have been given by inhalation in severe intractable cough (p.1112), including cough caused by malignant neoplasms.[1-4] Cough suppression is produced by an indirect peripheral action on sensory receptors, but as all protective pulmonary reflexes may be lost and bronchospasm may be induced, nebulised local anaesthetics should be used in controlled circumstances only; there may also be temporary loss of the swallowing reflex.

1. Howard P, *et al.* Lignocaine aerosol and persistent cough. *Br J Dis Chest* 1977; **71:** 19–24.
2. Stewart CJ, Coady TJ. Suppression of intractable cough. *BMJ* 1977; **i:** 1660–1.
3. Sanders RV, Kirkpatrick MB. Prolonged suppression of cough after inhalation of lidocaine in a patient with sarcoid. *JAMA* 1984; **252:** 2456–7.
4. Brown RC, Turton CWG. Cough and angiotensin converting enzyme inhibition. *BMJ* 1988; **296:** 1741.

**Endoscopy.** Local anaesthetics such as lidocaine are sometimes used before endoscopy to improve patient comfort and facilitate passage of the endoscope. As mentioned in the discussion on drugs used in endoscopy (see p.666) some consider that the use of local anaesthetics for procedures such as gastrointestinal endoscopy should probably be reserved for those patients who prefer not to be sedated as their use in addition to premedication with opioids or benzodiazepines appears to serve little purpose.

References.

1. Chuah SY, *et al.* Topical anaesthesia in upper gastrointestinal endoscopy. *BMJ* 1991; **303:** 695.
2. Jameson JS, *et al.* Topical anaesthesia improves toleration for upper gastrointestinal endoscopy. *Gut* 1992; **33** (suppl): S51.
3. Randell T, *et al.* Topical anaesthesia of the nasal mucosa for fibreoptic airway endoscopy. *Br J Anaesth* 1992; **68:** 164–7.

**Mouth ulceration.** For the role of local anaesthetics in the management of mouth ulceration, see p.1245.

**Pain.** Pain and its general management are discussed on p.2. Local anaesthetics are used in a variety of situations for the management of pain. They are usually given by local injection or applied topically but are sometimes used intravenously in techniques such as intravenous regional anaesthesia, which involves the continuous infusion of local anaesthetics such as lidocaine to produce general analgesia. However, the technique is potentially dangerous and seldom employed.

NERVE BLOCKS. Nerve blocks produce analgesia by interrupting the nervous transmission of pain signals either by temporary inhibition of conduction or by destruction of the nerve. Nerve blocks may be used alone or with analgesics in the management of acute or chronic pain associated with a well-defined anatomical site, especially when the pain is unresponsive to or not adequately controlled by conventional therapy. The route of administration and method employed depend on the site to be blocked but may include peripheral nerve block, autonomic nerve blocks such as sympathetic nerve blocks and coeliac plexus block, and central nerve blocks such as epidural (including caudal) and spinal block. **Local anaesthetics** are used when a temporary effect is required. **Neurolytics** such as phenol or alcohol or freezing of the nerve (cryoanalgesia) produce more prolonged block, but even so the effects may last no more than a few months, and the variable and non-selective neural damage produced correlates poorly with pain relief; some consider the risk of complications to outweigh the benefits obtained.[1]

The use of nerve blocks in the *management of cancer* (p.5) has declined following the refinement of the use of conventional analgesics. Some consider that their value may be limited to patients with a life expectancy of 3 months or less[2] and that the main benefit of nerve blocks in cancer is to produce maximum pain relief rapidly. However, others consider that chemical and thermal neurolysis can provide long-term control of severe cancer pain without a substantial incidence of adverse effects.[3] Neurolytic blocks may be of particular value in cancer pain syndromes involving the viscera or the torso, but are rarely applicable in the management of extremity pain.[4] Neuropathic pain is rarely helped by somatic neural block and may even be aggravated,[1] but block of the splanchnic nerves or coeliac plexus with alcohol or phenol is reputed to be effective in relieving severe intractable pain caused by cancer of the pancreas, stomach, small intestine, gallbladder, or other abdominal viscera, especially when the cancer has not spread to the parietal peritoneum.[5]

Similar neurolytic blocks preceded by a local anaesthetic have also been used in patients with *severe intractable pain* of chronic pancreatitis, postcholecystectomy syndrome, or other chronic abdominal visceral diseases unrelieved by medical or surgical therapy.

Central nerve blocks using local anaesthetics with or without **opioids** are used for the *management of acute pain* such as labour pain (p.6) and postoperative pain (p.4) including that in children (p.3); they are also sometimes used for cancer pain.[1,6]

Sympathetic nerve blocks using repeated injections of local anaesthetics or neurolytics have been used for sympathetically maintained pain. Intravenous regional sympathetic block is an alternative when a single limb is involved;[1] guanethidine is one of the drugs that has been used.[7]

Injections of local anaesthetics with or without **corticosteroids** are often used for blocks of localised painful joints. Nerve blocks are also used to block localised painful trigger areas[8] such as postoperative or post-traumatic neuroma formation and for focal muscle pain.

For the role of nerve blocks in the management of low back pain, see p.7.


1. Hanks GW, Justins DM. Cancer pain: management. *Lancet* 1992; **339:** 1031–6.
2. WHO. Cancer pain relief and palliative care: report of a WHO expert committee. *WHO Tech Rep Ser 804*, 1990.
3. American Society of Anesthesiologists Task Force on Pain Management, Cancer Pain Section. Practice guidelines for cancer pain management. *Anesthesiology* 1996; **84:** 1243–7.
4. Marshall KA. Managing cancer pain: basic principles and invasive treatments. *Mayo Clin Proc* 1996; **71:** 472–7.
5. Bonica JJ. Management of pain with regional analgesia. *Postgrad Med J* 1984; **60:** 897–904.
6. Hunt R, Massolino J. Spinal bupivacaine for the pain of cancer. *Med J Aust* 1989; **150:** 350.
7. Hannington-Kiff JG. Relief of causalgia in limbs by regional intravenous guanethidine. *BMJ* 1979; **2:** 367–8.
8. Foley KM. The treatment of cancer pain. *N Engl J Med* 1985; **313:** 84–95.


**Postherpetic neuralgia.** For the role of local anaesthetics in the management of postherpetic neuralgia, see p.7.

**Soft-tissue rheumatism.** For the adjunctive use of local anaesthetics in the management of soft-tissue rheumatism, see p.11.

**Spasticity.** The management of spasticity (p.1386) involves physiotherapy and the use of antispastic drugs. Other approaches to treatment include nerve blocks with local anaesthetics; these can improve spasticity but should generally only be used when further muscle relaxation would not increase disability.

## Local Anaesthetic Techniques

Local anaesthetics are employed in several techniques. In order of increasing level of anaesthesia they are: surface or topical anaesthesia; infiltration anaesthesia; and regional nerve block, including peripheral nerve block, sympathetic nerve block, and central nerve block which includes epidural and spinal (intrathecal or subarachnoid) block. Local anaesthetics may also be given intravenously for regional anaesthesia in the extremities.

### Infiltration anaesthesia

Infiltration anaesthesia is produced by injection of a local anaesthetic such as lidocaine or bupivacaine directly into and around the field of operation without attempting to identify individual nerves. The drug used should not be absorbed too rapidly otherwise the anaesthesia will wear off too quickly for practical use; some local anaesthetics require the addition of a vasoconstrictor in low concentrations, which can increase the duration of infiltration anaesthesia and reduce peak plasma concentrations of the local anaesthetic. Infiltration anaesthesia is extensively used in dentistry.

Anaesthesia of small areas by infiltration techniques requires a relatively large amount of local anaesthetic, which is not a problem for minor surgery but would be for more extensive areas that required anaesthesia. The amount of local anaesthetic used can be reduced and the duration of anaesthesia increased by blocking specific nerves that innervate the area. This may be carried out at several levels. In *field block* anaesthesia subcutaneous injection of a local anaesthetic close to the nerves around the area to be anaesthetised blocks sensory nerve paths. This is a form of infiltration anaesthesia, but the technique requires less drug for a given area to be anaesthetised.

### Intravenous regional anaesthesia

Intravenous regional anaesthesia (Bier's block) involves injection of a dilute solution of local anaesthetic into a suitable limb vein after exsanguination and application of a tourniquet, in order to produce anaesthesia distal to it. Arterial flow must remain occluded for at least 20 minutes after injection and adrenaline should not be used. Intravenous regional anaesthesia may be used for short procedures where postoperative pain is not marked, such as manipulation of fractures and minor surgical procedures to the limbs. Although a safe procedure when performed correctly, complications have arisen; there have been fatalities associated with the use of bupivacaine, and prilocaine is the drug of choice. Facilities for resuscitation should be available.

### Regional nerve block

Regional nerve block anaesthesia involves specific blocks at the levels of major nerves or spinal roots, and may include peripheral nerve block, sympathetic nerve block, and central nerve block including epidural and spinal block. For a discussion of the use of nerve blocks in the management of pain, see above.

**Central nerve block.** Central nerve block includes epidural and spinal block.

*Epidural block* (also referred to as *extradural* or *peridural block*) is widely used to provide analgesia or anaesthesia in surgical and obstetric procedures. It involves injecting a local anaesthetic such as lidocaine, bupivacaine, or ropivacaine, alone or with a small dose of an opioid analgesic into the epidural space in the lumbar, sacral (*caudal block*), thoracic, or cervical regions. Introduction of a cannula into the epidural space enables prolonged analgesia or anaesthesia (epidural anaesthesia) to be provided through the use of 'top-up' doses or continuous infusion of the drugs. A vasoconstrictor is sometimes added to reduce systemic exposure to the local anaesthetic. A test dose at the intended injection site is recommended before starting epidural anaesthesia to ensure that the main dose is not accidentally injected intravascularly or into the subarachnoid space.

*Spinal block* (also referred to as *subarachnoid* or *intrathecal block*) is produced by injecting a solution of a suitable drug such as bupivacaine within the spinal subarachnoid space, causing temporary paralysis of the nerves with which it comes into contact. It may be used, for example, to produce spinal anaesthesia in surgical procedures on the lower body. Vasoconstrictors have been added to prolong the duration of the block but the effect is not always clinically useful and there is a danger of restricting the blood supply to the spinal cord; therefore this practice is not recommended. The somatic level at which anaesthesia occurs depends on many factors including the specific gravity or baricity of the anaesthetic solution used and the positioning of the patient.

For the adverse effects of and precautions for central block, see above.

**Peripheral nerve block.** Peripheral nerve block anaesthesia involves injection into or around a peripheral nerve or plexus supplying the part to be anaesthetised; motor fibres may be blocked as well as sensory fibres. *Brachial plexus block* is widely used for procedures involving the arm; lower limb blocks are less simple although *sciatic* and *femoral blocks* may be combined to permit surgery below the knee. Other peripheral nerve blocks such as those for the head and neck, or *intercostal* or *paravertebral blocks* for local anaesthesia of the trunk, are mostly highly specialised techniques. Lidocaine, prilocaine, bupivacaine, or ropivacaine have all been widely employed for peripheral nerve blocks. Adrenaline is often added as a vasoconstrictor.

*Pudendal block* (usually with prilocaine) may be useful in obstetrics before forceps delivery, but as mentioned under Labour Pain on p.6, the technique of *paracervical local anaesthetic block* has largely fallen out of favour because of the high incidence of serious adverse effects on the fetus.

**Sympathetic nerve block.** Sympathetic nerve block such as *stellate ganglion blockade* and *lumbar sympathectomy* is used in the management of a range of painful conditions and vascular diseases (see under Complex Regional Pain Syndrome on p.5). Temporary block is obtained using local anaesthetics such as lidocaine or bupivacaine but permanent block may be produced with use of neurolytic agents such as phenol (see Pain, p.1188) or alcohol (see Pain, p.1167).

### Surface anaesthesia

Surface or topical anaesthesia blocks the sensory nerve endings in the skin or mucous membranes. Many local anaesthetics are effective surface anaesthetics, a notable exception being procaine. Penetration of intact skin by most local anaesthetics is poor whereas absorption through mucous membranes may be rapid. However, reliable percutaneous anaesthesia can be achieved by application of a eutectic mixture of lidocaine and prilocaine to intact skin (see under Surface Anaesthesia in Lidocaine, p.1380). Eutectic mixtures may be of value in providing surface anaesthesia for a number of minor medical or surgical procedures. Tetracaine also provides reliable percutaneous anaesthesia. Other methods of dermal delivery of local anaesthetics include a transdermal patch of lidocaine, and an iontophoretic drug delivery system incorporating lidocaine and adrenaline. Anaesthesia of the skin and subcutaneous tissues is also discussed under Infiltration Anaesthesia, below.

There are a number of special uses of topical anaesthesia including anaesthetising the cornea during ophthalmological procedures and the throat and larynx before intubation and bronchoscopy. Absorption from the respiratory tract is rapid and care is essential to avoid administering a toxic dose. Great care is also necessary when employing local anaesthetics to anaesthetise the urethra; if trauma has occurred, rapid absorption of the drug may occur and give rise to serious adverse effects.

Local anaesthetics have been included in topical preparations to relieve the pain of haemorrhoids (p.1243) but good evidence of their efficacy is lacking. Similar uses include pain relief in pruritus ani and anal fissure. Excessive application of local anaesthetics to the rectal mucosa should be avoided as absorption can occur; use for periods of no longer than a few days is recommended to prevent sensitisation of the anal skin. Local anaesthetics are sometimes included in topical preparations for the relief of pruritus (p.1137). However, they are only marginally effective and can very occasionally cause sensitisation. The use of local anaesthetics in rubefacient and topical analgesic preparations is mentioned on p.4.

## Amylocaine Hydrochloride *(BANM)*

Amilocaína, hidrocloruro de; Amyleinii Chloridum; Amylocain. Hydrochlor.; Chlorhydrate d'Amyléine. 1-(Dimethylaminomethyl)-1-methylpropyl benzoate hydrochloride.

$C_{14}H_{21}NO_2,HCl$ = 271.8.

*CAS — 532-59-2 (amylocaine hydrochloride); 644-26-8 (amylocaine hydrochloride).*

### Profile

Amylocaine, a benzoic acid ester, is a local anaesthetic (p.1367) used mainly as the hydrochloride in a range of preparations for application to the skin or mucous membranes. It has also been used in preparations for the relief of painful anorectal conditions and has been included in oral mixtures for the relief of coughs.

### Preparations

**Proprietary Preparations** (details are given in Part 3)
***Fr.:*** Dolodent.

**Multi-ingredient:** ***Belg.:*** Babygencal†; Dentophar; Dequalinium†; Rectovasol; ***Braz.:*** Fonergin; Hemodotti; Hermodotti†; ***Canad.:*** Pommade Midy†; Rhino-Mex†; ***Fr.:*** Amygdol†; Avenoc†; Campho-Pneumine†; Collustan†; Elenol; Frazoline†; Glottyl†; Parkipan; Pholcones†; Pulmoll; Sedaplaie†; ***Ital.:*** Dentinale; Proctosedyl; ***Mon.:*** Bronchodermine; ***Spain:*** Eucalyptospirine Lact†; Hemodren Compuesto; ***Thai.:*** Biochin; Izac; Lobacin†; Mybacin.

## Articaine Hydrochloride *(BANM, USAN, rINNM)*

40045; Articaini Hydrochloridum; Carticaine Hydrochloride; Hidrocloruro de articaína; Hoe-045. Methyl 4-methyl-3-(2-propylaminopropionamido)thiophene-2-carboxylate hydrochloride.

$C_{13}H_{20}N_2O_3S,HCl$ = 320.8.

*CAS — 23964-58-1 (articaine); 23964-57-0 (articaine hydrochloride).*

*ATC — N01BB08.*

**Pharmacopoeias.** In *Eur.* (see p.vi).

**Ph. Eur. 5.0** (Articaine Hydrochloride). A white or almost white crystalline powder. Freely soluble in water and in alcohol. A 1% solution in water has a pH of 4.2 to 5.2. Protect from light.

### Profile

Articaine hydrochloride is an amide local anaesthetic (p.1367). It has been used as a 1 or 2% solution with or without adrenaline for infiltration and regional anaesthesia. A 4% solution of articaine hydrochloride with adrenaline is used similarly in dentistry. A 5% hyperbaric solution of articaine hydrochloride with glucose has been used for spinal block.

**Porphyria.** Articaine hydrochloride is considered to be unsafe in patients with porphyria because it has been shown to be porphyrinogenic in *in-vitro* systems.

### Preparations

**Proprietary Preparations** (details are given in Part 3)
***Austria:*** Septanest; Ubistesin; Ultracain Dental; ***Braz.:*** Carbostesin†; Septanest†; ***Canad.:*** Astracaine; Ultracaine D-S†; ***Denm.:*** Septanest; Septocaine; ***Fin.:*** Ultracain D-Suprarenin; ***Fr.:*** Alphacaine; Predesic; ***Ger.:*** Ubistesin; Ultracain; Ultracain D-S; Ultracain hyperbar; Ultracain Suprarenin; ***Ital.:*** Alfacaina; Cartidont; Citocartin; Primacaine; Septanest; Ubistesin; Ultracain D-S†; ***Neth.:*** Ultracain D-S; Ultracain Hyperbaar†; ***Norw.:*** Septocaine; ***Spain:*** Articaina C/E; Ultracain; ***Switz.:*** Alphacaine; Rudocaine; Septanest; Ubistesin; Ultracaine D-S; ***UK:*** Septanest; ***USA:*** Septocaine.

## Benzocaine *(BAN, rINN)*

Anaesthesinum; Anesthamine; Benzocaína; Benzocainum; Ethoform; Éthoforme; Ethyl Aminobenzoate; Ethylis Aminobenzoas. Ethyl 4-aminobenzoate.

$C_9H_{11}NO_2$ = 165.2.

*CAS — 94-09-7.*

*ATC — C05AD03; D04AB04; N01BA05; R02AD01.*

**Pharmacopoeias.** In *Chin., Eur.* (see p.vi), *Int., Jpn, Pol.,* and *US.*

**Ph. Eur. 5.0** (Benzocaine). Colourless crystals or a white crystalline powder. M.p. 89° to 92°. Very slightly soluble in water; freely soluble in alcohol. Protect from light.

**USP 27** (Benzocaine). Small, white crystals or a white odourless crystalline powder. M.p. 88° to 92°. Soluble 1 in 2500 of water, 1 in 5 of alcohol, 1 in 2 of chloroform, 1 in 4 of ether, and 1 in 30 to 50 of almond oil or olive oil; dissolves in dilute acids.

### Adverse Effects and Treatment

As for Local Anaesthetics in general, p.1367.

**Hypersensitivity.** The incidence of positive reactions in patients patch tested with benzocaine has ranged from 3.3 to 5.9%.[1,2] Patch testing with benzocaine has been recommended by The International Contact Dermatitis Research Group as an indicator of contact hypersensitivity to local anaesthetics. However, it was found that of 40 patients who had had positive reactions to benzocaine with tetracaine and cinchocaine, 21 were not allergic to benzocaine alone.[3]


1. Rudzki E, Kleniewska D. The epidemiology of contact dermatitis in Poland. *Br J Dermatol* 1970; **83:** 543–5.
2. Bandmann H-J, *et al.* Dermatitis from applied medicaments. *Arch Dermatol* 1972; **106:** 335–7.
3. Beck MH, Holden A. Benzocaine—an unsatisfactory indicator of topical local anaesthetic sensitization for the UK. *Br J Dermatol* 1988; **118:** 91–4.


### Precautions

As for Local Anaesthetics in general, p.1368.

### Interactions

For interactions associated with local anaesthetics, see p.1368.

### Pharmacokinetics

See under Local Anaesthetics, p.1368.

### Uses and Administration

Benzocaine, a para-aminobenzoic acid ester, is a local anaesthetic used for surface anaesthesia (p.1370); it has low potency and low systemic toxicity. It is used, often with other drugs such as analgesics, antiseptics, antibacterials, antifungals, and antipruritics, for the temporary local relief of pain associated with dental conditions, oropharyngeal disorders, haemorrhoids, anal pruritus, and ear pain.

Lozenges containing benzocaine in usual doses of up to 10 mg are used for the relief of sore throat. Gels, pastes, solutions, and sprays containing benzocaine in concentrations of up to 20% have been used for surface anaesthesia of the mouth and throat.

Benzocaine is used in ear drops, creams, ointments, lotions, solutions, sprays, gels, and suppositories in concentrations up to 20% for topical analgesia and anaesthesia.

Benzocaine has also been used as the hydrochloride.

**Obesity.** It has been reported[1] that despite the inclusion of benzocaine in some over-the-counter appetite suppressants there is no good evidence of its value in obesity (p.1583).

1. Anonymous. A nasal decongestant and a local anesthetic for weight control? *Med Lett Drugs Ther* 1979; **21:** 65–6.

### Preparations

***USP 27:*** Antipyrine and Benzocaine Otic Solution; Antipyrine, Benzocaine, and Phenylephrine Hydrochloride Otic Solution; Benzocaine and Menthol Topical Aerosol; Benzocaine Cream; Benzocaine Gel; Benzocaine Lozenges; Benzocaine Ointment; Benzocaine Otic Solution; Benzocaine Topical Aerosol; Benzocaine Topical Solution; Benzocaine, Butamben, and Tetracaine Hydrochloride Gel; Benzocaine, Butamben, and Tetracaine Hydrochloride Ointment; Benzocaine, Butamben, and Tetracaine Hydrochloride Topical Aerosol; Benzocaine, Butamben, and Tetracaine Hydrochloride Topical Solution.

**Proprietary Preparations** (details are given in Part 3)

***Arg.:*** Cerax; Lanacaina; Lodoc; ***Austral.:*** Applicaine; ***Austria:*** Anaestherit; ***Braz.:*** Oragard Baby†; Solarcaine; ***Canad.:*** Anbesol Baby; Baby Orajel; Dexatrim; Johnson & Johnson Burn Cream†; Orajel; Outgro; Sirop Dentition†; Topicaine†; Zilactin Baby; Zilactin-B; ***Chile:*** Anbesol; Baby Orajel; BBdent Gel Topico; Dentispray; Foille; Kalmafta; Orajel; ***Ger.:*** Anaesthesin; Anaesthesin N; Flavamed Halstabletten; Kontakto Derm; Labocane; Subcutin N; Zahnerol N; ***Israel:*** Anadent; Baby Gel; Lanacane; Maintain; ***Ital.:*** Gengivarium†; ***Mex.:*** Auralyt; Garde Gomas; ***NZ:*** Applicaine†; Solarcaine; ***Port.:*** Dentispray; ***Spain:*** Dentispray; Gartricin; Hurricaine; Lanacane; Nani Pre Dental; ***Switz.:*** Orajel†; ***UK:*** AAA; Burneze; Lanacane; Orajel; Ultra Chloraseptic; Ultracare; ***USA:*** Americaine; Americaine Anesthetic; Americaine Otic; Baby Anbesol; Baby Orajel; Benzodent; Chigger-Tox; Dent's Extra Strength Toothache Gum; Dent's Maximum Strength Toothache Drops; Dermoplast; Detane; Diet Ayds†; Hurricaine; Lanacane; Mycinettes; Numzident; Orabase Baby; Orabase Gel; Orabase-B; Orajel; Otocain; SensoGARD; Slim Mint†; Spec-T†; Trocaine; Vicks Children's Chloraseptic; Zilactin-B Medicated.

**Multi-ingredient:** numerous preparations are listed in Part 3.

## Bupivacaine Hydrochloride

*(BANM, USAN, rINNM)*

AH-2250; Bupivacaini Hydrochloridum; Hidrocloruro de bupivacaína; LAC-43; Win-11318. (±)-(1-Butyl-2-piperidyl)formo-2′,6′-xylidide hydrochloride monohydrate.

$C_{18}H_{28}N_2O,HCl,H_2O$ = 342.9.

*CAS — 2180-92-9 (bupivacaine); 18010-40-7 (anhydrous bupivacaine hydrochloride); 14252-80-3 (bupivacaine hydrochloride monohydrate).*

*ATC — N01BB01.*

**Pharmacopoeias.** In *Chin., Eur.* (see p.vi), *Int., Pol.,* and *US.*

**Ph. Eur. 5.0** (Bupivacaine Hydrochloride). A white crystalline powder or colourless crystals. Soluble in water; freely soluble in alcohol. Protect from light.

**USP 27** (Bupivacaine Hydrochloride). A white, odourless, crystalline powder. Freely soluble in water and in alcohol; slightly soluble in acetone and in chloroform. A 1% solution in water has a pH of 4.5 to 6.0.

**Stability of solutions.** For a discussion of the effect that pH has on the stability of local anaesthetic solutions and the pain associated with their injection, see p.1369.

For reference to the stability of admixtures of bupivacaine and fentanyl in solution, with or without adrenaline, see under Fentanyl, p.40.

### Adverse Effects and Treatment

As for Local Anaesthetics in general, p.1367.

Bupivacaine appears to be more cardiotoxic than other local anaesthetics. Cardiac arrest due to bupivacaine can be resistant to electrical defibrillation and a successful outcome may require prolonged resuscitative efforts.

◊ For reference to the toxic threshold for bupivacaine plasma concentrations, see Absorption under Pharmacokinetics, below.

**Effects on the cardiovascular system.** Bupivacaine[1,2] and etidocaine[2] appear to be more cardiotoxic than most other commonly used local anaesthetics and marked cardiovascular depression may occur at plasma concentrations only slightly above those for CNS toxicity.[2] Fatalities have occurred. Simultaneous seizures and cardiovascular collapse may develop rapidly following inadvertent intravascular injection and even prompt oxygenation and blood pressure support might not prevent cardiac arrest.[2] Ventricular fibrillation which is very resistant to normal methods of defibrillation may develop. Since lidocaine and the other local anaesthetics have additive effects on the CNS bretylium may be preferable to lidocaine for the treatment of induced arrhythmias.[1] Seizures and life-threatening ventricular fibrillation have also been reported following systemic absorption of bupivacaine solutions in an adolescent patient undergoing wound debridement.[3] Fatal cardiotoxicity has occurred following the use of bupivacaine in intravenous regional anaesthesia, possibly due to leakage past the tourniquet, and the use of bupivacaine in this technique should be avoided.[1] Fatalities have also been associated with the use of 0.75% solutions for epidural anaesthesia in obstetric patients and this strength is no longer recommended for obstetric anaesthesia. See also Labour Pain under Uses and Administration, below.

1. Anonymous. Cardiotoxicity of local anaesthetic drugs. *Lancet* 1986; **ii:** 1192–4.
2. Albright GA. Cardiac arrest following regional anesthesia with etidocaine or bupivacaine. *Anesthesiology* 1979; **51:** 285–7.
3. Yan AC, Newman RD. Bupivacaine-induced seizures and ventricular fibrillation in a 13-year-old girl undergoing wound debridement. *Pediatr Emerg Care* 1998; **14:** 354–5.

**Effects on the eyes.** Bilateral retinal haemorrhages developed in a 47-year-old woman[1] after receiving a caudal block with bupivacaine 0.5%. The haemorrhages cleared and her usual vision returned by 3 months.

1. Ling C, *et al.* Bilateral retinal haemorrhages following epidural injection. *Br J Ophthalmol* 1993; **77:** 316–17.

**Prolonged block.** Reports of prolonged block following the use of bupivacaine in regional anaesthesia.[1,2]

1. Pathy GV, Rosen M. Prolonged block with recovery after extradural analgesia for labour. *Br J Anaesth* 1975; **47:** 520–2.
2. Brockway MS, *et al.* Prolonged brachial plexus block with 0.42% bupivacaine. *Br J Anaesth* 1989; **63:** 604–5.

### Precautions

As for Local Anaesthetics in general, p.1368.

Bupivacaine is contra-indicated for use in intravenous regional anaesthesia (Bier's block) and for paracervical block in obstetrics. The 0.75% solution is contra-indicated for epidural block in obstetrics.

**Renal impairment.** Spinal block after the administration of 3 mL bupivacaine 0.75% was reported to be more rapid in onset and of shorter duration in patients with chronic renal failure when compared with control patients.[1]

1. Orko R, *et al.* Subarachnoid anaesthesia with 0.75% bupivacaine in patients with chronic renal failure. *Br J Anaesth* 1986; **58:** 605–9.

### Interactions

For interactions associated with local anaesthetics, see p.1368.

**Antiarrhythmics.** There is an increased risk of myocardial depression when bupivacaine and antiarrhythmics are administered concomitantly.

**Beta blockers.** *Propranolol* reduced the clearance of bupivacaine by 35% in 6 healthy subjects.[1] There is a risk of increased bupivacaine toxicity if these drugs are used together.

1. Bowdle TA, *et al.* Propranolol reduces bupivacaine clearance. *Anesthesiology* 1987; **66:** 36–8.

**Calcium-channel blockers.** There is a theoretical risk that the adverse effects of bupivacaine on the heart might be enhanced in patients taking calcium-channel blockers, but evidence of a clinical problem is lacking.

**Histamine $H_2$-antagonists.** Studies of the effect of $H_2$-antagonists on the pharmacokinetics of bupivacaine have yielded variable results. While a group of workers[1] found that pretreatment with *cimetidine* decreased the clearance of bupivacaine, others have failed to find any significant pharmacokinetic effects.[2,3] Similarly, pretreatment with *ranitidine* has either increased plasma concentrations of bupivacaine[4] or had no significant effect.[3]

1. Noble DW, *et al.* Effects of H-2 antagonists on the elimination of bupivacaine. *Br J Anaesth* 1987; **59:** 735–7.
2. Pihlajamäki KK. Lack of effect of cimetidine on the pharmacokinetics of bupivacaine in healthy subjects. *Br J Clin Pharmacol* 1988; **26:** 403–6.
3. Flynn RJ, *et al.* Does pretreatment with cimetidine and ranitidine affect the disposition of bupivacaine? *Br J Anaesth* 1989; **62:** 87–91.
4. Wilson CM. Plasma bupivacaine concentrations associated with extradural anaesthesia for caesarean section: influence of pretreatment with ranitidine. *Br J Anaesth* 1986; **58:** 1330P–1331P.

**Local anaesthetics.** For reference to the effect of bupivacaine on the protein binding of lidocaine and mepivacaine, see p.1378 and p.1381, respectively.

### Pharmacokinetics

Bupivacaine is about 95% bound to plasma proteins. Reported half-lives are from 1.5 to 5.5 hours in adults and about 8 hours in neonates. It is metabolised in the liver and is excreted in the urine principally as metabolites with only 5 to 6% as unchanged drug.

Bupivacaine is distributed into breast milk in small quantities. It crosses the placenta but the ratio of fetal concentrations to maternal concentrations is relatively low. Bupivacaine also diffuses into the CSF.

See also under Local Anaesthetics, p.1368.

**Absorption.** The toxic threshold for bupivacaine plasma concentrations is considered by some[1] to lie in the range of 2 to 4 micrograms/mL and in the UK the maximum single recommended dose for anhydrous bupivacaine hydrochloride is 150 mg (equivalent to approximately 2 mg/kg). Administration of bupivacaine for *regional anaesthesia* of the head and neck in a mean total dose of 3.4 mg/kg has produced mean peak plasma concentrations of 3.56 and 4.95 micrograms/mL when administered with or without adrenaline, respectively without producing toxicity.[2] Similarly, *intrapleural* administration of bupivacaine 0.5% in a dose of 2.5 mg/kg has produced mean peak plasma concentrations of 2.57 and 3.22 micrograms/mL when given with or without adrenaline, respectively without producing toxicity.[3] A further study[4] in which a 72-hour interpleural infusion of bupivacaine hydrochloride with adrenaline was administered to cholecystectomy patients showed appreciable interpatient variability in steady-state plasma drug concentrations (range 1.3 to 3.2 micrograms/mL; mean 2.1 micrograms/mL); no patient suffered any adverse effects. Bilateral *intercostal* nerve blocks using bupivacaine 2 mg/kg have also produced concentrations within the presumed toxic range without adverse effects but the use of adrenaline with this block did not reliably reduce peak plasma-bupivacaine concentrations.[5]

*Stellate ganglion block* with bupivacaine 0.25% has produced a mean peak plasma concentration of 0.34 and 0.47 micrograms/mL after doses of 10 or 20 mL, respectively.[6] Administration of bupivacaine 0.5% in a dose of 3 mg/kg with or without adrenaline for *sciatic* and *femoral nerve block* produced mean peak plasma concentrations below 0.8 micrograms/mL.[7]

*Intra-articular* bupivacaine is rapidly absorbed from the synovial membrane of the knee during arthroscopy but plasma concentrations did not exceed 0.35 micrograms/mL after controlled pressure-irrigation with isotonic solutions containing up to 200 mg.[8] Although a group of workers found that the maximum plasma concentrations of bupivacaine after intra-articular injection of 30 mL of a 0.5% solution for arthroscopy was 0.875 micrograms/mL they suggested that adrenaline should probably be added to minimise absorption.[9]

1. Tucker GT. Pharmacokinetics of local anaesthetics. *Br J Anaesth* 1986; **58:** 717–31.
2. Neill RS, Watson R. Plasma bupivacaine concentrations during combined regional and general anaesthesia for resection and reconstruction of head and neck carcinomata. *Br J Anaesth* 1984; **56:** 485–92.
3. Gin T, *et al.* Effect of adrenaline on venous plasma concentrations of bupivacaine after interpleural administration. *Br J Anaesth* 1990; **64:** 662–6.
4. Kastrissios H, *et al.* The disposition of bupivacaine following a 72h interpleural infusion in cholecystectomy patients. *Br J Clin Pharmacol* 1991; **32:** 251–4.
5. Bodenham A, Park GR. Plasma concentrations of bupivacaine after intercostal nerve block in patients after orthotopic liver transplantation. *Br J Anaesth* 1990; **64:** 436–41.
6. Hardy PAJ, Williams NE. Plasma concentrations of bupivacaine after stellate ganglion block using two volumes of 0.25% bupivacaine plain solution. *Br J Anaesth* 1990; **65:** 243–4.
7. Misra U, *et al.* Plasma concentrations of bupivacaine following combined sciatic and femoral 3 in 1 nerve blocks in open knee surgery. *Br J Anaesth* 1991; **66:** 310–13.
8. Debruyne D, *et al.* Monitoring serum bupivacaïne levels during arthroscopy. *Eur J Clin Pharmacol* 1985; **27:** 733–5.
9. Butterworth JF, *et al.* Effect of adrenaline on plasma concentrations of bupivacaine following intra-articular injection of bupivacaine for knee arthroscopy. *Br J Anaesth* 1990; **65:** 537–9.

SURFACE ANAESTHESIA. Studies of the absorption of bupivacaine following surface application.

1. McBurney A, *et al.* Absorption of lignocaine and bupivacaine from the respiratory tract during fibreoptic bronchoscopy. *Br J Clin Pharmacol* 1984; **17:** 61–6.

**Pregnancy.** Bupivacaine crosses the placenta to a lesser degree than lidocaine or mepivacaine following maternal injection. Values of 0.2 to 0.4 have been reported[1,2] for the ratio of fetal to maternal concentrations for bupivacaine compared with values of 0.5 to 0.7 quoted[2,3] for lidocaine and mepivacaine. The greater degree of protein-binding of bupivacaine compared with these other drugs not only limits the amount of bupivacaine available to cross the placenta but also reduces the relative amount of free drug in the fetal circulation[2] (see also under Protein Binding, below). Addition of adrenaline to the injection does not appear to affect the placental transfer rate of bupivacaine.[4] Measurement of a beta-phase half-life of 25 hours in the neonate compared with 1.25 hours in mothers suggests that the neonate is less able to metabolise bupivacaine.[5]

1. Denson DD, *et al.* Serum bupivacaine concentrations in term parturients following continuous epidural analgesia for labor and delivery. *Ther Drug Monit* 1984; **6:** 393–8.
2. Blogg CE, Simpson BR. Obstetric analgesia and the newborn baby. *Lancet* 1974; **i:** 1283.
3. Poppers PJ. Evaluation of local anaesthetic agents for regional anaesthesia in obstetrics. *Br J Anaesth* 1975; **47:** 322–7.
4. Reynolds F, *et al.* Effect of time and adrenaline on the feto-maternal distribution of bupivacaine. *Br J Anaesth* 1989; **62:** 509–14.
5. Caldwell J, *et al.* Pharmacokinetics of local anaesthetic agents administered epidurally during childbirth. *Br J Clin Pharmacol* 1976; **3:** 956P–957P.

**Protein binding.** The two major binding proteins for bupivacaine in the blood are $\alpha_1$-acid glycoprotein, the influence of which is predominant at low concentrations, and albumin, which plays the major role at high concentrations. Reduction in pH from 7.4 to 7.0 decreases the affinity of the $\alpha_1$-acid glycoprotein for bupivacaine but has no effect on albumin affinity.[1] Binding of bupivacaine is reduced during pregnancy but it is considered that the increase in free bupivacaine concentrations is unlikely to cause a clinically significant increase in the risk of CNS or cardiovascular toxicity.[2]

As fetal plasma contains little $\alpha_1$-acid glycoprotein the binding capacity for bupivacaine is reduced and this may contribute to the difference between maternal and fetal plasma concentration at delivery[3] (see also under Pregnancy, above).

Ageing, uncomplicated by disease, does not affect the protein binding of bupivacaine.[4]

1. Denson D, *et al.* Alpha$_1$-acid glycoprotein and albumin in human serum bupivacaine binding. *Clin Pharmacol Ther* 1984; **35:** 409–15.
2. Denson DD, *et al.* Bupivacaine protein binding in the term parturient: effects of lactic acidosis. *Clin Pharmacol Ther* 1984; **35:** 702–9.
3. Petersen MC, *et al.* Relationship between the transplacental gradients of bupivacaine and $\alpha_1$-acid glycoprotein. *Br J Clin Pharmacol* 1981; **12:** 859–62.
4. Veering BT, *et al.* Age does not influence the serum protein binding of bupivacaine. *Br J Clin Pharmacol* 1991; **32:** 501–3.

## Uses and Administration

Bupivacaine hydrochloride is a local anaesthetic of the amide type with actions and uses similar to those described on p.1369. It has a slow onset and a long duration of action. The speed of onset and duration of action are increased by the addition of a vasoconstrictor, and absorption into the circulation from the site of injection is reduced. Slow accumulation occurs with repeated doses. It is used mainly for infiltration anaesthesia and regional nerve blocks, particularly epidural block, but is contra-indicated for obstetric paracervical block and for use in intravenous regional anaesthesia (Bier's block). The 0.75% solution is contra-indicated for epidural block in obstetrics. (Local anaesthetic techniques are discussed on p.1370.)

Bupivacaine is a racemic mixture but the *S*(−)-isomer levobupivacaine (see p.1377) is also used. The carbonated solution of bupivacaine is also available for injection in some countries (see p.1369).

In recommended doses bupivacaine produces complete sensory blockade but the concentration of bupivacaine solution used affects the extent of motor blockade achieved. A 0.25% solution generally produces incomplete motor block, a 0.5% solution will usually produce motor block and some muscle relaxation, and complete motor block and muscle relaxation can be achieved with a 0.75% solution.

The dosage of bupivacaine used depends on the site of injection and the procedure used, as well as the status of the patient. Bupivacaine is given as the hydrochloride monohydrate salt although doses are expressed in terms of the anhydrous hydrochloride; bupivacaine hydrochloride monohydrate 10.55 mg is approximately equivalent to anhydrous bupivacaine hydrochloride 10 mg. In the UK the suggested general **maximum single dose** of bupivacaine hydrochloride is 150 mg with or without adrenaline followed if necessary by doses of up to 50 mg every 2 hours. In the USA the recommended maximum single dose is 175 mg of the plain preparation or 225 mg when given with adrenaline; doses may be repeated at intervals of not less than 3 hours but the total daily dose should not exceed 400 mg. The dose should be reduced in the elderly, in children, in debilitated patients, and in cardiac or hepatic disease.

A test dose of bupivacaine, preferably with adrenaline, should be given before commencing epidural block to detect inadvertent intravascular administration. Subsequent doses should be given in small increments.

Solutions with or without adrenaline may be used for most **local anaesthetic techniques** and procedures apart from dental infiltration, when adrenaline is added to the solution (see below).

- For *infiltration anaesthesia* bupivacaine hydrochloride is typically used as a 0.25% solution in doses up to the recommended maximum (see above). When a longer duration of anaesthesia is required, as in dental or surgical procedures of the maxillary and mandibular area, a 0.5% solution with adrenaline 1 in 200 000 has been used but a total dose of 90 mg (18 mL) should not be exceeded over a single dental sitting.
- For *peripheral nerve block* the usual dose is 12.5 mg (5 mL) as a 0.25% solution or 25 mg (5 mL) as a 0.5% solution, although doses up to the recommended maximum single dose (see above) may also be given. A 0.75% solution has been used for *retrobulbar block* in ophthalmic surgery in a dose of 15 to 30 mg (2 to 4 mL).
- For *sympathetic nerve block* 50 to 125 mg (20 to 50 mL) as a 0.25% solution is recommended.
- For *lumbar epidural block* in surgery a 0.25% solution of bupivacaine hydrochloride may be used in a dose of 25 to 50 mg (10 to 20 mL) or as a 0.5% solution in a dose of 50 to 100 mg (10 to 20 mL). A 0.75% solution is also used for induction of lumbar epidural block in non-obstetric surgery in a single dose of 75 to 150 mg (10 to 20 mL). For *caudal block* in surgery 37.5 to 75 mg (15 to 30 mL) as a 0.25% solution or 75 to 150 mg (15 to 30 mL) as a 0.5% solution may be used. In the management of **acute pain** bupivacaine may be given as an epidural bolus or by continuous infusion. For analgesia during *labour*, doses of 15 to 30 mg (6 to 12 mL) as a 0.25% solution or 30 to 60 mg (6 to 12 mL) as a 0.5% solution have been recommended as a bolus for lumbar block. Alternatively, when given as an infusion, a dose of 10 to 15 mg (10 to 15 mL) per hour as a 0.1% solution or 10 to 15 mg (8 to 12 mL) per hour as a 0.125% solution has been recommended for lumbar block. Bupivacaine may also be given as a bolus caudal injection for labour pain; doses of 25 to 50 mg (10 to 20 mL) as a 0.25% solution or 50 to 100 mg (10 to 20 mL) as a 0.5% solution are recommended. For *postoperative pain* bupivacaine may be given as an epidural infusion in doses of 4 to 15 mg (4 to 15 mL) per hour as a 0.1% solution or 5 to 15 mg (4 to 12 mL) per hour as a 0.125% solution.
- Hyperbaric solutions of bupivacaine hydrochloride without adrenaline may be used for *spinal block*. Preparations containing 0.5% are available and are given in doses of 10 to 20 mg (2 to 4 mL).

**Action.** Addition of potassium chloride 0.2 mmol to 40 mL of bupivacaine 0.25% solution resulted in a more rapid onset of sensory loss than the same dose of plain bupivacaine in patients undergoing brachial plexus block for forearm or hand surgery.[1]

Hyaluronidase did not increase the speed of onset of brachial plexus block produced by bupivacaine 0.5%, with or without adrenaline, but did reduce the duration of anaesthesia.[2]

Administration of bupivacaine encapsulated in liposomes can prolong postsurgical analgesic action without motor block.[3,4]

For a comparison of the vasoactivity of bupivacaine and some other local anaesthetics, see p.1369.

1. Parris MR, Chambers WA. Effects of the addition of potassium to prilocaine or bupivacaine: studies on brachial plexus blockade. *Br J Anaesth* 1986; **58:** 297–300.
2. Keeler JF, *et al.* Effect of addition of hyaluronidase to bupivacaine during axillary brachial plexus block. *Br J Anaesth* 1992; **68:** 68–71.
3. Boogaerts S, *et al.* Epidural administration of liposomal bupivacaine for the management of postsurgical pain. *Br J Anaesth* 1993; **70:** (suppl 1): 104.
4. Boogaerts JG, *et al.* Pharmacokinetic-pharmacodynamic specific behaviour of liposome-associated bupivacaine in humans. *Br J Anaesth* 1995; **74** (suppl 1): 74.

**Administration in children.** Bupivacaine 0.25% injected intra-operatively up to a maximum dose of 1.5 mg/kg with adrenaline has been used in infants for the control of postoperative pain due to pyloromyotomy and appears to attenuate some of the cardiac and respiratory effects associated with the use of general anaesthesia alone.[1] Doses of 2.5 mg of bupivacaine per year of age, as a 0.5% solution, have been used for ilio-inguinal nerve block in children undergoing herniotomy.[2] A study[3] in infants undergoing abdominal surgery found that an epidural infusion of bupivacaine produced comparable analgesia to an intravenous infusion of morphine. It was considered that bupivacaine might be preferable to morphine in neonates and young infants who are particularly prone to respiratory depression, but older children might require additional sedation or analgesia to prevent postoperative restlessness.

1. McNicol LR, *et al.* Peroperative bupivacaine for pyloromyotomy pain. *Lancet* 1990; **335:** 54–5.
2. Smith BAC, Jones SEF. Analgesia after herniotomy in a paediatric day unit. *BMJ* 1982; **285:** 1466.
3. Wolf AR, Hughes D. Pain relief for infants undergoing abdominal surgery: comparison of infusions of IV morphine and extradural bupivacaine. *Br J Anaesth* 1993; **70:** 10–16.

**Labour pain.** For a discussion of the management of labour pain, including mention of the use of local anaesthetics, see p.6.

Early experience in nearly 1000 patients suggested that 8 mL of a 0.5% solution of bupivacaine with adrenaline was the optimum dose for epidural block during labour;[1] pain relief lasted for about 2 hours. Decreasing the concentration of the final dose to 0.25% reduced the persistence of sensory and motor nerve block after delivery. Others[2] found that bupivacaine 0.375% was the most suitable concentration for epidural analgesia when using a regimen of regular 'top-up' doses of 0.5 mg/kg about every 90 minutes. However, the use of low doses of bupivacaine 0.25% for epidural analgesia in primiparous women was associated with a lower incidence of forceps delivery and oxytocin augmentation.[3] Although an even lower concentration of bupivacaine (0.0625%) used with sufentanil[4] produced analgesia similar to that with 0.125% bupivacaine used alone, the duration of the second stage of labour and the incidence of instrumental and surgical delivery were not reduced. Similar results were obtained using bupivacaine 0.0625% with diamorphine 0.005%; in addition pruritus and drowsiness produced by diamorphine were considered to be troublesome in many patients.[5]

Intrathecal injections of bupivacaine with or without an opioid are sometimes used[6,7] with epidural injections to achieve a faster onset of analgesia and a reduced degree of motor block in the management of labour pain. Intrathecal injections containing bupivacaine have also been given alone[8,9] for the management of labour pain but the use of this route alone is usually associated with anaesthesia and management of postoperative pain in caesarean section. Bupivacaine has also been tried with lidocaine for epidural anaesthesia in caesarean section in order to reduce the dose of bupivacaine and minimise cardiotoxicity.[10]

1. Crawford JS. Lumbar epidural block in labour: a clinical analysis. *Br J Anaesth* 1972; **44:** 66–74.
2. Purdy G, *et al.* Continuous extradural analgesia in labour: comparison between "on demand" and regular "top-up" injections. *Br J Anaesth* 1987; **59:** 319–24.
3. Turner MJ, *et al.* Primiparous women using epidural analgesia. *BMJ* 1990; **300:** 123.
4. Auroy Y, Benhamou D. Extradural analgesia for labour: 0.125% bupivacaine vs 0.0625% bupivacaine with 0.2 micrograms $mL^{-1}$ sufentanil. *Br J Anaesth* 1995; **74** (suppl 1): 105–6.
5. Bailey CR, *et al.* Diamorphine-bupivacaine mixture compared with plain bupivacaine for analgesia. *Br J Anaesth* 1994; **72:** 58–61.
6. Stacey RGW, *et al.* Single space combined spinal-extradural technique for analgesia in labour. *Br J Anaesth* 1993; **71:** 499–502.
7. Collis RE, *et al.* Randomised comparison of combined spinal-epidural and standard epidural analgesia in labour. *Lancet* 1995; **345:** 1413–16.
8. Kestin IG, *et al.* Analgesia for labour and delivery using incremental diamorphine and bupivacaine via a 32-gauge intrathecal catheter. *Br J Anaesth* 1992; **68:** 244–7.
9. McHale S, *et al.* Continuous subarachnoid infusion of 0.125% bupivacaine for analgesia during labour. *Br J Anaesth* 1992; **69:** 634–6.
10. Howell P, *et al.* Comparison of four local extradural anaesthetic solutions for elective Caesarean section. *Br J Anaesth* 1990; **65:** 648–53.

## Preparations

***BP 2003:*** Bupivacaine and Adrenaline Injection; Bupivacaine Injection;
***USP 27:*** Bupivacaine Hydrochloride in Dextrose Injection; Bupivacaine Hydrochloride Injection.

**Proprietary Preparations** (details are given in Part 3)

***Arg.:*** Bupicaina; Bupinex; Caina G; Duracaine; ***Austral.:*** Marcain; ***Austria:*** Bucain; Carbostesin; Dolanaest; ***Belg.:*** Marcaine; ***Braz.:*** Bupiabbott; Bupiabbott Plus; Marcaina; Neocaina; ***Canad.:*** Marcaine; Sensorcaine; ***Chile:*** Duracaine; ***Denm.:*** Marcain; ***Fin.:*** Bicain; Marcain; ***Fr.:*** Marcaine; ***Ger.:*** Bucain; Carbostesin; Dolanaest; ***Gr.:*** Marcaine; ***Hong Kong:*** Marcaine; ***India:*** Marcain; Sensoricaine; ***Irl.:*** Marcain; ***Israel:*** Kamacaine; Marcaine; ***Ital.:*** Bupibil; Bupicain; Bupiforan; Bupisen; Bupisolver; Bupixamol; Bupyl†; Marcaina; ***Malaysia:*** Marcain; ***Mex.:*** Buvacaina; ***Neth.:*** Marcaine; ***Norw.:*** Marcain; ***NZ:*** Marcain; ***Port.:*** Bupinostrum Adrenalina; Marcaina; ***S.Afr.:*** Macaine; Regibloc†; ***Singapore:*** Marcain; ***Spain:*** Svedocain Sin Vasoconstr; ***Swed.:*** Marcain; ***Switz.:*** Carbostesin; Duracain; ***Thai.:*** Marcaine; ***UK:*** Marcain; ***USA:*** Marcaine; Sensorcaine.

**Multi-ingredient:** ***Austral.:*** Marcain with Fentanyl; Marcain with Pethidine; ***Fin.:*** Solomet c bupivacain hydrochlorid; ***NZ:*** Bupafen; Marcain with Fentanyl; Marcain with Pethidine†.

## Butacaine Sulfate *(rINNM)*

Butacain. Sulph.; Butacaine Sulphate *(BANM)*; Sulfato de butacaína.
3-Dibutylaminopropyl 4-aminobenzoate sulphate.

$(C_{18}H_{30}N_2O_2)_2,H_2SO_4 = 711.0.$

*CAS — 149-16-6 (butacaine); 149-15-5 (butacaine sulfate).*

### Profile

Butacaine, a para-aminobenzoic acid ester, is a local anaesthetic (p.1367) used for surface anaesthesia. It has been used topically, as the sulfate, in solutions for dental pain and in ear and nasal drops.

### Preparations

**Proprietary Preparations** (details are given in Part 3)

**Multi-ingredient:** ***Fr.:*** Relaxoddi†; ***Spain:*** Topicaina†.

## Butoxycaine Hydrochloride

Butoxicaína, hidrocloruro de; Butoxycaini Hydrochloridum. 2-Diethylaminoethyl-(p-butoxybenzoate) hydrochloride.

$C_{17}H_{27}NO_3,HCl = 329.9.$

*CAS — 3772-43-8 (butoxycaine); 2350-32-5 (butoxycaine hydrochloride).*

### Profile

Butoxycaine, a para-aminobenzoic acid ester, is a local anaesthetic (p.1367) that has been used as the base or hydrochloride for surface anaesthesia.

### Preparations

**Proprietary Preparations** (details are given in Part 3)
**Multi-ingredient: *Ger.:*** Bismolan; Hamo-ratiopharm†.

## Butyl Aminobenzoate

Butamben *(USAN)*; Butilaminobenzoato; Butoforme. Butyl 4-aminobenzoate.

$C_{11}H_{15}NO_2 = 193.2.$

*CAS — 94-25-7.*

**Pharmacopoeias.** In *Fr.* and *US.*

**USP 27** (Butamben). A white, odourless, crystalline powder. M.p. 57° to 59°. Soluble 1 in 7000 of water; soluble in alcohol, in ether, in chloroform, in fixed oils, and in dilute acids. It slowly hydrolyses when boiled with water.

## Butyl Aminobenzoate Picrate

Abbott-34842; Butamben Picrate *(USAN)*; Butilaminobenzoato, picrato de.

$(C_{11}H_{15}NO_2)_2,C_6H_3N_3O_7 = 615.6.$

*CAS — 577-48-0.*

### Profile

Butyl aminobenzoate, a para-aminobenzoic acid ester, is a local anaesthetic (p.1367) that has been used for surface anaesthesia of the skin and mucous membranes. It has also been used for relief of pain and pruritus associated with anorectal disorders. A suspension of butyl aminobenzoate 5 or 10% has been given epidurally.

Butyl aminobenzoate picrate is applied to the skin as a 1% ointment.

◊ References.


1. Korsten HH, *et al.* Long-lasting epidural sensory blockade by n-butyl-p-aminobenzoate in the terminally ill intractable cancer pain patient. *Anesthesiology* 1991; **75:** 950–60.
2. Armstrong DG, Kanat IO. Analgesic efficacy of topical butamben picrate. *J Am Podiatr Med Assoc* 1995; **85:** 738–40.
3. Shulman M, *et al.* Nerve blocks with 5% butamben suspension for the treatment of chronic pain syndromes. *Reg Anesth Pain Med* 1998; **23:** 395–401.


### Preparations

***USP 27:*** Benzocaine, Butamben, and Tetracaine Hydrochloride Gel; Benzocaine, Butamben, and Tetracaine Hydrochloride Ointment; Benzocaine, Butamben, and Tetracaine Hydrochloride Topical Aerosol; Benzocaine, Butamben, and Tetracaine Hydrochloride Topical Solution; Erythromycin Ethylsuccinate Injection.

**Proprietary Preparations** (details are given in Part 3)
***USA:*** Butesin Picrate†.

**Multi-ingredient: *Austral.:*** Butesin Picrate; ***Braz.:*** Nestosyl†; ***Fr.:*** Nestosyl; Preparation H; Tyrothricine Lafran†; ***India:*** Proctosedyl; ***Spain:*** Alvogil; Topicaina; ***Switz.:*** Alvogyl; ***USA:*** Cetacaine.

## Chloroprocaine Hydrochloride *(rINNM)*

Hidrocloruro de cloroprocaína. 2-Diethylaminoethyl 4-amino-2-chlorobenzoate hydrochloride.

$C_{13}H_{19}ClN_2O_2,HCl = 307.2.$

*CAS — 133-16-4 (chloroprocaine); 3858-89-7 (chloroprocaine hydrochloride).*

*ATC — N01BA04.*

**Pharmacopoeias.** In *US.*

**USP 27** (Chloroprocaine Hydrochloride). A white odourless crystalline powder. Soluble 1 in 20 of water and 1 in 100 of alcohol; very slightly soluble in chloroform; practically insoluble in ether. Solutions are acid to litmus.

**pH of solutions.** For a discussion of the effect that pH has on the stability of local anaesthetic solutions and the pain associated with their injection, see p.1369.

### Adverse Effects, Treatment, and Precautions

As for Local Anaesthetics in general, p.1367. Chloroprocaine is said to be unsuitable for intravenous regional anaesthesia (Bier's block) because of a high incidence of thrombophlebitis associated with such use. It is also contra-indicated in spinal anaesthesia due to potential neurotoxicity.

### Interactions

For interactions associated with local anaesthetics, see p.1368.

### Pharmacokinetics

Chloroprocaine is hydrolysed rapidly in the circulation by plasma cholinesterase. It has a half-life of 19 to 26 seconds in adults. It is excreted in the urine mainly as metabolites.

See also under Local Anaesthetics, p.1368.

### Uses and Administration

Chloroprocaine, a para-aminobenzoic acid ester, is a local anaesthetic with actions and uses similar to those described on p.1369. It has properties similar to those of procaine (p.1383). It has a rapid onset (6 to 12 minutes) and short duration (one hour) of action.

Chloroprocaine is used as the hydrochloride for infiltration, peripheral nerve block, and central nerve block including lumbar and caudal epidural blocks. It may be given, if necessary, with adrenaline 1 in 200 000 to delay absorption and reduce toxicity. Chloroprocaine is not an effective surface anaesthetic. It should not be used for spinal anaesthesia. (Local anaesthetic techniques are discussed on p.1370.)

The dosage of chloroprocaine used depends on the site of injection and the procedure used. In adults the **maximum single dose** of chloroprocaine hydrochloride without adrenaline should not exceed 800 mg; when given with adrenaline 1 in 200 000 the maximum single dose should not exceed 1 g. A test dose of chloroprocaine, preferably with adrenaline, should be given before starting epidural block to detect inadvertent intravascular injection. Doses for various procedures include:

- *mandibular nerve block*: 40 to 60 mg (2 to 3 mL) as a 2% solution.
- *infra-orbital nerve block*: 10 to 20 mg (0.5 to 1 mL) as a 2% solution.
- *brachial plexus block*: 600 to 800 mg (30 to 40 mL) as a 2% solution.
- *digital nerve block*: 30 to 40 mg (3 to 4 mL) as a 1% solution without adrenaline.
- in obstetrics a dose of 200 mg (10 mL) per side as a 2% solution is suggested for *pudendal block* and for a *paracervical block* a 1% solution in a dose of 30 mg (3 mL) at each of 4 sites.
- *lumbar epidural block*: 40 to 50 mg (2 to 2.5 mL) as a 2% solution or 60 to 75 mg (2 to 2.5 mL) as a 3% solution for each segment to be anaesthetised, the usual total dose being 300 to 750 mg with smaller repeat doses being given at intervals of 40 to 50 minutes.
- *caudal block*: 300 to 500 mg (15 to 25 mL) as a 2% solution or 450 to 750 mg (15 to 25 mL) as a 3% solution may be given and repeated at intervals of 40 to 60 minutes.

Dosages should be reduced in children, elderly or debilitated patients, and those with cardiac or liver disease. For children concentrations of 0.5 to 1% are suggested for infiltration and 1 to 1.5% for nerve block procedures.

### Preparations

***USP 27:*** Chloroprocaine Hydrochloride Injection.

**Proprietary Preparations** (details are given in Part 3)
***Canad.:*** Nesacaine; ***Switz.:*** Ivracain; Nesacain; ***USA:*** Nesacaine.

## Cinchocaine *(BAN, rINN)*

Cincainum; Cincocaína; Dibucaine. 2-Butoxy-N-(2-diethylaminoethyl)cinchoninamide; 2-Butoxy-N-(2-diethylaminoethyl)quinoline-4-carboxamide.

$C_{20}H_{29}N_3O_2 = 343.5.$

*CAS — 85-79-0.*

*ATC — C05AD04; D04AB02; N01BB06; S01HA06.*

**Pharmacopoeias.** In *US.*

**USP 27** (Dibucaine). A white to off-white powder, with a slight characteristic odour. M.p. 62.5° to 66°. Soluble 1 in 4600 of water, 1 in 0.7 of alcohol, 1 in 0.5 of chloroform, and 1 in 1.4 of ether; soluble in 1N hydrochloric acid. It darkens on exposure to light. Store in airtight containers. Protect from light.

## Cinchocaine Hydrochloride *(BANM, rINNM)*

Cincaini Chloridum; Cinchocaini Hydrochloridum; Dibucaine Hydrochloride; Dibucainium Chloride; Hidrocloruro de cincocaína; Percainum; Sovcainum.

$C_{20}H_{29}N_3O_2,HCl = 379.9.$

*CAS — 61-12-1.*

*ATC — C05AD04; D04AB02; N01BB06; S01HA06.*

NOTE. This compound was originally marketed under the name Percaine, but accidents occurred owing to the confusion of this name with procaine.

**Pharmacopoeias.** In *Eur.* (see p.vi), *Jpn,* and *US.*

**Ph. Eur. 5.0** (Cinchocaine Hydrochloride). A white or almost white, crystalline powder or colourless crystals; it is hygroscopic. It agglomerates very easily. Very soluble in water; freely soluble in alcohol, in acetone, and in dichloromethane. A 2% solution in water has a pH of 5.0 to 6.0. Store in airtight containers. Protect from light.

**USP 27** (Dibucaine Hydrochloride). Colourless or white to off-white crystals or white to off-white, crystalline powder. It is odourless, somewhat hygroscopic, and darkens on exposure to light. Freely soluble in water, in alcohol, in acetone, and in chloroform. Its solutions have a pH of about 5.5. Store in airtight containers. Protect from light.

### Profile

Cinchocaine is an amide local anaesthetic (p.1367) that is now generally only used for surface anaesthesia. It is one of the most potent and toxic of the long-acting local anaesthetics and its parenteral use was restricted to spinal anaesthesia.

For surface anaesthesia cinchocaine has been used, as the base or hydrochloride, in creams and ointments containing up to 1% and in suppositories for the temporary relief of pain and itching associated with skin and anorectal conditions. Cinchocaine benzoate has also been used topically.

**Action.** For a comparison of the vasoactivity of cinchocaine and some other local anaesthetics, see p.1369.

**Plasma cholinesterase deficiency.** For mention of the use of cinchocaine in the determination of plasma cholinesterase activity, see under Precautions of Suxamethonium Chloride, p.1408.

### Preparations

***USP 27:*** Dibucaine Cream; Dibucaine Hydrochloride Injection; Dibucaine Ointment.

**Proprietary Preparations** (details are given in Part 3)
***Austral.:*** Nupercaine Heavy†; ***Braz.:*** Nupercainal; ***Canad.:*** Nupercainal; ***Denm.:*** Cincain; ***Ger.:*** DoloPosterine N; ***India:*** Nupercainal; ***Swed.:*** Cincain; ***Switz.:*** Nupercainal†; ***UK:*** Nupercainal; ***USA:*** Nupercainal.

**Multi-ingredient: *Arg.:*** Anuar; Proctyl; Scheriproct; Ultraproct; ***Austral.:*** Proctosedyl; Rectinol HC; Scheriproct; Ultraproct; ***Austria:*** Ciloprin cum Anaesthetico; Scheriproct; Ultraproct; ***Belg.:*** Scheriproct; Tri-histalex; Ultraproct; ***Braz.:*** Proctil†; Proctyl; Senol; Ultraproct; ***Canad.:*** Nupercainal; Proctomyxin; Proctosedyl; Proctosone; ***Chile:*** Scheriproct; Ultraproct; ***Denm.:*** Proctosedyl; ***Fin.:*** Ciloprin cum Anaesthetico; Faktu; Proctosedyl; Scheriproct; ***Fr.:*** Anti-Hemorroidaires†; Deliproct; Ultraproct; ***Ger.:*** Anumedin; Faktu; Otobacid N; Procto-Kaban; Proctospre; Scheriproct; Ultraproct; ***Gr.:*** Scheriproct Neo; ***Hong Kong:*** Borraginol-N; Decatylen; Faktu; Proctosedyl; Proctosone; Protozone†; Ultraproct; ***India:*** Otogesic; ***Irl.:*** Proctosedyl; Scheriproct; Ultraproct; ***Israel:*** Proctosedyl†; ***Ital.:*** Ultraproct; ***Malaysia:*** Decatylen; Proctosedyl; ***Mex.:*** Proctoacid; Scheriproct; Ultraproct; ***Neth.:*** Proctosedyl; ***Norw.:*** Proctosedyl; Scheriproct; ***NZ:*** Proctosedyl; Ultraproct; ***Port.:*** Faktu; Scheriproct; ***S.Afr.:*** Cepacaine; Proctosedyl; Scheriproct; ***Singapore:*** Decatylen; Faktu; Proctosedyl; ***Spain:*** Anestesia Loc Braun S/A; Ruscus; Scheriproct; ***Swed.:*** Proctosedyl; Scheriproct N; ***Switz.:*** Ciloprine ca; Decatylene Neo; Faktu; Locaseptil-Neo; Proctospre†; Scheriproct; Ultraproct†; ***Thai.:*** Faktu†; Proctosedyl; Scheriproct; ***UAE:*** Supraproct-S; ***UK:*** Proctosedyl; Scheriproct; Ultraproct; Uniroid-HC; ***USA:*** Corticaine.

*Used as an adjunct in:* ***Austria:*** Butazolidin; ***Ger.:*** Butazolidin†; ***Switz.:*** Butazolidine†.

## Coca

Coca Leaves; Hoja de Coca.

### Profile

Coca is the dried leaves of *Erythroxylum coca* (Bolivian or Huanuco leaf) or of *E. truxillense* (Peruvian or Truxillo leaf) (Erythroxylaceae), indigenous to Bolivia and Peru and cultivated in Colombia and Indonesia.

Coca leaves contain about 0.7 to 1.5% of total alkaloids, of which cocaine, cinnamyl-cocaine, and α-truxilline are the most important.

Coca was formerly used for its stimulant action and for the relief of gastric pain, nausea, and vomiting, but it has no place in modern medicine. The practice of coca leaf chewing still continues in South America.

# Cocaine *(BAN)*

Cocaína; Methyl Benzoylecgonine. (1R,2R,3S,5S)-2-Methoxycarbonyltropan-3-yl benzoate.

$C_{17}H_{21}NO_4 = 303.4.$

*CAS — 50-36-2.*

*ATC — N01BC01; R02AD03; S01HA01; S02DA02.*

NOTE. The following names have also been used to describe various forms of cocaine: basuco, bazooka, bernice, blow, C, charlie, coke, crack, flake, freebase, girl, gold dust, her, lady, leaf, nose candy, pasta, rock, she, snow, space dust, toot, white girl, white lady.

**Pharmacopoeias.** In *Br.* and *US.*

**BP 2003** (Cocaine). It may be obtained from the leaves of *Erythroxylum coca* and other spp. of *Erythroxylum*, or by synthesis. Colourless crystals or a white, crystalline powder. It is slightly volatile. M.p. 96° to 98°. Practically insoluble in water; freely soluble in alcohol and in ether; very soluble in chloroform; soluble in arachis oil; slightly soluble in liquid paraffin.

**USP 27** (Cocaine). Colourless to white crystals or white, crystalline powder. M.p. 96° to 98°. Soluble 1 in 600 of water, 1 in 7 of alcohol, 1 in 1 of chloroform, 1 in 3.5 of ether, 1 in 12 of olive oil, and 1 in 80 to 100 of liquid paraffin. A saturated solution in water is alkaline to litmus. Protect from light.

## Cocaine Hydrochloride *(BANM)*

Chloridrato de Cocaína; Cocaína, hidrocloruro de; Cocaine Hydrochlor.; Cocaini Hydrochloridum; Cocainium Chloratum.

$C_{17}H_{21}NO_4,HCl = 339.8.$

*CAS — 53-21-4.*

*ATC — N01BC01; R02AD03; S01HA01; S02DA02.*

NOTE. CCN is a code approved by the BP 2003 for use on single unit doses of eye drops containing cocaine hydrochloride where the individual containers may be too small to bear all the appropriate labelling information.

**Pharmacopoeias.** In *Chin., Eur.* (see p.vi), *Jpn, Pol., US,* and *Viet.*

**Ph. Eur. 5.0** (Cocaine Hydrochloride). Hygroscopic, colourless crystals or a white crystalline powder. M.p. about 197° with decomposition. Very soluble in water; freely soluble in alcohol. Protect from moisture and light.

**USP 27** (Cocaine Hydrochloride). Colourless crystals or white, crystalline powder. Soluble 1 in 0.5 of water, 1 in 3.5 of alcohol, and 1 in 15 of chloroform; soluble in glycerol; insoluble in ether. Protect from light.

**Stability in solutions.** ALKALIS. Solutions of cocaine hydrochloride are adversely affected by alkalis.

PHENOL. A stability study[1] was conducted in response to queries over conflicting data on the incompatibility of cocaine hydrochloride solutions and phenol. Some pharmacists had reported that cocaine hydrochloride eye drops preserved with phenol had shown no sign of physical incompatibility. The BPC 1973 states that cocaine hydrochloride is incompatible with phenol but suggests that cocaine hydrochloride solutions may be preserved with chlorocresol. The study found that there was no sign of physical incompatibility in aqueous solutions containing cocaine hydrochloride 5% and phenol 0.5% stored for a year at temperatures of 0° to 37° but there was a fall in pH, greatest at the higher temperatures, which was suggestive of chemical change. It was recommended that such solutions should be stored in a cool place.

1. *PSGB Lab Report P/75/14* 1975.

## Adverse Effects

Because the therapeutic use of cocaine is now very restricted many reports of adverse effects occur in the context of abuse. However, both systemic and local effects have followed its use as a surface anaesthetic. Although some effects are similar to those of other local anaesthetics (p.1367), cocaine differs in that it acts as a potent indirect-acting sympathomimetic. It stimulates the CNS causing agitation, dilated pupils, tachycardia, hypertension, hallucinations, hypertonia, and hyperreflexia. Convulsions, coma, and metabolic acidosis may develop. Symptoms of CNS stimulation and sympathetic overactivity are very marked in overdosage with cocaine. A single oral dose of 1.2 g or less may be fatal, but some persons have a cocaine idiosyncrasy and severe toxicity may occur after doses of only 10 mg intravenously. Systemic absorption of small doses may slow the heart, but with increasing doses tachycardia, hypertension, and ventricular fibrillation occur.

High concentrations of cocaine should not be used topically as, in addition to risks of systemic toxicity following absorption, lasting local damage may occur.

Topical application of cocaine to the cornea can cause corneal damage with clouding, pitting, sloughing, and occasionally ulceration. Topical application to the nose or mouth has been reported to cause loss of smell and taste respectively.

Prolonged use of cocaine by nasal inhalation may cause mucosal damage or perforation of the nasal septum.

**Abuse.** Cocaine abuse and its effects have been discussed in a number of reviews.[1-5]

Cocaine abuse was once only in the form of chewing of coca leaves containing small amounts of cocaine, but processing of the leaves has led to abuse with a variety of more dangerous preparations containing higher concentrations of cocaine.[6] Coca paste, produced by maceration of the leaves with petrol and sulfuric acid, contains about 40 to 90% of cocaine sulfate and is smoked with tobacco or cannabis. Treatment of coca paste with hydrochloric acid produces cocaine hydrochloride, which is abused by intravenous injection, either alone or with diamorphine, or by sniffing to achieve nasal absorption. Alkaloidal cocaine (cocaine base; 'freebase'), which is abused by smoking, is produced by treating cocaine hydrochloride with alkali, followed either by heating (to form 'crack' cocaine) or by extracting the base from ether or another organic solvent. The route of administration of cocaine determines the rate and extent of its absorption, although once absorbed, the pharmacokinetics are independent of route. The route of administration rather than the form of cocaine used is important in determining the abuse potential; intravenous cocaine hydrochloride and smoked cocaine base have a greater potential for abuse than intranasal cocaine hydrochloride because of their greater rapidity and intensity of effects.

The psychological effects of cocaine abuse may be described by a cycle of initial euphoria followed by dysphoria and finally schizophreniform psychosis.[6,7] Euphoria may be accompanied by other symptoms of stimulation such as sexual arousal, anorexia, insomnia, hyperexcitability, loquacity, and grandiosity, and users may appear manic. After a short time these feelings are replaced by symptoms of dysphoria including considerable anxiety, fear, depression, apathy, irritability, and suspiciousness. Dysphoria may be ameliorated by repeated administration, so the user develops the need to take the drug continuously to feel relatively well, but repeated administration appears to diminish the intensity of the effects.[6] During euphoria and dysphoria users may experience a wide range of physical symptoms including palpitations, headache, dizziness, gastrointestinal effects, hyperhidrosis, tremors, tachycardia, hypertension, fever, and myoclonic jerks. Seizures can also occur following repeated use. In chronic abusers psychological deterioration may eventually occur, resulting in loss of mental function, compulsive disorders, suicidal ideation, psychopathic disorders, and ultimately a psychosis resembling acute paranoid schizophrenia similar to that seen with amfetamines.[6,7] Symptoms may include paranoia, stereotyped behaviour, delusions, loss of impulse control, violence, and visual, olfactory, auditory, gustatory, and tactile hallucinations. Overdosage can result in death due to status epilepticus, hyperthermia, ventricular tachycardia, and cardiac or respiratory arrest.[6]

For further details of the adverse effects of cocaine abuse, including effects due to use during pregnancy, see below.

1. Johanson C-E, Fischman MW. The pharmacology of cocaine related to its abuse. *Pharmacol Rev* 1989; **41:** 3–52.
2. Warner EA. Cocaine abuse. *Ann Intern Med* 1993: **119:** 226–35.
3. Strang J, *et al.* Cocaine in the UK—1991. *Br J Psychiatry* 1993; **162:** 1–13.
4. Das G. Cocaine abuse in North America: a milestone in history. *J Clin Pharmacol* 1993; **33:** 296–310.
5. Hatsukami DK, Fischman MW. Crack cocaine and cocaine hydrochloride: are the differences myth or reality? *JAMA* 1996; **276:** 1580–8.
6. Arif A, ed. *Adverse health consequences of cocaine abuse.* Geneva: WHO, 1987.
7. Leikin JB, *et al.* Clinical features and management of intoxication due to hallucinogenic drugs. *Med Toxicol Adverse Drug Exp* 1989; **4:** 324–50.

BREAST FEEDING. The American Academy of Pediatrics[1] has stated that, when used as a drug of abuse by breast-feeding mothers, cocaine has caused signs of intoxication in the infant, notably diarrhoea, vomiting, irritability, seizures, and tremulousness.

Acute intoxication has been reported in a breast-fed child whose mother was using cocaine intranasally.[2]

1. American Academy of Pediatrics. The transfer of drugs and other chemicals into human milk. *Pediatrics* 2001; **108:** 776–89. Correction. *ibid.*; 1029. Also available at: http://aappolicy.aappublications.org/cgi/content/full/pediatrics%3b108/3/776 (accessed 02/06/04)
2. Chasnoff IJ, *et al.* Cocaine intoxication in a breast-fed infant. *Pediatrics* 1987; **80:** 836–8.

EFFECTS ON THE BLOOD. References.

1. Leissinger CA. Severe thrombocytopenia associated with cocaine use. *Ann Intern Med* 1990; **112:** 708–10.

EFFECTS ON THE CARDIOVASCULAR SYSTEM. There appears to be no relationship between underlying heart disease and the risk of cocaine-induced cardiac effects and cardiac events can occur regardless of the route of abuse.[1] Cardiovascular toxicity due to cocaine may be related to individual sensitivity and therefore may not be predictable or dose dependent.[2] Patients with plasma cholinesterase deficiency are particularly at risk for sudden death.[3] Other risk factors for cardiovascular disease, such as cigarette smoking or pre-existing atherosclerosis, may exacerbate the cardiac toxicity of cocaine.[4-6] Cocaine blocks reuptake of catecholamines at adrenergic nerve endings and thus produces sympathetic stimulation of the cardiovascular system. Accumulation of catecholamines predisposes the myocardium to arrhythmias,[7] and sinus tachycardia, supraventricular or ventricular tachyarrhythmias, myocarditis, and sudden arrhythmic death may occur.[7-9] Severe hypertension can lead to cerebrovascular accidents and stroke has occurred even in young adults without other predisposing conditions.[10,11] Aortic dissection and rupture of the aorta have also occurred.[6] Up to 25% of emergency admissions to US urban hospitals with nontraumatic chest pain have detectable amounts of cocaine or its metabolites in their urine, but only a minority of these have myocardial infarction,[6] as chest pain without signs of myocardial infarction also commonly occurs.[8] Asymptomatic myocardial ischaemia manifesting as episodes of ST segment elevation has also been reported during withdrawal of cocaine.[12] The mechanism for these changes is probably multifactional, including increased myocardial oxygen demand, coronary vasoconstriction, and enhanced platelet aggregation and thrombus formation.[6] The immediate vasoconstrictor effect of cocaine may be followed by delayed or recurrent vasoconstriction due to its active metabolites, benzoylecgonine and ethyl methyl ecgonine.[6]

Vasoconstriction may also produce ischaemia in the fingers, toes, spinal cord,[8] kidneys,[13] spleen,[14] and intestines.[15] Other reported cardiovascular effects include dilated cardiomyopathy and premature atherosclerosis.[6]

1. VanDette JM, Cornish LA. Medical complications of illicit cocaine use. *Clin Pharm* 1989; **8:** 401–11.
2. Thadani PV. Cardiovascular toxicity of cocaine: underlying mechanisms. *J Appl Cardiol* 1990; **5:** 317–20.
3. Cregler LL, Mark H. Medical complications of cocaine abuse. *N Engl J Med* 1986; **315:** 1495–1500.
4. Moliterno DJ, *et al.* Coronary-artery vasoconstriction induced by cocaine, cigarette smoking, or both. *N Engl J Med* 1994; **330:** 454–9.
5. Higgins ST, *et al.* Influence of cocaine use on cigarette smoking. *JAMA* 1994; **272:** 1724.
6. Lange RA, Hillis LD. Cardiovascular complications of cocaine use. *N Engl J Med* 2001; **345:** 351–8. Correction. *ibid.*; 1432.
7. Loper KA. Clinical toxicology of cocaine. *Med Toxicol Adverse Drug Exp* 1989; **4:** 174–85.
8. Anonymous. Acute reactions to drugs of abuse. *Med Lett Drugs Ther* 1990; **32:** 92–4.
9. Bauman JL, *et al.* Cocaine-related sudden cardiac death: a hypothesis correlating basic science and clinical observations. *J Clin Pharmacol* 1994; **34:** 902–11.
10. Kaku DA, Lowenstein DH. Emergence of recreational drug abuse as a major risk factor for stroke in young adults. *Ann Intern Med* 1990; **113:** 821–7.
11. Levine SR, *et al.* Cerebrovascular complications of the use of the "crack" form of alkaloidal cocaine. *N Engl J Med* 1990; **323:** 699–704.
12. Nademanee K, *et al.* Myocardial ischemia during cocaine withdrawal. *Ann Intern Med* 1989; **111:** 876–80.
13. Sharff JA. Renal infarction associated with intravenous cocaine use. *Ann Emerg Med* 1984; **13:** 1145–7.
14. Novielli KD, Chambers CV. Splenic infarction after cocaine use. *Ann Intern Med* 1991; **114:** 251–2.
15. Freudenberger RS, *et al.* Intestinal infarction after intravenous cocaine administration. *Ann Intern Med* 1990; **113:** 715–16.

EFFECTS ON THE CNS. Severe CNS depression with deep coma has been seen in a few cocaine abusers after prolonged binges.[1]

1. Roberts JR, Greenberg MI. Cocaine washout syndrome. *Ann Intern Med* 2000; **132:** 679–80.

EFFECTS ON THE KIDNEYS. For reference to renal failure following rhabdomyolysis associated with cocaine abuse, see under Effects on the Muscles, below. There has been a report[1] of acute renal failure occurring in a 16-year-old girl secondary to cocaine abuse but without evidence of rhabdomyolysis.

For reference to renal ischaemia due to cocaine abuse, see under Effects on the Cardiovascular System, above.

1. Leblanc M, *et al.* Cocaine-induced acute renal failure without rhabdomyolysis. *Ann Intern Med* 1994; **121:** 721–2.

EFFECTS ON THE LUNGS. Smoking the free base has resulted in a range of pulmonary complications not previously encountered with other methods of abuse for cocaine. Associated adverse effects have included pulmonary oedema, hypersensitivity pneumonitis, pulmonary haemorrhage, obliterative bronchiolitis, abnormalities of pulmonary function, pneumomediastinum, and pneumothorax.[1] Severe or life-threatening exacerbations of asthma have also been reported.[2]

1. Ettinger NA, *et al.* A review of the respiratory effects of smoking cocaine. *Am J Med* 1989; **87:** 664–8.
2. Rubin RB, Neugarten J. Cocaine-associated asthma. *Am J Med* 1990; **88:** 438–9.

EFFECTS ON THE MOUTH. Gingival necrosis following the abuse of cocaine by local application to the gingivae has been reported.[1]

1. Parry J, *et al.* Mucosal lesions due to oral cocaine use. *Br Dent J* 1996; **180:** 462–4.

EFFECTS ON THE MUSCLES. Rhabdomyolysis, sometimes progressing to renal failure, has been associated with free-base smoking or injection of cocaine hydrochloride.[1-3]

1. Roth D, *et al.* Acute rhabdomyolysis associated with cocaine intoxication. *N Engl J Med* 1988; **319:** 673–7.
2. Herzlich BC, *et al.* Rhabdomyolysis related to cocaine abuse. *Ann Intern Med* 1988; **109:** 335–6.
3. Pogue VA, Nurse HM. Cocaine-associated acute myoglobinuric renal failure. *Am J Med* 1989; **86:** 183–6.

EFFECTS ON SEXUAL FUNCTION. While the initial euphoria of cocaine abuse may be accompanied by sexual arousal, sexual dysfunction can occur[1] and male infertility has been reported.[2] Priapism associated with cocaine abuse has also occurred.[3]

1. Cregler LL, Mark H. Medical complications of cocaine abuse. *N Engl J Med* 1986; **315:** 1495–1500.
2. Bracken MB, *et al.* Association of cocaine use with sperm concentration, motility, and morphology. *Fertil Steril* 1990; **53:** 315–22.
3. Altman AL, *et al.* Cocaine associated priapism. *J Urol* 1999; **161:** 1817–18.

EFFECTS ON THE SKIN. Urticarial vasculitis occurred in a young man following intranasal abuse of cocaine.[1]

1. Hofbauer GFL, *et al.* Uritcarial vasculitis following cocaine use. *Br J Dermatol* 1999; **141:** 600–601.

OVERDOSAGE. References to fatal overdosage from cocaine abuse.

1. Greenland VC, *et al.* Vaginally administered cocaine overdose in a pregnant woman. *Obstet Gynecol* 1989; **74:** 476–7.
2. Peretti FJ, *et al.* Cocaine fatality: an unexplained blood concentration in a fatal overdose. *Forensic Sci Int* 1990; **48:** 135–8.
3. Karch SB, *et al.* Relating cocaine blood concentrations to toxicity–an autopsy study of 99 cases. *J Forensic Sci* 1998; **43:** 41–5.

PREGNANCY. The effects of cocaine abuse during pregnancy have been reviewed.[1-3] Women who abuse cocaine during pregnancy appear to have an increased risk of spontaneous abortion,[4] abruptio placentae[5,6] and associated still-births,[7] premature labour,[8-10] and other birth complications.[8-10] These effects may be due to vasoconstriction by cocaine increasing maternal blood pressure and reducing placental blood flow.[11] Uterine rupture[12] during pregnancy and rupture of ectopic pregnancies[13] have also been associated with cocaine. Neonates born to mothers abusing cocaine have an increased risk of intra-uterine growth retardation and may have lower birth-weight, smaller head size, and shorter length.[5,7-9,14-16] Cocaine is possibly teratogenic and congenital abnormalities associated with abuse include cardiovascular abnormalities,[8,17,18] limb reduction defects,[19] intestinal atresia or infarction,[19] skull defects,[7] and genito-urinary tract anomalies.[20] Neurobehavioural impairment[21] and signs of transient CNS irritability[22] may also occur. Some workers[23,24] have found effects on cognition and motor delays while others have found effects on arousal and attention regulation rather than cognitive processes.[25] Cocaine can increase neonatal cerebral blood flow[26] and cerebral infarction and associated seizures have occurred in neonates whose mothers took cocaine near to the onset of labour.[27] Evidence on the risk of intraventricular haemorrhage is conflicting.[6,23]


1. Slutsker L. Risks associated with cocaine use during pregnancy. *Obstet Gynecol* 1992; **79:** 778–89.
2. Volpe JJ. Effects of cocaine use on the fetus. *N Engl J Med* 1992; **327:** 399–407. Correction. *ibid.*; 1039.
3. Wiggins RC. Pharmacokinetics of cocaine in pregnancy and effects on fetal maturation. *Clin Pharmacokinet* 1992; **22:** 85–93.
4. Chasnoff IJ, *et al.* Cocaine use in pregnancy. *N Engl J Med* 1985; **313:** 666–9.
5. Dombrowski MP, *et al.* Cocaine abuse is associated with abruptio placentae and decreased birth weight, but not shorter labor. *Obstet Gynecol* 1991; **77:** 139–41.
6. Dusick AM, *et al.* Risk of intracranial hemorrhage and other adverse outcomes after cocaine exposure in a cohort of 323 very low birth weight infants. *J Pediatr* 1993; **122:** 438–45.
7. Bingol N, *et al.* Teratogenicity of cocaine in humans. *J Pediatr* 1987; **110:** 93–6.
8. Little BB, *et al.* Cocaine abuse during pregnancy: maternal and fetal implications. *Obstet Gynecol* 1989; **73:** 157–60.
9. Mastrogiannis DS, *et al.* Perinatal outcome after recent cocaine usage. *Obstet Gynecol* 1990; **76:** 8–11.
10. Spence MR, *et al.* The relationship between recent cocaine use and pregnancy outcome. *Obstet Gynecol* 1991; **78:** 326–9.
11. Farrar HC, Kearns GL. Cocaine: clinical pharmacology and toxicology. *J Pediatr* 1989; **115:** 665–75.
12. Gonsoulin W, *et al.* Rupture of unscarred uterus in primigravid woman in association with cocaine abuse. *Am J Obstet Gynecol* 1990; **163:** 526–7.
13. Thatcher SS, *et al.* Cocaine use and acute rupture of ectopic pregnancies. *Obstet Gynecol* 1989; **74:** 478–9.
14. Zuckerman B, *et al.* Effects of maternal marijuana and cocaine use on fetal growth. *N Engl J Med* 1989; **320:** 762–8.
15. Chasnoff IJ, *et al.* Temporal patterns of cocaine use in pregnancy: perinatal outcome. *JAMA* 1989; **261:** 1741–4.
16. Little BB, Snell LM. Brain growth among fetuses exposed to cocaine in utero: asymmetrical growth retardation. *Obstet Gynecol* 1991; **77:** 361–4.
17. Lipshultz SE, *et al.* Cardiovascular abnormalities in infants prenatally exposed to cocaine. *J Pediatr* 1991; **118:** 44–51.
18. Shaw GM, *et al.* Maternal use of cocaine during pregnancy and congenital cardiac anomalies. *J Pediatr* 1991; **118:** 167–8.
19. Hoyme HE, *et al.* Prenatal cocaine exposure and fetal vascular disruption. *Pediatrics* 1990; **85:** 743–7.
20. Chávez GF, *et al.* Maternal cocaine use during early pregnancy as a risk factor for congenital urogenital anomalies. *JAMA* 1989; **262:** 795–8.
21. Singer LT, *et al.* Neurobehavioural sequelae of fetal cocaine exposure. *J Pediatr* 1991; **119:** 667–72.
22. Doberczak TM, *et al.* Neonatal neurologic and electroencephalographic effects of intrauterine cocaine exposure. *J Pediatr* 1988; **113:** 354–8.
23. Singer LT, *et al.* Increased incidence of intraventricular hemorrhage and developmental delay in cocaine-exposed, very low birth weight infants. *J Pediatr* 1994; **124:** 765–71.
24. Azuma SD, Chasnoff IJ. Outcome of children prenatally exposed to cocaine and other drugs: a path analysis of three-year data. *Pediatrics* 1993; **92:** 396–402.
25. Mayes LC, *et al.* Information processing and developmental assessments in 3-month-old infants exposed prenatally to cocaine. *Pediatrics* 1995; **95:** 539–45.
26. van der Bor M, *et al.* Increased cerebral blood flow velocity in infants of mothers who abuse cocaine. *Pediatrics* 1990; **85:** 733–6.
27. Chasnoff IJ, *et al.* Perinatal cerebral infarction and maternal cocaine use. *J Pediatr* 1986; **108:** 456–9.


## Treatment of Adverse Effects

As for Local Anaesthetics in general, p.1368.

**Cocaine overdosage.** In the emergency management of overdosage with cocaine the general aims are to establish adequate ventilation and support the circulation. If oral ingestion of a large amount is suspected the stomach should be emptied and activated charcoal administered.[1] A tourniquet may be applied to limit absorption if the drug was injected. Patients who have swallowed packages containing cocaine for the purpose of smuggling, may be given laxatives but surgical intervention may be required if signs of toxicity appear.[2]

Sedation with intravenous diazepam may be sufficient to manage the symptoms of cocaine overdose. Sedation with benzodiazepines may also be appropriate initial therapy for hypertension or tachyarrhythmias since the excessive sympathetic tone is largely centrally mediated.[3] Severe life-threatening arrhythmias may require treatment with intravenous propranolol although, following a report of paradoxical hypertension presumably due to unopposed α-adrenergic stimulation, a beta blocker with both α- and β-adrenergic effects such as labetalol is preferred by some if hypertension is also present;[2,4] sodium nitroprusside[3,4] or phentolamine[3,5] may also be used. Although labetalol can reduce the hypertension it does not alleviate cocaine-induced coronary vasoconstriction;[6] it has therefore been suggested that glyceryl trinitrate would be preferable for patients with cocaine-induced chest pain.[5,6] Chest pain may also be treated with aspirin. Calcium-channel blockers such as verapamil may also be of use as an antagonist for coronary artery vasoconstriction induced by cocaine.[5] There is concern about the use of lidocaine for the treatment of cocaine-induced arrhythmias as lidocaine may enhance toxicity.[5] Diazepam should be used to manage seizures[1,4] but if they cannot be controlled phenytoin can be used as an adjunct.[1] Hyperthermia should be treated with physical cooling but the use of dantrolene may also be necessary.[1] Control of anxiety and agitation with benzodiazepines when combined with rapid cooling may also have the effect of decreasing heat production in hyperthermic patients.[3] Metabolic acidosis should be monitored and treated where necessary.[1,4] Short-acting barbiturates or benzodiazepines may be used for dysphoric agitation but drugs that lower the seizure threshold or aggravate hyperthermia such as phenothiazines or haloperidol should be avoided.[1]


1. Loper KA. Clinical toxicology of cocaine. *Med Toxicol Adverse Drug Exp* 1989; **4:** 174–85.
2. Ramrakha P, Barton I. Drug smuggler's delirium. *BMJ* 1993; **306:** 470–1.
3. Anonymous. Acute reactions to drugs of abuse. *Med Lett Drugs Ther* 1996; **38:** 43–6.
4. Farrar HC, Kearns GL. Cocaine: clinical pharmacology and toxicology. *J Pediatr* 1989; **115:** 665–75.
5. Hollander JE. The management of cocaine-associated myocardial ischemia. *N Engl J Med* 1995; **333:** 1267–72.
6. Boehrer JD, *et al.* Influence of labetalol on cocaine-induced coronary vasoconstriction in humans. *Am J Med* 1993; **94:** 608–10.


**Withdrawal.** Cocaine can produce psychological dependence but does not produce a major physical withdrawal syndrome. The management of cocaine abuse and dependence has been reviewed.[1-3] There is no advantage to gradual withdrawal and it is best for the patient to discontinue the drug abruptly.[1,4] The three major psychiatric complications associated with cocaine withdrawal are dysphoric agitation, severe depression, and psychotic symptoms.[1] Such complications are initially managed with psychosocial treatments. However patients with more severe dependence or those who fail to respond to psychosocial treatments should be considered for drug therapies. Dysphoric agitation is best treated with diazepam; propranolol may also be used in more persistent cases. Depressive symptoms during the acute post-cocaine phase are usually transient and require no treatment other than close observation. Desipramine has been used with equivocal results; it appears to be of most benefit in patients who have antecedent or consequent symptoms of severe depression.[3] Trazodone and imipramine have also been tried but had more adverse effects than desipramine.[3] Antipsychotics such as chlorpromazine, haloperidol, and promazine have been used successfully to manage patients with psychotic symptoms associated with cocaine dependence.[1]

Several drugs have been tried in the maintenance of abstinence from cocaine.[1] Lithium may be useful in patients with bipolar disorder or cyclothymic personality. Methylphenidate may be helpful in patients with attention deficit disorders but has potential for abuse itself. Phenothiazine derivatives have been tried in the control of impulsive behaviour and to decrease cocaine craving, although adverse effects may limit their acceptability. Carbamazepine has been reported to suppress the craving for cocaine although this has not been supported by subsequent trials.[3] Buprenorphine has been investigated to suppress cocaine and opioid use in patients dependent on both drugs.[3] Anxiolytics or antidepressants are considered unlikely to be of benefit in maintaining abstinence.[3] MAOIs such as phenelzine have been used in a manner analogous to the use of disulfiram in alcohol abuse to provoke unpleasant reactions if patients relapse.[5]

There is evidence to suggest that cocaine use affects the dopaminergic modulation of CNS function, and several drugs that interact with the dopamine system have been tried in the treatment of cocaine abuse and dependence, but with mixed results.[3]


1. Arif A, ed. *Adverse health consequences of cocaine abuse.* Geneva: WHO, 1987.
2. Kleber HD. Pharmacotherapy, current and potential, for the treatment of cocaine dependence. *Clin Neuropharmacol* 1995; **18** (suppl 1): S96–S109.
3. Mendelson JH, Mello NK. Management of cocaine abuse and dependence. *N Engl J Med* 1996; **334:** 965–72.
4. DoH. *Drug misuse and dependence: guidelines on clinical management.* London: HMSO, 1999. Also available at: http://www.dh.gov.uk/assetRoot/04/07/81/98/04078198.pdf (accessed 02/06/04)
5. Brewer C. Cocaine and crack. *BMJ* 1989; **299:** 792.


## Precautions

As for Local Anaesthetics in general, p.1368.

Since some patients have a marked sensitivity to cocaine the administration of a test dose before use on mucous membranes has been suggested. Cocaine should not be applied to damaged mucosa because of the risk of systemic toxicity from enhanced absorption. Ophthalmic preparations of cocaine should not be applied to the eyes for prolonged periods as damage to the cornea may occur not only from the local action of cocaine, but also from loss of the protective eyelid reflexes. As with other mydriatics, there is also a risk of cocaine precipitating angle-closure glaucoma in patients predisposed to the condition. Patients receiving cocaine for surface anaesthesia should be monitored for possible cardiovascular effects. Cocaine should be used with great caution in patients with hypertension, cardiovascular disease, or thyrotoxicosis. It is not recommended for use during pregnancy or breast feeding.

**Abuse.** Cocaine is subject to abuse. See under Adverse Effects, above.

**Gilles de la Tourette's syndrome.** Gilles de la Tourette's syndrome, which had been well controlled for 10 years by haloperidol, was precipitated in a 27-year-old man following intranasal use of cocaine on one occasion.[1]


1. Mesulam M-M. Cocaine and Tourette's syndrome. *N Engl J Med* 1986; **315:** 398.


**Myasthenia gravis.** Report of a patient in whom cocaine abuse first unmasked and then exacerbated myasthenia gravis.[1]


1. Berciano J, *et al.* Myasthenia gravis unmasked by cocaine abuse. *N Engl J Med* 1991; **325:** 892.


**Porphyria.** Cocaine has been associated with acute attacks of porphyria and is considered unsafe in porphyric patients.

## Interactions

For interactions associated with local anaesthetics, see p.1368.

Cocaine and adrenaline enhance each other's sympathomimetic effects and should preferably not be used together. Caution is needed if cocaine is used with other drugs that may also potentiate the action of catecholamines such as guanethidine or MAOIs.

**Adrenaline.** In a report[1] of 3 cases of arrhythmias associated with the use of a paste containing cocaine 25% and adrenaline 0.18% for local anaesthesia of the nasal mucosa, the amount of cocaine applied to the nasal mucosa ranged from about 2.5 to 4.5 mg/kg. The maximum recommended dose of cocaine alone in healthy adults is 1.5 mg/kg.


1. Nicholson KEA, Rogers JEG. Cocaine and adrenaline paste: a fatal combination? *BMJ* 1995; **311:** 250–1.


**Alcohol.** In the presence of alcohol, cocaine is metabolised to its ethyl homologue cocaethylene.[1] Cocaethylene appears to have the same stimulant effects as cocaine but it has a longer half-life and *animal* studies suggest that it is more toxic than the parent drug. However, a review of the literature concluded that the use of cocaine with alcohol did not cause more cardiovascular problems than expected from the additive effects of each drug.[2]


1. Randall T. Cocaine, alcohol mix in body to form even longer lasting, more lethal drug. *JAMA* 1992; **267:** 1043–4.
2. Pennings EJM, *et al.* Effects of concurrent use of alcohol and cocaine. *Addiction* 2002; **97:** 773–83.


**Beta blockers.** *Propranolol* potentiated cocaine-induced coronary vasoconstriction following intranasal administration of cocaine in a placebo-controlled study.[1] Because of a possible risk of paradoxical hypertension associated with the use of propranolol to manage arrhythmias associated with cocaine overdosage some prefer the use of labetalol for this indication (see under Treatment of Adverse Effects, above).


1. Lange RA, *et al.* Potentiation of cocaine-induced coronary vasoconstriction by beta-adrenergic blockade. *Ann Intern Med* 1990; **112:** 897–903.


**Haloperidol.** For the effect of cocaine on haloperidol, see under Chlorpromazine, p.680.

## Pharmacokinetics

Cocaine may be slowly absorbed from some sites because of the vasoconstriction it produces, but absorption occurs from all sites of application, including mucous membranes and the gastrointestinal tract, and may be enhanced when there is inflammation. Cocaine is rapidly absorbed when smoked.

Cocaine is rapidly metabolised by plasma esterases and hepatic esterases to ecgonine methyl ester. Benzoylecgonine, another major metabolite of cocaine, may be produced by spontaneous hydrolysis. Cocaine is also demethylated to the active metabolite norcocaine which is not excreted but undergoes further metabolism. There is considerable interindividual variation in the plasma half-life of cocaine possibly due to differences in esterase activity.

Cocaine and its metabolites are excreted in the urine, about 10% appearing as unchanged drug; they may be detectable in urine for several days or even weeks after administration. Cocaine crosses the blood-brain barrier and accumulates within the CNS. It does not appear to undergo rapid metabolism within the brain and concentrations in the CNS following acute intoxication may greatly exceed those in plasma.

Cocaine crosses the placenta and the presence of its metabolites in neonatal hair has been used to indicate intra-uterine exposure. Cocaine is distributed into breast milk.

See also under Local Anaesthetics, p.1368.

◊ References.


1. Busto U, *et al.* Clinical pharmacokinetics of non-opiate abused drugs. *Clin Pharmacokinet* 1989; **16:** 1–26.
2. Graham K, *et al.* Determination of gestational cocaine exposure by hair analysis. *JAMA* 1989; **262:** 3328–30.
3. Burke WM, Ravi NV. Urinary excretion of cocaine. *Ann Intern Med* 1990; **112:** 548–9.

4. Ravi NV, Burke WM. Cocaine and traffic accident fatalities in New York City. *JAMA* 1990; **263:** 2887.
5. Schenker S, *et al.* The transfer of cocaine and its metabolites across the term human placenta. *Clin Pharmacol Ther* 1993; **53:** 329–39.

**Absorption.** Cocaine is rapidly absorbed from the pulmonary vasculature when smoked and the speed of onset of its effects is similar to that obtained after intravenous injection.[1] Absorption from mucous membranes is delayed by vasoconstriction and peak plasma concentrations of up to 474 nanograms/mL have been obtained 15 to 120 minutes after application of doses of 1.5 to 2 mg/kg to the nasal mucosa as a 10% cocaine hydrochloride solution;[2,3] cocaine may still be detectable in the nose several hours later and this may result in prolonged systemic absorption.[2] In a study it was estimated that only 5% of the total dose of cocaine hydrochloride used prior to nasal surgery was absorbed from the nasal mucosa following application of 500 mg of cocaine hydrochloride as a 25% paste with adrenaline or 200 mg as a 10% solution with adrenaline (Moffett's solution) and blood concentrations were well below those associated with toxicity[4] (but see also Adrenaline, under Interactions, above). Peak serum concentrations of cocaine have been obtained after 50 to 90 minutes following oral administration and are similar to those obtained after nasal application.[3]

1. Farrar HC, Kearns GL. Cocaine: clinical pharmacology and toxicology. *J Pediatr* 1989; **115:** 665–75.
2. Van Dyke C, *et al.* Cocaine: plasma concentrations after intranasal application in man. *Science* 1976; **191:** 859–61.
3. Van Dyke C, *et al.* Oral cocaine: plasma concentrations and central effects. *Science* 1978; **200:** 211–13.
4. Quiney RE. Intranasal topical cocaine: Moffett's method or topical cocaine paste? *J Laryngol Otol* 1986; **100:** 279–83.

## Uses and Administration

Cocaine, a benzoic acid ester, is a local anaesthetic with actions and uses similar to those described on p.1369. It is used as a surface anaesthetic but, because of systemic adverse effects and its abuse potential, its use is now almost entirely restricted to surgery of the ear, nose, and throat. It has been largely replaced by other drugs in ophthalmology because of its corneal toxicity, although it may still be useful in removal or debridement of the corneal epithelium. Cocaine also blocks the uptake of catecholamines at adrenergic nerve endings and potentiates the action of catecholamines. Its sympathomimetic actions cause tachycardia, peripheral vasoconstriction, a rise in blood pressure, and mydriasis. The use of cocaine with sympathomimetics such as adrenaline increases the risk of cardiac arrhythmias. Despite this hazard some use this combination in otolaryngology to improve the operative field and reduce absorption.

When applied to mucous membranes, surface anaesthesia develops rapidly and persists for 30 minutes or longer depending on the concentration of cocaine used, the dose, and on the vascularity of the tissue.

Cocaine hydrochloride is used for the administration of cocaine in aqueous solutions; cocaine hydrochloride 1.12 g is approximately equivalent to 1 g of cocaine. Solutions containing up to 4% have been used in ophthalmology (but see Precautions, above).

Solutions containing up to 10% of cocaine are applied to the nasal mucosa in otolaryngological procedures. Pastes containing up to 25% of cocaine have also been applied.

In order to avoid systemic effects, the usual maximum total dose recommended for application to the nasal mucosa in healthy adults is 1.5 mg/kg. It should be used only by those skilled in the precautions needed to minimise absorption and the consequent risk of arrhythmias.

Cocaine was used with diamorphine or morphine for the relief of severe pain, especially in terminal illness, but this use is now obsolete.

Cocaine solutions should *never* be given by injection; other local anaesthetics are equally effective and much safer.

◊ References.

1. Middleton RM, Kirkpatrick MB. Clinical use of cocaine: a review of the risks and benefits. *Drug Safety* 1993; **9:** 212–17.
2. Latorre F, Klimek L. Does cocaine still have a role in nasal surgery? *Drug Safety* 1999; **20:** 9–13.

### Preparations

***USP 27:*** Cocaine and Tetracaine Hydrochlorides and Epinephrine Topical Solution; Cocaine Hydrochloride Tablets for Topical Solution.

## Diperodon Hydrochloride *(BANM, rINNM)*

Diperocaine Hydrochloride; Hidrocloruro de diperodón. 3-Piperidinopropylene bis(phenylcarbamate) hydrochloride.

$C_{22}H_{27}N_3O_4,HCl = 433.9.$

*CAS — 101-08-6 (anhydrous diperodon); 51552-99-9 (diperodon monohydrate); 537-12-2 (diperodon hydrochloride).*

### Profile

Diperodon is a local anaesthetic (p.1367) that has been used as the base or the hydrochloride for surface anaesthesia.

### Preparations

**Proprietary Preparations** (details are given in Part 3)

**Multi-ingredient:** ***USA:*** Bactine First Aid Antibiotic Plus Anesthetic†.

## Dyclonine Hydrochloride *(BANM, rINNM)*

Dyclocaine Hydrochloride; Dyclocaini Chloridum; Hidrocloruro de diclonina. 4′-Butoxy-3-piperidinopropiophenone hydrochloride.

$C_{18}H_{27}NO_2,HCl = 325.9.$

*CAS — 586-60-7 (dyclonine); 536-43-6 (dyclonine hydrochloride).*

*ATC — N01BX02; R02AD04.*

**Pharmacopoeias.** In *US.*

**USP 27** (Dyclonine Hydrochloride). White crystals or white crystalline powder, with a slight odour. Soluble 1 in 60 of water, 1 in 24 of alcohol, and 1 in 2.3 of chloroform; soluble in acetone; practically insoluble in ether and in hexane. A 1% solution in water has a pH of 4.0 to 7.0. Store in airtight containers. Protect from light.

### Profile

Dyclonine hydrochloride is a local anaesthetic (p.1367) used topically for surface anaesthesia of the skin and mucous membranes in concentrations of 0.5 or 1%. Single doses in excess of 200 mg should generally not be used. Lozenges containing up to 3 mg have been used for the temporary relief of pain associated with sore throats or mouth irritation. It may cause irritation at the site of application and should not be given by injection or used in the eyes.

### Preparations

***USP 27:*** Dyclonine Hydrochloride Gel; Dyclonine Hydrochloride Topical Solution.

**Proprietary Preparations** (details are given in Part 3)

***Canad.:*** Sucrets; Sucrets for Kids; ***Israel:*** Childrens Cherry Sucrets; Sucrets Children's Formula; Sucrets Maximum Strength; ***USA:*** Dyclone†; Sucrets.

**Multi-ingredient:** ***Canad.:*** Skin Shield†; Tanac; ***USA:*** Cepacol Maximum Strength Sore Throat; Skin Shield; Tanac.

## Ethyl Chloride

Aethylium Chloratum; Chlorethyl; Cloruro de etilo; Ethylis Chloridum; Hydrochloric Ether; Monochlorethane. Chloroethane.

$C_2H_5Cl = 64.51.$

*CAS — 75-00-3.*

*ATC — N01BX01.*

**Pharmacopoeias.** In *Pol.* and *US.*

**USP 27** (Ethyl Chloride). A colourless, mobile, very volatile liquid at low temperatures or under pressure, with a characteristic ethereal odour. B.p. 12° to 13°. Slightly soluble in water; freely soluble in alcohol and in ether. Store in airtight containers, preferably hermetically sealed.

**Stability.** Ethyl chloride is highly flammable and mixtures of the gas with 5 to 15% of air are explosive.

### Adverse Effects and Precautions

As for Chloroform, p.1296.

Cutaneous sensitisation can occur rarely. Thawing of frozen tissue following surgery may be painful and prolonged spraying onto the skin can cause chemical frostbite. Freezing may also distort the histological structure of biopsy specimens. Ethyl chloride should not be applied to broken skin or mucous membranes.

### Uses and Administration

Owing to its low boiling-point and the intense cold produced by evaporation, ethyl chloride has been used as a local anaesthetic in minor surgery but such use is not generally recommended. It has also been used topically for the relief of pain and to test the effectiveness of regional anaesthesia. Ethyl chloride was formerly used as an inhalational anaesthetic but has no place in modern anaesthetic practice.

### Preparations

**Proprietary Preparations** (details are given in Part 3)

***Denm.:*** Kloraetyl†; ***Ger.:*** Chloraethyl "Dr Henning"; Holsten aktiv†; WariActiv; ***Hong Kong:*** WariActiv; ***Mex.:*** Traumazol; ***Spain:*** Cloretilo Chemirosa; ***Switz.:*** Chlorethyl; ***UK:*** Cryogesic.

**Multi-ingredient:** ***Ger.:*** Olbas; ***USA:*** Fluro-Ethyl.

## Ethyl *p*-Piperidinoacetylaminobenzoate

EPAB; *p*-Piperidinoacetilaminobenzoato de etilo; SA-7. 4-[(1-Piperidinylacetyl)amino]benzoic acid ethyl ester.

$C_{16}H_{22}N_2O_3 = 290.4.$

*CAS — 41653-21-8.*

### Profile

Ethyl *p*-piperidinoacetylaminobenzoate is an amide local anaesthetic (p.1367) that has been given by mouth for the symptomatic relief of gastritis.

### Preparations

**Proprietary Preparations** (details are given in Part 3)

***Jpn:*** Sulcain.

**Multi-ingredient:** ***Hong Kong:*** Sulcain; ***Singapore:*** Sulcain; ***Thai.:*** Sulcain.

## Etidocaine *(BAN, USAN, rINN)*

(±)-2-(*N*-Ethylpropylamino)-butyro-2′,6′-xylidide.

$C_{17}H_{28}N_2O = 276.4.$

*CAS — 36637-18-0.*

*ATC — N01BB07.*

## Etidocaine Hydrochloride *(BANM, rINNM)*

Hidrocloruro de etidocaína; W-19053.

$C_{17}H_{28}N_2O,HCl = 312.9.$

*CAS — 36637-19-1.*

*ATC — N01BB07.*

### Adverse Effects, Treatment, and Precautions

As for Local Anaesthetics in general, p.1367.

**Effects on the cardiovascular system.** For a discussion of the cardiotoxicity of etidocaine, see under the Adverse Effects of Bupivacaine Hydrochloride, p.1371.

**Porphyria.** Etidocaine is considered to be unsafe in patients with porphyria because it has been shown to be porphyrinogenic in *animals*.

### Interactions

For interactions associated with local anaesthetics, see p.1368.

### Pharmacokinetics

Etidocaine is rapidly absorbed into the circulation after parenteral injection and is about 95% bound to plasma proteins. It crosses the placenta but the ratio of fetal to maternal concentrations is relatively low. It also diffuses across the blood-brain barrier. Etidocaine is metabolised in the liver and its numerous metabolites are excreted in the urine; less than 10% of the drug is excreted unchanged. The plasma elimination half-life of etidocaine is 2 to 3 hours in adults.

See also under Local Anaesthetics, p.1368.

**Pregnancy.** Following maternal injection etidocaine rapidly crosses the placenta[1] but the degree of transfer is less than for other local anaesthetics including bupivacaine.[2] The ratio of fetal to maternal concentrations of etidocaine varies but values up to about 0.35 are usual.[1,2] Some metabolites appear to be transferred to a greater degree than the parent compound[1]. Etidocaine is highly protein bound but the fraction of unbound drug in plasma increases in pregnant women during delivery.[1] Protein binding of etidocaine is also reduced in fetal plasma.[3] Although neonates are able to metabolise etidocaine it appears that they are less able to do so than adults; a mean elimination half-life of 6.42 hours has been reported in neonates.[3]

1. Morgan DJ, *et al.* Disposition and placental transfer of etidocaine in pregnancy. *Eur J Clin Pharmacol* 1977; **12:** 359–65.
2. Poppers PJ. Evaluation of local anaesthetic agents for regional anaesthesia in obstetrics. *Br J Anaesth* 1975; **47:** 322–7.
3. Morgan D, *et al.* Pharmacokinetics and metabolism of the anilide local anaesthetics in neonates: 11: etidocaine. *Eur J Clin Pharmacol* 1978; **13:** 365–71.

### Uses and Administration

Etidocaine hydrochloride is a local anaesthetic of the amide type with actions and uses similar to those described on p.1369. It has a rapid onset and a long duration of action. Etidocaine has been used for infiltration anaesthesia, peripheral nerve block, and epidural block, usually with adrenaline 1 in 200 000. (Local anaesthetic techniques are discussed on p.1370.)

### Preparations

**Proprietary Preparations** (details are given in Part 3)

***Fr.:*** Duranest†; ***Ger.:*** Duranest†; ***USA:*** Duranest†.

## Fomocaine Hydrochloride *(BANM, rINNM)*

4-[3-(α-Phenoxy-*p*-tolyl)propyl]morpholine hydrochloride.

$C_{20}H_{25}NO_2,HCl = 347.9.$

*CAS — 17692-39-6 (fomocaine); 56583-43-8 (fomocaine hydrochloride).*

### Profile

Fomocaine is a local anaesthetic that has been included, as the hydrochloride, in mixed products intended for use in infected skin conditions.

### Preparations

**Proprietary Preparations** (details are given in Part 3)

**Multi-ingredient: Ger.:** Pellit dermal Wund- und Heilsalbe†.

### Ketocaine Hydrochloride *(rINNM)*

Chetocaina Cloridrata; Hidrocloruro de ketocaína. 2′-(2-Di-isopropylaminoethoxy)butyrophenone hydrochloride.

$C_{18}H_{29}NO_2,HCl = 327.9.$

*CAS — 1092-46-2 (ketocaine); 1092-47-3 (ketocaine hydrochloride).*

#### Profile

Ketocaine hydrochloride is a local anaesthetic (p.1367) that has been used as a surface anaesthetic in suppositories or ointments for anorectal disorders.

#### Preparations

**Proprietary Preparations** (details are given in Part 3)

**Multi-ingredient: Ital.:** Proctolyn.

## Levobupivacaine *(BAN, rINN)*

S(−)-Bupivacaine; Levobupivacaína; Lévobupivacaïne. (S)-1-Butyl-2-piperidylformo-2′,6′-xylidide.

$C_{18}H_{28}N_2O = 288.4.$

*CAS — 27262-47-1.*

*ATC — N01BB10.*

### Levobupivacaine Hydrochloride *(BANM, USAN, rINNM)*

Hidrocloruro de levobupivacaína.

$C_{18}H_{28}N_2O,HCl = 324.9.$

*CAS — 27262-48-2.*

*ATC — N01BB10.*

#### Adverse Effects, Treatment, and Precautions

As for Local Anaesthetics in general, p.1367.

Levobupivacaine is contra-indicated for use in intravenous regional anaesthesia (Bier's block) and for paracervical block in obstetrics. The 0.75% solution is also contra-indicated for epidural block in obstetrics.

**Effects on the cardiovascular system.** It has been suggested[1] that levobupivacaine may have a lower risk of causing cardiotoxicity than bupivacaine (for the effects of bupivacaine on the cardiovascular system see p.1371).

1. Mather LE, Chang DH. Cardiotoxicity with modern local anaesthetics: is there a safer choice? *Drugs* 2001; **61:** 333–42.

#### Interactions

For interactions associated with local anaesthetics, see p.1368. Plasma concentrations of levobupivacaine may be reduced by enzyme-inducing drugs such as rifampicin. Levobupivacaine is metabolised by the cytochrome P450 isoenzymes CYP3A4 and CYP1A2 and there is a theoretical possibility that substrates for or inhibitors of these isoenzymes may adversely alter plasma concentrations of levobupivacaine.

#### Pharmacokinetics

The pharmacokinetics of levobupivacaine are similar to those of the racemic form, bupivacaine (p.1371). Levobupivacaine is at least 97% bound to plasma proteins. After intravenous administration the mean half-life is about 80 minutes. Levobupivacaine is extensively metabolised and excreted as its metabolites mainly in the urine, with smaller amounts appearing in the faeces. 3-Hydroxylevobupivacaine is a major metabolite and its formation is mediated by the cytochrome P450 isoenzyme CYP1A2; the isoenzyme CYP3A4 is also involved in the metabolism of levobupivacaine.

#### Uses and Administration

Levobupivacaine is a local anaesthetic of the amide type with actions and uses similar to those described on p.1369. It is the S-enantiomer of bupivacaine (p.1371). Levobupivacaine is given as the hydrochloride for infiltration anaesthesia and regional nerve blocks including epidural block; however it is contra-indicated for obstetric paracervical block and for use in intravenous regional anaesthesia (Bier's block). The 0.75% solution is also contra-indicated for epidural blocks in obstetrics. (Local anaesthetic techniques are discussed on p.1370.)

Levobupivacaine hydrochloride is available in solutions containing the equivalent of 0.25 to 0.75% of levobupivacaine. The dosage depends on the site of injection and the procedure used as well as the status of the patient. The recommended **maximum single dose** is 150 mg. The total daily dose should not exceed 400 mg. A test dose of a suitable local anaesthetic, preferably with adrenaline, should be given before commencing epidural block with levobupivacaine to detect inadvertent intravascular administration. Subsequent doses of levobupivacaine should be given in small increments. Bupivacaine should be given in reduced doses to elderly, debilitated, or acutely ill patients.

- For **surgical anaesthesia** doses of levobupivacaine for *epidural block* are 50 to 100 mg (10 to 20 mL) as a 0.5% solution, or 75 to 150 mg (10 to 20 mL) as a 0.75% solution; for caesarean section, doses are 75 to 150 mg (15 to 30 mL) as a 0.5% solution. The dose for *spinal block* is 15 mg (3 mL) as a 0.5% solution.
- For *peripheral nerve blocks*, doses are 2.5 to 150 mg as a 0.25 or 0.5% solution; a volume of 40 mL should not be exceeded. Alternatively doses for peripheral block may be expressed on the basis of body-weight: 1 to 2 mg/kg (0.4 mL/kg) as a 0.25 or 0.5% solution.
- For *infiltration anaesthesia* up to 150 mg (60 mL) as a 0.25% solution may be used. For peribulbar block in *ophthalmic* procedures 37.5 to 112.5 mg (5 to 15 mL) as a 0.75% solution may be given. For ilioinguinal or iliohypogastric blocks in **children** under 12 years, doses of levobupivacaine are 1.25 to 2.5 mg/kg (0.25 to 0.5 mL/kg) as a 0.25 or 0.5% solution.
- In the management of **acute pain** it may be given as an epidural bolus or by continuous infusion. For pain relief during *labour* 15 to 50 mg (6 to 20 mL) as a 0.25% solution is given as a bolus. Alternatively, a 0.125% solution may be given as an infusion in a dose of 5 to 12.5 mg (4 to 10 mL) per hour, or a 0.0625% solution may be given in a dose of 5 to 12.5 mg (8 to 20 mL) per hour. For *postoperative pain* 10 to 25 mg (4 to 10 mL) per hour as a 0.25% solution, 12.5 to 18.75 mg (10 to 15 mL) per hour as a 0.125% solution, or 12.5 to 18.75 mg (20 to 30 mL) per hour as a 0.0625% solution may be given as an epidural infusion.

In some countries such as the UK, the manufacturers recommend that a lower concentration such as the 0.125% solution should be used if other analgesics are also given for pain relief; the US manufacturers specifically state that the 0.125% solution should only be used for adjunctive therapy with fentanyl or clonidine. When necessary, dilutions should be made with sodium chloride 0.9%.

◊ Reviews

1. Foster RH, Markham A. Levobupivacaine: a review of its pharmacology and use as a local anaesthetic. *Drugs* 2000; **59:** 551–79.

**Action.** A comparison[1] of epidural bupivacaine with levobupivacaine in women in labour found that levobupivacaine had 98% of the potency of the racemate, a clinically insignificant difference. However it was pointed out that whereas the concentration of bupivacaine solutions was expressed in terms of the hydrochloride, solutions of levobupivacaine had their strength expressed in terms of the free base. When calculations were made in terms of molar equivalents levobupivacaine appeared to be 13% less potent than racemic bupivacaine. The difference in expression should be borne in mind when evaluating comparative studies.

1. Lyons G, *et al.* Epidural pain relief in labour: potencies of levobupivacaine and racemic bupivacaine. *Br J Anaesth* 1998; **81:** 899–901.

#### Preparations

**Proprietary Preparations** (details are given in Part 3)

***Austral.:*** Chirocaine; ***Austria:*** Chirocaine; ***Belg.:*** Chirocaine; ***Braz.:*** Chirocaine†; Novabupi; ***Fin.:*** Chirocaine; ***Gr.:*** Chirocaine; ***Irl.:*** Chirocaine; ***Ital.:*** Chirocaine; ***Neth.:*** Chirocaine; ***NZ:*** Chirocaine; ***Swed.:*** Chirocaine; ***UK:*** Chirocaine; ***USA:*** Chirocaine.

## Lidocaine *(BAN, rINN)*

Lidocaína; Lidocainum; Lignocaine. 2-Diethylaminoaceto-2′,6′-xylidide.

$C_{14}H_{22}N_2O = 234.3.$

*CAS — 137-58-6.*

*ATC — C01BB01; C05AD01; D04AB01; N01BB02; R02AD02; S01HA07; S02DA01.*

**Pharmacopoeias.** In *Eur.* (see p.vi), *Int., Jpn, Pol.,* and *US.*

**Ph. Eur. 5.0** (Lidocaine). A white or almost white, crystalline powder. M.p. 66° to 70°. Practically insoluble in water; very soluble in alcohol and in dichloromethane.

**USP 27** (Lidocaine). A white to slightly yellow crystalline powder with a characteristic odour. M.p. 66° to 69°. Practically insoluble in water; very soluble in alcohol and in chloroform; freely soluble in ether and in benzene; dissolves in oils.

**Eutectic mixture.** Lidocaine forms a mixture with prilocaine that has a melting-point lower than that of either ingredient. This eutectic mixture is used in the preparation of topical dosage forms.

### Lidocaine Hydrochloride *(BANM, rINNM)*

Hidrocloruro de lidocaína; Lidocaini Hydrochloridum; Lignoc. Hydrochlor.; Lignocaine Hydrochloride.

$C_{14}H_{22}N_2O,HCl,H_2O = 288.8.$

*CAS — 73-78-9 (anhydrous lidocaine hydrochloride); 6108-05-0 (lidocaine hydrochloride monohydrate).*

*ATC — C01BB01; C05AD01; D04AB01; N01BB02; R02AD02; S01HA07; S02DA01.*

NOTE. LIDFLN is a code approved by the BP 2003 for use on single unit doses of eye drops containing lidocaine hydrochloride and fluorescein sodium where the individual container may be too small to bear all the appropriate labelling information.

**Pharmacopoeias.** In *Chin., Eur.* (see p.vi), *Int., Pol., US,* and *Viet.*

**Ph. Eur. 5.0** (Lidocaine Hydrochloride). A white crystalline powder. M.p. 74° to 79°. Very soluble in water; freely soluble in alcohol. A 0.5% solution in water has a pH of 4.0 to 5.5. Protect from light.

**USP 27** (Lidocaine Hydrochloride). A white, odourless, crystalline powder. M.p. 74° to 79°. Very soluble in water and in alcohol; soluble in chloroform; insoluble in ether.

**Incompatibility.** Lidocaine hydrochloride has been reported to be incompatible in solution with amphotericin B,[1] sulfadiazine sodium,[2] methohexital sodium,[2] cefazolin sodium,[3] or phenytoin sodium.[4]

Acid stable drugs such as adrenaline hydrochloride, noradrenaline acid tartrate, or isoprenaline may begin to deteriorate within several hours of admixture with lidocaine hydrochloride as lidocaine solutions may raise the pH of the final solution above the maximum pH for their stability. Such extemporaneous mixtures should be used promptly after preparation.[5]

1. Whiting DA. Treatment of chromoblastomycosis with high local concentrations of amphotericin B. *Br J Dermatol* 1967; **79:** 345–51.
2. Riley BB. Incompatibilities in intravenous solutions. *J Hosp Pharm* 1970; **28:** 228–40.
3. Kleinberg ML, *et al.* Stability of antibiotics frozen and stored in disposable hypodermic syringes. *Am J Hosp Pharm* 1980; **37:** 1087–8.
4. Kirschenbaum HL, *et al.* Stability and compatibility of lidocaine hydrochloride with selected large-volume parenterals and drug additives. *Am J Hosp Pharm* 1982; **39:** 1013–15.
5. Parker EA. Xylocaine hydrochloride 2% injection. *Am J Hosp Pharm* 1971; **28:** 805.

**pH of solutions.** For the effect pH has on the surface tension and administration of lidocaine solutions by infusion, see under Administration in Uses and Administration, p.1369. For its effect on the stability of local anaesthetic solutions and the pain associated with their injection, see p.1369.

**Stability.** Although there was no decrease in the lidocaine content of lidocaine hydrochloride and adrenaline injection during transport and storage under tropical conditions, the content of adrenaline fell to almost zero in some samples after several months; supply of the injection as a dry powder and separate solvent should be considered for the tropics.[1]

The lidocaine content of buffered cardioplegic solutions has been reported[2] to decrease when stored in PVC containers at ambient temperature, but not when stored at 4°. This loss appeared to result from pH-dependent sorption of lidocaine onto the plastic and did not occur when lidocaine solutions were stored in glass bottles.

1. Abu-Reid IO, *et al.* Stability of drugs in the tropics: a study in Sudan. *Int Pharm J* 1990; **4:** 6–10.
2. Lackner TE, *et al.* Lidocaine stability in cardioplegic solution stored in glass bottles and polyvinyl chloride bags. *Am J Hosp Pharm* 1983; **40:** 97–101.

#### Adverse Effects and Treatment

As for Local Anaesthetics in general, p.1367.

**Effects on the CNS.** A report[1] of suspected psychotic reactions associated with the use of lidocaine in 6 patients given intravenous lidocaine for the treatment of cardiac disorders.

For the suggestion that lidocaine may be associated with an increased risk of neurotoxic complications when used for spinal anaesthesia, see under Adverse Effects of Central Block, p.1367.

1. Turner WM. Lidocaine and psychotic reactions. *Ann Intern Med* 1982; **97:** 149–50.

**Effects on the skin.** Erythema and pigmentation of the upper lip in a child following local dental infiltration of lidocaine was attributed to a type of fixed drug eruption.[1] Erythema may also occur after topical administration of some lidocaine formulations, such as transdermal patches, while transient blanching of the skin is frequent after application of eutectic lidocaine/prilocaine mixtures to the skin.[2]

True hypersensitivity reactions, including dermatitis, are rare (see also p.1367) but can occur.[3]

1. Curley RK, *et al.* An unusual cutaneous reaction to lignocaine. *Br Dent J* 1987; **162:** 113–14.
2. Villada G, *et al.* Local blanching after epicutaneous application of EMLA cream: a double-blind randomized study among 50 healthy volunteers. *Dermatologica* 1990; **181:** 38–40.
3. Bircher AJ, *et al.* Delayed-type hypersensitivity to subcutaneous lidocaine with tolerance to articaine: confirmation by in vivo and in vitro tests. *Contact Dermatitis* 1996; **34:** 387–9.

**Overdosage.** The most serious effects of lidocaine intoxication are on the CNS and cardiovascular system and overdosage can result in severe hypotension, asystole, bradycardia, apnoea, seizures, coma, cardiac arrest, respiratory arrest, and death. Intoxication with lidocaine is relatively common and can occur as a result of acute overdosage following poor control of intravenous maintenance infusions or after accidental injection of concentrated solutions. However, it more commonly results from inadvertent intravascular administration during regional anaesthesia, or from too rapid injection of antiarrhythmic doses, particularly in patients with circulatory insufficiency, or when clearance is reduced due to heart failure, liver disease, old age, or through interaction with other drugs.[1] Seizures have also been reported after excessive doses administered subcutaneously.[2] Although the bioavailability of lidocaine is low it may be sufficient to result in significant toxicity when swallowed[1] and there have been reports of CNS toxicity, seizures, and death in children[3-7] and adults[8-10] following the ingestion of topical solutions and after the use of viscous preparations in the mouth. Death has also ensued after gargling with a 4% lidocaine solution.[11] Lidocaine is absorbed from mucous membranes and serious toxicity has been reported after urethral[12] or rectal[13] instillation of lidocaine preparations.

1. Denaro CP, Benowitz NL. Poisoning due to class 1B antiarrhythmic drugs: lignocaine, mexiletine and tocainide. *Med Toxicol Adverse Drug Exp* 1989; **4:** 412–28.
2. Pelter MA, *et al.* Seizure-like reaction associated with subcutaneous lidocaine injection. *Clin Pharm* 1989; **8:** 767–8.
3. Sakai RI, Lattin JE. Lidocaine ingestion. *Am J Dis Child* 1980; **134:** 323.
4. Rothstein P, *et al.* Prolonged seizures associated with the use of viscous lidocaine. *J Pediatr* 1982; **101:** 461–3.
5. Mofenson HC, *et al.* Lidocaine toxicity from topical mucosal application. *Clin Pediatr (Phila)* 1983; **22:** 190–2.
6. Giard MJ, *et al.* Seizures induced by oral viscous lidocaine. *Clin Pharm* 1983; **2:** 110.
7. Amitai Y, *et al.* Death following accidental lidocaine overdose in a child. *N Engl J Med* 1986; **314:** 182–3.
8. Parish RC, *et al.* Seizures following oral lidocaine for esophageal anesthesia. *Drug Intell Clin Pharm* 1985; **19:** 199–201.
9. Fruncillo RJ, *et al.* CNS toxicity after ingestion of topical lidocaine. *N Engl J Med* 1982; **306:** 426–7.
10. Geraets DR, *et al.* Toxicity potential of oral lidocaine in a patient receiving mexiletine. *Ann Pharmacother* 1992; **26:** 1380–1.
11. Zuberi BF, *et al.* Lidocaine toxicity in a student undergoing upper gastrointestinal endoscopy. *Gut* 2000; **46:** 435.
12. Dix VW, Tresidder GC. Collapse after use of lignocaine jelly for urethral anaesthesia. *Lancet* 1963; **i:** 890.
13. Pottage A, Scott DB. Safety of "topical" lignocaine. *Lancet* 1988; **i:** 1003.

**Pregnancy.** The overall effect of maternal epidural anaesthesia appears to be beneficial for the fetus (see under Labour Pain, p.6) but lidocaine may have transient effects on the neonatal auditory system.[1]

1. Bozynski MEA, *et al.* Effect of prenatal lignocaine on auditory brain stem evoked response. *Arch Dis Child* 1989; **64:** 934–8.

## Precautions

As for Local Anaesthetics in general, p.1368.

In general lidocaine should not be given to patients with hypovolaemia, heart block or other conduction disturbances, and should be used with caution in patients with congestive heart failure, bradycardia, or respiratory depression. Lidocaine is metabolised in the liver and must be given with caution to patients with hepatic impairment. The plasma half-life of lidocaine may be prolonged in conditions that reduce hepatic blood flow such as cardiac and circulatory failure. Metabolites of lidocaine may accumulate in patients with renal impairment.

The intramuscular injection of lidocaine may increase creatine phosphokinase concentrations that can interfere with the diagnosis of acute myocardial infarction.

**Breast feeding.** No adverse effects have been observed in breast-fed infants whose mothers were receiving lidocaine, and the American Academy of Pediatrics[1] considers that it is therefore usually compatible with breast feeding.

1. American Academy of Pediatrics. The transfer of drugs and other chemicals into human milk. *Pediatrics* 2001; **108:** 776–89. Correction. *ibid.*; 1029. Also available at: http://aappolicy.aappublications.org/cgi/content/full/pediatrics%3b108/3/776 (accessed 02/06/04)

**Cerebrovascular disorders.** Administration of lidocaine 5 mg/kg by intravenous infusion over 30 minutes was associated with a 12% reduction in cerebral blood flow in healthy subjects although it returned to normal within 60 minutes.[1] Cerebral blood flow in patients with diabetes was lower than in healthy subjects, but was unaffected by lidocaine infusion, indicating reduced cerebrovascular reactivity.

1. Kastrup J, *et al.* Intravenous lidocaine and cerebral blood flow: impaired microvascular reactivity in diabetic patients. *J Clin Pharmacol* 1990; **30:** 318–23.

**Porphyria.** Lidocaine is considered to be unsafe in patients with porphyria because it has been shown to be porphyrinogenic in *animals*.

**Renal impairment.** The pharmacokinetics of lidocaine and its metabolite monoethylglycinexylidide appear to be unaffected in patients with renal failure except that accumulation of the metabolite glycinexylidide may occur during infusions of 12 hours or more.[1] Data to predict the amount of lidocaine and glycinexylidide removed during haemodialysis have been provided.[2,3] Lidocaine does not appear to be removed during haemofiltration.[4]

1. Collinsworth KA, *et al.* Pharmacokinetics and metabolism of lidocaine in patients with renal failure. *Clin Pharmacol Ther* 1975; **18:** 59–64.
2. Gibson TP, Nelson HA. Drug kinetics and artificial kidneys. *Clin Pharmacokinet* 1977; **2:** 403–26.
3. Lee CC, Marbury TC. Drug therapy in patients undergoing haemodialysis: clinical pharmacokinetic considerations. *Clin Pharmacokinet* 1984; **9:** 42–66.
4. Saima S, *et al.* Negligible removal of lidocaine during arteriovenous hemofiltration. *Ther Drug Monit* 1990; **12:** 154–6.

**Smoking.** The effects of smoking on lidocaine therapy are unclear. Studies in a limited number of patients have found reduced systemic bioavailability suggestive of induction of drug-metabolising activity[1] and an inconsistent effect on protein binding.[2,3]

1. Huet P-M, Lelorier J. Effects of smoking and chronic hepatitis B on lidocaine and indocyanine green kinetics. *Clin Pharmacol Ther* 1980; **28:** 208–15.
2. McNamara PJ, *et al.* Effect of smoking on binding of lidocaine to human serum proteins. *J Pharm Sci* 1980; **69:** 749–51.
3. Davis D, *et al.* The effects of age and smoking on the plasma protein binding of lignocaine and diazepam. *Br J Clin Pharmacol* 1985; **19:** 261–5.

## Interactions

For interactions associated with local anaesthetics, see p.1368.

The clearance of lidocaine may be reduced by propranolol and cimetidine (see below). The cardiac depressant effects of lidocaine are additive with those of beta blockers and of other antiarrhythmics. Additive cardiac effects may also occur when lidocaine is given with intravenous phenytoin; however, the long-term use of phenytoin and other enzyme-inducers may increase dosage requirements of lidocaine (see below). Hypokalaemia produced by acetazolamide, loop diuretics, and thiazides antagonises the effect of lidocaine.

**Antiarrhythmics.** Lidocaine toxicity, arising from the use of an oral preparation containing lidocaine, has been reported[1] in a patient who was receiving *mexiletine*. There are individual reports of seizures or heart failure and cardiac arrest in patients who received lidocaine with *ajmaline*,[2] *amiodarone*,[3,4] or *tocainide*.[5] Delirium has been reported in a patient who received lidocaine with *procainamide*.[6]

1. Geraets DR, *et al.* Toxicity potential of oral lidocaine in a patient receiving mexiletine. *Ann Pharmacother* 1992; **26:** 1380–1.
2. Bleifeld W. Side effects of antiarrhythmic drugs. *Naunyn Schmiedebergs Arch Pharmacol* 1971; **269:** 282–97.
3. Siegmund JB, *et al.* Amiodarone interaction with lidocaine. *J Cardiovasc Pharmacol* 1993; **21:** 513–15.
4. Keidar S, *et al.* Sinoatrial arrest due to lidocaine injection in sick sinus syndrome during amiodarone administration. *Am Heart J* 1982; **104:** 1384–5.
5. Forrence E, *et al.* A seizure induced by concurrent lidocaine-tocainide therapy—is it just a case of additive toxicity? *Drug Intell Clin Pharm* 1986; 20: 56–9.
6. Ilyas M, *et al.* Delirium induced by a combination of anti-arrhythmic drugs. *Lancet* 1969; **ii:** 1368–9.

**Antiepileptics.** Studies in healthy subjects and patients with epilepsy[1,2] suggest that long-term use of drugs such as *phenytoin* or *barbiturates* may increase dosage requirements for lidocaine due to induction of drug-metabolising microsomal enzymes. Phenytoin can also increase plasma concentrations of $\alpha_1$-acid glycoprotein and thereby reduce the free fraction of lidocaine in plasma.[3]

The cardiac depressant effects of lidocaine may be dangerously enhanced by intravenous phenytoin.[4]

1. Heinonen J, *et al.* Plasma lidocaine levels in patients treated with potential inducers of microsomal enzymes. *Acta Anaesthesiol Scand* 1970; **14:** 89–95.
2. Perucca E, Richens A. Reduction of oral bioavailability of lignocaine by induction of first pass metabolism in epileptic patients. *Br J Clin Pharmacol* 1979; **8:** 21–31.
3. Routledge PA, *et al.* Lignocaine disposition in blood in epilepsy. *Br J Clin Pharmacol* 1981; **12:** 663–6.
4. Wood RA. Sinoatrial arrest: an interaction between phenytoin and lignocaine. *BMJ* 1971; **1:** 645.

**Beta blockers.** Significant increases in plasma-lidocaine concentrations have occurred with *propranolol*,[1-4] owing to a reduction in the clearance of lidocaine from plasma. A similar interaction has been observed with *nadolol*[3] and *metoprolol*,[2] although in another study[5] metoprolol did not alter the pharmacokinetics of lidocaine. The hepatic metabolism of lidocaine may be reduced as a result of a fall in hepatic blood flow associated with reduced cardiac output or it may be caused by direct inhibition of hepatic microsomal enzymes.[6] Significant impairment of lidocaine clearance would therefore be most likely to occur with those drugs that lack intrinsic sympathomimetic activity and have a greater effect on cardiac output or with the more lipid-soluble drugs that have greater effects on microsomal oxygenases. The reduction in clearance produced by propranolol seems to be mainly by direct inhibition of metabolism rather than by lowering of hepatic blood flow.[4]

1. Ochs HR, *et al.* Reduction in lidocaine clearance during continuous infusion and by coadministration of propranolol. *N Engl J Med* 1980; **303:** 373–7.
2. Conrad KA, *et al.* Lidocaine elimination: effects of metoprolol and of propranolol. *Clin Pharmacol Ther* 1983; **33:** 133–8.
3. Schneck DW, *et al.* Effects of nadolol and propranolol on plasma lidocaine clearance. *Clin Pharmacol Ther* 1984; **36:** 584–7.
4. Bax NDS, *et al.* The impairment of lignocaine clearance by propranolol—major contribution from enzyme inhibition. *Br J Clin Pharmacol* 1985; **19:** 597–603.
5. Miners JO, *et al.* Failure of 'therapeutic' doses of β-adrenoceptor antagonists to alter the disposition of tolbutamide and lignocaine. *Br J Clin Pharmacol* 1984; **18:** 853–60.
6. Tucker GT, *et al.* Effects of β-adrenoceptor antagonists on the pharmacokinetics of lignocaine. *Br J Clin Pharmacol* 1984; **17** (suppl 1): 21S–28S.

**$H_2$-antagonists.** There have been numerous studies[1-4] of the interaction between *cimetidine* and lidocaine but differences between the studies make interpretation of the overall clinical significance of the results difficult. Cimetidine appears to reduce the hepatic metabolism of lidocaine; it may also reduce its clearance by decreasing hepatic blood flow. Significant increases in plasma-lidocaine concentrations have been reported. Changes in protein binding are not generally important but patients with myocardial infarction who have increased levels of $\alpha_1$-acid glycoprotein may be partially protected from increases in concentrations of free lidocaine.[5] Since it is not possible to identify those patients at risk all patients receiving these drugs concurrently should be closely monitored for signs of toxicity. The use of other $H_2$-antagonists may be preferable. In studies in healthy subjects *ranitidine* either had no effect on lidocaine kinetics[6] or produced changes consistent with small reductions in hepatic blood flow.[7]

1. Feely J, *et al.* Increased toxicity and reduced clearance of lidocaine by cimetidine. *Ann Intern Med* 1982; **96:** 592–4.
2. Knapp AB, *et al.* The cimetidine-lidocaine interaction. *Ann Intern Med* 1983; **98:** 174–7.
3. Patterson JH, *et al.* Influence of a continuous cimetidine infusion on lidocaine plasma concentrations in patients. *J Clin Pharmacol* 1985; **25:** 607–9.
4. Bauer LA, *et al.* Cimetidine-induced decrease in lidocaine metabolism. *Am Heart J* 1984; **108:** 413–15.
5. Berk SI, *et al.* The effect of oral cimetidine on total and unbound serum lidocaine concentrations in patients with suspected myocardial infarction. *Int J Cardiol* 1987; **14:** 91–4.
6. Feely J, Guy E. Lack of effect of ranitidine on the disposition of lignocaine. *Br J Clin Pharmacol* 1983; **15:** 378–9.
7. Robson RA, *et al.* The effect of ranitidine on the disposition of lignocaine. *Br J Clin Pharmacol* 1985; **20:** 170–3.

**Local anaesthetics.** Although a number of drugs were shown to reduce the amount of lidocaine bound to $\alpha_1$-acid glycoprotein only the displacement produced by *bupivacaine* was considered to be of possible clinical significance.[1]

There is concern about the use of lidocaine to treat *cocaine*-induced arrhythmias as lidocaine may enhance toxicity.[2]

1. Goolkasian DL, *et al.* Displacement of lidocaine from serum $\alpha_1$-acid glycoprotein binding sites by basic drugs. *Eur J Clin Pharmacol* 1983; **25:** 413–17.
2. Hollander JE. The management of cocaine-associated myocardial ischemia. *N Engl J Med* 1995; **333:** 1267–72.

**Neuromuscular blockers.** The possible interaction between neuromuscular blockers and antiarrhythmics including lidocaine is discussed under Atracurium, p.1400.

**Oral contraceptives.** For mention of the effect of oral contraceptives on the protein binding of lidocaine, see under Protein Binding in Pharmacokinetics, below.

## Pharmacokinetics

Lidocaine is readily absorbed from the gastrointestinal tract, from mucous membranes, and through damaged skin. Absorption through intact skin is poor. It is rapidly absorbed from injection sites including muscle.

After an intravenous dose lidocaine is rapidly and widely distributed into highly perfused tissues followed by redistribution into skeletal muscle and adipose tissue. Lidocaine is bound to plasma proteins, including $\alpha_1$-acid glycoprotein (AAG). The extent of binding is variable but is about 66%. Plasma protein binding of lidocaine depends in part on the concentrations of both lidocaine and AAG. Any alteration in the concentration of AAG can greatly affect plasma concentrations of lidocaine (see under Protein Binding, below).

Plasma concentrations decline rapidly after an intravenous dose with an initial half-life of less than 30 minutes; the elimination half-life is 1 to 2 hours but may be prolonged if infusions are given for longer than 24 hours or if hepatic blood flow is reduced.

Lidocaine is largely metabolised in the liver and any alteration in liver function or hepatic blood flow can have a significant effect on its pharmacokinetics and dosage requirements. First-pass metabolism is extensive and bioavailability is about 35% after oral administration. Metabolism in the liver is rapid and about 90% of a given dose is dealkylated to form monoethylglycinexylidide and glycinexylidide. Both of these metabolites may contribute to the therapeutic and toxic effects of lidocaine and since their half-lives are longer than that of lidocaine, accumulation, particularly of glycinexylidide, may occur during prolonged infusions. Further metabolism occurs and metabolites are excreted in the urine with less than 10% of unchanged lidocaine. Reduced clearance of lidocaine has been found in patients with heart failure, alcoholic liver disease, or chronic or viral hepatitis. Concomitant therapy with drugs that alter hepatic blood flow or induce drug-metabolising microsomal enzymes can also affect the clearance of lidocaine (see under Interactions, above). Renal impairment does not affect the clearance of lidocaine but accumulation of its active metabolites can occur.

Lidocaine crosses the placenta and blood-brain barrier; it is distributed into breast milk.

See also under Local Anaesthetics, p.1368.

◊ References.

1. Nattel S, *et al.* The pharmacokinetics of lignocaine and β-adrenoceptor antagonists in patients with acute myocardial infarction. *Clin Pharmacokinet* 1987; **13:** 293–316.

**Absorption.** SURFACE APPLICATION. Serum-lidocaine concentrations were usually so low as to be unmeasurable in patients who gargled and expectorated 15 mL (300 mg) of a 2% viscous solution before endoscopy[1] and mean peak serum concentrations of lidocaine were below those associated with toxicity following endotracheal application of 100 mg of lidocaine by spray.[2] The relative bioavailability of lidocaine has been found to be higher when applied to the upper respiratory tract than after administration to the lower respiratory tract.[3] Acceptably low plasma-lidocaine concentrations were noted with the following regimen used before bronchoscopy: a 4% lidocaine solution gargled for 30 seconds, a 2% solution sprayed onto the oropharynx, a 2% jelly applied to the oropharynx and nasal passages, and a 1% solution injected through a bronchoscope.[4] However, a fatality has been reported following the use of lidocaine as a gargle (see Overdosage, above); the absorption of intranasal lidocaine can also be highly variable.[5] For bronchoscopy, inhalation of lidocaine from a nebuliser rather than a direct spray may result in lower peak serum concentrations.[6]

Absorption of lidocaine is generally poor through intact skin. However, there is some evidence that absorption may be greater following application to the skin of preterm infants.[7]

1. Fazio A, *et al.* Lidocaine serum concentrations following endoscopy. *Drug Intell Clin Pharm* 1987; **21:** 752–3.
2. Scott DB, *et al.* Plasma lignocaine concentrations following endotracheal spraying with an aerosol. *Br J Anaesth* 1976; **48:** 899–902.
3. McBurney A, *et al.* Absorption of lignocaine and bupivacaine from the respiratory tract during fibreoptic bronchoscopy. *Br J Clin Pharmacol* 1984; **17:** 61–6.
4. Ameer B, *et al.* Systemic absorption of topical lidocaine in elderly and young adults undergoing bronchoscopy. *Pharmacotherapy* 1989; **9:** 74–81.
5. Scavone JM, *et al.* The bioavailability of intranasal lignocaine. *Br J Clin Pharmacol* 1989; **28:** 722–4.
6. Labedzki L, *et al.* Reduced systemic absorption of intrabronchial lidocaine by high-frequency nebulization. *J Clin Pharmacol* 1990; **30:** 795–7.
7. Barrett DA, Rutter N. Percutaneous lignocaine absorption in newborn infants. *Arch Dis Child* 1994; **71:** F122–F124.

**Protein binding.** Lidocaine is markedly bound to $\alpha_1$-acid glycoprotein (AAG), a plasma protein which is increased after trauma, surgery, burns, myocardial infarction, in chronic inflammatory disorders such as Crohn's disease, and in cancer. Protein binding may therefore be greatly increased in these conditions and reduced in neonates, the nephrotic syndrome, and in liver disease when AAG concentrations are lower than normal. This can result in an eightfold variation in the free fraction of lidocaine between these conditions.[1] Measurement of free drug concentrations may be a better guide to dosage requirements than measurement of total plasma concentrations.[2] AAG concentrations may also be reduced by oestrogens[3] leading to a higher free fraction of lidocaine in women than in men and the free fraction is further increased during pregnancy and in women taking oral contraceptives.[3,4] Protein binding may also be affected by other concomitant drug therapy or smoking (for further details, see under Interactions, above and Precautions, Smoking, above).

1. Routledge PA. Pharmacological terms: protein binding. *Prescribers' J* 1988; **28:** 34–5.
2. Shand DG. $\alpha_1$-Acid glycoprotein and plasma lidocaine binding. *Clin Pharmacokinet* 1984; **9** (suppl 1): 27–31.
3. Routledge PA, *et al.* Sex-related differences in the plasma protein binding of lignocaine and diazepam. *Br J Clin Pharmacol* 1981; **11:** 245–50.
4. Wood M, Wood AJJ. Changes in plasma drug binding and $\alpha_1$-acid glycoprotein in mother and newborn infant. *Clin Pharmacol Ther* 1981; **29:** 522–6.

## Uses and Administration

Lidocaine is a local anaesthetic of the amide type with actions and uses similar to those described on p.1369. It is used for infiltration anaesthesia and regional nerve blocks. It has a rapid onset of action and anaesthesia is obtained within a few minutes depending on the site of administration; it has an intermediate duration of action. The speed of onset and duration of action of lidocaine are increased by the addition of a vasoconstrictor and absorption into the circulation from the site of injection is reduced. It is generally given as the hydrochloride. Lidocaine hydrochloride monohydrate 1.23 g or anhydrous lidocaine hydrochloride 1.16 g is approximately equivalent to 1 g of lidocaine. A carbonated solution of lidocaine is also available in some countries for injection (see p.1369). Lidocaine is also a useful surface anaesthetic but it may be rapidly and extensively absorbed following topical application to mucous membranes, and systemic effects may occur. Hyaluronidase (p.1698) has been added to preparations of lidocaine used for surface and infiltration anaesthesia but may enhance systemic absorption. (Local anaesthetic techniques are discussed on p.1370.)

Lidocaine is included in some injections, such as depot corticosteroids, to prevent pain, itching, and other local irritation. Lidocaine sodium has also been included in intramuscular injections of some antibacterials to reduce the pain on administration.

Lidocaine is also a class Ib antiarrhythmic used in the treatment of ventricular arrhythmias, especially after myocardial infarction. It has been given by intravenous infusion in the treatment of refractory status epilepticus.

USE IN LOCAL ANAESTHESIA.

The dose of lidocaine hydrochloride used for local anaesthesia depends on the site of injection and the procedure used. Specific licensed doses for individual procedures are not generally available in the UK, although US product information often includes them (see below). When given with adrenaline, the suggested general **maximum single dose** of lidocaine hydrochloride is 500 mg; without adrenaline, the recommended maximum single dose in the UK is 200 mg and in the USA, 300 mg, except for spinal anaesthesia (see below). Lidocaine hydrochloride solutions containing adrenaline 1 in 200 000 are used for infiltration anaesthesia and nerve blocks; higher concentrations of adrenaline are seldom necessary, except in dentistry, where solutions of lidocaine hydrochloride with adrenaline 1 in 80 000 are widely used. Doses should be reduced in children, the elderly, and in debilitated patients. A test dose, preferably with adrenaline, should be given before commencing epidural block to detect inadvertent intravascular or subarachnoid administration.

The following doses have been recommended for individual **local anaesthetic procedures** in the USA:

- For percutaneous *infiltration anaesthesia*, 5 to 300 mg (1 to 60 mL of a 0.5% solution, or 0.5 to 30 mL of a 1% solution).
- The dosage in *peripheral nerve block* depends on the route of administration. For brachial plexus block 225 to 300 mg (15 to 20 mL) as a 1.5% solution is used; for intercostal nerve block 30 mg (3 mL) is given as a 1% solution; for paracervical block a 1% solution is used in a dose of 100 mg (10 mL) on each side, repeated not more frequently than every 90 minutes; for paravertebral block a 1% solution may be used in doses of 30 to 50 mg (3 to 5 mL); a 1% solution is recommended for pudendal block in doses of 100 mg (10 mL) on each side; for retrobulbar block a 4% solution may be used in doses of 120 to 200 mg (3 to 5 mL).
- For *sympathetic nerve block* a 1% solution is recommended; doses are 50 mg (5 mL) for cervical block and 50 to 100 mg (5 to 10 mL) for lumbar block.
- For *epidural anaesthesia* 2 to 3 mL of solution is needed for each dermatome to be anaesthetised but usual total doses and recommended concentrations are: lumbar epidural 250 to 300 mg (25 to 30 mL) as a 1% solution for analgesia and 225 to 300 mg (15 to 20 mL) as a 1.5% solution or 200 to 300 mg (10 to 15 mL) as a 2% solution for anaesthesia, and for thoracic epidural a 1% solution may be used at doses of 200 to 300 mg (20 to 30 mL). In obstetric caudal analgesia up to 300 mg (30 mL) is used as a 0.5% or 1% solution and in surgical caudal analgesia a 1.5% solution may be used in doses of 225 to 300 mg (15 to 20 mL). For continuous epidural anaesthesia, the maximum doses should not be repeated more frequently than every 90 minutes.
- A hyperbaric solution of 1.5% or 5% lidocaine hydrochloride in glucose 7.5% solution is available for *spinal anaesthesia*; adrenaline should not be used. Doses of up to 50 mg (1 mL) as a 5% solution and 9 to 15 mg (0.6 to 1 mL) as a 1.5% solution have been used during labour for a normal vaginal delivery. Up to 75 mg (1.5 mL) as the 5% solution has been used for caesarean section and 75 to 100 mg (1.5 to 2 mL) for other surgical procedures.
- For *intravenous regional anaesthesia* a 0.5% solution without adrenaline has been used in doses of 50 to 300 mg (10 to 60 mL); a maximum dose of 4 mg/kg has been recommended for adults.

Lidocaine may be used in a variety of formulations for **surface anaesthesia**.

- Lidocaine ointment is used for *anaesthesia of skin and mucous membranes* with a maximum recommended total dose of 20 g of 5% ointment (equivalent to 1 g of lidocaine base) in 24 hours.
- Gels are used for *anaesthesia of the urinary tract* and the dose used varies in different countries. The manufacturers in the UK have suggested the following doses given as a 2% gel: in females 60 to 100 mg of lidocaine hydrochloride inserted into the urethra several minutes before examination; in males 200 mg instilled initially followed by 60 to 100 mg. A 1% gel may also be used. The doses used in the USA are similar: in females 60 to 100 mg of lidocaine hydrochloride as a 2% gel is inserted into the urethra several minutes before examination; in males 100 to 200 mg is used before catheterisation and 600 mg before sounding or cystoscopy.

  A gel may also be applied for the treatment of *major aphthae* in immunocompromised patients; a dose of 20 to 30 mg (2 to 3 mL) as a 1% gel or 40 to 60 mg (2 to 3 mL) as a 2% gel is used. A maximum volume of up to 15 mL is recommended within 24 hours.
- Topical solutions are used for *surface anaesthesia of mucous membranes of the mouth, throat, and upper gastrointestinal tract.* For painful conditions of the mouth and throat a 2% solution may be used: 300 mg (15 mL) may be rinsed and ejected or, for pharyngeal pain, the solution is gargled and swallowed if necessary; it should not be used more frequently than every 3 hours. The recommended maximum daily dose in the USA for topical oral solutions is 2.4 g. Doses of 40 to 300 mg as a 4% solution (1 to 7.5 mL) are used before bronchoscopy, bronchography, laryngoscopy, oesophagoscopy, endotracheal intubation, and biopsy in the mouth and throat. Lidocaine in a strength of 10% has also been used as a spray for application to mucous membranes for the prevention of pain during various procedures including use in otorhinolaryngology, den-

tistry, introduction of instruments into the respiratory and gastrointestinal tracts, and in obstetrics. The dose depends on the extent of the site to be anaesthetised; 10 to 50 mg is generally sufficient for dentistry and otorhinolaryngology; for other procedures, the maximum dose in a 24-hour period is 200 mg. For laryngotracheal anaesthesia 160 mg of lidocaine hydrochloride as a 4% solution is sprayed or instilled as a single dose into the lumen of the larynx and trachea.

- Lidocaine is used *rectally* as suppositories, sprays, ointments, and creams in the treatment of haemorrhoids and other painful perianal conditions.
- *Eye drops* containing lidocaine hydrochloride 4% with fluorescein are used in tonometry.
- A *eutectic mixture* containing lidocaine base 2.5% and prilocaine base 2.5% is applied as a cream under an occlusive dressing to produce *surface anaesthesia of the skin* before procedures requiring needle puncture, surgical treatment of localised lesions, and split skin grafting; it has been used similarly, but without an occlusive dressing, before removal of genital warts (see also under Surface Anaesthesia, below).
- Other methods of dermal delivery include a *transdermal patch* of lidocaine 5% for the treatment of pain associated with postherpetic neuralgia, and an *iontophoretic drug delivery system* incorporating lidocaine and adrenaline.

USE IN ARRHYTHMIAS.

For the treatment of **ventricular arrhythmias** lidocaine is given *intravenously* as the hydrochloride. It may be used in advanced cardiac life support for cardiac arrest due to ventricular fibrillation and pulseless ventricular tachycardia when direct current shocks (together with adrenaline) have failed to restore a normal rhythm. For adults, a dose of 1 to 1.5 mg/kg can be given and repeated after 3 to 5 minutes to a total dose of 3 mg/kg if necessary. The *endotracheal* route has been employed when intravenous access cannot be obtained, although doses should probably be larger than those employed intravenously; the precise endotracheal dose has not yet been established, however.

Lidocaine is also used in other ventricular arrhythmias in which the patient is in a more stable condition. In these circumstances lidocaine hydrochloride is usually given as a loading dose followed by an infusion. Usual doses are 50 to 100 mg or 1 to 1.5 mg/kg as a direct *intravenous injection* at a rate of 25 to 50 mg/minute. If no effect is seen within 5 to 10 minutes of this loading dose, it may be repeated once or twice to a maximum dose of 200 to 300 mg in 1 hour. A *continuous intravenous infusion* is usually commenced after loading, at a dose of 1 to 4 mg/minute. It is rarely necessary to continue this infusion for longer than 24 hours, but in the event that a longer infusion is required, the dose may need to be reduced to avoid potential toxicity resulting from an increase in the half-life. Dosage may need to be reduced in the elderly and in patients with heart failure or liver disorders.

In emergency situations, lidocaine hydrochloride has also been given for arrhythmias by *intramuscular* injection into the deltoid muscle in a dose of 300 mg, repeated if necessary after 60 to 90 minutes.

**Action.** For a comparison of the vasoactivity of lidocaine and some other local anaesthetics, see p.1369.

**Burns.** Lidocaine given intravenously has been reported to have produced pain relief in a few patients with second-degree burns.[1]

1. Jönsson A, *et al.* Inhibition of burn pain by intravenous lignocaine infusion. *Lancet* 1991; **338:** 151–2.

**Cardiac arrhythmias.** Lidocaine is classified as a class Ib antiarrhythmic drug (p.809) and may be used in the treatment of ventricular arrhythmias, including those associated with cardiac arrest and myocardial infarction. It is usually given intravenously (see above). Some forms of ventricular tachycardia may be terminated by the use of lidocaine; the overall treatment options are described under Cardiac Arrhythmias, p.816. Lidocaine may also be used during advanced cardiac life support (p.812).

Lidocaine has been considered for the *prophylaxis* of ventricular fibrillation in patients with proven or suspected myocardial infarction. However, while some studies have identified a protective effect,[1,2] in others this has not been shown to be accompanied by a reduction in mortality and might even have increased it.[3,4] Nevertheless, a review of the available evidence[5] concluded that lidocaine prophylaxis was a reasonable policy for patients at highest risk of ventricular fibrillation such as those with acute transmural infarction, under 65 years of age, and within 6 hours of the onset of infarction symptoms.

It has been suggested that the increased mortality sometimes seen with lidocaine might be associated with the duration of administration; a study[6] found that patients who received a bolus dose of lidocaine followed by a 40-hour continuous infusion for prophylaxis of ventricular arrhythmias experienced more episodes of heart failure than patients who received the bolus dose followed by an 8-hour infusion.

1. Horwitz RI, Feinstein AR. Improved observational method for studying therapeutic efficacy: suggestive evidence that lidocaine prophylaxis prevents death in acute myocardial infarction. *JAMA* 1981; **246:** 2455–9.
2. Koster RW, Dunning AJ. Intramuscular lidocaine for prevention of lethal arrhythmias in the prehospitalization phase of acute myocardial infarction. *N Engl J Med* 1985; **313:** 1105–10.
3. MacMahon S, *et al.* Effects of prophylactic lidocaine in suspected acute myocardial infarction: an overview of results from the randomized, controlled trials. *JAMA* 1988; **260:** 1910–16.
4. Hine LK, *et al.* Meta-analytic evidence against prophylactic use of lidocaine in acute myocardial infarction. *Ann Intern Med* 1989; **149:** 2694–8.
5. Nattel S, Arenal A. Antiarrhythmic prophylaxis after acute myocardial infarction: is lidocaine still useful? *Drugs* 1993; **45:** 9–14.
6. Pharand C, *et al.* Lidocaine prophylaxis for fatal ventricular arrhythmias after acute myocardial infarction. *Clin Pharmacol Ther* 1995; **57:** 471–8.

**Hiccup.** A protocol for the management of intractable hiccups may be found under Chlorpromazine, p.682. Lidocaine is one of a large number of drugs that has been tried in the treatment of hiccups without strong evidence of their efficacy. It has been given in the form of a 2% viscous solution taken by mouth. Nebulised lidocaine has also been tried.[1]

1. Neeno TA, Rosenow EC. Intractable hiccups: consider nebulized lidocaine. *Chest* 1996; **110:** 1129–30.

**Intubation.** Lidocaine has produced conflicting results when used to attenuate the pressor response and rise in intra-ocular pressure induced by procedures such as tracheal intubation.[1-5] For an overall discussion of this problem, see under Anaesthesia, p.1397.

1. Tam S, *et al.* Attenuation of circulatory responses to endotracheal intubation using intravenous lidocaine: a determination of the optimal time of injection. *Can Anaesth Soc J* 1985; **32:** S65.
2. Murphy DF, *et al.* Intravenous lignocaine pretreatment to prevent intraocular pressure rise following suxamethonium and tracheal intubation. *Br J Ophthalmol* 1986; **70:** 596–8.
3. Drenger B, Pe'er J. Attenuation of ocular and systemic responses to tracheal intubation by intravenous lignocaine. *Br J Ophthalmol* 1987; **71:** 546–8.
4. Miller CD, Warren SJ. IV lignocaine fails to attenuate the cardiovascular response to laryngoscopy and tracheal intubation. *Br J Anaesth* 1990; **65:** 216–19.
5. Mostafa SM, *et al.* Effects of nebulized lignocaine on the intraocular pressure responses to tracheal intubation. *Br J Anaesth* 1990; **64:** 515–17.

**Migraine and cluster headache.** Despite periodic interest, lidocaine has so far failed to find an accepted role in the management of migraine (p.464) or cluster headache (p.464). Lidocaine has been tried for the emergency parenteral treatment of migraine, but in a comparative study with dihydroergotamine or chlorpromazine it was found to be less effective than either.[1] Intranasal instillation of lidocaine has produced rapid relief of headache in some patients with acute migraine (though early relapse was common).[2] It has also been reported to be effective in aborting individual attacks of headache during cluster periods in patients with cluster headache.[3,4] However, most patients do not appear to obtain complete pain relief.

1. Bell R, *et al.* A comparative trial of three agents in the treatment of acute migraine headache. *Ann Emerg Med* 1990; **19:** 1070–82.
2. Maizels M, *et al.* Intranasal lidocaine for treatment of migraine: a randomized, double-blind, controlled trial. *JAMA* 1996; **276:** 319–21.
3. Kittrelle JP, *et al.* Cluster headache: local anesthetic abortive agents. *Arch Neurol* 1985; **42:** 496–8.
4. Robbins L. Intranasal lidocaine for cluster headache. *Headache* 1995; **35:** 83–4.

**Neuropathic pain syndromes.** Lidocaine may be useful in the management of some types of neuropathic pain syndromes (p.7). The pain of *postherpetic neuralgia* has been significantly reduced by the application of lidocaine 5% transdermal patches;[1,2] a eutectic mixture of lidocaine and prilocaine has also been of benefit (see Surface Anaesthesia below). Syndromes where intravenous lidocaine therapy has been tried include *diabetic neuropathy*[3] and *central neuropathic pain* associated with stroke or spinal cord injury.[4]

1. Rowbotham MC, *et al.* Lidocaine patch: double-blind controlled study of a new treatment method for post-herpetic neuralgia. *Pain* 1996; **65:** 39–44.
2. Comer AM, Lamb HM. Lidocaine patch 5%. *Drugs* 2000, **59:** 245–9.
3. Kastrup J, *et al.* Treatment of chronic painful diabetic neuropathy with intravenous lidocaine infusion. *BMJ* 1986; **292:** 173.
4. Attal N, *et al.* Intravenous lidocaine in central pain: a double-blind, placebo-controlled, psychophysical study. *Neurology* 2000; **54:** 564–74.

**Pleurodesis.** Lidocaine has been instilled intrapleurally as a 1% solution in doses of up to 300 mg to relieve the severe chest pain associated with the use of tetracycline for pleurodesis.[1-3] While the larger doses were significantly more effective[2] toxic plasma concentrations were less likely to occur if a dose of 3 mg/kg or less was used.[3]

1. Harbecke RG. Intrapleurally given tetracycline with lidocaine. *JAMA* 1980; **244:** 1899–1900.
2. Sherman S, *et al.* Optimum anesthesia with intrapleural lidocaine during chemical pleurodesis with tetracycline. *Chest* 1988; **93:** 533–6.
3. Wooten SA, *et al.* Systemic absorption of tetracycline and lidocaine following intrapleural instillation. *Chest* 1988; **94:** 960–3.

**Status epilepticus.** Lidocaine hydrochloride may be used to control status epilepticus (p.352) resistant to more conventional treatment, particularly in those with respiratory disease. It has a rapid onset of action but its effect is short-lived and continuous infusion may be necessary.[1] It should also be noted that doses producing high plasma concentrations of lidocaine can result in CNS toxicity including seizures.[1] Recurrence of seizures associated with the withdrawal of prolonged lidocaine therapy may be due to its accumulated metabolites exerting an excitatory effect on the nervous system when the inhibitory effect of lidocaine is being reduced.[2]

Lidocaine was used instead of diazepam for 42 episodes of status epilepticus in 36 patients who either had limited pulmonary reserve or who had not responded to intravenous diazepam.[3] Lidocaine 1.5 to 2 mg/kg (usually a dose of 100 mg) was administered as a single intravenous dose over 2 minutes. This dose was repeated once if there was no positive response to the first dose (11 episodes) or if the seizures recurred (19 episodes). Subsequently a continuous infusion of lidocaine at a rate of 3 to 4 mg/kg per hour was given in the 7 episodes that recurred after the second dose; 5 of these showed a positive response. The 11 episodes not responding to the first dose did not respond to the second dose or to a continuous infusion.

1. Bauer J, Elger CE. Management of status epilepticus in adults. *CNS Drugs* 1994; **1:** 26–44.
2. Wallin A, *et al.* Lidocaine treatment of neonatal convulsions, a therapeutic dilemma. *Eur J Clin Pharmacol* 1989; **36:** 583–6.
3. Pascual J, *et al.* Role of lidocaine (lignocaine) in managing status epilepticus. *J Neurol Neurosurg Psychiatry* 1992; **55:** 49–51.

**Surface anaesthesia.** EUTECTIC MIXTURES. A cream containing lidocaine 2.5% and prilocaine 2.5% as a eutectic mixture can produce local anaesthesia when applied topically to intact skin. It appears to be of value in minor medical or surgical procedures in *adults* and *children*,[1-3] such as venepuncture, intravenous or arterial cannulation, retrobulbar injections, lumbar puncture, curettage of molluscum contagiosum lesions, genital wart removal, split skin grafting, laser treatment, extracorporeal shock wave therapy, separation of preputial adhesions, and circumcision. It has also been tried as an anaesthetic for the ear drum in preparation for otological procedures such as myringotomy and grommet insertion but is potentially ototoxic and should not be used in the presence of a perforation. Postherpetic neuralgia (p.7) has also been treated with some success.[4,5]

The eutectic cream is usually applied to skin under an occlusive dressing for at least 60 minutes although it has been suggested that for children aged 1 to 5 years 30 minutes may be sufficient.[6] The manufacturers suggest a maximum application time of 5 hours. The onset and duration of the effect may be affected by the site of application.[2] When used for the removal of genital warts an occlusive dressing is not necessary and the application time recommended by the manufacturer is 5 to 10 minutes. The level of anaesthesia begins to decline after 10 to 15 minutes when applied to the genital mucosa and any procedure should be started immediately.

Eutectic mixtures of lidocaine and prilocaine have also been used in *neonates* to reduce the pain of puncture procedures[7] and for circumcision,[8] and appear to be safe and efficacious. There has been concern that excessive absorption (particularly of prilocaine) might lead to methaemoglobinaemia (see p.1367), and UK licensing information recommends that the eutectic cream not be used in children less than 1 year old. However, there seems to be little evidence of this, and the *British National Formulary* considers that it may be used under specialist supervision in infants over 1 month of age. Similarly, in other countries, including the USA, the cream is licensed for use in neonates provided that their gestational age is at least 37 weeks, and that methaemoglobin values are monitored in those aged 3 months or less; it should not be used in infants under 1 year who are receiving methaemoglobin-inducing drugs.

Systemic absorption of both drugs from the eutectic cream appears to be minimal across intact skin[6] even after prolonged or extensive use.[9] However, it should not be used on wounds or mucous membranes (except for genital warts in adults) and should not be used for atopic dermatitis. It should not be applied to or near the eyes because it causes corneal irritation, and it should not be instilled in the middle ear. It should be used with caution in patients with anaemia or congenital or acquired methaemoglobinaemia. Transient paleness, redness, and oedema may occur following application.

Some studies suggest that a topical gel formulation of tetracaine 4% can produce longer and more rapid anaesthesia than the above lidocaine with prilocaine cream (see Surface Anaesthesia, under Uses and Administration of Tetracaine, p.1385). It has also been suggested[10] that topical tetracaine may have practical advantages over the eutectic mixture of lidocaine and prilocaine, which has to be applied for at least one hour, and causes vasoconstriction at the site of application which can make venepuncture difficult.


1. Lee JJ, Rubin AP. Emla cream and its current uses. *Br J Hosp Med* 1993; **50:** 463–6.
2. Buckley MM, Benfield P. Eutectic lidocaine/prilocaine cream: a review of the topical anaesthetic/analgesic efficacy of a eutectic mixture of local anaesthetics (EMLA). *Drugs* 1993; **46:** 126–51.
3. Koren G. Use of the eutectic mixture of local anesthetics in young children for procedure-related pain. *J Pediatr* 1993; **122** (suppl): S30–S35.
4. Litman SJ, *et al.* Use of EMLA cream in the treatment of post-herpetic neuralgia. *J Clin Anesth* 1996; **8:** 54–7.
5. Kost RG, Straus SE. Postherpetic neuralgia—pathogenesis, treatment, and prevention. *N Engl J Med* 1996; **335:** 32–42.
6. Hanks GW, White I. Local anaesthetic creams. *BMJ* 1988; **297:** 1215–16.
7. Gourrier E, *et al.* Use of EMLA® cream in a department of neonatology. *Pain* 1996; **68:** 431–4.
8. Taddio A, *et al.* Efficacy and safety of lidocaine-prilocaine cream for pain during circumcision. *N Engl J Med* 1997; **336:** 1197–1201.
9. Scott DB. Topical anaesthesia of intact skin. *Br J Parenter Ther* 1986; **7:** 134–5.
10. Russell SCS, Doyle E. Paediatric anaesthesia. *BMJ* 1997; **314:** 201–3.


**Tinnitus.** Tinnitus is the perception of a noise that arises or appears to arise within the head.

Objective tinnitus may be audible to others and arises from lesions outside the auditory system. Subjective tinnitus (tinnitus aurium) originates from sites within the auditory system and is perceived only by the patient. A simple and remediable cause of tinnitus can be impacted ear wax. Tinnitus is often associated with head injury, vertigo, and hearing loss, including age-related and noise-induced hearing loss. It may also be a symptom of an underlying disorder such as Ménière's disease, may be associated with anxiety or depressive disorders, or may be a manifestation of drug toxicity (for example with aspirin or quinine). In such cases, treatment of the underlying disorder or removal of the offending drug can resolve the tinnitus.

Treatment of tinnitus is difficult although reassurance and counselling are often effective in helping patients to tolerate their condition. Maskers or, if the tinnitus is associated with hearing loss, hearing aids are also used; surgery is rarely indicated. Treatment with a wide variety of drugs has been tried. Intravenous lidocaine has proven to be effective in reducing or eliminating tinnitus but the effect only lasts for a few hours and is, therefore, impractical for most patients. Efforts to find an effective oral analogue of lidocaine have not, so far, been successful. Other drugs that have been tried include benzodiazepines such as alprazolam, the antiepileptics carbamazepine and phenytoin, tricyclic antidepressants, and the loop diuretic furosemide, but adverse effects limit their use. Ginkgo biloba has been tried but there are doubts about its value.

References.


1. Luxon LM. Tinnitus: its causes, diagnosis, and treatment. *BMJ* 1993; **306:** 1490–1.
2. Robson AK, Birchall JP. Management of tinnitus. *Prescribers' J* 1994; **34:** 1–7.
3. Coles RRA. Drug treatment of tinnitus in Britain. In: Reich GE, Vernon JA, eds. *Proceedings of the fifth international tinnitus seminar.* Portland: American Tinnitus Association, 1995.
4. Vesterager V. Tinnitus—investigation and management. *BMJ* 1997; **314:** 728–31.
5. Simpson JJ, Davies WE. Recent advances in the pharmacological treatment of tinnitus. *Trends Pharmacol Sci* 1999; **20:** 12–18.
6. Dobie RA. A review of randomized clinical trials in tinnitus. *Laryngoscope* 1999; **109:** 1202–11.
7. Lockwood AH, *et al.* Tinnitus. *N Engl J Med* 2002; **347:** 904–10.


## Preparations

***BP 2003:*** Lidocaine and Adrenaline Injection; Lidocaine and Chlorhexidine Gel; Lidocaine Gel; Lidocaine Injection; Lidocaine Ointment; Sterile Lidocaine Solution;
***USP 27:*** Lidocaine Hydrochloride and Dextrose Injection; Lidocaine Hydrochloride and Epinephrine Injection; Lidocaine Hydrochloride Injection; Lidocaine Hydrochloride Jelly; Lidocaine Hydrochloride Oral Topical Solution; Lidocaine Hydrochloride Topical Solution; Lidocaine Ointment; Lidocaine Oral Topical Solution; Lidocaine Topical Aerosol; Neomycin and Polymyxin B Sulfates and Lidocaine Cream; Neomycin and Polymyxin B Sulfates, Bacitracin Zinc, and Lidocaine Ointment; Neomycin and Polymyxin B Sulfates, Bacitracin, and Lidocaine Ointment.

**Proprietary Preparations** (details are given in Part 3)
***Arg.:*** Gobbicaina; Indican; Larjancaina; Regiocaina; Solvente Indoloro; Xylocaina; ***Austral.:*** Lignospan; Nurocain; Nurocain with Sympathin†; Stud 100†; Xylocaine; Xylocaine Special Adhesive; Xylocard; ***Austria:*** Lidocorit; Neo-Xylestesin; Neo-Xylestesin forte and Neo-Xylestesin special; Xylanaest; Xylocain; Xylocard; Xyloneural; ***Belg.:*** Linisol; Otoralgyl†; Xylocaine; Xylocaine Visqueuse; Xylocard; ***Braz.:*** Hypocaina†; Lidial; Lidocabbott; Lidocalm; Lidocord†; Lidogel; Lidogeyer; Lidojet; Lidospray; Lidoston; Xylestesin; Xylocaina; ***Canad.:*** Afterburn; Family Medicated Sunburn Relief†; Lidodan; Solarcaine Lidocaine; Xylocaine; Xylocard; Zilactin-L; ***Chile:*** Calmante De Denticion; Dentaliv; Dimecaina; Exido; Gelcain; Prolong; Solin; Xylocaina 2%; ***Denm.:*** Xylocain; ***Fin.:*** Lidocard; Xylocain; ***Fr.:*** Dynexan; Mesocaine; Otoralgyl†; Xylocaine; Xylocard; ***Ger.:*** Anaesthol†; Dynexan; Gelicain; Haemo-Exhirud Bufexamac; Heweneural; Licain; Lidesthesin; Lidocard; Lidocaton†; Lidoject; LidoPosterine; Neo-Lidocaton†; Nor-Anaesthol†; Rowo-629; Sagittaproct†; Xylestesin-A, Xylestesin centro; Xylestesin-S; Xylestesin; Xylestesin-F; Xylocain; Xylocain f.d. Kardiologie; Xylocitin; Xylocitin cor; Xyloneural; ***Gr.:*** Ecocain; Xylocaine; ***Hong Kong:*** Xylestin-A; Xylocaine; Xylocard; ***India:*** Gesicain; Tivision; Xylocaine; Xylocard; ***Irl.:*** Xylocaine; Xylocard†; ***Israel:*** After Burn; Esracain; Lidocadren; LidoPen; Stud 100; Xylocaine; ***Ital.:*** Basicaina; Ecocain; Lident Adrenalina; Lident Andrenor; Lidomol; Lidosen; Lidrian; Luan; Odontalg; Ortodermina; Xilo-Mynol†; Xylocaina; Xylonor; ***Jpn:*** Penles; ***Malaysia:*** Xylocaine; Xylocard; ***Mex.:*** Pisacaina; Rucaina†; Uvega; Xylocaina; ***Neth.:*** Dentinox; Otalgan; Xylocaine; Xylocard†; ***Norw.:*** Xylocain; Xylocard†; ***NZ:*** Nurocain†; Virasolve; Xylocaine; Xylocard; ***Port.:*** Lidonostrum; Lincaina; Xilonibsa; Xylocaina; Xylocard; ***S.Afr.:*** Lignospan Special; Peterkaien†; Remicaine; Remicard; Xylocaine; Xylotox; ***Singapore:*** Dube; Xylocaine; Xylocard†; ***Spain:*** Aeroderm; Curadent†; Dermovagisil; Llorentecaina Noradrenal†; Octocaine†; Xilonibsa; Xylocaina; Xylonor 2% Sin Vasoconst; Xylonor Especial; ***Swed.:*** Xylocain; Xylocard; ***Switz.:*** Kenergon; Lidocaton†; Lignospan; Lubogliss†; Neo-Sinedol; Neurodol Tissugel; Rapidocaine; Sedagul; Solarcaine; Xylesine; Xylestesin-F; Xylestesin-S "special"; Xylocain; Xylocard; Xyloneural; Xylonor†; ***Thai.:*** Docaine; Lido Spray; Lidocation; Lidocaton; Neo-Lidocaton; Xylocaine; Xylocard; ***UAE:*** Ecocain; ***UK:*** Dequaspray; Laryng-O-Jet; Lignostab-A; Premjact; Rinstead†; Stud; Vagisil; Xylocaine; Xylocaine 2% Plain†; Xylocard†; Xylotox; ***USA:*** Anestacon; Dentipatch; Dilocaine; Dr Scholl's Cracked Heel Relief; Duo-Trach Kit; L-M-X4; LidaMantle; Lidoderm; Lidoject†; LidoPen; Nervocaine; Octocaine; Xylocaine; Zilactin-L.

**Multi-ingredient:** numerous preparations are listed in Part 3.

# Mepivacaine Hydrochloride

*(BANM, rINNM)*

Hidrocloruro de mepivacaína; Mepivacaini Chloridum; Mepivacaini Hydrochloridum. (1-Methyl-2-piperidyl)formo-2′,6′-xylidide hydrochloride.

$C_{15}H_{22}N_2O,HCl$ = 282.8.
*CAS — 96-88-8 (mepivacaine); 22801-44-1 ((±)-mepivacaine); 1722-62-9 (mepivacaine hydrochloride).*
*ATC — N01BB03.*

**Pharmacopoeias.** In *Eur.* (see p.vi), *Jpn*, and *US*.

**Ph. Eur. 5.0** (Mepivacaine Hydrochloride). A white crystalline powder. Freely soluble in water and in alcohol; very slightly soluble in dichloromethane. A 2% solution in water has a pH of 4.0 to 5.0.

**USP 27** (Mepivacaine Hydrochloride). A white, odourless, crystalline solid. Freely soluble in water and in methyl alcohol; very slightly soluble in chloroform; practically insoluble in ether. A 2% solution in water has a pH of about 4.5.

**pH of solutions.** For a discussion of the effect that pH has on the stability of local anaesthetic solutions and the pain associated with their injection, see p.1369.

## Adverse Effects, Treatment, and Precautions

As for Local Anaesthetics in general, p.1367.

**Porphyria.** Mepivacaine is considered to be unsafe in patients with porphyria because it has been shown to be porphyrinogenic in *in-vitro* systems.

## Interactions

For interactions associated with local anaesthetics, see p.1368.

**Bupivacaine.** Studies *in vitro* showed that bupivacaine dramatically reduced the binding of mepivacaine to α-1-acid glycoprotein.[1]


1. Hartrick CT, *et al.* Influence of bupivacaine on mepivacaine protein binding. *Clin Pharmacol Ther* 1984; **36:** 546–50.


## Pharmacokinetics

Mepivacaine is about 78% bound to plasma proteins. The plasma half-life has been reported to be about 2 to 3 hours in adults and about 9 hours in neonates. It is rapidly metabolised in the liver and less than 10% of a dose is reported to be excreted unchanged in the urine. Over 50% of a dose is excreted as metabolites into the bile but these probably undergo enterohepatic circulation as only small amounts appear in the faeces. Several metabolites are also excreted via the kidneys and include glucuronide conjugates of hydroxy compounds and an *N*-demethylated compound, 2′,6′-pipecoloxylidide. Mepivacaine crosses the placenta.

See also under Local Anaesthetics, p.1368.

**Pregnancy.** There is considerable transfer of mepivacaine across the placenta following maternal administration and the ratio of fetal to maternal concentrations[1] is about 0.7. Although neonates have a very limited capacity to metabolise mepivacaine it appears they are able to eliminate the drug.[2]


1. Lurie AO, Weiss JB. Blood concentration of mepivacaine and lidocaine in mother and baby after epidural anesthesia. *Am J Obstet Gynecol* 1970; **106:** 850–6.
2. Meffin P, *et al.* Clearance and metabolism of mepivacaine in the human neonate. *Clin Pharmacol Ther* 1973; **14:** 218–25.


## Uses and Administration

Mepivacaine hydrochloride is a local anaesthetic of the amide type with actions and uses similar to those described on p.1369. It is mainly used for infiltration anaesthesia, peripheral nerve block, and epidural block. (Local anaesthetic techniques are discussed on p.1370.) Mepivacaine has a rapid onset and an intermediate duration of action. The speed of onset and duration of action are increased by the addition of a vasoconstrictor and absorption into the circulation from the site of injection is reduced.

The dosage of mepivacaine hydrochloride varies with the site of injection and the type of **local anaesthetic procedure**. In adults, the **maximum single dose** of mepivacaine hydrochloride should not generally exceed 400 mg and the total dose in 24 hours should not exceed 1 g. Doses should be reduced in the elderly, in debilitated patients, and in those with cardiac or hepatic impairment. Concentrations of less than 2% should be used in children under 3 years or weighing less than about 14 kg (30 pounds); the dose in children should not exceed 5 to 6 mg/kg.

- For *infiltration anaesthesia* up to 400 mg as a 1% (40 mL) or 0.5% (80 mL) solution is used. For *dental infiltration and nerve block* a 2% solution with a vasoconstrictor or a 3% plain solution is used. For anaesthesia at a single site in the jaw a dose of 36 mg (1.8 mL) as a 2% solution or 54 mg (1.8 mL) as a 3% solution is used. For anaesthesia of the entire oral cavity 180 mg (9 mL) as a 2% solution or 270 mg (9 mL) as a 3% solution is used. Some recommend that no more than 400 mg should be given at a single dental sitting.
- For *peripheral nerve blocks*, namely *cervical, brachial plexus, intercostal,* and *pudendal blocks*, 1 or 2% solutions may be used in doses of 50 to 400 mg (5 to 40 mL) as a 1% solution, or 100 to 400 mg (5 to 20 mL) as a 2% solution. For pudendal block half of the dose is injected on each side. For *paracervical block* a dose of up to 100 mg (10 mL) as a 1% solution on each side has been suggested allowing an interval of 5 minutes between sides. This may be repeated at an interval of not less than 90 minutes, and for a combined paracervical and pudendal block up to 150 mg (15 mL) as a 1% solution is injected on each side. For therapeutic nerve block in the management of pain 10 to 50 mg (1 to 5 mL) as a 1% solution or 20 to 100 mg (1 to 5 mL) as a 2% solution may be given.
- For *epidural block* usual doses are: 150 to 300 mg (15 to 30 mL) as a 1% solution, 150 to 375 mg (10 to 25 mL) as a 1.5% solution, or 200 to 400 mg (10 to 20 mL) as a 2% solution. Hyperbaric solutions of mepivacaine hydrochloride without adrenaline have also been used for *spinal block*.

Mepivacaine has been included in the intramuscular injections of other drugs to minimise the pain produced at the injection site.

Mepivacaine has also been used as a surface anaesthetic but other local anaesthetics such as lidocaine are more effective.

**Action.** For a comparison of the vasoactivity of mepivacaine and some other local anaesthetics, see p.1369.

## Preparations

***USP 27:*** Mepivacaine Hydrochloride and Levonordefrin Injection; Mepivacaine Hydrochloride Injection.

**Proprietary Preparations** (details are given in Part 3)
***Austral.:*** Carbocaine; Scandonest; ***Austria:*** Mepinaest; Scandicain; Scandonest; ***Belg.:*** Scandicaine; ***Braz.:*** Scandicaine†; Scandinor†; ***Canad.:*** Carbocaine; Polocaine; ***Denm.:*** Carbocain; Scandonest; ***Fr.:*** Carbocaine; ***Ger.:*** Meaverin; Meaverin "A" mit Adrenalin†; Meaverin "N" mit Noradrenaline†; Meaverin hyperbar†; Mecain; Mepicaton†; Mepihexal; Mepivastesin; Scandicain; ***Hong Kong:*** Mepivastesin; ***Israel:*** Tevacaine; ***Ital.:*** Carbocaina; Carbosen; Mepi-Mynol†; Mepibil; Mepicain; Mepident; Mepiforan; Mepisolver; Mepivamol; Mepivirgi; Mepyl†; Molcain; Optocain; Pericaina; Scandonest; ***Neth.:*** Scandicaine; ***Norw.:*** Carbocain; Scandonest; ***Port.:*** Scandinibsa; ***S.Afr.:*** Carbocaine; Scandonest; ***Spain:*** Isogaine; Scandinibsa; ***Swed.:*** Carbocain; ***Switz.:*** Mepicaton†; Scandicain; Scandonest; ***Thai.:*** Mepicaton; ***USA:*** Carbocaine; Carbocaine with Neo-Cobefrin; Isocaine; Polocaine.

**Multi-ingredient:** ***Ger.:*** Meaverin; Thesit.

*Used as an adjunct in:* ***Austria:*** Estradurin; ***Belg.:*** Estradurine; ***Denm.:*** Estradurin; ***Fin.:*** Estradurin; ***Ger.:*** Estradurin; ***Hong Kong:*** Nevramin; ***Jpn:*** Amasulin; Bestcall; Lilacillin; Pansporin; Takesulin; ***Malaysia:*** Nevramin; ***Mex.:*** Kedacillin; ***Neth.:*** Estradurin; ***Norw.:*** Estradurin; ***Port.:*** Linamin Plus; ***Singapore:*** Nevramin; ***Swed.:*** Estradurin; ***Switz.:*** Estradurin; ***Thai.:*** Nevramin.

# Myrtecaine *(rINN)*

Mirtecaína; Nopoxamine. 2-[2-(10-Norpin-2-en-2-yl)ethoxy]triethylamine.

$C_{17}H_{31}NO$ = 265.4.
*CAS — 7712-50-7.*

## Profile

Myrtecaine is a local anaesthetic (p.1367) used topically as the base or laurilsulfate in rubefacient preparations for the treatment of muscle and joint pain. Myrtecaine laurilsulfate is also used in preparations with antacids for the symptomatic relief of gastrointestinal disorders.

### Preparations

**Proprietary Preparations** (details are given in Part 3)

**Multi-ingredient: *Arg.:*** Algesal; Flexicamin Crema; ***Austria:*** Acidrine†; Algesal; Latesyl; Rheugesal; ***Belg.:*** Acidrine†; ***Chile:*** Sinacid; ***Fr.:*** Acidrine; Algesal Suractive†; ***Ger.:*** Acidrine; Algesal; Algesalona; ***Ital.:*** Acidrine; ***Mex.:*** Algesal; ***Neth.:*** Algesal Forte; ***Port.:*** Algesal; Latesil; ***Spain:*** Algesal; ***Switz.:*** Algesal; Algesalona.

## Octacaine Hydrochloride *(pINNM)*

Hidrocloruro de octacaína. 3-Diethylaminobutyranilide hydrochloride.

$C_{14}H_{22}N_2O,HCl = 270.8$.

*CAS — 13912-77-1 (octacaine); 59727-70-7 (octacaine hydrochloride).*

### Profile

Octacaine hydrochloride is a local anaesthetic (p.1367) that has been used for surface anaesthesia.

### Preparations

**Proprietary Preparations** (details are given in Part 3)

**Multi-ingredient: *Ger.:*** Batrax†; ***Switz.:*** Batramycine.

## Oxetacaine *(BAN, rINN)*

Oxetacaína; Oxethazaine *(USAN)*; Wy-806. 2,2′-(2-Hydroxyethylimino)bis[N-(αα-dimethylphenethyl)-N-methylacetamide].

$C_{28}H_{41}N_3O_3 = 467.6$.

*CAS — 126-27-2 (oxetacaine); 13930-31-9 (oxetacaine hydrochloride).*

*ATC — C05AD06.*

**Pharmacopoeias.** In *Br.* and *Jpn.*

**BP 2003** (Oxetacaine). A white or almost white powder. Practically insoluble in water; freely soluble in methyl alcohol; very soluble in chloroform; soluble in ethyl acetate.

### Profile

Oxetacaine is an amide anaesthetic (p.1367) that is stated to have a prolonged action. It is administered by mouth with antacids for the symptomatic relief of gastro-oesophageal reflux disease (p.1242). It has also been used as the hydrochloride in ointments and suppositories for the relief of pain associated with haemorrhoids.

### Preparations

**Proprietary Preparations** (details are given in Part 3)

***Hong Kong:*** Strocain; ***India:*** Tricaine-MPS; ***Ital.:*** Emoren; ***Jpn:*** Strocain; ***Singapore:*** Strocain; ***Thai.:*** Strocain.

**Multi-ingredient: *Arg.:*** Mucaine; ***Austral.:*** Mucaine; ***Austria:*** Tepilta; ***Belg.:*** Muthesa†; ***Braz.:*** Droxaine; ***Canad.:*** Mucaine; ***Chile:*** Mucaine; ***Fr.:*** Mutesa; ***Ger.:*** Tepilta; ***Gr.:*** Oxaine-M; ***Hong Kong:*** Gastrocaine; Milzine; Mucaine; Oxema Improved; ***India:*** Mucaine; Pepticaine; ***Irl.:*** Mucaine†; ***Ital.:*** Gastrodue; Magnesia Bisurata Aromatic Plus†; Mucoxin†; ***NZ:*** Mucaine; ***Port.:*** Betalgil†; ***S.Afr.:*** Mucaine; ***Singapore:*** Mucaine; ***Spain:*** Natrocitral; Roberfarin; Tepilta†; ***Switz.:*** Muthesa; ***Thai.:*** Mucaine; ***UK:*** Mucaine†.

## Oxybuprocaine Hydrochloride

*(BANM, rINNM)*

Benoxinate Hydrochloride; Hidrocloruro de oxibuprocaína; Oxybuprocaini Hydrochloridum. 2-Diethylaminoethyl 4-amino-3-butoxybenzoate hydrochloride.

$C_{17}H_{28}N_2O_3,HCl = 344.9$.

*CAS — 99-43-4 (oxybuprocaine); 5987-82-6 (oxybuprocaine hydrochloride).*

*ATC — D04AB03; S01HA02.*

NOTE. BNX is a code approved by the BP 2003 for use on single unit doses of eye drops containing oxybuprocaine hydrochloride where the individual container may be too small to bear all the appropriate labelling information.

**Pharmacopoeias.** In *Eur.* (see p.vi), *Jpn*, and *US.*

**Ph. Eur. 5.0** (Oxybuprocaine Hydrochloride). A white crystalline powder or colourless crystals. It exhibits polymorphism. Very soluble in water; freely soluble in alcohol. A 10% solution in water has a pH of 4.5 to 6.0. Protect from light.

**USP 27** (Benoxinate Hydrochloride). White or slightly off-white, crystals or crystalline powder, odourless or with a slight characteristic odour. Soluble 1 in 0.8 of water, 1 in 2.6 of alcohol, and 1 in 2.5 of chloroform; insoluble in ether. A 1% solution in water has a pH of 5.0 to 6.0.

### Adverse Effects, Treatment, and Precautions

As for Local Anaesthetics in general, p.1367.

**Effects on the eyes.** Fibrinous iritis and moderate corneal swelling occurred in 2 patients following the use of a 0.4% or 1% solution of oxybuprocaine hydrochloride for topical anaesthesia of the eye for minor surgery.[1] The effects may have been due to inadvertent entry of the drug into the anterior chamber of the eye.

1. Haddad R. Fibrinous iritis due to oxybuprocaine. *Br J Ophthalmol* 1989; **73:** 76–7.

### Interactions

For interactions associated with local anaesthetics, see p.1368.

### Uses and Administration

Oxybuprocaine, a para-aminobenzoic acid ester, is a local anaesthetic with actions and uses similar to those described on p.1369. It is used for surface anaesthesia (p.1370) and is reported to be less irritant than tetracaine when applied to the conjunctiva in therapeutic concentrations.

Oxybuprocaine is used as the hydrochloride in a 0.4% solution in short ophthalmological procedures. One drop instilled into the conjunctival sac anaesthetises the surface of the eye sufficiently to allow tonometry after 60 seconds and a further drop after 90 seconds provides adequate anaesthesia for the fitting of contact lenses. Three drops at 90-second intervals produces sufficient anaesthesia after 5 minutes for removal of a foreign body from the corneal epithelium, or for incision of a Meibomian cyst through the conjunctiva. The sensitivity of the cornea is normal again after about 1 hour.

A 1% solution of oxybuprocaine hydrochloride is used for surface anaesthesia of the ear nose, and throat.

### Preparations

***BP 2003:*** Oxybuprocaine Eye Drops;

***USP 27:*** Benoxinate Hydrochloride Ophthalmic Solution; Fluorescein Sodium and Benoxinate Hydrochloride Ophthalmic Solution.

**Proprietary Preparations** (details are given in Part 3)

***Arg.:*** Oftalmocaina; ***Austria:*** Novain; ***Belg.:*** Novesine†; Unicaine†; ***Braz.:*** Anestocil†; ***Fin.:*** Oftan Obucain; ***Fr.:*** Cebesine; Novesine; ***Ger.:*** Benoxinat SE; Conjuncain-EDO; Novesine; Oxbarukain; ***Hong Kong:*** Benoxinate; Novesin; ***India:*** Bendzon; ***Israel:*** Localin; ***Ital.:*** Novesina; ***Malaysia:*** Novesin; ***Port.:*** Anestocil; ***S.Afr.:*** Novesin; ***Singapore:*** Novesin; ***Spain:*** Benoxinato†; Prescaina; ***Switz.:*** Novesin; ***Thai.:*** Novesin.

**Multi-ingredient: *Austral.:*** Fluress; ***Austria:*** Flurekain; ***Belg.:*** Anesthesique Doublet†; ***Canad.:*** Fluress†; ***Fin.:*** Oftan Flurekain; ***Ger.:*** Thilorbin; ***Mex.:*** Mentalgina; ***NZ:*** Fluress; ***Port.:*** Fluotest; Mebocaina; ***Spain:*** Anestesi Doble; Fluotest; ***Swed.:*** Fluress; ***Switz.:*** Collu-Blache; Mebucaine; ***UAE:*** B-Cool; ***USA:*** Flu-Oxinate; Fluorox; Flurate; Fluress; Flurox.

## Parethoxycaine Hydrochloride *(rINNM)*

Hidrocloruro de paretoxicaína. 2-Diethylaminoethyl 4-ethoxybenzoate hydrochloride.

$C_{15}H_{23}NO_3,HCl = 301.8$.

*CAS — 94-23-5 (parethoxycaine); 136-46-9 (parethoxycaine hydrochloride).*

### Profile

Parethoxycaine hydrochloride, a para-aminobenzoic acid ester, is a local anaesthetic (p.1367) that has been used in pastilles for painful conditions of the mouth and throat.

### Preparations

**Proprietary Preparations** (details are given in Part 3)

***Fr.:*** Maxicaine†.

## Pramocaine Hydrochloride *(BANM, rINNM)*

Hidrocloruro de pramocaína; Pramoxine Hydrochloride; Pramoxinium Chloride. 4-[3-(4-Butoxyphenoxy)propyl]morpholine hydrochloride.

$C_{17}H_{27}NO_3,HCl = 329.9$.

*CAS — 140-65-8 (pramocaine); 637-58-1 (pramocaine hydrochloride).*

*ATC — C05AD07; D04AB07.*

**Pharmacopoeias.** In *US.*

**USP 27** (Pramoxine Hydrochloride). A white or almost white crystalline powder; it may have a faint aromatic odour. Freely soluble in water and in alcohol; soluble 1 in 35 of chloroform; very slightly soluble in ether. A 1% solution in water has a pH of about 4.5. Store in airtight containers.

### Profile

Pramocaine hydrochloride is a local anaesthetic (p.1367) used for surface anaesthesia. It is used alone or with corticosteroids and other drugs, usually in a concentration of 1%, in a wide range of formulations for the relief of pain and itching associated with minor skin conditions and anorectal disorders. Initial burning or stinging may occur following topical application. It should not be used for the nose or eyes. The base has been used similarly.

### Preparations

***USP 27:*** Neomycin and Polymyxin B Sulfates and Pramoxine Hydrochloride Cream; Pramoxine Hydrochloride Cream; Pramoxine Hydrochloride Jelly.

**Proprietary Preparations** (details are given in Part 3)

***Fr.:*** Tronothane; ***Israel:*** Anti Itch; ***Ital.:*** Tronotene; ***S.Afr.:*** Anugesic; ***Spain:*** Balsabit; Pramox; ***USA:*** Fleet Pain Relief; Prax; Proctofoam; Tronothane.

**Multi-ingredient: *Arg.:*** Anusol Duo; Anusol Duo S; Anusol-A; ***Belg.:*** Nestosyl†; ***Canad.:*** Anugesic-HC; Anusol Plus; Anuzinc HC Plus; Aveeno Anti-Itch; Hemorrhoid Ointment; Onguent Hemorrhoidal; PrameGel; Pramox HC; Proctodan-HC; Proctofoam-HC; Sarna-P; ***Chile:*** Caladryl Clear; ***Irl.:*** Anugesic-HC; Proctofoam-HC; ***Israel:*** Epifoam; Proctofoam-HC; ***Ital.:*** Proctofoam-HC; ***S.Afr.:*** Anugesic; Proctofoam; ***UK:*** Anugesic-HC; Proctocream HC†; Proctofoam-HC; ***USA:*** 1 + 1-F; AmLactin AP; Analpram-HC; Anusol; Aveeno Anti-Itch†; Bactine Pain Relieving Cleansing; Betadine Plus First Aid Antibiotics & Pain Reliever; Bite & Itch Lotion; Caladryl; Caladryl Clear; Cortane-B; Cortic; Cyotic; Enzone; Epifoam; Hemorid For Women; Itch-X; Neosporin + Pain Relief; Oti-Med; Otomar-HC; Phicon; Phicon-F; PrameGel; Pramosone; PramOtic; Proctofoam-HC; Tri-Biozene; Tri-Otic; Tronolane; Zone-A; Zoto-HC.

## Prilocaine *(BAN, USAN, rINN)*

Prilocainum. 2-Propylaminopropiono-o-toluidide.

$C_{13}H_{20}N_2O = 220.3$.

*CAS — 721-50-6.*

*ATC — N01BB04.*

**Pharmacopoeias.** In *Eur.* (see p.vi).

**Ph. Eur. 5.0** (Prilocaine). A white or almost white, crystalline powder. M.p. 36° to 39°. Slightly soluble in water; very soluble in alcohol and in acetone.

**Eutectic mixture.** Prilocaine forms a mixture with lidocaine that has a melting-point lower than that of either ingredient. This eutectic mixture is used in the preparation of topical dosage forms.

## Prilocaine Hydrochloride *(BANM, USAN, rINNM)*

Astra-1512; Hidrocloruro de prilocaína; L-67; Prilocaini Hydrochloridum; Propitocaine Hydrochloride.

$C_{13}H_{20}N_2O,HCl = 256.8$.

*CAS — 721-50-6 (prilocaine); 1786-81-8 (prilocaine hydrochloride).*

*ATC — N01BB04.*

**Pharmacopoeias.** In *Eur.* (see p.vi) and *US.*

**Ph. Eur. 5.0** (Prilocaine Hydrochloride). A white crystalline powder or colourless crystals. M.p. 168° to 171°. Freely soluble in water and in alcohol; very slightly soluble in acetone.

**USP 27** (Prilocaine Hydrochloride). A white odourless crystalline powder. M.p. 166° to 169°. Soluble 1 in 3.5 of water, 1 in 4.2 of alcohol, and 1 in 175 of chloroform; very slightly soluble in acetone; practically insoluble in ether.

**pH of solutions.** For a discussion of the effect that pH has on the stability of local anaesthetic solutions and the pain associated with their injection, see p.1369.

### Adverse Effects, Treatment, and Precautions

As for Local Anaesthetics in general, p.1367.

Prilocaine has relatively modest toxicity compared with most amide-type local anaesthetics. However, dose-related methaemoglobinaemia and cyanosis, attributed to the metabolite *o*-toluidine, appear to occur more frequently with prilocaine than with other local anaesthetics (see Methaemoglobinaemia, p.1367). Symptoms usually occur when doses of prilocaine hydrochloride exceed about 8 mg/kg but the very young may be more susceptible. Methaemoglobinaemia has been observed in neonates whose mothers received prilocaine shortly before delivery and it has also been reported after prolonged topical application of a prilocaine/lidocaine eutectic mixture in children. (See under Surface Anaesthesia in Lidocaine, p.1380 for precautions to be observed with such a eutectic mixture.) Methaemoglobinaemia may be treated by giving oxygen followed, if necessary, by an injection of methylthioninium chloride.

Prilocaine is contra-indicated for paracervical block in obstetrics.

Prilocaine should be avoided in patients with anaemia, congenital or acquired methaemoglobinaemia, cardiac or ventilatory failure, or hypoxia.

**Effects on the CNS.** For reference to the prilocaine serum concentrations associated with CNS toxicity, see under Absorption in Pharmacokinetics, below.

**Porphyria.** Prilocaine has been associated with acute attacks of porphyria and is considered unsafe in porphyric patients.

### Interactions

For interactions associated with local anaesthetics, see p.1368.

Methaemoglobinaemia may occur at lower doses of prilocaine in patients receiving therapy with other drugs known to cause such conditions (e.g. sulfonamides such as sulfamethoxazole in co-trimoxazole).

**Neuromuscular blockers.** For a possible interaction between *mivacurium* and prilocaine, see under Atracurium, p.1401.

## Pharmacokinetics

Prilocaine is reported to be 55% bound to plasma proteins. It is rapidly metabolised mainly in the liver and also in the kidneys and is excreted in the urine mainly as metabolites. One of the principal metabolites excreted in the urine is *o*-toluidine, which is believed to cause the methaemoglobinaemia observed after large doses. Prilocaine crosses the placenta and during prolonged epidural anaesthesia may produce methaemoglobinaemia in the fetus. It is distributed into breast milk.

See also under Local Anaesthetics, p.1368.

**Absorption.** Peak serum concentrations of prilocaine hydrochloride attained after the use of 8.5 mL of a 1% solution for retrobulbar and facial nerve block were well below the concentration of 20 micrograms/mL associated with CNS toxicity due to prilocaine.[1]

1. Goggin M, *et al.* Serum concentrations of prilocaine following retrobulbar block. *Br J Anaesth* 1990; **64:** 107–9.

## Uses and Administration

Prilocaine is a local anaesthetic of the amide type with actions and uses similar to those described on p.1369. It has a similar anaesthetic potency to lidocaine. However, it has a slower onset of action, less vasodilator activity, and a slightly longer duration of action; it is also less toxic. Prilocaine hydrochloride is used for infiltration anaesthesia and nerve blocks in solutions of 0.5%, 1%, and 2%; 1 or 2% solutions are used for epidural block and for analgesia, and for intravenous regional anaesthesia 0.5% solutions are used. A 3% solution with the vasoconstrictor felypressin (p.1324) or a 4% solution without are used for dental procedures. A 4% solution with adrenaline 1 in 200 000 is also used for dentistry in some countries. Carbonated solutions of prilocaine have also been tried in some countries in epidural and brachial plexus nerve blocks (see under Administration, p.1369). Prilocaine is used for surface anaesthesia in a eutectic mixture with lidocaine. (Local anaesthetic techniques are discussed on p.1370.)

The dosage used in various **local anaesthetic procedures** varies with the site of injection and the procedure used. The recommended **maximum single dose** in adults for prilocaine hydrochloride is 400 mg if used alone, or 300 mg if used with felypressin. Doses should be reduced in elderly or debilitated patients. The dose for children over 6 months of age is up to 5 mg/kg. For *dental infiltration* or *dental nerve blocks*, the usual adult dose of prilocaine hydrochloride without felypressin is 40 to 80 mg (1 to 2 mL) as a 4% solution; children under 10 years generally require about 40 mg (1 mL). Similar doses of the 4% solution with adrenaline (1:200 000) may be used for most routine dental procedures. The usual adult dose of prilocaine hydrochloride with felypressin 0.03 international units/mL is 30 to 150 mg (1 to 5 mL) as a 3% solution; children under 10 years generally require 30 to 60 mg (1 to 2 mL).

A eutectic mixture (see Surface Anaesthesia, p.1380) of prilocaine base 2.5% and lidocaine base 2.5% is applied as a cream under an occlusive dressing to produce *surface anaesthesia* of the skin before procedures requiring needle puncture, surgical treatment of localised lesions, and split skin grafting; it has been used similarly, but without an occlusive dressing, before removal of genital warts.

**Action.** For a comparison of the vasoactivity of prilocaine and some other local anaesthetics, see p.1369.

**Infiltration anaesthesia.** Addition of felypressin at a concentration of 0.03 international units/mL to prilocaine 3% injection did not reduce plasma concentrations of prilocaine after infiltration of a 60-mg dose into the upper premolar region.[1]

1. Cannell H, Whelpton R. Systemic uptake of prilocaine after injection of various formulations of the drug. *Br Dent J* 1986; **160:** 47–9.

### Preparations

***BP 2003:*** Prilocaine Injection;
***USP 27:*** Prilocaine and Epinephrine Injection; Prilocaine Hydrochloride Injection.

**Proprietary Preparations** (details are given in Part 3)
***Austral.:*** Citanest; Citanest Dental; ***Belg.:*** Citanest; ***Braz.:*** Citanest; Citocaina; ***Canad.:*** Citanest; ***Denm.:*** Citanest Octapressin; ***Fin.:*** Citanest Octapressin; Citanest†; ***Ger.:*** Xylonest; ***Irl.:*** Citanest with Octapressin†; Citanest†; ***Ital.:*** Citanest con Octapressin; ***Mex.:*** Citanest Octapresin; ***Neth.:*** Citanest; Citanest Octapressine†; ***Norw.:*** Citanest Octapressin; ***NZ:*** Citanest; Citanest with Octapressin; ***Port.:*** Citanest Octapressin†; ***Spain:*** Citanest; Citanest Octapressin; ***Swed.:*** Citanest; Citanest Octapressin; ***Switz.:*** Xylonest; Xylonest-Octapressin†; ***UK:*** Citanest; Citanest with Octapressin; ***USA:*** Citanest.

**Multi-ingredient:** ***Arg.:*** Emla; ***Austral.:*** Emla; ***Austria:*** Emla; ***Belg.:*** Emla; ***Braz.:*** Emla; Medicaina†; ***Canad.:*** Emla; ***Chile:*** Eutecaina; ***Denm.:*** Emla; ***Fin.:*** Citanest†; Emla; ***Fr.:*** Emla; Emlapatch; ***Ger.:*** Emla; ***Gr.:*** Emla; ***Hong Kong:*** Emla; ***Irl.:*** Emla; ***Israel:*** Emla; ***Ital.:*** Emla; ***Malaysia:*** Emla; ***Neth.:*** Emla; ***Norw.:*** Citanest†; Emla; ***NZ:*** Emla; ***Port.:*** Emla; ***S.Afr.:*** Emla; ***Singapore:*** Emla; ***Spain:*** Emla; ***Swed.:*** Emla; ***Switz.:*** Emla; ***Thai.:*** Emla; ***UK:*** Emla; ***USA:*** Emla.

---

## Procaine Hydrochloride *(BANM, rINNM)*

Allocaine; Ethocaine Hydrochloride; Hidrocloruro de procaína; Novocainum; Procaini Hydrochloridum; Procainii Chloridum; Procainium Chloride; Syncaine. 2-Diethylaminoethyl 4-aminobenzoate hydrochloride.

$C_{13}H_{20}N_2O_2,HCl = 272.8.$
*CAS — 59-46-1 (procaine); 51-05-8 (procaine hydrochloride).*
*ATC — C05AD05; N01BA02; S01HA05.*

**Pharmacopoeias.** In *Chin., Eur.* (see p.vi), *Int., Jpn, Pol., US,* and *Viet.*

**Ph. Eur. 5.0** (Procaine Hydrochloride). A white crystalline powder or colourless crystals. Very soluble in water; soluble in alcohol. A 2% solution in water has a pH of 5.0 to 6.5. Protect from light.

**USP 27** (Procaine Hydrochloride). Odourless, small, white crystals or white, crystalline powder. Soluble 1 in 1 of water and 1 in 15 of alcohol; slightly soluble in chloroform; practically insoluble in ether.

**Incompatibility.** Procaine hydrochloride has been reported to be incompatible with aminophylline, barbiturates, magnesium sulfate, phenytoin sodium, sodium bicarbonate, and amphotericin B.

**Stability of solutions.** Degradation of procaine in a cardioplegic solution containing magnesium, sodium, potassium, and calcium salts was found to be temperature dependent.[1] At a storage temperature of 6° the shelf-life of the solution was 5 weeks and this was increased to 9 weeks when the storage temperature was −10°. Using carbon dioxide instead of nitrogen in the head space did not affect stability of procaine.

1. Synave R, *et al.* Stability of procaine hydrochloride in a cardioplegic solution containing bicarbonate. *J Clin Hosp Pharm* 1985; **10:** 385–8.

### Adverse Effects, Treatment, and Precautions

As for Local Anaesthetics in general, p.1367.

**Effects on the cardiovascular system.** Severe hypotension leading to cardiac arrest and death developed in a patient following the infusion of 600 mg of procaine for malignant hyperthermia.[1]

1. MacLachlan D, Forrest AL. Procaine and malignant hyperthermia. *Lancet* 1974; **i:** 355.

**Hypersensitivity.** Of 600 persons with dermatitis or eczema submitted to patch testing with 2% aqueous solution of procaine hydrochloride, 4.8% gave a positive reaction.[1]

For reports of hypersensitivity including anaphylactic reactions associated with procaine and other local anaesthetics, see under Adverse Effects of Local Anaesthetics, p.1367.

1. Rudzki E, Kleniewska D. The epidemiology of contact dermatitis in Poland. *Br J Dermatol* 1970; **83:** 543–5.

**Systemic lupus erythematosus.** The limited theoretical risk from using procaine for local anaesthesia in patients who have had procainamide-induced systemic lupus erythematosus was aired some years ago.[1-3]

1. Dubois EL. Procaine anesthesia after procainamide-induced systemic erythematosus. *JAMA* 1977; **238:** 2201.
2. Alarcón-Segovia D. Procaine anesthesia after procainamide-induced systemic erythematosus. *JAMA* 1977; **238:** 2201.
3. Lee SL. Procaine anesthesia after procainamide-induced systemic erythematosus. *JAMA* 1977; **238:** 2201.

### Interactions

For interactions associated with local anaesthetics, see p.1368.

**Diuretics.** Concomitant administration of *acetazolamide* extends the plasma half-life of procaine.[1]

1. Calvo R, *et al.* Effects of disease and acetazolamide on procaine hydrolysis by red blood cell enzymes. *Clin Pharmacol Ther* 1980; **27:** 179–83.

### Pharmacokinetics

Procaine is poorly absorbed from mucous membranes and is usually given parenterally. It is rapidly hydrolysed by plasma cholinesterase to para-aminobenzoic acid and diethylaminoethanol; some may also be metabolised in the liver. Only about 6% is bound to plasma proteins. About 80% of the para-aminobenzoic acid is excreted unchanged or conjugated in the urine. About 30% of the diethylaminoethanol is excreted in the urine, the remainder being metabolised in the liver.

See also under Local Anaesthetics, p.1368.

### Uses and Administration

Procaine hydrochloride, a para-aminobenzoic acid ester, is a local anaesthetic with actions and uses similar to those described on p.1369. Because of its poor penetration of intact mucous membranes, procaine is ineffective for surface application and has been chiefly used by injection, although in general it has been replaced by lidocaine and other local anaesthetics. It has a slow onset of action and a short duration of action. It has vasodilator activity and therefore a vasoconstrictor may be added to delay absorption and increase the duration of action. Procaine has mainly been used for infiltration anaesthesia, peripheral nerve blocks, and spinal block. (Local anaesthetic techniques are discussed on p.1370.) It has also been used in cardioplegic solutions to protect the myocardium during cardiac surgery.

For *infiltration anaesthesia* 0.25 or 0.5% solutions of procaine hydrochloride have been used in doses of 350 to 600 mg.

For *peripheral nerve block* a usual dose of 500 mg of procaine hydrochloride has been given as a 0.5% (100 mL), 1% (50 mL), or 2% (25 mL) solution. Doses up to 1 g have been used. For infiltration and peripheral nerve block adrenaline has been added to solutions, in general to give a final concentration of 1 in 200 000 to 1 in 100 000.

Procaine hydrochloride has been used with propoxycaine in dentistry.

Procaine forms poorly soluble salts or conjugates with some drugs, for example penicillin, and is used to prolong their action after injection. It may also reduce the pain of injection.

Procaine-*N*-glucoside hydrochloride has been included in a preparation for gastrointestinal disorders, and procaine ascorbate has been included in a multivitamin preparation.

**Action.** For a comparison of the vasoactivity of procaine and some other local anaesthetics, see p.1369.

### Preparations

***USP 27:*** Procaine and Tetracaine Hydrochlorides and Levonordefrin Injection; Procaine Hydrochloride and Epinephrine Injection; Procaine Hydrochloride Injection; Propoxycaine and Procaine Hydrochlorides and Levonordefrin Injection; Propoxycaine and Procaine Hydrochlorides and Norepinephrine Bitartrate Injection.

**Proprietary Preparations** (details are given in Part 3)
***Arg.:*** Endocaina; Fadacaina; Procanest; ***Austria:*** Geroaslan H3; Gerovital H3; Novanaest; ***Canad.:*** Novocain; ***Ger.:*** Hewedolor Procain; Lophakomp-Procain N; Novocain; Pasconeural-Injektopas; Pasconeural-Injektopas 1%†; ***Hong Kong:*** Gerovital H3; ***Ital.:*** Lenident; ***Spain:*** Anestesia Loc Braun C/A†; Venocaina†; ***USA:*** Novocain.

**Multi-ingredient:** ***Arg.:*** 6 Copin; Dastonil; Gero H3 Aslan; Gingeron; Muco-Anestyl; Otalex G; Otonorthia; Sicadentol Plus; ***Austral.:*** Cardioplegia Concentrate; ***Austria:*** Aslavital; Biolecit H3†; Causat; Gerontin; KH3; Regenerin; ***Braz.:*** Algidente; Auditol†; Axol†; Bismu-Jet; Claudemor; Colutoide; Dordente†; Fonergin; Geri-Kan H3†; KLGH 3†; Malvosulfam†; Nahora†; Otobel; Otoloide; Otonax†; Oturga; Passaja†; Pradente†; Timpanol; Usedent†; Verlin†; ***Chile:*** Betonvit; Diltotal; KH3; KH3-Vit; Megavit; Pantiban; ***Denm.:*** Kardioplex; ***Fr.:*** Antiseptique-Calmante†; Novitan†; Otylol†; Rectophedrol†; X-Adene†; ***Ger.:*** Bismolan N; Cardioplegin N; Causat B12 N†; Causat N†; Dodecatol N†; Echtrovit-K†; Gero H3 Aslan; Hewedolor plus Coffein; Impletol†; KH3; NeyChondrin N (Revitorgan-Dilutionen N Nr 68); NeyPulpin N (Revitorgan-Dilutionen N Nr 10); Otalgan; Otodolor†; Polytamin; Procaneural; Revicain; Revicain comp; Revicain comp plus; Veno-Kattwiga N; ***Hong Kong:*** Cardioplegia; KH3; ***Israel:*** Bedodeka Antineuralgica; ***Ital.:*** Citroftalmina VC†; Citroftalmina†; Dentosedina; Ginvapast; Mios; Neo-Ustiol; Oftalzina†; Otalgan; Otomidone; Otopax; Rinantipiol; Ustiosan; ***Malaysia:*** Cardioplegia; ***NZ:*** KH3; ***Port.:*** Claudemor; Gramixina†; KH3†; Otalgan†; Otocalma; ***S.Afr.:*** Salusa; Universal Earache Drops†; ***Singapore:*** Cardioplegia; ***Spain:*** Anestesia Loc Braun S/A; Anestina Braun†; Co Bucal; Coliriocilina Adren Astr; Dentol Topico; Eupnol; Kanafosal; Kanafosal Predni; KH3 Powel†; Neocolan; Nulacin Fermentos; Oftalmol Dexa†; Oftalmol Ocular; Otalgan; Otonasal†; Otosedol; Tangenol; ***Switz.:*** Anaestalgin; Ginvapast; Otalgan; Otosan; ***Thai.:*** Cardioplegia; KH3; ***UK:*** KH3†; ***USA:*** Ravocaine and Novocain†.

*Used as an adjunct in:* ***Braz.:*** Cianotrat-Dexa; Dexa-Neuriberi; Dexador; Dexagil; Dexaneurin; Isacilin†; ***Chile:*** Dolo-Neurobionta; ***Ger.:*** Eukalisan N; Redox-Injektopas†; ***Ital.:*** Neuroftal; ***Malaysia:*** Alinamin B12; ***Singapore:*** Alinamin B12; ***Spain:*** Sulmetin; Sulmetin Papaverina; ***USA:*** Hemocyte†; Hytinic.

---

## Propanocaine Hydrochloride *(rINNM)*

467D$_3$; Hidrocloruro de propanocaína. 3-Diethylamino-1-phenylpropyl benzoate hydrochloride.

$C_{20}H_{25}NO_2,HCl = 347.9.$
*CAS — 493-76-5 (propanocaine); 1679-79-4 (propanocaine hydrochloride).*

### Profile

Propanocaine hydrochloride, a benzoic acid ester, is a local anaesthetic (p.1367) that has been used topically for surface anaesthesia.

### Preparations

**Proprietary Preparations** (details are given in Part 3)
**Multi-ingredient:** ***Fr.:*** Lelong Irritations†; ***Spain:*** Detraine.

---

## Propipocaine *(rINN)*

Propipocaína; Propoxypiperocaine. 3-Piperidino-4′-propoxypropiophenone.

$C_{17}H_{25}NO_2 = 275.4.$
*CAS — 3670-68-6.*

### Profile

Propipocaine is a local anaesthetic (p.1367) that has been used for surface anaesthesia.

### Preparations

**Proprietary Preparations** (details are given in Part 3)
**Multi-ingredient:** ***Ger.:*** Nifucin†.

---

**Propoxycaine Hydrochloride** *(rINNM)*

Hidrocloruro de propoxicaína; Propoxycainium Chloride. 2-Diethylaminoethyl 4-amino-2-propoxybenzoate hydrochloride.

$C_{16}H_{26}N_2O_3,HCl = 330.9.$

*CAS — 86-43-1 (propoxycaine); 550-83-4 (propoxycaine hydrochloride).*

**Pharmacopoeias.** In *US.*

**USP 27** (Propoxycaine Hydrochloride). A white odourless crystalline solid. It discolours on prolonged exposure to light and air. Soluble 1 in 2 of water, 1 in 10 of alcohol, and 1 in 80 of ether; practically insoluble in acetone and in chloroform. A 2% solution in water has a pH of about 5.4. Protect from light.

### Profile

Propoxycaine hydrochloride, a para-aminobenzoic acid ester, is a local anaesthetic (p.1367). It has been used in a concentration of 0.4% with procaine hydrochloride 2% solution and a vasoconstrictor for infiltration anaesthesia and nerve block in dental procedures. Propoxycaine has a more rapid onset and a longer duration of action than that of procaine.

### Preparations

***USP 27:*** Propoxycaine and Procaine Hydrochlorides and Levonordefrin Injection; Propoxycaine and Procaine Hydrochlorides and Norepinephrine Bitartrate Injection.

**Proprietary Preparations** (details are given in Part 3)
**Multi-ingredient:** ***USA:*** Ravocaine and Novocain†.

## Proxymetacaine Hydrochloride

*(BANM, rINNM)*

Hidrocloruro de proximetacaína; Proparacaine Hydrochloride. 2-Diethylaminoethyl 3-amino-4-propoxybenzoate hydrochloride.

$C_{16}H_{26}N_2O_3,HCl = 330.9.$

*CAS — 499-67-2 (proxymetacaine); 5875-06-9 (proxymetacaine hydrochloride).*

*ATC — S01HA04.*

NOTE. PROX is a code approved by the BP 2003 for use on single unit doses of eye drops containing proxymetacaine hydrochloride where the individual container may be too small to bear all the appropriate labelling information. PROXFLN is a similar code approved for eye drops containing proxymetacaine hydrochloride and fluorescein sodium.

**Pharmacopoeias.** In *Br.* and *US.*

**BP 2003** (Proxymetacaine Hydrochloride). A white or almost white, odourless or almost odourless, crystalline powder. Soluble in water and in chloroform; very soluble in dehydrated alcohol; practically insoluble in ether. A 1% solution in water has a pH of 5.7 to 6.4. Protect from light.

**USP 27** (Proparacaine Hydrochloride). A white to off-white, or faintly buff-coloured, odourless, crystalline powder. Soluble in water, in warm alcohol, and in methyl alcohol; insoluble in ether and in benzene.

### Adverse Effects, Treatment, and Precautions

As for Local Anaesthetics in general, p.1367.

A severe immediate-type corneal reaction to proxymetacaine may rarely occur. Allergic contact dermatitis has also been reported.

**Effects on the skin.** Exacerbation of Stevens-Johnson syndrome has been reported[1] in a woman after ophthalmic anaesthesia with proxymetacaine hydrochloride.

1. Ward B, *et al.* Dermatologic reaction in Stevens-Johnson syndrome after ophthalmic anesthesia with proparacaine hydrochloride. *Am J Ophthalmol* 1978; **86:** 133–5.

### Interactions

For interactions associated with local anaesthetics, see p.1368.

### Pharmacokinetics

See under Local Anaesthetics, p.1368.

### Uses and Administration

Proxymetacaine hydrochloride, a meta-aminobenzoic acid ester, is a local anaesthetic with actions and uses similar to those described on p.1369. It is used for surface anaesthesia (p.1370) in ophthalmology in a concentration of 0.5%. Proxymetacaine is of similar potency to tetracaine in equal concentrations and induces anaesthesia within about 20 seconds. The duration of action may be 15 minutes or longer. Instillation of 1 or 2 drops permits tonometry after 30 seconds. For removal of foreign bodies or sutures from the cornea 1 or 2 drops are instilled every 5 to 10 minutes for up to 3 applications, or 1 or 2 drops are instilled 2 to 3 minutes before the procedure. For deeper anaesthesia such as needed for cataract extraction 1 drop is instilled every 5 to 10 minutes to a total of 5 to 7 applications.

**Trigeminal neuralgia.** There have been anecdotal reports that proxymetacaine eye drops relieved trigeminal neuralgia (p.8) refractory to carbamazepine.[1,2] However, a controlled study failed to demonstrate any benefit.[3]

1. Zavon MR, Fichte CM. Trigeminal neuralgia relieved by ophthalmic anesthetic. *JAMA* 1991; **265:** 2807.
2. Zavon MR, Fichte CM. Trigeminal neuralgia relieved by optical anesthesia. *JAMA* 1991; **266:** 1649.
3. Kondziolka D, *et al.* The effect of single-application topical ophthalmic anesthesia in patients with trigeminal neuralgia: a randomized double-blind placebo-controlled trial. *J Neurosurg* 1994; **80:** 993–7.

### Preparations

***BP 2003:*** Proxymetacaine Eye Drops;
***USP 27:*** Fluorescein Sodium and Proparacaine Hydrochloride Ophthalmic Solution; Proparacaine Hydrochloride Ophthalmic Solution.

**Proprietary Preparations** (details are given in Part 3)
***Arg.:*** Anestalcon; Poen-Caina NF; ***Austral.:*** Alcaine; Ophthetic; ***Braz.:*** Anestalcon; Visonest; ***Canad.:*** Ak-Taine; Alcaine; Diocaine; Ophthetic; ***Chile:*** Anestalcon; ***Ger.:*** Chibro-Kerakain†; Proparakain-POS; ***Gr.:*** Alcaine; ***Hong Kong:*** Alcaine; ***Malaysia:*** Alcaine; ***Mex.:*** Alcaine; ***Norw.:*** Alcaine; ***NZ:*** Ophthetic; ***S.Afr.:*** Ophthetic†; ***Singapore:*** Alcaine; ***Switz.:*** Alcaine; ***USA:*** Ak-Taine; Alcaine; Ocu-Caine; Ophthetic; Parcaine.
**Multi-ingredient:** ***Canad.:*** Fluoracaine; ***USA:*** Fluoracaine; Fluorocaine.

**Quinisocaine Hydrochloride** *(BANM, rINNM)*

Chinisocainum Hydrochloride; Dimethisoquin Hydrochloride *(USAN)*; Dimethisoquinium Chloride; Hidrocloruro de quinisocaína. 2-(3-Butyl-1-isoquinolyloxy)-*NN*-dimethylethylamine hydrochloride.

$C_{17}H_{24}N_2O,HCl = 308.8.$

*CAS — 86-80-6 (quinisocaine); 2773-92-4 (quinisocaine hydrochloride).*

*ATC — D04AB05.*

### Profile

Quinisocaine hydrochloride is a local anaesthetic (p.1367) available in some countries for use as a surface anaesthetic in the form of an ointment or cream in a concentration of 0.5% or as suppositories. It is used for the relief of pruritus, anogenital or anorectal irritation, and minor skin conditions.

### Preparations

**Proprietary Preparations** (details are given in Part 3)
***Fr.:*** Quotane; ***Ger.:*** Haenal†; Isochinol; ***Switz.:*** Isochinol.
**Multi-ingredient:** ***Fr.:*** Rectoquotane.

## Ropivacaine Hydrochloride

*(BANM, rINNM)*

AL-281; Hidrocloruro de ropivacaína. (*S*)-2′,6′-Dimethyl-1-propylpiperidine-2-carboxanilide hydrochloride monohydrate.

$C_{17}H_{26}N_2O,HCl,H_2O = 328.9.$

*CAS — 84057-95-4 (ropivacaine); 98717-15-8 (anhydrous ropivacaine hydrochloride); 132112-35-7 (ropivacaine hydrochloride monohydrate).*

*ATC — N01BB09.*

### Adverse Effects, Treatment, and Precautions

As for Local Anaesthetics in general, p.1367.

Ropivacaine is contra-indicated for use in intravenous regional anaesthesia (Bier's block) and for paracervical block in obstetrics.

**Effects on the cardiovascular system.** Ropivacaine is structurally related to bupivacaine, but data from extensive *animal* studies suggest that ropivacaine may be less cardiotoxic than bupivacaine.[1] Results from a study[2] in 12 healthy male volunteers support these data; at doses producing CNS symptoms cardiovascular changes, such as depression of conduction and diastolic function, were less pronounced with ropivacaine than with bupivacaine.

1. Cederholm I. Preliminary risk-benefit analysis of ropivacaine in labour and following surgery. *Drug Safety* 1997; **16:** 391–402.
2. Knudsen K, *et al.* Central nervous and cardiovascular effects of i.v. infusions of ropivacaine, bupivacaine and placebo in volunteers. *Br J Anaesth* 1997; **78:** 507–14.

### Interactions

For interactions associated with local anaesthetics, see p.1368.

Administration of ropivacaine with general anaesthetics, opioid analgesics, or drugs structurally related to amide-type local anaesthetics (e.g. certain antiarrhythmics) may result in potentiation of adverse effects.

The metabolism of ropivacaine is mediated by the cytochrome P450 isoenzyme CYP1A2 and the potential exists for interactions between ropivacaine and other drugs that inhibit or act as a substrate for this isoenzyme. Prolonged administration of ropivacaine should be avoided in patients treated with potent CYP1A2 inhibitors, such as fluvoxamine. Plasma concentrations of ropivacaine may be reduced by enzyme-inducing drugs such as rifampicin.

### Pharmacokinetics

Ropivacaine is about 94% bound to plasma proteins. The terminal elimination half-life has been reported to be 1.8 hours. It is extensively metabolised in the liver, predominantly by aromatic hydroxylation which is mediated by the cytochrome P450 isoenzyme CYP1A2; the isoenzyme CYP3A4 plays a minor role in the metabolism of ropivacaine. The metabolites are excreted mainly in the urine; about 1% of a dose is excreted as unchanged drug. Some metabolites also have a local anaesthetic effect but less than that of ropivacaine. Ropivacaine crosses the placenta.

See also under Local Anaesthetics, p.1368.

### Uses and Administration

Ropivacaine hydrochloride is a local anaesthetic of the amide type with actions and uses similar to those described on p.1369. It is a long-acting local anaesthetic, although onset and duration of action are dependent upon the administration site; the presence of a vasoconstrictor such as adrenaline has no effect. Ropivacaine is used for epidural block, peripheral nerve block, and infiltration anaesthesia and field block. (Local anaesthetic techniques are discussed on p.1370.) At high doses ropivacaine produces surgical anaesthesia, whereas at lower doses it is used for the management of acute pain such as labour pain (p.6) and in postoperative analgesia (p.4).

Like bupivacaine (p.1371), ropivacaine has a differential blocking effect on nerve fibres and, at the lowest concentration used, there is good differentiation between sensory and motor block. The onset and duration of sensory block produced by ropivacaine is generally similar to that obtained with bupivacaine but the motor block is often slower in onset, shorter in duration, and less intense.

Ropivacaine hydrochloride is administered in concentrations of 0.2 to 1%. The dosage depends on the site of injection and the procedure used, as well as the status of the patient. The dose of ropivacaine should be reduced in the elderly, and in acutely ill or debilitated patients. A test dose of lidocaine with adrenaline should be given before commencing epidural block with ropivacaine to detect inadvertent intravascular administration.

- For **surgical anaesthesia**, doses of ropivacaine hydrochloride for *lumbar epidural block* are 75 to 150 mg (15 to 30 mL) as a 0.5% solution, or 112.5 to 187.5 mg (15 to 25 mL) as a 0.75% solution, or 150 to 200 mg (15 to 20 mL) as a 1% solution; for caesarean section, doses are 100 to 150 mg (20 to 30 mL) as a 0.5% solution or 112.5 to 150 mg (15 to 20 mL) as a 0.75% solution. Doses for *thoracic epidural block* to establish a block for postoperative pain relief are 25 to 75 mg (5 to 15 mL) as a 0.5% solution or 37.5 to 112.5 mg (5 to 15 mL) as a 0.75% solution; the actual dose used depends on the level of the injection.
- For *peripheral nerve block* of major nerves such as the brachial plexus, typical doses are 175 to 250 mg (35 to 50 mL) as a 0.5% solution; 225 to 300 mg (30 to 40 mL) as a 0.75% solution has also been recommended for brachial plexus block.
- For *infiltration anaesthesia* and *field block* up to 200 mg (40 mL) as a 0.5% solution or up to 225 mg (30 mL) as a 0.75% solution may be used.
- In the management of **acute pain** ropivacaine hydrochloride is used as a 0.2% solution for epidural block (0.5% solutions may be used for infiltration). Doses for *lumbar epidural block* are 20 to 40 mg (10 to 20 mL) as an initial bolus followed by 20 to 30 mg (10 to 15 mL) at intervals of not less than 30 minutes. Alternatively, 12 to 20 mg (6 to 10 mL) per hour may be given as a continuous epidural infusion;

if additional pain relief is required, doses of up to 28 mg (14 mL) per hour may be given. Doses for *thoracic epidural block* are 12 to 28 mg (6 to 14 mL) per hour as a continuous infusion.

- For *infiltration anaesthesia* doses are 2 to 200 mg (1 to 100 mL) as a 0.2% solution or 5 to 200 mg (1 to 40 mL) as a 0.5% solution.
- In children aged 1 year and over, ropivacaine hydrochloride may be used for the management of pre- and postoperative pain. A 0.2% solution is given in doses of 2 mg/kg (1 mL/kg) to achieve a *caudal epidural block*.

◊ References.


1. Markham A, Faulds D. Ropivacaine: a review of its pharmacology and therapeutic use in regional anaesthesia. *Drugs* 1996; **52:** 429–49.
2. McClure JH. Ropivacaine. *Br J Anaesth* 1996; **76:** 300–307.
3. Morton C. Ropivacaine. *Br J Hosp Med* 1997; **58:** 97–100.
4. Stienstra R. The place of ropivacaine in anesthesia. *Acta Anaesthesiol Belg* 2003; **54:** 141–8.


### Preparations

**Proprietary Preparations** (details are given in Part 3)
***Arg.:*** Naropin; ***Austral.:*** Naropin; ***Austria:*** Naropin; ***Belg.:*** Naropin; ***Braz.:*** Naropin; ***Canad.:*** Naropin; ***Chile:*** Naropin; ***Denm.:*** Naropin; ***Fin.:*** Naropin; ***Fr.:*** Naropeine; ***Ger.:*** Naropin; ***Gr.:*** Naropeine; ***Hong Kong:*** Naropin; ***Irl.:*** Naropin; ***Israel:*** Narop; ***Ital.:*** Naropina; ***Malaysia:*** Naropin; ***Mex.:*** Naropin; ***Neth.:*** Naropin; ***Norw.:*** Naropin; ***NZ:*** Naropin; ***Port.:*** Naropeine; ***S.Afr.:*** Naropin; ***Singapore:*** Naropin; ***Spain:*** Naropin; ***Swed.:*** Narop; ***Switz.:*** Naropin; ***Thai.:*** Naropin; ***UK:*** Naropin; ***USA:*** Naropin.

**Multi-ingredient:** ***Austral.:*** Naropin with Fentanyl; ***NZ:*** Naropin with Fentanyl.

---

## Tetracaine *(BAN, rINN)*

Amethocaine; Tetracaína. 2-Dimethylaminoethyl 4-butylaminobenzoate.

$C_{15}H_{24}N_2O_2$ = 264.4.
*CAS — 94-24-6.*
*ATC — C05AD02; D04AB06; N01BA03; S01HA03.*

**Pharmacopoeias.** In *US.*

**USP 27** (Tetracaine). A white or light yellow waxy solid. M.p. 41° to 46°. Very slightly soluble in water; soluble 1 in 5 of alcohol and 1 in 2 of chloroform or of ether; soluble in benzene. Store in airtight containers. Protect from light.

### Tetracaine Hydrochloride *(BANM, rINNM)*

Amethocaine Hydrochloride; Dicainum; Hidrocloruro de tetracaína; Tetracaini Hydrochloridum; Tetracainii Chloridum.

$C_{15}H_{24}N_2O_2,HCl$ = 300.8.
*CAS — 136-47-0.*
*ATC — C05AD02; D04AB06; N01BA03; S01HA03.*

NOTE. TET is a code approved by the BP 2003 for use on single unit doses of eye drops containing tetracaine hydrochloride where the individual container may be too small to bear all the appropriate labelling information.

**Pharmacopoeias.** In *Chin., Eur.* (see p.vi), *Int., Jpn, Pol., US,* and *Viet.*

**Ph. Eur. 5.0** (Tetracaine Hydrochloride). A white, slightly hygroscopic, polymorphic, crystalline powder. Freely soluble in water; soluble in alcohol. A 1% solution in water has a pH of 4.5 to 6.5. Protect from light.

**USP 27** (Tetracaine Hydrochloride). A fine, white, odourless, hygroscopic, polymorphic, crystalline powder. Very soluble in water; soluble in alcohol; insoluble in ether and in benzene. Its solutions are neutral to litmus. Store in airtight containers. Protect from light.

### Adverse Effects and Treatment

As for Local Anaesthetics in general, p.1367.

Tetracaine has high systemic toxicity. Absorption of tetracaine from mucous membranes is rapid and adverse reactions can occur abruptly without the appearance of prodromal signs or convulsions; fatalities have occurred.

A stinging sensation may occur when tetracaine is used in the eye. Mild erythema at the site of application is frequently seen with topical administration; slight oedema or pruritus occur less commonly. Blistering of the skin may occur.

**Urethral stricture.** There has been a report[1] of a sudden increase in the incidence of urethral stricture following transurethral surgery, which may have been due to an increase in the concentration of tetracaine hydrochloride in the lubricant gel from 0.[illegible] to 3%.

1. Pansadoro V. Role of local anaesthetics in urethral strictures after transurethral surgery. *Lancet* 1990; **336:** 64.

### Precautions

As for Local Anaesthetics in general, p.1368.

Tetracaine should not be applied to inflamed, traumatised, or highly vascular surfaces. It should not be used to provide anaesthesia for bronchoscopy or cystoscopy, as lidocaine is a safer alternative.

### Interactions

For interactions associated with local anaesthetics, see p.1368.

### Pharmacokinetics

See under Local Anaesthetics, p.1368. Tetracaine is reported to be about 15% bioavailable following application of a 4% gel to intact skin, with a mean absorption and elimination half-life of about 75 minutes.

### Uses and Administration

Tetracaine, a para-aminobenzoic acid ester, is a potent local anaesthetic with actions and uses similar to those described on p.1369. It is used for surface anaesthesia and spinal block; its use in other local anaesthetic techniques is restricted by its systemic toxicity.

Tetracaine is generally used as the hydrochloride in solutions and creams, and as the base in gels or ointments.

For *anaesthesia of the eye*, solutions containing 0.5 to 1% tetracaine hydrochloride and ointments containing 0.5% tetracaine have been used. Instillation of a 0.5% solution produces anaesthesia within 25 seconds that lasts for 15 minutes or longer and is suitable for use before minor surgical procedures.

For *topical anaesthesia*, a 1% cream or a 0.5% ointment has been used. These preparations have been used for painful conditions of the *anus or rectum*. A 4% gel is used as a *percutaneous local anaesthetic* before *venepuncture or venous cannulation*. The gel is applied to the centre of the area to be anaesthetised and covered with an occlusive dressing. Gel and dressing are removed after 30 minutes for venepuncture and after 45 minutes for venous cannulation. A single application generally provides anaesthesia for 4 to 6 hours. This method is not suitable for premature infants or those less than 1 month of age.

Tetracaine hydrochloride has also been used in the *mouth* in sprays and lozenges.

Tetracaine hydrochloride has also been used for *spinal block* usually as a 0.5% solution.

**Action.** For a comparison of the vasoactivity of tetracaine with some other local anaesthetics, see p.1369.

**Spinal block.** A study[1] in 40 patients indicated that for patients undergoing caesarean section with spinal anaesthesia (see Central Nerve Block, p.1370) doses of 12 or 14 mg of tetracaine provided better intraoperative analgesia than doses of 8 or 10 mg without leading to excessive spread of the block.

1. Hirabayashi Y, *et al.* Visceral pain during Caesarean section: effect of varying dose of spinal amethocaine. *Br J Anaesth* 1995; **75:** 266–8.

**Surface anaesthesia.** A topical gel formulation of tetracaine 4% appears to provide more rapid and prolonged surface anaesthesia (see p.1370) than a eutectic mixture of lidocaine and prilocaine.[1,2] In a double-blind placebo-controlled study[3] the tetracaine gel formulation was significantly better than the eutectic mixture in reducing pain caused by laser treatment of portwine stains. Similar findings were also seen in a comparative study in children requiring venous cannulation.[4] The same formulation appears to be equally effective when incorporated into a transdermal patch.[5]

There have been reports of seizures and death in children after the use of a mixture of tetracaine, adrenaline, and cocaine on mucosal surfaces;[6] application of preparations of tetracaine to highly vascular surfaces is contra-indicated. A gel containing a mixture of lidocaine, adrenaline, and tetracaine has been found to be an effective alternative to the cocaine-containing preparation.[7]

Tetracaine has also been incorporated into a mucosa-adhesive polymer film to relieve the pain of oral lesions resulting from radiation and antineoplastic therapy.[8] Liposome-encapsulated tetracaine has also been shown to provide adequate surface anaesthesia.[9]


1. McCafferty DF, *et al.* In vivo assessment of percutaneous local anaesthetic preparations. *Br J Anaesth* 1989; **62:** 17–21.
2. Rømsing J, *et al.* Tetracaine gel vs EMLA cream for percutaneous anaesthesia in children. *Br J Anaesth* 1999; **82:** 637–8.
3. McCafferty DF, *et al.* Effect of percutaneous local anaesthetics on pain reduction during pulse dye laser treatment of portwine stains. *Br J Anaesth* 1997; **78:** 286–9.
4. Arrowsmith J, Campbell C. A comparison of local anaesthetics for venepuncture. *Arch Dis Child* 2000; **82:** 309–10.
5. McCafferty DF, Woolfson AD. New patch delivery system for percutaneous local anaesthesia. *Br J Anaesth* 1993; **71:** 370–4.
6. Wong S, Hart LL. Tetracaine/adrenaline/cocaine for local anesthesia. *DICP Ann Pharmacother* 1990; **24:** 1181–3.
7. Ernst AA, *et al.* Lidocaine adrenaline tetracaine gel versus tetracaine adrenaline cocaine gel for topical anesthesia in linear scalp and facial lacerations in children aged 5 to 17 years. *Pediatrics* 1995; **95:** 255–8.
8. Yotsuyanagi T, *et al.* Mucosa-adhesive film containing local analgesic. *Lancet* 1985; **ii:** 613.
9. Fisher R, *et al.* Topical anaesthesia of intact skin: liposome-encapsulated tetracaine vs EMLA. *Br J Anaesth* 1998; **81:** 972–3.


### Preparations

***BP 2003:*** Tetracaine Eye Drops;
***USP 27:*** Benzocaine, Butamben, and Tetracaine Hydrochloride Gel; Benzocaine, Butamben, and Tetracaine Hydrochloride Ointment; Benzocaine, Butamben, and Tetracaine Hydrochloride Topical Aerosol; Benzocaine, Butamben, and Tetracaine Hydrochloride Topical Solution; Cocaine and Tetracaine Hydrochlorides and Epinephrine Topical Solution; Procaine and Tetracaine Hydrochlorides and Levonordefrin Injection; Tetracaine and Menthol Ointment; Tetracaine Hydrochloride Cream; Tetracaine Hydrochloride for Injection; Tetracaine Hydrochloride in Dextrose Injection; Tetracaine Hydrochloride Injection; Tetracaine Hydrochloride Ophthalmic Solution; Tetracaine Hydrochloride Topical Solution; Tetracaine Ointment; Tetracaine Ophthalmic Ointment.

**Proprietary Preparations** (details are given in Part 3)
***Arg.:*** Tray-Te; ***Braz.:*** Anestesico; ***Canad.:*** Ametop; Cepacol Viractin; Pontocaine; Supracaine†; ***Ger.:*** Ophtocain N; Oto-Flexiole N†; ***Hong Kong:*** Ametop; ***Irl.:*** Ametop; ***Israel:*** Pontocaine; ***NZ:*** Ametop; ***S.Afr.:*** Ametop†; Anethaine†; Covostet; ***Spain:*** Anest Compuesto†; Anestesia Topi Braun C/A; Anestesia Topi Braun S/A; Anestesico; Hemonet; ***UK:*** Ametop; Anethaine; ***USA:*** Cepacol Viractin Cold Sore Treatment; Pontocaine.

**Multi-ingredient:** ***Arg.:*** Clevosan; Drill; ***Austria:*** Dynexan; Herviros; Neocones; ***Belg.:*** Anesthesique Double†; ***Braz.:*** Anesdente do Bebe; Anestesiol; Hexomedine; Osmogenol†; Oto Betnovate; Oto-Biotic; UM Instante†; Um Minuto†; ***Canad.:*** Endospray; Panocaine†; ***Fr.:*** Amygdospray†; Aphtoral; Broncorinol maux de gorge; Cantalene; Codetricine vitamine C; Drill; Eludril; Hexomedine; Lysofon†; Oromedine; Oroseptol Lysozyme†; Otylol†; Solutricine Maux de Gorge; Solutricine Tetracaine; Tyrcine†; ***Ger.:*** Acoin; Gingicain D; Herviros; ***Hong Kong:*** Herviros†; Norgotin†; ***Israel:*** Anaesthetic Ear Drops; Otidin; ***Ital.:*** Corizzina; Donalg; Lasoproct†; Odongi; Recto-Reparil; Ruscoroid; ***Port.:*** Anucet; Colircusi Anestesico; Davicaina†; Drill; Hemofissural; Lubrificante Anestesico; Xilonibsa; ***S.Afr.:*** Dynexan; ***Spain:*** Anestesi Doble; Anestina Braun†; Blastoestimulina; Carbocaina; Dentikrisos; Neocones; Otogen Calmante; Resorborina; Topicaina; Vinciseptil Otico; ***Switz.:*** Adrectal†; Angidine; Dynexan†; Eludril; Tonex†; Tyrothricine + Gramicidine; ***UK:*** Eludril; ***USA:*** Cetacaine; Stypto-Caine.

---

## Tolycaine Hydrochloride *(BANM, rINNM)*

Hidrocloruro de tolicaína. Methyl 2-(2-diethylaminoacetamido)-*m*-toluate hydrochloride.

$C_{15}H_{22}N_2O_3,HCl$ = 314.8.
*CAS — 3686-58-6 (tolycaine); 7210-92-6 (tolycaine hydrochloride).*

### Profile

Tolycaine hydrochloride is an amide local anaesthetic (p.1367) included in some preparations to reduce the pain of injection.

### Preparations

**Proprietary Preparations** (details are given in Part 3)
*Used as an adjunct in:* ***Ger.:*** Tardocillin.

---

## Tricaine Mesilate

Metacaine Mesylate; Tricaína, mesilato de; Tricaine Mesylate; TS-222. Ethyl 3-aminobenzoate methanesulphonate.

$C_{10}H_{15}NO_5S$ = 261.3.
*CAS — 886-86-2.*

### Profile

Tricaine mesilate is a derivative of an isomer of benzocaine (see p.1370) and although it has been used as a local anaesthetic in human medicine it is now mainly used as an anaesthetic and tranquilliser for fish and other cold-blooded animals.

---

## Trimecaine Hydrochloride *(rINNM)*

Hidrocloruro de trimecaína; Trimecainium Chloratum. 2-Diethylamino-2′,4′,6′-trimethylacetanilide hydrochloride.

$C_{15}H_{24}N_2O,HCl$ = 284.8.
*CAS — 616-68-2 (trimecaine); 1027-14-1 (trimecaine hydrochloride).*

### Profile

Trimecaine hydrochloride is an amide local anaesthetic (p.1367) included in some preparations to reduce the pain of injection.

### Preparations

**Proprietary Preparations** (details are given in Part 3)
*Used as an adjunct in:* ***Austria:*** Ketazon; ***Ger.:*** Ketazon†.

# Muscle Relaxants

The muscle relaxants included in this chapter are used in the management of musculoskeletal and neuromuscular disorders. There are 2 main types:

- **centrally acting relaxants**—these generally have a selective action on the CNS and are principally used for relieving painful muscle spasms or spasticity occurring in musculoskeletal and neuromuscular disorders. Their mechanism of action may be due to their CNS-depressant activity. Baclofen and tizanidine are two examples.
- **directly acting relaxants**—dantrolene is a drug that has a direct action on skeletal muscle and is used for the relief of spasticity associated with a variety of conditions.

Also included in this chapter are miscellaneous drugs, such as botulinum toxins A and B, that inhibit the release of acetylcholine at the motor nerve terminals.

Some benzodiazepines are also used in the treatment of muscle spasms; further details may be found under Diazepam, p.690.

Other drugs that block transmission at the neuromuscular junction and are used as adjuncts to general anaesthesia are discussed in the chapter on Neuromuscular Blockers, p.1397.

Drugs used to relax *smooth muscle* include antimuscarinics, which are described in a separate chapter (p.475), and some gastrointestinal drugs such as mebeverine (p.1273).

### Muscle spasm

Spasm is a painful involuntary contraction of muscle which can cause involuntary movement, interfere with function, and cause distortion. It is a symptom of many muscular and other types of disorders and treatment should primarily be aimed at the underlying cause. Centrally acting muscle relaxants and benzodiazepines are used to treat muscle spasms such as *splinting* that occur in response to local trauma or musculoskeletal and joint disorders. Splinting is a reflex muscular spasm that produces muscular rigidity and acts as a protective mechanism to prevent movement and further damage of the affected part. Short courses of muscle relaxants may be considered in the management of acute low back pain (p.7).

**Cramps** are muscle spasms of abrupt onset that occur at rest and usually last for a few seconds or minutes. They are often precipitated by dehydration and hyponatraemia produced by vigorous exercise, excessive sweating, diarrhoea, and vomiting, or may be associated with drug therapy or haemodialysis. Pregnant women, the elderly, and those with peripheral vascular disease, appear to be particularly susceptible to night cramps of the feet or legs, the cause of which is not well understood.

The management of muscle cramps has been reviewed.[1,2] Quinine has traditionally been used for *nocturnal cramps* but there has been concern over its efficacy and potential for adverse effects, especially in the elderly. Meta-analyses[3,4] have indicated that although quinine was modestly effective in the treatment of nocturnal cramps in ambulatory patients the risk of serious adverse effects should be borne in mind; patients should be closely monitored over a period of at least 4 weeks while the efficacy of quinine was assessed. In the UK, it is recommended that treatment should be stopped every 3 months to see whether it is still needed.[5] In the USA, the FDA has ruled that quinine products should no longer be used for the management of nocturnal cramps.[6,7] There is little convincing evidence to support the use of other drugs.[1,2,6]

A systematic review[8] concluded that magnesium (as the lactate and citrate) is modestly effective in the treatment of *leg cramps in pregnancy*; calcium salts were ineffective, and although early evidence suggested benefit with sodium chloride, high doses were required with their attendant cardiovascular risks.

*Haemodialysis-induced cramp* (p.1221) is a common complication occurring during or after dialysis.[1,9] Its aetiology is not clear but response to blood volume expansion with hypertonic solutions such as glucose, mannitol, or saline suggests that hypovolaemia may be involved. Haemodialysis-induced cramp has also been reported to respond to quinine.


1. McGee SR. Muscle cramps. *Arch Intern Med* 1990; **150:** 511–18.
2. Butler JV, *et al.* Nocturnal leg cramps in older people. *Postgrad Med J* 2002; **78:** 596–8.
3. Man-Son-Hing M, Wells G. Meta-analysis of efficacy of quinine for treatment of nocturnal leg cramps in elderly people. *BMJ* 1995; **310:** 13–17.
4. Man-Son-Hing M, *et al.* Quinine for nocturnal leg cramps: a meta-analysis including unpublished data. *J Gen Intern Med* 1998; **13:** 600–606.
5. Anonymous. Quinine for nocturnal leg cramps? *Drug Ther Bull* 1996; **34:** 7–8.
6. FDA. Drug products for the treatment and/or prevention of nocturnal leg muscle cramps for over-the-counter human use. *Fed Regist* 1994; **59:** 43234–52.
7. Nightingale SL. Quinine for nocturnal leg cramps. *ACP J Club* 1995; **123:** 86.
8. Young GL, Jewell D. Interventions for leg cramps in pregnancy. Available in The Cochrane Library; Issue 2. Chichester: John Wiley; 2004.
9. Mujais SK. Muscle cramps during hemodialysis. *Int J Artif Organs* 1994; **17:** 570–2.


### Spasticity

The term spasticity has been loosely applied to various disorders of motor control resulting from CNS disease and marked by effects such as increased muscle tone, exaggerated stretch reflexes, impaired voluntary movement, weakness, loss of dexterity, abnormal posture, and often disturbed gait. In some patients muscle spasm and pain may be more distressing than impaired movement. Other complications may include contractures, pressure sores, and infection. Spasticity is a feature of neurological conditions such as multiple sclerosis, cerebral palsy, head injury, and stroke, particularly if there are spinal lesions.

Spasticity is disabling and difficult to treat when severe, but mild or moderate forms may be effectively managed by conservative treatment. Some patients may even use spasticity to provide a means of posture control and care should be taken that treatment does not lead to increased disability.

Various discussions on the management of spasticity have been published.[1-8] The mainstay of management is physiotherapy with antispastic drugs, although the evidence for the latter is rather scanty.[9,10] Baclofen, dantrolene, diazepam, and tizanidine are the drugs most often used. These 4 drugs act via different mechanisms, which are not fully understood.

*Baclofen* is thought to act at the spinal cord level but may also have supraspinal sites of action. It is a powerful neuronal depressant and may exert its inhibitory effects by acting as an agonist at GABA (gamma aminobutyric acid) receptors. *Diazepam* is also thought to act centrally by enhancing the response to GABA. In contrast, *dantrolene* acts directly on muscles, possibly by interfering with the release of calcium from muscular sarcoplasmic reticulum needed for contraction. *Tizanidine* is a centrally acting relaxant and α-adrenergic agonist; it is thought to act at spinal and supraspinal levels by inhibiting the presynaptic activity of excitatory interneurones.[7] It can produce additive effects with baclofen, allowing a reduction in the dosage of both drugs; use with benzodiazepines is not recommended because of the potential for interactions. All these are usually given by mouth but baclofen may also be given intrathecally in severe chronic spasticity.[11,12] Injection directly into the spinal subarachnoid space allows immediate delivery to the site of action in the spinal cord and the use of considerably lower doses than those given orally. It has been reported[13] that some patients receiving long-term intrathecal baclofen treatment have been able to stop their therapy without symptoms of spasticity re-appearing, and that others have been able to reduce the dosage required.

Other drugs that may produce some benefit or are being studied in spasticity include *other benzodiazepines, clonidine, gabapentin,* and *memantine.*

Alternative approaches to treatment include nerve blocks using *local anaesthetics*; they should generally only be used when further muscle relaxation would not increase disability. *Chemical neurolysis* using alcohol or phenol is only considered when there is intractable continuous pain. Local injections of *botulinum A toxin* have produced some encouraging results in the management of limb spasticity in post-stroke or spinal injury patients and in children with cerebral palsy;[14-16] its temporary effect may be an advantage over chemical neurolysis but the need for regular injections may limit acceptability in children.[14]

Nondrug treatments have included electrical stimulation techniques such as transcutaneous nerve stimulation and dorsal column stimulation; vibration applied to agonist spastic muscles to improve voluntary movement; cooling to decrease afferent inputs from peripheral receptors; and orthopaedic surgery or neurosurgery.


1. Young RR. Spasticity: a review. *Neurology* 1994; **44** (suppl 9): S12–S20.
2. Ko CK, Ward AB. Management of spasticity. *Br J Hosp Med* 1997; **58:** 400–5.
3. Kita M, Goodkin DE. Drugs used to treat spasticity. *Drugs* 2000; **59:** 487–95.
4. Anonymous. The management of spasticity. *Drug Ther Bull* 2000; **38:** 44–6.
5. Bhakta BB. Management of spasticity in stroke. *Br Med Bull* 2000; **56:** 476–85.
6. Burchiel KJ, Hsu FPK. Pain and spasticity after spinal cord injury: mechanisms and treatment. *Spine* 2001; **26** (suppl): S146–S160.
7. Ward AB. A summary of spasticity management – a treatment algorithm. *Eur J Neurol* 2002; **9** (suppl 1): 48–52.
8. Abbruzzese G. The medical management of spasticity. *Eur J Neurol* 2002; **9** (suppl 1): 30–4.
9. Taricco M, *et al.* Pharmacological interventions for spasticity following spinal cord injury. Available in The Cochrane Library; Issue 2. Chichester: John Wiley; 2004.
10. Shakespeare DT, *et al.* Anti-spasticity agents for multiple sclerosis. Available in The Cochrane Library; Issue 2. Chichester: John Wiley; 2004.
11. McLean BN. Intrathecal baclofen in severe spasticity. *Br J Hosp Med* 1993; **49:** 262–7.
12. Anonymous. Intrathecal baclofen for spasticity. *Med Lett Drugs Ther* 1994; **36:** 21–2.
13. Dressnandt J, Conrad B. Lasting reduction of severe spasticity after ending chronic treatment with intrathecal baclofen. *J Neurol Neurosurg Psychiatry* 1996; **60:** 168–73.
14. Neville B. Botulinum toxin in the cerebral palsies. *BMJ* 1994; **309:** 1526–7.
15. Fried GW, Fried KM. Spinal cord injury and use of botulinum toxin in reducing spasticity. *Phys Med Rehabil Clin N Am* 2003; **14:** 901–10.
16. Preiss RA, *et al.* The effects of botulinum toxin (BTX-A) on spasticity of the lower limb and on gait in cerebral palsy. *J Bone Joint Surg Br* 2003; **85:** 943–8.


## Afloqualone *(rINN)*

Aflocualona; HQ-495. 6-Amino-2-fluoromethyl-3-o-tolylquinazolin-4(3*H*)-one.

$C_{16}H_{14}FN_3O$ = 283.3.

*CAS — 56287-74-2.*

**Pharmacopoeias.** In *Jpn.*

### Profile

Afloqualone is a centrally acting skeletal muscle relaxant that has been given by mouth for the treatment of muscle spasm associated with musculoskeletal conditions. Photosensitivity reactions have been reported.

◊ References.


1. Ishikawa T, *et al.* Photoleukomelanodermatitis (Kobori) induced by afloqualone. *J Dermatol* 1994; **21:** 430–3.


## Baclofen *(BAN, USAN, rINN)*

Aminomethyl Chlorohydrocinnamic Acid; Ba-34647; Baclofeno; Baclofenum. β-Aminomethyl-p-chlorohydrocinnamic acid; (*RS*)-Amino-3-(4-chlorophenyl)butyric acid.

$C_{10}H_{12}ClNO_2$ = 213.7.

*CAS — 1134-47-0.*

*ATC — M03BX01.*

**Pharmacopoeias.** In *Eur.* (see p.vi), *Jpn, Pol.,* and *US.*

**Ph. Eur. 5.0** (Baclofen). A white or almost white powder. It exhibits polymorphism. Slightly soluble in water; very slightly soluble in alcohol; practically insoluble in acetone; dissolves in dilute mineral acids and in dilute solutions of alkali hydroxides.

**USP 27** (Baclofen). A white to off-white, odourless or practically odourless, crystalline powder. Slightly soluble in water; very slightly soluble in methyl alcohol; insoluble in chloroform. Store in airtight containers.

### Adverse Effects

Adverse effects associated with baclofen are often transient and dose-related. They may be minimised by increasing doses gradually or controlled by a reduction in dosage.

The most common side-effects include drowsiness, nausea, dizziness, lassitude, lightheadedness, confusion, fatigue, muscular pain and weakness, and hypotension. Other side-effects include euphoria, hallucinations, depression, headache, tinnitus, convulsions, paraesthesias, slurred speech, dry mouth, taste alterations, vomiting, diarrhoea or constipation, ataxia, nystagmus, tremors, insomnia, visual disturbances, skin rashes, pruritus, increased sweating, urinary disturbances, respiratory or cardiovascular depression, blood sugar changes, alterations in liver function values, and a paradoxical increase in spasticity. Problems with erection and ejaculation have also been reported with intrathecal baclofen; these are usually reversible on withdrawal of therapy.

Overdosage may lead to muscular hypotonia, drowsiness, respiratory depression, coma, and convulsions (see also below).

Abrupt withdrawal of baclofen may result in a withdrawal syndrome (see under Precautions, below).

**Effects on the nervous system.** Epilepsy, progressing to status epilepticus, has been associated with the use of baclofen in a patient who had had no previous history of seizures.[1] Baclofen had been given in a dose of 80 mg daily and symptoms had resolved following gradual withdrawal and the use of antiepileptics.

1. Rush JM, Gibberd FB. Baclofen-induced epilepsy. *J R Soc Med* 1990; **83:** 115–16.

## Treatment of Adverse Effects

Treatment of overdosage is symptomatic. Consideration should be given to gastric lavage and/or the use of activated charcoal in patients who have ingested more than 100 mg within an hour of presentation; activated charcoal is recommended in children who have taken more than 5 mg/kg or 100 mg within the last hour. Observation should continue for at least 6 hours after ingestion. For the use of physostigmine salicylate in the treatment of intrathecal baclofen overdosage, see below.

**Overdosage.** Atropine sulfate 600 micrograms intravenously[1] was used to treat a patient who had ingested 420 mg of baclofen and had failed to improve after gastric lavage and induced diuresis. Bradycardia, hypotension, hypothermia, and respiratory depression all improved and no further treatment was needed. The clinical course and management of acute intoxication in 8 adolescents, who ingested estimated amounts of baclofen ranging from 60 to more than 600 mg, has also been described.[2]

Accidental *intrathecal* overdosage has caused respiratory depression, decreased alertness, coma, muscle weakness, and vomiting.[3] Mild intrathecal bolus overdoses of baclofen in patients without cardiac compromise can be treated using physostigmine. Physostigmine salicylate is given intravenously in a dose of 1 to 2 mg over 5 minutes and may be repeated at intervals of 30 to 60 minutes.[3,4] Physostigmine was ineffective in a patient who accidentally received 10 mg of baclofen intrathecally;[5] in such severe overdosage, respiratory support and time to recover is needed.[4] A lumbar tap to remove about 30 to 50 mL of cerebrospinal fluid may help to reduce the intrathecal concentration of baclofen if implemented soon after the overdose.

1. Ferner RE. Atropine treatment for baclofen overdose. *Postgrad Med J* 1981; **57:** 580–1.
2. Perry HE, *et al.* Baclofen overdose: drug experimentation in a group of adolescents. *Pediatrics* 1998; **101:** 1045–8.
3. Müller-Schwefe G, Penn RD. Physostigmine in the treatment of intrathecal baclofen overdose. *J Neurosurg* 1989; **71:** 273–5.
4. Penn RD, Kroin JS. Failure of physostigmine in treatment of acute severe intrathecal baclofen intoxication. *N Engl J Med* 1990; **322:** 1533–4.
5. Saltuari L, *et al.* Failure of physostigmine in treatment of acute severe intrathecal baclofen intoxication. *N Engl J Med* 1990; **322:** 1533.

## Precautions

Baclofen stimulates gastric acid secretion and should be used with caution in patients with a history of peptic ulcer and avoided in those with active peptic ulcer disease. It should also be used with caution in patients with severe psychiatric disorders or epilepsy or convulsive disorders since these disorders may be exacerbated by baclofen. Liver function should be monitored in patients with liver disease; patients with renal impairment need a reduced dose. Baclofen should be used with caution in patients with respiratory impairment. Observations of increased blood sugar concentrations suggest caution in patients with diabetes mellitus. Care is also required in the elderly, in whom adverse effects may be more common, and in patients with cerebrovascular disease (who tolerate baclofen poorly). It should be used with caution in patients who use their spasticity to maintain posture or to increase function. Urine retention may be exacerbated in patients with hypertonic bladder sphincters. Baclofen may cause drowsiness; patients affected should not drive or operate machinery.

Abrupt withdrawal of baclofen may result in a withdrawal syndrome and exacerbation of spasticity; dosage should be reduced gradually over at least 1 to 2 weeks, or longer if symptoms occur.

**Anaesthesia.** Acute bradycardia and hypotension occurred following rib retraction in 3 patients given baclofen 30 mg by mouth 90 minutes before thoracic surgery under general anaesthesia, but not in a further 3 patients given placebo.[1] Giving atropine and ephedrine relieved bradycardia and hypotension in 2 patients, but a brief cardiac arrest occurred in 1. Baclofen may disturb autonomic control of the circulation during general anaesthesia and surgery.

1. Sill JC, *et al.* Bradycardia and hypotension associated with baclofen used during general anaesthesia. *Anesthesiology* 1986; **64:** 255–8.

**Breast feeding.** The concentrations of baclofen found in breast milk are small[1] and the UK manufacturer states that no undesirable effects are to be expected in breast-fed infants. The American Academy of Pediatrics also considers that baclofen is usually compatible with breast feeding; no adverse effects have been observed in breast-feeding infants whose mothers were receiving baclofen.[2]

1. Eriksson G, Swahn C-G. Concentrations of baclofen in serum and breast milk from a lactating woman. *Scand J Clin Lab Invest* 1981; **41:** 185–7.
2. American Academy of Pediatrics. The transfer of drugs and other chemicals into human milk. *Pediatrics* 2001; **108:** 776–89. Correction. *ibid.*; 1029. Also available at: http://aappolicy.aappublications.org/cgi/content/full/pediatrics%3b108/3/776 (accessed 23/06/04)

**Peptic ulcer.** Results of a study of baclofen-stimulated gastric acid secretion in 10 healthy subjects given 600 micrograms/kg intravenously suggested that patients on baclofen might be at risk from baclofen-induced hyperacidity.[1]

1. Pugh S, *et al.* Clinical and experimental significance of the newly discovered activity of baclofen (PCP-GABA) as a stimulant of gastric acid secretion. *Gut* 1985; **26:** A545.

**Porphyria.** Baclofen is considered to be unsafe in patients with porphyria because it has been shown to be porphyrinogenic in *in-vitro* systems.

**Pregnancy and the neonate.** Two successful pregnancies have been reported[1] in a woman receiving intrathecal baclofen; there was no evidence of teratogenicity, and neurodevelopmental outcome in the children seemed normal. However, convulsions were seen in a week-old infant whose mother had taken oral baclofen during pregnancy.[2] The convulsions, which were refractory to antiepileptics, lidocaine, and pyridoxine, ceased within 30 minutes of giving baclofen to the infant.

1. Calderón Muñoz F, *et al.* Pregnancy outcome in a woman exposed to continuous intrathecal baclofen infusion. *Ann Pharmacother* 2000; **34:** 956.
2. Ratnayaka BDM, *et al.* Neonatal convulsions after withdrawal of baclofen. *BMJ* 2001; **323:** 85.

**Renal impairment.** Reports of baclofen toxicity in patients with severe renal impairment.[1] Most patients had received 15 mg or more of baclofen daily although one patient who had received the manufacturer's suggested dose of 5 mg daily still developed toxic symptoms after only 4 days of treatment.

1. Chen K-S, *et al.* Baclofen toxicity in patients with severely impaired renal function. *Ann Pharmacother* 1997; **31:** 1315–20.

**Respiratory disorders.** Baclofen might precipitate bronchoconstriction in susceptible individuals. A patient with asthma developed symptomatic bronchoconstriction after taking baclofen on two separate occasions.[1] Another patient who had a history of exercise-induced dyspnoea and wheezing was found to have bronchial hyperresponsiveness to methacholine only after taking baclofen.

1. Dicpinigaitis PV, *et al.* Baclofen-induced bronchoconstriction. *Ann Pharmacother* 1993; **27:** 883–4.

**Withdrawal.** Psychiatric reactions including hallucinations, paranoia, delusions, psychosis, anxiety, confusion, and agitation have been reported[1-4] on abrupt withdrawal of oral baclofen; symptoms generally resolved on restarting. Convulsions have also been reported.[5] The abrupt withdrawal of intrathecal baclofen may also result in high fever, altered mental status, exaggerated rebound spasticity, and muscle rigidity which in rare cases has advanced to rhabdomyolysis, multiple organ failure, and death.[6-8]

Except for serious adverse reactions, the dose of oral baclofen should be gradually reduced: in the UK the Committee on Safety of Medicines recommends reduction over at least 1 to 2 weeks or longer if symptoms occur. Similarly, the FDA has advised against the abrupt withdrawal of intrathecal baclofen.[8]

1. Lees AJ, *et al.* Hallucinations after withdrawal of baclofen. *Lancet* 1977; **i:** 858.
2. Stein R. Hallucinations after sudden withdrawal of baclofen. *Lancet* 1977; **ii:** 44–5.
3. Harrison SA, Wood CA. Hallucinations after preoperative baclofen discontinuation in spinal cord injury patients. *Drug Intell Clin Pharm* 1985; **19:** 747–9.
4. Committee on Safety of Medicines/Medicines Control Agency. Severe withdrawal reactions with baclofen. *Current Problems* 1997; **23:** 3. Also available at: http://www.mca.gov.uk/ourwork/monitorsafequalmed/currentproblems/volume23.htm (accessed 23/06/04)
5. Barker I, Grant IS. Convulsions after abrupt withdrawal of baclofen. *Lancet* 1982; **ii:** 556–7.
6. Green LB, Nelson VS. Death after acute withdrawal of intrathecal baclofen: case report and literature review. *Arch Phys Med Rehabil* 1999; **80:** 1600–4.
7. Grenier B, *et al.* Hyperthermie grave liée à un sevrage brutal de baclofène administré de façon continue par voie intrathécale. *Ann Fr Anesth Reanim* 1996; **15:** 659–62.
8. Coffey RJ [Medtronic]. Important drug warning (issued April 2002). Available at: http://www.fda.gov/medwatch/SAFETY/2002/baclofen.pdf (accessed 23/06/04)

## Interactions

Alcohol and other CNS depressants may exacerbate the CNS effects of baclofen and should be avoided; severe aggravation of hyperkinetic symptoms may possibly occur in patients taking lithium. There may be increased weakness if baclofen is given to patients taking a tricyclic antidepressant and there may be an increased hypotensive effect if it is given to patients receiving antihypertensive therapy. Ibuprofen (see below) and other drugs that produce renal insufficiency may reduce baclofen excretion leading to toxicity.

**Dopaminergics.** For reports of patients with Parkinson's disease taking levodopa who have experienced adverse effects when given baclofen, see under Levodopa, on p.1208.

**NSAIDs.** There has been a report of an elderly patient who developed baclofen toxicity after concomitant ibuprofen therapy was started.[1] It appeared that acute renal insufficiency caused by ibuprofen had impaired baclofen excretion.

1. Dahlin PA, George J. Baclofen toxicity associated with declining renal clearance after ibuprofen. *Drug Intell Clin Pharm* 1984; **18:** 805–8.

## Pharmacokinetics

Baclofen is rapidly and almost completely absorbed from the gastrointestinal tract following an oral dose. Peak plasma concentrations occur about 0.5 to 3 hours after ingestion, but the rate and extent of absorption vary between patients, and may vary inversely with the dose. After oral doses some baclofen crosses the blood-brain barrier, with concentrations in CSF about 12% of those in the plasma. Approximately 30% of baclofen is bound to plasma proteins. About 70 to 80% of a dose is excreted in the urine mainly as unchanged drug; about 15% is metabolised in the liver. The elimination half-life of baclofen is about 3 to 4 hours in plasma and about 1 to 5 hours in the CSF. Baclofen crosses the placenta and is distributed into breast milk.

**Absorption.** A crossover study in 5 healthy subjects given baclofen 20 mg by mouth after an overnight fast or a standardised breakfast showed that baclofen was rapidly absorbed in both cases, and the rate and extent of absorption were not significantly altered by the presence of food.[1] There is no need to modify the current practice of giving baclofen with food to minimise gastrointestinal side-effects.

1. Peterson GM, *et al.* Food does not affect the bioavailability of baclofen. *Med J Aust* 1985; **142:** 689–90.

## Uses and Administration

Baclofen, an analogue of gamma-aminobutyric acid (p.1690), is a centrally acting skeletal muscle relaxant. It interferes with the release of excitatory neurotransmitters and inhibits monosynaptic and polysynaptic transmission at the spinal cord level. It may also act at supraspinal sites producing CNS depression. Baclofen is one of the drugs commonly used for the symptomatic relief of severe chronic spasticity associated with a variety of conditions.

Baclofen is given *by mouth* in divided doses, preferably with or after food or milk. The initial dose of baclofen is 5 mg three times daily for 3 days, increased to 10 mg three times daily for 3 days, then in similar increments and intervals until either a dose of 20 mg three times daily is reached or until the desired therapeutic effect is obtained. Higher doses have been used. Doses of more than 80 to 100 mg daily are not generally recommended although doses of up to 150 mg daily have been given to carefully supervised patients.

In the UK a dosage range of 0.75 to 2 mg/kg daily has been used for children; in children over 10 years a maximum daily dosage of 2.5 mg/kg may be given. It is usual to start with a low dose of 2.5 mg given four times daily, increased cautiously about every 3 days until the desired therapeutic effect is obtained. The recommended daily maintenance doses are: 12 months to 2 years, 10 to 20 mg; 2 to 6 years, 20 to 30 mg; 6 to 10 years, 30 to 60 mg.

Elderly patients should receive lower initial doses, although final maintenance doses may be in the same range as younger adults. For dosage in renal impairment, see below.

If no benefit is apparent within 6 weeks of achieving the maximum dosage, therapy should probably be gradually withdrawn.

Baclofen is also given *by continuous intrathecal infusion* in the treatment of spasticity in patients intolerant of or unresponsive to baclofen by mouth. Before beginning the intrathecal regimen any existing antispastic therapy should be gradually withdrawn to avoid overdosage or drug interactions. Intrathecal test doses are given initially to determine if there is going to be any benefit before implanting a controlled infusion pump. It is important that patients are monitored closely in experienced centres during screening and immediately following implantation of the infusion pump and that resuscitation equipment is available for immediate use.

Test doses start at 25 or 50 micrograms given over at least 1 minute and are increased by 25 micrograms every 24 hours until a dose of 100 micrograms is reached or a positive response of about 4 to 8 hours is obtained. Patients who fail to respond to a test dose of up to 100 micrograms are considered to be unsuitable for intrathecal treatment. For children aged 4 to 18 years with spasticity of cerebral origin an initial test dose of 25 micrograms is recommended. However, the manufacturers do not recommend the use of intrathecal baclofen in patients in this age group with spasticity of spinal origin.

For patients showing a positive response lasting for longer than 8 to 12 hours, the test dose that was required to produce the response can then be given as a 24-hour infusion; if the response to the test dose lasted 8 to 12 hours or less, then a dose equivalent to twice the test dose is given. Daily dosage can then be adjusted as required. Maintenance doses range from about 10 micrograms to 2 mg daily, depending on the cause of spasticity, with most patients being adequately maintained with 300 to 800 micrograms daily.

**Administration in renal impairment.** Doses of baclofen should be reduced in renal impairment or in patients undergoing chronic haemodialysis; 5 mg daily by mouth has been suggested (but see also under Precautions, above).

**Dystonias.** There have been reports of improvement in patients with various forms of dystonia (p.1209) treated with baclofen[1-5] although there has also been a report[6] of a patient whose condition deteriorated during baclofen therapy.

1. Narayan RK, *et al.* Intrathecal baclofen for intractable axial dystonia. *Neurology* 1991; **41:** 1141–2.
2. Greene PE, Fahn S. Baclofen in the treatment of idiopathic dystonia in children. *Mov Disord* 1992; **7:** 48–52.
3. van Hilten BJ, *et al.* Intrathecal baclofen for the treatment of dystonia in patients with reflex sympathetic dystrophy. *N Engl J Med* 2000; **343:** 625–30.
4. Albright AL, *et al.* Intrathecal baclofen for generalized dystonia. *Dev Med Child Neurol* 2001; **43:** 652–7.
5. Jaffe MS, Nienstedt LJ. Intrathecal baclofen for generalized dystonia: a case report. *Arch Phys Med Rehabil* 2001; **82:** 853–5.
6. Silbert PL, Stewart-Wynne EG. Increased dystonia after intrathecal baclofen. *Neurology* 1992; **42:** 1639–40.

**Gastro-oesophageal reflux disease.** Baclofen has been tried[1,2] in the treatment of gastro-oesophageal reflux disease (p.1242). It may control gastro-oesophageal reflux by inhibiting transient sphincter relaxation. Although both studies reported a reduction in the number of reflux episodes there was no effect on acid reflux symptoms. However, a subsequent study[3] has shown a positive effect on the symptoms of acid reflux.

1. Van Herwaarden MA, *et al.* The effect of baclofen on gastro-oesophageal reflux, lower oesophageal sphincter function and reflux symptoms in patients with reflux disease. *Aliment Pharmacol Ther* 2002; **16:** 1655–62.
2. Zhang Q, *et al.* Control of transient lower oesophageal sphincter relaxations and reflux by the $GABA_B$ agonist baclofen in patients with gastro-oesophageal reflux disease. *Gut* 2002; **50:** 19–24.
3. Ciccaglione AF, Marzio L. Effect of acute and chronic administration of the $GABA_B$ agonist baclofen on 24 hour pH metry and symptoms in control subjects and in patients with gastro-oesophageal reflux disease. *Gut* 2003; **52:** 464–70.

**Hiccup.** Baclofen has been given by mouth in daily divided doses ranging from 10 to 80 mg for the management of intractable hiccup (p.682) poorly controlled by other drugs.

References.

1. Burke AM, *et al.* Baclofen for intractable hiccups. *N Engl J Med* 1988; **319:** 1354.
2. Lance JW, Bassil GT. Familial intractable hiccup relieved by baclofen. *Lancet* 1989; **ii:** 276–7.
3. Yaqoob M, *et al.* Baclofen for intractable hiccups. *Lancet* 1989; **ii:** 562–3.
4. Ramirez FC, Graham DY. Treatment of intractable hiccup with baclofen: results of a double-blind randomized, controlled, cross-over study. *Am J Gastroenterol* 1992; **87:** 1789–91.
5. Ramirez FC, Graham DY. Hiccups, compulsive water drinking, and hyponatremia. *Ann Intern Med* 1993; **118:** 649.
6. Walker P, *et al.* Baclofen, a treatment for chronic hiccup. *J Pain Symptom Manage* 1998; **16:** 125–32.

**Migraine and cluster headache.** The efficacy of baclofen in conditions such as trigeminal neuralgia or various types of neuropathic pain suggested that it may be useful in migraine or cluster headache. Pilot studies confirmed these hypotheses with baclofen proving useful for prophylaxis[1] in migraine (p.464) and for treatment[2] in cluster headache (p.464).

1. Hering-Hanit R. Baclofen for prevention of migraine. *Cephalalgia* 1999; **19:** 589–91.
2. Hering-Hanit R, Gadoth N. The use of baclofen in cluster headache. *Curr Pain Headache Rep* 2001; **5:** 79–82.

**Pain.** Like some other muscle relaxants baclofen is used in the management of painful conditions associated with muscle spasm or spasticity (see below). The use of muscle relaxants for conditions such as acute low back pain is referred to on p.7. Baclofen does not appear to possess conventional analgesic activity[1] but may potentiate the analgesia produced by opioid analgesics,[2] and has been used as an adjuvant in neuropathic pain,[3,4] notably trigeminal neuralgia[5] (p.8).

1. Terrence CF, *et al.* Is baclofen an analgesic? *Clin Neuropharmacol* 1983; **6:** 241–5.
2. Panerai AE, *et al.* Baclofen prolongs the analgesic effect of fentanyl in man. *Br J Anaesth* 1985; **57:** 954–5.
3. Fromm GH. Baclofen as an adjuvant analgesic. *J Pain Symptom Manage* 1994; **9:** 500–9.
4. Slonimski M, *et al.* Intrathecal baclofen in pain management. *Reg Anesth Pain Med* 2004; **29:** 269–76.
5. Fromm GH, *et al.* Baclofen in the treatment of trigeminal neuralgia: double-blind study and long-term follow-up. *Ann Neurol* 1984; **15:** 240–4.

**Spasticity.** Baclofen is one of the main drugs used in the management of spasticity (see p.1386). It is used to reduce muscle spasm and pain especially in spinal cord lesions in conditions such as multiple sclerosis or paraplegia. Baclofen is also used for spasticity of cerebral origin.

Patients with severe spasticity often require high doses of baclofen by mouth before a response occurs and, consequently, some may fail to respond because adverse effects limit increases in dosage. Intrathecal baclofen is therefore sometimes tried as this produces much higher concentrations in the CNS than oral doses.[1,2] It may be given intrathecally by bolus injection or by continuous infusion; infusion is probably preferred[3] to minimise the risk of overdosage. There is a large interindividual variation in the dose required to produce improvement in spasticity:

- In patients with spasticity of spinal origin, maintenance doses have ranged from 12 micrograms to about 2 mg daily, with most adequately managed on 300 to 800 micrograms daily
- In patients with spasticity of cerebral origin, maintenance doses have ranged from 22 micrograms to 1.4 mg daily, with an average daily dose of 276 micrograms after 12 months and 307 micrograms after 24 months
- For children under the age of 12 years with spasticity of cerebral origin, maintenance doses have ranged from 24 micrograms to about 1.2 mg daily, with an average daily dose of 274 micrograms

An increased dose of baclofen may be given at night to prevent spasms that interfere with sleep.

Although reports of tolerance to the effect of intrathecal baclofen have raised doubt[4] over whether long-term benefit can be maintained, a number of workers have achieved long-term efficacy.[5-8] It has been reported[9] that some patients receiving long-term intrathecal baclofen treatment have been able to stop their therapy without symptoms of spasticity re-appearing and others have been able to reduce the dosage required.

1. McLean BN. Intrathecal baclofen in severe spasticity. *Br J Hosp Med* 1993; **49:** 262–7.
2. Anonymous. Intrathecal baclofen for spasticity. *Med Lett Drugs Ther* 1994; **36:** 21–2.
3. Penn RD, Kroin JS. Intrathecal baclofen. *N Engl J Med* 1989; **321:** 1414–15.
4. Lewis KS, Mueller WM. Intrathecal baclofen for severe spasticity secondary to spinal cord injury. *Ann Pharmacother* 1993; **27:** 767–74.
5. Penn RD, *et al.* Intrathecal baclofen for severe spinal spasticity. *N Engl J Med* 1989; **320:** 1517–21.
6. Azouvi P, *et al.* Intrathecal baclofen administration for control of severe spinal spasticity: functional improvement and long-term follow-up. *Arch Phys Med Rehabil* 1996; **77:** 35–9.
7. Dario A, *et al.* Long-term intrathecal baclofen infusion in supraspinal spasticity of adulthood. *Acta Neurol Scand* 2002; **105:** 83–7.
8. Campbell WM, *et al.* Long-term safety and efficacy of continuous intrathecal baclofen. *Dev Med Child Neurol* 2002; **44:** 660–5.
9. Dressnandt J, Conrad B. Lasting reduction of severe spasticity after ending chronic treatment with intrathecal baclofen. *J Neurol Neurosurg Psychiatry* 1996; **60:** 168–73.

**Stiff-man syndrome.** There have been anecdotal case reports[1] of benefit with intrathecal baclofen in a patient with stiff-man syndrome (see Muscle Spasm, p.696) inadequately controlled with other drugs or oral baclofen. However, in a double-blind placebo-controlled study[2] clinical improvement was evident in only 1 of 3 patients given intrathecal baclofen.

1. Stayer C, *et al.* Intrathecal baclofen therapy for stiff-man syndrome and progressive encephalomyelopathy with rigidity and myoclonus. *Neurology* 1997; **49:** 1591–7.
2. Silbert PL, *et al.* Intrathecal baclofen therapy in stiff-man syndrome: a double-blind, placebo-controlled trial. *Neurology* 1995; **45:** 1893–7.

**Tardive dyskinesia.** Baclofen is one of many drugs that have been tried in antipsychotic-induced tardive dyskinesia (see Extrapyramidal Disorders, p.677) but its efficacy is unclear. A systematic review[1] found the effects of baclofen, and other gamma-aminobutyric acid agonists to be inconclusive and unconvincing in the management of antipsychotic-induced tardive dyskinesia. The review also pointed out that the adverse effects caused by use of these drugs might outweigh any benefits.

1. Soares KVS, *et al.* Gamma-aminobutyric acid agonists for neuroleptic-induced tardive dyskinesia. Available in The Cochrane Library; Issue 2. Chichester: John Wiley; 2004.

**Tetanus.** The management of tetanus is described on p.1398 and p.149. Beneficial responses have been seen with baclofen by continuous intrathecal infusion,[1-5] usually in doses of 1 to 2 mg daily.[1,5] However, the therapeutic range of intrathecal baclofen in severe tetanus may be very narrow and deep coma with loss of spontaneous respiration and reflexes has been reported[6] following an increase in dosage from 1.2 mg to 2 mg daily. This adverse effect could be fatal in the absence of ventilatory support. To avoid the risk of secondary infection from an indwelling intraspinal catheter intermittent intrathecal baclofen has also been used.[7,8]

1. Müller H, *et al.* Intrathecal baclofen in tetanus. *Lancet* 1986; **i:** 317–18.
2. Dressnandt J, *et al.* Intrathecal baclofen in tetanus: four cases and a review of reported cases. *Intensive Care Med* 1997; **23:** 896–902.
3. Engrand N, *et al.* The efficacy of intrathecal baclofen in severe tetanus. *Anesthesiology* 1999; **90:** 1773–6.
4. Boots RJ, *et al.* The treatment of tetanus with intrathecal baclofen. *Anaesth Intensive Care* 2000; **28:** 438–42.
5. Santos ML, *et al.* Intrathecal baclofen for the treatment of tetanus. *Clin Infect Dis* 2004; **38:** 321–8.
6. Romijn JA, *et al.* Reversible coma due to intrathecal baclofen. *Lancet* 1986; **ii:** 696.
7. Demaziere J, *et al.* Intermittent intrathecal baclofen for severe tetanus. *Lancet* 1991; **337:** 427.
8. Saissy JM, *et al.* Treatment of severe tetanus by intrathecal injections of baclofen without artificial ventilation. *Intensive Care Med* 1992; **18:** 241–4.

**Tourette's syndrome.** Improvement was noted in children with Tourette's syndrome (see Tics, p.664) treated with baclofen compared with placebo in a small study.[1]

1. Singer HS, *et al.* Baclofen treatment in Tourette syndrome: a double-blind, placebo-controlled, crossover trial. *Neurology* 2001; **56:** 599–604.

**Urinary incontinence.** Baclofen has been used with some benefit in the management of urinary incontinence and retention (p.476) secondary to lesions of the spinal cord.

References.

1. Hachen HJ, Krucker V. Clinical and laboratory assessment of the efficacy of baclofen (Lioresal®) on urethral sphincter spasticity in patients with traumatic paraplegia. *Eur Urol* 1977; **3:** 237–40.
2. Leyson JFJ, *et al.* Baclofen in the treatment of detrusor-sphincter dyssynergia in spinal cord injury patients. *J Urol (Baltimore)* 1980; **124:** 82–4.
3. Kums JJM, Delhaas EM. Intrathecal baclofen infusion in patients with spasticity and neurogenic bladder disease. *World J Urol* 1991; **9:** 153–6.

## Preparations

***BP 2003:*** Baclofen Oral Solution; Baclofen Tablets;
***USP 27:*** Baclofen Tablets.

**Proprietary Preparations** (details are given in Part 3)

***Arg.:*** Lioresal; ***Austral.:*** Baclo; Baclohexal; Clofen; Lioresal; ***Austria:*** Lioresal; ***Belg.:*** Lioresal; ***Braz.:*** Lioresal; ***Canad.:*** Lioresal; Liotec; Nu-Baclo; ***Chile:*** Lioresyl; ***Denm.:*** Lioresal; ***Fin.:*** Baclon; Baclopar; Lioresal; ***Fr.:*** Lioresal; ***Ger.:*** Lebic; Lioresal; ***Gr.:*** Miorel; Vioridon; ***Hong Kong:*** Lioresal; ***India:*** Lioresal; ***Irl.:*** Baclopar; Lioresal; ***Israel:*** Baclosal; Lioresal; ***Ital.:*** Lioresal; ***Malaysia:*** Clofen; Lioresal; ***Neth.:*** Lioresal; ***Norw.:*** Lioresal; ***NZ:*** Lioresal†; Pacifen; ***Port.:*** Lioresal; ***S.Afr.:*** Lioresal; ***Singapore:*** Lioresal; ***Spain:*** Lioresal; ***Swed.:*** Lioresal; ***Switz.:*** Lioresal; ***Thai.:*** Baclosal; Lioresal; ***UK:*** Baclospas; Balgifen†; Lioresal; Lyflex; ***USA:*** Kemstro; Lioresal.

# Botulinum Toxins

Toxinas botulínicas.

*ATC — M03AX01.*

**Description.** Botulinum toxins A and B are neurotoxins produced by *Clostridium botulinum*. They are proteins comprising a heavy chain thought to be responsible for binding to the target cells and translocation of the toxin across the cell membrane, linked by a disulfide bond to a light chain responsible for the toxic activity.

## Botulinum A Toxin

Toxina botulínica A.

**Pharmacopoeias.** *Eur.* (see p.vi) includes the injection.

**Ph. Eur. 5.0** (Botulinum Toxin Type A for Injection; Toxinum Botulinicum Typum A ad Iniectabile). A dried preparation containing purified botulinum neurotoxin type A, which may be present in the form of a complex with haemagglutinins and non-toxic proteins, prepared from a suitable strain of *Clostridium botulinum* type A.

## Botulinum B Toxin

Toxina botulínica B.

### Units

The dose of preparations containing botulinum toxins A or B is expressed in terms of units, but the available preparations are used at different doses for the same indications, and the units of one preparation cannot be considered to apply to another.

◊ It has been suggested that the difference between botulinum A toxin preparations may not only be confined to just a numerical dosage adjustment.[1] Reviews of the literature have suggested that there may also be a difference in the incidence of adverse effects. The reported frequency of dysphagia for Dysport (28% and 44%) in patients with spasmodic torticollis was greater than that for Botox (9.5 to 17%). This variation might relate to differences in bioactivity not recognised by the mouse lethality bioassay which is used to determine the potency of preparations.

1. Borodic G. Therapeutic botulinum toxin. *Lancet* 1994; **344:** 1370.

### Adverse Effects

Injections of botulinum toxins have been associated with a transient burning sensation, bruising at the injection site, and local weakness. Deep or misplaced injections may paralyse nearby muscle groups and excessive doses may paralyse distant muscles. Overdosage can produce a widespread paralysis.

There have been occasional reports of hypersensitivity reactions such as skin rashes and flu-like symptoms. There have also been rare reports of cardiovascular adverse effects, including arrhythmia and myocardial infarction.

- The most common adverse effects **following injection into muscles around the eye**, such as in the management of blepharospasm, hemifacial spasm, or strabismus are ptosis, lachrymation, photophobia, and ocular irritation. Some patients may be unable to close the eyelid completely. Other adverse effects that have been reported include ectropion and entropion, and diplopia. Patients experience a reduction in blinking and this can lead to dry eye, keratitis, and corneal damage. Angle-closure glaucoma has been reported. Vertical deviation has also occurred in patients treated for horizontal strabismus. Needle penetrations of the eye during treatment of strabismus have resulted in vitreous and retrobulbar haemorrhages.
- Dysphagia is the most common adverse effect **following injection into neck muscles** in the treatment of spasmodic torticollis and there may be pooling of saliva with risk of aspiration in severely affected patients (*important*, see also under Precautions, below). Dry mouth, paralysis of the vocal cords, and weakness of the neck muscles may also occur. Generalised weakness, malaise, nausea, and visual disturbances have occasionally been reported. Other effects which have occurred rarely include drowsiness, numbness, stiffness, ptosis, and headache. Respiratory difficulties, associated with the use of large doses, have occurred on rare occasions.
- Adverse effects most frequently associated with **injection into the lower limbs** in the treatment of cerebral palsy include falling, leg pain, and local and general weakness; lethargy and leg cramps have also been reported.
- Common adverse effects **following injection into the upper limb** in the treatment of spasticity associated with stroke are arm pain, muscle weakness, and hypertonia. A perceived increase in non-axillary sweating, within one month of the injection, has been reported after treatment for hyperhidrosis of the axillae; rarely, mild transient weakness of the arms has also occurred.
- Headache is the most frequent adverse effect **following injection into the muscles around the forehead** in the treatment of glabellar (frown) lines. Other adverse effects frequently reported include ptosis, facial pain, muscle weakness, and nausea.

◊ Reviews.

1. Klein AW. Complications and adverse reactions with the use of botulinum toxin. *Dis Mon* 2002; **48:** 336–56.

**Angiosarcoma.** It has been suggested[1] that botulinum A toxin injection might have acted as a triggering factor in the initiation of angiosarcoma in a 66-year-old patient being treated for blepharospasm.

1. Kárpáti S, *et al.* Human herpesvirus type 8-positive facial angiosarcoma developing at the site of botulinum toxin injection for blepharospasm. *Br J Dermatol* 2000; **143:** 660–2.

**Antibody formation.** Neutralising antibodies that reduce or abolish the beneficial effects of treatment have been found after prolonged treatment with botulinum A toxin.[1] A review[2] in 1994 considered that there was growing concern over the development of antibodies after repeated injections, as many of the conditions for which botulinum toxin is indicated require indefinite treatment. Antibody formation was reported to be more common with high doses (as in spasmodic torticollis) than after low doses (as for blepharospasm). The occurrence of antibodies appeared to correlate with the dose per injection, the quantity of botulinum protein given per injection, the number of injections given, and the frequency of injections.

Antibodies have also developed following the use of botulinum B toxin. However, botulinum toxin B is antigenically distinct from botulinum A toxin, and may be of value in patients who develop resistance to treatment associated with antibody formation to type A toxin.[3] Botulinum F toxin is also antigenically distinct and is being studied in a similar way.

1. Hambleton P, *et al.* Antitoxins and botulinum toxin treatment. *BMJ* 1992; **304:** 959–60.
2. Borodic GE, Pearce LB. New concepts in botulinum toxin therapy. *Drug Safety* 1994; **11:** 145–52.
3. Brin MF, *et al.* Safety and efficacy of NeuroBloc (botulinum toxin type B) in type A-resistant cervical dystonia. *Neurology* 1999; **53:** 1431–8.

**Biliary colic.** A 43-year-old woman with no previous history of gallbladder disease experienced single episodes of biliary colic after each of 3 sessions of treatment with botulinum A toxin for blepharospasm.[1] Botulinum A toxin might have exerted a systemic effect to block acetylcholine release leading to gallbladder hypomotility with delayed emptying and stasis.

1. Schnider P, *et al.* Gallbladder dysfunction induced by botulinum A toxin. *Lancet* 1993; **342:** 811–12.

**Dysphagia.** By November 1993, the UK Committee on Safety of Medicines had received 4 reports of severe dysphagia with choking in patients who had received injections of botulinum A toxin into the neck muscles as a treatment for torticollis.[1] The dysphagia developed 5 to 7 days after the injection and in one patient it was persisting 6 weeks after the injection. The dysphagia led to aspiration of the stomach contents into the lungs and one patient with a history of poor lung function died from bronchopneumonia. Dysphagia is also reported to be a common adverse effect in patients with spasmodic torticollis being treated with Botulinum B toxin.[2]

See also under Units, above for further reference to dysphagia as an adverse effect.

1. Committee on Safety of Medicines/Medicines Control Agency. Reminder: botulinum type A toxin (Dysport)—severe dysphagia with unlicensed route of administration. *Current Problems* 1993; **19:** 11.
2. Lew MF, *et al.* The safety and efficacy of botulinum toxin type B in the treatment of patients with cervical dystonia: summary of three controlled clinical trials. *Neurology* 2000; **55** (suppl 5): S29–S35.

**Effects on the eyes.** Acute angle-closure glaucoma has been reported[1] in an 83-year-old woman after a series of injections of botulinum A toxin for the treatment of blepharospasm. Permanent extra-ocular muscle damage following botulinum A toxin injection into the left inferior rectus muscle has been reported[2] in a 70-year-old man.

1. Corridan P, *et al.* Acute angle-closure glaucoma following botulinum toxin injection for blepharospasm. *Br J Ophthalmol* 1990; **74:** 309–10.
2. Mohan M, *et al.* Permanent extraocular muscle damage following botulinum toxin injection. *Br J Ophthalmol* 1999; **83:** 1309–10.

### Treatment of Adverse Effects

The use of artificial tears may relieve keratitis and dry eye. In the event of overdosage general supportive care is required. The patient should be monitored for several days for signs of paralysis and artificial respiration may be necessary. Since the effects of botulinum toxins are irreversible once bound to nerve terminals, it is doubtful that specific botulinum antitoxin (p.1610) will be of value unless given very rapidly after overdosage.

### Precautions

Botulinum toxin is contra-indicated in generalised disorders of muscle activity such as myasthenia gravis. As with other biological products, the potential for botulinum toxin to cause anaphylaxis should be considered.

Botulinum toxins should only be used by appropriately qualified and trained specialists. Injections must be made with great care, especially those into the neck, to avoid unintended paralysis; the relevant anatomy, and any alterations due to previous surgery, must be understood before injection.

The effects of botulinum toxins in pregnancy are unknown; fetal malformations and abortion have been reported in *rabbits*, and the manufacturers recommend that botulinum toxins should not be given to pregnant women. Breast feeding is also considered a contra-indication: it is not clear whether the toxin is distributed into breast milk.

When **injected into the muscles around the eyes**, as for the treatment of blepharospasm, hemifacial spasm, or strabismus, reduced blinking can lead to corneal exposure, persistent epithelial defect, and corneal ulceration, especially in patients with seventh cranial nerve disorders. Corneal sensation should be carefully tested in previously treated eyes, injection into the lower eyelid area avoided, and any resulting epithelial defect vigorously treated.

**Handling.** Residual botulinum A toxin or spillages should be inactivated by autoclaving or use of a dilute hypochlorite solution (0.5%). Botulinum B toxin may be decontaminated in a similar manner; a strong caustic solution may also be used.

### Interactions

The effect of botulinum toxins may theoretically be potentiated by aminoglycosides or spectinomycin. Interactions may also occur with other drugs that have neuromuscular blocking activity, including lincosamides, polymyxins, tetracyclines, and muscle relaxants.

### Uses and Administration

Botulinum toxins cause neuromuscular blockade by inhibiting the calcium-ion mediated release of acetylcholine at the motor nerve terminals, resulting in a diminished endplate potential and subsequent flaccid paralysis of the affected muscles. The paralysis persists until new nerve terminals form, usually within 2 to 4 months.

Botulinum A toxin is given as a complex with haemagglutinin by local injection in the treatment of hemifacial spasm, blepharospasm, spasmodic torticollis, lower limb spasticity in children with cerebral palsy, and upper limb spasticity associated with stroke in adults. Botulinum A toxin is also used for the management of strabismus and hyperhidrosis, and has also been approved for the treatment of glabellar (frown) lines in adults up to 65 years of age. It is being investigated for use in the management of several other disorders. Botulinum B toxin is also used in the management of spasmodic torticollis and, being antigenically distinct, it has the potential for use in patients who develop resistance to treatment due to the development of antibodies to type A toxin.

Doses of botulinum toxins A and B are expressed in terms of units, which have not been standardised between preparations (see under Units, above). Doses are therefore specific to each individual preparation; details are given below.

*Botulinum F toxin* is under investigation for the treatment of similar neuromuscular disorders.

◊ Reviews.

1. Borodic GE, Pearce LB. New concepts in botulinum toxin therapy. *Drug Safety* 1994; **11:** 145–52.
2. Hughes AJ. Botulinum toxin in clinical practice. *Drugs* 1994; **48:** 888–93.

**Achalasia.** The treatment of choice for achalasia (see Oesophageal Motility Disorders, p.1246) is mechanical dilatation of the lower oesophageal sphincter, or if necessary surgery, but more recently injection of botulinum A toxin[1-3] has been found to be effective. However, one year after treatment only 7 of 22 (32%) patients who received botulinum A toxin were in symptomatic remission compared with 14 of 20 (70%) patients treated with mechanical dilatation.[4] It was recommended that its use would be better reserved for patients thought to be at risk from mechanical dilatation or surgery.[3-5] Another study[6] demonstrated that intrasphincteric injection of botulinum toxin A was safe and effective for the treatment of achalasia in the short and medium term, although only a weak correlation with dose emerged.

1. Pasricha PJ, *et al.* Intrasphincteric botulinum toxin for the treatment of achalasia. *N Engl J Med* 1995; **332:** 774–8. Correction. *ibid.*; **333:** 75.
2. Cuillière C, *et al.* Achalasia: outcome of patients treated with intrasphincteric injection of botulinum toxin. *Gut* 1997; **41:** 87–92.
3. da Silveira EBV, Rogers AI. Treatment of achalasia with botulinum A toxin. *Am J Ther* 2002; **9:** 157–61.
4. Vaezi MF, *et al.* Botulinum toxin versus pneumatic dilatation in the treatment of achalasia: a randomised trial. *Gut* 1999; **44:** 231–9.

5. Spiess AE, Kahrilas PJ. Treating achalasia: from whalebone to laparoscope. *JAMA* 1998; **280:** 638–42.
6. Annesse V, *et al.* A multicentre randomised study of intrasphincteric botulinum toxin in patients with oesophageal achalasia. *Gut* 2000; **46:** 597–600.

**Anal fissure.** Anal fissure is a superficial tear in the mucosa of the distal anal canal characterised by pain on defaecation, rectal bleeding, and spasm of the anal sphincter. Healing, which is usually uneventful, may be helped by conservative management with bran and bulk laxatives and topical local anaesthetics for pain relief. Surgical treatment has been used for patients who develop a chronic condition but since this has been associated with high rates of long-term incontinence and recurrence, alternative treatments are being investigated.[1] As hypertonicity of the internal anal sphincter may be involved in the pathophysiology of chronic anal fissure, local injections of botulinum A toxin have been used to produce paresis of this sphincter.[2-4] The duration of the effect appears to be long enough to allow complete healing of the fissure in most patients although some may relapse; a long-term, follow-up trial[5] involving 57 completely healed patients, noted a high recurrence rate (41.5%) once the effects of botulinum toxin disappeared. Temporary incontinence had been the only adverse effect reported during treatment. Although possibly less effective than botulinum toxin,[1,6] topical application of nitrates can relax the anal sphincter and a randomised controlled study[7] has produced encouraging results in the treatment of anal fissure using glyceryl trinitrate ointment. Follow-up[8] of patients treated with glyceryl trinitrate indicated that after 24 to 38 months most had not experienced further problems or had had occasional recurrences which in the majority of cases had responded to further topical treatment. Isosorbide dinitrate ointment has also been tried, and may be of benefit with botulinum A toxin.[9] Calcium antagonists may also be effective: nifedipine[10] and diltiazem[11] have both produced promising results in small studies, and the latter may be useful in patients resistant to topical nitrates.[12]

1. Cook TA, *et al.* The pharmacology of the internal anal sphincter and new treatments of ano-rectal disorders. *Aliment Pharmacol Ther* 2001; **15:** 887–98.
2. Jost WH, Schimrigk K. Botulinum toxin in therapy of anal fissure. *Lancet* 1995; **345:** 188–9.
3. Maria G, *et al.* A comparison of botulinum toxin and saline for the treatment of chronic anal fissure. *N Engl J Med* 1998; **338:** 217–20.
4. Jost WH. Ten years' experience with botulin toxin in anal fissure. *Int J Colorectal Dis* 2002; **17:** 298–302.
5. Minguez M, *et al.* Long-term follow-up (42 months) of chronic anal fissure after healing with botulinum toxin. *Gastroenterology* 2002; **123:** 112–17.
6. Brisinda G, *et al.* A comparison of injections of botulinum toxin and topical nitroglycerin ointment for the treatment of chronic anal fissure. *N Engl J Med* 1999; **341:** 65–9. Correction. *ibid.*; 624.
7. Lund JN, Scholefield JH. A randomised, prospective, double-blind, placebo-controlled trial of glyceryl trinitrate ointment in treatment of anal fissure. *Lancet* 1997; **349:** 11–14. Correction. *ibid.*: 656.
8. Lund JN, Scholefield JH. Follow-up of patients with chronic anal fissure treated with topical glyceryl trinitrate. *Lancet* 1998; **352:** 1681.
9. Lysy J, *et al.* Topical nitrates potentiate the effect of botulinum toxin in the treatment of patients with refractory anal fissure. *Gut* 2001; **48:** 221–4.
10. Cook TA, *et al.* Oral nifedipine reduces resting anal pressure and heals chronic anal fissure. *Br J Surg* 1999; **86:** 1269–73.
11. Jonas M, *et al.* A randomized trial of oral vs topical diltiazem for chronic anal fissures. *Dis Colon Rectum* 2001; **44:** 1074–8.
12. Jonas M, *et al.* Diltiazem heals glyceryl trinitrate-resistant chronic anal fissures: a prospective study. *Dis Colon Rectum* 2002; **45:** 1091–5.

**Anismus.** Anismus is a condition in which inappropriate contraction of the anal sphincters occurs when bowel evacuation is attempted; it seems to be a form of dystonia.

Treatment with botulinum A toxin was investigated in 7 patients with intractable constipation due mainly to anismus.[1] The toxin was injected bilaterally into the puborectalis muscle using an electromyographically guided needle; patients were allowed to continue with their laxatives throughout the study if required. Symptoms improved in all but one of the patients, although two patients could not be regarded as treatment successes because they developed faecal incontinence; four patients had an excellent clinical outcome. However, another study involving 24 patients found the clinical effectiveness of botulinum A toxin to be limited, and further trials are needed to determine its role in the treatment of anismus.[2]

1. Hallan RI, *et al.* Treatment of anismus in intractable constipation with botulinum A toxin. *Lancet* 1988; **ii:** 714–17.
2. Ron Y, *et al.* Botulinum toxin type-A in therapy of patients with anismus. *Dis Colon Rectum* 2001; **44:** 1821–6.

**Blepharospasm.** Blepharospasm is a focal dystonia characterised by repeated involuntary blinking caused by spasms of the orbicularis oculi muscle of the eye, and can result in functional blindness. Blepharospasm is often associated with other dystonias of the head and neck, such as Meige syndrome, in which patients also suffer from involuntary contractures of the muscles around the mouth. Oral drug treatment as used for dystonias in general (see p.1209) is usually ineffective, and surgery (facial nerve avulsion) is often followed by recurrent spasm.[1] Local injections of botulinum A toxin into the orbicularis oculi muscle mimic the effect of surgical denervation of the muscle and are reported[2-5] to have been effective in over 70% of patients. Symptomatic improvement has been reported to last from about 9 to 15 weeks; no increase in duration of effect is apparent following multiple injections. In one retrospective study in patients with blepharospasm and Meige syndrome, treatment with botulinum A toxin was still effective in most patients 11 years after the start of therapy.[4]

For blepharospasm botulinum A toxin is injected into the orbicularis oculi of the upper and lower lids; injection into additional sites in the brow area and upper facial area may be indicated if the spasms interfere with vision. Doses of botulinum A toxin are expressed in terms of units, which have not been standardised between preparations. Doses are therefore *specific to each individual preparation*:

- The preparation *Botox* (Allergan, UK) is injected intramuscularly in an initial dose of 1.25 to 2.5 units at each site to a total of up to 25 units per eye. An effect is usually obtained within 3 days and reaches a peak after 1 to 2 weeks; each treatment lasts for about 3 months. If the response lasts less than 2 months the dose may be increased up to 5 units at each site but the total dose given in a 12-week period should not exceed 100 units. Giving more often than every 3 months confers no additional benefit. *Botox* (Allergan) is also available in the USA and given in similar doses, although higher cumulative doses of up to 200 units are allowed in a 30-day period
- For the preparation *Dysport* (Ipsen, UK) the initial dose is a total of 120 units per eye given as subcutaneous injections of 20 and 40 units per site. Subsequently the total dose may need to be reduced to 60 to 80 units per eye. With this preparation the relief of symptoms may begin within 2 to 4 days with a maximum effect being obtained within 2 weeks. Injections of Dysport may need to be repeated every 8 weeks.

1. Kennedy RH, *et al.* Treatment of blepharospasm with botulinum toxin. *Mayo Clin Proc* 1989; **64:** 1085–90.
2. Grandas F. Blepharospasm: a review of 264 patients. *J Neurol Neurosurg Psychiatry* 1988; **51:** 767–72.
3. Elston JS. The management of blepharospasm and hemifacial spasm. *J Neurol* 1992; **239:** 5–8.
4. Mauriello JA, *et al.* Treatment selections of 239 patients with blepharospasm and Meige syndrome over 11 years. *Br J Ophthalmol* 1996; **80:** 1073–6.
5. Defazio G, Livrea P. Primary blepharospasm: diagnosis and management. *Drugs* 2004; **64:** 237–44.

**Cosmetic use.** Botulinum A toxin has been used for the cosmetic treatment of facial lines and wrinkles and age-related neck degeneration.[1-5]

For the temporary improvement in appearance of moderate to severe glabellar (frown) lines two doses of botulinum A toxin are injected into each of the corrugator muscles and one dose into the procerus muscle. Doses of botulinum A toxin are expressed in terms of units, which have not been standardised between preparations. Doses are therefore *specific to each individual preparation*: the preparation *Botox Cosmetic* (Allergan, USA) is injected intramuscularly, not closer than 1 cm above the central eyebrow. A dose of 4 units is given into each of 5 sites to a total dose of 20 units. An effect is obtained in 1 to 2 days which increases in intensity in the first week; each treatment lasts for about 3 to 4 months. More frequent dosing is not recommended as safety and effectiveness have not been evaluated.

1. Olver JM. Botulinum toxin A treatment of overactive corrugator supercilii in thyroid eye disease. *Br J Ophthalmol* 1998; **82:** 528–33.
2. Song KH. Botulinum toxin type A injection for the treatment of frown lines. *Ann Pharmacother* 1998 **32:** 1365–7.
3. Anonymous. Cosmetic use of botulinum toxin. *Med Lett Drugs Ther* 1999; **41:** 63–4.
4. Anonymous. Botulinum toxin (Botox Cosmetic) for frown lines. *Med Lett Drugs Ther* 2002; **44:** 47–8.
5. Carruthers A. Botulinum toxin type A: history and current cosmetic use in the upper face. *Dis Mon* 2002; **48:** 299–322.

**Gastric motility disorders.** Some benefit has been reported from the use of botulinum A toxin injection in gastric motility disorders (p.1241). In an open-label study[1] 6 diabetic patients with gastroparesis experienced an improvement in gastric emptying after treatment with botulinum A toxin.

1. Ezzeddine D, *et al.* Pyloric injection of botulinum toxin for treatment of diabetic gastroparesis. *Gastrointest Endosc* 2002; **55:** 920–3.

**Hand dystonia.** Hand dystonia, or hand cramp, is a type of focal dystonia (p.1209). It is more commonly reported in people who perform repetitive movements with their hands, such as writers, keyboard operators, and musicians. Treatment was traditionally with antimuscarinics, although with limited success, but botulinum toxin has increasingly become the first-line option.[1] A double-blind study reported that 8 out of 10 patients had greater subjective improvement in focal hand dystonia, compared with placebo, after treatment with botulinum A toxin given by the intramuscular route; objective improvement in muscle strength was seen in 6 patients.[2] However, pain and severe weakness in the shoulder region resembling neuralgic amyotrophy has been reported[3] in 2 patients injected with botulinum A toxin for writer's cramp. It was considered that if unexplained pain occurred in the shoulder or upper arm after a first injection of botulinum A toxin further injections were contra-indicated.

1. Karp BI. Botulinum toxin treatment of occupational and focal hand dystonia. *Mov Disord* 2004; **19** (suppl 8): S116–S119.
2. Cole R, *et al.* Double-blind trial of botulinum toxin for treatment of focal hand dystonia. *Mov Disord* 1995; **10:** 466–71.
3. Sheean GL, *et al.* Pain and remote weakness in limbs injected with botulinum toxin A for writer's cramp. *Lancet* 1995; **346:** 154–6.

**Headache.** The therapeutic effect of botulinum A toxin in headache was first observed as a coincidental side-effect in patients receiving the drug for hyperfunctional facial lines. A review[1] of subsequent studies concluded that efficacy could be demonstrated for the prophylaxis of migraine (p.464); a small number of patients who received treatment during the acute phase of a migraine attack also experienced pain relief. Contradictory results had been reported in the studies evaluating tension-type headache (p.465). However, it was emphasised that an important finding had been the need to inject botulinum A toxin at the site of the pain or trigger points and not on a standardised basis, and that this should be considered in future studies. Improvement had been noted in individual cases of cluster headache (p.464) and in some patients with headache attributed to disorders of the neck.

Some benefit has also been seen with botulinum B toxin in the treatment of migraine and tension-type headaches.[2]

1. Göbel H, *et al.* Evidence-based medicine: botulinum toxin A in migraine and tension-type headache. *J Neurol* 2001; **248** (suppl 1): 34–8.
2. Fadeyi MO, Adams QM. Use of botulinum toxin type B for migraine and tension headaches. *Am J Health-Syst Pharm* 2002; **59:** 1860–2.

**Hemifacial spasm.** Hemifacial spasm is characterised by involuntary unilateral synchronous contractions of muscles innervated by the facial nerve. The spasms usually begin with twitching of muscles around the eye or mouth but as the disease progresses their frequency increases and they spread to involve the rest of the facial muscles. Hemifacial spasm may be improved by surgery but there is a risk of irreversible paralysis. Few drugs are effective for hemifacial spasm but carbamazepine has been reported to have been of help on occasions. Reports suggest that injections of botulinum A toxin may be effective in relieving symptoms in about 75% of patients but there do not appear to be any studies comparing it against other treatments. Repeat injections are required by most patients every 3 to 4 months but long-term efficacy appears to be maintained. Dosage regimens of botulinum A toxin used in hemifacial spasm are similar to those used for blepharospasm (see above) although an electromyographically guided needle may be required to identify small muscles around the mouth.

References.

1. Elston JS. The management of blepharospasm and hemifacial spasm. *J Neurol* 1992; **239:** 5–8.
2. Chen R-S, *et al.* Botulinum toxin A injection in the treatment of hemifacial spasm. *Acta Neurol Scand* 1996; **94:** 207–11.
3. Boghen DR, Lesser RL. Blepharospasm and hemifacial spasm. *Curr Treat Options Neurol* 2000; **2:** 393–400.
4. Jost WH, Kohl A. Botulinum toxin: evidence-based medicine criteria in blepharospasm and hemifacial spasm. *J Neurol* 2001; **248** (suppl 1): 21–4.
5. Defazio G, *et al.* Botulinum toxin A treatment for primary hemifacial spasm: a 10-year multicenter study. *Arch Neurol* 2002; **59:** 418–20.

**Hyperhidrosis.** A number of drugs and surgical techniques have been used in the treatment of hyperhidrosis (p.1136). Botulinum A toxin is used in the management of focal hyperhidrosis because of its ability to block cholinergic transmission at nerve terminals innervating the sweat glands. Encouraging results have been obtained in patients with severe resistant focal hyperhidrosis using intradermal[1,2] or subcutaneous[3,4] injections and results from two larger multicentre studies[5,6] confirm that intradermal injection of botulinum A is effective and well-tolerated for the treatment of axillary hyperhidrosis. In the UK, it is given for this purpose as the preparation *Botox* (Allergan, UK), by intradermal injection in doses of 50 units to each axilla, evenly distributed in multiple sites approximately 1 to 2 cm apart. Clinical improvement generally occurs within a week of injection, and may last for 4 to 7 months; repeat injections may be given once the effects of the previous injection have subsided. Some workers[7] prefer to use intradermal injections for palmar hyperhidrosis in order to minimise the risk of reversible weakness of the small muscles of the hand reported with subcutaneous injection.

1. Naumann M, *et al.* Focal hyperhidrosis: effective treatment with intracutaneous botulinum toxin. *Arch Dermatol* 1998; **134:** 301–4.
2. Schnider P, *et al.* Treatment of focal hyperhidrosis with botulinum toxin type A: long-term follow-up in 61 patients. *Br J Dermatol* 2001; **145:** 289–93.
3. Schnider P, *et al.* Double-blind trial of botulinum A toxin for the treatment of focal hyperhidrosis of the palms. *Br J Dermatol* 1997; **136:** 548–52.
4. Schnider P, *et al.* Uses of botulinum toxin. *Lancet* 1997; **349:** 953.
5. Heckmann M, *et al.* Botulinum toxin A for axillary hyperhidrosis (excessive sweating). *N Engl J Med* 2001; **344:** 488–93.
6. Naumann M, *et al.* Botulinum toxin type A in treatment of bilateral primary axillary hyperhidrosis: randomised, parallel group, double blind, placebo controlled trial. *BMJ* 2001; **323:** 596–9.
7. Heckmann M, *et al.* Optimizing botulinum toxin therapy for hyperhidrosis. *Br J Dermatol* 1998; **138:** 553–4.

**Hyperlachrymation.** Botulinum A toxin may be of benefit[1,2] in the management of hyperlachrymation ('crocodile tears').

1. Riemann R, *et al.* Successful treatment of crocodile tears by injection of botulinum toxin into the lacrimal gland: a case report. *Ophthalmology* 1999; **106:** 2322–4.
2. Keegan DJ, *et al.* Botulinum toxin treatment for hyperlacrimation secondary to aberrant regenerated seventh nerve palsy or salivary gland transplantation. *Br J Ophthalmol* 2002; **86:** 43–6.

**Laryngeal dystonias.** Botulinum A toxin has been tried in the treatment of spasmodic dysphonia,[1,2] focal laryngeal dystonia,[3] and dysfunctional spasm following total laryngectomy.[4] Botulinum B toxin has also been used.[5]

1. Whurr R, *et al.* Meta-analysis of botulinum toxin treatment of spasmodic dysphonia: a review of 22 studies. *Int J Lang Commun Disord* 1998; **33** (suppl): 327–9.
2. Gibbs SR, Blitzer A. Botulinum toxin for the treatment of spasmodic dysphonia. *Otolaryngol Clin North Am* 2000; **33:** 879–94.
3. Marion M-H, *et al.* Stridor and focal laryngeal dystonia. *Lancet* 1992; **339:** 457–8.
4. Crary MA, *et al.* Using botulinum toxin A to improve speech and swallowing function following total laryngectomy. *Arch Otolaryngol Head Neck Surg* 1996; **122:** 760–3.
5. Sataloff RT, *et al.* Botulinum toxin type B for treatment of spasmodic dysphonia: a case report. *J Voice* 2002; **16:** 422–4.

**Micturition disorders.** Preliminary results[1] suggest that injection of botulinum A toxin into the detrusor muscle can increase functional bladder capacity and restore continence in patients with urinary incontinence (p.476) after spinal cord injury who are resistant to antimuscarinics.

Similar results[2] have been found in children with detrusor hyperreflexia caused by myelomeningocele. Botulinum A Toxin has also been tried in other bladder voiding dysfunctions.[3]

1. Schurch B, *et al.* Botulinum-A toxin for treating detrusor hyperreflexia in spinal cord injured patients: a new alternative to anticholinergic drugs? Preliminary results. *J Urol (Baltimore)* 2000; **164:** 692–7.
2. Schulte-Baukloh H, *et al.* Efficacy of botulinum-A toxin in children with detrusor hyperreflexia due to myelomeningocele: preliminary results. *Urology* 2002; **59:** 325–7.
3. Phelan MW, *et al.* Botulinum toxin urethral sphincter injection to restore bladder emptying in men and women with voiding dysfunction. *J Urol (Baltimore)* 2001; **165:** 1107–10.

**Nystagmus.** Surgery, corrective spectacles, and drug therapy have all been tried for the treatment of nystagmus (rapid involuntary movement of the eyeball). Retrobulbar injection of botulinum A toxin has produced improvement in patients with acquired or congenital nystagmus.[1-4] In 6 patients with acquired nystagmus visual acuity was improved, and the amplitude of the nystagmus was reduced, but the frequency was generally unchanged and the need for repeated injections and adverse effects such as diplopia limited patient acceptability.[1]

1. Repka MX, *et al.* Treatment of acquired nystagmus with botulinum neurotoxin A. *Arch Ophthalmol* 1994; **112:** 1320–4.
2. Carruthers J. The treatment of congenital nystagmus with Botox. *J Pediatr Ophthalmol Strabismus* 1995; **32:** 306–8.
3. Lennerstrand G, *et al.* Treatment of strabismus and nystagmus with botulinum toxin type A: an evaluation of effects and complications. *Acta Ophthalmol Scand* 1998; **76:** 27–37.
4. Stahl JS, *et al.* Medical treatment of nystagmus and its visual consequences. *J R Soc Med* 2002; **95:** 235–7.

**Ocular surgery.** Ptosis is a common adverse effect of botulinum A toxin (see Adverse Effects, above). Therapeutic ptosis induced with botulinum toxin has been described as a useful adjunct in the management of patients undergoing epikeratoplasty since it promoted stabilisation of the epithelium on the graft.[1]

1. Freegard T, *et al.* Therapeutic ptosis with botulinum toxin in epikeratoplasty. *Br J Ophthalmol* 1993; **77:** 820–2.

**Pain.** There have been anecdotal reports of the use of botulinum A toxin in the treatment of painful disorders such as postcholecystectomy pain associated with sphincter of Oddi dysfunction,[1] and relief of orofacial pain associated with temporomandibular joint dysfunction[2] and facial arthromyalgia.[3] Promising results have been obtained from an open study[4] investigating botulinum toxin as a treatment for chronic refractory tennis elbow in 14 patients. Its efficacy in relieving pain in other chronic conditions such as low back pain, and myofascial pain, in addition to improving function, has also been demonstrated in individual studies.[5] The general management of pain is discussed on p.2 with separate sections on biliary and renal colic (p.4), low back pain (p.7), orofacial pain (p.7), postoperative analgesia (p.4), and soft-tissue rheumatism (p.11).

1. Pasricha PJ, *et al.* Intrasphincteric injection of botulinum toxin for suspected sphincter of Oddi dysfunction. *Gut* 1994; **35:** 1319–21.
2. Girdler NM. Use of botulinum toxin to alleviate facial pain. *Br J Hosp Med* 1994; **52:** 363.
3. Girdler NM. Uses of botulinum toxin. *Lancet* 1997; **349:** 953.
4. Morré HHE, *et al.* Treatment of chronic tennis elbow with botulinum toxin. *Lancet* 1997; **349:** 1746.
5. Lang AM. Botulinum toxin therapy for myofascial pain disorders. *Curr Pain Headache Rep* 2002; **6:** 355–60.

**Spasmodic torticollis.** Spasmodic torticollis (cervical dystonia) is a focal dystonia (p.1209) characterised by spasmodic rotation of the head as a result of dystonic spasm of the neck muscles. The head may turn to one side (torticollis), extend (retrocollis), or flex (antecollis). Spasms may be repetitive or sustained. Response of spasmodic torticollis to drug therapy is usually poor and surgery has been associated with potentially serious complications. Intramuscular injections of botulinum toxins can be effective but dysphagia, which can have severe consequences (see under Adverse Effects, above) occurs in a significant number of patients. Other side-effects have included lethargy, local weakness, vertigo, and dysphonia.

When injecting botulinum toxins localisation of the involved muscles with electromyographic guidance may be useful. Multiple injection sites allow more uniform contact with the innervation areas of the dystonic muscle and are especially useful in larger muscles. Bilateral injection of the sternocleidomastoid muscle is not recommended as there is an increased risk of adverse effects, especially dysphagia. Reduced doses may be required for patients with reduced muscle mass.

Doses of botulinum toxins, which are expressed in terms of units, have not been standardised between preparations. Doses are therefore *specific to each individual preparation.*

In the UK the usual initial dose of botulinum A toxin as the preparation *Dysport* (Ipsen, UK) is 500 units injected in divided doses into the two or three most active neck muscles:

- for *rotational torticollis*, 350 units is given initially into the splenius capitis muscle (ipsilateral to the direction of the chin/head rotation) and 150 units into the sternocleidomastoid muscle (contralateral to rotation)
- for *laterocollis*, 350 units is given initially into the ipsilateral splenius capitis muscle and 150 units into the ipsilateral sternocleidomastoid muscle; if associated with *shoulder elevation*, ipsilateral trapezoid or levator scapulae muscles may also require treatment; if 3 muscles need treatment, 300 units are injected into the splenius capitis muscle, 100 units into the sternocleidomastoid muscle, and 100 units into the third muscle
- for *retrocollis*, 250 units is given into each of the splenius capitis muscles which may be followed after 6 weeks by bilateral trapezius injections in a dose of up to 250 units per muscle; bilateral splenii injections may increase the risk of neck muscle weakness

Subsequent doses may range from 250 to 1000 units, although the higher doses may be accompanied by an increase in adverse effects such as dysphagia; doses above 1000 units are not recommended. An initial effect is usually observed within 1 week; injections usually need to be repeated every 8 to 12 weeks.

Recommended doses in the UK for botulinum A toxin as the preparation *Botox* (Allergan, UK) are listed below but the manufacturer has stated that in practice the maximum total dose is not usually more than 200 units. No more than 50 units should be given at any one injection site; limiting the dose injected into the sternocleidomastoid muscle to less than 100 units may reduce the risk of dysphagia.

- *Type I* (head rotated toward side of shoulder elevation)—sternocleidomastoid muscle: total dosage of 50 to 100 units divided amongst at least 2 sites; levator scapulae: total of 50 units amongst 1 or 2 sites; scalene: total of 25 to 50 units amongst 1 or 2 sites; splenius capitis: total of 25 to 75 units amongst 1 to 3 sites; trapezius: total of 25 to 100 units amongst 1 to 8 sites
- *Type II* (head rotation only)—sternocleidomastoid muscle: total dosage of 25 to 100 units divided amongst at least 2 sites if more than 25 units is given
- *Type III* (head tilted toward side of shoulder elevation)—sternocleidomastoid muscle: total dosage of 25 to 100 units at posterior border divided amongst at least 2 sites if more than 25 units is given; levator scapulae: total of 25 to 100 units amongst at least 2 sites; scalene: total of 25 to 75 units amongst at least 2 sites; trapezius: total of 25 to 100 units amongst 1 to 8 sites
- *Type IV* (bilateral posterior cervical muscle spasm with elevation of the face)—splenius capitis and splenius cervicis: a total dosage of 50 to 200 units divided amongst 2 to 8 sites and which include both sides of the neck

Botulinum A toxin as the preparation Botox is also available in the USA for the treatment of spasmodic torticollis. The manufacturers (Allergan, USA) recommend that doses should be tailored to meet individual patient requirements.

In the UK the usual initial dose of botulinum B toxin as the preparation *NeuroBloc* (Elan Pharma, UK) is 5000 to 10 000 units given by intramuscular injection in divided doses into the two to four most affected muscles.

Botulinum B toxin as the preparation *Myobloc* is also available in the USA. The initial dose is 2500 to 5000 units given by intramuscular injection divided between the affected muscles. The manufacturers (Elan, USA) recommend that patients with no previous history of tolerating botulinum injections should be started on a lower initial dose.

References.

1. Blackie JD, Lees AJ. Botulinum toxin treatment in spasmodic torticollis. *J Neurol Neurosurg Psychiatry* 1990; **53:** 640–3.
2. Greene P, *et al.* Double-blind, placebo-controlled trial of botulinum toxin injections for the treatment of spasmodic torticollis. *Neurology* 1990; **40:** 1213–18.
3. Anderson TJ, *et al.* Botulinum toxin treatment of spasmodic torticollis. *J R Soc Med* 1992; **85:** 524–9.
4. Brans JWM, *et al.* Botulinum toxin versus trihexyphenidyl in cervical dystonia: a prospective, randomized, double-blind controlled trial. *Neurology* 1996; **46:** 1066–72.
5. Brin MF, *et al.* Safety and efficacy of NeuroBloc (botulinum toxin type B) in type A-resistant cervical dystonia. *Neurology* 1999; **53:** 1431–8.
6. Brashear A, *et al.* Safety and efficacy of NeuroBloc (botulinum toxin B) in type A-resistant cervical dystonia. *Neurology* 1999; **53:** 1439–46.
7. Velickovic M, *et al.* Cervical dystonia: pathophysiology and treatment options. *Drugs* 2001; **61:** 1921–43.
8. Figgitt DP, Noble S. Botulinum toxin B: a review of its therapeutic potential in the management of cervical dystonia. *Drugs* 2002; **62:** 705–22.
9. Dressler D, *et al.* Botulinum toxin type B in antibody-induced botulinum toxin type A therapy failure. *J Neurol* 2003; **250:** 967–9. Correction. *ibid.*; 1263–5.
10. Walker FO. Botulinum toxin therapy for cervical dystonia. *Phys Med Rehabil Clin N Am* 2003; **14:** 749–66.
11. Lew MF. Duration of effectiveness of botulinum toxin type B in the treatment of cervical dystonia. *Adv Neurol* 2004; **94:** 211–15.
12. Jankovic J. Treatment of cervical dystonia with botulinum toxin. *Mov Disord* 2004; **19** (suppl 8): S109–S115.

**Spasticity.** The mainstay of management of spasticity, as discussed on p.1386, is physiotherapy together with antispastic drugs. Chemical neurolysis should only be considered when there is intractable continuous pain. Local injections of botulinum A toxin, as an alternative to chemical neurolysis, have been used in the management of limb spasticity in post-stroke patients[1-4] and children with cerebral palsy.[5-10] Botulinum B toxin has also been tried.[10,11]

Doses of botulinum A toxin, which are expressed in terms of units, have not been standardised between preparations. Doses are therefore *specific to each individual preparation:* Botulinum A toxin is used in the management of dynamic equinus foot deformity associated with spasticity in children with cerebral palsy.

- For children over 2 years of age the recommended total dose of botulinum A toxin as the preparation *Botox* (Allergan, UK) is 4 units/kg injected into each of 2 sites in the medial and lateral heads of the gastrocnemius muscle. When both lower limbs are to be injected on the same occasion this total dose should be divided between the 2 limbs. Clinical improvement generally occurs within the first 2 weeks. Repeat doses should not be given more frequently than every 2 months
- For children over 2 years of age the recommended total dose of botulinum A toxin as the preparation *Dysport* (Ipsen, UK) is 10 to 30 units/kg divided between both calf muscles, primarily targeted to the gastrocnemius muscle. The maximum dose administered should not exceed 1000 units per patient. Clinical improvement generally occurs within the first 2 weeks. Repeat doses should not be given more frequently than every 8 weeks
- In the treatment of upper limb spasticity associated with stroke, the exact dosage and number of injection sites of botulinum A toxin *as the preparation Botox* (Allergan, UK) should be tailored to the individual based on the muscles involved, the severity of the spasticity, and the presence of local weakness. The manufacturer recommends a total dose of 50 units into the flexor digitorum profundus, the flexor digitorum sublimis, the flexor carpi radialis, or the flexor carpi ulnaris, and a total dose of 20 units into the adductor pollicis or flexor pollicis longus. In clinical trials, cumulative doses did not exceed 360 units at any treatment session.

1. Simpson DM, *et al.* Botulinum toxin type A in the treatment of upper extremity spasticity: a randomized, double-blind, placebo-controlled trial. *Neurology* 1996; **46:** 1306–10.
2. Bhakta BB, *et al.* Use of botulinum toxin in stroke patients with severe upper limb spasticity. *J Neurol Neurosurg Psychiatry* 1996; **61:** 30–5.
3. Burbaud P, *et al.* A randomised, double blind, placebo controlled trial of botulinum toxin in the treatment of spastic foot in hemiparetic patients. *J Neurol Neurosurg Psychiatry* 1996; **61:** 265–9.
4. Brashear A, *et al.* Intramuscular injection of botulinum toxin for the treatment of wrist and finger spasticity after a stroke. *N Engl J Med* 2002; **347:** 395–400.
5. Zelnik N, *et al.* The role of botulinum toxin in the treatment of lower limb spasticity in children with cerebral palsy—a pilot study. *Isr J Med Sci* 1997; **33:** 129–33.
6. Carr LJ, *et al.* Position paper on the use of botulinum toxin in cerebral palsy. *Arch Dis Child* 1998; **79:** 271–3.
7. Fehlings D, *et al.* An evaluation of botulinum-A toxin injections to improve upper extremity function in children with hemiplegic cerebral palsy. *J Pediatr* 2000; **137:** 331–7.
8. Ubhi T, *et al.* Randomised double blind placebo controlled trial of the effect of botulinum toxin on walking in cerebral palsy. *Arch Dis Child* 2000; **83:** 481–7.
9. Koman LA, *et al.* Botulinum toxin type A neuromuscular blockade in the treatment of equinus foot deformity in cerebral palsy: a multicenter, open-label clinical trial. *Pediatrics* 2001; **108:** 1062–71.
10. Berweck S, Heinen F. Use of botulinum toxin in pediatric spasticity (cerebral palsy). *Mov Disord* 2004; **19** (suppl 8): S162–S167.
11. Brashear A, *et al.* Botulinum toxin type B in upper-limb post-stroke spasticity: a double-blind, placebo-controlled trial. *Arch Phys Med Rehabil* 2004; **85:** 705–9.

**Stiff-man syndrome.** A patient with stiff-man syndrome (see Muscle Spasm, p.696) had marked improvement of ambulation and cessation of pain after injection of botulinum A toxin into affected paraspinal muscles.[1] In another case-report, improvement in rigidity and muscle spasm was reported[2] in 2 patients after botulinum treatment; muscle spasms reduced within 3 days of treatment. It was also found that there was an increase in the duration of effect of botulinum A toxin after each subsequent injection and only a gradual return of painful spasm.

1. Davis D, Jabbari B. Significant improvement of stiff-person syndrome after paraspinal injection of botulinum toxin A. *Mov Disord* 1993; **8:** 371–3.
2. Liguori R, *et al.* Botulinum toxin A improves muscle spasms and rigidity in stiff-person syndrome. *Mov Disord* 1997; **12:** 1060–3.

**Strabismus.** Botulinum A toxin has been used to weaken overactive extra-ocular muscles as an alternative or adjunct to surgery in the correction of strabismus (p.1487). Not all patients respond to botulinum A toxin and many patients who do respond require more than one injection to maintain improvement. Botulinum A toxin does not appear to offer a better degree of correction than traditional surgery, and it has been suggested that it should be reserved for use in patients unresponsive to, or unsuitable for, surgery. In the USA botulinum A toxin as the preparation *Botox* (Allergan, USA) is indicated for the treatment of strabismus in patients 12 years of age or older. Depending on the direction and degree of deviation to be corrected the recommended initial dose of Botox to be injected into any one extra-ocular muscle ranges from 1.25 to 5 units. Paralysis is usually seen within the first 2 days and increases in intensity during the first week. The paralysis lasts for 2 to 6 weeks and gradually resolves over a further 2 to 6 weeks. It is recommended that patients are re-examined 7 to 14 days after injection to assess the effect of the dose given. If treatment is required for residual or recurrent strabismus, patients are either given treatment at the previous dosage if response was judged to have been adequate or up to twice the previous dose if paralysis had been incomplete. Repeat injections should not be given until the effects of the previous dose have dissipated. No more than 25 units should be injected into any one muscle; the manufacturer recommends that the cumulative dose in a 30-day period should not exceed 200 units. Injections should be diluted with unpreserved 0.9% sodium chloride solution so that the volume administered per muscle is between 0.05 mL and 0.15 mL. Injections should also be made using an electromyographically guided needle to aid location of the target muscle.

References.


1. Biglan AW, *et al.* Management of strabismus with botulinum A toxin. *Ophthalmology* 1989; **96:** 935–43.
2. Carruthers JDA, *et al.* Botulinum vs adjustable suture surgery in the treatment of horizontal misalignment in adult patients lacking fusion. *Arch Ophthalmol* 1990; **108:** 1432–5.
3. Lyons CJ, *et al.* Botulinum toxin therapy in dysthyroid strabismus. *Eye* 1990; **4:** 538–42.
4. McNeer KW. An investigation of the clinical use of botulinum toxin A as a postoperative adjustment procedure in the therapy of strabismus. *J Pediatr Ophthalmol Strabismus* 1990; **27:** 3–9.
5. Scott AB, *et al.* Botulinum treatment of childhood strabismus. *Ophthalmology* 1990; **97:** 1434–8.
6. Petitto VB, Buckley EG. Use of botulinum toxin in strabismus after retinal detachment surgery. *Ophthalmology* 1991; **98:** 509–13.
7. Elston J. Is botulinum toxin helpful in squint management? *Br J Ophthalmol* 1998; **82:** 105.
8. Tejedor J, Rodríguez JM. Early retreatment of infantile esotropia: comparison of reoperation and botulinum toxin. *Br J Ophthalmol* 1999; **83:** 783–7.


**Stuttering.** Botulinum toxin may be of benefit in the treatment of stuttering (p.702).[1,2]


1. Brin MF, *et al.* Laryngeal botulinum toxin injections for disabling stuttering in adults. *Neurology* 1994; **44:** 2262–6.
2. Cordivari C, *et al.* New therapeutic indications for botulinum toxins. *Mov Disord* 2004; **19** (suppl 8): S157–S161.


**Tourette's syndrome.** Improvement in tics was noted in patients with Tourette's syndrome (see Tics, p.664) treated with botulinum A toxin.[1,2]


1. Kwak CH, *et al.* Botulinum toxin in the treatment of tics. *Arch Neurol* 2000; **57:** 1190–3.
2. Marras C, *et al.* Botulinum toxin for simple motor tics: a randomized, double-blind, controlled clinical trial. *Neurology* 2001; **56:** 605–10.


**Tremor.** Local injection of botulinum A toxin[1-4] has been tried in patients with essential tremor (p.872) that fails to respond to conventional treatment. Botulinum A toxin injection has also been successfully used to treat essential palatal tremor[5-7] and associated symptoms such as uncomfortable ear clicking.


1. Henderson JM, *et al.* Botulinum toxin A in non-dystonic tremors. *Eur Neurol* 1996; **36:** 29–35.
2. Jankovic J, *et al.* A randomized, double-blind, placebo-controlled study to evaluate botulinum toxin type A in essential hand tremor. *Mov Disord* 1996; **11:** 250–6.
3. Pacchetti C, *et al.* Botulinum toxin treatment for functional disability induced by essential tremor. *Neurol Sci* 2000; **21:** 349–53.
4. Brin MF, *et al.* A randomized, double masked, controlled trial of botulinum toxin type A in essential hand tremor. *Neurology* 2001; **56:** 1523–8.
5. Deuschl G, *et al.* Ear click in palatal tremor: its origin and treatment with botulinum toxin. *Neurology* 1991; **41:** 1677–9.
6. Jamieson DRS, *et al.* Ear clicks in palatal tremor caused by activity of the levator veli palatini. *Neurology* 1996; **46:** 1168–9.
7. Cho JW, *et al.* Case of essential palatal tremor: atypical features and remarkable benefit from botulinum toxin injection. *Mov Disord* 2001; **16:** 779–82.


**Vaginismus.** Report[1] of one patient who had relief of vaginismus (painful involuntary spasm of the vaginal or perianal muscles severe enough to prevent intercourse) for more than 24 months after injection of botulinum toxin into the vaginal wall muscles.


1. Brin MF, Vapnek JM. Treatment of vaginismus with botulinum toxin injections. *Lancet* 1997; **349:** 252–3.


## Preparations

**Ph. Eur.:** Botulinum Toxin Type A for Injection.

**Proprietary Preparations** (details are given in Part 3)
***Arg.:*** Botox; ***Austral.:*** Botox; Dysport; ***Austria:*** Botox; Dysport; ***Belg.:*** Botox; Dysport; ***Braz.:*** Botox; Dysport; ***Canad.:*** Botox; ***Denm.:*** Botox; Dysport; ***Fin.:*** Botox; Dysport; ***Fr.:*** Botox; Dysport; NeuroBloc; Vistabel; ***Ger.:*** Botox; Dysport; NeuroBloc; ***Gr.:*** Botox; Dysport; ***Hong Kong:*** Botox; Dysport; ***Irl.:*** Botox; Dysport; NeuroBloc; ***Israel:*** Botox; Dysport; ***Ital.:*** Botox; Dysport; NeuroBloc; ***Jpn:*** Botox; ***Malaysia:*** Botox; Dysport; ***Mex.:*** Botox; ***Norw.:*** Botox; ***NZ:*** Botox; Dysport; ***Port.:*** Botox; NeuroBloc; ***S.Afr.:*** Botox; ***Singapore:*** Botox; Dysport; ***Spain:*** Botox; Dysport; NeuroBloc; ***Swed.:*** Botox; Dysport; ***Switz.:*** Botox; Dysport; ***Thai.:*** Botox; ***UK:*** Botox; Dysport; NeuroBloc; ***USA:*** Botox; Myobloc.

---

## Carisoprodol *(BAN, rINN)*

Carisoprodolum; Isopropylmeprobamate. 2-Methyl-2-propyltrimethylene carbamate isopropylcarbamate.

$C_{12}H_{24}N_2O_4$ = 260.3.
*CAS — 78-44-4.*
*ATC — M03BA02.*

**Pharmacopoeias.** In *Eur.* (see p.vi) and *US.*

**Ph. Eur. 5.0** (Carisoprodol). A white or almost white fine powder. M.p. 92° to 95°. Very slightly soluble in water; freely soluble in alcohol, in acetone, and in dichloromethane.

**USP 27** (Carisoprodol). A white crystalline powder having a mild characteristic odour. M.p. 91° to 94°. Soluble 1 in 2083 of water, 1 in 2.5 of alcohol and of acetone, and 1 in 2.3 of chloroform. Store in airtight containers.

### Adverse Effects, Treatment, and Precautions

As for Meprobamate, p.706.

An idiosyncratic reaction may occur within minutes of a dose in patients who have not previously received carisoprodol. The symptoms, which include severe weakness and central disturbances, usually subside over several hours. There may be a short-lived quadriplegia. Cross reactivity can occur with its metabolite meprobamate.

Overdosage may result in stupor, coma, shock, respiratory depression, and rarely death.

Carisoprodol should be used with caution in patients with impaired hepatic or renal function. It may cause drowsiness, and patients affected should not drive or operate machinery.

**Breast feeding.** Carisoprodol is distributed into breast milk, achieving concentrations 2 to 4 times those in maternal plasma; the UK manufacturer and the *British National Formulary* recommend that it is best avoided in women who are breast feeding.

**Dependence.** There are reports of carisoprodol dependence, probably due to its metabolism to meprobamate.[1,2] In one case the patient experienced symptoms of meprobamate withdrawal which resolved with a dose-reducing schedule of meprobamate.

Dependence may occur more often when carisoprodol is given in high doses and for prolonged periods, especially in patients with a history of alcohol or drug dependence or in those with marked personality disorders. One group[2] found that patients with a history of substance abuse were twice as likely to use carisoprodol in larger doses to those prescribed than those with no such history.


1. Luehr JG, *et al.* Mail-order (veterinary) drug dependence. *JAMA* 1990; **263:** 657.
2. Reeves RR, *et al.* Carisoprodol (Soma): abuse potential and physician unawareness. *J Addict Dis* 1999; **18:** 51–6.


**Porphyria.** Carisoprodol has been associated with acute attacks of porphyria and is considered unsafe in porphyric patients.

### Interactions

The CNS effects of carisoprodol may be potentiated by alcohol or other CNS depressants.

### Pharmacokinetics

Carisoprodol is absorbed from the gastrointestinal tract. It is metabolised in the liver and excreted in urine as metabolites, including meprobamate. It is distributed in substantial amounts into breast milk.

◊ References.


1. Olsen H, *et al.* Carisoprodol elimination in humans. *Ther Drug Monit* 1994; **16:** 337–40.


### Uses and Administration

Carisoprodol is a centrally acting skeletal muscle relaxant whose mechanism of action is not completely understood but may be related to its sedative actions. After doses by mouth its effects begin within about 30 minutes and last for 4 to 6 hours. It is used as an adjunct in the short-term symptomatic treatment of painful muscle spasm (p.1386) associated with musculoskeletal conditions. A usual dose is 350 mg given three or four times daily by mouth. Half the usual dose or less is recommended in elderly patients. It is also given with analgesics in compound preparations.

### Preparations

***USP 27:*** Carisoprodol and Aspirin Tablets; Carisoprodol Tablets; Carisoprodol, Aspirin, and Codeine Phosphate Tablets.

**Proprietary Preparations** (details are given in Part 3)
***Arg.:*** Listaflex; ***Canad.:*** Soma; ***Denm.:*** Somadril; ***Ger.:*** Sanoma†; ***India:*** Carisoma; ***Mex.:*** Somacid; ***Norw.:*** Somadril; ***Spain:*** Mio Relax; ***Swed.:*** Somadril; ***Thai.:*** Myolax; ***UK:*** Carisoma; ***USA:*** Soma.

**Multi-ingredient:** ***Arg.:*** Algiseda; Flexicamin; Flexicamin A; Flexicamin B12; Flogiatrin; Flogiatrin B12; Ketazon Flex; Mefenix Relax; Naprontag Flex; Rumisedan Fuerte; Solocalm Plus; Solocalm-Flex; ***Braz.:*** Algi-Butazolon; Algi-Tanderil; Beserol; Diclofetamol; Dorilax; Dorpinol†; Dorserol†; Mio-Citalgan; Mioflex; Mionevrix; Paceflex; Sedilax; Somaflex†; Tandene; Tanderalgin; Tandriflan; Tandrilax; Torsilax; Trilax; ***Fin.:*** Somadril Comp; ***India:*** Carisoma Compound; Somaflam; ***Ital.:*** Flexidone†; Soma Complex; ***Mex.:*** Blocacid; Dolaren; Duoflex; Naxodol; Somalgesic; ***Spain:*** Flexagil; Relaxibys; ***Swed.:*** Somadril Comp; ***Thai.:*** Alaxan; Asialax; Cariso-Co; Carisoma Compound; Caritasone; Muscelax; Myophen; Polixan; ***USA:*** Sodol Compound; Soma Compound; Soma Compound with Codeine.

---

## Chlorphenesin Carbamate *(BANM, USAN, pINNM)*

Carbamato de clorfenesina; U-19646. 3-(4-Chlorophenoxy)propane-1,2-diol 1-carbamate.

$C_{10}H_{12}ClNO_4$ = 245.7.
*CAS — 104-29-0 (chlorphenesin); 886-74-8 (chlorphenesin carbamate).*

**Pharmacopoeias.** In *Jpn.*

### Adverse Effects and Precautions

Chlorphenesin carbamate produces drowsiness and dizziness. There may also be nausea, headache, weakness, confusion, agitation, and insomnia. Hypersensitivity reactions have been reported. There are rare reports of blood disorders.

It should be used with caution in patients with hepatic impairment. Patients affected by drowsiness should not drive or operate machinery.

### Interactions

The CNS effects of chlorphenesin carbamate may be potentiated by alcohol or other CNS depressants.

### Pharmacokinetics

Chlorphenesin carbamate is readily and completely absorbed from the gastrointestinal tract and partly metabolised in the liver. It is excreted in the urine, mainly as the glucuronide metabolite.

### Uses and Administration

Chlorphenesin carbamate is a centrally acting skeletal muscle relaxant related to mephenesin (p.1394). Its mode of action may be related to general depressant effects on the CNS. It is used as an adjunct in the symptomatic treatment of painful muscle spasm (p.1386) associated with musculoskeletal conditions. The usual initial dose is 800 mg three times daily given by mouth reduced to 400 mg four times daily or less once a response has been achieved. It has been recommended that chlorphenesin carbamate should not be given for longer than 8 weeks.

Chlorphenesin base (p.396) is used as an antifungal.

### Preparations

**Proprietary Preparations** (details are given in Part 3)
***USA:*** Maolate.

---

## Chlorzoxazone *(BAN, rINN)*

Chlorobenzoxazolinone; Clorzoxazona. 5-Chlorobenzoxazol-2(3*H*)-one.

$C_7H_4ClNO_2$ = 169.6.
*CAS — 95-25-0.*
*ATC — M03BB03.*

**Pharmacopoeias.** In *US.*

**USP 27** (Chlorzoxazone). A white or practically white, practically odourless, crystalline powder. Slightly soluble in water; sparingly soluble in alcohol, in isopropyl alcohol, and in methyl alcohol; soluble in solutions of alkali hydroxides and ammonia. Store in airtight containers.

### Adverse Effects and Treatment

The most common side-effects of chlorzoxazone are drowsiness and dizziness. There may occasionally also be gastrointestinal irritation and gastrointestinal bleeding has been reported rarely. Other effects that have occurred are headache, overstimulation, and rarely sensitivity reactions including skin rashes, petechiae, ecchymoses, urticaria and pruritus; very rarely, angioedema or anaphylactoid reactions may occur. Some patients taking chlorzoxazone have developed jaundice and liver damage suspected to be caused by the drug.

Following overdosage there may be gastrointestinal disturbances, drowsiness, dizziness, headache, malaise, and sluggishness followed by marked loss of muscle tone, hypotension, and respiratory depression. Emptying the stomach by lavage should be considered, followed by administration of activated charcoal and supportive therapy.

**Effects on the liver.** Hepatotoxicity, sometimes fatal, has been associated with chlorzoxazone treatment.[1]


1. Powers BJ, *et al.* Chlorzoxazone hepatotoxic reactions: an analysis of 21 identified or presumed cases. *Arch Intern Med* 1986; **146:** 1183–6.


**Overdosage.** Overdosage and coma occurred on 2 occasions in a patient taking chlorzoxazone; on the second occasion, the patient responded to intravenous flumazenil.[1]


1. Roberge RJ, *et al.* Two chlorzoxazone (Parafon forte) overdoses and coma in one patient: reversal with flumazenil. *Am J Emerg Med* 1998; **16:** 393–5.


**Torticollis.** There has been a report of a patient with a spasmodic torticollis-like syndrome, consisting of tonic deviation of the head to the right, clenching of the teeth, and dysarthria, which developed repeatedly within 2 hours of ingesting chlorzoxazone for low back pain.[1] Intravenous injection of benzatropine mesilate 1 mg gave rapid relief of symptoms.


1. Rosin MA. Chlorzoxazone-induced spasmodic torticollis. *JAMA* 1981; **246:** 2575.


### Precautions

Chlorzoxazone should not be given to patients with impaired liver function and should be discontinued if signs of liver toxicity appear. Patients should be advised to report to their doctor any signs or symptoms of possible liver toxicity such as fever, rash, jaundice, dark urine, anorexia, nausea, vomiting, or right upper quadrant pain. Chlorzoxazone may cause drowsiness; patients affected should not drive or operate machinery.

The urine of patients taking chlorzoxazone may be coloured orange or reddish-purple by a phenolic metabolite.

**Porphyria.** Chlorzoxazone has been associated with acute attacks of porphyria and is considered unsafe in porphyric patients.

### Interactions

The CNS effects of chlorzoxazone may be enhanced by alcohol and other CNS depressants.

**Disulfiram.** A study[1] of the efficacy of disulfiram as an inhibitor of the cytochrome P450 isoenzyme CYP2E1 (an enzyme involved in the metabolism of chlorzoxazone) found that a single 500-mg dose of disulfiram reduced plasma clearance of chlorzoxazone by 85%, resulting in a doubling of peak plasma concentrations and prolongation of chlorzoxazone's elimination half-life from a mean of 0.92 to 5.1 hours.

1. Kharasch ED, *et al.* Single-dose disulfiram inhibition of chlorzoxazone metabolism: a clinical probe for P450 2E1. *Clin Pharmacol Ther* 1993; **53:** 643–50.

**Isoniazid.** Isoniazid inhibited the clearance of chlorzoxazone by 56% when given to 10 slow acetylator subjects resulting in an increase in sedation, headache, and nausea.[1] Two days after discontinuation of isoniazid there had been a rebound increase in the clearance of chlorzoxazone by 56% over the pre-isoniazid clearance value. Similar but less pronounced effects have also been reported[2] in rapid acetylators with chlorzoxazone's pharmacokinetic parameters returning to baseline values in 2 days.

1. Zand R, *et al.* Inhibition and induction of cytochrome P4502E1-catalyzed oxidation by isoniazid in humans. *Clin Pharmacol Ther* 1993; **54:** 142–9.
2. O'Shea D, *et al.* Modulation of CYP2E1 activity by isoniazid in rapid and slow N-acetylators. *Br J Clin Pharmacol* 1997; **43:** 99–103.

### Pharmacokinetics

Chlorzoxazone is reported to be completely absorbed after oral doses and peak plasma concentrations are achieved after 1 to 2 hours. It is rapidly metabolised in the liver via the cytochrome P450 isoenzyme CYP2E1, mainly to 6-hydroxychlorzoxazone, and excreted in the urine primarily as the glucuronide metabolite. The elimination half-life of chlorzoxazone is about 1 hour.

### Uses and Administration

Chlorzoxazone is a centrally acting skeletal muscle relaxant with sedative properties. It is claimed to inhibit muscle spasm by exerting an effect primarily at the level of the spinal cord and subcortical areas of the brain. Its effects begin within an hour of an oral dose and last for 3 to 4 hours.

It is used as an adjunct in the symptomatic treatment of painful muscle spasm (p.1386) associated with musculoskeletal conditions. The usual initial dose is 500 mg three or four times daily by mouth; the dose can often be reduced subsequently to 250 mg three or four times daily, although doses of up to 750 mg three or four times daily may be given if necessary. Chlorzoxazone is also given with analgesics in compound preparations.

### Preparations

***USP 27:*** Chlorzoxazone Tablets.

**Proprietary Preparations** (details are given in Part 3)
***Chile:*** Fenarol-S; ***Denm.:*** Paraflex; ***Hong Kong:*** Solaxin; ***India:*** Parafon DSC; ***Swed.:*** Paraflex; ***Thai.:*** Chlorzox; ***USA:*** Paraflex; Parafon Forte DSC; Remular-S.

**Multi-ingredient:** ***Arg.:*** Ibupirac Flex; Paraflex AN; Paraflex Plus; Rucaten Forte; ***Austria:*** Parafon; ***Braz.:*** Paralon; ***Canad.:*** Acetazone Forte; Acetazone Forte C8; Back-Aid; Gin Pain; Parafon Forte; Parafon Forte C8†; Tylenol Aches & Strains; ***Chile:*** Beserol-S; Brevex; Desdol; Flectadol; Tonoflex; Winasorb Flex; ***Fin.:*** Paraflex comp; ***Hong Kong:*** Relaxin-P; ***India:*** Duodil; Fenaplus-MR; Flamar-MX; Myospaz; Myospaz Forte; Osteoflam-MR; Parafon; Systaflam; ***Malaysia:*** Paras; ***Mex.:*** Parafon Forte; Reumophan; ***Swed.:*** Paraflex comp; ***Switz.:*** Zafor†; ***Thai.:*** Cezox; Parafon; ***USA:*** Flexaphen.

## Cyclobenzaprine Hydrochloride *(USAN, rINNM)*

Hidrocloruro de ciclobenzaprina; MK-130 (cyclobenzaprine); Proheptatriene Hydrochloride; Ro-4-1557 (cyclobenzaprine); RP-9715 (cyclobenzaprine). 3-(5*H*-Dibenzo[*a*,*d*]cyclohepten-5-ylidene)-*NN*-dimethylpropylamine hydrochloride.

$C_{20}H_{21}N,HCl = 311.8.$

*CAS — 303-53-7 (cyclobenzaprine); 6202-23-9 (cyclobenzaprine hydrochloride).*

*ATC — M03BX08.*

**Pharmacopoeias.** In *US.*

**USP 27** (Cyclobenzaprine Hydrochloride). A white to off-white, odourless, crystalline powder. Freely soluble in water, in alcohol, and in methyl alcohol; sparingly soluble in isopropyl alcohol; slightly soluble in chloroform and in dichloromethane; insoluble in hydrocarbons.

### Adverse Effects, Treatment, and Precautions

Cyclobenzaprine is structurally related to the tricyclic antidepressants and shares their adverse effects and precautions (see Amitriptyline, p.281). Cyclobenzaprine should be used with caution in the elderly and patients with hepatic impairment; use in moderate to severe hepatic impairment is not recommended.

It may cause drowsiness; patients affected should not drive or operate machinery.

**The elderly.** Symptoms of toxicity[1] (hallucinations, insomnia, and restlessness) were seen in a 76-year-old patient taking cyclobenzaprine at therapeutic doses. The US manufacturer states that the elderly may be more likely to experience adverse effects such as hallucinations and confusion..

In another study[2] the mean elimination half-life of cyclobenzaprine in the elderly was longer than in younger subjects and clearance was reduced. It was suggested that it should be used in a reduced dose or frequency in the elderly.

1. Douglass MA, Levine DP. Hallucinations in an elderly patient taking recommended doses of cyclobenzaprine. *Arch Intern Med* 2000; **160:** 1373.
2. Winchell GA, *et al.* Cyclobenzaprine pharmacokinetics, including the effects of age, gender, and hepatic insufficiency. *J Clin Pharmacol* 2002; **42:** 61–9.

**Neuroleptic malignant syndrome.** Report of a neuroleptic malignant-like syndrome associated with cyclobenzaprine in a 36-year-old man.[1] It was not clear whether the syndrome was due to an idiosyncratic reaction or to an overdose.

1. Theoharides TC, *et al.* Neuroleptic malignant-like syndrome due to cyclobenzaprine. *J Clin Psychopharmacol* 1995; **15:** 79–81.

**Overdosage.** Treatment of cyclobenzaprine overdose is mainly symptomatic and supportive. A large retrospective study[1] found that cyclobenzaprine hydrochloride overdoses of up to 1 g rarely present with the serious cardiovascular and neurological effects seen with tricyclic antidepressant overdoses. There were no reports of seizures, life-threatening arrhythmias, or fatalities. However, 150 patients required treatment in the intensive care unit, 13 patients needed assisted ventilation, and 8 were unresponsive to stimuli. It was noted that observation may be sufficient for overdoses of under 50 mg in children.

1. Spiller HA, *et al.* Five-year multicentre retrospective review of cyclobenzaprine toxicity. *J Emerg Med* 1995; **13:** 781–5.

### Interactions

Cyclobenzaprine is structurally related to the tricyclic antidepressants and may be subject to similar interactions (see Amitriptyline, p.284). The CNS effects of cyclobenzaprine may be enhanced by alcohol or other CNS depressants.

**Antidepressants.** Report[1] of a patient with QT prolongation associated with use of cyclobenzaprine and *fluoxetine*. The patient developed torsade de pointes, progressing into ventricular fibrillation, when given *droperidol* as premedication prior to surgery. QT abnormalities resolved on stopping cyclobenzaprine.

1. Michalets EL, *et al.* Torsade de pointes resulting from the addition of droperidol to an existing cytochrome P450 drug interaction. *Ann Pharmacother* 1998; **32:** 761–5.

**Antipsychotics.** For a report of an interaction between cyclobenzaprine and *droperidol*, see under Antidepressants above.

### Pharmacokinetics

Cyclobenzaprine hydrochloride is readily and almost completely absorbed from the gastrointestinal tract, although plasma concentrations vary considerably among individuals given the same dose. About 93% is bound to plasma proteins and has a reported effective half-life of 8 to 37 hours. It is extensively metabolised, principally to glucuronide conjugates, and excreted in the urine. Cytochrome P450 isoenzymes CYP3A4, CYP1A2, and to a lesser extent CYP2D6 mediate its demethylation. Some unchanged drug appears in the bile and is excreted in the faeces.

◊ References.

1. Winchell GA, *et al.* Cyclobenzaprine pharmacokinetics, including the effects of age, gender, and hepatic insufficiency. *J Clin Pharmacol* 2002; **42:** 61–9.

### Uses and Administration

Cyclobenzaprine hydrochloride is a centrally acting skeletal muscle relaxant, related to the tricyclic antidepressants. It acts mainly at the brain stem to decrease tonic somatic motor activity influencing both alpha and gamma motor systems. Additional activity at spinal cord sites may be involved. Effects begin within 1 hour of a dose by mouth; the effects of a single dose have been reported to last as long as 12 to 24 hours.

It is used as an adjunct in the symptomatic treatment of painful muscle spasm (p.1386) associated with musculoskeletal conditions. The usual dose is 5 mg three times daily given by mouth, increased if necessary to 10 mg three times daily. Treatment for more than 2 or 3 weeks is not recommended. A starting dose of 5 mg with less frequent dosing is recommended for elderly patients. For doses in patients with hepatic impairment, see below.

**Administration in hepatic impairment.** A starting dose of 5 mg of cyclobenzaprine hydrochloride by mouth, and perhaps less frequent dosing (see above), is recommended for those with mild hepatic impairment; use in moderate to severe hepatic impairment is not recommended.

**Back pain.** A meta-analysis[1] of 14 studies concluded that cyclobenzaprine hydrochloride, in the short term, improves low back pain (p.7). Doses given to patients were titrated and ranged from 10 to 60 mg daily with a median dose of 30 mg daily. Patients improved moderately in the first 4 days of treatment, with the effects of cyclobenzaprine hydrochloride gradually declining with time although there was some evidence of continued improvement at two weeks. Further studies are needed to determine the optimal length of use in the management of acute back pain. Adverse effects were common with at least one occurring in 53% of patients.

1. Browning R, *et al.* Cyclobenzaprine and back pain: a meta-analysis. *Arch Intern Med* 2001; **161:** 1613–20.

**Fibromyalgia.** Studies of the efficacy of cyclobenzaprine in the management of fibromyalgia, a painful musculoskeletal disorder which usually responds poorly to analgesics, have produced conflicting results but a meta-analysis[1] of 5 such studies suggested that cyclobenzaprine had some modest benefit in the condition. Patients were more likely to report overall improvement and moderate reductions in individual symptoms, particularly sleep, while taking the drug.

1. Tofferi JK, *et al.* Treatment of fibromyalgia with cyclobenzaprine: a meta-analysis. *Arthritis Rheum* 2004; **51:** 9–13.

### Preparations

***USP 27:*** Cyclobenzaprine Hydrochloride Tablets.

**Proprietary Preparations** (details are given in Part 3)
***Braz.:*** Miosan; ***Canad.:*** Flexeril; Flexitec; Novo-Cycloprine; ***Chile:*** Ciclamil; Masterelax; Medarex; Nostaden; Reflexan; Relexil; Tensamon; Tensiomax; Tensodox; Tonalgen; ***Ital.:*** Flexiban; ***Port.:*** Flexiban; ***Spain:*** Yurelax; ***USA:*** Flexeril.

**Multi-ingredient:** ***Arg.:*** Dorixina Relax.

## Dantrolene Sodium *(BANM, USAN, rINNM)*

Dantroleno sódico; F-440; F-368 (dantrolene). The hemiheptahydrate of the sodium salt of 1-[5-(4-nitrophenyl)furfurylideneamino]imidazolidine-2,4-dione.

$C_{14}H_9N_4NaO_5,3\frac{1}{2}H_2O = 399.3.$

*CAS — 7261-97-4 (dantrolene); 14663-23-1 (anhydrous dantrolene sodium); 24868-20-0 (dantrolene sodium, hemiheptahydrate).*

*ATC — M03CA01.*

**Pharmacopoeias.** In *Jpn.*

### Adverse Effects

Adverse effects associated with dantrolene sodium tend to occur at the start of treatment, but are often short lived and can be controlled by adjusting the dose. The most common side-effects are drowsiness, dizziness, fatigue, weakness, and general malaise. Diarrhoea may be severe enough to require withdrawal. If diarrhoea recurs on reintroduction of dantrolene, then treatment should probably be stopped permanently. Other side-effects reported include nausea and vomiting, anorexia, constipation, abdominal cramps, gastrointestinal bleeding, tachycardia, unstable blood pressure, dyspnoea, rashes (often acneform), pruritus, chills and fever, headache, myalgia, nervousness, insomnia, confusion, visual disturbances, mental depression, dysphagia and speech disturbances, and seizures. Haematuria, crystalluria, urinary frequency and retention, and incontinence may occur. Rare but serious adverse effects include hepatotoxicity which may be fatal (see below) and pleural effusion with pericarditis.

Serious side-effects do not appear to be a problem with the short-term use of intravenous dantrolene sodium in the treatment of malignant hyperthermia.

**Effects on the liver.** Dantrolene has caused hepatotoxicity with raised liver enzyme values, jaundice, and hepatitis;[1-3] fatalities have been reported.[1,3] Not all patients experienced symptoms such as anorexia, nausea, or abdominal discomfort before the onset of disease and the severity of hepatic injury was unrelated to clinical presentation. In the first report[1] the 14 fatalities occurred with doses in excess of 200 mg daily; a later review[3] found the mean dose associated with 27 fatalities to be 582 mg daily, while reports of non-fatal liver toxicity (95 cases) were associated with a mean dose of 263 mg daily. The onset of hepatic injury was usually between 1 and 6 months after starting treatment and fatalities were not reported in the first 2 months. Only rarely did injury develop before 45 days of treatment. Females appeared to be at greater risk of serious liver injury and the severity of reaction appeared to be age-related with most fatalities occurring in patients over 30 years of age. The liver injury was usually hepatocellular and might include ascending cholangitis; there was little evidence of hypersensitivity.

1. Utili R, *et al.* Dantrolene-associated hepatic injury: incidence and character. *Gastroenterology* 1977; **72:** 610–16.
2. Wilkinson SP, *et al.* Hepatitis from dantrolene sodium. *Gut* 1979; **20:** 33–6.
3. Chan CH. Dantrolene sodium and hepatic injury. *Neurology* 1990; **40:** 1427–32.

**Effects on the lungs.** Pulmonary oedema associated with heart failure,[1] and pleural effusions with eosinophilia[2,3] have been reported rarely in patients receiving dantrolene. These reactions generally resolve on withdrawal of the drug but resolution may take several months; corticosteroid therapy may be of benefit in dantrolene-related eosinophilic pleural effusion.[3]

1. Robillart A, *et al.* Insuffisance cardiaque par surdosage en dantrolène. *Ann Fr Anesth Reanim* 1986; **5:** 617–19.
2. Mahoney JM, Bachtel MD. Pleural effusion associated with chronic dantrolene administration. *Ann Pharmacother* 1994; **28:** 587–9.
3. Felz MW, Haviland-Foley DJ. Eosinophilic pleural effusion due to dantrolene: resolution with steroid therapy. *South Med J* 2001; **94:** 502–4.

**Lymphomas.** A case of fatal lymphocytic lymphoma was associated with prolonged dantrolene therapy (600 mg daily) for progressive spastic paraplegia.[1]

1. Wan HH, Tucker JS. Dantrolene and lymphocytic lymphoma. *Postgrad Med J* 1980; **56:** 261–2.

### Precautions

It is recommended that dantrolene sodium should not be given to patients with active liver disease. Liver-function tests should be performed in all patients before and during treatment; if abnormal values are found, treatment should generally be stopped. The risk of liver injury may be increased in patients over 30 years of age, in females (especially those taking oestrogens), in those with a prior history of liver disease, and with doses above 400 mg daily (see under Effects on the Liver, above). Dantrolene sodium should be used with caution in patients with cardiac or pulmonary disorders. It should not be given to patients who use their spasticity to maintain posture or function or to patients with acute muscle spasm.

Dantrolene sodium may cause drowsiness; patients affected should not drive or operate machinery.

## Interactions

The CNS effects of dantrolene sodium may be enhanced by alcohol or other CNS depressants. Use with other potentially hepatotoxic drugs such as oestrogens may possibly increase the risk of liver damage and should be avoided.

**Calcium-channel blockers.** Severe hyperkalaemia and myocardial depression occurred with intravenous dantrolene for prophylaxis of malignant hyperthermia in a patient also taking verapamil for angina.[1] The peak serum-potassium concentration was 7.1 mmol/litre 2.5 hours after the dantrolene infusion. Nifedipine was substituted for verapamil in a subsequent operation and only a small increase in serum potassium occurred after dantrolene. Ventricular fibrillation and cardiovascular collapse associated with hyperkalaemia have been seen with this combination in *animal* studies, and the manufacturers recommend that calcium-channel blockers and intravenous dantrolene should not be used together.

1. Rubin AS, Zablocki AD. Hyperkalaemia, verapamil, and dantrolene. *Anesthesiology* 1987; **66:** 246–9.

## Pharmacokinetics

Dantrolene sodium is slowly and almost completely absorbed from the gastrointestinal tract after oral doses. It is metabolised in the liver mainly to the hydroxylated metabolite, which is nearly as potent as dantrolene sodium, and the acetamide metabolite which has weak muscle relaxant activity. It is excreted in the urine, mainly as metabolites with a small amount of unchanged dantrolene; some is excreted in the bile. Dantrolene is bound extensively to plasma proteins. The elimination half-life of oral dantrolene is about 9 hours, although half-lives of up to 12 hours have been reported after intravenous use.

## Uses and Administration

Dantrolene sodium is a muscle relaxant with a direct action on skeletal muscle. It uncouples muscular contraction from excitation, probably by interfering with the release of calcium from the sarcoplasmic reticulum.

It has an important role when given by mouth, for the symptomatic relief of chronic, severe spasticity (p.1386). It is also given, usually by intravenous injection, for the treatment of malignant hyperthermia.

For **spasticity**, the initial dose is 25 mg daily by mouth increased gradually as necessary, at 7-day intervals, over about 7 weeks to a maximum dose of 100 mg four times daily. If no response is achieved within 45 days treatment should be stopped. In the UK dantrolene is not recommended for use in children, but in the USA a suggested dose for children is 0.5 mg/kg once daily, increased gradually if necessary to 2 mg/kg three times daily; dosage four times daily may be necessary for some children but a dose of 100 mg four times daily should not be exceeded.

In the treatment of **malignant hyperthermia**, dantrolene sodium is given, with supportive measures, in an initial dose of 1 mg/kg by rapid intravenous injection, repeated, if necessary, to a total dose of 10 mg/kg. An average dose of 2.5 mg/kg is usually effective. If a relapse or recurrence occurs, dantrolene should be given again at the last effective dose. In the USA, doses of 1 to 2 mg/kg by mouth four times daily have been recommended for up to 3 days after the crisis to prevent recurrence, and similar doses have been given for 1 to 2 days before surgery in individuals thought to be at risk of developing the syndrome. Prophylactic doses may also be given intravenously; 2.5 mg/kg has been recommended, infused over about 60 minutes, starting about 75 minutes before anticipated anaesthesia, with further doses during anaesthesia and surgery if signs of malignant hyperthermia develop.

**Hyperthermia.** Dantrolene is used in the treatment of hyperthermia associated with muscle rigidity and fulminant hypermetabolism of skeletal muscle, which occurs in the neuroleptic malignant syndrome (see below and p.677) and in malignant hyperthermia (see below). There is also anecdotal evidence that dantrolene may produce beneficial effects for the treatment of similar symptoms resulting from poisoning with various agents such as carbon monoxide,[1] MAOIs,[2] and ethyltenamfetamine.[3] However, following suggestions that it might also be of use in cocaine intoxication, the manufacturers[4] warned physicians that they should not regard dantrolene as an effective treatment for all types of hyperthermia and rigidity accompanying poisoning.

Dantrolene has been tried as part of treatment for heat stroke (see under Fever and Hyperthermia, p.8) but does not appear to affect outcome.[5]

1. Ten Holter JBM, Schellens RLLAM. Dantrolene sodium for treatment of carbon monoxide poisoning. *BMJ* 1988; **296:** 1772–3.
2. Kaplan RF, *et al.* Phenelzine overdose treatment with dantrolene sodium. *JAMA* 1986; **255:** 642–4.
3. Tehan B. Ecstasy and dantrolene. *BMJ* 1993; **306:** 146.
4. Fox AW. More on rhabdomyolysis associated with cocaine intoxication. *N Engl J Med* 1989; **321:** 1271.
5. Bouchama A, Knochel JP. Heat stroke. *N Engl J Med* 2002; **346:** 1978–88.

MALIGNANT HYPERTHERMIA. Malignant hyperthermia (malignant hyperpyrexia) is a rare but potentially fatal syndrome associated with general anaesthesia, in which a sudden increase in the concentration of calcium in muscle cytoplasm initiates a series of metabolic disturbances. The disorder appears to be genetically determined and is more common in males. In susceptible individuals a reaction may be induced by inhalation anaesthetics (mainly halogenated hydrocarbons), suxamethonium, prolonged anaesthesia, pre-operative exercise, muscle trauma, fever, or anxiety. However, many reactions occur in individuals who have had uneventful general anaesthesia previously. Early signs and symptoms of the syndrome include tachycardia, unstable blood pressure, hypercapnia, rising temperature, and hyperventilation followed by metabolic acidosis and hyperkalaemia. Muscle rigidity develops in many patients and later there may be evidence of muscle damage including raised serum concentrations of creatine phosphokinase and other enzymes, myoglobinaemia, and myoglobinuria. Hyperthermia develops relatively late. Other late complications may include renal failure, intravascular coagulopathy, and pulmonary oedema.

Treatment should be started as soon as possible after symptoms appear with dantrolene being given by rapid intravenous injection until symptoms disappear.[1-3] Supportive treatment must also be given including immediate withdrawal of anaesthesia, administration of oxygen, correction of acidosis with sodium bicarbonate, control of hyperkalaemia with insulin, and cooling procedures (see p.8).

The incidence of reactions in susceptible individuals can be reduced by avoiding triggering agents. Dantrolene has also been given prophylactically, but a high incidence of adverse effects has been reported,[4] and such use is not generally recommended.[3] Susceptibility to malignant hyperthermia can be detected by histological examination of muscle fibres obtained by biopsy and study of their response to caffeine and/or halothane *in vitro*.

Dantrolene has been suggested[5] for use as a secondary drug in the treatment of a related and potentially fatal syndrome that has developed in some children following induction of anaesthesia with halothane and suxamethonium (see also Children, under Precautions of Suxamethonium, p.1407).

1. Britt BA. Dantrolene. *Can Anaesth Soc J* 1984; **31:** 61–75.
2. Ward A, *et al.* Dantrolene: a review of its pharmacodynamic and pharmacokinetic properties and therapeutic use in malignant hyperthermia, the neuroleptic malignant syndrome and an update of its use in muscle spasticity. *Drugs* 1986; **32:** 130–68.
3. Krause T, *et al.* Dantrolene—a review of its pharmacology, therapeutic use and new developments. *Anaesthesia* 2004; **59:** 364–73.
4. Wedel DJ, *et al.* Clinical effects of intravenously administered dantrolene. *Mayo Clin Proc* 1995; **70:** 241–6.
5. Rosenberg H, Gronert GA. Intractable cardiac arrest in children given succinylcholine. *Anesthesiology* 1992; **77:** 1054.

**Neuroleptic malignant syndrome.** Dantrolene has been used, usually alone or with bromocriptine, in the treatment of neuroleptic malignant syndrome (p.677), although some workers have not found it to be of use,[1] and evidence from controlled trials in lacking.[2] Doses reported for dantrolene have varied greatly.[3,4] For those patients unable to swallow and when rapid control of symptoms is required, doses of 1 mg/kg or more have been given initially by intravenous injection. Up to 600 mg has been given daily by mouth in divided doses.

1. Rosebush PI, *et al.* The treatment of neuroleptic malignant syndrome: are dantrolene and bromocriptine useful adjuncts to supportive care? *Br J Psychiatry* 1991; **159:** 709–12.
2. Krause T, *et al.* Dantrolene—a review of its pharmacology, therapeutic use and new developments. *Anaesthesia* 2004; **59:** 364–73.
3. Ward A, *et al.* Dantrolene: a review of its pharmacodynamic and pharmacokinetic properties and therapeutic use in malignant hyperthermia, the neuroleptic malignant syndrome and an update of its use in muscle spasticity. *Drugs* 1986; **32:** 130–68.
4. Harpe C, Stoudemire A. Aetiology and treatment of neuroleptic malignant syndrome. *Med Toxicol* 1987; **2:** 166–76.

**Tetanus.** Dantrolene has effectively controlled muscle spasms in the treatment of tetanus (see p.1398). It has also been used as an adjunct[1] to neuromuscular blockade; there are conflicting reports[2,3] of its value in avoiding mechanical ventilation.

1. Tidyman M, *et al.* Adjunctive use of dantrolene in severe tetanus. *Anesth Analg* 1985; **64:** 538–40.
2. Checketts MR, White RJ. Avoidance of intermittent positive pressure ventilation in tetanus with dantrolene therapy. *Anaesthesia* 1993; **48:** 969–71.
3. Possamai C, *et al.* Dantrolene infusion in severe tetanus. *Anaesthesia* 1997; **52:** 610.

## Preparations

**Proprietary Preparations** (details are given in Part 3)
***Austral.:*** Dantrium; ***Austria:*** Dantamacrin; ***Belg.:*** Dantrium; ***Braz.:*** Dantrolen; ***Canad.:*** Dantrium; ***Denm.:*** Dantrium; ***Fr.:*** Dantrium; ***Ger.:*** Dantamacrin; ***Gr.:*** Dantrolen; ***Hong Kong:*** Dantrium; ***Irl.:*** Dantrium; ***Israel:*** Dantrium; ***Ital.:*** Dantrium; ***Neth.:*** Dantrium; ***NZ:*** Dantrium; ***Port.:*** Dantrium; ***S.Afr.:*** Dantrium; ***Switz.:*** Dantamacrin; ***UK:*** Dantrium; ***USA:*** Dantrium.

## Eperisone Hydrochloride *(rINNM)*

Hidrocloruro de eperisona. 4′-Ethyl-2-methyl-3-piperidinopropiophenone hydrochloride.

$C_{17}H_{25}NO,HCl = 295.8.$
*CAS — 64840-90-0 (eperisone).*

### Profile

Eperisone is a centrally acting skeletal muscle relaxant that has been used in the symptomatic treatment of muscle spasm (p.1386) and spasticity (p.1386). It may also have a vasodilator action. Eperisone hydrochloride has been given by mouth in usual doses of 50 mg three times daily after food.

**Effects on the skin.** A non-pigmenting fixed drug eruption developed in a 42-year-old woman after taking oral diclofenac sodium and eperisone hydrochloride.[1] There was no residual hyperpigmentation and the rash and accompanying itching and burning sensation resolved within 7 days after stopping both drugs. On rechallenge with eperisone, an erythematous plaque developed at the same site within a couple of hours. The lesion disappeared within 5 days with no sequelae.

1. Choonhakarn C. Non-pigmenting fixed drug eruption: a new case due to eperisone hydrochloride. *Br J Dermatol* 2001; **144:** 1288–9.

### Preparations

**Proprietary Preparations** (details are given in Part 3)
***Jpn:*** Myonal; ***Malaysia:*** Myonal; ***Singapore:*** Myonal; ***Thai.:*** Myonal.

## Idrocilamide *(rINN)*

Idrocilamida; LCB-29. *N*-(2-Hydroxyethyl)cinnamamide.

$C_{11}H_{13}NO_2 = 191.2.$
*CAS — 6961-46-2.*

### Adverse Effects

When given by mouth idrocilamide was reported to produce abdominal pain, nausea, and drowsiness. Excitement, euphoria and hallucinations, and depression may occur.

### Uses and Administration

Idrocilamide is a centrally acting muscle relaxant. It is reported to have local muscle relaxant and anti-inflammatory effects and is now mainly used topically.

### Preparations

**Proprietary Preparations** (details are given in Part 3)
***Belg.:*** Srilane; ***Fr.:*** Srilane; ***Hong Kong:*** Srilane; ***Switz.:*** Talval.

## Mephenesin *(BAN, rINN)*

Cresoxydiol; Glykresin; Mefenesina. 3-(*o*-Tolyloxy)propane-1,2-diol.

$C_{10}H_{14}O_3 = 182.2.$
*CAS — 59-47-2.*
*ATC — M03BX06.*

NOTE. The name tolynol has been applied to both mephenesin and *p*,α-dimethylbenzyl alcohol (p.1680).

**Pharmacopoeias.** In *It.*

### Profile

Mephenesin is a centrally acting skeletal muscle relaxant used for the symptomatic treatment of painful muscle spasm (p.1386) associated with musculoskeletal conditions. Its clinical usefulness is considered to be limited by its brief duration of action. It is given by mouth in doses of 1.5 to 3 g daily in divided doses. It is also applied topically, usually with rubefacients.

**Porphyria.** Mephenesin is considered to be unsafe in patients with porphyria because it has been shown to be porphyrinogenic in *in-vitro* systems.

### Preparations

**Proprietary Preparations** (details are given in Part 3)
***Fr.:*** Decontractyl; ***Ger.:*** DoloVisano M.

**Multi-ingredient:** ***Belg.:*** Algipan; Decontractyl†; ***Fr.:*** Algipan; Decontractyl; Traumalgyl; ***India:*** Acks; Flamar; Medicreme; Relaxyl; ***Ital.:*** Relaxar; ***S.Afr.:*** Spasmend.

## Mephenoxalone (rINN)

AHR-233; Methoxadone; OM-518. 5-(2-Methoxyphenoxymethyl)oxazolidin-2-one.

$C_{11}H_{13}NO_4$ = 223.2.

*CAS — 70-07-5.*

*ATC — N05BX01.*

### Profile

Mephenoxalone has actions similar to those of meprobamate (p.706). It has been given by mouth in a dose of 400 mg three times daily as a muscle relaxant in the treatment of muscle spasm (p.1386). It has also been given for the treatment of anxiety.

### Preparations

**Proprietary Preparations** (details are given in Part 3)
***Neth.:*** Dorsiflex.

## Metaxalone (BAN, USAN, rINN)

AHR-438; Metaxalona. 5-(3,5-Xylyloxymethyl)oxazolidin-2-one.

$C_{12}H_{15}NO_3$ = 221.3.

*CAS — 1665-48-1.*

### Adverse Effects, Treatment, and Precautions

As for Chlorzoxazone, p.1392.

Metaxalone may cause drowsiness; patients affected should not drive or operate machinery.

Patients taking metaxalone excrete in the urine a metabolite which gives a false positive reaction to copper sulfate-based tests for glycosuria.

### Interactions

The CNS effects of metaxalone may be enhanced by alcohol and other CNS depressants.

### Pharmacokinetics

Metaxalone is absorbed from the gastrointestinal tract, metabolised in the liver, and excreted in urine as metabolites. The plasma elimination half-life is about 2 to 3 hours.

### Uses and Administration

Metaxalone is a centrally acting skeletal muscle relaxant. Its mode of action may be related to its sedative properties.

It is used as an adjunct in the symptomatic treatment of painful muscle spasm (p.1386) associated with musculoskeletal conditions. The usual dose is 800 mg three or four times daily by mouth.

### Preparations

**Proprietary Preparations** (details are given in Part 3)
***USA:*** Skelaxin.

## Methocarbamol (BAN, rINN)

Guaiphenesin Carbamate; Metocarbamol. 2-Hydroxy-3-(2-methoxyphenoxy)propyl carbamate.

$C_{11}H_{15}NO_5$ = 241.2.

*CAS — 532-03-6.*

*ATC — M03BA03.*

**Pharmacopoeias.** In *US.*

**USP 27** (Methocarbamol). A white powder, odourless or having a slight characteristic odour. M.p. about 94° or, if previously ground to a fine powder, about 90°. Soluble 1 in 40 of water at 20°; sparingly soluble in chloroform; soluble in alcohol only with heating; insoluble in *n*-hexane and in benzene. Store in airtight containers.

### Adverse Effects

Side-effects reported with methocarbamol include nausea, vomiting, anorexia, lightheadedness, dizziness, lassitude, drowsiness, restlessness, anxiety, confusion, tremor, vertigo, blurred vision, fever, headache, convulsions, and hypersensitivity reactions including rashes, pruritus, urticaria, angioedema, and conjunctivitis with nasal congestion.

After injection patients may experience flushing and a metallic taste; incoordination, diplopia, nystagmus, vertigo, syncope, hypotension, bradycardia, and anaphylaxis have been reported. There may be sloughing and thrombophlebitis at the site of injection.

### Precautions

Methocarbamol is contra-indicated in coma or pre-coma states, brain damage, myasthenia gravis, or in patients with a history of epilepsy. Caution is advisable in renal or hepatic impairment. Methocarbamol may cause drowsiness; patients affected should not drive or operate machinery.

Preparations for injection may contain, as a solvent, a macrogol which could increase existing acidosis and urea retention in patients with renal impairment; such preparations should not be used in patients with known or suspected renal disease.

**Abnormal coloration.** Methocarbamol has been reported to cause brown to black or green discoloration of the urine on standing.[1]

1. Baran RB, Rowles B. Factors affecting coloration of urine and feces. *J Am Pharm Assoc* 1973; **NS13:** 139–42.

### Interactions

The CNS effects of methocarbamol may be potentiated by alcohol or other CNS depressants. Methocarbamol has also been reported to potentiate the effect of anorectics and antimuscarinics, and to inhibit the effect of pyridostigmine.

### Pharmacokinetics

Methocarbamol is rapidly and almost completely absorbed from the gastrointestinal tract after oral doses. Its plasma half-life is reported to be about 1 to 2 hours. It is metabolised by dealkylation and hydroxylation and is excreted in urine primarily as the glucuronide and sulfate conjugates of its metabolites. A small amount is excreted in faeces.

### Uses and Administration

Methocarbamol is a centrally acting skeletal muscle relaxant whose action may be due to general depressant effects on the CNS.

Methocarbamol is used as an adjunct in the short-term symptomatic treatment of painful muscle spasm (p.1386) associated with musculoskeletal conditions. It is sometimes given with analgesics in compound preparations for the treatment of musculoskeletal pain.

The usual initial dose by mouth for muscle spasm is 1.5 g four times daily, reduced to a maintenance dose of about 4 g daily after 2 to 3 days. A dose of 750 mg three times daily may be sufficient for a therapeutic effect. Half the maximum daily dose or less may be sufficient for elderly patients.

Methocarbamol has also been given intravenously at a rate of not more than 300 mg/minute, by slow injection or by infusion in sodium chloride 0.9% or glucose 5% injection. The parenteral route should not be used for more than 3 consecutive days and the dose should not exceed 3 g daily. The patient should remain lying down during, and for 10 to 15 minutes after, intravenous doses. The US manufacturers state that the injection is hypertonic and extravasation should be avoided. However, it may also be given by intramuscular injection in a dose of up to 500 mg into each gluteal region at intervals of 8 hours.

### Preparations

***USP 27:*** Methocarbamol Injection; Methocarbamol Tablets.

**Proprietary Preparations** (details are given in Part 3)
***Canad.:*** Robaxin; ***Fin.:*** Robaxin†; ***Fr.:*** Lumirelax; ***Ger.:*** Ortoton; ***Hong Kong:*** Robaxin; ***India:*** Robinax; ***Mex.:*** Labycarbol†; Remisol; Rexivin; Robaxin†; ***S.Afr.:*** Robaxin; ***Spain:*** Robaxin; ***Swed.:*** Robaxin†; ***Thai.:*** Laxan; Mebaxin†; Musxan; Myocin; Myomethol; Robaxin; ***UK:*** Robaxin; ***USA:*** Robaxin.

**Multi-ingredient:** ***Canad.:*** Aspirin Backache; Dodds Back Ease; Methoxacet; Methoxacet-C; Methoxisal; Methoxisal-C; Muscle & Back Pain Relief; Muscle & Back Pain Relief-8; Muscle Relaxant and Analgesic; Obusforme; Relaxophen; Robaxacet; Robaxacet-8; Robaxisal; Robaxisal-C; Spasmhalt; Spasmhalt-ASA; ***Ger.:*** Ortoton Plus; ***India:*** Ibugesic-M; Robiflam; Robinaxol; ***Irl.:*** Robaxisal†; ***Mex.:*** Artridol; Carbager-Plus; Carbamox; Malival Compuesto; Morlan FB 25; Remisol-PLS; Robaxifen; Robaxisal; Vengesic; ***S.Afr.:*** Robaxisal; ***Spain:*** Robaxisal; Robaxisal Compuesto; ***Swed.:*** Robaxisal Forte†; ***Thai.:*** Sancago†; ***USA:*** Robaxisal†.

## Pridinol Mesilate (rINNM)

C-238 (pridinol); Mesilato de pridinol; Pridinol Mesylate. 1,1-Diphenyl-3-piperidinopropan-1-ol methanesulphonate.

$C_{20}H_{25}NO,CH_3SO_3H$ = 391.5.

*CAS — 511-45-5 (pridinol); 968-58-1 (pridinol hydrochloride); 6856-31-1 (pridinol mesilate).*

*ATC — M03BX03.*

### Profile

Pridinol mesilate is a centrally acting muscle relaxant used in the symptomatic treatment of muscle spasm (p.1386). The usual initial dose by mouth is 2 to 8 mg three times daily, reduced to 4 to 8 mg daily for maintenance treatment. It is also given by intramuscular injection or rectally, and has been applied in compound topical preparations.

Pridinol has been used as the hydrochloride for its antimuscarinic properties in the management of parkinsonism (p.1196).

### Preparations

**Proprietary Preparations** (details are given in Part 3)
***Ger.:*** Myoson; Parks; ***Hong Kong:*** Konlax; ***Ital.:*** Lyseen; ***Thai.:*** Konlax†.

**Multi-ingredient:** ***Arg.:*** Blokium Flex; Diclogesic Relax; Diclomar Flex; Dioxaflex Plus; Metaflex Plus NF; Oxa Sport; Oxadisten; Rodinac Flex; Vesalion Flex; Voltaren Flex; Xedenol Flex; ***Ital.:*** Algolisina.

## Thiocolchicoside (rINN)

Tiocolchicósido. 3,10-Di(demethoxy)-3-glucopyranosyloxy-10-methylthiocolchicine.

$C_{27}H_{33}NO_{10}S$ = 563.6.

*CAS — 602-41-5.*

*ATC — M03BX05.*

**Pharmacopoeias.** In *Fr.*

### Profile

Thiocolchicoside is a muscle relaxant which has been claimed to possess GABA-mimetic and glycinergic actions. It is used in the symptomatic treatment of painful muscle spasm (p.1386). The usual initial dose is 16 mg daily by mouth. It has also been given intramuscularly, in doses up to 8 mg daily, or applied as cream or ointment. Photosensitivity reactions may occur.

### Preparations

**Proprietary Preparations** (details are given in Part 3)
***Braz.:*** Coltrax; ***Fr.:*** Coltramyl; Miorel; Myoplege; ***Gr.:*** Musco-ril; Thiacomin; ***Ital.:*** Decontril; Miotens; Muscoflex; Muscoril; Sciomir; Strialisin; Tiorilene; Tioside; ***Port.:*** Coltramyl; Relmus.

**Multi-ingredient:** ***Ital.:*** Tioscina†; ***Mex.:*** Neuroflax; ***Port.:*** Adalgur N; Relmus Compositum; ***Spain:*** Adalgur; Liviane Compuesto†.

## Tizanidine Hydrochloride (BANM, USAN, rINNM)

AN-021; DS-103-282; DS-103-282-ch; Hidrocloruro de tizanidina. 5-Chloro-*N*-(2-imidazolin-2-yl)-2,1,3-benzothiadiazol-4-ylamine hydrochloride.

$C_9H_8ClN_5S,HCl$ = 290.2.

*CAS — 51322-75-9 (tizanidine); 64461-82-1 (tizanidine hydrochloride).*

*ATC — M03BX02.*

### Adverse Effects and Precautions

Tizanidine hydrochloride may cause drowsiness; patients affected should not drive or operate machinery. Other adverse effects include dry mouth, fatigue, dizziness or vertigo, muscle pain and weakness, insomnia, anxiety, headache, bradycardia, nausea, and gastrointestinal disturbances. Hallucinations have occurred on rare occasions. Many adverse effects have been found to be dose related and slow titration of doses appears to reduce the frequency of occurrence. Hypotension may occur.

Increases in liver enzymes and rarely acute hepatitis have been associated with tizanidine and it is contra-indicated in patients with severe hepatic dysfunction. In the UK it is recommended that liver function should be monitored monthly in all patients for the first 4 months and in those who develop symptoms suggestive of hepatic dysfunction; similarly, in the USA baseline assessment and monitoring at 1, 3, and 6 months is advised. Treatment should be stopped if liver enzymes are persistently raised.

Caution is required in the elderly and in patients with renal insufficiency.

### Interactions

The CNS effects of tizanidine may be enhanced by alcohol or other CNS depressants. There may be an additive hypotensive effect when tizanidine is used in patients receiving antihypertensive therapy; bradycardia may also be enhanced if given with beta blockers or digoxin. Caution should be exercised when tizanidine is given with drugs known to increase the QT interval. The clearance of tizanidine has been reported to be lower in women receiving hormonal contraceptives.

**Antiepileptics.** For reference to an interaction between tizanidine and phenytoin, see p.374.

### Pharmacokinetics

Tizanidine is absorbed from the gastrointestinal tract and peak plasma concentrations occur about 1 to 2 hours after doses by mouth. Tizanidine undergoes extensive first-pass metabolism in the liver and is excreted mainly in the urine as inactive metabolites. Elimination half-lives of 2 to 4 hours have been reported.

### Uses and Administration

Tizanidine hydrochloride is a centrally acting skeletal muscle relaxant. It is an $\alpha_2$-adrenergic agonist structurally related to clonidine (p.885) and acts mainly at spinal and supraspinal levels to inhibit excitatory interneurones. It is used for the symptomatic relief of spasticity associated with multiple sclerosis or with spinal cord injury or disease. It is also used in the symptomatic treatment of painful muscle spasm (p.1386) associated with musculoskeletal conditions.

Tizanidine hydrochloride is usually given in divided doses by mouth; doses are expressed in terms of the base. Tizanidine hydrochloride 1.14 mg is equivalent to 1 mg tizanidine base. The usual initial daily dose in the UK in the management of spasticity is the equivalent of 2 mg of the base given as a single dose. The dose may be increased thereafter according to response in steps of 2 mg at intervals of at least 3 to 4 days, usually up to 24 mg daily given in 3 or 4 divided doses. A similar schedule, with an initial daily dose of 4 mg, increased as required in steps of 2 to 4 mg, is used in the USA. The maximum recommended dose is 36 mg daily. Maintenance doses have been given in some countries in the form of modified-release preparations. For dosage in renal impairment, see below.

In the treatment of painful muscle spasm tizanidine hydrochloride is given in doses equivalent to 2 to 4 mg of the base three times daily.

**Administration in renal impairment.** In the UK, the manufacturer recommends that in patients with renal insufficiency, treatment with tizanidine hydrochloride should be started with the equivalent of 2 mg of the base once daily; thereafter they advise a slow increase in the once-daily dose before increasing the frequency of administration. Similar recommendations are made by the US manufacturer.

**Headache.** Results from an open-label study[1] and a later controlled study[2] suggested that tizanidine might be of value in the prophylaxis of chronic daily headache. However, an earlier controlled study[3] failed to demonstrate any significant advantage over placebo in the treatment of chronic tension-type headache. In another study[4] tizanidine was also effective when given with a long-acting NSAID as part of a detoxification regimen for patients with chronic daily headaches induced by analgesic overuse.

1. Saper JR, *et al.* An open-label dose-titration study of the efficacy and tolerability of tizanidine hydrochloride tablets in the prophylaxis of chronic daily headache. *Headache* 2001; **41:** 357–68.
2. Saper JR, *et al.* Chronic daily headache prophylaxis with tizanidine: a double-blind, placebo-controlled, multicenter outcome study. *Headache* 2002; **42:** 470–82.
3. Murros K, *et al.* Modified-release formulation of tizanidine in chronic tension-type headache. *Headache* 2000; **40:** 633–7.
4. Smith TR. Low-dose tizanidine with nonsteroidal anti-inflammatory drugs for detoxification from analgesic rebound headache. *Headache* 2002; **42:** 175–7.

**Premedication.** The value of tizanidine as a premedicant is being studied.[1] A dose of tizanidine 12 mg appears to have sedative and sympatholytic effects comparable with clonidine 150 micrograms.

1. Meittinen TJ, *et al.* The sedative and sympatholytic effects of oral tizanidine in healthy volunteers. *Anesth Analg* 1996; **82:** 817–20.

**Spasticity.** The efficacy of tizanidine for spasticity (p.1386) associated with cerebral and spinal disorders[1-3] has been demonstrated in several placebo-controlled studies and in comparative studies it has produced similar improvements in muscle tone to baclofen or diazepam. Carefully titrated doses of tizanidine and baclofen used together may have additive beneficial effects[1,2] but use with benzodiazepines is not recommended because of potential interactions.[1] It was considered that tizanidine might have the advantage of being better tolerated than baclofen.

1. Wagstaff AJ, Bryson HM. Tizanidine: a review of its pharmacology, clinical efficacy and tolerability in the management of spasticity associated with cerebral and spinal disorders. *Drugs* 1997; **53:** 435–52.
2. Anonymous. Tizanidine for spasticity. *Med Lett Drugs Ther* 1997; **39:** 62–3.
3. Gelber DA, *et al.* Open-label dose-titration safety and efficacy study of tizanidine hydrochloride in the treatment of spasticity associated with chronic stroke. *Stroke* 2001; **32:** 1841–6.

## Preparations

**Proprietary Preparations** (details are given in Part 3)
***Arg.:*** Sirdalud; ***Austria:*** Sirdalud; ***Belg.:*** Sirdalud; ***Braz.:*** Sirdalud; ***Canad.:*** Zanaflex; ***Chile:*** Sirdalud; ***Denm.:*** Sirdalud; ***Fin.:*** Sirdalud; ***Ger.:*** Sirdalud; ***Gr.:*** Sirdalud; ***India:*** Sirdalud; ***Irl.:*** Zanaflex; ***Ital.:*** Sirdalud; ***Mex.:*** Sirdalud; ***Neth.:*** Sirdalud; ***Port.:*** Sirdalud; ***Spain:*** Sirdalud; ***Switz.:*** Sirdalud; ***Thai.:*** Sirdalud; ***UK:*** Zanaflex; ***USA:*** Zanaflex.

## Tolperisone Hydrochloride *(BANM, rINNM)*

Hidrocloruro de tolperisona; N-553. 2,4′-Dimethyl-3-piperidinopropiophenone hydrochloride.

$C_{16}H_{23}NO,HCl = 281.8.$

*CAS — 728-88-1 (tolperisone); 3644-61-9 (tolperisone hydrochloride).*

*ATC — M03BX04.*

**Pharmacopoeias.** In *Jpn.*

### Profile

Tolperisone hydrochloride is a centrally acting muscle relaxant that has been used for the symptomatic treatment of spasticity (p.1386) and muscle spasm (p.1386), in usual doses of 50 to 150 mg three times daily by mouth. It has also been given by injection.

## Preparations

**Proprietary Preparations** (details are given in Part 3)
***Arg.:*** Miodom; ***Ger.:*** Mydocalm; ***Hong Kong:*** Mydocalm; ***Switz.:*** Mydocalm; ***Thai.:*** Biocalm; Musocalm; Mydocalm; Mydosone; Myolax†; Myoxan; Risocalm; Shiwalax; Soneriper; Spamus; Tanderon.

**Multi-ingredient:** ***Mex.:*** Mydocalm-A.

# Neuromuscular Blockers

Anaesthesia, p.1397
Intensive care, p.1398
Tetanus, p.1398

Neuromuscular blockers (myoneuronal blockers) affect transmission at the neuromuscular junction and are used as adjuncts to general anaesthesia, particularly to enable adequate muscle relaxation to be achieved with light anaesthesia. There are 2 main types of neuromuscular blockers: competitive (non-depolarising neuromuscular blockers) and depolarising neuromuscular blockers (see Table 1, below).

**Table 1.** Classification of neuromuscular blockers.

| Competitive | | Depolarising |
|---|---|---|
| *Aminosteroidal* | *Benzylisoquinolinium* | Suxamethonium |
| Pancuronium | Alcuronium | |
| Pipecuronium | Atracurium | |
| Rapacuronium | Cisatracurium | |
| Rocuronium | Doxacurium | |
| Vecuronium | Gallamine | |
| | Metocurine | |
| | Mivacurium | |
| | Tubocurarine | |

- **Competitive neuromuscular blockers** act by competing with acetylcholine for receptors on the motor end-plate. Their action can be opposed by increasing the local concentration of acetylcholine, for example by giving an anticholinesterase such as neostigmine (p.1492). Tubocurarine (p.1409) was formerly the standard reference drug of this type but its use has declined, therefore details of the actions and uses of competitive neuromuscular blockers are discussed under Atracurium, p.1399.
- **Depolarising neuromuscular blockers** act by depolarising the motor end-plate to prevent the normal response to acetylcholine; their action is not reversed by anticholinesterases. Suxamethonium (p.1406) is the standard reference drug of this type.

Other drugs that have muscle relaxant properties and which are used in the management of musculoskeletal and neuromuscular disorders are discussed in the chapter on Muscle Relaxants, p.1386.

◊ General references.

1. Agoston S, *et al.* Clinical pharmacokinetics of neuromuscular blocking drugs. *Clin Pharmacokinet* 1992; **22:** 94–115.
2. Book WJ, *et al.* Adverse effects of depolarising neuromuscular blocking agents: incidence, prevention and management. *Drug Safety* 1994; **10:** 331–49.
3. Abel M, *et al.* Adverse effects of nondepolarising neuromuscular blocking agents: incidence, prevention and management. *Drug Safety* 1994; **10:** 420–38.
4. Hunter JM. New neuromuscular blocking drugs. *N Engl J Med* 1995; **332:** 1691–9.
5. Naguib M, Magboul MMA. Adverse effects of neuromuscular blockers and their antagonists. *Drug Safety* 1998; **18:** 99–116.
6. Guay J, *et al.* Clinical pharmacokinetics of neuromuscular relaxants in pregnancy. *Clin Pharmacokinet* 1998; **34:** 483–96.
7. Atherton DPL, Hunter JM. Clinical pharmacokinetics of the newer neuromuscular blocking drugs. *Clin Pharmacokinet* 1999; **36:** 169–89.
8. Sparr HJ, *et al.* Newer neuromuscular blocking agents: how do they compare with established agents? *Drugs* 2001; **61:** 919–42.
9. McManus MC. Neuromuscular blockers in surgery and intensive care, part 2. *Am J Health-Syst Pharm* 2001; **58:** 2381–95.
10. Brandom BW, Fine GF. Neuromuscular blocking drugs in pediatric anesthesia. *Anesthesiol Clin North America* 2002; **20:** 45–58.

## Anaesthesia

Neuromuscular blockers are used in general anaesthesia for their muscle relaxant effects to facilitate intubation at induction and to provide continued relaxation during maintenance. Their use is determined partly by their onset and duration of action (see Table 2), but both onset and duration are dose-dependent and can therefore vary. Generally, *competitive neuromuscular blockers*, due to their slower onset and longer duration of action, are used in major operations, while the *depolarising neuromuscular blockers* (usually suxamethonium), with a much faster onset and shorter duration, are used for minor operations or manipulations and particularly for intubation. Following suxamethonium to aid intubation, a longer-acting competitive drug may then be given to maintain muscle relaxation throughout the operation. Competitive neuromuscular blockers with a short to intermediate duration of action, such as atracurium and vecuronium, are more widely used than those with a longer duration of action such as pancuronium.

Suxamethonium has been widely used following the induction of anaesthesia to aid **intubation**; however, because of the adverse effects such as myalgia associated with suxamethonium (see also below), alternative neuromuscular blockers have been investigated for intubation and some now question the use of suxamethonium for *elective* procedures,[1] especially in day-case patients.[2] Some competitive blockers such as vecuronium have a relatively rapid onset of action and have been used for intubation during routine, planned surgery. However, they act too slowly to enable rapid intubation in an *emergency*, when suxamethonium remains the drug of choice. Although rocuronium, a competitive blocker, is only slightly slower in onset, and may be suitable in emergencies if suxamethonium is contra-indicated,[3-5] it has a much longer duration of action, and needs to be given with an opioid such as alfentanil,[6] or with propofol,[5] to obtain equivalent intubating conditions.

In attempting to create more favourable conditions for rapid intubation with competitive neuromuscular blockers and thus provide an alternative to suxamethonium, anaesthetists have tried using large doses[4] or combinations[7] of competitive blockers. Other methods tried include the administration of competitive neuromuscular blockers in divided doses in an attempt to shorten the onset to paralysis.[4,8] This so-called *priming principle* involves administration of a small initial dose, termed the priming dose, followed by a large paralysing dose. Priming may be with 2 doses of the same competitive relaxant or a combination of 2 different relaxants which may then exhibit synergism. However, some consider[8] that priming techniques are associated with unacceptable adverse effects such as muscle weakness and aspiration, and that they are not safe especially in the elderly.[4] In another technique, a single large dose of a neuromuscular blocker is administered followed by the induction anaesthetic as soon as the patient complains of weakness.[4] This is called the *timing principle* and although it has been successfully used with some neuromuscular blockers, problems such as perceived muscle weakness or shortness of breath may occur if the anaesthetic is not injected at the right moment.

The use of anaesthetic regimens that avoid or reduce the need for a neuromuscular blocker during intubation has also been investigated. The anaesthetic propofol with a short-acting opioid such as alfentanil has often been tried. In addition to its use alone, such a regimen has been combined successfully with low doses of suxamethonium[9] or rocuronium,[10] or standard doses of vecuronium,[11] to produce suitable conditions for intubation.

Procedures such as intubation can cause **complications**: an undesirable pressor response may occur, resulting in increased heart rate and arterial blood pressure. There may also be an increase in intracranial pressure and intra-ocular pressure. Furthermore, the use of suxamethonium to facilitate intubation is itself associated with a transient increase in intra-ocular pressure. Small doses of a competitive neuromuscular blocker have been given before suxamethonium[12] to prevent this rise in intra-ocular pressure, although some consider such a measure ineffective.[13] Opioids such as alfentanil and fentanyl appear to be effective in attenuating both the pressor response[14-16] and the rise in intra-ocular pressure[17,18] associated with intubation, but the use of lidocaine has produced conflicting results.[19-23] Many anaesthetics, with the exception of ketamine, reduce intra-ocular pressure to some extent and prior administration of thiopental may help to counteract the effect of suxamethonium.[24]

Other drugs that have been used or tried in the prevention of the haemodynamic response to intubation include magnesium sulfate[25] and propofol.[26,27]

Competitive neuromuscular blockers are usually used to provide muscle relaxation during **maintenance** anaesthesia. Patients given a neuromuscular blocker generally require less anaesthetic permitting a state of 'lighter anaesthesia' and hence reducing the adverse effects of the anaesthetic. At the end of the procedure any residual block should be reversed with an anticholinesterase and the patient should be monitored until spontaneous respiration has resumed. For further details see Anaesthesia under Uses of General Anaesthetics, p.1296.

**Table 2.** Relative speed of onset and duration of action of neuromuscular blockers.

| Neuromuscular blocker | Onset* | Duration† |
|---|---|---|
| Alcuronium | Intermediate | Intermediate |
| Atracurium | Intermediate | Short/Intermediate |
| Cisatracurium | Intermediate | Short/Intermediate |
| Doxacurium | Slow | Long |
| Gallamine | Rapid | Intermediate |
| Mivacurium | Intermediate | Short |
| Pancuronium | Rapid | Long |
| Pipecuronium | Intermediate | Intermediate/Long |
| Rocuronium | Rapid | Intermediate |
| Suxamethonium | Ultra-rapid | Ultra-short |
| Tubocurarine | Intermediate/Slow | Intermediate |
| Vecuronium | Rapid | Intermediate |

| **Onset:* | *†Duration:* |
|---|---|
| Ultra-rapid, less than 1 minute | Ultra-short, less than 8 minutes |
| Rapid, 1 to 2 minutes | Short, 8 to 20 minutes |
| Intermediate, 2 to 4 minutes | Intermediate, 20 to 50 minutes |
| Slow, more than 4 minutes | Long, more than 50 minutes |

*Onset and duration of action are dose-dependent*

1. Steyn M, Morton NS. Tracheal intubation without neuromuscular block. *Br J Anaesth* 1994; **73:** 862.
2. Cartwright DP. Suxamethonium in day-case anaesthesia. *Br J Anaesth* 1993; **71:** 918–19.
3. Hunter JM. Rocuronium: the newest aminosteroid neuromuscular blocking drug. *Br J Anaesth* 1996; **76:** 481–3.
4. Sparr HJ. Choice of the muscle relaxant for rapid-sequence induction. *Eur J Anaesthesiol* 2001; **18** (suppl 23): 71–6.
5. Perry JJ, *et al.* Are intubation conditions using rocuronium equivalent to those using succinylcholine. *Acad Emerg Med* 2002; **9:** 813–23.
6. Sparr HJ, *et al.* Influence of induction technique on intubating conditions after rocuronium in adults: comparison with rapid-sequence induction using thiopentone and suxamethonium. *Br J Anaesth* 1996; **77:** 339–42.
7. Naguib M, *et al.* Comparison of suxamethonium and different combinations of rocuronium and mivacurium for rapid tracheal intubation in children. *Br J Anaesth* 1997; **79:** 450–5.
8. Jones RM. The priming principle: how does it work and should we be using it? *Br J Anaesth* 1989; **63:** 1–3.
9. Nimmo SM, *et al.* Effectiveness and sequelae of very low-dose suxamethonium for nasal intubation. *Br J Anaesth* 1995; **74:** 31–4.
10. Barclay K, *et al.* Low-dose rocuronium improves conditions for tracheal intubation after induction of anaesthesia with propofol and alfentanil. *Br J Anaesth* 1997; **78:** 92–4.
11. Groener R, Moyes DG. Rapid tracheal intubation with propofol, alfentanil and a standard dose of vecuronium. *Br J Anaesth* 1997; **79:** 384–5.
12. Chiu CL, *et al.* The effect of mivacurium pretreatment on intra-ocular pressure changes induced by suxamethonium. *Anaesthesia* 1998; **53:** 501–505.
13. Book WJ, *et al.* Adverse effects of depolarising neuromuscular blocking agents: incidence, prevention and management. *Drug Safety* 1994; **10:** 331–49.
14. Crawford DC, *et al.* Effects of alfentanil on the pressor and catecholamine responses to tracheal intubation. *Br J Anaesth* 1987: **59:** 707–12.
15. Scheinin B, *et al.* Alfentanil obtunds the cardiovascular and sympathoadrenal responses to suxamethonium-facilitated laryngoscopy and intubation. *Br J Anaesth* 1989; **62:** 385–92.
16. Chung F, Evans D. Low-dose fentanyl: haemodynamic response during induction and intubation in geriatric patients. *Can Anaesth Soc J* 1985; **32:** 622–8.
17. Mostafa SM, *et al.* Comparison of effects of fentanyl and alfentanil on intra-ocular pressure. *Anaesthesia* 1986; **41:** 493–8.
18. Sweeney J, *et al.* Modification by fentanyl and alfentanil of the intraocular pressure response to suxamethonium and tracheal intubation. *Br J Anaesth* 1989; **63:** 688–91.
19. Tam S, *et al.* Attenuation of circulatory responses to endotracheal intubation using intravenous lidocaine: a determination of the optimal time of injection. *Can Anaesth Soc J* 1985; **32:** S65.
20. Miller CD, Warren SJ. I.V. lignocaine fails to attenuate the cardiovascular response to laryngoscopy and tracheal intubation. *Br J Anaesth* 1990; **65:** 216–19.
21. Murphy DF, *et al.* Intravenous lignocaine pretreatment to prevent intraocular pressure rise following suxamethonium and tracheal intubation. *Br J Ophthalmol* 1986; **70:** 596–8.
22. Drenger B, Pe'er J. Attenuation of ocular and systemic responses to tracheal intubation by intravenous lignocaine. *Br J Ophthalmol* 1987; **71:** 546–8.
23. Mostafa SM, *et al.* Effects of nebulized lignocaine on the intraocular pressure responses to tracheal intubation. *Br J Anaesth* 1990; **64:** 515–17.
24. Holloway KB. Control of the eye during general anaesthesia for intraocular surgery. *Br J Anaesth* 1980; **52:** 671–9.
25. Ashton WB, *et al.* Attenuation of the pressor response to tracheal intubation by magnesium sulphate with and without alfentanil in hypertensive proteinuric patients undergoing caesarean section. *Br J Anaesth* 1991; **67:** 741–7.
26. Brossy MJ, *et al.* Haemodynamic and catecholamine changes after induction of anaesthesia with either thiopentone or propofol with suxamethonium. *Br J Anaesth* 1994; **72:** 596–8.
27. Gin T, *et al.* Plasma catecholamines and neonatal condition after induction of anaesthesia with propofol or thiopentone at caesarean section. *Br J Anaesth* 1993; **70:** 311–116.

**Intensive care**

The use of neuromuscular blockers in patients requiring mechanical ventilation as part of intensive care has been discussed in a number of reviews[1-3] and guidelines.[4] Neuromuscular blockers are used to provide additional relaxation and facilitate ventilatory support in patients who fail to respond to sedation alone. It is important to ensure that such patients are adequately sedated and relatively pain free before these drugs are used. Patients who are considered most likely to benefit are those with spontaneous respiration that is counterproductive to mechanical ventilation. Patients with little inherent respiratory muscle activity are less likely to obtain an improvement in oxygenation. Neuromuscular blockers may also improve control of intracranial pressure in patients with intracranial hypertension, including prevention of rises in intracranial pressure associated with routine tracheobronchial suction.

Pancuronium has been widely used as a neuromuscular blocker in intensive care because of its tendency to increase arterial pressure and the majority of patients requiring a neuromuscular blocker can be adequately managed with pancuronium; however, its long duration of action may be a problem in some circumstances, and its vagolytic activity can also produce tachycardia. Vecuronium, atracurium, and cisatracurium have relatively few cardiovascular effects, but there has been some concern over the ability of the atracurium metabolite laudanosine to accumulate in the CNS (see under Pharmacokinetics, p.1402). Atracurium and cisatracurium may also be more suitable in patients with hepatic or renal impairment as their metabolism does not lead to the accumulation of active metabolites. Other neuromuscular blockers that have been used in intensive care include doxacurium, pipecuronium, and rocuronium.

Close monitoring of neuromuscular blockade is recommended since the pharmacodynamics and pharmacokinetics of neuromuscular blockers may be altered in patients in intensive care;[1-4] this should also allow the lowest effective neuromuscular blocking dose to be used, and reduce adverse events. Prolonged neuromuscular blockade has been related to dosage.

Other factors which may potentiate neuromuscular blockade include drug interactions, electrolyte imbalance, hypothermia, or changes in acid-base balance.[1,3] Conversely, dosage requirements may be increased in patients with burns or in those receiving prolonged therapy. Tachyphylaxis has occurred with some neuromuscular blockers, but may resolve on switching to another blocker.

Prolonged neuromuscular blockade has been associated with adverse effects and should be avoided when possible. Recovery following withdrawal of prolonged treatment may be longer than pharmacologically predicted due to the accumulation of active metabolites; this is a particular problem for neuromuscular blockers with a long duration of action and for patients with hepatic or renal impairment. An acute myopathy has also followed prolonged use, most commonly with aminosteroid neuromuscular blockers; there are case reports suggesting that concomitant use of corticosteroids might increase the risk.[4,5]

When rapid reversal of paralysis is necessary an anticholinesterase such as neostigmine may be used, but relatively little is known about the efficacy of anticholinesterases in reversing prolonged paralysis.[6]

**Neonatal intensive care.** Neuromuscular blockers such as pancuronium bromide are used in neonatal intensive care to obtain muscle relaxation during mechanical ventilation in infants with severe pulmonary disease, especially in those whose respiratory efforts are out of phase with the ventilator.[7] They are only used in infants at high risk of complications such as *pneumothorax* or *intraventricular haemorrhage*; their routine use in all ventilated neonates is not recommended.[8]

Abolition of spontaneous respiration during mechanical ventilation has had variable effects on the incidence of *pneumothorax* in infants with respiratory distress syndrome. Although a reduced incidence was found in one study[9] involving infants of less than 33 weeks' gestation, in another study[10] the incidence was reduced only in infants with a gestational age of 27 to 32 weeks; no reduction was obtained in those below 26 weeks' gestation. Paralysis also failed to reduce the incidence of pneumothorax or interstitial emphysema in a study[11] of infants with hyaline membrane disease but did appear to speed recovery of lung function.

The aetiology of *intraventricular haemorrhage* remains obscure but there is a well recognised association with gestational age;[12] less mature neonates are more susceptible and the incidence decreases sharply after 30 weeks' gestation. There appears to be an association between fluctuating cerebral blood-flow velocity in the first day of life and subsequent development of intraventricular haemorrhage.[13] Respiratory paralysis from the first day of life until 72 hours of age has been reported[14] to stabilise both cerebral and arterial blood-flow velocity and to produce a decrease in the incidence and severity of intraventricular haemorrhage in infants with respiratory distress syndrome. However, respiratory paralysis has also been reported to have no effect on the development of intraventricular haemorrhage.[9,10]

The use of neuromuscular blockers in the newborn is not without complications. Multiple joint contractures, possibly potentiated by concomitant use of aminoglycosides or phenobarbital, have been reported[15,16] in infants given pancuronium, and regular passive limb movements should be performed during paralysis. Marked oedema, severe disturbances of fluid balance, and renal failure followed by death have been reported in 2 neonates.[17] Hypoxaemia may develop following induction of paralysis unless a significant increase in ventilator support is made;[9,13,18] hypotension may also occur.[19] Drugs such as pancuronium which are metabolised in the liver and excreted in the urine have a prolonged action in premature infants.[7] As with adults (see above), continuous use of neuromuscular blockers in neonates has been associated with prolonged neuromuscular block on discontinuation.[20]


1. Coursin DB, *et al.* Muscle relaxants in critical care. *Curr Opin Anaesthesiol* 1993; **6:** 341–6.
2. Elliot JM, Bion JF. The use of neuromuscular blocking drugs in intensive care practice. *Acta Anaesthesiol Scand* 1995; **39** (suppl 106): 70–82.
3. Lewis KS, Rothenberg DM. Neuromuscular blockade in the intensive care unit. *Am J Health-Syst Pharm* 1999; **56:** 72–5.
4. Murray MJ, *et al.* Clinical practice guidelines for sustained neuromuscular blockade in the adult critically ill patient. *Am J Health-Syst Pharm* 2002; **59:** 179–95.
5. Fischer JR, Baer RK. Acute myopathy associated with combined use of corticosteroids and neuromuscular blocking agents. *Ann Pharmacother* 1996; **30:** 1437–45.
6. Watling SM, Dasta JF. Prolonged paralysis in intensive care unit patients after the use of neuromuscular blocking agents: a review of the literature. *Crit Care Med* 1994; **22:** 884–93.
7. Levene MI, Quinn MW. Use of sedatives and muscle relaxants in newborn babies receiving mechanical ventilation. *Arch Dis Child* 1992; **67:** 870–3.
8. Cools F, Offringa M. Neuromuscular paralysis for newborn infants receiving mechanical ventilation. Available in The Cochrane Library; Issue 2. Chichester: John Wiley; 2004.
9. Greenough A, *et al.* Pancuronium prevents pneumothoraces in ventilated premature babies who actively expire against positive pressure inflation. *Lancet* 1984; **i:** 1–3.
10. Cooke RWI, Rennie JM. Pancuronium and pneumothorax. *Lancet* 1984; **i:** 286–7.
11. Pollitzer MJ, *et al.* Pancuronium during mechanical ventilation speeds recovery of lungs of infants with hyaline membrane disease. *Lancet* 1981; **i:** 346–8.
12. Miall-Allen VM, *et al.* Blood pressure fluctuation and intraventricular hemorrhage in the preterm infant of less than 31 weeks' gestation. *Pediatrics* 1989; **83:** 657–61.
13. Perlman JM, *et al.* Fluctuating cerebral blood-flow velocity in respiratory distress syndrome. *N Engl J Med* 1983; **309:** 204–9.
14. Perlman JM, *et al.* Reduction in intraventricular hemorrhage by elimination of fluctuating cerebral blood-flow velocity in preterm infants with respiratory distress syndrome. *N Engl J Med* 1985; **312:** 1353–7.
15. Sinha SK, Levene MI. Pancuronium bromide induced joint contractures in the newborn. *Arch Dis Child* 1984; **59:** 73–5.
16. Fanconi S, *et al.* Effects of paralysis with pancuronium bromide on joint mobility in premature infants. *J Pediatr* 1995; **127:** 134–6.
17. Reynolds EOR, *et al.* Muscle relaxation and periventricular hemorrhage. *N Engl J Med* 1985; **313:** 955–6.
18. Philips JB, *et al.* Hypoxaemia in ventilated neonates after pancuronium paralysis. *Lancet* 1979, **i:** 877.
19. McIntosh N. Hypotension associated with pancuronium use in the newborn. *Lancet* 1985; **ii:** 279.
20. Björklund LJ. Use of sedatives and muscle relaxants in newborn babies receiving mechanical ventilation. *Arch Dis Child* 1993; **69:** 544.


**Tetanus**

The clinical manifestations of tetanus following infection with *Clostridium tetani* are caused by the highly potent neurotoxin tetanospasmin produced by its germinating spores.

The muscular symptoms of generalised tetanus include trismus (lockjaw), glottal spasm, generalised muscle spasm, opisthotonus (spasm of the back muscles resulting in backward arching of the body), respiratory spasm, and paralysis. Other complications include electrolyte disturbances and autonomic dysfunction leading to cardiovascular effects such as hypertension, tachycardia, and peripheral vasoconstriction. Patients may have a milder form in which the twitching and muscle spasms are limited to the area near the site of the injury, but such localised tetanus is rare and can progress to the generalised form.

Treatment aims to destroy the causative organism and/or neutralise any unbound toxin in the body, to control rigidity and muscle spasms, and to control autonomic dysfunction. For the **antibacterial treatment and prevention** of tetanus and neutralisation of tetanospasmin, see p.149.

Following antibacterial therapy the mainstay of treatment of **rigidity and spasms** is sedation with *benzodiazepines* such as diazepam or midazolam; they may also reduce patient anxiety. *Opioid analgesics* can be added to treatment to provide analgesia and additional sedation; in addition, *morphine* may control autonomic overactivity. *Antiepileptics*, particularly phenobarbital, may also provide additional sedation. *Chlorpromazine* is sometimes used with benzodiazepines to minimise rigidity and muscle spasms. Sedation with *propofol* may also control spasms and rigidity without the need for an additional relaxant; however, mechanical ventilation is required. Centrally acting muscle relaxants have also been tried to control muscle spasms. *Baclofen* has been given by the intrathecal route, but its therapeutic range in severe tetanus may be very narrow and deep coma and loss of spontaneous respiration has been reported. *Dantrolene* has also been reported to be effective. When muscle spasms are severe or interfere with respiration, *competitive neuromuscular blockers* have been used in addition to benzodiazepine sedation, to control spasms and to induce therapeutic paralysis so mechanical ventilation can be initiated.

Control of **autonomic overactivity** may be achieved with sedation; benzodiazepines, antiepileptics, and morphine have all been used (see above). *Beta blockers* such as propranolol have also been used; however, they are no longer recommended because of the potential for severe cardiovascular effects. Labetalol has both alpha- and beta-blocking activity but offers no advantage over propranolol. More recently, *esmolol*, a short-acting beta blocker, has been used. *Magnesium sulfate* has been found to minimise autonomic disturbance in ventilated patients and controls spasms in non-ventilated patients, but there is need for further investigation. **Electrolyte disturbance** is corrected with calcium and magnesium salts.

References.


1. Attygalle D, Karalliedde L. Unforgettable tetanus. *Eur J Anaesthesiol* 1997; **14:** 122–33.
2. Ernst ME, *et al.* Tetanus: pathophysiology and management. *Ann Pharmacother* 1997; **31:** 1507–13.
3. Farrar JJ, *et al.* Tetanus. *J Neurol Neurosurg Psychiatry* 2000; **69:** 292–301.
4. Cook TM, *et al.* Tetanus: a review of the literature. *Br J Anaesth* 2001; **87:** 477–87.


## Alcuronium Chloride *(BAN, USAN, rINN)*

Alcuronii Chloridum; Allnortoxiferin Chloride; Cloruro de alcuronio; Diallylnortoxiferine Dichloride; Diallyltoxiferine Chloride; Ro-4-3816. NN′-Diallylbisnortoxiferinium dichloride.

$C_{44}H_{50}Cl_2N_4O_2$ = 737.8.

*CAS — 23214-96-2 (alcuronium); 15180-03-7 (alcuronium chloride).*

*ATC — M03AA01.*

**Pharmacopoeias.** In *Eur.* (see p.vi) and *Int.*

**Ph. Eur. 5.0** (Alcuronium Chloride). A white or slightly greyish-white, crystalline powder. Freely soluble in water and in methyl alcohol; soluble in alcohol; practically insoluble in cyclohexane. Store under nitrogen in an airtight container. Protect from light.

### Profile

Alcuronium chloride is a benzylisoquinolinium competitive neuromuscular blocker (see Atracurium, p.1399) that is used for endotracheal intubation and to provide muscle relaxation in general anaesthesia for surgical procedures (see Anaesthesia, p.1397). It can induce histamine release to some degree. Anaphylactoid reactions have been associated with the use of alcuronium. It has some vagolytic action and may produce tachycardia; hypotension may also occur.

Doses of neuromuscular blockers need to be carefully titrated for individual patients according to response, and may vary with the procedure, the other drugs given, and the state of the patient; monitoring of the degree of block is recommended in order to reduce the risk of overdosage. An initial dose of 150 to 250 micrograms/kg has been given intravenously. Muscle relaxation occurs after about 2 minutes and the effect lasts for about 20 to 30 minutes. Supplementary doses of 30 micrograms/kg have been given to provide additional periods of muscle relaxation.

**Porphyria.** Alcuronium is considered to be unsafe in patients with porphyria because it has been shown to be porphyrinogenic in *animals*.

**Pregnancy.** Alcuronium crosses the placenta. No evidence of neuromuscular block was seen in any of the neonates born to 12 women who received alcuronium 15 to 30 mg by intravenous injection, 5.0 to 10.5 minutes before delivery[1] but caution was advised if alcuronium was given in obstetrics in high doses or for a prolonged period.


1. Ho PC, *et al.* Caesarean section and placental transfer of alcuronium. *Anaesth Intensive Care* 1981; **9:** 113–18.


**Renal impairment.** Alcuronium is excreted mainly by the kidneys and accumulation, with prolonged paralysis, may therefore be expected in patients with renal impairment given large or repeated doses. A prolonged elimination half-life has been reported in anuria.[1] However, doses of 160 micrograms/kg have been used without any problems in patients with chronic renal failure undergoing renal transplantation.[2] The average duration of action of this dose was 37 minutes and any residual neuromuscular blockade at the end of surgery was successfully reversed using atropine and neostigmine.

1. Raaflaub J, Frey P. Zur Pharmakokinetik von Diallyl-nor-toxiferin beim Menschen. *Arzneimittelforschung* 1972; **22:** 73–8.
2. Kaushik S, *et al.* Use of alcuronium in patients undergoing renal transplantation. *Br J Anaesth* 1984; **56:** 1229–33.

### Preparations

**Proprietary Preparations** (details are given in Part 3)
***Austria:*** Alloferin; ***Braz.:*** Alloferine; ***Ger.:*** Alloferin; ***Hong Kong:*** Alloferin; ***Israel:*** Alloferin†; ***Malaysia:*** Alloferin; ***S.Afr.:*** Alloferin; ***Singapore:*** Alloferin; ***Thai.:*** Alloferin†.

## Atracurium Besilate *(BAN, rINN)*

33A74; Atracurium Besylate *(USAN)*; Besilato de atracurio; BW-33A. 2,2′-(3,11-Dioxo-4,10-dioxatridecamethylene)bis(1,2,3,4-tetrahydro-6,7-dimethoxy-2-methyl-1-veratrylisoquinolinium) di(benzenesulphonate).

$C_{53}H_{72}N_2O_{12},2C_6H_5O_3S = 1243.5.$

*CAS — 64228-81-5.*

*ATC — M03AC04.*

**Pharmacopoeias.** In *Br., It.,* and *US.*

**BP 2003** (Atracurium Besilate). A white to pale yellow hygroscopic powder or flaky crystals. It contains about 58% of the *cis-cis* isomer, about 36% of the *cis-trans* isomer, and about 6% of the *trans-trans* isomer. Soluble in water; very soluble in acetonitrile and in chloroform; practically insoluble in ether. A 1% solution in water has a pH of 3.5 to 5.0. Store in airtight containers at a temperature of 2° to 8°. Protect from light.

**USP 27** (Atracurium Besylate). A white to off-white solid. It contains not less than 5.0% and not more than 6.5% of the *trans-trans* isomer, not less than 34.5% and not more than 38.5% of the *cis-trans* isomer, and not less than 55.0% and not more than 60.0% of the *cis-cis* isomer. It is unstable at room temperature. Store in airtight containers at a temperature not exceeding 8°. Protect from light.

### Cisatracurium Besilate *(BAN, rINN)*

Bésilate de Cisatracurium; Besilato de cisatracurio; BW-51W (cisatracurium); BW-51W89 (cisatracurium); Cisatracurium Besylate; 51W89 (cisatracurium). (1R,1′R,2R,2′R)-2,2′-(3,11-Dioxo-4,10-dioxatridecamethylene)bis(1,2,3,4-tetrahydro-6,7-dimethoxy-2-methyl-1-veratrylisoquinolinium) dibenzenesulfonate.

*CAS — 96946-42-8.*

*ATC — M03AC11.*

**Incompatibility.** Neuromuscular blockers are generally incompatible with alkaline solutions, for example barbiturates such as thiopental sodium. It is good practice not to administer neuromuscular blockers in the same syringe, or simultaneously through the same needle, as other drugs.

The manufacturers state that cisatracurium is incompatible with ketorolac trometamol or propofol emulsion; in addition, lactated Ringer's injection with glucose 5% or lactated Ringer's solution should not be used as a diluent when preparing solutions of cisatracurium for infusion.

**Stability.** In a stability study,[1] solutions of cisatracurium (as the besilate) in concentrations of 2 or 10 mg/mL were stable for at least 90 days when stored in the original vials at 4° either exposed to or protected from light; similar solutions stored at 23° were stable for at least 45 days. Solutions of 2 mg/mL stored in plastic syringes at 4° or 23° were stable for at least 30 days. Solutions of 0.1, 2, or 5 mg/mL in 5% glucose injection or 0.9% sodium chloride injection in PVC minibags were stable for at least 30 days stored at 4°; the 5 mg/mL solution was also stable for at least 30 days stored at 23°.

1. Xu QA, *et al.* Stability of cisatracurium besylate in vials, syringes, and infusion admixtures. *Am J Health-Syst Pharm* 1998; **55:** 1037–41.

### Adverse Effects

The adverse effects of competitive neuromuscular blockers are generally similar although they differ in their propensity to cause histamine release and associated cardiovascular effects. The latter appear to be rare with the aminosteroidal blockers and the benzylisoquinolinium blocker cisatracurium (see below). Competitive neuromuscular blockers with vagolytic activity may produce tachycardia and a rise in blood pressure. The use of blockers which lack an effect on the vagus will not counteract the bradycardia produced during anaesthesia by the other drugs employed or by vagal stimulation. Reduction in blood pressure with compensatory tachycardia may occur with some competitive neuromuscular blockers due in part to sympathetic ganglion blockade or the release of histamine. Reduction in gastrointestinal motility and tone may occur as a result of ganglionic blockade.

Histamine release may also lead to wheal-and-flare effects at the site of injection, flushing, occasionally bronchospasm, and rarely anaphylactoid reactions.

Malignant hyperthermia has been associated rarely with competitive neuromuscular blockers.

Some competitive neuromuscular blockers such as pancuronium, tubocurarine, and vecuronium can cause a decrease in the partial thromboplastin time and prothrombin time.

In overdosage there is prolonged apnoea due to paralysis of the intercostal muscles and diaphragm, with cardiovascular collapse and the effects of histamine release.

*Atracurium and its isomer cisatracurium* have no significant vagal or ganglionic blocking activity at recommended doses. Unlike atracurium, cisatracurium does not induce histamine release and is therefore associated with greater cardiovascular stability.

For possible risks from their major metabolite laudanosine, see under Pharmacokinetics, below.

**Effects on body temperature.** Competitive neuromuscular blockers are not considered to be a trigger factor for malignant hyperthermia; however, there have been rare case reports of apparent association. Two cases of mild malignant hyperthermia have been reported[1] where tubocurarine was probably the triggering drug. Each episode developed in a member of a known malignant hyperthermia family despite preventive measures such as prophylactic cooling, and avoidance of potent inhalation anaesthetics and depolarising neuromuscular blockers. Another case[2] was associated with the use of pancuronium.

1. Britt BA, *et al.* Malignant hyperthermia induced by curare. *Can Anaesth Soc J* 1974; **21:** 371–5.
2. Waterman PM, *et al.* Malignant hyperthermia: a case report. *Anesth Analg* 1980; **59:** 220–1.

**Effects on the muscles.** For reference to acute myopathy and prolonged muscle weakness after withdrawal of long-term continuous infusions of competitive neuromuscular blockers, see under Intensive Care, p.1398.

**Hypersensitivity.** There have been reports of severe anaphylactoid reactions following administration of atracurium[1,2] or cisatracurium.[3,4] For a discussion of hypersensitivity reactions associated with neuromuscular blockers, see under Suxamethonium Chloride, p.1407.

1. Stirton-Hopkins C. Life-threatening reaction to atracurium. *Br J Anaesth* 1988; **60:** 597–8.
2. Oh TE, Horton JM. Adverse reactions to atracurium. *Br J Anaesth* 1989; **62:** 467–8.
3. Briassoulis G, *et al.* Persistent anaphylactic reaction after induction with thiopentone and cisatracurium. *Paediatr Anaesth* 2000; **10:** 429–34.
4. Legros CB, *et al.* Severe anaphylactic reaction to cisatracurium in a child. *Anesth Analg* 2001; **92:** 648–9.

### Treatment of Adverse Effects

It is essential to maintain assisted respiration in patients who have received a competitive neuromuscular blocker until spontaneous breathing is fully restored; in addition a cholinesterase inhibitor such as neostigmine is usually given intravenously, with atropine or glycopyrronium, to hasten reversal of the neuromuscular block. Patients need to be closely monitored after reversal of block to ensure that muscle relaxation does not return.

Severe hypotension may require intravenous fluid replacement and cautious use of a pressor agent; the patient should be positioned to facilitate venous return from the muscles.

Giving an antihistamine before induction of neuromuscular blockade may help to prevent histamine-induced adverse effects in patients with asthma or those susceptible to bronchospasm.

**Reversal of neuromuscular blockade.** For a discussion of the use of anticholinesterases for reversal of residual neuromuscular block produced by intermediate- or short-acting blockers after surgical or similar procedures, see under Neostigmine, p.1493.

### Precautions

Patients who have received a neuromuscular blocker should always have their respiration assisted or controlled until the drug has been inactivated or antagonised.

Atracurium and other competitive neuromuscular blockers should be used with great care, if at all, in respiratory insufficiency or pulmonary disease and in the dehydrated or severely ill patient. The response to neuromuscular blockers is often unpredictable in patients with neuromuscular disorders and they should be used with great care in these patients (see below). Caution is also needed in patients with a history of conditions such as asthma where release of histamine would be a hazard. Care is also required in patients with a history of hypersensitivity to any neuromuscular blocker.

Resistance to the effects of competitive neuromuscular blockers may occur in patients with burns (see below). The effect of competitive neuromuscular blockers may vary in patients with hepatic impairment: resistance appears to occur to some, such as doxacurium, metocurine, pancuronium, and tubocurarine, while dosage of others, including mivacurium and rocuronium, may need to be reduced because of a prolonged action.

Competitive neuromuscular blockers excreted mainly in the urine should be used with caution in renal impairment; a reduction in dosage may be necessary. Doses may need to be reduced in infants and neonates because of increased sensitivity to competitive muscle relaxants. Doses in obese patients should usually be based upon the patient's ideal body-weight rather than actual body-weight.

The effects of competitive neuromuscular blockers are increased by metabolic or respiratory acidosis and hypokalaemia, hypermagnesaemia, hypocalcaemia, and hypophosphataemia and dehydration. Competitive neuromuscular blockade may also be enhanced by raised body temperature and reduced in hypothermia.

In contrast to other competitive neuromuscular blockers, reduction in body temperature may necessitate a dosage reduction for *atracurium and its isomer cisatracurium* since cooling reduces the rate of inactivation of atracurium and cisatracurium, but physiological variations in body temperature and pH will not significantly affect their action.

**Burns.** The dose requirements of competitive neuromuscular blockers are increased in patients with burns,[1-3] the dose correlating with both the extent of the burn and time after injury. This resistance is usually not seen in patients with less than 10% body-surface burns but if more than 40% of the body-surface is affected the dose of competitive blocker may need to be up to five times higher than in patients without burns. Resistance peaks about 2 weeks after injury, persists for many months in patients with major burns, and decreases gradually with healing of the burn. The mechanism of resistance is multifactorial but may be partly explained by increased protein binding, increased volume of distribution, and increased numbers of acetylcholine receptors at the motor end-plate requiring more muscle relaxant to produce a given effect. Despite the high doses of competitive relaxants that are required, recovery from neuromuscular blockade is not seriously impaired and their effects can be reversed with usual doses of an anticholinesterase.

1. Martyn J, *et al.* Clinical pharmacology of muscle relaxants in patients with burns. *J Clin Pharmacol* 1986; **26:** 680–5.
2. Anonymous. Neuromuscular blockers in patients with burns. *Lancet* 1988; **ii:** 1003–4.
3. Tschida SJ, *et al.* Resistance to nondepolarizing neuromuscular blocking agents. *Pharmacotherapy* 1996; **16:** 409–18.

**Cardiopulmonary bypass.** The effect of cardiopulmonary bypass on the pharmacokinetics and pharmacodynamics of competitive neuromuscular blockers can be complex but generally their dosage may need to be reduced. Although the intensity of neuromuscular blockade of most competitive neuromuscular blockers is reduced by hypothermia[1] used during cardiopulmonary bypass, their administration during this procedure is associated with rises in plasma concentrations, reduced clearance, and prolongation of the elimination half-life.[2-6] Various mechanisms, including reduced distribution to highly perfused tissues such as the lungs, have been proposed to explain this effect.[2] For atracurium, it appears that it is a reduction in the temperature-dependent inactivation by Hofmann elimination during hypothermia which enables lower doses to be used.[7]

1. Buzello W, *et al.* Unequal effects of cardiopulmonary bypass-induced hypothermia on neuromuscular blockade from constant infusion of alcuronium, d-tubocurarine, pancuronium, and vecuronium. *Anesthesiology* 1987; **66:** 842–6.
2. Walker JS, *et al.* Alcuronium kinetics in patients undergoing cardiopulmonary bypass surgery. *Br J Clin Pharmacol* 1983; **15:** 237–44.
3. Walker JS, *et al.* Altered d-tubocurarine disposition during cardiopulmonary bypass surgery. *Clin Pharmacol Ther* 1984; **35:** 686–94.
4. Wierda JMKH, Agoston S. Pharmacokinetics of vecuronium during hypothermic bypass. *Br J Anaesth* 1989; **63:** 627P–628P.

5. Smeulers NJ, *et al.* Hypothermic cardiopulmonary bypass influences the concentration-response relationship and the biodisposition of rocuronium. *Eur J Anaesthesiol* 1995; **12** (suppl 11): 91–4.
6. Asokumar B, *et al.* Pharmacokinetics of doxacurium during normothermic and hypothermic cardiopulmonary bypass surgery. *Can J Anaesth* 1998; **45:** 515–20.
7. Flynn PJ, *et al.* Use of atracurium in cardiac surgery involving cardiopulmonary bypass with induced hypothermia. *Br J Anaesth* 1984; **56:** 967–72.

**Hepatic impairment.** The effect of competitive neuromuscular blockers may vary in patients with hepatic impairment (see Precautions, above) but alterations in the pharmacokinetics of atracurium and cisatracurium in patients with hepatic impairment (see under Biotransformation, in Pharmacokinetics, below) do not appear to be clinically significant and a reduction in dosage is not generally recommended.

**Neuromuscular disorders.** Caution is needed if competitive neuromuscular blockers are given to patients with neuromuscular disease since severe complications have been reported.[1] Increased response may be seen in patients with paraplegia or quadriplegia, but resistance has been reported in patients with hemiplegia. Increased response also may occur in patients with amyotrophic lateral sclerosis, neurofibromatosis, and poliomyelitis; this is of little concern unless the respiratory muscles are involved when prolonged apnoea may occur. Patients with myasthenia gravis usually show increased sensitivity to competitive neuromuscular blockers although small doses have been given without complications. During remission of myasthenia gravis a normal response is usual but since remission is often incomplete, small intermittent doses are advised. A significantly greater exaggeration of response is seen in patients with the myasthenic syndrome. Both normal and increased responses have been reported in patients with myotonias or muscular dystrophies but exquisite sensitivity occurs in patients with ocular muscular dystrophy. A normal response to competitive relaxants may be expected in patients with multiple sclerosis, muscular denervation, Parkinson's disease, and tetanus.

1. Azar I. The response of patients with neuromuscular disorders to muscle relaxants: a review. *Anesthesiology* 1984; **61:** 173–87.

**Pregnancy.** A review[1] of the pharmacokinetics of neuromuscular blockers in pregnancy concluded that atracurium and mivacurium are the best choice in pregnancy since their actions are predictable; their duration of action is either unchanged or only slightly prolonged. Atracurium also has a low umbilical to maternal vein concentration (uv/mv) ratio. In general, it is advisable[1] to choose a neuromuscular blocker with a low uv/mv ratio and a short duration of action, and to inject the lowest dose required to produce adequate surgical conditions.

Atracurium 300 micrograms/kg given to 26 women undergoing caesarean section, with subsequent incremental doses of 100 or 200 micrograms/kg if necessary, produced good surgical relaxation in all patients without any complications.[2] Of the 26 neonates delivered, respiration was established within 90 seconds in 21, with an Apgar score of 10 at 5 minutes. The remaining 5 neonates were delivered by caesarean section because of fetal distress and were slower to start breathing.

A study[3] of 22 women in the immediate postpartum period found the onset and duration of cisatracurium to be significantly shorter when compared with nonpregnant patients.

1. Guay J, *et al.* Clinical pharmacokinetics of neuromuscular relaxants in pregnancy. *Clin Pharmacokinet* 1998; **34:** 483–96.
2. Frank M, *et al.* Atracurium in obstetric anaesthesia: a preliminary report. *Br J Anaesth* 1983; **55:** 113S-114S.
3. Pan PH, Moore C. Comparison of cisatracurium-induced neuromuscular blockade between immediate postpartum and nonpregnant patients. *J Clin Anesth* 2001; **13:** 112–7.

**Renal impairment.** Although some differences in the pharmacokinetics of atracurium and cisatracurium have been reported in patients with renal impairment (see under Pharmacokinetics, below), duration of their neuromuscular blocking action is not significantly dependent on renal function and usual doses may be given to such patients.[1,2] Atracurium has been given by infusion to patients with end-stage renal failure[3] when the initial dose required for induction of neuromuscular block was 37% higher than that required by patients without renal impairment. The increase could be explained by the larger extracellular fluid volume in patients with chronic renal failure.

Although the pharmacokinetics of atracurium and cisatracurium are not appreciably different in renal impairment, those of their metabolites may be (see under Pharmacokinetics, below) and therefore it has been suggested that neuromuscular function should be monitored during use of atracurium.[4]

1. Hunter JM, *et al.* Use of the muscle relaxant atracurium in anephric patients: preliminary communication. *J R Soc Med* 1982; **75:** 336–340.
2. Boyd AH, *et al.* Pharmacodynamics of the 1R cis-1′R cis isomer of atracurium (51W89) in health and chronic renal failure. *Br J Anaesth* 1995; **74:** 400–404.
3. Gramstad L. Atracurium, vecuronium and pancuronium in end-stage renal failure: dose-response properties and interactions with azathioprine. *Br J Anaesth* 1987; **59:** 995–1003.
4. Vandenbrom RHG, *et al.* Pharmacokinetics and neuromuscular blocking effects of atracurium besylate and two of its metabolites in patients with normal and impaired renal function. *Clin Pharmacokinet* 1990; **19:** 230–40.

**Resistance.** The aetiology of resistance to competitive blockers is not clear but might be due to pharmacodynamic or pharmacokinetic alterations associated with disease states such as burn injuries (see above) or hepatic impairment (see Precautions, above) or concomitant drug therapy (see Interactions, below). One review[1] noted that there had been numerous case reports of resistance to competitive neuromuscular blockers; most had been associated with use of single doses or short-term intermittent therapy, but more recent reports had documented resistance during continuous infusions in 9 patients of whom 7 had received atracurium and 2 rocuronium. Resistance to atracurium had followed 2 different patterns. Patients had required either usual or raised doses for initial control but both groups had subsequently required progressive increases. Most patients with resistance to atracurium were successfully managed by transfer to pancuronium or doxacurium.

1. Tschida SJ, *et al.* Resistance to nondepolarizing neuromuscular blocking agents. *Pharmacotherapy* 1996; **16:** 409–18.

**Tourniquets.** Atracurium might be unsuitable for neuromuscular blockade of a limb which has been isolated with a tourniquet in order to provide a bloodless field for surgery.[1] Atracurium undergoes non-enzymatic degradation in plasma and would therefore continue to degrade locally leading to a loss of blockade in the limb, which could not be corrected by further doses unless the tourniquet was deflated.

1. Shannon PF. Neuromuscular block and tourniquets. *Br J Anaesth* 1994; **73:** 726.

## Interactions

A number of drugs may influence neuromuscular transmission and thus interfere with the action of both competitive and depolarising neuromuscular blockers, resulting in potentiation or antagonism of neuromuscular block. Some interactions may be advantageous, such as the reversal of competitive neuromuscular block by anticholinesterases. In general, adverse interactions are potentially more serious in patients with impaired neuromuscular function (see Neuromuscular Disorders, above, and under Suxamethonium Chloride, p.1408).

Drug interactions affecting neuromuscular blockers of either type (competitive and depolarising) as well as those specific for competitive neuromuscular blockers are discussed below. For drug interactions specific to depolarising neuromuscular blockers see under Interactions in Suxamethonium Chloride, p.1408.

◊ Reviews.

1. Feldman S, Karalliedde L. Drug interactions with neuromuscular blockers. *Drug Safety* 1996; **15:** 261–73.
2. Cammu G. Interactions of neuromuscular blocking drugs. *Acta Anaesthesiol Belg* 2001; **52:** 357–63.

**Antiarrhythmics.** Lidocaine, procainamide, quinidine, and verapamil all have some neuromuscular blocking activity and may enhance the block produced by neuromuscular blockers. Large doses of *lidocaine* may reduce the release of acetylcholine and act directly on the muscle membrane. *Quinidine* has a curare-like action at the neuromuscular junction and depresses the muscle action potential. If given during recovery from neuromuscular block it can result in muscle weakness and apnoea and it should be avoided, if possible, in the immediate postoperative period. For details regarding interactions with calcium-channel blockers, see below.

**Antibacterials.** Some antibacterials in very high concentration can produce a muscle paralysis that may be additive to or synergistic with that produced by neuromuscular blockers. The neuromuscular block produced by antibacterials may be enhanced in patients with intracellular potassium deficiency, low plasma-calcium concentration, neuromuscular disease, or a tendency to a high plasma-antibacterial concentration, for example following large doses or in renal impairment. The interaction appears to be more important for competitive neuromuscular blockers. The antibacterials most commonly implicated are aminoglycosides, lincosamides, polymyxins, and, more rarely, tetracyclines.

The *aminoglycosides* diminish release of, and sensitivity to, acetylcholine and their effect can be reversed, at least in part, by calcium, fampridine, or an anticholinesterase. The interaction can occur with most routes of aminoglycoside administration. There are reports of potentiation of neuromuscular blockade occurring with many different aminoglycoside-neuromuscular blocker combinations[1-6] and all aminoglycosides should be used with extreme caution during surgery and in the postoperative period.

The *lincosamides* (*clindamycin* and *lincomycin*) can prolong the action of muscle relaxants producing a neuromuscular block that may be difficult to reverse with calcium or anticholinesterases.[7-9] Patients should be monitored for prolonged paralysis.

There have been reports of prolonged apnoea[2,5,8] following the use of *polymyxins* (*colistin, polymyxin B*) with a neuromuscular blocker. The block is difficult to reverse; calcium may be partially successful, but neostigmine may increase the block.

*Tetracyclines* have weak neuromuscular blocking properties; potentiation of neuromuscular block has been reported in patients with myasthenia gravis.[2] Reversal of the block may be partly achieved with calcium, but the value of anticholinesterases is questionable.

The *ureidopenicillins* (*azlocillin* and *mezlocillin*), and the closely related *piperacillin*, are reported to prolong the block produced by vecuronium.[10,11]

*Vancomycin* has been reported to increase neuromuscular blockade by vecuronium.[12] Prolonged paralysis and apnoea has occurred in a patient recovering from suxamethonium-induced blockade after being given vancomycin.[13]

1. Hall DR, *et al.* Gentamicin, tubocurarine, lignocaine and neuromuscular blockade. *Br J Anaesth* 1972; **44:** 1329–32.
2. Pittinger CB, *et al.* Antibiotic-induced paralysis. *Anesth Analg Curr Res* 1970; **49:** 487–501.
3. Waterman PM, Smith RB. Tobramycin-curare interaction. *Anesth Analg Curr Res* 1977; **56:** 587–8.
4. Regan AG, Perumbetti PPV. Pancuronium and gentamicin interaction in patients with renal failure. *Anesth Analg* 1980; **59:** 393.
5. Giala MM, Paradelis AG. Two cases of prolonged respiratory depression due to interaction of pancuronium with colistin and streptomycin. *J Antimicrob Chemother* 1979; **5:** 234–5.
6. Jedeikin R, *et al.* Prolongation of neuromuscular blocking effect of vecuronium by antibiotics. *Anaesthesia* 1987; **42:** 858–60.
7. Booij LHD, *et al.* Neostigmine and 4-aminopyridine antagonism of lincomycin-pancuronium neuromuscular blockade in man. *Anesth Analg* 1978; **57:** 316–21.
8. de Gouw NE, *et al.* Interaction of antibiotics on pipecuronium-induced neuromuscular blockade. *J Clin Anesth* 1993; **5:** 212–15.
9. Sloan PA, Rasul M. Prolongation of rapacuronium neuromuscular blockade by clindamycin and magnesium. *Anesth Analg* 2002; **94:** 123–4.
10. Tryba M. Wirkungsverstäkung nicht-depolarisierender Muskelrelaxantien durch Acylaminopenicilline: Untersuchungen am Beispiel von Vecuronium. *Anaesthesist* 1985; **34:** 651–5.
11. Tryba M, Klemm D. Wechselwirkungen zwischen Acylaminopenicillinen und nicht depolarisierenden Muskelrelaxantien. *Fortschr Antimikrob Antineoplast Chemother* 1985; **4-7:** 1827–33.
12. Huang KC, *et al.* Vancomycin enhances the neuromuscular blockade of vecuronium. *Anesth Analg* 1990; **70:** 194–6.
13. Albrecht RF, Lanier WL. Potentiation of succinylcholine-induced phase II block by vancomycin. *Anesth Analg* 1993; **77:** 1300–2.

**Anticholinesterases.** Anticholinesterases, including *ecothiopate, edrophonium, galantamine, neostigmine, pyridostigmine, rivastigmine*, and possibly *donepezil*, antagonise the effect of competitive neuromuscular blockers. Some anticholinesterases such as neostigmine inhibit both acetylcholinesterase and plasma cholinesterase, and are used clinically to antagonise competitive neuromuscular blockade. Conversely, anticholinesterases enhance the action of depolarising muscle relaxants such as suxamethonium thus prolonging neuromuscular block, although suxamethonium-induced phase II block can be reversed with an anticholinesterase. See also Interactions in Suxamethonium Chloride, p.1408.

**Antiepileptics.** Resistance to competitive neuromuscular blockers has been reported in patients receiving chronic treatment with *carbamazepine*[1,2] or *phenytoin*[3,4] and rapid recovery from neuromuscular block may occur. In addition, children on chronic antiepileptic drugs (carbamazepine and/or phenytoin) were found to recover quicker from rocuronium-induced paralysis than those not on antiepileptics[5]. In a study[6] with cisatracurium, faster recovery rates were also recorded in patients receiving acute or chronic treatment with unspecified antiepileptics. However, atracurium[1] and mivacurium[7] appear to be unaffected by chronic carbamazepine therapy and the effect of chronic phenytoin treatment on atracurium has usually been minimal.[3] Although one study[8] did report that epileptic patients receiving one or more antiepileptics had significantly shorter times to recovery from atracurium, the authors pointed out that the patient populations were different from those in the previous studies.[1,3]

A report of sensitivity to vecuronium[9] has suggested that acute administration of phenytoin may increase rather than decrease the effect of competitive neuromuscular blockers.

1. Ebrahim Z, *et al.* Carbamazepine therapy and neuromuscular blockade with atracurium and vecuronium. *Anesth Analg* 1988; **67:** S55.
2. Whalley DG, Ebrahim Z. Influence of carbamazepine on the dose-response relationship of vecuronium. *Br J Anaesth* 1994; **72:** 125–6.
3. Ornstein E, *et al.* The effect of phenytoin on the magnitude and duration of neuromuscular block following atracurium or vecuronium. *Anesthesiology* 1987; **67:** 191–6.
4. Hernández-Palazón J, *et al.* Rocuronium-induced neuromuscular blockade is affected by chronic phenytoin therapy. *J Neurosurg Anesthesiol* 2001; **13:** 79–81.
5. Soriano SG, *et al.* Onset and duration of action of rocuronium in children receiving chronic anticonvulsant therapy. *Paediatr Anaesth* 2000; **10:** 133–6.
6. Koenig HM, Edwards TL. Cisatracurium-induced neuromuscular blockade in anticonvulsant treated neurosurgical patients. *J Neurosurg Anesthesiol* 2000; **12:** 314–18.
7. Spacek A, *et al.* Chronic carbamazepine therapy does not influence mivacurium-induced neuromuscular block. *Br J Anaesth* 1996; **77:** 500–502.
8. Tempelhoff R, *et al.* Resistance to atracurium-induced neuromuscular blockade in patients with intractable seizure disorders treated with anticonvulsants. *Anesth Analg* 1990; **71:** 665–9.
9. Baumgardner JE, Bagshaw R. Acute versus chronic phenytoin therapy and neuromuscular blockade. *Anaesthesia* 1990; **45:** 493–4.

**Antineoplastics.** It has been recommended that atracurium should be used with care in patients receiving anti-oestrogenic drugs,[1] following a case of prolonged neuromuscular blockade with atracurium in a patient receiving *tamoxifen*. See also under Interactions in Suxamethonium Chloride, p.1408.

1. Naguib M, Gyasi HK. Antiestrogenic drugs and atracurium—a possible interaction? *Can Anaesth Soc J* 1986; **33:** 682–3.

**Aprotinin.** Following reports of apnoea, caution has been advised when aprotinin is used with neuromuscular blockers.[1,2]


1. Chasapakis G, Dimas C. Possible interaction between muscle relaxants and the kallikrein-trypsin inactivator "Trasylol". *Br J Anaesth* 1966; **38:** 838–9.
2. Marcello B, Porati U. Trasylol e blocco neuromuscolare: nota preventiva. *Minerva Anestesiol* 1967; **33:** 814–5.


**Benzodiazepines.** There are conflicting reports of the effect of *diazepam* on neuromuscular blockers; potentiation,[1,2] or antagonism[1] of neuromuscular block, and a lack of interaction[3-5] have all been reported.


1. Feldman SA, Crawley BE. Interaction of diazepam with the muscle-relaxant drugs. *BMJ* 1970; **2:** 336–8.
2. Yuan H-B, *et al.* The interaction of diazepam with vecuronium: a clinical study. *Chin Med J* 1994; **54:** 259–64.
3. Bradshaw EG, Maddison S. Effect of diazepam at the neuromuscular junction. *Br J Anaesth* 1979; **51:** 955–60.
4. Asbury AJ, *et al.* Effect of diazepam on pancuronium-induced neuromuscular blockade maintained by a feedback system. *Br J Anaesth* 1981; **53:** 859–63.
5. Driessen JJ, *et al.* Benzodiazepines and neuromuscular blocking drugs in patients. *Acta Anaesthesiol Scand* 1986; **30:** 642–6.


**Beta blockers.** There is conflicting evidence for the effect of beta blockers on the activity of neuromuscular blockers. Lack of effect on depolarising neuromuscular block[1] and antagonism[2,3] or enhancement[4,5] of both competitive and depolarising block have been reported. The exact mechanism of interaction is not clear. There have also been reports of some neuromuscular blockers such as atracurium[6,7] and alcuronium[8] increasing the hypotension and bradycardia associated with the use of anaesthesia in patients receiving beta blockers; these include reports in patients using beta blockers in eye drops for glaucoma.


1. McCammon RL, *et al.* The effect of esmolol on the onset and duration of succinylcholine-induced neuromuscular blockade. *Anesthesiology* 1985; **63:** A317.
2. Varma YS, *et al.* Effect of propranolol hydrochloride on the neuromuscular blocking action of d-tubocurarine and succinylcholine in man. *Indian J Med Res* 1972; **60:** 266–72.
3. Varma YS, *et al.* Comparative effect of propranolol, oxprenolol and pindolol on neuromuscular blocking action of d-tubocurarine in man. *Indian J Med Res* 1973; **61:** 1382–6.
4. Rozen MS, Whan FM. Prolonged curarization associated with propranolol. *Med J Aust* 1972; **1:** 467–8.
5. Murthy VS, *et al.* Cardiovascular and neuromuscular effects of esmolol during induction of anesthesia. *J Clin Pharmacol* 1986; **26:** 351–7.
6. Glynne GL. Drug Interaction? *Anaesthesia* 1984; **39:** 293.
7. Rowlands DE. Drug Interaction? *Anaesthesia* 1984; **39:** 1252.
8. Yate B, Mostafa SM. Drug Interaction? *Anaesthesia* 1984; **39:** 728.


**Botulinum A toxin.** The neuromuscular block induced by botulinum toxins (p.1389) is enhanced by competitive neuromuscular blockers.

**Calcium-channel blockers.** Calcium-channel blockers such as diltiazem, nicardipine, nifedipine, and verapamil enhance the effect of competitive neuromuscular blockers.[1-6] *Verapamil* may interfere with the release of acetylcholine and prolonged administration may lead to a reduction in intracellular calcium concentration. Potentiation of neuromuscular blockade has been reported[1,6] and the block may be resistant to reversal with neostigmine; edrophonium may be required. The dose requirement for vecuronium was reduced by as much as 50% in surgical patients receiving *diltiazem*.[2,3] A similar effect was seen with *nicardipine*,[4] which reduced the requirement for vecuronium in a dose-dependent fashion. The interaction of vecuronium with diltiazem appeared to be due to a pharmacodynamic mechanism[2] but nicardipine also reduced the plasma clearance of vecuronium, indicating a partial pharmacokinetic mechanism as well.[4] *Nifedipine* also caused an increase in the intensity and duration of action of atracurium and vecuronium when given during anaesthesia.[5]


1. van Poorten JF, *et al.* Verapamil and reversal of vecuronium neuromuscular blockade. *Anesth Analg* 1984; **63:** 155–7.
2. Sumikawa K, *et al.* Reduction in vecuronium infusion dose requirements by diltiazem in humans. *Anesthesiology* 1992; **77:** A939.
3. Takasaki Y, *et al.* Diltiazem potentiates the neuromuscular blockade by vecuronium in humans. *Jpn J Anesthesiol* 1995; **44:** 503–7.
4. Kawabata K, *et al.* Decrease in vecuronium infusion dose requirements by nicardipine in humans. *Anesth Analg* 1994; **79:** 1159–64.
5. Jelen-Esselborn S, Blobner M. Wirkungsverstärkung von nichtdepolarisierenden Muskelrelaxanzien durch Nifedipin i.v. in Inhalationsanaesthesie. *Anaesthesist* 1990; **39:** 173–8.
6. Jones RM, *et al.* Verapamil potentiation of neuromuscular blockade: failure of reversal with neostigmine but prompt reversal with edrophonium. *Anesth Analg* 1985; **64:** 1021–5.


**Cardiac inotropes.** Pancuronium or suxamethonium may interact with *cardiac glycosides*[1] resulting in an increased incidence of arrhythmias; the interaction is more likely with pancuronium.


1. Bartolone RS, Rao TLK. Dysrhythmias following muscle relaxant administration in patients receiving digitalis. *Anesthesiology* 1983; **58:** 567–9.


**Corticosteroids.** Antagonism of the neuromuscular blocking effects of pancuronium[1] and vecuronium[2] has been reported in patients taking corticosteroids. This interaction may occur only with long-term corticosteroid treatment and may be expected with all competitive neuromuscular blockers.

For reference to a suggestion that concomitant use of corticosteroids might increase the risk of acute myopathy associated with prolonged use of neuromuscular blockers, see under Intensive Care, p.1398.


1. Azar I, *et al.* Resistance to pancuronium in an asthmatic patient treated with aminophylline and steroids. *Can Anaesth Soc J* 1982; **29:** 280–2.
2. Parr SM, *et al.* Betamethasone-induced resistance to vecuronium: a potential problem in neurosurgery? *Anaesth Intensive Care* 1991; **19:** 103–5.


**Diuretics.** *Furosemide*, and possibly *mannitol*, have been reported to enhance tubocurarine neuromuscular block in patients with renal failure,[1] but antagonism of tubocurarine by furosemide has also occurred.[2] Small doses of furosemide (less than 100 micrograms/kg) may inhibit protein kinase, which inhibits muscle contraction and potentiates neuromuscular blockade, whereas high doses inhibit phosphodiesterase, increasing cAMP activity and resulting in antagonism of neuromuscular blockade. The potassium-depleting effect of diuretics may enhance the effect of competitive neuromuscular blockers.


1. Miller RD, *et al.* Enhancement of d-tubocurarine neuromuscular blockade by diuretics in man. *Anesthesiology* 1976; **45:** 442–5.
2. Azar I, *et al.* Furosemide facilitates recovery of evoked twitch response after pancuronium. *Anesth Analg* 1980; **59:** 55–7.


**Ganglion blockers.** Prolonged neuromuscular blockade has been reported[1,2] in patients receiving neuromuscular blockers and *trimetaphan*. Trimetaphan may have direct neuromuscular blocking activity and some activity against plasma cholinesterase.


1. Wilson SL, *et al.* Prolonged neuromuscular blockade associated with trimethaphan: a case report. *Anesth Analg Curr Res* 1976; **55:** 353–6.
2. Poulton TH, *et al.* Prolonged apnea following trimethaphan and succinylcholine. *Anesthesiology* 1979; **50:** 54–6.


**General anaesthetics.** Neuromuscular blockers are potentiated in a dose-dependent manner by inhalation anaesthetics.[1-5] The dose of neuromuscular blocker may need to be reduced by up to 70%[1] depending on the anaesthetic used and its concentration, and on the choice of blocker; the interaction is of greater clinical importance with competitive blockers. *Isoflurane, enflurane, desflurane*, and *sevoflurane* produce the greater potentiation, followed by *halothane* and *cyclopropane*. Reversal of competitive block with an anticholinesterase has been reported to be reduced.[6,7] See also under Interactions in Suxamethonium Chloride, p.1408.

Potentiation of the neuromuscular blocking effects of tubocurarine[8] and atracurium[9] has been reported following the intravenous administration of *ketamine*. Results from studies *in vitro* suggest that ketamine decreases sensitivity to acetylcholine and it would therefore be expected to potentiate all neuromuscular blockers, but no interaction was reported for pancuronium.[8] Early data[10] suggesting that ketamine potentiates suxamethonium-induced blockade have not been confirmed by later studies.[8,11]

For incompatibility between neuromuscular blockers and alkaline solutions such as thiopental sodium, see under Incompatibility, above.


1. Cannon JE, *et al.* Continuous infusion of vecuronium: the effect of anesthetic agents. *Anesthesiology* 1987; **67:** 503–6.
2. Swen J, *et al.* Interaction between nondepolarizing neuromuscular blocking agents and inhalation anesthetics. *Anesth Analg* 1989; **69:** 752–5.
3. Ghourin AF, White PF. Comparative effects of desflurane and isoflurane on vecuronium-induced neuromuscular blockade. *J Clin Anesth* 1992; **4:** 34–8.
4. Vanlinthout LEM, *et al.* Effect of isoflurane and sevoflurane on the magnitude and time course of neuromuscular block produced by vecuronium, pancuronium and atracurium. *Br J Anaesth* 1996; **76:** 389–95.
5. Wulf H, *et al.* Augmentation of the neuromuscular blocking effects of cisatracurium during desflurane, sevoflurane, isoflurane or total i.v. anaesthesia. *Br J Anaesth* 1998; **80:** 308–12.
6. Delisle S, Bevan DR. Impaired neostigmine antagonism of pancuronium during enflurane anaesthesia in man. *Br J Anaesth* 1982; **54:** 441–5.
7. Gill SS, *et al.* Edrophonium antagonism of atracurium during enflurane anaesthesia. *Br J Anaesth* 1990; **64:** 300–5.
8. Johnston RR, *et al.* The interaction of ketamine with d-tubocurarine, pancuronium, and succinylcholine in man. *Anesth Analg Curr Res* 1974; **53:** 496–501.
9. Toft P, Helbo-Hansen S. Interaction of ketamine with atracurium. *Br J Anaesth* 1989; **62:** 319–20.
10. Bovill JG, *et al.* Current status of ketamine anaesthesia. *Lancet* 1971; **i:** 1285–8.
11. Helbo-Hansen HS, *et al.* Ketamine does not affect suxamethonium-induced neuromuscular blockade in man. *Eur J Anaesthesiol* 1989; **6:** 419–23.


**Histamine $H_2$-antagonists.** There are conflicting reports of the effects of histamine $H_2$-antagonists on neuromuscular blockade. *Cimetidine* has been variously reported to prolong suxamethonium-induced paralysis[1] or to have no effect.[2] *Famotidine* and *ranitidine* have been reported[2] not to interact with suxamethonium. Cimetidine, but not ranitidine, has been reported[3] to delay recovery from vecuronium-induced neuromuscular block. Neither drug appeared to affect recovery after the use of atracurium.


1. Kambam JR, *et al.* Effect of cimetidine on duration of action of succinylcholine. *Anesth Analg* 1987; **66:** 191–2.
2. Turner DR, *et al.* Neuromuscular block by suxamethonium following treatment with histamine type 2 antagonists or metoclopramide. *Br J Anaesth* 1989; **63:** 348–50.
3. McCarthy G, *et al.* Effect of H2-receptor antagonist pretreatment on vecuronium- and atracurium-induced neuromuscular blockade. *Br J Anaesth* 1991; **66:** 713–15.


**Immunosuppressants.** Antagonism of the neuromuscular blocking effects of competitive neuromuscular blockers has been reported with *azathioprine*,[1] although the effect may not be clinically important. Azathioprine probably inhibits phosphodiesterase activity at the motor nerve terminal resulting in increased release of acetylcholine. There have been reports of prolonged neuromuscular blockade with atracurium, pancuronium, and vecuronium in some patients receiving *ciclosporin* intravenously.[2,3] This effect has been attributed to an interaction with polyethoxylated castor oil used as the solvent for intravenous ciclosporin but a similar reaction has been reported in a patient receiving ciclosporin by mouth.[4]


1. Gramstad L. Atracurium, vecuronium and pancuronium in end-stage renal failure: dose-response properties and interaction with azathioprine. *Br J Anaesth* 1987; **59:** 995–1003.
2. Crosby E, Robblee JA. Cyclosporine-pancuronium interaction in a patient with a renal allograft. *Can J Anaesth* 1988; **35:** 300–2.
3. Sidi A, *et al.* Prolonged neuromuscular blockade and ventilatory failure after renal transplantation and cyclosporine. *Can J Anaesth* 1990; **37:** 543–8.
4. Ganjoo P, Tewari P. Oral cyclosporine-vecuronium interaction. *Can J Anaesth* 1994; **41:** 1017.


**Lithium.** There have been isolated reports of prolonged neuromuscular blockade following the use of neuromuscular blockers in patients receiving lithium.[1,2]


1. Borden H, *et al.* The use of pancuronium bromide in patients receiving lithium carbonate. *Can Anaesth Soc J* 1974; **21:** 79–82.
2. Hill GE, *et al.* Potentiation of succinylcholine neuromuscular blockade by lithium carbonate. *Anesthesiology* 1976; **44:** 439–42.


**Local anaesthetics.** Healthy subjects who had undergone regional anaesthesia of the forearm experienced symptoms suggestive of local anaesthetic toxicity on deflation of the tourniquet cuff when mivacurium and *prilocaine* had been used together for anaesthesia;[1] administration of prilocaine or mivacurium alone did not produce such an effect. The suggestion that mivacurium may alter vascular permeability, allowing a more rapid diffusion of prilocaine back into the blood from the tissues, should be investigated.[2]

The interaction between neuromuscular blockers and *lidocaine* is discussed under Antiarrhythmics above.


1. Torrance JM, *et al.* Low-dose mivacurium supplementation of prilocaine i.v. regional anaesthesia. *Br J Anaesth* 1997; **78:** 222–3.
2. Torrance JM, *et al.* Interactions between mivacurium and prilocaine. *Br J Anaesth* 1997; **78:** 262.


**Magnesium salts.** Parenteral magnesium salts may potentiate the effects of competitive and depolarising neuromuscular blockers;[1] the neuromuscular block is deepened and prolonged and a reduction in the dose of the blocker may be needed. Magnesium salts should be used with caution in the postoperative period, as use shortly after recovery from neuromuscular block can lead to recurarisation.[2] Magnesium salts reduce release of and sensitivity to acetylcholine, thus contributing to neuromuscular blockade.


1. Ghoneim MM, Long JP. The interaction between magnesium and other neuromuscular blocking agents. *Anesthesiology* 1970; **32:** 23–7.
2. Fuchs-Buder T, Tassonyi E. Magnesium sulphate enhances residual neuromuscular block induced by vecuronium. *Br J Anaesth* 1996; **76:** 565–6.


**MAOIs.** There appears to be a theoretical hazard with pancuronium in patients receiving MAOIs since it releases stored adrenaline;[1] alcuronium, atracurium, or vecuronium would appear to be suitable alternatives.


1. Stack CG, *et al.* Monoamine oxidase inhibitors and anaesthesia: a review. *Br J Anaesth* 1988; **60:** 222–7.


**Neuromuscular blockers.** A competitive neuromuscular blocker given shortly before a depolarising blocker such as suxamethonium antagonises the depolarising neuromuscular block. This interaction has been used clinically to reduce muscle fasciculations caused by suxamethonium (see Anaesthesia, p.1397 and Effects on the Muscles, p.1406) and tried for other adverse effects associated with suxamethonium (see Effects on Plasma-potassium Concentration, p.1407). To achieve this antagonism a small non-paralysing dose of a competitive blocker is given before suxamethonium. If a paralysing dose of a competitive blocker is followed some time later with a dose of suxamethonium, for example to facilitate abdominal closure, the resulting neuromuscular block is influenced by the competitive blocker used, the depth of residual block, the dose of suxamethonium, and whether an anticholinesterase is given; antagonism, enhancement, and a combination of the two have been seen.[1,2]

A competitive blocker is often given following the short-acting suxamethonium to maintain neuromuscular blockade during long procedures. The action of the competitive blocker has been reported to be considerably potentiated and prolonged in these circumstances,[3,4] and reduction in the dose of the competitive blocker may be appropriate.

Combination of competitive blockers may have additive or synergistic effects and the interaction may differ depending on which blocker is given first. Caution is needed if a small dose of a shorter-acting blocker is given near the end of an operation in which a long-acting blocker has been given previously, since the resulting block may be greater than expected and much longer than desired.[5-7]


1. Scott RPF, Norman J. Effect of suxamethonium given during recovery from atracurium. *Br J Anaesth* 1988; **61:** 292–6.
2. Black AMS. Effect of suxamethonium given during recovery from atracurium. *Br J Anaesth* 1989; **62:** 348–9.

3. d'Hollander AA, *et al.* Clinical and pharmacological actions of a bolus injection of suxamethonium: two phenomena of distinct duration. *Br J Anaesth* 1983; **55:** 131–4.
4. Ono K, *et al.* Influence of suxamethonium on the action of subsequently administered vecuronium or pancuronium. *Br J Anaesth* 1989; **62:** 324–6.
5. Rashkovsky OM, *et al.* Interaction between pancuronium bromide and vecuronium bromide. *Br J Anaesth* 1985; **57:** 1063–6.
6. Middleton CM, *et al.* Use of atracurium or vecuronium to prolong the action of tubocurarine. *Br J Anaesth* 1989; **62:** 659–63.
7. Kim KS, *et al.*Interactions between mivacurium and pancuronium. *Br J Anaesth* 1997; **79:** 19–23.

**Sex hormones.** Resistance to the neuromuscular blocking effects of suxamethonium and vecuronium in a patient was attributed to previous long-term therapy with *testosterone*,[1] although the exact mechanism could not be explained. See also under Interactions in Suxamethonium Chloride, p.1408.

1. Reddy P, *et al.* Resistance to muscle relaxants in a patient receiving prolonged testosterone therapy. *Anesthesiology* 1989; **70:** 871–3.

**Smoking.** Preliminary work suggests that smoking might affect the dose requirements for neuromuscular blockers. One study[1] found that smokers needed more vecuronium than non-smokers; it was considered that the effect might be explained at the receptor level, although increased metabolism of vecuronium could not be excluded. In contrast, an earlier study[2] found the amount of atracurium required was reduced in smokers.

1. Teiriä H, *et al.* Effect of smoking on dose requirements for vecuronium. *Br J Anaesth* 1996; **76:** 154–5.
2. Kroeker KA, *et al.* Neuromuscular blockade in the setting of chronic nicotine exposure. *Anesthesiology* 1994; **81:** A1120.

**Sympathomimetics.** Intravenous *salbutamol* has been reported to enhance the blockade obtained with pancuronium and vecuronium.[1] See also under Interactions in Suxamethonium Chloride, p.1408.

1. Salib Y, Donati F. Potentiation of pancuronium and vecuronium neuromuscular blockade by intravenous salbutamol. *Can J Anaesth* 1993; **40:** 50–3.

**Xanthines.** Resistance to neuromuscular block with pancuronium, requiring an increase in dosage or transfer to vecuronium, has been reported in patients receiving *aminophylline* with[1] or without[2] corticosteroid therapy. It was suggested that this effect might be due to inhibition of phosphodiesterase by aminophylline resulting in increased release of acetylcholine at the nerve terminal.

1. Azar I, *et al.* Resistance to pancuronium in an asthmatic patient treated with aminophylline and steroids. *Can Anaesth Soc J* 1982; **29:** 280–2.
2. Daller JA, *et al.* Aminophylline antagonizes the neuromuscular blockade of pancuronium but not vecuronium. *Crit Care Med* 1991; **19:** 983–5.

## Pharmacokinetics

Following intravenous injection both atracurium besilate and cisatracurium besilate undergo spontaneous degradation via Hofmann elimination (a non-enzymatic breakdown process occurring at physiological pH and temperature) to produce laudanosine and other metabolites. There is also ester hydrolysis by non-specific plasma esterases. The metabolites have no neuromuscular blocking activity.

About 80% of atracurium besilate is bound to plasma proteins. Atracurium besilate and its metabolites cross the placenta in clinically insignificant amounts. Excretion of atracurium and cisatracurium is in urine and bile, mostly as metabolites. The elimination half-life has been reported to be about 20 minutes for atracurium and 22 to 29 minutes for cisatracurium but laudanosine has an elimination half-life of about 3 to 6 hours.

◊ Reviews.

1. Kisor DF, Schmith VD. Clinical pharmacokinetics of cisatracurium besilate. *Clin Pharmacokinet* 1999; **36:** 27–40.
2. Atherton DPL, Hunter JM. Clinical pharmacokinetics of the newer neuromuscular blocking drugs. *Clin Pharmacokinet* 1999; **36:** 169–89.
3. Booij LHDJ, Vree TB. Skeletal muscle relaxants: pharmacodynamics and pharmacokinetics in different patient groups. *Int J Clin Pract* 2000; **54:** 526–34.

**Biotransformation.** Atracurium and cisatracurium are degraded by Hofmann elimination and metabolised by non-specific plasma esterases. Hofmann elimination is generally believed to be the main route of degradation but *in-vitro* work suggests ester hydrolysis is more important.[1] Both routes are independent of renal and hepatic function and no dosage reduction is recommended for elderly patients or those with impaired renal or hepatic function. However, the elimination half-life of atracurium has been found to be slightly longer in elderly patients[2] and in those with hepatic cirrhosis[3] compared with young and healthy patients, although others[4] have found no change in the pharmacokinetics of atracurium in the elderly. Renal and hepatic involvement in the metabolism of atracurium[2] may help to explain any tendency to reduced elimination but this does not appear to be clinically significant. Although clearance of cisatracurium has been reported to be reduced in patients with renal failure[5] this appears to have little significant effect on its pharmacodynamics.[6] Differences in the pharmacokinetics of cisatracurium in patients with hepatic impairment have been reported to be minor.[7]

The major biotransformation product of atracurium and cisatracurium is *laudanosine*; it has no clinical neuromuscular blocking activity but has been associated with CNS stimulation in *animal* studies. It is more lipid soluble than atracurium and cisatracurium and has a half-life of around 3 hours compared with one of approximately 20 minutes for atracurium. Higher plasma-laudanosine concentrations have been reported in patients with renal failure[5,8,9] than in patients with normal renal function. The elimination half-life of laudanosine was found to be significantly greater in patients with hepatic cirrhosis[3] and in elderly patients[2] compared with healthy and young patients respectively. High plasma-laudanosine concentrations were also observed in 10 critically ill patients with acute respiratory distress syndrome;[10] no adverse effects were noted.

Laudanosine crosses the blood-brain barrier in man. The concentration of laudanosine in the CSF increases during an infusion of atracurium and the CSF-to-plasma ratio gradually increases. A ratio of 0.14 was found at 125 to 140 minutes[11] during an infusion of atracurium at a mean rate of 510 micrograms/kg per hour. No evidence of CNS stimulation has been reported in man although patients given atracurium[12] had a 20% higher mean arterial-thiopental concentration at awakening compared with patients given vecuronium, suggesting that laudanosine may have had a minor stimulatory effect on the CNS. The blood-brain barrier appears to be effective in preventing a very high concentration of laudanosine from reaching the CNS and it is considered unlikely[13] that concentrations great enough to provoke seizures will be reached. Cisatracurium may be associated with the production of less laudanosine than atracurium.[14]

1. Stiller RL, *et al.* In vitro degradation of atracurium in human plasma. *Br J Anaesth* 1985; **57:** 1085–8.
2. Kent AP, *et al.* Pharmacokinetics of atracurium and laudanosine in the elderly. *Br J Anaesth* 1989; **63:** 661–6.
3. Parker CJR, Hunter JM. Pharmacokinetics of atracurium and laudanosine in patients with hepatic cirrhosis. *Br J Anaesth* 1989; **62:** 177–83.
4. d'Hollander AA, *et al.* Clinical evaluation of atracurium besylate requirement for a stable muscle relaxation during surgery: lack of age-related effects. *Anesthesiology* 1983; **59:** 237–40.
5. Eastwood NB, *et al.* Pharmacokinetics of 1R-cis 1'R-cis atracurium besylate (51W89) and plasma laudanosine concentrations in health and chronic renal failure. *Br J Anaesth* 1995; **75:** 431–5.
6. Boyd AH, *et al.* Pharmacodynamics of the 1R cis-1'R cis isomer of atracurium (51W89) in health and chronic renal failure. *Br J Anaesth* 1995; **74:** 400–404.
7. De Wolf AM, *et al.* Pharmacokinetics and pharmacodynamics of cisatracurium in patients with end-stage liver disease undergoing liver transplantation. *Br J Anaesth* 1996; **76:** 624–8.
8. Fahey MR, *et al.* Effect of renal failure on laudanosine excretion in man. *Br J Anaesth* 1985; **57:** 1049–51.
9. Vandenbrom RHG, *et al.* Pharmacokinetics and neuromuscular blocking effects of atracurium besylate and two of its metabolites in patients with normal and impaired renal function. *Clin Pharmacokinet* 1990; **19:** 230–40.
10. Farenc C, *et al.* Pharmacokinetic-pharmacodynamic modeling of atracurium in intensive care patients. *J Clin Pharmacol* 2001; **41:** 44–50.
11. Eddleston JM, *et al.* Concentrations of atracurium and laudanosine in cerebrospinal fluid and plasma during intracranial surgery. *Br J Anaesth* 1989; **63:** 525–30.
12. Beemer GH, *et al.* Production of laudanosine following infusion of atracurium in man and its effects on awakening. *Br J Anaesth* 1989; **63:** 76–80.
13. Yate PM, *et al.* Clinical experience and plasma laudanosine concentrations during the infusion of atracurium in the intensive therapy unit. *Br J Anaesth* 1987; **59:** 211–17.
14. Boyd AH, *et al.* Comparison of the pharmacokinetics and pharmacodynamics of an infusion of cis-atracurium (51W89) or atracurium in critically ill patients undergoing mechanical ventilation in an intensive therapy unit. *Br J Anaesth* 1996; **76:** 382–8.

## Uses and Administration

Competitive neuromuscular blockers act by competing with acetylcholine for receptors on the motor end-plate of the neuromuscular junction to produce blockade. The muscles that produce fine rapid movements such as those of the face are the first to be affected followed by those of the limbs and torso; the last to be affected are those of the diaphragm. The paralysis is reversible with recovery occurring in reverse order. Restoration of normal neuromuscular function can be hastened by increasing the concentration of acetylcholine at the motor end-plate by giving an anticholinesterase such as neostigmine.

Atracurium and cisatracurium are competitive benzylisoquinolinium neuromuscular blockers. The commercial preparation of atracurium is a mixture of 10 stereoisomers of which cisatracurium constitutes about 15%. Cisatracurium, the *R-cis,1'R-cis*-isomer of atracurium, is about 3 times more potent than the mixture of isomers of atracurium. Following an intravenous dose of atracurium, muscle relaxation begins in about 2 minutes and lasts for 15 to 35 minutes; onset may be slightly slower for cisatracurium.

Atracurium besilate and cisatracurium besilate are used for endotracheal intubation and to provide muscle relaxation in general anaesthesia for surgical procedures (see Anaesthesia, p.1397) and to aid controlled ventilation (see Intensive Care, p.1398).

Doses of neuromuscular blockers need to be carefully titrated for individual patients according to response, and may vary with the procedure, the other drugs given, and the state of the patient; monitoring of the degree of block is recommended in order to reduce the risk of overdosage.

For **atracurium besilate**, the usual initial dose for adults and children over 1 month of age is 300 to 600 micrograms/kg by intravenous injection. Subsequent doses of 100 to 200 micrograms/kg may be given as necessary, typically every 15 to 25 minutes for maintenance in prolonged procedures. It is recommended that in patients with cardiovascular disease the initial dose should be administered over a period of 60 seconds.

Atracurium besilate may also be given by continuous intravenous infusion at a rate of 5 to 10 micrograms/kg per minute to maintain neuromuscular block during prolonged procedures. Somewhat higher infusion rates may be used in patients undergoing controlled ventilation in intensive care.

**Cisatracurium** is given as the besilate but doses are expressed as the base. Cisatracurium 1 mg is approximately equivalent to 1.34 mg of cisatracurium besilate. The usual initial dose for adults is 150 micrograms/kg. The neuromuscular block may be extended with a maintenance dose of 30 micrograms/kg about every 20 minutes. The usual initial dose for children aged 1 month and over is 150 micrograms/kg. The neuromuscular block may be extended in children between 2 and 12 years of age with a maintenance dose of 20 micrograms/kg about every 9 minutes.

Cisatracurium besilate may also be given by continuous intravenous infusion to adults and children over 2 years of age at an initial rate equivalent to cisatracurium 3 micrograms/kg per minute followed by a rate of 1 to 2 micrograms/kg per minute after stabilisation.

◊ Reviews.

1. Hughes R. Atracurium—the first years. *Clin Anaesthesiol* 1985; **3:** 331–45.
2. Bryson HM, Faulds D. Cisatracurium besilate: a review of its pharmacology and clinical potential in anaesthetic practice. *Drugs* 1997; **53:** 848–66.

**Administration in infants and children.** Children generally require larger doses of competitive neuromuscular blockers on a weight basis than adolescents or adults to achieve similar degrees of neuromuscular blockade and may recover more quickly. In contrast, neonates and infants under 1 year of age are more sensitive and usual doses may produce prolonged neuromuscular blockade.

References.

1. Brandom BW, Fine GF. Neuromuscular blocking drugs in pediatric anesthesia. *Anesthesiol Clin North America* 2002; **20:** 45–58.

**Electroconvulsive therapy.** Competitive neuromuscular blockers have been used to reduce the intensity of muscle contractions and minimise trauma in patients receiving ECT, but suxamethonium (p.1409) is generally preferred because of its short duration of action.

**Intravenous regional anaesthesia.** Competitive neuromuscular blockers and/or opioid analgesics have been added to the local anaesthetic used in intravenous regional anaesthesia (p.1370) to improve the quality of anaesthesia. However atracurium (see Tourniquets under Precautions, above) and mivacurium (see Tourniquets, p.1404) might be unsuitable for such use.

**Shivering.** Various drugs have been tried in the treatment of postoperative shivering (p.1295). There are reports of neuromuscular blockers being used to treat shivering after cardiac surgery in order to reduce cardiovascular stress;[1] one study[2] has suggested that vecuronium might be preferable to pancuronium as it does not increase myocardial work and may be associated with fewer complications.

1. Cruise C, *et al.* Comparison of meperidine and pancuronium for the treatment of shivering after cardiac surgery. *Can J Anaesth* 1992; **39:** 563–8.
2. Dupuis J-Y, *et al.* Pancuronium or vecuronium for the treatment of shivering after cardiac surgery. *Anesth Analg* 1994; **79:** 472–81.

**Tetanus.** For a comment on the role of competitive neuromuscular blockers in the management of muscle spasms caused by tetanus, see p.1398.

### Preparations

**USP 27:** Atracurium Besylate Injection.

**Proprietary Preparations** (details are given in Part 3)
***Arg.:*** Gelolagar; Nimbex; Tracrium; Tracurix; Tracuron; ***Austral.:*** Nimbex; Tracrium; ***Austria:*** Nimbex; Tracrium; ***Belg.:*** Nimbex; Tracrium; ***Braz.:*** Abbottracurium; Atracur†; Nimbium; Sitrac; Tracrium; Tracur; ***Canad.:*** Nimbex; Tracrium†; ***Chile:*** Nimbex; Tracrium; ***Denm.:*** Nimbex; Tracrium; ***Fin.:*** Nimbex; Tracrium†; ***Fr.:*** Nimbex; Tracrium; ***Ger.:*** Nimbex; Tracrium; ***Gr.:*** Nimbex; Tracrium; ***Hong Kong:*** Nimbex; Tracrium; ***India:*** Tracrium; ***Irl.:*** Nimbex; Tracrium; ***Israel:*** Mycurium; Tracrium; ***Ital.:*** Nimbex; Tracrium; ***Malaysia:*** Nimbex; Tracrium; ***Mex.:*** Ifacur; Nimbex; Relatrac; Trablok; Tracrium; ***Neth.:*** Nimbex; Tracrium; ***Norw.:*** Nimbex; Tracrium†; ***NZ:*** Tracrium; ***Port.:*** Faulcurium; Nimbex; Tracrium†; ***S.Afr.:*** Nimbex; Tracrium; ***Singapore:*** Nimbex; Tracrium; ***Spain:*** Laurak; Nimbex; Tracrium; ***Swed.:*** Nimbex; Tracrium; ***Switz.:*** Nimbex; Tracrium; ***Thai.:*** Nimbex; Tracrium; ***UK:*** Nimbex; Tracrium; ***USA:*** Nimbex; Tracrium.

## Doxacurium Chloride *(BAN, USAN, rINN)*

BW-A938U; Cloruro de doxacurio. A mixture of the (1*R*,1′*S*,2*S*,2′*R*), (1*R*,1′*R*,2*S*,2′*S*), and (1*S*,1′*S*,2*R*,2′*R*) stereoisomers (a *meso* isomer and two enantiomers respectively) of 1,1′,2,2′,3,3′,4,4′-octahydro-6,6′,7,7′,8,8′-hexamethoxy-2,2′-dimethyl-1,1′-bis(3,4,5-trimethoxybenzyl)-2,2′-[butanedioylbis(oxytrimethylene)]di-isoquinolinium dichloride, all of which are in a *trans* configuration at the 1 and 2 positions of the isoquinolinium rings.

$C_{56}H_{78}Cl_2N_2O_{16}$ = 1106.1.

*CAS — 133814-18-3 (doxacurium); 106819-53-8 (doxacurium chloride, meso isomer); 83348-52-1 (doxacurium chloride, total racemate).*

*ATC — M03AC07.*

### Adverse Effects, Treatment, and Precautions

As for competitive neuromuscular blockers in general (see Atracurium, p.1399). Doxacurium has little histamine-releasing activity and causes negligible vagal or sympathetic blockade so that significant cardiovascular side-effects are not a problem.

**Renal impairment.** Although the duration of neuromuscular block and speed of recovery following the use of doxacurium were found to be prolonged in patients with renal failure when compared with patients with normal renal function, the differences were not significant.[1]

1. Cashman JN, *et al.* Neuromuscular block with doxacurium (BW A938U) in patients with normal or absent renal function. *Br J Anaesth* 1990; **64:** 186–92.

### Interactions

For interactions associated with competitive neuromuscular blockers, see Atracurium, p.1400.

### Pharmacokinetics

Following intravenous administration, doxacurium chloride is excreted mainly unchanged in the urine and bile. The elimination half-life is reported to be about 2 hours.

◊ Reviews.

1. Atherton DPL, Hunter JM. Clinical pharmacokinetics of the newer neuromuscular blocking drugs. *Clin Pharmacokinet* 1999; **36:** 169–89.

### Uses and Administration

Doxacurium chloride is a benzylisoquinolinium competitive neuromuscular blocker (see Atracurium, p.1402). It is used for endotracheal intubation and to provide muscle relaxation in general anaesthesia for surgical procedures (see Anaesthesia, p.1397) and to aid controlled ventilation (see under Intensive Care, below).

Doses of neuromuscular blockers need to be carefully titrated for individual patients according to response, and may vary with the procedure, the other drugs given, and the state of the patient; monitoring of the degree of block is recommended in order to reduce the risk of overdosage. Doxacurium is given as the chloride although doses are expressed in terms of the equivalent amount of doxacurium base. The usual initial dose is 50 micrograms/kg intravenously; maintenance doses of 5 to 10 micrograms/kg are employed. At the above dose muscle relaxation occurs within about 5 minutes and the effect lasts for about 100 minutes. For longer procedures an initial dose of 80 micrograms/kg may be used, which produces muscle relaxation in about 4 minutes and the effects last for about 2½ hours.

◊ Reviews.

1. Mirakhur RK. Newer neuromuscular blocking drugs: an overview of their clinical pharmacology and therapeutic use. *Drugs* 1992; **44:** 182–99.

**Administration in the elderly.** Several studies have shown that the duration of action of doxacurium is prolonged in the elderly, although the precise mechanism for this is subject to debate.[1-3] Since both the onset of action and recovery are delayed, some consider[4] that doxacurium may not be suitable for use in the elderly for surgical procedures of less than one hour.

1. Levy G. Effect of advanced age on the pharmacodynamics of doxacurium. *Clin Pharmacol Ther* 1994; **55:** 359.
2. Varin F, *et al.* Effect of advanced age on the pharmacodynamics of doxacurium. *Clin Pharmacol Ther* 1994; **55:** 359–60.
3. Schmith VD, *et al.* Effect of advanced age on the pharmacodynamics of doxacurium. *Clin Pharmacol Ther* 1994; **55:** 360–2.
4. Martlew RA, Harper NJN. The clinical pharmacology of doxacurium in young adults and in elderly patients. *Anaesthesia* 1995; **50:** 779–82.

**Administration in infants and children.** As for some other neuromuscular blockers, children over 2 years of age have been found to require more doxacurium per kg body-weight than adults to achieve a similar degree of neuromuscular blockade,[1] and the dosage requirement may be almost twice as great as that for adults.[2] Children may also recover more quickly.[1] However, the sensitivity of infants under one year of age appears to be increased.[2]

1. Goudsouzian NG, *et al.* Neuromuscular and cardiovascular effects of doxacurium in children anaesthetized with halothane. *Br J Anaesth* 1989; **62:** 263–8.
2. Taivainen T, Meretoja OA. Doxacurium in infants, children and adolescents during balanced anaesthesia. *Br J Anaesth* 1995; **74** (suppl 1): 98–9.

**Intensive care.** Experience of the use of doxacurium to facilitate mechanical ventilation in patients in intensive care (see p.1398) is relatively limited. It appears to offer prolonged neuromuscular block without the tachycardia associated with pancuronium; recovery after prolonged use may also be faster than with pancuronium.[1] There has been an anecdotal report of the successful management with doxacurium of 4 patients who had developed tachyphylaxis to long-term administration of atracurium.[2]

1. Murray MJ, *et al.* Double-blind, randomized multicenter study of doxacurium vs. pancuronium in intensive care unit patients who require neuromuscular-blocking agents. *Crit Care Med* 1995; **23:** 450–8.
2. Coursin DB, *et al.* Doxacurium infusion in critically ill patients with atracurium tachyphylaxis. *Am J Health-Syst Pharm* 1995; **52:** 635–9.

### Preparations

**Proprietary Preparations** (details are given in Part 3)
***Canad.:*** Nuromax; ***USA:*** Nuromax.

## Gallamine Triethiodide *(BANM, rINN)*

Benzcurine Iodide; Gallamini Triethiodidum; Gallamone Triethiodide; Trietioduro de galamina. 2,2′,2″-(Benzene-1,2,3-triyltrioxy)tris(tetraethylammonium) tri-iodide.

$C_{30}H_{60}I_3N_3O_3$ = 891.5.

*CAS — 153-76-4 (gallamine); 65-29-2 (gallamine triethiodide).*

*ATC — M03AC02.*

**Pharmacopoeias.** In *Eur.* (see p.vi), *Int.*, and *US.*

**Ph. Eur. 5.0** (Gallamine Triethiodide). A white, or almost white, hygroscopic powder. Very soluble in water; slightly soluble in alcohol; practically insoluble in dichloromethane. Store in airtight containers. Protect from light.

**USP 27** (Gallamine Triethiodide). A white, hygroscopic, odourless, amorphous powder. Very soluble in water; sparingly soluble in alcohol; very slightly soluble in chloroform. pH of a 2% solution in water is between 5.3 and 7.0. Store in airtight containers. Protect from light.

### Adverse Effects, Treatment, and Precautions

As for competitive neuromuscular blockers in general (see Atracurium, p.1399). Tachycardia often develops due to the vagolytic action of gallamine triethiodide and blood pressure may be raised. It has a small histamine-releasing effect; occasional anaphylactoid reactions have been reported. It should be avoided in patients hypersensitive to iodine and in severe renal impairment. Although competitive muscle relaxants have been given with great care to patients with myasthenia gravis (see Neuromuscular Disorders, p.1400), the manufacturer of gallamine triethiodide recommends that it should not be used in such patients.

**Cardiopulmonary bypass.** Alterations in the pharmacokinetics of competitive neuromuscular blockers in patients undergoing surgery involving cardiopulmonary bypass usually necessitate the use of reduced doses (see p.1399). However, the pharmacokinetics of gallamine in patients undergoing cardiopulmonary bypass appear not to differ significantly from those in control patients.[1]

1. Shanks CA, *et al.* Gallamine disposition in open-heart surgery involving cardiopulmonary bypass. *Clin Pharmacol Ther* 1983; **33:** 792–9.

**Renal impairment.** Gallamine triethiodide is excreted unchanged in the urine and the manufacturers consider that it should be avoided in severe renal impairment since prolonged paralysis may occur. Significantly prolonged elimination half-life and reduced clearance have been reported[1] in patients with chronic renal failure given gallamine triethiodide in initial doses of 2 mg/kg intravenously.

1. Ramzan MI, *et al.* Gallamine disposition in surgical patients with chronic renal failure. *Br J Clin Pharmacol* 1981; **12:** 141–7.

### Interactions

For interactions associated with competitive neuromuscular blockers, see Atracurium, p.1400.

### Pharmacokinetics

Following intravenous administration gallamine triethiodide is distributed throughout body tissues. It is not metabolised, and is excreted in the urine as unchanged drug.

### Uses and Administration

Gallamine triethiodide is a benzylisoquinolinium competitive neuromuscular blocker (see Atracurium, p.1402). Muscle relaxation occurs within about 1 to 2 minutes following intravenous injection and lasts for about 20 to 30 minutes. It is used to provide muscle relaxation in general anaesthesia for surgical procedures (see Anaesthesia, p.1397) and to aid controlled ventilation (see Intensive Care, p.1398).

Doses of neuromuscular blockers need to be carefully titrated for individual patients according to response, and may vary with the procedure, the other drugs given, and the state of the patient; monitoring of the degree of block is recommended in order to reduce the risk of overdosage. An initial test dose of 20 mg may be given intravenously to the patient before anaesthesia to determine undue sensitivity. In the UK, initial doses of 80 to 120 mg by intravenous injection have been recommended, with further doses of 20 to 40 mg as required. In children, a dose of 1.5 mg/kg has been recommended, reduced to 600 micrograms/kg for neonates.

In the USA and some other countries lower doses have generally been used; an initial dose of 1 mg/kg intravenously, up to a maximum of 80 mg, with additional doses of 0.5 to 1 mg/kg after about 50 to 60 minutes if required.

Gallamine triethiodide has also been given intramuscularly, with or without hyaluronidase.

### Preparations

**BP 2003:** Gallamine Injection;
**USP 27:** Gallamine Triethiodide Injection.

**Proprietary Preparations** (details are given in Part 3)
***Austral.:*** Flaxedil†; ***Braz.:*** Flaxedil†; ***Canad.:*** Flaxedil†; ***Denm.:*** Relaxan†; ***Neth.:*** Flaxedil†; ***Spain:*** Miowas G†; ***UK:*** Flaxedil.

## Metocurine Iodide *(USAN)*

Dimethyl Tubocurarine Iodide; (+)-*O*,*O*′-Dimethylchondrocurarine Di-iodide; Dimethyltubocurarine Iodide; Dimetiltubocurarinio, ioduro de; Trimethyltubocurarine Iodide. (+)-6,6′,7′,12′-Tetramethoxy-2,2,2′,2′-tetramethyltubocuraranium di-iodide.

$C_{40}H_{48}I_2N_2O_6$ = 906.6.

*CAS — 5152-30-7 (metocurine); 7601-55-0 (metocurine iodide).*

*ATC — M03AA04.*

### Profile

Metocurine iodide is a benzylisoquinolinium competitive neuromuscular blocker (see Atracurium, p.1402) that has been used to provide muscle relaxation in surgical and other procedures.

Metocurine iodide has a moderate risk of inducing histamine release; it also has some ganglion blocking activity.

### Preparations

**Proprietary Preparations** (details are given in Part 3)
***Canad.:*** Metubine†; ***USA:*** Metubine†.

## Mivacurium Chloride *(BAN, USAN, rINN)*

BW-B1090U; Cloruro de mivacurio. A mixture of the stereoisomers of (*E*)-1,1′,2,2′,3,3′,4,4′-octahydro-6,6′,7,7′-tetramethoxy-2,2′-dimethyl-1,1′-bis(3,4,5-trimethoxybenzyl)-2,2′-[oct-4-enedioylbis(oxytrimethylene)]di-isoquinolinium dichloride.

$C_{58}H_{80}Cl_2N_2O_{14}$ = 1100.2.

*CAS — 106861-44-3 (mivacurium chloride, total racemate).*

*ATC — M03AC10.*

**Incompatibility.** See under Atracurium, p.1399 for details regarding the incompatibility of neuromuscular blockers.

### Adverse Effects, Treatment, and Precautions

As for competitive neuromuscular blockers in general (see Atracurium, p.1399). Mivacurium chloride has no significant vagal or ganglion blocking activity at recommended doses. It may induce histamine release especially when given in large doses rapidly.

Mivacurium should be used with caution, if at all, in patients with plasma cholinesterase deficiency, since its duration of action will be prolonged in such patients.

**Burns.** In common with other competitive muscle relaxants patients with burns may develop resistance to mivacurium and require increased doses (see under Atracurium, p.1399). However, as these patients may also have reduced plasma cholinesterase activity dosage requirements could also be reduced. The manufacturer recommends that such patients should be given a test dose of 15 to 20 micrograms/kg with subsequent dosage adjustments being guided by monitoring of the block.

**Neuromuscular disorders.** Neuromuscular blockade was successfully achieved with mivacurium in an obese elderly patient with myasthenia gravis requiring surgery.[1] Only about half the usual dose was required and even then recovery was delayed. See Atracurium, p.1400 for a discussion of the use of competitive neuromuscular blockers in patients with neuromuscular disorders.

1. Seigne RD, Scott RPF. Mivacurium chloride and myasthenia gravis. *Br J Anaesth* 1994; **72:** 468–9.

**Plasma cholinesterase deficiency.** There have been reports of prolonged neuromuscular block produced by mivacurium in patients with plasma cholinesterase deficiency.[1-4] Time to full recovery had varied; a patient required up to 8 hours.

1. Goudsouzian NG, *et al.* Prolonged neuromuscular block from mivacurium in two patients with cholinesterase deficiency. *Anesth Analg* 1993; **77:** 183–5.
2. Sockalingam I, Green DW. Mivacurium-induced prolonged neuromuscular block. *Br J Anaesth* 1995; **74:** 234–6.
3. Fox MH, Hunt PCW. Prolonged neuromuscular block associated with mivacurium. *Br J Anaesth* 1995; **74:** 237–8.
4. Zimmer S. Mivacurium and prolonged neuromuscular block. *Br J Anaesth* 1995; **75:** 823.

**Tourniquets.** Mivacurium might be unsuitable for neuromuscular blockade of a limb which has been isolated with a tourniquet in order to provide a bloodless field for surgery.[1] It is largely inactivated by the enzymatic action of plasma cholinesterase and would therefore continue to degrade locally leading to a loss of blockade in the limb, which could not be corrected by further doses unless the tourniquet was deflated. However, as for other competitive neuromuscular blockers, the use of mivacurium to supplement regional anaesthesia has produced prolonged muscle weakness well beyond cuff deflation.[2] This suggests that mivacurium is not broken down in the ischaemic limb and that recovery is not dependent on plasma concentrations of mivacurium.
See also Local Anaesthetics, under Interactions in Atracurium, p.1401, for a report of symptoms suggestive of local anaesthetic toxicity when prilocaine and mivacurium were used together.

1. Shannon PF. Neuromuscular block and tourniquets. *Br J Anaesth* 1994; **73:** 726.
2. Torrance JM, *et al.* Low-dose mivacurium supplementation of prilocaine i.v. regional anaesthesia. *Br J Anaesth* 1997; **78:** 222–3.

## Interactions

For interactions associated with competitive neuromuscular blockers, see Atracurium, p.1400.

**Metoclopramide.** Metoclopramide, an inhibitor of plasma cholinesterase, was found to significantly prolong the duration of action of mivacurium in patients undergoing surgery, although in this study only marginal inhibition of plasma cholinesterase by metoclopramide occurred.

1. Skinner HJ, *et al.* Influence of metoclopramide on plasma cholinesterase and duration of action of mivacurium. *Br J Anaesth* 1999; **82:** 542–5.

## Pharmacokinetics

Mivacurium is a mixture of 3 stereoisomers, 2 of which (*cis-trans* and *trans-trans*) are considered to account for most of the neuromuscular blocking effect. All 3 isomers are inactivated by plasma cholinesterase. Renal and hepatic mechanisms are involved in their elimination with excretion in urine and bile.

◊ Reviews.

1. Atherton DPL, Hunter JM. Clinical pharmacokinetics of the newer neuromuscular blocking drugs. *Clin Pharmacokinet* 1999; **36:** 169–89.

## Uses and Administration

Mivacurium chloride is a benzylisoquinolinium competitive neuromuscular blocker (see Atracurium, p.1402).

Following intravenous injection muscle relaxation occurs within 1.5 to 2.5 minutes, depending on the dose with a duration of action of about 10 to 20 minutes. It is used for endotracheal intubation and to provide muscle relaxation in general anaesthesia for surgical procedures (see Anaesthesia, p.1397) and to aid controlled ventilation (see Intensive Care, p.1398).

Doses of neuromuscular blockers need to be carefully titrated for individual patients according to response, and may vary with the procedure, the other drugs given, and the state of the patient; monitoring of the degree of block is recommended in order to reduce the risk of overdosage. Mivacurium is given as the chloride although doses are expressed in terms of mivacurium base. The initial dose by intravenous injection is 70 to 250 micrograms/kg. Doses up to 150 micrograms/kg may be administered over 5 to 15 seconds but higher doses should be given over 30 seconds. In patients with asthma or cardiovascular disease, or those who are sensitive to falls in arterial blood pressure, administration should be over 60 seconds. To give a dose of 250 micrograms/kg for tracheal intubation, an injection of 150 micrograms/kg may be followed 30 seconds later by an injection of 100 micrograms/kg. Maintenance doses of 100 micrograms/kg may be given at intervals of 15 minutes. In children aged 2 to 6 months an initial dose of 150 micrograms/kg has been given; in children aged 7 months to 12 years, an initial dose of 200 micrograms/kg has been given. A maintenance dose of 100 micrograms/kg may be given every 6 to 9 minutes for children aged 2 months to 12 years. Mivacurium chloride may also be given by continuous intravenous infusion for maintenance of block. For adults the initial rate is 8 to 10 micrograms/kg per minute adjusted every 3 minutes if necessary by increments of 1 microgram/kg per minute to a usual rate of 6 to 7 micrograms/kg per minute; in children aged 2 months to 12 years the usual dose is 11 to 14 micrograms/kg per minute.

Reduced doses may be required in the elderly and in patients with hepatic or renal impairment (see below). For obese patients weighing more than 30% over their ideal body-weight the manufacturer recommends that the initial dose should be based upon their ideal body-weight and not actual body-weight.

◊ Reviews.

1. Mirakhur RK. Newer neuromuscular blocking drugs: an overview of their clinical pharmacology and therapeutic use. *Drugs* 1992; **44:** 182–99.
2. Frampton JE, McTavish D. Mivacurium: a review of its pharmacology and therapeutic potential in general anaesthesia. *Drugs* 1993; **45:** 1066–89.
3. Feldman S. Mivacurium. *Br J Hosp Med* 1997; **57:** 199–201.

**Action.** Mivacurium has a shorter duration of action than most other competitive neuromuscular blockers. Studies[1-3] suggest that it is a useful alternative to suxamethonium for the production of neuromuscular block of short duration and has the advantage that its block can be reversed with an anticholinesterase. For a discussion of the choice of anticholinesterase for reversal of neuromuscular block produced by short-acting blockers such as mivacurium, see under Neostigmine, p.1493. Although its onset of action may be accelerated by giving a priming dose,[4] mivacurium has a slower onset than suxamethonium and so may not be a suitable alternative[5] when rapid intubation is required. For a general review of neuromuscular blockers, see Anaesthesia, p.1397.

1. Brandom BW, *et al.* Comparison of mivacurium and suxamethonium administered by bolus and infusion. *Br J Anaesth* 1989; **62:** 488–93.
2. Caldwell JE, *et al.* Comparison of the neuromuscular block induced by mivacurium, suxamethonium or atracurium during nitrous oxide-fentanyl anaesthesia. *Br J Anaesth* 1989; **63:** 393–9.
3. Goldberg ME, *et al.* Comparison of tracheal intubating conditions and neuromuscular blocking profiles after intubating doses of mivacurium chloride or succinylcholine in surgical outpatients. *Anesth Analg* 1989; **69:** 93–9.
4. Haxby EJ, *et al.* Mivacurium priming intervals. *Br J Anaesth* 1994; **72:** 485P.
5. Anonymous. Mivacurium—a new neuromuscular blocker. *Med Lett Drugs Ther* 1992; **34:** 82.

**Administration in the elderly.** In a study[1] comparing the effects of mivacurium in elderly and young adults, the duration of neuromuscular effects was prolonged in elderly patients by about 30%. The mean infusion requirement in elderly patients was 3.67 micrograms/kg per minute compared with 5.5 micrograms/kg per minute in young adults.
The manufacturers state that elderly patients may require decreased infusion rates or smaller or less frequent maintenance bolus doses.

1. Maddineni VR, *et al.* Neuromuscular and haemodynamic effects of mivacurium in elderly and young adult patients. *Br J Anaesth* 1994; **73:** 608–12.

**Administration in hepatic or renal impairment.** The pharmacokinetics of mivacurium have been studied in patients with renal[1-3] or hepatic impairment.[1,4,5] The duration of relaxation produced by mivacurium was about 1.5 times greater than normal in patients with end-stage renal disease and up to about 3 times greater than normal in patients with end-stage liver disease. Reduced plasma-cholinesterase activity in the patients with hepatic impairment may have played an important part in this effect. Although an anticholinesterase such as neostigmine hastens recovery by only a few minutes in healthy subjects, its use may be indicated in patients in whom recovery is delayed.[2]
The manufacturers recommend that, in patients with end-stage renal or liver disease, the dose should be adjusted according to individual clinical response.

1. Cook DR, *et al.* Pharmacokinetics of mivacurium in normal patients and in those with hepatic or renal failure. *Br J Anaesth* 1992; **69:** 580–5.
2. Phillips BJ, Hunter JM. Use of mivacurium chloride by constant infusion in the anephric patient. *Br J Anaesth* 1992: **68:** 492–8.
3. Head-Rapson AG, *et al.* Pharmacokinetics and pharmacodynamics of the three isomers of mivacurium in health, in end-stage renal failure and in patients with impaired renal function. *Br J Anaesth* 1995; **75:** 31–6.
4. Devlin JC, *et al.* Pharmacodynamics of mivacurium chloride in patients with hepatic cirrhosis. *Br J Anaesth* 1993; **71:** 227–31.
5. Head-Rapson AG, *et al.* Pharmacokinetics of the three isomers of mivacurium and pharmacodynamics of the chiral mixture in hepatic cirrhosis. *Br J Anaesth* 1994; **73:** 613–18.

## Preparations

**Proprietary Preparations** (details are given in Part 3)
**Arg.:** Mivacron; **Austral.:** Mivacron; **Austria:** Mivacron; Novacrium; **Belg.:** Mivacron; **Braz.:** Mivacron; **Canad.:** Mivacron; **Chile:** Mivacron; **Denm.:** Mivacron; **Fin.:** Mivacron; **Fr.:** Mivacron; **Ger.:** Mivacron; **Gr.:** Mivacron; **Hong Kong:** Mivacron; **Irl.:** Mivacron; **Israel:** Mivacron; **Ital.:** Mivacron; **Malaysia:** Mivacron; **Mex.:** Mivacron†; **Neth.:** Mivacron; **Norw.:** Mivacron; **NZ:** Mivacron; **Port.:** Mivacron†; **S.Afr.:** Mivacron; **Singapore:** Mivacron; **Spain:** Mivacron; **Swed.:** Mivacron; **Switz.:** Mivacron; **Thai.:** Mivacron†; **UK:** Mivacron; **USA:** Mivacron.

# Pancuronium Bromide *(BAN, USAN, rINN)*

Bromuro de pancuronio; NA-97; Org-NA-97; Pancuronii Bromidum. 1,1′-(3α,17β-Diacetoxy-5α-androstan-2β,16β-ylene)bis(1-methylpiperidinium) dibromide.

$C_{35}H_{60}Br_2N_2O_4$ = 732.7.
*CAS — 15500-66-0.*
*ATC — M03AC01.*

**Pharmacopoeias.** In *Eur.* (see p.vi) and *Jpn.*
**Ph. Eur. 5.0** (Pancuronium Bromide). White or almost white, hygroscopic crystalline powder. Very soluble to freely soluble in water; freely soluble in alcohol; very soluble in dichloromethane. Store in airtight containers. Protect from light.

## Adverse Effects, Treatment, and Precautions

As for competitive neuromuscular blockers in general (see Atracurium, p.1399).

Pancuronium has vagolytic and sympathomimetic action which may cause tachycardia and hypertension, but does not produce ganglionic blockade. It has little histamine-releasing effect. Hypersensitivity reactions are relatively rare but bradycardia, bronchospasm, hypotension, and cardiovascular collapse have been reported. Pancuronium has been associated with excessive salivation in some patients.

Pancuronium should be used with caution in patients with raised catecholamine concentrations, or in those who are receiving drugs with sympathomimetic effects, as cardiovascular side-effects are more likely in these patients.

**Effects on the ears.** A study[1] found that neonates who survived congenital diaphragmatic hernia were more likely to suffer from sensorineural hearing loss after prolonged administration of pancuronium bromide during the neonatal period. However, the authors commented that the association is not necessarily causal and that further investigation is required.

1. Cheung P-Y, *et al.* Prolonged use of pancuronium bromide and sensorineural hearing loss in childhood survivors of congenital diaphragmatic hernia. *J Pediatr* 1999; **135:** 233–9.

**Hypersensitivity.** Reports of anaphylactoid or anaphylactic reactions associated with pancuronium bromide.
See also under Suxamethonium Chloride, p.1407.

1. Brauer FS, Ananthanarayan CR. Histamine release by pancuronium. *Anesthesiology* 1978; **49:** 434–5.
2. Patriarca G, *et al.* Pancuronium allergy: a case report. *Br J Anaesth* 1989; **62:** 210–12.
3. Moneret-Vautrin DA, *et al.* Simultaneous anaphylaxis to thiopentone and a neuromuscular blocker: a study of two cases. *Br J Anaesth* 1990; **64:** 743–5.
4. Sanchez-Guerrero IM, *et al.* Anaphylactoid reaction induced by pancuronium during general anaesthesia. *Eur J Anaesthesiol* 1998; **15:** 613–14.

**Postoperative complications.** Because of its prolonged duration of action, pancuronium may be more likely than other neuromuscular blockers to produce residual neuromuscular block; such residual block is associated with an increased incidence of postoperative respiratory complications.[1,2]

1. Berg H, *et al.* Residual neuromuscular block is a risk factor for postoperative pulmonary complications: a prospective, randomised, and blinded study of postoperative pulmonary complications after atracurium, vecuronium and pancuronium. *Acta Anaesthesiol Scand* 1997; **41:** 1095–1103.
2. Bissinger U, *et al.* Postoperative residual paralysis and respiratory status: a comparative study of pancuronium and vecuronium. *Physiol Res* 2000; **49:** 455–62.

## Interactions

For interactions associated with competitive neuromuscular blockers, see Atracurium, p.1400.

## Pharmacokinetics

Following intravenous injection pancuronium bromide is rapidly distributed into body tissues; about 80% may be bound to plasma proteins. A small proportion is metabolised in the liver to metabolites with weak neuromuscular blocking activity. It is largely excreted in urine as unchanged drug and metabolites; a small amount is excreted in bile. The plasma elimination half-life is about 2 hours. It crosses the placenta in small amounts.

**Pregnancy.** In 15 patients undergoing caesarean section[1] given pancuronium bromide 100 micrograms/kg intravenously with other agents, mean maternal arterial and umbilical venous serum concentrations of pancuronium bromide and metabolites were

520 and 120 nanograms/mL, respectively at delivery (mean of 13 minutes after injection), giving a fetal to maternal ratio of 0.23.

1. Wingard LB, *et al.* Modified fluorometric quantitation of pancuronium bromide and metabolites in human maternal and umbilical serums. *J Pharm Sci* 1979; **68:** 914–15.

## Uses and Administration

Pancuronium bromide is an aminosteroidal competitive neuromuscular blocker (see Atracurium, p.1402). Muscle relaxation occurs within about 1.5 to 2 minutes of intravenous administration and lasts for about 45 to 60 minutes.

Pancuronium bromide is used for endotracheal intubation and to provide muscle relaxation in general anaesthesia for surgical procedures (see Anaesthesia, p.1397) and to aid controlled ventilation (see Intensive Care, p.1398).

Doses of neuromuscular blockers need to be carefully titrated for individual patients according to response, and may vary with the procedure, the other drugs given, and the state of the patient; monitoring of the degree of block is recommended in order to reduce the risk of overdosage. The initial dose for intubation is usually 50 to 100 micrograms/kg by intravenous injection, with maintenance doses of 10 to 20 micrograms/kg. Children may be given similar doses. Some manufacturers recommend a reduction in the initial dose to 20 to 60 micrograms/kg when pancuronium is given following suxamethonium. Doses of 30 to 40 micrograms/kg initially have been suggested in neonates, with maintenance doses of 10 to 20 micrograms/kg as necessary; in the USA, dosage based on an initial test dose of 20 micrograms/kg has been advocated for the neonate.

Adult patients under intensive care who require assisted ventilation for conditions such as intractable status asthmaticus or tetanus may be given 60 micrograms/kg intravenously every 1 to 1½ hours or less frequently.

Care should be taken when giving pancuronium to patients with hepatic or renal impairment, see below.

**Administration in hepatic impairment.** Prolonged neuromuscular blockade may occur in patients with liver disease given pancuronium bromide since increased elimination half-life with increased volume of distribution and reduced clearance has been reported.[1] However, the expanded distribution volume may necessitate an increase in the dose of pancuronium in these patients[1,2] and may be interpreted as resistance to the neuromuscular blocking effects of pancuronium.

1. Duvaldestin P, *et al.* Pancuronium pharmacokinetics in patients with liver cirrhosis. *Br J Anaesth* 1978; **50:** 1131–6.
2. Ward ME, *et al.* Althesin and pancuronium in chronic liver disease. *Br J Anaesth* 1975; **47:** 1199–1204.

**Administration in renal impairment.** Prolonged neuromuscular blockade may occur following administration of pancuronium to patients with severe renal impairment. Pancuronium distributes rapidly into extracellular fluid following intravenous injection and the initial neuromuscular blockade produced will depend upon the peak drug concentration in this fluid. Since extracellular fluid volume is increased in chronic renal failure such patients may require a larger initial dose of pancuronium and a 45% increase in dose requirement has been reported[1] in patients with end-stage renal failure. Renal excretion is the main route of elimination and prolonged elimination half-life with reduced clearance may be expected in renal failure; total dose requirements may be reduced. The main infusion rate of pancuronium to maintain 90% blockade in patients with end-stage renal failure was reported to be 61.5% less than for patients with normal renal function.

1. Gramstad L. Atracurium, vecuronium and pancuronium in end-stage renal failure. *Br J Anaesth* 1987; **59:** 995–1003.

**Fetal paralysis.** Pancuronium bromide 100 micrograms/kg of the estimated fetal-weight, and administered into the umbilical vein, produced fetal paralysis for about 40 minutes during intravascular exchange transfusion.[1] A dose of 200 to 300 micrograms/kg produced fetal paralysis for about 1 to 8 hours for more complicated transfusion procedures.[2] No adverse effects were reported.

1. Copel JA, *et al.* The use of intravenous pancuronium bromide to produce fetal paralysis during intravascular transfusion. *Am J Obstet Gynecol* 1988; **158:** 170–1.
2. Moise KJ, *et al.* Intravenous pancuronium bromide for fetal neuromuscular blockade during intrauterine transfusion for red-cell alloimmunization. *Obstet Gynecol* 1989; **74:** 905–8.

**Neuroleptic malignant syndrome.** Pancuronium is one of several drugs for which there have been isolated reports[1] of success in the management of neuroleptic malignant syndrome (p.677).

1. Sangal R, Dimitrijevic R. Neuroleptic malignant syndrome: successful treatment with pancuronium. *JAMA* 1985; **254:** 2795–6.

### Preparations

***BP 2003:*** Pancuronium Injection.

**Proprietary Preparations** (details are given in Part 3)
***Arg.:*** Bemicin; Pancuron; Pavulon; Plumger; ***Austral.:*** Pavulon; ***Austria:*** Pavulon†; ***Braz.:*** Pancuron†; Pavulon; ***Canad.:*** Pavulon†; ***Chile:*** Pavulon; ***Denm.:*** Pavulon; ***Fin.:*** Pavulon; ***Fr.:*** Pavulon; ***Gr.:*** Pavulon; ***Hong Kong:*** Pavulon; ***India:*** Panconium; ***Irl.:*** Pavulon; ***Israel:*** Pavulon; ***Ital.:*** Pavulon; ***Malaysia:*** Pavulon; ***Mex.:*** Bromurex; Minoprest†; Panlem; Parulon†; Pavulon†; ***Neth.:*** Pavulon; ***Norw.:*** Pavulon; ***Port.:*** Pancurox; Pavulon; ***S.Afr.:*** Curon-B†; Pavulon; ***Singapore:*** Pavulon; ***Spain:*** Pavulon; ***Swed.:*** Pavulon; ***Switz.:*** Pavulon; ***Thai.:*** Pavulon; ***UK:*** Pavulon†; ***USA:*** Pavulon.

## Pipecuronium Bromide *(BAN, USAN, rINN)*

Bromuro de pipecuronio; Pipecurium Bromide; RGH-1106. 1,1,1′,1′-Tetramethyl-4,4′-(3α,17β-diacetoxy-5α-androstan-2β,16β-diyl)dipiperazinium dibromide.
$C_{35}H_{62}Br_2N_4O_4$ = 762.7.
*CAS — 52212-02-9 (anhydrous pipecuronium bromide); 68399-57-5 (pipecuronium bromide dihydrate).*
*ATC — M03AC06.*

### Profile

Pipecuronium bromide is an aminosteroidal competitive neuromuscular blocker (see Atracurium, p.1399). Pipecuronium is reported to have no significant cardiovascular adverse effects or histamine-related effects. Following intravenous injection muscle relaxation occurs within 2.5 to 3 minutes with a duration of action of about 30 minutes to 2 hours, depending on the dose.

Pipecuronium bromide has been used for endotracheal intubation and to provide muscle relaxation in general anaesthesia for surgical procedures (see Anaesthesia, p.1397) and to aid mechanical ventilation (see Intensive Care, p.1398).

Doses of neuromuscular blockers need to be carefully titrated for individual patients according to response, and may vary with the procedure, the other drugs given, and the state of the patient; monitoring of the degree of block is recommended in order to reduce the risk of overdosage. Initial doses of 80 to 100 micrograms/kg intravenously have been recommended, with subsequent doses of 10 to 20 micrograms/kg. Lower initial doses are given following suxamethonium or in patients at high risk: 50 to 60 micrograms/kg has been recommended, or 35 micrograms/kg for caesarean section.

◊ Reviews.

1. Mirakhur RK. Newer neuromuscular blocking drugs: an overview of their clinical pharmacology and therapeutic use. *Drugs* 1992; **44:** 182–99.

### Preparations

**Proprietary Preparations** (details are given in Part 3)
***Austria:*** Arpilon; ***Ital.:*** Arduan†; ***USA:*** Arduan†.

## Rapacuronium Bromide *(BAN, USAN, rINN)*

Bromuro de rapacuronio; Org-9487. 1-(3α-Acetoxy-2β-piperidino-17β-propionyloxy-5α-androstan-16β-yl)-1-allylpiperidinium bromide; 1-Allyl-1-(3α,17β-dihydroxy-2β-piperidino-5α-androstan-16β-yl)piperidinium bromide, 3-acetate 17-propionate.
$C_{37}H_{61}BrN_2O_4$ = 677.8.
*CAS — 156137-99-4.*

### Profile

Rapacuronium bromide, an analogue of vecuronium (p.1409), is an aminosteroidal competitive neuromuscular blocker (see Atracurium, p.1402). It was used to provide muscle relaxation in general anaesthesia for surgical procedures and for endotracheal intubation, but was withdrawn from the market following reports of severe bronchospasm, including fatalities.

◊ Reviews.

1. Wight WJ, Wright PMC. Pharmacokinetics and pharmacodynamics of rapacuronium bromide. *Clin Pharmacokinet* 2002; **41:** 1059–76.

### Preparations

**Proprietary Preparations** (details are given in Part 3)
***USA:*** Raplon†.

# Rocuronium Bromide *(BAN, USAN, rINN)*

Bromuro de rocuronio; Org-9426. 1-Allyl-1-(3α,17β-dihydroxy-2β-morpholino-5α-androstan-16β-yl)pyrrolidinium bromide 17-acetate; 1-(17β-Acetoxy-3α-hydroxy-2β-morpholino-5α-androstan-16β-yl)-1-allylpyrrolidinium bromide.
$C_{32}H_{53}BrN_2O_4$ = 609.7.
*CAS — 119302-91-9.*
*ATC — M03AC09.*

## Adverse Effects, Treatment, and Precautions

As for competitive neuromuscular blockers in general (see Atracurium, p.1399). Rocuronium is reported to have minimal cardiovascular and histamine-releasing effects. High doses (greater than 900 micrograms/kg of rocuronium bromide) have mild vagolytic activity. It should be used with caution in patients with biliary disease or hepatic or renal impairment.

**Hepatic impairment.** There have been conflicting reports of the pharmacokinetics and pharmacodynamics of rocuronium in patients with hepatic impairment. In contrast to earlier studies[1,2] one group of workers[3] found a significant reduction in the plasma clearance of rocuronium in patients with cirrhosis. The elimination half-life has been variously reported to be unchanged[1] or prolonged[2,3] with delayed recovery.[3] Some studies[2,3] found that the onset of action was not affected while one group of workers[1] reported a delay.

The manufacturers recommend that care should be taken when giving rocuronium to patients with clinically significant hepatic impairment, see under Uses and Administration, below.

1. Khalil M, *et al.* Pharmacokinetics and pharmacodynamics of rocuronium in patients with cirrhosis. *Anesthesiology* 1994; **80:** 1241–7.
2. Magorian T, *et al.* The pharmacokinetics and neuromuscular effects of rocuronium bromide in patients with liver disease. *Anesth Analg* 1995; **80:** 754–9.
3. van Miert MM, *et al.* The pharmacokinetics and pharmacodynamics of rocuronium in patients with hepatic cirrhosis. *Br J Clin Pharmacol* 1997; **44:** 139–44.

**Hypersensitivity.** Although rocuronium is considered to have minimal histamine-releasing effects, histaminoid reactions have been reported[1] on induction of anaesthesia in 3 patients who had been given rocuronium. An increased incidence of severe hypersensitivity reactions (particularly anaphylactic shock) has been reported with rocuronium compared with other neuromuscular blockers available in France.[2] Fatalities have occurred.[3]

See also the discussion of the relative risks of hypersensitivity associated with neuromuscular blockers, under Suxamethonium Chloride, p.1407.

1. Neal SM, *et al.* Histaminoid reactions associated with rocuronium. *Br J Anaesth* 2000; **84:** 108–11.
2. Mayer M. Information importante de pharmacovigilance: Esméron® et manifestations allergiques. Available at: http://agmed.sante.gouv.fr/htm/10/filltrpsc/letesmer.pdf (accessed 28/05/04)
3. Baillard C, *et al.* Anaphylaxis to rocuronium. *Br J Anaesth* 2002; **88:** 600–602.

**Pain on administration.** Severe transient burning pain associated with injection of rocuronium was considered[1] to be responsible for the spontaneous movement sometimes seen in the arm or wrist into which rocuronium is given. It is recommended that rocuronium should be given only when a deep stage of unconsciousness has been achieved.

1. Borgeat A, Kwiatkowski D. Spontaneous movements associated with rocuronium: is pain on injection the cause? *Br J Anaesth* 1997; **79:** 382–3.

**Renal impairment.** In a study[1] of the pharmacokinetics and neuromuscular effects of rocuronium, the clearance of rocuronium was reduced in patients with renal failure when compared with healthy patients, but the accompanying increase in duration of clinical relaxation did not reach statistical significance. However, it was recommended that rocuronium should be used with caution in the presence of renal failure as there were large inter-patient variations in both clinical response and pharmacokinetic parameters. It has been suggested[2] that chronic renal failure may have played a role in the prolongation of neuromuscular blockade in a 47-year-old woman given rocuronium 1 mg/kg. Although this dose is within the recommended adult dose range, it was criticised[3] as being excessive for a patient with renal impairment.

The manufacturer recommends that care should be taken when giving rocuronium to patients with renal failure, see under Uses and Administration, below.

1. Cooper RA, *et al.* Time course of neuromuscular effects and pharmacokinetics of rocuronium bromide (ORG 9426) during isoflurane anaesthesia in patients with and without renal failure. *Br J Anaesth* 1993; **71:** 222–6.
2. Lewis KS, *et al.* Prolonged neuromuscular blockade associated with rocuronium. *Am J Health-Syst Pharm* 1999; **56:** 1114–18.
3. Cozanitis DA, Booij HD. Muscle relaxants and renal failure. *Am J Health-Syst Pharm* 2000; **57:** 1713–14.

## Interactions

For interactions associated with competitive neuromuscular blockers, see Atracurium, p.1400.

## Pharmacokinetics

Following intravenous administration plasma concentrations of rocuronium follow a three compartment open model. There is an initial distribution phase with a half-life of 1 to 2 minutes followed by a slower distribution phase with a half-life of 14 to 18 minutes. It is reported to be about 30% bound to plasma proteins. The elimination half-life is about 1.2 to 1.4 hours. Up to 40% of a dose may be excreted in the urine within 24 hours; rocuronium is also excreted in the bile. The main metabolite of rocuronium, 17-desacetylrocuronium, is reported to have a weak neuromuscular blocking effect.

◊ References.

1. Khuenl-Brady KS, Sparr H. Clinical pharmacokinetics of rocuronium bromide. *Clin Pharmacokinet* 1996; **31:** 174–83.
2. McCoy EP, *et al.* Pharmacokinetics of rocuronium after bolus and continuous infusion during halothane anaesthesia. *Br J Anaesth* 1996; **76:** 29–33.
3. Wierda JMKH, *et al.* Pharmacokinetics and pharmacokinetic-dynamic modelling of rocuronium in infants and children. *Br J Anaesth* 1997; **78:** 690–5.
4. Atherton DPL, Hunter JM. Clinical pharmacokinetics of the newer neuromuscular blocking drugs. *Clin Pharmacokinet* 1999; **36:** 169–89.
5. Proost JH, *et al.* Urinary, biliary and faecal excretion of rocuronium in humans. *Br J Anaesth* 2000; **85:** 717–23.

**Intensive care.** The pharmacokinetics of rocuronium appear to differ between intensive care patients receiving prolonged administration and surgical patients.[1] The volume of distribution at steady state may be increased, the plasma clearance decreased, and the terminal half-life prolonged. Recovery time on discontinuation may also be longer.

1. Sparr HJ, *et al.* Pharmacodynamics and pharmacokinetics of rocuronium in intensive care patients. *Br J Anaesth* 1997; **78:** 267–73.

**Pregnancy.** The mean concentration of rocuronium in venous plasma of 32 patients given a dose of 600 micrograms/kg before undergoing caesarean section was 2412 nanograms/mL at delivery;[1] the ratio of mean concentrations of rocuronium in umbilical venous plasma to maternal venous plasma at this time was 0.16. In 12 of these patients the mean concentration of rocuronium in umbilical arterial plasma was 271 nanograms/mL giving a ratio of 0.62 for the mean concentration of rocuronium in arterial to venous umbilical plasma. The concentration of 17-desacetylrocuronium in maternal venous plasma was 178 nanograms/mL and was less than 25 nanograms/mL in umbilical plasma.

1. Abouleish E, *et al.* Rocuronium (Org 9426) for Caesarean section. *Br J Anaesth* 1994; **73:** 336–41.

## Uses and Administration

Rocuronium bromide is an aminosteroidal competitive neuromuscular blocker (see Atracurium, p.1402). Following intravenous injection it produces muscle relaxation within 1 to 2 minutes with a duration of about 30 to 50 minutes. Rocuronium bromide is used for endotracheal intubation and to provide muscle relaxation in general anaesthesia for surgical procedures (see Anaesthesia, p.1397) and to aid controlled ventilation (see Intensive Care, p.1398).

Doses of neuromuscular blockers need to be carefully titrated for individual patients according to response, and may vary with the procedure, the other drugs given, and the state of the patient; monitoring of the degree of block is recommended in order to reduce the risk of overdosage. A usual initial dose is 600 micrograms/kg by intravenous injection with maintenance doses of 150 micrograms/kg by injection; maintenance may also be by infusion at a rate of 300 to 600 micrograms/kg per hour although higher rates have been used in the USA. Similar doses to those used in adults have been used in the UK in infants and children older than one month but maintenance doses may be required more frequently. In the USA, rocuronium is licensed for use in children aged 3 months and over; again doses are similar to those used in adults.

For obese patients weighing more than 30% over their ideal body-weight the UK manufacturer recommends that doses should be calculated according to lean body-mass; in the USA the manufacturer recommends that dosage should be based on actual body-weight. The UK manufacturer also recommends reduced maintenance doses of 75 to 100 micrograms/kg by injection in the elderly. For doses in hepatic or renal impairment, see below.

◊ Reviews and discussions.

1. Mirakhur RK. Newer neuromuscular blocking drugs: an overview of their clinical pharmacology and therapeutic use. *Drugs* 1992; **44:** 182–9.
2. Hunter JM. Rocuronium: the newest aminosteroid neuromuscular blocking drug. *Br J Anaesth* 1996; **76:** 481–3.

**Administration in children.** In a study involving 70 children, conditions for intubation were judged to be good to excellent within one minute of intravenous administration of rocuronium 600 or 900 micrograms/kg, with a trend to better conditions with the higher dose.[1]

1. Fuchs-Buder T, Tassonyi E. Intubating conditions and time course of rocuronium-induced neuromuscular block in children. *Br J Anaesth* 1996; **77:** 335–8.

INTRAMUSCULAR ROUTE. Intramuscular injection of rocuronium 1 mg/kg into the deltoid muscle permitted tracheal intubation to be carried out in lightly anaesthetised infants after 2.5 minutes.[1] In children a dose of 1.8 mg/kg enabled tracheal intubation after 3 minutes. However, the mean time to initial recovery after these large doses was 57 minutes in infants and 70 minutes in children. This prolonged duration of action may limit intramuscular use for brief procedures, particularly in children.

1. Reynolds LM, *et al.* Intramuscular rocuronium in infants and children: dose-ranging and tracheal intubating conditions. *Anesthesiology* 1996; **85:** 231–9.

**Administration in hepatic or renal impairment.** The UK manufacturer recommends a reduced maintenance dose of 75 to 100 micrograms/kg in patients with hepatic or biliary-tract disease, or renal failure. Initial doses remain unaltered.

## Preparations

**Proprietary Preparations** (details are given in Part 3)
***Arg.:*** Zemuron; ***Austral.:*** Esmeron; ***Austria:*** Esmeron; ***Belg.:*** Esmeron; ***Braz.:*** Esmeron; ***Canad.:*** Zemuron; ***Chile:*** Esmeron; ***Denm.:*** Esmeron; ***Fin.:*** Esmeron; ***Fr.:*** Esmeron; ***Ger.:*** Esmeron; ***Gr.:*** Esmeron; ***Hong Kong:*** Esmeron; ***Irl.:*** Esmeron; ***Israel:*** Esmeron; ***Ital.:*** Esmeron; ***Malaysia:*** Esmeron; ***Neth.:*** Esmeron; ***Norw.:*** Esmeron; ***NZ:*** Esmeron; ***Port.:*** Esmeron; ***S.Afr.:*** Esmeron; ***Singapore:*** Esmeron; ***Spain:*** Esmeron; ***Swed.:*** Esmeron; ***Switz.:*** Esmeron; ***Thai.:*** Esmeron; ***UK:*** Esmeron; ***USA:*** Zemuron.

# Suxamethonium Chloride *(BAN, pINN)*

Choline Chloride Succinate; Cloruro de suxametonio; Succicurarium Chloride; Succinylcholine Chloride; Suxamethonii Chloridum; Suxametonklorid. 2,2′-Succinyldioxybis(ethyltrimethylammonium) dichloride dihydrate.

$C_{14}H_{30}Cl_2N_2O_4,2H_2O$ = 397.3.

*CAS — 306-40-1 (suxamethonium); 55-94-7 (suxamethonium bromide); 71-27-2 (anhydrous suxamethonium chloride); 6101-15-1 (suxamethonium chloride dihydrate); 541-19-5 (suxamethonium iodide).*

*ATC — M03AB01.*

**Pharmacopoeias.** In *Chin., Eur.* (see p.vi), *Int., Jpn, Pol.,* and *US.*

**Ph. Eur. 5.0** (Suxamethonium Chloride). A white or almost white, hygroscopic, crystalline powder. Freely soluble in water; slightly soluble in alcohol. A 0.5% solution in water has a pH of 4.0 to 5.0. Protect from light.

**USP 27** (Succinylcholine Chloride). A white, odourless, crystalline powder. The anhydrous form is hygroscopic. Soluble 1 in 1 of water and 1 in 350 of alcohol; slightly soluble in chloroform; practically insoluble in ether. Its solutions in water have a pH of about 4. Store in airtight containers at a temperature of 25°, excursions permitted between 15° and 30°.

**Incompatibility.** Incompatibilities of neuromuscular blockers are discussed under Atracurium, p.1399.

**Stability.** A study of the loss of potency of suxamethonium chloride 20 mg/mL in water indicated that decomposition occurred at a considerably higher rate at 40° than at 25° and that the pH range of maximum stability was 3.75 to 4.50 for unbuffered solutions.[1] Assuming the usual conditions of manufacturing, transit, and storage the total loss of potency was estimated to be 7% and 9% respectively for injections kept at room temperature for 4 and 6 weeks. If unbuffered, suxamethonium chloride injection complying with USP 27 pH limits (3.0 to 4.5) must be stored at room temperature; it should not be kept for longer than 4 weeks.

1. Boehm JJ, *et al.* Shelf life of unrefrigerated succinylcholine chloride injection. *Am J Hosp Pharm* 1984; **41:** 300–2.

## Adverse Effects

The neuromuscular blocking action of suxamethonium chloride is terminated by the enzyme plasma cholinesterase and prolonged apnoea may occur in patients with an atypical enzyme or with low enzyme activity. Apnoea may also occur following development of phase II block (see Uses and Administration, below) after high or repeated doses of suxamethonium chloride, although tachyphylaxis may also occur with repeated doses.

Transient fasciculations occur during the onset of depolarising block. Rhabdomyolysis, myoglobinaemia, and myoglobinuria have been reported and may be associated with muscle damage following fasciculations. Postoperative muscle pain occurs in some patients but is not directly related to the degree of fasciculation. A transient rise in intra-gastric pressure may occur secondary to fasciculation of abdominal muscles. A transient increase in intra-ocular pressure often occurs. Depolarisation of skeletal muscle produces an immediate increase in plasma-potassium concentration and this can have serious consequences in some patients (see below).

Stimulation of the vagus nerve and parasympathetic ganglia by suxamethonium chloride may be followed by bradycardia, other arrhythmias, and hypotension, and may be exacerbated by the raised plasma-potassium concentration; cardiac arrest has been reported. Tachycardia and an increase in blood pressure due to stimulation of sympathetic ganglia have also been reported.

Suxamethonium chloride may cause an increase in salivary, bronchial, and gastric secretion and other muscarinic effects. Salivary gland enlargement has occurred.

Direct release of histamine from mast cells occurs but this is not the main mechanism of hypersensitivity reactions (see Hypersensitivity, below). Flushing, skin rash, bronchospasm, and shock have been reported.

Other reported effects include prolonged respiratory depression and apnoea.

Suxamethonium chloride is implicated in the development of malignant hyperthermia (p.1394) in those patients with a genetic predisposition to the syndrome.

◊ Reviews of the adverse effects of suxamethonium.

1. Book WJ, *et al.* Adverse effects of depolarising neuromuscular blocking agents: incidence, prevention and management. *Drug Safety* 1994; **10:** 331–49.
2. Orebaugh SL. Succinylcholine: adverse effects and alternatives in emergency medicine. *Am J Emerg Med* 1999; **17:** 715–21.

**Effects on intra-ocular pressure.** Doses of suxamethonium are often followed 20 to 30 seconds later by a transient increase in intra-ocular pressure, which may be due in part to contracture of extra-ocular muscles. If suxamethonium is used during eye surgery after incision of the eyeball or to patients with a penetrating eye injury, there is a theoretical risk that any increase in intra-ocular pressure may result in extrusion of ocular contents and loss of sight. However, there appear to be few reports of vitreous extrusion associated with suxamethonium,[1] and a large retrospective study[2] has failed to find any evidence that suxamethonium caused additional eye damage in patients with penetrating eye injuries. Furthermore, the procedure of intubation itself is associated with a greater increase in intra-ocular pressure than that seen with suxamethonium. Nonetheless, some suggest that a rapid competitive neuromuscular blocker would be preferable to aid intubation in patients with penetrating eye injuries, after incision of the eyeball, and in glaucoma, although others consider that the risk of a transient rise of intra-ocular pressure in these situations should be weighed against the need for rapid intubation.[1,3] For a discussion on the use of various drugs to counteract the rise in intra-ocular pressure associated with suxamethonium and intubation in general, see under Anaesthesia, p.1397.

1. Book WJ, *et al.* Adverse effects of depolarising neuromuscular blocking agents: incidence, prevention and management. *Drug Safety* 1994; **5:** 331–49.
2. Libonati MM, *et al.* The use of succinylcholine in open eye surgery. *Anesthesiology* 1985; **62:** 637–40.
3. Edmondson L. Intraocular pressure and suxamethonium. *Br J Anaesth* 1997; **79:** 146.

**Effects on the muscles.** Muscle fasciculations and postoperative muscle pain commonly follow use of suxamethonium. Fasciculations (generalised and desynchronised contractions of skeletal muscle fibres) occur during the onset of depolarising block in almost all patients given suxamethonium and may cause muscle damage. They are seen especially in the 'fine' muscles of the hands and face, and can be useful as an indication that suxamethonium is working. Attempts have been made to prevent their development with the aim of reducing postoperative muscle pain. However, there appears to be no direct correlation between the extent of visible fasciculations and muscle pain.[1,2] Slow infusion of suxamethonium[3] or administration in divided doses[4] reduces fasciculations but not muscle pain.

Postoperative muscle pain is one of the most common side-effects of suxamethonium and has been noted in about 50% of patients, although the reported incidence varies widely from around 1.5 to about 90%.[2] It usually occurs on the first postoperative day and lasts for 2 or 3 days, and most commonly affects muscles of the neck, shoulders, and upper abdomen.[2] The incidence and severity of muscle pain is increased in patients who are mobile soon after surgery and in females, but it occurs less often in children, pregnant women, and the elderly.[2]

The mechanism of suxamethonium-induced muscle pain is not fully understood; there have been many attempts to prevent it. Pretreatment with a small dose of a competitive neuromuscular blocker reduces both visible fasciculations and the incidence and severity of muscle pain,[1,2,5-8] but may delay the onset and reduce the intensity of subsequent suxamethonium block[9] and impair conditions for intubation[1,9] (see Neuromuscular Blockers, under Interactions in Atracurium, p.1401). In addition, larger doses of suxamethonium are required;[10] consequently the practice is considered controversial by some authors.[10,11] Pretreatment with a small dose (10 mg) of suxamethonium in a 'self-taming' technique appears to offer no protection against muscle pain.[1,2] The choice of anaesthetic induction agent has been suggested to be significant, as has the timing of administration, but despite claims for benefit with, for example, propofol, this remains questionable.[2] Pretreatment with benzodiazepines or NSAIDs has produced conflicting results.[2] Other drugs that have been tried include lidocaine, calcium gluconate, and vitamin C; there is some evidence that lidocaine may be the most effective pretreatment.[2] Not all methods have concentrated on drug treatment. A simple regimen of stretching exercises before premedication has reduced the incidence of both fasciculations and postoperative muscle pain.[12]

Suxamethonium may also produce an increase in jaw tension (masseter spasm or trismus)[13] in both adults[14] and children[15,16] during the onset of neuromuscular blockade. Tracheal intubation is greatly hindered in affected patients. It is not possible to predict which patients will show this response and the mechanism is unknown, although in about 50% of patients it may indicate the onset of malignant hyperthermia. Pretreatment with a paralysing dose of a competitive neuromuscular blocker prevents the response[16] but it is not known whether this is clinically useful.


1. O'Sullivan EP, *et al.* Differential effects of neuromuscular blocking agents on suxamethonium-induced fasciculations and myalgia. *Br J Anaesth* 1988; **60:** 367–71.
2. Wong SF, Chung F. Succinylcholine-associated postoperative myalgia. *Anaesthesia* 2000; **55:** 144–52.
3. Feingold A, Velazquez JL. Suxamethonium infusion rate and observed fasciculations: a dose-response study. *Br J Anaesth* 1979; **51:** 241–5.
4. Wilson DB, Dundee JW. Failure of divided doses of succinylcholine to reduce the incidence of muscle pains. *Anesthesiology* 1980; **52:** 273–5.
5. Bennetts FE, Khalil KI. Reduction of post-suxamethonium pains by pretreatment with four non-depolarising agents. *Br J Anaesth* 1981; **53:** 531–6.
6. Erkola O, *et al.* Five non-depolarizing muscle relaxants in precurarization. *Acta Anaesthesiol Scand* 1983; **27:** 427–32.
7. Sosis M, *et al.* Comparison of atracurium and d-tubocurarine for prevention of succinylcholine myalgia. *Anesth Analg* 1987; **66:** 657–9.
8. Findlay GP, Spittal MJ. Rocuronium pretreatment reduces suxamethonium-induced myalgia: comparison with vecuronium. *Br J Anaesth* 1996; **76:** 526–9.
9. Pauca AL, *et al.* Inhibition of suxamethonium relaxation by tubocurarine and gallamine pretreatment during induction of anaesthesia in man. *Br J Anaesth* 1975; **47:** 1067–73.
10. McManus CM. Neuromuscular blockers in surgery and intensive care, part 2. *Am J Health-Syst Pharm* 2001; **58:** 2381–99.
11. Mencke T, *et al.* Pretreatment before succinylcholine for outpatient anesthesia? *Anesth Analg* 2002; **94:** 573–6.
12. Magee DA, Robinson RJS. Effect of stretch exercises on suxamethonium induced fasciculations and myalgia. *Br J Anaesth* 1987; **59:** 596–601.
13. Saddler JM. Jaw stiffness—an ill understood condition. *Br J Anaesth* 1991; **67:** 515–16.
14. Leary NP, Ellis FR. Masseteric muscle spasm as a normal response to suxamethonium. *Br J Anaesth* 1990; **64:** 488–92.
15. Van Der Spek AFL, *et al.* Changes in resistance to mouth opening induced by depolarizing and non-depolarizing neuromuscular relaxants. *Br J Anaesth* 1990; **64:** 21–7.
16. Smith CE, *et al.* Pretreatment with non-depolarizing neuromuscular blocking agents and suxamethonium-induced increases in resting jaw tension in children. *Br J Anaesth* 1990; **64:** 577–81.


**Effects on plasma-potassium concentration.** Suxamethonium causes depolarisation of motor end-plates in skeletal muscle, resulting in an immediate increase in plasma-potassium concentration. The rise is usually small, being about 0.5 mmol or less per litre, but suxamethonium is best avoided in patients whose plasma-potassium concentration is already high, such as those with renal impairment. An exaggerated response, with severe hyperkalaemia resulting in ventricular fibrillation and cardiac arrest, has been reported in patients with burns,[1,2] massive trauma, closed head injury, neuromuscular disease (see Neuromuscular Disorders, in Precautions, below), and severe long-lasting sepsis.[3] See also Children, in Precautions, below for reference to fatal cardiac arrest associated with hyperkalaemia in children. With burns or trauma the period of greatest risk is from about 10 to 90 days after the injury, but may be further prolonged if there is delayed healing or persistent infection. These patients may still react abnormally to suxamethonium 2 years after the injury. In neuromuscular disease the greatest risk period is usually from 3 weeks to 6 months after onset, but severe hyperkalaemia may occur after 24 to 48 hours or later than 6 months. Patients with severe sepsis for more than a week should be considered at risk of hyperkalaemia and suxamethonium should not be given until the infection has cleared. The mechanism of this hyperkalaemic response appears to be a supersensitivity of acetylcholine receptors in which the entire muscle fibre membrane, rather than discrete motor end-plate sites, becomes directly excitable by depolarising drugs. Depolarisation by suxamethonium thus results in release of potassium over the entire muscle fibre membrane and hyperkalaemia results.

Various methods have been tried to attenuate the hyperkalaemia, including pretreatment with a small dose of a competitive neuromuscular blocker[3,4] or with suxamethonium itself.[5,6] No method is reliable enough to be used clinically.

Anaesthetics such as thiopental and halothane can increase the hyperkalaemic response.[4]


1. Martyn J, *et al.* Clinical pharmacology of muscle relaxants in patients with burns. *J Clin Pharmacol* 1986; **26:** 680–5.
2. Anonymous. Neuromuscular blockers in patients with burns. *Lancet* 1988; **ii:** 1003–4.
3. Kohlschütter B, *et al.* Suxamethonium-induced hyperkalaemia in patients with severe intra-abdominal infections. *Br J Anaesth* 1976; **48:** 557–62.
4. Dhanaraj VJ, *et al.* A study of the changes in serum potassium concentration with suxamethonium using different anaesthetic agents. *Br J Anaesth* 1975; **47:** 516–19.
5. Magee DA, Gallagher EG. "Self-taming" of suxamethonium and serum potassium concentration. *Br J Anaesth* 1984; **56:** 977–9.
6. Plötz J, Schreiber W. Side effects induced by suxamethonium on the skeletal muscle and their prevention. *Br J Anaesth* 1985; **57:** 1044–5.


**Hypersensitivity.** Hypersensitivity reactions to neuromuscular blockers occur more commonly in women than in men,[1,2] in atopic patients and those who have a history of asthma or allergy,[2] and in patients who have had a previous reaction to anaesthetic drugs.[2] Circulatory collapse, flushing, skin rash, urticaria, and bronchospasm have occurred in hypersensitivity reactions associated with suxamethonium;[1,3,4] deaths have been reported.[3,5] The exact mechanism by which neuromuscular blockers produce hypersensitivity reactions is still uncertain; they all have a direct effect on mast cells, releasing histamine without immunological involvement, and could cause anaphylactoid reactions. Histamine release associated with use of aminosteroidal blockers is rare compared with the benzylisoquinolinium blockers.[6] Tubocurarine is considered to be the most potent releaser of histamine, with pancuronium and vecuronium having only very weak activity. Suxamethonium is considered to have only 1% of the histamine-releasing activity of tubocurarine but is more likely to produce serious hypersensitivity reactions. Data from intradermal testing has been used to qualify the risk of allergic reactions associated with the neuromuscular blockers.[7] The benzylisoquinolinium blockers alcuronium and tubocurarine and the depolarising blocker suxamethonium were considered to be associated with the highest risk. Benzylisoquinolinium blockers atracurium, cisatracurium, gallamine and mivacurium and the aminosteroid rocuronium presented an intermediate risk. The aminosteroids pancuronium and vecuronium were considered to have the lowest risk.

A type I immediate hypersensitivity reaction involving IgE antibodies is considered to be the mechanism of most hypersensitivity reactions associated with neuromuscular blockers.[2,5,8,9] Antibodies reacting with neuromuscular blockers, including suxamethonium, have been demonstrated.[5,9] The antibodies appear to be directed against quaternary or tertiary ammonium-ion groups which are present in neuromuscular blockers; such groups are also found in other drugs, cosmetics, disinfectants, and foods. This may help explain the cross-reactivity reported between different neuromuscular blockers[1,2,5,9,10] and how sensitisation occurs without prior exposure to any neuromuscular blocker.[2,5] At least 50% of patients sensitive to one neuromuscular blocker will react to one or more others[11] with some patients sensitive to most.[1] Intradermal skin tests are used to investigate and predict sensitivity to neuromuscular blockers, but their interpretation is controversial and it cannot be concluded that all patients with positive skin tests will have clinical sensitivity.[1,11] Although radioallergosorbent tests can detect antibodies to suxamethonium, alcuronium, and thiopental[3,12] some consider that their routine use is not justified as reactions could be avoided by taking an adequate patient history.[13]


1. Youngmen PR, *et al.* Anaphylactoid reactions to neuromuscular blocking agents: a commonly undiagnosed condition? *Lancet* 1983; **ii:** 597–9.
2. Fisher MM, Munro I. Life-threatening anaphylactoid reactions to muscle relaxants. *Anesth Analg* 1983; **62:** 559–64.
3. Brahams D. Fatal reaction to suxamethonium: case for screening by radioallergosorbent test? *Lancet* 1989; **i:** 1400–1.
4. Moneret-Vautrin DA, *et al.* Simultaneous anaphylaxis to thiopentone and a neuromuscular blocker: a study of two cases. *Br J Anaesth* 1990; **64:** 743–5.
5. Fisher M, Baldo B. Adverse reactions to alcuronium: an Australian disease? *Med J Aust* 1983; **1:** 630–2.
6. Naguib M, *et al.* Histamine-release haemodynamic changes produced by rocuronium, vecuronium, mivacurium, atracurium and tubocurarine. *Br J Anaesth* 1995; **75:** 588–92.
7. Rose M, Fisher M. Rocuronium: high risk for anaphylaxis? *Br J Anaesth* 2001; **86:** 678–82.
8. Vervloet D. Anaphylactoid reactions to suxamethonium. *Lancet* 1983; **ii:** 1197.
9. Harle DG, *et al.* Detection of IgE antibodies to suxamethonium after anaphylactoid reactions during anaesthesia. *Lancet* 1984; **I:** 930–2.
10. Harle DG, *et al.* Cross-reactivity of metocurine, atracurium, vecuronium and fazadinium with IgE antibodies from patients unexposed to these drugs but allergic to other myoneural blocking drugs. *Br J Anaesth* 1985; **57:** 1073–6.
11. Withington DE. Relevance of histamine to the anaesthetist. *Br J Hosp Med* 1988; **40:** 264–70.
12. Assem ESK. Anaphylactic anaesthetic reactions: the value of paper radioallergosorbent tests for IgE antibodies to muscle relaxants and thiopentone. *Anaesthesia* 1990; **45:** 1032–8.
13. Noble DW, Yap PL. Screening for antibodies to anaesthetics. *BMJ* 1989; **299:** 2.


## Treatment of Adverse Effects

Following administration of suxamethonium chloride assisted respiration should be maintained until spontaneous respiration has been fully restored. Transfusion of fresh frozen plasma or other source of plasma cholinesterase will help the destruction of the suxamethonium when prolonged paralysis is a result of atypical or low serum concentrations of plasma cholinesterase. Anticholinesterases should not normally be used since they potentiate the usual phase I block (see under Uses and Administration, below). If the neuromuscular block ceases to be depolarising in type and acquires some features of a competitive block (phase II block) the cautious use of an anticholinesterase may be considered. A short-acting anticholinesterase such as edrophonium may be given intravenously and if an obvious improvement is maintained for several minutes, neostigmine may be given with atropine.

Severe hypersensitivity reactions should be treated promptly with supportive and symptomatic measures.

If malignant hyperthermia develops, it may be treated as described on p.1394.

The muscarinic effects of suxamethonium chloride, such as bradycardia and excessive salivary secretion, may be reduced by giving an antimuscarinic such as atropine before suxamethonium. A small dose of a competitive neuromuscular blocker given before suxamethonium has been used to reduce some of the adverse effects of suxamethonium on the muscles (see Effects on the Muscles, above).

## Precautions

Patients who have received a neuromuscular blocker should always have their respiration assisted or controlled until the drug has been inactivated or antagonised.

Suxamethonium chloride is contra-indicated in patients with atypical plasma cholinesterase and should be used with caution in patients with reduced plasma cholinesterase activity (see below), which may occur in certain disease states and following exposure to certain drugs. Plasma cholinesterase concentrations fall during pregnancy and the puerperium and therefore maternal paralysis may be mildly prolonged. Suxamethonium is contra-indicated in patients with burns, massive trauma, renal impairment with a raised plasma-potassium concentration, severe long-lasting sepsis, and severe hyperkalaemia, since suxamethonium-induced rises in plasma-potassium concentration can have serious consequences in such patients; patients who have been immobilised for prolonged periods may be at similar risk. It is contra-indicated in patients with a history of hypersensitivity to the drug and, because of the possibility of cross-sensitivity (see above), should be used with caution when hypersensitivity to any neuromuscular blocker has previously occurred. Suxamethonium should be avoided in patients with a penetrating eye injury, raised intra-ocular pressure or glaucoma, or those about to undergo incision of the eyeball in eye surgery, because of the risks from increased intra-ocular pressure (although see under Adverse Effects, above). Suxamethonium chloride produces muscle contractions before relaxation and should therefore be used with caution in patients with bone fractures. It is contra-indicated in patients with a personal or family history of malignant hyperthermia.

The response to suxamethonium chloride is often unpredictable in patients with neuromuscular disorders and it should be used with great caution in these patients (see below). Caution is also needed if it is given to a patient with cardiac or respiratory disease. Children may be at special risk from cardiac arrest associated with hyperkalaemia (see below).

Hypothermia may enhance the neuromuscular blocking effects of suxamethonium chloride and an increase in body temperature may reduce them.

**Children.** Reports of fatal cardiac arrests[1,2] in apparently healthy children and adolescents, who were subsequently found to have had undiagnosed myopathies, led to restrictions in the USA on the use of suxamethonium in this age group. Suxamethonium was contra-indicated except for emergency tracheal intubation or where an immediate securing of an airway was essential. Many anaesthetists disagreed[2] with this contra-indication and an FDA Committee advised[3] that it should be replaced by a warning about the possibility of cardiac arrest associated with hyperkalaemia with special attention being paid to male children who are considered to be at the highest risk. One British anaesthetist who questioned the rationale behind restricting the elective use of suxamethonium pointed out that alternatives to suxamethonium had not been demonstrated to be as safe or effective for airway management.[4] The rare occurrence of cardiac arrest in children might be further reduced by taking a careful family history to exclude undiagnosed myopathies and by using an intravenous as opposed to inhalation induction when suxamethonium is to be used.[4] A survey had found that most cases of cardiac arrest in children in the UK associated with the use of suxamethonium had been caused by vagal overactivity in non-atropinised patients.

1. Rosenberg H, Gronert GA. Intractable cardiac arrest in children given succinylcholine. *Anesthesiology* 1992; **77:** 1054.
2. Book WJ, *et al.* Adverse effects of depolarising neuromuscular blocking agents: incidence, prevention and management. *Drug Safety* 1994; **10:** 331–49.
3. *FDC Reports Pink Sheet* 1994; June 13: 16.
4. Hopkins PM. Use of suxamethonium in children. *Br J Anaesth* 1995; **75:** 675–7.

**Neuromuscular disorders.** Caution is needed if suxamethonium is to be given to patients with neuromuscular disease, since severe complications have been reported.[1] Hyperkalaemia and cardiac arrhythmias or cardiac arrest have been reported following administration of suxamethonium to patients with hemiplegia, diffuse intracranial lesions (head injury, encephalitis, ruptured cerebral aneurysm), tetanus, paraplegia, acute anterior horn cell disease, and muscular dystrophies. An exaggerated response to suxamethonium has been reported in the myasthenic syndrome but resistance may occur in patients with neurofibromatosis. Resistance may also occur in patients with myasthenia gravis, but uneventful administration has also been reported, although early onset of phase II block is possible in these patients. Muscle contractures and hyperkalaemia may be expected in amyotrophic lateral sclerosis and muscular denervation. Suxamethonium should be avoided in patients with myotonias, as response is unpredictable. It is recommended that suxamethonium is also avoided in hemiplegia, paraplegia, muscular denervation, and muscular dystrophies.

1. Azar I. The response of patients with neuromuscular disorders to muscle relaxants: a review. *Anesthesiology* 1984; **61:** 173–87.

**Plasma cholinesterase deficiency.** Suxamethonium is normally rapidly hydrolysed by plasma cholinesterase and the clinical effects usually last for only several minutes. Activity of the enzyme varies between individuals and prolonged paralysis following suxamethonium is commonly due to a hereditary or acquired reduction in plasma cholinesterase activity. The genes involved in the control of plasma cholinesterase production are termed usual, atypical (dibucaine-resistant), fluoride-resistant, and silent. About 96% of the population are homozygous for the usual gene. The commonest variant in western populations is the atypical form with about 3 to 4% of the population being heterozygous for this variant. They exhibit a slightly prolonged response to suxamethonium. Homozygotes for the atypical variant have a frequency of about 0.04%. They exhibit markedly prolonged apnoea following a standard dose of suxamethonium but can be readily identified by biochemical tests. The fluoride-resistant and silent variants occur very rarely. A measure of plasma cholinesterase activity can be obtained from the percentage inhibition of the enzyme by the local anaesthetic cinchocaine (commonly known in this context by its American name, dibucaine) to give the dibucaine number. Most normal people have a dibucaine number of about 80.

Acquired plasma cholinesterase deficiency is clinically less important than genetically determined deficiency. The enzyme is synthesised in the liver and **severe liver impairment** or malnutrition may cause abnormally low enzyme levels with some prolongation of suxamethonium activity. Reduced enzyme activity may also be found in severe anaemia, burns, cancer, collagen diseases, severe dehydration, severe infections, malnutrition, myocardial infarction, myxoedema, and renal impairment; plasmapheresis or plasma exchange removes significant amounts of plasma cholinesterase.

During **pregnancy** there is a rapid fall in plasma cholinesterase concentration which persists throughout pregnancy and for up to several weeks into the puerperium. The concentration of atypical plasma cholinesterase is also reduced in pregnancy and the puerperium. A number of **drugs** reduce plasma cholinesterase synthesis or activity and may prolong suxamethonium paralysis as discussed under Interactions, below.

References.

1. Wood GJ, Hall GM. Plasmapheresis and plasma cholinesterase. *Br J Anaesth* 1978; **50:** 945–9.
2. Evans RT, Wroe JM. Plasma cholinesterase changes during pregnancy: their interpretation as a cause of suxamethonium-induced apnoea. *Anaesthesia* 1980; **35:** 651–4.
3. Lumley J. Prolongation of suxamethonium following plasma exchange. *Br J Anaesth* 1980; **52:** 1149–50.
4. Williams FM. Clinical significance of esterases in man. *Clin Pharmacokinet* 1985; **10:** 392–403.
5. Robson N, *et al.* Plasma cholinesterase changes during the puerperium. *Anaesthesia* 1986; **41:** 243–9.
6. Cherala SR, *et al.* Placental transfer of succinylcholine causing transient respiratory depression in the newborn. *Anaesth Intensive Care* 1989; **17:** 202–4.

**Renal impairment.** Suxamethonium chloride may be given in usual doses to patients with renal failure[1,2] although it is usually recommended that it should be avoided if hyperkalaemia is also present (see Effects on Plasma-potassium Concentration above). However, in a retrospective review[3] of 38 patients with serum potassium levels greater than 5.5 mmol/litre given a standard intubation dose of suxamethonium, there were no reports of dysrhythmias or unexpected admissions to the intensive care unit.

Patients with renal failure given repeated doses of suxamethonium did not show an excessive increase in serum potassium; however sinus bradycardia commonly occurred and it was recommended that repeated injections should be avoided in such patients.[2] If necessary, pretreatment with glycopyrrolate or atropine to protect against bradycardia should be considered.

1. Ryan DW. Preoperative serum cholinesterase concentration in chronic renal failure. *Br J Anaesth* 1977; **49:** 945–9.
2. Thapa S, Brull SJ. Succinylcholine-induced hyperkalemia in patients with renal failure: an old question revisited. *Anesth Analg* 2000; **91:** 237–41.
3. Schow AJ, *et al.* Can succinylcholine be used safely in hyperkalemic patients? *Anesth Analg* 2002; **95:** 119–22.

## Interactions

A number of drugs may interact with depolarising neuromuscular blockers such as suxamethonium. The mechanisms of interaction can include a direct effect on neuromuscular transmission or an alteration of enzyme activity and may result in potentiation or antagonism of neuromuscular block. In general, such interactions are potentially more serious in patients with impaired neuromuscular function or reduced activity of plasma cholinesterase, who are more sensitive to suxamethonium's effects.

Interactions common to competitive and depolarising neuromuscular blockers are covered under Atracurium, p.1400 whereas those specific for depolarising blockers are discussed below.

**Antiarrhythmics.** See under Atracurium, p.1400.

**Antibacterials.** See under Atracurium, p.1400.

**Anticholinesterases.** The action of suxamethonium may be markedly prolonged in patients using eye drops containing *ecothiopate*, a long-acting anticholinesterase that inhibits both acetylcholinesterase and plasma cholinesterase. Following systemic absorption of ecothiopate, plasma cholinesterase activity may rapidly be reduced to 5% or less of normal and prolonged apnoea after use of suxamethonium has occurred. On discontinuing ecothiopate, enzyme activity remains depressed for 1 to 2 months. If a patient has used ecothiopate eye drops in the previous 2 months, suxamethonium should not be given unless normal plasma cholinesterase activity can be demonstrated; a competitive neuromuscular blocker is preferable. Exposure to *organophosphorus insecticides* may also reduce plasma cholinesterase activity resulting in prolonged paralysis after use of suxamethonium; enzyme activity may be totally abolished. Anticholinesterases including *edrophonium, neostigmine, pyridostigmine, rivastigmine, tacrine,* and possibly *donepezil* enhance the action of suxamethonium, although suxamethonium-induced phase II block can be reversed with an anticholinesterase. Care should be taken if there is a need to use suxamethonium for urgent short procedures after a competitive-neuromuscular-induced block has been antagonised with an anticholinesterase, as the resulting block may be greatly prolonged.[1]

1. Fleming NW, *et al.* Neuromuscular blocking action of suxamethonium after antagonism of vecuronium by edrophonium, pyridostigmine or neostigmine. *Br J Anaesth* 1996; **77:** 492–5.

**Antiepileptics.** The mean time to recovery from suxamethonium-induced neuromuscular block was 14.3 minutes in 9 patients receiving chronic treatment with phenytoin and/or carbamazepine compared with 10.0 minutes in 9 patients not receiving antiepileptics.[1]

1. Melton AT, *et al.* Prolonged duration of succinylcholine in patients receiving anticonvulsants: evidence for mild upregulation of acetylcholine receptors? *Can J Anaesth* 1993; **40:** 939–42.

**Antineoplastics.** *Cyclophosphamide* has been reported to prolong the neuromuscular block produced by suxamethonium through reduction of plasma cholinesterase activity, possibly by alkylation of the enzyme.[1] Since enzyme activity may be reduced by up to 70% for several days to several weeks, it was suggested[2] that suxamethonium should be avoided if possible in patients receiving cyclophosphamide. A more recent case report[3] would also support this suggestion. Other alkylating agents also reported to reduce plasma cholinesterase activity include *chlormethine, thiotepa,* and *tretamine*.[2]

1. Walker IR, *et al.* Cyclophosphamide, cholinesterase and anaesthesia. *Aust N Z J Med* 1972; **3:** 247–51.
2. Zsigmond EK, Robins G. The effect of a series of anti-cancer drugs on plasma cholinesterase activity. *Can Anaesth Soc J* 1972; **19:** 75–82.
3. Koseoglu V, *et al.* Acquired pseudocholinesterase deficiency after high-dose cyclophosphamide. *Bone Marrow Transplant* 1999; **24:** 1367–8.

**Aprotinin.** See under Atracurium, p.1401.

**Benzodiazepines.** See under Atracurium, p.1401.

**Beta blockers.** See under Atracurium, p.1401.

**Cardiac inotropes.** See under Atracurium, p.1401.

**Ganglion blockers.** See under Atracurium, p.1401.

**General anaesthetics.** Tachyphylaxis and phase II block (see below) develop earlier, and after smaller total doses of suxamethonium, when inhalation anaesthetics are used. Halothane may increase the incidence of arrhythmias associated with suxamethonium and can potentiate suxamethonium-induced muscle damage.[1] Suxamethonium should be used with caution with other drugs that might produce additive cardiovascular effects. Severe bradycardia and asystole have occurred when used in anaesthetic regimens with propofol and opioids such as fentanyl. See also under Interactions in Atracurium, p.1401.

1. Laurence AS, Henderson P. Serum myoglobin after suxamethonium administration to children: effect of pretreatment before iv and inhalation induction. *Br J Anaesth* 1986; **58:** 126P.

**Histamine $H_2$ antagonists.** See under Atracurium, p.1401.

**Lithium.** See under Atracurium, p.1401.

**Local anaesthetics.** *Procaine, cocaine,* and *chloroprocaine* are ester-type local anaesthetics which are hydrolysed by plasma cholinesterase and may competitively enhance the neuromuscular blocking activity of suxamethonium. See also Antiarrhythmics under Atracurium, p.1400.

**Magnesium salts.** See under Atracurium, p.1401.

**MAOIs.** Reduction of plasma cholinesterase activity by *phenelzine* has been reported[1] to cause significant prolongation of suxamethonium paralysis. Enzyme activity may be reduced to 10% of normal and recovery can take up to a month. The dosage of suxamethonium may need to be substantially reduced or a competitive neuromuscular blocker used.

1. Bodley PO, *et al.* Low serum pseudocholinesterase levels complicating treatment with phenelzine. *BMJ* 1969; **3:** 510–12.

**Metoclopramide.** Dose-dependent prolongation of suxamethonium-induced neuromuscular blockade has been reported in patients given metoclopramide.[1,2] The potent inhibitory effect of metoclopramide on plasma cholinesterase may account for this interaction.

1. Turner DR, *et al.* Neuromuscular block by suxamethonium following treatment with histamine type 2 antagonists or metoclopramide. *Br J Anaesth* 1989; **63:** 348–50.
2. Kao YJ, *et al.* Dose-dependent effect of metoclopramide on cholinesterases and suxamethonium metabolism. *Br J Anaesth* 1990; **65:** 220–4.

**Neuromuscular blockers.** See under Atracurium, p.1401.

**Sex hormones.** *Oestrogens* and oestrogen-containing *oral contraceptives* reduce plasma cholinesterase activity[1] possibly due to suppression of hepatic synthesis of the enzyme, but little prolongation of suxamethonium paralysis may be expected since activity is reduced by only about 20%. See also under Atracurium, p.1402.

1. Robertson GS, Aberd MB. Serum protein and cholinesterase changes in association with contraceptive pills. *Lancet* 1967; **i:** 232–5.

**Sympathomimetics.** *Bambuterol* can inhibit plasma cholinesterase activity and so prolong the activity of suxamethonium.[1] Phase II block has been reported in some patients with abnormal plasma cholinesterase.[2]

1. Staun P, *et al.* The influence of 10 mg and 20 mg bambuterol on the duration of succinylcholine-induced neuromuscular blockade. *Acta Anaesthesiol Scand* 1990; **34:** 498–500.
2. Bang U, *et al.* The effect of bambuterol on plasma cholinesterase activity and suxamethonium-induced neuromuscular blockade in subjects heterozygous for abnormal plasma cholinesterase. *Acta Anaesthesiol Scand* 1990; **34:** 600–4.

## Pharmacokinetics

After injection, suxamethonium is rapidly hydrolysed by plasma cholinesterase. One molecule of choline is split off rapidly to form succinylmonocholine which is then slowly hydrolysed to succinic acid and choline. About 10% of suxamethonium is excreted unchanged in the urine. Succinylmonocholine has weak muscle-relaxant properties mainly of a competitive nature.

The gene responsible for the expression of plasma cholinesterase exhibits polymorphism and enzyme activity varies between individuals (see under Precautions, above).

Small amounts of suxamethonium cross the placenta.

◊ Reviews.

1. Booij LHDJ, Vree TB. Skeletal muscle relaxants: pharmacodynamics and pharmacokinetics in different patient groups. *Int J Clin Pract* 2000; **54:** 526–34.

## Uses and Administration

Suxamethonium is a depolarising neuromuscular blocker used to produce muscle relaxation. It combines with cholinergic receptors of the motor end-plate to produce depolarisation but is resistant to breakdown by acetylcholinesterase. This prevents repolarisation and subsequent depolarisation, and a flaccid muscle paralysis occurs. This initial depolarisation block is commonly known as a **phase I block.** The muscles that produce fine rapid movements such as those of the face are the first to be affected followed by those of the limbs, abdomen, and chest; the diaphragm is affected last. Recovery occurs in reverse order. When excessive amounts of suxamethonium accumulate at the neuromuscular junction, for example following high or prolonged dosage, the nature of the block may change to one with characteristics similar to competitive block.

This is commonly termed **phase II block** or **dual block** and may be associated with prolonged neuromuscular blockade and apnoea.

Following intravenous injection suxamethonium chloride acts in about 30 to 60 seconds and has a duration of action of about 2 to 6 minutes. Following intramuscular injection it acts in 2 to 3 minutes and has a duration of action of about 10 to 30 minutes.

Suxamethonium is used in surgical and other procedures in which a rapid onset and brief duration of muscle relaxation is needed (see Anaesthesia, p.1397), including intubation, endoscopies, and ECT. It is used as suxamethonium chloride, and is normally given by intravenous injection. The content of preparations of suxamethonium chloride may be described in terms of either the dihydrate or the anhydrous form, depending on the country of origin, and this should be borne in mind when evaluating the literature although the differences are small (anhydrous suxamethonium chloride 1 mg is approximately equivalent to 1.1 mg of the dihydrate).

Suxamethonium should be given after induction of general anaesthesia because paralysis is usually preceded by painful muscle fasciculations. A competitive neuromuscular blocker may sometimes be given before suxamethonium to try to reduce some of the adverse effects on the muscles (see under Effects on the Muscles, above). Premedication with an antimuscarinic may be of value in reducing bradycardia and excessive salivation. Assisted respiration is necessary.

An initial test dose of 100 micrograms/kg of suxamethonium chloride may be given intravenously if increased sensitivity is suspected. Doses of neuromuscular blockers need to be carefully titrated for individual patients according to response, and may vary with the procedure, the other drugs given, and the state of the patient; monitoring of the degree of block is recommended in order to reduce the risk of overdosage. The response to suxamethonium varies considerably and the usual single dose of suxamethonium chloride for an adult is 0.3 to 1.1 mg/kg by intravenous injection. Supplementary doses of 50 to 100% of the initial dose may be given at 5 to 10 minute intervals if required but the total dose given by repeated intravenous injection or continuous infusion (see below) should not exceed 500 mg/hour. Infants and children are more resistant to suxamethonium than adults. A recommended intravenous dose for infants under one year of age is 2 mg/kg; a dose of 1 mg/kg is recommended for children 1 to 12 years old.

When a suitable vein is inaccessible suxamethonium chloride has been given by intramuscular injection in a dose of 3 to 4 mg/kg to a maximum total dose of 150 mg. The intramuscular dose for infants is up to 4 to 5 mg/kg and for older children up to 4 mg/kg to a maximum total dose of 150 mg.

For prolonged procedures in adults sustained relaxation may be obtained by continuous intravenous infusion of a 0.1 to 0.2% solution. A rate of 2.5 to 4 mg/minute is usually adequate but may be adjusted as necessary. The total dose given by repeated intravenous injection (see above) or continuous infusion should not exceed 500 mg/hour.

Suxamethonium bromide and suxamethonium iodide have also been used.

**Electroconvulsive therapy.** Suxamethonium chloride is used to decrease the muscular contractions associated with electrically induced convulsions. It temporarily paralyses muscles during ECT, preventing violent muscle contractions which can potentially result in broken bones and fractures.

Suxamethonium chloride remains the most commonly used neuromuscular blocker in ECT. However, patients with a history of malignant hyperthermia, neuroleptic malignant syndrome, catatonic schizophrenia, and organophosphate poisoning are more susceptible to side-effects.[1] Mivacurium has been used, with satisfactory results, in at-risk-patients, although histamine release and hypotension may be a problem. Other competitive neuromuscular blockers tried include atracurium and vecuronium.

1. Ding Z, White PF. Anesthesia for electroconvulsive therapy. *Anesth Analg* 2002; **94:** 1351–64.

### Preparations

***BP 2003:*** Suxamethonium Chloride Injection;
***USP 27:*** Succinylcholine Chloride for Injection; Succinylcholine Chloride Injection.

**Proprietary Preparations** (details are given in Part 3)
***Arg.:*** Fosfitone; Succi; ***Austral.:*** Scoline; ***Austria:*** Lysthenon; ***Belg.:*** Myoplegine; ***Braz.:*** Quelicin; ***Canad.:*** Anectine†; Quelicin; ***Fin.:*** Sukolin; ***Fr.:*** Celocurine; ***Ger.:*** Lysthenon; Pantolax; Succicuran†; ***Gr.:*** Lycitrope; ***India:*** Midarine; ***Irl.:*** Anectine; ***Israel:*** Succinyl; ***Ital.:*** Midarine; Myotenlis; ***Malaysia:*** Ethicoline; Succinyl; ***Mex.:*** Anectine; Ectinex†; Uxicolin; ***Norw.:*** Curacit; ***NZ:*** Ethicholine; ***Port.:*** Mioflex; ***S.Afr.:*** Scoline; ***Singapore:*** Ethicholine; ***Spain:*** Anectine; Mioflex; ***Swed.:*** Celocurin; ***Switz.:*** Lysthenon; Midarine; Succinolin; ***Thai.:*** Succinyl; ***UK:*** Anectine; ***USA:*** Anectine; Quelicin.

## Tubocurarine Chloride *(BAN, rINN)*

Cloruro de tubocurarina; *d*-Tubocurarine Chloride; (+)-Tubocurarine Chloride Hydrochloride Pentahydrate; Tubocurarini Chloridum. (+)-7′,12′-Dihydroxy-6,6′-dimethoxy-2,2′,2′-trimethyltubocuraranium dichloride pentahydrate.

$C_{37}H_{42}Cl_2N_2O_6,5H_2O$ = 771.7.
*CAS — 57-95-4 (tubocurarine); 57-94-3 (anhydrous tubocurarine chloride); 6989-98-6 (tubocurarine chloride, pentahydrate).*
*ATC — M03AA02.*

**Pharmacopoeias.** In *Chin., Eur.* (see p.vi), *Int., Jpn,* and *US.*
**Ph. Eur. 5.0** (Tubocurarine Chloride). A white or slightly yellowish crystalline powder. Soluble in water and in alcohol; practically insoluble in acetone; dissolves in solutions of alkali hydroxides. A 1% solution in water has a pH of 4.0 to 6.0. Store in airtight containers.
**USP 27** (Tubocurarine Chloride). A white or yellowish-white to greyish-white, crystalline powder. Soluble 1 in 20 of water and 1 in 45 of alcohol. Store in airtight containers.

### Adverse Effects, Treatment, and Precautions

As for competitive neuromuscular blockers in general (see Atracurium, p.1399). A transient fall in blood pressure commonly occurs, due in part to ganglionic blockade and the release of histamine; there may be an increase in heart rate. Tubocurarine has a greater propensity to cause histamine release than other competitive neuromuscular blockers in clinical use. Tubocurarine should be used with caution in patients with renal impairment. Resistance to the effect of tubocurarine may occur in patients with hepatic impairment.

### Interactions

For interactions associated with competitive neuromuscular blockers, see Atracurium, p.1400.

### Pharmacokinetics

Tubocurarine chloride is a quaternary ammonium compound and absorption from the gastrointestinal tract is extremely poor. Absorption is slow and irregular when given intramuscularly. Following intravenous injection tubocurarine is widely distributed throughout body tissues; less than 50% is bound to plasma proteins. Following a single dose extensive redistribution to tissues is responsible for the termination of activity, but after a large single dose or repeated small doses tissue saturation occurs and renal excretion becomes the main determinant of duration. When given in usual doses it does not pass the blood-brain barrier, and does not appear to cross the placenta in significant amounts. Up to 75% of a dose is excreted unchanged in the urine in 24 hours, and up to 12% in bile. Biliary excretion is increased in renal impairment. A small proportion of a dose is metabolised in the liver.

### Uses and Administration

Tubocurarine is a benzylisoquinolinium competitive neuromuscular blocker (see Atracurium, p.1402). It may be obtained from extracts of the stems of *Chondodendron tomentosum* (Menispermaceae) and is one of the active principles of curare, by which name it is sometimes referred to in anaesthetic literature. Tubocurarine chloride is the chloride of (+)-tubocurarine. Following intravenous injection of tubocurarine chloride neuromuscular block appears within 1 minute and lasts for about 30 minutes; the maximum effect is attained within 2 to 5 minutes.

Tubocurarine chloride has been used similarly to other competitive neuromuscular blockers to produce muscle relaxation in various procedures but has largely been replaced by other drugs with fewer cardiovascular effects and a lower potential for histamine release.

Doses used have varied according to the degree of muscle relaxation required. Doses of neuromuscular blockers need to be carefully titrated for individual patients according to response, and may vary with the procedure, the other drugs given, and the state of the patient; monitoring of the degree of block is recommended in order to reduce the risk of overdosage. An initial dose of 6 to 9 mg intravenously has been suggested followed by 3 to 4.5 mg after 3 to 5 minutes if necessary; additional doses of 3 mg may be given as required for prolonged procedures. Higher doses have been given in some countries. It has also been given intramuscularly but absorption is slow and erratic. Tubocurarine should be given with caution in reduced doses to patients with renal impairment; if large or repeated doses are given neuromuscular block may be prolonged.

Tubocurarine chloride has also been used to control the muscle spasms of tetanus (p.1398).

### Preparations

***USP 27:*** Tubocurarine Chloride Injection.

**Proprietary Preparations** (details are given in Part 3)
***Arg.:*** Decurin; ***Israel:*** Curarine; Tubarine; ***Spain:*** Curarina Miro†.

## Vecuronium Bromide *(BAN, USAN, rINN)*

Bromuro de vecuronio; Org-NC-45. 1-(3α,17β-Diacetoxy-2β-piperidino-5α-androstan-16β-yl)-1-methylpiperidinium bromide.

$C_{34}H_{57}BrN_2O_4$ = 637.7.
*CAS — 50700-72-6.*
*ATC — M03AC03.*

**Incompatibility.** A solution containing vecuronium bromide 1 mg/mL was found to be visually incompatible with furosemide.[1] For incompatibilities of competitive neuromuscular blockers in general, see under Atracurium on p.1399.

1. Chiu MF, Schwartz ML. Visual compatibility of injectable drugs used in the intensive care unit. *Am J Health-Syst Pharm* 1997; **54:** 64–5.

### Adverse Effects, Treatment, and Precautions

As for competitive neuromuscular blockers in general (see Atracurium, p.1399).

Vecuronium bromide has little histamine-releasing activity although a local reaction at the site of injection has been reported; bronchospasm and anaphylactoid reactions have been rarely reported. It also has little vagolytic or ganglion-blocking activity and produces no significant adverse cardiovascular effects at usual doses.

Caution may be needed in patients with hepatic or renal impairment (see under Uses and Administration, below); dosage adjustments may be required in renal failure.

**Elderly.** It has been recommended that neuromuscular function should be monitored in elderly patients receiving vecuronium since there may be a risk of prolonged block.[1]

1. Slavov V, *et al.* Comparison of duration of neuromuscular blocking effect of atracurium and vecuronium in young and elderly patients. *Br J Anaesth* 1995; **74:** 709–11.

**Pregnancy.** The proportion of vecuronium crossing the placenta following doses of 60 to 80 micrograms/kg was considered clinically insignificant and its use during obstetric anaesthesia was considered safe for the newborn.[1]

1. Demetriou M, *et al.* Placental transfer of Org NC 45 in women undergoing caesarean section. *Br J Anaesth* 1982; **54:** 643–5.

### Interactions

For interactions associated with competitive neuromuscular blockers, see Atracurium, p.1400.

### Pharmacokinetics

Following intravenous administration vecuronium is rapidly distributed. It is taken up by the liver and partly metabolised; the metabolites have some neuromuscular blocking activity. It is excreted mainly in bile as unchanged drug and metabolites; some is also excreted in urine. The plasma elimination half-life is reported to range from about 30 to 80 minutes.

### Uses and Administration

Vecuronium bromide is an aminosteroidal competitive neuromuscular blocker (see Atracurium, p.1402).

Following intravenous injection muscle relaxation occurs within about 1.5 to 2 minutes and lasts for about 20 to 30 minutes.

Vecuronium bromide is used for endotracheal intubation and to provide muscle relaxation in general anaesthesia for surgical procedures (see Anaesthesia, p.1397) and to aid controlled ventilation (see Intensive Care, p.1398).

Doses of neuromuscular blockers need to be carefully titrated for individual patients according to response, and may vary with the procedure, the other drugs given, and the state of the patient; monitoring of the degree of block is recommended in order to reduce the risk of overdosage. The usual initial dose for intubation is 80 to 100 micrograms/kg by intravenous injection, although reduced initial doses of 30 to 50 micrograms/kg are suggested following the use of suxamethonium. Higher initial doses ranging from 150 to 300 micrograms/kg have sometimes been used for other procedures. However, it is recommended that the dose should not exceed 100 micrograms/kg in caesarean section or neonatal surgery. Maintenance doses of 20 to 30 micrograms/kg may be given as required during prolonged procedures; in the USA a lower maintenance dose of 10 to 15 micrograms/kg is recommended. Neuromuscular blockade may also be maintained with an intravenous infusion given at a rate of 0.8 to 1.4 micrograms/kg per minute but should be preceded by an initial bolus injection of 40 to 100 micrograms/kg. The UK manufacturers recommend that in obese patients the dosage of vecuronium should be reduced taking into account lean body-mass. Children older than 5 months can be given adult doses but children up to 1 year may have a more rapid response and the high initial dose for intubation may not be necessary. Neonates and infants below 5 months of age may be more sensitive to vecuronium and it is recommended that they should be given an initial test dose of 10 to 20 micrograms/kg, followed by increments according to response. The duration of action and recovery is longer in neonates and infants than in children and adults and they may require smaller maintenance doses given less frequently.

**Administration in hepatic impairment.** Although the manufacturers make no specific recommendations for dosage reduction in hepatic impairment, the duration of action of vecuronium was reported to be significantly prolonged in patients with cholestasis[1] or cirrhosis with oesophageal varices[2] given a dose of 200 micrograms/kg intravenously. Plasma clearance was significantly reduced and the elimination half-life significantly increased from a mean of 58 to 98 minutes.[1] A dose of 150 micrograms/kg was found to have a similar onset and duration of action in patients with hepatic impairment and healthy controls,[2] but a dose of 100 micrograms/kg had a slower onset and slightly shorter duration of action in those with liver disturbance.[3] Following a dose of vecuronium, rapid and extensive hepatic uptake occurs, which largely determines its short duration of action. However, as the dose increases this mechanism becomes saturated, and hepatic elimination becomes more important in terminating activity. This would help to explain the variation in results seen with the different doses. Caution is needed if large single doses or repeated doses are given to patients with hepatic impairment.


1. Lebrault C, *et al.* Pharmacokinetics and pharmacodynamics of vecuronium in patients with cholestasis. *Br J Anaesth* 1986; **58:** 983–7.
2. Hunter JM, *et al.* The use of different doses of vecuronium in patients with liver dysfunction. *Br J Anaesth* 1985; **57:** 758–64.
3. Bell CF, *et al.* Use of atracurium and vecuronium in patients with oesophageal varices. *Br J Anaesth* 1985; **57:** 160–8.


**Administration in renal impairment.** A small proportion of vecuronium bromide is excreted in urine and it may be given in usual doses to patients with renal failure.[1,2] No clinically significant difference in elimination half-life, clearance, or duration of action were reported[1] between patients with renal failure and those with normal renal function. The onset of neuromuscular block may be slightly slower in renal failure[2] and these patients may require an increase of around 20% in the initial dose of vecuronium.[3] However, the dosage requirement for maintenance of neuromuscular block may be reduced by about 20%[3] and slight prolongation of block may occur if dosage is not adjusted, but reversal of residual block with neostigmine is prompt and effective.[2]

Resistance to vecuronium has been reported[2] in 2 anephric patients. Total doses of 620 and 660 micrograms/kg produced maximum neuromuscular block of 77% and 36%, respectively but, despite the high doses used, there were no adverse effects or residual curarisation.


1. Fahey MR, *et al.* Pharmacokinetics of Org NC 45 (Norcuron) in patients with and without renal failure. *Br J Anaesth* 1981; **53:** 1049–53.
2. Hunter JM, *et al.* Comparison of vecuronium, atracurium and tubocurarine in normal patients and in patients with no renal function. *Br J Anaesth* 1984; **56:** 941–51.
3. Gramstad L. Atracurium, vecuronium and pancuronium in end-stage renal failure: dose-response properties and interactions with azathioprine. *Br J Anaesth* 1987; **59:** 995–1003.


## Preparations

**Proprietary Preparations** (details are given in Part 3)

***Arg.:*** Galaren; Norcuron; Rivecrum; Vecural; Vecuron; ***Austral.:*** Norcuron; ***Austria:*** Norcuron; ***Belg.:*** Norcuron; ***Braz.:*** Norcuron; ***Canad.:*** Norcuron; ***Chile:*** Norcuron; ***Denm.:*** Norcuron†; ***Fin.:*** Norcuron; ***Fr.:*** Norcuron; ***Ger.:*** Norcuron; ***Gr.:*** Norcuron; ***Hong Kong:*** Norcuron; ***India:*** Norcuron; ***Irl.:*** Norcuron; ***Israel:*** Norcuron; ***Ital.:*** Norcuron; ***Malaysia:*** Norcuron; ***Mex.:*** Curlem; Norcuron†; ***Neth.:*** Norcuron; ***Norw.:*** Norcuron; ***NZ:*** Norcuron; ***Port.:*** Norcuron; ***S.Afr.:*** Norcuron; ***Singapore:*** Norcuron; ***Spain:*** Norcuron; ***Swed.:*** Norcuron; ***Switz.:*** Norcuron; ***Thai.:*** Norcuron; ***UK:*** Norcuron; ***USA:*** Norcuron.

# Nonionic Surfactants

A surfactant is a compound that can reduce the interfacial tension between 2 immiscible phases. This is due to the molecule containing 2 localised regions, one being hydrophilic in nature and the other hydrophobic.

The properties of nonionic surfactants are largely dependent on the proportions of these 2 groups in the molecule. Hydrophilic groups include the oxyethylene group ($-O.CH_2.CH_2-$) and the hydroxyl group ($-OH$). By varying the number of these groups in a hydrophobic molecule, such as a fatty acid, substances are obtained which range from strongly hydrophobic and water-insoluble compounds, such as glyceryl monostearate, to strongly hydrophilic and water-soluble compounds, such as the macrogols. These 2 extreme types are not satisfactory as emulsifying agents, though they are useful stabilisers in the presence of efficient emulsifying agents. Between these extremes are the nonionic emulsifying agents in which the proportions of hydrophilic and hydrophobic groups are more evenly balanced; these include some of the macrogol esters and ethers, and sorbitan derivatives. By virtue of the processes used in their manufacture, nonionic surfactants are usually mixtures of related compounds; the properties of a particular material may vary from one manufacturer to another and there may be variation in batches from an individual source.

Nonionic surfactants differ from anionic surfactants (p.1574) by the absence of charge on, or ionisation of, the molecule; they are generally less irritant than anionic or cationic surfactants.

In addition to their use as emulsifiers some nonionic surfactants are also used in pharmacy as solubilising and wetting agents. Nonionic surfactants have applications in the food, cosmetic, paint, pesticide, and textile industries as well as being used as oil slick dispersants. Some macrogol ethers such as nonoxinol 9 are used as spermicides.

Since nonionic surfactants do not ionise to any great extent in solution, they are generally compatible with both anionic and cationic substances, but they reduce the antimicrobial action of many preservatives.

Nonionic surfactants may be classified according to their hydrophilic-lipophilic balance (HLB). This is an arbitrary scale of values denoting the relative affinity of the surfactant for oil and water. Lipophilic surfactants have low HLB values (less than 10) and are generally used as antifoaming agents, water-in-oil emulsifying agents, and as wetting agents; hydrophilic surfactants have higher HLB values (greater than 10) and are generally used as oil-in-water emulsifying agents and solubilising agents.

The range of nonionic surfactants used in pharmaceutical practice is large and their classification can be varied and complex. The principal groups of nonionic surfactants are outlined below.

**Glycol and glycerol esters** are a group of nonionic surfactants consisting of fatty acid esters of glycols and glycerol. Hydrophobic properties predominate and these compounds are poor emulsifying agents if used alone, though they are useful stabilisers for both oil-in-water and water-in-oil emulsions. If a small amount of soap, sulfated fatty alcohol, or other surfactant is added to the esters, a 'self-emulsifying' product is formed, which is capable of producing satisfactory oil-in-water emulsions. **Acetoglycerides** are mixed glyceryl esters in which the glycerol is esterified partly with a fatty acid and partly with acetic acid.

**Macrogol esters** are polyoxyethylene esters of fatty acids, mainly stearates. The hydrophilic properties of the oxyethylene group are weaker than those of the hydroxyl group but by introducing a sufficient number into a fatty acid molecule, substances are produced in which the hydrophilic and hydrophobic properties are sufficiently well balanced for the esters to act as efficient oil-in-water emulsifying agents. They may also be used as wetting and solubilising agents. Since the ester linkage is prone to hydrolysis, these compounds are less resistant to acids and alkalis than the macrogol ethers.

**Macrogol ethers** are condensation products prepared by reaction between fatty alcohols or alkylphenols and ethylene oxide. The ether linkage confers good stability to acids and alkalis. Macrogol ethers are widely used in the preparation of oil-in-water emulsions and as wetting and solubilising agents.

**Sorbitan derivatives** are derivatives of the cyclic mono- or di-anhydrides of sorbitol. They consist of *sorbitan esters*, which are prepared by esterification of one or more of the hydroxyl groups in the anhydrides with a fatty acid such as stearic, palmitic, oleic, or lauric acid, and *polysorbates*, which are polyoxyethylene derivatives of the sorbitan esters. Sorbitan esters are oil-soluble, water-dispersible, nonionic surfactants and are effective water-in-oil emulsifiers. Polysorbates are more hydrophilic, water-soluble compounds and are used as oil-in-water emulsifying agents. By varying the number of oxyethylene groups in the molecule, and the type of fatty acid in the sorbitan ester, surfactants with a wide range of properties may be obtained.

**Poloxamers** are copolymers of polyoxyethylene and polyoxypropylene. They are used as oil-in-water emulsifiers and as solubilising and wetting agents in a variety of pharmaceutical preparations intended for internal use.

Other nonionic compounds with surface activity such as the higher fatty alcohols are covered in the chapter on Paraffins and Similar Bases (p.1479).

---

## Diacetylated Monoglycerides

Monoglicéridos diacetilados.

**Pharmacopoeias.** In *USNF.*

**USNF 22** (Diacetylated Monoglycerides). Consists of glycerol esterified with edible fat-forming fatty acids and acetic acid. A clear liquid. Very soluble in alcohol 80%, in vegetable oils, and in mineral oils; sparingly soluble in alcohol 70%. Store in airtight containers. Protect from light.

### Profile

Diacetylated monoglycerides have been used as plasticisers.

---

## Diethylene Glycol Monopalmitostearate

Diethylene Glycol Monostearate; Diéthylène Glycol (Stéarate de); Diethylenglycoli Monopalmitostearas; Diethyleni Glycoli Stearas; Diglycol Stearate.

*CAS — 106-11-6 (diethylene glycol monostearate); 36381-62-1 (diethylene glycol monopalmitate).*

**Pharmacopoeias.** In *Eur.* (see p.vi). *USNF* includes Diethylene Glycol Stearates.

**Ph. Eur. 5.0** (Diethylene Glycol Monopalmitostearate). A mixture of diethylene glycol mono- and di-esters of stearic and palmitic acids. It contains not less than 45.0% of monoesters produced from the condensation of diethylene glycol and stearic acid of vegetable or animal origin and not more than 8% of free diethylene glycol. A white or almost white, waxy solid. Practically insoluble in water; soluble in hot alcohol and in acetone. M.p. 43° to 50°. Protect from light.

**USNF 22** (Diethylene Glycol Stearates). A mixture of diethylene glycol mono- and di-esters of stearic and palmitic acids. It contains not less than 45.0% of monoesters produced from the condensation of ethylene glycol and stearic acid of vegetable or animal origin. A white or almost white, waxy solid. Practically insoluble in water; soluble in hot alcohol and in acetone. M.p. 43° to 50°. Store in airtight containers at a temperature not exceeding 40°. Protect from light. Do not allow to freeze.

### Profile

Diethylene glycol monopalmitostearate has similar properties and uses to glyceryl monostearate or self-emulsifying glyceryl monostearate (see below). Diethylene glycol monolaurate and mono-oleate have also been used.

---

## *p*-Di-isobutyl-phenoxypolyethoxyethanol

*p*-Diisobutilfenoxipolietoxietanol.

### Profile

*p*-Di-isobutyl-phenoxypolyethoxyethanol has been used as a spermicide.

### Preparations

**Proprietary Preparations** (details are given in Part 3)
***Canad.:*** Ortho-Gynol†; ***NZ:*** Ortho-Gynol.

---

## Ethylene Glycol Monopalmitostearate

Ethylene Glycol Monostearate; Ethylene Glycol Stearate; Éthylène Glycol (Stéarate d'); Ethylenglycoli Monopalmitostearas; Ethylenglycoli Monostearas; Ethyleni Glycoli Stearas; Monopalmitoestearato de etilenglicol.

*CAS — 111-60-4 (ethylene glycol monostearate); 4219-49-2 (ethylene glycol monopalmitate).*

**Pharmacopoeias.** In *Eur.* (see p.vi). *USNF* includes Ethylene Glycol Stearates.

**Ph. Eur. 5.0** (Ethylene Glycol Monopalmitostearate). A mixture of ethylene glycol mono- and di-esters of stearic and palmitic acids. It contains not less than 50% of monoesters produced from the condensation of ethylene glycol and stearic acid and not more than 5% of free ethylene glycol. A white or almost white, waxy solid. Practically insoluble in water; soluble in hot alcohol and in acetone. M.p. 54° to 60°. Protect from light.

**USNF 22** (Ethylene Glycol Stearates). A mixture of ethylene glycol mono- and di-esters of stearic and palmitic acids. It contains not less than 50% of monoesters produced from the condensation of ethylene glycol and stearic acid of vegetable or animal origin. A white or almost white, waxy solid. Practically insoluble in water; soluble in hot alcohol and in acetone. M.p. 54° to 60°. Store in airtight containers. Avoid temperatures above 40°. Do not allow to freeze.

### Profile

Ethylene glycol monopalmitostearate has similar properties and uses to glyceryl monostearate or self-emulsifying glyceryl monostearate (below). Ethylene glycol monolaurate and mono-oleate have also been used.

---

## Glyceryl Behenate

Behenato de glicerilo.

**Pharmacopoeias.** In *USNF. Eur.* (see p.vi) includes Glycerol Dibehenate.

**Ph. Eur. 5.0** (Glycerol Dibehenate; Glyceroli Dibehenas). A mixture of diacylglycerols, mainly dibehenoylglycerol, together with variable quantities of mono- and triacylglycerols. It contains 13 to 21% of monoacylglycerols, 40 to 60% of diacylglycerols, and 21 to 35% of triacylglycerols, obtained by esterification of glycerol and behenic acid. A hard, waxy mass or powder or white or almost white, unctuous flakes. Insoluble in water; partly soluble in hot alcohol; soluble in dichloromethane. M.p. 65° to 77°.

**USNF 22** (Glyceryl Behenate). A mixture of glycerides of fatty acids, mainly behenic acid. A fine powder with a faint odour. M.p. about 70°. Practically insoluble in water and in alcohol; soluble in chloroform. Store in airtight containers at a temperature not exceeding 35°.

### Profile

Glyceryl behenate is used as a lubricant and binder in tablet-making.

---

## Glyceryl Distearate

Glycerol Distearate; Glyceroli Distearas.

*CAS — 1323-83-7.*

**Pharmacopoeias.** In *Eur.* (see p.vi). Also in *USNF.*

**Ph. Eur. 5.0** (Glycerol Distearate). A mixture of diacylglycerols, mainly distearoylglycerol, together with variable quantities of mono- and triacylglycerols. It contains 8 to 22% of monoacylglycerols, 40 to 60% of diacylglycerols, and 25 to 35% of triacylglycerols, obtained by partial glycerolysis of vegetable oils containing triacylglycerols of palmitic or stearic acid or by esterification of glycerol with stearic acid 50 (type I), stearic acid 70 (type II), or stearic acid 95 (type III). The fatty acids may be of vegetable or animal origin.

A hard, waxy mass or powder, or white or almost white, unctuous flakes. Insoluble in water; partly soluble in hot alcohol; soluble in dichloromethane. M.p. 50° to 60° (types I and II) or 50° to 70° (type III).

**USNF 22** (Glyceryl Distearate). A mixture of diglycerides, mainly glyceryl distearate, together with variable quantities of monoglycerides and triglycerides. It contains 8 to 22% of monoglycerides, 40 to 60% of diglycerides, and 25 to 35% of triglycerides. It is obtained by partial glycerolysis of vegetable oil that consists mainly of triglycerides of palmitic or stearic acid or by esterification of glycerol with stearic acid. The fatty acids may be of vegetable or animal origin.

Hard, waxy mass or powder, or white or almost white flakes. Insoluble in water; partly soluble in hot alcohol; soluble in dichloromethane and in tetrahydrofuran. Store in airtight containers at a temperature not exceeding 40°. Protect from light. Do not allow to freeze.

### Profile

Glyceryl distearate is used as an emulsifying and/or solubilising agent.

## Glyceryl Monolinoleate

Glycerol Monolinoleate; Glyceroli Monolinoleas; Monolinolein.
*CAS — 26545-74-4.*

**Pharmacopoeias.** In *Eur.* (see p.vi). Also in *USNF.*

**Ph. Eur. 5.0** (Glycerol Monolinoleate). A mixture of monoacylglycerols, mainly mono-oleoylglycerol and monolinoleoylglycerol, together with variable quantities of di- and triacylglycerols. It contains 32 to 52% of monoacylglycerols, 40 to 55% of diacylglycerols, and 5 to 20% of triacylglycerols, obtained by partial glycerolysis of vegetable oils mainly containing triacylglycerols of linoleic acid. A suitable antoxidant may be added.
Amber, oily liquids which may be partially solidified at room temperature. Practically insoluble in water; freely soluble in dichloromethane. Store in airtight containers. Protect from light.

**USNF 22** (Glyceryl Monolinoleate). A mixture of monoglycerides, mainly glyceryl mono-oleate and glyceryl monolinoleate, together with variable quantities of diglycerides and triglycerides. It is obtained by partial glycerolysis of vegetable oil that consists mainly of triglycerides of linoleic acid. It contains 32 to 52% of monoglycerides, 40 to 55% of diglycerides, and 5 to 20% of triglycerides. A suitable antoxidant may be added.
Amber, oily liquids that may be partially solidified at room temperature. Practically insoluble in water; freely soluble in dichloromethane; soluble in tetrahydrofuran. Store in airtight containers at a temperature not exceeding 40°. Protect from light. Do not allow to freeze.

### Profile

Glyceryl monolinoleate is used as an emulsifying and/or solubilising agent.

## Glyceryl Mono-oleate

Monolein; Monooleato de glicerilo.
*CAS — 25496-72-4.*

**Pharmacopoeias.** In *Eur.* (see p.vi). Also in *USNF.*

**Ph. Eur. 5.0** (Glycerol Mono-oleates). Mixtures of monoacylglycerols, mainly mono-oleoylglycerol, together with variable quantities of di- and triacylglycerols. They are defined by the nominal content of monoacylglycerols and obtained by partial glycerolysis of vegetable oils mainly containing triacylglycerols of oleic acid, or by esterification of glycerol by oleic acid. A suitable antoxidant may be added.
Amber, oily liquids which may be partially solidified at room temperature. Practically insoluble in water; freely soluble in dichloromethane. Store in airtight containers. Protect from light.

**USNF 22** (Glyceryl Monooleate). A mixture of monoglycerides, mainly glyceryl mono-oleate, together with variable quantities of di- and triglycerides. It is obtained by partial glycerolysis of vegetable oil that consists mainly of triglycerides of oleic acid, or by esterification of glycerol with oleic acid of vegetable or animal origin. It is defined by the nominal content of monoglycerides. A suitable antoxidant may be added.
Amber, oily liquids that may be partially solidified at room temperature. Practically insoluble in water; freely soluble in dichloromethane; soluble in tetrahydrofuran. Store in airtight containers at a temperature not exceeding 40°. Protect from light. Do not allow to freeze.

### Profile

Glyceryl mono-oleate has similar properties to glyceryl monostearate or self-emulsifying glyceryl monostearate (below).

## Glyceryl Monostearate

Glycérol (Monostéarate de); Glyceroli Monostearas; GMS; Monoestearato de glicerilo; Monostearin.
*CAS — 31566-31-1 (glyceryl monostearate); 26657-96-5 (glyceryl monopalmitate).*

**Pharmacopoeias.** In *Eur.* (see p.vi), *Int.*, *Jpn*, and *Pol.* Also in *USNF.*

**Ph. Eur. 5.0** (Glycerol Monostearate 40-55). A mixture of monoacylglycerols, mainly monostearoylglycerol, together with variable quantities of di- and triacylglycerols. It contains 40 to 55% of monoacylglycerols, 30 to 45% of diacylglycerols, and 5 to 15% of triacylglycerols, obtained by partial glycerolysis of vegetable oils mainly containing triacylglycerols of palmitic or stearic acid, or by esterification of glycerol with stearic acid.
A white or almost white, hard, waxy mass or unctuous powder or flakes. Practically insoluble in water; soluble in alcohol at 60°. M.p. 54° to 64°.

**USNF 22** (Glyceryl Monostearate). It contains not less than 90% of monoglycerides of saturated fatty acids, chiefly glyceryl monostearate ($C_{21}H_{42}O_4 = 358.6$) and glyceryl monopalmitate ($C_{19}H_{38}O_4 = 330.5$). It may contain a suitable antoxidant.
A white wax-like solid, beads, or flakes with a slight, agreeable, fatty odour. M.p. not below 55°. Insoluble in water but may be dispersed in hot water with the aid of a small amount of soap or other suitable surfactant; soluble 1 in 10 of chloroform, 1 in 100 of ether and of methyl alcohol, 1 in 33 of isopropyl alcohol; dissolves in hot organic solvents such as alcohol, acetone, mineral or fixed oils, and benzene. Store in airtight containers. Protect from light.

## Self-emulsifying Glyceryl Monostearate

Monoestearato de glicerilo autoemulsionable; Monostearin Emulsificans; Self-emulsifying Mono- and Diglycerides of Food Fatty Acids; Self-emulsifying Monostearin.

**Pharmacopoeias.** In *Br.*

**BP 2003** (Self-emulsifying Glyceryl Monostearate). A mixture consisting principally of mono-, di-, and triglycerides of stearic and palmitic acids, and of minor proportions of other fatty acids; it may also contain free fatty acids, free glycerol, and soap. It contains not less than 30% of monoglycerides, not more than 7% of free glycerol, and not more than 6% of soap, calculated as sodium oleate, all calculated with reference to the anhydrous substance.
A white to cream-coloured, hard, waxy solid with a faint fatty odour. Dispersible in hot water; soluble in hot dehydrated alcohol and in hot liquid paraffin; soluble in hot vegetable oils, but may give turbid solutions at concentrations below 20%.

**Incompatibility.** Because of the presence of soap, self-emulsifying glyceryl monostearate is incompatible with acids and high concentrations of ionisable salts, hard water, calcium compounds, zinc oxide, and oxides of heavy metals.

### Profile

Glyceryl monostearate is a poor water-in-oil emulsifying agent but it is a useful stabiliser of water-in-oil and oil-in-water emulsions in preparations for internal and external use. It has emollient properties. Glyceryl monostearate is also used in the food and cosmetic industries.

It is usual to add a small amount of soap, sulfated fatty alcohol, or other surfactant, to glyceryl monostearate, which has the effect of making the product self-emulsifying and capable of producing satisfactory oil-in-water emulsions. Self-emulsifying glyceryl monostearate is used as an emulsifying agent for oils, fats, solvents, and waxes in the preparation of bases of the non-emulsified, emulsified, and vanishing-cream types. It is not intended for inclusion in preparations for internal use.

Aqueous preparations containing self-emulsifying glyceryl monostearate should contain a preservative to prevent fungal or bacterial growth.

## Macrogol Cetostearyl Ethers

Éteres cetoestearílicos de macrogol; Macrogoli Aether Cetostearylicus.

**Pharmacopoeias.** In *Eur.* (see p.vi).

**Ph. Eur. 5.0** (Macrogol Cetostearyl Ether). A mixture of ethers of mixed macrogols with linear fatty alcohols, mainly cetostearyl alcohol. It may contain some free macrogols and it contains various amounts of free cetostearyl alcohol. The amount of ethylene oxide reacted with cetostearyl alcohol is from 2 to 33 units per molecule (nominal value). White or yellowish-white waxy, unctuous mass, pellets, microbeads, or flakes. Macrogol cetostearyl ether with low numbers of ethylene oxide units per molecule is practically insoluble in water; soluble in alcohol and in dichloromethane. Macrogol cetostearyl ether with higher numbers of ethylene oxide units per molecule is dispersible or soluble in water; soluble in alcohol and in dichloromethane. Macrogol cetostearyl ether solidifies at 32° to 52°. Store in airtight containers. The labelling states the amount of ethylene oxide reacted with cetostearyl alcohol (nominal value).

## Cetomacrogol 1000 *(BAN, rINN)*

Polyethylene Glycol 1000 Monocetyl Ether; Polyoxyethylene Glycol 1000 Monocetyl Ether.
*CAS — 9004-95-9; 68439-49-6.*

**Description.** Cetomacrogol 1000 is a macrogol ether containing 20 to 24 oxyethylene groups in the polyoxyethylene chain. It is represented by the formula $CH_3.[CH_2]_m.[O.CH_2.CH_2]_n.OH$, where *m* may be 15 or 17 and *n* may be 20 to 24.

**Pharmacopoeias.** In *Int.*

**Incompatibility.** Cetomacrogol has been reported to be incompatible with phenols and to reduce the antibacterial activity of quaternary ammonium compounds. Cetomacrogol may separate from solutions in the presence of a high concentration of electrolytes.

## Polyoxyl 20 Cetostearyl Ether

Éter cetoestearílico de polioxil 20.

**Pharmacopoeias.** In *USNF.*

**USNF 22** (Polyoxyl 20 Cetostearyl Ether). A mixture of the monocetostearyl (mixed hexadecyl and octadecyl) ethers of mixed macrogols, the average polymer length being equivalent to 17.2 to 25.0 oxyethylene units. A cream-coloured waxy unctuous mass, melting, when heated, to a clear brownish-yellow liquid. Soluble in water, in alcohol, and in acetone; insoluble in petroleum spirit. A 10% solution in water has a pH of 4.5 to 7.5. Store at a temperature of 8° to 15° in airtight containers.

### Profile

Macrogol cetostearyl ethers are used as surfactants and emulsifiers. Macrogol cetostearyl ether (22) is used with cetostearyl alcohol (for example, in the form of Cetomacrogol Emulsifying Wax BP 2003) as an emulsifying agent for making oil-in-water emulsions that are unaffected by moderate concentrations of electrolytes and that are stable over a wide pH range. It is also used to disperse volatile oils in water to form transparent sols.

### Preparations

***BP 2003:*** Cetomacrogol Emulsifying Wax.

## Macrogol 15 Hydroxystearate

Macrogoli 15 Hydroxystearas.

**Pharmacopoeias.** In *Eur.* (see p.vi).

**Ph. Eur. 5.0** (Macrogol 15 Hydroxystearate). A mixture of mainly mono- and di-esters of 12-hydroxystearic acid and macrogols obtained by ethoxylation of 12-hydroxystearic acid. The number of moles of ethylene oxide reacted per mole of 12-hydroxystearic acid is 15 (nominal value). It contains free macrogols. A yellowish, waxy mass. It solidifies at about 25°. Very soluble in water; soluble in alcohol; insoluble in liquid paraffin. Store in airtight containers.

### Profile

Macrogol 15 hydroxystearate is a nonionic surfactant used as a solubilising agent.

## Macrogol Lauril Ethers

α-Dodecyl-ω-hydroxypoly(oxyethylene); Éteres láuricos de macrogol; Laureth Compounds; Lauromacrogols; Macrogol Lauryl Ethers; Macrogoli Aether Laurilicum; Polyoxyl Lauryl Ethers.
*CAS — 9002-92-0.*

**Description.** Macrogol lauril ethers have the general formula $C_{12}H_{25}(OCH_2CH_2)_nOH$.

**Pharmacopoeias.** In *Eur.* (see p.vi) and *Jpn.* Also in *USNF.*

**Ph. Eur. 5.0** (Macrogol Lauryl Ether). A mixture of ethers of mixed macrogols with fatty alcohols, mainly $C_{12}H_{26}O$. It contains a variable amount of free $C_{12}H_{26}O$ and it may contain free macrogols. The number of moles of ethylene oxide reacted per mole of $C_{12}H_{26}O$ is 3 to 23 (nominal value). Macrogol lauril ether with 3 to 5 units of ethylene oxide per molecule is a colourless liquid. Practically insoluble in water and in petroleum spirit; soluble or dispersible in alcohol. Macrogol lauril ether with 9 to 23 units of ethylene oxide per molecule is a white, waxy mass. Soluble or dispersible in water; soluble in alcohol; practically insoluble in petroleum spirit. Macrogol lauril ether should be stored in airtight containers.

**USNF 22** (Polyoxyl Lauryl Ether). A mixture of the monolauril ethers of mixed polyethylene glycols, the average polymer length being equivalent to not less than 3 and not more than 23 oxyethylene units (nominal value). It contains various amounts of free lauril alcohol, and it may contain some free polyethylene glycols. Store in airtight containers in a dry place at a temperature of 8° to 15°.

## Laureth 4 *(USAN)*

*CAS — 9002-92-0.*

**Description.** A mixture of monolauril ethers of macrogols where the average value of *n* in the formula given above is 4.

## Lauromacrogol 400 *(rINN)*

Laureth 9 *(USAN)*; Polidocanol.
*CAS — 9002-92-0; 3055-99-0.*
*ATC — C05BB02.*

**Description.** Lauromacrogol 400 is a mixture of monolauril ethers of macrogols where the average value of *n* in the formula given above is 9. It has sometimes, however, been erroneously described as containing 8, rather than 9, oxyethylene groups.

### Adverse Effects

There have been occasional reports of allergic skin reactions following the topical application of preparations containing laureth compounds.

◊ A 63-year-old man developed pulmonary oedema, a dramatic fall in heart rate, transient left pyramidal syndrome and died following sclerotherapy with lauromacrogol 400 to control gastric variceal bleeding;[1] the fatality was attributed to the action of the drug that had passed into the systemic circulation. Another patient has been described[2] who suffered a reversible ischaemic neurological deficit after sclerotherapy with lauromacrogol 400 for varicose veins of the leg.

1. Paterlini A, *et al.* Heart failure and endoscopic sclerotherapy of variceal bleeding. *Lancet* 1984; **i:** 1241.
2. Van der Plas JPL, *et al.* Reversible ischaemic neurological deficit after sclerotherapy of varicose veins. *Lancet* 1994; **343:** 428.

### Uses and Administration

Macrogol lauril ethers (laureth compounds) have been used as surfactants and spermicides. Lauromacrogol 400 is used as a sclerosant in the treatment of oesophageal and gastric varices (p.1716) and varicose veins (p.1717), and has been used as a local anaesthetic and antipruritic (see p.1137) in combination topical preparations.

### Preparations

**Proprietary Preparations** (details are given in Part 3)

***Arg.:*** Aet; Aetoxy Sklerol; ***Austral.:*** Aethoxysclerol; ***Austria:*** Aethoxysklerol; ***Belg.:*** Aethoxysklerol; ***Braz.:*** Aethoxysclerol; ***Denm.:*** Aethoxysklerol; ***Fin.:*** Aethoxysklerol; ***Fr.:*** Aetoxisclerol; ***Ger.:*** Aethoxysklerol; Anaesthesulf; Hamo-Europuran N†; Recessan; ***Ital.:*** Atossisclerol Kreussler; ***Mex.:*** Farmaflebon; ***Neth.:*** Aethoxysklerol; ***Spain:*** Etoxisclerol; ***Swed.:*** Aethoxysklerol; ***Switz.:*** Aethoxysklerol; ***Thai.:*** Aethoxysklerol.

**Multi-ingredient:** ***Arg.:*** Solcoseryl Dental; ***Austral.:*** TAGG†; ***Austria:*** Balneum Plus; Dentinox; Gingivan; Optiderm†; Paididont; Prurimix; Solcoseryl Dental; Vonum; ***Belg.:*** Cose-Anal; Neo-Alcos-Anal†; ***Braz.:*** Nene Dent N; ***Ger.:*** Acoin; Alcos-Anal; Balneum Plus; Brand- u. Wundgel-Medice N; Collomack; Corti-Dynexan; Dentinox N; Haemo-Exhirud; Hexamon; Inflam; Meaverin; Medigel; Optiderm; Rectosellan H†; Sagittaproct S†; Solcoseryl Dental; Tamposit N; Thesit; Thesit P†; Varitan N†; Vivisun†; ***Hong Kong:*** Balneum Intensiv Plus; Collomack; Solcoseryl Dental; ***Irl.:*** Balneum Plus; ***Israel:*** Balneum Plus; Derma-Care; ***Ital.:*** Optiderm; ***Malaysia:*** Balneum Intensiv Plus; Collomack; Solcoseryl Dental; ***Mex.:*** Nene Dent; ***Norw.:*** Alcos-Anal; ***Port.:*** Anacal; Hidratante VV; Optiderme†; ***Singapore:*** Balneum Intensiv Plus; Collomack; ***Switz.:*** Balneum Hermal Plus; Decasept N; Dentinox†; Optiderm; Oxydermine; Prurimed; Ralur; Remexal; Sclerovein; Solcoseryl Dental; Sportusal; Sportusal Spray sine heparino; Venucreme; Venugel; ***Thai.:*** Balneum Intensiv Plus; Collomack; Solcoseryl Dental; ***UK:*** Anacal; Balneum Plus; E45 Itch Relief.

## Macrogol Monomethyl Ethers

Éteres monometílicos de macrogol; Polyethylene Glycol Monomethyl Ethers. α-Methyl-ω-hydroxypoly(oxyethylene).

*CAS — 9004-74-4.*

**Pharmacopoeias.** In *USNF.*

**USNF 22** (Polyethylene Glycol Monomethyl Ether). Addition polymers of ethylene oxide and methyl alcohol, represented by the formula $CH_3(OCH_2CH_2)_nOH$, where *n* represents the average number of oxyethylene groups. The name is usually designated by a number that corresponds approximately to its average molecular weight.

As the average molecular weight increases, the water solubility, vapour pressure, hygroscopicity, and solubility in organic solvents decrease while congealing temperature, specific gravity, flash-point, and viscosity increase. Liquid grades occur as clear to slightly hazy, colourless or practically colourless, slightly hygroscopic, viscous liquids with a slight characteristic odour. Solid grades occur as practically odourless, white, waxy, plastic material with a consistency similar to beeswax, or as creamy white flakes, beads, or powders. Liquid grades are miscible with water; solid grades are freely soluble in water; all grades are soluble in alcohol, in acetone, in chloroform, in ethyl acetate, in ethylene glycol monoethyl ether, and in toluene; all grades are insoluble in ether and in hexane. Store in airtight containers.

### Profile

Macrogol monomethyl ethers may be used as ointment bases, solvents, and plasticisers.

## Macrogol Oleyl Ethers

Éteres oleílicos de macrogol; Macrogoli Aether Oleicum.

**Pharmacopoeias.** In *Eur.* (see p.vi).

**Ph. Eur. 5.0** (Macrogol Oleyl Ether). A mixture of ethers of mixed macrogols with linear fatty alcohols, mainly oleyl alcohol. It may contain some free macrogols and it contains various amounts of free oleyl alcohol. Macrogol oleyl ether with 2 to 5 units of ethylene oxide per molecule is a yellow liquid. Practically insoluble in water and in petroleum spirit; soluble in alcohol. Macrogol oleyl ether with 10 to 20 units of ethylene oxide per molecule is a yellowish-white, waxy mass. Dispersible or soluble in water; soluble in alcohol; practically insoluble in petroleum spirit. Macrogol oleyl ethers should be stored in airtight containers. Protect from light.

## Polyoxyl 10 Oleyl Ether

Éter oleílico de polioxil 10; Polyethylene Glycol Mono-oleyl Ether.

*CAS — 9004-98-2.*

**Pharmacopoeias.** In *USNF.*

**USNF 22** (Polyoxyl 10 Oleyl Ether). A mixture of the monooleyl ethers of mixed macrogols, the average polymer length being equivalent to 8.6 to 10.4 oxyethylene units. It may contain suitable stabilisers.

A soft white semisolid or pale yellow liquid with a bland odour. Soluble in water and in alcohol; dispersible in liquid paraffin and in propylene glycol with possible separation on standing. Store at a temperature of 8° to 15° in airtight containers.

### Profile

Macrogol oleyl ethers such as polyoxyl 10 oleyl ether are used as surfactants.

## Macrogol Stearates

Ésteres del macrogol; Macrogoli Stearas; Polyoxyethylene Glycol Stearates; Polyoxyethylene Stearates; Polyoxyl Stearates.

*CAS — 9004-99-3.*

**Nomenclature.** There are two systems of nomenclature used for these compounds; these substances have the general formula $C_{17}H_{35}COO.[O.CH_2CH_2]_n.H$. In the systems used by *BAN* and *USAN* the numbers in the names refer to the approximate polymer length in oxyethylene units whereas in the system used by *INN* the number refers to the average molecular weight of the polymer chain. Thus, the names Macrogol 8 Stearate (*BAN*), Polyoxyl 8 Stearate (*USAN*), and Macrogol Stearate 400 (*rINNM*) all describe the same compound and similarly Macrogol 40 Stearate (*BAN*), Polyoxyl 40 Stearate (*USAN*), and Macrogol Stearate 2000 (*rINNM*) all refer to another.

**Pharmacopoeias.** In *Eur.* (see p.vi).

*USNF* includes a monograph for macrogol stearate with 40 oxyethylene units.

**Ph. Eur. 5.0** (Macrogol Stearate). A mixture of the mono- and di-esters of mainly stearic acid and/or palmitic acid and macrogols. It may be obtained by ethoxylation or by esterification of macrogols with stearic acid 50 (type I) or stearic acid 95 (type II). The average polymer length is equivalent to 6 to 100 ethylene oxide units per molecule (nominal value). It may contain free macrogols. White or slightly yellowish waxy mass. Soluble in alcohol and in isopropyl alcohol. Compounds containing 6 to 9 units of ethylene oxide per molecule are practically insoluble but freely dispersible in water; miscible with fatty oils and with waxes. Compounds containing 20 to 100 units of ethylene oxide per molecule are soluble in water; practically insoluble in fatty oils and in waxes. Store in airtight containers.

**USNF 22** (Polyoxyl 40 Stearate). A mixture of the mono- and di-esters of stearic acid and mixed macrogols, the average polymer length being about 40 oxyethylene units. It contains not less than 17% and not more than 27% of free macrogols. It is a waxy, white to light tan solid, odourless or with a faint fat-like odour. Congealing range 37° to 47°. Soluble in water, in alcohol, in acetone, and in ether; insoluble in liquid paraffin and in vegetable oils. Store in airtight containers.

**Incompatibility.** Macrogol stearates have been reported to be generally stable with electrolytes and weak acids or bases although strong acids or bases may cause hydrolysis and saponification. Discoloration or precipitation may occur with phenolic substances and complexation with preservatives. Decrease in the antimicrobial activity of bacitracin, chloramphenicol, phenoxymethylpenicillin, and tetracycline has been stated to occur with concentrations of macrogol stearates exceeding 5%.

### Profile

Macrogol stearates are macrogol esters that are used as emulsifying and solubilising agents.

## Menfegol *(rINN)*

Menphegol. α-[*p*-(*p*-Menthyl)phenyl]-ω-hydroxypoly(oxyethylene).

*CAS — 57821-32-6.*

### Profile

Menfegol consists of menthylphenyl ethers of macrogols represented by the formula $C_{16}H_{23}(OCH_2CH_2)_nOH$. It is a nonionic surfactant used as a spermicide.

### Preparations

**Proprietary Preparations** (details are given in Part 3)

***Hong Kong:*** Neo Sampoon; ***Malaysia:*** Neo Sampoon; ***Singapore:*** Neo Sampoon.

## Mono- and Di-glycerides

E471 (mono- and di-glycerides of fatty acids); Mono y diglicéridos.

**Pharmacopoeias.** In *USNF.*

**USNF 22** (Mono- and Di-glycerides). A mixture of glycerol mono- and di-esters, with minor amounts of tri-esters, of fatty acids from edible oils. It contains not less than 40% of monoglycerides. It may contain suitable stabilisers. Store in airtight containers. Protect from light.

### Profile

Mono- and di-glycerides is used as an emulsifying agent.

## Nonoxinols

Macrogol Nonylphenyl Ethers; Nonoxinoles; Nonoxynols. α-(4-Nonylphenyl)-ω-hydroxypoly(oxyethylene).

*CAS — 26027-38-3.*

**Nomenclature.** Nonoxinols are a series of nonylphenyl ethers of macrogols of differing chain lengths, represented by the formula $C_{15}H_{23}.[O.CH_2.CH_2]_n.OH$.

Nonoxinol is *BAN* and *rINN.* The name may be followed by a figure indicating the approximate number of oxyethylene groups in the polyoxyethylene chain. *USAN* specifies Nonoxynol 4, Nonoxynol 9, Nonoxynol 15, and Nonoxynol 30.

## Nonoxinol 9 *(BAN, rINN)*

Nonoxinolum 9; Nonoxynol 9 *(USAN).* α-(4-Nonylphenyl)-ω-hydroxynona(oxyethylene).

$C_{33}H_{60}O_{10}$ (nominal) = 616.8.

**Pharmacopoeias.** In *Eur.* (see p.vi), *Int.*, and *US.*

**Ph. Eur. 5.0** (Nonoxinol 9). A mixture consisting mainly of mononnonylphenyl ethers of macrogols corresponding to the formula: $C_{15}H_{23}.(O.CH_2.CH_2)_n.OH$ where the average value of *n* is 9. A clear, colourless to light yellow, viscous liquid. Miscible with water, with alcohol, and with vegetable oils. Store in airtight containers.

**USP 27** (Nonoxynol 9). An anhydrous liquid mixture consisting chiefly of monononylphenyl ethers of macrogols corresponding to the formula $C_{15}H_{23}.[O.CH_2.CH_2]_n.OH$, in which the average value of *n* is about 9. A clear, colourless to light yellow, viscous liquid. Soluble in water, in alcohol, and in maize oil. Store in airtight containers.

## Nonoxinol 10 *(BAN, rINN)*

Nonoxynol 10. α-(4-Nonylphenyl)-ω-hydroxydeca(oxyethylene).

$C_{35}H_{64}O_{11}$ (nominal) = 660.9.

## Nonoxinol 11 *(BAN, rINN)*

Nonoxynol 11. α-(4-Nonylphenyl)-ω-hydroxyundeca(oxyethylene).

$C_{37}H_{68}O_{12}$ (nominal) = 704.9.

### Adverse Effects and Precautions

Nonoxinols used as vaginal spermicides may cause local irritation.

**Pregnancy.** Maternal use of spermicidal contraceptives has been linked to an increased frequency of congenital abnormalities, including trisomy, but it has been suggested that such studies may be flawed by recall bias.[1] Meta-analysis of 9 studies also supported the view that peri- and postconceptual maternal use of spermicides was not associated with adverse fetal outcome.[2]

1. Mishell DR. Contraception. *N Engl J Med* 1989; **320:** 777–87.
2. Einarson TR, *et al.* Maternal spermicide use and adverse reproductive outcome: a meta-analysis. *Am J Obstet Gynecol* 1990; **162:** 655–60.

**Toxic shock syndrome.** Toxic shock syndrome has been associated with the use of a vaginal contraceptive sponge impregnated with nonoxinol 9. A review[1] of 13 cases reported in the USA up to November 1984 found that in 4 of the cases there were other predisposing conditions: postpartum use, use during menstruation, and prolonged retention.

1. Faich G, *et al.* Toxic shock syndrome and the vaginal contraceptive sponge. *JAMA* 1986; **255:** 216–18.

**Urinary-tract infection.** Use of spermicidal foam or jelly containing nonoxinol 9 may disturb the normal vaginal flora and predispose to colonisation with *Escherichia coli* and the development of bacteriuria.[1] An increased risk of acute *E. coli* urinary-tract infection has been reported[2] associated with the use of condoms coated with nonoxinol 9.

1. Hooton TM, *et al.* Escherichia coli bacteriuria and contraceptive method. *JAMA* 1991; **265:** 64–9.
2. Fihn SD, *et al.* Association between use of spermicide-coated condoms and Escherichia coli urinary tract infection in young women. *Am J Epidemiol* 1996; **144:** 512–20.

### Uses

Nonoxinols have surface active properties and may be used as solubilising agents. Nonoxinol 9 is used as a spermicide for contraception (p.1535).

**Antimicrobial activity.** Nonoxinol 9 has activity *in vitro* against a number of bacteria and viruses and it was hoped[1,2] that use of spermicidal contraceptives containing nonoxinol 9 might provide some protection against sexually transmitted diseases, including chlamydial, gonococcal, and HIV infection. However, controlled studies involving HIV-negative female sex workers or other high-risk women have found that use of nonoxinol 9 does not reduce the rate of new HIV,[3,4] or gonorrhoea or chlamydia infection;[3,5] meta-analyses,[6,7] including these and other studies, have come to similar conclusions. Furthermore, nonoxinol 9 has an irritant action and may increase the risk of genital ulceration, leading to an increased risk of infection by HIV. The United Nations[8] and WHO[9] have therefore advised against its use by women at high risk.

1. North BB. Vaginal contraceptives: effective protection from sexually transmitted diseases for women? *J Reprod Med* 1988; **33:** 307–311.
2. Anonymous. Multipurpose spermicides. *Lancet* 1992; **340:** 211–13.
3. Roddy RE, *et al.* A controlled trial of nonoxynol 9 film to reduce male-to-female transmission of sexually transmitted diseases. *N Engl J Med* 1998; **339:** 504–10.
4. Van Damme L, *et al.* Effectiveness of COL-1492, a nonoxynol-9 vaginal gel, on HIV-1 transmission in female sex workers: a randomised controlled trial. *Lancet* 2002; **360:** 971–7. Correction. *ibid.*; 1892.
5. Roddy RE, *et al.* Effect of nonoxynol-9 gel on urogenital gonorrhea and chlamydial infection: a randomized controlled trial. *JAMA* 2002; **287:** 1117–22.
6. Wilkinson D, *et al.* Nonoxynol-9 for preventing vaginal acquisition of HIV infection by women from men. Available in The Cochrane Library; Issue 2. Chichester: John Wiley; 2004.

7. Wilkinson D, *et al.* Nonoxynol-9 for preventing vaginal acquisition of sexually transmitted infections by women from men. Available in The Cochrane Library; Issue 2. Chichester: John Wiley; 2004.
8. Anonymous. UN warns against use of spermicide. *BMJ* 2000; **321:** 194.
9. Anonymous. Nonoxinol 9 ineffective in preventing HIV infection. *WHO Drug Inf* 2002; **16:** 120–1.

### Preparations

**Proprietary Preparations** (details are given in Part 3)
***Arg.:*** Delfen; ***Austral.:*** Delfen†; Lubarol; Ortho-Creme†; ***Austria:*** Delfen; Patentex; ***Belg.:*** Gynintim Film†; Patentex†; ***Braz.:*** Espermicida Preserv; Pessarios Profilaticos Rendell; ***Canad.:*** Advantage 24; Comfort†; Delfen; Encare†; K-Y Plus Spermicidal Lubricant; Lifestyles; Ortho Shields†; Ortho-Gynol II; Ramses; Sheik; Shields; Titan†; Trojan; ***Chile:*** Impidol; Supoviol; VCF; ***Fin.:*** Patentex; ***Fr.:*** Patentex†; ***Ger.:*** Ortho-Gel†; Patentex; Patentex Oval; ***Hong Kong:*** VCF†; ***India:*** Delfen; ***Irl.:*** Delfen; Gynol II; Ortho-Creme; Orthoforms†; ***Israel:*** Delfen; ***Ital.:*** C-Film†; ***Mex.:*** Lorophyn; Preforms†; ***NZ:*** Rendells Plus; ***Port.:*** Delfen; Rendells; ***S.Afr.:*** Delfen; ***Spain:*** Lineafarm†; Nacha; Nobliten†; Yadalan†; ***Switz.:*** C-Film; Delfen; Patentex Oval N; Syn-A-Gen; ***UK:*** C-Film†; Delfen; Double Check†; Duracreme†; Duragel; Gynol II; Ortho-Creme; Orthoforms; Prelude; Today†; ***USA:*** Advantage 24; Because†; Delfen; Emko†; Encare; Gynol; Koromex†; Ramses†; Semicid; Sheik Elite; Shur-Seal; VCF.

**Multi-ingredient:** ***Arg.:*** Lorophyn; ***Canad.:*** Protectaid; ***Ger.:*** A-gen 53; ***Hong Kong:*** Protectaid; ***Israel:*** Glovan; ***Ital.:*** Betaform Habitat†; Florigien†; Vironox†; ***Spain:*** Lavolen; ***UK:*** Protectaid.

## Octoxinols

Macrogol Tetramethylbutylphenyl Ethers; Octoxinoles; Octoxynols; Octylphenoxy Polyethoxyethanol. α-[4-(1,1,3,3-Tetramethylbutyl)phenyl]-ω-hydroxypoly(oxyethylene).
*CAS — 9002-93-1.*

**Nomenclature.** Octoxinols are a series of tetramethylbutylphenyl ethers of macrogols of differing chain lengths, represented by the formula $C_{14}H_{21}.[O.CH_2.CH_2]_n.OH$.
Octoxinol is *BAN* and *rINN*. The name may be followed by a figure indicating the approximate number of oxyethylene groups in the polyoxyethylene chain. *USAN* specifies Octoxynol 9.

## Octoxinol 9 *(BAN, rINN)*

Octoxynol 9 *(USAN).*
$C_{32}H_{58}O_{10}$ (nominal) = 602.8.

**Pharmacopoeias.** In *USNF.*
**USNF 22** (Octoxynol 9). An anhydrous liquid mixture consisting chiefly of mono-octylphenyl ethers of macrogols, corresponding to the formula $C_{14}H_{21}.[O.CH_2.CH_2]_n.OH$, in which the average value of *n* is about 9. A clear, pale yellow, viscous liquid with a faint odour. Miscible with water, with alcohol, and with acetone; soluble in toluene and in benzene; practically insoluble in petroleum spirit. Store in airtight containers.

## Octoxinol 10 *(BAN, rINN)*

$C_{34}H_{62}O_{11}$ (nominal) = 646.8.
**Pharmacopoeias.** In *Eur.* (see p.vi).
**Ph. Eur. 5.0** (Octoxinol 10). A mixture consisting mainly of mono-octylphenyl ethers of macrogols corresponding to the formula: $C_{14}H_{21}.(O.CH_2.CH_2)_n.OH$ where the average value of *n* is 10. A clear, colourless or light yellow, viscous liquid. Miscible with water, with alcohol, and with vegetable oils. Store in airtight containers.

### Profile

Octoxinols have surface active properties and may be used as solubilising agents. They are also used as spermicides.

### Preparations

**Proprietary Preparations** (details are given in Part 3)
***Austral.:*** Ortho-Gynol; Summers Eve Disposable†; Summers Eve Feminine†; ***USA:*** Koromex†; Ortho-Gynol; Vagi-Gard Medicated Disposable Douche.

**Multi-ingredient:** ***Austral.:*** Summers Eve Feminine†; ***Canad.:*** Aseptone Quat†; ***Chile:*** Summer's Eve Hierbas; ***USA:*** Feminique; Massengill; Massengill Disposable; Summers Eve Disposable.

## Poloxamers

Poloxamera; Poloxámeros; Polyethylene-polypropylene glycol. α-Hydro-ω-hydroxypoly(oxyethylene)poly(oxypropylene)poly-(oxyethylene) block copolymer.
*CAS — 9003-11-6.*

**Nomenclature.** Poloxamer is *BAN* and *rINN*. The name is followed by a figure, the first 2 digits of which, when multiplied by 100, correspond to the approximate average molecular weight of the polyoxypropylene portion and the third digit, when multiplied by 10, corresponds to the percentage by weight of the polyoxyethylene portion. *USAN* specifies Poloxamer 182D, Poloxamer 182LF, Poloxamer 188, Poloxamer 188LF, and Poloxamer 331.
Poloxalene (*BAN, USAN, rINN*) is also a poloxamer.

**Pharmacopoeias.** In *Eur.* (see p.vi). Also in *USNF.*
**Ph. Eur. 5.0** (Poloxamers). A synthetic block copolymer of ethylene oxide and propylene oxide represented by the general formula: $HO(C_2H_4O)_a(C_3H_6O)_b(C_2H_4O)_aH$. It may contain a suitable antioxidant. Poloxamer 124 is a colourless or almost colourless liquid. Poloxamer 188, poloxamer 237, poloxamer 338, and poloxamer 407 are white or almost white, waxy powders, microbeads or flakes; m.p. about 50°. All poloxamers are very soluble in water and in alcohol; practically insoluble in petroleum spirit (50° to 70°). pH of a 10% solution in water is 5.0 to 7.5. Store in airtight containers.
**USNF 22** (Poloxamer). A synthetic block copolymer of ethylene oxide and propylene oxide with the general formula $HO(C_2H_4O)_a(C_3H_6O)_b(C_2H_4O)_aH$. It may contain a suitable antoxidant. Poloxamer 124 is a colourless liquid with a mild odour. Poloxamers 188, 237, 338, and 407 are white, prilled or cast solids, odourless or with a mild odour. All poloxamers are freely soluble in water and in alcohol. Poloxamers 124 and 407 are freely soluble in isopropyl alcohol and in propylene glycol; poloxamer 237 is sparingly soluble in isopropyl alcohol and in xylene; poloxamer 338 is sparingly soluble in propylene glycol; poloxamer 124 is freely soluble in xylene. A 2.5% solution in water has a pH of 5.0 to 7.5. Store in airtight containers.

**Incompatibility.** Poloxamers have been reported to be incompatible with phenols.

## Poloxalene *(BAN, USAN, rINN)*

Poloxaleno; SKF-18667.

**Pharmacopoeias.** In *US* for veterinary use only.
**USP 27** (Poloxalene). A synthetic block copolymer of ethylene oxide and propylene oxide. A colourless or pale yellow liquid. Soluble in water, in chloroform, and in ethylene dichloride. A 2.5% solution in water has a pH of 5.0 to 7.5. Store in airtight containers at a temperature of 8° to 15°. Protect from light.

## Poloxamer 188 *(BAN, USAN, rINN)*

Poloxalkol; Poloxámero 188.

NOTE. Compounded preparations of poloxamer 188 may be represented by the following names:

- Co-danthramer *x/y* (*BAN*)—where *x* and *y* are the strengths in milligrams of dantron and poloxamer respectively.

**Pharmacopoeias.** In *Eur.* (see p.vi). Also in *USNF.*
**Ph. Eur. 5.0** (Poloxamers). Poloxamer 188 is a poloxamer in which *a* in the general formula given above is 75 to 85 and *b* is 25 to 30; it has an average molecular weight of 7680 to 9510. It is a white or almost white, waxy powder, microbeads, or flakes. M.p. about 50°. Very soluble in water and in alcohol; practically insoluble in petroleum spirit (50° to 70°). pH of a 10% solution is 5.0 to 7.5. Store in airtight containers.
**USNF 22** (Poloxamer). Poloxamer 118 is a poloxamer in which *a* in the general formula averages 80 and *b* averages 27; it has an average molecular weight of 7680 to 9510. A white prilled or cast solid, odourless or with a very mild odour. M.p. about 52°. Freely soluble in water and in alcohol. Store in airtight containers.

## Poloxamer 407 *(BAN, rINN)*

Poloxámero 407.

**Pharmacopoeias.** In *Eur.* (see p.vi). Also in *USNF.*
**Ph. Eur. 5.0** (Poloxamers). Poloxamer 407 is a poloxamer in which *a* in the general formula given above is 95 to 105 and *b* is 54 to 60; it has an average molecular weight of 9840 to 14 600. It is a white or almost white, waxy powder, microbeads, or flakes. M.p. about 50°. Very soluble in water and in alcohol; practically insoluble in petroleum spirit (50° to 70°). pH of a 10% solution in water is 5.0 to 7.5. Store in airtight containers.
**USNF 22** (Poloxamer). Poloxamer 407 is a poloxamer in which *a* in the general formula averages 101 and *b* averages 56; it has an average molecular weight of 9840 to 14 600. A white, prilled or cast solid, odourless or with a very mild odour. M.p. about 56°. Freely soluble in water, in alcohol, and in isopropyl alcohol. Store in airtight containers.

### Precautions

Poloxamers may increase the absorption of liquid paraffin and other fat-soluble substances.

### Uses and Administration

Poloxamers are used as emulsifying agents for intravenous fat emulsions, as solubilising agents to maintain clarity in elixirs and syrups, and as wetting agents for antibacterials. They may also be used in ointment or suppository bases and as tablet binders or coaters.

Poloxamer 188 is used as a wetting agent in the treatment of constipation. It is usually given with a laxative such as dantron. Poloxamer 188 has also been used as an emulsifying agent in fluorocarbon blood substitutes. Poloxamer 188 has been investigated for its ability to improve blood flow in sickle-cell crisis; it has also been tried in myocardial infarction. Other investigational uses include the treatment of burns.

Poloxamer 407 is used in solutions for contact lens care, as is poloxamer 338.

Poloxalene is used as a defoaming agent in the treatment of bloat in ruminants.

◊ References.

1. Orringer EP, *et al.* Purified poloxamer 188 for treatment of acute vaso-occlusive crisis of sickle cell disease: a randomized controlled trial. *JAMA* 2001; **286:** 2099–2106.
2. Gibbs WJ, Hagemann TM. Purified poloxamer 188 for sickle cell vaso-occlusive crisis. *Ann Pharmacother* 2004; **38:** 320–4.

### Preparations

**Proprietary Preparations** (details are given in Part 3)
***Austral.:*** Clerz†; Coloxyl; Pliagel; ***Braz.:*** Pliagel†; ***Canad.:*** Clerz; ***Fr.:*** Alkenide; Idrocol†; ***NZ:*** Coloxyl; Pliagel†.

**Multi-ingredient:** ***Austria:*** Actizyme†; ***Irl.:*** Ailax; Codalax; Cotron; ***NZ:*** Codalax; Conthram; ***UK:*** Ailax†; Codalax; Danlax; ***USA:*** Baby Orajel Tooth and Gum Cleanser; ControlRx.

## Polyoxyl Castor Oils

Aceites de ricino polioxietilenados; Macrogolglycerol Ricinoleate; Macrogolglyceroli Ricinoleas; Polyethoxylated Castor Oils; Polyoxyethylene Castor Oils.

**Pharmacopoeias.** In *Eur.* (see p.vi).
**Ph. Eur. 5.0** (Macrogolglycerol Ricinoleate; Polyoxyl Castor Oil BP 2003). It contains mainly ricinoleyl glycerol ethoxylated with 30 to 50 molecules of ethylene oxide (nominal value), with small amounts of macrogol ricinoleate and of the corresponding free glycols. It results from the reaction of castor oil with ethylene oxide. A clear, yellow, viscous liquid or semi-solid. Relative density about 1.05; viscosity, at 25°, 500 to 800 mPa s. Freely soluble in water and in alcohol; very soluble in dichloromethane. Protect from light.

## Polyoxyl 35 Castor Oil

Aceite de ricino polioxil 35.

**Pharmacopoeias.** In *USNF.*
**USNF 22** (Polyoxyl 35 Castor Oil). A mixture of the triricinoleate ester of ethoxylated glycerol with smaller amounts of macrogol ricinoleate and the corresponding free glycols. It is produced by reacting 1 mole of glycerol ricinoleate with about 35 moles of ethylene oxide.
A yellow oily liquid with a faint characteristic odour. Sp. gr. 1.05 to 1.06; viscosity, at 25°, 650 to 850 mPa s. Very soluble in water, producing a practically odourless and colourless solution; soluble in alcohol and in ethyl acetate; insoluble in mineral oils. Store in airtight containers.

**Incompatibility.** Polyethoxylated castor oils are reported to affect polyvinyl chloride containers and apparatus adversely.

### Adverse Effects

Polyoxyl castor oils (such as Cremophor EL), used as vehicles in various intravenous injections, have been associated with severe anaphylactoid reactions, hyperlipidaemias, alterations in blood viscosity, and erythrocyte aggregation. They may also lead to adverse effects due to alterations in the pharmacokinetics of the formulated drug.

◊ References.

1. Bagnarello AG, *et al.* Unusual serum lipoprotein abnormality induced by the vehicle of miconazole. *N Engl J Med* 1977; **296:** 497–9.
2. Forrest ARW, *et al.* Long-term Althesin infusion and hyperlipidaemia. *BMJ* 1977; **2:** 1357–8.
3. Dye D, Watkins J. Suspected anaphylactic reaction to Cremophor EL. *BMJ* 1980; **280:** 1353.
4. Howrie DL, *et al.* Anaphylactoid reactions associated with parenteral cyclosporine use: possible role of Cremophor EL. *Drug Intell Clin Pharm* 1985; **19:** 425–7.
5. Chapuis B, *et al.* Anaphylactic reaction to intravenous cyclosporine. *N Engl J Med* 1985; **312:** 1259.
6. Siddall SJ, *et al.* Anaphylactic reactions to teniposide. *Lancet* 1989; **i:** 394.
7. ten Tije AJ, *et al.* Pharmacological effects of formulation vehicles: implications for cancer chemotherapy. *Clin Pharmacokinet* 2003; **42:** 665–85.

### Uses

Polyoxyl castor oils are macrogol esters used as emulsifying and solubilising agents. Polyoxyl 35 castor oil has been used as a solvent in vehicles for various intravenous injections.

## Polyoxyl Hydrogenated Castor Oils

Aceites de ricino hidrogenados y polioxietilenados; Macrogolglycerol Hydroxystearate; Macrogolglyceroli Hydroxystearas.

**Pharmacopoeias.** In *Eur.* (see p.vi).
**Ph. Eur. 5.0** (Macrogolglycerol Hydroxystearate; Hydrogenated Polyoxyl Castor Oil BP 2003). It contains mainly trihydroxystearyl glycerol ethoxylated with 7 to 60 molecules of ethylene oxide (nominal value), with small amounts of macrogol hydroxystearate and of the corresponding free glycols. It results from the reaction of hydrogenated castor oil with ethylene oxide. Polyoxyl hydrogenated castor oil with less than 10 units of ethylene oxide per molecule is a yellowish, turbid, viscous liquid. Practically insoluble in water; dispersible in alcohol; soluble in acetone. Polyoxyl hydrogenated castor oil with more than 20 units of ethylene oxide per molecule is a white or yellowish, semi-liquid or pasty mass. Freely soluble in water, in alcohol, and in acetone; practically insoluble in petroleum spirit.

## Polyoxyl 40 Hydrogenated Castor Oil

Aceite de ricino hidrogenado polioxil 40.

**Pharmacopoeias.** In *USNF.*
**USNF 22** (Polyoxyl 40 Hydrogenated Castor Oil). A mixture of mainly the trihydroxystearate ester of ethoxylated glycerol, with smaller amounts of macrogol trihydroxystearate and the corres-

ponding free glycols. It is produced by reacting 1 mole of glycerol trihydroxystearate with about 40 to 45 moles of ethylene oxide.

A white to yellowish paste or pasty liquid with a faint odour. Congealing range 20° to 30°. Very soluble in water, producing an odourless, colourless solution; soluble in alcohol and in ethyl acetate; insoluble in liquid paraffin. Store in airtight containers.

### Profile

Polyoxyl hydrogenated castor oils are used as surfactants.

## Polysorbates

Polisorbatos.

**Description.** A series of mixtures of fatty acid esters of sorbitol and its anhydrides copolymerised with approximately 20 moles of ethylene oxide for each mole of sorbitol and its anhydrides.

**Incompatibility.** Polysorbates have been reported to be stable with electrolytes and weak acids and bases although saponification may occur in the presence of strong acids and bases. Discoloration or precipitation may occur with phenolic substances. The oleic acid esters are sensitive to oxidation. For reference to the possible incompatibility of polysorbate 80 with hydroxybenzoates, see p.1184.

## Polysorbate 20 *(BAN, USAN, rINN)*

E432; Polisorbato 20; Polyoxyethylene 20 Sorbitan Monolaurate; Polysorbatum 20; Sorbimacrogol Laurate 300; Sorboxaethenum Laurinicum.

$C_{58}H_{114}O_{26}$ (approximate).

*CAS — 9005-64-5.*

**Pharmacopoeias.** In *Eur.* (see p.vi) and *Int.* Also in *USNF.*

**Ph. Eur. 5.0** (Polysorbate 20). A mixture of partial esters of fatty acids, mainly lauric acid, with sorbitol and its anhydrides ethoxylated with approximately 20 moles of ethylene oxide for each mole of sorbitol and its anhydrides. A clear or slightly opalescent yellowish to brownish-yellow oily liquid. Relative density about 1.10. Soluble in water, in dehydrated alcohol, in ethyl acetate, and in methyl alcohol; practically insoluble in liquid paraffin and in fatty oils. Store in airtight containers. Protect from light.

**USNF 22** (Polysorbate 20). A laurate ester of sorbitol and its anhydrides copolymerised with approximately 20 moles of ethylene oxide for each mole of sorbitol and its anhydrides. A lemon to amber liquid with a faint characteristic odour. Soluble in water, in alcohol, in dioxan, in ethyl acetate, and in methyl alcohol; insoluble in liquid paraffin. Store in airtight containers.

## Polysorbate 40 *(BAN, USAN, rINN)*

E434; Polisorbato 40; Polyoxyethylene 20 Sorbitan Monopalmitate; Polysorbatum 40; Sorbimacrogol Palmitate 300.

$C_{62}H_{122}O_{26}$ (approximate).

*CAS — 9005-66-7.*

**Pharmacopoeias.** In *Eur.* (see p.vi). Also in *USNF.*

**Ph. Eur. 5.0** (Polysorbate 40). Mixture of partial esters of fatty acids, mainly palmitic acid, with sorbitol and its anhydrides ethoxylated with approximately 20 moles of ethylene oxide for each mole of sorbitol and sorbitol anhydrides. An oily, viscous, yellowish or brownish-yellow liquid. Relative density about 1.10. Miscible with water, with dehydrated alcohol, with ethyl acetate, and with methyl alcohol; practically insoluble in fatty oils and in liquid paraffin. Store in airtight containers. Protect from light.

**USNF 22** (Polysorbate 40). A palmitate ester of sorbitol and its anhydrides copolymerised with approximately 20 moles of ethylene oxide for each mole of sorbitol and its anhydrides. A yellow liquid with a faint characteristic odour. Soluble in water and in alcohol; insoluble in liquid paraffin and in vegetable oils. Store in airtight containers.

## Polysorbate 60 *(BAN, USAN, rINN)*

E435; Polisorbato 60; Polyoxyethylene 20 Sorbitan Monostearate; Polysorbatum 60; Sorbimacrogol Stearate 300; Sorboxaethenum Stearinicum.

$C_{64}H_{126}O_{26}$ (approximate).

*CAS — 9005-67-8.*

**Pharmacopoeias.** In *Eur.* (see p.vi), *Int.*, and *Pol.* Also in *USNF.*

**Ph. Eur. 5.0** (Polysorbate 60). A mixture of partial esters of fatty acids, mainly stearic acid 50, with sorbitol and its anhydrides ethoxylated with approximately 20 moles of ethylene oxide for each mole of sorbitol and its anhydrides. A yellowish-brown gelatinous mass which becomes a clear liquid at temperatures above 25°. Relative density about 1.10. Soluble in water, in dehydrated alcohol, in ethyl acetate, and in methyl alcohol; practically insoluble in liquid paraffin and in fatty oils. Store in airtight containers. Protect from light.

**USNF 22** (Polysorbate 60). A mixture of stearate and palmitate esters of sorbitol and its anhydrides copolymerised with approximately 20 moles of ethylene oxide for each mole of sorbitol and its anhydrides. A lemon to orange-coloured oily liquid or semi-gel with a faint characteristic odour. Soluble in water, in ethyl acetate, and in toluene; insoluble in liquid paraffin and in vegetable oils. Store in airtight containers.

## Polysorbate 80 *(BAN, USAN, rINN)*

E433; Olethytan 20; Polisorbato 80; Polyäthylenglykol-Sorbitanoleat; Polyoxyethylene 20 Sorbitan Mono-oleate; Polysorbatum 80; Polysorbitanum 80 Oleinatum; Sorbimacrogol Oleate 300; Sorboxaethenum Oleinicum; Sorethytan 20 Mono-oleate.

$C_{64}H_{124}O_{26}$ (approximate).

*CAS — 9005-65-6.*

**Pharmacopoeias.** In *Chin., Eur.* (see p.vi), *Int., Jpn*, and *Pol.* Also in *USNF.*

**Ph. Eur. 5.0** (Polysorbate 80). A mixture of partial esters of fatty acids, mainly oleic acid, with sorbitol and its anhydrides ethoxylated with approximately 20 moles of ethylene oxide for each mole of sorbitol and its anhydrides. A clear yellowish or brownish-yellow oily liquid. Relative density about 1.10. Miscible with water, with dehydrated alcohol, with ethyl acetate, and with methyl alcohol; practically insoluble in liquid paraffin and in fatty oils. Store in airtight containers. Protect from light.

**USNF 22** (Polysorbate 80). An oleate ester of sorbitol and its anhydrides copolymerised with approximately 20 moles of ethylene oxide for each mole of sorbitol and its anhydrides. A lemon to amber-coloured oily liquid with a faint characteristic odour. Sp. gr. between 1.06 and 1.09; viscosity, at 25°, between 300 and 500 mPa s. Very soluble in water, producing an odourless and practically colourless solution; soluble in alcohol and in ethyl acetate; insoluble in liquid paraffin. Store in airtight containers.

## Polysorbate 85 *(BAN, USAN, rINN)*

Polisorbato 85; Polyoxyethylene 20 Sorbitan Trioleate; Sorbimacrogol Trioleate 300.

$C_{100}H_{188}O_{28}$ (approximate).

*CAS — 9005-70-3.*

**Description.** A mixture of mainly trioleate esters of sorbitol and its anhydrides copolymerised with approximately 20 moles of ethylene oxide for each mole of sorbitol and its anhydrides.

### Adverse Effects and Precautions

Polysorbates may increase the absorption of fat-soluble substances.

There have been occasional reports of hypersensitivity following topical application of preparations containing polysorbates.

Fatalities in low-birth-weight infants associated with the injection of a polysorbate-containing preparation are discussed below.

Polysorbates used as excipients may also lead to adverse effects due to alterations in the pharmacokinetics of the formulated drug.

◊ References.

1. ten Tije AJ, *et al.* Pharmacological effects of formulation vehicles: implications for cancer chemotherapy. *Clin Pharmacokinet* 2003; **42:** 665–85.

**Effects in infants.** Following the introduction in the USA of an intravenous preparation of vitamin E (E-Ferol) there were a number of reports of unusual liver and kidney disorders with 38 deaths being reported among treated low-birth-weight infants. Affected infants had unexplained hypotension, thrombocytopenia, renal dysfunction, hepatomegaly, cholestasis, ascites, and metabolic acidosis;[1-3] the preparation was subsequently withdrawn from the market in April 1984 about 5 months after it was introduced. *In-vitro* evidence was produced demonstrating that E-Ferol suppressed the response of human lymphocytes to phytohaemagglutinin. However, it was the mixture of polysorbates, polysorbate 20 and in particular polysorbate 80, that was shown to be responsible for this suppression rather than the α-tocopherol acetate component. Despite this *in-vitro* data, overwhelming infection was not a feature in the affected infants.[2] Large doses of polysorbates were unavoidably injected when E-Ferol was used and it was suggested that polysorbates may accumulate as a result of an alteration in the metabolism by low-birth-weight infants; polysorbate-induced alteration of membrane fluidity in cells of vessel walls may have led to changes in structure and function.[2]

1. Alade SL, *et al.* Polysorbate 80 and E-Ferol toxicity. *Pediatrics* 1986; **77:** 593–7.
2. Balistreri WF, *et al.* Lessons from the E-Ferol tragedy. *Pediatrics* 1986; **78:** 503–6.
3. Golightly LK, *et al.* Pharmaceutical excipients: adverse effects associated with inactive ingredients in drug products. *Med Toxicol* 1988; **3:** 128–65 and 209–240.

**Hypersensitivity.** Local inflammatory reactions following intramuscular injection of a vitamin A preparation were considered[1] to be due to a hypersensitivity reaction to polysorbate 80, included as an excipient.

1. Shelley WB, *et al.* Polysorbate 80 hypersensitivity. *Lancet* 1995; **345:** 1312–13.

### Uses

Polysorbates are hydrophilic nonionic surfactants that are used as emulsifying agents for the preparation of stable oil-in-water emulsions in pharmaceutical products; they are frequently used with a sorbitan ester in varying proportions to produce products with a range of texture and consistency. Polysorbates have also been used in the formulation of insecticide and herbicide sprays, industrial detergents, and cosmetic products. They are also used as emulsifiers in the food industry.

Polysorbates are used as solubilising agents for a variety of substances including essential oils and oil-soluble vitamins such as vitamins A, D, and E, and as wetting agents in the formulation of oral and parenteral suspensions. However, see Adverse Effects and Precautions, above.

Polysorbates may also be used for their surfactant properties in preparations for the removal of ear wax, and for the management of dry eyes and upper respiratory-tract disorders.

### Preparations

**Proprietary Preparations** (details are given in Part 3)

***Belg.:*** Oleosorbate†; ***Canad.:*** Diopteras; Tears Encore; ***Fr.:*** Cerumenol; ***USA:*** Viva-Drops.

**Multi-ingredient:** ***Arg.:*** Balsan; Otoclean Gotas Oticas; ***Austria:*** Expigen; Nasimild†; ***Fin.:*** Expigen; ***Fr.:*** Fluisedal; Fluisedal sans promethazine; Paroplak; Prorhinel; ***Norw.:*** Expigent†; ***S.Afr.:*** Dilinct; Expigen; ***Switz.:*** Prorhinel; Rhinocure Simplex†; Rhinocure†.

## Propylene Glycol Diacetate

Diacetato de propilenglicol. Propanediol diacetate.

$C_7H_{12}O_4$ = 160.2.

*CAS — 623-84-7 (1,2-isomer); 628-66-0 (1,3-isomer).*

### Profile

Propylene glycol diacetate is an emulsifying and/or solubilising agent, and a solvent. It is included in some external preparations for ear infection.

### Preparations

**Proprietary Preparations** (details are given in Part 3)

***Austral.:*** VoSoL†.

**Multi-ingredient:** ***Canad.:*** VoSoL; VoSoL HC; ***NZ:*** VoSoL; ***USA:*** AA-HC Otic†; Acetasol; Acetasol HC; VoSoL; VoSoL HC.

## Propylene Glycol Laurate

E477 (propylene glycol esters of fatty acids).

## Propylene Glycol Dilaurate

E477 (propylene glycol esters of fatty acids); Propylene Dilaurate; Propylenglycoli Dilauras.

*CAS — 22788-19-8.*

**Pharmacopoeias.** In *Eur.* (see p.vi).

**Ph. Eur. 5.0** (Propylene Glycol Dilaurate). A mixture of the propylene glycol mono- and di-esters of lauric acid. It contains a minimum of 70% of di-esters and a maximum of 30% of mono-esters. The content of free propylene glycol is not more than 2%. A colourless or slightly yellow, clear oily liquid at 20°. Practically insoluble in water; very soluble in alcohol, in methyl alcohol, and in dichloromethane. Protect from moisture.

## Propylene Glycol Monolaurate

E477 (propylene glycol esters of fatty acids); Propylenglycoli Monolauras.

**Pharmacopoeias.** In *Eur.* (see p.vi).

**Ph. Eur. 5.0** (Propylene Glycol Monolaurate). A mixture of the propylene glycol mono- and di-esters of lauric acid. It contains 45 to 70% of mono-esters and 30 to 55% of di-esters (type I) or a minimum of 90% of mono-esters and a maximum of 10% of di-esters (type II). The content of free propylene glycol is not more than 5% (type I) or not more than 1% (type II). A colourless or slightly yellow, clear oily liquid at 20°. Practically insoluble in water; very soluble in alcohol, in methyl alcohol, and in dichloromethane. Protect from moisture.

### Profile

Propylene glycol mono- and dilaurate have similar properties to propylene glycol monopalmitostearate (below) and are used as emulsifying and solubilising agents.

## Propylene Glycol Monopalmitostearate

E477 (propylene glycol esters of fatty acids); Monopalmitoestearato de propilenglicol; Propylene Glycol Monostearate; Propylene Glycol Stearate; Propylèneglycol (Stéarate de); Propylenglycoli Monopalmitostearas; Propylenglycoli Monostearas; Prostearin.

*CAS — 1323-39-3 (propylene glycol monostearate); 29013-28-3 (propylene glycol monopalmitate).*

**Pharmacopoeias.** In *Eur.* (see p.vi). Also in *USNF.*

**Ph. Eur. 5.0** (Propylene Glycol Monopalmitostearate). A mixture of the propylene glycol mono- and di-esters of stearic and palmitic acids. It contains a minimum of 50% of mono-esters produced from the condensation of propylene glycol and stearic acid 50. A white or almost white, waxy solid. M.p. 33° to 40°. Practically insoluble in water; soluble in hot alcohol and in acetone. Protect from light.

**USNF 22** (Propylene Glycol Monostearate). A mixture of the propylene glycol mono- and di-esters of stearic and palmitic acids. It contains not less than 90% of mono-esters of saturated fatty acids, chiefly propylene glycol monostearate and propylene glycol monopalmitate. A white, wax-like solid, beads, or flakes, with a slight agreeable fatty odour. Congealing temperature not less than 45°. Insoluble in water but it may be dispersed in hot water with the aid of a small amount of soap or other suitable surfactant; soluble in organic solvents such as alcohol, acetone, ether, benzene, and fixed or mineral oils.

### Profile

Propylene glycol monopalmitostearate is obtainable commercially in the pure, non-dispersible form, or in the self-emulsifying form containing a small proportion of soap or other primary emulsifying agent. It is used as a stabiliser or emulsifier similarly to glyceryl monostearate or self-emulsifying glyceryl monostearate (p.1412).

## Quillaia

E999 (quillaia extract); Panama Wood; Quillaia Bark; Quillaiae Cortex; Quillay; Seifenrinde; Soap Bark.
*CAS — 631-01-6 (quillaic acid).*

**Pharmacopoeias.** In *Br.*, *Fr.*, and *Swiss.*

**BP 2003** (Quillaia). The dried inner part of the bark of *Quillaja saponaria* and other species of *Quillaja* containing not less than 22% of alcohol (45%)-soluble extractive. It is odourless or almost odourless, but the dust or powder is strongly sternutatory.

### Adverse Effects

Quillaia taken by mouth has been reported to produce gastrointestinal irritation. It has been suggested that the ingestion of large amounts may produce liver damage, respiratory failure, convulsions, and coma.

### Uses

Quillaia contains 2 amorphous saponin glycosides, quillaic acid and quillaiasapotoxin. It is used as an emulsifying agent and frothing agent; it is often used with tragacanth mucilage or another thickening agent. Quillaia is also used for its surfactant properties in preparations for skin and respiratory-tract disorders.

### Preparations

***BP 2003:*** Quillaia Liquid Extract; Quillaia Tincture.

**Proprietary Preparations** (details are given in Part 3)

**Multi-ingredient:** ***Braz.:*** Bluderm; ***Chile:*** Fitotos; Notosil; Sedotus; ***Fin.:*** Kvilla; ***Fr.:*** Coaltar Saponine le Beuf†; ***Hong Kong:*** Pectoral; ***Ital.:*** Soluzione Composta Alcoolica Saponosa di Coaltar†; ***Swed.:*** Quilla simplex; ***Switz.:*** Expectoran Codein.

## Sorbitan Esters

Ésteres del sorbitán.

**Description.** A series of mixtures of the partial esters of sorbitol and its mono- and di-anhydrides with fatty acids.

## Sorbitan Laurate *(BAN, rINN)*

E493; Laurato de sorbitán; Sorbitan Monolaurate *(USAN)*; Sorbitani Lauras.
$C_{18}H_{34}O_6$ (approximate).
*CAS — 1338-39-2.*

**Pharmacopoeias.** In *Eur.* (see p.vi). Also in *USNF.*

**Ph. Eur. 5.0** (Sorbitan Laurate). A mixture of the partial esters of sorbitol and its mono- and di-anhydrides with lauric acid. A brownish-yellow viscous liquid. Relative density about 0.98. Practically insoluble but dispersible in water; miscible with alcohol; slightly soluble in cottonseed oil. Protect from light.

**USNF 22** (Sorbitan Monolaurate). A partial ester of sorbitol and its mono- and di-anhydrides with lauric acid. A yellow to amber oily liquid with a bland characteristic odour. Insoluble in water; soluble in liquid paraffin; slightly soluble in cottonseed oil and in ethyl acetate. Store in airtight containers.

## Sorbitan Oleate *(BAN, rINN)*

E494; NSC-406239; Oleato de sorbitán; Sorbitan Monooleate *(USAN)*; Sorbitan Mono-oleate; Sorbitani Oleas.
$C_{24}H_{44}O_6$ (approximate).
*CAS — 1338-43-8.*

**Pharmacopoeias.** In *Eur.* (see p.vi). Also in *USNF.*

**Ph. Eur. 5.0** (Sorbitan Oleate). A mixture usually obtained by esterification of 1 mole of sorbitol and its mono- and di-anhydrides per mole of oleic acid. A suitable antoxidant may be added. A brownish-yellow viscous liquid. Relative density about 0.99. Practically insoluble but dispersible in water; miscible with alcohol; soluble in fatty oils producing a hazy solution. Protect from light.

**USNF 22** (Sorbitan Monooleate). A partial oleate ester of sorbitol and its mono- and di-anhydrides. A yellow to amber-coloured, viscous, oily liquid with a bland characteristic odour. Insoluble in water and in propylene glycol; miscible with mineral and vegetable oils. Store in airtight containers.

## Sorbitan Palmitate *(BAN, rINN)*

E495; Palmitato de sorbitán; Sorbitan Monopalmitate *(USAN)*; Sorbitani Palmitas.
$C_{22}H_{42}O_6$ (approximate).
*CAS — 26266-57-9.*

**Pharmacopoeias.** In *Eur.* (see p.vi). Also in *USNF.*

**Ph. Eur. 5.0** (Sorbitan Palmitate). A mixture of the partial esters of sorbitol and its mono- and di-anhydrides with palmitic acid. A yellowish or yellow powder, waxy flakes, or hard masses. M.p. 44° to 51°. Practically insoluble in water; slightly soluble in alcohol; soluble in fatty oils. Protect from light.

**USNF 22** (Sorbitan Monopalmitate). A partial ester of sorbitol and its mono- and di-anhydrides with palmitic acid. A cream-coloured, waxy solid with a faint fatty odour. Insoluble in water; soluble in warm dehydrated alcohol; soluble with haze in warm liquid paraffin and in warm arachis oil.

## Sorbitan Sesquioleate *(BAN, USAN, rINN)*

Sesquioleato de sorbitán; Sorbitani Sesquioleas.
$C_{33}H_{60}O_{6.5}$ (approximate).
*CAS — 8007-43-0.*

**Pharmacopoeias.** In *Eur.* (see p.vi) and *Jpn.* Also in *USNF.*

**Ph. Eur. 5.0** (Sorbitan Sesquioleate). A mixture usually obtained by esterification of 2 moles of sorbitol and its mono- and di-anhydrides per 3 moles of oleic acid. A suitable antoxidant may be added. Relative density about 0.99. A pale yellow or slightly brownish-yellow paste, which becomes a viscous, oily, brownish-yellow liquid at about 25°. Dispersible in water; slightly soluble in dehydrated alcohol; soluble in fatty oils. Protect from light.

**USNF 22** (Sorbitan Sesquioleate). A partial oleate ester of sorbitol and its mono- and di-anhydrides. A yellow to amber-coloured, oily viscous liquid. Insoluble in water and in propylene glycol; soluble in alcohol, in isopropyl alcohol, in cottonseed oil, and in liquid paraffin. Store in airtight containers.

## Sorbitan Stearate *(BAN, rINN)*

E491; Estearato de sorbitán; Sorbitan Monostearate *(USAN)*; Sorbitani Stearas.
$C_{24}H_{46}O_6$ (approximate).
*CAS — 1338-41-6.*

**Pharmacopoeias.** In *Eur.* (see p.vi). Also in *USNF.*

**Ph. Eur. 5.0** (Sorbitan Stearate). A mixture of the partial esters of sorbitol and its mono- and di-anhydrides with stearic acid. A pale yellow, waxy solid. M.p. 50° to 55°. Practically insoluble but dispersible in water; slightly soluble in alcohol. Protect from light.

**USNF 22** (Sorbitan Monostearate). A partial ester of sorbitol and its mono- and di-anhydrides with stearic acid. A cream-coloured to tan, hard, waxy solid with a bland odour. Insoluble in cold water and in acetone; dispersible in warm water; soluble, with haze, above 50° in ethyl acetate and in liquid paraffin.

## Sorbitan Trioleate *(BAN, USAN, rINN)*

Sorbitani Trioleas; Trioleato de sorbitán.
$C_{60}H_{108}O_8$ (approximate).
*CAS — 26266-58-0.*

**Pharmacopoeias.** In *Eur.* (see p.vi). Also in *USNF.*

**Ph. Eur. 5.0** (Sorbitan Trioleate). A mixture usually obtained by esterification of 1 mole of sorbitol and its mono- and di-anhydrides per 3 moles of oleic acid. A suitable antoxidant may be added. A pale yellow, light yellowish or brown solid which becomes a brownish-yellow, viscous, oily liquid at about 25°. Relative density about 0.98. Practically insoluble but dispersible in water; slightly soluble in alcohol; soluble in fatty oils. Protect from light.

**USNF 22** (Sorbitan Trioleate). A tri-ester of sorbitol and its mono- and di-anhydrides with oleic acid. A yellow to amber-coloured, oily liquid. Insoluble in water, in ethylene glycol, and in propylene glycol; soluble in alcohol, in isopropyl alcohol, in methyl alcohol, in maize oil, in cottonseed oil, and in liquid paraffin. Store in airtight containers.

## Sorbitan Tristearate *(BAN, USAN, rINN)*

E492; Triestearato de sorbitán.
$C_{60}H_{114}O_8$ (approximate).
*CAS — 26658-19-5.*

**Description.** A mixture of the partial tri-esters of sorbitol and its mono- and di-anhydrides with stearic acid.

### Adverse Effects

There have been occasional reports of hypersensitive skin reactions following the topical application of creams containing sorbitan esters.

**Hypersensitivity.** References.


1. Finn OA, Forsyth A. Contact dermatitis due to sorbitan monolaurate. *Contact Dermatitis* 1975; **1:** 318.
2. Hannuksela M, *et al.* Allergy to ingredients of vehicles. *Contact Dermatitis* 1976; **2:** 105–10.
3. Austad J. Allergic contact dermatitis to sorbitan monooleate (Span 80). *Contact Dermatitis* 1982; **8:** 426–7.
4. Boyle J, Kennedy CTC. Contact urticaria and dermatitis to Alphaderm. *Contact Dermatitis* 1984; **10:** 178.


### Uses

Sorbitan esters are lipophilic nonionic surfactants that are used as emulsifying agents in the preparation of emulsions, creams, and ointments for pharmaceutical and cosmetic use. When used alone they produce stable water-in-oil emulsions but they are frequently used with a polysorbate in varying proportions to produce water-in-oil or oil-in-water emulsions or creams with a variety of different textures and consistencies. Sorbitan esters are also used as emulsifiers and stabilisers in food.

## Sucrose Esters

E473 (sucrose esters of fatty acids); Ésteres de sacarosa.

### Profile

Sucrose esters are nonionic compounds with surface-active properties produced by esterification of 1 or more hydroxyl groups in sucrose with a fatty acid such as stearic or palmitic acid. Commercial sucrose esters are mixtures of the mono-, di-, and tri-esters of palmitic and stearic acids with sucrose; various grades are available. Sucrose esters are used as dispersing and emulsifying agents in food and cosmetic preparations.

## Tyloxapol *(BAN, USAN, rINN)*

Superinone; Tiloxapol.
*CAS — 25301-02-4.*
*ATC — R05CA01.*

**Pharmacopoeias.** In *US.*

**USP 27** (Tyloxapol). A polymer of 4-(1,1,3,3-tetramethylbutyl)phenol with ethylene oxide and formaldehyde. A viscous amber liquid, sometimes slightly turbid, with a slight aromatic odour. Slowly but freely miscible with water; soluble in chloroform, in glacial acetic acid, in carbon disulfide, in carbon tetrachloride, in toluene, and in benzene. A 5% solution has a pH of 4.0 to 7.0. Tyloxapol should not be allowed to come into contact with metals. Store in airtight containers.

### Adverse Effects

Slight inflammation of the eyelids has been reported after prolonged use of aqueous inhalations of tyloxapol. It has been reported that occasional febrile reactions may occur.

### Uses and Administration

Tyloxapol is a nonionic surfactant of the alkyl aryl polyether alcohol type. It is used in solutions for cleansing contact lenses and artificial eyes. Aqueous solutions have been used for inhalation as a mucolytic for tenacious bronchopulmonary secretions. Tyloxapol has also been used as a vehicle for aerosol medication and for antibacterials administered in irrigation solutions for pyogenic bone or joint infections.

### Preparations

**Proprietary Preparations** (details are given in Part 3)

***Austria:*** Tacholiquin; ***Canad.:*** Enuclene; ***Fr.:*** Translight†; ***Ger.:*** Enuclen; Tacholiquin; ***NZ:*** Enuclene; ***Spain:*** Lacermucin†; ***USA:*** Enuclene.

**Multi-ingredient:** ***Ger.:*** Complete†; ***Israel:*** Complete All-In-One†.

# Nutritional Agents and Vitamins

Dietary Modification, p.1417
Enteral and Parenteral Nutrition, p.1418
Trace Elements, p.1419
Vitamins, p.1419

The principal constituents of food are carbohydrates, fats, minerals, proteins, vitamins, indigestible fibre, and water. Energy is provided by the metabolism of carbohydrates, fats, surplus protein, and alcohol.

**Carbohydrates** found in foods may be classified according to their degree of polymerisation into three main groups, namely sugars, oligosaccharides, and polysaccharides; all of these are made up only of carbon, hydrogen, and oxygen. Sugars can be further subdivided into *monosaccharides* (single-molecule sugars), such as fructose and glucose, *disaccharides* (whose molecules consist of two monosaccharides joined together), such as lactose and sucrose, and *sugar alcohols* (polyols) such as sorbitol and mannitol. *Oligosaccharides* typically consist of 3 to 9 monosaccharides joined together, and include malto-oligosaccharides such as maltodextrins. *Polysaccharides* consist of many monosaccharides joined together and include starches and non-starch polysaccharides such as cellulose. Non-starch polysaccharides are the major fraction of dietary fibre, and many authorities now consider this term is preferable to dietary fibre.

**Fats** have the same elemental composition as carbohydrates, but with a lower proportion of oxygen. Dietary fat is usually in the form of triglycerides, esters of glycerol with three fatty acid molecules. Essential fatty acids are ones that cannot be made in the body and which must be supplied by the food.

**Proteins** are made up of carbon, hydrogen, oxygen, and nitrogen; most proteins also contain sulfur and some contain phosphorus. They are required for the regulation of body processes such as growth and tissue maintenance. Excess protein can be converted into carbohydrate and used to provide energy.

Proteins consist of chains of **amino acids** of which there are *essential* and *non-essential* types. Essential amino acids (indispensable amino acids) cannot be synthesised in sufficient amounts in the body and must therefore be present in food; non-essential amino acids can be synthesised in the body. There are eight essential amino acids: isoleucine, leucine, lysine, methionine, phenylalanine, threonine, tryptophan, and valine. Arginine and histidine are also essential for infant growth while synthesis of cysteine, taurine, and tyrosine may be inadequate in premature infants.

Several inorganic elements, or minerals, are essential dietary constituents; those which are required in relatively small amounts are known as **trace elements** (see below). Their main function is to act as essential cofactors in various enzyme systems.

**Vitamins** and their general role in health are described below.

## Dietary Modification

Infants, children, elderly people, and pregnant or lactating women have particular nutritional requirements, but in most cases, provided that they are in good general health, adjustment to intake is all that is required rather than extensive modification or supplementation.

Dietary modification is important in the management of a variety of disorders. Calorie restriction is fundamental to the management of obesity, although it may be difficult to motivate patients to accept long-term changes to their eating habits, and some fashionable diets are at best of little value.

The role of diet in the aetiology of cardiovascular disorders (such as salt intake in hypertension and fat intake in ischaemic heart disease) is recognised to be of importance and has lead to public health campaigns for healthier eating patterns.

Dietary modification is also an accepted part of the management of diabetes mellitus, while protein restriction is important in the management of uraemia or hepatic encephalopathy.

There are also various metabolic disorders such as phenylketonuria, or forms of intolerance to dietary components, such as coeliac disease, in which the diet must be modified to exclude or drastically reduce certain food components.

**Amino acid metabolic disorders.** Various inborn errors of amino-acid metabolism are known. They are not common but their consequences are often serious or fatal. Although in some cases there is no effective treatment, early diagnosis is important as some conditions can be managed by dietary modification and/or the use of vitamins. Two of the better known syndromes, homocystinuria and phenylketonuria, are discussed briefly below. Cystinosis, another disorder of amino acid metabolism, is discussed on p.1712. Urea cycle disorders are discussed under Hyperammonaemia on p.1421.

**Homocystinuria**. Homocystinuria in its classical form is an autosomal recessive disorder due to a genetic deficiency of the enzyme cystathionine synthetase, resulting in accumulation of homocysteine (oxidised extracellularly to homocystine).[1] Manifestations may include mental retardation, atherosclerosis, thromboembolism, osteoporosis, and ocular symptoms including lens dislocation, glaucoma, cataract, and retinal detachment. Dietary restriction of methionine and cystine supplements have been used for treatment; some patients may respond to treatment with B vitamins (pyridoxine, cobalamins, and folic acid),[1,2] or to betaine.[3-6]

**Phenylketonuria**. Phenylketonuria is an autosomal recessive disorder that is usually due to a defect in the enzyme phenylalanine hydroxylase. This results in raised blood concentrations of phenylalanine in the neonate, and if untreated produces a syndrome of skin rash, depigmentation, hypertonia, seizures, and severe mental retardation. The disease is controlled by use of a synthetic diet very low in phenylalanine,[7-11] and if started early this can permit relatively normal intellectual development. High-dose tyrosine does not appear to be an effective alternative to a diet low in phenylalanine.[12,13]

1. Isherwood DM. Homocystinuria. *BMJ* 1996; **313:** 1025–6.
2. Schuh S, *et al.* Homocystinuria and megaloblastic anemia responsive to vitamin $B_{12}$ therapy. *N Engl J Med* 1984; **310:** 686–90.
3. Smolin LA, *et al.* The use of betaine for the treatment of homocystinuria. *J Pediatr* 1981; **99:** 467–72.
4. Wilcken DEL, *et al.* Homocystinuria—the effects of betaine in the treatment of patients not responsive to pyridoxine. *N Engl J Med* 1983; **309:** 448–53.
5. Holme E, *et al.* Betaine for treatment of homocystinuria caused by methylenetetrahydrofolate reductase deficiency. *Arch Dis Child* 1989; **64:** 1061–4.
6. Anonymous. Betaine for homocystinuria. *Med Lett Drugs Ther* 1997; **39:** 12.
7. Rylance G. Outcome of early detected and early treated phenylketonuria patients. *Postgrad Med J* 1989; **65** (suppl 2): S7–9.
8. Link R. Phenylketonuria diet in adolescents— energy and nutrient intake—is it adequate? *Postgrad Med J* 1989; **65** (suppl 2): S21–4.
9. American Academy of Pediatrics Committee on Genetics. Maternal phenylketonuria. *Pediatrics* 1991; **88:** 1284–5.
10. Thompson GN, *et al.* Pregnancy in phenylketonuria: dietary treatment aimed at normalising maternal plasma phenylalanine concentration. *Arch Dis Child* 1991; **66:** 1346–9.
11. Medical Research Council. Report of the Medical Research Council Working Party on Phenylketonuria. Recommendations on the dietary management of phenylketonuria. *Arch Dis Child* 1993; **68:** 426–7.
12. Pietz J, *et al.* Effect of high-dose tyrosine supplementation on brain function in adults with phenylketonuria. *J Pediatr* 1995; **127:** 936–43.
13. Smith ML, *et al.* Randomised controlled trial of tyrosine supplementation on neuropsychological performance in phenylketonuria. *Arch Dis Child* 1998; **78:** 116–21.

**Cardiovascular disease.** Modification of the diet may be helpful in patients with, or at risk of, cardiovascular disease. In patients with hypertension (p.825), reduction in salt intake may be tried before commencing drug therapy or used as an adjunct to such therapy. Reduction in the total intake of dietary fat, and in particular of saturated fatty acids, is considered important for both the general population and those considered at high risk of ischaemic heart disease (see Cardiovascular Risk Reduction, p.819). An increased intake of long chain n-3 polyunsaturated fatty acids has been recommended and also a restriction on *trans* fatty acids. Dietary cholesterol should be restricted although it may make less of a contribution to plasma cholesterol levels than dietary saturates.[1,2]

For discussion of the possibility that antoxidant vitamins may reduce the risk of ischaemic heart disease see under Vitamins, below. The link between folic acid, homocysteine, and ischaemic heart disease is discussed on p.1429.

1. DoH. Nutritional aspects of cardiovascular disease. *Report on health and social subjects 46.* London: HMSO, 1994. [COMA report.]
2. Krauss RM, *et al.* AHA Dietary Guidelines: revision 2000: a statement for healthcare professionals from the Nutrition Committee of the American Heart Association. *Circulation* 2000; **102:** 2284–99. Also available at: http://circ.ahajournals.org/cgi/reprint/102/18/2284.pdf (accessed 20/05/04)

**Coeliac disease.** Coeliac disease (gluten-sensitive enteropathy; coeliac sprue) is an inflammatory disorder of the small intestine that results from an immunological reaction to the gliadin fraction of gluten (p.1694). The inflammation leads to mucosal atrophy with subsequent malabsorption, although the extent and severity of mucosal inflammation varies widely, and some patients are asymptomatic. In adults, anaemia and mild gastrointestinal symptoms that may be confused with irritable bowel syndrome are the usual symptoms. In infants and children there may be growth retardation or failure to thrive, and gastrointestinal symptoms may be more marked. Other nutritional deficiencies, including calcium malabsorption leading to osteopenia, may also occur, and mouth ulcers are also common.

Treatment of coeliac disease involves a strict, life-long, gluten-free diet. Nutritional supplements may be necessary at the start of treatment but can usually be stopped once mucosal recovery has occurred. Diagnosis is confirmed by normalisation of the mucosa on repeat biopsy after 3 to 4 months. Dermatitis herpetiformis (p.1134) is a non-gastrointestinal manifestation of coeliac disease. Patients may have no gastrointestinal symptoms, although mucosal abnormalities are generally apparent on biopsy. These patients also respond to a gluten-free diet.

Coeliac disease is associated with a number of auto-immune diseases, including type 1 diabetes, thyroid disease, and IgA deficiency. Patients with coeliac disease have an increased incidence of small-bowel lymphoma and a slight increase in the incidence of some other gastrointestinal cancers. There is some evidence that this incidence is reduced in patients maintaining a strict diet.

Reviews.

1. Duggan JM. Recent developments in our understanding of adult coeliac disease. *Med J Aust* 1997; **166:** 312–15.
2. Ferguson A. Coeliac disease. *Prescribers' J* 1997; **37:** 206–12.
3. Mäki M, Collin P. Coeliac disease. *Lancet* 1997; **349:** 1755–9.
4. Barr GD, Grehan MJ. Coeliac disease. *Med J Aust* 1998; **169:** 109–14.
5. Branski D, Troncone R. Celiac disease: a reappraisal. *J Pediatr* 1998; **133:** 181–7.
6. Feighery C. Coeliac disease. *BMJ* 1999; **319:** 236–9.
7. Farrell RJ, Kelly CP. Celiac sprue. *N Engl J Med* 2002; **346:** 180–8.
8. Green PHR, Jabri B. Coeliac disease. *Lancet* 2003; **362:** 383–91.

**Diabetes mellitus.** Dietary control is important in both type 1 and type 2 diabetes mellitus (p.324). The goals of dietary modification are to maintain glucose concentrations in the normal range or as close to normal as possible, and a lipid and lipoprotein profile and blood pressure that reduce the risk of macrovascular disease.

**Fish odour syndrome.** Fish odour syndrome (trimethylaminuria) is an inherited metabolic disorder in which there is impaired hepatic *N*-oxidation of trimethylamine. Trimethylamine is formed in the intestine by bacterial degradation of foods rich in choline and carnitine, and is readily absorbed from the gut. If not oxidised in the liver, it is excreted in the breath, urine, sweat, and vaginal secretions. It smells of rotting fish, and has a high olfactory potency. Treatment involves dietary modification to avoid choline-rich foods such as eggs, liver, peas, soya beans, and sea fish. Short-term treatments to reduce the intestinal flora, and thereby decrease the production of trimethylamine, are occasionally used; examples include metronidazole, neomycin, and lactulose.

References.

1. Pike MG, *et al.* Lactulose in trimethylaminuria, the fish-odour syndrome. *Helv Paediatr Acta* 1988; **43:** 345–8.
2. Rehman HU. Fish odour syndrome. *Postgrad Med J* 1999; **75:** 451–2.
3. Mitchell SC, Smith RL. Trimethylaminuria: the fish malodor syndrome. *Drug Metab Dispos* 2001; **29:** 517–21.

**Hepatic encephalopathy.** Restriction of dietary protein intake is a mainstay of the treatment of hepatic encephalopathy, but care is required to avoid malnutrition (see p.1243).

**Inflammatory bowel disease.** In inflammatory bowel diseases (p.1243) dietary modification or supplementation may often be necessary to maintain the nutritional status of the patient. Such supplementation may be oral, nasogastric, or parenteral.

Enteral feeding, particularly with elemental diets has been shown to be effective in the treatment of active Crohn's disease,[1] but is probably less effective than corticosteroids.[2-4] The terminology surrounding the use of these diets has been elucidated.[5] The term elemental diet was originally coined to describe diets containing free amino acids and glucose and was often prefixed by the phrase 'chemically defined'. However, it came to embrace diets whose nitrogen sources included peptides and were often also called predigested diets. It was suggested[5] that the term elemental diet could be used for either type but that for those with an amino acid nitrogen source the term chemically defined elemental diet should be used whereas for those with a peptide nitrogen source predigested elemental diet was suitable. The term polymeric diet should be used for those diets with a whole protein nitrogen source.

1. Teahon K, *et al.* Ten years' experience with an elemental diet in the management of Crohn's disease. *Gut* 1990; **31:** 1133–7.

2. Griffiths AM, *et al.* Meta-analysis of enteral nutrition as a primary treatment of active Crohn's disease. *Gastroenterology* 1995; **108:** 1056–67.
3. Messori A, *et al.* Defined-formula diets versus steroids in the treatment of active Crohn's disease: a meta-analysis. *Scand J Gastroenterol* 1996; **31:** 267–72.
4. Zachos M, *et al.* Enteral nutritional therapy for induction of remission in Crohn's disease. Available in The Cochrane Library; Issue 2. Chichester: John Wiley; 2004.
5. Payne-James JJ, Silk DBA. Use of elemental diets in the treatment of Crohn's disease by gastroenterologists. *Gut* 1990; **31:** 1424.

**Malignant neoplasms.** For a discussion of the possible link between an increased intake of antoxidant vitamins and a reduced risk of developing malignancies, see under Vitamins, below.

**Obesity.** Obesity is relatively common in the developed world, and is accompanied by an increased risk of cardiovascular disease, diabetes, and other disorders. Methods such as dietary modification, behaviour therapy, and exercise with adjunctive drug therapy, where indicated (see p.1583) can produce weight loss, but the essence of treatment is a reduction in calorific intake, usually by about 300 to 500 kcal daily in patients with a body-mass index (BMI) of 27 to 35, and 500 to 1000 kcal in those with a BMI greater than 35. This would be expected to produce a weight loss of about 0.25 to 1 kg weekly. Very low calorie diets (less than 600 to 800 kcal daily) should only be considered after the failure of determined attempts to lose weight by conventional calorie restriction. For weight loss to be achieved and sustained, eating behaviour must be permanently modified, which may pose difficulties. The proportion of calories from fat in particular, and also alcohol and sugars should be reduced and those from high carbohydrate foods increased. It is obviously important to maintain an adequate intake of essential nutrients.

Artificial sweeteners or other non-sucrose sweeteners are often used as part of weight-reducing diets.

**Renal failure.** Low-protein diets may be of value in preventing or slowing the progression of chronic renal failure (p.1222). Patients with renal failure who adopt a protein-restricted diet have fewer symptoms of uraemia than those on a normal diet.[1] Some results have also suggested that protein restriction can slow the progression of renal failure,[2] but the value of low-protein diets in delaying the onset of end-stage renal disease has been the subject of much controversy. Two large multicentre studies provided little evidence of a substantial benefit,[3,4] but a systematic review[5] provided support for dietary protein restriction. It has been suggested that the benefit of other interventions such as the use of ACE inhibitors,[6] as well as the difficulties in obtaining patient compliance with such a restrictive diet,[7] may have limited the benefits to be obtained from protein restriction, but there is also evidence that response and outcome vary depending on the cause of renal failure.[4,8]

1. Klahr S. Chronic renal failure: management. *Lancet* 1991; **338:** 423–7.
2. Mallick NP. Dietary protein and progression of chronic renal disease. *BMJ* 1994; **309:** 1101–2.
3. Locatelli F, *et al.* Prospective, randomised, multicentre trial of effect of protein restriction on progression of chronic renal insufficiency. *Lancet* 1991; **337:** 1299–1304.
4. Klahr S, *et al.* The effects of dietary protein restriction and blood-pressure control on the progression of chronic renal disease. *N Engl J Med* 1994; **330:** 877–84.
5. Fouque D, *et al.* Low protein diets for chronic renal failure in non diabetic adults. Available in The Cochrane Library; Issue 2. Chichester: John Wiley; 2004.
6. Shiigai T, *et al.* Dietary protein restriction and blood-pressure control in chronic renal insufficiency. *N Engl J Med* 1994; **331:** 405.
7. Barsotti G, Giovannetti S. Low-protein diet and chronic renal failure. *Lancet* 1991; **338:** 442.
8. Locatelli F, *et al.* Low-protein diet and chronic renal failure. *Lancet* 1991; **338:** 442–3.

## Enteral and Parenteral Nutrition

Malnutrition of varying degrees is not uncommon in hospitalised patients, and some form of nutritional support is important in patients who cannot eat an adequate normal diet. Such support should provide for the patient's requirements for energy, in the form of carbohydrate and fat, nitrogen as amino acids or protein, water and electrolytes; where appropriate, vitamins and trace elements should also be supplied. The decision to initiate nutritional support depends on the patient's clinical condition: indications may include unconsciousness, obstruction or inability to swallow, inflammatory bowel disease, fistula, short bowel syndrome, and weakness and malnutrition associated with trauma, surgery, or malignant disease. If possible, nutritional support should be by the enteral route; it is easier, more physiological, and less prone to complications than the parenteral route.

**Enteral nutrition** includes feeding by mouth, by nasogastric or nasoenteric tube, or directly into a gastrostomy or other enterostomy. It may be supplemental, if normal food intake is possible but inadequate, or total. Individual patients vary in their requirements according to age, size, and metabolic state, but a diet supplying 2000 to 3000 kcal of energy and 10 to 15 g of nitrogen (as 60 to 90 g of protein) in 2 to 3 litres of fluid is fairly typical; because absorption from the gastrointestinal tract is incomplete requirements are higher than by the parenteral route. Preparations containing whole protein (often derived from milk or soya) are generally preferred; elemental diets, in which nitrogen is supplied as amino acids or oligopeptides, are less well tolerated and less palatable, although they may have a role in impaired digestion or when a zero-residue diet is desired.

Although preferred to parenteral nutrition, enteral feeding is not without complications. Patients may be at risk of oesophagitis, aspiration, and regurgitation as a result of the tube insertion; other potential problems include diarrhoea, nausea and vomiting, gastric retention, hyperglycaemia, fluid and electrolyte disturbances, and microbial contamination of the feed regimen.

**Parenteral nutrition** is reserved for situations in which it is impossible to meet nutritional requirements by the enteral route. Like enteral nutrition it may be given supplementally or as the sole source of body requirements (total parenteral nutrition or TPN). The normal route of administration is via a dedicated central venous catheter. However, peripheral administration is increasingly used for short-term feeding. This reduces some complications and insertion is less complex, but because of the risk of thrombophlebitis feeds used should have low osmolality and neutral pH. Other measures to delay the development of peripheral thrombophlebitis are mentioned under Adverse Effects and Precautions, below.

The formulation of the nutritional solution must be adjusted according to the patient's requirements. The solution should supply sufficient energy to allow for the resting energy expenditure (around 25 kcal/kg in the average adult) but must also take into account any increased energy expenditure of illness. Conversely, starvation can reduce resting metabolism and energy requirements. Various formulae exist for the calculation of energy expenditure in patients. Energy is best supplied in the form of carbohydrate (at least 30%, and preferably 60% of energy requirements should be in this form) and fat. Glucose is the optimal carbohydrate energy source, while fat is supplied as a lipid emulsion, often of soya oil. Nitrogen is supplied as amino acids, but to ensure that these are used for protein synthesis rather than as sources of energy it is important to control the ratio of non-protein energy to nitrogen in the solution. A ratio of 150 to 200 kcal per g of nitrogen is usually considered optimal but in hypercatabolic patients (e.g. in sepsis) lower ratios of 120 kcal per g or less may be appropriate. All essential amino acids are supplied although there is some variation between solutions as to which non-essential amino acids are present.

Parenteral nutrition must also supply the patient's requirements for fluid, essential electrolytes such as sodium, potassium, magnesium, bicarbonate, and calcium (as well as phosphate, since glucose infusion may provoke hypophosphataemia), and, particularly if treatment is prolonged, vitamins and trace elements. If glucose loading produces signs of hyperglycaemia insulin may be added to correct it.

The major complication of parenteral nutrition is bacterial colonisation of the catheter, which can lead to septicaemia. Other problems may include venous thrombosis or air embolism, extravasation due to misplacement of the catheter tip, and metabolic disturbances. Adverse effects of overfeeding include respiratory and hepatic dysfunction. Complications of long-term total parenteral nutrition include gallbladder sludging, gallstones, cholestasis, and abnormal liver function tests.

**Stability and compatibility.** The complex nature of solutions for parenteral nutrition renders them susceptible to compatibility problems.[1-13] Stability is dependent upon several factors including pH and relative concentrations of the components. Amino acids exert a buffering effect on the overall pH of mixed solutions containing amino acids, glucose, and fat emulsions but amino acids with glucose undergo the Maillard reaction (browning) and the life of combined solutions is therefore limited. Solutions containing electrolytes, particularly divalent cations, are not stable, and aggregation will eventually occur. Additives should be added only if there is known compatibility, and any additions performed aseptically before the start of the infusion.

1. Allwood MC. Compatibility and stability of TPN mixtures in big bags. *J Clin Hosp Pharm* 1984; **9:** 181–98.
2. Niemiec PW, Vanderveen TW. Compatibility considerations in parenteral nutrient solutions. *Am J Hosp Pharm* 1984; **41:** 893–911.
3. Parry VA, *et al.* Effect of various nutrient ratios on the emulsion stability of total nutrient admixtures. *Am J Hosp Pharm* 1986; **43:** 3017–22.
4. Hardy G. Ten years of TPN with 3 litre bags. *Pharm J* 1987; **239:** HS26–HS28.
5. Johnson OL, *et al.* The destabilization of parenteral feeding emulsions by heparin. *Int J Pharmaceutics* 1989; **53:** 237–40.
6. Takagi J, *et al.* Sterility of total parenteral nutrient solutions stored at room temperature for seven days. *Am J Hosp Pharm* 1989; **46:** 973–7.
7. Tripp MG, *et al.* Stability of total nutrient admixtures in a dual-chamber flexible container. *Am J Hosp Pharm* 1990; **47:** 2496–503.
8. Vaughan LM, *et al.* Incompatibility of iron dextran and a total nutrient admixture. *Am J Hosp Pharm* 1990; **47:** 1745–6.
9. Washington C. The stability of intravenous fat emulsions in total parenteral nutrition mixtures. *Int J Pharmaceutics* 1990; **66:** 1–21.
10. Manning RJ, Washington C. Chemical stability of total parenteral nutrition mixtures. *Int J Pharmaceutics* 1992; **81:** 1–20.
11. Neuzil J, *et al.* Oxidation of parenteral lipid emulsion by ambient and phototherapy lights: potential toxicity of routine parenteral feeding. *J Pediatr* 1995; **126:** 785–90.
12. Trissel LA, *et al.* Compatibility of parenteral nutrient solutions with selected drugs during simulated Y-site administration. *Am J Health-Syst Pharm* 1997; **54:** 1295–1300.
13. Allwood MC. Pharmaceutical aspects of parenteral nutrition: from now to the future. *Nutrition* 2000; **16:** 615–8.

**Adverse effects and precautions.** ENTERAL NUTRITION. Reviewing the complications of enteral nutrition it was noted[1] that many of the problems encountered could be avoided by using a fine bore tube, administering the feed by continuous infusion, and by careful monitoring of the patient for metabolic abnormalities. Positioning the tube in the small bowel rather than the stomach has been suggested to reduce the incidence of aspiration,[2] although few studies have been done comparing intraduodenal and intragastric feeding in terms of clinical outcomes, and there are concerns about appropriate placement, infection, and reflux.[3] Prokinetic drugs such as metoclopramide, or erythromycin, have been used to promote gastric emptying and reduce residual gastric volumes.[2,3]

Complexation of the nutrients with aluminium-containing antacids, also given via the tube, may occur and this deposition of solid masses may cause oesophageal obstruction.[4]

Diarrhoea in patients receiving enteral nutrition may not necessarily be caused by the tube feeding itself;[5,6] malabsorption, infections and microbial contamination, underlying disease, and concomitant drug therapy can be possible contributors.[7] However, enteral feeding has been shown to be associated with increased colonic secretion, which can be reversed by infusion of short-chain fatty acids.[8]

While enteral tube feeding and the presence of a nasogastric tube are risk factors for infection, optimal nourishment through enteral feeding in high-risk patients unable to tolerate oral nutrition may also improve their immune status.[9]

1. Bastow MD. Complications of enteral nutrition. *Gut* 1986; **21** (suppl 1): 51–5.
2. McClave SA, Dryden GW. Critical care nutrition: reducing the risk of aspiration. *Semin Gastrointest Dis* 2003; **14:** 2–10.
3. MacLaren R. Intolerance to intragastric enteral nutrition in critically ill patients: complications and management. *Pharmacotherapy* 2000; **20:** 1486–98.
4. Valli C, *et al.* Interaction of nutrients with antacids: a complication during enteral tube feeding. *Lancet* 1986; **i:** 747–8.
5. Edes TE, *et al.* Diarrhea in tube-fed patients: feeding formula not necessarily the cause. *Am J Med* 1990; **88:** 91–3.
6. Heimburger DC. Diarrhea with enteral feeding: will the real cause please stand up? *Am J Med* 1990; **88:** 89–90.
7. Eisenberg P. An overview of diarrhea in the patient receiving enteral nutrition. *Gastroenterol Nurs* 2002; **25:** 95–104.
8. Bowling TE, *et al.* Reversal by short-chain fatty acids of colonic fluid secretion induced by enteral feeding. *Lancet* 1993; **342:** 1266–8.
9. Marion ND, Rupp ME. Infection control issues of enteral feeding systems. *Curr Opin Clin Nutr Metab Care* 2000; **3:** 363–6.

PARENTERAL NUTRITION. A common complication of parenteral nutrition is infection of the intravenous feeding catheter site[1] which can lead to septicaemia. Infection and colonisation of central venous catheters may be reduced if the catheter is tunnelled through subcutaneous tissue before emerging through the skin.[2] Strict aseptic techniques should be used[1] for changing the dressing or bags containing the nutrient fluids.

Thrombophlebitis can occur following the use of either peripheral or central veins. Although it has been suggested that infusion of hyperosmolar solutions via a central line is less likely to produce thrombophlebitis, because the feed is immediately diluted by a large volume of blood, major thrombotic complications such as pulmonary embolism and right atrial thrombosis could be more common than hitherto recognised in children and adolescents receiving long term parenteral nutrition via central catheters.[3,4] The use of a fine-bore silicone catheter peripherally may avoid the need for central vein cannulation[5] and there is a lower incidence of thrombophlebitis when fine-bore silicone catheters rather than teflon ones are used for peripheral administration of parenteral nutrition.[6] The use of administration sets with filters may decrease thrombophlebitis during peripheral infusion.[7] The addition of heparin to the feed, and the use of local hydrocortisone and glyceryl trinitrate, has also been reported to prolong the survival of peripheral infusion sites.[8] Extravasation may also be a problem, particularly with hyperosmolar solutions, and has led to severe tissue damage; hyaluronidase or thiomucase may be used in the treatment of such extravasation.[9]

Parenteral nutrition may be associated with atrophic changes in the mucosal structure and enzymic activity of the intestine, leading to increased permeability with a possible increased risk of bacteraemia and endotoxaemia. These changes, which have been attributed to lack of glutamine (which is unstable in solution), can reportedly be prevented by addition of glutamine-releasing dipeptides to solutions for total parenteral nutrition—see p.1433. Some have questioned the extent of this mucosal atrophy or bacterial translocation associated with parenteral feeding.[10,11]

Prolonged parenteral nutrition has been associated with hepatobiliary complications, especially in children;[12] cholelithiasis and cholestasis have been reported, with the latter sometimes progressing to liver failure.[13] Although the aetiology is considered multifactorial,[13] contamination of the solution with aluminium has been suggested as one possible cause of the cholestasis.[14]


1. Attar A, Messing B. Evidence-based prevention of catheter infection during parenteral nutrition. *Curr Opin Clin Nutr Metab Care* 2001; **4:** 211–18.
2. de Cicco M, *et al.* Source and route of microbial colonisation of parenteral nutrition catheters. *Lancet* 1989; **ii:** 1258–61.
3. Dollery CM, *et al.* Thrombosis and embolism in long-term central venous access for parenteral nutrition. *Lancet* 1994; **344:** 1043–5.
4. Dollery CM. Pulmonary embolism in parenteral nutrition. *Arch Dis Child* 1996; **74:** 95–8.
5. Kohlhardt SR, Smith RC. Fine bore silicone catheters for peripheral intravenous nutrition in adults. *BMJ* 1989; **299:** 1380–1.
6. Madan M, *et al.* Influence of catheter type on occurrence of thrombophlebitis during peripheral intravenous nutrition. *Lancet* 1992; **339:** 101–103.
7. Bethune K, *et al.* Use of filters during the preparation and administration of parenteral nutrition: position paper and guidelines prepared by a British pharmaceutical nutrition group working party. *Nutrition* 2001; **17:** 403–8.
8. Moclair AE, *et al.* Total parenteral nutrition via a peripheral vein: a comparison of heparinised and non-heparinised regimens. *Int J Pharm Pract* 1991; **1:** 38–40.
9. Gil M-E, Mateu J. Treatment of extravasation from parenteral nutrition solution. *Ann Pharmacother* 1998; **32:** 51–5.
10. MacFie J. Enteral versus parenteral nutrition: the significance of bacterial translocation and gut-barrier function. *Nutrition* 2000; **16:** 606–11.
11. Jeejeebhoy KN. Total parenteral nutrition: potion or poison? *Am J Clin Nutr* 2001; **74:** 160–3.
12. Kaufman SS. Prevention of parenteral nutrition-associated liver disease in children. *Pediatr Transplant* 2002; **6:** 37–42.
13. Btaiche IF, Khalidi N. Parenteral nutrition-associated liver complications in children. *Pharmacotherapy* 2002; **22:** 188–211.
14. Arnold CJ, *et al.* Parenteral nutrition-associated cholestasis in neonates: the role of aluminum. *Nutr Rev* 2003; **61:** 306–10.


**Uses.** Parenteral and enteral nutrition now have an established place either for supplemental use or for providing total nutritional requirements in many conditions. General reviews as well as those pertaining to special groups of patients or disorders have been published.[1-15]


1. ASPEN Board of Directors. Guidelines for the use of parenteral and enteral nutrition in adult and pediatric patients. *J Parenter Enteral Nutr* 1993; **17** (suppl): 1SA–52SA.
2. Elia M. Changing concepts of nutrient requirements in disease: implications for artificial nutritional support. *Lancet* 1995; **345:** 1279–84.
3. Mattox TW, *et al.* Recent advances: parenteral nutrition support. *Ann Pharmacother* 1995; **29:** 174–80.
4. American Gastroenterological Association. Guidelines for the use of enteral nutrition. *Gastroenterology* 1995; **108:** 1280.
5. Souba WW. Nutritional support. *N Engl J Med* 1997; **336:** 41–8.
6. Cerra FB, *et al.* Applied nutrition in ICU patients: a consensus statement of the American College of Chest Physicians. *Chest* 1997; **111:** 769–78.
7. Heyland DK, *et al.* Total parenteral nutrition in the critically ill patient: a meta-analysis. *JAMA* 1998; **280:** 2013–19.
8. Jolliet P, *et al.* Enteral nutrition in intensive care patients: a practical approach. *Clin Nutr* 1999; **18:** 47–56.
9. Pinchasik D. From TPN to breast feeding—feeding the premature infant—2000: part I: parenteral nutrition. *Am J Perinatol* 2001; **18:** 59–72.
10. Heine RG, Bines JE. New approaches to parenteral nutrition in infants and children. *J Paediatr Child Health* 2002; **38:** 433–7.
11. Atten MJ, *et al.* Part IV: enteral nutrition support. *Dis Mon* 2002; **48:** 751–90.
12. Schattner M. Enteral nutritional support of the patient with cancer: route and role. *J Clin Gastroenterol* 2003; **36:** 297–302.
13. Hoffer LJ. Protein and energy provision in critical illness. *Am J Clin Nutr* 2003; **78:** 906–11.
14. Howard L, Ashley C. Nutrition in the perioperative patient. *Annu Rev Nutr* 2003; **23:** 263–82.
15. Anderson ADG, *et al.* Peripheral parenteral nutrition. *Br J Surg* 2003; **90:** 1048–54.


## Trace Elements

Trace elements are inorganic substances found in small amounts in the tissues and required for various metabolic processes; together with the vitamins (see below) they are sometimes referred to as micronutrients. The elements considered essential are chromium, copper, fluorine, iodine, iron, manganese, molybdenum, selenium, and zinc. Iron, in the form of haem, plays an essential role in oxygen transport while iodine is required by the thyroid for the formation of thyroid hormones; most of the other essential trace elements are cofactors for various enzymes. Boron, nickel, silicon, and vanadium may also be essential, and it has been suggested on the basis of *animal* studies that there might be a requirement for tin.

Well-defined deficiency syndromes exist for copper, iodine, iron, selenium, and zinc; although deficiency of other trace elements is possible, their deficiency syndromes are not well defined because of their ubiquity in the diet. Guidance concerning the intake of various trace elements has been published—see also Human Requirements under Vitamins, below.

◊ References.


1. WHO. *Trace elements in human nutrition and health.* Geneva: WHO, 1996.


## Vitamins

Vitamins are organic substances required by the body in small amounts for various metabolic processes. Most are not synthesised in the body, or are synthesised in small or insufficient quantities. Vitamins are sometimes classified as fat soluble or water soluble. Substances in the vitamin A, D, E, and K groups are generally fat soluble, and biotin, folic acid, niacin, pantothenic acid, vitamins $B_1$, $B_2$, $B_6$, and $B_{12}$, and vitamin C substances are generally water soluble.

Vitamin deficiency may result from an inadequate diet, perhaps due to increased requirements such as during pregnancy, or may be induced by disease or drugs. Vitamins may be used clinically for the prevention and treatment of specific vitamin deficiency states and details of these uses are provided under the individual drug monographs.

Large doses of vitamins (megavitamin therapy) have been proposed for a variety of disorders, but adequate evidence of their value is lacking. Excessive intakes of most water-soluble vitamins have little effect due to their rapid excretion in urine, but excessive intakes of fat-soluble vitamins accumulate in the body and are potentially dangerous.

**Stability.** Water-soluble vitamins are liable to degrade in solution especially if exposed to light. Addition of vitamin mixtures to infusion solutions for parenteral nutrition should therefore be carried out as soon as possible before infusion. Solutions should be used within 24 hours of preparation and be protected from light.

**Human requirements.** Vitamins and trace elements are essential nutrients and in many countries guidance has been published concerning their intake.

In the UK various terms are used to define intake:[1]

- estimated average requirement (EAR) is used for the requirements of energy, proteins, vitamins, or minerals of a group of people and usually about half will need more and half less than the specified figure
- lower reference nutrient intake (LRNI) is applied to proteins, vitamins, or minerals and is that amount that is enough for only a few people who have low needs
- reference nutrient intake (RNI) is also applied to proteins, vitamins, or minerals and is an amount that is enough, or more than enough, for about 97% of people in a group
- a safe intake is used to indicate an intake or range of intakes where there is not enough information to estimate EAR, LRNI, or RNI, but rather it is an amount enough for almost everyone but is not so large as to cause undesirable effects
- dietary reference value (DRV) is used to cover EAR, LRNI, RNI, and safe intake.

It is emphasised in the report that these intakes are not meant to be recommendations for any individual or group; they do not reflect either a recommendation that such an amount should be taken daily in the diet or as a supplement. They are intended rather as yardsticks for the assessment of dietary surveys and food supply statistics; to provide guidance on appropriate dietary composition and meal provision; or for food labelling purposes in which case it is envisaged that an EAR will be used.

In the USA the National Academy of Sciences has traditionally set recommended dietary allowances (RDAs),[2] defined as the levels of intake of essential nutrients that, on the basis of scientific knowledge, are judged to be adequate to meet the known nutrient needs of practically all healthy persons. The allowances are amounts that are intended to be consumed as part of a normal diet. However, new dietary reference intakes (DRIs) have been developed,[3] which include 3 reference values in addition to the traditional RDA as follows:

- the estimated average requirement is the intake that meets the needs of half the individuals in a group
- the adequate intake is the mean intake level that appears to sustain a desired marker of health, and will be set when there is insufficient evidence to establish an RDA
- the tolerable upper intake level is the maximum intake that is not likely to adversely affect health.

Information pertaining to the requirements of specific vitamins and minerals is provided under the individual monographs.


1. DoH. Dietary reference values for food energy and nutrients for the United Kingdom: report of the panel on dietary reference values of the committee on medical aspects of food policy. *Report on health and social subjects 41.* London: HMSO, 1991.
2. Subcommittee on the tenth edition of the RDAs, Food and Nutrition Board, Commission on Life Sciences, National Research Council. *Recommended dietary allowances.* 10th ed. Washington, DC: National Academy Press, 1989.
3. Standing Committee on the Scientific Evaluation of Dietary Reference Intakes of the Food and Nutrition Board. *Dietary Reference Intakes: applications in dietary assessment.* Washington DC: National Academy Press, 2001. Also available at: http://www.nap.edu/catalog/9956.html (accessed 20/05/04)


**Supplementation.** An adequate dietary intake of vitamins is necessary for good health but whether vitamin supplementation in the absence of any demonstrable deficiency is beneficial or even worthwhile remains debatable.

It is generally considered that healthy persons eating a normal balanced diet should have no need for vitamin supplementation.[1,2] A review of the topic[1] pointed out that the vitamins that people chose for self medication are often not the ones that are actually present in inadequate amounts in their diets and that the commercial preparations available often do not make it clear whether the amounts they contain are near the physiological requirements or many times greater. Supplementation should concentrate on groups of people at risk of deficiency such as neonates, who need vitamin K; pregnant and lactating women, who need calcium, folic acid, and iron; and certain groups who need vitamin D; vegans and their infants may require vitamin $B_{12}$ supplements. A multivitamin supplement might be considered for some groups such as the elderly and those with reduced calorie intake. However, one might have difficulty in finding a good multivitamin preparation containing all 13 vitamins but no non-vitamins. Also with many of the multivitamin preparations the doses and ratios varied inexplicably.

A review[3] of supplementation specifically in children concluded that, provided schoolchildren and adolescents eat a wide variety of foods, there was no need for vitamin supplementation. However, it was recommended that supplementation with vitamins A, C, and D should be given to those between the ages of 6 months and 2 years and preferably up to the age of 5 years. Several authorities in different countries have set upper safety limits for vitamins; these vary considerably.[4]


1. Truswell S. Who should take vitamin supplements? *BMJ* 1990; **301:** 135–6. Correction. *ibid.*; 354.
2. Waine C. Vitamin and mineral supplements. *Pharm J* 2001; **267:** 352–4.
3. Kendall HE. Vitamin and mineral supplements for children. *Pharm J* 1990; **245:** 460–2.
4. Mason P. Upper safety limits for vitamins—why have different authorities set different guidance? *Pharm J* 2003; **271:** 55–7.


MENTAL FUNCTION. Administration of vitamin and mineral supplements to children was reported in 1988 to increase non-verbal intelligence[1] and the topic has since remained highly controversial. In the following two years more studies were published but these failed to substantiate the earlier possible effect and concluded that vitamin supplementation did not improve mental functioning or reasoning in children.[2,3] Suggestions were made shortly after these publications that there might be a subset of children with poor nutritional status who would receive some benefit[4] but this again was disputed.[5]

In 1991 another study was published,[6] this time coinciding with the launch of the proprietary product used in the study, with the publication of a book on the subject, and with the showing on British television of a documentary concerning the study. This study purported to demonstrate that supplementation with exactly the recommended dietary allowances of vitamins improved the IQ of children, a finding that was said not to occur significantly with other quantities of vitamin supplementation. This view attracted extremely harsh criticism[7-9] from physicians, nutritionists, psychologists, and epidemiologists.


1. Benton D, Roberts G. Effect of vitamin and mineral supplementation on intelligence of a sample of schoolchildren. *Lancet* 1988; **i:** 140–3.
2. Naismith DJ, *et al.* Can children's intelligence be increased by vitamin and mineral supplements? *Lancet* 1988; **ii:** 335.
3. Crombie IK, *et al.* Effect of vitamin and mineral supplementation on verbal and non-verbal reasoning of schoolchildren. *Lancet* 1990; **335:** 744–7.
4. Benton D, Buts J-P. Vitamin/mineral supplementation and intelligence. *Lancet* 1990; **335:** 1158–60.
5. Crombie IK, *et al.* Vitamin/mineral supplementation and intelligence. *Lancet* 1990; **336:** 175.
6. Schoenthaler SJ, *et al.* Controlled trial of vitamin-mineral supplementation: effects on intelligence and performance. *Personality Indiv Diff* 1991; **12:** 351–62.
7. Whitehead RG. Vitamins, minerals, schoolchildren, and IQ. *BMJ* 1991; **302:** 548.
8. Peto R. Vitamins and IQ. *BMJ* 1991; **302:** 906.
9. Anonymous. Brains and vitamins. *Lancet* 1991; **337:** 587–8.

PROPHYLAXIS OF ISCHAEMIC HEART DISEASE. Hypercholesterolaemia is a major risk factor for the development of atherosclerosis and consequently ischaemic heart disease. Since oxidation of lipids, particularly low-density-lipoprotein (LDL) cholesterol,[1] has been proposed as a factor in atherogenesis, the possibility of preventing atherosclerosis by the use of dietary antioxidants such as vitamins E and C and betacarotene has been investigated. A six-year trial of supplementation with vitamins C and E in hypercholesterolaemic patients showed a slowing of atherosclerotic progression, especially in men.[2] Prospective epidemiological studies have revealed a reduced risk of ischaemic heart disease in individuals taking vitamin E supplements,[3,4] and those with a high carotene intake (particularly smokers).[3] In a further prospective cohort study,[5] dietary vitamin E consumption, but not vitamin E supplementation, was associated with decreased risk of death from ischaemic heart disease. Intake of vitamin C, however, did not appear to be associated with a decreased risk of ischaemic heart disease in these studies,[3-5] although another study[6] found a significantly lower risk in those taking vitamin C supplements. Data from some studies assessing serum or fat concentrations also provide evidence that high betacarotene concentrations are associated with decreased cardiovascular disease.[7-9]

However, despite these promising results, randomised placebo-controlled trials have failed to find any benefit for betacarotene supplements in the primary or secondary prevention of ischaemic heart disease, and those for vitamin E supplements are inconclusive. In the Alpha Tocopherol, Beta Carotene Cancer Prevention (ATBC) study, which monitored cardiovascular disease as a secondary end-point, vitamin E was not associated with a decreased incidence of ischaemic heart disease, and betacarotene was associated with a small increased risk.[10] In further analyses, neither supplement appreciably altered the incidence of angina pectoris,[11] nor showed any beneficial effect on cardiovascular deaths in the subset of men with previous myocardial infarction.[12] It has been suggested that the lack of effect of vitamin E in this study may be due to an insufficiently high dose of tocopherol. Similarly, neither the Betacarotene and Retinol Efficacy Trial (CARET)[13] nor the Skin Cancer Prevention Study[9] found an effect for betacarotene supplementation on the risk of death from cardiovascular disease.

In studies specifically on cardiovascular end-points, no benefit from betacarotene supplements was seen in a large, randomised, placebo-controlled study[14] in healthy men. Studies of supplementation with high-dose vitamin E in patients with evidence of ischaemic heart disease,[15] or after myocardial infarction,[16] failed to show any beneficial effect on cardiovascular deaths, although in one study[15] there was a reduction in non-fatal myocardial infarction and major cardiovascular events. The Heart Outcomes Prevention Evaluation (HOPE) study also showed that vitamin E treatment for 4 to 6 years had no effect on cardiovascular events in high-risk patients.[17] Another large-scale study, the Heart Protection Study, assessed the effect of a 'cocktail' of vitamin E, vitamin C, and betacarotene on the development of ischaemic heart disease in high-risk subjects, and again found no evidence of benefit.[18] Another study[19] using a similar cocktail in patients with established heart disease found no effect on clinical outcome. In view of the lack of evidence of benefit with vitamin supplements, it has been recommended that the emphasis should instead be on consuming a balanced diet including antioxidant-rich fruits, vegetables, and whole grains rather than vitamin supplements;[20] authors of a meta-analysis[21] of trials of antioxidant vitamins for the prevention of cardiovascular disease concluded that, in view of a possibly harmful effect of betacarotene and inefficacy of vitamin E, the use of these supplements be discouraged.

For a discussion of the possibility that folic acid may reduce ischaemic heart disease through its homocysteine-lowering effect, see p.1429.


1. Jha P, *et al.* The antioxidant vitamins and cardiovascular disease: a critical review of epidemiologic and clinical trial data. *Ann Intern Med* 1995; **123:** 860–72. Correction. *ibid.* 1996; **124:** 934.
2. Salonen RM, *et al.* Six-year effect of combined vitamin C and E supplementation on atherosclerotic progression: the antioxidant supplementation in atherosclerosis prevention (ASAP) study. *Circulation* 2003; **107:** 947–53.
3. Rimm EB, *et al.* Vitamin E consumption and the risk of coronary heart disease in men. *N Engl J Med* 1993; **328:** 1450–6.
4. Stampfer MJ, *et al.* Vitamin E consumption and the risk of coronary disease in women. *N Engl J Med* 1993; **328:** 1444–9.
5. Kushi LH, *et al.* Dietary antioxidant vitamins and death from coronary heart disease in postmenopausal women. *N Engl J Med* 1996; **334:** 1156–62.
6. Osganian SK, *et al.* Vitamin C and risk of coronary heart disease in women. *J Am Coll Cardiol* 2003; **42:** 246–52.
7. Morris DL, *et al.* Serum carotenoids and coronary heart disease: the Lipid Research Clinics Coronary Primary Prevention Trial and Follow-up Study. *JAMA* 1994; **272:** 1439–41.
8. Kardinaal AFM, *et al.* Antioxidants in adipose tissue and risk of myocardial infarction: the EURAMIC study. *Lancet* 1993; **342:** 1379–84.
9. Greenberg ER, *et al.* Mortality associated with low plasma concentration of beta carotene and the effect of oral supplementation. *JAMA* 1996; **275:** 699–703.
10. The Alpha-Tocopherol, Beta-Carotene Cancer Prevention Study Group. The effect of vitamin E and beta carotene on the incidence of lung cancer and other cancers in male smokers. *N Engl J Med* 1994; **330:** 1029–35.
11. Rapola JM, *et al.* Effect of vitamin E and beta carotene on the incidence of angina pectoris. *JAMA* 1996; **275:** 693–8. Correction. *ibid.* 1998; **279:** 1528.
12. Rapola JM, *et al.* Randomised trial of α-tocopherol and β-carotene supplements on incidence of major coronary events in men with previous myocardial infarction. *Lancet* 1997; **349:** 1715–20.
13. Omenn GS, *et al.* Effects of a combination of beta carotene and vitamin A on lung cancer and cardiovascular disease. *N Engl J Med* 1996; **334:** 1150–5.
14. Hennekens CH, *et al.* Lack of effect of long-term supplementation with beta carotene on the incidence of malignant neoplasms and cardiovascular disease. *N Engl J Med* 1996; **334:** 1145–9.
15. Stephens NG, *et al.* Randomised controlled trial of vitamin E in patients with coronary disease: Cambridge Heart Antioxidant Study (CHAOS). *Lancet* 1996; **347:** 781–6.
16. GISSI-Prevenzione Investigators (Gruppo Italiano per lo Studio della Sopravvivenza nell'Infarto miocardico). Dietary supplementation with n-3 polyunsaturated fatty acids and vitamin E after myocardial infarction: results of the GISSI-Prevenzione trial. *Lancet* 1999; **354:** 447–55. Correction. *ibid.* 2001; **357:** 642.
17. The Heart Outcomes Prevention Evaluation Study Investigators. Vitamin E supplementation and cardiovascular events in high-risk patients. *N Engl J Med* 2000; **342:** 154–60.
18. Heart Protection Study Collaborative Group. MRC/BHF Heart Protection Study of antioxidant vitamin supplementation in 20 536 high-risk individuals: a randomised placebo-controlled trial. *Lancet* 2002; **360:** 23–33.
19. Brown BG, *et al.* Simvastatin and niacin, antioxidant vitamins, or the combination for the prevention of coronary disease. *N Engl J Med* 2001; **345:** 1583–92.
20. Tribble DL. Antioxidant consumption and risk of coronary heart disease: emphasis on vitamin C, vitamin E, and β-carotene: a statement for healthcare professionals from the American Heart Association. *Circulation* 1999; **99:** 591–5.
21. Vivekananthan DP, *et al.* Use of antioxidant vitamins for the prevention of cardiovascular disease: meta-analysis of randomised trials. *Lancet* 2003; **361:** 2017–23. Correction. *ibid.*; **362:** 922.


PROPHYLAXIS OF MALIGNANT NEOPLASMS. There is evidence that a diet rich in fruit and vegetables is associated with a lower incidence of malignant disease, particularly of the respiratory and digestive tracts.[1] It has been hypothesised that some of the benefits of such a diet derive from the role of antioxidant vitamins such as the carotenoids and vitamins C and E in scavenging free radicals.[2,3] However, it is by no means certain that these are the only, or necessarily the most important, dietary components responsible for benefit, since components such as dietary fibre may also play a role. In addition, different antioxidants may vary in their properties and efficacy,[3,4] and the appropriate dosage remains largely conjectural, and perhaps as a result the evidence of benefit is often conflicting.

Several clinical trials of the use of **vitamin A** or **betacarotene** in the secondary or primary prevention of malignancy have been reported. Prolongation of disease-free interval in patients with various malignant neoplasms was reported in 1 study of betacarotene,[5] and others reported remission of oral leucoplakia in patients treated with betacarotene and vitamin A,[6,7] or betacarotene alone.[8] Vitamin A alone was reported to reduce the incidence of primary tobacco-related neoplasms in a study of patients treated surgically for lung cancer.[9] In a prospective, cohort study,[10] vitamin A intake, including preformed vitamin A and carotenoids, was associated with a reduced risk of breast cancer among smokers. However, other results have largely failed to substantiate any benefit for secondary prevention. No reduction in the incidence of new skin cancers,[11-13] or in malignant transformation of cervical dysplasia,[14] or in new colorectal adenomas[15] was reported in other studies. In a primary prevention study, a combination of betacarotene, vitamin E, and selenium was associated with a reduction in stomach and oesophageal cancers in a population at high risk of these cancers and with a diet low in micronutrients in China.[16] In contrast, other primary prevention studies have failed to show any benefit, and possibly some harm, from betacarotene supplements in well-nourished populations. A study in smokers[17-19] showed an increase in lung cancer and associated mortality in those receiving betacarotene (20 mg daily), but not those receiving vitamin E (50 mg daily). Similarly, an increased risk of lung cancer was noted in recipients of betacarotene (30 mg daily) with vitamin A (25 000 units daily) in another study in individuals at high risk of lung cancer, and this study was stopped early as a result.[20,21] A third study in healthy men found no benefit or harm for betacarotene supplements (50 mg on alternate days) in terms of incidence of malignant neoplasms, including those of the lung;[22] a subgroup analysis of this study suggested that supplementation may reduce the risk of prostate cancer in those men with low baseline betacarotene levels.[23]

**Vitamin C** has also been proposed for prevention of malignancy but there is no real evidence to justify it. It certainly appears to be ineffective as adjuvant therapy in the treatment of advanced malignancy,[24] and combination with betacarotene and vitamin E failed to show any effect in preventing colorectal adenoma.[15] At physiological concentrations vitamin C is an important antioxidant,[3] but supplementation is unlikely to be justified in anyone eating a balanced diet.[1]

**Vitamin E substances** are also known to play an important antioxidant role in the body. Animal studies have suggested that they should inhibit tumour production, and the Chinese study mentioned above found combined antioxidant therapy including vitamin E to be of benefit in the primary prevention of stomach and oesophageal cancers.[16] Other studies in western populations have generally been disappointing; vitamin E had no effect on lung cancer incidence in those at risk,[17,18] and did not prevent the development of new colorectal adenomas.[15] However, further analysis of the lung-cancer study[25] suggests that vitamin E may have protected against prostate cancer. There is preliminary evidence that selenium (see p.1444) or vitamin E supplementation may reduce the risk of prostate cancer, and a large randomised study is underway to further investigate this.

Results from the Nurses' Health Study have indicated that prolonged use of multivitamins was associated with reduced risk of developing cancer of the colon.[26] This effect was thought to be due to the **folate** component and could be demonstrated after 15 years of use, but not after shorter-term ingestion. Dietary folate was also associated with a modest reduction in risk for colon cancer.

While a diet involving frequent consumption of fruits and vegetables is likely to be beneficial,[1] others have also suggested that these associations may have been overstated, and that weight control and regular exercise should be prioritised; in addition, folic acid intake might reduce the risk of cancer, especially in those regularly consuming alcohol.[27]


1. Austoker J. Diet and cancer. *BMJ* 1994; **308:** 1610–14.
2. Hennekens CH. Antioxidant vitamins and cancer. *Am J Med* 1994; **97** (suppl 3A): 2S–4S.
3. Halliwell B. Free radicals, antioxidants, and human disease: curiosity, cause, or consequence? *Lancet* 1994; **344:** 721–4.
4. Hankinson SE, Stampfer MJ. All that glitters is not beta carotene. *JAMA* 1994; **272:** 1455–6.
5. Santamaria L, *et al.* First clinical report (1980-1988) of cancer chemoprevention with betacarotene plus canthaxanthin supplemented to patients after radical treatment. *Boll Chim Farm* 1988; **127:** 57S–60S.
6. Stich HF, *et al.* Remission of oral leukoplakias and micronuclei in tobacco/betel quid chewers treated with beta-carotene and with beta-carotene plus vitamin A. *Int J Cancer* 1988; **42:** 195–9.
7. Sankaranarayanan R, *et al.* Chemoprevention of oral leukoplakia with vitamin A and beta carotene: an assessment. *Oral Oncol* 1997; **33:** 231–6.
8. Garewal HS, *et al.* β-Carotene produces sustained remissions in patients with oral leukoplakia. *Arch Otolaryngol Head Neck Surg* 1999; **125:** 1305–10.
9. Pastorino U, *et al.* Adjuvant treatment of stage I lung cancer with high-dose vitamin A. *J Clin Oncol* 1993; **11:** 1216–22.
10. Cho E, *et al.* Premenopausal intakes of vitamins A, C, and E, folate, and carotenoids, and risk of breast cancer. *Cancer Epidemiol Biomarkers Prev* 2003; **12:** 713–20.
11. Greenberg ER, *et al.* A clinical trial of beta carotene to prevent basal-cell and squamous-cell cancers of the skin. *N Engl J Med* 1990 **323:** 789–95.
12. Green A, *et al.* Daily sunscreen application and betacarotene supplementation in prevention of basal-cell and squamous-cell carcinomas of the skin: a randomised controlled trial. *Lancet* 1999; **354:** 723–9. Correction. *ibid.*; 1038.
13. Frieling UM, *et al.* A randomized, 12-year primary-prevention trial of beta carotene supplementation for nonmelanoma skin cancer in the Physicians' Health Study. *Arch Dermatol* 2000; **136:** 179–84.
14. de Vet HCW, *et al.* The effect of beta-carotene on the regression and progression of cervical dysplasia: a clinical experiment. *J Clin Epidemiol* 1991; **44:** 273–83.
15. Greenberg ER, *et al.* A clinical trial of antioxidant vitamins to prevent colorectal adenoma. *N Engl J Med* 1994; **331:** 141–7.
16. Blot WJ, *et al.* Nutrition intervention trials in Linxian, China: supplementation with specific vitamin/mineral combinations, cancer incidence, and disease-specific mortality in the general population. *J Natl Cancer Inst* 1993; **85:** 1483–92.
17. The Alpha-Tocopherol, Beta-Carotene Cancer Prevention Study Group. The effect of vitamin E and beta carotene on the incidence of lung cancer and other cancers in male smokers. *N Engl J Med* 1994; **330:** 1029–35.
18. Albanes D, *et al.* α-Tocopherol and β-carotene supplements and lung cancer incidence in the alpha-tocopherol, beta-carotene cancer prevention study: effects of base-line characteristics and study compliance. *J Natl Cancer Inst* 1996; **88:** 1560–70.
19. The ATBC Study Group. Incidence of cancer and mortality following α-tocopherol and β-carotene supplementation: a postintervention follow-up. *JAMA* 2003; **290:** 476–85.
20. Omenn GS, *et al.* Effects of a combination of beta carotene and vitamin A on lung cancer and cardiovascular disease. *N Engl J Med* 1996; **334:** 1150–5.
21. Omenn GS, *et al.* Risk factors for lung cancer and for intervention effects in CARET, the Beta-Carotene and Retinol Efficacy Trial. *J Natl Cancer Inst* 1996; **88:** 1550–9.
22. Hennekens CH, *et al.* Lack of effect of long-term supplementation with beta carotene on the incidence of malignant neoplasms and cardiovascular disease. *N Engl J Med* 1996; **334:** 1145–9.
23. Cook NR, *et al.* β-Carotene supplementation for patients with low baseline levels and decreased risks of total and prostate carcinoma. *Cancer* 1999; **86:** 1783–92.
24. Moertel CG, *et al.* High-dose vitamin C versus placebo in the treatment of patients with advanced cancer who have had no prior chemotherapy: a randomized double-blind comparison. *N Engl J Med* 1985; **312:** 137–41.
25. Heinonen OP, *et al.* Prostate cancer and supplementation with α-tocopherol and β-carotene: incidence and mortality in a controlled trial. *J Natl Cancer Inst* 1998; **90:** 440–6.
26. Giovannucci E, *et al.* Multivitamin use, folate, and colon cancer in women in the Nurses' Health Study. *Ann Intern Med* 1998; **129:** 517–24.
27. Willett WC. Diet and cancer: one view at the start of the millennium. *Cancer Epidemiol Biomarkers Prev* 2001; **10:** 3–8.


## Acesulfame Potassium *(BANM, rINNM)*

Acesulfame K; Acesulfamo potásico; Acesulfamum Kalicum; E950; H73-3293; Hoe-095K. 6-Methyl-1,2,3-oxathiazin-4(3*H*)-one 2,2-dioxide potassium.

$C_4H_4KNO_4S$ = 201.2.

*CAS* — *55589-62-3.*

**Pharmacopoeias.** In *Eur.* (see p.vi).

**Ph. Eur. 5.0** (Acesulfame Potassium). A white, crystalline powder or colourless crystals. Soluble in water; very slightly soluble in alcohol and in acetone.

### Profile

Acesulfame potassium is an intense sweetener about 200 times as sweet as sucrose. It is used in foods and does not appear to be affected by cooking.

### Preparations

**Proprietary Preparations** (details are given in Part 3)
**Multi-ingredient:** ***Arg.:*** Genser Sweet; ***Chile:*** Marco Sweet Light.

## Alanine *(USAN, rINN)*

A; Ala; Alanina; L-Alanine; Alaninum. L-2-Aminopropionic acid.
$C_3H_7NO_2$ = 89.09.
*CAS — 56-41-7.*

**Pharmacopoeias.** In *Chin., Eur.* (see p.vi), and *US.*
**Ph. Eur. 5.0** (Alanine). A white or almost white crystalline powder or colourless crystals. Freely soluble in water; very slightly soluble in alcohol. Protect from light.
**USP 27** (Alanine). White, odourless, crystals or crystalline powder. Freely soluble in water; slightly soluble in 80% alcohol; insoluble in ether. pH of a 5% solution in water is between 5.5 and 7.0. Store in airtight containers.

### Profile

Alanine is an aliphatic amino acid. It is used as a dietary supplement. The dipeptide *N*(2)-L-alanyl-L-glutamine is used similarly.

**Hypoglycaemia.** References to the investigational use of alanine in the management of insulin-induced hypoglycaemia.[1-3]

1. Wiethop BV, Cryer PE. Glycemic actions of alanine and terbutaline in IDDM. *Diabetes Care* 1993; **16:** 1124–30.
2. Wiethop BV, Cryer PE. Alanine and terbutaline in treatment of hypoglycemia in IDDM. *Diabetes Care* 1993; **16:** 1131–6.
3. Saleh TY, Cryer PE. Alanine and terbutaline in the prevention of nocturnal hypoglycemia in IDDM. *Diabetes Care* 1997; **20:** 1231–6.

### Preparations

**Proprietary Preparations** (details are given in Part 3)
***Arg.:*** Dipeptiven; ***Austria:*** Dipeptiven; ***Braz.:*** Dipeptiven†; ***Denm.:*** Dipeptiven; ***Fin.:*** Dipeptiven; ***Fr.:*** Dipeptiven; ***Ger.:*** Dipeptamin; ***Gr.:*** Dipeptiven; ***Ital.:*** Dipeptiven; ***Mex.:*** Dipeptiven; ***Norw.:*** Dipeptiven; ***Port.:*** Dipeptiven; ***Spain:*** Dipeptiven; ***Swed.:*** Dipeptiven; ***Switz.:*** Dipeptiven; ***Thai.:*** Dipeptiven; ***UK:*** Dipeptiven.
**Multi-ingredient:** ***Arg.:*** Normoprost Compuesto; ***Port.:*** Tebetane Composto†; ***Spain:*** Tebetane Compuesto; ***UK:*** Amino MS†.

## Arginine *(rINN)*

Arg; Arginina; L-Arginine; Argininum; R. L-2-Amino-5-guanidinovaleric acid.
$C_6H_{14}N_4O_2$ = 174.2.
*CAS — 74-79-3.*

**Pharmacopoeias.** In *Eur.* (see p.vi) and *US.*
**Ph. Eur. 5.0** (Arginine). A white or almost white crystalline powder, or colourless crystals. Freely soluble in water; very slightly soluble in alcohol. Protect from light.
**USP 27** (Arginine). White, practically odourless crystals. Freely soluble in water; sparingly soluble in alcohol; insoluble in ether.

### Arginine Aspartate

Arginini Aspartas; Aspargininum. (2*S*)-2-Amino-5-guanidinopentanoic acid (2*S*)-2-aminobutanedioate.
$C_{10}H_{21}N_5O_6$ = 307.3.
*CAS — 7675-83-4.*

**Pharmacopoeias.** In *Eur.* (see p.vi).
**Ph. Eur. 5.0** (Arginine Aspartate). White granules or powder. Very soluble in water, practically insoluble in alcohol and in methylene chloride.

### Arginine Glutamate *(BAN, USAN, rINNM)*

Glutamato de arginina. L-Arginine L-glutamate.
$C_6H_{14}N_4O_2,C_5H_9NO_4$ = 321.3.
*CAS — 4320-30-3.*
*ATC — A05BA01.*

### Arginine Hydrochloride *(USAN, rINNM)*

L-Arginine Monohydrochloride; Arginini Hydrochloridum; Hidrocloruro de arginina.
$C_6H_{14}N_4O_2,HCl$ = 210.7.
*CAS — 1119-34-2.*
*ATC — B05XB01.*

**Pharmacopoeias.** In *Chin., Eur.* (see p.vi), *Jpn,* and *US.*
**Ph. Eur. 5.0** (Arginine Hydrochloride). A white or almost white crystalline powder, or colourless crystals. Freely soluble in water; very slightly soluble in alcohol. Protect from light.
**USP 27** (Arginine Hydrochloride). White, practically odourless, crystals or crystalline powder. Freely soluble in water.

### Adverse Effects and Precautions

Nausea, vomiting, flushing, headache, numbness, and local venous irritation may occur if arginine solutions are infused too rapidly. Elevated plasma-potassium concentrations have been reported in uraemic patients and arginine should therefore be used with caution in patients with renal disease or anuria. Arginine hydrochloride should be given cautiously to patients with electrolyte disturbances as its high chloride content could lead to the development of hyperchloraemic acidosis.

**Extravasation.** A report[1] of necrosis after extravasation of a 10% solution of arginine hydrochloride. Both osmotic and local hyperkalaemic effects had been proposed as a mechanism for the injury.

1. Bowlby HA, Elanjian SI. Necrosis caused by extravasation of arginine hydrochloride. *Ann Pharmacother* 1992; **26:** 263–4.

**Hyperkalaemia.** Two alcoholic patients with severe liver disease and moderate renal insufficiency developed severe hyperkalaemia after administration of arginine hydrochloride and one died.[1] Both patients had received a total dose of 300 mg of spironolactone some time before arginine hydrochloride, but the contribution of spironolactone to the hyperkalaemia was not known. In a study to investigate the mechanism of metabolic changes due to arginine, plasma potassium concentrations were found to be significantly higher in diabetic subjects than those for normal subjects, leading the authors to suppose that while arginine-induced hyperkalaemia may be promoted by low insulin blood levels, it could not be attributed to glucagon, pH changes, or aldosterone inhibition.[2]

In another fatal case due to an overdose of arginine,[3] a 21-month-old girl developed an acute metabolic acidosis and transient, but severe, hyponatraemia, and irreversible brain death; no hyperkalaemia was observed. Unlike the previously reported case, the patient had normal renal function, and the authors supposed the absence of hyperkalaemia to be due to a rapid increase in renal potassium excretion.

1. Bushinsky DA, Gennari FJ. Life-threatening hyperkalemia induced by arginine. *Ann Intern Med* 1978; **89:** 632–4.
2. Massara F, *et al.* The risk of pronounced hyperkalaemia after arginine infusion in the diabetic subject. *Diabete Metab* 1981; **7:** 149–53.
3. Gerard JM, Luisiri A. A fatal overdose of arginine hydrochloride. *J Toxicol Clin Toxicol* 1997; **35:** 621–5.

**Hypersensitivity.** A 10-year-old boy experienced an anaphylactic reaction 5 minutes after the start of an infusion of a 5% arginine hydrochloride solution in a test for growth-hormone output.[1] This was considered to be a very rare event and only one other apparent allergic reaction had been reported to the manufacturers.

1. Tiwary CM, *et al.* Anaphylactic reaction to arginine infusion. *N Engl J Med* 1973; **288:** 218.

### Uses and Administration

Arginine is a polar aliphatic amino acid that is essential for infant growth. It is used as a dietary supplement.

Arginine stimulates the release of growth hormone by the pituitary gland and may be used instead of, or in addition to, other tests such as insulin-induced hypoglycaemia, for the evaluation of growth disorders; false-positive and false-negative results are relatively common and evaluation therefore should not be made on the basis of a single arginine test. It is used as a 10% solution of the hydrochloride in usual doses of 30 g by intravenous infusion given over 30 minutes; children should be given 500 mg/kg.

Arginine is used in certain conditions accompanied by hyperammonaemia; for further details see below.

Arginine hydrochloride has also been used as an acidifying agent. In severe metabolic alkalosis intravenous doses have been calculated by the formula:

$$\text{intravenous dose (in grams)} = \text{desired decrease in plasma-bicarbonate concentration (mEq or mmol/litre)} \times [\text{patient's body-weight (in kg)}/9.6]$$

In forced acid diuresis to hasten drug elimination after overdose a suggested dose has been 10 g intravenously over 30 minutes. However, this has the potential to cause myoglobinuria with acute renal failure, and is rarely used.

Arginine may also be used in the form of the acetylasparaginate, aspartate, citrate, glutamate, oxoglurate, tidiacicate (thiazolidine-2,4-dicarboxylate), and timonacicate (thiazolidine-4-carboxylate). Formulation as an arginine salt is used to improve the solubility of a number of drugs, notably analgesics and antibiotics.

**Hyperammonaemia.** Hyperammonaemia is a characteristic feature of inborn errors of the urea cycle, caused by defects in the enzymes carbamyl phosphate synthetase (CPS), ornithine transcarbamylase (OTC), argininosuccinate synthetase (ASS), argininosuccinate lyase (ASL), arginase (hyperargininaemia), or *N*-acetylglutamate synthase (NAGS).[1] During the urea cycle, waste ammonia, in the form of the ammonium ion, is normally condensed with bicarbonate and ATP to form carbamoyl phosphate which undergoes several more reactions, including one leading to the synthesis of arginine, and ultimate transformation to urea for excretion. Thus, in defects of this cycle ammonia accumulates and arginine synthesis is deficient. Hyperammonaemia is often associated with respiratory alkalosis in patients with urea cycle disorders.[2]

The basis of treatment is dietary protein restriction, to decrease the requirement for waste nitrogen synthesis,[3] and the use of drugs to stimulate alternative pathways of waste nitrogen excretion.[4,5] These include arginine, citrulline, sodium benzoate, sodium phenylacetate, and sodium phenylbutyrate. In the initial management of severe hyperammonaemia, haemodialysis is preferred over peritoneal dialysis because it is more effective.[2]

Arginine supplements are given except in hyperargininaemia,[4] although citrulline may be used in some cases instead; it may be useful for CPS and OTC deficiency, but it is not recommended for patients with ASS or ASL deficiency, as levels of citrulline are already elevated.[4,6] For the treatment of acute hyperammonaemia, a loading dose of arginine 600 mg/kg over 90 minutes has been recommended pending definitive diagnosis.[2,6] A dose of 200 mg/kg or 4 g/m² has been advocated for CPS or OTC deficiency,[5,6] and 600 mg/kg or 12 g/m² for ASS or ASL deficiency.[5,6] The same dose as the loading dose is then given over 24 hours, as a constant maintenance infusion,[5,6] until conversion to oral medication is made.[6] For long-term management, doses of arginine 400 to 700 mg/kg daily have been recommended.[5,6]

Patients also receive concomitant treatment with sodium benzoate and sodium phenylacetate[5,6] or sodium phenylbutyrate[4,5] unless suffering from ASL deficiency, which can usually be managed with protein restriction and arginine alone.[5,7] When sodium benzoate is conjugated with glycine and excreted as hippuric acid it provides an alternative pathway of nitrogen excretion, while sodium phenylacetate and sodium phenylbutyrate provide a second and even more effective pathway by conjugation with glutamine.[5,6]

The usual initial doses of sodium benzoate and sodium phenylacetate in affected infants are 250 mg/kg or 5.5 g/m² of each drug by intravenous infusion over 90 minutes, followed by a further 250 mg/kg (or 5.5 g/m²) daily by constant maintenance infusion. Infusion is continued until the drugs can be taken orally; although earlier oral protocols were based on sodium benzoate, sodium phenylbutyrate is now preferred at a dosage of 450 to 600 mg/kg daily.[5,6] It has been suggested that carnitine supplementation should be added to minimise neurological symptoms and toxicity, but its value is uncertain.[3,8]

Liver transplantation (p.1346) may achieve long-term correction of urea cycle disorders, even in the very young patient, and gene replacement therapy is under investigation.[9]

Hyperammonaemia and hepatic encephalopathy (p.1243) can also arise from a variety of other causes[8] for which arginine may not be advocated. Carglumic acid (p.1668) is the treatment of choice for patients with hyperammonaemia arising from NAGS deficiency.

1. Summar M, Tuchman M. Proceedings of a consensus conference for the management of patients with urea cycle disorders. *J Pediatr* 2001; **138** (suppl): S6–S10.
2. The Urea Cycle Disorders Conference Group. Consensus statement from a conference for the management of patients with urea cycle disorders. *J Pediatr* 2001; **138** (suppl): S1–S5.
3. Leonard JV. The nutritional management of urea cycle disorders. *J Pediatr* 2001; **138** (suppl): S40–S45.
4. Berry GT, Steiner RD. Long-term management of patients with urea cycle disorders. *J Pediatr* 2001; **138** (suppl): S56–S61.
5. Batshaw ML, *et al.* Alternative pathway therapy for urea cycle disorders: twenty years later. *J Pediatr* 2001; **138** (suppl): S46–S55.
6. Summar M. Current strategies for the management of neonatal urea cycle disorders. *J Pediatr* 2001; **138** (suppl): S30–S39.
7. Brusilow SW, *et al.* Treatment of episodic hyperammonemia in children with inborn errors of urea synthesis. *N Engl J Med* 1984; **310:** 1630–4.
8. Leonard JV, Morris AAM. Inborn errors of metabolism around time of birth. *Lancet* 2000; **356:** 583–7.
9. Lee B, Goss J. Long-term correction of urea cycle disorders. *J Pediatr* 2001; **138** (suppl): S62–S71.

**Hypotensive action.** Arginine is the physiological precursor of nitric oxide and this has been suggested as an explanation for the hypotensive effect that has been reported in healthy subjects[1-3] and hypertensive patients[1,4] given infusions of arginine, although effects of arginine unrelated to nitric oxide generation cannot be excluded.[4] Decrease in plasma-cholesterol concentrations has also been reported in 2 hypercholesterolaemic patients given arginine infusions.[5] It has even been suggested that arginine might be suitable for the short-term control of hypertension,[3] although in the absence of controlled studies of its effect this must be considered speculative. Because of apparent improvement in endothelial function with arginine, some interest has surrounded its potential role in other cardiovascular diseases, such as coronary artery disease and heart failure.[6]

1. Nakaki T, *et al.* L-arginine-induced hypotension. *Lancet* 1990; **336:** 696.
2. Hishikawa K, *et al.* L-arginine-induced hypotension. *Lancet* 1991; **337:** 683–4.
3. Petros AJ, *et al.* L-arginine-induced hypotension. *Lancet* 1991; **337:** 1044–5.
4. Pedrinelli R, *et al.* Pressor, renal and endocrine effects of L-arginine in essential hypertensives. *Eur J Clin Pharmacol* 1995; **48:** 195–201.

5. Korbut R, *et al.* Effect of L-arginine on plasminogen-activator inhibitor in hypertensive patients with hypercholesterolemia. *N Engl J Med* 1993; **328:** 287–8.
6. Cheng JWM, Balwin SN. L-arginine in the management of cardiovascular diseases. *Ann Pharmacother* 2001; **35:** 755–64.

### Preparations

***BP 2003:*** Arginine Hydrochloride Intravenous Infusion;
***USP 27:*** Arginine Hydrochloride Injection.

**Proprietary Preparations** (details are given in Part 3)
***Arg.:*** Inteligen; Laclorene; ***Austria:*** Sangenor; ***Belg.:*** Dynamisan†; ***Braz.:*** Desfatigan†; Reforgan; Targifor; ***Fr.:*** Dynamisan; Energitum; Eucol†; Pargine; Sargenor; Tiadilon†; ***Ger.:*** Eubiol; ***Israel:*** Carginine; ***Ital.:*** Bioarginina; Dynamisan; Sargenor; Sulfile; ***Mex.:*** Fertibion†; ***Port.:*** Asparten; Bio-Energol Plus; Dynamisan†; Sargenor; Sulfile; ***Spain:*** Hepacitol†; Livercrom†; Potenciator; Sargenor; Sorbenor; ***Switz.:*** Dynamisan; ***USA:*** R-Gene.

**Multi-ingredient:** ***Arg.:*** Inteligen Ginseng; ***Austria:*** Leberinfusion; Rocmaline; ***Braz.:*** Necroplex†; Ornihepat; Ornitargin; Targifor C; ***Fr.:*** Arginotri-B; Arnilose†; Citrarginine; Epuram; Fastenyl; Hepagrume; Hepargitol; Rocmaline; Sargenor a la Vitamine C; ***Ger.:*** Glutarsin E; Infumal†; Polilevo N; ***Ital.:*** Calciofix; Glutargin; Ipoazotal; Ipoazotal Complex; Isoram; Polilevo; Somatron; Tonoplus; Vitasprint Complex; ***Spain:*** Dynamogen; Sanieb; ***Switz.:*** Activital; Arginotri-B; Vitasprint Complex.

## Arrowroot

Amylum Marantae; Araruta; Maranta.

### Profile

Arrowroot consists of the starch granules of the rhizomes of *Maranta arundinacea* (Marantaceae). It has the general properties of starch (p.1449). It has been used as a suspending agent in the preparation of barium meals and has sometimes been used in place of starch in tablet manufacture.

## Asparagine Monohydrate

L-Asparagine Monohydrate; Asparaginum Monohydricum; N (asparagine). (2S)-2,4-Diamino-4-oxobutanoic acid monohydrate.

$C_4H_8N_2O_3,H_2O = 150.1.$
*CAS — 70-47-3 (anhydrous asparagine).*

**Pharmacopoeias.** In *Eur.* (see p.vi).

**Ph. Eur. 5.0** (Asparagine Monohydrate). A white crystalline powder or colourless crystals. Slightly soluble in water; practically insoluble in alcohol and in dichloromethane. A 2% solution in water has a pH of 4.0 to 6.0.

### Profile

Asparagine is a non-essential amino acid.

### Preparations

**Proprietary Preparations** (details are given in Part 3)
**Multi-ingredient:** ***Ital.:*** Acutil Fosforo; ***Spain:*** Agudil.

## Aspartame *(BAN, USAN, rINN)*

APM; Aspartamo; Aspartamum; E951; SC-18862. Methyl *N*-L-α-aspartyl-L-phenylalaninate; 3-Amino-*N*-(α-methoxycarbonylphenethyl)succinamic acid; *N*-L-α-aspartyl-L-phenylalanine, 1-methyl ester.

$C_{14}H_{18}N_2O_5 = 294.3.$
*CAS — 22839-47-0.*

**Pharmacopoeias.** In *Chin.* and *Eur.* (see p.vi). Also in *USNF.*

**Ph. Eur. 5.0** (Aspartame). A white, slightly hygroscopic, crystalline powder. Sparingly or slightly soluble in water and in alcohol; practically insoluble in dichloromethane and in *n*-hexane. Store in airtight containers.

**USNF 22** (Aspartame). White, odourless, crystalline powder having a sweet taste. Sparingly soluble in water; slightly soluble in alcohol. pH of a 0.8% solution in water is about 5.

**Stability.** In the presence of moisture aspartame hydrolyses to form aspartylphenylalanine and a diketopiperazine derivative, with a resulting loss of sweetness.

### Adverse Effects and Precautions

Excessive use of aspartame should be avoided by patients with phenylketonuria since one of its metabolic products is phenylalanine. Aspartame's sweetness is lost during prolonged cooking.

◊ The safety and side-effects of aspartame as a pharmaceutical excipient have been reviewed.[1,2]

Aspartame is hydrolysed in the gastrointestinal tract to methyl alcohol aspartic acid, and phenylalanine. However, even with extraordinary consumption, methyl alcohol toxicity stemming from aspartame use is extremely unlikely. Aspartate concentrations in blood do not rise significantly following a very large dose (50 to 100 mg/kg) and therefore toxicity related to aspartate is also not expected to occur. Despite the similarity of aspartate to glutamate, studies in glutamate-sensitive persons have shown that they are not affected by aspartame consumption. Plasma concentrations of phenylalanine are also unlikely to be markedly elevated following modest consumption of aspartame by healthy persons but persons with phenylketonuria should avoid or limit their use of aspartame.

A number of adverse effects have been reported[1,2] following the use of aspartame, either as spontaneously recorded complaints from consumers or as published case reports in the medical literature. Most frequently reported problems have been headache, neuropsychiatric or behavioural symptoms, seizures, gastrointestinal symptoms, and hypersensitivity or dermatological symptoms. Available data do not provide evidence for serious widespread health consequences attendant upon the use of aspartame but it would appear that certain individuals may have an unusual sensitivity to the product. A safety review[3] by the European Commission Scientific Committee on Food (ECSCF) concluded that no causal link could be established between the consumption of aspartame and the occurrence of epilepsy or seizures, or cognition, mood and behaviour; this included individuals considered sensitive to aspartame.

Studies have confirmed aspartame's lack of effect on children's behaviour or cognitive function.[4,5]

An increased incidence of brain cancer was postulated to be related to aspartame use in a recent report;[6] however, the FDA[7] and the ECSCF[3] maintain that the available evidence does not support an association.

1. Golightly LK, *et al.* Pharmaceutical excipients: adverse effects associated with 'inactive' ingredients in drug products (part II). *Med Toxicol* 1988; **3:** 209–40.
2. American Academy of Pediatrics. "Inactive" ingredients in pharmaceutical products: update. *Pediatrics* 1997; **99:** 268–78.
3. European Commission Health and Consumer Protection Directorate-General. Opinion of the Scientific Committee on Food: update on the safety of aspartame (expressed on 4 December 2002). Available at: http://europa.eu.int/comm/food/fs/sc/scf/out155_en.pdf (accessed 14/05/04)
4. Shaywitz BA, *et al.* Aspartame, behavior, and cognitive function in children with attention deficit disorder. *Pediatrics* 1994; **93:** 70–5.
5. Wolraich ML, *et al.* Effects of diets high in sucrose or aspartame on the behavior and cognitive performance of children. *N Engl J Med* 1994; **330:** 301–7.
6. Olney JW, *et al.* Increasing brain tumor rates: is there a link to aspartame? *J Neuropathol Exp Neurol* 1996; **55:** 1115–23.
7. Anonymous. Aspartame: no apparent link with brain tumours. *WHO Drug Inf* 1997; **11:** 18–19.

**Breast feeding.** Aspartame 50 mg/kg given orally to lactating healthy women resulted in small but significant increases in breast milk aspartate, phenylalanine, and tyrosine concentrations.[1] However, it was noted that these levels were similar to postprandial milk samples and were unlikely to impact upon total amounts of amino acids ingested by the infant. Furthermore, the dose of aspartame given in the study was considerably higher than the projected intake of about 7.5 to 8.5 mg/kg daily, assuming all sucrose intake were replaced by aspartame, and no aspartame abuse. Nonetheless, the American Academy of Pediatrics[2] considers that caution is required when aspartame is ingested by lactating mothers where either the mother or infant has phenylketonuria.

1. Stegink LD, *et al.* Plasma, erythrocyte and human milk levels of free amino acids in lactating women administered aspartame or lactose. *J Nutr* 1979; **109:** 2173–81.
2. American Academy of Pediatrics. The transfer of drugs and other chemicals into human milk. *Pediatrics* 2001; **108:** 776–89. Correction. *ibid.*; 1029. Also available at: http://aappolicy.aappublications.org/cgi/content/full/pediatrics%3b108/3/776 (accessed 14/05/04)

### Pharmacokinetics

Aspartame is hydrolysed in the gastro intestinal tract to its 3 primary constituents, methyl alcohol, aspartic acid, and phenylalanine.

### Uses

Aspartame is an intense sweetening agent about 180 to 200 times as sweet as sucrose. It is used in foods, beverages, and pharmaceuticals. Each g provides approximately 17 kJ (4 kcal).

**Sickle-cell disease.** There is some preliminary evidence that aspartame may have beneficial effects in sickle-cell disease.[1]

1. Manion CV, *et al.* Aspartame effect in sickle cell anemia. *Clin Pharmacol Ther* 2001; **69:** 346–55.

### Preparations

**Proprietary Preparations** (details are given in Part 3)
***Arg.:*** Nutrasweet; Slap; ***Braz.:*** Dietacil; Dietamina†; Doce Vida; Finn; Stetic†; Sucret†; ***Chile:*** Marco Sweett; Modellsweet; Naturalist; Ridersweet; Valsweet; ***Fr.:*** D Sucril†; ***Ital.:*** Aspartina; Dolcor†; Futura; Suaviter; Sweet Touch†; Vantaggio†; Weight Watchers Punto†; ***Mex.:*** Canderel†; ***NZ:*** Equal; ***Port.:*** Canderel†; Dolcevita; Neo Dulceril†; ***Thai.:*** Equal; Espar; Sweetabb†.

**Multi-ingredient:** ***Arg.:*** Genser Sweet; ***Chile:*** Marco Sweet Light; Nutrasweet; ***Ital.:*** Weight Watchers Punto†.

## Aspartame Acesulfame

L-Phenylalanine, L-α-aspartyl-2-methyl ester, compound with 6-methyl-1,2,3-oxathiazin-4(3*H*)-one 2,2-dioxide (1:1).

$C_{18}H_{23}O_9N_3S = 457.5.$
*CAS — 106372-55-8.*

**Pharmacopoeias.** In *USNF.*

**USNF 22** (Aspartame Acesulfame). White, odourless, crystalline powder. Slightly soluble in water and in alcohol. It contains not less than 63.0% and not more than 66.0% of aspartame, calculated on the dried basis, and not less than 34.0% and not more than 37.0% of acesulfame, calculated as the acid form on the dried basis.

### Profile

Aspartame acesulfame is a compound of aspartame (above) and acesulfame (p.1420), and is used similarly in foods. It is an intense sweetener about 350 times as sweet as sucrose.

## Aspartic Acid *(USAN, rINN)*

Ácido aspártico; Acidum Asparticum; Asp; L-Aspartic Acid; D. L-Aminosuccinic acid.

$C_4H_7NO_4 = 133.1.$
*CAS — 56-84-8.*

**Pharmacopoeias.** In *Chin., Eur.* (see p.vi), and *US.*

**Ph. Eur. 5.0** (Aspartic Acid). A white or almost white crystalline powder, or colourless crystals. Slightly soluble in water; practically insoluble in alcohol. It dissolves in dilute solutions of alkali hydroxides and in dilute mineral acids. Protect from light.

**USP 27** (Aspartic Acid). A white or almost white crystalline powder, or colourless crystals. Slightly soluble in water; practically insoluble in alcohol and in ether; soluble in dilute solutions of alkali hydroxides and in dilute mineral acids. Protect from light.

### Profile

Aspartic acid is an aliphatic acidic amino acid. It is used as a dietary supplement.

# Betacarotene *(rINN)*

all-*trans*-β-Carotene; Beta Carotene *(USAN)*; Betacaroteno; Betacarotenum; E160(a); Provitamin A. β,β-Carotene; (*all-E*)-1,1′-(3,7,12,16-Tetramethyl-1,3,5,7,9,11,13,15,17-octadecanonaene-1,18-diyl)bis[2,6,6-trimethylcyclohexene].

$C_{40}H_{56} = 536.9.$
*CAS — 7235-40-7.*
*ATC — A11CA02; D02BB01.*

**Description.** Carotene exists in 3 isomeric forms, all of which are converted to some extent into vitamin A in the livers of man and animals. Of the 3 isomers of carotene, the *beta* compound is more active than the *alpha-* or *gamma-*isomers. The vitamin A activity of plants is due to the presence of *alpha-, beta-,* and *gamma*-carotenes and to kryptoxanthine; that of animal tissues is due to both vitamin A and carotene, while fish-liver oils contain vitamin A but no carotene.

**Pharmacopoeias.** In *Eur.* (see p.vi) and *US.*

**Ph. Eur. 5.0** (Betacarotene). A brown-red or brownish-red crystalline powder. Practically insoluble in water and in dehydrated alcohol; slightly soluble in cyclohexane. It is sensitive to air, heat and light, especially in solution. Store in airtight containers at a temperature not exceeding 25°. Protect from light.

**USP 27** (Beta Carotene). Red or reddish-brown to violet-brown crystals or crystalline powder. Insoluble in water, in acids, and in alkalis; practically insoluble in alcohol and in methyl alcohol; soluble in carbon disulfide, in chloroform, and in benzene; sparingly soluble in ether, in petroleum spirit, and in vegetable oils. Store in airtight containers. Protect from light.

## Units

Vitamin A activity in foods is expressed in terms of retinol equivalents: 6 micrograms of betacarotene represents 1 retinol equivalent (or 10 of the former International units for provitamin A—see p.1451).

## Adverse Effects and Precautions

Loose stools may occasionally occur during treatment with betacarotene and the skin may assume a slightly yellow discoloration. Bruising and arthralgia have been reported rarely.

Excessive intake of betacarotene does not result in hypervitaminosis A (see Pharmacokinetics, below).

**Carcinogenicity.** For reference to the finding of an increased incidence of lung cancers in individuals receiving betacarotene supplements, compared with those receiving placebo, in studies investigating the ability of betacarotene to protect against malignancy, see under Prophylaxis of Malignant Neoplasms, p.1420.

**Effects on the skin.** Yellow pigmentation of the skin may result from an unusually high consumption of carrots or other source of carotene,[1] or from a defect in the enzyme that normally metabolises betacarotene to vitamin A.[2] Hypercarotenaemia can be distinguished from jaundice by the fact that the sclerae retain their normal white colour. Pigmentation occurs first on the palms and soles and may extend to the nasolabial folds. Although it has been stated that the condition is harmless as the body converts carotene to retinol only as required,[1] others consider that long-standing hypercarotenaemia can have clinical sequelae;[2] neutropenia[3] and amenorrhoea[4] have been reported to be associated with the condition.

1. Sharman IM. Hypercarotenaemia. *BMJ* 1985; **290:** 95.
2. Vaughan Jones SA, Black MM. Metabolic carotenaemia. *Br J Dermatol* 1994; **131:** 145.
3. Shoenfeld Y, *et al.* Neutropenia induced by hypercarotenaemia. *Lancet* 1982; **i:** 1245.
4. Kemmann E, *et al.* Amenorrhoea associated with carotenemia. *JAMA* 1983; **249:** 926–9.

## Pharmacokinetics

Gastrointestinal absorption of betacarotene depends on the presence of bile and is increased by dietary fat. About 20 to 60% of betacarotene is metabolised to retinol in the intestinal wall, and a small amount is converted to vitamin A in the liver. The proportion of betacarotene converted to vitamin A decreases as the intake of betacarotene increases, and high doses of betacarotene do not lead to abnormally high serum concentrations of vitamin A. Unchanged betacarotene is distributed to various tissues including fat, the adrenal glands, and ovaries.

◊ References.


1. Wang X-D. Review: absorption and metabolism of β-carotene. *J Am Coll Nutr* 1994; **13:** 314–25.


## Human Requirements

Carotenes, of which betacarotene has the highest activity, are major dietary sources of vitamin A—see p.1452.

## Uses and Administration

Betacarotene is a carotenoid precursor of vitamin A (p.1451). It is used for the prevention of vitamin A deficiency at a dose of 6 to 15 mg daily for adults and 3 to 6 mg daily for children. In the treatment of vitamin A deficiency, vitamin A is preferred to betacarotene.

Betacarotene may be given by mouth to reduce the severity of photosensitivity reactions in patients with erythropoietic protoporphyria (see also below). Doses are in the range of 30 to 300 mg daily for adults and 30 to 150 mg daily for children, depending upon severity; they may be taken as either single daily doses or divided doses but should preferably be taken with meals. The protection offered by betacarotene is not total and generally 2 to 6 weeks of treatment resulting in a yellow coloration of palms and soles is necessary before patients should attempt to increase their exposure to sunlight.

Betacarotene and other carotenoids (alphacarotene and gammacarotene) are used as colouring agents for foods.

Betacarotene has antoxidant activity and has been studied for its possible protective benefit in a number of disorders.

**Age-related macular degeneration.** A study in patients with age-related macular degeneration indicated that the risk of developing this disorder (a leading cause of irreversible blindness among elderly persons) was markedly decreased amongst those with the highest dietary carotenoid intake;[1] in particular, lutein and zeaxanthin, or green leafy vegetables (which contain high concentrations of these carotenoids) were associated with a lower risk. Increasing the dietary intake of these carotenoids may be of benefit in reducing the development of this disorder. However, systematic reviews found that there is no evidence that antoxidant vitamin and mineral supplementation would either prevent the onset[2] or delay the progression[3] of macular degeneration in those without the condition or with just early signs. However, there was one study that showed modest benefit from vitamin C, vitamin E, betacarotene, and zinc supplementation in those with moderate to severe signs of the disease.


1. Seddon JM, *et al.* Dietary carotenoids, vitamins A, C, and E, and advanced age-related macular degeneration. *JAMA* 1994; **272:** 1413–20.
2. Evans JR, Henshaw K. Antioxidant vitamin and mineral supplementation for preventing age-related macular degeneration. Available in The Cochrane Library; Issue 2. Chichester: John Wiley; 2004.
3. Evans JR. Antioxidant vitamin and mineral supplements for age-related macular degeneration. Available in The Cochrane Library; Issue 2. Chichester: John Wiley; 2004.


**Deficiency states.** A study in Senegalese children suffering from vitamin A deficiency as defined by abnormal results on eye cytology found that supplementation with betacarotene (in a single dose equivalent to 200 000 units of vitamin A) was as effective as a single 200 000 unit dose of vitamin A palmitate in reversing the ocular changes.[1] Since betacarotene is less toxic than vitamin A itself it would have some advantages for vitamin A supplementation, either as an oral supplement or by encouraging the consumption of carotenoid-rich fruit and vegetables. A study in Indonesian women found that a betacarotene supplement improved vitamin A status, whereas an additional daily portion of dark-green leafy vegetables containing a similar amount of betacarotene did not.[2] However, others contended that consumption of food sources of carotenoids were effective in improving vitamin A status in deficiency states,[3,4] and that it might not be appropriate to extrapolate these findings to vitamin A deficient children.[3,5] WHO policy was to promote dietary adjustment wherever vitamin A deficiency was endemic.[5]

For further discussion of vitamin A deficiency and the value of supplementation in various disease states, see under Vitamin A Substances, p.1453.


1. Carlier C, *et al.* A randomised controlled trial to test equivalence between retinyl palmitate and β carotene for vitamin A deficiency. *BMJ* 1993; **307:** 1106–10.
2. de Pee S, *et al.* Lack of improvement in vitamin A status with increased consumption of dark-green leafy vegetables. *Lancet* 1995; **346:** 75–81.
3. Reddy V. Vitamin A status and dark green leafy vegetables. *Lancet* 1995; **346:** 1634–5.
4. Underwood BA. Vitamin A status and dark green leafy vegetables. *Lancet* 1995; **346:** 1635.
5. WHO. Vitamin A status: is dietary replacement practicable. *WHO Drug Inf* 1995; **9:** 141.


**Ischaemic heart disease.** There are results from epidemiological studies suggesting the potential benefits of dietary betacarotene in preventing ischaemic heart disease, particularly in smokers; however, randomised placebo-controlled studies of betacarotene supplements have returned negative results, as discussed on p.1420.

**Malignant neoplasms.** Some evidence from epidemiological studies suggested that higher dietary intakes of carotenoids and especially betacarotene had a protective effect against cancer. Consequently several randomised placebo-controlled trials examining the use of betacarotene supplements in the primary or secondary prevention of malignancy were instigated. However, the results of studies so far published have generally been disappointing. Moreover, some results suggest that supplementation with betacarotene may actually be harmful: an increase in lung cancer was seen in those at risk for this malignancy (see p.1420).

**Porphyria.** Despite a lack of robust evidence, betacarotene is the most widely used systemic drug for the management of erythropoietic protoporphyria,[1,2] a non-acute porphyria characterised by cutaneous photosensitivity (p.1040). It is often administered with canthaxanthin to reduce the skin discoloration caused by betacarotene alone.


1. Todd DJ. Erythropoietic protoporphyria. *Br J Dermatol* 1994; **131:** 751–66.
2. Todd DJ. Therapeutic options for erythropoietic protoporphyria. *Br J Dermatol* 2000; **142:** 826.


## Preparations

***USP 27:*** Beta Carotene Capsules.

**Proprietary Preparations** (details are given in Part 3)
***Arg.:*** B-Caroteno; ***Austral.:*** B-Tene†; ***Austria:*** Carotaben; ***Braz.:*** Vitcaroten; Zirvit Beta; ***Canad.:*** Betatene; ***Ger.:*** BellaCarotin mono†; Carotaben; ***Ital.:*** Tannisol; ***Neth.:*** Carotaben†; ***Switz.:*** Carotaben; ***UK:*** Arocin†; Biocarotine; Pervita†.

**Multi-ingredient:** ***Arg.:*** Bronsul; Sol Bronce Vital; ***Austral.:*** Antioxidant Forte Tablets†; Antioxidant Tablets†; Beta A-C†; Beta-Ace Tablets†; Cold Sore Tablets†; Eye Health Herbal Plus Formula 4†; Lifesystem Herbal Plus Formula 5 Eye Relief†; Lifesystem Herbal Plus Formula 8 Echinacea†; Odourless Garlic†; Sinus and Hayfever†; ***Austria:*** Oleovit A; Oleovit A + D; ***Braz.:*** Purpuralin; ***Chile:*** Unitone; ***Fr.:*** Difrarel; Phenoro†; ***Ger.:*** Carotin; Sonnenbraun†; ***Hong Kong:*** Purpuralin; ***Ital.:*** Aclon Lievit†; Agedin Plus; Angstrom Viso; Ecamannan; Keratolip; Levudin; Mirtilene; Solecin; Tannidin Plus; ***Mex.:*** Unitone; ***Port.:*** Rilastil Dermo Solar; ***Spain:*** Aceite Acalorico; Mirtilus; ***Switz.:*** Apotrin†; Linola gras; Visaline; ***USA:*** Antiox†.

---

## Biotin *(rINN)*

Biotina; Biotinum; Coenzyme R; Vitamin H. *cis*-5-(Hexahydro-2-oxo-1*H*-thieno[3,4-*d*]imidazol-4-yl)valeric acid.

$C_{10}H_{16}N_2O_3S$ = 244.3.
*CAS — 58-85-5.*
*ATC — A11HA05.*

**Pharmacopoeias.** In *Eur.* (see p.vi) and *US.*

**Ph. Eur. 5.0** (Biotin). A white crystalline powder or colourless crystals. Very slightly soluble in water and in alcohol; practically insoluble in acetone. It dissolves in dilute solutions of alkali hydroxides. Protect from light.

**USP 27** (Biotin). A practically white crystalline powder. Very slightly soluble in water and in alcohol; insoluble in other common organic solvents. Store in airtight containers.

### Profile

Biotin is traditionally considered to be a vitamin B substance. It is an essential coenzyme in fat metabolism and in other carboxylation reactions. Biotin deficiency may result in the urinary excretion of organic acids and changes in skin and hair. Deficiency of biotin is very unlikely in man because of its widespread distribution in food. Egg-yolk and offal are especially good sources. Biotin deficiency has been reported however during long-term parenteral nutrition and in patients with biotinidase deficiency, an inherited metabolic disorder.

Biotin combines with avidin, a glycoprotein present in raw egg-white, to form an inactive compound.

**Adverse effects.** For reference to life-threatening pleuropericarditis in a patient receiving biotin and pantothenic acid see p.1443.

**Deficiency states.** Biotin has been used to treat deficiency of biotinidase or holocarboxylase synthetase, enzymes responsible for the recycling and incorporation of biotin.

References.


1. McVoy JRS, *et al.* Partial biotinidase deficiency: clinical and biochemical features. *J Pediatr* 1990; **116:** 78–83.
2. Lara EB, *et al.* Biotinidase deficiency in black children. *J Pediatr* 1990; **116:** 750–2.
3. Baumgartner ER, Suormala T. Multiple carboxylase deficiency: inherited and acquired disorders of biotin metabolism. *Int J Vitam Nutr Res* 1997; **67:** 377–84.
4. Thuy LP, *et al.* Prenatal diagnosis of holocarboxylase synthetase deficiency by assay of the enzyme in chorionic villus material followed by prenatal treatment. *Clin Chim Acta* 1999; **284:** 59–68.
5. Wolf B. Biotinidase deficiency: new directions and practical concerns. *Curr Treat Options Neurol* 2003; **5:** 321–8.


**Human requirements.** In the UK neither a reference nutrient intake (RNI) nor an estimated average requirement (EAR—see p.1419) has been set for biotin although it was considered that an intake of between 10 and 200 micrograms daily was both safe and adequate.[1] Similarly in the USA an adequate intake of 30 micrograms daily has been set for adults.[2]


1. DoH. Dietary reference values for food energy and nutrients for the United Kingdom: report of the panel on dietary reference values of the committee on medical aspects of food policy. *Report on health and social subjects 41.* London: HMSO, 1991.
2. Standing Committee on the Scientific Evaluation of Dietary Reference Intakes of the Food and Nutrition Board. *Dietary Reference Intakes for thiamin, riboflavin, niacin, vitamin $B_6$, folate, vitamin $B_{12}$, pantothenic acid, biotin, and choline.* Washington, DC: National Academy Press, 2000. Also available at: http://www.nap.edu/catalog/6015.html (accessed 21/05/04)


### Preparations

**Proprietary Preparations** (details are given in Part 3)
***Austria:*** Bio-H-Tin; Curatin; Medobiotin; Merzbiotin; ***Ger.:*** Bio-H-Tin; Biokur; Biotin-Asmedic; Deacura; Gabunat; Medobiotin; Natuderm; Priorin Biotin†; Rombellin; ***Ital.:*** Biodermatin; Diathynil; Nebiotin; ***Spain:*** Medebiotin; ***Switz.:*** Bio-H-Tin; Rombellin; ***USA:*** Appearex.

**Multi-ingredient:** ***Arg.:*** Megaplus; Tersoderm Anticaspa; ***Fr.:*** Arbum; Forcapil; Zeniac; Zeniac LP; ***Ger.:*** Carotin; Sonnenbraun†; ***Ital.:*** Herbavit†; ***Spain:*** Doctodermis; Lacerdermol.

---

## Calcium Fluoride

Cálcico, fluoruro.

$CaF_2$ = 78.07.
*CAS — 7789-75-5.*

**Pharmacopoeias.** In *Ger.*

### Profile

Calcium fluoride is used as a fluoride supplement (see Sodium Fluoride, p.1444) for the prevention of dental caries. Calcium fluoride is also used as a source of calcium.

Native calcium fluoride (Calcarea Fluorica; Calc. Fluor.) is used in homoeopathic medicine.

### Preparations

**Proprietary Preparations** (details are given in Part 3)
***Denm.:*** Bifluorid; ***Fr.:*** Calcifluor.

**Multi-ingredient:** ***Fr.:*** Fluopate†; ***India:*** Calcinol; ***Ital.:*** Bifluorid; ***Spain:*** Calcio Geve D y C†; ***Swed.:*** Bifluorid.

---

## Carnitine *(rINN)*

Carnitina; ST-198; Vitamin $B_T$. (3-Carboxy-2-hydroxypropyl)trimethylammonium hydroxide, inner salt; 3-Hydroxy-4-trimethylammoniobutyrate.

$C_7H_{15}NO_3$ = 161.2.
*CAS — 461-06-3.*

## Levocarnitine *(BAN, USAN, rINN)*

L-Carnitine; Levocarnitina; Levocarnitinum. (*R*)-(3-Carboxy-2-hydroxypropyl)trimethylammonium hydroxide, inner salt; (*R*)-3-Hydroxy-4-trimethylammoniobutyrate.

$C_7H_{15}NO_3$ = 161.2.
*CAS — 541-15-1.*
*ATC — A16AA01.*

**Pharmacopoeias.** In *Eur.* (see p.vi) and *US.*

**Ph. Eur. 5.0** (Levocarnitine). A white, hygroscopic, crystalline powder or colourless crystals. Freely soluble in water; soluble in warm alcohol; practically insoluble in acetone. A 5% solution in water has a pH of 6.5 to 8.5. Store in airtight containers.

**USP 27** (Levocarnitine). White, hygroscopic, crystals or crystalline powder. Freely soluble in water and in hot alcohol; practically insoluble in acetone, in ether, and in benzene. pH of a 5% solution in water is between 5.5 and 9.5. Store in airtight containers.

## Adverse Effects and Precautions

Gastrointestinal disturbances such as nausea, vomiting, diarrhoea, and abdominal cramps have been reported following the administration of levocarnitine. Body odour has also been noticed in some patients, possibly due to the formation of the metabolite trimethylamine (see Fish Odour Syndrome, p.1417). Seizures have been reported.

Patients with severe renal impairment should not be given high doses of levocarnitine by mouth for long periods, because of the accumulation of the metabolites trimethylamine and trimethylamine-*N*-oxide. This is said not to occur to the same extent after intravenous administration. Diabetic patients administered carnitine while receiving insulin or hypoglycaemic drugs should be monitored for hypoglycaemia.

**Renal impairment.** Of 30 patients given DL-carnitine intravenously after dialysis sessions 3 developed myasthenia-like symptoms but when these 3 were given only levocarnitine the symptoms did not occur.[1] It was considered that in anuric uraemic patients the D-isomer was not excreted adequately and that accumulation had blocked neuromuscular transmission. It was therefore suggested that levocarnitine, rather than the DL-form, should be used. (High and prolonged oral doses of levocarnitine should, however, be avoided—see above.)

1. Bazzato G, *et al.* Myasthenia-like syndrome after DL but not L-carnitine. *Lancet* 1981; **i:** 1209.

## Pharmacokinetics

Oral doses of levocarnitine are absorbed slowly and incompletely from the small intestine. Plasma concentrations after oral doses represent the sum of endogenous and exogenous material. Levocarnitine does not appear to bind to plasma proteins. It is mainly eliminated by the kidneys, undergoing extensive tubular reabsorption. After intravenous administration, levocarnitine appears to undergo minimal metabolism. Levocarnitine given orally may undergo degradation in the gastrointestinal tract, leading to the formation of metabolites such as trimethylamine-*N*-oxide and γ-butyrobetaine, recovered in the urine and faeces, respectively.

◊ References.

1. Evans AM, Fornasini G. Pharmacokinetics of L-carnitine. *Clin Pharmacokinet* 2003; **42:** 941–67.

## Uses and Administration

Carnitine is an amino acid derivative which is an essential cofactor of fatty acid metabolism.

Carnitine is used in the treatment of primary carnitine deficiency and in carnitine deficiency secondary to a variety of defects of intermediary metabolism or other conditions such as haemodialysis. Both the L- and the DL-isomers have been used, but it is believed that only levocarnitine is effective and in addition, that DL-carnitine supplementation can lead to carnitine deficiency.

In the UK, depending on the condition, up to 200 mg/kg daily of levocarnitine is given by mouth, administered in 2 to 4 divided doses. Rarely, higher doses of up to 400 mg/kg daily may be needed. In the USA, lower doses of about 1 to 3 g daily are recommended for adults; the dose given for infants and children is 50 to 100 mg/kg daily in divided doses, to a maximum of 3 g daily.

When administered intravenously, up to 100 mg/kg daily is given in 3 to 4 divided doses by slow intravenous injection over 2 to 3 minutes. Higher intravenous doses have been given, but are associated with an increased incidence of adverse effects.

In patients with carnitine deficiency secondary to haemodialysis, the recommended dose of levocarnitine is 10 to 20 mg/kg intravenously after each dialysis session, adjusted according to plasma-carnitine concentrations. A maintenance dose of 1 g daily by mouth may be considered (but see Adverse Effects and Precautions, above).

Levocarnitine is under investigation for the treatment of zidovudine-induced mitochondrial myopathy.

Carnitine hydrochloride, carnitine orotate, and bicarnitine chloride have also been used.

**Carnitine supplementation.** Carnitine, which has been the subject of several reviews,[1-4] occurs as distinct L- and D-isomers although naturally-occurring carnitine is almost exclusively the L-isomer. In higher animals carnitine is an essential co-factor of fatty acid metabolism in the heart, liver, and skeletal muscle. It is normally synthesised in the liver, brain, and kidneys in sufficient quantities to meet human requirements but dietary sources such as meat and dairy products also provide carnitine. In plasma and tissues carnitine is present in the free form and as acylcarnitine esters of which acetylcarnitine (see p.1646) is the most abundant.

Although DL-carnitine is the form often present in over-the-counter preparations and dietary supplements, levocarnitine should be preferred, as the two isomers differ in their actions. Levocarnitine acts as a substrate for carnitine acetyltransferase while D-carnitine acts as a competitive inhibitor; also, levocarnitine-induced stimulation of palmitate oxidation is competitively inhibited by D-palmitoylcarnitine. Such differences are believed to account for findings of benefit only with the L-isomer, or unwanted effects when D-carnitine or DL-carnitine was administered.[1,3]

Primary carnitine deficiency is a disorder of the membrane transport of carnitine and patients have presented with hypoglycaemia and encephalopathy, skeletal myopathy, and cardiomyopathy. Therapy with carnitine in these primary deficiency states is considered to have a rational basis.[1,2] Secondary carnitine deficiency occurs in many inherited metabolic disorders, especially in the organic acidurias and disorders of beta-oxidation, but the value of carnitine for these conditions is controversial.[2,5-9]

Carnitine deficiency may also arise during the long-term use of drugs such as valproic acid,[1,10] pivampicillin,[11,12] or pivmecillinam,[11] which are conjugated with carnitine. Whether carnitine supplementation can prevent or reverse this type of deficiency is unclear: treatment with carnitine, although it raised plasma-carnitine concentrations, had no more effect than placebo on the well-being of children receiving valproic acid therapy in one study,[13] but others have found levocarnitine supplementation of value in attenuating valproate-induced hyperammonaemia after a protein-rich meal,[14] and some paediatric neurologists consider supplementation justified in selected children with epilepsy,[15] including those with, or at risk of, valproate-induced hepatotoxicity.

Since carnitine supplementation has been associated with a reduction[16,17] in the incidence of haemodialysis-induced cramps it has been suggested that these cramps might be due in part to carnitine deficiency.

There is also some evidence[1,18] that carnitine supplements may be of benefit to low birth-weight preterm infants, but a double-blind study[19] failed to confirm this effect. However, premature infants at particular risk of carnitine deficiency, such as those on long-term parenteral nutrition, may benefit.[4,20] Some consider that carnitine supplements may be advisable in full-term infants receiving formula feeds.[21]

Low concentrations of carnitine have also been reported to occur in a variety of other conditions and there is some evidence that carnitine supplementation may exert a cardioprotective role. Benefit in patients with cardiomyopathies,[1,22,23] reduction of infarct size and prevention of arrhythmias in patients with myocardial infarction,[1,2] increased exercise tolerance in patients with angina[1,2] or intermittent claudication,[2] and protection from the cardiotoxicity of the anthracycline antineoplastics[1] have all been described in patients given carnitine supplementation. However, the use of carnitine in healthy subjects in an attempt to improve athletic performance is controversial.[24]

There is some suggestion that carnitine supplementation may be of benefit in alleviating chemotherapy-induced fatigue.[25]

One case report has described a dramatic response of long-standing leg ulcers to carnitine therapy in a patient with sickle-cell disease.[26]

1. Goa KL, Brogden RN. L-Carnitine: a preliminary review of its pharmacokinetics, and its therapeutic use in ischaemic cardiac disease and primary and secondary carnitine deficiencies in relationship to its role in fatty acid metabolism. *Drugs* 1987; **34:** 1–24.
2. Anonymous. Carnitine deficiency. *Lancet* 1990; **335:** 631–3.
3. Li Wan Po A. Carnitine: a scientifically exciting molecule. *Pharm J* 1990; **245:** 388–9.
4. Walter JH. L-carnitine. *Arch Dis Child* 1996; **74:** 475–8.
5. Anonymous. Medium chain acyl CoA dehydrogenase deficiency. *Lancet* 1991; **338:** 544–5.
6. Rinaldo P, *et al.* Effect of treatment with glycine and L-carnitine in medium-chain acyl-coenzyme A dehydrogenase deficiency. *J Pediatr* 1993; **122:** 580–4.
7. Winter SC, *et al.* Carnitine deficiency. *Lancet* 1990; **335:** 981–2.
8. Chalmers RA, *et al.* Carnitine deficiency. *Lancet* 1990; **335:** 982.
9. Evangeliou A, Vlassopoulos D. Carnitine metabolism and deficit when supplementation is necessary? *Curr Pharm Biotechnol* 2003; **4:** 211–9.
10. Raskind JY, El-Chaar GM. The role of carnitine supplementation during valproic acid therapy. *Ann Pharmacother* 2000; **34:** 630–8.
11. Holme E, *et al.* Carnitine deficiency induced by pivampicillin and pivmecillinam therapy. *Lancet* 1989; **ii:** 469–73.
12. Melegh B. Carnitine supplementation in pivampicillin treatment. *Lancet* 1989; **ii:** 1096.
13. Freeman JM, *et al.* Does carnitine administration improve the symptoms attributed to anticonvulsant medications?: a double-blinded, crossover study. *Pediatrics* 1994; **93:** 893–5.
14. Gidal BE, *et al.* Diet- and valproate-induced transient hyperammonemia: effect of L-carnitine. *Pediatr Neurol* 1997; **16:** 301–5.
15. De Vivo DC, *et al.* L-carnitine supplementation in childhood epilepsy: current perspectives. *Epilepsia* 1998; **39:** 1216–25.
16. Ahmad S, *et al.* Multicenter trial of L-carnitine in maintenance hemodialysis patients II: clinical and biochemical effects. *Kidney Int* 1990; **38:** 912–8.
17. Sakurauchi Y, *et al.* Effects of L-carnitine supplementation on muscular symptoms in hemodialyzed patients. *Am J Kidney Dis* 1998; **32:** 258–64.
18. Shortland GJ, Walter JH. L-carnitine. *Lancet* 1990; **335:** 1215.
19. Shortland GJ, *et al.* Randomised controlled trial of L-carnitine as a nutritional supplement in preterm infants. *Arch Dis Child Fetal Neonatal Ed* 1998; **78:** F185–F188.
20. Sulkers EJ, *et al.* L-carnitine. *Lancet* 1990; **335:** 1215.
21. Giovannini M, *et al.* Is carnitine essential in children? *J Int Med Res* 1991; **19:** 88–102.
22. Helton E, *et al.* Metabolic aspects of myocardial disease and a role for L-carnitine in the treatment of childhood cardiomyopathy. *Pediatrics* 2000; **105:** 1260–70. Correction. *ibid.*; **106:** 623.
23. Rizos I. Three-year survival of patients with heart failure caused by dilated cardiomyopathy and L-carnitine administration. *Am Heart J* 2000; **139** (suppl): S120–S123.
24. Tonda ME, Hart LL. N,N-dimethylglycine and L-carnitine as performance enhancers in athletes. *Ann Pharmacother* 1992; **26:** 935–7.
25. Graziano F, *et al.* Potential role of levocarnitine supplementation for the treatment of chemotherapy-induced fatigue in non-anaemic cancer patients. *Br J Cancer* 2002; **86:** 1854–7.
26. Harrell HL. L-Carnitine for leg ulcers. *Ann Intern Med* 1990; **113:** 412.

## Preparations

***USP 27:*** Levocarnitine Injection; Levocarnitine Oral Solution; Levocarnitine Tablets.

**Proprietary Preparations** (details are given in Part 3)

***Arg.:*** Albicar; ***Braz.:*** Levocarnin; ***Canad.:*** Carnitor; ***Chile:*** Carnicor; ***Fr.:*** Levocarnil; ***Ger.:*** Biocarn; L-Carn; Nefrocarnit; ***Hong Kong:*** Carnitene; Carnitor; ***Ital.:*** Anetin†; Briocor†; Cardimet†; Cardiobil; Cardiogen; Carnicor†; Carnitene; Carnitolo; Carnitop; Carnovis; Carnum; Carrier; Carvis†; Carvit†; Elleci; Eucar; Eucarnil; Farnitin; Framil†; Karrer; Kernit; Lefcar; Levocarvit; Medocarnitin; Megavis; Metina; Miocardin; Miocor; Miotonal; Neo Cardiol; Transfert; ***Mex.:*** Cardispan; ***Port.:*** Disocor; ***Spain:*** Carnicor; Secabiol; ***UK:*** Carnitor; Elcarn†; ***USA:*** Carnitor; VitaCarn.

**Multi-ingredient:** ***Arg.:*** Enlinea; Garcinol Max; Herbaccion Diet; Tonekin Plus; ***Braz.:*** Hepanisan†; Pepsivit; ***Chile:*** Grisetin Con Carnitina; ***Fr.:*** Arkotonic†; ***Ital.:*** Biocarnil; Carfosid; Carpantin; Co-Carnetina B12; Memorandum; ***Mex.:*** Lipovitasi-Or; ***Spain:*** Hepadif; Malandil; Pranzo.

## Choline Bitartrate

Bitartarato de Colina; Choline Acid Tartrate; Cholinii Tartras. 2-Hydroxyethyltrimethylammonium hydrogen tartrate.

$C_9H_{19}NO_7$ = 253.2.

*CAS — 87-67-2.*

**Pharmacopoeias.** In *US.*

**USP 27** (Choline Bitartrate). A white, hygroscopic, crystalline powder; odourless or with a faint trimethylamine odour. Clear and colourless in solution. Freely soluble in water; slightly soluble in alcohol; insoluble in chloroform and in ether. pH of a 10% solution in water is between 3.0 and 4.0.

## Choline Chloride *(rINN)*

Cholinii Chloridum; Cloruro de colina. 2-Hydroxyethyltrimethylammonium chloride.

$C_5H_{14}ClNO$ = 139.6.

*CAS — 62-49-7 (choline); 67-48-1 (choline chloride).*

**Pharmacopoeias.** In *Fr.* and *US.*

**USP 27** (Choline Chloride). Hygroscopic, colourless or white crystals or crystalline powder, usually having a slight odour of trimethylamine. Clear and colourless in solution. Soluble in water and in alcohol. pH of a 10% solution in water is between 4.0 and 7.0.

## Profile

Choline is an acetylcholine precursor. It is involved in lipid metabolism and acts as a methyl donor in various other metabolic processes. Choline has traditionally been considered to be a vitamin B substance although its functions do not justify its classification as a vitamin. Choline can be synthesised in the body. However, its absence in total parenteral nutrition causes hepatic steatosis, and it is also thought to be a requirement in the diet of neonates. Sources of choline, which occurs mostly as lecithin, include egg-yolk and vegetable and animal fat.

Choline is used as a dietary supplement and has been used to treat liver disorders such as fatty liver and cirrhosis. It has been tried in the management of Alzheimer's disease (see Dementia, p.1484) but without success. Choline is used as the bitartrate, dihydrogen citrate, and orotate salts as well as the chloride.

**Human requirements.** In the USA, an adequate intake (see p.1419) of 550 mg daily in men and 425 mg daily in women has been determined for choline.[1] The tolerable upper intake level for adults is 3.5 g daily.[1]

1. Standing Committee on the Scientific Evaluation of Dietary Reference Intakes of the Food and Nutrition Board. *Dietary Reference Intakes for thiamin, riboflavin, niacin, vitamin $B_6$, folate, vitamin $B_{12}$, pantothenic acid, biotin, and choline.* Washington, DC: National Academy Press, 2000. Also available at: http://www.nap.edu/catalog/6015.html (accessed 24/05/04)

## Preparations

**Proprietary Preparations** (details are given in Part 3)

***Ger.:*** neurotropan; ***Hong Kong:*** Athero†.

**Multi-ingredient:** ***Arg.:*** Bil 13; ***Austral.:*** Gingo A†; Liv-Detox†; ***Austria:*** Orocholin; ***Belg.:*** Sulfarlem Choline†; ***Braz.:*** Alcafelol; Aminotox; Anekron; B-Vesil; Betaliver; Biofigado†; Biohepax; Boldobeba†; Colagotil†; Colinvintol†; Cynatrop†; Enterofigon†; Epacrosil†; Epativan B6; Epocler; Ergohepat B12†; Eviepar†; Extrato Hepatico Composto; Extrato Hepatico Vitaminado; Figadobil†; Hecrosine B12†; Hepachofril Solution†; Hepachofril†; Hepacitron†; Hepalin†; Hepasedan†; Hepationina†; Hepatobe†; Hepatocler†; Hepatotris; Hepofilina†; Hormo Hepatico; Infiltran B12†; Jecohepat†; Jurubileno†; Lisotox†; Litrison†; Mesitol†; Metiocolin B12; Metiocolin Composto; Metionina Composta†; Necro B-6; Necrohepat†; Neofarmotox†; Olocynan†; Olohepat†; Panvitrop†; Scolybil†; Vesibil†; Xantina B12; Xantinon B12; Xantinon Complex; ***Chile:*** Hepabil; ***Fr.:*** Citrocholine; Cysticholt†; Desintex-Choline; Hepacholine; Hepagrume; Kalicitrine†; Phosphocholine†; Romarinex-Choline†; ***Ger.:*** Hepalipon N†; Hepatofalk Neu†; Hepatofalk†; Lipovitan; ***Hong Kong:*** Bilsan; Hepatofalk; ***India:*** Delphicol; Mecolin; Sorbiline; ***Ital.:*** Epa-Treis†; ***Port.:*** Metionina†; ***S.Afr.:*** Hepavite; Prohep; ***Spain:*** Antibioflus†; Hepato Fardi; ***Thai.:*** Liporon; Proheparum†; ***UK:*** Fat-Solv†; Lipotropic Factors; ***USA:*** Ilopan-Choline†.

## Chondroitin Sulfate–Iron Complex

Chondroitin Sulphate–Iron Complex; Ferropolichondrum; Hierro y sulfato de condroitina, complejo de.

*CAS — 54391-57-0.*

*ATC — B03AB07.*

### Profile

Chondroitin sulfate-iron complex is used as a source of iron (p.1434) for iron-deficiency anaemia (p.733). It is given by mouth in doses of up to 900 mg daily, equivalent to up to 90 mg of iron daily.

### Preparations

**Proprietary Preparations** (details are given in Part 3)
***Ital.:*** Condrofer; Isairon.

## Chromium

Cromo.

Cr = 51.9961.

## Chromium Trichloride

Chromic Chloride; Cromo, tricloruro de.

$CrCl_3,6H_2O$ = 266.4.

*CAS — 10025-73-7 (anhydrous chromium trichloride); 10060-12-5 (chromium trichloride hexahydrate).*

**Pharmacopoeias.** In *US.*

**USP 27** (Chromic Chloride). Dark green, odourless, slightly deliquescent crystals. Soluble in water and in alcohol; slightly soluble in acetone; practically insoluble in ether. Store in airtight containers.

## Chromium Tripicolinate

Chromium Picolinate; Cromo, picolinato de.

$C_{18}H_{12}N_3O_6Cr$ = 418.3.

**Pharmacopoeias.** In *USNF.*

**USNF 22** (Chromium Picolinate). Store in airtight containers.

### Adverse Effects

Trivalent salts of chromium, such as chromium trichloride, are generally considered to produce few adverse effects. However, hexavalent forms of chromium are notably toxic (see under Chromium Trioxide, p.1670).

**Effects on the kidneys.** Two cases of renal failure were attributed to ingestion of excessive doses of chromium tripicolinate in women with no previous history of renal dysfunction.[1,2] For mention of decreases in glomerular filtration rate in children receiving chromium-supplemented total parenteral nutrition, see below.

1. Wasser WG, *et al.* Chronic renal failure after ingestion of over-the-counter chromium picolinate. *Ann Intern Med* 1997; **126:** 410.
2. Cerulli J, *et al.* Chromium picolinate toxicity. *Ann Pharmacother* 1998; **32:** 428–31.

**Effects on the skin.** There have been rare reports[1,2] of cutaneous reactions to oral chromium tripicolinate, including one of acute generalised exanthematous pustulosis.

1. Fowler JF. Systemic contact dermatitis caused by oral chromium picolinate. *Cutis* 2000; **65:** 116.
2. Young PC, *et al.* Acute generalized exanthematous pustulosis induced by chromium picolinate. *J Am Acad Dermatol* 1999; **41:** 820–3.

### Uses and Administration

Chromium is an essential trace element that potentiates insulin action and thus influences carbohydrate, lipid, and protein metabolism. Dietary sources rich in chromium include brewers' yeast, meat, whole grains, and nuts. Chromium trichloride has been given as a chromium supplement in total parenteral nutrition. Chromium tripicolinate is used as a chromium supplement, and is being investigated for improving glycaemic control in patients with diabetes mellitus.

**Diabetes mellitus.** A review[1] of trivalent chromium as an adjunct in the management of diabetes mellitus (p.324).

1. Ryan GJ, *et al.* Chromium as adjunctive treatment for type 2 diabetes. *Ann Pharmacother* 2003; **37:** 876–85.

**Human requirements.** In the UK neither a reference nutrient intake (RNI) nor an estimated average requirement (EAR—see p.1419) has been set for chromium although a safe and adequate intake was believed to be above 25 micrograms daily for adults.[1] Similarly, in the USA a recommended dietary allowance has not been published but the adequate intake was estimated to be 35 micrograms daily for young men and 25 micrograms daily for young women.[2] WHO considers that the minimum population mean intake likely to meet normal needs for chromium might be approximately 33 micrograms daily, and that supplementation of this element should not exceed 250 micrograms daily until more is known.[3]

1. DoH. Dietary reference values for food energy and nutrients for the United Kingdom: report of the panel on dietary reference values of the committee on medical aspects of food policy. *Report on health and social subjects 41.* London: HMSO, 1991.
2. Standing Committee on the Scientific Evaluation of Dietary Reference Intakes of the Food and Nutrition Board. *Dietary Reference Intakes for vitamin A, vitamin K, arsenic, boron, chromium, copper, iodine, iron, manganese, molybdenum, nickel, silicon, vanadium, and zinc.* Washington DC: National Academy Press, 2001. Also available at: http://www.nap.edu/catalog/10026.html (accessed 24/05/04)
3. WHO. Chromium. In: *Trace elements in human nutrition and health.* Geneva: WHO, 1996: 155–60.

**Supplementation.** Although a daily chromium intake of 200 nanograms/kg has been suggested in children receiving total parenteral nutrition (TPN), a study in 15 children[1] receiving long-term parenteral nutrition found that supplementation at about this level was associated with serum-chromium concentrations 4 to 42 times higher than the mean value in 15 children not receiving TPN. Raised serum-chromium concentrations were associated with a decrease in glomerular filtration rate; one year after discontinuing chromium supplementation, which reduced intake to 50 nanograms/kg daily (as contaminants of water and TPN solutions), chromium concentrations, although lower, were still higher than controls and renal function had not altered. The authors subsequently discontinued chromium supplementation in both children and adults, since chromium contamination of TPN solutions appeared adequate to prevent deficiency, although it was acknowledged that signs of chromium deficiency might take some years to appear. Chromium contamination in various preparations used in paediatric parenteral nutrition has been studied.[2]

1. Moukarzel AA, *et al.* Excessive chromium intake in children receiving total parenteral nutrition. *Lancet* 1992; **339:** 385–8.
2. Hak EB, *et al.* Chromium and zinc contamination of parenteral nutrient solution components commonly used in infants and children. *Am J Health-Syst Pharm* 1998; **55:** 150–4.

### Preparations

***USP 27:*** Chromic Chloride Injection.

**Proprietary Preparations** (details are given in Part 3)
***Arg.:*** Tonekin; ***Austral.:*** Chrome†; ***Canad.:*** Bio-Chrome; Micro Cr†; ***Chile:*** Edul K-200; ***Ital.:*** Croben; ***Mex.:*** Cromifusin; ***USA:*** Chroma-Pak.

**Multi-ingredient:** ***Arg.:*** Cholesterol Reducing Plan; Herbaccion Diet; Tonekin Plus; ***Austral.:*** Bio-Chromium†; Bioglan 3B Beer Belly Buster†; Citri Slim+Trim†; Digestaid†; Pro-Shape†; ***Canad.:*** Formula Cl†; ***Fr.:*** Bio-Chrome†.

## Citrulline

$N^5$-(Aminocarbonyl)-L-ornithine; $N^\delta$-Carbamylornithine; Citrulina. α-Amino-δ-ureidovaleric acid.

$C_6H_{13}N_3O_3$ = 175.2.

*CAS — 372-75-8.*

### Profile

Citrulline is an amino acid that is involved in the urea cycle. Citrulline and citrulline malate are used as dietary supplements.

**Hyperammonaemia.** Citrulline has been given as an alternative to arginine in the management of hyperammonaemia due to urea cycle disorders (p.1421).

Lysinuric protein intolerance is another condition associated with hyperammonaemia and similar neurological sequelae. In this condition there is no deficiency of urea-cycle enzymes but a deficiency of urea-cycle substrate, such as ornithine, which results in reduced synthesis of citrulline. Supplements of citrulline given with meals have been reported to have resulted in a substantial increase in protein tolerance, striking acceleration in linear growth, and an increase in bone mass in a child with this disorder who presented with osteoporosis.[1]

1. Carpenter TO, *et al.* Lysinuric protein intolerance presenting as childhood osteoporosis: clinical and skeletal response to citrulline therapy. *N Engl J Med* 1985; **312:** 290–4.

### Preparations

**Proprietary Preparations** (details are given in Part 3)
***Fr.:*** Stimol; ***Port.:*** Dynergum.

**Multi-ingredient:** ***Braz.:*** Necroplex†; Ornihepat; Ornitargin; ***Fr.:*** Epuram; ***Ger.:*** Polilevo N; ***Ital.:*** Ideolider†; Ipoazotal; Ipoazotal Complex; Polilevo.

## Cod-liver Oil *(BAN)*

Aceite de Hígado de Bacalao; Cod Liver Oil; Huile de Foie de Morue; Iecoris Aselli Oleum; Lebertran; Ol. Morrh.; Óleo de Bacalhau; Oleum Jecoris Aselli; Oleum Morrhuae; Olio di Fegato di Merluzzo.

*CAS — 8001-69-2.*

**Pharmacopoeias.** In *Chin., Eur.* (see p.vi), *Jpn, Pol.,* and *US.*

**Ph. Eur. 5.0** (Cod-liver Oil (Type A) and Cod-liver Oil (Type B)). Purified fatty oils obtained from the fresh livers of *Gadus morhua* and other species of Gadidae, solid substances being removed by cooling and filtering. The oils contain not less than 600 units (180 micrograms) and not more than 2500 units (750 micrograms) of vitamin A per g and not less than 60 units (1.5 micrograms) and not more than 250 units (6.25 micrograms) of vitamin $D_3$ (colecalciferol) per g. Authorised antioxidants in concentrations not exceeding those prescribed by the competent authority may be added.

Clear yellowish viscous liquids. Practically insoluble in water; slightly soluble in alcohol; miscible with petroleum spirit. Store in well-filled airtight containers. Store under an inert gas if no antoxidant is added. Protect from light.

**USP 27** (Cod Liver Oil). The partially destearinated fixed oil obtained from the fresh livers of *Gadus morrhua* and other species of Gadidae. It contains not less than 600 units (180 micrograms) and not more than 2500 units (750 micrograms) of vitamin A per g and not less than 60 units (1.5 micrograms) and not more than 250 units (6.25 micrograms) of vitamin D per g. It may be flavoured by the addition of not more than 1% of a suitable flavour or a mixture of flavours. A suitable antioxidant may be added.

A thin, oily liquid, having a characteristic, slightly fishy but not rancid odour. Slightly soluble in alcohol; freely soluble in carbon disulfide, in chloroform, in ether, and in ethyl acetate. Store in airtight containers. It may be bottled or packaged in containers from which air has been expelled by the production of a vacuum or by an inert gas.

### Profile

Cod-liver oil is a rich source of vitamin D (p.1461) and a good source of vitamin A (p.1451). It also contains several essential fatty acids.

Cod-liver oil dressings or ointment have been advocated to accelerate healing in burns, ulcers, pressure sores, and superficial wounds, but controlled observations have failed to substantiate claims of their value.

### Preparations

***USNF 22:*** Cod Liver Oil Capsules.

**Proprietary Preparations** (details are given in Part 3)
***Austral.:*** Hypol†; ***Austria:*** Adecaps; Vitapan; ***Belg.:*** Surmoruine†; ***Ger.:*** Gelovital; Unguentolan; ***Hong Kong:*** Scott's Emulsion; ***Ital.:*** Dermovitamina; ***Spain:*** Aceite Geve Concentrado; ***Switz.:*** Morrhulan.

**Multi-ingredient:** ***Arg.:*** Atomoderma A-D; Atomoderma Plus; Hipoglos con Hidrocortisona; ***Austral.:*** Desitin Nappy Rash Ointment; Hypol†; ***Austria:*** Dermilon; Dermowund; Desitin; Leukichtan; Linobion-Globuli†; Mirfulan; Nuri-Kapseln; Pudan-Lebertran-Zinksalbe; Vulpuran; ***Belg.:*** Mitosyl; Newderm; Polyseptol; Pyal†; Vitamorrhuine†; ***Braz.:*** AD-Furp†; Blumen; Calciumvit Infantil; Dermoglos†; Hiposan; Preparado H†; Topiglos; Topo Worth†; Vitacolor†; ***Canad.:*** Caldesene†; Desitin; ***Chile:*** Cikavit; Deltisan; Dulinas; Pediaderm; ***Fr.:*** Eryteal†; Halivite; Magalite; ***Ger.:*** Dermilon; Desitin; Leukona-Wundsalbe; Mirfulan; Mirfulan Spray N; Mitosyl; Zinksalbe; ***Hong Kong:*** Desitin; Scott's Emulsion Orange; ***Irl.:*** Caldease; Morhulin; ***Israel:*** Desitin; Rekasitin; Zincod; ***Ital.:*** Fosfarsile Junior; Idustatin†; Neo-Ustiol; Steril Zeta; Trofo 5; Viocidina†; ***Mex.:*** Desitin; Glossderm; Sutin; ***Norw.:*** Aselli; ***Port.:*** Pomaglos†; ***S.Afr.:*** Achromide; Daromide; Ung Vernleigh; ***Singapore:*** Desitin; ***Spain:*** Avril; Recto Menaderm†; Siete Mares Higado Bacal†; ***Switz.:*** Keroderm; Perles d'huile de foie de morue du Dr Geistlich†; Phlogidermil†; Vita-Hexin; ***UK:*** Clogar; M & M; Morhulin; Scott's Emulsion†; Woodwards Nappy Rash Ointment†; ***USA:*** A and D Medicated; Caldesene; Clocream; Desitin; Diaper Rash; Dyprotex.

## Copper

Cobre.

Cu = 63.546.

*CAS — 7440-50-8.*

**Pharmacopoeias.** *Eur.* (see p.vi) includes Copper for Homoeopathic Preparations.

**Ph. Eur. 5.0** (Copper for Homoeopathic Preparations; Cuprum ad Praeparationes Homoeopathicae). A reddish-brown powder. Practically insoluble in water and in alcohol; soluble in hydrochloric acid and in nitric acid.

## Calcium Copperedetate

Cuproedetato cálcico. Calcium [ethylenediaminetetra-acetato(4—)-*N,N′,O,O′*]copper (II) dihydrate.

$C_{10}H_{12}CaCuN_2O_8,2H_2O$ = 427.9.

*CAS — 66317-91-7 (anhydrous calcium copperedetate).*

**Pharmacopoeias.** In *BP(Vet).*

**BP(Vet) 2003** (Calcium Copperedetate). A blue, odourless or almost odourless, crystalline powder. It contains 9.1 to 9.7% of Ca and 14.4 to 15.3% of Cu. Freely soluble in water, the solution gradually precipitating the tetrahydrate; practically insoluble in alcohol.

## Copper Chloride

Cobre, cloruro de; Cupric Chloride.

$CuCl_2,2H_2O$ = 170.5.

*CAS — 7447-39-4 (anhydrous copper chloride); 10125-13-0 (copper chloride dihydrate).*

**Pharmacopoeias.** In *US.*

**USP 27** (Cupric Chloride). Bluish-green, deliquescent crystals. Freely soluble in water; soluble in alcohol; slightly soluble in ether. Store in airtight containers at a temperature of 25°, excursions permitted between 15° and 30°.

## Copper Gluconate

Cobre, gluconato de. Copper D-gluconate (1:2); Bis(D-gluconato-$O^1$,$O^2$) copper.

$C_{12}H_{22}CuO_{14}$ = 453.8.

*CAS — 527-09-3.*

**Pharmacopoeias.** In *US.*

## Copper Sulfate

Cobre, sulfato de; Copper Sulph.; Copper Sulphate; Cuivre (Sulfate de); Cupri Sulfas; Cupri Sulphas; Cupric Sulfate; Kupfersulfat; Sulfato de Cobre. Copper (II) sulphate pentahydrate.

$CuSO_4,5H_2O$ = 249.7.

*CAS — 7758-98-7 (anhydrous copper sulfate); 7758-99-8 (copper sulfate pentahydrate).*

*ATC — V03AB20.*

NOTE. Crude copper sulfate is sometimes known as 'blue copperas', 'blue stone', and 'blue vitriol'.

**Pharmacopoeias.** In *Eur.* (see p.vi), *US*, and *Viet.*

*Eur.* and *Viet.* also include anhydrous copper sulfate.

**Ph. Eur. 5.0** (Copper Sulphate Pentahydrate). A blue crystalline powder or transparent blue crystals. Freely soluble in water; practically insoluble in alcohol; soluble in methyl alcohol.

**Ph. Eur. 5.0** (Copper Sulphate, Anhydrous). A greenish-grey, very hygroscopic, powder. Freely soluble in water; practically insoluble in alcohol; slightly soluble in methyl alcohol. Store in airtight containers.

**USP 27** (Cupric Sulfate). Deep blue, triclinic crystals, or blue, crystalline granules or powder. It effloresces slowly in dry air. Soluble 1 in 3 of water, 1 in 0.5 of boiling water, 1 in 500 of alcohol, and 1 in 3 of glycerol. Its solutions are acid to litmus. Store in airtight containers at a temperature of 25°, excursions permitted between 15° and 30°.

### Adverse Effects and Treatment

Adverse effects from copper have tended to arise following absorption of the metal from cooking utensils and during dialysis. Ingestion of copper from cooking utensils is associated mainly with hepatotoxicity. Dialysis procedures may supply copper through the water supply or from parts of the equipment and when this happens patients may suffer haemolysis and other haematological reactions with kidney involvement as well as hepatotoxicity; the toxicity is generally a result of poor equipment maintenance.

Adverse effects attributed to copper have been reported in women with copper-containing intra-uterine devices. There have been isolated case reports of various effects such as allergy and endometrial changes. However, with these devices it is difficult to separate those adverse effects that are due to the device from those due solely to the copper.

The symptoms of Wilson's disease (hepatolenticular degeneration) (see p.1049) are due to an accumulation of copper in various parts of the body.

Copper salts if ingested can produce severe gastrointestinal effects and there may be systemic absorption of copper leading to the effects discussed above. The use of sprays of copper salts in agriculture has been associated with lung changes. Treatment of copper poisoning is symptomatic and may involve the use of a chelating agent to remove any absorbed metal. Dialysis has been tried.

**Effects on the liver.** A report of cirrhosis and acute liver failure attributable to chronic excessive copper supplement ingestion.[1]

1. O'Donohue J, *et al.* Micronodular cirrhosis and acute liver failure due to chronic copper self-intoxication. *Eur J Gastroenterol Hepatol* 1993; **5:** 561–2.

### Interactions

Large doses of zinc supplements may inhibit the gastrointestinal absorption of copper.

### Uses and Administration

Copper is an essential trace element although severe copper deficiency, which is associated with anaemia, neutropenia, and bone demineralisation, is rare in humans. Copper sulfate is added to parenteral feeds as a source of copper in the prophylaxis and treatment of deficiency states. Doses that have been used for prophylaxis range from 0.5 to 1.5 mg (7.9 to 23.6 micromoles) of copper daily although up to 3 mg daily has been suggested in established deficiency; infants have received 20 micrograms/kg (0.3 micromol/kg) of copper daily. The dose should be governed by the serum-copper concentration which in healthy adults ranges between 0.7 and 1.6 micrograms/mL (0.01 to 0.025 micromol/mL).

Copper sulfate and other soluble salts of copper have an astringent action on mucous surfaces and in strong solutions they are corrosive.

Copper has a contraceptive effect (p.1535) when present in the uterus, and is added to some intra-uterine contraceptive devices; such devices are considered to be effective and safe for several years after insertion, and may be the most effective method for emergency contraception (p.1536). Copper is also reported to have an antimicrobial action.

Copper sulfate has been used to prevent the growth of algae in reservoirs, ponds, and swimming pools and as a molluscicide in the control of fresh-water snails that act as intermediate hosts in the life-cycle of the parasites causing schistosomiasis.

Reagents containing copper sulfate are used in tests for reducing sugars.

In veterinary medicine calcium copperedetate, copper methionate, copper oxide, and cuproxoline are used for the prevention and treatment of copper deficiency.

Copper bracelets are worn as a folk remedy for rheumatic disorders: there is no good evidence to justify such a practice.

Copper (Cuprum Metallicum; Cuprum Met.) is used in homoeopathic medicine.

**Deficiency states.** Acquired copper deficiency is very rare and the small number of cases have usually involved patients on total parenteral nutrition or long-term enteral nutrition.[1]

Menkes' disease is an X-linked genetic disorder associated with a defect in copper transport, which almost invariably results in death due to progressive cerebral degeneration by the age of 3 years. Early initiation of treatment with copper-histidine complex may be of benefit in such children.[2,3]

1. Masugi J, *et al.* Copper deficiency anemia and prolonged enteral feeding. *Ann Intern Med* 1994; **121:** 386.
2. Sarkar B, *et al.* Copper-histidine therapy for Menkes' disease. *J Pediatr* 1993; **123:** 828–30.
3. Cox DW. Disorders of copper transport. *Br Med Bull* 1999; **55:** 544–55.

**Human requirements.** In the UK dietary reference values (see p.1419) have been published for copper.[1] Although an estimated average requirement (EAR) could not be derived a reference nutrient intake (RNI) of 1.2 mg (19 micromoles) daily was set for adults; RNIs of lower values were also specified for infants and children.[1]

In the USA the recommended dietary allowance (RDA) for copper is 900 micrograms daily in adults, and the tolerable upper intake level is 10 mg daily.[2]

WHO has estimated a minimum population mean intake of 1.2 mg daily for women and 1.3 mg daily for men, and safe upper limits of population mean intakes of 10 mg daily for women and 12 mg daily for men;[3] values are also estimated for infants and children.

1. DoH. Dietary reference values for food energy and nutrients for the United Kingdom: report of the panel on dietary reference values of the committee on medical aspects of food policy. *Report on health and social subjects 41.* London: HMSO, 1991.
2. Standing Committee on the Scientific Evaluation of Dietary Reference Intakes of the Food and Nutrition Board. *Dietary Reference Intakes for vitamin A, vitamin K, arsenic, boron, chromium, copper, iodine, iron, manganese, molybdenum, nickel, silicon, vanadium, and zinc.* Washington DC: National Academy Press, 2001. Also available at: http://www.nap.edu/catalog/10026.html (accessed 24/05/04)
3. WHO. Copper. In: *Trace elements in human nutrition and health.* Geneva: WHO, 1996: 123–43.

**Schistosomiasis.** Although most control programmes for schistosomiasis (p.100) use niclosamide as a molluscicide, and copper salts have largely been abandoned for snail control, WHO noted in 1993 that copper sulfate was still used for this purpose in Egypt.[1]

1. WHO. The control of schistosomiasis: second report of the WHO expert committee. *WHO Tech Rep Ser 830* 1993.

### Preparations

***BPC 1973:*** Compound Ferrous Sulphate Tablets;
***USP 27:*** Cupric Chloride Injection; Cupric Sulfate Injection.

**Proprietary Preparations** (details are given in Part 3)
***Austral.:*** Multiload; ***Braz.:*** Multiload; ***Canad.:*** Gyne-T; Micro Cu†; ***Chile:*** Diuprotect; Multiload; ***Denm.:*** CuNova T†; Gyne-T†; Multiload; ***Fr.:*** Gyne-T†; Gynefix†; Gynelle 375; Ionarthrol; Metacuprol; ML Cu 250†; ML Cu 375†; Multiload; Remoplexe†; UT 380; ***Ger.:*** Gyne-T†; Multiload; ***Hong Kong:*** Gyne-T†; Multiload; ***Irl.:*** Multiload†; Ortho Gyne-T†; ***Israel:*** Anticon; Gyne-T†; Mona-Lisa†; Multiload; ***Ital.:*** Gravigard; Mini-Gravigard†; Multiload; No-Gravid; Telo Cypro; ***Malaysia:*** Multiload; ***Mex.:*** Cuprifusin; Multiload; Protec T†; ***Mon.:*** Sertalia; ***Neth.:*** Multiload; ***NZ:*** Multiload; ***Port.:*** Multiload; ***S.Afr.:*** Cuprocept CCL; Dalcept; Multiload; Tricept; ***Singapore:*** Multiload; Sof-T; ***Switz.:*** Fincoid†; Multiload; Sof-T†; ***Thai.:*** Multiload; ***UK:*** Gyne-T†; Gynefix; Multiload; ***USA:*** Paragard T380A.

**Multi-ingredient:** ***Arg.:*** Dermalibour; ***Austral.:*** APR Cream; Ascoxal†; ***Braz.:*** Belagin; Micotox†; Sulfato Ferroso Composto; Sulfatofer; ***Canad.:*** Nova-T; ***Chile:*** Agua Sulfatada Picrica; Nova-T; ***Fin.:*** Ascoxal; ***Fr.:*** Bioceanat†; Cicalfate; Dermalibour; Dermo-Sulfuryl; Dermocreme†; Dermocuivre; Eryase; Femiplexe†; Nova-T; Oligoderm; Oligorhine; Ramet Dalibour†; Ramet Pain†; Ruboderm†; Sanoformine†; Septalibour; ***Ger.:*** Nova-T; ***Hong Kong:*** Aderma Dermalibour; Nova-T; ***India:*** Hepatoglobine; ***Irl.:*** Ferrotab; ***Israel:*** Nova-T; ***Ital.:*** Cuprosodio; Cuprosodio Plus; Emmenoiasi; Nova-T; Sterimar Cu; ***Malaysia:*** Nova-T; ***Mex.:*** Ascoxal; Dalidome; Nova-T; ***Neth.:*** Nova-T; ***Norw.:*** Ascoxal; ***NZ:*** Nova-T; ***S.Afr.:*** Nova-T; ***Singapore:*** Ferromex†; Neogobion; Nova-T; ***Spain:*** Acnosan†; ***Swed.:*** Ascoxal; ***Switz.:*** Nova-T; ***Thai.:*** Nova-T; ***UK:*** Foresight Iron Formula; Nova-T†; ***USA:*** ORA5.

## Cyclamic Acid *(BAN, USAN)*

Ciclámico, ácido; Cyclam. Acid; E952; Hexamic Acid. *N*-Cyclohexylsulphamic acid.

$C_6H_{13}NO_3S$ = 179.2.

*CAS — 100-88-9.*

## Calcium Cyclamate

Calc. Cyclam.; Calcium Cyclohexanesulfamate; Ciclamato de calcio; Cyclamate Calcium; E952. Calcium *N*-cyclohexylsulphamate dihydrate.

$C_{12}H_{24}CaN_2O_6S_2,2H_2O$ = 432.6.

*CAS — 139-06-0 (anhydrous calcium cyclamate); 5897-16-5 (calcium cyclamate dihydrate).*

## Sodium Cyclamate *(BAN, rINN)*

Ciclamato de sodio; Cyclamate Sodium; E952; Natrii Cyclamas; Sod. Cyclam.; Sodium Cyclohexanesulphamate. Sodium *N*-cyclohexylsulphamate.

$C_6H_{12}NNaO_3S$ = 201.2.

*CAS — 139-05-9.*

**Pharmacopoeias.** In *Chin.* and *Eur.* (see p.vi).

**Ph. Eur. 5.0** (Sodium Cyclamate). A white crystalline powder or colourless crystals. Freely soluble in water; slightly soluble in alcohol. A 10% solution in water has a pH of 5.5 to 7.5.

### Profile

Cyclamic acid and its calcium and sodium salts are intense sweetening agents. In dilute solutions (up to about 0.17%) sodium cyclamate is about 30 times as sweet as sucrose but this factor decreases at higher concentrations. When the concentration approaches 0.5%, a bitter taste becomes noticeable. It is stable to heat.

The use of cyclamates as artificial sweeteners in food, soft drinks, and artificial sweetening tablets was at one time prohibited in Great Britain and some other countries because of concern about the metabolite cyclohexylamine. However, after reappraisal their use is now allowed.

### Preparations

**Proprietary Preparations** (details are given in Part 3)
***Arg.:*** Kaldil Diet; ***Braz.:*** Sucaryl†; ***Canad.:*** Sucaryl.

**Multi-ingredient:** ***Arg.:*** Chuker; ***Austral.:*** Sucaryl†; ***Braz.:*** Adocante Docura†; Adocyl C†; Belpen†; Finn Cristal; ***Chile:*** Sucaryl; Sukar-Sin; ***Fr.:*** Sucaryl; ***Israel:*** Sucrin; ***Ital.:*** Diet Sucaryl; ***NZ:*** Sucaryl; ***Port.:*** Dulceril.

## Cysteine *(rINN)*

C; Cisteína; Cys; L-Cysteine; E920. L-2-Amino-3-mercaptopropionic acid.

$C_3H_7NO_2S$ = 121.2.

*CAS — 52-90-4.*

**Pharmacopoeias.** In *Ger.*

## Cysteine Hydrochloride *(rINNM)*

Cys Hydrochloride; L-Cysteine Hydrochloride Monohydrate; Cysteini Hydrochloridum Monohydricum; Hidrocloruro de cisteína. L-2-Amino-3-mercaptopropionic acid hydrochloride monohydrate.

$C_3H_7NO_2S,HCl,H_2O$ = 175.6.

*CAS — 52-89-1 (anhydrous L-cysteine hydrochloride); 7048-04-6 (L-cysteine hydrochloride monohydrate).*

**Pharmacopoeias.** In *Chin.*, *Eur.* (see p.vi), and *US*.

**Ph. Eur. 5.0** (Cysteine Hydrochloride Monohydrate; Cysteine Hydrochloride BP 2003). A white crystalline powder or colourless crystals. Freely soluble in water; slightly soluble in alcohol. Protect from light.

**USP 27** (Cysteine Hydrochloride). White crystals or crystalline powder. Soluble in water, in alcohol, and in acetone.

### Profile

Cysteine is a polar aliphatic amino acid. Cysteine and cysteine hydrochloride are used as dietary supplements.

Cysteine and cysteine hydrochloride are included in preparations used in ophthalmology; eye drops have been used to prevent corneal ulceration after chemical burns.

**Precautions.** Cysteine, like other sulfhydryl-containing drugs, could produce a false-positive result in the nitroprusside test for ketone bodies used in diabetes and suspected hepatocellular injury.[1]

1. Csako G, Elin RJ. Unrecognized false-positive ketones from drugs containing free-sulfhydryl group(s). *JAMA* 1993; **269:** 1634.

### Preparations

***USP 27:*** Cysteine Hydrochloride Injection.

**Proprietary Preparations** (details are given in Part 3)

**Multi-ingredient:** ***Fr.:*** Lobamine-Cysteine; Phakan; ***Ger.:*** Hepatofalk Neu†; ***Hong Kong:*** Hepatofalk; ***Port.:*** Phakan; ***S.Afr.:*** Prohep; ***Switz.:*** Lobamine-Cysteine†; Phakolen; ***Thai.:*** Proheparum†.

## Cystine *(USAN, rINN)*

Cistina; L-Cystine; Cystinum; Di(α-aminopropionic)-β-disulphide; β,β′-Dithiodialanine. L-3,3′-Dithiobis(2-aminopropionic acid).

$C_6H_{12}N_2O_4S_2$ = 240.3.

*CAS — 56-89-3.*

**Pharmacopoeias.** In *Chin.* and *Eur.* (see p.vi).

**Ph. Eur. 5.0** (Cystine). A white crystalline powder. Practically insoluble in water and in alcohol. It dissolves in dilute solutions of alkali hydroxides. Protect from light.

### Profile

Cystine is an aliphatic amino acid. It is used as a dietary supplement.

Low-methionine diets with cystine supplementation have been used in the treatment of congenital homocystinuria (see Amino Acid Metabolic Disorders, p.1417).

### Preparations

**Proprietary Preparations** (details are given in Part 3)
***Fr.:*** Gelucystine; ***Ital.:*** Cistidil; Mavigen Sebo; ***Spain:*** Crecil.

**Multi-ingredient:** ***Arg.:*** Lohp; Megacistin; Megaplus; ***Austria:*** Gelacet; ***Canad.:*** Amino-Cerv; ***Fr.:*** Cysticho†; Cystine $B_6$; Forcapil; Solacy; ***Ger.:*** Gelacet N; Gerontamin†; Pantovigar N; ***Switz.:*** Gelacet; ***USA:*** Amino-Cerv.

## Dectaflur *(USAN, rINN)*

SKF-38094. 9-Octadecenylamine hydrofluoride.

$C_{18}H_{38}NF$ = 287.5.

*CAS — 36505-83-6 (nonstereospecific); 1838-19-3 (9-octadecenylamine).*

### Profile

Dectaflur is used as a source of fluoride (see Sodium Fluoride, p.1444) in the prevention of dental caries.

### Preparations

**Proprietary Preparations** (details are given in Part 3)

**Multi-ingredient:** ***Austria:*** Elmex; ***Belg.:*** Elmex; ***Fin.:*** Elmex; ***Ger.:*** Elmex; Lawefluor N; Multifluorid; ***Israel:*** Elmex; ***Ital.:*** Elmex; ***Neth.:*** Elmex; ***S.Afr.:*** Elmex†; ***Spain:*** Elmex†; ***Switz.:*** Elmex.

## Dextrin *(BAN)*

British Gum; Dextrina; Dextrinum; Dextrinum Album; Starch Gum.

$[C_6H_{10}O_5]_n.xH_2O$.

*CAS — 9004-53-9.*

**Pharmacopoeias.** In *Chin., Eur.* (see p.vi), and *Jpn.* Also in *USNF.*

**Ph. Eur. 5.0** (Dextrin). Maize, potato, or cassava starch partially hydrolysed and modified by heating with or without the presence of acids, alkalis, or pH control agents. A white or almost white, free-flowing powder. Very soluble in boiling water forming a mucilaginous solution; slowly soluble in cold water; practically insoluble in alcohol. A 5% dispersion in water has a pH of 2.0 to 8.0.

**USNF 22** (Dextrin). It is starch, or partially hydrolysed starch, modified by heating in a dry state, with or without acids, alkalis, or pH control agents. A white, yellow, or brown free-flowing powder. Its solubility in water varies; it is usually very soluble, but often contains an insoluble portion.

## Icodextrin *(BAN, USAN, rINN)*

Icodextrina.

$[C_6H_{10}O_5]_n$.

*CAS — 9004-53-9; 337376-15-5.*

### Profile

Dextrin, a glucose polymer, is (1→4)-α-D-glucan with a weight-average molecular weight of about 20 000 and more than 85% of its molecules with molecular weights between 1640 and 45 000. It is a source of carbohydrate sometimes used in oral dietary supplements and tube feeding. Glucose is rapidly released in the gastrointestinal tract but because of the high average molecular weight of dextrin, solutions have a lower osmolarity than isocaloric solutions of glucose. Additionally, preparations based on dextrin and intended for dietary supplementation usually have a low electrolyte content and are free of lactose and sucrose. These properties make such preparations suitable for dietary supplementation in a variety of diseases including certain gastrointestinal disorders where malabsorption is a problem, in disaccharide intolerance (without isomaltose intolerance), and in acute and chronic hepatic and renal diseases where protein, mineral, and fluid restriction are often necessary.

Dextrin is also used as a tablet and capsule diluent, and as a binding, suspending, and viscosity-increasing agent. It has also been used as an adhesive and stiffening agent for surgical dressings.

Dextrin sulfate intravaginal gel is under investigation in the prophylaxis of HIV infection and AIDS.

Icodextrin is used in dialysis fluids as an alternative to glucose-based solutions (see also below). Icodextrin-based fluids are used as vehicles for administration of drugs via the peritoneal cavity. They may also be instilled intraperitoneally to reduce adhesions after abdominal surgery.

**Dialysis.** Glucose-based solutions are commonly used in dialysis solutions for continuous ambulatory peritoneal dialysis (CAPD). However, there is rapid absorption of glucose across the peritoneal membrane, reducing the duration of ultrafiltration and leading to long-term metabolic complications such as hyperglycaemia, hyperinsulinaemia, hyperlipidaemia and obesity. Other osmotic agents have been investigated. One study reported results in 11 patients[1] receiving CAPD who had suffered repeated fluid overload from glucose-based dialysis solutions, and suggested that replacement of glucose with dextrin as the osmotic agent could reverse fluid overload and possibly reduce the frequency of exchange. However, others[2] considered that the proposed frequency of exchange would not provide adequate removal of urea, and that in addition to underdialysis there would be an accumulation of poorly-metabolisable glucose polymers in the blood.

Icodextrin is another alternative.[3] It is a glucose polymer, given in iso-osmolar solution. Studies supported by the manufacturers have found that it can be used in ultrafiltration for up to 12 hours, with lower transperitoneal absorption and potential calorie load than glucose solutions.[4,5] It can also be metabolised by amylases in the blood, so is less likely to accumulate than other glucose polymers if absorbed,[5] although the resultant concentrations of maltose (the primary metabolite) have resulted in falsely elevated blood-glucose measurements with some test methods.[6,7] In a study in CAPD patients, icodextrin was well-tolerated and produced at least equivalent ultrafiltration to glucose solutions.[4]


1. Stein A, *et al.* Glucose polymer for ultrafiltration failure in CAPD. *Lancet* 1993; **341:** 1159.
2. Martis L, *et al.* CAPD with dialysis solution containing glucose polymer. *Lancet* 1993; **342:** 176–7.
3. Frampton JE, Plosker GL. Icodextrin: a review of its use in peritoneal dialysis. *Drugs* 2003; **63:** 2079–2105.
4. Mistry CD, *et al.* A randomized multicenter clinical trial comparing isosmolar icodextrin with hyperosmolar glucose solutions in CAPD. *Kidney Int* 1994; **46:** 496–503.
5. Peers E, Gokal R. Icodextrin provides long dwell peritoneal dialysis and maintenance of intraperitoneal volume. *Artif Organs* 1998; **22:** 8–12.
6. Riley SG, *et al.* Spurious hyperglycaemia and icodextrin in peritoneal dialysis fluid. *BMJ* 2003; **327:** 608–9.
7. Medicines and Healthcare products Regulatory Agency. Medical device alert: ref MDA/2003/011 issued 16 April 2003. Available at: http://devices.mhra.gov.uk/mda/mdawebsitev2.nsf/e8be0ee313c493aa80256bbb00307b2e/78eb05af8601ccc38025 6d0a0047994e/$FILE/MDA-2003-011.pdf (accessed 14/05/04)


**Hypersensitivity.** Skin reactions, sometimes severe and generalised, have occurred in patients receiving icodextrin.[1-4] Reactions have sometimes been delayed up to about 2 weeks after administration.[3]


1. Fletcher S, *et al.* Icodextrin allergy in a peritoneal dialysis patient. *Nephrol Dial Transplant* 1998; **13:** 2656–8.
2. Goldsmith D, *et al.* Allergic reactions to the polymeric glucose-based peritoneal dialysis fluid icodextrin in patients with renal failure. *Lancet* 2000; **355:** 897.
3. Queffeulou G, *et al.* Allergy to icodextrin. *Lancet* 2000; **356:** 75.
4. Al-Hoqail IA, Crawford RI. Acute generalized exanthematous pustulosis induced by icodextrin. *Br J Dermatol* 2001; **145:** 1026–7.


### Preparations

***USNF 22:*** Liquid Glucose.

**Proprietary Preparations** (details are given in Part 3)

***Austral.:*** Poly-Joule; ***Fr.:*** Caloreen; ***Gr.:*** Caloreen; ***Irl.:*** Caloreen†; ***S.Afr.:*** Caloreen†; ***UK:*** Adept; Caloreen; Dexemel.

**Multi-ingredient:** ***Fr.:*** Picot.

## Ferric Ammonium Citrate

381; Ammonium Ferric Citrate; Citrato amónico férrico; Ferricum Citricum Ammoniatum; Iron and Ammonium Citrate.

*CAS — 1185-57-5.*

*ATC — V08CA07.*

**Pharmacopoeias.** In *US.*

**USP 27** (Ferric Ammonium Citrate). It contains between 16.5% and 18.5% of iron. Store in airtight containers at a temperature of 8° to 15°. Protect from light.

### Profile

Ferric ammonium citrate is given by mouth as a source of iron (see p.1434) for iron-deficiency anaemia (p.733). It is also used as a food additive, as an acidity regulator, anticaking agent, or source of iron. It has been used as a colouring agent.

### Preparations

***USP 27:*** Ferric Ammonium Citrate for Oral Solution.

**Proprietary Preparations** (details are given in Part 3)

***Braz.:*** Vinho Ferruginoso; Vinho Tonificante†; ***India:*** Rubraplex; ***Ital.:*** Ferriseltz†; Sciroppo Fenoglio; ***Port.:*** Cobalti; ***Spain:*** Ferriseltz.

**Multi-ingredient:** ***Arg.:*** ITE B12 Forte; ***Austria:*** Ferrovin-Chinaeisenwein; ***Belg.:*** Ferrifol B12†; ***Braz.:*** Anemokol†; Carneferrol†; Cobalplex†; Emotonico†; Ferroben; Ferrotrat B12; Gladiaton†; Hematiase B12; Hepavitose; Regulador Xavier n-2†; Rubrobion; Tonico Prata†; Tonosai†; Veafer†; ***Canad.:*** Geritol; Heparos†; Maltlevol; ***Ger.:*** Praefeminon plus; ***Hong Kong:*** Nutroplex; ***India:*** Blosyn; Dexorange; Ferradol; Ferrochelate; Globac-Z; Haem Up; Hepatoglobine; ***Ital.:*** Emopon; ***Malaysia:*** Nutroplex; ***Singapore:*** Nutroplex; ***UK:*** Ironorm; Lexpec with Iron; Lexpec with Iron-M; ***USA:*** Geritol; Geritonic.

## Ferric Pyrophosphate

Férrico, pirofosfato; Iron Pyrophosphate.

$Fe_4(P_2O_7)_3$ = 745.2.

*CAS — 10058-44-3.*

### Profile

Ferric pyrophosphate is given by mouth as a source of iron (see p.1434) for iron-deficiency anaemia (p.733).

### Preparations

**Proprietary Preparations** (details are given in Part 3)

**Multi-ingredient:** ***Austral.:*** Incremin Iron†; ***Chile:*** Incremin; ***Mex.:*** Incremin Con Hierro; ***USA:*** Kovitonic†; Vitafol; Vitalize.

## Ferritin

Ferritina.

### Profile

Ferritin is the major iron storage protein of vertebrates found mainly in the liver, spleen, intestinal mucosa, and bone marrow and consisting of a soluble protein shell (apoferritin) with a core of crystalline ferric hydroxyphosphate complex. It has been given by mouth as a source of iron (p.1434) in iron-deficiency anaemias (p.733).

### Preparations

**Proprietary Preparations** (details are given in Part 3)

***Ital.:*** Femit†; Profer†; ***Mex.:*** Ferroprotina†; ***Spain:*** Ferroprotina; Hierco; Kilor; Profer; Tedec Profer†.

## Ferrocholinate *(rINN)*

Ferrocolinato.

$C_{11}H_{20}FeNO_9,2H_2O$ = 402.2.

*CAS — 1336-80-7.*

### Profile

Ferrocholinate is a chelate prepared by reacting equimolar quantities of freshly precipitated ferric hydroxide with choline dihydrogen citrate. It is given by mouth as a source of iron (see p.1434) for iron-deficiency anaemia (p.733).

### Preparations

**Proprietary Preparations** (details are given in Part 3)

***Spain:*** Podertonic.

## Ferrous Ascorbate

Ferroso, ascorbato.

$C_{12}H_{14}FeO_{12}$ = 406.1.

*CAS — 24808-52-4.*

*ATC — B03AA10.*

### Profile

Ferrous ascorbate is used as a source of iron (see p.1434) for iron-deficiency anaemia (p.733). It is given by mouth as the anhydrous form in usual dose units of 245 mg and as a hydrated form in usual dose units of 275 mg; both forms provide about 33 mg of iron per dose unit; the total dose is usually up to the equivalent of 200 mg of iron daily.

### Preparations

**Proprietary Preparations** (details are given in Part 3)

***Canad.:*** Ascofer†; ***Fr.:*** Ascofer; ***Spain:*** Ferro Semar†.

**Multi-ingredient:** ***Austria:*** China-Eisenwein.

## Ferrous Aspartate

Ferroso, aspartato.

$C_8H_{12}FeN_2O_8,4H_2O$ = 392.1.

*ATC — B03AA09.*

### Profile

Ferrous aspartate is used as a source of iron (see p.1434) for iron-deficiency anaemia (p.733). It is given by mouth in usual doses of up to 750 mg daily (equivalent to about 100 mg of iron daily).

### Preparations

**Proprietary Preparations** (details are given in Part 3)

***Belg.:*** Spartocine; ***Fin.:*** Spartocine; ***Ger.:*** Spartocine N.

## Ferrous Chloride

Ferroso, cloruro. Iron (II) chloride tetrahydrate.

$FeCl_2,4H_2O$ = 198.8.

*CAS — 7758-94-3 (anhydrous ferrous chloride); 13478-10-9 (ferrous chloride tetrahydrate).*

*ATC — B03AA05.*

### Profile

Ferrous chloride is used as a source of iron (see p.1434) for iron-deficiency anaemia (p.733). It is given by mouth in usual doses of about 350 to 700 mg daily in divided doses (equivalent to about 100 to 200 mg of iron daily).

### Preparations

**Proprietary Preparations** (details are given in Part 3)

***Fr.:*** Fer UCB; ***Ger.:*** Ferro 66†; Vitaferro; ***Switz.:*** Ferrascorbin.

**Multi-ingredient:** ***Switz.:*** Ferrascorbin.

# Ferrous Fumarate

Ferrosi Fumaras; Ferroso, fumarato.

$C_4H_2FeO_4$ = 169.9.

*CAS — 141-01-5.*

*ATC — B03AA02; B03AD02.*

**Pharmacopoeias.** In *Chin., Eur.* (see p.vi), *Int., US,* and *Viet.*

**Ph. Eur. 5.0** (Ferrous Fumarate). A fine, reddish-orange or reddish-brown powder. Slightly soluble in water; very slightly soluble in alcohol. Store in airtight containers. Protect from light.

**USP 27** (Ferrous Fumarate). A reddish-orange to red-brown, odourless powder, which may contain soft lumps that produce a yellow streak when crushed. Slightly soluble in water; very slightly soluble in alcohol. Its solubility in dilute hydrochloric acid is limited by the separation of fumaric acid.

## Profile

Ferrous fumarate is used as a source of iron (see p.1434) for iron-deficiency anaemia (p.733). It is given by mouth in usual doses of up to 600 mg daily (equivalent to about 200 mg of iron daily); doses of up to 1.2 g daily (equivalent to about 400 mg of iron daily) may be used if necessary.

### Preparations

**BP 2003:** Ferrous Fumarate and Folic Acid Tablets; Ferrous Fumarate Capsules; Ferrous Fumarate Oral Suspension; Ferrous Fumarate Tablets; **USP 27:** Ferrous Fumarate and Docusate Sodium Extended-release Tablets; Ferrous Fumarate Tablets.

**Proprietary Preparations** (details are given in Part 3)
***Arg.:*** Hemoferrol; ***Austria:*** Ferretab; Ferrobet; ***Belg.:*** Ferrum Hausmann†; Ferumat†; ***Braz.:*** Ferrin†; ***Canad.:*** Neo-Fer; Novo-Fumar†; Palafer; ***Fr.:*** Fumafer; ***Ger.:*** Ferrokapsul; Ferrum Hausmann; Rulofer N; ***Hong Kong:*** Ferosoft†; Triniscon†; ***Irl.:*** Galfer; ***Ital.:*** Ferro-12†; ***Malaysia:*** Firon; ***Mex.:*** Biofuroso; Croferron; Fernadin; Ferro-Terapina; Ferval; Fumavit; Gestaferron†; Medifer; Regufer†; Reufirron†; ***Norw.:*** Nycoplus Neo-Fer; ***Swed.:*** Erco-Fer; ***Switz.:*** Ferretab†; Ferrum Hausmann; ***Thai.:*** F-Tab; Ferdek; Fermasian; Fermate; ***UK:*** Fersaday; Fersamal; Galfer; ***USA:*** Femiron; Feostat; Ferretts; Ferro-Dok; Hemaspan; Hemocyte; Nephro-Fer; Vitron-C.

**Multi-ingredient:** ***Arg.:*** Anemidox-Ferrum; Autrinic Compuesto; Ferretab Compuesto; Ferrocebrina; Hematon; ***Austral.:*** Blackmores for Women Bio Iron†; Children's Calcium With Minerals†; Extralife PMS-Care†; Medinat PMT-Eze†; ***Austria:*** Ferretab comp; ***Belg.:*** Gestiferrol; ***Braz.:*** Betozone; Iloban; Renutrin†; Rubralong; ***Canad.:*** Appedrine; Caltrate + Iron & Vitamin D†; Dexatrim†; Fortiplex; Palafer CF; Prevencal & D & Fer†; ***Chile:*** Cronoferril; Ferranim; Ferro Vitaminico; Folifer; Microfemin; Orlon; ***Fin.:*** Matrifolin; ***Ger.:*** Blutquick Forte S†; Ferrodix; ***Hong Kong:*** Fortifer; ***India:*** Anemidox; Autrin; Elferri-Z; Fervit; Globac-Z; Hemsi; Hepasules; Hepatoglobine; Livogen; Probofex; Siderfol; ***Irl.:*** BC 500 with Iron†; Ferrocap F; Folex†; Galfer FA; Givitol; ***Israel:*** Folex; Foric; ***Malaysia:*** Odiron-C; ***Mex.:*** Autrin; Ferlor AF; Ferrotemp; Fumarol; ***S.Afr.:*** Autrin; Pregamal; Trinsicon†; ***Singapore:*** Odiron-C; Wanse; ***Spain:*** Foliferron; ***Swed.:*** Erco-Fer vitamin†; ***Switz.:*** Duofer; Duofer Fol; ***Thai.:*** Adnemic; Adnemic F; Biocalron; FBC; FBC Plus; FBIC; Ferli-6; Ferplus-B; Ferropro; Hemarate; Hemolax; Intricon; Obimin-AZ; Polycolvit; Polyvit; Trinsicon; ***UK:*** Folex†; Galfer FA; Givitol†; Meterfolic; Pregaday; ***USA:*** ABC to Z; Anemagen; Anemagen OB; Berocca Plus; Berplex†; Caltrate + Iron & Vitamin D; Certagen; Cevi-Fer; Chromagen; Chromagen FA; Chromagen Forte; Contrin; Estrostep Fe; Ferotrinsic; Ferrogels Forte; Fetrin; Formula B Plus; Fumatinic; Geriot; Gevral T; Hem Fe; Hematinic; Hematinic Plus; Hemocyte Plus; Hemocyte-F; Junel Fe; Livitrinsic-f; Loestrin Fe; Nephro-Fer Rx; Parvlex; Pronemia Hematinic; Thera Hematinic; Theragenerix-H; Tolfrinic; TriHEMIC; Trinsicon; Vitafol; Yelets; Zodeac.

## Ferrous Gluceptate

Ferroso, gluceptato; Ferrous Glucoheptonate.
$Fe(C_7H_{13}O_8)_2$ = 506.2.
*CAS — 25126-38-9.*

### Profile

Ferrous gluceptate is given by mouth as a source of iron (see p.1434) for iron-deficiency anaemia (p.733).

### Preparations

**Proprietary Preparations** (details are given in Part 3)
***Chile:*** Unifer.
**Multi-ingredient:** ***Spain:*** Clamarvit; Normovite Antianemico.

# Ferrous Gluconate

E579; Eisen(II)-Gluconat; Ferrosi Gluconas; Ferroso, gluconato. Iron (II) di(D-gluconate).
$C_{12}H_{22}FeO_{14},xH_2O$.
*CAS — 299-29-6 (anhydrous ferrous gluconate); 12389-15-0 (ferrous gluconate dihydrate).*
*ATC — B03AA03.*

**Pharmacopoeias.** In *Eur.* (see p.vi).
*Chin., Pol.,* and *US* specify the dihydrate.

**Ph. Eur. 5.0** (Ferrous Gluconate). A greenish-yellow to grey powder or granules. It contains not less than 11.8% and not more than 12.5% of ferrous iron calculated with reference to the dried substance. Freely but slowly soluble in water producing a greenish-brown solution, more readily soluble in hot water; practically insoluble in alcohol. A 10% solution in water has a pH of 4.0 to 5.5 three to four hours after preparation. Protect from light.

**USP 27** (Ferrous Gluconate). A yellowish-grey or pale greenish-yellow, fine powder or granules having a slight odour resembling that of burnt sugar. Soluble 1 in 5 of water; practically insoluble in alcohol. A 5% solution in water is acid to litmus. Store in airtight containers.

### Profile

Ferrous gluconate is used as a source of iron (see p.1434) for iron-deficiency anaemia (p.733). It is given by mouth in doses of up to 1.8 g daily (equivalent to up to 210 mg of iron daily).

### Preparations

**BP 2003:** Ferrous Gluconate Tablets; **USP 27:** Ferrous Gluconate Capsules; Ferrous Gluconate Elixir; Ferrous Gluconate Tablets.

**Proprietary Preparations** (details are given in Part 3)
***Austral.:*** Fergon; ***Austria:*** Ferro-Agepha; Losferron; ***Belg.:*** Fernore†; Losferron; ***Braz.:*** Ferrin†; ***Canad.:*** Fertinic†; Novo-Ferrogluc; ***Chile:*** Glucoferro K; ***Ger.:*** Eisen-Sandoz; Ferrum Verla; Losan Fe†; Losferron; Rulofer G; Vitaferro; ***Irl.:*** Fergon†; ***Israel:*** Ferro; ***Ital.:*** Auxofer; Bioferal; Bioglufer; Blizer; Blustark; Crom 80; Cromatonferro; Emonorm; Emoxiron; Eriglobin; Eritropiu; Ferig; Ferrematos†; Ferro Complex; Ferrogyn; Flexifer; Glucoferro; Ironax†; Losferron; Megafer; Monoferro; Prontoferro; Sidervim; Sustemial; ***Neth.:*** Losferron; ***NZ:*** Fergon; ***Port.:*** Anemital; Bioferro; Hemototal; Losferron; ***Switz.:*** Loesfer; ***USA:*** Fergon.

**Multi-ingredient:** ***Austria:*** Losferron-Fol; ***Braz.:*** Apefer†; ***Fr.:*** Tot'Hema; Triogene†; ***Ger.:*** Biovital Aktiv; Blutquick Forte S†; Blutquick Forte†; Ferro-C-Calcium; Ferrodix; Floradix Krauterblut; Folsana†; ***India:*** Elferri; Gynae-CVP; JP Tone; Pentavite; ***Malaysia:*** Sangobion; ***Port.:*** Tot'Hema; ***S.Afr.:*** Kiddie Vite; ***Singapore:*** Neogobion; Sangobion; ***Spain:*** Clamarvit; ***Switz.:*** Duofer; Duofer Fol; Ferrascorbin; Loesfer + acide folique†; ***Thai.:*** Ferro-Be-Sian; Glufer-C; Sangobion†; ***UK:*** Ferfolic SV; Foresight Iron Formula; ***USA:*** Compete; Ferralet Plus; Hemocyte-V†; Hemocyte†; Hytinic; Iromin-G; Mission Surgical Supplement.

## Ferrous Glycine Sulfate

Ferroso de glicina, sulfato; Ferrous Aminoacetosulphate; Ferrous Glycine Sulphate.
*CAS — 14729-84-1.*

### Profile

Ferrous glycine sulfate is a chelate of ferrous sulfate and glycine used as a source of iron (see p.1434) for iron-deficiency anaemia (p.733). It is given by mouth in doses containing the equivalent of up to 150 mg of iron daily.

### Preparations

**Proprietary Preparations** (details are given in Part 3)
***Braz.:*** Neutrofer; ***Denm.:*** Glycifer; ***Fin.:*** Obsidan; ***Ger.:*** Ferro sanol; Ferro sanol duodenal; ***Irl.:*** Plesmet; ***Port.:*** Ferrocutid; ***Spain:*** Glutaferro; ***Swed.:*** Niferex; ***Switz.:*** Ferrosanol duodenal; ***UK:*** Plesmet.

**Multi-ingredient:** ***Braz.:*** Neutrofer Folico; ***Fin.:*** Obsidan comp; ***India:*** Fecontin-F; Fecontin-Z.

## Ferrous Lactate

E585; Ferroso, lactato; Iron Lactate.
$C_6H_{10}FeO_6,3H_2O$ = 288.0.
*CAS — 5905-52-2 (anhydrous ferrous lactate); 6047-24-1 (ferrous lactate trihydrate).*

### Profile

Ferrous lactate is used as a source of iron (see p.1434) for iron-deficiency anaemia (p.733).

### Preparations

**Proprietary Preparations** (details are given in Part 3)
***Arg.:*** Cromatonbic Ferro; ***S.Afr.:*** Ferro Drops L; ***Spain:*** Cromatonbic Ferro.

## Ferrous Oxalate

Ferroso, oxalato; Ferrum Oxalicum Oxydulatum; Iron Protoxalate.
$C_2FeO_4,2H_2O$ = 179.9.
*CAS — 516-03-0 (anhydrous ferrous oxalate); 6047-25-2 (ferrous oxalate dihydrate).*

### Profile

Ferrous oxalate has been used as a source of iron (see p.1434).

### Preparations

**Proprietary Preparations** (details are given in Part 3)
**Multi-ingredient:** ***Fr.:*** Disulone.

## Ferrous Succinate

Ferroso, succinato.
$C_4H_4FeO_4$ = 171.9.
*CAS — 10030-90-7.*
*ATC — B03AA06.*

### Profile

Ferrous succinate is used as a source of iron (see p.1434) for iron-deficiency anaemia (p.733). It is given by mouth in doses of up to about 600 mg daily (equivalent to up to about 200 mg of iron daily).

### Preparations

**Proprietary Preparations** (details are given in Part 3)
***Arg.:*** Ferdromaco; ***Canad.:*** Cerevon†; ***Denm.:*** Ferromyn†; ***Fr.:*** Inofer†; ***Ger.:*** Ferrlecit 2; ***Swed.:*** Ferromyn S.
**Multi-ingredient:** ***Belg.:*** Ferrifol†; ***India:*** Hematrine.

# Ferrous Sulfate

Eisen(II)-Sulfat; Ferreux (Sulfate); Ferrosi Sulfas Heptahydricus; Ferroso, sulfato; Ferrous Sulphate; Ferrum Sulfuricum Oxydulatum; Iron (II) Sulphate Heptahydrate; Iron Sulphate.
$FeSO_4,7H_2O$ = 278.0.
*CAS — 7720-78-7 (anhydrous ferrous sulfate); 7782-63-0 (ferrous sulfate heptahydrate).*
*ATC — B03AA07; B03AD03.*

NOTE. Crude ferrous sulfate is known as Green Vitriol or Green Copperas.

**Pharmacopoeias.** In *Chin., Eur.* (see p.vi), *Int., Jpn, US,* and *Viet.*
*Swiss* also includes ferrous sulfate sesquihydrate.

**Ph. Eur. 5.0** (Ferrous Sulphate Heptahydrate). A light green crystalline powder or bluish-green crystals, efflorescent in air. It is oxidised in moist air, becoming brown. Freely soluble in water; very soluble in boiling water; practically insoluble in alcohol. A 5% solution in water has a pH of 3.0 to 4.0. Store in airtight containers.

**USP 27** (Ferrous Sulfate). Pale bluish-green, odourless, crystals or granules. It is efflorescent in dry air and oxidises readily in moist air to form brownish-yellow basic ferric sulfate. Soluble 1 in 1.5 of water and 1 in 0.5 of boiling water; insoluble in alcohol. A 10% solution in water is acid to litmus, having a pH of about 3.7. Store in airtight containers.

## Dried Ferrous Sulfate *(USAN)*

Dried Ferrous Sulphate; Exsiccated Ferrous Sulphate; Ferrosi Sulfas Exsiccatus; Ferroso desecado, sulfato.
*CAS — 13463-43-9.*

**Pharmacopoeias.** In *Br., Int., US,* and *Viet.*

**BP 2003** (Dried Ferrous Sulphate). Ferrous sulfate deprived of part of its water of crystallisation by drying at 40°. It contains 86.0 to 90.0% of $FeSO_4$. A greyish white powder. It dissolves slowly, but almost completely, in freshly boiled and cooled water.

**USP 27** (Dried Ferrous Sulfate). A greyish-white to buff-coloured powder consisting primarily of ferrous sulfate monohydrate with varying amounts of ferrous sulfate tetrahydrate. It contains 86.0 to 89.0% of $FeSO_4$. Slowly soluble in water; insoluble in alcohol.

### Profile

Ferrous sulfate is used as a source of iron (see p.1434) for iron-deficiency anaemia (p.733). It is given by mouth and the dried form is frequently used in solid dosage forms and the heptahydrate in liquid dosage forms. Usual doses of dried ferrous sulfate are up to 600 mg daily (equivalent to 180 to 195 mg of iron daily, this figure being somewhat variable depending on the purity and water content of the salt).

Ferrous sulfate oxidised with nitric and sulfuric acids yields ferric subsulfate solution, also known as Monsel's solution, which has been used as a haemostatic.

### Preparations

**BP 2003:** Ferrous Sulphate Tablets; Paediatric Ferrous Sulphate Oral Solution; Prolonged-release Ferrous Sulphate Tablets;
**BPC 1973:** Compound Ferrous Sulphate Tablets;
**USP 27:** Ferric Subsulfate Solution; Ferrous Sulfate Oral Solution; Ferrous Sulfate Syrup; Ferrous Sulfate Tablets.

**Proprietary Preparations** (details are given in Part 3)
***Arg.:*** Eurofer; Factofer; Fer-In-Sol; Ferlea; Ferrocebrina; Ferromas; Ferrometion; Hemoferrol; Iberol; Siderblut; Vitaferro; ***Austral.:*** Ferro-Gradumet; Ferrograd C; ***Austria:*** Ferro-Gradumet; Ferrograd C; Infa-Tardyferon; Tardyferon; ***Belg.:*** Fero-Grad; Fero-Gradumet; Resoferon†; ***Braz.:*** Cimefer; Fer-In-Sol; Ferroklinge; Ferronil; Ferrototal; Ferrotron; Iberol; Ironfer; Lomfer; Sulfatofer; Sulfer Plus; Sulferro; Sulferrol; ***Canad.:*** Fer-In-Sol; Fero-Grad; Ferodan; Novo-Ferrosulfate†; Slow-Fe; ***Chile:*** Ferinsol; Ferrigot; Ferromalt; Iberol Simple; ***Denm.:*** Ferro; ***Fin.:*** Duroferon; Retafer; ***Fr.:*** Fero-Grad vitamine C; Timoferol; ***Ger.:*** Aktiferrin N; Ceferro; Dreisafer; Eisen-Diasporal†; Eisendragees-ratiopharm; Eryfer; Ferrogamma; FERROinfant N; Haemoprotect; Hamatopan; Kendural C; Plastufer; Tardyferon; Vitaferro; ***Gr.:*** Fer-In-Sol; Microfer; Resoferon; Tardyferon; ***Hong Kong:*** Feospan; Fer-In-Sol†; Sorbifer†; ***Irl.:*** Feospan; Fer-In-Sol; Ferrograd; Ferrograd C; ***Israel:*** Ferro-Gradumet; Slow-Fe; ***Ital.:*** Fer-In-Sol; Ferrograd; Ferrograd C; ***Malaysia:*** Feospan; ***Mex.:*** Elfer†; Fer-In-Sol; Ferifer; Forcil†; Hemobion; Hemofer†; Ifersol†; Reguce†; Sulfafer†; Tardyferon†; Valdefer; ***Neth.:*** Fero-Gradumet; Liquifer; ***Norw.:*** Duroferon; Ferro-Retard†; Ferromax; ***NZ:*** Ferro-Gradumet; Ferrograd C; ***Port.:*** Ferro-Gradumet; Tardyferon; ***S.Afr.:*** Fero-Grad; ***Singapore:*** Feospan; Retafer†; ***Spain:*** Fero-Gradumet; Tardyferon; ***Swed.:*** Duroferon; ***Switz.:*** Ferro-Gradumet; Resoferon; ***Thai.:*** Fer-In-Sol; Ferrotabs; Pediron; ***UAE:*** Kdiron; ***UK:*** Feospan; Ferrograd; Ferrograd C; Ironorm; Slow-Fe; ***USA:*** Ed-in-Sol; Fe[50]; Feosol; Fer-gen-sol; Fer-In-Sol; Fer-Iron; Feratab; Fero-Grad; Irospan; Slow-Fe.

**Multi-ingredient:** ***Arg.:*** Factofer B12; Fefol; Ferro Folic; Iberol; Rubiron; Sideralce; ***Austral.:*** Fefol; FGF Tabs; Irontona†; ***Austria:*** Aktiferrin; Aktiferrin compositum; Ferrograd Fol; Ferrum-Quarz; Kephalodoron; Tardyferon-Fol; ***Braz.:*** Anemix; Anemofer; Betozone; Biotonico Fontoura†; Ceviron†; Cobaldoze; Combiron; Coraben; Dobiron; Ferroben†; Ferrocomplex; Ferrofran†; Ferroplex; Ferrotonico; Ferrotonico B12; Ferrotrat; Fortonal†; Fosfotonico†; Hemo-Ped†; Iberin Folico; Iberol; Novofer; Rubiron B12†; Rubragil; Sulfato Ferroso Composto; Sulfatofer; Teutonico†; Tonico Blumen; Tonico No 1†; Trifacta†; ***Canad.:*** Iberet; Slow-Fe Folic; ***Chile:*** Ferranem; Ferro F-500 Gradumet; Iberol; Iberol Folico; ***Fr.:*** Tardyferon; Tardyferon $B_9$; ***Ger.:*** Biovital Aktiv; Biovital N†; Eisenkapseln; Eryfer comp; Ferro sanol comp; Ferro sanol gyn; Ferro-Folgamma; Ferro-Folsan; Hamatopan F; Kendural-Fol-500; Kendural-Plus†; Plastulen N; Tardyferon-Fol; ***Gr.:*** Feofol; Fero-folic-500; Gyno-Tardyferon; ***Hong Kong:*** Iberet; Iberet-Folic; ***India:*** Conviron-TR; Fefol; Fefol-Z; Ferrochelate-Z; Fesovit; Iberol; Plastules; ***Irl.:*** Fefol; Ferrograd Folic; Ferrotab; Fesovit†; ***Israel:*** Aktiferrin-F; Ferrograd Folic; Slow-Fe Folic; ***Ital.:*** Cura†; Ferrograd Folic; ***Malaysia:*** Iberet; Iberet-Folic; ***Mex.:*** Ferro Folico; Iberet; Iberol; Orafer Comp†; ***Norw.:*** Pregnifer†; ***NZ:*** Ferrograd Folic; ***Port.:*** Ferro-Folsan; Ferrograd Folico; Folifer; Tardyferon-Fol; ***S.Afr.:*** Fefol; Fero-Folic; Fo-liglobin; Iberet†; ***Singapore:*** Fefol†; Ferromex†; Iberet; Iberet-Folic; Tardyferon $B_9$; ***Spain:*** Iberet†; Pildoras Ferrug Sanatori†; Vitagama Fluor Complex†; ***Switz.:*** Actiferrine; Actiferrine-F Nouvelle formule; Fero-Folic; Gyno-Tardyferon; Kendural; Tardyferon; ***Thai.:*** Iberet; ***UAE:*** Folicron; ***UK:*** Fefol; Ferrograd Folic; Ironorm; Pregnavite Forte F†; Slow-Fe Folic; ***USA:*** Aqua Ban Plus; Fero-Folic; Generet; Gerivites; Iberet; Iberet-Folic; Slow Fe with Folic Acid.

## Ferrous Tartrate

Ferrosi Tartras; Ferroso, tartrato.

$C_4H_4FeO_6,2\frac{1}{2}H_2O$ = 249.0.

*CAS — 2944-65-2 (anhydrous ferrous tartrate).*

*ATC — B03AA08.*

### Profile

Ferrous tartrate has been used as a source of iron (see p.1434) for iron-deficiency anaemia (p.733).

---

# Folic Acid *(BAN, rINN)*

Ácido fólico; Acidum Folicum; Folacin; Folinsyre; PGA; Pteroylglutamic Acid; Pteroylmonoglutamic Acid; Vitamin $B_9$; Vitamin $B_{11}$. *N*-[4-(2-Amino-4-hydroxypteridin-6-ylmethylamino)benzoyl]-L(+)-glutamic acid.

$C_{19}H_{19}N_7O_6$ = 441.4.

*CAS — 59-30-3 (folic acid); 6484-89-5 (sodium folate).*

*ATC — B03BB01.*

**Pharmacopoeias.** In *Chin., Eur.* (see p.vi), *Int., Jpn, Pol.,* and *US.*

**Ph. Eur. 5.0** (Folic Acid). A yellowish or orange crystalline powder. Practically insoluble in water and in most organic solvents. It dissolves in dilute acids and in alkaline solutions. Protect from light.

**USP 27** (Folic Acid). A yellow, yellow-brownish, or yellowish-orange, odourless crystalline powder. Very slightly soluble in water; insoluble in alcohol, in acetone, in chloroform, and in ether. It readily dissolves in dilute solutions of alkali hydroxides and carbonates; soluble in hot, 3N hydrochloric acid and in hot, 2N sulfuric acid; soluble in hydrochloric acid and in sulfuric acid, yielding pale yellow solutions. Protect from light.

### Adverse Effects

Folic acid is generally well tolerated. Gastrointestinal disturbances and hypersensitivity reactions have been reported rarely.

### Precautions

Folic acid should never be given alone or with inadequate amounts of vitamin $B_{12}$ for the treatment of undiagnosed megaloblastic anaemia, since folic acid may produce a haematopoietic response in patients with a megaloblastic anaemia due to vitamin $B_{12}$ deficiency without preventing aggravation of neurological symptoms. This masking of the true deficiency state can lead to serious neurological damage, such as subacute combined degeneration of the spinal cord (see also below).

**Breast feeding.** Folic acid is excreted into breast milk. No adverse effects have been observed in breast-fed infants whose mothers were receiving folic acid, and the American Academy of Pediatrics considers that it is therefore usually compatible with breast feeding.[1]

1. American Academy of Pediatrics. The transfer of drugs and other chemicals into human milk. *Pediatrics* 2001; **108:** 776–89. Correction. *ibid.*; 1029. Also available at: http://aappolicy.aappublications.org/cgi/content/full/pediatrics%3b108/3/776 (accessed 14/05/04)

**Vitamin $B_{12}$ deficiency.** The issue of fortification of food with folic acid to reduce the number of infants born with neural tube defects (see below) has created debate[1-5] on the amount of fortification and on the risks of masking vitamin $B_{12}$ deficiency, particularly in the elderly. As mentioned in Precautions, above, it is accepted that folic acid should not be used in megaloblastic anaemia due to vitamin $B_{12}$ deficiency, because it will not prevent the neurological manifestations of this deficiency, and may delay the diagnosis. Masking of vitamin $B_{12}$ deficiency has been noted with daily doses of folic acid of 5 mg, and it is generally considered that very low doses do not have this effect. It has also been stated that folic acid may precipitate the neurological manifestations of vitamin $B_{12}$ deficiency; however, a review of the evidence suggests this is unlikely.[6]

Nevertheless, concerns regarding neurological effects of vitamin $B_{12}$ deficiency in the elderly have led to adoption of a level of folic acid fortification in the USA that is accepted will not provide optimum protection against neural tube defects, but that is hoped will minimise any risks.[7] It has been suggested that concomitant fortification with vitamin $B_{12}$ might also be a solution.

1. Mills JL. Fortification of foods with folic acid—how much is enough? *N Engl J Med* 2000; **342:** 1442–5.
2. Wharton B, Booth I. Fortification of flour with folic acid: a controlled field trial is needed. *BMJ* 2001; **323:** 1198–9.
3. Wald NJ, *et al.* Quantifying the effect of folic acid. *Lancet* 2001; **358:** 2068–73. Correction. *ibid.* 2002; **359:** 630.
4. Oakley GP. Delaying folic acid fortification of flour: governments that do not ensure fortification are committing public health malpractice. *BMJ* 2002; **324:** 1348–9. Correction. *ibid.*; **325:** 259.
5. Reynolds EH. Benefits and risks of folic acid to the nervous system. *J Neurol Neurosurg Psychiatry* 2002; **72:** 567–71.
6. Dickinson CJ. Does folic acid harm people with vitamin $B_{12}$ deficiency? *Q J Med* 1995; **88:** 357–64.
7. Tucker KL, *et al.* Folic acid fortification of the food supply: potential benefits and risks for the elderly population. *JAMA* 1996; **276:** 1879–85. Correction. *ibid.* 1997; **277:** 714.

### Interactions

Folate deficiency states may be produced by a number of drugs including antiepileptics, oral contraceptives, antituberculous drugs, alcohol, and folic acid antagonists such as methotrexate, pyrimethamine, triamterene, trimethoprim, and sulfonamides. In some instances, such as during methotrexate or antiepileptic therapy, replacement therapy with folinic acid or folic acid may become necessary in order to prevent megaloblastic anaemia developing; folate supplementation has reportedly decreased serum-phenytoin concentrations in a few cases (see Interactions, Vitamins, p.375) and there is a possibility that such an effect could also occur with barbiturate antiepileptics.

Antiepileptic-associated folate deficiency is discussed further under Adverse Effects of Phenytoin, p.370.

◊ References.

1. Lambie DG, Johnson RH. Drugs and folate metabolism. *Drugs* 1985; **30:** 145–55.

### Pharmacokinetics

Folic acid is rapidly absorbed from the gastrointestinal tract, mainly from the duodenum and jejunum. Dietary folates are stated to have about half the bioavailability of crystalline folic acid. The naturally occurring folate polyglutamates are largely deconjugated and reduced by dihydrofolate reductase in the intestines to form 5-methyltetrahydrofolate, which appears in the portal circulation, where it is extensively bound to plasma proteins. Folic acid given therapeutically enters the portal circulation largely unchanged, since it is a poor substrate for reduction by dihydrofolate reductase. It is converted to the metabolically active form 5-methyltetrahydrofolate in the plasma and liver.

The principal storage site of folate is the liver; it is also actively concentrated in the CSF.

Folate undergoes enterohepatic circulation. Folate metabolites are eliminated in the urine and folate in excess of body requirements is excreted unchanged in the urine. Folate is distributed into breast milk. Folic acid is removed by haemodialysis.

### Human Requirements

Body stores of folate in healthy persons have been reported as being between 5 to 10 mg, but may be much higher. In the UK about 150 to 200 micrograms of folate daily is considered a suitable average intake for all healthy persons except women of child-bearing potential and pregnant women who require additional folic acid to protect against neural tube defects in their offspring (see below). In the US the recommended dietary allowance is 400 micrograms of dietary folate equivalents (see below) in both men and women. Folate is present, chiefly combined with several L(+)-glutamic acid moieties, in many foods, particularly liver, kidney, yeast, nuts, and leafy green vegetables. The vitamin is readily oxidised to unavailable forms and is easily destroyed during cooking.

**UK and US recommended dietary intake.** In the UK dietary reference values (see p.1419) have been published for folate.[1] In the USA recommended dietary allowances (RDAs) had been set, and have recently been reviewed[2] under the programme to set Dietary Reference Intakes (see p.1419). Differing amounts are recommended for infants and children of varying ages, for adult males and females, and for pregnant and lactating women. In the UK the Reference Nutrient Intake (RNI) for adult males and females is 200 micrograms daily and the Estimated Average Requirement (EAR) is 150 micrograms daily. In the USA the RDA is expressed in terms of dietary folate equivalents (DFEs) where 1 microgram DFE is equivalent to 1 microgram folate from natural sources, 0.5 micrograms of a folic acid supplement taken on an empty stomach, or 0.6 micrograms of folic acid from fortified food or as a supplement taken with meals. An RDA of 400 micrograms DFE daily for adult men and women has been set; the EAR is 320 micrograms DFE daily and the tolerable upper intake level is 1 mg daily.

Folate requirements are increased during pregnancy; an RNI of 300 micrograms daily has been suggested for pregnant women in the UK and an RDA of 600 micrograms daily in the USA. In view of the value of folate in preventing neural tube defects, it is now recommended that women planning a pregnancy receive supplemental folic acid before conception and during the first trimester (see Neural Tube Defects, below). To increase the intake in women of child-bearing age, folic acid fortification of grain-based foods has been adopted in the USA, and advocated in other countries including the UK. However, there remains some debate over the appropriate level of fortification to optimise prevention of neural tube defects and to minimise the risks of masking underlying vitamin $B_{12}$ deficiency in the elderly (see Vitamin $B_{12}$ deficiency, above).

1. DoH. Dietary reference values for food energy and nutrients for the United Kingdom: report of the panel on dietary reference values of the committee on medical aspects of food policy. *Report on health and social subjects 41.* London: HMSO, 1991.
2. Standing Committee on the Scientific Evaluation of Dietary Reference Intakes of the Food and Nutrition Board. *Dietary Reference Intakes for thiamin, riboflavin, niacin, vitamin $B_6$, folate, vitamin $B_{12}$, pantothenic acid, biotin, and choline.* Washington, DC: National Academy Press, 2000. Also available at: http://www.nap.edu/catalog/6015.html (accessed 24/05/04)

### Uses and Administration

Folic acid is a member of the vitamin B group. Folic acid is reduced in the body to tetrahydrofolate, which is a coenzyme for various metabolic processes including the synthesis of purine and pyrimidine nucleotides, and hence in the synthesis of DNA; it is also involved in some amino-acid conversions, and in the formation and utilisation of formate. Deficiency, which can result in megaloblastic anaemia (p.734), develops when the dietary intake is inadequate (as in malnutrition), when there is malabsorption (as in sprue), increased utilisation (as in pregnancy or conditions such as haemolytic anaemia), increased loss (as in haemodialysis), or as a result of the administration of folate antagonists and other drugs that interfere with normal folate metabolism (see Interactions, above).

Folic acid is used in the treatment and prevention of the folate deficiency state. It does not correct folate deficiency due to dihydrofolate reductase inhibitors; calcium folinate (p.1431) is used for this purpose. Folic acid is also used in women of child-bearing potential and pregnant women to protect against neural tube defects in their offspring. This is discussed in more detail in Neural Tube Defects, below.

For the treatment of folate-deficient megaloblastic anaemia it is recommended in the UK that folic acid is given orally in doses of 5 mg daily for 4 months; up to 15 mg daily may be necessary in malabsorption states. Continued oral administration of folic acid 5 mg every 1 to 7 days may be necessary in chronic haemolytic states such as thalassaemia major or sickle-cell anaemia, depending on the diet and rate of haemolysis; similar doses may be necessary in some patients receiving renal dialysis in order to prevent deficiency.

In the USA the usual recommended therapeutic dose for folate deficiency is lower; folic acid 0.25 to 1 mg daily by mouth is suggested until a haematopoietic response has been obtained, although some patients require higher doses, especially in malabsorption states. The usual maintenance dose is 400 micrograms daily.

In the prophylaxis of megaloblastic anaemia of pregnancy, the usual dose is 200 to 500 micrograms daily in the UK.

For women of child-bearing potential at high risk of having a pregnancy affected by neural tube defect, the dose of folic acid is 4 or 5 mg daily starting before pregnancy (in the USA the recommendation is 4 weeks before) and continued through the first trimester. For other women of child-bearing potential the dose is 400 micrograms daily.

Folic acid may also be given by intramuscular, intravenous, or subcutaneous injection as the sodium salt.

**Deficiency states.** Reviews of the use of folic acid in conditions associated with folate deficiency.

1. Davis RE. Clinical chemistry of folic acid. *Clin Chem* 1986; **25:** 233–94.
2. Crellin R, *et al.* Folates and psychiatric disorders: clinical potential. *Drugs* 1993; **45:** 623–36.
3. Wickramasinghe SN. Folate and vitamin $B_{12}$ deficiency and supplementation. *Prescribers' J* 1997; **37:** 88–95.
4. Mason P. Folic acid—new roles for a well known vitamin. *Pharm J* 1999; **263:** 673–7.

**Ischaemic heart disease.** Elevated blood-homocysteine concentrations may be an independent risk factor for atherosclerosis and ischaemic heart disease (p.815),[1,2] and there is evidence that they are inversely related to blood-folate concentrations.[3] Epidemiological studies[4-6] indicate that individuals with a high intake of folate or vitamin $B_6$, from vitamin supplements or food, are at lower risk of ischaemic heart disease or stroke. Furthermore, meta-analyses suggest that folic acid reduces blood-homocysteine levels,[3,7] and that vitamin $B_{12}$, but not $B_6$, may have an additional effect.[7] However, a large cohort study[8] found no evidence of an independent association between folate or vitamin $B_{12}$ concentrations and death from cardiovascular disease.

Folic acid supplementation has been found to improve arterial endothelial function in a small study of healthy adults,[9] and has been associated with a trend towards improved endothelial function in patients with coronary artery disease in another.[10] However, a large open-label study[11] found that, while folic acid supplementation significantly reduced plasma homocysteine concentrations, it did not reduce recurrence of cardiovascular events in patients with stable coronary artery disease. While patients already using vitamin B supplementation on their own initiative were not ineligible, exclusion of these patients did not alter results. Most patients had been treated with lipid-lowering therapy, and the authors state that this may have overshadowed any potential beneficial effects of folic acid. Thus, there is growing interest in the results of ongoing prospective randomised trials to assess the effect of folic acid in the primary or secondary prevention of ischaemic heart disease. The American Heart Association has stated that until the results of these trials become available routine testing of plasma-homocysteine concentrations cannot be justified.[12] However, all patients should be encouraged to consume the recommended[12] dietary allowance (RDA) of folate, vitamin $B_6$ and vitamin $B_{12}$. A meta-analysis has also indicated that the relationship between hyperhomocysteinaemia and ischaemic heart disease and stroke risk in healthy individuals may not be as strong as has been suggested, and that the results of these trials may elucidate the relevance of homocysteine levels.[13]

In a small study[14] in renal transplant recipients with hyperhomocysteinaemia, vitamin $B_6$ was effective in reducing post-methionine-loading plasma homocysteine concentrations, and folic acid plus vitamin $B_{12}$ was effective in lowering fasting plasma-homocysteine concentrations. The authors concluded that all three of these B-group vitamins may have a role in reducing atherosclerotic outcomes in this patient group.[14]


1. Welch GN, Loscalzo J. Homocysteine and atherothrombosis. *N Engl J Med* 1998; **338:** 1042–50.
2. Mangoni AA, Jackson SHD. Homocysteine and cardiovascular disease: current evidence and future prospects. *Am J Med* 2002; **112:** 556–65.
3. Boushey CJ, *et al.* A quantitative assessment of plasma homocysteine as a risk factor for vascular disease: probable benefits of increasing folic acid intakes. *JAMA* 1995; **274:** 1049–57.
4. Morrison HI, *et al.* Serum folate and risk of fatal coronary heart disease. *JAMA* 1996; **275:** 1893–6.
5. Rimm EB, *et al.* Folate and vitamin $B_6$ from diet and supplements in relation to risk of coronary heart disease among women. *JAMA* 1998; **279:** 359–64.
6. Bazzano LA, *et al.* Dietary intake of folate and risk of stroke in US men and women: NHANES I Epidemiologic Follow-up Study. *Stroke* 2002; **33:** 1183–9.
7. Homocysteine Lowering Trialists' Collaboration. Lowering blood homocysteine with folic acid based supplements: meta-analysis of randomised trials. *BMJ* 1998; **316:** 894–8.
8. Hung J, *et al.* Folate and vitamin B-12 and risk of fatal cardiovascular disease: cohort study from Busselton, Western Australia. *BMJ* 2003; **326:** 131–4.
9. Woo KS, *et al.* Long-term improvement in homocysteine levels and arterial endothelial function after 1-year folic acid supplementation. *Am J Med* 2002; **112:** 535–9.
10. Thambyrajah J, *et al.* A randomized double-blind placebo-controlled trial of the effect of homocysteine-lowering therapy with folic acid on endothelial function in patients with coronary artery disease. *J Am Coll Cardiol* 2001; **37:** 1858–63.
11. Liem A, *et al.* Secondary prevention with folic acid: effects on clinical outcomes. *J Am Coll Cardiol* 2003; **41:** 2105–13.
12. Malinow MR, *et al.* Homocyst(e)ine, diet, and cardiovascular diseases: a statement for healthcare professionals from the Nutrition Committee, American Heart Association. *Circulation* 1999; **99:** 178–82. Also available at: http://circ.ahajournals.org/cgi/reprint/99/1/178.pdf (accessed 21/05/04)
13. The Homocysteine Studies Collaboration. Homocysteine and risk of ischemic heart disease and stroke: a meta-analysis. *JAMA* 2002; **288:** 2015–22.
14. Bostom AG, *et al.* Treatment of hyperhomocysteinemia in renal transplant recipients. *Ann Intern Med* 1997; **127:** 1089–92.


**Neural tube defects.** Failure of the fetal neural tube to fuse normally during the first 4 weeks of pregnancy may result in one of several congenital defects. These include anencephaly (absence of the brain and cranial vault) and spina bifida (failure of the vertebrae to fuse).[1] The latter ranges from spina bifida occulta, where neurological abnormalities are rare, to meningocoele or meningomyelocoele, where the meninges, or meninges and spinal cord, herniate outwards through the vertebral defect and which may be associated with hydrocephalus and paralysis of the lower limbs and sphincters.

The reasons for this failure in normal development are not well understood and appear to include both environmental and genetic factors. The risk is increased in certain geographical areas, and in the offspring of parents with previous children who had neural tube defects, or of parents who themselves suffer from the condition.[1]

A defect in the methylenetetrahydrofolate reductase gene has been identified, which is estimated to occur in about 5 to 15% of white populations, and appears to result in an increased requirement for folates, and an increased risk of recurrent early pregnancy loss and neural tube defects.[2,3] Since the 1960s there has been some evidence that the mother's folate status was significant, and in the early 1980s two groups published evidence for claims that the oral administration of folic acid, with or without other vitamins, in the period around conception, reduced the incidence of neural tube defect in the offspring of mothers who had previously borne children with the defect.[4,5]

Although criticised on several grounds, the conclusions of these studies were borne out by a large multicentre study initiated by the Medical Research Council (MRC) of the UK.[6] This study was terminated early because of overwhelming evidence that folic acid 4 mg daily taken from before conception until the twelfth week of gestation by women with a history of a previous pregnancy affected by a neural tube defect reduced the incidence of such defect by about two-thirds. Other studies and systematic reviews have since confirmed the benefits of supplementation.[7,8] Multivitamins alone (A, D, $B_1$, $B_2$, nicotinamide, $B_6$, and C) did not demonstrate a similar benefit.

**Prevention of recurrence.** In the light of the MRC study, it is recommended in the UK that in couples with spina bifida or a history of previous offspring with neural tube defect, all those women who may become pregnant should receive folic acid 5 mg daily (in the absence of a commercially-available 4-mg dosage form) until the twelfth week of pregnancy.[9] In the USA, recommendations are 4 mg of folic acid daily from at least four weeks before conception through the first 3 months of pregnancy.[10] It must be borne in mind that only about 60 to 70% of neural tube defects appear to be folate-sensitive, and parents should be counselled appropriately.

The investigators in the MRC trial acknowledged that a 4-mg dose may not be optimal, and both early[4,5] and later[11] studies imply that much lower doses of folic acid may reduce the risk of recurrence, but this has yet to be clearly demonstrated. Furthermore, the optimum length of time that supplements should be given to these women before conception is unknown.

**Prevention of occurrence.** First occurrences of neural tube defects account for about 95% of cases, and there are obvious public health implications if the benefits of folate in mothers known to be at risk can be extended to the general population. A study in Hungary[12] indicated that folic acid 800 micrograms daily with multivitamins, taken for at least one month before conception and until the third month of gestation decreased the incidence of first occurrence of neural tube defects. A case control study in the USA[13] (where the normal incidence of neural tube defect is much lower than Hungary) suggested that a periconceptional folic acid intake of as little as 400 micrograms daily reduced the occurrence of the disorder by 60%.

With such results in mind the US Public Health Service has recommended that all women of child-bearing age who are capable of pregnancy should receive folic acid 400 micrograms daily although care should be taken to keep folate consumption below 1 mg daily except under medical supervision.[1,14] Such universal coverage would allow for the problem of unplanned pregnancies but would be difficult to achieve, other than by fortification of dietary staples with folate. Food fortification has therefore been adopted in the USA, at a level of 140 micrograms of folic acid per 100 g of cereal-grain product. While this amount will probably be insufficient to provide maximum reduction in the incidence of neural tube defects,[15,16] there is some evidence of benefit,[17] and it was chosen to minimise the risk of masking vitamin $B_{12}$ deficiency in the elderly.[18] Efforts to increase the use of folic acid supplements in women of child-bearing potential are still advocated.

In the UK, the current recommendation is that all women planning a pregnancy should take an extra 400 micrograms of folic acid daily before conception and during the first twelve weeks of pregnancy, bringing the average folate intake to about 600 micrograms daily.[9] In unplanned pregnancies, supplementation should begin as soon as pregnancy is suspected. Some, however, consider this amount to be too low.[19] As in the USA, food fortification has been considered, and the Committee on Medical Aspects of Food and Nutrition Policy concluded that universal fortification of flour at 240 micrograms of folic acid per 100 g in food would significantly reduce the number of neural tube defects.[20] However, mandatory fortification awaits further evidence,[21] a decision that has been criticised,[22] and debate continues as to the amount, if any, of fortification necessary.[19,23-25] Patients receiving antiepileptic drugs are at increased risk of neural tube defect and it has been suggested that folic acid supplementation for such patients should be at the level used for prevention of recurrence,[26] i.e. 4 or 5 mg daily.

The mechanism by which folic acid protects against neural tube defects is unknown, but various theories have been postulated including a positive effect in promoting neural tube closure,[27] or a selective abortifacient effect on affected fetuses (terathanasia),[28] although the latter has been disputed.[29] There is some evidence that low maternal vitamin $B_{12}$ concentrations are an independent risk factor for neural tube defects,[30,31] perhaps indicating a role for methionine synthase in their aetiology, and suggesting that additional supplementation with cobalamins may be warranted, or that methionine supplements could be investigated as an alternative to folic acid.[32,33] Interestingly, the results from the Hungarian programme[34,35] and from other studies[36,37] suggest that multivitamin supplements (including folic acid) may also reduce the occurrence of other congenital abnormalities.


1. Botto LD, *et al.* Neural-tube defects. *N Engl J Med* 1999; **341:** 1509–19.
2. Molloy AM, *et al.* Thermolabile variant of 5,10-methylenetetrahydrofolate reductase associated with low red-cell folates: implications for folate intake recommendations. *Lancet* 1997; **349:** 1591–3.
3. Nelen WLDM, *et al.* Recurrent early pregnancy loss and genetic-related disturbances in folate and homocysteine metabolism. *Br J Hosp Med* 1997; **58:** 511–13.
4. Smithells RW, *et al.* Apparent prevention of neural tube defects by periconceptional vitamin supplementation. *Arch Dis Child* 1981; **56:** 911–18.
5. Laurence KM, *et al.* Double-blind randomised controlled trial of folate treatment before conception to prevent recurrence of neural tube defects. *BMJ* 1981; **282:** 1509–11.
6. MRC Vitamin Study Research Group. Prevention of neural tube defects: results of the Medical Research Council vitamin study. *Lancet* 1991; **338:** 131–7.
7. Berry RJ, *et al.* Prevention of neural-tube defects with folic acid in China. *N Engl J Med* 1999; **341:** 1485–90. Correction. *ibid.*; 1864.
8. Lumley J, *et al.* Periconceptional supplementation with folate and/or multivitamins for preventing neural tube defects. Available in The Cochrane Library; Issue 2. Chichester: John Wiley; 2004.
9. DoH. *Folic acid and the prevention of neural tube defects: report from an expert advisory group.* London: Department of Health, 1992.
10. Centers for Disease Control. Use of folic acid for prevention of spina bifida and other neural tube defects—1983-1991. *MMWR* 1991; **40:** 513–16.
11. Kirke PN, *et al.* A randomised trial of low dose folic acid to prevent neural tube defects. *Arch Dis Child* 1992; **67:** 1442–6.
12. Czeizel AE, Dudás I. Prevention of the first occurrence of neural-tube defects by periconceptional vitamin supplementation. *N Engl J Med* 1992; **327:** 1832–5.
13. Werler MM, *et al.* Periconceptional folic acid exposure and risk of occurrent neural tube defects. *JAMA* 1993; **269:** 1257–61.
14. Centers for Disease Control. Recommendations for use of folic acid to reduce number of spina bifida cases and other neural tube defects. *JAMA* 1993; **269:** 1233–8.
15. Daly S, *et al.* Minimum effective dose of folic acid for food fortification to prevent neural-tube defects. *Lancet* 1997; **350:** 1666–9.
16. Brown JE, *et al.* Predictors of red cell folate level in women attempting pregnancy. *JAMA* 1997; **277:** 548–52.
17. Honein M, *et al.* Impact of folic acid fortification of the US food supply on the occurrence of neural tube defects. *JAMA* 2001; **285:** 2981–6.
18. Tucker KL, *et al.* Folic acid fortification of the food supply: potential benefits and risks for the elderly population. *JAMA* 1996; **276:** 1879–85. Correction. *ibid.* 1997; **277:** 714.
19. Wald NJ, *et al.* Quantifying the effect of folic acid. *Lancet* 2001; **358:** 2069–73. Correction. *ibid.* 2002; **359:** 630.
20. DoH. Consultation by the UK health departments and the Food Standards Agency on the report of the Committee on Medical Aspects of Food and Nutrition Policy on folic acid and the prevention of disease. Available at: http://www.dh.gov.uk/assetRoot/04/01/44/29/04014429.pdf (accessed 14/05/04)
21. Food Standards Agency. Extract from the minutes of the Food Standards Agency board meeting of 9 May 2002: item 4: folic acid and the prevention of disease (Paper FSA 02/05/02). Available at: http://www.foodstandards.gov.uk/multimedia/pdfs/folicacid_disease_annexc.pdf (accessed 19/05/04)
22. Oakley GP. Delaying folic acid fortification of flour: governments that do not ensure fortification are committing public health malpractice. *BMJ* 2002; **324:** 1348–9. Correction. *ibid.*; **325:** 259.
23. Mills JL. Fortification of foods with folic acid — how much is enough? *N Engl J Med* 2000; **342:** 1442–5.
24. Wharton B, Booth I. Fortification of flour with folic acid: a controlled field trial is needed. *BMJ* 2001; **323:** 1198–9.
25. Reynolds E. Fortification of flour with folic acid: fortification has several potential risks. *BMJ* 2002; **324:** 918.
26. Girling JC, Shennan AH. Epilepsy and pregnancy. *BMJ* 1993; **307:** 937.
27. Zhao Q, *et al.* Prenatal folic acid treatment suppresses acrania and meroanencephaly in mice mutant for the Cart1 homeobox gene. *Nat Genet* 1996; **13:** 275–83.
28. Hook EB, Czeizel AE. Can terathanasia explain the protective effect of folic-acid supplementation on birth defects? *Lancet* 1997; **350:** 513–15.
29. Burn J, Fisk NM. Terathanasia, folic acid, and birth defects. *Lancet* 1997; **350:** 1322–3.
30. Kirke PN, *et al.* Maternal plasma folate and vitamin $B_{12}$ are independent risk factors for neural tube defects. *Q J Med* 1993; **86:** 703–8.
31. Mills JL, *et al.* Homocysteine metabolism in pregnancies complicated by neural-tube defects. *Lancet* 1995; **345:** 149–51.
32. Klein NW. Folic acid and prevention of spina bifida. *JAMA* 1996; **275:** 1636.
33. Lewis DP, *et al.* Drug and environmental factors associated with adverse pregnancy outcomes: Part III: folic acid: pharmacology, therapeutic recommendations, and economics. *Ann Pharmacother* 1998; **32:** 1087–95.
34. Czeizel AE. Prevention of congenital abnormalities by periconceptional multivitamin supplementation. *BMJ* 1993; **306:** 1645–8.
35. Czeizel AE. Reduction of urinary tract and cardiovascular defects by periconceptional multivitamin supplementation. *Am J Med Genet* 1996; **62:** 179–83.
36. Shaw GM, *et al.* Risks of orofacial clefts in children born to women using multivitamins containing folic acid periconceptionally. *Lancet* 1995; **346:** 393–6.
37. Botto LD, *et al.* Periconceptional multivitamin use and the occurrence of conotruncal heart defects: results from a population-based, case-control study. *Pediatrics* 1996; **98:** 911–17.


**Prophylaxis of malignant neoplasms.** For reference to an epidemiological study suggesting that long-term use of folate-containing multivitamin supplements may be associated with a reduced risk of colon cancer, see p.1420.

## Preparations

***BP 2003:*** Ferrous Fumarate and Folic Acid Tablets; Folic Acid Tablets;
***USP 27:*** Folic Acid Injection; Folic Acid Tablets.

**Proprietary Preparations** (details are given in Part 3)
***Arg.:*** Acifol; Conacid; ***Austral.:*** Megafol; ***Austria:*** Folsan; ***Belg.:*** Folavit; ***Braz.:*** Acfol; Acifolico†; Afopic; Endofolin; Folacin; Folin; Neo Folico; ***Canad.:*** Folvite†; Novo-Folacid†; ***Chile:*** Folacid; Folisanin; ***Denm.:*** Folimet; ***Fin.:*** Folvite; ***Fr.:*** Speciafoldine; ***Ger.:*** DreisaFol; Fol-Asmedic; Folarell; Fol-

cur; Folgamma Mono†; Folsan; Folverlan; Gravi-Fol; Lafol; RubieFol; ***Gr.:*** Filicine; ***Hong Kong:*** Foliamin†; Triniscon†; ***India:*** Ingafol; Rubraplex; ***Irl.:*** Cardioguard; Clonfolic; ***Ital.:*** Folina; Folingrav; Serengrav; ***Mex.:*** AF; Folitab†; Precileucin†; ***Port.:*** Acfol; Folicil; ***Spain:*** Acfol; ***Swed.:*** Folacin; ***Switz.:*** Andreafol; Foli-Rivo; Folvite; ***Thai.:*** Foliamin; Folivit; ***UAE:*** Folicum; ***UK:*** Folatine†; Folicare; Lexpec; Preconceive; ***USA:*** Folvite.

**Multi-ingredient:** ***Arg.:*** Anemidox-Ferrum; Blastop; Factofer B12; Fefol; Ferranin Complex; Ferretab Compuesto; Ferro Folic; Ferrocebrina; Hierroquick; ITE B12 Forte; Rubiron; Sideralce; Yectafer Complex; ***Austral.:*** Antioxidant Forte Tablets†; Children's Calcium With Minerals†; Fefol; FGF Tabs; Pre Natal†; Vita-Preg†; ***Austria:*** Aktiferrin compositum; Beneuran compositum; Ferretab comp; Ferrograd Fol; Losferron-Fol; Tardyferon-Fol; ***Belg.:*** Ferrifol B12†; Ferrifol†; Gestiferrol; ***Braz.:*** Anemofer; Betozone; Cobalplex†; Coraben; Ferroplex; Ferrotonico B12; Ferrotrat; Ferrumvit; Fol Sang; Folacin; Folifer; Foliper†; Iberin Folico; Iloban; Neutrofer Folico; Noripurum Folico; Vi-Ferrin; ***Canad.:*** Folacin 12†; Palafer CF; Slow-Fe Folic; ***Chile:*** Cronoferril; Ferranem; Ferranim; Ferro F-500 Gradumet; Ferro Vitaminico; Folifer; Iberol Folico; Maltofer Fol; ***Fin.:*** Obsidan comp; ***Fr.:*** Gynosoja; Tardyferon $B_9$; ***Ger.:*** $B_{12}$ Fol-Vicotrat; Eryfer comp; Ferro sanol comp; Ferro sanol gyn; Ferro-Folgamma; Ferro-Folsan; Folgamma; Folicombin; Folsana†; Hamatopan F; Hepagrisevit Forte-N; Kendural-Fol-500; Medivitan N; Medyn; MerSol; Plastulen N; Selectafer N; Tardyferon-Fol; ***Hong Kong:*** Epargriseovit†; Hepatofalk; Iberet-Folic; ***India:*** Anemidox; Blosyn; Conviron-TR; Dexorange; Elferri-Z; Fecontin-F; Fecontin-Z; Fefol; Fefol-Z; Ferrochelate; Ferrochelate-Z; Fervit; Fesovit; Globac-Z; Hepasules; Hepatoglobine; Jectocos Plus; Livogen; Plastules; Probofex; Raricap; Tonoferon; ***Irl.:*** Fefol; Ferrocap F; Ferrograd Folic; Folex†; Galfer FA; Givitol; ***Israel:*** Aktiferrin-F; Ferrifol-3; Ferrograd Folic; Folex; Foric; Slow-Fe Folic; ***Ital.:*** Efargen†; Epargriseovit; Evafer; Ferrograd Folic; Folepar B12; Oro B12†; ***Malaysia:*** Iberet-Folic; Sangobion; ***Mex.:*** Ferlor AF; Ferranina Fol; Ferro Folico; Orafer Comp†; ***Norw.:*** Pregnifer†; ***NZ:*** Ferrograd Folic; ***Port.:*** Ferro-Folsan; Ferrograd Folico; Ferrum Fol; Folifer; Tardyferon-Fol; ***S.Afr.:*** Fefol; Fero-Folic; Ferrimed; Foliglobin; Hepabionta†; Pregamal; Trinsicon†; ***Singapore:*** Fefol†; Iberet-Folic; Neogobion; Sangobion; Tardyferon $B_9$; Wanse; ***Spain:*** Foli Doce; Foliferron; Hepa Factor; Normovite Antianemico; ***Switz.:*** Actiferrine-F Nouvelle formule; Duofer Fol; Fero-Folic; Gyno-Tardyferon; Loesfer + acide folique†; Maltofer Fol; ***Thai.:*** Adnemic F; Cilfer-12-F†; Ferli-6; Sangobion†; Trinsicon; ***UAE:*** Folicron; ***UK:*** Fefol; Ferfolic SV; Ferrograd Folic; Folex†; Folic Plus†; Galfer FA; Givitol†; Hematinic; Ironorm; Lexpec with Iron; Lexpec with Iron-M; Meterfolic; Pregaday; Pregnavite Forte F†; Slow-Fe Folic; ***USA:*** ABC to Z; Berocca Plus; Berplex†; Bevitamel; Centurion A–Z; Certagen; Cevi-Fer; Chromagen FA; Chromagen Forte; Compete; Contrin; Fe-Tinic Forte; Feocyte; Fero-Folic; Ferotrinsic; Ferralet Plus; Ferrex Forte; Ferrex Forte Plus; Ferrogels Forte; FOLTX; Formula B Plus; Geriot; Geritol Complete; Gevral T; Hematinic; Hematinic Plus; Hemocyte Plus; Hemocyte-F; Iberet-Folic; Icar-C Plus; Ircon-FA; Iromin-G; Kovitonic†; Livitrinsic-f; Nephro-Fer Rx; Niferex Forte; Nu-Iron Plus†; Nu-Iron V; Parvlex; Poly-Iron Forte; PremesisRx; Pronemia Hematinic; Slow Fe with Folic Acid; Thera Hematinic; Theragenerix-H; Theravee Hematinic; Tri-HEMIC; Trinsicon; Vitafol; Yelets; Zodeac.

---

# Folinic Acid

Citrovorum Factor; Folínico, ácido; Leucovorin. 5-Formyltetrahydropteroylglutamic acid; N-[4-(2-Amino-5-formyl-5,6,7,8-tetrahydro-4-hydroxypteridin-6-ylmethylamino)benzoyl]-L(+)-glutamic acid.

$C_{20}H_{23}N_7O_7$ = 473.4.

*CAS — 58-05-9.*

## Calcium Folinate *(BAN, rINN)*

Calcii Folinas; Calcium Folinate-SF; Calcium Leucovorin; Folinato cálcico; Leucovorin Calcium; NSC-3590. The calcium salt of folinic acid (1:1).

$C_{20}H_{21}CaN_7O_7$ = 511.5.

*CAS — 1492-18-8 (anhydrous calcium folinate); 41927-89-3 (calcium folinate pentahydrate); 6035-45-6 (calcium folinate pentahydrate).*

*ATC — V03AF03.*

**Pharmacopoeias.** In *Eur.* (see p.vi), *Int., Jpn,* and *US.*

*Chin.* includes the pentahydrate.

**Ph. Eur. 5.0** (Calcium Folinate). A white or light yellow, amorphous or crystalline powder. Sparingly soluble in water; practically insoluble in alcohol and in acetone. A 2.5% solution in water has a pH of 6.8 to 8.0. Store in airtight containers. Protect from light.

**USP 27** (Leucovorin Calcium). A yellowish-white or yellow, odourless, powder. Very soluble in water; practically insoluble in alcohol. Protect from light.

**Incompatibility.** Calcium folinate and fluorouracil, with or without 5% glucose, were incompatible when mixed in various ratios and stored in polyvinyl chloride containers at various temperatures.[1]

1. Trissel LA, *et al.* Incompatibility of fluorouracil with leucovorin calcium or levoleucovorin calcium. *Am J Health-Syst Pharm* 1995; **52:** 710–15.

## Calcium Levofolinate *(BAN, rINN)*

Calcii Levofolinas Pentahydricus; Levofolinate; Levofolinato de calcio; Levoleucovorin Calcium *(USAN)*. The calcium salt of the isomer of S-folinic acid (1:1).

$C_{20}H_{21}CaN_7O_7,5H_2O$ = 601.6.

*CAS — 80433-71-2 (anhydrous calcium levofolinate).*

*ATC — V03AF04.*

**Pharmacopoeias.** In *Eur.* (see p.vi).

**Ph. Eur. 5.0** (Calcium Levofolinate Pentahydrate). A white or light yellow, amorphous or crystalline, hygroscopic powder. Slightly soluble in water; practically insoluble in alcohol and in acetone. A 0.8% solution in water has a pH of 7.5 to 8.5. Store in airtight containers. Protect from light.

## Adverse Effects

Occasional hypersensitivity, including anaphylactic reactions, has been reported; pyrexia has occurred rarely after injections.

## Precautions

As for Folic Acid, p.1429.

## Interactions

As for Folic Acid, p.1429.

Folinic acid should not be used with a folic acid antagonist such as methotrexate as this may nullify the effect of the antagonist. Folinic acid enhances the toxicity, as well as the antineoplastic action, of fluorouracil, especially on the gastrointestinal tract.

## Pharmacokinetics

Calcium folinate is well absorbed after oral and intramuscular administration and, unlike folic acid (p.1429), is rapidly converted to biologically active folates. Folate is concentrated in the liver and CSF although distribution occurs to all body tissues. Folates are mainly excreted in the urine, with small amounts in the faeces.

◊ References.

1. McGuire BW, *et al.* Pharmacokinetics of leucovorin calcium after intravenous, intramuscular, and oral administration. *Clin Pharm* 1988; **7:** 52–8.
2. Wolfrom C, *et al.* Pharmacokinetic study of methotrexate, folinic acid and their serum metabolites in children treated with high-dose methotrexate and leucovorin rescue. *Eur J Clin Pharmacol* 1990; **39:** 377–83.
3. Zittoun J, *et al.* Pharmacokinetic comparison of leucovorin and levoleucovorin. *Eur J Clin Pharmacol* 1993; **44:** 569–73.
4. Mader RM, *et al.* Pharmacokinetics of rac-leucovorin vs [S]-leucovorin in patients with advanced gastrointestinal cancer. *Br J Clin Pharmacol* 1994; **37:** 243–8.
5. Schmitz JC, *et al.* Disposition of folic acid and its metabolites: a comparison with leucovorin. *Clin Pharmacol Ther* 1994; **55:** 501–8.

## Uses and Administration

Folinic acid is the 5-formyl derivative of tetrahydrofolic acid, the active form of folic acid. Folinic acid is used principally as an antidote to folic acid antagonists, such as methotrexate (p.570), which block the conversion of folic acid to tetrahydrofolate by binding the enzyme dihydrofolate reductase. It does not block the antimicrobial action of folate antagonists such as trimethoprim or pyrimethamine, but may reduce their haematological toxicities.

Folinic acid is given as calcium folinate, although doses are stated in terms of folinic acid. It can be given by mouth, by intramuscular injection, or by intravenous injection or infusion. Intravenous injections should be given over several minutes because of their calcium content; the maximum recommended rate is equivalent to folinic acid 160 mg/minute when used as an antidote to folic acid antagonists. It has been recommended that oral doses should not be greater than 50 mg, since absorption is saturable. Calcium levofolinate, the active laevo-isomer, which is used similarly to calcium folinate, is given in doses half those recommended for the racemic form.

In cases of inadvertent **overdosage of a folic acid antagonist**, folinic acid should be given as soon as possible and preferably within the first hour. Doses equal to or greater than the dose of methotrexate have been recommended. Alternatively it has been stated that for large doses or overdoses of methotrexate, calcium folinate may be given by intravenous infusion in a dose equivalent to 75 mg of folinic acid within 12 hours, followed by 12 mg intramuscularly every 6 hours for 4 doses. Although vincristine is not a folic acid antagonist, folinic acid has also been proposed for some manifestations of vincristine toxicity overdosage—see p.592.

Folinic acid is used with high-dose methotrexate antineoplastic therapy to reduce the toxicity of the methotrexate (**'folinic acid rescue'**; 'calcium leucovorin rescue'). Folinic acid is given after an appropriate interval, usually 24 hours, has elapsed for methotrexate to exert its antineoplastic effect and the objective is to maintain plasma concentrations of reduced folates at a level equivalent to or greater than the plasma-methotrexate concentration. Dosage must therefore be adapted according to the methotrexate regimen, and the patient's ability to clear the antineoplastic. In general, doses of up to 120 mg have been given over 12 to 24 hours, by intramuscular injection or intravenous injection or infusion, followed by 12 to 15 mg intramuscularly, or 15 mg by mouth, every 6 hours for the next 48 to 72 hours. With doses of methotrexate below 100 mg, folinic acid 15 mg by mouth every 6 hours for 48 to 72 hours may suffice.

Folinic acid is also used **with fluorouracil** to enhance the cytotoxic effect in advanced colorectal cancer. Both high-dose regimens (typically doses of folinic acid 200 mg/m$^2$, followed by fluorouracil) and low-dose regimens (20 mg/m$^2$) have been used—for details, see Uses and Administration of Fluorouracil, p.555. Sodium folinate has been used similarly, or may also be given by intravenous infusion over 2 hours at a dose equivalent to folinic acid 500 mg/m$^2$. An intravenous injection of fluorouracil 600 mg/m$^2$ is administered one hour after the start of the folinate infusion. Treatment is given weekly for 6 weeks, and may then be repeated after a 2-week interval.

Folinic acid, like folic acid, is effective in the treatment of folate-deficient **megaloblastic anaemia** (see p.734). Doses of 15 mg daily by mouth have been suggested. If given intramuscularly a dose of up to 1 mg daily has been recommended on the grounds that higher doses have not been proven to be any more effective. It is unsuitable for megaloblastic anaemia secondary to vitamin-$B_{12}$ deficiencies.

Folinic acid has been used in the form of calcium mefolinate.

**HIV infection and AIDS.** Calcium folinate has been used to reduce the toxicity of pyrimethamine and trimethoprim in patients with HIV infection. However, adjunctive administration of oral calcium folinate to patients with AIDS receiving co-trimoxazole for the treatment of *Pneumocystis carinii* pneumonia (PCP) was associated with a higher rate of therapeutic failure and a decrease in survival and did not reduce the frequency of dose-limiting co-trimoxazole toxicity.[1] Calcium folinate did not reduce the toxicity of co-trimoxazole being used for the primary prophylaxis of PCP.[2] Vitamin $B_{12}$ and folinic acid supplementation in patients with HIV infection did not prevent or reduce zidovudine-induced myelosuppression.[3]

1. Safrin S, *et al.* Adjunctive folinic acid with trimethoprim-sulfamethoxazole for Pneumocystis carinii pneumonia in AIDS patients is associated with an increased risk of therapeutic failure and death. *J Infect Dis* 1994; **170:** 912–17.
2. Bozzette SA, *et al.* The tolerance for zidovudine plus thrice weekly or daily trimethoprim-sulfamethoxazole with and without leucovorin for primary prophylaxis in advanced HIV disease. *Am J Med* 1995; **98:** 177–82.
3. Falguera M, *et al.* Study of the role of vitamin $B_{12}$ and folinic acid supplementation in preventing hematologic toxicity of zidovudine. *Eur J Haematol* 1995; **55:** 97–102.

## Preparations

***BP 2003:*** Calcium Folinate Injection; Calcium Folinate Tablets;
***USP 27:*** Leucovorin Calcium Injection; Leucovorin Calcium Tablets.

**Proprietary Preparations** (details are given in Part 3)

***Arg.:*** Asovorin; Cromatonbic Folinico; Elvefocal; Estroquin; Folinfabra; Leucocalcin; Rontafor; ***Austria:*** Cehafolin†; Isovorin; Levorin†; Rescuvolin; Ribofolin; ***Belg.:*** Elvorine; Ledervorin; ***Braz.:*** Calfolin†; Folicorin; Isovorin; Legifol CS; Levorin; Nyrin; Prevax; Rescuvolin; Tecnovorin; ***Chile:*** Covorit; ***Denm.:*** Isovorin; Rescuvolin; ***Fin.:*** Antrex; Isovorin; Rescuvolin; ***Fr.:*** Elvorine; Folinoral; Lederfoline; Osfolate†; Perfolate†; ***Ger.:*** DeGalin; FOLI-cell; Lederfolat; Neofolin; O-folin; Rescuvolin; Ribofolin; VoriNa; ***Gr.:*** Buateron; Calcifolin; Fedolen; Foliment; Folinato; Folmigor; Foxolin; Isovorin; Reotan; Rescuvolin; Veravorin; ***Irl.:*** Isovorin; Lederfolin; ***Israel:*** Rescuvolin†; ***Ital.:*** Biofolic; Calcifolin; Calfolex; Calinat; Citofolin; Divical; Ecofol; Emovis; Folaren; Foliben; Folicalgyn; Folidar; Folinac; Folinvit; Foliplus; Folix†; Furoic; Lederfolin; Levofolene; Osfolato; Perfolin†; Prefolic; Resfolin; Sanifolin; Sulton; Tonofolin; ***Malaysia:*** Nyrin; Rescuvolin; ***Mex.:*** Dalisol; Flynoken A; Folcane†; Ifavor; Lenovor†; Medsavorina; Tecfoline†; ***Neth.:*** Isovorin†; Ledervorin†; ***Norw.:*** Isovorin; Rescuvolin; ***NZ:*** Rescuvolin; ***Port.:*** Folinovo; Isovorin; Lederfoline; Medifolin; Raycept; ***S.Afr.:*** Isovorin; Refolinon†; Rescuvolin; ***Singapore:*** Rescuvolin; ***Spain:*** Cromatonbic Folinico; Folaxin; Folidan; Isovorin; Lederfolin; ***Swed.:*** Citrec†; Isovorin; Rescuvolin; ***Switz.:*** Isovorin†; Osfolate†; ***Thai.:*** Rescuvolin; ***UK:*** Isovorin; Lederfolin; Refolinon; Sodiofolin; ***USA:*** Wellcovorin†.

**Multi-ingredient:** ***Braz.:*** Fisifer Folico†; ***Ital.:*** Carfosid; Emazian B12; Emoantitossina; Emopon; Eparmefolin; Ferritin Complex; Ferrofolin; For Liver†; Hepa-Factor; Idropan B; Ipavit.

---

# Fructose

Fructosa; D-Fructose; Fructosum; Fruit Sugar; Laevulose; Laevulosum; Levulose. D-(−)-Fructopyranose.

$C_6H_{12}O_6$ = 180.2.

*CAS — 57-48-7.*

*ATC — V06DC02.*

**Pharmacopoeias.** In *Eur.* (see p.vi), *Jpn*, and *US*.
**Ph. Eur. 5.0** (Fructose). A white crystalline powder with a very sweet taste. Very soluble in water; soluble in alcohol.
**USP 27** (Fructose). Colourless crystals or a white crystalline powder. Is odourless and has a sweet taste. Freely soluble in water; soluble 1 in 15 of alcohol and 1 in 14 of methyl alcohol.

### Adverse Effects

Large doses of fructose given by mouth may cause flatulence, abdominal pain, and diarrhoea. Lactic acidosis and hyperuricaemia may follow intravenous infusions; fatalities have occurred.

**Hypersensitivity.** Urticaria in a patient associated with the ingestion of certain foods was found to be caused by D-psicose, a minor constituent of high-fructose syrup, which is used as a sweetening agent.[1]

1. Nishioka K, *et al.* Urticaria induced by D-psicose. *Lancet* 1983; **ii:** 1417–18.

### Precautions

Fructose should not be given to patients with hereditary fructose intolerance.

It should be given with caution to patients with impaired kidney function or severe liver damage.

**Intravenous administration.** Reiterations of the view that the use of intravenous infusions containing fructose and sorbitol, which remained popular in some countries, should be abandoned.[1,2] Not only can they lead to life-threatening build-up of lactic acid, they have led to fatalities in patients with undiagnosed hereditary fructose intolerance.

1. Collins J. Time for fructose solutions to go. *Lancet* 1993; **341:** 600.
2. Committee on Safety of Medicines/Medicines Control Agency. Reminder: fructose and sorbitol containing parenteral solutions should not be used. *Current Problems* 2001; **27:** 13. Also available at: http://www.mca.gov.uk/ourwork/monitorsafequalmed/currentproblems/cpaug2001.pdf (accessed 21/05/04)

### Pharmacokinetics

Fructose is absorbed from the gastrointestinal tract but more slowly than glucose. It is metabolised more rapidly than glucose, mainly in the liver where it is phosphorylated and a part is converted to glucose; other metabolites include lactic acid and pyruvic acid. Although the metabolism of fructose is not dependent on insulin, and insulin is not considered necessary for its removal from the blood, glucose is a metabolic product of fructose and requires the presence of insulin for its further metabolism.

### Uses and Administration

Fructose is sweeter than sucrose or sorbitol. It is used as a sweetener in foods for diabetics; in the UK it has been advised that the intake of fructose be limited to 25 g daily in persons with diabetes mellitus.

Fructose has been employed as an alternative to glucose in parenteral nutrition but its use is not recommended because of the risk of lactic acidosis. Use by intravenous infusion in the treatment of severe alcohol poisoning is also no longer recommended.

Solutions of fructose with glucose have been used in the treatment of nausea and vomiting (p.1245) including vomiting of pregnancy.

### Preparations

***BP 2003:*** Fructose Intravenous Infusion;
***USP 27:*** Fructose and Sodium Chloride Injection; Fructose Injection.

**Proprietary Preparations** (details are given in Part 3)
***Austria:*** Laevoral; Laevosan†; ***Fr.:*** Fruxucre†; ***Ital.:*** Fructal; Fructan; Fructofin; Fructopiran; Fructosil; Laevosan; ***Spain:*** Fleboplast Levulosa†; Levulosado; Suero Levulosado Vitulia†; ***UK:*** Levugen†.

**Multi-ingredient:** ***Austral.:*** Emetrol; ***Braz.:*** Dramin B-6 DL; ***Fr.:*** Arnilose†; Filigel; ***Israel:*** Peptical; ***Ital.:*** Eparema-Levul; Giflorex; Liozim; Weight Watchers Punto†; ***Norw.:*** Invertos†; ***Spain:*** Levulosalino Isot†; Levusalino†; ***USA:*** Emetrol; Formula EM.

---

## Gleptoferron *(BAN, USAN, rINN)*

Gleptoferrón.
$C_7H_{14}O_8.(C_6H_{10}O_5)_n.FeOOH$.
*CAS — 57680-55-4.*

### Profile

Gleptoferron is a macromolecular complex of ferric hydroxide and dextran-glucoheptonic acid. It has been employed for iron-deficiency anaemia in veterinary medicine. It is given by intramuscular injection.

---

## Glucose

Glucosa.
*ATC — B05CX01; V04CA02; V06DC01.*

### Anhydrous Glucose

Anhydrous Dextrose; Anhydrous Glucose; Dextrosum Anhydricum; Glucosa anhidra; D-Glucose; Glucosum Anhydricum. D-(+)-Glucopyranose.
$C_6H_{12}O_6$ = 180.2.
*CAS — 50-99-7.*

**Pharmacopoeias.** In *Chin.*, *Eur.* (see p.vi), *Int.*, *Jpn*, *Pol.*, *US*, and *Viet.*
Some pharmacopoeias include anhydrous glucose and/or glucose monohydrate as separate monographs whereas others permit the anhydrous and/or monohydrate under a single monograph.
**Ph. Eur. 5.0** (Glucose, Anhydrous). A white crystalline powder with a sweet taste. Freely soluble in water; sparingly soluble in alcohol.
The BP 2003 directs that when Glucose Intravenous Infusion is required as a diluent for official injections or intravenous infusions, Glucose Intravenous Infusion 5% should be used.
**USP 27** (Dextrose). It contains one molecule of water of hydration or is anhydrous. Colourless crystals or white, crystalline or granular powder. It is odourless and has a sweet taste. Soluble 1 in 1 of water and 1 in 100 of alcohol; very soluble in boiling water; soluble in boiling alcohol.

### Glucose Monohydrate

Dextrosum Monohydridicum; Glucosa monohidrato; D-Glucose Monohydrate; Glucosum Monohydridicum; Glycosum; Grape Sugar. D-(+)-Glucopyranose monohydrate.
$C_6H_{12}O_6,H_2O$ = 198.2.
*CAS — 5996-10-1.*

**Pharmacopoeias.** In *Chin.*, *Eur.* (see p.vi), *Int.*, *US*, and *Viet.*
Some pharmacopoeias include anhydrous glucose and/or glucose monohydrate as separate monographs whereas others permit the anhydrous and/or monohydrate under a single monograph.
*Eur.* includes Glucose, Liquid and Glucose, Liquid, Spray-dried.
*USNF* includes Dextrose Excipient and Liquid Glucose.
**Ph. Eur. 5.0** (Glucose Monohydrate; Glucose BP 2003). A white crystalline powder with a sweet taste. Freely soluble in water; sparingly soluble in alcohol.
**Ph. Eur. 5.0** (Glucose, Liquid). A clear, colourless, or brown viscous liquid containing a mixture of glucose, oligosaccharides, and polysaccharides obtained by hydrolysis of starch, in aqueous solution. It contains not less than 70.0% of dry matter. Miscible with water. It may partly or totally solidify at room temperature, liquefying again on heating to 50°.
**Ph. Eur. 5.0** (Glucose, Liquid, Spray-dried). A white or almost white, slightly hygroscopic powder or granules. Freely soluble in water.
**USP 27** (Dextrose). It contains one molecule of water of hydration or is anhydrous. Colourless crystals or white, crystalline or granular powder. It is odourless and has a sweet taste. Soluble 1 in 1 of water and 1 in 100 of alcohol; very soluble in boiling water; soluble in boiling alcohol.
**USNF 22** (Liquid Glucose). It is obtained by incomplete hydrolysis of starch; it consists chiefly of glucose, dextrins, maltose, and water. It is a colourless or yellowish, thick, syrupy, odourless or nearly odourless liquid. Miscible with water; sparingly soluble in alcohol.

### Adverse Effects and Precautions

Intravenous glucose solutions (particularly hyperosmotic solutions, which also have a low pH) may cause local pain, vein irritation, and thrombophlebitis, and tissue necrosis if extravasation occurs. Some of these reactions may be due to degradation products present after autoclaving or to poor administration technique. Intravenous infusion can lead to the development of fluid and electrolyte disturbances including hypokalaemia, hypomagnesaemia, and hypophosphataemia. Prolonged administration or rapid infusion of large volumes of iso-osmotic solutions may cause oedema or water intoxication; conversely, prolonged or rapid administration of hyperosmotic solutions may result in dehydration as a consequence of the induced hyperglycaemia.

The use of hyperosmotic glucose solutions is contra-indicated in patients with anuria, intracranial or intraspinal haemorrhage, and in delirium tremens where there is dehydration.

It has been suggested that glucose solutions should not be used after acute ischaemic strokes as hyperglycaemia has been implicated in increasing cerebral ischaemic brain damage and in impairing recovery.

Glucose solutions should not be given through the same infusion equipment as whole blood as haemolysis and clumping can occur.

**Pregnancy.** Glucose solutions are commonly employed as hydrating fluids and as vehicles for the administration of other drugs. It has been suggested that if used during labour the glucose load on the mother may lead to fetal hyperglycaemia, hyperinsulinaemia, and acidosis, with subsequent neonatal hypoglycaemia and jaundice.[1,2] Others[3] have found no evidence of such an effect, especially if the fetus is well-oxygenated,[4] and note that the number of patients included in such reports is often small and the selection criteria not homogeneous.

1. Kenepp NB, *et al.* Fetal and neonatal hazards of maternal hydration with 5% dextrose before caesarean section. *Lancet* 1982; **i:** 1150–2.
2. Singhi S, *et al.* Hazards of maternal hydration with 5% dextrose. *Lancet* 1982; **ii:** 335–6.
3. Piquard F, *et al.* Does fetal acidosis develop with maternal glucose infusion during normal labor? *Obstet Gynecol* 1989; **74:** 909–14.
4. Cerri V, *et al.* Intravenous glucose infusion in labor does not affect maternal and fetal acid-base balance. *J Matern Fetal Med* 2000; **9:** 204–8.

**Stroke.** Hyperglycaemia may be caused by physiological stress during ischaemic stroke, and this worsens cerebral ischaemic damage and impairs recovery. During cerebral ischaemia, cellular hypoxia causes a shift from aerobic to anaerobic metabolism of glucose leading to intracellular lactic acidosis, which is toxic to the cell. Hyperglycaemia provides more glucose for anaerobic metabolism, further worsening intracellular acidosis. Blood-glucose concentrations should therefore be monitored and hyperglycaemia avoided or treated. Glucose infusions should not be used routinely after ischaemic stroke, unless specifically indicated. Hypoglycaemia must also be avoided and for patients who do require glucose, it should be administered by continuous infusion, avoiding large infusions or boluses that can cause hyperglycaemia.[1]

1. Wass CT, Lanier WL. Glucose modulation of ischemic brain injury: review and clinical recommendations. *Mayo Clin Proc* 1996; **71:** 801–12.

### Pharmacokinetics

Glucose is rapidly absorbed from the gastrointestinal tract. Peak plasma concentrations of glucose occur about 40 minutes after oral administration to hypoglycaemic patients. It is metabolised via pyruvic or lactic acid to carbon dioxide and water with the release of energy. All body cells are capable of oxidising glucose and it forms the principal source of energy in cellular metabolism.

### Uses and Administration

Glucose, a monosaccharide, is administered by mouth or by intravenous infusion in the treatment of carbohydrate and fluid depletion. It is the preferred source of carbohydrate in parenteral nutrition regimens (p.1418) and is used in oral rehydration solutions (p.1222) for the prevention and treatment of dehydration due to acute diarrhoeal diseases (p.1241).

Glucose is also used in the treatment of hypoglycaemia (see below) and is given orally in the glucose tolerance test as a diagnostic aid for diabetes mellitus (see p.324).

The way in which the strengths of glucose solutions for intravenous use are expressed varies in different countries. Both Glucose Intravenous Infusion (BP 2003) and Dextrose Injection (USP 27) may be prepared from either anhydrous glucose or glucose monohydrate. However, the potency of the BP 2003 preparation is expressed in terms of anhydrous glucose whereas that of the USP 27 is expressed in terms of glucose monohydrate. Anhydrous glucose 0.9 g is approximately equivalent to glucose monohydrate 1 g. Thus, the term glucose 5% may represent, depending on origin, either 50 g/litre of anhydrous glucose (equivalent to about 55 g/litre of glucose monohydrate) or 50 g/litre of glucose monohydrate (equivalent to about 45 g/litre of anhydrous glucose). As the manner in which such preparations are referred to in the medical literature is sometimes ambiguous, it has not always been possible to state clearly in *Martindale* whether the strengths of glucose solutions mentioned relate to the anhydrous or hydrated form; however, in *Martindale*, unless otherwise specified, glucose injection is a 5% solution to distinguish it from more concentrated forms. For many practical purposes it is probably less important to know the exact way in which the strength of a given concentration is expressed than to avoid confusion between completely different strengths such as 5, 10, and 50% as the more concentrated forms are associated with particular adverse effects and precautions.

Solutions of glucose in water are iso-osmotic with blood at a concentration of anhydrous glucose 5.05% or glucose monohydrate 5.51%. Glucose solution 5% is therefore the strength often employed for fluid depletion; it may be administered via a peripheral vein. Glucose solutions with a concentration greater than 5% are hyperosmotic and are generally used as a carbohydrate source; a 50% solution is often employed in the treatment of severe hypoglycaemia (but see also Hypoglycaemia, below). Hyperosmotic solutions should generally be administered via a central vein although the *American Hospital Formulary Service* suggests that concentrations up to 10% may be administered via a peripheral vein for short periods provided the site is alternated regularly. In the emergency treatment of hypoglycaemia it may be necessary to use a peripheral vein but the solution should be given slowly; a suggested rate for glucose 50% in such circumstances is 3 mL/minute.

The dose of glucose is variable and is dependent on individual patient requirements; serum-glucose concentrations may need to be carefully monitored. The maximum rate of glucose utilisation has been estimated to be about 500 to 800 mg/kg per hour.

Strongly hyperosmotic glucose solutions (25 to 50%) have also been used to reduce cerebrospinal pressure (p.833) and cerebral oedema caused by delirium tremens or acute alcohol intoxication (p.1166) although they do not appear to be widely employed. Glucose solution 50% has also been used as a sclerosing agent in the treatment of varicose veins (p.1717) and as an irritant to produce adhesive pleuritis in the management of pleural effusions and pneumothorax.

**Ectopic pregnancy.** Ectopic pregnancy is now recognised at earlier stages as a result of improved diagnostic techniques. Surgery remains the mainstay of treatment, but although conservative surgical techniques may be used in an attempt to preserve fertility, nonsurgical methods have been increasingly investigated. The best established therapy is with methotrexate (p.572), but hyperosmolar glucose solutions have also been used. Local instillation of 5 to 20 mL of glucose 50% into the gestational sac (salpingocentesis) has been described.[1] It was reported to be more effective than expectant management of early tubal pregnancy[2] but another study was discontinued because of a higher failure rate with glucose than local methotrexate.[3]

1. Natofsky JG, *et al.* Ultrasound-guided injection of ectopic pregnancy. *Clin Obstet Gynecol* 1999; **42:** 39–47.
2. Lang PFJ, *et al.* Laparoscopic instillation of hyperosmolar glucose vs. expectant management of tubal pregnancies with serum hCG≤2500 mIU/mL. *Acta Obstet Gynecol Scand* 1997; **76:** 797–800.
3. Sadan O, *et al.* Methotrexate versus hyperosmolar glucose in the treatment of extrauterine pregnancy. *Arch Gynecol Obstet* 2001; **265:** 82–4.

**Glycogen storage disease type I.** Starch may be a more acceptable alternative to glucose in the control of the hypoglycaemia of type I glycogen storage disease, see p.1449.

**Haemodialysis-induced cramp.** Suggestions that haemodialysis-induced cramps (p.1221) are due to hypovolaemia (see p.1386) are supported by the efficacy of volume expansion with hypertonic solutions in the management of such cramps. Intravenous infusion of 50 mL of glucose 50% solution has been used as an effective alternative to infusion of sodium chloride or mannitol.[1,2]

1. Milutinovich J, *et al.* Effect of hypertonic glucose on the muscular cramps of hemodialysis. *Ann Intern Med* 1979; **90:** 926–8.
2. Canzanello VJ, *et al.* Comparison of 50% dextrose water, 25% mannitol, and 23.5% saline for the treatment of hemodialysis-associated muscle cramps. *Trans Am Soc Artif Intern Organs* 1991; **37:** 649–52.

**Hyperkalaemia.** Insulin, together with glucose to prevent hypoglycaemia, is given to stimulate the cellular uptake of potassium in the emergency treatment of moderate to severe hyperkalaemia (p.1219). Usually, 50 mL of glucose 50% is administered.

**Hypoglycaemia.** Glucose is used to correct insulin-induced hypoglycaemia, as discussed on p.335, either by mouth or by infusion of a hypertonic solution (20 or 50%). Glucose 5 or 10% may be used but larger volumes are required. Although 50% glucose solution has been generally used to correct hypoglycaemia in children, some consider that so concentrated a solution is associated with unacceptable morbidity and possible mortality, and that it should be replaced by the 10% solution for this purpose.[1] A 5 or 10% solution is used to prevent the hypoglycaemia associated with insulin infusion for the treatment of diabetic ketoacidosis, once blood-glucose concentrations have fallen below 12.5 mmol/litre (see p.328).

1. Winrow AP, *et al.* Paediatric resuscitation: don't use 50% dextrose. *BMJ* 1993; **306:** 1612.

**Myocardial infarction.** Some results in diabetic and nondiabetic patients have suggested that the value of a glucose, insulin, and potassium combination in patients with myocardial infarction should be further investigated (see p.342).

**Pain.** Oral glucose solution has been used similarly to sucrose solution (p.1450) to alleviate mild pain in neonates,[1-3] and there is some suggestion it may be more effective than topically applied local anaesthetic.[4]

1. Skogsdal Y, *et al.* Analgesia in newborns given oral glucose. *Acta Paediatr Scand* 1997; **86:** 217–20.
2. Carbajal R, *et al.* Randomised trial of analgesic effects of sucrose, glucose, and pacifiers in term neonates. *BMJ* 1999; **319:** 1393–7.
3. Carbajal R, *et al.* Crossover trial of analgesic efficacy of glucose and pacifier in very preterm neonates during subcutaneous injections. *Pediatrics* 2002; **110:** 389–93.
4. Gradin M, *et al.* Pain reduction at venipuncture in newborns: oral glucose compared with local anesthetic cream. *Pediatrics* 2002; **110:** 1053–7.

## Preparations

***BP 2003:*** Glucose Intravenous Infusion; Glucose Irrigation Solution; Potassium Chloride and Glucose Intravenous Infusion; Potassium Chloride, Sodium Chloride and Glucose Intravenous Infusion; Sodium Chloride and Glucose Intravenous Infusion;
***Ph. Eur.:*** Anticoagulant Acid-Citrate-Glucose Solutions (ACD); Anticoagulant Citrate-Phosphate-Glucose Solution (CPD);
***USNF 22:*** Dextrose Excipient; Liquid Glucose;
***USP 27:*** Alcohol in Dextrose Injection; Anticoagulant Citrate Dextrose Solution; Anticoagulant Citrate Phosphate Dextrose Adenine Solution; Anticoagulant Citrate Phosphate Dextrose Solution; Dextrose and Sodium Chloride Injection; Dextrose Injection; Half-strength Lactated Ringer's and Dextrose Injection; Lactated Ringer's and Dextrose Injection; Multiple Electrolytes and Dextrose Injection Type 1; Multiple Electrolytes and Dextrose Injection Type 2; Multiple Electrolytes and Dextrose Injection Type 4; Potassium Chloride in Dextrose and Sodium Chloride Injection; Potassium Chloride in Dextrose Injection; Potassium Chloride in Lactated Ringer's and Dextrose Injection; Ringer's and Dextrose Injection; Sodium Chloride and Dextrose Tablets.

**Proprietary Preparations** (details are given in Part 3)
***Arg.:*** Glucotem; Nutrosa; ***Austral.:*** Insta-Glucose; ***Braz.:*** Glicosado†; ***Canad.:*** Glucodex; ***Fin.:*** Glucosteril; ***Ger.:*** Glucosteril; ***Irl.:*** Hycal†; ***Ital.:*** Energen; ***Mex.:*** Dextralpha†; ***Port.:*** Glucosada†; Glucosado; Glucosteril; ***Spain:*** Apir Glucoibys†; Apir Glucosado; Apiroflex Glucosada†; Flebobag Glucosa; Fleboplast Glucosa; Glucosmon; Plast Apyr Glucosado; Suero Glucosado Vitulia; ***USA:*** Dex4 Glucose; Glutose; Insulin Reaction.

**Multi-ingredient:** numerous preparations are listed in Part 3.

---

## Glutamic Acid *(USAN, rINN)*

Ácido glutámico; Acidum Glutamicum; E; E620; Glu; L-Glutamic Acid; Glutaminic Acid. L-(+)-2-Aminoglutaric acid.

$C_5H_9NO_4$ = 147.1.
*CAS — 56-86-0.*

**Pharmacopoeias.** In *Chin.* and *Eur.* (see p.vi).

**Ph. Eur. 5.0** (Glutamic Acid). A white crystalline powder or colourless crystals. Freely soluble in boiling water; slightly soluble in cold water; practically insoluble in alcohol, in acetic acid, and in acetone. Protect from light.

## Glutamic Acid Hydrochloride *(rINNM)*

Aciglumin; Glu Hydrochloride; Hidrocloruro del ácido glutámico. L-(+)-2-Aminoglutaric acid hydrochloride.

$C_5H_9NO_4,HCl$ = 183.6.
*CAS — 138-15-8.*
*ATC — A09AB01.*

**Pharmacopoeias.** In *Ger.*

## Glutamine *(USAN, rINN)*

Gln; L-Glutamine; Levoglutamida; Levoglutamide; Q. L-Glutamic acid 5-amide; L-(+)-2-Aminoglutaramic acid.

$C_5H_{10}N_2O_3$ = 146.1.
*CAS — 56-85-9.*
*ATC — A16AA03.*

**Pharmacopoeias.** In *Ger.* and *US.*

**USP 27** (Glutamine). White crystals or crystalline powder. Soluble in water; practically insoluble in alcohol and in ether. Store at a mean temperature not exceeding 25°.

### Profile

Glutamic acid is an aliphatic acidic amino acid which is degraded readily in the body to form glutamine (levoglutamide). Glutamic acid and glutamine are used as dietary supplements. The dipeptides *N*(2)-L-alanyl-L-glutamine (Ala-Gln) and glycyl-L-glutamine (Gly-Gln) are used similarly.

Glutamic acid hydrochloride, which releases hydrochloric acid in the stomach, has been used in the symptomatic treatment of achlorhydria or hypochlorhydria in usual doses by mouth of 250 to 750 mg with meals.

A glutamine-based oral suspension is under investigation for the treatment of oral mucositis.

**Antineoplastic toxicity.** Vincristine neurotoxicity has been reduced by the use of oral glutamic acid (see Administration Error, p.592).

Oral supplementation with glutamine may also have a role in alleviating the diarrhoea associated with irinotecan (see Effects on the gastrointestinal system, p.564).

A glutamine-based oral suspension is under investigation for the treatment of oral mucositis associated with cancer chemotherapy (p.497).

**Parenteral and enteral nutrition.** Evidence that glutamine is involved in the regulation of muscle protein synthesis, maintenance of gut mucosal barrier function, and possibly enhanced immunological response has led to studies of supplementation with glutamine or more stable peptide derivatives in parenteral and enteral nutrition regimens for patients with injury and infection.[1]

Supplementation of parenteral nutrition regimens with glutamine has been shown to reduce clinical infection in patients who have undergone bone marrow transplantation[2] or who have suffered multiple trauma.[3] Improved survival has been reported among intensive-care patients given parenteral feeds supplemented with glutamine,[4,5] although a larger study found it difficult to demonstrate benefit.[6] A systematic review,[7] including these studies, inferred that seriously ill patients, with gastrointestinal failure and receiving parenteral nutrition, should receive glutamine supplements for at least 6 days and at a dose of greater than 200 mg/kg daily, in order to derive maximum benefit.

In patients undergoing major uncomplicated surgery on the lower gastrointestinal tract, a significantly better postoperative nitrogen balance was achieved in those whose total parenteral nutrition regimen had been supplemented with about 20 g daily of glutamine coupled with alanine (L-alanyl-L-glutamine) (equivalent to about 12 g daily of glutamine) when compared with a control group.[8] Others[9] have shown that supplementation of total parenteral nutrition solutions with a glutamine dipeptide (glycyl-L-glutamine), in quantities equivalent to 230 mg/kg of glutamine daily, prevented the increased intestinal permeability and atrophic changes in the intestinal mucosa associated with unsupplemented solutions. Supplementation of total parenteral nutrition with α-ketoglutarate or a dipeptide, ornithine-α-ketoglutarate, reduced muscle protein depletion in one study,[10] suggesting that this may be a more physiological way of providing glutamine.

1. Sacks GS. Glutamine supplementation in catabolic patients. *Ann Pharmacother* 1999; **33:** 348–54.
2. Ziegler TR, *et al.* Clinical and metabolic efficacy of glutamine-supplemented parenteral nutrition after bone marrow transplantation: a randomized, double-blind, controlled study. *Ann Intern Med* 1992; **116:** 821–8.
3. Houdijk APJ, *et al.* Randomised trial of glutamine-enriched enteral nutrition on infectious morbidity in patients with multiple trauma. *Lancet* 1998; **352:** 772–6.
4. Griffiths RD, *et al.* Six-month outcome of critically ill patients given glutamine-supplemented parenteral nutrition. *Nutrition* 1997; **13:** 295–302.
5. Goeters C, *et al.* Parenteral L-alanyl-L-glutamine improves 6-month outcome in critically ill patients. *Crit Care Med* 2002; **30:** 2032–7.
6. Powell-Tuck J, *et al.* A double blind, randomised, controlled trial of glutamine supplementation in parenteral nutrition. *Gut* 1999; **45:** 82–8.
7. Novak F, *et al.* Glutamine supplementation in serious illness: a systematic review of the evidence. *Crit Care Med* 2002; **30:** 2022–9.
8. Stehle P, *et al.* Effect of parenteral glutamine peptide supplements on muscle glutamine loss and nitrogen balance after major surgery. *Lancet* 1989; **i:** 231–3.
9. van der Hulst RRWJ, *et al.* Glutamine and the preservation of gut integrity. *Lancet* 1993; **334:** 1363–5.
10. Wernerman J, *et al.* α-Ketoglutarate and postoperative muscle catabolism. *Lancet* 1990; **335:** 701–3.

## Preparations

**Proprietary Preparations** (details are given in Part 3)
***Arg.:*** Dipeptiven; ***Austria:*** Dipeptiven; Neuroglutamin; ***Braz.:*** Dipeptiven†; ***Denm.:*** Dipeptiven; ***Fin.:*** Dipeptiven; Hypochylin; ***Fr.:*** Dipeptiven; ***Ger.:*** Dipeptamin; Glutamin; Gluti-Agil mono; Pepsaletten N; ***Gr.:*** Dipeptiven; ***Ital.:*** Dipeptiven; Glutacerebro; Glutaven; Memoril; ***Mex.:*** Dipeptiven; ***Norw.:*** Dipeptiven; Glutacid†; ***Port.:*** Cebrotex; Dipeptiven; ***Spain:*** Dipeptiven; ***Swed.:*** Dipeptiven; Hypochylin; ***Switz.:*** Dipeptiven; ***Thai.:*** Dipeptiven; ***UK:*** Dipeptiven.

**Multi-ingredient:** ***Arg.:*** Normoprost Compuesto; ***Austral.:*** Aspartatol†; Bioglan Digestive Zyme†; Liv-Detox†; Prozyme†; ***Austria:*** Aslavital; Pansan†; ***Braz.:*** Espasmo Novozyme†; Taludon; ***Chile:*** Glutacyl Vitaminado; Hexalectol; ***Fr.:*** Phakan; Vita-Dermacide; YSE Glutamique; ***Ger.:*** Glutarsin E; Vitasprint $B_{12}$; ***Hong Kong:*** Esafosfina Glutammica; ***Ital.:*** Acutil Fosforo; Briogen; Esaglut; Fosfo Plus; Glutamin Fosforo; Memoserina S†; Memovit B12; Vitasprint; Vitasprint Complex; ***Port.:*** Espasmo Canulase; Phakan; Relavit Fosforo; Tebetane Composto†; ***S.Afr.:*** Lentogesic; Spasmo-Canulase; ***Spain:*** Agudil; Gammamida Complex†; Gastro Gobens†; Gastroglutal; Jorkil†; Mederebro Compuesto†; Nucleserina; Tebetane Compuesto; ***Switz.:*** Phakolen; Spasmo-Canulase; Vitasprint Complex; ***UK:*** Amino MS†; Fat-Solv†.

---

## Glycine *(rINN)*

Aminoacetic Acid; E640 (glycine or glycine sodium); G; Glicina; Gly; Glycinum; Glycocoll; Sucre de Gélatine.

$C_2H_5NO_2$ = 75.07.
*CAS — 56-40-6.*
*ATC — B05CX03.*

**Pharmacopoeias.** In *Chin.*, *Eur.* (see p.vi), *Jpn*, and *US.*

**Ph. Eur. 5.0** (Glycine). A white or almost white crystalline powder. It exhibits polymorphism. Freely soluble in water; very slightly soluble in alcohol. A 5% solution in water has a pH of 5.9 to 6.4.

**USP 27** (Glycine). A white, odourless crystalline powder. Soluble 1 in 4 of water at 25°, 1 in 2.6 at 50°, 1 in 1.9 at 75°, and 1 in

1.5 at 100°; soluble 1 in 1254 of alcohol; very slightly soluble in ether. Its solutions are acid to litmus.

### Adverse Effects and Precautions

Systemic absorption of glycine irrigation solutions can lead to disturbances of fluid and electrolyte balance and cardiovascular and pulmonary disorders.

Glycine irrigation should be used cautiously in patients with hepatic impairment since any absorption and consequent metabolism may cause hyperammonaemia. The possible effects on fluid and electrolyte balance warrant cautious use in patients with cardiopulmonary or renal dysfunction; glycine irrigation is contraindicated in anuric patients.

◊ Reports and discussions concerning adverse effects, including disturbances of fluid and electrolyte balance, after the use of glycine irrigation solutions, and precautions to be observed.


1. Ovassapian A, *et al.* Visual disturbances: an unusual symptom of transurethral prostatic resection reaction. *Anesthesiology* 1982; **57:** 332–4.
2. Sinclair JF, *et al.* Absorption of 1.5% glycine after percutaneous ultrasonic lithotripsy for renal stone disease. *BMJ* 1985; **291:** 691–2.
3. Goble NM, *et al.* Absorption of 1.5% glycine after percutaneous ultrasonic lithotripsy for renal stone disease. *BMJ* 1985; **291:** 966–7.
4. Miller RA, Whitfield HN. Absorption of 1.5% glycine after percutaneous ultrasonic lithotripsy for renal stone disease. *BMJ* 1985; **291:** 967.
5. Hahn RG, Rundgren M. Vasopressin and amino acid concentrations in serum following absorption of irrigating fluid containing glycine and ethanol. *Br J Anaesth* 1989; **63:** 337–9.
6. Baumann R, *et al.* Absorption of glycine irrigating solution during transcervical resection of endometrium. *BMJ* 1990; **300:** 304–5.
7. Boto TCA, *et al.* Absorption of irrigating fluid during transcervical resection of endometrium. *BMJ* 1990; **300:** 748.
8. Rao PN. Absorption of irrigating fluid during transcervical resection of endometrium. *BMJ* 1990; **300:** 748–9.
9. Wiener J, Gregory L. Absorption of irrigating fluid during transcervical resection of endometrium. *BMJ* 1990; **300:** 749.
10. Magos AL, *et al.* Absorption of irrigating fluid during transcervical resection of endometrium. *BMJ* 1990; **300:** 1079.
11. Istre O, *et al.* Postoperative cerebral oedema after transcervical endometrial resection and uterine irrigation with 1.5% glycine. *Lancet* 1994; **344:** 1187–9.
12. Beutler JJ, Koomans HA. Safety and transcervical endometrial resection. *Lancet* 1995; **345:** 55.
13. Hahn RG, Persson P-G. Acute myocardial infarction after prostatectomy. *Lancet* 1996; **347:** 355.


### Uses and Administration

Glycine is the simplest of the amino acids. It is used as a dietary supplement.

Glycine is sometimes used with antacids in the treatment of gastric hyperacidity. It is also used as an ingredient of some aspirin preparations with the object of reducing gastric irritation.

Sterile solutions of glycine 1.5% in water, which are hypotonic and non-conductive, are used as urogenital irrigation solutions during certain surgical procedures, particularly transurethral resection of the prostate.

Glycine hydrochloride has also been used.

### Preparations

***BP 2003:*** Glycine Irrigation Solution;
***USP 27:*** Glycine Irrigation.

**Proprietary Preparations** (details are given in Part 3)
***Fr.:*** Derm Hydralin; Gyn-Hydralin; Uro 3000†; ***Hong Kong:*** Hydralin; ***Mex.:*** Glisuret.

**Multi-ingredient:** ***Arg.:*** Normoprost Compuesto; ***Austral.:*** Cal Alkyline†; ***Austria:*** Centramin; ***Braz.:*** B-Vesil; ***Chile:*** Dolotol 12; ***Fr.:*** Cristopal; Item Alphazole; Phakan; Pruriced; ***India:*** Cotaryl; ***Ital.:*** Detoxicon; Digestivo Antonetto; ***Mex.:*** Segel; ***Mon.:*** Magnesium Glycocolle Lafarge; ***Port.:*** Phakan; Tebetane Composto†; ***Spain:*** Sanieb; Tebetane Compuesto; ***Switz.:*** Phakolen.

*Used as an adjunct in:* ***Austral.:*** Cardiprin; Disprin Direct; ***Fr.:*** Juvepirine†; Sargepirine†; ***Ger.:*** Godamed; Praecineural; ***Hong Kong:*** Cardiprin; ***Israel:*** Lysoprin; ***Ital.:*** Aspiglicina; Geyfritz; ***Malaysia:*** Cardiprin; Glyprin; ***NZ:*** Cardiprin; ***Singapore:*** Cardiprin; ***Thai.:*** Caparin; Cardiprin; ***UK:*** Beechams Lemon Tablets†.

## Halibut-liver Oil

Aceite de hígado de fletán; Aceite de Higado de Hipogloso; Heilbuttleberöl; Ol. Hippogloss.; Oleum Hippoglossi; Oleum Jecoris Hippoglossi.

*CAS — 8001-46-5.*

**Pharmacopoeias.** In *Br.*

**BP 2003** (Halibut-liver Oil). The fixed oil extracted from the fresh or suitably preserved liver of the halibut species belonging to the genus *Hippoglossus*. It contains not less than 30 000 units of vitamin A activity per g. Wt per mL 0.915 to 0.925 g. A pale to golden yellow liquid with a fishy, but not rancid, odour and taste. Practically insoluble in alcohol; miscible with chloroform, with ether and with petroleum spirit. Store in well-filled containers. Protect from light.

### Profile

Halibut-liver oil is used as a means of administering vitamins A (p.1451) and D (p.1461); the proportion of vitamin A to vitamin D is usually greater in halibut-liver oil than in cod-liver oil (p.1425). It is usually given in capsules.

### Preparations

***BP 2003:*** Halibut-liver Oil Capsules.

**Proprietary Preparations** (details are given in Part 3)
***Arg.:*** Pancutan Base; ***Canad.:*** Nutrol A; ***Switz.:*** Halibut.

**Multi-ingredient:** ***Arg.:*** Pancutan; ***Austria:*** Nuri-Kapseln; Vitawund; ***Chile:*** Hipoglos; Mintaglos; Nistaglos; ***Fr.:*** Eryteal†; Preparation H; ***Port.:*** Halibut; ***Switz.:*** A Vogel Capsules polyvitaminees; Perles d'huile de foie de morue du Dr Geistlich†.

## Hetaflur *(BAN, USAN, rINN)*

Cetylamine Hydrofluoride; GA-242; SKF-2208. Hexadecylamine hydrofluoride.

$C_{16}H_{35}N,HF = 261.5.$

*CAS — 3151-59-5.*

### Profile

Hetaflur is used as a source of fluoride (see Sodium Fluoride, p.1444) in the prevention of dental caries.

### Preparations

**Proprietary Preparations** (details are given in Part 3)
**Multi-ingredient:** ***Israel:*** Elmex.

## Histidine *(USAN, rINN)*

H; His; Histidina; L-Histidine; Histidinum. L-2-Amino-3-(1*H*-imidazol-4-yl)propionic acid.

$C_6H_9N_3O_2 = 155.2.$

*CAS — 71-00-1.*

**Pharmacopoeias.** In *Chin., Eur.* (see p.vi), and *US.*

**Ph. Eur. 5.0** (Histidine). Colourless crystals or a white crystalline powder. Soluble in water; very slightly soluble in alcohol. Protect from light.

**USP 27** (Histidine). White, odourless crystals. Soluble in water; very slightly soluble in alcohol; insoluble in ether. pH of a 2% solution in water is between 7.0 and 8.5.

## Histidine Hydrochloride

Histidine Monohydrochloride; Histidini Hydrochloridum Monohydricum; Histidinium Chloride. L-Histidine hydrochloride monohydrate.

$C_6H_9N_3O_2,HCl,H_2O = 209.6.$

*CAS — 645-35-2 (anhydrous histidine hydrochloride).*

**Pharmacopoeias.** In *Chin.* and *Eur.* (see p.vi).

**Ph. Eur. 5.0** (Histidine Hydrochloride Monohydrate). A white, crystalline powder or colourless crystals. Freely soluble in water; slightly soluble in alcohol. A 5% solution in water has a pH of 3.0 to 5.0. Protect from light.

### Profile

Histidine is a heterocyclic amino acid which is essential for infant growth and which may be essential for some other groups, such as patients with uraemia. Histidine and histidine hydrochloride are used as dietary supplements.

Histidine, like glycine, is sometimes used with antacids in the treatment of gastric hyperacidity.

## Purified Honey

Clarified Honey; Gereinigter Honig; Mel Depuratum; Mel Despumatum; Miel Blanc; Miel purificada; Purified Honey; Strained Honey.

**Pharmacopoeias.** In *Br., Chin., Fr., Ger.,* and *Jpn.*

**BP 2003** (Purified Honey). It is obtained by purification of the honey from the comb of the bee, *Apis mellifera* and other species of Apis. A thick, syrupy, translucent, pale yellow or yellowish-brown liquid with a pleasant, characteristic odour, and a sweet, characteristic taste which varies according to the floral origin.

### Profile

Honey, which contains about 70 to 80% of glucose and fructose, is used as a demulcent and sweetening agent, especially in linctuses and cough mixtures (p.1112).

**Precautions.** Honey has been identified as a source of *Clostridium botulinum* spores and thus recommendations have been made that honey should not be given to infants under 1 year because of the risk of causing infant botulism.[1,2]


1. Arnon SS, *et al.* Honey and other environmental risk factors for infant botulism. *J Pediatr* 1979; **94:** 331–6.
2. Tanzi MG, Gabay MP. Association between honey consumption and infant botulism. *Pharmacotherapy* 2002; **22:** 1479–83.


**Wounds.** Anecdotal reports and traditional usage dating back to Ancient Egypt suggest that honey may be of some value as a wound dressing (p.1139). Its antibacterial properties are attributed both to high osmolality and the liberation of hydrogen peroxide, but may vary with the source:[1-3] in Europe, some of the best activity has been seen with lime-flower honey.[2] A group from India[4] has reported that these properties offer a potentially simple and cheap means of preserving skin grafts in developing countries, with 100% uptake of reconstituted grafts stored for up to 6 weeks and 80% uptake of those stored for 7 to 12 weeks. In comparison with silver sulfadiazine, occlusive honey dressings were found to be more effective for the treatment of superficial partial thickness thermal burns.[5] Sterilised manuka honey (p.1709) was also reported to heal a leg ulcer infected with meticillin-resistant *Staphylococcus aureus*.[6] However, concern has been expressed since honey may contain not only chemical contaminants but clostridial spores (see also above), and it has been suggested[2] that to be medically acceptable, honey must be sterile, residue-free, and of measured antibacterial activity.

Sugar (p.1450) has been used similarly to honey in treating wounds.


1. Greenwood D. Honey for superficial wounds and ulcers. *Lancet* 1993; **341:** 90–1.
2. Postmes T, *et al.* Honey for wounds, ulcers, and skin graft preservation. *Lancet* 1993; **341:** 756–7.
3. Molan PC. Re-introducing honey in the management of wounds and ulcers - theory and practice. *Ostomy Wound Manage* 2002; **48:** 28–40.
4. Subrahmanyam M. Storage of skin grafts in honey. *Lancet* 1993; **341:** 63–4.
5. Subrahmanyam M. A prospective randomised clinical and histological study of superficial burn wound healing with honey and silver sulfadiazine. *Burns* 1998; **24:** 157–61.
6. Natarajan S, *et al.* Healing of an MRSA-colonized, hydroxyurea-induced leg ulcer with honey. *J Dermatol Treat* 2001; **12:** 33–6.


### Preparations

**Proprietary Preparations** (details are given in Part 3)
***Ital.:*** Oramil; ***Neth.:*** Melrosum.

**Multi-ingredient:** ***Austral.:*** Logicin Natural Lozenges; ***Austria:*** Anifer Fenchelhonig; Thierry†; ***Braz.:*** Blumel†; Broncmel†; Calmatoss; Elixir de Inhame†; Expectomel; Mel de Jatahy†; Melagriao†; Melxi; Pectoral†; ***Canad.:*** Herbal Cough Expectorant†; Mielocol; ***Chile:*** Jarabe Palto Compuesto Con Miel; Paltomiel; Paltomiel Plus; Pulmosina; ***Fr.:*** Feromiel; Taido; ***Irl.:*** Venos Honey & Lemon; ***Ital.:*** Alvear con Ginseng; Apiserum con Telergon 1; Bebimix; Bioton; Biovigor†; Cocktail Reale†; Fon Wan Eleuthero; Fon Wan Ginsenergy; Fon Wan Pocket Energy†; Fon Wan Pollen†; Liozim; Miegel†; Nerex; Nutrigel; Pollingel Ginseng; ***Mex.:*** Guayalin-Plus; ***NZ:*** Lemsip Dry Cough; Robitussin Honey Cough; ***Switz.:*** Neo-Angin au miel et citron; ***UK:*** Adult Meltus for Chesty Coughs & Catarrh†; Beehive Balsam; Buttercup Syrup (Honey and Lemon flavour); Herb and Honey Cough Elixir; Honey & Molasses; Jackson's Lemon Linctus; Jackson's Troublesome Coughs; Lemsip Cough & Cold Dry Cough; Lockets; Lockets Medicated Linctus; M & M; Meltus Expectorant; Meltus Honey & Lemon; Potters Children's Cough Pastilles; Potters Gees Linctus; Regina Royal Five; Sanderson's Throat Specific; Throaties Pastilles; Venos Honey & Lemon; Zubes Honey & Lemon.

## Invert Sugar

Azúcar invertido.

*CAS — 8013-17-0.*
*ATC — C05BB03.*

**Pharmacopoeias.** *Br.* and *US* include preparations of invert sugar.

### Profile

Invert sugar is an equimolecular mixture of glucose and fructose which may be prepared by the hydrolysis of sucrose with a suitable mineral acid such as hydrochloric acid. Invert sugar has similar actions and uses to those of glucose (p.1432) and fructose (p.1431). It has been used as a 5 or 10% solution as an alternative to glucose in parenteral nutrition but, as with fructose, such use cannot be recommended.

A syrup of invert sugar is used as a stabilising agent; when mixed with suitable proportions of sucrose-based syrup it will help to prevent crystallisation of the sucrose.

### Preparations

***BP 2003:*** Invert Syrup;
***USP 27:*** Invert Sugar Injection; Multiple Electrolytes and Invert Sugar Injection Type 1; Multiple Electrolytes and Invert Sugar Injection Type 2; Multiple Electrolytes and Invert Sugar Injection Type 3.

**Proprietary Preparations** (details are given in Part 3)
**Multi-ingredient:** ***Norw.:*** Travert†; ***S.Afr.:*** Emex; ***USA:*** Travert.

## Iron

Ferrum; Hierro.

$Fe = 55.845.$

*CAS — 7439-89-6.*

**Pharmacopoeias.** *Eur.* (see p.vi) includes a form for homoeopathic preparations.

**Ph. Eur. 5.0** (Iron for Homoeopathic Preparations; Ferrum ad Praeparationes Homoeopathicae). A fine, blackish-grey powder, without metallic lustre, obtained by reduction or sublimation. Practically insoluble in water and in alcohol; it dissolves with heating in dilute mineral acids.

### Adverse Effects

The astringent action of **oral** iron preparations sometimes produces gastrointestinal irritation and abdominal pain with nausea and vomiting. These irritant adverse effects are usually related to the amount of elemental iron taken rather than the type of preparation. Other gastrointestinal effects may include either diarrhoea or constipation. Adverse effects may be reduced by giving it with or after food (rather than on an empty stomach) or by beginning therapy with a small dose and increasing gradually. Modified-release products are claimed to produce fewer side-effects but this may only reflect the lower availability of iron from these preparations. Oral liquid preparations containing iron salts may blacken the teeth and should be drunk through a straw. The faeces of patients taking iron salts may be coloured black.

The adverse effects associated with iron given **parenterally** are described under iron dextran (see p.1436).

Since absorbed iron is conserved by the body, **iron overload**, with increased storage of iron in various tissues (haemosiderosis), may occur as a result of excessive or mistaken therapy, especially parenteral therapy. Patients with pre-existing iron storage or absorption diseases are also at risk.

Acute iron **overdosage** can be divided into four stages.

- In the first phase, which occurs up to 6 hours after oral ingestion, gastrointestinal toxicity, notably vomiting and diarrhoea, predominates. Other effects may include cardiovascular disorders such as hypotension and tachycardia, metabolic changes including acidosis and hyperglycaemia, and CNS depression ranging from lethargy to coma. Patients with only mild to moderate poisoning do not generally progress past this first phase.
- The second phase may occur at 6 to 24 hours after ingestion and is characterised by a temporary remission or clinical stabilisation.
- In the third phase gastrointestinal toxicity recurs together with shock, metabolic acidosis, convulsions, coma, hepatic necrosis and jaundice, hypoglycaemia, coagulation disorders, oliguria or renal failure, and pulmonary oedema.
- The fourth phase may occur several weeks after ingestion and is characterised by gastrointestinal obstruction and possibly late hepatic damage.

Relatively small amounts of iron may produce symptoms of toxicity. It has been stated that more than the equivalent of 20 mg/kg of iron could lead to some symptoms of toxicity and that in a young child the equivalent of about 60 mg/kg of iron should be regarded as extremely dangerous. Estimates of acute lethal dosages have ranged from the equivalent of 150 mg/kg of iron upwards. Serum-iron concentrations have also been used as an indication of the severity of overdosage: a peak concentration of 5 micrograms/mL or more is reportedly associated with severe poisoning in many patients.

**Effects on the cardiovascular system.** For a suggestion that iron overload may contribute to ischaemic heart disease, see under Precautions, below.

**Effects on growth.** Iron supplementation in iron-replete children has been reported to adversely affect their growth—see below, under Precautions.

**Iron overload.** Because the body lacks a mechanism for the excretion of excess iron, abnormally high absorption or repeated blood transfusion will result in iron overload (p.1035), leading eventually to haemochromatosis. The consequences of haemochromatosis include pigment deposition in skin and other organs, mild liver dysfunction, endocrine dysfunction (failure of the adolescent growth spurt, hypogonadism, sometimes diabetes and hypothyroidism), and heart disease (pericarditis, heart failure, and arrhythmias). If unchecked, the iron build-up can lead to death, mainly through heart failure or arrhythmia. Where the increased iron intake cannot be avoided (as in patients receiving regular transfusions for β-thalassaemia—see p.735) treatment with the iron chelator desferrioxamine is used to retard accumulation.

## Treatment of Adverse Effects

In treating acute iron poisoning, speed is essential to reduce absorption of iron from the gastrointestinal tract. Gastric lavage should be considered and serum-iron concentrations may be an aid to estimating the severity of poisoning. Chelation therapy with desferrioxamine (p.1034) may be necessary.

Other measures include the symptomatic management and therapy of metabolic and cardiovascular disorders.

◊ General references.


1. Proudfoot AT, *et al.* Management of acute iron poisoning. *Med Toxicol* 1986; **i:** 83–100.
2. Mann KV, *et al.* Management of acute iron overdose. *Clin Pharm* 1989; **8:** 428–40.
3. Mills KC, Curry SC. Acute iron poisoning. *Emerg Med Clin North Am* 1994; **12:** 397–413.
4. Fine JS. Iron poisoning. *Curr Probl Pediatr* 2000; **30:** 71–90.


**Overdosage.** References highlighting the specific problem of iron overdose in children.[1-3] Child-resistant packaging and warning labels may be helpful in reducing the problem.


1. Anonymous. Iron-containing drugs and supplements: accidental poisoning. *WHO Drug Inf* 1995; **9:** 159–60.
2. Fitzpatrick R, Murray V. Iron toxicity: dietary supplements. *Pharm J* 1996; **256:** 666.
3. Committee on Safety of Medicines/Medicines Control Agency. Oral iron supplements: accidental overdose may be fatal in children. *Current Problems* 2001; **27:** 14. Also available at: http://www.mca.gov.uk/ourwork/monitorsafequalmed/currentproblems/cpaug2001.pdf (accessed 21/05/04)


**Overdosage in pregnancy.** Limited data on the treatment of iron overdose in pregnancy from the UK National Teratology Information Service, suggested that treatment with desferrioxamine should not be withheld if clinically indicated.[1-3] Most pregnancies had a normal outcome.


1. McElhatton PR, *et al.* The consequences of iron overdose and its treatment with desferrioxamine in pregnancy. *Hum Exp Toxicol* 1991; **10:** 251–9.
2. McElhatton PR, *et al.* Outcome of pregnancy following deliberate iron overdose by the mother. *Hum Exp Toxicol* 1993; **12:** 579.
3. McElhatton PR, *et al.* The outcome of pregnancy following iron overdose by the mother. *Br J Clin Pharmacol* 1998; **45:** 212P–213P.


## Precautions

Iron compounds should not be given to patients receiving repeated blood transfusions or to patients with anaemias not produced by iron deficiency unless iron deficiency is also present. Oral and parenteral iron therapy should not be used together. Care should be taken in patients with iron-storage or iron-absorption diseases such as haemochromatosis, haemoglobinopathies, or existing gastrointestinal diseases such as inflammatory bowel disease, intestinal strictures and diverticulae.

Liquid preparations containing iron salts should be well diluted with water and swallowed through a straw to prevent discoloration of the teeth.

**Effects in non-deficient subjects.** There has been concern about the potential consequences of iron supplementation in individuals and groups who are not actually iron-deficient. Apart from the suggestion that certain populations may be at somewhat increased risk of microbial *infection* following supplementation (see Infections, below), there is some evidence that supplementation in non-iron-deficient children may *retard their growth*.[1] It has also been proposed that iron may be associated with *ischaemic heart disease*, by modifying low-density lipoprotein in ways which increase its atherogenic potential and by sensitising the myocardium to ischaemic injury.[2,3] However, conclusions of a cohort study[4] and a systematic review[5] did not support any correlation between iron status and coronary heart disease.


1. Idjradinata P, *et al.* Adverse effect of iron supplementation on weight gain of iron-replete young children. *Lancet* 1994; **343:** 1252–4.
2. Burt MJ, *et al.* Iron and coronary heart disease: iron's role is undecided. *BMJ* 1993; **307:** 575–6.
3. Sullivan JL. Iron and coronary heart disease: iron makes myocardium vulnerable to ischaemia. *BMJ* 1993; **307:** 1066–7.
4. Sempos CT, *et al.* Serum ferritin and death from all causes and cardiovascular disease: the NHANES II Mortality Study. *Ann Epidemiol* 2000; **10:** 441–8.
5. Danesh J, Appleby P. Coronary heart disease and iron status: meta-analyses of prospective studies. *Circulation* 1999; **99:** 852–4.


INFECTIONS. Iron is not only an essential element for humans but is also essential for many micro-organisms. Thus, it has been suggested that persons with either adequate iron stores or iron overload may provide optimum conditions for microbial growth and therefore be susceptible to an increased incidence and severity of infection; conversely, iron-deficiency anaemia may offer some protection against infections. The topic has been reviewed[1] and although there is no evidence that small amounts of iron supplements or iron-fortified food in normal people will render them more prone to infection[2] there is some evidence that in populations with a high prevalence of endemic infectious disease such as malaria, iron therapy may be followed by a higher incidence of infectious complications or by a flare-up of existing low-grade disease. Therefore, the routine use of iron supplements in such communities has been questioned;[3,4] however, an increasing number of studies have failed to demonstrate a detrimental effect.[5-8] A subsequent systematic review[9] concluded that, while iron supplementation slightly increases the risk of developing diarrhoea, it has no apparent harmful effect on the overall incidence of infectious illnesses in children.


1. Hershko C, *et al.* Iron and infection. *BMJ* 1988; **296:** 660–4.
2. Bullen JJ, Ward CG. Iron and infection. *BMJ* 1988; **296:** 1539.
3. Oppenheimer SJ, *et al.* Iron supplementation increases prevalence and effects of malaria: report on clinical studies in Papua New Guinea. *Trans R Soc Trop Med Hyg* 1986; **80:** 603–12.
4. Smith AW, *et al.* The effects on malaria of treatment of iron-deficiency anaemia with oral iron in Gambian children. *Ann Trop Paediatr* 1989; **9:** 17–23.
5. Harvey PWJ, *et al.* The effect of iron therapy on malarial infection in Papua New Guinean schoolchildren. *Am J Trop Med Hyg* 1989; **40:** 12–18.
6. Boele van Hensbroek M, *et al.* Iron, but not folic acid, combined with effective antimalarial therapy promotes haematological recovery in African children after acute falciparum malaria. *Trans R Soc Trop Med Hyg* 1995; **89:** 672–6.
7. van den Hombergh J, *et al.* Does iron therapy benefit children with severe malaria-associated anaemia? A clinical trial with 12 weeks supplementation of oral iron in young children from the Turiani Division, Tanzania. *J Trop Pediatr* 1996; **42:** 220–7.
8. Menendez C, *et al.* Randomised placebo-controlled trial of iron supplementation and malaria chemoprophylaxis for prevention of severe anaemia and malaria in Tanzanian infants. *Lancet* 1997; **350:** 844–50.
9. Gera T, Sachdev HPS. Effect of iron supplementation on incidence of infectious illness in children: systematic review. *BMJ* 2002; **325:** 1142.


**Interference with diagnostic tests.** Although studies *in vitro* demonstrated that iron (ferrous sulfate) caused a false-positive result in the Hemoccult test for blood in faeces, this did not occur *in vivo* in persons receiving oral iron therapy.[1,2] An explanation for the difference in these findings was that hydrogen peroxide in the Hemoccult developer converted ferrous ions in solution to ferric ions, which caused oxidation in the test, whereas *in vivo* the iron was probably eliminated in the faeces in the form of non-reactive insoluble iron precipitates.[2]


1. Kulbaski MJ, *et al.* Oral iron and the Hemoccult test: a controversy on the teaching wards. *N Engl J Med* 1989; **320:** 1500.
2. McDonnell M, Elta G. More on oral iron and the Hemoccult test. *N Engl J Med* 1989; **321:** 1684.


**Porphyria.** Erythropoietic protoporphyria was exacerbated by oral iron therapy in 4 patients;[1] a further patient had a variable reaction to iron, being able to tolerate it on some occasions but suffering from exacerbation of porphyria on others.[2]


1. Milligan A, *et al.* Erythropoietic protoporphyria exacerbated by oral iron therapy. *Br J Dermatol* 1988; **119:** 63–6.
2. McClements BM, *et al.* Erythropoietic protoporphyria and iron therapy. *Br J Dermatol* 1990; **122:** 423–6.


## Interactions

Iron salts are not well absorbed by mouth, and administration with food may further impair their absorption.

Compounds containing calcium and magnesium, including antacids and mineral supplements, and bicarbonates, carbonates, oxalates, or phosphates, may also impair the absorption of iron by the formation of insoluble complexes. Similarly the absorption of both iron salts and tetracyclines is diminished when taken together by mouth. If treatment with both drugs is required, a time interval of about 2 to 3 hours should be allowed between them. A suitable interval is also advised if an iron supplement is required in patients receiving trientine. Zinc salts may decrease the absorption of iron.

Some agents, such as ascorbic acid and citric acid, may actually increase the absorption of iron.

The response to iron may be delayed in patients receiving systemic chloramphenicol.

Iron salts can also decrease the absorption of other drugs and thus reduce their bioavailability and clinical effect. Drugs so affected include bisphosphonates, entacapone, fluoroquinolones, levodopa, methyldopa, mycophenolate mofetil, and penicillamine. Iron salts may reduce the efficacy of levothyroxine (p.1601).

Interactions with parenteral iron are mentioned under Iron Dextran, p.1437.

◊ Reviews.


1. Campbell NRC, Hasinoff BB. Iron supplements: a common cause of drug interactions. *Br J Clin Pharmacol* 1991; **31:** 251–5.


## Pharmacokinetics

Iron is irregularly and incompletely absorbed from the gastrointestinal tract, the main sites of absorption being the duodenum and jejunum. Absorption is aided by the acid secretion of the stomach and by some dietary acids (such as ascorbic acid) and is more readily effected when the iron is in the ferrous state or is part of the haem complex (haem-iron). Absorption is also increased in conditions of iron deficiency or in the fasting state but is decreased if the body stores are overloaded. Only about 5 to 15% of the iron ingested in food is normally absorbed.

Following absorption the majority of iron is bound to transferrin and transported to the bone marrow where it is incorporated into haemoglobin; the remainder is contained within the storage forms, ferritin (p.1427) or haemosiderin, or as myoglobin, with smaller amounts occurring in haem-containing enzymes or in plasma bound to transferrin.

Only very small amounts of iron are excreted as the majority released after the destruction of the haemoglobin molecule is re-used. This conservation of body iron, and lack of an excretory mechanism for excess iron, is the reason for the development of iron overload with excessive iron therapy or repeated transfusions.

◊ General references.

1. Harju E. Clinical pharmacokinetics of iron preparations. *Clin Pharmacokinet* 1989; **17:** 69–89.

## Human Requirements

The body contains about 4 g of iron most of which is present as haemoglobin.

Apart from haemorrhage, iron is mainly lost from the body in the faeces, urine, from skin, and sweat, but the total loss is very small. Iron is also lost in small amounts in breast milk and in menstrual blood. In healthy men and postmenopausal women the loss is replaced by the absorption of about 1 mg of iron daily; about 1.5 to 2 mg needs to be absorbed daily by premenopausal women. In childhood and adolescence, the need is proportionately greater because of growth. Iron absorption is variable but is usually between 5 and 15% and therefore a dietary allowance containing the equivalent of about 10 mg of iron daily is usually sufficient for men and postmenopausal women; up to 15 mg daily may be necessary for premenopausal women with normal menstrual blood losses; some authorities recommend higher amounts or supplements during pregnancy. For further details concerning dietary requirements, see below and for a discussion of prophylactic iron given during pregnancy, see Iron-deficiency Anaemia, under Uses and Administration, below.

Good dietary sources of haem-iron are animal products such as meat and fish; non-haem-iron is also found in animal products and in vegetable products such as legumes and some leafy vegetables, but some vegetable products with a high iron content also contain phosphates or phytates which inhibit absorption by the formation of unabsorbable complexes.

**UK and US recommended dietary intake.** In the UK, dietary reference values (DRV)[1] and in the USA, recommended dietary allowances (RDA)[2] have been published for iron.

In the UK the estimated average requirement (EAR) for adult males and postmenopausal females is 6.7 mg daily and the reference nutrient intake (RNI) is 8.7 mg daily; for premenopausal females, but without heavy menstrual blood losses, the EAR and RNI are 11.4 and 14.8 mg daily respectively. Amounts for infants, children, and adolescents, which are proportionately higher than those for adults, are also given. No increase is considered necessary during pregnancy or lactation.[1]

In the USA the RDA for adult males and postmenopausal females is 8 mg daily and that for premenopausal women is 18 mg. The tolerable upper intake level is 45 mg daily. Amounts for infants, children, and adolescents, again proportionately higher than for adults, are also provided. The RDA for pregnant women is 27 mg daily. An RDA of 9 mg for lactating adult women has been estimated from the EAR of non-menstruating women plus the average iron content of human milk.[2]

The Food and Agriculture Organization of the United Nations and the World Health Organization have together published guidelines concerning iron requirements and these take into account many factors including bioavailability of iron in the diet.[3]

For the definitions of DRV, EAR, RNI, and RDA, see under Vitamins, p.1419.

1. DoH. Dietary reference values for food energy and nutrients for the United Kingdom: report of the panel on dietary reference values of the committee on medical aspects of food policy. *Report on health and social subjects 41.* London: HMSO, 1991.
2. Standing Committee on the Scientific Evaluation of Dietary Reference Intakes of the Food and Nutrition Board. *Dietary reference intakes for vitamin A, vitamin K, arsenic, boron, chromium, copper, iodine, iron, manganese, molybdenum, nickel, silicon, vanadium, and zinc.* Washington DC: National Academy Press, 2001. Also available at http://www.nap.edu/catalog/10026.html (accessed 24/05/04)
3. FAO/WHO. *Requirements of vitamin A, iron, folate and vitamin* $B_{12}$: report of a joint FAO/WHO expert consultation. Rome: Food and Agriculture Organization of the United Nations, 1988.

## Uses and Administration

Iron is an essential constituent of the body, being necessary for haemoglobin formation and for the oxidative processes of living tissues. Iron deficiency results in defective erythropoiesis and anaemia. Iron and iron salts should only be given for the treatment or prophylaxis of iron-deficiency anaemias (see below). They should not be given for the treatment of other types of anaemia except where iron deficiency is also present. Iron-deficiency anaemias respond readily to iron therapy but the underlying cause of the anaemia should be determined and treated.

The preferred route for the administration of iron is by mouth, usually as soluble ferrous salts, which are better absorbed than ferric salts. The usual adult dose for the treatment of iron-deficiency anaemia is 100 to 200 mg of iron daily in divided doses. The usual adult prophylactic dose is 60 to 120 mg of iron daily. There are various recommendations for children's doses and up to 2 mg/kg of iron three times daily for treatment and 1 mg/kg daily for prophylaxis of iron-deficiency anaemia has been employed. Therapy is generally continued until haemoglobin concentrations reach normal values, which may take some weeks, and then for a further 3 months or more to restore body-iron stores.

Further information concerning the dosage of iron salts and compounds used is provided in the individual monographs; this information, however, tends to reflect the amounts of iron contained in different salts or available commercial preparations and therefore, in some instances, may not be within the general range of iron dosages as quoted above.

The iron content of various iron salts is tabulated in Table 1, below.

Modified-release dosage forms of iron are claimed to result in reduced gastrointestinal side-effects and have the advantage of once-daily dosing. The preparations are designed to release the iron gradually along the gut but in some instances the iron may not be released until the preparation reaches a part of the gut where absorption is poor thus resulting in sub-optimal dosing.

Iron can also be given parenterally in circumstances where oral therapy cannot be undertaken and such use is typified by iron dextran (see p.1436).

**Anoxic seizures.** Reductions in the frequency of breath-holding episodes in children treated with iron,[1] and especially in those with iron-deficiency anaemia,[2] suggest that there might be a relationship between anoxic seizures (p.478) and iron deficiency.[3]

1. Daoud AS, *et al.* Effectiveness of iron therapy on breath-holding spells. *J Pediatr* 1997; **130:** 547–50.
2. Mocan H, *et al.* Breath holding spells in 91 children and response to treatment with iron. *Arch Dis Child* 1999; **81:** 261–2.
3. Hannon DW. Breath-holding spells: waiting to inhale, waiting for systole, or waiting for iron therapy? *J Pediatr* 1997; **130:** 510–12.

**Cough.** In a small study[1] of 19 patients, iron supplementation with ferrous sulfate successfully reduced the cough associated with ACE inhibitors (see p.843). The authors hypothesised that this effect was due to the inhibition by iron of nitric oxide synthase. However, there are some concerns[2] about the effect of giving a nitric oxide synthase inhibitor to hypertensive patients, as it has been found to increase blood pressure in *animal* studies.

1. Lee S-C, *et al.* Iron supplementation inhibits cough associated with ACE inhibitors. *Hypertension* 2001; **38:** 166–70.
2. Lev I, Rian AJJT. Iron supplementation in ACE inhibition as a treatment for cough: is it really inoffensive? *Hypertension* 2001; **38:** e38.

**Iron-deficiency anaemia.** Iron deficiency eventually results in anaemia (p.733), usually of a microcytic, hypochromic type, and because iron requirements are increased during infancy, puberty, pregnancy, and menstruation, such anaemias are most common in women and children.[1] Although any underlying cause for the iron deficiency should be sought and treated, most iron-deficiency anaemias respond well to treatment with oral iron.[2] The usual dose is sufficient of a ferrous salt to supply about 100 to 200 mg of elemental iron daily, with the aim of increasing haemoglobin concentrations by 0.1 to 0.2 g per 100 mL per day or 2 g per 100 mL over 3 to 4 weeks.[2] Treatment is continued for about 3 months once haemoglobin concentrations have returned to the normal range, in order to aid replenishment of iron stores. Parenteral iron therapy is rarely indicated. Prophylactic administration may be justifiable in certain groups, such as in pregnancy and in pre-school children, but there is some debate as to its value, and its use in the former has declined.[3-7] (For the possible problems associated with iron supplementation in those who are not deficient, see Effects in Non-deficient subjects, under Precautions, above.) Usual prophylactic doses provide about 60 to 120 mg of elemental iron daily. Intermittent iron supplementation is under study.[8]

1. World Health Organization. *Iron deficiency anaemia assessment, prevention, and control: a guide for programme managers.* Geneva: WHO, 2001. Available at: http://www.who.int/nut/documents/ida_assessment_prevention_control.pdf (accessed 19/05/04)
2. Smith AG. Prescribing iron. *Prescribers' J* 1997; **37:** 82–7.
3. Hibbard BM. Iron and folate supplements during pregnancy: supplementation is valuable only in selected patients. *BMJ* 1988; **297:** 1324 and 1326.
4. Horn E. Iron and folate supplements during pregnancy: supplementing everyone treats those at risk and is cost effective. *BMJ* 1988; **297:** 1325 and 1327.
5. US Preventive Services Task Force. Routine iron supplementation during pregnancy: policy statement. *JAMA* 1993; **270:** 2846–8.
6. US Preventive Services Task Force. Routine iron supplementation during pregnancy: review article. *JAMA* 1993; **270:** 2848–54.
7. Anonymous. Routine iron supplements in pregnancy are unnecessary. *Drug Ther Bull* 1994; **32:** 30–1.
8. Cook JD. Iron supplementation: is less better? *Lancet* 1995; **346:** 587.

**Table 1.** Approximate amounts of different iron salts that supply 60mg of elemental iron.

| Iron salt | Amount |
|---|---|
| Ferrous ascorbate (anhydrous) | 437 mg |
| Ferrous aspartate (tetrahydrate) | 422 mg |
| Ferrous chloride (tetrahydrate) | 214 mg |
| Ferrous fumarate (anhydrous) | 183 mg |
| Ferrous gluconate (dihydrate) | 518 mg |
| Ferrous succinate (anhydrous) | 185 mg |
| Ferrous sulfate (dried) | 186 mg |
| Ferrous sulfate (heptahydrate) | 300 mg |

## Preparations

**Proprietary Preparations** (details are given in Part 3)

***Austria:*** Liquifer; ***Israel:*** Ferrocal; ***Ital.:*** Liquifer; Normofer†; ***Jpn:*** Ferromia; ***Malaysia:*** Ferrocyte; ***Mex.:*** Unifer; ***Singapore:*** Ferrocyte; ***Spain:*** Glutaferro; ***Switz.:*** Liquifer†; ***Thai.:*** Ferrocyte; ***USA:*** Icar; Ircon.

**Multi-ingredient:** ***Arg.:*** Hierroquick; ***Austral.:*** Clements Iron†; ***Austria:*** China Eisenwein†; China-Eisenwein; ***Braz.:*** Ferlis B12†; Ferrocitol†; Ferrumvit; Folifer; Folipet†; Hemofer†; Nervoforcan†; Norden†; Olohepat†; Sadol; Sangotone; Vi-Ferrin; ***Denm.:*** Ferroplex-frangula; ***Ger.:*** Biovital Classic; Biovital N†; Blutquick Forte S†; Ferrodix; Folicombin; ***India:*** Raricap; Raricap L; ***Ital.:*** Carfosid; Evafer; ***Singapore:*** Memoloba; ***Thai.:*** Cilfer-12-F†; Hemo-Cyto-Serum; ***UK:*** Hematinic; ***USA:*** Centurion A–Z; Feocyte; FeoGen; Geritol Complete; I-L-X; Icar-C Plus; Ircon-FA; Theravee Hematinic; Ultra-Natal.

# Iron Dextran

Hierro dextrano; Iron-Dextran Complex.

*CAS — 9004-66-4.*

**Pharmacopoeias.** *Br., Chin.,* and *US* include injections.

**BP 2003** (Iron Dextran Injection). A sterile colloidal solution containing a complex of ferric hydroxide and dextrans of weight average molecular weight between 5000 and 7000. It contains 4.75 to 5.25% of iron and 17.0 to 23.0% of dextrans. pH 5.2 to 6.5.

**USP 27** (Iron Dextran Injection). A sterile colloidal solution of ferric hydroxide in complex with partially hydrolysed dextran of low molecular weight. It may contain not more than 0.5% of phenol as a preservative. pH 5.2 to 6.5.

## Adverse Effects and Treatment

Severe anaphylactoid reactions may occur with iron dextran and fatalities have been reported. It is therefore recommended that it be given where there are facilities for the emergency treatment of such reactions, that certain precautions be observed, and that test doses be employed (see Precautions, below).

Intravenous use may be associated with peripheral vascular flushing, tachycardia, and hypotension and syncope; thrombophlebitis may also occur at the site of injection, although the incidence can be reduced by giving iron dextran in sodium chloride 0.9% rather than glucose 5%. Intramuscular injection is associated with local reactions, pain, and staining at the site of injection; leakage along the injection track may occur unless the proper administration technique is used (see Uses and Administration, below). Other immediate reactions with either route include nausea, vomiting, and taste disturbance.

Patients may also experience delayed reactions 1 to 2 days after administration of iron dextran, such as arthralgia, myalgia, regional lymphadenopathy, chills, fever, paraesthesia, dizziness, malaise, headache, nausea, vomiting, and haematuria.

Overdose of parenteral iron is unlikely to be associated with any acute manifestations. Unwarranted parenteral iron therapy will result in iron overload and excess storage of iron (haemochromatosis) in the long term. The consequences of this include liver and endocrine dysfunction and heart disease (see Iron Overload, p.1435), and possibly an increased risk of infection (see Infections, under Precautions for Iron, p.1435). Iron overload may require chelation therapy with desferrioxamine (p.1034).

Intramuscular injection of iron complexes such as iron dextran has resulted in sarcomas at the injection site in *animals*. There is some evidence that this may occur in humans.

**Effects on the blood.** A 1-year-old girl with Down's syndrome and iron-deficiency anaemia was given three intramuscular injections of iron dextran over 6 days (to a total of 30 mg/kg). Pancytopenia developed subsequently, which reappeared when challenged with iron dextran. Tests indicated an allergic pathogenesis for the pancytopenia.[1] For further discussion of hypersensitivity reactions to iron dextran, see under Hypersensitivity, below.

Thrombocytopenia has also been reported after iron dextran therapy.[2]

1. Hurvitz H, *et al.* Pancytopenia caused by iron-dextran. *Arch Dis Child* 1986; **61:** 194–6.
2. Go RS, *et al.* Thrombocytopenia after iron dextran administration in a patient with severe iron deficiency anemia. *Ann Intern Med* 2000; **132:** 925.

**Hypersensitivity.** The Boston Collaborative Drug Surveillance Program monitored consecutively 32 812 medical inpatients. Drug-induced anaphylaxis occurred in 1 of 169 patients given iron dextran (route of administration not stated).[1]

An investigation of 481 persons who received a total of 2099 intravenous injections of iron dextran found 3 life-threatening immediate anaphylactoid reactions; 8 severe delayed reactions were also observed, and many reactions of a less serious nature.[2] In a more recent series,[3] 10 of 573 patients experienced anaphylactoid reactions after intravenous iron dextran. Other serious reactions included 1 case of cardiac arrest, and 3 cases of dyspnoea, hypertension, or chest pain.

In a report of a lupus-like disorder associated with use of iron dextran,[4] the illness resolved with appropriate treatment but recurred on rechallenge.

For discussion of pancytopenia believed to have an underlying allergic pathogenesis, see under Effects on the Blood, above.

1. Porter J, Jick H. Drug-induced anaphylaxis, convulsions, deafness, and extrapyramidal symptoms. *Lancet* 1977; **i:** 587–8.
2. Hamstra RD, *et al.* Intravenous iron dextran in clinical medicine. *JAMA* 1980; **243:** 1726–31.
3. Fishbane S, *et al.* The safety of intravenous iron dextran in hemodialysis patients. *Am J Kidney Dis* 1996; **28:** 529–34.
4. Oh VMS. Iron dextran and systemic lupus erythematosus. *BMJ* 1992; **305:** 1000.

**Overdosage.** A 29-year-old woman was given 32 mL iron dextran (Imferon) intravenously. Twenty-four hours later she developed muscle cramps, bilateral frontal headaches, with subsequent neck stiffness, and marked opisthotonia with photophobia.[1] The haemoglobin concentration did not rise following the infusion of iron which indicated there had been no iron deficiency. Thus, abnormally high concentrations of free iron had followed the iron therapy and this free iron was able to cross into the CSF and was responsible for the meningitic symptoms.

1. Shuttleworth D, *et al.* Meningism due to intravenous iron dextran. *Lancet* 1983; **ii:** 453.

## Precautions

Iron dextran is contra-indicated in patients with severe liver damage or acute kidney infection. It is also contra-indicated in persons with a history of hypersensitivity to the preparation. Teratogenicity has been demonstrated in non-anaemic *animals* given the equivalent of about three times the maximum human dose and its use should be avoided in pregnancy if possible.

Additionally, iron dextran should be given with caution to patients with a history of allergic disorders or asthma and in these patients the intramuscular, and not the intravenous, route should be used. Patients with rheumatoid arthritis may experience a worsening of symptoms when given iron dextran intravenously. Patients with other inflammatory disorders such as lupus erythematosus may be at increased risk of delayed reactions. Large doses of iron dextran by infusion may lead to serum discoloration; this should not be mistaken as evidence of haemolysis. Oral iron salts should be discontinued before administration of parenteral iron.

A test dose should be given before administration of a full therapeutic dose (see Uses and Administration, below) and emergency measures for the treatment of allergic reactions should be available (see Anaphylactic Shock, p.855). Patients should be kept under observation for at least 1 hour after administration of a test dose or following intravenous administration.

Iron dextran formulated with phenol as a preservative is intended for administration by the intramuscular route only.

## Interactions

As for Iron, p.1435.

**Enalapril.** Enalapril may possibly potentiate the adverse systemic reactions seen with intravenous iron therapy.[1]

1. Rolla G, *et al.* Systemic reactions to intravenous iron therapy in patients receiving angiotensin-converting enzyme inhibitor. *J Allergy Clin Immunol* 1994; **93:** 1074–5.

## Pharmacokinetics

After intramuscular injection iron dextran is absorbed primarily through the lymphatic system: about 60% is absorbed after 3 days and up to 90% after 1 to 3 weeks. The reticuloendothelial cells gradually separate iron from the iron-dextran complex; the distribution and elimination of iron is described on p.1435. Absorption of drug inadvertently deposited in subcutaneous tissue may take months or even years.

◊ References.

1. Spruill WJ. Timing iron dextran doses when plasmapheresis is required. *Clin Pharm* 1990; **9:** 419–20.

## Uses and Administration

Iron dextran is given by injection, and should be used only in the treatment of proven iron-deficiency anaemia (p.733) where oral therapy, as described on p.1436, is ineffective or impracticable. Before commencing therapy, all patients should receive a test dose administered via the intended route, and should be observed for adverse reactions (see Precautions, above).

For iron-deficiency anaemia, total dosage is calculated according to the haemoglobin concentration and bodyweight of the patient; allowance is also made for additional iron to replenish iron stores. Iron dextran injection is usually supplied with a table from which the recommended dose can be obtained for patients of different weights and haemoglobin (Hb) status. There may be variations between countries in the doses obtained from such tables. Doses can also be calculated from various formulae. Typical formulae used for a preparation containing the equivalent of 50 mg/mL of iron are as follows:

$$\text{Dose in mL} = \{0.0476 \times \text{body-weight (kg)} \times [14.8 - \text{Hb level (g/100 mL)}]\} + \text{1 mL per 5 kg body-weight, to a maximum of 14 mL}$$

$$\text{Dose in mL for children up to 15 kg} = \{0.0476 \times \text{body-weight (kg)} \times [12 - \text{Hb level (g/100 mL)}]\} + \text{1 mL per 5 kg body-weight.}$$

Using these formulae a 70-kg man with a haemoglobin value of 5.9 g per 100 mL would be given a total of 2.2 g of iron (44 mL of the iron dextran preparation). An alternative formula is:

$$\text{Dose in mL} = \{0.0442 \times \text{body-weight (kg)} \times [\text{desired Hb level (g/100 mL)} - \text{measured Hb level}]\} + (0.26 \times \text{body-weight})$$

In adults, the calculated lean body-weight should normally be used in this formula rather than the actual body-weight. Note that doses obtained from tables or the above formulae are for iron-deficiency anaemia, and are not suitable for iron replacement for simple blood loss.

The total dose requirement may be administered as a series of **intramuscular** injections daily or once or twice weekly. It is given by deep intramuscular injection into the upper outer quadrant of the buttock; to prevent leakage along the injection track, the subcutaneous tissue is drawn to one side before the needle is inserted. Before the first therapeutic dose, a test dose should be given: a dose of 0.2 mL (10 mg) has been suggested for children weighing less than 10 kg, 0.3 mL (15 mg) for those weighing 10 to 20 kg, and 0.5 mL (25 mg) for adults. A suggested therapeutic dosage per intramuscular injection for children is: less than 5 kg, up to 0.5 mL (25 mg); 5 to 9 kg, up to 1 mL (50 mg). Adults and larger children normally receive 2 mL (100 mg).

Iron dextran is also given **intravenously** either by total-dose infusion (TDI) or as divided injections. In total-dose infusion, the total dose calculated according to the haemoglobin concentration (as outlined above) is given by slow intravenous infusion in about 500 mL of sodium chloride 0.9% or glucose 5%; sodium chloride may be preferable due to the reduced incidence of thrombophlebitis. The test dose should be given from the prepared infusion. The first 25 mg of iron should be infused over 15 minutes, and if no adverse reaction has occurred the rate of infusion may be increased progressively to 45 to 60 drops/minute; the infusion usually takes 4 to 6 hours. Recommendations for the rate of administration for both the test dose and the remainder of the infusion may vary.

For divided intravenous administration, the total dose is also calculated according to the haemoglobin concentration. A test dose of 0.5 mL (25 mg) of the iron dextran preparation should be given by slow intravenous injection. If, after an observation period of about 1 hour, this test dose has been well tolerated, the remainder of the total dose may be given in divided doses of up to 2 mL (100 mg) daily, until the total dose has been reached. The injection should be given at a rate not exceeding the equivalent of 50 mg iron (1 mL) per minute. Alternatively, the individual doses may be diluted in 10 to 20 mL of sodium chloride 0.9% or glucose 5% for slow intravenous injection, or in 100 mL for infusion over at least 30 minutes. Recommendations for the observation period, dilution, and rate of administration may vary. Patients given iron dextran intravenously should be observed closely for at least one hour after administration.

**Anaemia of chronic renal failure.** US guidelines for the treatment of anaemia of chronic renal failure[1] recommend the regular use of small intravenous doses of iron dextran, iron sucrose, or sodium ferric gluconate complex to prevent iron deficiency and promote improved erythropoiesis; oral iron is usually insufficient to maintain adequate iron stores in these patients, particularly when also treated with erythropoietin.

1. National Kidney Foundation. K/DOQI clinical practice guidelines for anemia of chronic kidney disease. *Am J Kidney Dis* 2001; **37** (suppl 1): S182–S238. Also available at: http://www.kidney.org/professionals/kdoqi/guidelines_updates/doqi_upex.html (accessed 19/05/04)

## Preparations

***BP 2003:*** Iron Dextran Injection;
***USP 27:*** Iron Dextran Injection.

**Proprietary Preparations** (details are given in Part 3)
***Arg.:*** Fexiron; ***Belg.:*** Fercayl†; ***Canad.:*** Dexiron; Infufer; ***Ger.:*** Cosmofer; ***Gr.:*** Cosmofer; ***Hong Kong:*** Cosmofer; ***India:*** Imferon; ***Mex.:*** Driken; Ferrocel†; Ferroin; Imferon†; ***Spain:*** Imferon; ***Switz.:*** Ferrum Hausmann; ***UK:*** Cosmofer; ***USA:*** DexFerrum; INFeD.

---

## Iron Polymaltose

Ferromaltose; Ferrum Polyisomaltose; Hierro polimaltosa.

## Profile

Iron polymaltose is a complex of ferric hydroxide and isomaltose. It is used as a source of iron (p.1434) for iron-deficiency anaemia (p.733). It is given by mouth in usual doses containing the equivalent of 100 mg of iron daily although up to 300 mg daily has been given in some countries. It is also given parenterally, the total dose being calculated and given by intravenous infusion or, preferably, as a series of intramuscular injections containing the equivalent of up to 200 mg of iron in a single day; injections are usually given only every few days. For further information relating to the parenteral use of iron, see Iron Dextran, p.1436.

## Preparations

**Proprietary Preparations** (details are given in Part 3)
***Arg.:*** Ferranin; ***Austral.:*** Ferrosig; Ferrum H; ***Austria:*** Ferrum Hausmann; ***Braz.:*** Noripurum; ***Chile:*** Maltofer; ***Fin.:*** Colleofer†; Maltofer; ***Fr.:*** Maltofer; ***Ger.:*** Ferrum Hausmann; ***Gr.:*** Ferrum Hausmann; Hemafer; ***Hong Kong:*** Ferrum Hausmann; ***India:*** Phosfomin Iron; ***Irl.:*** Ferrum; ***Israel:*** Ferripel-3; ***Ital.:*** Intrafer; ***Malaysia:*** Maltofer; ***Mex.:*** Ferranina; ***NZ:*** Ferrum H; ***Port.:*** Ferrum Hausmann; ***S.Afr.:*** Ferrimed; Ferrimed DS; ***Singapore:*** Ferrum Hausmann; ***Switz.:*** Ferrum Hausmann; Maltofer.

**Multi-ingredient:** ***Arg.:*** Ferranin Complex; ***Braz.:*** Noripurum Folico; Noripurum Vitaminado; ***Chile:*** Maltofer Fol; ***Gr.:*** Ferrum Fol Hausmann; Hemafer fol; ***Israel:*** Ferrifol-3; ***Mex.:*** Ferranina Fol; ***Port.:*** Ferrum Fol; ***S.Afr.:*** Ferrimed; ***Switz.:*** Maltofer Fol.

## Iron Sorbitol

Astra-1572; Hierro sorbitol; Iron Sorbitex *(USAN)*; Iron-Sorbitol-Citric Acid Complex.

*CAS — 1338-16-5.*

**Pharmacopoeias.** *Br.* and *US* include injections.

**BP 2003** (Iron Sorbitol Injection). A sterile colloidal solution of a complex of ferric iron, sorbitol, and citric acid, stabilised with dextrin and sorbitol. It contains 4.75 to 5.25% of iron. pH 7.2 to 7.9. Store at a temperature not exceeding 25°. It should not be stored at a low temperature. Do not allow to freeze.

**USP 27** (Iron Sorbitex Injection). A sterile solution of a complex of iron, sorbitol, and citric acid that is stabilised with the aid of dextrin and an excess of sorbitol. pH 7.2 to 7.9.

### Adverse Effects, Treatment, and Precautions

As for Iron Dextran, p.1436.

There may be severe systemic reactions, and cardiac complications, such as complete atrioventricular block, ventricular tachycardia, or ventricular fibrillation, may be fatal. The urine of patients treated with iron sorbitol may become dark on standing.

Iron sorbitol should not be administered intravenously. It should preferably be avoided in patients with pre-existing cardiac abnormalities.

◊ A description of adverse events in 3 patients with the malabsorption syndrome treated with intramuscular injections of iron sorbitol.[1] Two patients died; in one, findings were consistent with anaphylaxis and in the other cardiac toxicity was considered to be due to a direct effect. In the third patient direct cardiac toxicity was also implicated.

1. Karhunen P, *et al.* Reaction to iron sorbitol injection in three cases of malabsorption. *BMJ* 1970; **2:** 521–2.

### Interactions

As for Iron Dextran, p.1437.

### Pharmacokinetics

About 66% of iron sorbitol is absorbed within 3 hours of intramuscular injection, most of it directly into the blood circulation, and some via the lymphatic system. Almost all is absorbed within about 10 days. Clearance of iron sorbitol from the plasma is rapid, and is mainly via the reticuloendothelial system, as described for Iron Dextran, p.1437.

### Uses and Administration

Iron sorbitol should be used only in the treatment of proven iron-deficiency anaemia (p.733) where oral therapy, as described on p.1436, is ineffective or impracticable.

It is given by deep intramuscular injection into the upper outer quadrant of the buttock; to prevent leakage along the injection track, the subcutaneous tissue is drawn to one side before the needle is inserted.

Total dosage is calculated according to body-weight and the haemoglobin concentration of the blood, and tables are usually provided with iron sorbitol injections for this purpose. The recommended single dose is the equivalent of 1.5 mg/kg of iron up to a maximum of 100 mg daily; these doses are then given daily or every other day until the total dosage has been achieved. Iron sorbitol is not recommended in children under 3 kg in body-weight.

Iron sorbitol should not be given intravenously.

### Preparations

***BP 2003:*** Iron Sorbitol Injection;
***USP 27:*** Iron Sorbitex Injection.

**Proprietary Preparations** (details are given in Part 3)
***Arg.:*** Yectafer; ***Austria:*** Jectofer; ***Canad.:*** Jectofer; ***Denm.:*** Jectofer†; ***Ger.:*** Jectofer; ***India:*** Jectocos; ***Irl.:*** Jectofer; ***Neth.:*** Jectofer†; ***Norw.:*** Jectofer; ***Spain:*** Yectofer†; ***Swed.:*** Jectofer†; ***UK:*** Jectofer†.

**Multi-ingredient:** ***Arg.:*** Yectafer Complex; ***India:*** Jectocos Plus.

## Iron Succinyl-Protein Complex

Complejo de hierro succinil-proteína; Iron Proteinsuccinylate; ITF-282.

*CAS — 93615-44-2.*

### Profile

Iron succinyl-protein complex is a source of iron (p.1434) used for iron-deficiency anaemia (p.733). It is given by mouth in doses of up to 1.6 g daily (equivalent to up to 80 mg of iron daily).

◊ References.

1. Köpcke W, Sauerland MC. Meta-analysis of efficacy and tolerability data on iron proteinsuccinylate in patients with iron deficiency anemia of different severity. *Arzneimittelforschung* 1995; **45:** 1211–16.

### Preparations

**Proprietary Preparations** (details are given in Part 3)
***Arg.:*** Ferplex; ***Braz.:*** Fisiofer; ***Chile:*** Fisiofer; Legofer; ***Gr.:*** Fysiofer; Legofer; ***Ital.:*** Ferlatum; Ferplex; Ferremon; Ferrofolin Simplex†; Folinemic Ferro; Legofer; Pernexin; Proteoferrina; Rekord Ferro; ***Mex.:*** Ferxal; ***Port.:*** Fervit; Fetrival; Legofer; ***Spain:*** Ferplex; Ferrocur; Lactoferrina.

**Multi-ingredient:** ***Braz.:*** Fisifer Folico†; ***Ital.:*** Ferrofolin.

## Iron Sucrose *(BAN, USAN)*

Eisenzucker; Ferric Hydroxide Sucrose; Ferric Oxide, Saccharated; Ferrum Oxydatum Saccharatum; Hierro sacarosa; Iron (III) hydroxide-sucrose complex; Iron Saccharate; Oxyde de Fer Sucré; Saccharated Iron Oxide; XI-921.

*CAS — 8047-67-4.*
*ATC — B03AB02; B03AC02.*

**Pharmacopoeias.** In *Swiss.*
*US* includes an injection.

**USP 27** (Iron Sucrose Injection). A sterile, colloidal solution of ferric hydroxide in complex with sucrose in water for injection. Sodium hydroxide may be added to adjust the pH. It contains no antimicrobial agent, chelating agent, dextran, gluconate, or other added substances. pH 10.5 to 11.1 at 20°. It is intended for intravenous use only. When administered by intravenous infusion, it should be diluted with 0.9% sodium chloride injection to a concentration of 0.5 to 2.0 mg of elemental iron/mL. Do not allow to freeze.

### Adverse Effects, Treatment, and Precautions

For parenteral iron, see Iron Dextran, p.1436. Iron sucrose injection is strongly alkaline and must not be administered subcutaneously or intramuscularly. The injection should be used with caution in patients with a history of asthma, eczema, anaphylaxis, or other allergic disorders.

### Pharmacokinetics

Iron sucrose is rapidly cleared from the plasma after intravenous injection with a terminal half-life of about 6 hours. A competitive exchange of iron takes place from the iron sucrose complex to the iron-binding protein transferrin. About 5% of a dose is eliminated via the kidneys in the first 4 hours after administration.

### Uses and Administration

Iron sucrose is used as a source of iron (p.1434) for iron-deficiency anaemia (p.733). It is given when oral iron therapy is ineffective or impractical, by slow intravenous injection or intravenous infusion in sodium chloride 0.9%. The dose is calculated according to body-weight and iron deficit, a usual dose being the equivalent of 100 mg of iron administered not more than 3 times weekly. The maximum single dose is 200 mg of iron. A small test dose should be administered initially. Iron sucrose has also been given by mouth.

**Anaemia of chronic renal failure.** For guidelines referring to the use of iron sucrose in patients with anaemia of chronic renal failure, see under Iron Dextran, p.1437.

Further references.

1. Silverberg DS, *et al.* Intravenous ferric saccharate as an iron supplement in dialysis patients. *Nephron* 1996; **72:** 413–7.
2. Sunder-Plassmann G, Horl WH. Safety of intravenous injection of iron saccharate in haemodialysis patients. *Nephrol Dial Transplant* 1996; **11:** 1797–1802.
3. Charytan C, *et al.* Efficacy and safety of iron sucrose for iron deficiency in patients with dialysis-associated anemia: North American clinical trial. *Am J Kidney Dis* 2001; **37:** 300–7.
4. Stoves J, *et al.* A randomized study of oral vs intravenous iron supplementation in patients with progressive renal insufficiency treated with erythropoietin. *Nephrol Dial Transplant* 2001; **16:** 967–74.

### Preparations

***USP 27:*** Iron Sucrose Injection.

**Proprietary Preparations** (details are given in Part 3)
***Chile:*** Venofer; ***Denm.:*** Venofer; ***Fr.:*** Venofer; ***Ger.:*** FERROinfant Neu; Venofer; ***Gr.:*** Venofer; ***Hong Kong:*** Venofer; ***Israel:*** Venofer; ***Ital.:*** Ferroven†; Ferrum Hausmann; Unifer; ***Mex.:*** Venoferrum; ***Norw.:*** Venofer; ***Port.:*** Venofer; ***S.Afr.:*** Venofer; ***Singapore:*** Venofer; ***Spain:*** Venofer; ***Swed.:*** Venofer; ***Switz.:*** Venofer; ***Thai.:*** Venofer†; ***UK:*** Venofer; ***USA:*** Venofer.

**Multi-ingredient:** ***Austria:*** Ferrovin-Eisenelixier; ***Ger.:*** Hicoton; Junisana; Selectafer N.

## Isoleucine *(USAN, rINN)*

I; Ile; Isoleucina; L-Isoleucine; Isoleucinum. L-2-Amino-3-methylvaleric acid.

$C_6H_{13}NO_2$ = 131.2.
*CAS — 73-32-5.*

**Pharmacopoeias.** In *Chin.*, *Eur.* (see p.vi), *Jpn*, and *US*.

**Ph. Eur. 5.0** (Isoleucine). A white or almost white, crystalline powder or flakes. Sparingly soluble in water; slightly soluble in alcohol. It dissolves in dilute mineral acids and in dilute solutions of alkali hydroxides. Protect from light.

**USP 27** (Isoleucine). White, practically odourless crystals. Soluble in water; slightly soluble in hot alcohol; insoluble in ether. pH of a 1% solution in water is between 5.5 and 7.0.

### Profile

Isoleucine is a branched-chain amino acid that is an essential constituent of the diet. It is used as a dietary supplement. It is also an ingredient of several preparations that have been promoted for disorders of the liver.

### Preparations

**Proprietary Preparations** (details are given in Part 3)

**Multi-ingredient:** ***Ger.:*** Bramin-hepa; Falkamin; ***Ital.:*** Falkamin; Isobranch; Isoram.

## Isomalt *(BAN)*

Bay-i-3930; E953; Isomalta; Isomaltitol; Isomaltum; Palatinit.

*CAS — 64519-82-0.*

**Pharmacopoeias.** In *Eur.* (see p.vi).

**Ph. Eur. 5.0** (Isomalt). A mixture of 6-*O*-α-D-glucopyranosyl-D-glucitol ($C_{12}H_{24}O_{11}$ = 344.3) and 1-*O*-α-D-glucopyranosyl-D-mannitol dihydrate ($C_{12}H_{24}O_{11}$,$2H_2O$ = 380.3) and neither of the two components is less than 3%, calculated with reference to the anhydrous substance. A white or almost white powder or granules. Freely soluble in water; practically insoluble in dehydrated alcohol.

### Profile

Isomalt is a sugar alcohol (polyol) used as a bulk sweetener in foods. The ingestion of large quantities may produce flatulence and have a laxative effect.

◊ Isomalt is partly metabolised in the small intestine to glucose, mannitol, and sorbitol and the remaining isomalt is completely metabolised by the flora of the large intestine.[1] The Australian manufacturers have commented that the hydrolysis and absorption is minimal and does not significantly affect blood-sugar or insulin concentrations; they consider isomalt to be suitable for use by diabetic patients.[2]

1. FAO/WHO. Evaluation of certain food additives and contaminants: twenty-ninth report of the joint FAO/WHO expert committee on food additives. *WHO Tech Rep Ser 733* 1986.
2. Barnes JA. Martindale and isomalt. *Aust J Pharm* 1994; **75:** 183.

## Lactose

Lactosa; Lactosum; Lattosio; Milk Sugar; Saccharum Lactis.

*CAS — 63-42-3 (anhydrous lactose); 5989-81-1 (lactose monohydrate); 10039-26-6 (lactose monohydrate, cyclic); 64044-51-5 (lactose monohydrate, open form).*

**Description.** Lactose is a disaccharide obtained from the whey of milk. It may exist in a number of distinct forms depending upon the crystallisation and drying processes employed. The forms can vary in the contents of crystalline and amorphous lactose, the amounts of α-lactose (*O*-β-D-galactopyranosyl-(1→4)-α-D-glucopyranose) and β-lactose (*O*-β-D-galactopyranosyl-(1→4)-β-D-glucopyranose), and in their hydration states. The α-form of lactose exists in either the anhydrous ($C_{12}H_{22}O_{11}$ = 342.3) or monohydrate ($C_{12}H_{22}O_{11}$,$H_2O$ = 360.3) state whereas the β-form exists only in the anhydrous state. Commercial lactose is mainly the α-monohydrate.

**Pharmacopoeias.** In *Chin.*, *Eur.* (see p.vi), *Int.*, *Jpn*, *Pol.*, and *Viet.* Also in *USNF.* Some pharmacopoeias include separate monographs for anhydrous lactose and lactose monohydrate.

**Ph. Eur. 5.0** (Lactose, Anhydrous). It is β-lactose or a mixture of α-lactose and β-lactose. A white or almost white, crystalline powder. Freely but slowly soluble in water; practically insoluble in alcohol.

**Ph. Eur. 5.0** (Lactose Monohydrate; Lactose BP 2003). It is the monohydrate of α-lactose. It may be modified as to its physical characteristics and may contain varying proportions of amorphous lactose. A white or almost white, crystalline powder. Freely but slowly soluble in water; practically insoluble in alcohol. Store in airtight containers.

**USNF 22** (Anhydrous Lactose). It is primarily β-lactose or a mixture of α- and β-lactose. It is a white or almost white powder. Freely soluble in water; practically insoluble in alcohol.

**USNF 22** (Lactose Monohydrate). It is a natural disaccharide, obtained from milk, which consists of one glucose and one galactose moiety. It may be modified as to its physical characteristics, and may contain varying proportions of amorphous lactose. It is a white, free-flowing powder. Freely, but slowly soluble in water; practically insoluble in alcohol. Store in airtight containers.

### Adverse Effects and Precautions

Lactose intolerance occurs due to a deficiency of the intestinal enzyme lactase. Ingestion of lactose by patients with lactase deficiency leads to a clinical syndrome of abdominal pain, diarrhoea, distension, and flatulence; symptoms may also occur in persons without such a deficiency who have ingested excessive amounts of lactose.

Lactose is contra-indicated in patients with galactosaemia, the glucose-galactose malabsorption syndrome, or lactase deficiency.

**Lactose intolerance.** A review of lactose intolerance.[1] The capacity of the infant intestine to produce lactase, the enzyme responsible for digesting lactose, is retained into adulthood only by a minority of the world's population, mostly of north European descent; in Africa and Asia more than 90% of the population are lactase deficient. Because of the ubiquity of lactose in the diet and the consequent frequency of abdominal symptoms, attempts have been made to treat lactose intolerance by dietary exclusion (which need not be complete since lactase deficiency is rarely absolute). An alternative is enzyme replacement therapy with β-galactosidase from micro-organisms (see Tilactase, p.1756), but the role of such therapy has yet to be fully determined. The findings of one study[2] suggested that, in adults with lactose intolerance, the use of lactose-digestive aids is unnecessary if lactose intake is limited to the equivalent of 240 mL of milk or less daily.

There has been concern that lactose might be contaminated with protein from milk, and it has been recommended that children with cows' milk allergy avoid lactose-containing foods. However, a small study[3] found that children allergic to cows' milk could still tolerate lactose.

For the use of soya in infants intolerant to cows' milk, see p.1448.


1. Anonymous. Lactose intolerance. *Lancet* 1991; **338:** 663–4.
2. Suarez FL, *et al.* A comparison of symptoms after the consumption of milk or lactose-hydrolysed milk by people with self-reported severe lactose intolerance. *N Engl J Med* 1995; **333:** 1–4.
3. Fiocchi A, *et al.* Clinical tolerance to lactose in children with cows' milk allergy. *Pediatrics* 2003; **112:** 359–62.


## Pharmacokinetics

Lactose is hydrolysed by lactase in the small intestine to glucose and galactose, which are then absorbed.

## Uses and Administration

Lactose, the carbohydrate component of milk, is less sweet than sucrose.

Lactose is widely used in pharmaceutical manufacturing. In the production of capsules or tablets it may be employed as a diluent, bulking agent, filler, or excipient and in powders as a bulking agent. Lactose is also used as a carrier for drugs in dry powder inhalers. Characteristics such as particle size make different grades of lactose suitable for different applications.

### Preparations

**Proprietary Preparations** (details are given in Part 3)
***Austria:*** Vitawund Baby; ***Canad.:*** Novo-Plus†.

**Multi-ingredient:** ***Austria:*** Ichth-Oestren; ***Braz.:*** Lacto-Purga†.

---

## Leucine *(USAN, rINN)*

α-Aminoisocaproic Acid; L; Leu; Leucina; L-Leucine; Leucinum. L-2-Amino-4-methylvaleric acid.

$C_6H_{13}NO_2$ = 131.2.
*CAS — 61-90-5.*

**Pharmacopoeias.** In *Chin., Eur.* (see p.vi), *Jpn,* and *US.*

**Ph. Eur. 5.0** (Leucine). A white or almost white, crystalline powder or shiny flakes. Sparingly soluble in water; practically insoluble in alcohol. It dissolves in dilute mineral acids and in dilute solutions of alkali hydroxides. Protect from light.

**USP 27** (Leucine). White, practically odourless crystals. Sparingly soluble in water; insoluble in ether. pH of a 1% solution in water is between 5.5 and 7.0.

### Profile

Leucine is a branched-chain amino acid that is an essential constituent of the diet. It is used as a dietary supplement. It is also an ingredient of several preparations that have been promoted for disorders of the liver.

### Preparations

**Proprietary Preparations** (details are given in Part 3)

**Multi-ingredient:** ***Fr.:*** Revitalose; ***Ger.:*** Bramin-hepa; Falkamin; ***Ital.:*** Falkamin; Isobranch; Isoram.

---

## Lysine *(USAN, rINN)*

K; Lisina; Lys; L-Lysine. L-2,6-Diaminohexanoic acid.

$C_6H_{14}N_2O_2$ = 146.2.
*CAS — 56-87-1.*
*ATC — B05XB03.*

**Pharmacopoeias.** In *Ger.* as the monohydrate.

## Lysine Acetate *(rINNM)*

Acetato de lisina; Lys Acetate; L-Lysine Monoacetate; Lysini Acetas. L-2,6-Diaminohexanoic acid acetate.

$C_6H_{14}N_2O_2,C_2H_4O_2$ = 206.2.
*CAS — 57282-49-2.*

**Pharmacopoeias.** In *Chin., Eur.* (see p.vi), and *US.*

**Ph. Eur. 5.0** (Lysine Acetate). A white or almost white, crystalline powder or colourless crystals. It exhibits polymorphism. Freely soluble in water; very slightly soluble in alcohol. Protect from light.

**USP 27** (Lysine Acetate). White, odourless crystals or crystalline powder. Freely soluble in water.

## Lysine Hydrochloride *(USAN, rINNM)*

Hidrocloruro de lisina; Lys Hydrochloride; L-Lysine Monohydrochloride; Lysini Hydrochloridum. L-2,6-Diaminohexanoic acid hydrochloride.

$C_6H_{14}N_2O_2,HCl$ = 182.6.
*CAS — 657-27-2.*

**Pharmacopoeias.** In *Chin., Eur.* (see p.vi), *Jpn,* and *US.*

**Ph. Eur. 5.0** (Lysine Hydrochloride). A white crystalline powder or colourless crystals. Freely soluble in water; slightly soluble in alcohol. Protect from light.

**USP 27** (Lysine Hydrochloride). A white, odourless powder. Freely soluble in water.

### Profile

Lysine is an aliphatic amino acid that is an essential constituent of the diet. Lysine and lysine hydrochloride are used as dietary supplements.

### Preparations

**Proprietary Preparations** (details are given in Part 3)
***Port.:*** Incremin.

**Multi-ingredient:** ***Austral.:*** Cold Sore Relief†; Cold Sore Tablets†; Vitaline†; ***Fr.:*** Acti 5†; Curasten; Revitalose; ***India:*** Ferrochelate; Logical; Tonoferon; ***Ital.:*** Biocarnil; Calciofix; ***Mex.:*** Corpotasin CL; ***Spain:*** Acticinco†; Calcioretard†; Euzymina Lisina I; Euzymina Lisina II; Malandil; Pranzo; ***UK:*** Amino MS†; ***USA:*** Klorvess.

---

## Maize Oil

Aceite de maíz; Corn Oil; Huile de Maïs; Ol. Mayd.; Oleum Maydis.

**Pharmacopoeias.** In *Eur* (see p.vi) and *Jpn.* Also in *USNF.*

**Ph. Eur. 5.0** (Maize Oil, Refined; Maydis Oleum Raffinatum). The refined fatty oil obtained from the seeds of *Zea mays.* A clear, light yellow or yellow oil. Practically insoluble in water and in alcohol; miscible with dichloromethane and with petroleum spirit (b.p.: 40° to 60°). Store at a temperature not exceeding 25°. Protect from light.

**USNF 22** (Corn Oil). The refined fixed oil obtained from the embryos of *Zea mays* (Gramineae). A clear, light yellow, oily liquid having a faint characteristic odour. Slightly soluble in alcohol; miscible with chloroform, with ether, with petroleum spirit, and with benzene. Store in airtight containers at a temperature not exceeding 40°. Protect from light.

### Profile

Maize oil has a high content of unsaturated acids and has been used in patients with familial hypercholesterolaemia and as a high-calorie nutritional supplement. It is also used as an oily vehicle.

### Preparations

**Proprietary Preparations** (details are given in Part 3)

**Multi-ingredient:** ***USA:*** Lipomul.

---

## Malt Extract

Extracto de malta; Extractum Bynes.

### Profile

Malt extract contains 50% or more of maltose, with dextrin, glucose, and small amounts of other carbohydrates, and protein. It is prepared from malted grain of barley (*Hordeum distichon, H. vulgare*) or a mixture of this with not more than 33% of malted grain of wheat (*Triticum aestivum* or *T. turgidum*).

Malt extract has nutritive properties. It is chiefly used as a vehicle in preparations containing cod-liver oil (p.1425) and halibut-liver oil (p.1434). It is a useful flavouring agent for masking bitter tastes.

A product known as malt soup extract, obtained from barley grains, and containing 73% maltose with 12% other polymeric carbohydrates as well as small amounts of proteins, electrolytes, and vitamins, is sometimes used as a laxative.

### Preparations

**Proprietary Preparations** (details are given in Part 3)
***USA:*** Maltsupex.

**Multi-ingredient:** ***Braz.:*** Anemokol†; Pinosil†; ***Fr.:*** Elixir Contre La Toux Weleda†; Galactogil; ***Switz.:*** Optilax†; ***USA:*** Syllamalt†.

---

## Maltitol *(BAN)*

E965; Hydrogenated Maltose; D-Maltitol; Maltitolum. α-D-Glucopyranosyl-1,4-D-glucitol.

$C_{12}H_{24}O_{11}$ = 344.3.
*CAS — 585-88-6.*

**Pharmacopoeias.** In *Eur.* (see p.vi).

**Ph. Eur. 5.0** (Maltitol). A white crystalline powder. Very soluble in water; practically insoluble in dehydrated alcohol.

## Maltitol Syrup

E965; Hydrogenated Glucose Syrup; Hydrogenated High Maltose-glucose Syrup; Liquid Maltitol; Maltitol, jarabe de; Maltitol Solution; Maltitolum Liquidum.

**Pharmacopoeias.** In *Eur.* (see p.vi). Also in *USNF.*

**Ph. Eur. 5.0** (Maltitol, Liquid). An aqueous solution of a hydrogenated, part hydrolysed starch, containing not less than 68.0% w/w and not more than 85.0% w/w of anhydrous substance composed of a mixture of mainly D-maltitol with D-sorbitol and hydrogenated oligo- and polysaccharides. It contains not less than 50.0% w/w of D-maltitol and not more than 8.0% w/w of D-sorbitol, both calculated with reference to the anhydrous substance. A clear, colourless, syrupy liquid. Miscible with water and with glycerol.

**USNF 22** (Maltitol Solution). A water solution containing, on the anhydrous basis, not less than 50.0% of D-maltitol (w/w) and not more than 8.0% of D-sorbitol (w/w). Do not store at a temperature below 20°.

**Nomenclature.** Hydrogenated glucose syrup is a generic term encompassing products of widely varying composition and it was concluded that such products containing up to 90% of maltitol should more properly be called maltitol syrup.[1] This was subsequently amended to include products containing up to 98% maltitol.[2] Preparations containing a minimum of 98% of maltitol were assigned the title maltitol.


1. FAO/WHO. Evaluation of certain food additives and contaminants: thirty-third report of the joint FAO/WHO expert committee on food additives. *WHO Tech Rep Ser 776* 1989.
2. FAO/WHO. Evaluation of certain food additives and contaminants: forty-first report of the joint FAO/WHO expert committee on food additives. *WHO Tech Rep Ser 837* 1993.


### Profile

Maltitol and maltitol syrup are bulk sweeteners used in foods; they are considered to be less cariogenic than sucrose. The ingestion of large quantities may produce flatulence and diarrhoea.

### Preparations

***USNF 22:*** Maltitol Solution.

---

## Maltodextrin

Maltodextrina; Maltodextrinum.

**Pharmacopoeias.** In *Eur.* (see p.vi). Also in *USNF.*

**Ph. Eur. 5.0** (Maltodextrin). A mixture of glucose, disaccharides, and polysaccharides, obtained by the partial hydrolysis of starch. The degree of hydrolysis, expressed as dextrose equivalent (DE) is not more than 20 (nominal value). A white or almost white, slightly hygroscopic powder or granules. Freely soluble in water.

**USNF 22** (Maltodextrin). A nonsweet, nutritive saccharide mixture of polymers that consists of D-glucose units with a dextrose equivalent of less than 20. It is prepared by the partial hydrolysis of food grade starch with suitable acids and/or enzymes. White, hygroscopic powder or granules. Freely soluble or readily dispersible in water; slightly soluble to insoluble in dehydrated alcohol. pH of a 20% solution in water is between 4.0 and 7.0. Store in airtight containers at a temperature not exceeding 30° and a relative humidity not exceeding 50%.

### Profile

Maltodextrin, a malto-oligosaccharide, is a source of carbohydrate often used in oral dietary supplements and tube feeding. It rapidly releases glucose in the gastrointestinal tract but because of the high average molecular weight of maltodextrin, solutions have a lower osmolarity than isocaloric solutions of glucose. Additionally, preparations based on maltodextrin and intended for dietary supplementation usually have a low electrolyte content and are free of other sugars such as fructose, galactose, lactose, and sucrose. These properties make such preparations suitable for dietary supplementation in a variety of diseases including certain gastrointestinal disorders where malabsorption is a problem, in disaccharide intolerance (without isomaltose intolerance), and in acute and chronic hepatic and renal diseases where protein, mineral, and fluid restriction are often necessary.

Maltodextrin is also employed as a pharmaceutical excipient.

### Preparations

**Proprietary Preparations** (details are given in Part 3)
***Arg.:*** MC Modulo Calorico; ***Austral.:*** Maxijul†; ***Braz.:*** Oligossac; ***Canad.:*** Moducal; ***Chile:*** Modulo Calorico; ***Fin.:*** Fantomalt; ***Irl.:*** Fibrosine†; ***Israel:*** Maxijul†; ***Ital.:*** Energen; Fantomalt; Maltovis; Nidex; ***NZ:*** Moducal; ***Port.:*** Fantomalt; Fibrosine†.

**Multi-ingredient:** ***Austral.:*** Moducal†; ***Braz.:*** Nidex; ***Chile:*** Nutrasweet; ***Fr.:*** Gumilk; ***Ital.:*** Giflorex.

## Maltose

Maltosa. 4-*O*-α-D-Glucopyranosyl-β-D-glucopyranose.

$C_{12}H_{22}O_{11}$ = 342.3.

*CAS — 69-79-4 (anhydrous maltose); 6363-53-7 (maltose monohydrate).*

**Pharmacopoeias.** In *Jpn.* Also in *USNF*, which permits the anhydrous and monohydrate forms.

**USNF 22** (Maltose). It contains one molecule of water of hydration or is anhydrous. A white, odourless, crystalline powder that has a sweet taste. Freely soluble in water; very soluble in dehydrated alcohol; practically insoluble in ether; slightly soluble in methyl alcohol. pH of a 10% solution in water is between 3.7 and 4.7 (anhydrous form) and between 4.0 and 5.5 (monohydrate form).

### Profile

Maltose, a disaccharide composed of two glucose molecules, is less sweet than sucrose. It is obtained from starch by hydrolysis with amylase. The hydration of maltose depends on the solvent from which it is crystallised. Maltose is often present with other sugars in mixtures used as carbohydrate sources. It is also used as a pharmaceutical excipient.

**Adverse effects.** Hyponatraemia developed in a patient with acute renal failure after liver transplantation following intravenous infusion of normal immunoglobulin in 10% maltose.[1] The effect, which recurred on each of four successive infusions, resembled that of hyperglycaemia and was thought to be due to accumulation of maltose and other osmotically active metabolites in the extracellular fluid.

1. Palevsky PM, *et al.* Maltose-induced hyponatremia. *Ann Intern Med* 1993; **118:** 526–8.

**Precautions.** Preparations containing maltose may interfere with glucose test results. Incidents, including one fatality, have occurred where overestimation of glucose results masked hypoglycaemia, resulting in the inappropriate administration of insulin.[1]

1. Medicines and Healthcare products Regulatory Agency. Medical device alert: ref MDA/2003/011 issued 16 April 2003. Available at: http://devices.mhra.gov.uk/mda/mdawebsitev2.nsf/e8be0ee313c493aa80256bbb00307b2e/78eb05af8601ccc380256d0a0047994e/$FILE/MDA-2003-011.pdf (accessed 19/05/04)

### Preparations

***USNF 22:*** Liquid Glucose.

**Proprietary Preparations** (details are given in Part 3)
***Jpn:*** Martos-10.

**Multi-ingredient:** ***Fr.:*** Picot.

## Manganese

Manganeso.

Mn = 54.938049.

*CAS — 7439-96-5.*

## Manganese Chloride

Manganeso, cloruro de.

$MnCl_2.4H_2O$ = 197.9.

*CAS — 7773-01-5 (anhydrous manganese chloride); 13446-34-9 (manganese chloride tetrahydrate).*

**Pharmacopoeias.** In *US.*

**USP 27** (Manganese Chloride). Large, irregular, pink, odourless, translucent crystals. Soluble in water and in alcohol; insoluble in ether. Store in airtight containers. pH of a 5% solution in water is between 3.5 and 6.0.

## Manganese Gluconate

Manganeso, gluconato de. Bis(D-gluconato-$O^1$,$O^2$) manganese; Manganese D-gluconate.

$C_{12}H_{22}MnO_{14}$ = 445.2.

**Pharmacopoeias.** In *US.*

**USP 27** (Manganese Gluconate). It is either the anhydrous or dihydrate form.

## Manganese Sulfate

Manganese Sulphate; Manganeso, sulfato de; Mangani Sulfas Monohydricum. Manganese (II) sulphate monohydrate.

$MnSO_4,H_2O$ = 169.0.

*CAS — 7785-87-7 (anhydrous manganese sulfate); 10034-96-5 (manganese sulfate monohydrate); 10101-68-5 (manganese sulfate tetrahydrate).*

**Pharmacopoeias.** In *Eur.* (see p.vi) and *US. Br.* and *Fr.* also include the tetrahydrate.

**BP 2003** (Manganese Sulphate). The tetrahydrate occurs as pale pink, odourless or almost odourless, crystals or crystalline powder. Freely soluble in water; practically insoluble in alcohol.

**Ph. Eur. 5.0** (Manganese Sulphate Monohydrate). It occurs as a pale pink, slightly hygroscopic, crystalline powder. Freely soluble in water; practically insoluble in alcohol.

**USP 27** (Manganese Sulfate). The monohydrate occurs as pale red, slightly efflorescent crystals, or as a purple, odourless powder. Soluble in water; insoluble in alcohol. Store in airtight containers at a temperature of 25°, excursions permitted between 15° and 30°.

### Adverse Effects and Precautions

Acute poisoning due to ingestion of manganese or manganese salts is rare. The main symptoms of chronic poisoning, either from injection or usually inhalation of manganese dust or fumes in air, include extrapyramidal effects which may be followed by progressive deterioration in the CNS. Parenteral manganese should be used cautiously in patients with reduced biliary excretion, especially in cholestatic liver disease. When the duration of total parenteral nutrition is likely to exceed 1 month, serum-manganese concentration and liver function should be checked before commencing treatment and regularly during treatment; additives containing manganese should be discontinued if serum-manganese concentrations are raised or cholestasis develops.

**Accumulation.** Cholestatic liver disease, and possibly changes in the basal ganglia, have been reported to be associated with hypermanganesaemia in children receiving long-term parenteral nutrition;[1,2] manganese accumulation may be secondary to impaired biliary excretion.[3] Manganese supplementation in such patients requires re-appraisal and whole blood manganese concentrations should be monitored regularly. A low-dose regimen of not more than 1 microgram/kg (0.018 micromol/kg) daily has been suggested,[2,3] a dose that was also recommended by the American Society of Clinical Nutrition.[4] Hypermanganesaemia and basal ganglia manganese deposition resolved over time in 2 children when the manganese dose in their parenteral nutrition was reduced.[5] Manganese accumulation in the basal ganglia has been observed in patients with liver cirrhosis,[6,7] and may be associated with parkinsonism.[7,8]

1. Reynolds AP, *et al.* Manganese in long term paediatric parenteral nutrition. *Arch Dis Child* 1994; **71:** 527–8.
2. Fell JME, *et al.* Manganese toxicity in children receiving long-term parenteral nutrition. *Lancet* 1996; **347:** 1218–21.
3. Beath SV, *et al.* Manganese toxicity and parenteral nutrition. *Lancet* 1996; **347:** 1773–4. Correction. *ibid.* **348:** 416.
4. Greene HL, *et al.* Guidelines for the use of vitamins, trace elements, calcium, magnesium, and phosphorus in infants and children receiving total parenteral nutrition: report of the Subcommittee on Pediatric Parenteral Nutrient Requirements from the Committee on Clinical Practice Issues of The American Society for Clinical Nutrition. *Am J Clin Nutr* 1988; **48:** 1324–42.
5. Kafritsa Y, *et al.* Long term outcome of brain manganese deposition in patients on home parenteral nutrition. *Arch Dis Child* 1998; **79:** 263–5.
6. Krieger D, *et al.* Manganese and chronic hepatic encephalopathy. *Lancet* 1995; **346:** 270–4.
7. Burkhard PR, *et al.* Chronic Parkinsonism associated with cirrhosis. *Arch Neurol* 2003; **60:** 521–8.
8. Zatta P, *et al.* The role of metals in neurodegenerative processes: aluminum, manganese, and zinc. *Brain Res Bull* 2003; **62:** 15–28.

### Pharmacokinetics

Absorption of manganese from the gastrointestinal tract is variable, ranging from 3 to 50%. There is some evidence that the amount absorbed decreases as intake increases, suggesting a homoeostatic response. In the circulation, manganese is bound to transmanganin, a beta-1-globulin. Manganese is stored in the brain, kidneys, pancreas, and liver. It is excreted in bile, and undergoes enterohepatic circulation.

### Uses and Administration

Manganese is an essential trace element and small amounts of a salt such as the chloride or sulfate are sometimes added to solutions for total parenteral nutrition. Suggested doses are 275 micrograms (5 micromoles) elemental manganese daily for adults and children over 40 kg, and 1 microgram/kg (0.0182 micromol/kg) daily for infants and children to a maximum of 15 micrograms (see also Accumulation, above).

Manganese compounds or salts that have been used in therapeutics in addition to those mentioned above include manganese amino acid chelate, manganese dioxide, manganese gluconate, and manganese hydrogen citrate.

**Human requirements.** In the UK neither a reference nutrient intake (RNI) nor an estimated average requirement (EAR) (see p.1419) has been set for manganese although a safe intake for adults was believed to lie above 1.4 mg (26 micromoles) daily.[1] Similarly, in the USA a recommended dietary allowance has not been published, although an adequate intake has been estimated to be 2.3 mg daily for men and 1.8 mg daily for women.[2] A tolerable upper intake level of 11 mg has also been set.[2] WHO has not proposed a safe range of mean population intakes for manganese since neither intakes resulting in deficiency nor threshold toxicity levels have been established.[3] Diets high in unrefined cereals, nuts, leafy vegetables, and tea will be high in manganese.

1. DoH. Dietary reference values for food energy and nutrients for the United Kingdom: report of the panel on dietary reference values of the committee on medical aspects of food policy. *Report on health and social subjects 41.* London: HMSO, 1991.
2. Standing Committee on the Scientific Evaluation of Dietary Reference Intakes of the Food and Nutrition Board. *Dietary Reference Intakes for vitamin A, vitamin K, arsenic, boron, chromium, copper, iodine, iron, manganese, molybdenum, nickel, silicon, vanadium, and zinc.* Washington DC: National Academy Press, 2001. Also available at: http://www.nap.edu/catalog/10026.html (accessed 24/05/04)
3. WHO. Manganese. In: *Trace elements in human nutrition and health.* Geneva: WHO, 1996; 163–7.

### Preparations

***BPC 1973:*** Compound Ferrous Sulphate Tablets;
***USP 27:*** Manganese Chloride for Oral Solution; Manganese Chloride Injection; Manganese Sulfate Injection.

**Proprietary Preparations** (details are given in Part 3)
***Canad.:*** Micro Mn†; ***Fr.:*** Mangaplexe; ***Mex.:*** MN-Fusin.

**Multi-ingredient:** ***Austral.:*** Bio Magnesium†; Bio-Chromium†; Bioglan Joint Mobility†; Natures Way Total Zinc†; ***Braz.:*** Eviprostat†; Xantina B12; Xantinon B12; ***Fr.:*** Oligoderm; ***Hong Kong:*** Eviprostat†; ***Irl.:*** Ferrotab; ***Singapore:*** Eviprostat; Ferromex†; Neogobion.

## Medium-chain Triglycerides

Triglicéridos de cadena media; Triglycerida Saturata Media.

**Pharmacopoeias.** In *Eur.* (see p.vi). Also in *USNF.*

**Ph. Eur. 5.0** (Triglycerides, Medium-chain). They are obtained from the oil extracted from the hard, dried fraction of the endosperm of *Cocos nucifera* or from the dried endosperm of *Elaeis guineensis*. They consist of a mixture of triglycerides of saturated fatty acids, mainly of octanoic acid and of capric acid ($C_{10}H_{20}O_2$ = 172.3). They contain not less than 95% of saturated fatty acids with 8 and 10 carbon atoms. A colourless or slightly yellowish, oily liquid. Practically insoluble in water; miscible with alcohol, with dichloromethane, with petroleum spirit, and with fatty oils. Store in well-filled containers. Protect from light.

**USNF 22** (Medium-Chain Triglycerides). They are obtained from the oil extracted from the hard, dried fraction of the endosperm of *Cocos nucifera* or from the dried endosperm of *Elaeis guineensis*. They consist of a mixture of triglycerides of saturated fatty acids, mainly of octanoic acid and of capric acid ($C_{10}H_{20}O_2$ = 172.3). They contain not less than 95% of saturated fatty acids with 8 and 10 carbon atoms. A colourless or slightly yellowish, oily liquid. Practically insoluble in water; miscible with alcohol, with dichloromethane, with petroleum spirit, and with fatty oils. Store in airtight containers at a temperature not exceeding 25°. Protect from light.

### Profile

Medium-chain triglycerides are used for enteral and parenteral nutrition (p.1418) in conditions associated with malabsorption of fat, such as cystic fibrosis, enteritis, and steatorrhoea, and following intestinal resection. Medium-chain triglycerides are more readily hydrolysed than long-chain triglycerides and are not dependent upon biliary or pancreatic secretions for absorption from the gastrointestinal tract. They provide 35 kJ (8.3 kcal) per g. They do not provide essential fatty acids.

Medium-chain triglycerides have also been used as bases for pharmaceutical preparations.

### Preparations

**Proprietary Preparations** (details are given in Part 3)
***Arg.:*** Teceeme; ***Austral.:*** Liquigen; MCT Oil; ***Canad.:*** MCT Oil; ***Fin.:*** Liquigen; MCT Oljy; ***Fr.:*** Liquigen; ***Israel:*** MCT; ***Ital.:*** MCT; Mytic 810; ***Malaysia:*** MCT Oil; ***NZ:*** Liquigen; MCT Oil; ***Port.:*** MCT Oil; ***Singapore:*** Liquigen†; MCT; ***Thai.:*** MCT Oil†; ***UK:*** Alembicol D; ***USA:*** MCT.

**Multi-ingredient:** ***Arg.:*** Lipofundin MCT/LCT; Lipofundin MCT/LCT-E; Otocalmia; ***Austral.:*** Caprilon; ***Austria:*** Lipofundin mit MCT; Structolipid; ***Belg.:*** Medialipide; ***Chile:*** Lipofundin MCT/LCT; ***Denm.:*** Structolipid; ***Fin.:*** Nutriflex Lipid; Structolipid; Vasolipid; ***Fr.:*** Liprocil; Medialipide; Structolipide; ***Ger.:*** Gleitgelen; Lipofundin MCT; Lipovenos MCT; ***Gr.:*** Lipofundin MCT/LCT; Structolipid; ***Hong Kong:*** Lipofundin MCT/LCT; ***Irl.:*** Caprilon; Liquigen; MCT Duocal; ***Israel:*** Lipofundin MCT/LCT; ***Ital.:*** Caprilon; Lipofundin MCT; Nutriperi Lipid; Nutriplus Lipid; Nutrispecial Lipid; ***Mex.:*** Lipovenoes MCT; ***Norw.:*** Nutriflex Lipid; Structolipid; Vasolipid; ***NZ:*** Structolipid; ***Port.:*** Lipofundina MCT/LCT; Nutribraun; Structolipid; ***S.Afr.:*** Lipofundin MCT/LCT; ***Singapore:*** Lipofundin MCT/LCT; ***Spain:*** Lipofundina MCT/LCT; Structolipid; ***Swed.:*** Structolipid; Vasolipid; ***Switz.:*** Lipofundin MCT; Structolipid; ***Thai.:*** Lipofundin MCT/LCT; ***UK:*** Caprilon; Imuderm; Lipofundin MCT/LCT; Liquigen; MCT Duocal; MCT Oil; Structolipid.

## Molybdenum

Molibdeno.

Mo = 95.94.

## Ammonium Molybdate

Molibdato de amonio. Hexaammonium molybdate tetrahydrate.

$(NH_4)_6Mo_7O_{24},4H_2O$ = 1235.9.

*CAS — 12054-85-2.*

**Pharmacopoeias.** In *US.*

**USP 27** (Ammonium Molybdate). Colourless or slightly greenish or yellowish crystals. Soluble in water; practically insoluble in alcohol. Store in airtight containers.

## Sodium Molybdate

Molibdato de sodio; Natrii Molybdas Dihydricus.

$Na_2MoO_4,2H_2O$ = 241.9.

**Pharmacopoeias.** In *Eur.* (see p.vi). *Ger.* also includes a monograph for the anhydrous substance.

**Ph. Eur. 5.0** (Sodium Molybdate Dihydrate). It occurs as a white powder or colourless crystals. Freely soluble in water.

### Adverse Effects

Very high intakes of molybdenum, and associated increases in xanthine oxidase activity, may result in hyperuricaemia, and possibly gout. Molybdenum intoxication may impair the utilisation of copper.

**Uses and Administration**

Molybdenum is an essential trace element and small amounts, in the form of ammonium molybdate or sodium molybdate, are sometimes added to solutions for total parenteral nutrition. A suggested dose is about 20 to 120 micrograms (0.2 to 1.2 micromoles) elemental molybdenum daily.

Ammonium molybdate is used in veterinary medicine to treat copper poisoning in sheep.

**Human requirements.** In the UK neither a reference nutrient intake (RNI) nor an estimated average requirement (EAR) (see p.1419) has been set for molybdenum although a safe intake was believed to be between 50 and 400 micrograms (0.5 and 4 micromoles) daily for adults.[1] In the USA, the recommended dietary allowance is 45 micrograms daily for adults.[2] The tolerable upper intake level is 2 mg daily.[2] WHO make the suggestion that the adult basal requirement for molybdenum could be about 25 micrograms daily,[3] corresponding to approximately 400 nanograms/kg.

Foods contributing to dietary molybdenum include milk, beans, breads, and cereals; however, extreme regional variations occur in molybdenum contents of food crops due to soil differences.


1. DoH. Dietary reference values for food energy and nutrients for the United Kingdom: report of the panel on dietary reference values of the committee on medical aspects of food policy. *Report on health and social subjects 41*. London: HMSO, 1991.
2. Standing Committee on the Scientific Evaluation of Dietary Reference Intakes of the Food and Nutrition Board. *Dietary Reference Intakes for vitamin A, vitamin K, arsenic, boron, chromium, copper, iodine, iron, manganese, molybdenum, nickel, silicon, vanadium, and zinc*. Washington DC: National Academy Press, 2001. Also available at: http://www.nap.edu/catalog/10026.html (accessed 24/05/04)
3. WHO. Molybdenum. In: *Trace elements in human nutrition and health*. Geneva: WHO, 1996; 144–54.


**Preparations**

***USP 27:*** Ammonium Molybdate Injection.

**Proprietary Preparations** (details are given in Part 3)
***Fr.:*** Molybdene Injectable; ***USA:*** Molypen.

## Monosodium Glutamate

Chinese Seasoning; E621; Glutamato monosódico; MSG; Natrii Glutamas; Sodium Glutamate. Sodium hydrogen L-(+)-2-aminoglutarate monohydrate.

$C_5H_8NNaO_4,H_2O = 187.1.$
*CAS — 142-47-2 (anhydrous monosodium glutamate).*

**Pharmacopoeias.** In *Chin.* Also in *USNF.*

**USNF 22** (Monosodium Glutamate). White, practically odourless, free-flowing crystals or crystalline powder. It may have either a slightly sweet or slightly salty taste. Freely soluble in water; sparingly soluble in alcohol. pH of a 5% solution in water is between 6.7 and 7.2. Store in airtight containers.

**Profile**

Monosodium glutamate is widely used as a flavour enhancer and imparts a meaty flavour.

In susceptible individuals, ingestion of foods containing monosodium glutamate may result in flushing, facial pressure, chest pain, headache, and nausea. The symptoms tend to occur within an hour of eating 3 g or more of monosodium glutamate on an empty stomach.

**Preparations**

**Proprietary Preparations** (details are given in Part 3)
**Multi-ingredient: *Chile:*** Glutacyl Vitaminado; ***Thai.:*** Hemo-Cyto-Serum.

## Neotame

N-[N-(3,3-Dimethylbutyl)-L-α-aspartyl]-L-phenylalanine 1-methyl ester.

**Profile**

Neotame is an intense sweetener used in foods and beverages. It has between 7000 and 13 000 times the sweetening power of sucrose and is stable to heat.

◊ References.


1. Anonymous. Neotame—a new artificial sweetener. *Med Lett Drugs Ther* 2002; **44:** 73–4.


# Nicotinic Acid *(rINN)*

375; Ácido nicotínico; Acidum Nicotinicum; Niacin; Nikotinsäure. Pyridine-3-carboxylic acid.

$C_6H_5NO_2 = 123.1.$
*CAS — 59-67-6.*
*ATC — C04AC01; C10AD02.*

NOTE. Some published sources use the term niacin as a generic term to include both nicotinic acid and nicotinamide.

**Pharmacopoeias.** In *Chin., Eur.* (see p.vi), *Int., Jpn, US,* and *Viet.*

**Ph. Eur. 5.0** (Nicotinic Acid). A white, crystalline powder. Sparingly soluble in water; soluble in boiling water and in boiling alcohol. It dissolves in dilute solutions of alkali hydroxides and carbonates. Protect from light.

**USP 27** (Niacin). White crystals or crystalline powder, odourless or has a slight odour. Soluble 1 in 60 of water; freely soluble in boiling water, in boiling alcohol, and in solutions of alkali hydroxides and carbonates; practically insoluble in ether.

## Nicotinamide *(rINN)*

Niacinamide; Nicotinamida; Nicotinamidum; Nicotinic Acid Amide; Nicotylamide; Vitamin $B_3$; Vitamin PP. Pyridine-3-carboxamide.

$C_6H_6N_2O = 122.1.$
*CAS — 98-92-0.*
*ATC — A11HA01.*

**Pharmacopoeias.** In *Chin., Eur.* (see p.vi), *Int., Jpn, Pol., US,* and *Viet.*

**Ph. Eur. 5.0** (Nicotinamide). A white crystalline powder or colourless crystals. Freely soluble in water and in dehydrated alcohol. A 5% solution in water has a pH of 6.0 to 7.5.

**USP 27** (Niacinamide). A white crystalline powder, odourless or practically so. Soluble 1 in 1.5 of water, 1 in 10 of boiling water, and 1 in 5.5 of alcohol; soluble in glycerol. Its solutions are neutral to litmus. Store in airtight containers.

## Adverse Effects and Treatment

Nicotinic acid has a vasodilator action and when given by mouth or by injection in therapeutic doses it may cause flushing, a sensation of heat, faintness, and a pounding in the head. These symptoms are transient and various strategies have been proposed to reduce them (see below). Nicotinamide does not have a vasodilator action.

Other adverse effects that have been reported, especially following high doses of nicotinic acid, include dryness of the skin, pruritus, hyperpigmentation, abdominal cramps, diarrhoea, nausea and vomiting, anorexia, activation of peptic ulcer, amblyopia, jaundice and impairment of liver function, decrease in glucose tolerance, hyperglycaemia, and hyperuricaemia. Most of these effects subside on withdrawal of the drug.

Topical nicotinamide may cause dryness of the skin and, less frequently, pruritus, erythema, burning sensation, and irritation. Frequency of application should be reduced if these effects occur.

**Incidence of adverse effects.** Nicotinic acid produces frequent adverse effects, but they are not usually serious, tend to decrease with time, and some can be minimised by following appropriate instructions for use.[1,2] Dermal and gastrointestinal reactions are most common. Truncal and facial flushing are reported in 90 to 100% of treated patients in large clinical trials; they appear to be prostaglandin-mediated and can be reduced with aspirin 75 mg or 325 mg given shortly before nicotinic acid administration, or simply by giving the nicotinic acid with food, and by starting therapy with a low dose and gradually increasing this. Flushing may be less common with modified-release formulations.[2]


1. Knodel LC, Talbert RL. Adverse effects of hypolipidaemic drugs. *Med Toxicol* 1987; **2:** 10–32.
2. American Society of Health-System Pharmacists. ASHP therapeutic position statement on the safe use of niacin in the management of dyslipidemias. *Am J Health-Syst Pharm* 1997; **54:** 2815–19.


**Effects on the eyes.** Retrospective survey of hyperlipidaemic patients suggested that dry eyes (sicca syndromes), blurred vision, and swollen eyelids might be associated with nicotinic acid therapy in some patients.[1] The effects appeared to be dose-related and reversible. In 2 patients treatment was discontinued because of symptoms suggestive of cystoid macular oedema. Three other cases of nicotinic acid maculopathy have been reported.[2]


1. Fraunfelder FW, *et al.* Adverse ocular effects associated with niacin therapy. *Br J Ophthalmol* 1995; **79:** 54–6.
2. Callanan D, *et al.* Macular edema associated with nicotinic acid (niacin). *JAMA* 1998; **279:** 1702.


**Effects on glucose tolerance.** Nicotinic acid can reduce glucose tolerance, and this may be problematic in patients with diabetes mellitus,[1,2] although nicotinamide has been investigated in the prevention of diabetes mellitus (see below).


1. American Society of Health-System Pharmacists. ASHP therapeutic position statement on the safe use of niacin in the management of dyslipidemias. *Am J Health-Syst Pharm* 1997; **54:** 2815–19.
2. Kreisberg RA. Niacin: a therapeutic dilemma—"one man's drink is another's poison". *Am J Med* 1994; **97:** 313–16.


**Effects on the liver.** Hepatotoxicity may occur with nicotinic acid.[1-6] Significant elevations of liver enzymes are occasionally seen with nicotinic acid therapy. They are more common in patients given large dosage increases over short periods of time, and in patients treated with modified-release formulations. It has been suggested[7] that since effects on liver function may in some instances lead to hepatic failure and are more common with modified-release dosage forms the use of crystalline immediate-release preparations should be preferred, a view shared by other commentators.[8] However, although studies appear to confirm a more frequent association of hepatotoxicity with modified-release dosage forms[6,9,10] it should be borne in mind that these effects can also occur with the immediate-release preparations, especially at high doses. Some manufacturers of modified-release preparations have stated that cases of severe hepatotoxicity, including fulminant hepatic necrosis, have occurred when patients have substituted modified-release dosage forms for immediate-release crystalline preparations at equivalent doses. There is also a suggestion that not all modified-release preparations are alike in their effects.[11]


1. Mullin GE, *et al.* Fulminant hepatic failure after ingestion of sustained-release nicotinic acid. *Ann Intern Med* 1989; **iii:** 253–5.
2. Knopp RH. Niacin and hepatic failure. *Ann Intern Med* 1989; **iii:** 769.
3. Henkin Y, *et al.* Rechallenge with crystalline niacin after drug-induced hepatitis from sustained-release niacin. *JAMA* 1990; **264:** 241–3.
4. Hodis HN. Acute hepatic failure associated with the use of low-dose sustained-release niacin. *JAMA* 1990; **264:** 181.
5. Etchason JA, *et al.* Niacin-induced hepatitis: a potential side effect with low-dose time-release niacin. *Mayo Clin Proc* 1991; **66:** 23–8.
6. Rader JI, *et al.* Hepatic toxicity of unmodified and time-release preparations of niacin. *Am J Med* 1992; **92:** 77–81.
7. Palumbo PJ. Rediscovery of crystalline niacin. *Mayo Clin Proc* 1991; **66:** 112–13.
8. Kreisberg RA. Niacin: a therapeutic dilemma—"one man's drink is another's poison". *Am J Med* 1994; **97:** 313–16.
9. McKenney JM, *et al.* A comparison of the efficacy and toxic effects of sustained- vs immediate-release niacin in hypercholesterolemic patients. *JAMA* 1994; **271:** 672–7.
10. Gray DR, *et al.* Efficacy and safety of controlled-release niacin in dyslipoproteinemic veterans. *Ann Intern Med* 1994; **121:** 252–8.
11. Lavie CJ, Milani RV. Safety and side-effects of sustained-release niacin. *JAMA* 1994; **272:** 513–14.


**Effects on the muscles.** Myopathy has been noted with nicotinic acid.[1,2] Rhabdomyolysis has occurred when nicotinic acid was given with lovastatin (see Lipid Regulating Drugs, under Interactions of Simvastatin, p.999).


1. Litin SC, Anderson CF. Nicotinic-acid associated myopathy: a report of three cases. *Am J Med* 1989; **86:** 481–3.
2. Gharavi AG, *et al.* Niacin-induced myopathy. *Am J Cardiol* 1994; **74:** 841–2.


**Hyperuricaemia.** Nicotinic acid decreases urinary excretion of uric acid, which may result in elevation of serum uric acid and exacerbation of pre-existing gout.[1]


1. American Society of Health-System Pharmacists. ASHP therapeutic position statement on the safe use of niacin in the management of dyslipidemias. *Am J Health-Syst Pharm* 1997; **54:** 2815–19.


## Precautions

Nicotinic acid should be given cautiously to patients with a history of peptic ulcer disease, and to those with diabetes mellitus, gout, or hepatic impairment. Modified-release preparations should not be substituted for equivalent doses of immediate-release crystalline nicotinic acid preparations, as cases of severe hepatotoxicity, including fulminant hepatic necrosis, have occurred. Liver function tests and plasma glucose should be frequently monitored.

## Interactions

There may be an increased risk of myopathy or rhabdomyolysis when nicotinic acid is used with statins (see Lipid Regulating Drugs, under Interactions of Simvastatin, p.999). Nicotinic acid may increase the requirements for insulin or oral hypoglycaemics. Aspirin may reduce the clearance of nicotinic acid. *In vitro* studies suggest that colestipol and colestyramine may reduce the availability of nicotinic acid, and some manufacturers recommend an interval of at least 4 to 6 hours between administration of nicotinic acid and bile-acid binding resins.

**Antiepileptics.** For the effect of nicotinamide on *carbamazepine*, see Vitamins, p.357.

**Nicotine.** In a patient receiving nicotinic acid as part of her regular medication, addition of therapy with transdermal nicotine patches was followed by flushing and dizziness after usual doses of nicotinic acid.[1] The patient had experienced such reactions 3 years previously on commencing nicotinic acid therapy, but not subsequently, and it was suggested that on this occasion an interaction might have been responsible.


1. Rockwell KA. Potential interaction between niacin and transdermal nicotine. *Ann Pharmacother* 1993; **27:** 1283–4.


## Pharmacokinetics

Nicotinic acid and nicotinamide are readily absorbed from the gastrointestinal tract following oral administration and widely distributed in the body tissues. Nicotinic acid appears in breast milk. The main route of metabolism is their conversion to *N*-methylnicotinamide and the 2-pyridone and 4-pyridone derivatives; nicotinuric acid is also formed. Small amounts of nicotinic acid and nicotinamide are excreted unchanged in urine following therapeutic doses; however the amount excreted unchanged is increased with larger doses.

◊ References.

1. Pieper JA. Overview of niacin formulations: differences in pharmacokinetics, efficacy, and safety. *Am J Health-Syst Pharm* 2003; **60** (Suppl 2): S9–14.

## Human Requirements

The daily human requirement of nicotinic acid, though not definitely known, is probably about 15 to 20 mg. Yeast, meat, fish, potatoes, green vegetables, and wholemeal cereals are good sources of nicotinic acid and nicotinamide. However they may be present in a bound, unabsorbable form in cereals, especially maize. Nicotinic acid can also be obtained from the conversion of tryptophan in the body, 60 mg of dietary tryptophan being considered equivalent to 1 mg of dietary nicotinic acid, so requirements are influenced by dietary protein intake and if protein intake is adequate there is little need for any preformed vitamin in the diet. There is generally little loss of nicotinic acid from foods during cooking.

**UK and US recommended dietary intake.** In the UK dietary reference values (see p.1419) have been published for nicotinic acid[1] and in the USA recommended dietary allowances (RDAs) have been set.[2] In the UK the reference nutrient intake (RNI) is 6.6 mg niacin equivalent per 1000 kcal daily and the estimated average requirement (EAR) is 5.5 mg niacin equivalent per 1000 kcal daily for adult males and females. One niacin equivalent is equal to 1 mg of dietary nicotinic acid or 60 mg of dietary tryptophan. In the US the RDAs are also expressed in niacin equivalents and are 16 mg daily for adult males and 14 mg daily for adult females; the EAR is 12 mg daily in males and 11 mg daily in females. The tolerable upper intake level for adults is 35 mg daily.[2]

1. DoH. Dietary reference values for food energy and nutrients for the United Kingdom: report of the panel on dietary reference values of the committee on medical aspects of food policy. *Report on health and social subjects 41*. London: HMSO, 1991.
2. Standing Committee on the Scientific Evaluation of Dietary Reference Intakes of the Food and Nutrition Board. *Dietary Reference Intakes for thiamin, riboflavin, niacin, vitamin $B_6$, folate, vitamin $B_{12}$, pantothenic acid, biotin, and choline*. Washington, DC: National Academy Press, 2000. Also available at: http://www.nap.edu/catalog/6015.html (accessed 24/05/04)

## Uses and Administration

Nicotinic acid and nicotinamide, the form which occurs naturally in the body, are water-soluble vitamin B substances which are converted to nicotinamide adenine dinucleotide (Nadide, p.1719) and nicotinamide adenine dinucleotide phosphate (NADP). These coenzymes are involved in electron transfer reactions in the respiratory chain.

Nicotinic acid deficiency develops when the dietary intake is inadequate. Deficiency leads to the development of a syndrome known as pellagra, characterised by skin lesions, especially on areas exposed to sunlight, with hyperpigmentation and hyperkeratinisation. Other symptoms include diarrhoea, abdominal pain, glossitis, stomatitis, loss of appetite, headache, lethargy, and mental and neurological disturbances. Nicotinic acid deficiency may occur with other vitamin B-complex deficiency states, for example in alcoholism.

Nicotinic acid and nicotinamide are used in the treatment and prevention of nicotinic acid deficiency. Nicotinamide is preferred as it does not cause vasodilatation. They are usually given by mouth, the preferred route, but may also be given by the intramuscular route or by slow intravenous administration. Doses of up to 500 mg daily (of either compound) in divided doses have been recommended.

Nicotinic acid has been employed for its vasodilator action in the treatment of a variety of disorders; its value is not considered to be established.

In high doses, nicotinic acid has beneficial effects on blood lipid profiles, and has been used, with dietary modification and often with other lipid regulating drugs, in hyperlipidaemias (see below). For the immediate-release preparations, up to 600 mg daily by mouth in 3 divided doses has been given initially, gradually increased over 2 to 4 weeks to doses of up to 6 g daily; side-effects may be a limiting factor. Alternatively, initial doses of 375 or 500 mg at night have been given as a modified-release preparation and gradually increased according to response to a maintenance dose of 1 to 2 g at bedtime. The daily dose should not be increased by more than 500 mg in any 4-week period.

Topical nicotinamide is used in the treatment of mild to moderate inflammatory acne (see below), typically as a 4% gel applied twice daily.

Nicotinamide has been shown to inhibit the destruction of pancreatic beta cells *in vitro* and is therefore being investigated in the prevention and treatment of type 1 diabetes mellitus (see below).

**Acne.** Topical nicotinamide may be used in the treatment of inflammatory acne (p.1133); nicotinamide 4% was as effective as clindamycin 1% when applied topically twice daily for 8 weeks.[1]

1. Shalita AR, *et al.* Topical nicotinamide compared with clindamycin gel in the treatment of inflammatory acne vulgaris. *Int J Dermatol* 1995; **34:** 434–7.

**Diabetes mellitus.** Nicotinic acid can affect glucose tolerance and should be used with care in established diabetes (see under Adverse Effects and Treatment, above). However, the drug has been used successfully in patients with diabetes. Nicotinamide has been reported to induce remission in patients with newly diagnosed type 1 diabetes mellitus (p.324), and may delay the onset of disease.[1,2] However, a randomised trial found modified-release nicotinamide at 1.2 g/m$^2$ daily (to a maximum of 3 g daily) to be ineffective in preventing the onset of diabetes mellitus in first-degree relatives of patients with the disease.[3] Nicotinic acid can also raise high-density lipoprotein (HDL)-cholesterol concentrations (see below);[4,5] changes in glucose tolerance were mild enough for the drug to be considered as an alternative to statins and fibrates in diabetic patients.

1. Elliott RB, Chase HP. Prevention or delay of type 1 (insulin-dependent) diabetes mellitus in children using nicotinamide. *Diabetologia* 1991; **34:** 362–5.
2. Pozzilli P, *et al.* Meta-analysis of nicotinamide treatment in patients with recent-onset IDDM. *Diabetes Care* 1996; **19:** 1357–63.
3. European Nicotinamide Diabetes Intervention Trial Group. European Nicotinamide Diabetes Intervention Trial (ENDIT): a randomised controlled trial of intervention before the onset of type I diabetes. *Lancet* 2004; **363:** 925–31.
4. Elam MB, *et al.* Effect of niacin on lipid and lipoprotein levels and glycemic control in patients with diabetes and peripheral arterial disease: the ADMIT study: a randomized trial. *JAMA* 2000; **284:** 1263–70.
5. Grundy SM, *et al.* Efficacy, safety, and tolerability of once-daily niacin for the treatment of dyslipidemia associated with type 2 diabetes: results of the assessment of diabetes control and evaluation of the efficacy of Niaspan trial. *Arch Intern Med* 2002; **162:** 1568–76.

**Hyperlipidaemias.** Nicotinic acid is reported to have a favourable effect on blood-lipid profiles, raising high-density lipoprotein (HDL)-cholesterol and lowering low-density lipoprotein (LDL)-cholesterol. Immediate-release preparations exhibit this effect to a greater degree than modified-release preparations (although modified-release preparations may be better at lowering LDL-cholesterol).[1,2] Nicotinic acid was less effective than lovastatin at reducing LDL-cholesterol in patients with primary hypercholesterolaemia, but more effective at increasing HDL-cholesterol; lovastatin was better tolerated.[3] Some have recommended that nicotinic acid be substituted for a statin to lower LDL-cholesterol when patients cannot tolerate a statin, or used with a statin when the reduction in LDL-cholesterol is insufficient.[2,4] The first-line treatment for hyperlipidaemias remains dietary and lifestyle modification; where this fails, drug therapy may be considered (p.823). Nicotinic acid is used particularly in familial hypertriglyceridaemia, or in familial combined hyperlipidaemia when both triglyceride and cholesterol concentrations are similarly elevated.

1. McKenney JM, *et al.* A comparison of the efficacy and toxic effects of sustained- vs immediate-release niacin in hypercholesterolemic patients. *JAMA* 1994; **271:** 672–7.
2. McKenney J. Niacin for dyslipidemia: considerations in product selection. *Am J Health-Syst Pharm* 2003; **60:** 995–1005.
3. Illingworth DR, *et al.* Comparative effects of lovastatin and niacin in primary hypercholesterolemia: a prospective trial. *Arch Intern Med* 1994; **154:** 1586–95.
4. Miller M. Niacin as a component of combination therapy for dyslipidemia. *Mayo Clin Proc* 2003; **78:** 735–42.

**Pemphigus.** Oral treatment with nicotinamide and a tetracycline[1-6] has controlled lesions in pemphigus and pemphigoid (p.1137), including persistent pemphigoid gestationis,[5] and ocular cicatricial pemphigoid.[6]

1. Sawai T, *et al.* Pemphigus vegetans with oesophageal involvement: successful treatment with minocycline and nicotinamide. *Br J Dermatol* 1995; **132:** 668–70.
2. Kolbach DN, *et al.* Bullous pemphigoid successfully controlled by tetracycline and nicotinamide. *Br J Dermatol* 1995; **133:** 88–90.
3. Reiche L, *et al.* Combination therapy with nicotinamide and tetracyclines for cicatricial pemphigoid: further support for its efficacy. *Clin Exp Dermatol* 1998; **23:** 254–7.
4. Goon ATJ, *et al.* Tetracycline and nicotinamide for the treatment of bullous pemphigoid: our experience in Singapore. *Singapore Med J* 2000; **41:** 327–30.
5. Amato L, *et al.* Successful treatment with doxycycline and nicotinamide of two cases of persistent pemphigoid gestationis. *J Dermatol Treat* 2002; **13:** 143–6.
6. Dragan L, *et al.* Tetracycline and niacinamide: treatment alternatives in ocular cicatricial pemphigoid. *Cutis* 1999; **63:** 181–3.

## Preparations

***BP 2003:*** Nicotinamide Tablets; Nicotinic Acid Tablets; Vitamins B and C Injection;
***BPC 1973:*** Compound Vitamin B Tablets; Strong Compound Vitamin B Tablets;
***USP 27:*** Niacin Injection; Niacin Tablets; Niacinamide Injection; Niacinamide Tablets.

**Proprietary Preparations** (details are given in Part 3)
***Austral.:*** Papulex†; ***Austria:*** Direktan; Nicovitol; ***Belg.:*** Ucemine PP; ***Canad.:*** Papulex†; ***Chile:*** Cotina; Niacex; Vectidan; ***Fr.:*** Nicobion; ***Ger.:*** Nicobion; ***Hong Kong:*** Nicobid†; ***Irl.:*** Papulex†; ***Mex.:*** Hipocol; Nacro†; Nicotinoid†; Pepevit; ***Swed.:*** Nicangin; ***Thai.:*** Natinate†; Nicotabs; ***UK:*** Niaspan; Nicam; Papulex†; ***USA:*** Niacor†; Niaspan; Nicotinex†; Slo-Niacin.

**Multi-ingredient:** ***Arg.:*** Antikatarata; Parencias; ***Austral.:*** Bio-Chromium†; Bioglan Cirflo†; Bioglan Fingers & Toes†; Chilblain Formula†; Gingo A†; Prochol†; Silybum Complex†; ***Austria:*** Beneuran Vit B-Komplex; Cosaldon†; Diligan; Pertrombon; Spasmocor; ***Belg.:*** Trihistalex; Vitapantol†; ***Braz.:*** Gaba; Hepato-Flux†; Necrohepat†; Nicopaverina; Nicopaverina B6; ***Chile:*** Perfungol; Ureadin Forte; ***Fin.:*** Neurovitan; Vertipam; ***Fr.:*** Bio-Chrome†; Glutamag Vitamine†; TTD-$B_3$-$B_4$; Vita-Dermacide; Vitaphakol†; Vitarutine; ***Ger.:*** Antisklerosin S†; Eukalisan forte†; Eukalisan N; Hepagrisevit Forte-N; MerSol; Peteha; Telbibur N; Vitreolent plus†; ***Hong Kong:*** Epargriseovit†; ***India:*** Diligan; Hepa-Merz; Sioneuron; Unienzyme c MPS; ***Israel:*** Babyzim; ***Ital.:*** Efargen†; Emazian B12; Emoantitossina; Emopon; Epargriseovit; Flar†; Folepar B12; For Liver†; Fosforilasi; Neuroftal; Solvobil; Vit-Porphyrin; ***Port.:*** Diligan; Ureadin Forte; Vitaphakol†; ***S.Afr.:*** Cosaldon; ***Spain:*** Depurativo Richelet; Espasmo Digestomen†; Euzymina Lisina I; Euzymina Lisina II; Vitaphakol; ***Swed.:*** Histilos†; Theranyl; ***Switz.:*** Vitaphakol†; ***UK:*** Crampex; Epopa†; Quiet Life; S.P.H.P.; ***USA:*** Advicor.

---

## Olaflur *(BAN, USAN, rINN)*

Amine Fluoride 297; GA-297; SKF-38095. 2,2′-(3-[*N*-(2-Hydroxyethyl)octadecylamino]propylimino)diethanol dihydrofluoride.
$C_{27}H_{60}F_2N_2O_3$ = 498.8.
*CAS — 6818-37-7.*
*ATC — A01AA03.*

### Profile

Olaflur is used as a source of fluoride (see Sodium Fluoride, p.1444) in the prevention of dental caries.

### Preparations

**Proprietary Preparations** (details are given in Part 3)
***Fr.:*** Elmex; Elmex Sensitive; ***Israel:*** Elmex.

**Multi-ingredient:** ***Austria:*** Elmex; ***Belg.:*** Elmex; ***Fin.:*** Elmex; ***Fr.:*** Elmex; Elmex Sensitive; Meridol; ***Ger.:*** Elmex; Lawefluor N; Multifluorid; ***Israel:*** Elmex; Meridol; ***Ital.:*** Elmex; ***Neth.:*** Elmex; ***Port.:*** Meridol†; ***S.Afr.:*** Elmex†; ***Spain:*** Elmex†; ***Switz.:*** Elmex.

---

## Ornithine *(rINN)*

α,δ-Diaminovaleric Acid; L-Ornithine; Ornitina. L-2,5-Diaminovaleric acid.
$C_5H_{12}N_2O_2$ = 132.2.
*CAS — 70-26-8.*

**Pharmacopoeias.** *Ger.* includes Ornithine Aspartate and Ornithine Hydrochloride.

### Profile

Ornithine is an aliphatic amino acid. It is used as a dietary supplement.

The aspartate, hydrochloride, and oxoglurate (ornithine ketoglutarate) have been used in various indications including the treatment of hyperammonaemia (p.1421) and hepatic encephalopathy (p.1243).

◊ References.

1. Kircheis G, *et al.* Therapeutic efficacy of L-ornithine-L-aspartate infusions in patients with cirrhosis and hepatic encephalopathy: results of a placebo-controlled, double-blind study. *Hepatology* 1997; **25:** 1351–60.
2. Stauch S, *et al.* Oral L-ornithine-L-aspartate therapy of chronic hepatic encephalopathy: results of a placebo-controlled double-blind study. *J Hepatol* 1998; **28:** 856–64.
3. Rapport L, Lockwood B. Ornithine ketoglutarate. *Pharm J* 2001; **266:** 688–90.

### Preparations

**Proprietary Preparations** (details are given in Part 3)
***Austria:*** Cere; Hepa; Ornicetil; ***Braz.:*** Hepa-Merz†; ***Chile:*** Hepa-Merz; ***Fr.:*** Cetornan; Ornicetil; ***Ger.:*** Hepa-Merz; Hepa-Merz KT; Hepa-Vibolex; ***Hong Kong:*** Hepa-Merz; ***India:*** Hepa-Merz; ***Ital.:*** Ornicetil; Ornicetil S†; Ornil; Ornil KGF; ***Spain:*** Ornicetil†; ***Switz.:*** Ornicetil†.

**Multi-ingredient:** ***Braz.:*** Necroplex†; Ornihepat; Ornitargin; ***Fr.:*** Arnilose†; Epuram; Ornitaine; ***Ger.:*** Polilevo N; ***India:*** Hepa-Merz; ***Ital.:*** Ipoazotal; Ipoazotal Complex; Polilevo; Somatron.

---

## Pantothenic Acid *(BAN)*

Pantoténico, ácido; Vitamin $B_5$. (+)-(*R*)-3-(2,4-Dihydroxy-3,3-dimethylbutyramido)propionic acid.
$C_9H_{17}NO_5$ = 219.2.
*CAS — 79-83-4 (D-pantothenic acid); 599-54-2 (DL-pantothenic acid).*
*ATC — A11HA31; D03AX04.*

## Calcium Pantothenate *(BANM, rINN)*

Calcii Pantothenas; Dextro Calcium Pantothenate; Pantotenato de calcio.
$(C_9H_{16}NO_5)_2Ca$ = 476.5.
*CAS — 137-08-6 (calcium D-pantothenate); 6381-63-1 (calcium DL-pantothenate);.*
*ATC — A11HA31; D03AX04.*

**Pharmacopoeias.** In *Chin., Eur.* (see p.vi), *Jpn, Pol., US,* and *Viet.*

*US* also has a monograph for Racemic Calcium Pantothenate.

*Ger.* also includes Sodium Pantothenate.

**Ph. Eur. 5.0** (Calcium Pantothenate). A white, slightly hygroscopic powder. Freely soluble in water; slightly soluble in alcohol. A 5% solution has a pH of 6.8 to 8.0. Store in airtight containers.

**USP 27** (Calcium Pantothenate). The calcium salt of the dextrorotatory isomer of pantothenic acid. A white, odourless, slightly hygroscopic powder. Soluble 1 in 3 of water; practically insoluble in alcohol, in chloroform, and in ether; soluble in glycerol. Store in airtight containers.

**USP 27** (Racemic Calcium Pantothenate). A mixture of the calcium salts of the dextrorotatory and laevorotatory isomers of pantothenic acid. The physiological activity of Racemic Calcium Pantothenate is approximately one-half that of Calcium Pantothenate. A white, slightly hygroscopic powder, having a faint characteristic odour. Freely soluble in water; practically insoluble in alcohol, in chloroform, and in ether; soluble in glycerol. Its solutions are neutral or alkaline to litmus. Store in airtight containers.

### Adverse Effects

Pantothenic acid is reported to be generally non-toxic.

◊ A report of life-threatening eosinophilic pleuropericarditis associated with the use of biotin and pantothenic acid.[1] Symptoms resolved on discontinuation of the vitamins.

1. Debourdeau PM, *et al.* Life-threatening eosinophilic pleuropericardial effusion related to vitamins $B_5$ and H. *Ann Pharmacother* 2001; **35:** 424–6.

### Pharmacokinetics

Pantothenic acid is readily absorbed from the gastrointestinal tract following oral administration. It is widely distributed in the body tissues and appears in breast milk. About 70% of pantothenic acid is excreted unchanged in the urine and about 30% in the faeces.

### Human Requirements

Pantothenic acid is widely distributed in foods. Meat, legumes, and whole grain cereals are particularly rich sources; other good sources include eggs, milk, vegetables, and fruits.

**UK and US recommended dietary intake.** In the UK neither a reference nutrient intake (RNI) nor an estimated average requirement (EAR) has been set (see p.1419) for pantothenic acid although an intake of 3 to 7 mg daily for adults was believed to be adequate.[1] Similarly, in the USA a recommended dietary allowance has not been published but an adequate intake for adults was believed to be 5 mg daily, increased to 6 mg in pregnancy and 7 mg during lactation.[2]

1. DoH. Dietary reference values for food energy and nutrients for the United Kingdom: report of the panel on dietary reference values of the committee on medical aspects of food policy. *Report on health and social subjects 41.* London: HMSO, 1991.
2. Standing Committee on the Scientific Evaluation of Dietary Reference Intakes of the Food and Nutrition Board. *Dietary Reference Intakes for thiamin, riboflavin, niacin, vitamin $B_6$, folate, vitamin $B_{12}$, pantothenic acid, biotin, and choline.* Washington, DC: National Academy Press, 2000. Also available at: http://www.nap.edu/catalog/6015.html (accessed 24/05/04)

### Uses and Administration

Pantothenic acid is traditionally considered to be a vitamin B substance. It is a component of coenzyme A which is essential in the metabolism of carbohydrate, fat, and protein.

Deficiency of pantothenic acid is unlikely in man because of its widespread distribution in food.

Pantothenic acid has no accepted therapeutic uses in human medicine, though it has been administered by mouth as a nutritional supplement, often as the calcium salt and usually with other vitamins of the B group.

### Preparations

***USP 27:*** Calcium Pantothenate Tablets.

**Proprietary Preparations** (details are given in Part 3)
***Arg.:*** Cidermex; ***Austral.:*** Pantonate†; ***Canad.:*** Calpan†; ***Ger.:*** Kerato Biciron; ***Switz.:*** Pantothen; ***UK:*** Cantopal†.

**Multi-ingredient:** ***Arg.:*** Bifena; Megaplus; ***Austral.:*** Bioglan Zn-A-C†; Hair and Skin Formula†; ***Austria:*** Lemuval; Salbei-Halspastillen; ***Belg.:*** Vitapantol†; ***Braz.:*** Gaba; Luftgaz†; Pantevit; Varizol; ***Chile:*** Foltene Research Anticaspa; Hydrating B5 Gel; Modane; ***Fr.:*** Forcapil; Modane; Thiopon Pantothenique†; ***Ger.:*** Azupanthenol; Carotin; Pantovigar N; Potsilo N; Regepithel; Sonnenbraun†; ***Hong Kong:*** Regepithel; ***India:*** Sioneuron; ***Ital.:*** Esaglut; Lasonil H†; Lasoproct†; Nuleron; Silisan; Vitecaf; ***Mex.:*** Espaven; Modaton; ***Spain:*** Calcio 20 Complex; Hubergrip; Lacerdermol; Lupidon; Pantenil; Pulmofasa; Pulmofasa Antihist†; Tri Hachemina; ***Switz.:*** Cortifluid N; Decasept N; Osa†; Sili-Met-San; ***Thai.:*** Chinta†.

## Phenylalanine *(USAN, rINN)*

α-Aminohydrocinnamic Acid; F; Fenilalanina; Phe; L-Phenylalanine; Phenylalaninum. L-2-Amino-3-phenylpropionic acid.

$C_9H_{11}NO_2$ = 165.2.

*CAS — 63-91-2.*

**Pharmacopoeias.** In *Chin., Eur.* (see p.vi), *Jpn,* and *US.*

**Ph. Eur. 5.0** (Phenylalanine). A white or almost white, crystalline powder, or shiny, white flakes. Sparingly soluble in water; very slightly soluble in alcohol. It dissolves in dilute mineral acids and in dilute solutions of alkali hydroxides. Protect from light.

**USP 27** (Phenylalanine). White, odourless crystals. Sparingly soluble in water; very slightly soluble in alcohol, in methyl alcohol, and in dilute mineral acids. pH of a 1% solution in water is between 5.4 and 6.0.

### Profile

Phenylalanine is an aromatic amino acid which is an essential constituent of the diet. It is used as a dietary supplement.

Phenylalanine intake should be restricted in patients with phenylketonuria (see Amino Acid Metabolic Disorders, p.1417).

**Vitiligo.** There is no totally effective treatment for vitiligo (localised hypopigmentation, p.1137). Oral or topical photochemotherapy with psoralens is generally considered to be the best available treatment, but experimental therapy includes UVA phototherapy with phenylalanine. Use of phenylalanine in doses of up to 100 mg/kg by mouth with UVA/sunlight led to beneficial results in more than 90% of 200 patients with vitiligo.[1] Optimal repigmentation of the vitiliginous macules was noted in early disease, but prolonged use still induced repigmentation in long-standing cases. Repigmentation occurred mainly in areas rich in follicles. Such therapy is contra-indicated in phenylketonuria and in pregnancy.

Similarly a further open study reported responses in 94 of 149 patients receiving 50 to 100 mg/kg daily of phenylalanine plus twice weekly UVA treatment.[2] However, only 22% of responders had repigmentation in more than 60% of the affected area. Higher doses did not seem to be more effective than 50 mg/kg daily. Another group reported on 6 years' experience of treatment of vitiligo using 50 or 100 mg/kg daily of phenylalanine, with application of 10% phenylalanine gel and daily sun exposure.[3] Although not ideal, they considered the treatment useful, especially for its ability to rapidly repigment the face. The same group performed an open trial, adding topical 0.025% clobetasol propionate, and ultraviolet exposure during autumn and winter; 65.5% of patients achieved 100% repigmentation on the face.[4]

1. Cormane RH, *et al.* Treatment of vitiligo with L-phenylalanine and light. *Br J Dermatol* 1986; **115:** 587.
2. Siddiqui AH, *et al.* L-Phenylalanine and UVA irradiation in the treatment of vitiligo. *Dermatology* 1994; **188:** 215–18.
3. Camacho F, Mazuecos J. Treatment of vitiligo with oral and topical phenylalanine: 6 years of experience. *Arch Dermatol* 1999; **135:** 216–17.
4. Camacho F, Mazuecos J. Oral and topical L-phenylalanine, clobetasol propionate, and UVA/sunlight - a new study for the treatment of vitiligo. *J Drugs Dermatol* 2002; **2:** 127–31.

### Preparations

**Proprietary Preparations** (details are given in Part 3)
**Multi-ingredient:** ***Arg.:*** KLB6 Fruit Diet; ***Fr.:*** Revitalose.

## Polysaccharide-Iron Complex

Complejo polisacárido hierro.

### Profile

Polysaccharide-iron complex is used as a source of iron (p.1434) for iron-deficiency anaemia (p.733). It is given by mouth in doses containing the equivalent of up to 300 mg of iron daily.

### Preparations

**Proprietary Preparations** (details are given in Part 3)
***Belg.:*** Ferricure; ***Canad.:*** Niferex†; ***Chile:*** Niferex; ***Hong Kong:*** Niferex; ***UK:*** Niferex; ***USA:*** Fe-Tinic; Ferrex; Ferrex Plus; Hytinic; Niferex; Nu-Iron; Poly-Iron.

**Multi-ingredient:** ***USA:*** Fe-Tinic Forte; Ferrex Forte; Ferrex Forte Plus; Ferrex PC; Hemocyte-F; Niferex Forte; Nu-Iron Plus†; Nu-Iron V; Poly-Iron Forte.

## Proline *(USAN, rINN)*

P; Pro; Prolina; L-Proline; Prolinum. L-Pyrrolidine-2-carboxylic acid.

$C_5H_9NO_2$ = 115.1.

*CAS — 147-85-3.*

**Pharmacopoeias.** In *Chin., Eur.* (see p.vi), and *US.*

**Ph. Eur. 5.0** (Proline). A white or almost white, crystalline powder or colourless crystals. Very soluble in water; freely soluble in alcohol. Protect from light.

**USP 27** (Proline). White, odourless crystals. Freely soluble in water and in dehydrated alcohol; insoluble in butyl alcohol, in ether, and in isopropyl alcohol.

### Profile

Proline is a heterocyclic amino acid. It is used as a dietary supplement.

### Preparations

**Proprietary Preparations** (details are given in Part 3)
**Multi-ingredient:** ***Port.:*** Creme Laser Hidrante.

## Saccharin

Benzoic Acid Sulphimide; Benzoic Sulfimide; Benzosulphimide; E954; Gluside; Sacarina; Saccarina; Saccharinum; o-Sulfobenzimide; Zaharina. 1,2-Benzisothiazolin-3-one 1,1-dioxide.

$C_7H_5NO_3S$ = 183.2.

*CAS — 81-07-2.*

**Pharmacopoeias.** In *Eur.* (see p.vi). Also in *USNF.*

**Ph. Eur. 5.0** (Saccharin). A white, crystalline powder or colourless crystals. Slightly soluble in cold water; sparingly soluble in boiling water and in alcohol. It dissolves in dilute solutions of alkali hydroxides and carbonates. A saturated solution, prepared without heating, is acid to litmus.

**USNF 22** (Saccharin). White crystals or white, crystalline powder. Is odourless or has a faint, aromatic odour. In dilute solutions, it is intensely sweet. Soluble 1 in 290 of water, 1 in 25 of boiling water, and 1 in 31 of alcohol; slightly soluble in chloroform and in ether; is readily dissolved by dilute solutions of ammonia, by solutions of alkali hydroxides, and by solutions of alkali carbonates with the evolution of carbon dioxide. Its solutions are acid to litmus.

## Saccharin Calcium

Calcium Benzosulphimide; Calcium Saccharin; E954; Sacarina cálcica.

$C_{14}H_8CaN_2O_6S_2,3\frac{1}{2}H_2O$ = 467.5.

*CAS — 6485-34-3 (anhydrous saccharin calcium); 6381-91-5 (hydrated saccharin calcium).*

**Pharmacopoeias.** In *US.*

**USP 27** (Saccharin Calcium). White crystals or white, crystalline powder. Is odourless, or has a faint, aromatic odour, and has an intensely sweet taste, even in dilute solutions. Its dilute solution is about 300 times as sweet as sucrose. Soluble 1 in 2.6 of water and 1 in 4.7 of alcohol.

## Saccharin Sodium

E954; Sacarina sódica; Saccharin Sod.; Saccharinnatrium; Saccharinum Natricum; Saccharoidum Natricum; Sodium Benzosulphimide; Sodium Saccharin; Soluble Gluside; Soluble Saccharin.

$C_7H_4NNaO_3S$ = 205.2.

*CAS — 128-44-9 (anhydrous saccharin sodium); 6155-57-3 (saccharin sodium dihydrate).*

**Pharmacopoeias.** In *Chin., Eur.* (see p.vi), *Int., Jpn,* and *US.*

Some pharmacopoeias specify the dihydrate but it may contain a variable quantity of water as a result of efflorescence.

**Ph. Eur. 5.0** (Saccharin Sodium). A white crystalline powder or colourless crystals. It may contain a variable quantity of water. Efflorescent in dry air. Freely soluble in water; sparingly soluble in alcohol. Store in airtight containers.

**USP 27** (Saccharin Sodium). White crystals or white, crystalline powder. Is odourless, or has a faint, aromatic odour, and has an intensely sweet taste, even in dilute solutions. Its dilute solution is about 300 times as sweet as sucrose. When in powdered form, it usually contains about one-third the theoretical amount of water of hydration as a result of efflorescence. Soluble 1 in 1.5 of water and 1 in 50 of alcohol.

### Adverse Effects

There have been rare reports of hypersensitivity and photosensitivity reactions with saccharin.

Saccharin-associated bladder tumours in *rats* given high doses have been the cause of much concern and investigation. However, it is now generally accepted that these findings are not relevant to the use of saccharin as a sweetener in man.

**Effects on the liver.** Elevated liver enzyme values in an elderly woman followed administration of two different medications sweetened with saccharin sodium.[1] Findings resolved on discontinuation of all preparations containing saccharin, and were subsequently found to recur on rechallenge with a small amount of saccharin sodium.

1. Negro F, *et al.* Hepatotoxicity of saccharin. *N Engl J Med* 1994; **331:** 134–5.

### Pharmacokinetics

Saccharin is readily absorbed from the gastrointestinal tract. It is almost all excreted unchanged in the urine within 24 to 48 hours.

### Uses and Administration

Saccharin and its salts are intense sweeteners, a dilute solution having about 300 times the sweetening power of sucrose. They are used in pharmaceuticals and in foods and beverages and are heat stable. They have no food value. The salts are more often used than saccharin itself as they are considered to be more palatable.

### Preparations

***USP 27:*** Saccharin Sodium Oral Solution; Saccharin Sodium Tablets.

**Proprietary Preparations** (details are given in Part 3)
***Braz.:*** Sukir†; ***Chile:*** Sukar-Sin; ***Fr.:*** Sucredulcor; ***NZ:*** Sactabs; Sweetex†.

**Multi-ingredient:** ***Arg.:*** Chuker; Semble; Sucaryl; Suimel; ***Austral.:*** Sucaryl†; ***Braz.:*** Adocante Docura†; Adocyl C†; Belpen†; Finn Cristal; ***Chile:*** Sucaryl; Sukar-Sin; ***Fr.:*** Sucaryl; ***Israel:*** Sucrin; ***Ital.:*** Diet Sucaryl; ***NZ:*** Sucaryl; ***Port.:*** Dulceril.

## Safflower Oil

Aceite de cártamo; Carthami Oleum Raffinatum.

**Pharmacopoeias.** In *Eur.* (see p.vi) and *US.*

*Chin.* and *Jpn* include Safflower, the flower of *Carthamus tinctorius.*

**Ph. Eur. 5.0** (Safflower Oil, Refined). The fatty oil obtained from seeds of *Carthamus tinctorius* (type I) or from seeds of hybrids of *Carthamus tinctorius* (type II), by expression and/or extraction followed by refining. Type II refined safflower oil is rich in oleic acid. It may contain a suitable antoxidant. A clear, viscous, yellow to pale yellow liquid. Relative density about 0.922 (type

I) and about 0.914 (type II). Practically insoluble in alcohol; miscible with petroleum spirit (b.p.: 40° to 60°). Store in well-filled airtight containers. Protect from light.
**USP 27** (Safflower Oil). The refined fixed oil yielded from the seed of *Carthamus tinctorius* (Compositae). A light yellow oil. It thickens and becomes rancid on prolonged exposure to air. Insoluble in water; miscible with chloroform and with ether. Store in airtight containers. Protect from light.

## Profile

Safflower oil is the refined fixed oil obtained from the seeds of the safflower, or false (bastard) saffron, *Carthamus tinctorius* (Compositae). It contains about 75% of linoleic acid as well as various saturated fatty acids.

Safflower oil has similar actions and uses to those of soya oil, p.1447. Emulsions containing a mixture of safflower oil 5% and soya oil 5%, or 10% and 10% respectively, are given as part of total parenteral nutrition regimens.

**Adverse effects.** For reference to the association of lipid emulsion administration, as part of a parenteral nutrition regimen, with the development of sinus bradycardia, see Effects on the Cardiovascular System, under Soya Oil, p.1447.

## Preparations

**Proprietary Preparations** (details are given in Part 3)
***Arg.:*** Lipidos.
**Multi-ingredient:** ***Canad.:*** GLA-130†; Microlipid; ***Chile:*** Liposyn; ***Denm.:*** Liposyn; ***Fin.:*** Liposyn; Novamix†; ***Ger.:*** Abbolipid; ***Israel:*** Liposyn; ***Ital.:*** Liposyn; ***Mex.:*** Liposyn; ***Swed.:*** Liposyn; Novamix†; ***Switz.:*** A Vogel Capsules polyvitaminees; ***UK:*** Efamol Safflower & Linseed†; Epopa†; Exzem Oil†; ***USA:*** Liposyn II; Microlipid.

# Selenium

Selenio.
Se = 78.96.

## Selenious Acid

Selenioso ácido. Monohydrated selenium dioxide.
$H_2SeO_3$ = 129.0.
*CAS — 7783-00-8.*

**Pharmacopoeias.** In *US.*
**USP 27** (Selenious Acid). Store in airtight containers.

## Potassium Selenate

Selenato potásico.
$K_2SeO_4$ = 221.2.
*CAS — 7790-59-2.*

**Pharmacopoeias.** In *BP(Vet).*
**BP(Vet) 2003** (Potassium Selenate). Colourless, odourless or almost odourless crystals or a white crystalline powder. Freely soluble in water.

## Sodium Selenate

Disodium Selenate; Natriumseleniat; NSC 378348; Sodium Selenium Oxide.
$Na_2SeO_4$ = 188.9.
*CAS — 13410-01-0.*
*ATC — A12CE01.*

## Sodium Selenite

Natrii Selenis Pentahydricus; Selenito sódico.
$Na_2SeO_3,5H_2O$ = 263.0.
*CAS — 10102-18-8.*
*ATC — A12CE02.*

**Pharmacopoeias.** In *Eur.* (see p.vi).
**Ph. Eur. 5.0** (Sodium Selenite Pentahydrate). A white, hygroscopic, crystalline powder. Freely soluble in water; practically insoluble in alcohol. Store in airtight containers.

## Adverse Effects

Overdosage of selenium has been associated with loss of hair, nail changes, diarrhoea, dermatitis, garlic odour of breath, fatigue, and peripheral neuropathy.

◊ References.

1. Clark RF, *et al.* Selenium poisoning from a nutritional supplement. *JAMA* 1996; **275:** 1087–8.

## Pharmacokinetics

Selenium compounds are generally readily absorbed from the gastrointestinal tract. Selenium is stored in red blood cells, the liver, spleen, heart, and nails. It is converted in tissues to its metabolically active forms. Selenium is excreted in the urine, and to a lesser extent in the faeces.

## Uses and Administration

Selenium is an essential trace element and is an integral part of the enzyme system glutathione peroxidase; this enzyme protects intracellular structures against oxidative damage. Deficiency of selenium has been associated with an endemic form of cardiomyopathy, Keshan disease, seen in certain areas of China. Selenium is present in foods mainly as the amino acids selenomethionine and selenocysteine and derivatives.

Selenious acid and its sodium salt, sodium selenite, are used as a source of selenium, especially for patients with deficiency states following prolonged parenteral nutrition. Suggested doses for addition to total parenteral nutrition are 31.5 micrograms elemental selenium daily for adults and children greater than 40 kg, and 2 micrograms/kg daily for infants and children to a maximum of 30 micrograms daily. Sodium selenate has also been used.

Selenate and selenite salts are used for selenium deficiency states in veterinary medicine.

◊ References.

1. Rayman MP. The importance of selenium to human health. *Lancet* 2000; **356:** 233–41.

**Administration in neonates.** The low selenium plasma concentrations in preterm neonates have been suggested to be a potential risk factor for neonatal respiratory disorders and retinopathy of prematurity. A systematic review[1] found that supplementation with selenium did not reduce the incidence of these complications, nor is it associated with improved survival. However, it is associated with benefit in terms of reduction in the number of episodes of late-onset sepsis in very preterm infants. There was evidence that recommended doses in this group might be inadequate for some populations.

1. Darlow BA, Austin NC. Selenium supplementation to prevent short-term morbidity in preterm neonates. Available in The Cochrane Library; Issue 2. Chichester: John Wiley; 2004.

**Human requirements.** In the UK dietary reference values (see p.1419)[1] and in the USA recommended dietary allowances (RDA)[2] have been published for selenium. In the UK the reference nutrient intake for adults is 75 and 60 micrograms daily respectively; values are also given for infants and children of varying ages and for lactating women. The UK report also noted that there was no convincing evidence that high intakes protected against cancer or cardiovascular disease; indeed, there was even some evidence that high intakes disturbed selenium homoeostasis and it was recommended that the maximum safe intake from all sources should be set at 450 micrograms daily for adult males. In the USA, the RDA for adult males and females is 55 micrograms daily, and again values are also given for infants and children as well as pregnant and lactating women. The tolerable upper intake level is 400 micrograms daily.[2] WHO have recommended a lower limit of the safe range of population mean intakes of dietary selenium of 40 micrograms daily for adult males and 30 micrograms daily for adult females.[3] A maximum daily safe dietary selenium intake of 400 micrograms was suggested for adults.

1. DoH. Dietary reference values for food energy and nutrients for the United Kingdom: report of the panel on dietary reference values of the committee on medical aspects of food policy. *Report on health and social subjects 41.* London: HMSO, 1991.
2. Standing Committee on the Scientific Evaluation of Dietary Reference Intakes of the Food and Nutrition Board. *Dietary Reference Intakes for vitamin C, vitamin E, selenium, and carotenoids.* Washington DC: National Academy Press, 2000. Also available at: http://www.nap.edu/catalog/9810.html (accessed 24/05/04)
3. WHO. Selenium. In: *Trace elements in human nutrition and health.* Geneva: WHO, 1996; 105–22.

**Prophylaxis of malignant neoplasms.** Selenium supplementation did not protect against the development of new basal or squamous cell carcinomas of the skin in a study of patients with a history of these cancers.[1] However, analysis of secondary end-points indicated a reduced incidence of various other cancers in this study group.[1] Subsequent study has suggested, in particular, an association between low selenium intake and the risk of prostate cancer; incidence was reduced by 63% in patients receiving the supplement.[2] Further follow-up confirmed this inverse association, but found that only men with low baseline selenium concentrations were likely to benefit;[3] trials of selenium supplementation with prostate cancer detection as primary end-points are ongoing. Another group has also reported an inverse correlation between surrogate measurements of long-term selenium intake and the risk of advanced prostate cancer.[4]

1. Clark LC, *et al.* Effects of selenium supplementation for cancer prevention in patients with carcinoma of the skin: a randomized controlled trial. *JAMA* 1996; **276:** 1957–63. Correction. *ibid.* 1997; **277:** 1520.
2. Clark LC, *et al.* Decreased incidence of prostate cancer with selenium supplementation: results of a double-blind cancer prevention trial. *Br J Urol* 1998; **81:** 730–4.
3. Duffield-Lillico AJ, *et al.* Selenium supplementation, baseline plasma selenium status and incidence of prostate cancer: an analysis of the complete treatment period of the Nutritional Prevention of Cancer Trial. *BJU Int* 2003; **91:** 608–12.
4. Yoshizawa K, *et al.* Study of prediagnostic selenium level in toenails and the risk of advanced prostate cancer. *J Natl Cancer Inst* 1998; **90:** 1219–24.

## Preparations

***USP 27:*** Selenious Acid Injection.

**Proprietary Preparations** (details are given in Part 3)
***Arg.:*** Selebound; ***Austria:*** Selen; Selenase; ***Canad.:*** Micro Se†; ***Fr.:*** Celnium†; Plexium; Selenion; ***Ger.:*** Cefasel; Selemun; Selenase; Selit†; Seltrans; ***Hong Kong:*** Selepen; ***Mex.:*** Selefusin; ***Switz.:*** Selenase; ***USA:*** Sele-Pak; Selepen.

**Multi-ingredient:** ***Austral.:*** Vitaglow Selemite B†; ***Canad.:*** Selenium Plus; Vita-E Plus Selenium†; ***Fr.:*** Bio-Selenium; Selenium-ACE; ***Ital.:*** Fosfarsile Forte; Influ-Zinc; Longevital; Neomyrt Plus; Selenium-ACE; Tannidin Plus; ***Port.:*** Rilastil Dermo Solar; Selenium-ACE; ***UK:*** Se-Power; Selenium-ACE†; ***USA:*** Beta Prostate.

## Serine *(USAN, rINN)*

β-Hydroxyalanine; S; Ser; Serina; L-Serine; Serinum. L-2-Amino-3-hydroxypropionic acid.
$C_3H_7NO_3$ = 105.1.
*CAS — 56-45-1.*

**Pharmacopoeias.** In *Chin., Eur.* (see p.vi), and *US.*
**Ph. Eur. 5.0** (Serine). White or almost white crystalline powder or colourless crystals. Freely soluble in water; practically insoluble in alcohol. Protect from light.
**USP 27** (Serine). White, odourless crystals. Soluble in water; practically insoluble in dehydrated alcohol and in ether.

## Profile

Serine is an aliphatic amino acid. It is used as a dietary supplement.

## Sodium Feredetate *(BAN, rINN)*

Feredetato sódico; Sodium Ironedetate. The monohydrated iron chelate of the monosodium salt of ethylenediamine-*NNN′N′*-tetra-acetic acid; Iron (III) sodium ethylenediaminetetra-acetate monohydrate.
$C_{10}H_{12}FeN_2NaO_8,H_2O$ = 385.1.
*CAS — 15708-41-5 (anhydrous sodium feredetate).*
*ATC — B03AB03.*

**Pharmacopoeias.** In *Br.*
**BP 2003** (Sodium Feredetate). A yellow or yellowish brown, hygroscopic, crystalline powder. A 1% solution in water has a pH of 4.0 to 6.5. Store in airtight containers.

## Profile

Sodium feredetate is used as a source of iron (p.1434) for iron-deficiency anaemia (p.733). It is given by mouth in doses of up to 1.42 g daily (equivalent to up to about 205 mg of iron daily).

## Preparations

***BP 2003:*** Sodium Feredetate Oral Solution.

**Proprietary Preparations** (details are given in Part 3)
***Fr.:*** Ferrostrane; ***UK:*** Sytron.

## Sodium Ferric Gluconate Complex *(USAN)*

D-Gluconic acid, iron (3+) sodium salt; Ferric Sodium Gluconate; Iron Gluconate; Natrii ferrigluconas; Sodium Ferric Gluconate; Sodium ferrigluconate; Sodium-Iron(III) Gluconate Complex.
$[NaFe_2O_3(C_6H_{11}O_7)(C_{12}H_{22}O_{11})_5]_x$.
*CAS — 34089-81-1.*

NOTE. Distinguish from Ferrous Gluconate.

## Profile

Sodium ferric gluconate complex is used as a source of iron (p.1434) for iron-deficiency anaemia (p.733).

**Anaemia of chronic renal failure.** For guidelines referring to the use of sodium ferric gluconate complex in patients with chronic renal failure, see under Iron Dextran, p.1437.

## Preparations

**Proprietary Preparations** (details are given in Part 3)
***Ger.:*** Ferrlecit; ***Israel:*** Ferrlecit; ***Ital.:*** Actiferro; Emoferrina†; Epaplex 40; Extrafer; Ferlixit; Ferri-Emina; Ferritin Oti; Ferrosprint; Fevital Simplex; Fisiofer†; Gibifer†; Hemocromo; Inferil; Ipocromo†; Lisiofer†; Rossepar; Rubroferrina; Sanifer; ***USA:*** Ferrlecit.
**Multi-ingredient:** ***Ital.:*** Ferritin Complex.

# Sodium Fluoride

Fluoruro sódico; Natrii Fluoridum; Natrium Fluoratum.
NaF = 41.99.
*CAS — 7681-49-4.*
*ATC — A01AA01; A12CD01.*

**Pharmacopoeias.** In *Eur.* (see p.vi), *Pol.*, and *US.*
**Ph. Eur. 5.0** (Sodium Fluoride). A white powder or colourless crystals. Soluble in water; practically insoluble in alcohol.
**USP 27** (Sodium Fluoride). A white, odourless powder. Soluble 1 in 25 of water; insoluble in alcohol.

## Adverse Effects and Treatment

In the controlled amounts recommended for fluoridation of drinking water and at the recommended doses used in dentistry for caries prophylaxis, sodium fluoride has not been shown to have significant side-effects.

In acute poisoning, sodium fluoride taken by mouth is corrosive, forming hydrofluoric acid in the stomach. Effects include hypocalcaemia, hyperkalaemia, tremors, hyperreflexia, paraesthesia, tetany, convulsions, cardiac arrhythmias, shock, respiratory arrest, and cardiac failure. Death may occur within 2 to 4 hours. Although there is much interindividual variation, a single oral dose of 5 to 10 g of sodium fluoride would be considered lethal in an untreated adult by most authorities.

However, dangerous poisoning has been reported after oral doses of less than 1 g, and the minimum dose that can cause possibly fatal toxicity in children has been suggested to be 5 mg/kg of fluoride ion.

Treatment of acute poisoning involves gastric lavage with lime water or a weak solution of another calcium salt to precipitate fluoride, maintenance of high urine output, slow intravenous injections of calcium gluconate 10% for hypocalcaemia and tetany, and symptomatic and supportive measures. Magnesium sulfate, or aluminium hydroxide may also reduce fluoride absorption. Haemodialysis may be considered.

Chronic fluoride poisoning may result in skeletal fluorosis, manifestations of which include increased density and coarsened trabeculation of bone and calcification in ligaments, tendons, and muscle insertions. Clinical signs are bone pain, stiffness, limited movement, and in severe cases, crippling deformities. Prolonged excessive intake by children during the period of tooth development before eruption can result in dental fluorosis characterised by mottled enamel. At fluoride concentrations in drinking water of 1 to 2 ppm (1 to 2 mg/litre) dental fluorosis is mild with white opaque flecks on the teeth. At higher concentrations, enamel defects become more severe with brown to black staining and the teeth have a pitted corroded appearance.

The fluoridation of water has been a subject of considerable controversy. Suggestions that it increases the incidence of thyroid disorders, chromosome aberrations, and cancer have not been substantiated.

◊ Reviews of the toxic effects of fluoride salts.

1. Fluorine and Fluorides. *Environmental Health Criteria 36*. Geneva: WHO, 1984. Available at: http://www.inchem.org/documents/ehc/ehc/ehc36.htm (accessed 21/05/04)
2. Whitford GM. The physiological and toxicological characteristics of fluoride. *J Dent Res* 1990; **69** (Spec Iss): 539–49.
3. Whitford GM. The metabolism and toxicity of fluoride. *Monogr Oral Sci* 1996; **16:** 1–153.
4. Fluorides. *Environmental Health Criteria 227*. Geneva: WHO, 2002. Available at: http://www.inchem.org/documents/ehc/ehc/ehc227.htm (accessed 21/05/04)

**Carcinogenicity.** Based on comparisons of cancer mortality rates for communities residing in fluoridated and non-fluoridated cities, it was alleged that artificial fluoridation of water might be associated with an increased risk of cancer.[1] Re-examination of this data by others did not confirm the relationship, nor did further studies in a number of countries.[2] In Great Britain, the Working Party on Fluoridation of Water and Cancer[3] found nothing that could lead them to conclude that either fluoride occurring naturally in water, or fluoride added to water supplies, was capable of inducing cancer, or of increasing the mortality from cancer. In this respect, fluoridation of drinking water was considered safe. Further study in *animal* models by the USA National Toxicology Programme[4] found no evidence of carcinogenicity in female *rats* or in *mice* of either sex. A small number of osteosarcomas was found in male *rats* in the medium- and high-dose groups, although the association between sodium fluoride administration and the tumour was uncertain.

1. Yiamouyiannis J, Burk D. Fluoridation and cancer: age-dependence of cancer mortality related to artificial fluoridation. *Fluoride* 1977; **10**: 102–25S.
2. Clemmesen J. The alleged association between artificial fluoridation of water supplies and cancer: a review. *Bull WHO* 1983; **61:** 871–83.
3. DHSS. *Fluoridation of water and cancer: a review of the epidemiological evidence: report of the working party.* London: HMSO, 1985.
4. Public Health Service report on fluoride benefits and risks. *JAMA* 1991; **266:** 1061–2, 1066–7.

**Effects on bone and joints.** Exacerbation of rheumatoid arthritis in a 68-year-old woman was attributed to sodium fluoride given in a dose equivalent to 22 mg of fluorine daily for osteoporosis.[1] An increased risk of hip fracture in the elderly has been suggested as being associated with fluoridated water;[2] another study[3] reported that this association was confined to fluoride concentrations of more than 110 micrograms/litre. However, a large case-control study[4] found no increase in the risk of hip fracture for people ingesting fluoridated water at concentrations of about 1 mg/litre (1 ppm). Similarly, a large prospective study[5] in older white women found no increase in the risk of fractures with long-term exposure to fluoridated drinking water, and even a suggestion of a reduction in the risk of fractures of the hip and vertebrae, due to increased bone mineral density of the femoral neck and lumbar spine, in those women continuously exposed to fluoridation. Use of fluoride, particularly in doses of 40 mg or more daily, may be associated with a peripheral pain syndrome, usually manifested as bone pain in the distal lower limbs, but sometimes involving the upper limbs and axial skeleton. The cause is uncertain: both stress fractures and increased bone growth at the site of pain have been proposed.[6] For comment on the influence of therapeutic doses of fluoride on the incidence of fractures, see below under Osteoporosis in Uses and Administration.

1. Duell PB, Chesnut CH. Exacerbation of rheumatoid arthritis by sodium fluoride treatment of osteoporosis. *Arch Intern Med* 1991; **151:** 783–4.
2. Danielson C, *et al.* Hip fractures and fluoridation in Utah's elderly population. *JAMA* 1992; **268**: 746–8.
3. Jacqmin-Gadda H, *et al.* Fluorine concentration in drinking water and fractures in the elderly. *JAMA* 1995; **273:** 775–6.
4. Hillier S, *et al.* Fluoride in drinking water and risk of hip fracture in the UK: a case-control study. *Lancet* 2000; **355:** 265–9.
5. Phipps KR, *et al.* Community water fluoridation, bone mineral density, and fractures: prospective study of effects in older women. *BMJ* 2000; **321:** 860–4.
6. Jones G, Sambrook PN. Drug-induced disorders of bone metabolism: incidence, management and avoidance. *Drug Safety* 1994; **10:** 480–9.

**Effects on the kidneys.** Nephrotoxicity has been associated with high plasma concentrations of fluoride during anaesthesia with fluorine-containing anaesthetics such as methoxyflurane (p.1304). Elevated fluoride ion concentrations have also been noted in the plasma of patients receiving enflurane or isoflurane, although no clinical effect on renal function was found (see p.1298 and p.1301).

**Fluorosis.** Discussions of chronic fluorosis.[1-3] In a 1994 report, WHO considered that in temperate climates, teeth seemed not to be affected if fluoride concentrations in drinking water were not greatly above 1 ppm; fluorosis affecting bone had not been detected at concentrations of 4 to 8 ppm in temperate regions, although it could occur at concentrations of more than 6 ppm in tropical areas.[4] However, a later systematic review[5] of the effects of water fluoridation, which included 214 studies worldwide, considered that at a concentration of 1 ppm, an estimated 12.5% of exposed people would develop sufficient fluorosis of their teeth to cause aesthetic concern. Swallowing of fluoridated toothpaste by infants may be related to fluorosis of permanent incisors,[6] as may prolonged ingestion of infant formula feeds reconstituted with fluoridated water.[3]

1. Anonymous. Chronic fluorosis. *BMJ* 1981; **282:** 253–4.
2. Mason JO. A message to health professionals about fluorosis. *JAMA* 1991; **265**: 2939.
3. Horowitz HS. Proper use of fluoride products in fluoridated communities. *Lancet* 1999; **353:** 1462.
4. WHO. Fluorides and oral health: report of a WHO expert committee on oral health status and fluoride use. *WHO Tech Rep Ser 846* 1994.
5. McDonagh MS, *et al.* Systematic review of water fluoridation. *BMJ* 2000; **321:** 855–9.
6. Rock WP, Sabieha AM. The relationship between reported toothpaste usage in infancy and fluorosis of permanent incisors. *Br Dent J* 1997; **183:** 165–70.

**Hypersensitivity.** Rash and other hypersensitivity reactions have been reported following use of oral sodium fluoride preparations including fluoride-containing toothpastes and drinking water.[1]

1. Mummery RV. Claimed fluoride allergy. *Br Dent J* 1984; **157:** 48.

**Overdosage.** References.

1. McIvor ME. Acute fluoride toxicity: pathophysiology and management. *Drug Safety* 1990; **5:** 79–85.
2. Gessner BD, *et al.* Acute fluoride poisoning from a public water system. *N Engl J Med* 1994; **330:** 95–9.
3. Arnow PM, *et al.* An outbreak of fatal fluoride intoxication in a long-term hemodialysis unit. *Ann Intern Med* 1994; **121:** 339–44.

## Precautions

When considering fluoride supplementation, allowance should be made for fluorides ingested from other sources; fluoride supplements in children are not generally recommended when the fluoride content of drinking water is over 0.7 ppm (0.6 ppm in the USA) (see also Uses and Administration, below). Care should be taken to prevent children swallowing excessive fluoride after topical application to teeth.

Patients with impaired renal function may be particularly susceptible to fluorosis. Regular dialysis with fluoridated water may result in additional fluoride absorption; a maximum concentration of 0.2 ppm of fluoride in the dialysate has been recommended. Dialysis patients not using deionised water are at risk from changes in the fluoride content of the water supply.

## Interactions

Aluminium, calcium, and magnesium salts may decrease the absorption of fluoride.

## Pharmacokinetics

Sodium fluoride and other soluble fluorides are readily absorbed from the gastrointestinal tract. Inhaled fluorides (from industrial fumes and dusts) are absorbed through the lungs. Fluoride is deposited predominantly in the bones and teeth. It is principally excreted in the urine but small amounts may also be excreted in faeces and sweat. It readily crosses the placenta and is present in saliva, nails, and hair. There is some evidence of distribution into breast milk.

## Uses and Administration

Sodium fluoride is used to prevent dental caries and may be used to increase bone density in osteoporosis (see below). Sodium fluoride is used as a source of fluoride in total parenteral nutrition.

The content of sodium fluoride is usually expressed in terms of the fluoride; 2.2 mg of sodium fluoride is approximately equivalent to 1 mg of fluoride. Each g provides approximately 23.8 mmol of sodium and fluoride.

For **dental caries prophylaxis**, sodium fluoride is used as an adjunct to diet and oral hygiene. It may render the enamel of teeth more resistant to acid, promote remineralisation, or reduce microbial acid production. Fluoride may be administered through fluoridation of the public water supply to achieve a usual fluoride concentration of 1 ppm in temperate regions. The concentration may vary from 0.6 to 1.2 ppm depending on the climatic temperature with the lower concentrations being used in hotter regions where more water is likely to be consumed. Fluoridation of salt at a minimum concentration of 200 mg of fluoride per kg of salt is an alternative.

Alternatively, sodium fluoride may be administered as an oral supplement to children considered to be at high risk of caries. The daily dosage should be adjusted for the fluoride content of the drinking water, for fluorides ingested from other sources such as the diet, and for the age of the child. Guidelines in the USA and the UK both suggest that, where the drinking water contains less than 0.3 ppm of fluoride, children aged 6 months to 3 years may be given sodium fluoride 0.55 mg (equivalent to 0.25 mg of fluoride) daily; those aged 3 to 6 years, 1.1 mg (equivalent to 0.5 mg of fluoride) daily; and those aged 6 years and over, 2.2 mg (equivalent to 1 mg of fluoride) daily. Supplements are not recommended for infants under 6 months of age. When drinking water contains 0.3 to 0.7 ppm (0.3 to 0.6 ppm in the USA) of fluoride lower doses should be considered. Specifically, it is recommended that no additional fluoride should be given to children less than 3 years of age and for older children the above doses should be halved. If the water contains more than 0.7 ppm (0.6 ppm in the USA) of fluoride, supplementation is not recommended. Tablets should be sucked or chewed before swallowing since the topical action of fluoride on enamel and plaque is considered to be more important than the systemic effect. The value of giving fluoride during pregnancy, to benefit the child, is not established. Dental benefits from the use of dietary fluoride supplements by adults are unsubstantiated.

After tooth eruption, local fluoride application is effective. Daily mouth-rinses of sodium fluoride 0.05% (about 225 ppm fluoride) or weekly mouth-rinses of sodium fluoride 0.2% (900 ppm) may be used, but are not recommended for children aged under 6 years because they are unable to effectively spit the rinse out after use. Sodium fluoride 2% (about 9090 ppm) solution is available for topical use, under professional supervision. Fluoridated toothpastes are now widely available and are a convenient source of fluoride. In the UK, the maximum permitted fluoride level in conventional toothpastes is sodium fluoride 0.32% (0.15% or 1500 ppm fluoride); higher concentrations of sodium fluoride 0.619% (2800 ppm fluoride) are available under professional supervision. Low-dose formulations for children under 7 years of age usually contain sodium fluoride 0.11% (500 ppm), and their use should be supervised to avoid excessive use or ingestion. Sodium fluoride has also been applied topically as a varnish under professional supervision. Alternatively, sodium fluoride solutions or gels acidified with phosphoric acid and commonly known as acidulated phosphate fluoride preparations may be used. These preparations are considered to increase the fluoride uptake by the enamel and protect the enamel from demineralisation. For maximum benefit, eating, drinking, or rinsing should be avoided for at least 15 to 30 minutes after topical fluoride application.

Other fluoride compounds used in oral hygiene products and toothpastes include aluminium fluoride, ammonium fluoride, calcium fluoride (p.1423), dectaflur (p.1427), olaflur (p.1442), potassium fluoride, sodium monofluorophosphate (p.1446), and stannous fluoride (p.1448). Other fluorides used in the fluoridation of water supplies include sodium silicofluoride (p.1446).

Sodium fluoride has also been used, like some other fluoride compounds, in rodenticides and insecticides.

**Human requirements.** In the USA dietary reference intakes have been set for fluoride. These propose an adequate intake (see p.1419) for dental caries prevention to be 4 mg daily in adult men and 3 mg in women;[1] lower values are suggested in children and adolescents, depending on age. The tolerable upper intake level is 10 mg daily in adults.[1]


1. Standing Committee on the Scientific Evaluation of Dietary Reference Intakes of the Food and Nutrition Board. *Dietary Reference Intakes for calcium, phosphorus, magnesium, vitamin D, and fluoride*. Washington, DC: National Academy Press, 1999. Also available at: http://www.nap.edu/catalog/5776.html (accessed 24/05/04)


**Dental caries prophylaxis.** References.


1. WHO. Fluorides and oral health: report of a WHO expert committee on oral health status and fluoride use. *WHO Tech Rep Ser 846* 1994.
2. Lewis DW, *et al.* Periodic health examination, 1995 update: 2: prevention of dental caries. *Can Med Assoc J* 1995; **152:** 836–46.
3. American Academy of Pediatrics, Committee on Nutrition. Fluoride supplementation for children: interim policy recommendations. *Pediatrics* 1995; **95:** 777.
4. Holt RD, *et al.* British Society of Paediatric Dentistry: a policy document on fluoride dietary supplements and fluoride toothpastes for children. *Int J Paediatr Dent* 1996; **6:** 139–42.
5. Anonymous. Fluoride supplement dosage: a statement by the British Dental Association, the British Society of Paediatric Dentistry and the British Association for the Study of Community Dentistry. *Br Dent J* 1997; **182:** 6–7.
6. Craig GC. Fluorides and the prevention of dental decay: a statement from the Representative Board of the British Dental Association. *Br Dent J* 2000; **188:** 654.
7. Centers for Disease Control and Prevention. Recommendations for using fluoride to prevent and control dental caries in the United States. *MMWR* 2001; **50** (RR-14): 1–42.
8. Marinho VCC, *et al.* Fluoride gels for preventing dental caries in children and adolescents. Available in The Cochrane Library; Issue 2. Chichester: John Wiley; 2004.
9. Marinho VCC, *et al.* Fluoride toothpastes for preventing dental caries in children and adolescents. Available in The Cochrane Library: Issue 2. Chichester: John Wiley; 2004.
10. Marinho VCC, *et al.* Fluoride varnishes for preventing dental caries in children and adolescents. Available in The Cochrane Library: Issue 2. Chichester: John Wiley; 2004.


**Osteoporosis.** Fluoride has been used in the treatment of osteoporosis (p.763) to improve bone strength by inducing subclinical fluorosis. The predominant effect of fluoride on the skeleton is to stimulate osteoblasts and increase trabecular bone mass. Because antiresorptive drugs cannot restore lost bone mass, this is potentially valuable in the treatment of osteoporosis. However, too much fluoride can increase bone fragility, and the overall effect of sodium fluoride on the incidence of fracture has not been established.

A controlled study in patients with postmenopausal osteoporosis[1] found that sodium fluoride 75 mg daily with a calcium supplement increased trabecular bone mass of the spine but did not reduce the incidence of vertebral fractures. Patients given sodium fluoride also had a higher incidence of nonvertebral fractures. An extension and reanalysis of the study,[2] however, showed that gradual increases in bone mass observed in patients receiving lower doses of sodium fluoride (down to about 40 mg daily) were associated with a decrease in the incidence of fractures. A previous study[3] had reported a beneficial effect in vertebral fracture rate in patients with primary osteoporosis and at least one vertebral crush fracture. In this study sodium fluoride was given in a daily dose of 50 mg; calcium and vitamin D were also given. Interim analysis of a subsequent study using a slow-release formulation of sodium fluoride 50 mg daily taken intermittently with a regular calcium supplement showed a decrease in vertebral fractures of 50% at 2.5 years.[4] At 4 years the beneficial effect was sustained, the main effect being seen in a reduced incidence of new vertebral fractures;[5] no reduction was seen in the incidence of recurrent fractures but this study found no evidence of an increase in nonvertebral fractures. Some consider that low-dose fluoride can be of benefit in established postmenopausal osteoporosis, but the therapeutic window is narrow, and calcium and vitamin D must be given concomitantly to meet the calcium demand and avoid resorption of established bone.[6] A further double-blind study failed to demonstrate a reduction in vertebral fracture rates in women with osteoporosis treated with fluoride, and calcium and vitamin D compared with women who received only calcium and vitamin D.[7] This was despite a significant increase in bone mass density of the spine in the fluoride-treated groups. Fluoride regimens consisted of 50 mg enteric-coated sodium fluoride daily, or 150 or 200 mg sodium monofluorophosphate daily. In contrast, a further 4-year study found a decrease in vertebral fracture rates in women with moderate osteoporosis treated with sodium monofluorophosphate 156 mg daily plus calcium compared with those receiving calcium alone.[8]

A systematic review of 11 studies concluded that fluoride can increase bone mineral density at the lumbar spine, but this does not reduce the rate of vertebral fractures.[9] The authors of this review considered that fluoride should not be used in the first-line therapy of postmenopausal osteoporosis.


1. Riggs BL, *et al.* Effect of fluoride treatment on the fracture rate in postmenopausal women with osteoporosis. *N Engl J Med* 1990; **322:** 802–9.
2. Riggs BL, *et al.* Clinical trial of fluoride therapy in postmenopausal osteoporotic women: extended observations and additional analysis. *J Bone Miner Res* 1994; **9:** 265–75.
3. Mamelle N, *et al.* Risk-benefit ratio of sodium fluoride treatment in primary vertebral osteoporosis. *Lancet* 1988; **ii:** 361–5.
4. Pak CYC, *et al.* Slow-release sodium fluoride in the management of postmenopausal osteoporosis: a randomized controlled trial. *Ann Intern Med* 1994; **120:** 625–32.
5. Pak CYC, *et al.* Treatment of postmenopausal osteoporosis with slow-release sodium fluoride: final report of a randomized controlled trial. *Ann Intern Med* 1995; **123:** 401–8.
6. Anonymous. New drugs for osteoporosis. *Med Lett Drugs Ther* 1996; **38:** 1–3.
7. Meunier PJ, *et al.* Fluoride salts are no better at preventing new vertebral fractures than calcium-vitamin D in postmenopausal osteoporosis: the FAVOStudy. *Osteoporosis Int* 1998; **8:** 4–12.
8. Reginster JY, *et al.* The effect of sodium monofluorophosphate plus calcium on vertebral fracture rate in postmenopausal women with moderate osteoporosis: a randomized, controlled trial. *Ann Intern Med* 1998; **129:** 1–8.
9. Haguenauer D, *et al.* Fluoride for treating postmenopausal osteoporosis. Available in The Cochrane Library; Issue 2. Chichester: John Wiley; 2004.


## Preparations

***BP 2003:*** Sodium Fluoride Mouthwash; Sodium Fluoride Oral Drops; Sodium Fluoride Tablets;
***USP 27:*** Sodium Fluoride and Acidulated Phosphate Topical Solution; Sodium Fluoride and Phosphoric Acid Gel; Sodium Fluoride and Phosphoric Acid Topical Solution; Sodium Fluoride Oral Solution; Sodium Fluoride Tablets.

**Proprietary Preparations** (details are given in Part 3)
***Arg.:*** Fluordent; Fluorogel; Naf Buches; Nafluor; Pentafresh; ***Austral.:*** Fluor†; Flurets†; Neutrafluor; Orofluor†; Phos-Flur†; ***Austria:*** Duraphat; Fluodont; Osteofluor†; Zymafluor; ***Belg.:*** Procal; ***Braz.:*** Fluocaril†; Fluodel†; Fluornatrium; Fluotrat; Novodentin†; Primafluor; ***Canad.:*** Duraflor†; Fluor-A-Day; Fluoridrops; Fluorinse; Fluoritabs; Fluorosol; Fluotic; Karidium; Oral-B Anti-Cavity Dental Rinse; Oro-NaF; PDF; Pedi-Dent†; Solu-Flur†; ***Chile:*** Caristop; Fluocaril Bi-Fluore; Gengisyl; Vitaflur; ***Denm.:*** Bifluorid; Duraphat; Fluorette; ***Fin.:*** Duraphat; Fludent; Fluorilette; ***Fr.:*** Fluodontyl; Fluogum; Fluoplexe; Fluor Microsol; Fluor†; Fluorex; Osteofluor†; Sanogyl; Zymafluor; ***Ger.:*** Duraphat; Fluoretten; Fluoros; Koreberon†; NaFril; Ospur F†; Ossin; Zymafluor; ***India:*** Otoflour; ***Irl.:*** Reach Junior Fluoride†; ***Israel:*** Denticare; Duraphat; Fluden; Fluvium; Teeth Tough; Zymafluor; ***Ital.:*** AZ Verde; Dentosan Extra Fluor; Eburdent; Fluodent†; Fluor Verde; Fluor-In; Fluordent†; Fluorigard†; Fluorvitin†; Oral-B Collutorio Protezione Anti-Carie Fluorinse; Oralsan†; Zymafluor; ***Mex.:*** Audifluor; ***Neth.:*** Dagra Fluor†; Davitamon fluor†; Zymafluor; ***Norw.:*** Duraphat; Fluorette; Flux; ***Port.:*** Fluor-In†; Fluorigard Ortho†; Medusit; Oratol F; Zymafluor; ***S.Afr.:*** Listerfluor†; Zymafluor; ***Spain:*** Fluodontyl; Fluor; Zymafluor; ***Swed.:*** Dentan; Duraphat; Fludent; Fluorette; Top dent fluor; ***Switz.:*** Fluocaril; Fluortop†; Ossin; Ossofluor; Zymafluor; ***Thai.:*** Zymafluor; ***UK:*** Duraphat; En-De-Kay; Fluor-A-Day; Fluorigard; ***USA:*** ACT; APF; Denta Plus; DentaGel; EtheDent; Fluorigard; Fluorinse; Fluoritab; Flura; Karidium; Karigel; Karigel-N; Luride; Minute-Gel; MouthKote F/R†; NeutraGard Advanced; OrthoWash; Pediaflor; Pharmaflur; Phos-Flur; Point-Two; Prevident; SF Gel; Thera-Flur.

**Multi-ingredient:** ***Arg.:*** ADC Fluor; Cal-C-Vita Fluor; Esmedent con Fluor; Fluorexidina; Odol Control Sarro; Odol Med Antiplaca; Odol Tratamiento de Encias; Oral-B Dientes Sensibles con Fluor; Oral-B Enjuague Bucal; Sens-Out; Squam; Tri-Vi-Fluor; ***Austral.:*** Macleans Sensitive†; Oral-B Sensitive†; ***Austria:*** Elmex; Ossiplex; ***Belg.:*** Elmex; ***Braz.:*** Calcigenol Irradiado†; Malvatricin; Poly-Vi-Fluor; Proplax†; Sensodyne Antitartaro; Sensodyne C/Bicarbonato de Sodio; Sensodyne Fresh Mint; Sensodyne Protecao Total; Tri-Vi-Fluor; ***Canad.:*** Cepacol with Fluoride; Oral Plan; Oral-B Anti-Bacterial with Fluoride; Poly-Vi-Flor†; Sensodyne-F; Tri-Vi-Flor; Tri-Vi-Sol with Fluoride; ***Chile:*** Caristop; Kariax; Listermint Con Fluor; Oralgene; Sensaid con Fluor; ***Fin.:*** Elmex; Xerodent; ***Fr.:*** Elmex; Elmex Sensitive; Fluocaril Bi-Fluore; Fluocaril dents sensibles; Fluocaril Junior and Fluocaril Kids; Fluogel; Fluopate†; Fluoselgine; Fluosept†; Parogencyl anti-age gencives; Paroplak; Sanoformine†; Sanogyl; Sanogyl Fluo; Sanogyl Junior; Zymaduo; ***Ger.:*** D-Fluoretten; Elmex; Fluor-Vigantoletten; Lawefluor N; Multifluorid; Natabec F; Ossiplex; Zymafluor D; ***Irl.:*** Listermint with Fluoride†; ***Israel:*** Elmex; ***Ital.:*** Actifluor; Actisens; Aqua Emoform; AZ Junior†; AZ Protezione Completa†; AZ Protezione Gengive; AZ Tartar Control; Benodent; Bifluorid; Broxo al Fluoro; Broxodin; Clorexident Ortodontico†; Dentosan Junior; Dentosan Placca & Carie; Dentosan Sensibile; Eburdent F; Elmex; Emoform-Tat; Eudent con Glysan; Fluocaril; Fluocaril Bi-Fluore; Lacalut; Merfluan Sali Dentali†; Oral-B Collutorio per la Protezione di Denti e Gengive; Ossiplex; Otofluor; Plax; Pronto Emoform†; Ridiodent; Tetrafluor†; Valda F3†; ***Mex.:*** Fluoxytil; ***Neth.:*** Davitamon AD Fluor†; Elmex; ***NZ:*** Luborant†; ***Port.:*** Bexident; Biofluor; Biofluor Sensitive; ***S.Afr.:*** Elmex†; Ossiplex; ***Spain:*** Elmex†; Vitagama Fluor; ***Swed.:*** Bifluorid; Xerodent; ***Switz.:*** Elmex; ***Thai.:*** Poly-Vi-Flor; ***UK:*** Dentyl pH; Listermint with Fluoride; Macleans Mouthguard; Saliva Orthana; Sensodyne Mint; Sensodyne-F; ***USA:*** Adeflor M; Apatate with Fluoride; ControlRx; Florical; Florvite; Mulvidren-F Softab; Poly-Vi-Flor; Polytabs-F; Sensitivity Protection Crest; Soluvite; Tri Vit with Fluoride; Tri-Vi-Flor; Trivitamin Fluoride Drops; Vi-Daylin/F.

---

# Sodium Monofluorophosphate

MFP Sodium; Monofluorofosfato sódico; Natrii Monofluorophosphas; Sodium Fluorophosphate. Disodium phosphorofluoridate.

$Na_2PO_3F$ = 143.9.
*CAS — 10163-15-2.*
*ATC — A01AA02; A12CD02.*

**Pharmacopoeias.** In *US.*

**USP 27** (Sodium Monofluorophosphate). A white to slightly grey, odourless powder. Freely soluble in water. pH of a 2% solution in water is between 6.5 and 8.0.

## Profile

Sodium monofluorophosphate is used as a source of fluoride (see Sodium Fluoride, p.1444) in toothpastes for the prevention of dental caries. It may also be given by mouth in the management of osteoporosis.

In the UK, the maximum permitted fluoride level in toothpastes is 1.14% of sodium monofluorophosphate (0.15% or 1500 ppm of fluoride). Low-dose formulations for children under 7 years of age typically contain sodium monofluorophosphate 0.38% (500 ppm fluoride), and their use should be supervised to avoid excessive use or ingestion.

Other monofluorophosphate salts permitted for use in oral hygiene products and dentifrices include ammonium monofluorophosphate, calcium monofluorophosphate, and potassium monofluorophosphate.

**Osteoporosis.** For reference to the use of fluorides, including sodium monofluorophosphate, in the treatment of osteoporosis, see under Uses of Sodium Fluoride, p.1446.

## Preparations

**Proprietary Preparations** (details are given in Part 3)
***Arg.:*** Osteomar; ***Austral.:*** Fluorocare†; ***Austria:*** Osteopro; ***Braz.:*** Unique Plus; ***Chile:*** Fluocaril Bi-Fluore; Gengisyl; ***Ger.:*** Mono-Tridin; ***Ital.:*** Neo Emoform; Neo Fluostomygen; Oralsan†.

**Multi-ingredient:** ***Arg.:*** Fluocalcic; Hexiben Plus; Negaporosis; Odol Med Antiplaca; Squam; ***Austral.:*** Thermodent†; ***Austria:*** Fluocalcic; ***Belg.:*** Fluocalcic; ***Braz.:*** Fluomint; ***Canad.:*** Sensodyne-F; Viadent; ***Chile:*** Caristop; Gingilacer; Sensilacer; ***Fr.:*** Architex†; Emoform Sensibles; Fluocalcic†; Fluocaril Bi-Fluore; Fluocaril blancheur; Fluocaril Junior and Fluocaril Kids; Fluorocalciforte†; Parogencyl anti-age gencives; Sanogyl; Sanogyl Fluo; Sanogyl Junior; ***Ger.:*** Calcivit F; Fluoril; Tridin; Tridin Forte; ***Ital.:*** Aqua Emoform; Biogreen; Broxo al Fluoro; Broxodin; Calcitridin; Cepacol†; Dentosan Carie & Alito; Dentosan Junior; Emoform-Tat; Eudent con Glysan; Fluocaril Bi-Fluore; Formedico; Neo-Stomygen; Orosanyl; Periogard Plus; Periogard†; Pronto Emoform†; Sanogyl Bianco†; Stomygen; Tetrafluor†; ***Mex.:*** Dentsiblen; Fluoxytil; Periodentyl; ***Port.:*** Periogard†; Sensitive Care†; ***Switz.:*** Emoform-F au fluor; Fluo-calc; ***USA:*** Optimoist; Sensodyne-F.

---

# Sodium Silicofluoride

Fluosilicato sódico; Sodium Fluorosilicate; Sodium Fluosilicate; Sodium Hexafluorosilicate.

$Na_2SiF_6$ = 188.1.
*CAS — 16893-85-9.*

## Profile

Sodium silicofluoride is used as a source of fluoride (see Sodium Fluoride, p.1444) for the fluoridation of drinking water. It has also been considered for inclusion in oral hygiene products.

Other silicofluoride (fluorosilicate) salts permitted for use in oral hygiene products include ammonium silicofluoride, magnesium silicofluoride, and potassium silicofluoride.

Sodium silicofluoride has also been used in insecticides.

---

# Sorbitol

E420; D-Sorbitol; Sorbitolum. D-Glucitol.

$C_6H_{14}O_6$ = 182.2.
*CAS — 50-70-4.*
*ATC — A06AG07; B05CX02; V04CC01; A06AD18.*

**Pharmacopoeias.** In *Chin., Eur.* (see p.vi), *Jpn, Pol.,* and *Viet.* Also in *USNF.*
*US* includes only Sorbitol Solution.

**Ph. Eur. 5.0** (Sorbitol). A white or almost white crystalline powder. It exhibits polymorphism. Very soluble in water; practically insoluble in alcohol.

**USNF 22** (Sorbitol). White, odourless, hygroscopic powder, granules, or crystalline masses having a sweet taste with a cold sensation. Soluble 1 in 0.45 of water; sparingly soluble in alcohol; practically insoluble in solvent ether. pH of a 10% w/w solution in water is between 3.5 and 7.0.

**Incompatibility.** For reference to the incompatibility of sorbitol with hydroxybenzoates, see p.1184.

## Adverse Effects and Precautions

As for Fructose, p.1432.

**Effects on electrolyte balance.** Sorbitol is employed as a vehicle in some proprietary preparations of activated charcoal intended to reduce drug absorption after poisoning; the sorbitol increases the palatability of the preparation and also produces an osmotic diarrhoea that facilitates elimination of the activated charcoal and adsorbed drug. Repeated doses of such preparations are often advocated but a case report has described a patient with end-stage renal failure in whom profuse watery diarrhoea and subsequent hypernatraemia was induced by the sorbitol.[1] For debate about such multiple dose therapy see Poisoning, under Activated Charcoal, p.1031.


1. Gazda-Smith E, Synhavsky A. Hypernatraemia following treatment of theophylline toxicity with activated charcoal and sorbitol. *Arch Intern Med* 1990; **150:** 689 and 692.


**Effects on the gastrointestinal tract.** Sorbitol is often used as a sweetener in sugar-free liquid preparations and the risk of sorbitol-induced diarrhoea associated with such products has been highlighted.[1-3] Chronic sorbitol-induced diarrhoea with associated pneumatosis intestinalis has been reported in a child receiving 21.7 g sorbitol daily in liquid medications.[4]

Colonic necrosis in a renal transplant recipient who received sodium polystyrene sulfonate suspension in sorbitol enemas for hyperkalaemia has been attributed to the sorbitol component.[5] It was subsequently pointed out that the manufacturers' instructions to give a cleansing enema both before and after the resin enema had not been followed and that this complication had never been reported when the product was administered properly.[6] It has also been suggested that sorbitol contributed to the morbidity in a patient who developed septicaemia as a complication of intestinal pseudo-obstruction, following the use of charcoal with sorbitol to treat self-poisoning with theophylline.[7] It was suggested that gaseous distension following bacterial metabolism of sorbitol had rendered the bowel wall ischaemic, facilitating passage of bacteria or of endotoxin into the systemic circulation.


1. Brown AM, Masson E. 'Hidden' sorbitol in proprietary medicines - a cause for concern? *Pharm J* 1990; **245:** 211.
2. Edes TE, *et al.* Diarrhea in tube-fed patients: feeding formula not necessarily the cause. *Am J Med* 1990; **88:** 91–3.
3. Johnston KR, *et al.* Gastrointestinal effects of sorbitol as an additive in liquid medications. *Am J Med* 1994; **97:** 185–91.
4. Duncan B, *et al.* Medication-induced pneumatosis intestinalis. *Pediatrics* 1997; **99:** 633–6.
5. Wootton FT, *et al.* Colonic necrosis with Kayexalate-Sorbitol enemas after renal transplantation. *Ann Intern Med* 1989; **111:** 947–9.
6. Shepard KV. Cleansing enemas after sodium polystyrene sulfonate enemas. *Ann Intern Med* 1990; **112:** 711.
7. Longdon P, Henderson A. Intestinal pseudo-obstruction following the use of enteral charcoal and sorbitol and mechanical ventilation with papaveretum sedation for theophylline poisoning. *Drug Safety* 1992; **7:** 74–7.


## Pharmacokinetics

Sorbitol is poorly absorbed from the gastrointestinal tract following oral or rectal administration. It is metabolised mainly in the liver, to fructose (see p.1432), a reaction catalysed by the enzyme sorbitol dehydrogenase. Some sorbitol may be converted directly to glucose by the enzyme aldose reductase.

## Uses and Administration

Sorbitol is a polyhydric sugar alcohol (polyol) with half the sweetening power of sucrose. It occurs naturally in many fruits and vegetables and is prepared commercially by the reduction of glucose.

It has been employed as a 30% solution as an alternative to glucose in parenteral nutrition (p.1418) but its use is not recommended because of the risk of lactic acidosis.

Sorbitol may be administered by mouth or rectally as an osmotic laxative in the management of constipation (p.1240); doses of 20 to 50 g have been suggested.

Solutions containing about 3% of sorbitol are used as irrigating fluids in transurethral surgical procedures.

Sorbitol was formerly given intravenously as a 50% solution as an osmotic diuretic.

Sorbitol also acts as a bulk sweetening agent. It is used in limited quantities as a sweetener in energy-reduced diabetic food products. It is also used as an alternative to sucrose in many sugar-free oral liquid preparations and in sugar-free foods as it is less likely to cause dental caries.

Sorbitol also has humectant and stabilising properties and is used in various pharmaceutical and cosmetic products including toothpaste.

## Preparations

***Ph. Eur.:*** Sorbitol, Liquid (Crystallising); Sorbitol, Liquid (Non-crystallising); Sorbitol, Liquid, Partially Dehydrated;
***USNF 22:*** Noncrystallizing Sorbitol Solution;
***USP 27:*** Sorbitol Solution.

**Proprietary Preparations** (details are given in Part 3)
***Arg.:*** Progras; ***Austral.:*** Sorbilax; ***Belg.:*** Syn MD†; ***Braz.:*** Minilax; ***Swed.:*** Cystosol; Resulax; Sorbitur†; ***Switz.:*** Syn MD†.

**Multi-ingredient:** ***Arg.:*** Humectante Bucal; ***Austral.:*** Aquae; Carbosorb S; Fleet Micro-Enema; Medevac; Microlax; ***Austria:*** Glandosane; Lemazol; Microklist; Naturaform Fruchtewurfel mit Manna; Resectal; Trommgallol; Yal; ***Belg.:*** Bilagol†; Microlax; ***Braz.:*** Anekron; Biliflux; Biofigado†; Colachofra; Hepalin†; Hepatobe†; Hormo Hepatico; Jecohepat†; Scolybil†; ***Canad.:*** Charac Tol; Charcodote; Microlax; Moi-Stir; Salivart; ***Chile:*** Salivart; Secand; Tabletas Phillips; ***Denm.:*** Klyx; ***Fin.:*** Klyx; Microlax; Somanol + Ethanol; ***Fr.:*** Apilaxe; Arnilose†; Artisial; Exova; Hepacholine; Hepagrume; Hepargitol; Megabyl†; Microlax; Nivabetol; Norbiline†; Ornitaine; Parapsyllium; Schoum; Spagulax au Sorbitol; SST; Vitaphakol†; ***Ger.:*** Artisial†; Dr. Hotz Vollbad†; Flacar; Freka-Drainjet Purisole; Glandosane; Klysma Sorbit; Microklist; Tutofusin S; Yal; ***Hong Kong:*** Aquae; Microlax; Salivart; ***India:*** Alkasol-P; Mecolin; Sorbiline; ***Irl.:*** Luborant†; ***Israel:*** Charcodote; Glandosane; ***Ital.:*** Citroepatina; Macrolax; Magisbile; Norbiline†; Novilax; Si-Cliss†; Sorbiclis; Weight Watchers Punto†; ***Malaysia:*** Microlax; ***Mex.:*** Clyss-Go; ***Neth.:*** Microlax; ***Norw.:*** Klyx; Microlax; ***NZ:*** Carbosorb S; Medevac; Microlax; ***Port.:*** Clyss-Go; Glandosane; Purisole; Vitaphakol†; ***S.Afr.:*** Agofell; Microlax; ***Spain:*** Levaliver†; Polisilan Gel†; Primperan Complex†; Sualyn†; Sugarbil; Sugarceton†; Vitaphakol; ***Swed.:*** Klyx; Microlax; Somanol†; Vi-Siblin S; ***Switz.:*** Agarol Soft; Cital; Glandosane; Microklist; Microlax†; Purisole†; Pursana; Vitaphakol†; Yal; ***Thai.:*** Glandosane; ***UK:*** Glandosane; Luborant; Relaxit; SST; ***USA:*** Actidose with Sorbitol; Glandosane†; Moi-Stir; Salivart.

# Soya Bean

Habas de soja; Soja Bean; Soyabean; Soybean.

**Description.** Soya bean is the seed of the soya plant *Glycine max* (*G. hispida*) or *G. soja*. It is a source of soya oil and soya protein.

## Soya Oil

Aceite de soja; Soja Bean Oil; Sojae Oleum; Soyabean Oil; Soyabean Oil; Soybean Oil.

**Pharmacopoeias.** In *Chin.*, *Jpn*, and *US*.

*Eur.* (see p.vi) includes both hydrogenated and refined oils. *Ger.* also includes a partially hydrogenated oil. *USNF* includes the hydrogenated oil.

**Ph. Eur. 5.0** (Soya-bean Oil, Refined; Soiae Oleum Raffinatum). It is the fatty oil obtained from seeds of *Glycine soja* and *G. max* (*G. hispida*) by extraction and subsequent refining. It may contain a suitable antioxidant and is a clear, pale yellow liquid. Practically insoluble in alcohol; miscible with petroleum spirit. Store in well-filled containers at a temperature not exceeding 25°. Protect from light.

The BP 2003 directs that when Soya Oil, Soyabean Oil, or Soyabean Oil is demanded, Refined Soya Oil shall be supplied.

**Ph. Eur. 5.0** (Soya-bean Oil, Hydrogenated; Soiae Oleum Hydrogenatum). It is obtained by refining, bleaching, hydrogenation, and deodorisation of soya oil. It consists mainly of triglycerides of palmitic and stearic acids and is a white mass or powder which melts to a clear, pale yellow liquid when heated. Practically insoluble in water; very slightly soluble in alcohol; freely soluble in dichloromethane, in petroleum spirit after heating, and in toluene. Protect from light.

**USP 27:** (Soybean Oil). The refined fixed oil obtained from the seeds of the soya plant *Glycine max* (Fabaceae). A clear, pale yellow, oily liquid having a characteristic odour. Insoluble in water; miscible with chloroform and with ether. Store in airtight containers at a temperature not exceeding 40°. Protect from light.

**USNF 22** (Hydrogenated Soybean Oil). The product obtained by refining, bleaching, hydrogenation, and deodorisation of oil obtained from seeds of the soya plant, *Glycine max* (Fabaceae). It consists mainly of triglycerides of palmitic and stearic acids. A white mass or powder that melts to a clear, pale yellow liquid when heated. M.p. between 66° and 72°. Practically insoluble in water; very slightly soluble in alcohol; freely soluble in dichloromethane, in petroleum spirit after heating, and in toluene. Store in airtight containers. Avoid temperatures above 40°. Do not allow to freeze. Protect from light and moisture.

**Incompatibility.** For mention of the compatibility and stability of solutions and emulsions for parenteral nutrition see under Enteral and Parenteral Nutrition, p.1418.

## Adverse Effects

Hypersensitivity reactions including fever and chills have been reported after the infusion of soya oil emulsion although they are considered to be fairly rare. Other rare immediate reactions include dyspnoea, cyanosis, nausea, vomiting, headache, and chest and back pain.

Prolonged or too rapid infusion of soya oil emulsion or its use in patients with impaired fat metabolism has been associated with the 'overload syndrome'. This is manifested by blood disorders such as bone-marrow depression, anaemia, thrombocytopenia, and spontaneous bleeding, hepatosplenomegaly, raised liver enzyme values, hyperlipidaemia, seizures, and shock. Pigmentation of tissues after prolonged therapy with lipid emulsion infusions has also been reported.

Soya protein-based infant feeds can be antigenic and cause gastrointestinal adverse effects in sensitive individuals.

**Bacteraemia.** A strong association has been demonstrated between the administration of lipids through peripheral venous catheters made of Teflon and development of coagulase-negative staphylococcal bacteraemia in neonates.[1] It was suggested that investigation of catheters made of other materials, or other delivery systems, might reduce the opportunity for coagulase-negative staphylococci to adhere and come into contact with nutrient-rich growth media in the form of lipid emulsions. Others also took the view that this work should not lead to the abandonment of parenteral lipids in premature infants.[2]


1. Freeman J, *et al.* Association of intravenous lipid emulsion and coagulase-negative staphylococcal bacteremia in neonatal intensive care units. *N Engl J Med* 1990; **323:** 301–8.
2. Klein JO. From harmless commensal to invasive pathogen: coagulase-negative staphylococci. *N Engl J Med* 1990; **323:** 339–40.


**Effects on the cardiovascular system.** Sinus bradycardia has been reported in a patient receiving total parenteral nutrition that included soya oil-based emulsion via a central line.[1] The authors suggested that it might be wise to administer fat emulsion only through a peripheral vein. However, sinus bradycardia has been reported after a safflower oil-based emulsion given via a peripheral vein as part of a TPN regimen.[2]


1. Sternberg A, *et al.* Intralipid-induced transient sinus bradycardia. *N Engl J Med* 1981; **304:** 422–3.
2. Traub SL, *et al.* Sinus bradycardia associated with peripheral lipids and total parenteral nutrition. *J Parenter Enteral Nutr* 1985; **9:** 358–60.


**Effects on the endocrine system.** Soya bean is a rich source of phytoestrogens including isoflavones, and it has been demonstrated that infants fed soya-based formula have high serum concentrations of these substances.[1] It has been suggested that these may be sufficient to exert biological effects, bringing the safety of soya-based formulae into question. As yet, effects have not been observed clinically, but further studies are needed to assess the short- and long-term effects of soya-based products.[2]


1. Setchell KDR, *et al.* Exposure of infants to phyto-oestrogens from soy-based infant formula. *Lancet* 1997; **350:** 23–7.
2. Essex C. Phytoestrogens and soy based infant formula. *BMJ* 1996; **313:** 507–8.


**Effects on the nervous system.** CNS disorders in 2 patients receiving infusions of fractionated soya emulsion included convulsions, coma, and cortical blindness in one young woman.[1] A similar case was attributed to fat embolism,[2] but, occurring after what the manufacturers pointed out was a faster than recommended infusion,[3] may perhaps have represented a fat-overload syndrome.


1. Jellinek EH. Dangers of intravenous fat infusions. *Lancet* 1976; **ii:** 967.
2. Estebe JP, Malledant Y. Fat embolism after lipid emulsion infusion. *Lancet* 1991; **337:** 673.
3. McCracken M. Fat embolism after lipid emulsion infusion. *Lancet* 1991; **337:** 983.


**Hypersensitivity.** Urticaria has been reported in 2 patients following the administration intravenously of soya oil emulsions.[1,2] In one case the patient had previously received the emulsion for 19 days without ill-effect.[1]

Anaphylactic reactions have been documented after the ingestion of several foods or foodstuffs containing, or prepared from, soya beans, although the exact allergen remains unknown. In one patient who suffered anaphylactic attacks after eating such products a specific IgE-antibody response to the allergen Kunitz soybean trypsin inhibitor was demonstrated.[3] This was not, however, the only allergen present in soya beans as other patients who had a negative response to this allergen had positive responses in whole soya bean tests.

IgE antibodies to soya bean antigens have also been found in workers who suffered from asthma after handling soya beans[4,5] leading to the suggestion that an allergic mechanism had been responsible; the asthma was believed to have been due to the dust released during the handling of the beans.


1. Kamath KR, *et al.* Acute hypersensitivity reaction to Intralipid. *N Engl J Med* 1981; **304:** 360.
2. Hiyama DT, *et al.* Hypersensitivity following lipid emulsion infusion in an adult patient. *J Parenter Enteral Nutr* 1989; **13:** 318–20.
3. Moroz LA, Yang WH. Kunitz soybean trypsin inhibitor: a specific allergen in food anaphylaxis. *N Engl J Med* 1980; **302:** 1126–8.
4. Sunyer J, *et al.* Case-control study of serum immunoglobulin-E antibodies reactive with soybean in epidemic asthma. *Lancet* 1989; **i:** 179–82.
5. Hernando L, *et al.* Asthma epidemics and soybean in Cartagena (Spain). *Lancet* 1989; **i:** 502.


**Pulmonary fat emboli.** Pulmonary fat emboli or microemboli, sometimes fatal, have occurred in several infants who received infusions of fat emulsions based on soya oil.[1-3]

In one case[3] the patient's serum, which contained a high concentration of C-reactive protein, agglutinated the fat emulsion and this finding was considered to support the hypothesis that microemboli are formed by agglutination of fat emulsion in the blood by C-reactive protein. The authors of this report did not consider the precise pathogenesis to be clear, nor did they know whether the condition was preventable, but did suggest that it may be prudent either to ensure that the C-reactive protein concentration was normal (less than 10 mg/litre) or to perform a creaming test to determine which babies may embolise the infused fat emulsion. However, other studies,[4] while not excluding a role of C-reactive protein in agglutination, have failed to find any correlation between raised concentrations of this protein and the rate of agglutination.


1. Barson AJ, *et al.* Fat embolism in infancy after intravenous fat infusions. *Arch Dis Child* 1978; **53:** 218–23.
2. Levene MI, *et al.* Pulmonary fat accumulation after Intralipid infusion in the preterm infant. *Lancet* 1980; **ii:** 815–8.
3. Hulman G, Levene M. Intralipid microemboli. *Arch Dis Child* 1986; **61:** 702–3.
4. Zagara G, *et al.* C-reactive protein and serum agglutination in vivo of intravenous fat emulsions. *Lancet* 1989; **i:** 733.


## Precautions

Intravenous soya oil emulsion should not be given to patients with severe liver disease, acute shock, or severe or pathological hyperlipidaemia, or when the ability to metabolise fat may otherwise be impaired. Caution has also been advised in patients with pulmonary disease, renal insufficiency, uncompensated diabetes mellitus, hyperthyroidism, sepsis, and some disorders of blood coagulation. If given to such patients, the elimination of fat should be monitored daily.

Intravenous soya oil emulsion may interfere with some laboratory tests if blood is taken before fat has adequately cleared; this may take 4 to 6 hours.

Egg-yolk phospholipids may be used as emulsifiers in some preparations, which should not be given to patients with severe egg allergy.

Fat emulsions may extract phthalate plasticisers from administration bags and sets and non-phthalate containing equipment should be used wherever possible.

Soya-based infant feeds should be avoided in infants with documented cows' milk protein-induced enteropathy or enterocolitis, as these infants are frequently also sensitive to soya protein.

**Neonatal hyperbilirubinaemia.** In neonates with hyperbilirubinaemia, intravenous lipid emulsions should be used with caution because of the risk of displacing bilirubin from albumin. The risk appears to be higher in preterm infants,[1] at higher doses,[1] and with intermittent rather than continuous dosing.[2]

1. Spear ML, *et al.* The effect of 15-hour fat infusions of varying dosage on bilirubin binding to albumin. *J Parenter Enteral Nutr* 1985; **9:** 144–7.
2. Brans YW, *et al.* Influence of intravenous fat emulsion on serum bilirubin in very low birthweight neonates. *Arch Dis Child* 1987; **62:** 156–60.

## Uses and Administration

Emulsions of fractionated soya oil containing 10, 20, or 30% are given by slow intravenous infusion as part of total parenteral nutrition regimens (p.1418), usually with amino acid and carbohydrate solutions. The solutions and emulsions may be administered at separate sites, given at the same site through a Y-connector, or combined in one admixture. Fat emulsions provide a high energy intake in a relatively small volume. They may also be used to prevent or correct essential fatty acid deficiency. When used as a calorie source the dose of the emulsion is determined by the energy requirements and clinical status of the patient; the amount, generally, should not comprise more than 60% of patients' total calorie intake. For the prevention and correction of fatty acid deficiency about 5 to 10% of total calorific intake should be as an intravenous fat emulsion.

The composition and dosage recommendations of commercial preparations do differ slightly but they should be started slowly. Suggested initial rates for the 10% and 20% products are 1 mL/minute and 0.5 mL/minute respectively for 15 to 30 minutes. The rate may then be increased and up to about 500 mL (or 10 mL/kg) of 10% or 250 mL (or 5 mL/kg) of 20% emulsion may be given on the first day. The total daily dosage may then be increased gradually on subsequent days; suggested daily dose ranges are 500 to 1500 mL of a 10% or 500 to 1000 mL of a 20% emulsion and suggested rates of administration are 500 mL of a 10% emulsion over a period of not less than 3 hours, and 500 mL of a 20% emulsion over not less than 5 hours. Where a 30% emulsion is used, a dose of 333 mL or about 4.75 mL/kg has been recommended, given over 5 hours or more; the first dose should not exceed 3 mL/kg.

Soya oil also has emollient properties and is used as a bath additive in the treatment of dry skin conditions.

Preparations made from whole soya beans, containing soya oil and soya protein, are used as the basis of lactose-free vegetable milks for infants and patients with lactose or similar disaccharide intolerance or with an allergy to cows' milk protein (see also below).

**Administration.** It has been suggested[1] that it is the concentration of phospholipid solubilisers, and particularly the excess present as free phospholipid liposomes, that determines the effect of lipid emulsions on plasma-lipid concentrations. In 20 premature infants requiring parenteral nutrition, infusion of up to 4 g/kg of fat daily as a 20% emulsion (twice the usual maximum dose) had less effect on plasma lipid concentrations than 2 g/kg daily as a 10% emulsion; the difference was thought to be due to the fact that the 20% emulsion was relatively liposome-poor, with a ratio of phospholipids to triglycerides of 0.06, whereas the liposome-rich 10% emulsion had a ratio of 0.12. The authors suggested that the 10% emulsion should not be used in preterm infants. Others noted similar results;[2] a 10% lipid emulsion with a reduced phospholipid content has, however, been reported to be relatively well tolerated in premature infants.[3]

For mention of the risk of kernicterus if lipid infusions are given to hyperbilirubinaemic neonates, see under Precautions, above.

1. Haumont D, *et al.* Effect of liposomal content of lipid emulsions on plasma lipid concentrations in low birth weight infants receiving parenteral nutrition. *J Pediatr* 1992; **121:** 759–63.
2. Cairns PA, *et al.* Tolerance of mixed lipid emulsion in neonates: effect of concentration. *Arch Dis Child Fetal Neonatal Ed* 1996; **75:** F113–F116.
3. Gohlke BC, *et al.* Serum lipids during parenteral nutrition with a 10% lipid emulsion with reduced phospholipid emulsifier content in premature infants. *J Pediatr Endocrinol Metab* 1997; **10:** 505–9.

**Food intolerance.** The American Academy of Pediatrics has recommended[1] that soya-based infant feeds are appropriate for use in galactosaemia and hereditary lactase deficiency, and documented allergy to cows' milk protein. However, infants with documented cows' milk protein enteropathy or enterocolitis should receive hydrolysed protein formula, as they are likely to be sensitive to soya protein. They concluded that soya-based infant feeds have no proven role in the prevention of atopic disease or in the management of infantile colic.

The FDA has warned against the use of soya-based drinks intended for adults as the sole source for nutrition for infants.[2] It was stated that soya drinks can lead to severe protein and calorie malnutrition, multiple vitamin and mineral deficiency, and death in infants who receive no other source of nourishment, and should not be confused with soya-based infant formulas, which are specially formulated to meet the nutritional needs of infants.

For reference to the use of soya-based foods themselves causing allergic reactions, see under Hypersensitivity, above.

1. American Academy of Pediatrics. Soy protein-based formulas: recommendations for use in infant feeding. *Pediatrics* 1998; **101:** 148–53.
2. Nightingale S. Warnings issued about practices, products: soy drink warning. *JAMA* 1985; **254:** 1428.

**Hyperlipidaemias.** Soya protein has been tried in the treatment of hyperlipidaemia (p.823). Soya isoflavones such as genistein (p.1692) and daidzein are able to mimic oestrogen and may therefore have a beneficial effect on blood lipids.[1,2] Other constituents of soya protein, including fytic acid and saponins may also contribute to this, and some authorities consider that intact soya protein will provide the maximum cholesterol-lowering effect.[2] A meta-analysis of controlled trials found that the substitution of soya protein for animal protein in the diet resulted in significant decreases in serum total cholesterol, low-density lipoprotein (LDL)-cholesterol, and triglyceride concentrations.[3] A subsequent systematic review of studies reached similar conclusions,[1] and the FDA considers that a low-fat diet including 25 g daily of soya protein may reduce the risk of ischaemic heart disease.[2] Soya protein does not appear to have a cholesterol-lowering effect in subjects with normal cholesterol concentrations,[2] although a small study found it to be beneficial in type 2 diabetes patients with near-normal lipid concentrations.[4]

1. Costa RL, Summa MA. Soy protein in the management of hyperlipidemia. *Ann Pharmacother* 2000; **34:** 931–5.
2. Erdman JW. Soy protein and cardiovascular disease: a statement for healthcare professionals from the Nutrition Committee of the AHA. *Circulation* 2000; **102:** 2555–9.
3. Anderson JW, *et al.* Meta-analysis of the effects of soy protein intake on serum lipids. *N Engl J Med* 1995; **333:** 276–82.
4. Hermansen K, *et al.* Beneficial effects of a soy-based dietary supplement on lipid levels and cardiovascular risk markers in type 2 diabetic subjects. *Diabetes Care* 2001; **24:** 228–33.

**Menopausal disorders.** Soya contains isoflavones, in particular genistein (p.1692) and daidzein, which have been investigated for their oestrogen-modulating effects in the treatment of menopausal symptoms (p.1540).[1] A small reduction in the incidence of hot flushes has been noted.[2] Isoflavones may have a beneficial effect on cholesterol and lipid concentrations (see above). Some epidemiological studies and *animal* data suggest that they may also provide protection against breast cancer.[1] However, phytoestrogens could also stimulate breast tumour growth due to oestrogenic activity. These stimulating and inhibitory effects may be concentration-dependent; soya products contain only small amounts of phytoestrogens and it may be difficult to consume enough soy to have any beneficial effect on breast cancer growth.[3] A few small studies have shown that soya isoflavones can decrease bone turnover, leading to speculation that they could be used to prevent osteoporosis (p.763).[1] The effects of these isoflavones should be investigated in larger trials before they can be recommended as alternatives to conventional HRT.[3,4]

1. Vincent A, Fitzpatrick LA. Soy isoflavones: are they useful in menopause? *Mayo Clin Proc* 2000; **75:** 1174–84.
2. Upmalis DH, *et al.* Vasomotor symptom relief by soy isoflavone extract tablets in postmenopausal women: a multicenter, double-blind, randomized, placebo-controlled study. *Menopause* 2000; **7:** 236–42. Correction. *ibid.*; 422.
3. de Lemos ML. Effects of soy phytoestrogens genistein and daidzein on breast cancer growth. *Ann Pharmacother* 2001; **35:** 1118–21.
4. Anonymous. The role of isoflavones in menopausal health: consensus opinion of the North American Menopause Society. *Menopause* 2000; **7:** 215–29.

## Preparations

**Proprietary Preparations** (details are given in Part 3)
***Arg.:*** Lipofundin N; Lipovenos; Sojar Men; Sojar Pro; Soyacal; ***Austral.:*** Intralipid; Ivelip; ***Austria:*** Balneum; Elolipid; Intralipid; Lipofundin; Lipovenos; Olbad Cordes; Solipid†; ***Belg.:*** Intralipid†; Ivelip†; Lipovenoes†; ***Braz.:*** Endolipid; Lipofundin S†; Lipovenos†; ***Canad.:*** Intralipid; ***Chile:*** Lipofundin; ***Denm.:*** Intralipid; Lipofundin†; Lipovenos†; Vasolipid†; ***Fin.:*** Intralipid; ***Fr.:*** Endolipide; Gydrelle Phyto; Gynalpha; Intralipide; Ivelip; Lipoven†; ***Ger.:*** Allergika; Balneoconzen N; Balneovit; Balneum; Deltalipid; Eucerin Omega Fettsauren Olbad; Hoecutin Olbad†; Intralipid; Kneipp Neurodermatitis-Bad†; Lipofundin N; Lipopharm; Lipovenos; Olbad Cordes; Penatoel; salvilipid; ***Gr.:*** Clinomel; Lipovenoes; Nutriflex Lipid; ***Hong Kong:*** Intralipid; Lipofundin N; Phyto-Care; ***Irl.:*** Balneum; Intralipid; Lipofundin S†; ***Israel:*** Balneum; Intralipid; Ivelip; ***Ital.:*** Balneum Hermal; Elolipid; Intralipid; Ivelip; Lipofundin S; Lipovenos; Soyacal; ***Jpn:*** Intrafat; ***Malaysia:*** Intralipid; ***Mex.:*** Ivelip; Lipovenoes; ***Mon.:*** Evestrel; ***Neth.:*** Intralipid; ***Norw.:*** Intralipid; Lipovenos†; ***NZ:*** Intralipid; ***Port.:*** Balneum†; Banholeum; Emulsao de Lipidos; Intralipid; Lipovenoes; ***S.Afr.:*** Intralipid†; ***Singapore:*** Intralipid; Intralipos; ***Spain:*** Flavodrei; Ivelip; Lipovenos; Soyacal; ***Swed.:*** Intralipid; Lipovenos; ***Switz.:*** Balneum Hermal; Intralipid; Lipidem†; Lipovenos; ***Thai.:*** Intralipid; Lipofundin S; Lipovenoes; ***UK:*** Balneum; Intralipid; Ivelip; Lipofundin; Lipovenos†; ***USA:*** Intralipid; Liposyn III.

**Multi-ingredient:** ***Arg.:*** Clinoleic; Derrumal; Lipofundin MCT/LCT; Lipofundin MCT/LCT-E; ***Austral.:*** Bioglan Mens Super Soy/Clover†; Bioglan Soy Power Plus†; Extralife Meno-Care†; Hypol†; Lifechange Menopause Formula†; Phytolife†; Soy Forte with Block Cohosh†; ***Austria:*** Badeol; Balneum mit Teer; Balneum Plus; Clinoleic; Clinomel; Compleven; Gesamtnahrlosung; KabiMix; Kabiven; Lipofundin mit MCT; Nutriflex Lipid; Olbad Cordes comp; Oleosint; PE-Mix; Structolipid; TriMix; ***Belg.:*** Clinoleic†; Clinomel†; Medialipide; ***Braz.:*** Piascledine; ***Chile:*** Lipofundin MCT/LCT; Liposyn; ***Denm.:*** Clinoleic; Kabiven; Liposyn; Vitrimix; ***Fin.:*** Clinoleic; Compleven; KabiMix Basal†; Kabiven; Liposyn; Novamix†; Nutriflex Lipid; Structolipid; Vamin Glukos Combi; Vasolipid; ***Fr.:*** Biopause; Clinoleic; Clinomel; Gynosoja; Ivemix†; KabiMix; Kabiven; Medialipide; Nutriflex Lipide; Oliclinomel; Perikabiven; Piascledine; Structolipide; Trive†; Vitrimix KV; ***Ger.:*** Abbolipid; Balneum Plus; Clinoleic; Clinomel; Compleven; Lipofundin MCT; Lipovenos MCT; Nutriflex Lipid; Oleobal; Sulfo-Olbad Cordes; Windol Basisbad; ***Gr.:*** Clinoleic; Lipofundin MCT/LCT; ***Hong Kong:*** Lipofundin MCT/LCT; Palmetto Plus; Phytoestrin; Sawmetto Vivo-Livo; Vitrimix KV; ***Irl.:*** Balneum Plus; Balneum with Tar†; Vitrimix KV; ***Israel:*** Balneum Plus; Clinoleic; Lipofundin MCT/LCT; Liposyn; ***Ital.:*** Climil Complex; Climil Gel; Climil-80; Clinoleic; Clinomel; Fitogen; Ginil; KabiMix; Kabiven; Lipofundin MCT; Liposyn; Nutriperi Lipid; Nutriplus Lipid; Nutrispecial Lipid; Piascledine; Pulsalux; Soymen; Trivemil; ***Malaysia:*** Vitrimix KV; ***Mex.:*** Clinoleic; Liposyn; Lipovenoes MCT; Soyaloid; Soydex; ***Neth.:*** KabiMix; Vitrimix KV; ***Norw.:*** Ivamix; KabiMix; Kabiven; Nutriflex Lipid; Vasolipid; Vitrimix; ***Port.:*** Banholeum Composto; Banholeum Gel; Lipofundina MCT/LCT; Nutribraun; Structolipid; Vitrimix; ***S.Afr.:*** Clinomel; Lipofundin MCT/LCT; Lipovenoes†; ***Singapore:*** Kabiven; Lipofundin MCT/LCT; Vitrimix KV†; ***Spain:*** Clinoleic; Clinomel; KabiMix; Kabiven; Lipofundina MCT/LCT; Nutriplasmal; Oliclinomel; Structolipid; Trive†; ***Swed.:*** Clinoleic; Clinomel; Compleven; KabiMix; Kabiven; Liposyn; Novamix†; Nutriflex Lipid N; Structolipid; Vasolipid; Vitrimix; ***Switz.:*** Antidry; Balneum Hermal Plus; Clinoleic; Demosvelte N†; Lipofundin MCT; Melisol†; Structolipid; Vitrimix†; ***Thai.:*** Lipofundin MCT/LCT; Trive†; Vitrimix; ***UK:*** Balneum Plus; Clinoleic; Clinomel†; Compleven; KabiMix†; Kabiven; Lipofundin MCT/LCT; OlioClinomel; Phytolife Plus; Structolipid; Vitrimix KV; ***USA:*** Anusol; Liposyn II.

---

## Stannous Fluoride

Fluoruro estañoso; Stannosi Fluoridum. Tin fluoride.

$SnF_2$ = 156.7.

*CAS — 7783-47-3.*

*ATC — A01AA04.*

**Pharmacopoeias.** In *US.*

**USP 27** (Stannous Fluoride). A white crystalline powder. Freely soluble in water; practically insoluble in alcohol, in chloroform, and in ether. pH of a freshly prepared 0.4% solution in water is between 2.8 and 3.5.

**Stability.** Aqueous solutions of stannous fluoride decompose within a few hours with the formation of a white precipitate; they slowly attack glass.

### Profile

Stannous fluoride is used as a source of fluoride (see Sodium Fluoride, p.1444) for the prophylaxis of dental caries. Dental gels containing concentrations of stannous fluoride 0.4% are available for daily use. Higher concentrations have been applied under professional supervision. Stannous fluoride has also been used in dentifrices and mouth rinses.

Stannous fluoride has an unpleasant taste.

### Preparations

***USP 27:*** Stannous Fluoride Gel.

**Proprietary Preparations** (details are given in Part 3)
***Fr.:*** Emoform; ***Ital.:*** Gel-Kam; ***Port.:*** Gel Kam†; ***UK:*** Fluorigard Gel-Kam; Stop†; ***USA:*** Gel Kam; Gel-Kam; Gel-Tin; PerioMed; Stop.

**Multi-ingredient:** ***Fr.:*** Meridol; ***Israel:*** Meridol; ***Ital.:*** Actifluor; ***Port.:*** Meridol†.

---

## Stanol Esters

Estanol, ésteres de.

### Profile

Stanol esters are formed by the esterification of plant stanols with unsaturated fatty acids. Sitostanol, the main plant stanol used, is produced by the saturation of sitosterol (p.982) derived from wood pulp. Stanol esters reduce plasma levels of total cholesterol and low-density lipoprotein (LDL)-cholesterol by inhibiting the intestinal absorption of cholesterol. They are incorporated into foods such as margarine, which are used as part of a cholesterol-lowering diet in the management of hyperlipidaemias (p.823).

◊ References.

1. Miettinen TA, *et al.* Reduction of serum cholesterol with sitostanol-ester margarine in a mildly hypercholesterolemic population. *N Engl J Med* 1995; **333:** 1308–12.

2. Gylling H, *et al.* Reduction of serum cholesterol in postmenopausal women with previous myocardial infarction and cholesterol malabsorption induced by dietary sitostanol ester margarine: women and dietary sitostanol. *Circulation* 1997; **96:** 4226–31.
3. Nguyen TT, *et al.* Cholesterol-lowering effect of stanol ester in a US population of mildly hypercholesterolemic men and women: a randomized controlled trial. *Mayo Clin Proc* 1999; **74:** 1198–1206.
4. Hallikainen MA, Uusitupa MIJ. Effects of 2 low-fat stanol ester-containing margarines on serum cholesterol concentrations as part of a low-fat diet in hypercholesterolemic subjects. *Am J Clin Nutr* 1999; **69:** 403–10.
5. Vuorio AF, *et al.* Stanol ester margarine alone and with simvastatin lowers serum cholesterol in families with familial hypercholesterolemia caused by the FH-North Karelia mutation. *Arterioscler Thromb Vasc Biol* 2000; **20:** 500–506.
6. Law M. Plant sterol and stanol margarines and health. *BMJ* 2000; **320:** 861–4.
7. Tammi A, *et al.* Plant stanol ester margarine lowers serum total and low-density lipoprotein cholesterol concentrations of healthy children: the STRIP project. *J Pediatr* 2000; **136:** 503–10.
8. Hallikainen MA, *et al.* Plant stanol esters affect serum cholesterol concentrations of hypercholesterolemic men and women in a dose-dependent manner. *J Nutr* 2000; **130:** 767–76.
9. Lichtenstein AH, Deckelbaum RJ. AHA Science Advisory: stanol/sterol ester-containing foods and blood cholesterol levels: a statement for healthcare professionals from the Nutrition Committee of the Council on Nutrition, Physical Activity, and Metabolism of the American Heart Association. *Circulation* 2001; **103:** 1177–9. Also available at: http://circ.ahajournals.org/cgi/reprint/103/8/1177.pdf (accessed 25/05/04)
10. Homma Y, *et al.* Decrease in plasma low-density lipoprotein cholesterol, apolipoprotein B, cholesteryl ester transfer protein, and oxidized low-density lipoprotein by plant stanol ester-containing spread: a randomized, placebo-controlled trial. *Nutrition* 2003; **19:** 369–74.
11. Katan MB, *et al.* Efficacy and safety of plant stanols and sterols in the management of blood cholesterol levels. *Mayo Clin Proc* 2003; **78:** 965–78.
12. Naumann E, *et al.* Changes in serum concentrations of noncholesterol sterols and lipoproteins in healthy subjects do not depend on the ratio of plant sterols to stanols in the diet. *J Nutr* 2003; **133:** 2741–7.


### Preparations

**Proprietary Preparations** (details are given in Part 3)
**Multi-ingredient:** ***UK:*** Kolestop; Lestrin.

## Starch

Almidón; Amido; Amidon; Amilo; Amylum; Stärke.
*CAS — 9005-25-8 (starch); 9005-82-7 (α-amylose); 9004-34-6 (β-amylose); 9037-22-3 (amylopectin).*

**Description.** Starch consists of polysaccharide granules obtained from the caryopsis of maize, *Zea mays*, rice, *Oryza sativa*, wheat, *Triticum aestivum* (*T. vulgare*), from the tubers of potato, *Solanum tuberosum* or from the rhizomes of cassava, *Manihot utilissima*. Maize starch is also known as corn starch. Starch contains amylose and amylopectin, both polysaccharides based on α-glucose.

**Pharmacopoeias.** Some or all of the starches described are included in *Chin., Eur.* (see p.vi), *Int., Jpn,* and *Pol.* Also in *USNF. Chin.* and *Eur.* also include Pregelatinised Starch, *USNF* also includes Pregelatinized Starch, and *US* includes Absorbable Dusting Powder and Topical Starch.

**Ph. Eur. 5.0** (Maize Starch; Maydis Amylum). It is obtained from the caryopsis of *Zea mays*. It is a tasteless, matt, white to slightly yellowish, very fine powder which creaks when pressed between the fingers. The presence of granules with cracks or irregularities on the edge is exceptional. Practically insoluble in cold water and in alcohol. Store in airtight containers.

**Ph. Eur. 5.0** (Potato Starch; Solani Amylum). It is obtained from the tuber of *Solanum tuberosum*. It is a very fine, white powder which creaks when pressed between the fingers. It does not contain starch grains of any other origin but may contain a minute quantity, if any, of fragments of the tissue of the original plant. Practically insoluble in cold water and in alcohol. The pH of a 20% mixture in water after 15 minutes is 5.0 to 8.0. Store in airtight containers.

**Ph. Eur. 5.0** (Rice Starch; Oryzae Amylum). It is obtained from the caryopsis of *Oryza sativa*. It is a tasteless, very fine, white powder which creaks when pressed between the fingers. The presence of granules with cracks or irregularities on the edge is exceptional. Practically insoluble in cold water and in alcohol. Store in airtight containers.

**Ph. Eur. 5.0** (Wheat Starch; Tritici Amylum). It is obtained from the caryopsis of *Triticum aestivum* (*T. vulgare*). It is a very fine, white powder which creaks when pressed between the fingers. It does not contain starch grains of any other origin but may contain a minute quantity, if any, of fragments of the tissue of the original plant. Practically insoluble in cold water and in alcohol. The pH of a 20% mixture in water after 15 minutes is 4.5 to 7.0. Store in airtight containers.

**Ph. Eur. 5.0** (Pregelatinised Starch; Amylum Pregelificatum). It is prepared from maize starch, potato starch, or rice starch by mechanical processing in the presence of water, with or without heat, to rupture all or part of the starch granules, and subsequent drying. It contains no added substances but it may be modified to render it compressible and to improve its flow characteristics. It is a white or yellowish white powder that swells in cold water.

**BP 2003** (Tapioca Starch). It is obtained from the rhizomes of *Manihot utilssima*. It is a very fine powder which creaks when pressed between the fingers. Practically insoluble in cold water and in alcohol. Store in airtight containers.

The BP 2003 gives Cassava Starch as an approved synonym.

The BP 2003 directs that when starch is specified and the type is not indicated, Maize Starch, Potato Starch, Rice Starch, Wheat Starch, or in tropical countries where these are not available, Tapioca Starch may be supplied or used.

**USNF 22** (Starch). Granules separated from the mature grain of corn, *Zea mays* (Gramineae) or of wheat, *Triticum aestivum* (Gramineae), or from tubers of the potato, *Solanum tuberosum* (Solanaceae). Irregular, angular, odourless, white masses or fine powder. Insoluble in cold water and in alcohol. A 20% slurry in water after 5 minutes of continuous agitation has a pH of 4.5 to 7.0 (corn and wheat starch) and 5.0 to 8.0 (potato starch).

**USNF 22** (Tapioca Starch). Granules separated from the tubers of tapioca (cassava), *Manihot utilissima* (Euphorbiaceae). Irregular, angular, white to pale yellow masses or fine powder. Insoluble in cold water and in alcohol. A 20% slurry in water after 5 minutes of continuous agitation has a pH of 4.5 to 7.0.

**USNF 22** (Pregelatinized Starch). It is starch that has been chemically and/or mechanically processed to rupture all or part of the granules in the presence of water and subsequently dried. It may be modified to render it compressible and flowable.

### Adverse Effects

◊ The use of starch glove powders by surgeons has resulted in contamination of surgical wounds by starch and in the development of complications such as inflammation, adhesions, and granulomatous lesions. In addition, glove starch powder may be a risk factor in the development of latex allergy, and may act as a vector for bacterial pathogens. Because of these risks, it has been proposed that the use of powder in latex gloves be banned.[1,2]


1. Haglaund U, Junghanns K, eds. Glove powder—the hazards which demand a ban. *Eur J Surg* 1997; **163** (suppl 579): 1–55.
2. AAAAI and ACAAI joint statement concerning the use of powdered and non-powdered natural latex gloves. *Ann Allergy Asthma Immunol* 1997; **79:** 487.


**Effects of cassava.** In 1985 WHO added malnutrition-related diabetes (which included the type previously known as tropical diabetes) to its classification of diabetes mellitus.[1] Epidemiological evidence had suggested an association between fibrocalculous pancreatic diabetes (a subclass of malnutrition-related diabetes) and the consumption of cassava root (tapioca, manioc), which for many people living in tropical developing countries, where protein intake was low, was the main source of food energy. Cassava root contains several cyanogenic substances and although food preparation and processing could reduce the cyanide content, there was the possibility that in persons with an inadequate protein intake, particularly if deficient in sulfur-containing amino acids which are involved in detoxification pathways, accumulation of cyanides might occur. WHO, however, did consider that further research was necessary to firmly establish any relation between this type of diabetes and high levels of cassava consumption. In a review which appeared in the following year[2] the cassava/malnutrition hypothesis was thought to be attractive, but unproven; also there was strong evidence against it being the only cause.

WHO deleted malnutrition-related diabetes from its most recent report on the classification of diabetes.[3] Fibrocalculous pancreatic diabetes is now fibrocalculous pancreatopathy, a disease which may cause diabetic mellitus but is not considered a form of diabetes.

Neurotoxicity including spastic paraparesis[4] and optic neuropathy[5] caused by exposure to cyanide after ingestion of cassava root has been reported.


1. WHO. Diabetes mellitus: report of a WHO study group. *WHO Tech Rep Ser 727* 1985.
2. Abu-Bakare A, *et al.* Tropical or malnutrition-related diabetes: a real syndrome? *Lancet* 1986; **i:** 1135–8.
3. Alberti KGMM, Zimmet PZ. Definition, diagnosis, and classification of diabetes mellitus and its complications. Part I: diagnosis and classification of diabetes mellitus. Provisional report of a WHO consultation. *Diabet Med* 1998; **15:** 539–53.
4. Cliff J, *et al.* Association of high cyanide and low sulphur intake in cassava-induced spastic paraparesis. *Lancet* 1985; **ii:** 1211–3.
5. Freeman AG. Optic neuropathy and chronic cyanide toxicity. *Lancet* 1986; **i:** 441–2.


### Uses and Administration

Starch is absorbent and is widely used in dusting powders, either alone or mixed with zinc oxide or other similar substances. Starch is used as a surgical glove powder, but such use has been discouraged (see above). It is incorporated in many tablets as a disintegrating agent. Pregelatinised starch is used similarly as a tablet binder.

A starch mucilage is given by mouth in the treatment of iodine poisoning.

Rice-based solutions may be used in the prevention and treatment of dehydration due to acute diarrhoeal diseases (p.1241) and may have advantages under certain circumstances over conventional oral rehydration solutions.

**Glycogen storage disease type I.** Type I glycogen storage disease is an autosomal recessive metabolic disorder in which glucose-6-phosphatase is not expressed, resulting in hypoglycaemia due to lack of glucose production. Accumulation of glycogen and other metabolic derangements can lead to complications including renal impairment, hepatomegaly and hepatic adenoma, hyperuricaemia, hyperlipidaemias, and lactic acidosis. The condition has been successfully managed by continuous nocturnal nasogastric infusion of glucose and frequent daytime feedings. However, such a regimen requires good patient compliance and monitoring of the night-time infusions.[1] As an alternative, a more standard diet together with uncooked corn starch suspensions prepared with tap water at room temperature and taken every 6 hours in doses of 1.75 to 2.5 g/kg have been reported[2] to be very satisfactory in maintaining normoglycaemia. In one infant, in whom starch was not satisfactory, the lack of response was considered to be due to inadequate pancreatic amylase activity and although it was subsequently reported[3] that addition of a pancreatic enzyme concentrate had produced some improvement, the response was still inadequate to maintain normoglycaemia for more than 2 hours. It was considered that other amylase preparations should be identified for possible use in such patients. A small study of 7 young adults with glycogen storage disease type I found that a single dose of uncooked corn starch maintained plasma glucose concentrations for 7 hours in 5 of the patients.[4] A long-term study of the effects of corn starch therapy found that complications were less among patients with near normal metabolic control and in those having started therapy at a younger age, but other factors appeared to be involved in the pathogenesis.[5] Corn starch therapy has nonetheless been reported to have caused the amelioration of proximal renal tubular dysfunction in 3 patients who had previously only received frequent daytime feeding as therapy. In 16 other patients who had previously received treatment with corn starch or glucose infusions such renal dysfunction was not identified and it was considered that the rapid response to therapy may explain why renal tubular dysfunction is not found more frequently in these patients.[6]

For a brief description of glycogen storage disease type II, see under Acid Alpha Glucosidase, p.1646.


1. Goldberg T, Slonim AE. Nutrition therapy for hepatic glycogen storage diseases. *J Am Diet Assoc* 1993; **93:** 1423–30.
2. Chen Y-T, *et al.* Cornstarch therapy in type 1 glycogen-storage disease. *N Engl J Med* 1984; **310:** 171–5.
3. Chen Y-T, Sidbury JB. Cornstarch therapy in type 1 glycogen-storage disease. *N Engl J Med* 1984; **311:** 128–9.
4. Wolfsdorf JI, Crigler JF. Cornstarch regimens for nocturnal treatment of young adults with type I glycogen storage disease. *Am J Clin Nutr* 1997; **65:** 1507–11.
5. Weinstein DA, Wolfsdorf JI. Effect of continuous glucose therapy with uncooked cornstarch on the long-term clinical course of type 1a glycogen storage disease. *Eur J Pediatr* 2002; **161** (suppl): S35–S39.
6. Chen Y-T, *et al.* Amelioration of proximal renal tubular dysfunction in type I glycogen storage disease with dietary therapy. *N Engl J Med* 1990; **323:** 590–3.


### Preparations

***BP 2003:*** Compound Zinc Paste; Dithranol Paste; Talc Dusting Powder;
***USP 27:*** Absorbable Dusting Powder; Topical Starch.

**Proprietary Preparations** (details are given in Part 3)
***Austral.:*** Karicare Food Thickener†; ***Fr.:*** Pyoralene†; ***Mex.:*** Panaline; ***NZ:*** Karicare Food Thickener.

**Multi-ingredient:** ***Austral.:*** Nucolox; ZSC; ***Austria:*** Myrtilen; ***Braz.:*** Talco Alivio; ***Fr.:*** Magic Mix; ***Israel:*** Baby Paste; ***Ital.:*** Lenipasta; ***NZ:*** Nucolox; Odor Eze; ***Port.:*** Cuidaderma; ***UK:*** Herbheal Ointment; Psorasolv; Skin Clear; ***USA:*** Balmex Baby; Desitin with Zinc Oxide; Diaparene Corn Starch; Mexsana; Norforms; Yeast-X.

## Stevioside

Esteviósido; Eupatorin; Rebaudin; Stevin; Steviosin.
$C_{38}H_{60}O_{18}$ = 804.9.
*CAS — 57817-89-7.*

**Pharmacopoeias.** In *Chin.*

### Profile

Stevioside is a glycoside extracted from the leaves of yerba dulce, *Stevia rebaudiana* (Compositae). It has about 300 times the sweetness of sucrose and has been used as a sweetening agent in foods. An extract of the leaves of *Stevia rebaudiana* which contains stevioside as well as other glycosides including rebaudioside A, has been used similarly.

◊ References.


1. Hanson JR, De Oliveira BH. Stevioside and related sweet diterpenoid glycosides. *Nat Prod Rep* 1993; **10:** 301–9.


**Hypertension.** The antihypertensive action of stevioside has been investigated. A dose of 250 mg three times daily was found to lower blood pressure in patients with mild to moderate hypertension,[1] and 500 mg three times daily decreased blood pressure and the incidence of left ventricular hypertrophy in patients with mild hypertension.[2]


1. Chan P, *et al.* A double-blind placebo-controlled study of the effectiveness and tolerability of oral stevioside in human hypertension. *Br J Clin Pharmacol* 2000; **50:** 215–20.
2. Hsieh M-H, *et al.* Efficacy and tolerability of oral stevioside in patients with mild essential hypertension: a two-year, randomized, placebo-controlled study. *Clin Ther* 2003; **25:** 2797–2808.

## Sucralose *(BAN)*

Sucralosa; TGS; Trichlorogalactosucrose. 1,6-Dichloro-1,6-dideoxy-β-D-fructofuranosyl 4-chloro-4-deoxy-α-D-galactopyranoside.

$C_{12}H_{19}Cl_3O_8$ = 397.6.
*CAS — 56038-13-2.*

**Pharmacopoeias.** In *USNF.*

**USNF 22** (Sucralose). A white to off-white, crystalline powder. Freely soluble in water, in alcohol, and in methyl alcohol; slightly soluble in ethyl acetate. Store in a cool, dry place at a temperature not exceeding 21°.

### Profile

Sucralose is used as a sweetening agent in foods and beverages. It has between about 300 and 1000 times the sweetening power of sucrose and is stable to heat. It has no food value.

◊ References.


1. Anonymous. Sucralose—a new artificial sweetener. *Med Lett Drugs Ther* 1998; **40:** 67–8.


## Sucrose

Azúcar; Cane Sugar; Refined Sugar; Sacarosa; Saccharose; Saccharum; Sucre; Sucrosum; Zucker. β-D-Fructofuranosyl-α-D-glucopyranoside.

$C_{12}H_{22}O_{11}$ = 342.3.
*CAS — 57-50-1.*

**Description.** Sucrose is obtained from sugar-cane, *Saccharum officinarum* (Gramineae), sugar-beet, *Beta vulgaris* (Chenopodiaceae), and other sources.

**Pharmacopoeias.** In *Chin., Eur.* (see p.vi), *Jpn, Pol.,* and *Viet.* Also in *USNF.*

*Br.* also contains Compressible Sugar.

*Eur.* also includes Sugar Spheres.

*USNF* also includes Compressible Sugar, Confectioner's Sugar, and Sugar Spheres.

**Ph. Eur. 5.0** (Sucrose). A white or almost white, crystalline powder or shiny, colourless or white or almost white crystals. Very soluble in water; slightly soluble in alcohol; practically insoluble in dehydrated alcohol.

**USNF 22** (Sucrose). A sugar obtained from *Saccharum officinarum* (Gramineae), *Beta vulgaris* (Chenopodiaceae), and other sources. White, crystalline powder or lustrous, dry, colourless or white crystals. Soluble 1 in 0.5 of water, 1 in 0.2 of boiling water, and 1 in 170 of alcohol; practically insoluble in dehydrated alcohol.

**Incompatibility.** Sucrose may be contaminated by traces of heavy metals or sulfites and this may lead to incompatibility with other ingredients when it is used as a pharmaceutical excipient. Syrup preserved with hydroxybenzoates has been reported to be incompatible with a range of compounds.

### Adverse Effects and Precautions

Sucrose consumption increases the incidence of dental caries.

Sucrose use should be avoided in patients with the glucose-galactose malabsorption syndrome, fructose intolerance, or sucrase-isomaltase deficiency. The intake of sucrose from dietary and other sources must be controlled in patients with diabetes mellitus.

**Dietary sugar.** Conclusions and recommendations of the Panel on Dietary Sugars after reviewing the evidence relating to sugars in the diet and the health of the population in the UK.[1]

No evidence was found that the consumption of most sugars naturally incorporated into the cellular structure of foods (intrinsic sugars) represented a threat to health and consideration was therefore mainly directed towards the dietary use of sugars not so incorporated (extrinsic sugars), of which sucrose was the principal non-milk extrinsic sugar.

There was extensive evidence suggesting that sugars were the most important dietary factor in the cause of dental caries and it was recommended that consumption of non-milk extrinsic sugars should be decreased.

It was considered that dietary sugars may contribute to the development of obesity, a condition which plays an important part in the aetiology of a number of diseases. For the majority of the population, who had normal plasma lipids and normal glucose tolerance, the consumption of sugars within the present range carried no special metabolic risks but those persons consuming more than about 200 g daily should replace the excess with starch. It was, however, recommended that those with special medical problems such as diabetes or hypertriglyceridaemia should restrict non-milk extrinsic sugar to less than about 20 to 50 g daily unless otherwise instructed by their own physician or dietitian. It was also concluded that current consumption of sugars, particularly sucrose, played no direct causal role in the development of cardiovascular (atherosclerotic coronary, peripheral, or cerebral vascular) disease, essential hypertension, or diabetes mellitus, and also had no significant specific effects on behaviour or psychological function. Although links between sucrose intake and certain other diseases (such as colorectal cancer, renal and biliary calculi, and Crohn's disease) had been proposed it was not felt that the evidence was adequate to justify any general dietary recommendations.

The conclusions of a joint FAO/WHO consultation on carbohydrates in human nutrition[2] were broadly in agreement with the above. However, they note that the terms intrinsic and extrinsic sugars have not gained wide acceptance, either in the UK or other countries in the world, and they recommended against the use of these terms.


1. DoH. Dietary sugars and human disease: report of the panel on dietary sugars of the committee on medical aspects of food policy. *Report on health and social subjects 37.* London: HMSO, 1989.
2. FAO/WHO. *Carbohydrates in human nutrition: report of a joint FAO/WHO expert consultation. FAO Food and Nutrition 66.* Rome: Food and Agriculture Organization of the United Nations, 1998.


**Effects on the kidneys.** Acute renal failure with severe hyponatraemia has followed the use of granulated sugar to treat an infected pneumonectomy wound cavity.[1] It was noted that intravenous sucrose had long been known to be nephrotoxic in both animal models and man and that mild renal insufficiency before sucrose intoxication might have contributed to the nephrosis. Others, however, considered that the nephrotoxicity might have been caused by gentamicin, a solution of which had been used to irrigate the cavity prior to packing the wound.[2] Intravenous immunoglobulin preparations containing sucrose (as a stabilising agent) have also caused acute renal failure.[3,4]


1. Debure A, *et al.* Acute renal failure after use of granulated sugar in deep infected wound. *Lancet* 1987; **i:** 1034–5.
2. Archer H, *et al.* Toxicity of topical sugar. *Lancet* 1987; **i:** 1485–6.
3. Ahsan N, *et al.* Intravenous immunoglobulin-induced osmotic nephrosis. *Arch Intern Med* 1994; **154:** 1985–7.
4. Zhang R, Szerlip HM. Reemergence of sucrose nephropathy: acute renal failure caused by high-dose intravenous immune globulin therapy. *South Med J* 2000; **93:** 901–4.


### Pharmacokinetics

Sucrose is hydrolysed in the small intestine by the enzyme sucrase to glucose and fructose, which are then absorbed. Sucrose is excreted unchanged in the urine when given intravenously.

### Uses and Administration

Sucrose, a disaccharide, is used as a sweetening agent. It is commonly used as household sugar. If the sweetness of sucrose is taken as 100, fructose has a value of about 173, glucose 74, maltose 32, galactose 32, and lactose 16.

Sucrose is used as a tablet excipient and lozenge basis, and as a suspending and viscosity-increasing agent. Syrups prepared from concentrated solutions of sucrose form the basis of many linctuses.

**Cough.** Sucrose syrups are used as demulcents in linctuses used for treating cough (p.1112).

**Diagnostic test for gastrointestinal damage.** Sucrose is not absorbed from the healthy gastrointestinal tract. It has been proposed that the absorption of sucrose could be used as a diagnostic test of gastric damage.[1-3]


1. Sutherland LR, *et al.* A simple non-invasive marker of gastric damage: sucrose permeability. *Lancet* 1994; **343:** 998–1000.
2. Meddings JB, *et al.* Sucrose permeability: a novel means of detecting gastroduodenal damage noninvasively. *Am J Ther* 1995; **2:** 843–9.
3. Kawabata H, *et al.* Sucrose permeability as a means of detecting diseases of the upper digestive tract. *J Gastroenterol Hepatol* 1998; **13:** 1002–6.


**Gastrointestinal spasm.** For mention of a beneficial effect of sucrose solution in infant colic, see p.1242.

**Glycogen storage disease type V.** Sucrose 75 g by mouth improved exercise tolerance in patients with type V glycogen storage disease (McArdle's disease), an autosomal recessive disorder characterised by mutations in the gene for myophosphorylase, an enzyme essential for glycogenolysis.[1]


1. Vissing J, Haller RG. The effect of oral sucrose on exercise tolerance in patients with McArdle's disease. *N Engl J Med* 2003; **349:** 2503–9.


**Hiccup.** Administration of a teaspoon of dry granulated sugar resulted in the immediate cessation of hiccup in 19 of 20 patients;[1] 12 of the patients had suffered from hiccup for less than 6 hours but in the remaining 8 persistent hiccup had been present for 24 hours to 6 weeks. The effect may be due to stimulation of the pharynx. A protocol for the treatment of intractable hiccup (p.682) suggests that swallowing dry granulated sugar is one of the first treatments that should be tried.


1. Engleman EG, *et al.* Granulated sugar as treatment for hiccups in conscious patients. *N Engl J Med* 1971; **285:** 1489.


**Pain.** A systematic review[1] concluded that sucrose solutions could reduce physiological and behavioural indicators of stress and pain in neonates undergoing painful procedures although there had been some doubt expressed[2] over whether this indicated effective analgesia. The review[1] was unable to determine an optimal dose, but 1 mL of a 25% solution or 2 mL of a 50% solution has been reported to reduce crying time in premature[3] and full-term[4] infants, respectively, when given 2 minutes before heel prick sampling. Similarly, 2 mL of a 75% sucrose solution by mouth reduced crying time in infants receiving intramuscular vaccines.[5] A literature review[6] has suggested that a dose of 500 mg sucrose provides effective analgesia for neonates. However, a randomised trial found pacifiers (dummies) to have a better analgesic effect than 2 mL of a 30% sucrose solution; a synergistic effect was found with a combination of sucrose and pacifiers.[7] The route of administration of the sucrose solution may also be important: a reduced pain response was only noted after intraoral administration; administration via a nasogastric tube was ineffective.[8]

A trial in preterm infants found that, while there were no differences on neurobehavioural developmental outcomes between infants given repeated sucrose analgesia or placebo, higher number of doses of sucrose predicted lower scores in motor development, vigour, alertness and orientation. The authors postulated that repeated stimulation by sucrose may interfere with normal functioning and maturation of the preterm infant's endogenous opiate system, and cautioned against the routine use of sucrose analgesia in this population.[9] For choice of analgesic in children, see p.3.


1. Stevens B, *et al.* Sucrose for analgesia in newborn infants undergoing painful procedures. Available in The Cochrane Library; Issue 2. Chichester: John Wiley; 2004.
2. Anonymous. Pacifiers, passive behaviour, and pain. *Lancet* 1992; **339:** 275–6.
3. Ramenghi LA, *et al.* Reduction of pain response in premature infants using intraoral sucrose. *Arch Dis Child* 1996; **74:** F126–F128.
4. Haouari N, *et al.* The analgesic effect of sucrose in full term infants: a randomised controlled trial. *BMJ* 1995; **310:** 1498–1500.
5. Lewindon PJ, *et al.* Randomised controlled trial of sucrose by mouth for the relief of infant crying after immunisation. *Arch Dis Child* 1998; **78:** 453–6.
6. Masters-Harte LD, Abdel-Rahman SM. Sucrose analgesia for minor procedures in newborn infants. *Ann Pharmacother* 2001; **35:** 947–52.
7. Carbajal R, *et al.* Randomised trial of analgesic effects of sucrose, glucose, and pacifiers in term neonates. *BMJ* 1999; **319:** 1393–7.
8. Ramenghi LA, *et al.* "Sucrose analgesia": absorptive mechanism or taste perception. *Arch Dis Child Fetal Neonatal Ed* 1999; **80:** F146–F147.
9. Johnston CC, *et al.* Routine sucrose analgesia during the first week of life in neonates younger than 31 weeks' postconceptional age. *Pediatrics* 2002; **110:** 523–8.


**Wound healing.** Sugar, either in the form of granulated sugar[1,2] or pastes composed of caster sugar and icing sugar,[3,4] has been used successfully in the treatment of a variety of wounds (p.1139) including open mediastinitis after cardiac surgery,[1] large abscesses and bed sores,[3,4] and diabetic ulcers.[2] Debridement of the wound is believed to be due partly to the osmotic effect of sugar and partly to the mechanical cleansing action but it is not known how sugar stimulates granulation tissue to form.[3,4] Once granulation tissue is well established and the wound is shrinking, an alternative wound preparation, such as an alginate, hydrocolloid, or hydrogel, should be used as sugar pastes cause bleeding.[5] Sugar is also effective at deodorising malodorous wounds. The use of the combined caster and icing sugar pastes, of which details of the formulas used are provided in the original publications,[3,4] has been advocated as a way to overcome the problems of possible non-sterility and contamination of commercial granulated sugar.[3,4]

Honey (p.1434) has been used similarly.


1. Trouillet JL, *et al.* Use of granulated sugar in treatment of open mediastinitis after cardiac surgery. *Lancet* 1985; **ii:** 180–4.
2. Quatraro A, *et al.* Sugar and wound healing. *Lancet* 1985; **ii:** 664.
3. Gordon H, *et al.* Sugar and wound healing. *Lancet* 1985; **ii:** 663–4.
4. Middleton KR, Seal D. Sugar as an aid to wound healing. *Pharm J* 1985; **235:** 757–8.
5. Seal DV, Middleton K. Healing of cavity wounds with sugar. *Lancet* 1991; **338:** 571–2.


### Preparations

**BP 2003:** Compressible Sugar; Syrup;
**Ph. Eur.:** Sugar Spheres;
**USNF 22:** Compressible Sugar; Confectioner's Sugar; Sugar Spheres; Syrup.

**Proprietary Preparations** (details are given in Part 3)

**Multi-ingredient:** ***Arg.:*** Semble; ***Fr.:*** Gelodiet; ***Jpn:*** U-Pasta; ***S.Afr.:*** Emetrol.

## Sucrose Polyesters

Poliésteres de la sacarosa.

### Profile

A sucrose polyester that is a mixture of hexa-, hepta-, and octa-fatty acid esters of sucrose is used as a nondigestible fat substitute by the food industry. Fat substitutes have been promoted as part of a strategy to reduce fat and calories in the diet to aid body-weight control.

Possible adverse effects of sucrose polyesters are flatulence, anal leakage, abdominal cramps, and loose bowel movements. They may also reduce the absorption of fat-soluble vitamins.

◊ References.


1. Cotton JR, *et al.* Replacement of dietary fat with sucrose polyester: effects on energy intake and appetite control in non-obese males. *Am J Clin Nutr* 1996; **63:** 891–6.

2. Goldman P. Olestra: assessing its potential to interact with drugs in the gastrointestinal tract. *Clin Pharmacol Ther* 1997; **61:** 613–18.
3. Cheskin LJ, *et al.* Gastrointestinal symptoms following consumption of olestra or regular triglyceride potato chips: a controlled comparison. *JAMA* 1998; **279:** 150–2.
4. Sandler RS, *et al.* Gastrointestinal symptoms in 3181 volunteers ingesting snack foods containing olestra or triglycerides. *Ann Intern Med* 1999; **130:** 253–61.

## Sunflower Oil

Aceite de girasol; Helianthi Annui Oleum; Huile de Tournesol; Oleum Helianthi; Sunflowerseed Oil.

**Pharmacopoeias.** In *Eur.* (see p.vi).

**Ph. Eur. 5.0** (Sunflower Oil, Refined; Helianthi Annui Oleum Raffinatum). The fatty oil obtained from the seeds of *Helianthus annuus* by mechanical expression or by extraction and then refined. A suitable antoxidant may be added. A clear, light yellow liquid. Practically insoluble in water and in alcohol; miscible with petroleum spirit (b.p.: 40° to 60°). Store in well-filled airtight containers. Protect from light.

### Profile

Sunflower oil is used in pharmaceutical preparations. It is rich in linoleic acid (p.1690).

**Multiple sclerosis.** As discussed on p.646, the role of dietary lipids in multiple sclerosis remains to be proven,[1] although many patients modify their diets and take supplements of sunflower and other oils. Some studies have shown a reduction in severity and duration of relapse in patients taking linoleic acid supplements (as sunflower oil)[2] and another[3] has reported benefit in patients who limit their intake of dietary saturated fatty acids and supplement their diet with polyunsaturated fatty acids.

1. Anonymous. Lipids and multiple sclerosis. *Lancet* 1990; **336:** 25–6.
2. Millar JHD, *et al.* Double-blind trial of linoleate supplementation of the diet in multiple sclerosis. *BMJ* 1973; **1:** 765–8.
3. Swank RL, Dugan BB. Effect of low saturated fat diet in early and late cases of multiple sclerosis. *Lancet* 1990; **336:** 37–9.

### Preparations

**Proprietary Preparations** (details are given in Part 3)
***Port.:*** Oleoban.

**Multi-ingredient:** ***Arg.:*** Alofresh; ***Austria:*** Pelsana Med; Piniment; ***Fr.:*** Oropur; ***Ger.:*** derma-loges N†; ***NZ:*** Snorenz; ***Port.:*** Oleoban Composto; Oleoban Gel; ***Switz.:*** Huile de millepertuis A. Vogel (huile de St. Jean); Pelsano; ***UK:*** Goodnight StopSnore; Snor-Away; Snorenz†.

## Thaumatin *(BAN)*

E957; Katemfe; Taumatina.

*CAS — 53850-34-3.*

### Profile

Thaumatin is a mixture in the ratio of 2:1 of two polypeptides thaumatin I and thaumatin II, each consisting of 207 amino acid residues and having a molecular weight of about 22 000, derived from the fruit of *Thaumatococcus daniellii* (Scitamineae). It is an odourless, cream-coloured, proteinaceous powder with an intensely sweet taste.

Thaumatin is a protein whose amino-acid range excludes histidine. It produces an intense sweetness that builds up gradually but persists for up to an hour, and is considered to be by far the sweetest of such compounds in use. It is approved as a sweetener and flavour modifier in foods and drinks.

## Threonine *(USAN, rINN)*

β-Methylserine; T; Thr; L-Threonine; Threoninum; Treonina. L-2-Amino-3-hydroxybutyric acid.

$C_4H_9NO_3$ = 119.1.

*CAS — 72-19-5.*

**Pharmacopoeias.** In *Chin.*, *Eur.* (see p.vi), *Jpn*, and *US.*

**Ph. Eur. 5.0** (Threonine). A white, crystalline powder or colourless crystals. Soluble in water; practically insoluble in alcohol. A 2.5% solution in water has a pH of 5.0 to 6.5. Protect from light.

**USP 27** (Threonine). White, odourless crystals. Freely soluble in water; insoluble in dehydrated alcohol, in chloroform, and in ether. pH of a 5% solution in water is between 5.0 and 6.5.

### Profile

Threonine is an aliphatic amino acid which is an essential constituent of the diet. It is used as a dietary supplement.

Threonine has been investigated for the treatment of various spastic disorders.

### Preparations

**Proprietary Preparations** (details are given in Part 3)
**Multi-ingredient:** ***Ital.:*** Stimolfit.

## Tyrosine *(USAN, rINN)*

Tirosina; Tyr; L-Tyrosine; Tyrosinum; Y. L-2-Amino-3-(4-hydroxyphenyl)propionic acid.

$C_9H_{11}NO_3$ = 181.2.

*CAS — 60-18-4.*

**Pharmacopoeias.** In *Chin.*, *Eur.* (see p.vi), and *US.*

**Ph. Eur. 5.0** (Tyrosine). A white crystalline powder or colourless crystals. Very slightly soluble in water; practically insoluble in alcohol. It dissolves in dilute mineral acids and in dilute solutions of alkali hydroxides. Protect from light.

**USP 27** (Tyrosine). White, odourless crystals or crystalline powder. Very slightly soluble in water; insoluble in alcohol and in ether.

### Profile

Tyrosine is an aromatic amino acid. It is used as a dietary supplement.

**Phenylketonuria.** Tyrosine was not an effective alternative to a diet low in phenylalanine in patients with phenylketonuria, see under Amino Acid Metabolic Disorders, p.1417.

### Preparations

**Proprietary Preparations** (details are given in Part 3)
**Multi-ingredient:** ***Arg.:*** Refrane Bronce; ***Austral.:*** Aussie Tan Pre-Tan†; Bioglan Zellulean with Escin†; Tyroseng†; ***India:*** Placentrex; ***Port.:*** Rilastil Dermo Solar; ***UK:*** Amino MS†.

## Valine *(USAN, rINN)*

α-Aminoisovaleric Acid; V; Val; Valina; L-Valine; Valinum. (*S*)-2-Amino-3-methylbutanoic acid.

$C_5H_{11}NO_2$ = 117.1.

*CAS — 72-18-4.*

**Pharmacopoeias.** In *Chin.*, *Eur.* (see p.vi), *Jpn*, and *US.*

**Ph. Eur. 5.0** (Valine). A white or almost white, crystalline powder or colourless crystals. Soluble in water; very slightly soluble in alcohol. Protect from light.

**USP 27** (Valine). White, odourless crystals. Soluble in water; practically insoluble in alcohol, in acetone, and in ether. pH of a 5% solution in water is between 5.5 and 7.0.

### Profile

Valine is a branched-chain amino acid which is an essential constituent of the diet. It is used as a dietary supplement. It is also an ingredient of several preparations that have been promoted for disorders of the liver.

### Preparations

**Proprietary Preparations** (details are given in Part 3)
**Multi-ingredient:** ***Fr.:*** Revitalose; ***Ger.:*** Bramin-hepa; Falkamin; ***Ital.:*** Falkamin; Isobranch; Isoram.

# Vitamin A *(USAN)*

Retinol *(BAN, rINN)*; Antixerophthalmic Vitamin; Axerophtholum; Oleovitamin A; Vitamin A Alcohol; Vitaminum A. 15-Apo-β-carotén-15-ol; 3,7-Dimethyl-9-(2,6,6-trimethylcyclohex-1-enyl)nona-2,4,6,8-tetraen-1-ol.

$C_{20}H_{30}O$ = 286.5.

*CAS — 68-26-8.*

*ATC — D10AD02; R01AX02; S01XA02.*

**Description.** Vitamin A is generally used in the form of esters, such as the acetate, palmitate, and propionate.

Vitamin A Acetate. Retinol Acetate; Retinyl Acetate; $C_{22}H_{32}O_2$ = 328.5; CAS — 127-47-9

Vitamin A Palmitate. Retinol Palmitate; Retinyl Palmitate; $C_{36}H_{60}O_2$ = 524.9; CAS — 79-81-2

Vitamin A Propionate. Retinol Propionate; Retinyl Propionate; $C_{23}H_{34}O_2$ = 342.5; CAS — 7069-42-3.

**Pharmacopoeias.** In *Eur.* (see p.vi), *US*, and *Viet.*, which permit retinol or its esters.

*Chin.* includes a monograph for the acetate. *Jpn* and *Pol.* include monographs for the acetate and the palmitate.

*Br.* includes a monograph for a natural ester concentrate.

*Eur.* also includes monographs for synthetic concentrates in an oily form, a powder form, and a solubilisate/emulsion.

*Int.* includes an oily concentrated form.

The BP 2003 states that the term 'Retinol' is used within BP titles for preparations containing synthetic ester(s) and the term 'Vitamin A' within the BP title for the preparation containing material of natural origin.

**Ph. Eur. 5.0** (Vitamin A). Under the name Vitamin A are included a number of substances of very similar structure (including (*Z*)-isomers) found in animal tissues and possessing similar activity. The principal and biologically most active substance is all-(*E*) retinol.

Vitamin A is generally used in the form of esters such as the acetate, propionate, and palmitate. Synthetic retinol ester refers to an ester of synthetic retinol (acetate, propionate, or palmitate) or a mixture of synthetic retinol esters.

Retinol acetate occurs as pale yellow crystals. M.p. about 60°; once melted it tends to yield a supercooled melt. Retinol propionate occurs as a reddish-brown oily liquid. Retinol palmitate occurs as a fat-like, light yellow solid, or as a yellow oily liquid, if melted. M.p. about 26°. All retinol esters are practically insoluble in water; soluble or partly soluble in dehydrated alcohol; miscible with organic solvents. Vitamin A and its esters are sensitive to the action of air, oxidising agents, acids, light, and heat. Store in well-filled airtight containers. Protect from light. Once the container has been opened, its contents should be used as soon as possible and any part of the contents not used should be protected by an atmosphere of inert gas.

**Ph. Eur. 5.0** (Vitamin A Concentrate (Oily Form), Synthetic; Vitaminum A Densatum Oleosum; Synthetic Retinol Concentrate (Oily Form) BP 2003). It is prepared from synthetic retinol ester as is or by dilution with a suitable vegetable oil. It contains not less than 500 000 units of vitamin A per g. It is a yellow or brownish-yellow, oily liquid; practically insoluble in water; soluble or partly soluble in dehydrated alcohol; miscible with organic solvents. Partial crystallisation may occur in highly concentrated solutions. Store in well-filled airtight containers. Protect from light. Once the container has been opened, its contents should be used as soon as possible and any part of the contents not used at once should be protected by an atmosphere of inert gas.

**Ph. Eur. 5.0** (Vitamin A Concentrate (Powder Form), Synthetic; Vitaminum A Pulvis; Synthetic Retinol Concentrate (Powder Form) BP 2003). It is obtained by dispersing a synthetic retinol ester in a matrix of gelatin or acacia or other suitable material. It contains not less than 250 000 units of vitamin A per g. It is a yellowish powder usually in the form of particles of almost uniform size. Practically insoluble in water or may swell or form an emulsion, depending on formulation. Store in well-filled airtight containers. Protect from light. Once the container has been opened, its contents should be used as soon as possible and any part of the contents not used at once should be protected by an atmosphere of inert gas.

**Ph. Eur. 5.0** (Vitamin A Concentrate (Solubilisate/Emulsion), Synthetic; Vitaminum A in Aqua Dispergibile; Synthetic Retinol Concentrate, Solubilisate/Emulsion BP 2003). It is a liquid form (water is generally used as solvent) of synthetic retinol ester and a suitable solubiliser. It contains not less than 100 000 units of vitamin A per g. It is a yellow or yellowish liquid of variable opalescence and viscosity. Highly concentrated solutions may become cloudy at low temperatures or take the form of a gel. A mixture of 1 g with 10 mL of water previously warmed to 50° gives after cooling to 20°, a uniform, slightly opalescent and slightly yellow dispersion. Store in airtight containers. Protect from light. Once the container has been opened, its contents should be used as soon as possible and any part of the contents not used at once should be protected by an atmosphere of inert gas.

**BP 2003** (Natural Vitamin A Ester Concentrate). It consists of a natural ester or a mixture of natural esters of retinol or of a solution of the ester or mixture of esters in arachis oil or other suitable vegetable oil. It contains not less than 485 000 units of vitamin A per g. It is a yellow oil or a mixture of oil and crystalline material, with a faint odour. Practically insoluble in water; soluble or partly soluble in alcohol; miscible with chloroform, with ether, and with petroleum spirit. Store in airtight containers at 8° to 15°. Protect from light.

**USP 27** (Vitamin A). It may consist of retinol or its esters formed from edible fatty acids, principally acetic and palmitic acids. In liquid form, it is a light yellow to red oil that may solidify upon refrigeration. In solid form, has the appearance of any diluent that has been added. It may be practically odourless or may have a mild fishy odour but no rancid odour or taste. It is unstable in air and light. In liquid form, it is insoluble in water and in glycerol; soluble in dehydrated alcohol and in vegetable oils; very soluble in chloroform and in ether. In solid form, may be dispersible in water. Store in airtight containers, preferably under an atmosphere of inert gas. Protect from light.

## Units

The International Standards for vitamin A and for provitamin A were discontinued in 1954 and 1956 respectively but the International units for these substances have continued to be widely used. In 1960–1, the WHO Expert Committee on Biological Standardization stated that the International unit for vitamin A is equivalent to the activity of 0.000344 mg of pure all-*trans* vitamin A acetate and the International unit for provitamin A is equivalent to the activity of 0.0006 mg of pure all-*trans* β-carotene.

The activity of one International unit is contained in 0.0003 mg of all-*trans* retinol, in 0.00055 mg of all-*trans* retinol palmitate, and in 0.000359 mg of all-*trans* retinol propionate.

The USP 27 defines 1 USP unit as equal to the biological activity of 0.0003 mg of the all-*trans* isomer of retinol, and is equivalent to the International unit.

Vitamin A activity in foods is currently expressed in terms of retinol equivalents: 1 retinol equivalent is defined as 1 microgram of all-*trans* retinol, 6 micrograms of all-*trans* beta carotene, or 12 micrograms of other provitamin A carotenoids.

## Adverse Effects and Precautions

The administration of excessive amounts of vitamin A substances over long periods can lead to toxicity. Rarely, acute toxicity may also occur with very high doses.

- Hypervitaminosis A (chronic toxicity) is characterised by fatigue, irritability, anorexia and loss of weight, vomiting and other gastrointestinal disturbances, low-grade fever, hepatosplenomegaly, skin changes (yellowing, dryness, sensitivity to sunlight), alopecia, dry hair, cracking and bleeding lips, anaemia, headache, hypercalcaemia, subcutaneous swelling, nocturia, and pains in bones and joints. Symptoms of chronic toxicity may also include raised intracranial pressure and papilloedema mimicking brain tumours, tinnitus, and visual disturbances which may be severe. Symptoms usually clear on withdrawal of vitamin A, but in children premature closure of the epiphyses of the long bones may result in arrested bone growth.
- Acute vitamin A intoxication is characterised by sedation, dizziness, nausea and vomiting, erythema, pruritus, desquamation, and increased intracranial pressure (resulting in bulging fontanelle in infants).

Hypervitaminosis A does not appear to be a problem with large doses of carotenoids (see Pharmacokinetics under Betacarotene, p.1423).

Enhanced susceptibility to the effects of vitamin A may be seen in children and in patients with liver disease.

Excessive doses of vitamin A should be avoided in pregnancy because of potential teratogenic effects; for further details see Pregnancy, below.

Gastrointestinal absorption of vitamin A may be impaired in cholestatic jaundice and fat-malabsorption conditions.

**Benign intracranial hypertension.** High doses of vitamin A cause increased intracranial pressure, and, in infants, this is manifested as bulging of the fontanelle. In one study,[1] 11.5% of infants receiving 3 doses of 50 000 units of vitamin A at monthly intervals had bulging fontanelle, compared with 1% of infants receiving placebo. The bulging lasted between 24 and 72 hours and subsided without treatment,[1] and did not appear to be associated with any physical or developmental abnormalities on long-term follow-up.[2] In another study in neonates, bulging fontanelle occurred in 4.6% of recipients of vitamin A 50 000 units and 2.7% of placebo recipients 24 hours after administration.[3] In contrast, less than 1% of infants given 3 doses of 25 000 units of vitamin A at monthly intervals had bulging fontanelle in a further study.[4]


1. de Francisco A, *et al.* Acute toxicity of vitamin A given with vaccines in infancy. *Lancet* 1993; **342:** 526–7.
2. van Dillen J, *et al.* Long-term effect of vitamin A with vaccines. *Lancet* 1996; **347:** 1705.
3. Agoestina T, *et al.* Safety of one 52 micromol (50 000 IU) oral dose of vitamin A administered to neonates. *Bull WHO* 1994; **72:** 859–68.
4. WHO/CHD Immunisation-Linked Vitamin A Supplementation Study Group. Randomised trial to assess benefits and safety of vitamin A supplementation linked to immunisation in early infancy. *Lancet* 1998; **352:** 1257–63. Correction. *ibid.* 1999; **353:** 154.


**Carcinogenicity.** For mention of the *increased* risk of lung cancer in high-risk individuals receiving betacarotene and vitamin A, when compared with placebo, in a study investigating vitamins in lung cancer prevention, see Prophylaxis of Malignant Neoplasms, p.1420.

**Effects on the blood.** Normochromic macrocytic anaemia developed in a patient who had been receiving vitamin A 150 000 units daily by mouth for several months.[1] The patient's haemoglobin returned to normal when vitamin A was discontinued, and the accompanying symptoms of perioral dermatitis and glossitis also disappeared. Similarly, normochromic normocytic anaemia and thrombocytopenia in an infant given 62 000 units daily for 80 days, resolved upon discontinuation of the vitamin A.[2]


1. White JM. Vitamin-A-induced anaemia. *Lancet* 1984; **ii:** 573.
2. Perrotta S, *et al.* Infant hypervitaminosis A causes severe anemia and thrombocytopenia: evidence of a retinol-dependent bone marrow cell growth inhibition. *Blood* 2002; **99:** 2017–22.


**Effects on bone.** Excessive dietary intake of vitamin A may be associated with osteoporosis. In an epidemiological study,[1] a dietary intake of retinol greater than 1500 micrograms daily (5000 units) doubled the risk of hip fracture compared with an intake of less than 500 micrograms daily (about 1670 units) in women (odds ratio, 2.1; 95% confidence interval 1.1 to 4.0). These data were confirmed by the Nurses' Health Study,[2] which found that postmenopausal women with the highest vitamin A and retinol intakes were at increased risk for hip fracture, irrespective of whether the intakes were from food plus supplements, or food alone. Women with daily retinol intakes of more than 1500 micrograms had a relative risk for hip fracture of 1.64 compared with those consuming less than 500 micrograms daily. Betacarotene intake, however, did not correlate significantly with an increased risk of fracture. A large cohort study[3] of men found that the overall risk of any fracture, including hip fractures, was substantially increased among men with the highest concentrations of serum retinol; there was no association between serum betacarotene levels and the risk of fracture. Subsequently, routine supplementation and the fortification of food with vitamin A in Western countries has been questioned.[4]


1. Melhus H, *et al.* Excessive dietary intake of vitamin A is associated with reduced bone mineral density and increased risk for hip fracture. *Ann Intern Med* 1998; **129:** 770–8.
2. Feskanich D, *et al.* Vitamin A intake and hip fractures among postmenopausal women. *JAMA* 2002; **287:** 47–54.
3. Michaëlsson K, *et al.* Serum retinol levels and the risk of fracture. *N Engl J Med* 2003; **348:** 287–94.
4. Lips P. Hypervitaminosis A and fractures. *N Engl J Med* 2003; **348:** 347–9.


**Effects on the immune system.** Vitamin A deficiency is generally associated with impaired immunity, and treatment of deficiency results in reductions in morbidity and mortality from a number of infectious diseases (see under Deficiency States, below). However, a few studies have shown increased prevalence of diarrhoea and/or respiratory-tract infections with high doses of vitamin A. There is a possibility that high single doses of vitamin A may temporarily attenuate the immune response in non-deficient children.[1] For mention that high-dose vitamin A supplements have been associated with a reduced response to measles vaccine in some studies, see p.1623.


1. Anonymous. Childhood morbidity, immunity and micronutrients. *WHO Drug Inf* 1996; **10:** 12–16.


**Effects on the liver.** Vitamin A is stored in the Dissë space of liver cells and excess administration can lead to fibrosis and obstruction of sinusoidal blood flow, causing non-cirrhotic portal hypertension and hepatocellular dysfunction.[1] Although hepatotoxicity has typically been reported with habitual ingestion of doses of vitamin A greater than 50 000 units daily, a case of severe hepatic fibrosis, with jaundice and hepatomegaly, has been reported in a patient who had been taking 25 000 units daily for at least 6 years in a multivitamin supplement.[2]


1. Sherlock S. The spectrum of hepatotoxicity due to drugs. *Lancet* 1986; **ii:** 440–4.
2. Kowalski TE, *et al.* Vitamin A hepatotoxicity: a cautionary note regarding 25,000 IU supplements. *Am J Med* 1994; **97:** 523–8.


**Hypersensitivity.** Local inflammatory reactions and severe anaphylactoid reactions have occurred in patients receiving vitamin A injections, and are usually attributed to solubilisers such as polyoxyl castor oils (p.1414), and, less commonly, polysorbates (p.1415).

A case of cutaneous hypersensitivity to retinol palmitate, and not other injection ingredients, has been described.[1]


1. Shelley WB, *et al.* Hypersensitivity to retinol palmitate injection. *BMJ* 1995; **311:** 232.


**Pregnancy.** The fact that synthetic vitamin A derivatives such as isotretinoin are teratogenic (p.1150) has prompted concern about the potential teratogenicity of high doses of vitamin A.

A prospective cohort study found that a total daily intake of vitamin A from all sources of greater than 15 000 units during early pregnancy was associated with a significantly increased risk of birth defects of structures arising from the cranial neural crest.[1] When vitamin A intake from supplements was analysed separately, an apparent vitamin A threshold dose for the development of birth defects of 10 000 units daily was suggested. However, this study has been criticised[2,3] and some suggest the data allows for a higher threshold dose.[3] A further study found no significant difference in birth defect rates between women consuming greater than 8000 or 10 000 units of vitamin A daily in the period around conception (as supplements and fortified cereals) and those consuming less than 5000 units daily.[4]

Following earlier case reports in the USA suggesting that large doses of vitamin A (equivalent to about ten times the daily recommended dietary allowance of 2250 units) taken in early pregnancy may cause birth defects, the UK Chief Medical Officer cautioned women against the use of vitamin A supplements except under medical supervision.[5] Additionally, advice was given that liver or liver products should not be eaten because high concentrations of vitamin A had been detected in some samples of animal liver. However, others thought that the avoidance of liver or liver products might result in inadequate nutrition in some and that a less alarmist view might have been to suggest a limitation on intake rather than total prohibition.[6,7]

The American College of Obstetricians and Gynecologists has recommended that women who are pregnant or planning pregnancy should ensure that any vitamin supplements they take contain a daily dose of vitamin A of no more than 5000 units.[8] The Australian Adverse Drug Reactions Advisory Committee has advised women in this category to avoid vitamin A supplements and to not exceed the recommended daily allowance of 2500 units from all sources.[9]


1. Rothman KJ, *et al.* Teratogenicity of high vitamin A intake. *N Engl J Med* 1995; **333:** 1369–73.
2. Werler MM, *et al.* Teratogenicity of high vitamin A intake. *N Engl J Med* 1996; **334:** 1195–6.
3. Watkins M, *et al.* Teratogenicity of high vitamin A intake. *N Engl J Med* 1996; **334:** 1196.
4. Mills JL, *et al.* Vitamin A and birth defects. *Am J Obstet Gynecol* 1997; **177:** 31–6.
5. Department of Health. *Women cautioned: watch your vitamin A intake.* London: Department of Health, 1990 (18 October).
6. Nelson M. Vitamin A, liver consumption, and risk of birth defects. *BMJ* 1990; **301:** 1176.
7. Sanders TAB. Vitamin A and pregnancy. *Lancet* 1990; **336:** 1375.
8. American College of Obstetricians and Gynecologists. Vitamin A supplementation during pregnancy. *Int J Gynecol Obstet* 1993; **40:** 175.
9. Adverse Drug Reactions Advisory Committee. Vitamin A and birth defects. *Aust Adverse Drug React Bull* 1996; **15:** 14–15. Also available at: http://www.tga.health.gov.au/docs/html/aadrbltn/aadr9611.htm (accessed 21/05/04)


## Interactions

Absorption of vitamin A from the gastrointestinal tract may be reduced by the presence of neomycin, colestyramine, or liquid paraffin.

There is an increased risk of hypervitaminosis A if vitamin A is given with synthetic retinoids such as acitretin, isotretinoin, and tretinoin.

There is conflicting evidence regarding the effect of vitamin A on the response to measles vaccine (see p.1623).

## Pharmacokinetics

Vitamin A substances are readily absorbed from the gastrointestinal tract but absorption may be reduced in the presence of fat malabsorption, low protein intake, or impaired liver or pancreatic function. Vitamin A esters are hydrolysed by pancreatic enzymes to retinol, which is then absorbed and re-esterified. Some retinol is stored in the liver. It is released from the liver bound to a specific $\alpha_1$-globulin (retinol-binding protein) in the blood. The retinol not stored in the liver undergoes glucuronide conjugation and subsequent oxidation to retinal and retinoic acid; these and other metabolites are excreted in urine and faeces. Vitamin A does not readily diffuse across the placenta (but see Pregnancy, above), but is present in breast milk.

◊ References.


1. Hartmann D, *et al.* Pharmacokinetic modelling of the plasma concentration-time profile of the vitamin retinyl palmitate following intramuscular administration. *Biopharm Drug Dispos* 1990; **11:** 689–700.


## Human Requirements

Dietary vitamin A is derived from 2 sources, *preformed retinoids* from animal sources such as liver, kidney, dairy produce, and eggs (fish-liver oils are the most concentrated natural source), and *provitamin carotenoids* which can be obtained from many plants; the latter are converted to retinol in the body but are less effectively utilised. Carotenes (α, β, and γ) are major sources and of these, β-carotene (betacarotene—see p.1422) has the highest vitamin A activity and is the most plentiful in food. Variable amounts of β-carotenes are found in carrots and dark green or yellow vegetables. Red palm oil is a good source of α- and β-carotenes.

**UK and US recommended dietary intake.** In the UK dietary reference values (see p.1419) have been published[1] for vitamin A and similarly in the USA recommended dietary allowances (RDAs) have been set.[2] Differing amounts are recommended for infants and children of varying ages, for adult males and females, and for pregnant and lactating women (but see Pregnancy, above). In the UK the reference nutrient intake (RNI) for adult males and females is 700 and 600 micrograms retinol equivalents (about 2330 and 2000 units) daily, respectively and the estimated average requirement (EAR) is 500 and 400 micrograms retinol equivalents (approximately 1660 and 1330 units) daily, respectively. This UK report[1] also highlighted the toxicity associated with large doses of vitamin A and recommended that regular intakes should not exceed 9000 micrograms (30 000 units) daily in adult men and 7500 micrograms (25 000 units) daily in adult women. Figures were also given for infants and children who were said to be more sensitive to the effects of vitamin A. These limits did not apply to therapeutic doses of vitamin A used under medical supervision.[1] In pregnancy the RNI is 700 micrograms retinol equivalents (2330 units) daily and in nursing mothers 950 micrograms (3160 units) daily. In the USA the RDA for adults is 900 micrograms daily for men and 700 micrograms daily for women.[2] The tolerable upper intake level is 3000 micrograms daily.


1. DoH. Dietary reference values for food energy and nutrients for the United Kingdom: report of the panel on dietary reference values of the committee on medical aspects of food policy. *Report on health and social subjects 41.* London: HMSO, 1991.
2. Standing Committee on the Scientific Evaluation of Dietary Reference Intakes of the Food and Nutrition Board. *Dietary Reference Intakes for vitamin A, vitamin K, arsenic, boron, chromium, copper, iodine, iron, manganese, molybdenum, nickel, silicon, vanadium, and zinc.* Washington DC: National Academy Press, 2001. Also available at: http://www.nap.edu/catalog/10026.html (accessed 24/05/04)

## Uses and Administration

Vitamin A, a fat-soluble vitamin, is essential for growth, for the development and maintenance of epithelial tissue, and for vision, particularly in dim light. Vitamin A deficiency develops when the dietary intake is inadequate and is seen more frequently in young children than in adults. It is rare in developed countries but remains a major problem in many developing countries. Prolonged deficiency leads to xerophthalmia or 'dry eye', the initial symptom of which is night blindness which may progress to severe eye lesions and blindness. Other symptoms include changes in the skin and mucous membranes.

Vitamin A is used in the treatment and prevention of vitamin A deficiency. It may be given by mouth in an oil- or water-based form, the oil-based generally being the preferred type. It can also be administered by intramuscular injection of a water-miscible form; oil-miscible preparations of vitamin A are poorly absorbed from injection sites after intramuscular injection and are not usually given by this route. For further details concerning vitamin A supplementation, including doses for the treatment and prophylaxis of xerophthalmia, see below.

Vitamin A supplements are often given to patients with primary biliary cirrhosis or chronic cholestatic liver disease as deficiencies are common in these disorders. An intramuscular dose of 100 000 units every 2 to 4 months has been suggested.

Vitamins A and D have been used together as cream or ointment in the treatment of minor skin disorders including abrasions. Vitamin A has also been used alone to treat various skin disorders including acne and psoriasis. It has been tried in patients with retinitis pigmentosa to retard the decline in retinal function.

**Deficiency states.** Vitamin A deficiency is relatively rare in developed countries and is usually only seen in certain medical conditions such as biliary cirrhosis or cholestatic jaundice. However, it is a continuing problem in many developing countries and children appear to be particularly vulnerable.

In the developing countries where dietary intake may often be less than desirable, infections such as measles, acute respiratory diseases, and diarrhoea can be major precipitating factors of vitamin A deficiency. Thus WHO have targeted elimination of vitamin A deficiency as an important strategy in child health,[1,2] and as part of the Expanded Programme on Immunization. They recommend the use of vitamin A supplements in the treatment of vitamin A deficiency and to prevent vitamin A deficiency where the periodic administration of supplements is determined to be the most feasible and effective method of improving vitamin A status. In universal distribution programmes,[2,3] supplemental doses are given to all children up to the age of 5 at a dose of 200 000 units every 4 to 6 months, with infants between the ages of 6 and 12 months receiving half this dose. Infants aged less than 6 months may receive 50 000 units if they are not breast fed or if they are breast fed and their mothers have not received supplemental vitamin A. If clinical signs of vitamin A deficiency are evident at the time of routine supplementation, treatment should be given as described under Xerophthalmia, below. Mothers should receive 200 000 units within 6 weeks of delivery of a child. Targeted distribution programmes involve vitamin A supplementation to children and pregnant women in specific high-risk areas.[2] Doses used in children are similar to those used in universal programmes, but doses used in pregnant women should not exceed 10 000 units daily, or 25 000 units weekly.[2]

A number of studies have indicated that general supplementation with vitamin A decreases both mortality rates and morbidity among children in developing countries with a high prevalence of vitamin A deficiency.[4-7] Although not all studies have confirmed these findings,[8,9] two meta-analyses concur that the effect is likely to be genuine especially as regards measles infection,[10,11] (see Measles, below) and researchers and commentators have agreed that overall improvement of vitamin A status is worthwhile and necessary.[8,12-14] Supplementation with vitamin A 23 300 units weekly, or the equivalent amount of betacarotene, in women of child-bearing age reduced pregnancy-related mortality.[15] Some studies have evaluated mortality specifically in infants less than 6 months of age. In one study there was no overall benefit on early infant mortality with a tendency for the relative risk of mortality to increase with improved nutritional status,[16] whereas others reported decreases in mortality at 6 months[17] and 1 year[18] of age. A further study found no sustained benefit of vitamin A supplements on vitamin A status or morbidity beyond the age of 6 months, in infants receiving supplements with immunisation at 6, 10, and 14 weeks.[19] A study in vitamin-A-deficient children has demonstrated abnormalities in T-cell subsets which are corrected by vitamin A supplementation,[20] and it has been proposed that the apparent effects of vitamin A on morbidity and mortality may be due to modulation of immune function (see also Effects on the Immune System, above).

In countries in which vitamin A deficiency is not widespread some form of supplementation may still be considered. In the UK, the Department of Health has recommended for children aged 1 to 5 years routine supplementation with 700 units of vitamin A daily, with ascorbic acid and vitamin D; some breast-fed infants from 1 or 6 months of age may also benefit. Preterm infants have low vitamin A status at birth, which may increase their risk of developing chronic lung disease.[21] A meta-analysis of trials in low birth-weight infants found that vitamin A supplementation was associated with a reduced requirement for oxygen at 36 weeks postmenstrual age.[21] While trials of vitamin A supplementation to prevent chronic lung disease in very low birth-weight infants have had conflicting results,[22,23] some have commented that differences in patient population, postnatal therapies, and dosage of vitamin A could explain these discrepancies, and consider optimal supplementation necessary.[24]


1. Potter AR. Reducing vitamin A deficiency: could save the eyesight and lives of countless children. *BMJ* 1997; **314:** 317–18.
2. WHO/UNICEF/IVACG Task Force. *Vitamin A supplements: a guide to their use in the treatment and prevention of vitamin A deficiency and xerophthalmia.* 2nd ed. Geneva: WHO, 1997.
3. WHO. Integration of vitamin A supplementation with immunization. *Wkly Epidem Rec* 1999; **74:** 1–6.
4. Rahmathullah L, *et al.* Reduced mortality among children in southern India receiving a small weekly dose of vitamin A. *N Engl J Med* 1990; **323:** 929–35.
5. West KP, *et al.* Efficacy of vitamin A in reducing preschool child mortality in Nepal. *Lancet* 1991; **338:** 67–71.
6. Daulaire NMP, *et al.* Childhood mortality after a high dose of vitamin A in a high risk population. *BMJ* 1992; **304:** 207–10.
7. Ghana VAST Study Team. Vitamin A supplementation in northern Ghana: effects on clinic attendances, hospital admissions, and child mortality. *Lancet* 1993; **342:** 7–12.
8. Vijayaraghavan K, *et al.* Effect of massive dose of vitamin A on morbidity and mortality in Indian children. *Lancet* 1990; **336:** 1342–5.
9. Herrera MG, *et al.* Vitamin A supplementation and child survival. *Lancet* 1992; **340:** 267–71.
10. Glasziou PP, Mackerras DEM. Vitamin A supplementation in infectious diseases: a meta-analysis. *BMJ* 1993; **306:** 366–70.
11. Fawzi WW, *et al.* Vitamin A supplementation and child mortality: a meta-analysis. *JAMA* 1993; **269:** 898–903.
12. Anonymous. Vitamin A and malnutrition/infection complex in developing countries. *Lancet* 1990; **336:** 1349–51.
13. Humphrey JH, Rice AL. Vitamin A supplementation of young infants. *Lancet* 2000; **356:** 422–4.
14. Villamor E, Fawzi WW. Vitamin A supplementation: implications for morbidity and mortality in children. *J Infect Dis* 2000; **182** (suppl): S122–S133.
15. West KP, *et al.* Double blind, cluster randomised trial of low dose supplementation with vitamin A or β carotene on mortality related to pregnancy in Nepal. *BMJ* 1999; **318:** 570–5. Correction. *ibid.*; 1386.
16. West KP, *et al.* Mortality of infants <6 mo of age supplemented with vitamin A: a randomized double-masked trial in Nepal. *Am J Clin Nutr* 1995; **62:** 143–8.
17. Rahmathullah L, *et al.* Impact of supplementing newborn infants with vitamin A on early infant mortality: community based randomised trial in southern India. *BMJ* 2003; **327:** 254–7.
18. Humphrey JH, *et al.* Impact of neonatal vitamin A supplementation on infant morbidity and mortality. *J Pediatr* 1996; **128:** 489–96.
19. WHO/CHD Immunisation-Linked Vitamin A Supplementation Study Group. Randomised trial to assess benefits and safety of vitamin A supplementation linked to immunisation in early infancy. *Lancet* 1998; **352:** 1257–63. Correction. *ibid.* 1999; **353:** 154.
20. Semba RD, *et al.* Abnormal T-cell subset proportions in vitamin-A-deficient children. *Lancet* 1993; **341:** 5–8.
21. Darlow BA, Graham PJ. Vitamin A supplementation for preventing morbidity and mortality in very low birthweight infants. Available in The Cochrane Library; Issue 2. Chichester: John Wiley; 2004.
22. Tyson JE, *et al.* Vitamin A supplementation for extremely-low-birth-weight infants. *N Engl J Med* 1999; **340:** 1962–8.
23. Wardle SP, *et al.* Randomised controlled trial of oral vitamin A supplementation in preterm infants to prevent chronic lung disease. *Arch Dis Child Fetal Neonatal Ed* 2001; **84:** F9–F13.
24. Shenai JP. Vitamin A supplementation in very low birth weight neonates: rationale and evidence. *Pediatrics* 1999; **104:** 1369–74.


ANAEMIA. A study among pregnant Indonesian women with nutritional anaemia (p.733) demonstrated a beneficial effect for vitamin A on haemoglobin when given with iron supplementation.[1] Vitamin A is considered essential for haematopoiesis; it has been suggested that vitamin A is required for the mobilisation and utilisation of iron for haemoglobin synthesis.[2]


1. Suharno D, *et al.* Supplementation with vitamin A and iron for nutritional anaemia in pregnant women in West Java, Indonesia. *Lancet* 1993; **342:** 1325–8.
2. van den Broek N. Anaemia and micronutrient deficiencies. *Br Med Bull* 2003; **67:** 149–60.


DIARRHOEA. Although oral rehydration therapy remains the mainstay of the management of diarrhoea (p.1241) once it develops, it has been suggested that vitamin A supplementation may be of use in reducing the incidence and mortality of diarrhoea during childhood. Several large mortality trials reported that vitamin A supplementation was associated with reduced mortality attributed to diarrhoea,[1-3] but one did not.[4] The effect on morbidity from diarrhoea is even less clear. A reduction in the severity, but not the incidence, of diarrhoea has been noted in two studies.[5,6] However, in one study in children with subclinical vitamin A deficiency, there was an increased prevalence of diarrhoea for 2 weeks after vitamin A supplementation,[7] and in another study, vitamin A increased the incidence of diarrhoea in children aged less than 30 months.[8] A meta-analysis[9] concluded that vitamin A supplementation has no consistent overall protective effect on the incidence of diarrhoea. While severity was not examined, they noted that the decrease in diarrhoea mortality rates but not incidence can be reconciled if vitamin A reduces diarrhoea severity and not susceptibility to infection. One group[10] proposed that the inconsistent findings on morbidity of vitamin A supplementation may be due to co-existing micronutrient deficiencies, such as zinc deficiency, that affect the bioavailability of vitamin A. They found combined zinc and vitamin A supplementation to be more effective in reducing persistent diarrhoea and dysentery than either zinc or vitamin A alone.


1. West KP, *et al.* Efficacy of vitamin A in reducing preschool child mortality in Nepal. *Lancet* 1991; **338:** 67–71.
2. Daulaire NMP, *et al.* Childhood mortality after a high dose of vitamin A in a high risk population. *BMJ* 1992; **304:** 207–10.
3. Ghana VAST Study Team. Vitamin A supplementation in northern Ghana: effects on clinic attendances, hospital admissions, and child mortality. *Lancet* 1993; **342:** 7–12.
4. Vijayaraghavan K, *et al.* Effect of massive dose of vitamin A on morbidity and mortality in Indian children. *Lancet* 1990; **336:** 1342–5.
5. Barreto ML, *et al.* Effect of vitamin A supplementation on diarrhoea and acute lower-respiratory-tract infections in young children in Brazil. *Lancet* 1994; **344:** 228–31.
6. Bhandari N, *et al.* Impact of massive dose of vitamin A given to preschool children with acute diarrhoea on subsequent respiratory and diarrhoeal morbidity. *BMJ* 1994; **309:** 1404–7.
7. Stansfield SK, *et al.* Vitamin A supplementation and increased prevalence of childhood diarrhoea and acute respiratory infections. *Lancet* 1993; **342:** 578–82.
8. Dibley MJ, *et al.* Vitamin A supplementation fails to reduce incidence of acute respiratory illness and diarrhea in preschool-age Indonesian children. *J Nutr* 1996; **126:** 434–42.
9. Grotto I, *et al.* Vitamin A supplementation and childhood morbidity from diarrhea and respiratory infections: a meta-analysis. *J Pediatr* 2003; **142:** 297–304.
10. Rahman MM, *et al.* Simultaneous zinc and vitamin A supplementation in Bangladeshi children: randomised double blind controlled trial. *BMJ* 2001; **323:** 314–18.


HIV INFECTION AND AIDS. A study in Malawi found that the rates of vertical transmission of HIV infection (birth of seropositive infants to seropositive mothers) were inversely related to maternal vitamin A status;[1] vitamin A deficiency during pregnancy was associated with a threefold to fourfold increased risk of mother-to-child transmission of HIV. This was not incompatible with the role of vitamin A in immunity and maintenance of mucosal surfaces, and since both HIV infection and pregnancy are risk factors for vitamin A deficiency, it was suggested that nutritional intervention to reduce vitamin A deficiency might help combat mother-to-child transmission. However, another study[2] in Tanzania, for which vertical transmission data were not available, found no evidence of an effect of vitamin A on birth outcomes in HIV-infected women and the authors pointed out that serum concentrations of vitamin A might be a marker of the stage of HIV disease rather than being causally related to outcome. The study did however find that multivitamin supplements reduced the risk of low birth-weight and size for age, and of premature birth, in the offspring of these women.[2] Similarly, a South African study[3] supplementing HIV-infected pregnant women with vitamin A and betacarotene found that this did not reduce the overall risk of vertical transmission to neonates. Supplementation did reduce the incidence of preterm births, and among these neonates, risk of perinatal HIV transmission was lower in those whose mothers had been supplemented. Vitamin A supplementation increased the risk of HIV transmission through breast feeding, with no effect on mortality at 24 months, in a Tanzanian trial.[4] However, the same group found that vitamin A supplementation reduced mortality in infants and children infected with HIV;[5] the authors caution that these beneficial effects are not generalisable to communities with access to antiretroviral therapy and good nutrition. Means of reducing the risk of HIV infection in neonates are discussed under HIV Infection Prophylaxis, p.623.


1. Semba RD, *et al.* Maternal vitamin A deficiency and mother-to-child transmission of HIV-1. *Lancet* 1994; **343:** 1593–7.
2. Fawzi WW, *et al.* Randomised trial of effects of vitamin supplements on pregnancy outcomes and T-cell counts in HIV-1-infected women in Tanzania. *Lancet* 1998; **351:** 1477–82.
3. Coutsoudis A, *et al.* Randomized trial testing the effect of vitamin A supplementation on pregnancy outcomes and early mother-to-child HIV-1 transmission in Durban, South Africa. *AIDS* 1999; **13:** 1517–24.
4. Fawzi WW, *et al.* Randomized trial of vitamin supplements in relation to transmission of HIV-1 through breastfeeding and early child mortality. *AIDS* 2002; **16:** 1935–44.
5. Fawzi WW, *et al.* A randomized trial of vitamin A supplements in relation to mortality among human immunodeficiency virus-infected and uninfected children in Tanzania. *Pediatr Infect Dis J* 1999; **18:** 127–33.


MEASLES. Vitamin A supplementation has an important role in the prevention of complications from measles.[1,2] Two studies specifically addressing vitamin A status and measles have found that complications such as pneumonia and diarrhoea were less common in children who had received supplements at the time of diagnosis than in those given a placebo.[3,4] A systematic review of randomised trials concluded that a dose of 200 000 units of vitamin A given on two consecutive days reduced mortality in children with measles.[5] WHO has recommended treating children in populations where vitamin A deficiency is common with high-dose vitamin A supplements during episodes of measles.[6] A dose of 200 000 units should be given on two consecutive days to all children over 12 months of age. This should be followed by a further dose at least 2 weeks later. Infants less than 6 months of age should receive doses of 50 000 units and those between 6 and 12 months should be given 100 000 units. Studies in the USA have indicated that even among well-nourished children from a developed country, vitamin A deficiency in measles patients is not uncommon,[7,8] and vitamin A supplementation needs to be considered in children at risk.[9]


1. Glasziou PP, Mackerras DEM. Vitamin A supplementation in infectious diseases: a meta-analysis. *BMJ* 1993; **306:** 366–70.
2. Fawzi WW, *et al.* Vitamin A supplementation and child mortality: a meta-analysis. *JAMA* 1993; **269:** 898–903.
3. Barclay AJG, *et al.* Vitamin A supplements and mortality related to measles: a randomised clinical trial. *BMJ* 1987; **294:** 294–6.
4. Hussey GD, Klein M. A randomized, controlled trial of vitamin A in children with severe measles. *N Engl J Med* 1990; **323:** 160–4.
5. D'Souza RM, D'Souza R. Vitamin A for treating measles in children. Available in The Cochrane Library; Issue 2. Chichester: John Wiley; 2004.
6. WHO/UNICEF/IVACG Task Force. *Vitamin A supplements: a guide to their use in the treatment and prevention of vitamin A deficiency and xerophthalmia.* 2nd ed. Geneva: WHO, 1997.
7. Arrieta AC, *et al.* Vitamin A levels in children with measles in Long Beach, California. *J Pediatr* 1992; **121:** 75–8.
8. Butler JC, *et al.* Measles severity and serum retinol (vitamin A) concentration among children in the United States. *Pediatrics* 1993; **91:** 1176–81.
9. Committee on Infectious Diseases of the American Academy of Pediatrics. Vitamin A treatment of measles. *Pediatrics* 1993; **91:** 1014–15.


RESPIRATORY-TRACT INFECTIONS. Mortality trials did not show a consistent impact for vitamin A supplementation on death from non-measles-related respiratory infections.[1-3] Similarly, other studies have found no benefit of vitamin A on subsequent respiratory morbidity.[4-6] A meta-analysis of trials reporting pneumonia morbidity and mortality found no overall benefit or harm from vitamin A supplementation.[7] However, an increased prevalence of symptoms of respiratory infections associated with vitamin A supplementation has been noted in two studies,[8,9] particularly in children with adequate nutritional status. A meta-analysis of the effect of vitamin A supplementation on childhood morbidity found an increased incidence of respiratory-tract infections; since most trials had excluded children with overt vitamin A deficiency, the authors commented that high-dose vitamin A administered to children with adequate vitamin A stores might cause a temporary decline in immune status, increasing their susceptibility to infection.[10]

Vitamin A was not effective for the treatment of childhood non-measles-related lower respiratory-tract infections[11] or pneumonia.[12] Similarly, there was no benefit from vitamin A in the treatment of respiratory syncytial virus infection in children in two studies.[13,14] In one of these studies there was a tendency for vitamin A to improve outcomes in the subgroup of severely ill children,[13] and in the other there was a slight increase in duration of hospitalisation in low-risk children receiving vitamin A.[14]


1. West KP, *et al.* Efficacy of vitamin A in reducing preschool child mortality in Nepal. *Lancet* 1991; **338:** 67–71.
2. Daulaire NMP, *et al.* Childhood mortality after a high dose of vitamin A in a high risk population. *BMJ* 1992; **304:** 207–10.
3. Ghana VAST Study Team. Vitamin A supplementation in northern Ghana: effects on clinic attendances, hospital admissions, and child mortality. *Lancet* 1993; **342:** 7–12.
4. Barreto ML, *et al.* Effect of vitamin A supplementation on diarrhoea and acute lower-respiratory-tract infections in young children in Brazil. *Lancet* 1994; **344:** 228–31.
5. Bhandari N, *et al.* Impact of massive dose of vitamin A given to preschool children with acute diarrhoea on subsequent respiratory and diarrhoeal morbidity. *BMJ* 1994; **309:** 1404–7.
6. Kartasasmita CB, *et al.* Plasma retinol level, vitamin A supplementation and acute respiratory infections in children of 1-5 years old in a developing country. *Tubercle Lung Dis* 1995; **76:** 563–9.
7. The Vitamin A and Pneumonia Working Group. Potential interventions for the prevention of childhood pneumonia in developing countries: a meta-analysis of data from field trials to assess the impact of vitamin A supplementation on pneumonia morbidity and mortality. *Bull WHO* 1995; **73:** 609–19.
8. Stansfield SK, *et al.* Vitamin A supplementation and increased prevalence of childhood diarrhoea and acute respiratory infections. *Lancet* 1993; **342:** 578–82.
9. Dibley MJ, *et al.* Vitamin A supplementation fails to reduce incidence of acute respiratory illness and diarrhea in preschool-age Indonesian children. *J Nutr* 1996; **126:** 434–42.
10. Grotto I, *et al.* Vitamin A supplementation and childhood morbidity from diarrhea and respiratory infections: a meta-analysis. *J Pediatr* 2003; **142:** 297–304.
11. Kjolhede CL, *et al.* Clinical trial of vitamin A as adjuvant treatment for lower respiratory tract infections. *J Pediatr* 1995; **126:** 807–12.
12. Nacul LC, *et al.* Randomised, double blind, placebo controlled clinical trial of efficacy of vitamin A treatment in non-measles childhood pneumonia. *BMJ* 1997; **315:** 505–10.
13. Dowell SF, *et al.* Treatment of respiratory syncytial virus infection with vitamin A: a randomised placebo-controlled trial in Santiago, Chile. *Pediatr Infect Dis J* 1996; **15:** 782–6.
14. Bresee JS, *et al.* Vitamin A therapy for children with respiratory syncytial virus infection: a multicenter trial in the United States. *Pediatr Infect Dis J* 1996; **15:** 777–82.


SHIGELLOSIS. A single high-dose vitamin A supplement, given with standard antibacterial treatment, reduced the severity of acute shigellosis in children in Bangladesh.[1]


1. Hossain S, *et al.* Single dose vitamin A treatment in acute shigellosis in Bangladeshi children: randomised double blind controlled trial. *BMJ* 1998; **316:** 422–6.


XEROPHTHALMIA. Vitamin A deficiency is responsible in many developing countries for visual problems which may culminate in xerophthalmia and blindness. Supplementation with vitamin A as recommended by WHO and discussed under Deficiency states, above, will raise the vitamin A status of the individual and act prophylactically against the development of xerophthalmia. For the treatment of xerophthalmia (which includes night blindness, conjunctival xerosis with Bitot's spots, corneal xerosis, corneal ulceration, and keratomalacia) WHO have stated that oral doses of vitamin A, preferably in an oil-based preparation, are the treatment of choice and should be given immediately the disorder is recognised.[1] All patients over 1 year of age (with the exception of women of reproductive age) should receive 200 000 units by mouth immediately on diagnosis; infants aged 6 to 12 months should receive 100 000 units, and those aged less than 6 months, 50 000 units. The dose should be repeated the next day, and again at least 2 weeks later. In women of reproductive age there is a need to balance the possible teratogenic effects of vitamin A should they be pregnant (see Pregnancy, above) with the serious consequences of xerophthalmia. WHO recommend that when there are severe signs of active xerophthalmia (i.e. acute corneal lesions) high-dose vitamin A treatment should be given as described above for those aged over 1 year. When only less severe signs are present (night blindness, Bitot's spots), women of reproductive age should receive a daily oral dose of 5000 to 10 000 units for at least 4 weeks. Alternatively, a weekly dose of not more than 25 000 units may be substituted.

Although xerophthalmia is far less common in developed countries, vitamin A deficiency should be considered in all patients with recurrent conjunctival or corneal disorders associated with gastrointestinal or liver disease.[2]


1. WHO/UNICEF/IVACG Task Force. *Vitamin A supplements: a guide to their use in the treatment and prevention of vitamin A deficiency and xerophthalmia.* 2nd ed. Geneva: WHO, 1997.
2. Watson NJ, *et al.* Vitamin A deficiency and xerophthalmia in the United Kingdom. *BMJ* 1995; **310:** 1050–1. Correction. *ibid.:* 1320.


**Malignant neoplasms.** Epidemiological studies suggest that antoxidant vitamins such as the vitamin A substances may play a role in preventing the development of malignancy but there is currently little evidence from prospective studies to support this (see p.1420). Conversely, synthetic retinoids such as tretinoin (all-*trans*-retinoic acid) have an established role in treating some cancers (see p.1161).

**Retinitis pigmentosa.** Retinitis pigmentosa is the name applied to a group of slowly progressive hereditary degenerative diseases of the retina that often results in blindness in adulthood. The rod and cone photoreceptors in the retina are primarily affected and initial symptoms include night blindness and intolerance to light. Later signs include infiltration of pigment from the retinal pigmentary epithelium into the retinal layers. Various treatments have been tried but none appear to have any proven benefit. Results of one large double-blind study[1] suggest that whereas treatment with vitamin A might slow the decline in visual acuity treatment with vitamin E appears to have a deleterious effect on the rate of decline. Vitamin E did appear to delay the rate of vision decline in 3 patients with retinitis pigmentosa and a defect in α-tocopherol-transfer protein associated with vitamin E deficiency.[2] Transplantation of the retina is being investigated as a treatment for retinitis pigmentosa.[3]


1. Berson EL, *et al.* A randomized trial of vitamin A and vitamin E supplementation for retinitis pigmentosa. *Arch Ophthalmol* 1993; **111:** 761–2.
2. Yokota T, *et al.* Retinitis pigmentosa and ataxia caused by a mutation in the gene for the α-tocopherol-transfer protein. *N Engl J Med* 1996; **335:** 1770–1.
3. Anonymous. Transplantation as a therapy for retinitis pigmentosa? *Br J Ophthalmol* 1997; **81:** 430.


## Preparations

***BP 2003:*** Paediatric Vitamins A, C and D Oral Drops;
***BPC 1973:*** Vitamins A and D Capsules;
***USP 27:*** Oleovitamin A and D; Oleovitamin A and D Capsules; Vitamin A Capsules.

**Proprietary Preparations** (details are given in Part 3)

***Arg.:*** A-Vitel; Amenite A; Andrioderma; Arovit; Atomoderma A; Bagovit A; Cazmar; Fiosen-A; Flavostat; Masivol; Metabolite-A; Midermus; Rogadermis; Skinderm A; ***Austral.:*** Dermalife†; Ungvita; ***Austria:*** Arcavit A; Avitol; Oleovit A; ***Belg.:*** Dagravit A†; Vitamuruine; ***Braz.:*** Arovit; Lacrigel A; Nalfan†; Retinar; ***Canad.:*** A-Mulsion†; Arovit; ***Chile:*** Bagovit-A; ***Denm.:*** A-vitamin; ***Fin.:*** A-Vitamiini; ***Fr.:*** A 313; Arovit; Avibon; ***Ger.:*** A-Mulsin; A-Vicotrat; Augenkraft†; Oculotect; Oculotect sine; Ophtol-A†; Ophtosan†; Solan-M; Vitadral; Vitafluid; Vitagel; ***Hong Kong:*** Aquasol A†; ***Israel:*** Avipur; ***Ital.:*** Akeral†; Arovit; Euvitol; Repervit; Vit-A-N; ***Malaysia:*** Fairy ADE; ***Mex.:*** A Grin; A-Vicon; A-Vitex†; Acon; Avinal-Ex†; Microvita; Pertamin†; ***Neth.:*** Dagravit A Forte; ***NZ:*** Dermalife; Ro-A-Vit†; Ungvita; ***Port.:*** A-Vite; Vitaminoftalmina; ***S.Afr.:*** Arovit; ***Spain:*** Auxina A Masiva; Biominol A; Dif Vitamin A Masivo; Ido A 50†; Mulsal A Megadosis†; Rinocusi Vitaminico; ***Swed.:*** Arovit; ***Switz.:*** Arovit; Oculotect; ***UK:*** Biovit-A; ***USA:*** Aquasol A; Del-Vi-A†; Palmitate-A; Pedi-Vit-A; Retinol-A.

**Multi-ingredient: *Arg.:*** A-D-C; A-Vitel E; AD Shock; Adermicina; Adermicina A; Atomoderma A-D; Atomoderma A-E; Aulo Gelio Pie; Bagovit A Plus; Bagovit Avant Piel; Celuvital; Crema de Ordene; Derivoco; Herbaccion Nutriderm; Hipoglos; Hipoglos con Hidrocortisona; Masivol Urea; Medicreme; Nemegel; O-Biol; Palan; Panoxi; Platsul-A; Redoxon A; Salvicutan; Sulfadiazina de Plata; Sulfaplat; Ulcevarin; Vagicural; Vitapelen; Zoodermina Cream; ***Austral.:*** Althaea Complex†; Arthriforte†; Bioglan Micelle A plus E†; Bioglan Zn-A-C†; Dermalife Plus; ER Cream; Garlic, Horseradish, A & C Capsules†; Hydrastis Complex†; John Plunketts Protective Day Cream†; Macro Natural Vitamin E Cream; Natures Way Total Zinc†; Proyeast†; Sambucus Complex†; Trifolium Complex†; Verbascum Complex†; ***Austria:*** A-E-Mulsin; Arcavit A/E; Coldistop; Gelacet; Gerogelat; Lemuval; Oleovit; Oleovit A; Oleovit A + D; Regenerin; Rovigon; Ultren; Vasovitol; ***Belg.:*** AD-Vitan†; Dagravit A-E†; Neo-Cutigenol; Neo-Debiol AD3†; Newderm; Rovigon; Vita-Mefren; Vitaminic A-D†; Vitamorrhuine†; Vitapantol†; ***Braz.:*** AD-Furp†; AD-Til; ADE 2 (Adedois); Adeforte; Aderofix D3†; Aderogil D3; Belglos†; Dermalisan; Epitezan; Gaduol; Gotil-AD†; Hipoderme; Hipodermon; Hipodex; Hipoglos; Hipoglos Oftalmico†; Licovit; Natural Wealth Beta†; Preparado H†; Regenom; Solemil†; Vitadesan; ***Canad.:*** A & D; A & D Ointment; Antiseptic Skin Cream; Aquasol A†; Le Stick a Levres; Nutrol A D; ***Chile:*** Brexon; Dermaglos; Dermaglos Plus; Droxel; Panthoderm-A; Pediaderm; Platsul A; Pomada Vitaminica; Povin; Rovigon; Sanoderm; ***Fin.:*** A-Vita; Aesol; Oftan A-Pant; Wicarba; Wicnevit; ***Fr.:*** Alpha 5 DS; Auxergyl $D_3$†; Calmoroide†; Cirkan a la Prednacinolone; Dermocalm†; Pommade Lelong; Rovigon; Solacy; ***Ger.:*** A + D + E-Vicotrat†; A + $D_3$-Vicotrat†; A + E Thilo; A-E-Mulsin; Coldastop; Corti-Flexiole†; Cosaldon A†; duraultra; Gelacet N; Golden Star†; Hewekzem novo N; Kollateral A + E†; Kwim; Magopsor†; Oculotect; Regepithel; Remederm; Rovigon G; Salus Augenschutz-Kapseln NA; Unguentacid; ***Gr.:*** Aquasol A+D; Eviol-A; ***Hong Kong:*** Aderma Epitheliale; Hypotears; Regepithel; ***India:*** Medithane; Ossivite; Rovigon; Sclerobion; Sharkomalt; Sharkovit; ***Israel:*** Aquitol; Aronal Forte; Oleovit A + $D_3$; Vita-Merfen NF; Vitamidyne A and D; ***Ital.:*** AD Pabyrn; Adiboran AD†; Adisterolo; Aminotril†; Babysteril; Derman-Oil; Dermana Pasta; Dicalcium; Evitex; Granoleina; Lasonil H†; Lasoproct†; Midium; NeoCeuticals Spot Treatment; Provitamin A-E; Retinovit; Rinopanteina; Rovigon; Tocalfa; ***Mex.:*** Adekon; Adekon C; Adeloren; Adibal; Hipoglos Plus; Kamiloderm; Microka; Quinoret; Sutin; Vitalorange; ***Neth.:*** Dagravit A-E Forte; Davitamon AD Fluor†; Davitamon AD†; Dohyfral Vitamine AD3†; Halitran; ***NZ:*** Dermalife Plus†; Ungvita†; ***Port.:*** Esclerobion; Rovigon; Synchrovit; Zelderme†; ***S.Afr.:*** Vandol; ***Spain:*** Adiod; Antihemorroidal; Auxina A + E; Biominol A D; Bronquimar Vit A†; Calcio 20 Complex; Cicatral; Dermo Halibut Infantil; Dimayon†; Epitelizante; Evitex A E Fuerte; Gramoce A; Grietalgen; Grietalgen Hidrocort; Halibut; Halibut Hidrocortisona; Hubergrip; Lacerdermol; Lacerdermol Complex; Mastiol; Mitosyl; Poli ABE†; Queratil†; Ravigona†; Trivitan†; Vicomin A C; Vitaber A E; Wobenzimal; ***Swed.:*** AD-vitamin; ***Switz.:*** Alphastria; Antikeloides Creme; Carbamide Creme; Coldistop; Gelacet; Kamillosan†; Leniderm; Malvedrin; Oravil; Riccomycine†; Riccovitan; Rovigon; Sanhelios Capsules a la vitamine A; Unatol; Vita-Hexin; Vita-Merfen; ***Thai.:*** Rovigon†; ***UK:*** S.P.H.P.; Se-Power; ***USA:*** A and D Medicated; Aloe Grande; Clocream; Comfortine†; Diaper Guard; Lazercreme; Lobana Derm-Aide; Lobana Peri-Garde; Phicon.

---

# Vitamin B Substances

Vitaminas B.

The B vitamin group includes the $B_1$ substances (thiamine and its derivatives), $B_2$ (riboflavin), $B_6$ (pyridoxine and derivatives), and $B_{12}$ (the cobalamins). In addition, nicotinic acid and its derivatives (p.1441) and folic acid (p.1429) are held to be part of the group, as is pantothenic acid (p.1442), but these latter substances are not generally referred to by their traditional B nomenclature.

## Preparations

**Proprietary Preparations** (details are given in Part 3)

**Multi-ingredient: *Braz.:*** Plex B; Xantina B12; Xantinon B12; ***India:*** Elferri; Hycibex; JP Tone; Livogen; Lupizyme; Terramycin SF; Toniazol; Vitexid; ***Malaysia:*** Luckyhepa.

---

# Vitamin $B_1$ Substances

Vitaminas $B_1$.

### Acetiamine Hydrochloride *(rINNM)*

Acethiamine Hydrochloride; Diacethiamine Hydrochloride; Hidrocloruro de acetiamina. *N*-(5-Acetoxy-3-acetylthiopent-2-en-2-yl)-*N*-(4-amino-2-methylpyrimidin-5-ylmethyl)formamide hydrochloride monohydrate.

$C_{16}H_{22}N_4O_4S,HCl,H_2O = 420.9.$
*CAS — 299-89-8 (acetiamine).*

### Benfotiamine *(rINN)*

Benfotiamina; *S*-Benzoylthiamine *O*-Monophosphate. *N*-(4-Amino-2-methylpyrimidin-5-ylmethyl)-*N*-(2-benzoylthio-4-dihydroxyphosphinyloxy-1-methylbut-1-enyl)formamide.

$C_{19}H_{23}N_4O_6PS = 466.4.$
*CAS — 22457-89-2.*

### Bisbentiamine *(rINN)*

*O*-Benzoylthiamine Disulphide; Bisbentiamina. *NN'*-{Dithiobis[2-(2-benzoyloxyethyl)-1-methylvinylene]}bis[*N*-(4-amino-2-methylpyrimidin-5-ylmethyl)formamide].

$C_{38}H_{42}N_8O_6S_2 = 770.9.$
*CAS — 2667-89-2.*

### Cycotiamine *(rINN)*

CCT; Cicotiamina; Cyclocarbothiamine. *N*-(4-Amino-2-methylpyrimidin-5-ylmethyl)-*N*-[1-(2-oxo-1,3-oxathian-4-ylidene)ethyl]formamide.

$C_{13}H_{16}N_4O_3S = 308.4.$
*CAS — 6092-18-8.*

### Fursultiamine *(rINN)*

Fursultiamina; Thiamine Tetrahydrofurfuryl Disulphide; TTFD. *N*-(4-Amino-2-methylpyrimidin-5-ylmethyl)-*N*-[4-hydroxy-1-methyl-2-(tetrahydrofurfuryldithio)but-1-enyl]formamide.

$C_{17}H_{26}N_4O_3S_2 = 398.5.$
*CAS — 804-30-8.*

### Octotiamine *(rINN)*

Octotiamina; TATD; Thioctothiamine. *N*-[2-(3-Acetylthio-7-methoxycarbonylheptyldithio)-4-hydroxy-1-methylbut-1-enyl]-*N*-(4-amino-2-methylpyrimidin-5-ylmethyl)formamide.

$C_{23}H_{36}N_4O_5S_3$ = 544.8.

*CAS — 137-86-0.*

### Prosultiamine *(rINN)*

DTPT; Prosultiamina; Thiamine Propyl Disulphide. *N*-(4-Amino-2-methylpyrimidin-5-ylmethyl)-*N*-(4-hydroxy-1-methyl-2-propyldithiobut-1-enyl)formamide.

$C_{15}H_{24}N_4O_2S_2$ = 356.5.

*CAS — 59-58-5.*

### Sulbutiamine *(rINN)*

Bisibutiamine; *O*-Isobutyrylthiamine Disulphide; Sulbutiamina. *NN'*-{Dithiobis[2-(2-isobutyryloxyethyl)-1-methylvinylene]}bis[*N*-(4-amino-2-methylpyrimidin-5-ylmethyl)formamide].

$C_{32}H_{46}N_8O_6S_2$ = 702.9.

*CAS — 3286-46-2.*

*ATC — A11DA02.*

### Thiamine Hydrochloride *(BANM, rINNM)*

Aneurine Hydrochloride; Hidrocloruro de tiamina; Thiamin Hydrochloride; Thiamine Chloride; Thiamini Hydrochloridum; Thiaminii Chloridum; Vitamin $B_1$. 3-(4-Amino-2-methylpyrimidin-5-ylmethyl)-5-(2-hydroxyethyl)-4-methylthiazolium chloride hydrochloride.

$C_{12}H_{17}ClN_4OS,HCl$ = 337.3.

*CAS — 59-43-8 (thiamine); 67-03-8 (thiamine hydrochloride).*

*ATC — A11DA01.*

**Pharmacopoeias.** In *Chin., Eur.* (see p.vi), *Int., Jpn, Pol., US,* and *Viet.*

Thiamine hydrobromide is included in *Int.*

**Ph. Eur. 5.0** (Thiamine Hydrochloride). A white or almost white, crystalline powder or colourless crystals. Freely soluble in water; slightly soluble in alcohol; soluble in glycerol. A 2.5% solution in water has a pH of 2.7 to 3.3. Store in nonmetallic containers. Protect from light.

**USP 27** (Thiamine Hydrochloride). White crystals or crystalline powder, usually having a slight, characteristic odour. When exposed to air, the anhydrous product rapidly absorbs about 4% of water. Soluble 1 in 1 of water and 1 in 170 of alcohol; insoluble in ether and in benzene; soluble in glycerol. pH of a 1% solution in water is between 2.7 and 3.4. Store in airtight containers. Protect from light.

**Stability.** Sterile thiamine hydrochloride solutions of pH 4 or less lose activity only very slowly but neutral or alkaline solutions deteriorate rapidly, especially in contact with air.

### Thiamine Nitrate *(BANM, rINNM)*

Aneurine Mononitrate; Nitrato de tiamina; Thiamine Mononitrate; Thiamini Nitras; Vitamin $B_1$ Mononitrate. 3-(4-Amino-2-methylpyrimidin-5-ylmethyl)-5-(2-hydroxyethyl)-4-methylthiazolium nitrate.

$C_{12}H_{17}N_5O_4S$ = 327.4.

*CAS — 532-43-4.*

*ATC — A11DA01.*

**Pharmacopoeias.** In *Chin., Eur.* (see p.vi), *Int., Jpn, Pol., US,* and *Viet.*

**Ph. Eur. 5.0** (Thiamine Nitrate). A white or almost white, crystalline powder or small, colourless crystals. Sparingly soluble in water; freely soluble in boiling water; slightly soluble in alcohol and in methyl alcohol. A 2% solution in water has a pH of 6.8 to 7.6. Store in nonmetallic containers. Protect from light.

**USP 27** (Thiamine Mononitrate). White crystals or crystalline powder, usually having a slight characteristic odour. Soluble 1 in 44 of water; slightly soluble in alcohol; very slightly soluble in chloroform. pH of a 2% solution in water is between 6.0 and 7.5. Store in airtight containers. Protect from light.

## Adverse Effects and Precautions

Adverse effects seldom occur following administration of thiamine, but hypersensitivity reactions have occurred, mainly after parenteral administration. These reactions have ranged in severity from very mild to, very rarely, fatal anaphylactic shock (see below).

**Breast feeding.** Supplementation did not significantly affect thiamine concentration in breast milk of healthy, well-nourished, lactating women when compared with those not given thiamine; the authors supposed that absorptive capacity of the mammary gland may be saturable.[1] Based on this, the American Academy of Pediatrics considers its use to be usually compatible with breast feeding.[2]


1. Nail PA, *et al.* The effect of thiamin and riboflavin supplementation on the level of those vitamins in human breast milk and urine. *Am J Clin Nutr* 1980; **33:** 198–204.
2. American Academy of Pediatrics. The transfer of drugs and other chemicals into human milk. *Pediatrics* 2001; **108:** 776–89. Correction. *ibid.*; 1029. Also available at: http://aappolicy.aappublications.org/cgi/content/full/pediatrics%3b108/3/776 (accessed 19/05/04)


**Hypersensitivity.** The UK Committee on Safety of Medicines had received, between 1970 and July 1988, 90 reports of adverse reactions associated with the use of an injection containing high doses of vitamins B and C. The most frequent reactions were anaphylaxis (41 cases, including 2 fatalities), dyspnoea or bronchospasm (13 cases), and rash or flushing (22 cases); 78 of the reactions occurred during, or shortly after, intravenous injection and the other 12 after intramuscular injection.[1] They recommended that parenteral treatment be used only when essential, and that, when given, facilities for treating anaphylaxis should be available. They also recommended that, when the intravenous route was used, the injection be given slowly (over 10 minutes). Various authors[2,3] have noted that parenteral treatment is *essential* for the prophylaxis and treatment of Wernicke's encephalopathy (see below).


1. Committee on Safety of Medicines. Parentrovite & allergic reactions. *Current Problems 24* 1989.
2. Wrenn KD, Slovis CM. Is intravenous thiamine safe? *Am J Emerg Med* 1992; **10:** 165.
3. Thomson AD, Cook CCH. Parenteral thiamine and Wernicke's encephalopathy: the balance of risks and concerns. *Alcohol Alcohol* 1997; **32:** 207–9.


## Pharmacokinetics

Small amounts of thiamine are well absorbed from the gastrointestinal tract following oral administration, but the absorption of doses larger than about 5 mg is limited. It is also rapidly absorbed following intramuscular administration. It is widely distributed to most body tissues, and appears in breast milk. Within the cell thiamine is mostly present as the diphosphate. Thiamine is not stored to any appreciable extent in the body and amounts in excess of the body's requirements are excreted in the urine as unchanged thiamine or as metabolites.

◊ References.


1. Weber W, *et al.* Nonlinear kinetics of the thiamine cation in humans: saturation of nonrenal clearance and tubular reabsorption. *J Pharmacokinet Biopharm* 1990; **18:** 501–23.
2. Tallaksen CME, *et al.* Kinetics of thiamin and thiamin phosphate esters in human blood, plasma and urine after 50 mg intravenously or orally. *Eur J Clin Pharmacol* 1993; **44:** 73–8.


## Human Requirements

Thiamine requirements are directly related to the carbohydrate intake and the metabolic rate. A daily dietary intake of about 0.9 to 1.5 mg of thiamine is recommended for healthy men and about 0.8 to 1.1 mg for healthy women. Cereals, nuts, peas, beans, and yeast are rich sources of thiamine. Pork and some other meats especially liver, heart, or kidneys, and also fish, contain significant amounts. Flour and bakery products are often enriched with thiamine. Considerable losses of thiamine may result from cooking processes.

**UK and US recommended dietary intake.** In the UK dietary reference values (see p.1419) have been published for thiamine[1] and similarly in the USA recommended dietary allowances (RDAs) have been set.[2] In the UK for adult males and females the reference nutrient intake (RNI) is 0.4 mg per 1000 kcal daily and the estimated average requirement (EAR) is 0.3 mg per 1000 kcal daily. In the USA an RDA of 1.2 mg daily in adult males and 1.1 mg daily in females is recommended.


1. DoH. Dietary reference values for food energy and nutrients for the United Kingdom: report of the panel on dietary reference values of the committee on medical aspects of food policy. *Report on health and social subjects 41.* London: HMSO, 1991.
2. Standing Committee on the Scientific Evaluation of Dietary Reference Intakes of the Food and Nutrition Board. *Dietary Reference Intakes for thiamin, riboflavin, niacin, vitamin $B_6$, folate, vitamin $B_{12}$, pantothenic acid, biotin, and choline.* Washington, DC: National Academy Press, 2000. Also available at: http://www.nap.edu/catalog/6015.html (accessed 24/05/04)


## Uses and Administration

Thiamine is a water-soluble vitamin, although some of its derivatives have greater lipophilicity. It is an essential coenzyme for carbohydrate metabolism in the form of the diphosphate (thiamine pyrophosphate, cocarboxylase). Thiamine deficiency develops when the dietary intake is inadequate; severe deficiency leads to the development of a syndrome known as beri-beri. Chronic 'dry' beri-beri is characterised by peripheral neuropathy, muscle wasting and muscle weakness, and paralysis. Acute 'wet' beri-beri is characterised by cardiac failure and oedema. Wernicke-Korsakoff syndrome (demyelination of the CNS) may develop in severe cases of thiamine deficiency. Severe thiamine deficiency, characterised by lactic acidosis and neurological deterioration, has been reported within a relatively short time of the initiation of thiamine-free total parenteral nutrition; some deaths have occurred.

Thiamine is used in the treatment and prevention of thiamine deficiency. It is given by mouth, the preferred route, or if necessary by the intramuscular or intravenous routes (but see Hypersensitivity, above); intravenous injections should be given slowly over 10 minutes. In the treatment of mild chronic thiamine deficiency usual doses of 10 to 25 mg daily by mouth, in single or divided doses, have been recommended. In severe thiamine deficiency doses of up to 300 mg daily are given, and even higher daily doses may be employed in Wernicke-Korsakoff syndrome by the intravenous route.

Thiamine is usually given as either the hydrochloride or nitrate salts although other salts such as the dicamsylate, disulfide, monophosphate (monophosphothiamine) or pyrophosphate may be employed.

Other compounds that possess vitamin $B_1$ activity and may be used as alternatives to thiamine include benfotiamine, cycotiamine, octotiamine, prosultiamine, and sulbutiamine. Acetiamine, bisbentiamine, and fursultiamine have also been used.

**Wernicke-Korsakoff syndrome.** The Wernicke-Korsakoff syndrome is a manifestation of thiamine deficiency seen particularly in alcoholics, but which may accompany other conditions including starvation or prolonged fasting, or persistent vomiting. It was originally classified as two separate disorders, Wernicke's encephalopathy and Korsakoff's syndrome, but these are now thought to represent aspects of a single pathological process.

Classical Wernicke's symptoms comprise confusion, ataxia, ophthalmoplegia, and nystagmus. Ophthalmoplegia and ataxia may precede the mental symptoms by some days. Hypothermia may be seen, and collapse and sudden death may occur in some patients. The manifestations of Korsakoff's syndrome are short-term memory loss, learning deficits, and confabulation. The conditions are associated with demyelination and glial proliferation, as well as haemorrhagic lesions, mainly in the periventricular regions of the brain; characteristic biochemical abnormalities include raised serum-pyruvate concentration, which has been postulated as a cause of encephalopathy.[1]

Early recognition and treatment is important, both because of the risk of collapse and sudden death,[2] and to prevent irreversible damage to the CNS. Korsakoff symptoms respond less well to treatment than those associated with Wernicke's encephalopathy,[3] and may indeed only become evident on treatment.

Treatment is with parenteral thiamine, preferably intravenously, to ensure adequate absorption; any risks of parenteral treatment are considered justifiable.[4] Although as little as 2 or 3 mg may be enough to reverse the ocular symptoms, which generally begin to improve in 1 to 6 hours, doses of at least 100 mg should be given initially. (In practice a typical dose is 500 mg given intravenously with other vitamins every 8 hours, for 2 days if symptoms persist, and followed by 100 mg twice daily by mouth, or 250 mg daily intravenously until the patient can take oral thiamine.[4,5]) The ataxia and acute confusional state may also resolve dramatically although improvement may not be noted for days or months. The effects of the syndrome on memory are much harder to reverse. Some 25% of patients make a full, and 50% a partial, recovery.[3]


1. Petrie WM, Ban TA. Vitamins in psychiatry: do they have a role? *Drugs* 1985; **30:** 58–65.
2. Reuler JB, *et al.* Wernicke's encephalopathy. *N Engl J Med* 1985; **312:** 1035–9.
3. Anonymous. Korsakoff's syndrome. *Lancet* 1990; **336:** 912–13.
4. Cook CCH, Thomson AD. B-complex vitamins in the prophylaxis and treatment of Wernicke-Korsakoff syndrome. *Br J Hosp Med* 1997; **57:** 461–5.
5. Chataway J, Hardman E. Thiamine doses for alcohol withdrawal. *Br J Hosp Med* 1994; **51:** 615.


## Preparations

***BP 2003:*** Thiamine Injection; Thiamine Tablets; Vitamins B and C Injection;

***BPC 1973:*** Compound Vitamin B Tablets; Strong Compound Vitamin B Tablets;

***USP 27:*** Thiamine Hydrochloride Elixir; Thiamine Hydrochloride Injection; Thiamine Hydrochloride Tablets; Thiamine Mononitrate Elixir.

**Proprietary Preparations** (details are given in Part 3)

***Arg.:*** Megastene; ***Austral.:*** Beta-Sol; Betamin; ***Austria:*** Beneuran; Bevitol; Diclo-B; ***Belg.:*** Aneurol†; Benerva; Beneurol; Betamine; ***Braz.:*** Arcalion; Becaps†; Benerva; Proton†; ***Canad.:*** Betaxin; Bewon†; ***Chile:*** Betamin; ***Fin.:*** Neuramin; Vita-B1; ***Fr.:*** Arcalion; Benerva; Bevitine; ***Ger.:*** Aneurin; B1-ASmedic; $B_1$ Vicotrat; Betabion; Imilgamma†; Lophakomp-B1†; milgamma mono; ***Gr.:*** Benerva; ***Hong Kong:*** Arcalion; ***India:*** Arcalion; Benalgis; ***Irl.:*** Benerva; ***Ital.:*** Benerva; Betabion†; Bivitasi; ***Jpn:*** Alinamin-F; Neuvita; ***Malaysia:*** Arcalion; ***Mex.:*** Benal; Benerva; Carzilasa; TTC†; X-2; ***Port.:*** Arcalion; Trifosfaneurina; ***Singapore:*** Arcalion; ***Spain:*** Arcalion; Benerva; Neurostop; Surmenalit; ***Swed.:*** Benerva; Betabion; ***Switz.:*** Arcalion; Benerva; **Thai.:** Alinamin-F; Arcalion; Menamin; **UAE:** Thiavit; **UK:** Benerva.

**Multi-ingredient: Arg.:** Algio Nervomax; Algio Nervomax Fuerte; Co-Tioctan; Cobenexol Forte; Cobenexol Fuerte; CVP B1 B6 B12; Dexabion; Dolo Nervobion; Dolo Nervobion 10000; Dorixina B1 B6 B12; Dr Calm; Klosidol B1 B6 B12; Nervobion Fuerte; Nervomax TB12; Venostasin; **Austral.:** Berberis Complex†; **Austria:** Ambene N; Arca-Be; Beneuran compositum; Beneuran Vit B-Komplex; Calcisan B + C; Cellobexon; Diclovit; Dilaescol; Dolo-Neurobion; Neurobion; Neuromerck; Neuromultivit; Noxenur†; Pronerv; **Belg.:** Betapyr; Neurobion; Vioneurin; **Braz.:** Aminocid; Betinjectol†; Bituelve†; Boldobeba†; Ceviron†; Cianotrat-Dexa; Citoneurin; Copena†; Dexa-Citoneurin; Dexa-Cronobe; Dexa-Neuriberi; Dexacobal; Dexador; Dexadoze; Dexagil; Dexaneurin; Dexanevral; Doxal; Dozeneurin; Espasmocron; Fol Sang; Lisan; Rubizuel†; Sulfato Ferroso Composto; Sulfatofer; Thiaminose; Trinalgen†; Trinevral†; Trirubin; Venofortan; Vibetrat Dexa†; Vibetrat†; Vipirim†; Vitaneuron; **Canad.:** Penta-3B; Penta-3B + C; Penta-Thion; **Chile:** Betonvit; Dolotol 12; Nefersil B; Neurobionta; Neurocam; Tol 12; **Fin.:** Neurobion; Neurovitan; **Fr.:** Algo-Nevriton†; Enuretine†; Hexaquine; **Ger.:** $B_{1/6}$ Effekton†; Bevit Forte; Discmigon†; Dolo-Neurobion forte; Dolo-Neurobion N; Hewedolor neuro; Medivitan N Neuro; milgamma; milgamma N; milgamma-NA; Milneuron NA; Neuralysan S; Neuro; Neuro uno; Neuro-AS N; neuro-B forte; Neuro-Effekton B; Neuro-Lichtenstein; Neuro-Lichtenstein N; Neuro-ratiopharm; Neuro-ratiopharm N; Neuro-Vibolex; Neurobion; Neurobion N; Neurogrisevit N†; Neurotrat S; Neurotrat†; Novirell B Duo; Novirell B†; Pantovigar N; Pleomix-B; Recatol N†; Regepithel; Vitaject; Vitamin B duo; Vitobasan N†; **Hong Kong:** 3B; Alinamin-F; Childrens Coltalin with Vit $B_1$; Coltalin with Vit $B_1$; Magesto; Neuro B1-6-12; Neurobion; Neurorubine; Nevramin; Princi-B Fort; Regepithel; Tonterin; Vida Neurotab; Vidaclofen-Plus; **India:** Sioneuron; Vitneurin; **Israel:** Betrivit†; Calmanervin; Tribemin; **Ital.:** Adenobeta; Adenoplex Forte; Adenovit; Antiadiposo; Benexol B12; Dobetin con Vitamina B1; Dobetin Totale; Emazian B12; Emoantitossina; Emopon; Esaglut; Fibronevrina; Firmavit†; Folepar B12; For Liver†; Fosforilasi; Fosfoutipi Vitaminico; Menalgon B6†; Menalgon†; Mionevrasi; Neuraben; Neurobiontat†; Neurofta1; Nevril†; Novaneurina B12†; Odontalgico Dr. Knapp con Vit. B1; OH B12 B1†; Pungino†; Rubjovit; Sinevrile†; Triferon†; Trinevrina B6; **Jpn:** Neurovitan; **Malaysia:** 3B; Alinamin B12; Flavettes Neuroforte; Neuro B; Neurobion; Neurorubine; Neurovit; Nevramin; Princi-B Fort; **Mex.:** B1-12-15; Bedocil; Benexol B12; Cobotiaxina; Dexabion; Dolo-Neurobion; Dolo-Pangavit; Dolo-Tiaminal; Duciclon; Ferrotemp; Lipovitasi-Or; Neuralin; Neurobion; Pangavit Hypak; Pangavit Pediatrico; Selectadoce; Tiabexol; Tiamidexal; Tiaminal $B_{12}$; Tiaminal $B_{12}$ Trivalente; Tribedoxyl; **Neth.:** Princi B1 + B6; **Port.:** Linamin Plus; Neurobion; Tridocemine†; **S.Afr.:** Kiddie Vite; Neurobion; **Singapore:** 3B†; Alinamin B12; Alinamin-F; Neurobion; Neurodex; Neuroforte; Neurorubine; Neurovit; Nevramin; Princi-B Fort; **Spain:** Acetuber; Antineurina; Benexol B1 B6 B12; Bester Complex; Calmante Vitaminado P G; Calmante Vitaminado PG Efervescente; Calmante Vitaminado Rinver; Dalamon; Epixian†; Gammamida Complex†; Hidroxil B12 B6 B1; Inzitan; Mederebro; Mederebro Compuesto†; Meloka; Menalgil B6; Nervobion; Neuromade; Neurostop Complex; Pazbronquial; Quimpedor; Refulgin†; Sugarceton†; Teovit†; Viadetres; **Swed.:** Neurobion; **Switz.:** Neurotrat†; Tribeton†; **Thai.:** 3B; Alinamin B12; Alinamin-F; Beromin; Cydoxmine-B; Cyriamine; Diasgest; Digestin; Douzabox; Endogest; Genavit; Hemolax; Mesto-Of; Neubee; Neurobex; Neurobion; Nevramin; Nuvit; Princi-B; Tribesian; Trivit-B; Vioneurin†; Vita-B; Vitamedin; Vitron; **UAE:** 3V; **UK:** Labiton; Quiet Life.

# Vitamin $B_2$ Substances

Vitaminas $B_2$.

## Riboflavin *(BAN, rINN)*

E101; Lactoflavin; Riboflavina; Riboflavine; Riboflavinum; Vitamin $B_2$; Vitamin G. 7,8-Dimethyl-10-(1′-D-ribityl)isoalloxazine; 3,10-Dihydro-7,8-dimethyl-10-(D-*ribo*-2,3,4,5-tetrahydroxypentyl)benzopteridine-2,4-dione.

$C_{17}H_{20}N_4O_6$ = 376.4.
*CAS — 83-88-5.*
*ATC — A11HA04.*

**Pharmacopoeias.** In *Chin., Eur.* (see p.vi), *Int., Jpn, Pol., US,* and *Viet.*

**Ph. Eur. 5.0** (Riboflavin). A yellow or orange-yellow crystalline powder. It exhibits polymorphism. Very slightly soluble in water; practically insoluble in alcohol. Store in airtight containers. Protect from light. Solutions deteriorate on exposure to light, especially in the presence of alkali.

**USP 27** (Riboflavin). A yellow to orange-yellow crystalline powder, having a slight odour. When dry, it is not appreciably affected by diffused light, but in solution light induces quite rapid deterioration, especially in the presence of alkalis. Very slightly soluble in water, in alcohol, and in isotonic sodium chloride solution; insoluble in chloroform and in ether; soluble in dilute solutions of alkalis. Its saturated solution in water is neutral to litmus. Store in airtight containers. Protect from light.

## Riboflavin Sodium Phosphate *(BANM, rINNM)*

Fosfato sódico de riboflavina; Riboflavin 5′-Phosphate Sodium; Riboflavine Phosphate (Sodium Salt); Riboflavine Sodium Phosphate; Riboflavini Natrii Phosphas; Vitamin $B_2$ Phosphate. The sodium salt of riboflavine 5′-phosphate.

$C_{17}H_{20}N_4NaO_9P$ = 478.3.
*CAS — 130-40-5.*

**Pharmacopoeias.** In *Eur.* (see p.vi) and *Jpn.*
*Chin.* and *US* specify the dihydrate salt.

**Ph. Eur. 5.0** (Riboflavin Sodium Phosphate). A yellow or orange-yellow, hygroscopic, crystalline powder. Soluble in water; very slightly soluble in alcohol. A 1% solution in water has a pH of 5.0 to 6.5. Store in airtight containers. Protect from light.

**USP 27** (Riboflavin 5′-Phosphate Sodium). A fine, orange-yellow, hygroscopic, crystalline powder, having a slight odour. When dry, it is not affected by diffused light, but when in solution light induces rapid deterioration. Sparingly soluble in water. pH of a 1% solution in water is between 5.0 and 6.5. Store in airtight containers. Protect from light.

## Adverse Effects and Precautions

Large doses of riboflavin result in a bright yellow discoloration of the urine which may interfere with certain laboratory tests.

**Breast feeding.** Supplementation significantly increased riboflavin concentration in the breast milk of lactating women compared with those not given riboflavin. Significant differences between the two groups decreased over the period from 1 to 6 weeks postpartum; both groups of women had breast milk concentrations above previously reported normal values, and the authors concluded that supplementation was not necessary in healthy, well-nourished women.[1] The American Academy of Pediatrics considers the use of riboflavin to be usually compatible with breast feeding.[2]

1. Nail PA, *et al.* The effect of thiamin and riboflavin supplementation on the level of those vitamins in human breast milk and urine. *Am J Clin Nutr* 1980; **33:** 198–204.
2. American Academy of Pediatrics. The transfer of drugs and other chemicals into human milk. *Pediatrics* 2001; **108:** 776–89. Correction. *ibid.*; 1029. Also available at: http://aappolicy.aappublications.org/cgi/content/full/pediatrics%3b108/3/776 (accessed 19/05/04)

## Pharmacokinetics

Riboflavin is absorbed from the gastrointestinal tract. Although riboflavin is widely distributed to body tissues little is stored in the body.

Riboflavin is converted in the body to the coenzyme flavine mononucleotide (FMN; riboflavin 5′-phosphate) and then to another coenzyme flavine adenine dinucleotide (FAD). About 60% of FMN and FAD are bound to plasma proteins. Riboflavin is excreted in urine, partly as metabolites. As the dose increases, larger amounts are excreted unchanged. Riboflavin crosses the placenta and is distributed into breast milk.

## Human Requirements

The riboflavin requirement is often related to the energy intake but it appears to be more closely related to resting metabolic requirements. A daily dietary intake of about 1.1 to 1.7 mg of riboflavin is recommended. Liver, kidney, fish, eggs, milk, cheese, yeast, and some green vegetables such as broccoli and spinach are the richest sources of riboflavin. In general, little loss of riboflavin occurs during cooking, but considerable losses may occur if foods, especially milk, are exposed to sunlight.

**UK and US recommended dietary intake.** In the UK dietary reference values (see p.1419) have been published for riboflavin[1] and similarly in the USA recommended dietary allowances (RDAs) have been set.[2] Differing amounts are recommended for infants and children of varying ages, for adult males and females of varying ages, and for pregnant and lactating women; the differences between age groups are intended to reflect the changes in caloric intakes at these ages. In the UK the reference nutrient intake (RNI) is 1.3 mg daily and 1.1 mg daily for adult males and females respectively; the estimated average requirement (EAR) is 1.0 mg daily and 0.9 mg daily respectively. In the USA the RDAs for adult males and females are 1.3 and 1.1 mg daily respectively.

1. DoH. Dietary reference values for food energy and nutrients for the United Kingdom: report of the panel on dietary reference values of the committee on medical aspects of food policy. *Report on health and social subjects 41.* London: HMSO, 1991.
2. Standing Committee on the Scientific Evaluation of Dietary Reference Intakes of the Food and Nutrition Board. *Dietary Reference Intakes for thiamin, riboflavin, niacin, vitamin $B_6$, folate, vitamin $B_{12}$, pantothenic acid, biotin, and choline.* Washington, DC: National Academy Press, 2000. Also available at: http://www.nap.edu/catalog/6015.html (accessed 24/05/04)

## Uses and Administration

Riboflavin, a water-soluble vitamin, is essential for the utilisation of energy from food. The active, phosphorylated forms, flavine mononucleotide (FMN) and flavine adenine dinucleotide (FAD), are involved as coenzymes in oxidative/reductive metabolic reactions. Riboflavin is also necessary for the functioning of pyridoxine and nicotinic acid.

Riboflavin deficiency develops when the dietary intake is inadequate. Deficiency leads to the development of a well-defined syndrome known as ariboflavinosis, characterised by cheilosis, angular stomatitis, glossitis, keratitis, surface lesions of the genitalia, and seborrhoeic dermatitis. There may also be normocytic anaemia and ocular symptoms including itching and burning of the eyes, photophobia, and corneal vascularisation. Some of these symptoms may, in fact, be due to other vitamins such as pyridoxine or nicotinic acid which do not function correctly in the absence of riboflavin. Riboflavin deficiency may also occur in association with other vitamin B-complex deficiency states such as pellagra.

Riboflavin is used in the treatment and prevention of riboflavin deficiency. It is usually given in doses of 1 or 2 mg by mouth for prophylaxis, and doses of up to 30 mg daily in divided doses are used for treatment. Riboflavin, as the sodium phosphate, is also a component of intramuscular or intravenous vitamins B and C injections; riboflavin sodium phosphate 1.27 g is approximately equivalent to 1 g of riboflavin.

Riboflavin tetrabutyrate has also been used.

Riboflavin is also used as a colouring agent for food.

**Migraine.** Results from an open pilot study[1] and a placebo-controlled trial[2] have suggested that riboflavin in high doses (400 mg daily) might be of some benefit in the prophylaxis of migraine attacks (p.464).

1. Schoenen J, *et al.* High-dose riboflavin as a prophylactic treatment of migraine: results of an open pilot study. *Cephalalgia* 1994; **14:** 328–9.
2. Schoenen J, *et al.* Effectiveness of high-dose riboflavin in migraine prophylaxis: a randomized controlled trial. *Neurology* 1998; **50:** 466–70.

## Preparations

**BP 2003:** Vitamins B and C Injection;
**BPC 1973:** Compound Vitamin B Tablets; Strong Compound Vitamin B Tablets;
**USP 27:** Riboflavin Injection; Riboflavin Tablets.

**Proprietary Preparations** (details are given in Part 3)
**Belg.:** Berivine; Ribon; **Fin.:** Vita-B2; **Fr.:** Beflavine; **Ger.:** B2-ASmedic; **Hong Kong:** Hibon; **Thai.:** Boflavin.

**Multi-ingredient: Austral.:** Antioxidant Forte Tablets†; Antioxidant Tablets†; Extralife Eye-Care†; Liv-Detox†; **Austria:** Beneuran Vit B-Komplex; **Braz.:** Sulfatofer; Vipirim†; **Fr.:** Glutamag Vitamine†; **Ger.:** Golden Star†; Kwim; **Hong Kong:** Alinamin-F; **India:** Hepa-Merz; **Ital.:** Emazian B12; Emoantitossina; Facovit; For Liver†; Fosforilasi; Neurofta1; **Jpn:** Neurovitan; **Mex.:** Pangavit Pediatrico; **Singapore:** Alinamin-F; **Spain:** Aftasone B C; Balneogel†; **Thai.:** Alinamin-F; **UK:** Quiet Life; Se-Power.

# Vitamin $B_6$ Substances

Vitaminas $B_6$.

Vitamin $B_6$ is usually available as pyridoxine but the term is also used to refer to the related compounds, pyridoxal and pyridoxamine.

## Metadoxine

Pyridoxine Pidolate. Pyridoxine L-5-oxopyrrolidine-2-carboxylate.

$C_8H_{11}NO_3, C_5H_7NO_3$ = 298.3.
*CAS — 74536-44-0.*

## Pyridoxal Phosphate

Codecarboxylase; Pyridoxal 5-Phosphate. 3-Hydroxy-5-hydroxymethyl-2-methylpyridine-4-carboxaldehyde 5′-phosphate.

$C_8H_{10}NO_6P$ = 247.1.
*CAS — 54-47-7.*
*ATC — A11HA06.*

## Pyridoxamine Hydrochloride

Pyridoxamine Dihydrochloride. 4-Aminomethyl-5-hydroxy-6-methyl-3-pyridinemethanol hydrochloride.

$C_8H_{12}N_2O_2$,2HCl = 241.1.
*CAS — 524-36-7.*

## Pyridoxine Hydrochloride *(BANM, rINNM)*

Adermine Hydrochloride; Hidrocloruro de piridoxina; Piridossina Cloridrato; Pyridoxini Hydrochloridum; Pyridoxinii Chloridum; Pyridoxinium Chloride; Pyridoxol Hydrochloride; Vitamin $B_6$. 3-Hydroxy-4,5-bis(hydroxymethyl)-2-picoline hydrochloride.

$C_8H_{11}NO_3$,HCl = 205.6.
*CAS — 65-23-6 (pyridoxine); 58-56-0 (pyridoxine hydrochloride).*
*ATC — A11HA02.*

**Pharmacopoeias.** In *Chin., Eur.* (see p.vi), *Int., Jpn, Pol., US,* and *Viet.*

**Ph. Eur. 5.0** (Pyridoxine Hydrochloride). A white or almost white, crystalline powder. Freely soluble in water; slightly soluble in alcohol. A 5% solution in water has a pH of 2.4 to 3.0. Protect from light.

**USP 27** (Pyridoxine Hydrochloride). White or practically white crystals or crystalline powder. Soluble 1 in 5 of water and 1 in 115 of alcohol; insoluble in ether. Its solutions in water have a pH of about 3. Store in airtight containers. Protect from light.

## Adverse Effects and Precautions

Long-term administration of large doses of pyridoxine is associated with the development of severe peripheral neuropathies; the dose at which these occur is controversial (see below).

**Breast feeding.** Vitamin $B_6$ is excreted into breast milk.[1,2] While some have expressed concern over the inhibition of breast milk secretion by pyridoxine,[3] others have cautioned that pyridoxine deficiency may cause seizures in the neonate.[4] The American Academy of Pediatrics considers the use of pyridoxine to be usually compatible with breast feeding.[5]


1. West KD, Kirksey A. Influence of vitamin $B_6$ intake on the content of the vitamin in human milk. *Am J Clin Nutr* 1976; **29:** 961–9.
2. Roepke JLB, Kirksey A. Vitamin $B_6$ nutriture during pregnancy and lactation: 1. Vitamin $B_6$ intake, levels of the vitamin in biological fluids, and condition of the infant at birth. *Am J Clin Nutr* 1979; **32:** 2249–56.
3. Greentree LB. Dangers of vitamin $B_6$ in nursing mothers. *N Engl J Med* 1979; **300:** 141–2.
4. Lande NI. More on dangers of vitamin $B_6$ in nursing mothers. *N Engl J Med* 1979; **300:** 926–7.
5. American Academy of Pediatrics. The transfer of drugs and other chemicals into human milk. *Pediatrics* 2001; **108:** 776–89. Correction. *ibid.*; 1029. Also available at: http://aappolicy.aappublications.org/cgi/content/full/pediatrics%3b108/3/776 (accessed 19/05/04)


**Effects on the nervous system.** Severe sensory neuropathy has been described in patients receiving large doses of pyridoxine (2 to 6 g daily) for periods of 2 to 40 months.[1] It has, however, been debated as to whether smaller doses may produce such effects. Some contend that amounts of pyridoxine below this level are unlikely to produce toxic effects[2,3] although there have been some case reports[4,5] with amounts up to about 500 mg daily. Following a review of the possible toxicity associated with lower doses of pyridoxine, proposals were put forward in the UK to limit the dose freely available in dietary supplements to 10 mg daily; products supplying up to 50 mg daily would continue to be available from pharmacies and higher doses would only be available on prescription.[6] These proposals have been heavily contested.[6,7] An upper limit of 100 mg daily has been suggested in the USA.[7]


1. Schaumburg H, *et al.* Sensory neuropathy from pyridoxine abuse: a new megavitamin syndrome. *N Engl J Med* 1983; **309:** 445–8.
2. Pauling L. Sensory neuropathy from pyridoxine abuse. *N Engl J Med* 1984; **310:** 197.
3. Baker H, Frank O. Sensory neuropathy from pyridoxine abuse. *N Engl J Med* 1984; **310:** 197.
4. Berger A, Schaumburg HH. More on neuropathy from pyridoxine abuse. *N Engl J Med* 1984; **311:** 986.
5. Waterston JA, Gilligan BS. Pyridoxine neuropathy. *Med J Aust* 1987; **146:** 640–2.
6. Collier J. Vitamin B-6: food or medicine? *BMJ* 1998; **317:** 92–3.
7. Anonymous. Still time for rational debate about vitamin $B_6$. *Lancet* 1998; **351:** 1523.


## Interactions

Pyridoxine reduces the effects of levodopa (see p.1208), but this does not occur if a dopa decarboxylase inhibitor is also given. Pyridoxine reduces the activity of altretamine. It has also been reported to decrease serum concentrations of phenobarbital (p.369) and phenytoin (p.375). Many drugs may increase the requirements for pyridoxine; such drugs include hydralazine, isoniazid, penicillamine, and oral contraceptives.

## Pharmacokinetics

Pyridoxine, pyridoxal, and pyridoxamine are readily absorbed from the gastrointestinal tract following oral administration and are converted to the active forms pyridoxal phosphate and pyridoxamine phosphate. They are stored mainly in the liver where there is oxidation to 4-pyridoxic acid and other inactive metabolites which are excreted in the urine. As the dose increases, proportionally greater amounts are excreted unchanged in the urine. Pyridoxal crosses the placenta and is distributed into breast milk.

## Human Requirements

For adults, the daily requirement of pyridoxine is probably about 1.5 to 2 mg and this amount is present in most normal diets. The requirement tends to increase as protein intake increases due to the role of the vitamin in amino acid metabolism. Meats, especially chicken, kidney, and liver, cereals, eggs, fish, and certain vegetables and fruits are good sources of pyridoxine.

**UK and US recommended dietary intake.** In the UK[1] dietary reference values (see p.1419) have been published for vitamin $B_6$ and similarly in the USA recommended dietary allowances (RDAs) have been set.[2] Differing amounts are recommended for infants and children of varying ages, for adult males and females, and during pregnancy and lactation. In the UK the reference nutrient intake (RNI) is 15 micrograms per g of protein daily for adult males and females and the estimated average requirement (EAR) is 13 micrograms per g of protein daily for the same group. In the USA the RDA for adult men ranges from 1.3 to 1.7 mg daily and that for adult women ranges from 1.3 to 1.5 mg daily.[2] The tolerable upper intake level is 100 mg daily.[2]


1. DoH. Dietary reference values for food energy and nutrients for the United Kingdom: report of the panel on dietary reference values of the committee on medical aspects of food policy. *Report on health and social subjects 41*. London: HMSO, 1991.
2. Standing Committee on the Scientific Evaluation of Dietary Reference Intakes of the Food and Nutrition Board. *Dietary Reference Intakes for thiamin, riboflavin, niacin, vitamin $B_6$, folate, vitamin $B_{12}$, pantothenic acid, biotin, and choline.* Washington, DC: National Academy Press, 2000. Also available at: http://www.nap.edu/catalog/6015.html (accessed 24/05/04)


## Uses and Administration

Pyridoxine, a water-soluble vitamin, is involved principally in amino acid metabolism, but is also involved in carbohydrate and fat metabolism. It is also required for the formation of haemoglobin.

Deficiency of pyridoxine is rare in humans because of its widespread distribution in foods. Pyridoxine deficiency may however be drug-induced and can occur, for instance, during isoniazid therapy. Inadequate utilisation of pyridoxine may result from certain inborn errors of metabolism. Pyridoxine deficiency may lead to sideroblastic anaemia, dermatitis, cheilosis, and neurological symptoms such as peripheral neuritis, and convulsions.

Pyridoxine is used in the treatment and prevention of pyridoxine deficiency states. It is usually given by mouth, the preferred route, but may also be given by the subcutaneous, intramuscular, or intravenous routes. Doses of pyridoxine hydrochloride up to 150 mg daily are used in general deficiency states; higher doses of up to 400 mg daily are used in the treatment of sideroblastic anaemias (see below); and similar doses have been used to treat certain metabolic disorders such as homocystinuria (see Amino Acid Metabolic Disorders, below) or primary hyperoxaluria (below). Pyridoxine has also been used to treat seizures due to hereditary syndromes of pyridoxine deficiency or dependency in infants.

Pyridoxine has also been tried in a wide variety of other disorders, including the treatment of depression and other symptoms associated with the premenstrual syndrome (see below) and the use of oral contraceptives, although its efficacy has been questioned.

Pyridoxine is usually administered as the hydrochloride although other salts such as the citrate, oxoglurate, phosphate, and phosphoserinate, have also been employed. Metadoxine, the pidolate, has been investigated in alcoholism (see below).

For the use of pyridoxine in the prophylaxis of isoniazid-induced peripheral neuritis and for the treatment of acute isoniazid toxicity, see under Isoniazid, p.223.

Pyridoxal phosphate may be used to treat vitamin $B_6$ deficiency. Pyridoxamine has also been given.

◊ Reviews.


1. Bender DA. Non-nutritional uses of vitamin $B_6$. *Br J Nutr* 1999; **81:** 7–20.


**Alcoholism and alcohol poisoning.** Pyridoxine and its pidolate, known as metadoxine, have been tried in the treatment of alcohol poisoning and alcoholism.[1] One study showed pyridoxine to be ineffective in acute alcohol poisoning[2] but another[3] suggested that the pidolate might be of benefit as an adjunct in the management of alcohol withdrawal (p.1166). In patients treated for alcoholic fatty liver, liver function returned to normal more quickly with metadoxine, even in patients who did not completely abstain from alcohol.[4]


1. Addolorato G, *et al.* Metadoxine in the treatment of acute and chronic alcoholism: a review. *Int J Immunopathol Pharmacol* 2003; **16:** 207–14.
2. Mardel S, *et al.* Intravenous pyridoxine in acute ethanol intoxication. *Hum Exp Toxicol* 1994; **13:** 321–3.
3. Rizzo A, *et al.* Uso terapeutico della metadoxina nell'alcolismo cronico: studio clinico in doppio cieco su pazienti ricoverati in un reparto di medicina generale. *Clin Ter* 1993; **142:** 243–50.
4. Caballería J, *et al.* Metadoxine accelerates fatty liver recovery in alcoholic patients: results of a randomized double-blind, placebo-control trial. *J Hepatol* 1998; **28:** 54–60.


**Amino acid metabolic disorders.** Pyridoxine has been used in various inborn errors of amino acid metabolism, such as homocystinuria (p.1417), with or without cobalamins and folate. For the use of pyridoxine in primary hyperoxaluria, another inherited metabolic disorder, see below.

**Anaemias.** Some patients with acquired or hereditary sideroblastic anaemia (p.734) that is severe enough to require treatment will respond to high doses (up to 400 mg daily) of pyridoxine, and a trial is considered worthwhile in all patients.

**Carpal tunnel syndrome.** Pyridoxine has been advocated by some[1] for patients with carpal tunnel syndrome (see Soft-tissue Rheumatism, p.11), but evidence of efficacy is considered to be limited.[2]


1. Lewis PJ. Pyridoxine supplements may help patients with carpal tunnel syndrome. *BMJ* 1995; **310:** 1534.
2. O'Connor D, *et al.* Non-surgical treatment (other than steroid injection) for carpal tunnel syndrome. Available in The Cochrane Library; Issue 2. Chichester: John Wiley; 2004.


**Epilepsy.** Pyridoxine-dependent epilepsy is an autosomal recessive disorder associated with decreased central γ-aminobutyric acid (GABA) concentrations and elevated cerebral glutamate concentrations. Untreated patients suffer from progressive encephalopathy, mental retardation, and intractable epilepsy; lifelong supplementation with pyridoxine can control epileptic symptoms but mental retardation may still develop. Test doses of pyridoxine intravenously, repeated at intervals of 10 minutes up to a total of 500 mg if necessary, have been suggested in the diagnosis of pyridoxine-dependent epilepsy; if the patient responds then a daily oral dose of 5 mg/kg is suggested although there is no real consensus on the appropriate dosage.[1] A study in one patient[2] found that although pyridoxine 5 mg/kg reduced glutamate concentrations in cerebrospinal fluid from their untreated value of 200 times normal limits, it did so only to 10 times the normal value, despite remission of symptoms. Doses of 10 mg/kg daily were required to normalise CSF glutamate, and it was suggested that this was a more appropriate target for therapy. An epidemiological study[3] defined cases as those children with recurrent seizures that ceased within 7 days of oral pyridoxine at a usual dose of 30 mg/kg daily (minimum dose 15 mg/kg daily; maximum dose 1000 mg/kg daily), or within 30 minutes of intravenous pyridoxine (usual dose 100 mg; minimum dose 50 mg), that recurred when supplementation was withdrawn, and ceased again upon dosage as before. The study found that, despite their rarity, pyridoxine-dependent seizures frequently present atypically, and the author suggested that pyridoxine be given to all children with intractable seizures beginning before 3 years of age, including neonates with suspected hypoxic-ischaemic encephalopathy.


1. Gospe SM. Current perspectives on pyridoxine-dependent seizures. *J Pediatr* 1998; **132:** 919–23.
2. Baumeister FAM, *et al.* Glutamate in pyridoxine-dependent epilepsy: neurotoxic glutamate concentration in the cerebrospinal fluid and its normalization by pyridoxine. *Pediatrics* 1994; **94:** 318–21.
3. Baxter P. Epidemiology of pyridoxine dependent and pyridoxine responsive seizures in the UK. *Arch Dis Child* 1999; **81:** 431–3.


**Ischaemic heart disease.** For mention of the possible link between vitamin $B_6$, hyperhomocysteinaemia, and atherosclerosis and ischaemic heart disease, see under Folic Acid, p.1429.

**Palmar-plantar erythrodysesthesia syndrome.** Pyridoxine, in doses of 100 to 300 mg daily, has been used successfully[1] for treating and preventing palmar-plantar erythrodysesthesia syndrome associated with antineoplastic therapy (see p.495).


1. Nagore E, *et al.* Antineoplastic therapy-induced palmar plantar erythrodysesthesia ('hand-foot') syndrome: incidence, recognition and management. *Am J Clin Dermatol* 2000; **1:** 225–34.


**Premenstrual syndrome.** Pyridoxine has been widely used in the premenstrual syndrome (p.1551) despite controversy over its effectiveness. Some consider that depressive symptoms may be provoked by pyridoxine deficiency because of its role as a coenzyme in the production of certain neurotransmitters, but it is difficult to attribute any of the other symptoms of the premenstrual syndrome to pyridoxine deficiency and doses of 50 mg are no more effective than a placebo.[1] A systematic review found that although treatment with pyridoxine was more effective than placebo, there was insufficient high-quality evidence to recommend its routine use in premenstrual syndrome.[2] If pyridoxine is used, the dosage should be restricted (see Effects on the Nervous System, above) because of concerns about neurotoxicity.[3]


1. West CP. The premenstrual syndrome. *Prescribers' J* 1987; **27** (2): 9–15.
2. Wyatt KM, *et al.* Efficacy of vitamin B-6 in the treatment of premenstrual syndrome: systematic review. *BMJ* 1999; **318:** 1375–81.
3. Severino SK, Moline ML. Premenstrual syndrome: identification and management. *Drugs* 1995; **49:** 71–82.


**Primary hyperoxaluria.** Primary hyperoxaluria (as distinct from the various forms secondary to other disorders) is a genetic disorder characterised by excessive synthesis and urinary excretion of oxalic acid. Two forms are known, type I (hyperglycolic aciduria) and type II (L-glyceric aciduria), associated with different enzyme defects. They are marked by recurrent calcium oxalate kidney stones, or nephrocalcinosis, leading to renal failure, together with extrarenal deposition of calcium oxalate and frequently severe peripheral vascular insufficiency. Treatment with high doses of pyridoxine may help decrease oxalate excretion particularly in type I disease,[1,2] although response is variable.[3] A few patients may respond to lower (physiological) doses.[4] Such treatment can be used with an oral orthophosphate supplement, which helps reduce renal deposition of calcium oxalate, and the combination appears to preserve renal function.[5] Therapy with magnesium salts, potassium citrate, and thiazide diuretics has also been suggested.[2] In patients in whom renal failure develops, the results of kidney transplantation have been disappointing, due to deposition of calcium oxalate in the new kidney, although concomitant liver transplantation can correct the enzyme defect.[1,6] Pre-emptive liver transplantation, performed before renal failure or systemic oxalosis has occurred, may be an option.[2]


1. Cochat P, Basmaison O. Current approaches to the management of primary hyperoxaluria. *Arch Dis Child* 2000; **82:** 470–3.
2. Marangella M, *et al.* The primary hyperoxalurias. *Contrib Nephrol* 2001; **136:** 11–32.
3. Toussaint C. Pyridoxine-responsive PH1: treatment. *J Nephrol* 1998; **11** (suppl 1): 49–50.
4. Yendt ER, Cohanim M. Response to a physiologic dose of pyridoxine in type I primary hyperoxaluria. *N Engl J Med* 1985; **312:** 953–7.
5. Milliner DS, *et al.* Results of long-term treatment with orthophosphate and pyridoxine in patients with primary hyperoxaluria. *N Engl J Med* 1994; **331:** 1553–8.
6. Watts RWE, *et al.* Combined hepatic and renal transplantation in primary hyperoxaluria type I: clinical report of nine cases. *Am J Med* 1991; **90:** 179–88.


## Preparations

***BP 2003:*** Pyridoxine Tablets; Vitamins B and C Injection;
***BPC 1973:*** Strong Compound Vitamin B Tablets;
***USP 27:*** Pyridoxine Hydrochloride Injection; Pyridoxine Hydrochloride Tablets.

**Proprietary Preparations** (details are given in Part 3)

***Arg.:*** Benadon; ***Austral.:*** Pyroxin; Vita B6†; ***Austria:*** Benadon†; Diclo-B; Reisevit; ***Belg.:*** Bedoxine; ***Braz.:*** Fonto-Vit B6; Neuri B6; Seis-B; ***Canad.:*** Carthamex; Hi Potency KIB$_6$; ***Chile:*** Metadoxil; Vitabe; ***Fin.:*** Heksavit; Vita-B6; ***Fr.:*** Becilan; Dermo 6; ***Ger.:*** B6-ASmedic; B$_6$ Vicotrat; Bonasanit; Hexobion; Lophakomp-B6†; ***Gr.:*** Besix; ***India:*** Pyricontin; ***Irl.:*** Benadon†; Complement Continus; ***Israel:*** Anacrodyne; B Six; ***Ital.:*** Benadon; Memosprint; Metadoxil; Xanturenasi; ***Mex.:*** Benadon†; Metasin; ***Norw.:*** AFI-B$_6$†; ***Port.:*** Benadon; Metadoxil; ***S.Afr.:*** Lactosec; ***Spain:*** Bequlinina†; Benadon; Conductasa; Godabion B6; Serfoxide†; ***Swed.:*** Benadon; ***Switz.:*** Benadon; Complement Continus; ***Thai.:*** B-6; Metadoxil; ***UK:*** Complement Continus†; Orovite Complement B$_6$†; Woman Kind†; ***USA:*** Vitelle Nestrex.

**Multi-ingredient:** ***Arg.:*** 6 Copin; Algio Nervomax; Algio Nervomax Fuerte; Blastop; Cadencial Plus; Cobenexol Forte; Cobenexol Fuerte; CVP B1 B6 B12; Dexabion; Dolo Nervobion; Dolo Nervobion 10000; Dorixina B1 B6 B12; Flexicamin B12; Flogiatrin B12; Holomagnesio B6; KLB6 Fruit Diet; Klosidol B1 B6 B12; Lohp; Magnebe; Megacistin; Megaplus; Nervobion Fuerte; Nervomax TB12; Neuronal Vascular; Sindrolen; ***Austral.:*** Bio Magnesium†; Extralife Flow-Care†; Extralife Fluid-Care†; Extralife PMS-Care†; Extralife Uri-Care†; Liv-Detox†; Mag-Orot†; Medinat PMT-Eze†; Natures Way Total Zinc†; Zinc Zenith†; ***Austria:*** Arca-Be; Aslavital; Astronautal; Beneuran compositum; Beneuran Vit B-Komplex; Contravert B$_6$; Diclovit; Dolo-Neurobion; Echnatol B$_6$; Neurobion; Neuromerck; Neuromultivit; Pronerv; Sigmalin B$_6$; Sigmalin B$_6$ forte; Sigmalin B$_6$ ohne Coffein; Vertirosan Vitamin B$_6$; ***Belg.:*** Betapyr; Neurobion; Postadoxine†; R Calm + B6†; Vioneurin; ***Braz.:*** Alergo Filinal; Aminocid; Aminotox; Anekron; Benistina†; Betaliver; Betinjectol†; Biofigado†; Biohepax; Bronquitos; Cianotrat-Dexa; Citoneurin; Colinvintol†; Dexa-Citoneurin; Dexa-Cronobe; Dexa-Neuriberi; Dexacobal; Dexador; Dexadoze; Dexagil; Dexaneurin; Dexanevral; Diagrin†; Doxal; Dramavit B6; Dramin B-6; Dramin B-6 DL; Emetrol; Enterofigon†; Epacrosil†; Epativan B6; Epocler; Estac; Eviepar†; Extrato Hepatico Composto†; Figadobil†; Gabax; Hepacitron†; Hepalin†; Hepatobe†; Hormo Hepatico; Jecohepat†; Levordiol; Lisosmalen†; Megestran; Monotrean B6†; Nausicalm; Nausilon B6†; Necro B-6; Nicopaverina B6; Pantevit; Plagon†; Plasonil†; Trinalgen†; Trinevral†; Trirubin; Vibetrat Dexa†; Vibetrat†; Vipirim†; Vominil; Vomistop†; Xantinon Complex; ***Canad.:*** Diclectin; Formula Gyn†; Penta-3B; Penta-3B + C; ProstGard; ***Chile:*** Activator; Betonvit; Dolotol 12; Ferro Vitaminico; Gamalate B6; Glutacyl Vitaminado; Hexalectol; Nefersil B; Neurobionta; Neurocam; Tol 12; ***Fin.:*** Neurobion; Neurovitan; Wicnecarb; Wicnevit; ***Fr.:*** Alphane†; Antebor B$_6$†; Arbum; Catarstat; Cysti-Z; Cystine B$_6$; Forcapil; Lyso-6; Magne-B$_6$; Osteogen†; Phakan; Uvimag B$_6$; ***Ger.:*** AntiFocal N; B$_{1/6}$ Effekton†; Bevit Forte; Bramin-hepa; Dolo-Neurobion forte; Dolo-Neurobion N; Hepagrisevit Forte-N; Hewedolor neuro; Medivitan N; Medivitan N Neuro; Medyn; milgamma; milgamma N; milgamma-NA; Milneuron NA; Neuralysan S; Neuro; Neuro uno; Neuro-AS N; neuro-B forte; Neuro-Effekton B; Neuro-Lichtenstein; Neuro-Lichtenstein N; Neuro-ratiopharm; Neuro-ratiopharm N; Neuro-Vibolex; Neurobion; Neurobion N; Neurogrisevit N†; Neurotrat S; Neurotrat†; Nifurantin B 6; Novirell B Duo; Novirell B†; Pleomix-B; Recatol N†; Reisegold; Telbibur N; Vitaject; Vitamin B duo; Vitobasan N†; ***Hong Kong:*** 3B; C-Sik; Navidoxine; Neuro B1-6-12; Neurobion; Neurorubine; Nevramin; Princi-B Fort; Vida Neurotab; Vidaclofen-Plus; ***India:*** Blosyn; Conviron-TR; Cx-3; Cx-4; Cx-5; Eternex; Gocox Compound; Ipcacin Kid; Ipcazide; Isokin-300; Rifa; Rifa E; Sclerobion; Sioneuron; Vitneurin; Wokex-2; Wokex-3; Wokex-4; ***Irl.:*** Optimax†; ***Israel:*** Betrivit†; Calmanervin; Tribemin; ***Ital.:*** Acutil Fosforo; Adenoplex Forte; Adenovit; Alcalosio; Antemesyl†; Antimicotico†; Benexol B12; Coxanturenasi; Dobetin Totale; Efargen†; Emoantitossina; Esaglut; Firmavit†; For Liver†; Fosforil Calcium†; Fosforilasi; Furanvit†; Lozione Same AS†; Menalgon B6†; Miazide B6; Midium; Mionevrasi; Neo-Geynevral†; Neuraben; Neurobionta†; Sedofit; Triferont†; Trinevrina B6; ***Jpn:*** Neurovitan; ***Malaysia:*** 3B; Becoloxin; Flavettes Neuroforte; Navidoxine; Neuro B; Neurobion; Neurorubine; Neurovit; Nevramin; Princi-B Fort; ***Mex.:*** Benexol B12; Bonadoxina; Bonazin; Cobotiaxina; Dexabion; Dolo-Neurobion; Dolo-Pangavit; Dolo-Tiaminal; Duciclon; Emediba; Lecifar-K; Liatriz; Meclifar; Neuralin; Neurobion; Pangavit Hypak; Pangavit Pediatrico; Selectadoce; Tiamidal B$_{12}$ Trivalente; Tribedoxyl; Vo-Remi; ***Neth.:*** Emesafene; Princi B1 + B6; ***Port.:*** Detoxergon; Esclerobion; Linamin Plus; Nausefe; Neurobion; Phakan; Tridocemine†; ***S.Afr.:*** Asic; Neurobion; Nicene†; Vomifene; ***Singapore:*** 3B†; Navidoxine; Neurobion; Neurodex; Neuroforte; Neurorubine; Neurovit; Nevramin; Princi-B Fort; ***Spain:*** Acetuber; Aftasone B C; Agudil; Antineurina; Benexol B1 B6 B12; Bester Complex; Biodramina Cafeina; Cariban; Cefabol; Dalamon; Dorken; Duplicalcio 150†; Epixian†; Gamalate B6; Gammamida Complex†; Hidroxil B12 B6 B1; Levaliver†; Mederebro; Mederebro Compuesto†; Menalgil B6; Nervobion; Neuromade; Neurostop Complex; Nucleserina; Pazbronquial; Pleocortex B6†; Poli ABE†; Quimpedor; Redutona; Relaxedans†; Sirodina; Taurobetina; Teovit†; Tepazepan; Trivitan†; Trofi Milinat†; ***Swed.:*** Neurobion; ***Switz.:*** Acne Gel; Antemin compositum; Catarstat; Demodenal compositum†; Itinerol B$_6$; Linervidol; Lyso-6; Magnesplus†; Medramine retard†; Medramine-B$_6$ Rectocaps†; Neurotrat†; Phakolen; Suracton; Tribeton†; ***Thai.:*** 3B; Beromin; Cydoxmine-B; Cyriamine; Douzabox; Ferli-6; Genavit; Hemolax; Neubee; Neurobex; Neurobion; Nevramin; Nuvit; Princi-B; Tribesian; Tricortin; Trivit-B; Vita-B; Vitamedin; Vitron; ***UAE:*** 3V; ***UK:*** Fat-Solv†; HealthAid Boldo-Plus; Kelp Plus 3; Rapi-snooze†; ***USA:*** Beelith; FOLTX; KLB6; Lurline PMS; Marlyn Formula 50; PremesisRx; Releaf for PMS.

*Used as an adjunct in:* ***Ger.:*** Isozid comp N; tebesium; ***Ital.:*** Etanicozid B6; ***Spain:*** Cemidon B6; Isoetam†; Tisobrif.

# Vitamin B$_{12}$ Substances

Vitaminas B$_{12}$.

Vitamin B$_{12}$ is the name generally used for a group of related cobalt-containing compounds, also known as cobalamins, of which cyanocobalamin and hydroxocobalamin are the principal forms in clinical use.

## Cyanocobalamin *(BAN, rINN)*

Cianocobalamina; Cobamin; Cyanocobalaminum; Cycobemin.
*Coα-[α-(5,6-Dimethylbenzimidazolyl)]-Coβ-cyanocobamide.*
$C_{63}H_{88}CoN_{14}O_{14}P$ = 1355.4.
*CAS — 68-19-9.*
*ATC — B03BA01.*

**Pharmacopoeias.** In *Chin., Eur.* (see p.vi), *Int., Jpn, Pol., US,* and *Viet.*

**Ph. Eur. 5.0** (Cyanocobalamin). A dark red, crystalline powder or dark red crystals. The anhydrous substance is very hygroscopic. Sparingly soluble in water and in alcohol; practically insoluble in acetone. Store in airtight containers. Protect from light.

**USP 27** (Cyanocobalamin). Dark red crystals or amorphous or crystalline red powder. In the anhydrous form it is very hygroscopic and when exposed to air it may absorb about 12% of water. Soluble 1 in 80 of water; soluble in alcohol; insoluble in acetone, in chloroform, and in ether. Store in airtight containers. Protect from light.

## Hydroxocobalamin *(BAN, USAN, rINN)*

Hidroxicobalamina; Hydroxocobalaminum; Idrossocobalamina.
*Coα-[α-(5,6-Dimethylbenzimidazolyl)]-Coβ-hydroxocobamide.*
$C_{62}H_{89}CoN_{13}O_{15}P$ = 1346.4.
*CAS — 13422-51-0.*
*ATC — B03BA03; V03AB33.*

NOTE. The hydrated form of hydroxocobalamin has been referred to as aquocobalamin.

**Pharmacopoeias.** In *Int.* and *US.*
*Jpn* also includes mecobalamin.
*Chin.* includes cobamamide.

**USP 27** (Hydroxocobalamin). Dark red crystals or red crystalline powder. Is odourless or has not more than a slight acetone odour. The anhydrous form is very hygroscopic. Soluble 1 in 50 of water and 1 in 100 of alcohol; practically insoluble in acetone, in chloroform, in ether, and in benzene; sparingly soluble in methyl alcohol. pH of a 2% solution in water is between 8.0 and 10.0. Store in airtight containers at a temperature of 8° to 15°. Protect from light.

## Hydroxocobalamin Acetate *(BANM, rINNM)*

Acetatocobalamin; Hydroxocobalamini acetas.
$C_{64}H_{93}CoN_{13}O_{17}P$ = 1406.4.
*CAS — 22465-48-1.*

**Pharmacopoeias.** In *Eur.* (see p.vi), *Jpn,* and *Viet.*

**Ph. Eur. 5.0** (Hydroxocobalamin Acetate). A dark red, very hygroscopic, crystalline powder or dark red crystals. Soluble in water. Some decomposition may occur on drying. Store at a temperature between 2° and 8° in airtight containers. Protect from light.

## Hydroxocobalamin Chloride *(BANM, rINNM)*

Hydroxocobalamini Chloridum.
$C_{62}H_{90}ClCoN_{13}O_{15}P$ = 1382.8.

**Pharmacopoeias.** In *Eur.* (see p.vi), *Int.,* and *Viet.*

**Ph. Eur. 5.0** (Hydroxocobalamin Chloride). A dark red, very hygroscopic, crystalline powder or dark red crystals. Soluble in water. Some decomposition may occur on drying. Store at a temperature between 2° and 8° in airtight containers. Protect from light.

## Hydroxocobalamin Sulfate *(BANM, rINNM)*

Hydroxocobalamin Sulphate; Hydroxocobalamini Sulfas.
$C_{124}H_{180}Co_2N_{26}O_{34}P_2S$ = 2790.8.

**Pharmacopoeias.** In *Eur.* (see p.vi), *Int.,* and *Viet.*

**Ph. Eur. 5.0** (Hydroxocobalamin Sulphate). A dark red, very hygroscopic, crystalline powder or dark red crystals. Soluble in water. Some decomposition may occur on drying. Store at a temperature between 2° and 8° in airtight containers. Protect from light.

## Adverse Effects and Precautions

Allergic hypersensitivity reactions have occurred rarely following the parenteral administration of the vitamin B$_{12}$ compounds cyanocobalamin and hydroxocobalamin. Antibodies to hydroxocobalamin-transcobalamin II complex have developed during hydroxocobalamin therapy.

Arrhythmias secondary to hypokalaemia have occurred at the beginning of parenteral treatment with hydroxocobalamin.

Intranasal cyanocobalamin may cause rhinitis, nausea, and headache.

Cyanocobalamin or hydroxocobalamin should, if possible, not be given to patients with suspected vitamin B$_{12}$ deficiency without first confirming the diagnosis. Regular monitoring of the blood is advisable. Use of doses greater than 10 micrograms daily may produce a haematological response in patients with folate deficiency; indiscriminate use may mask the precise diagnosis. Conversely, folate may mask vitamin B$_{12}$ deficiency (see p.1429).

Cyanocobalamin should not be used for Leber's disease or tobacco amblyopia since these optic neuropathies may degenerate further.

**Breast feeding.** Vitamin B$_{12}$ is distributed into breast milk.[1] The American Academy of Pediatrics considers its use to be usually compatible with breast feeding.[2]


1. Samson RR, McClelland DBL. Vitamin B$_{12}$ in human colostrum and milk. *Acta Paediatr Scand* 1980; **69:** 93–9.
2. American Academy of Pediatrics. The transfer of drugs and other chemicals into human milk. *Pediatrics* 2001; **108:** 776–89. Correction. *ibid.*; 1029. Also available at: http://aappolicy.aappublications.org/cgi/content/full/pediatrics%3b108/3/776 (accessed 19/05/04)


**Hypersensitivity.** Analysis, by the Boston Collaborative Drug Surveillance Program, of data on 15 438 patients hospitalised between 1975 and 1982 detected 3 allergic skin reactions attributed to cyanocobalamin among 168 recipients of the drug.[1] For the purposes of the study, reactions were defined as being generalised morbilliform exanthems, urticaria, or generalised pruritus only.

In a patient with a generalised pruritic reaction to hydroxocobalamin (with subsequent urticaria, bronchospasm, and oropharyngeal angioedema), cyanocobalamin was relatively well-tolerated, with only one episode of delayed urticaria.[2]


1. Bigby M, *et al.* Drug-induced cutaneous reactions: a report from the Boston Collaborative Drug Surveillance Program on 15 438 consecutive inpatients, 1975 to 1982. *JAMA* 1986; **256:** 3358–63.
2. Heyworth-Smith D, Hogan PG. Allergy to hydroxycobalamin, with tolerance of cyanocobalamin. *Med J Aust* 2002; **177:** 162–3.


## Interactions

Absorption of vitamin B$_{12}$ from the gastrointestinal tract may be reduced by neomycin, aminosalicylic acid, histamine H$_2$-antagonists, and colchicine. Serum concentrations may be decreased by concurrent administration of oral contraceptives. Many of these interactions are unlikely to be of clinical significance but should be taken into account when performing assays for blood concentrations. Parenteral chloramphenicol may attenuate the effect of vitamin B$_{12}$ in anaemia.

## Pharmacokinetics

Vitamin B$_{12}$ substances bind to intrinsic factor, a glycoprotein secreted by the gastric mucosa, and are then actively absorbed from the gastrointestinal tract. Absorption is impaired in patients with an absence of intrinsic factor, with a malabsorption syndrome or with disease or abnormality of the gut, or after gastrectomy. Absorption from the gastrointestinal tract can also occur by passive diffusion; little of the vitamin present in food is absorbed in this manner although the process becomes increasingly important with larger amounts such as those used therapeutically. After intranasal administration, peak plasma concentrations of cyanocobalamin have been reached in 1 to 2 hours. The bioavailability of the intranasal preparation is about 7 to 11% of that by intramuscular injection.

Vitamin B$_{12}$ is extensively bound to specific plasma proteins called transcobalamins; transcobalamin II appears to be involved in the rapid transport of the cobalamins to tissues. Vitamin B$_{12}$ is stored in the liver, excreted in the bile, and undergoes extensive enterohepatic recycling; part of a dose is excreted in the urine, most of it in the first 8 hours; urinary excretion, however, accounts for only a small fraction in the reduction of total body stores acquired by dietary means. Vitamin B$_{12}$ diffuses across the placenta and also appears in breast milk.

**Retention in the body.** After injection of cyanocobalamin a large proportion is excreted in the urine within 24 hours; the body retains only 55% of a 100-microgram dose and 15% of a 1000-microgram dose. Body stores of vitamin B$_{12}$ amount to

2000 to 3000 micrograms which is believed to be enough for 3 to 4 years. If 1000 micrograms is injected monthly, the 150 micrograms retained lasts for about 1 month. Hydroxocobalamin is better retained than cyanocobalamin; 90% of a 100-microgram dose and 30% of a 1000-microgram dose are retained and that range is believed to be enough for 2 to 10 months.[1]

1. Anonymous. Time to drop cyanocobalamin? *Drug Ther Bull* 1984; **22:** 43.

## Human Requirements

For adults, the daily requirement of vitamin $B_{12}$ is probably about 1 to 2 micrograms and this amount is present in most normal diets. Vitamin $B_{12}$ occurs only in animal products; it does not occur in vegetables, therefore strict vegetarian (vegan) diets that exclude dairy products may provide an inadequate amount although it has been said that many years of vegetarianism are necessary before a deficiency is produced, if at all. Meats, especially liver and kidney, milk, eggs, and other dairy products, and fish are good sources of vitamin $B_{12}$.

**UK and US recommended dietary intake.** In the UK[1] dietary reference values (see p.1419) have been published for vitamin $B_{12}$ and similarly in the USA recommended dietary allowances (RDAs) have been set.[2] Differing amounts are recommended for infants and children of varying ages, adults and pregnant and lactating women. In the UK the reference nutrient intake (RNI) is 1.5 micrograms daily for adult males and females and the estimated average requirement (EAR) is 1.25 micrograms daily. In the USA the RDA for adults is 2.4 micrograms daily.

1. DoH. Dietary reference values for food energy and nutrients for the United Kingdom: report of the panel on dietary reference values of the committee on medical aspects of food policy. *Report on health and social subjects 41*. London: HMSO, 1991.

2. Standing Committee on the Scientific Evaluation of Dietary Reference Intakes of the Food and Nutrition Board. *Dietary Reference Intakes for thiamin, riboflavin, niacin, vitamin $B_6$, folate, vitamin $B_{12}$, pantothenic acid, biotin, and choline*. Washington, DC: National Academy Press, 2000. Also available at: http://www.nap.edu/catalog/6015.html (accessed 24/05/04)

## Uses and Administration

Vitamin $B_{12}$, a water-soluble vitamin, occurs in the body mainly as methylcobalamin (mecobalamin) and as adenosylcobalamin (cobamamide) and hydroxocobalamin. Mecobalamin and cobamamide act as coenzymes in nucleic acid synthesis. Mecobalamin is also closely involved with folic acid in several important metabolic pathways.

Vitamin $B_{12}$ deficiency can occur in strict vegetarians with an inadequate dietary intake, although it may take many years before a deficiency is produced. Deficiency is more likely in patients with malabsorption syndromes or metabolic disorders, nitrous oxide-induced megaloblastosis, or following gastrectomy or extensive ileal resection. Deficiency leads to the development of megaloblastic anaemias and demyelination and other neurological damage. A specific anaemia known as pernicious anaemia develops in patients with an absence of the intrinsic factor necessary for good absorption of the vitamin from dietary sources.

Vitamin $B_{12}$ preparations are used in the treatment and prevention of vitamin $B_{12}$ deficiency. It is essential to identify the exact cause of deficiency, preferably before starting therapy. Hydroxocobalamin is generally preferred to cyanocobalamin; it binds more firmly to plasma proteins and is retained in the body longer (see under Pharmacokinetics, above). Cyanocobalamin and hydroxocobalamin are generally given by the intramuscular route, although cyanocobalamin may be given by mouth or intranasally (see also under Administration, below). Oral cyanocobalamin may be used in treating or preventing vitamin $B_{12}$ deficiency of dietary origin.

In the UK, recommended doses for pernicious anaemia and other macrocytic anaemias without neurological involvement are hydroxocobalamin (or cyanocobalamin) 250 to 1000 micrograms intramuscularly on alternate days for 1 to 2 weeks, then 250 micrograms weekly until the blood count returns to normal. Maintenance doses of 1000 micrograms of hydroxocobalamin are given every 2 to 3 months (or monthly for cyanocobalamin). If there is neurological involvement, hydroxocobalamin or cyanocobalamin may be given in doses of 1000 micrograms on alternate days and continued for as long as improvement occurs. For the prophylaxis of anaemia associated with vitamin $B_{12}$ deficiency resulting from gastrectomy or malabsorption syndromes hydroxocobalamin may be given in doses of 1000 micrograms intramuscularly every 2 or 3 months or cyanocobalamin in doses of 250 to 1000 micrograms intramuscularly each month. For vitamin $B_{12}$ deficiency of dietary origin, cyanocobalamin 50 to 150 micrograms may be taken daily by mouth between meals.

Lower doses of both cyanocobalamin and hydroxocobalamin are recommended in the USA. For the treatment of deficiency, the usual intramuscular dose of cyanocobalamin is 100 micrograms daily for 7 days, then on alternate days for 7 further doses, then every 3 to 4 days for 2 to 3 weeks. For hydroxocobalamin the dose is 30 to 50 micrograms daily for 5 to 10 days. For maintenance, both cyanocobalamin and hydroxocobalamin are given at a dose of 100 to 200 micrograms monthly, based on haematological monitoring. An intranasal preparation of cyanocobalamin is also available for maintenance therapy, the recommended dose being 500 micrograms once weekly. Oral doses of up to 1000 micrograms of cyanocobalamin have also been used. In patients with normal gastrointestinal absorption, doses of 1 to 25 micrograms daily are considered sufficient as a dietary supplement.

Treatment usually results in rapid haematological improvement and a striking clinical response. However, neurological symptoms respond more slowly and in some cases remission may not be complete.

Hydroxocobalamin may also be given in the treatment of tobacco amblyopia and Leber's optic atrophy; initial doses are 1000 micrograms daily for 2 weeks intramuscularly followed by 1000 micrograms twice weekly for as long as improvement occurs. Thereafter, 1000 micrograms is administered every 1 to 3 months.

Cyanocobalamin and hydroxocobalamin are also used in the Schilling test to investigate vitamin $B_{12}$ absorption and deficiency states. They are administered in a non-radioactive form together with cyanocobalamin radioactively-labelled with cobalt-57 (p.1523) or cobalt-58 (p.1523) and the amount of radioactivity excreted in the urine can be used to assess absorption status. A differential Schilling test, in which the forms of cyanocobalamin are given under different conditions can provide information concerning the cause of the malabsorption. Cobamamide and mecobalamin may also be used for vitamin $B_{12}$ deficiency.

**Administration.** The small amounts of vitamin $B_{12}$ present in the diet are absorbed from the gastrointestinal tract by an active process which involves binding with intrinsic factor. As intrinsic factor is absent in patients who have developed pernicious anaemia it has often been assumed that oral treatment with vitamin $B_{12}$ preparations will therefore be ineffective. However, about 1% of an oral dose is absorbed by passive diffusion, and with large doses this amount may be sufficient for therapy. Thus attention has been given again to the use of oral cobalamins for the treatment of pernicious anaemia.[1-3] Oral cyanocobalamin 2000 micrograms daily was as effective as intramuscular therapy in patients with vitamin $B_{12}$ deficiency in a comparative study.[4] Some now consider that oral doses of 1000 micrograms daily,[3] or every 2 weeks for children,[5] are a suitable alternative to injections given at monthly or so intervals; others still deem oral administration to be unjustified on the grounds of negligible oral absorption.[6] A review[7] concluded that, while there is substantial evidence to support the use of 1000 to 2000 micrograms daily of oral cobalamin as maintenance therapy, parenteral therapy is preferable for initial treatment of those with neurological symptoms. Cyanocobalamin is also effective when given intranasally,[8] with peak plasma concentrations greater than those achievable orally, and this may offer another alternative to injection. The intranasal absorption of hydroxocobalamin has been studied.[9,10] Cobalamin has also been administered sublingually.[11]

1. Lederle FA. Oral cobalamin for pernicious anemia: medicine's best kept secret? *JAMA* 1991; **265:** 94–5.

2. Hathcock JN, Troendle GJ. Oral cobalamin for treatment of pernicious anemia? *JAMA* 1991; **265:** 96–7.

3. Elia M. Oral or parenteral therapy for B12 deficiency. *Lancet* 1998; **352:** 1721–2.

4. Kuzminski AM, *et al.* Effective treatment of cobalamin deficiency with oral cobalamin. *Blood* 1998; **92:** 1191–8.

5. Çetin M, Altay C. Efficacy of oral vitamin $B_{12}$ treatment in children. *J Pediatr* 2001; **139:** 754.

6. Van der Kuy P-HM, *et al.* Bioavailability of oral hydroxocobalamin. *Br J Clin Pharmacol* 2000; **49:** 395P–396P.

7. Lane LA, Rojas-Fernandez C. Treatment of Vitamin $B_{12}$-deficiency anemia: oral versus parenteral therapy. *Ann Pharmacother* 2002; **36:** 1268–72.

8. Romeo VD, *et al.* Intranasal cyanocobalamin. *JAMA* 1992; **268:** 1268–9.

9. van Asselt DZB, *et al.* Nasal absorption of hydroxocobalamin in healthy elderly adults. *Br J Clin Pharmacol* 1998; **45:** 83–6.

10. Slot WB, *et al.* Normalization of plasma vitamin B12 concentration by intranasal hydroxocobalamin in vitamin B12-deficient patients. *Gastroenterology* 1997; **113:** 430–3.

11. Delpre G, *et al.* Sublingual therapy for cobalamin deficiency as an alternative to oral and parenteral cobalamin supplementation. *Lancet* 1999; **354:** 740–1.

**Amino acid metabolic disorders.** References to the use of hydroxocobalamin in the treatment of inborn errors of vitamin $B_{12}$ metabolism.[1-7] Some patients with homocystinuria (p.1417) or methylmalonic aciduria have responded to cobalamins.

1. Schuh S, *et al.* Homocystinuria and megaloblastic anemia responsive to vitamin $B_{12}$ therapy. *N Engl J Med* 1984; **310:** 686–90.

2. Hoffbrand AV, *et al.* Hereditary abnormal transcobalamin II previously diagnosed as congenital dihydrofolate reductase deficiency. *N Engl J Med* 1984; **310:** 789–90.

3. Shinnar S, Singer HS. Cobalamin C mutation (methylmalonic aciduria and homocystinuria) in adolescence. *N Engl J Med* 1984; **311:** 451–4.

4. Bhatt HR, *et al.* Treatment of hydroxocobalamin-resistant methylmalonic acidaemia with adenosylcobalamin. *Lancet* 1986; **ii:** 465.

5. van der Meer SB, *et al.* Prenatal treatment of a patient with vitamin $B_{12}$-responsive methylmalonic acidemia. *J Pediatr* 1990; **117:** 923–6.

6. Andersson HC, Shapira E. Biochemical and clinical response to hydroxocobalamin versus cyanocobalamin treatment in patients with methylmalonic acidemia and homocystinuria (cblC). *J Pediatr* 1998; **132:** 121–4.

7. Linnell JC, Bhatt HR. Inherited errors of cobalamin metabolism and their management. *Baillieres Clin Haematol* 1995; **8:** 567–601.

**Cyanide toxicity.** Hydroxocobalamin combines with cyanide to form cyanocobalamin, and thus may be used as an antidote to cyanide toxicity (p.1506). Hydroxocobalamin is reported to be effective in controlling cyanide toxicity due to nitroprusside infusion,[1] and after exposure to inhaled combustion products in residential fires.[2]

1. Zerbe NF, Wagner BKJ. Use of vitamin B12 in the treatment and prevention of nitroprusside-induced cyanide toxicity. *Crit Care Med* 1993; **21:** 465–7.

2. Houeto P, *et al.* Relation of blood cyanide to plasma cyanocobalamin concentration after a fixed dose of hydroxocobalamin in cyanide poisoning. *Lancet* 1995; **346:** 605–8.

**Deficiency states.** The emergence of newer metabolic assays for homocysteine and methylmalonic acid has led to the identification of subtle vitamin $B_{12}$ deficiency[1,2] without the overt manifestations of megaloblastic anaemia (p.734) or neurological disease; this condition appears to be particularly common in the elderly.[1] At present, there is no clear clinical rationale for treating subtle deficiency.[1,3] However, preliminary findings from a study suggested it may be linked to some immunological impairment, identified as impaired antibody responses to pneumococcal vaccine.[4] Moreover, raised homocysteine concentrations have been identified as a risk factor for atherosclerosis and ischaemic heart disease, and there is increasing interest in the potential of B vitamins, including $B_{12}$, to reduce homocysteine concentrations and therefore atherosclerotic outcomes (see Ischaemic Heart Disease, under Uses of Folic Acid, p.1429).

Dietary vitamin $B_{12}$ deficiency in infants may lead to developmental abnormalities.[5,6]

The issue of fortification of food with folic acid to reduce the number of infants born with neural tube defects has created debate on the risks of masking vitamin $B_{12}$ deficiency, see under Folic Acid, p.1429.

1. Carmel R. Subtle cobalamin deficiency. *Ann Intern Med* 1996; **124:** 338–40.

2. Green R. Screening for vitamin $B_{12}$ deficiency: caveat emptor. *Ann Intern Med* 1996; **124:** 509–11.

3. Metz J. What's the use of oral vitamin $B_{12}$? A neglected but valid treatment route may have new uses in the future. *Med J Aust* 1999; **170:** 407.

4. Fata FT, *et al.* Impaired antibody responses to pneumococcal polysaccharide in elderly patients with low serum vitamin $B_{12}$ levels. *Ann Intern Med* 1996; **124:** 299–304.

5. Emery ES, *et al.* Vitamin B12 deficiency: a cause of abnormal movements in infants. *Pediatrics* 1997; **99:** 255–6.

6. von Schenck U, *et al.* Persistence of neurological damage induced by dietary vitamin B-12 deficiency in infancy. *Arch Dis Child* 1997; **77:** 137–9.

**Ischaemic heart disease.** For mention of the possible link between vitamin $B_{12}$, hyperhomocysteinaemia, and atherosclerosis and ischaemic heart disease, see under Folic Acid p.1429.

**Neural tube defects.** There is abnormality in homocysteine metabolism in many women who give birth to children with neural tube defects (p.1430); the enzyme methionine synthase, which converts homocysteine to methionine, requires both folate and vitamin $B_{12}$ as cofactors, and low maternal vitamin $B_{12}$ concentrations may be an independent risk factor for neural tube defects.[1] If confirmed, this would suggest that additional supplementation with cobalamins may be warranted.

1. Mills JL, *et al.* Homocysteine metabolism in pregnancies complicated by neural-tube defects. *Lancet* 1995; **345:** 149–51.

## Preparations

***BP 2003:*** Cyanocobalamin Tablets; Hydroxocobalamin Injection;
***USP 27:*** Cyanocobalamin Injection; Hydroxocobalamin Injection.

**Proprietary Preparations** (details are given in Part 3)

***Arg.:*** Benzoral; Lisoneurin B12; Methycobal; Reedvit; Vitam Doce; ***Austral.:*** Cytamen; Neo-Cytamen; ***Austria:*** Diclo-B; Erycytol; Hepavit; ***Belg.:*** Forta B; Novobedouze†; ***Braz.:*** Bedozil; Cianon B12; Cronobe; Enzicoba; Methycobal†; Rubranova; Xantox†; Zinabol†; ***Canad.:*** Bedoz; Rubion†; Rubramin†; ***Denm.:*** Behepan†; Betolvex; Vibeden; ***Fin.:*** Betolvex; Cohemin; ***Fr.:*** Cobanzyme; Cyanokit; Dodecavit; Epithea; Indusil T†; ***Ger.:*** Ambe 12; Aquo-Cytobion; B 12-L 90; B12 Depot-Rotexmedica; B12 Ehrl†; B12 Rotexmedica; B12 Steigerwald; B12-Horfervit†; $B_{12}$ Ankermann; $B_{12}$ Depot-Hevert; $B_{12}$ Depot-Vicotrat†; $B_{12}$ Vicotrat; $B_{12}$-ASmedic; Cytobion; Hamo-Vibolex; Lophakomp-B 12; Lophakomp-B 12 Depot; Neurotrat $B_{12}$†; Novidroxin; Novirell B Mono; Vicapan N; Vita-Brachont†; ***Gr.:*** Articlox; ***Hong Kong:*** Cobamin; Cyanokit; Methycobal; Triniscon†; ***India:*** Methycobal; ***Irl.:*** Cytacon; Cytamen; Neo-Cytamen; ***Israel:*** Bedodeka; Nascobal; ***Ital.:*** Cobaforte; Dobetin; Eritrovit B12; Indusil; Neo-Cytamen; OH B12; Reticulogen†; ***Jpn:*** Methycobal; ***Malaysia:*** Methycobal; ***Mex.:*** Axofor; Biocobal; Biotrefon L; Compensal; Doprit†; Droxivit; Duradoce; Exorvit; Hidrowil†; Lentorem†; Leo-Doce; Maxibol; Nebal†; Neribax; Neurofor; Parol†; Rubrina; Sanovit; Valamin 12; Vidavit†; ***Neth.:*** Hydrocobamine; ***Norw.:*** Betolvex; ***NZ:*** Neo-Cytamen; ***Port.:*** Bedoze; Co-Vibedoze; Cobamet; Cobaxid; Jaba $B_{12}$; Made B12†; OH B12; Permadoze; Tridocemine; ***S.Afr.:*** Betolvex†; Cobalatec; Norivite-12†; ***Singapore:*** Hidomin; Methycobal; Neuromethyn; ***Spain:*** Ambritan†; Asimil B12†; Cromatonbic B12; Isopto B 12; Lifaton B12†; Megamilbedoce; Optovite B12; Reticulogen Fortificado; Zimadoce; ***Swed.:*** Behepan; Betolvex; Betolvidon; ***Switz.:*** Betolvex; Vitarubin; ***Thai.:*** Ampavit; Hitocobamin; Methycobal; Neuromet; Redisol; Sicobal; ***UAE:*** Cynovit; ***UK:*** Cemac B12†; Cobalin-H; Cytacon; Cytamen; Neo-Cytamen; ***USA:*** Crystamine; Crysti 1000; Cyanoject†; Cyomin; Ener-B†; Hydro Cobex; Hydro-Crysti-12; LA-12; Nascobal.

**Multi-ingredient:** ***Arg.:*** Algio Nervomax; Algio Nervomax Fuerte; Anemidox-Ferrum; Bioneural B12; Blastop; Blokium B12; Buta Rut B12; Cobenexol Forte; Cobenexol Fuerte; Corteroid Gesic; CVP B1 B6 B12; Dastonil; Delta Tomanil B12; Dexabion; Dioxaflex B12; Dolo Nervobion; Dolo Nervobion 10000; Dorixina B1 B6 B12; Factofer B12; Ferranin Complex; Ferrocebrina; Flexicamin B12; Flogiatrin B12; ITE B12 Forte; Klosidol B1 B6 B12; Nervobion Fuerte; Nervomax TB12; Nucleo CMP; Oxa B12; Rubiron; Sindrolen; Tunik B12; Vesalion B12; Virobron B12 NF; Xedenol B12; Yectafer Complex; ***Austral.:*** Medinat PMT-Eze†; ***Austria:*** Ambene; Ambene N; Arca-Be; Beneuran compositum; Diclovit; Neurobion; Neuromerck; Neuromultivit; Pronerv; Rheumesser; ***Belg.:*** Ferrifol B12†; Neurobion; Vioneurin; ***Braz.:*** Aminocid; Anemofer; Betinjectol†; Bituelve†; Cianotrat-Dexa; Citoneurin; Cobactin; Cobaglobal; Cobavital; Coraben; Dexa-Citoneurin; Dexa-Cronobe; Dexa-Neuriberi; Dexacobal; Dexador; Dexadoze; Dexagil; Dexalgen; Dexaneurin; Dexanevral; Dozeneurin; Ergohepat B12†; Ferroplex; Ferrotrat; Fol Sang; Hematiase B12; Hepasedan†; Hepatotris; Iloban; Infiltran B12†; Lisan; Lisotox†; Metiocolin B12; Metiocolin Composto; Nucleo CMP; Rubizuel†; Trinalgen†; Trinevral†; Trirubin; Vi-Ferrin; Vibetrat Dexa†; Vibetrat†; Vipirim†; Vitaneuron; Xantinon Complex; ***Canad.:*** Acti-$B_{12}$; Folacin 12†; Fortiplex; Heparos†; Penta-3B; Penta-3B + C; ***Chile:*** Betonvit; Citoneuron; Cronoferril; Dolotol 12; Ferranem; Ferranim; Folifer; Nefersil B; Neurobionta; Neurocam; Tol 12; ***Fin.:*** Neurobion; Neurovitan; ***Fr.:*** Forcapil; Nuclevit $B_{12}$†; Vibalgan†; ***Ger.:*** Ambene Comp; AntiFocal N; $B_{12}$ Fol-Vicotrat; Causat B12 N†; Dodecatol N†; Dolo-Neurobion forte; Eryfer comp; Eukalisan forte†; Eukalisan N; Ferro sanol comp; Ferro-Folgamma; Folgamma; Hepagrisevit Forte-N; Hepatofalk†; Medivitan N; Medyn; milgamma N; Neuro-Lichtenstein; Neuro-ratiopharm; Neuro-Vibolex; Neurobion; Neurotrat†; NeyNormin N (Revitorgan-Dilutionen N Nr 65); NeyTumorin N (Revitorgan-Dilutionen N Nr 66); Novirell B†; Pernaemyl†; Selectafer N; Telbibur N; Vitaject; Vitasprint $B_{12}$; ***Hong Kong:*** 3B; Epargriseovit†; Hepatofalk†; Neuro B1-6-12; Neurobion; Neurorubine; Nevramin; Princi-B Fort; Trabit†; Vida Neurotab; Vidaclofen-Plus; ***India:*** Anemidox; Blosyn; Calcinol; Conviron-TR; Delphicol; Dexorange; Elferri-Z; Ferrochelate; Fervit; Globac-Z; Hepasules; Hepatoglobine; Jectocos Plus; Macalvit; Ostocalcium B-12; Plastules; Sioneuron; Tonoferon; Vitneurin; ***Israel:*** Betrivit†; Tribemin; ***Ital.:*** Adenobeta; Adenoplex Forte; Adenovit; Benexol B12; Betascor B12†; Briogen; Calcio Dobetin; Co-Carnetina B12; Dobetin con Vitamina B1; Dobetin Totale; Efargen†; Emazian B12; Emoantitossina; Emopon; Epargriseovit; Eparmefolin; Fibronevrina; Firmavit†; Folepar B12; For Liver†; Fosfo Plus; Fosfoutipi Vitaminico; Gluta Complex; Glutamin Fosforo; Hepa-Factor; Hepatos B12; Memoserina S†; Memovisus; Memovit B12; Menalgon B6†; Menalgon†; Mionevrasi; Neo-Eparbiol; Neo-Geynevral†; Neuraben; Neurobionta†; Nevril†; Novaneurina B12†; OH B12 B1†; Oro B12†; Porfirin 12; Sinevrile†; Tonogen; Tricortin; Triferon†; Trinevrina B6; Vitasprint; Vitasprint Complex; ***Jpn:*** Neurovitan; ***Malaysia:*** 3B; Alinamin B12; Flavettes Neuroforte; Neuro B; Neurobion; Neurorubine; Neurovit; Nevramin; Princi-B Fort; Sangobion; ***Mex.:*** B1-12-15; Bedocil; Benexol B12; Ciprolisina; Cobotiaxina; Dexabion; Dolo-Neurobion; Dolo-Pangavit; Dolo-Tiaminal; Duciclon; Gonakor; Iodarsolo B12; Milbeta; Neuralin; Neurobion; Neuroflax; Orafer Comp†; Pangavit Hypak; Pangavit Pediatrico; Selectadoce; Tiabexol; Tiamidexal; Tiaminal $B_{12}$; Tiaminal $B_{12}$ Trivalente; Tribedoxyl; ***Port.:*** Linamin Plus; Neurobion; Tridocemine†; ***S.Afr.:*** Foliglobin; Neurobion; Prohep; Revaton†; Trinsicon†; ***Singapore:*** 3B†; Alinamin B12; Neogobion; Neurobion; Neurodex; Neuroforte; Neurorubine; Neurovit; Nevramin; Princi-B Fort; Sangobion; Wanse; ***Spain:*** Antineurina; Benexol B1 B6 B12; Bester Complex; Calcio 20 Complex; Covitasa B12; Dalamon; Duplicalcio B12; Enoton; Foli Doce; Gammamida Complex†; Hepa Factor; Hidroxil B12 B6 B1; Inzitan; Malandil; Mederebro; Mederebro Compuesto†; Menalgil B6; Meneparol†; Metabolicum†; Milbedoce Anabolico†; Nervobion; Neuromade; Neurostop Complex; Prodessal†; Refulgin†; Rubrocortin; Sugarceton†; Taurobetina; Teovit†; Tonico Juventus; Trofalgon; Trofi Milina†; Viadetres; Vitafardi C B12; ***Swed.:*** Neurobion; ***Switz.:*** Neurotrat†; Tribeton†; Vitasprint Complex; ***Thai.:*** 3B; Alinamin B12; Beromin; Cilfer-12-F†; Cydoxmine-B; Cyriamine; Douzabox; Genavit; Hemolax; Neubee; Neurobex; Neurobion; Nevramin; Nuvit; Ostone-B12; Princi-B; Sangobion†; Trabit; Tribesian; Tricortin; Trinsicon; Trivit-B; Vioneurin†; Vita-B; Vitamedin; Vitron; ***UAE:*** 3V; ***UK:*** Dicopac; Hematinic; ***USA:*** Anemagen; Bevitamel; Chromagen; Chromagen FA; Chromagen Forte; Contrin; Fe-Tinic Forte; FeoGen; Ferotrinsic; Ferralet Plus; Ferrex Forte; Ferrex Forte Plus; Ferrogels Forte; Fetrin; FOLTX; Fumatinic; Hem Fe; Hemocyte-F; Icar-C Plus; Livitrinsic-f; Niferex Forte; Nu-Iron Plus†; Poly-Iron Forte; PremesisRx; Pronemia Hematinic; Tolfrinic; TriHEMIC; Trinsicon.

# Vitamin C Substances

Vitaminas C.

Several substances have vitamin C activity, notably ascorbic acid and its calcium and sodium salts. Natural products with a high vitamin C content include black currant (p.1661), lemon (p.1706), sweet orange (p.1724), and rose fruit (p.1740).

## Ascorbic Acid *(BAN, rINN)*

Ácido ascórbico; Acidum Ascorbicum; L-Ascorbic Acid; Cevitamic Acid; E300; Vitamin C. The enolic form of 3-oxo-L-gulofuranolactone; 2,3-Didehydro-L-*threo*-hexono-1,4-lactone.

$C_6H_8O_6$ = 176.1.

*CAS — 50-81-7.*

*ATC — A11GA01; G01AD03; S01XA15.*

**Pharmacopoeias.** In *Chin., Eur.* (see p.vi), *Int., Jpn, Pol., US,* and *Viet.*

**Ph. Eur. 5.0** (Ascorbic Acid). A white or almost white crystalline powder or colourless crystals becoming discoloured on exposure to air and moisture. Freely soluble in water; soluble in alcohol. A 5% solution in water has a pH of 2.1 to 2.6. Store in nonmetallic containers. Protect from light.

**USP 27** (Ascorbic Acid). White or slightly yellow crystals or powder. On exposure to light, it gradually darkens. In the dry state, is reasonably stable in air, but in solution rapidly oxidises. Soluble 1 in 3 of water and 1 in 40 of alcohol; insoluble in chloroform, in ether, and in benzene. Store in airtight containers. Protect from light.

## Calcium Ascorbate *(BANM, rINNM)*

Ascorbato cálcico; Calcii Ascorbas; E302.

$(C_6H_7O_6)_2Ca,2H_2O$ = 426.3.

*CAS — 5743-27-1.*

**Pharmacopoeias.** In *Chin., Eur.* (see p.vi), and *US.*

**Ph. Eur. 5.0** (Calcium Ascorbate). A white or slightly yellowish crystalline powder. Freely soluble in water; practically insoluble in alcohol. A 10% solution in water has a pH between 6.8 and 7.4. Store in nonmetallic containers. Protect from light.

**USP 27** (Calcium Ascorbate). A white to slightly yellow, practically odourless, powder. Freely soluble in water (about 1 in 2); slightly soluble in alcohol; insoluble in ether. pH of a 10% solution in water is between 6.8 and 7.4. Store in airtight containers. Protect from light.

## Sodium Ascorbate *(BANM, rINN)*

Ascorbato de sodio; E301; Monosodium L-Ascorbate; Natrii Ascorbas. 3-Oxo-L-gulofuranolactone sodium enolate.

$C_6H_7NaO_6$ = 198.1.

*CAS — 134-03-2.*

**Pharmacopoeias.** In *Chin., Eur.* (see p.vi), and *US.*

**Ph. Eur. 5.0** (Sodium Ascorbate). A white or yellowish crystalline powder or crystals. Freely soluble in water; sparingly soluble in alcohol; practically insoluble in dichloromethane. A 10% solution in water has a pH of 7.0 to 8.0. Store in nonmetallic containers. Protect from light.

**USP 27** (Sodium Ascorbate). White or very faintly yellow, odourless or practically odourless, crystals or crystalline powder. On exposure to light it gradually darkens. Soluble 1 in 1.3 of water; very slightly soluble in alcohol; insoluble in chloroform and in ether. pH of a 10% solution in water is between 7.0 and 8.0. Store in airtight containers. Protect from light.

## Adverse Effects and Precautions

Ascorbic acid is usually well tolerated. Large doses are reported to cause diarrhoea and other gastrointestinal disturbances. It has also been stated that large doses may result in hyperoxaluria and the formation of renal calcium oxalate calculi and ascorbic acid should therefore be given with care to patients with hyperoxaluria (see Effects on the Kidneys, below). Tolerance may be induced with prolonged use of large doses, resulting in symptoms of deficiency when intake is reduced to normal.

Large doses of ascorbic acid have resulted in haemolysis in patients with G6PD deficiency (see Effects on the Blood, below).

**Effects on the blood.** There are reports of haemolysis in patients with G6PD deficiency following large doses of ascorbic acid either intravenously[1,2] or in soft drinks.[3] There has also been a report[4] of a patient with paroxysmal nocturnal haemoglobinuria suffering haemolysis following the ingestion of large amounts of ascorbic acid in a soft drink. There is concern that the large quantities of vitamin C in feeds for premature neonates may have a pro-oxidant effect, and lead to haemolysis. However, a double-blind study found no increase in erythrocyte destruction or hyperbilirubinaemia in premature neonates receiving vitamin C.[5]


1. Campbell GD, *et al.* Ascorbic acid-induced hemolysis in G-6-PD deficiency. *Ann Intern Med* 1975; **82:** 810.
2. Rees DC, *et al.* Acute haemolysis induced by high dose ascorbic acid in glucose-6-phosphate dehydrogenase deficiency. *BMJ* 1993; **306:** 841–2.
3. Mehta JB, *et al.* Ascorbic-acid-induced haemolysis in G-6-PD deficiency. *Lancet* 1990; **336:** 944.
4. Iwamoto N, *et al.* Haemolysis induced by ascorbic acid in paroxysmal nocturnal haemoglobinuria. *Lancet* 1994; **343:** 357.
5. Doyle J, *et al.* Does vitamin C cause hemolysis in premature newborn infants? Results of a multicenter double-blind, randomized, controlled trial. *J Pediatr* 1997; **130:** 103–9.


**Effects on the kidneys.** Although renal impairment associated with excessive oxalate excretion has been reported following the administration of large doses of ascorbic acid[1-3] it has been considered that healthy persons can ingest large amounts of ascorbic acid with relatively small increases in oxalate excretion[4-6] and without an increased risk of oxalate stone formation.


1. Reznik VM, *et al.* Does high-dose ascorbic acid accelerate renal failure? *N Engl J Med* 1980; **302:** 1418–19.
2. Swartz RD, *et al.* Hyperoxaluria and renal insufficiency due to ascorbic acid administration during total parenteral nutrition. *Ann Intern Med* 1984; **100:** 530–1.
3. Balcke P, *et al.* Ascorbic acid aggravates secondary hyperoxalemia in patients on chronic hemodialysis. *Ann Intern Med* 1984; **101:** 344–5.
4. Tsao CS. Ascorbic acid administration and urinary oxalate. *Ann Intern Med* 1984; **101:** 405–6.
5. Wandzilak TR, *et al.* Effect of high dose vitamin C on urinary oxalate levels. *J Urol (Baltimore)* 1994; **151:** 834–7.
6. Curhan GC, *et al.* Intake of vitamins B6 and C and the risk of kidney stones in women. *J Am Soc Nephrol* 1999; **10:** 840–5.


**Effects on the teeth.** A report of dental enamel erosion which was attributed to the daily ingestion of chewable ascorbic acid tablets over a period of 3 years.[1] The tablets lowered the pH of the saliva to a level at which calcium was lost from the tooth enamel.


1. Giunta JL. Dental erosion resulting from chewable vitamin C tablets. *J Am Dent Assoc* 1983; **107:** 253–6.


**Interference with laboratory tests.** Ascorbic acid, a strong reducing agent, interferes with laboratory tests involving oxidation and reduction reactions. Falsely-elevated or false-negative test results may be obtained from plasma, faeces, or urine samples depending on such factors as the dose of ascorbic acid and specific method employed.

## Interactions

For the effect of ascorbic acid on various drugs see under desferrioxamine (p.1034), hormonal contraceptives (p.1535), fluphenazine (under Chlorpromazine, p.680), and warfarin (p.1027). Ascorbic acid may increase the absorption of iron in iron-deficiency states.

## Pharmacokinetics

Ascorbic acid is readily absorbed from the gastrointestinal tract and is widely distributed in the body tissues. Plasma concentrations of ascorbic acid rise as the dose ingested is increased until a plateau is reached with doses of about 90 to 150 mg daily. Body stores of ascorbic acid in health are about 1.5 g although more may be stored at intakes above 200 mg daily. The concentration is higher in leucocytes and platelets than in erythrocytes and plasma. In deficiency states the concentration in leucocytes declines later and at a slower rate, and has been considered to be a better criterion for the evaluation of deficiency than the concentration in plasma.

Ascorbic acid is reversibly oxidised to dehydroascorbic acid; some is metabolised to ascorbate-2-sulfate, which is inactive, and oxalic acid which are excreted in the urine. Ascorbic acid in excess of the body's needs is also rapidly eliminated unchanged in the urine; this generally occurs with intakes exceeding 200 mg daily. Ascorbic acid crosses the placenta and is distributed into breast milk. It is removed by haemodialysis.

## Human Requirements

A daily dietary intake of about 30 to 100 mg of vitamin C has been recommended for adults. There is, however, wide variation in individual requirements. Humans are unable to form their own ascorbic acid and so a dietary source is necessary. Most dietary ascorbic acid is obtained from fruit and vegetable sources; only small amounts are present in milk and animal tissues. Relatively rich sources include rose hips (rose fruit), black currant, citrus fruits, leafy vegetables, tomatoes, potatoes, and green and red peppers.

Ascorbic acid is readily destroyed during cooking processes. Considerable losses may also occur during storage.

**UK and US recommended dietary intake.** In the UK[1] dietary reference values (see p.1419) have been published for vitamin C and similarly in the USA recommended dietary allowances (RDAs) have been set.[2] Differing amounts are recommended for infants and children of varying ages, for adult males and females, and for pregnant and lactating women. In the UK the reference nutrient intake (RNI) is 40 mg daily for adult males and females and the estimated average requirement (EAR) is 30 mg daily. In general the amount recommended in the USA for all ages and groups is higher than that set in the UK; the RDA is 90 mg daily for men and 75 mg daily for women.[2] The RDA is increased in smokers by 35 mg daily. The tolerable upper intake level is 2 g daily.[2] The EAR is 75 mg daily for men and 60 mg daily for women.

1. DoH. Dietary reference values for food energy and nutrients for the United Kingdom: report of the panel on dietary reference values of the committee on medical aspects of food policy. *Report on health and social subjects 41.* London: HMSO, 1991.
2. Standing Committee on the Scientific Evaluation of Dietary Reference Intakes of the Food and Nutrition Board. *Dietary Reference Intakes for vitamin C, vitamin E, selenium, and carotenoids.* Washington DC: National Academy Press, 2000. Also available at: http://www.nap.edu/catalog/9810.html (accessed 24/05/04)

## Uses and Administration

Vitamin C, a water-soluble vitamin, is essential for the synthesis of collagen and intercellular material. Vitamin C deficiency develops when the dietary intake is inadequate. It is rare in adults, but may occur in infants, alcoholics, or the elderly. Deficiency leads to the development of a well-defined syndrome known as scurvy. This is characterised by capillary fragility, bleeding (especially from small blood vessels and the gums), normocytic or macrocytic anaemia, cartilage and bone lesions, and slow healing of wounds.

Vitamin C is used in the treatment and prevention of deficiency. It completely reverses symptoms of deficiency. It is usually given by mouth, the preferred route, as ascorbic acid, and has been given to children in the form of a suitable fruit juice such as orange juice or as black currant or rose hip syrups. Ascorbic acid or sodium ascorbate may be administered parenterally, preferably by the intramuscular route, but also by the intravenous or subcutaneous routes. Doses of 25 to 75 mg daily in the prevention of deficiency, and 250 mg or more daily in divided doses for the treatment of deficiency, have been recommended.

Ascorbic acid 100 to 200 mg daily may be given with desferrioxamine in the treatment of patients with thalassaemia, to improve the chelating action of desferrioxamine, thereby increasing the excretion of iron (see p.1034). In iron deficiency states ascorbic acid may increase gastrointestinal iron absorption and ascorbic acid or ascorbate salts are therefore included in some oral iron preparations. Ascorbic acid or sodium ascorbate have been used in treating methaemoglobinaemia. Ascorbic acid has been used to acidify urine. It has also been tried in the treatment of many other disorders (see below) but there is little evidence of beneficial effect.

Eye drops containing potassium ascorbate have been used for the treatment of chemical burns. Potassium ascorbate 10% is used alternately with sodium citrate 10%; it is believed that the ascorbate works by mopping up free oxygen radicals thus aiding in the prevention of corneal epithelial damage.

Ascorbic acid and calcium and sodium ascorbates are used as antioxidants in pharmaceutical manufacturing and in the food industry.

◊ A beneficial effect of vitamin C therapy has been claimed for an extraordinary number of conditions, including Alzheimer's disease (see Dementia, under Vitamin E, p.1465), atherosclerosis (see Prophylaxis of Ischaemic Heart Disease, p.1420), cancer (see Prophylaxis of Malignant Neoplasms, p.1420), the common cold (p.618), idiopathic thrombocytopenic purpura (p.1082), and pre-eclampsia (see Hypertension, p.825). Other conditions claimed to benefit include asthma, wound healing, psychiatric disorders, infections due to abnormal leucocyte function, infertility, osteogenesis imperfecta, pain in Paget's disease, and opioid withdrawal. Generally there are few properly controlled studies to substantiate these claims.

## Preparations

***BP 2003:*** Ascorbic Acid Injection; Ascorbic Acid Tablets; Paediatric Vitamins A, C and D Oral Drops; Vitamins B and C Injection;
***USP 27:*** Ascorbic Acid Injection; Ascorbic Acid Oral Solution; Ascorbic Acid Tablets.

**Proprietary Preparations** (details are given in Part 3)
***Arg.:*** Cebion; Cewin; Redoxon; Vicenrik; ***Austral.:*** Bioglan Cal C†; Cecon†; Pro-C†; Redoxon†; Sugarless C†; Supa C†; Vita C†; ***Austria:*** Ascorbin; Bioagil†; C-Vit; Calcascorbin; Ce-Limo; Cebion; Cetebe; Cevitol; Iroviton-Irocovit-C; Mel-C; Redoxon; Tetesept Vitamin C; Vicedent†; ***Belg.:*** C-Dose; C-Will; Cenol†; Cetamine; Cevi-drops; Redoxon; Upsa C; Upsavit C; ***Braz.:*** Active C; Ascortil†; Cebion; Ceklin; Cenevit; Cetozone; Cevita; Ceviton; Cewin; Citron†; Citroplex; Citrovit; Energil C; Fonto-Vit C; Lento C†; Redoxon; Vi-Ce; Vitabase Vitamina C; Vitacitrus; Vitafran†; Vitageyer C; Vitascorb†; Vitax†; ***Canad.:*** Action; Apo-C†; Ascorbex; Balanced C Complex; C Forte†; C-1000†; C-3000†; Ester-C; Kamu Jay; Kyolic Formula 103; Nutrol C; Ortic C†; Proflavanol C; Redoxon; Revitalose C; Super C; Timed Release C; Vita-C; ***Chile:*** Cebion; Crevet; Esvit C; Mintavit-C; Necta C; Redoxon; Vitac; Vitaseve; ***Fin.:*** Ascorbin; Bio-C-Vitamin; C-Poretta†; C-Tabs; C-vimin; Ceerexin; Cevi-Tabs; Poremax-C; Puru-C; Vita-C; ***Fr.:*** Arkovital C†; Laroscorbine; Midy Vitamine C; Vitascorbol; ***Ger.:*** Ascorell; Ascorvit; ASS OPT†; C-L90; Cebion; Cebion N; Cetebe; Hermes Cevitt; Synum C; Vagi-C; ***Gr.:*** Cebion; ***Hong Kong:*** C Rose Hips†; C-1000†; Cecap; Cegrovit; Celin; Cetrinets; Chewies†; Delrosa; Flavettes; Redoxon; Vicemex; Vorange; ***India:*** Cecon; Celin; Limcee; ***Irl.:*** Redoxon; Rubex; ***Israel:*** C500; Cereon; Redoxon; Vi-C; Vitascarbol†; ***Ital.:*** Acidylina†; Addivita; Agrumina; Agruvit; Ascomed†; Bio-Ci; C Monovit; C-Lisa; C-Tard; Cebion; Cecon†; Duo-C; Dynaphos-C; Ergofit†; Grumivit; Lemonvit†; Redoxon; Vici; Vicitina†; Zig C†; ***Malaysia:*** Ascorbin; Cecap; Ceelin; Cetrinets; Chewette C; Citrex; Dumovit C; Upha C; Vita C; ***Mex.:*** Cemina; Cevalin; Dermoskin C; Infa-C-Vit†; Redoxon; ***Neth.:*** C-Will; Redoxon; ***Norw.:*** AFI-C†; Bio-C; ***NZ:*** Citravite; Redoxon†; ***Port.:*** Anti-rugas C; C'Nergil; Cebiolon; Cebion†; Cecrisina; Citavi; Prevegyne; Redoxon; Vivin C†; ***S.Afr.:*** Chewy C; Redoxon†; Rovit C; Scorbex; ***Singapore:*** Ascorbin; Cetrinets; Dancimin-C; Dumovit C; Flavettes; Redoxon†; Vorange; ***Spain:*** Caramelos Vit C†; Cebion; Citrolider†; Citrovit; Ledovit C†; Redoxon; Unimicebrina; Upsa C†; ***Swed.:*** C-vimin; Ido-C; ***Switz.:*** C-Naryl†; Cegrovit; Cetebe; Demovit C; Redoxon; Vicemex; Vita-Ce; ***Thai.:*** Bio-C; C Mon; C-Will; Hicee; Mita-c; Mymin C†; Redoxon†; Teddy-C; Vitacimin; ***UK:*** Buffered C; Buffered C 500; Haliborange Halibonbons; Redoxon; ***USA:*** Ascor; Cebid†; Cecon; Cenolate; Cevi-Bid; Dull-C; N'ice Vitamin C; Sunkist; Vita-C.

**Multi-ingredient:** numerous preparations are listed in Part 3.

---

# Vitamin D Substances

Vitaminas D.

The term vitamin D is used for a range of closely related sterol compounds including alfacalcidol, calcifediol, calcitriol, colecalciferol, dihydrotachysterol, and ergocalciferol. Newer vitamin D analogues include doxercalciferol, falecalcitriol, maxacalcitol, and paricalcitol.

## Alfacalcidol *(BAN, rINN)*

Alfacalcidolum; EB-644; 1α-Hydroxycholecalciferol; 1α-Hydroxyvitamin $D_3$; 1α-OHD$_3$. (5Z,7E)-9,10-Secocholesta-5,7,10(19)-triene-1α,3β-diol.

$C_{27}H_{44}O_2$ = 400.6.
*CAS — 41294-56-8.*
*ATC — A11CC03.*

**Pharmacopoeias.** In *Eur.* (see p.vi).

**Ph. Eur. 5.0** (Alfacalcidol). White or almost white crystals which are sensitive to air, heat, and light. Practically insoluble in water; freely soluble in alcohol; soluble in fatty oils. Reversible isomerisation to pre-alfacalcidol takes place in solution, depending on temperature and time. Activity is due to both compounds. Store at 2° to 8° under an atmosphere of nitrogen in airtight containers. The contents of an opened container should be used immediately. Protect from light.

## Calcifediol *(BAN, USAN, rINN)*

Calcidiol; Calcifediolum; 25-Hydroxycholecalciferol; 25-Hydroxyvitamin $D_3$; 25-(OH)$D_3$; U-32070E. (5Z,7E)-9,10-Secocholesta-5,7,10(19)-triene-3β,25-diol monohydrate.

$C_{27}H_{44}O_2,H_2O$ = 418.7.
*CAS — 19356-17-3 (anhydrous calcifediol); 63283-36-3 (calcifediol monohydrate).*
*ATC — A11CC06.*

**Pharmacopoeias.** In *Eur.* (see p.vi), *Pol.*, and *US.*

**Ph. Eur. 5.0** (Calcifediol). White or almost white crystals which are sensitive to air, heat, and light. Practically insoluble in water; freely soluble in alcohol; soluble in fatty oils. Reversible isomerisation to pre-calcifediol takes place in solution, depending on temperature and time. The activity is due to both compounds. Store at 2° to 8° under an atmosphere of nitrogen in airtight containers. The contents of an opened container should be used immediately. Protect from light.

**USP 27** (Calcifediol). Store in airtight containers. Protect from light.

## Calcitriol *(BAN, USAN, rINN)*

Calcitriolum; 1,25-Dihydroxycholecalciferol; 1α,25-Dihydroxycholecalciferol; 1α,25-Dihydroxyvitamin $D_3$; 1α,25(OH)$_2D_3$; Ro-21-5535. (5Z,7E)-9,10-Secocholesta-5,7,10(19)-triene-1α,3β,25-triol.

$C_{27}H_{44}O_3$ = 416.6.
*CAS — 32222-06-3.*
*ATC — A11CC04; D05AX03.*

**Pharmacopoeias.** In *Eur.* (see p.vi).

**Ph. Eur. 5.0** (Calcitriol). White or almost white crystals. Practically insoluble in water; freely soluble in alcohol; soluble in fatty oils. It is sensitive to air, heat, and light. A reversible isomerisation to pre-calcitriol takes place in solution, depending on temperature and time. The activity is due to both compounds. Store at 2° to 8° under an atmosphere of nitrogen in airtight containers. The contents of an opened container should be used immediately. Protect from light.

## Colecalciferol *(BAN, rINN)*

Activated 7-Dehydrocholesterol; Cholecalciferol; Cholecalciferolum; Vitamin $D_3$. (5Z,7E)-9,10-Secocholesta-5,7,10(19)-trien-3β-ol.

$C_{27}H_{44}O$ = 384.6.
*CAS — 67-97-0.*
*ATC — A11CC05.*

**Description.** Colecalciferol is the naturally occurring form of vitamin D. It is produced from 7-dehydrocholesterol, a sterol present in mammalian skin, by ultraviolet irradiation.

**Pharmacopoeias.** In *Chin., Eur.* (see p.vi), *Int., Jpn, Pol., US,* and *Viet.*

*Eur.* also includes monographs for concentrates in an oily form, a powder form, and a water-dispersible form. *US* also includes a solution.

**Ph. Eur. 5.0** (Cholecalciferol; Colecalciferol BP 2003). White or almost white crystals which are sensitive to air, heat, and light. Practically insoluble in water; freely soluble in alcohol; soluble in fatty oils. Solutions in volatile solvents are unstable and should be used immediately. A reversible isomerisation to pre-colecalciferol takes place in solution, depending on temperature and time. The activity is due to both compounds. Store under nitrogen in airtight containers at a temperature of 2° to 8°. The contents of an opened container should be used immediately. Protect from light.

The BP 2003 directs that when calciferol or vitamin D is prescribed or demanded, Colecalciferol or Ergocalciferol shall be dispensed or supplied.

**Ph. Eur. 5.0** (Cholecalciferol Concentrate (Oily Form); Cholecalciferolum Densatum Oleosum; Colecalciferol Concentrate (Oily Form) BP 2003). A solution of colecalciferol in a suitable vegetable oil. It contains not less than 500 000 units/g. It may contain suitable stabilisers such as antioxidants. A clear, yellow liquid. Practically insoluble in water; slightly soluble in dehydrated alcohol; miscible with solvents of fats. Partial solidification may occur, depending on the temperature. Store in well-filled airtight containers. Protect from light. The contents of an opened container are to be used as soon as possible; any unused part is to be protected by an atmosphere of nitrogen.

**Ph. Eur. 5.0** (Cholecalciferol Concentrate (Powder Form); Cholecalciferoli Pulvis; Colecalciferol Concentrate (Powder Form) BP 2003). It is obtained by dispersing an oily solution of colecalciferol in an appropriate matrix which is usually based on a combination of gelatin and carbohydrates of suitable quality. It contains not less than 100 000 units/g. It may contain suitable stabilisers such as antioxidants. White or yellowish-white, small particles. Depending on their formulation, it may be practically insoluble in water or may swell or form a dispersion. Store in well-filled airtight containers. Protect from light. The contents of an opened container are to be used as soon as possible; any unused part is to be protected by an atmosphere of nitrogen.

**Ph. Eur. 5.0** (Cholecalciferol Concentrate (Water-dispersible Form); Cholecalciferolum in Aqua Dispergibile; Colecalciferol Concentrate (Water-dispersible Form) BP 2003). A solution of colecalciferol in a suitable vegetable oil to which suitable solubilisers have been added. It contains not less than 100 000 units/g. It may contain suitable stabilisers such as antioxidants. A slightly yellowish liquid of variable opalescence and viscosity. Highly concentrated solutions may become cloudy at low temperatures or form a gel at room temperature. Store in well-filled airtight containers. Protect from light. The contents of an opened container are to be used as soon as possible; any unused part is to be protected by an atmosphere of inert gas.

**USP 27** (Cholecalciferol). White, odourless crystals. Insoluble in water; soluble in alcohol, in chloroform, and in fatty oils. M.p. about 85°. It is affected by air and light. Store under nitrogen in hermetically sealed containers at a temperature of 8° to 15°. Protect from light.

**USP 27** (Cholecalciferol Solution). A solution of colecalciferol in an edible vegetable oil, in polysorbate 80, or in propylene glycol. Store in airtight containers. Protect from light.

## Dihydrotachysterol *(BAN, rINN)*

Dichysterol; Dihidrotaquisterol. (5E,7E,22E)-10α-9,10-Secoergosta-5,7,22-trien-3β-ol.

$C_{28}H_{46}O$ = 398.7.
*CAS — 67-96-9.*
*ATC — A11CC02.*

**Pharmacopoeias.** In *US.*

**USP 27** (Dihydrotachysterol). Colourless or white, odourless crystals, or white, odourless, crystalline powder. Practically insoluble in water; soluble in alcohol; freely soluble in chloroform and in ether; sparingly soluble in vegetable oils. Store in hermetic glass containers from which the air has been displaced by an inert gas. Protect from light.

**Doxercalciferol** *(USAN, rINN)*

1α-Hydroxyergocalciferol; 1α-Hydroxyvitamin $D_2$; 1α-OH-$D_2$. (5Z,7E,22E)-9,10-Secoergosta-5,7,10(19),22-tetraene-1α,3β-diol.

$C_{28}H_{44}O_2$ = 412.6.
*CAS — 54573-75-0.*

**Ergocalciferol** *(BAN, rINN)*

Calciferol; Ergocalciferolum; Irradiated Ergosterol; Viosterol; Vitamin $D_2$. (5Z,7E,22E)-9,10-Secoergosta-5,7,10(19),22-tetraen-3β-ol.

$C_{28}H_{44}O$ = 396.6.
*CAS — 50-14-6.*
*ATC — A11CC01.*

**Description.** Ergocalciferol is an antirachitic substance obtained from ergosterol, a sterol present in fungi and yeasts, by ultraviolet irradiation.

**Pharmacopoeias.** In *Chin., Eur.* (see p.vi), *Int., Jpn, US,* and *Viet.*

**Ph. Eur. 5.0** (Ergocalciferol). White or almost white, crystals or white or slightly yellowish crystalline powder. It is sensitive to air, heat, and light. Practically insoluble in water; freely soluble in alcohol; soluble in fatty oils. Solutions in volatile solvents are unstable and should be used immediately. A reversible isomerisation to pre-ergocalciferol takes place in solution, depending on temperature and time. The activity is due to both compounds. Store under nitrogen in airtight containers at a temperature of 2° to 8°. The contents of an opened container should be used immediately. Protect from light.

The BP 2003 directs that when calciferol or vitamin D is prescribed or demanded, Ergocalciferol or Colecalciferol shall be dispensed or supplied.

**USP 27** (Ergocalciferol). White, odourless crystals. It is affected by air and light. Insoluble in water; soluble in alcohol, in chloroform, in ether, and in fatty oils. Store in hermetically sealed containers under nitrogen at a temperature of 8° to 15°. Protect from light.

**Falecalcitriol** *(rINN)*

Flocalcitriol; Hexafluorocalcitriol; Ro 23-4194; ST 630. (+)-(5Z,7E)-26,26,26,27,27,27-Hexafluoro-9,10-secocholesta-5,7,10(19)-triene-1α,3β,25-triol.

$C_{27}H_{38}F_6O_3$ = 524.6.
*CAS — 83805-11-2.*

**Maxacalcitol** *(USAN, rINN)*

1α,25-Dihydroxy-22-oxavitamin $D_3$; OCT; 22-Oxacalcitriol; Sch-209579. (+)-(5Z,7E,20S)-20-(3-Hydroxy-3-methylbutoxy)-9,10-secopregna-5,7,10(19)-triene-1α,3β-diol.

$C_{26}H_{42}O_4$ = 418.6.
*CAS — 103909-75-7.*

**Paricalcitol** *(USAN, rINN)*

ABT-358; Compound 49510; Paracalcin. (7E,22E)-19-Nor-9,10-secoergosta-5,7,22-triene-1α,3β,25-triol.

$C_{27}H_{44}O_3$ = 416.6.
*CAS — 131918-61-1.*

**Pharmacopoeias.** In *US.*

**USP 27** (Paricalcitol). A white to almost white powder. Insoluble in water; soluble in alcohol. Store under argon in airtight containers at a temperature of −25° to −10°.

## Units

The Second International Standard Preparation (1949) of vitamin D consisted of bottles containing approximately 6 g of a solution of colecalciferol in vegetable oil (1000 units/g). This standard has now been discontinued.

NOTE. One unit of vitamin D is contained in 25 nanograms of colecalciferol or ergocalciferol (i.e. 1 mg of colecalciferol or ergocalciferol is equivalent to 40 000 units of vitamin D as determined by bioassay in *rats*).

## Adverse Effects and Treatment

Excessive intake of vitamin D leads to the development of hypercalcaemia and its associated effects including hypercalciuria, ectopic calcification, and renal and cardiovascular damage (for a discussion of vitamin-D mediated hypercalcaemia and its treatment, see p.1218). Symptoms of overdosage include anorexia, lassitude, nausea and vomiting, diarrhoea, polyuria, sweating, headache, thirst, and vertigo. Interindividual tolerance to vitamin D varies considerably; infants and children are generally more susceptible to its toxic effects. The vitamin should be withdrawn if toxicity occurs. It has been stated that vitamin D dietary supplementation may be detrimental in persons already receiving an adequate intake through diet and exposure to sunlight, since the difference between therapeutic and toxic concentrations is relatively small.

The most potent forms of vitamin D, such as alfacalcidol and calcitriol, might reasonably be expected to pose a greater risk of toxicity; however, their effects are reversed rapidly on withdrawal.

Hypersensitivity reactions have occurred.

◊ Vitamin D is the most likely of all vitamins to cause overt toxicity. Doses of 60 000 units daily can cause hypercalcaemia, with muscle weakness, apathy, headache, anorexia, nausea and vomiting, bone pain, ectopic calcification, proteinuria, hypertension, and cardiac arrhythmias. Chronic hypercalcaemia can lead to generalised vascular calcification, nephrocalcinosis, and rapid deterioration of renal function.[1] A number of reports of accidental overdosage, leading to hypercalcaemia or nephrocalcinosis, occurred in the UK following introduction of a concentrated alfacalcidol oral solution that was 10 times stronger than the former presentation.[2]

Hypercalcaemia has been reported in one person following brief industrial exposure to colecalciferol.[3]

A study in children treated for renal osteodystrophy has provided some evidence that hypercalcaemia may occur more frequently with calcitriol than with ergocalciferol.[4] Another such study has suggested that vitamin D has nephrotoxic properties independent of the degree of induced hypercalcaemia, and that the decline in renal function may be more marked with calcitriol.[5]

Topical calcitriol may affect calcium homoeostasis, and hypercalcaemia has been reported in some studies.[6] For mention of the effect of other vitamin D analogues used in psoriasis on calcium homoeostasis, see p.1144.

1. Anonymous. Toxic effects of vitamin overdosage. *Med Lett Drugs Ther* 1984; **26:** 73–4.
2. Committee on Safety of Medicines/Medicines Control Agency. Accidental overdose with alfacalcidol (One-Alpha drops). *Current Problems* 2001; **27:** 3. Also available at: http://www.mca.gov.uk/ourwork/monitorsafequalmed/currentproblems/cpfeb2001.pdf (accessed 21/05/04)
3. Jibani M, Hodges NH. Prolonged hypercalcaemia after industrial exposure to vitamin $D_3$. *BMJ* 1985; **290:** 748–9.
4. Hodson EM, *et al.* Treatment of childhood renal osteodystrophy with calcitriol or ergocalciferol. *Clin Nephrol* 1985; **24:** 192–200.
5. Chan JCM, *et al.* A prospective, double-blind study of growth failure in children with chronic renal insufficiency and the effectiveness of treatment with calcitriol versus dihydrotachysterol. *J Pediatr* 1994; **124:** 520–8.
6. Bourke JF, *et al.* Vitamin D analogues in psoriasis: effects on systemic calcium homeostasis. *Br J Dermatol* 1996; **135:** 347–54.

## Precautions

Vitamin D should not be given to patients with hypercalcaemia. It should be used with caution in infants, who may have increased sensitivity to its effects, and patients with renal impairment or calculi, or heart disease, who might be at increased risk of organ damage if hypercalcaemia occurred. Plasma phosphate concentrations should be controlled during vitamin D therapy to reduce the risk of ectopic calcification.

It is advised that patients receiving pharmacological doses of vitamin D should have their plasma-calcium concentration monitored at regular intervals, especially initially or if symptoms suggest toxicity (see above). Similar monitoring is recommended in infants if they are breast fed by mothers receiving pharmacological doses of vitamin D (see below).

**Breast feeding.** Vitamin D is distributed into breast milk,[1] and its concentration appears to correlate with vitamin D levels in the serum of exclusively breast-fed infants.[2] The American Academy of Pediatrics considers the use of vitamin D to be usually compatible with breast feeding,[3] although they and others[4] recommend that the infant be closely monitored for hypercalcaemia or clinical manifestations of vitamin D toxicity if the mother is receiving pharmacological doses of vitamin D.

1. Rothberg AD, *et al.* Maternal-infant vitamin D relationships during breast-feeding. *J Pediatr* 1982; **101:** 500–503.
2. Cancela L, *et al.* Relationship between the vitamin D content of maternal milk and the vitamin D status of nursing women and breast-fed infants. *J Endocrinol* 1986; **110:** 43–50.
3. American Academy of Pediatrics. The transfer of drugs and other chemicals into human milk. *Pediatrics* 2001; **108:** 776–89. Correction. *ibid.*; 1029. Also available at: http://aappolicy.aappublications.org/cgi/content/full/pediatrics%3b108/3/776 (accessed 19/05/04)
4. Greer FR, *et al.* High concentrations of vitamin $D_2$ in human milk associated with pharmacologic doses of vitamin $D_2$. *J Pediatr* 1984; **105:** 61–4.

**Pregnancy.** Hypercalcaemia during pregnancy may produce congenital disorders in the offspring, and neonatal hypoparathyroidism. However, the risks to the fetus of untreated maternal hypoparathyroidism are considered greater than the risks of hypercalcaemia due to vitamin D therapy. Indeed, one report noted increased requirements for vitamin D preparations during pregnancy for the treatment of hypoparathyroidism;[1] the doses tended to need increasing during the second half of pregnancy. In one woman in whom the dose of calcitriol was kept at the increased level after delivery (in an attempt to allow for the calcium loss involved in breast feeding) hypercalcaemia developed; this did not occur in 2 women who did not breast feed and in whom the dose of the vitamin D preparations was reduced soon after delivery.[1]

1. Caplan RH, Beguin EA. Hypercalcemia in a calcitriol-treated hypoparathyroid woman during lactation. *Obstet Gynecol* 1990; **76:** 485–9.

## Interactions

There is an increased risk of hypercalcaemia if vitamin D is given with thiazide diuretics and calcium. Plasma-calcium concentrations should be monitored in such situations. Some antiepileptics may increase vitamin D requirements (e.g. carbamazepine, phenobarbital, phenytoin, and primidone). Rifampicin and isoniazid may reduce the effectiveness of vitamin D.

**Danazol.** A report of hypercalcaemia associated with danazol in a patient maintained on alfacalcidol therapy for hypoparathyroidism.[1] Introduction of danazol appeared to reduce the maintenance requirement for alfacalcidol.

1. Hepburn NC, *et al.* Danazol-induced hypercalcaemia in alphacalcidol-treated hypoparathyroidism. *Postgrad Med J* 1989; **65:** 849–50.

**Levothyroxine.** Three patients receiving dihydrotachysterol and calcium for postoperative hypoparathyroidism, following thyroidectomy, developed hypercalcaemia when their concomitant levothyroxine therapy was discontinued before a radioiodine scan.[1] The dose of dihydrotachysterol should be reduced and serum-calcium concentrations should be monitored when thyroid treatment is interrupted, since elimination of dihydrotachysterol may be delayed in hypothyroidism.

1. Lamberg B-A, Tikkanen MJ. Hypercalcaemia due to dihydrotachysterol treatment in patients with hypothyroidism after thyroidectomy. *BMJ* 1981; **283:** 461–2.

## Pharmacokinetics

Vitamin D substances are well absorbed from the gastrointestinal tract. The presence of bile is essential for adequate intestinal absorption; absorption may be decreased in patients with decreased fat absorption.

Vitamin D and its metabolites circulate in the blood bound to a specific α-globulin. Vitamin D can be stored in adipose and muscle tissue for long periods of time. It is slowly released from such storage sites and from the skin where it is formed in the presence of sunlight or ultraviolet light. Ergocalciferol and colecalciferol have a slow onset and a long duration of action; calcitriol and its analogue alfacalcidol, however, have a more rapid action and shorter half-lives.

Colecalciferol and ergocalciferol are hydroxylated in the liver by the enzyme vitamin D 25-hydroxylase to form 25-hydroxycholecalciferol (calcifediol) and 25-hydroxyergocalciferol respectively. These compounds undergo further hydroxylation in the kidneys by the enzyme vitamin D 1-hydroxylase to form the active metabolites 1,25-dihydroxycholecalciferol (calcitriol) and 1,25-dihydroxyergocalciferol respectively. Further metabolism also occurs in the kidneys, including the formation of the 1,24,25-trihydroxy derivatives. Of the synthetic analogues, alfacalcidol is converted rapidly in the liver to calcitriol, and dihydrotachysterol is hydroxylated, also in the liver, to its active form 25-hydroxydihydrotachysterol.

Vitamin D compounds and their metabolites are excreted mainly in the bile and faeces with only small amounts appearing in urine; there is some enterohepatic recycling but it is considered to have a negligible contribution to vitamin D status. Certain vitamin D substances may be distributed into breast milk.

## Human Requirements

The daily requirements of vitamin D in adults are small and may be met mainly by exposure to sunlight and/or obtained from the diet. A daily dietary intake of about 200 to 400 units (5 to 10 micrograms of colecalciferol or ergocalciferol) of vitamin D is generally considered adequate for healthy adults. In comparison with older adults (in the age range of 25 years upwards) the requirements per kg body-weight are greater in infants, children, and young adults and during pregnancy and lactation. Requirements may also be higher in people who are not exposed to adequate sunlight such as the elderly or housebound.

Vitamin D is present in few foods. Fish-liver oils, especially cod-liver oil, are good sources of vitamin D. Other sources, which contain much smaller amounts, include butter, eggs, and liver. Some foods are fortified with vitamin D, and milk and margarine may therefore also supply the vitamin. Cooking processes do not appear to affect the activity of vitamin D.

**UK and US recommended dietary intake.** In the UK dietary reference values (see p.1419) for vitamin D have only been published for selected groups of the population.[1] In the USA recommended dietary allowances had been set, and have recently been replaced by dietary reference intakes[2] (see p.1419). Differing amounts are recommended for infants and children of varying ages, for adults, and for pregnant and lactating women. In the UK a dietary intake was considered unnecessary for adults living a normal lifestyle who were being exposed to solar radiation; for those confined indoors a reference nutrient intake (RNI) of 10 micrograms (400 units) [as colecalciferol or ergocalciferol] daily was set. This RNI of 10 micrograms daily was also considered to be applicable to all persons aged 65 years or more and to pregnant and lactating women. RNIs were set for children up to the age of 3 years; dietary intake was considered unnecessary for older children. Mention was made that in order to achieve the above reference nutrient intakes, supplementation of the diet may actually be required and supplementation was also recommended for Asian [i.e. from the Indian subcontinent] women and children in the UK. In the USA,[2] adequate intakes for vitamin D are: 5 micrograms (200 units) daily (as colecalciferol) for all persons from birth through to age 50 years, including pregnant or lactating women; 10 micrograms daily for adults aged 51 to 70 years; and 15 micrograms daily for those aged greater than 70 years. The tolerable upper intake level is 50 micrograms daily.

1. DoH. Dietary reference values for food energy and nutrients for the United Kingdom: report of the panel on dietary reference values of the committee on medical aspects of food policy. *Report on health and social subjects 41*. London: HMSO, 1991.
2. Standing Committee on the Scientific Evaluation of Dietary Reference Intakes of the Food and Nutrition Board. *Dietary Reference Intakes for calcium, phosphorus, magnesium, vitamin D, and fluoride*. Washington, DC: National Academy Press, 1999. Also available at: http://www.nap.edu/catalog/5776.html (accessed 24/05/04)

## Uses and Administration

Vitamin D compounds are fat-soluble sterols, sometimes considered to be hormones or hormone precursors, which are essential for the proper regulation of calcium and phosphate homoeostasis and bone mineralisation.

Vitamin D deficiency develops when there is inadequate exposure to sunlight or a lack of the vitamin in the diet. Deficiency generally takes a long time to develop due to slow release of the vitamin from body stores. It may occur in some infants who are breast fed without supplemental vitamin D or exposure to sunlight, in the elderly whose mobility and thus exposure to light may be impaired, and in persons with fat malabsorption syndromes; certain disease states such as renal failure may also affect the metabolism of vitamin D substances to metabolically active forms and thus result in deficiency. Deficiency leads to the development of a syndrome characterised by hypocalcaemia, hypophosphataemia, undermineralisation or demineralisation of bone, bone pain, bone fractures, and muscle weakness, known in adults as osteomalacia (see below). In children, in whom there may be growth retardation and skeletal deformity, especially of the long bones, it is known as rickets.

Vitamin D compounds are used in the treatment and prevention of vitamin D deficiency states and hypocalcaemia in disorders such as hypoparathyroidism and secondary hyperparathyroidism, as indicated by the cross-references given below.

A variety of forms and analogues of vitamin D are available, and the choice of agent depends on the cause of the condition to be treated and the relative properties of the available agents. Colecalciferol and ergocalciferol are equal in potency, and have a slow onset and relatively prolonged duration of action. Dihydrotachysterol has relatively weak antirachitic activity, but its actions are faster in onset and less persistent than those of the calciferols and it does not require renal hydroxylation. Calcifediol, an intermediate metabolite, has some action of its own but is also converted to the more potent 1,25-dihydroxycholecalciferol (calcitriol); calcitriol and its analogue alfacalcidol are the most potent and rapidly acting of the vitamin D substances.

- For the treatment of simple nutritional deficiencies **colecalciferol** or **ergocalciferol** are generally preferred. They are usually given by mouth, but may also be administered by intramuscular injection. A dose of 10 micrograms (400 units) daily is generally sufficient in adults for the prevention of simple deficiency states; in the UK, 20 micrograms (800 units) daily is recommended in some ethnic groups consuming unleavened bread, and in the elderly living alone. Deficiency due to malabsorption states or liver disease often requires higher doses for treatment, of up to 1 mg (40 000 units) daily. Doses of up to 2.5 mg (100 000 units) daily may be used in the treatment of hypocalcaemia due to hypoparathyroidism.
- Where large doses are required it may be preferable to use one of the more potent derivatives. In particular, when renal function is impaired as in secondary hyperparathyroidism associated with chronic renal failure, with consequent reduction in the conversion of calciferols to their active metabolites, then a drug such as alfacalcidol, calcitriol, doxercalciferol, maxacalcitol, or paricalcitol, which does not require renal hydroxylation, should be given. **Calcitriol** is given by mouth or by intravenous injection. Usual initial adult doses of 250 nanograms daily or on alternate days are given by mouth, increased if necessary, in steps of 250 nanograms at intervals of 2 to 4 weeks, to a usual dose of 0.5 to 1 microgram daily. Initial doses intravenously are usually 500 nanograms three times a week increased if necessary in steps of 250 to 500 nanograms at intervals of 2 to 4 weeks, to a usual dose of 0.5 to 3 micrograms three times a week. For moderate to severe secondary hyperparathyroidism in dialysis patients initial doses of 0.5 to 4 micrograms have been given three times a week, increased if necessary in steps of 250 to 500 nanograms at intervals of 2 to 4 weeks to a maximum of 8 micrograms given three times a week. Alternatively, **alfacalcidol** is given in initial doses of 1 microgram daily by mouth, or 500 nanograms for elderly patients. Doses of 0.25 to 1 microgram daily may be given for maintenance. Suggested doses for children under 20 kg are 50 nanograms/kg daily and for premature infants and neonates a dose of 50 to 100 nanograms/kg daily. Doses of alfacalcidol may also be given by intravenous injection over 30 seconds. **Doxercalciferol** is given by mouth or intravenous injection. The initial oral dose is 10 micrograms three times weekly at dialysis, increased by increments of 2.5 micrograms after 8 weeks if necessary. The maximum recommended dose by mouth is 20 micrograms three times weekly. The initial intravenous dose is 4 micrograms given three times weekly, and increased after 8 weeks in increments of 1 to 2 micrograms if required.

  **Maxacalcitol** is given intravenously at a dose of 2.5 to 10 micrograms three times weekly; the dose may be gradually increased if necessary, to a maximum of 20 micrograms three times weekly. **Paricalcitol** is given intravenously at a dose of 40 to 100 nanograms/kg on alternate days or less frequently. The dose may be increased if necessary by 2 to 4 micrograms at intervals of 2 to 4 weeks.
- Of the other available forms, **calcifediol**, the 25-hydroxylated metabolite of colecalciferol, is given in usual adult doses of 50 to 100 micrograms daily or 100 to 200 micrograms on alternate days by mouth. For hypocalcaemic tetany due to hypoparathyroidism, **dihydrotachysterol** is given in initial adult doses of 250 to 2500 micrograms daily by mouth, depending on severity, for three days. Maintenance doses have ranged from 250 micrograms weekly to 1000 micrograms daily.

When vitamin D substances are given in pharmacological doses, dosage must be individualised for each patient, and should be based on regular monitoring of plasma-calcium concentrations (initially weekly, and then every 2 to 4 weeks), to optimise clinical response and avoid hypercalcaemia.

Vitamin D, usually in the form of calcitriol, may be used in the treatment of osteoporosis (see below). In established postmenopausal osteoporosis, calcitriol 0.25 micrograms twice daily is recommended. Vitamin D and calcium supplements are often given as adjuncts to other therapies in osteoporosis.

Calcitriol has been used in the management of psoriasis (see below).

Calciferol derivatives are used as a rodenticide.

◊ General references.

1. Fraser DR. Vitamin D. *Lancet* 1995; **345:** 104–7.
2. van der Wielen RPJ, *et al.* Serum vitamin D concentrations among elderly people in Europe. *Lancet* 1995; **346:** 207–10.
3. Gloth FM, *et al.* Vitamin D deficiency in homebound elderly persons. *JAMA* 1995; **274:** 1683–6.
4. Nellen JFJB, *et al.* Hypovitaminosis D in immigrant women: slow to be diagnosed. *BMJ* 1996; **312:** 570–2.
5. Thomas MK, *et al.* Hypovitaminosis D in medical inpatients. *N Engl J Med* 1998; **338:** 777–83.
6. Compston JE. Vitamin D deficiency: time for action. *BMJ* 1998; **317:** 1466–7.

**Hyperparathyroidism.** Vitamin D has been employed for certain forms of hyperparathyroidism. The secondary hyperparathyroidism of renal osteodystrophy (p.764) may respond to oral or intravenous treatment with calcitriol, or its analogue alfacalcidol,[1-3] which do not require renal hydroxylation for activation. Newer analogues for this indication include paricalcitol,[4,5] doxercalciferol,[6] falecalcitriol,[7] and maxacalcitol.[8,9] However, doses capable of suppressing parathyroid hormone secretion may lead to hypercalcaemia[3] and a decline in renal function[10] (see also under Adverse Effects, above).

1. Andress DL, *et al.* Intravenous calcitriol in the treatment of refractory osteitis fibrosa of chronic renal failure. *N Engl J Med* 1989; **321:** 274–9.
2. Argilés À, *et al.* High-dose alfacalcidol for anaemia in dialysis. *Lancet* 1993; **342:** 378–9.
3. Quarles LD, *et al.* Prospective trial of pulse oral versus intravenous calcitriol treatment of hyperparathyroidism in ESRD. *Kidney Int* 1994; **45:** 1710–21.
4. Martin KJ, *et al.* Therapy of secondary hyperparathyroidism with 19-nor-1α,25-dihydroxyvitamin $D_2$. *Am J Kidney Dis* 1998; **32** (suppl 2): S61–6.
5. Teng M, *et al.* Survival of patients undergoing hemodialysis with paricalcitol or calcitriol therapy. *N Engl J Med* 2003; **349:** 446–56.
6. Frazão JM, *et al.* Intermittent doxercalciferol (1α-hydroxyvitamin $D_2$) therapy for secondary hyperparathyroidism. *Am J Kidney Dis* 2000; **36:** 550–61.
7. Akiba T, *et al.* Controlled trial of falecalcitriol versus alfacalcidol in suppression of parathyroid hormone in hemodialysis patients with secondary hyperparathyroidism. *Am J Kidney Dis* 1998; **32:** 238–46.
8. Akizawa T, *et al.* Long-term effect of 1,25-dihydroxy-22-oxavitamin D(3) on secondary hyperparathyroidism in haemodialysis patients: one-year administration study. *Nephrol Dial Transplant* 2002; **17** (suppl 10): 28–36.
9. Yasuda M, *et al.* Multicenter clinical trial of 22-oxa-1,25-dihydroxyvitamin D3 for chronic dialysis patients. *Am J Kidney Dis* 2003; **41** (suppl 1): S108–S111.
10. Chan JCM, *et al.* A prospective, double-blind study of growth failure in children with chronic renal insufficiency and the effectiveness of treatment with calcitriol versus dihydrotachysterol. *J Pediatr* 1994; **124:** 520–8.

**Hypoparathyroidism.** Although parenteral calcium salts may be given acutely for hypocalcaemic tetany, long-term treatment of hypoparathyroidism (p.765) usually aims at correction of associated hypocalcaemia with oral vitamin D compounds, which increase the intestinal absorption of calcium. If dietary calcium is inadequate these may be combined with calcium supplementation.

Hypoparathyroidism in *pregnancy* poses severe risks of fetal hyperparathyroidism with neonatal hypocalcaemic rickets, which may be fatal. Treatment with calcium and either colecalciferol or ergocalciferol in doses of 1.25 to 2.5 mg daily, or dihydrotachysterol 0.25 to 1.0 mg daily is essential.[1] Calcitriol, in doses of between 0.25 to 3 micrograms daily, with calcium supplementation, has also been suggested; the dosage is adjusted to physiological requirements during pregnancy.[2]

1. Hague WM. Treatment of endocrine diseases. *BMJ* 1987; **294:** 297–300.
2. Callies F, *et al.* Management of hypoparathyroidism during pregnancy - report of twelve cases. *Eur J Endocrinol* 1998; **139:** 284–9.

**Malignant neoplasms.** The active form of vitamin D, calcitriol (1,25-dihydroxycholecalciferol) has been found to promote tissue differentiation and to inhibit cellular proliferation *in vitro*. These findings have prompted workers to investigate the potential role and efficacy of vitamin D metabolites or analogues (sometimes referred to as deltanoids) in malignant neoplasms and in other disorders of cell growth such as psoriasis (see below).

*Animal* and *in vitro* studies with alfacalcidol have led to the suggestion that evaluation should be undertaken in malignant disease of the human breast.[1] A study in humans has been performed with the calcitriol derivative calcipotriol (p.1144); in this trial calcipotriol used topically in advanced or cutaneous metastatic breast cancer was considered to exert some positive effects and further investigation was considered warranted.[2] Regression of T-cell lymphoma of the skin (mycosis fungoides, p.511) has been reported following application of calcipotriol,[3] and following systemic treatment with calcitriol and a retinoid in a patient who failed to respond to topical calcipotriol.[4] However, 3 other patients with cutaneous T-cell lymphoma failed to respond to calcitriol and isotretinoin,[5] which may have been because of the phenotype or stage of the disease.[6]

1. Colston KW, *et al.* Possible role for vitamin D in controlling breast cancer cell proliferation. *Lancet* 1989; **i:** 188–91.
2. Bower M, *et al.* Topical calcipotriol treatment in advanced breast cancer. *Lancet* 1991; **337:** 701–2. Correction. *ibid.*; 1618.
3. Scott-Mackie P, *et al.* Calcipotriol and regression in T-cell lymphoma of skin. *Lancet* 1993; **342:** 172.
4. French LE, *et al.* Remission of cutaneous T-cell lymphoma with combined calcitriol and acitretin. *Lancet* 1994; **344:** 686–7.
5. Thomsen K. Cutaneous T-cell lymphoma and calcitriol and isotretinoin treatment. *Lancet* 1995; **345:** 1583.
6. French LE, Saurat J-H. Treatment of cutaneous T-cell lymphoma by retinoids and calcitriol. *Lancet* 1995; **346:** 376–7.

**Osteomalacia.** Treatment of osteomalacia (p.762) primarily aims at correcting any underlying deficiency states, and vitamin D substances, calcium, or phosphate supplements may be given by mouth as necessary. Where rickets is due to impaired synthesis of calcitriol (type I pseudodeficiency) or receptor resistance (type II pseudodeficiency) replacement therapy with calcitriol may be indicated (in the latter case with very high dose calcium),[1] while X-linked hypophosphataemic rickets is generally treated with phosphate supplementation and calcitriol, although vitamin D alone is also effective.[2] The use of single large doses of a vitamin D substance (stosstherapie), for the prophylaxis of rickets, is highly controversial because of problems with toxicity, although it may be effective in patients with rickets due to proven vitamin D deficiency.[3] Factors contributing to reported resurgences in rickets[4-6] include increased breast feeding without sufficient vitamin D supplementation, and less exposure to sunlight. In the UK, renewed public health campaigns have been called for, along with supplementation of infants from high-risk groups with 400 units of vitamin D daily,[5] while in the USA, the American Academy of Pediatrics has recommended that all infants have a minimum intake of 200 units daily.[7] Others have commented that even 200 units daily may not be enough as a preventive measure,[8] and that, in those children with good exposure to sunlight, calcium supplementation may also be necessary.[9]


1. Hochberg Z, *et al.* Calcium therapy for calcitriol-resistant rickets. *J Pediatr* 1992; **121:** 803–8.
2. Seikaly MG, *et al.* The effect of phosphate supplementation on linear growth in children with X-linked hypophosphatemia. *Pediatrics* 1994; **94:** 478–81.
3. Shah BR, Finberg L. Single-day therapy for nutritional vitamin D-deficiency rickets: a preferred method. *J Pediatr* 1994; **125:** 487–90.
4. Kreiter SR, *et al.* Nutritional rickets in African American breast-fed infants. *J Pediatr* 2000; **137:** 153–7.
5. Shaw NJ, Pal BR. Vitamin D deficiency in UK Asian families: activating a new concern. *Arch Dis Child* 2002; **86:** 147–9.
6. Welch TR, *et al.* Vitamin D-deficient rickets: the reemergence of a once-conquered disease. *J Pediatr* 2000; **137:** 143–5.
7. Gartner LM, *et al.* Prevention of rickets and vitamin D deficiency: new guidelines for vitamin D intake. *Pediatrics* 2003; **111:** 908–10.
8. Greer FR. Vitamin D deficiency—it's more than rickets. *J Pediatr* 2003; **143:** 422–3.
9. Bishop N. Rickets today—children still need milk and sunshine. *N Engl J Med* 1999; **341:** 602–4.


PREGNANCY AND THE NEONATE. It has been supposed that most infants receive adequate calcium and vitamin D during pregnancy and during breast feeding or bottle feeding to prevent the development of rickets. However, this has been disputed,[1] and it is accepted that there are certain groups of women whose infants may be at special risk of neonatal rickets; these include those suffering economic deprivation, those living at high latitudes, and Asian immigrants [i.e. from the Indian subcontinent] in northern Europe, especially in winter. It is therefore suggested that pregnant women in such circumstances should receive supplements as the diet and sunshine exposure may not be providing adequate calcium (1 to 1.2 g daily) or vitamin D (400 units daily).[2] Alternatively, 1000 units vitamin D daily during the third trimester, or a single dose of 100 000 to 200 000 units of ergocalciferol during the sixth or seventh month, has been proposed.[3] Furthermore, routine vitamin D supplementation of infants in high-risk groups has been recommended (see Osteomalacia, above).


1. Welch TR, *et al.* Vitamin D-deficient rickets: the reemergence of a once-conquered disease. *J Pediatr* 2000; **137:** 143–5.
2. Misra R, Anderson DC. Providing the fetus with calcium. *BMJ* 1990; **300:** 1220–1.
3. Shaw NJ, Pal BR. Vitamin D deficiency in UK Asian families: activating a new concern. *Arch Dis Child* 2002; **86:** 147–9.


**Osteopetrosis.** For mention of the use of high-dose calcitriol in the management of osteopetrosis, see under Corticosteroids, p.1085.

**Osteoporosis.** Studies using vitamin D in pharmacological[1-3] or supplemental[4-6] doses for the treatment of osteoporosis (p.763) have produced conflicting results.[1-7] However, in patients over 75 years of age, in whom dietary deficiencies are common, calcium and vitamin D supplements are recommended. Supplementation is also recommended in elderly institutionalised patients.[8]

Vitamin D may be used in the prevention of corticosteroid-induced osteoporosis (see Effects on Bones and Joints, p.1069).


1. Ott SM, Chesnut CH. Calcitriol treatment is not effective in postmenopausal osteoporosis. *Ann Intern Med* 1989; **110:** 267–74.
2. Gallagher JC, Goldgar D. Treatment of postmenopausal osteoporosis with high doses of synthetic calcitriol: a randomized controlled study. *Ann Intern Med* 1990; **113:** 649–55.
3. Tilyard MW, *et al.* Treatment of postmenopausal osteoporosis with calcitriol or calcium. *N Engl J Med* 1992; **326:** 357–62.
4. Chapuy MC, *et al.* Effect of calcium and cholecalciferol treatment for three years on hip fractures in elderly women. *BMJ* 1994; **308:** 1081–2.
5. Lips P, *et al.* Vitamin D supplementation and fracture incidence in elderly persons. *Ann Intern Med* 1996; **124:** 400–6.
6. Dawson-Hughes B, *et al.* Effect of calcium and vitamin D supplementation on bone density in men and women 65 years of age or older. *N Engl J Med* 1997; **337:** 670–6.
7. Gillespie WJ, *et al.* Vitamin D and vitamin D analogues for preventing fractures associated with involutional and post-menopausal osteoporosis. Available in The Cochrane Library; Issue 2. Chichester: John Wiley; 2004.
8. Anonymous. Lifestyle advice for fracture prevention. *Drug Ther Bull* 2002; **40:** 83–6.


**Psoriasis.** A vitamin D analogue, calcipotriol (p.1144), is often used as an alternative to more traditional topical drugs in the initial management of mild to moderate psoriasis (p.1137). Another vitamin D analogue, tacalcitol (p.1158), is used similarly, and maxacalcitol[1] and falecalcitriol[2] have been investigated. Calcitriol itself has been tried, both topically[3-5] and orally.[6]


1. Barker JNWN, *et al.* Topical maxacalcitol for the treatment of psoriasis vulgaris: a placebo-controlled, double-blind, dose-finding study with active comparator. *Br J Dermatol* 1999; **141:** 274–8.
2. Durakovic C, *et al.* Rationale for use and clinical responsiveness of hexafluoro-1,25-dihydroxyvitamin $D_3$ for the treatment of plaque psoriasis: a pilot study. *Br J Dermatol* 2001; **144:** 500–506.
3. Sips AJAM, *et al.* Topically applied low-dose calcitriol has no calciotropic effect in patients with stable plaque psoriasis. *J Am Acad Dermatol* 1994; **30:** 966–9.
4. Langner A, *et al.* A long-term multicentre assessment of the safety and tolerability of calcitriol ointment in the treatment of chronic plaque psoriasis. *Br J Dermatol* 1996; **135:** 385–9.
5. Ring J, *et al.* Calcitriol 3 μg $g^{-1}$ ointment in combination with ultraviolet B phototherapy for the treatment of plaque psoriasis: results of a comparative study. *Br J Dermatol* 2001; **144:** 495–9.
6. Perez A, *et al.* Safety and efficacy of oral calcitriol (1,25-dihydroxyvitamin $D_3$) for the treatment of psoriasis. *Br J Dermatol* 1996; **134:** 1070–8.


**Renal osteodystrophy.** See under Hyperparathyroidism, above.

**Rickets.** See Osteomalacia, above.

## Preparations

***BP 2003:*** Calcitriol Capsules; Calcium and Colecalciferol Tablets; Calcium and Ergocalciferol Tablets; Colecalciferol Injection; Colecalciferol Tablets; Ergocalciferol Injection; Ergocalciferol Tablets; Paediatric Vitamins A, C and D Oral Drops;
***BPC 1973:*** Calcium with Vitamin D Tablets; Vitamins A and D Capsules;
***USP 27:*** Calcifediol Capsules; Calcium with Vitamin D Tablets; Dihydrotachysterol Capsules; Dihydrotachysterol Oral Solution; Dihydrotachysterol Tablets; Ergocalciferol Capsules; Ergocalciferol Oral Solution; Ergocalciferol Tablets; Oleovitamin A and D; Oleovitamin A and D Capsules; Paricalcitol Injection.

**Proprietary Preparations** (details are given in Part 3)
***Arg.:*** Alfa Calcimax; Alpha D3; Dexiven; Ostelin; Raquiferol; Rexamat; Silcor; ***Austral.:*** AT 10†; Calcijex; Citrihexal; Kosteo; Ostelin; Rocaltrol; Sitriol; ***Austria:*** AT 10; Bocatriol; Calcijex; Etalpha; Laevovit $D_3$; Oleovit $D_3$; Rocaltrol; Silkis; Vi-$De_3$; ***Belg.:*** 1-Alpha; AT 10; D-Cure†; Dedrogyl; Dihydral†; Rocaltrol; Silkis; ***Braz.:*** Alfad; Calcijex; Rocaltrol; Sigmatriol†; Silkis; ***Canad.:*** Calcijex†; D-Tabs†; D-Vi-Sol; Drisdol; Hectorol; Hytakerol; One-Alpha; Ostoforte; Rocaltrol; ***Chile:*** Acuode; Alfa D; Etalpha; Genevis; Genevis D2; Rocaltrol; ***Denm.:*** Dygratyl; Etalpha; Rocaltrol; ***Fin.:*** Calcijex; Deetipat; Devitol; Dygratyl; Etalpha; Jekovit; Silkis; ***Fr.:*** Adrigyl; Dedrogyl; Rocaltrol; Silkis; Sterogyl; Un-Alfa; Uvedose; Uvesterol D; Zyma-D2; ***Ger.:*** AT 10; Bocatriol; Bondiol; D-Mulsin†; D-Tracetten†; $D_3$ Vicotrat; Decostriol; Dedrei; Dedrogyl; Dekristol; Doss; EinsAlpha; Ospur $D_3$; Osteotriol; Rocaltrol; Silkis; Tachystin; Vigantol; Vigantoletten; Vigorsan†; ***Gr.:*** Abbocalcijex; Alpha D3; Dedrogyl; One-Alpha; Ostelin; Sterogyl; ***Hong Kong:*** Alfarol†; Alpha D3; Calcijex; One-Alpha; Rocaltrol; ***India:*** Alpha D3; Arachitol; Calcirol; Rolsical; ***Irl.:*** Calcijex; One-Alpha; Rocaltrol; ***Israel:*** Alpha D3; Calcijex; One-Alpha; Osteo D†; ***Ital.:*** Alpha D3; Atiten; Calcijex; Dediol; Deril; Didrogyl; Difix; Diseon; Diserinal; Geniad; Ostelin; Ostidil-D3; Rocaltrol; Sefal; Tridelta; ***Jpn:*** Alfarol; Onealfa; Oxarol; Rocaltrol; ***Malaysia:*** Fairy ADE; One-Alpha; ***Mex.:*** Alfad; Calcijex†; Doferol†; Genevis D2†; Lemytriol; Rocaltrol; Tirocal; Vita-D-Grin†; ***Neth.:*** Devaron; Dihydral; Etalpha; Neo Dohyfral†; Rocaltrol; Silkis; ***Norw.:*** AFI-$D_2$; Calcijex; Etalpha; Rocaltrol; ***NZ:*** One-Alpha; Rocaltrol; ***Port.:*** Dedrogyl; Etalpha; Rocaltrol; Vigantol; ***S.Afr.:*** One-Alpha; Rocaltrol; ***Singapore:*** Alpha D3; Bon-One; Bongreen; Calcijex; One-Alpha; Rocaltrol; Roical; ***Spain:*** Alfadelta†; Calcijex; Etalpha; Hidroferol; Rocaltrol; ***Swed.:*** Calcijex; Detrixin†; Devitre; Dygratyl; Etalpha; Rocaltrol; ***Switz.:*** AT 10; Bocatriol; Calcijex; Rocaltrol; Silkis; Vi-$De_3$; ***Thai.:*** Alpha D3; Bon-One; One-Alpha; Rocaltrol; ***UK:*** AlfaD†; AT 10; Calcijex; One-Alpha; Rocaltrol; Silkis; ***USA:*** Calciferol; Calcijex; Calderol; Delta-D; DHT; Drisdol; Hectorol; Hytakerol; Rocaltrol; Zemplar.

**Multi-ingredient: *Arg.:*** A-D-C; AD Shock; Adermicina; Anartrit; Atomoderma A-D; Calcimax D3; Calcio Cit; Calcio Masticable; Calcium D; Caltrate + D; Cavirox; Citramar D; Dr Selby; Ostram D3; Regucal D; Sinamida Cicatrizante; Taxus; Vitapelen; ***Austral.:*** Bio Magnesium†; Caltrate + Vitamin D; Caltrate Plus; Children's Calcium With Minerals†; FAB Tri-Cal†; Lifesystem Mineral Plus Formula 10 Osteoporosis†; Natures Way Total Calcium Plus†; Osteoporosis Mineral Plus Formula 9†; Prosteo†; Red Seal Liquid Calcium†; Soy Forte with Block Cohosh†; ***Austria:*** Cacit mit Vitamin $D_3$; Cal-D-or; Cal-D-Vita; Cal-De; Calcipot $D_3$; Calcisan D; Calcium-D-Sandoz; Maxi-Kalz Vit D3; Oleovit A + D; Osteocur; Ostram-Vit $D_3$; Ruticalzon; ***Belg.:*** AD-Vitan†; Cacit Vitamine $D_3$; D-Vital; Neo-Debiol AD3†; Newderm; Pyal†; Sandoz Ca-D; Steovit D3; Topcal D3; Vitaminic A-D†; Vitamorrhuine†; ***Braz.:*** AD-Furp†; AD-Til; ADE 2 (Adedois); Adeforte; Aderofix D3†; Aderogil D3; Belglos†; Calcio Day D†; Caltrate + D; Caltrate + M; Dermalisan; Gaduol; Gotil-AD†; Hipoderme; Hipodermon; Hipodex; Hipoglos; Hipoglos Oftalmico†; Hormoginase†; Miocalven D; Natecal D; Natural Wealth Beta†; Normagrin†; Os-Cal + D; Ossocal-D; Solemil†; Vitadesan; ***Canad.:*** A & D; A & D Ointment; Antiseptic Skin Cream; Cal D; Calburst; Calcite D; Calcium D; Calcium Magnesium Plus; Caltrate + Iron & Vitamin D†; Caltrate Plus; Caltrate with D; Mega Cal Calcium; Neo Cal D; Nutrol A D; Os-Cal D; Prevencal & D & Fer†; Prevencal & D & Magnesium†; Prevencal & D†; Viactiv; ***Chile:*** Aplical-D; Brexon; Cadevit; Calcefor D; Calcigran; Calcio Day D; Calcio Nil Forte; Calciovit Puro; Calcium Forte D; Calcium-Sandoz Forte D; Calcivorin D; Caldar-D; Caldeval; Caprimida D; Dermaglos; Dermaglos Plus; Dical-D; Elcal-D; Levucal D; Natecal D; Ostram D3; Pediaderm; Platsul A; Pomada Vitaminica; Povin; Sanoderm; ***Denm.:*** Calcichew $D_3$; CaviD; Ideos; ***Fin.:*** Calcichew $D_3$; D-Calsor; Ideos; Kalcipos-D; Ostram-Vit $D_3$; ***Fr.:*** Auxergyl $D_3$†; Cacit Vitamine $D_3$; Calcidose Vitamine D; Calciprat $D_3$; Calcos Vitamine $D_3$; Calperos $D_3$; Caltrate Vitamine $D_3$; Densical vitamine $D_3$; Fixical Vitamine $D_3$; Frubiose Vitamine D; Ideos; Metocalcium; Osseans D3; Osteocal D3; Ostram Vitamine $D_3$; Zymaduo; ***Ger.:*** A + D + E-Vicotrat†; A + $D_3$-Vicotrat†; Calcigen D; Calcilac KT; Calcimagon-D3; Calcimed $D_3$; Calcium $D_3$; Calcium Verla D; Calcium-D-Sandoz; Calcium-dura Vit $D_3$; Calcivit D; calcivitase; D-Fluoretten; Fluor-Vigantoletten; Frubiase Calcium forte 500; Ideos; Ossofortin; Ossofortin forte; Osspulvit S; Sandocal-D; Strafortin; Zymafluor D; ***Gr.:*** Calcioral D3; ***Hong Kong:*** Bone Plus†; Calcichew $D_3$; Calcioday-D; Calperos $D_3$; Caltrate + D; Caltrate Plus; Citracal + D; Mega-Cal with Vit D; Os-Cal + D; Osteocare; Tri-Cal†; ***India:*** Anemidox; Cal-Aid; Calcinol; Incad; Kalzana; Kemicetine Antiozena; Logical; Macalvit; Omilcal; Ossivite; Ostocalcium; Ostocalcium B-12; Sharkomalt; Sharkovit; Styptocid; Trical-D; ***Irl.:*** Bio-Calcium + $D_3$; Bio-Calcium + $D_3$ + K; Calcichew $D_3$; Calvidin; Chocovite; Decal; Ideos; Osteofos D3; ***Israel:*** Aquitol; Caltrate + Vit D; Caltrate Plus; Oleovit A + $D_3$; Vitamidyne A and D; ***Ital.:*** AD Pabyrn; Adiboran AD†; Adisterolo; Cacit Vitamina D3; Calcidon; Calciovit Urto†; Calciozim; Calcium-D3-Sandoz; Calisvit; CalplusD3; Caltrate; Dicalcium; Effercal D3; Eurocal D3; Fitogen; Foscald3; Fosforil Calcium†; Fruttocal†; Granoleina; Ideos; Kalaz D3; Metocal Vitamina D; Natecal; Orotre; Osteofos D3; Ostram $D_3$; ***Malaysia:*** Adult Citrex Cal-Mag-D3; Calcioday-D; Caltrate + D; Citracal + D; Dumocalcin; Junior Citrex Cal-Mag-D3; Os-Cal + D; ***Mex.:*** Adekon; Adekon C; Adeloren; Adibal; Caltrate + D; Caltrec; Dical; Posture D; Sutin; Vitalorange; ***Mon.:*** Orocal $D_3$; ***Neth.:*** CaD; Davitamon AD Fluor†; Davitamon AD†; Dohyfral Vitamine AD3†; Halitran; Zwitsavit-D†; ***Norw.:*** Calcigran; Ideos; ***NZ:*** Oscal D†; ***Port.:*** Calcigenol; Calcitab D; Calcium 600; Calcium-D-Sandoz; Caltrate Plus; Caltrate Plus Mastigavel; Decalcit; Densical D; Frucalde†; Ideos; Zelderme†; ***S.Afr.:*** Vandol; ***Singapore:*** Cal-D3; Calcioday-D; Caltrate + Vit D; Caltrate Plus; Cavit-D3; Dumocalcin; Os-Cal + D; Procal-D†; ***Spain:*** Adiod; Biominol A D; Calcio 20 Complex; Calcio 20 Fuerte; Calcio Geve D y C†; Calcio Vitam D3†; Calcium-Sandoz Forte D; Caosina D; Carbocal D; Cicatral; Cimascal D; Creacal; Disnal; Duplicalcio†; Grietalgen; Grietalgen Hidrocort; Ideos; Mencalisvit; Mitosyl; Natecal D; Osteomerck; Ostine; Osvical D; Osvical†; Queratil†; Redoxon Calciovit; Veriscal D; ***Swed.:*** AD-vitamin; Cal-D-Vita; Calcichew $D_3$; Ideos; Kalcipos-D; Ostram-Vit $D_3$†; ***Switz.:*** Cal-De; Calcimagon-D3; Calciplus†; Calcium D Sauter; Calcivit; Calperos $D_3$; Decalcit; Frubiose Calcium†; Linola gras; Malvedrin; Riccomycine†; Riccovitan; ***Thai.:*** Cal-D-Vita; Calcioday-D; Caltrate + D; Caltrate Plus; Combi-Cal; Effcal; Ostone-B12; Prima-Cal Plus Vit D; ***UK:*** Adcal-$D_3$; Cacit D3; Calceos; Calcichew $D_3$; Calcium and Ergocalciferol Tablets; Calfovit D3; Caltrate Plus; Caltrate†; Chocovite†; Crampex; Folic Plus†; Haliborange Calcium Plus Vitamin D; Osteocare; Porosis D†; S.P.H.P.; ***USA:*** A and D Medicated; Calcarb with Vitamin D; Calcet; Calcium 600; Calel-D; Caltrate + Iron & Vitamin D; Caltrate + Vitamin D; Caltrate Plus; Citracal + D; Citracal Plus with Magnesium; Clocream; Desert Pure Calcium; Diaper Guard; FemCal†; Lobana Derm-Aide; Lobana Peri-Garde; Os-Cal + D; Oyster Calcium with Vitamin D; Posture-D.

---

# Vitamin E Substances

Vitaminas E.

NOTE. The food additive number E306 is used for tocopherols.

Vitamin E is a generic term applied to a large number of natural or synthetic compounds. The most important substances are the **tocopherols** of which **alpha tocopherols** are the most active and widely distributed in nature; other naturally occurring tocopherols include beta, gamma, and delta tocopherols, but these are not used in therapeutics. The other group of compounds with vitamin E activity are the tocotrienols.

Alpha tocopherols occur naturally in the *d* optical isomer form, which is more active than the synthetic racemic *dl* form; for further details concerning the comparative activities of the different forms and isomers of vitamin E compounds, see under Units, below.

## d-Alpha Tocopherol

Natural Alpha Tocopherol; Natural α-Tocopherol; *d*-α-tocoferol; *RRR*-α-Tocopherol; *d*-α-Tocopherol; *RRR*-α-Tocopherolum. (+)-2,5,7,8-Tetramethyl-2-(4,8,12-trimethyltridecyl)chroman-6-ol.

$C_{29}H_{50}O_2$ = 430.7.
*CAS — 59-02-9.*

**Pharmacopoeias.** In *Eur.* (see p.vi). *US* allows it under the title Vitamin E.

**Ph. Eur. 5.0** (*RRR*-α-Tocopherol; *RRR*-Alpha-Tocopherol BP 2003). A clear, colourless, or yellowish-brown viscous oily liquid. Practically insoluble in water; freely soluble in dehydrated alcohol, in acetone, in dichloromethane, and in fatty oils. Store under an inert gas in airtight containers. Protect from light.

**USP 27** (Vitamin E). A clear, yellow, or greenish-yellow, practically odourless, viscous oil. It is unstable to air and light, particularly in alkaline media. Insoluble in water; soluble in alcohol; miscible with acetone, with chloroform, with ether, and with vegetable oils. Store under an inert gas in airtight containers. Protect from light.

## dl-Alpha Tocopherol

all-*rac*-α-Tocopherol; Alpha Tocopherol; E307; int-*rac*-α-Tocopherolum; Synthetic Alpha Tocopherol; Synthetic α-Tocopherol; *dl*-α-Tocoferol; α-Tocopherol; *dl*-α-Tocopherol; α-Tocopherolum. (±)-2,5,7,8-Tetramethyl-2-(4,8,12-trimethyltridecyl)chroman-6-ol.

$C_{29}H_{50}O_2$ = 430.7.
*CAS — 10191-41-0.*

**Pharmacopoeias.** In *Eur.* (see p.vi) and *Jpn*. *US* allows it under the title Vitamin E.

**Ph. Eur. 5.0** (all-*rac*-α-Tocopherol; Alpha Tocopherol BP 2003). A clear, colourless or yellowish-brown viscous oily liquid. Practically insoluble in water; freely soluble in dehydrated alcohol, in acetone, in dichloromethane, and in fatty oils. Store under an inert gas. Protect from light.

**USP 27** (Vitamin E). A clear, yellow, or greenish-yellow, practically odourless, viscous oil. It is unstable to air and light, particularly in alkaline media. Insoluble in water; soluble in alcohol; miscible with acetone, with chloroform, with ether, and with vegetable oils. Store under an inert gas in airtight containers. Protect from light.

### *d*-Alpha Tocoferil Acetate

*d*-Alpha Tocopheryl Acetate; *d*-α-tocoferilo, acetato de; *RRR*-α-Tocopheroli Acetas; *RRR*-α-Tocopheryl Acetate; *d*-α-Tocopheryl Acetate. (+)-α-Tocopherol acetate.

$C_{31}H_{52}O_3$ = 472.7.

*CAS — 58-95-7.*

**Pharmacopoeias.** In *Eur.* (see p.vi). *US* allows it under the title Vitamin E.

**Ph. Eur. 5.0** (*RRR*-α-Tocopheryl Acetate; *RRR*-Alpha-Tocopheryl Acetate BP 2003). A clear, pale greenish-yellow, viscous oily liquid. Practically insoluble in water; soluble in alcohol; freely soluble in dehydrated alcohol, in acetone, and in fatty oils. Protect from light.

**USP 27** (Vitamin E). A clear, yellow, or greenish-yellow, practically odourless, viscous oil. It may solidify in the cold. It is stable to air and light, but unstable to alkali. Insoluble in water; soluble in alcohol; miscible with acetone, with chloroform, with ether, and with vegetable oils. Store in airtight containers. Protect from light.

### *dl*-Alpha Tocoferil Acetate

all-*rac*-α-Tocopheryl Acetate; Alpha Tocopheryl Acetate; *dl*-Alpha Tocopheryl Acetate; int-*rac*-α-Tocopherylis Acetas; *dl*-α-tocoferilo, acetato de; α-Tocopherol Acetate; α-Tocopheroli Acetas; *dl*-α-Tocopheryl Acetate. (±)-α-Tocopherol acetate.

$C_{31}H_{52}O_3$ = 472.7.

*CAS — 7695-91-2.*

**Pharmacopoeias.** In *Chin., Eur.* (see p.vi), *Jpn*, and *Pol. US* allows it under the title Vitamin E.

*Eur.* also has a monograph for the concentrated powdered form.

**Ph. Eur. 5.0** (all-*rac*-α-Tocopheryl Acetate; Alpha Tocopheryl Acetate BP 2003). A clear, colourless or slightly greenish-yellow, viscous, oily liquid. Practically insoluble in water; freely soluble in dehydrated alcohol, in acetone, and in fatty oils. Protect from light.

**Ph. Eur. 5.0** (α-Tocopherol Acetate Concentrate (Powder Form); α-Tocopheroli Acetatis Pulvis; Alpha Tocopheryl Acetate Concentrate (Powder Form) BP 2003). It prepared either by finely dispersing *dl*-alpha tocoferil acetate in a suitable carrier (e.g. gelatin, acacia, carbohydrates, lactoproteins, or a mixture of these) or by adsorbing *dl*-alpha tocoferil acetate on to silicic acid. The concentrate contains not less than 25% of *dl*-alpha tocoferil acetate. Almost white, yellowish, or light-brown small particles. Depending on the formulation, the powder may be practically insoluble in water or may swell or form a dispersion. Store in well-filled airtight containers. Protect from light.

**USP 27** (Vitamin E). A clear, yellow, or greenish-yellow, practically odourless, viscous oil. It is stable to air and light, but unstable to alkali. Insoluble in water; soluble in alcohol; miscible with acetone, with chloroform, with ether, and with vegetable oils. Store in airtight containers. Protect from light.

### *d*-Alpha Tocoferil Acid Succinate

*d*-Alpha Tocopheryl Acid Succinate; *d*-α-tocoferilo, succinato ácido; *RRR*-α-Tocopheroli Hydrogenosuccinas; *d*-α-Tocopheryl Acid Succinate; *RRR*-α-Tocopheryl Hydrogen Succinate. (+)-α-Tocopherol hydrogen succinate.

$C_{33}H_{54}O_5$ = 530.8.

*CAS — 4345-03-3.*

**Pharmacopoeias.** In *Eur.* (see p.vi). *US* allows it under the title Vitamin E. *USNF* also includes Vitamin E Polyethylene Glycol Succinate, a mixture formed by the esterification of *d*-alpha tocoferil acid succinate with a macrogol.

**Ph. Eur. 5.0** (*RRR*-α-Tocopheryl Hydrogen Succinate; *RRR*-Alpha Tocopheryl Hydrogen Succinate BP 2003). A white or almost white crystalline powder. Practically insoluble in water; soluble in dehydrated alcohol and in acetone; very soluble in dichloromethane. Protect from light.

**USP 27** (Vitamin E). A white, practically odourless, powder. M.p. about 75°; it is unstable when held molten. It is stable to air and light, but unstable to alkali. Insoluble in water; soluble in alcohol, in acetone, in ether, and in vegetable oils; very soluble in chloroform; slightly soluble in alkaline solution. Store in airtight containers. Protect from light.

### *dl*-Alpha Tocoferil Acid Succinate

*dl*-Alpha Tocopheryl Acid Succinate; Alpha Tocopheryl Hydrogen Succinate; *dl*-α-tocoferilo, succinato ácido; DL-α-Tocopheroli Hydrogenosuccinas; *dl*-α-Tocopheryl Acid Succinate; DL-α-Tocopheryl Hydrogen Succinate. (±)-α-Tocopherol hydrogen succinate.

$C_{33}H_{54}O_5$ = 530.8.

*CAS — 17407-37-3.*

**Pharmacopoeias.** In *Eur.* (see p.vi). *US* allows it under the title Vitamin E.

**Ph. Eur. 5.0** (DL-α-Tocopheryl Hydrogen Succinate; Alpha Tocopheryl Hydrogen Succinate BP 2003). A white or almost white, crystalline powder. Practically insoluble in water; soluble in dehydrated alcohol and in acetone; very soluble in dichloromethane. Protect from light.

**USP 27** (Vitamin E). A white, practically odourless, powder. M.p. about 70°; it is unstable when held molten. It is stable to air and light, but unstable to alkali. Insoluble in water; soluble in alcohol, in acetone, in ether, and in vegetable oils; very soluble in chloroform; slightly soluble in alkaline solution. Store in airtight containers. Protect from light.

## Units

Though the potency of preparations of vitamin E is still sometimes expressed in units, the International Standard for vitamin E was discontinued in 1956. The International Unit was the activity contained in 1 mg of a standard preparation of α-tocoferil acetate. Past editions of the USP have stated that in expressing vitamin E activity of tocopherol products, the following equivalents of 1 mg were to be used:

- *dl*-alpha tocoferil acetate, 1 unit
- *dl*-alpha tocoferil acid succinate, 0.89 unit
- *dl*-alpha tocopherol, 1.1 units
- *d*-alpha tocoferil acetate, 1.36 units
- *d*-alpha tocopherol, 1.49 units
- *d*-alpha tocoferil acid succinate, 1.21 units.

For dietary purposes, vitamin-E activity may now be expressed in terms of alpha tocopherol equivalents (α-TEs). One α-TE is the activity contained in 1 mg of *d*-alpha tocopherol (natural alpha tocopherol; *RRR*-α-tocopherol), 1.4 mg *dl*-alpha tocopherol, 1.1 mg *d*-alpha tocoferil acetate, 1.5 mg *dl*-alpha tocoferil acetate, 1.2 mg *d*-alpha tocoferil acid succinate, or 1.7 mg *dl*-alpha tocoferil acid succinate.

## Adverse Effects and Precautions

Vitamin E is usually well tolerated. Large doses may cause diarrhoea, abdominal pain, and other gastrointestinal disturbances, and have also been reported to cause blurred vision, dizziness, fatigue and weakness. Contact dermatitis has occurred following topical application.

Large doses of vitamin E have been reported to increase bleeding tendency in vitamin-K deficient patients such as those taking oral anticoagulants. However, it has also been suggested that it may increase the risk of thrombosis in some patients, such as those taking oestrogens. The clinical significance of these effects is not known.

A higher incidence of necrotising enterocolitis has been noted in premature infants weighing less than 1.5 kg treated with vitamin E.

◊ For a review and discussion of liver and kidney toxicity in premature neonates associated with an intravenous preparation of vitamin E (E-Ferol) and attributed to the inclusion of polysorbates, see p.1415.

## Interactions

Various drugs may interfere with the absorption of vitamin E including colestyramine, colestipol, and orlistat. High doses of vitamin E may increase the effects of oral anticoagulants.

## Pharmacokinetics

Absorption of vitamin E from the gastrointestinal tract is dependent on the presence of bile and on normal pancreatic function. The amount of vitamin E absorbed varies widely between about 20% and 80% and appears to decrease as the dose is increased. It enters the blood via the chylomicrons in the lymph and is bound to beta lipoproteins. It is widely distributed to all tissues, and stored in adipose tissue. Some vitamin E is metabolised in the liver to glucuronides of tocopheronic acid and its γ-lactone. Some is excreted in the urine, but most of a dose is slowly excreted in the bile. Vitamin E appears in breast milk but is poorly transferred across the placenta.

## Human Requirements

The daily requirement of vitamin E has not been clearly defined but is probably about 3 to 12 mg of *d*-alpha tocopherol or the equivalent of other vitamin E substances. Requirements increase with increased dietary amounts of polyunsaturated fatty acids. There appears to be no evidence that supplements are required in subjects on balanced diets.

Vitamin E is widely distributed in food. The richest sources are vegetable oils especially wheat-germ oil, sunflower oil, and cottonseed oil; cereals and eggs are also good sources. It does not appear to be destroyed by cooking processes.

**UK and US recommended dietary intake.** In the UK neither a reference nutrient intake (RNI—see p.1419) nor an estimated average requirement (EAR) has been set for vitamin E although daily intakes of 4 mg and 3 mg α-tocopherol equivalents (see under Units, above) were considered adequate for men and women, respectively.[1]

In the USA the recommended dietary allowance for adults is 15 mg daily of alpha tocopherol, and the tolerable upper intake level is 1000 mg daily.[2]

1. DoH. Dietary reference values for food energy and nutrients for the United Kingdom: report of the panel on dietary reference values of the committee on medical aspects of food policy. *Report on health and social subjects 41*. London: HMSO, 1991.
2. Standing Committee on the Scientific Evaluation of Dietary Reference Intakes of the Food and Nutrition Board. *Dietary Reference Intakes for vitamin C, vitamin E, selenium, and carotenoids*. Washington DC: National Academy Press, 2000. Also available at: http://www.nap.edu/catalog/9810.html (accessed 24/05/04)

## Uses and Administration

Vitamin E, a fat-soluble vitamin, prevents the oxidation of polyunsaturated fatty acids. It reacts with free radicals, which are the cause of oxidative damage to cell membranes, without the formation of another free radical in the process.

Vitamin E deficiency is rare but develops when the dietary intake is inadequate. In children with cystic fibrosis or biliary atresia, malabsorption of fat may lead to a vitamin E deficiency; deficiency may also occur in children with abnormalities of lipid transport, as in abetalipoproteinaemia. Low vitamin E concentrations are also found in premature, very low birth-weight infants. In previously healthy adults malabsorption and low intake of vitamin E must continue for a number of years before signs of deficiency appear. The major signs of vitamin E deficiency are the development of myopathic and neurological disorders.

Vitamin E is used in the treatment and prevention of vitamin E deficiency. It is usually given by mouth, generally the preferred route, but may also be given by intramuscular or intravenous routes. It may be given as *d*- or *dl*-alpha tocopherol or as the respective acetates or acid succinates.

Recommended doses vary, in part because of differences in the activity of different preparations; however, a daily dose of several times the recommended dietary allowance (RDA), or around 40 to 50 mg of *d*-alpha tocopherol, has been suggested for deficiency syndromes; somewhat higher daily doses have been given in cystic fibrosis (100 to 200 mg of *dl*-alpha tocoferil acetate, or about 67 to 135 mg of *d*-alpha tocopherol) and much higher daily doses in abetalipoproteinaemia (50 to 100 mg/kg of *dl*-alpha tocoferil acetate, or about 33 to 67 mg/kg *d*-alpha tocopherol).

Vitamin E has also been tried in retinopathy of prematurity and intraventricular haemorrhage in neonates (see Perinatal Disorders, below), and in a wide variety of other disorders, for which the evidence of value is generally lacking (see Prophylaxis of Ischaemic Heart Disease, p.1420, and Prophylaxis of Malignant Neoplasms, p.1420).

Other substances with vitamin-E activity which have been used include *dl*-alpha tocoferil palmitate and tocofersolan (tocophersolan), a water-soluble substance which is *d*-alpha tocoferil acid succinate combined with a macrogol. Wheat-germ oil is also widely used as a source of vitamin E.

Vitamin E is also often used as an antoxidant in pharmaceutical manufacturing.

◊ General references.

1. Meydani M. Vitamin E. *Lancet* 1995; **345:** 170–5.

**Dementia.** A hypothesis that free radicals may initiate and maintain mechanisms responsible for neurodegeneration in Alzheimer's disease (p.1484) has prompted the investigation of various drugs for antoxidant therapy. Preliminary studies[1] have suggested that alpha tocopherol might possibly slow progression. A prospective cohort study found that self-administration of combined vitamin C and vitamin E was associated with a lower risk of vascular dementia in elderly men,[2] although no significant protective effect was seen against Alzheimer's disease.

However, other studies have suggested that high intake of vitamins C and E, whether from diet[3] or supplements,[4] may reduce the risk of Alzheimer's disease. Yet another study suggested that dietary vitamin E, but not vitamin C, intake reduced the risk of Alzheimer's disease;[5] a population-based study found vitamin E intake from food and supplements to be associated with reduced cognitive decline.[6] US guidelines have suggested[7] that vitamin E 1000 units twice daily by mouth be considered in patients with Alzheimer's disease in an attempt to slow progression of the disease.


1. Sano M, *et al.* A controlled trial of selegiline, alpha-tocopherol, or both as treatment for Alzheimer's disease. *N Engl J Med* 1997; **336:** 1216–22.
2. Masaki KH, *et al.* Association of vitamin E and C supplement use with cognitive function and dementia in elderly men. *Neurology* 2000; **54:** 1265–72.
3. Engelhart MJ, *et al.* Dietary intake of antioxidants and risk of Alzheimer disease. *JAMA* 2002; **287:** 3223–9.
4. Zandi PP, *et al.* Reduced risk of Alzheimer disease in users of antioxidant vitamin supplements: the Cache County study. *Arch Neurol* 2004; **61:** 82–8.
5. Morris MC, *et al.* Dietary intake of antioxidant nutrients and the risk of incident Alzheimer disease in a biracial community study. *JAMA* 2002; **287:** 3230–7.
6. Morris MC, *et al.* Vitamin E and cognitive decline in older persons. *Arch Neurol* 2002; **59:** 1125–32.
7. Doody RS, *et al.* Practice parameter: management of dementia (an evidence-based review). Report of the Quality Standards Subcommittee of the American Academy of Neurology. *Neurology* 2001; **56:** 1154–66. Also available at: http://www.neurology.org/cgi/reprint/56/9/1154.pdf (accessed 19/05/04)


**Ischaemic heart disease.** For a discussion of studies involving vitamin E in the prophylaxis of ischaemic heart disease, see p.1420.

**Malignant neoplasms.** For a discussion of studies involving vitamin E in the prophylaxis of malignant neoplasms, see p.1420.

**Muscle spasm.** Vitamin E is one of a number of drugs that have been tried in the management of nocturnal cramps (p.1386) but there is little convincing evidence to support its use.[1,2] It has also been tried for haemodialysis-induced cramp.[3]


1. Connolly PS, *et al.* Treatment of nocturnal leg cramps: a crossover trial of quinine vs vitamin E. *Arch Intern Med* 1992; **152:** 1877–80.
2. FDA. Drug products for the treatment and/or prevention of nocturnal leg muscle cramps for over-the-counter human use. *Fed Regist* 1994; **59:** 43234–52.
3. Roca AO, *et al.* Dialysis leg cramps: efficacy of quinine versus vitamin E. *ASAIO J* 1992; **38:** M481–M485.


**Muscular dystrophies.** Vitamin E substances have been used in some countries in the management of muscular dystrophies, but controlled studies[1] have failed to demonstrate any benefit.


1. Örndahl G, *et al.* Functional deterioration and selenium-vitamin E treatment in myotonic dystrophy: a placebo-controlled study. *J Intern Med* 1994; **235:** 205–10.


**Parkinsonism.** Vitamin E has been tried (as *dl*-alpha tocopherol) in an attempt to slow neurodegeneration in patients with Parkinson's disease (p.1196) but has proved ineffective.[1]


1. The Parkinson Study Group. Effects of tocopherol and deprenyl on the progression of disability in early Parkinson's disease. *N Engl J Med* 1993; **328:** 176–83.


**Perinatal disorders.** The primary biological action of vitamin E is known to be the protection of polyunsaturated fatty acids, and thus membranes, from oxidation. Two disorders that may particularly affect premature and very low birth-weight infants are *retinopathy of prematurity* (below) and *intraventricular haemorrhage* (p.740) and as both may have some association with the occurrence of excess oxygen or oxidant stress, interest has been shown in the possible role vitamin E may have in their prevention.

**Retinopathy of prematurity.** Retinopathy of prematurity (retrolental fibroplasia) is a disease associated with immature vascularisation of the retina. Formation of retinal lesions may interfere with normal development, resulting in neovascularisation and fibrovascular proliferation. Some cases regress spontaneously but advanced cases can lead to tractional retinal detachment and loss of vision. The pathogenesis of retinopathy of prematurity is not clearly understood, but is likely to be multifactorial.[1,2]

Following the acknowledgement of a link between retinopathy of prematurity and oxygen therapy, the use of oxygen was reduced and the incidence of this disorder declined. A subsequent rise in incidence probably reflected the increased survival rate of extremely premature infants due to improved neonatal care, and certainly, variations in incidence between countries, or indeed areas, may reflect varying levels of available postnatal care.[2] Despite extensive research (see p.1237), a safe concentration of arterial oxygen has not been defined and antioxidants such as vitamin E have been used prophylactically for several decades. However, this use is controversial. Studies assessing the efficacy of vitamin E prophylaxis have not produced clear results. Some considered that vitamin E prophylaxis had a beneficial effect and recommended[3] routine prophylaxis as soon as possible after birth for infants less than 1.5 kg. However, others feel that there is no data to support prophylaxis with vitamin E[4,5] and that antioxidants cannot be recommended for routine use.[1] The various studies have been re-evaluated by meta-analysis, the results of which suggest that vitamin E may reduce the incidence of stage 3+ retinopathy of prematurity.[6] The authors recommended that a well-controlled trial should be conducted.

Other agents suggested for prophylaxis include penicillamine and antenatal dexamethasone, with some suggestion of benefit.[7,8] Reduction in ambient-light exposure did not alter the incidence of retinopathy of prematurity.[9,10]


1. Holmström G. Retinopathy of prematurity. *BMJ* 1993; **307:** 694–5.
2. Wheatley CM, *et al.* Retinopathy of prematurity: recent advances in our understanding. *Arch Dis Child Fetal Neonatal Ed* 2002; **87:** F78–F82.
3. Johnson L, *et al.* Effect of sustained pharmacologic vitamin E levels on incidence and severity of retinopathy of prematurity: a controlled clinical trial. *J Pediatr* 1989; **114:** 827–38.
4. Law MR, *et al.* Is routine vitamin E administration justified in very low-birthweight infants? *Dev Med Child Neurol* 1990; **32:** 442–50.
5. Ehrenkranz RA. Vitamin E and retinopathy of prematurity: still controversial. *J Pediatr* 1989; **114:** 801–3.
6. Raju TNK, *et al.* Vitamin E prophylaxis to reduce retinopathy of prematurity: a reappraisal of published trials. *J Pediatr* 1997; **131:** 844–50.
7. Higgins RD, *et al.* Antenatal dexamethasone and decreased severity of retinopathy of prematurity. *Arch Ophthalmol* 1998; **116:** 601–5.
8. Phelps DL, *et al.* D-Penicillamine for preventing retinopathy of prematurity in preterm infants. Available in The Cochrane Library; Issue 2. Chichester: John Wiley; 2004.
9. Reynolds JD, *et al.* Lack of efficacy of light reduction in preventing retinopathy of prematurity. *N Engl J Med* 1998; **338:** 1572–6.
10. Phelps DL, Watts JL. Early light reduction for preventing retinopathy of prematurity in very low birth weight infants. Available in The Cochrane Library; Issue 2. Chichester: John Wiley; 2004.


**Tardive dyskinesia.** Reviews[1,2] on the use of vitamin E in the management of antipsychotic-induced tardive dyskinesia (see under Extrapyramidal Disorders, p.677) concluded that evidence of benefit has generally come from small studies with methodological problems. One review[1] concluded that whereas vitamin E may protect against deterioration of tardive dyskinesia there was no evidence that it produced symptomatic improvement. It was suggested[2] that vitamin E therapy may be most beneficial in those patients with tardive dyskinesia of less than 5-years duration. Further large-scale studies are required to establish its place in treatment.


1. Soares KVS, McGrath JJ. Vitamin E for neuroleptic-induced tardive dyskinesia. Available in The Cochrane Library; Issue 2. Chichester: John Wiley; 2004.
2. Boomershine KH, *et al.* Vitamin E in the treatment of tardive dyskinesia. *Ann Pharmacother* 1999; **33:** 1195–1202.


## Preparations

***BP 2003:*** Alpha Tocopheryl Succinate Tablets;
***USNF 22:*** Tocopherols Excipient;
***USP 27:*** Vitamin E Capsules; Vitamin E Preparation.

**Proprietary Preparations** (details are given in Part 3)

***Arg.:*** Ephynal; Etec; Evion; Risordan; Senexon E; Tonovital E; ***Austral.:*** Alpha Keri Silky Smooth†; Bio E†; Bio Enhaced Natural E†; Bioglan Micelle E†; Bioglan Natural E†; Bioglan Water Soluble E†; Chew-E†; Dal-E†; Macro E†; Mega E†; Vita E†; ***Austria:*** Avigilen; Ephynal; Etocoderm; Etocovit; Evit; Evitol; Optovit E; Tetefit Vitamin E; Tocovenos; Vitactiv E; ***Belg.:*** Ephynal; Optovit E; ***Braz.:*** E Plus; E Radicaps; E-Mil; Efherol; Ephynal; Fonto-Vit E; Tesurene†; Vieta; Vita-E; Vitabase†; Zirvit E; ***Canad.:*** Aquasol E; Kyolic Formula 106; Novo E; Nutrol E; Organex; Vita-E†; ***Chile:*** Egogyn; Etec 1000; ***Fin.:*** Bio-E-Vitamin; Equiday; Esol; Ido-E; Tokovitan; Vita-E; ***Fr.:*** Dermorelle; Ephynal; Toco; Tocolion; Tocomine†; Tocopa; ***Ger.:*** Antioxidans E; Biogenis One-a-Day†; Biopto-E; Biosan E; Detulin; E-Mulsin; E-Tonil; E-Vicotrat; Elex E; Embial; Ephynal; Eplonat; Equiday E†; Eusovit; Evion; Evit†; Flexal Vitamin E; Malton E; Mowivit; Optovit; Pexan E†; Puncto E; Sanavitan S; Spondyvit; Tocorell; Tocovenos†; Tocovital; Togasan; Uno-Vit; Vibolex E; Vita-E; Vitagutt Vitamin E; Vitazell E; ***Hong Kong:*** Myra 300-E; Natopherol; Topher-E; ***India:*** Evion; ***Irl.:*** Ephynal; ***Israel:*** Ephynal†; Evitex; Evitol; ***Ital.:*** E-Vitum; Ephynal; Evasen Crema; Evion; Evitina†; Na-To-Caps†; Natovit; Rigentex; Sursum; Tocogen†; ***Malaysia:*** Citrex Vitamin E; Fairy ADE; Juvela; Natopherol; ***Mex.:*** Bacferol; Ekanin†; Elibet†; Ephynal†; Eugerminal; Vitalle; ***Neth.:*** Davitamon E†; ***Norw.:*** AFI-E†; Bio-E-Vitamin; Ido-E; ***NZ:*** Micelle E; ***Port.:*** Ephynal; Oxivite†; Ve; ***S.Afr.:*** Ephynal; ***Singapore:*** Juvela†; Myra 300-E; Natopherol; ***Spain:*** Auxina E; Ephynal; ***Swed.:*** E-vidon; E-vimin; Ido-E; ***Switz.:*** Ephynal; Evit; Optovit; ***Thai.:*** Bio-E; Chew-E†; E-Drops; ***UK:*** Bio E†; Ephynal; Prairie Gold; Vita-E; ***USA:*** Amino-Opti-E†; Aquasol E†; Aquavit-E; E-Gems; Nutr-E-Sol; Vita-Plus E; Vitec.

**Multi-ingredient: *Arg.:*** A-Vitel E; Acilac; Atomoderma A-E; Brunavera; Cardiax; Lipofundin MCT/LCT-E; Redudiet; ***Austral.:*** Althaea Complex†; Antioxidant Forte Tablets†; Antioxidant Tablets†; Arthriforte†; Beta A-C†; Beta-Ace Tablets†; Bioglan Bioage Peripheral†; Bioglan Fingers & Toes†; Bioglan Maxepa†; Bioglan Micelle A plus E†; Bioglan Primrose-E†; Curash Baby Wipes†; Curash Babycare; Echinacea & Antioxidants†; Epo + Maxepa + Vitamin E Herbal Plus Formula 8†; ER Cream; Eye Health Herbal Plus Formula 4†; Ginkgo Complex†; Ginzing E†; Hair and Skin Formula†; Lifechange Circulation Aid†; Lifesystem Herbal Plus Formula 5 Eye Relief†; Lifesystem Herbal Plus Formula 8 Echinacea†; Lifesystem Herbal Plus Formula 9 Fatty Acids And Vitamin E†; Macro Natural Vitamin E Cream; ML 20†; Sambucus Complex†; Selenium E†; Serenoa Complex†; Trillium Complex†; Viburnum Complex†; ***Austria:*** A-E-Mulsin; Arcavit A/E; Colagain†; Coldistop; Dr Schmidgall Halsweh; Droxaryl; Gerogelat; Lecivital; Magnesium Tonil Vitamin E; Mamellin; Pasuma-Dragees; Regenerin; Rovigon; Ulcurilen; Vasovitol; ***Belg.:*** Dagravit A-E†; Rovigon; ***Braz.:*** Adeforte; Gerosenil†; Ioimbina Composta†; Licovit; Neurofitol†; Renovator†; Sexormom†; ***Canad.:*** Bionagre plus E; Bye Bye Burn†; Super Gamma Oil with Vitamin E†; Vita-E Plus Selenium†; ***Chile:*** Dermaglos Plus; Rovigon; Salonpas; ***Fin.:*** Aesol; Cellavie; ***Fr.:*** Alpha 5 DS; Arkotonic†; Bio-Selenium; Cicatryl; Circularine†; Cirkan a la Prednacinolone; Difrarel E; Enuretine†; Ophtadil; Parogencyl anti-age gencives; Rovigon; Topialyse; Trisolvit†; ***Ger.:*** A + D + E-Vicotrat†; A + E Thilo; A-E-Mulsin; Alsicur†; Alsiroyal†; anabol-loges; Antimyopikum†; Biogenis†; Buer Vitamin E + Magnesium†; Coldastop; Dr. Hotz Vollbad†; Dynef; E-Vicotrat + Magnesium†; Elex†; Hewekzem novo N; Kollateral A + E†; Lasar†; Lipidavit; Lipovitan; Magium E†; Magnesium Tonil; Magnesium-Plus-Hevert; Magopsor†; Mapurit; NeyChondrin N (Revitorgan-Dilutionen N Nr 68); NeyNormin N (Revitorgan-Dilutionen N Nr 65); NeyPulpin N (Revitorgan-Dilutionen N Nr 10); NeyTumorin N (Revitorgan-Dilutionen N Nr 66); Protecor; Remederm; Rovigon G; RubieMag + E; Salus Herz-Schutz-Kapseln; Ulcurilen N; Unguentacid; Ureata S; Vaso-E-Bion; ***Gr.:*** Eviol-A; ***Hong Kong:*** Aderma Epitheliale; Difrarel E; E-Prime; Haemosol†; Karoyan S†; ***India:*** Cadvion; Rovigon; Sclerobion; Vitexid; ***Ital.:*** Angstrom Viso; Babysteril; Capill; Derman-Oil; Dermana Pasta; Ecamannan; Efagel; Emortrofine; Ener-E; Eurogel; Forticrin; Granoleina; Ictom 3; Midium; Mirtilene; Pasta Dicofarm; Provitamin A-E; Retinovit; Rovigon; Royal E; Rutisan CE; Tannidin Plus; Tocalfa; Ultravisin; Vasopt; Vit Eparin; ***Malaysia:*** Balance Elastin E; Boots Antenatal Massage Cream; Natopherol Dermal-Day; Salonpas; ***Mex.:*** Aveendix; Periodentyl; ***Mon.:*** Tocogestan†; ***Neth.:*** Dagravit A-E Forte; ***NZ:*** Chap Stick; ***Port.:*** Antiestrias; Creme Laser Hidrante; Disoderme†; Esclerobion; Nutraisdin; Rilastil Dermo Solar; Rovigon; Synchrorose; Synchrovit; ***Singapore:*** Desitin Creamy; ***Spain:*** Auxina A + E; Difrarel E†; Poli ABE†; Ravigona†; Trivitan†; Vitaber A E; Wobenzimal; ***Switz.:*** Acne-Med Wolff Simplex; Alphastria; Coldistop; Leniderm; Linola gras; Oravil; Rovigon; Visaline; ***Thai.:*** Men Hormone; Rovigon†; Siduol; ***UK:*** Efatime†; Exzem Oil†; Octacosanol; Se-Power; ***USA:*** Aloe Grande; Anusol; Comfortine†; Diaper Guard; Lactinol-E; Lazercreme; Lobana Derm-Aide; Lobana Peri-Garde; Phicon; Ze Caps.

---

# Vitamin K Substances

Vitaminas K.

The term vitamin K is used for a range of naphthoquinone compounds which include acetomenaphthone, menadiol, menadione, menatetrenone, and phytomenadione.

## Acetomenaphthone *(BAN)*

Acetomenadione; Acetomenaftona; Acetomenaph.; Menadiol Diacetate; Vitamin $K_4$ Diacetate. 2-Methyl-1,4-naphthylene diacetate.

$C_{15}H_{14}O_4$ = 258.3.
*CAS — 573-20-6.*

**Pharmacopoeias.** In *Chin.*

## Menadiol Sodium Phosphate *(BANM)*

Menadiol, fosfato sódico de; Menadiol Sodium Diphosphate; Menadiolum Solubile; Vitamin $K_4$ Sodium Phosphate. 2-Methylnaphthalene-1,4-diyl bis(disodium phosphate) hexahydrate.

$C_{11}H_8Na_4O_8P_2,6H_2O$ = 530.2.
*CAS — 481-85-6 (menadiol); 131-13-5 (anhydrous menadiol sodium phosphate); 6700-42-1 (menadiol sodium phosphate hexahydrate); 84-98-0 (menadiol diphosphate).*

NOTE. Menadiol Potassium Sulfate (Potassium Menaphthosulfate) is *BAN* and Menadiol Sodium Sulfate is *rINN*.

**Pharmacopoeias.** In *Br.* and *US.*

**BP 2003** (Menadiol Sodium Phosphate). A white to pink, hygroscopic, crystalline powder with a characteristic odour. Very soluble in water; practically insoluble in alcohol.

**USP 27** (Menadiol Sodium Diphosphate). A white to pink, hygroscopic, powder having a characteristic odour. Very soluble in water; insoluble in alcohol. Its solutions in water are neutral or slightly alkaline to litmus having a pH of about 8. Store in airtight containers at a temperature not exceeding 8°. Protect from light.

## Menadione *(BAN)*

Menadiona; Menadionum; Menaph.; Menaphthene; Menaphthone; Methylnaphthochinonum; Vitamin $K_3$. 2-Methyl-1,4-naphthoquinone.

$C_{11}H_8O_2$ = 172.2.
*CAS — 58-27-5.*
*ATC — B02BA02.*

**Pharmacopoeias.** In *Eur.* (see p.vi) and *US.*

**Ph. Eur. 5.0** (Menadione). A pale yellow crystalline powder. It is unstable in light. Practically insoluble in water; sparingly soluble in alcohol and in methyl alcohol; freely soluble in toluene. Protect from light.

**USP 27** (Menadione). A bright yellow, practically odourless, crystalline powder. It is affected by sunlight. Practically insoluble in water; soluble 1 in 60 of alcohol, 1 in 50 of vegetable oils, and 1 in 10 of benzene; sparingly soluble in chloroform. Store at a temperature of 25°, excursions permitted between 15° and 30°. Protect from light.

**Handling.** Menadione powder is irritating to the respiratory tract and to the skin. The alcoholic solution has vesicant properties.

## Menadione Sodium Bisulfite *(rINN)*

Bisulfito sódico de menadiona; Kavitanum; Menadione Sodium Bisulphite *(BANM)*; Menaph. Sod. Bisulphite; Menaphthone Sodium Bisulphite; Methylnaphthochinonumnatrium Bisulfurosum; Vikasolum; Vitamin $K_3$ Sodium Bisulphite. Sodium 1,2,3,4-tetrahydro-2-methyl-1,4-dioxonaphthalene-2-sulphonate trihydrate.

$C_{11}H_8O_2NaHSO_3,3H_2O$ = 330.3.
*CAS — 130-37-0 (anhydrous menadione sodium bisulfite); 6147-37-1 (menadione sodium bisulfite trihydrate).*

**Pharmacopoeias.** In *Chin.* and *Pol.*

### Menatetrenone

E3100; Ea-0167; Menaquinone-4; Menaquinone 4; Menaquinone K4; Menatetren; Menatetrenona; Menatetrenonum; MK4; Vitamin $K_{2(20)}$; Vitamin MK 4. 2-Methyl-3-(3,7,11,15-tetramethyl-2,6,10,14-hexadeca-tetraenyl)-1,4-naphthoquinone.

$C_{31}H_{40}O_2$ = 444.6.
*CAS — 863-61-6.*

**Pharmacopoeias.** In *Jpn.*

### Phytomenadione *(BAN, rINN)*

Fitomenadiona; Methylphytylnaphthochinonum; Phylloquinone; Phytomenad.; Phytomenadionum; Phytonadione; Vitamin $K_1$. 2-Methyl-3-[3,7,11,15-tetramethylhexadec-2-enyl] naphthalene-1,4-dione.

$C_{31}H_{46}O_2$ = 450.7.
*CAS — 84-80-0.*
*ATC — B02BA01.*

**Pharmacopoeias.** In *Chin., Eur.* (see p.vi), *Int., Jpn, US,* and *Viet.*

**Ph. Eur. 5.0** (Phytomenadione). A mixture of the *trans* (*E*) and *cis* (*Z*) isomers. It contains not less than 75% of *trans*-phytomenadione, and also allows not more than 4% of *trans*-epoxyphytomenadione.

A clear, intense yellow, viscous, oily liquid, which decomposes on exposure to actinic light. Practically insoluble in water; sparingly soluble in alcohol; miscible with fatty oils. Protect from light.

**USP 27** (Phytonadione). A mixture of the *E* and *Z* isomers. It contains not more than 21% of the *Z* isomer. A clear, yellow to amber, very viscous, odourless or practically odourless, liquid. It is stable in air, but decomposes on exposure to sunlight. Insoluble in water; slightly soluble in alcohol; soluble in dehydrated alcohol, in chloroform, in ether, in vegetable oils, and in benzene. Store in airtight containers. Protect from light.

**Stability.** A polyethoxylated castor oil formulation of phytomenadione was stable for at least 30 days at room temperature when repackaged in amber glass dropper bottles.[1] When refrigerated at 4° to 8°, it was stable in both plastic and amber glass bottles.

1. Wong VK, Ho PC. Stability of Konakion repacked in dropper bottles for oral administration. *Aust J Hosp Pharm* 1996; **26:** 641–4.

## Adverse Effects and Precautions

Intravenous administration of *phytomenadione* has caused severe reactions resembling hypersensitivity or anaphylaxis. Symptoms have included facial flushing, sweating, chest constriction and chest pain, dyspnoea, cyanosis, and cardiovascular collapse; fatalities have been reported. Anaphylactic reactions have generally been associated with an overly rapid rate of infusion but have also been reported even when the solution was diluted and infused slowly. They are generally thought to be due to polyethoxylated castor oil which is present as a surfactant in some parenteral formulations; reports of such reactions with formulations that do not contain polyethoxylated castor oil are rare.

Pain, swelling, and phlebitis may occur at the injection site when phytomenadione is given. Localised skin reactions including atrophy or necrosis have been reported following intramuscular or subcutaneous injection of phytomenadione.

Phytomenadione formulations solubilised with lecithin and a bile salt should be given with caution to patients with severely impaired liver function and to premature neonates weighing less than 2.5 kg, since the bile salt may displace bilirubin.

Administration of *menadione* and *menadiol sodium phosphate* to neonates, especially premature infants, or to the mother during late pregnancy has been associated with the development in the infant of haemolytic anaemia, hyperbilirubinaemia, and kernicterus, and such use is not recommended. Phytomenadione has a lower risk of haemolysis. Menadione and menadiol sodium phosphate have also been reported to cause haemolysis in patients with G6PD deficiency or vitamin E deficiency.

**Breast feeding.** Vitamin K is variably distributed into breast milk; a study found phytomenadione concentrations in the first 10 mL of expressed milk ("fore milk") to be lower than those in the last 10 mL ("hind milk"). These changes may be related to the lipid concentration, which is higher in hind milk. Lipid composition also changes over the course of lactation, with pronounced changes in the first week, and the authors proposed that a mechanism exists whereby vitamin K concentration in milk is higher in the first few days of life so as to meet the neonate's nutritional requirements at a time when vitamin K status is precarious.[1] The American Academy of Pediatrics considers[2] that, as no adverse effects have been observed in breast-fed infants whose mothers were receiving phytomenadione, its use is therefore usually compatible with breast feeding.

1. von Kries R, *et al.* Vitamin $K_1$ content of maternal milk: influence of the stage of lactation, lipid composition, and vitamin $K_1$ supplements given to the mother. *Pediatr Res* 1987; **22:** 513–17.
2. American Academy of Pediatrics. The transfer of drugs and other chemicals into human milk. *Pediatrics* 2001; **108:** 776–89. Correction. *ibid.*; 1029. Also available at: http://aappolicy.aappublications.org/cgi/content/full/pediatrics%3b108/3/776 (accessed 19/05/04)

**Carcinogenicity.** A case-control study from the UK[1] suggested an increased risk of cancer in children who had received vitamin K at birth for the prevention of vitamin K deficiency bleeding (see below). A further study[2] by the same authors indicated that this risk was associated with intramuscular, but not oral, administration, and was strongest for childhood leukaemia. In response to these data, the British Paediatric Association recommended that the oral route be preferred for prophylaxis,[3] whereas the American Academy of Pediatrics continued to advocate the intramuscular route.[4]

Subsequent studies from the USA,[5] Sweden,[6] Denmark,[6,7] Germany,[8] and England[9] did not confirm an increased risk of childhood cancer, including leukaemias, after the use of intramuscular vitamin K. More recently, 4 further studies were published.[10-13] Two of the reports, a case-control study in Scotland[10] and an ecological study in Britain,[11] showed no increased risk of any cancers with the use of intramuscular vitamin K. A third case-control study in England and Wales[12] found a borderline association between intramuscular vitamin K and cancers, particularly leukaemia. In the fourth study, a case-control study in northern England,[13] there was an increased risk (odds ratio 1.79) of acute lymphoblastic leukaemia developing 1 to 6 years after birth in children who had received intramuscular vitamin K. In 1998 an expert working group formed by the UK Committee on Safety of Medicines reviewed all the available studies.[14] They concluded that there was no increased risk of solid tumours with vitamin K, and that, although an increased risk of leukaemia could not be excluded, observed results were compatible with chance. Moreover, they could not identify a plausible mechanism for a carcinogenic effect of vitamin K. The UK Department of Health[15] advocates either oral or intramuscular prophylaxis, and recommends that the parents should be involved in the decision on which route of administration is used.

1. Golding J, *et al.* Factors associated with childhood cancer in a national cohort study. *Br J Cancer* 1990; **62:** 304–8.
2. Golding J, *et al.* Childhood cancer, intramuscular vitamin K, and pethidine given during labour. *BMJ* 1992; **305:** 341–6.
3. British Paediatric Association. *Vitamin K prophylaxis in infancy.* London, 1992: British Paediatric Association.
4. American Academy of Pediatrics Vitamin K Ad Hoc Task Force. Controversies concerning vitamin K and the newborn. *Pediatrics* 1993; **91:** 1001–3.
5. Klebanoff MA, *et al.* The risk of childhood cancer after neonatal exposure to vitamin K. *N Engl J Med* 1993; **329:** 905–8.
6. Ekelund H, *et al.* Administration of vitamin K to newborn infants and childhood cancer. *BMJ* 1993; **307:** 89–91.
7. Olsen JH, *et al.* Vitamin K regimens and incidence of childhood cancer in Denmark. *BMJ* 1994; **308:** 895–6.
8. von Kries R, *et al.* Vitamin K and childhood cancer: a population based case-control study in Lower Saxony, Germany. *BMJ* 1996; **313:** 199–203.
9. Ansell P, *et al.* Childhood leukaemia and intramuscular vitamin K: findings from a case-control study. *BMJ* 1996; **313:** 204–5.
10. McKinney PA, *et al.* Case-control study of childhood leukaemia and cancer in Scotland: findings for neonatal intramuscular vitamin K. *BMJ* 1998; **316:** 173–7.
11. Passmore SJ, *et al.* Ecological studies of relation between hospital policies on neonatal vitamin K administration and subsequent occurrence of childhood cancer. *BMJ* 1998; **316:** 184–9.
12. Passmore SJ, *et al.* Case-control studies of relation between childhood cancer and neonatal vitamin K administration. *BMJ* 1998; **316:** 178–184.
13. Parker L, *et al.* Neonatal vitamin K administration and childhood cancer in the north of England: retrospective case-control study. *BMJ* 1998; **316:** 189–93.
14. Committee on Safety of Medicines/Medicines Control Agency. Safety of intramuscular vitamin K (Konakion). *Current Problems* 1998; **24:** 3–4. Also available at: http://www.mca.gov.uk/ourwork/monitorsafequalmed/currentproblems/volume24a.htm (accessed 21/05/04)
15. Department of Health. *Vitamin K for newborn babies.* London, 1998: Department of Health. Also available at: http://www.dh.gov.uk/assetRoot/04/01/34/96/04013496.pdf (accessed 21/05/04)

**Effects on the blood.** Cerebral arterial thrombosis developed in 2 patients with malabsorption syndromes due to coeliac disease during treatment with vitamin K for severe deficiency of vitamin-K-dependent coagulation factors. An increased tendency to thrombotic events had previously been reported to be present in patients with intestinal inflammatory disorders. It was suggested that if bleeding did occur in such patients treatment should be with plasma infusions or small doses of vitamin K but that vitamin K deficiency should not be specifically treated since a gluten-free diet or corticosteroids given for the gastrointestinal disorder will result in a gradual correction.[1]

1. Florholmen J, *et al.* Cerebral thrombosis in two patients with malabsorption syndrome treated with vitamin K. *BMJ* 1980; **281:** 541.

## Interactions

Vitamin K decreases the effects of oral anticoagulants (see p.1027), and is used to counteract excessive effects of these drugs, see below. Vitamin K may reduce the response to resumed therapy with anticoagulants for a week or more.

## Pharmacokinetics

The fat-soluble vitamin K compounds phytomenadione and menadione require the presence of bile for their absorption from the gastrointestinal tract; the water-soluble derivatives of menadione can be absorbed in the absence of bile. Vitamin K accumulates mainly in the liver but is stored in the body only for short periods of time. Vitamin K does not appear to cross the placenta readily and it is variably distributed into breast milk. Phytomenadione is rapidly metabolised to more polar metabolites and is excreted in bile and urine as glucuronide and sulfate conjugates.

**Absorption.** Absorption of phytomenadione from the colloidal (micellar) preparation was more irregular and unpredictable after intramuscular than intravenous administration in healthy adults;[1] when used as an antidote to anticoagulant drugs, this formulation should be given intravenously. In neonates, plasma phytomenadione concentrations were within or above the adult fasting plasma range 24 days after receiving a single dose of the colloidal preparation either orally (3 mg) or intramuscularly (1.5 mg).[2]

1. Soedirman JR, *et al.* Pharmacokinetics and tolerance of intravenous and intramuscular phylloquinone (vitamin $K_1$) mixed micelles formulation. *Br J Clin Pharmacol* 1996; **41:** 517–23.
2. Schubiger G, *et al.* Vitamin $K_1$ concentration in breast-fed neonates after oral or intramuscular administration of a single dose of a new mixed-micellar preparation of phylloquinone. *J Pediatr Gastroenterol Nutr* 1993; **16:** 435–9.

## Human Requirements

The minimum daily requirements of vitamin K are not clearly defined but an intake of about 1 microgram/kg daily appears to be adequate. Vitamin K requirements in normal adults can be met from the average diet and from the synthesis of menaquinones (also known as vitamin $K_2$) by bacterial action in the intestine. Vitamin K occurs naturally as phytomenadione (vitamin $K_1$), which is present in many foods, especially leafy green vegetables such as cabbage and spinach, and is also present in liver, cows' milk, egg-yolk, and some cereals.

**UK and US recommended dietary intake.** In the UK neither a reference nutrient intake (RNI) nor an estimated average requirement (EAR—see p.1419) has been set for vitamin K although an intake of 1 microgram/kg daily was considered to be both safe and adequate for adults; a higher intake of 10 micrograms daily (about 2 micrograms/kg daily) was believed to be justified in infants because of the absence of hepatic menaquinones in early life and reliance on dietary vitamin K alone. It was stated that all babies should receive prophylactic vitamin K at birth[1] and for further details concerning neonatal use, see Vitamin K Deficiency Bleeding, below.

In the USA, adequate intake levels have been determined to be 120 micrograms daily for adult men and 90 micrograms daily for adult women.[2]

1. DoH. Dietary reference values for food energy and nutrients for the United Kingdom: report of the panel on dietary reference values of the committee on medical aspects of food policy. *Report on health and social subjects 41.* London: HMSO, 1991.
2. Standing Committee on the Scientific Evaluation of Dietary Reference Intakes of the Food and Nutrition Board. *Dietary Reference Intakes for vitamin A, vitamin K, arsenic, boron, chromium, copper, iodine, iron, manganese, molybdenum, nickel, silicon, vanadium, and zinc.* Washington DC: National Academy Press, 2001. Also available at: http://www.nap.edu/catalog/10026.html (accessed 24/05/04)

## Uses and Administration

Vitamin K is an essential cofactor in the hepatic synthesis of prothrombin (factor II) and other blood clotting factors (factors VII, IX, and X, and proteins C and S) and in the function of proteins such as osteocalcin important for bone development.

Vitamin K deficiency may develop in neonates, but is uncommon in adults, although it may occur in patients with malabsorption syndromes, obstructive jaundice or hepatic disease. Deficiency leads to the development of hypoprothrombinaemia, in which the clotting time of the blood is prolonged and spontaneous bleeding can occur. Coumarin anticoagulants interfere with vitamin K metabolism, and their effects can be antagonised by giving vitamin K.

Vitamin K compounds are used in the treatment and prevention of haemorrhage associated with vitamin K deficiency. The dose of vitamin K should be carefully controlled by prothrombin-time estimations.

Phytomenadione is a naturally occurring vitamin K substance. It is the only vitamin K compound used to reverse hypoprothrombinaemia and haemorrhage caused by anticoagulant therapy. It is not effective as a heparin antidote. For over-anticoagulation, the dose depends on the international normalised ratio (INR) and the degree of haemorrhage. Typical doses of phytomenadione are 0.5 to 5 mg by slow intravenous injection or up to 5 mg orally (see also Over-anticoagulation, below). Depending on the solubilising agents used, some formulations of phytomenadione are more suitable for intravenous use than others, and administration details vary. Phytomenadione has also been used in hypoprothrombinaemia due to certain cephalosporins (see Cefamandole, Adverse Effects, p.169).

In the treatment of vitamin K deficiency bleeding in neonates, phytomenadione may be given in a dose of 1 mg intravenously or intramuscularly; further doses may be given if necessary. As a prophylactic measure, a single dose of 0.5 to 1 mg may be given intramuscularly to the newborn infant, or 2 mg orally followed by a second dose of 2 mg after 4 to 7 days; for further details see below.

Menadiol sodium phosphate is a water-soluble derivative of menadione, a synthetic lipid-soluble vitamin K analogue. It may be used for the prevention of vitamin K deficiency in patients with malabsorption syndromes in whom oral phytomenadione may be inefficiently absorbed. It is given in usual doses equivalent to 10 to 40 mg of menadiol phosphate daily by mouth.

Menadiol dibutyrate and menatetrenone have also been used and the latter has been used in the management of osteoporosis. Acetomenaphthone has been used in preparations promoted for the relief of chilblains.

**Action.** References to the action of vitamin K and the role of vitamin K-dependent coagulation proteins and carboxyglutamate-containing proteins such as osteocalcin.


1. Friedman PA. Vitamin K-dependent proteins. *N Engl J Med* 1984; **310:** 1458–60.
2. Rick ME. Protein C and protein S: vitamin K-dependent inhibitors of blood coagulation. *JAMA* 1990; **263:** 701–3.
3. Shearer MJ. Vitamin K. *Lancet* 1995; **345:** 229–34.


**Neonatal intraventricular haemorrhage.** Vitamin K crosses the placenta slowly and to a limited extent,[1,2] but sufficiently to warrant studies to assess whether antenatal administration of phytomenadione to the mother may reduce the incidence or severity of intraventricular haemorrhage (p.740) in the preterm neonate. Two studies did find that such antenatal administration had a beneficial outcome[3,4] but this finding was not confirmed by a subsequent study.[5] Moreover, a larger randomised controlled study failed to find any benefit from vitamin K prophylaxis.[6] A systematic review of trials concluded that vitamin K did not significantly prevent periventricular haemorrhage, and could not be recommended for routine clinical use.[7]


1. Yang Y-M, *et al.* Maternal-fetal transport of vitamin $K_1$ and its effects on coagulation in premature infants. *J Pediatr* 1989; **115:** 1009–13.
2. Kazzi NJ, *et al.* Placental transfer of vitamin $K_1$ in preterm pregnancy. *Obstet Gynecol* 1990; **75:** 334–7.
3. Pomerance JJ, *et al.* Maternally administered antenatal vitamin $K_1$: effect on neonatal prothrombin activity, partial thromboplastin time, and intraventricular hemorrhage. *Obstet Gynecol* 1987; **70:** 235–41.
4. Morales WJ, *et al.* The use of antenatal vitamin K in the prevention of early neonatal intraventricular hemorrhage. *Am J Obstet Gynecol* 1988; **159:** 774–9.
5. Kazzi NJ, *et al.* Maternal administration of vitamin K does not improve the coagulation profile of preterm infants. *Pediatrics* 1989; **84:** 1045–50.
6. Thorp JA, Antepartum vitamin K and phenobarbital for preventing intraventricular hemorrhage in the premature newborn: a randomized, double-blind, placebo-controlled trial. *Obstet Gynecol* 1994; **83:** 70–6.
7. Crowther CA, Henderson-Smart DJ. Vitamin K prior to preterm birth for preventing neonatal periventricular haemorrhage. Available in The Cochrane Library; Issue 2. Chichester: John Wiley; 2004.


**Over-anticoagulation.** Doses of vitamin K for over-anticoagulation with warfarin have traditionally been large, and this continues to be reflected in manufacturers' literature for these products, where recommended oral or parenteral doses range from 2.5 to 10 mg up to 25 mg initially, with a maximum dose of 40 to 50 mg. However, large doses of vitamin K may result in over-correction, and increase the delay before resumed anticoagulant therapy becomes effective. In addition, the time to onset of action is a minimum of 1 to 2 hours, irrespective of dose. There is increasing evidence that lower doses of vitamin K are effective in over-anticoagulation.[1,2] The British Society of Haematology currently recommends doses of phytomenadione of 5 mg by slow intravenous injection for patients with major bleeding, and 0.5 mg intravenously or 5 mg orally for those with risk factors for bleeding (see Treatment of Adverse Effects of Warfarin, p.1023).


1. Weibert RT, *et al.* Correction of excessive anticoagulation with low-dose oral vitamin $K_1$. *Ann Intern Med* 1997; **125:** 959–62.
2. Fetrow CW, *et al.* Antagonism of warfarin-induced hypoprothrombinemia with use of low-dose subcutaneous vitamin $K_1$. *J Clin Pharmacol* 1997; **37:** 751–7.


**Vitamin K deficiency bleeding.** Vitamin K deficiency bleeding (VKDB; haemorrhagic disease of the newborn; HDN), of which 3 types have been recognised, is associated with a clotting defect due to vitamin K deficiency.

- In early VKDB bleeding occurs at the time of delivery or during the first 24 hours of life and is typically seen in infants whose mothers have taken drugs that affect vitamin K metabolism such as warfarin, some antiepileptics, rifampicin, or isoniazid.
- Classic VKDB, the most common type, usually occurs at 2 to 5 days of age and breast feeding is an important factor as human breast milk has a much lower content of vitamin K than either cow's milk or infant formulas.
- Late VKDB presents frequently as intracranial haemorrhage in infants over one month of age. The vitamin-K deficiency in these cases can be either idiopathic (usually in breast-fed infants who did not receive vitamin K at birth) and/or can be a secondary manifestation of other disorders such as chronic diarrhoea, cystic fibrosis or other malabsorption syndromes, biliary atresia, or $\alpha_1$-antitrypsin deficiency.[1]

Treatment of VKDB involves use of parenteral phytomenadione, usually 1 mg initially with further doses depending on response. More immediate treatment, in the form of blood transfusion or blood clotting factors, may be needed to compensate for severe blood loss and delayed response to vitamin K. VKDB, particularly the late type, carries a high risk of morbidity or death; therefore, the emphasis has been on prevention. It has long been known that administration of vitamin K to the neonate soon after birth can reduce the incidence of VKDB. Menadiol sodium phosphate was formerly used, but reports in the 1950s of jaundice and kernicterus in infants given this vitamin K analogue caused concern, and led to the preferential use of phytomenadione either intramuscularly or orally. Administration of phytomenadione, usually as a single intramuscular injection, has been standard practice for neonates considered at high risk of VKDB, such as those who had a complicated delivery, those born prematurely, and those whose mothers were receiving antiepileptic therapy. Since it is not possible to selectively identify all neonates that are at risk for VKDB, the routine use of phytomenadione in all neonates has been advocated. However, such practice has been controversial, particularly as regards the route.[2,3] Some have considered that oral administration is less invasive and more acceptable to parents.[3] However, there has also been concern about the adequacy of absorption of orally administered phytomenadione, and the lack of a suitable oral formulation. In addition, there was some evidence[4-6] to suggest that a single intramuscular dose was more effective than a single oral dose in preventing late VKDB, and that repeated oral doses might be required, which may be less convenient and carry the risk of poor compliance. More recently, a possible increased risk of childhood cancer in neonates treated with intramuscular, but not oral, phytomenadione has been reported (see Carcinogenicity, above). Although the association remains controversial, it led to recommendations for the preferential use of oral vitamin K in neonates at low-risk of VKDB in some countries, including the UK[7] and Germany,[8] whereas other countries, including the USA,[9,10] still preferred the intramuscular route for all neonates.

There is still no agreement on the most effective oral dose and its frequency of administration, and study of this has been complicated by the lack of a suitable oral preparation of phytomenadione.[11,12] Options currently available for oral administration include the polyethoxylated castor oil and polysorbate-80 containing preparations (unlicensed for oral use) and the colloidal, micelle formulation (licensed for oral use in some countries). These preparations are packaged in glass ampoules, therefore are unsuitable for parents to administer at home. The colloidal preparation may be absorbed more reliably (see under Pharmacokinetics, above).

The 1992 recommendations of the British Paediatric Society[7] for oral use of the polyethoxylated castor oil formulation suggested a single dose of 500 micrograms on the day of birth. For breast-fed babies, additional doses of 500 micrograms at 7 to 10 days and at 4 to 6 weeks, or 200 micrograms at weekly intervals for 26 weeks, or 50 micrograms daily for 26 weeks, were recommended. Current UK doses[13] for the colloidal preparation in healthy term neonates are 2 mg soon after birth, then 2 mg at 4 to 7 days. Exclusively breast-fed infants should be given a third oral dose of 2 mg one month after birth. Further monthly doses of 2 mg have been recommended while the infant remains exclusively breast-fed. A report[14] of the failure of prophylaxis in 3 breast-fed babies (2 of whom had unidentified cholestatic liver disease) who received 2 doses of this formulation, as recommended in Switzerland, emphasises the importance of the third, and possibly, other, follow-up doses. Plasma vitamin K concentrations in breast-fed infants receiving 3 oral doses of this formulation were at least equal to concentrations in those receiving a single intramuscular dose.[15] A study in Germany, however, found the mixed micellar oral formulation to be no more efficacious than older vitamin K preparations,[16] and a pharmacokinetic study found its absorption to be unreliable in infants with conjugated hyperbilirubinaemia;[17] the authors suggest that even 3 oral doses may not provide sufficient protection against VKDB in infants with latent cholestasis. The most recent advice from the UK Department of Health[13] advocates that all newborn infants should receive vitamin K prophylaxis, both oral and intramuscular administration should be available, and that parents should be involved in the decision on which route of administration is used.

Various other oral regimens have been investigated or are in use. In the Netherlands a regimen of 1 mg orally or intramuscularly at birth, followed by 25 micrograms daily or 1 mg weekly by mouth from 1 week to 3 months of age has been found satisfactory.[18,19] In Germany[8,19] and Australia[19] the suggested oral regimen for the polyethoxylated castor oil formulation was 1 mg at birth, at 3 to 10 days and at weeks 3 to 6, although some failures have been reported in babies receiving this regimen,[8] and the Australian data confirm it is less effective than a single intramuscular dose.[19] One hospital in the USA has satisfactorily used, for many years, a single 2-mg dose administered via nasogastric tube to neonates after birth,[20] although the American Academy of Pediatrics still advocates use of the intramuscular route.[10] In Denmark, a 2-mg dose at birth followed by a weekly dose of 1 mg during the first 3 months of life has effectively prevented any late VKDB in healthy breast-fed babies.[21]

Although phytomenadione crosses the placenta slowly and to a limited extent, it is nevertheless recommended that pregnant women receiving drugs that are vitamin K antagonists (particularly antiepileptics) should receive phytomenadione 10 to 20 mg daily from 36 weeks gestation.[22] This is in addition to the requirement that their neonates, who are at high risk of VKDB, receive intramuscular phytomenadione soon after birth. Maternal phytomenadione administration has been investigated as a means of improving vitamin K status in breast-fed neonates. In 1 study,[23] 5 mg daily for 12 weeks was effective for this purpose.


1. Hathaway WE. Haemostatic disorders in the newborn. In: Bloom AL, Thomas DP, eds. *Haemostasis and thrombosis*. 2nd ed. Edinburgh: Churchill Livingstone, 1987: 554–69.
2. Tripp JH, McNinch AW. Haemorrhagic disease and vitamin K. *Arch Dis Child* 1987; **62:** 436–7.
3. Brown SG, *et al.* Should intramuscular vitamin K prophylaxis for haemorrhagic disease of the newborn be continued? A decision analysis. *N Z Med J* 1989; **102:** 3–5.
4. Clarkson PM, James AG. Parenteral vitamin $K_1$: the effective prophylaxis against haemorrhagic disease for all newborn infants. *N Z Med J* 1990; **103:** 95–6.
5. McNinch AW, Tripp JH. Haemorrhagic disease of the newborn in the British Isles: two year prospective study. *BMJ* 1991; **303:** 1105–9.
6. Von Kries R. Neonatal vitamin K. *BMJ* 1991; **303:** 1083–4.
7. British Paediatric Association. *Vitamin K prophylaxis in infancy*. London, 1992: British Paediatric Association.
8. von Kries R, *et al.* Repeated oral vitamin K prophylaxis in West Germany: acceptance and efficacy. *BMJ* 1995; **310:** 1097–8.
9. American Academy of Pediatrics Vitamin K Ad Hoc Task Force. Controversies concerning vitamin K and the newborn. *Pediatrics* 1993; **91:** 1001–3.
10. American Academy of Pediatrics Committee on Fetus and Newborn. Controversies concerning vitamin K and the newborn. *Pediatrics* 2003; **112:** 191–2.
11. Barton JS, *et al.* Neonatal vitamin K prophylaxis in the British Isles: current practice and trends. *BMJ* 1995; **310:** 632–3.
12. Rennie JM, Kelsall AWR. Vitamin K prophylaxis in the newborn—again. *Arch Dis Child* 1994; **70:** 248–51.
13. Department of Health. *Vitamin K for newborn babies*. London, 1998: Department of Health.
14. Baenziger O, *et al.* Oral vitamin K prophylaxis for newborn infants: safe enough? *Lancet* 1996; **348:** 1456.
15. Greer FR, *et al.* A new mixed micellar preparation for oral vitamin K prophylaxis: randomised controlled comparison with an intramuscular formulation in breast fed infants. *Arch Dis Child* 1998; **79:** 300–5.
16. von Kries R, *et al.* Oral mixed micellar vitamin K for prevention of late vitamin K deficiency bleeding. *Arch Dis Child Fetal Neonatal Ed* 2003; **88:** F109–F112.
17. Pereira SP, *et al.* Intestinal absorption of mixed micellar phylloquinone (vitamin $K_1$) is unreliable in infants with conjugated hyperbilirubinaemia: implications for oral prophylaxis of vitamin K deficiency bleeding. *Arch Dis Child Fetal Neonatal Ed* 2003; **88:** F113–F118.
18. Cornelissen M, Hirasing R. Vitamin K for neonates. *BMJ* 1994; **309:** 1441–2.
19. Cornelissen M, *et al.* Prevention of vitamin K deficiency bleeding: efficacy of different multiple oral dose schedules of vitamin K. *Eur J Pediatr* 1997; **156:** 126–30.
20. Clark FI, James EJP. Twenty-seven years of experience with oral vitamin $K_1$ therapy in neonates. *J Pediatr* 1995; **127:** 301–4.
21. Nørgaard Hansen K, Ebbesen F. Neonatal vitamin K prophylaxis in Denmark: three years' experience with oral administration during the first three months of life compared with one oral administration at birth. *Acta Paediatr Scand* 1996; **85:** 1137–9.
22. Delgado-Escueta AV, Janz D. Consensus guidelines: preconception counseling, management, and care of the pregnant woman with epilepsy. *Neurology* 1992; **42** (suppl 5): 149–60.
23. Greer FR, *et al.* Improving the vitamin K status of breastfeeding infants with maternal vitamin K supplements. *Pediatrics* 1997; **99:** 88–92.


## Preparations

***BP 2003:*** Menadiol Phosphate Injection; Menadiol Phosphate Tablets; Phytomenadione Injection; Phytomenadione Tablets;
***USP 27:*** Menadiol Sodium Diphosphate Injection; Menadiol Sodium Diphosphate Tablets; Menadione Injection; Phytonadione Injection; Phytonadione Tablets.

**Proprietary Preparations** (details are given in Part 3)
***Arg.:*** K1; Konakion; Mestil-Ka; ***Austral.:*** K Thrombin; Konakion; ***Austria:*** Kavitol; Konakion; Vikaman†; ***Belg.:*** Konakion; Vitamon K; ***Braz.:*** Kanakion; Kavit; Vikatron; ***Chile:*** Auriderm Corps; Konakion MM; ***Denm.:*** Konakion; ***Fin.:*** Konakion; ***Ger.:*** Kanavit; Konakion; Pertix-Solo†; ***Gr.:*** Konakion; ***Hong Kong:*** Konakion; ***India:*** Kenadion; ***Irl.:*** Konakion; ***Israel:*** Konakion; ***Ital.:*** Konakion; ***Jpn:*** Glakay; Kaytwo; ***Mex.:*** K-50; Konakion; ***Neth.:*** Konakion; ***Norw.:*** Konakion Novum; ***NZ:*** K-Thrombin;

Konakion; **Port.:** Kanakion; **S.Afr.:** Konakion; **Singapore:** Konakion†; **Spain:** Kaergona Hidrosoluble; Konakion; **Swed.:** Konakion; **Switz.:** Konakion; **Thai.:** Glakay; Konakion; KP; **UK:** Konakion; Synkavit†; **USA:** Aquamephyton; Mephyton.

**Multi-ingredient: Arg.:** Antidiar; Estreptocarbocaftiazol; Kacerutin; **Austral.:** Chilblain Formula†; **Braz.:** Enteromicina†; Frenovex†; **Chile:** Hepabil; Katin; **Fr.:** Bilkaby†; **Hong Kong:** Haemosol†; **India:** Cadisper C; K5 Hair Tincture; Kalpastic; Siochrome; Styptocid; **Irl.:** Bio-Calcium + $D_3$ + K; **Mex.:** Hemosin-K; Microka; **Spain:** Caprofides Hemostatico; Cromoxin K; Quercetol K†; Vitaendil C K P†; **Thai.:** Siduol.

## Xylitol *(BAN)*

E967; Xilitol; Xylit; *meso*-Xylitol; Xylitolum.

$C_5H_{12}O_5$ = 152.1.

*CAS — 87-99-0 (xylitol); 16277-71-7 (D-xylitol).*

**Pharmacopoeias.** In *Eur.* (see p.vi) and *Jpn.* Also in *USNF.*

**Ph. Eur. 5.0** (Xylitol). White crystals or crystalline powder. M.p. 92° to 96°. Very soluble in water; sparingly soluble in alcohol.

**USNF 22** (Xylitol). White crystals or crystalline powder. Crystalline xylitol has a melting range between 92° and 96°. It has a sweet taste and produces a cooling sensation in the mouth. Soluble 1 in about 0.65 of water; sparingly soluble in alcohol.

### Adverse Effects

Large amounts taken by mouth may cause diarrhoea and flatulence. Ingestion of xylitol is not likely to lead to hyperoxaluria which can occur with intravenous infusion. Hyperuricaemia, changes in liver-function tests, and acidosis (including lactic acidosis) have occurred after intravenous infusion.

### Uses and Administration

Xylitol is a polyhydric alcohol (polyol) related to the pentose sugar, xylose (p.1766). It is used as a bulk sweetener in foods. Xylitol is also used as a sweetening agent in sugar-free preparations as it is non-cariogenic and is less likely to cause dental caries than sucrose. It is under investigation for the prevention of dental caries and acute otitis media. It was formerly considered as a substitute for glucose in intravenous nutrition but such use has generally been abandoned due to adverse effects.

**Dental caries.** Chewing-gum containing xylitol appears to have a useful role in the prevention of dental caries (p.136).[1-3]

1. Edgar WM. Sugar substitutes, chewing gum and dental caries—a review. *Br Dent J* 1998; **184:** 29–32.
2. Gales MA, Nguyen T-M. Sorbitol compared with xylitol in prevention of dental caries. *Ann Pharmacother* 2000; **34:** 98–100.
3. Maguire A, Rugg-Gunn AJ. Xylitol and caries prevention—is it a magic bullet? *Br Dent J* 2003; **194:** 429–36.

**Otitis media.** It has been suggested that xylitol chewing gum[1,2] and xylitol syrup[2,3] may have a preventative effect against acute otitis media (p.138). However, a randomised trial[4] found xylitol to be ineffective when given only during an acute respiratory-tract infection.

1. Uhari M, *et al.* Xylitol chewing gum in prevention of acute otitis media: double blind randomised trial. *BMJ* 1996; **313:** 1180–4.
2. Uhari M, *et al.* A novel use of xylitol sugar in preventing acute otitis media. *Pediatrics* 1998; **102:** 879–84.
3. Uhari M, *et al.* Xylitol in preventing acute otitis media. *Vaccine* 2001; **19:** S144–S147.
4. Tapiainen T, *et al.* Xylitol administered only during respiratory infections failed to prevent acute otitis media. Abstract: *Pediatrics* 2002; **109:** 302. Full version: http://pediatrics.aappublications.org/cgi/content/full/109/2/e19 (accessed 19/05/04)

### Preparations

**Proprietary Preparations** (details are given in Part 3)
**Canad.:** Trident; **Ger.:** Xylit; **Irl.:** Oralbalance†.

**Multi-ingredient: Arg.:** Periobacter; Periodent; **Braz.:** Mentoval†; **Chile:** Oralgene; **Fr.:** Exova; **Ger.:** Cardioplegin N; Duocal†; Kalium-Magnesium-Asparaginat; Kaloplasmal†; salvi CAL GX†; **Mex.:** Dentsiblen; Fluoxytil; Periodentyl; Perioxidin; **UK:** Biotene Oralbalance; BioXtra; Saliva Orthana; Salivace†; **USA:** Optimoist.

## Dried Yeast

Brewers' Yeast; Cerevisiae Fermentum Siccatum; Faex Siccata; Fermento de Cerveja; Levadura desecada; Levedura Sêca; Levure de Bière; Saccharomyces Siccum; Trockenhefe.

**Pharmacopoeias.** In *Jpn.*

### Profile

Dried yeast consists of unicellular fungi belonging to the family Saccharomycetaceae, dried by a process which avoids decomposition of the vitamins present. The chief species are *Saccharomyces cerevisiae, S. carlsbergensis,* and *S. monacensis.* Dried yeast contains thiamine, nicotinic acid, riboflavin, pyridoxine, pantothenic acid, biotin, folic acid, cyanocobalamin, aminobenzoic acid, inositol, and chromium.

Dried yeast is a rich source of vitamins of the B group. It has been used for the prevention and treatment of vitamin B deficiency in doses of 1 to 8 g daily by mouth. Yeast is an ingredient of some preparations for treating haemorrhoids, and some preparations intended to restore normal gastrointestinal flora. Yeast is widely used in brewing.

**Antibiotic-associated colitis.** Although other organisms, including *Candida* spp., have been implicated in antibiotic-associated diarrhoea, colonisation of the colon with *Clostridium difficile,* a toxin-producing Gram-positive anaerobe, is the most common identifiable cause of antibiotic-associated colitis (p.128) and pseudomembranous colitis. There are reports of benefit with dried yeast in patients with *C. difficile*-associated diarrhoea;[1,2] commercially available brewers' yeast tablets were used, at a dose of 3 tablets three times daily (strength unspecified), in 3 patients refractory to standard treatment,[1] or as adjunctive therapy in 11 patients, using the same dose.[2]

1. Schellenberg D, *et al.* Treatment of Clostridium difficile diarrhoea with brewer's yeast. *Lancet* 1994; **343:** 171–2.
2. Barthram J, *et al.* Further research warranted. *Pharm J* 1997; **259:** 371.

### Preparations

**Proprietary Preparations** (details are given in Part 3)
**Belg.:** Preparation H Sperti†; **Braz.:** Bioflorin; Diarril†; Florax; Ginoflorax; **Fr.:** Microlev; **Ger.:** Faexojodan†; Furunkulosin; Levurinetten N; **India:** Laviest; **Ital.:** Lievitovit 300†; Nutrivit; Zimocel; **Mex.:** Cervekanin†; Levadin†; Levifusa; Leza†; **Port.:** Lio-Levedura; **Thai.:** Brewers Yeast; **UK:** Bio-Strath.

**Multi-ingredient: Austral.:** Bio-Chromium†; ML 20†; Plantiodine Plus†; Preparation H†; Vitaglow Selemite B†; **Austria:** Levurinetten; Sperti Preparation H; **Braz.:** Carbo-Levedo†; Composto Emagrecedor; Emagrevit; Manolio†; Preparado H†; Staphylase†; **Canad.:** Preparation H; **Chile:** Sperti (Preparation H); **Fr.:** Actisoufre; Calciforte; Carbolevure; Carbophagix†; Fluorocalciforte†; Levure Or; Phytophanere; Preparation H; Solacy; Spasmag; **Ger.:** Haut-Vital N†; Imbak†; Pantovigar N; Sperti Preparation H; **India:** Elferri; Livogen; Medithane; Plastules; **Irl.:** Preparation H; **Israel:** Preparation H; **Ital.:** Aclon Lievit†; Alvear Complex†; Bifilact; Bio-Real†; Eurogel; Florelax; Lactisporin; Lactivis; Lactolife; Lactovit†; Levudin; Lievistar†; Lievitosohn; Lievitovit; Preparazione H; Sillix; Sillix C; Vigogel†; **Neth.:** Sperti Preparation H; **Port.:** Bioregime Fort; Sperti Preparacao H; **S.Afr.:** Revaton†; **Singapore:** Preparation H; **Spain:** Preparacion H; **Switz.:** A Vogel Capsules polyvitaminees; Carbolevure; Sperti Preparation H; **UK:** B Complex†; Bio-Strath Artichoke Formula; Bio-Strath Valerian Formula; Bio-Strath Willow Formula; Brewers Yeast; Brewers Yeast with Garlic†; Preparation H; Tonic Yeast; Yeast Vite; **USA:** Medicone; Preparation H; Rectagene Medicated Balm; Wyanoids Relief Factor.

## Zinc

Zn = 65.409.

*CAS — 7440-66-6.*

## Zinc Acetate

E650; Zinc, acetato de; Zinci Acetas Dihydricus.

$(CH_3CO_2)_2Zn,2H_2O$ = 219.5.

*CAS — 557-34-6 (anhydrous zinc acetate); 5970-45-6 (zinc acetate dihydrate).*

*ATC — A16AX05.*

NOTE. Zinc Acetate, Basic is *rINN.*

**Pharmacopoeias.** In *Eur.* (see p.vi) and *US.*

**Ph. Eur. 5.0** (Zinc Acetate Dihydrate; Zinc Acetate BP 2003). A white crystalline powder or leaflets. Freely soluble in water; soluble in alcohol. A 5% solution in water has a pH of 5.8 to 7.0. Store in nonmetallic containers.

**USP 27** (Zinc Acetate). White crystals or granules having a slight acetous odour. Is slightly efflorescent. Soluble 1 in 2.5 of water and 1 in 30 of alcohol; freely soluble in boiling alcohol. pH of a 5% solution in water is between 6.0 and 8.0. Store in airtight containers.

## Zinc Chloride

Zinc, cloruro de; Zinci Chloridum; Zincum Chloratum.

$ZnCl_2$ = 136.3.

*CAS — 7646-85-7.*

*ATC — B05XA12.*

**Pharmacopoeias.** In *Eur.* (see p.vi), *Jpn, Pol.,* and *US.*

**Ph. Eur. 5.0** (Zinc Chloride). A white, deliquescent, crystalline powder or cast in white sticks. Very soluble in water; freely soluble in alcohol and in glycerol. An approximately 10% solution in water has a pH of 4.6 to 5.5. Store in nonmetallic containers.

**USP 27** (Zinc Chloride). A white or practically white, odourless, crystalline powder, or white or practically white crystalline granules. May also be in porcelain-like masses or moulded into cylinders. It is very deliquescent. Soluble 1 in 0.5 of water, 1 in 1.5 of alcohol, and 1 in 2 of glycerol. Its solution in water or in alcohol is usually slightly turbid, but the turbidity disappears when a small quantity of hydrochloric acid is added. A 10% solution in water is acid to litmus. Store in airtight containers.

**Turbidity.** Zinc chloride almost always contains some oxychloride which produces a slightly turbid aqueous solution. Turbid solutions, except when intended for ophthalmic use, may be cleared by adding gradually a small amount of dilute hydrochloric acid. Solutions of zinc chloride should be filtered through asbestos or sintered glass, since they dissolve paper and cotton wool.

## Zinc Gluconate

Zinc, gluconato de.

$C_{12}H_{22}O_{14}Zn$ = 455.7.

*CAS — 4468-02-4.*

*ATC — A12CB02.*

**Pharmacopoeias.** In *Chin.* and *US.*

**USP 27** (Zinc Gluconate). White or practically white powder or granules. Soluble in water; very slightly soluble in alcohol. pH of a 1% solution in water is between 5.5 and 7.5.

## Zinc Sulfate

Zinc, sulfato de; Zinc Sulphate; Zinci Sulfas; Zincum Sulfuricum.

$ZnSO_4,7H_2O$ = 287.6.

*CAS — 7733-02-0 (anhydrous zinc sulfate); 7446-20-0 (zinc sulfate heptahydrate).*

*ATC — A12CB01.*

NOTE. 'White vitriol' or 'white copperas' is crude zinc sulfate. ZSU is a code approved by the BP 2003 for use on single unit doses of eye drops containing zinc sulfate where the individual container may be too small to bear all the appropriate labelling information.

**Pharmacopoeias.** In *Chin., Eur.* (see p.vi), *Jpn, Pol.,* and *Viet. Eur.* also includes the hexahydrate.

*US* includes the monohydrate and the heptahydrate in one monograph.

**Ph. Eur. 5.0** (Zinc Sulphate Heptahydrate; Zinci Sulfas Heptahydricus). Colourless, transparent, crystals or as a white crystalline powder; efflorescent. Very soluble in water; practically insoluble in alcohol. A 5% solution in water has a pH of 4.4 to 5.6. Store in nonmetallic airtight containers.

**Ph. Eur. 5.0** (Zinc Sulphate Hexahydrate; Zinci Sulfas Hexahydricus). Colourless, transparent, crystals or a white crystalline powder; efflorescent. Very soluble in water; practically insoluble in alcohol. A 5% solution in water has a pH of 4.4 to 5.6. Store in nonmetallic airtight containers.

**USP 27** (Zinc Sulfate). It contains one or seven molecules of water of hydration. Colourless, transparent, prisms, or small needles. May occur as a white, granular, crystalline powder. It is odourless and is efflorescent in dry air. Very soluble in water (heptahydrate); freely soluble in water (monohydrate); practically insoluble in alcohol (monohydrate); insoluble in alcohol (heptahydrate); freely soluble in glycerol (heptahydrate). Its solutions are acid to litmus. Store in airtight containers.

### Adverse Effects, Treatment, and Precautions

The most frequent adverse effects of zinc salts (the gluconate and sulfate) administered by mouth are gastrointestinal and include abdominal pain, dyspepsia, nausea, vomiting, diarrhoea, gastric irritation, and gastritis. These are particularly common if zinc salts are taken on an empty stomach, and may be reduced by administration with meals.

In acute overdosage zinc salts are corrosive, due to the formation of zinc chloride by stomach acid; treatment consists of administration of milk or alkali carbonates and activated charcoal. The use of emetics or gastric lavage should be avoided.

Prolonged administration of high doses of zinc supplements by mouth or parenterally leads to copper deficiency with associated sideroblastic anaemia and neutropenia. Zinc toxicity has occurred after the use of contaminated water in haemodialysis solutions. High serum zinc concentrations may be reduced by using a chelating drug such as sodium calcium edetate (p.1051).

Metal fume fever is an occupational disease associated with inhalation of freshly-oxidised metal fumes, most commonly from zinc, iron or copper. It is characterised by fever, nausea, dyspnoea, and chest pain, and is generally self-limiting and does not appear to be associated with long-term sequelae.

**Effects on the blood.** There have been reports[1,2] of anaemia and neutropenia in patients consuming excessive amounts of zinc supplements for acne.

1. Porea TJ, *et al.* Zinc-induced anemia and neutropenia in an adolescent. *J Pediatr* 2000; **136:** 688–90.
2. Igic PG, *et al.* Toxic effects associated with consumption of zinc. *Mayo Clin Proc* 2002; **77:** 713–16.

**Parenteral nutrition.** Zinc was found to be a common contaminant of various components used for total parenteral nutrition (TPN), and rubber stoppers or glass may have been the source.[1] Levels of zinc found may exceed daily requirements even before the addition of supplementary zinc. The authors suggested it may be important to routinely monitor zinc status in patients receiving long-term TPN, particularly infants and children.

1. Hak EB, *et al.* Chromium and zinc contamination of parenteral nutrient solution components commonly used in infants and children. *Am J Health-Syst Pharm* 1998; **55:** 150–4.

### Interactions

The absorption of zinc may be reduced by iron supplements, penicillamine, phosphorus-containing preparations, and tetracyclines. Zinc supplements reduce the absorption of copper, fluoroquinolones (see Antacids and Metal Ions, under Interactions of Ciprofloxacin, p.190), iron, penicillamine, and tetracyclines (p.267).

### Pharmacokinetics

Zinc is incompletely absorbed from the gastrointestinal tract, and absorption is reduced in the presence of some dietary constituents such as phytates. Bioavailability of dietary zinc varies widely between different sources, but is about 20 to 30%. Zinc is distributed throughout the body with the highest concentrations found in muscle, bone, skin, and prostatic fluids. It is primarily excreted in the faeces, and regulation of faecal losses is important in zinc homoeostasis. Small amounts are lost in urine and perspiration.

### Uses and Administration

Zinc is an essential element of nutrition and traces are present in a wide range of foods. It is a constituent of many enzyme systems and is present in all tissues. Features of zinc deficiency include growth retardation and defects of rapidly-dividing tissues such as the skin, the immune system, and the intestinal mucosa. Water-soluble zinc salts are used as supplements to correct zinc deficiency; for example, in malabsorption syndromes, during parenteral feeding, in conditions with increased body losses (trauma, burns, and protein-losing states), and in acrodermatitis enteropathica (a rare genetic disorder characterised by severe zinc deficiency). They have been tried in the treatment of a large number of conditions that may be related to zinc deficiency.

Doses of zinc salts are usually expressed in terms of elemental zinc, and the following salts contain approximately 50 mg of zinc:

- zinc acetate (dihydrate) 168 mg
- zinc chloride 104 mg
- zinc gluconate 348 mg
- zinc sulfate (heptahydrate) 220 mg

The approximate number of millimoles of zinc contained in these salts are:

- 4.6 mmol in 1 g zinc acetate (dihydrate)
- 7.3 mmol in 1 g zinc chloride
- 2.2 mmol in 1 g zinc gluconate
- 3.5 mmol in 1 g zinc sulfate (heptahydrate)

In deficiency states, zinc is usually given by mouth as the sulfate, the sulfate monohydrate, or the gluconate, in doses of up to 50 mg of elemental zinc three times daily. When intravenous supplements are required, zinc chloride or zinc sulfate may be given; a suggested dose for parenteral nutrition is 6.5 mg of elemental zinc (100 micromoles) daily.

Oral zinc salts, commonly the acetate, may be used as copper absorption inhibitors in Wilson's disease (p.1049).

Zinc sulfate is used topically in a variety of skin conditions mainly for its astringent properties. The insoluble zinc salts, commonly the oxide (p.1163), are used similarly. A 1.2% solution of zinc acetate is used topically in combination with erythromycin in the treatment of acne vulgaris (p.1133). Zinc sulfate is also used as an astringent in eye drops. Zinc chloride has been used for its powerful caustic and astringent properties, usually in very dilute solution, in, for example, mouthwashes.

**Age-related macular degeneration.** High doses of dietary supplements such as betacarotene, vitamin C, vitamin E, and zinc are being promoted for preservation of vision in the elderly but there are no data to suggest any benefit for patients who do not have age-related macular degeneration or have only mild disease and such treatment is not necessarily harmless.[1] For further details see under Betacarotene, p.1423.

1. Anonymous. Antioxidant vitamins and zinc for macular degeneration. *Med Lett Drugs Ther* 2003; **45:** 45–46.

**Common cold.** Zinc salts, in the form of lozenges, have been tried in the treatment of the common cold (p.618) with variable results.[1-6] A systematic review of randomised trials found that there was no strong evidence to recommend their use.[7] Intranasal preparations of zinc sulfate or zinc gluconate have generally proven ineffective.[8,9]

1. Al-Nakib W, *et al.* Prophylaxis and treatment of rhinovirus colds with zinc gluconate lozenges. *J Antimicrob Chemother* 1987; **20:** 893–901.
2. Douglas RM, *et al.* Failure of effervescent zinc acetate lozenges to alter the course of upper respiratory tract infections in Australian adults. *Antimicrob Agents Chemother* 1987; **31:** 1263–5.
3. Smith DS, *et al.* Failure of zinc gluconate in treatment of acute upper respiratory tract infections. *Antimicrob Agents Chemother* 1989; **33:** 646–8.
4. Mossad SB, *et al.* Zinc gluconate lozenges for treating the common cold: a randomized, double-blind, placebo-controlled study. *Ann Intern Med* 1996; **125:** 81–8.
5. Macknin ML, *et al.* Zinc gluconate lozenges for treating the common cold in children: a randomized controlled trial. *JAMA* 1998; **279:** 1962–7.
6. Prasad AS, *et al.* Duration of symptoms and plasma cytokine levels in patients with the common cold treated with zinc acetate: a randomized, double-blind, placebo-controlled trial. *Ann Intern Med* 2000; **133:** 245–52.
7. Marshall I. Zinc for the common cold. Available in The Cochrane Library; Issue 2. Chichester: John Wiley; 2004.
8. Belongia EA, *et al.* A randomized trial of zinc nasal spray for the treatment of upper respiratory illness in adults. *Am J Med* 2001; **111:** 103–8.
9. Turner RB. Ineffectiveness of intranasal zinc gluconate for prevention of experimental rhinovirus colds. *Clin Infect Dis* 2001; **33:** 1865–70.

**Deficiency states.** General references.

1. Bryce-Smith D. Zinc deficiency—the neglected factor. *Chem Br* 1989; **25:** 783–6.
2. Prasad AS. Zinc deficiency: has been known of for 40 years but ignored by global health organisations. *BMJ* 2003; **326:** 409–10.

DIAGNOSIS AND TESTING. A loss of taste acuity is a sign of zinc deficiency (see below) and this has been used as a test for the condition: patients who do not immediately perceive a strong flavour on tasting a dilute (typically 0.1 or 0.2%) solution of zinc sulfate are considered likely to benefit from supplementation. However, a study in pregnant women failed to confirm that the ability to taste such a solution was related to zinc deficiency.[1]

1. Mahomed K, *et al.* Failure to taste zinc sulphate solution does not predict zinc deficiency in pregnancy. *Eur J Obstet Gynecol Reprod Biol* 1993; **48:** 169–75.

DIARRHOEA. Chronic diarrhoea can be a sign of zinc deficiency, and diarrhoea can lead to excessive zinc losses and zinc deficiency when dietary zinc is inadequate. Zinc supplements have been shown to reduce the incidence, intensity, or duration of acute diarrhoea (p.1241) in children in developing countries.[1-4] A pooled analysis of 10 trials performed in developing countries found that zinc supplementation was associated with a 25% reduction in prevalence of diarrhoea.[5]

1. Sazawal S, *et al.* Zinc supplementation in young children with acute diarrhea in India. *N Engl J Med* 1995; **333:** 839–44.
2. Roy SK, *et al.* Randomised controlled trial of zinc supplementation in malnourished Bangladeshi children with acute diarrhoea. *Arch Dis Child* 1997; **77:** 196–200.
3. Ruel MT, *et al.* Impact of zinc supplementation on morbidity from diarrhea and respiratory infections among rural Guatemalan children. *Pediatrics* 1997; **99:** 808–13.
4. Penny ME, *et al.* Randomized, community-based trial of the effect of zinc supplementation, with and without other micronutrients on the duration of persistent childhood diarrhea in Lima, Peru. *J Pediatr* 1999; **135:** 208–17.
5. Bhutta ZA, *et al.* Prevention of diarrhea and pneumonia by zinc supplementation in children in developing countries: pooled analysis of randomized controlled trials. *J Pediatr* 1999; **135:** 689–97.

GROWTH RETARDATION. Growth retardation (p.1314) in a group of short Japanese children without endocrine abnormalities was found to be associated with mild to moderate zinc deficiency; supplementation with zinc sulfate 5 mg/kg daily by mouth over 6 months resulted in an improvement in growth velocity despite unchanged growth hormone production.[1] Similarly, supplementation with 10 mg zinc daily for 6 days of each week, for 6 months, increased the growth rate of stunted Ethiopian infants; weight also increased in both stunted and non-stunted children, and the authors commented that these effects were at least partly due to improvements in appetite, and reduced morbidity from infection.[2]

1. Nakamura T, *et al.* Mild to moderate zinc deficiency in short children: effect of zinc supplementation on linear growth velocity. *J Pediatr* 1993; **123:** 65–9.
2. Umeta M, *et al.* Zinc supplementation and stunted infants in Ethiopia: a randomised controlled trial. *Lancet* 2000; **355:** 2021–6.

TASTE DISORDERS. Zinc appears to be effective for the treatment of taste disturbances (p.682) associated with zinc deficiency but there is insufficient evidence to determine its efficacy for taste dysfunction secondary to conditions that do not involve low serum zinc concentrations.[1]

1. Heyneman CA. Zinc deficiency and taste disorders. *Ann Pharmacother* 1996; **30:** 186–7.

**Human requirements.** In the UK dietary reference values (DRV)[1] and in the USA recommended dietary allowances (RDA)[2] have been published for zinc (see p.1419 for an explanation of these terms). In the UK the reference nutrient intake (RNI) for adult males and females is 9.5 and 7.0 mg daily respectively; values are also given for infants and children of varying ages and for lactating women. In the USA the RDA for adults is 11 mg daily for men and 8 mg daily for women.[2] The tolerable upper intake level is 40 mg daily. WHO recommend lower limits of the safe ranges of population mean intakes of dietary zinc for 3 categories of diets based on high, moderate, and low zinc bioavailability: values are 4.0, 6.5, and 13.1 mg dietary zinc daily for women, and 5.6, 9.4, and 18.7 mg dietary zinc daily for men, respectively.[3] They recommend an upper limit of the safe range of population mean intakes of zinc of 35 mg daily for women, and 45 mg daily for men.

1. DoH. Dietary reference values for food energy and nutrients for the United Kingdom: report of the panel on dietary reference values of the committee on medical aspects of food policy. *Report on health and social subjects 41.* London: HMSO, 1991.
2. Standing Committee on the Scientific Evaluation of Dietary Reference Intakes of the Food and Nutrition Board. *Dietary Reference Intakes for vitamin A, vitamin K, arsenic, boron, chromium, copper, iodine, iron, manganese, molybdenum, nickel, silicon, vanadium, and zinc.* Washington DC: National Academy Press, 2001. Also available at: http://www.nap.edu/catalog/10026.html (accessed 24/05/04)
3. WHO. Zinc. In: *Trace elements in human nutrition and health.* Geneva: WHO, 1996: 72–104.

**Wilson's disease.** References.

1. Anderson LA, *et al.* Zinc acetate treatment in Wilson's disease. *Ann Pharmacother* 1998; **32:** 78–87.

## Preparations

***BP 2003:*** Zinc Sulphate Eye Drops; Zinc Sulphate Lotion;
***USP 27:*** White Lotion; Zinc Chloride Injection; Zinc Sulfate Injection; Zinc Sulfate Ophthalmic Solution.

**Proprietary Preparations** (details are given in Part 3)

***Arg.:*** Z-Kraft; ***Austral.:*** Bioglan Zinc Chelate†; Zincaps; ***Austria:*** Solvezink; Zinkamin; ***Braz.:*** Zincopan; ZN Xampu; ***Canad.:*** Anu-Aide; Anusol; Anuzinc; Egozinc; Fisherman's Friend Zinc; Micro Zn†; PMS-Egozinc†; Rivasol; ***Chile:*** Biolane; Num-Zit; ***Denm.:*** Solvezink†; ***Fin.:*** Solvezink†; ***Fr.:*** Rubozinc; Vitazinc†; Zymizinc; ***Ger.:*** Biolectra Zink; Biosan Zink; Cefazink; Curazink; Nefro-Zinc; Ophtopur-Z; Solvezink; Unizink; Virudermin; Zink beta; Zink Verla; Zink-D Longoral; Zink-Ratiopharm; Zink-Sandoz; Zinkamin; Zinkbrause; Zinkit; Zinkorot; zinkotase; ***Hong Kong:*** Anuzinc†; Egozinc; Zincaps; ***Israel:*** Avazinc; Zincol; ***Ital.:*** Pontefix; ***Mex.:*** Metazinc†; Zn-Fusin; ***Norw.:*** Solvezink; ***NZ:*** Elemental Zinc; Zincaps; ***S.Afr.:*** ZN 220†; ***Swed.:*** Solvezink; ***Switz.:*** Collazin; Virudermin; ***Thai.:*** Zincaps; Zinctab; ***UK:*** Cold-Gard†; Solvazinc; Tartar Control Listerine; Z Span†; Zincosol; ***USA:*** Eye-Sed†; Halls Zinc Defense; Ivy Dry; Orazinc; Verazinc; Zinca-Pak; Zincate.

**Multi-ingredient:** ***Arg.:*** Caladryl Incoloro; Callicida; Cicatrina; Clean-AC; Cleanance; Crema de Ordene; Dermalibour; Kelual Zinc; Lacto-Cev Zn; Lactocrem Bebe; Lagrimas de Santa Lucia; Litiofarm; Megaplus; Negacne; Ninderm; ***Austral.:*** Antioxidant Forte Tablets†; Antioxidant Tablets†; APR Cream; Beta A-C†; Beta-Ace Tablets†; Bio-Chromium†; Bioglan Joint Mobility†; Bioglan The Blue One†; Bioglan Zn-A-C†; Caprilate†; Children's Calcium With Minerals†; Cold and Flu Relief†; Cold Sore Relief†; Cold Sore Tablets†; Echinacea & Antioxidants†; Echinacea 4000†; Echinacea ACE + Zinc†; Echinacea ACE Plus Zinc†; Echinacea Complex†; Echinacea Herbal Plus Formula†; Extralife Eye-Care†; Extralife Flow-Care†; Galium Complex†; Goodnight Formula†; Horse Radish and Garlic Tablets†; In A Wink†; Lifechange Mens Complex with Saw Palmetto†; Lifesystem Herbal Plus Formula 8 Echinacea†; Logicin Natural Lozenges; Natures Way Total Zinc†; Odourless Garlic†; Prefrin Z†; Proyeast†; Serenoa Complex†; Sinus and Hayfever†; Strepsils Zinc Cold Relief†; Trifolium Complex†; Urapro†; Visine Allergy†; Vita-Minis Cold & Flu†; Z-Acne†; ZBM†; Zinc + C250†; Zinc C Plus†; Zinc Plus†; Zinc Supplement†; Zinc Zenith†; Zincfrin; Zinvit C†; Zinvit G†; Zinvit†; ***Austria:*** Efalith; Ophtaguttal; Zeller-Augenwasser; ***Belg.:*** Zincfrin; Zincfrin Antihistaminicum; Zineryt; ***Braz.:*** Antiseptin†; Babyglos†; Belagin; Borato de Sodio†; Colirio Blumen†; Colirio Helios†; Colirio Legrand; Colirio Moura Brasil†; Colirio Teuto; Colirio Vima†; Dexa-Vastrictol†; Efederm†; Fluo-Vaso; Kalloplast†; Mirabel; Mirorroidin; Neo Vastrictol†; Pomada Blumen†; Pomada Martel†; Vastrictol†; Verlin†; Visiplex; Visolon†; Visual; Zincolok; ***Canad.:*** Anodan-HC; Anugesic-HC; Anusol Plus; Anusol-HC; Anuzinc HC; Anuzinc HC Plus; Beminal Z†; Hemcort HC; Hemorrhoid Ointment; Lipactin; Listerine Antisptic Tartar Control; Onguent Hemorrhoidal; Orajel Mouth Aid; PMS-Egozinc-HC; Proctodan-HC; ProstGard; Rectogel; Rectogel HC; Rivasol HC; Visine Allergy; Zinc Plus; Zincfrin; Zincfrin-A; ***Chile:*** Agua Sulfatada Picrica; Caladryl Clear; Clean-AC; Cleanance; Deltisan; Gingilacer; Oculosan; Orajel Compuesto; Pomada Antihemorroidal; Primacy C+AHA; ***Denm.:*** Zincfrin; ***Fin.:*** Wicnelact; Zincfrin; Zincfrin-A; ***Fr.:*** Aftagel; Alphane†; Arbum; Cicalfate; Cystel Shampooing Antiseborrheique; Cysti-Z; Dermalibour; Dermo-Sulfuryl; Femiplexe†; Kelual Zinc; Keralac Plus; Keraliss 14†; Ramet Dalibour†; Ramet Pain†; Ruboderm†; Septalibour; Serozinc; Visiolyre†; Vitasedine†; YSE; YSE Glutamique; Zeniac; Zeniac LP; ***Ger.:*** Baran-mild N†; Efadermin; Gehwol Nagelpilz; Lipactin; Oculosan N; Zincfrin; Zineryt; ***Hong Kong:*** Aderma Dermalibour; Chelated Zinc†; Hemcort HC; Oculosan; Osteocare; Visine Allergy Relief; ***India:*** Andre; Elferri-Z; Fecontin-Z; Fefol-Z; Ferrochelate-Z; New Eye Lotion; Ocurest-Z; Zad-G; Zinco Sulpha; ***Irl.:*** Efalith; Zineryt; ***Israel:*** Hemo; Visine AC; ***Ital.:*** Acnesan; Bagno Oculare; Cuprosodio; Cuprosodio Plus; Emmenoiasi; Forbrand; Formedico; Ginsana Ton; Indaco; Influ-Zinc; Influ-Zinc Gola; Lozione Same AS†; Meziv; Zinc-Imizol; Zincometil; Zineryt; ***Malaysia:*** Adult Citrex; Oculosan; Zincfrin; ***Mex.:*** Afazol Z; Dalidome; Exastrin; Periodentyl; Z Frin; ***Neth.:*** Zineryt; ***NZ:*** Clear Eyes ACR; Efalith†; Listerine Tartar Control; Prefrin Z†; Redoxon Double Action; Zinc Defence; Zincfrin; ***Port.:*** Bioclin Sebo Care; Kemphor; Mentofenol†; Oralbiotico; Oratol; Zineryt; ***S.Afr.:*** Nazene; Oculoforte; Oculosan; ***Singapore:*** New Daigaku; Redoxon Double Action; Vita Calmag Zn; ***Spain:*** Acnosan†; Buco Regis; Cilinavagin Neomicina†; Clo Zinc†; Cloram Zinc; Coliriocilina Adren Astr; Dexa Vasoc†; Fluo Vasoc†; Mirantal†; Odamida; Odontocromil c Sulfamida; Vasocon Ant†; Vasoconstr†; Zincfrin; Zineryt; ***Swed.:*** Mezinc; Zincfrin; ***Switz.:*** Acne Lotion; Bonactin†; Collypan; Efalith; Hima-Pasta nouvelle formule; Lipactin; Oculosan; Oculosan forte†; Rocanal Permanent Gangrene†; Rocanal Permanent Vital†; Zincfrin†; ***Thai.:*** Oculosan; Opplin; Visotone; Zincfrin†; ***UK:*** Brushtox†; Ceezinc†; Dispello; Efalith†; Flavo-Zinc; Lypsyl Cold Sore Gel; Osteocare; Redoxon Double Action; Se-Power; Strepsils Zinc Defence; Vicks Vital; Zineryt; ***USA:*** Amerigel; Benadryl Itch; Caladryl Clear; Clear Eyes ACR; Dermasept Antifungal; Gets-It; Nasal-Ease; Orajel Mouth Aid; Sulpho-Lac; Super Ivy Dry; VasoClear A; Visine Allergy Relief; Ze Caps; Zincfrin.

# Organic Solvents

Most of the solvents described in this chapter have no specific therapeutic use. Additional solvents used in pharmacy and described in other chapters include alcohols, chlorinated hydrocarbons such as chloroform and trichloroethylene, fixed oils, glycols, paraffins, and water.

Organic solvents are widely used in industry and toxicity may follow acute or chronic exposure. Adverse effects may occur due to inhalation, ingestion, or absorption through the skin. Organic solvents are irritant to the skin and mucous membranes, and also commonly affect the CNS. They may sensitise the myocardium to catecholamines and cardiac arrhythmias may occur. Chronic exposure may lead to central and peripheral neurotoxicity, as well as to renal toxicity and hepatotoxicity.

◊ References.


1. White RF, Proctor SP. Solvents and neurotoxicity. *Lancet* 1997; **349:** 1239–43.


**Abuse.** Since they are volatile liquids and have CNS effects many organic solvents are implicated in volatile substance abuse. Clinical features of intoxication are similar to those of alcohol intoxication, with initial CNS stimulation followed by CNS depression, which may progress to delirium, convulsions, coma, and death. Sudden death due to cardiac arrhythmias has also been reported.

References.


1. Proceedings of a meeting on substance abuse. *Hum Toxicol* 1989; **8:** 253–334.
2. Ashton CH. Solvent abuse. *BMJ* 1990; **300:** 135–6.


## Acetone

Acetona; Acetonum; Dimethyl Ketone; 2-Propanone.

$C_3H_6O$ = 58.08.

*CAS — 67-64-1.*

**Pharmacopoeias.** In *Eur.* (see p.vi). Also in *USNF.*

**Ph. Eur. 5.0** (Acetone). A volatile, clear, colourless liquid; the vapour is flammable. Miscible with water and with alcohol. Protect from light.

**USNF 22** (Acetone). A transparent, colourless, mobile, volatile, very flammable liquid, having a characteristic odour. Sp. gr. not more than 0.789. Miscible with water, with alcohol, with chloroform, with ether, and with most volatile oils. A 50% solution in water is neutral to litmus. Store in airtight containers remote from fire.

### Adverse Effects and Treatment

Inhalation of acetone vapour causes excitement followed by CNS depression with headache, restlessness, fatigue, and possibly convulsions, leading to coma and respiratory depression in severe cases. Vomiting and haematemesis may occur. There may be a latent period before the onset of symptoms of acetone poisoning. Similar symptoms may be seen after ingestion of acetone although hyperglycaemia has also been reported. The vapour is irritant to mucous membranes in high concentrations.

Acetone is commonly implicated in volatile substance abuse (see above).

Treatment of adverse effects consists of removal from exposure and general supportive and symptomatic measures; activated charcoal may be given if the patient presents within 1 hour of ingestion.

◊ For the possible effect of acetone on the metabolism of acetonitrile, see under Acetonitrile, below.

### Pharmacokinetics

Acetone is absorbed through the lungs following inhalation. Some absorption occurs from the gastrointestinal tract. It is mostly excreted unchanged, predominantly through the lungs and also in the urine.

### Uses

Acetone is widely used as an industrial, pharmaceutical, and domestic solvent; it is also used as an extraction solvent in food processing.

## Acetonitrile

Acetonitrilo; Ethanenitrile; Methyl Cyanide.

$C_2H_3N$ = 41.05.

*CAS — 75-05-8.*

**Description.** Acetonitrile is a colourless liquid with an aromatic odour. Wt per mL about 0.79 g. B.p. about 81°. It emits highly toxic fumes of hydrogen cyanide when heated to decomposition or when reacted with acids or oxidising agents. Store in airtight containers.

### Adverse Effects and Treatment

As for cyanides (see Hydrocyanic Acid, p.1506).

◊ Cyanide poisoning, including a fatality, has been reported[1,2] in a number of infants following ingestion of artificial nail removers containing acetonitrile. As acetonitrile is slowly metabolised to cyanide, serious toxic effects may not occur until several hours after ingestion and there is the danger that these products may be confused with acetone-based nail polish removers which are less toxic. In a report[3] of an adult who died after ingestion of acetonitrile, the onset of symptoms was delayed for 24 hours. It was considered that concomitant ingestion of acetone had slowed the metabolism of acetonitrile.


1. Caravati EM, Litovitz TL. Pediatric cyanide intoxication and death from an acetonitrile-containing cosmetic. *JAMA* 1988; **260:** 3470–3.
2. Losek JD, *et al.* Cyanide poisoning from a cosmetic nail remover. *Pediatrics* 1991; **88:** 337–40.
3. Boggild MD, *et al.* Acetonitrile ingestion: delayed onset of cyanide poisoning due to concurrent ingestion of acetone. *Postgrad Med J* 1990; **66:** 40–1.


### Pharmacokinetics

Acetonitrile is absorbed by inhalation, ingestion, and through the skin. It undergoes metabolism to cyanide, which is responsible for the toxicity of acetonitrile.

### Uses

Acetonitrile is used as an industrial solvent. It may also be present in artificial nail removers.

## Amyl Acetate

Acetato de amilo.

$C_7H_{14}O_2$ = 130.2.

*CAS — 123-92-2 (iso-amyl acetate); 53496-15-4 (sec-amyl acetate); 628-63-7 (n-amyl acetate).*

**Description.** Amyl acetate is a mixture of isomers, principally *iso-*, *sec-*, and *n*-amyl acetate. *iso*-Amyl acetate is a clear colourless liquid with a sharp, fruity odour. Wt per mL about 0.87 g. B.p. about 140°. Slightly soluble in water; miscible with alcohol and with ether. Store in airtight containers.

### Adverse Effects and Treatment

Prolonged exposure to amyl acetate may produce headache, fatigue, and depression of the CNS. Irritation of mucous membranes may also occur.

Treatment of adverse effects consists of removal from exposure and general supportive and symptomatic measures; activated charcoal may be given if the patient presents within 1 hour of ingestion.

**Effects on the heart.** A 27-year-old man developed headache, nausea, and vomiting after using a paint containing amyl acetate as the solvent in an unventilated room.[1] Some days later chest pain and dyspnoea developed; he was admitted to hospital 2 weeks after exposure with heart failure which slowly responded to treatment.


1. Weissberg PL, Green ID. Methyl-cellulose paint possibly causing heart failure. *BMJ* 1979; **ii:** 1113–14.


### Uses

Amyl acetate is used as a pharmaceutical and industrial solvent.

## Amylene Hydrate

Aethyldimethylmethanolum; Dimethylethyl Carbinol; Hidrato de amileno; Tertiary Amyl Alcohol. 2-Methylbutan-2-ol.

$C_5H_{12}O$ = 88.15.

*CAS — 75-85-4.*

**Pharmacopoeias.** In *USNF.*

**USNF 22** (Amylene Hydrate). A clear, colourless liquid having a camphoraceous odour. Sp. gr. 0.803 to 0.807. Distilling range 97° to 103°. Freely soluble in water; miscible with alcohol, with chloroform, with ether, and with glycerol. Its solutions are neutral to litmus. Store in airtight containers.

### Adverse Effects

Amylene hydrate is irritant and has a depressant effect on the CNS.

### Uses

Amylene hydrate is used as a pharmaceutical solvent. It was formerly used as a hypnotic.

## Aniline

Anilina; Phenylamine.

$C_6H_7N$ = 93.13.

*CAS — 62-53-3.*

**Description.** Aniline is a colourless or pale yellow oily liquid with a characteristic odour, readily darkening to brown on exposure to air and light. Wt per mL about 1.02 g. B.p. about 183°. Store in airtight containers. Protect from light.

### Adverse Effects, Treatment, and Precautions

Inhalation, ingestion, or cutaneous absorption of aniline results in methaemoglobinaemia, with cyanosis, headache, weakness, stupor, convulsions, and coma. Irritation of the skin or mucous membranes, nausea and vomiting, and cardiac arrhythmias may occur. Haemolysis has been reported and may give rise to renal damage or jaundice. Death is usually a result of cardiovascular collapse.

Treatment may involve oxygen, methylthioninium chloride (p.1043), transfusions, or possibly haemodialysis. Gastric aspiration or activated charcoal may be considered in patients who present within 1 hour of ingestion.

Bladder papillomas have been reported in workers previously exposed to aniline. Commercial aniline may be contaminated with β-naphthylamine, a potential carcinogen.

**Handling.** Suitable precautions should be taken to avoid skin contact with aniline as it can penetrate skin and produce systemic toxicity.

### Uses

Aniline is a solvent with wide industrial applications.

## Benzene

Benceno; Phenyl Hydride.

$C_6H_6$ = 78.11.

*CAS — 71-43-2.*

NOTE. Benzene may be known as 'benzina', 'benzol', 'benzole', or 'benzolum'. However, 'benzol' is also used to describe a mixture of hydrocarbons and 'benzin' or 'benzine' is used as a name for a petroleum distillate (see also Petroleum Spirit, p.1476).

**Description.** Benzene is a clear colourless flammable liquid with a characteristic aromatic odour. Wt per mL about 0.88 g. B.p. about 80°. Store in airtight containers.

### Adverse Effects, Treatment, and Precautions

Symptoms of acute poisoning following inhalation or ingestion of benzene include initial excitement or euphoria followed by CNS depression with headache, dizziness, blurred vision, and ataxia, which in severe cases may progress to coma (accompanied by hyperactive reflexes), convulsions, and death from respiratory failure. Other symptoms include nausea and irritation of the mucous membranes; ventricular arrhythmias may occur. Direct skin contact with liquid benzene may result in marked irritation, and dermatitis may develop on prolonged or repeated exposure.

Prolonged industrial exposure to benzene vapour has been associated with adverse effects on the gastrointestinal tract and the CNS but in particular with marked effects on the bone marrow and blood. Decreases in the numbers of red or white blood cells or of platelets may occur, producing symptoms of headache, fatigue, anorexia, pallor, and petechiae. In severe cases pancytopenia or aplastic anaemia may develop. Leukaemia, particularly acute myeloid leukaemia, has also developed, often many years after exposure to benzene has ceased. These effects have been reported in workers exposed to relatively high concentrations of the vapour (around 200 ppm or more) but reduced red blood cell counts and anaemia have also been reported at lower concentrations. Chromosome abnormalities have been observed after prolonged exposure to benzene, particularly at the higher concentrations associated with blood dyscrasias; however, the significance of these abnormalities in the development of leukaemia is unclear.

Treatment of poisoning consists of symptomatic and supportive measures. Gastric lavage may be performed for acute intoxication if the patient presents within 1 hour of ingestion but care must be taken to avoid aspiration. Activated charcoal may be given. In chronic poisoning, repeated blood transfusions may be necessary. Adrenaline and other sympathomimetics should be avoided because of the risk of precipitating cardiac arrhythmias.

◊ Reviews.


1. Health and Safety Executive. Benzene. *Toxicity Review 4.* London: HMSO, 1982.
2. Benzene. *Environmental Health Criteria 150.* Geneva: WHO, 1993. Available at: http://www.inchem.org/documents/ehc/ehc/ehc150.htm (accessed 29/06/04)


**Malignant neoplasms.** Epidemiological data support an association between benzene exposure and acute myeloid leukaemia, but the risk following low levels of exposure (1 to 10 ppm) is less clear.[1] However, a large cohort study[2] suggested that there is an increased risk of acute myeloid leukaemia and of non-Hodgkin's lymphoma with benzene exposure at levels below 10 ppm.


1. Austin H, *et al.* Benzene and leukemia: a review of the literature and a risk assessment. *Am J Epidemiol* 1988; **127:** 419–39.
2. Hayes RB, *et al.* Benzene and the dose-related incidence of hematologic neoplasms in China. *J Natl Cancer Inst* 1997; **89:** 1065–71.


**Pregnancy.** An evaluation of the USA National Natality and Fetal Mortality Survey noted that maternal or paternal occupational exposure to agents such as benzene was associated with an increased risk of still-birth and that paternal exposure to benzene increased the risk of low-birth-weight infants.[1]


1. Savitz DA, *et al.* Effect of parents' occupational exposures on risk of stillbirth, preterm delivery, and small-for-gestational-age infants. *Am J Epidemiol* 1989; **129:** 1201–18.

#### Pharmacokinetics

Benzene is absorbed after inhalation and ingestion, but is not significantly absorbed through the skin. Some is excreted unchanged from the lungs. Oxidation to phenol and related quinol compounds occurs, the metabolites being excreted in the urine as conjugates of sulfuric or glucuronic acid.

#### Uses

Benzene was formerly applied as a pediculicide. Its use as an industrial solvent is decreasing.

## Butyl Acetate

Acetato de butilo. *n*-Butyl acetate.

$C_6H_{12}O_2$ = 116.2.

*CAS — 123-86-4.*

**Description.** Butyl acetate is a clear, colourless flammable liquid with a strong fruity odour. Wt per mL about 0.88 g. B.p. 123° to 126°. Slightly soluble in water; miscible with alcohol. Store in airtight containers.

#### Adverse Effects

Butyl acetate is irritant. High concentrations may cause CNS depression.

#### Uses

Butyl acetate is used as an industrial solvent and as an extraction solvent in food processing.

## Butyl Alcohol

Alcohol butílico; *n*-Butanol; *n*-Butyl Alcohol. Butan-1-ol.

$C_4H_{10}O$ = 74.12.

*CAS — 71-36-3.*

**Pharmacopoeias.** In *USNF.*

**USNF 22** (Butyl Alcohol). A clear, colourless, mobile liquid having a characteristic, penetrating vinous odour. Sp. gr. 0.807 to 0.809. It distils within a range of 1.5°, including 117.7°. Soluble in water; miscible with alcohol, with ether, and with many other organic solvents. Store in airtight containers at a temperature not exceeding 40°.

#### Adverse Effects and Precautions

Butyl alcohol may be irritant and may cause mild CNS depression with headache, dizziness, and drowsiness.

◊ References to the toxicity of butyl alcohol.


1. Butanols—four isomers: 1-butanol, 2-butanol, tert-butanol, isobutanol. *Environmental Health Criteria 65.* Geneva: WHO, 1987. Available at: http://www.inchem.org/documents/ehc/ehc/ehc65.htm (accessed 29/06/04)
2. 1-Butanol health and safety guide. *IPCS Health and Safety Guide 3.* Geneva: WHO, 1987. Available at: http://www.inchem.org/documents/hsg/hsg/hsg003.htm (accessed 29/06/04)


**Handling.** Suitable precautions should be taken to avoid skin contact with butyl alcohol as it can penetrate skin and produce systemic toxicity.

#### Uses

Butyl alcohol is used as an industrial and pharmaceutical solvent and as an extraction solvent in food processing.

## Butylamine

Butilamina; *n*-Butylamine.

$C_4H_{11}N$ = 73.14.

*CAS — 109-73-9.*

**Description.** Butylamine is a colourless to pale yellow flammable liquid with an ammoniacal odour. Wt per mL about 0.744 g. B.p. about 78°. Miscible with water, with alcohol, and with ether. Store in airtight containers.

#### Adverse Effects and Precautions

Butylamine is irritant. Symptoms of CNS depression may be observed after exposure to high concentrations of the vapour.

**Handling.** Suitable precautions should be taken to avoid skin contact with butylamine as it can penetrate skin and produce systemic toxicity.

#### Uses

Butylamine is used as a solvent.

## Carbon Disulfide

Carbon Bisulphide; Carbon Disulphide; Carbonei Sulfidum; Carboneum Bisulfuratum; Carboneum Sulfuratum; Disulfuro de carbono; Schwefelkohlenstoff.

$CS_2$ = 76.14.

*CAS — 75-15-0.*

**Description.** Carbon disulfide is a clear, colourless, volatile, flammable liquid with a chloroform-like odour. Commercial grades have an unpleasant odour described by some as being reminiscent of decaying radishes. Wt per mL about 1.26 g. B.p. about 46°. Store in airtight containers.

**Stability.** The vapour of carbon disulfide when mixed with air in the proportions of 1 to 50% is highly explosive.

#### Adverse Effects, Treatment, and Precautions

Carbon disulfide is irritant. Toxic effects may occur as a result of inhalation, ingestion, or absorption through the skin.

Acute poisoning may result in gastrointestinal disturbances and euphoria, followed by CNS depression. Symptoms include headache, dizziness, mood changes, and in severe cases, manic psychoses, delirium, hallucinations, coma, convulsions, and death due to respiratory failure.

Chronic poisoning has been associated with occupational exposure to carbon disulfide vapour for prolonged periods. It is characterised by peripheral neuropathies; CNS effects such as headache, fatigue, insomnia, tremor, emotional lability, extrapyramidal disorders, bipolar disorder, and encephalopathy; gastrointestinal effects including anorexia, dyspepsia, and ulcerative changes; and effects on the eye. Occupational exposure to carbon disulfide has been shown to be associated with an increased incidence of mortality from coronary heart disease. The action of carbon disulfide on endocrine function has resulted in menstrual irregularities, an increased incidence of spontaneous abortions and premature births, loss of libido, sperm abnormalities, and decreased serum-thyroxine concentrations; there is limited evidence of impaired glucose tolerance.

Treatment consists of removal from exposure and general supportive and symptomatic measures. Gastric lavage may be performed if the patient presents within 1 hour of ingestion; activated charcoal may be given. Adrenaline and other sympathomimetics should be avoided because of the risk of precipitating cardiac arrhythmias. Peripheral neuropathies may be only slowly reversible.

◊ Reviews of the toxicity of carbon disulfide.


1. Carbon Disulfide. *Environmental Health Criteria 10.* Geneva: WHO, 1979. Available at: http://www.inchem.org/documents/ehc/ehc/ehc010.htm (accessed 29/06/04)
2. WHO. Recommended health-based limits in occupational exposure to selected organic solvents. *WHO Tech Rep Ser 664* 1981.
3. Health and Safety Executive. Carbon disulphide. *Toxicity Review 3.* London: HMSO, 1981.


**Effects on endocrine function.** The effects of exposure to carbon disulfide were studied retrospectively in 265 female workers in the rayon industry exposed for at least 1 year, and 291 non-exposed female workers.[1] Levels of exposure varied over the study period from 0.7 to 30.6 mg/m³. Women exposed to carbon disulfide had a higher risk of menstrual disturbances than non-exposed women. However, there was no difference between the 2 groups in incidence of toxaemia, emesis gravidarum, spontaneous abortion, premature or overdue delivery, or congenital malformation.


1. Zhou SY, *et al.* Effects of occupational exposure to low-level carbon disulfide ($CS_2$) on menstruation and pregnancy. *Ind Health* 1988; **26:** 203–14.


**Effects on the heart.** An increased incidence of mortality from cardiovascular disease has been found in workers occupationally exposed to carbon disulfide.[1-3] The evidence suggests that the risk decreases after cessation of exposure.


1. Nurminen M, Hernberg S. Effects of intervention on the cardiovascular mortality of workers exposed to carbon disulphide: a 15 year follow up. *Br J Ind Med* 1985; **42:** 32–5.
2. Sweetnam PM, *et al.* Exposure to carbon disulphide and ischaemic heart disease in a viscose rayon factory. *Br J Ind Med* 1987; **44:** 220–7.
3. MacMahon B, Monson RR. Mortality in the US rayon industry. *J Occup Med* 1988; **30:** 698–705.


**Handling.** Suitable precautions should be taken to avoid skin contact with carbon disulfide as it can penetrate skin and produce systemic toxicity.

#### Pharmacokinetics

Carbon disulfide is rapidly absorbed after inhalation and ingestion, and is also absorbed through intact skin. It is excreted unchanged through the lungs and in the urine predominantly as metabolites.

#### Uses

Carbon disulfide is used as an industrial solvent and has been used, in the vapour form, as an insecticide.

## Carbon Tetrachloride

Tetracloruro de carbono. Tetrachloromethane.

$CCl_4$ = 153.8.

*CAS — 56-23-5.*

**Description.** Carbon tetrachloride is a clear, colourless, mobile, liquid with a chloroform-like odour. Sp. gr. 1.588 to 1.590. B.p. 76° to 78°. Practically insoluble in water; miscible with alcohol, chloroform, ether, petroleum spirit, and fixed and volatile oils. Store in airtight containers at a temperature not exceeding 30°. Protect from light.

**Handling.** Avoid contact with carbon tetrachloride; the vapour and liquid are poisonous. Care should be taken not to vaporise carbon tetrachloride in the presence of a flame because of the production of harmful gases, mainly phosgene.

#### Adverse Effects

Individual response to carbon tetrachloride varies widely; inhalation or ingestion of a few mL of carbon tetrachloride has proved fatal and its toxicity appears to be increased by alcohol. Symptoms of poisoning follow inhalation, ingestion, or topical application but develop more rapidly after inhalation.

Carbon tetrachloride is irritant; repeated application of carbon tetrachloride to the skin may result in dermatitis. Aspiration may result in pulmonary oedema.

Adverse effects after acute exposure from any route include gastrointestinal disturbances such as nausea, vomiting, and abdominal pain, and CNS disturbances such as headache, dizziness, and drowsiness, with progression to convulsions, coma, and death from respiratory depression or circulatory collapse. Death may also occur as a result of ventricular arrhythmia. Hepatic and renal cellular necrosis can occur and are associated with free radical production; symptoms usually begin a few days or up to 2 weeks after acute exposure to carbon tetrachloride. Renal damage may present as oliguria, progressing to proteinuria, anuria, weight gain, and oedema. Symptoms of hepatic damage include anorexia, jaundice, and hepatomegaly. If hepatorenal necrosis is not fatal recovery is eventually complete.

Symptoms of chronic poisoning are similar to those of acute poisoning; in addition, paraesthesias, visual disturbances, anaemia, and aplastic anaemia have occurred. Carcinogenicity has been demonstrated in *animals.*

◊ References.


1. Melamed E, Lavy S. Parkinsonism associated with chronic inhalation of carbon tetrachloride. *Lancet* 1977; **i:** 1015.
2. Johnson BP, *et al.* Cerebellar dysfunction after acute carbon tetrachloride poisoning. *Lancet* 1983; **ii:** 968.
3. Perez AJ, *et al.* Acute renal failure after topical application of carbon tetrachloride. *Lancet* 1987; **i:** 515–6.
4. Health and Safety Executive. Carbon tetrachloride, chloroform. *Toxicity Review 23.* London: HMSO, 1992.
5. Manno M, Rezzadore M. Critical role of ethanol abuse in carbon tetrachloride poisoning. *Lancet* 1994; **343:** 232.
6. Carbon tetrachloride health and safety guide. *IPCS Health and Safety Guide 108.* Geneva: WHO, 1998. Available at: http://www.inchem.org/documents/hsg/hsg/hsg108.htm (accessed 29/06/04)


#### Treatment of Adverse Effects

If carbon tetrachloride vapour has been inhaled the patient should be removed to the fresh air. Clothing contaminated by liquid should be removed and the skin washed. If carbon tetrachloride has been ingested gastric lavage may be performed if the patient presents within 1 hour and activated charcoal may be given.

The usual symptomatic and supportive measures should be instituted. Hepatic and renal function should be monitored closely. Haemodialysis or peritoneal dialysis may be needed if renal function is impaired. Adrenaline or other sympathomimetics should be avoided because of the risk of precipitating cardiac arrhythmias.

Acetylcysteine (p.1114) may be given to patients recently exposed to carbon tetrachloride in an attempt to prevent or modify hepatic and renal damage.

◊ Experimental studies and anecdotal reports suggest that hyperbaric oxygen therapy is of potential benefit in the treatment of carbon tetrachloride poisoning.[1]


1. Burkhart KK, *et al.* Hyperbaric oxygen treatment for carbon tetrachloride poisoning. *Drug Safety* 1991; **6:** 332–8.


#### Pharmacokinetics

Carbon tetrachloride is readily absorbed after inhalation and ingestion. It is also absorbed through the skin. Metabolism to reactive free radicals is thought to account for the hepatorenal toxicity of carbon tetrachloride.

Carbon tetrachloride is slowly excreted from the body via the lungs and the urine.

#### Uses

Carbon tetrachloride is employed in industry as a solvent and degreaser. It was formerly used in certain types of fire extinguisher and as an industrial and domestic dry cleaner but has been largely replaced for this purpose by less toxic substances. Carbon tetrachloride has also been used for the fumigation of cereals.

Carbon tetrachloride was formerly given by mouth as an anthelmintic but it has been superseded by equally effective and less toxic drugs.

## Cyclohexane

Ciclohexano; Hexahydrobenzene; Hexamethylene.

$C_6H_{12}$ = 84.16.

*CAS — 110-82-7.*

**Description.** Cyclohexane is a colourless, flammable liquid. Wt per mL about 0.78 g. B.p. about 81°. Store in airtight containers.

#### Adverse Effects

Cyclohexane is irritant, and may also have effects on the CNS.

◊ Reviews of the toxicity of cyclohexane.


1. Health and Safety Executive. Cyclohexane, cumene, para-dichlorobenzene (p-DCB), chlorodifluoromethane (CFC 22). *Toxicity Review 25.* London: HMSO, 1991.


#### Uses

Cyclohexane is used as an industrial solvent.

## Dichloromethane

Diclorometano; Methylene Chloride; Methyleni Chloridum.

$CH_2Cl_2$ = 84.93.

*CAS — 75-09-2.*

**Pharmacopoeias.** In *Eur.* (see p.vi). Also in *USNF.*

**Ph. Eur. 5.0** (Methylene Chloride; Dichloromethane BP 2003). A clear, colourless, volatile liquid. Relative density 1.320 to 1.332. It may contain not more than 2% of alcohol and/or not more than 0.03% of 2-methylbut-2-ene as stabiliser. Sparingly soluble in water; miscible with alcohol. Store in airtight containers. Protect from light.

**USNF 22** (Methylene Chloride). A clear, colourless, mobile liquid having an odour resembling chloroform. Sp. gr. 1.318 to 1.322. Miscible with alcohol, with ether, and with fixed and volatile oils. Store in airtight containers.

**Stability.** Phosgene is produced on heating of dichloromethane.

### Adverse Effects and Treatment

Acute exposure to dichloromethane vapour may depress the CNS; symptoms progress from headache and dizziness to coma and death in severe cases. Pulmonary oedema has been reported. Significant exposure may result in raised blood concentrations of carboxyhaemoglobin and symptoms of carbon monoxide poisoning. Cardiovascular effects have been attributed to hypoxia secondary to carboxyhaemoglobinaemia. There has been a report of haemolysis following acute ingestion of dichloromethane.

Chronic occupational exposure to dichloromethane vapour has produced gastrointestinal disturbances in addition to symptoms observed after acute poisoning. Dichloromethane is a common constituent of paint strippers and may be implicated in volatile substance abuse (p.1471).

The liquid is irritant and high concentrations of the vapour are irritant to the eyes.

Treatment of acute poisoning consists of removal from exposure and supportive and symptomatic measures. Carboxyhaemoglobinaemia should be managed as for carbon monoxide poisoning (p.1235) by administration of 100% oxygen; hyperbaric oxygen may be indicated. Activated charcoal may be given following ingestion. Adrenaline and other sympathomimetics should be avoided because of the risk of precipitating cardiac arrhythmias.

◊ References.


1. Methylene Chloride. *Environmental Health Criteria 32.* Geneva: WHO, 1984. Available at: http://www.inchem.org/documents/ehc/ehc/ehc32.htm (accessed 29/06/04)
2. Health and Safety Executive. Dichloromethane (methylene chloride). *Toxicity Review 12.* London: HMSO, 1985.
3. Methylene chloride health and safety guide. *IPCS Health and Safety Guide 6.* Geneva: WHO, 1987. Available at: http://www.inchem.org/documents/hsg/hsg/hsg006.htm (accessed 29/06/04)
4. Rioux JP, Myers RAM. Methylene chloride poisoning: a paradigmatic review. *J Emerg Med* 1988; **6:** 227–38.
5. Manno M, *et al.* Double fatal inhalation of dichloromethane. *Hum Exp Toxicol* 1992; **11:** 540–5.


### Pharmacokinetics

Dichloromethane is rapidly absorbed following inhalation and is also absorbed after ingestion and slowly through intact skin. It appears to be partially metabolised to carbon dioxide and carbon monoxide which are exhaled, although significant blood-carboxyhaemoglobin concentrations may be attained. Some unchanged dichloromethane is exhaled and small amounts are excreted in the urine.

### Uses

Dichloromethane is used as a pharmaceutical and industrial solvent. It is also employed as an extraction solvent in food processing.

Dichloromethane is widely used in paint strippers.

## Dichloropropane

Dicloropropano; Propylene Dichloride. 1,2-Dichloropropane.

$C_3H_6Cl_2$ = 113.0.

*CAS — 78-87-5.*

**Description.** Dichloropropane is a colourless, mobile, flammable liquid. Wt per mL about 1.16 g. B.p. about 96°. Store in airtight containers.

### Adverse Effects

Dichloropropane is irritant; high concentrations may result in CNS depression.

◊ Acute renal failure, haemolytic anaemia, acute liver disease, and disseminated intravascular coagulation has been reported[1] following intentional inhalation of a stain remover containing dichloropropane; the patient recovered following blood transfusions and haemodialysis.


1. Locatelli F, Pozzi C. Relapsing haemolytic-uraemic syndrome after organic solvent sniffing. *Lancet* 1983; **ii:** 220.


### Uses

Dichloropropane is used as an industrial solvent, dry cleaning agent, and agricultural defumigant.

## Diethyl Phthalate

Diethylis Phthalas; Ethyl Phthalate; Ftalato de dietilo. Benzene-1,2-dicarboxylic acid diethyl ester.

$C_{12}H_{14}O_4$ = 222.2.

*CAS — 84-66-2.*

**Pharmacopoeias.** In *Eur.* (see p.vi) and *Viet.* Also in *USNF.*

**Ph. Eur. 5.0** (Diethyl Phthalate). A clear, colourless or very slightly yellow, oily liquid. Relative density 1.117 to 1.121. Practically insoluble in water; miscible with alcohol. Store in airtight containers.

**USNF 22** (Diethyl Phthalate). A colourless, practically odourless, oily liquid. Sp. gr. 1.118 to 1.122 at 20°. Insoluble in water; miscible with alcohol, with ether, and with other usual organic solvents. Store in airtight containers.

### Adverse Effects

Diethyl phthalate is irritant and, in high concentrations, causes CNS depression. There has been concern about potential toxicity resulting from exposure to phthalates used as plasticisers.

◊ References.


1. Health and Safety Executive. Review of the toxicity of the esters of o-phthalic acid (phthalate esters). *Toxicity Review 14.* London: HMSO, 1986.
2. Kamrin MA, Mayor GH. Diethyl phthalate: a perspective. *J Clin Pharmacol* 1991; **31:** 484–9.
3. Shea KM, *et al.* Pediatric exposure and potential toxicity of phthalate plasticizers. *Pediatrics* 2003; **111:** 1467–74.


### Uses

Diethyl phthalate is used as a denaturant of alcohol, for example in surgical spirit, and as a solvent and plasticiser.

### Preparations

***BP 2003:*** Surgical Spirit.

## Dimethyl Sulfoxide *(BAN, USAN, rINN)*

Dimethyl Sulphoxide; Dimethylis Sulfoxidum; Dimetil sulfóxido; DMSO; Methyl Sulphoxide; NSC-763; SQ-9453; Sulphinylbismethane.

$C_2H_6OS$ = 78.13.

*CAS — 67-68-5.*

*ATC — G04BX13; M02AX03.*

**Pharmacopoeias.** In *Eur.* (see p.vi) and *US.*

**Ph. Eur. 5.0** (Dimethyl Sulfoxide). A colourless hygroscopic liquid or crystals. F.p. not lower than 18.3°. Relative density 1.100 to 1.104. Miscible with water and with alcohol. Store in airtight glass containers. Protect from light.

**USP 27** (Dimethyl Sulfoxide). A clear, colourless, odourless, hygroscopic liquid. M.p. about 18.4°. Sp. gr. 1.095 to 1.097. Soluble in water; practically insoluble in alcohol, in acetone, in chloroform, in ether, and in benzene. Store in airtight containers. Protect from light.

### Adverse Effects and Treatment

High concentrations of dimethyl sulfoxide applied to the skin may cause burning discomfort, itching, erythema, vesiculation, and urticaria. Continued use may result in scaling.

Systemic effects, including gastrointestinal disturbances, drowsiness, headache, and hypersensitivity reactions, may occur after administration by any route. A garlic-like odour on the breath and skin is attributed to the formation of dimethyl sulfide (see Pharmacokinetics, below). Intravascular haemolysis has been reported following intravenous administration. Local discomfort and spasm may occur when given by bladder instillation.

Treatment of adverse effects consists of symptomatic and supportive measures. Gastric lavage may be helpful after acute ingestion, although it should be remembered that absorption is rapid.

◊ Reviews.


1. Brobyn RD. The human toxicology of dimethyl sulfoxide. *Ann N Y Acad Sci* 1975; **243:** 497–506.
2. Willhite CC, Katz PI. Toxicology updates: dimethyl sulfoxide. *J Appl Toxicol* 1984; **4:** 155–60.


◊ Dimethyl sulfoxide given by intravenous infusion for spinal cord injury to 14 patients caused transient haemolysis and haemoglobinuria.[1] Infusion strengths greater than 10% were associated with grossly discoloured urine but there was no evidence of renal damage. In 2 patients, raised liver and muscle enzyme concentrations, mild jaundice, and evidence of haemolysis developed after receiving dimethyl sulfoxide intravenously for arthritis.[2] One also developed acute renal tubular necrosis, deterioration in level of consciousness, and evidence of cerebral infarction. Acute, reversible neurological deterioration in a patient has been associated with intravenous dimethyl sulfoxide.[3]

Serum hyperosmolality[4] has been reported in a patient who had pre-existing diabetes insipidus after receiving haematopoietic stem cells cryopreserved in dimethyl sulfoxide following chemotherapy for a malignant germ-cell tumour; symptoms included severe headache, confusion, and abdominal pain.


1. Muther RS, Bennett WM. Effects of dimethyl sulfoxide on renal function in man. *JAMA* 1980; **244:** 2081–3.
2. Yellowlees P, *et al.* Dimethylsulphoxide-induced toxicity. *Lancet* 1980; **ii:** 1004–6.
3. Bond GR, *et al.* Dimethylsulphoxide-induced encephalopathy. *Lancet* 1989; **i:** 1134–5.
4. Thomé S, *et al.* Dimethylsulphoxide-induced serum hyperosmolality after cryopreserved stem-cell graft. *Lancet* 1994; **344:** 1431–2.


### Precautions

When used as a penetrating basis for other drugs applied topically, dimethyl sulfoxide may enhance their toxic effects.

Since dimethyl sulfoxide has been associated with lens changes in *animals*, the manufacturers recommend assessment of ophthalmic function every 6 months during long-term treatment of cystitis with intravesical instillation of dimethyl sulfoxide. Hepatic and renal function should also be assessed at intervals of 6 months. Bladder instillation may be harmful in patients with urinary-tract malignancy because of vasodilatation.

### Interactions

◊ For mention of an interaction between dimethyl sulfoxide and *sulindac*, see p.92.

### Pharmacokinetics

Dimethyl sulfoxide is readily absorbed after administration by all routes. It is metabolised by oxidation to dimethyl sulfone and by reduction to dimethyl sulfide. Dimethyl sulfoxide and the sulfone metabolite are excreted in the urine and faeces. Dimethyl sulfide is excreted through the lungs and skin and is responsible for the characteristic odour from patients.

### Uses and Administration

Dimethyl sulfoxide is a highly polar substance with exceptional solvent properties for both organic and inorganic chemicals, and is widely used as an industrial solvent.

It has been reported to have a wide spectrum of pharmacological activity including membrane penetration, anti-inflammatory effects, local analgesia, weak bacteriostasis, diuresis, vasodilatation, dissolution of collagen, and free-radical scavenging.

The principal use of dimethyl sulfoxide is as a vehicle for drugs such as idoxuridine (p.637); it aids penetration of the drug into the skin, and so may enhance the drug's effect. It is also used as a 50% aqueous solution for bladder instillation for the symptomatic relief of interstitial cystitis; doses of 50 mL are instilled and allowed to remain for 15 minutes. Treatment is repeated every 2 weeks initially.

Dimethyl sulfoxide has been administered orally, intravenously, or topically for a wide range of indications including cutaneous and musculoskeletal disorders, but evidence of beneficial effects is limited.

Dimethyl sulfoxide is used as a cryoprotectant for various human tissues.

◊ Reviews.


1. Trice JM, Pinals RS. Dimethyl sulfoxide: a review of its use in the rheumatic disorders. *Semin Arthritis Rheum* 1985; **15:** 45–60.
2. Swanson BN. Medical use of dimethyl sulfoxide (DMSO). *Rev Clin Basic Pharm* 1985; **5:** 1–33.


**Cryopreservation.** Dimethyl sulfoxide is used as a cryoprotectant in various assisted conception techniques.[1] Adverse effects have been reported in patients receiving haematopoietic stem cells cryopreserved in dimethyl sulfoxide (see under Adverse Effects, above).


1. Trounson AO. Cryopreservation. *Br Med Bull* 1990; **46:** 695–708.


**Extravasation of antineoplastics.** Several reports have suggested a role for topical dimethyl sulfoxide in the treatment of anthracycline extravasation.[1-4] The problem of antineoplastic extravasation and its management is discussed further on p.496.


1. Lawrence HJ, Goodnight SH. Dimethyl sulfoxide and extravasation of anthracycline agents. *Ann Intern Med* 1983; **98:** 1025.
2. Olver IN, *et al.* A prospective study of topical dimethyl sulfoxide for treating anthracycline extravasation. *J Clin Oncol* 1988; **6:** 1732–5.
3. Rospond RM, Engel LM. Dimethyl sulfoxide for treating anthracycline extravasation. *Clin Pharm* 1993; **12:** 560–1.
4. Bertelli G, *et al.* Dimethylsulphoxide and cooling after extravasation of antitumour agents. *Lancet* 1993; **341:** 1098.


**Gallstones.** For mention of the use of dimethyl sulfoxide to dissolve gallstones, see Methyl *tert*-Butyl Ether, p.1476.

**Interstitial cystitis.** Interstitial cystitis is an inflammatory condition of the bladder of unknown aetiology. Symptoms include pain, urinary frequency, urinary urgency, and nocturia. Many treatments have been tried, including local and systemic drug therapy and surgery.

Bladder instillations of a 50% aqueous solution of dimethyl sulfoxide appear to alleviate symptoms.[1,2] The chief effect of dimethyl sulfoxide may be on sensory nerves since there appears to be no significant alteration in the endoscopic or morphological appearance of the bladder after treatment.[3] Treatment has successfully been repeated at relapse.[3]

Oral administration of pentosan polysulfate sodium may also provide some relief of symptoms.


1. Fowler JE. Prospective study of intravesical dimethyl sulfoxide in treatment of suspected early interstitial cystitis. *Urology* 1981; **18:** 21–6.
2. Perez-Marrero R, *et al.* A controlled study of dimethyl sulfoxide in interstitial cystitis. *J Urol (Baltimore)* 1988; **140:** 36–9.
3. Ryan PG, Wallace DMA. Are we making progress in the drug treatment of disorders of the bladder, prostate, and penis? *J Clin Pharm Ther* 1990; **15:** 1–12.


**Raised intracranial pressure.** Intravenous osmotic diuretics, particularly mannitol, are used to lower raised intracranial pressure (p.833). Small preliminary studies[1,2] indicated that intravenous administration of dimethyl sulfoxide could control raised intracranial pressure refractory to other treatments but some workers[1] encountered problems with fluid overload and difficulties with administration.

1. Marshall LF, *et al.* Dimethyl sulfoxide for the treatment of intracranial hypertension: a preliminary trial. *Neurosurgery* 1984; **14:** 659–63.
2. Karaca M, *et al.* Dimethyl sulphoxide lowers ICP after closed head trauma. *Eur J Clin Pharmacol* 1991; **40:** 113–14.

### Preparations

***USP 27:*** Dimethyl Sulfoxide Irrigation.

**Proprietary Preparations** (details are given in Part 3)
***Canad.:*** Kemsol; Rimso; ***Ger.:*** Rheumabene; ***UK:*** Rimso; ***USA:*** Rimso.

**Multi-ingredient: *Austria:*** Dolobene; ***Braz.:*** Dolobene; ***Ger.:*** Dolobene; Verrumal; ***Hong Kong:*** Dolobene; Verrumal; ***Israel:*** Verrumal; Verucid; ***Malaysia:*** Verrumal; ***Singapore:*** Verrumal; ***Spain:*** Artrodesmol Extra; ***Switz.:*** Dolo Demotherm; Dolobene; Histalgane; Histalgane mite; Remexal; Roll-bene†; Sportusal; Sportusal Spray sine heparino; Venucreme; Venugel; Verra-med; Verrumal; ***Thai.:*** Verrumal.

## Dimethylacetamide

Acetyldimethylamine; Dimethylacetamidum; Dimetilacetamida; DMAC. *NN*-Dimethylacetamide.

$C_4H_9NO = 87.12.$
*CAS — 127-19-5.*

**Pharmacopoeias.** In *Eur.* (see p.vi).

**Ph. Eur. 5.0** (Dimethylacetamide). A clear, colourless, slightly hygroscopic liquid. Relative density 0.941 to 0.944. B.p. about 165°. Miscible with water, with alcohol, and with most common organic solvents. Store in airtight containers. Protect from light.

### Adverse Effects and Precautions

As for Dimethylformamide (below), although a disulfiram-like reaction with alcohol has not been reported.

◊ A review[1] of the toxicology of dimethylacetamide with reference to its use as a vehicle for antineoplastics.

1. Kim S-N. Preclinical toxicology and pharmacology of dimethylacetamide, with clinical notes. *Drug Metab Rev* 1988; **19:** 345–68.

**Handling.** Suitable precautions should be taken to avoid skin contact with dimethylacetamide as it can penetrate skin and produce systemic toxicity.

### Uses

Dimethylacetamide is used as an industrial and pharmaceutical solvent.

## Dimethylformamide

Dimetilformamida; DMF. *NN*-Dimethylformamide.

$C_3H_7NO = 73.09.$
*CAS — 68-12-2.*

**Description.** Dimethylformamide is a colourless liquid. Wt per mL about 0.95 g. B.p. about 153°.

### Adverse Effects and Precautions

Dimethylformamide is irritant. Gastrointestinal effects including nausea, vomiting, loss of appetite, and abdominal pain, CNS effects such as headache, dizziness, and weakness, and liver damage have been reported in workers occupationally exposed to the liquid or vapour. Some workers exposed to dimethylformamide have experienced a disulfiram-like effect after consumption of alcohol.

◊ Reviews of the adverse effects of dimethylformamide.

1. Dimethylformamide. *Environmental Health Criteria 114.* Geneva: WHO, 1991. Available at: http://www.inchem.org/documents/ehc/ehc/ehc114.htm (accessed 30/06/04)

**Effects on the liver.** Exposure to dimethylformamide was considered to be the most likely cause of elevated liver enzyme values in 36 of 58 (62%) workers in a fabric coating factory.[1] Symptoms reported were generally mild and included anorexia, abdominal pain, nausea, headache, dizziness, and a disulfiram-type reaction to alcohol.

Hepatotoxicity has occurred following acute poisoning with a veterinary drug formulated in dimethylformamide. There were only minor increases in liver enzyme values in a patient who was treated early with acetylcysteine.[2]

1. Redlich CA, *et al.* Liver disease associated with occupational exposure to the solvent dimethylformamide. *Ann Intern Med* 1988; **108:** 680–6.
2. Buylaert W, *et al.* Hepatotoxicity of N,N-dimethylformamide (DMF) in acute poisoning with the veterinary euthanasia drug T-61. *Hum Exp Toxicol* 1996; **15:** 607–11.

**Handling.** Suitable precautions should be taken to avoid skin contact with dimethylformamide as it can penetrate skin and produce systemic toxicity.

**Malignant neoplasms.** There have been reports of testicular cancer in men occupationally exposed to dimethylformamide.[1] Such an association could not, however, be substantiated by epidemiological data[2] on 3859 male employees exposed to dimethylformamide between 1950 and 1970 and followed up to 1984. It has been suggested that although dimethylformamide may not itself be carcinogenic, it may increase absorption through the skin of heavy metal carcinogens, possibly including chromates.[3]

1. Levin SM, *et al.* Testicular cancer in leather tanners exposed to dimethylformamide. *Lancet* 1987; **ii:** 1153.
2. Chen JL, Kennedy GL. Dimethylformamide and testicular cancer. *Lancet* 1988; **i:** 55.
3. Ducatman AM. Dimethylformamide, metal dyes, and testicular cancer. *Lancet* 1989; **i:** 911.

### Pharmacokinetics

Dimethylformamide is absorbed after inhalation and through intact skin. It is excreted mainly in the urine as metabolites.

### Uses

Dimethylformamide is used as an industrial solvent.

## Dioxan

Diethylene Dioxide; Diethylene Ether; Dioxane; Dioxano. 1,4-Dioxane.

$C_4H_8O_2 = 88.11.$
*CAS — 123-91-1.*

NOTE. Do not confuse dioxan and dioxin (p.1681).

**Description.** Dioxan is a colourless flammable liquid with an ethereal odour. Wt per mL about 1.03 g. B.p. about 101°. Store in airtight containers.

**Stability.** It is dangerous to distil or evaporate dioxan unless precautions have been taken to remove explosive peroxides.

### Adverse Effects, Treatment, and Precautions

Dioxan vapour is irritant to mucous membranes. High concentrations may cause nausea and vomiting, and CNS depression with headache, dizziness, drowsiness, and in severe cases unconsciousness. On repeated exposure, severe hepatic and renal damage, including necrotic changes, can occur and may be fatal. Direct contact with liquid dioxan can result in dermatitis. Dioxan has been shown to be carcinogenic in *animals.*

Treatment consists of removal from exposure and general supportive and symptomatic measures.

**Handling.** Suitable precautions should be taken to avoid skin contact with dioxan as it can penetrate skin and produce systemic toxicity.

### Pharmacokinetics

Dioxan is absorbed after inhalation and through the skin. It is metabolised by oxidation to β-hydroxyethoxy-acetic acid.

### Uses

Dioxan is used as an industrial solvent.

## Epichlorohydrin

Epiclorhidrina. 1-Chloro-2,3-epoxypropane.

$C_3H_5ClO = 92.52.$
*CAS — 106-89-8.*

**Description.** Epichlorohydrin is a colourless, flammable liquid. Wt per mL about 1.18 g. B.p. 115° to 118°. Store in airtight containers.

**Stability.** The vapour of epichlorohydrin forms explosive mixtures with air. Harmful gases including phosgene are liberated on heating of epichlorohydrin.

### Adverse Effects and Precautions

Epichlorohydrin is irritant. It has been shown to be carcinogenic in *animals.*

◊ References to the toxicity of epichlorohydrin.

1. Epichlorohydrin. *Environmental Health Criteria 33.* Geneva: WHO, 1984. Available at: http://www.inchem.org/documents/ehc/ehc/ehc33.htm (accessed 30/06/04)
2. Epichlorohydrin health and safety guide. *IPCS Health and Safety Guide 8.* Geneva: WHO, 1987. Available at: http://www.inchem.org/documents/hsg/hsg/hsg008.htm (accessed 30/06/04)
3. Health and Safety Executive. Ammonia, 1-chloro-2,3-epoxypropane (epichlorohydrin), carcinogenicity of cadmium and its compounds. *Toxicity Review 24.* London: HMSO, 1991.

**Handling.** Suitable precautions should be taken to avoid skin contact with epichlorohydrin as it can penetrate skin and produce systemic toxicity.

### Uses

Epichlorohydrin is used as an industrial solvent.

## Solvent Ether

Aether; Aether Aethylicus; Aether Solvens; Diethyl Ether; Eter; Éter disolvente; Ether; Éther rectifié; Ethyl Ether; Ethyl Oxide.

$(C_2H_5)_2O = 74.12.$
*CAS — 60-29-7.*

NOTE. Solvent ether is not intended for anaesthesia; only ether of a suitable quality (see p.1298) should be so used.

**Pharmacopoeias.** In *Eur.* (see p.vi), *Jpn, Pol.,* and *US.*

**Ph. Eur. 5.0** (Ether). A colourless, clear, volatile, highly flammable liquid. It may contain a suitable non-volatile antioxidant at a suitable concentration. Relative density 0.714 to 0.716. Distillation range 34° to 35°. Soluble in water; miscible with alcohol, with dichloromethane, and with fatty oils. Store at 8° to 15° in airtight containers. Protect from light.

**USP 27** (Ether). A colourless, mobile, volatile, flammable liquid, having a characteristic sweet, pungent odour. It is slowly oxidised by the action of air and light, with the formation of peroxides. B.p. about 35°. Sp. gr. 0.713 to 0.716. Soluble 1 in 12 of water; miscible with alcohol, with chloroform, with dichloromethane, with petroleum spirit, with benzene, and with fixed and volatile oils; soluble in hydrochloric acid. Store in partly filled airtight containers at a temperature not exceeding 30° and remote from fire. Protect from light.

**Stability.** Though ether is one of the lightest of liquids, its vapour is very heavy, being $2\frac{1}{2}$ times heavier than air.

Ether is very volatile and flammable and mixtures of its vapour with oxygen, nitrous oxide, or air at certain concentrations are explosive. It should not be used in the presence of an open flame or any electrical apparatus liable to produce a spark; precautions should be taken against the production of static electrical discharge. Explosive peroxides are generated by the atmospheric oxidation of solvent ether and it is dangerous to distil a sample which contains peroxides.

### Adverse Effects

As for Anaesthetic Ether, p.1299. Ingestion of 30 to 60 mL may be fatal.

### Uses

Solvent ether is widely used as a pharmaceutical and industrial solvent, and is used as an extraction solvent in food processing.

### Preparations

**Proprietary Preparations** (details are given in Part 3)
**Multi-ingredient: *Belg.:*** Solution Antiseptique; ***S.Afr.:*** Famstim†.

## Ethyl Acetate

Acetato de etilo; Acetic Ether; Aethylis Acetas; Aethylium Aceticum; Ethyl Ethanoate; Ethylis Acetas.

$C_4H_8O_2 = 88.11.$
*CAS — 141-78-6.*

**Pharmacopoeias.** In *Eur.* (see p.vi) and *Pol.* Also in *USNF.*

**Ph. Eur. 5.0** (Ethyl Acetate). A colourless, clear, volatile liquid. Relative density 0.898 to 0.902. B.p. 76° to 78°. Soluble in water; miscible with alcohol, with acetone, and with dichloromethane. Store at a temperature not exceeding 30°. Protect from light.

**USNF 22** (Ethyl Acetate). A transparent, colourless, flammable liquid having a fragrant, refreshing, slightly acetous odour. Sp. gr. 0.894 to 0.898. Soluble in water; miscible with alcohol, with ether, and with fixed and volatile oils. Store in airtight containers at a temperature not exceeding 40°.

### Adverse Effects

Ethyl acetate is irritant to mucous membranes. High concentrations may cause CNS depression. Ethyl acetate may be implicated in volatile substance abuse (p.1471).

◊ For discussion of neurotoxicity after occupational exposure to solvents and the absence of such an effect with ethyl acetate, see under Toluene, p.1477.

### Uses

Ethyl acetate is used as a flavour and solvent in pharmaceutical preparations. It is also employed in industry as a solvent and is used as an extraction solvent in food processing.

## Formamide

Carbamaldehyde; Formamida; Methanamide.

$CH_3NO = 45.04.$
*CAS — 75-12-7.*

**Description.** Formamide is a colourless, oily liquid. B.p. 210°. Wt per mL, about 1.13 g.

### Profile

Formamide is used as an industrial solvent. It is reported to be irritant.

## Glycofurol

Glicofurol; Glycofurol 75; Tetrahydrofurfuryl Alcohol Polyethylene Glycol Ether. α-(Tetrahydrofuranyl)-ω-hydroxypoly(oxyethylene).

$C_5H_9O.(C_2H_4O)_n.OH.$
*CAS — 9004-76-6; 31692-85-0.*

**Description.** Glycofurol is a clear, colourless, almost odourless liquid. Wt per mL about 1.08 g. B.p. 80° to 100°. Incompatible with oxidising agents. Store under nitrogen in airtight containers. Protect from light.

### Profile

Glycofurol is used as a pharmaceutical solvent for injections.

## Hexachloroethane

Hexacloroetano.

$C_2Cl_6 = 236.7.$
*CAS — 67-72-1.*

### Profile

Hexachloroethane is a chlorinated hydrocarbon used in industry as a solvent. Eye irritation and photophobia have resulted from industrial exposure to the vapour. It was formerly used in veterinary medicine as an anthelmintic, but has been superseded by less toxic drugs.

## n-Hexane

n-Hexano.

$C_6H_{14}$ = 86.18.

*CAS — 110-54-3.*

**Description.** *n*-Hexane is a colourless, flammable, volatile liquid with a faint odour. Wt per mL about 0.66 g. B.p. about 69°. Store in airtight containers.

### Adverse Effects

*n*-Hexane is irritant. Acute exposure to the vapour may result in CNS depression with headache, drowsiness, dizziness, and in severe cases unconsciousness. Chronic occupational exposure and abuse of *n*-hexane have been associated with the development of peripheral neuropathies. *n*-Hexane is a constituent of some adhesives and may be implicated in volatile substance abuse (p.1471). Some adverse effects of petrol have been attributed to its content of *n*-hexane.

◊ References.

1. Health and Safety Executive. *n*-Hexane. *Toxicity Review 18.* London: HMSO, 1987.
2. *n*-Hexane. *Environmental Health Criteria 122.* Geneva: WHO, 1991. Available at: http://www.inchem.org/documents/ehc/ehc/ehc122.htm (accessed 30/06/04)
3. *n*-Hexane health and safety guide. *IPCS Health and Safety Guide 59.* Geneva: WHO, 1991. Available at: http://www.inchem.org/documents/hsg/hsg/hsg059.htm (accessed 30/06/04)

**Effects on the nervous system.** There have been many reports of peripheral neuropathy attributed to the abuse of, and occupational exposure to, *n*-hexane, although symptoms tend to be milder in the latter.[1] Tetraplegia has occurred in severe cases. There is typically a clinical deterioration several weeks after exposure followed by a slow recovery which, in severe cases, may not be complete. It has been suggested that methyl ethyl ketone potentiates the peripheral neuropathy induced by *n*-hexane. Occupational exposure to *n*-hexane has also been associated with cranial nerve neuropathy.

Parkinsonism in a leather worker, possibly associated with exposure to solvents, predominantly *n*-hexane, has been noted.[2]

For further discussion of neurotoxicity after occupational exposure to solvents including *n*-hexane, see under Toluene, p.1477.

1. Lolin Y. Chronic neurological toxicity associated with exposure to volatile substances. *Hum Toxicol* 1989; **8:** 293–300.
2. Pezzoli G, *et al.* Parkinsonism due to n-hexane exposure. *Lancet* 1989; **ii:** 874.

### Pharmacokinetics

*n*-Hexane is absorbed after inhalation and to a limited extent through the skin. Oxidative metabolites, including 2,5-hexanedione are excreted in the urine largely as conjugates. Some unchanged *n*-hexane is excreted via the lungs.

### Uses

*n*-Hexane is widely used as an industrial solvent, as a solvent in glues, and as an extraction solvent in food processing.

### Preparations

**Proprietary Preparations** (details are given in Part 3)

**Multi-ingredient:** ***Austral.:*** Sacsol†.

## Isobutyl Alcohol

Alcohol isobutílico; Isobutanol.

$C_4H_{10}O$ = 74.12.

*CAS — 78-83-1.*

### Profile

Isobutyl alcohol is used as an industrial solvent. It is also used as an anaesthetic in the American lobster, *Homarus americanus*.

◊ References.

1. Butanols—four isomers: 1-butanol, 2-butanol, tert-butanol, isobutanol. *Environmental Health Criteria 65.* Geneva: WHO, 1987. Available at: http://www.inchem.org/documents/ehc/ehc/ehc65.htm (accessed 30/06/04)
2. Isobutanol health and safety guide. *IPCS Health and Safety Guide 9.* Geneva: WHO, 1987. Available at: http://www.inchem.org/documents/hsg/hsg/hsg009.htm (accessed 30/06/04)

## Kerosene

Kerosine; 'Paraffin'; Queroseno.

*CAS — 8008-20-6.*

**Description.** Kerosene is a mixture of hydrocarbons, chiefly members of the alkane series, distilled from petroleum. It is a clear, colourless liquid with a characteristic odour. Sp. gr. about 0.8 g. B.p. 180° to 300°. An odourless grade is available. Store in airtight containers.

### Adverse Effects

The chief danger from ingestion of kerosene is pneumonitis and attendant pulmonary complications resulting from aspiration. Spontaneous or induced vomiting increases the risk of aspiration. Ingestion of kerosene results in a burning sensation in the mouth and throat, gastrointestinal disturbances, and possibly cough, dyspnoea, and transient cyanosis. There may be excitation followed by CNS depression, with weakness, dizziness, drowsiness, confusion, incoordination, and restlessness progressing to convulsions, coma, and respiratory depression in severe cases. Cardiac arrhythmias have been reported.

The course of poisoning from inhalation is similar to that following ingestion although CNS and cardiac effects are more likely. Kerosene is irritant.

**Abuse.** A case of volatile substance abuse (p.1471) involving inhalation and ingestion of kerosene has been reported.[1]

1. Das PS, *et al.* Kerosene abuse by inhalation and ingestion. *Am J Psychiatry* 1992; **149:** 710.

### Treatment of Adverse Effects

Treatment of kerosene poisoning is supportive and symptomatic. Every precaution should be taken to avoid aspiration of kerosene into the lungs. Most authorities agree that gastric lavage should generally be avoided unless a very large amount of kerosene or an additional toxin such as a pesticide has been ingested. Activated charcoal may be given. Adrenaline and other sympathomimetics should be avoided because of the risk of precipitating cardiac arrhythmias.

### Uses

Kerosene is used as a degreaser and cleaner and as an illuminating and fuel oil in kerosene ('paraffin') lamps and stoves. The odourless grade has been used as a solvent in the preparation of some insecticide sprays.

## 2-Methoxyethanol

Ethylene Glycol Monomethyl Ether; 2-Metoxietanol.

$C_3H_8O_2$ = 76.09.

*CAS — 109-86-4.*

**Description.** 2-Methoxyethanol is a clear, colourless to slightly yellow liquid. Wt per mL about 0.96 g. B.p. about 125°. Miscible with water, with alcohol, with acetone, with dimethylformamide, with ether, and with glycerol. Store in airtight containers.

### Adverse Effects and Precautions

2-Methoxyethanol is irritant to mucous membranes. Ingestion may result in CNS depression with confusion, weakness, and in severe cases coma and death from respiratory depression. Nausea, metabolic acidosis, and renal damage may also occur. Prolonged industrial exposure to the vapour has been associated with severe effects on the CNS characterised by headache, dizziness, lethargy, weakness, ataxia, tremor, disorientation, mental changes, weight loss, and visual disturbances. Anaemia has also been reported.

◊ References to the toxicity of 2-methoxyethanol and other glycol ethers.

1. Health and Safety Executive. Glycol ethers. *Toxicity Review 10.* London: HMSO, 1985.
2. 2-Methoxyethanol, 2-ethoxyethanol, and their acetates. *Environmental Health Criteria 115.* Geneva: WHO, 1990. Available at: http://www.inchem.org/documents/ehc/ehc/ehc115.htm (accessed 30/06/04)
3. Browning RG, Curry SC. Clinical toxicology of ethylene glycol monoalkyl ethers. *Hum Exp Toxicol* 1994; **13:** 325–35.

**Handling.** Suitable precautions should be taken to avoid skin contact with 2-methoxyethanol as it can penetrate skin and produce systemic toxicity.

### Uses

2-Methoxyethanol is used as an industrial solvent.

## Methyl Alcohol

Metanol; Methanol.

$CH_3OH$ = 32.04.

*CAS — 67-56-1.*

**Pharmacopoeias.** In *Br.* and *Ger.* Also in *USNF.*

**BP 2003** (Methanol). A colourless, clear, hygroscopic liquid. B.p. 65°. Relative density 0.791 to 0.793. Miscible with water, with dehydrated alcohol, and with ether. Store at a temperature not exceeding 25°. Protect from moisture.

**USNF 22** (Methyl Alcohol). A clear, colourless, flammable liquid having a characteristic odour. Miscible with water, with alcohol, with ether, with benzene, and with most other organic solvents. Store in airtight containers remote from heat, sparks, and open flames.

### Adverse Effects

Immediate signs of acute poisoning following ingestion of methyl alcohol resemble those of ethanol (alcohol; ethyl alcohol) intoxication (see p.1166), but are milder. Characteristic symptoms of methyl alcohol poisoning are caused by toxic metabolites and develop after a latent period of about 12 to 24 hours, or longer if taken with ethanol. The outstanding features of poisoning are metabolic acidosis with rapid, shallow breathing, visual disturbances which often proceed to irreversible blindness, and severe abdominal pain. Other symptoms include headache, gastrointestinal disturbances, pain in the back and extremities, and coma which in severe cases may terminate in death due to respiratory failure or, rarely, to circulatory collapse. Mania and convulsions occasionally occur. Individual response to methyl alcohol varies widely. Ingestion of 30 mL is considered to be potentially fatal.

Absorption of methyl alcohol through the skin or inhalation of the vapour may also lead to toxic systemic effects.

◊ References to the adverse effects of methyl alcohol.

1. Jacobsen D, McMartin KE. Methanol and ethylene glycol poisonings: mechanism of toxicity, clinical course, diagnosis and treatment. *Med Toxicol* 1986; **1:** 309–34.
2. Anderson TJ, *et al.* Neurologic sequelae of methanol poisoning. *Can Med Assoc J* 1987; **136:** 1177–9.
3. Cavalli A, *et al.* Severe reversible cardiac failure associated with methanol intoxication. *Postgrad Med J* 1987; **63:** 867–8.
4. Shapiro L, *et al.* Unusual case of methanol poisoning. *Lancet* 1993; **341:** 112.

**Handling.** Suitable precautions should be taken to avoid skin contact with methyl alcohol as it can penetrate skin and produce systemic toxicity.

### Treatment of Adverse Effects

Gastric lavage may be considered if the patient presents within 1 hour of ingesting methyl alcohol. Activated charcoal is probably of little use as it does not absorb significant amounts of methyl alcohol. Metabolic acidosis (p.1217) should be corrected immediately with intravenous sodium bicarbonate. Treatment with ethanol, which delays the oxidation of methyl alcohol to its toxic metabolites formaldehyde and formic acid, should also be initiated, the dosage being adjusted to achieve and maintain a blood-ethanol concentration of 1 to 1.5 mg/mL. An oral dose of about 50 g (equivalent to 150 mL of 40% v/v ethanol) for an adult of around 70 kg body-weight has been suggested; the ethanol should be well diluted before administration. If required, an ethanol infusion may then be given for which the following doses have been used:

- for an average adult, 110 mg/kg per hour (1.38 mL/kg per hour of 10% ethanol, or 2.76 mL/kg per hour of 5% ethanol)
- for a non-drinker or child, 66 mg/kg per hour (0.825 mL/kg per hour of 10% ethanol, or 1.65 mL/kg per hour of 5% ethanol)
- for a chronic drinker, 153.78 mg/kg per hour (1.95 mL/kg per hour of 10% ethanol, or 3.9 mL/kg per hour of 5% ethanol)

Fomepizole (p.1039), an inhibitor of alcohol dehydrogenase, is also used; it inhibits the metabolism of methyl alcohol to its toxic metabolites.

Haemodialysis may be indicated to increase the removal of methyl alcohol and its toxic metabolites. Peritoneal dialysis has been used but is less efficient. Some authorities recommend initiation of haemodialysis if the amount of methyl alcohol ingested exceeds 30 mL (equivalent to about 24 g), if the blood-methyl alcohol concentration is greater than 500 micrograms/mL, or if severe metabolic acidosis or visual complications develop. If haemodialysis is used, a constant blood-ethanol concentration may be ensured either by increasing the ethanol infusion rate or by addition of ethanol to the dialysate fluid. Treatment should not be discontinued prematurely since oxidation and excretion of methyl alcohol may continue for several days; patients should, therefore, be closely observed and monitored. Suitable supportive treatment should be carried out as required.

Folinic acid and folic acid have been given in the treatment of methyl alcohol toxicity because they may enhance the metabolism of formic acid.

◊ References.

1. Barceloux DG, *et al.* American Academy of Clinical Toxicology Ad Hoc Committee on the Treatment Guidelines for Methanol Poisoning. American Academy of Clinical Toxicology practice guidelines on the treatment of methanol poisoning. *J Toxicol Clin Toxicol* 2002; **40:** 415–46.

### Pharmacokinetics

Methyl alcohol is readily absorbed from the gastrointestinal tract and distributed throughout the body fluids. It may also be absorbed after inhalation or through large areas of skin. Oxidation by alcohol dehydrogenase with formation of formaldehyde and formic acid takes place mainly in the liver and also in the kidneys. These metabolites are thought to be largely responsible for the characteristic symptoms of methyl alcohol poisoning. Metabolism is much slower than for ethanol, which competitively inhibits the metabolism of methyl alcohol. Oxidation and excretion may continue for several days after ingestion. Elimination of unchanged methyl alcohol via the lungs and in the urine is a minor route of excretion.

### Uses

Methyl alcohol is used as a pharmaceutical and industrial solvent. It is also used as 'wood naphtha' to denature ethanol in the preparation of industrial methylated spirits. Methyl alcohol is also used as an extraction solvent in food processing.

### Preparations

**Proprietary Preparations** (details are given in Part 3)

**Multi-ingredient:** ***Ger.:*** Acarex; ***India:*** Methazil.

## Methyl tert-Butyl Ether

Éter metilterbutílico; Methyl Terbutyl Ether; Methyl Tertiary Butyl Ether; MTBE. 2-Methoxy-2-methylpropane.

$C_5H_{12}O$ = 88.15.

*CAS — 1634-04-4.*

**Description.** Methyl *tert*-butyl ether is a volatile, flammable liquid. Wt per mL about 0.74 g. B.p. about 55°. Store in airtight containers.

**Stability.** Explosive peroxides may be generated by the atmospheric oxidation of methyl tert-butyl ether, but the risk is lower than with solvent ether.

### Adverse Effects

Methyl *tert*-butyl ether is irritant and may cause CNS depression. Adverse effects that have been reported after use as a gallstone solvent are described under Uses and Administration, below.

### Uses and Administration

Methyl *tert*-butyl ether is a solvent that has been used for the rapid dissolution of cholesterol gallstones.

**Gallstones.** An alternative to bile acid therapy in patients with gallstones (p.1761) who are not considered suitable for surgery is direct instillation of a solvent into the gallbladder.

Methyl *tert*-butyl ether has been used to dissolve cholesterol gallstones; stones rich in calcium or pigments are not dissolved.[1] Unfortunately incomplete dissolution and residual debris can lead to recurrence of stone formation.[2] The solvent is most commonly instilled via a percutaneous transhepatic catheter,[1,3] although other routes have been used.[4] Gallbladder stones were treated in 75 patients with continuous infusion and aspiration of methyl *tert*-butyl ether 4 to 6 times per minute for an average of 5 hours daily for 1 to 3 days.[1] At least 95% of the stone mass was dissolved in 72 patients. Gallbladder stones recurred in 4 patients between 6 and 16 months after the procedure; 7 of 51 patients with residual stone fragments had an episode of biliary colic during 6 to 42 months of follow-up. Nausea, sometimes with emesis, occurred in about one-third of patients. Overflow of solvent from the gallbladder can result in absorption from the gastrointestinal tract; methyl *tert*-butyl ether is detected on the breath and sedation can occur. One patient in whom overflow occurred developed ulcerative duodenitis and intravascular haemolysis. Coma and acute renal failure have also complicated treatment and have been attributed to leakage alongside the catheter rather than overflow of solvent.[5] Other workers[6,7] have obtained similar results for the dissolution of gallstones. One group[6] found that nausea and vomiting could be reduced if the treatment time was kept short and the perfusion volume was kept as low as possible; they also managed to prevent bile leakage and haemorrhage using a tissue adhesive or subcutaneous administration of ceruletide to contract the gallbladder. Dissolution of gallbladder stones with methyl *tert*-butyl ether is likely to remain confined to specialist centres for use in patients unsuitable for surgical treatment.[1] A combination of litholytic modalities such as dissolution with solvents or bile acids, or lithotripsy may overcome some of the disadvantages of individual treatments.[8]

Methyl *tert*-butyl ether has been instilled via a nasobiliary catheter to dissolve stones in the common bile duct. Although effective in some cases,[9] further study has indicated disappointing overall results.[1,10]

Various combinations of drugs have been investigated to dissolve pigment-rich or mixed stones. For common bile-duct stones these include a cocktail of dimethyl sulfoxide 60%, methyl *tert*-butyl ether 20%, and sodium bicarbonate 20%, and a regimen of alternating infusions of pentyl ether and edetic acid-urea 10%.[11] A similar regimen of methyl hexyl ether and edetic acid-urea has been used successfully in 2 patients with calcified gallbladder stones.[12]


1. Bouchier IAD. Gall stones. *BMJ* 1990; **300:** 592–7.
2. Maudgal DP, Northfield TC. A practical guide to the nonsurgical treatment of gallstones. *Drugs* 1991; **41:** 185–92.
3. Thistle JL, *et al.* Dissolution of cholesterol gallbladder stones by methyl *tert*-butyl ether administered by percutaneous transhepatic catheter. *N Engl J Med* 1989; **320:** 633–9.
4. Foerster E-Ch, *et al.* Direct dissolution of gallbladder stones. *Lancet* 1989; **i:** 954.
5. Ponchon T, *et al.* Renal failure during dissolution of gallstones by methyl-*tert*-butyl ether. *Lancet* 1988; **ii:** 276–7.
6. Hellstern A, *et al.* Gall stone dissolution with methyl tert-butyl ether: how to avoid complications. *Gut* 1990; **31:** 922–5.
7. McNulty J, *et al.* Dissolution of cholesterol gall stones using methyltertbutyl ether: a safe effective treatment. *Gut* 1991; **32:** 1550–3.
8. Salen G, Tint GS. Nonsurgical treatment of gallstones. *N Engl J Med* 1989; **320:** 665–6.
9. Murray WR, *et al.* Choledocholithiasis—in vivo stone dissolution using methyl tertiary butyl ether (MTBE). *Gut* 1988; **29:** 143–5.
10. Neoptolemos JP, *et al.* How good is methyl tert-butyl (MTBE) for common bile duct (CBD) stone dissolution? *Gut* 1989; **30:** A736–7.
11. Anonymous. Gallstones, bile acids, and the liver. *Lancet* 1989; **ii:** 249–51.
12. Swobodnik W, *et al.* Dissolution of calcified gallbladder stones by treatment with methyl-hexyl ether and urea-EDTA. *Lancet* 1988; **ii:** 216.


## Methyl Butyl Ketone

2-Hexanone; Methyl *n*-Butyl Ketone; Metilbutilcetona. Hexan-2-one.

$C_6H_{12}O$ = 100.2.

*CAS — 591-78-6.*

**Description.** Methyl butyl ketone is a colourless, volatile liquid. Wt per mL about 0.82 g. B.p. about 127°. Store in airtight containers.

## Methyl Isobutyl Ketone

Hexone; Isopropylacetone; Metilisobutilcetona; MIBK. 4-Methylpentan-2-one.

$C_6H_{12}O$ = 100.2.

*CAS — 108-10-1.*

**Pharmacopoeias.** In *USNF.*

**USNF 22** (Methyl Isobutyl Ketone). A transparent, colourless, mobile, volatile liquid having a faint ketonic and camphoraceous odour. Sp. gr. not more than 0.799. Distilling range 114° to 117°. Slightly soluble in water; miscible with alcohol, with ether, and with benzene. Store in airtight containers.

### Adverse Effects and Precautions

Methyl butyl ketone and methyl isobutyl ketone may depress the CNS in high concentrations. Their vapours are irritating to mucous membranes. Methyl isobutyl ketone may be implicated in volatile substance abuse (p.1471).

◊ References.


1. Methyl isobutyl ketone. *Environmental Health Criteria 117.* Geneva: WHO, 1990. Available at: http://www.inchem.org/documents/ehc/ehc/ehc117.htm (accessed 30/06/04)
2. Methyl isobutyl ketone health and safety guide. *IPCS Health and Safety Guide 58.* Geneva: WHO, 1991. Available at: http://www.inchem.org/documents/hsg/hsg/hsg058.htm (accessed 30/06/04)


**Effects on the nervous system.** Peripheral neuropathy[1] has occurred following occupational exposure to methyl butyl ketone, particularly an outbreak of neuropathy in a printing plant after the replacement of methyl isobutyl ketone by methyl butyl ketone in a solvent mixture with methyl ethyl ketone. Methyl ethyl ketone may have potentiated the neurotoxicity induced by methyl butyl ketone.

For further discussion of neurotoxicity after occupational exposure to solvents including methyl butyl ketone, see under Toluene, p.1477.


1. Lolin Y. Chronic neurological toxicity associated with exposure to volatile substances. *Hum Toxicol* 1989; **8:** 293–300.


**Handling.** Suitable precautions should be taken to avoid skin contact with methyl butyl ketone or methyl isobutyl ketone as they can penetrate skin and produce systemic toxicity.

### Uses

Methyl isobutyl ketone is used as an industrial and pharmaceutical solvent and also as an alcohol denaturant. Methyl butyl ketone is used as an industrial solvent.

## Methyl Chloride

Cloruro de metilo; Monochloromethane. Chloromethane.

$CH_3Cl$ = 50.49.

*CAS — 74-87-3.*

**Description.** Methyl chloride is a colourless gas compressed to a colourless liquid with an ethereal odour. B.p. about –24°. Store in airtight containers.

### Adverse Effects and Treatment

Symptoms of methyl chloride intoxication often appear after a latent period of several hours and are similar after acute or chronic exposure to the vapour. Symptoms include gastrointestinal disturbances such as nausea, vomiting, and abdominal pain, and signs of CNS depression including headache, weakness, drowsiness, confusion, visual disturbances, and incoordination progressing to convulsions, coma, and death from respiratory depression in severe cases. There have been a few reports of hepatic and renal damage.

Treatment consists of removal from exposure and supportive and symptomatic measures. Neurological effects may persist for many months.

◊ References to the toxicity of methyl chloride.


1. Repko JD, Lasley SM. Behavioral, neurological, and toxic effects of methyl chloride: a review of the literature. *CRC Crit Rev Toxicol* 1979; **6:** 283–302.


### Uses

Methyl chloride is used as an industrial solvent. It has been used as an aerosol propellant and refrigerant and was formerly used as a local anaesthetic.

## Methyl Ethyl Ketone

Ethyl Methyl Ketone; MEK; Metiletilcetona. Butan-2-one.

$C_4H_8O$ = 72.11.

*CAS — 78-93-3.*

**Description.** Methyl ethyl ketone is a colourless flammable liquid with an acetone-like odour. Wt per mL about 0.81 g. B.p. 79° to 81°. Soluble in water; miscible with alcohol and with ether. Store in airtight containers.

### Adverse Effects

Methyl ethyl ketone is irritant. Inhalation may result in mild CNS effects including headache and dizziness; nausea and vomiting may also occur.

Methyl ethyl ketone may be implicated in volatile substance abuse (p.1471).

◊ References.


1. Methyl ethyl ketone. *Environmental Health Criteria 143.* Geneva: WHO, 1992. Available at: http://www.inchem.org/documents/ehc/ehc/ehc143.htm (accessed 30/06/04)


**Effects on the nervous system.** There are isolated reports of neurotoxicity produced by methyl ethyl ketone alone.[1] These include 1 of retrobulbar neuritis and 1 of peripheral neuropathy. It has been suggested, however, that methyl ethyl ketone potentiates the peripheral neuropathy induced by methyl butyl ketone and *n*-hexane.

For further discussion of neurotoxicity after occupational exposure to solvents including methyl ethyl ketone, see under Toluene, p.1477.


1. Lolin Y. Chronic neurological toxicity associated with exposure to volatile substances. *Hum Toxicol* 1989; **8:** 293–300.


### Uses

Methyl ethyl ketone is used as an industrial solvent and as an extraction solvent in food processing.

## Octyldodecanol

Octildodecanol; Octyldodecanolum.

$C_{20}H_{42}O$ = 298.5.

**Pharmacopoeias.** In *Eur.* (see p.vi). Also in *USNF.*

**Ph. Eur. 5.0** (Octyldodecanol). A condensation product of saturated liquid fatty alcohols. It contains not less than 90% of (*RS*)-2-octyldodecan-1-ol, the remainder consisting mainly of related alcohols. A clear, colourless to yellowish, oily liquid. Relative density 0.830 to 0.850. Practically insoluble in water; miscible with alcohol. Protect from light.

**USNF 22** (Octyldodecanol). It contains not less than 90% of 2-octyldodecanol, the remainder consisting chiefly of related alcohols. A clear, water-white, free-flowing liquid. Insoluble in water; soluble in alcohol and in ether. Store in airtight containers.

### Profile

Octyldodecanol is used as a pharmaceutical solvent.

## Petroleum Spirit

Éter de petróleo; Light Petroleum; Petroleum Benzin; Petroleum Ether; Solvent Hexane.

**Description.** Petroleum spirit is a purified distillate of petroleum, consisting of a mixture of the lower members of the paraffin series of hydrocarbons. It is a colourless, transparent, very volatile, highly flammable liquid with a characteristic odour. It is available in a variety of boiling ranges.

**Pharmacopoeias.** In *Ger., Jpn.*, and *Pol.* Various boiling ranges are specified.

*Swiss* describes Benzinum Medicinale, consisting mainly of hexane and heptane.

◊ NOTE. The motor fuel termed 'petrol' in the UK and 'gasoline' in the USA is a mixture of volatile hydrocarbons of variable composition containing paraffins (alkanes), olefins (alkenes), cycloparaffins, and aromatic compounds.

### Adverse Effects and Treatment

As for Kerosene, p.1475. Petroleum spirit and petrol, being more volatile and of lower viscosity than kerosene, are more likely to be inhaled and to cause aspiration pneumonitis. The toxicity of petrol varies with its composition; some adverse effects have been attributed to lead additives or to the content of *n*-hexane or benzene. Petrol may be implicated in volatile solvent abuse (p.1471).

◊ References to the toxicity of petroleum spirit.[1-3]

For discussion of neurotoxicity after occupational exposure to solvents including petrol, see under Toluene, p.1477.


1. Selected petroleum products. *Environmental Health Criteria 20.* Geneva: WHO, 1982. Available at: http://www.inchem.org/documents/ehc/ehc/ehc020.htm (accessed 30/06/04)
2. Daniels AM, Latcham RW. Petrol sniffing and schizophrenia in a Pacific island paradise. *Lancet* 1984; **i:** 389.
3. Eastwell HD. Elevated lead levels in petrol "sniffers". *Med J Aust* 1985; **143** (suppl): S63–4.


### Uses

Petroleum spirit and other petroleum distillates are used as pharmaceutical solvents.

## Propylene Carbonate

Carbonato de propileno. 4-Methyl-1,3-dioxolan-2-one.

$C_4H_6O_3$ = 102.1.

*CAS — 108-32-7.*

**Description.** Propylene carbonate is a clear colourless mobile liquid. Freely soluble in water; miscible with alcohol and with chloroform; practically insoluble in petroleum spirit.

**Pharmacopoeias.** In *USNF.*

**USNF 22** (Propylene Carbonate). Sp. gr. 1.203 to 1.210 at 20°. Store in airtight containers.

### Profile

Propylene carbonate is used as a solvent in oral and topical pharmaceuticals and for cellulose-based polymers and plasticisers. It has been used as a nonvolatile, stabilising liquid carrier in hard gelatin capsules.

## Tetrachloroethane

Acetylene Tetrachloride; Tetracloroetano. 1,1,2,2-Tetrachloroethane.

$C_2H_2Cl_4$ = 167.8.

*CAS — 79-34-5.*

**Description.** Tetrachloroethane is a colourless liquid with a chloroform-like odour. B.p. about 146°. Wt per mL about 1.59 g. Store in airtight containers.

### Adverse Effects and Treatment

As for Carbon Tetrachloride, p.1472. Tetrachloroethane is probably the most toxic of the chlorinated hydrocarbons. Poisoning can occur through percutaneous absorption as well as after ingestion or inhalation.

**Handling.** Suitable precautions should be taken to avoid skin contact with tetrachloroethane as it can penetrate skin and produce systemic toxicity.

### Uses

Tetrachloroethane is used as an industrial solvent.

## Tetrachloroethylene

Perchloroethylene; Tetrachloroethene; Tetrachloroethylenum; Tetracloroetileno.

$C_2Cl_4$ = 165.8.

*CAS — 127-18-4.*

### Adverse Effects and Treatment

As for Carbon Tetrachloride, p.1472. Symptoms, especially following ingestion, are less severe with tetrachloroethylene than with carbon tetrachloride.

The vapour or liquid may be irritating to skin or mucous membranes.

Tetrachloroethylene may be implicated in volatile substance abuse (p.1471). Dependence may follow habitual inhalation of small quantities of tetrachloroethylene vapour.

◊ References to adverse effects of tetrachloroethylene.


1. Bagnell PC, Ellenberger HA. Obstructive jaundice due to a chlorinated hydrocarbon in breast milk. *Can Med Assoc J* 1977; **117:** 1047–8.
2. Tetrachloroethylene. *Environmental Health Criteria 31.* Geneva: WHO, 1984. Available at: http://www.inchem.org/documents/ehc/ehc/ehc31.htm (accessed 30/06/04)
3. Tetrachloroethylene health and safety guide. *IPCS Health and Safety Guide 10.* Geneva: WHO, 1987. Available at: http://www.inchem.org/documents/hsg/hsg/hsg010.htm (accessed 30/06/04)
4. Health and Safety Executive. Tetrachloroethylene (tetrachloroethene, perchloroethylene). *Toxicity Review 17.* London: HMSO, 1987.
5. Mutti A, *et al.* Nephropathies and exposure to perchloroethylene in dry-cleaners. *Lancet* 1992; **340:** 189–93.


### Pharmacokinetics

Tetrachloroethylene is slightly absorbed from the gastrointestinal tract; absorption is increased in the presence of alcohol and fats or oils. It is absorbed following inhalation and after direct contact with the skin. It is excreted unchanged in expired air; initial elimination is rapid but a proportion may be retained and excreted slowly.

Metabolites of tetrachloroethylene, mainly trichloroacetic acid, have been found in the urine.

### Uses and Administration

Tetrachloroethylene is a chlorinated hydrocarbon widely used as a solvent in industry. It was formerly given by mouth as an anthelmintic, but has been superseded by equally effective and less toxic drugs.

## Toluene

Methylbenzene; Phenylmethane; Tolueno; Toluol; Toluole.

$C_7H_8$ = 92.14.

*CAS — 108-88-3.*

**Description.** Toluene is a colourless, volatile, flammable liquid with a characteristic odour. Wt per mL about 0.87 g. B.p. about 111°. Store in airtight containers.

### Adverse Effects, Treatment, and Precautions

Toluene has similar acute toxicity to benzene (p.1471) but is a less serious industrial hazard. Adverse effects are treated similarly to benzene. It is a common constituent of adhesives and is frequently implicated in volatile substance abuse (p.1471). Commercial toluene may contain benzene, and this may perhaps influence the pattern of adverse effects. In addition to acute toxic effects, toluene abuse has been associated with damage to the nervous system, kidneys, liver, heart, and lungs (see below). Chronic poisoning caused by occupational exposure to toluene has resulted mainly in nervous system disorders.

◊ Reviews.


1. WHO. Recommended health-based limits in occupational exposure to selected organic solvents. *WHO Tech Rep Ser 664* 1981.
2. Toluene. *Environmental Health Criteria 52.* Geneva: WHO, 1985. Available at: http://www.inchem.org/documents/ehc/ehc/ehc52.htm (accessed 30/06/04)
3. Health and Safety Executive. Toluene. *Toxicity Review 20.* London: HMSO, 1989.


◊ The non-neurological toxicity following volatile substance abuse has been reviewed.[1] Chronic toluene abuse may result in damage to the *kidneys*; renal tubular acidosis and glomerulonephritis have been described, although evidence for the latter is only circumstantial. Renal tubular acidosis has been regarded as reversible; however, there are reports suggesting that damage to renal tubules is permanent.

The few reports linking chronic toluene abuse with *liver* damage cover hepatomegaly and hepatorenal failure. Effects on the *heart* are usually acute; sudden death has resulted from ventricular arrhythmias. Chronic myocarditis with fibrosis has been reported. Chronic toluene inhalation can cause damage to the *lungs.* Autopsies in a few patients have shown changes indicative of emphysema.

*Nervous system* toxicity has also been reviewed.[2] Cerebellar dysfunction has occurred after toluene abuse; an acute intoxication phase, which usually subsides within weeks of abstinence, is followed by a chronic phase which may be permanent. Diffuse CNS disease such as encephalopathy, dementia, and multifocal brain injury may also develop. An association between toluene abuse and peripheral neuropathy has not been confirmed; muscle weakness may be a result of electrolyte and fluid disturbances. The review cites individual reports of choreoathetosis, epilepsy, and optic atrophy with anosmia and deafness after toluene abuse. Some of these neurological effects, particularly cerebellar effects and diffuse CNS disease have also occurred after occupational exposure to toluene.

Some studies have noted an excess mortality from motor neurone diseases among leather workers,[3] although this has not been confirmed by others.[4] Occupational exposure to solvents has been postulated as the cause.[3] Of the many agents currently used in leather work, those with known or probable neurotoxic effects are *n*-hexane, methyl butyl ketone, toluene, and methyl ethyl ketone. Ethyl acetate is commonly used but has no recognised neurological side-effects.[3] A Swedish study of workers in a range of occupations has found some support for an increased risk of amyotrophic lateral sclerosis after occupational exposure to solvents, probably toluene and petrol.[5] Another Swedish study found an association between multiple sclerosis and occupational exposure to solvents, especially white spirit and petrol.[5]


1. Marjot R, McLeod AA. Chronic non-neurological toxicity from volatile substance abuse. *Hum Toxicol* 1989; **8:** 301–6.
2. Lolin Y. Chronic neurological toxicity associated with exposure to volatile substances. *Hum Toxicol* 1989; **8:** 293–300.
3. Hawkes CH, *et al.* Motoneuron disease: a disorder secondary to solvent exposure? *Lancet* 1989; **i:** 73–6.
4. Martyn CN. Motoneuron disease and exposure to solvents. *Lancet* 1989; **i:** 394.
5. Gunnarsson L-G, Lindberg G. Amyotrophic lateral sclerosis in Sweden 1970-83 and solvent exposure. *Lancet* 1989; **i:** 958.


**Handling.** Suitable precautions should be taken to avoid skin contact with toluene as it can penetrate skin and produce systemic toxicity.

**Pregnancy.** Retrospective surveys of pregnancies in mothers with a history of solvent abuse suggested that toluene abuse during pregnancy can cause preterm delivery and perinatal death. It was suggested that toluene may be teratogenic as intra-uterine exposure was associated with prenatal and postnatal growth retardation, microcephaly, impairment of mental development, and facial dysmorphia.[1-3] It is uncertain if these results can be extrapolated to cover occupational exposure. Although some studies of occupational exposure to solvents during pregnancy have suggested an association,[4,5] exposure is usually to a number of solvents[5] and there is little consistent evidence to link exposure to any particular one with spontaneous abortion, retarded fetal development, still-birth, or congenital malformation.[6]


1. Wilkins-Haug L, Gabow PA. Toluene abuse during pregnancy: obstetric complications and perinatal outcomes. *Obstet Gynecol* 1991; **77:** 504–9.
2. Pearson MA, *et al.* Toluene embryopathy: delineation of the phenotype and comparison with fetal alcohol syndrome. *Pediatrics* 1994; **93:** 211–15.
3. Arnold GL, *et al.* Toluene embryopathy: clinical delineation and developmental follow-up. *Pediatrics* 1994; **93:** 216–20.
4. McDonald JC, *et al.* Chemical exposures at work in early pregnancy and congenital defect: a case-referent study. *Br J Ind Med* 1987; **44:** 527–33.
5. Khattak S, *et al.* Pregnancy outcome following gestational exposure to organic solvents: a prospective controlled study. *JAMA* 1999; **281:** 1106–9.
6. Scott A. *BMJ* 1992; **304:** 369.


### Pharmacokinetics

Toluene is absorbed after inhalation and ingestion, and to some extent through the skin. It is rapidly metabolised mainly by oxidation to benzoic acid which is excreted in the urine largely as the glycine conjugate hippuric acid; *o*-, *m*-, and *p*-cresol are minor urinary metabolites. Some unchanged toluene is excreted through the lungs.

### Uses

Toluene is widely used as an industrial solvent.

## Tri-*n*-butyl Phosphate

Tributyl Phosphate; Tri-*n*-butylis Phosphas; Tri(*n*-butyl)phosphate. Phosphoric acid tributyl ester.

$C_{12}H_{27}O_4P$ = 266.3.

*CAS — 126-73-8.*

**Pharmacopoeias.** In *Eur.* (see p.vi).

**Ph. Eur. 5.0** (Tri-*n*-butyl Phosphate). A clear, colourless to pale yellow liquid. Slightly soluble in water; miscible with alcohol. Protect from light.

### Profile

Tri-*n*-butyl phosphate is an organophosphate that is used as a solvent and plasticiser.

◊ References.


1. Tri-*n*-butyl phosphate. *Environmental Health Criteria 112.* Geneva: WHO, 1991. Available at: http://www.inchem.org/documents/ehc/ehc/ehc112.htm (accessed 29/06/04)


## Trichloroethane

Methylchloroform; α-Trichloroethane; Tricloroetano. 1,1,1-Trichloroethane.

$C_2H_3Cl_3$ = 133.4.

*CAS — 71-55-6.*

**Description.** Trichloroethane is a colourless, slightly hygroscopic liquid. Sp. gr. about 1.31. B.p. about 74°. Practically insoluble in water; miscible with alcohol, with chloroform, and with ether. Non-flammable. Store in airtight containers.

### Adverse Effects and Treatment

Acute intoxication with trichloroethane may result in initial excitement followed by CNS depression with dizziness, drowsiness, headache, lightheadedness, and ataxia, progressing to coma and death from respiratory depression in severe cases. Death may also occur from ventricular arrhythmias. Fatalities have occurred following accidental exposure to high concentrations of trichloroethane in confined spaces. Trichloroethane is commonly used in dry cleaning, typewriter correction fluids, and as a solvent for plaster removal and is frequently implicated in volatile substance abuse (p.1471).

Nausea, vomiting, and diarrhoea have been reported following ingestion. Trichloroethane is a mild irritant.

Treatment of adverse effects consists of removal from exposure and general supportive and symptomatic measures. Activated charcoal may be given. Adrenaline and other sympathomimetics should be avoided because of the risk of precipitating cardiac arrhythmias.

◊ Reviews.


1. Health and Safety Executive. 1,1,1-Trichloroethane. *Toxicity Review 9.* London: HMSO, 1984.
2. 1,1,1-Trichloroethane. *Environmental Health Criteria 136.* Geneva: WHO, 1992. Available at: http://www.inchem.org/documents/ehc/ehc/ehc136.htm (accessed 30/06/04)


**Effects on the heart.** Effects on the heart of trichloroethane abuse were considered usually to be acute, and sudden death from ventricular arrhythmias had occurred in abusers. There have, however, been a few cases of chronic cardiac toxicity after both abuse and occupational exposure.[1]


1. Marjot R, McLeod AA. Chronic non-neurological toxicity from volatile substance abuse. *Hum Toxicol* 1989; **8:** 301–6.


**Effects on the liver.** According to a brief review of non-neurological toxicity from volatile substance abuse,[1] there were no reports of damage to the liver after the abuse of trichloroethane. There was a report of hepatotoxicity following acute occupational exposure, but this might have been a hypersensitivity reaction. There was another report[2] of fatty liver disease in 4 patients with a history of occupational exposure to trichloroethane although there has been some debate over the validity of the association for 2 of these cases.[3,4]


1. Marjot R, McLeod AA. Chronic non-neurological toxicity from volatile substance abuse. *Hum Toxicol* 1989; **8:** 301–6.
2. Hodgson MJ, *et al.* Liver disease associated with exposure to 1,1,1-trichloroethane. *Arch Intern Med* 1989; **149:** 1793–8.
3. Guzelian PS. 1,1,1-Trichloroethane and the liver. *Arch Intern Med* 1991; **151:** 2321–2.
4. Hodgson MJ, Vanthiel DH. 1,1,1-Trichloroethane and the liver. *Arch Intern Med* 1991; **151:** 2322 and 2325–6.


**Effects on the skin.** Scleroderma has been reported[1] in 3 patients occupationally exposed to trichloroethylene and, in 2 cases, also to trichloroethane.


1. Flindt-Hansen H, Isager H. Scleroderma after occupational exposure to trichlorethylene and trichlorethane. *Acta Derm Venereol (Stockh)* 1987; **67:** 263–4.


### Pharmacokinetics

Trichloroethane is absorbed after inhalation and ingestion, and through intact skin. Small amounts are metabolised to trichloroethanol and trichloroacetic acid and excreted in the urine, but it is largely excreted unchanged through the lungs over a period of days.

### Uses

Trichloroethane has wide applications as an industrial solvent. It is commonly used in dry cleaning, typewriter correction fluids, and as a solvent for plaster removal.

### Preparations

**Proprietary Preparations** (details are given in Part 3)
**UK:** Zoff.
**Multi-ingredient: *Austral.*:** Sacsol NF†.

## White Spirit

Stoddard Solvent; Trementina.

*CAS — 64742-82-1 (white spirit type 1); 64741-92-0 (white spirit type 2); 64742-48-9 (white spirit type 3); 64742-88-7 (white spirit type 0); 8052-41-3 (Stoddard solvent).*

**Description.** White spirit is a mixture of hydrocarbons available as a colourless liquid. Store in airtight containers.

### Adverse Effects and Treatment

As for Kerosene, p.1475.

◊ References to the toxicity of white spirit.[1]

For discussion of neurotoxicity after occupational exposure to solvents including white spirit, see under Toluene, p.1477.

1. Selected petroleum products. *Environmental Health Criteria 20.* Geneva: WHO, 1982. Available at: http://www.inchem.org/documents/ehc/ehc/ehc020.htm (accessed 30/06/04)

### Uses

White spirit is used as an industrial solvent. It is available in various grades. One grade available in the USA is known as Stoddard solvent.

## Xylene

Dimethylbenzene; Xileno; Xylol; Xylole.

$C_8H_{10}$ = 106.2.

*CAS — 1330-20-7; 108-38-3 (m-xylene); 95-47-6 (o-xylene); 106-42-3 (p-xylene).*

**Description.** Xylene is a mixture of the *o*-, *m*-, and *p*-isomers in which the *m*-isomer predominates. It is a colourless, volatile, flammable liquid. Wt per mL about 0.86 g. B.p. about 138° to 142°. Store in airtight containers.

### Adverse Effects, Treatment, and Precautions

The acute toxicity of xylene is similar to that of benzene (p.1471) but is less marked. Adverse effects are treated similarly to benzene.

Xylene has been implicated in volatile substance abuse (p.1471). Commercial xylene may contain benzene, and this may perhaps influence the pattern of adverse effects.

Xylene should not be used to dissolve ear wax if the tympanic membrane is perforated.

◊ References.

1. WHO. Recommended health-based limits in occupational exposure to selected organic solvents. *WHO Tech Rep Ser 664* 1981.
2. Health and Safety Executive. Xylenes. *Toxicity Review 26.* London: HMSO, 1992.
3. Xylenes. *Environmental Health Criteria 190.* Geneva: WHO, 1997. Available at: http://www.inchem.org/documents/ehc/ehc/ehc190.htm (accessed 30/06/04)

**Effects on the eyes.** Eye injuries due to accidental contact with paints containing xylene have been reported.[1] The injuries resembled alkali burns and were treated in a similar manner.

1. Ansari EA. Ocular injury with xylene - a report of two cases. *Hum Exp Toxicol* 1997; **16:** 273–5.

**Effects on the nervous system.** References to the adverse effects of xylene on the nervous system.

1. Arthur LJH, Curnock DA. Xylene-induced epilepsy following innocent glue sniffing. *BMJ* 1982; **284:** 1787.
2. Roberts FP, *et al.* Near-pure xylene causing reversible neuropsychiatric disturbance. *Lancet* 1988; **ii:** 273.

**Handling.** Suitable precautions should be taken to avoid skin contact with xylene as it can penetrate skin and produce systemic toxicity.

### Pharmacokinetics

Xylene is absorbed after inhalation, ingestion, and to some extent through the skin. It is rapidly metabolised by oxidation to the corresponding *o*-, *m*-, or *p*-methylbenzoic (toluic) acids and excreted in the urine largely as the glycine conjugate, methylhippuric acid (toluric acid). Xylenols are minor metabolites and are excreted in the urine as the glucuronide and sulfate conjugates. Some unchanged xylene is excreted through the lungs.

### Uses

Xylene is used as an industrial and pharmaceutical solvent and in preparations to dissolve ear wax.

### Preparations

**Proprietary Preparations** (details are given in Part 3)
***Fr.*:** Cerulyse; ***Ital.*:** Cerulisina; ***Switz.*:** Novo-Cerusol.

# Paraffins and Similar Bases

This chapter includes a number of substances used mainly as bases for the preparation of creams, ointments, other topical preparations, and suppositories. They are used either as inert carriers for drugs or for their various emulsifying and emollient properties. Some are also used to improve the texture, stability, or water repellent properties of the final preparation. The bases discussed include petroleum hydrocarbons, animal fats and waxes, vegetable oils, and silicones. Other substances used in the preparation of bases can be found in Soaps and other Anionic Surfactants (p.1574) and in Nonionic Surfactants (p.1411).

## Hard Paraffin

Hartparaffin; Paraff. Dur.; Paraffin; Paraffin Wax; Paraffinum Durum; Paraffinum Solidum; Parafina sólida.

*CAS — 8002-74-2.*

**Pharmacopoeias.** In *Chin., Eur.* (see p.vi), *Int., Jpn,* and *Pol.* Also in *USNF.*

*USNF* also includes Synthetic Paraffin.

**Ph. Eur. 5.0** (Paraffin, Hard). A purified mixture of solid saturated hydrocarbons, generally obtained from petroleum. M.p. 50° to 61°. It is a colourless or white mass. The melted substance is free from fluorescence in daylight. Practically insoluble in water and in alcohol; freely soluble in dichloromethane. Protect from light.

**USNF 22** (Paraffin). A purified mixture of solid hydrocarbons obtained from petroleum. It is a colourless or white, odourless, more or less translucent mass showing a crystalline structure, and is slightly greasy to the touch. It has a congealing range of 47° to 65°. Insoluble in water and in alcohol; slightly soluble in dehydrated alcohol; freely soluble in chloroform, in ether, in volatile oils, and in most warm fixed oils. An alcoholic extract is neutral to litmus. Store at a temperature not exceeding 40°.

**USNF 22** (Synthetic Paraffin). A very hard odourless white wax containing mostly long-chain, unbranched, saturated hydrocarbons, with a small amount of branched hydrocarbons. The average molecular weight may range from 400 to 1400. Insoluble in water; very slightly soluble in aliphatic, oxygenated, and halogenated hydrocarbon solvents; slightly soluble in aromatic and normal paraffinic solvents.

### Profile

Hard paraffin is employed principally as a stiffening ingredient in ointment bases. It is also used in creams, and as a coating for capsules and tablets.

A variety of hard paraffin (m.p. 43° to 46°) is employed in physiotherapy in the form of paraffin-wax baths for the relief of pain in inflamed joints and sprains.

The injection of paraffins may produce granulomatous reactions.

### Preparations

***BP 2003:*** Paraffin Ointment; Simple Ointment; Wool Alcohols Ointment.

**Proprietary Preparations** (details are given in Part 3)

**Multi-ingredient: *Fr.:*** Grassolind Neutral; ***UK:*** Melrose.

## Liquid Paraffin

905 (mineral hydrocarbons); Dickflüssiges Paraffin; Heavy Liquid Petrolatum; Huile de Vaseline Épaisse; Liquid Petrolatum; Mineral Oil; Oleum Petrolei; Oleum Vaselini; Paraffinum Liquidum; Paraffinum Subliquidum; Parafina líquida; Vaselinöl; Vaselinum Liquidum; White Mineral Oil.

*CAS — 8012-95-1.*
*ATC — A06AA01.*

**Pharmacopoeias.** In *Chin., Eur.* (see p.vi), *Jpn, Pol.,* and *US.*

**Ph. Eur. 5.0** (Paraffin, Liquid). A purified mixture of liquid saturated hydrocarbons obtained from petroleum. It is a transparent, colourless, oily liquid, free from fluorescence in daylight. Relative density 0.827 to 0.890. Viscosity 110 to 230 mPa s. Practically insoluble in water; slightly soluble in alcohol; miscible with hydrocarbons. Protect from light.

**USP 27** (Mineral Oil). A mixture of liquid hydrocarbons obtained from petroleum. It may contain a suitable stabiliser. It is a transparent, colourless, odourless or almost odourless, oily liquid, free, or practically free, from fluorescence. Insoluble in water and in alcohol; soluble in volatile oils; miscible with fixed oils (except castor oil). Store in airtight containers.

## Light Liquid Paraffin

Dünnflüssiges Paraffin; Huile de Vaseline Fluide; Light Liquid Petrolatum; Light Mineral Oil; Light White Mineral Oil; Paraff. Liq. Lev.; Paraffinum Liquidum Leve; Paraffinum Liquidum Tenue; Paraffinum Perliquidum; Spray Paraffin; Vaselina líquida.

*ATC — A06AA01.*

**Pharmacopoeias.** In *Eur.* (see p.vi) and *Jpn.* Also in *USNF. US* also includes Topical Light Mineral Oil .

**Ph. Eur. 5.0** (Paraffin, Light Liquid). A purified mixture of liquid saturated hydrocarbons obtained from petroleum. It is a transparent, colourless, oily liquid, free from fluorescence in daylight. Relative density 0.810 to 0.875. Viscosity 25 to 80 mPa s. Practically insoluble in water; slightly soluble in alcohol; miscible with hydrocarbons. Protect from light.

**USNF 22** (Light Mineral Oil). A mixture of liquid hydrocarbons obtained from petroleum. It may contain a suitable stabiliser. It has similar characteristics to Mineral Oil but a lower kinematic viscosity. Store in airtight containers.

### Adverse Effects and Precautions

Excessive dosage by mouth, or rectum, may result in anal seepage and irritation. Liquid paraffin is absorbed to a slight extent and may give rise to foreign-body granulomatous reactions. Similar reactions have followed the injection of liquid paraffin and may be considerably delayed in onset. Injection may also cause vasospasm and prompt surgical removal may be required to prevent severe damage. Lipoid pneumonia has been reported following the aspiration of liquid paraffin.

Chronic ingestion of liquid paraffin may rarely be associated with impaired absorption of fat-soluble vitamins and possibly other compounds. It should not be used when abdominal pain, nausea, or vomiting is present. Prolonged use should be avoided. The UK Committee on Safety of Medicines considers that it should not be used in children under 3 years of age.

◊ Haematological changes and deposition of food grade liquid paraffins in the liver, spleen, and lymph nodes has occurred during feeding studies in *rats.*[1]

1. FAO/WHO. Evaluation of certain food additives and contaminants: forty-fourth report of the joint FAO/WHO expert committee on food additives. *WHO Tech Rep Ser 859* 1995.

**Granuloma.** References.

1. Bloem JJ, van der Waal I. Paraffinoma of the face: a diagnostic and therapeutic problem. *Oral Surg* 1974; **38:** 675–80.
2. Albers DD, *et al.* Oil granuloma of the ureter. *J Urol (Baltimore)* 1984; **132:** 114.

**Lipoid pneumonia.** References.

1. Varkey B, Kutty AVP. Lipoid pneumonia with lipoid granulomata in scalene node. *Ann Intern Med* 1976; **84:** 176–7.
2. Anonymous. Case records of the Massachusetts general hospital. *N Engl J Med* 1977; **296:** 1105–11.
3. Becton DL, *et al.* Lipoid pneumonia in an adolescent girl secondary to use of lip gloss. *J Pediatr* 1984; **105:** 421–3.
4. Beermann B, *et al.* Lipoid pneumonia: an occupational hazard of fire eaters. *BMJ* 1984; **289:** 1728–9.

### Uses and Administration

Taken internally, liquid paraffin acts as a lubricant and, since it keeps the stools soft, it has been used in the symptomatic treatment of constipation (p.1240), although it should be used with caution because of its adverse effects. Up to 45 mL has been given daily by mouth, usually in the evening although it should not be taken immediately before going to bed. Liquid paraffin is an ingredient of several preparations that contain other laxatives such as cascara, magnesium hydroxide, or phenolphthalein. It has also been given as an enema in a usual dose of 120 mL.

Externally, liquid paraffin may be used as an ingredient of ointment bases, as an emollient and cleanser in certain skin conditions, and as an ophthalmic lubricant in the management of dry eye (p.1576).

Light liquid paraffin has similar uses to liquid paraffin.

### Preparations

***BP 2003:*** Cetomacrogol Emulsifying Ointment; Cetrimide Emulsifying Ointment; Emulsifying Ointment; Light Liquid Paraffin Eye Drops; Liquid Paraffin and Magnesium Hydroxide Oral Emulsion; Liquid Paraffin Oral Emulsion; Simple Eye Ointment; Wool Alcohols Ointment;
***USP 27:*** Bland Lubricating Ophthalmic Ointment; Mineral Oil Emulsion; Mineral Oil, Rectal; Topical Light Mineral Oil.

**Proprietary Preparations** (details are given in Part 3)

***Arg.:*** Babix; Lansoyl; Laxuave Enteral; Lexavite; Lubritina Franklin; Modaton NI; Oilatum; ***Austral.:*** Agarol; Oilatum Bar; Oilatum Emollient; Oilatum Shower Gel; ***Belg.:*** Lansoyl; ***Braz.:*** Nujol; Oilatum†; Purol†; ***Canad.:*** Fleet Enema Mineral Oil; Lansoyl; Nujol; Skin Conditioner & Bath Oil†; Therapeutic Bath Oil†; ***Fr.:*** Lansoyl; Laxamalt; Lubentyl; Nujol†; Nutra Nutraderme†; Oilatum Emollient; Oilatum Soap; Oleatum Bar†; Oleatum Emollient†; Oleatum Gel†; Restrical; ***Ger.:*** Agarol N; Obstinol M; Oleatum†; ***Gr.:*** Agarol Plain; Nujol; Paragel; ***Hong Kong:*** Agarol; Body Wash; Keri; Oilatum Bar; Oilatum Emollient; Oilatum Gel; Vigarol; ***Irl.:*** Alcoderm; Oilatum Gel†; ***Ital.:*** Agarol CM; Duratirs; ***Malaysia:*** Balneum; Laxaron; Oilatum; ***Mon.:*** Parlax; ***NZ:*** Fleet Mineral Enema; Oilatum; ***Singapore:*** Balneum; Nutraderm; Oilatum Bar; Oilatum Emollient; Oilatum Gel; ***Spain:*** Emuliquen Simple; Hodernal; ***Switz.:*** Lansoyl†; Laxamalt†; Paragol N; ***Thai.:*** Nutraderm†; Oilatum Bar; Oilatum Emollient; Oilatum Gel; ***UK:*** Cetraben Bath Oil; Dermamist; Keri; Oilatum Bath Formula; Oilatum Fragrance Free; Oilatum Gel; Oilatum Junior; Oilatum Skin Therapy†; Oilatum Soap; Zerobase; ***USA:*** Kondremul; Liqui-Doss; Milkinol†.

**Multi-ingredient: *Arg.:*** Agarol; Aqualane; Cold Cream Naturel; Mil-Par; Usar Fibras; ***Austral.:*** Alpha Keri; Alpha Keri Tar†; DermaVeen Shower & Bath†; Dermeze†; Duratears; E45†; Egozite Baby Cream; Granugen; Hamilton Body Lotion; Hamilton Cleansing Lotion; Hamilton Dry Skin; Lacri-Lube; Oilatum Plus; Parachoc; Pinetarsol; Rikoderm; Soov Prickly Heat; ***Austria:*** Balneum F; ***Belg.:*** Duratears; Lacrytube; Tulle Vaseline; ***Braz.:*** Agarol; Balmex; Fenogar†; Laxantil†; Manon†; ***Canad.:*** Agarol Plain; Agarol†; Akwa Tears; Alpha Keri; Duolube; Duratears; Episec; Huile de Bain Therapeutique; Hypotears; Lacri-Lube; Laxarol†; Lubriderm; Magnolax; Oculube†; Optilube; Penederm; Puralube; Stancare†; Therapeutic Bath Oil; Therapeutic Skin Lotion; Ti-Lub; ***Chile:*** Acnaid; Acnoxyl Jabon; Cold Cream Avene; Durasolets; Duratears; Lacri-Lube; ***Denm.:*** Ojensalve Neutral†; ***Fr.:*** Balmex†; Balneum surgras†; Cerat Inalterable; Cold Cream Naturel; Dexeryl; Lubentyl a la Magnesie; Melaxose; Oilatum Body Oil; Oilatum Cream; Parapsyllium; Transitol†; Transulose; ***Ger.:*** Allergika; Balneum F; Befelka-Oel; Coliquifilm; Gleitgelen; Hoecutin Olbad F†; Oleobal; Parfenac Basisbad; Windol Basisbad; ***Gr.:*** Duratears; ***Hong Kong:*** Alpha Keri; Balneum Hermal; Duratears; Ego Skin Cream; Egozite Baby Cream; Hydromol; Oilatum Cream; Oilatum Plus; Polytar Emollient; Soov Prickly Heat; ***India:*** Agarol; Cetraben; Cremaffin; ***Irl.:*** Agarol†; Diprobath†; Emulsiderm; Hydromol; Lacri-Lube; Oilatum Emollient; Oilatum Junior Flare-Up†; Oilatum Plus; Petrolagar No. 2†; Petrolagar with Phenolphthalein†; Polytar Emollient; ***Israel:*** Balneum F; Duratears; Emulsiderm; Hypotears†; Lacri-Lube†; Lacrimol; ***Ital.:*** Balneum Hermal Forte; Duolaxan; Lacrilube; ***Malaysia:*** Balneum; Duratears Naturale; Egozite Baby Cream; Lacrilube; Oilatum Plus Antibacterial; Soov Prickly Heat; ***Mex.:*** Acuafil; Milpar; ***Norw.:*** Simplex; ***NZ:*** Alpha Keri; BK; DP; DP Lotion - HC; Duratears†; E45†; Ego Skin Cream; Egozite Baby; Hydroderm; Karicare Baby Bath Oil†; Karicare Breast and Body Cream; Karicare Mother and Baby†; Lacrilube; Oilatum Plus; Pharmacycare Bath Oil†; Pharmacycare Hand & Body†; Poly-Visc; Polytar Emollient; ***Port.:*** Balmex†; Banholeum Gel; Oleoban Gel; ***S.Afr.:*** Agarol†; Lacrilube†; Millypar†; Oilatum Plus; ***Singapore:*** Alpha Keri†; Balneum; DermaVeen Shower & Bath; Duratears; Egozite Baby Cream; Lacrilube; Lubrifilm†; Oilatum Plus; QV Flare Up; Soov Prickly Heat; ***Spain:*** Aceite Acalorico; Agarol†; Emuliquen Laxante; Lubrifilm; Vaselatum; ***Switz.:*** Agarol†; Antidry; Balmandol; Balneum Hermal F; Coliquifilm; Duratears†; Melisol†; Paragar; ***Thai.:*** Agarol; Balneum; Duratears; Emulax; Oilatum Cream; Oilatum Plus; ***UK:*** 50:50; Agarol†; Alpha Keri; Ashbourne Emollient Medicinal Bath Oil; Cetraben; Dermalo; Dermol; Diprobase; Diprobath; Doublebase; Emulsiderm; Epaderm; Hydromol; Imuderm; Infaderm; Lacri-Lube; Lubri-Tears; Mil-Par; Oilatum Cream; Oilatum Emollient; Oilatum Junior; Oilatum Junior Flare-Up; Oilatum Plus; Polytar Emollient; ***USA:*** Agoral; Akwa Tears; Alpha Keri; Desitin Creamy; Dry Eyes; Duratears Naturale; Haley's M-O; Hemorid For Women; Hydrocerin; Hypotears; Lacri-Gel; Lacri-Lube; Lacticare; LubriTears; Puralube; Refresh PM; Tears Again; Tears Renewed; Throat Discs; Vagisil; ZBT†.

## White Soft Paraffin

905 (mineral hydrocarbons); Paraff. Moll. Alb.; Paraffinum Molle Album; Vaselina Branca; Vaselina filante; Vaseline Officinale; White Petrolatum; White Petroleum Jelly.

**Pharmacopoeias.** In *Chin., Eur.* (see p.vi), *Int., Jpn, Pol., US,* and *Viet.*

Many pharmacopoeias use the title Vaselinum Album; in Great Britain the name 'Vaseline' is a trade-mark.

**Ph. Eur. 5.0** (Paraffin, White Soft). Purified and wholly or nearly decolorised mixture of semi-solid hydrocarbons, obtained from petroleum. It may contain a suitable antioxidant. It is not suitable for oral use. A white or almost white, translucent, soft unctuous mass, slightly fluorescent in daylight when melted. Drop point 35° to 70°. Practically insoluble in water, in alcohol, and in glycerol; soluble in dichloromethane. Protect from light.

The BP 2003 gives White Petroleum Jelly as an approved synonym.

**USP 27** (White Petrolatum). A purified mixture of semisolid hydrocarbons obtained from petroleum, and wholly or nearly decolorised. It may contain a suitable stabiliser. A white or faintly yellowish unctuous mass, transparent in thin layers even after cooling to 0°. Insoluble in water; slightly soluble in cold or hot alcohol and in cold dehydrated alcohol; freely soluble in chloroform, in benzene, and in carbon disulfide; soluble in ether, in petroleum spirit, and in most fixed and volatile oils.

## Yellow Soft Paraffin

Paraff. Moll. Flav.; Paraffinum Molle Flavum; Petrolatum; Petroleum Jelly; Vaselina Amarela; Vaselina amarilla; Yellow Petrolatum; Yellow Petroleum Jelly.

*CAS — 8009-03-8.*

**Pharmacopoeias.** In *Chin., Eur.* (see p.vi), *Jpn, Pol.,* and *US.*

Many pharmacopoeias use the title Vaselinum Flavum; in Great Britain the name 'Vaseline' is a trade-mark.

**Ph. Eur. 5.0** (Paraffin, Yellow Soft). A purified mixture of semi-solid hydrocarbons obtained from petroleum. A yellow, translucent, unctuous mass, slightly fluorescent in daylight when melted. It has a drop point of 40° to 60°. Practically insoluble in water, in alcohol, and in glycerol; soluble in dichloromethane. Protect from light.

**USP 27** (Petrolatum). A purified mixture of semi-solid hydrocarbons obtained from petroleum. It may contain a suitable stabiliser. It is an unctuous yellowish to light amber mass, having not more than a slight fluorescence even after being melted. It is transparent in thin layers. It is free or practically free from odour. M.p. 38° to 60°. Insoluble in water; practically insoluble in cold or hot alcohol and in cold dehydrated alcohol; freely soluble in benzene, in carbon disulfide, in chloroform, and in turpentine oil; soluble in ether, in petroleum spirit, and in most fixed and volatile oils.

### Adverse Effects

Adverse effects of soft paraffin are rare when used in topical preparations, but sensitivity reactions and acne have been reported following topical use. Granulomatous reactions following absorption or injection and lipoid pneumonia following aspiration have occurred.

◊ Burns to the scalp, face, and hands have been reported[1] in 5 patients who accidentally ignited their hair following the application of paraffin-based hair grease. Four patients suffered inhalation injury, 2 of whom required intubation.

1. Bascom R, *et al.* Inhalation injury related to use of petrolatum-based hair grease. *J Burn Care Rehabil* 1984; **5:** 327–30.

**Hypersensitivity.** The allergenicity of soft paraffin products has been investigated.[1-3] Considering their widespread use there are very few reports of sensitivity; white soft paraffin is generally less sensitising than yellow soft paraffin, although allergenicity differs from product to product. The allergenic components are probably polycyclic aromatic hydrocarbons present as impurities and quantities found in a particular paraffin depend on the source and purification method. Only the purest forms should be used in pharmaceuticals, cosmetics, and for patch testing, and highly purified white soft paraffin is preferred to yellow soft paraffin.

1. Dooms-Goossens A, Degreef H. Contact allergy to petrolatums (I). Sensitising capacity of different brands of yellow and white petrolatums. *Contact Dermatitis* 1983; **9:** 175–85.
2. Dooms-Goossens A, Degreef H. Contact allergy to petrolatums (II). Attempts to identify the nature of the allergens. *Contact Dermatitis* 1983; **9:** 247–56.
3. Dooms-Goossens A, Dooms M. Contact allergy to petrolatums (III). Allergenicity prediction and pharmacopoeial requirements. *Contact Dermatitis* 1983; **9:** 352–9.

### Uses and Administration

Soft paraffin is used as an ointment basis and as an emollient in the management of skin disorders. It is not readily absorbed by the skin. Sterile dressings containing soft paraffin are used for wound dressing and as a packing material. Soft paraffin is also included in ointments used as ophthalmic lubricants in the management of dry eye (p.1576). Application of soft paraffin has also been used for the eradication of pubic lice from the eyelashes (see Pediculosis, p.1499).

### Preparations

***BP 2003:*** Cetomacrogol Emulsifying Ointment; Cetrimide Emulsifying Ointment; Emulsifying Ointment; Paraffin Ointment; Simple Eye Ointment; Simple Ointment; Wool Alcohols Ointment;
***USP 27:*** Bland Lubricating Ophthalmic Ointment; Hydrophilic Ointment; Hydrophilic Petrolatum; Petrolatum Gauze; White Ointment; Yellow Ointment.

**Proprietary Preparations** (details are given in Part 3)
***Austral.:*** Jelonet; Uni Salve; Unitulle; ***Braz.:*** Vaselina; ***Canad.:*** Aquaphor†; Vaseline; ***Fr.:*** Jelonet; Unitulle†; Vaselitulle; ***Ital.:*** Adaptic; Jelonet; Lomatuell H; ***Mex.:*** Lubrilin†; ***S.Afr.:*** Jelonet; ***Spain:*** Lacrilube; ***UK:*** Dermamist; Jelonet; Paratulle; Vaseline; ***USA:*** Ocu-Lube.

**Multi-ingredient:** ***Arg.:*** Aqualane; ***Austral.:*** Blistex Medicated Lip Conditioner†; DermaVeen Moisturising†; Dermeze†; E45†; Gold Cross Skin Basics Zinc Cream; Lacri-Lube; Poly Visc; ***Austria:*** Tiroler Steinol; ***Belg.:*** Duratears; Lacrytube; Tulle Vaseline; ***Canad.:*** Akwa Tears; Chapstick Medicated Lip Balm; Diaper Guard†; Duolube; Duratears; Hydrophil; Hypotears; Lacri-Lube; Moisturel; Oculube†; Optilube; Prevex; Puralube; ***Chile:*** Chapstick Medicated; Durasolets; Duratears; Lacri-Lube; Pasta Lassar; ***Denm.:*** Ojensalve Neutral†; ***Fr.:*** Dexeryl; Grassolind Neutral; Ictyane; Oilatum Cream; Transitol†; Transulose; ***Ger.:*** Allergika; Coliquifilm; ***Gr.:*** Duratears; ***Hong Kong:*** Balneum Hermal; Duratears; Dyprotex; Oilatum Cream; ***India:*** Cetraben; ***Irl.:*** Lacri-Lube; ***Israel:*** Duratears; Hypotears†; Kamil Blue; Lacri-Lube†; Lacrimol; ***Ital.:*** Lacrilube; ***Malaysia:*** Balneum; Duratears Naturale; Lacrilube; ***Norw.:*** Simplex; ***NZ:*** Duratears†; Lacrilube; Poly-Visc; ***S.Afr.:*** Lacrilube†; ***Singapore:*** Balneum; Duratears; Lacrilube; Lubrifilm†; ***Spain:*** Lubrifilm; Tears Lubricante; Vaselina Boricada; Vaselina Mentolada; ***Switz.:*** Coliquifilm; ***Thai.:*** Balneum; Duratears; Oilatum Cream; ***UK:*** 50:50; Cetraben; Diprobase; Epaderm; Hewletts; Hydromol; Imuderm; Lacri-Lube; Lubri-Tears; Melrose; Oilatum Cream; Oilatum Junior; ***USA:*** Akwa Tears; Bottom Better; Chapstick Medicated Lip Balm; Desitin Creamy; Diaper Guard; Dry Eyes; Duratears Naturale; Formulation R; Hemorid For Women; Hydrocerin; Hypotears; Lacri-Gel; Lacri-Lube; LubriTears; Puralube; Refresh PM; Tears Again; Tears Renewed.

## Alkyl Benzoate

Alkyl (C12-15) Benzoate; Benzoato de alquilo.

**Pharmacopoeias.** In *USNF.*

**USNF 22** (Alkyl (C12-15) Benzoate). It consists of esters of a mixture of $C_{12}$ to $C_{15}$ primary and branched alcohols and benzoic acid. It is a clear, practically colourless, oily liquid. Insoluble in water, in glycerol, and in propylene glycol; soluble in alcohol, in acetone, in ethyl acetate, in isopropyl alcohol, in isopropyl myristate, in isopropyl palmitate, in liquid paraffin, in vegetable oils, in volatile silicones, and in wool fat. Store in airtight containers. Protect from light.

### Profile

Alkyl benzoate has emollient properties. It may be used as an oily vehicle.

## White Beeswax

Cera Alba; Cera Blanca; Cêra Branca; Cera de abejas; Cire Blanche; E901; Gebleichtes Wachs; White Wax.
*CAS — 8012-89-3.*

**Pharmacopoeias.** In *Eur.* (see p.vi), *Jpn,* and *Pol.* Also in *USNF.*

**Ph. Eur. 5.0** (Beeswax, White). It is bleached yellow beeswax. It occurs as white or yellowish-white pieces or plates, translucent when thin, with an odour similar to that of yellow beeswax, though fainter and never rancid, and with a fine-grained, matt and non-crystalline fracture, becoming soft and malleable when warmed in the hand. Drop point 61° to 66°. Practically insoluble in water; partially soluble in hot alcohol; completely soluble in fatty and essential oils.

**USNF 22** (White Wax). It is bleached and purified yellow beeswax. A yellowish-white solid, somewhat translucent in thin layers. It has a faint characteristic odour and is free from rancidity. M.p. 62° to 65°. Insoluble in water; sparingly soluble in cold alcohol; boiling alcohol dissolves the cerotic acid and a portion of the myricin that are constituents of the wax; completely soluble in chloroform, in ether, in fixed oils, and in volatile oils; partly soluble in cold benzene and in cold carbon disulfide; completely soluble in these liquids at about 30°.

## Yellow Beeswax

Cêra Amarela; Cera Amarilla; Cera de abejas amarilla; Cera Flava; Cire Jaune; E901; Gelbes Wachs; Yellow Wax.
*CAS — 8012-89-3.*

**Pharmacopoeias.** In *Chin., Eur.* (see p.vi), *Jpn,* and *Pol.* Also in *USNF.*

**Ph. Eur. 5.0** (Beeswax, Yellow). The wax obtained by melting with hot water the walls of the honeycomb of the bee, *Apis mellifera,* and removing the foreign matter. It occurs as yellow or light brown pieces or plates with a faint and characteristic odour of honey, and with a fine-grained, matt and non-crystalline fracture, becoming soft and malleable when warmed in the hand. Drop point 61° to 66°. Practically insoluble in water; partially soluble in hot alcohol; completely soluble in fatty and essential oils.

**USNF 22** (Yellow Wax). The purified wax from the honeycomb of the bee, *Apis mellifera* (Apidae). It is a solid, varying in colour from yellow to greyish-brown with an agreeable honey-like odour, somewhat brittle when cold, pliable when warmed in the hand, and presenting a dull, granular, noncrystalline fracture when broken. M.p. 62° to 65°. Insoluble in water; sparingly soluble in cold alcohol; boiling alcohol dissolves the cerotic acid and a portion of the myricin that are constituents of the wax; completely soluble in chloroform, in ether, in fixed oils, and in volatile oils; partly soluble in cold benzene and in cold carbon disulfide; completely soluble in these liquids at about 30°.

### Profile

Yellow beeswax is used as a stiffening agent in ointments and creams, and enables water to be incorporated to produce water-in-oil emulsions. White beeswax has similar uses; it is occasionally used to adjust the melting-point of suppositories.

A sterile preparation of white beeswax, hard paraffin, and isopropyl palmitate (Sterile Surgical Bone Wax) has been used to control bleeding from damaged bone in orthopaedic surgery. It should not be confused with Aseptic Surgical Wax (BPC 1949), also known as Horsley's Wax, which contained yellow beeswax, olive oil, and phenol in a mercuric chloride solution and was used to control haemorrhage in bone or cranial surgery.

Hypersensitivity to beeswax has been reported.

### Preparations

***BP 2003:*** Paraffin Ointment;
***USP 27:*** Rose Water Ointment; White Ointment; Yellow Ointment.

**Proprietary Preparations** (details are given in Part 3)
**Multi-ingredient:** ***Arg.:*** Aqualane; Cold Cream Naturel; Zoodermina Cream; ***Austria:*** Tiroler Steinol; ***Braz.:*** Balmex; ***Chile:*** Cold Cream Avene; ***Fr.:*** Balmex†; Cerat Inalterable; Cold Cream Naturel; ***Port.:*** Balmex†.

## Candelilla Wax

E902.
*CAS — 8006-44-8.*

**Pharmacopoeias.** In *USNF.*

**USNF 22** (Candelilla Wax). The purified wax from the leaves of the plant *Euphorbia antisyphilitica.* It is a hard, yellowish-brown, opaque to translucent wax. M.p.between 68.5° and 72.5°. Insoluble in water; soluble in chloroform and in toluene. Protect from moisture. Avoid excessive heat and freezing.

### Profile

Candelilla wax is used as a pharmaceutical excipient and in the food industry.

## Cetostearyl Alcohol

Alcohol cetoestearílico; Alcohol Cetylicus et Stearylicus; Alcool Cetostearilico; Cetearyl Alcohol; Cetostearyl Alc.; Cetylstearylalkohol.
*CAS — 8005-44-5; 67762-27-0.*

**Pharmacopoeias.** In *Eur.* (see p.vi), *Int.,* and *Pol.* Also in *USNF.*

**Ph. Eur. 5.0** (Cetostearyl Alcohol). A mixture of solid aliphatic alcohols. It contains not less than 90% of stearyl plus cetyl alcohols and not less than 40% of stearyl alcohol. A white or pale yellow wax-like mass, plates, flakes, or granules. M.p. 49° to 56°. Practically insoluble in water; soluble in alcohol and in petroleum spirit. When melted, it is miscible with fatty oils, with liquid paraffin, and with melted wool fat.

**Ph. Eur. 5.0** (Cetostearyl Alcohol (Type A), Emulsifying; Alcohol Cetylicus et Stearylicus Emulsificans A). A mixture containing not less than 80% cetostearyl alcohol and not less than 7% sodium cetostearyl sulfate, both calculated with reference to the anhydrous substance. A suitable buffer may be added. White or pale yellow, wax-like mass, plates, flakes, or granules. Soluble in hot water giving an opalescent solution; practically insoluble in cold water; slightly soluble in alcohol.

**Ph. Eur. 5.0** (Cetostearyl Alcohol (Type B), Emulsifying; Alcohol Cetylicus et Stearylicus Emulsificans B). A mixture containing not less than 80% cetostearyl alcohol and not less than 7% sodium laurilsulfate, both calculated with reference to the anhydrous substance. A suitable buffer may be added. White or pale yellow, wax-like mass, plates, flakes, or granules. Soluble in hot water giving an opalescent solution; practically insoluble in cold water; slightly soluble in alcohol.

**USNF 22** (Cetostearyl Alcohol). It contains not less than 40% of stearyl alcohol ($C_{18}H_{38}O = 270.5$) and the sum of the stearyl alcohol content and the cetyl alcohol ($C_{16}H_{34}O = 242.4$) content is not less than 90%. Unctuous, white flakes or granules, having a faint, characteristic odour. M.p. 48° to 55°. Insoluble in water; soluble in alcohol and in ether.

### Profile

Cetostearyl alcohol is used in creams, ointments, and other topical preparations as a stiffening agent and emulsion stabiliser. Used with suitable hydrophilic substances, as in Emulsifying Wax, it produces oil-in-water emulsions that are stable over a wide pH range. It is also used to improve the emollient properties of paraffin ointments.

Cetostearyl alcohol can cause hypersensitivity.

### Preparations

***BP 2003:*** Cetomacrogol Emulsifying Wax; Cetrimide Emulsifying Ointment; Emulsifying Wax;
***USNF 22:*** Emulsifying Wax.

## Cetyl Alcohol

Alcohol cetílico; Alcohol Cetylicus; Álcool Cetílico; Cetanol; 1-Hexadecanol; Hexadecyl Alcohol.
*CAS — 36653-82-4; 124-29-8.*

**Pharmacopoeias.** In *Eur.* (see p.vi), *Int., Jpn,* and *Pol.* Also in *USNF.*

**Ph. Eur. 5.0** (Cetyl Alcohol). A mixture of solid alcohols consisting mainly of cetyl alcohol ($C_{16}H_{33}OH = 242.4$). It occurs as a white unctuous mass, powder, flakes, or granules. M.p. 46° to 52°. Practically insoluble in water; freely to sparingly soluble in alcohol; miscible when melted with animal and vegetable oils, with liquid paraffin, and with melted wool fat.

**USNF 22** (Cetyl Alcohol). A mixture containing not less than 90% of cetyl alcohol ($C_{16}H_{34}O = 242.4$), the remainder consisting chiefly of related alcohols. White unctuous flakes, cubes, granules, or castings, with a faint characteristic odour. M.p. 45° to 50°. Insoluble in water; soluble in alcohol and in ether, the solubility increasing with increasing temperature.

### Profile

Cetyl alcohol is used in topical preparations for its emollient, water absorptive, stiffening, and weak emulsifying properties. It may be incorporated into suppositories to raise the melting-point and may be used in the coating of modified-release solid dose forms.

Cetyl alcohol can cause hypersensitivity.

### Preparations

**Proprietary Preparations** (details are given in Part 3)
**Multi-ingredient:** ***Hong Kong:*** Ego Skin Cream; ***NZ:*** Ego Skin Cream.

## Cetyl Esters Wax

Cera de ésteres cetílicos; Synthetic Spermaceti.

**Pharmacopoeias.** In *Int.* Also in *USNF.*

**USNF 22** (Cetyl Esters Wax). A mixture consisting primarily of esters of saturated fatty alcohols ($C_{14}$ to $C_{18}$) and saturated fatty acids ($C_{14}$ to $C_{18}$). White to off-white somewhat translucent flakes with a crystalline structure and a pearly lustre when caked; it has a faint odour and is free from rancidity. M.p. 43° to 47°. Insoluble in water; practically insoluble in cold alcohol; soluble in boiling alcohol, in chloroform, in ether, and in fixed and volatile oils; slightly soluble in cold petroleum spirit. Store in a dry place at a temperature not exceeding 40°.

### Profile

Cetyl esters wax is used as a stiffening agent and emollient in creams and ointments as a replacement for natural spermaceti obtained from the sperm whale and the bottle-nosed whale.

### Preparations

***USP 27:*** Rose Water Ointment.

**Proprietary Preparations** (details are given in Part 3)
**Multi-ingredient:** ***Arg.:*** Cold Cream Naturel.

## Cholesterol

Cholesterin; Cholesterolum; Colesterol. Cholest-5-en-3β-ol.
$C_{27}H_{46}O = 386.7.$
*CAS — 57-88-5.*

**Pharmacopoeias.** In *Eur.* (see p.vi), *Jpn,* and *Pol.* Also in *USNF.*

**Ph. Eur. 5.0** (Cholesterol). A white or almost white, crystalline powder. It is sensitive to light. M.p. 147° to 150°. Practically insoluble in water; sparingly soluble in alcohol and in acetone. Protect from light.

**USNF 22** (Cholesterol). White or faintly yellow, practically odourless, pearly leaflets, needles, powder, or granules. It acquires a yellow to pale tan colour on prolonged exposure to light. M.p. 147° to 150°. Insoluble in water; slowly soluble 1 in 100 of alcohol; soluble 1 in 50 of dehydrated alcohol; soluble in acetone, in chloroform, in dioxan, in ether, in ethyl acetate, in petroleum spirit, and in vegetable oils. Protect from light.

### Profile

Cholesterol imparts water-absorbing power to ointments and is used as an emulsifying agent. It has emollient activity.

Cholesteryl benzoate has been used as an ingredient in dermatological preparations.

### Preparations

**Proprietary Preparations** (details are given in Part 3)
**Multi-ingredient:** ***Chile:*** Perfungol.

## Coconut Oil

Aceite de coco; Coconut Butter; Oleum Cocois; Oleum Cocos Raffinatum; Oleum Cocosis.
*CAS — 8001-31-8.*

**Pharmacopoeias.** In *Eur.* (see p.vi) and *Jpn.*

**Ph. Eur. 5.0** (Coconut Oil, Refined). The refined fatty oil obtained from the dried, solid part of the endosperm of *Cocos nucifera*. A white or almost white, unctuous mass. M.p. 23° to 26°. Practically insoluble in water; very slightly soluble in alcohol; freely soluble in dichloromethane and in petroleum spirit (b.p. 65° to 70°). Store in well-filled containers. Protect from light.

### Profile

Coconut oil forms a readily absorbable ointment basis. It is also used in food manufacturing. Topical preparations have been used for pediculosis.

Fractionated coconut oil (thin vegetable oil) is used as a source of medium-chain triglycerides (p.1440).

### Preparations

**Proprietary Preparations** (details are given in Part 3)
***Ger.:*** Aesculo Gel L; ***UK:*** Nitlotion.
**Multi-ingredient:** ***Arg.:*** Tersoderm Cabellos Grasos; ***Malaysia:*** Palmer's Cocoa Butter Formula; Palmer's Cocoa Butter Formula Nappy Rash; Palmer's Cocoa Butter Formula Nursing; ***Mex.:*** Nutegen G; ***NZ:*** Mr Nits.

## Emulsifying Wax

Anionic Emulsifying Wax; Cera Emulsificans; Cera emulsionante; Cetylanum; Emulsif. Wax.
*CAS — 8014-38-8.*

**Pharmacopoeias.** In *Br.* Also in *USNF.*

**BP 2003** (Emulsifying Wax). It is prepared from 9 parts of cetostearyl alcohol and 1 part of sodium laurilsulfate or sodium salts of similar sulfated higher primary aliphatic alcohols. An almost white or pale yellow, waxy solid or flakes, becoming plastic when warmed, with a faint characteristic odour. Practically insoluble in water, forming an emulsion; partly soluble in alcohol.

**USNF 22** (Emulsifying Wax). It is prepared from cetostearyl alcohol containing a polyoxyethylene derivative of a fatty acid ester of sorbitan. M.p. 50° to 54°. It is a creamy-white, wax-like solid, with a mild characteristic odour. Insoluble in water; soluble in alcohol; freely soluble in chloroform, in ether, in most hydrocarbon solvents, and in aerosol propellants.

### Profile

Emulsifying wax added to fatty or paraffin bases facilitates the preparation of oil-in-water emulsions which are absorbed and are nongreasy when rubbed into the skin. It is a constituent of many hydrophilic ointment bases for so-called 'washable' ointments.

**Sunscreen activity.** Emulsifying ointment, which contains emulsifying wax with white soft paraffin and liquid paraffin, was found to have major sunscreen activity in clinically normal skin.[1] It should not be used before phototherapy or in phototesting procedures.

1. Cox NH, Sharpe G. Emollients, salicylic acid, and ultraviolet erythema. *Lancet* 1990; **335:** 53–4.

### Preparations

***BP 2003:*** Aqueous Cream; Emulsifying Ointment.
**Proprietary Preparations** (details are given in Part 3)
**Multi-ingredient:** ***UK:*** Epaderm; Hydromol.

## Hard Fat

Adeps Neutralis; Adeps Solidus; Glycérides Semi-synthétiques Solides; Grasa sólida; Hartfett; Massa Estearínica; Neutralfett.

**Pharmacopoeias.** In *Eur.* (see p.vi), *Int.*, and *Pol.* Also in *USNF.*

**Ph. Eur. 5.0** (Hard Fat). A mixture of triglycerides, diglycerides, and monoglycerides obtained either by esterification of fatty acids of natural origin with glycerol or by transesterification of natural fats. A white or almost white, waxy, brittle mass. M.p. 30° to 45°; it does not differ by more than 2° from the nominal value. Practically insoluble in water; slightly soluble in dehydrated alcohol. When heated to 50°, it melts giving a colourless or slightly yellowish liquid. Protect from light and heat.

**USNF 22** (Hard Fat). A mixture of glycerides of saturated fatty acids. A white mass, almost odourless and free from rancid odour, and greasy to the touch. M.p. is between 27° and 44° and does not differ by more than 2° from the nominal value. The melted substance is colourless or slightly yellowish and forms a white emulsion when shaken with an equal amount of hot water. Practically insoluble in water; slightly soluble in alcohol; freely soluble in ether. Store in airtight containers at a temperature 5° or more below the melting-point.

### Profile

The name Hard Fat is applied to a range of bases with varying degrees of hardness and differing melting ranges used for the preparation of suppositories.

## Isopropyl Myristate

Isopropylis Myristas; Miristato de isopropilo. Tetradecanoic acid 1-methylethyl ester; Isopropyl tetradecanoate.
$C_{17}H_{34}O_2$ = 270.5.
*CAS — 110-27-0.*

**Pharmacopoeias.** In *Eur.* (see p.vi). Also in *USNF.*

**Ph. Eur. 5.0** (Isopropyl Myristate). A clear, colourless, oily liquid. Relative density about 0.853. Immiscible with water; miscible with alcohol, with dichloromethane, with fatty oils, and with liquid paraffin. Protect from light.

**USNF 22** (Isopropyl Myristate). A clear practically colourless, almost odourless, oily liquid; congeals at about 5°. Insoluble in water, in glycerol and in propylene glycol; freely soluble in alcohol. Miscible with most organic solvents and with fixed oils. Store in airtight containers. Protect from light.

**Incompatibility.** Isopropyl myristate is incompatible with hard paraffin.

### Profile

Isopropyl myristate is resistant to oxidation and hydrolysis and does not become rancid. It is absorbed fairly readily by the skin and is used as a basis for relatively nongreasy emollient ointments and creams. It is also used as a solvent for many substances applied externally.

Other isopropyl fatty acid esters, including di-isopropyl adipate, isopropyl laurate, isopropyl linoleate, and isopropyl palmitate (below) have similar properties and are used for similar purposes to those of isopropyl myristate.

### Preparations

**Proprietary Preparations** (details are given in Part 3)
***Spain:*** Nucoa†.
**Multi-ingredient:** ***Hong Kong:*** Hydromol; ***Irl.:*** Diprobath†; Emulsiderm; Hydromol; ***Israel:*** Emulsiderm; ***UK:*** Dermol; Diprobath; Doublebase; Emulsiderm; Hydromol.

## Isopropyl Palmitate

Isopropylis Palmitas; Palmitato de isopropilo. Hexadecanoic acid 1-methylether ester; Isopropyl hexadecanoate.
$C_{19}H_{38}O_2$ = 298.5.
*CAS — 142-91-6.*

**Pharmacopoeias.** In *Eur.* (see p.vi). Also in *USNF.*

**Ph. Eur. 5.0** (Isopropyl Palmitate). A clear, colourless, oily liquid. Relative density about 0.854. Immiscible with water; miscible with alcohol, with dichloromethane, with fatty oils, and with liquid paraffin. Protect from light.

**USNF 22** (Isopropyl Palmitate). A colourless, mobile, liquid with a very slight odour. Insoluble in water, in glycerol, and in propylene glycol; soluble in alcohol, in acetone, in castor oil, in chloroform, in cottonseed oil, in ethyl acetate, and in mineral oil. Store in airtight containers. Protect from light.

### Profile

Isopropyl palmitate has properties and uses similar to those of isopropyl myristate (above).

### Preparations

**Proprietary Preparations** (details are given in Part 3)
**Multi-ingredient:** ***Chile:*** Fotoprotector Isdin Extrem.

## Laurocapram *(USAN, rINN)*

Azone; N-0252. 1-Dodecylazacycloheptan-2-one; 1-Dodecylhexahydro-2*H*-azepin-2-one.
$C_{18}H_{35}NO$ = 281.5.
*CAS — 59227-89-3.*

**Pharmacopoeias.** In *Chin.*

### Profile

Laurocapram has been investigated for enhancing the penetration of drugs through the skin.

## Microcrystalline Wax

Cera microcristalina; E905.

**Pharmacopoeias.** In *USNF.*

**USNF 22** (Microcrystalline Wax). A mixture of straight-chain, branched-chain, and cyclic hydrocarbons, obtained by solvent fractionation of the still bottom fraction of petroleum by suitable dewaxing or de-oiling means. A white or cream-coloured odourless waxy solid. Melting range 54° to 102°. Insoluble in water; sparingly soluble in dehydrated alcohol; soluble in chloroform, in ether, in volatile oils, and in most warm fixed oils. Store in airtight containers.

### Profile

Microcrystalline wax is used as a stiffening agent in creams and ointments and as a tablet and capsule coating agent.

## Oleic Acid

Acidum Oleicum; Oleico, ácido; Ölsäure.
*CAS — 112-80-1* ($C_{18}H_{34}O_2$).

**Pharmacopoeias.** In *Eur.* (see p.vi). Also in *USNF.*

**Ph. Eur. 5.0** (Oleic Acid). It contains 65 to 88% of (*Z*)-octadec-9-enoic acid [$C_{18}H_{34}O_2$ = 282.5] together with varying amounts of saturated and other unsaturated fatty acids. It may contain a suitable antioxidant. It is a clear, yellowish or brownish, oily liquid. Practically insoluble in water; miscible with alcohol and with dichloromethane. Store in well-filled airtight containers. Protect from light.

**USNF 22** (Oleic Acid). It is manufactured from fats and oils derived from edible sources, animal or vegetable, and consists chiefly of (*Z*)-9-octadecenoic acid [$CH_3.(CH_2)_7.CH{:}CH.(CH_2)_7.COOH$ = 282.5]. It may contain suitable stabilisers. Oleic acid solely for external use is exempt from the requirement that it be prepared from edible sources. It is a colourless to pale yellow oily liquid when freshly prepared with a characteristic lard-like odour. On exposure to air it gradually absorbs oxygen and darkens in colour. When strongly heated in air, it is decomposed with the production of acid vapours. Congealing point between 3° and 10° for oleic acid from animal sources and between 10° and 16° for oleic acid from vegetable sources. Practically insoluble in water; miscible with alcohol, with chloroform, with ether, with benzene and with fixed and volatile oils. Store in airtight containers.

### Profile

Oleic acid forms soaps with alkaline substances and is used as an emulsifying or solubilising agent. It occurs in edible fats and oils which are used as foods or food components and has been used as a choleretic.

### Preparations

***BP 2003:*** Chloroxylenol Solution; White Liniment.
**Proprietary Preparations** (details are given in Part 3)
**Multi-ingredient:** ***Braz.:*** Gamaline-V; Glavit; Primoris; ***Chile:*** Acnoxyl Jabon; ***Fr.:*** Relaxoddi†.

## Oleyl Alcohol

Alcohol oleico; Alcohol Oleicus.
*CAS — 143-28-2.*

**Pharmacopoeias.** In *Eur.* (see p.vi). Also in *USNF.*

**Ph. Eur. 5.0** (Oleyl Alcohol). A mixture of unsaturated and saturated long-chain fatty alcohols consisting mainly of octadec-9-enol (oleyl alcohol and elaidyl alcohol; $C_{18}H_{36}O$ = 268.5). It may be of vegetable or animal origin. A colourless or light yellow liquid.

**USNF 22** (Oleyl Alcohol). A mixture of unsaturated and saturated high molecular weight fatty alcohols consisting chiefly of oleyl alcohol ($C_{18}H_{36}O$ = 268.5). A clear, colourless to light yellow, oily liquid with a faint characteristic odour. Insoluble in water; soluble in alcohol, in ether, in isopropyl alcohol, and in light liquid paraffin. Store in well-filled airtight containers at a temperature not exceeding 25°.

### Profile

Oleyl alcohol is used as an emollient and as an emulsifying and solubilising agent. The acetate has also been used.

## Fractionated Palm Kernel Oil

Aceite de palma refinado.

**Pharmacopoeias.** In *Br.*

**BP 2003** (Fractionated Palm Kernel Oil). It is obtained by expression of the natural oil from the kernels of *Elaeis guineensis* followed by selective solvent fractionation and hydrogenation. A white, odourless or almost odourless, solid, brittle fat. M.p. 31° to 36°. Practically insoluble in water and in alcohol; miscible with chloroform, with ether, and with petroleum spirit (boiling range, 40° to 60°). Store at a temperature not exceeding 25°.

### Profile

Fractionated palm kernel oil is used as a basis for suppositories. It has also been used in food manufacturing. The unfractionated oil has been used as an emollient and as an ointment basis.

## Shea Butter

Manteca de Karité.

### Profile

Shea butter is a natural fat obtained from the kernel of the fruit of *Butyrospermum parkii* (Sapotaceae) indigenous to West Africa. It is used as an ointment and cream basis.

---

## Silicones

Siliconas.

*ATC — A03AX13.*

**Description.** Silicones are polymers with a structure consisting of alternate atoms of silicon and oxygen, with organic groups attached to the silicon atoms. As the degree of polymerisation increases, the products become more viscous and the various grades are distinguished by a number, approximately corresponding to the viscosity of the particular grade. Silicones may be fluids, greases, waxes, resins, or rubbers depending on the degree of polymerisation.

## Cyclomethicone

$(C_2H_6OSi)_n$.

*CAS — 69430-24-6.*

**Pharmacopoeias.** In *USNF.*

**USNF 22** (Cyclomethicone). A fully methylated cyclic siloxane containing repeating units of the formula $[-(CH_3)_2SiO-]_n$, in which *n* is 4, 5, or 6, or a mixture of them. Store in airtight containers.

## Dimeticone *(BAN, rINN)*

Dimethicone *(USAN)*; Dimethyl Silicone Fluid; Dimethylpolysiloxane; Dimethylsiloxane; Dimeticonas; Dimeticonum; E900; Huile de Silicone; Methyl Polysiloxane; Permethylpolysiloxane; Silicone Oil; Siliconum Liquidum. Poly(dimethylsiloxane).

$CH_3.[Si(CH_3)_2.O]_nSi(CH_3)_3$.

*CAS — 9006-65-9.*

*ATC — A03AX13.*

**Description.** Dimeticones are fluid silicones in which the organic group is a methyl radical.

Simeticone (activated dimeticone), a mixture of liquid dimeticones with silicon dioxide, is described on p.1289.

**Pharmacopoeias.** In *Chin.* and *Eur.* (see p.vi). Also in *USNF.*

**Ph. Eur. 5.0** (Dimeticone). The degree of polymerisation is such that the kinematic viscosities are nominally between 20 and 1300 mm²/second; dimeticones with a nominal viscosity of 50 mm²/second or lower are intended for external use only. Dimeticones are clear, colourless, liquids of various viscosities. Practically insoluble in water; very slightly soluble to practically insoluble in dehydrated alcohol; miscible with ethyl acetate, with methyl ethyl ketone, and with toluene.

**USNF 22** (Dimethicone). A mixture of fully methylated linear siloxane polymers containing repeating units of the formula $[-(CH_3)_2SiO-]_n$, stabilised with trimethylsiloxy end-blocking units of the formula $[(CH_3)_3SiO-]$, wherein *n* has an average value such that the corresponding nominal viscosity is in a discrete range between 20 and 30 000 centistokes. It is a clear colourless, odourless liquid. Insoluble in water, in alcohol, in acetone, and in methyl alcohol; very slightly soluble in isopropyl alcohol; soluble in amyl acetate, in chlorinated hydrocarbons, in ether, in *n*-hexane, in petroleum spirit, in benzene, in toluene, and in xylene. Store in airtight containers.

### Adverse Effects and Precautions

Adverse effects from the clinical use of silicones appear to be rare. Foreign-body reactions have been reported following their use as joint implants. Other implants, notably breast implants used for reconstruction following mastectomy or for cosmetic purposes, carry the risk of migration of silicone with cyst formation and other complications; accidental intravascular injection has been fatal. Late adverse ocular effects can follow the intravitreal injection of liquid silicone in the management of retinal detachment (see below).

**Breast feeding.** Concern has been raised regarding the possible effects on infants of mothers with silicone breast implants who breast feed. Oesophageal dysfunction has been reported in a number of such children,[1] although this finding has not been confirmed by subsequent reports. The American Academy of Pediatrics therefore states[2] that the current evidence does not justify classifying silicone implants as a contra-indication to breast feeding.


1. Levine JJ, Ilowite NT. Sclerodermalike esophageal disease in children breast-fed by mothers with silicone breast implants. *JAMA* 1994; **271:** 213–6. Correction. *ibid.*; **272:** 770.
2. American Academy of Pediatrics. The transfer of drugs and other chemicals into human milk. *Pediatrics* 2001; **108:** 776–89. Correction. *ibid.*; 1029. Also available at: http://aappolicy.aappublications.org/cgi/content/full/pediatrics%3b108/3/776 (accessed 01/07/04)


**Connective tissue disorders.** Since the introduction of silicone breast implants in the early 1960s there have been numerous anecdotal reports of various connective tissue disorders occurring in women who have undergone breast reconstruction or augmentation with these implants. Scleroderma has been the most frequently reported disorder; others have included systemic lupus erythematosus, rheumatoid arthritis, and inflammatory myopathies. A syndrome of vague musculoskeletal symptoms, fever, and fatigue has also been reported. These cases led the FDA to call for a moratorium in the US on the use of silicone breast implants in January 1992. However, with the exception of one study of self-reported symptoms which showed only a small increase in risk,[1] large epidemiological studies,[2-5] meta-analyses,[6] and a review by the Medical Devices Agency in the UK have so far failed to show any association between silicone breast implants and connective tissue disorders.


1. Hennekens CH, *et al.* Self-reported breast implants and connective-tissue diseases in female health professionals: a retrospective cohort study. *JAMA* 1996; **275:** 616–21.
2. Gabriel SE, *et al.* Risk of connective-tissue diseases and other disorders after breast implantation. *N Engl J Med* 1994; **330:** 1697–1702.
3. Sánchez-Guerrero J, *et al.* Silicone breast implants and the risk of connective-tissue diseases and symptoms. *N Engl J Med* 1995; **332:** 1666–70.
4. Silverman BG, *et al.* Reported complications of silicone gel breast implants: an epidemiologic review. *Ann Intern Med* 1996; **124:** 744–56.
5. Nyrén O, *et al.* Risk of connective tissue disease and related disorders among women with breast implants: a nation-wide retrospective cohort study in Sweden. *BMJ* 1998; **316:** 417–22.
6. Janowsky EC, *et al.* Meta-analyses of the relation between silicone breast implants and the risk of connective-tissue diseases. *N Engl J Med* 2000; **342:** 781–90.


### Uses and Administration

Dimeticones and other silicones are water-repellent and have a low surface tension. They are used in topical barrier preparations for protecting the skin against water-soluble irritants. Creams, lotions, and ointments containing a dimeticone are employed for the prevention of bedsores and napkin rash and to protect the skin against trauma due to incontinence or stoma discharge. Silicone preparations should not be applied where free drainage is necessary or to inflamed or abraded skin. Silicones, usually a dimeticone, are also used topically as wound dressings.

Silicones have also been used for arthroplasty in rheumatic disorders, by intravitreal injection for retinal detachment, and by subcutaneous injection or implantation in reconstructive or cosmetic surgery.

Dimeticones, in particular simeticone (activated dimeticone) (p.1289), are used in the treatment of flatulence.

**Retinal detachment.** Retinal detachment is separation of the retina from the underlying retinal pigmentary epithelium and usually requires surgical repair. Intravitreal injection of liquid silicone has been used for retinal tamponade with or after surgery in complicated or persistent detachment of the retina.[1,2] Late complications following its use may include cataract, glaucoma, and keratopathy.


1. Chan C, Okun E. The question of ocular tolerance to intravitreal liquid silicone: a long-term analysis. *Ophthalmology* 1986; **93:** 651–60.
2. Gray RH, *et al.* Fluorescein angiographic findings in three patients with long-term intravitreal liquid silicone. *Br J Ophthalmol* 1989; **73:** 991–5.


### Preparations

**Proprietary Preparations** (details are given in Part 3)

***Arg.:*** Aerogal; Atoderm; Europiel; Kurapel; ***Austral.:*** Egozite Protective Baby Lotion; Instru-Safe†; Rosken Skin Repair; Silic 15; ***Canad.:*** Barrier Cream; Barriere; Protecto-Derm†; ***Chile:*** Cadinol; Lomprax; Neogasol; ***Fr.:*** Cica-Care; Ophtasiloxane; ***Ger.:*** Jaikin N; Symadal M; ***Hong Kong:*** Egozite Protective Baby Lotion; Silic 15; Skin Repair; ***Israel:*** Adato-Sil Ol; ***Ital.:*** Cica-Care; Mepiform; Mepitel; Radioced†; ***Malaysia:*** Egozite Protective Baby Lotion; Silic 15; ***NZ:*** Aquim; DP Barrier Cream; Egozite Protective Baby Lotion; Pharmacycare Barrier†; Silicare; ***Singapore:*** DP†; Egozite Protective Baby Lotion; Silic 15; Skin Repair; ***UK:*** Cica-Care; Dermatix; Silgel; ***USA:*** Mentholatum Softlips; Pro-Q.

**Multi-ingredient:** ***Austral.:*** Dermalife Plus; Dimethicream; Eczema Cream; Egozite Baby Cream; Hamilton Skin Repair; Nappy-Mate†; Silcon; ***Austria:*** Ceolat Compositum; Evalgan; ***Braz.:*** Balmex; ***Canad.:*** Blistex Lip Balm; Blistex Lip Tone; Complex 15; Diaper Guard†; Moisturel; Prevex; Soft Lips; Zilactin-Lip; ***Chile:*** Aero Itan; Balsamo Analgesico con Fenilbutazona; Blisprotex; Neopankreoflat; Xeragel; ***Denm.:*** Silan; ***Fr.:*** Balmex†; ***Hong Kong:*** Dyprotex; Egozite Baby Cream; Hamilton Skin Repair; ***India:*** Siloderm; Tinidafyl Plus; ***Irl.:*** Conotrane; Siopel; Sprilon; Vasogen; ***Israel:*** Kamil Blue; Kelo-Cote; ***Ital.:*** Angstrom Viso; Rikospray; ***Malaysia:*** Egozite Baby Cream; ***Mon.:*** Dermo Silanols; ***NZ:*** Dermalife Plus†; E45†; Egoderm; Egozite Baby; Karicare Barrier Cream; Rosken Skin Repair; Silic; Ungvita†; ***Port.:*** Balmex†; ***S.Afr.:*** Arola Rosebalm; Siopel†; ***Singapore:*** Egozite Baby Cream; Scarfade; ***Spain:*** Dermo Halibut Infantil; Proskin; Silidermil; Tegunal†; ***Swed.:*** Silon; ***UK:*** Conotrane; Cymex; Silastic†; Siopel; Sprilon; Vasogen; ***USA:*** Blistex Lip Balm; ControlRx; Diaper Guard; Dyprotex; Maxilube; Mentholatum Cherry Ice; Mentholatum Natural Ice; Mentholatum Softlips Lipbalm; Mentholatum Softlips Lipbalm (UV).

---

## Squalane

Cosbiol; Dodecahydrosqualene; Escualano; Perhydrosqualène; Spinacane; Squalanum. 2,6,10,15,19,23-Hexamethyltetracosane.

$C_{30}H_{62}$ = 422.8.

*CAS — 111-01-3.*

**Pharmacopoeias.** In *Eur.* (see p.vi). Also in *USNF.*

**Ph. Eur. 5.0** (Squalane). A clear, colourless, oily liquid. Relative density about 0.815. It may be of vegetable (unsaponifiable matter of olive oil) or animal (shark liver oil) origin. Practically insoluble in water and in alcohol; freely soluble in acetone and in cyclohexane; miscible with most fats and oils.

**USNF 22** (Squalane). A saturated hydrocarbon obtained by hydrogenation of squalene, an aliphatic triterpene occurring in some fish oils. It is a colourless, almost odourless, transparent oil. Insoluble in water; very slightly soluble in dehydrated alcohol; miscible with chloroform and with ether; slightly soluble in acetone. Store in airtight containers.

### Profile

Squalane is a saturated derivative of squalene, a constituent of human sebum. It is miscible with human sebum and is included in topical preparations to increase skin permeability. It is also used as an emollient.

### Preparations

**Proprietary Preparations** (details are given in Part 3)

**Multi-ingredient:** ***Arg.:*** Cremisona; ***Port.:*** Creme Laser Hidrante; Lactonico.

---

## Stearyl Alcohol

Alcohol estearílico; Alcohol Stearylicus; Alcool Stéarylique; 1-Octadecanol; Octadecyl Alcohol.

*CAS — 112-92-5.*

**Pharmacopoeias.** In *Eur.* (see p.vi), *Jpn*, and *Pol.* Also in *USNF.*

**Ph. Eur. 5.0** (Stearyl Alcohol). A mixture of solid alcohols; it contains not less than 95.0% of stearyl alcohol ($C_{18}H_{38}O$ = 270.5). White, unctuous flakes, granules, or mass. M.p. 57° to 60°. Practically insoluble in water; soluble in alcohol. When melted, it is miscible with fatty oils, with liquid paraffin, and with melted wool fat.

**USNF 22** (Stearyl Alcohol). It contains not less than 90% of stearyl alcohol ($C_{18}H_{38}O$ = 270.5), the remainder consisting chiefly of related alcohols. White unctuous flakes or granules with a faint characteristic odour. M.p. 55° to 60°. Insoluble in water; soluble in alcohol and in ether.

### Profile

Stearyl alcohol is used to thicken ointments and creams and to increase their water-holding capacity; it has emollient and weak emulsifying properties. It is also used in modified-release solid dose formulations.

Stearyl alcohol can cause hypersensitivity.

### Preparations

**Proprietary Preparations** (details are given in Part 3)

***USA:*** SFC Lotion.

---

## Theobroma Oil

Beurre de Cacao; Burro di Cacao; Butyrum Cacao; Cacao Butter; Cocoa Butter; Kakaobutter; Manteca de cacao; Manteiga de Cacau; Ol. Theobrom.; Oleum Cacao; Oleum Theobromatis.

*CAS — 8002-31-1.*

**Pharmacopoeias.** In *Br.*, *Fr.*, *Ger.*, *Jpn*, and *Pol.* Also in *USNF.*

**BP 2003** (Theobroma Oil). The solid fat obtained from the roasted seeds of *Theobroma cacao*. A yellowish-white, somewhat brittle, solid fat, with a slight odour of cocoa. M.p. 31° to 34°. Slightly soluble in alcohol; freely soluble in chloroform, in ether, and in petroleum spirit (boiling range, 40° to 60°). Store at a temperature not exceeding 25°.

**USNF 22** (Cocoa Butter). A fat obtained from the seeds of *Theobroma cacao* (Sterculiaceae). It is a yellowish-white, usually brittle solid with a faint agreeable odour. M.p. 31° to 35°. Slightly soluble in alcohol; soluble in boiling dehydrated alcohol; freely soluble in chloroform and in ether.

### Profile

Theobroma oil is used as a basis for suppositories. If it is heated to more than 36° during preparation the solidification point will be appreciably lowered due to the formation of metastable states, leading to subsequent difficulty in setting. It is a major ingredient of chocolate.

---

## Wool Alcohols

Alcoholes Adipis Lanae; Alcoholes de lana; Alcoholia Lanae; Alcolanum; Lanalcolum; Lanolin Alcohols; Wollwachsalkohole; Wool Wax Alcohols.

*CAS — 8027-33-6.*

**Pharmacopoeias.** In *Eur.* (see p.vi). Also in *USNF.*

**Ph. Eur. 5.0** (Wool Alcohols). A mixture of sterols and higher aliphatic alcohols obtained from wool fat and containing not less than 30.0% of cholesterol. It may contain not more than 200 ppm of butylated hydroxytoluene. A pale yellow to brownish-yellow, brittle mass becoming plastic on heating. M.p. not lower than 58°. Practically insoluble in water; slightly soluble in alcohol (90%); soluble in boiling dehydrated alcohol, and in dichloromethane. Store in well-filled containers. Protect from light.

**USNF 22** (Lanolin Alcohols). A mixture of sterols, aliphatic alcohols, and triterpenoid alcohols obtained by the hydrolysis of wool fat. It may contain not more than 0.1% of a suitable antioxidant. It is a hard, waxy amber solid with a characteristic odour. M.p. not below 56°. Insoluble in water; slightly soluble in alcohol; freely soluble in chloroform, in ether, and in petroleum spirit. Store at a temperature not exceeding 25°. Protect from light.

**Incompatibility.** Wool alcohols is incompatible with coal tar, ichthammol, resorcinol, and phenol.

### Profile

Wool alcohols is an emulsifying agent and emulsion stabiliser used in the preparation of water-in-oil creams and ointments. It increases the water absorbing capacity of hydrocarbon mixtures; the addition of 5% of wool alcohols permits a threefold increase in the amount of water that can be incorporated in soft paraffin and such emulsions are not 'cracked' by the addition of weak acids.

It has an emollient action on the skin and is used in preparations for dry skin and dry eyes.

Derivatives of wool alcohols with similar uses include acetylated wool alcohols and ethoxylated wool alcohols.

Wool alcohols may cause hypersensitivity.

### Preparations

***BP 2003:*** Wool Alcohols Ointment.

**Proprietary Preparations** (details are given in Part 3)

**Multi-ingredient:** ***Arg.:*** Macoderm; ***Canad.:*** Lacri-Lube; ***Ger.:*** Coliquifilm; ***Irl.:*** Oilatum Emollient; ***Israel:*** Adinol; ***Ital.:*** Lacrilube; ***NZ:*** Lacrilube; ***S.Afr.:*** Lacrilube†; ***Switz.:*** Coliquifilm; ***UK:*** Ashbourne Emollient Medicinal Bath Oil; Dermalo; Lacri-Lube; Oilatum Emollient; ***USA:*** Hydrocerin; Refresh PM.

## Wool Fat

Adeps Lanae; Anhydrous Lanolin; Cera Lanae; Graisse de Suint Purifiée; Lanoléine; Lanolin; Lanolina; Lanolina anhidra; Purified Lanolin; Refined Wool Fat; Suarda; Wollfett; Wollwachs.

*CAS — 8006-54-0.*

**Pharmacopoeias.** In *Chin., Eur.* (see p.vi), *Int., Jpn, Pol., US,* and *Viet.* Some pharmacopoeias include Hydrous Wool Fat which is prepared by the addition of water to wool fat.

*Eur.* also includes Hydrogenated Wool Fat.

*US* also includes Modified Lanolin.

**Ph. Eur. 5.0** (Wool Fat). A purified, anhydrous, waxy material obtained from the wool of the sheep (*Ovis aries*). It may contain not more than 200 ppm of butylated hydroxytoluene. A yellow, unctuous substance. When melted, it is a clear or almost clear, yellow liquid. Drop point 38° to 44°. 10 g absorbs not less than 20 mL of water. Practically insoluble in water; slightly soluble in boiling dehydrated alcohol; it forms an opalescent solution in petroleum spirit. Store at a temperature not exceeding 25°.

**Ph. Eur. 5.0** (Wool Fat, Hydrogenated; Adeps Lanae Hydrogenatus). A mixture of higher aliphatic alcohols and sterols obtained from the direct, high-pressure, high-temperature hydrogenation of anhydrous wool fat during which the esters and acids present are reduced to corresponding alcohols. It may contain butylated hydroxytoluene. A white or pale yellow, unctuous substance. M.p. 45° to 55°. Practically insoluble in water; soluble in boiling alcohol and in petroleum spirit. Store in well-filled containers. Protect from light.

**Ph. Eur. 5.0** (Wool Fat, Hydrous; Adeps Lanae Cum Aqua). A mixture of 75% of wool fat and 25% of water. It may contain not more than 150 ppm of butylated hydroxytoluene. A pale yellow, unctuous substance. Drop point 38° to 44°. Store at a temperature not exceeding 25°.

**USP 27** (Lanolin). A purified wax-like substance obtained from the wool of the sheep, *Ovis aries* (Bovidae). It is a yellow tenacious unctuous mass with a slight characteristic odour. Melting range 38° to 44°. It contains not more than 0.25% of water. It may contain not more than 0.02% of a suitable antoxidant. Insoluble in water, but mixes without separation with about twice its weight of water; sparingly soluble in cold alcohol; more soluble in hot alcohol; freely soluble in chloroform and in ether. Store at a temperature preferably between 15° and 30°.

**USP 27** (Modified Lanolin). It is Lanolin that has been processed to reduce the contents of free lanolin alcohols and detergent and pesticide residues. It contains not more than 0.25% of water. It may contain not more than 0.02% of a suitable antoxidant. Store in airtight, preferably rust-proof, containers and preferably at a temperature of 15° to 30°.

### Profile

Wool fat is used in the formulation of water-in-oil creams and ointments. When mixed with a suitable vegetable oil or with soft paraffin it gives emollient creams that penetrate the skin. It can absorb about 30% of water.

Derivatives and modifications of wool fat include hydrogenated wool fat (hydrogenated lanolin), hydrous wool fat (hydrous lanolin), poloxyl lanolin (ethoxylated lanolin), isopropyl lanolate, lanolin oil, and lanolin wax.

Wool fat can cause sensitivity reactions.

◊ General reviews.

1. Barnett G. Lanolin and derivatives. *Cosmet Toilet* 1986; **101** (Mar): 23–44.

**Hypersensitivity.** Treatment of wool fat to remove both detergent and natural free fatty alcohols reduced the incidence of hypersensitivity in lanolin-sensitive patients to almost zero.[1]

1. Clark EW, *et al.* Lanolin with reduced sensitizing potential. *Contact Dermatitis* 1977; **3:** 69–74.

**Pesticide residues.** Reports of pesticide residues in wool fat and comments on risks.

1. Copeland CA, *et al.* Pesticide residue in lanolin. *JAMA* 1989; **261:** 242.
2. Cade PH. Pesticide in lanolin. *JAMA* 1989; **262:** 613.
3. Copeland CA, Wagner SL. Pesticide in lanolin. *JAMA* 1989; **262:** 613.

### Preparations

***BP 2003:*** Simple Eye Ointment; Simple Ointment;
***USP 27:*** Modified Lanolin.

**Proprietary Preparations** (details are given in Part 3)
***Austral.:*** Lansinoh; ***Port.:*** Multi-Mam Lanolina; ***S.Afr.:*** Duratears.

**Multi-ingredient:** ***Arg.:*** Dr Selby; Ninderm; Quem Plus; ***Austral.:*** Alpha Keri; Alpha Keri Tar†; Duratears; E45†; Lacri-Lube; Poly Visc; Rikoderm; Silcon; Soothe'n Heal†; ***Austria:*** Tiroler Steinol; ***Belg.:*** Duratears; Lacrytube; ***Canad.:*** Akwa Tears; Alpha Keri; Duratears; Huile de Bain Therapeutique; Lubriderm; Optilube; Stancare†; Therapeutic Bath Oil; Therapeutic Skin Lotion; ***Chile:*** Duratears; Lacri-Lube; Pasta Lassar; ***Fr.:*** Grassolind Neutral; ***Gr.:*** Duratears; ***Hong Kong:*** Alpha Keri; Balneum Hermal; Duratears; ***Irl.:*** Lacri-Lube; ***Israel:*** Duratears; Kamil Blue; Lacrimol; Pedisol; ***Malaysia:*** Balneum; Duratears Naturale; Lacrilube; ***Mex.:*** Acuafil; ***NZ:*** Alpha Keri; BK; DP; DP Lotion - HC; Hydroderm; Karicare Baby Bath Oil†; Karicare Mother and Baby†; Oralife Peppermint; Pharmacycare Bath Oil†; Pharmacycare Hand & Body†; ***Singapore:*** Alpha Keri†; Balneum; Duratears; Lacrilube; Lubrifilm†; ***Spain:*** Lubrifilm; Tears Lubricante; ***Switz.:*** Duratears†; ***Thai.:*** Balneum; Duratears; ***UK:*** Alpha Keri; Hewletts; Lubri-Tears; Melrose; ***USA:*** Akwa Tears; Alpha Keri; Bottom Better; Dry Eyes; Duratears Naturale; Lacri-Gel; Lacri-Lube; LubriTears.

# Parasympathomimetics

Dementia, p.1484
Eaton-Lambert myasthenic syndrome, p.1485
Glaucoma and ocular hypertension, p.1485
Myasthenia gravis, p.1486
Reversal of mydriasis, p.1487
Strabismus, p.1487

Parasympathomimetics may be classified into 2 distinct pharmacological groups:

- cholinergic agonists, such as bethanechol, carbachol, methacholine, and pilocarpine which act directly on effector cells to mimic the effects of acetylcholine. They are sometimes referred to as cholinomimetics or true parasympathomimetics; some such as bethanechol, carbachol, and methacholine are choline esters
- anticholinesterases (cholinesterase inhibitors) which inhibit the enzymic hydrolysis of acetylcholine by acetylcholinesterase and other cholinesterases, thereby prolonging and enhancing its actions in the body. They may be classified by the length of time taken to restore active enzyme following binding of enzyme to drug. The 'reversible' anticholinesterases such as ambenonium, neostigmine, physostigmine, and pyridostigmine generally produce enzyme inhibition for a few hours, whereas 'irreversible' anticholinesterases such as dyflos and ecothiopate produce extremely prolonged inhibition, and return of cholinesterase activity depends on synthesis of new enzyme. Centrally acting reversible anticholinesterases include donepezil, galantamine, rivastigmine, and tacrine.

Parasympathomimetics may be used topically for their miotic action in glaucoma and strabismus, given systemically to reverse the neuromuscular blockade of neuromuscular blockers, or may be used in myasthenia gravis and for dementia of the Alzheimer's type. Other uses have included treatment of paralytic ileus or other disorders of decreased gastrointestinal motility (p.1241), and postoperative urinary retention (p.476).

Drugs such as fampridine and guanidine, which enhance the release of acetylcholine from nerve terminals, are also discussed in this chapter.

## Dementia

Dementia is a syndrome in which impairment of cortical or subcortical function leads to deterioration of cognitive processes or intellectual abilities including memory, judgement, language, communication, and abstract thinking. Unlike delirium there is no gross clouding of consciousness. There may be changes in personality and behaviour disturbances. Dementia is usually progressive, though not always irreversible, and loss of social and other skills often leads to complete dependence on others.

Although dementia is more prevalent in the elderly it is not an inevitable consequence of ageing. Dementia can result from many conditions including:

- *neurodegenerative diseases*: Alzheimer's disease, Pick's disease, Huntington's chorea, Parkinson's disease, Lewy-body disease, multiple sclerosis, progressive supranuclear palsy
- *vascular diseases*: multiple cerebral infarcts, occlusion of carotid artery, cranial arteritis
- *trauma*: subdural haematoma
- *neoplasms*
- *CNS infections*: encephalitis, syphilis, toxoplasmosis, AIDS, Creutzfeldt-Jakob disease
- *endocrine/metabolic disorders*: hypothyroidism, uraemia, hepatic failure, cardiac failure, respiratory failure, hypoxia
- *toxic insults*: alcohol, solvents, heavy metals, drug therapy
- *hydrocephalus*
- *nutritional deficiency*: vitamin $B_{12}$, folic acid, thiamine
- *depression*

Alzheimer's disease is the most common cause of dementia and accounts for over half of all patients; about one-third of dementia cases are due to vascular disease.

Treatment of dementia can be broadly divided into control of disturbed behaviour (p.665) and attempts to improve or preserve cognitive function (see below). Although many drugs have been tried in the management of cognitive impairment most have produced little or no benefit.

**Alzheimer's disease** is a progressive degenerative condition affecting mainly patients over 60 years of age. The rare early-onset form of Alzheimer's disease (familial Alzheimer's disease) is sometimes referred to as pre-senile dementia. Death usually occurs within 10 years of onset. Apart from age other risk factors include Down's syndrome and a family history of Alzheimer's disease. Presence of the ε4 allele of apolipoprotein E is another risk factor; it correlates with prevalence and age of onset in some forms of Alzheimer's disease but use for routine clinical or predictive testing is controversial. Elevated levels of plasma homocysteine have also been linked with the development of dementia and Alzheimer's disease. Dialysis dementia, an irreversible condition which has occurred in dialysis patients, has been associated with excess aluminium in the dialysing fluid but the role of aluminium in Alzheimer's disease, if any, is unclear.

Deficiencies in numerous neurotransmitters have been found in patients with Alzheimer's disease but reduced choline acetyltransferase activity leading to reduced synthesis of acetylcholine remains the most consistent defect correlating with the severity of the condition. Attempts to increase acetylcholine concentrations in the brain have included use of *acetylcholine precursors*, *cholinesterase inhibitors*, *enhancers of acetylcholine release*, and *cholinergic agonists*. However, none replace lost cholinergic neurones and therefore none affect overall progression of the disease.

Treatments using *precursors of acetylcholine* such as lecithin or choline alone are not generally considered to produce useful improvements, although it has been suggested that choline alfoscerate may be of some benefit.

Donepezil, galantamine, rivastigmine, and tacrine are the main *cholinesterase inhibitors*. All have produced modest improvement in cognition and global clinical impression in patients with mild to moderately severe disease; but there is a lack of long-term studies and little evidence of their effectiveness in advanced disease. Tacrine is often poorly tolerated and may cause serious hepatotoxicity; for these reasons it is rarely used now. Donepezil, galantamine, and rivastigmine may be more acceptable to patients. UK guidelines recommend use of these drugs under specialist supervision for patients with mild to moderate dementia; benefit should be assessed 2 to 4 months after reaching maintenance dosage, and every 6 months thereafter, and treatment only continued if there is evidence of benefit. Other cholinesterase inhibitors which have been tried or are under study for use in Alzheimer's disease include metrifonate and physostigmine.

Fampridine, which *enhances acetylcholine release from nerve terminals* has also been tried in Alzheimer's disease but there is little evidence of clinical benefit.

Limited improvement has been reported with some *cholinergic agonists* but pilocarpine may exacerbate the dementia. Muscarinic $M_1$ agonists such as cevimeline and xanomeline have been investigated on the basis that muscarinic $M_1$ receptors appear to be preserved throughout the course of Alzheimer's disease. However, these drugs have not been successful in improving symptoms of the disease. An alternative line of investigation is the *stimulation of nicotinic receptors* using nicotine.

A hypothesis that free radicals may initiate and maintain mechanisms responsible for neurodegeneration in Alzheimer's disease has prompted the investigation of drugs such as vitamin E (e.g. α-tocopherol), ginkgo biloba, idebenone, and selegiline for *antoxidant* therapy but their value remains to be confirmed. However, US guidelines suggest consideration of vitamin E supplementation in an attempt to slow progression of the disease; selegiline is considered to have a less favourable risk-benefit ratio.

*Neurotropic or nootropic drugs* such as piracetam have also been tried in Alzheimer's disease and other dementias but there is little convincing evidence of clinical usefulness.

The *N-methyl-D-aspartate (NMDA) receptor antagonist* memantine has shown some benefit in various dementias and is used in the treatment of moderately severe to severe Alzheimer's disease; it is thought to act through modulation of the effects of the neurotransmitter glutamate.

Many drugs with *vasodilator activity* were originally tried in dementia when it was believed that the condition was due to 'cerebrovascular insufficiency' (p.820), but overall there is little convincing evidence of benefit. Ergot derivatives such as co-dergocrine mesilate and nicergoline have been the most commonly used; however, any effectiveness is now attributed to their action as metabolic enhancers or nootropic drugs and their place in therapy has still to be established.

The *calcium-channel blocker* nimodipine has been of benefit in dementia of various aetiologies but its role in therapy remains unclear.

Observations have suggested that *oestrogens* may reduce the risk and delay the onset of Alzheimer's disease in postmenopausal women receiving HRT. However, a large controlled study found that combined HRT increased the risk of substantial decline in global cognitive function, did not prevent the development of mild cognitive impairment, and doubled the risk of dementia. A beneficial effect of oestrogens on cognitive function in postmenopausal women who already have mild or moderate Alzheimer's disease has not been demonstrated in controlled studies (see p.1540). Some retrospective studies also indicate an inverse association between the use of *anti-inflammatory drugs* such as NSAIDs and the risk of developing Alzheimer's disease. The possibility of an association between *statin* therapy and a reduced risk of developing dementia has also been mooted.

A vaccine for Alzheimer's disease is being investigated.

**Vascular dementia** is a syndrome produced by ischaemic, hypoxic, or haemorrhagic brain lesions. Vessel occlusion is the most common cause of vascular dementia and produces a variety of cognitive deficits depending on the site of ischaemia. Among the major forms of dementia recognised are those due to multiple infarcts, single strategic infarcts, and subcortical white matter ischaemia (Binswanger's disease). Vascular dementia has a more acute onset than dementia due to Alzheimer's disease and in contrast to the continuous progression of Alzheimer's disease often has a stepwise progression. Risk factors for vascular dementia parallel those for stroke (p.836) and similar methods for prevention and treatment may be of use but there is a lack of evidence from adequately controlled trials.

**Lewy-body dementia** is distinguished from other types of dementia by a state of fluctuating cognitive impairment and confusion; hallucinations, paranoid delusions, a tendency to fall for no apparent reason, and transient clouding or loss of consciousness are also characteristic symptoms. In addition, mild extrapyramidal symptoms may be present and there is increased susceptibility to the extrapyramidal adverse effects of antipsychotics (see the Elderly, under Precautions of Chlorpromazine on p.678). Severe cholinergic deficits in patients with Lewy-body dementia have prompted treatment with cholinesterase inhibitors. *Donepezil* and *rivastigmine* have been shown to be well tolerated and effective, but further trials are needed to establish their role.

References.

1. Cummings JL. Dementia: the failing brain. *Lancet* 1995; **345:** 1481–4. Correction. *ibid.*; 1551.
2. Fleming KC, *et al.* Dementia: diagnosis and evaluation. *Mayo Clin Proc* 1995; **70:** 1093–1107.
3. Gooch MD, Stennett DJ. Molecular basis of Alzheimer's disease. *Am J Health-Syst Pharm* 1996; **53:** 1545–57.
4. Amar K, Wilcock G. Vascular dementia. *BMJ* 1996; **312:** 227–31.
5. Konno S, *et al.* Classification, diagnosis and treatment of vascular dementia. *Drugs Aging* 1997; **11:** 361–73.
6. Parnetti L, *et al.* Cognitive enhancement therapy for Alzheimer's disease: the way forward. *Drugs* 1997; **53:** 752–68.
7. American Psychiatric Association. Practice guideline for the treatment of patients with Alzheimer's disease and other dementias of late life. *Am J Psychiatry* 1997; **154** (suppl): 1–39. Also available at: http://www.psych.org/psych_pract/treatg/pg/pg_dementia_32701.cfm (accessed 15/06/04)
8. Benzi G, Moretti A. Is there a rationale for the use of acetylcholinesterase inhibitors in the therapy of Alzheimer's disease? *Eur J Pharmacol* 1998; **346:** 1–13.
9. Small GW. Treatment of Alzheimer's disease: current approaches and promising developments. *Am J Med* 1998; **104** (suppl 4A): 32S–38S.
10. Eccles M, *et al.* North of England evidence based guidelines development project: guideline for the primary care management of dementia. *BMJ* 1998; **317:** 802–8.
11. Sachdev PS, *et al.* Vascular dementia: diagnosis, management and possible prevention. *Med J Aust* 1999; **170:** 81–5.
12. Flynn BL. Pharmacologic management of Alzheimer disease: Part I: hormonal and emerging investigational drug therapies. *Ann Pharmacother* 1999; **33:** 178–87.
13. Flynn BL, Ranno AE. Pharmacologic management of Alzheimer disease: Part II: antioxidants, antihypertensives, and ergoloid derivatives. *Ann Pharmacother* 1999; **33:** 188–97.
14. Flicker L. Acetylcholinesterase inhibitors for Alzheimer's disease. *BMJ* 1999; **318:** 615–6.
15. Krall WJ, *et al.* Cholinesterase inhibitors: a therapeutic strategy for Alzheimer disease. *Ann Pharmacother* 1999; **33:** 441–50.
16. Mayeux R, Sano M. Treatment of Alzheimer's disease. *N Engl J Med* 1999; **341:** 1670–9.

17. Sramek JJ, *et al.* Mild cognitive impairment: emerging therapeutics. *Ann Pharmacother* 2000; **34:** 1179–88.
18. Praticò D, Delantry N. Oxidative injury in diseases of the central nervous system: focus on Alzheimer's disease. *Am J Med* 2000; **109:** 577–85.
19. Korczyn AD. Muscarinic M(1) agonists in the treatment of Alzheimer's disease. *Expert Opin Invest Drugs* 2000; **9:** 2259–67.
20. Grutzendler J, Morris JC. Cholinesterase inhibitors for Alzheimer's disease. *Drugs* 2001; **61:** 41–52.
21. Brodaty H, *et al.* Pharmacological treatment of cognitive deficits in Alzheimer's disease. *Med J Aust* 2001; **175:** 324–9. Correction. *ibid.* **176:** 297–8.
22. Doody RS, *et al.* Practice parameter: management of dementia (an evidence-based review). Report of the Quality Standards Subcommittee of the American Academy of Neurology. *Neurology* 2001; **56:** 1154–66. Also available at: http://www.aan.com/professionals/practice/pdfs/gl0012.pdf (accessed 15/06/04)
23. National Institute for Clinical Excellence. Guidance on the use of donepezil, rivastigmine and galantamine for the treatment of Alzheimer's disease (issued January 2001). Available at: http://www.nice.org.uk/pdf/ALZHEIMER_full_guidance.pdf (accessed 15/06/04)
24. Seshadri S, *et al.* Plasma homocysteine as a risk factor for dementia and Alzheimer's disease. *N Engl J Med* 2002; **346:** 476–83.
25. McKeith IG. Dementia with Lewy bodies. *Br J Psychiatry* 2002; **180:** 144–7.
26. Swanberg MM, Cummings JL. Benefit-risk considerations in the treatment of dementia with Lewy bodies. *Drug Safety* 2002; **25:** 511–23.
27. Clark CM, Karlawish JHT. Alzheimer disease: current concepts and emerging diagnostic and therapeutic strategies. *Ann Intern Med* 2003; **138:** 400–10.
28. Boustani M, *et al.* Screening for dementia in primary care: a summary of the evidence for the U.S. Preventive Services Task Force. *Ann Intern Med* 2003; **138:** 927–37.
29. Scott HD, Laake K. Statins for the prevention of Alzheimer's disease. Available in The Cochrane Library; Issue 2. Chichester: John Wiley; 2004.

## Eaton-Lambert myasthenic syndrome

Eaton-Lambert myasthenic syndrome is a rare auto-immune disease of the neuromuscular junction. Unlike myasthenia gravis (below), in which autoantibodies affect acetylcholine receptors, antibodies in Eaton-Lambert syndrome act presynaptically to reduce release of acetylcholine. Weakness mostly affects the proximal muscles, particularly those of the limbs; respiratory and ocular muscles are usually spared. Autonomic symptoms including dry mouth, constipation, and impotence are common. Over half of patients also develop small cell carcinoma of the lung. Response to treatment with *anticholinesterases* alone is poor; treatment with *3,4-diaminopyridine*, which increases acetylcholine release, appears to be more effective, particularly when given with *pyridostigmine*. The use of similar drugs such as *guanidine* and *fampridine* is limited by severe adverse effects. Low-dose guanidine has been tried with pyridostigmine where 3,4-diaminopyridine is not readily available. Although there has been some improvement with the combination, the incidence of side-effects, especially gastrointestinal reactions, is still high. Some patients may obtain additional benefit when anticholinesterases are used in addition to 3,4-diaminopyridine. Immunosuppressants are also used, and unlike myasthenia gravis, treatment with *corticosteroids* does not appear to induce an initial exacerbation of symptoms. Plasma exchange or high-dose intravenous normal immunoglobulin have been tried in patients with severe weakness.

References.

1. Newsom-Davis J. Myasthenia gravis and the Lambert-Eaton myasthenic syndrome. *Prescribers' J* 1993; **33:** 205–12.
2. Oh SJ, *et al.* Low-dose guanidine and pyridostigmine: relatively safe and effective long-term symptomatic therapy in Lambert-Eaton myasthenic syndrome. *Muscle Nerve* 1997; **20:** 1146–52.
3. Seneviratne U, de Silva R. Lambert-Eaton myasthenic syndrome. *Postgrad Med J* 1999; **75:** 516–20.
4. Pascuzzi RM. Myasthenia gravis and Lambert-Eaton syndrome. *Ther Apher* 2002; **6:** 57–68.

## Glaucoma and ocular hypertension

Intra-ocular pressure rises when there is an imbalance between production and drainage of aqueous humour in the eye. Aqueous humour is secreted by the ciliary body and flows into the posterior chamber of the eye. It then passes through the pupil into the anterior chamber from where about 75% drains from the eye through the trabecular meshwork into Schlemm's canal and then into the episcleral veins. The remainder is removed by the uveoscleral route, passing through the ciliary muscle and finally into the episcleral tissues.

The term **ocular hypertension** is used to describe intra-ocular pressure above an upper normal value of 21 mmHg when there are no signs of optic nerve damage. The term **glaucoma** is used to describe a group of conditions characterised by cupping (excavation) of the optic disc and damage of the optic nerve leading to gradual visual loss. Raised intra-ocular pressure is an important risk factor for glaucoma, and as it is the only one that can be altered, current therapy for glaucoma is directed at lowering it. The aim is not just to reduce intra-ocular pressure to a normal value but to a level at which damage to the optic nerve ceases.[1-4] Some patients may have raised intra-ocular pressure for many years without evidence of glaucoma. Whether these patients would receive long-term benefit from a reduction in intra-ocular pressure is under study but many ophthalmologists consider that therapy is indicated if the intra-ocular pressure is higher than 30 mmHg. Glaucoma can also occur and progress in patients with an intra-ocular pressure within the normal range (normal tension glaucoma).

Raised intra-ocular pressure associated with glaucoma is usually due to reduced outflow of aqueous humour from the eye. Glaucoma is described as open-angle or angle-closure depending on the mechanism of the obstruction of drainage and may be acute or chronic. Glaucoma may also be referred to as primary or secondary. Primary glaucoma is usually associated with a direct disturbance of aqueous outflow whereas secondary glaucoma develops as a consequence of a number of diseases or of trauma.

The most common form of glaucoma is **chronic open-angle glaucoma** (simple glaucoma; wide-angle glaucoma) which is due to blockage in drainage through the trabecular meshwork. Intra-ocular pressure increases gradually, and the condition is usually asymptomatic until well advanced and severe damage has occurred. Usually, both eyes are affected. Risk factors include old age, diabetes, Afro-Caribbean race, a family history of glaucoma, and myopia. A 'steroid glaucoma' may be produced, after a few weeks of treatment with eye drops containing corticosteroids, in patients predisposed to open-angle glaucoma; the risk with systemic corticosteroids appears to be less.

In contrast, **angle-closure glaucoma** (closed-angle glaucoma; narrow-angle glaucoma) usually occurs as an acute emergency. Patients present with a painful red eye, sweating, and nausea and vomiting as a result of a rapid rise in intra-ocular pressure. This can result from blockage of the flow of aqueous humour into the anterior chamber. The resulting rise in intra-ocular pressure bows the iris against the trabecular meshwork restricting aqueous outflow and thereby further raising intra-ocular pressure. It usually occurs in patients with hypermetropia who have a shallow anterior chamber and a narrow filtration angle. The use of mydriatics in such patients is contra-indicated as dilatation of the pupil can precipitate an acute attack of angle-closure glaucoma.

ANTIGLAUCOMA DRUGS.

Although many drugs are effective in reducing intra-ocular pressure there is little data on their long-term effect on visual field changes in glaucoma.[2,5] Drugs used in the treatment of glaucoma lower intra-ocular pressure by a variety of mechanisms and their effects are often additive. Their use has been discussed in a number of reviews.[1,3,6-9]

- *Beta blockers* inhibit beta receptors in the ciliary epithelium and thereby reduce the secretion of aqueous humour. They have traditionally been the drugs of first choice for initial and maintenance treatment of open-angle and other chronic glaucomas and of ocular hypertension; other drugs are used with them when further reductions in intra-ocular pressure are required. They are better tolerated than miotics but can produce systemic effects, and their safety, particularly in the elderly, has been questioned.[10,11] Studies suggest that individual topical beta blockers are probably equally effective in reducing intra-ocular pressure but if a nonselective beta blocker is used an additional reduction in pressure may not be obtained with adrenaline (see below).
- *Prostaglandin analogues* such as latanoprost, bimatoprost, and travoprost lower intra-ocular pressure by increasing uveoscleral outflow. They are increasingly a first choice, alone or as adjuncts, in the treatment of ocular hypertension or open-angle glaucoma. They appear to be well-tolerated but may cause a potentially irreversible increase in brown pigmentation of the iris; the long-term significance of this effect is unknown. Unoprostone is also used in some countries.
- *Parasympathomimetic miotics* facilitate trabecular drainage by constricting the pupil and pulling open the trabecular meshwork. However, this can cause blurred vision and browache, especially in younger patients, and the small pupil may cause problems if central vision is already limited. Parasympathomimetic miotics also reduce uveoscleral outflow and this can cause a paradoxical increase in intra-ocular pressure in patients with a recessed anterior angle. They should not be used in the presence of inflammation as adhesions may form between the pupil and the lens (posterior synechiae). Pilocarpine is the miotic most frequently employed and is indicated in the treatment of open-angle glaucoma and other chronic glaucomas. It is often added to treatment with other drugs when further reductions in intra-ocular pressure are required. It requires frequent instillation and this may lead to problems with compliance. Carbachol is sometimes used when resistance or intolerance to pilocarpine develops. Physostigmine is more potent than pilocarpine but is poorly tolerated and is rarely used now; it was used with pilocarpine but rarely alone. Stronger or longer-acting anticholinesterase miotics such as demecarium and ecothiopate can cause pupillary block and induce angle-closure glaucoma. They are usually only used in patients refractory to other antiglaucoma treatment or in those in whom the lens of the eye has been removed (aphakic patients). Pilocarpine is also used in the emergency treatment of angle-closure glaucoma before surgery or laser therapy.
- *Sympathomimetics* such as dipivefrine increase outflow of aqueous humour through the trabecular meshwork and the uveoscleral route and may also reduce its rate of production. They are used in open-angle glaucoma and other chronic glaucomas usually when further reductions in intra-ocular pressure are required in patients receiving beta blockers (but may not produce an additive effect if used with a nonselective beta blocker).[12] As they produce pupillary dilatation they can induce an acute attack if used in angle-closure glaucoma. Adrenaline can cause eye irritation and produce systemic effects; it is now rarely used. Dipivefrine is converted into adrenaline by corneal esterases and ocular adverse effects are usually less than with adrenaline itself. Guanethidine, an adrenergic neurone blocker, reduces aqueous secretion and is used either alone or in combination to enhance and prolong the effect of adrenaline; prolonged use can cause fibrosis and corneal changes. The $alpha_2$-adrenoceptor agonist clonidine has also been used in some countries, while more recent introductions include apraclonidine and brimonidine. $Alpha_2$-adrenoceptor agonists lower intra-ocular pressure by reducing production of aqueous humour. Apraclonidine is used alone or as an adjunct to other drugs in the control of intra-ocular pressure associated with ocular surgery or in the short-term to delay laser treatment or surgery for patients with glaucoma not adequately controlled with other drugs; tachyphylaxis and ocular irritation limit its long-term use. Brimonidine is another $alpha_2$-adrenoceptor agonist used similarly.
- *Carbonic anhydrase inhibitors* such as acetazolamide, reduce production of aqueous humour by a mechanism independent of their diuretic action. They are used as part of the emergency treatment of angle-closure glaucoma to produce a rapid reduction in intra-ocular pressure before surgery or laser therapy. Systemic doses may be added to treatment in open-angle glaucoma and other chronic glaucomas in patients refractory to standard treatment but many patients are unable to tolerate prolonged therapy. Topical carbonic anhydrase inhibitors, such as dorzolamide or brinzolamide, have a lower potential to produce adverse effects. They are used similarly to other topical drugs either alone or as an adjunct in patients resistant to or intolerant of first-line drugs.
- *Osmotic diuretics* reduce vitreous volume and can produce a marked reduction in intra-ocular pressure. They are used in the short-term management of glaucoma when a rapid reduction in intra-ocular pressure is required before surgery. Mannitol and urea are both given intravenously and have a faster onset than glycerol or isosorbide given orally.
- *Several other drugs* are used topically in glaucoma and ocular hypertension. The alpha-adrenergic antagonist dapiprazole is used in some countries.

DIAGNOSIS OF GLAUCOMA.

*Open-angle glaucoma* is asymptomatic in its early stages and the use of screening methods for detecting early disease is of great importance.[13] Measurement of intra-ocular pressure alone is a poor diagnostic tool and a combination of direct examination of the optic nerve together with visual field examination and intra-ocular pressure tonometry is considered to be more reliable.[3] Provocative tests such as placing the patient prone in a dark room are sometimes used to identify eyes suffering from or at risk of *angle-closure glaucoma*. Short-acting mydriatics have also been used but are not without risk. Long-term follow-up of patients whose treatment had been determined by the use of a provocative test using phenylephrine with pilocarpine has suggested that this test is neither sensitive nor specific.[14]

TREATMENT OF GLAUCOMA.

*Open-angle glaucoma* is frequently treated first with a topical beta blocker or a prostaglandin analogue. It may be necessary to combine these drugs or add others such as a miotic, a sympathomimetic, or a topical carbonic anhydrase inhibitor to control intra-ocular pressure. It has been suggested that each type of drug should be tried alone first before resorting to combination therapy. If further reduction of intra-ocular pressure is required a systemic carbonic anhydrase inhibitor may be used but long-term treatment is poorly tolerated. If this is unsuccessful, surgery (trabeculectomy) or laser treatment (trabeculoplasty) is usually indicated. Laser treatment appears to be as effective as topical drug therapy[15] although its effects may be short-lived.[16] It has been suggested that it might be of use in the initial treatment of older patients who cannot use eye drops or when surgery needs to be postponed or is contra-indicated.[3] However, the early use of surgery is now often advocated in Europe, especially for younger patients, although this is still a subject of debate in the USA. Some consider that there is an unnecessary risk of continuing visual loss while drug treatment is being evaluated, and they advocate surgery as the primary treatment.[17] The earlier use of surgical intervention is supported by evidence that long-term drug therapy[18] or laser treatment[3] may have a deleterious effect on the outcome of subsequent surgery and by evidence that surgery is more effective than drug or laser treatment in producing long-term intra-ocular pressure control.[16]

It is essential to start treatment for an *acute attack of angle-closure glaucoma* within 24 to 48 hours. If treatment is delayed adhesions may form between the iris and the cornea (peripheral anterior synechiae) and the trabecular meshwork may be damaged. *Chronic angle-closure glaucoma* may then develop with permanently raised intra-ocular pressure which ultimately leads to total loss of vision (absolute glaucoma). The initial treatment aims to produce a rapid reduction in intra-ocular pressure. A miotic such as pilocarpine is used topically to constrict the pupil while a carbonic anhydrase inhibitor such as acetazolamide is given by mouth or by intravenous injection. Osmotic diuretics such as mannitol or urea given intravenously or glycerol or isosorbide given orally may also be used. When intra-ocular pressure has been reduced sufficiently, laser therapy or surgery is performed on both eyes to increase drainage of aqueous humour. If further topical treatment is required after surgery, treatment is usually as for open-angle glaucoma. Beta blockers, with or without adrenaline, are preferred to pilocarpine as there is a risk of posterior synechiae forming when pilocarpine is used.

Glaucoma filtering surgery such as trabeculectomy can be highly effective in reducing intra-ocular pressure, but in some groups of patients, such as children, Afro-Caribbeans, or those who have had previous ocular surgery, there is a high failure rate, usually due to formation of scar tissue.[19] The scar formation is associated with proliferation of fibroblasts and the subconjunctival injection of antiproliferative drugs such as fluorouracil has been shown to reduce the failure rate of surgery but at a cost of increased epithelial toxicity and conjunctival wound leaks.[19] A study group[20] reporting on the long-term follow-up of patients treated with fluorouracil recommended that fluorouracil should still be used in the surgical management of glaucoma in patients with a history of ocular surgery, but in view of the increased incidence of late-onset conjunctival wound leaks, suggested caution in its use in eyes with good prognoses at the dosage they employed. The use of a single intraoperative topical application of mitomycin has been investigated as an alternative to the regimen of multiple injections required with fluorouracil. Rates of success comparable with those for fluorouracil have been achieved but a plea for caution has been made[21] over the risk of adverse effects that could affect vision and the need to determine long-term safety of antiproliferative drugs. Other drugs are also being studied as antiproliferative agents. Whether the use of antiproliferative drugs is of benefit to all patients undergoing glaucoma surgery is under study.[10]

*Postoperative ocular hypertension* may occur following surgery on the anterior chamber of the eye or procedures such as trabeculoplasty. Acetylcholine or carbachol instilled directly into the anterior chamber of the eye (intracameral instillation) are used intra-operatively to reduce early postoperative rises in intra-ocular pressure in procedures such as cataract extraction. The short action of acetylcholine can be an advantage as prolonged miosis is associated with severe postoperative pain. However, some consider carbachol to be the more effective drug;[22,23] standard antiglaucoma drugs including beta blockers, pilocarpine, apraclonidine, and carbonic anhydrase inhibitors have also been used for prophylaxis of postoperative ocular hypertension.


1. Quigley HA. Open-angle glaucoma. *N Engl J Med* 1993; **328:** 1097–1106.
2. Liesegang TJ. Glaucoma: changing concepts and future directions. *Mayo Clin Proc* 1996; **71:** 689–94.
3. Anonymous. The management of primary open angle glaucoma. *Drug Ther Bull* 1997; **35:** 4–6.
4. Coleman AL. Glaucoma. *Lancet* 1999; **354:** 1803–10.
5. Rossetti L, *et al.* Randomized clinical trials on medical treatment of glaucoma: are they appropriate to guide clinical practice? *Arch Ophthalmol* 1993; **111:** 96–103.
6. Taniguchi T, Kitazawa Y. A risk-benefit assessment of drugs used in the management of glaucoma. *Drug Safety* 1994; **11:** 68–74.
7. Alward WLM. Medical management of glaucoma. *N Engl J Med* 1998; **339:** 1298–1307.
8. Hoyng PFJ, van Beek LM. Pharmacological therapy for glaucoma. *Drugs* 2000; **59:** 411–34.
9. Khaw PT, *et al.* Glaucoma—2: Treatment. *BMJ* 2004; **328:** 156–8.
10. Diggory P, Franks W. Medical treatment of glaucoma—a reappraisal of the risks. *Br J Ophthalmol* 1996; **80:** 85–9.
11. O'Donoghue E. β Blockers and the elderly with glaucoma: are we adding insult to injury? *Br J Ophthalmol* 1995; **79:** 794–6.
12. Sorensen SJ, Abel SR. Comparison of the ocular beta-blockers. *Ann Pharmacother* 1996; **30:** 43–54.
13. Khaw PT, *et al.* Glaucoma—1: Diagnosis. *BMJ* 2004; **328:** 97–9. Correction. *ibid.*; 762.
14. Wishart PK. Does the pilocarpine phenylephrine provocative test help in the management of acute and subacute angle closure glaucoma? *Br J Ophthalmol* 1991; **75:** 284–7.
15. Glaucoma Laser Trial Research Group. The glaucoma laser trial (GLT) and glaucoma laser trial follow-up study: 7. results. *Am J Ophthalmol* 1995; **120:** 718–31.
16. Migdal C, *et al.* Long-term functional outcome after early surgery compared with laser and medicine in open-angle glaucoma. *Ophthalmology* 1994; **101:** 1651–7.
17. Hitchings RA. Primary surgery for primary open angle glaucoma—justified or not? *Br J Ophthalmol* 1993; **77:** 445–8.
18. Broadway D, *et al.* Adverse effects of topical antiglaucomatous medications on the conjunctiva. *Br J Ophthalmol* 1993; **77:** 590–6.
19. Khaw PT, *et al.* 5-Fluorouracil and beyond. *Br J Ophthalmol* 1991; **75:** 577–8.
20. The Fluorouracil Filtering Surgery Study Group. Five-year follow-up of the Fluorouracil Filtering Surgery Study. *Am J Ophthalmol* 1996; **121:** 349–66.
21. Khaw PT. Antiproliferative agents and the prevention of scarring after surgery: friend or foe? *Br J Ophthalmol* 1995; **79:** 627.
22. Ruiz RS, *et al.* Effects of carbachol and acetylcholine on intraocular pressure after cataract extraction. *Am J Ophthalmol* 1989; **107:** 7–10.
23. Hollands RH, *et al.* Control of intraocular pressure after cataract extraction. *Can J Ophthalmol* 1990; **25:** 128–32.


## Myasthenia gravis

Myasthenia gravis is an auto-immune disorder characterised by defective neuromuscular transmission and consequent muscular weakness. It is caused by the formation of autoantibodies specific for nicotinic acetylcholine receptors. The thymus appears to be involved in many patients and some have a thymoma. There appear to be several types of myasthenia. Classifications based on the distribution and severity of symptoms include ocular myasthenia, where the disease is clinically confined to the extra-ocular muscles and mild or moderate generalised myasthenia, also affecting muscles other than the extra-ocular muscles; acute fulminating myasthenia; and late severe myasthenia. Another classification, based on the age of onset and the presence, or absence of thymoma, divides patients into those with thymoma; those without thymoma and onset before age of 40; and those without thymoma and onset after 40 years of age. Other types of myasthenia include transient neonatal myasthenia due to transplacental passage of receptor antibodies, which may persist for 1 to 6 weeks in the infants of myasthenic mothers, penicillamine-induced myasthenia, and congenital myasthenia (see under 3,4-Diaminopyridine, p.1489).

DIAGNOSIS OF MYASTHENIA GRAVIS.

Although all patients have circulating antibodies to acetylcholine receptors they are undetectable by radio-immunoassay in about 15% of patients who are described as having seronegative myasthenia. Patients may often be tested first for their reaction to an anticholinesterase. Intravenous edrophonium preceded by atropine (Tensilon test) is the most commonly used anticholinesterase test because of its rapid onset and short duration of action. Severe adverse effects can occasionally occur so testing should only be undertaken when facilities for endotracheal intubation and controlled ventilation are immediately available. A positive result is considered to be a rapid but temporary increase in muscle strength. Repetitive nerve stimulation is also used as a diagnostic test but, like the anticholinesterase test, is not specific for myasthenia gravis.

TREATMENT OF MYASTHENIA GRAVIS.

- Symptomatic treatment is with an *anticholinesterase*; pyridostigmine and neostigmine are those most commonly used. Most patients prefer pyridostigmine as it produces less muscarinic adverse effects and has a longer duration of action, although the quicker onset of action of neostigmine may offer an advantage at the beginning of the day. The dose must be adjusted to give the optimum therapeutic response but muscle strength may not be restored to normal and some patients must live with a degree of disability. The effect may vary for different muscles and the dosage should be adjusted so that the bulbar and respiratory muscles receive optimum treatment. Overdosage may lead to a 'cholinergic crisis' (see Adverse Effects of Neostigmine, p.1492). Edrophonium may be employed to establish whether the patient is underdosed or overdosed.
- *Corticosteroids* are the main immunosuppressive drugs used for treatment. They are also useful in patients with ocular myasthenia, who as a group respond poorly to anticholinesterases and to thymectomy, provided that their disability is severe enough to warrant long-term corticosteroid treatment with its attendant side-effects. Many start with low doses such as 5 to 20 mg of prednisolone daily or on alternate days, to reduce the risk of steroid-induced exacerbations of weakness, and increase the dose slowly thereafter according to response; an improvement is usually seen after a few weeks. Others use more aggressive regimens to obtain a more rapid response and start with large doses such as 60 to 80 mg of prednisolone daily. Whichever method is used, once clinical benefit has been obtained the regimen should be modified to alternate-day dosage, with the dose being slowly tapered when the patient is in remission. Patients taking corticosteroids require less anticholinesterase therapy and, if the dosage of the anticholinesterase is not reduced, an initial deterioration in the myasthenia may occur in the first few weeks of treatment (see also under Interactions of Neostigmine, p.1493). It is rarely possible to withdraw corticosteroids completely but some patients may be maintained satisfactorily on as little as 10 mg on alternate days. If remission cannot be maintained on low-dose prednisolone, addition of azathioprine at a dosage of 2 to 3 mg/kg daily may be considered.
- Addition of *azathioprine* to treatment may allow a reduction in the dose of both corticosteroids and anticholinesterases. Azathioprine may also be of use when corticosteroids are contra-indicated or when response to corticosteroids alone is insufficient, but it has a much slower onset of action than corticosteroids and is not usually used alone. *Ciclosporin* is effective in some patients unresponsive to anticholinesterases and corticosteroids but serious adverse effects including nephrotoxicity may limit its use; the time to response is similar to that with corticosteroids. Other drugs such as *cyclophosphamide* and *methotrexate* have also been tried and benefit has been reported with *mycophenolate mofetil*.
- Plasma exchange provides a dramatic but short-lived improvement and is useful as a short-term measure in myasthenic crisis to improve ill patients while other therapies take effect, but there is no evidence that repeated plasma exchange combined with immunosuppression is superior to immunosuppression alone. A similar short-term benefit has been seen from the use of high-dose intravenous *normal immunoglobulins*.
- Thymectomy may be offered to all patients sufficiently fit to undergo surgery unless they have minimal symptoms, purely ocular disease, or late onset or seronegative disease. Thymectomy is usually avoided in prepubertal children because of concern over the effect on growth and the developing immune system; it has been suggested that symptomatic treatment with anticholinesterases should be continued until adolescence, when the disease often improves spontaneously. After thymectomy, remission or improvement may be expected in about 80% of patients without thymomas, although this may take some years; the response is poorer in those with thymomas.

References.


1. Evoli A, *et al.* A practical guide to the recognition and management of myasthenia gravis. *Drugs* 1996; **52:** 662–70.
2. Yi Q, Lefvert AK. Current and future therapies for myasthenia gravis. *Drugs Aging* 1997; **11:** 132–9.
3. Newsom-Davis J. Myasthenia gravis. *Prescribers' J* 2000; **40:** 93–8.
4. Vincent A, *et al.* Myasthenia gravis. *Lancet* 2001; **357:** 2122–8.
5. Pascuzzi RM. Myasthenia gravis and Lambert-Eaton syndrome. *Ther Apher* 2002; **6:** 57–68.
6. Vincent A, Drachman DB. Myasthenia gravis. *Adv Neurol* 2002; **88:** 159–88.

### Reversal of mydriasis

Topical miotics (mydriolytics) are sometimes used to reverse the effects of mydriatics following surgery or ophthalmoscopic examination but do not appear to be in routine clinical use. *Pilocarpine* can counteract the mydriatic effect of topical sympathomimetics, such as phenylephrine and hydroxyamfetamine, but is ineffective against mydriasis produced by antimuscarinics, such as homatropine, and may impair vision further when used with tropicamide. Furthermore, there is also the risk that pilocarpine might precipitate angle-closure glaucoma in susceptible patents. *Dapiprazole* appears to be safer than pilocarpine when used to reverse sympathomimetic-induced mydriasis and is effective to some degree against tropicamide-induced mydriasis. It also appears to enhance recovery of accommodation after the use of cycloplegics.

The rate of reversal of mydriasis is generally slower in patients with dark irides than in those with lighter irides.

### Strabismus

Strabismus, sometimes referred to as a squint or cast, is a lack of coordination of the visual axes of the eyes so that the eyes are usually either turned towards (convergent strabismus) or away (divergent strabismus) from each other. It can arise from a physical defect of the attachment of the extra-ocular muscles to the eye or from paralysis, spasms, or overactivity affecting the extra-ocular muscles of one of the eyes. In young children strabismus or other conditions which prevent a clear image being formed on the retina can result in visual impairment (amblyopia) in the affected eye if not treated.

Treatment for strabismus often consists of eye exercises, and methods to force preferential use of the affected eye by restricting vision through the healthy eye. This is accomplished either by using an eye patch or by penalisation with glasses or the cycloplegic drug *atropine*. However, as prolonged use of atropine eye drops may be required there is a risk of systemic toxicity. Surgery may sometimes be necessary. Extra-ocular injection of *botulinum A toxin* has been used to weaken an overactive extra-ocular eye muscle as an aid to eye realignment; repeated injections may be required. Long-acting parasympathomimetic miotics such as *demecarium*, *dyflos*, and *ecothiopate* have been used in the diagnosis and management of convergent strabismus (esotropia) due to excessive accommodation. Centrally-acting drugs such as levodopa and citicoline have also been investigated. With any form of treatment care has to be taken not to induce amblyopia in the healthy eye.

References.

1. Chatzistefanou KI, Mills MD. The role of drug treatment in children with strabismus and amblyopia. *Paediatr Drugs* 2000; **2:** 91–100.

---

## Aceclidine Hydrochloride *(rINNM)*

Hidrocloruro de aceclidina. 3-Acetoxyquinuclidine hydrochloride; 3-Quinuclidinyl acetate hydrochloride.

$C_9H_{15}NO_2,HCl$ = 205.7.

*CAS — 827-61-2 (aceclidine); 6109-70-2 (aceclidine hydrochloride).*

*ATC — S01EB08.*

NOTE. Aceclidine is *USAN*.

### Adverse Effects, Treatment, and Precautions

As for Neostigmine, p.1492. For adverse effects and precautions of miotics, see also Pilocarpine, p.1495.

### Uses and Administration

Aceclidine hydrochloride is a parasympathomimetic miotic that is a cholinergic agonist. It is used in eye drops to lower intra-ocular pressure in patients with glaucoma (p.1485).

### Preparations

**Proprietary Preparations** (details are given in Part 3)

***Belg.:*** Glaucocare†; ***Fr.:*** Glaucostat†; ***Ger.:*** Glaucotat†; ***Gr.:*** Glaucostat; ***Ital.:*** Glaunorm; ***Neth.:*** Glaucocare†; ***Port.:*** Glaucostat; ***Spain:*** Glaucostat†; ***Switz.:*** Glaucostat†.

**Multi-ingredient:** ***Belg.:*** Glaucofrin†; ***Fr.:*** Glaucadrine†; ***Ital.:*** Glautimol; ***Neth.:*** Glaucofrin†; ***Switz.:*** Glaucadrine†.

---

## Acetylcholine Chloride *(BAN, rINN)*

Acetylcholini Chloridum; Cloruro de acetilcolina. (2-Acetoxyethyl)trimethylammonium chloride.

$C_7H_{16}ClNO_2$ = 181.7.

*CAS — 51-84-3 (acetylcholine); 60-31-1 (acetylcholine chloride).*

*ATC — S01EB09.*

**Pharmacopoeias.** In *Eur.* (see p.vi) and *US.*

*Jpn* includes Acetylcholine Chloride for Injection.

**Ph. Eur. 5.0** (Acetylcholine Chloride). A very hygroscopic, white or almost white crystalline powder or colourless crystals. Very soluble in water; freely soluble in alcohol; slightly soluble in dichloromethane. Protect from light.

**USP 27** (Acetylcholine Chloride). White or off-white crystals or crystalline powder. Very soluble in water; freely soluble in alcohol; insoluble in ether. It is decomposed by hot water and by alkalis. Store in airtight containers.

### Adverse Effects

Because it is rapidly hydrolysed in the body by cholinesterases the toxicity of acetylcholine is normally relatively low.

Adverse effects of the choline esters include nausea and vomiting, abdominal pain, flushing, sweating, salivation, lachrymation, rhinorrhoea, eructation, diarrhoea, urinary frequency, headache, difficulty in visual accommodation, bradycardia, peripheral vasodilatation leading to hypotension, and bronchoconstriction.

### Treatment of Adverse Effects

Atropine sulfate may be given intravenously, intramuscularly, or subcutaneously to control the muscarinic and most nicotinic effects of the choline esters. Supportive treatment may be required.

### Precautions

Choline esters are generally contra-indicated for systemic use in intestinal or urinary obstruction or where increased muscular activity of the urinary or gastrointestinal tract is liable to be harmful. They are also contra-indicated in asthma and obstructive airways disease, in cardiovascular disorders including bradycardia or heart block and recent myocardial infarction, and in hypotension, vagotonia, epilepsy, parkinsonism, hyperthyroidism, peptic ulceration, and pregnancy.

Although acetylcholine is normally rapidly hydrolysed in the body, systemic effects have followed topical application of choline esters to the eye, and caution is advisable in the above conditions.

### Interactions

As for Neostigmine, p.1492. Acetylcholine is hydrolysed in the body by cholinesterase and its effects are markedly prolonged and enhanced by prior administration of anticholinesterases.

**Beta blockers.** A report[1] of severe bronchospasm with subsequent pulmonary oedema after intra-ocular injection of acetylcholine chloride in a patient also receiving *metoprolol* by mouth.

1. Rasch D, *et al.* Bronchospasm following intraocular injection of acetylcholine in a patient taking metoprolol. *Anesthesiology* 1983; **59:** 583–5.

**NSAIDs.** According to the manufacturers of acetylcholine chloride ophthalmic preparations, there have been reports that acetylcholine and carbachol were ineffective when used in patients treated with topical (ophthalmic) NSAIDs.

### Uses and Administration

Acetylcholine is an endogenous chemical transmitter with a very wide range of actions in the body; it is a powerful quaternary ammonium parasympathomimetic but its action is transient as it is rapidly destroyed by cholinesterase. It is released from postganglionic parasympathetic nerves and also from some postganglionic sympathetic nerves to produce peripheral actions which correspond to those of muscarine. It is accordingly a vasodilator and cardiac depressant, a stimulant of the vagus and the parasympathetic nervous system, and it has a tonic action on smooth muscle. It also increases lachrymal, salivary, and other secretions. All the muscarinic actions of acetylcholine are abolished by atropine.

Acetylcholine also has actions which correspond to those of nicotine and is accordingly a stimulant of skeletal muscle, the autonomic ganglia, and the adrenal medulla. The nicotinic actions of acetylcholine on skeletal muscle are blocked by competitive neuromuscular blockers; they are also inhibited by massive doses or discharge of acetylcholine itself, which has clinical application in relation to the mode of action of suxamethonium (p.1408).

Acetylcholine chloride is used as a miotic to reduce postoperative rises in intra-ocular pressure associated with cataract surgery, penetrating keratoplasty, iridectomy, and other anterior segment surgery (see p.1485) but is ineffective when applied topically as it is hydrolysed more rapidly than it can penetrate the cornea. Doses of 0.5 to 2 mL of a freshly prepared 1% solution of acetylcholine chloride are therefore instilled directly into the anterior chamber of the eye (intracameral instillation). Miosis occurs within seconds and lasts for about 20 minutes.

**Diagnosis and testing.** AUTONOMIC FAILURE. Acetylcholine has been used in a sweat-spot test for autonomic neuropathy in diabetic patients.[1] An area on the dorsum of the foot is painted with iodine and starch, followed by intradermal injection of acetylcholine into the centre of the area. Sweat produced in response to acetylcholine reacts with the iodine and starch to produce fine black dots corresponding to the pores of the sweat glands; a normal response is indicated by a uniform distribution of dark spots whereas in diabetic autonomic neuropathy this pattern is lost to a varying degree. A similar test has been carried out[2] to assess sympathetic nerve function and therefore predict the success of lumbar sympathectomy in patients with critical limb ischaemia.

1. Ryder REJ, *et al.* Acetylcholine sweatspot test for autonomic denervation. *Lancet* 1988; **i:** 1303–5.
2. Altomare DF. Acetylcholine sweat test: an effective way to select patients for lumbar sympathectomy. *Lancet* 1994; **344:** 976–8.

### Preparations

***USP 27:*** Acetylcholine Chloride for Ophthalmic Solution.

**Proprietary Preparations** (details are given in Part 3)

***Austral.:*** Miochol; ***Belg.:*** Miochol†; ***Braz.:*** Miochol-E†; ***Canad.:*** Miochol; Miochol-E; ***Chile:*** Miochol-E; ***Fin.:*** Miochol-E; ***Fr.:*** Miochole; ***Ger.:*** Miochol-E; ***Gr.:*** Miochol-E; ***Hong Kong:*** Miochol-E; ***Irl.:*** Miochol; ***Israel:*** Miochol; Miochol-E; ***Ital.:*** Miochol-E; Miovisin; ***NZ:*** Miochol; ***S.Afr.:*** Covochol; Miochol; ***Singapore:*** Miochol-E; ***Swed.:*** Miochol†; ***Switz.:*** Miochol; ***Thai.:*** Miochol; ***UK:*** Miochol; ***USA:*** Miochol.

---

## Ambenonium Chloride *(BAN, rINN)*

Ambestigmini Chloridum; Cloruro de ambenonio; Win-8077.

*N,N′*-Oxalylbis(*N*-2-aminoethyl-*N*-2-chlorobenzyldiethylammonium) dichloride.

$C_{28}H_{42}Cl_4N_4O_2$ = 608.5.

*CAS — 7648-98-8 (ambenonium); 115-79-7 (anhydrous ambenonium chloride); 52022-31-8 (ambenonium chloride tetrahydrate).*

*ATC — N07AA30.*

**Pharmacopoeias.** In *Jpn.*

### Adverse Effects, Treatment, and Precautions

As for Neostigmine, p.1492.

Ambenonium produces fewer muscarinic side-effects than neostigmine. As there is only slight warning of overdosage, routine use of atropine with ambenonium is contra-indicated because the muscarinic symptoms of overdosage may be suppressed leaving only the more serious nicotinic effects (fasciculation and paralysis of voluntary muscle).

### Pharmacokinetics

Ambenonium chloride is poorly absorbed from the gastrointestinal tract. It does not appear to be hydrolysed by cholinesterases.

### Uses and Administration

Ambenonium is a quaternary ammonium compound that is a reversible inhibitor of cholinesterase activity with actions similar to those of neostigmine (p.1493), but of longer duration. Ambenonium chloride is given by mouth in the treatment of myasthenia gravis (p.1486) in usual doses of 5 to 25 mg three or four times daily, adjusted according to individual response. It may be of value in patients who cannot tolerate neostigmine or pyridostigmine.

### Preparations

**Proprietary Preparations** (details are given in Part 3)

***Fr.:*** Mytelase; ***Gr.:*** Mytelase; ***Swed.:*** Mytelase; ***USA:*** Mytelase.

---

## Bethanechol Chloride *(BAN)*

Betanecol, cloruro de; Carbamylmethylcholine Chloride. (2-Carbamoyloxypropyl)trimethylammonium chloride.

$C_7H_{17}ClN_2O_2$ = 196.7.

*CAS — 674-38-4 (bethanechol); 590-63-6 (bethanechol chloride).*

*ATC — N07AB02.*

**Pharmacopoeias.** In *Jpn* and *US.*

**USP 27** (Bethanechol Chloride). Colourless or white crystals, or white crystalline powder, usually having a slight, amine-like odour. It is hygroscopic and exhibits polymorphism. Freely soluble in water and in alcohol; insoluble in chloroform and in ether. pH of a 1% solution in water is between 5.5 and 6.5. Store in airtight containers.

**Stability.** References to the stability of oral liquid preparations of bethanechol chloride prepared extemporaneously from tablets.

1. Schlatter JL, Saulnier J-L. Bethanechol chloride oral solutions: stability and use in infants. *Ann Pharmacother* 1997; **31:** 294–6.
2. Allen LV, Erickson MA. Stability of bethanechol chloride, pyrazinamide, quinidine sulfate, rifampin, and tetracycline hydrochloride in extemporaneously compounded oral liquids. *Am J Health-Syst Pharm* 1998; **55:** 1804–9.

**Sterilisation.** The US manufacturers state that solutions of bethanechol chloride may be autoclaved at 120° for 20 minutes without discoloration or loss of potency.

### Adverse Effects and Treatment

As described for choline esters under Acetylcholine Chloride, p.1487.

### Precautions

As described for choline esters under Acetylcholine Chloride, p.1487.

Bethanechol should not be given by the intravenous or intramuscular routes as very severe muscarinic adverse effects are liable to occur, calling for emergency use of atropine.

**Autonomic neuropathy.** Patients with autonomic neuropathy might be more susceptible to the adverse effects of bethanechol and they should be started on low-dosage regimens and observed closely for signs of toxicity.[1]

1. Caraco Y, *et al.* Bethanechol-induced cholinergic toxicity in diabetic neuropathy. *DICP Ann Pharmacother* 1990; **24:** 327–8.

### Interactions

As for Neostigmine, p.1492.

**Pharmacokinetics**

Bethanechol chloride is poorly absorbed from the gastrointestinal tract. It is not hydrolysed by cholinesterases. At standard doses bethanechol does not cross the blood-brain barrier.

**Uses and Administration**

Bethanechol chloride, a choline ester, is a quaternary ammonium parasympathomimetic that mainly exhibits the muscarinic actions of acetylcholine (p.1487). It is not inactivated by cholinesterases so its actions are more prolonged than those of acetylcholine. Bethanechol chloride has little if any nicotinic activity and is used for its actions on the bladder and gastrointestinal tract. It has been used as an alternative to catheterisation in the treatment of urinary retention and has also been used for gastric atony and retention, abdominal distension following surgery, congenital megacolon, and gastro-oesophageal reflux disease.

Bethanechol chloride is given in usual doses of 5.15 mg subcutaneously or 10 to 50 mg by mouth, both up to 4 times daily, but dosage must be adjusted individually. Oral doses should be taken on an empty stomach. The effects usually occur within 5 to 15 minutes of a subcutaneous dose, or 30 to 90 minutes of an oral dose, and disappear within about 1 to 2 hours depending on the dose and route. However, large oral doses (300 to 400 mg) may produce effects for up to six hours. For a warning to avoid intravenous or intramuscular use, see under Precautions, above.

**Decreased gastrointestinal motility.** Parasympathomimetics such as bethanechol enhance gastric contractions and increase intestinal motility and form just one of many treatments that have been used in conditions associated with decreased gastrointestinal motility (p.1241).

**Gastro-oesophageal reflux disease.** Prokinetic drugs such as bethanechol have been tried in gastro-oesophageal reflux disease (p.1242) but their value is not clear.

References.

1. Thanick KD, *et al.* Reflux esophagitis: effect of oral bethanechol on symptoms and endoscopic findings. *Ann Intern Med* 1980; **93:** 805–8.
2. Saco LS, *et al.* Double-blind controlled trial of bethanechol and antacid versus placebo and antacid in the treatment of erosive esophagitis. *Gastroenterology* 1982; **82:** 1369–73.
3. Thanick K, *et al.* Bethanechol or cimetidine in the treatment of symptomatic reflux esophagitis: a double-blind control study. *Arch Intern Med* 1982; **142:** 1479–81.
4. Strickland AD, Chang JHT. Results of treatment of gastro-esophageal reflux with bethanechol. *J Pediatr* 1983; **103:** 311–15.

**Stuttering.** A double-blind placebo-controlled study[1] in 10 patients with stuttering (p.702) on the whole failed to confirm an earlier report[2] of benefit using bethanechol although 2 patients who did respond elected to continue treatment after the study.

1. Kampman K, Brady JP. Bethanechol in the treatment of stuttering. *J Clin Psychopharmacol* 1993; **13:** 284–5.
2. Hays P. Bethanechol chloride in treatment of stuttering. *Lancet* 1987; **i:** 271.

**Urinary incontinence and retention.** Bethanechol is one of the parasympathomimetics that have been given to increase detrusor activity in patients with overflow incontinence, but there have been doubts about the effectiveness of such treatment (see p.476). Bethanechol was also one of the parasympathomimetics used in the management of postoperative urinary retention but they have generally been superseded by catheterisation.

References.

1. Finkbeiner AE. Is bethanechol chloride clinically effective in promoting bladder emptying: a literature review. *J Urol (Baltimore)* 1985; **134:** 443–9.
2. Kemp B, *et al.* Prophylaxis and treatment of bladder dysfunction after Wertheim-Meigs operation: the positive effect of early postoperative detrusor stimulation using the cholinergic drug betanecholchloride. *Int Urogynecol J Pelvic Floor Dysfunct* 1997; **8:** 138–41.
3. Riedl CR, *et al.* Electromotive administration of intravesical bethanechol and the clinical impact on acontractile detrusor management: introduction of a new test. *J Urol (Baltimore)* 2000; **164:** 2108–11.

**Preparations**

***USP 27:*** Bethanechol Chloride Injection; Bethanechol Chloride Tablets.

**Proprietary Preparations** (details are given in Part 3)

***Arg.:*** Miotonachol; ***Austral.:*** Urecholine†; Urocarb; ***Austria:*** Myocholine; ***Belg.:*** Muscaran†; ***Braz.:*** Liberan; ***Canad.:*** Duvoid; Myotonachol; Urecholine†; ***Ger.:*** Myocholine; ***India:*** Urotonine; ***Israel:*** Urecholine; ***Ital.:*** Urecholine†; ***S.Afr.:*** Urecholine†; ***Spain:*** Myo Hermes†; ***Switz.:*** Myocholine; ***Thai.:*** Ucholine; Urecholine; ***UK:*** Myotonine; ***USA:*** Duvoid†; Myotonachol; Urecholine.

## Carbachol *(BAN, rINN)*

Carbach.; Carbacholine; Carbacholum; Carbacholum Chloratum; Carbacol; Choline Chloride Carbamate. *O*-Carbamoylcholine chloride; (2-Carbamoyloxyethyl)trimethylammonium chloride.

$C_6H_{15}ClN_2O_2$ = 182.6.

*CAS — 51-83-2.*

*ATC — N07AB01; S01EB02.*

NOTE. CAR is a code approved by the BP 2003 for use on single unit doses of eye drops containing carbachol where the individual container may be too small to bear all the appropriate labelling information.

**Pharmacopoeias.** In *Eur.* (see p.vi), *Pol.*, and *US.*

**Ph. Eur. 5.0** (Carbachol). A white, crystalline, hygroscopic powder. Very slightly soluble in water; sparingly soluble in alcohol; practically insoluble in acetone. Store in airtight containers. Protect from light.

**USP 27** (Carbachol). Store in airtight containers.

**Incompatibility.** Chlorocresol (0.025 to 0.1%) and chlorobutanol (0.5%) were both found to be incompatible with a solution of carbachol (0.8%) and sodium chloride (0.69%), very slight precipitates forming on heating and increasing on standing.[1]

1. *PSGB Lab Report No.911* 1962.

**Adverse Effects and Treatment**

As described for choline esters under Acetylcholine Chloride, p.1487. Carbachol has substantial nicotinic activity which may be unmasked by the use of atropine to counteract muscarinic effects. Carbachol also produces adverse effects similar to those of other miotics such as pilocarpine (p.1495) when used in the eye but may produce more ciliary spasm than pilocarpine.

**Effects on the gastrointestinal tract.** A report[1] of fatal oesophageal rupture after subcutaneous injection of carbachol to relieve urinary retention.

1. Cochrane P. Spontaneous oesophageal rupture after carbachol therapy. *BMJ* 1973; **1:** 463–4.

**Overdosage.** Life-threatening attacks of profuse sweating, intestinal cramps, explosive defaecation, hypothermia, hypotension, and bradycardia occurred in a 36-year-old man after deliberate poisoning with 30 to 40 mg of carbachol.[1] The patient's 10-year-old son had died after poisoning with a similar dose of carbachol.

1. Sangster B, *et al.* Two cases of carbachol intoxication. *Neth J Med* 1979; **22:** 27–8.

**Precautions**

As described for choline esters under Acetylcholine Chloride, p.1487. For precautions when used as a miotic see under Pilocarpine, p.1495. Carbachol should not be given by the intravenous or intramuscular routes as very severe muscarinic adverse effects are liable to occur, calling for emergency treatment with atropine.

**Interactions**

**NSAIDs.** According to the manufacturers of acetylcholine chloride ophthalmic preparations, there have been reports that acetylcholine and carbachol were ineffective when used in patients treated with topical (ophthalmic) NSAIDs.

**Uses and Administration**

Carbachol, a choline ester, is a quaternary ammonium parasympathomimetic with the muscarinic and nicotinic actions of acetylcholine (p.1487). It is not inactivated by cholinesterases so its actions are more prolonged than those of acetylcholine.

Carbachol has a miotic action and eye drops containing 0.75 to 3% are sometimes used up to four times daily to lower intra-ocular pressure in glaucoma, usually with other miotics (see below). Miosis occurs within 10 to 20 minutes of instillation of carbachol eye drops and lasts for 4 to 8 hours; reduction in intra-ocular pressure lasts for 8 hours.

Carbachol is also given intra-ocularly, up to 0.5 mL of a 0.01% solution being instilled into the anterior chamber of the eye (intracameral instillation), to produce miosis in ocular surgery and to reduce postoperative rises in intra-ocular pressure. The maximum degree of miosis is usually obtained within 2 to 5 minutes of intra-ocular instillation and miosis lasts for 24 to 48 hours.

Carbachol has been used for the treatment of urinary retention (p.476) in a dose of 2 mg given three times daily by mouth on a empty stomach, although catheterisation is generally preferred. For the acute symptoms of postoperative urinary retention, doses of 250 micrograms have been given subcutaneously, repeated twice if necessary at 30-minute intervals. For a warning to avoid intravenous or intramuscular use, see under Precautions, above. Carbachol has also been used in some countries for the treatment of decreased gastrointestinal motility (p.1241).

**Dry mouth.** Carbachol has been used as an alternative to pilocarpine in the treatment of radiation-induced xerostomia.[1] The overall treatment of dry mouth is discussed on p.1576.

1. Joensuu H. Treatment for post-irradiation xerostomia. *N Engl J Med* 1994; **330:** 141–2.

**Glaucoma and ocular hypertension.** Carbachol is sometimes used as an alternative to pilocarpine in the management of glaucoma (p.1485) when resistance or intolerance to pilocarpine develops. It is also instilled into the anterior chamber of the eye (intracameral instillation) to minimise postoperative rises in intra-ocular pressure associated with ocular surgery, and some[1,2] have found it to be more effective than acetylcholine.

1. Ruiz RS, *et al.* Effects of carbachol and acetylcholine on intraocular pressure after cataract extraction. *Am J Ophthalmol* 1989; **107:** 7–10.
2. Hollands RH, *et al.* Control of intraocular pressure after cataract extraction. *Can J Ophthalmol* 1990; **25:** 128–32.

**Preparations**

***USP 27:*** Carbachol Intraocular Solution; Carbachol Ophthalmic Solution.

**Proprietary Preparations** (details are given in Part 3)

***Arg.:*** Miostat; ***Austral.:*** Miostat; ***Belg.:*** Miostat; ***Canad.:*** Carbastat; Miostat; ***Fin.:*** Doryl; ***Ger.:*** Carbamann; Doryl; Jestryl; ***Hong Kong:*** Miostat; ***Israel:*** Miostat; ***Ital.:*** Mioticol; ***Malaysia:*** Miostat; ***NZ:*** Miostat†; ***S.Afr.:*** Miosys; ***Singapore:*** Miostat; ***Swed.:*** Isopto Karbakolin; ***Switz.:*** Doryl; Miostat; Spersacarbachol†; ***Thai.:*** Miostat; ***USA:*** Carbastat; Miostat.

**Multi-ingredient:** ***Ital.:*** Mios.

## Cevimeline Hydrochloride *(USAN, rINNM)*

AF-102; AF-102B; FKS-508; Hidrocloruro de cevimelina; SND-5008; SNI-2011; SNK-508. (±)-*cis*-2-Methylspiro[1,3-oxathiolane-5,3′-quinuclidine] hydrochloride hemihydrate.

$C_{10}H_{17}NOS,HCl,\frac{1}{2}H_2O$ = 244.8.

*CAS — 107233-08-9 (cevimeline); 153504-70-2 (cevimeline hydrochloride).*

**Adverse Effects, Treatment, and Precautions**

As for Neostigmine, p.1492.

Sweating is a common problem with cevimeline; patients who sweat excessively should be advised to drink extra fluids to avoid dehydration. The manufacturer recommends that cevimeline should not be given when miosis is undesirable such as in patients with acute iritis or angle-closure glaucoma. Blurred vision may affect the performance of skilled tasks. In addition cevimeline should be given with care to those with renal calculi or with biliary-tract disorders. It should also be used with caution in patients deficient in the cytochrome P450 isoenzyme CYP2D6 who may be at a higher risk of adverse effects.

**Interactions**

As for Neostigmine, p.1492.

Drugs which inhibit cytochrome P450 isoenzymes CYP2D6, CYP3A3, or CYP3A4 inhibit the metabolism of cevimeline.

**Pharmacokinetics**

After oral doses cevimeline is absorbed from the gastrointestinal tract; peak concentrations are reached in 1.5 to 2 hours. The rate and extent of absorption are decreased when given with food. Cevimeline is less than 20% bound to plasma proteins. It is metabolised in the liver by cytochrome P450 isoenzymes CYP2D6, CYP3A3, and CYP3A4. Cevimeline is primarily excreted in the urine, mainly as metabolites; about 0.5% of a dose is excreted in the faeces.

**Uses and Administration**

Cevimeline is a selective muscarinic $M_1$ agonist used to improve the symptoms of dry mouth (see p.1576) in patients with Sjögren's syndrome. It is given as the hydrochloride although doses are expressed in terms of the base; 36.8 mg of cevimeline hydrochloride, equivalent to 30 mg of cevimeline base, is given three times daily by mouth.

**Dementia.** Muscarinic $M_1$ agonists such as cevimeline have proved unsuccessful in relieving the symptoms of Alzheimer's disease (see p.1484).

**Preparations**

**Proprietary Preparations** (details are given in Part 3)

***USA:*** Evoxac.

## Choline Alfoscerate *(rINN)*

Alfoscerato de colina; Choline Glycerophosphate; L-α-Glycerylphosphorylcholine. Choline hydroxide, (*R*)-2,3-dihydroxypropyl hydrogen phosphate, inner salt.

$C_8H_{20}NO_6P$ = 257.2.

*CAS — 28319-77-9.*

*ATC — N07AX02.*

**Profile**

Choline alfoscerate is reported to be a precursor of acetylcholine and has been tried in the treatment of Alzheimer's disease and other dementias (below).

**Dementia.** Treatment with precursors of acetylcholine is not generally thought to be of benefit in dementia (p.1484). However, in an analysis of 8 controlled clinical trials the use of choline alfoscerate in patients with dementia of the Alzheimer's type, vascular dementia, or acute cerebrovascular disease was claimed to be of some benefit. Results of a further 3 uncontrolled trials in the same review suggested that it might favour functional recovery in patients with cerebral stroke.

1. Parnetti L, *et al.* Choline alphoscerate in cognitive decline and in acute cerebrovascular disease: an analysis of published clinical data. *Mech Ageing Dev* 2001; **122:** 2041–55.

**Preparations**

**Proprietary Preparations** (details are given in Part 3)

***Arg.:*** Gliatilin; ***Ital.:*** Brezal; Delecit; Gliatilin.

## Demecarium Bromide *(BAN, rINN)*

BC-48; Bromuro de demecario. *N,N′*-Decamethylenebis(*N,N,N*-trimethyl-3-methylcarbamoyloxyanilinium) dibromide.

$C_{32}H_{52}Br_2N_4O_4$ = 716.6.

*CAS — 56-94-0.*

*ATC — S01EB04.*

**Pharmacopoeias.** In *US.*

**USP 27** (Demecarium Bromide). A white or slightly yellow, slightly hygroscopic, crystalline powder. Freely soluble in water and in alcohol; sparingly soluble in acetone; soluble in ether. pH of a 1% solution in water is between 5.0 and 7.0. Store in airtight containers. Protect from light.

**Adverse Effects**

As for Neostigmine, p.1492 and Ecothiopate Iodide, p.1490. For adverse effects of miotics, see also Pilocarpine, p.1495.

#### Treatment of Adverse Effects

As for Ecothiopate Iodide, p.1490.

Pralidoxime has been reported to be more active in counteracting the effects of dyflos and ecothiopate than of demecarium.

#### Precautions

As for Neostigmine, p.1492 and Ecothiopate Iodide, p.1490. For precautions of miotics, see also Pilocarpine, p.1495.

#### Interactions

As for Ecothiopate Iodide, p.1490.

#### Uses and Administration

Demecarium is a quaternary ammonium compound that is a reversible inhibitor of cholinesterase with a long duration of action similar to that of ecothiopate iodide (p.1490). Its miotic action begins within about 15 to 60 minutes of its application and may persist for a week or more. It causes a reduction in intra-ocular pressure that is maximal in 24 hours and may persist for 9 days or more.

Demecarium bromide has been used in the treatment of open-angle glaucoma (p.1485), particularly in aphakic patients and when other drugs have proved inadequate. The dosage varies, 1 or 2 drops of a 0.125% or 0.25% solution being instilled from twice weekly, preferably at bedtime, to twice daily. Demecarium bromide has also been used in the diagnosis and management of accommodative convergent strabismus (p.1487).

#### Preparations

*USP 27:* Demecarium Bromide Ophthalmic Solution.

**Proprietary Preparations** (details are given in Part 3)
*USA:* Humorsol.

## 3,4-Diaminopyridine

3,4-Diaminopiridina.

#### Profile

3,4-Diaminopyridine has similar actions and uses to fampridine (p.1491) but is reported to be more potent in enhancing the release of acetylcholine from nerve terminals. It is used in the Eaton-Lambert myasthenic syndrome (below) and other myasthenic conditions (below). It has been tried in multiple sclerosis (below) and in botulism. There have been isolated reports of seizures and 3,4-diaminopyridine is therefore contra-indicated in patients with epilepsy.

**Congenital myasthenia.** Congenital or hereditary myasthenia is a heterogeneous group of rare disorders associated with various defects in neuromuscular transmission including presynaptic impairment of acetylcholinesterase release, postsynaptic abnormality of acetylcholine receptors, or a deficiency of acetylcholinesterase.[1] Symptoms may be similar to those of myasthenia gravis (p.1486) but there are no immunological abnormalities. Although some forms may respond to anticholinesterases, therapy is usually unsatisfactory. Experience in 16 patients[2] has suggested that 3,4-diaminopyridine used alone or with anticholinesterases may be of benefit. Clinical improvement was seen in 5 of 11 patients with congenital myasthenia who were given 3,4-diaminopyridine as part of a placebo-controlled trial; 3 of the 11 responded to placebo.[3] There have also been reports of benefit from the use of quinidine sulfate in patients with the slow-channel congenital myasthenic syndrome.[4]

1. Engel AG. Congenital myasthenic syndromes. *Neurol Clin North Am* 1994; **12:** 401–37.
2. Palace J, *et al.* 3,4-Diaminopyridine in the treatment of congenital (hereditary) myasthenia. *J Neurol Neurosurg Psychiatry* 1991; **54:** 1069–72.
3. Anlar B, *et al.* 3,4-Diaminopyridine in childhood myasthenia: double-blind, placebo-controlled trial. *J Child Neurol* 1996; **11:** 458–61.
4. Harper CM, Engel AG. Quinidine sulfate therapy for the slow-channel congenital myasthenic syndrome. *Ann Neurol* 1998; **43:** 480–4.

**Eaton-Lambert myasthenic syndrome.** Daily doses of up to 100 mg of 3,4-diaminopyridine by mouth have been found[1] to be effective in the treatment of both the motor and autonomic deficits of patients with Eaton-Lambert syndrome (p.1485). A usual starting dose of 10 mg given three or four times daily increasing if necessary to a maximum of 20 mg given five times daily has been used.[2] However, some workers have recommended limiting the dose to 80 mg daily because of the increased risk of seizures with higher doses.[3] Adverse effects appear to be mainly mild and dose related,[1] although there is a report of cardiac arrest following toxicity.[4] Most patients experience some form of paraesthesia up to 60 minutes after a dose.[1-3] 3,4-Diaminopyridine can produce mild excitatory effects and some patients may experience difficulty in sleeping.

1. McEvoy KM, *et al.* 3,4-Diaminopyridine in the treatment of Lambert-Eaton myasthenic syndrome. *N Engl J Med* 1989; **321:** 1567–71.
2. Newsom-Davis J. Myasthenia gravis and the Lambert-Eaton myasthenic syndrome. *Prescribers' J* 1993; **33:** 205–212.
3. Sanders DB, *et al.* A randomized trial of 3,4-diaminopyridine in Lambert-Eaton myasthenic syndrome. *Neurology* 2000; **54:** 603–7.
4. Boerma CE, *et al.* Cardiac arrest following an iatrogenic 3,4-diaminopyridine intoxication in a patient with Lambert-Eaton myasthenic syndrome. *J Toxicol Clin Toxicol* 1995; **33:** 249–51.

**Multiple sclerosis.** 3,4-Diaminopyridine has been tried in the management of multiple sclerosis (p.646). In a crossover study[1] involving 36 patients with multiple sclerosis, 3,4-diaminopyridine given in a dosage of up to 100 mg daily improved symptoms of leg weakness to a greater extent than placebo but paraesthesia and abdominal pain which occurred in most patients were dose-limiting in some. A systematic review[2] of the use of aminopyridines for symptomatic management of multiple sclerosis was unable to come to any conclusion, and commented on the problem of publication bias in this area.

1. Bever CT, *et al.* Treatment with oral 3,4-diaminopyridine improves leg strength in multiple sclerosis patients: results of a randomized, double-blind, placebo-controlled, crossover trial. *Neurology* 1996; **47:** 1457–62.
2. Solari A, *et al.* Aminopyridines for symptomatic treatment in multiple sclerosis. Available in The Cochrane Library; Issue 2. Chichester: John Wiley; 2004.

## Distigmine Bromide *(BAN, rINN)*

BC-51; Bispyridostigmine Bromide; Bromuro de distigmina; Hexamarium Bromide. 3,3′-[*N*,*N*′-Hexamethylenebis(methylcarbamoyloxy)]bis(1-methylpyridinium bromide).

$C_{22}H_{32}Br_2N_4O_4$ = 576.3.

*CAS — 15876-67-2.*

*ATC — N07AA03.*

**Pharmacopoeias.** In *Jpn.*

#### Adverse Effects, Treatment, and Precautions

As for Neostigmine, p.1492. The anticholinesterase action of distigmine, and hence its adverse effects, may be prolonged, and if treatment with atropine is required it should be maintained for at least 24 hours. Distigmine may stimulate uterine contractions and the UK manufacturer has advised that it should be avoided in pregnancy.

#### Interactions

As for Neostigmine, p.1492.

#### Pharmacokinetics

Distigmine is poorly absorbed from the gastrointestinal tract.

#### Uses and Administration

Distigmine is a quaternary ammonium compound that is a reversible inhibitor of cholinesterase activity with actions similar to those of neostigmine (p.1493) but more prolonged. Maximum inhibition of plasma cholinesterase occurs 9 hours after a single intramuscular dose, and persists for about 24 hours. It is one of several drugs that have been used in the prevention and treatment of postoperative gastrointestinal atony (see Decreased Gastrointestinal Motility, p.1241). It has also been used in postoperative urinary retention (p.476), although it has been superseded by catheterisation. A dose of 500 micrograms of distigmine bromide was injected intramuscularly about 24 to 72 hours after surgery and repeated at intervals of 1 to 3 days until normal function was restored. Alternatively it has been given by mouth in a dose of 5 mg daily thirty minutes before breakfast. A similar dose by mouth, given daily or on alternate days, has been employed in the management of neurogenic bladder.

Distigmine bromide may also be given by mouth with short-acting parasympathomimetics for the treatment of myasthenia gravis (p.1486), but patients being treated with parasympathomimetics tend to prefer pyridostigmine. The initial dose is 5 mg daily before breakfast, increased at intervals of 3 to 4 days if necessary to a maximum of 20 mg daily; children may be given up to 10 mg daily according to age.

#### Preparations

**Proprietary Preparations** (details are given in Part 3)
***Austria:*** Ubretid; ***Fin.:*** Ubretid; ***Ger.:*** Ubretid; ***Gr.:*** Ubretid; ***Hong Kong:*** Ubretid; ***Neth.:*** Ubretid; ***NZ:*** Ubretid†; ***Port.:*** Tonus; ***S.Afr.:*** Ubretid†; ***Singapore:*** Ubretid; ***Switz.:*** Ubretid; ***UK:*** Ubretid.

# Donepezil Hydrochloride

*(BANM, USAN, rINNM)*

BNAG; E-2020; ER-4111 (donepezil); Hidrocloruro de donepezilo. (±)-2-[(1-Benzyl-4-piperidyl)methyl]-5,6-dimethoxy-1-indanone hydrochloride.

$C_{24}H_{29}NO_3,HCl$ = 416.0.

*CAS — 120014-06-4 (donepezil); 142057-79-2 (donepezil); 120011-70-3 (donepezil hydrochloride); 142057-77-0 (donepezil hydrochloride).*

*ATC — N06DA02.*

#### Adverse Effects and Treatment

Adverse effects of acetylcholinesterase inhibitors such as donepezil notably include nausea, vomiting, anorexia, diarrhoea, fatigue, and dizziness. Other common adverse effects include abdominal pain, dyspepsia, headache, somnolence, muscle cramps, insomnia, sweating, tremor, and syncope; upper-respiratory-tract and urinary-tract infections have been noted. Rare cases of angina, sinoatrial and atrioventricular blocks, bradycardia, peptic ulcers, gastrointestinal haemorrhage, extrapyramidal symptoms, and seizures have been observed. Psychiatric disturbances, including depression, hallucinations, agitation, aggressive behaviour, and confusion have also been reported. There is a potential for bladder outflow obstruction. Minor increases in plasma-creatine kinase have also occurred with donepezil.

Hepatotoxicity has occurred with tacrine, and has limited its use (see Tacrine, Precautions, p.1497); individual cases of increased liver transaminases have been noted with other acetylcholinesterase inhibitors.

The use of acetylcholinesterase inhibitors has been associated with weight loss and consequently some manufacturers have recommended that a patient's weight is monitored during treatment. Female patients have been found to be more susceptible to nausea, vomiting, anorexia, and weight loss.

Overdosage with cholinesterase inhibitors may result in 'cholinergic crisis', the details of which are described under Adverse Effects of Neostigmine, p.1492.

◊ Review of the safety profile of donepezil.

1. Committee on Safety of Medicines/Medicines Control Agency. Donepezil (Aricept). *Current Problems* 1999; **25:** 7. Also available at: http://www.mca.gov.uk/ourwork/monitorsafequalmed/currentproblems/volume25mar.htm (accessed 21/05/04)

**Effects on the nervous system.** Restless legs, mumbling, and stuttering developed in an elderly patient after increasing the dose of donepezil to 10 mg daily.[1] Symptoms resolved when donepezil was withdrawn and recurred on rechallenge.

1. Amouyal-Barkate K, *et al.* Abnormal movements with donepezil in Alzheimer disease. *Ann Pharmacother* 2000; **34:** 1347.

**Effects on the skin.** A report[1] of purpuric rash associated with donepezil.

1. Bryant CA, *et al.* Purpuric rash with donepezil treatment. *BMJ* 1998; **317:** 787.

**Effects on the urinary tract.** Urinary incontinence is a recognised adverse effect of the older anticholinesterases such as neostigmine; not unexpectedly there have also been cases associated with donepezil.[1]

1. Hashimoto M, *et al.* Urinary incontinence: an unrecognised adverse effect with donepezil. *Lancet* 2000; **356:** 568.

#### Precautions

Donepezil and other acetylcholinesterase inhibitors should be used with caution, if at all, in patients with gastrointestinal or urinary-tract obstruction; their use is not recommended in patients recovering from bladder or gastrointestinal surgery. Care is also required in patients with a history of asthma, obstructive pulmonary disease, Parkinson's disease, or epilepsy and in those at risk of developing peptic ulcer disease. Patients with cardiovascular conduction disorders such as sick-sinus syndrome may be susceptible to the vagotonic effects of the acetylcholinesterase inhibitors.

#### Interactions

As for Neostigmine, p.1492. Hepatic metabolism of donepezil via the cytochrome P450 system has been demonstrated; plasma concentrations of donepezil may be raised by drugs that inhibit the isoenzyme CYP3A4 such as ketoconazole, itraconazole, and erythromycin and by those that inhibit the isoenzyme CYP2D6 such as fluoxetine and quinidine. Plasma concentrations may be reduced by enzyme inducers such as rifampicin, phenytoin, carbamazepine, and alcohol.

#### Pharmacokinetics

Donepezil hydrochloride is well absorbed from the gastrointestinal tract, maximum plasma concentrations being achieved within 3 to 4 hours. It is about 95% bound to plasma proteins. Donepezil undergoes partial metabolism via the cytochrome P450 system to 4 major metabolites. About 11% of a dose is present in plasma as 6-*O*-desmethyl donepezil, which has similar activity to the parent compound. Over 10 days, about 57% of a dose is recovered from the urine as unchanged drug and metabolites, and about 15% from the faeces; 28% remains unrecovered suggesting accumulation. The elimination half-life is about 70 hours. Steady-state concentrations are achieved within 3 weeks of the start of therapy.

◊ References.

1. Tiseo PJ, *et al.* Metabolism and elimination of $^{14}$C-donepezil in healthy volunteers: a single-dose study. *Br J Clin Pharmacol* 1998; **46** (suppl 1): 19–24.

### Uses and Administration

Donepezil hydrochloride, a piperidine derivative, is a reversible and specific inhibitor of acetylcholinesterase with actions similar to those of neostigmine (p.1493). It is highly selective for the CNS and is used for the symptomatic treatment of mild to moderately severe dementia in Alzheimer's disease (below). Donepezil hydrochloride is given in an initial dose of 5 mg by mouth once daily in the evening and increased if necessary after 4 to 6 weeks to a maximum of 10 mg once daily. Clinical benefit should be reassessed on a regular basis.

**Dementia.** Donepezil hydrochloride is used in the symptomatic treatment of mild to moderately severe dementia in *Alzheimer's disease* (see Dementia, p.1484). In individual trials, it appears to produce modest benefits in some patients.[1-3] These findings are also supported by a systematic review[4] which concluded that, for treatment periods of up to 1 year, donepezil produces modest improvements in cognitive function and global clinical state. Although there are no comparative studies of donepezil and tacrine it has been suggested[5-7] that donepezil may prove preferable as it appears to be better tolerated and hepatotoxicity has not been reported to be a problem (but see Adverse Effects, above). UK guidelines recommend that treatment with donepezil should be under specialist supervision, that benefit should be assessed 2 to 4 months after reaching maintenance dosage, and every 6 months thereafter, and treatment only continued if there is evidence of benefit.[8]

Benefit has also been reported in patients with more severe dementia.[4,9]

Donepezil may also be effective in the treatment of *vascular dementia*. Results from a randomised, controlled trial[10] have shown an improvement in cognition and global function in patients with probable or possible vascular dementia. A systematic review also concluded that donepezil improved mild to moderate vascular cognitive impairment in the short term.[11]


1. Rogers SL, *et al.* A 24-week, double-blind, placebo-controlled trial of donepezil in patients with Alzheimer's disease. *Neurology* 1998; **50:** 136–45.
2. Mohs RC, *et al.* A 1-year, placebo-controlled preservation of function survival study of donepezil in AD patients. *Neurology* 2001; **57:** 481–8.
3. Winblad B, *et al.* A 1-year, randomized, placebo-controlled study of donepezil in patients with mild to moderate AD. *Neurology* 2001; **57:** 489–95.
4. Birks JS, Harvey R. Donepezil for dementia due to Alzheimer's disease. Available in The Cochrane Library; Issue 2. Chichester: John Wiley; 2004.
5. American Psychiatric Association. Practice guideline for the treatment of patients with Alzheimer's disease and other dementias of late life. *Am J Psychiatry* 1997; **154** (suppl): 1–39.
6. Shintani EY, Uchida KM. Donepezil: an anticholinesterase inhibitor for Alzheimer's disease. *Am J Health-Syst Pharm* 1997; **54:** 2805–10.
7. Barner EL, Gray SL. Donepezil use in Alzheimer disease. *Ann Pharmacother* 1998; **32:** 70–7.
8. National Institute for Clinical Excellence. Guidance on the use of donepezil, rivastigmine, and galantamine for the treatment of Alzheimer's disease (issued January 2001). Available at: http://www.nice.org.uk/pdf/ALZHEIMER_full_guidance.pdf (accessed 15/06/04)
9. Feldman H, *et al.* A 24-week, randomized, double-blind study of donepezil in moderate to severe Alzheimer's disease. *Neurology* 2001; **57:** 613–20.
10. Black S, *et al.* Efficacy and tolerability of donepezil in vascular dementia: positive results of a 24-week, multicenter, international, randomized, placebo-controlled clinical trial. *Stroke* 2003; **34:** 2323–30.
11. Malouf R, Birks J. Donepezil for vascular cognitive impairment. Available in The Cochrane Library; Issue 2. Chichester: John Wiley; 2004.


### Preparations

**Proprietary Preparations** (details are given in Part 3)
***Arg.:*** Alzaimax; Cristaclar; Eranz; Onefin; Valpex; ***Austral.:*** Aricept; ***Austria:*** Aricept; ***Belg.:*** Aricept; ***Braz.:*** Eranz; ***Canad.:*** Aricept; ***Chile:*** Dozolin; Eranz; Evimal; ***Denm.:*** Aricept; ***Fin.:*** Aricept; ***Fr.:*** Aricept; ***Ger.:*** Aricept; ***Gr.:*** Aricept; ***Hong Kong:*** Aricept; ***Irl.:*** Aricept; ***Israel:*** Aricept; Asenta; ***Ital.:*** Aricept; Memac; ***Jpn:*** Aricept; ***Malaysia:*** Aricept; ***Mex.:*** Eranz; ***Norw.:*** Aricept; ***NZ:*** Aricept; ***Port.:*** Aricept; ***S.Afr.:*** Aricept; ***Singapore:*** Aricept; ***Spain:*** Aricept; ***Swed.:*** Aricept; ***Switz.:*** Aricept; ***Thai.:*** Aricept; ***UK:*** Aricept; ***USA:*** Aricept.

## Dyflos *(BAN)*

DFP; Difluorophate; Di-isopropyl Fluorophosphate; Di-isopropylfluorophosphonate; Fluostigmine; Isoflurofato; Isoflurophate. Di-isopropyl phosphorofluoridate.

$C_6H_{14}FO_3P$ = 184.1.
*CAS — 55-91-4.*
*ATC — S01EB07.*

**Pharmacopoeias.** In *US.*

**USP 27** (Isoflurophate). A clear, colourless, or faintly yellow liquid. Specific gravity about 1.05. Sparingly soluble in water; soluble in alcohol and in vegetable oils. It is decomposed by moisture with the evolution of hydrogen fluoride. Store at 8° to 15° in sealed containers.

**Handling.** The vapour of dyflos is very toxic. The eyes, nose, and mouth should be protected when handling dyflos, and contact with the skin should be avoided. Dyflos can be removed from the skin by washing with soap and water. Contaminated material should be immersed in a 2% aqueous solution of sodium hydroxide for several hours.

### Adverse Effects

As for Neostigmine, p.1492 and Ecothiopate Iodide, p.1490. For adverse effects of miotics, see also Pilocarpine, p.1495.

The anticholinesterase action of dyflos, and hence its adverse effects, may be prolonged. Its vapour is extremely irritating to the eye and mucous membranes.

Systemic toxicity also occurs after inhalation of the vapour. Prolonged use of dyflos in the eye may cause slowly reversible depigmentation of the lid margins in dark-skinned patients.

### Treatment of Adverse Effects

As for Ecothiopate Iodide, p.1490.

### Precautions

As for Neostigmine, p.1492 and Ecothiopate Iodide, p.1490. For precautions of miotics, see also Pilocarpine, p.1495.

### Interactions

As for Ecothiopate Iodide, p.1490.

### Pharmacokinetics

Dyflos is readily absorbed from the gastrointestinal tract, from skin and mucous membranes, and from the lungs. Dyflos interacts with cholinesterases producing stable phosphonylated and phosphorylated derivatives which are then hydrolysed and excreted mainly in the urine.

### Uses and Administration

Dyflos is an irreversible inhibitor of cholinesterases with actions similar to those of ecothiopate iodide (p.1490). Dyflos has a powerful miotic action which begins within 5 to 10 minutes and may persist for up to 4 weeks; it causes a reduction in intra-ocular pressure which is maximal in 24 hours and may persist for a week.

Dyflos has been used mainly in the treatment of open-angle glaucoma (p.1485), particularly in aphakic patients and when other drugs have proved inadequate. It was also employed in the diagnosis and management of accommodative convergent strabismus (p.1487).

Dyflos is applied locally usually as a 0.025% ophthalmic ointment.

### Preparations

***USP 27:*** Isoflurophate Ophthalmic Ointment.

## Ecothiopate Iodide *(BAN, rINN)*

Echothiophate Iodide; Ecostigmine Iodide; Ioduro de ecotiopato; MI-217. (2-Diethoxyphosphinylthioethyl)trimethylammonium iodide.

$C_9H_{23}INO_3PS$ = 383.2.
*CAS — 6736-03-4 (ecothiopate); 513-10-0 (ecothiopate iodide).*
*ATC — S01EB03.*

**Pharmacopoeias.** In *Jpn* and *US.*

**USP 27** (Echothiophate Iodide). A white, crystalline, hygroscopic solid having a slight mercaptan-like odour. Soluble 1 in 1 of water, 1 in 25 of dehydrated alcohol, and 1 in 3 of methyl alcohol; practically insoluble in other organic solvents. Its solutions in water have a pH of about 4. Store in airtight containers preferably at a temperature below 0°. Protect from light.

### Adverse Effects

As for Neostigmine, p.1492. For adverse effects of miotics, see also Pilocarpine, p.1495.

Ecothiopate is an irreversible cholinesterase inhibitor; its action, and hence its adverse effects, may be prolonged.

Plasma and erythrocyte cholinesterases may be diminished by treatment with eye drops of ecothiopate or other long-acting anticholinesterases, and systemic toxicity occurs more frequently than with shorter-acting miotics. Acute iritis, retinal detachment, or precipitation of acute glaucoma may occasionally occur, and iris cysts (especially in children) or lens opacities may develop on prolonged treatment.

### Treatment of Adverse Effects

In systemic poisoning, atropine sulfate may be given parenterally with pralidoxime chloride as for intoxication with organophosphorus insecticides (see p.1050); subconjunctival injection of pralidoxime has been employed to reverse severe ocular adverse effects. Supportive treatment, including assisted ventilation, should be given as necessary.

To prevent or reduce development of iris cysts in patients receiving ecothiopate eye drops, phenylephrine eye drops may be given simultaneously.

### Precautions

As for Neostigmine, p.1492. For precautions of miotics, see also under Pilocarpine, p.1495. In general ecothiopate, in common with other long-acting anticholinesterases, should be used only where therapy with other drugs has proved ineffective. Ecothiopate iodide should not be used in patients with iodine hypersensitivity.

### Interactions

As for Neostigmine, p.1492. The possibility of an interaction remains for a considerable time after stopping long-acting anticholinesterases such as ecothiopate.

### Uses and Administration

Ecothiopate is an irreversible inhibitor of cholinesterase with actions similar to those of neostigmine (p.1493), but much more prolonged. Its miotic action begins within 10 to 30 minutes of its application and may persist for 1 to 4 weeks; it causes a reduction in intra-ocular pressure which is maximal after 24 hours and may persist for days or weeks.

Ecothiopate iodide is used mainly in the treatment of open-angle glaucoma (p.1485), particularly in aphakic patients and when other drugs have proved inadequate. It is given as drops of a 0.03 to 0.25% solution. The manufacturers recommend 2 daily doses to allow for diurnal variations in intra-ocular pressure, although it has also been given once daily or on alternate days. It is advisable to give the single dose or one of the 2 daily doses at bedtime.

Ecothiopate iodide eye drops are also used in the diagnosis and management of accommodative convergent strabismus (p.1487).

### Preparations

***USP 27:*** Echothiophate Iodide for Ophthalmic Solution.

**Proprietary Preparations** (details are given in Part 3)
***Austral.:*** Phospholine Iodide; ***Canad.:*** Phospholine Iodide†; ***Fr.:*** Phospholine Iodide†; ***Israel:*** Phospholine Iodide†; ***UK:*** Phospholine Iodide†; ***USA:*** Phospholine Iodide.

## Edrophonium Chloride *(BAN, rINN)*

Cloruro de edrofonio; Edrophonii Chloridum. Ethyl(3-hydroxyphenyl)dimethylammonium chloride.

$C_{10}H_{16}ClNO$ = 201.7.
*CAS — 312-48-1 (edrophonium); 116-38-1 (edrophonium chloride).*

**Pharmacopoeias.** In *Eur.* (see p.vi), *Int., Jpn,* and *US.*

**Ph. Eur. 5.0** (Edrophonium Chloride). A white or almost white crystalline powder. Very soluble in water; freely soluble in alcohol; practically insoluble in dichloromethane. A 10% solution in water has a pH of 4.0 to 5.0. Protect from light.

**USP 27** (Edrophonium Chloride). A white odourless crystalline powder. Soluble 1 in 0.5 of water and 1 in 5 of alcohol; insoluble in chloroform and in ether. A 10% solution in water is practically colourless and the pH is between 4.0 and 5.0.

### Adverse Effects, Treatment, and Precautions

As for Neostigmine, p.1492.

### Interactions

As for Neostigmine, p.1492.

### Uses and Administration

Edrophonium is a quaternary ammonium compound that is a reversible inhibitor of cholinesterase activity. It has actions similar to those of neostigmine (p.1493) but its effect on skeletal muscle is claimed to be particularly prominent. Its action is rapid in onset and of short duration. In patients with myasthenia gravis, there is immediate subjective improvement and muscle strength increases. This effect usually lasts only for about 5 to 15 minutes, after which time the typical signs and symptoms return; because of its brief action the drug is not suitable for the routine treatment of myasthenia gravis.

Edrophonium chloride is used in **myasthenia gravis** (p.1486) both diagnostically and to distinguish between under- or over-treatment with other anticholinesterases.

- The usual *diagnostic procedure* is to inject 2 mg intravenously and, if no adverse reaction occurs within 30 to 45 seconds, to continue with the injection of a further 8 mg. In the UK the recommended total dose for children is 100 micrograms/kg, one-fifth of the dose being given initially, followed 30 seconds later by the remainder if no adverse effects develop. In the USA the manufacturers recommend a total dose of 5 mg for children weighing less than 34 kg and 10 mg for heavier children with one-fifth of the dose being given initially followed by increments of 1 mg every 30 to 45 seconds; the recommended total dose for infants is 0.5 mg.

  When intravenous injection is difficult edrophonium chloride may be given by intramuscular injection; the usual dose in adults is 10 mg while children below 34 kg in weight may be given 2 mg and heavier children 5 mg; a suggested dose for infants is 0.5 to 1 mg given intramuscularly or subcutaneously. Atropine should always be available when the test is carried out in order to treat any severe muscarinic reactions that may occur.
- To *detect under- or over-treatment*, test doses of 1 to 2 mg of edrophonium chloride are given intravenously to distinguish severe symptoms of myasthenia gravis due to inadequate therapy from the effects of overdosage with anticholinesterase drugs. If treatment has been inadequate, edrophonium chloride will produce an immediate amelioration of symptoms, whereas in cholinergic crises due to over-treatment the symptoms will be temporarily aggravated. The manufacturers suggest testing one hour after the last dose of treatment but the *British National Formulary* recommends testing just before the next dose is due. Testing should only be undertaken when facilities for endotracheal intubation and controlled ventilation are immediately available.

Edrophonium chloride was originally introduced for the **reversal of neuromuscular blockade** in anaesthesia. In the UK, the recommended dose for the reversal of the effects of competitive neuromuscular blockers is 500 to 700 micrograms/kg given by intravenous injection over several minutes either with or after atropine sulfate 600 micrograms; in the USA a dose of 10 mg of edrophonium chloride is given over 30 to 45 seconds and repeated as required up to a maximum of 40 mg. The brevity of its action limits its value. Where prolonged apnoea occurs in a patient treated with a depolarising neuromuscular blocker, such as suxamethonium, edrophonium 10 mg may be given intravenously with atropine to determine the presence of phase II block (see p.1408).

Edrophonium bromide has been used similarly to edrophonium chloride.

**Reversal of neuromuscular blockade.** For a discussion of whether edrophonium might be more suitable than neostigmine for reversal of residual block after the use of the shorter-acting competitive neuromuscular blockers, see under Uses and Administration of Neostigmine, p.1493.

**Snake bite.** For the use of anticholinesterases in the treatment of snake bite, see under Uses and Administration of Neostigmine, p.1493.

**Tetrodotoxin poisoning.** Management of poisoning due to tetrodotoxin, a heat stable neuromuscular blocking toxin found in various marine animals, such as puffer fish, is mainly symptomatic and supportive. Reports[1,2] on the effectiveness of intravenous anticholinesterases such as edrophonium or neostigmine in reversing muscle weakness in tetrodotoxin poisoning have been conflicting. Although it appears that anticholinesterases may only be effective during partial block produced by tetrodotoxin, some consider[3] that, as there is no specific antidote, any measure that brings about improvement may be tried.

1. Chew SK, *et al.* Anticholinesterase drugs in the treatment of tetrodotoxin poisoning. *Lancet* 1984; **ii:** 108.
2. Tibballs J. Severe tetrodotoxic fish poisoning. *Anaesth Intensive Care* 1988; **16:** 215–17.
3. Karalliedde L. Management of puffer fish poisoning. *Br J Anaesth* 1995; **75:** 500.

## Preparations

***BP 2003:*** Edrophonium Injection;
***USP 27:*** Edrophonium Chloride Injection.

**Proprietary Preparations** (details are given in Part 3)
***Canad.:*** Enlon; Tensilon†; ***S.Afr.:*** Tensilon†; ***Spain:*** Anticude; ***USA:*** Enlon; Enlon-Plus; Reversol; Tensilon.

## Eptastigmine *(rINN)*

*N*-Demethyl-*N*-heptylphysostigmine; Eptastigmina. (3a*S*,8a*R*)-1,2,3,3a,8,8a-Hexahydro-1,3a,8-trimethylpyrrolo[2,3-*b*]indol-5-yl heptylcarbamate.

$C_{21}H_{33}N_3O_2$ = 359.5.
*CAS — 101246-68-8.*

### Profile

Eptastigmine is a long-acting inhibitor of cholinesterase activity; it is a lipophilic derivative of physostigmine (p.1494). It has been studied in the oral treatment of Alzheimer's disease (see Dementia, p.1484) but development was stopped after reports of aplastic anaemia.

## Eseridine Salicylate *(rINNM)*

Eserine Aminoxide Salicylate; Eserine Oxide Salicylate; Physostigmine Aminoxide Salicylate; Physostigmine *N*-Oxide Salicylate; Salicilato de eseridina. (4a*S*,9a*S*)-2,3,4,4a,9,9a-Hexahydro-2,4a,9-trimethyl-1,2-oxazino[6,5-*b*]indol-6-ylmethylcarbamate salicylate.

$C_{15}H_{21}N_3O_3,C_7H_6O_3$ = 429.5.
*CAS — 25573-43-7 (eseridine); 5995-96-0 (eseridine salicylate).*

### Profile

Eseridine salicylate, a derivative of physostigmine, is an inhibitor of cholinesterase activity that has been given by mouth in preparations for dyspepsia and other gastric disorders.

### Preparations

**Proprietary Preparations** (details are given in Part 3)
***Fr.:*** Geneserine.

## Fampridine *(USAN, rINN)*

EL-970; Fampridina. 4-Aminopyridine; 4-Pyridinamine.

$C_5H_6N_2$ = 94.11.
*CAS — 504-24-5.*

### Profile

Fampridine enhances the release of acetylcholine from nerve terminals and has been used intravenously to reverse the effects of competitive neuromuscular blockers. It has also been tried by mouth and intravenously in the management of a number of neurological disorders including Eaton-Lambert myasthenic syndrome (p.1485), multiple sclerosis (p.646), spinal cord injury, and Alzheimer's disease (see Dementia, p.1484), and for the reversal of neuromuscular blockade in patients with botulism (p.1611).

Fampridine has also been considered as a specific antidote in poisoning with calcium-channel blockers such as verapamil (p.1019).

Adverse effects, especially seizures, may limit its use.

◊ References.

1. Ter Wee PM, *et al.* 4-Aminopyridine and haemodialysis in the treatment of verapamil intoxication. *Hum Toxicol* 1985; **4:** 327–9.
2. Davidson M, *et al.* 4-Aminopyridine in the treatment of Alzheimer's disease. *Biol Psychiatry* 1988; **23:** 485–90.
3. Hansebout RR, *et al.* 4-Aminopyridine in chronic spinal cord injury: a controlled, double-blind, crossover study in eight patients. *J Neurotrauma* 1993; **10:** 1–18.

**Multiple sclerosis.** Fampridine has potassium-channel blocking activity and has been tried in the treatment of multiple sclerosis to improve conduction in demyelinated fibres. Improvements have been reported in walking, dexterity, and vision, but only small numbers of patients have been studied. A systematic review[1] was unable to come to a conclusion about its safety and efficacy, noting that publication bias posed a problem in this area.

1. Solari A, *et al.* Aminopyridines for symptomatic treatment in multiple sclerosis. Available in The Cochrane Library; Issue 2. Chichester: John Wiley; 2004.

# Galantamine Hydrobromide

*(BANM, USAN, rINNM)*

Galanthamine Hydrobromide; Galanthamini Hydrobromidum; Hidrobromuro de galantamina. (4a*S*,6*R*,8a*S*)-4a,5,9,10,11,12-Hexahydro-3-methoxy-11-methyl-6*H*-benzofuro[3a,3,2-*ef*][2]benzazepin-6-ol hydrobromide.

$C_{17}H_{21}NO_3,HBr$ = 368.3.
*CAS — 357-70-0 (galantamine); 1953-04-4 (galantamine hydrobromide).*
*ATC — N06DA04.*

**Description.** The hydrobromide of galantamine, an alkaloid which has been obtained from the Caucasian snowdrop (Voronov's snowdrop), *Galanthus woronowii* (Amaryllidaceae), and related species.

**Pharmacopoeias.** In *Chin.*

## Adverse Effects, Treatment, and Precautions

As for Donepezil, p.1489. Galantamine is contra-indicated in patients with severe renal or severe hepatic impairment; also it should not be given to patients with both significant hepatic and renal impairment. For details regarding dose adjustments in moderate hepatic impairment, see under Uses and Administration, below. Patients with galactose intolerance, the Lapp lactase deficiency, or glucose-galactose malabsorption should not take galantamine.

## Interactions

As for Neostigmine, p.1492. The bioavailability of galantamine may be increased by drugs that inhibit the cytochrome P450 isoenzyme CYP2D6, such as quinidine, fluoxetine, fluvoxamine, and paroxetine, and by those that inhibit the isoenzyme CYP3A4, such as ketoconazole and ritonavir. Dose reduction of galantamine may be required when given with such drugs.

## Pharmacokinetics

Galantamine is absorbed from the gastrointestinal tract; maximum concentrations are reached in about 1 hour. The presence of food delays the rate of absorption and reduces maximum concentrations although the extent of absorption is not affected. Protein binding is low. Galantamine is partially metabolised by the cytochrome P450 isoenzymes CYP2D6 and CYP3A4; a number of active metabolites are formed. The elimination half-life is about 7 to 8 hours. After 7 days, the majority of a single oral dose is recovered in the urine with up to about 6% detected in the faeces. Clearance is reported to be 20% lower in females than in males.

## Uses and Administration

Galantamine hydrobromide is a reversible inhibitor of acetylcholinesterase activity, with actions similar to those of neostigmine (p.1493). It also has an intrinsic action on nicotinic receptors. It is used in the symptomatic treatment of mild to moderately severe dementia in Alzheimer's disease (below).

Galantamine is given as the hydrobromide although doses are expressed in terms of the base; 5.1 mg of galantamine hydrobromide is approximately equivalent to 4 mg of galantamine base. An initial dose of 4 mg is given twice daily with food for four weeks, then increased to 8 mg twice daily. This dose should be maintained for at least four weeks; thereafter, according to individual patient response and tolerability, the dose may be further increased to 12 mg twice daily. The clinical benefit of galantamine should be reassessed on a regular basis. Reductions in dose may be necessary in patients with hepatic impairment (see below) or in those also taking certain cytochrome P450 isoenzyme inhibitors (see Interactions, above).

Galantamine hydrobromide has also been used in various neuromuscular disorders, and to curtail the muscle relaxation produced by competitive neuromuscular blockers.

**Administration in hepatic impairment.** No dose adjustment is necessary in mild hepatic impairment. Patients with moderate impairment should begin with a dose of 4 mg once daily, preferably taken in the morning, for at least one week; thereafter the dose may be increased to 4 mg twice daily for at least 4 weeks, with subsequent increases up to a maximum of 8 mg twice daily. Galantamine is contra-indicated in severe hepatic impairment.

**Dementia.** Reviews[1-3] suggest that galantamine is of benefit in patients with mild to moderate symptoms of *Alzheimer's disease* (see Dementia, p.1484); evidence in more severely impaired subjects is lacking. In the UK, guidelines recommend the use of galantamine in such patients under specialist supervision, with benefits assessed 2 to 4 months after achieving maintenance dosage, and every 6 months thereafter; treatment should only continue where there is evidence of benefit.[4]

Galantamine may also be effective in the treatment of *vascular dementia.* Results from a randomised, controlled trial[5] have shown a trend towards improved cognition in patients with probable vascular dementia, although patients numbers were too small for this to be significant.

1. Scott LJ, Goa KL. Galantamine: a review of its use in Alzheimer's disease. *Drugs* 2000; **60:** 1095–1122.

2. Olin J, Schneider L. Galantamine for dementia due to Alzheimer's disease. Available in The Cochrane Library; Issue 2. Chichester: John Wiley; 2004.
3. Pearson VE. Galantamine: a new Alzheimer drug with a past life. *Ann Pharmacother* 2001; **35:** 1406–13.
4. National Institute for Clinical Excellence. Guidance on the use of donepezil, rivastigmine and galantamine for the treatment of Alzheimer's disease (issued January 2001). Available at: http://www.nice.org.uk/pdf/ALZHEIMER_full_guidance.pdf (accessed 15/06/04)
5. Erkinjuntti T, *et al.* Efficacy of galantamine in probable vascular dementia and Alzheimer's disease combined with cerebrovascular disease: a randomised trial. *Lancet* 2002; **359:** 1283–90.

## Preparations

**Proprietary Preparations** (details are given in Part 3)
***Arg.:*** Numencial; Reminyl; ***Austral.:*** Reminyl; ***Austria:*** Nivalin†; Reminyl; ***Belg.:*** Reminyl; ***Braz.:*** Reminyl; Trezor†; ***Canad.:*** Reminyl; ***Denm.:*** Reminyl; ***Fin.:*** Reminyl; ***Fr.:*** Reminyl; ***Ger.:*** Reminyl; ***Gr.:*** Reminyl; ***Irl.:*** Reminyl; ***Ital.:*** Reminyl; ***Norw.:*** Reminyl; ***NZ:*** Reminyl; ***S.Afr.:*** Reminyl; ***Singapore:*** Reminyl; ***Spain:*** Reminyl; ***Swed.:*** Reminyl; ***Switz.:*** Reminyl; ***Thai.:*** Reminyl; ***UK:*** Reminyl; ***USA:*** Reminyl.

## Guanidine Hydrochloride

Carbamidine Hydrochloride; Guanidina, hidrocloruro de; Iminourea Hydrochloride.

$CH_5N_3,HCl$ = 95.53.

*CAS — 113-00-8 (guanidine); 50-01-1 (guanidine hydrochloride).*

### Profile

Guanidine hydrochloride enhances the release of acetylcholine from nerve terminals. It has been given by mouth to reverse neuromuscular blockade in patients with botulism (p.1611), but its efficacy has not been established. Guanidine hydrochloride has also been tried in Eaton-Lambert myasthenic syndrome (p.1485) and other neurological disorders, but its use has been associated with bone-marrow suppression in some patients.

◊ References.

1. Kaplan JE, *et al.* Botulism, type A, and treatment with guanidine. *Ann Neurol* 1979; **6:** 69–71.
2. Critchley EMR, *et al.* Outbreak of botulism in North West England and Wales. *Lancet* 1989; **ii:** 849–53.
3. Neal KR, Dunbar EM. Improvement in bulbar weakness with guanoxan in type B botulism. *Lancet* 1990; **335:** 1286–7.
4. Oh SJ, *et al.* Low-dose guanidine and pyridostigmine: relatively safe and effective long-term symptomatic therapy in Lambert-Eaton myasthenic syndrome. *Muscle Nerve* 1997; **20:** 1146–52.

## Methacholine Chloride *(BAN, rINN)*

Acetyl-β-methylcholine Chloride; Amechol Chloride; Cloruro de metacolina; Methacholinium Chloratum. (2-Acetoxypropyl)trimethylammonium chloride.

$C_8H_{18}ClNO_2$ = 195.7.

*CAS — 55-92-5 (methacholine); 62-51-1 (methacholine chloride).*

**Pharmacopoeias.** In *Fr., Swiss,* and *US.*

**USP 27** (Methacholine Chloride). Colourless or white crystals, or a white crystalline powder. It is odourless or has a slight odour, and is very hygroscopic. Soluble 1 in 1.2 of water, 1 in 1.7 of alcohol, and 1 in 2.1 of chloroform. Its solutions are neutral to litmus. Store in airtight containers.

### Adverse Effects and Treatment

As for Acetylcholine Chloride, p.1487. Severe adverse cholinergic effects have followed the oral and parenteral use of methacholine and these routes are no longer used.

### Precautions

As for Neostigmine, p.1492.

Methacholine has the potential to produce severe bronchoconstriction and it should not be used for inhalation challenge tests in patients with clinically apparent asthma, wheezing, or poor pulmonary function.

Methacholine should not be given orally or parenterally.

### Interactions

As for Neostigmine, p.1492. Methacholine is slowly hydrolysed by acetylcholinesterase, and its effects are markedly enhanced if used after anticholinesterases.

### Uses and Administration

Methacholine is a quaternary ammonium parasympathomimetic with the muscarinic actions of acetylcholine (p.1487). It is hydrolysed by acetylcholinesterase at a considerably slower rate than acetylcholine and is more resistant to hydrolysis by non-specific cholinesterases so that its actions are more prolonged.

Inhalation of nebulised solutions of methacholine chloride are used to provoke bronchoconstriction in the diagnosis of bronchial airway hypersensitivity (but see Precautions, above).

Methacholine chloride has been used in eye drops as a miotic.

## Preparations

**Proprietary Preparations** (details are given in Part 3)
***Canad.:*** Provocholine; ***Ger.:*** Provokit; ***USA:*** Mecholyl; Provocholine.
**Multi-ingredient:** ***Braz.:*** Frixodont†; Pomalgex†.

## Neostigmine *(BAN)*

Neostigmina. 3-(Dimethylcarbamoyloxy)trimethylanilinium ion.

$C_{12}H_{19}N_2O_2$ = 223.3.

*CAS — 59-99-4.*

*ATC — N07AA01; S01EB06.*

## Neostigmine Bromide *(BANM, pINN)*

Bromuro de neostigmina; Neostig. Brom.; Neostigmini Bromidum; Neostigminii Bromidum; Neostigminum Bromatum; Synstigminium Bromatum.

$C_{12}H_{19}BrN_2O_2$ = 303.2.

*CAS — 114-80-7.*

*ATC — N07AA01; S01EB06.*

**Pharmacopoeias.** In *Chin., Eur.* (see p.vi), *Int.,* and *US.*

**Ph. Eur. 5.0** (Neostigmine Bromide). Hygroscopic, colourless crystals or a white crystalline powder. Very soluble in water; freely soluble in alcohol. Protect from light.

**USP 27** (Neostigmine Bromide). Store in airtight containers.

**Stability.** References.

1. Porst H, Kny L. Kinetics of the degradation of neostigmine bromide in aqueous solution. *Pharmazie* 1985; **40:** 713–17.

## Neostigmine Metilsulfate

Neostig. Methylsulph.; Neostigmina, metilsulfato de; Neostigmine Methylsulfate; Neostigmine Methylsulphate *(BANM)*; Neostigmini Metilsulfas; Proserinum.

$C_{13}H_{22}N_2O_6S$ = 334.4.

*CAS — 51-60-5.*

*ATC — N07AA01; S01EB06.*

**Pharmacopoeias.** In *Chin., Eur.* (see p.vi), *Int., Jpn, Pol.,* and *US.*

**Ph. Eur. 5.0** (Neostigmine Metilsulfate). Hygroscopic, colourless crystals or a white crystalline powder. Very soluble in water; freely soluble in alcohol. Store in airtight containers. Protect from light.

**USP 27** (Neostigmine Methylsulfate). Store in airtight containers.

### Adverse Effects

The side-effects of neostigmine are chiefly due to excessive cholinergic stimulation and most commonly include increased salivation, nausea and vomiting, abdominal cramps, and diarrhoea. Allergic reactions have been reported; rashes have been associated with the use of the bromide salt. Neostigmine penetrates the blood-brain barrier poorly and CNS effects are usually only seen with high doses.

Overdosage may lead to a 'cholinergic crisis', characterised by both muscarinic and nicotinic effects. These effects may include excessive sweating, lachrymation, increased peristalsis, involuntary defaecation and urination or desire to urinate, miosis, ciliary spasm, nystagmus, bradycardia and other arrhythmias, hypotension, muscle cramps, fasciculations, weakness and paralysis, tight chest, wheezing, and increased bronchial secretion combined with bronchoconstriction. CNS effects include ataxia, convulsions, coma, slurred speech, restlessness, agitation, and fear. Death may result from respiratory failure, due to a combination of the muscarinic, nicotinic and central effects, or cardiac arrest.

It has been reported that a paradoxical increase in blood pressure and heart rate may result from nicotinic stimulation of sympathetic ganglia, especially where atropine has been given to reverse the muscarinic effects (see under Treatment of Adverse Effects, below).

In patients with myasthenia gravis, in whom other symptoms of overdosage may be mild or absent, the major symptom of cholinergic crisis is increased muscular weakness, which must be differentiated from the muscular weakness caused by an exacerbation of the disease itself (myasthenic crisis).

The adverse effects of parasympathomimetics applied topically for their miotic action are discussed under Pilocarpine on p.1495.

### Treatment of Adverse Effects

If a life-threatening amount of neostigmine has been taken by mouth and the patient presents within 1 hour, the stomach may be emptied by lavage; giving activated charcoal to decrease absorption should also be considered. When necessary maintenance of respiration should take priority. Atropine sulfate should be given in usual doses of 1 to 2 mg, preferably intravenously, or else intramuscularly and repeated as necessary to control the muscarinic effects; doses of up to 4 mg have been suggested. Nicotinic effects, including muscle weakness and paralysis, are not antagonised by atropine; small doses of a competitive neuromuscular blocker have been suggested for the control of muscle twitching. Use of the cholinesterase reactivator pralidoxime as an adjunct to atropine has also been suggested (see p.1050). Further supportive treatment should be given as required.

### Precautions

Neostigmine is contra-indicated in patients with mechanical intestinal or urinary-tract obstruction, or peritonitis. It should be used with extreme caution in patients who have undergone recent intestinal or bladder surgery and in patients with bronchial asthma. It should be used with caution in patients with cardiovascular disorders including arrhythmias, bradycardia, recent myocardial infarction, and hypotension, as well as in patients with vagotonia, epilepsy, hyperthyroidism, parkinsonism, renal impairment, or peptic ulcer disease. When neostigmine is given by injection, atropine should always be available to counteract any excessive muscarinic reactions; atropine may also be given before, or with, neostigmine to prevent or minimise muscarinic side-effects but this may mask the initial symptoms of overdosage and lead to cholinergic crisis.

The UK manufacturer has advised that as the severity of myasthenia gravis often fluctuates considerably during pregnancy, particular care is needed to avoid cholinergic crisis caused by overdosage; it has also been reported that neonatal myasthenia may follow large doses during pregnancy. The amount of neostigmine distributed into breast milk is very small but breast-fed infants need to be monitored.

Large doses of neostigmine by mouth should be avoided in conditions where there may be increased absorption from the gastrointestinal tract. It should be avoided in patients known to be hypersensitive to neostigmine; the bromide ion from neostigmine bromide may contribute to the allergic reaction.

The precautions of parasympathomimetics applied topically for their miotic action are discussed under Pilocarpine on p.1495.

**Neuromuscular disorders.** Residual non-depolarising neuromuscular block in a patient with dystrophia myotonica was only partly reversed by neostigmine and atropine, and following a second dose of both drugs complete neuromuscular block developed.[1] In a second patient, with a history of progressive muscle dystrophy, the use of neostigmine to reverse residual non-depolarising blockade gave rise to a tonic response in the indirectly stimulated muscle. The type and degree of the response to neostigmine, and probably other anticholinesterases, cannot be predicted in patients with neuromuscular disease.

A patient with sero-negative ocular myasthenia gravis had exaggerated responses to both vecuronium and neostigmine.[2] The dose of neuromuscular blockers and their antagonists used in patients with myasthenia gravis should be titrated carefully regardless of the severity of the condition.

1. Buzello W, *et al.* Hazards of neostigmine in patients with neuromuscular disorders: report of two cases. *Br J Anaesth* 1982; **54:** 529–34.
2. Kim J-M, Mangold J. Sensitivity to both vecuronium and neostigmine in a sero-negative myasthenic patient. *Br J Anaesth* 1989; **63:** 497–500.

### Interactions

Drugs with neuromuscular blocking activity, such as the aminoglycosides, clindamycin, colistin, cyclopropane, and the halogenated inhalational anaesthetics, may antagonise the effects of neostigmine. A number of drugs, including quinine, chloroquine, hydroxychloroquine, quinidine, procainamide, propafenone, lithium, and the beta blockers, that have the potential to aggravate myasthenia gravis can reduce the effectiveness of treatment with parasympathomimetics. Prolonged bradycardia has also occurred in patients receiving beta blockers when given neostigmine. Anticholinesterases, such as neostigmine, can inhibit the metabolism of suxamethonium and enhance and prolong its action.

Ophthalmic use of anticholinesterases, such as ecothiopate, should be undertaken with care in patients receiving neostigmine systemically for myasthenia gravis, because of possible additive toxicity.

Antimuscarinics such as atropine antagonise the muscarinic effects of neostigmine.

**Beta blockers.** There have been several reports of bradycardia and hypotension when neostigmine or physostigmine were given to patients receiving beta blockers[1-4] but no significant changes in heart rate were noted in a study of pyridostigmine given to 8 patients taking beta blockers.[5] Beta blockers have the potential to aggravate the symptoms of myasthenia gravis and may therefore reduce the effectiveness of parasympathomimetic treatment.

1. Sprague DH. Severe bradycardia after neostigmine in a patient taking propranolol to control paroxysmal atrial tachycardia. *Anesthesiology* 1975; **42:** 208–10.
2. Seidl DC, Martin DE. Prolonged bradycardia after neostigmine administration in a patient taking nadolol. *Anesth Analg* 1984; **63:** 365–7.
3. Baraka A, Dajani A. Severe bradycardia following physostigmine in the presence of beta-adrenergic blockade: a case report. *Middle East J Anesthesiol* 1984; **7:** 291–3.
4. Eldor J, *et al.* Prolonged bradycardia and hypotension after neostigmine administration in a patient receiving atenolol. *Anaesthesia* 1987; **42:** 1294–7.
5. Arad M, *et al.* Safety of pyridostigmine in hypertensive patients receiving beta blockers. *Am J Cardiol* 1992; **69:** 518–22.

**Calcium-channel blockers.** Use of calcium-channel blockers such as verapamil with neuromuscular blockers may produce an enhanced muscle block which is resistant to reversal with neostigmine[1] but which can be reversed by edrophonium.[2]

1. van Poorten JF, *et al.* Verapamil and reversal of vecuronium neuromuscular blockade. *Anesth Analg* 1984; **63:** 155–7.
2. Jones RM, *et al.* Verapamil potentiation of neuromuscular blockade: failure of reversal with neostigmine but prompt reversal with edrophonium. *Anesth Analg* 1985; **64:** 1021–5.

**Corticosteroids.** Although use of glucocorticoids alone may improve strength in myasthenic patients, use of methylprednisolone in patients receiving neostigmine or pyridostigmine has exacerbated symptoms and produced profound weakness needing assisted ventilation.[1] Since the adverse effects of combined therapy usually occur before any expected benefits it has been suggested that the glucocorticoid should be given on alternate days in small doses which are increased gradually until the optimal effect is achieved.[2]

1. Brunner NG, *et al.* Corticosteroids in management of severe, generalized myasthenia gravis: effectiveness and comparison with corticotrophin therapy. *Neurology* 1972; **22:** 603–10.
2. Jubiz W, Meikle AW. Alterations of glucocorticoid actions by other drugs and disease states. *Drugs* 1979; **18:** 113–21.

## Pharmacokinetics

Neostigmine is a quaternary ammonium compound and, as the bromide, is poorly absorbed from the gastrointestinal tract. After parenteral doses as the metilsulfate, neostigmine is rapidly eliminated and is excreted in the urine both as unchanged drug and metabolites. Neostigmine undergoes hydrolysis by cholinesterases and is also metabolised in the liver. Protein binding to human serum albumin is reported to range from 15 to 25%. Penetration into the CNS is poor. Neostigmine crosses the placenta and very small amounts are distributed into breast milk.

◊ Neostigmine appears to be poorly and variably absorbed when given by mouth. In 3 myasthenic patients peak plasma concentrations were obtained 1 to 2 hours after a single 30-mg dose by mouth and the mean plasma half-life was 0.87 hours; bioavailability was estimated to be 1 to 2%.[1] Mean plasma half-lives of 0.89 and 1.20 hours have been obtained following intravenous[1] and intramuscular[2] injections of neostigmine metilsulfate respectively, although again only a few patients were studied. Metabolism and biliary excretion may play significant roles in the elimination of neostigmine.[2] About 80% of a dose may be excreted in the urine within 24 hours: about 50% of a dose as unchanged drug and 15% as 3-hydroxyphenyltrimethylammonium.[2] Mean plasma elimination half-lives for neostigmine have been found to be shorter in infants (0.65 hours) and children (0.80 hours) compared with adults (1.12 hours) but this does not appear to be related to its duration of effect in antagonising neuromuscular blockade.[3] For the half-life in anephric patients, see Administration in Renal Impairment, below.

1. Aquilonius S-M, *et al.* A pharmacokinetic study of neostigmine in man using gas chromatography–mass spectrometry. *Eur J Clin Pharmacol* 1979; **15:** 367–71.
2. Somani SM, *et al.* Kinetics and metabolism of intramuscular neostigmine in myasthenia gravis. *Clin Pharmacol Ther* 1980; **28:** 64–8.
3. Fisher DM, *et al.* The neuromuscular pharmacology of neostigmine in infants and children. *Anesthesiology* 1983; **59:** 220–5.

## Uses and Administration

Neostigmine is a quaternary ammonium compound that inhibits cholinesterase activity and thus prolongs and intensifies the physiological actions of acetylcholine (p.1487). It probably also has direct effects on skeletal muscle fibres. The anticholinesterase actions of neostigmine are reversible.

Neostigmine is used in the treatment of myasthenia gravis, and has been used as an alternative to edrophonium in the diagnosis of myasthenia gravis (p.1486). It is used in anaesthesia to reverse the neuromuscular blockade produced by competitive neuromuscular blockers (see below). It is also used in the management of paralytic ileus. Neostigmine has been used in the management of postoperative urinary retention (p.476) but has generally been superseded by catheterisation. It is sometimes used to lower intra-ocular pressure in the management of glaucoma (p.1485) and to reduce rises in intra-ocular pressure associated with ophthalmic surgery, although other parasympathomimetics are usually used when such miotics are required.

Neostigmine is given as the bromide and as the metilsulfate. Neostigmine bromide is given by mouth and has been used topically as eye drops; the metilsulfate is given by intramuscular, intravenous, or subcutaneous injection.

The manufacturers state that 0.5 mg of neostigmine metilsulfate by intravenous injection is approximately equivalent in effect to 1 to 1.5 mg of neostigmine metilsulfate by intramuscular or subcutaneous injection, or 15 mg of neostigmine bromide by mouth.

In the treatment of **myasthenia gravis**, neostigmine bromide is given by mouth in a total daily dose usually between 75 and 300 mg, divided throughout the day, and if necessary the night, according to individual response; larger portions of the total dose may be given at times of greater fatigue. The maximum daily dose that most patients can tolerate is 180 mg. A usual total daily dose in children is 15 to 90 mg by mouth. In patients in whom oral therapy is impractical neostigmine metilsulfate may be given in doses of 0.5 to 2.5 mg by intramuscular or subcutaneous injection at intervals, giving a total daily dose usually in the range 5 to 20 mg. Single doses in children have ranged from 200 to 500 micrograms.

In the treatment of neonatal myasthenia gravis doses in the range 50 to 250 micrograms of the metilsulfate by intramuscular or subcutaneous injection, or 1 to 5 mg of the bromide by mouth, have been given usually every 4 hours; treatment is rarely needed beyond 8 weeks of age.

To **reverse neuromuscular blockade** produced by competitive neuromuscular blockers, the usual adult dose in the UK is 50 to 70 micrograms/kg given by intravenous injection over a period of 60 seconds; in the USA lower doses of 0.5 to 2 mg are used. Additional neostigmine may be given until the muscle power is normal but a total of 5 mg should not be exceeded. The patient should be well ventilated until complete recovery of normal respiration is assured. To counteract any muscarinic effects 0.6 to 1.2 mg of atropine sulfate is given by intravenous injection with or before the dose of neostigmine; it has been suggested that in the presence of bradycardia atropine sulfate should be given several minutes before neostigmine. Glycopyrronium bromide has been used as an alternative to atropine sulfate.

In the treatment of paralytic **ileus** and postoperative **urinary retention**, doses of 15 to 30 mg of the bromide by mouth, or more usually 0.5 mg of the metilsulfate by subcutaneous or intramuscular injection, have been used.

**Administration in renal impairment.** The dosage of neostigmine may need to be adjusted in patients with renal impairment. The mean serum elimination half-life of 79.8 minutes obtained in patients with normal renal function was found to be prolonged to 181.1 minutes in anephric patients.[1]

1. Cronnelly R, *et al.* Renal function and the pharmacokinetics of neostigmine in anesthetized man. *Anesthesiology* 1979; **51:** 222–6.

**Decreased gastrointestinal motility.** Parasympathomimetics enhance gastric contractions and increase intestinal motility and have been used in conditions associated with decreased gastrointestinal motility (p.1241). Good results have been reported with intravenous neostigmine in the treatment of acute colonic pseudo-obstruction,[1,2] a condition that appears to be due to parasympathomimetic dysfunction. These results have been confirmed in a randomised double-blind study.[3] It has therefore been suggested that parasympathomimetics should be tried before colonic decompression or surgery when conservative management has failed or a rapid resolution is required.[3] Neostigmine has also been used in the treatment of severe constipation due to disrupted intestinal motility.[4,5]

1. Hutchinson R, Griffiths C. Acute colonic pseudo-obstruction: a pharmacological approach. *Ann R Coll Surg Engl* 1992; **74:** 364–7.
2. Stephenson BM, *et al.* Parasympathomimetic decompression of acute colonic pseudo-obstruction. *Lancet* 1993; **342:** 1181–2.
3. Ponec RJ, *et al.* Neostigmine for the treatment of acute colonic pseudo-obstruction. *N Engl J Med* 1999; **341:** 137–41.
4. Miller LS. Neostigmine for severe constipation with spinal cord lesions. *Ann Intern Med* 1984; **101:** 279.
5. Thurtle OA, *et al.* Intractable constipation in malignant phaeochromocytoma: combined treatment with adrenergic blockade and cholinergic drugs. *J R Soc Med* 1984; **77:** 327–8.

**Reversal of neuromuscular blockade.** Anticholinesterases have often been used after surgery to antagonise residual neuromuscular block induced by long-acting competitive neuromuscular blockers. However, there has been continuing debate[1-3] on whether anticholinesterases can be used in reduced doses or even omitted for intermediate-acting blockers such as atracurium and vecuronium and shorter-acting blockers such as mivacurium.

Decreasing the anticholinesterase dose may reduce adverse effects. Although it is not clear whether omitting neostigmine reversal reduces nausea and vomiting,[3,4] it avoids any adverse effects neostigmine may have on gut anastomoses. One commentator[1] considered that the wide variation in recovery time with aminosteroid blockers such as rocuronium was an indication for always using at least a small dose of anticholinesterase when these drugs were used. However, it was suggested that, if the block was being carefully monitored and recovery was established, a reduced dose of 1.25 mg of neostigmine might be preferable following a benzylisoquinolinium blocker such as atracurium or mivacurium. In children, smaller doses of an anticholinesterase could be used, even after an aminosteroid blocker, and after a blocker such as mivacurium, they might not be needed at all.

Others have preferred to reserve neostigmine reversal for cases where it was deemed clinically necessary: in a study[4] employing such a protocol, 68% of those receiving rocuronium were given neostigmine, against 10% of those receiving mivacurium.

It has been suggested that because of its shorter duration of action edrophonium might be more suitable than neostigmine to antagonise residual block for neuromuscular blockers with shorter actions and in particular, that edrophonium might be more appropriate than neostigmine for use with mivacurium. Neostigmine inhibits the plasma cholinesterase responsible for the metabolism of mivacurium and its use can in theory delay rather than speed recovery, although in practice there is considered to be little evidence for such an effect.[1] Edrophonium also has lesser effects on the vagus, a more rapid onset of action, and may be associated with a lower incidence of nausea and vomiting than neostigmine.[5] Neostigmine can cause clinically significant neuromuscular blockade if it is given to a patient who has already recovered a large degree of neuromuscular function[6,7] but edrophonium appears not to have this effect.[8] However, the antagonism produced by edrophonium is not adequately and reliably sustained especially following profound block.[9,10]

1. Hunter JM. Is it always necessary to antagonize residual neuromuscular block? Do children differ from adults? *Br J Anaesth* 1996; **77:** 707–9.
2. Fawcett WJ. Neuromuscular block in children. *Br J Anaesth* 1997; **78:** 627.
3. Fuchs-Buder T, Mencke T. Use of reversal agents in day care procedures (with special reference to postoperative nausea and vomiting). *Eur J Anaesthesiol* 2001; **18** (suppl 23): 53–9.
4. Joshi GP, *et al.* The effects of antagonizing residual neuromuscular blockade by neostigmine and glycopyrrolate on nausea and vomiting after ambulatory surgery. *Anesth Analg* 1999; **89:** 628–31.
5. Watcha MF, *et al.* Effect of antagonism of mivacurium-induced neuromuscular block on postoperative emesis in children. *Anesth Analg* 1995; **80:** 713–17.
6. Hughes R, *et al.* Neuromuscular blockade by neostigmine. *Br J Anaesth* 1979; **51:** 568P.
7. Payne JP, *et al.* Neuromuscular blockade by neostigmine in anaesthetized man. *Br J Anaesth* 1980; **52:** 69–75.
8. Astley BA, *et al.* Electrical and mechanical responses after neuromuscular blockade with vecuronium, and subsequent antagonism with neostigmine or edrophonium. *Br J Anaesth* 1987; **59:** 983–8.
9. Caldwell JE, *et al.* Antagonism of profound neuromuscular blockade induced by vecuronium or atracurium: comparison of neostigmine with edrophonium. *Br J Anaesth* 1986; **58:** 1285–9.
10. Mirakhur RK, *et al.* Antagonism of vecuronium-induced neuromuscular blockade with edrophonium or neostigmine. *Br J Anaesth* 1987; **59:** 473–7.

**Snake bite.** The general management of snake bites is discussed on p.1639. Numerous reports from India have claimed benefit for anticholinesterases in the treatment of neurotoxic envenoming from snake bites but failure to distinguish between cobra and krait bites, lack of controls, and inadequate information about other therapy vitiate the claims.[1] However, edrophonium has been shown in 2 double-blind studies to be more effective than placebo[2] and antivenom[3] in the treatment of snake bite due to the Philippine cobra (*Naja naja philippinensis*). Neostigmine has also been reported[4] to have been effective in reversing paralysis in 2 patients bitten by *Micrurus frontalis* (a coral snake). Similarly, another patient made a remarkable recovery when treated with neostigmine after being bitten by an Asiatic cobra (*Naja naja kaouthia*).[5] Anticholinesterases would be expected to be of little value for bites from snakes whose venom contains neurotoxins which act presynaptically, including the Asian krait, the Australian tiger snake, and the taipan[6] and, although beneficial results have been reported in individual patients,[7] overall results are considered to be inconsistent.[2,8] However, it is recommended that a test dose of edrophonium preceded by atropine should be given to patients with neurological signs following a snake bite by any species and if improvement occurs, a longer acting anticholinesterase such as neostigmine can be given.[2,3]


1. Reid HA. Venoms and antivenoms. *Trop Dis Bull* 1983; **80:** 23.
2. Watt G, *et al.* Positive response to edrophonium in patients with neurotoxic envenoming by cobras (Naja naja philippinensis). *N Engl J Med* 1986; **315:** 1444–8.
3. Watt G, *et al.* Comparison of Tensilon® and antivenom for the treatment of cobra-bite paralysis. *Trans R Soc Trop Med Hyg* 1989; **83:** 570–3.
4. Vital Brazil O, Vieira RJ. Neostigmine in the treatment of snake accidents caused by Micrurus frontalis: report of two cases. *Rev Inst Med Trop Sao Paulo* 1996; **38:** 61–7.
5. Gold BS. Neostigmine for the treatment of neurotoxicity following envenomation by the Asiatic cobra. *Ann Emerg Med* 1996; **28:** 87–9.
6. Brophy T, Sutherland SK. Use of neostigmine after snake bite. *Br J Anaesth* 1979; **51:** 264–5.
7. Warrell DA, *et al.* Severe neurotoxic envenoming by the Malayan krait Bungarus candidus (Linnaeus): response to antivenom and anticholinesterase. *BMJ* 1983 **286:** 678–80.
8. Trevett AJ, *et al.* Failure of 3,4-diaminopyridine and edrophonium to produce significant clinical benefit in neurotoxicity following the bite of Papuan taipan (Oxyuranus scutellatus carini). *Trans R Soc Trop Med Hyg* 1995; **89:** 444–6.


**Tetrodotoxin poisoning.** For reference to the use of neostigmine in the treatment of tetrodotoxin poisoning caused by eating puffer fish, see under Uses and Administration of Edrophonium Chloride, p.1491.

## Preparations

**BP 2003:** Neostigmine Injection; Neostigmine Tablets;
**USP 27:** Neostigmine Bromide Tablets; Neostigmine Methylsulfate Injection.

**Proprietary Preparations** (details are given in Part 3)
***Arg.:*** Fadastigmina; Prostigmin; ***Austral.:*** Prostigmin; ***Austria:*** Normastigmin; Prostigmin; ***Belg.:*** Prostigmine†; Robinul-Neostigmine; ***Braz.:*** Prostigmine; ***Canad.:*** Prostigmin; ***Chile:*** Prostigmine; ***Denm.:*** Robinul-Neostigmin; ***Fin.:*** Glycostigmin; Robinul-Neostigmin; ***Fr.:*** Prostigmine; ***Ger.:*** Neostig-Reu†; ***Gr.:*** Prostigmine; ***Hong Kong:*** Prostigmin; ***India:*** Tilstigmin; ***Irl.:*** Prostigmin†; Robinul-Neostigmine†; ***Israel:*** Prostigmine†; ***Ital.:*** Intrastigmina; Prostigmina; ***Malaysia:*** Prostigmin; ***Mex.:*** Prostigmine; ***Neth.:*** Prostigmin; ***Norw.:*** Prostigmin†; Robinul-Neostigmin; ***Port.:*** Prostigmine; ***Spain:*** Prostigmine; ***Swed.:*** Robinul-Neostigmin; ***Switz.:*** Prostigmine; Robinul-Neostigmine; ***Thai.:*** Prostigmin; ***UK:*** Robinul-Neostigmine; ***USA:*** Neostigmine Min-I-Mix; Prostigmin.

**Multi-ingredient:** ***Austria:*** Normastigmin mit Pilocarpin; Pilostigmin Puroptal; ***Ger.:*** Syncarpin-N.

---

## Paraoxon

E-600. Diethyl *p*-nitrophenyl phosphate.
$C_{10}H_{14}NO_6P$ = 275.2.
*CAS — 311-45-5.*
*ATC — S01EB10.*

### Profile

Paraoxon is a potent inhibitor of cholinesterase activity which has been used with other miotics in the treatment of glaucoma. It is the active metabolite of the organophosphorus insecticide parathion (p.1508) and therefore produces similar toxicity but with a faster onset.

### Preparations

**Proprietary Preparations** (details are given in Part 3)
**Multi-ingredient:** ***Ital.:*** Mios.

---

## Physostigmine *(BAN)*

Eserine; Fisostigmina. (3a*S*,8a*R*)-1,2,3,3a,8,8a-Hexahydro-1,3a,8-trimethylpyrrolo[2,3-*b*]indol-5-yl methylcarbamate.
$C_{15}H_{21}N_3O_2$ = 275.3.
*CAS — 57-47-6.*
*ATC — S01EB05; V03AB19.*

**Description.** An alkaloid obtained from the calabar bean (ordeal bean; chopnut), the seed of *Physostigma venenosum* (Leguminosae).

**Pharmacopoeias.** In *US.*

**USP 27** (Physostigmine). An alkaloid usually obtained from the dried ripe seed of *Physostigma venenosum* (Leguminosae). It is a white, odourless, microcrystalline powder which acquires a red tint on exposure to heat, light, or air, or on contact with traces of metals. M.p. not lower than 103°. Slightly soluble in water; freely soluble in alcohol; very soluble in chloroform and in dichloromethane; soluble in fixed oils and in benzene. Store in airtight containers. Protect from light.

## Physostigmine Salicylate *(BANM)*

Eserine Salicylate; Eserini Salicylas; Fisostigmina, salicilato de; Physostig. Sal.; Physostigmine Monosalicylate; Physostigmini Salicylas.
$C_{15}H_{21}N_3O_2,C_7H_6O_3$ = 413.5.
*CAS — 57-64-7.*
*ATC — S01EB05; V03AB19.*

**Pharmacopoeias.** In *Eur.* (see p.vi), *Int., Pol.,* and *US.*

**Ph. Eur. 5.0** (Physostigmine Salicylate). Colourless or almost colourless crystals. It becomes red on exposure to air and light; the colour develops more quickly in the presence of moisture. Sparingly soluble in water; soluble in alcohol. A 0.9% solution in water has a pH of 5.1 to 5.9. Store in airtight containers. Protect from light. Aqueous solutions are unstable.

**USP 27** (Physostigmine Salicylate). White, shining, odourless, crystals or white powder. It acquires a red tint on exposure to heat, light, or air, or on contact with traces of metals for long periods. Soluble 1 in 75 of water, 1 in 16 of alcohol, 1 in 6 of chloroform, and 1 in 250 of ether. Store in airtight containers at a temperature of 25°, excursions permitted between 15° and 30°. Protect from light.

**Stability.** See below.

## Physostigmine Sulfate

Eserine Sulphate; Eserini Sulfas; Fisostigmina, sulfato de; Physostig. Sulph.; Physostigmine Sulphate *(BANM)*; Physostigmini Sulfas.
$(C_{15}H_{21}N_3O_2)_2,H_2SO_4$ = 648.8.
*CAS — 64-47-1.*
*ATC — S01EB05; V03AB19.*

**Pharmacopoeias.** In *Eur.* (see p.vi) and *US.*

**Ph. Eur. 5.0** (Physostigmine Sulphate). A white or almost white, hygroscopic crystalline powder. It becomes red on exposure to air and light; the colour develops more quickly in the presence of moisture. Very soluble in water; freely soluble in alcohol. A 1% solution in water has a pH of 3.5 to 5.5. Store in well-filled airtight glass containers. Protect from light. Aqueous solutions are unstable.

**USP 27** (Physostigmine Sulfate). A white, odourless, microcrystalline powder. It is deliquescent in moist air, and acquires a red tint on exposure to heat, light, or air, or on contact with traces of metals for long periods. Soluble 1 in 4 of water, 1 in 0.4 of alcohol, and 1 in 1200 of ether. Store in airtight containers. Protect from light.

**Stability.** In aqueous solutions physostigmine is hydrolysed to eseroline and subsequently oxidised to the red compound rubreserine and other coloured products. Solutions for injection should not be used if more than slightly discoloured.

### Adverse Effects, Treatment, and Precautions

Systemic effects as for Neostigmine, p.1492. For adverse effects and precautions for topical miotics see also under Pilocarpine, p.1495.

Systemic toxic effects of physostigmine are usually more severe than those occurring with neostigmine. Physostigmine crosses the blood-brain barrier and may therefore produce CNS effects. Physostigmine is not well tolerated when used in the eyes for long periods and may produce follicles in the conjunctiva; hypersensitivity reactions are also common. Prolonged use of ophthalmic ointments containing physostigmine may cause depigmentation of the lid margins in dark-skinned patients.

**Overdosage.** Symptomatic and supportive treatment, including the use of diazepam and atropine where necessary, is generally recommended for systemic toxicity due to physostigmine. However, in an early report, the use of atropine in a patient who had taken 1 g of physostigmine had to be abandoned after it produced tachycardia and multifocal ventricular ectopic beats.[1] In a similar case of severe poisoning a slow intravenous injection of propranolol 5 mg reduced the high pulse rate and controlled pulse irregularities despite frequent intravenous doses of atropine.[2]


1. Cumming G, *et al.* Treatment and recovery after massive overdosage of physostigmine. *Lancet* 1968; **ii:** 147–9.
2. Valero A. Treatment of severe physostigmine poisoning. *Lancet* 1968; **ii:** 459–60.


### Interactions

As for Neostigmine, p.1492.

### Pharmacokinetics

Physostigmine is readily absorbed from the gastrointestinal tract, subcutaneous tissues, and mucous membranes. It is largely destroyed in the body by hydrolysis of the ester linkage by cholinesterases; a parenteral dose is claimed to be destroyed within 2 hours. It crosses the blood-brain barrier. Little is excreted in the urine.

◊ Small studies suggest marked interindividual differences in the absorption and metabolism of physostigmine salicylate after doses of up to 4 mg by mouth, perhaps because of saturable presystemic metabolism.[1-3] Oral bioavailability ranged from 5.2 to 11.7% in 3 of 5 subjects.[3]

In a study[4] of a single application of a physostigmine (base) transdermal system in 6 subjects, the mean absolute bioavailability was 36% (range 12.6 to 53.2%); the interindividual variability in absolute bioavailability was decreased by about 30% in comparison with an oral solution of physostigmine salicylate. There was continued absorption of physostigmine following removal of the transdermal system, indicating a drug reservoir in the skin.

In a study[5] of 9 patients with Alzheimer's disease, a mean elimination half-life for physostigmine of 16.4 minutes was reported with intravenous physostigmine salicylate. Cholinesterase inhibition was more prolonged than suggested by its elimination half-life.


1. Gibson M, *et al.* Physostigmine concentrations after oral doses. *Lancet* 1985; **i:** 695–6.
2. Sharpless NS, Thal LJ. Plasma physostigmine concentrations after oral administration. *Lancet* 1985; **i:** 1397–8.
3. Whelpton R, Hurst P. Bioavailability of oral physostigmine. *N Engl J Med* 1985; **313:** 1293–4.
4. Walker K, *et al.* Pharmacokinetics of physostigmine in man following a single application of a transdermal system. *Br J Clin Pharmacol* 1995; **39:** 59–63.
5. Asthana S, *et al.* Clinical pharmacokinetics of physostigmine in patients with Alzheimer's disease. *Clin Pharmacol Ther* 1995; **58:** 299–309.


### Uses and Administration

Physostigmine is a reversible tertiary amine inhibitor of cholinesterase activity with actions similar to those of neostigmine (p.1493). Physostigmine has been used, alone or more usually with other miotics such as pilocarpine, to decrease intra-ocular pressure in glaucoma (p.1485). It is a more potent miotic than pilocarpine but is rarely tolerated for prolonged periods. When it is used in glaucoma physostigmine has usually been given as eye drops containing 0.25 or 0.5% of the salicylate or as an ophthalmic ointment containing 0.25% of the sulfate.

Physostigmine crosses the blood-brain barrier and has been used to reverse the central as well as the peripheral effects of agents with antimuscarinic actions following overdosage but such treatment is not usually recommended. Physostigmine is also under investigation in the management of Alzheimer's disease (below).

**Antimuscarinic poisoning.** As physostigmine penetrates the blood-brain barrier it has been used to reverse the central effects of poisoning with agents that have antimuscarinic actions including tricyclic antidepressants, antihistamines, some antiemetics, some antiparkinsonian drugs, and phenothiazines. However, reviewers agree that in general such a use is inappropriate and hazardous. Physostigmine does not appear to affect the mortality rate in tricyclic antidepressant poisoning[1] and its use can lead to severe cardiac[2,3] and respiratory effects[2,3] and to convulsions.[3,4]


1. Aquilonius S-M, Hedstrand U. The use of physostigmine as an antidote in tricyclic anti-depressant intoxication. *Acta Anaesthesiol Scand* 1978; **22:** 40–5.
2. Caine ED. Anticholinergic toxicity. *N Engl J Med* 1979; **300:** 1278.
3. Newton RW. Physostigmine salicylate in the treatment of tricyclic antidepressant overdosage. *JAMA* 1975; **231:** 941–3.
4. Knudsen K, Heath A. Effects of self poisoning with maprotiline. *BMJ* 1984; **288:** 601–3.


**Baclofen overdosage.** For references to the use of physostigmine in the treatment of baclofen overdosage, see p.1387.

**Cerebellar ataxias.** Double-blind controlled studies indicate that physostigmine[1,2] can produce symptomatic improvement in some patients with cerebellar ataxia including those with hereditary forms of spinocerebellar degeneration such as Friedreich's ataxia.


1. Rodriguez-Budelli MM, *et al.* Action of physostigmine on inherited ataxias. *Adv Neurol* 1978; **21:** 195–202.
2. Aschoff JC, *et al.* Physostigmin in der Behandlung von Kleinhirnataxien. *Nervenarzt* 1996; **67:** 311–18.


**Dementia.** Physostigmine has been studied in the symptomatic management of Alzheimer's disease (see Dementia, p.1484). However, a systematic review concluded that the evidence of its effectiveness was limited and the benefits shown were not convincing.[1] Small early studies with oral physostigmine in Alzheimer's disease were inconclusive; a larger multicentre study[2] using controlled-release physostigmine found that it produced some improvement in cognitive and global function, but gastrointestinal adverse effects were common and led to a high drop-out rate.


1. Coelho Filho JM, Birks J. Physostigmine for dementia due to Alzheimer's disease. Available in The Cochrane Library; Issue 2. Chichester: John Wiley; 2004.
2. Thal LJ, *et al.* A 24-week randomized trial of controlled-release physostigmine in patients with Alzheimer's disease. *Neurology* 1999; **52:** 1146–52.


### Preparations

**USP 27:** Physostigmine Salicylate Injection; Physostigmine Salicylate Ophthalmic Solution; Physostigmine Sulfate Ophthalmic Ointment.

**Proprietary Preparations** (details are given in Part 3)
***Austria:*** Anticholium; ***Ger.:*** Anticholium; ***USA:*** Antilirium.

**Multi-ingredient:** ***Belg.:*** Miotic Double†; ***Braz.:*** Enterotonus†; ***Ger.:*** Isopto Pilomin†; Pilo-Eserin†; ***India:*** Bi-Miotic.

---

## Pilocarpine *(BAN)*

Pilocarpina. (3*S*,4*R*)-3-Ethyldihydro-4-[(1-methyl-1*H*-imidazol-5-yl)methyl]furan-2(3*H*)-one.
$C_{11}H_{16}N_2O_2$ = 208.3.
*CAS — 92-13-7.*
*ATC — N07AX01; S01EB01.*

**Description.** An alkaloid obtained from the leaves of jaborandi, *Pilocarpus microphyllus* (Rutaceae) and other species of *Pilocarpus.*

**Pharmacopoeias.** In *US.*

**USP 27** (Pilocarpine). A viscous, exceedingly hygroscopic, oily liquid or crystals. M.p. about 34°. Soluble in water, in alcohol, and in chloroform; sparingly soluble in ether and in benzene; practically insoluble in petroleum spirit. Store in airtight containers at a temperature not exceeding 8°. Protect from light.

### Pilocarpine Borate

Pilocarpina, borato de.

$C_{11}H_{16}N_2O_2,xBH_3O_3$.

*CAS — 16509-56-1.*

*ATC — N07AX01; S01EB01.*

### Pilocarpine Hydrochloride *(BANM)*

Pilocarp. Hydrochlor.; Pilocarpina, hidrocloruro de; Pilocarpine Monohydrochloride; Pilocarpini Chloridum; Pilocarpini Hydrochloridum; Pilocarpinium Chloratum.

$C_{11}H_{16}N_2O_2,HCl = 244.7$.

*CAS — 54-71-7.*

*ATC — N07AX01; S01EB01.*

NOTE. PIL is a code approved by the BP 2003 for use on single unit doses of eye drops containing pilocarpine hydrochloride where the individual container may be too small to bear all the appropriate labelling information.

**Pharmacopoeias.** In *Eur.* (see p.vi), *Int., Jpn, Pol.,* and *US.*

**Ph. Eur. 5.0** (Pilocarpine Hydrochloride). Hygroscopic, colourless crystals or white or almost white crystalline powder. Very soluble in water and in alcohol. A 5% solution in water has a pH of 3.5 to 4.5. Store in airtight containers. Protect from light.

**USP 27** (Pilocarpine Hydrochloride). Colourless, translucent, odourless, hygroscopic crystals. Soluble 1 in 0.3 of water, 1 in 3 of alcohol, and 1 in 360 of chloroform; insoluble in ether. Its solutions are acid to litmus. Store in airtight containers. Protect from light.

**Stability.** Pilocarpine hydrochloride oral solution, prepared from powder or eye drops and buffered at pH 5.5, was found[1] to be stable for 60 days at 25° and for 90 days at 4°.

1. Fawcett JP, *et al.* Formulation and stability of pilocarpine oral solution. *Int J Pharm Pract* 1994; **3:** 14–18.

### Pilocarpine Nitrate *(BANM)*

Pilocarp. Nit.; Pilocarpina, nitrato de; Pilocarpine Mononitrate; Pilocarpini Nitras; Pilocarpinii Nitras; Pilocarpinium Nitricum.

$C_{11}H_{16}N_2O_2,HNO_3 = 271.3$.

*CAS — 148-72-1.*

*ATC — N07AX01; S01EB01.*

NOTE. PIL is a code approved by the BP 2003 for use on single unit doses of eye drops containing pilocarpine nitrate where the individual container may be too small to bear all the appropriate labelling information.

**Pharmacopoeias.** In *Chin., Eur.* (see p.vi), *Int., US,* and *Viet.*

**Ph. Eur. 5.0** (Pilocarpine Nitrate). Colourless crystals, or white or almost white crystalline powder. Freely soluble in water; sparingly soluble in alcohol. A 5% solution in water has a pH of 3.5 to 4.5. Protect from light.

**USP 27** (Pilocarpine Nitrate). Shining white crystals. Soluble 1 in 4 of water and 1 in 75 of alcohol; insoluble in chloroform and in ether. Its solutions are acid to litmus. Store in airtight containers. Protect from light.

## Adverse Effects, Treatment, and Precautions

Systemic effects and cautions are as for Neostigmine, p.1492.

With the *oral* use of pilocarpine, sweating is noted as a common problem; caution is needed to avoid dehydration in patients who may sweat excessively and who cannot maintain an adequate fluid intake. Paradoxical hypertension and constipation, confusion, and increased urinary frequency are also specifically included among the adverse effects reported. The manufacturer recommends that it should not be given when miosis is undesirable such as in patients with acute iritis or angle-closure glaucoma. Blurred vision may affect the performance of skilled tasks. In addition pilocarpine should be given with care to those with cognitive or psychiatric disturbances, with renal calculi or renal impairment, or with biliary-tract disorders. Dosage should be reduced in patients with hepatic impairment (see Administration in Hepatic Impairment, below).

After *ocular* use pilocarpine is usually better tolerated than the anticholinesterases, but in common with other miotics may produce ciliary spasm, ocular pain and irritation, blurred vision, lachrymation, myopia, and browache. Conjunctival vascular congestion, superficial keratitis, vitreous haemorrhage, and increased pupillary block have been reported. Lens opacities have occurred following prolonged use. Treatment with miotics should be stopped if symptoms of systemic toxicity develop.

Miotics are contra-indicated in conditions where pupillary constriction is undesirable such as acute iritis, acute uveitis, anterior uveitis, and some forms of secondary glaucoma. They should be avoided in acute inflammatory disease of the anterior segment of the eye. If possible, treatment with long-acting miotics should be stopped before surgery on the eye as there is an increased risk of hyphaema. Miotics should be used with extreme caution in patients with a history of retinal detachment and in young patients with myopia. Care is also needed in patients with corneal or conjunctival damage. Miosis may cause blurred vision and difficulty with dark adaptation and caution is necessary with night driving or when hazardous tasks are undertaken in poor illumination. Miotics should not be used by patients wearing soft contact lenses.

**Alzheimer's disease.** In patients with dementia of Alzheimer type, CNS symptoms may be induced or exacerbated by the use of pilocarpine eye drops.[1,2]

1. Reyes PF, *et al.* Mental status changes induced by eye drops in dementia of the Alzheimer type. *J Neurol Neurosurg Psychiatry* 1987; **50:** 113–15.
2. Fraunfelder FT, Morgan R. The aggravation of dementia by pilocarpine. *JAMA* 1994; **271:** 1742–3.

**Asthma.** A reminder that topical miotics can precipitate bronchospasm in susceptible patients.[1] However, the severity of bronchospasm induced by carbachol has been reported to be less than that produced by timolol. Bronchospastic complications are much less likely to occur with pilocarpine but have nevertheless been reported. As inhalations of methacholine are used to induce bronchospasm in the diagnosis of latent asthma, the risk of exacerbating asthma should be considered before methacholine is used in the eye.

1. Prakash UBS, *et al.* Pulmonary complications from ophthalmic preparations. *Mayo Clin Proc* 1990; **65:** 521–9.

**Glaucoma.** Miotics usually lower intra-ocular pressure by decreasing the resistance to outflow of aqueous humour from the anterior chamber through the trabecular network. However, they appear to reduce uveoscleral outflow and this may cause a paradoxical rise in intra-ocular pressure in patients with severely compromised trabecular outflow as was reported in a patient with post-traumatic angle-recession glaucoma.[1] It has been recommended that pilocarpine should be avoided after drainage operations for glaucoma because its miotic effect can increase the occurrence of posterior pupillary synechiae; a topical beta blocker is usually adequate if control of intra-ocular pressure is required.[2] Pilocarpine-induced miosis was shown to cause a significant deterioration in visual field in patients with chronic open-angle glaucoma in one study.[3] It was suggested that this should be an important consideration when choosing therapy for glaucoma, particularly in cases where field loss approaches the permitted legal minimum for driving. Of 53 patients receiving long-term therapy with pilocarpine gel, 15 developed a corneal haze, which persisted for at least 2 years in 13; although the patients remained asymptomatic the long-term effects were unknown.[4] Many patients using the gel also developed superficial punctate keratitis which usually cleared spontaneously during treatment.

1. Bleiman BS, Schwartz AL. Paradoxical intraocular pressure response to pilocarpine: a proposed mechanism and treatment. *Arch Ophthalmol* 1979; **97:** 1305–6.
2. Phillips CI, *et al.* Posterior synechiae after glaucoma operations: aggravation by shallow anterior chamber and pilocarpine. *Br J Ophthalmol* 1987; **71:** 428–32.
3. Webster AR, *et al.* The effect of pilocarpine on the glaucomatous visual field. *Br J Ophthalmol* 1993; **77:** 721–5.
4. Johnson DH, *et al.* Corneal changes during pilocarpine gel therapy. *Am J Ophthalmol* 1986; **101:** 13–15.

**Hypersensitivity.** Contact urticaria involving the eyelids has been reported[1] in a patient following treatment with pilocarpine eye drops for glaucoma.

1. O'Donnell BF, Foulds IS. Contact allergic dermatitis and contact urticaria due to topical ophthalmic preparations. *Br J Ophthalmol* 1993; **77:** 740–1.

**Retinal detachment.** The use of miotics has been implicated in numerous reports as a cause of retinal detachment but reviews of the subject have concluded that there is little factual evidence to support the association.[1,2] However, there is circumstantial evidence that retinal detachment is more likely to occur with strong miotics. Furthermore, patients with myopia or pre-existing retinal damage appear to be at greater risk and there is the possibility that even low concentrations of relatively mild miotics such as 1% pilocarpine might precipitate retinal detachment.

1. Alpar JJ. Miotics and retinal detachment: a survey and case report. *Ann Ophthalmol* 1979; **11:** 395–401.
2. Beasley H, Fraunfelder FT. Retinal detachments and topical ocular miotics. *Ophthalmology* 1979; **86:** 95–8.

**Systemic absorption.** Systemic adverse effects after the ophthalmic use of pilocarpine are thought to be rare and reports of toxicity appear to involve elderly patients treated for acute angle-closure glaucoma prior to surgery and who received 2 to 5 times the usual daily dose of pilocarpine in a few hours.[1]

1. Everitt DE, Avorn J. Systemic effects of medications used to treat glaucoma. *Ann Intern Med* 1990; **112:** 120–5.

## Interactions

As for Neostigmine, p.1492.

## Pharmacokinetics

Mean elimination half-lives for pilocarpine have been reported to be 0.76 and 1.35 hours after oral doses of 5 and 10 mg of the hydrochloride respectively. Inactivation of pilocarpine is thought to occur at neuronal synapses and probably in plasma. Pilocarpine and its inactive metabolites, including pilocarpic acid, are excreted in the urine.

## Uses and Administration

Pilocarpine is a tertiary amine direct-acting parasympathomimetic with primarily the muscarinic effects of acetylcholine (p.1487). It is used mainly in the treatment of glaucoma (p.1485) and in the treatment of dry eye (p.1576) or dry mouth (below); it has also been used as a diaphoretic in diagnostic tests for cystic fibrosis and leprosy (below). Topical application of pilocarpine to the eye produces miosis (pupil constriction) by contraction of the iris sphincter muscle; contraction of the ciliary muscle results in increased accommodation. Constriction of the pupil also pulls open the trabecular meshwork in the eye and this in turn facilitates drainage of aqueous humour and reduction of intra-ocular pressure. Following the use of eye drops, miosis occurs in about 10 to 30 minutes and lasts 4 to 8 hours while peak reduction in intra-ocular pressure occurs within 75 minutes and the reduction usually persists for 4 to 14 hours.

Pilocarpine is used in the treatment of open-angle **glaucoma** (but see also Adverse Effects, above) and is commonly given with topical beta blockers or sympathomimetic drugs. It is used as the hydrochloride or the nitrate, usually as 0.5 to 4% eye drops given 4 times daily, the dose being adjusted individually. Solutions containing 0.25 to 10% of the hydrochloride are also available and the higher strengths may sometimes be required in patients with heavily pigmented irides. A modified-release system inserted into the conjunctival sac and releasing 20 or 40 micrograms of pilocarpine per hour for 7 days, and a 4% ophthalmic gel have also been used. Pilocarpine may also be used as part of the emergency treatment of acute attacks of angle-closure glaucoma prior to surgery.

The miotic action of pilocarpine has been used to antagonise the effects of sympathomimetic mydriatics on the eye and in surgical procedures on the eye. Pilocarpine borate has been used similarly in ophthalmology to the hydrochloride and nitrate.

Pilocarpine hydrochloride is used in the treatment of **dry mouth** following radiotherapy for malignant neoplasms of the head and neck. It increases salivary flow only in patients with residual salivary gland function. The initial dose is 5 mg by mouth three times daily with or immediately after meals, increased gradually if necessary after 4 to 8 weeks until an adequate response is obtained, up to a maximum of 10 mg three times daily. Doses of 5 mg by mouth four times daily are used to treat **dry eye** or mouth in patients with Sjögren's syndrome; this dose may be increased to a maximum of 30 mg daily. Treatment should be stopped if no improvement is obtained after 3 months of use.

**Administration in hepatic impairment.** The UK manufacturers recommend that daily doses of *oral* pilocarpine should be reduced in patients with moderate to severe cirrhosis. The dose may gradually be increased to 5 mg three times daily if tolerated.

**Diagnosis and testing.** CYSTIC FIBROSIS. The fact that individuals with cystic fibrosis have abnormally high concentrations of sodium and chloride in their sweat has been used in the diagnosis of this condition and pilocarpine iontophoresis has been used to promote sweating as part of that test.[1]

1. Gibson LE, Cooke RE. A test for concentration of electrolytes in sweat in cystic fibrosis of the pancreas utilizing pilocarpine by iontophoresis. *Pediatrics* 1959; **23:** 545–9.

LEPROSY. The induction of sweat secretion by intradermal injection of pilocarpine nitrate has been used to assess the functional status of dermal nerves in patients with leprotic skin lesions.[1]

1. Joshi PB. Pilocarpine test in assesment of therapeutic efficacy in maculoanaesthetic leprosy. *Lepr India* 1976; **48:** 55–60.

**Dry mouth.** Pilocarpine is used as a sialogogue in the treatment of dry mouth (p.1576) following radiotherapy for head and neck cancer. It is also used as a treatment for dry mouth and dry eye in the auto-immune disease, Sjögren's syndrome.[1-3]


1. Wiseman LR, Faulds D. Oral pilocarpine: a review of its pharmacological properties and clinical potential in xerostomia. *Drugs* 1995; **49:** 143–55.
2. Nelson JD, *et al.* Oral pilocarpine for symptomatic relief of keratoconjunctivitis sicca in patients with Sjögren's syndrome. *Adv Exp Med Biol* 1998; **438:** 979–83.
3. Vivino FB, *et al.* Pilocarpine tablets for the treatment of dry mouth and dry eye symptoms in patients with Sjögren syndrome: a randomized, placebo-controlled, fixed-dose, multicenter trial. *Arch Intern Med* 1999; **159:** 174–81.


**Reversal of mydriasis.** Pilocarpine has been used to reverse the effects of mydriatics following surgery or ophthalmoscopic examination but other miotics may be preferred (see p.1487). It counteracts the mydriatic effects of sympathomimetics, such as phenylephrine and hydroxyamfetamine,[1] but is ineffective against mydriasis produced by antimuscarinics, such as homatropine,[1] and may impair vision further when used with tropicamide.[2] Furthermore, there is also the risk of pilocarpine precipitating angle-closure glaucoma in susceptible patients (see Glaucoma, under Precautions, above).


1. Anastasi LM, *et al.* Effect of pilocarpine in counteracting mydriasis. *Arch Ophthalmol* 1968; **79:** 710–15.
2. Nelson ME, Orton HP. Counteracting the effects of mydriatics: does it benefit the patient? *Arch Ophthalmol* 1987; **105:** 486–9.


## Preparations

***BP 2003:*** Pilocarpine Hydrochloride Eye Drops; Pilocarpine Nitrate Eye Drops;
***USP 27:*** Pilocarpine Hydrochloride Ophthalmic Solution; Pilocarpine Nitrate Ophthalmic Solution; Pilocarpine Ocular System.

**Proprietary Preparations** (details are given in Part 3)
***Arg.:*** Alvis; Gel Carpina; Isopto Carpina; Klonocarpina; Pilocarpol; Pilomed; Sonadryl; Tensiocap; Wetol; Xao Pil; ***Austral.:*** Isopto Carpine; Ocusert†; Pilopt; PV Carpine; ***Austria:*** Pilax; Piloftal; Pilogel; Salagen; ***Belg.:*** Isopto Carpine; Pilo; ***Braz.:*** Isopto Carpine; ***Canad.:*** Diocarpine; Isopto Carpine; Miocarpine; Pilopine HS; Salagen; ***Chile:*** Pilogel; ***Fin.:*** Isopto Carpine; Salagen; ***Fr.:*** Chibro-Pilocarpine†; Pilo; Salagen; ***Ger.:*** Asthenopin†; Borocarpin-S; Pilo-Stulln; Pilocarpol; Pilogel†; Pilomann; Pilomann-Öl; Pilopos; Salagen; Spersacarpin; Vistacarpin†; ***Gr.:*** Dispercarpine; Isopto Carpine; Pilocollyre; Pilotina; Salagen; ***Hong Kong:*** Isopto Carpine; Pilogel HS; Spersacarpine; ***India:*** Carpo-Miotic; Pilocar; ***Irl.:*** Isopto Carpine; Pilogel; Salagen; ***Israel:*** Glaucocarpine; Isopto Carpine; Mi-Pilo; Pilogel; Salagen; ***Ital.:*** Dropilton; Liocarpina†; Pilogel; Pilotonina; Salagen; ***Malaysia:*** Isopto Carpine; Pilo; Spersacarpine; ***Mex.:*** Pilo; Pilof Nicolich†; ***Neth.:*** Salagen; ***Norw.:*** Isopto Carpine; Pilo; ***NZ:*** Isopto Carpine†; Ocusert†; Pilopt; PV Carpine†; ***Port.:*** Pilocarcil; Piloplex; Salagen; ***S.Afr.:*** Isopto Carpine; Pilogel; ***Singapore:*** Isopto Carpine; Pilogel; Spersacarpine†; ***Spain:*** Isopto Carpina; ***Swed.:*** Licarpin†; Salagen; ***Switz.:*** Isopto Carpine†; Pilo†; Pilogel HS†; Spersacarpine; ***Thai.:*** Isopto Carpine; Pilogel†; Pilomann†; ***UK:*** Isopto Carpine†; Ocusert†; Pilogel; Salagen; ***USA:*** Adsorbocarpine; Akarpine; Isopto Carpine; Ocu-Carpine; Ocusert; Pilagan†; Pilocar; Pilopine HS; Piloptic; Pilopto-Carpine; Pilostat; Salagen.

**Multi-ingredient:** ***Arg.:*** Amplus; Glaucocin; Glaucotensil; Ofal P; Pilotim; Timpilo; ***Austral.:*** Timpilo; ***Austria:*** Betacarpin; Fotil; Normastigmin mit Pilocarpin; Pilostigmin Puroptal; Thiloadren; Timpilo; ***Belg.:*** Carteopil; Miotic Double†; Normoglaucon; ***Canad.:*** E-Pilo†; Timpilo; ***Denm.:*** Fotil; Timpilo; ***Fin.:*** Fotil; Timpilo; ***Fr.:*** Carpilo; Montavon†; Timpilo; ***Ger.:*** Fotil; Glauko Biciron; Isopto Pilomin†; Normoglaucon; Pilo-Eserin†; Syncarpin-N; Thiloadren N; Timpilo; TP-Ophtal; ***Gr.:*** Thilocombin; ***Hong Kong:*** Timpilo; ***India:*** Bi-Miotic; ***Israel:*** Timpilo; ***Ital.:*** Equiton; Mios; Pilobloc; Pilodren; Ripix; Timicon; ***Malaysia:*** Normoglaucon; Timpilo; ***Mex.:*** Timpilo†; ***Neth.:*** Normoglaucon; Timpilo; ***Norw.:*** Fotil; Timpilo; ***NZ:*** Timpilo; ***Port.:*** Normoglaucon; Timoglau Plus; ***Singapore:*** Normoglaucon; Timpilo; ***Swed.:*** Fotil; Timpilo; ***Switz.:*** Arteopilo; Fotil; Ripix; Timpilo; ***Thai.:*** Fotil; Normoglaucon; ***USA:*** E-Pilo.

---

# Pyridostigmine Bromide *(BAN, rINN)*

Bromuro de piridostigmina; Pyridostig. Brom.; Pyridostigmini Bromidum. 3-Dimethylcarbamoyloxy-1-methylpyridinium bromide.

$C_9H_{13}BrN_2O_2 = 261.1.$

*CAS — 155-97-5 (pyridostigmine); 101-26-8 (pyridostigmine bromide).*

*ATC — N07AA02.*

**Pharmacopoeias.** In *Chin., Eur.* (see p.vi), *Int., Jpn,* and *US.*

**Ph. Eur. 5.0** (Pyridostigmine Bromide). A white or almost white deliquescent crystalline powder. Very soluble in water and in alcohol. Store in airtight containers. Protect from light.

**USP 27** (Pyridostigmine Bromide). A white or practically white, hygroscopic, crystalline powder, having an agreeable characteristic odour. Freely soluble in water, in alcohol, and in chloroform; practically insoluble in ether; slightly soluble in petroleum spirit. Store in airtight containers.

## Adverse Effects, Treatment, and Precautions

As for Neostigmine, p.1492. It has been stated that muscarinic adverse effects occur less frequently with pyridostigmine treatment than with neostigmine.

**Breast feeding.** Pyridostigmine was present in breast milk from 2 nursing mothers receiving maintenance therapy for myasthenia gravis in a concentration between 36 and 113% of that in maternal plasma,[1] but in both cases the dose ingested per kg body-weight by the nursing infant was 0.1% or less of that ingested by the mother. Maternal medication with pyridostigmine should be no obstacle to breast feeding, at least with doses in the range of 180 to 300 mg daily. On the basis of this study, the American Academy of Pediatrics considers[2] that pyridostigmine is usually compatible with breast feeding.


1. Hardell L-I, *et al.* Pyridostigmine in human breast milk. *Br J Clin Pharmacol* 1982; **14:** 565–7.
2. American Academy of Pediatrics. The transfer of drugs and other chemicals into human milk. *Pediatrics* 2001; **108:** 776–89. Correction. *ibid.*; 1029. Also available at: http://aappolicy.aappublications.org/cgi/content/full/pediatrics%3b108/3/776 (accessed 15/06/04)


**Psychosis.** Postoperative psychosis in a patient with myasthenia gravis who received large doses of pyridostigmine bromide was attributed to bromide intoxication,[1] but this diagnosis has been challenged.[2]


1. Rothenberg DM, *et al.* Bromide intoxication secondary to pyridostigmine bromide therapy. *JAMA* 1990; **263:** 1121–2.
2. Senecal P-E, Osterloh J. Confusion from pyridostigmine bromide: was there bromide intoxication? *JAMA* 1990; **264:** 454–5.


**Renal impairment.** In patients receiving pyridostigmine for the reversal of neuromuscular blockade produced by competitive neuromuscular blockers, pyridostigmine kinetics were not significantly different in 5 following renal transplantation from those in 5 with normal renal function. However, in 4 anephric patients the elimination half-life was significantly increased and the plasma clearance significantly decreased.[1] It appeared that approximately 75% of the plasma clearance of pyridostigmine depended on renal function.


1. Cronnelly R, *et al.* Pyridostigmine kinetics with and without renal function. *Clin Pharmacol Ther* 1980; **28:** 78–81.


## Interactions

As for Neostigmine, p.1492.

## Pharmacokinetics

Pyridostigmine bromide is poorly absorbed from the gastrointestinal tract. It undergoes hydrolysis by cholinesterases and is also metabolised in the liver. Pyridostigmine is excreted mainly in the urine as unchanged drug and metabolites. Pyridostigmine crosses the placenta and very small amounts are distributed into breast milk (see Breast Feeding, above). Penetration into the CNS is poor.

◊ It has been suggested[1] that data from pharmacokinetic studies of pyridostigmine might have varied because of the analytical methods used or inappropriate storage conditions of plasma samples; it was recommended that samples should be acidified and stored at −75°. Mean terminal elimination half-life was 200 minutes in 11 healthy subjects given 60 mg of pyridostigmine by mouth; maximum plasma concentrations were obtained 1 to 5 hours after dosing. The mean terminal elimination half-life after a 4-mg intravenous infusion in 10 of these subjects was 97 minutes.[1] Oral bioavailability was calculated to vary from 11.5 to 18.9%. In an earlier study food did not appear to affect bioavailability but did delay the time taken to achieve peak plasma concentrations.[2] It appears that 75% of the plasma clearance of pyridostigmine depends on renal function.[3] 3-Hydroxy-*N*-methylpyridinium has been identified as one of the 3 metabolites isolated from the urine of patients taking pyridostigmine.[4]


1. Breyer-Pfaff U, *et al.* Pyridostigmine kinetics in healthy subjects and patients with myasthenia gravis. *Clin Pharmacol Ther* 1985; **37:** 495–501.
2. Aquilonius S-M, *et al.* Pharmacokinetics and oral bioavailability of pyridostigmine in man. *Eur J Clin Pharmacol* 1980; **18:** 423–8.
3. Cronnelly R, *et al.* Pyridostigmine kinetics with and without renal function. *Clin Pharmacol Ther* 1980: **28:** 78–81.
4. Somani SM, *et al.* Pyridostigmine in man. *Clin Pharmacol Ther* 1972; **13:** 393–9.


## Uses and Administration

Pyridostigmine is a quaternary ammonium compound that is a reversible inhibitor of cholinesterase activity with actions similar to those of neostigmine (p.1493), but is slower in onset and of longer duration. It is given as the bromide.

Pyridostigmine is mainly used in the treatment of myasthenia gravis (p.1486). It has also been used in the treatment of paralytic ileus. Pyridostigmine is sometimes used to reverse the neuromuscular blockade produced by competitive neuromuscular blockers but is generally considered less satisfactory than neostigmine. It has also been used as prophylaxis against the neuromuscular effects of nerve gas poisoning (see also below). Pyridostigmine has been used in the management of postoperative urinary retention (p.476) but has generally been superseded by catheterisation.

For **myasthenia gravis**, total daily doses in the UK may range from 0.3 to 1.2 g by mouth; however, the *British National Formulary* states that daily doses of 450 mg should not be exceeded in order to avoid receptor downregulation. It also notes that patients receiving pyridostigmine in doses over 360 mg daily may need more aggressive therapy. In the USA, licensed doses are somewhat higher, ranging up to 1.5 g daily.

The dose should be divided throughout the day and, if necessary, the night according to the response of the patient; larger portions of the total daily dose may be given at times of greater fatigue.

A suggested dose in the US for children is 7 mg/kg daily in 5 or 6 divided doses. An alternative regimen used in the UK is an initial dose of 30 mg for children under 6 years or 60 mg for those aged 6 to 12 years. This is increased gradually by increments of 15 to 30 mg daily until a satisfactory response is obtained, which is usually within the dosage range of 30 to 360 mg daily.

Pyridostigmine has also been given as modified-release tablets, usually once or twice daily but these offer less flexibility of dosage. If necessary it has also been given by intramuscular injection or in severe cases by very slow intravenous injection. However, the intravenous route is hazardous and, if used, atropine must be available to counteract any severe muscarinic reactions.

In the treatment of neonatal myasthenia doses in the range of 50 to 150 micrograms/kg by intramuscular injection or 5 to 10 mg by mouth (30 to 60 minutes before feeds) have been given every 4 to 6 hours; however, neostigmine has generally been preferred. Treatment is rarely needed beyond 8 weeks of age.

To **reverse neuromuscular blockade** produced by *competitive neuromuscular blockers*, doses of 10 to 20 mg have been given intravenously, with or preceded by atropine sulfate 0.6 to 1.2 mg to counteract any muscarinic effects. Glycopyrronium bromide has been used as an alternative to atropine.

In the USA pyridostigmine is licensed for prophylaxis against the neuromuscular effects of the nerve gas poison *soman* in military combat use only; the recommended dose is 30 mg by mouth every 8 hours started at least several hours before exposure to soman. If nerve gas poisoning occurs, pyridostigmine should be stopped and the patient should be treated with atropine and pralidoxime immediately.

In the treatment of paralytic **ileus** and postoperative **urinary retention** pyridostigmine bromide has been given by mouth in doses of 60 to 240 mg.

**Decreased gastrointestinal motility.** Parasympathomimetics such as pyridostigmine enhance gastric contractions and increase intestinal motility and form one of many treatments that have been used in a variety of conditions associated with decreased gastrointestinal motility (p.1241).

Pyridostigmine, generally in doses of 60 mg up to 3 times daily, has been used to relieve severe constipation in patients with impaired intestinal motility due to Parkinson's disease.[1]


1. Sadjadpour K. Pyridostigmine bromide and constipation in Parkinson's disease. *JAMA* 1983; **249:** 1148.


**Growth hormone deficiency.** Although the value of stimulated growth hormone secretion tests has been questioned (see Growth Retardation, p.1314) pyridostigmine with somatorelin has been found to be a potent and reproducible test for distinguishing patients with severe growth hormone deficiency from normal subjects.[1] However, the combination is not effective in patients over 55 years of age,[2] and somatorelin with arginine is generally preferred where an alternative to the gold standard of the insulin-tolerance test is required.[1]


1. Ghigo E, *et al.* Diagnostic and therapeutic uses of growth hormone-releasing substances in adult and elderly subjects. *Baillieres Clin Endocrinol Metab* 1998; **12:** 341–58.
2. Vierhapper H, *et al.* The use of the pyridostigmine growth hormone-releasing hormone stimulation test to detect growth hormone deficiency in patients with pituitary adenomas. *Metabolism* 2002; **51:** 34–7.


**Nerve gas poisoning.** Pyridostigmine has been used prophylactically to protect soldiers against attack with nerve gas agents (p.1719) that inhibit acetylcholinesterase.[1] Pyridostigmine binds reversibly to acetylcholinesterase and provides a protected store from which acetylcholinesterase is later released.[1-3] Prophylaxis with pyridostigmine greatly enhances the efficacy of treatment with atropine and pralidoxime against exposure to soman but it is not effective alone and may not be uniformly effective against other nerve agents.[1] Giving 30 mg of pyridostigmine every 8 hours provides the optimum level of protection[2] and, although adverse effects are common at this dosage, the performance of military duties is not impaired.[4] However, neurological symptoms in veterans suffering the so-called Gulf War Syndrome appear to be more common in those who reported exposure to a range of potentially toxic substances which include pyridostigmine.[5] It has been suggested that these symptoms may be evidence of organophosphate-induced polyneuropathy resulting from exposure to a combination of organophosphorus compounds and other cholinesterase inhibitors such as pyridostigmine.[6] A study in *hens*[7] (a species susceptible to anticholinesterases) has also found symptoms of enhanced neurotoxicity when pyridostigmine, the insect repellent diethyltoluamide, and the pyrethroid insecticide permethrin were used together.


1. United States Army. *Medical Management of Chemical Casualties Handbook*, 3rd ed. Aberdeen, Maryland: Medical Research Institute of Chemical Defense; 1999. Also available at: http://www.vnh.org/CHEMCASU/titlepg.html (accessed 15/06/04)
2. Ministry of Defence. *Medical manual of defence against chemical agents*. London: HMSO, 1987. (JSP312).
3. Anonymous. Prevention and treatment of injury from chemical warfare agents. *Med Lett Drugs Ther* 2002; **44:** 1–4.
4. Keeler JR, *et al.* Pyridostigmine used as a nerve agent pretreatment under wartime conditions. *JAMA* 1991; **266:** 693–5.
5. The Iowa Persian Gulf Study Group. Self-reported illness and health status among gulf war veterans: a population-based study. *JAMA* 1997; **277:** 238–45.
6. Haley RW, Kurt TL. Self-reported exposure to neurotoxic chemical combinations in the gulf war: a cross-sectional epidemiologic study. *JAMA* 1997; **277:** 231–7.
7. Abou-Donia MB, *et al.* Neurotoxicity resulting from coexposure to pyridostigmine bromide, DEET, and permethrin: implications of gulf war chemical exposure. *J Toxicol Environ Health* 1996; **48:** 35–56.


**Post-poliomyelitis syndrome.** Pyridostigmine has been reported to be of benefit in reducing fatigue associated with post-poliomyelitis syndrome.[1] A suggested[2] dose is 30 mg daily increased gradually to about 60 mg three times daily but side-effects are common.


1. Trojan DA, Cashman NR. Anticholinesterases in post-poliomyelitis syndrome. *Ann N Y Acad Sci* 1995; **753:** 285–95.
2. Thorsteinsson G. Management of postpolio syndrome. *Mayo Clin Proc* 1997; **72:** 627–38.


## Preparations

***BP 2003:*** Pyridostigmine Tablets;
***USP 27:*** Pyridostigmine Bromide Injection; Pyridostigmine Bromide Syrup; Pyridostigmine Bromide Tablets.

**Proprietary Preparations** (details are given in Part 3)
***Arg.:*** Mestinon; ***Austral.:*** Mestinon; ***Austria:*** Mestinon; ***Belg.:*** Mestinon†; ***Braz.:*** Mestinon; ***Canad.:*** Mestinon; Regonol†; ***Chile:*** Mestinon; ***Denm.:*** Mestinon; ***Fin.:*** Mestinon; ***Fr.:*** Mestinon; ***Ger.:*** Kalymin; Mestinon; ***Gr.:*** Mestinon; ***Hong Kong:*** Mestinon; ***India:*** Distinon; ***Irl.:*** Mestinon; ***Israel:*** Mestinon; ***Ital.:*** Mestinon; ***Malaysia:*** Mestinon; ***Mex.:*** Mestinon; ***Neth.:*** Mestinon; ***Norw.:*** Mestinon; ***NZ:*** Mestinon; ***Port.:*** Mestinon; ***S.Afr.:*** Mestinon; ***Singapore:*** Mestinon; ***Spain:*** Mestinon; ***Swed.:*** Mestinon; ***Switz.:*** Mestinon; ***Thai.:*** Mestinon; ***UK:*** Mestinon; ***USA:*** Mestinon; Regonol†.

# Rivastigmine *(BAN, USAN, rINN)*

ENA-713 (rivastigmine or rivastigmine hydrochloride tartrate); SDZ-212-713; SDZ-ENA-713 (rivastigmine or rivastigmine hydrochloride tartrate). (−)-*m*-[(*S*)-1-(Dimethylamino)ethyl]phenyl ethylmethylcarbamate.

$C_{14}H_{22}N_2O_2$ = 250.3.
*CAS — 123441-03-2.*
*ATC — N06DA03.*

## Rivastigmine Hydrogen Tartrate *(BANM, rINNM)*

ENA-713 (rivastigmine or rivastigmine hydrogen tartrate); Hidrogenotartrato de rivastigmina; Rivastigmine Bitartrate; Rivastigmine Tartrate; SDZ-ENA-713 (rivastigmine or rivastigmine hydrogen tartrate).

$C_{14}H_{22}N_2O_2.C_4H_6O_6$ = 400.4.
*CAS — 129101-54-8.*
*ATC — N06DA03.*

## Adverse Effects, Treatment, and Precautions

As for Donepezil, p.1489. Rivastigmine is not recommended for use in patients with severe hepatic impairment.

## Interactions

As for Neostigmine, p.1492.

## Pharmacokinetics

Rivastigmine is readily absorbed from the gastrointestinal tract and peak plasma concentrations are reached in about one hour. Food delays absorption by about 1.5 hours and reduces maximum plasma concentrations. Rivastigmine is about 40% bound to plasma proteins and readily crosses the blood-brain barrier. It is rapidly and extensively metabolised, primarily by cholinesterase-mediated hydrolysis to the weakly active decarbamylated metabolite. The plasma half-life of rivastigmine is about one hour and more than 90% of a dose is excreted in the urine within 24 hours. Less than 1% of a dose appears in the faeces.

## Uses and Administration

Rivastigmine is a carbamate type reversible acetylcholinesterase inhibitor; it is also an inhibitor of butyrylcholinesterase. Rivastigmine is selective for the CNS and is used for the symptomatic treatment of mild to moderately severe dementia in Alzheimer's disease (below). It is given as the hydrogen tartrate but doses are expressed in terms of the base; 2.4 mg of rivastigmine hydrogen tartrate is approximately equivalent to 1.5 mg of rivastigmine base. An initial dose is 1.5 mg given twice daily with food. Thereafter, the dose may be increased according to response by increments of 1.5 mg twice daily at intervals of at least 2 weeks to a maximum dose of 6 mg twice daily. If treatment is interrupted for more than a few days, it should be re-initiated at 1.5 mg twice daily, and then increased, if required, as described above. Clinical benefit should be reassessed on a regular basis.

**Dementia.** Studies[1-3] and a systematic review[4] indicate that rivastigmine may be of benefit in the management of patients with mild to moderate *Alzheimer's disease* (see Dementia, p.1484). UK guidelines[5] recommend its use in such patients under specialist supervision, with benefits assessed 2 to 4 months after achieving maintenance dosage and every 6 months thereafter; treatment should only continue where there is evidence of benefit. Rivastigmine given in titrated doses of up to 6 mg twice daily was also found to be well tolerated, and to produce some improvement in behavioural and psychiatric symptoms, in a group of patients with *Lewy-body dementia*.[6]


1. Anand R, *et al.* Efficacy and safety results of the early phase studies with Exelon™ (ENA-713) in Alzheimer's disease: an overview. *J Drug Dev Clin Pract* 1996; **8:** 109–116.
2. Agid Y, *et al.* Efficacy and tolerability of rivastigmine in patients with dementia of the Alzheimer type. *Curr Ther Res* 1998; **59:** 837–45.
3. Rösler M, *et al.* Efficacy and safety of rivastigmine in patients with Alzheimer's disease: international randomised controlled trial. *BMJ* 1999; **318:** 633–8. Correction. *ibid.* 2001; **322:** 1456.
4. Birks J, *et al.* Rivastigmine for Alzheimer's disease. Available in The Cochrane Library; Issue 2. Chichester: John Wiley; 2004.
5. National Institute for Clinical Excellence. Guidance on the use of donepezil, rivastigmine and galantamine for the treatment of Alzheimer's disease (issued January 2001). Available at: http://www.nice.org.uk/pdf/ALZHEIMER_full_guidance.pdf (accessed 15/06/04)
6. McKeith I, *et al.* Efficacy of rivastigmine in dementia with Lewy bodies: a randomised, double-blind, placebo-controlled international study. *Lancet* 2000; **356:** 2031–36.


## Preparations

**Proprietary Preparations** (details are given in Part 3)
***Arg.:*** Exelon; ***Austral.:*** Exelon; ***Austria:*** Exelon; ***Belg.:*** Exelon; ***Braz.:*** Exelon; Prometax; ***Canad.:*** Exelon; ***Chile:*** Exelon; ***Denm.:*** Exelon; ***Fin.:*** Exelon; ***Fr.:*** Exelon; ***Ger.:*** Exelon; ***Gr.:*** Exelon; ***Hong Kong:*** Exelon; ***India:*** Exelon; ***Irl.:*** Exelon; ***Israel:*** Exelon; ***Ital.:*** Exelon; Prometax; ***Malaysia:*** Exelon; ***Mex.:*** Exelon; ***Neth.:*** Exelon; ***Norw.:*** Exelon; ***NZ:*** Exelon; ***Port.:*** Exelon; Prometax; ***S.Afr.:*** Exelon; ***Singapore:*** Exelon; ***Spain:*** Exelon; Prometax; ***Swed.:*** Exelon; ***Switz.:*** Exelon; ***Thai.:*** Exelon; ***UK:*** Exelon; ***USA:*** Exelon.

# Tacrine Hydrochloride

*(BANM, USAN, rINNM)*

CI-970; Hidrocloruro de tacrina; Tetrahydroaminoacridine Hydrochloride; THA. 1,2,3,4-Tetrahydroacridin-9-ylamine hydrochloride.

$C_{13}H_{14}N_2,HCl$ = 234.7.
*CAS — 321-64-2 (tacrine); 1684-40-8 (tacrine hydrochloride).*
*ATC — N06DA01.*

**Pharmacopoeias.** In *US* as the monohydrate.

**USP 27** (Tacrine Hydrochloride). The monohydrate occurs as a white powder. Freely soluble in water, in alcohol, in dimethyl sulfoxide, in methyl alcohol, in propylene glycol, and in 0.1N hydrochloric acid; sparingly soluble in linoleic acid and in macrogol 400.

## Adverse Effects and Treatment

As for Donepezil, p.1489. Hepatotoxicity is common, and may be severe.

**Effects on the CNS.** A report of tonic or tonic-clonic seizures in 6 of 78 patients given tacrine for mild or moderate dementia of the Alzheimer's type.[1]


1. Lebert F, *et al.* Convulsive effects of tacrine *Lancet* 1996; **347:** 1339–40.


**Effects on the liver.** Examination of data from 2446 patients aged at least 50 years who received tacrine for Alzheimer's disease suggested that raised serum-alanine aminotransferase (ALT) concentrations are likely to occur in about 50% of patients.[1] Most cases developed within the first 12 weeks of therapy,[1] but an asymptomatic increase in ALT concentrations has been reported in a patient after more than 80 weeks of therapy.[2] The increase is usually asymptomatic and mild, and resolves upon dosage reduction or discontinuation of treatment. However, a small percentage of patients may develop unpredictable life-threatening hepatotoxicity although frequent monitoring of ALT concentrations during the first 12 weeks of therapy can identify susceptible individuals. No significant correlation has been found between plasma-tacrine concentrations and hepatotoxicity.[3]

For guidelines on the monitoring of ALT concentrations during tacrine therapy, see Precautions, below.


1. Watkins PB, *et al.* Hepatotoxic effects of tacrine administration in patients with Alzheimer's disease. *JAMA* 1994; **271:** 992–8.
2. Terrell PS, *et al.* Late-onset alanine aminotransferase increase with tacrine. *Ann Pharmacother* 1996; **30:** 301.
3. Ford JM, *et al.* Serum concentrations of tacrine hydrochloride predict its adverse effects in Alzheimer's disease. *Clin Pharmacol Ther* 1993; **53:** 691–5.


## Precautions

As for Donepezil, p.1489. Tacrine should be used with care in patients with impaired liver function or who have a history of such impairment.

Serum-alanine aminotransferase (ALT) concentrations should be monitored in patients receiving continuous treatment with tacrine. Monitoring should be carried out every other week from at least week 4 to week 16 of therapy, and then every 3 months thereafter. Weekly monitoring is recommended in patients with ALT concentrations that are greater than twice the upper limit of the normal range.

If signs of liver involvement worsen, the dose should be reduced or the drug withdrawn. If a threefold to fivefold increase of ALT concentrations occurs, a reduction in the dose by 40 mg daily is recommended. For greater increases in ALT, tacrine should be withdrawn. Treatment with tacrine may be reconsidered once signs of liver dysfunction return to normal; more frequent monitoring of liver enzyme values will be required. Withdrawal is also imperative should jaundice develop, confirmed by elevated total bilirubin levels. Patients who develop jaundice should not be treated again with tacrine.

Abruptly stopping tacrine therapy, or a large reduction in the dose, may be associated with behavioural disturbances and a decline in cognitive function.

## Interactions

As for Neostigmine, p.1492. Since tacrine is metabolised in the liver by the cytochrome P450 enzyme system (principally CYP1A2), drugs that either inhibit or induce the same isoenzymes may raise or lower plasma concentrations of tacrine, respectively. Tacrine may competitively inhibit the metabolism of other drugs that are also metabolised by the cytochrome P450 isoenzyme CYP1A2.

**Antidepressants.** *Fluvoxamine*, an inhibitor of the cytochrome P450 isoenzyme CYP1A2, has increased plasma concentrations and reduced oral clearance of tacrine.[1]


1. Becquemont L, *et al.* Influence of the CYP1A2 inhibitor fluvoxamine on tacrine pharmacokinetics in humans. *Clin Pharmacol Ther* 1997; **61:** 619–27.


**$H_2$-antagonists.** *Cimetidine*, a non-specific inhibitor of the cytochrome P450 enzyme system, has been shown to inhibit the metabolism of tacrine resulting in reduced oral clearance and an increase in plasma concentrations.[1,2]


1. de Vries TM. Effect of cimetidine and low-dose quinidine on tacrine pharmacokinetics in humans. *Pharm Res* 1993; **10:** S337.
2. Forgue ST, *et al.* Inhibition of tacrine oral clearance by cimetidine. *Clin Pharmacol Ther* 1996; **59:** 444–9.


**HRT.** HRT with estradiol and levonorgestrel significantly increased tacrine plasma concentrations in all but one person in a study involving 10 healthy female subjects.[1] Metabolism of tacrine via the cytochrome P450 isoenzyme CYP1A2 was said to have been inhibited by the HRT.


1. Laine K, *et al.* Plasma tacrine concentrations are significantly increased by concomitant hormone replacement therapy. *Clin Pharmacol Ther* 1999; **66:** 602–8.


**Tobacco smoking.** Cigarette smoking can markedly reduce plasma-tacrine concentrations.[1]


1. Welty D, *et al.* The effect of smoking on the pharmacokinetics and metabolism of Cognex® in healthy volunteers. *Pharm Res* 1993; **10:** S334.


**Xanthines.** For the effect of tacrine on the metabolism of *theophylline*, see p.803.

## Pharmacokinetics

Tacrine is rapidly absorbed from the gastrointestinal tract but large interindividual variations in oral bioavailability and the time to achieve peak plasma concentrations have been reported. Food reduces the absorption of tacrine by about 30 to 40%. Tacrine is subject to an extensive first-pass effect in the liver, and is metabolised by the cytochrome P450 system (principally CYP1A2) to several metabolites, the main one of which is the 1-hydroxy metabolite velnacrine. Tacrine is 55% bound to plasma proteins. Little unchanged drug is excreted in urine.

◊ In 3 studies in a total of 21 patients peak plasma concentrations of tacrine hydrochloride were achieved 0.5 to 3 hours after oral doses of 25 or 50 mg and oral bioavailability ranged from less than 5% to up to 36%.[1-3] Mean elimination half-lives were 1.37 and 1.59 hours after the 25 mg dose and 2.14 and 3.2 hours after the 50 mg dose. Tacrine's elimination appears to be mainly by metabolism in the liver and less than 3% of a dose was recovered unchanged in the urine of one patient.[1] Plasma concentrations of tacrine's main metabolite 1-hydroxy-9-aminotetrahydroacridine (velnacrine) rapidly exceed those of the parent compound and elimination half-lives of 43 and 81 minutes were found for this metabolite in 2 patients studied.[2] Tacrine's pharmacokinetics have been reviewed.[4]

1. Forsyth DR, *et al.* Pharmacokinetics of tacrine hydrochloride in Alzheimer's disease. *Clin Pharmacol Ther* 1989; **46:** 634–41.
2. Hartvig P, *et al.* Clinical pharmacokinetics of intravenous and oral 9-amino-1,2,3,4-tetrahydroacridine, tacrine. *Eur J Clin Pharmacol* 1990; **38:** 259–63.
3. Sitar DS, *et al.* Bioavailability and pharmacokinetic disposition of tacrine HCl in elderly patients with Alzheimer's disease. *Clin Pharmacol Ther* 1995; **57:** 198.
4. Madden S, *et al.* Clinical pharmacokinetics of tacrine. *Clin Pharmacokinet* 1995; **28:** 449–57.

## Uses and Administration

Tacrine hydrochloride is a centrally acting reversible cholinesterase inhibitor used in the treatment of mild to moderately severe dementia in Alzheimer's disease (below).

The initial dose of tacrine hydrochloride, expressed in terms of tacrine, is 10 mg four times a day for a minimum of 4 weeks. Dosage should not be increased during this period because the potential exists for a delay in onset of increased liver enzyme concentrations. Serum-alanine aminotransferase concentrations should be monitored regularly (see Precautions, above) and, if there is no significant increase, the daily dose may be increased by 40 mg at four-week intervals until a satisfactory response is obtained, up to a maximum of 160 mg daily in four divided doses. Tacrine should be taken on an empty stomach to improve absorption, although it can be taken with food by patients in whom gastrointestinal adverse effects may be a problem.

Tacrine has been used to antagonise competitive neuromuscular blockers and as a postoperative respiratory stimulant.

**Dementia.** Tacrine is used in the symptomatic management of Alzheimer's disease (see Dementia, p.1484). It may delay cognitive decline in some patients with mild or moderate Alzheimer's disease but many cannot tolerate the dosage required and have to stop treatment because of gastrointestinal effects or signs of hepatotoxicity. There have been numerous studies of the use of tacrine in Alzheimer's disease and a meta-analysis[1] found tacrine to have a small beneficial effect on both cognition and global clinical impression, although it was considered that the clinical relevance of these findings was unclear and that there were no data from long-term controlled studies. Some have considered[2-6] that a cautious trial of tacrine may be warranted in patients with mild to moderately severe Alzheimer's disease (although alternative drugs are now available) and various guidelines on its use have been issued.[5,6] The metabolite velnacrine has also been tried but does not appear to be effective, and is also associated with hepatotoxicity.[7]

1. Qizilbash N, *et al.* Cholinesterase inhibition for Alzheimer disease: a meta-analysis of the tacrine trials. *JAMA* 1998; **280:** 1777–82.
2. Crimson ML. Tacrine: first drug approved for Alzheimer's disease. *Ann Pharmacother* 1994; **28:** 744–51.
3. Davis KL, Powchik P. Tacrine. *Lancet* 1995; **345:** 625–30.
4. Samuels SC, Davis KL. A risk-benefit assessment of tacrine in the treatment of Alzheimer's disease. *Drug Safety* 1997; **16:** 66–77.
5. Lyketsos CG, *et al.* Guidelines for the use of tacrine in Alzheimer's disease: clinical application and effectiveness. *J Neuropsychiatr Clin Neurosci* 1996; **8:** 67–73.
6. American Psychiatric Association. Practice guideline for the treatment of patients with Alzheimer's disease and other dementias of late life. *Am J Psychiatry* 1997; **154** (suppl): 1–39. Also available at: http://www.psych.org/psych_pract/treatg/pg/pg_dementia_32701.cfm (accessed 15/06/04)
7. Birks J, Wilcock GGW. Velnacrine for Alzheimer's disease. Available in The Cochrane Library; Issue 2. Chichester: John Wiley; 2004.

## Preparations

***USP 27:*** Tacrine Capsules.

**Proprietary Preparations** (details are given in Part 3)

***Arg.:*** Cognitiv; ***Austral.:*** Cognex†; THA; ***Austria:*** Cognex†; ***Belg.:*** Cognex†; ***Braz.:*** Cognex†; Tacrinal; ***Fr.:*** Cognex†; ***Ger.:*** Cognex†; ***Gr.:*** Cognex; ***Hong Kong:*** Cognex†; ***Israel:*** Cognex†; ***NZ:*** Cognex†; ***Port.:*** Cognex†; ***Spain:*** Cognex; ***Swed.:*** Cognex†; ***Switz.:*** Cognex†; ***USA:*** Cognex.

## Xanomeline *(USAN, rINN)*

LY-246708; Xanomelina. 3-[4-(Hexyloxy)-1,2,5-thiadiazol-3-yl]-1,2,5,6-tetrahydro-1-methylpyridine.

$C_{14}H_{23}N_3OS = 281.4.$

*CAS — 131986-45-3.*

## Profile

Xanomeline is a selective muscarinic $M_1$ agonist. Xanomeline tartrate has been studied in the management of Alzheimer's disease but drugs of this type have not generally produced benefit.

◊ References.

1. Sramek JJ, *et al.* The safety and tolerance of xanomeline tartrate in patients with Alzheimer's disease. *J Clin Pharmacol* 1995; **35:** 800–806.
2. Bodick NC, *et al.* Effects of xanomeline, a selective muscarinic receptor agonist, on cognitive function and behavioral symptoms in Alzheimer disease. *Arch Neurol* 1997; **54:** 465–73.

# Pesticides and Repellents

Pediculosis, p.1499
Scabies, p.1499
Vector control, p.1500

This chapter describes compounds used as pesticides and as insect repellents. The term pesticide covers fungicides, herbicides, insecticides (including acaricides), molluscicides, and rodenticides, among others. Most of the pesticides included here are used in clinical or veterinary practice or in vector control against human or animal disease. Some are used primarily in an agricultural or horticultural setting and are included because of their potential toxicity.

Pesticides can be absorbed during application, by consumption of treated or contaminated products or by accidental contamination, and they may be stored or retained in the tissues. International regulations and controls operate to reduce the risk to both public and user. Values for acceptable daily intakes of pesticides have been published by the Food and Agriculture Organization of the United Nations and the World Health Organization (WHO) through the WHO Technical Report series of publications or through *Pesticides Residues in Food: yearly evaluations*, FAO Plant Production and Protection Papers, Rome.

Classification of the main pesticides included in this chapter is given in Table 1, below.

The **fungicides** included in this chapter are some of those used in the management of plant disease.

**Herbicides** are used for weed control both in the domestic setting and professionally in agriculture and horticulture. Those here have been included primarily because they are toxic and have been associated with many cases of poisoning.

**Insect repellents** can help to avoid insect bites and the unpleasant reactions they may produce. Perhaps more importantly, the correct use of insect repellents plays a major role in personal protection against a number of communicable diseases transmitted by insect vectors. Examples are babesiosis (ticks), Lyme disease (ticks), malaria (mosquitoes), relapsing fevers (lice and ticks), spotted fevers (ticks), and typhus fever (fleas, lice, and mites). Some compounds, such as diethyltoluamide and dimethyl phthalate, are effective as repellents while others, such as benzyl benzoate and some of the pyrethroids, are effective both as repellents and as insecticides.

**Insecticides** have numerous applications. They are used in the treatment of ectoparasitic infections such as pediculosis (lice infections) (below) and in the vector control (below) of a number of communicable diseases that are spread by insects. Acaricides are used to treat scabies (mite infections) (see, below) and are included within the broad classification of insecticides, although acari (mites) are not, technically, insects. Insecticides are also widely used in veterinary practice and in agriculture and horticulture.

The insecticides used in veterinary practice are often classified as topical or systemic ectoparasiticides. Topical ectoparasiticides are applied topically to the host animal (such as dogs or cats) to kill its ectoparasites (such as fleas). In the case of systemic ectoparasiticides the term 'systemic' refers to the ingestion of the insecticide by the ectoparasite from the host's blood; the insecticide may be present in the host's blood either as a result of absorption through the skin after topical application or after systemic administration.

**Molluscicides** are used in agriculture or horticulture or in the domestic garden to control snail and slug pests. Additionally, molluscicides such as niclosamide (described in the Anthelmintics chapter on p.110) are used against the freshwater snail vector *Bulinus* in the control of schistosomiasis.

**Rodenticides** may be used to exterminate rats and mice which may be vectors for diseases such as leptospirosis, plague, rat-bite fever, and some haemorrhagic fevers. Many rodenticides are anticoagulants. Warfarin (p.1022) is a commonly used rodenticide.

**Table 1.** Classification of pesticides.

| | |
|---|---|
| Fungicides | Benomyl, cicloheximide, hexachlorobenzene, pentachlorophenol |
| Herbicides | Dichlorophenoxyacetic acid, dinitro-*o*-cresol, dinitrophenol, diquat, glyphosate, paraquat, pentachlorophenol, trichlorophenoxyacetic acid |
| Insect repellents | Butopyronoxyl, dibutyl phthalate, diethyltoluamide, dimethyl phthalate, dioctyl adipate, ethohexadiol, piperonal |
| Insecticides | |
| Carbamate | Bendiocarb, carbaryl, carbosulfan, methomyl, propoxur |
| Chlorinated | Chlordane, clofenotane, dieldrin, endosulfan, endrin, heptachlor, lindane, methoxychlor |
| Organophosphorus | Azamethiphos, bromophos, chlorpyrifos, clofenvinfos, coumafos, cythioate, dichlorvos, dimethoate, dimpylate, dioxation, ethion, famphur, fenitrothion, fenthion, heptenophos, iodofenphos, malathion, naled, parathion, phosmet, phoxim, pirimiphos-methyl, propetamphos, pyraclofos, temefos |
| Pyrethroid | Alpha-cypermethrin, bioallethrin, cyfluthrin, cyhalothrin, cypermethrin, deltamethrin, esdepallethrine, etofenprox, fenvalerate, flumethrin, permethrin, phenothrin, pyrethrum flower, resmethrin, tetramethrin |
| Miscellaneous | Amitraz, benzyl benzoate, chloropicrin, copper oleate, cymiazole, cyromazine, diflubenzuron, emamectin, ethylene dibromide, ethylene dichloride, fipronil, fluazuron, fluvalinate, lufenuron, methoprene, methyl bromide, pyriproxyfen, rotenone, sulfiram, triflumuron |
| Molluscicides | Endod, metaldehyde, pentachlorophenol |
| Rodenticides | Aluminium phosphide, antu, brodifacoum, bromadiolone, chloralose, chlorophacinone, coumatetralyl, difenacoum, diphenadione, flocoumafen, fluoroacetamide, norbormide, red squill, sodium fluoroacetate |

## Clinical Uses of Pesticides and Repellents

### Pediculosis

Two species of louse cause pediculosis in man; these are *Pediculus humanus* with its two varieties, *Pediculus humanus capitis* (the head louse) and *Pediculus humanus humanus* (the body louse), and *Pthirus pubis* (*Phthirus pubis*) (the pubic or crab louse). Unlike the head louse, the body louse is an important vector for a number of infections including epidemic typhus (p.152), trench fever (p.150), and relapsing fever (p.143).

Insecticides used in the treatment of pediculosis include malathion, and some pyrethroids such as bioallethrin, permethrin, phenothrin, and tetramethrin. Carbaryl is also effective, although there has been some concern over a theoretical risk of carcinogenicity. Lindane has been used for pubic lice, but many strains of head lice are resistant.

In the UK it has been common for the recommended drugs for the treatment of head lice to be rotated periodically to reduce the emergence of resistance, a problem observed with the newer pyrethroids as well as older insecticides such as lindane, although the value of such rotation policies is debatable. Lotions are preferred to shampoos for head lice since contact time with the insecticide is longer and treatment is thus more effective. Treatment is usually repeated after 7 days. Egg cases ('nits') can be removed by combing the wet hair with a fine tooth comb. A head louse repellent containing piperonal is available.

Malathion has also been suggested for treatment of infestation of the eye lashes and brows with pubic lice (pthiriasis or phthiriasis palpebrarum). Other treatments have included the application of a thick layer of yellow soft paraffin or application of yellow mercuric oxide 1% eye ointment twice daily for about 7 or 8 days or a single application of fluorescein eye drops.

Clothing and bed linen of persons with body lice should be washed in hot water or dry cleaned and ironed.

Topical or systemic antimicrobials should be given as necessary for secondary infections.

References.

1. Burgess IF. Human lice and their management. *Adv Parasitol* 1995; **36:** 271–342.
2. Chosidow O. Scabies and pediculosis. *Lancet* 2000; **355:** 819–26.
3. Roos TC, *et al.* Pharmacotherapy of ectoparasitic infections. *Drugs* 2001; **61:** 1067–88.
4. Dodd CS. Interventions for treating headlice. Available in The Cochrane Library; Issue 1. Chichester: John Wiley; 2004.

### Scabies

Scabies is a parasitic infection of the skin by the mite *Sarcoptes scabiei*. The predominant symptom is pruritus, which is caused by an allergic reaction to the parasite and may not occur until several weeks after infection for the first time. Subsequent infections usually result in pruritus after a few days. Pruritus may persist for some months after effective treatment with an acaricide, but is not necessarily an indication for further acaricidal treatment; rather, antipruritics should be used. A severe crusted form (Norwegian scabies) may occur rarely, particularly in immunocompromised or incapacitated patients.

Treatment is with the acaricides permethrin or malathion applied, preferably as aqueous lotions, to clean, cool, dry skin over the entire body and left on for 8 to 24 hours, depending upon the preparation. The preparation should be reapplied to the hands whenever they are washed during this period. In adults, it is not usually necessary to treat the face and scalp, but these areas should be treated in young children or patients with atypical or crusted scabies. A single treatment is usually effective, but treatment may be repeated after 7 to 10 days if necessary. Close family and personal contacts should be treated at the same time. Other drugs used topically in the treatment of scabies include benzyl benzoate, crotamiton, lindane, and sulfur; sulfiram is used in combination with benzyl benzoate. A single oral dose of ivermectin may be effective.

In addition to treatment with an acaricide, symptomatic treatment of the itching with crotamiton, calamine lotion, or systemic antihistamines or corticosteroids may be required.

References.


1. Elgart ML. A risk-benefit assessment of agents used in the treatment of scabies. *Drug Safety* 1996; **14:** 386–93.
2. Chosidow O. Scabies and pediculosis. *Lancet* 2000; **355:** 819–26.
3. Roos TC, *et al.* Pharmacotherapy of ectoparasitic infections. *Drugs* 2001; **61:** 1067–88.
4. Walker GJA, Johnstone PW. Interventions for treating scabies. Available in The Cochrane Library; Issue 1. Chichester: John Wiley; 2004.


## Vector control

Many pests are involved in the transmission of communicable diseases, and vector control[1,2] is an important part of the fight against such diseases. Insecticides are used in the control of filariasis (p.100) (*Aedes, Anopheles, Culex,* and *Mansonia* mosquitoes);[3] leishmaniasis (p.597) (*Phlebotomus* or *Lutzomyia* sandflies);[4] malaria (p.444) (*Anopheles* mosquitoes);[5-8] onchocerciasis (p.100) (*Simulium* blackflies);[9] African trypanosomiasis (p.599) (*Glossina* tsetse flies);[10] and American trypanosomiasis (p.600) (*Triatoma* bugs).[11] The insecticide temefos is useful in dracunculiasis (p.98) (crustacean host to the guinea worm larvae). In some cases, as in filariasis or onchocerciasis, the insecticides used act primarily against the larval stage of the insect vector, whereas in other situations, as in malaria, activity is against the adult insect; in trypanosomiasis, activity is directed against both adult and immature stages. The majority of the experience gained in insecticidal vector control has probably been in malaria, and, for instance, a positive effect seen in the control of leishmaniasis has been considered to be mainly a byproduct of the concomitant malaria control programmes.

Insect repellents can provide personal protection against many insect vectors. For example, in malaria, insect repellents as well as the use of insecticides are important in preventing mosquito bites.

Molluscicides are used in the control of schistosomiasis (p.100) (*Bulinus* snails).[12]

Rodenticides are also extremely valuable in the vector control of some diseases such as leptospirosis (p.133), plague (p.141), rat-bite fever (p.121), and some haemorrhagic fevers (p.618).


1. Chavasse DC, Yap HH, eds. *Chemical methods for the control of vectors and pests of public health importance.* Geneva: WHO, 1997.
2. Rozendaal JA. *Vector control: methods for use by individuals and communities.* Geneva: WHO, 1997.
3. WHO. Lymphatic filariasis: the disease and its control. *WHO Tech Rep Ser 821* 1992.
4. WHO. Control of the leishmaniases. *WHO Tech Rep Ser 793* 1990.
5. WHO. Vector control for malaria and other mosquito-borne diseases. *WHO Tech Rep Ser 857* 1995.
6. WHO. *Malaria vector control: insecticides for indoor residual spraying.* Geneva: WHO, 2001.
7. WHO. *International travel and health.* Geneva: WHO, 2003.
8. Lengeler C. Insecticide-treated bednets and curtains for preventing malaria. Available in The Cochrane Library; Issue 1. Chichester: John Wiley; 2004.
9. WHO. Report of a WHO expert committee on onchocerciasis control. *WHO Tech Rep Ser 852* 1995.
10. WHO. Control and surveillance of African trypanosomiasis: report of a WHO expert committee. *WHO Tech Rep Ser 881* 1998.
11. WHO. Control of Chagas disease: second report of the WHO expert committee. *WHO Tech Rep Ser 905* 2002.
12. WHO. The control of schistosomiasis: second report of the WHO expert committee. *WHO Tech Rep Ser 830* 1993.


## Aluminium Phosphide

Aluminum Phosphide; Fosfuro de aluminio.

AlP = 57.96.

*CAS — 20859-73-8 (aluminium phosphide); 7803-51-2 (phosphine); 1314-84-7 (zinc phosphide).*

### Profile

Aluminium phosphide is used for the fumigation of grain and as a rodenticide. It releases phosphine ($PH_3$) in the presence of moisture and this accounts for its pesticidal activity. Phosphine gas has a garlic-like odour repulsive to man and domestic animals but apparently not to *rats.* Zinc phosphide is used similarly.

◊ References to poisoning associated with aluminium phosphide.


1. Wilson R, *et al.* Acute phosphine poisoning aboard a grain freighter. *JAMA* 1980; **244:** 148–50.
2. Singh S, *et al.* Aluminium phosphide ingestion. *BMJ* 1985; **290:** 1110–11.
3. Anger F, *et al.* Fatal aluminium phosphide poisoning. *J Anal Toxicol* 2000; **24:** 90–2.
4. Nocera A, *et al.* Dangerous bodies: a case of fatal aluminium phosphide poisoning. *Med J Aust* 2000; **173:** 133–5.
5. Popp W, *et al.* Phosphine poisoning in a German office. *Lancet* 2002; **359:** 1574.


## Amitraz *(BAN, USAN, pINN)*

U-36059. *N,N'*-[(Methylimino)dimethylidyne]di-2,4-xylidine.

$C_{19}H_{23}N_3$ = 293.4.

*CAS — 33089-61-1.*

**Pharmacopoeias.** In *BP(Vet).* Also in *US* for veterinary use only.

**BP(Vet) 2003** (Amitraz). A white to buff powder. Practically insoluble in water; decomposes slowly in alcohol; freely soluble in acetone.

### Profile

Amitraz is used as a topical ectoparasiticide in veterinary practice. It is effective against various lice, mites, and ticks.

◊ References to poisoning with amitraz.


1. Jorens PG, *et al.* An unusual poisoning with the unusual pesticide amitraz. *Hum Exp Toxicol* 1997; **16:** 600–1.
2. Aydin K, *et al.* Amitraz poisoning in children: clinical and laboratory findings of eight cases. *Hum Exp Toxicol* 1997; **16:** 680–2.
3. Leung VK, *et al.* Amitraz poisoning in humans. *J Toxicol Clin Toxicol* 1999; **37:** 513–14.
4. Yaramis A, *et al.* Amitraz poisoning in children. *Hum Exp Toxicol* 2000; **19:** 431–3.
5. Yilmaz HL, Yildizdas DR. Amitraz poisoning, an emerging problem: epidemiology, clinical features, management, and preventive strategies. *Arch Dis Child* 2003; **88:** 130–4.


## Antu

1-(1-Naphthyl)-2-thiourea; α-Naphthylthiourea.

$C_{11}H_{10}N_2S$ = 202.3.

*CAS — 86-88-4.*

### Profile

Antu was formerly used as a rodenticide. The carcinogenic risk from naphthylamine impurities restricted its use.

## Azamethiphos *(BAN)*

Azametifós; CGA-18809; OMS-1825. S-[(6-Chloro-2,3-dihydro-2-oxo-1,3-oxazolo[4,5-*b*]pyridin-3-yl)methyl] *O,O*-dimethyl phosphorothioate.

$C_9H_{10}ClN_2O_5PS$ = 324.7.

*CAS — 35575-96-3.*

### Profile

Azamethiphos is an organophosphorus insecticide (p.1507) used in veterinary practice for the control of sea-lice infestation in salmon and for the control of ectoparasites in the environment.

## Bendiocarb

2,3-Isopropylidenedioxyphenyl methylcarbamate.

$C_{11}H_{13}NO_4$ = 223.2.

*CAS — 22781-23-3.*

### Profile

Bendiocarb is a carbamate insecticide (p.1501) for agricultural and household use.

## Benomyl

Benomilo. Methyl 1-(butylcarbamoyl)benzimidazol-2-ylcarbamate.

$C_{14}H_{18}N_4O_3$ = 290.3.

*CAS — 17804-35-2.*

### Profile

Benomyl is a fungicide used for the treatment and control of fungal plant diseases.

◊ References.


1. Benomyl. *Environmental Health Criteria 148.* Geneva: WHO, 1993. Available at: http://www.inchem.org/documents/ehc/ehc/ehc148.htm (accessed 23/04/04)
2. Benomyl health and safety guide. *IPCS Health and Safety Guide 81.* Geneva: WHO, 1993. Available at: http://www.inchem.org/documents/hsg/hsg/hsg81_e.htm (accessed 23/04/04)


**Toxicity.** Although experimental evidence in *animals* has suggested a possible link between benomyl and congenital eye defects (anophthalmia) the association could not be substantiated in humans.[1-4]


1. Gilbert R. "Clusters" of anophthalmia in Britain. *BMJ* 1993; **307:** 340–1.
2. Bianchi F, *et al.* Clusters of anophthalmia. *BMJ* 1994; **308:** 205.
3. Kristensen P, Irgens LM. Clusters of anophthalmia. *BMJ* 1994; **308:** 205–6.
4. Castilla EE. Clusters of anophthalmia. *BMJ* 1994; **308:** 206.


## Benzyl Benzoate

Benzoato de bencilo; Benzoato de Benzilo; Benzoesäurebenzylester; Benzyl Benz.; Benzylis Benzoas.

$C_6H_5.CO.O.CH_2.C_6H_5$ = 212.2.

*CAS — 120-51-4.*

*ATC — P03AX01.*

**Pharmacopoeias.** In *Eur.* (see p.vi), *Int., Jpn,* and *US.*

**Ph. Eur. 5.0** (Benzyl Benzoate). Colourless or almost colourless crystals, or a colourless or almost colourless oily liquid. F.p. is not below 17°. Practically insoluble in water; miscible with alcohol, with dichloromethane, and with fatty and essential oils. Store in well-filled airtight containers. Protect from light.

**USP 27** (Benzyl Benzoate). A clear, colourless, oily liquid with a slight aromatic odour. Practically insoluble in water and in glycerol; miscible with alcohol, with chloroform, and with ether. Store at a temperature not exceeding 40° in well-filled airtight containers. Protect from light.

### Adverse Effects and Treatment

Benzyl benzoate is irritant to the eyes and mucous membranes and it may be irritant to the skin. Hypersensitivity reactions have been reported. If ingested, benzyl benzoate may cause stimulation of the CNS and convulsions. Systemic symptoms have been reported following excessive topical use. Gastric lavage should be considered after ingestion of very large amounts if the patient presents within 1 hour. For poisoning associated with topical use the skin should be washed. Appropriate symptomatic measures should also be instituted.

### Uses and Administration

Benzyl benzoate is an acaricide used in the treatment of scabies (p.1499) although other treatments are generally preferred. A 25% emulsion is applied to the whole body, usually from the neck down; if the application is thorough, one treatment may suffice, although the possibility of failure is lessened by a second application within 5 days. Alternatively, three applications at 12-hour intervals, without bathing, may be made, followed by bathing 12 hours after the last application. Another alternative regimen recommended by the *British National Formulary* is one application to the whole body, repeated, without bathing, on the next day, and washed off 24 hours later; a third application may sometimes be necessary. Benzyl benzoate is not generally recommended for infants and children, but if used the application should be diluted to minimise the risk of irritation, although this also reduces efficacy.

Benzyl benzoate has also been used as a pediculicide.

Benzyl benzoate is also used as a solubilising agent.

### Preparations

***BP 2003:*** Benzyl Benzoate Application;
***USP 27:*** Benzyl Benzoate Lotion.

**Proprietary Preparations** (details are given in Part 3)
***Austral.:*** Ascabiol; Benzemul; ***Braz.:*** Acarsan; Benzibel; Benzoax; Benzoben; Benzocan; Benzotizan; Miticocan; Parasimed; Pruridol; Sarnaton; Sarnigal†; Sarnisan†; Sarnodex; Scabenzil; Scabioid; Zilaben; ***Ger.:*** Acaril; Acarosan; Antiscabiosum; ***Irl.:*** Ascabiol; ***Israel:*** Scabiex; ***Ital.:*** Mom Lozione Preventiva; ***Mex.:*** Ansar; Escacin†; ***Port.:*** Acarilbial; Neo-Acarina; ***S.Afr.:*** Ascabiol; ***UK:*** Ascabiol.

**Multi-ingredient:** ***Arg.:*** Anusol Duo S; Anusol-A; Arnecrem; Detebencil; Perbel; Permecil; Sapucai; Scabioderm; ***Austral.:*** Anusol; ***Belg.:*** Pulmex; Pulmex Baby; ***Braz.:*** Anusol-HC; Benzilol†; ***Fr.:*** Allerbiocid S; Ascabiol; Sanytol; ***Hong Kong:*** Anusol-HC†; ***Irl.:*** Anugesic-HC; Anusol-HC; Sudocrem†; ***Ital.:*** Antiscabbia Candioli al DDT Terapeutico; Dekar 2; Mom Zanzara†; ***Malaysia:*** Anusol; ***Mex.:*** Scabisan Plus; ***NZ:*** Anusol; ***S.Afr.:*** Anugesic; Anusol-HC†; ***Singapore:*** Anusol; ***Spain:*** Tulgrasum Cicatrizante; Yacutin; ***Swed.:*** Tenutex; ***Thai.:*** Anusol; ***UK:*** Anugesic-HC; Anusol-HC, Plus HC; Sudocrem; ***USA:*** Anumed; Anumed HC; Hemril.

## Bioallethrin *(BAN)*

Allethrin I; Bioaletrina; Depallethrin. (*RS*)-3-Allyl-2-methyl-4-oxocyclopent-2-enyl (1*R*,3*R*)-2,2-dimethyl-3-(2-methylprop-1-enyl)cyclopropanecarboxylate.

$C_{19}H_{26}O_3$ = 302.4.

*CAS — 584-79-2 (RS-bioallethrin); 28434-00-6 (S-bioallethrin).*

*ATC — P03AC02.*

### Profile

Bioallethrin is a pyrethroid insecticide (see Pyrethrum Flower, p.1509). It is used topically, with the synergist piperonyl butoxide (p.1509), in the treatment of pediculosis (p.1499). It is also used in anti-mosquito devices and for the control of household insect pests.

◊ References.


1. Allethrins. *Environmental Health Criteria 87.* Geneva: WHO, 1989. Available at: http://www.inchem.org/documents/ehc/ehc/ehc87.htm (accessed 23/04/04)
2. Allethrins health and safety guide. *IPCS Health and Safety Guide 24.* Geneva: WHO, 1989. Available at: http://www.inchem.org/documents/hsg/hsg/hsg024.htm (accessed 23/04/04)


### Preparations

**Proprietary Preparations** (details are given in Part 3)
***UK:*** Actomite.

**Multi-ingredient:** ***Arg.:*** Limpacid; Para Piojicida; Scabioderm; ***Austral.:*** Paralice; ***Belg.:*** Para; ***Braz.:*** Sarnapen; ***Canad.:*** Para; ***Denm.:*** Para†; ***Fr.:*** Para Special Poux; ***Ger.:*** Jacutin N; Spregal; ***Israel:*** Monocide†; ***Ital.:*** Cruzzy; ***Neth.:*** Para-Speciaal.

## Brodifacoum

Brodifacum; WBA-8119. 3-[3-(4'-Bromobiphenyl-4-yl)-1,2,3,4-tetrahydro-1-naphthyl]-4-hydroxycoumarin.

$C_{31}H_{23}BrO_3$ = 523.4.

*CAS — 56073-10-0.*

### Profile

Brodifacoum is an anticoagulant rodenticide. It is reported to be effective in warfarin-resistant strains of rodents.

◊ References.

1. Anticoagulant rodenticides. *Environmental Health Criteria 175.* Geneva: WHO, 1995. Available at: http://www.inchem.org/documents/ehc/ehc/ehc175.htm (accessed 23/04/04)
2. Brodifacoum health and safety guide. *IPCS Health and Safety Guide 93.* Geneva: WHO, 1995. Available at: http://www.inchem.org/documents/hsg/hsg/hsg093.htm (accessed 23/04/04)

**Toxicity.** Brodifacoum, a second-generation anticoagulant rodenticide, inhibits prothrombin synthesis to cause bleeding that may be occult.[1] It is absorbed from the gastrointestinal tract; dermal absorption is possible. Poisons containing 100 mg in each kg of bait are not hazardous to man; more concentrated forms are particularly hazardous and their availability should be restricted. Baits, which should be prepared only by trained personnel, should contain a suitable marker-dye.

There have been reports of poisoning with brodifacoum.[2-7]

1. WHO. Safe use of pesticides: ninth report of the WHO expert committee on vector biology and control. *WHO Tech Rep Ser 720* 1985.
2. Watts RG, *et al.* Accidental poisoning with a superwarfarin compound (brodifacoum) in a child. *Pediatrics* 1990; **86:** 883–7.
3. Ross GS, *et al.* An acquired hemorrhagic disorder from long-acting rodenticide ingestion. *Arch Intern Med* 1992; **152:** 410–12.
4. Kruse JA, Carlson RW. Fatal rodenticide poisoning with brodifacoum. *Ann Emerg Med* 1992; **21:** 331–6.
5. Tecimer C, Yam LT. Surreptitious superwarfarin poisoning with brodifacoum. *South Med J* 1997; **90:** 1053–5.
6. Corke PJ. Superwarfarin (brodifacoum) poisoning. *Anaesth Intensive Care* 1997; **25:** 707–9.
7. La Rosa FG, *et al.* Brodifacoum intoxication with marijuana smoking. *Arch Pathol Lab Med* 1997; **121:** 67–9.

## Bromadiolone

Bromadiolona. 3-[3-(4′-Bromobiphenyl-4-yl)-3-hydroxy-1-phenylpropyl]-4-hydroxycoumarin.

$C_{30}H_{23}BrO_4$ = 527.4.

*CAS — 28772-56-7.*

### Profile

Bromadiolone is an anticoagulant rodenticide.

◊ References.

1. Anticoagulant rodenticides. *Environmental Health Criteria 175.* Geneva: WHO, 1995. Available at: http://www.inchem.org/documents/ehc/ehc/ehc175.htm (accessed 23/04/04)
2. Bromadiolone health and safety guide. *IPCS Health and Safety Guide 94.* Geneva: WHO, 1995. Available at: http://www.inchem.org/documents/hsg/hsg/hsg094.htm (accessed 23/04/04)

**Toxicity.** Bromadiolone, a second-generation anticoagulant rodenticide, inhibits prothrombin synthesis to cause bleeding that may be occult.[1] It is absorbed from the gastrointestinal tract; dermal absorption is possible. Poisons containing 100 mg in each kg of bait are not hazardous to man; more concentrated forms are particularly hazardous and their availability should be restricted. Baits, which should be prepared only by trained personnel, should contain a suitable marker-dye.

There have been reports of poisoning with bromadiolone.[2]

1. WHO. Safe use of pesticides: ninth report of the WHO expert committee on vector biology and control. *WHO Tech Rep Ser 720* 1985.
2. Greeff MC, *et al.* "Superwarfarin" (bromodialone) poisoning in two children resulting in prolonged anticoagulation. *Lancet* 1987; **ii:** 1269.

## Bromophos

Bromofós; OMS-658. O-4-Bromo-2,5-dichlorophenyl O,O-dimethyl phosphorothioate.

$C_8H_8BrCl_2O_3PS$ = 366.0.

*CAS — 2104-96-3.*

### Profile

Bromophos is an organophosphorus insecticide (p.1507) used in veterinary practice for the control of ectoparasites in the environment. It has also been used as an agricultural insecticide.

## Butopyronoxyl

Butopiroxinilo; Indalone. Butyl 3,4-dihydro-2,2-dimethyl-4-oxo-2*H*-pyran-6-carboxylate.

$C_{12}H_{18}O_4$ = 226.3.

*CAS — 532-34-3.*

### Profile

Butopyronoxyl has been used as an insect repellent.

## Carbamate Insecticides

Insecticidas del grupo de los carbamatos.

**Description.** The carbamate insecticides are *N*-substituted esters of carbamic acid.

◊ References.

1. WHO. Carbamate pesticides: a general introduction. *Environmental Health Criteria 64.* Geneva: WHO, 1986.

### Adverse Effects

As for Organophosphorus Insecticides, p.1507.

The carbamates are cholinesterase inhibitors, differing from the organophosphorus insecticides in that the inhibition they produce is generally less intense and more rapidly reversible. In addition, they do not appear to enter the CNS as readily and severe central effects are therefore uncommon.

### Treatment of Adverse Effects

If substantial amounts of carbamate insecticides have been ingested the use of gastric lavage should be considered if the patient presents within 1 hour. Contaminated clothing should be removed and the skin washed with soap and water. Treatment is largely symptomatic and supportive and includes atropine, but this may not always be necessary due to the rapidly reversible nature of the cholinesterase inhibition produced. Pralidoxime has usually been contra-indicated as some *animal* studies have suggested that it may increase the toxicity of carbamates. However, the evidence is not conclusive and some authorities state that it may be given in severe cases unresponsive to atropine and supportive care.

◊ References.

1. WHO. Safe use of pesticides: fourteenth report of the WHO expert committee on vector biology and control. *WHO Tech Rep Ser 813* 1991.
2. Proudfoot A, ed. *Pesticide poisoning: notes for the guidance of medical practitioners.* 2nd ed. London: DoH, The Stationery Office, 1996.

## Carbaryl *(BAN)*

Carbaril *(pINN)*; Carbarilo; OMS-29. 1-Naphthyl methylcarbamate.

$C_{12}H_{11}NO_2$ = 201.2.

*CAS — 63-25-2.*

**Pharmacopoeias.** In *Br.*

**BP 2003** (Carbaryl). A white to off-white or light grey powder which darkens on exposure to light. Very slightly soluble in water; soluble in alcohol and in acetone. Store at a temperature not exceeding 25°. Protect from light.

### Adverse Effects and Treatment

As for Carbamate Insecticides, above. Carbaryl may be absorbed following ingestion, inhalation, or skin contamination.

Carbaryl has been reported to produce neoplasms in *mice* and *rats* and in late 1995 the UK Department of Health advised that it would be prudent to consider carbaryl as a potential human carcinogen; its medicinal use was limited to prescription only. However, the Department of Health emphasised that the risk was a theoretical one and that any risk from the intermittent use of head lice preparations was likely to be very small.

### Uses and Administration

Carbaryl is a carbamate insecticide (above). It is used as a 0.5 or 1.0% lotion or shampoo in the treatment of head and pubic pediculosis (p.1499). Lotions are generally preferred to shampoos as the contact time is longer. Aqueous lotions are preferred to treat pubic lice because alcoholic lotions are irritant to excoriated skin and the genitalia; aqueous lotions may also be preferable in asthmatic subjects or children to avoid alcoholic fumes. Skin or hair treated with an alcohol-based preparation should be allowed to dry naturally.

Carbaryl is also used as a topical ectoparasiticide in veterinary practice and as an agricultural, horticultural, and household insecticide.

◊ References.

1. Carbaryl health and safety guide. *IPCS Health and Safety Guide 78.* Geneva: WHO, 1993. Available at: http://www.inchem.org/documents/hsg/hsg/hsg78_e.htm (accessed 23/04/04)
2. Carbaryl. *Environmental Health Criteria 153.* Geneva: WHO, 1994. Available at: http://www.inchem.org/documents/ehc/ehc/ehc153.htm (accessed 23/04/04)

### Preparations

***BP 2003:*** Carbaryl Lotion.

**Proprietary Preparations** (details are given in Part 3)

***Irl.:*** Carylderm†; Derbac-C†; ***Israel:*** Carbacide†; Hafif; ***UK:*** Carylderm; Mitchell Expel Anti Lice Spray†.

**Multi-ingredient:** ***Fr.:*** Acarcid perles†.

## Carbosulfan

Carbosulfán. 2,3-Dihydro-2,2-dimethylbenzofuran-7-yl (dibutylaminothio)methylcarbamate.

$C_{20}H_{32}N_2O_3S$ = 380.5.

### Profile

Carbosulfan is a carbamate insecticide (p.1501) used in agriculture and for the larvicidal treatment of rivers in the control of onchocerciasis (p.100).

## Chloralose *(rINN)*

Alphachloralose; Chloralosane; α-Chloralose; Cloralosa; Glucochloral. (*R*)-1,2-*O*-(2,2,2-Trichloroethylidene)-α-D-glucofuranose.

$C_8H_{11}Cl_3O_6$ = 309.5.

*CAS — 15879-93-3.*

### Profile

Chloralose has general properties similar to those of cloral hydrate (p.684), of which it is a derivative. It is used as a rodenticide. It was formerly used for its hypnotic properties.

## Chlordane

Clordano. 1,2,4,5,6,7,8,8-Octachloro-2,3,3a,4,7,7a-hexahydro-4,7-methanoindene.

$C_{10}H_6Cl_8$ = 409.8.

*CAS — 57-74-9.*

### Profile

Chlordane is a chlorinated insecticide (p.1501). Its use is limited, or even prohibited, in some countries because of toxicity due to its persistent nature.

◊ References.

1. Kutz FW, *et al.* A fatal chlordane poisoning. *J Toxicol Clin Toxicol* 1983; **20:** 167–74.
2. Olanoff LS, *et al.* Acute chlordane intoxication. *J Toxicol Clin Toxicol* 1983; **20:** 291–306.
3. Chlordane. *Environmental Health Criteria 34.* Geneva: WHO, 1984. Available at: http://www.inchem.org/documents/ehc/ehc/ehc34.htm (accessed 23/04/04)
4. Chlordane health and safety guide. *IPCS Health and Safety Guide 13.* Geneva: WHO, 1988. Available at: http://www.inchem.org/documents/hsg/hsg/hsg013.htm (accessed 23/04/04)

## Chlorinated Insecticides

Insecticidas clorados.

### Adverse Effects

Chlorinated or organochlorine insecticides form a very wide group and the toxicity of individual members varies considerably. In general these insecticides produce symptoms consistent with CNS stimulation. They may be absorbed through the respiratory and gastrointestinal tracts and through the skin.

Symptoms of acute poisoning include nausea and vomiting, paraesthesia, giddiness, tremors, convulsions, coma, and respiratory failure. Liver, kidney, and myocardial toxicity have been reported. Effects on the blood include agranulocytosis and aplastic anaemia. Symptoms may be complicated by the effects of the solvent.

Chlorinated insecticides have been reported to enhance microsomal hepatic enzyme activity. Skin reactions can occur after contact.

*Polychlorinated biphenyl* (PCB) and terphenyl compounds were formerly used as insecticides in many countries. They accumulate in body fat and are not readily excreted, although they are distributed into breast milk and possibly cross the placenta; because of this and because of accidental contamination they remain a cause for concern. The related polybrominated biphenyl compounds (PBB), which have no insecticidal uses, have also been absorbed by humans following accidental contamination of the food chain.

Some chlorinated insecticides have weak oestrogenic effects; it has been proposed that exposure may increase the risk of breast cancer.

### Treatment of Adverse Effects

If chlorinated insecticides have been ingested gastric lavage may be considered if more than 2 g has been taken and the patient presents within 1 hour. Contaminated clothing should be removed and the skin washed with soap and water. Treatment is largely symptomatic and supportive with treatment of CNS stimulation such as hyperactivity and convulsions.

◊ References.

1. WHO. Safe use of pesticides: fourteenth report of the WHO expert committee on vector biology and control. *WHO Tech Rep Ser 813* 1991.
2. Proudfoot A, ed. Pesticide poisoning: notes for the guidance of medical practitioners. 2nd ed. London: DoH, The Stationery Office, 1996.

### Uses

The chlorinated or organochlorine insecticides were widely used but, because of persistence in man, many have been banned or restricted.

◊ References.

1. WHO. Polychlorinated biphenyls and terphenyls. *Environmental Health Criteria 140.* Geneva: WHO, 1992. Available at: http://www.inchem.org/documents/ehc/ehc/ehc140.htm (accessed 28/05/04)
2. Polychlorinated biphenyls and polychlorinated terphenyls (PCBs and PCTs) health and safety guide. *IPCS Health and Safety Guide 68.* Geneva: WHO, 1992. Available at: http://www.inchem.org/documents/hsg/hsg/hsg68.htm (accessed 28/05/04)

## Chlorophacinone

Clorofacinona; LM-91. 2-[2-(4-Chlorophenyl)-2-phenylacetyl]indane-1,3-dione.

$C_{23}H_{15}ClO_3$ = 374.8.

*CAS — 3691-35-8.*

### Profile

Chlorophacinone is an indanedione derivative used as an anticoagulant rodenticide. It is also reported to uncouple oxidative phosphorylation with consequent stimulation of cellular metabolism which may contribute to its toxicity.

◊ References.


1. Burucoa C, *et al.* Chlorophacinone intoxication: biological and toxicological study. *J Toxicol Clin Toxicol* 1989; **27:** 79–89.
2. Anticoagulant rodenticides. *Environmental Health Criteria 175.* Geneva: WHO, 1995. Available at: http://www.inchem.org/documents/ehc/ehc/ehc175.htm (accessed 28/05/04)


## Chloropicrin

Cloropicrina; Nitrochloroform. Trichloronitromethane.

$CCl_3NO_2$ = 164.4.

*CAS — 76-06-2.*

### Profile

Chloropicrin is a lachrymatory agent with an intense odour. It is intensely irritating to the skin and mucous membranes. It is an insecticide and is used for fumigating stored grain and soil. Chloropicrin is also added to other fumigants as a warning gas.

## Chlorpyrifos *(BAN)*

Clorpirifós. *O,O*-Diethyl *O*-3,5,6-trichloro-2-pyridyl phosphorothioate.

$C_9H_{11}Cl_3NO_3PS$ = 350.6.

*CAS — 2921-88-2.*

### Profile

Chlorpyrifos is an organophosphorus insecticide (p.1507) used in agriculture.

## Cicloheximide *(rINN)*

Cicloheximida; Cycloheximide *(USAN)*; U-4527. 3-{(2*R*)-2-[(1*S*,3*S*,5*S*)-3,5-Dimethyl-2-oxocyclohexyl]-2-hydroxyethyl}glutarimide.

$C_{15}H_{23}NO_4$ = 281.3.

*CAS — 66-81-9.*

### Profile

Cicloheximide is an antimicrobial substance produced by strains of *Streptomyces griseus*. It has antifungal properties and has been used for the treatment and control of certain mycotic plant diseases.

## Clofenotane *(rINN)*

Chlorofenotano; Chlorophenothane; Chlorphenothanum; Clofenotano; DDT; Dichlorodiphenyltrichloroethane; Dichophanum; Dicophane. 1,1,1-Trichloro-2,2-bis(4-chlorophenyl)ethane.

$C_{14}H_9Cl_5$ = 354.5.

*CAS — 50-29-3.*

*ATC — P03AB01.*

**Pharmacopoeias.** In *It.*

### Adverse Effects and Treatment

As for Chlorinated Insecticides, p.1501.

◊ References.


1. DDT and its derivatives. *Environmental Health Criteria 9.* Geneva: WHO, 1979. Available at: http://www.inchem.org/documents/ehc/ehc/ehc009.htm (accessed 28/05/04)
2. DDT and its derivatives—environmental aspects. *Environmental Health Criteria 83.* Geneva: WHO, 1989. Available at: http://www.inchem.org/documents/ehc/ehc/ehc83.htm (accessed 28/05/04)


**Carcinogenicity.** Some small epidemiological studies have suggested that certain organochlorines, namely 1,1-dichloro-2,2-bis(*p*-chlorophenyl)ethylene (DDE), a metabolite of clofenotane, and polychlorinated biphenyls (PCBs), might increase the risk of breast cancer in women. However, re-analysis[1,2] of the available data indicated that an association with breast cancer was unlikely for clofenotane; there was no evidence for an association with the PCBs. Any link between exposure to clofenotane and the development of testicular cancer in men was also refuted[3] following long-term monitoring of populations in Scandinavia.


1. Key T, Reeves G. Organochlorines in the environment and breast cancer. *BMJ* 1994; **308:** 1520–1.
2. van't Veer P, *et al.* DDT (dicophane) and postmenopausal breast cancer in Europe: case-control study. *BMJ* 1997; **315:** 81–5.
3. Ekbom A, *et al.* DDT and testicular cancer. *Lancet* 1996; **347:** 553–4.


**Effects on fertility.** A metabolite of clofenotane, 1,1-dichloro-2,2-bis(*p*-chlorophenyl)ethylene (DDE), was reported[1] to have anti-androgenic properties in *rats* and exposure to clofenotane might account for a previously reported decline in male fertility and an increase in male reproductive abnormalities.


1. Keke WR, *et al.* Persistent DDT metabolite p,p′-DDE is a potent androgen receptor antagonist. *Nature* 1995; **375:** 581–5.


**Effects on the nervous system.** A retrospective study[1] found that retired malaria workers exposed long-term to clofenotane did less well in neurobehavioural tests than a control group, and had an increase in neuropsychological and psychiatric symptoms.


1. van Wendel de Joode B, *et al.* Chronic nervous-system effects of long-term occupational exposure to DDT. *Lancet* 2001; **357:** 1014–16.


**Pregnancy.** In a large prospective study[1] of children born between 1959 and 1966, an association was found between preterm births and small-for-gestational-age babies, and maternal concentrations of a metabolite of clofenotane, 1,1-dichloro-2,2-bis(*p*-chlorophenyl)ethylene (DDE) measured in serum samples which had been stored during pregnancy.


1. Longnecker MP, *et al.* Association between maternal serum concentration of the DDT metabolite DDE and preterm and small-for-gestational-age babies at birth. *Lancet* 2001; **358:** 110–14.


### Pharmacokinetics

Clofenotane may be absorbed after ingestion or inhalation or through the skin. Clofenotane is stored in the body, particularly in body fat, and is very slowly eliminated. It crosses the placenta and appears in breast milk. It is metabolised in the body to the ethylene derivative, 1,1-dichloro-2,2-bis(*p*-chlorophenyl)ethylene (DDE); the acetic acid derivative (DDA) also appears in the urine.

### Uses

Clofenotane is a chlorinated insecticide (p.1501). It is a stomach and contact poison and retains its activity for long periods under a variety of conditions. It is effective against disease vectors such as fleas, lice, and mosquitoes and has been applied topically for pediculosis (p.1499) and scabies (p.1499), although more suitable alternatives exist.

Because of the extreme persistence of clofenotane, concern over its effect in the environment, and the problem of resistance, the widespread use of clofenotane is now generally discouraged. It is no longer used in some countries while in others its use is limited.

◊ Despite reservations regarding the use of clofenotane for vector control, many countries have relied on it for the control of both malaria and visceral leishmaniasis. WHO has concluded[1,2] that clofenotane might be used provided that all the following conditions were met: that it was used only for indoor spraying; that it was known to be effective; that it was manufactured to WHO's specifications; and that the necessary safety precautions were taken in its use and disposal. However, they recommended further investigation of the effects of clofenotane in breast milk and of suspected carcinogenicity, as well as clarification of the significance of the reduced density of muscarinic receptors caused by clofenotane.


1. WHO. Vector control for malaria and other mosquito-borne diseases. *WHO Tech Rep Ser 857* 1995.
2. WHO. WHO expert committee on malaria: twentieth report. *WHO Tech Rep Ser 892* 2000.


### Preparations

**Proprietary Preparations** (details are given in Part 3)

**Multi-ingredient:** ***Ital.:*** Antiscabbia Candioli al DDT Terapeutico.

## Clofenvinfos *(BAN, rINN)*

Chlorfenvinphos; Clofenvinfós. 2-Chloro-1-(2,4-dichlorophenyl)vinyl diethyl phosphate.

$C_{12}H_{14}Cl_3O_4P$ = 359.6.

*CAS — 470-90-6.*

### Profile

Clofenvinfos is an organophosphorus insecticide (p.1507) used in agriculture.

## Copper Oleate

Cobre, oleato de.

$Cu(C_{18}H_{33}O_2)_2$ = 626.5.

*CAS — 1120-44-1.*

### Profile

Copper oleate has been used topically as an insecticide for the treatment of pediculosis (p.1499).

### Preparations

**Proprietary Preparations** (details are given in Part 3)

**Multi-ingredient:** ***Arg.:*** Plus & Plus.

## Coumafos *(BAN, rINN)*

Bayer-21199; Coumaphos; Cumafós. *O*-3-Chloro-4-methyl-7-coumarinyl *O,O*-diethyl phosphorothioate.

$C_{14}H_{16}ClO_5PS$ = 362.8.

*CAS — 56-72-4.*

### Profile

Coumafos is an organophosphorus insecticide (p.1507) used as a topical ectoparasiticide in veterinary practice.

## Coumatetralyl

Cumatetralilo. 4-Hydroxy-3-(1,2,3,4-tetrahydro-1-naphthyl)coumarin.

$C_{19}H_{16}O_3$ = 292.3.

*CAS — 5836-29-3.*

### Profile

Coumatetralyl is an anticoagulant rodenticide.

◊ References.


1. Anticoagulant rodenticides. *Environmental Health Criteria 175.* Geneva: WHO, 1995. Available at: http://www.inchem.org/documents/ehc/ehc/ehc175.htm (accessed 28/05/04)


## Cyfluthrin *(BAN)*

Bay-VI-1704; Ciflutrina; Cyfluthin. (*RS*)-α-Cyano-4-fluoro-3-phenoxybenzyl (1*RS*,3*RS*;1*RS*,3*SR*)-3-(2,2-dichlorovinyl)-2,2-dimethylcyclopropanecarboxylate.

$C_{22}H_{18}Cl_2FNO_3$ = 434.3.

*CAS — 68359-37-5.*

*ATC — P03BA01.*

### Profile

Cyfluthrin is a pyrethroid insecticide (see Pyrethrum Flower, p.1509) used in agriculture and veterinary practice, and in the vector control of malaria (p.444).

### Preparations

**Proprietary Preparations** (details are given in Part 3)

***Ital.:*** Responsar; Solfac.

## Cyhalothrin *(BAN)*

Cihalotrina; PP-563. (*RS*)-α-Cyano-3-phenoxybenzyl (*Z*)-(1*RS*,3*RS*)-3-(2-chloro-3,3,3-trifluoropropenyl)-2,2-dimethylcyclopropanecarboxylate.

$C_{23}H_{19}ClF_3NO_3$ = 449.9.

*CAS — 68085-85-8.*

### Profile

Cyhalothrin is a pyrethroid insecticide (see Pyrethrum Flower, p.1509) that is used, particularly as a mixture of the (*Z*)-(1*R*,3*R*) *S* ester and the (*Z*)-(1*S*,3*S*) *R* ester (known as lambda-cyhalothrin), for the control of insect pests in public health. It has also been used in agriculture and in veterinary practice.

◊ References.


1. Cyhalothrin. *Environmental Health Criteria 99.* Geneva: WHO, 1990. Available at: http://www.inchem.org/documents/ehc/ehc/ehc99.htm (accessed 23/04/04)
2. Cyhalothrin and lambda-cyhalothrin health and safety guide. *IPCS Health and Safety Guide 38.* Geneva: WHO, 1990. Available at: http://www.inchem.org/documents/hsg/hsg/hsg038.htm (accessed 23/04/04)


## Cymiazole

CGA-50439; CGA-192357 (cymiazole hydrochloride); Cimiazol; Xymiazole. 2,4-Dimethyl-*N*-(3-methyl-2(3*H*)-thiazolylidene)benzenamine.

$C_{12}H_{14}N_2S$ = 218.3.

*CAS — 61676-87-7 (cymiazole); 121034-85-3 (cymiazole hydrochloride).*

### Profile

Cymiazole is a pesticide used in beekeeping.

## Cypermethrin *(BAN)*

Cipermetrina; NRDC-149. (*RS*)-α-Cyano-3-phenoxybenzyl (1*RS*,3*RS*)-(1*RS*,3*RS*)-3-(2,2-dichlorovinyl)-2,2-dimethylcyclopropanecarboxylate.

$C_{22}H_{19}Cl_2NO_3$ = 416.3.

*CAS — 52315-07-8.*

*ATC — P03BA02.*

## Alpha-cypermethrin *(BAN)*

(*SR*)-α-Cyano-3-phenoxybenzyl (1*RS*,3*RS*)-3-(2,2-dichlorovinyl)-2,2-dimethylcyclopropanecarboxylate.

$C_{22}H_{19}Cl_2NO_3$ = 416.3.

*CAS — 67375-30-8.*

### Profile

Cypermethrin, an isomeric mixture containing alpha-cypermethrin, is a pyrethroid insecticide (see Pyrethrum Flower, p.1509) used in veterinary practice as a topical ectoparasiticide and to control sea-lice infestation in salmon. It is also used in agriculture. Zeta-cypermethrin is also used. Alpha-cypermethrin is used in agriculture and for vector control in the management of malaria (p.444).

◊ References.


1. Cypermethrin. *Environmental Health Criteria 82.* Geneva: WHO, 1989. Available at: http://www.inchem.org/documents/ehc/ehc/ehc82.htm (accessed 23/04/04)

2. Cypermethrin health and safety guide. *IPCS Health and Safety Guide 22*. Geneva: WHO, 1989. Available at: http://www.inchem.org/documents/hsg/hsg/hsg022.htm (accessed 23/04/04)
3. Alpha-cypermethrin. *Environmental Health Criteria 142*. Geneva: WHO, 1992. Available at: http://www.inchem.org/documents/ehc/ehc/ehc142.htm (accessed 23/04/04)

## Cyromazine (BAN, rINN)

CGA-72662; Ciromazina. N-Cyclopropyl-1,3,5-triazine-2,4,6-triamine.

$C_6H_{10}N_6$ = 166.2.
*CAS — 66215-27-8.*

### Profile

Cyromazine is used as a topical ectoparasiticide in veterinary practice.

## Cythioate (BAN)

Citioato. *O,O*-Dimethyl *O*-(4-sulphamoylphenyl) phosphorothioate.

$C_8H_{12}NO_5PS_2$ = 297.3.
*CAS — 115-93-5.*

### Profile

Cythioate is an organophosphorus insecticide (p.1507) used as a systemic ectoparasiticide in veterinary practice; it is administered by mouth to the host animal.

## Daminozide

Daminozida. *N*-Dimethylaminosuccinamic acid.

$C_6H_{12}N_2O_3$ = 160.2.
*CAS — 1596-84-5.*

### Profile

Daminozide is a plant growth regulator that has been used in pesticides to improve fruit crops. There have been concerns about residues of the chemical in the fruit.

## Deltamethrin (BAN)

Decamethrin; Deltametrina; NRDC-161. (*S*)-α-Cyano-3-phenoxybenzyl (1*R*,3*R*)-3-(2,2-dibromovinyl)-2,2-dimethylcyclopropanecarboxylate.

$C_{22}H_{19}Br_2NO_3$ = 505.2.
*CAS — 52918-63-5.*
*ATC — P03BA03.*

**Pharmacopoeias.** In *BP(Vet)*.

**BP(Vet) 2003** (Deltamethrin). A white to buff-coloured crystalline powder. Insoluble in water; soluble in alcohol and in acetone.

### Profile

Deltamethrin is a pyrethroid insecticide (see Pyrethrum Flower, p.1509) used in the vector control of malaria (p.444). It is also used as a topical ectoparasiticide in veterinary practice and as an agricultural and household insecticide.

◊ References.

1. Deltamethrin health and safety guide. *IPCS Health and Safety Guide 30*. Geneva: WHO, 1989. Available at: http://www.inchem.org/documents/hsg/hsg/hsg030.htm (accessed 26/04/04)
2. Deltamethrin. *Environmental Health Criteria 97*. Geneva: WHO, 1990. Available at: http://www.inchem.org/documents/ehc/ehc/ehc97.htm (accessed 26/04/04)

### Preparations

**Proprietary Preparations** (details are given in Part 3)
**Braz.:** Del-Lend; Deltacid; Deltamitren; Deltapio; Deotrin; Hexafen; Piro-li-N†; **Mex.:** Difexon.
**Multi-ingredient: Arg.:** Capitis; Deca-Scab; Hexa-Defital NF; Nopucid Compuesto; **Braz.:** Deltacid Plus; Nopucid Composto†; **Chile:** Launol.

## Dibromochloropropane

Dibromocloropropano. 1,2-Dibromo-3-chloropropane.

$C_3H_5Br_2Cl$ = 236.3.
*CAS — 96-12-8.*

### Profile

Dibromochloropropane has been used as a pesticide. Low sperm counts and evidence of testicular damage have occurred in workers exposed to dibromochloropropane.

## Dibutyl Phthalate

Butyl Phthalate; DBP; Dibutylis Phthalas; Ftalato de dibutilo. Dibutyl benzene-1,2-dicarboxylate.

$C_{16}H_{22}O_4$ = 278.3.
*CAS — 84-74-2.*

**Pharmacopoeias.** In *Eur.* (see p.vi). Also in *USNF.*

**Ph. Eur. 5.0** (Dibutyl Phthalate). A clear, oily, colourless or very slightly yellow liquid. Practically insoluble in water; miscible with alcohol. Store in airtight containers.

**USNF 22** (Dibutyl Phthalate). A clear, oily, colourless or very slightly yellow liquid. Practically insoluble in water; miscible with alcohol and with ether. Store in airtight containers. Avoid temperatures above 40°. Do not allow to freeze. Protect from moisture.

### Adverse Effects and Precautions

Dibutyl phthalate has occasionally caused hypersensitivity reactions. As with other phthalates contact with plastics should be avoided.

### Uses and Administration

Dibutyl phthalate has been used as an insect repellent although it is slightly less effective than dimethyl phthalate (p.1504). It is less volatile and less easily removed by washing than dimethyl phthalate, and its chief use therefore has been for the impregnation of clothing.

Dibutyl phthalate has also been used as a plasticiser.

◊ References.

1. Di-*n*-butyl phthalate. *Environmental Health Criteria 189*. Geneva: WHO, 1997. Available at: http://www.inchem.org/documents/ehc/ehc/ehc189.htm (accessed 26/04/04)

### Preparations

**Proprietary Preparations** (details are given in Part 3)
**Multi-ingredient: S.Afr.:** Mylol.

## Dichlorophenoxyacetic Acid

2,4-D; Diclorofenoxiacético, ácido. 2,4-Dichlorophenoxyacetic acid.

$C_8H_6Cl_2O_3$ = 221.0.
*CAS — 94-75-7.*

### Adverse Effects, Treatment, and Precautions

Most cases of poisoning with dichlorophenoxyacetic acid have involved its ingestion with other herbicides; the solvent may also play a part in any toxicity. There is little pattern to the range of adverse effects that may occur following ingestion, inhalation, or topical exposure.

Adverse effects have involved the central and peripheral nervous system, muscles, and the cardiovascular system. Gastrointestinal effects are common with poisoning. Hepatotoxicity, nephrotoxicity, and pulmonary disorders have occurred but it is not clear that dichlorophenoxyacetic acid contributed to the toxicity. The role of phenoxyacetic acids in cancer is discussed under trichlorophenoxyacetic acid (p.1510).

Gastric lavage should be considered after ingestion of substantial amounts if the patient presents within 1 hour. Contaminated clothing should be removed and the skin washed with soap and water. Forced alkaline diuresis or haemodialysis has been reported to be effective in removing dichlorophenoxyacetic acid. Further treatment is symptomatic.

◊ References.

1. 2,4-Dichlorophenoxyacetic acid (2,4-D). *Environmental Health Criteria 29*. Geneva: WHO, 1984. Available at: http://www.inchem.org/documents/ehc/ehc/ehc29.htm (accessed 26/04/04)
2. 2,4-Dichlorophenoxyacetic (2,4-D) health and safety guide. *IPCS Health and Safety Guide 5*. Geneva: WHO, 1987. Available at: http://www.inchem.org/documents/hsg/hsg/hsg005.htm (accessed 26/04/04)
3. 2,4-Dichlorophenoxyacetic acid (2,4-D)—environmental aspects. *Environmental Health Criteria 84*. Geneva: WHO, 1989. Available at: http://www.inchem.org/documents/ehc/ehc/ehc84.htm (accessed 26/04/04)
4. Bradberry SM, *et al.* Mechanisms of toxicology, clinical features, and management of acute chlorophenoxy herbicide poisoning: a review. *J Toxicol Clin Toxicol* 2000; **38:** 111–22.

### Uses

Dichlorophenoxyacetic acid is a herbicide widely used for weed control in cereals and other crops. It is usually used as its salts or esters in combination with other herbicides.

## Dichlorvos (BAN, USAN, rINN)

DDVP; Diclorvós; NSC-6738; OMS-14; SD-1750. 2,2-Dichlorovinyl dimethyl phosphate.

$C_4H_7Cl_2O_4P$ = 221.0.
*CAS — 62-73-7.*

**Pharmacopoeias.** In *Fr.* for veterinary use.

### Profile

Dichlorvos is an organophosphorus insecticide (p.1507) of short persistence, effective against a wide range of insects. It is sometimes used as a fumigant. It has been used for the extermination of insects in aircraft (disinsection). It is also used as a topical ectoparasiticide and as an anthelmintic in veterinary practice. Concern has been expressed over its possible carcinogenicity.

◊ References.

1. Dichlorvos health and safety guide. *IPCS Health and Safety Guide 18*. Geneva: WHO, 1988. Available at: http://www.inchem.org/documents/hsg/hsg/hsg018.htm (accessed 26/04/04)
2. Dichlorvos. *Environmental Health Criteria 79*. Geneva: WHO, 1989. Available at: http://www.inchem.org/documents/ehc/ehc/ehc79.htm (accessed 26/04/04)

## Dieldrin (BAN, pINN)

Dieldrina.

*CAS — 60-57-1 (HEOD).*

**Description.** Dieldrin contains about 85% of (1*R*,4*S*,5*S*,8*R*)-1,2,3,4,10,10-hexachloro-6,7-epoxy-1,4,4a,5,6,7,8,8a-octahydro-1,4:5,8-dimethanonaphthalene (HEOD), $C_{12}H_8Cl_6O$ = 380.9. The remaining 15% is mainly chlorinated organic compounds related to HEOD.

### Adverse Effects and Treatment

As for Chlorinated Insecticides, p.1501.

Dieldrin is more toxic than clofenotane (p.1502) and is readily absorbed through the skin.

◊ References.

1. Aldrin and dieldrin. *Environmental Health Criteria 91*. Geneva: WHO, 1989. Available at: http://www.inchem.org/documents/ehc/ehc/ehc91.htm (accessed 26/04/04)
2. Aldrin and dieldrin health and safety guide. *IPCS Health and Safety Guide 21*. Geneva: WHO, 1989. Available at: http://www.inchem.org/documents/hsg/hsg/hsg021.htm (accessed 26/04/04)
3. Høyer AP, *et al.* Organochlorine exposure and risk of breast cancer. *Lancet* 1998; **352:** 1816–20.

### Uses

Dieldrin is a chlorinated insecticide (p.1501) formerly used as a sheepdip. Its use is now limited to a few specified purposes such as termite control.

## Diethyltoluamide (BAN, rINN)

DEET; *N,N*-Diethyl-3-methylbenzamide; Diethyltoluamidum; Dietiltoluamida; Dietiltoluamida. *NN*-Diethyl-*m*-toluamide.

$C_{12}H_{17}NO$ = 191.3.
*CAS — 134-62-3.*
*ATC — P03BX01.*

**Pharmacopoeias.** In *Int.* and *US.*

**USP 27** (Diethyltoluamide). A colourless liquid with a faint pleasant odour. Practically insoluble in water and in glycerol; miscible with alcohol, with carbon disulfide, with chloroform, with ether, and with isopropyl alcohol. Store in airtight containers.

### Adverse Effects and Precautions

Occasional hypersensitivity to diethyltoluamide has been reported. Diethyltoluamide should not be applied near the eyes, to mucous membranes, to broken skin, or to areas of skin flexion, as irritation or blistering may occur. Systemic toxicity has been reported following application of large topical doses, particularly in children.

◊ Hypersensitivity and anaphylaxis has been described in a patient after exposure to diethyltoluamide.[1] Toxic encephalopathy has been noted in children who received liberal applications of this compound;[2] seizures have also been reported,[3] and there have been cases of manic psychosis[4] and cardiovascular toxicity (sinus bradycardia and orthostatic hypotension)[5] associated with topical application. An assessment[6] of both published and unpublished data concluded that there had been remarkably few problems considering the widespread use of diethyltoluamide and that the encephalopathy in children had not been substantiated by detailed surveillance; however, another case analysis[7] did find an association with encephalopathy in children.

Toxic reactions, including death, have been reported following the ingestion of large amounts of diethyltoluamide-containing insect repellents.[8]

1. Miller JD. Anaphylaxis associated with insect repellent. *N Engl J Med* 1982; **307:** 1341–2.
2. Roland EH, *et al.* Toxic encephalopathy in a child after brief exposure to insect repellents. *Can Med Assoc J* 1985; **132:** 155–6.
3. Anonymous. Seizures temporally associated with use of DEET insect repellent—New York and Connecticut. *Arch Dermatol* 1989; **125:** 1619–20.
4. Snyder JW, *et al.* Acute manic psychosis following the dermal application of N,N-diethyl-m-toluamide (DEET) in an adult. *J Toxicol Clin Toxicol* 1986; **24:** 429–39.
5. Clem JR, *et al.* Insect repellent (N,N-diethyl-m-toluamide) cardiovascular toxicity in an adult. *Ann Pharmacother* 1993; **27:** 289–93.
6. Goodyer L, Behrens RH. Short report: the safety and toxicity of insect repellents. *Am J Trop Med Hyg* 1998; **59:** 323–4.
7. Briassoulis G, *et al.* Toxic encephalopathy associated with use of DEET insect repellents: a case analysis of its toxicity in children. *Hum Exp Toxicol* 2001; **20:** 8–14.
8. Tenenbein M. Severe toxic reactions and death following the ingestion of diethyltoluamide-containing insect repellents. *JAMA* 1987; **258:** 1509–11.

### Uses

Diethyltoluamide is an insect repellent that is effective against mosquitoes as well as blackflies, harvest-bugs or chiggers, midges, ticks, and fleas. It is considered to be of value for personal protection against malaria (p.444). It has also been used as a repellent against leeches. It may be applied to skin and clothing.

### Preparations

**USP 27:** Diethyltoluamide Topical Solution.

**Proprietary Preparations** (details are given in Part 3)
**Fr.:** Insect Ecran; Item Antipoux; Moskizol†; **Ger.:** Autan†; **S.Afr.:** Mylol; **UK:** Bens; Bug Guards†; Jungle Formula Insect Repellent; Mijex; Ultrathon†.

**Multi-ingredient: Canad.:** Muskol; **Fr.:** Tiq'Aouta; **Hong Kong:** Pellit; **Israel:** Yatushan Plus; **Ital.:** Entom†; Sinezan; **S.Afr.:** Mylol; No-Bite; **Thai.:** Pellit; **UK:** Jungle Formula Insect Repellent Plus U.V. Sunscreens†.

## Difenacoum

Difenacum. 3-(3-Biphenyl-4-yl-1,2,3,4-tetrahydro-1-naphthyl)-4-hydroxycoumarin.
$C_{31}H_{24}O_3$ = 444.5.
*CAS — 56073-07-5.*

### Profile

Difenacoum is an anticoagulant rodenticide.

◊ References.

1. Anticoagulant rodenticides. *Environmental Health Criteria 175.* Geneva: WHO, 1995. Available at: http://www.inchem.org/documents/ehc/ehc/ehc175.htm (accessed 26/04/04)
2. Difenacoum health and safety guide. *IPCS Health and Safety Guide 95.* Geneva: WHO, 1995. Available at: http://www.inchem.org/documents/hsg/hsg/hsg095.htm (accessed 26/04/04)

**Toxicity.** Difenacoum, a second-generation anticoagulant rodenticide inhibits prothrombin synthesis to cause bleeding that may be occult.[1] It is absorbed from the gastrointestinal tract; dermal absorption is possible. Poisons containing 100 mg in each kg of bait are not hazardous to man; more concentrated forms are particularly hazardous and their availability should be restricted. Baits, which should be prepared only by trained personnel, should contain a suitable marker-dye.

There have been reports of poisoning with difenacoum.[2-4]

1. WHO. Safe use of pesticides: ninth report of the WHO expert committee on vector biology and control. *WHO Tech Rep Ser 720* 1985.
2. Barlow AM, *et al.* Difenacoum (Neosorexa) poisoning. *BMJ* 1982; **285:** 541.
3. Butcher GP, *et al.* Difenacoum poisoning as a cause of haematuria. *Hum Exp Toxicol* 1992; **11:** 553–4.
4. McCarthy PT, *et al.* Covert poisoning with difenacoum: clinical and toxicological observations. *Hum Exp Toxicol* 1997; **16:** 166–70.

## Diflubenzuron

1-(4-Chlorophenyl)-3-(2,6-difluorobenzoyl)urea.
$C_{14}H_9ClF_2N_2O_2$ = 310.7.
*CAS — 35367-38-5.*

### Profile

Diflubenzuron is an insecticide and larvicide that acts as a growth regulator by interfering with the formation of cuticle. It is used in agriculture and for the control of disease vectors.

Diflubenzuron possesses residual activity against mosquito larvae.

◊ References.

1. Diflubenzuron. health and safety guide. *IPCS Health and Safety Guide 99.* Geneva: WHO, 1995. Available at: http://www.inchem.org/documents/hsg/hsg/hsg099.htm (accessed 26/04/04)
2. Diflubenzuron. *Environmental Health Criteria 184.* Geneva: WHO, 1996. Available at: http://www.inchem.org/documents/ehc/ehc/ehc184.htm (accessed 26/04/04)

## Dimethoate

Dimetoato; Fosfamid. *O,O*-Dimethyl *S*-methylcarbamoylmethyl phosphorodithioate.
$C_5H_{12}NO_3PS_2$ = 229.3.
*CAS — 60-51-5.*

### Profile

Dimethoate is an organophosphorus insecticide (p.1507) used in agriculture.

◊ References.

1. Dimethoate health and safety guide. *IPCS Health and Safety Guide 20.* Geneva: WHO, 1988. Available at: http://www.inchem.org/documents/hsg/hsg/hsg020.htm (accessed 28/05/04)
2. Dimethoate. *Environmental Health Criteria 90.* Geneva: WHO, 1989. Available at: http://www.inchem.org/documents/ehc/ehc/ehc90.htm (accessed 28/05/04)
3. Jovanović D, *et al.* A case of unusual suicidal poisoning by the organophosphorus insecticide dimethoate. *Hum Exp Toxicol* 1990; **9:** 49–51.

## Dimethyl Phthalate

DMP; Ftalato de dimetilo; Methyl Phthalate. Dimethyl benzene-1,2-dicarboxylate.
$C_{10}H_{10}O_4$ = 194.2.
*CAS — 131-11-3.*

**Pharmacopoeias.** In *Br.* and *Fr.*

**BP 2003** (Dimethyl Phthalate). A colourless or faintly coloured liquid, odourless or almost odourless. Slightly soluble in water; miscible with alcohol, with ether, and with most organic solvents.

### Adverse Effects and Precautions

Dimethyl phthalate may cause temporary smarting and should not be applied near the eyes or to mucous membranes. As with other phthalates contact with plastics should be avoided.

### Uses

Dimethyl phthalate is an insect repellent.

### Preparations

**Proprietary Preparations** (details are given in Part 3)

**Multi-ingredient: Fr.:** SVR Creme Antimoustique; Tiq'Aouta; **Hong Kong:** Pellit; **Israel:** Yatushan Plus; **S.Afr.:** Mylol; **Thai.:** Pellit.

## Dimpylate *(BAN, rINN)*

Diazinon; Dimpilato. *O,O*-Diethyl *O*-(2-isopropyl-6-methylpyrimidin-4-yl) phosphorothioate.
$C_{12}H_{21}N_2O_3PS$ = 304.3.
*CAS — 333-41-5.*

**Pharmacopoeias.** In *BP(Vet).*

**BP(Vet) 2003** (Dimpylate). A clear, yellowish-brown, slightly viscous liquid. Practically insoluble in water; miscible with alcohol, with ether, and with most organic solvents.

### Profile

Dimpylate is an organophosphorus insecticide (p.1507) used as a systemic ectoparasiticide in veterinary practice; it is applied topically to the host animal. It is also employed as an insecticide in agriculture and horticulture.

◊ References.

1. Wagner SL, Orwick DL. Chronic organophosphate exposure associated with transient hypertonia in an infant. *Pediatrics* 1994; **94:** 94–7.

## Dinitro-o-cresol

DNOC. 4,6-Dinitro-o-cresol.
$C_7H_6N_2O_5$ = 198.1.
*CAS — 534-52-1.*

### Profile

Dinitro-*o*-cresol is a dinitrophenol formerly used as an insecticide and herbicide. It increases metabolism by uncoupling oxidative phosphorylation and was also formerly used in obesity. Fatal poisoning has occurred.

◊ References.

1. Dinitro-ortho-cresol. *Environmental Health Criteria 220.* Geneva: WHO, 2000. Available at: http://www.inchem.org/documents/ehc/ehc/ehc220.htm (accessed 26/04/04)

## Dinitrophenol

Dinitrofenol. 2,4-Dinitrophenol.
$C_6H_4N_2O_5$ = 184.1.
*CAS — 51-28-5.*

### Profile

Dinitrophenol has been used as a herbicide. Since dinitrophenol increases metabolism by uncoupling oxidative phosphorylation it was formerly used in the treatment of obesity. Fatal poisoning has occurred.

## Dioctyl Adipate

Adipato de dioctilo; DEHA; Di-(2-ethylhexyl)adipate.
$C_{22}H_{42}O_4$ = 370.6.

### Profile

Dioctyl adipate is used as an insect repellent. It is also used as a plasticiser by the plastics industry; concern about the migration of this and other plasticisers into foodstuffs from polythene films used to wrap them ('cling film') have led to its use at lower concentrations.

### Preparations

**Proprietary Preparations** (details are given in Part 3)
**UK:** Protec.

## Dioxation *(BAN, rINN)*

Dioxathion; Dioxatión. It consists mainly of *cis* and *trans* isomers of *S,S'*-1,4-dioxan-2,3-diyl bis(*O,O*-diethyl phosphorodithioate).
$C_{12}H_{26}O_6P_2S_4$ = 456.5.
*CAS — 78-34-2.*

### Profile

Dioxation is an organophosphorus insecticide (p.1507) that has been used in agriculture and as a topical ectoparasiticide in veterinary practice.

## Diphenadione *(BAN, pINN)*

Difenadiona; Diphacinone. 2-(Diphenylacetyl)indan-1,3-dione.
$C_{23}H_{16}O_3$ = 340.4.
*CAS — 82-66-6.*
*ATC — B01AA10.*

### Profile

Diphenadione is used as an anticoagulant rodenticide.

## Diquat Dibromide

Dibromuro de diquat. 9,10-Dihydro-8a,10a-diazoniaphenanthrene dibromide; 1,1'-Ethylene-2,2'-bipyridyldiylium dibromide.
$C_{12}H_{12}Br_2N_2$ = 344.0.
*CAS — 2764-72-9 (diquat); 85-00-7 (diquat dibromide).*

### Profile

Diquat dibromide is a contact herbicide used in agriculture and horticulture. It has similar adverse effects to those of paraquat (p.1508).

◊ References.

1. Paraquat and diquat. *Environmental Health Criteria 39.* Geneva: WHO, 1984. Available at: http://www.inchem.org/documents/ehc/ehc/ehc39.htm (accessed 26/04/04)
2. Diquat health and safety guide. *IPCS Health and Safety Guide 52.* Geneva: WHO, 1991. Available at: http://www.inchem.org/documents/hsg/hsg/hsg052.htm (accessed 26/04/04)
3. Proudfoot A, ed. Pesticide poisoning: notes for the guidance of medical practitioners. 2nd ed. London: DoH, The Stationery Office, 1996.
4. Jones GM, Vale JA. Mechanisms of toxicity, clinical features, and management of diquat poisoning: a review. *J Toxicol Clin Toxicol* 2000; **38:** 123–8.

## Emamectin

Emamectina. A mixture of (4"-*R*)-5-*O*-Demethyl-4"-deoxy-4"-(methylamino)avermectin $A_{1a}$ and (4"-*R*)-5-*O*-Demethyl-25-de(1-methylpropyl)-4"-deoxy-4"-(methylamino)-25-(1-methylethyl)avermectin $A_{1a}$ in the ratio of 9:1.
*CAS — 121124-29-6 (major component); 121424-52-0 (minor component); 137335-79-6.*

### Profile

Emamectin is an avermectin insecticide used for the control of sea-lice infestation in salmon.

## Endod

### Profile

Endod is obtained from the dried fruits of *Phytolacca dodecandra* (Phytolaccaceae) and has molluscicidal properties. It has been investigated for the control of the snail vector of schistosomiasis.

## Endosulfan

Endosulfán. 1,4,5,6,7,7-Hexachloro-8,9,10-trinorborn-5-en-2,3-ylenebismethylene sulphite.
$C_9H_6Cl_6O_3S$ = 406.9.
*CAS — 115-29-7.*

### Profile

Endosulfan is a chlorinated insecticide (p.1501) used in agriculture.

◊ References.

1. Endosulfan. *Environmental Health Criteria 40.* Geneva: WHO, 1984. Available at: http://www.inchem.org/documents/ehc/ehc/ehc40.htm (accessed 26/04/04)
2. Endosulfan health and safety guide. *IPCS Health and Safety Guide 17.* Geneva: WHO, 1988. Available at: http://www.inchem.org/documents/hsg/hsg/hsg017.htm (accessed 26/04/04)
3. Blanco-Coronado JL, *et al.* Acute intoxication by endosulfan. *J Toxicol Clin Toxicol* 1992; **30:** 575–83.
4. Boereboom FT, *et al.* Nonaccidental endosulfan intoxication: a case report with toxicokinetic calculations and tissue concentrations. *J Toxicol Clin Toxicol* 1998; **36:** 345–52.
5. Chugh SN, *et al.* Endosulfan poisoning in Northern India: a report of 18 cases. *Int J Clin Pharmacol Ther* 1998; **36:** 474–7.

## Endrin

Endrín. (1*R*,4*S*,4a*S*,5*S*,6*S*,7*R*,8*R*,8a*R*)-1,2,3,4,10,10-Hexachloro-1,4,4a,5,6,7,8,8a-octahydro-6,7-epoxy-1,4:5,8-dimethanonaphthalene.
$C_{12}H_8Cl_6O$ = 380.9.
*CAS — 72-20-8.*

### Profile

Endrin is a chlorinated insecticide (p.1501), but its use was prohibited, at least in some countries, because of toxicity and persistence in the environment.

◊ General references to endrin,[1-4] including reports of poisoning.[2,3]

1. Anonymous. Acute convulsions associated with endrin poisoning—Pakistan. *JAMA* 1985; **253:** 334–5.

2. Runhaar EA, *et al.* A case of fatal endrin poisoning. *Hum Toxicol* 1985; **4:** 241–7.
3. Endrin health and safety guide. *IPCS Health and Safety Guide 60.* Geneva: WHO, 1991. Available at: http://www.inchem.org/documents/hsg/hsg/hsg060.htm (accessed 26/04/04)
4. Endrin. *Environmental Health Criteria 130.* Geneva: WHO, 1992. Available at: http://www.inchem.org/documents/ehc/ehc/ehc130.htm (accessed 26/04/04)

## Esdepallethrine

Esdepaletrina. (*S*)-3-Allyl-2-methyl-4-oxocyclopent-2-enyl (1*R*,3*R*)-2,2-dimethyl-3-(2-methylprop-1-enyl)-cyclopropanecarboxylate.

$C_{19}H_{26}O_3$ = 302.4.
*CAS — 28434-00-6.*

### Profile

Esdepallethrine is a pyrethroid insecticide (see Pyrethrum Flower, p.1509). It is used as an acaricide with piperonyl butoxide (p.1509) in the topical treatment of scabies (p.1499).

Esdepallethrine is also used in devices and sprays to control insects, including mosquitoes.

### Preparations

**Proprietary Preparations** (details are given in Part 3)

**Multi-ingredient: *Arg.:*** Acardust; ***Braz.:*** Vapio†; ***Canad.:*** Scabene; ***Fr.:*** A-Par; Acardust; Spregal; ***Israel:*** Acardust; ***Ital.:*** Acardust†; ***S.Afr.:*** Spregal; ***Switz.:*** Acardust†.

## Ethion

Diethion; Etión. *O,O,O',O'*-Tetraethyl *S,S'*-methylenediphosphorodithioate.

$C_9H_{22}O_4P_2S_4$ = 384.5.
*CAS — 563-12-2.*

### Profile

Ethion is an organophosphorus insecticide used as a topical ectoparasiticide in veterinary practice.

## Ethohexadiol

Ethylhexanediol; Etohexadiol. 2-Ethylhexane-1,3-diol.

$C_8H_{18}O_2$ = 146.2.
*CAS — 94-96-2.*

### Profile

Ethohexadiol is an insect repellent. It may be applied topically to the skin and to clothing. It has been used with dimethyl phthalate.

### Preparations

**Proprietary Preparations** (details are given in Part 3)

***Fr.:*** Insect Ecran.

## Ethylene Dibromide

Dibromuro de etileno; EDB. 1,2-Dibromoethane.

$C_2H_4Br_2$ = 187.9.
*CAS — 106-93-4.*

### Profile

Ethylene dibromide is an insecticidal fumigant and a lead scavenger used in the petroleum industry. Its use has been restricted in certain areas because of carcinogenicity in *animals* and because of evidence of persistence in fruit and cereals that have undergone fumigation.

Ethylene dibromide is more toxic than carbon tetrachloride or ethylene dichloride. It is irritant to the eyes, skin, and mucous membranes. Inhalation leads to drowsiness, CNS depression, and possibly pulmonary oedema. Contact with the skin causes blistering and it is readily absorbed. Kidney and liver damage may occur.

◊ Reports of poisoning due to ethylene dibromide.

1. Letz GA, *et al.* Two fatalities after acute occupational exposure to ethylene dibromide. *JAMA* 1984; **252:** 2428–31.
2. Singh S, *et al.* Non-fatal ethylene dibromide ingestion. *Hum Exp Toxicol* 2000; **19:** 152–3.
3. Mehrotra P, *et al.* Two cases of ethylene dibromide poisoning. *Vet Hum Toxicol* 2001; **43:** 91–2.

## Ethylene Dichloride

Brocide; Dicloruro de etileno; Dutch Liquid. 1,2-Dichloroethane.

$C_2H_4Cl_2$ = 98.96.
*CAS — 107-06-2.*

### Profile

Ethylene dichloride is an insecticidal fumigant. It is also used in the petroleum industry and as an industrial solvent. Exposure to the vapour may cause lachrymation and corneal clouding, nasal irritation, and vertigo due to the depressant effect on the CNS. Contact with the skin may cause dermatitis. Kidney and liver damage, hypotension and cardiac impairment, gastrointestinal disturbances, haemorrhage, coma, and pulmonary oedema may follow absorption after inhalation, topical application, or ingestion.

Ethylene dichloride has been reported to be carcinogenic in *animals.*

◊ References.

1. 1,2 Dichloroethane. *Environmental Health Criteria 62.* Geneva: WHO, 1987. Available at: http://www.inchem.org/documents/ehc/ehc/ehc62.htm (accessed 26/04/04)
2. 1,2-Dichloroethane health and safety guide. *IPCS Health and Safety Guide 55.* Geneva: WHO, 1991. Available at: http://www.inchem.org/documents/hsg/hsg/hsg055.htm (accessed 26/04/04)
3. Proudfoot A, ed. Pesticide poisoning: notes for the guidance of medical practitioners. 2nd ed. London: DoH, The Stationery Office, 1996.

## Etofenprox (*rINN*)

α-[(*p*-Ethoxy-β,β-dimethylphenethyl)oxy]-*m*-phenoxytoluene.

$C_{25}H_{28}O_3$ = 376.5.
*CAS — 80844-07-1.*

### Profile

Etofenprox is a pyrethroid insecticide (see Pyrethrum Flower, p.1509) used in the vector control of malaria (p.444).

## Famphur

Famfur; Famophos.

$C_{10}H_{16}NO_5PS_2$ = 325.3.
*CAS — 52-85-7.*

### Profile

Famphur is an organophosphorus insecticide (p.1507) used as a systemic ectoparasiticide in veterinary practice; it is applied topically to the host animal.

## Fenitrothion (*BAN*)

Fenitrotión. *O,O*-Dimethyl *O*-4-nitro-*m*-tolyl phosphorothioate.

$C_9H_{12}NO_5PS$ = 277.2.
*CAS — 122-14-5.*

### Profile

Fenitrothion is an organophosphorus insecticide (p.1507) used as a topical ectoparasiticide in veterinary practice. It is also used as an agricultural insecticide.

◊ References.

1. Fenitrothion health and safety guide. *IPCS Health and Safety Guide 65.* Geneva: WHO, 1991. Available at: http://www.inchem.org/documents/hsg/hsg/hsg065.htm (accessed 26/04/04)
2. Fenitrothion. *Environmental Health Criteria 133.* Geneva: WHO, 1992. Available at: http://www.inchem.org/documents/ehc/ehc/ehc133.htm (accessed 26/04/04)
3. Bouma MJ, Nesbit R. Fenitrothion intoxication during spraying operations in the malaria programme for Afghan refugees in North West Frontier Province of Pakistan. *Trop Geogr Med* 1995; **47:** 12–14.

## Fenthion (*BAN*)

Bayer-29493; Fentión; S-752. *O,O*-Dimethyl *O*-4-methylthio-*m*-tolyl phosphorothioate.

$C_{10}H_{15}O_3PS_2$ = 278.3.
*CAS — 55-38-9.*

**Pharmacopoeias.** In *BP(Vet).*

**BP(Vet) 2003** (Fenthion). A yellowish-brown oily substance. Immiscible with water; miscible with alcohol and with chloroform.

### Profile

Fenthion is an organophosphorus insecticide (p.1507) used as a systemic ectoparasiticide in veterinary practice; it is applied topically to the host animal. Fenthion has also been used in agriculture.

**Toxicity.** Macular changes have been detected in the eyes of workers regularly exposed to fenthion.[1] It was considered that there was a need for long-term studies on subjects exposed to different organophosphorus compounds to assess their role in producing macular changes.

1. Misra UK, *et al.* Some observations on the macula of pesticide workers. *Hum Toxicol* 1985; **4:** 135–45.

## Fenvalerate (*BAN*)

Fenvalerato; OMS-2000; Pydrin; S-5602; SD-43775; WL-43775. (*RS*)-α-Cyano-3-phenoxybenzyl (*RS*)-2-(4-chlorophenyl)-3-methylbutyrate.

$C_{25}H_{22}ClNO_3$ = 419.9.
*CAS — 51630-58-1.*

### Profile

Fenvalerate is a pyrethroid insecticide (see Pyrethrum Flower, p.1509) used as a topical ectoparasiticide in veterinary practice. It has also been used as an insecticide in agriculture and horticulture.

Esfenvalerate, one of the stereoisomers of fenvalerate, is also used as an agricultural insecticide.

◊ References.

1. Fenvalerate health and safety guide. *IPCS Health and Safety Guide 34.* Geneva: WHO, 1989. Available at: http://www.inchem.org/documents/hsg/hsg/hsg034.htm (accessed 26/04/04)
2. Fenvalerate. *Environmental Health Criteria 95.* Geneva: WHO, 1990. Available at: http://www.inchem.org/documents/ehc/ehc/ehc95.htm (accessed 26/04/04)

## Fipronil (*BAN*)

Fipronilo; MB-46030; RM-1601. (*RS*)-5-Amino-1-(2,6-dichloro-4-trifluoromethylphenyl)-4-(trifluoromethylsulfinyl)pyrazole-3-carbonitrile.

$C_{12}H_4Cl_2F_6N_4OS$ = 437.1.
*CAS — 120068-37-3.*

### Profile

Fipronil is used as a topical ectoparasiticide in veterinary practice. It has also been investigated for the treatment of head lice.

## Flocoumafen

Flocoumafene; Flocumafeno; OMS-3047. 4-Hydroxy-3-[1,2,3,4-tetrahydro-3-[4-(4-trifluoromethylbenzyloxy)phenyl]-1-naphthyl]coumarin.

$C_{33}H_{25}F_3O_4$ = 542.5.
*CAS — 90035-08-8.*

### Profile

Flocoumafen is a coumarin derivative used as an anticoagulant rodenticide. It is said to be effective in rodents resistant to other anticoagulant rodenticides.

◊ References.

1. Anticoagulant rodenticides. *Environmental Health Criteria 175.* Geneva: WHO, 1995. Available at: http://www.inchem.org/documents/ehc/ehc/ehc175.htm (accessed 26/04/04)

## Fluazuron (*rINN*)

CGA-157419; Fluazurón. 1-(4-Chloro-3-{[3-chloro-5-(trifluoromethyl)-2-pyridyl]oxy}phenyl)-3-(2,6-difluorobenzoyl)urea.

$C_{20}H_{10}Cl_2F_5N_3O_3$ = 506.2.
*CAS — 86811-58-7.*

### Profile

Fluazuron is used as a topical ectoparasiticide in veterinary practice.

## Flumethrin (*BAN*)

Flumetrina. α-Cyano-4-fluoro-3-phenoxybenzyl 3-(β,4-dichlorostyryl)-2,2-dimethylcyclopropanecarboxylate.

$C_{28}H_{22}Cl_2FNO_3$ = 510.4.
*CAS — 69770-45-2.*

### Profile

Flumethrin is a pyrethroid insecticide (see Pyrethrum Flower, p.1509) used as a topical ectoparasiticide in veterinary practice.

◊ Reports of poisoning with flumethrin.

1. Box SA, Lee MR. A systemic reaction following exposure to a pyrethroid insecticide. *Hum Exp Toxicol* 1996; **15:** 389–90.

## Fluoroacetamide

Compound 1081; Fluoroacetamida.

$FCH_2.CONH_2$ = 77.06.
*CAS — 640-19-7.*

### Profile

Fluoroacetamide is a rodenticide and produces adverse effects similar to those of sodium fluoroacetate (p.1510).

## Fluvalinate

Fluvalinato; ZR-3210. Cyano(3-phenoxyphenyl)methyl ester of *N*-[2-chloro-4-(trifluoromethyl)phenyl]-DL-valine.

$C_{26}H_{22}ClF_3N_2O_3$ = 502.9.
*CAS — 69409-94-5.*

### Profile

Fluvalinate is a pesticide used in beekeeping.

## Glyphosate

Glifosato. *N*-(Phosphonomethyl)glycine.

$C_3H_8NO_5P$ = 169.1.
*CAS — 1071-83-6.*

### Profile

Glyphosate is used as a herbicide.

◊ References.

1. Glyphosate. *Environmental Health Criteria 159.* Geneva: WHO, 1994. Available at: http://www.inchem.org/documents/ehc/ehc/ehc159.htm (accessed 26/04/04)

**Toxicity.** Reports of poisoning with glyphosate products[1-3] and guidelines for treatment[4] have been published. The toxicity has been believed to be largely due to the inclusion of a surfactant, polyoxyethyleneamine, in the herbicide (Roundup) formulation.


1. Sawada Y, *et al.* Probable toxicity of surface-active agent in commercial herbicide containing glyphosate. *Lancet* 1988; **i:** 299.
2. Talbot AR, *et al.* Acute poisoning with a glyphosate-surfactant herbicide ('Roundup'): a review of 93 cases. *Hum Exp Toxicol* 1991; **10:** 1–8.
3. Menkes DB, *et al.* Intentional self-poisoning with glyphosate-containing herbicides. *Hum Exp Toxicol* 1991; **10:** 103–7.
4. Proudfoot A, ed. *Pesticide poisoning: notes for the guidance of medical practitioners.* 2nd ed. London: DoH, The Stationery Office, 1996.


## Heptachlor

Heptacloro. 1,4,5,6,7,8,8-Heptachloro-3a,4,7,7a-tetrahydro-4,7-methanoindene.

$C_{10}H_5Cl_7$ = 373.3.

*CAS — 76-44-8.*

### Profile

Heptachlor is a chlorinated insecticide (p.1501), but its use was prohibited, at least in some countries, because of its persistent nature.

◊ References.


1. Heptachlor. *Environmental Health Criteria 38.* Geneva: WHO, 1984. Available at: http://www.inchem.org/documents/ehc/ehc/ehc38.htm (accessed 26/04/04)
2. Heptachlor health and safety guide. *IPCS Health and Safety Guide 14.* Geneva: WHO, 1988. Available at: http://www.inchem.org/documents/hsg/hsg/hsg014.htm (accessed 26/04/04)


## Heptenophos

Heptenofós; Hoe-02982. 7-Chlorobicyclo[3.2.0]hepta-2,6-dien-6-yl dimethyl phosphate.

$C_9H_{12}ClO_4P$ = 250.6.

*CAS — 23560-59-0.*

### Profile

Heptenophos is an organophosphorus insecticide (p.1507) that has been used in veterinary practice for the control of ectoparasites. It is also used in agriculture.

## Hexachlorobenzene

HCB; Hexaclorobenceno.

$C_6Cl_6$ = 284.8.

*CAS — 118-74-1.*

NOTE. Hexachlorobenzene should not be confused with gamma benzene hexachloride (lindane).

### Profile

Hexachlorobenzene has been used as an agricultural fungicide. It is not biodegradable to any significant extent and hexachlorobenzene residues in food have arisen as a result of its occurrence in industrial wastes as well as its use as a fungicide; its use is banned in some countries.

Hexachlorobenzene is reported to be distributed into breast milk.

◊ References.


1. Hexachlorobenzene. *Environmental Health Criteria 195.* Geneva: WHO, 1997. Available at: http://www.inchem.org/documents/ehc/ehc/ehc195.htm (accessed 26/04/04)
2. Hexachlorobenzene health and safety guide. *IPCS Health and Safety Guide 107.* Geneva: WHO, 1998. Available at: http://www.inchem.org/documents/hsg/hsg/hsg107.htm (accessed 26/04/04)


**Toxicity.** Porphyria cutanea tarda[1] and parkinsonism[2] have both been reported in subjects who had ingested seed crops treated with hexachlorobenzene. In a further report the symptoms of porphyria in some patients have been said to persist for many years.[3]


1. Cam C, Nigogosyan G. Acquired toxic porphyria cutanea tarda due to hexachlorobenzene. *JAMA* 1963; **183:** 88–91.
2. Chapman LJ, *et al.* Parkinsonism and industrial chemicals. *Lancet* 1987; **i:** 332–3.
3. Cripps DJ, *et al.* Porphyria turcica due to hexachlorobenzene: a 20 to 30 year follow-up study on 204 patients. *Br J Dermatol* 1984; **111:** 413–22.


## Hydrocyanic Acid

Cianhídrico, ácido; Prussic Acid.

*CAS — 74-90-8.*

**Description.** Hydrocyanic acid is an aqueous solution containing hydrogen cyanide, HCN = 27.03. A colourless liquid with a characteristic almond odour.

### Adverse Effects and Precautions

Hydrocyanic acid and its vapour are intensely poisonous. Cyanides interfere with the oxygen uptake of cells by inhibition of cytochrome oxidase, an enzyme necessary for cellular oxygen transport.

Poisoning by cyanides may occur from inhalation of the vapour, ingestion, or absorption through the skin. Poisoning may arise from cyanide pesticides, industrial accidental exposure, or the inhalation of fumes from some burning plastics. Poisoning may also occur from cyanide-containing plants or fruits.

When large doses of hydrocyanic acid are taken, unconsciousness occurs within a few seconds and death within a few minutes. With smaller toxic doses the symptoms, which occur within a few minutes, may include constriction of the throat, nausea, vomiting, giddiness, headache, palpitation, hyperpnoea then dyspnoea, bradycardia (although initially there may be tachycardia), unconsciousness, and violent convulsions, followed by death. The characteristic smell of bitter almonds may not be obvious and not all individuals can detect it. Cyanosis is not prominent. Similar but usually slower effects occur with cyanide salts.

The fatal dose of hydrocyanic acid for man is considered to be about 50 mg and of the cyanides about 250 mg.

### Treatment of Adverse Effects

Treatment must be given rapidly but should not involve the use of antidotes unless it is certain that cyanide has been absorbed and poisoning is severe.

Cyanide is absorbed very rapidly on inhalation and the poisoned patient should be removed from the area and given oxygen. Steps should be taken to ensure that the airway is adequate. Contaminated clothing should be removed and skin washed. If the patient is conscious, amyl nitrite may be inhaled for up to 30 seconds in every minute but the value of this practice is questionable. Should the patient be unconscious or nearly so, then in the UK and some other countries it is the practice to give dicobalt edetate (p.1036) by injection since it forms a stable complex with the cyanide ion. However, cyanide poisoning should be confirmed, as absence of cyanide puts the patient at risk from the adverse effects of dicobalt edetate. The recommended dose of dicobalt edetate is 300 mg given intravenously over about 1 to 5 minutes, depending on the severity of the poisoning, and repeated once or twice depending on the response. It is customary to give 50 mL of glucose 50% intravenously after each injection, although the value of this has been questioned. An alternative treatment is to inject, as soon as possible, 10 mL of sodium nitrite injection (3%) intravenously over 5 to 20 minutes, then, using the same needle and vein, to continue with an injection of 12.5 g of sodium thiosulfate (50 mL of a 25% solution or 25 mL of a 50% solution) administered over a period of about 10 minutes. Sodium nitrite converts haemoglobin to methaemoglobin which competes with cytochrome oxidase for cyanide, with the formation of cyanmethaemoglobin; sodium thiosulfate aids the conversion or inactivation of cyanide from cyanmethaemoglobin to thiocyanate. If toxic symptoms recur, the injections of nitrite and thiosulfate may be repeated at half the initial doses. Appropriate measures should be instituted to correct hypotension and acidosis.

Hydroxocobalamin may be used for the management of cyanide toxicity. The usual dose is 70 mg/kg by intravenous infusion, repeated once or twice according to severity.

If cyanide has been ingested, one of the above procedures should be instituted. Activated charcoal or gastric lavage may be considered if the patient presents within 1 hour.

◊ Some references concerning the management of cyanide poisoning.[1-3] The use of solutions A and B (15.8% ferrous sulfate in 0.3% citric acid, and 6% sodium carbonate respectively) as so called oral antidotes in persons exposed to cyanide has been condemned as ineffective and lacking scientific evidence.[2]


1. Langford RM, Armstrong RF. Algorithm for managing injury from smoke inhalation. *BMJ* 1989; **299:** 902–5.
2. Koizumi A. Fighting myths. *Lancet* 1994; **344:** 559–60.
3. Proudfoot A, ed. *Pesticide poisoning: notes for the guidance of medical practitioners.* 2nd ed. London: DoH, The Stationery Office, 1996.


### Uses

Cyanides have various industrial applications. Hydrocyanic acid and cyanide salts produce hydrogen cyanide, which has been used as a gas for the eradication of rabbits, rodents, and some other pests. Cyanide salts that might be encountered include calcium cyanide, mercuric cyanide, potassium cyanide, potassium ferricyanide, potassium sodium cyanide, and sodium cyanide.

### Preparations

**Proprietary Preparations** (details are given in Part 3)

**Multi-ingredient:** ***Spain:*** Oftalmol Dexa†; Oftalmol Ocular.

## Imidacloprid

Bay-NTN-33893. 1-[(6-Chloro-3-pyridinyl)methyl]-4,5-dihydro-*N*-nitro-1*H*-imidazol-2-amine.

$C_9H_{10}ClN_5O_2$ = 255.7.

*CAS — 105827-78-9; 138261-41-3.*

### Profile

Imidacloprid is used as a topical ectoparasiticide in veterinary practice, and as an insecticide in agriculture. It has also been investigated for use in the treatment of head lice.

## Iodofenphos (BAN)

Iodofenfós; Jodfenphos. *O*-2,5-Dichloro-4-iodophenyl *O,O*-dimethyl phosphorothioate.

$C_8H_8Cl_2IO_3PS$ = 413.0.

*CAS — 18181-70-9.*

### Profile

Iodofenphos is an organophosphorus insecticide (p.1507) used in veterinary practice for the control of ectoparasites in the environment. It has also been used as an agricultural insecticide. It is an effective mosquito larvicide.

## Lindane (BAN, USAN, rINN)

666; Benhexachlor; Gamma Benzene Hexachloride; Gamma-BHC; Gamma-HCH; HCH; Hexicide; Lindano; Lindanum. 1α,2α,3β,4α,5α,6β-Hexachlorocyclohexane.

$C_6H_6Cl_6$ = 290.8.

*CAS — 58-89-9.*

*ATC — P03AB02.*

**Pharmacopoeias.** In *Chin., Eur.* (see p.vi), *Int.,* and *US.*

**Ph. Eur. 5.0** (Lindane). A white or almost white crystalline powder. Practically insoluble in water; soluble in dehydrated alcohol; freely soluble in acetone. Protect from light.

**USP 27** (Lindane). A white, crystalline powder with a slight musty odour. Practically insoluble in water; soluble in dehydrated alcohol; freely soluble in chloroform; sparingly soluble in ether; slightly soluble in ethylene glycol.

### Adverse Effects, Treatment, and Precautions

As for Chlorinated Insecticides, p.1501.

There has been some concern over the application of higher than normal concentrations of lindane to the skin in the treatment of scabies and pediculosis and therefore lindane should not be used as a first-line treatment; children are considered to be particularly at risk. Resistance has limited its use in pediculosis, so children with that infection tend not to be exposed to it anyway. However, use has continued in scabies and here treatment should be avoided in young children and in women who are breast feeding or are pregnant, and in patients with skin disease. Lindane should also be avoided in patients who have a body-weight less than 50 kg or a history of epilepsy.

◊ Seizures have been reported following the topical use of lindane.[1] In reply, one of the manufacturers stated that up to the end of 1983 they were aware of 21 cases of convulsive disorders apparently associated with the use of their product; it had been used by over 40 million people. Of the 21 cases, the seizures were definitely or probably caused by the product in 11, but in 9 the seizures were associated with ingestion or excessive use.[2]

Isolated reports of adverse effects associated with lindane include disseminated intravascular coagulation and subsequent death after oral ingestion[3] and aplastic anaemia after prolonged topical exposure (twice daily application for 3 weeks).[4]


1. Etherington JD. Major epileptic seizures and topical gammabenzene hexachloride. *BMJ* 1984; **289:** 228.
2. Kelly VT. Major epileptic seizures and topical gammabenzene hexachloride. *BMJ* 1984; **289:** 837.
3. Rao CVSR, *et al.* Disseminated intravascular coagulation in a case of fatal lindane poisoning. *Vet Hum Toxicol* 1988; **30:** 132–4.
4. Rauch AE, *et al.* Lindane (Kwell)-induced aplastic anemia. *Arch Intern Med* 1990; **150:** 2393–5.


### Uses and Administration

Lindane is a chlorinated insecticide (p.1501). It has been used topically in a concentration of 1% for scabies (p.1499) in selected patients and has also been used in pediculosis (p.1499), but use for head lice is restricted by resistance.

Lindane has been used for the control of disease vectors including mosquitoes, lice, and fleas, but resistance has developed. It has also been used as an agricultural and a horticultural insecticide, but its use is prohibited or restricted in many countries.

◊ References.


1. Lindane. *Environmental Health Criteria 124.* Geneva: WHO, 1991. Available at: http://www.inchem.org/documents/ehc/ehc/ehc124.htm (accessed 26/04/04)
2. Lindane health and safety guide. *IPCS Health and Safety Guide 54.* Geneva: WHO, 1991. Available at: http://www.inchem.org/documents/hsg/hsg/hsg054.htm (accessed 26/04/04)


### Preparations

***USP 27:*** Lindane Cream; Lindane Lotion; Lindane Shampoo.

**Proprietary Preparations** (details are given in Part 3)

***Arg.:*** Gamma-Scab; Hexa-Defital; ***Austria:*** Jacutin; ***Belg.:*** Quellada†; ***Braz.:*** Escabin†; Escabron; Lendianon†; Lindanoxil†; Pediletan; Pilensar; Piodrex; Pioletal; Pionax†; Plurisan†; Pruritrat†; Sarpiol†; ***Canad.:*** Hexit; Kwellada†; ***Chile:*** Plomurol; Scabexyl; ***Fr.:*** Aphtiria†; Elentol†; Scabecid; ***Ger.:*** Delitex N; Jacutin; Quellada H†; ***India:*** Ascabiol; Gab; ***Irl.:*** Quellada; ***Israel:*** Bicide; ***Malaysia:*** Jacutin; ***Mex.:*** Escarbicida†; Herklin; Scabene†; Scabisan; War Lin†; ***NZ:*** Benhex; ***Port.:*** Musside; Sarcoderma; ***S.Afr.:*** Gambex; Quellada†; ***Singapore:*** Jacutin; ***Switz.:*** Jacutin; ***Thai.:*** Jacutin; ***USA:*** G-well†.

**Multi-ingredient:** ***Arg.:*** Gamma-Scab; Hexa-Defital; ***Braz.:*** Lindanoxil†; ***Fr.:*** Elenol; ***India:*** Emscab; Scabine; ***Mex.:*** Herklin; Scabisan Plus; ***Spain:*** Sudosin†; Yacutin.

## Lufenuron (BAN, rINN)

CGA-184699; Lufenurón. 1-[2,5-Dichloro-4-(1,1,2,3,3,3-hexafluoropropoxy)phenyl]-3-(2,6-difluorobenzoyl)urea; (RS)-N-[2,5-Dichloro-4-(1,1,2,3,3,3-hexafluoropropoxy)phenylcarbamoyl]-2,6-difluorobenzamide.

$C_{17}H_8Cl_2F_8N_2O_3$ = 511.2.

*CAS — 103055-07-8.*

### Profile

Lufenuron is used as a systemic ectoparasiticide in veterinary practice; it is given by mouth or injection to the host animal.

## Malathion (BAN)

Carbofos; Compound 4047; Malathionum; Malatión; OMS-1. Diethyl 2-(dimethoxyphosphinothioylthio)succinate.

$C_{10}H_{19}O_6PS_2$ = 330.4.

*CAS — 121-75-5.*

*ATC — P03AX03.*

**Pharmacopoeias.** In *Eur.* (see p.vi) and *US.*

**Ph. Eur. 5.0** (Malathion). A clear, colourless or slightly yellowish liquid. It freezes at about 3°. Slightly soluble in water; miscible with alcohol, with acetone, with cyclohexane, and with vegetable oils. Store in airtight containers. Protect from light.

**USP 27** (Malathion). A yellow to deep brown liquid with a characteristic odour. Congeals at about 2.9°. Slightly soluble in water; miscible with alcohols, with ethers, with esters, with ketones, with aromatic and alkylated aromatic hydrocarbons, and with vegetable oils. Store in airtight containers. Protect from light.

**Stability.** The manufacturers have reported that malathion is sensitive to heat and is degraded at temperatures above 30°.

### Adverse Effects and Treatment

As for Organophosphorus Insecticides, p.1507.

Malathion is one of the safer organophosphorus insecticides but its toxicity may be increased by the presence of impurities.

◊ Acute renal insufficiency has been described in a patient associated with excessive exposure to a malathion spray.[1] The condition resolved without specific treatment. Renal toxicity had not previously been associated with organophosphorus pesticides. In a second case of acute poisoning,[2] due to ingestion of malathion, mild transient renal insufficiency and proteinuria with several other late complications including cardiac arrhythmias, pulmonary oedema, diffuse interstitial fibrosis, and muscle weakness due to peripheral neuropathy, were seen subsequent to recovery from the initial cholinergic toxicity.

1. Albright RK, *et al.* Malathion exposure associated with acute renal failure. *JAMA* 1983; **250:** 2469.
2. Dive A, *et al.* Unusual manifestations after malathion poisoning. *Hum Exp Toxicol* 1994; **13:** 271–4.

### Uses and Administration

Malathion is an organophosphorus insecticide (p.1507). It is used in the treatment of head and pubic pediculosis (p.1499) and in scabies (p.1499); lotions of 0.5% and shampoos of 1% are commonly available. Lotions are generally preferred to shampoos as the contact time is longer. Aqueous lotions are preferred to treat pubic lice and scabies because alcoholic lotions are irritant to excoriated skin and the genitalia; aqueous lotions may also be preferable in asthmatic subjects or children to avoid alcoholic fumes. Skin or hair treated with an alcohol-based preparation should be allowed to dry naturally.

Malathion is also used in veterinary practice, agriculture, and horticulture. It is widely used for adult and larval mosquito control although resistance occurs.

### Preparations

***USP 27:*** Malathion Lotion.

**Proprietary Preparations** (details are given in Part 3)

***Austral.:*** Cleensheen†; Lice Rid; ***Belg.:*** Prioderm; Radikal; ***Denm.:*** Prioderm; ***Fin.:*** Prioderm; ***Fr.:*** Prioderm; ***Gr.:*** Sicaril; Specifthir; ***Irl.:*** Derbac-M; Prioderm; ***Israel:*** Prioderm; ***Ital.:*** Aftir Gel; ***Neth.:*** Noury Hoofdlotion†; Prioderm; ***Norw.:*** Prioderm; ***NZ:*** Derbac-M; Prioderm; ***Port.:*** Olicide; ***Singapore:*** A-Lices; ***Swed.:*** Prioderm; ***Switz.:*** Lusap; Prioderm; ***UK:*** Derbac-M; Prioderm; Quellada M; Suleo-M; ***USA:*** Ovide.

**Multi-ingredient:** ***Arg.:*** Aero Helpp Forte; Para Plus; ***Belg.:*** Para Plus; ***Fr.:*** Para Plus; ***Gr.:*** Para-plus; ***Israel:*** Para Plus; ***NZ:*** Para Plus.

## Metaldehyde

Metaldehído.

$(C_2H_4O)_x$.

*CAS — 9002-91-9.*

**Description.** Metaldehyde is a cyclic polymer of acetaldehyde.

### Adverse Effects and Treatment

Symptoms of poisoning by metaldehyde, which may be delayed, include vomiting and diarrhoea, fever, drowsiness, convulsions, and coma. Death from respiratory failure may occur within 48 hours. Kidney and liver damage may occur.

Treatment is symptomatic, although lavage may be considered if more than 50 mg/kg has been ingested within the preceding hour.

◊ References.

1. Longstreth WT, Pierson DJ. Metaldehyde poisoning from slug bait ingestion. *West J Med* 1982; **137:** 134–7.
2. Proudfoot A, ed. *Pesticide poisoning: notes for the guidance of medical practitioners.* 2nd ed. London: DoH, The Stationery Office, 1996.

### Uses

Metaldehyde is a molluscicide used in pellets against slugs and snails. It is an ingredient of some firelighters.

'Meta' is compressed metaldehyde which has been used as a solid fuel burning with a non-luminous carbon-free flame.

## Methomyl

Metomilo. S-Methyl N-(methylcarbamoyloxy)thioacetimidate.

$C_5H_{10}N_2O_2S$ = 162.2.

*CAS — 16752-77-5.*

### Profile

Methomyl is a carbamate insecticide (p.1501) that has been used in agriculture.

◊ References.

1. Methomyl health and safety guide. *IPCS Health and Safety Guide 97.* Geneva: WHO, 1995. Available at: http://www.inchem.org/documents/hsg/hsg/hsg097.htm (accessed 26/04/04)
2. Methomyl. *Environmental Health Criteria 178.* Geneva: WHO, 1996. Available at: http://www.inchem.org/documents/ehc/ehc/ehc178.htm (accessed 26/04/04)

◊ Reports of poisoning with methomyl and its management.

1. Martinez-Chuecos J, *et al.* Management of methomyl poisoning. *Hum Exp Toxicol* 1990; **9:** 251–4.
2. Buchholz U, *et al.* An outbreak of food-borne illness associated with methomyl-contaminated salt. *JAMA* 2002; **288:** 604–10.

## Methoprene (rINN)

Metopreno; ZR-515. Isopropyl 11-methoxy-3,7,11-trimethyldodeca-2(E),4(E)-dienoate.

$C_{19}H_{34}O_3$ = 310.5.

*CAS — 40596-69-8.*

### Profile

Methoprene is an insect growth regulator which mimics the action of insect juvenile hormones and, if it is applied at the appropriate period of sensitivity, it causes death by preventing the transformation of larva to pupa. It is used against a variety of insects including fleas and mosquitoes. It is used in veterinary practice for the control of ectoparasites in the environment, rather than being applied to the animals themselves. It is also used in agriculture.

### Preparations

**Proprietary Preparations** (details are given in Part 3)

**Multi-ingredient:** ***Fr.:*** Acarcid perles†.

## Methoxychlor

Methoxy-DDT. 1,1,1-Trichloro-2-2-bis(p-methoxyphenyl)-ethane.

$C_{16}H_{15}Cl_3O_2$ = 345.6.

*CAS — 72-43-5.*

### Profile

Methoxychlor is a chlorinated insecticide (p.1501) used in agriculture, horticulture, and veterinary practice.

## Methyl Bromide

Bromuro de metilo. Bromomethane; Monobromomethane.

$CH_3Br$ = 94.94.

*CAS — 74-83-9.*

### Adverse Effects, Treatment, and Precautions

Methyl bromide is a vesicant. Toxic effects after inhalation or percutaneous absorption are mainly due to neurotoxicity and include dizziness, headache, vomiting, blurred vision, weakness, ataxia, confusion, mania, hallucinations, mental depression, convulsions, pulmonary oedema, and coma. Renal and hepatic toxicity may also occur and death may be due to circulatory collapse or respiratory failure. Onset of symptoms may be preceded by a latent period. Concentrations of 1% or more are irritant to the eyes. Treatment is symptomatic although dimercaprol or acetylcysteine therapy has been tried.

Rubber absorbs and retains methyl bromide and should not therefore be used in protective clothing.

◊ References to toxicity of methyl bromide including reports of poisoning.

1. Chavez CT, *et al.* Methyl bromide optic atrophy. *Am J Ophthalmol* 1985; **99:** 715–19.
2. Langard S, *et al.* Fatal accident resulting from methyl bromide poisoning after fumigation of a neighbouring house: leakage through sewage pipes. *J Appl Toxicol* 1996; **16:** 445–8.
3. De Haro L, *et al.* Central and peripheral neurotoxic effects of chronic methyl bromide intoxication. *J Toxicol Clin Toxicol* 1997; **35:** 29–34.
4. Michalodimitrakis MN, *et al.* Death following intentional methyl bromide poisoning: toxicological data and literature review. *Vet Hum Toxicol* 1997; **39:** 30–4.
5. Horowitz BZ, *et al.* An unusual exposure to methyl bromide leading to fatality. *J Toxicol Clin Toxicol* 1998; **36:** 353–7.
6. Lifshitz M, Gavrilov V. Central nervous system toxicity and early peripheral neuropathy following dermal exposure to methyl bromide. *J Toxicol Clin Toxicol* 2000; **38:** 799–801.
7. Yamano Y, *et al.* Three cases of acute methyl bromide poisoning in a seedling farm family. *Ind Health* 2001; **39:** 353–8.
8. Hoizey G, *et al.* An unusual case of methyl bromide poisoning. *J Toxicol Clin Toxicol* 2002; **40:** 817–21.

### Uses

Methyl bromide has been used as an insecticidal fumigant for soil and some foodstuffs.

When supplied for fumigation it usually contains chloropicrin as a lachrymatory warning agent.

Methyl bromide has been used as a gaseous disinfectant; it has low antimicrobial activity but good penetrating power.

Methyl bromide was formerly used with carbon tetrachloride in some fire extinguishers. It has also been used as a refrigerant.

◊ General references.

1. Methyl bromide (bromoethane) health and safety guide. *IPCS Health and Safety Guide 86.* Geneva: WHO, 1994. Available at: http://www.inchem.org/documents/hsg/hsg/hsg86_e.htm (accessed 26/04/04)
2. Methyl bromide. *Environmental Health Criteria 166.* Geneva: WHO, 1995. Available at: http://www.inchem.org/documents/ehc/ehc/ehc166.htm (accessed 26/04/04)

## Naled

Bromchlophos. Dimethyl 1,2-dibromo-2,2-dichloroethyl phosphate.

$C_4H_7Br_2Cl_2O_4P$ = 380.8.

*CAS — 300-76-5.*

### Profile

Naled is an organophosphorus insecticide used as a topical ectoparasiticide in veterinary practice.

## Naphthalene

Naftaleno; Naphthalin.

$C_{10}H_8$ = 128.2.

*CAS — 91-20-3.*

### Adverse Effects, Treatment, and Precautions

Ingestion of naphthalene can produce headache, nausea and vomiting, diarrhoea, profuse sweating, dysuria, coma, and convulsions. Doses as low as 2 g have proved fatal to the small child. Treatment is symptomatic and includes emptying the stomach by lavage. The vapour is irritating to the eyes; chronic exposure has led to cataract formation. Haemolytic anaemia and haematuria leading to acute renal failure may occur particularly in persons with G6PD deficiency. Blood transfusions may be required.

**Pregnancy.** Haemolytic anaemia in a neonate has been attributed to inhalation of naphthalene by the mother during the twenty-eighth week of pregnancy.[1]

1. Athanasion M, *et al.* Hemolytic anemia in a female newborn infant whose mother inhaled naphthalene before delivery. *J Pediatr* 1997; **130:** 680–1.

### Uses

Naphthalene has been used in lavatory deodorant discs and in mothballs. It has also been used as a soil fumigant.

## Norbormide

McN-1025; Norbormida. 5-[α-Hydroxy-α-(2-pyridyl)benzyl]-7-[α-(2-pyridyl)benzylidene]-8,9,10-trinorborn-5-ene-2,3-dicarboximide.

$C_{33}H_{25}N_3O_3$ = 511.6.

*CAS — 991-42-4.*

### Profile

Norbormide is a selective rodenticide effective against most species of *rats,* in which it produces extreme irreversible peripheral vasoconstriction. It is not very toxic to other rodents.

## Organophosphorus Insecticides

Insecticidas organofosforados.

**Description.** The organophosphorus or organophosphate insecticides may be esters, amides, or thiol derivatives of phosphoric, phosphonic, phosphorothioic, or phosphonothioic acids.

◊ References.

1. WHO. Organophosphorus insecticides: a general introduction. *Environmental Health Criteria 63.* Geneva: WHO, 1986. Available at: http://www.inchem.org/documents/ehc/ehc/ehc63.htm (accessed 19/07/04)

### Adverse Effects

Organophosphorus insecticides are potent cholinesterase inhibitors and can be very toxic. This inhibition results in both muscarinic and nicotinic effects with some central involvement.

Toxic effects may include abdominal cramps, nausea, vomiting, diarrhoea, pancreatitis, urinary incontinence, miosis or mydriasis, weakness, respiratory disturbances, lachrymation, increased salivation and sweating, bradycardia or tachycardia, hypotension or hypertension, cyanosis, muscular twitching, and convulsions.

Some organophosphorus compounds cause delayed neuropathy. CNS symptoms include restlessness, anxiety, dizziness, confusion, coma, and depression of the respiratory or cardiovascular system. Patients may experience mental disturbances. Inhalation or external contact can cause local as well as systemic effects.

Repeated exposure may have a cumulative effect though the organophosphorus insecticides are, in contrast to the chlorinated insecticides, rapidly metabolised and excreted and are not appreciably stored in body tissues.

◊ References to the adverse effects and poisoning encountered with organophosphorus compounds such as insecticides (including sheepdips).


1. Minton NA, Murray VSG. A review of organophosphate poisoning. *Med Toxicol* 1988; **3:** 350–75.
2. Karalliedde L, Senanayake N. Organophosphorus insecticide poisoning. *Br J Anaesth* 1989; **63:** 736–50.
3. Öztürk MA, *et al.* Anticholinesterase poisoning in Turkey—clinical, laboratory and radiologic evaluation of 269 cases. *Hum Exp Toxicol* 1990; **9:** 273–9.
4. WHO. Safe use of pesticides: fourteenth report of the WHO expert committee on vector biology and control. *WHO Tech Rep Ser 813* 1991.
5. Casey P, Vale JA. Deaths from pesticide poisoning in England and Wales: 1945–1989. *Hum Exp Toxicol* 1994; **13:** 95–101.
6. Eyer P. Neuropsychopathological changes by organophosphorus compounds—a review. *Hum Exp Toxicol* 1995; **14:** 857–64.
7. Proudfoot A, ed. *Pesticide poisoning: notes for the guidance of medical practitioners.* 2nd ed. London: DoH, The Stationery Office, 1996.
8. Steenland K. Chronic neurological effects of organophosphate pesticides. *BMJ* 1996; **312:** 1312–13.
9. Brown AA, Brix KA. Review of health consequences from high-, intermediate- and low-level exposure to organophosphorus nerve agents. *J Appl Toxicol* 1998; **18:** 393–408.
10. Koksal N, *et al.* Organophosphate intoxication as a consequence of mouth-to-mouth breathing from an affected case. *Chest* 2002; **122:** 740–1.


### Treatment of Adverse Effects

Rapid treatment for poisoning with organophosphorus insecticides is essential. Use of gastric lavage may be considered if a substantial amount has been ingested within 1 to 2 hours of presentation. Contaminated clothing should be removed and the skin, including any areas contaminated by vomiting or hypersecretion, should receive copious and prolonged washing with soap and water. Contamination of the eye is treated by washing of the conjunctiva. The patient should be treated with atropine (see Poisoning, p.478) and either pralidoxime (p.1050) or obidoxime (p.1046) and symptomatic treatment should be instituted. Diazepam is sometimes given; it may be necessary to give it parenterally in moderate to severe poisoning to control muscle fasciculations and convulsions; oral administration in mild poisoning may be helpful in relieving anxiety. The patient should be observed for signs of deterioration due to delayed absorption.

## Paraquat

1,1′-Dimethyl-4,4′-bipyridyldiylium ion.

$C_{12}H_{14}N_2$ = 186.3.

*CAS — 4685-14-7.*

## Paraquat Dichloride

Dicloruro de paraquat.

$C_{12}H_{14}Cl_2N_2$ = 257.2.

*CAS — 1910-42-5.*

### Adverse Effects

Concentrated solutions of paraquat may cause irritation, inflammation, and possibly blistering of the skin, cracking and shedding of the nails, and delayed healing of cuts and wounds. It is not significantly absorbed from undamaged skin. A few fatalities have occurred following skin contact, but these appear to have been associated with prolonged contact and concentrated solutions.

Splashes in the eye cause severe inflammation, which may be delayed for 12 to 24 hours, corneal oedema, reduced visual acuity, and extensive superficial stripping of the corneal and conjunctival epithelium, which usually slowly heals. Inhalation of dust or spray may cause nasal bleeding.

Paraquat weedkillers available for use in domestic gardens contain 2.5% w/v paraquat, sometimes in association with other herbicides such as diquat. While this strength of paraquat can cause nausea and vomiting as well as some respiratory changes when ingested, it is not considered to be a lethal form.

Most of the cases of severe poisoning follow the ingestion or sometimes injection of the concentrated forms of paraquat herbicide (20% w/v), the distribution of which is restricted to agriculturalists and horticulturalists. In many cases this ingestion is intentional. It is considered that patients who ingest 20 to 40 mg/kg suffer moderate to severe poisoning; most, but not all, die up to about 2 or 3 weeks after ingestion. Severe acute poisoning occurs with ingestion of higher doses. The irritant effects of paraquat are reflected in oesophageal ulceration and gastrointestinal effects. There is widespread organ damage, most notably involving the kidneys and lungs. In such poisoning death is virtually certain and occurs rapidly.

Preparations of paraquat may contain an emetic or a laxative and some contain a malodorous agent to deter ingestion.

◊ General references concerning paraquat toxicity and its treatment.


1. Paraquat and diquat. *Environmental Health Criteria 39.* Geneva: WHO, 1984. Available at: http://www.inchem.org/documents/ehc/ehc/ehc39.htm (accessed 26/04/04)
2. Bismuth C, *et al.* Paraquat poisoning. *Drug Safety* 1990; **5:** 243–51.
3. Pond SM. Manifestations and management of paraquat poisoning. *Med J Aust* 1990; **152:** 256–9.
4. Paraquat health and safety guide. *Health and Safety Guide 51.* Geneva: WHO, 1991. Available at: http://www.inchem.org/documents/hsg/hsg/hsg051.htm (accessed 26/04/04)
5. WHO. Safe use of pesticides: fourteenth report of the WHO expert committee on vector biology and control. *WHO Tech Rep Ser 813* 1991.
6. Proudfoot A, ed. *Pesticide poisoning: notes for the guidance of medical practitioners.* 2nd ed. London: DoH, The Stationery Office, 1996.


### Treatment of Adverse Effects

Following contact with paraquat, contaminated clothing should be removed and the skin washed with soap and water. The eyes, if splashed, should be irrigated; later topical therapy may involve the symptomatic use of antibacterials or corticosteroids.

There is no specific treatment for paraquat poisoning and the immediate aim is to remove or inactivate the paraquat. If the patient presents less than 6 hours after ingestion the initial management involves the oral administration of an adsorbent, preferably activated charcoal given in a dose of 100 g and followed by 50 g every 2 hours for up to 6 hours post ingestion. Fuller's earth (often as a 15% suspension) and bentonite (as a 7% suspension) are alternative oral adsorbents and are given in similar doses to those of charcoal. When none of these adsorbents is available, a suspension of clay or of uncontaminated soil should be considered if medical attention is likely to be delayed. An osmotic laxative may be used with the first dose of the adsorbent in order to hasten bowel evacuation and prevent obstruction due to the adsorbent. Patients may require intensive supportive therapy, but oxygen should not be given initially as it appears to enhance the pulmonary toxicity of paraquat; however, it may be needed in later stages as part of palliative care.

Methods aimed at hastening elimination such as forced diuresis, peritoneal dialysis, haemodialysis, and haemoperfusion have been tried but the first three appear to be ineffective and results with the last method have varied; no method is of proven value.

◊ For some general references concerning the treatment of paraquat toxicity, see under Adverse Effects, above.

Once paraquat has been absorbed, moderate to severe poisoning may result in acute renal failure, hepatitis, and pulmonary fibrosis; death may occur after 2 to 3 weeks. Pulse therapy with cyclophosphamide and methylprednisolone might be of benefit in such patients but not in those with fulminant poisoning.[1,2]


1. Lin J-L, *et al.* Pulse therapy with cyclophosphamide and methylprednisolone in patients with moderate to severe paraquat poisoning: a preliminary report. *Thorax* 1996; **51:** 661–3.
2. Lin J-L, *et al.* A prospective clinical trial of pulse therapy with glucocorticoid and cyclophosphamide in moderate to severe paraquat poisoned patients. *Am J Respir Crit Care Med* 1999; **159:** 357–60. Correction to the dose of cyclophosphamide. *ibid.* 2001; **163:** 292.


### Uses

Paraquat is a contact herbicide widely used as the dichloride in agriculture and horticulture. Liquid concentrates are supplied in the UK only to approved users.

## Parathion

Paratión. O,O-Diethyl O-4-nitrophenyl phosphorothioate.

$C_{10}H_{14}NO_5PS$ = 291.3.

*CAS — 56-38-2.*

### Profile

Parathion is an organophosphorus insecticide (p.1507) that has been used in agriculture and horticulture. Its metabolite diethyl nitrophenyl phosphate (paraoxon, p.1494) contributes to its toxicity.

◊ References.


1. Parathion health and safety guide. *IPCS Health and Safety Guide 74.* Geneva: WHO, 1992. Available at: http://www.inchem.org/documents/hsg/hsg/hsg74.htm (accessed 26/04/04)


◊ Reports of poisoning with parathion.


1. Anastassiades CJ, Ioannides M. Organophosphate poisoning and auricular fibrillation. *BMJ* 1984; **289:** 290.
2. Golsousidis H, Kokkas V. Use of 19 590 mg of atropine during 24 days of treatment, after a case of unusually severe parathion poisoning. *Hum Toxicol* 1985; **4:** 339–40.
3. Clifford NJ, Nies AS. Organophosphate poisoning from wearing a laundered uniform previously contaminated with parathion. *JAMA* 1989; **262:** 3035–6.
4. Wang M-H, *et al.* Q-T interval prolongation and pleomorphic ventricular tachyarrhythmia ('Torsade de pointes') in organophosphate poisoning: report of a case. *Hum Exp Toxicol* 1998; **17:** 587–90.


## Pentachlorophenol

PCP; Penta; Pentaclorofenol.

$C_6HCl_5O$ = 266.3.

*CAS — 87-86-5.*

NOTE. The name PCP has also been used as a synonym for phencyclidine hydrochloride.

### Adverse Effects, Treatment, and Precautions

Pentachlorophenol may be absorbed in toxic amounts through the skin or by inhalation, as well as by ingestion. Pentachlorophenol and its aqueous solutions are irritant to the eyes, mucous membranes, and to the skin, and may produce caustic burns. The systemic effects are due to uncoupling of oxidative phosphorylation with consequent stimulation of cellular metabolism. Acute poisoning with pentachlorophenol increases metabolic rate, leading to raised temperature with copious sweating and thirst, restlessness, fatigue, increased rate and depth of respiration, and tachycardia. There may be abdominal pain and nausea, and death has occurred from respiratory failure. Symptoms of subacute or chronic poisoning include hyperpyrexia and CNS, haematological, renal, reproductive, respiratory, and skin disorders.

Treatment is symptomatic. Raised body temperature should be treated by physical means; the use of antipyretics is not recommended since they can increase toxicity.

◊ Reviews of the toxicity of pentachlorophenol.


1. Health and Safety Executive. Pentachlorophenol. *Toxicity Review 5.* London: HMSO, 1982.
2. Pentachlorophenol. *Environmental Health Criteria 71.* Geneva: WHO, 1987. Available at: http://www.inchem.org/documents/ehc/ehc/ehc71.htm (accessed 26/04/04)
3. Pentachlorophenol health and safety guide. *Health and Safety Guide 19.* Geneva: WHO, 1989. Available at: http://www.inchem.org/documents/hsg/hsg/hsg019.htm (accessed 26/04/04)
4. Jorens PG, Schepens PJC. Human pentachlorophenol poisoning. *Hum Exp Toxicol* 1993; **12:** 479–95.


◊ There have been reports of malignant neoplasms,[1,2] aplastic anaemia,[3] pancreatitis,[4] intravascular haemolysis,[5] and urticaria[6] associated with exposure to pentachlorophenol.


1. Greene MH, *et al.* Familial and sporadic Hodgkin's disease associated with occupational wood exposure. *Lancet* 1978; **ii:** 626–7.
2. Hardell L. Malignant lymphoma of histiocytic type and exposure to phenoxyacetic acids or chlorophenols. *Lancet* 1979; **i:** 55–6.
3. Roberts HJ. Aplastic anemia due to pentachlorophenol. *N Engl J Med* 1981; **305:** 1650–1.
4. Cooper RG, Macaulay MB. Pentachlorophenol pancreatitis. *Lancet* 1982; **i:** 517.
5. Hassan AB, *et al.* Intravascular haemolysis induced by pentachlorophenol. *BMJ* 1985; **291:** 21–2.
6. Kentor PM. Urticaria from contact with pentachlorophenate. *JAMA* 1986; **256:** 3350.


### Pharmacokinetics

Pentachlorophenol may be absorbed after ingestion or inhalation or through the skin. Following ingestion, the majority of a dose is eliminated in the urine as unchanged pentachlorophenol and its glucuronide, with small amounts appearing in the faeces.

### Uses

Pentachlorophenol has been used mainly as the sodium salt ($C_6Cl_5NaO$ = 288.3), as a preservative for a wide range of industrial and agricultural products, including wood and other building materials, textiles, glues, and starch. It has also been used for the control of slime and algae, and as a molluscicide, fungicide, and herbicide.

## Permethrin *(BAN, USAN, rINN)*

Permetrina. 3-Phenoxybenzyl (1RS,3RS)-(1RS,3SR)-3-(2,2-dichlorovinyl)-2,2-dimethylcyclopropanecarboxylate.

$C_{21}H_{20}Cl_2O_3$ = 391.3.

*CAS — 52645-53-1.*

*ATC — P03AC04.*

### Profile

Permethrin is a pyrethroid insecticide (see Pyrethrum Flower, p.1509). It is used in the treatment of head pediculosis (p.1499) as a 1% application; there have been signs of resistance. It is also employed as an acaricide in the treatment of scabies (p.1499) as a 5% cream.

Permethrin is also used as a topical ectoparasiticide in veterinary practice and as an agricultural, horticultural, and household insecticide.

Permethrin is active against mosquitoes and is widely used for the impregnation of bednets and curtains in the control of malaria (p.444). It is also active against blackflies in the adult and larval stages and is used for the larvicidal treatment of rivers in the control of onchocerciasis (p.100). It is also active against tsetse flies.

Permethrin is suitable for aircraft disinsection.

◊ References.


1. Permethrin health and safety guide. *IPCS Health and Safety Guide 33.* Geneva: WHO, 1989. Available at: http://www.inchem.org/documents/hsg/hsg/hsg033.htm (accessed 26/04/04)
2. Permethrin. *Environmental Health Criteria 94.* Geneva: WHO, 1990. Available at: http://www.inchem.org/documents/ehc/ehc/ehc94.htm (accessed 26/04/04)


### Preparations

**Proprietary Preparations** (details are given in Part 3)

**Arg.:** Blum; Capitis; Dermoper; Duncankil; Fripi; Hairclin; Helpp; Kinderval; Kwell; Lumat; Nopucid; Pelo Libre; Percapyl; Sapucai; Witty; ***Austral.:***

Lyclear; Nix†; Pyrifoam; Quellada; **Belg.:** Nix; Zalvor; **Braz.:** Clean Hair; Kwell; Lendrex; Nedax; Nedax Plus; Permetel; Permetrix†; Piolhol Plus; Piosan†; Piosol†; Piostop; Toppyc; Wellcid; **Canad.:** Kwellada-P; Nix; **Chile:** Assy Espuma; Kilnits; **Denm.:** Nix; **Fin.:** Nix; **Fr.:** Insect Ecran; Modul'Aid; Moskizol†; Nix; **Ger.:** Delixi†; InfectoPedicul; **Gr.:** Nix; **Hong Kong:** Quellada; **India:** Perlice; **Irl.:** Lyclear; **Israel:** Lyclear; Mite-X; Nok; Zehu-Ze; **Ital.:** Nix; Pre Clean Mom; **Mex.:** Novo-Herklin 2000; **Neth.:** Loxazol; **Norw.:** Nix; **NZ:** Lyclear†; Lyderm; Pyrifoam; Quellada P†; **Port.:** Desintan P†; Nix; **S.Afr.:** Lyclear; **Spain:** Sarcop; **Swed.:** Nix; **Switz.:** Loxazol; **UK:** Bug Proof†; Lyclear; Residex P55; **USA:** Acticin; Elimite; Nix.

**Multi-ingredient: Arg.:** Aero Helpp Forte; Arnecrem; Detebencil; Para Plus; Pedicrem; Perbel; Permecil; Sapucai; **Belg.:** Para Plus; Shampoux†; **Braz.:** Piolhol; **Fr.:** Acarcid perles†; Anti-Ac; Charlieu Anti-Poux; Para Plus; Pyreflor; Sanytol; **Gr.:** Para-plus; **Israel:** Para Plus; **NZ:** Para Plus; **S.Afr.:** Nitagon.

## Phenothrin *(BAN, rINN)*

Fenotrina; S-2539. 3-Phenoxybenzyl (1*RS*,3*RS*)-(1*RS*,3*SR*)-2,2-dimethyl-3-(2-methylprop-1-enyl)cyclopropanecarboxylate.

$C_{23}H_{26}O_3$ = 350.5.
*CAS — 26002-80-2.*
*ATC — P03AC03.*

### Profile

Phenothrin is a pyrethroid insecticide (see Pyrethrum Flower, below). It is used for the treatment of head and pubic pediculosis (p.1499) as a 0.2% alcoholic or 0.5% aqueous lotion, or as a 0.5% alcoholic foam; as with permethrin there have been signs of resistance.

Phenothrin is also used in veterinary practice as a topical ectoparasiticide, as a household insecticide, and for the disinsection of public areas and aircraft.

◊ References.


1. d-Phenothrin health and safety guide. *IPCS Health and Safety Guide 32*. Geneva: WHO, 1989. Available at: http://www.inchem.org/documents/hsg/hsg/hsg032.htm (accessed 26/04/04)
2. d-Phenothrin. *Environmental Health Criteria 96*. Geneva: WHO, 1990. Available at: http://www.inchem.org/documents/ehc/ehc/ehc96.htm (accessed 26/04/04)


**Aircraft disinsection.** References.


1. Russell RC, Paton R. In-flight disinsection as an efficacious procedure for preventing international transport of insects of public health importance. *Bull WHO* 1989; **67:** 543–7.


### Preparations

**Proprietary Preparations** (details are given in Part 3)
**Arg.:** Nopucid MC; Sumo; **Fr.:** Itax Antipoux; Item Antipoux; Parasidose; **Gr.:** Ivaliten; Sitem; **Irl.:** Headmaster; **Israel:** Sof-Sof; **Ital.:** Cruzzy Shampoo Potenziato alla Sumitrina; Mediker; Mom Gel; Mom Shampoo Schiuma; Ottocid; **Mon.:** Hegor Antipoux; **NZ:** Full Marks; Parasidose; **UK:** Full Marks; **USA:** Pronto.

**Multi-ingredient: Fr.:** Itax Antipoux†; Sanytol; **Gr.:** Cif Candioli; **Ital.:** Mom Shampoo Antiparassitario; Neo Mom.

## Phosmet *(BAN)*

Fosmet. *O,O*-Dimethyl phthalimidomethyl phosphorodithioate.

$C_{11}H_{12}NO_4PS_2$ = 317.3.
*CAS — 732-11-6.*

### Profile

Phosmet is an organophosphorus insecticide (p.1507) used as a systemic ectoparasiticide in veterinary practice; it is applied topically to the host animal. It has also been used in agriculture and horticulture.

## Phoxim *(BAN)*

Bayer-9053; Foxim. 2-(Diethoxyphosphinothioyloxyimino)-2-phenylacetonitrile.

$C_{12}H_{15}N_2O_3PS$ = 298.3.
*CAS — 14816-18-3.*

### Profile

Phoxim is an organophosphorus insecticide (p.1507) used as a topical ectoparasiticide in veterinary practice. It is also used for the larvicidal treatment of rivers in the control of onchocerciasis (p.100).

### Preparations

**Proprietary Preparations** (details are given in Part 3)
**Ital.:** Baythion EC.

## Piperonal

Heliotropin; Piperonylaldehyde. 1,3-Benzodioxole-5-carboxaldehyde.

$C_8H_6O_3$ = 150.1.
*CAS — 120-57-0.*

### Profile

Piperonal is used as an insect repellent against head lice (p.1499).

### Preparations

**Proprietary Preparations** (details are given in Part 3)
**Fr.:** Para Repulsif; **UK:** Rappell.

## Piperonyl Butoxide *(BAN)*

Butóxido de piperonilo. 5-[2-(2-Butoxyethoxy)ethoxymethyl]-6-propyl-1,3-benzodioxole.

$C_{19}H_{30}O_5$ = 338.4.
*CAS — 51-03-6.*

**Pharmacopoeias.** In *BP(Vet)*.

**BP(Vet) 2003** (Piperonyl Butoxide). A yellow or pale brown oily liquid with a faint characteristic odour. Very slightly soluble in water; miscible with alcohol, with chloroform, with ether, and with petroleum oils.

### Profile

Piperonyl butoxide is used as a synergist for pyrethrin and pyrethroid insecticides. Mixtures of piperonyl butoxide and pyrethrins or pyrethroids are used in the treatment of pediculosis (p.1499).

Piperonyl butoxide is considered to cause a variety of gastrointestinal effects as well as mild CNS depression.

### Preparations

**Proprietary Preparations** (details are given in Part 3)

**Multi-ingredient: Arg.:** Acardust; Aero Helpp Forte; Capitis; Deca-Scab; Hexa-Defital NF; Limpacid; Nopucid Compuesto; Para Piojicida; Para Plus; Quitoso; Scabioderm; **Austral.:** Banlice; Lyban†; Paralice; Sundown with Insect Repellent†; **Belg.:** Para; Para Plus; Shampoux†; **Braz.:** Deltacid Plus; Nopucid Composto†; Piolhol; Sarnapen; Vapio†; **Canad.:** Licetrol; Para; Pronto; R & C; Scabene; **Chile:** Launol; **Denm.:** Para†; **Fr.:** A-Par; Acarcid perles†; Acardust; Anti-Ac; Charlieu Anti-Poux; Itax Antipoux†; Para Plus; Para Special Poux; Pyreflor; Spray-Pax; Spregal; **Ger.:** Goldgeist; Jacutin N; Quellada P†; Spregal; **Gr.:** Para-plus; Runde; **Israel:** A-200; Acardust; Kin Soff; Para Plus; **Ital.:** Acardust†; Baygon; Cruzzy; Cruzzy Antiparassitario†; Entom†; Mafu†; Milice; Mom Piretro Emulsione; Sinezan; **Neth.:** Para-Speciaal; **Norw.:** Rinsoderm†; **NZ:** Para Plus; **Port.:** Para-Pio; Quitoso; **S.Afr.:** Nitagon; Spregal; **Swed.:** Crinopex†; **Switz.:** Acardust†; **UK:** Buzpel†; Fortefog; Patriot†; Prevent; **USA:** Barc†; Blue; Clear Total Lice Elimination System†; End Lice†; InnoGel Plus†; Licide; Pronto; Pyrinex†; Pyrinyl II; Pyrinyl Plus; R & C†; RID; Tegrin-LT†; Tisit; Triple X†.

## Pirimiphos-Methyl

Metilpirimifós. *O*-2-Diethylamino-6-methylpyrimidin-4-yl *O,O*-dimethyl phosphorothioate.

$C_{11}H_{20}N_3O_3PS$ = 305.3.
*CAS — 29232-93-7.*

### Profile

Pirimiphos-methyl is an organophosphorus insecticide (p.1507). It is used in agriculture and domestically.

### Preparations

**Proprietary Preparations** (details are given in Part 3)

**Multi-ingredient: Fr.:** Anti-Ac.

## Propetamphos *(BAN)*

Propetamfós. Isopropyl (*E*)-3-[(ethylamino)(methoxy)phosphinothio-oxy]but-2-enoate.

$C_{10}H_{20}NO_4PS$ = 281.3.
*CAS — 31218-83-4.*

### Profile

Propetamphos is an organophosphorus insecticide (p.1507) used as a topical ectoparasiticide in veterinary practice.

## Propoxur *(BAN)*

2-Isopropoxyphenyl methylcarbamate.

$C_{11}H_{15}NO_3$ = 209.2.
*CAS — 114-26-1.*

### Profile

Propoxur is a carbamate insecticide (p.1501) used as a topical ectoparasiticide in veterinary practice. It is also used as a fumigant in agriculture.

### Preparations

**Proprietary Preparations** (details are given in Part 3)
**Ital.:** Pulvis-3†.

**Multi-ingredient: Ital.:** Baygon.

## Pyraclofos

Piraclofós. (*RS*)-[*O*-1-(4-Chlorophenyl)pyrazol-4-yl *O*-ethyl *S*-propyl phosphorothioate].

$C_{14}H_{18}ClN_2O_3PS$ = 360.8.
*CAS — 77458-01-6.*

### Profile

Pyraclofos is an organophosphorus insecticide (p.1507) used for the larvicidal treatment of rivers in the control of onchocerciasis (p.100).

## Pyrethrum Flower

Chrysanthème Insecticide; Dalmatian Insect Flowers; Flor del pelitre; Insect Flowers; Insektenblüten; Piretro; Pyrethri Flos.

*CAS — 8003-34-7 (pyrethrum); 121-21-1 (pyrethrin I); 121-29-9 (pyrethrin II); 25402-06-6 (cinerin I); 121-20-0 (cinerin II).*
*ATC — P03AC01.*

**Pharmacopoeias.** In *BP(Vet)*, which also includes the extract. *US* includes only the extract.

**BP(Vet) 2003** (Pyrethrum Flower). The dried flowerheads of *Chrysanthemum cinerariaefolium* containing not less than 1% of pyrethrins of which not less than one-half consists of pyrethrin I. It has a faint but characteristic odour.

**BP(Vet) 2003** (Pyrethrum Extract). An extract prepared from Pyrethrum Flower. It contains 24.5 to 25.5% of pyrethrins, of which not less than half consists of pyrethrin I. A dark olive green or brown viscous liquid or, if decolourised, a pale amber liquid. Store in a well-filled container. Protect from light. It should be thoroughly stirred before use.

**USP 27** (Pyrethrum Extract). A mixture of three naturally occurring, closely related insecticidal esters of chrysanthemic acid (pyrethrins I: jasmolin I, cinerin I, and pyrethrin I) and three closely related esters of pyrethric acid (pyrethrins II: jasmolin II, cinerin II, and pyrethrin II). The ratio of pyrethrins I to pyrethrins II is not less than 0.8 and not more than 2.8. It may contain pigments characteristic of chrysanthemum species, triglyceride oils, terpenoids, and carotenoid. It may also contain suitable solvents and antioxidants. It contains no other added substances. It is a pale yellow liquid having a bland, flowery odour. Insoluble in water; soluble in liquid paraffin and in most organic solvents. Store in airtight containers. Protect from light.

### Adverse Effects and Precautions

Pyrethrum is irritant to the eyes and mucosa. Hypersensitivity reactions have been reported.

### Uses

Pyrethrum flower is mainly used for the preparation of pyrethrum extracts containing a mixture of chrysanthemic acid and pyrethric acid esters (pyrethrins I and II).

Pyrethrins in the form of pyrethrum extract have a long history of use as insecticides. Pyrethrum is rapidly toxic to many insects. It has a much quicker knock-down effect than clofenotane or lindane, but it is less persistent and less stable. Its action can be enhanced by certain substances such as piperonyl butoxide (p.1509), and pyrethrins with piperonyl butoxide are used clinically in the treatment of pediculosis (p.1499).

Pyrethroid insecticides (synthetic analogues of pyrethrins), such as permethrin and phenothrin, are also used clinically; deltamethrin and permethrin are among those used for the vector control of malaria.

Pyrethrum, pyrethrins, and pyrethroids are also used as topical ectoparasiticides in veterinary practice and as agricultural, horticultural, and household insecticides.

### Preparations

**Proprietary Preparations** (details are given in Part 3)

**Multi-ingredient: Arg.:** Quitoso; **Austral.:** Banlice; Lyban†; Sundown with Insect Repellent†; **Canad.:** Licetrol; Pronto; R & C; **Fr.:** Spray-Pax; **Ger.:** Goldgeist; Quellada P†; **Israel:** A-200; Kin Soff; **Ital.:** Cruzzy Antiparassitario†; Entom†; Milice; Sinezan; **Norw.:** Rinsoderm†; **Port.:** Para-Pio; Quitoso; **Swed.:** Crinopex†; **UK:** Buzpel†; Fortefog; Patriot†; Prevent; Savlon Natural First Aid for Insect Bites & Stings; **USA:** Barc†; Blue; Clear Total Lice Elimination System†; End Lice†; InnoGel Plus†; Licide; Pronto; Pyrinex†; Pyrinyl II; Pyrinyl Plus; R & C†; RID; Tegrin-LT†; Tisit; Triple X†.

## Pyriproxyfen

Piriproxifeno; S-9318; S-31183. 2-[1-Methyl-2-(4-phenoxyphenoxy)ethoxy]pyridine.

$C_{20}H_{19}NO_3$ = 321.4.
*CAS — 95737-68-1.*

### Profile

Pyriproxyfen is used as a topical ectoparasiticide in veterinary practice.

## Red Squill

Esquila.

*CAS — 507-60-8 (scilliroside).*

### Profile

Red squill is a red variety of *Urginea maritima*, which contains, in addition to cardiac glycosides, an active principle, scilliroside. It is very toxic to *rats* and has been incorporated in rat poisons; it has neurotoxic and cardiotoxic properties.

## Resmethrin

Resmetrina. 5-Benzyl-3-furylmethyl (1*RS*,3*RS*)-(1*RS*,3*SR*)-2,2-dimethyl-3-(2-methylprop-1-enyl)cyclopropanecarboxylate.

$C_{22}H_{26}O_3$ = 338.4.
*CAS — 10453-86-8.*

### Profile

Resmethrin is a pyrethroid insecticide (see Pyrethrum Flower, p.1509) used in veterinary practice for the control of ectoparasites in the environment. Resmethrin is also used as an agricultural, horticultural, and household insecticide, but is not synergised by pyrethrum synergists such as piperonyl butoxide (p.1509).

◊ References.

1. Resmethrins. *Environmental Health Criteria 92*. Geneva: WHO, 1989. Available at: http://www.inchem.org/documents/ehc/ehc/ehc092.htm (accessed 26/04/04)
2. Resmethrins health and safety guide. *IPCS Health and Safety Guide 25*. Geneva: WHO, 1989. Available at: http://www.inchem.org/documents/hsg/hsg/hsg025.htm (accessed 26/04/04)

## Rotenone

Rotenona; Rotenonum. (2*R*,6a*S*,12a*S*)-1,2,6,6a,12,12a-Hexahydro-2-isopropenyl-8,9-dimethoxychromeno[3,4-*b*]furo[2,3-*h*]chromen-6-one.

$C_{23}H_{22}O_6$ = 394.4.

*CAS — 83-79-4.*

### Profile

Rotenone is a non-systemic insecticide used in agriculture and in horticulture.

Rotenone is the active ingredient of derris (the dried rhizome and roots of *Derris elliptica*; also known as tuba root or aker-tuba) and of lonchocarpus (the dried root of *Lonchocarpus utilis*; also known as cube root, timbo, or barbusco). Powdered forms of derris and of lonchocarpus have been used as insecticides and fish poisons.

◊ References.

1. Rotenone health and safety guide. *IPCS Health and Safety Guide 73*. Geneva: WHO, 1992. Available at: http://www.inchem.org/documents/hsg/hsg/hsg073.htm (accessed 26/04/04)

## Sodium Fluoroacetate

Compound 1080; Fluoroacetato sódico; Sodium Monofluoroacetate.

$FCH_2.CO_2Na$ = 100.0.

*CAS — 62-74-8.*

### Adverse Effects, Treatment, and Precautions

Sodium fluoroacetate is highly toxic, the lethal dose if ingested being about 1 to 5 mg/kg. Toxic effects may be delayed for several hours after absorption by mouth or inhalation, and include nausea and vomiting, apprehension, muscle twitching, cardiac irregularities, convulsions, respiratory failure, coma, and death usually due to ventricular fibrillation.

Treatment is generally supportive and symptomatic.

◊ References to sodium fluoroacetate toxicity.

1. Chi CH, *et al.* Clinical presentation and prognostic factors in sodium monofluoroacetate intoxication. *J Toxicol Clin Toxicol* 1996; **34:** 707–12.
2. Chi CH, *et al.* Hemodynamic abnormalities in sodium monofluoroacetate intoxication. *Hum Exp Toxicol* 1999; **18:** 351–3.

### Uses

Sodium fluoroacetate is a highly effective rodenticide but must be used with great caution because of its toxicity to other animals and to man.

## Sulfiram *(BAN, rINN)*

Monosulfiram; Sulfiramum. Tetraethylthiuram monosulphide.

$C_{10}H_{20}N_2S_3$ = 264.5.

*CAS — 95-05-6.*

### Adverse Effects and Precautions

An erythematous rash has occasionally been reported. Sulfiram produces effects similar to those of disulfiram (p.1681) if ingested with alcohol. As there may be a risk of absorption following the application of sulfiram to the whole body, patients are advised to abstain from alcohol for at least 48 hours.

◊ The reactions to alcohol occasionally reported in patients who have applied sulfiram solution[1,2] resemble those seen with disulfiram. Analysis has shown that sulfiram solutions exposed to room light undergo photochemical conversion to disulfiram, and that the concentration of disulfiram, and the ability of the solution to inhibit aldehyde dehydrogenase and hence the metabolism of alcohol, increases with the duration of such storage.[3,4] Whether patients who have applied sulfiram solution should avoid direct light immediately afterwards remains to be elucidated.[4]

1. Blanc D, Deprez P. Unusual adverse reaction to an acaricide. *Lancet* 1990; **335:** 1291–2.
2. Burgess I. Adverse reactions to monosulfiram. *Lancet* 1990; **336:** 873.
3. Mays DC, *et al.* Photolysis of monosulfiram: a mechanism for its disulfiram-like reaction. *Clin Pharmacol Ther* 1994; **55:** 191.
4. Lipsky JJ, *et al.* Monosulfiram, disulfiram, and light. *Lancet* 1994; **343:** 304.

### Uses and Administration

Sulfiram is a pesticide that has been used as an acaricide, either alone or in conjunction with benzyl benzoate, in the treatment of scabies (p.1499), although other treatments are now preferred. Sulfiram has also been used as a pesticide in veterinary practice.

### Preparations

**Proprietary Preparations** (details are given in Part 3)

***Braz.:*** Sulfitrat; Tetmosol; Tiosol†; Valfiran; ***India:*** Tetmosol; ***Mex.:*** Tetmosol; ***Port.:*** Thiosan; ***S.Afr.:*** Tetmosol; ***Singapore:*** Tetmosol.

**Multi-ingredient:** ***Fr.:*** Ascabiol.

## Temefos *(USAN, rINN)*

27165; Temefós; Temephos. *O,O'*-(Thiodi-*p*-phenylene) *O,O,O',O'*-tetramethyl bis(phosphorothioate).

$C_{16}H_{20}O_6P_2S_3$ = 466.5.

*CAS — 3383-96-8.*

### Profile

Temefos is an organophosphorus insecticide (p.1507). It is effective against the larvae of mosquitoes, blackflies, and other insects, and is used for the larvicidal treatment of rivers in the control of onchocerciasis (p.100). It is also effective against the crustacean host to the larvae of the guinea worm and is used in the control of dracunculiasis (p.98); treatment of drinking water is both effective and acceptable.

## Tetrachlorvinphos

ENT-25841; SD-8447; Tetraclorvinfós. 2-Chloro-1-(2,4,5-trichlorophenyl)vinyl dimethyl phosphate.

$C_{10}H_9Cl_4O_4P$ = 366.0.

*CAS — 961-11-5; 22248-79-9 (Z-tetrachlorvinphos); 22350-76-1 (E-tetrachlorvinphos).*

### Profile

Tetrachlorvinphos is an organophosphorus insecticide (p.1507) used as an ectoparasiticide in veterinary practice.

## Tetramethrin *(rINN)*

Tetrametrina. Cyclohex-1-ene-1,2-dicarboximidomethyl (1*RS*,3*RS*)-(1*RS*,3*SR*)-2,2-dimethyl-3-(2-methylprop-1-enyl)cyclopropanecarboxylate.

$C_{19}H_{25}NO_4$ = 331.4.

*CAS — 7696-12-0.*

*ATC — P03BA04.*

### Profile

Tetramethrin is a pyrethroid insecticide (see Pyrethrum Flower, p.1509) used in the treatment of pediculosis (p.1499). It is also used in veterinary practice for the control of ectoparasites in the environment and as a household insecticide.

◊ References.

1. Tetramethrin health and safety guide. *IPCS Health and Safety Guide 31*. Geneva: WHO, 1989. Available at: http://www.inchem.org/documents/hsg/hsg/hsg031.htm (accessed 26/04/04)
2. Tetramethrin. *Environmental Health Criteria 98*. Geneva: WHO, 1990. Available at: http://www.inchem.org/documents/ehc/ehc/ehc98.htm (accessed 26/04/04)

### Preparations

**Proprietary Preparations** (details are given in Part 3)

**Multi-ingredient:** ***Fr.:*** Itax Antipoux†; ***Gr.:*** Cif Candioli; Runde; ***Ital.:*** Baygon; Mafu†; Mom Piretro Emulsione; Mom Shampoo Antiparassitario; Neo Mom.

## Trichlorophenoxyacetic Acid

2,4,5-T; Triclorofenoxiacético, ácido. 2,4,5-Trichlorophenoxyacetic acid.

$C_8H_5Cl_3O_3$ = 255.5.

*CAS — 35915-18-5.*

### Profile

Trichlorophenoxyacetic acid is a selective herbicide with similar actions to dichlorophenoxyacetic acid (p.1503). It is usually used in ester formulations. It was used with dichlorophenoxyacetic acid as a defoliating agent in the Vietnam war.

**Toxicity.** The phenoxy herbicides were used for defoliation in Vietnam as Agent Orange, which consisted of a mixture of dichlorophenoxyacetic acid, trichlorophenoxyacetic acid, and the impurity TCDD (dioxin), and concern has been expressed that they may have contributed to an increased incidence of cancer among exposed subjects as well as an adverse effect on the offspring of those subjects. This has been a matter of considerable debate,[1] prompting a series of biennial reassessments of the health effects of Agent Orange by the US National Academy of Sciences' Institute of Medicine.[2] To date the Institute has concluded[3] that there is evidence of increased incidence of chronic lymphocytic leukaemia, soft tissue sarcoma, Hodgkin's disease, non-Hodgkin's lymphoma, and chloracne, with phenoxy herbicides.

1. McCarthy M. Agent Orange. *Lancet* 1993; **342:** 362.
2. Stephenson J. New IOM report links Agent Orange exposure to risk of birth defect in Vietnam vets' children. *JAMA* 1996; **275:** 1066–7.
3. Institute of Medicine. *Veterans and Agent Orange: update 2002 (2003)*. Washington: The National Academies Press. Also available at: http://www.nap.edu/books/0309086167/html (accessed 26/04/04)

## Triflumuron

Triflumurón; Trifluron. 2-Chloro-*N*-([{4-(trifluoromethoxy)phenyl}amino]carbonyl)benzamide.

$C_{15}H_{10}ClF_3N_2O_3$ = 358.7.

*CAS — 64628-44-0.*

### Profile

Triflumuron is an insecticide used in agriculture and as a topical ectoparasiticide in veterinary practice.

### Preparations

**Proprietary Preparations** (details are given in Part 3)

***Ital.:*** Baycidal.

# Prostaglandins

The prostaglandins, along with thromboxanes and leukotrienes, are all derived from 20-carbon polyunsaturated fatty acids and are collectively termed *eicosanoids*. In man, the most common precursor is arachidonic acid (eicosatetraenoic acid) whereas eicosapentaenoic acid is a predominant precursor in fish and marine animals.

Arachidonic acid is released from cell-membrane phospholipids by the enzyme phospholipase $A_2$ and is then rapidly metabolised by several enzymes, the major ones being cyclo-oxygenase (prostaglandin synthetase) and lipoxygenase (see Figure 1, below). The prostaglandins, thromboxanes, and prostacyclin (sometimes collectively termed *prostanoids*) all contain ring structures and are products of arachidonic acid oxidation by cyclo-oxygenase, an enzyme with 2 isoforms (COX-1 or COX-2) widely distributed in cell membranes. The leukotrienes are products of the lipoxygenase pathway; arachidonic acid is metabolised by lipoxygenases to hydroperoxyeicosatetraenoic acids, which are then further metabolised to leukotrienes. The initial step in the cyclo-oxygenase pathway is the formation of cyclic endoperoxide prostaglandin $G_2$ ($PGG_2$) which is then reduced to the endoperoxide prostaglandin $H_2$ ($PGH_2$). Prostaglandin $H_2$ is then converted to the primary prostaglandins prostaglandin $D_2$, prostaglandin $E_2$, and prostaglandin $F_{2\alpha}$, to thromboxane $A_2$ ($TXA_2$) via the enzyme thromboxane synthetase, or to prostacyclin ($PGI_2$) via the enzyme prostacyclin synthetase. These products are further metabolised and rapidly inactivated in the body. The secondary prostaglandins, prostaglandin $A_2$ ($PGA_2$), prostaglandin $B_2$ ($PGB_2$), and prostaglandin $C_2$ ($PGC_2$) are derived from prostaglandin $E_2$, but are formed during extraction and probably do not occur biologically.

The prostaglandins are all derivatives of the carbon skeleton 7-(2-octilcyclopentyl)heptanoic acid (also known as prostanoic acid). All natural prostaglandins have a double bond at position 1,2 and a hydroxyl group at position 3 of the octil side-chain. Depending on the substitutions on the cyclopentane ring, the main series of prostaglandins are distinguished by the letters A, B, C, D, E, and F; the members of each series are further subdivided by subscript numbers which indicate the degree of unsaturation in the side-chains—hence, those derived from eicosatrienoic acid (dihomo-γ-linolenic acid) have the subscript 1, those derived from arachidonic acid have the subscript 2, and those derived from eicosapentaenoic acid have the subscript 3. In man, only prostaglandins of the '2' series appear to be of physiological importance. Thromboxane $A_2$ has an oxane rather than a cyclopentane ring; it is chemically unstable and breaks down to thromboxane $B_2$. Prostacyclin has a double-ring structure and breaks down to 6-keto-prostaglandin $F_{1\alpha}$.

Endogenous prostaglandins are autacoids; they can be formed by virtually all tissues and cells in response to a variety of stimuli, have a wide range of **actions**, and are involved in the regulation of virtually all biological functions. Prostaglandins appear to act through various receptor-mediated mechanisms. Some of their effects are mediated within cells by activation or inhibition of adenylate cyclase and the regulation of cyclic adenosine monophosphate production. At one time prostaglandin $E_2$ and prostaglandin $F_{2\alpha}$ were thought to be of paramount importance, but with the discovery of thromboxane $A_2$, prostacyclin, and the leukotrienes it was realised that these primary prostaglandins belong to a large family of physiologically active eicosanoids. Thromboxane $A_2$ induces platelet aggregation and constricts arterial smooth muscle whereas prostacyclin causes vasodilatation and prevents platelet aggregation; the balance between these opposing actions has an important role in the regulation of intravascular platelet aggregation and thrombus formation. The leukotrienes are important mediators of inflammation.

The pharmacological properties of prostaglandins are wide-ranging and include contraction or relaxation of smooth muscle in the blood vessels, bronchi, uterus, and gastrointestinal tract; inhibition of gastric acid secretion; and effects on platelet aggregation, the endocrine system, and metabolic processes.

Individual prostaglandins vary greatly in their activities and potencies; their actions also depend on the animal species, on the tissues in which they are acting, and on the concentration present, and entirely opposite actions may be elicited with very small structural changes in the molecule.

The diverse **clinical applications** of prostaglandins reflect their wide-ranging physiological and pharmacological properties. Synthetic analogues have been developed with the aim of obtaining compounds that are more stable, have a longer duration of action, and a more specific effect. Applications include:

- softening and dilating the cervix and for uterine stimulation, e.g. dinoprost (prostaglandin $F_{2\alpha}$) (p.1514) and its analogue carboprost (p.1514); dinoprostone (prostaglandin $E_2$) (p.1515) and its analogue sulprostone (p.1520); and gemeprost (p.1518) and misoprostol (p.1519), analogues of prostaglandin $E_1$
- vasodilators and inhibitors of platelet aggregation, e.g. alprostadil (prostaglandin $E_1$) (p.1512) and its analogue limaprost (p.1519); and epoprostenol (prostacyclin) (p.1516) and its analogue iloprost (p.1518)
- inhibition of gastric acid secretion and protection of the gastrointestinal mucosa, e.g. misoprostol (p.1519)
- glaucoma treatment, e.g. bimatoprost (p.1514), latanoprost (p.1519), travoprost (p.1521), and unoprostone (p.1521)
- as luteolytics (causing regression of the corpus luteum in the ovary) in veterinary medicine, e.g. synthetic analogues of prostaglandin $F_{2\alpha}$.


◊ References.

1. Moncada S, Vane JR. Arachidonic acid metabolites and the interactions between platelets and blood-vessel walls. *N Engl J Med* 1979; **300:** 1142–7.
2. Higgs GA, Vane JR. Inhibition of cyclo-oxygenase and lipoxygenase. *Br Med Bull* 1983; **39:** 265–70.
3. Halushka PV, *et al.* Thromboxane, prostaglandin and leukotriene receptors. *Annu Rev Pharmacol Toxicol* 1989; **29:** 213–39.
4. Smith WL, *et al.* Prostaglandin and thromboxane biosynthesis. *Pharmacol Ther* 1991; **49:** 153–79.
5. O'Neill C. The biochemistry of prostaglandins: a primer. *Aust N Z J Obstet Gynaecol* 1994; **34:** 332–7.
6. Wu KK. Molecular regulation and augmentation of prostacyclin biosynthesis. *Agents Actions Suppl* 1995; **45:** 11–17.


**Figure 1.** Prostaglandin biosynthesis.

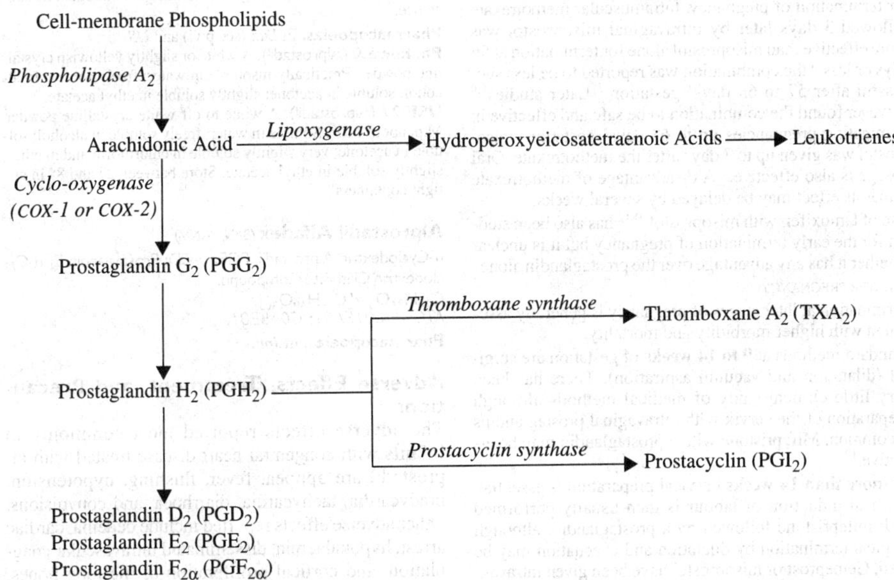


### Labour induction and augmentation

The uterus is normally spontaneously contractile but during pregnancy various physiological mechanisms maintain it in a quiescent state; retention of the fetus is also aided by a firm and contracted cervix. During the final 4 to 5 weeks of pregnancy the cervix normally undergoes a 'ripening' process in which it becomes softened and dilated, so that at parturition it is not a barrier to delivery of the fetus. Endogenous prostaglandins play an important role in this process, and also sensitise the uterus in preparation for labour.

- Labour usually begins spontaneously but in some cases it may be necessary to induce labour, for example in pregnancies that go beyond term, or where premature rupture of the membranes occurs or there are other maternal or fetal indications for early delivery.[1]
- Once labour has started, augmentation of uterine activity may be necessary if contractions fail to progress satisfactorily. A process of active management of labour, where augmentation is begun at an early stage, has been advocated; however, a study[2] in nulliparous women found no reduction in the rate of caesarean section when active management was used.

Various techniques are available for **induction of labour**. Before pharmacological methods are used, women may be offered sweeping of the membranes.[3] This can avoid the use of drugs in some cases, but it is associated with increased maternal discomfort, irregular contractions, and bleeding.[4] When formal induction of labour is required, prostaglandins are preferred to oxytocin in all women with intact membranes, but either may be used in women who have ruptured membranes, as neither method then offers any particular advantage.[3]

Dinoprostone (prostaglandin $E_2$) is the most widely used prostaglandin and has been given by various routes. It is usually given intravaginally as gel, vaginal tablets, or pessaries. Although some have found the gel to be more effective,[5] a systematic review[6] considered the clinical benefits equivalent, and UK guidelines favour use of vaginal tablets.[3] Dinoprostone given this way produces similar results to oxytocin infusions[7] but with lower rates of neonatal jaundice and postpartum haemorrhage. It is also less invasive and, as its effects are more akin to spontaneous labour, it is more popular with the mother than oxytocin. The intravenous and oral routes have been associated with frequent adverse, particularly gastrointestinal, effects[8,9] and intravaginal dosage is now preferred. The intracervical route is no more effective than the intravaginal route, and is no longer recommended.[3]

Oxytocin should not be started for 6 hours after use of vaginal prostaglandins.[3] Whenever possible, amniotomy (deliberate rupture of the fetal membranes) should be performed in women with intact membranes before giving oxytocin.[3] Oxytocin is given by slow intravenous infusion. UK guidelines favour a starting dose of 1 to 2 milliunits/minute, increased at intervals of 30 minutes, and titrated against contractions.[3] However, there have been conflicting findings about the dose. Some have used low doses effectively[10-12] (e.g. starting at 0.5 or 0.7 milliunits/minute) and found them to be as effective as higher doses and to cause less uterine hyperstimulation.[11] In contrast, a double-blind study[13] reported that high doses of oxytocin (starting at 4.5 milliunits/minute) were associated with a shorter duration of labour without a demonstrable increase in adverse fetal or neonatal effects. Others also found that the failure of induction was less frequent with higher doses (starting at 6 milliunits/minute), although there was a higher rate of caesarean section for fetal distress.[14]

Misoprostol has also been investigated. Most studies have used the intravaginal route and have suggested it may be more effective than standard methods of labour induction.[15] Oral dosage may also be effective, although less so than intravaginal.[16] However, the risk of uterine hyperstimulation may be increased with misoprostol and there is as yet insufficient evidence of its safety to recommend routine use.

The antiprogestogen mifepristone also produces cervical dilatation and stimulates uterine contraction and has been tried for cervical ripening and for induction of labour. A systematic review of trials found that it may be effective, but its place in therapy has yet to be established.[17]

In pregnancies at term, premature rupture of the fetal membranes (i.e. before labour begins) might increase the risk of both maternal and fetal infection.[18] The usual practice in such situations has often been to induce labour immediately, either with oxytocin intravenously or dinoprostone vaginally. Some have suggested expectant management as an alternative to immediate induction,[19] but this has been criticised.[18]

Oxytocin or a prostaglandin may also be used for **labour augmentation**. Doses of oxytocin are similar to those used for induction. Low-dose regimens, starting at 1 milliunit/minute intravenously, have proved successful[20,21] and are increasingly used, although higher doses starting at 6 milliunits/minute[22] have been given. Comparison of the two approaches[14] found that high doses led to shorter labour, fewer forceps deliveries, and a lower incidence of caesarean section for dystocia, but more commonly resulted in uterine hyperstimulation.

Dinoprostone is the prostaglandin most often used for augmentation of labour. As with its use for induction, dinoprostone results in less neonatal jaundice and postpartum haemorrhage, and is more popular with mothers than oxytocin. It is usually given intravaginally as a gel or pessaries. A gel may be given intracervically, but this is a more invasive route. Oral dinoprostone tablets have been used despite their gastrointestinal side-effects, and are considered to be more useful for augmentation than for induction.

Once delivery has successfully been initiated, management of the third stage of labour may be considered to reduce the risks of postpartum haemorrhage (see p.1684).


1. Chamberlain G, Zander L. ABC of labour care: induction. *BMJ* 1999; **318:** 995–8. Correction. *ibid.*; 1584.
2. Frigoletto FD, *et al.* A clinical trial of active management of labor. *N Engl J Med* 1995; **333:** 745–50.
3. Royal College of Obstetricians and Gynaecologists. Induction of labour: evidence-based clinical guideline number 9 (issued June 2001). Available at: http://www.nice.org.uk/pdf/inductionoflabourrcogrep.pdf (accessed 23/06/04)
4. Boulvain M, *et al.* Membrane sweeping for induction of labour. Available in The Cochrane Library; Issue 2. Chichester: John Wiley; 2004.
5. Mahmood TA. A prospective comparative study on the use of prostaglandin $E_2$ gel (2 mg) and prostaglandin $E_2$ tablet (3 mg) for the induction of labour in primigravid women with unfavourable cervices. *Eur J Obstet Gynecol Reprod Biol* 1989; **33:** 169–75.
6. Kelly AJ, *et al.* Vaginal prostaglandin (PGE2 and PGF2a) for induction of labour at term. Available in The Cochrane Library; Issue 2. Chichester: John Wiley; 2004.
7. Silva-Cruz A, *et al.* Prostaglandin $E_2$ gel compared to oxytocin for medically-indicated labour induction at term: a controlled clinical trial. *Pharmatherapeutica* 1988; **5:** 228–32.
8. Luckas M, Bricker L. Intravenous prostaglandin for induction of labour. Available in The Cochrane Library; Issue 2. Chichester: John Wiley; 2004.
9. French L. Oral prostaglandin E2 for induction of labour. Available in The Cochrane Library; Issue 2. Chichester: John Wiley; 2004.
10. Blakemore KJ, *et al.* A prospective comparison of hourly and quarter-hourly oxytocin dose increase intervals for the induction of labor at term. *Obstet Gynecol* 1990; **75:** 757–61.
11. Mercer B, *et al.* Labor induction with continuous low-dose oxytocin infusion: a randomized trial. *Obstet Gynecol* 1991; **77:** 659–63.
12. Wein P. Efficacy of different starting doses of oxytocin for induction of labor. *Obstet Gynecol* 1989; **74:** 863–8.
13. Merrill DC, Zlatnik FJ. Randomized, double-masked comparison of oxytocin dosage in induction and augmentation of labor. *Obstet Gynecol* 1999; **94:** 455–63.
14. Satin AJ, *et al.* High- versus low-dose oxytocin for labor stimulation. *Obstet Gynecol* 1992; **80:** 111–16.
15. Hofmeyr GJ, Gülmezoglu AM. Vaginal misoprostol for cervical ripening and induction of labour. Available in The Cochrane Library; Issue 2. Chichester: John Wiley; 2004.
16. Alfirevic Z. Oral misoprostol for induction of labour. Available in The Cochrane Library; Issue 2. Chichester: John Wiley; 2004.
17. Neilson JP. Mifepristone for induction of labour. Available in The Cochrane Library; Issue 2. Chichester: John Wiley; 2004.
18. Duff P. Premature rupture of the membranes at term. *N Engl J Med* 1996; **334:** 1053–4.
19. Hannah ME, *et al.* Induction of labor compared with expectant management for prelabor rupture of the membranes at term. *N Engl J Med* 1996; **334:** 1005–10.
20. Seitchik J, Castillo M. Oxytocin augmentation of dysfunctional labor I: clinical data. *Am J Obstet Gynecol* 1982; **144:** 899–905.
21. Seitchik J, Castillo M. Oxytocin augmentation of dysfunctional labor III: multiparous patients. *Am J Obstet Gynecol* 1983; **145:** 777–80.
22. Akoury HA, *et al.* Oxytocin augmentation of labor and perinatal outcome in nulliparas. *Obstet Gynecol* 1991; **78:** 227–30.


### Termination of pregnancy

Termination of pregnancy can be achieved medically or surgically. One of the main factors influencing the choice of method is the stage of gestation.[1,2]

• EARLY PREGNANCY

Surgical methods are commonly used in early pregnancy.[2,3] Menstrual extraction (menstrual regulation), which usually involves aspiration of the uterine cavity and induction of uterine bleeding is sometimes used when menstruation is no more than **14 days** overdue. Dilatation and vacuum aspiration has been widely used at up to **63 days** of amenorrhoea although other methods may be preferred before 49 days since most failures occur during this period. Cervical preparation is sometimes performed, commonly with prostaglandins; isosorbide mononitrate has also been tried.[4]

Medical methods of termination are also effective at this stage[3,5] and usually involve oral mifepristone followed by a prostaglandin. Mifepristone blocks the effects of progesterone on the uterus, leading to uterine contractions; it may also increase the myometrial sensitivity to prostaglandins. Prostaglandins soften and dilate the cervix and stimulate uterine contractions. Although both mifepristone and prostaglandins have been used alone, mifepristone is probably not sufficiently effective as a single agent,[5] while the doses of prostaglandins required are associated with adverse effects. Mifepristone is given orally, followed 36 to 48 hours later by a low dose of prostaglandin. Gemeprost, given intravaginally, is often used; misoprostol, orally or vaginally, is an alternative.[2] Sulprostone has been used but has to be given by intravenous infusion.

The antimetabolite methotrexate has a role in the management of ectopic pregnancy and has also been investigated for termination of pregnancy. Intramuscular methotrexate followed 3 days later by intravaginal misoprostol was more effective than misoprostol alone for termination at 56 days or less;[6] the combination was reported to be less successful after 57 to 63 days' gestation.[7] Later studies[8,9] however found the combination to be safe and effective in terminating pregnancies up to 63 days' gestation; misoprostol was given up to 7 days after the methotrexate. Oral dosage is also effective.[5] A disadvantage of methotrexate is that its effect may be delayed by several weeks.

Use of tamoxifen with misoprostol[10-12] has also been studied for the early termination of pregnancy but it is unclear whether it has any advantage over the prostaglandin alone.

• LATER PREGNANCY

Termination at later stages of pregnancy is generally associated with higher morbidity and mortality.

Standard methods at **9 to 14 weeks** of gestation are surgical (dilatation and vacuum aspiration). There has been very little clinical study of medical methods although preparation of the cervix with intravaginal prostaglandins is common. Mifepristone with a prostaglandin may be effective.[13]

At **more than 14 weeks** cervical preparation is essential. Medical induction of labour is then usually performed with mifepristone followed by a prostaglandin, although surgical termination by dilatation and evacuation may be used. Gemeprost or misoprostol have been given intravaginally, but usually in repeated doses; carboprost may be given intramuscularly or sulprostone intravenously. Intra-amniotic dinoprost or extra-amniotic dinoprostone have been used when none of the above prostaglandins were available but these routes carry additional risks. Adverse effects with prostaglandins are generally more frequent with intra-amniotic than with extra-amniotic administration. Other methods have included the intra-amniotic administration of hypertonic sodium chloride and the intra-amniotic administration of hyperosmolar urea augmented with dinoprost.


1. WHO. Medical methods for termination of pregnancy: report of a WHO scientific group. *WHO Tech Rep Ser 871* 1997.
2. Royal College of Obstetricians and Gynaecologists. The care of women requesting induced abortion. Available at: http://www.rcog.org.uk/guidelines.asp?PageID=108&GuidelineID=31 (accessed 23/06/04)
3. Bygdeman M, Danielsson KG. Options for early therapeutic abortion: a comparative review. *Drugs* 2002; **62:** 2459–70.
4. Thomson AJ, *et al.* Randomised trial of nitric oxide donor versus prostaglandin for cervical ripening before first-trimester termination of pregnancy. *Lancet* 1998; **352:** 1093–6.
5. Christin-Maitre S, *et al.* Medical termination of pregnancy. *N Engl J Med* 2000; **342:** 946–56.
6. Creinin MD, Vittinghoff E. Methotrexate and misoprostol vs misoprostol alone for early abortion: a randomized controlled trial. *JAMA* 1994; **272:** 1190–5.
7. Creinin MD. Methotrexate and misoprostol for abortion at 57–63 days gestation. *Contraception* 1994; **50:** 511–15.
8. Hausknecht RU. Methotrexate and misoprostol to terminate early pregnancy. *N Engl J Med* 1995; **333:** 537–40.
9. Creinin MD, *et al.* A randomized trial comparing misoprostol three and seven days after methotrexate for early abortion. *Am J Obstet Gynecol* 1995; **173:** 1578–84.
10. Mishell DR, *et al.* A medical method of early pregnancy termination using tamoxifen and misoprostol. *Contraception* 1998; **58:** 1–6.
11. Wiebe ER. Tamoxifen compared to methotrexate when used with misoprostol for abortion. *Contraception* 1999; **59:** 265–70.
12. Jain JK, *et al.* A comparison of tamoxifen and misoprostol to misoprostol alone for early pregnancy termination. *Contraception* 1999; **60:** 353–6.
13. Stewart P, *et al.* Report from the Faculty of Family Planning and Reproductive Health Care AGM, May 2003: medical termination of pregnancy in the late first trimester. *J Fam Plann Reprod Health Care* 2003; **29:** 243–4.


---

## Alfaprostol *(BAN, USAN, rINN)*

K-11941; Ro-22-9000. Methyl (*Z*)-7-{(1*R*,2*S*,3*R*,5*S*)-2-[(3*S*)-5-cyclohexyl-3-hydroxypent-1-ynyl]-3,5-dihydroxycyclopentyl}hept-5-enoate.

$C_{24}H_{38}O_5$ = 406.6.

*CAS — 74176-31-1.*

### Profile

Alfaprostol is a synthetic analogue of dinoprost (prostaglandin $F_{2\alpha}$). It is used as a luteolytic in veterinary medicine.

---

## Alprostadil *(BAN, USAN, rINN)*

Alprostadilum; $PGE_1$; Prostaglandin $E_1$; U-10136. (*E*)-(8*R*,11*R*,12*R*,15*S*)-11,15-Dihydroxy-9-oxoprost-13-enoic acid; 7-{(1*R*,2*R*,3*R*)-3-Hydroxy-2-[(*E*)-(3*S*)-3-hydroxyoct-1-enyl]-5-oxocyclopentyl}heptanoic acid.

$C_{20}H_{34}O_5$ = 354.5.

*CAS — 745-65-3.*

*ATC — C01EA01; G04BE01.*

NOTE. In *Martindale* the term alprostadil is used for the exogenous substance and prostaglandin $E_1$ for the endogenous substance.

**Pharmacopoeias.** In *Eur.* (see p.vi) and *US.*

**Ph. Eur. 5.0** (Alprostadil). A white or slightly yellowish crystalline powder. Practically insoluble in water; freely soluble in alcohol; soluble in acetone; slightly soluble in ethyl acetate.

**USP 27** (Alprostadil). A white to off-white crystalline powder. M.p. about 110°. Soluble in water; freely soluble in alcohol; soluble in acetone; very slightly soluble in chloroform and in ether; slightly soluble in ethyl acetate. Store between 2° and 8° in airtight containers.

### Alprostadil Alfadex *(BAN, rINNM)*

α-Cyclodextrin Alprostadil; $PGE_1$ α-CD; Prostaglandin $E_1$ α-Cyclodextrin Clathrate Compound.

$C_{20}H_{34}O_5,x[C_{36}H_{60}O_{30}]$.

*ATC — C01EA01; G04BE01.*

**Pharmacopoeias.** In *Jpn.*

### Adverse Effects, Treatment, and Precautions

The adverse effects reported most commonly in **infants** with congenital heart disease treated with alprostadil are apnoea, fever, flushing, hypotension, bradycardia, tachycardia, diarrhoea, and convulsions. Other adverse effects reported include oedema, cardiac arrest, hypokalaemia, disseminated intravascular coagulation, and cortical proliferation of the long bones. Weakening of the wall of the ductus arteriosus and pulmonary artery may occur following prolonged infusion. Alprostadil should be avoided in neonates with respiratory distress syndrome and should be used with caution in those with bleeding tendencies; blood pressure and respiratory status should be monitored during infusion.

Adverse effects reported in **adults** given alprostadil have included headache, flushing, hypotension, diarrhoea, and pain and inflammation at the infusion site.

Following intracavernosal or intra-urethral alprostadil for the treatment of erectile dysfunction, the most frequently reported adverse effect is pain during erection. Local reactions including penile fibrosis, fibrotic nodules, and Peyronie's disease have been reported. Priapism may occur (see below). Systemic effects are less common but hypotension and other adverse effects have been reported. Intracavernosal or intra-urethral use should be avoided in patients with complicating penile deformities or with sickle-cell disease, myeloma, leukaemias, or other conditions predisposing to prolonged erection.

◊ A review[1] of adverse effects associated with alprostadil in infants with congenital heart disease.

1. Lewis AB, *et al.* Side effects of therapy with prostaglandin $E_1$ in infants with critical congenital heart disease. *Circulation* 1981; **64:** 893–8.

**Effects on the bones.** Periosteal or cortical hyperostosis has been reported in infants following therapy with alprostadil for cyanotic congenital heart disease.[1-4] A retrospective review of 30 infants[2] treated with alprostadil revealed radiographic signs of periosteal reactions in 5. Changes could be detected after even short courses of therapy; 3 developed relatively mild periosteal changes in the ribs after infusions ranging from 9 to 205 hours and one had involvement of the left femur after infusion for 71 hours. Resolution of lesions had occurred in most bones 6 to 12 months later. In a further study,[5] radiological evidence of cortical hyperostosis was found in 53 of 86 infant heart transplant recipients who had received alprostadil infusion pre-operatively. Of 53 of the infants who had received alprostadil for less than 30 days, 21 were affected (2 severely). Correspondingly, of those treated for 30 to 60 days, 18 of 22 were affected (13 severely). All 14 infants treated for more than 60 days were affected (7 severely). Since the associated bone changes may persist for months after discontinuation of alprostadil, caution should be exercised to avoid misdiagnosis.

1. Ueda K, *et al.* Cortical hyperostosis following long-term administration of prostaglandin $E_1$ in infants with cyanotic congenital heart disease. *J Pediatr* 1980; **97:** 834–6.
2. Ringel RE, *et al.* Periosteal changes secondary to prostaglandin administration. *J Pediatr* 1983; **103:** 251–3.
3. Williams JL. Periosteal hyperostosis resulting from prostaglandin therapy. *Eur J Radiol* 1986; **6:** 231–2.
4. Kalloghlian AK, *et al.* Cortical hyperostosis simulating osteomyelitis after short-term prostaglandin $E_1$ infusion. *Eur J Pediatr* 1996; **155:** 173–4.
5. Woo K, *et al.* Cortical hyperostosis: a complication of prolonged prostaglandin infusion in infants awaiting cardiac transplantation. *Pediatrics* 1994; **93:** 417–20.

**Effects on the gastrointestinal tract.** Hyperplasia of the gastric mucosa, resulting in gastric outlet obstruction, has been reported in several neonates receiving alprostadil infusion.[1-3] It was suggested that this effect was dose-dependent.[1] Regression of the obstruction usually occurred after cessation of therapy.

For a report of necrotising enterocolitis in infants receiving alprostadil for congenital heart disease, see Dinoprostone, p.1515.

1. Peled N, *et al.* Gastric-outlet obstruction induced by prostaglandin therapy in neonates. *N Engl J Med* 1992; **327:** 505–10.
2. Merkus PJFM, *et al.* Prostaglandin E1 and gastric outlet obstruction in infants. *Lancet* 1993; **342:** 747.
3. Kobayashi N, *et al.* Acute gastric outlet obstruction following the administration of prostaglandin: an additional case. *Pediatr Radiol* 1997; **27:** 57–9.

**Effects on the metabolism.** Severe hyperglycaemia with apparent ketoacidosis occurred during postoperative infusion of alprostadil in the infant of a diabetic mother.[1] The manufacturers had received reports of hyperglycaemia associated with alprostadil in 5 infants, one of whom had a diabetic mother. Hypoglycaemia has also been reported in a few infants.[2]

1. Cohen MH, Nihill MR. Postoperative ketotic hyperglycaemia during prostaglandin $E_1$ infusion in infancy. *Pediatrics* 1983; **71:** 842–4.
2. Lewis AB, *et al.* Side effects of therapy with prostaglandin $E_1$ in infants with critical congenital heart disease. *Circulation* 1981; **64:** 893–8.

**Effects on the skin.** A 63-year-old man with Peyronie's disease[1] developed toxic pustuloderma (acute generalised exanthematous pustulosis) 6 days after receiving a single intracavernosal injection of alprostadil to define the penile morphology. He was treated with antihistamines and topical corticosteroids and the condition resolved completely within a week.

1. Gallego I, *et al.* Toxic pustuloderma induced by intracavernous prostaglandin $E_1$. *Br J Dermatol* 1997; **136:** 975–6.

**Priapism.** If priapism occurs following the use of alprostadil for erectile dysfunction, its treatment should not be delayed more than 6 hours. Initial therapy is by penile aspiration. If aspiration is unsuccessful a sympathomimetic with action on alpha-adrenergic receptors is given by cautious intracavernosal injection, with continuous monitoring of blood pressure and pulse. Extreme caution is necessary in patients with coronary heart disease, hypertension, cerebral ischaemia, or if taking an antidepressant. Low doses and dilute solutions are recommended as follows:

- intracavernosal injection of phenylephrine 100 to 200 micrograms (0.5 to 1 mL of a 200 micrograms/mL solution) every 5 to 10 minutes; maximum total dose 1 mg

*alternatively*

- intracavernosal injection of adrenaline 10 to 20 micrograms (0.5 to 1 mL of a 20 micrograms/mL solution) every 5 to 10 minutes; maximum total dose 100 micrograms

*alternatively*

- intracavernosal injection of metaraminol may be used, but it should be noted that fatal hypertensive crises have been reported; metaraminol 100 micrograms (5 mL of a 20 micrograms/mL solution) may be given by careful slow injection every 15 minutes; a maximum total dose of up to 1 mg has been suggested.

If necessary the sympathomimetic injections can be followed by further penile aspiration. If sympathomimetics are unsuccessful, urgent surgical referral is required.

## Pharmacokinetics

Following infusion alprostadil is rapidly metabolised by oxidation during passage through the pulmonary circulation. It is excreted in the urine as metabolites within about 24 hours. Systemic absorption of alprostadil occurs following intracavernosal injection.

◊ References.

1. Cox JW, *et al.* Pulmonary extraction and pharmacokinetics of prostaglandin $E_1$ during continuous intravenous infusion in patients with adult respiratory distress syndrome. *Am Rev Respir Dis* 1988; **137:** 5–12.
2. Cawello W, *et al.* Dose proportional pharmacokinetics of alprostadil (prostaglandin $E_1$) in healthy volunteers following intravenous infusion. *Br J Clin Pharmacol* 1995; **40:** 273–6.
3. Lea AP, *et al.* Intracavernous alprostadil: a review of its pharmacodynamic and pharmacokinetic properties and therapeutic potential in erectile dysfunction. *Drugs Aging* 1996; **8:** 56–74.

## Uses and Administration

Alprostadil is a prostaglandin (p.1511) that causes vasodilatation and prevents platelet aggregation. The endogenous substance is termed prostaglandin $E_1$. Alprostadil is used mainly in congenital heart disease and in erectile dysfunction (p.1745).

Alprostadil is used to maintain the patency of the ductus arteriosus in neonates with **congenital heart disease** until surgery is possible. It is given by continuous intravenous infusion beginning with doses of 50 to 100 nanograms/kg per minute; doses should be reduced as soon as possible to the minimum necessary to maintain response. Lower starting doses may be effective in some patients. The dose can be increased to 400 nanograms/kg per minute but, in general, higher infusion rates do not improve effect. Alprostadil may also be given by continuous infusion through an umbilical artery catheter placed at the ductal opening.

In the management of **erectile dysfunction**, alprostadil is given by intracavernosal injection; preparations may contain alprostadil or alprostadil alfadex, but the dose is expressed in terms of the base. Alprostadil may also be given as an intra-urethral application.

By *intracavernosal injection*, the initial dose is 2.5 micrograms, increased incrementally until a suitable dose is established. The usual dose range is 5 to 20 micrograms and the maximum recommended dose is 60 micrograms. Normally, the second dose should be 5 micrograms if some response to the first dose is observed, or 7.5 micrograms if there is no response; increments should then be of 5 to 10 micrograms until an effective dose is reached. In cases of erectile dysfunction of neurogenic origin secondary to spinal cord injury the initial dose is 1.25 micrograms, with a second dose of 2.5 micrograms, and third dose and subsequent increments of 2.5 to 5 micrograms. While finding a suitable dose, the interval between doses should be at least 1 day if there has been a partial response. If there is no response however, the next, higher dose may be given within 1 hour. Once established, the optimal dose should be given not more than once daily and not more than three times per week.

Alprostadil may also be injected intracavernosally in the diagnosis of erectile dysfunction in doses ranging from 5 to 20 micrograms.

By *intra-urethral (transurethral) application*, the initial dose is 250 micrograms. The dose may be increased incrementally to 500 or 1000 micrograms or decreased to 125 micrograms according to response. The optimal dose should be given not more than twice daily or seven times per week. A dose of 500 micrograms may be used diagnostically.

Alprostadil is also available in some countries as a *topical* formulation for the treatment of erectile dysfunction. There is also ongoing investigation of the use of topical formulations for female sexual dysfunction.

**Ergotamine poisoning.** Alprostadil[1,2] is one of many drugs that have been used to treat the circulatory disturbances in ergotamine poisoning (p.467).

1. Levy JM, *et al.* Prostaglandin $E_1$ for alleviating symptoms of ergot intoxication: a case report. *Cardiovasc Intervent Radiol* 1984; **7:** 28–30.
2. Horstmann R, *et al.* Kritische extremitätenischämie durch ergotismus. *Dtsch Med Wochenschr* 1993; **118:** 1067–71.

**Haemorrhagic cystitis.** Bladder irrigation with alprostadil produced resolution of severe haemorrhagic cystitis in 5 of 6 children who had undergone bone marrow transplantation.[1] Alprostadil was given via a catheter and retained for 1 hour each day for at least 7 consecutive days.

1. Trigg ME, *et al.* Prostaglandin $E_1$ bladder instillations to control severe hemorrhagic cystitis. *J Urol (Baltimore)* 1990; **143:** 92–4.

**Hepatic disorders.** Benefit has been reported in patients with *viral hepatitis* (p.618) given intravenous alprostadil alone or followed by oral dinoprostone or misoprostol.[1,2] Prostaglandins were studied because they had previously been shown to have a cytoprotective effect in experimentally induced hepatitis or in isolated hepatocytes, but the mechanism by which they exerted a beneficial effect was uncertain.

Combined intravenous therapy with glucagon, insulin, and alprostadil formulated in lipid microspheres has also been found effective in preventing *acute fulminant hepatic failure* after hepatic arterial infusion of antineoplastic chemotherapy.[3]

1. Sinclair SB, *et al.* Biochemical and clinical response of fulminant viral hepatitis to administration of prostaglandin E: a preliminary report. *J Clin Invest* 1989; **84:** 1063–9.
2. Flowers M, *et al.* Prostaglandin E in the treatment of recurrent hepatitis B infection after orthotopic liver transplantation. *Transplantation* 1994; **58:** 183–92.
3. Ikegami T, *et al.* Randomized control trial of lipo-prostaglandin $E_1$ in patients with acute liver injury induced by Lipiodol-targeted chemotherapy. *Clin Pharmacol Ther* 1995; **57:** 582–9.

**Peripheral vascular disease.** Various prostaglandins, including alprostadil,[1-7] have been used in the treatment of peripheral vascular disease (p.831), particularly in severe Raynaud's syndrome, but do not constitute mainline therapy.

1. Clifford PC, *et al.* Treatment of vasospastic disease with prostaglandin $E_1$. *BMJ* 1980; **281:** 1031–4.
2. Telles GS, *et al.* Prostaglandin $E_1$ in severe lower limb ischaemia: a double-blind controlled trial. *Br J Surg* 1984; **71:** 506–8.
3. Mohrland JS, *et al.* A multiclinic, placebo-controlled, double-blind study of prostaglandin $E_1$ in Raynaud's syndrome. *Ann Rheum Dis* 1985; **44:** 754–60.
4. Sethi GK, *et al.* Intravenous infusion of prostaglandin $E_1$ ($PGE_1$) in management of limb ischemia. *Am Surg* 1986; **52:** 474–8.
5. Langevitz P, *et al.* Treatment of refractory ischemic skin ulcers in patients with Raynaud's phenomenon with $PGE_1$ infusions. *J Rheumatol* 1989; **16:** 1433–5.
6. The ICAI Study Group. Prostanoids for chronic critical leg ischemia: a randomized, controlled, open-label trial with prostaglandin $E_1$. *Ann Intern Med* 1999; **130:** 412–21.
7. Bartolone S, *et al.* Efficacy evaluation of prostaglandin E1 against placebo in patients with progressive systemic sclerosis and significant Raynaud's phenomenon. *Minerva Cardioangiol* 1999; **47:** 137–43.

## Preparations

***USP 27:*** Alprostadil Injection.

**Proprietary Preparations** (details are given in Part 3)

***Arg.:*** Cardiobron; Caverject; Prolisina VR; Prostavasin; ***Austral.:*** Caverject; Muse; Prostin VR; ***Austria:*** Alprostapint; Caverject; Minprog; Muse; Prostavasin; ***Belg.:*** Caverject; Prostin VR; ***Braz.:*** Apilcav; Caverject; Muse; Prostavasin; ***Canad.:*** Caverject; Muse; Prostin VR; ***Chile:*** Caverject; Prostin Pediatrico; ***Denm.:*** Caverject; Muse; Prostivas; Rigidur†; Viridal†; ***Fin.:*** Caverject; Muse; Prostivas; Rigidur†; ***Fr.:*** Caverject; Edex; Muse; Prostine VR; ***Ger.:*** Caverject; Minprog; Muse; Prostavasin; Viridal; ***Gr.:*** Caverject; Prostin VR; ***Hong Kong:*** Caverject; Muse†; Prostavasin; Prostin VR; ***India:*** Prostin VR; ***Irl.:*** Caverject; Muse; Viridal; ***Israel:*** Alprostapint; Caverject; Muse; Prostin VR; ***Ital.:*** Alprostar; Caverject; Prostavasin; Prostin VR; Viridal; ***Jpn:*** Liple; Prostandin; ***Malaysia:*** Caverject; Prostin VR; ***Mex.:*** Caverject; Muse; ***Neth.:*** Caverject; Prostin VR; ***Norw.:*** Bondil; Caverject; Prostivas; ***NZ:*** Caverject; Muse; Prostin VR; ***Port.:*** Caverject; Prostin VR; Vasoprost; ***S.Afr.:*** Caverject; Muse; Prostin VR; ***Singapore:*** Caverject; Eglandin; Muse†; ***Spain:*** Caverject; Muse†; Sugiran; ***Swed.:*** Bondil; Caverject; Prostivas; Rigidur Duo†; ***Switz.:*** Caverject; Muse; Prostin VR; ***Thai.:*** Caverject; Muse; Prostin VR; ***UK:*** Caverject; Muse; Prostin VR; Viridal; ***USA:*** Caverject; Edex; Muse; Prostin VR.

### Beraprost Sodium *(USAN, rINNM)*

Beraprost sódico; ML-1129; ML-1229 (beraprost); TRK-100. Sodium (±)-(1R,2R,3aS,8bS)-2,3,3a,8b-tetrahydro-2-hydroxy-1-[(E)-(3S,4RS)-3-hydroxy-4-methyl-1-octen-6-ynyl]-1H-cyclopenta[b]benzofuran-5-butyrate.

$C_{24}H_{29}NaO_5$ = 420.5.

*CAS — 88430-50-6 (beraprost); 88475-69-8 (beraprost sodium).*

*ATC — B01AC19.*

#### Profile

Beraprost is a synthetic analogue of epoprostenol (prostacyclin) that causes vasodilatation and prevents platelet aggregation. It is given by mouth as the sodium salt in the management of pulmonary hypertension (p.832) and peripheral vascular disease (p.831).

In primary pulmonary hypertension, beraprost sodium is given in an initial dose of 60 micrograms daily in three divided doses; this may be increased gradually if necessary to 180 micrograms daily in three or four divided doses. For peripheral vascular disease a dose of 120 micrograms daily in three divided doses is used.

Adverse effects of beraprost include headache, flushing, nausea, diarrhoea, and increased liver enzyme, bilirubin, and triglyceride concentrations.

**Cardiovascular disorders.** References to the use of beraprost for pulmonary hypertension or intermittent claudication;[1-6] results of studies for the latter indication have been conflicting.

1. Nagaya N, *et al.* Effect of orally active prostacyclin analogue on survival of outpatients with primary pulmonary hypertension. *J Am Coll Cardiol* 1999; **34:** 1188–92.
2. Lievre M, *et al.* Oral beraprost sodium, a prostaglandin $I_2$ analogue, for intermittent claudication: a double-blind, randomized, multicenter controlled trial. *Circulation* 2000; **102:** 426–31.
3. Melian EB, Goa KL. Beraprost: a review of its pharmacology and therapeutic efficacy in the treatment of peripheral arterial disease and pulmonary arterial hypertension. *Drugs* 2002; **62:** 107–33.
4. Galiè N, *et al.* Effects of beraprost sodium, an oral prostacyclin analogue, in patients with pulmonary arterial hypertension: a randomized, double-blind, placebo-controlled trial. *J Am Coll Cardiol* 2002; **39:** 1496–1502.
5. Mohler ER, *et al.* Treatment of intermittent claudication with beraprost sodium, an orally active prostaglandin $I_2$ analogue: a double-blinded, randomized, controlled trial. *J Am Coll Cardiol* 2003; **41:** 1679–86.
6. Barst RJ, *et al.* Beraprost therapy for pulmonary arterial hypertension. *J Am Coll Cardiol* 2003; **41:** 2119–25.

#### Preparations

**Proprietary Preparations** (details are given in Part 3)
***Jpn:*** Dorner; ***Thai.:*** Dorner.

---

### Bimatoprost *(BAN, USAN, rINN)*

AGN-192024. (Z)-7-{(1R,2R,3R,5S)-3,5-Dihydroxy-2-[(1E,3S)-3-hydroxy-5-phenyl-1-pentenyl]cyclopentyl}-N-ethyl-5-heptenamide.

$C_{25}H_{37}NO_4$ = 415.6.

*CAS — 155206-00-1.*

*ATC — S01EE03.*

#### Adverse Effects and Precautions

As for Latanoprost, p.1519. Ocular pruritus is common. Hypertension and headache also commonly occur.

#### Pharmacokinetics

Small amounts of bimatoprost are absorbed from eye drops, with peak blood concentrations seen within 10 minutes of dosing. Bimatoprost is metabolised by oxidation, de-ethylation and glucuronidation and is excreted in the urine and faeces. The elimination half-life is 45 minutes.

#### Uses and Administration

Bimatoprost is a synthetic prostaglandin analogue that is structurally related to dinoprost (prostaglandin $F_{2\alpha}$). It is used to reduce intra-ocular pressure in the treatment of open-angle glaucoma and ocular hypertension (p.1485). It is given once daily as a 0.03% ophthalmic solution.

◊ References.

1. Sherwood M, *et al.* Six-month comparison of bimatoprost once-daily and twice-daily with timolol twice-daily in patients with elevated intraocular pressure. *Surv Ophthalmol* 2001; **45** (suppl 4): S361–S368.
2. Brandt JD, *et al.* Comparison of once- or twice-daily bimatoprost with twice-daily timolol in patients with elevated IOP: a 3-month clinical trial. *Ophthalmology* 2001; **108:** 1023–31.
3. Whitcup SM, *et al.* A randomised, double masked, multicentre clinical trial comparing bimatoprost and timolol for the treatment of glaucoma and ocular hypertension. *Br J Ophthalmol* 2003; **87:** 57–62.

#### Preparations

**Proprietary Preparations** (details are given in Part 3)
***Arg.:*** Lumigan; ***Austral.:*** Lumigan; ***Braz.:*** Lumigan; ***Chile:*** Lumigan; ***Ger.:*** Lumigan; ***Irl.:*** Lumigan; ***Ital.:*** Lumigan; ***Norw.:*** Lumigan; ***Spain:*** Lumigan; ***Thai.:*** Lumigan; ***UK:*** Lumigan; ***USA:*** Lumigan.

---

## Carboprost *(BAN, USAN, rINN)*

15-Me-PGF$_{2\alpha}$; Methyldinoprost; (15S)-15-Methylprostaglandin $F_{2\alpha}$; U-32921. (5Z,13E)-(8R,9S,11R,12R,15S)-9,11,15-Trihydroxy-15-methylprosta-5,13-dienoic acid; (Z)-7-{(1R,2R,3R,5S)-3,5-Dihydroxy-2-[(E)-(3S)-3-hydroxy-3-methyloct-1-enyl]cyclopentyl}hept-5-enoic acid.

$C_{21}H_{36}O_5$ = 368.5.

*CAS — 35700-23-3.*

*ATC — G02AD04.*

### Carboprost Methyl *(BANM, USAN, rINNM)*

Metil carboprost; U-36384. The methyl ester of carboprost.

$C_{22}H_{38}O_5$ = 382.5.

*CAS — 35700-21-1.*

*ATC — G02AD04.*

**Pharmacopoeias.** In *Chin.*

### Carboprost Trometamol *(BANM, rINNM)*

Carboprost trometamol; Carboprost Tromethamine *(USAN)*; U-32921E.

$C_{21}H_{36}O_5,C_4H_{11}NO_3$ = 489.6.

*CAS — 58551-69-2.*

*ATC — G02AD04.*

**Description.** Carboprost trometamol is a compound of carboprost with trometamol in a ratio of 1:1.

**Pharmacopoeias.** In *US.*

**USP 27** (Carboprost Tromethamine). A white to off-white powder. Soluble in water. Store at –25° to –10°.

### Adverse Effects and Precautions

As for Dinoprostone, p.1515.

Carboprost may cause bronchospasm and, less frequently, dyspnoea and pulmonary oedema. Patients with cardiopulmonary disorders should be monitored for reductions in arterial-oxygen content.

Once a prostaglandin has been given to terminate pregnancy it is essential that termination take place; if the prostaglandin is unsuccessful other measures should be used.

### Uses and Administration

Carboprost is a synthetic 15-methyl analogue of dinoprost (prostaglandin $F_{2\alpha}$). It is a uterine stimulant with a more prolonged action than dinoprost; the presence of the methyl group delays inactivation by enzymic dehydrogenation.

Carboprost is used for the termination of pregnancy (p.1512) and for the treatment of refractory postpartum haemorrhage due to uterine atony (p.1684) and not controlled by oxytocin and ergot preparations. It is usually given intramuscularly as the trometamol salt but doses are expressed in terms of carboprost. Carboprost trometamol 1.3 micrograms is approximately equivalent to 1 microgram of carboprost.

For the termination of second trimester pregnancy (between 13 and 20 weeks of gestation) the equivalent of 250 micrograms of carboprost is given by deep intramuscular injection and repeated every 1½ to 3½ hours depending on the uterine response; if necessary the dose may be increased to 500 micrograms, but the total dose given should not exceed 12 mg. If preferred, a test dose of 100 micrograms may be given initially. Carboprost trometamol has also been given intra-amniotically in a dose equivalent to 2.5 mg of carboprost over five minutes; this dose may be repeated after 24 hours if termination has not occurred and the membranes are intact.

Carboprost methyl given as vaginal pessaries has been tried for termination of pregnancy in the second trimester.

For the treatment of postpartum haemorrhage the equivalent of 250 micrograms of carboprost is given by deep intramuscular injection as the trometamol salt at intervals of about 90 minutes; the interval may be reduced if necessary, but should not be less than 15 minutes. A total dose of 2 mg should not be exceeded.

**Haemorrhagic cystitis.** Carboprost trometamol instilled into the bladder successfully controlled cyclophosphamide-induced haemorrhagic cystitis (p.540) in 15 of 24 bone marrow transplant patients.[1] The dose consisted of 50 mL of solutions containing 2 to 10 micrograms/mL instilled four times daily for 7 days.

1. Ippoliti C, *et al.* Intravesicular carboprost for the treatment of hemorrhagic cystitis after marrow transplantation. *Urology* 1995; **46:** 811–15.

### Preparations

***USP 27:*** Carboprost Tromethamine Injection.

**Proprietary Preparations** (details are given in Part 3)
***Belg.:*** Prostin/15M; ***Denm.:*** Prostinfenem; ***Hong Kong:*** Hemabate†; ***India:*** Prostodin; ***Neth.:*** Prostin/15M; ***NZ:*** Prostin/15M; ***Swed.:*** Prostinfenem; ***UK:*** Hemabate; ***USA:*** Hemabate.

---

### Cloprostenol Sodium *(BANM, USAN, rINNM)*

Cloprostenol sódico; ICI-80996. Sodium (±)-(Z)-7-{(1R,2R,3R,5S)-2-[(E)-(3R)-4-(3-chlorophenoxy)-3-hydroxybut-1-enyl]-3,5-dihydroxycyclopentyl}hept-5-enoate.

$C_{22}H_{28}ClNaO_6$ = 446.9.

*CAS — 40665-92-7 (cloprostenol); 55028-72-3 (cloprostenol sodium).*

**Pharmacopoeias.** In *BP(Vet).*

**BP(Vet) 2003** (Cloprostenol Sodium). A white or almost white amorphous hygroscopic powder. Freely soluble in water, in alcohol, and in methyl alcohol; practically insoluble in acetone. Protect from light and moisture.

#### Profile

Cloprostenol is a synthetic analogue of dinoprost (prostaglandin $F_{2\alpha}$). The sodium salt is used as a luteolytic in veterinary medicine.

---

### Dinoprost *(BAN, USAN, rINN)*

PGF$_{2\alpha}$; Prostaglandin $F_{2\alpha}$; U-14583. (5Z,13E)-(8R,9S,11R,12R,15S)-9,11,15-Trihydroxyprosta-5,13-dienoic acid; (Z)-7-{(1R,2R,3R,5S)-3,5-Dihydroxy-2-[(E)-(3S)-3-hydroxyoct-1-enyl]cyclopentyl}hept-5-enoic acid.

$C_{20}H_{34}O_5$ = 354.5.

*CAS — 551-11-1.*

*ATC — G02AD01.*

NOTE. In *Martindale* the term dinoprost is used for the exogenous substance and prostaglandin $F_{2\alpha}$ for the endogenous substance.

**Pharmacopoeias.** In *Jpn.*

### Dinoprost Trometamol *(BANM, rINNM)*

Dinoprost trometamol; Dinoprost Tromethamine *(USAN)*; Dinoprostum Trometamoli; PGF$_{2\alpha}$ THAM; Prostaglandin $F_{2\alpha}$ Trometamol; U-14583E.

$C_{20}H_{34}O_5,C_4H_{11}NO_3$ = 475.6.

*CAS — 38562-01-5.*

*ATC — G02AD01.*

**Pharmacopoeias.** In *Eur.* (see p.vi) and *US.*

**Ph. Eur. 5.0** (Dinoprost Trometamol). A white or almost white powder. Very soluble in water; freely soluble in alcohol; practically insoluble in acetonitrile.

**USP 27** (Dinoprost Tromethamine). A white to off-white crystalline powder. Very soluble in water; slightly soluble in chloroform; freely soluble in dimethylformamide; soluble in methyl alcohol. Store in airtight containers.

#### Adverse Effects and Precautions

As for Dinoprostone, p.1515.

Dinoprost can cause bronchoconstriction, and bronchospasm with wheezing and dyspnoea has occurred, especially in asthmatic patients.

Once a prostaglandin has been given to terminate pregnancy it is essential that termination take place; if the prostaglandin is unsuccessful other measures should be used.

#### Interactions

◊ A severe reaction was reported following the use of oxytocin, methylergometrine, and dinoprost (see under Dinoprostone, p.1516).

#### Uses and Administration

Dinoprost is a prostaglandin of the F series (p.1511) with actions on smooth muscle; the endogenous substance is termed prostaglandin $F_{2\alpha}$ and is rapidly metabolised in the body. It induces contraction of uterine muscle at any stage of pregnancy and is reported to act predominantly as a vasoconstrictor on blood vessels and as a bronchoconstrictor on bronchial muscle.

Dinoprost is used principally for the termination of pregnancy (p.1512). It may also be used for missed abortion, hydatidiform mole, and fetal death *in utero*. Dinoprost has also been given for the induction of labour but has a higher incidence of adverse effects than dinoprostone, and is no longer routinely recommended; more appropriate treatment is discussed on p.1511.

Dinoprost is usually given intra-amniotically for termination of pregnancy. It has been given intravenously, but with a high incidence of adverse effects. The extra-amniotic route has also been used. Dinoprost is given as the trometamol salt, doses being expressed in terms of the equivalent amount of dinoprost; dinoprost trometamol 1.3 mg is approximately equivalent to 1 mg of dinoprost. It should not be given continuously for more than 2 days.

For the termination of pregnancy during the second trimester 40 mg of dinoprost is given intra-amniotically by slowly injecting 8 mL of a solution containing 5 mg/mL into the amniotic sac. A further dose of 10 to 40 mg after 24 hours may be given if the membranes are still intact.

**Ileus.** Ileus induced by vinca alkaloids in 3 patients with carcinoma of the lung was successfully relieved by the intravenous infusion of dinoprost 300 to 500 nanograms/kg per minute for 2 hours twice daily.[1]

1. Saito H, *et al.* Prostaglandin $F_{2\alpha}$ in the treatment of vinca alkaloid-induced ileus. *Am J Med* 1993; **95:** 549–51.

### Preparations

***BP 2003:*** Dinoprost Injection.

**Proprietary Preparations** (details are given in Part 3)
***Austral.:*** Prostin F2 Alpha; ***Fr.:*** Prostine $F_2$ Alpha†; ***Ger.:*** Minprostin $F_2\alpha$; ***Gr.:*** Enzaprost; ***Hong Kong:*** Prostin F2 Alpha; ***Irl.:*** Prostin F2; ***Israel:*** Prostin F2 Alpha; ***NZ:*** Prostin F2 Alpha; ***S.Afr.:*** Prostin F2 Alpha.

## Dinoprostone *(BAN, USAN, rINN)*

Dinoprostona; Dinoprostonum; $PGE_2$; Prostaglandin $E_2$; U-12062. (5*Z*,13*E*)-(8*R*,11*R*,12*R*,15*S*)-11,15-Dihydroxy-9-oxoprosta-5,13-dienoic acid; (*Z*)-7-{(1*R*,2*R*,3*R*)-3-Hydroxy-2-[(*E*)-(3*S*)-3-hydroxyoct-1-enyl]-5-oxocyclopentyl}hept-5-enoic acid.
$C_{20}H_{32}O_5$ = 352.5.
*CAS — 363-24-6.*
*ATC — G02AD02.*

NOTE. In *Martindale* the term dinoprostone is used for the exogenous substance and prostaglandin $E_2$ for the endogenous substance.

**Pharmacopoeias.** In *Eur.* (see p.vi) and *US.*

**Ph. Eur. 5.0** (Dinoprostone). A white or almost white, crystalline powder or colourless crystals. Practically insoluble in water; freely soluble in alcohol; very soluble in methyl alcohol. Store at a temperature not exceeding −15°.

**USP 27** (Dinoprostone). A white to off-white, crystalline powder. Freely soluble in alcohol, in acetone, in dichloromethane, in ether, in ethyl acetate, in isopropyl alcohol, in methyl alcohol; soluble in diisopropyl ether and in toluene; practically insoluble in hexanes. Protect from light.

### Adverse Effects

The incidence and severity of adverse reactions to dinoprostone are dose-related and also depend to some extent on the route; the intravenous route has been associated with a high incidence of adverse effects. Nausea, vomiting, diarrhoea, and abdominal pain are common by all routes. Back pain and rash can occur. Transient cardiovascular symptoms have included flushing, shivering, headache, dizziness, and hypotension; there have been rare reports of sudden cardiovascular collapse. Hypertension has also been reported. Convulsions and EEG changes have occurred rarely. Local tissue irritation and erythema, as well as pyrexia and raised white cell count, may follow intravenous doses but generally revert to normal after termination of the infusion. Transient pyrexia and raised white cell count may also occur following intravaginal use. Local infection may follow intra- or extra-amniotic therapy. Excessive uterine activity may occur and there have been occasional reports of uterine rupture following the use of prostaglandins to terminate pregnancy or induce labour; fetal distress and, rarely, fetal death have occurred during induction.

Dinoprostone, although generally acting as a bronchodilator, may cause bronchoconstriction in some individuals. Hypersensitivity reactions have occurred.

**Incidence of adverse effects.** Side-effects were evaluated in 626 patients[1] undergoing abortion (usually in the second trimester), using extra-amniotic or intra-amniotic dinoprost or dinoprostone, often with oxytocin. Vomiting occurred in 291, diarrhoea in 28, pyrexia in 34, transient hypotension (fall in systolic blood pressure of at least 20 mmHg) in 25, transient bronchospasm in 2 patients given extra-amniotic dinoprost, and blood loss exceeding 250 mL in 68 (38 lost more than 500 mL). No patients had convulsions even though 8 were epileptics receiving antiepileptics. Three patients sustained lacerations to the cervix. Five patients complained of breast soreness or lactation; these symptoms may have been under-reported. Overall 14 patients were readmitted; 13 because of excessive vaginal bleeding and 1 because of pelvic infection.

A later report describes the cumulative experience in 3313 pregnancies[2] in which dinoprostone gel was used for induction of term labour or cervical ripening. Adverse effects were rare. Vomiting, fever, and diarrhoea occurred in approximately 0.2% of mothers and were difficult to distinguish from the effects of concurrent drug therapy. Detectable myometrial activity was dose-related and more common after intravaginal than after intracervical use. Myometrial activity was reported in 0.6 to 6% of patients following intravaginal application and hyperstimulation was virtually non-existent at an intracervical dose of 500 micrograms. Fetal effects were negligible in the absence of uterine hyperstimulation.

1. MacKenzie IZ, *et al.* Prostaglandin-induced abortion: assessment of operative complications and early morbidity. *BMJ* 1974; **4:** 683–6.
2. Rayburn WF. Prostaglandin $E_2$ gel for cervical ripening and induction of labor: a critical analysis. *Am J Obstet Gynecol* 1989; **160:** 529–34.

**Effects on the bones.** Reversible periosteal reactions of the long bones and bone thickening have occurred in infants receiving long-term therapy with prostaglandins of the E series (see Alprostadil, p.1513). In addition, reversible widening of cranial sutures was reported[1] in 2 neonates given dinoprostone intravenously for 95 and 97 days respectively.

1. Hoevels-Guerich H, *et al.* Widening of cranial sutures after long-term prostaglandin $E_2$ therapy in two newborn infants. *J Pediatr* 1984; **105:** 72–4.

**Effects on the cardiovascular system.** Cardiovascular adverse effects are most common following intravenous dinoprostone but may also occur with other routes. Severe cardiovascular disorders reported with the intra-amniotic or intravaginal use of dinoprost or dinoprostone have included: cardiac arrhythmias in 3 patients,[1,2] fatal in 2 of them;[2] hypotension, tachypnoea, and tachycardia in 3 patients[3,4] with associated pyrexias in 2 patients;[3] and fatal myocardial infarction in a patient who had several high-risk factors for ischaemic heart disease.[5]

Severe hypertension occurred in a patient[6] who received dinoprostone by direct myometrial injection and by intravenous infusion concomitantly for postpartum haemorrhage.

1. Burt RL, *et al.* Hypokalemia and cardiac arrhythmia associated with prostaglandin-induced abortion. *Obstet Gynecol* 1977; **50:** 45S–46S.
2. Cates W, Jordaan HVF. Sudden collapse and death of women obtaining abortions induced with prostaglandin $F_{2\alpha}$. *Am J Obstet Gynecol* 1979; **133:** 398–400.
3. Phelan JP, *et al.* Dramatic pyrexic and cardiovascular response to intravaginal prostaglandin $E_2$. *Am J Obstet Gynecol* 1978; **132:** 28–32.
4. Cameron IT, Baird DT. Sudden collapse after intra-amniotic prostaglandin $E_2$ injection. *Lancet* 1984; **ii:** 1046.
5. Patterson SP, *et al.* A maternal death associated with prostaglandin $E_2$. *Obstet Gynecol* 1979; **54:** 123–4.
6. Veber B, *et al.* Severe hypertension during postpartum haemorrhage after i.v. administration of prostaglandin E2. *Br J Anaesth* 1992; **68:** 623–4.

**Effects on the fetus.** A woman who failed to abort despite receiving carboprost intravaginally 7 weeks after conception gave birth at 34 weeks' gestation to an infant with hydrocephalus and abnormal digits.[1]

For reports of adverse effects on the fetus due to hyperstimulation of the uterus during labour, see under Effects on the Uterus, below.

1. Collins FS, Mahoney MJ. Hydrocephalus and abnormal digits after failed first-trimester prostaglandin abortion attempt. *J Pediatr* 1983; **102:** 620–1.

**Effects on the gastrointestinal system.** Necrotising enterocolitis has been associated with the use of intravenous[1] or oral[2] dinoprostone, or intravenous alprostadil,[2] in infants with symptomatic congenital heart disease. It has been suggested that induced hypotension and apnoea may be responsible,[1] although others[3] did not support this view, or that pulmonary vasodilatation may produce systemic to pulmonary shunting, rendering the gastrointestinal tract relatively ischaemic.[2]

1. Leung MP, *et al.* Necrotizing enterocolitis in neonates with symptomatic congenital heart disease. *J Pediatr* 1988; **113:** 1044–6.
2. Singh GK, *et al.* Study of low dosage prostaglandin—usages and complications. *Eur Heart J* 1994; **15:** 377–81.
3. Miller MJS, Clark DA. Congenital heart disease and necrotizing enterocolitis. *J Pediatr* 1989; **115:** 335–6.

**Effects on the neonate.** Aspiration of the undissolved remnants of a dinoprostone vaginal tablet caused neonatal respiratory distress due to mechanical obstruction of the airways: there was no evidence to suggest absorption of dinoprostone from the tablet matrix.[1]

1. Andersson S, *et al.* Neonatal respiratory distress caused by aspiration of a vaginal tablet containing prostaglandin. *BMJ* 1987; **295:** 25–6.

**Effects on the nervous system.** Convulsions and EEG changes have been occasionally reported during the use of prostaglandins for termination of pregnancy. Convulsions occurred[1] in 5 of 320 women after intra-amniotic dinoprost, but in other large series[2-4] of patients given dinoprost or dinoprostone by various routes no problems occurred despite the inclusion of patients with a history of epilepsy. However, convulsions were reported[5] in 3 of 4 epileptic patients given sulprostone intramuscularly.

1. Lyneham RC, *et al.* Convulsions and electroencephalogram abnormalities after intra-amniotic prostaglandin $F_{2\alpha}$. *Lancet* 1973; **ii:** 1003–5.
2. MacKenzie IZ, *et al.* Convulsions and prostaglandin-induced abortion. *Lancet* 1973; **ii:** 1323.
3. Thiery M, *et al.* Prostaglandins and convulsions. *Lancet* 1974; **i:** 218.
4. Fraser IS, Gray C. Electroencephalogram changes after prostaglandin. *Lancet* 1974; **i:** 360.
5. Brandenburg H, *et al.* Convulsions in epileptic women after administration of prostaglandin $E_2$ derivative. *Lancet* 1990; **336:** 1138.

**Effects on the uterus.** Use of prostaglandins to induce labour or to terminate pregnancy is associated with an increased risk of hyperstimulation of the uterus. Uterine rupture has occurred with carboprost,[1] dinoprost or dinoprostone,[2-7] gemeprost,[8-10] misoprostol,[11] and sulprostone.[12-14] These effects have been reported with both parenteral and local administration. The risk of rupture and associated complications is increased in grand multiparae[4] and those with uterine scarring from previous caesarean section.[5,7] Studies have reported relative risks of between 6 and 10 times those of spontaneous labour following labour induction with dinoprostone in the latter group.[5,7] In addition to rupture, with the risk of potentially fatal maternal haemorrhage, hyperstimulation has been associated with fetal distress and death,[15-17] and maternal death due to amniotic fluid embolism.[15,18]

1. Vergote I, *et al.* Uterine rupture due to 15-methyl prostaglandin $F_{2\alpha}$. *Lancet* 1982; **ii:** 1402.
2. Claman P, *et al.* Uterine rupture with the use of vaginal prostaglandin $E_2$ for induction of labor. *Am J Obstet Gynecol* 1984; **150:** 889–90.
3. Keller F, Joyce TH. Uterine rupture associated with the use of vaginal prostaglandin $E_2$ suppositories. *Can Anaesth Soc J* 1984; **31:** 80–2.
4. Larsen JV, *et al.* Uterine hyperstimulation and rupture after induction of labour with prostaglandin $E_2$. *S Afr Med J* 1984; **65:** 615–16.
5. Ravasia DJ, *et al.* Uterine rupture during induced trial of labor among women with previous cesarean delivery. *Am J Obstet Gynecol* 2000; **183:** 1176–9.
6. Rabl M, *et al.* A randomized trial of vaginal prostaglandin $E_2$ for induction of labor: insert vs tablet. *J Reprod Med* 2002; **47:** 115–19.
7. Taylor DR, *et al.* Uterine rupture with the use of $PGE_2$ vaginal inserts for labor induction in women with previous cesarean sections. *J Reprod Med* 2002; **47:** 549–54.
8. Thavarasah AS, Achanna KS. Uterine rupture with the use of Cervagem (prostaglandin E1) for induction of labour on account of intrauterine death. *Singapore Med J* 1988; **29:** 351–2.
9. Byrne P, Onyekwuluje T. Uterine rupture after termination of pregnancy with gemeprost. *BMJ* 1991; **302:** 852.
10. Vine SJ, *et al.* Transverse posterior cervicoisthmic rupture after gemeprost pessaries for termination. *BMJ* 1992; **305:** 1332.
11. Blanchette HA, *et al.* Comparison of the safety and efficacy of intravaginal misoprostol (prostaglandin $E_1$) with those of dinoprostone (prostaglandin $E_2$) for cervical ripening and induction of labor in a community hospital. *Am J Obstet Gynecol* 1999; **180:** 1551–9.
12. Larue L, *et al.* Rupture d'un utérus sain lors d'une interruption de grossesse par prostaglandines au deuxième trimestre. *J Gynecol Obstet Biol Reprod (Paris)* 1991; **20:** 269–72.
13. Prasad RNV, Ratnam SS. Uterine rupture after induction of labour for intrauterine death using the prostaglandin $E_2$ analogue sulprostone. *Aust N Z J Obstet Gynaecol* 1992; **32:** 282–3.
14. de Boer MA, *et al.* Low dose sulprostone for termination of second and third trimester pregnancies. *Eur J Obstet Gynecol Reprod Biol* 2001; **99:** 244–8.
15. Stronge J, *et al.* A neonatal and maternal death following the administration of intravaginal prostaglandin. *J Obstet Gynaecol* 1987; **7:** 271–2.
16. Quinn MA, Murphy AJ. Fetal death following extra-amniotic prostaglandin gel: report of two cases. *Br J Obstet Gynaecol* 1981; **88:** 650–1.
17. Simmons K, Savage W. Neonatal death associated with induction of labour with intravaginal prostaglandin $E_2$: case report. *Br J Obstet Gynaecol* 1984; **91:** 598–9.
18. Less A, *et al.* Vaginal prostaglandin $E_2$ and fatal amniotic fluid embolus. *JAMA* 1990; **263:** 3259–60.

**Overdosage.** Severe adverse effects associated with intra-amniotic prostaglandins have been attributed to absorption into the systemic circulation of doses higher than would normally be given systemically. Rigors, vomiting, severe abdominal pain, and an intense desire to urinate and defaecate occurred[1] in 3 patients given dinoprostone intra-amniotically for mid-trimester abortion; one patient had peripheral vasoconstriction and a rapid low-volume pulse, with hypotension, and another had peripheral cyanosis. It was suggested[2] that this might have been due to displacement of the needle or cannula outside the amniotic sac. In 2 of the patients prior use of urea may have increased the rate of absorption of prostaglandins from the amniotic cavity. In a further report[3] flushing, severe headache, and nausea immediately after a test dose of dinoprost 2.5 mg was also thought to be due to incorrect positioning of the needle and consequent injection into the systemic circulation; at least part of the dose might have been injected into the peritoneal cavity.[4]

Severe reactions have also been reported with prostaglandins given to abort hydatidiform moles. A 20-year-old woman given 20 mg of dinoprostone by injection into the uterine cavity developed profound hypotension, bradycardia, and rigors, followed by nausea, vomiting, suprapubic pain, an increased pulse rate, pyrexia, and generalised flushing.[5] Since there are no fetal membranes in a molar pregnancy, intra-uterine administration is similar to extra-amniotic administration and the dose used was 100 times higher than the usual extra-amniotic dose.[4] However, in a similar patient[6] 'extra-amniotic' instillation of dinoprostone 200 micrograms was followed immediately by nausea, retching, severe abdominal pain, dizziness, difficulty in breathing and the production of frothy blood-stained sputum, an imperceptible pulse, and hypotension; the dinoprostone had probably been injected directly into the maternal circulation.

1. Ross AH, Whitehouse WL. Adverse reactions to intra-amniotic urea and prostaglandin. *BMJ* 1974; **1:** 642.
2. Craft I, Bowen-Simpkins P. Adverse reactions to intra-amniotic urea and prostaglandin. *BMJ* 1974; **2:** 446.
3. Brown R. Adverse reactions to intra-amniotic prostaglandin. *BMJ* 1974; **2:** 382.
4. Karim SMM. Adverse reactions to intra-amniotic prostaglandin. *BMJ* 1974; **3:** 347.

5. Smith AM. Adverse reactions to intra-amniotic prostaglandin. *BMJ* 1974; **2:** 382–3.
6. McNicol E, Gray H. Adverse reaction to extra-amniotic prostaglandin $E_2$. *Br J Obstet Gynaecol* 1977; **84:** 229–30.

## Precautions

Dinoprostone should not be given to patients in whom oxytocic drugs are generally contra-indicated (see Oxytocin, p.1336), or in those with a history of pelvic inflammatory disease. Since prostaglandins enhance the effects of oxytocin use of the 2 drugs together or in sequence should be carefully monitored.

Dinoprostone is contra-indicated in active cardiac, pulmonary, renal, or hepatic disease. It should be used with caution in patients with glaucoma or raised intra-ocular pressure, asthma or a history of asthma, epilepsy or a history of epilepsy, hepatic or renal impairment, or cardiovascular disease.

In the induction of labour cephalopelvic relationships should be carefully evaluated before use. During use uterine activity, fetal status, and the progress of cervical dilatation should be carefully monitored to detect adverse responses, such as hypertonus, sustained uterine contractions, or fetal distress. In patients with a history of hypertonic uterine contractility or tetanic uterine contractions, uterine activity and the state of the fetus should be continuously monitored throughout labour. Where high-tone myometrial contractions are sustained the possibility of uterine rupture should be considered.

Dinoprostone should not be given by the myometrial route, since there is a possible association with cardiac arrest in severely ill patients. The extra-amniotic route should not be used in patients with cervicitis or vaginal infections. Vaginal preparations of dinoprostone should not be used in the induction of labour once the membranes are ruptured. In some countries, intravenous prostaglandins are considered to be contra-indicated in women who smoke.

In the therapeutic termination of pregnancy, fetal damage has been observed in cases of incomplete termination and the appropriate treatment for complete evacuation of the uterus should therefore be instituted whenever termination is unsuccessful or incomplete. Dinoprostone should not be used for termination in patients with pelvic infection, unless adequate treatment has already been started.

**Administration.** For the hazards of unintentional systemic absorption of prostaglandins following intra-uterine use for the termination of pregnancy and abortion of hydatidiform moles, see Overdosage in Adverse Effects, above.

## Interactions

Dinoprostone enhances the effects of oxytocin on the uterus.

◊ Marked hypertension, vomiting, and severe dyspnoea occurred following the sequential use of oxytocin, methylergometrine, and dinoprost within the space of 10 minutes to a woman with postpartum haemorrhage.[1]

1. Cohen S, *et al.* Severe systemic reactions following administration of different ureotonic [uterotonic] drugs. *N Y State J Med* 1983; **83:** 1060–1.

## Uses and Administration

Dinoprostone is a prostaglandin of the E series (p.1511) with actions on smooth muscle; the endogenous substance is termed prostaglandin $E_2$ and is rapidly metabolised in the body. It induces contraction of uterine muscle at any stage of pregnancy and is reported to act mainly as a vasodilator and as a bronchodilator. In the UK, dinoprostone is used principally in the induction of labour (p.1511); it may also be used for the termination of pregnancy (p.1512), missed abortion, hydatidiform mole, and fetal death *in utero*.

Dinoprostone is usually given vaginally. It may also be given intravenously, extra-amniotically, or by mouth, but the intravenous route has been associated with a high incidence of adverse effects and is generally only used for missed abortion or hydatidiform mole; continuous use for more than 2 days is not recommended.

For the **induction of labour** dinoprostone is used to ripen (soften and dilate) the cervix before the membranes are ruptured and to induce labour at term. The cervical gel used for cervical ripening contains 500 micrograms in 2.5 mL, whereas the vaginal gel used for induction of labour contains 1 or 2 mg per 2.5 mL; the vaginal gel should not be used in the cervical canal. Pessaries containing 3 mg are also available for labour induction. These are not bioequivalent to the vaginal gel and their dosage is different.

To soften and dilate the cervix before induction of labour dinoprostone 500 micrograms is given as *cervical gel*. This dose may be repeated after 6 hours if there was no response to the initial dose; in some cases a third dose may be used to a maximum cumulative dose of 1.5 mg in 24 hours. For induction of labour the dose as *vaginal gel* is 1 mg (or 2 mg in primigravid patients with unfavourable induction features) followed, if necessary, by a further 1 or 2 mg after 6 hours; a total dose of 3 mg (or 4 mg in unfavourable primigravid patients) should not be exceeded. Alternatively a *vaginal pessary* containing 3 mg may be used and this may be followed, if necessary, by a further 3 mg after 6 to 8 hours; a total dose of 6 mg should not be exceeded.

A *modified-release pessary* delivering 5 mg over 12 hours can be used for cervical ripening and subsequent labour induction. If satisfactory cervical ripening does not occur within 8 to 12 hours then it should be removed and a second and final modified-release pessary inserted and retained for not more than 12 hours.

Dinoprostone may be given *by mouth* for the induction of labour in an initial dose of 500 micrograms, repeated hourly, and increased if necessary to 1 mg hourly until an adequate response is achieved; single doses of 1.5 mg should not be exceeded. Oral use has, however, generally been replaced by intravaginal dosage since the latter is associated with fewer gastrointestinal side-effects.

Dinoprostone has been given *intravenously* for the induction of labour but is no longer recommended for routine use by most authorities. A suggested intravenous dosage has been 250 nanograms/minute infused as a solution containing 1.5 micrograms/mL for 30 minutes, the dose being subsequently maintained or increased according to the patient's response; in fetal death *in utero* higher doses may be required and an initial rate of 500 nanograms/minute has been used with increases at intervals of not less than 1 hour.

For the **termination of pregnancy** in the second trimester 1 mL of a solution containing dinoprostone 100 micrograms/mL may be instilled *extra-amniotically* through a suitable Foley catheter, with subsequent doses of 1 or 2 mL given at intervals usually of 2 hours, according to response. Dinoprostone has also been given *intravenously* for the termination of pregnancy and for missed abortion or hydatidiform mole. A solution containing 5 micrograms/mL may be infused at a rate of 2.5 micrograms/minute for 30 minutes, thereafter, the infusion being maintained or increased to a rate of 5 micrograms/minute; this rate should be maintained for at least 4 hours before making further increases.

In the USA dinoprostone pessaries are used for the termination of second trimester pregnancy, a dose of 20 mg being given *intravaginally* and repeated every 3 to 5 hours according to response for up to 2 days; a total dose of 240 mg should not be exceeded. Pessaries are also used in the USA in missed abortion, fetal death *in utero*, and benign hydatidiform mole.

Dinoprostone is used in some centres to maintain the patency of the ductus arteriosus (see below).

**Haemorrhagic cystitis.** Dinoprostone instilled into the bladder for 4 hours and repeated for 4 days successfully improved severe cyclophosphamide-induced haemorrhagic cystitis (p.540) in a bone marrow transplant recipient.[1] Similar results were obtained in another series of 10 patients.[2]

1. Mohiuddin J, *et al.* Treatment of cyclophosphamide-induced cystitis with prostaglandin $E_2$. *Ann Intern Med* 1984; **101:** 142.
2. Laszlo D, *et al.* Prostaglandin E2 bladder instillation for the treatment of hemorrhagic cystitis after allogeneic bone marrow transplantation. *Haematologica* 1995; **80:** 421–5.

**Hepatic disorders.** See under Alprostadil, p.1513, for reference to the use of prostaglandins, including dinoprostone, in the treatment of viral hepatitis.

**Patent ductus arteriosus.** Prostaglandins, particularly alprostadil (p.1513) and dinoprostone, may be used to maintain the patency of the ductus arteriosus in infants with congenital heart disease until surgery can be performed to correct the malformation. Treatment for a longer period, especially with oral dinoprostone, may facilitate later surgery by allowing growth of the infants and their pulmonary arteries.

Beneficial responses to long-term use of dinoprostone have been reported.[1,2] Dinoprostone has been given orally in an initial dose of 20 to 25 micrograms/kg hourly, decreasing the frequency of doses after the first week; it was suggested that treatment should be continued for up to 4 weeks initially and a decision then made whether to proceed with surgery or to plan a longer course of treatment to encourage further growth. When gastrointestinal absorption is expected to be poor or when oral treatment is ineffective, dinoprostone has been given by intravenous infusion, beginning with a dose of 3 nanograms/kg per minute, adjusted according to response. Doses as high as 10 to 20 nanograms/kg per minute have been used but are reported to be exceptional, and severe adverse effects were encountered[2] in 4 of 11 infants given dinoprostone by intravenous infusion at an initial dose of 50 nanograms/kg per minute.

1. Silove ED, *et al.* Evaluation of oral and low dose intravenous prostaglandin $E_2$ in management of ductus dependent congenital heart disease. *Arch Dis Child* 1985; **60:** 1025–30.
2. Thanopoulos BD, *et al.* Prostaglandin $E_2$ administration in infants with ductus-dependent cyanotic congenital heart disease. *Eur J Pediatr* 1987; **146:** 279–82.

**Pemphigus.** Erosive oral lesions in 3 patients[1] with pemphigus vulgaris (p.1137), that had previously been refractory to standard corticosteroid therapy, resolved on sucking oral dinoprostone tablets 1.5 to 3 mg daily. Symptoms recurred within weeks of ceasing dinoprostone but could be controlled by courses of 0.5 to 1 mg daily for 1 to 2 weeks, when required.

1. Morita H, *et al.* Clinical trial of prostaglandin $E_2$ on the oral lesions of pemphigus vulgaris. *Br J Dermatol* 1995; **132:** 165–6.

**Peripheral vascular disease.** Various prostaglandins have been used in the treatment of peripheral vascular disease (p.831), particularly in severe Raynaud's syndrome (p.833), but do not constitute mainline therapy.

**Postpartum haemorrhage.** Dinoprostone and other prostaglandins have been used to control severe postpartum haemorrhage (p.1684) unresponsive to ergometrine and oxytocin.

Beneficial response to continuous intra-uterine irrigation with dinoprostone solution 1.5 micrograms/mL was seen in 22 patients with postpartum haemorrhage unresponsive to other treatment.[1] Postpartum haemorrhage was controlled in another patient using a dinoprostone 3-mg vaginal suppository held against the uterine wall.[2]

1. Peyser MR, Kupfermine MJ. Management of severe postpartum hemorrhage by intrauterine irrigation with prostaglandin $E_2$. *Am J Obstet Gynecol* 1990; **162:** 694–6.
2. Markos AR. Prostaglandin $E_2$ intrauterine suppositories in the treatment of secondary postpartum hemorrhage. *J R Soc Med* 1989; **82:** 504–5.

## Preparations

**Proprietary Preparations** (details are given in Part 3)
***Arg.:*** Prolisina E2; ***Austral.:*** Cervidil; Prostin E2; ***Austria:*** Prepidil; Propess; Prostin E2; ***Belg.:*** Prepidil; Prostin E2; ***Canad.:*** Cervidil; Prepidil; Prostin E2; ***Denm.:*** Minprostin; Propess†; ***Fin.:*** Minprostin; Propess; ***Fr.:*** Prepidil; Propess; Prostine $E_2$; ***Ger.:*** Cerviprost†; Minprostin $E_2$; Prepidil; Propess; ***Gr.:*** Propess; Prostin E2; ***Hong Kong:*** Prepidil†; Propess†; Prostin E2; ***India:*** Cerviprime; Primiprost; ***Irl.:*** Prepidil†; Prostin E2; ***Israel:*** Prepidil; Propess; Prostin E2; ***Ital.:*** Prepidil; Propess; Prostin E2; ***Malaysia:*** Prostin E2; ***Mex.:*** Prepidil; Propess†; ***Neth.:*** Prepidil; Propess; Prostin E2; ***Norw.:*** Minprostin; ***NZ:*** Prepidil†; Prostin E2; ***Port.:*** Propess; Prostin E2; ***S.Afr.:*** Prandin $E_2$; Prepidil; Propess; Prostin E2; ***Singapore:*** Prostin; ***Spain:*** Gravidex†; Prepidil; Propess; ***Swed.:*** Minprostin; Propess; ***Switz.:*** Prepidil; Propess; Prostin E2; ***Thai.:*** Prostin E2; ***UK:*** Prepidil†; Propess; Prostin E2; ***USA:*** Cervidil; Prepidil; Prostin E2.

---

# Epoprostenol *(USAN, rINN)*

$PGI_2$; PGX; Prostacyclin; Prostaglandin $I_2$; Prostaglandin X; U-53217. (5Z,13E)-(8R,9S,11R,12R,15S)-6,9-Epoxy-11,15-dihydroxyprosta-5,13-dienoic acid; (Z)-5-{(3aR,4R,5R,6aS)-5-Hydroxy-4-[(E)-(3S)-3-hydroxyoct-1-enyl]perhydrocyclopenta[b]furan-2-ylidene}valeric acid.

$C_{20}H_{32}O_5$ = 352.5.
*CAS — 35121-78-9.*
*ATC — B01AC09.*

NOTE. In *Martindale* the term epoprostenol is used for the exogenous substance and prostacyclin for the endogenous substance.

## Epoprostenol Sodium *(BAN, USAN, rINNM)*

Epoprostenol sódico; U-53217A.
$C_{20}H_{31}NaO_5$ = 374.4.
*CAS — 61849-14-7.*
*ATC — B01AC09.*

**Stability in solution.** Epoprostenol is unstable at physiological pH and solutions for infusion are prepared in an alkaline glycine buffer at pH 10.5. The half-life in aqueous solution of pH 7.4 has been reported[1] to be less than 3 minutes at 37°, but increased stability has been reported in plasma, albumin, or whole blood.[1,2]


1. El Tahir KEH, *et al.* Stability of prostacyclin in human plasma. *Clin Sci* 1980; **59:** 28P–29P.
2. Mikhailidis DP, *et al.* Infusion of prostacyclin (epoprostenol). *Lancet* 1982; **ii:** 767.


## Adverse Effects and Precautions

The incidence of adverse reactions to epoprostenol is dose-related. Side-effects during intravenous infusion commonly include hypotension, increased heart rate, flushing, and headache. Dosage should be reduced or the epoprostenol infusion stopped if excessive hypotension occurs. Bradycardia with pallor, sweating, nausea, and abdominal discomfort may occur. Erythema over the intravenous infusion site has been noted. Other side-effects reported have included nausea and vomiting, diarrhoea, jaw pain or non-specific musculoskeletal pain, anxiety, nervousness, tremor, flu-like symptoms, hyperglycaemia, drowsiness, and chest pain.

Coagulation of blood in the dialysis circuit has been reported rarely in patients given epoprostenol but no conventional anticoagulant. The use of epoprostenol for pulmonary hypertension is contra-indicated in patients with congestive heart failure due to severe left ventricular systolic dysfunction, and in patients who develop pulmonary oedema during dose-ranging. Sudden withdrawal of epoprostenol should be avoided because of the risk of rebound pulmonary hypertension. Haematological and cardiovascular monitoring is required in patients receiving epoprostenol infusions. Care should be taken to avoid extravasation.

◊ A study in 24 healthy subjects investigated the incidence of adverse effects with intravenous infusions of epoprostenol of up to 10 nanograms/kg per minute for up to 100 minutes.[1] Subjects varied in their susceptibility to epoprostenol but the same sequence of events was usually present. A change in pre-ejection period and facial flushing was often apparent at an infusion rate of 2 to 2.5 nanograms/kg per minute. A rise in heart rate and change in other cardiovascular variables was present when the infusion rate had increased to 4 to 5 nanograms/kg per minute; headache, generally the dose-limiting factor, was usually present at this dose and increased as the dose was raised, as did the other effects. Erythema over the vein and 'vagal reflex' only appeared after at least 1 hour of infusion; 'vagal reflex' took only a few seconds to develop.

Early studies showing that high doses were well tolerated had been conducted using a form of epoprostenol probably only half as potent as the commercially available product. It was proposed that 4 nanograms/kg per minute should in general be the maximum infusion rate for prolonged infusions, although higher rates could be tolerated in anaesthetised patients. Careful attention to infusion technique is necessary and monitoring of the heart rate is advisable in view of the suddenness with which the 'vagal reflex' can occur. Most of the adverse effects reported here have responded to a reduction in dosage.


1. Pickles H, O'Grady J. Side effects occurring during administration of epoprostenol (prostacyclin, $PGI_2$), in man. *Br J Clin Pharmacol* 1982; **14:** 177–85.


**Effects on the blood.** Reports of rebound platelet activation during continuous epoprostenol infusion.[1,2]


1. Yardumian DA, Machin SJ. Altered platelet function in patients on continuous infusion of epoprostenol. *Lancet* 1984; **i:** 1357.
2. Sinzinger H, *et al.* Rebound platelet activation during continuous epoprostenol infusion. *Lancet* 1984; **ii:** 759.


**Effects on the cardiovascular system.** Evidence that epoprostenol and its analogue iloprost can induce myocardial ischaemia in patients with coronary artery disease.[1]


1. Bugiardini R, *et al.* Myocardial ischemia induced by prostacyclin and iloprost. *Clin Pharmacol Ther* 1985; **38:** 101–8.


**Effects on mental state.** Symptoms of depression were associated with intravenous epoprostenol therapy in 4 patients.[1]


1. Ansell D, *et al.* Depression and prostacyclin infusion. *Lancet* 1986; **ii:** 509.


**Hypersensitivity.** Severe erythroderma occurred in a woman with undifferentiated connective tissue disease who was treated with epoprostenol for pulmonary hypertension.[1] Diffuse erythema, pruritus, and scaling, with chills, nausea, vomiting, and diarrhoea, developed about 2 months after starting therapy, and resolved with epoprostenol withdrawal and corticosteroid treatment.


1. Ahearn GS, *et al.* Severe erythroderma as a complication of continuous epoprostenol therapy. *Chest* 2002; **122:** 378–80.


## Interactions

Since epoprostenol is a potent vasodilator and inhibitor of platelet aggregation, care should be taken in patients receiving other vasodilators or anticoagulants. Epoprostenol may slightly increase serum concentrations of digoxin, and may reduce the thrombolytic effect of alteplase by increasing its hepatic clearance. The hypotensive effects of epoprostenol may be exacerbated by using acetate in dialysis fluids.

## Pharmacokinetics

Endogenous prostacyclin is a product of arachidonic acid metabolism with a very short half-life. Following intravenous infusion epoprostenol is hydrolysed rapidly to the more stable but much less active 6-keto-prostaglandin $F_{1\alpha}$ (6-oxo-prostaglandin $F_{1\alpha}$). A second metabolite, 6,15-diketo-13,14-dihydro-prostaglandin $F_{1\alpha}$, is formed by enzymatic degradation. Unlike many other prostaglandins, epoprostenol is not inactivated in the pulmonary circulation.

## Uses and Administration

Epoprostenol is a prostaglandin (p.1511) that causes vasodilatation and prevents platelet aggregation. The endogenous substance is termed prostacyclin. It is used mainly in extracorporeal procedures and in pulmonary hypertension.

Epoprostenol is given as the sodium salt and doses are expressed in terms of the base; 1.06 nanograms of epoprostenol sodium is equivalent to about 1 nanogram of epoprostenol. The drug is unstable in solution at physiological pH and also has a very short duration of action because of its rapid hydrolysis *in vivo*. It must therefore be given by continuous infusion. Great care must be taken in preparing a suitably diluted solution for infusion and only diluent as supplied by the manufacturer should be used to reconstitute epoprostenol.

Epoprostenol is used to **prevent platelet aggregation** when blood is brought into contact with nonbiological surfaces in procedures such as extracorporeal circulation, especially in renal dialysis patients. It is indicated for use when heparin carries a high risk of causing or exacerbating bleeding, or is otherwise contra-indicated. Epoprostenol is given by continuous intravenous infusion or into the blood supplying the extracorporeal circulation. The usual dose for renal dialysis is 4 nanograms/kg per minute intravenously before dialysis, then 4 nanograms/kg per minute into the arterial inlet of the dialyser during dialysis.

In the long-term treatment of primary **pulmonary hypertension** a dose-ranging procedure is performed first, in order to establish the maximum infusion rate that can be tolerated. Epoprostenol is then given by continuous infusion through a central venous catheter, the initial rate being 4 nanograms/kg per minute *less than* the maximum-tolerated infusion rate; if the maximum-tolerated infusion rate is less than 5 nanograms/kg per minute, then the initial rate should be one-half of this maximum rate. The maintenance dose is subsequently adjusted according to the patient's response. If symptoms recur or if adverse effects occur the dosage may be increased or decreased by steps of 1 to 2 nanograms/kg per minute at intervals of at least 15 minutes until a new maintenance dose is established.

**Action.** The discovery, properties, and clinical applications of prostacyclin have been reviewed.[1] Prostacyclin is the main product of arachidonic acid in vascular tissues, endothelial cells from vessel walls being the most active producers. It is a strong hypotensive agent through vasodilatation of vascular beds, including the pulmonary and cerebral circulations, and is also a potent endogenous inhibitor of platelet aggregation. Inhibition of aggregation is achieved by stimulation of adenylate cyclase, leading to an increase in cyclic adenosine monophosphate (cAMP) levels in the platelets. By inhibiting several steps in the activation of the arachidonic acid metabolic cascade, prostacyclin exerts an overall control of platelet aggregability.

Endogenous prostacyclin and thromboxane $A_2$ may be of more physiological and pathological importance[2] than the more classical prostanoids prostaglandin $E_2$ and prostaglandin $F_{2\alpha}$. They have directly opposing pharmacological actions in many systems, such as on platelet function, vascular smooth muscle, bronchopulmonary function, and gastrointestinal integrity. Thus prostanoid-mediated control of cellular and tissue function may reflect an interactive modulation between prostacyclin and thromboxane $A_2$ with imbalance resulting in dysfunction, for example in platelet and vascular disorders. Thromboxane $A_2$ has both bronchoconstrictor and pulmonary irritant actions and has brought about marked changes in respiratory function in experimental models; prostacyclin may oppose these effects on both the pulmonary vasculature and bronchial smooth muscle. Thromboxane $A_2$ has induced marked renal vasoconstriction *in vitro* whereas renal vasodilatation and stimulation of the release of renin has followed the administration of epoprostenol [exogenous prostacyclin] in *animals*. In contrast to the pro-ulcerogenic actions of thromboxane $A_2$, epoprostenol and its analogues, like other prostaglandins, have potent gastrointestinal anti-ulcer properties which can be disassociated from their gastric antisecretory properties. The term 'cytoprotection' has been used to describe this ability of exogenous prostaglandins to prevent gastrointestinal damage; endogenous prostaglandins might have a similar protective role. Epoprostenol also has a cytoprotective effect against experimental damage in the gastric mucosa, myocardium, and liver whereas thromboxane $A_2$ has a cytolytic effect.


1. Vane JR, Botting RM. Pharmacodynamic profile of prostacyclin. *Am J Cardiol* 1995; **75:** 3A–10A.
2. Whittle BJR, Moncada S. Pharmacological interactions between prostacyclin and thromboxanes. *Br Med Bull* 1983; **39:** 232–8.


**Acute respiratory distress syndrome.** Encouraging results[1-3] have been seen with inhaled epoprostenol in the treatment of acute respiratory distress syndrome (p.1075).


1. Walmrath D, *et al.* Aerosolised prostacyclin in adult respiratory distress syndrome. *Lancet* 1993; **342:** 961–2.
2. Walmrath D, *et al.* Direct comparison of inhaled nitric oxide and aerosolized prostacyclin in acute respiratory distress syndrome. *Am J Respir Crit Care Med* 1996; **153:** 991–6.
3. van Heerden PV, *et al.* Dose-response to inhaled aerosolized prostacyclin for hypoxemia due to ARDS. *Chest* 2000; **117:** 819–27.


**Heart failure.** Epoprostenol has been investigated for the treatment of heart failure but development was abandoned due to an increase in mortality associated with long-term use.[1,2]


1. Phillips BB, Gandhi AJ. Epoprostenol in the treatment of congestive heart failure. *Am J Health-Syst Pharm* 1997; **54:** 2613–15.
2. Califf RM, *et al.* A randomized controlled trial of epoprostenol therapy for severe congestive heart failure: the Flolan International Randomized Survival Trial (FIRST). *Am Heart J* 1997; **134:** 44–54.


**Peripheral vascular disease.** Various prostaglandins including epoprostenol have been used for their vasodilating effect in the treatment of peripheral vascular disease (p.831), particularly in severe Raynaud's syndrome (p.833), but do not constitute mainline therapy.

References.


1. Szczeklik A, *et al.* Successful therapy of advanced arteriosclerosis obliterans with prostacyclin. *Lancet* 1979; **i:** 1111–14.
2. Belch JJF, *et al.* Intermittent epoprostenol (prostacyclin) infusion in patients with Raynaud's syndrome: a double-blind controlled trial. *Lancet* 1983; **i:** 313–15.
3. Belch JJF, *et al.* Epoprostenol (prostacyclin) and severe arterial disease: a double-blind trial. *Lancet* 1983; **i:** 315–17.
4. De San Lazaro C, *et al.* Prostacyclin in severe peripheral vascular disease. *Arch Dis Child* 1985; **60:** 370–84.
5. Leaker B, *et al.* Treatment of acute renal failure, symmetrical peripheral gangrene, and septicaemia with plasma exchange and epoprostenol. *Lancet* 1987; **i:** 156.
6. Negus D, *et al.* Intra-arterial prostacyclin compared to Praxilene in the management of severe lower limb ischaemia: a double-blind trial. *J Cardiovasc Surg* 1987; **28:** 196–9.
7. Kingma K, *et al.* Double-blind, placebo controlled study of intravenous prostacyclin on hemodynamics in severe Raynaud's phenomenon: the acute vasodilatory effect is not sustained. *J Cardiovasc Pharmacol* 1995; **26:** 388–93.
8. Denton CP, Black CM. Raynaud's phenomenon and scleroderma. In: Snaith ML, ed. *ABC of rheumatology.* 3rd ed. London: BMJ Publishing Group, 2004: 87–91.


**Pulmonary hypertension.** Epoprostenol was originally introduced into the management of primary pulmonary hypertension (p.832) to sustain patients long enough for them to have heart-lung transplantation. However, long-term therapy may also have a role as an alternative to transplantation; sustained clinical improvement and improved survival have been reported[1-3] in some patients given long-term intravenous therapy using portable infusion pumps. Epoprostenol infusion may also have a role in patients with secondary pulmonary hypertension.[4,5]

Inhaled epoprostenol, a method of administration that may overcome some of the adverse effects associated with the parenteral route, has been used with some success in adults[6,7] with primary or secondary pulmonary hypertension and in neonates[8,9] with persistent pulmonary hypertension.


1. Higenbottam T, *et al.* Long term intravenous prostaglandin (epoprostenol or iloprost) for treatment of severe pulmonary hypertension. *Heart* 1998; **80:** 151–5.
2. Herner SJ, Mauro LS. Epoprostenol in primary pulmonary hypertension. *Ann Pharmacother* 1999; **33:** 340–7.
3. McLaughlin VV, *et al.* Survival in primary pulmonary hypertension: the impact of epoprostenol therapy. *Circulation* 2002; **106:** 1477–82.
4. McLaughlin VV, *et al.* Compassionate use of continuous prostacyclin in the management of secondary pulmonary hypertension: a case series. *Ann Intern Med* 1999; **130:** 740–3.
5. Badesch DB, *et al.* Continuous intravenous epoprostenol for pulmonary hypertension due to the scleroderma spectrum of disease: a randomized, controlled trial. *Ann Intern Med* 2000; **132:** 425–34.
6. Olschewski H, *et al.* Aerosolized prostacyclin and iloprost in severe pulmonary hypertension. *Ann Intern Med* 1996; **124:** 820–4.

7. Mikhail G, *et al.* An evaluation of nebulized prostacyclin in patients with primary and secondary pulmonary hypertension. *Eur Heart J* 1997; **18:** 1499–1504.
8. Bindl L, *et al.* Aerosolised prostacyclin for pulmonary hypertension in neonates. *Arch Dis Child Fetal Neonatal Ed* 1994; **71:** F214–F216.
9. Kelly LK, *et al.* Inhaled prostacyclin for term infants with persistent pulmonary hypertension refractory to inhaled nitric oxide. *J Pediatr* 2002; **141:** 830–2.

**Stroke.** Results with epoprostenol in patients with acute stroke have been inconclusive and a systematic review of randomised studies concluded that too few patients had been studied for the effect of epoprostenol on survival to be determined.[1]

1. Bath PMW, Bath FJ. Prostacyclin and analogues for acute ischaemic stroke. Available in The Cochrane Library; Issue 2. Chichester: John Wiley; 2004.

**Thrombotic microangiopathies.** Platelet aggregation has a major role in the pathogenesis of thrombotic thrombocytopenic purpura and the related disorder, haemolytic-uraemic syndrome (p.758). Prostacyclin deficiency has been demonstrated in both conditions, but case reports of epoprostenol treatment have indicated variable results.[1-7]

1. Webster J, *et al.* Prostacyclin deficiency in haemolytic-uraemic syndrome. *BMJ* 1980; **281:** 271.
2. Beattie TJ, *et al.* Prostacyclin infusion in haemolytic-uraemic syndrome of children. *BMJ* 1981; **283:** 470.
3. Johnson JE, *et al.* Ineffective epoprostenol therapy for thrombotic thrombocytopenic purpura. *JAMA* 1983; **250:** 3089–91.
4. Payton CD, *et al.* Successful treatment of thrombotic thrombocytopenic purpura by epoprostenol infusion. *Lancet* 1985; **i:** 927–8.
5. Tardy B, *et al.* Intravenous prostacyclin in thrombotic thrombocytopenic purpura: case report and review of the literature. *J Intern Med* 1991; **230:** 279–82.
6. Bobbio-Pallavicini E, *et al.* Intravenous prostacyclin (as epoprostenol) infusion in thrombotic thrombocytopenic purpura: four case reports and review of the literature. *Haematologica* 1994; **79:** 429–37.
7. Series C, *et al.* Interet de la prostacycline dans le traitement du syndrome hémolytique et urémique: à propos d'un cas. *Rev Med Interne* 1996; **17:** 76–8.

### Preparations

**Proprietary Preparations** (details are given in Part 3)
***Austral.:*** Flolan; ***Austria:*** Flolan; ***Belg.:*** Flolan; ***Canad.:*** Flolan; ***Denm.:*** Flolan; ***Fr.:*** Flolan; ***Irl.:*** Flolan; ***Israel:*** Flolan; ***Ital.:*** Flolan; ***Neth.:*** Flolan; ***Norw.:*** Flolan; ***Singapore:*** Flolan; ***Spain:*** Flolan; ***Switz.:*** Flolan; ***UK:*** Flolan; ***USA:*** Flolan.

## Etiproston Trometamol *(rINNM)*

Etiprostón trometamol; Etiproston Tromethamine. Trometamol salt of (*Z*)-7-[(1*R*, 2*R*,3*R*,5*S*)-3,5-dihydroxy-2-[(*E*)-2-[2-(phenoxymethyl)-1,3-dioxolan-2-yl]vinyl]cyclopentyl]-5-heptenoic acid.

$C_{24}H_{32}O_7,C_4H_{11}NO_3 = 553.6.$
*CAS — 59619-81-7 (etiproston).*

### Profile

Etiproston trometamol is a synthetic analogue of dinoprost (prostaglandin $F_{2\alpha}$). It is used as a luteolytic in veterinary medicine.

## Gemeprost *(BAN, USAN, rINN)*

16,16-Dimethyl-*trans*-$\Delta^2$-prostaglandin $E_1$ methyl ester; ONO-802; SC-37681. Methyl (2*E*,13*E*)-(8*R*,11*R*,12*R*,15*R*)-11,15-dihydroxy-16,16-dimethyl-9-oxoprosta-2,13-dienoate; Methyl (*E*)-7-{(1*R*,2*R*,3*R*)-3-hydroxy-2-[(*E*)-(3*R*)-3-hydroxy-4,4-dimethyloct-1-enyl]-5-oxocyclopentyl}hept-2-enoate.

$C_{23}H_{38}O_5 = 394.5.$
*CAS — 64318-79-2.*
*ATC — G02AD03.*

### Adverse Effects and Precautions

Gemeprost is given vaginally as pessaries and systemic adverse effects such as nausea, vomiting, and diarrhoea are relatively mild. Other reported side-effects have included headache, muscle weakness, dizziness, flushing, chills, backache, dyspnoea, chest pain, palpitations, and mild pyrexia. Vaginal bleeding and mild uterine pain may occur.

Uterine rupture has been reported rarely, most commonly in multiparous women and in those with a history of uterine surgery. There have also been rare reports of severe hypotension and coronary spasm with subsequent myocardial infarction.

The effects of gemeprost on the fetus are not known. Once a prostaglandin has been given to terminate pregnancy it is essential that termination take place; if the prostaglandin is unsuccessful other measures should be used.

Gemeprost should be used with caution in patients with obstructive airways disease, cardiovascular disease, raised intra-ocular pressure, cervicitis, or vaginitis. Blood pressure and pulse rate should be monitored after use; when given with mifepristone monitoring for 6 hours is recommended.

**Incidence of adverse effects.** The incidence of vomiting (19 or 35%) and diarrhoea (12 or 19%) in 2 studies of patients treated with gemeprost pessaries was similar to that seen with other prostaglandins, but gemeprost was reported to cause less uterine pain.[1,2] Like other prostaglandins used for termination of pregnancy it may occasionally produce hyperstimulation and uterine rupture (see Effects on the Uterus, under Dinoprostone, p.1515).

1. Cameron IT, Baird DT. The use of 16,16-dimethyl-trans-$\Delta^2$ prostaglandin $E_1$ methyl ester (gemeprost) vaginal pessaries for the termination of pregnancy in the early second trimester: a comparison with extra-amniotic prostaglandin $E_2$. *Br J Obstet Gynaecol* 1984; **91:** 1136–40.
2. Andersen LF, *et al.* Termination of second trimester pregnancy with gemeprost vaginal pessaries and intra-amniotic $PGF_{2\alpha}$: a comparative study. *Eur J Obstet Gynecol Reprod Biol* 1989; **31:** 1–7.

**Effects on the cardiovascular system.** Periods of ventricular standstill of up to 6 seconds were observed in a patient during treatment with gemeprost vaginal pessaries.[1] The patient required temporary cardiac pacing, but no persistent cardiac rhythm disturbances were detected on follow-up. Severe cardiogenic shock due to vasospasm, and subsequent stroke, has been reported in a patient who had received gemeprost pessaries some hours earlier; myocardial infarction ensuing from coronary spasm was reported in a second patient.[2]

1. Kalra PA, *et al.* Cardiac standstill induced by prostaglandin pessaries. *Lancet* 1989; **i:** 1460–1.
2. Lauer M, Berentelg J. Schwere kardiovaskuläre Komplikationen im Zusammenhang mit Gemeprost. *Zentralbl Gynakol* 2000; **122:** 324–7.

### Uses and Administration

Gemeprost is a synthetic analogue of alprostadil (prostaglandin $E_1$). It is used to soften and dilate the cervix and as a uterine stimulant in the termination of pregnancy (p.1512). In the first trimester, a pessary containing gemeprost 1 mg is inserted into the vagina 3 hours before surgery to ripen the cervix. Gemeprost may also be used for termination of pregnancy in the second trimester when a 1-mg pessary is inserted every 3 hours to a maximum of 5 pessaries. Should this course be ineffective one further course may be given after an interval of 24 hours. In the case of intra-uterine fetal death only one course of five pessaries should be given. Vaginal gemeprost is also used after oral mifepristone (p.1560) in the termination of pregnancy.

### Preparations

**Proprietary Preparations** (details are given in Part 3)
***Austral.:*** Cervagem; ***Denm.:*** Cervagem; ***Fin.:*** Cervagem; ***Fr.:*** Cervageme; ***Ger.:*** Cergem; ***Hong Kong:*** Cervagem; ***Ital.:*** Cervidil; ***Jpn:*** Preglandin; ***Malaysia:*** Cervagem; ***Norw.:*** Cervagem; ***NZ:*** Cervagem; ***Singapore:*** Cervagem; ***Swed.:*** Cervagem.

## Iloprost *(BAN, rINN)*

Ciloprost; ZK-36374. (*E*)-(3a*S*,4*R*,5*R*,6a*S*)-Hexahydro-5-hydroxy-4-[(*E*)-(3*S*,4*RS*)-3-hydroxy-4-methyl-1-octen-6-ynyl]-$\Delta^{2(1H),\delta}$-pentalenevaleric acid.

$C_{22}H_{32}O_4 = 360.5.$
*CAS — 73873-87-7; 78919-13-8.*
*ATC — B01AC11.*

## Iloprost Trometamol *(BANM, rINNM)*

Ciloprost Tromethamine; Iloprost trometamol; Iloprost Tromethamine.

$C_{22}H_{32}O_4,C_4H_{11}NO_3 = 481.6.$
*ATC — B01AC11.*

### Adverse Effects and Precautions

As for Epoprostenol, p.1517. Inhaled iloprost may cause cough.

**Effects on the cardiovascular system.** Hypotension was observed[1] in 2 of 6 patients given iloprost. Both patients recovered rapidly when iloprost was stopped, although one required intravenous atropine to correct sinus bradycardia.

Evidence of myocardial ischaemia was reported in 4 of 33 patients with coronary artery disease during iloprost infusion.[2] The same authors[3] noted a similar effect in 4 of 28 patients with stable angina in a subsequent study. According to one study,[4] there might be an increased risk of thromboembolism in some patients given iloprost, due to platelet activation and enhanced coagulation.

1. Upward JW, *et al.* Hypotension in response to iloprost, a prostacyclin analogue. *Br J Clin Pharmacol* 1986; **21:** 241–3.
2. Bugiardini R, *et al.* Myocardial ischemia induced by prostacyclin and iloprost. *Clin Pharmacol Ther* 1985; **38:** 101–8.
3. Bugiardini R, *et al.* Effects of iloprost, a stable prostacyclin analog, on exercise capacity and platelet aggregation in stable angina pectoris. *Am J Cardiol* 1986; **58:** 453–9.
4. Kovacs IB, *et al.* Infusion of a stable prostacyclin analogue, iloprost, to patients with peripheral vascular disease: lack of antiplatelet effect but risk of thromboembolism. *Am J Med* 1991; **90:** 41–6.

### Interactions

Iloprost may increase the effect of other vasodilators and antihypertensives. The use of iloprost with other inhibitors of platelet aggregation may increase the risk of bleeding.

### Pharmacokinetics

Following intravenous infusion iloprost is rapidly cleared from the plasma by oxidation. About 80% of the metabolites are excreted in the urine and 20% in the bile.

### Uses and Administration

Iloprost, a vasodilator and platelet aggregation inhibitor, is a stable analogue of the prostaglandin epoprostenol (prostacyclin). It is given as the trometamol salt in the treatment of peripheral vascular disease and pulmonary hypertension but doses are described in terms of iloprost; 1.3 nanograms of iloprost trometamol is equivalent to about 1 nanogram of iloprost.

The usual dose for peripheral vascular disease is the equivalent of iloprost 0.5 to 2 nanograms/kg per minute for 6 hours daily by intravenous infusion. The course of treatment may be up to 4 weeks. For pulmonary hypertension, the dose is 1 to 8 nanograms/kg per minute for 6 hours daily; alternatively, iloprost may be given by nebulised solution at a dose of 2.5 or 5 micrograms inhaled 6 to 9 times daily. Doses should be reduced in patients with hepatic or renal impairment (see below). Administration of iloprost by mouth is under investigation.

◊ Reviews.

1. Grant SM, Goa KL. Iloprost: a review of its pharmacodynamic and pharmacokinetic properties, and therapeutic potential in peripheral vascular disease, myocardial ischaemia and extracorporeal circulation procedures. *Drugs* 1992; **43:** 889–924.

**Administration in hepatic or renal impairment.** The dose of intravenous iloprost should be reduced, and may need to be halved, in patients with liver cirrhosis or renal impairment requiring dialysis. In hepatic impairment, the initial dose of inhaled iloprost should be 2.5 micrograms given at intervals of at least 3 hours to a maximum of 6 times daily; the dose may be cautiously increased or given more frequently according to patient response.

**Peripheral vascular disease.** Prostaglandins, including iloprost,[1-10] have been used in the treatment of peripheral vascular disease (p.831), particularly in severe Raynaud's syndrome (p.833), but do not constitute mainline therapy. Systematic review[10] suggests that intravenous iloprost produces prolonged benefit in Raynaud's phenomenon secondary to scleroderma. The benefits of oral iloprost are less clear. It is also unclear whether iloprost infusion is of benefit in occlusive peripheral arterial disease due to atherosclerosis: although a meta-analysis of (conflicting) controlled trials did suggest an effect,[6] firm conclusions are difficult.

1. Waller PC, *et al.* Placebo controlled trial of iloprost in patients with stable intermittent claudication. *Br J Clin Pharmacol* 1986; **21:** 562P–563P.
2. Rademaker M, *et al.* Comparison of intravenous infusions of iloprost and oral nifedipine in treatment of Raynaud's phenomenon in patients with systemic sclerosis: a double blind randomised study. *BMJ* 1989; **298:** 561–4.
3. Fiessinger JN, Schäfer M. Trial of iloprost versus aspirin treatment for critical limb ischaemia of thromboangiitis obliterans. *Lancet* 1990; **335:** 555–7.
4. Zahavi J, *et al.* Ischaemic necrotic toes associated with antiphospholipid syndrome and treated with iloprost. *Lancet* 1993; **342:** 862.
5. Tait IS, *et al.* Management of intra-arterial injection injury with iloprost. *Lancet* 1994; **343:** 419.
6. Loosemore TM, *et al.* A meta-analysis of randomized placebo control trials in Fontaine stages III and IV peripheral occlusive arterial disease. *Int Angiol* 1994; **13:** 133–42.
7. Wigley FM, *et al.* Oral iloprost treatment in patients with Raynaud's phenomenon secondary to systemic sclerosis: a multicenter, placebo-controlled, double-blind study. *Arthritis Rheum* 1998; **41:** 670–7.
8. Black CM, *et al.* Oral iloprost in Raynaud's phenomenon secondary to systemic sclerosis: a multicentre, placebo-controlled, dose-comparison study. *Br J Rheumatol* 1998; **37:** 952–60.
9. Scorza R, *et al.* Effects of long-term cyclic iloprost therapy in systemic sclerosis with Raynaud's phenomenon: a randomized, controlled study. *Clin Exp Rheumatol* 2001; **19:** 503–8.
10. Pope J, *et al.* Iloprost and cisaprost for Raynaud's phenomenon in progressive systemic sclerosis. Available in The Cochrane Library: Issue 2. Chichester: John Wiley; 2004.

**Pulmonary hypertension.** Epoprostenol is an accepted part of the management of pulmonary hypertension (p.832) and the use of iloprost, a stable analogue, has been studied. Inhaled iloprost was found[1] to improve walking-test distances, reduce severity of heart failure, and stabilise haemodynamic measures in a 12-week study of patients with severe primary pulmonary hypertension. Long-term treatment of at least 1 year has been reported to have sustained beneficial effects.[2] There are also reports of effective combination therapy using inhaled iloprost with intravenous epoprostenol[3] or oral sildenafil.[4] Continuous intravenous infusion[5] has also been tried with beneficial results.

1. Olschewski H, *et al.* Inhaled iloprost for severe pulmonary hypertension. *N Engl J Med* 2002; **347:** 322–9.
2. Hoeper MM, *et al.* Long-term treatment of primary pulmonary hypertension with aerosolized iloprost, a prostacyclin analogue. *N Engl J Med* 2000; **342:** 1866–70.
3. Petkov V, *et al.* Aerosolised iloprost improves pulmonary haemodynamics in patients with primary pulmonary hypertension receiving continuous epoprostenol treatment. *Thorax* 2001; **56:** 734–6.
4. Ghofrani HA, *et al.* Combination therapy with oral sildenafil and inhaled iloprost for severe pulmonary hypertension. *Ann Intern Med* 2002; **136:** 515–22.
5. Higenbottam TW, *et al.* Treatment of pulmonary hypertension with the continuous infusion of a prostacyclin analogue, iloprost. *Heart* 1998; **79:** 175–9.

#### Preparations

**Proprietary Preparations** (details are given in Part 3)
***Arg.:*** Ilomedine; ***Austria:*** Ilomedin; ***Denm.:*** Ilomedin; ***Fin.:*** Ilomedin; ***Fr.:*** Ilomedine; ***Ger.:*** Ilomedin; ***Gr.:*** Ilomedin; ***Hong Kong:*** Ilomedin; ***Israel:*** Ilomedin; ***Ital.:*** Endoprost; Ilomedin†; ***Neth.:*** Ilomedine; ***Norw.:*** Ilomedin; ***NZ:*** Ilomedin; ***Port.:*** Ilomedin; ***Spain:*** Ilocit†; Ilomedin; ***Swed.:*** Ilomedin; ***Switz.:*** Ilomedin; ***UK:*** Ventavis.

## Latanoprost *(BAN, USAN, rINN)*

PhXA-41; XA-41. Isopropyl (Z)-7-{(1R,2R,3R,5S)-3,5-dihydroxy-2-[(3R)-3-hydroxy-5-phenylpentyl]cyclopentyl}-5-heptenoate.

$C_{26}H_{40}O_5$ = 432.6.

*CAS — 130209-82-4.*

*ATC — S01EE01.*

### Adverse Effects and Precautions

Latanoprost eye drops may produce a gradual increase in the amount of brown pigment in the iris, due to increased melanin content of melanocytes. This change in eye colour is most evident in patients with mixed colour irises, and may be permanent in some patients. Darkening, thickening, and lengthening of eye lashes may occur and darkening of the palpebral skin has been reported rarely. Ocular irritation, conjunctival hyperaemia, and eyelid oedema may occur; there have also been rare reports of iritis and/or uveitis, and macular oedema.

**Effects on the eyes.** Latanoprost has been associated with various adverse effects on the eyes, including case reports of cystoid macular oedema[1] and bilateral optic disc oedema.[2] The manufacturers have stated that reports of macular oedema have mainly occurred in aphakic patients, in pseudophakic patients with torn posterior lens capsule or anterior chamber lenses, or in patients with risk factors for cystoid macular oedema such as those with diabetic retinopathy or retinal vein occlusion.

Herpes simplex dendritic keratitis developed in 2 patients during latanoprost therapy.[3] The author suggested that the biochemical changes in the cornea caused by latanoprost may predispose to herpes keratitis.

1. Wardrop DRA, Wishart PK. Latanoprost and cystoid macular oedema in a pseudophake. *Br J Ophthalmol* 1998; **82:** 843–4.
2. Stewart O, *et al.* Bilateral optic disc oedema associated with latanoprost. *Br J Ophthalmol* 1999; **83:** 1092–3.
3. Ekatomatis P. Herpes simplex dendritic keratitis after treatment with latanoprost for primary open angle glaucoma. *Br J Ophthalmol* 2001; **85:** 1008–9.

**Systemic effects.** The use of latanoprost eye drops has been associated with systemic adverse reactions. In a case report[1] of 2 patients with latanoprost-associated hypertension the authors mentioned that other events including peripheral and facial oedema, dyspnoea, exacerbation of asthma, tachycardia, and chest pain or angina pectoris had been reported. Another case report[2] also referred to exacerbation of angina. Although a study[3] involving 24 stable asthmatics found that latanoprost eye drops had no effect on pulmonary function or asthma symptoms the UK manufacturer urges caution in patients with severe or brittle asthma.

1. Peak AS, Sutton BM. Systemic adverse effects associated with topically applied latanoprost. *Ann Pharmacother* 1998; **32:** 504–5.
2. Mitra M, *et al.* Exacerbation of angina associated with latanoprost. *BMJ* 2001; **323:** 783.
3. Hedner J, *et al.* Latanoprost and respiratory function in asthmatic patients: randomized, double-masked, placebo-controlled crossover evaluation. *Arch Ophthalmol* 1999; **117:** 1305–9.

### Uses and Administration

Latanoprost is a synthetic analogue of dinoprost (prostaglandin $F_{2\alpha}$) that is used topically to reduce intraocular pressure in patients with open-angle glaucoma and ocular hypertension (p.1485). One drop of a 0.005% ophthalmic solution is instilled once daily in the evening.

◊ References.

1. Patel SS, Spencer CM. Latanoprost: a review of its pharmacological properties, clinical efficacy and tolerability in the management of primary open-angle glaucoma and ocular hypertension. *Drugs Aging* 1996; **9:** 363–78.
2. Eisenberg DL, Camras CB. A preliminary risk-benefit assessment of latanoprost and unoprostone in open-angle glaucoma and ocular hypertension. *Drug Safety* 1999; **20:** 505–14.
3. Einarson TR, *et al.* Meta-analysis of the effect of latanoprost and brimonidine on intraocular pressure in the treatment of glaucoma. *Clin Ther* 2000; **22:** 1502–15.
4. Zhang WY, *et al.* Meta-analysis of randomised controlled trials comparing latanoprost with timolol in the treatment of patients with open angle glaucoma or ocular hypertension. *Br J Ophthalmol* 2001; **85:** 983–90.
5. Feldman RM. An evaluation of the fixed-combination of latanoprost and timolol for use in open-angle glaucoma and ocular hypertension. *Expert Opin Pharmacother* 2004; **5:** 909–21.

#### Preparations

**Proprietary Preparations** (details are given in Part 3)
***Arg.:*** Louten; Ocuprost; Xalatan; ***Austral.:*** Xalatan; ***Austria:*** Xalatan; ***Belg.:*** Xalatan; ***Braz.:*** Xalatan; ***Canad.:*** Xalatan; ***Chile:*** Latof; Louten; Xalatan; ***Denm.:*** Xalatan; ***Fin.:*** Xalatan; ***Fr.:*** Xalatan; ***Ger.:*** Xalatan; ***Gr.:*** Xalatan; ***Hong Kong:*** Xalatan; ***Irl.:*** Xalatan; ***Israel:*** Xalatan; ***Ital.:*** Xalatan; ***Malaysia:*** Xalatan; ***Mex.:*** Xalatan; ***Neth.:*** Xalatan; ***Norw.:*** Xalatan; ***NZ:*** Xalatan; ***Port.:*** Xalatan; ***S.Afr.:*** Xalatan; ***Singapore:*** Xalatan; ***Spain:*** Xalatan; ***Swed.:*** Xalatan; ***Switz.:*** Xalatan; ***Thai.:*** Xalatan; ***UK:*** Xalatan; ***USA:*** Xalatan.

**Multi-ingredient:** ***Austral.:*** Xalacom; ***Belg.:*** Xalacom; ***Chile:*** Latof-T; Xalacom; ***Denm.:*** Xalcom; ***Fin.:*** Xalcom; ***Fr.:*** Xalacom; ***Ger.:*** Xalacom; ***Irl.:*** Xalacom; ***Ital.:*** Xalacom; ***Neth.:*** Xalacom; ***Norw.:*** Xalcom; ***Port.:*** Xalacom; ***Singapore:*** Xalacom; ***Spain:*** Xalacom; ***Swed.:*** Xalcom; ***Switz.:*** Xalacom; ***UK:*** Xalacom.

## Limaprost *(rINN)*

ONO-1206; OP-1206. (E)-7-{(1R,2R,3R)-3-Hydroxy-2-[(E)-(3S,5S)-3-hydroxy-5-methyl-1-nonenyl]-5-oxocyclopentyl}-2-heptenoic acid.

$C_{22}H_{36}O_5$ = 380.5.

*CAS — 74397-12-9 (limaprost); 88852-12-4 (limaprost alfadex).*

### Profile

Limaprost is a synthetic analogue of alprostadil (prostaglandin $E_1$) used in the management of peripheral vascular disease (p.831). It is given by mouth as limaprost alfadex, in a dose equivalent to limaprost 15 to 30 micrograms daily in three divided doses.

◊ References.

1. Shono T, Ikeda K. Rapid effect of oral limaprost in Raynaud's disease in childhood. *Lancet* 1989; **i:** 908.
2. Murai C, *et al.* Oral limaprost for Raynaud's phenomenon. *Lancet* 1989; **ii:** 1218.
3. Aoki Y, *et al.* Possible participation of a prostaglandin E1 analogue in the aggravation of diabetic nephropathy. *Diabetes Res Clin Pract* 1992; **16:** 233–8.
4. Sato Y, *et al.* Effect of oral administration of prostaglandin E1 on erectile dysfunction. *Br J Urol* 1997; **80:** 772–5.

#### Preparations

**Proprietary Preparations** (details are given in Part 3)
***Jpn:*** Opalmon.

## Luprostiol *(BAN, rINN)*

(±)-(Z)-7-{(1S,2R,3R,5S)-2-[(2S)-3-(3-Chlorophenoxy)-2-hydroxypropylthio]-3,5-dihydroxycyclopentyl}hept-5-enoic acid.

$C_{21}H_{29}ClO_6S$ = 445.0.

*CAS — 67110-79-6.*

### Profile

Luprostiol is a synthetic analogue of dinoprost (prostaglandin $F_{2\alpha}$). It is used as a luteolytic in veterinary medicine.

## Meteneprost *(USAN, rINN)*

9-Deoxo-16,16-dimethyl-9-methylene-prostaglandin $E_2$; U-46785. (5Z,13E)-(8R,11R,12R,15R)-11,15-Dihydroxy-16,16-dimethyl-9-methyleneprosta-5,13-dienoic acid; (Z)-7-{(1R,2R,3R)-3-Hydroxy-2-[(E)-(3R)-3-hydroxy-4,4-dimethyloct-1-enyl]-5-methylenecyclopentyl}hept-5-enoic acid.

$C_{23}H_{38}O_4$ = 378.5.

*CAS — 61263-35-2.*

### Profile

Meteneprost is a synthetic derivative of dinoprostone (prostaglandin $E_2$). It is a uterine stimulant and has been studied for the termination of pregnancy.

◊ References.

1. Takkar D, *et al.* Early abortion by mifepristone (RU 486) followed by vaginal gel (meteneprost) versus oral (misoprostol) prostaglandin. *Adv Contracept* 1999; **15:** 163–73.
2. An ICMR Task Force Study. A multicentre randomized comparative clinical trial of 200 mg RU486 (mifepristone) single dose followed by either 5 mg 9-methylene $PGE_2$ gel (meteneprost) or 600 μg oral $PGE_1$ (misoprostol) for termination of early pregnancy within 28 days of missed menstrual period. *Contraception* 2000; **62:** 125–30.

## Misoprostol *(BAN, USAN, rINN)*

SC-29333. (±)-Methyl 7-{(1R,2R,3R)-3-hydroxy-2-[(E)-(4RS)-4-hydroxy-4-methyloct-1-enyl]-5-oxocyclopentyl}heptanoate; (±)-Methyl (13E)-11,16-dihydroxy-16-methyl-9-oxoprost-13-enoate.

$C_{22}H_{38}O_5$ = 382.5.

*CAS — 59122-46-2.*

*ATC — A02BB01.*

### Adverse Effects

The commonest adverse effect of misoprostol is diarrhoea. Other gastrointestinal effects include abdominal pain, dyspepsia, flatulence, and nausea and vomiting. Increased uterine contractility and abnormal vaginal bleeding (including menorrhagia and intermenstrual bleeding) have been reported. Other adverse effects include skin rashes, headache, and dizziness. Hypotension is rarely seen at doses recommended for peptic ulcer disease.

**Incidence of adverse effects.** A summary of data on misoprostol presented to the FDA.[1] During controlled studies the most common adverse effect was diarrhoea (8.2% compared with 3.1% for placebo); it was dose-related but usually mild, only 8 of 2003 subjects receiving misoprostol having withdrawn because of incapacitating diarrhoea. Headaches and abdominal discomfort were also reported. The effects of misoprostol on the uterus and the potential risks of uterine bleeding or abortion in pregnant women were of more concern. In nonpregnant women taking part in the controlled studies there were menstrual complaints in 15 of 410 (3.7%) receiving misoprostol compared with 2 of 115 (1.7%) given placebo. In a study in pregnant women who had elected to undergo first trimester abortion, all 6 who had a spontaneous expulsion of the uterine contents had received 1 or 2 doses of misoprostol 400 micrograms the previous evening, while none of those given placebo aborted spontaneously; overall 25 of the 56 women receiving misoprostol experienced uterine bleeding compared with only 2 of 55 on placebo.

For reference to uterine rupture in women receiving misoprostol see under Dinoprostone, p.1515.

1. Lewis JH. Summary of the 29th meeting of the Gastrointestinal Drugs Advisory Committee, Food and Drug Administration—June 10, 1985. *Am J Gastroenterol* 1985; **80:** 743–5.

**Effects on the fetus.** For reports of congenital malformations possibly associated with the misuse of misoprostol, see under Termination of Pregnancy in Uses and Administration, below.

### Precautions

Misoprostol should not be used to treat peptic ulcer disease in patients who are pregnant or who may become pregnant because it can cause uterine contraction. It should be used with caution in patients in whom hypotension might cause severe complications.

**Inflammatory bowel disease.** Life-threatening diarrhoea was reported in a patient with unrecognised Crohn's disease following six doses of misoprostol.[1]

1. Kornbluth A, *et al.* Life-threatening diarrhea after short-term misoprostol use in a patient with Crohn ileocolitis. *Ann Intern Med* 1990; **113:** 474–5.

### Pharmacokinetics

Misoprostol is reported to be rapidly absorbed and metabolised to its active form (misoprostol acid; SC-30695) after oral doses; peak plasma concentrations of misoprostol acid occur after about 15 to 30 minutes. Food reduces the rate but not the extent of absorption. Misoprostol acid is further metabolised by oxidation in a number of body organs and is excreted mainly in the urine. The plasma elimination half-life is reported to be between 20 and 40 minutes.

◊ References.

1. Schoenhard G, *et al.* Metabolism and pharmacokinetic studies of misoprostol. *Dig Dis Sci* 1985; **30** (suppl): 126S–128S.
2. Karim A, *et al.* Effects of food and antacid on oral absorption of misoprostol, a synthetic prostaglandin $E_1$ analog. *J Clin Pharmacol* 1989; **29:** 439–43.
3. Foote EF, *et al.* Disposition of misoprostol and its active metabolite in patients with normal and impaired renal function. *J Clin Pharmacol* 1995; **35:** 384–9.
4. Zieman M, *et al.* Absorption kinetics of misoprostol with oral or vaginal administration. *Obstet Gynecol* 1997; **90:** 88–92.
5. Khan RU, El-Refaey H. Pharmacokinetics and adverse-effect profile of rectally administered misoprostol in the third stage of labor. *Obstet Gynecol* 2003; **101:** 968–74.

### Uses and Administration

Misoprostol is a synthetic analogue of alprostadil (prostaglandin $E_1$).

It is used in the treatment of benign gastric and duodenal ulceration including that associated with NSAIDs. The usual dose by mouth is 800 micrograms daily in two to four divided doses with food.

Misoprostol is also used prophylactically with NSAIDs to prevent NSAID-induced ulcers. The usual dose is 200 micrograms two to four times daily. A dose of 100 micrograms four times daily may be used in patients not tolerating the higher dose. Some preparations of NSAIDs contain misoprostol in an attempt to limit their adverse effects on the gastrointestinal mucosa.

Misoprostol may be used for termination of pregnancy at up to 49 days of amenorrhoea, in a single dose of 400 micrograms by mouth given 36 to 48 hours after mifepristone. It has also been used for induction of labour and in the management of postpartum haemorrhage (see below).

◊ General reviews.


1. Walley TJ. Misoprostol. *Prescribers' J* 1993; **33:** 78–82.
2. Goldberg AB, *et al.* Misoprostol and pregnancy. *N Engl J Med* 2000; **344:** 38–47.


**Labour induction and augmentation.** Prostaglandins are well established for the induction of labour (p.1511) and misoprostol has been widely investigated for this indication. A systematic review[1] of studies of misoprostol given *vaginally* found that it increased cervical ripening and induced labour. It was more effective than vaginal or intracervical prostaglandins, reducing the need for oxytocin augmentation and improving the rate of vaginal delivery achieved within 24 hours. It was also found to be more effective than intravenous oxytocin. Most studies used misoprostol tablets in a dose of 50 micrograms vaginally every 4 hours, but reported doses have varied from 25 micrograms every 2 to 3 hours, to 100 micrograms every 6 to 12 hours. Low doses of misoprostol resulted in more use of oxytocin, but caused less uterine hyperstimulation. Although unlicensed, misoprostol is reported to be used outside clinical trials particularly in the USA, and the American College of Obstetricians and Gynecologists has recommended a dose of 25 micrograms intravaginally every 3 to 6 hours.[2] Misoprostol has also been given *orally* but this route is less well established. A wide range of doses have been reported but most studies have used 50 micrograms every 4 hours. Oral misoprostol appears to be less effective than vaginal, but it is not clear that it causes fewer adverse effects, and its use cannot be recommended based on this limited information.[2,3] The risk of uterine hyperstimulation may be increased with misoprostol by either route, particularly at higher doses, and it should not be used in women with scarred uteri from previous caesarean delivery or uterine surgery[2] (see also Effects on the Uterus, under Adverse Effects of Dinoprostone, p.1515). There has also been some limited investigation of misoprostol given *sublingually*.[4,5]

Misoprostol has also been tried for active management of the third stage of labour (see Postpartum Haemorrhage, below).


1. Hofmeyr GJ, Gülmezoglu AM. Vaginal misoprostol for cervical ripening and induction of labour. Available in The Cochrane Library; Issue 2. Chichester: John Wiley; 2004.
2. Wing DA. A benefit-risk assessment of misoprostol for cervical ripening and labour induction. *Drug Safety* 2002; **25:** 665–76.
3. Alfirevic Z. Oral misoprostol for induction of labour. Available in The Cochrane Library; Issue 2. Chichester: John Wiley; 2004.
4. Shetty A, *et al.* Sublingual misoprostol for the induction of labor at term. *Am J Obstet Gynecol* 2002; **186:** 72–6.
5. Shetty A, *et al.* Sublingual compared with oral misoprostol in term labour induction: a randomised controlled trial. *Br J Obstet Gynaecol* 2002; **109:** 645–50.


**Organ and tissue transplantation.** Misoprostol 200 micrograms four times daily improved renal function in ciclosporin-treated recipients of renal transplants.[1] The number of patients who had acute graft rejection was lower in the misoprostol group than in the placebo group. However, another study[2] did not indicate any difference in the incidence of rejection episodes or in renal function when misoprostol was added to immunosuppressant regimens for kidney transplantation, and misoprostol does not appear to have gained a role in the usual management of renal transplantation (p.1346).


1. Moran M, *et al.* Prevention of acute graft rejection by the prostaglandin $E_1$ analogue misoprostol in renal-transplant recipients treated with cyclosporine and prednisone. *N Engl J Med* 1990; **322:** 1183–8.
2. Pouteil-Noble C, *et al.* Misoprostol in renal transplant recipients: a prospective, randomized, controlled study on the prevention of acute rejection episodes and cyclosporin A nephrotoxicity. *Nephrol Dial Transplant* 1994; **9:** 552–5.


**Peptic ulcer disease.** Misoprostol is used in the prophylaxis and treatment of peptic ulceration (p.1246) in patients taking NSAIDs. There is good evidence that misoprostol can reduce the risk of gastric and duodenal ulcer formation in patients on long-term NSAID treatment,[1-4] and it appears more effective in this respect than histamine $H_2$-antagonists,[1] for which evidence of benefit against gastric injury is less persuasive. However, misoprostol's abdominal adverse effects, particularly diarrhoea and abdominal cramps, may limit its usefulness and patient acceptability. Omeprazole, which is equally effective in preventing NSAID-induced ulceration, is better tolerated.[3] Improved formulations, in which the active isomer of misoprostol is bound to a polymer, may reduce adverse effects.[5]


1. Koch M, *et al.* Prevention of nonsteroidal anti-inflammatory drug-induced gastrointestinal mucosal injury: a meta-analysis of randomized controlled clinical trials. *Arch Intern Med* 1996; **156:** 2321–32.
2. Champion GD, *et al.* NSAID-induced gastrointestinal damage: epidemiology, risk and prevention, with an evaluation of the role of misoprostol: an Asia-Pacific perspective and consensus. *Drugs* 1997; **53:** 6–19.
3. Hawkey CJ, *et al.* Omeprazole compared with misoprostol for ulcers associated with nonsteroidal antiinflammatory drugs. *N Engl J Med* 1998; **338:** 727–34.
4. Rostom A, *et al.* Prevention of NSAID-induced gastroduodenal ulcers. Available in The Cochrane Library; Issue 2. Chichester: John Wiley; 2004.
5. Chen D, *et al.* Stabilization and sustained-release effect of misoprostol with methacrylate copolymer. *Int J Pharmaceutics* 2000; **203:** 141–8.


**Postpartum haemorrhage.** Prostaglandins, usually given parenterally, have an accepted role in the management of established postpartum haemorrhage (p.1684) not controlled by oxytocin and ergot preparations, and there have been reports[1,2] of the successful use of rectal misoprostol to control postpartum haemorrhage.

Misoprostol has also been given immediately after delivery in the active management of third-stage labour. It has been argued that it may be particularly useful in preventing postpartum haemorrhage in developing countries where there is limited access to health-care facilities and parenteral oxytocics.[3,4] In a study[5] of more than 18 500 women, which compared oral misoprostol 600 micrograms with intramuscular or intravenous oxytocin, a higher proportion of women who received misoprostol had blood loss of at least 1000 mL and required additional oxytocics. Misoprostol was also associated with significantly more shivering and pyrexia. Systematic reviews[6,7] dominated by these results concluded that oral misoprostol was less effective than injectable oxytocics in reducing blood loss and the use of additional oxytocics. There was uncertainty as to whether misoprostol (oral or rectal) was more effective than placebo or no treatment and it was suggested that there was insufficient evidence to justify its prophylactic use even if other uterotonics were unavailable.[7]


1. O'Brien P, *et al.* Rectally administered misoprostol for the treatment of postpartum hemorrhage unresponsive to oxytocin and ergometrine: a descriptive study. *Obstet Gynecol* 1998; **92:** 212–4.
2. Lokugamage AU, *et al.* A randomized study comparing rectally administered misoprostol versus Syntometrine combined with an oxytocin infusion for the cessation of primary post partum hemorrhage. *Acta Obstet Gynecol Scand* 2001; **80:** 835–9.
3. Darney PD. Misoprostol: a boon to safe motherhood...or not? *Lancet* 2001; **358:** 682–3.
4. Shannon C, Winikoff B. Use of misoprostol in third stage of labour. *Lancet* 2002; **359:** 709.
5. Gülmezoglu AM, *et al.* WHO multicentre randomised trial of misoprostol in the management of the third stage of labour. *Lancet* 2001; **358:** 689–95.
6. Villar J, *et al.* Systematic review of randomized controlled trials of misoprostol to prevent postpartum hemorrhage. *Obstet Gynecol* 2002; **100:** 1301–12.
7. Gülmezoglu AM, *et al.* Prostaglandins for prevention of postpartum haemorrhage. Available in The Cochrane Library; Issue 2. Chichester: John Wiley; 2004.


**Termination of pregnancy.** Prostaglandins are widely used for the termination of pregnancy (p.1512) and misoprostol has been studied both for cervical preparation and for inducing uterine contractions.

Vaginal misoprostol is effective for cervical ripening before surgical termination in the first trimester.[1] Oral misoprostol given after oral mifepristone is effective in terminating early pregnancy of up to 63 days and especially so at up to 49 days.[2,3] Misoprostol can also be given vaginally.[4-6] Use of vaginal misoprostol with intramuscular[7-9] or oral[10-12] methotrexate has also been studied.

Misoprostol on its own is only a weak abortifacient and is often ineffective when used alone for the termination of pregnancy, although it has been widely misused for this purpose in some countries, notably Brazil.[13-15] Anecdotal reports[15-17] and one small controlled study[18] have associated such misuse during the first trimester of pregnancy with congenital malformations, particularly of the skull, though the manufacturers had found no evidence of teratogenicity in *animals*.[19]

Intravaginal misoprostol has been reported to be as effective as dinoprostone for termination of pregnancy during the second trimester.[20]


1. El-Refaey H, *et al.* Cervical priming with prostaglandin E1 analogues, misoprostol and gemeprost. *Lancet* 1994; **343:** 1207–9. Correction. *ibid.*; 1650.
2. Peyron R, *et al.* Early termination of pregnancy with mifepristone (RU 486) and the orally active prostaglandin misoprostol. *N Engl J Med* 1993; **328:** 1509–13.
3. Spitz IM, *et al.* Early pregnancy termination with mifepristone and misoprostol in the United States. *N Engl J Med* 1998; **338:** 1241–7.
4. El-Refaey H, *et al.* Induction of abortion with mifepristone (RU 486) and oral or vaginal misoprostol. *N Engl J Med* 1995; **332:** 983–7.
5. Ashok PW, *et al.* Termination of pregnancy at 9-13 weeks' amenorrhoea with mifepristone and misoprostol. *Lancet* 1998; **52:** 542–3.
6. Schaff EA, *et al.* Vaginal misoprostol administered 1, 2, or 3 days after mifepristone for early medical abortion: a randomized trial. *JAMA* 2000; **284:** 1948–53.
7. Creinin MD, Vittinghoff E. Methotrexate and misoprostol vs misoprostol alone for early abortion: a randomized controlled trial. *JAMA* 1994; **272:** 1190–5.
8. Hausknecht RU. Methotrexate and misoprostol to terminate early pregnancy. *N Engl J Med* 1995; **333:** 537–40.
9. Creinin MD, *et al.* A randomized trial comparing misoprostol three and seven days after methotrexate for early abortion. *Am J Obstet Gynecol* 1995; **173:** 1578–84.
10. Creinin MD. Oral methotrexate and vaginal misoprostol for early abortion. *Contraception* 1996; **54:** 15–18.
11. Creinin MD, *et al.* Medical abortion with oral methotrexate and vaginal misoprostol. *Obstet Gynecol* 1997; **90:** 611–16.
12. Carbonell JLL, *et al.* Oral methotrexate and vaginal misoprostol for early abortion. *Contraception* 1998; **57:** 83–8.
13. Costa SH, Vessey MP. Misoprostol and illegal abortion in Rio de Janeiro, Brazil. *Lancet* 1993; **341:** 1258–61.
14. Coêlho HLL, *et al.* Misoprostol and illegal abortion in Fortaleza, Brazil. *Lancet* 1993; **341:** 1261–3. Correction. *ibid.*; 1486.
15. Fonseca W, *et al.* Misoprostol and congenital malformations. *Lancet* 1991; **338:** 56.
16. Shepard TH. Möbius syndrome after misoprostol: a possible teratogenic mechanism. *Lancet* 1995; **346:** 780.
17. Gonzalez CH, *et al.* Congenital abnormalities in Brazilian children associated with misoprostol misuse in first trimester of pregnancy. *Lancet* 1998; **351:** 1624–7.
18. Pastuszak AL, *et al.* Use of misoprostol during pregnancy and Möbius' syndrome in infants. *N Engl J Med* 1998; **338:** 1881–5.
19. Downie WW. Misuse of misoprostol. *Lancet* 1991; **338:** 247.
20. Jain JK, Mishell DR. A comparison of intravaginal misoprostol with prostaglandin $E_2$ for termination of second-trimester pregnancy. *N Engl J Med* 1994; **331:** 290–3.


## Preparations

**Proprietary Preparations** (details are given in Part 3)

***Austral.:*** Cytotec; ***Austria:*** Cyprostol; ***Belg.:*** Cytotec; ***Braz.:*** Cytotec; ***Canad.:*** Cytotec; ***Chile:*** Misotrol; ***Denm.:*** Cytotec; ***Fin.:*** Cytotec; ***Fr.:*** Cytotec; ***Ger.:*** Cytotec; ***Gr.:*** Cytotec; ***Hong Kong:*** Cytotec; ***India:*** Cytolog; ***Irl.:*** Cytotec; ***Israel:*** Cytotec; ***Ital.:*** Cytotec; Misodex; ***Malaysia:*** Cytotec; ***Mex.:*** Cytotec; ***Neth.:*** Cytotec; ***Norw.:*** Cytotec; ***NZ:*** Cytotec; ***Port.:*** Cytotec; ***S.Afr.:*** Cytotec; ***Singapore:*** Cytotec†; ***Spain:*** Corrigast†; Cytotec; Glefos; Menpros†; ***Swed.:*** Cytotec; ***Switz.:*** Cytotec; ***Thai.:*** Cytotec; ***UK:*** Cytotec; ***USA:*** Cytotec.

*Used as an adjunct in:* ***Arg.:*** Oxaprost; ***Austral.:*** Arthrotec; ***Austria:*** Arthrotec; ***Belg.:*** Arthrotec; ***Canad.:*** Arthrotec; ***Denm.:*** Arthrotec; ***Fin.:*** Arthrotec; ***Fr.:*** Artotec; ***Ger.:*** Arthotec; ***Hong Kong:*** Arthrotec; ***Irl.:*** Arthrotec; ***Israel:*** Arthrotec; ***Ital.:*** Artrotec; Misofenac; ***Mex.:*** Artrenac Pro; Artrotec; ***Neth.:*** Arthrotec; ***Norw.:*** Arthrotec; ***Port.:*** Arthrotec; Diclotec; ***S.Afr.:*** Arthrotec; ***Singapore:*** Arthrotec†; ***Spain:*** Artrotec; Normulen; ***Swed.:*** Arthrotec; ***Switz.:*** Arthrotec; ***Thai.:*** Arthrotec; ***UK:*** Arthrotec; Condrotec†; Napratec; ***USA:*** Arthrotec.

## Nocloprost *(rINN)*

(Z)-7-[(1R,2R,3R,5R)-5-Chloro-3-hydroxy-2-[(E)-(3R)-3-hydroxy-4,4-dimethyl-1-octenyl]cyclopentyl]-5-heptenoic acid.

$C_{22}H_{37}ClO_4$ = 401.0.

*CAS — 79360-43-3.*

### Profile

Nocloprost is a synthetic analogue of dinoprostone (prostaglandin $E_2$) that has been investigated in the treatment of peptic ulcer disease.

◊ References.


1. Täuber U, *et al.* Pharmacokinetics of nocloprost in human volunteers and its relation to dose. *Eur J Clin Pharmacol* 1993; **44:** 497–500.
2. Konturek JW, *et al.* Epidermal growth factor in gastric ulcer healing by nocloprost, a stable prostaglandin E2 derivative. *Scand J Gastroenterol* 1997; **32:** 980–4.


## Ornoprostil *(rINN)*

Ornoprostilo; OU-1308. Methyl (−)-(1R,2R,3R)-3-hydroxy-2-[(E)-(3S,5S)-3-hydroxy-5-methyl-1-nonenyl]-ε,5-dioxocyclopentaneheptanoate.

$C_{23}H_{38}O_6$ = 410.5.

*CAS — 70667-26-4.*

### Profile

Ornoprostil is a synthetic prostaglandin analogue that has been used in the treatment of peptic ulcer disease.

## Sulprostone *(USAN, rINN)*

CP-34089; 16-Phenoxy-ω-17,18,19,20-tetranor-prostaglandin $E_2$-methylsulfonylamide; SHB-286; Sulprostona; ZK-57671. (Z)-7-{(1R,2R,3R)-3-Hydroxy-2-[(E)-(3R)-3-hydroxy-4-phenoxybut-1-enyl]-5-oxocyclopentyl}-N-(methylsulphonyl)hept-5-enamide.

$C_{23}H_{31}NO_7S$ = 465.6.

*CAS — 60325-46-4.*

*ATC — G02AD05.*

### Adverse Effects and Precautions

As for Dinoprostone, p.1515. Use of sulprostone is contra-indicated in smokers or those who have smoked in the last 2 years.

Once a prostaglandin has been given to terminate pregnancy it is essential that termination take place; if the prostaglandin is unsuccessful other measures should be used.

**Effects on the cardiovascular system.** A 31-year-old woman died from cardiovascular shock during an abortion induced by mifepristone followed by sulprostone. She had 12 children, one previous abortion, and was a heavy cigarette smoker.[1] Four other deaths with sulprostone had not been associated with abortion.


1. Anonymous. A death associated with mifepristone/sulprostone. *Lancet* 1991; **337:** 969–70.


**Effects on the nervous system.** For a report of convulsions in epileptic patients given sulprostone, see under Dinoprostone, p.1515.

**Effects on the uterus.** For reference to hyperstimulation and uterine rupture following use of prostaglandins, including sulprostone, for termination of pregnancy or induction of labour, see p.1515.

### Uses and Administration

Sulprostone is a synthetic derivative of dinoprostone (prostaglandin $E_2$). It is a uterine stimulant and is used for dilatation of the cervix before surgical termination of pregnancy in the first trimester and for the termination of pregnancy in the second trimester (p.1512). It is also used to control postpartum haemorrhage (p.1684). Sulprostone is given by intravenous infusion. A dose of 500 micrograms over 3 to 6 hours is used for cervical dilatation in the first trimester and a similar dose over about 2 hours is given for postpartum haemorrhage. For termination of pregnancy in the second trimester sulprostone is infused at a rate of 100 micrograms/hour for up to 10 hours; if necessary the infusion rate may be increased to up to 500 micrograms/hour, to a maximum total dose of 1.5 mg. If unsuccessful the course may be repeated once, 12 to 24 hours later. Sulprostone has also been given extra-amniotically and locally into the cervix. It has also been given by the intramuscular route, but this is no longer recommended.

### Preparations

**Proprietary Preparations** (details are given in Part 3)
***Austria:*** Nalador; ***Fin.:*** Nalador; ***Fr.:*** Nalador; ***Ger.:*** Nalador; ***Hong Kong:*** Nalador; ***Ital.:*** Nalador; ***Neth.:*** Nalador; ***Port.:*** Nalador; ***Singapore:*** Nalador†; ***Switz.:*** Nalador; ***Thai.:*** Nalador.

## Tiaprost Trometamol *(BANM, rINNM)*

Tiaprost trometamol. Trometamol salt of (±)-(*Z*)-7-{(1*R*,2*R*,3*R*,5*S*)-3,5-dihydroxy-2-[(*E*)-(3*RS*)-3-hydroxy-4-(3-thienyloxy)but-1-enyl]cyclopentyl}hept-5-enoic acid.

$C_{20}H_{28}O_6S,C_4H_{11}NO_3$ = 517.6.

*CAS — 71116-82-0 (tiaprost).*

### Profile

Tiaprost trometamol is a synthetic analogue of dinoprost (prostaglandin $F_{2\alpha}$). It is used as a luteolytic in veterinary medicine.

## Travoprost *(BAN, USAN, rINN)*

AL-6221. Isopropyl (*Z*)-7-((1*R*,2*R*,3*R*,5*S*)-3,5-dihydroxy-2-{(1*E*,3*R*)-3-hydroxy-4-[(α,α,α-trifluoro-*m*-tolyl)oxy]-1-butenyl}cyclopentyl)-5-heptenoate.

$C_{26}H_{35}F_3O_6$ = 500.5.

*CAS — 157283-68-6.*

*ATC — S01EE04.*

### Adverse Effects and Precautions

As for Latanoprost, p.1519.

### Uses and Administration

Travoprost is a synthetic analogue of dinoprost (prostaglandin $F_{2\alpha}$). It is used topically in the treatment of open-angle glaucoma and ocular hypertension (p.1485), as a 0.004% ophthalmic solution once daily in the evening.

### Preparations

**Proprietary Preparations** (details are given in Part 3)
***Arg.:*** Travatan; ***Austral.:*** Travatan; ***Braz.:*** Travatan; ***Chile:*** Travatan; ***Denm.:*** Travatan; ***Fr.:*** Travatan; ***Ger.:*** Travatan; ***Hong Kong:*** Travatan; ***Irl.:*** Travatan; ***Ital.:*** Travatan; ***Norw.:*** Travatan; ***Port.:*** Travatan; ***Singapore:*** Travatan; ***Spain:*** Travatan; ***Thai.:*** Travatan; ***UK:*** Travatan; ***USA:*** Travatan.

## Treprostinil *(USAN, rINN)*

LRX-15; Treprostinol; 15AU81; U-62840; UT-15. ({(1*R*,2*R*,3a*S*,9a*S*)-2,3,3a,4,9,9a-Hexahydro-2-hydroxy-1-[(3*S*)-3-hydroxyoctyl]-1*H*-benz[*f*]inden-5-yl}oxy)acetic acid.

$C_{23}H_{34}O_5$ = 390.5.

*CAS — 81846-19-7.*

## Treprostinil Sodium *(rINNM)*

$C_{23}H_{33}NaO_5$ = 412.5.

*CAS — 289480-64-4.*

### Profile

Treprostinil, a vasodilator and platelet aggregation inhibitor, is an analogue of the prostaglandin epoprostenol (prostacyclin). Treprostinil sodium is given by continuous subcutaneous infusion in the treatment of pulmonary hypertension (p.832); doses are calculated in terms of treprostinil. Treprostinil sodium 1.32 nanograms is approximately equivalent to 1.25 nanograms of treprostinil. The infusion is started with a dose equivalent to treprostinil 1.25 nanograms/kg per minute; if this is not tolerated the dose should be halved. The infusion rate can be increased according to patient response, by increments of up to 1.25 nanograms/kg per minute each week for the first 4 weeks, followed by increases of up to 2.5 nanograms/kg per minute each week. There is limited experience with doses above 40 nanograms/kg per minute. Treprostinil, given intravenously, has been investigated in the treatment of intermittent claudication.

Infusion site pain and reactions, including erythema, induration, and rash, are the most common adverse effects reported during subcutaneous infusion of treprostinil. Other effects include headache, nausea and vomiting, restlessness, and anxiety. Abrupt cessation of the infusion should be avoided, because symptoms of pulmonary hypertension may worsen.

◊ References.


1. Moller ER, *et al.* Trial of a novel prostacyclin analog, UT-15, in patients with severe intermittent claudication. *Vasc Med* 2000; **5:** 231–7.
2. Simonneau G, *et al.* Continuous subcutaneous infusion of treprostinil, a prostacyclin analogue, in patients with pulmonary arterial hypertension: a double-blind, randomized placebo-controlled trial. *Am J Respir Crit Care Med* 2002; **165:** 800–804.
3. Vachiéry J-L, *et al.* Transitioning from IV epoprostenol to subcutaneous treprostinil in pulmonary arterial hypertension. *Chest* 2002; **121:** 1561–5.
4. Wade M, *et al.* Pharmacokinetics of treprostinil sodium administered by 28-day chronic continuous subcutaneous infusion. *J Clin Pharmacol* 2004; **44:** 503–9.
5. Vachiéry JL, Naeije R. Treprostinil for pulmonary hypertension. *Expert Rev Cardiovasc Ther* 2004; **2:** 183–91.


### Preparations

**Proprietary Preparations** (details are given in Part 3)
***Israel:*** Remodulin; ***USA:*** Remodulin.

## Unoprostone Isopropyl *(rINNM)*

Isopropyl Lunoprostone; Isopropyl Unoprostone; UF-021; Unoprostona de isopropilo. Isopropyl (+)-(*Z*)-7-[(1*R*,2*R*,3*R*,5*S*)-3,5-Dihydroxy-2-(3-oxodecyl)cyclopentyl]-5-heptenoate.

$C_{25}H_{44}O_5$ = 424.6.

*CAS — 120373-36-6 (unoprostone); 120373-24-2 (unoprostone isopropyl).*

*ATC — S01EE02.*

### Adverse Effects and Precautions

As for Latanoprost, p.1519.

### Uses and Administration

Unoprostone is a synthetic analogue of dinoprost (prostaglandin $F_{2\alpha}$) that is used topically as the isopropyl ester for the treatment of glaucoma and ocular hypertension (p.1485). One drop of a solution containing unoprostone isopropyl 0.12 or 0.15% is instilled twice daily.

◊ References.


1. Yamamoto T, *et al.* Clinical evaluation of UF-021 (Rescula; isopropyl unoprostone). *Surv Ophthalmol* 1997; **41** (suppl 2): S99–S103.
2. Eisenberg DL, Camras CB. A preliminary risk-benefit assessment of latanoprost and unoprostone in open-angle glaucoma and ocular hypertension. *Drug Safety* 1999; **20:** 505–14.
3. de Arruda Mello PA, *et al.* Safety of unoprostone isopropyl as mono- or adjunctive therapy in patients with primary open-angle glaucoma or ocular hypertension. *Drug Safety* 2002; **25:** 583–97.
4. Chiba T, *et al.* Comparison of iridial pigmentation between latanoprost and isopropyl unoprostone: a long term prospective comparative study. *Br J Ophthalmol* 2003; **87:** 956–9.
5. Stewart WC, *et al.* The safety and efficacy of unoprostone 0.15% versus brimonidine 0.2%. *Acta Ophthalmol Scand* 2004; **82:** 161–5.


### Preparations

**Proprietary Preparations** (details are given in Part 3)
***Arg.:*** Rescula; ***Braz.:*** Rescula; ***Chile:*** Rescula; ***Jpn:*** Rescula; ***Mex.:*** Rescula; ***Singapore:*** Rescula; ***Switz.:*** Rescula; ***Thai.:*** Rescula; ***USA:*** Rescula.

# Radiopharmaceuticals

Radioactive compounds are used in medicine as sources of radiation for radiotherapy and for diagnostic purposes. They have numerous uses in research and industry.

Sealed radioactive sources are bonded or encapsulated to prevent the escape of the radioactive material and are used as supplied. Unsealed sources, on the other hand, are radioactive materials usually in liquid, particulate, or gaseous form that are removed from their containers for application. Radiopharmaceuticals come within this category.

The aim of this chapter is to provide background information on the radionuclides that are used as radiopharmaceuticals. Care is required in the preparation, handling, use, and disposal of these compounds; they are thus best dealt with by those with suitable experience and training.

## Atomic Structure

An atom is composed of a central positively charged nucleus around which negatively charged electrons revolve in orbits. The electrons are arranged round the atomic nucleus in a series of 'shells' in each of which is a limited number of orbits.

The nucleus consists of 2 main kinds of particles known as protons, each of unit positive charge, and neutrons, which are uncharged; the total number of these particles in the nucleus is known as the *mass number*.

Each electron carries a negative charge which is of the same size as the positive charge of the proton, so that in the neutral atom the number of electrons is equal to the number of protons in the nucleus.

The number of protons in the nucleus is known as the *atomic number*, and this determines the number of electrons in the extranuclear structure. All the atoms of a particular chemical element have the same atomic number, but while the number of protons is constant, the number of neutrons in the atoms, and thus their masses (mass numbers), may vary. These different forms of the same element are known as isotopes of the element and these isotopes differ in some of their physical properties.

Some isotopes may be stable, the differences between them arising solely from their difference in mass; others may be radioactive (*radioisotopes*), their nuclei changing spontaneously and emitting particles or electromagnetic waves, or both.

Most of the naturally occurring isotopes are stable, though there are a number which are unstable and therefore radioactive, for example, uranium-235. In addition, artificial radionuclides are prepared by converting stable nuclei into unstable forms and even naturally occurring radionuclides may be prepared by artificial means.

The symbol used for a nuclide is a development of the chemical symbol for the atom, with the mass number as a superscript and the atomic number as a subscript; thus the symbols for the 3 hydrogen isotopes—common hydrogen, deuterium, and tritium—are ${}^{1}_{1}H$, ${}^{2}_{1}H$, and ${}^{3}_{1}H$, and the symbols for the 3 naturally occurring uranium isotopes are ${}^{234}_{92}U$, ${}^{235}_{92}U$, and ${}^{238}_{92}U$; as the atomic number can be inferred from the chemical symbol it is the usual practice to omit the subscript. It is also common practice to write out the full name of the element followed by the mass number, e.g. chromium-51 for ${}^{51}Cr$.

## Emissions from Radioisotopes

The 3 main types of emission from radioactive substances are *alpha particles, beta particles,* and *gamma-rays.* Most sources emit more than one type of radiation.

*Alpha particles* are positively charged particles (helium nuclei), each consisting of 2 protons and 2 neutrons.

*Beta particles* ($\beta^-$ or $\beta^+$) are identical to electrons or positrons but arise from the nucleus. They are emitted with great velocity and their energies are spread over a spectrum. Positrons are similar to electrons, having a similar mass but a positive charge.

*Gamma-rays* are electromagnetic radiations or *photons* with wavelengths much shorter than those of light.

In certain cases, e.g. chromium-51, *electron capture* (EC) occurs, an electron from an inner shell being absorbed by the nucleus with the production of an *X-ray* characteristic of the daughter atom or emission of an *Auger electron*.

The type of emission from a radionuclide largely determines its usefulness in medicine. Those emitting alpha particles are very little used partly because detection and measurement are difficult. Positron-emitters, such as carbon-11, fluorine-18, nitrogen-13, and oxygen-15, have become more popular in recent years and are used in positron-emission tomography (PET) where the radiation is measured from within the body, as opposed to computed tomography (CT) where the energy is supplied from an external source. Single photon emission tomography (SPECT) is another technique like positron-emission tomography that provides views of slices through the body and this technique employs gamma-ray emitting radionuclides which are the most accessible and the most common radiation source in radiopharmaceuticals.

## Decay of Radionuclides

A radionuclide will consist of atoms in several forms, including: unstable atoms, which will at some time undergo an energy change with the emission of ionising radiation; those which are actually undergoing this change; and those which have undergone the change. In quantitative terms this transition occurs at a rate that is characteristic of the radionuclide and it is expressed as its half-life—the time required for the activity to fall by one-half. Many radionuclides have complex decay characteristics with several possible energies of emitted particles and radiation. Some radionuclides may be in an excited or metastable state denoted by the suffix m attached to the mass number (e.g. technetium-99m) and undergo *isomeric transition* (IT) with the release of gamma-rays.

The activity of radionuclides is measured in terms of the rate of transformation or disintegration. The unit is the becquerel (Bq) = 1 transformation/second; the curie (Ci) was formerly used as the unit of activity; $1\ Ci = 3.7 \times 10^{10}$ Bq.

## Supply, Preparation, and Control

A wide range of radionuclides and specially formulated radiopharmaceuticals is available from specialised manufacturers. However, there are national controls on the use, transport, storage, and disposal of such compounds. Authority and guidance should be sought from the relevant bodies and authorities before using such compounds.

Generators are special features in the supply of radionuclides. They are receptacles containing a parent and daughter nuclide in equilibrium and from which the daughter nuclide, which usually has a short half-life, may be eluted. Generators are available for the production of indium-113m, krypton-81m, and technetium-99m. Generators are also available for some positron-emitters.

Storage conditions for radiopharmaceuticals should be such as to prevent the inadvertent emission of radioactivity as well as to meet the storage requirements for the pharmaceutical that has been labelled. Thus due account still has to be paid, for instance, to the effects of temperature and light. Radiopharmaceuticals are liable to decomposition by self-irradiation effects which may cause degradation of solvent, preservative, or other compounds. There can also be a continuous formation of oxidising and reducing chemical species arising from the effect of the radioactivity on any chemical substances present in the radiopharmaceutical, even in minute amounts.

## Adverse Effects

The internal irradiation of tissues following the administration of radionuclides carries similar dangers to exposure to ionising radiation from an external source, and local high irradiation doses may arise if these nuclides are specifically localised in a tissue. The most serious danger is genetic damage prior to and during the reproductive period. Tissues whose cells are in a continuous state of multiplication are particularly sensitive to the effects of radiation.

Untoward effects of exposure to the larger doses of irradiation include leucopenia, anaemia, inflammation of the skin, radiation sickness, and neoplasms.

In considering the effect of a given radionuclide it is usual to calculate the dose to the organ most critically affected, and also the dose to the whole body.

In considering the adverse effects of radiopharmaceuticals one should not forget the effects that might arise from the carrier or from contaminants.

## General Uses

Radiopharmaceuticals are used widely in many branches of medicine and surgery, mainly for the diagnosis and sometimes for the treatment of disease. They can provide information not available using other diagnostic techniques such as contrast media, ultrasound, and computed tomography or other external irradiation. Interesting developments have followed the tagging of monoclonal antibodies with radionuclides.

Many investigations involve the oral or parenteral administration of radionuclides or labelled compounds followed usually by an imaging procedure. Some investigations involve the measurement of radioactive concentrations in organs, tissues, blood, urine, or faeces. The quantities used are always the smallest that will give the desired accuracy of image or of measurement.

◊ Reviews.


1. Schwaiger M, Melin J. Cardiological applications of nuclear medicine. *Lancet* 1999; **354:** 661–6.
2. Corstens FHM, van der Meer JWM. Nuclear medicine's role in infection and inflammation. *Lancet* 1999; **354:** 765–70.
3. Eary JF. Nuclear medicine in cancer diagnosis. *Lancet* 1999; **354:** 853–7.
4. Chatal J-F, Hoefnagel CA. Radionuclide therapy. *Lancet* 1999; **354:** 931–5.
5. Krag D, Moffat F. Nuclear medicine and the surgeon. *Lancet* 1999; **354:** 1019–22.
6. Costa DC, *et al.* Nuclear medicine in neurology and psychiatry. *Lancet* 1999; **354:** 1107–1111.


## Radiological Terms

- Alpha particles–nuclei of helium atoms emitted by radioactive atomic nuclei
- annihilation–the interaction and disappearance of a positive and a negative electron with the conversion of their energy into electromagnetic radiation
- atomic number (Z)–the number of protons in the atomic nucleus
- Auger effect–the emission of an electron from an atom due to the filling of a vacancy in an inner electron shell
- becquerel (Bq)–the SI unit of activity, defined as 1 transformation/second. The curie was formerly used as the unit of activity. $1\ Bq = 2.7 \times 10^{-11}$ Ci
- beta particles–electrons or positrons emitted by radioactive atomic nuclei
- carrier-free–a preparation in which substantially all the atoms of the activated element present are radioactive. Material of high specific activity is often loosely referred to as 'carrier-free'
- curie (Ci)–now superseded as a unit of activity by the becquerel. A curie (Ci) represented $3.7 \times 10^{10}$ transformations/second. $1\ Ci = 3.7 \times 10^{10}$ Bq
- daughter–of a given nuclide, any nuclide that originates from it by radioactive decay
- electron capture (EC)–a mode of radioactivity decay involving the capture of an orbital electron by its nucleus

- gamma-radiation–electromagnetic radiation emitted in the process of a change in configuration of a nucleus or particle annihilation and having wavelengths shorter than those of X-rays
- gray (Gy)–the SI unit of absorbed dose, defined as 1 J/kg. The rad was formerly used as the unit of absorbed dose. 1 Gy = 100 rads
- isomeric transition (IT)–the decay of one isomer to another having a lower energy state. The transition is accompanied by the emission of gamma-radiation
- isomers–nuclides with the same mass number and atomic number but with nuclei having different energy states
- isotopes–nuclides with the same atomic number but different mass numbers
- nuclide–a species of atom having a specific mass number, atomic number, and nuclear energy state
- photon–a quantum of electromagnetic radiation
- positron–a positive beta particle
- rad (radiation absorbed dose)–now superseded as a unit of absorbed dose by the gray. A rad is equal to $10^{-2}$ J/kg. The röntgen and the rad in soft tissue are approximately equivalent in magnitude for moderate energies. 1 rad = $10^{-2}$ Gy
- radioactive decay–the spontaneous change of a nucleus resulting in the emission of a particle or a photon
- radioactivity–the property of certain nuclides of spontaneously emitting particles or photons or of undergoing spontaneous fission
- radioisotope–an isotope that is radioactive
- radionuclide–a nuclide that is radioactive
- rem (röntgen-equivalent-man)–now superseded as a unit of dose equivalent by the sievert (Sv). A rem is numerically equal to the absorbed dose in rads multiplied by the appropriate quality factor defining the biological effect and by any other modifying factors. The sievert is the joule/kg (J $kg^{-1}$) equal to 100 rem
- röntgen (R)–a unit of exposure of X- or gamma-radiation, equal to $2.58 \times 10^{-4}$ coulombs/kg in air; superseded by the SI unit of exposure, the coulomb/kg (C $kg^{-1}$). 1 C $kg^{-1}$ = $3.876 \times 10^3$ R
- sievert (Sv)–the SI unit of dose equivalent numerically equal to the absorbed dose in grays multiplied by the appropriate quality factor defining the biological effect and by any other modifying factors expressed in J/kg
- specific activity–the activity per unit mass of a material containing a radioactive substance
- X-rays–electromagnetic radiation other than annihilation radiation originating in the extranuclear part of the atom and having wavelengths much shorter than those of visible light

## Carbon-11

Carbono 11.

*CAS — 14333-33-6.*

**Half-life.** 20.4 minutes.

### Profile

Carbon-11 is a positron-emitter that is used in positron-emission tomography (see Emissions from Radioisotopes, p.1522). Compounds that have been labelled with carbon-11 include L-methionine for the detection of malignant neoplasms, acetic and palmitic acids for the study of myocardial metabolism, raclopride and mespiperone for the study of CNS dopaminergic $D_2$ receptors, and flumazenil for the study of GABA receptors. Labelled carbon monoxide may be used to assess blood volume.

### Preparations

***Ph. Eur.:*** L-Methionine (($^{11}$C)Methyl) Injection; Flumazenil (*N*-($^{11}$C)Methyl) Injection; Raclopride (($^{11}$C)Methoxy) Injection; Sodium Acetate ((1-$^{11}$C)) Injection;
***USP 27:*** Carbon Monoxide C 11; Flumazenil C 11 Injection; Mespiperone C 11 Injection; Methionine C 11 Injection; Raclopride C 11 Injection; Sodium Acetate C 11 Injection.

## Carbon-14

Carbono 14.

*CAS — 14762-75-5.*

**Half-life.** 5730 years.

### Profile

Carbon-14 has been used to label many organic compounds that may be employed in breath tests.

Urea (p.1162) labelled with carbon-14 is used in a breath test to detect *Helicobacter pylori* as an aid in the diagnosis of peptic ulcer disease (p.1246).

### Preparations

***USP 27:*** Urea C 14 Capsules.

**Proprietary Preparations** (details are given in Part 3)
***USA:*** Pytest.

## Chromium-51

Cromo 51.

*CAS — 14392-02-0.*
*ATC — V09CX04 (chromium edetate ($^{51}$Cr)).*

**Half-life.** 27.7 days.

### Profile

Chromium-51, as sodium chromate ($^{51}$Cr), is used to label red blood cells so that red cell survival and red cell volume can be measured. Chromium-51 activity in the faeces can be used to estimate gastrointestinal blood losses. Red blood cells labelled with chromium-51 and damaged by heat before re-injection have been used for spleen scanning.

As chromium edetate ($^{51}$Cr) given intravenously, chromium-51 is used in the determination of the glomerular filtration rate.

As chromic chloride ($^{51}$Cr), chromium-51 has been given intravenously for the determination of loss of serum protein into the gastrointestinal tract.

### Preparations

***Ph. Eur.:*** Chromium($^{51}$Cr) Edetate Injection; Sodium Chromate($^{51}$Cr) Sterile Solution;
***USP 27:*** Chromium Cr 51 Edetate Injection; Sodium Chromate Cr 51 Injection.

## Cobalt-57

Cobalto 57.

*CAS — 13981-50-5.*
*ATC — V09XX01 (cobalt cyanocobalamin ($^{57}$Co)).*

**Half-life.** 271 days.

### Profile

Cobalt-57, in the form of an aqueous solution or capsules of cyanocobalamin ($^{57}$Co), is given by mouth for the measurement of absorption of vitamin $B_{12}$ in the diagnosis of pernicious anaemia and other malabsorption syndromes. It is also used with cyanocobalamin ($^{58}$Co), see below.

### Preparations

***Ph. Eur.:*** Cyanocobalamin($^{57}$Co) Capsules; Cyanocobalamin($^{57}$Co) Solution;
***USP 27:*** Cyanocobalamin Co 57 Capsules; Cyanocobalamin Co 57 Oral Solution.

**Proprietary Preparations** (details are given in Part 3)
**Multi-ingredient:** ***UK:*** Dicopac.

## Cobalt-58

Cobalto 58.

*CAS — 13981-38-9.*
*ATC — V09XX02 (cobalt cyanocobalamin ($^{58}$Co)).*

**Half-life.** 70.8 days.

### Profile

Cobalt-58, in the form of an aqueous solution or capsules of cyanocobalamin ($^{58}$Co), is given by mouth for the measurement of absorption of vitamin $B_{12}$ in the diagnosis of pernicious anaemia and other malabsorption syndromes.

The different energies of cobalt-57 and cobalt-58 facilitate separation of the isotopes in a mixture. Advantage is taken of this to differentiate between failure of absorption due to lack of intrinsic factor (pernicious anaemia) and that due to ileal malabsorption by the simultaneous administration of free cyanocobalamin ($^{58}$Co) and cyanocobalamin ($^{57}$Co) bound to intrinsic factor. A dual isotope kit has been used for this purpose.

### Preparations

***Ph. Eur.:*** Cyanocobalamin($^{58}$Co) Capsules; Cyanocobalamin($^{58}$Co) Solution;
***USP 27:*** Cyanocobalamin Co 58 Capsules.

**Proprietary Preparations** (details are given in Part 3)
**Multi-ingredient:** ***UK:*** Dicopac.

## Erbium-169

*CAS — 15840-13-8.*
*ATC — V10AX04 (erbium citrate colloid ($^{169}$Er)).*

### Profile

Erbium-169 is a radionuclide that has been used in the treatment of arthritic conditions particularly of the small joints.

## Fluorine-18

Flúor 18.

*CAS — 13981-56-1.*
*ATC — V09AX02 (fludeoxyglucose ($^{18}$F)).*

**Half-life.** 110 minutes.

### Profile

Fluorine-18 is a positron-emitting radionuclide that is used in positron-emission tomography (see Emissions from Radioisotopes, p.1522).

Fludeoxyglucose ($^{18}$F) (2-deoxy-2-fluoro-$^{18}$F-α-D-glucopyranose; $^{18}$F-fluorodeoxyglucose) is given by intravenous injection for the assessment of cerebral and myocardial glucose metabolism in various physiological or pathological states including stroke and myocardial ischaemia. It is also used for the detection of malignant tumours including those of the brain, liver, lung, and thyroid gland. Fluorodopa ($^{18}$F) is also used in cerebral imaging. Sodium fluoride ($^{18}$F) is used in bone scanning.

### Preparations

***Ph. Eur.:*** Fludeoxyglucose ($^{18}$F) Injection; Sodium Fluoride ($^{18}$F) Injection;
***USP 27:*** Fludeoxyglucose F 18 Injection; Fluorodopa F 18 Injection; Sodium Fluoride F 18 Injection.

**Proprietary Preparations** (details are given in Part 3)
***Austria:*** 18F-FDG.

## Gallium-67

Galio 67.

*CAS — 14119-09-6.*
*ATC — V09HX01 (gallium citrate ($^{67}$Ga)).*

**Half-life.** 3.26 days.

### Profile

Gallium-67 is used in the form of an intravenous injection of gallium citrate ($^{67}$Ga).

Gallium citrate ($^{67}$Ga) is concentrated in some malignant tumours of the lymphatic system, as well as in some other tissues, and is used for tumour visualisation. Concentration also occurs in inflammatory lesions and the injection is therefore used for the localisation of focal inflammatory sites, such as may occur in abscesses, osteomyelitis, or sarcoidosis. Gallium scans have proved useful for the detection of the various infections and malignancies that may be encountered in patients with AIDS.

**Breast feeding.** The American Academy of Pediatrics has stated[1] that temporary cessation of breast feeding is required following exposure to gallium-67 since radioactivity has been reported to be present in breast milk for 2 weeks.

1. American Academy of Pediatrics. The transfer of drugs and other chemicals into human milk. *Pediatrics* 2001; **108:** 776–89. Correction. *ibid.*; 1029. Also available at: http://aappolicy.aappublications.org/cgi/content/full/pediatrics%3b108/3/776 (accessed 01/07/04)

### Preparations

***Ph. Eur.:*** Gallium($^{67}$Ga) Citrate Injection;
***USP 27:*** Gallium Citrate Ga 67 Injection.

## Gold-198

Oro 198.

*CAS — 10043-49-9.*
*ATC — V10AX06 (colloidal gold ($^{198}$Au)).*

**Half-life.** 65 hours (2.7 days).

### Profile

Gold-198, as colloidal gold ($^{198}$Au) with most of the activity associated with particles of diameter 5 to 20 nm, has been used by intrapleural or intraperitoneal injection in the treatment of malignant ascites and malignant pleural effusion, and by intravenous injection for the measurement of liver blood flow, in liver scanning, and for general investigations of the reticuloendothelial system. Since the gamma-ray energies are not particularly good for scanning and the radiation dose to the patient is relatively high, it has generally been superseded by more suitable agents such as technetium-99m-labelled compounds.

## Indium-111

Indio 111.

*CAS — 15750-15-9.*
*ATC — V09AX01 (indium pentetate ($^{111}$In)); V09GX02 (indium imciromab ($^{111}$In)); V09HB01 (indium oxinate labelled cells ($^{111}$In)); V09HB02 (indium tropolonate labelled cells ($^{111}$In)); V09IB01 (indium pentetreotide ($^{111}$In)); V09IB02 (indium satumomab pendetide ($^{111}$In)); V09IB03 (indium antiovariumcarcinoma antibody ($^{111}$In)); V09IB04 (indium capromab pendetide ($^{111}$In)).*

**Half-life.** 67 hours (2.8 days).

### Profile

Indium-111 as indium ($^{111}$In) complexed with pentetic acid (pentetate) is used diagnostically in CSF studies.

Leucocytes labelled with indium ($^{111}$In) hydroxyquinoline are used for the location of inflammatory lesions; applications have been the detection or localisation of abscesses, infections (including those occurring in patients with AIDS), inflammatory bowel diseases such as Crohn's disease or ulcerative colitis, and transplant rejection. Platelets have been similarly labelled and used for the detection of thrombi and for the investigation of thrombocytopenia. Labelled erythrocytes have been used to investigate gastrointestinal haemorrhage.

Colloids have been prepared using indium chloride ($^{111}$In) and have been used for investigation of the lymphatic system. Indium ($^{111}$In) bleomycin has been given by intravenous injection for the detection of tumours. Indium ($^{111}$In) pentetreotide is used for the detection and localisation of tumours originating from neuroendocrine cells.

Several different monoclonal antibodies, such as altumomab pentetate, capromab pendetide, ibritumomab tiuxetan, imciromab pentetate, and satumomab pendetide, have been labelled with indium-111. Uses include the detection, diagnosis, and evaluation of malignant neoplasms of the colon, rectum, prostate, and ovaries as well as the detection and localisation of myocardial infarction.

**Breast feeding.** The American Academy of Pediatrics has stated[1] that temporary cessation of breast feeding is required following exposure to indium-111 since a very small amount of radioactivity has been reported to be present in breast milk for 20 hours.

1. American Academy of Pediatrics. The transfer of drugs and other chemicals into human milk. *Pediatrics* 2001; **108:** 776–89. Correction. *ibid.*; 1029. Also available at: http://aappolicy.aappublications.org/cgi/content/full/pediatrics%3b108/3/776 (accessed 01/07/04)

### Preparations

***Ph. Eur.:*** Indium($^{111}$In) Chloride Solution; Indium($^{111}$In) Oxine Solution; Indium($^{111}$In) Pentetate Injection;
***USP 27:*** Indium In 111 Capromab Pentetide Injection; Indium In 111 Chloride Solution; Indium In 111 Ibritumomab Tiuxetan Injection; Indium In 111 Oxyquinoline Solution; Indium In 111 Pentetate Injection; Indium In 111 Pentetreotide Injection; Indium In 111 Satumomab Pendetide Injection.

**Proprietary Preparations** (details are given in Part 3)
***Austria:*** Octreoscan; ***Braz.:*** OncoScint†; ***Israel:*** Prostascint Kit; ***Ital.:*** Myoscint†; Octreoscan; OncoScint CR 103†; ***Spain:*** OncoScint CR 103; ***USA:*** Octreoscan; OncoScint CR/OV.

## Indium-113m

Indio 113m.
*CAS — 14885-78-0 (indium-113).*

**Half-life.** 99.5 minutes.

### Profile

Indium-113m is a daughter of tin-113 ($^{113}$Sn, half-life 115 days) and because of its short half-life is normally prepared just before use by elution from a sterile generator consisting of tin-113 adsorbed on an ion-exchange material contained in a column.

Indium-113m may be used for labelling a variety of materials with differing physical properties including particles and colloids suited to scanning procedures for various organs and tissues. Chelates with pentetic acid have also been used. The short half-life of indium-113m and its lack of beta-emission have allowed large doses to be given with a small radiation dose to the patient. High count rates for scanning are therefore achieved.

## Iodine-123

Iodo 123.
*CAS — 15715-08-9.*
*ATC — V09AB01 (iodine iofetamine ($^{123}$I)); V09AB02 (iodine iolopride ($^{123}$I)); V09AB03 (iodine ioflupane ($^{123}$I)); V09IX01 (iobenguane ($^{123}$I)); V09CX01 (sodium iodohippurate ($^{123}$I)); V09FX02 (sodium iodide ($^{123}$I)).*

**Half-life.** 13.2 hours.

### Profile

Iodine-123 has similar adverse effects and precautions to those of iodine-131 (see below).

Its principal use is in thyroid uptake tests and thyroid imaging when it is given by mouth or intravenous injection as sodium iodide ($^{123}$I).

Sodium iodohippurate ($^{123}$I) is given intravenously in tests of renal function and in renal imaging.

Iobenguane ($^{123}$I) (*m*-iodobenzylguanidine ($^{123}$I)) is given intravenously for the localisation of certain tumours, for example phaeochromocytomas, and for the evaluation of neuroblastoma. It is also used for functional studies of the adrenal medulla and myocardium.

Ioflupane ($^{123}$I) is given intravenously to detect loss of functioning dopaminergic neurones in the differential diagnosis of tremor and parkinsonism.

Various monoclonal antibodies have been labelled with iodine-123; potential applications include the detection of malignant neoplasms.

**Breast feeding.** The American Academy of Pediatrics has stated[1] that temporary cessation of breast feeding is required following exposure to iodine-123 since radioactivity has been reported to be present in breast milk for up to 36 hours.

1. American Academy of Pediatrics. The transfer of drugs and other chemicals into human milk. *Pediatrics* 2001; **108:** 776–89. Correction. *ibid.*; 1029. Also available at: http://aappolicy.aappublications.org/cgi/content/full/pediatrics%3b108/3/776 (accessed 01/07/04)

### Preparations

***Ph. Eur.:*** Sodium Iodide($^{123}$I) Injection; Sodium Iodohippurate($^{123}$I) Injection;
***USP 27:*** Iobenguane I 123 Injection; Iodohippurate Sodium I 123 Injection; Sodium Iodide I 123 Capsules; Sodium Iodide I 123 Solution.

**Proprietary Preparations** (details are given in Part 3)
***Ital.:*** DaTSCAN; ***UK:*** DaTSCAN.

## Iodine-125

Iodo 125.
*CAS — 14158-31-7.*
*ATC — V09CX03 (sodium iotalamate ($^{125}$I)); V09GB01 (fibrinogen ($^{125}$I)); V09GB02 (iodinated human albumin ($^{125}$I)); V09IX03 (iodine CC49 monoclonal antibody ($^{125}$I)).*

**Half-life.** 60.1 days.

### Profile

Iodine-125 has similar adverse effects and precautions to those of iodine-131 (see below).

Iodine-125 is not very suitable for the external counting of radioactivity in the thyroid gland because its gamma-energy is weak and tissue absorption is high. However, it is very suitable for radio-immunoassays *in vitro* and because it has a long half-life it is preferred as a label for many compounds to detect and estimate drugs and hormones in body fluids.

Iodine-125 has been used orally as sodium iodide ($^{125}$I) in the diagnosis of thyroid disorders.

Sodium iotalamate ($^{125}$I) has been used intravenously in the determination of glomerular filtration rate and sodium iodohippurate ($^{125}$I) intravenously for the measurement of effective renal plasma flow.

Iodine-125, as iodinated ($^{125}$I) human fibrinogen, has been used intravenously to demonstrate and locate deep-vein thrombosis of the leg. Iodinated ($^{125}$I) fibrinogen has also been used in the measurement of fibrinogen metabolism in certain disturbances of blood coagulation.

Human albumin iodinated with iodine-125 has been used for the determination of blood or plasma volume.

Iodine-125 implants have been used for the local treatment of cancers. Titanium capsules containing iodine-125 adsorbed onto a silver rod have been used in the treatment of cancers of the head and neck, lung, pancreas, and prostate. Brain tumours have been treated with titanium capsules containing iodine-125 adsorbed onto anion exchange resin spheres.

**Breast feeding.** The American Academy of Pediatrics has stated[1] that temporary cessation of breast feeding is required following exposure to iodine-125 since radioactivity has been reported to be present in breast milk for 12 days.

1. American Academy of Pediatrics. The transfer of drugs and other chemicals into human milk. *Pediatrics* 2001; **108:** 776–89. Correction. *ibid.*; 1029. Also available at: http://aappolicy.aappublications.org/cgi/content/full/pediatrics%3b108/3/776 (accessed 01/07/04)

### Preparations

***Ph. Eur.:*** Human Albumin Injection, Iodinated ($^{125}$I);
***USP 27:*** Iodinated I 125 Albumin Injection; Iothalamate Sodium I 125 Injection.

**Proprietary Preparations** (details are given in Part 3)
***Austral.:*** OncoSeeds; Rapid Strand; ***USA:*** Glofil.

## Iodine-131

Iodo 131.
*CAS — 10043-66-0.*
*ATC — V09IX02 (iobenguane ($^{131}$I)); V09CX02 (sodium iodohippurate ($^{131}$I)); V09FX03 (sodium iodide ($^{131}$I)); V10XA02 (iobenguane ($^{131}$I)); V10XA01 (sodium iodide ($^{131}$I)); V09XA03 (iodinated human albumin ($^{131}$I)); V09XA01 (iodine norcholesterol ($^{131}$I)); V09XA02 (iodocholesterol ($^{131}$I)); V10XA53 (iodine tositumomab ($^{131}$I)).*

**Half-life.** 8.04 days.

### Adverse Effects

A percentage of patients treated with iodine-131 for hyperthyroidism become hypothyroid each year, depending on the dose given, and eventually most patients will require thyroid replacement therapy. Hypoparathyroidism has also been reported. Radiation thyroiditis with soreness may develop shortly after treatment. There may be severe and potentially dangerous swelling of the thyroid especially in patients with large goitres and this has on rare occasions produced asphyxiation. Leukaemia and carcinoma of the thyroid have occasionally been reported, particularly in young patients. Retrospective studies have shown an increased incidence of thyroid cancer in adults after iodine-131 treatment for hyperthyroidism. However, the absolute risk of thyroid cancer is small and the underlying thyroid disease may play a role.

In the treatment of thyroid carcinoma, the larger doses of radioactive iodine sometimes cause nausea and vomiting a few days after ingestion, which may be due to gastritis as iodine-131 is also concentrated in gastric mucosa. Large doses depress the bone marrow.

◊ References.


1. Ron E, *et al.* Cancer mortality following treatment for adult hyperthyroidism. *JAMA* 1998; **280:** 347–55.
2. Franklyn JA, *et al.* Cancer incidence and mortality after radioiodine treatment for hyperthyroidism: a population-based cohort study. *Lancet* 1999; **353:** 2111–15.
3. Rivkees SA, Cornelius EA. Influence of iodine-131 dose on the outcome of hyperthyroidism in children. *Pediatrics* 2003; **111:** 745–9.


### Precautions

The use of sodium iodide ($^{131}$I) is contra-indicated, even in diagnostic doses, during pregnancy. Sodium iodide ($^{131}$I) should not be given to patients with large toxic nodular goitres or to patients with severe thyrotoxic heart disease. There is some controversy as to whether radio-iodine therapy exacerbates Graves' ophthalmopathy (see Hyperthyroidism, p.1594).

Many drugs have been reported to interfere with thyroid- or other organ-function studies and checks should be made on any treatment the patient might be receiving before any estimations are carried out.

**Breast feeding.** The American Academy of Pediatrics has stated[1] that temporary cessation of breast feeding is required following exposure to iodine-131 since radioactivity has been reported to be present in breast milk for 2 to 14 days; high doses used for the treatment of thyroid cancer may prolong exposure to the infant.

1. American Academy of Pediatrics. The transfer of drugs and other chemicals into human milk. *Pediatrics* 2001; **108:** 776–89. Correction. *ibid.*; 1029. Also available at: http://aappolicy.aappublications.org/cgi/content/full/pediatrics%3b108/3/776 (accessed 01/07/04)

### Uses and Administration

Iodine radioisotopes are mainly used in studies of thyroid function and in the treatment of hyperthyroidism (p.1594) and some forms of thyroid carcinoma (p.523).

Iodine radioisotopes can be incorporated into many compounds including liothyronine and levothyroxine, triglycerides and fatty acids, such as triolein and oleic acid, and proteins, such as iodinated human albumin, with varying degrees of stability and with little or no change in the biological activity of the labelled molecule. It is common practice to saturate the thyroid with non-radioactive iodine when uptake of radiation by the gland is not desired (see Radiation Protection, p.1599).

Sodium iodide ($^{131}$I) is given by mouth and by intravenous injection in studies of thyroid function, particularly in measurements of the uptake of iodine by the thyroid, and in thyroid scanning. It is also used in the treatment of hyperthyroidism and in the treatment of malignant neoplasms of the thyroid.

Injections containing iobenguane ($^{131}$I) (*m*-iodobenzylguanidine ($^{131}$I)) may be used for the localisation and treatment of phaeochromocytoma (p.831) and neuroblastoma (p.524).

Human albumin iodinated with iodine-131 is used in the determination of the blood or plasma volume.

Sodium iodohippurate ($^{131}$I) is used intravenously for renal-function tests and for renal imaging.

Rose bengal sodium ($^{131}$I) has been given intravenously in tests of liver function.

Iodinated ($^{131}$I) norcholesterol (6β-iodomethyl-19-norcholest-5(10)-en-3β-ol ($^{131}$I)) has been used for adrenal scintigraphy by slow intravenous injection.

Various monoclonal antibodies labelled with iodine-131 are used for the detection of malignant neoplasms and some are used for therapeutic purposes, such as iodine ($^{131}$I) tositumomab for non-Hodgkin's lymphoma.

### Preparations

***Ph. Eur.:*** Iobenguane($^{131}$I) Injection for Diagnostic Use; Iobenguane($^{131}$I) Injection for Therapeutic Use; Iodinated($^{131}$I) Norcholesterol Injection; Sodium Iodide($^{131}$I) Capsules for Diagnostic Use; Sodium Iodide($^{131}$I) Solution; Sodium Iodide($^{131}$I) Solution for Radiolabelling; Sodium Iodohippurate($^{131}$I) Injection;
***USP 27:*** Iobenguane I 131 Injection; Iodinated I 131 Albumin Aggregated Injection; Iodinated I 131 Albumin Injection; Iodohippurate Sodium I 131 Injection; Rose Bengal Sodium I 131 Injection; Sodium Iodide I 131 Capsules; Sodium Iodide I 131 Solution.

**Proprietary Preparations** (details are given in Part 3)
***UK:*** Theracap; ***USA:*** Bexxar; Iodotope.

## Iron-59

Hierro 59.
*CAS — 14596-12-4.*
*ATC — V09XX04 (ferric citrate ($^{59}$Fe)).*

**Half-life.** 44.6 days.

### Profile

Iron-59, in the form of ferrous citrate ($^{59}$Fe) or ferric citrate ($^{59}$Fe), has been used by intravenous injection in the measurement of iron absorption and utilisation. Ferric chloride ($^{59}$Fe) has been given for the same purpose.

## Krypton-81m

Criptón 81m.
*CAS — 15678-91-8.*
*ATC — V09EX01 (krypton gas ($^{81m}$Kr)).*

**Half-life.** 13.1 seconds.

### Profile

Krypton-81m is a daughter of rubidium-81 ($^{81}$Rb, half-life 4.58 hours), and is prepared immediately before use by elution from a generator containing rubidium-81 adsorbed on a suitable ion-exchange column using air or oxygen as the eluent. Krypton-81m is used as a gas in lung ventilation studies. Such ventilation studies can be combined with lung perfusion studies to diagnose pulmonary embolism.

### Preparations

***Ph. Eur.:*** Krypton($^{81m}$Kr) Inhalation Gas;
***USP 27:*** Krypton Kr 81m.

## Nitrogen-13

Nitrógeno 13.
*CAS — 13981-22-1.*

**Half-life.** 9.96 minutes.

### Profile

Nitrogen-13 is a positron-emitting radionuclide that is used in positron-emission tomography (see Emissions from Radioisotopes, p.1522). In the form of ammonia ($^{13}$N) it is given intravenously for imaging blood flow in organs such as the heart, brain, and liver. Nitrogen gas ($^{13}$N) may be used for pulmonary ventilation studies.

### Preparations

***Ph. Eur.:*** Ammonia($^{13}$N) Injection;
***USP 27:*** Ammonia N 13 Injection.

## Oxygen-15

Oxígeno 15.
*CAS — 13982-43-9.*

**Half-life.** 2 minutes.

### Profile

Oxygen-15 is a positron-emitting radionuclide used in positron-emission tomography (see Emissions from Radioisotopes, p.1522). It is used in the form of water ($^{15}$O) and is given intravenously to study cerebral and myocardial perfusion.

Oxygen gas, carbon dioxide, and carbon monoxide have also been labelled with oxygen-15.

### Preparations

***Ph. Eur.:*** Carbon Monoxide($^{15}$O); Oxygen($^{15}$O); Water($^{15}$O) Injection;
***USP 27:*** Water O 15 Injection.

## Phosphorus-32

Fósforo 32.
*CAS — 14596-37-3.*
*ATC — V10XX01 (sodium phosphate ($^{32}$P)); V10AX01 (phosphorus chromic phosphate colloid ($^{32}$P)).*

**Half-life.** 14.3 days.

### Profile

Phosphorus-32, given as sodium phosphate ($^{32}$P), is used intravenously in the treatment of polycythaemia vera (p.508). Phosphorus-32 is taken up by the rapidly proliferating haematopoietic cells sufficiently to reduce their reproduction. Sodium phosphate ($^{32}$P) has also been used intravenously in the treatment of chronic myeloid (p.507) and chronic lymphocytic leukaemia (p.507) and in the palliative treatment of bone metastases.

Chromic phosphate ($^{32}$P) is given intraperitoneally or intrapleurally in the treatment of malignant effusions (p.512); it may also be given by interstitial injection for the treatment of ovarian (p.520) or prostatic carcinoma (p.521).

### Preparations

***Ph. Eur.:*** Sodium Phosphate($^{32}$P) Injection;
***USP 27:*** Chromic Phosphate P 32 Suspension; Sodium Phosphate P 32 Solution.

**Proprietary Preparations** (details are given in Part 3)
***USA:*** Phosphocol.

## Rhenium-186

Renio 186.
*CAS — 14998-63-1.*
*ATC — V10BX03 (rhenium etidronate ($^{186}$Re)); V10AX05 (rhenium sulfide colloid ($^{186}$Re)).*

**Half-life.** 90.6 hours.

### Profile

Rhenium-186 has been used in colloidal form for the treatment of arthritic joint conditions. Rhenium ($^{186}$Re) etidronate is used for the palliation of painful bone metastases of prostate cancer. Monoclonal antibodies labelled with rhenium-186 have been investigated for the treatment of various malignant neoplasms.

### Preparations

**Proprietary Preparations** (details are given in Part 3)
***Switz.:*** Re-BONE.

## Rubidium-82

Rubidio 82.
*CAS — 14391-63-0.*

**Half-life.** 75 seconds.

### Profile

Rubidium-82 is a positron-emitting radionuclide that is used in positron-emission tomography (see Emissions from Radioisotopes, p.1522). Rubidium chloride ($^{82}$Rb) is administered intravenously for cardiac imaging.

### Preparations

***USP 27:*** Rubidium Chloride Rb 82 Injection.

## Samarium-153

Samario 153.
*CAS — 15766-00-4.*
*ATC — V10BX02 (samarium lexidronam ($^{153}$Sm)); V10AX02 (samarium hydroxyapatite colloid ($^{153}$Sm)).*

**Half-life.** 47 hours.

### Profile

Samarium-153, in the form of samarium ($^{153}$Sm) lexidronam (samarium ($^{153}$Sm) EDTMP) is used for the palliative treatment of painful bone metastases (p.513). It is given by intravenous injection.

### Preparations

***USP 27:*** Samarium Sm 153 Lexidronam Injection.

**Proprietary Preparations** (details are given in Part 3)
***Austral.:*** Quadramet; ***Fr.:*** Quadramet; ***Ital.:*** Quadramet; ***Port.:*** Quadramet; ***Spain:*** Quadramet; ***UK:*** Quadramet; ***USA:*** Quadramet.

## Selenium-75

Selenio 75.
*CAS — 14265-71-5.*
*ATC — V09DX01 (selenium tauroselcholic acid ($^{75}$Se)); V09XX03 (selenium norcholesterol ($^{75}$Se)).*

**Half-life.** 118.5 days.

### Profile

Selenium-75 in the form of tauroselcholic acid ($^{75}$Se) ($^{75}$SeHCAT) is used orally in the measurement of bile acid absorption for the assessment of ileal function.

Selenium-75 in the form of 6β-[(methyl[$^{75}$Se]seleno)methyl]-19-norcholest-5(10)-en-3β-ol (selenonorcholestenol ($^{75}$Se)) has been used intravenously in adrenal scintigraphy.

### Preparations

**Proprietary Preparations** (details are given in Part 3)
***UK:*** Scintadren.

## Strontium-89

Estroncio 89.
*CAS — 14158-27-1.*
*ATC — V10BX01 (strontium chloride ($^{89}$Sr)).*

**Half-life.** 50.5 days.

### Profile

Strontium-89, in the form of strontium chloride ($^{89}$Sr), is used for the palliation of pain in patients with bone metastases (p.513); it is given intravenously.

◊ References.

1. Robinson RG, *et al.* Strontium 89 therapy for the palliation of pain due to osseous metastases. *JAMA* 1995; **274:** 420–4.

### Preparations

***Ph. Eur.:*** Strontium($^{89}$Sr) Chloride Injection;
***USP 27:*** Strontium Chloride Sr 89 Injection.

**Proprietary Preparations** (details are given in Part 3)
***Austral.:*** Metastron; ***Austria:*** Metastron; ***Canad.:*** Metastron†; ***Fr.:*** Metastron; ***Ital.:*** Metastron; ***Spain:*** Metastron; ***UK:*** Metastron; ***USA:*** Metastron.

## Technetium-99m

Tecnecio 99m.
*CAS — 14133-76-7 (technetium-99).*
*ATC — V09AA01 (technetium exametazime ($^{99m}$Tc)); V09AA02 (technetium bicisate ($^{99m}$Tc)); V09BA01 (technetium oxidronate ($^{99m}$Tc)); V09BA02 (technetium medronate ($^{99m}$Tc)); V09BA03 (technetium pyrophosphate ($^{99m}$Tc)); V09BA04 (technetium butedronate ($^{99m}$Tc)); V09CA01 (technetium pentetate ($^{99m}$Tc)); V09CA02 (technetium succimer ($^{99m}$Tc)); V09CA03 (technetium mertiatide ($^{99m}$Tc)); V09CA04 (technetium gluceptate ($^{99m}$Tc)); V09CA05 (technetium gluconate ($^{99m}$Tc)); V09DA01 (technetium disofenin ($^{99m}$Tc)); V09DA02 (technetium etifenin ($^{99m}$Tc)); V09DA03 (technetium lidofenin ($^{99m}$Tc)); V09DA04 (technetium mebrofenin ($^{99m}$Tc)); V09DA05 (technetium galtifenin ($^{99m}$Tc)); V09DB01 (technetium nanocolloid ($^{99m}$Tc)); V09DB02 (technetium microcolloid ($^{99m}$Tc)); V09DB03 (technetium millimicrospheres ($^{99m}$Tc)); V09DB04 (technetium tin colloid ($^{99m}$Tc)); V09DB05 (technetium sulfur colloid ($^{99m}$Tc)); V09DB06 (technetium rhenium sulfide colloid ($^{99m}$Tc)); V09DB07 (technetium phytate ($^{99m}$Tc)); V09EA01 (technetium pentetate ($^{99m}$Tc)); V09EA02 (technetium technegas ($^{99m}$Tc)); V09EA03 (technetium nanocolloid ($^{99m}$Tc)); V09EB01 (technetium macrosalb ($^{99m}$Tc)); V09EB02 (technetium microspheres ($^{99m}$Tc)); V09FX01 (technetium pertechnetate ($^{99m}$Tc)); V09GA01 (technetium sestamibi ($^{99m}$Tc)); V09GA02 (technetium tetrofosmin ($^{99m}$Tc)); V09GA03 (technetium teboroxime ($^{99m}$Tc)); V09GA04 (technetium human albumin ($^{99m}$Tc)); V09GA05 (technetium furifosmin ($^{99m}$Tc)); V09GA06 (technetium stannous agent labelled cells ($^{99m}$Tc)); V09GA07 (technetium apcitide ($^{99m}$Tc)); V09HA01 (technetium human immunoglobulin ($^{99m}$Tc)); V09HA02 (technetium exametazime labelled cells ($^{99m}$Tc)); V09HA03 (technetium antigranulocyte antibody ($^{99m}$Tc)); V09HA04 (technetium sulesomab ($^{99m}$Tc)); V09IA01 (technetium antiCEA antibody ($^{99m}$Tc)); V09IA02 (technetium antimelanoma antibody ($^{99m}$Tc)); V09IA03 (technetium pentavalent succimer ($^{99m}$Tc)); V09IA04 (technetium votumumab ($^{99m}$Tc)); V09IA05 (technetium depreotide ($^{99m}$Tc)); V09IA06 (technetium arcitumomab ($^{99m}$Tc)).*

**Half-life.** 6.02 hours.

### Adverse Effects and Precautions

Hypersensitivity reactions have been reported with technetium-99m preparations.

**Breast feeding.** The American Academy of Pediatrics has stated[1] that temporary cessation of breast feeding is required following exposure to technetium-99m since radioactivity has been reported to be present in breast milk for 15 to 72 hours.

1. American Academy of Pediatrics. The transfer of drugs and other chemicals into human milk. *Pediatrics* 2001; **108:** 776–89. Correction. *ibid.*; 1029. Also available at: http://aappolicy.aappublications.org/cgi/content/full/pediatrics%3b108/3/776 (accessed 01/07/04)

### Uses and Administration

Technetium-99m is a daughter of molybdenum-99 ($^{99}$Mo, half-life 66.2 hours) and because of its short half-life is normally prepared just before use by elution from a sterile generator consisting of molybdenum-99 adsorbed onto alumina in a glass column. Technetium-99m as pertechnetate ($^{99m}TcO_4^-$) is obtained by elution with a sterile solution of sodium chloride 0.9%. Radiopharmaceuticals of technetium-99m are prepared shortly after elution to reduce loss by decay.

Because it has a short half-life and can be administered in relatively large doses, and because the energy of its gamma-emission is readily detected, technetium-99m is very widely used, either as the pertechnetate or in the form of various labelled compounds, particles, and colloids for scanning bone and organs such as the brain, heart, kidney, liver, lung, spleen, and thyroid.

Sodium pertechnetate ($^{99m}$Tc) is used intravenously for angiography and for imaging blood pools, brain, salivary glands, and thyroid gland; the oral route may also be used for brain and thyroid imaging. Topical application to the eye is used for studying nasolachrymal drainage and the intraurethral route for imaging the urinary tract. Potassium perchlorate may be given before administration of the pertechnetate to prevent uptake in the thyroid or choroid plexus and thus enhance visualisation in other organs.

Macroaggregates of human albumin labelled with technetium-99m [macrosalb ($^{99m}$Tc)] are used in lung scanning for the detection of abnormal lung perfusion patterns; following the intravenous injection of a suspension of suitable particle size, usually 10 to 100 micrometres, the particles become trapped in the lung capillaries enabling ischaemic areas to be defined. Labelled albumin microspheres of particle size 10 to 50 micrometres are used similarly. Labelled macroaggregates of albumin have also been used in venography for the detection of deep-vein thrombosis of the legs. Technetium ($^{99m}$Tc) apcitide is a labelled peptide that binds to the glycoprotein IIb/IIIa receptor of activated platelets, and is also used for imaging of deep-vein thrombosis.

When technetium-99m bound to human serum albumin is given intravenously it becomes evenly distributed in the circulation and highly vascular organs or pools of blood may be readily located. Such a preparation is used in the examination of the heart.

Technetium-99m in the form of a colloid, such as albumin, sulfur, antimony sulfide, or tin, is used intravenously for the examination of the liver, spleen, and bone marrow. Sulfur colloid ($^{99m}$Tc) may be given orally for oesophageal and gastrointestinal scanning. Albumin colloid ($^{99m}$Tc) may be given subcutaneously for scanning of the lymphatic system. Colloidal rhenium sulfide ($^{99m}$Tc) has been used for sentinel lymph node detection in patients with malignancies.

Technetium-99m complexes of iminodiacetic acid derivatives, such as disofenin, etifenin, lidofenin, and mebrofenin are used intravenously in the investigation of hepatic function and in the imaging of the hepatobiliary system.

Agents used intravenously in both brain and renal imaging are technetium-99m-labelled gluconate, gluceptate, and pentetate. Other technetium-99m-labelled compounds are used in brain and kidney scanning; for instance, labelled bicisate and exametazime have been used in brain imaging and betiatide, mertiatide, and succimer have been used in kidney studies. The pentetate is also given by inhalation for lung ventilation imaging, and orally for studies of gastro-oesophageal reflux and gastric emptying.

For bone scanning various labelled phosphate compounds may be used and include medronate, oxidronate, and pyrophosphate, all given intravenously. Technetium-99m as the pyrophosphate is also used in cardiac scintigraphy. Technetium-99m as the medronate and pyrophosphate are also used to label red blood cells for use in blood pool scintigraphy, cardiac scintigraphy, detection of gastrointestinal bleeding, and testicular scintigraphy.

Compounds used intravenously in cardiac imaging include technetium-99m-labelled sestamibi, teboroxime, and tetrofosmin. Technetium ($^{99m}$Tc) sestamibi is also used for breast imaging.

Technetium-99m-labelled leucocytes (prepared using exametazime) are used for localisation of sites of inflammation or infection.

Monoclonal antibodies labelled with technetium-99m, such as arcitumomab and nofetumomab merpentan, are used for the detection and localisation of malignant neoplasms. Labelled sulesomab is used in the detection of osteomyelitis. Technetium ($^{99m}$Tc) depreotide is a labelled peptide used intravenously for imaging of pulmonary malignancy.

Many other technetium-99m-labelled compounds have been prepared and used in different clinical studies for the examination of different organs or systems. Use with other radionuclides includes subtraction scanning with thallium-201 to detect parathyroid tumours.

### Preparations

**Ph. Eur.:** Sodium Pertechnetate($^{99m}$Tc) Injection (Fission); Sodium Pertechnetate($^{99m}$Tc) Injection (Non-fission); Technetium($^{99m}$Tc) Colloidal Rhenium Sulphide Injection; Technetium($^{99m}$Tc) Colloidal Sulphur Injection; Technetium($^{99m}$Tc) Colloidal Tin Injection; Technetium($^{99m}$Tc) Etifenin Injection; Technetium($^{99m}$Tc) Exametazime Injection; Technetium($^{99m}$Tc) Gluconate Injection; Technetium($^{99m}$Tc) Human Albumin Injection; Technetium($^{99m}$Tc) Macrosalb Injection; Technetium($^{99m}$Tc) Medronate Injection; Technetium($^{99m}$Tc) Mertiatide Injection; Technetium($^{99m}$Tc) Microspheres Injection; Technetium($^{99m}$Tc) Pentetate Injection; Technetium($^{99m}$Tc) Sestamibi Injection; Technetium($^{99m}$Tc) Succimer Injection; Technetium($^{99m}$Tc) Tin Pyrophosphate Injection;
**USP 27:** Sodium Pertechnetate Tc 99m Injection; Technetium Tc 99m (Pyro- and trimeta-) Phosphates Injection; Technetium Tc 99m Albumin Aggregated Injection; Technetium Tc 99m Albumin Colloid Injection; Technetium Tc 99m Albumin Injection; Technetium Tc 99m Apcitide Injection; Technetium Tc 99m Arcitumomab Injection; Technetium Tc 99m Bicisate Injection; Technetium Tc 99m Depreotide Injection; Technetium Tc 99m Disofenin Injection; Technetium Tc 99m Etidronate Injection; Technetium Tc 99m Exametazime Injection; Technetium Tc 99m Gluceptate Injection; Technetium Tc 99m Lidofenin Injection; Technetium Tc 99m Mebrofenin Injection; Technetium Tc 99m Medronate Injection; Technetium Tc 99m Mertiatide Injection; Technetium Tc 99m Nofetumomab Merpentan Injection; Technetium Tc 99m Oxidronate Injection; Technetium Tc 99m Pentetate Injection; Technetium Tc 99m Pyrophosphate Injection; Technetium Tc 99m Red Blood Cells Injection; Technetium Tc 99m Sestamibi Injection; Technetium Tc 99m Succimer Injection; Technetium Tc 99m Sulfur Colloid Injection; Technetium Tc 99m Tetrofosmin Injection.

**Proprietary Preparations** (details are given in Part 3)
***Austral.:*** Ceretec; Myoview; ***Austria:*** Cardiolite; Ceretec; TechneScan MAG3; ***Belg.:*** Cardiolite; Neurolite; ***Braz.:*** Amerscan Hepatate†; TCK-21†; TechneScan DMSA†; TechneScan DTPA†; TechneScan Enxofre†; TechneScan HDP†; TechneScan MAA†; TechneScan MAG3†; TechneScan MDB†; TechneScan PYP†; TechneScan Q12†; ***Canad.:*** Choletec†; ***Fr.:*** Cardiolite; Ceretec†; Myoview; Neurolite; ***Irl.:*** Cardiolite; ***Ital.:*** CEA-Scan; Ceretec; LeukoScan; Myoview; TechneScan MAG3; ***Spain:*** Cardiolite; CEA-Scan; Ceretec; Myoview; Neospect; Neurolite; TechneScan HDP; TechneScan MAG3; ***UK:*** Amerscan DMSA; Amerscan Hepatate; Amerscan Medronate; Amerscan Pentetate; Amerscan Pulmonate; Amerscan Stannous; Amertec; Angiocis; Cardiolite; CEA-Scan; Ceretec; Cholecis; Medrocis; Myoview; Nanocoll; Osteocis; Pentacis; Pulmocis; Renocis; ***USA:*** AcuTect; Cardiolite; CEA-Scan; Miraluma; NeoTect; TechneScan HDP.

## Thallium-201

Talio 201.
*CAS — 15064-65-0.*
*ATC — V09GX01 (thallium chloride ($^{201}$Tl)).*

**Half-life.** 73.1 hours.

### Profile

Thallium-201, in the form of thallous chloride ($^{201}$Tl), is given by intravenous injection for scanning the myocardium in the investigation of acute myocardial infarction. It is also used for myocardial perfusion imaging in cardiac stress testing of patients with ischaemic heart disease. Adenosine (p.852), dipyridamole (p.903), or dobutamine (p.906) may be used to induce pharmacological stress in those patients unable to tolerate exercise.

Other uses include muscle perfusion scintigraphy in peripheral vascular disorders, visualisation of brain and thyroid tumours and metastases, and the localisation of parathyroid adenomas and hyperplasia by thallium-201 and technetium-99m subtraction scanning.

### Preparations

**Ph. Eur.:** Thallous($^{201}$Tl) Chloride Injection;
**USP 27:** Thallous Chloride Tl 201 Injection.

## Tritium

Hydrogen-3; Tritio.
*CAS — 10028-17-8.*

**Half-life.** 12.3 years.

### Profile

Tritium, in the form of tritiated water, has been used to determine the total body water by a dilution technique.

### Preparations

**Ph. Eur.:** Tritiated($^{3}$H) Water Injection.

## Xenon-127

Xenón 127.
*CAS — 13994-19-9.*
*ATC — V09EX02 (xenon gas ($^{127}$Xe)).*

**Half-life.** 36.41 days.

### Profile

Xenon-127 has similar physical properties to those of xenon-133 (see below) and is also used by inhalation for pulmonary function studies and lung imaging.

### Preparations

**USP 27:** Xenon Xe 127.

## Xenon-133

Xenón 133.
*CAS — 14932-42-4.*
*ATC — V09EX03 (xenon gas ($^{133}$Xe)).*

**Half-life.** 5.25 days.

### Profile

Xenon-133 is an inert gas with relatively low solubility in plasma. In the gaseous form, it is mixed with air or oxygen in a bag or in a closed or open circuit spirometer. When the administration of gas is stopped, xenon-133 is excreted promptly and completely through the lungs. It is used by inhalation in pulmonary function studies and lung imaging as well as in cerebral blood flow studies. It has also been used for these purposes in the form of an injection in sodium chloride 0.9%.

### Preparations

**Ph. Eur.:** Xenon($^{133}$Xe) Injection;
**USP 27:** Xenon Xe 133; Xenon Xe 133 Injection.

## Yttrium-90

Itrio 90.
*CAS — 10098-91-6.*
*ATC — V10AA01 (yttrium citrate colloid ($^{90}$Y)); V10AA02 (yttrium ferrihydroxide colloid ($^{90}$Y)); V10AA03 (yttrium silicate colloid ($^{90}$Y)).*

**Half-life.** 64.1 hours.

Yttrium-90 conjugated to ibritumomab tiuxetan is used in the treatment of non-Hodgkin's lymphoma. Conjugates with various other monoclonal antibodies and compounds are also under investigation for malignant neoplasms.

Yttrium-90, in the form of a colloidal suspension of yttrium silicate ($^{90}$Y) has been used for instillation into pleural or peritoneal cavities in the treatment of malignant pleural effusion (p.512) or malignant ascites.

Yttrium-90, as either yttrium citrate ($^{90}$Y) or yttrium silicate ($^{90}$Y), has also been used in the treatment of arthritic conditions of joints.

Yttrium-90 enclosed in glass microspheres has been used for the local treatment of malignant neoplasms of the liver.

### Preparations

**USP 27:** Yttrium Y 90 Ibritumomab Tiuxetan Injection.

**Proprietary Preparations** (details are given in Part 3)
***UK:*** Ytracis.

# Sex Hormones

The male and female sex organs, the adrenal cortex, and the placenta produce steroidal hormones which influence the development and maintenance of structures directly and indirectly associated with reproduction. The secretion of these sex hormones is controlled by gonadotrophic hormones of the anterior lobe of the pituitary gland; the secretion of these gonadotrophic hormones is in turn influenced by the hypothalamus and also by the concentration of circulating sex hormones. There are 3 groups of endogenous sex hormones, androgens, oestrogens, and progestogens, all of which are derived from the same steroidal precursors. The progestogenic hormone, progesterone, is formed from pregnenolone, and both of these compounds may be converted to androgen precursors such as androstenedione. Androstenedione is converted to the androgenic hormone testosterone by hydroxysteroid dehydrogenases. Oestrogenic hormones are synthesised from androstenedione (and also from testosterone) by the action of aromatase.

**Testosterone** is the main androgenic hormone formed in the interstitial (Leydig) cells of the testes. A small proportion of circulating testosterone is also derived from the metabolism of less potent androgens secreted by the adrenal cortex and ovaries. In many target tissues testosterone is then converted to the more active dihydrotestosterone by 5α-reductase. Some testosterone also undergoes peripheral conversion to oestradiol.

Testosterone controls the development and maintenance of the male sex organs and the male secondary sex characteristics. It also produces systemic anabolic effects, such as increased retention of nitrogen, calcium, sodium, potassium, chloride, and phosphate. This leads to an increase in water retention and bone growth. The skin becomes more vascular and less fatty and erythropoiesis is increased.

Numerous derivatives of testosterone have been developed. Alkylation at the 17α position results in derivatives that are orally active (e.g. methyltestosterone, stanozolol) and esterification of the 17β-hydroxyl group increases lipid solubility and is used to prepare long-acting intramuscular preparations (e.g. testosterone enantate). Removal of the 19-methyl group is reported to improve the anabolic to androgenic ratio (e.g. nandrolone). The derivatives also vary in their plasma protein binding affinity, and degree of conversion to dihydrotestosterone and aromatic conversion to oestrogen. Numerous other structural modifications have been made.

**Oestradiol** is the most active of the naturally occurring oestrogens formed from androgen precursors in the ovarian follicles of premenopausal women. In men and postmenopausal women (and to an insignificant extent in premenopausal women) oestrogens are also formed in adipose tissue from adrenal androgens.

Oestrogens control the development and maintenance of the female sex organs, secondary sex characteristics, and mammary glands as well as certain functions of the uterus and its accessory organs (particularly the proliferation of the endometrium, the development of the decidua, and the cyclic changes in the cervix and vagina). Large amounts of oestradiol are also formed in the placenta; in late pregnancy, this increases the spontaneous activity of the uterine muscle and its response to oxytocic drugs. The additional activity of progesterone is essential for the complete biological function of the female sex organs.

A number of oestrogens are used therapeutically. Ethinyl substitution at the C17 position has led to the development of synthetic oestrogens such as ethinylestradiol and mestranol, which have greatly improved potency and oral activity. Oral activity of natural oestrogens is improved by esterification (e.g. estradiol valerate) or by conjugation (e.g. estrone sulfate). Esterification also increases solubility in lipid vehicles and is used to prepare long-acting intramuscular preparations.

A number of nonsteroidal oestrogens, including broparestrol, chlorotrianisene, dienestrol, and diethylstilbestrol, have also been used.

**Progesterone** is the main hormone secreted by the corpus luteum. It acts on the endometrium by converting the proliferative phase induced by oestrogen to a secretory phase thereby preparing the uterus to receive the fertilised ovum. Progesterone has a catabolic action and causes a slight rise in basal body temperature during the secretory phase of menstruation. During pregnancy the placenta produces large quantities of progesterone, which suppresses uterine motility and is responsible for the further development of the breasts.

Progestogens (gestagens, progestagens, progestins) are synthetic compounds with actions similar to those of progesterone. They are either progesterone derivatives or 19-nortestosterone analogues. The 19-nortestosterone analogues (such as norethisterone and norgestrel) possess some androgenic activity, but some newer norgestrel derivatives (desogestrel, gestodene, and norgestimate) have little androgenic activity. The progesterone derivatives dydrogesterone, hydroxyprogesterone, and medroxyprogesterone are less androgenic than the 19-nortestosterone analogues. The progesterone derivatives chlormadinone, and particularly cyproterone, have anti-androgenic activity.

The principal natural and synthetic sex hormones covered in this chapter are thus:

- **androgens and anabolic steroids**, typified by testosterone (p.1569)
- **oestrogens**, typified by estradiol (p.1550)
- **progestogens**, typified by progesterone (p.1566)

Other related substances also described in this chapter are:

- drugs with predominantly **weak androgenic** properties such as danazol and gestrinone
- drugs that combine **oestrogenic and progestogenic** properties such as tibolone
- drugs with predominantly **anti-androgenic** properties. These include the progesterone derivative cyproterone acetate, the nonsteroidal 5α-reductase inhibitor finasteride, and the plant extract saw palmetto. Those anti-androgens used principally in the hormonal treatment of prostate cancer are covered in the Antineoplastics chapter; they include the nonsteroidal drugs bicalutamide (p.530), flutamide (p.556), and nilutamide (p.576)
- drugs with predominantly **anti-oestrogenic** properties. These include the nonsteroidal anti-oestrogens clomifene, cyclofenil, and the more selective nonsteroidal anti-oestrogens ormeloxifene and raloxifene. Those anti-oestrogens used principally in the hormonal treatment of breast cancer are covered in the Antineoplastics chapter; they include the oestrogen receptor antagonists tamoxifen (p.584) and toremifene (p.589), and various aromatase inhibitors such as formestane (p.557) and anastrozole (p.528)
- drugs with predominantly **antiprogestogenic** properties such as the progestogen derivative mifepristone

The activity of endogenous sex hormones can be modulated by gonadotrophins, and gonadorelin and its analogues, and these are discussed in Hypothalamic and Pituitary Hormones, beginning on p.1312.

The therapeutic applications of sex hormones and related substances are broad and cover many circumstances where hormonal manipulation is desirable. Major applications are the use of oestrogens and progestogens for **contraception** (p.1535) and for the alleviation of **menopausal symptoms** (p.1540). A physiological application is the use of an androgen or an oestrogen in the management of **delayed puberty** and **hypogonadism**, (see Testosterone, p.1571 or Estradiol, p.1551). Other clinical applications include the management of **benign prostatic hyperplasia** (p.1555), **endometriosis** (p.1546), **gynaecomastia** (p.1546), **hirsutism** (p.1545), **infertility** (p.1316), **mastalgia** (p.1546), **menorrhagia** (p.1567), and **premenstrual syndrome** (p.1551). Hormonal manipulation also has an important role in the treatment of **malignant neoplasms** of the breast (p.514), prostate (p.521), and endometrium (p.516).

---

## Hormonal Contraceptives

Anticonceptivos hormonales.

### Types of Contraceptive

Hormonal contraceptives are currently only available for women although preparations for men are being evaluated. Oral hormonal contraceptives for women are divided into 2 main types: 'combined' (containing an oestrogen and a progestogen) and 'progestogen-only'. Parenteral preparations have also been developed and include subcutaneous implants and depot intramuscular injections. Progestogen-releasing intra-uterine devices and a combined hormonal contraceptive vaginal ring are available. A combined hormonal transdermal patch has also been developed.

Parenteral progestogen-only contraceptives provide reliable suppression of ovulation by suppressing the necessary mid-cycle surge of luteinising hormone. However, the low doses in progestogen-only oral contraceptives do not suppress it reliably in all cycles. Contraceptive efficacy is instead achieved by thickening the cervical mucus so that it is not readily penetrated by sperm, and by preventing proliferation of the endometrium so that it remains unfavourable for implantation of any fertilised ova. Intra-uterine progestogen-only devices act similarly; the physical presence of the system in the uterus may also contribute to overall contraceptive efficacy.

Oestrogens inhibit ovulation by suppressing the mid-cycle release of follicle-stimulating hormone. They act synergistically with progestogens in combined oral contraceptives to provide regular and consistent suppression of ovulation.

Oral preparations are also available for *emergency contraception* after unprotected coitus; they prevent implantation of any fertilised ova.

### Adverse Effects

Many reports have been published of adverse effects associated with the use of **combined oral contraceptives**. The data have mostly been gained retrospectively and often involve older preparations containing higher doses of oestrogen and progestogen than are used currently.

There may be gastrointestinal side-effects such as nausea or vomiting, chloasma (melasma) and other skin or hair changes, headache, water retention, weight gain, breast tenderness, and changes in libido.

Menstrual irregularities such as spotting, breakthrough bleeding, or amenorrhoea can occur during treatment. These effects may result from the relative balance of oestrogenic and progestogenic effects of particular products and their incidence may be reduced by changing to a different product. For example, early or mid-cycle spotting or absence of withdrawal bleeding may require a preparation with a greater oestrogen to progestogen ratio, or less progestogen as in multiphasic preparations, or temporary supplementation with an oestrogen.

Intolerance to contact lenses has been reported and vision may deteriorate in myopic patients. Some patients may experience depression and other mental changes. Preparations containing a progestogen with androgenic properties such as levonorgestrel or norgestrel may be associated with increased oiliness of the skin and acne. Conversely, acne may be improved with progestogens such as norgestimate or desogestrel.

There is an increased risk of cardiovascular disease and associated mortality related, at least in part, to the oestrogen content of combined oral contraceptives. The incidence of cardiovascular side-effects is probably less with the newer lower-dose preparations than with the older higher-dose preparations. Increased mortality from myocardial infarction is much greater with increased age and in cigarette smokers, although some evidence suggests that healthy women aged over 35 years who do not smoke are not at increased risk. Other risk factors include a family history of arterial disease, diabetes mellitus, hypertension, obesity, and migraine. Thrombosis may be more common when factor V Leiden is present or in patients with blood groups A, B, or AB. Specific risk factors for venous thromboembolism include a family history of venous thromboembolism, varicose veins, long-term immobilisation and, again obesity. Recent evidence has also indicated that the risk of venous thromboembolism varies according to the progestogen component of combined oral contraceptives; a higher incidence has been associated with desogestrel and gestodene than with levonorgestrel, norethisterone, and etynodiol. For further discussion see Venous Thromboembolism, below.

Combined oral contraceptives may cause hypertension and there may be reduced glucose tolerance and changes in lipid metabolism. Liver function can be impaired, although jaundice is rare. There appears to be a marked increase (though the incidence is still very low) in the relative risk of benign liver tumours. Malignant liver tumours have also been reported.

Combined oral contraceptives are reported to slightly increase the risk of cervical cancer (although other factors may be involved) and breast cancer, but to protect against ovarian cancer and endometrial cancer. For further discussion, see Carcinogenicity, below.

As with combined oral contraceptives, **progestogen-only contraceptives** may cause nausea, vomiting, headache, breast discomfort, depression, skin disorders, and weight gain. Menstrual irregularities such as amenorrhoea, breakthrough bleeding, spotting, and menorrhagia are more common with progestogen-only contraceptives, and are particularly common with parenteral preparations. Available progestogen-only contraceptives carry less risk of thromboembolic and cardiovascular disease than combined oral contraceptives.

**Carcinogenicity.** Concern has often been expressed as to whether the use of hormonal contraceptives by normally healthy women may either cause or increase the risk of developing malignant neoplasms. To investigate any possible link between such use and cancer, two main types of study have been employed by epidemiologists, namely the prospective study and the case-control study. Many factors have made direct comparison of results difficult and such factors include the type and composition of oral contraceptive used (which has changed over the years), the age of the patient, the age at which use first began, and the sexual and obstetric history of the patient. Overall the evidence indicates that combined oral contraceptives in fact exert a protective effect against the development of endometrial and ovarian carcinoma. However, there is a small increase in risk of breast cancer during use and for 10 years after discontinuation. In addition, there does appear to be a slight risk of cervical cancer with the prolonged use of combined oral contraceptives and a negligible risk of liver cancer. For further details concerning the effects on individual organs, see the following sections. It should be noted that even where the relative risk has been shown to be substantially increased this will not translate into many new cases of a rare cancer, and this contributes to the difficulties of assessing clinical relevance. It is also worthy of note that two large prospective cohort studies (the Nurses' Health Study and the Royal College of General Practitioners' study) found no evidence of a difference in overall mortality between women who had used oral contraceptives and those who had not.[1,2] Some general reviews on hormonal contraceptives and cancer are cited below.[3-5]

1. Colditz GA, *et al.* Oral contraceptive use and mortality during 12 years of follow-up: the Nurses' Health Study. *Ann Intern Med* 1994; **120:** 821–6.
2. Beral V, *et al.* Mortality associated with oral contraceptive use: 25 year follow up of cohort of 46 000 women from Royal College of General Practitioners' oral contraception study. *BMJ* 1999; **318:** 96–100.
3. WHO. Oral contraceptives and neoplasia: report of a WHO scientific group. *WHO Tech Rep Ser 817* 1992.
4. La Vecchia C, *et al.* Oral contraceptives and cancer: a review of the evidence. *Drug Safety* 1996; **14:** 260–72.
5. La Vecchia C, *et al.* Oral contraceptives and cancer: an update. *Drug Safety* 2001; **24:** 741–54.

BREAST. Numerous epidemiological studies have been published on the potential link between hormonal contraceptives and breast cancer. Most of these data relate to **combined oral contraceptives**, which are the most widely used form. The breast cancer risk from use of these contraceptives will require monitoring for some time to come as the first users of oral contraceptives continue to age, and because of the changing patterns of use.

Early studies from the 1980s variously failed to show any significant increase in risk of breast cancer in women who had ever used hormonal contraceptives compared with those who had never done so,[1-4] or showed an increase in risk,[5] or identified a risk in specific sub-groups of users.[6-12] Potential identified risk factors, for which much of the evidence was conflicting, included current use,[10] duration of use,[7,11] age at first use,[6] duration of use before a first full-term pregnancy,[7,8] nulliparity,[9] high-dose preparations,[11] and family history of breast cancer.[12] It was also reported that use of oral contraceptives might lead to an accelerated presentation of breast cancer,[13] or an increased risk of invasive cancer.[4]

In response to these studies, the UK Committee on Safety of Medicines,[14] the FDA in the USA,[15] and the International Committee for Research in Reproduction[16] issued advice that the available evidence did not require a change in prescribing practice. This advice has not been subsequently changed, although patients should be informed of the possible small increase in risk of breast cancer, which has to be weighed against established benefits of therapy.[17]

A Collaborative Group on Hormonal Factors in Breast Cancer was set up to re-analyse all the worldwide epidemiological evidence on breast cancer risk and hormonal contraceptives. The group identified individual data on 53 297 women with breast cancer, and 100 239 controls (women without breast cancer) from 54 studies, and published a summary of their findings,[18] and a further detailed review.[19] They reported that women currently using oral contraceptives have a slight increase in the relative risk of breast cancer (1.24; 95% confidence intervals 1.15 to 1.33), and that this risk decreases after stopping use, and is no longer significant after 10 or more years. There was a weak trend towards an increase in risk with increasing duration of use. Thus, it appears that the risk of breast cancer

- increases soon after first exposure
- does not increase with duration of exposure
- returns to normal 10 years after cessation of exposure.[18]

Reviews[20,21] of major studies published between 1990 and 2000, including that of the Collaborative Group, have also indicated that, in general, there is some excess breast cancer risk in current or recent users of oral contraceptives, but that excess risk does not persist in the long term after cessation of oral contraceptive use, regardless of duration of use.

The Collaborative Group found that cancers diagnosed in those who had ever used hormonal contraceptives were clinically less advanced than in those who had never done so.[18] Further information is required on whether this is related to earlier diagnosis or a biological effect of the hormones. In addition, data on breast cancer mortality are required.

When analysed by *age at first use*, the risk was largest in those women who started use as teenagers. Because of the trend towards earlier use, further review of long-term data is required.[18] The most important risk factor is, however, the *age at which women discontinue* the contraceptive; the greater the age at stopping, the more breast cancers are diagnosed.[17]

There was no difference in risk with *parity* when comparing nulliparous women, parous women who began use of oral contraceptives before their first child, and parous women who began use of oral contraceptives after the birth of their first child.[18]

*Low-dose* oral contraceptives were not associated with a decreased risk of breast cancer.[18] When preparations were grouped according to oestrogen dose (<50 micrograms, 50 micrograms, and >50 micrograms), there was, if anything, a decrease in breast cancer risk with increasing dose among women who had stopped use 10 or more years before, largely due to a reduction in breast cancer risk in those who had used the highest dose preparations.

The Collaborative Group's analysis did not note any difference in risk according to *family history*.[18] However, a subsequent cohort study found an increased risk of breast cancer among women with a strong family history of the disease who used earlier formulations of oral contraceptives.[22] It is not known whether this risk applies to newer lower-dosage formulations, or whether it is correlated with mutations in the BRCA1 or BRCA2 genes. These findings are of concern because women with BRCA1 or BRCA2 mutations are often encouraged to take oral contraceptives to reduce their risk of ovarian cancer.

There are far fewer data on risk of breast cancer with **progestogen-only contraceptives**, which are less frequently used than combined preparations.

A WHO study published in 1991 indicated that, overall, depot medroxyprogesterone acetate did not increase the risk of breast cancer (relative risk compared with never users 1.21; 95% confidence intervals 0.96 to 1.53) and that risk did not increase with duration of use.[23] However, there appeared to be a slight increase in risk within the first 4 years of use, especially in women under 35 years of age. These findings agreed with those of a smaller study[24] in which women who had used depot medroxyprogesterone acetate for 2 years or longer before the age of 25 had a relative risk of 4.6. Pooled analysis of these 2 studies indicated that current or recent use was the key factor.[25] The relative risk of breast cancer in women who had used medroxyprogesterone acetate in the last 5 years was 2.0, and there was no increased risk in women who had ceased use more than 5 years previously, regardless of their duration of use.

The Collaborative Group on Hormonal Factors in Breast Cancer reported that there was some evidence of an increased risk of breast cancer for use of oral or injectable progestogens in the previous 5 years (relative risk 1.17), and no risk 10 or more years after stopping use.[18] These findings were broadly similar to those for combined preparations. As for combined preparations, the most important factor is the *age at discontinuation*. For women who stop by age 30 after 5 years use of a progestogen-only preparation there would be an estimated increase from 44 to 46 or 47 cases per 10 000 compared with those who have never used a hormonal contraceptive. For 5 years use stopping by age 40 there would be an estimated increase from 160 to 170 cases diagnosed in the following 10 years.[17]

1. Ellery C, *et al.* A case-control study of breast cancer in relation to the use of steroid contraceptive agents. *Med J Aust* 1986; **144:** 173–6.
2. Paul C, *et al.* Oral contraceptives and breast cancer: a national study. *BMJ* 1986; **293:** 723–6.
3. The Cancer and Steroid Hormone Study of the Centers for Disease Control and the National Institute of Child Health and Human Development. Oral-contraceptive use and the risk of breast cancer. *N Engl J Med* 1986; **315:** 405–11.
4. Stanford JL, *et al.* Oral contraceptives and breast cancer: results from an expanded case-control study. *Br J Cancer* 1989; **60:** 375–81.
5. Miller DR, *et al.* Breast cancer before age 45 and oral contraceptive use: new findings. *Am J Epidemiol* 1989; **129:** 269–80.
6. Pike MC, *et al.* Breast cancer in young women and use of oral contraceptives: possible modifying effect of formulation and age at use. *Lancet* 1983; **ii:** 926–30.
7. Meirik O, *et al.* Oral contraceptive use and breast cancer in young women: a joint national case-control study in Sweden and Norway. *Lancet* 1986; **ii:** 650–4.
8. McPherson K, *et al.* Early oral contraceptive use and breast cancer: results of another case-control study. *Br J Cancer* 1987; **56:** 653–60.
9. Meirik O, *et al.* Breast cancer and oral contraceptives: patterns of risk among parous and nulliparous women—further analysis of the Swedish-Norwegian material. *Contraception* 1989; **39:** 471–5.
10. Romieu I, *et al.* Prospective study of oral contraceptive use and risk of breast cancer in women. *J Natl Cancer Inst* 1989; **81:** 1313–21.
11. UK National Case-Control Study Group. Oral contraceptive use and breast cancer risk in young women. *Lancet* 1989; **i:** 973–82.
12. UK National Case-Control Study Group. Oral contraceptive use and breast cancer risk in young women: subgroup analyses. *Lancet* 1990; **335:** 1507–9.
13. Kay CR, Hannaford PC. Breast cancer and the pill—a further report from the Royal College of General Practitioners' oral contraception study. *Br J Cancer* 1988; **58:** 675–80.
14. Committee on Safety of Medicines. Oral contraceptives and carcinoma of the breast. *Current Problems 26* 1989.
15. Anonymous. Cancer risks of oral contraception. *Lancet* 1989; **i:** 84.
16. International Committee for Research in Reproduction. Oral contraceptives and breast cancer. *JAMA* 1989; **262:** 206–7.
17. Committee on Safety of Medicines/Medicines Control Agency. Oral contraceptives and breast cancer. *Current Problems* 1998; **24:** 2–3. Available at: http://www.mca.gov.uk/ourwork/monitorsafequalmed/currentproblems/volume24a.htm (accessed 06/07/04)
18. Collaborative Group on Hormonal Factors in Breast Cancer. Breast cancer and hormonal contraceptives: collaborative reanalysis of individual data on 53 297 women with breast cancer and 100 239 women without breast cancer from 54 epidemiological studies. *Lancet* 1996; **347:** 1713–27.
19. Collaborative Group on Hormonal Factors in Breast Cancer. Breast cancer and hormonal contraceptives: further results. *Contraception* 1996; **54** (suppl): 1S–106S.
20. La Vecchia C, *et al.* Oral contraceptives and cancer: a review of the evidence. *Drug Safety* 1996; **14:** 260–72.
21. La Vecchia C, *et al.* Oral contraceptives and cancer: an update. *Drug Safety* 2001; **24:** 741–54.
22. Grabrick DM, *et al.* Risk of breast cancer with oral contraceptive use in women with a family history of breast cancer. *JAMA* 2000; **284:** 1791–8.
23. WHO Collaborative Study of Neoplasia and Steroid Contraceptives. Breast cancer and depot-medroxyprogesterone acetate: a multinational study. *Lancet* 1991; **338:** 833–8.
24. Paul C, *et al.* Depot medroxyprogesterone (Depo-Provera) and risk of breast cancer. *BMJ* 1989; **299:** 759–62.
25. Skegg DCG, *et al.* Depot medroxyprogesterone acetate and breast cancer: a pooled analysis of the World Health Organization and New Zealand studies. *JAMA* 1995; **273:** 799–804.

CERVIX. It is often considered difficult to carry out satisfactory epidemiological studies on the relationship between hormonal contraceptives and cervical cancer because of the many known variables that can influence the development of this type of neoplasm. For example, sexual activity *per se,* and multiple sexual partners (both of the woman and her partner) increase the risk, while the use of other non-hormonal barrier methods of contraception may offer some protection against cervical neoplasia. Nevertheless, there have been some suggestions that the use of oral contraceptives may be associated with an increased risk.

Two UK cohort studies from the 1980s revealed an increased risk of cervical cancer in women receiving oral contraceptives that was shown to increase with increasing duration of use.[1,2]

In 1992, WHO reviewed[3] these cohort data, and data from 18 case-controlled studies carried out up to 1990. They concluded that use of oral contraceptives for more than 5 years was associated with a modest increase in the relative risk of cervical squamous cell carcinoma (in the order of 1.3 to 1.8). Additional potential risk factors included recent or current use and high oestrogen dose. Of known risk factors for cervical cancer, women with multiple sexual partners, genital infection, or high parity had enhanced risks associated with oral contraceptives.[3] A later review came to similar conclusions.[4]

Most cervical cancers are squamous cell carcinomas, but it has been proposed that oral contraceptive use might be a particular risk factor for the rarer adenocarcinoma of the cervix, the incidence of which has risen in younger women. Reviewing studies up to 1990, WHO concluded that data were insufficient to draw firm conclusions on links between oral contraceptives and the risk of cervical adenocarcinoma.[3] A case-controlled study from 1994 found an increased risk of adenocarcinoma of the cervix in users of oral contraceptives.[5] Any use of oral contraceptives was associated with an approximate doubling of risk, and use for more than 12 years was associated with a relative risk 4.4 times greater than that in women who never used an oral contraceptive. In 1996, a WHO study reported that the strength of the observed relationship for cervical adenocarcinomas and adenosquamous carcinomas and oral contraceptives was about the same as that for invasive squamous cell cervical carcinomas.[6]

Human papilloma virus (HPV) has a role in the aetiology of cervical cancer and women who are HPV positive and using oral contraceptives may be at increased risk of cervical neoplasm.[7,8] A pooled analysis of 8 case-control studies in women who tested positive for HPV DNA suggested risk of invasive squamous cervical cancer or carcinoma *in situ* was increased about threefold in those who used oral contraceptives for 5 years or more.[9]

Data on the risk of cervical cancer with **progestogen-only contraceptives** are limited. WHO have investigated any possible link between the use of medroxyprogesterone acetate as a long-acting injectable contraceptive and cervical neoplasia. Analysis showed a small non-significant elevated risk (1.11; 95% confidence interval 0.9 to 1.29), and no clear association with duration of use.[10]


1. Vessey MP, *et al.* Neoplasia of the cervix uteri and contraception: a possible adverse effect of the pill. *Lancet* 1983; **ii:** 930–4.
2. Beral V, *et al.* Oral contraceptive use, and malignancies of the genital tract: results from the Royal College of General Practitioners' oral contraception study. *Lancet* 1988; **ii:** 1331–5.
3. WHO. Oral contraceptives and neoplasia: report of a WHO scientific group. *WHO Tech Rep Ser 817* 1992.
4. Moodley J. Combined oral contraceptives and cervical cancer. *Curr Opin Obstet Gynecol* 2004; **16:** 27–9.
5. Ursin G, *et al.* Oral contraceptive use and adenocarcinoma of cervix. *Lancet* 1994; **344:** 1390–4.
6. Thomas DB, Ray RM. Oral contraceptives and invasive adenocarcinomas and adenosquamous carcinomas of the uterine cervix. *Am J Epidemiol* 1996; **144:** 281–9.
7. La Vecchia C, *et al.* Oral contraceptives and cancer: a review of the evidence. *Drug Safety* 1996; **14:** 260–72.
8. La Vecchia C, *et al.* Oral contraceptives and cancer: an update. *Drug Safety* 2001; **24:** 741–54.
9. Moreno V, *et al.* Effect of oral contraceptives on risk of cervical cancer in women with human papillomavirus infection: the IARC multicentric case-control study. *Lancet* 2002; **359:** 1085–92.
10. WHO Collaborative Study of Neoplasia and Steroid Contraceptives. Depot-medroxyprogesterone acetate (DMPA) and risk of invasive squamous cell cervical cancer. *Contraception* 1992; **45:** 299–312.


ENDOMETRIUM. It has been reliably demonstrated that **combined oral contraceptives** decrease the risk of endometrial cancer. WHO analysed data from case-control and cohort studies published up to 1990,[1] including data from the large Cancer and Steroid Hormone Study (CASH) in the USA,[2] and reported that there was a highly significant trend of decreasing risk of endometrial cancer with increasing duration of use of combined oral contraceptives. The reduction in risk was estimated to be 20% after 1 year and 50% after 4 years' use.[1] The protective effect was observed for endometrial cancer with and without squamous elements,[1,2] and was found to persist for at least 15 years after cessation of use.[2] More recent studies with longer term follow-up have indicated that the protection persists for at least 20 years.[3,4] Further follow-up is required to determine the true duration of protection although data from one study[4] suggest that any protective effect may no longer be present 30 years after stopping combined oral contraceptive use.

The results of the WHO Collaborative Study on Neoplasia and Steroid Contraceptives suggested that protection may be greater with preparations containing high-dose progestogen.[5] However, a more recent study found that risk of endometrial cancer was unrelated to progestogen potency of the oral contraceptive, although this study also reported no protective effect for less than 5 years' use.[6]

Unopposed menopausal oestrogen replacement therapy is known to increase the risk of endometrial cancer (see p.1537), and there is some evidence[3,6] that it reduces the protective effect of previous oral contraception.

There are limited data on the effect of **progestogen-only contraceptives** on the risk of endometrial cancer, although they would be expected to be protective. Results from the WHO Collaborative Study[7] suggest that depot medroxyprogesterone acetate reduced the risk of endometrial cancer; the estimated relative risk in users was 0.21. However, many of the women in this study received supplemental oestrogen to control menstrual irregularity, and were therefore technically taking a form of combined therapy.[8] There was some evidence that the protective effect of medroxyprogesterone acetate was greater in women who had not received oestrogen,[8] and this requires further study.


1. WHO. Oral contraceptives and neoplasia: report of a WHO scientific group. *WHO Tech Rep Ser 817* 1992.
2. The Cancer and Steroid Hormone Study of the Centers for Disease Control and the National Institute of Child Health and Human Development. Combination oral contraceptive use and the risk of endometrial cancer. *JAMA* 1987; **257:** 796–800.
3. Stanford JL, *et al.* Oral contraceptives and endometrial cancer: do other risk factors modify the association? *Int J Cancer* 1993; **54:** 243–8.
4. Weiderpass E, *et al.* Use of oral contraceptives and endometrial cancer risk (Sweden). *Cancer Causes Control* 1999; **10:** 277–84.
5. Rosenblatt KA, *et al.* Hormonal content of combined oral contraceptives in relation to the reduced risk of endometrial carcinoma. *Int J Cancer* 1991; **49:** 870–4.
6. Voigt LF, *et al.* Recency, duration, and progestin content of oral contraceptives in relation to the incidence of endometrial cancer. *Cancer Causes Control* 1994; **5:** 227–33.
7. WHO Collaborative Study of Neoplasia and Steroid Contraceptives. Depot-medroxyprogesterone acetate (DMPA) and risk of endometrial cancer. *Int J Cancer* 1991; **49:** 186–90.
8. Szarewski A, Guillebaud J. Safety of DMPA. *Lancet* 1991; **338:** 1157–8.


GASTROINTESTINAL TRACT. A link between female sex hormones and the risk of colorectal cancer has been postulated. Epidemiological studies have variously shown a possible increased risk of rectal cancer,[1] a possible decreased risk of colorectal cancer[2] in women ever having used oral contraceptives, and no association between past oral contraceptive use and colorectal cancer.[3] A meta-analysis,[4] which included these 3 studies, found a reduction in the risk of colorectal cancer for women who had ever used oral contraceptives. Duration of use was not related to risk reduction, but the effect was apparently stronger for recent contraceptive use although this was based on limited data. (See also under Hormone Replacement Therapy, p.1537.)


1. Kune GA, *et al.* Oral contraceptive use does not protect against large bowel cancer. *Contraception* 1990; **41:** 19–25.
2. Fernandez E, *et al.* Oral contraceptives, hormone replacement therapy and the risk of colorectal cancer. *Br J Cancer* 1996; **73:** 1431–5.
3. Troisi R, *et al.* Reproductive factors, oral contraceptive use, and risk of colorectal cancer. *Epidemiology* 1997; **8:** 75–9.
4. Fernandez E, *et al.* Oral contraceptives and colorectal cancer risk: a meta-analysis. *Br J Cancer* 2001; **84:** 722–7.


LIVER. The use of **combined oral contraceptives** has been rarely associated with liver tumours, both benign (hepatic adenomas and focal nodular hyperplasia)[1] and malignant (hepatocellular carcinoma).[1,2]

Early studies of *hepatic adenoma* found that risk increased with the duration of use of oral contraceptives, and appeared to be higher in women who had used preparations with a high oestrogen content.[1] There are also case reports of adenoma that has regressed after stopping oral contraceptive use.[3] However, a study[4] in the 1990s found no increase in risk associated with contraceptive use, and the authors considered that lower doses of oestrogens might explain the different findings. The association between oral contraceptive use and *focal nodular hyperplasia* has also been studied. One case-control study[4] found a slight increase in risk associated with use for 10 years or more. Another study[5] which followed a series of patients for approximately 2 years after diagnosis found no correlation between oral contraceptive use and lesion size or number, and no increase in lesion size in those patients who continued to use hormonal contraception.

*Hepatocellular carcinomas* are associated with hepatitis B, and are relatively common in countries where this is endemic but rare elsewhere. Case-control studies in populations at high risk for hepatocellular carcinoma suggest that the use of oral contraceptives does not significantly affect the risk, although long-term data are scanty.[6,7] In contrast, case-control studies in countries where the prevalence of hepatitis B is low have shown an increased risk of hepatocellular carcinoma among users of oral contraceptives, particularly after long-term use (reviewed by WHO[1] and La Vecchia[2,8]). However, because the malignancy is so rare, this increased risk may be negligible.[2] For example, there has been no increase in mortality from liver cancer in young women in the UK since the introduction and use of oral contraceptives.[9] Similar findings have been reported for the USA and Sweden.[10]

There are limited data specifically on **progestogen-only contraceptives**. Results from a WHO study[11] provided no evidence that use of medroxyprogesterone acetate as a long-acting injectable contraceptive altered the risk of developing liver cancer but the power of the study to detect small alterations in risk was low.


1. WHO. Oral contraceptives and neoplasia: report of a WHO scientific group. *WHO Tech Rep Ser 817* 1992.
2. La Vecchia C, *et al.* Oral contraceptives and cancer: a review of the evidence. *Drug Safety* 1996; **14:** 260–72.
3. Aseni P, *et al.* Rapid disappearance of hepatic adenoma after contraceptive withdrawal. *J Clin Gastroenterol* 2001; **33:** 234–6.
4. Heinemann LAJ, *et al.* Modern oral contraceptive use and benign liver tumors: the German benign liver tumor case—control study. *Eur J Contracept Reprod Health Care* 1998; **3:** 194–200.
5. Mathieu D, *et al.* Oral contraceptive use and focal nodular hyperplasia of the liver. *Gastroenterology* 2000; **118:** 560–4.
6. The WHO Collaborative Study of Neoplasia and Steroid Contraceptives. Combined oral contraceptives and liver cancer. *Int J Cancer* 1989; **43:** 254–9.
7. Kew MC, *et al.* Contraceptive steroids as a risk factor for hepatocellular carcinoma: a case/control study in South African black women. *Hepatology* 1990; **11:** 298–302.
8. La Vecchia C, *et al.* Oral contraceptives and cancer: an update. *Drug Safety* 2001; **24:** 741–54.
9. Mant JWF, Vessey MP. Trends in mortality from primary liver cancer in England and Wales 1975-1992: influence of oral contraceptives. *Br J Cancer* 1995; **72:** 800–3.
10. Waetjen LE, Grimes DA. Oral contraceptives and primary liver cancer: temporal trends in three countries. *Obstet Gynecol* 1996; **88:** 945–9.
11. Anonymous. Depot-medroxyprogesterone acetate (DMPA) and cancer: memorandum from a WHO meeting. *Bull WHO* 1986; **64:** 375–82.


OVARY. There is convincing evidence that **combined oral contraceptives** reduce the risk of ovarian cancer,[1,2] possibly as a function of their inhibition of ovulation. Relative risks for ovarian cancer have variously been reported as 0.4 to 0.8 in those who have ever used oral contraceptives, and decrease with increasing duration of use. There is evidence that there may be a delay of several years before the protective effect becomes apparent,[3] but that it persists for as long as 20 or 30 years after cessation of use.[3,4] The protective effect has been noted for both malignant and borderline malignant tumours, and for each of the major histological subtypes of epithelial ovarian cancer.

It has been suggested that newer lower-dose oestrogen preparations may be slightly less protective than higher-dose preparations.[5] The relative risk for use of high-dose preparations was 0.68, and for low-dose preparations was 0.81, but it was noted that this difference could have occurred by chance. A later study[4] reported that risk reduction was not affected by oral contraceptive formulation.

The protective effect against ovarian cancer may have significant implications for public health. For example, it was estimated that oral contraceptive use may have prevented nearly one-quarter of deaths expected to occur due to ovarian cancer in 1986 in women aged 54 years or less in England and Wales.[6]

There are few data on the effects of **progestogen-only contraceptives** on the risk of ovarian cancer. WHO have investigated the effect of depot medroxyprogesterone acetate on ovarian cancer, and found that it was not associated with either a decrease or increase in risk (relative risk 1.07; 95% confidence interval 0.6 to 1.8).[7] This is perhaps surprising since the preparation, like combined oral contraceptives, inhibits ovulation.


1. Franceschi S, *et al.* Pooled analysis of 3 European case-control studies of epithelial ovarian cancer III: oral contraceptive use. *Int J Cancer* 1991; **49:** 61–5.
2. Whittemore AS, *et al.* Characteristics relating to ovarian cancer risk: collaborative analysis of 12 US case-control studies II: invasive epithelial ovarian cancers in white women. *Am J Epidemiol* 1992; **136:** 1184–1203.
3. Rosenberg L, *et al.* A case-control study of oral contraceptive use and invasive epithelial ovarian cancer. *Am J Epidemiol* 1994; **139:** 654–61.
4. Ness RB, *et al.* Risk of ovarian cancer in relation to estrogen and progestin dose and use characteristics of oral contraceptives. *Am J Epidemiol* 2000; **152:** 233–41.
5. Rosenblatt KA, *et al.* High-dose and low-dose combined oral contraceptives: protection against epithelial ovarian cancer and the length of the protective effect. *Eur J Cancer* 1992; **28A:** 1872–6.
6. Villard-Mackintosh L, *et al.* The effects of oral contraceptives and parity on ovarian cancer trends in women under 55 years of age. *Br J Obstet Gynaecol* 1989; **96:** 783–8.
7. WHO Collaborative Study of Neoplasia and Steroid Contraceptives. Depot-medroxyprogesterone acetate (DMPA) and risk of epithelial ovarian cancer. *Int J Cancer* 1991; **49:** 191–5.


SKIN. Although there have been some suggestions of a possible association between the use of oral contraceptives and the development of malignant melanoma[1-3] most studies, including analyses of relatively large numbers of women suffering from malignant melanoma, found no such association with either current or prior use of oral contraceptive preparations.[4-9] A meta-analysis of 18 case-control studies confirmed the lack of association.[10]


1. Beral V, *et al.* Malignant melanoma and oral contraceptive use among women in California. *Br J Cancer* 1977; **36:** 804–9.
2. Lerner AB, *et al.* Effects of oral contraceptives and pregnancy on melanomas. *N Engl J Med* 1979; **301:** 47.
3. Beral V, *et al.* Oral contraceptive use and malignant melanoma in Australia. *Br J Cancer* 1984; **50:** 681–5.
4. Bain C, *et al.* Oral contraceptive use and malignant melanoma. *J Natl Cancer Inst* 1982; **68:** 537–9.
5. Helmrich SP, *et al.* Lack of an elevated risk of malignant melanoma in relation to oral contraceptive use. *J Natl Cancer Inst* 1984; **72:** 617–20.
6. Green A, Bain C. Hormonal factors and melanoma in women. *Med J Aust* 1985; **142:** 446–8.
7. Østerlind A, *et al.* The Danish case-control study of cutaneous malignant melanoma III: hormonal and reproductive factors in women. *Int J Cancer* 1988; **42:** 821–4.
8. Palmer JR, *et al.* Oral contraceptive use and risk of cutaneous malignant melanoma. *Cancer Causes Control* 1992; **3:** 547–54.
9. Holly EA, *et al.* Cutaneous melanoma in women III: reproductive factors and oral contraceptive use. *Am J Epidemiol* 1995; **141:** 943–50.
10. Gefeller O, *et al.* Cutaneous malignant melanoma in women and the role of oral contraceptives. *Br J Dermatol* 1998; **138:** 122–4.


**Ectopic pregnancy.** Pregnancies in users of oral (but not parenteral) **progestogen-only contraceptives** are more likely to be ectopic than are pregnancies occurring in the general population. Oral progestogen-only contraceptives do not reliably inhibit ovulation and therefore offer less protection against ectopic pregnancy than against intra-uterine pregnancy. Early references to this effect are cited below.[1-5] Since parenteral progestogen-only contraceptives provide reliable suppression of ovulation, like combined oral contraceptives, they protect against both ectopic pregnancies and functional ovarian cysts. In the case of the levonorgestrel-releasing progestogen-only implant the risk of ectopic pregnancy is believed to be reduced overall, but the proportion of ectopic to intra-uterine pregnancies is increased among the very few pregnancies that do occur.

A small number of cases of ectopic pregnancy following failure of **emergency contraception** (mainly with the Yuzpe regimen) have been reported.[6]


1. Bonnar J. Progestagen-only contraception and tubal pregnancies. *Lancet* 1974; **i:** 170–1.
2. Bonnar J. Progestogen-only contraceptive and tubal pregnancies. *BMJ* 1974; **1:** 287.
3. Huntington KM. Progestagen-only contraception and tubal pregnancies. *Lancet* 1974; **i:** 360.
4. Liukko P, Erkkola R. Low-dose progestogens and ectopic pregnancy. *BMJ* 1976; **2:** 1257.
5. Corcoran R, Howard R. Low-dose progestagens and ectopic pregnancy. *Lancet* 1977; **i:** 98–9.
6. Nielsen CL, Miller L. Ectopic gestation following emergency contraceptive pill administration. *Contraception* 2000; **62:** 275–6.


**Effects on carbohydrate metabolism.** The potential effects of oral contraceptives on carbohydrate metabolism are of concern because impaired glucose tolerance, hyperinsulinism, and insulin resistance contribute to atherogenesis and cardiovascular disease.[1] Early studies suggested that the prevalence of abnormal glucose tolerance in oral contraceptive users was increased from about 4 to 35%.[2] This decreased glucose tolerance was found to be related to oestrogen dose, particularly those greater than 75 micrograms daily, and to the type of progestogen. Marked hyperglycaemia has been associated with contraceptives containing high doses of oestrogen but is not seen with combined oral contraceptives used currently, which contain lower doses of oestrogen.[1] Progestogens have little effect on glucose tolerance, but are associated with hyperinsulinaemia. This effect is dose-dependent, and levonorgestrel has the most potent effect, with desogestrel, gestodene, and norethindrone reported to have less effect.[1] Combined oral contraceptives can also induce insulin resistance;[1] it is believed that the oestrogen is responsible and that the progestogen modifies this effect.[3]

Despite evidence of these effects, more recent studies of lower-dose preparations containing desogestrel, levonorgestrel, or norethindrone have found little or no effect on various measurements of carbohydrate metabolism.[4,5] Also, data from the Nurses' Health Study indicate that oral contraceptive use does not appear to increase the risk of developing type 2 diabetes mellitus.[6,7] However, a study in the USA of breast-feeding women of Hispanic origin who had experienced recent gestational diabetes, suggested that the use of progestogen-only, but not combined, contraceptives was associated with an increased risk of developing type 2 diabetes mellitus in this group.[8]


1. Crook D, Godsland I. Safety evaluation of modern oral contraceptives: effects on lipoprotein and carbohydrate metabolism. *Contraception* 1998; **57:** 189–201.
2. Hurel SJ, Taylor R. Drugs and glucose tolerance. *Adverse Drug React Bull* 1995; (Oct.): 659–62.
3. Godsland IF, *et al.* Insulin resistance, secretion, and metabolism in users of oral contraceptives. *J Clin Endocrinol Metab* 1992; **74:** 64–70.
4. Troisi RJ, *et al.* Oral contraceptive use and glucose metabolism in a national sample of women in the United States. *Am J Obstet Gynecol* 2000; **183:** 389–95.
5. Knopp RH, *et al.* Comparison of the lipoprotein, carbohydrate, and hemostatic effects of phasic oral contraceptives containing desogestrel or levonorgestrel. *Contraception* 2001; **63:** 1–11.
6. Rimm EB, *et al.* Oral contraceptive use and the risk of type 2 (non-insulin-dependent) diabetes mellitus in a large prospective study of women. *Diabetologia* 1992; **35:** 967–72.
7. Chasan-Taber L, *et al.* A prospective study of oral contraceptives and NIDDM among US women. *Diabetes Care* 1997; **20:** 330–5.
8. Kjos SL, *et al.* Contraception and the risk of type 2 diabetes mellitus in Latina women with prior gestational diabetes mellitus. *JAMA* 1998; **280:** 533–8.


**Effects on the cardiovascular system.** Soon after their introduction in the 1960s it became apparent that **combined oral contraceptives** were associated with an increased risk of cardiovascular effects including *hypertension, venous thromboembolism, myocardial infarction,* and *stroke.* Consequently, there are a number of contra-indications and precautions relating to their use in women with risk factors for cardiovascular disease (see under Precautions, below).

Changing patterns of use, and a progressive reduction in doses, have meant a continued need to evaluate the risks associated with oral contraceptives.

Current use of lower-dose combined oral contraceptives (less than 50 micrograms oestrogen) increases blood pressure in many women, and also results in a small but significant increased risk of venous thromboembolism. Any increased risk of myocardial infarction and stroke is low in women aged less than 35 years who do not smoke and who do not have pre-existing hypertension. Further details of these adverse effects are covered in the sections below.

The effect of progestogens on the cardiovascular risk profile of oral contraceptives has not been established. Some of the newer progestogens have been reported to have more favourable effects on plasma lipids (see Effects on Lipids, below) and there is some suggestion that they may have a lower risk of myocardial infarction, but there are insufficient data to confirm or refute this. Recently, however, it has been reported that desogestrel and gestodene are associated with 1.5 to 2 times the risk of venous thromboembolism than older progestogens.

The Nurses' Health Study found no association between ever having used oral contraceptives and death from cardiovascular disease.[1] The Royal College of General Practitioners' study reported an increase in death from cerebrovascular disease with current or recent (within 10 years) use of oral contraceptives, but not for past use (greater than 10 years).[2]

Some general reviews are cited below.[3-7]


1. Colditz GA, *et al.* Oral contraceptive use and mortality during 12 years of follow-up: the Nurses' Health Study. *Ann Intern Med* 1994; **120:** 821–6.
2. Beral V, *et al.* Mortality associated with oral contraceptive use: 25 year follow up of cohort of 46 000 women from Royal College of General Practitioners' oral contraception study. *BMJ* 1999; **318:** 96–100.
3. WHO. WHO Scientific Group Meeting on Cardiovascular Disease and Steroid Hormone Contraceptive: summary of conclusions. *Wkly Epidem Rec* 1997; **72:** 361–3.
4. Chasan-Taber L, Stampfer MJ. Epidemiology of oral contraceptives and cardiovascular disease. *Ann Intern Med* 1998; **128:** 467–77.
5. WHO. Cardiovascular disease and steroid hormone contraception. *WHO Tech Rep Ser 877* 1998.
6. Hannaford P. Cardiovascular events associated with different combined oral contraceptives: a review of current data. *Drug Safety* 2000; **22:** 361–71.
7. Godsland IF, *et al.* Occlusive vascular diseases in oral contraceptive users: epidemiology, pathology and mechanisms. *Drugs* 2000; **60:** 721–869.


HYPERTENSION. In a one-year prospective multicentre study[1] involving 704 women under the age of 35 using a **combined oral contraceptive** containing levonorgestrel 250 micrograms and ethinylestradiol 50 micrograms and 703 women using a non-hormonal intra-uterine contraceptive device, those using the oral contraceptive developed higher systolic and diastolic blood pressures (systolic pressures were 3.6 to 5.0 mmHg higher, diastolic pressures were 1.9 to 2.7 mmHg higher). Only 4 women receiving oral contraceptives developed hypertension. A similar increase in blood pressure was noted in a study[2] involving 222 users of combined oral contraceptives containing 30 micrograms ethinylestradiol. There was a greater increase in blood pressure for those preparations containing 250 micrograms levonorgestrel than those containing 150 micrograms levonorgestrel.

More recently, data from the Nurses' Health Study[3] showed an increased risk (relative risk 1.8) for the development of hypertension in women taking lower-dose combined oral contraceptives. Increasing doses of progestogen were positively associated with hypertension, and the lowest risk occurred in women receiving triphasic preparations, which have the lowest total dose of progestogen. A UK study[4] found a small increase in blood pressure of 2.3/1.6 mmHg associated with the use of combined oral contraceptives. In this study, oral **progestogen-only contraceptives** were not associated with an increase in blood pressure.


1. WHO Task Force on Oral Contraceptives. The WHO multicentre trial of the vasopressor effects of combined oral contraceptives 1: comparisons with IUD. *Contraception* 1989; **40:** 129–45.
2. Khaw K-T, Peart WS. Blood pressure and contraceptive use. *BMJ* 1982; **285:** 403–7.
3. Chasan-Taber L, *et al.* Prospective study of oral contraceptives and hypertension among women in the United States. *Circulation* 1996; **94:** 483–9.
4. Dong W, *et al.* Blood pressure in women using oral contraceptives: results from the Health Survey for England 1994. *J Hypertens* 1997; **15:** 1063–8.


MYOCARDIAL INFARCTION. Case-control studies from the 1970s and early 1980s revealed an increased risk of acute myocardial infarction in users of oral contraceptives (generally of the high-dose type) relative to those never having used them.[1,2] Several large cohort studies have provided similar findings.[3-6] Among current users the reported[1-3,5,6] relative risk of myocardial infarction has varied between about 1.8 and 6.4, whereas in women having used oral contraceptives in the past the reported[2-5] relative risk has varied between about 0.8 and 2.5. Women who *smoke* while using oral contraceptives are at a greatly increased risk,[1,5,7] those smoking more than 15 to 25 cigarettes per day having at least a twentyfold increased risk of myocardial infarction compared with non-smoking non-oral contraceptive users.[1,5]

More recently, data on combined oral contraceptives that have lower oestrogen doses have revealed at most small and non-significant increases in risk of acute myocardial infarction associated with oral contraceptive use,[8-11] although case-control studies have suggested that again, there may be a greatly increased risk in women who smoke more than 20 to 25 cigarettes per day.[10,12]

These studies have principally been from the USA or the UK. The WHO Collaborative Study of Cardiovascular Disease and Steroid Hormone Contraception has reported the findings of an international multicentre case-control study.[13] The overall odds ratio for acute myocardial infarction in current users of combined oral contraceptives was 5.01 in Europe and 4.78 in Africa, Asia, and Latin America. This increase in risk reflected use in women who had coexistent risk factors such as smoking, and who had not had their blood pressure checked before use. Thus, when the background incidence of acute myocardial infarction is taken into account, use of combined oral contraceptives in non-smoking women aged less than 35 years is associated with an excess of 3 per million women-years, and this is likely to be lower in those women who have their blood pressure screened before and during use. However, in older women who smoke, the excess risk associated with the use of combined oral contraceptives is substantial (400 per million women-years). There was no increase in risk associated with past use of oral contraceptives irrespective of duration of use.

There has been interest in the effect of different progestogen components on the risk of myocardial infarction. Limited data from the WHO study[13] and from the USA[14] and the UK[10] suggest no difference in risk between desogestrel or gestodene compared with levonorgestrel. Analysis of European data[15] suggests a reduction in risk with gestodene- and desogestrel-containing products compared with other progestogens (0.28; 95% confidence intervals 0.09 to 0.86). A WHO Scientific Group meeting concluded that available data did not allow the conclusion that risk of myocardial infarction is related to progestogen type.[16] Moreover, there is probably a small increased risk of venous thromboembolism associated with desogestrel or gestodene (see below).


1. Shapiro S, *et al.* Oral-contraceptive use in relation to myocardial infarction. *Lancet* 1979; **i:** 743–7.
2. Slone D, *et al.* Risk of myocardial infarction in relation to current and discontinued use of oral contraceptives. *N Engl J Med* 1981; **305:** 420–4.
3. Royal College of General Practitioners' Oral Contraception Study. Further analyses of mortality in oral contraceptive users. *Lancet* 1981; **i:** 541–6.
4. Stampfer MJ, *et al.* A prospective study of past use of oral contraceptive agents and risk of cardiovascular diseases. *N Engl J Med* 1988; **319:** 1313–17.
5. Croft P, Hannaford PC. Risk factors for acute myocardial infarction in women: evidence from the Royal College of General Practitioners' oral contraception study. *BMJ* 1989; **298:** 165–8.
6. Vessey MP, *et al.* Mortality among oral contraceptive users: 20 year follow up of women in a cohort study. *BMJ* 1989; **299:** 1487–91.
7. Goldbaum GM, *et al.* The relative impact of smoking and oral contraceptive use on women in the United States. *JAMA* 1987; **258:** 1339–42.
8. Thorogood M, *et al.* Is oral contraceptive use still associated with an increased risk of fatal myocardial infarction? Report of a case-control study. *Br J Obstet Gynaecol* 1991; **98:** 1245–53.
9. Sidney S, *et al.* Myocardial infarction and use of low-dose oral contraceptives: a pooled analysis of 2 US studies. *Circulation* 1998; **98:** 1058–63.
10. Dunn N, *et al.* Oral contraceptives and myocardial infarction: results of the MICA case-control study. *BMJ* 1999; **318:** 1579–83.
11. Tanis BC, *et al.* Oral contraceptives and the risk of myocardial infarction. *N Engl J Med* 2001; **345:** 1787–93.
12. Rosenberg L, *et al.* Low-dose oral contraceptive use and the risk of myocardial infarction. *Arch Intern Med* 2001; **161:** 1065–70.
13. WHO Collaborative Study of Cardiovascular Disease and Steroid Hormone Contraception. Acute myocardial infarction and combined oral contraceptives: results of an international multicentre case-control study. *Lancet* 1997; **349:** 1202–9.
14. Jick H, *et al.* Risk of acute myocardial infarction and low-dose combined oral contraceptives. *Lancet* 1996; **347:** 627–8.
15. Lewis MA, *et al.* The use of oral contraceptives and the occurrence of acute myocardial infarction in young women: results from the transnational study on oral contraceptives and the health of young women. *Contraception* 1997; **56:** 129–40.
16. WHO. WHO Scientific Group Meeting on Cardiovascular Disease and Steroid Hormone Contraceptives: summary of conclusions. *Wkly Epidem Rec* 1997; **72:** 361–3.


STROKE. Current use of **combined oral contraceptives** has been associated with an increased risk of stroke, with most data relating to older high-dose oestrogen preparations. In general this association has been strongest for ischaemic stroke, and relatively weak for haemorrhagic stroke.[1] A Danish study found that low-dose oral contraceptives (30 to 40 micrograms of oestrogen) were associated with a lower risk of cerebral thromboembolism than preparations containing 50 micrograms oestrogen.[2]

Data on 2198 cases of stroke (haemorrhagic, ischaemic, and unclassified) and 6086 controls have been reported from the WHO Collaborative Study of Cardiovascular Disease and Steroid Hormone Contraception.[3,4] For all strokes combined, odds ratios for the current use of lower-dose (less than 50 micrograms oestrogen) and higher-dose preparations were, respectively, 1.41 (95% confidence intervals 0.90 to 2.20) and 2.71 (1.70 to 4.32) in Europe, and 1.86 (1.49 to 2.33) and 1.92 (1.48 to 2.50) in Africa, Asia, and Latin America. In Europe, it was estimated that the incidence rate of stroke in women aged 20 to 44 years was 4.8 per 100 000 women-years, and that this was increased to 6.7 per 100 000 in users of lower-dose preparations and 12.9 per 100 000 in users of higher-dose preparations.[3]

The risk of haemorrhagic stroke was significant only in women aged greater than 35 years, those who had a history of hypertension, and those who were current smokers.[3]

The overall odds ratio for ischaemic stroke was 2.99 (1.65 to 5.40) in Europe and 2.93 (2.15 to 4.00) in Africa, Asia, and Latin America.[4] Odds ratios were lower in women aged less than 35 years, those who did not smoke, those with no history of hypertension, and those who reported that their blood pressure had been checked before use. Duration of current use and past use were unrelated to risk.[4] Similar findings to those of the WHO study have also been published from the USA.[5] Low-dose preparations (less than 50 micrograms oestrogen) were associated with a non-significant increase in ischaemic stroke; the odds ratio was 1.18 (0.54 to 2.59); a later meta-analysis considered the association between low-dose combined oral contraceptives and stroke to be tenuous at best, and possibly non-existent.[6]

A meta-analysis[7] of studies of ischaemic stroke found that there was an overall increased risk associated with the current use of oral contraceptives. However, the risk was less elevated with lower oestrogen doses, and in studies that controlled for smoking and hypertension.

As regards the effect of the type of progestogen on risk of stroke, one case-control study[8] reported that there was no significant difference in risk of ischaemic stroke between low-dose oral contraceptives containing second generation progestogens and those containing desogestrel, gestodene, or norgestimate. However, another study[9] found that levonorgestrel- or norgestimate-containing preparations were associated with a higher risk of cerebral thrombosis than preparations containing desogestrel or gestodene. A reanalysis of the WHO data led to the cautious conclusion that the risk for stroke between second and third generation progestogens was similar,[10] and this was also supported by analysis of the General Practice Research Database.[11] A meta-analysis[7] also found no significant difference between progestogen generations in the risk of ischaemic stroke.

Data for **progestogen-only contraceptives** are limited. The Danish study reported no increase in cerebral thromboembolic attacks in users of oral progestogen-only contraceptives; the odds ratio was 0.9 (0.4 to 2.4).[2]


1. Vessey MP, *et al.* Oral contraceptives and stroke: findings in a large prospective study. *BMJ* 1984; **289:** 530–1.
2. Lidegaard Ø. Oral contraception and risk of a cerebral thromboembolic attack: results of a case-control study. *BMJ* 1993; **306:** 956–63.
3. WHO Collaborative Study of Cardiovascular Disease and Steroid Hormone Contraception. Haemorrhagic stroke, overall stroke risk, and combined oral contraceptives: results of an international, multicentre, case-control study. *Lancet* 1996; **348:** 505–10.
4. WHO Collaborative Study of Cardiovascular Disease and Steroid Hormone Contraception. Ischaemic stroke and combined oral contraceptives: results of an international, multicentre, case-control study. *Lancet* 1996; **348:** 498–505.
5. Petitti DB, *et al.* Stroke in users of low-dose oral contraceptives. *N Engl J Med* 1996; **335:** 8–15.
6. Chan W-S, *et al.* Risk of stroke in women exposed to low-dose oral contraceptives: a critical evaluation of the evidence. *Arch Intern Med* 2004; **164:** 741–7.
7. Gillum LA, *et al.* Ischemic stroke risk with oral contraceptives: a meta-analysis. *JAMA* 2000; **284:** 72–8.
8. Heinemann LAJ, *et al.* Case-control study of oral contraceptives and risk of thromboembolic stroke: results from international study on oral contraceptives and health of young women. *BMJ* 1997; **315:** 1502–4.
9. Lidegaard Ø, Kreiner S. Cerebral thrombosis and oral contraceptives: a case-control study. *Contraception* 1998; **57:** 303–14.
10. Poulter NR, *et al.* Effect on stroke of different progestagens in low oestrogen dose oral contraceptives. *Lancet* 1999; **354:** 301–2.
11. Jick SS, *et al.* Risk of idiopathic cerebral haemorrhage in women on oral contraceptives with differing progestagen components. *Lancet* 1999; **354:** 302–3.


VENOUS THROMBOEMBOLISM. Use of **combined oral contraceptives** has long been known to be associated with an increased risk of venous thromboembolic events, particularly deep-vein thrombosis and pulmonary embolism. This increased risk applies both to idiopathic events and events associated with surgery or trauma, is limited to current users and is probably highest in the first year of use. Most early data relate to high-dose combined preparations, and it has been suggested by some studies,[1] but not others,[2,3] that preparations containing lower doses of oestrogen may be associated with a lower risk. More recently, reports have identified an increased risk of cerebral-vein thrombosis with oral contraceptives.[4,5]

The WHO Collaborative Study of Cardiovascular Disease and Steroid Hormone Contraception reported data from over 10 times more cases than any previous study.[6] The increased risk of idiopathic deep-vein thrombosis and/or pulmonary embolism associated with current use of combined oral contraceptives was 4.15 (95% confidence intervals 3.09 to 5.57) in Europe and 3.25 (2.59 to 4.08) in Africa, Asia, and Latin America. The increased risk was apparent within 4 months of starting use, was unaffected by duration of use, and had disappeared within 3 months of stopping use. Risk was unaffected by age, hypertension, or smoking (in contrast to myocardial infarction, see above), but was increased in those with a body-mass index greater than 25 kg/m$^2$ and in those with a history of hypertension of pregnancy. Of preparations containing progestogens of the norethisterone or norgestrel type, risk was non-significantly less with lower-dose oestrogen than with high-dose oestrogen.

The progestogen component has generally been considered to be unrelated to thromboembolic events; therefore, it came as a surprise when WHO found a higher risk in combined oral contraceptives containing *desogestrel* or *gestodene* than in those containing older progestogens.[6] These risk data were the subject of a separate report,[7] and were subsequently confirmed by 3 further case-control studies.[8-10] The increased risk varied from 4.8 to 9.1 compared with non-users, and was found to be 1.5 to 2.6 times higher than for preparations containing levonorgestrel or other progestogens. The incidence of venous thromboembolic disease has been estimated to be 25 per 100 000 users per year for desogestrel- and gestodene-containing products and 15 per 100 000 users per year for products containing low-dose oestrogen with other progestogens, compared with 5 per 100 000 per year for non-users. The risk was especially high in women with the factor V Leiden mutation,[9] who are at increased risk of thrombosis, but screening to exclude these women from using oral contraceptives was not considered necessary.[11,12] Despite much debate about possible bias and confounding in these results,[13,14] and the ambiguous or contradictory results of subsequent studies,[15-17] many sources seem now to agree with the 1997 conclusion of a WHO scientific group meeting[18] that there is a modestly increased risk of venous thromboembolism associated with the use of products containing desogestrel or gestodene, compared with levonorgestrel. It is unclear to what extent products containing *cyproterone* are associated with increased risk.[19,20]

Regulatory agencies have reacted in different ways to these data. The UK Committee on Safety of Medicines has advised caution in prescribing of these products (see Cardiovascular Disease under Precautions, below), as have some other European authorities.

The mechanism behind differences in thrombotic potential is not known, but there is evidence that oral contraceptives may increase concentrations of prothrombin and factor VIII, and induce a resistance to the blood's natural anticoagulation system.[12] These effects may be greater with products containing desogestrel and gestodene compared with older progestogens.[12]


1. Vessey M, *et al.* Oral contraceptives and venous thromboembolism: findings in a large prospective study. *BMJ* 1986; **292:** 526.
2. Kierkegaard A. Deep vein thrombosis and the oestrogen content in oral contraceptives—an epidemiological analysis. *Contraception* 1985; **31:** 29–41.
3. Helmrich SP, *et al.* Venous thromboembolism in relation to oral contraceptive use. *Obstet Gynecol* 1987; **69:** 91–5.
4. de Bruijn SFTM, *et al.* Case-control study of risk of cerebral sinus thrombosis in oral contraceptive users and in carriers of hereditary prothrombotic conditions. *BMJ* 1998; **316:** 589–92. Correction. *ibid.*: 822.
5. Martinelli I, *et al.* High risk of cerebral-vein thrombosis in carriers of a prothrombin-gene mutation and in users of oral contraceptives. *N Engl J Med* 1998; **338:** 1793–7.
6. WHO Collaborative Study Group. Venous thromboembolic disease and combined oral contraceptives: results of international multicentre case-control study. *Lancet* 1995; **346:** 1575–82.
7. WHO Collaborative Study Group. Effect of different progestagens in low oestrogen oral contraceptives on venous thromboembolic disease. *Lancet* 1995; **346:** 1582–8.
8. Jick H, *et al.* Risk of idiopathic cardiovascular death and nonfatal venous thromboembolism in women using oral contraceptives with differing progestagen components. *Lancet* 1995; **346:** 1589–93.
9. Bloemenkamp KWM, *et al.* Enhancement by factor V Leiden mutation of risk of deep-vein thrombosis associated with oral contraceptives containing a third-generation progestagen. *Lancet* 1995; **346:** 1593–6.
10. Spitzer WO, *et al.* Third generation oral contraceptives and risk of venous thromboembolic disorders: an international case-control study. *BMJ* 1996; **312:** 83–8.
11. Vandenbroucke JP, *et al.* Factor V Leiden: should we screen oral contraceptive users and pregnant women? *BMJ* 1996; **313:** 1127–30.
12. Vandenbroucke JP, *et al.* Oral contraceptives and the risk of venous thrombosis. *N Engl J Med* 2001; **344:** 1527–35.
13. Lewis MA, *et al.* The increased risk of venous thromboembolism and the use of third generation progestagens: role of bias in observational research. *Contraception* 1996; **54:** 5–13.
14. Farley TMM, *et al.* Oral contraceptives and thrombotic diseases: impact of new epidemiologic studies. *Contraception* 1996; **54:** 193–5.
15. Farmer RDT, *et al.* Population-based study of risk of venous thromboembolism associated with various oral contraceptives. *Lancet* 1997; **349:** 83–8.
16. Farmer RDT, *et al.* Effect of 1995 pill scare on rates of venous thromboembolism among women taking combined oral contraceptives: analysis of General Practice Research Database. *BMJ* 2000; **321:** 477–9.
17. Jick H, *et al.* Risk of venous thromboembolism among users of third generation oral contraceptives compared with users of oral contraceptives with levonorgestrel before and after 1995: cohort and case-control analysis. *BMJ* 2000; **321:** 1190–5. Correction. *ibid.* 2001; **322:** 28.
18. WHO. WHO Scientific Group Meeting on Cardiovascular Disease and Steroid Hormone Contraceptives: summary of conclusions. *Wkly Epidem Rec* 1997; **72:** 361–3.
19. Savage R. Venous thromboembolism with Diane 35™ and Estelle 35™. Available at: http://www.medsafe.govt.nz/Profs/PUarticles/VTEwithCPA.htm (accessed 08/07/02)
20. Spitzer WO. Cyproterone acetate with ethinylestradiol as a risk factor for venous thromboembolism: an epidemiological evaluation. *J Obstet Gynaecol Can* 2003; **25:** 1011–18.


**Effects on the ears.** In the Royal College of General Practitioners' study of oral contraception in the UK,[1] by 1981 there had been 13 cases of newly occurring otosclerosis in each of the groups of oral contraceptive users (101 985 woman-years) and controls (146 534 woman-years); this showed a non-significant relative risk of 1.29. Although, by analogy with pregnancy, it may be prudent to suppose that oral contraceptives could exacerbate pre-existing otosclerosis, the data do not support the view that the condition is associated with their use.


1. Kay CR, Wingrave SJ. Oral contraceptives and otosclerosis. *BMJ* 1984; **288:** 1164.


**Effects on the eyes.** Analysis of data from 2 large UK cohort studies suggested that oral contraceptive use does not increase the risk of eye disease, with the possible exception of retinal vascular lesions.[1]


1. Vessey MP, *et al.* Oral contraception and eye disease: findings in two large cohort studies. *Br J Ophthalmol* 1998; **82:** 538–42.


**Effects on fertility.** Following the discontinuation of hormonal contraceptives some patients may experience amenorrhoea, anovulation, and infertility. This infertility, however, has been shown by most studies to be only temporary.

Data from the Oxford Family Planning Association study[1] have indicated that impairment of fertility after oral contraceptives was only very slight and short-lived in women who had previously had a baby. In nulliparous women aged 25 to 29 years impairment of fertility was more severe but the effect had almost entirely disappeared after 48 months. In nulliparous women aged 30 to 34 years there was even more impairment of fertility but this was not permanent as by 72 months after stopping oral contraceptive use the numbers of women who had not conceived were similar to a group who had previously used non-hormonal methods of contraception. In contrast to women using intra-uterine devices, in whom long-term use was associated with greater impairment of fertility than short-term (less than 42 months) use, there appears to be no association between fertility and duration of oral contraceptive use.[2]

After injectable progestogen-only contraceptives, smaller studies have again indicated that there are no long-lasting effects on fertility;[3] but it has also been suggested that a return to ovulation occurs significantly earlier in prior norethisterone enantate users than in medroxyprogesterone users.[4]

Infertility may also be related to the presence of pelvic inflammatory disease; for further details concerning the role of oral contraceptives in this disorder, see Pelvic Inflammatory Disease, below.


1. Anonymous. "Pill" use appears to impair fertility in a certain group of women. *Pharm J* 1986; **236:** 227.
2. Doll H, *et al.* Return of fertility in nulliparous women after discontinuation of the intrauterine device: comparison with women discontinuing other methods of contraception. *Br J Obstet Gynaecol* 2001; **108:** 304–14.
3. Fotherby K, *et al.* Return of ovulation and fertility in women using norethisterone enanthate. *Contraception* 1984; **29:** 447–55.
4. Garza-Flores J, *et al.* Return to ovulation following the use of long-acting injectable contraceptives: a comparative study. *Contraception* 1985; **31:** 361–6.


**Effects on the gallbladder.** Data from the Royal College of General Practitioners' (RCGP) oral contraception study accumulated up to December 1979 revealed no overall increased risk of gallbladder disease in the long-term, despite the indications of earlier data and other studies relating to short-term use.[1] Further studies[2,3] have identified an increased risk of gallbladder disease in oral contraceptive users under the age of 30 or 20 respectively. The latest data from the RCGP study show an increase in risk of mild hepatitis during the first 4 years of oral contraceptive use, possibly reflecting gallstone-associated cholestasis.[4] This risk then decreased to less than that seen in women who had never used oral contraceptives.


1. Wingrave SJ, Kay CR. Oral contraceptives and gallbladder disease: Royal College of General Practitioners' oral contraception study. *Lancet* 1982; **ii:** 957–9.
2. Scragg RKR, *et al.* Oral contraceptives, pregnancy, and endogenous oestrogen in gall stone disease—a case-control study. *BMJ* 1984; **288:** 1795–9.
3. Strom BL, *et al.* Oral contraceptives and other risk factors for gallbladder disease. *Clin Pharmacol Ther* 1986; **39:** 335–41.
4. Hannaford PC, *et al.* Combined oral contraceptives and liver disease. *Contraception* 1997; **55:** 145–51.


**Effects on the gastrointestinal tract.** Several studies,[1-3] and a meta-analysis,[4] have shown a weak association between oral contraceptive use and the onset of Crohn's disease or ulcerative colitis. However, the suggestion that oral contraceptives have an aetiological role in chronic inflammatory bowel disease cannot be regarded as established.

The rate of relapse of Crohn's disease in women taking oral contraceptives has also been studied. Although one study[5] reported an increased risk of relapse in women who had taken oral contraceptives in the past, both this study and another prospective cohort study[6] found no increase in risk in current users. These results may have been influenced by smoking, or changes in oestrogen dose and progestogen content.


1. Rhodes JM, *et al.* Colonic Crohn's disease and use of oral contraception. *BMJ* 1984; **288:** 595–6.
2. Entrican JH, Sircus W. Chronic inflammatory bowel disease, cigarette smoking, and use of oral contraceptives. *BMJ* 1986; **292:** 1464.
3. Corrao G, *et al.* Risk of inflammatory bowel disease attributable to smoking, oral contraception and breastfeeding in Italy: a nationwide case-control study. *Int J Epidemiol* 1998; **27:** 397–404.
4. Godet PG, *et al.* Meta-analysis of the role of oral contraceptive agents in inflammatory bowel disease. *Gut* 1995; **37:** 668–73.
5. Timmer A, *et al.* Oral contraceptive use and smoking are risk factors for relapse in Crohn's disease. *Gastroenterology* 1998; **114:** 1143–50.
6. Cosnes J, *et al.* Oral contraceptive use and the clinical course of Crohn's disease: a prospective cohort study. *Gut* 1999; **45:** 218–22.


**Effects on lipids.** Combined oral contraceptives have been reported to be associated with an excess risk of various adverse cardiovascular events (see above). Because other epidemiological evidence suggests that the composition of blood lipids may be one of several factors involved in the aetiology of some of these disorders, many workers have investigated the biochemical profiles of women taking various formulations of oral contraceptives. Results have often been conflicting as the net effect is the result of opposing actions of the oestrogen and the progestogen components, and depends on the ratio between these. In general, the oestrogen component increases triglycerides, but decreases low-density lipoproteins, whereas the progestogen component tends to decrease high-density lipoproteins and increase low-density lipoproteins, particularly if it is androgenic (19-nortestosterone-derived progestogens). Newer non-androgenic progestogens such as desogestrel and gestodene appear to have a less detrimental effect on serum lipids. However, the contribution of these lipid changes to the incidence of cardiovascular disease in oral contraceptive users is uncertain. In particular, contrary to expectations, desogestrel and gestodene appear to be associated with a higher risk of venous thromboembolism than older progestogens (see above).

Some references to the effects of various oral contraceptives on serum lipid profiles are given below.[1,2]

For further details concerning the proposed role of the various serum lipids and subfractions in the aetiology of cardiovascular disease, see Hyperlipidaemias, p.823.

For reports of pancreatitis secondary to hyperlipidaemia associated with the use of combined oral contraceptives, see below.


1. Crook D, Godsland I. Safety evaluation of modern oral contraceptives: effects on lipoprotein and carbohydrate metabolism. *Contraception* 1998; **57:** 189–201. Correction. *ibid.*: 420.
2. Knopp RH, *et al.* Comparison of the lipoprotein, carbohydrate, and hemostatic effects of phasic oral contraceptives containing desogestrel or levonorgestrel. *Contraception* 2001; **63:** 1–11.


**Effects on the liver.** The use of combined oral contraceptives has been rarely associated with the benign liver tumours, hepatic adenoma and focal nodular hyperplasia (see under Carcinogenicity, above).

**Effects on mental state.** A review of drug-induced mental depression concluded that since mood disturbance is common during the menstrual cycle, and particularly in the premenstrual phase, it is difficult to evaluate the possible association of depression with oral contraceptives.[1] The evidence, however, suggests that the incidence is a little greater than with control subjects but it is still only 4 to 6%. A later review[2] came to a similar conclusion that in a number of surveys in which oral contraceptives have been compared with either placebo or an intra-uterine device no increase in depression or other nervous symptoms has been found.

Cohort studies of injectable[3] and implantable[4] progestogen-only contraceptives found no overall change in depressive symptom score. A small increase in depressive score noted at the 2-year follow-up of implant users was found to occur in women who also experienced a decrease in relationship satisfaction, which the authors concluded was independent of contraceptive use.


1. Tyrer PJ. Drug-induced depression. *Prescribers' J* 1981; **21:** 237–42.
2. King DJ. Drug-induced psychiatric syndromes. *Prescribers' J* 1986; **26:** 50–8.
3. Westhoff C, *et al.* Depressive symptoms and Depo-Provera®. *Contraception* 1998; **57:** 237–40.
4. Westhoff C, *et al.* Depressive symptoms and Norplant® contraceptive implants. *Contraception* 1998; **57:** 241–5.


**Effects on the musculoskeletal system.** BONE DENSITY. Combined oral contraceptives are generally considered not to have a detrimental effect on bone mineral density, and may exert a positive effect although data are scanty.[1] Studies of oral contraceptive exposure in pre- and postmenopausal women have found improvement, as well as no change, in bone mineral density compared with no exposure.[1,2] However, a decrease in bone mineral density in premenopausal women has also been reported.[3] In a case-control study, oral contraceptive use late in reproductive life appeared to reduce the risk of hip fracture.[4]

In contrast, users of the progestogen-only contraceptive medroxyprogesterone acetate may have reductions in bone mineral density, although these appear to be reversible on discontinuation of the drug.[5] A small study has prospectively analysed the effect of combined oral contraceptives and parenteral progestogen-only contraceptives on bone mass in adolescents.[6] After 1 year of use, bone mineral density decreased by 1.5% in users of depot medroxyprogesterone acetate, but increased in users of combined oral contraceptives or levonorgestrel implants, and in control subjects. Some cross-sectional studies have reported no significant effect of medroxyprogesterone acetate on bone mineral density.[7,8] Others,[9-11] however, have reported reductions in bone mineral density, and that younger women and long-term users may be most affected. Whether this influences fracture risk has not been determined.


1. Cromer BA. Effects of hormonal contraceptives on bone mineral density. *Drug Safety* 1999; **20:** 213–22.
2. Pasco JA, *et al.* Oral contraceptives and bone mineral density: a population-based study. *Am J Obstet Gynecol* 2000; **182:** 265–9.
3. Prior JC, *et al.* Oral contraceptive use and bone mineral density in premenopausal women: cross-sectional, population-based data from the Canadian Multicentre Osteoporosis Study. *Can Med Assoc J* 2001; **165:** 1023–9.
4. Michaëlsson K, *et al.* Oral-contraceptive use and risk of hip fracture: a case-control study. *Lancet* 1999; **353:** 1481–4.
5. Cundy T, *et al.* Recovering of bone density in women who stop using medroxyprogesterone acetate. *BMJ* 1994; **308:** 247–8.
6. Cromer BA, *et al.* A prospective comparison of bone density in adolescent girls receiving depot medroxyprogesterone acetate (Depo-Provera), levonorgestrel (Norplant), or oral contraceptives. *J Pediatr* 1996; **129:** 671–6.
7. Gbolade B, *et al.* Bone density in long term users of depot medroxyprogesterone acetate. *Br J Obstet Gynaecol* 1998; **105:** 790–4.
8. Perrotti M, *et al.* Forearm bone density in long-term users of oral combined contraceptives and depot medroxyprogesterone acetate. *Fertil Steril* 2001; **76:** 469–73.
9. Cundy T, *et al.* Spinal bone density in women using depot medroxyprogesterone contraception. *Obstet Gynecol* 1998; **92:** 569–73.
10. Scholes D, *et al.* Bone mineral density in women using depot medroxyprogesterone acetate for contraception. *Obstet Gynecol* 1999; **93:** 233–8.
11. Ott SM, *et al.* Effects of contraceptive use on bone biochemical markers in young women. *J Clin Endocrinol Metab* 2001; **86:** 179–85.


RHEUMATOID ARTHRITIS. While reviews[1] have commented on the rare reports of arthritis or arthropathies attributed to oral contraceptives some large studies have investigated the incidence of rheumatoid arthritis in oral contraceptive users. A negative association between the use of oral contraceptives and the development of rheumatoid arthritis has been reported in four studies[2-5] thus giving rise to the suggestion that oral contraceptive use may, in fact, have some sort of protective role. These findings were not, however, substantiated by other workers[6-8] who found no association, either beneficial or detrimental, between the use of oral contraceptives and the later development of rheumatoid arthritis. A meta-analysis found no conclusive evidence of a protective effect of oral contraceptives on rheumatoid arthritis risk.[9]


1. Hart FD. Drug-induced arthritis and arthralgia. *Drugs* 1984; **28:** 347–54.
2. Wingrave SJ, Kay CR. Reduction in incidence of rheumatoid arthritis associated with oral contraceptives: Royal College of General Practitioners' oral contraception study. *Lancet* 1978; **i:** 569–71.
3. Vandenbroucke JP, *et al.* Oral contraceptives and rheumatoid arthritis: further evidence for a preventive effect. *Lancet* 1982; **ii:** 839–42.
4. Hazes JMW, *et al.* Reduction of the risk of rheumatoid arthritis among women who take oral contraceptives. *Arthritis Rheum* 1990; **33:** 173–9.
5. Spector TD, *et al.* The pill, parity, and rheumatoid arthritis. *Arthritis Rheum* 1990; **33:** 782–9.
6. Linos A, *et al.* Case-control study of rheumatoid arthritis and prior use of oral contraceptives. *Lancet* 1983; **i:** 1299–1300.
7. del Junco DJ, *et al.* Do oral contraceptives prevent rheumatoid arthritis? *JAMA* 1985; **254:** 1938–41.
8. Hannaford PC, *et al.* Oral contraceptives and rheumatoid arthritis: new data from the Royal College of General Practitioners' oral contraception study. *Ann Rheum Dis* 1990; **49:** 744–6.
9. Pladevall-Vila M, *et al.* Controversy of oral contraceptives and risk of rheumatoid arthritis: meta-analysis of conflicting studies and review of conflicting meta-analyses with special emphasis on analysis of heterogeneity. *Am J Epidemiol* 1996; **144:** 1–14.


**Effects on the nervous system.** Chorea has been reported in women using combined oral contraceptives. Reviews of the literature have reported the onset of chorea to range from 1 week to 11 months,[1] with an average of 3 months,[2] and resolution of symptoms after discontinuing the contraceptive to occur after 1 week to 5 months[1] or an average of 5 weeks.[2] The mechanism of this effect is unclear. Some cases occurred in patients with no history of neurological disease,[1,2] but others had a history of rheumatic fever, often with Sydenham chorea, or chorea gravidarum, chorea secondary to other conditions, or congenital heart disease.[2] There is some evidence that chorea could be mediated by the production of antiphospholipid antibodies, as either a primary antiphospholipid syndrome or secondary to systemic lupus erythematosus.[3,4] It has been suggested that the production of these antibodies could be aggravated by the oestrogen component of combined oral contraceptives.[3]

It is generally advised that combined oral contraceptives should be used with caution or avoided in women with antiphospholipid antibodies because they are at increased risk of venous thromboembolism, see Cardiovascular Disease, under Precautions, below.


1. Wadlington WB, *et al.* Chorea associated with the use of oral contraceptives: report of a case and review of the literature. *Clin Pediatr (Phila)* 1981; **20:** 804–6.
2. Galimberti D. Chorea induced by the use of oral contraceptives: report of a case and review of the literature. *Ital J Neurol Sci* 1987; **8:** 383–6.
3. Omdal R, Roalsø S. Chorea gravidarum and chorea associated with oral contraceptives—diseases due to antiphospholipid antibodies? *Acta Neurol Scand* 1992; **86:** 219–20.
4. Cervera R, *et al.* Chorea in the antiphospholipid syndrome: clinical, radiologic, and immunologic characteristics of 50 patients from our clinics and the recent literature. *Medicine (Baltimore)* 1997; **76:** 203–12.


**Effects on the pancreas.** There have been reports of pancreatitis secondary to hyperlipidaemia associated with the use of combined oral contraceptives.[1,2]


1. Parker WA. Estrogen-induced pancreatitis. *Clin Pharm* 1983; **2:** 75–9.
2. Stuyt PMJ, *et al.* Pancreatitis induced by oestrogen in a patient with type I hyperlipoproteinaemia. *BMJ* 1986; **293:** 734.


**Effects on the skin.** Oral contraceptives may cause chloasma, and those containing androgenic progestogens may cause or aggravate acne and hirsutism. More rarely, oral contraceptives have been implicated in photosensitivity reactions[1] and photosensitivity associated with drug-induced lupus erythematosus.[2] A survey of people using UV-A sunbeds at commercial premises in the UK revealed that the prevalence of pruritus, nausea, and skin rashes as side-effects to the sunbeds was higher in women taking oral contraceptives than in women receiving no medication.[3] There has been a report of hidradenitis suppurativa, a condition resulting in the recurrence of boils at the axillary apocrine sweat glands, anogenital region, and breasts, occurring in 7 women using oral contraceptives.[4]

For mention of the refuted association between oral contraceptives and malignant melanoma, see Skin under Carcinogenicity above.


1. Cooper SM, George S. Photosensitivity reaction associated with use of the combined oral contraceptive. *Br J Dermatol* 2001; **144:** 641–2.
2. Smith AG. Drug-induced photosensitivity. *Adverse Drug React Bull* 1989; (Jun.): 508–11.
3. Diffey BL. Use of UV-A sunbeds for cosmetic tanning. *Br J Dermatol* 1986; **115:** 67–76.
4. Stellon AJ, Wakeling M. Hidradenitis suppurativa associated with use of oral contraceptives. *BMJ* 1989; **298:** 28–9.


**Effects on the uterus.** The Oxford Family Planning Association study found that the risk of developing uterine leiomyomas (uterine fibroids) was reduced by the use of oral contraceptives.[1] The observed reduction in risk was approximately 17% with each five years of oral contraceptive use, and was not thought to be due to selective prescribing.[2,3] The authors hypothesised that unopposed oestrogen may be a risk factor for uterine fibroids, and that the reduced risk with oral contraceptives might be analogous to the reduction in endometrial carcinoma seen with these drugs (see above).[1] However, another case-control study involving 390 women with leiomyomas failed to find a protective (or detrimental) effect with oral contraceptive use.[4]


1. Ross RK, *et al.* Risk factors for uterine fibroids: reduced risk associated with oral contraceptives. *BMJ* 1986; **293:** 359–62.
2. Ratner H. Risk factors for uterine fibroids: reduced risk associated with oral contraceptives. *BMJ* 1986; **293:** 1027.
3. Ross RK, *et al.* Risk factors for uterine fibroids: reduced risk associated with oral contraceptives. *BMJ* 1986; **293:** 1027.
4. Parazzini F, *et al.* Oral contraceptive use and risk of uterine fibroids. *Obstet Gynecol* 1992; **79:** 430–3.


**Pelvic inflammatory disease.** It has been suggested that oral contraceptives protect against pelvic inflammatory disease. However, although oral contraceptives are thought to reduce the risk of developing acute pelvic inflammatory disease, higher rates of infection of the lower genital tract by *Chlamydia trachomatis*,[1] and, more tentatively, *Neisseria gonorrhoeae*,[2] have been reported. Other studies[3,4] have suggested that oral contraceptive use is associated with reduced symptom severity, but absence of symptoms is not the same as absence of disease: oral contraceptives might reduce the inflammatory reaction to infection, resulting in unrecognised disease and subsequent complications such as tubal infertility and ectopic pregnancy.[5] There is evidence that users of older oral contraceptives containing more than 50 micrograms of oestrogen may have been at increased risk of tubal infertility, particularly if first used before 20 years of age.[6] No increased risk, or an active decrease in risk (depending on age at first use) was reported for formulations containing 50 micrograms or less of oestrogen, which are now favoured.


1. Washington AE, *et al.* Oral contraceptives, Chlamydia trachomatis infection, and pelvic inflammatory disease: a word of caution about protection. *JAMA* 1985; **253:** 2246–50.
2. Louv WC, *et al.* Oral contraceptive use and the risk of chlamydial and gonococcal infections. *Am J Obstet Gynecol* 1989; **160:** 396–402.
3. Wølner-Hanssen P, *et al.* Decreased risk of symptomatic chlamydial pelvic inflammatory disease associated with oral contraceptive use. *JAMA* 1990; **263:** 54–9.
4. Ness RB, *et al.* Hormonal and barrier contraception and risk of upper genital tract disease in the PID Evaluation and Clinical Health (PEACH) study. *Am J Obstet Gynecol* 2001; **185:** 121–7.
5. Henry-Suchet J. Hormonal contraception and pelvic inflammatory disease. *Eur J Contracept Reprod Health Care* 1997; **2:** 263–7.
6. Cramer DW, *et al.* The relationship of tubal infertility to barrier method and oral contraceptive use. *JAMA* 1987; **257:** 2446–50.


## Precautions

Before hormonal contraceptives are given the woman should undergo an appropriate medical examination and her medical history should be carefully evaluated. Regular examination is recommended during use. The contraceptive effectiveness of combined and progestogen-only preparations may be reduced during episodes of vomiting or diarrhoea and extra contraceptive measures may be necessary during and for 7 days after recovery. For precautions to be observed if a 'pill' is missed, see under Uses and Administration, below.

**Combined oral contraceptives** are *contra-indicated* in women with markedly impaired liver function or cholestasis, the Dubin-Johnson or Rotor syndromes, hepatic adenoma, oestrogen-dependent neoplasms such as breast or endometrial cancer, cardiovascular disease (see also below) including previous or current thromboembolic disorders or high risk of them, and arterial disease or multiple risk factors for it, disorders of lipid metabolism, undiagnosed vaginal bleeding, possible pregnancy, or a history during pregnancy of pruritus or cholestatic jaundice, chorea, herpes gestationis, pemphigoid gestationis, or deteriorating otosclerosis. They are also contra-indicated in severe or focal migraine (or where there are other risk factors for cardiovascular disease) and should be used with caution in other forms of migraine (for further details, see below). They should be *given with caution* to women with a history of clinical depression, gallbladder disease, sickle-cell disease, or conditions influenced by fluid retention. They should also be used with caution in those with varicose veins (and should be avoided where the restrictions outlined under Venous Thromboembolism apply, see Cardiovascular Disease, below). Where not actually contra-indicated, they should also be used with caution in those with a risk factor for cardiovascular disease such as diabetes mellitus, smoking, obesity, hypertension, or a family history of cardiovascular disorders (see also below). Current opinion is that low-dose combined oral contraceptives may be used in women over the age of 35 years provided they do not smoke and have no other risk factors for cardiovascular disease, but that they should be avoided over the age of 50 years. Use by those undergoing surgery or prolonged bed rest may increase the risk of thromboembolic episodes and it is generally recommended that combined oral contraceptives should be stopped 4 to 6 weeks before major elective surgery (see also below). Combined oral contraceptives should not be used after recent evacuation of a hydatidiform mole until urine and plasma gonadotrophin concentrations have returned to normal. Contact lenses may irritate. The use of combined oral contraceptives may influence the results of certain laboratory tests including liver, thyroid, adrenal, and renal-function tests, plasma concentrations of binding proteins and lipid/lipoprotein fractions, and fibrinolysis and coagulation parameters.

Combined oral contraceptives should be *stopped immediately*, and appropriate investigations and treatment carried out, if any of the following occur:

- sudden severe chest pain, sudden breathlessness, or severe pain/swelling in calf of one leg (possibly indicative of thromboembolic complications)
- unusual, severe, prolonged headache, sudden disturbances of vision or hearing or other perceptual disorders, collapse, marked numbness or weakness affecting one side of the body, or other signs or symptoms suggestive of cerebrovascular accident
- a first unexplained epileptic seizure
- hepatitis, jaundice, generalised itching, liver enlargement, severe upper abdominal pain
- onset of severe depression
- significant rise in blood pressure (above 160 mmHg systolic or 100 mmHg diastolic)
- clear exacerbation of other conditions known to be capable of deteriorating during oral contraception or pregnancy.

**Progestogen-only contraceptives**, whether oral or injectable, may be used when oestrogen-containing preparations are contra-indicated but certain contra-indications and precautions must still be observed. They are contra-indicated in women with undiagnosed vaginal bleeding, possible pregnancy, severe arterial disease, hormone-dependent neoplasms, and severe liver disease such as hepatic adenoma.

Like combined oral contraceptives they should not be used after recent evacuation of a hydatidiform mole. Progestogen-only contraceptives should be used with caution in women with heart disease, malabsorption syndromes, liver dysfunction including recurrent cholestatic jaundice, or a history of jaundice in pregnancy. Oral progestogen-only contraceptives should also be used with caution in past ectopic pregnancy (see above) or functional ovarian cysts. Despite unsatisfactory evidence of hazard, other suggested cautions for progestogen-only contraceptives include diabetes mellitus, hypertension, migraine, and thromboembolic disorders.

**Breast feeding.** Combined oral contraceptives may diminish the volume of breast milk and the *British National Formulary* recommends that they should be avoided until weaning (or for at least 6 months after birth). Progestogen-only oral contraceptives do not affect lactation, but should not be given until 3 weeks after birth to avoid an increased risk of breakthrough bleeding. Similarly, progestogen-only parenteral contraceptives should not be given until 6 weeks after birth if a woman is breast feeding; they may be started within 5 days if she is not breast feeding, provided she is warned that heavy or prolonged bleeding may occur. Very small amounts of both oestrogens and progestogens are distributed into the breast milk.

The American Academy of Pediatrics[1] reviewed the use of hormonal contraceptives during lactation, commenting that early information was based on the use of high-dose contraceptives. It was noted that there might be a decrease in milk production, but that there was insufficient information to confirm that there was any alteration in the composition of breast milk, and that although there had been rare cases of gynaecomastia in breast-fed infants of mothers who received high-dose contraceptives, there was no consistent evidence of long-term adverse effects on the infant. A later study[2] of 48 children whose mothers had received high-dose combined oral contraceptives during breast feeding found no effect on these children compared with controls, up to 8 years of age. The Academy therefore considers[3] that combined oral contraceptives are usually compatible with breast feeding. Reviews[1,4] of progestogen-only contraceptives consider that they have no effect on milk production or composition, or on the infant.


1. American Academy of Pediatrics Committee on Drugs. Breast-feeding and contraception. *Pediatrics* 1981; **68:** 138–40.
2. Nilsson S, *et al.* Long-term follow-up of children breast-fed by mothers using oral contraceptives. *Contraception* 1986; **34:** 443–57.
3. American Academy of Pediatrics. The transfer of drugs and other chemicals into human milk. *Pediatrics* 2001; **108:** 776–89. Correction. *ibid.*; 1029. Also available at: http://aappolicy.aappublications.org/cgi/content/full/pediatrics%3b108/3/776 (accessed 16/06/04)
4. Fraser IS. A review of the use of progestogen-only minipills for contraception during lactation. *Reprod Fertil Dev* 1991; **3:** 245–54.


**Cardiovascular disease.** Combined oral contraceptives are associated with a number of arterial and venous risks. Progestogen-only contraceptives are associated with fewer risks, although they still need to be avoided when arterial disease is severe.

ARTERIAL DISEASE. In the UK the *British National Formulary* has recommended that combined oral contraceptives may be used with **caution** if any **one** of the following factors are present, but should be **avoided** if **two or more** factors are present:

- *family history of arterial disease* in first-degree relative aged under 45 years (avoid if there is also an atherogenic lipid profile)
- *diabetes mellitus* (avoid if diabetic complications are present)
- *hypertension* (avoid if blood pressure is above 160/100 mmHg)
- *smoking* (avoid if 40 or more cigarettes are smoked daily)
- *age over 35 years* (avoid if over 50 years)
- *obesity*—body-mass index above 30 kg/m$^2$ (avoid if body-mass index exceeds 39 kg/m$^2$)
- *migraine,* see under Migraine, below.

VENOUS THROMBOEMBOLISM. Combined oral contraceptives increase the risk of venous thromboembolism and should not be used in women with a personal history of venous or arterial thrombosis. In addition they should be used with **caution** if any **one** of the following risk factors are present, but should be **avoided** if **two or more** factors are present:

- *family history of venous thromboembolism* in first-degree relative aged under 45 years (avoid if there is a known prothrombotic coagulation abnormality such as antiphospholipid antibodies, which may occur in patients with systemic lupus erythematosus, or factor V Leiden)
- *long-term immobilisation* such as wheelchair use (avoid if confined to bed or with a leg in plaster)
- *varicose veins* (avoid during sclerosing treatment)
- *obesity*—body-mass index above 30 kg/m$^2$ (avoid if body-mass index greater than 39 kg/m$^2$).

The *British National Formulary* also advises that women taking combined oral contraceptives may be at an increased risk of deep-vein thrombosis during *travel* involving prolonged periods of immobility (over 5 hours). The risk may be reduced by appropriate exercise during the journey, and possibly by wearing elastic hosiery.

In the light of evidence indicating an increased risk of venous thromboembolism with combined oral contraceptives containing *desogestrel* or *gestodene* (see Venous Thromboembolism, under Effects on the Cardiovascular System, above), the UK Committee on Safety of Medicines (CSM) advised additional precautions for these products. As well as the usual precautions, it was initially advised they should not be used by obese women (body-mass index greater than 30 kg/m$^2$), those with varicose veins, or those with a history of thrombosis of any cause. Moreover, it was also recommended that they should be used only by women who were intolerant of other combined oral contraceptives and who were prepared to accept an increased risk of venous thromboembolism. Subsequently the CSM[1] has modified its advice as follows: they recommend that these products should be avoided in women with known risk factors for venous thromboembolism. However, in women without contra-indications, the type of combined contraceptive is considered a matter of clinical judgement and personal choice, as long as the woman is fully informed of the small excess risk associated with desogestrel- and gestodene-containing products.


1. Committee on Safety of Medicines/Medicines Control Agency. Combined oral contraceptives containing desogestrel or gestodene and the risk of venous thromboembolism. *Current Problems* 1999; **25:** 12. Also available at: http://www.mca.gov.uk/ourwork/monitorsafequalmed/currentproblems/volume25jun.htm (accessed 06/07/04)


**Lupus erythematosus.** Systemic lupus erythematosus (SLE) is an auto-immune disease which is far more common in women than in men, and usually has a peak onset for women in their 20s and 30s. There is some evidence to suggest that oral contraceptive use may be associated with a slightly increased risk in the onset of SLE. There are also reports and studies of the effect of contraceptives on disease exacerbation, although there has been an apparent reduction in reports which has coincided with the lowering of oestrogen content in contraceptive preparations. Patients with major disease, such as lupus nephritis, could be at greater risk of exacerbation. It is also generally advised that combined oral contraceptives should be avoided in women with antiphospholipid antibodies (which includes about a third of all patients with SLE) because they are at increased risk of venous thromboembolism.

References.


1. Petri M. Exogenous estrogen in systemic lupus erythematosus: oral contraceptives and hormone replacement therapy. *Lupus* 2001; **10:** 222–6.
2. Mok CC, *et al.* Use of exogenous estrogens in systemic lupus erythematosus. *Semin Arthritis Rheum* 2001; **30:** 426–35.


**Migraine.** In the UK the *British National Formulary* has recommended that combined oral contraceptives be **contra-indicated** in: migraine with typical focal aura; severe migraine regularly lasting longer than 72 hours despite treatment; and migraine treated with an ergot derivative. It also recommends **caution** in migraine without focal aura and migraine controlled with a serotonin (5-$HT_1$) agonist. A woman receiving a combined oral contraceptive should report any increase in headache frequency or the onset of focal symptoms. If focal neurological symptoms not typical of aura persist for longer than one hour the combined oral contraceptive should be discontinued and the woman referred urgently to a neurologist.

**Porphyria.** Oral contraceptives have been associated with acute attacks of porphyria and are considered unsafe in porphyric patients. The progestogen content is considered more hazardous than the oestrogen content. A progestogen-only contraceptive may be used with extreme caution if non-hormonal contraception is inappropriate and potential benefit outweighs the risk. The risk of an acute attack is greatest in women who have had a previous attack or are under 30 years of age. Long-acting progestogen preparations should never be used in those at risk.

**Pregnancy.** In contrast to the numerous cases of congenital malformations reported after the use of high doses of sex hormones for hormonal pregnancy tests, there have been only a few suggestions that continued use of oral contraceptives during early pregnancy may result in congenital limb reduction deformities,[1-3] and one case of neonatal choreoathetosis following prenatal exposure to oral contraceptives.[4]

Many studies, conversely, have shown no evidence that the use of oral contraceptives is associated with congenital malformations or teratogenic effects, whether past use (discontinued before conception), use after the last menstrual period, or known use in early pregnancy.[5-10] A meta-analysis[11] of some of these, plus other studies, confirmed this. The relative risk for all malformations with use of oral contraceptives was estimated to be 0.99 (95% confidence intervals 0.83 to 1.19). The use of oral contraceptives in early pregnancy also appears unlikely to increase the risk of hypospadia in male fetuses (see also under Precautions of Estradiol, p.1550).[12] For a discussion of the ectopic pregnancy risk in users of hormonal contraceptives, see above.


1. Janerich DT, *et al.* Oral contraceptives and congenital limb reduction defects. *N Engl J Med* 1974; **291:** 697–700.
2. McCredie J, *et al.* Congenital limb defects and the pill. *Lancet* 1983; **ii:** 623.
3. Kricker A, *et al.* Congenital limb reduction deformities and use of oral contraceptives. *Am J Obstet Gynecol* 1986; **155:** 1072–8.
4. Profumo R, *et al.* Neonatal choreoathetosis following prenatal exposure to oral contraceptives. *Pediatrics* 1990; **86:** 648–9.
5. Robinson SC. Pregnancy outcome following oral contraceptives. *Am J Obstet Gynecol* 1971; **109:** 354–8.
6. Royal College of General Practitioners' Oral Contraception Study. The outcome of pregnancy in former oral contraceptive users. *Br J Obstet Gynaecol* 1976; **83:** 608–16.
7. Rothman KJ, Louik C. Oral contraceptives and birth defects. *N Engl J Med* 1978; **299:** 522–4.
8. Vessey M, *et al.* Outcome of pregnancy in women using different methods of contraception. *Br J Obstet Gynaecol* 1979; **86:** 548–56.
9. Linn S, *et al.* Lack of association between contraceptive usage and congenital malformations in offspring. *Am J Obstet Gynecol* 1983; **147:** 923–8.
10. Källén B. Maternal use of oral contraceptives and Down syndrome. *Contraception* 1989; **39:** 503–6.
11. Bracken MB. Oral contraception and congenital malformations in offspring: a review and meta-analysis of the prospective studies. *Obstet Gynecol* 1990; **76:** 552–7.
12. Raman-Wilms L, *et al.* Fetal genital effects of first trimester sex hormone exposure: a meta-analysis. *Obstet Gynecol* 1995; **85:** 141–9.


**Sickle-cell disease.** *Sickle-cell disease* and oral contraceptive use are both associated with an increased risk of thrombosis but it is by no means certain that the two risks are additive. Study of a small number of women with sickle-cell disease found that combined and progestogen-only contraceptives had no effect on red cell deformability.[1] Some manufacturers have specifically warned against the use of combined oral contraceptives in sickle-cell disease but it has also been considered that there is no contra-indication to the use of low-dose combined preparations,[2,3] or that a progestogen-only pill[4] or depot injection of medroxyprogesterone acetate[5] be used.

For *sickle-cell trait* there is no increased risk of thrombosis and no contra-indication to the use of a combined or progestogen-only preparation. Many women with sickle-cell trait have, unnecessarily, been denied the use of oral contraceptives in the mistaken belief that advice for sickle-cell disease applies to the trait.[4]


1. Yoong WC, *et al.* Red cell deformability in oral contraceptive pill users with sickle cell anaemia. *Br J Haematol* 1999; **104:** 868–70.
2. Freie HMP. Sickle cell diseases and hormonal contraception. *Acta Obstet Gynecol Scand* 1983; **62:** 211–17.
3. Howard RJ, *et al.* Contraceptives, counselling, and pregnancy in women with sickle cell disease. *BMJ* 1993; **306:** 1735–7.

4. Evans DIK. Should patients who say that they have "sickle cells" be prescribed the contraceptive pill? *BMJ* 1984; **289:** 425.
5. Guillebaud J. Sickle cell disease and contraception. *BMJ* 1993; **307:** 506–7.

**Surgery.** Case reports and epidemiological studies showing an increased risk of idiopathic deep-vein thrombosis and pulmonary embolism in young women taking **combined oral contraceptives** (see above) led to the widespread belief that oral contraceptives may predispose to deep-vein thrombosis postoperatively. In consequence, the advice commonly given in the UK has been that, if possible, combined oral contraceptives should be stopped 4 weeks before major elective surgery and all surgery of the legs, and that prophylactic heparin should be considered where this was not possible.[1] They can normally be started again at the first menses occurring at least 2 weeks after full mobilisation. However, estimates of the size of the risk are variable;[2-5] one report[2] found that the incidence of deep-vein thrombosis postoperatively in young women taking combined oral contraceptives was about twice that of women not taking contraceptives but the difference was not statistically significant. Some have considered[6] that the risk to young women of becoming pregnant after stopping oral contraceptives, or of developing side-effects from prophylaxis, may be greater than the risk of developing postoperative deep-vein thrombosis. This is in line with the views of the Thromboembolic Risk Factors (THRIFT) Consensus Group.[7] They suggested that unless there were other risk factors there was insufficient evidence to support a policy of routinely stopping combined oral contraceptives before major surgery. Additionally, there was insufficient evidence to support routine specific thromboembolic prophylaxis in women without additional risk factors. A review[8] has subsequently recommended that women for whom major elective surgery was planned should continue taking the combined oral contraceptive but should receive thromboprophylaxis in the perioperative period. It has also been pointed out[9,10] that for patients awaiting surgery who require contraception, a progestogen-only oral contraceptive or an injection of medroxyprogesterone acetate may be suitable since neither preparation increases the risk of thrombosis.

1. Guillebaud J. Surgery and the pill. *BMJ* 1985; **291:** 498–9.
2. Vessey M, *et al.* Oral contraceptives and venous thromboembolism: findings in a large prospective study. *BMJ* 1986; **292:** 526.
3. Tso SC, *et al.* Deep vein thrombosis and changes in coagulation and fibrinolysis after gynaecological operations in Chinese: the effect of oral contraceptives and malignant disease. *Br J Haematol* 1980; **46:** 603–12.
4. Gallus AS, *et al.* Oral contraceptives and surgery: reduced antithrombin and antifactor XA levels without postoperative venous thrombosis in low-risk patients. *Thromb Res* 1984; **35:** 513–26.
5. Sagar S, *et al.* Oral contraceptives, antithrombin III activity, and postoperative deep-vein thrombosis. *Lancet* 1976; **i:** 509–11.
6. Sue-Ling H, Hughes LE. Should the pill be stopped preoperatively? *BMJ* 1988; **296:** 447–8.
7. Thromboembolic Risk Factors (THRIFT) Consensus Group. Risk of and prophylaxis for venous thromboembolism in hospital patients. *BMJ* 1992; **305:** 567–74.
8. Anonymous. Drugs in the peri-operative period: hormonal contraceptives and hormone replacement therapy. *Drug Ther Bull* 1999; **37:** 78–80.
9. Guillebaud J. Should the pill be stopped preoperatively? *BMJ* 1988; **296:** 786–7.
10. Guillebaud J, Robinson GE. Stopping the pill. *BMJ* 1991; **302:** 789.

**Travel.** For a warning that women taking oral contraceptives may be at increased risk of deep-vein thrombosis from travel involving prolonged immobility see under Cardiovascular Disease, above.

## Interactions

Enzyme-inducing drugs may cause failure of combined oral contraceptives by increasing their metabolism and clearance. This effect is well established for a number of *antiepileptics, griseofulvin*, and *rifamycin antibacterials*, and has also been suggested for some *antivirals* and for *modafinil*. Although less well documented, these interactions would also be expected to apply to progestogen-only contraceptives. Orally administered *retinoids* may cause failure of low-dose progestogen-only contraceptives. Rarely, *broad-spectrum antibacterials* have been associated with combined oral contraceptive failure, possibly by reducing enterohepatic recycling of the oestrogen component. As the doses of oestrogen and progestogen in oral contraceptives have decreased, reports of menstrual irregularities and unintended pregnancies attributed to these drug interactions have increased. Further details of drugs affecting hormonal contraceptives are given below under specific headings.

Oral contraceptives may, as well as being affected themselves by drug interactions, *affect other drugs*. Compounds undergoing oxidative metabolism can have their plasma concentration raised by oral contraceptives through an inhibitory action. Conversely, oral contraceptives appear to induce glucuronidation of some drugs thus reducing their plasma concentration. Oral contraceptives can also antagonise the actions of a number of drugs. Drugs affected include the following:

- some analgesics (increased clearance of paracetamol and morphine)
- anticoagulants (increased and decreased effects reported; see p.1027)
- some antidepressants (reduced effectiveness, but also increased toxicity; see p.285)
- antidiabetics (antagonism of effect)
- antihypertensives (antagonism of effect)
- benzodiazepines (increased or decreased clearance; see p.694)
- ciclosporin (increased toxicity; see p.1356)
- clofibrate (increased clearance and antagonism of effect)
- corticosteroids (reduced clearance and enhanced effect; see p.1073)
- lidocaine (increased free fraction due to altered protein binding; see Protein Binding, under Pharmacokinetics, p.1379)
- selegiline (decreased clearance; see p.1214)
- levothyroxine (reduced free fraction due to increased binding globulin concentration; see p.1601)
- xanthines (decreased clearance; see p.803).

◊ Reviews.

1. Back DJ, Orme ML'E. Pharmacokinetic drug interactions with oral contraceptives. *Clin Pharmacokinet* 1990; **18:** 472–84.
2. Shenfield GM. Oral contraceptives: are drug interactions of clinical significance? *Drug Safety* 1993; **9:** 21–37.
3. Quereux C, Bory JP. Interaction médicamenteuse et contraception orale. *Contracept Fertil Sex* 1998; **26:** 129–31.
4. Schwartz JB. Oral contraceptive therapy in women: drug interactions and unwanted outcomes. *J Gend Specif Med* 1999; **2:** 26–9.
5. Elliman A. Interactions with hormonal contraception. *Br J Fam Plann* 2000; **26:** 109–11. Correction. *ibid.*; 151.

**Antibacterials.** An interaction between the *rifamycins (rifampicin* and *rifabutin)* and oral contraceptives is well established (see Rifamycins, below) and alternative contraceptive measures are necessary. A variety of *broad-spectrum antibacterials* have been reported to decrease oral contraceptive efficacy. Some studies have pointed to interference with intestinal flora involved in enterohepatic circulation of oestrogens as being a likely mechanism for this interaction. Although up until 1985 there had been 32 reports[1] of unintended pregnancies in women receiving *penicillins* (25 of them with *ampicillin*) the ability of antibacterials to inhibit oral contraceptive efficacy remains unproven. The data are consistent, however, with the supposition that efficacy is occasionally impaired.[2] Several cases of unintended pregnancies have been reported following the use of *tetracyclines*. It is recommended that additional contraceptive precautions should be used while taking, and for 7 days after stopping, a short course of any broad-spectrum antibacterial. If these 7 days run into the last 7 days of the cycle, then the tablet-free interval (or the 7 inert tablets) should be omitted and the next cycle of tablets started immediately. If the course of antibacterial exceeds 3 weeks the intestinal flora develop resistance and additional precautions become unnecessary.

With regard to other antibacterials, in theory any one with significant effects on intestinal flora could affect contraceptive efficacy. Isolated cases of pregnancy have been reported following the use of *cephalosporins, chloramphenicol, dapsone, isoniazid, nitrofurantoin, sulfonamides*, and *co-trimoxazole* but it is impossible to determine which, if any, of these interactions is real.

1. Back DJ, *et al.* Evaluation of Committee on Safety of Medicines yellow card reports on oral contraceptive-drug interactions with anticonvulsants and antibiotics. *Br J Clin Pharmacol* 1988; **25:** 527–32.
2. Dickinson BD, *et al.* Drug interactions between oral contraceptives and antibiotics. *Obstet Gynecol* 2001; **98:** 853–60.

RIFAMYCINS. *Rifampicin* regularly results in menstrual irregularities and occasionally in unintended pregnancies in women receiving oral contraceptives. It is a potent enzyme inducer and considerably enhances the metabolism of oral contraceptives. For short courses of rifampicin, additional contraceptive precautions should be taken during the course and for at least 4 weeks after stopping. A non-hormonal method of contraception such as an intra-uterine device is recommended during, and for 4 to 8 weeks after stopping, long-term rifampicin therapy.

Similar precautions are recommended during *rifabutin* therapy.

TROLEANDOMYCIN. Severe pruritus and jaundice may occur if oral contraceptives and troleandomycin are given together.[1] It has been suggested that their hepatic effects may be additive or synergistic, and that concurrent use should be avoided.

1. Miguet J-P, *et al.* Jaundice from troleandomycin and oral contraceptives. *Ann Intern Med* 1980; **92:** 434.

**Antidepressants.** *Hypericum* may decrease blood concentrations of oral contraceptives by enzyme induction. There have been reports of intermenstrual bleeding and altered menstrual bleeding in women on long-term oral contraceptives who started taking hypericum.[1] Two cases of pregnancy have also been reported.[2]

1. Yue Q-Y, *et al.* Safety of St. John's wort (Hypericum perforatum). *Lancet* 2000; **355:** 576–7.
2. Medical Products Agency (Sweden). St John's wort may influence other medication. Available at: http://www.mpa.se/eng/news/2002/020206_stjohnswort.shtml (accessed 16/06/04)

**Antidiabetics.** *Troglitazone* is an enzyme inducer and increases the clearance of oestrogens and progestogens. A high-dose oral contraceptive, or an alternative method of contraception should be considered in women receiving troglitazone and requiring contraception.[1]

1. Loi C-M, *et al.* Effect of troglitazone on the pharmacokinetics of an oral contraceptive agent. *J Clin Pharmacol* 1999; **39:** 410–17.

**Antiepileptics.** Oral contraceptive failure and breakthrough bleeding have been reported in numerous cases during antiepileptic therapy.[1,2] *Phenytoin*, barbiturates such as *phenobarbital* and *primidone*, and *carbamazepine* have been most frequently implicated, and *oxcarbazepine, felbamate*, and *topiramate* may interact similarly.[3] These drugs increase clearance of oral contraceptives by enzyme induction, so diminishing their effect. In women receiving such antiepileptics use of non-hormonal contraceptives such as the intra-uterine device should be considered. If these are unsuitable, an oral contraceptive with an increased oestrogen content of 50 micrograms or more is generally recommended. The use of a monophasic preparation for 3 or 4 cycles without a break followed by a tablet-free interval of 4 days (tricycling) has also been suggested. Switching to a non-interacting antiepileptic such as valproate could be considered.

1. Mattson RH, Cramer JA. Epilepsy, sex hormones, and antiepileptic drugs. *Epilepsia* 1985; **26** (suppl 1): S40–S51.
2. Back DJ, *et al.* Evaluation of Committee on Safety of Medicines yellow card reports on oral contraceptive-drug interactions with anticonvulsants and antibiotics. *Br J Clin Pharmacol* 1988; **25:** 527–32.
3. Wilbur K, Ensom MHH. Pharmacokinetic drug interactions between oral contraceptives and second-generation anticonvulsants. *Clin Pharmacokinet* 2000; **38:** 355–65.

**Antifungals.** Menstrual irregularities and pregnancies have been reported in women receiving oral contraceptives and *griseofulvin*[1,2] and more studies are needed to confirm the existence of the interaction and the mechanism of action involved. Additional contraceptive measures should be considered in women using both drugs (and for at least 4 weeks after stopping griseofulvin). There have also been anecdotal reports[3-5] of menstrual irregularities and contraceptive failure with *fluconazole, itraconazole*, and *ketoconazole*, and similar advice applies to these if pregnancy is to be avoided with certainty.

1. van Dijke CPH, Weber JCP. Interaction between oral contraceptives and griseofulvin. *BMJ* 1984; **288:** 1125–6.
2. Back DJ, *et al.* Evaluation of Committee on Safety of Medicines yellow card reports on oral contraceptive-drug interactions with anticonvulsants and antibiotics. *Br J Clin Pharmacol* 1988; **25:** 527–32.
3. Pillans PI, Sparrow MJ. Pregnancy associated with a combined oral contraceptive and itraconazole. *N Z Med J* 1993; **106:** 436.
4. Meyboom RHB, *et al.* Disturbance of withdrawal bleeding during concomitant use of itraconazole and oral contraceptives. *N Z Med J* 1997; **110:** 300.
5. van Puijenbroek EP, *et al.* Verstoring van de pilcyclus tijdens het gelijktijdig gebruik van itraconazol en orale anticonceptiva. *Ned Tijdschr Geneeskd* 1998; **142:** 146–9.

**Antivirals.** A number of antivirals are likely to accelerate the metabolism of oestrogens and progestogens; theoretically therefore, they may decrease the efficacy of hormonal contraceptives. This has been suggested for *HIV-protease inhibitors* such as *nelfinavir* and *ritonavir*,[1] and for *nevirapine*. An alternative form of contraception should be considered.

Conversely, the area under the plasma-concentration-time curve for ethinylestradiol is reported to be increased by *efavirenz* although the clinical implications are unknown.

1. Ouellet D, *et al.* Effect of ritonavir on the pharmacokinetics of ethinyl oestradiol in healthy female volunteers. *Br J Clin Pharmacol* 1998; **46:** 111–16.

**Retinoids.** One woman taking an oral progestogen-only contraceptive (levonorgestrel 30 micrograms daily) showed a significant increase in plasma-progestogen while receiving *acitretin*, which indicated ovulation had occurred.[1] However, progestogen-only contraceptives do not suppress ovulation in all cycles, and this is not thought to be their primary mechanism of contraceptive efficacy (see p.1527). Nevertheless, because it is imperative that women receiving retinoids do not conceive, some have concluded that oral progestogen-only contraceptives are not suitable for use with retinoids.[2]

The anti-ovulatory efficacy of combined oral contraceptives was not affected by acitretin in 8 women in the study above,[1] or by *etretinate* in a study[3] in 12 women, and plasma concentrations of ethinylestradiol and levonorgestrel were not significantly changed by *isotretinoin* in another study in 9 women.[4] It has been concluded that, unless otherwise contra-indicated, oral combined contraceptives are the contraceptive method of choice for women undergoing retinoid treatment.[2]

Both isotretinoin and combined oral contraceptives can have adverse effects on plasma lipids;[5] it has therefore been recommended that plasma lipids should be monitored during concurrent retinoid and oral contraceptive therapy, and that an oral contraceptive containing a non-androgenic progestogen is preferred,[2] since these have less detrimental effects on lipids (p.1531).

1. Berbis P, *et al.* Acitretin (RO10-1670) and oral contraceptives: interaction study. *Arch Dermatol Res* 1988; **280:** 388–9.

2. Lehucher Ceyrac D, *et al.* Retinoids and contraception. *Dermatology* 1992; **184:** 161–70.
3. Berbis P, *et al.* Study on the influence of etretinate on biologic activity of oral contraceptives. *J Am Acad Dermatol* 1987; **17:** 302–3.
4. Orme M, *et al.* Isotretinoin and contraception. *Lancet* 1984; **ii:** 752–3.
5. Chen Y, *et al.* Elevation of serum triglyceride and cholesterol levels from isotretinoin therapy with concomitant oral contraceptives. *Pharmacoepidemiol Drug Safety* 1995; **4:** 91–6.


**Stimulants.** *Modafinil* induces hepatic enzymes and may reduce the efficacy of oral contraceptives. The UK manufacturer of modafinil has suggested that when oral contraceptives are also needed, a preparation containing at least 50 micrograms of ethinylestradiol should be used.

**Vitamins.** Large supplements of *vitamin C* have been reported to increase serum ethinylestradiol concentrations in women taking oral contraceptives,[1] but a further study showed no effect.[2]


1. Back DJ, *et al.* Interaction of ethinyloestradiol with ascorbic acid in man. *BMJ* 1981; **282:** 1516.
2. Zamag NM, *et al.* Absence of an effect of high vitamin C dosage on the systemic availability of ethinyl estradiol in women using a combination oral contraceptive. *Contraception* 1993; **48:** 377–91.


## Pharmacokinetics

For a discussion of the pharmacokinetics of oestrogens and progestogens, see Estradiol, p.1550 and Progesterone, p.1567, respectively. The extent of binding of progestogens to serum sex-hormone binding globulin may be altered when they are given with an oestrogen. Oestrogens increase serum concentrations of sex-hormone binding globulin, and progestogens differ in their ability to suppress this effect.

◊ Reference to the effects of hormonal contraceptives on binding proteins.[1]


1. Fotherby K. Interactions of contraceptive steroids with binding proteins and the clinical implications. *Ann N Y Acad Sci* 1988; **538:** 313–20.


## Uses and Administration

The main use of hormonal contraceptives is for contraception, but combined oral contraceptives are also commonly used in menstrual disorders such as dysmenorrhoea (p.6), premenstrual syndrome (p.1551), and menorrhagia (p.1567), particularly where contraception is also required. Combined oral contraceptives are also used in polycystic ovary syndrome (p.1317) and Turner's syndrome (p.1317), and may be used in endometriosis (p.1546); those containing non-androgenic progestogens may be used in acne (p.1133) and hirsutism (p.1545).

**Combined oral contraceptives** containing both an oestrogen and a progestogen are the most effective type of oral contraceptive for general use. The synthetic ethinyl derivatives ethinylestradiol and mestranol are the oestrogens typically used in such preparations. The progestogenic component is usually a 19-nortestosterone derivative such as desogestrel, etynodiol diacetate, gestodene, levonorgestrel, lynestrenol, norethisterone, norethisterone acetate, norgestimate, or norgestrel. Preparations may be *monophasic* (containing a fixed dose of oestrogen and progestogen), or *biphasic* or *triphasic* (when the dose of progestogen, or both the progestogen and oestrogen, are varied through the cycle). Phased preparations are designed to mimic more closely the pattern of endogenous hormone secretion and may provide better cycle control than monophasic preparations. More rarely, *sequential* preparations are used, which contain an oestrogen alone for part of the cycle. Combined oral contraceptives are taken for 21 days (or occasionally 22 days) followed by an interval of 7 days (or 6 days) when menstrual bleeding will occur. Some preparations include 21 (or 22) active tablets plus 7 (or 6) inert tablets to remove the need for counting days ('every day' preparations). Long- or extended-cycle preparations may be taken continuously for 84 days, followed by an interval of 7 days. The oestrogen content of most preparations is currently in the range of 20 to 50 micrograms daily although higher doses were often formerly used. Preparations containing ethinylestradiol in a lower dose of 15 micrograms, taken daily for 24 days followed by a 4-day interval, have recently become available. A formulation containing the lowest dose of oestrogen compatible with good cycle control should be chosen, considering the following:

- *low-strength* preparations (ethinylestradiol 20 micrograms) are most appropriate for women with risk factors for cardiovascular disease (see Precautions, above), provided a combined oral contraceptive is considered otherwise suitable
- *standard-strength* preparations (ethinylestradiol 30 or 35 micrograms or mestranol 50 micrograms if monophasic, or 30 to 40 micrograms if phased) are appropriate for most other women
- *high-strength* preparations (ethinylestradiol 50 micrograms) are generally used only in circumstances where bioavailability of the oestrogen is reduced, such as concomitant use of some enzyme-inducing drugs (see Interactions, above).

When first **starting** combined oral contraceptives, if the first tablet is taken on the first day of the menstrual cycle (the first day of bleeding) additional contraceptive precautions are unnecessary. If the first tablet is taken on the fourth day of the cycle or later, additional contraceptive precautions should be undertaken for 7 days (or 14 days for 'every day' preparations in case the inert tablets are inadvertently taken first). If amenorrhoea is present and pregnancy has been excluded, combined oral contraceptives may be started on any day, but additional precautions should be used for the first 7 days. In the case of abortion or miscarriage combined oral contraceptives should be started on the same day. In women not breast feeding, they may be started 3 weeks postpartum; progestogen-only contraceptives are preferred in breast-feeding women (see under Precautions, above).

When **changing** to a combined preparation containing a different progestogen, the new preparation should be started on the day following the last active tablet of the old preparation. If a tablet-free interval is taken then extra contraceptive precautions are necessary for the first 7 days of the new preparation. In the case of 'every day' preparations, to allow for the fact that the inert tablets may inadvertently be taken first, extra contraceptive precautions are necessary during the first 14 days. Meticulous regularity of dosage is essential and contraceptive protection may be lost if a dose is not taken at the proper time or is missed, especially if the missed dose is at the beginning or end of a cycle.

If a tablet is **missed** it should be taken as soon as possible (if more than one is missed, just the most recent dose should be taken and the others omitted); the remainder of the course should be taken as normal. If the gap in dosage is more than 12 hours, then extra contraceptive measures are required for the next 7 days. If these 7 days run into the last 7 days of the cycle, then the tablet-free interval (or the 7 inert tablets) should be omitted and the next cycle of tablets started immediately. Similarly, extra contraceptive measures are advised during, and for 7 days after recovery from, vomiting or diarrhoea.

**Progestogen-only oral contraceptives** are suitable for women when an oestrogen component is contra-indicated. They are taken continuously, usually **starting** on day one of the menstrual cycle, with no interval during menstrual bleeding. They may be associated with a higher failure rate than the combined preparations. Regularity in taking the doses is even more important with this type of preparation; contraceptive efficacy is reduced if a dose is delayed by more than 3 hours. Commonly used progestogens include the 19-nortestosterone derivatives etynodiol diacetate, levonorgestrel or norgestrel, and norethisterone.

When **changing** from a combined oral contraceptive preparation to an oral progestogen-only contraceptive, the new tablets should be started immediately with no tablet-free interval (or, in the case of 'every day' preparations, omitting the inert tablets). If there is a gap in administration of active ingredients, then extra contraceptive precautions are required for 7 days.

If a **missed tablet** is delayed by more than 3 hours, it should be taken as soon as possible and the next tablet taken at the correct time. Additional contraceptive methods should be used for the next 7 days. Additional contraceptive methods are also required during, and for 7 days after recovery from, vomiting and diarrhoea.

Progestogens are also used alone as **parenteral contraceptives** and provide a very high level of contraceptive efficacy. They are usually given within the first 5 days of the menstrual cycle. Injectable contraceptives are usually used to provide short-term protection or are used in women unable to use other methods. Medroxyprogesterone acetate is given by intramuscular injection as a long-acting depot preparation to provide contraception for up to 3 months. Norethisterone enantate is used similarly to provide protection for up to 2 months. Levonorgestrel is used in the form of a subcutaneous implant providing contraception for 5 years. A contraceptive implant containing etonogestrel, effective for 3 years, is also available. A combined parenteral contraceptive containing the oestrogen estradiol cipionate with medroxyprogesterone acetate, and given monthly by intramuscular injection, has been developed.

Hormonal **intra-uterine contraceptive devices** are also available. One such device releases progesterone to provide contraception for 1 year; another releases levonorgestrel for 5 years. These are usually inserted within 7 days of the onset of menstruation. A contraceptive **vaginal ring**, which releases ethinylestradiol and etonogestrel, is retained in the vagina for 3 weeks; it is then removed for a one-week interval after which a new ring is inserted.

A contraceptive **transdermal patch**, which releases ethinylestradiol and norelgestromin, has been developed. A new patch is applied each week for 3 weeks, followed by a one-week patch-free interval.

**Postcoital hormonal contraceptives** (emergency contraception) should be taken within 72 hours after unprotected intercourse to be most effective (for details see below). A single oral dose of levonorgestrel 1.5 mg may be given within 72 hours of intercourse, or it may be given as a dose of 750 micrograms within 72 hours of intercourse followed by a second dose 12 hours later. An alternative preparation available for such use consists of tablets each containing ethinylestradiol 50 micrograms and norgestrel 500 micrograms or levonorgestrel 250 micrograms. Two tablets should be taken within 72 hours and a further 2 tablets 12 hours later. If vomiting occurs within 3 hours of any dose it can be repeated, possibly with a suitable antiemetic.

**Contraception.** Contraception is used for fertility control, and some methods have additional non-contraceptive health benefits. There are a wide variety of regular methods including periodic abstinence (natural family planning), male and female barrier methods, intra-uterine devices (IUDs), female hormonal contraceptives, and female or male sterilisation. In addition, female hormonal contraceptives and copper IUDs are available for emergency (postcoital) contraception. The methods employed for contraceptive purposes can be grouped into three categories: those that prevent ovulation, those that prevent fertilisation of the ovum, and those that prevent implantation of the fertilised ovum. None of the available contraceptive methods are effective once implantation of a fertilised ovum has occurred, i.e. they are not abortifacients.

A large number of factors will influence the choice of contraceptive method. Those relating to the woman include age (and therefore likely fertility), parity, medical disorders, risk of sexually transmitted diseases, smoking status, breast feeding, and cultural and religious considerations. Those relating to the method include its failure rate, reversibility, ease of use, mechanism of action, adverse effects, and non-contraceptive benefits.

The most reliable reversible methods for contraception are those for which there can be no 'user' failure such as *progestogen injections* and *implants*, and progestogen or copper *intra-uterine devices* (IUDs). These methods have reported failure rates of between 0.09 and 2% during the first year of use. The duration of action of the various progestogen injections is up to 2 or 3 months, whereas progestogen implants and progestogen IUDs can be effective for 1 to 5 years, depending on the preparation. These long-acting progestogen preparations thicken cervical mucus, so preventing sperm penetration, and suppress the endometrium, so preventing implantation. In addition, they suppress ovulation; the degree of suppression is complete for injectable preparations, about 50% for implants, and low for the progestogen IUDs. Copper IUDs were traditionally thought to act by preventing implantation, but it is now thought that the biochemical changes which they produce in the uterus also prevent fertilisation. They are effective and have a prolonged action (up to 5 or 10 years), but they have been associated with an increased rate of pelvic inflammatory disease and ectopic pregnancy. Copper IUDs are generally unsuitable for nulliparous women and those at increased risk of sexually transmitted diseases.

Of methods subject to 'user' failure, *combined oral contraceptives* are the most effective. They have a reported failure rate during the first year of 0.1% if used perfectly, but 3% in typical practice. Their principal mechanism of action is to prevent ovulation, and they also decrease the chances of fertilisation and implantation. Combined oral contraceptives offer the non-contraceptive advantages of avoidance of dysmenorrhoea, premenstrual tension, and iron-deficiency anaemia, and in the long-term they protect against endometrial and ovarian cancer. However, they do not protect against sexually transmitted diseases, they are unsuitable for older women who smoke, and long-term use carries a slight increased risk of breast cancer. Other forms of combined contraceptive which have been developed recently include *monthly injection*, *vaginal ring*, and *transdermal patch*.

*Progestogen-only oral contraceptives* have a 0.5% failure rate during the first year of use if taken correctly, which is slightly higher than that for combined preparations; in practice, failure rates of from 1 to 10% have been reported. Regularity in taking them is essential; a dose should not be delayed for more than 3 hours. They act primarily to decrease the chance of fertilisation and implantation since they prevent ovulation in only 14 to 40% of cycles. They are useful for women who are breast feeding, for those who smoke and are more than 35 years of age, and if medical conditions contra-indicate the use of oestrogens.

*Barrier methods*, including both male and female condoms, vaginal sponges containing spermicide, and diaphragms and cervical caps used with spermicide, act as a mechanical barrier to prevent fertilisation, and inactivate sperm. Barrier methods decrease the risk of sexually transmitted diseases and a shift towards their use has occurred since the emergence of HIV infection in particular. However, barrier methods are not as effective in preventing conception as hormonal contraception and copper IUDs. Even when used correctly, failure rates in the first year of use vary from 3% for the male condom to 11.5% with the cervical cap plus spermicide. Spermicides, such as nonoxinol 9, may be used as foam or as dissolvable vaginal tablets or pessaries, or as a spermicide-containing polyvinyl alcohol film placed over the cervix. However, they are generally considered relatively ineffective when used as the sole method of contraception, and such use is not recommended.

*Natural family planning methods* such as periodic abstinence using the calendar, temperature, cervical mucus ('Billings') or sympto-thermal methods require high motivation to learn and practice effectively. However, they may be the only acceptable method to some people. More recently, daily measurement of urine hormone concentrations has been used as a predictor of the timing of ovulation and hence the risk of becoming pregnant; on 'unsafe' days abstinence or barrier methods are required. Traditional methods such as withdrawal (coitus interruptus) are widely used in some areas, but are considered relatively ineffective.

Various other methods of contraception are under investigation including the use of gonadorelin analogues, selective sex-hormone receptor modulators, and contraceptive vaccines. There has also been some investigation of **male contraception**. Weekly intramuscular injection of high-dose testosterone or nandrolone to produce azoospermia has been investigated with some success, but development of an oral contraceptive dosage form for males has been slow. Use of a progestogen with testosterone is being studied, as is the use of implants of synthetic androgens such as trestolone (7-α-methyl-19-nortestosterone; MENT).

The available irreversible methods of contraception are surgical male or female *sterilisation*. The use of mepacrine for non-surgical female sterilisation has been attempted but has proved extremely controversial.

References.


1. WHO. Facts about once-a-month injectable contraceptives: memorandum from a WHO meeting. *Bull WHO* 1993; **71:** 677–89.
2. Matlin SA. Prospects for pharmacological male contraception. *Drugs* 1994; **48:** 851–63.
3. Baird DT, Glasier AF. Hormonal contraception. *N Engl J Med* 1993; **328:** 1543–9.
4. Flemming CF. Oral contraception. *Prescribers' J* 1994; **34:** 227–34.
5. Weisberg E. Prescribing oral contraceptives. *Drugs* 1995; **49:** 224–31.
6. Anonymous. Long-acting progestogen-only contraception. *Drug Ther Bull* 1996; **34:** 93–6.
7. Anonymous. Choice of contraceptives. *Med Lett Drugs Ther* 1995; **37:** 9–12. Additional note. *ibid.*: 36.
8. WHO. *Contraceptive Method Mix: guidelines for policy and service delivery.* Geneva: World Health Organization, 1994.
9. Belfield T. *FPA Contraceptive Handbook: a guide for family planning and other health professionals.* 3rd ed. London: Family Planning Association, 1999.
10. Rowlands S. Contraception beyond the millennium. *Pharm J* 1998; **261:** 666–8.
11. Baird DT, Glasier AF. Contraception. *BMJ* 1999; **319:** 969–72.
12. Baird DT. Overview of advances in contraception. *Br Med Bull* 2000; **56:** 704–16.
13. Anderson RA. Hormonal contraception in the male. *Br Med Bull* 2000; **56:** 717–28.
14. Lähteenmäki P, Jukarainen H. Novel delivery systems in contraception. *Br Med Bull* 2000; **56:** 739–48.
15. Kubba A, *et al.* Contraception. *Lancet* 2000; **356:** 1913–19.


EMERGENCY CONTRACEPTION. Emergency contraception (postcoital contraception)[1–4] can be used after unprotected intercourse but before a fertilised ovum has been implanted. Methods that act after implantation are considered abortifacients. The two most commonly used emergency contraceptives are *oral contraceptives* and *copper IUDs*.

Oral contraceptive regimens (the so-called 'morning after pill') have historically employed a preparation containing high-dose oestrogen with a progestogen, taken within 72 hours of intercourse, and repeated 12 hours later (the Yuzpe regimen). This preparation is thought to act by a variety of mechanisms, which may depend on when in the menstrual cycle it is used. It may prevent implantation, prevent or delay ovulation, disrupt ovum transport, and alter corpus luteum function. Reported efficacy rates vary between 75 and 80%. However, levonorgestrel alone (without an oestrogen) is now widely recommended as an emergency contraceptive. A large WHO multicentre study found that levonorgestrel 750 micrograms alone within 72 hours of intercourse and repeated after 12 hours was more effective than the Yuzpe regimen and better tolerated.[5] Both regimens were most effective when given within 24 hours of intercourse.[5,6] A small observational study[7] of the Yuzpe method used between 72 and 120 hours after unprotected intercourse reported a trend towards decrease in effectiveness. A further large study[8] by WHO found that for up to 120 hours after intercourse, a single dose of levonorgestrel 1.5 mg was as effective as two doses of 750 micrograms given 12 hours apart, with a pregnancy rate of about 1.5%.

Copper, but not progestogen, IUDs can be inserted up to 120 hours after unprotected intercourse for postcoital contraception. They have a failure rate of less than 1% when used for emergency contraception. Thus, when efficacy is a priority the IUD is the emergency contraceptive method of choice.

Drugs under investigation for use as emergency contraceptives include *mifepristone*. When taken as a single 600-mg dose within 72 hours of unprotected intercourse this has been reported to be 100% effective.[9] Subsequently, a very low dose of 10 mg was shown to be similar in efficacy to the 600-mg dose.[10] A single dose of 10 mg was also found to be as effective as levonorgestrel 1.5 mg (in a single dose or 2 divided doses) for up to 120 hours after intercourse.[8] Although mifepristone is also effective after implantation (5 to 7 days after fertilisation), its action as an emergency contraceptive appears to depend on inhibiting ovulation or, if ovulation has occurred, preventing implantation.


1. Glasier A. Emergency postcoital contraception. *N Engl J Med* 1997; **337:** 1058–64.
2. Kubba A, Wilkinson C. Emergency contraception update. *Br J Fam Plann* 1998; **23:** 135–7.
3. Glasier A. Emergency contraception. *Br Med Bull* 2000; **56:** 729–38.
4. Cheng L, *et al.* Interventions for emergency contraception. Available in The Cochrane Library; Issue 2. Chichester: John Wiley; 2004.
5. Task Force on Postovulatory Methods of Fertility Regulation. Randomised controlled trial of levonorgestrel versus the Yuzpe regimen of combined oral contraceptives for emergency contraception. *Lancet* 1998; **352:** 428–33.
6. Piaggio G, *et al.* Timing of emergency contraception with levonorgestrel or the Yuzpe regimen. *Lancet* 1999; **353:** 721.
7. Rodrigues I, *et al.* Effectiveness of emergency contraceptive pills between 72 and 120 hours after unprotected sexual intercourse. *Am J Obstet Gynecol* 2001; **184:** 531–7.
8. von Hertzen H, *et al.* Low dose mifepristone and two regimens of levonorgestrel for emergency contraception: a WHO multicentre randomised trial. *Lancet* 2002; **360:** 1803–10.
9. Glasier A, *et al.* Mifepristone (RU 486) compared with high-dose estrogen and progestogen for emergency postcoital contraception. *N Engl J Med* 1992; **327:** 1041–4.
10. Task Force on Postovulatory Methods of Fertility Regulation. Comparison of three single doses of mifepristone as emergency contraception: a randomised trial. *Lancet* 1999; **353:** 697–702.


# Hormone Replacement Therapy

Tratamiento hormonal sustitutivo.

## The Menopause

The menopause is defined as the permanent cessation of cyclical menstruation due to loss of ovarian follicular activity. It is therefore determined in retrospect, conventionally after a period of 1 year without menstruation. In the few years prior to the menopause (the menopausal transition), ovarian oestradiol secretion declines, sometimes in a fluctuating manner, and there is a resultant increase in pituitary follicle-stimulating hormone (FSH) secretion. The menopausal transition may be characterised by irregular menstrual cycles and dysfunctional uterine bleeding, and fertility is much reduced compared with the early reproductive years. The term perimenopause is used to cover the menopausal transition and the first year after the menopause, and may last 3 to 5 years. It has sometimes been referred to as the climacteric. Oestrogen concentrations reach their minimum and FSH concentrations their maximum about 4 years after the menopause. After the menopause the ovaries may continue to produce some androgens, which together with adrenal androgens are converted to oestrogens (predominantly oestrone) in the periphery, but oestrogen concentrations are much lower than in premenopausal women. The median age for the natural menopause is about 51 years. If the menopause occurs in women aged 40 years or less, it is considered premature. The menopause may be induced by surgical removal of both ovaries, or sometimes by antineoplastic drugs or radiotherapy.

The decline in oestrogen concentrations during the perimenopause may be associated with both acute and long-term effects. However, some of these may be difficult to differentiate from the effects of ageing, and the incidence varies geographically. Established *acute symptoms* can include vasomotor instability, manifesting as hot flushes and night sweats, and vaginal atrophy and dyspareunia. Non-specific symptoms include palpitations, headache, backache, and psychological symptoms such as tiredness, lack of concentration, loss of libido, irritability, insomnia, and depression. Insomnia may occur secondary to night sweats. There is little evidence that depressive illness is disproportionately increased at the menopause. Urinary problems are common in ageing women, and may occur in the perimenopause, but the extent that these are due to lack of oestrogens has not been determined. An established *long-term consequence* of the decline in oestrogen concentrations is an increased risk of bone fractures resulting from an increase in the rate of bone resorption. In addition, decline in oestrogen concentrations is associated with adverse effects on blood lipoproteins, and this may be a risk factor for cardiovascular disease.

Acute and longer term effects of the menopause may be managed by using hormone replacement therapy (HRT) with oestrogens, with or without progestogens.

## Adverse Effects of HRT

When oestrogens are used for menopausal HRT, adverse effects include nausea and vomiting, abdominal cramps and bloating, weight changes, breast enlargement and tenderness, premenstrual-like syndrome, sodium and fluid retention, altered blood lipids, changes in liver function, cholestatic jaundice, rashes and chloasma (melasma), changes in libido, migraine, dizziness, depression, headache, leg cramps, and decreased tolerance of contact lenses. Transdermal delivery systems may cause contact sensitisation (possibly severe hypersensitivity reactions on continued exposure), and nasal sprays may cause local irritation, rhinorrhoea, and epistaxis. Headache has been reported on vigorous exercise. Use of oestrogen without a progestogen results in endometrial hyperplasia and an increased risk of endometrial carcinoma (see below). The addition of a progestogen for 10 to 14 days of a 28-day cycle reduces this risk but results in regular withdrawal bleeding towards the end of the progestogen. Use of continuous progestogen and oestrogen avoids withdrawal bleeding, but may result in irregular breakthrough bleeding, particularly in the early stages of therapy, or if used within 12 months of the last menstrual period. Current use of menopausal HRT is associated with an increased risk of venous thromboembolism and breast cancer (see below).

◊ Reviews.


1. Winship KA. Unopposed oestrogens. *Adverse Drug React Acute Poisoning Rev* 1987; **1:** 37–66.
2. Evans MP, *et al.* Hormone replacement therapy: management of common problems. *Mayo Clin Proc* 1995; **70:** 800–5.


**Carcinogenicity.** Use of unopposed oestrogen as menopausal HRT in women with a uterus increases the risk of endometrial cancer, irrespective of the route of administration. This risk is reduced, although possibly not eliminated completely, by the concomitant use of a progestogen. There is also evidence that use of HRT, as oestrogen alone or with a progestogen, increases the risk of breast cancer.

Because of continuing modifications in regimens for HRT there is a continuing need to monitor the incidence of various cancers in users of this therapy.

BREAST. Early age at menarche and late age at menopause increase the risk of breast cancer, and surgical oophorectomy at an early age decreases the risk of breast cancer. In addition, higher concentrations of unbound endogenous oestrogens in postmenopausal women appear to increase the risk of developing breast cancer.[1] Such risk factors have prompted concerns that menopausal HRT might be associated with an increased risk of breast cancer.

Reviews and analyses[2-4] of studies published during the 1970s and/or 1980s on the use of **unopposed oestrogen** replacement therapy in postmenopausal women have generally shown that there is an associated moderate increase in the risk of breast cancer; figures for overall relative risk compared with non-oestrogen users ranged from under 1 to up to 2. One of these,[3] a meta-analysis of studies from 1976 to 1989, further showed that although the relative risk of breast cancer rose to 1.3 after 15 years of oestrogen use, it did not appear to rise at all until after 5 years' use. A similar meta-analysis[4] differentiated between low-dose oestrogens and high-dose oestrogens; those taking 0.625 mg daily of conjugated oestrogens had a risk of breast cancer 1.08 times higher than non-oestrogen users, whereas the relative risk in those taking 1.25 mg daily or more was up to 2. A subsequent meta-analysis[5] differentiated between current use of HRT, duration of use, and use at any time. The highest relative risk of breast cancer was associated with current use (1.4); use for 10 years or more was associated with a relative risk of about 1.2, and having ever used HRT was not associated with an increased risk. In 1997 the Collaborative Group on Hormonal Factors in Breast Cancer reanalysed about 90% of the worldwide evidence on breast cancer and the use of HRT.[6] They reported that the relative risk of having breast cancer diagnosed was increased by a factor of 1.023 for each year of use, being 1.35 for 5 or more years of use. However, this effect was reduced on cessation of use, and had largely disappeared after about 5 years. In women who started therapy at age 50, the cumulative excess number of breast cancers diagnosed per 1000 women between age 50 and 70 were estimated to be 2, 6, and 12 for 5, 10, and 15 years use, respectively, from a baseline of 45 per 1000 in never-users.[6] In contrast, the arm of the Women's Health Initiative[7] that compared conjugated oestrogens with placebo over an average of about 7 years found a trend towards a reduction in breast cancer risk with HRT; extended follow-up is yet to be reported.

Most data relate to the use of unopposed oestrogen. There has been speculation both that the concomitant use of progestogen in HRT could reduce the risk of breast cancer and that it might increase it. Bergkvist *et al.*[8] suggested an increased relative risk of 4.4 in the small subgroup using long-term **combined therapy**, but because of the large confidence intervals they considered these results inconclusive. Analysis of the Nurses' Health Study cohort has provided evidence that current use of oestrogen and progestogen is associated with a similar increased relative risk of breast cancer to that of unopposed oestrogen (1.4 versus 1.3).[9] The Collaborative Group on Hormonal Factors in Breast Cancer[6] found no evidence of marked differences between preparations containing oestrogens alone and those containing oestrogens and progestogens. However, in a randomised trial, oestrogen plus progestogen was associated with greater increases in radiographic breast density than unopposed oestrogen.[10] The results of further cohort studies[11,12] and a case-control study[13] also suggest that the risk of breast cancer may be higher for current or recent use of combined HRT compared with oestrogen alone, and a cohort study[14] of over 1 million women (the Million Women Study) found relative risks of 1.3 for users of oestrogen alone, and 2.0 for combined HRT, compared with never-users. After an average follow-up of about 5 years the Women's Health Initiative,[15] comparing combined HRT with placebo in more than 16 000 women, was stopped early because of an increased rate of invasive breast cancer in women given HRT.

The public health perspective on the **implications** of any increased risk of breast cancer will depend on the background risk. This is high in western countries, so a small increased relative risk would equate to a large absolute increase in number of cases.[16]

If menopausal oestrogen therapy increases the risk of breast cancer, there is a need to ascertain whether these cancers can be detected early, how aggressive they are, and what the mortality rate from them is. Currently, there are limited data on these points.

- There is evidence[17,18] that the use of HRT decreases the sensitivity and specificity of screening mammography (resulting in more false positives and more false negatives), apparently because it increases radiographic breast density,[19] so decreasing the ability to interpret the mammogram. This is of concern for the success of screening programmes, and has been suggested as a factor in the increased detection of interval cancers (those detected between screening appointments).[20] In addition, HRT-associated increases in radiographic breast density could actually be a marker for risk of breast cancer.[10,21]
- Some data suggest that breast cancers in women on HRT may be of better prognostic grade.[22,23] The Collaborative Group on Hormonal Factors in Breast Cancer reported that breast cancers were more likely to be localised in current or recent users of HRT, but that there was evidence of an increased risk of metastasis with increasing duration of use.[6] However, the Women's Health Initiative[21] did not confirm previous findings of favourable prognosis, and found breast cancers in HRT users to be larger, more likely to be node positive, and at a more advanced stage at diagnosis.
- Follow-up of most studies is currently insufficient to give a clear indication of mortality risk with long-term use. Early data from a UK cohort study[24] suggested a decreased risk of breast cancer mortality, but after further follow-up the risk was no longer reduced.[25] Similarly, a study in 2614 women with breast cancer followed up for up to 22 years found that the use of HRT at the time of diagnosis was associated with a reduction in mortality, but the effect waned over time.[26] In contrast, data[9] from the Nurses' Health Study cohort suggest an increase in risk of death from breast cancer in women who have currently used HRT for 5 years or more (1.45). Similarly, although mortality was lower overall, a trend towards an increased risk of death from breast cancer (1.9; 95% confidence interval 0.4 to 8.4) was seen in a study of long-term use (mean of 17 years).[27]

The risk of breast cancer may be increased further by the use of HRT in women who are already at an increased risk. Although a recent study found a modest increase in risk in these women, it was not significantly higher, and there was a reduced total mortality rate.[28] It is unclear whether use of HRT in breast cancer survivors increases the risk of subsequent recurrence and associated mortality (see also under Precautions, below).


1. Toniolo PG, *et al.* A prospective study of endogenous estrogens and breast cancer in postmenopausal women. *J Natl Cancer Inst* 1995; **87:** 190–7.
2. Henderson BE. The cancer question: an overview of recent epidemiologic and retrospective data. *Am J Obstet Gynecol* 1989; **161:** 1859–64.
3. Steinberg KK, *et al.* A meta-analysis of the effect of estrogen replacement therapy on the risk of breast cancer. *JAMA* 1991; **265:** 1985–90.
4. Dupont WD, Page DL. Menopausal estrogen replacement therapy and breast cancer. *Arch Intern Med* 1991; **151:** 67–72.
5. Colditz GA, *et al.* Hormone replacement therapy and risk of breast cancer: results from epidemiologic studies. *Am J Obstet Gynecol* 1993; **168:** 1473–80.
6. Collaborative Group on Hormonal Factors in Breast Cancer. Breast cancer and hormone replacement therapy: collaborative reanalysis of data from 51 epidemiological studies of 52 705 women with breast cancer and 108 411 women without breast cancer. *Lancet* 1997; **350:** 1047–59. Correction. *ibid.*; 1484.
7. The Women's Health Initiative Steering Committee. Effects of conjugated equine estrogen in postmenopausal women with hysterectomy: the Women's Health Initiative randomized controlled trial. *JAMA* 2004; **291:** 1701–12.
8. Bergkvist L, *et al.* The risk of breast cancer after estrogen and estrogen—progestin replacement. *N Engl J Med* 1989; **321:** 293–7.
9. Colditz GA, *et al.* The use of estrogens and progestins and the risk of breast cancer in postmenopausal women. *N Engl J Med* 1995; **332:** 1589–93.
10. Greendale GA, *et al.* Effects of estrogen and estrogen-progestin on mammographic parenchymal density. *Ann Intern Med* 1999; **130:** 262–9.
11. Schairer C, *et al.* Menopausal estrogen and estrogen-progestin replacement therapy and breast cancer risk. *JAMA* 2000; **283:** 485–91.
12. Colditz GA, Rosner B. Cumulative risk of breast cancer to age 70 years according to risk factor status: data from The Nurses' Health Study. *Am J Epidemiol* 2000; **152:** 950–64.
13. Ross RK, *et al.* Effect of hormone replacement therapy on breast cancer risk: estrogen versus estrogen plus progestin. *J Natl Cancer Inst* 2000; **92:** 328–32.
14. Million Women Study Collaborators. Breast cancer and hormone-replacement therapy in the Million Women Study. *Lancet* 2003; **362:** 419–27. Correction. *ibid.*; 1160.
15. Writing Group for the Women's Health Initiative Investigators. Risks and benefits of estrogen plus progestin in healthy postmenopausal women: principal results from the Women's Health Initiative randomized controlled trial. *JAMA* 2002; **288:** 321–33.
16. WHO. Research on the menopause in the 1990s: report of a WHO scientific group. *WHO Tech Rep Ser 866* 1996.
17. Laya MB, *et al.* Effect of estrogen replacement therapy on the specificity and sensitivity of screening mammography. *J Natl Cancer Inst* 1996; **88:** 643–9.
18. Kavanagh AM, *et al.* Hormone replacement therapy and accuracy of mammographic screening. *Lancet* 2000; **355:** 270–4.
19. Rutter CM, *et al.* Changes in breast density associated with initiation, discontinuation, and continuing use of hormone replacement therapy. *JAMA* 2001; **285:** 171–6.
20. Cohen EL. Effect of hormone replacement therapy on cancer detection by mammography. *Lancet* 1997; **349:** 1624.
21. Chlebowski RT, *et al.* Influence of estrogen plus progestin on breast cancer and mammography in healthy postmenopausal women: the Women's Health Initiative randomized trial. *JAMA* 2003; **289:** 3243–53.
22. Harding C, *et al.* Hormone replacement therapy and tumour grade in breast cancer: prospective study in screening unit. *BMJ* 1996; **312:** 1646–7. Correction. *ibid.*; **313:** 198.
23. Gapstur SM, *et al.* Hormone replacement therapy and risk of breast cancer with a favorable histology: results of the Iowa Women's Health Study. *JAMA* 1999; **281:** 2091–7.
24. Hunt K, *et al.* Long-term surveillance of mortality and cancer incidence in women receiving hormone replacement therapy. *Br J Obstet Gynaecol* 1987; **94:** 620–35.
25. Hunt K, *et al.* Mortality in a cohort of long-term users of hormone replacement therapy: an updated analysis. *Br J Obstet Gynaecol* 1990; **97:** 1080–6.
26. Schairer C, *et al.* Estrogen replacement therapy and breast cancer survival in a large screening study. *J Natl Cancer Inst* 1999; **91:** 264–70.
27. Ettinger B, *et al.* Reduced mortality associated with long-term postmenopausal estrogen therapy. *Obstet Gynecol* 1996; **87:** 6–12.
28. Sellers TA, *et al.* The role of hormone replacement therapy in the risk for breast cancer and total mortality in women with a family history of breast cancer. *Ann Intern Med* 1997; **127:** 973–80.


CERVIX. Studies of the effect of HRT on cervical cancer risk are likely to be subject to the potential confounding of other risk factors such as sexual activity. There are few data on this risk, but study suggests oestrogens do not increase, and may decrease, the risk of cervical cancer.[1] Therapy with combined HRT did not significantly affect the incidence of cytological abnormalities found in annual cervical smears in women in the Heart and Estrogen/progestin Replacement Study (HERS).[2]


1. Parazzini, F, *et al.* Case-control study of oestrogen replacement therapy and risk of cervical cancer. *BMJ* 1997; **315:** 85–8.
2. Sawaya GF, *et al.* The positive predictive value of cervical smears in previously screened postmenopausal women: the Heart and Estrogen/progestin Replacement Study (HERS). *Ann Intern Med* 2000; **133:** 942–50.


ENDOMETRIUM. The increased incidence of endometrial hyperplasia and risk of cancer in women receiving unopposed oestrogen replacement therapy is well established. An analysis of case control studies published during the 1970s and 1980s revealed a relative risk of developing endometrial cancer of 1.4 to 7.6 in women who had ever used oestrogen, and a relative risk of 3.1 to 15 in long-term users, compared with nonusers.[1] Risk was also increased with higher doses of oestrogens. In general, endometrial cancer in oestrogen users was of a better prognostic stage, and survival rates were better, than in nonusers.[1] An elevated risk of endometrial cancer persists for a number of years after stopping unopposed oestrogen therapy.[2]

Addition of a progestogen to oestrogen replacement therapy reduces the incidence of endometrial hyperplasia[3] and cancer. However, the extent to which this alters the risks and benefits of oestrogen replacement therapy, and the optimum progestogen type, and dose and duration, have not been fully elucidated.

As regards risk of endometrial cancer, preliminary data from a cohort study revealed that the addition of cyclical progestogen to oestrogen therapy reduced this risk compared with oestrogen therapy alone.[4] A further case-control study confirmed that progestogens decreased the relative risk, and that the reduction in risk was greater when progestogens were used for 10 or more days per month than when they were used for less than 10 days per month.[5] Two much larger case-control studies have confirmed these findings.[6,7] However, 1 of these studies[6] reported that in long-term users the addition of a progestogen did not reduce the risk of endometrial cancer to that seen in nonusers—after 5 years of use, the relative risk of endometrial cancer with HRT containing 10 or more days of progestogen per month was 2.5 (95% confidence intervals 1.1 to 5.5). This finding remains to be confirmed.

Use of progestogens for 10 days of an 84-day cycle (long cycle) has been suggested to improve acceptability of combined HRT. However one study of a long-cycle regimen was discontinued because of an increased risk of endometrial hyperplasia and atypia compared with a conventional monthly cycle regimen.[8]

Some newer regimens of HRT employ continuous low-doses of progestogen with oestrogen, which avoid withdrawal bleeding. Data on the incidence of endometrial hyperplasia from randomised trials of these regimens have been reassuring.[3,9,10] Continuous norethisterone plus ethinylestradiol,[9] and continuous medroxyprogesterone plus conjugated oestrogens,[10] protected the endometrium against the hyperplasia seen with the oestrogen alone. Continuous therapy was as effective as cyclical therapy containing 12 days' progestogen,[10] and there is a suggestion from meta-analysis[3] that continuous therapy may even be more effective than sequential when given over a prolonged period, although this remains to be confirmed. The first data on endometrial cancer risk from continuous combined HRT suggest that it is as protective as sequential therapy with the progestogen administered for 10 or more days per month (odds ratio 1.07 per 5 years of use for both regimens).[7]

It is unclear whether use of HRT in endometrial cancer survivors increases the risk of subsequent recurrence and associated mortality (see also under Precautions, below).


1. Henderson BE. The cancer question: an overview of recent epidemiologic and retrospective data. *Am J Obstet Gynecol* 1989; **161:** 1859–64.
2. Rubin GL, *et al.* Estrogen replacement therapy and the risk of endometrial cancer: remaining controversies. *Am J Obstet Gynecol* 1990; **162:** 148–54.
3. Lethaby A, *et al.* Hormone replacement therapy in postmenopausal women: endometrial hyperplasia and irregular bleeding. Available in The Cochrane Library; Issue 2. Chichester: John Wiley; 2004.
4. Persson I, *et al.* Risk of endometrial cancer after treatment with oestrogens alone or in conjunction with progestogens: results of a prospective study. *BMJ* 1989; **298:** 147–51.
5. Voigt LF, *et al.* Progestagen supplementation of exogenous oestrogens and risk of endometrial cancer. *Lancet* 1991; **338:** 274–7.
6. Beresford S, *et al.* Risk of endometrial cancer in relation to use of oestrogen combined with cyclic progestagen therapy in postmenopausal women. *Lancet* 1997; **349:** 458–61.
7. Pike MC, *et al.* Estrogen-progestin replacement therapy and endometrial cancer. *J Natl Cancer Inst* 1997; **89:** 1110–16.
8. Cerin A, *et al.* Adverse endometrial effects of long-cycle estrogen and progestogen replacement therapy. *N Engl J Med* 1996; **334:** 668–9.
9. Speroff L, *et al.* The comparative effect on bone density, endometrium, and lipids of continuous hormones as replacement therapy (CHART Study). *JAMA* 1996; **276:** 1397–1403.
10. The Writing Group for the PEPI trial. Effects of hormone replacement therapy on endometrial histology in postmenopausal women. *JAMA* 1996; **275:** 370–5.


GASTROINTESTINAL TRACT. Evidence of an effect of oestrogen replacement therapy on colorectal cancer is ambiguous, since studies have reported both an increased and a decreased incidence; a meta-analysis in 1995 suggested no overall effect.[1] However, subsequent cohort studies did suggest a lower incidence of colon cancer in those who had received oestrogens.[2,3] This was most pronounced in current users in whom the relative risk was about one-third to one-half of that for women who had never taken oestrogen. Similarly, a large case-control study also reported a significant reduction in colon cancer, but not rectal cancer.[4] A later meta-analysis[5] concluded that the risk of colon cancer might be decreased among women who have recently used HRT, and that the risk of death from colon cancer might also be reduced. The Women's Health Initiative,[6] a placebo-controlled trial of combined HRT in more than 16 000 women, found that those taking HRT had a decreased risk of developing colorectal cancer, but that at diagnosis there was greater lymph node involvement and it was at a more advanced stage.


1. MacLennan SC, *et al.* Colorectal cancer and oestrogen replacement therapy: a meta-analysis of epidemiological studies. *Med J Aust* 1995; **162:** 491–3.
2. Calle EE, *et al.* Estrogen replacement therapy and risk of fatal colon cancer in a prospective cohort of postmenopausal women. *J Natl Cancer Inst* 1995; **87:** 517–23.
3. Grodstein F, *et al.* Postmenopausal hormone use and risk for colorectal cancer and adenoma. *Ann Intern Med* 1998; **128:** 705–12.
4. Newcomb PA, Storer BE. Postmenopausal hormone use and risk of large-bowel cancer. *J Natl Cancer Inst* 1995; **87:** 1067–71.
5. Nanda K, *et al.* Hormone replacement therapy and the risk of colorectal cancer: a meta-analysis. *Obstet Gynecol* 1999; **93:** 880–8.
6. Chlebowski RT, *et al.* Estrogen plus progestin and colorectal cancer in postmenopausal women. *N Engl J Med* 2004; **350:** 991–1004.


OVARY. There was no clear evidence that the use of oestrogen replacement therapy altered the risk of invasive ovarian cancer in various case-control studies reviewed by the Collaborative Ovarian Cancer Group.[1] However, subsequent study of a large cohort has suggested that long-term oestrogen replacement therapy may increase the risk of fatal ovarian cancer.[2,3] Similarly, a meta-analysis indicated an increased risk for invasive epithelial ovarian cancer, especially after long-term use of HRT.[4]


1. Whittemore AS, *et al.* Characteristics relating to ovarian cancer risk: collaborative analysis of 12 US case-control studies. *Am J Epidemiol* 1992; **136:** 1184–1203.
2. Rodriguez C, *et al.* Estrogen replacement therapy and fatal ovarian cancer. *Am J Epidemiol* 1995; **141:** 828–35.
3. Rodriguez C, *et al.* Estrogen replacement therapy and ovarian cancer mortality in a large prospective study of US women. *JAMA* 2001; **285:** 1460–5.
4. Garg PP, *et al.* Hormone replacement therapy and the risk of epithelial ovarian carcinoma: a meta-analysis. *Obstet Gynecol* 1998; **92:** 472–9.


**Effects on the cardiovascular system.** Various facts support the theory that oestrogens may be cardioprotective. For example, mortality rates for cardiovascular disease in women are lower than those in men at all ages. In addition, women who have a surgically induced menopause at a young age are at increased risk of ischaemic heart disease compared with women who have a natural menopause.

Conversely, use of high doses of oestrogens for malignant disease is associated with an increased risk of cardiovascular events. Similarly, use of oestrogens in combined oral contraceptives carries a small increased risk of cardiovascular disease (see p.1530). Moreover, an early study in men surviving a myocardial infarction found that high doses of conjugated oestrogens (5 mg daily) were associated with a higher incidence of subsequent coronary events than placebo (see Effects on the Cardiovascular System, in Conjugated Oestrogens, p.1543).

In practice, a number of large observational studies found a decreased risk of ischaemic heart disease and mortality in women receiving menopausal HRT compared with those who have never received this therapy (see below). The reduction in risk was estimated as 30 to 50%, but biases such as the healthy user effect seem to play a part in this estimate; unfortunately, results from controlled studies have cast doubt on the extent of any reduction in risk. There is also evidence to show that HRT *increases* the risk of stroke (see below) and venous thromboembolism (see below).

The mechanisms by which oestrogen exerts its cardiovascular effects are not fully understood.[1] Oestrogen has beneficial effects on lipoproteins, but adverse effects on triglycerides (see below). Similarly, it has beneficial effects on some, and adverse effects on other, mediators of thrombosis. Oestrogen may also have a direct beneficial effect on the coronary vasculature. Progestogens may reduce the beneficial effects of oestrogens on some lipids, although observational data has suggested that this is not sufficient to reverse potential benefit.


1. Mendelsohn ME, Karas RH. The protective effects of estrogen on the cardiovascular system. *N Engl J Med* 1999; **340:** 1801–11.


HYPERTENSION. Although high doses of oestrogens have been associated with increased blood pressure, use of menopausal HRT in normotensive women has little effect on blood pressure or may be associated with a small decrease. An observational study[1] of normotensive postmenopausal women also found that, over time, the average increase in systolic blood pressure was significantly less in women who were taking HRT. Similarly, there is some evidence that use of HRT in hypertensive women does not alter blood pressure[2] and may even reduce it.[3]


1. Scuteri A, *et al.* Hormone replacement therapy and longitudinal changes in blood pressure in postmenopausal women. *Ann Intern Med* 2001; **135:** 229–38.
2. Lip GYH, *et al.* Hormone replacement therapy and blood pressure in hypertensive women. *J Hum Hypertens* 1994; **8:** 491–4.
3. Affinito P, *et al.* Effects of hormonal replacement therapy in postmenopausal hypertensive patients. *Maturitas* 2001; **40:** 75–83.


ISCHAEMIC HEART DISEASE. In 1991, Stampfer and Colditz reviewed 31 case-control and cohort studies on the risk of ischaemic heart disease in women using menopausal HRT.[1] Four studies showed an adverse trend, 2 showed no effect on risk, and 25 showed a trend to **reduction in risk** or a significant reduction in risk. The summary relative risk was 0.56, with estimated 95% confidence intervals of 0.50 to 0.61. Other reviews have reported similar reductions in risk.[2,3] Much of the data relate to the use of unopposed oestrogen, which is no longer recommended in women with a uterus because of the risk of endometrial cancer (see above).

There has been concern that the **addition of progestogen** might negate or reduce the cardiovascular benefits of oestrogens by reducing the oestrogen-induced rise in serum high-density-lipoprotein cholesterol concentrations. It has been postulated that this may be particularly true for progestogens derived from nortestosterone rather than progesterone. Results from the Postmenopausal Estrogen/Progestin Interventions Trial (PEPI) indicated that the beneficial effects on blood lipoproteins and fibrinogen, although greatest with unopposed oestrogen, were still present when combined with medroxyprogesterone or micronised progesterone (micronised progesterone was preferable to medroxyprogesterone).[4] Moreover, the UK Medical Research Council Study reported a fairly even balance between possibly beneficial and adverse effects on lipid concentrations and coagulability when conjugated oestrogens alone were compared with conjugated oestrogens plus norgestrel (a nortestosterone derivative).[5] Similar results were reported in the CHART study for ethinylestradiol with or without norethisterone.[6] Although reassuring, these 3 studies provide information only on surrogate endpoints.

Data from the Nurses' Health Study cohort[7] showed a greater reduction in the risk of major ischaemic heart disease among women receiving an oestrogen plus a progestogen (relative risk 0.4) than those receiving an oestrogen alone (0.6), as compared with the risk in women not using hormones. *In-vitro* data suggest that progestogens may actually protect against atherosclerosis via inhibition of smooth muscle cell proliferation.[8]

As regards **duration of HRT use**, it appears that current use is the most important factor for cardiovascular risk reduction. Users with coronary risk factors appear to derive greater benefit from HRT than those at low risk of coronary artery disease.[9] Of concern, the Nurses' Health Study reported that the apparent benefit from HRT decreased with increasing duration of use beyond 10 years because of an increase in mortality from breast cancer.[9]

However, a number of studies have found **no beneficial effect** on risk of heart disease. In contrast to previous findings, a retrospective case-control study[10] did not find a decreased risk of myocardial infarction in women currently using combined HRT or oestrogens alone. The authors of this study suggested that the benefit of HRT may not be as large as has been estimated in some qualitative overviews, and emphasised the need for data from randomised trials.[10] This has been confirmed by results[11] of the Heart and Estrogen/Progestin Replacement Study, a randomised placebo-controlled trial in women with established ischaemic heart disease. Combined HRT with conjugated oestrogens plus medroxyprogesterone produced no overall reduction in the occurrence of myocardial infarction or death due to ischaemic heart disease in these women. This overall lack of effect was due to an initial increase in cardiac events during the first year, with a later beneficial effect in years 3 to 5. During unblinded follow-up[12] of 2.7 years, these late beneficial effects did not persist and the risk of cardiovascular events was not reduced. Observational data from the Nurses' Health Study cohort[13] also noted a trend towards an initial increase in cardiac events followed by a decrease in risk with long-term use of HRT, in women with a history of ischaemic heart disease. Another study, the Estrogen Replacement and Atherosclerosis trial, found that HRT did not affect the progression of existing coronary atherosclerosis as measured by angiography.[14] Oestrogen therapy for 2 years also had no effect on the risk of further cardiac events in postmenopausal women who had survived a myocardial infarction.[15] There is also some evidence that the risks and benefits of HRT may vary according to the presence or absence of particular prothrombotic mutations.[16] These worrying results have suggested that HRT should not be used for secondary prevention in women with heart disease, in contrast to some earlier suggestions (see also under Uses and Administration, below).

In women without pre-existing heart disease, observational data from the Nurses' Health Study[17] showed a reduced risk of major coronary events in users of HRT, compared with never-users. However, there were increased rates of coronary events at an average follow-up of about 5 years in the Women's Health Initiative,[18] a primary prevention trial comparing combined HRT with placebo in over 16 000 women. The risk was highest in the first year of HRT but decreased to a smaller non-significant excess risk in the following years.[19] The arm of the Women's Health Initiative that compared unopposed conjugated oestrogens with placebo in more than 10 000 women with prior hysterectomy found that over an average of almost 7 years there was no difference in the risk of ischaemic heart disease.[20] These results suggest that HRT should also not be used for primary prevention of ischaemic heart disease.


1. Stampfer MJ, Colditz GA. Estrogen replacement therapy and coronary heart disease: a quantitative assessment of the epidemiologic evidence. *Prev Med* 1991; **20:** 47–63.
2. Grady D, *et al.* Hormone therapy to prevent disease and prolong life in postmenopausal women. *Ann Intern Med* 1992; **117:** 1016–37.
3. Barrett-Connor E, Bush TL. Estrogen and coronary heart disease in women. *JAMA* 1991; **265:** 1861–7.
4. The Writing Group for the PEPI Trial. Effects of estrogen or estrogen/progestin regimens on heart disease risk factors in postmenopausal women: the Postmenopausal Estrogen/Progestin Interventions (PEPI) Trial. *JAMA* 1995; **273:** 199–208. Correction. *ibid.*; **274:** 1676.
5. Medical Research Council's General Practice Research Framework. Randomised comparison of oestrogen versus oestrogen plus progestogen hormone replacement therapy in women with hysterectomy. *BMJ* 1996; **312:** 473–8.
6. Speroff L, *et al.* The comparative effect on bone density, endometrium, and lipids of continuous hormones as replacement therapy (CHART Study): a randomized controlled trial. *JAMA* 1996; **276:** 1397–1403.
7. Grodstein F, *et al.* Postmenopausal estrogen and progestin use and the risk of cardiovascular disease. *N Engl J Med* 1996; **335:** 453–61. Correction. *ibid.*; 1046.
8. Lee W-S, *et al.* Progesterone inhibits arterial smooth muscle cell proliferation. *Nature Med* 1997; **3:** 1005–1008.
9. Grodstein F, *et al.* Postmenopausal hormone therapy and mortality. *N Engl J Med* 1997; **336:** 1769–75.
10. Sidney S, *et al.* Myocardial infarction and the use of estrogen and estrogen-progestogen in postmenopausal women. *Ann Intern Med* 1997; **127:** 501–8.
11. Hulley S, *et al.* Randomized trial of estrogen plus progestin for secondary prevention of coronary heart disease in postmenopausal women. *JAMA* 1998; **280:** 605–13.
12. Grady D, *et al.* Cardiovascular disease outcomes during 6.8 years of hormone therapy: Heart and Estrogen/Progestin Replacement Study follow-up (HERS II). *JAMA* 2002; **288:** 49–57. Correction. *ibid.*; 1064.
13. Grodstein F, *et al.* Postmenopausal hormone use and secondary prevention of coronary events in the Nurses' Health Study: a prospective, observational study. *Ann Intern Med* 2001; **135:** 1–8.
14. Herrington DM, *et al.* Effects of estrogen replacement on the progression of coronary-artery atherosclerosis. *N Engl J Med* 2000; **343:** 522–9.
15. The ESPRIT team. Oestrogen therapy for prevention of reinfarction in postmenopausal women: a randomised placebo controlled trial. *Lancet* 2002; **360:** 2001–8.
16. Psaty BM, *et al.* Hormone replacement therapy, prothrombotic mutations, and the risk of incident nonfatal myocardial infarction in postmenopausal women. *JAMA* 2001; **285:** 906–13.
17. Grodstein F, *et al.* A prospective, observational study of postmenopausal hormone therapy and primary prevention of cardiovascular disease. *Ann Intern Med* 2000; **133:** 933–41.
18. Writing Group for the Women's Health Initiative Investigators. Risks and benefits of estrogen plus progestin in healthy postmenopausal women: principal results from the Women's Health Initiative randomized controlled trial. *JAMA* 2002; **288:** 321–33.
19. Manson JE, *et al.* Estrogen plus progestin and the risk of coronary heart disease. *N Engl J Med* 2003; **349:** 523–34.
20. The Women's Health Initiative Steering Committee. Effects of conjugated equine estrogen in postmenopausal women with hysterectomy: the Women's Health Initiative randomized controlled trial. *JAMA* 2004; **291:** 1701–12.


STROKE. The Framingham Study suggested a more than twofold increased risk of stroke in women using menopausal HRT.[1] However, subsequent studies reporting risk of stroke separately from other cardiovascular events showed either no effect on risk[2] or a decreased risk in the order of 30 to 50%.[3,4]

Data from the Nurses' Health Study cohort[5] revealed little association between the risk of stroke of any type and current use of unopposed oestrogens or oestrogen plus progestogen. However, they reported a trend towards an increased risk of stroke in current users of high-dose oestrogen therapy (1.25 mg or higher). Similarly, a large Danish case-control study found that unopposed oestrogens or oestrogen plus progestogen had no effect on the risk of non-fatal haemorrhagic or thromboembolic stroke,[6] and data from the Heart and Estrogen/Progestin Replacement Study indicated that combined HRT in women with pre-existing ischaemic heart disease had no effect on risk of stroke.[7,8] In contrast to these results, the Women's Health Initiative, a placebo-controlled trial of over 16 000 healthy women, found that combined HRT increased the risk of ischaemic stroke, and that the increase in risk became apparent after about 1 year of starting HRT.[9] Furthermore, the arm of the Women's Health Initiative that compared unopposed conjugated oestrogens with placebo in more than 10 000 women with prior hysterectomy also found an increased risk of stroke.[10]

In a controlled study in postmenopausal women who had recently had a stroke or transient ischaemic attack, the use of unopposed oestrogen had no significant effect on mortality or the recurrence of stroke.[11]


1. Wilson PWF, *et al.* Postmenopausal estrogen use, cigarette smoking, and cardiovascular morbidity in women over 50: the Framingham study. *N Engl J Med* 1985; **313:** 1038–43.
2. Stampfer MJ, *et al.* Postmenopausal estrogen therapy and cardiovascular disease: ten-year follow-up from the Nurses' Health Study. *N Engl J Med* 1991; **325:** 756–62.
3. Paganini-Hill A, *et al.* Postmenopausal oestrogen treatment and stroke: a prospective study. *BMJ* 1988; **297:** 519–22.
4. Finucane FF, *et al.* Decreased risk of stroke among postmenopausal hormone users: results from a national cohort. *Arch Intern Med* 1993; **153:** 73–9.
5. Grodstein F, *et al.* Postmenopausal estrogen and progestin use and the risk of cardiovascular disease. *N Engl J Med* 1996; **335:** 453–61. Correction. *ibid.*; 1406.
6. Tønnes Pedersen A, *et al.* Hormone replacement therapy and risk of non-fatal stroke. *Lancet* 1997; **350:** 1277–83.
7. Simon JA, *et al.* Postmenopausal hormone therapy and risk of stroke: the Heart and Estrogen-progestin Replacement Study (HERS). *Circulation* 2001; **103:** 638–42.
8. Grady D, *et al.* Cardiovascular disease outcomes during 6.8 years of hormone therapy: Heart and Estrogen/Progestin Replacement Study follow-up (HERS II). *JAMA* 2002; **288:** 49–57. Correction. *ibid.*; 1064.
9. Wassertheil-Smoller S, *et al.* Effect of estrogen plus progestin on stroke in postmenopausal women: the Women's Health Initiative: a randomized trial. *JAMA* 2003; **289:** 2673–84.
10. The Women's Health Initiative Steering Committee. Effects of conjugated equine estrogen in postmenopausal women with hysterectomy: the Women's Health Initiative randomized controlled trial. *JAMA* 2004; **291:** 1701–12.
11. Viscoli CM, *et al.* A clinical trial of estrogen-replacement therapy after ischemic stroke. *N Engl J Med* 2001; **345:** 1243–9.

VENOUS THROMBOEMBOLISM. Traditionally it has been assumed that, unlike combined oral contraceptives, menopausal HRT is not associated with an increased risk of venous thromboembolism.

However, observational studies have provided substantial evidence that there is an increased risk of deep-vein thrombosis and/or pulmonary embolism in women receiving HRT.[1-4] The relative risk of venous thromboembolism was found to be 2.1 to 3.6 in current users compared with past-users or those who had never received HRT. This equates to an excess of 16 to 23 cases per 100 000 women per year. One study found that the increase in risk was restricted to the first year of use.[4] Another reported an increased risk with increasing oestrogen dose.[2]

Evidence from randomised placebo-controlled trials[5-8] supports the findings of the observational studies above. The UK Committee on Safety of Medicines considers that the absolute risk of venous thromboembolism in all women using HRT is higher than was originally suggested, and that the risks are higher particularly in older women and in women with predisposing factors, such as a history of venous thromboembolism.[9]

1. Daly E, *et al.* Risk of venous thromboembolism in users of hormone replacement therapy. *Lancet* 1996; **348:** 977–80.
2. Jick H, *et al.* Risk of hospital admission for idiopathic venous thromboembolism among users of postmenopausal oestrogens. *Lancet* 1996; **348:** 981–83.
3. Grodstein F, *et al.* Prospective study of exogenous hormones and risk of pulmonary embolism in women. *Lancet* 1996; **348:** 983–7.
4. Pérez Gutthann S, *et al.* Hormone replacement therapy and risk of venous thromboembolism: population based case-control study. *BMJ* 1997; **314:** 796–800.
5. Grady D, Furberg C. Venous thromboembolic events associated with hormone replacement therapy. *JAMA* 1997; **278:** 477.
6. Grady D, *et al.* Postmenopausal hormone therapy increases risk for venous thromboembolic disease: the Heart and Estrogen/progestin Replacement Study. *Ann Intern Med* 2000; **132:** 689–96. Correction. *ibid.* 2001; **134:** 81.
7. Hulley S, *et al.* Noncardiovascular disease outcomes during 6.8 years of hormone therapy: Heart and Estrogen/Progestin Replacement Study follow-up (HERS II). *JAMA* 2002; **288:** 58–66.
8. Writing Group for the Women's Health Initiative Investigators. Risks and benefits of estrogen plus progestin in healthy postmenopausal women: principal results from the Women's Health Initiative randomized controlled trial. *JAMA* 2002; **288:** 321–33.
9. Committee on Safety of Medicines/Medicines Control Agency. New product information for hormone replacement therapy. *Current Problems* 2002; **28:** 1–2. Also available at: http://www.mca.gov.uk/ourwork/monitorsafequalmed/currentproblems/cpapril2002.pdf (accessed 16/06/04)

**Effects on the gallbladder.** The use of HRT is reported to increase the risk of gallstone formation and cholecystectomy in postmenopausal women.[1-3]

1. Uhler ML, *et al.* Estrogen replacement therapy and gallbladder disease in postmenopausal women. *Menopause* 2000; **7:** 162–7.
2. Simon JA, *et al.* Effect of estrogen plus progestin on risk for biliary tract surgery in postmenopausal women with coronary artery disease: the Heart and Estrogen/progestin Replacement Study. *Ann Intern Med* 2001; **135:** 493–501.
3. Hulley S, *et al.* Noncardiovascular disease outcomes during 6.8 years of hormone therapy: Heart and Estrogen/Progestin Replacement Study follow-up (HERS II). *JAMA* 2002; **288:** 58–66.

**Effects on lipids.** Oestrogens increase serum high-density-lipoprotein cholesterol and decrease low-density-lipoprotein cholesterol concentrations, effects that are considered favourable and may be a mechanism behind their apparent reduction in ischaemic heart disease in postmenopausal women, although controlled studies have not found combined HRT to reduce coronary events (see Effects on the Cardiovascular System, above). Oestrogens may also increase serum triglyceride concentrations, which is undesirable. Severe hypertriglyceridaemia and pancreatitis have occurred in women with hypertriglyceridaemia treated with oestrogens.[1,2] Use of concomitant progestogen reduces oestrogen-induced hypertriglyceridaemia.[2]

1. Glueck CJ, *et al.* Severe hypertriglyceridemia and pancreatitis when estrogen replacement therapy is given to hypertriglyceridemic women. *J Lab Clin Med* 1994; **123:** 59–64.
2. Isley WL, Oki J. Estrogen-induced pancreatitis after discontinuation of concomitant medroxyprogesterone therapy. *Am J Med* 1997; **102:** 416–17.

**Effects on mental function.** For results suggesting that HRT may increase the risk of developing dementia see under Uses and Administration, below.

**Pancreatitis.** Unopposed oestrogen has been associated with pancreatitis in women with hypertriglyceridaemia (see Effects on Lipids, above).

## Precautions

Before menopausal HRT is given the woman should undergo an appropriate medical examination and her medical history should be carefully evaluated. Regular examination is recommended during use.

HRT should be avoided in women with active thrombophlebitis or thromboembolic disease; it should not be given to those with a history of recurrent thromboembolism unless they are already receiving anticoagulant treatment.

HRT should not be given to those with undiagnosed abnormal vaginal bleeding, and abnormal vaginal bleeding during therapy should be investigated (see below). HRT is also contra-indicated in women with oestrogen-dependent neoplasms such as those of the breast or endometrium, and is usually considered contra-indicated in women with a history of these conditions although this has been debated (see below). Active liver disease, Dubin-Johnson or Rotor syndromes, severe cardiac disease, and severe diabetes with vascular changes are also generally considered to be contra-indications.

Prolonged exposure to unopposed oestrogens increases the risk of endometrial cancer whatever the route of administration (see above). HRT should be used with caution in women with antiphospholipid antibodies or predisposing factors to thromboembolism (see also Venous Thromboembolism, above), and in migraine, a history of breast nodules or fibrocystic disease, uterine fibroids, or a history of endometriosis. Consideration should be given to temporarily stopping HRT 4 to 6 weeks prior to elective surgery (but see also below).

HRT should be stopped immediately, and appropriate investigations and treatment carried out, if any of the following occur:

- sudden severe chest pain, sudden breathlessness, or severe pain/swelling in calf of one leg (possibly indicative of thromboembolic complications)
- unusual, severe, prolonged headache, sudden disturbances of vision or hearing or other perceptual disorders, collapse, marked numbness or weakness affecting one side of the body, or other signs or symptoms suggestive of cerebrovascular accident
- a first unexplained epileptic seizure
- hepatitis, jaundice, generalised itching, liver enlargement, severe upper abdominal pain
- onset of severe depression
- significant rise in blood pressure (above 160 mmHg systolic or 100 mmHg diastolic)
- clear exacerbation of other conditions known to be capable of deteriorating during HRT or pregnancy.

Although evidence is in many cases less well established, HRT should perhaps also be used with caution in diseases which may be exacerbated during pregnancy or oestrogen therapy including diabetes, asthma, epilepsy, hypertension, cardiac or renal disease, sickle-cell disease, melanoma, otosclerosis, multiple sclerosis, systemic lupus erythematosus, and chorea.

Doses of oestrogen in HRT are insufficient to provide contraception. HRT is contra-indicated in known or suspected pregnancy, and in women who are breast feeding.

**Endometriosis.** Endometriosis may be reactivated by unopposed oestrogen use in postmenopausal women. This has occurred, even in women who have previously undergone hysterectomy and bilateral oophorectomy for endometriosis.[1,2] Reactivation of endometriosis can result in ureteric obstruction and consequent renal damage.[1,2] Use of combined HRT rather than unopposed oestrogen has been advocated for women who have had radical surgery for endometriosis.[1]

1. Manyonda IT, *et al.* Obstructive uropathy from endometriosis after hysterectomy and oophorectomy; two case reports. *Eur J Obstet Gynecol Reprod Biol* 1989; **31:** 195–8.
2. Brough RJ, O'Flynn K. Recurrent pelvic endometriosis and bilateral ureteric obstruction associated with hormone replacement therapy. *BMJ* 1996; **312:** 1221–2.

**Lupus erythematosus.** Systemic lupus erythematosus (SLE) is an auto-immune disease which is far more common in women than in men, and usually has a peak onset for women in their 20s and 30s. There is some evidence to suggest that HRT use may be associated with a slightly increased risk in the onset of SLE, but there are few reports and studies of disease exacerbation in postmenopausal patients with SLE. However, women with antiphospholipid antibodies (which includes about a third of all patients with SLE) may be at increased risk of venous thromboembolism associated with HRT.

References.

1. Petri M. Exogenous estrogen in systemic lupus erythematosus: oral contraceptives and hormone replacement therapy. *Lupus* 2001; **10:** 222–6.
2. Mok CC, *et al.* Use of exogenous estrogens in systemic lupus erythematosus. *Semin Arthritis Rheum* 2001; **30:** 426–35.

**Malignant neoplasms.** HRT is usually avoided in women who have been treated for breast cancer because of the concern that oestrogen will stimulate cancer recurrence, although there is a lack of clinical evidence to substantiate this concern.[1] A retrospective observational study[2] and a retrospective case-control study[3] among women diagnosed with breast cancer did not find any evidence of an adverse effect in those who began HRT after diagnosis. A systematic review[4] of studies of HRT in breast cancer survivors reached a similar conclusion, but also noted that these studies were small, not randomised, and many were uncontrolled. It has been suggested that such therapy should not necessarily be withheld from these patients provided that the possible risks are understood.[1] Short-term continuous combined HRT in selected women with severe menopausal symptoms has been suggested.[5] Others suggest that HRT should be combined with tamoxifen in such patients.[6,7] More recently, however, an open randomised study[8] was stopped early when it was found that 2 years of HRT increased the risk of breast cancer (local recurrence, contralateral cancer, or distant metastases); this has cast doubt on the safety of HRT in these patients.

Similarly, HRT is usually avoided in patients who have been treated for endometrial cancer, because of the theoretical risk of stimulating tumour recurrence.[9] There is a lack of well-designed studies on this subject, but some data suggest that HRT might not increase the rate of recurrence or death.[10]

1. Cobleigh MA, *et al.* Estrogen replacement therapy in breast cancer survivors: a time for change. *JAMA* 1994; **272:** 540–5.
2. Durna EM, *et al.* Hormone replacement therapy after a diagnosis of breast cancer: cancer recurrence and mortality. *Med J Aust* 2002; **177:** 347–51.
3. O'Meara ES, *et al.* Hormone replacement therapy after a diagnosis of breast cancer in relation to recurrence and mortality. *J Natl Cancer Inst* 2001; **93:** 754–62.
4. Col NF, *et al.* Hormone replacement therapy after breast cancer: a systematic review and quantitative assessment of risk. *J Clin Oncol* 2001; **19:** 2357–63.
5. Eden JA. Estrogen replacement therapy in survivors of breast cancer: a risk-benefit assessment. *Drugs Aging* 1996; **8:** 127–33.
6. Powles TJ, *et al.* Hormone replacement after breast cancer. *Lancet* 1993; **342:** 60–1.
7. Powles TJ, Hickish T. Breast cancer response to hormone replacement therapy withdrawal. *Lancet* 1995; **345:** 1442.
8. Holmberg L, Anderson H. HABITS (hormonal replacement therapy after breast cancer—is it safe?), a randomised comparison: trial stopped. *Lancet* 2004; **363:** 453–5.
9. Committee on Gynecologic Practice. ACOG committee opinion: hormone replacement therapy in women treated for endometrial cancer (number 235, May 2000). *Int J Gynecol Obstet* 2001; **73:** 283–4.
10. Suriano KA, *et al.* Estrogen replacement therapy in endometrial cancer patients: a matched control study. *Obstet Gynecol* 2001; **97:** 555–60.

**Porphyria.** HRT should be used with caution in patients with porphyria.

**Surgery.** A review[1] recommended that women receiving HRT and due to have major elective surgery or leg surgery should continue taking the HRT and should routinely receive thromboprophylaxis (e.g. subcutaneous low-molecular-weight heparins and the use of graduated elastic compression stockings) in the perioperative period. Similar management was proposed when undergoing emergency surgery but prophylaxis was considered unnecessary with minor surgery. These conclusions were based on the advice of specialist groups but it was noted that there was some conflict with recommendations of manufacturers and those of the *British National Formulary*. The *British National Formulary* states that it may be prudent to stop HRT a month before surgery; failing that, prophylaxis as above is recommended.

1. Anonymous. Drugs in the peri-operative period: hormonal contraceptives and hormone replacement therapy. *Drug Ther Bull* 1999; **37:** 78–80.

**Vaginal bleeding.** Menopausal HRT is contra-indicated in patients with undiagnosed abnormal vaginal bleeding, which may be a symptom of endometrial carcinoma. The causes of abnormal vaginal bleeding in women receiving HRT and guidelines on their investigation and treatment have been reviewed.[1,2]

1. Good AE. Diagnostic options for assessment of postmenopausal bleeding. *Mayo Clin Proc* 1997; **72:** 345–9.
2. Spencer CP, *et al.* Management of abnormal bleeding in women receiving hormone replacement therapy. *BMJ* 1997; **315:** 37–42.

## Interactions

Drugs that increase the hepatic metabolism of oestrogens and progestogens have been associated with failure of the combined oral contraceptive (see p.1534). Important examples include rifamycins, some antiepileptics, and griseofulvin. It is not unreasonable to assume that these drugs would also be associated with decreased effectiveness of HRT, but there appears to be little information on this (for one report, see Antiepileptics, below).

Although oral contraceptives may antagonise or reduce the effects of a number of drugs (see p.1534), the lower doses of oestrogens used in HRT are considered less likely to induce interactions, although the possibility remains.

**Alcohol.** Acute ingestion of an alcoholic beverage led to a threefold increase in circulating estradiol in women on menopausal HRT.[1] The authors suggest that drinking habits may need to be considered when deciding on an appropriate dose of HRT.

1. Ginsburg ES, *et al.* Effects of alcohol ingestion on estrogens in postmenopausal women. *JAMA* 1996; **276:** 1747–51.

**Antiepileptics.** *Phenytoin* was reported to diminish the effect of conjugated oestrogens in a menopausal woman.[1]

1. Notelovitz M, *et al.* Interaction between estrogen and Dilantin in a menopausal woman. *N Engl J Med* 1981; **304:** 788–9.

**Levothyroxine.** Increased doses of levothyroxine may be needed in hypothyroid women who receive oestrogens for postmenopausal HRT—see p.1601.

## Pharmacokinetics

For a discussion of the pharmacokinetics of oestrogens and progestogens, see Estradiol, p.1550 and Progesterone, p.1567, respectively. The extent of binding of progestogens to serum sex-hormone binding globulin may be altered when they are administered with an oestrogen. Oestrogens increase serum concentrations of sex-hormone binding globulin, and progestogens differ in their ability to suppress this effect.

## Uses and Administration

The most commonly used oestrogens in menopausal HRT are natural oestrogens such as estradiol, and conjugated oestrogens. Dosages of oestrogens used in HRT are generally lower than those used in combined oral contraceptives, and do not therefore provide contraception.

Various dosage forms of the different oestrogenic compounds used for HRT are available, including oral tablets, intranasal sprays, subcutaneous implants, topical applications for vulvovaginal use, intravaginal rings, and transdermal skin patches and gels. Generally, if prolonged therapy (for more than 2 to 4 weeks) with an oestrogen by any route is envisaged in a woman with an intact uterus, a progestogen is required to prevent endometrial proliferation. This may be given by mouth cyclically for 10 to 14 days per cycle or continuously; transdermal preparations are now also available. Both progesterone derivatives such as medroxyprogesterone and dydrogesterone, and 19-nortestosterone analogues such as norethisterone, norgestrel, and levonorgestrel are used. Doses of progestogens for HRT are similar to those used in combined oral contraceptives.

**Administration.** In a discussion of the relative merits of oral and transdermal oestrogen therapy[1] it was suggested that there was circumstantial and theoretical evidence to suppose that transdermal therapy might be preferable in women who smoke, who suffer from migraine, hepatobiliary disease, or hypertriglyceridaemia, or who have a history of thromboembolism. In contrast, oral HRT might be preferable in patients with hypercholesterolaemia. However, studies to examine these suppositions were needed. Various alternatives to oral oestrogen therapy have been reviewed.[2,3] For reviews of estradiol implants or given transdermally, see p.1551.

1. Lufkin EG, Ory SJ. Relative value of transdermal and oral estrogen therapy in various clinical situations. *Mayo Clin Proc* 1994; **69:** 131–5.
2. Baker VL. Alternatives to oral estrogen replacement: transdermal patches, percutaneous gels, vaginal creams and rings, implants, and other methods of delivery. *Obstet Gynecol Clin North Am* 1994; **21:** 271–97.
3. Jewelewicz R. New developments in topical estrogen therapy. *Fertil Steril* 1997; **67:** 1–12.

**Cardiovascular disorders.** Observational studies have shown a decreased risk of ischaemic heart disease and consequent mortality in women receiving menopausal HRT and oestrogens are known to have some beneficial effects on the plasma lipid profile (see Effects on Lipids, above). Data from a randomised crossover study[1] showed that both simvastatin and continuous conjugated oestrogens plus medroxyprogesterone had beneficial effects on plasma lipoprotein concentrations, although simvastatin was more effective. (In addition, the hormones increased, whereas simvastatin decreased, triglyceride concentrations.) However, results from randomised placebo-controlled studies of combined HRT for primary or secondary prevention of ischaemic heart disease have shown no overall benefit from HRT, and possibly an increased risk of coronary events (see Ischaemic Heart Disease, under Adverse Effects, above). It has therefore been recommended that HRT should not be used for prevention of cardiovascular disease.[2] Cardiovascular risk reduction, including management of blood lipids, is discussed on p.819.

Some observational studies have reported that women receiving HRT have better survival rates after revascularisation procedures (p.834) than women not receiving this therapy.[3,4]

1. Darling GM, *et al.* Estrogen and progestin compared with simvastatin for hypercholesterolemia in postmenopausal women. *N Engl J Med* 1997; **337:** 595–601.
2. Mosca L, *et al.* Evidence-based guidelines for cardiovascular disease prevention in women. *Circulation* 2004; **109:** 672–93.
3. O'Keefe JH, *et al.* Estrogen replacement therapy after coronary angioplasty in women. *J Am Coll Cardiol* 1997; **29:** 1–5.
4. Sullivan JM, *et al.* Effect on survival of estrogen replacement therapy after coronary artery bypass grafting. *Am J Cardiol* 1997; **79:** 847–50.

**Dementia.** Several observational studies[1-3] have suggested that oestrogens can reduce the risk and delay the onset of Alzheimer's disease (p.1484) in postmenopausal women receiving HRT. However, subsequent meta-analyses[4,5] concluded that studies conducted so far had substantial methodological problems and that results were conflicting. A further observational study[6] has also reported improved global cognition, and a slower rate of decline over 3 years in women receiving HRT. This study also found[7] that previous HRT use reduced the risk of developing dementia, but that current HRT use had no effect unless it was taken for more than 10 years. Any apparent benefits of HRT have been thrown into question, however, by the results of two large controlled studies of women who received conjugated oestrogens with medroxyprogesterone, or placebo, for about 4 years. At the end of the Heart and Estrogen/Progestin Replacement Study of women with coronary disease, there was no difference in cognitive function tests between those receiving HRT or placebo.[8] In the Women's Health Initiative Memory Study of over 4000 women aged 65 years and older, HRT had no clinically significant effect on global cognitive function, but the risk of suffering a substantial decline was higher for the HRT group.[9] Also, HRT did not prevent the development of mild cognitive impairment, and actually doubled the risk of dementia.[10] The absolute risk of dementia is small, however, and this increase is equivalent to 45 cases of dementia per year for every 10 000 women taking HRT compared with 22 cases for placebo.

Some reports[11-13] suggest that treatment with oestrogens may be of benefit in women who already have Alzheimer's disease. However, in a controlled trial in women with mild to moderate Alzheimer's disease, oestrogen replacement therapy for one year did not slow the progression of disease or improve global, cognitive, or functional outcomes.[14]

1. Tang M-X,*et al.* Effect of oestrogen during menopause on risk and age at onset of Alzheimer's disease. *Lancet* 1996; **348:** 429–32.
2. Paganini-Hill A, Henderson VW. Estrogen replacement therapy and risk of Alzheimer disease. *Arch Intern Med* 1996; **156:** 2213–17.
3. Kawas C, *et al.* A prospective study of estrogen replacement therapy and the risk of developing Alzheimer's disease: the Baltimore Longitudinal Study of Aging. *Neurology* 1997; **48:** 1517–21.
4. Yaffe K, *et al.* Estrogen therapy in postmenopausal women: effects on cognitive function and dementia. *JAMA* 1998; **279:** 688–95.
5. LeBlanc ES, *et al.* Hormone replacement therapy and cognition: systematic review and meta-analysis. *JAMA* 2001; **285:** 1489–99.
6. Carlson MC, *et al.* Hormone replacement therapy and reduced cognitive decline in older women: the Cache county study. *Neurology* 2001; **57:** 2210–16.
7. Zandi PP, *et al.* Hormone replacement therapy and incidence of Alzheimer disease in older women: the Cache county study. *JAMA* 2002; **288:** 2123–9.
8. Grady D, *et al.* Effect of postmenopausal hormone therapy on cognitive function: the Heart and Estrogen/progestin Replacement Study. *Am J Med* 2002; **113:** 543–8.
9. Rapp SR, *et al.* Effect of estrogen plus progestin on global cognitive function in postmenopausal women: the Women's Health Initiative Memory Study: a randomized controlled trial. *JAMA* 2003; **289:** 2663–72.
10. Shumaker SA, *et al.* Estrogen plus progestin and the incidence of dementia and mild cognitive impairment in postmenopausal women: the Women's Health Initiative Memory Study: a randomized controlled trial. *JAMA* 2003; **289:** 2651–62.
11. Ohkura T, *et al.* Long-term estrogen replacement therapy in female patients with dementia of the Alzheimer type: 7 case reports. *Dementia* 1995; **6:** 99–107.
12. Schneider LS, *et al.* Potential role for estrogen replacement in the treatment of Alzheimer's dementia. *Am J Med* 1997; **103** (suppl 3A): 46S–50S.
13. Asthana S, *et al.* High-dose estradiol improves cognition for women with AD: results of a randomized study. *Neurology* 2001; **57:** 605–12.
14. Mulnard RA, *et al.* Estrogen replacement therapy for treatment of mild to moderate Alzheimer disease: a randomized controlled trial. *JAMA* 2000; **283:** 1007–15. Correction. *ibid.*; **284:** 2597.

**Hyperparathyroidism.** The effects of HRT have been studied in postmenopausal women with mild primary hyperparathyroidism (p.765). Oestrogens have been reported to reduce the rate of bone turnover and plasma-concentrations of calcium in these patients, as well as increase bone mineral density.[1-4]

1. Marcus R, *et al.* Conjugated estrogens in the treatment of postmenopausal women with hyperparathyroidism. *Ann Intern Med* 1984; **100:** 633–40.
2. Selby PL, Peacock M. Ethinyl estradiol and norethindrone in the treatment of primary hyperparathyroidism in postmenopausal women. *N Engl J Med* 1986; **314:** 1481–5.
3. Grey AB, *et al.* Effect of hormone replacement therapy on bone mineral density in postmenopausal women with mild primary hyperparathyroidism: a randomized, controlled trial. *Ann Intern Med* 1996; **125:** 360–8.
4. Orr-Walker BJ, *et al.* Effects of hormone replacement therapy on bone mineral density in postmenopausal women with primary hyperparathyroidism: four-year follow-up and comparison with healthy postmenopausal women. *Arch Intern Med* 2000; **160:** 2161–6.

**Menopausal disorders.** ACUTE MENOPAUSAL SYMPTOMS. Where symptoms are severe enough to warrant treatment, HRT with oestrogens is the mainstay of treatment for *vasomotor symptoms and atrophic vaginitis*. Commentators[1-3] have suggested that there are few absolute contra-indications to the treatment of women with acute symptoms, although undiagnosed vaginal bleeding, before or during therapy, should always be investigated, as it can be a sign of endometrial cancer. In addition, women with active thrombophlebitis or thromboembolic disorders should not receive HRT, and the risk-benefit should be considered carefully in women with predisposing risk factors for venous thromboembolism (see also Precautions, above). HRT should also not be used in women with oestrogen-dependent cancer, although some have suggested that short-term HRT need not necessarily be withheld in women who have survived breast cancer if menopausal symptoms are severe and unresponsive to other measures (see also Malignant Neoplasms under Precautions, above).

If the woman is in the perimenopause she is potentially fertile, and HRT does not provide contraception. It is now considered that, in women under 50 years of age and free of all risk factors for venous and arterial disease, a low-oestrogen dose combined oral contraceptive (p.1535) can be used to provide both relief of menopausal symptoms and contraception.[4] If HRT is used in perimenopausal women, then non-hormonal contraceptive measures should be used if required (see p.1535).

Perimenopausal women with a uterus should also receive a cyclical progestogen, which will cause regular withdrawal bleeding. An alternative is the levonorgestrel intra-uterine device with concomitant oral or transdermal oestrogen.[5] In women with a uterus who are postmenopausal (more than 12 months) continuous combined HRT may be used, which induces an atrophic endometrium. An alternative is the hormonal agent tibolone, which does not require concomitant progestogen. Women without a uterus, and who have not had endometriosis, may receive continuous oestrogen alone. For a discussion of the risks of endometrial cancer with HRT, see under Adverse Effects, above.

- In women experiencing solely *vaginal symptoms*, HRT administered just for a few weeks may be sufficient. This may be administered vaginally.
- Mild *vasomotor symptoms* may be adequately managed with lifestyle changes such as maintaining a lower core body temperature, physical activity, and relaxation techniques.[6] Moderate to severe symptoms can be controlled with HRT, usually given orally or transdermally.[6,7] The lowest dose that controls symptoms is given short term, generally for no more than 5 years. Alternative hormonal therapies include the progestogens megestrol and medroxyprogesterone. Non-hormonal therapies have also been tried although evidence for the efficacy of these is less conclusive than that for HRT. The antidepressants fluoxetine, paroxetine, and venlafaxine have shown some benefit in small trials, and low doses of gabapentin have been reported to be effective. Clonidine or veralipride may be considered when HRT is not suitable, but the use of these can be limited by adverse effects. Various other therapies have been used to manage vasomotor symptoms based on anecdotal reports of benefit, but they have generally not been effective when studied in placebo-controlled trials. These include isoflavones from soya or red clover, evening primrose oil, cimicifuga (black cohosh), and vitamin E.
- *Non-specific symptoms* may also improve in women administered HRT. For example, oestrogens have reduced the incidence of urinary-tract infections,[8] and dysuria and incontinence (see below), although good evidence is somewhat scanty. Similarly, many women report improved mood and well-being when given oestrogens, although it is unclear to what extent this is due to relief of other symptoms. Two large controlled studies[9,10] have found that combined HRT improved some quality of life measures in postmenopausal women with vasomotor symptoms, but that asymptomatic women in general received no benefit. True depression needs to be identified and treated appropriately.[1] Moreover, the addition of progestogens carries some risk of adverse effects on mood such as depression, anxiety, and irritability. Androgens such as testosterone are sometimes used as adjuncts to HRT to improve psychological well-being and libido.[1,2]

LONG-TERM EFFECTS. There are extensive data from observational studies on the beneficial effects on fracture rates and cardiovascular disease, on the risks for development of breast cancer and endometrial cancer, and on the possible effects on overall mortality. However, the women receiving HRT in these studies may differ from women not receiving HRT, and the extent of any bias resulting from this is unclear.[11] Randomised prospective studies have confirmed the increased risk of breast cancer, venous thromboembolism, and stroke associated with combined HRT (see under Adverse Effects, above). Contrary to the anticipated benefits for preventing ischaemic heart disease, these studies also found an increase in coronary events. These results have led to recommendations that HRT should not be used long term solely for the prevention of chronic disease in generally healthy postmenopausal women.[12-15]

- It is generally agreed that all women who have had a *premature natural or induced menopause* should receive HRT until the age of 50 years, unless there are specific contra-indications to therapy (mentioned in the discussion of acute symptoms above). Considerations as to how long they need to continue HRT after the usual age for the menopause are probably the same as for other women.
- Some women who have, or who are at risk of developing, *osteoporosis* may receive long-term HRT (but other treatments are now preferred—see also below). Risk factors for osteoporosis include familial predisposition, sedentary lifestyle, cigarette smoking, low body-weight, corticosteroid therapy, and a subnormal peak bone mass, for example, due to a calcium-deficient diet in childhood and adolescence. Where possible, treatment should be combined with adequate dietary calcium, weight-bearing exercise, and cessation of smoking.
- Women who have, or are at risk of developing, *ischaemic heart disease* had also been considered likely to benefit from HRT but such use is not now recommended (see above).

- Women who are at high risk of *breast cancer* should probably not receive long-term HRT (see also Malignant Neoplasms under Precautions, above). Those with a family history of breast cancer may be at particular risk.

Long-term HRT is given orally or transdermally. As mentioned above, oestrogens alone are suitable for women without a uterus who have not had endometriosis. In other women, a progestogen is also required to reduce the risk of endometrial hyperplasia and carcinoma (see also Carcinogenicity under Adverse Effects, above) or recurrence of endometriosis. This may be administered cyclically in perimenopausal women, but continuous administration is likely to be preferred in women who have been postmenopausal for more than 1 year since it avoids withdrawal bleeding. Tibolone is an alternative in women who have been postmenopausal for more than 1 year. Non-hormonal options for osteoporosis prophylaxis or treatment include bisphosphonates, as discussed on p.763. The selective oestrogen-receptor modulator raloxifene is also available.


1. Greendale GA, *et al.* The menopause. *Lancet* 1999; **353:** 571–80.
2. McKinney KA, Thompson W. A practical guide to prescribing hormone replacement therapy. *Drugs* 1998; **56:** 49–57.
3. McNagny SE. Prescribing hormone replacement therapy for menopausal symptoms. *Ann Intern Med* 1999; **131:** 605–16.
4. The North American Menopause Society. Clinical challenges of perimenopause: consensus opinion of the North American Menopause Society. *Menopause* 2000; **7:** 5–13.
5. Anonymous. Hormone replacement therapy. *Drug Ther Bull* 1996; **34:** 81–4.
6. Anonymous. Treatment of menopause-associated vasomotor symptoms: position statement of The North American Menopause Society. *Menopause* 2004; **11:** 11–33.
7. Shanafelt TD, *et al.* Pathophysiology and treatment of hot flashes. *Mayo Clin Proc* 2002; **77:** 1207–18.
8. Raz R, Stamm WE. A controlled trial of intravaginal estriol in postmenopausal women with recurrent urinary tract infections. *N Engl J Med* 1993; **329:** 753–6.
9. Hlatky MA, *et al.* Quality-of-life and depressive symptoms in postmenopausal women after receiving hormone therapy: results from the Heart and Estrogen/Progestin Replacement Study (HERS) trial. *JAMA* 2002; **287:** 591–7.
10. Hays J, *et al.* Effects of estrogen plus progestin on health-related quality of life. *N Engl J Med* 2003; **348:** 1839–54.
11. Grodstein F, *et al.* Understanding the divergent data on postmenopausal hormone therapy. *N Engl J Med* 2003; **348:** 645–50.
12. U.S. Preventive Services Task Force. Postmenopausal hormone replacement therapy for primary prevention of chronic conditions: recommendations and rationale. *Ann Intern Med* 2002; **137:** 834–9.
13. Rymer J, *et al.* Making decisions about hormone replacement therapy. *BMJ* 2003; **326:** 322–6.
14. Solomon CG, Dluhy RG. Rethinking postmenopausal hormone therapy. *N Engl J Med* 2003; **348:** 579–80.
15. Baber RJ, *et al.* Hormone replacement therapy: to use or not to use? *Med J Aust* 2003; **178:** 630–3.


**Osteoporosis.** Oestrogens may be used in selected patients for the treatment and prevention of postmenopausal osteoporosis (p.763). They have a direct antiresorptive effect on bone, and will increase bone mass density (BMD). However, data from the Heart and Estrogen/Progestin Replacement Study (HERS) have called into question the benefit of HRT in reducing the incidence of fractures.[1,2] A meta-analysis[3] including the initial HERS data,[1] most of which were from women without osteoporosis, consequently found only non-significant reduction in fracture risk in older women although overall the risk of fracture was reduced by between 20 and 30%. Subsequent results from the Women's Health Initiative[4] showed that, contrary to the results of this meta-analysis, combined HRT did reduce the risk of fracture in healthy postmenopausal women.

Despite the probable benefits, there is substantial evidence to show that HRT is associated with an increased risk of cancer, particularly breast cancer (see Breast under Carcinogenicity, above), and some cardiovascular diseases such as stroke and venous thromboembolism (see Effects on the Cardiovascular System, above). It is now generally recommended by authorities, such as the UK Committee on Safety of Medicines (CSM),[5] that the risk to benefit ratio of HRT is unfavourable for the prevention of osteoporosis as first-line therapy, and that it should not be used in this way for women over 50 years of age. HRT does, however, remain an option when other osteoporosis prevention therapies are unsuitable. Younger women who have experienced premature menopause may be given HRT for menopausal symptoms and to prevent osteoporosis until the age of 50, after which its use should be reviewed and considered a second-line choice.

Suggested minimum daily doses are 0.625 mg of conjugated oestrogens by mouth, 2 mg of estradiol by mouth or 50 micrograms transdermally, and 15 micrograms of ethinylestradiol by mouth; lower doses may also be effective,[6-9] and a transdermal patch supplying 14 micrograms of estradiol daily is licensed for the prevention of osteoporosis in the USA. Addition of a progestogen (required to prevent endometrial hyperplasia in women with a uterus) does not impair the beneficial effect of oestrogens on BMD, whether administered cyclically or continuously,[10,11] and may provide a further reduction in risk of fractures.[12] Although current, long-term use of HRT can increase BMD and reduce fracture risk, unresolved issues are the duration of therapy required to prevent fractures in old age, and the ideal age to start therapy to obtain the maximum benefits to the bone with the minimum risk of breast cancer.[12-14]

Oestrogens may also be used in women to reduce the risk of corticosteroid-induced osteoporosis (see Effects on Bones and Joints, p.1069).


1. Cauley JA, *et al.* Effects of hormone replacement therapy on clinical fractures and height loss: the Heart and Estrogen/Progestin Replacement Study (HERS). *Am J Med* 2001; **110:** 442–50.
2. Hulley S, *et al.* Noncardiovascular disease outcomes during 6.8 years of hormone therapy: Heart and Estrogen/Progestin Replacement Study follow-up (HERS II). *JAMA* 2002; **288:** 58–66.
3. Torgerson DJ, Bell-Syer SEM. Hormone replacement therapy and prevention of nonvertebral fractures: a meta-analysis of randomized trials. *JAMA* 2001; **285:** 2891–7.
4. Cauley JA, *et al.* Effects of estrogen plus progestin on risk of fracture and bone mineral density: the Women's Health Initiative randomized trial. *JAMA* 2003; **290:** 1729–38.
5. Further advice on safety of HRT: risk:benefit unfavourable for first-line use in prevention of osteoporosis—Epinet message from Professor G Duff, Chairman of Committee on Safety of Medicines (CSM) (issued December 2003). Available at: http://medicines.mhra.gov.uk/ourwork/monitorsafequalmed/safetymessages/hrtepinet_31203.pdf (accessed 16/06/04)
6. Recker RR, *et al.* The effect of low-dose continuous estrogen and progesterone therapy with calcium and vitamin D on bone in elderly women: a randomized, controlled trial. *Ann Intern Med* 1999; **130:** 897–904.
7. Prestwood KM, *et al.* The effect of low dose micronized 17β-estradiol on bone turnover, sex hormone levels, and side effects in older women: a randomized, double blind, placebo-controlled study. *J Clin Endocrinol Metab* 2000; **85:** 4462–9.
8. Bjarnason NH, *et al.* Low doses of estradiol in combination with gestodene to prevent early postmenopausal bone loss. *Am J Obstet Gynecol* 2000; **183:** 550–60.
9. Lees B, Stevenson JC. The prevention of osteoporosis using sequential low-dose hormone replacement therapy with estradiol-17β and dydrogesterone. *Osteoporosis Int* 2001; **12:** 251–8.
10. The Writing Group for the PEPI trial. Effects of hormone therapy on bone mineral density: results from the Postmenopausal Estrogen/Progestin Interventions (PEPI) trial. *JAMA* 1996; **276:** 1389–96.
11. Speroff L, *et al.* The comparative effect on bone density, endometrium, and lipids of continuous hormones as replacement therapy (CHART Study): a randomized controlled trial. *JAMA* 1996; **276:** 1397–1403.
12. Michaëlsson K, *et al.* Hormone replacement therapy and risk of hip fracture: population based case-control study. *BMJ* 1998; **316:** 1858–63.
13. Schneider DL, *et al.* Timing of postmenopausal estrogen for optimal bone mineral density: the Rancho Bernardo study. *JAMA* 1997; **277:** 543–7.
14. Cauley JA, *et al.* Timing of estrogen replacement therapy for optimal osteoporosis prevention. *J Clin Endocrinol Metab* 2001; **86:** 5700–5.


**Urinary incontinence.** Urinary incontinence (p.476) may be one of a number of acute symptoms associated with a decline in oestrogen levels at the menopause (see Menopausal Disorders, above). Studies[1,2] suggest that oestrogens used with alpha-adrenoceptor agonists are effective in the management of female stress incontinence and this combination has been advocated for use in postmenopausal patients with mild symptoms. Unfortunately addition of a progestogen to treatment to reduce the risk of endometrial carcinoma in women with an intact uterus might exacerbate the incontinence.[3] The value of oestrogens used without an alpha-adrenoceptor agonist in urinary incontinence is less clear. One study[4] reported that the combination of oestrogen therapy and pelvic floor exercises for 18 months was more effective than exercises alone in women with mild stress incontinence. However, a placebo-controlled study[5] found no improvement after 6 months of oestrogen therapy. Some[6] consider that oestrogens may be of use for symptoms of urgency, frequency, and nocturia in postmenopausal patients with urge incontinence; it has been suggested that hypoestrogenism may reduce the sensory threshold of the bladder.[7] A meta-analysis of 23 studies concluded that oestrogen therapy subjectively improved urinary incontinence in postmenopausal women but many of the studies examined were considered to be deficient in some respect.[8] Later well-designed studies[9,10] of women with stress, urge, or mixed incontinence found that HRT did not improve, or even worsened, measures of incontinence, although there was the possibility that concomitant progestogen therapy might have affected efficacy.


1. Walter S, *et al.* Stress urinary incontinence in postmenopausal women treated with oral estrogen (estriol) and an alpha-adrenoceptor-stimulating agent (phenylpropanolamine): a randomized double-blind placebo-controlled study. *Int Urogynecol J* 1990; **1:** 74–9.
2. Hilton P, *et al.* Oral and intravaginal estrogens alone and in combination with alpha-adrenergic stimulation in genuine stress incontinence. *Int Urogynecol J* 1990; **1:** 80–6.
3. Benness C, *et al.* Do progestogens exacerbate urinary incontinence in women on HRT? *Neurourol Urodyn* 1991; **10:** 316–17.
4. Ishiko O, *et al.* Hormone replacement therapy plus pelvic floor muscle exercise for postmenopausal stress incontinence: a randomized, controlled trial. *J Reprod Med* 2001; **46:** 213–20.
5. Jackson S, *et al.* The effect of oestrogen supplementation on post-menopausal urinary stress incontinence: a double-blind placebo-controlled trial. *Br J Obstet Gynaecol* 1999; **106:** 711–18.
6. Cardozo L. Role of estrogens in the treatment of female urinary incontinence. *J Am Geriatr Soc* 1990; **38:** 326–8.
7. Fantl JA, *et al.* Postmenopausal urinary incontinence: comparison between non-estrogen-supplemented and estrogen-supplemented women. *Obstet Gynecol* 1988; **71:** 823–8.
8. Fantl JA *et al.* Estrogen therapy in the management of urinary incontinence in postmenopausal women: a meta-analysis: first report of the hormones and urogenital therapy committee. *Obstet Gynecol* 1994; **83:** 12–18.
9. Fantl JA, *et al.* Efficacy of estrogen supplementation in the treatment of urinary incontinence. *Obstet Gynecol* 1996; **88:** 745–9.
10. Grady D, *et al.* Postmenopausal hormones and incontinence: the Heart and Estrogen/Progestin Replacement Study. *Obstet Gynecol* 2001; **97:** 116–20.


## Algestone Acetophenide *(USAN, rINNM)*

Acetofenido de algestona; Alphasone Acetophenide; Dihydroxyprogesterone Acetophenide; SQ-15101. 16α,17α-(1-Phenylethylidenedioxy)pregn-4-ene-3,20-dione; 16α,17α-Isopropylidenedioxypregn-4-ene-3,20-dione.

$C_{29}H_{36}O_4$ = 448.6.

*CAS — 595-77-7 (algestone); 24356-94-3 (algestone acetophenide).*

### Profile

Algestone acetophenide is a progestogen (see Progesterone, p.1566) that is given by intramuscular injection in monthly doses of 150 mg, with estradiol enantate, as a hormonal contraceptive (see p.1527). It has also been applied topically in the treatment of acne.

◊ References.


1. Martínez GH, *et al.* Vaginal bleeding patterns in users of Perlutal®, a once-a-month injectable contraceptive consisting of 10 mg estradiol enanthate combined with 150 mg dihydroxyprogesterone acetophenide: a trial of 5462 woman-months. *Contraception* 1998; **58:** 21–7.


### Preparations

**Proprietary Preparations** (details are given in Part 3)

**Multi-ingredient: *Arg.:*** Atrimon; Perlutal; ***Braz.:*** Ciclovular†; Evitas†; Femineo; Perlutan; Uno-Ciclo; ***Chile:*** Agurin; Unalmes†; ***Hong Kong:*** Progestrol†; ***Mex.:*** Anafertin; Ginoplan; Patector; Perlutal; Yectames; ***Port.:*** Cicnor; ***Spain:*** Topasel.

## Allylestrenol *(BAN, rINN)*

Alilestrenol; Allyloestrenol. 17α-Allylestr-4-en-17β-ol.

$C_{21}H_{32}O$ = 300.5.

*CAS — 432-60-0.*

*ATC — G03DC01.*

### Profile

Allylestrenol is a progestogen (see Progesterone, p.1566) structurally related to progesterone that has been given in threatened and recurrent miscarriage, and to prevent premature labour. However, with the exception of proven progesterone deficiency, such use is no longer recommended. In threatened miscarriage in progesterone-deficient women a suggested dose is 5 mg three times daily by mouth for 5 to 7 days.

**Pregnancy.** A case-control study of allylestrenol use in pregnancy during 1980 to 1984 in Hungary indicated that it was not teratogenic.[1]


1. Czeizel A, Huiskes N. A case-control study to evaluate the risk of congenital anomalies as a result of allylestrenol therapy during pregnancy. *Clin Ther* 1988; **10:** 725–39.


### Preparations

**Proprietary Preparations** (details are given in Part 3)

***Braz.:*** Orageston†; ***Hong Kong:*** Turinal; ***India:*** Maintane; Profar; ***Malaysia:*** Turinal; ***Mex.:*** Crestanon†; Gestanon†; ***Singapore:*** Turinal.

## Altrenogest *(BAN, USAN, rINN)*

A-35957; A-41300; RH-2267; RU-2267. 17α-Allyl-17β-hydroxy-19-norandrosta-4,9,11-trien-3-one; 17β-Hydroxy-19,21,24-trinorchola-4,9,11,22-tetraen-3-one.

$C_{21}H_{26}O_2$ = 310.4.

*CAS — 850-52-2.*

### Profile

Altrenogest is a progestogen (see Progesterone, p.1566) used in veterinary medicine.

## Androstanolone *(BAN, rINN)*

Androstanolo; Dihydrotestosterone; Stanolone. 17β-Hydroxy-5α-androstan-3-one.

$C_{19}H_{30}O_2$ = 290.4.

*CAS — 521-18-6.*

*ATC — A14AA01; G03BB02.*

### Profile

Androstanolone is formed naturally in the body from testosterone (p.1569) by the action of 5α-reductase, and is more active than the parent compound. It has anabolic and androgenic properties and is applied topically in the form of a 2.5% gel for male hypogonadism, gynaecomastia, and for lichen sclerosus in both men and women.

**Lichen sclerosus.** For references to the use of androgens such as androstanolone in lichen sclerosus, see under Testosterone, p.1572.

### Preparations

**Proprietary Preparations** (details are given in Part 3)

***Belg.:*** Andractim; ***Fr.:*** Andractim; ***Spain:*** Gelovit†; ***Thai.:*** Andractim.

## Androstenedione

Androstenodiona. Androst-4-ene-3,17-dione.
$C_{19}H_{26}O_2$ = 286.4.
*CAS — 63-05-8.*

### Profile

Androstenedione is a naturally occurring adrenal androgen that is a precursor of androgens and oestrogens (see p.1527). It has been employed in an attempt to enhance athletic performance and as hormone replacement for men.

**Action.** The effects of androstenedione have been studied in groups of young (under 40 years of age) and older (35 to 65 years) men with normal testosterone levels.[1-3] Testosterone levels were reported to remain unchanged[1] as well as increase,[2,3] although levels returned to baseline in the longer study of 12 weeks.[3] In all 3 trials, levels of oestrogens (oestradiol and oestrone) increased. Changes in lipid profiles were also noted, particularly a decrease in high-density lipoprotein (HDL) cholesterol.[1,3] Androstenedione did not enhance the effects of resistance training.[1,3]


1. King DS, *et al.* Effect of oral androstenedione on serum testosterone and adaptations to resistance training in young men: a randomized controlled trial. *JAMA* 1999; **281:** 2020–8.
2. Leder BZ, *et al.* Oral androstenedione administration and serum testosterone concentrations in young men. *JAMA* 2000; **283:** 779–82.
3. Broeder CE, *et al.* The Andro Project: physiological and hormonal influences of androstenedione supplementation in men 35 to 65 years old participating in a high-intensity resistance training program. *Arch Intern Med* 2000; **160:** 3093–3104.


### Preparations

**Proprietary Preparations** (details are given in Part 3)
**Multi-ingredient:** ***Thai.:*** Metharmon-F.

## Broparestrol *(rINN)*

α-Bromo-β-(4-ethylphenyl)stilbene.
$C_{22}H_{19}Br$ = 363.3.
*CAS — 479-68-5.*

### Profile

Broparestrol is a synthetic nonsteroidal oestrogen (see Diethylstilbestrol, p.1548) that has been used as an ingredient of preparations promoted for topical use in acne and similar skin disorders.

## Chlormadinone Acetate *(BANM, USAN, rINNM)*

Acetato de clormadinona; NSC-92338. 6-Chloro-17-hydroxypregna-4,6-diene-3,20-dione acetate.
$C_{23}H_{29}ClO_4$ = 404.9.
*CAS — 1961-77-9 (chlormadinone); 302-22-7 (chlormadinone acetate).*
*ATC — G03DB06.*

**Pharmacopoeias.** In *Chin., Fr.,* and *Jpn.*

### Adverse Effects and Precautions

As for progestogens in general (see Progesterone, p.1566).

**Effects on the skin.** A report of auto-immune dermatitis in one patient associated with chlormadinone acetate.[1]


1. Katayama I, Nishioka K. Autoimmune progesterone dermatitis with persistent amenorrhoea. *Br J Dermatol* 1985; **112:** 487–91.


### Interactions

As for progestogens in general (see Progesterone, p.1567).

### Uses and Administration

Chlormadinone acetate is a progestogen structurally related to progesterone (p.1567) that may have some anti-androgenic activity. It is given by mouth either alone or with an oestrogen in the treatment of menstrual disorders such as menorrhagia (p.1567) and endometriosis (p.1546) at doses of 2 to 10 mg daily either cyclically or continuously. It may also be used as the progestogen component of combined oral contraceptives (see p.1535) at a dose of 1 to 2 mg daily, particularly in women with androgen-dependent conditions such as acne and hirsutism. Chlormadinone acetate has been used in some countries in the management of prostatic hyperplasia and prostate cancer; doses of 25 or 50 mg respectively have been given twice daily.

### Preparations

**Proprietary Preparations** (details are given in Part 3)
***Fr.:*** Luteran; ***Ger.:*** Gestafortin; ***Jpn:*** Prostal; ***Mex.:*** Lutoral; Nidal†.

**Multi-ingredient:** ***Chile:*** Belara; ***Ger.:*** Belara; Gestamestrol N; Neo-Eunomin; Ovosiston; ***Mex.:*** Lutoral E; Secuentex-21; ***Switz.:*** Belara; Neo-Eunomine†.

## Chlorotrianisene *(BAN, rINN)*

Clorotrianiseno; NSC-10108; Tri-*p*-anisylchloroethylene. Chlorotris(4-methoxyphenyl)ethylene.
$C_{23}H_{21}ClO_3$ = 380.9.
*CAS — 569-57-3.*
*ATC — G03CA06.*

**Pharmacopoeias.** In *Chin.*

### Profile

Chlorotrianisene is a synthetic nonsteroidal oestrogen structurally related to diethylstilbestrol (p.1548). It has a prolonged action, and has been given by mouth for the treatment of menopausal symptoms, female hypogonadism, and prostatic carcinoma.

### Preparations

**Proprietary Preparations** (details are given in Part 3)
***Mex.:*** Estregur†.

## Clomifene Citrate *(BANM, rINNM)*

Chloramiphene Citrate; Citrato de clomifeno; Clomifeni Citras; Clomiphene Citrate *(USAN)*; MER-41; MRL-41; NSC-35770. A mixture of the *E* and *Z* isomers of 2-[4-(2-chloro-1,2-diphenylvinyl)phenoxy]triethylamine dihydrogen citrate.
$C_{26}H_{28}ClNO,C_6H_8O_7$ = 598.1.
*CAS — 911-45-5 (clomifene); 15690-57-0 ((E)-clomifene); 15690-55-8 ((Z)-clomifene); 50-41-9 (clomifene citrate); 7599-79-3 ((E)-clomifene citrate); 7619-53-6 ((Z)-clomifene citrate).*
*ATC — G03GB02.*

NOTE. Clomifene may be separated into its *Z* and *E* isomers, zuclomifene and enclomifene.

**Pharmacopoeias.** In *Chin., Eur.* (see p.vi), *Int., Jpn,* and *US.*
**Ph. Eur. 5.0** (Clomifene Citrate). A white or pale yellow, crystalline powder. It contains 30 to 50% of the *Z* isomer. Slightly soluble in water; sparingly soluble in alcohol. Protect from light.
**USP 27** (Clomiphene Citrate). A white to pale yellow, essentially odourless powder. It contains 30 to 50% of the *Z* isomer. Slightly soluble in water and in chloroform; sparingly soluble in alcohol; insoluble in ether; freely soluble in methyl alcohol.

### Adverse Effects

The incidence and severity of adverse effects of clomifene citrate tend to be related to the dose used. The most commonly reported adverse effects are reversible ovarian enlargement and cyst formation, vasomotor flushes resembling menopausal symptoms, and abdominal or pelvic discomfort or pain, sometimes with nausea or vomiting. Ovarian hyperstimulation syndrome has occurred. Breast tenderness, abnormal uterine bleeding, weight gain, headache, and endometriosis have also been reported. Transient visual disturbances such as after-images and blurring of vision may occur, and there have been rare reports of cataracts and optic neuritis. Skin reactions such as allergic rashes and urticaria have occasionally been reported and reversible hair loss has been reported rarely. CNS disturbances have included convulsions, dizziness, lightheadedness, nervous tension, fatigue, vertigo, insomnia, and depression. Abnormalities in liver function tests and jaundice have sometimes been reported. Following therapy with clomifene citrate there is an increased risk of multiple births, but rarely more than twins. There is also an increased risk of ectopic pregnancy. Although there have been reports of congenital disorders such as neural tube defects or Down's syndrome in infants born to women treated with clomifene the role of the drug in the causation of these defects has not been established and the incidence is reported to be similar to that for the general population.

**Carcinogenicity.** There have been a number of reports suggesting an association between drug therapy to treat infertility by stimulating ovulation and the subsequent development of ovarian cancer.[1-5] Concern has focussed in particular on the use of clomifene citrate and gonadotrophins, and a study has reported an increased risk of ovarian cancer in women who had prolonged clomifene therapy (for one year or more) although not in those who received the drug for a shorter period.[6] No association between gonadotrophin therapy and ovarian cancer was noted in this study. The conclusions of this study were only tentative, since the numbers who developed ovarian cancer were small; it has been pointed out that a successfully achieved pregnancy may reduce the risk of some other cancers, and that the risks and benefits of the procedure are not easy to balance.[7] A review[8] of epidemiological and cohort studies concluded that clomifene was not associated with any increase in the risk of ovarian cancer when used for less than 12 cycles, but noted conflicting results, limitations of the data, and the need to control for infertility and nulliparity as risk factors for ovarian cancer. A further cohort study[9] found no association between the use of clomifene and ovarian cancer. As a matter of prudence the UK Committee on Safety of Medicines has recommended that clomifene should not normally be used for more than 6 cycles.[10] However, the UK guidelines[11] on the treatment of infertility considered that the limit of 6 cycles related to one course of treatment only. In practice many women required more than one course and it was considered that benefit may be derived from use of up to 12 cycles.


1. Fishel S, Jackson P. Follicular stimulation for high tech pregnancies: are we playing it safe? *BMJ* 1989; **299:** 309–11.
2. Kulkarni R, McGarry JM. Follicular stimulation and ovarian cancer. *BMJ* 1989; **299:** 740.
3. Dietl J. Ovulation and ovarian cancer. *Lancet* 1991; **338:** 445.
4. Willemsen W, *et al.* Ovarian stimulation and granulosa-cell tumour. *Lancet* 1993; **341:** 986–8.
5. Tewari K, *et al.* Fertility drugs and malignant germ-cell tumour of ovary in pregnancy. *Lancet* 1998; **351:** 957–8.
6. Rossing MA, *et al.* Ovarian tumors in a cohort of infertile women. *N Engl J Med* 1994; **331:** 77–6.
7. Whittemore AS. The risk of ovarian cancer after treatment for infertility. *N Engl J Med* 1994; **331:** 805–6.
8. Duckitt K, Templeton AA. Cancer in women with infertility. *Curr Opin Obstet Gynecol* 1998; **10:** 199–203.
9. Potashnik G, *et al.* Fertility drugs and the risk of breast and ovarian cancers: results of a long-term follow-up study. *Fertil Steril* 1999; **71:** 853–9.
10. Committee on Safety of Medicines/Medicines Control Agency. Clomiphene (Clomid, Serophene): possible association with ovarian cancer. *Current Problems* 1995; **21:** 7.
11. National Collaborating Centre for Women's and Children's Health. Fertility: assessment and treatment for people with fertility problems. February 2004. Available at: http://www.rcog.org.uk/resources/Public/Fertility_full.pdf (accessed 16/06/04)


**Effects on the CNS.** Convulsions occurred when clomifene citrate was given to an infertile woman;[1] only five other cases had been reported since 1963.


1. Rimmington MR, *et al.* Convulsions after clomiphene citrate. *BMJ* 1994; **309:** 512.


**Effects on the eyes.** As mentioned above, clomifene may cause visual disturbances, which resolve on cessation of treatment. However, visual symptoms have persisted in a few cases.[1]


1. Purvin VA. Visual disturbance secondary to clomiphene citrate. *Arch Ophthalmol* 1995; **113:** 482–4.


**Effects on the fetus.** Discussions and individual reports of congenital disorders after treatment of the mother with clomifene,[1-10] plus evidence that the incidence of fetal disorders is not increased following infertility treatment.[11-14]


1. Dyson JL, Kohler HG. Anencephaly and ovulation stimulation. *Lancet* 1973; **i:** 1256–7.
2. Field B, Kerr C. Ovulation stimulation and defects of neural-tube closure. *Lancet* 1974; **ii:** 1511.
3. Singh M, Singhi S. Possible relationship between clomiphene and neural tube defects. *J Pediatr* 1978; **93:** 152.
4. Halal F, *et al.* Méga-urètre, hypospadias et anus imperforé chez un nouveau-né: rôle possible du clomiphène pris par la mère. *Can Med Assoc J* 1980; **122:** 1159–60.
5. Cornel MC, *et al.* Ovulation induction and neural tube defects. *Lancet* 1989; **i:** 1386.
6. Czeizel A. Ovulation induction and neural tube defects. *Lancet* 1989; **ii:** 167.
7. Cuckle H, Wald N. Ovulation induction and neural tube defects. *Lancet* 1989; **ii:** 1281.
8. Cornel MC, *et al.* Ovulation induction, in-vitro fertilisation, and neural tube defects. *Lancet* 1989; **ii:** 1530.
9. Vollset SE. Ovulation induction and neural tube defects. *Lancet* 1990; **337:** 178.
10. White L, *et al.* Neuroectodermal tumours in children born after assisted conception. *Lancet* 1990; **336:** 1577.
11. Mills JL, *et al.* Risk of neural tube defects in relation to maternal fertility and fertility drug use. *Lancet* 1990; **336:** 103–4.
12. Rosa F. Ovulation induction and neural tube defects. *Lancet* 1990; **336:** 1327.
13. Werler MM, *et al.* Ovulation induction and risk of neural tube defects. *Lancet* 1994; **344:** 445–6.
14. Whiteman D, *et al.* Reproductive factors, subfertility, and risk of neural tube defects: a case-control study based on the Oxford Record Linkage Study Register. *Am J Epidemiol* 2000; **152:** 823–8.


### Precautions

Clomifene is contra-indicated in patients with liver disease and the potential for toxicity should be considered in patients with a history of liver dysfunction. It should not be used in pregnancy, or in patients with undiagnosed abnormal uterine bleeding; some sources suggest it should also be avoided in patients with hormone-dependent tumours, and in those with pre-existing mental depression or thrombophlebitis because of the risk of exacerbation. The cause of infertility should be investigated. The patient should be warned of the possibility of multiple births.

Patients taking clomifene, particularly those with polycystic ovaries, should receive the lowest doses possible to minimise ovarian enlargement or cyst formation. The patient should be instructed to report any abdominal or pelvic pain as this may indicate the presence or enlargement of ovarian cysts. They should also be evaluated for the presence of ovarian cysts before each cycle of treatment. If abnormal enlargement occurs, clomifene should not be given until the ovaries have returned to pre-treatment size, and subsequent doses should be reduced. Clomifene should be used with caution in patients with uterine fibroids, due to the potential for enlargement of the fibroids.

Treatment should be stopped if visual disturbances develop and the patient warned that this might affect their ability to drive or operate machinery. Long-term cyclic therapy is not recommended, because of the uncertainty regarding increased risk of ovarian cancer: a maximum of 6 cycles of treatment has generally been advised but see also under Carcinogenicity, above.

## Pharmacokinetics

Clomifene citrate is absorbed from the gastrointestinal tract. It is metabolised in the liver and slowly excreted via the bile. Unchanged drug and metabolites are excreted in the faeces. The biological half-life is reported to be 5 days although traces are found in the faeces for up to 6 weeks. Enterohepatic recirculation takes place. The *E*-isomer is reported to be less well absorbed and more rapidly eliminated than the *Z*-isomer.

◊ References.

1. Szutu M, *et al.* Pharmacokinetics of intravenous clomiphene isomers. *Br J Clin Pharmacol* 1989; **27:** 639–40.

## Uses and Administration

Clomifene is a nonsteroidal compound which has both oestrogenic and anti-oestrogenic properties, the latter residing principally in the *E*-isomer. Its action in stimulating ovulation is believed to be related to its anti-oestrogenic properties. It stimulates the secretion of pituitary gonadotrophic hormones, probably by blocking the negative feedback effect of oestrogens at receptor sites in the hypothalamus and pituitary.

Clomifene is the most widely used drug in the treatment of anovulatory infertility (p.1316). Therapy with clomifene will not be successful unless the woman, though anovulatory, is capable of ovulation and her partner is fertile. It is ineffective in primary pituitary or primary ovarian failure. The usual dose by mouth is 50 mg of clomifene citrate daily for 5 days, starting on or about the 5th day of the menstrual cycle or at any time if there is amenorrhoea. If ovulation does not occur, a course of 100 mg daily for 5 days may be given starting as early as 30 days after the previous one. Women should be examined for pregnancy and ovarian enlargement or cysts between treatment cycles. In general, 3 courses of therapy are adequate to assess whether ovulation is obtainable. If ovulation has not occurred, the diagnosis should be re-evaluated. Once ovulation is established, each treatment cycle of clomifene should be started on or about the 5th day of the menstrual cycle. If pregnancy has not occurred after a total of about 6 treatment cycles, some consider further clomifene therapy is not recommended (but see also under Carcinogenicity, above).

Clomifene has also been used with gonadotrophins and in *in-vitro* fertilisation programmes.

Clomifene has also been used in the treatment of male infertility due to oligospermia to stimulate gonadotrophin release and enhance spermatogenesis.

**Infertility.** Systematic reviews have indicated that clomifene therapy was effective in the management of unexplained subfertility[1] or oligo-amenorrhoea[2] in women, although the absolute treatment effect was small in the former case, and concerns about the adverse effects remained. Another such review, originally issued in 1996, considered that evidence of improved fertility following clomifene treatment in men with idiopathic oligospermia or asthenospermia was lacking,[3] although treatment appeared to have a beneficial effect on some endocrine outcomes.

1. Hughes E, *et al.* Clomiphene citrate for unexplained subfertility in women. Available in The Cochrane Library; Issue 2. Chichester: John Wiley; 2004.
2. Hughes E, *et al.* Clomiphene citrate for ovulation induction in women with oligo-amenorrhoea. Available in The Cochrane Library; Issue 2. Chichester: John Wiley; 2004.
3. Vandekerckhove P, *et al.* Clomiphene or tamoxifen for idiopathic oligo/asthenospermia. Available in The Cochrane Library; Issue 2. Oxford: Update Software; 2002.

## Preparations

***BP 2003:*** Clomifene Tablets;
***USP 27:*** Clomiphene Citrate Tablets.

**Proprietary Preparations** (details are given in Part 3)
***Arg.:*** Genozym; Serofene; ***Austral.:*** Clomhexal; Clomid; Serophene; ***Austria:*** Clomid†; Serophene; ***Belg.:*** Clomid; ***Braz.:*** Clomid; Serofene; ***Canad.:*** Clomid; Serophene; ***Chile:*** Serofene; Zimaquin; ***Denm.:*** Clomivid†; Pergotime; ***Fin.:*** Clomifen; ***Fr.:*** Clomid; Pergotime; ***Ger.:*** Clomhexal; Clostilbegyt†; Dyneric†; ***Gr.:*** Serpafar; ***Hong Kong:*** Arcafen†; Clomid; Clostilbegyt; Duinum; Fertilan; Ova-Mit; Serophene; ***India:*** Clofert; Fertomid; Ovipreg; Ovofar; Siphene; ***Irl.:*** Clomid; Serophene†; ***Israel:*** Ikaclomin; ***Ital.:*** Clomid; Prolifen; Serofene; ***Malaysia:*** Clomid; Clostilbegyt; Duinum; Ova-Mit; Ovinum; Phenate; Serophene; ***Mex.:*** Omifin; Serophene; ***Neth.:*** Clomid; Serophene; ***Norw.:*** Clomivid†; Pergotime; ***NZ:*** Clomid†; Phenate; ***Port.:*** Dufine; ***S.Afr.:*** Clomid; Clomihexal; Fertomid; Serophene; ***Singapore:*** Clomid; Clostilbegyt; Duinum†; Ova-Mit; Ovinum; Phenate; Serophene; ***Spain:*** Clomifeno†; Omifin; ***Swed.:*** Clomivid†; Pergotime; ***Switz.:*** Clomid; Serophene; ***Thai.:*** Clomid; Duinum; Omicite†; Ova-Mit; Ovinum; Serophene; ***UK:*** Clomid; Serophene†; ***USA:*** Clomid; Serophene.

## Clostebol Acetate *(BAN, rINNM)*

Acetato de clostebol; 4-Chlorotestosterone Acetate; Chlortestosterone Acetate. 4-Chloro-3-oxoandrost-4-en-17β-yl acetate; 4-Chloro-17β-hydroxyandrost-4-en-3-one acetate.

$C_{21}H_{29}ClO_3$ = 364.9.

*CAS — 1093-58-9 (clostebol); 855-19-6 (clostebol acetate).*

### Profile

Clostebol acetate has anabolic properties (see Testosterone, p.1569) and is given in doses of 30 mg weekly by intramuscular injection, or 15 mg 2 or 3 times daily by mouth, for 3 weeks followed by a 3-week pause. It has also been applied topically to wounds and ulcers, and has been used as an ophthalmological preparation.

### Preparations

**Proprietary Preparations** (details are given in Part 3)
***Chile:*** Trofodermin; ***Ger.:*** Megagrisevit; ***Mex.:*** Trofodermin-S†.

**Multi-ingredient:** ***Braz.:*** Infepan†; Novaderm; Trofodermin; ***Chile:*** Trofodermin Neomicina; ***Ital.:*** Trofodermin; ***Thai.:*** Trofodermin.

# Conjugated Oestrogens

Conjugated Estrogens; Estrogeni Coniuncti; Estrógenos conjugados.

*ATC — G03CA57.*

**Pharmacopoeias.** In *Eur.* (see p.vi) and *US.*

**Ph. Eur. 5.0** (Estrogens, Conjugated). A mixture of various conjugated forms of oestrogens obtained from the urine of pregnant mares or by synthesis, dispersed in a suitable powdered diluent. It contains two principal components, 52.5 to 61.5% of sodium estrone sulfate and 22.5 to 30.5% of sodium equilin sulfate; the total of the combined two is 79.5 to 88.0%. It also contains 2.5 to 9.5% of sodium 17α-estradiol sulfate, 13.5 to 19.5% of sodium 17α-dihydroequilin sulfate, and 0.5 to 4.0% of sodium 17β-dihydroequilin sulfate. All percentages are related to the labelled content.

An almost white brownish amorphous powder.

**USP 27** (Conjugated Estrogens). A mixture of sodium estrone sulfate and sodium equilin sulfate, derived wholly or in part from equine urine or synthetically from estrone and equilin. It contains other conjugated oestrogenic substances of the type excreted by pregnant mares. It contains 52.5 to 61.5% of sodium estrone sulfate and 22.5 to 30.5% of sodium equilin sulfate; the total of the two combined should comprise 79.5 to 88.0% of the labelled content of conjugated oestrogens. It should contain, as sulfate conjugates, 13.5 to 19.5% of 17α-dihydroequilin, 2.5 to 9.5% of 17α-estradiol, and 0.5 to 4.0% of 17β-dihydroequilin, relative to the labelled content of conjugated oestrogens.

If it is obtained from natural sources it is a buff-coloured amorphous powder which is odourless or has a slight characteristic odour; the synthetic form is a white to light buff-coloured crystalline or amorphous powder, odourless or with a slight odour. Store at a temperature of 25°, excursions permitted between 15° and 30°.

## Adverse Effects and Precautions

As for oestrogens in general (see Estradiol, p.1550). See also under Hormone Replacement Therapy, p.1536.

**Effects on the cardiovascular system.** In a study of postmenopausal women with ischaemic heart disease, there was an increase in adverse cardiac events in the first year of use of HRT containing 0.625 mg conjugated oestrogens.[1] An increase in cardiac events has also been reported in healthy postmenopausal women after an average follow-up of about 5 years treatment with a similar regimen.[2] Again, the highest risk was in the first year of HRT[3] (see also p.1538).

In an early study of *men* with a previous myocardial infarction, treatment with conjugated oestrogens 5 mg daily was stopped, again because of a higher incidence of subsequent coronary events.[4] Moreover, treatment with the lower 2.5 mg dose was later also stopped because of suggestions of adverse trends including a greater incidence of venous thromboembolism.[5]

1. Hulley S, *et al.* Randomized trial of estrogen plus progestin for secondary prevention of coronary heart disease in postmenopausal women. *JAMA* 1998; **280:** 605–13.
2. Writing Group for the Women's Health Initiative Investigators. Risks and benefits of estrogen plus progestin in healthy postmenopausal women: principal results from the Women's Health Initiative randomized controlled trial. *JAMA* 2002; **288:** 321–33.
3. Manson JE, *et al.* Estrogen plus progestin and the risk of coronary heart disease. *N Engl J Med* 2003; **349:** 523–34.
4. Coronary Drug Project Research Group. The Coronary Drug Project: initial findings leading to modifications of its research protocol. *JAMA* 1970; **214:** 1303–13.
5. Coronary Drug Project Research Group. The Coronary Drug Project: findings leading to discontinuation of the 2.5-mg/day estrogen group. *JAMA* 1973; **226:** 652–7.

**Effects on the gallbladder.** In a study[1] of postmenopausal women with ischaemic heart disease, combined HRT containing conjugated oestrogens was associated with a slight increase in the risk of biliary tract surgery. Analysis of data obtained during the Coronary Drug Project indicated a significant increase in the development of gallbladder disease among men treated with conjugated oestrogens 2.5 and 5 mg daily, compared with those treated with placebo.[2]

1. Simon JA, *et al.* Effect of estrogen plus progestin on risk for biliary tract surgery in postmenopausal women with coronary artery disease: the Heart and Estrogen/progestin Replacement Study. *Ann Intern Med* 2001; **135:** 493–501.
2. The Coronary Drug Project Research Group. Gallbladder disease as a side effect of drugs influencing lipid metabolism: experience in the Coronary Drug Project. *N Engl J Med* 1977; **296:** 1185–90.

**Effects on the nervous system.** Reversible chorea developed in a 57-year-old woman receiving conjugated oestrogens and norgestrel;[1] the woman had a history of migraine and Sydenham's chorea.

1. Steiger MJ, Quinn NP. Hormone replacement therapy induced chorea. *BMJ* 1991; **302:** 762.

**Hypersensitivity.** A report of an anaphylactic reaction after intravenous conjugated oestrogens.[1]

1. Searcy CJ, *et al.* Anaphylactic reaction to intravenous conjugated estrogens. *Clin Pharm* 1987; **6:** 74–6.

## Interactions

See under Hormone Replacement Therapy, p.1539.

## Pharmacokinetics

Conjugated oestrogens taken by mouth are hydrolysed by enzymes present in the intestine that remove the sulfate group and allow absorption of the unconjugated oestrogen. Metabolism occurs primarily in the liver; there is some enterohepatic recycling (see also under Estradiol, p.1550).

## Uses and Administration

Conjugated oestrogens have actions and uses similar to those described for estradiol (see p.1551).

When used as menopausal HRT (p.1540) doses of 0.3 to 1.25 mg daily are given by mouth either cyclically or continuously, with a progestogen either cyclically or continuously in women with a uterus. Topical vaginal therapy may be used specifically for menopausal atrophic vaginitis; 0.5 to 2 g of a 0.0625% cream may be employed daily for 3 weeks of a 4-week cycle. If used long-term in a woman with a uterus, cyclical progestogen is required.

When given as replacement therapy on a cyclical basis, doses of 1.25 mg daily by mouth are used for primary ovarian failure and doses of 0.3 to 0.625 mg daily are used for female hypogonadism, although higher doses were formerly used.

For the palliative treatment of prostatic carcinoma (p.521), a dose of 1.25 to 2.5 mg three times daily by mouth has been used. A dose of 10 mg three times daily for at least 3 months has been used for palliative treatment of breast carcinoma in men and postmenopausal women (p.514).

Abnormal uterine bleeding has been treated acutely by giving 25 mg of conjugated oestrogens by slow intravenous injection, repeated if required after 6 to 12 hours; the intramuscular route has also been used.

Synthetic conjugated oestrogens are derived from plant material, and are not a generic equivalent of conjugated oestrogens described in USP 27 (see above). Synthetic conjugated oestrogens, A, contains a mixture of nine derivatives of estrone, equilin, estradiol, and equilenin. It is used in doses of 0.45 to 1.25 mg daily by mouth for the relief of vasomotor symptoms associated with the menopause. A dose of 0.3 mg daily may be used for menopausal vulvar and vaginal atrophy, but an alternative topical therapy should be considered if this is the only symptom being treated. Synthetic conjugated oestrogens, B, contains a mixture of ten derivatives of estrone, equilin, estradiol, and equilenin. It is used in doses of 0.625 to 1.25 mg daily by mouth for the relief of vasomotor symptoms associated with the menopause.

**Haemorrhagic disorders.** Some references to the use of high-dose intravenous or oral conjugated oestrogens in the management of haemorrhagic disorders associated with renal failure.[1-6]

1. Liu YK, *et al.* Treatment of uraemic bleeding with conjugated oestrogen. *Lancet* 1984; **ii:** 887–90.

2. Livio M, *et al.* Conjugated estrogens for the management of bleeding associated with renal failure. *N Engl J Med* 1986; **315:** 731–5.
3. Bronner MH, *et al.* Estrogen-progesterone therapy for bleeding gastrointestinal telangiectasias in chronic renal failure: an uncontrolled trial. *Ann Intern Med* 1986; **105:** 371–4.
4. Seth S, Geier TM. Use of conjugated estrogens to control gastrointestinal tract bleeding in two patients with chronic renal failure. *Clin Pharm* 1988; **7:** 906–9.
5. Shemin D, *et al.* Oral estrogens decrease bleeding time and improve clinical bleeding in patients with renal failure. *Am J Med* 1990; **89:** 436–40.
6. Heunisch C, *et al.* Conjugated estrogens for the management of gastrointestinal bleeding secondary to uremia of acute renal failure. *Pharmacotherapy* 1998; **18:** 210–7.

## Preparations

*USP 27:* Conjugated Estrogens Tablets.

**Proprietary Preparations** (details are given in Part 3)

***Arg.:*** Belestar; Livomarin; Premarin; ***Austral.:*** Premarin; ***Austria:*** Conjugen; Oestro-Feminal; Premarin; ***Belg.:*** Premarin; ***Braz.:*** Estrogenon; Estroplus; Menosedan; Premarin; Repogen; ***Canad.:*** CES; Congest; Premarin; ***Chile:*** Climatrol E; Conpremin; Estrarona; Profemina; ***Denm.:*** Premarin; ***Fin.:*** Premarin; ***Fr.:*** Premarin; ***Ger.:*** Climarest; Conjugen†; Femavit; Oestrofeminal; Transannon; ***Gr.:*** Premarin; ***Hong Kong:*** Equin; Premarin; ***India:*** Premarin; ***Irl.:*** Premarin; ***Israel:*** Premaril; Prevagin-Premaril; ***Ital.:*** Emopremarin; Premarin; ***Malaysia:*** Premarin; ***Mex.:*** Premarin; Sultrona; Terapova; ***Neth.:*** Dagynil; Premarin; ***NZ:*** Premarin; ***S.Afr.:*** Premarin; ***Singapore:*** Premarin; ***Spain:*** Carentil†; Equin; Premarin; ***Swed.:*** Premarina; ***Switz.:*** Conjugen†; Premarin; Transannon; ***Thai.:*** Premarin; ***UK:*** Premarin; ***USA:*** Cenestin; Premarin.

**Multi-ingredient:** ***Arg.:*** Periofem Ciclico; Periofem Continuo; Premelle Ciclico; Premelle Continuo; ***Austral.:*** Menoprem; Premia; Premia Continuous; Premia Low; Provelle; ***Austria:*** Cyclo-Premarin-MPA†; Perennia; Premarin compositum; Premarin MPA†; Premarin Plus; Sequennia; ***Belg.:*** Premelle; Premplus; ***Braz.:*** Ero Test†; Menosedan Ciclo; Menosedan Fase; Menosedan MPA; Menostress†; Menotensil; Premarin MPA; Premelle; Premelle Ciclo; Prempro Bifasico; Prempro Monofasico; Repogen Ciclo; Repogen Conti; ***Canad.:*** Premplus; ***Chile:*** Climatrol Ht; Climatrol Ht Continuo; Conpremin Pak; Conpremin Pak Plus; Novafac; Novafac 30; Novafac CC; Prempak; Profemina CC; Profemina MP; ***Ger.:*** Climopax; Climopax Cyclo; ***Gr.:*** Premelle; ***Hong Kong:*** Premelle; Premelle Cycle; Prempak; ***Irl.:*** Premique; Premique Cycle; Prempak-C; ***Israel:*** Premaril MP; Premaril Plus MP; ***Ital.:*** Premelle C; Premelle S; Premelle Sequenziale; Prempak; ***Malaysia:*** Plentiva; Plentiva Cycle 5; Premelle; Prempak; ***Mex.:*** Premarin Pak†; Premelle; ***Neth.:*** Premarin Plus; Premelle; Premelle Cycle; Prempak-C; ***NZ:*** Menoprem; Premia; Premia Continuous; Prempak-C; Provette Continuous†; Provette Sequential†; ***Port.:*** Premarin Plus; Premelle; Premelle Cycle; ***S.Afr.:*** Premelle; Prempak N; ***Singapore:*** Premelle; Premelle Cycle; Prempak-C; ***Spain:*** Premelle; Premelle Ciclico; ***Swed.:*** Premelle; Premelle Sekvens; ***Switz.:*** Cyclo-Premella ST; Cyclo-Premella†; Premarin Plus; Premella; ***Thai.:*** Premelle; Premelle Cycle; Prempak†; ***UK:*** Premique; Premique Cycle; Prempak-C; ***USA:*** Premarin with Methyltestosterone†; Premphase; Prempro.

---

## Cyclofenil *(BAN, rINN)*

Ciclofenilo; F-6066; H-3452; ICI-48213. 4,4′-(Cyclohexylidenemethylene)bis(phenyl acetate).

$C_{23}H_{24}O_4$ = 364.4.

*CAS — 2624-43-3.*

*ATC — G03GB01.*

### Profile

Cyclofenil is a nonsteroidal anti-oestrogen that has been used in the treatment of menstrual disturbances and anovulatory infertility due to hypothalamic-pituitary dysfunction.

It has been given by mouth in doses of 200 mg three times daily for 5 days, in a cyclical regimen for 3 to 4 cycles. It has also been given for menopausal symptoms.

### Preparations

**Proprietary Preparations** (details are given in Part 3)

***Braz.:*** Fertodur†; Menopax; ***Ital.:*** Neoclym; ***Mex.:*** Fertodur.

---

# Cyproterone Acetate *(BANM, USAN, rINNM)*

Acetato de ciproterona; Cyproteroni Acetas; NSC-81430; SH-714; SH-881 (cyproterone). 6-Chloro-1β,2β-dihydro-17α-hydroxy-3′H-cyclopropa[1,2]pregna-1,4,6-triene-3,20-dione acetate.

$C_{24}H_{29}ClO_4$ = 416.9.

*CAS — 2098-66-0 (cyproterone); 427-51-0 (cyproterone acetate).*

*ATC — G03HA01.*

NOTE. Compounded preparations of cyproterone acetate may be represented by the following names:

- Co-cyprindiol *(BAN)*—cyproterone acetate 2000 parts and ethinylestradiol 35 parts (w/w).

**Pharmacopoeias.** In *Eur.* (see p.vi).

**Ph. Eur. 5.0** (Cyproterone Acetate). A white or almost white, crystalline powder. Practically insoluble in water; sparingly soluble in dehydrated alcohol; freely soluble in acetone; very soluble in dichloromethane; soluble in methyl alcohol. Protect from light.

## Adverse Effects

When given to men cyproterone inhibits spermatogenesis, reduces the volume of ejaculate, and causes infertility; these effects are slowly reversible. Abnormal spermatozoa may be produced. Gynaecomastia is common and permanent enlargement of the mammary glands may occur; galactorrhoea and benign nodules have been reported rarely. There may be initial sedation and depressive mood changes. Patients may experience alterations in hair pattern, skin reactions and rarely rashes or hypersensitivity, weight changes, and anaemia. Osteoporosis may occur rarely. Altered liver function and breathlessness may occur. There have also been reports of hepatitis, jaundice, and hepatic failure, sometimes fatal, developing usually after several months of high-dose cyproterone therapy, but its association with liver cancer is uncertain.

When low-dose cyproterone is given with ethinylestradiol to women, adverse effects associated with combined oral contraceptives (see p.1527) may occur.

**Carcinogenicity.** See Effects on the Liver, below.

**Effects on the cardiovascular system.** Combined oral contraceptives are associated with a small increased risk of cardiovascular disease (see p.1530). Deep-vein thrombosis associated with antibodies to cyproterone acetate in women using oral contraceptives containing cyproterone acetate and ethinylestradiol has been reported.[1,2] The risk of venous thromboembolism may also be increased for women taking contraceptives containing cyproterone compared with levonorgestrel;[3] a review by the authorities in New Zealand considered the risk to be at least as great as with third-generation oral contraceptives.[4] Others have questioned the association,[5] but the UK Committee on Safety of Medicines[6] has also warned that preparations containing cyproterone and ethinylestradiol should not be used solely for contraception, but for treatment of severe acne and hirsutism, and that they should be withdrawn 3 or 4 cycles after the treated condition has completely resolved.

1. Leroy O, *et al.* Deep venous thrombosis and antibodies to cyproterone acetate. *Lancet* 1990; **336:** 509.
2. Beaumont V, Beaumont J-L. Thrombosis and antibodies to cyproterone acetate. *Lancet* 1991; **337:** 113.
3. Vasilakis-Scaramozza C, Jick H. Risk of venous thromboembolism with cyproterone or levonorgestrel contraceptives. *Lancet* 2001; **358:** 1427–9.
4. Savage R. Venous thromboembolism with Diane 35™ and Estelle 35™. Available at: http://www.medsafe.govt.nz/Profs/PUarticles/VTEwithCPA.htm (accessed 08/07/02)
5. Spitzer WO. Cyproterone acetate with ethinylestradiol as a risk factor for venous thromboembolism: an epidemiological evaluation. *J Obstet Gynaecol Can* 2003; **25:** 1011–18.
6. Committee on Safety of Medicines/Medicines Control Agency. Cyproterone acetate (Dianette): risk of venous thromboembolism (VTE). *Current Problems* 2002; **28:** 9–10. Also available at: http://www.mca.gov.uk/ourwork/monitorsafequalmed/currentproblems/cpoct2002.pdf (accessed 12/05/04)

**Effects on the eyes.** Bilateral optic atrophy in one elderly male patient was thought to be associated with cyproterone.[1] The authors could find no other cases from the published literature or the manufacturers' records.

1. Markus H, *et al.* Visual loss and optic atrophy associated with cyproterone acetate. *BMJ* 1992; **305:** 159.

**Effects on the liver.** There have been numerous reports of hepatic reactions associated with cyproterone acetate. In February 1995, the UK Committee on Safety of Medicines noted that it had received 96 reports of reactions including hepatitis, cholestatic jaundice, and hepatic failure, following cyproterone treatment;[1] 33 cases had led to fatalities. Nearly all cases (91 of 96) were in elderly men typically receiving high doses (300 mg) for prostatic cancer, and toxicity usually developed after several months of treatment. In view of this it was recommended that the use of cyproterone acetate in prostatic cancer be restricted to short courses for the testosterone flare associated with the commencement of gonadorelin analogue therapy, or for hot flushes after surgical or chemical castration, or for patients unresponsive to, or intolerant of, other treatments.

Although there is little doubt of the risk of hepatotoxicity, suggestions of an association between cyproterone therapy and the development of liver cancer remain contentious. There are individual reports of hepatocellular carcinoma developing in patients receiving cyproterone,[2,3] and some evidence *in vitro* of the formation of DNA adducts in exposed hepatocytes,[4] but there does not seem to be clinical evidence to support any association between use of cyproterone acetate and the development of liver tumours.[4,5]

1. Committee on Safety of Medicines/Medicines Control Agency. Hepatic reactions with cyproterone acetate (Cyprostat, Androcur). *Current Problems* 1995; **21:** 1.
2. Watanabe S, *et al.* Three cases of hepatocellular carcinoma among cyproterone users. *Lancet* 1994; **344:** 1567–8.
3. Rüdiger T, *et al.* Hepatocellular carcinoma after treatment with cyproterone acetate combined with ethinyloestradiol. *Lancet* 1995; **345:** 452–3.
4. Lewis S. Warning on cyproterone. *Lancet* 1995; **345:** 247.
5. Rabe T, *et al.* Liver tumours in women on oral contraceptives. *Lancet* 1994; **344:** 1568–9.

## Precautions

When used for hypersexuality, cyproterone is contra-indicated in men with liver diseases or malignant or wasting diseases. In addition, it should not be given to men with severe chronic depression, severe diabetes with vascular changes, sickle-cell anaemia, or to those with a history of thromboembolic disorders. It may delay bone maturation and testicular development and so should not be given to immature youths. When used for prostate cancer, there are no absolute contra-indications to the use of cyproterone, but the above conditions should prompt cautious consideration of the risks and benefits.

In men treated with cyproterone, liver function should be monitored before treatment, and whenever any symptoms or signs suggestive of hepatotoxicity occur. If cyproterone-induced hepatotoxicity occurs, treatment should be withdrawn. In men with prostate cancer, it may be advisable to limit the duration of treatment (see Effects on the Liver, above). Men with diabetes require careful monitoring of diabetic control. Since anaemia has been observed, regular blood counts are recommended during treatment. Adrenocortical suppression has been reported and function should be monitored regularly during treatment. Patients should be advised that the initial sedative effects may interfere with driving and the operation of machinery.

When cyproterone is given with ethinylestradiol to women the precautions for combined oral contraceptives (see p.1532) should be observed.

**Pregnancy.** Use of cyproterone during pregnancy might carry a risk of feminisation of a male fetus. However, there are a few case reports of healthy male infants born to mothers who had inadvertently taken a combination of cyproterone acetate and ethinylestradiol during the early stages of pregnancy,[1,2] and of a male fetus that was found to have no malformations after abortion was induced.[3] For further information on oral contraceptive use in pregnancy, see p.1533.

1. Statham BN, *et al.* Conception during 'Diane' therapy—a successful outcome. *Br J Dermatol* 1985; **113:** 374.
2. Bye P. Comments on 'conception during "Diane" therapy—a successful outcome'. *Br J Dermatol* 1986; **114:** 516.
3. Bergh T, Bakos O. Exposure to antiandrogen during pregnancy: case report. *BMJ* 1987; **294:** 677–8.

## Interactions

The manufacturers state that alcohol may reduce the effectiveness of cyproterone acetate as it is ineffective in chronic alcoholics.

When given with ethinylestradiol to women, interactions similar to those for combined oral contraceptives (see p.1534) might be anticipated.

## Pharmacokinetics

Cyproterone acetate is slowly absorbed from the gastrointestinal tract with peak plasma concentrations being achieved in 3 to 4 hours. It is about 96% bound to plasma proteins. The terminal elimination half-life is about 38 hours. Cyproterone is metabolised in the liver; about 35% of a dose is excreted in urine as free and conjugated metabolites, the remainder being excreted in the bile. The principal metabolite, 15β-hydroxycyproterone, has anti-androgenic activity.

**The elderly.** In a study[1] of healthy men, a decrease in hepatic clearance of cyproterone acetate was found in elderly men and thought to be due to an age-related reduction in liver volume.

1. Kuhnz W, *et al.* Investigation into the age-dependence of the pharmacokinetics of cyproterone acetate in healthy male volunteers. *Eur J Clin Pharmacol* 1997; **53:** 75–80.

## Uses and Administration

Cyproterone acetate is a progestogen with anti-androgenic properties.

It is used for the control of libido in severe hypersexuality or sexual deviation in adult males (see Disturbed Behaviour, p.665). The usual dose by mouth is 50 mg twice daily after meals.

It is also used in males for the palliative treatment of prostatic carcinoma (p.521) where other drugs are ineffective or not tolerated, to control disease flare or hot flushes associated with gonadorelin analogue therapy, and to control hot flushes associated with orchidectomy. The usual initial dose for disease flare or palliation is 300 mg daily in 2 or 3 divided doses after meals and maintenance treatment is continued with doses of 200 to 300 mg daily, but there is a risk of hepatotoxicity with long-term therapy. For the treatment of hot flushes, a dose of 50 mg daily is used; this may be increased up to 150 mg daily in 3 divided doses if necessary.

Cyproterone acetate may be used with ethinylestradiol in females for the control of acne (see below) and hirsutism (see below), and also provides contraception in these women. The usual doses are 2 mg of cyproterone acetate with 35 micrograms of ethinylestradiol given daily for 21 days of each menstrual cycle; the first treatment course is started on the first day of the menstrual cycle and each subsequent course is started after 7 tablet-free days have followed the preceding course. Treatment should be withdrawn 3 or 4 cycles after the condition has completely resolved.

Cyproterone acetate has also been given by depot intramuscular injection.

**Acne.** Comparisons of cyproterone acetate 2 mg with either 35 or 50 micrograms of ethinylestradiol in the treatment of refractory acne (p.1133) in women[1-3] have shown that, in general, both combinations were effective but that the lower dose of oestrogen was considered more acceptable for long-term therapy.

1. Colver GB, *et al.* Cyproterone acetate and two doses of oestrogen in female acne; a double-blind comparison. *Br J Dermatol* 1988; **118:** 95–9.
2. Fugère P, *et al.* Cyproterone acetate/ethinyl estradiol in the treatment of acne: a comparative dose-response study of the estrogen component. *Contraception* 1990; **42:** 225–34.
3. Anonymous. Dianette for women with acne. *Drug Ther Bull* 1990; **28:** 15–16.

**Hidradenitis suppurativa.** Some reports[1-3] of a beneficial response to cyproterone acetate with ethinylestradiol in women with hidradenitis suppurativa, an androgen-dependent disorder of the skin and hair in the pubic and axillary regions.

1. Mortimer PS, *et al.* A double-blind controlled cross-over trial of cyproterone acetate in females with hidradenitis suppurativa. *Br J Dermatol* 1986; **115:** 263–8.
2. Sawers RS, *et al.* Control of hidradenitis suppurativa in women using combined antiandrogen (cyproterone acetate) and oestrogen therapy. *Br J Dermatol* 1986; **115:** 269–74.
3. Mortimer PS, *et al.* Mediation of hidradenitis suppurativa by androgens. *BMJ* 1986; **292:** 961.

**Hirsutism.** Hirsutism is an abnormal growth in females of coarse pigmented terminal hair in an adult male pattern, and is one of the clinical expressions of hyperandrogenism. Most women with hirsutism have increased concentrations of circulating androgens from the ovaries associated with polycystic ovary syndrome (p.1317).[1] In rare cases, the adrenal gland is the primary source of increased androgens, for example, in congenital adrenal hyperplasia (p.1078). In a few cases, severe hirsutism is associated with frank virilisation due to massively increased circulating androgen concentrations from an androgen-secreting tumour.[2] Hirsutism is an adverse effect of androgenic progestogens, such as norgestrel, used in hormonal contraceptives and HRT. Androgens and anabolic steroids may also cause hirsutism in females.

**Treatment** for hirsutism employs topical cosmetic treatments such as bleaching, shaving, plucking, and electrolysis, and in the mildest cases this may be all that is required. However, such mechanical means of treatment are more usually combined with drug therapy to prevent further conversion of vellus to terminal hair, and to slow the regrowth of terminal hair, which may become lighter and softer. Because the growth cycle of hair is long, a response to therapy may not be seen for 6 to 12 months.

The mainstay of drug therapy for hirsutism is an anti-androgen, the most commonly used being the steroidal anti-androgens *cyproterone acetate* and *spironolactone*. To increase efficacy (by suppressing ovarian androgen production) and minimise the chance of conception (because of the risk of feminisation of a male fetus), cyclical *ethinylestradiol* is commonly used with cyproterone acetate, while combined (nonandrogenic) *hormonal contraceptives* are commonly used with spironolactone, which has no progestogenic activity. Cyproterone acetate may be used in a low-dose combined preparation containing cyproterone acetate 2 mg with ethinylestradiol 35 micrograms.[1,2] In more severe hirsutism, the two drugs may be prescribed separately in a 'reversed sequential regimen', with cyproterone acetate 50 to 150 mg given on days 5 to 15 of the menstrual cycle and ethinylestradiol 30 to 50 micrograms on days 5 to 26.[1-3] When a satisfactory response has been achieved, the cyproterone dosage is gradually reduced, and eventually the low-dose combination preparation may be sufficient.

In some countries spironolactone is the drug of choice for the treatment of hirsutism, particularly if there is associated obesity and hypertension; doses of up to 300 mg daily have been given initially, with the aim of reducing the dose when hair growth has been controlled.[3] Despite its wide use, however, evidence of benefit is considered scanty.[4] *Flutamide, finasteride,* and *leuprorelin* have also been shown to be effective, although some consider finasteride to be less active.[5] The condition has also been reported to respond to *ketoconazole*. *Eflornithine* is used topically for the reduction of facial hair. It is thought to slow hair growth by the inhibition of ornithine decarboxylase in hair follicles.

Although non-androgenic oral contraceptives have a role in reducing hyperandrogenism in polycystic ovary syndrome and corticosteroids have a role in congenital adrenal hyperplasia, neither is generally considered sufficient to reduce the hirsutism associated with these diseases, and an anti-androgen is usually added to the therapy.[2,5] Combination with a corticosteroid may however produce more prolonged response in appropriate patients (see also p.1098).

1. Conway GS, Jacobs HS. Hirsutism. *BMJ* 1990; **301:** 619–20.
2. Rittmaster RS. Hirsutism. *Lancet* 1997; **349:** 191–5.
3. Delahunt JW. Hirsutism: practical therapeutic guidelines. *Drugs* 1993; **45:** 223–31.
4. Farquhar C, *et al.* Spironolactone versus placebo or in combination with steroids for hirsutism and/or acne. Available in The Cochrane Library; Issue 2. Chichester: John Wiley; 2004.
5. Carmina E. A risk-benefit assessment of pharmacological therapies for hirsutism. *Drug Safety* 2001; **24:** 267–76.

## Preparations

***BP 2003:*** Cyproterone Tablets.

**Proprietary Preparations** (details are given in Part 3)
***Arg.:*** Androcur; Androstat; Asisdun; Asoteron; Ceprater; Ciclamil; Ciproferma; Ciproplex; CPD; Omnigeriat; Purfilx; Rubidox; ***Austral.:*** Androcur; Cyprone; Cyprostat; Procur; ***Austria:*** Andro-Diane; Androcur; Curandron; ***Belg.:*** Androcur; ***Braz.:*** Androcur; Androsteron†; Bioterona; Cetoteron; ***Canad.:*** Alti-CPA; Androcur; ***Chile:*** Ciproviron; ***Denm.:*** Androcur; ***Fin.:*** Androcur; ***Fr.:*** Androcur; ***Ger.:*** Androcur; Virilit; ***Gr.:*** Androcur; ***Hong Kong:*** Androcur; ***Irl.:*** Androcur; ***Israel:*** Androcur; Andromocur; Cypron; ***Ital.:*** Androcur; ***Malaysia:*** Androcur; ***Mex.:*** Androcur; ***Neth.:*** Androcur; ***Norw.:*** Androcur; ***NZ:*** Androcur; Siterone; ***Port.:*** Androcur; ***S.Afr.:*** Androcur; ***Singapore:*** Androcur; ***Spain:*** Androcur; ***Swed.:*** Androcur; ***Switz.:*** Androcur; ***Thai.:*** Androcur; ***UK:*** Androcur; Cyprostat.

**Multi-ingredient:** ***Arg.:*** Climene; Diane; ***Austral.:*** Brenda-35 ED; Climen; Diane-35 ED; Juliet; ***Austria:*** Climen; Diane; Minerva; Sterignyon; ***Belg.:*** Climen; Diane; ***Braz.:*** Climene; Diane; Elamax; Selene; ***Canad.:*** Diane; ***Chile:*** Anuar; Climene; Diane; Dixi-35; Drina; Evilin; Lady-Ten 35; ***Denm.:*** Climen; Diane; ***Fin.:*** Diane; Femilar; ***Fr.:*** Climene; Diane; Holgyeme; Minerva; ***Ger.:*** Climen; Diane; ***Gr.:*** Gynofen 35; ***Hong Kong:*** Climen; Diane; ***Irl.:*** Dianette; ***Israel:*** Diane; ***Ital.:*** Climen; Diane; Pausene; ***Malaysia:*** Climen; Diane; ***Mex.:*** Climene; Diane; ***Neth.:*** Climene; Diane; ***Norw.:*** Climen; Diane; ***NZ:*** Diane; Estelle; ***Port.:*** Climen; Diane; ***S.Afr.:*** Climen; Diane; Minerva; ***Singapore:*** Climen; Diane; ***Spain:*** Climen; Climen; Diane; ***Swed.:*** Diane; ***Switz.:*** Climen; Diane; ***Thai.:*** Climen; Diane; Lady-35; Preme; Sucee; Tina†; ***UK:*** Dianette.

# Danazol *(BAN, USAN, pINN)*

Win-17757. 17α-Pregna-2,4-dien-20-yno[2,3-*d*]isoxazol-17β-ol.
$C_{22}H_{27}NO_2$ = 337.5.
*CAS — 17230-88-5.*
*ATC — G03XA01.*

**Pharmacopoeias.** In *Chin.* and *US.*

**USP 27** (Danazol). A white to pale yellow crystalline powder. Practically insoluble or insoluble in water and in petroleum spirit; sparingly soluble in alcohol and in benzene; soluble in acetone; freely soluble in chloroform; slightly soluble in ether. Store in airtight containers. Protect from light.

## Adverse Effects

Side-effects of danazol that reflect inhibition of the pituitary-ovarian axis include menstrual disturbances and amenorrhoea (occasionally persistent), hot flushes, sweating, reduction in breast size, changes in libido, vaginal dryness and irritation, emotional lability, and nervousness.

Side-effects attributable to androgenic activity include acne, oily skin or hair, mild hirsutism, oedema, weight gain, deepening of the voice, androgenic alopecia, and rarely clitoral hypertrophy. Testicular atrophy and a reduction in spermatogenesis may occur.

Other side-effects include gastrointestinal disturbances, increased or decreased blood cell counts, thrombotic events, headache, backache, dizziness, tremor, depression, fatigue, sleep disorders, muscle spasm or cramp, skin rash, hyperglucagonaemia, abnormal glucose tolerance, decreased serum high-density-lipoprotein cholesterol, increased serum low-density-lipoprotein cholesterol, and elevation of liver-function test values and rarely cholestatic jaundice. Some patients may experience tachycardia and hypertension. Benign intracranial hypertension and visual disturbances have occurred.

**Effects on carbohydrate metabolism.** Diabetes mellitus developed in a patient receiving danazol 400 mg twice daily for endometriosis.[1] The diabetes developed 8 weeks after starting danazol therapy and resolved completely after the drug was discontinued.

1. Seifer DB, *et al.* Insulin-dependent diabetes mellitus associated with danazol. *Am J Obstet Gynecol* 1990; **162:** 474–5.

**Effects on the liver.** As with other 17α-alkylated steroids (see p.1570), cholestasis, peliosis hepatis, and hepatic adenomas have been associated with danazol.[1-6]

1. Ohsawa T, Iwashita S. Hepatitis associated with danazol. *Drug Intell Clin Pharm* 1986; **20:** 889.
2. Boue F, *et al.* Danazol and cholestatic hepatitis. *Ann Intern Med* 1986; **105:** 139–40.
3. Fermand JP, *et al.* Danazol-induced hepatocellular adenoma. *Am J Med* 1990; **88:** 529–30.
4. Bray GP, *et al.* Resolution of danazol-induced cholestasis with S-adenosylmethionine. *Postgrad Med J* 1993; **69:** 237–9.
5. Makdisi WJ, *et al.* Fatal peliosis of the liver and spleen in a patient with agnogenic myeloid metaplasia treated with danazol. *Am J Gastroenterol* 1995; **90:** 317–8.
6. Bork K, *et al.* Hepatocellular adenomas in patients taking danazol for hereditary angio-oedema. *Lancet* 1999; **353:** 1066–7.

**Effects on the skin.** Erythema multiforme developed in two patients receiving danazol for profuse bleeding.[1]

1. Gately LE, Andes WA. Danazol and erythema multiforme. *Ann Intern Med* 1988; **109:** 85.

**Pancreatitis.** There have been reports of pancreatitis in patients receiving danazol.[1,2]

1. Chevalier X, *et al.* Danazol induced pancreatitis and hepatitis. *Clin Rheumatol* 1990; **9:** 239–41.
2. Balasch J, *et al.* Acute pancreatitis associated with danazol treatment for endometriosis. *Hum Reprod* 1994; **9:** 1163–5.

## Precautions

Danazol should be used with caution in conditions which may be adversely affected by fluid retention, such as in cardiovascular, hepatic, and renal disorders, migraine, and epilepsy; it should be avoided in marked cardiac, hepatic, or renal dysfunction. It should also be used with care in patients with diabetes mellitus or polycythaemia. Danazol should not be given to patients with undiagnosed genital bleeding or androgen-dependent tumours. As with other 17α-alkylated compounds, there is an increased risk of liver disorders and liver function should be monitored during therapy. It should not be used in patients with a thromboembolic disorder or a history of thrombosis.

Danazol should not be given during pregnancy because of a possible androgenic effect on the female fetus (see below), and non-hormonal contraception is recommended during treatment. Caution is required in children and adolescents since precocious sexual development may occur in boys and virilisation in girls, and premature epiphyseal closure may occur in both sexes.

In the event of androgenic effects, danazol should be withdrawn, as they may prove irreversible on continued use.

**Breast feeding.** The manufacturers warn that danazol should be avoided in breast-feeding women because of the theoretical potential for androgenic effects in the infant.

**Porphyria.** Danazol has been associated with acute attacks of porphyria and is considered unsafe in porphyric patients.

**Pregnancy.** Reports of masculinisation of female infants born to mothers who had received danazol during pregnancy.[1-3]

1. Shaw RW, Farquhar JW. Female pseudohermaphroditism associated with danazol exposure in utero: case report. *Br J Obstet Gynaecol* 1984; **91:** 386–9.
2. Kingsbury AC. Danazol and fetal masculinization: a warning. *Med J Aust* 1985; **143:** 410–11.
3. Brunskill PJ. The effects of fetal exposure to danazol. *Br J Obstet Gynaecol* 1992; **99:** 212–15.

## Interactions

Therapy with danazol may inhibit the hepatic metabolism of a number of drugs including carbamazepine (see p.356), ciclosporin (see p.1356), warfarin (see p.1027), and possibly tacrolimus (see p.1365). Introduction of danazol appeared to reduce the maintenance requirement for alfacalcidol (see p.1462).

**Lovastatin.** For reference to rhabdomyolysis attributed to use of danazol with lovastatin, see p.999.

## Pharmacokinetics

Danazol is absorbed from the gastrointestinal tract and metabolised in the liver; absorption is markedly increased if it is taken with food. A plasma elimination half-life of 3 to 6 hours has been reported following a single dose, but is increased to about 26 hours with repeated dosing. Ethisterone, 2-hydroxymethylethisterone, and 17-hydroxymethylethisterone are described as the major metabolites, though none have pituitary inhibiting activity. Danazol and its metabolites may undergo enterohepatic circulation. Metabolites are excreted in the urine and faeces.

## Uses and Administration

Danazol suppresses the pituitary-ovarian axis by inhibiting pituitary output of gonadotrophins. It has weak androgenic activity.

Danazol has been given by mouth in the treatment of a variety of conditions including endometriosis, some benign breast disorders such as mastalgia and fibrocystic breast disease, gynaecomastia, menorrhagia associated with dysfunctional uterine bleeding, and prevention of hereditary angioedema. It may also be employed for the pre-operative thinning of the endometrium prior to hysteroscopic endometrial ablation, and has been tried in a variety of other conditions including pubertal or pre-pubertal breast hypertrophy and various blood disorders.

When given to women, treatment with danazol should be started on day 1 of the menstrual cycle or after pregnancy has been otherwise excluded.

In **endometriosis** the usual dose is 200 to 800 mg daily in 2 to 4 divided doses, adjusted according to the response. Therapy is given for 3 to 6 months or continued for up to 9 months if necessary.

In the treatment of **benign breast disorders** the usual initial dose is 100 to 400 mg daily in 2 divided doses, adjusted according to response, and continued for 3 to 6 months. For **gynaecomastia** 200 mg daily has been given to male adolescents, increased after 2 months to 400 mg daily if no response occurs; adult men have been given 400 mg daily initially, in up to 4 divided doses. Therapy is usually tried for 6 months.

In dysfunctional uterine bleeding manifesting as **menorrhagia** doses of 200 mg daily have been given and treatment is reviewed after 3 months.

In the management of **hereditary angioedema** initial doses of 200 mg two or three times daily are given, and then reduced according to the patient's response.

For **pre-operative thinning** of the endometrium danazol has been given in a dose of 400 to 800 mg daily in up to 4 divided doses, for 3 to 6 weeks.

**Blood disorders.** While danazol may produce thrombocytopenia and leucopenia its use has also been investigated in some blood disorders. Early reports[1,2] of a potential to increase plasma concentrations of factor VIII and factor IX in patients with the *haemophilias* (p.737) were not substantiated,[3,4] but increased platelet counts have been reported[5-9] in patients with *idiopathic thrombocytopenic purpura* (p.1082), although in one study[7] 7 of 10 patients derived no benefit. A study on its action in this disorder[10] indicated that danazol may influence the number of available binding sites for monomeric immunoglobulin G (Fc receptors) on monocytes. Another study[11] showed that sex, age (in women only), and the status of the spleen influenced the response of auto-immune thrombocytopenia to danazol. *Thrombocytopenia associated with rheumatic disorders*, such as systemic lupus erythematosus, the antiphospholipid antibody syndrome, and rheumatoid arthritis has also been reported to respond to treatment with danazol.[12] For mention of the use of danazol in *Henoch-Schönlein purpura* see Hypersensitivity Vasculitis, p.1081.

Additionally there have been reports of response to danazol therapy in patients with *auto-immune haemolytic anaemia*,[13,14] *paroxysmal nocturnal haemoglobinuria*,[15] *hereditary haemorrhagic telangiectasia*,[16] and *Evan's syndrome* due to systemic lupus erythematosus,[17] and conflicting reports in patients with *myelodysplastic syndromes*.[18-20]


1. Gralnick HR, Rick ME. Danazol increases factor VIII and factor IX in classic hemophilia and Christmas disease. *N Engl J Med* 1983; **308:** 1393–5.
2. Gralnick HR, *et al.* Benefits of danazol treatment in patients with hemophilia A (classic hemophilia). *JAMA* 1985; **253:** 1151–3.
3. Garewal HS, *et al.* Effect of danazol on coagulation parameters and bleeding in hemophilia. *JAMA* 1985; **253:** 1154–6.
4. Kasper CK, Boylen AL. Poor response to danazol in hemophilia. *Blood* 1985; **65:** 211–13.
5. Ahn YS, *et al.* Danazol for the treatment of idiopathic thrombocytopenic purpura. *N Engl J Med* 1983; **308:** 1396–9.
6. Buelli M, *et al.* Danazol for the treatment of idiopathic thrombocytopenic purpura. *Acta Haematol (Basel)* 1985; **74:** 97–8.
7. McVerry BA, *et al.* The use of danazol in the management of chronic immune thrombocytopenic purpura. *Br J Haematol* 1985; **61:** 145–8.
8. Mylvaganam R, *et al.* Very low dose danazol in idiopathic thrombocytopenic purpura and its role as an immune modulator. *Am J Med Sci* 1989; **298:** 215–20.
9. Edelmann DZ, *et al.* Danazol in non-splenectomised patients with refractory idiopathic thrombocytopenic purpura. *Postgrad Med J* 1990; **66:** 827–30.
10. Schreiber AD, *et al.* Effect of danazol in immune thrombocytopenic purpura. *N Engl J Med* 1987; **316:** 503–8.
11. Ahn YS, *et al.* Long-term danazol therapy in autoimmune thrombocytopenia: unmaintained remission and age-dependent response in women. *Ann Intern Med* 1989; **111:** 723–9.
12. Blanco R, *et al.* Successful therapy with danazol in refractory autoimmune thrombocytopenia associated with rheumatic diseases. *Br J Rheumatol* 1997; **36:** 1095–9.
13. Ahn YS, *et al.* Danazol therapy for autoimmune hemolytic anemia. *Ann Intern Med* 1985; **102:** 298–301.
14. Tan AM, *et al.* Danazol for treatment of refractory autoimmune hemolytic anaemia. *Ann Acad Med Singapore* 1989; **18:** 707–9.
15. Harrington WJ, *et al.* Danazol for paroxysmal nocturnal hemoglobinuria. *Am J Hematol* 1997; **54:** 149–54.
16. Haq AU, *et al.* Hereditary hemorrhagic telangiectasia and danazol. *Ann Intern Med* 1988; **109:** 171.
17. Aranegui P, *et al.* Danazol for Evan's syndrome due to SLE. *DICP Ann Pharmacother* 1990; **24:** 641–2.
18. Wattel E, *et al.* Androgen therapy in myelodysplastic syndromes with thrombocytopenia: a report on 20 cases. *Br J Haematol* 1994; **87:** 205–8.
19. Chabannon C, *et al.* A review of 76 patients with myelodysplastic syndromes treated with danazol. *Cancer* 1994; **73:** 3073–80.
20. Letendre L, *et al.* Myelodysplastic syndrome treatment with danazol and cis-retinoic acid. *Am J Hematol* 1995; **48:** 233–6.


**Endometriosis.** Endometriosis is a condition affecting women in their reproductive years,[1] in which endometrial tissue develops outside the uterine cavity. It occurs most often in the pelvic peritoneal cavity and occasionally elsewhere such as the thoracic cavity.[2] The aetiology is uncertain, although it is widely believed that retrograde flow of menstrual tissue introduces endometrial cells into the pelvic cavity, and that an immunological deficiency allows these cells to implant and grow; there may also be a degree of genetic susceptibility.[1] The advent of laparoscopy has indicated that the condition is more common than was previously thought, and not all women with endometriosis are symptomatic.[3]

The most common symptom is pain, usually manifesting as secondary dysmenorrhoea, dyspareunia, or cyclical back or pelvic pain. Pain may occur on micturition or defaecation if endometriosis affects the bladder or bowel; fibrosis and adhesions can develop. Endometriosis is also strongly associated with infertility. Severe endometriosis can distort the pelvic anatomy and thereby reduce fecundity, but how minimal and mild disease might affect fertility is unclear. Management will depend in part on the presenting complaint, the extent of disease, and whether fertility is an issue.[1,4-8] Minimal asymptomatic disease may resolve spontaneously.

Where **infertility** is the presenting symptom drug therapy has not been shown to be of direct value.[1,8-10] Conservative surgery may be of benefit in mild disease,[10] and is generally recommended in more severe cases.[1,8] Assisted reproductive techniques (see Infertility, p.1316) offer the best chance of conception in more severe disease[1,8,10] but the extent of benefit in mild or moderate endometriosis is less clear.[10]

For patients whose primary symptom is **pain**, drug treatments are effective and are the mainstay of treatment. For more extensive disease the most commonly used initial treatment is conservative surgery, followed by drugs to suppress the endometriosis if pain was the principal complaint or if removal of endometriotic deposits was incomplete. Because available drugs also tend to suppress ovulation they are potentially contraceptive, and their use will defer opportunities for conception in women wishing to conceive.[9]

One of the most widely used treatments is *danazol*, which has been shown to produce subjective improvement in symptoms of pain and reduction of some pelvic abnormalities and tissue implants.[11] Its androgenic effects can be a problem and there is concern about its effect on blood lipids, therefore therapy is restricted to 6 months, or rarely up to 9 months. *Gestrinone* has been shown to be equally effective and may be a useful alternative.[12] *Progestogens* such as medroxyprogesterone acetate, dydrogesterone, or norethisterone acetate are also commonly used. They appear to be as effective as danazol in relieving pain symptoms[12] and tend to be better tolerated.[1,4]

*Combined oral contraceptives* have been used in a continuous fashion, but such use is associated with a high incidence of breakthrough bleeding. However, it is now apparent that the usual cyclical use of combined oral contraceptives is associated with a decreased incidence of endometriosis,[13] and cyclical use is being investigated as a treatment although evidence of benefit remains scanty.[14]

The other major group of drugs that are used in endometriosis are *gonadorelin* and its analogues such as buserelin, goserelin, leuprorelin, nafarelin, and triptorelin. They are as effective as danazol[15] and their adverse effects, which resemble menopausal symptoms, may be better tolerated than the androgenic effects of danazol.[16] Long-term use is limited by the risk of osteoporosis, but concomitant low-dose oestrogen and progestogen HRT[1,7,15] or tibolone[17] ('add-back' therapy) can be used to prevent this. Parathyroid hormone[18] may also be effective for 'add-back' therapy. Gonadorelin analogues may also be used to facilitate laparoscopic procedures.[6]

Investigational drugs include the *antiprogestogens* such as mifepristone.[5]

There is a relatively high recurrence rate of endometriosis after conservative surgery and drug therapy. In women who can accept loss of child-bearing potential, definitive therapy is surgical oophorectomy and hysterectomy with complete excision or ablation of endometrial deposits. Oestrogen replacement therapy is given, but carries a risk of recurrence of the disease; some have suggested that combined HRT may be preferable (see p.1539).


1. Child TJ, Tan SL. Endometriosis: aetiology, pathogenesis and treatment. *Drugs* 2001; **61:** 1735–50.
2. Joseph J, Sahn SA. Thoracic endometriosis syndrome: new observations from an analysis of 110 cases. *Am J Med* 1996; **100:** 164–70.
3. Anonymous. Endometriosis: time for re-appraisal. *Lancet* 1992; **340:** 1073.
4. Lu PY, Ory SJ. Endometriosis: current management. *Mayo Clin Proc* 1995; **70:** 453–63.
5. Kettel LM, Hummel WP. Modern medical management of endometriosis. *Obstet Gynecol Clin North Am* 1997; **24:** 361–73.
6. Adamson GD, Nelson HP. Surgical treatment of endometriosis. *Obstet Gynecol Clin North Am* 1997; **24:** 375–409.
7. Anonymous. Managing endometriosis. *Drug Ther Bull* 1999; **37:** 25–9.
8. Olive DL, Pritts EA. Treatment of endometriosis. *N Engl J Med* 2001; **345:** 266–75.
9. Hughes E, *et al.* Ovulation suppression for endometriosis. Available in The Cochrane Library; Issue 2. Chichester: John Wiley; 2004.
10. Olive DL, Pritts EA. The treatment of endometriosis: a review of the evidence. *Ann N Y Acad Sci* 2002; **955:** 360–72.
11. Selak V, *et al.* Danazol for pelvic pain associated with endometriosis. Available in The Cochrane Library; Issue 2. Chichester: John Wiley; 2004.
12. Prentice A, *et al.* Progestagens and anti-progestagens for pain associated with endometriosis. Available in The Cochrane Library; Issue 2. Chichester: John Wiley; 2004.
13. Vessey MP, *et al.* Epidemiology of endometriosis in women attending family planning clinics. *BMJ* 1993; **306:** 182–4.
14. Moore J, *et al.* Modern combined oral contraceptives for pain associated with endometriosis. Available in The Cochrane Library; Issue 2. Chichester: John Wiley; 2004.
15. Prentice A, *et al.* Gonadotrophin-releasing hormone analogues for pain associated with endometriosis. Available in The Cochrane Library; Issue 2. Chichester: John Wiley; 2004.
16. Anonymous. Gonadotropin releasing hormone analogues for endometriosis. *Drug Ther Bull* 1993; **31:** 21–2.
17. Lindsay PC, *et al.* The effect of add-back treatment with tibolone (Livial) on patients treated with the gonadotropin-releasing hormone agonist triptorelin (Decapetyl). *Fertil Steril* 1996; **65:** 342–8.
18. Finkelstein JS, *et al.* Parathyroid hormone for the prevention of bone loss induced by estrogen deficiency. *N Engl J Med* 1994; **331:** 1618–23.


**Gynaecomastia.** Gynaecomastia is a benign glandular enlargement of the male breast, caused either by increased oestrogenic activity or decreased androgenic activity. Examples of gynaecomastia caused by increased oestrogenic activity include oestrogen-secreting malignancies, increased aromatisation of androgens into oestrogens (associated with an increase in adipose tissue), and exposure to drugs with oestrogenic activity such as digitoxin. Neonatal and pubertal gynaecomastia (the former due to exposure to maternal oestrogens, the latter because oestrogen levels increase before androgens do) come into this category. Examples of gynaecomastia caused by decreased androgenic activity include the various forms of hypogonadism, increased metabolism of androgens (for example in alcoholism), and exposure to drugs with anti-androgenic properties such as spironolactone, cimetidine, ketoconazole, cyproterone acetate, or flutamide. Some systemic disorders may also be associated with gynaecomastia, including cirrhosis of the liver, hyperthyroidism, and renal failure; it may also occur on refeeding after starvation.

Gynaecomastia has a high rate of spontaneous regression, and specific therapy (other than the removal of any cause) need only be considered if the enlarged breast tissue causes sufficient pain, embarrassment, or emotional discomfort to interfere with the patient's daily life.[1] Drug therapy is only likely to be of benefit while tissue is still proliferating; once glandular tissue has become inactive and fibrotic (usually after more than 12 months) a complete response is unlikely.

Testosterone itself is unlikely to be of benefit (and may be aromatised to oestradiol, exacerbating the situation), but a non-aromatisable androgen such as *androstanolone* (dihydrotestosterone) may produce some benefit.[1,2] *Danazol* has produced marked responses in some patients.[2] Quite good responses have also been reported with *tamoxifen*,[2,3] and this has been recommended as a drug of choice.[1] Aromatase inhibitors such as *anastrozole* are under investigation.[2] *Clomifene*[4,5] and *testolactone*,[6] have also been tried. Where drug therapy is unsuccessful, or the breast enlargement is long-standing, surgical removal of breast tissue is advocated.[1]


1. Braunstein GD. Gynecomastia. *N Engl J Med* 1993; **328:** 490–5.
2. Gruntmanis U, Braunstein GD. Treatment of gynecomastia. *Curr Opin Investig Drugs* 2001; **2:** 643–9.
3. McDermott MT, *et al.* Tamoxifen therapy for painful idiopathic gynecomastia. *South Med J* 1990; **83:** 1283–5.
4. LeRoith D, *et al.* The effect of clomiphene citrate on pubertal gynaecomastia. *Acta Endocrinol (Copenh)* 1980; **95;** 177–80.
5. Plourde PV, *et al.* Clomiphene in the treatment of adolescent gynecomastia: clinical and endocrine studies. *Am J Dis Child* 1983; **137:** 1080–2.
6. Zachmann M, *et al.* Treatment of pubertal gynaecomastia with testolactone. *Acta Endocrinol (Copenh)* 1986; **279** (suppl): 218–26.


**Hereditary angioedema.** Danazol has been used successfully[1,2] to prevent attacks of hereditary angioedema (p.761). Patients with lupus erythematosus-like syndromes associated with hereditary angioedema have also benefited from danazol therapy.[3-5]


1. Farkas H, *et al.* The efficacy of short-term danazol prophylaxis in hereditary angioedema patients undergoing maxillofacial and dental procedures. *J Oral Maxillofac Surg* 1999; **57:** 404–8.
2. Farkas H, *et al.* Danazol therapy for hereditary angio-oedema in children. *Lancet* 1999; **354:** 1031–2.
3. Masse R, *et al.* Reversal of lupus-erythematosus-like disease with danazol. *Lancet* 1980; **ii:** 651.
4. Donaldson VH, Hess EV. Effect of danazol on lupus-erythematosus-like disease in hereditary angioneurotic oedema. *Lancet* 1980; **ii:** 1145.
5. Duhra P, *et al.* Discoid lupus erythematosus associated with hereditary angioneurotic oedema. *Br J Dermatol* 1990; **123:** 241–4.


**Mastalgia.** Mastalgia is often associated with nodularity or other fibrocystic changes in the female breast, and is sometimes divided into cyclical mastalgia, which accounts for about two-thirds of all cases, non-cyclical mastalgia, and chest-wall or costochondral pain (Tietze's syndrome). Cyclical mastalgia is most common in the third decade of life, following a chronic relapsing course thereafter, and usually resolving at the menopause. Non-cyclical mastalgia tends to present later in life and the duration of symptoms is usually shorter, with spontaneous resolution occurring in 50% of cases; it tends to be more refractory to drug treatment.

Once clear pathological causes of pain have been excluded most patients can be managed by simple reassurance.[1-5] Drug treatment should rarely be considered unless pain has been present for about 6 months.[2] Patients who are receiving an oral contraceptive or HRT may find that symptoms improve on stopping treatment.[1,2,4] It has been suggested that reducing the intake of saturated fat in the diet may be worthwhile, and there is evidence that a low-fat diet reduces symptoms of tenderness and swelling.[6]

*Danazol* is probably the most effective drug for mastalgia,[3] and produces the most rapid response;[2,5] open studies suggest that it is of benefit in about 70% or more of patients with cyclical mastalgia,[1-4] and somewhat fewer with the non-cyclical form.[1,3,4] However, adverse effects may require dosage reduction. Danazol given only during the luteal phase (days 14 to 28) has been reported to be effective in cyclical mastalgia, and to cause few adverse effects.[7] *Gestrinone* has also been reported to be effective in cyclical mastalgia.[5]

Other drugs for cyclical mastalgia are *bromocriptine* or *gamolenic acid* (as evening primrose oil in most cases). Both are reported to produce a response in about 50% of cases, and appear to be equally effective.[1-3] However, gamolenic acid produces fewer adverse effects.[1,2,4,5] Again these drugs are less effective in non-cyclical mastalgia.[1,3] A small study[8] has reported that *lisuride* was effective in cyclical mastalgia.

A good response to danazol or bromocriptine would be expected within 2 months; gamolenic acid may take 3 to 4 months to show an effect.[1,4,5] When a response is achieved, therapy is withdrawn after 6 months to see if continued treatment is needed; even if pain recurs it may be less severe and therapy may be unnecessary.[1,2,5]

In refractory cyclical or non-cyclical mastalgia *tamoxifen*[9,10] has been shown to be effective; however, the concept of using tamoxifen in otherwise healthy premenopausal women has produced some concern.[11-13] *Goserelin* has also been shown to be effective.[14] Injection of a *local anaesthetic* with a *corticosteroid* has proved effective for the pain of non-cyclical mastalgia.[15]

*Other drugs* that have been used for cyclical mastalgia include antibiotics, diuretics, pyridoxine, and the progestogens, but there is no evidence that they are any better than placebo.[1,2,5]


1. Gateley CA, Mansel RE. Management of the painful and nodular breast. *Br Med Bull* 1991; **47:** 284–94.
2. Anonymous. Cyclical breast pain—what works and what doesn't. *Drug Ther Bull* 1992; **30:** 1–3.
3. Gateley CA, *et al.* Drug treatments for mastalgia: 17 years experience in the Cardiff mastalgia clinic. *J R Soc Med* 1992; **85:** 12–15.
4. Mansel RE. Breast pain. *BMJ* 1994; **309:** 866–8.
5. Holland PA, Gateley CA. Drug therapy of mastalgia: what are the options. *Drugs* 1994; **48:** 709–16.
6. Boyd NF, *et al.* Effect of a low fat high-carbohydrate diet on symptoms of cyclical mastopathy. *Lancet* 1988; **ii:** 128–32.
7. O'Brien PMS, Abukhalil IEH. Randomized controlled trial of the management of premenstrual syndrome and premenstrual mastalgia using luteal phase-only danazol. *Am J Obstet Gynecol* 1999; **180:** 18–23.
8. Kaleli S, *et al.* Symptomatic treatment of premenstrual mastalgia in premenopausal women with lisuride maleate: a double-blind placebo-controlled randomized study. *Fertil Steril* 2001; **75:** 718–23.
9. Fentiman IS, *et al.* Double-blind controlled trial of tamoxifen therapy for mastalgia. *Lancet* 1986; **i:** 287–8.
10. Fentiman IS, *et al.* Studies of tamoxifen in women with mastalgia. *Br J Clin Pract* 1989; **43** (suppl 68): 34–6.
11. Anonymous. Tamoxifen for benign breast disease. *Lancet* 1986; **i:** 305.
12. Smallwood JA, Taylor I. Tamoxifen for mastalgia. *Lancet* 1986; **i:** 680–1.
13. Fentiman IS, *et al.* Tamoxifen for mastalgia. *Lancet* 1986; **i:** 681.
14. Hamed H, *et al.* LHRH analogue for treatment of recurrent and refractory mastalgia. *Ann R Coll Surg Engl* 1990; **72:** 221–4.
15. Khan HN, *et al.* Local anaesthetic and steroid combined injection therapy in the management of non-cyclical mastalgia. *Breast* 2004; **13:** 129–32.


**Menorrhagia.** Danazol is effective in the treatment of menorrhagia (p.1567) but it is only used short term because of its adverse effects.

References.


1. Bonduelle M, *et al.* A comparative study of danazol and norethisterone in dysfunctional uterine bleeding presenting as menorrhagia. *Postgrad Med J* 1991; **67:** 833–6.
2. Need JA, *et al.* Danazol in the treatment of menorrhagia: the effect of a 1 month induction dose (200 mg) and 2 month's maintenance therapy (200 mg, 100 mg, 50 mg or placebo). *Aust N Z J Obstet Gynaecol* 1992; **32:** 346–52.
3. Higham JM, Shaw RW. A comparative study of danazol, a regimen of decreasing doses of danazol, and norethindrone in the treatment of objectively proven unexplained menorrhagia. *Am J Obstet Gynecol* 1993; **169:** 1134–9.
4. Fraser IS, *et al.* Depot goserelin and danazol pre-treatment before rollerball endometrial ablation for menorrhagia. *Obstet Gynecol* 1996; **87:** 544–50.
5. Erian MM, *et al.* The effects of danazol after endometrial resection—results of a randomized, placebo-controlled, double-blind study. *Aust N Z J Obstet Gynaecol* 1998; **38:** 210–4.
6. Beaumont H, *et al.* Danazol for heavy menstrual bleeding. Available in The Cochrane Library; Issue 2. Chichester: John Wiley; 2004.


**Premenstrual syndrome.** Danazol may be useful[1-3] in the management of the premenstrual syndrome (p.1551), but some have found it to be of value only for cyclical mastalgia rather than for general symptoms,[4] and in any case adverse effects limit its long-term use.


1. Halbreich U, *et al.* Elimination of ovulation and menstrual cyclicity (with danazol) improves dysphoric premenstrual syndromes. *Fertil Steril* 1991; **56:** 1066–9.
2. Deeny M, *et al.* Low dose danazol in the treatment of the premenstrual syndrome. *Postgrad Med J* 1991; **67:** 450–4.
3. Hahn PM, *et al.* A randomized, placebo-controlled, crossover trial of danazol for the treatment of premenstrual syndrome. *Psychoneuroendocrinology* 1995; **20:** 193–209.
4. O'Brien PMS, Abukhalil IEH. Randomized controlled trial of the management of premenstrual syndrome and premenstrual mastalgia using luteal phase-only danazol. *Am J Obstet Gynecol* 1999; **180:** 18–23.


**Skin disorders.** A patient with a skin condition involving cholinergic pruritus, erythema, and urticaria that was unresponsive to treatment with antihistamines and anti-inflammatory drugs was successfully treated with danazol 600 mg daily.[1] This dose of danazol also resolved a case of chronic actinic dermatitis.[2] In both of these patients, the skin disorder had been associated with low plasma concentrations of antiprotease.


1. Berth-Jones J, Graham-Brown RAC. Cholinergic pruritus, erythema and urticaria: a disease spectrum responding to danazol. *Br J Dermatol* 1989; **121:** 235–7.
2. Humbert P, *et al.* Chronic actinic dermatitis responding to danazol. *Br J Dermatol* 1991; **124:** 195–7.


## Preparations

***USP 27:*** Danazol Capsules.

**Proprietary Preparations** (details are given in Part 3)
***Arg.:*** Ladogal; ***Austral.:*** Azol; Danocrine; ***Austria:*** Danokrin; ***Belg.:*** Danatrol; ***Braz.:*** Ladogal; ***Canad.:*** Cyclomen; ***Chile:*** Danogar; ***Denm.:*** Danocrine; ***Fin.:*** Danocrine; ***Fr.:*** Danatrol; ***Ger.:*** Winobanin†; ***Gr.:*** Danatrol; ***Hong Kong:*** Anargil; Danazant†; Danocrine; ***India:*** Danogen; Gonablok; Zendol; ***Irl.:*** Danazant; Danol; ***Israel:*** Danocrine; ***Ital.:*** Danatrol; ***Malaysia:*** Anargil; Azol; Ladogal; Vabon; ***Mex.:*** Danalem; Kendazol†; Ladogal; Lisigon†; Norciden†; Zoldan-A; ***Neth.:*** Danatrol; ***Norw.:*** Danocrine; ***NZ:*** D-Zol; Danocrine; ***Port.:*** Danatrol; Mastodanatrol; ***S.Afr.:*** Danogen; Ladazol; ***Singapore:*** Azol; Ladogal; ***Spain:*** Danatrol; ***Swed.:*** Danocrine; ***Switz.:*** Danatrol; ***Thai.:*** Anargil; Ectopal; Ladogal; Vabon; ***UK:*** Danol; ***USA:*** Danocrine.

# Delmadinone Acetate *(BANM, USAN, rINNM)*

Acetato de delmadinona; RS-1301. 6-Chloro-17α-hydroxypregna-1,4,6-triene-3,20-dione acetate.

$C_{23}H_{27}ClO_4$ = 402.9.

*CAS — 15262-77-8 (delmadinone); 13698-49-2 (delmadinone acetate).*

## Profile

Delmadinone acetate is a progestogen with anti-androgenic and anti-oestrogenic activity. It is used as an anti-androgen in veterinary practice.

# Demegestone *(rINN)*

Demegestona; R-2453. 17α-Methyl-19-norpregna-4,9-diene-3,20-dione.

$C_{21}H_{28}O_2$ = 312.4.

*CAS — 10116-22-0.*

*ATC — G03DB05.*

## Profile

Demegestone is a progestogen structurally related to progesterone (p.1566). It has been given cyclically or continuously for its progestogenic effects.

## Preparations

**Proprietary Preparations** (details are given in Part 3)
***Fr.:*** Lutionex†.

# Desogestrel *(BAN, USAN, rINN)*

Org-2969. 13β-Ethyl-11-methylene-18,19-dinor-17α-pregn-4-en-20-yn-17β-ol.

$C_{22}H_{30}O$ = 310.5.

*CAS — 54024-22-5.*

*ATC — G03AC09.*

**Pharmacopoeias.** In *Br.*

**BP 2003** (Desogestrel). A white, crystalline powder. Practically insoluble in water; slightly soluble in alcohol and in ethyl acetate; sparingly soluble in *n*-hexane.

## Adverse Effects and Precautions

As for progestogens in general (see Progesterone, p.1566). See also under Hormonal Contraceptives, p.1527. Desogestrel is reported to have few androgenic effects, and to have less adverse effect on the serum lipid profile than older 19-nortestosterone derivatives. However, there is some evidence that desogestrel-containing combined oral contraceptives are associated with a small increased risk of venous thromboembolism (see p.1531, and for precautions, see p.1533).

## Interactions

As for progestogens in general (see Progesterone, p.1567). See also under Hormonal Contraceptives, p.1534.

## Pharmacokinetics

After oral doses, desogestrel undergoes oxidative transformation to its active metabolite 3-keto-desogestrel (see also Etonogestrel, p.1554) in the intestinal mucosa and liver. In the blood, about 32% of 3-keto-desogestrel is bound to sex hormone binding globulin, and 66% to albumin.

◊ References.


1. Madden S, *et al.* Metabolism of the contraceptive steroid desogestrel by the intestinal mucosa. *Br J Clin Pharmacol* 1989; **27:** 295–9.
2. Madden S, *et al.* Metabolism of the contraceptive steroid desogestrel by human liver in vitro. *J Steroid Biochem* 1990; **35:** 281–8.
3. Kuhnz W, *et al.* Protein binding of the contraceptive steroids gestodene, 3-keto-desogestrel and ethinyloestradiol in human serum. *J Steroid Biochem* 1990; **35:** 313–18.


## Uses and Administration

Desogestrel is a progestogen (see Progesterone, p.1567) structurally related to levonorgestrel that is used as a hormonal contraceptive (see p.1535). A typical daily dose of 150 micrograms is used as the progestogenic component of monophasic combined oral contraceptive preparations. Doses of 50 to 150 micrograms daily may be used in triphasic combined preparations. A dose of 75 micrograms daily by mouth is used as a progestogen-only contraceptive; unlike traditional progestogen-only contraceptives, desogestrel is said to reliably inhibit ovulation.

**Contraception.** The effects of a progestogen-only contraceptive containing desogestrel have been reported.[1,2] Desogestrel has also been investigated as a male contraceptive in combination with low-dose intramuscular[3] or transdermal[4] testosterone.


1. Collaborative study group on the desogestrel-containing progestogen-only pill. A double-blind study comparing the contraceptive efficacy, acceptability and safety of two progestogen-only pills containing desogestrel 75 micrograms/day or levonorgestrel 30 micrograms/day. *Eur J Contracept Reprod Health Care* 1998; **3:** 169–78.
2. Rice CF, *et al.* A comparison of the inhibition of ovulation achieved by desogestrel 75 μg and levonorgestrel 30 μg daily. *Hum Reprod* 1999; **14:** 982–5.
3. Wu FCW, *et al.* Oral progestogen combined with testosterone as a potential male contraceptive: additive effects between desogestrel and testosterone enanthate in suppression of spermatogenesis, pituitary-testicular axis, and lipid metabolism. *J Clin Endocrinol Metab* 1999; **84:** 112–22.
4. Hair WM, *et al.* A novel male contraceptive pill-patch combination: oral desogestrel and transdermal testosterone in the suppression of spermatogenesis in normal men. *J Clin Endocrinol Metab* 2001; **86:** 5201–9.


## Preparations

**Proprietary Preparations** (details are given in Part 3)
***Arg.:*** Cerazette; ***Belg.:*** Cerazette; ***Braz.:*** Cerazette; ***Chile:*** Arlette 28; Cerazette; ***Denm.:*** Cerazette; ***Fin.:*** Cerazette; ***Fr.:*** Cerazette; ***Ger.:*** Cerazette; ***Ital.:*** Cerazette; ***Mex.:*** Cerazette; ***Neth.:*** Cerazette; ***NZ:*** Cerazette; ***Port.:*** Cerazette; ***Spain:*** Cerazet; ***Swed.:*** Cerazette; ***Switz.:*** Cerazette; ***UK:*** Cerazette.

**Multi-ingredient:** ***Arg.:*** Marvelon; Mercilon; ***Austral.:*** Marvelon; ***Austria:*** Gracial; Laurina; Liseta; Marvelon; Mercilon; ***Belg.:*** Gracial; Marvelon; Mercilon; Ovidol; ***Braz.:*** Femina; Gracial; Mercilon; Microdiol; Minian; Primera; ***Canad.:*** Marvelon; Ortho-Cept; ***Chile:*** Ciclidon; Dal; Desoren; Gracial; Gynostat; Marvelon; Midalet; Neolette; ***Denm.:*** Desorelle; Gracial; Marvelon; Mercilon; Novynette; ***Fin.:*** Gracial; Marvelon; Mercilon; ***Fr.:*** Cycleane; Mercilon; Varnoline; ***Ger.:*** Biviol; Cyclosa; Desmin; Lamuna; Lovelle; Lovina†; Marvelon; Novial; Oviol; ***Gr.:*** Gracial; Marvelon; Mercilon; ***Hong Kong:*** Gracial; Marvelon; Mercilon; Novynette; ***India:*** Novelon; ***Irl.:*** Marviol; Mercilon; ***Israel:*** Mercilon; Microdiol; ***Ital.:*** Dueva; Gracial; Mercilon; Planum; Practil; Securgin; ***Malaysia:*** Marvelon; Mercilon; Novynette; ***Mex.:*** Marvelon; Mercilon; ***Neth.:*** Gracial; Marvelon; Mercilon; Ovidol; ***Norw.:*** Marvelon; ***NZ:*** Marvelon; Mercilon; ***Port.:*** Gracial; Marvelon; Mercilon; ***S.Afr.:*** Marvelon; Mercilon; ***Singapore:*** Marvelon; Mercilon; ***Spain:*** Gracial; Microdiol; Suavuret; ***Swed.:*** Desolett; Mercilon; Trimiron; ***Switz.:*** Gracial; Marvelon; Mercilon; Ovidol†; ***Thai.:*** Marvelon; Mercilon; ***UK:*** Marvelon; Mercilon; ***USA:*** Apri; Cyclessa; Desogen; Kariva; Mircette; Ortho-Cept.

# Dienestrol *(BAN, rINN)*

Dehydrostilbestrol; Dienestrolum; Dienoestrol; Dienoestrolum; Oestrodienolum. *(E,E)*-4,4′-[Di(ethylidene)ethylene]diphenol; 4,4′-(1,2-Diethylidene-1,2-ethanediyl)bisphenol.

$C_{18}H_{18}O_2$ = 266.3.

*CAS — 84-17-3 (dienestrol); 13029-44-2 ((E,E)-dienestrol).*

*ATC — G03CB01.*

**Pharmacopoeias.** In *Eur.* (see p.vi) and *US.*

**Ph. Eur. 5.0** (Dienestrol). A white or almost white, crystalline powder. Practically insoluble in water; freely soluble in alcohol and in acetone; dissolves in dilute solutions of alkali hydroxides. Protect from light.

**USP 27** (Dienestrol). Colourless, white, or practically white needle-like crystals, or white or practically white crystalline powder. It is odourless. Practically insoluble in water; soluble in alcohol, in acetone, in ether, in methyl alcohol, in propylene glycol, and in solutions of alkali hydroxides; slightly soluble in chloroform and in fatty oils.

### Profile

Dienestrol is a synthetic nonsteroidal oestrogen structurally related to diethylstilbestrol (p.1548). It is used as a 0.01% cream in the treatment of menopausal atrophic vaginitis. If used on a long-term basis in women with a uterus a progestogen is required.

Dienestrol diacetate has been used as an ingredient of topical preparations for skin disorders.

**Porphyria.** Dienestrol is considered to be unsafe in patients with porphyria because it has been shown to be porphyrinogenic in *animals* or *in-vitro* systems.

### Preparations

*USP 27:* Dienestrol Cream.

**Proprietary Preparations** (details are given in Part 3)
***Belg.:*** Ortho-Dienoestrol†; ***Denm.:*** Sexadien; ***Irl.:*** Ortho†; ***Israel:*** Ortho-Dienoestrol†; ***UK:*** Ortho-Dienoestrol†; ***USA:*** Ortho-Dienestrol.

## Dienogest *(BAN, USAN, rINN)*

STS-557. 17-Hydroxy-3-oxo-19-nor-17α-pregna-4,9-diene-21-nitrile.

$C_{20}H_{25}NO_2$ = 311.4.
*CAS — 65928-58-7.*

### Profile

Dienogest is a nonethinylated progestogen (see Progesterone, p.1566) structurally related to nortestosterone. It is reported to have anti-androgenic properties. Dienogest is used as the progestogen component of some combined oral contraceptives (see p.1527); a typical daily dose is 2 mg. It is also used as the progestogen component in HRT (see p.1536) in a daily dose of 2 mg.

◊ Reviews.

1. Foster RH, Wilde MI. Dienogest. *Drugs* 1998; **56:** 825–33.
2. Wellington K, Perry CM. Estradiol valerate/dienogest. *Drugs* 2002; **62:** 491–504.

### Preparations

**Proprietary Preparations** (details are given in Part 3)
**Multi-ingredient: *Denm.:*** Climodien; ***Ger.:*** Climodien; Valette; ***Norw.:*** Climodien; ***Port.:*** Climodien; ***Spain:*** Climodien; Mevaren; ***Swed.:*** Climodien.

# Diethylstilbestrol *(BAN, rINN)*

DES; Diethylstilbestrolum; Diethylstilboestrol; Dietilestilbestrol; NSC-3070; Stilbestrol; Stilboestrol. (*E*)-αβ-Diethylstilbene-4-4′-diol.

$C_{18}H_{20}O_2$ = 268.4.
*CAS — 56-53-1.*
*ATC — G03CB02; L02AA01.*

**Pharmacopoeias.** In *Chin., Eur.* (see p.vi), and *US.*

**Ph. Eur. 5.0** (Diethylstilbestrol). A white or almost white crystalline powder. Practically insoluble in water; freely soluble in alcohol; dissolves in solutions of alkali hydroxides. Protect from light.

**USP 27** (Diethylstilbestrol). A white, odourless, crystalline powder. Practically insoluble in water; soluble in alcohol, in chloroform, in ether, in fatty oils, and in dilute alkali hydroxides. Store in airtight containers. Protect from light.

## Diethylstilbestrol Dipropionate *(BANM, rINNM)*

Dipropionato de dietilestilbestrol; Stilboestrol Dipropionate. (*E*)-αβ-Diethylstilbene-4,4′-diol dipropionate.

$C_{24}H_{28}O_4$ = 380.5.
*CAS — 130-80-3.*
*ATC — G03CB02; L02AA01.*

## Adverse Effects and Precautions

Dose-related adverse effects of diethylstilbestrol include nausea, fluid retention, and arterial and venous thrombosis, and these effects are common at the doses used for palliation of cancer. Impotence and gynaecomastia occur in men, and withdrawal bleeding may occur in women, as may hypercalcaemia and bone pain in women treated for breast cancer. Diethylstilbestrol should be used with caution in those with cardiovascular disease or renal or hepatic impairment. Use of diethylstilbestrol is contra-indicated if pregnancy is suspected.

Adverse effects and precautions of oestrogens in general (steroidal compounds) are covered under Estradiol, on p.1550.

*Historically,* high doses of diethylstilbestrol and related substances were used for 'hormonal support' in pregnant women to try to prevent miscarriages and preterm births, most commonly in the USA. This practice was later shown to be ineffective. Adverse effects on the genito-urinary tract of offspring of these women have been noted. In particular, an increased incidence of changes in the cervix and vagina including adenosis and rarely clear-cell adenocarcinoma has been seen in postpubertal daughters of women who received diethylstilbestrol or related substances during pregnancy (see below). A possible increased incidence of abnormalities of the genital tract and of abnormal spermatozoa has been reported in male offspring similarly exposed (see below). The recipients themselves appear to be at a small increased risk of breast cancer (see below).

**Carcinogenicity.** BREAST. No statistically significant difference in the incidence of breast cancer was found among a group of 693 women who had received diethylstilbestrol during pregnancy 25 years earlier compared with a control group of 668 who had not.[1] This finding was, however, criticised[2] on the basis that the study lacked the statistical power to reject the null hypothesis. In another study[3] the incidence of breast cancer in 3033 women who had taken diethylstilbestrol in pregnancy during the period 1940 to 1960 was compared with the incidence in a comparable group of unexposed women. This study involved over 85 000 women-years of follow-up in each group and it was found that the incidence of breast cancer per 100 000 women-years was 134 in the exposed group and 93 in the unexposed group (a relative risk of 1.4). The authors concluded that in those women given diethylstilbestrol there was a moderately increased incidence of breast cancer but that some unrecognised concomitant of exposure could not be excluded as a possibility for the increase. Although this study suggested that the risk increased over time, subsequent follow-up,[4] while confirming a modest increase in risk overall, did not confirm a higher risk in these women as time went on. Two cases of breast cancer[5] in premenopausal women exposed to diethylstilbestrol *in utero* have raised the possibility that the risk of breast cancer may be increased in these women, in addition to the known genito-urinary risk (see below under Pregnancy, Effects on Female Offspring). However, a cohort study[6] involving 4536 women exposed *in utero* found no increased risk of other cancers overall, and did not show an increased risk of breast cancer (relative risk 1.18; 95% confidence intervals 0.56 to 2.49). Nonetheless, since these women were relatively young, continued follow-up was considered necessary.

1. Bibbo M, *et al.* A twenty-five-year follow-up study of women exposed to diethylstilbestrol during pregnancy. *N Engl J Med* 1978; **298:** 763–7.
2. Clark LC, Portier KM. Diethylstilbestrol and the risk of cancer. *N Engl J Med* 1979; **300:** 263–4.
3. Greenberg ER, *et al.* Breast cancer in mothers given diethylstilbestrol in pregnancy. *N Engl J Med* 1984; **311:** 1393–8.
4. Colton T, *et al.* Breast cancer in mothers prescribed diethylstilbestrol in pregnancy. *JAMA* 1993; **269:** 2096–2100.
5. Huckell C, *et al.* Premenopausal breast cancer after in-utero exposure to stilboestrol. *Lancet* 1996; **348:** 331.
6. Hatch EE, *et al.* Cancer risk in women exposed to diethylstilbestrol in utero. *JAMA* 1998; **280:** 630–4.

GENITO-URINARY TRACT. See below under Pregnancy, Effects on Female Offspring.

KIDNEY. Renal carcinoma was associated with the long-term use of diethylstilbestrol for prostate cancer in 2 men.[1]

1. Nissenkorn I, *et al.* Oestrogen-induced renal carcinoma. *Br J Urol* 1979; **51:** 6–9.

LIVER. Hepatic angiosarcoma developed in a 76-year-old man who had received diethylstilbestrol 3 mg daily for 12 years.[1] Hepatoma developed in another elderly man who had received a similar dose for 4.5 years.[2]

1. Hoch-Ligeti C. Angiosarcoma of the liver associated with diethylstilbestrol. *JAMA* 1978; **240:** 1510–11.
2. Brooks JJ. Hepatoma associated with diethylstilbestrol therapy for prostate carcinoma. *J Urol (Baltimore)* 1982; **128:** 1044–5.

**Effects on the blood.** Adverse haematological effects reported with diethylstilbestrol include severe bone-marrow changes in a 71-year-old man given diethylstilbestrol in a massive dose of 150 mg daily for 7 years[1] and fatal immune haemolytic anaemia in a 69-year-old man given weekly infusions of diethylstilbestrol 1 g for 9 weeks.[2] The latter reaction was due to an IgG antibody specific for diethylstilbestrol.

1. Anderson AL, Lynch EC. Myelodysplastic syndrome associated with diethylstilbestrol therapy. *Arch Intern Med* 1980; **140:** 976–7.
2. Rosenfeld CS, *et al.* Diethylstilbestrol-associated hemolytic anemia with a positive direct antiglobulin test result. *Am J Med* 1989; **86:** 617–18.

**Pregnancy.** EFFECTS ON FEMALE OFFSPRING. The DESAD (Diethylstilbestrol and Adenosis) Project carried out by the National Cancer Institute in the USA led to several reports linking exposure to diethylstilbestrol *in utero* to adverse genital-tract effects.[1-3] It was reported that of nearly 300 young females with clear-cell adenocarcinoma of the genital tract, more than 80% had been exposed *in utero* to diethylstilbestrol-type hormones.[1] Patients had been aged 7 to 28 years at the time of diagnosis. Doses and duration of treatment varied widely; 1.5 mg of diethylstilbestrol daily throughout pregnancy or varying amounts for a week or more during the first trimester had shown an association. Vaginal adenosis, rare in unexposed young women, was present in about a third of those exposed in the first 4 months of pregnancy, and cervical ectropion in more than two-thirds. Vaginal epithelial changes were most closely associated with early exposure to diethylstilbestrol, with the total dose, and with the duration of exposure; their incidence decreased with age. The risk of cancer in the first 25 years after exposure was small.[2] Fertility did not appear to be impaired in women who had been exposed *in utero* to diethylstilbestrol but the relative risk of an unfavourable outcome of pregnancy in such a group was 1.69. However, of the women who became pregnant, 81% of those exposed to diethylstilbestrol and 95% of control subjects had at least one full-term live birth.[3] In a review of vaginal adenosis and its association with maternal diethylstilbestrol ingestion during pregnancy[4] it was noted that the link between diethylstilbestrol and particularly the benign changes in the vagina and cervix (adenosis) seemed well established. The association between this drug and the development of genital malignancies was less clear, and the very low incidence in the prospective studies in the USA supported this concept. The size of the problem in the UK was small, but clinicians should be aware that it existed. Cases of vaginal adenosis in young women should be investigated and screened appropriately, and preferably referred to centres where colposcopic expertise is available. Treatment of simple vaginal adenosis should be avoided.

Later reviews[5,6] have highlighted the fact that adverse effects were still emerging in women who had been exposed to diethylstilbestrol *in utero* several decades ago. The need for thorough medical screening of such women was emphasised; genital-tract examination was particularly important. It was pointed out[6] that many women exposed to diethylstilbestrol *in utero* were in the reproductive stage of their lives and warranted special observation since a diethylstilbestrol-damaged genital tract posed a potential problem during pregnancy.[5,6] It has also been suggested, for example, that such women are at increased risk of developing pre-eclampsia.[7] There is limited data from one cohort study[8] to suggest that the *male offspring of these exposed women* may in turn be at increased risk of hypospadias, although the absolute risk remains small.

Further information on the adverse effects of diethylstilbestrol in females exposed to the drug *in utero* can be obtained from the references listed below.[9-19] For mention of the possible increased risk of breast cancer in these women, see Carcinogenicity, above.

1. Professional and Public Relations Committee of the DESAD (Diethylstilbestrol and Adenosis) Project of the Division of Cancer Control and Rehabilitation. Exposure in utero to diethylstilbestrol and related synthetic hormones: association with vaginal and cervical cancers and other abnormalities. *JAMA* 1976; **236:** 1107–9.
2. O'Brien PC, *et al.* Vaginal epithelial changes in young women enrolled in the National Cooperative Diethylstilbestrol Adenosis (DESAD) Project. *Obstet Gynecol* 1979; **53:** 300–8.
3. Barnes AB, *et al.* Fertility and outcome of pregnancy in women exposed in utero to diethylstilbestrol. *N Engl J Med* 1980; **302:** 609–13.
4. Emens M. Vaginal adenosis and diethylstilboestrol. *Br J Hosp Med* 1984; **31:** 42–8.
5. Anonymous. Diethylstilboestrol—effects of exposure in utero. *Drug Ther Bull* 1991; **29:** 49–50.
6. Wingfield M. The daughters of stilboestrol. *BMJ* 1991; **302:** 1414–15.
7. Mittendorf R, Williams MA. Stilboestrol exposure in utero and risk of pre-eclampsia. *Lancet* 1995; **345:** 265–6.
8. Klip H, *et al.* Hypospadias in sons of women exposed to diethylstilbestrol in utero: a cohort study. *Lancet* 2002; **359:** 1102–7.
9. Herbst AL, *et al.* Prenatal exposure to stilbestrol: a prospective comparison of exposed female offspring with unexposed controls. *N Engl J Med* 1975; **292:** 334–9.
10. Herbst AL, *et al.* Age-incidence and risk of diethylstilbestrol-related clear cell adenocarcinoma of the vagina and cervix. *Am J Obstet Gynecol* 1977; **128:** 43–50.
11. Kaufman RH, *et al.* Upper genital tract changes associated with in-utero exposure to diethylstilbestrol. *Am J Obstet Gynecol* 1977; **128:** 51.
12. Fowler WC, Edelman DA. In utero exposure to DES: evaluation and followup of 199 women. *Obstet Gynecol* 1978; **51:** 459–63.
13. Anderson B, *et al.* Development of DES-associated clear-cell carcinoma: the importance of regular screening. *Obstet Gynecol* 1979; **53:** 293–9.
14. Noller KL, *et al.* Maturation of vaginal and cervical epithelium in women exposed in utero to diethylstilbestrol (DESAD project). *Am J Obstet Gynecol* 1983; **146:** 279–85.
15. Robboy SJ, *et al.* Increased incidence of cervical and vaginal dysplasia in 3980 diethylstilbestrol-exposed young women: experience of the National Collaborative Diethylstilbestrol Adenosis Project. *JAMA* 1984; **252:** 2979–83.
16. Kaufman RH, *et al.* Upper genital tract changes and infertility in diethylstilbestrol-exposed women. *Am J Obstet Gynecol* 1986; **154:** 1312–18.
17. Melnick S, *et al.* Rates and risks of diethylstilbestrol-related clear-cell adenocarcinoma of the vagina and cervix—an update. *N Engl J Med* 1987; **316:** 514–16.
18. Helmerhorst TJM, *et al.* Colposcopic findings and intraepithelial neoplasia in diethylstilbestrol-exposed offspring: the Dutch experience. *Am J Obstet Gynecol* 1989; **161:** 1191–4.
19. Giusti RM, *et al.* Diethylstilbestrol revisited: a review of the long-term health effects. *Ann Intern Med* 1995; **122:** 778–88.

EFFECTS ON MALE OFFSPRING. The effects of exposure to diethylstilbestrol *in utero* have been studied in male offspring.[1-4] Problems in passing urine and abnormalities of the penile urethra were found to be more common in young males exposed to diethylstilbestrol *in utero* than in controls in one study.[1] In another,[2] genital tract abnormalities such as epididymal cysts, capsular induration, and defective testicles occurred in 41 of 163 diethylstilbestrol-exposed men compared with 11 of 168 controls; sperm counts and motility were also reduced in exposed males. In contrast, comparison of 828 men exposed to diethylstilbestrol *in utero* with 676 unexposed men suggested that, overall, diethylstilbestrol exposure did not result in an increased risk of genito-urinary abnormalities, infertility, or testicular cancer.[3] It was suggested that previously reported increased frequencies of such abnormalities may have resulted from a selection bias and/or from a difference in diethylstilbestrol usage. Another study[4] in 253 exposed men found that although there was an increased incidence of congenital malformations of the genitalia (18 cases compared with 5 of 241 controls), this was not associated with any decrease in fertility or impairment of sexual function.

Isolated reports of adverse effects occurring in young men who were exposed to diethylstilbestrol *in utero* have included seminoma and epididymal cysts in one man.[5]

For reference to possible effects on the male *grandchildren* of women who took diethylstilbestrol (the offspring of women exposed *in utero*) see above.

1. Henderson BE, *et al.* Urogenital tract abnormalities in sons of women treated with diethylstilbestrol. *Pediatrics* 1976; **58:** 505–7.
2. Anonymous. Offspring of women given DES remains under study. *JAMA* 1977; **238:** 932.
3. Leary FJ, *et al.* Males exposed in utero to diethylstilbestrol. *JAMA* 1984; **252:** 2984–9.
4. Wilcox AJ, *et al.* Fertility in men exposed prenatally to diethylstilbestrol. *N Engl J Med* 1995; **332:** 1411–16.
5. Conley GR, *et al.* Seminoma and epididymal cysts in a young man with known diethylstilbestrol exposure in utero. *JAMA* 1983; **249:** 1325–6.

**Veterinary use.** In the European Union, the use of diethylstilbestrol or other stilbenes in veterinary medicine is banned unless prior steps are taken to ensure the treated animal and its products are not available for human or animal consumption.

### Pharmacokinetics

Diethylstilbestrol is readily absorbed from the gastrointestinal tract. It is slowly metabolised in the liver and excreted in the urine and faeces, mainly as the glucuronide.

### Uses and Administration

Diethylstilbestrol is a synthetic nonsteroidal oestrogen that has been used in the palliation of breast and prostate cancer.

Daily doses of 10 to 20 mg are occasionally used by mouth in the palliative treatment of malignant neoplasms of the breast in postmenopausal women (p.514). The usual dose in carcinoma of the prostate (p.521) is 1 to 3 mg daily by mouth; higher doses were formerly given. Diethylstilbestrol has also been used in the treatment of prostatic carcinoma in the form of its diphosphate salts (see Fosfestrol, p.1555).

Diethylstilbestrol has been used as pessaries in the short-term management of menopausal atrophic vaginitis at a dose of 1 mg daily.

### Preparations

***BP 2003:*** Diethylstilbestrol Pessaries; Diethylstilbestrol Tablets;
***USP 27:*** Diethylstilbestrol Injection; Diethylstilbestrol Tablets.

**Proprietary Preparations** (details are given in Part 3)
***Braz.:*** Destilbenol; ***Fr.:*** Distilbene; ***Irl.:*** Boestrol.

**Multi-ingredient:** ***Braz.:*** Calmovarin†; ***Spain:*** Cilinavagin Neomicina†; ***UK:*** Tampovagan†.

---

## Drospirenone *(BAN, USAN, rINN)*

Dihydrospirenone; Drospirenona; ZK-30595. (6R,7R,8R,9S,-10R,13S,14S,15S,16S,17S)-1,3′,4′,6,6a,7,8,9,10,11,12,13,14,15,-15a,16-Hexadecahydro-10,13-dimethylspiro-[17*H*-dicyclopropa[6,7:15,16]cyclopenta[*a*]phenanthrene-17,2′(5′*H*)-furan]-3,5′(2*H*)-dione.

$C_{24}H_{30}O_3$ = 366.5.
*CAS — 67392-87-4.*

### Adverse Effects and Precautions

As for progestogens in general (see Progesterone, p.1566). See also under Hormonal Contraceptives, p.1527. Drospirenone has antimineralocorticoid activity and therefore should not be used in patients at risk of hyperkalaemia, such as those with renal or hepatic impairment or adrenal insufficiency.

**Effects on the cardiovascular system.** As with combined oral contraceptives containing other progestogens, there are reports[1,2] of thrombotic and ischaemic events in patients taking a preparation of ethinylestradiol and drospirenone.

1. Vayá A, *et al.* Transient ischaemic attack associated with the new contraceptive Yasmin. *Thromb Res* 2003; **112:** 121.
2. van Grootheest K, Vrieling T. Thromboembolism associated with the new contraceptive Yasmin. *BMJ* 2003; **326:** 257.

### Interactions

As for progestogens in general (see Progesterone, p.1567). See also under Hormonal Contraceptives, p.1534. Because drospirenone has antimineralocorticoid activity, it may potentially exacerbate the effects of drugs that can increase serum potassium, such as ACE inhibitors, angiotensin II receptor antagonists, aldosterone antagonists, potassium-sparing diuretics, or NSAIDs.

### Pharmacokinetics

After oral doses, drospirenone is about 97% bound to plasma proteins, though it does not bind to sex hormone binding globulin or corticosteroid binding globulin. It is extensively metabolised with a terminal half-life of about 30 hours. The metabolites are excreted in the urine and faeces.

### Uses and Administration

Drospirenone is a progestogen (see Progesterone, p.1567) with antimineralocorticoid and anti-androgenic activity, that is used as the progestogenic component of a combined oral contraceptive (see p.1535) in doses of 3 mg daily. It has also been used as the progestogenic component of menopausal HRT (see p.1540) in a dose of 2 mg daily.

◊ References.

1. Huber J, *et al.* Efficacy and tolerability of a monophasic oral contraceptive containing ethinylestradiol and drospirenone. *Eur J Contracept Reprod Health Care* 2000; **5:** 25–34.
2. Foidart JM. The contraceptive profile of a new oral contraceptive with antimineralocorticoid and antiandrogenic effects. *Eur J Contracept Reprod Health Care* 2000; **5** (suppl 3): 25–33.
3. Oelkers W, *et al.* Effect of an oral contraceptive containing drospirenone on the renin-angiotensin-aldosterone system in healthy female volunteers. *Gynecol Endocrinol* 2000; **14:** 204–13.
4. Krattenmacher R. Drospirenone: pharmacology and pharmacokinetics of a unique progestogen. *Contraception* 2000; **62:** 29–38.

### Preparations

**Proprietary Preparations** (details are given in Part 3)
**Multi-ingredient:** ***Austral.:*** Yasmin; ***Austria:*** Yasmin; Yirala; ***Belg.:*** Yasmin; ***Denm.:*** Yasmin; ***Fr.:*** Jasmine; ***Ger.:*** Petibelle; Yasmin; ***Irl.:*** Yasmin; ***Israel:*** Yasmin; ***Norw.:*** Yasmin; ***Port.:*** Yasmin; ***Swed.:*** Yasmin; ***UK:*** Yasmin; ***USA:*** Yasmin.

---

## Dutasteride *(BAN, USAN, rINN)*

Dutasterida; GG-745; GI-198745; GI-198745X. α,α,α,α′,α′,α′-Hexafluoro-3-oxo-4-aza-5α-androst-1-ene-17β-carboxy-2′,5′-xylidide; 3-Oxo-2′,5′-bis(trifluoromethyl)-4-aza-5α-androst-1-ene-17β-carboxanilide.

$C_{27}H_{30}F_6N_2O_2$ = 528.5.
*CAS — 164656-23-9.*
*ATC — G04CB02.*

### Adverse Effects and Precautions

As for Finasteride, p.1554.

### Pharmacokinetics

Dutasteride is absorbed from the gastrointestinal tract, reaching a peak serum concentration in 1 to 3 hours, with a bioavailability of about 60%. It is highly bound to plasma proteins. Dutasteride is metabolised by the cytochrome P450 isoenzymes CYP3A4 and CYP3A5, and most of a dose is excreted as metabolites in the faeces. At steady state the elimination half-life is about 3 to 5 weeks.

### Uses and Administration

Dutasteride, like finasteride, p.1554 is an inhibitor of 5α-reductase. Unlike finasteride, it is claimed to inhibit both the type-1 and type-2 isoforms of the enzyme. It is used in the treatment of benign prostatic hyperplasia in doses of 500 micrograms daily by mouth. It has also been investigated in the treatment of alopecia.

◊ References.

1. Roehrborn CG, *et al.* Efficacy and safety of a dual inhibitor of 5-alpha-reductase types 1 and 2 (dutasteride) in men with benign prostatic hyperplasia. *Urology* 2002; **60:** 434–41.
2. Andriole GL, Kirby R. Safety and tolerability of the dual 5alpha-reductase inhibitor dutasteride in the treatment of benign prostatic hyperplasia. *Eur Urol* 2003; **44:** 82–8.
3. Roehrborn CG, *et al.* Efficacy and safety of dutasteride in the four-year treatment of men with benign prostatic hyperplasia. *Urology* 2004; **63:** 709–15.

### Preparations

**Proprietary Preparations** (details are given in Part 3)
***Fr.:*** Avodart; ***UK:*** Avodart; ***USA:*** Avodart.

---

## Dydrogesterone *(BAN, USAN, rINN)*

Dehydroprogesterone; 6-Dehydro-*retro*-progesterone; 6-Dehydro-9β,10α-progesterone; Didrogesteron; Didrogesterona; Isopregnenone; NSC-92336. 9β,10α-Pregna-4,6-diene-3,20-dione.

$C_{21}H_{28}O_2$ = 312.4.
*CAS — 152-62-5.*
*ATC — G03DB01.*

**Pharmacopoeias.** In *Br., Jpn,* and *US.*

**BP 2003** (Dydrogesterone). A white or almost white crystalline powder; odourless or almost odourless. Practically insoluble in water; sparingly soluble in alcohol and in methyl alcohol; soluble in acetone; freely soluble in chloroform; slightly soluble in ether and in fixed oils. Protect from light.

**USP 27** (Dydrogesterone). A white to pale yellow crystalline powder. Practically insoluble in water; soluble 1 in 40 of alcohol, 1 in 2 of chloroform, and 1 in 200 of ether.

### Adverse Effects and Precautions

As for progestogens in general (see Progesterone, p.1566).

**Porphyria.** Dydrogesterone has been associated with acute attacks of porphyria and is considered unsafe in porphyric patients.

**Pregnancy.** Anomalies (non-virilising) of the genito-urinary tract were found in a 4-month-old baby whose mother had taken dydrogesterone 20 mg daily from the eighth to twentieth week of pregnancy and 10 mg daily from then until term.[1] She had also been given hydroxyprogesterone caproate 250 mg by intramuscular injection weekly from the eighth to the twentieth week.

1. Roberts IF, West RJ. Teratogenesis and maternal progesterone. *Lancet* 1977; **ii:** 982.

### Interactions

As for progestogens in general (see Progesterone, p.1567).

### Uses and Administration

Dydrogesterone is a progestogen structurally related to progesterone (p.1567). It does not have oestrogenic or androgenic properties.

Dydrogesterone is given by mouth in the treatment of menstrual disorders such as menorrhagia (p.1567), usually in a dose of 10 mg twice daily in a cyclical regimen, and for the treatment of endometriosis (p.1546) in a dose of 10 mg two or three times daily cyclically or continuously. It is also given cyclically in doses of 10 mg once or twice daily, or continuously in doses of 5 mg daily, for endometrial protection during menopausal HRT (p.1536).

In threatened miscarriage suggested doses have been 40 mg initially followed by 10 mg or more every 8 hours, continued for a week after symptoms cease. In recurrent miscarriage suggested doses have been 10 mg twice daily. However, such use is not recommended unless there is proven progesterone deficiency. Cyclical dydrogesterone has also been used in infertility (p.1316) in doses of 10 mg twice daily.

### Preparations

***BP 2003:*** Dydrogesterone Tablets;
***USP 27:*** Dydrogesterone Tablets.

**Proprietary Preparations** (details are given in Part 3)
***Austral.:*** Duphaston; ***Austria:*** Duphaston; ***Belg.:*** Duphaston; ***Chile:*** Duphaston; ***Fin.:*** Terolut; ***Fr.:*** Duphaston; ***Ger.:*** Duphaston; ***Gr.:*** Duphaston; ***Hong Kong:*** Duphaston; ***India:*** Duphaston; ***Irl.:*** Duphaston; ***Israel:*** Biphaston; ***Ital.:*** Dufaston; ***Malaysia:*** Duphaston; ***Neth.:*** Duphaston; ***NZ:*** Duphaston; ***Port.:*** Duphaston; ***S.Afr.:*** Duphaston; ***Singapore:*** Duphaston; ***Spain:*** Duphaston†; ***Swed.:*** Duphaston; ***Switz.:*** Duphaston; ***Thai.:*** Duphaston; ***UK:*** Duphaston.

**Multi-ingredient:** ***Austral.:*** Femoston; ***Austria:*** Femoston; Femoston Conti; Femphascyl; Femphascyl conti; ***Belg.:*** Femoston; Femoston Conti; ***Fin.:*** Femoston; Femoston Conti; ***Fr.:*** Climaston; ***Ger.:*** Femoston; ***Gr.:*** Femaston; ***Hong Kong:*** Femoston; ***Irl.:*** Femoston; Femoston Conti; ***Ital.:*** Femoston; Femoston Conti; ***Malaysia:*** Femoston; ***Mex.:*** Lutalmin; ***Neth.:*** Femoston; ***Port.:*** Femoston; Femoston 1/5; ***Singapore:*** Femoston; ***Switz.:*** Femoston; Femoston Conti; ***UK:*** Femapak; Femoston; Femoston Conti.

---

## Elcometrine

16-Methylene-17-alpha-acetoxy-19 Norprogesterone; ST-1435.

$C_{23}H_{30}O_4$ = 370.5.
*CAS — 7759-35-5.*

### Profile

Elcometrine is a synthetic progestogen that is being developed for use in contraception and menopausal HRT, and in the management of endometriosis.

### Preparations

**Proprietary Preparations** (details are given in Part 3)
***Braz.:*** Elmetrin†.

---

## Equilin

Equilina. 3-Hydroxyestra-1,3,5(10),7-tetraen-17-one.

$C_{18}H_{20}O_2$ = 268.4.
*CAS — 474-86-2.*

**Pharmacopoeias.** In *US.*

**USP 27** (Equilin). Store in airtight containers. Protect from light.

### Profile

Equilin is a natural oestrogenic hormone found in horses. Sodium equilin sulfate is one of the components of both conjugated oestrogens (p.1543) and esterified oestrogens (see below) used for menopausal HRT.

---

## Esterified Oestrogens

Esterified Estrogens; Estrógenos esterificados.

**Pharmacopoeias.** In *US.*

**USP 27** (Esterified Estrogens). A mixture of the sodium salts of the sulfate esters of the oestrogenic substances, principally estrone. It contains 75 to 85% of sodium estrone sulfate and 6 to 15% of sodium equilin sulfate, in such a proportion that the total of these two components is not less than 90%, of the labelled amount of esterified oestrogens. A white or buff-coloured amorphous powder; odourless or having a slight characteristic odour. Store in airtight containers.

### Profile

Esterified oestrogens have actions and uses similar to those described for estradiol (see below). They are used for the same purposes (principally menopausal HRT), and in a similar dosage by mouth, as conjugated oestrogens (see p.1543), although higher cyclical doses of 2.5 to 7.5 mg daily are still licensed for use in female hypogonadism.

### Preparations

**USP 27:** Esterified Estrogens Tablets.

**Proprietary Preparations** (details are given in Part 3)
**Arg.:** Menest; **Chile:** Femibel; **Switz.:** Oestro-Feminal; **USA:** Estratab; Menest.

**Multi-ingredient: Chile:** Delitan; Feminova-T; **USA:** Estratest; Menogen†.

## Estradiol *(BAN, rINN)*

Beta-oestradiol; Dihydrofolliculin; Dihydrotheelin; Dihydroxyoestrin; Estradiolum; NSC-9895; NSC-20293 (alpha-estradiol); Oestradiol. Estra-1,3,5(10)-triene-3,17β-diol.

$C_{18}H_{24}O_2$ = 272.4.
*CAS — 50-28-2 (anhydrous estradiol).*
*ATC — G03CA03.*

NOTE. In *Martindale* the term oestradiol is used for the endogenous substance.

**Pharmacopoeias.** In *Chin.* and *US.*
*Eur.* (see p.vi) includes the hemihydrate.

**Ph. Eur. 5.0** (Estradiol Hemihydrate). A white or almost white crystalline powder or colourless crystals. Practically insoluble in water; sparingly soluble in alcohol; soluble in acetone; slightly soluble in dichloromethane.

**USP 27** (Estradiol). White or creamy-white, odourless, hygroscopic small crystals or crystalline powder. Practically insoluble in water; soluble 1 in 28 of alcohol, 1 in 435 of chloroform, and 1 in 150 of ether; soluble in acetone, in dioxan, and in solutions of fixed alkali hydroxides; sparingly soluble in vegetable oils. Store in airtight containers at a temperature of 25°, excursions permitted between 15° and 30°. Protect from light.

### Estradiol Benzoate *(BANM, rINN)*

Benzoato de estradiol; Beta-oestradiol Benzoate; Dihydroxyoestrin Monobenzoate; Estradioli Benzoas; NSC-9566; Oestradiol Benzoate. Estra-1,3,5(10)-triene-3,17β-diol 3-benzoate.

$C_{25}H_{28}O_3$ = 376.5.
*CAS — 50-50-0.*
*ATC — G03CA03.*

**Pharmacopoeias.** In *Chin., Eur.* (see p.vi), *Jpn,* and *Pol.*

**Ph. Eur. 5.0** (Estradiol Benzoate). An almost white crystalline powder or colourless crystals. It exhibits polymorphism. Practically insoluble in water; sparingly soluble in acetone; freely soluble in dichloromethane; slightly soluble in methyl alcohol.

### Estradiol Cipionate *(BANM, rINNM)*

Cipionato de estradiol; Estradiol Cypionate; Oestradiol Cyclopentylpropionate; Oestradiol Cypionate. Estra-1,3,5(10)-triene-3,17β-diol 17-(3-cyclopentylpropionate).

$C_{26}H_{36}O_3$ = 396.6.
*CAS — 313-06-4.*
*ATC — G03CA03.*

**Pharmacopoeias.** In *US.*

**USP 27** (Estradiol Cypionate). A white to practically white crystalline powder, odourless or has a slight odour. Insoluble in water; soluble 1 in 40 of alcohol, 1 in 7 of chloroform, and 1 in 2800 of ether; soluble in acetone and in dioxan; sparingly soluble in vegetable oils. Store in airtight containers. Protect from light.

### Estradiol Dipropionate *(BANM, rINNM)*

Dihydroxyoestrin Dipropionate; Dipropionato de estradiol; Oestradiol Dipropionate. Estra-1,3,5(10)-triene-3,17β-diol dipropionate.

$C_{24}H_{32}O_4$ = 384.5.
*CAS — 113-38-2.*
*ATC — G03CA03.*

### Estradiol Enantate *(BANM, rINNM)*

Enantato de estradiol; Estradiol Enanthate *(USAN)*; Oestradiol Enanthate; Oestradiol 17-Heptanoate; SQ-16150. Estra-1,3,5(10)-triene-3,17β-diol 17-heptanoate.

$C_{25}H_{36}O_3$ = 384.6.
*CAS — 4956-37-0.*
*ATC — G03CA03.*

### Estradiol Hexahydrobenzoate *(BANM, rINNM)*

Hexahidrobenzoato de estradiol; Oestradiol Hexahydrobenzoate. Estra-1,3,5(10)-triene-3,17β-diol 17-cyclohexanecarboxylate.

$C_{25}H_{34}O_3$ = 382.5.
*CAS — 15140-27-9.*
*ATC — G03CA03.*

### Estradiol Phenylpropionate *(BANM, rINNM)*

Fenilpropionato de estradiol; Oestradiol Phenylpropionate. Estra-1,3,5(10)-triene-3,17β-diol 17-(3-phenylpropionate).

$C_{27}H_{32}O_3$ = 404.5.
*ATC — G03CA03.*

### Estradiol Valerate *(BANM, rINN)*

Estradioli Valeras; NSC-17590; Oestradiol Valerate; Valerato de estradiol. Estra-1,3,5(10)-triene-3,17β-diol 17-valerate.

$C_{23}H_{32}O_3$ = 356.5.
*CAS — 979-32-8.*
*ATC — G03CA03.*

**Pharmacopoeias.** In *Chin., Eur.* (see p.vi), and *US.*

**Ph. Eur. 5.0** (Estradiol Valerate). A white or almost white, crystalline powder or colourless crystals. Practically insoluble in water; soluble in alcohol. Protect from light.

**USP 27** (Estradiol Valerate). A white crystalline powder which is usually odourless or may have a faint fatty odour. Practically insoluble in water; soluble in benzyl benzoate, in dioxan, in methyl alcohol, and in castor oil; sparingly soluble in arachis oil and in sesame oil. Store in airtight containers. Protect from light.

### Adverse Effects

The adverse effects of estradiol and other oestrogens are related, in part, to dose and duration of therapy, and to the gender and age of the recipient. In addition, adverse effects may be modified by a progestogen in combined oral contraceptives or menopausal HRT. Whether adverse effects of natural and synthetic oestrogens differ, and whether the route of administration has an effect, is less clear.

The adverse effects of oestrogens used in hormonal contraceptives are considered in detail starting on p.1527. Those of oestrogens used in HRT are considered in detail starting on p.1536.

The use of oestrogens in girls may cause premature closure of the epiphyses resulting in decreased final adult height.

Large doses of oestrogens used in palliation of cancers have also been associated with nausea, fluid retention, venous and arterial thrombosis, and cholestatic jaundice. In men, they cause impotence and feminising effects such as gynaecomastia. In women, they may cause withdrawal bleeding, and, when used for breast cancer, they have caused hypercalcaemia and bone pain.

**Effects on the skin.** There is some evidence[1] that transdermal patches in which estradiol is dissolved in the adhesive matrix cause fewer skin reactions than those employing release of estradiol from an alcoholic reservoir.

1. Ross D. Randomised crossover comparison of skin irritation with two transdermal oestradiol patches. *BMJ* 1997; **315:** 288.

### Precautions

The precautions for the use of estradiol and other oestrogens used as menopausal HRT are considered in detail starting on p.1539. Those for oestrogens used in hormonal contraceptives are considered in detail starting on p.1532.

High doses of oestrogen used in treating malignant disease should be used cautiously in patients with cerebrovascular disorders, coronary artery disease, or venous thromboembolism. They may exacerbate hypercalcaemia of malignancy.

Oestrogens should be used with caution in children because premature closure of the epiphyses may occur resulting in inhibited linear growth and small stature.

Oestrogens have been reported to interfere with some diagnostic tests such as those for thyroid function and glucose tolerance.

**Breast feeding.** Estradiol has been detected in breast milk following the use of pessaries containing 50 or 100 mg of estradiol.[1] The American Academy of Pediatrics considers that estradiol is usually compatible with breast feeding.[2]

1. Nilsson S, *et al.* Transfer of estradiol to human milk. *Am J Obstet Gynecol* 1978; **132:** 653–7.
2. American Academy of Pediatrics. The transfer of drugs and other chemicals into human milk. *Pediatrics* 2001; **108:** 776–89. Correction. *ibid.*; 1029. Also available at: http://aappolicy.aappublications.org/cgi/content/full/pediatrics%3b108/3/776 (accessed 13/08/02)

**Cosmetic use.** Use of cosmetic products containing oestrogens has led to adverse effects such as precocious puberty in children and gynaecomastia or postmenopausal bleeding in adults.[1]

1. Anonymous. Estrogens in cosmetics. *Med Lett Drugs Ther* 1985; **27:** 54–5.

**Porphyria.** Oestrogens are considered to be unsafe in patients with porphyria although there is conflicting experimental evidence of porphyrinogenicity.

**Pregnancy.** Although gross abnormalities of the genito-urinary tract have been reported in the male offspring of women who took diethylstilbestrol during pregnancy there is conflicting evidence as to whether the oestrogen produced an increased risk of abnormalities, infertility, or testicular cancer in such offspring (see p.1548). The male fetus is normally protected from the feminising effects of the natural oestrogens in the uterine environment by the early development of the testes and the secretion of male hormones.[1] However, there has been considerable concern about a rising incidence of disorders of the male reproductive tract, and a reduction in sperm counts, which has been noted in the last 20 to 30 years. It has been hypothesised that overexposure of male fetuses to environmental oestrogens derived from pollutants such as pesticides and plastics may be responsible for this decline,[2,3] although some dispute this.[4]

For discussion of the lack of effects of hormonal contraceptives on the fetus, including evidence that they are unlikely to increase the risk of hypospadia in the male fetus, see Pregnancy, under Precautions of Hormonal Contraceptives, p.1533.

1. Mittwoch U, *et al.* Male sexual development in "a sea of oestrogen". *Lancet* 1993; **342:** 123–4.
2. Sharpe RM, Skakkebaek NE. Are oestrogens involved in falling sperm counts and disorders of the male reproductive tract? *Lancet* 1993; **341:** 1392–5.
3. de Kretser DM. Declining sperm counts. *BMJ* 1996; **312:** 457–8.
4. Thomas JA. Falling sperm counts. *Lancet* 1995; **346:** 635.

**Veterinary use.** An FAO/WHO expert committee considered it unnecessary to establish an acceptable daily intake or acceptable residual level in food for endogenous hormones.[1] Residues resulting from the use of estradiol as a growth promotor in accordance with good animal husbandry practice were thought unlikely to pose a hazard to human health. However, it should be noted that in the European Union the use of steroidal hormones such as oestrogens in veterinary practice is restricted, and their use as growth promotors is banned.

There is concern about the effect of environmental oestrogens on male fertility and development, see Pregnancy, above.

1. FAO/WHO. Evaluation of certain veterinary drug residues in food: thirty-second report of the joint FAO/WHO expert committee on food additives. *WHO Tech Rep Ser 763* 1988.

### Interactions

Interactions involving estradiol and other oestrogens used in menopausal HRT are covered on p.1539. Interactions for oestrogens used in hormonal contraceptives are covered on p.1534.

### Pharmacokinetics

In general, estradiol and other oestrogens are readily absorbed from the gastrointestinal tract and through the skin or mucous membranes. However, the natural unconjugated oestrogens such as estradiol undergo extensive first-pass metabolism in the gastrointestinal tract and liver after oral doses. They are, therefore, generally not orally active, although a micronised preparation of estradiol has sufficient bioavailability (3 to 5%) to be orally active. Estradiol is metabolised in part to less active oestrogens such as estriol and estrone. Synthetic oestrogens produced by alkylation of the C17 position, such as ethinylestradiol, are more slowly metabolised and are therefore orally active. Conjugated oestrogens, which are essentially oestrogen metabolites, are also orally active because they are hydrolysed by enzymes in the lower gastrointestinal tract allowing absorption of the active oestrogen. Vaginal, transdermal, intranasal, or parenteral administration of oestrogens also avoids first-pass hepatic metabolism. Plasma-estradiol concentrations are reported to reach a peak 1.5 to 2 hours after a dose by mouth, and again at about 8 hours due to enterohepatic recycling. Estradiol esters are rapidly hydrolysed to free estradiol when given by mouth. After intramuscular injection of the esters, absorption is prolonged.

Oestrogens are extensively bound to plasma proteins. Naturally occurring oestrogens such as estradiol are principally bound to sex-hormone binding globulin. Conversely, ethinylestradiol is mostly bound to albumin.

Oestrogens are metabolised in the liver. A variety of sulfate and glucuronide conjugates are formed, and these are excreted in the urine and the bile. Those excreted in the bile undergo enterohepatic recycling or are excreted in the faeces.

◊ References to the pharmacokinetics of estradiol[1-4] and other oestrogens.[5,6]


1. Kuhnz W, *et al.* Pharmacokinetics of estradiol, free and total estrone, in young women following single intravenous and oral administration of 17β-estradiol. *Arzneimittelforschung* 1993; **43:** 966–73.
2. Schubert W, *et al.* Pharmacokinetic evaluation of oral 17β-oestradiol and two different fat soluble analogues in ovariectomized women. *Eur J Clin Pharmacol* 1993; **44:** 563–8.
3. Baker VL. Alternatives to oral estrogen replacement: transdermal patches, percutaneous gels, vaginal creams and rings, implants, other methods of delivery. *Obstet Gynecol Clin North Am* 1994; **21:** 271–9.
4. Price TM, *et al.* Single-dose pharmacokinetics of sublingual versus oral administration of micronized 17β-estradiol. *Obstet Gynecol* 1997; **89:** 340–5.
5. Stumpf PG. Pharmacokinetics of estrogen. *Obstet Gynecol* 1990; **75** (suppl): 9S–14S.
6. O'Connell MB. Pharmacokinetic and pharmacologic variation between different estrogen products. *J Clin Pharmacol* 1995; **35** (suppl): 18S–24S.


## Uses and Administration

Estradiol is the most active of the naturally occurring oestrogens (for further details, see p.1527). Estradiol and its semisynthetic esters and other natural oestrogens are primarily used as menopausal HRT (see p.1540) whereas synthetic derivatives such as ethinylestradiol and mestranol have a major role as components of combined oral contraceptives (see Hormonal Contraceptives, p.1535). Estradiol may also be used as replacement therapy for female hypogonadism or primary ovarian failure (p.1317). Replacement therapy ('add-back' therapy) may also be given to women in whom the pituitary-ovarian axis is suppressed by therapy with gonadorelin or its analogues.

Estradiol hemihydrate 1.03 mg is approximately equivalent to 1 mg of the anhydrous substance.

For **menopausal HRT** oral preparations of estradiol are commonly used, as are transdermal patches. Transdermal gels, subcutaneous implants, and a nasal spray are also available. Intramuscular injections were formerly used. In women with a uterus, a progestogen is also required, given cyclically or continuously, usually by mouth although some transdermal preparations are available. Local vaginal estradiol preparations are used specifically for the treatment of menopausal atrophic vaginitis; these are generally recommended for short-term use only, if given without a progestogen in women with a uterus, although specific recommendations vary between products.

For use by mouth estradiol or estradiol valerate are normally given; doses are 1 to 2 mg daily cyclically or more often continuously.

Estradiol may be used topically as transdermal skin patches to provide a systemic effect; a variety of patches are available which release between 25 and 100 micrograms of estradiol every 24 hours. A low-dose patch supplying 14 micrograms daily is also available. Depending on the preparation, patches are replaced once or twice weekly. Each new patch is applied to a different area of skin in rotation, usually below the waistline; patches should not be applied on or near the breasts. Topical gel preparations are also applied for systemic effect: the usual dose is 0.5 to 1.5 mg of estradiol daily. The gel should not be applied on or near the breasts or on the vulval region. A topical emulsion is also available, and a dose of estradiol hemihydrate 8.7 mg is applied daily. A nasal spray is also available, delivering 150 micrograms of estradiol hemihydrate per spray. The usual initial dose is 300 micrograms daily; maintenance doses are 150 to 600 micrograms daily.

In order to prolong the duration of action subcutaneous implants of estradiol may be used. The dose of estradiol is generally 25 to 100 mg with a new implant being given after about 4 to 8 months according to oestrogen concentrations.

Estradiol may be used locally either as 25-microgram vaginal tablets, at an initial dose of one tablet daily for 2 weeks followed by a maintenance dose of one tablet twice a week, or as a 0.01% vaginal cream, in initial amounts of 2 to 4 g of cream daily for 1 to 2 weeks followed by half the initial dose for a similar period, then a maintenance dose of 1 g up to 3 times weekly. A local delivery system using a 3-month vaginal ring contains 2 mg of estradiol hemihydrate, and delivers about 7.5 micrograms of estradiol per 24 hours. Another 3-month vaginal ring system, which contains estradiol acetate, releases either 50 or 100 micrograms of estradiol daily, and is used for the relief of both local and systemic postmenopausal symptoms.

Intramuscular injections of estradiol benzoate or valerate esters have been used as oily depot solutions, usually given once every 3 to 4 weeks. The cipionate, dipropionate, enantate, hexahydrobenzoate, phenylpropionate, and undecylate esters have been used similarly. The enantate and cipionate esters are used as the oestrogen component of combined injectable **contraceptives**.

Estradiol and other oestrogens have sometimes been used in higher doses for palliative treatment in **prostate cancer** (p.521) and **breast cancer** in men and postmenopausal women (p.514).

**Administration.** IMPLANTS. There may be a striking interpatient variation in blood-estradiol concentrations in women receiving estradiol implants,[1] and symptoms of oestrogen deficiency have re-appeared in some patients even though serum-estradiol concentrations were within or above the physiological range.[2] Following debate on the appropriateness of using serum concentrations of estradiol as a guide to implant administration, rather than symptoms,[3-7] it is now recommended that estradiol concentration should be monitored during therapy.

Cyclical progestogen may be required for a prolonged period after discontinuation of estradiol implants in women with a uterus.[7]


1. Guirgis RR. Oestradiol implants: what dose, how often? *Lancet* 1987; **ii:** 856.
2. Gangar K, *et al.* Symptoms of oestrogen deficiency associated with supraphysiological plasma oestradiol concentrations in women with oestradiol implants. *BMJ* 1989; **299:** 601–2.
3. Ginsburg J, Hardiman P. Oestrogen deficiency and oestradiol implants. *BMJ* 1989; **299:** 1031.
4. Studd J, *et al.* Symptoms of oestrogen deficiency in women with oestradiol implants. *BMJ* 1989; **299:** 1400–1.
5. Swyer GIM. Symptoms of oestrogen deficiency in women with oestradiol implants. *BMJ* 1989; **299:** 854.
6. Tobias JH, Chambers TJ. Symptoms of oestrogen deficiency in women with oestradiol implants. *BMJ* 1989; **299:** 854.
7. Wardle P, Fox R. Symptoms of oestrogen deficiency in women with oestradiol implants. *BMJ* 1989; **299:** 1102.


INTRANASAL ADMINISTRATION. The intranasal route for estradiol HRT has been reviewed.[1] It appears to be comparable in efficacy to oral[2] or transdermal use[3] in the treatment of menopausal symptoms. As with transdermal application, the intranasal route avoids intestinal and hepatic first-pass metabolism.


1. Dooley M, *et al.* Estradiol-intranasal: a review of its use in the management of menopause. *Drugs* 2001; **61:** 2243–62.
2. Studd J, *et al.* Efficacy and acceptability of intranasal 17β-oestradiol for menopausal symptoms: randomised dose-response study. *Lancet* 1999; **353:** 1574–8. Correction. *ibid.*; **354:** 780.
3. Lopes P, *et al.* Randomized comparison of intranasal and transdermal estradiol. *Obstet Gynecol* 2000; **96:** 906–12.


SUBLINGUAL ADMINISTRATION. A pharmacokinetic study[1] of micronised estradiol found the sublingual route to result in more rapid absorption, a higher peak concentration, and rapid elimination, compared with oral administration. Sublingual micronised estradiol has been studied for the management of postpartum depression.[2]


1. Price TM, *et al.* Single-dose pharmacokinetics of sublingual versus oral administration of micronized 17 β-estradiol. *Obstet Gynecol* 1997; **89:** 340–5.
2. Ahokas A, *et al.* Estrogen deficiency in severe postpartum depression: successful treatment with sublingual physiologic 17β-estradiol: a preliminary study. *J Clin Psychiatry* 2001; **62:** 332–6.


TRANSDERMAL ADMINISTRATION. Transdermal estradiol given via patches applied to the skin has been reviewed.[1-3] This method of delivery has certain advantages over the oral route in that gastrointestinal and hepatic first-pass metabolism is avoided, liver enzymes are not stimulated (although this may also mean that beneficial effects on serum lipids are absent), and the prolonged drug release from the patch means less frequent application is necessary and hence patient compliance may be improved. For oestrogen replacement in menopausal and postmenopausal women estradiol patches are used continuously or in a cyclical manner, with added progestogen for part of the cycle in those women with an intact uterus. This does not lead to drug accumulation and produces blood-estradiol concentrations and estradiol to estrone ratios similar to those normally observed in premenopausal women. The patch is well tolerated with skin irritation being the main problem. Patches are as effective as oral oestrogens in treating menopausal and postmenopausal symptoms such as flushing and vaginal atrophy and in preventing osteoporosis.


1. Balfour JA, Heel RC. Transdermal estradiol: a review of its pharmacodynamic and pharmacokinetic properties, and therapeutic efficacy in the treatment of menopausal complaints. *Drugs* 1990; **40:** 561–82.
2. Cheang A, *et al.* A risk-benefit appraisal of transdermal estradiol therapy. *Drug Safety* 1993; **9:** 365–79.
3. Jewelewicz R. New developments in topical estrogen therapy. *Fertil Steril* 1997; **67:** 1–12.


**Depression.** The use of oestrogen therapy in the treatment of postnatal depression has been shown to be effective.[1,2] However, although such therapy could be a useful adjunct after failure of conventional treatment (see Depression, p.279), the risk of serious adverse effects including thrombosis is likely to limit its value.[3] There is also some evidence that oestrogen replacement therapy with transdermal estradiol can relieve depressive mood symptoms in perimenopausal women,[4,5] although whether any benefit is maintained with combination HRT is unclear, and antidepressants remain the standard of care in perimenopausal or postmenopausal women with clinical depression.


1. Gregoire AJP, *et al.* Transdermal oestrogen for treatment of severe postnatal depression. *Lancet* 1996; **347:** 930–3.
2. Ahokas A, *et al.* Estrogen deficiency in severe postpartum depression: successful treatment with sublingual physiologic 17β-estradiol: a preliminary study. *J Clin Psychiatry* 2001; **62:** 332–6.
3. Lawrie TA, *et al.* Oestrogens and progestogens for preventing and treating postnatal depression. Available in the Cochrane Library; Issue 2. Chichester: John Wiley; 2004.
4. Schmidt PJ, *et al.* Estrogen replacement in perimenopause-related depression: a preliminary report. *Am J Obstet Gynecol* 2000; **183:** 414–20.
5. Soares C de N, *et al.* Efficacy of estradiol for the treatment of depressive disorders in perimenopausal women. *Arch Gen Psychiatry* 2001; **58:** 529–34.


**Gender reassignment.** Oestrogens such as ethinylestradiol and conjugated oestrogens are used in male-to-female transsexuals to develop and maintain secondary sexual characteristics. There is some evidence that this use improves vascular function.[1]


1. New G, *et al.* Long-term estrogen therapy improves vascular function in male to female transsexuals. *J Am Coll Cardiol* 1997; **29:** 1437–44.


**Growth disorders.** Early researchers found that supraphysiological doses of oestrogens inhibited somatic growth and from this experience oestrogens, such as ethinylestradiol in oral doses of over 200 micrograms daily, came to be used for the treatment of acromegaly and for the arrest of growth in tall girls.[1] One study has reported that treatment with conjugated oestrogens 7.5 to 11.25 mg daily resulted in an average decrease of about 5 cm from final predicted height.[2] However, treatment with physiological doses causes growth stimulation, not inhibition, and such physiological doses have been used to promote growth in girls with conditions such as female hypogonadism and Turner's syndrome (see p.1317). Oestrogen therapy has occasionally been used in girls with delayed puberty (see p.1314).


1. Rosenfield RL. Toward optimal estrogen-replacement therapy. *N Engl J Med* 1983; **309:** 1120–1.
2. Weimann E, *et al.* Oestrogen treatment of constitutional tall stature: a risk-benefit ratio. *Arch Dis Child* 1998; **78:** 148–51.


**Haemorrhagic disorders.** Limited evidence supports the use of oestrogens in various bleeding disorders such as hereditary haemorrhagic telangiectasia, haemorrhagic cystitis, and those associated with chronic renal failure and gastrointestinal vascular malformations.

References.


1. Vase P. Estrogen treatment of hereditary hemorrhagic telangiectasia. *Acta Med Scand* 1981; **209:** 393–6.
2. Livio M, *et al.* Conjugated estrogens for the management of bleeding associated with renal failure. *N Engl J Med* 1986; **315:** 731–5.
3. van Cutsem E, *et al.* Treatment of bleeding gastrointestinal vascular malformations with oestrogen-progesterone. *Lancet* 1990; **335:** 953–5.
4. Ordemann R, *et al.* Encouraging results in the treatment of haemorrhagic cystitis with estrogen - report of 10 cases and review of the literature. *Bone Marrow Transplant* 2000; **25:** 981–5.


**Lactation inhibition.** Synthetic oestrogens (e.g. quinestrol) and nonsteroidal oestrogens (e.g. diethylstilbestrol) were historically employed to suppress lactation (p.1317). However, such use is now considered inappropriate because of an increased risk of puerperal thromboembolism.

**Premenstrual syndrome.** Premenstrual syndrome (PMS) presents as a variable combination of psychological and somatic symptoms occurring during the luteal phase of the menstrual cycle, which resolve during, and immediately following, menstruation.[1,2] Another term, premenstrual dysphoric disorder, has been proposed to cover severe cyclical mood disorder that is functionally incapacitating.[2,3] Whereas about 20 to 30% of women have complaints that may be classified as PMS, only 3 to 5% meet criteria for premenstrual dysphoric disorder.[3] The term premenstrual tension (PMT) has sometimes been applied to the psychological symptoms. Many symptoms of PMS are the same as normal premenstrual symptoms, but are more severe. Premenstrual syndrome is not fully understood although it is thought to be due to the effects of the normal luteal phase release of progesterone on CNS neurotransmitter function; the syndrome is abolished by surgical or medical suppression of ovarian function. A recent study has shown that oestrogens, as well as progestogens, can induce symptoms.[4] Findings from another study demonstrated that women with PMS may metabolise progesterone differently to those without PMS.[5]

Initial management includes non-medical interventions such as education and support, counselling, stress management, relaxation techniques, and exercise; caffeine and salt restriction are of unproven benefit. The herbal remedy agnus castus has been found to be of benefit.[6] For patients with moderate to severe symptoms, a number of drugs have been tried with varying degrees of success; objective assessment of efficacy has been hampered by varying diagnostic criteria, a marked placebo response, and difficulties in obtaining reproducible responses. Treatment may be aimed at modifying the menstrual cycle or treating specific symptoms.[2]

In women with predominantly psychological symptoms, *SSRIs* can be helpful.[7-10] Fluoxetine and sertraline have been shown in controlled trials to alleviate both the psychological and somatic symptoms in women with premenstrual syndrome. *Clomipramine*, a nonselective serotonin reuptake inhibitor, has also been tried with some success. The anxiolytic *alprazolam* has also been used, but use of this and other benzodiazepines should be restricted to the luteal phase of the cycle in selected patients to minimise the risk of dependence and tolerance.[2,7]

Abdominal bloating and swelling associated with PMS has traditionally been thought to be due to sodium and water retention. However, in most women with these symptoms there is no evidence of an increase in body-weight or in body sodium or total water, and use of *diuretics* is therefore not justified.[1] Nevertheless, in women with appreciable weight gain in the luteal phase, diuretics may be useful.[1,7] Another symptom of PMS, cyclical mastalgia, is discussed on p.1546.

*Pyridoxine* has been tried on the basis that it is a cofactor in neurotransmitter (specifically serotonin) synthesis, and has been found to relieve depression induced by oral contraceptives in selected patients. However, its efficacy in premenstrual syndrome is equivocal, and high daily doses have been associated with neurotoxicity.[2,7,8,11] *Calcium* supplementation may relieve symptoms of PMS.[12]

Treatments that modify the menstrual cycle have often been used in women with PMS. In general, drugs with proven efficacy such as danazol, oestrogen implants, and gonadorelin analogues are reserved for women with severe PMS unresponsive to other treatments, because of their adverse effects. *Progestogen* therapy was once popular, but beneficial responses have not been universally achieved and the theory that progesterone was necessary to correct a hormone imbalance is now losing ground. In addition, a systematic review[13] of clinical trials found no evidence to support the use of progesterone or progestogens for premenstrual syndrome. Combined oral contraceptives have met with limited success[1,2,7,9] and in some women, PMS is caused or exacerbated by them. Young women with severe symptoms and women approaching the menopause may benefit from *oestrogen* delivered either as implants or transdermal patches. In women with a uterus, administration with a cyclical progestogen is required to avoid endometrial hyperplasia which unfortunately, may be associated with the return of symptoms, although they may be milder.[1,2] *Danazol* can be useful, but there is concern over its adverse effects on lipids during long-term use and over the risk of masculinisation of a female fetus should pregnancy occur. For patients with severe symptoms not amenable to other treatments, gonadorelin analogues such as *goserelin* can be used to eliminate ovarian function, 'add-back' treatment with oestrogen plus progestogen being given to protect against the side-effects of oestrogen deficiency including osteoporosis. This treatment is very effective for both physical and psychological symptoms. Short-term use (3 months) of a gonadorelin analogue alone has been used to confirm the diagnosis of PMS, or to predict the response to bilateral oophorectomy.[1,2] Immunological control using an analogue of *luteinising hormone-releasing hormone* (LHRH) to raise antibodies against natural LHRH and thus suppress ovarian function has also been proposed.


1. O'Brien PMS. Helping women with premenstrual syndrome. *BMJ* 1993; **307:** 1471–5.
2. Severino SK, Moline ML. Premenstrual syndrome: identification and management. *Drugs* 1995; **49:** 71–82.
3. Gold JH. Premenstrual dysphoric disorder. *JAMA* 1997; **278:** 1024–5.
4. Schmidt PJ, *et al.* Differential behavioral effects of gonadal steroids in women with and those without premenstrual syndrome. *N Engl J Med* 1998; **338:** 209–16.
5. Rapkin AJ, *et al.* Progesterone metabolite allopregnanolone in women with premenstrual syndrome. *Obstet Gynecol* 1997; **90:** 709–14.
6. Schellenberg R. Treatment for the premenstrual syndrome with agnus castus fruit extract: prospective, randomised, placebo controlled study. *BMJ* 2001; **322:** 134–7.
7. Mortola JF. A risk-benefit appraisal of drugs used in the management of premenstrual syndrome. *Drug Safety* 1994; **10:** 160–9.
8. Barnhart KT, *et al.* A clinician's guide to the premenstrual syndrome. *Med Clin North Am* 1995; **79:** 1457–72.
9. Steiner M. Premenstrual syndromes. *Annu Rev Med* 1997; **48:** 447–55.
10. Dimmock PW, *et al.* Efficacy of selective serotonin-reuptake inhibitors in premenstrual syndrome: a systematic review. *Lancet* 2000; **356:** 1131–6.
11. Wyatt KM, *et al.* Efficacy of vitamin B-6 in the treatment of premenstrual syndrome: systematic review. *BMJ* 1999; **318:** 1375–81.
12. Thys-Jacobs S, *et al.* Calcium carbonate and the premenstrual syndrome: effects on premenstrual and menstrual symptoms. *Am J Obstet Gynecol* 1998; **179:** 444–52.
13. Wyatt K, *et al.* Efficacy of progesterone and progestogens in management of premenstrual syndrome: systematic review. *BMJ* 2001; **323:** 776–80.


## Preparations

***BP 2003:*** Estradiol Injection; Estradiol Transdermal Patches;
***USP 27:*** Estradiol Cypionate Injection; Estradiol Injectable Suspension; Estradiol Pellets; Estradiol Tablets; Estradiol Vaginal Cream; Estradiol Valerate Injection.

**Proprietary Preparations** (details are given in Part 3)
***Arg.:*** Aerodiol; Climaderm; Estraderm; Estreva; Estring; Estrofem; Etrosteron; Eutocol; Evorel; Fem 7; Ginatex; Hormodiol; Lindisc; Progynon; Replasyn; Ronfase; Rontagel; Transdiol; Trial Gel; Trial Sat; ***Austral.:*** Aerodiol; Climara; Dermestril; Estraderm; Estring†; Estrofem; Femtran; Menorest; Primogyn Depot; Progynova; Sandrena; Vagifem; Zumenon; ***Austria:*** Climara; Cycloderm; Dermestril; Estracutan; Estraderm; Estramon; Estring; Estrofem; Estrogel; FemSeven; FemSieben; Klimapur; Klimareduct; Linoladiol; Menorest; Merimono; Oesclim; Progynon; Progynova; Sandrena; Sterigin; Systen; Vagifem; Zerella; Zumenon; ***Belg.:*** Aerodiol; Climara; Dermestril; Estraderm; Estreva; Estrofem; Feminova; Meno-Implant; Oestrogel; Progynova; Systen; Vagifem; Zumenon; ***Braz.:*** Aerodiol; Benzo-Ginoestril; Climaderm; Estradelle; Estraderm; Estreva; Estrofem; Fem 7; Ginedisc; Hormodose; Lindisc; Menorest; Merimono; Oesclim†; Oestrogel; Primogyna; Reglovar†; Riselle; Sandrena; Systen; ***Canad.:*** Climara; Delestrogen; Estrace; Estraderm; Estradot; Estring; Estrogel; Femogex†; Oesclim; Vivelle; ***Chile:*** Climaderm; Dermatrans; Enadiol; Epiestrol; Estranova E; Estreva; Farlutes; Fem 7; Femalon; Femiderm; Ginoderm; Mirion; Oesclim; Primaquin; Primofol Depot; Primogyna; Sandrena; Transvital; ***Denm.:*** Aerodiol; Climara; Divigel; Estraderm; Estring; Estrofem; Estrogel; Evorel; Femanest; FemSeven†; Menorest†; Progynon; Sandrena; Vagifem; ***Fin.:*** Climara; Dermestril; Divigel; Estraderm; Estrena; Estring; Estrofem; Estrogel; Evorel; FemSeven; Menorest; Merimono; Progynova; Vagifem; Zumenon; ***Fr.:*** Aerodiol; Benzo-Gynoestryl†; Climara; Delidose; Dermestril; Estraderm; Estrapatch; Estrofem; Evafilm; Femsept; Menorest; Oesclim; Oestrodose; Oestrogel; Oromone; Progynova; Provames; Systen; Thais; ***Ger.:*** Aerodiol; Cerella; Cutanum; Dermestril; Ephelia; Estrabeta; Estraderm; Estramon; Estreva; Estrifam; Estring; Estronorm; Evorel; Fem 7; Femoston mono; Gynokadin; GynPolar; Linoladiol N; Menorest; Merimono; Pantostin; Progynon Depot 10; Progynova; Sandrena; Sisare mono; Tradelia; Vagifem; ***Gr.:*** Dermestril; Estraderm TTS; Menorest; Oestrogel; Vagifem; ***Hong Kong:*** Aerodiol; Bisteron†; Dermestril; Estraderm; Estreva; Estrofem; Fem 7; Oestrogel; Progynova; ***India:*** Estraderm; ***Irl.:*** Climara; Dermestril; Divigel; Epiestrol; Estraderm; Estradot; Estramon†; Estrofem; Evorel; Fematab; Fematrix†; Menorest; Oestrogel; Vagifem; ***Israel:*** Climara†; Dermestril; Estraderm; Estrofem; Evorel; Meno-Patch; Oestrodose; Oestrogel; Progynova; Vagifem; ***Ital.:*** Aerodiol; Armonil; Climara; Dermestril; Ephelia; Epiestrol; Esclima; Estraderm; Estroclim; Estrodose; Estrofem; FemSeven; Gelestra; Menorest; Progynon Depot†; Progynova; Sandrena; Sprediol; Systen; Vagifem; Zerella; ***Malaysia:*** Divigel; Estrofem; Oestrogel; Progynova; Trisequens; ***Mex.:*** Benzo-Ginestryl; Climaderm; Estraderm; Evorel; Fem 7; Ginedisc; Oestrogel; Primogyn; Sandrena; Systen; ***Mon.:*** Estreva; ***Neth.:*** Aerodiol; Climara; Dermestril; Estraderm; Estring; Estrofem; Fem 7; Meno-Implant; Menorest; Progynon Depot 10; Progynova; Sandrena; Systen; Vagifem; Zumenon; ***Norw.:*** Climara; Estraderm; Estradot; Estring; Evorel; Menorest†; Progynova; Vagifem; ***NZ:*** Climara; Estraderm; Estring†; Estrofem; Femtran; Progynova; Sandrena; Vagifem; ***Port.:*** Climara; Dermestril; Estraderm; Estradot; Estrofem; Estronar; Menorest; Vagifem; Zumenon; ***S.Afr.:*** Climara; Estraderm; Estring; Estro-Pause; Estrofem; Evorel; Femigel; Primogyn Depot; Progynova; Vagifem; ***Singapore:*** Divigel; Estraderm; Estrofem; Fem 7; Oestrogel; Progynova; Vagifem; ***Spain:*** Absorlent; Alcis; Cliogan; Dermestril; Endomina; Esotran†; Estraderm; Evopad; Menorest; Meriestra; Oestraclin; Oestrodose; Progynon Depot†; Progynova; Vagifem; ***Swed.:*** Climara; Divigel; Estraderm; Evorel; Femanest; FemSeven; Menorest; Oesclim; Oestring; Progynon; Vagifem; ***Switz.:*** Cerina; Climara; Dermestril; Divigel; Epiestrol; Estraderm; Estramon; Estring; Estrofem N; FemSeven; Menorest; Oestrogel; Progynon Depot 10†; Progynova; Sandrena; Systen; Vagifem; Zumenon; ***Thai.:*** Climara; Divigel; Estrofem; Oestrogel; Progynon; Progynova; Vagifem; ***UK:*** Adgyn Estro†; Aerodiol; Climaval; Dermestril†; Elleste-Solo; Estraderm; Estring; Evorel; Fematrix; FemSeven; FemTab; Menorest†; Menoring; Oestrogel; Progynova; Sandrena; Vagifem; Zumenon; ***USA:*** Alora; Climara; Delestrogen; depGynogen; Depogen; Esclim; Estrace; Estraderm; Estrasorb; Estring; EstroGel; FemPatch; Femring; Gynodiol; Vagifem; Valergen; Vivelle.

**Multi-ingredient:** ***Arg.:*** Activelle; Atrimon; Ciclocur; Climene; Cristerona; Dilena; Dos Dias N; Estracomb; Estragest; Evorel Conti; Evorel Sequi; Farludiol; Farludiol Ciclo; Gynodian Depot; Hosterona; Kliogest; Lubriderm; Menstrogen; Mesigyna; Perlutal; Plenifem; Prefest; Primosiston; Supligol; Trial Combi; Trial Gest; Trial Pack; Trisequens; ***Austral.:*** Climen; Divina†; Estalis Continuous; Estalis Sequi; Estracombi; Estrapak†; Femoston; Kliogest; Kliovance; Trisequens; ***Austria:*** Activelle; Climabelle; Climen; Cyclacur; Estalis; Estalis Sequens; Estracomb; Estragest†; Femipak; Femoston; Femoston Conti; Femphascyl; Femphascyl conti; FemSeven Combi; Filena; Gravibinon†; Gynodian Depot; Ichth-Oestren; Kliogest; Liseta; Mericomb; Merigest; Perikliman; Totelle cyclo; Tri-Filena†; Trisequens; ***Belg.:*** Activelle; Climen; Cyclocur; Dimenformon; Diviplus; Diviva; Estracombi; Feminova Plus; Femoston; Femoston Conti; Kliogest; Totelle; Trisequens; Trivina; ***Braz.:*** Activelle; Cicloprimogyna; Ciclovular†; Cliane; Climene; Cyclofemina; Dilena; Elamax; Estalis; Estandron P; Estracomb; Estragest; Evitas†; Femineo; Gestadinona; Ginecoside; Ginedisc 50 Plus; Hormoginase†; Kliogest; Lindisc Duo; Mericomb; Merigest; Mesigyna; Normomensil; Perlutan; Postoval; Prefest; Progest†; Suprema; Trinestril; Trisequens; Uno-Ciclo; ***Canad.:*** Climacteron; Estalis; Estalis Sequi; Estracomb; ***Chile:*** Activelle; Agurin; Cliane; Climene; Cyclofem; Enadiol CC; Enadiol MP; Estandron Prolongado; Estracomb; Estragest; Estranova 30 Simple; Estranova CC; Farlupost; Fem 7 Combi; Gravidinona; Gynodian Depot; Kilios; Kliogest; Mesigyna; Novafem; Postoval; Primaquin MP; Primaquin MP Continuo; Progyluton; Totelle; Trisequens; Unalmes†; ***Denm.:*** Activelle; Climen; Climodien; Cyclo-Progynon; Divina; Divina Plus; Estracomb; Evo-Conti; Evo-Sequi; Femanor; Femasekvens; Indivina; Klimalet; Klimaxil; Kliogest; Nuvelle; Ostranorm; Totelle; Trevina; Trinorm; Trisekvens; ***Fin.:*** Activelle; Climara Duo; Cyclabil; Divina; Divitren; Estalis; Estalis Sekvens; Estracomb; Evorel Conti; Evorel Sequi; Femilar; Femoston; Femoston Conti; Indivina; Kliogest; Mericomb; Merigest; Senikolp; Totelle Sekvens; Trisekvens; ***Fr.:*** Activelle; Avadene; Climaston; Climene; Divina; Diviseq; Duova; Kliogest; Novofemme; Successia; Trisequens; ***Ger.:*** Activelle; Aknefug-Emulsion; Alpicort F; Androfemon; Climen; Climodien; Crinohermal fem; Cyclo-Menorette; Cyclo-Progynova; CycloOstrogynal; CycloPolar†; Ell-Cranell†; Estalis Sequi; Estracomb; Estrafemol; Estragest; Fem 7 Combi; Femoston; Gianda; Gravibinon; Gynamon; Gynodian Depot; Indivina; Jephagynon; Klimonorm; Kliogest N; Linoladiol-H N; Mericomb; Merigest; NeoOstrogynal; NeyNormin N (Revitorgan-Dilutionen N Nr 65); Novofem; Osmil; Ostronara; Procyclo; Sisare; Syngynon; Trisequens; ***Gr.:*** Activelle; Estopause; Estracomb TTS; Femaston; Kliogest; Trisequens; ***Hong Kong:*** Activelle; Climen; Dilena; Estracomb; Femoston; Hormonin; Klimonorm; Kliogest; Progestrol†; Trisequens; ***India:*** Kemicetine Antiozena; Mixogen; ***Irl.:*** Activelle; Diviseq; Estalis; Estalis Sequi; Estracombi; Estrapak; Evorel Conti; Femoston; Femoston Conti; Femplan-MA†; Indivina; Kliogest; Novofem; Nuvelle; Tridestra†; Trisequens; ***Israel:*** Activelle; Evorel Conti; Evorel Sequi; Kliogest; Meno-MPA; Meno-Net; Progyluton; Trisequens; ***Ital.:*** Activelle; Biormon; Climen; Combiseven; Duo-Ormogyn†; Estalis Sequi; Estracomb; Femoston; Femoston Conti; Filena; Gravibinan; Gynodian Depot; Kliogest; Menovis; Nuvelle; Nuvelle TS; Pausene; Tesor-C†; Totelle; Trisequens; ***Malaysia:*** Activelle; Climen; Femoston; Klimonorm; Kliogest; Progyluton; ***Mex.:*** Anafertin; Binodian; Cliane; Climene; Cyclofemina; Damax; Despamen; Dilena; Estracomb; Estrapak†; Evorelconti; Ginoplan; Gravidinona; Lutalmin; Lutoginestryl F; Mesigyna; Metrigen Fuerte; Ominol; Patector; Perlutal; Primosiston; Progediol; Proger-F; Progyluton; Yectames; ***Mon.:*** FemseptCombi; ***Neth.:*** Activelle; Climene; Cyclocur; Divina; Estracomb; Fem 7 Sequi; Femoston; Kliogest; Trisequens; ***Norw.:*** Activelle; Climen; Climodien; Cyclabil; Diviseq; Estalis; Estalis Sekvens; Estracomb†; Indivina; Kliogest; Novofem; Trisekvens; ***NZ:*** Cliane; Estrapak; Kliogest; Kliovance; Nuvelle; Trisequens; ***Port.:*** Activelle; Cicnor; Climara Duo; Climen; Climodien; Dilena; Emmenovis; Estalis; Estalis Sequi; Estracomb; Femoston; Femoston 1/5; Kliogest; Nuvelle; Progyluton; Trisequens; ***S.Afr.:*** Activelle; Climen; Divina; Estracombi; Evorel Conti; Evorel Sequi; Kliogest; Mixogen; Postoval; Prefesta; Primodian Depot; Trisequens; Trivina; ***Singapore:*** Activelle; Climen; Estracomb; Femoston; Kliogest; Progyluton; Trisequens; ***Spain:*** Absorlent Plus; Activelle; Auroclim; Climen; Climodien; Clisin; Estalis; Estalis Sequi; Estracomb; Gynodian Depot†; Merigest; Merigest Sequi; Mevaren; Nuvelle; Perifem; Progyluton; Topasel; Trisequens; ***Swed.:*** Activelle; Climodien; Cyclabil; Divina; Divina Plus; Estalis; Estalis Sekvens; Estracomb; Evorel Micronor; Femanor; Femasekvens; Indivina; Kliogest; Totelle Sekvens; Trisekvens; Trivina; ***Switz.:*** Activelle; Alpicort F; Climen; Cyclacur; Diviseq; Estalis; Estalis Sequi; Estracomb; Estragest; Fem 7 Combi; Femoston; Femoston Conti; Gynodian Depot; Indivina; Kliogest N; Linoladiol; Mericomb; Merigest; OestroTabs Plus Cyclic; Primosiston; Systen Conti; Systen Sequi; Triaval; Trisequens; ***Thai.:*** Activelle; Climen; Cyclo-Progynova; Duoton; Indivina; Klimonorm†; Kliogest†; Primodian Depot; Trisequens†; ***UK:*** Adgyn Combi†; Climagest; Climesse; Cyclo-Progynova 1 mg; Cyclo-Progynova 2 mg; Elleste Duet Conti; Elleste-Duet; Estracombi; Estrapak†; Evorel Conti; Evorel Pak; Evorel Sequi; Femapak; Femoston; Femoston Conti; FemSeven Conti; FemSeven Sequi; FemTab Continuous; FemTab Sequi; Hormonin; Indivina; Kliofem; Kliovance; Novofem; Nuvelle; Nuvelle Continuous; Nuvelle TS†; Tridestra; Trisequens; ***USA:*** Activella; ClimaraPro; CombiPatch; depAndrogyn†; Depo-Testadiol; Depotestogen; Duo-Cyp†; Duratestrin†; Lunelle; Prefest; Test-Estro†; Valertest†.

## Estrapronicate *(rINN)*

Estrapronicato. Oestradiol 17-nicotinate 3-propionate.

$C_{27}H_{31}NO_4$ = 433.5.
*CAS — 4140-20-9.*

### Profile

Estrapronicate is a derivative of estradiol (p.1550) with nicotinic acid. It has been used as an ingredient of a combined preparation with an anabolic steroid and a progestogen for osteoporosis.

## Estriol *(BAN)*

Estriolum; Follicular Hormone Hydrate; Oestriol; Theelol. Estra-1,3,5(10)-triene-3,16α,17β-triol.

$C_{18}H_{24}O_3$ = 288.4.
*CAS — 50-27-1.*
*ATC — G03CA04.*

**Pharmacopoeias.** In *Eur.* (see p.vi), *Jpn*, and *US.*

**Ph. Eur. 5.0** (Estriol). A white or almost white crystalline powder. Practically insoluble in water; sparingly soluble in alcohol.

**USP 27** (Estriol). A white or practically white, odourless, crystalline powder. Insoluble in water; sparingly soluble in alcohol; soluble in acetone, in chloroform, in dioxan, in ether, and in vegetable oils. Store in airtight containers.

## Estriol Sodium Succinate *(BAN, rINNM)*

Oestriol Sodium Succinate; Succinato sódico de estriol. Disodium 3-hydroxyestra-1,3,5(10)-triene-16α,17β-diyl disuccinate.

$C_{26}H_{30}Na_2O_9$ = 532.5.
*CAS — 113-22-4.*
*ATC — G03CA04.*

## Estriol Succinate *(BAN, rINN)*

Oestriol Succinate; Succinato de estriol. 3-Hydroxyestra-1,3,5(10)-triene-16α,17β-diyl di(hydrogen succinate).

$C_{26}H_{32}O_9$ = 488.5.
*CAS — 514-68-1.*
*ATC — G03CA04.*

### Profile

Estriol is a naturally occurring oestrogen with actions and uses similar to those described for estradiol (p.1550). It is claimed to have only a mild proliferative effect on the endometrium.

It is used for menopausal HRT (p.1536). When oestrogens are given to women with a uterus, a progestogen is required, particularly if used long-term. For short-term treatment, doses of estriol by mouth have been 500 micrograms to 3 mg daily given for one month followed by 500 micrograms to 1 mg daily. Estriol has also been given with other natural oestrogens such as estradiol and estrone (p.1553); usual doses of estriol have ranged from about 250 micrograms to 2 mg daily. It is also given intravaginally for the short-term treatment of menopausal atrophic vaginitis as a 0.01% or 0.1% cream or as pessaries containing 500 micrograms.

Estriol succinate has also been given by mouth in the treatment of menopausal disorders. The sodium succinate salt has been used parenterally in the treatment of haemorrhage and thrombocytopenia.

### Preparations

**Proprietary Preparations** (details are given in Part 3)
***Arg.:*** Orgestriol; ***Austral.:*** Ovestin; ***Austria:*** Ortho-Gynest; Ovestin; Styptanon; ***Belg.:*** Aacifemine; Ortho-Gynest; ***Braz.:*** Ovestrion; Styptanon; ***Chile:*** Ovestin; Sinapause; ***Denm.:*** Ovestin; ***Fin.:*** Ovestin; Pausanol; ***Fr.:*** Gydrelle; Physiogine; Trophicreme; ***Ger.:*** Cordes Estriol; Gynasan; OeKolp; Oestro-Gynaedron M; Ortho-Gynest; Ovestin; Ovo-Vinces†; Synapause E; Xapro; ***Gr.:*** Ovestin; ***Hong Kong:*** Ovestin; ***India:*** Evalon; ***Irl.:*** Ortho-Gynest; Ovestin†; ***Israel:*** Ortho-Gynest; Ovestin; ***Ital.:*** Colpogyn; Ortho Gynest Depot; Ovestin; Trofogin; ***Mex.:*** Ortho-Gynest; Ovestin; Sinapause; ***Neth.:*** Synapause-E₃; ***Norw.:*** Ovesterin; ***NZ:*** Ovestin; ***Port.:*** Ovestin; Pausigin; Synapausa; ***S.Afr.:*** Synapause; ***Singapore:*** Ovestin†; ***Spain:*** Ovestinon; Synapause†; ***Swed.:*** Ovesterin;

***Switz.:*** Oestro-Gynaedron Nouveau; Ortho-Gynest; Ovestin; ***Thai.:*** Ovestin; ***UK:*** Ortho-Gynest; Ovestin.

**Multi-ingredient:** ***Arg.:*** Tropivag Plus; ***Austria:*** Gynoflor; ***Belg.:*** Gynoflor; ***Fr.:*** Florgynal; Trophigil; ***Ger.:*** Cyclo-Menorette; CycloOstrogynal; Gynoflor; NeoOstrogynal; Oestrugol N; ***Hong Kong:*** Gyno-Flor E†; Hormonin; ***Switz.:*** Gynoflor; ***UK:*** Hormonin.

---

## Estrone *(BAN, rINN)*

Estrona; Follicular Hormone; Folliculin; Ketohydroxyoestrin; Oestrone. 3-Hydroxyestra-1,3,5(10)-trien-17-one.

$C_{18}H_{22}O_2$ = 270.4.
*CAS — 53-16-7.*
*ATC — G03CA07.*

**Pharmacopoeias.** In *US.*

**USP 27** (Estrone). Odourless, small white crystals or white to creamy-white crystalline powder. Practically insoluble in water; soluble 1 in 250 of alcohol and 1 in 110 of chloroform at 15°; soluble 1 in 50 of boiling alcohol, 1 in 33 of boiling acetone, 1 in 145 of boiling benzene, and 1 in 80 of boiling chloroform; soluble 1 in 50 of acetone at 50°; soluble in dioxan and in vegetable oils; slightly soluble in solutions of fixed alkali hydroxides. Store in airtight containers at a temperature of 25°, excursions permitted between 15° and 30°. Protect from light.

### Profile

Estrone is a naturally occurring oestrogen with actions and uses similar to those described for estradiol (see p.1550).

For menopausal HRT (see p.1536) estrone has been given by mouth at a dose of 1.4 to 2.8 mg daily in a cyclical or continuous regimen, as a combination product with estradiol and estriol. Estrone has also been given by intramuscular injection in oily solutions and aqueous suspensions. When used specifically for menopausal atrophic vaginitis, estrone has been given vaginally. If used in women with a uterus, estrone by any route should be given with a progestogen.

### Preparations

***USP 27:*** Estrone Injectable Suspension; Estrone Injection.

**Proprietary Preparations** (details are given in Part 3)
***Canad.:*** Oestrilin†; ***USA:*** Kestrone.

**Multi-ingredient:** ***Braz.:*** Gineburno; ***Fin.:*** Senikolp; ***Fr.:*** Synergon; ***Hong Kong:*** Hormonin; ***Spain:*** Cicatral; Grietalgen; Grietalgen Hidrocort; ***Thai.:*** Metharmon-F; ***UK:*** Hormonin.

---

## Estropipate *(BAN)*

Estropipato; Piperazine Estrone Sulfate; Piperazine Oestrone Sulphate. Piperazine 17-oxoestra-1,3,5-(10)-trien-3-yl hydrogen sulphate.

$C_{18}H_{22}O_5S,C_4H_{10}N_2$ = 436.6.
*CAS — 7280-37-7.*

**Pharmacopoeias.** In *Br.* and *US.*

**BP 2003** (Estropipate). A white or almost white crystalline powder. Very slightly soluble in water, in alcohol, in chloroform, and in ether.

**USP 27** (Estropipate). A white to yellowish-white fine crystalline powder, odourless or may have a slight odour. Very slightly soluble in water, in alcohol, in chloroform, and in ether; soluble 1 in 500 of warm alcohol; soluble in warm water. Store in airtight containers.

### Adverse Effects and Precautions

As for oestrogens in general (see Estradiol, p.1550). See also under Hormone Replacement Therapy, p.1536.

### Interactions

See under Hormone Replacement Therapy, p.1539.

### Uses and Administration

Estropipate is a semisynthetic conjugate of estrone with piperazine that is used for menopausal HRT (see p.1536). Its action is due to estrone (p.1553) to which it is hydrolysed in the body.

Estropipate is given by mouth for the short-term treatment of menopausal symptoms; suggested doses have ranged from 0.75 to 6 mg daily, given cyclically or continuously. When used longer term for the prevention of postmenopausal osteoporosis a daily dose of 0.75 or 1.5 mg is given cyclically or continuously. In women with a uterus estropipate should be used with a progestogen. Estropipate has also been used short term for menopausal atrophic vaginitis as a vaginal cream containing 0.15%; 2 to 4 g of cream is applied daily. It is also given by mouth in the treatment of female hypogonadism, castration, and primary ovarian failure in doses of 1.5 to 9 mg daily, in a cyclical regimen.

### Preparations

***BP 2003:*** Estropipate Tablets;
***USP 27:*** Estropipate Tablets; Estropipate Vaginal Cream.

**Proprietary Preparations** (details are given in Part 3)
***Austral.:*** Genoral; Ogen; ***Braz.:*** Ogenest†; ***Canad.:*** Ogen; ***Irl.:*** Harmogen; ***Mex.:*** Ogen†; ***S.Afr.:*** Ortho-Est; ***UK:*** Harmogen; ***USA:*** Ogen; Ortho-Est.

---

## Ethinylestradiol *(BAN, rINN)*

Aethinyloestradiolum; Ethinyl Estradiol; Ethinylestradiolum; Ethinyloestradiol; Etinilestradiol; NSC-10973. 17α-Ethynylestra-1,3,5(10)-triene-3,17β-diol; 19-Nor-17α-pregna-1,3,5(10)-trien-20-yne-3,17β-diol.

$C_{20}H_{24}O_2$ = 296.4.
*CAS — 57-63-6.*
*ATC — G03CA01; L02AA03.*

NOTE. Compounded preparations of ethinylestradiol may be represented by the following names:

- Co-cyprindiol (*BAN*)—ethinylestradiol 35 parts and cyproterone acetate 2000 parts (w/w).

**Pharmacopoeias.** In *Chin., Eur.* (see p.vi), *Int., Jpn, Pol.,* and *US.*

**Ph. Eur. 5.0** (Ethinylestradiol). A white to slightly yellowish-white, crystalline powder. Practically insoluble in water; freely soluble in alcohol; dissolves in dilute alkaline solutions. Protect from light.

**USP 27** (Ethinyl Estradiol). A white to creamy white, odourless, crystalline powder. Insoluble in water; soluble in alcohol, in chloroform, in ether, in vegetable oils, and in solutions of fixed alkali hydroxides. Store in nonmetallic airtight containers. Protect from light.

### Adverse Effects and Precautions

As for oestrogens in general (see Estradiol, p.1550). See also under Hormonal Contraceptives, p.1527.

**Effects on calcium homoeostasis.** Two patients with metastatic breast cancer given ethinylestradiol developed rapidly progressive irreversible and fatal hypercalcaemia, considered to be due to stimulation of osteolysis by the oestrogen.[1]

1. Cornbleet M, *et al.* Fatal irreversible hypercalcaemia in breast cancer. *BMJ* 1977; **1:** 145.

**Effects on the liver.** Cholestasis and pruritus developed in a liver transplant recipient receiving ethinylestradiol at a dose of 50 micrograms daily for the treatment of menorrhagia.[1] Symptoms subsided on withdrawal of ethinylestradiol but returned on its re-introduction.

1. Fedorkow DM, *et al.* Cholestasis induced by oestrogen after liver transplantation. *BMJ* 1989; **299:** 1080–1.

### Interactions

See under Hormonal Contraceptives, p.1534.

### Pharmacokinetics

Ethinylestradiol is rapidly and well absorbed from the gastrointestinal tract. The presence of an ethinyl group at the 17-position greatly reduces hepatic first-pass metabolism compared with estradiol, enabling the compound to be much more active by mouth, but there is some initial conjugation by the gut wall, and the systemic bioavailability is only about 40%. Ethinylestradiol is highly protein bound, but unlike naturally occurring oestrogens, which are mainly bound to sex-hormone binding globulin, it is principally bound to albumin. It is metabolised in the liver, and excreted in urine and faeces. Metabolites undergo enterohepatic recycling.

◊ References.

1. Back DJ, *et al.* The gut wall metabolism of ethinyloestradiol and its contribution to the pre-systemic metabolism of ethinyloestradiol in humans. *Br J Clin Pharmacol* 1982; **13:** 325–30.

### Uses and Administration

Ethinylestradiol is a synthetic oestrogen with actions similar to those of estradiol (see p.1551).

It is frequently used as the oestrogenic component of combined oral contraceptive preparations; a typical daily dose is 20 to 40 micrograms (for guidance on appropriate dose, see p.1535). Ethinylestradiol is also used as an emergency contraceptive (p.1536) combined with levonorgestrel or norgestrel. A combined preparation of ethinylestradiol with the anti-androgen cyproterone (p.1544) is used for the hormonal treatment of acne (p.1133) and hirsutism (p.1545), particularly when contraception is also required. Ethinylestradiol is also used as the oestrogenic component of a combined contraceptive transdermal patch. A dose of 20 micrograms ethinylestradiol is released daily with norelgestromin. A new patch is applied each week for 3 weeks of a 4-week cycle.

Ethinylestradiol has also been used for menopausal HRT (p.1536); doses of 10 to 20 micrograms daily were given (with a progestogen in women with a uterus), but natural oestrogens are usually preferred.

For the treatment of female hypogonadism, 50 micrograms has been given up to three times daily for 14 consecutive days in every 4 weeks, followed by a progestogen for the next 14 days. Lower doses of 10 to 50 micrograms daily on a cyclical basis have also been used.

For the palliative treatment of malignant neoplasms of the prostate (p.521) doses of 150 micrograms to 3 mg have been given daily. For palliation of malignant neoplasms of the breast (p.514) in postmenopausal women doses of 100 micrograms to 1 mg three times daily have been used.

### Preparations

***BP 2003:*** Ethinylestradiol Tablets; Levonorgestrel and Ethinylestradiol Tablets;
***USP 27:*** Ethinyl Estradiol Tablets; Ethynodiol Diacetate and Ethinyl Estradiol Tablets; Levonorgestrel and Ethinyl Estradiol Tablets; Norethindrone Acetate and Ethinyl Estradiol Tablets; Norethindrone and Ethinyl Estradiol Tablets; Norgestrel and Ethinyl Estradiol Tablets.

**Proprietary Preparations** (details are given in Part 3)
***Austral.:*** Estigyn†; ***Austria:*** Progynon C; ***Canad.:*** Estinyl†; ***Ger.:*** Progynon C; Turisteron; ***India:*** Lynoral; ***Israel:*** Progynon C; ***Neth.:*** Lynoral; ***Norw.:*** Etifollin†; ***S.Afr.:*** Estinyl; ***USA:*** Estinyl.

**Multi-ingredient:** ***Arg.:*** April; Cilest; Diane; Dos Dias N; Evelea; Femexin; Femiane; Ginelea; Ginelea T; Gynovin; Harmonet; Lindiol; Lutogynestryl; Marvelon; Mercilon; Microgynon; Microvlar; Minesse; Minulet; Miranova; Mirelle; Neogynon; Nordette; Nordiol; Norgestrel Plus; Ovral; Secret 28; Tridestan N; Tridette; Trinordiol; Triquilar; ***Austral.:*** Biphasil; Brenda-35 ED; Brevinor; Diane-35 ED; Femoden ED; Improvil; Juliet; Levlen ED; Loette; Logynon ED; Marvelon; Microgynon; Microlevlen ED; Minulet; Monofeme; Nordette; Nordiol; Norimin; Sequilar ED; Synphasic; Tri-Minulet; Trifeme; Trioden; Triphasil; Triquilar; Yasmin; ***Austria:*** Cileste; Diane; FemHRT; Gracial; Gynovin; Harmonette; Laurina; Levlen†; Liogynon†; Loette; Lyndiol†; Marvelon; Meliane; Mercilon; Microgynon; Minerva; Minesse; Minulet; Mirelle; Monogestin†; Myvlar†; Neo-Stediril; Neogynon; Ovanon†; Ovranette; Ovysmen; Perikursal; Primosiston; Sequilar; Stediril D; Sterigynon; Tri-Minulet; TriCilest; Trigynon; Trinordiol; Trinovum; Triodena; Triogestena†; Triogestin†; Vivelle; Yasmin; Yermonil; Yirala; ***Belg.:*** Binordiol; Cilest; Conova†; Diane; Femodene; Fysioquens†; Gracial; Harmonet; Lyndiol†; Marvelon; Meliane; Mercilon; Microgynon; Minestril; Ministat†; Minulet; Mirelle; Neo-Stediril; Neogynon; Ovanon†; Ovidol; Ovostat†; Ovysmen; Stediril 30; Stediril D; Tri-Minulet; Trigynon; Trinordiol; Trinovum; Triodene; Yasmin; ***Braz.:*** Anacyclin; Anfertil; Ciclo; Ciclomestril†; Ciclon; Ciclovulon; Diane; Diminut; Evanor; Femiane; Femina; Gestinol; Gestrelan; Ginesse; Gracial; Gynera; Harmonet; Karin†; Levordiol; Lovelle; Mercilon; Microdiol; Micropil; Microvlar; Minesse; Minian; Minulet; Mirelle; Neovlar; Nociclin; Nordette; Normamor; Normex†; Ovoresta; Primera; Primosiston; Primovlar†; Progest†; Selene; Tamisa; Trinordiol; Trinovum; Triquilar; Unidose†; ***Canad.:*** Alesse; Brevicon; Cyclen; Demulen; Diane; FemHRT; Loestrin 1.5/30; Marvelon; Min-Ovral; Minestrin; Ortho 0.5/35; Ortho 1/35; Ortho 10/11†; Ortho 7/7/7; Ortho-Cept; Ovral; Select 1/35; Synphasic; Tri-Cyclen; Triphasil; Triquilar; ***Chile:*** Anovulatorio Micro-Dosis; Anuar; Anulette; Belara; Careza; Ciclidon; Ciclomex; Dal; Desoren; Diane; Dixi-35; Drina; Evilin; Farlutal Estrogeno; Feminol; Gracial; Gynera; Gynostat; Harmonet; Innova Cd; Lady-Ten 35; Loette; Mactex; Marvelon; Microfemin; Microgen; Microgynon; Midalet; Minesse; Minulet; Mirelle; Modutrol; Neofam; Neolette; Nordette; Nordiol; Norvetal; Orlon; Primosiston; Tri-Ciclomex; Tri-Mactex; Trifas; Trinordiol; Triquilar; Trolit; ***Denm.:*** Cilest; Conova†; Desorelle; Diane; Dystrol†; Econ; Fironetta; Gracial; Gynatrol; Gynera; Harmonet; Lyndiol†; Marvelon; Meloden; Mercilon; Microgyn; Milvane; Minulet; Neogentrol; Neogynon; Novynette; NuvaRing; Tetragynon; Tri-Minulet; Trinordiol; Trinovum; Triquilar; Yasmin; ***Fin.:*** Cilest; Diane; Femoden; Gracial; Harmonet; Marvelon; Meliane; Mercilon; Microgynon; Minulet; Mirelle; Neo-Primovlar; Tri-Femoden; Tri-Minulet; Trikvilar; Trinordiol; ***Fr.:*** Adepal; Cilest; Cycleane; Daily; Diane; Effiprev; Evra; Harmonet; Holgyeme; Jasmine; Ludeal; Meliane; Melodia; Mercilon; Milli Anovlar†; Minerva; Minesse; Minidril; Miniphase; Minulet; Moneva; Ortho-Novum 1/35; Ovanon†; Phaeva; Physiostat†; Planor; Stediril; Tetragynon; Tri-Minulet; Triella; Trinordiol; Varnoline; ***Ger.:*** Anacyclin†; Belara; Biviol; Cilest; Conceplan M; Cyclosa; Desmin; Diane; Eve; Femigoa; Femovan; Femranette mikro; Gravistat; Lamuna; Leios; Lovelle; Lovina†; Lyn-ratiopharm-Sequenz; Lyn-ratiopharm†; Lyndiol†; Marvelon; Microgynon; Minisiston; Minulet; Miranova; MonoStep; Neo-Eunomin; Neo-Stediril; Neogynon; Neorlest†; Non-Ovlon; Nora-ratiopharm; NovaStep; Novial; Nuriphasic†; Ostro-Primolut; Ovanon†; Oviol; Ovoresta M; Ovoresta†; Ovysmen; Perikursal; Petibelle; Pramino; Pregnon L†; Primosiston; Prosiston; Sequilar; Sequostat; Sinovula; Stediril; Stediril 30; Stediril D; Synphasec; Tetragynon; Triette; Trigoa; Trinordiol; Trinovum; Triquilar; Trisiston; TriStep; Valette; Yasmin; Yermonil†; ***Gr.:*** Gracial; Gynera; Gynofen 35; Harmonette; Marvelon; Meliane; Mercilon; Minulet; Neogynon; Nordette; Nordiol-21; Ovral; Tri-Minulet; Trigynera; Trinordiol; Triquilar; ***Hong Kong:*** Brevinor; Diane; Duoluton†; Eugynon; Gerivit†; Gracial; Gynera; Harmonet; Lyndiol†; Marvelon; Meliane; Mercilon; Microgynon; Minulet; Neogynon; Nordette; Nordiol†; Norimin; Novynette; Ovral†; Rigevidon; Synphase; Tri-Regol; Trinordiol; Trinovum; Triquilar; ***India:*** Duoluton-L; Mixogen; Novelon; Ovral; Triquilar; ***Irl.:*** Binovum†; Brevinor; Cilest; Dianette; Femodene; Logynon; Marviol; Mercilon; Microgynon 30; Microlite; Minesse†; Minulet; Normin†; NuvaRing; Ovran; Ovran 30†; Ovranette; Ovysmen†; Tri-Minulet; Trinordiol; Trinovum†; Triodene; Yasmin; ***Israel:*** Diane; Gynera; Harmonet; Logynon; Meliane; Mercilon; Microdiol; Microgynon; Minesse; Minulet; Neogynon; Nordette; Ortho Cyclen; Trinordiol; Yasmin; ***Ital.:*** Arianna; Diane; Dueva; Egogyn 30; Eugynon; Evanor-D; Fedra; Ginoden; Gracial; Harmonet; Loette; Mercilon; Microgynon; Milvane; Minesse; Minulet; Miranova; Novogyn; Ovranet; Planum; Practil; Securgin; Tri-Minulet; Trigynon; Trinordiol; Trinovum†; ***Jpn:*** Ange; ***Malaysia:*** Diane; Gynera; Loette; Marvelon; Meliane; Mercilon; Microgynon 30; Minulet; Nordette; Novynette; Rigevidon; Tri-Regol; Trinordiol; Triquilar; ***Mex.:*** Cilest; Diane; Gynovin; Marvelon; Mercilon; Microgynon; Minulet; Neogynon; Nordet; Nordiol; Ortho-Novum 1/35†; Ovral; Trinordiol; Triquilar; ***Neth.:*** Binordiol†; Cilest; Diane; Femodeen; Fysioquens; Gracial; Harmonet; Marvelon; Meliane; Mercilon; Microgynon; Mini Pregnon; Ministat; Minulet; Modicon; Neo-Stediril†; Neocon; Neogynon; Ovanon; Ovidol; Ovostat; Stediril 30, Stediril D; Tri-Minulet; Trigynon; Trinordiol; Trinovum; Triodeen; ***Norw.:*** Diane; Eugynon†; Follimin; Marvelon; Microgynon; Synfase; Tetragynon; Trinordiol; Trionetta; Yasmin; ***NZ:*** Biphasil†; Brevinor; Diane; Estelle; Femodene; Levlen ED; Loette; Marvelon; Melodene; Mercilon; Microgynon; Minulet; Monofeme; Nordette; Nordiol; Norimin; Ovral; Synphasic; Trifeme; Triphasil; Triquilar; ***Port.:*** Diane; Gracial; Gynera; Harmonet; Marvelon;

Mercilon; Microgeste; Microginon; Minigeste; Minulet; Miranova; Neomonovar; Tetragynon†; Tri-Gynera; Tri-Minulet; Trinordiol; Triquilar; Yasmin; ***S.Afr.:*** Biphasil; Brevinor†; Cilest; Diane; E-Gen-C; Femodene ED; Loette; Logynon ED; Marvelon; Melodene; Menoflush; Menoflush + ¼†; Mercilon; Minerva; Minesse; Minulette; Mirelle; Nordette; Nordiol; Normovlar ED†; Ovostat†; Ovral; Tri-Minulet; TriCilest; Trinovum; Triodene; Triphasil; ***Singapore:*** Diane; Gynera; Loette; Marvelon; Meliane; Mercilon; Microgynon; Minulet; Nordette; Trinordiol; Triquilar; ***Spain:*** Diane; Gracial; Gynovin; Harmonet; Loette; Meliane; Melodene 15; Microdiol; Microgynon; Minesse; Minulet; Neo Lyndiol†; Neogynona; Ovoplex; Primosiston†; Suavuret; Tri-Minulet; Triagynon; Triciclor; Trigynovin; ***Swed.:*** Cilest; Desolett; Diane; Follimin; Follinett; Lyndiolett†; Mercilon; Neovletta; Orthonett Novum; Regunon†; Restovar; Synfase; Trimiron; Trinordiol; Trinovum; Trionetta; Yasmin; ***Switz.:*** Belara; Binordiol; Cilest; Diane; Gracial; Gynera; Harmonet; Marvelon; Meloden; Mercilon; Microgynon; Milvane; Minesse; Minulet; Mirelle; Neo-Eunomine†; Neo-Stediril†; Neogynon; Normophasic†; Ologyn; Ovanon†; Ovidol†; Ovysmen; Primosiston; Sequilar†; Stediril 30; Stediril D; Tetragynon; Tri-Minulet; Trinordiol; Trinovum; Triquilar; Yermonil†; ***Thai.:*** Anna; Diane; Eugynon 250; FMP; Gynera; Hormone Multicap; Horon; Lady-35; Lyndiol; Marvelon; Meliane; Mercilon; Microgest; Microgynon; Minulet; Nordette; Nordiol†; Ovral†; Preme; R-Den; Riget; Rigevidon; Sucee; Tina†; Trinordiol†; Triquilar; ***UK:*** Binovum; Brevinor; Cilest; Dianette; Eugynon 30; Evra; Femodene; Femodette; Loestrin; Logynon; Marvelon; Mercilon; Microgynon 30; Minulet; Norimin; Ovran 30; Ovran†; Ovranette; Ovysmen; Schering PC4†; Synphase; Tri-Minulet; Triadene; Trinordiol; Trinovum; Yasmin; ***USA:*** Alesse; Apri; Aviane; Brevicon; Cryselle; Cyclessa; Demulen; Desogen; Enpresse; Estrostep; Estrostep Fe; FemHRT; Genora 0.5/35 and 1/35†; Jenest†; Junel Fe; Kariva; Lessina; Levlen; Levlite; Levora; Lo/Ovral; Loestrin; Loestrin Fe; Mircette; Modicon; Necon 10/11; Necon 0.5/35, 1/35; NEE 1/35; Nelova 0.5/35E and 1/35E†; Nelova 10/11†; Nordette; Norethin 1/35E†; Norinyl 1 + 35; NuvaRing; Ortho Cyclen; Ortho Evra; Ortho Tri-Cyclen; Ortho-Cept; Ortho-Novum 1/35; Ortho-Novum 10/11; Ortho-Novum 7/7/7; Ovcon 35; Ovcon 50; Ovral; Portia; Preven; Previfem; Seasonale; Sprintec; Tri-Levlen; Tri-Norinyl; Tri-Sprintec; TriNessa; Triphasil; Trivora; Yasmin; Zovia.

---

## Ethylestrenol *(BAN, USAN, rINN)*

Ethyloestrenol; Etilestrenol. 17α-Ethylestr-4-en-17β-ol; 19-Nor-17α-pregn-4-en-17β-ol.

$C_{20}H_{32}O$ = 288.5.

*CAS — 965-90-2.*

*ATC — A14AB02.*

### Profile

Ethylestrenol is a 17α-alkylated anabolic steroid (see Testosterone, p.1569) with little androgenic effect and slight progestational activity. It has been used for the promotion of growth in boys with short stature or delayed bone growth. It is used in veterinary medicine.

---

## Etonogestrel *(BAN, USAN, rINN)*

3-keto-Desogestrel; Org-3236. 13-Ethyl-17-hydroxy-11-methylene-18,19-dinor-17α-pregn-4-en-20-yn-3-one; 17β-Hydroxy-11-methylene-18-homo-19-nor-17α-pregn-4-en-20-yn-3-one.

$C_{22}H_{28}O_2$ = 324.5.

*CAS — 54048-10-1.*

*ATC — G03AC08.*

### Adverse Effects and Precautions

As for progestogens in general (see Progesterone, p.1566). See also under Hormonal Contraceptives, p.1527.

**Breast feeding.** Etonogestrel was found in the breast milk of 42 women who received a contraceptive etonogestrel implant. Over the 4-month study, compared with a group who were given an intra-uterine non-hormonal device, etonogestrel did not affect the volume or composition of breast milk, or the growth of the breast-fed infants.[1]

1. Reinprayoon D, *et al.* Effects of the etonogestrel-releasing contraceptive implant (Implanon®) on parameters of breastfeeding compared to those of an intrauterine device. *Contraception* 2000; **62:** 239–46.

**Vaginal bleeding.** Prolonged vaginal bleeding, of 2 to 26 weeks' duration, has been reported with the use of etonogestrel subdermal implants. Blood transfusion was needed in the management of 1 patient.[1]

1. Adverse Drug Reactions Advisory Committee (ADRAC). Implanon and vaginal bleeding. *Aust Adverse Drug React Bull* 2003; **22:** 11–12. Also available at: http://www.tga.gov.au/adr/aadrb/aadr0306.htm (accessed 13/05/04)

### Pharmacokinetics

Etonogestrel is highly bound to plasma proteins. It is metabolised by the cytochrome P450 isoenzyme CYP3A4, and both metabolites and unchanged drug are excreted in the urine and faeces. The elimination half-life is about 25 to 30 hours. Etonogestrel is distributed into breast milk.

◊ References.

1. Timmer CJ, Mulders TMT. Pharmacokinetics of etonogestrel and ethinylestradiol released from a combined contraceptive vaginal ring. *Clin Pharmacokinet* 2000; **39:** 233–42.

### Uses and Administration

Etonogestrel, the active metabolite of desogestrel (p.1547), is used as a hormonal contraceptive (see p.1535). A progestogen-only contraceptive containing 68 mg of etonogestrel, as a subdermal implant, is effective for 3 years. Etonogestrel is also used as the progestogen component of a combined contraceptive delivered via a vaginal ring device. The ring releases an average of 120 micrograms daily of etonogestrel and 15 micrograms daily of ethinylestradiol and remains in the vagina for 3 weeks; it is then removed for a one-week break after which a new ring is inserted.

Etonogestrel is under investigation as a male contraceptive, given orally or by implant, together with testosterone implants or injections.

◊ References.

1. Edwards JE, Moore A. Implanon: a review of clinical studies. *Br J Fam Plann* 1999; **24:** 3–16.
2. Le J, Tsourounis C. Implanon: a critical review. *Ann Pharmacother* 2001; **35:** 329–36.

### Preparations

**Proprietary Preparations** (details are given in Part 3)
***Arg.:*** Implanon; ***Austral.:*** Implanon; ***Austria:*** Implanon; ***Belg.:*** Implanon; ***Braz.:*** Implanon; ***Chile:*** Implanon; ***Denm.:*** Implanon; ***Fin.:*** Implanon; ***Fr.:*** Implanon; ***Ger.:*** Implanon; ***Irl.:*** Implanon; ***Ital.:*** Implanon; ***Malaysia:*** Implanon; ***Mex.:*** Implanon; ***Neth.:*** Implanon; ***Norw.:*** Implanon; ***Port.:*** Implanon; ***Spain:*** Implanon; ***Swed.:*** Implanon; ***Switz.:*** Implanon; ***Thai.:*** Implanon; ***UK:*** Implanon.

**Multi-ingredient:** ***Denm.:*** NuvaRing; ***Irl.:*** NuvaRing; ***USA:*** NuvaRing.

---

## Etynodiol Diacetate *(BANM, pINNM)*

Aethynodiolum Diaceticum; Diacetato de etinodiol; Ethynodiol Diacetate *(USAN)*; SC-11800. 19-Nor-17α-pregn-4-en-20-yne-3β,17β-diol diacetate.

$C_{24}H_{32}O_4$ = 384.5.

*CAS — 1231-93-2 (etynodiol); 297-76-7 (etynodiol diacetate).*

*ATC — G03DC06.*

**Pharmacopoeias.** In *Br., Pol.,* and *US.*

**BP 2003** (Etynodiol Diacetate). A white or almost white, odourless or almost odourless, crystalline powder. Very slightly soluble in water; soluble in alcohol; freely soluble in chloroform and in ether. Protect from light.

**USP 27** (Ethynodiol Diacetate). A white, odourless, crystalline powder. Insoluble in water; soluble in alcohol; very soluble in chloroform; freely soluble in ether; sparingly soluble in fixed oils. Protect from light.

### Adverse Effects and Precautions

As for progestogens in general (see Progesterone, p.1566). See also under Hormonal Contraceptives, p.1527.

**Pregnancy.** Fetal adrenal cytomegaly in a 17-week-old fetus was associated with the maternal ingestion of an oral contraceptive containing etynodiol diacetate 2 mg and mestranol 100 micrograms from the sixth to the fourteenth week of pregnancy.[1]

1. Gau GS, Bennett MJ. Fetal adrenal cytomegaly. *J Clin Pathol* 1979; **32:** 305–6.

### Interactions

As for progestogens in general (see Progesterone, p.1567). See also under Hormonal Contraceptives, p.1534.

### Pharmacokinetics

Etynodiol diacetate is readily absorbed from the gastrointestinal tract and rapidly metabolised, largely to norethisterone (p.1562). About 60% of a dose is stated to be excreted in urine and about 30% in faeces; the half-life in plasma is about 25 hours.

### Uses and Administration

Etynodiol diacetate is a progestogen (see Progesterone, p.1567) that is used as the progestogenic component of combined oral contraceptives and also alone as an oral progestogen-only contraceptive (see p.1535); typical daily doses are 1 to 2 mg in combination products and 500 micrograms for progestogen-only contraceptives.

### Preparations

***USP 27:*** Ethynodiol Diacetate and Ethinyl Estradiol Tablets; Ethynodiol Diacetate and Mestranol Tablets.

**Proprietary Preparations** (details are given in Part 3)
***Fr.:*** Lutometrodiol†; ***Israel:*** Femulen; ***NZ:*** Femulen; ***UK:*** Femulen.

**Multi-ingredient:** ***Arg.:*** Soluna; ***Belg.:*** Conova†; ***Braz.:*** Normex†; Unidose†; ***Canad.:*** Demulen; ***Denm.:*** Conova†; ***USA:*** Demulen; Zovia.

---

## Finasteride *(BAN, USAN, rINN)*

Finasterida; Finasteridum; MK-906; MK-0906. *N-tert*-Butyl-3-oxo-4-aza-5α-androst-1-ene-17β-carboxamide.

$C_{23}H_{36}N_2O_2$ = 372.5.

*CAS — 98319-26-7.*

*ATC — D11AX10; G04CB01.*

**Pharmacopoeias.** In *Eur.* (see p.vi) and *US.*

**Ph. Eur. 5.0** (Finasteride). A white or almost white crystalline powder. It exhibits polymorphism. Practically insoluble in water; freely soluble in dehydrated alcohol and in dichloromethane. Protect from light.

**USP 27** (Finasteride). A white to off-white crystalline solid. Very slightly soluble in water; freely soluble in alcohol and in chloroform. Store in airtight containers.

### Adverse Effects

The most commonly reported adverse effects of finasteride are decreased libido, impotence, ejaculation disorders, and reduced volume of ejaculate.

Breast tenderness and enlargement (gynaecomastia) may occur, and there have been reports of hypersensitivity reactions such as swelling of the lips and face, pruritus, urticaria, and rashes. Testicular pain has also been reported.

**Incidence of adverse effects.** In a study using prescription event monitoring data,[1] the most commonly reported adverse effects of finasteride in 14 772 patients were impotence or ejaculatory failure (2.1% of patients), reduced libido (1%), and breast disorders such as gynaecomastia (0.4%). Adverse effects reported in a single patient each, and verified on rechallenge, were exfoliative dermatitis, perioral numbness, and swollen glands. Finasteride appeared to be associated with ataxia in 1 patient and wheeziness in another.

1. Wilton L, *et al.* The safety of finasteride used in benign prostatic hypertrophy: a non-interventional observational cohort study in 14 772 patients. *Br J Urol* 1996; **78:** 379–84.

**Effects on the breast.** Gynaecomastia was the adverse effect of finasteride most frequently reported to the FDA between June 1992 and February 1995 (a total of 214 reports).[1] The onset after therapy ranged from 14 days to 2.5 years, and the condition could be unilateral or bilateral. Mastectomy was performed in 12 men. Of the 86 men for whom information after discontinuation was available, partial or complete remission of gynaecomastia occurred in 80%, and no change occurred in 20%. In 2 of the cases, primary intraductal breast carcinoma was subsequently found, although 1 probably had breast cancer before finasteride therapy. Continued surveillance of the relationship between finasteride and breast cancer is required.

1. Green L, *et al.* Gynecomastia and breast cancer during finasteride therapy. *N Engl J Med* 1996; **335:** 823.

### Precautions

Finasteride should be used with caution in hepatic impairment. When used for benign prostatic hyperplasia, finasteride should be used with caution in men at risk of obstructive uropathy. Patients should be evaluated for prostatic carcinoma before and during therapy. Use of finasteride decreases concentrations of serum markers of prostate cancer such as prostate specific antigen (PSA) by up to 50% even when cancer is present, and reference values should be adjusted accordingly; the ratio of free to total PSA (percent free PSA) remains constant.

Studies in *animals* suggest finasteride could produce feminisation (hypospadia) of a male fetus if used in pregnant women; therefore, its use is contra-indicated in women who are or may become pregnant. In addition, it is recommended that women in this category should not handle crushed or broken finasteride tablets. Finasteride has been detected in semen, therefore use of a condom is recommended if the patient's sexual partner is, or may become, pregnant.

### Pharmacokinetics

Finasteride is absorbed following oral administration, and peak plasma concentrations are achieved in 1 to 2 hours. The mean bioavailability has variously been reported as 63% and 80%. It is about 90% bound to plasma protein. Finasteride is metabolised in the liver and excreted in urine and faeces as metabolites. The mean terminal half-life is about 6 hours in patients under 60 years of age but may be prolonged to about 8 hours in those 70 years of age or older.

◊ References.

1. Steiner JF. Clinical pharmacokinetics and pharmacodynamics of finasteride. *Clin Pharmacokinet* 1996; **30:** 16–27.

### Uses and Administration

Finasteride is an azasteroid that inhibits the type-2 isoform of 5α-reductase, the enzyme responsible for conversion of testosterone to the more active dihydrotestosterone, and therefore has anti-androgenic properties. It is given by mouth in a dose of 5 mg daily in the management of benign prostatic hyperplasia to cause regression of the enlarged prostate and to improve symptoms; it may reduce the incidence of acute urinary retention and the need for surgery. Response may be delayed and treatment for 6 months or more may be required to assess whether benefit has been achieved.

In the treatment of male-pattern baldness (alopecia androgenetica) in men, finasteride is given by mouth in a dose of 1 mg daily. In general, use for 3 months or more is required before benefit is seen, and effects are reversed within 12 months of ceasing therapy.

**Alopecia.** In men with male-pattern baldness (alopecia—see p.1134), treatment with oral finasteride for 12 months resulted in an 11% increase in vertex hair count, which was maintained in those who continued therapy.[1] Extension of this study to 5 years found that long-term treatment with finasteride maintained beneficial effects, or at least slowed hair loss.[2] The use of oral finasteride for this purpose has been reviewed.[3,4] Some efficacy has also been found with topical finasteride.[5]


1. Kaufman KD, *et al.* Finasteride in the treatment of men with androgenetic alopecia. *J Am Acad Dermatol* 1998; **39:** 578–89.
2. The finasteride male pattern hair loss study group. Long-term (5-year) multinational experience with finasteride 1 mg in the treatment of men with androgenetic alopecia. *Eur J Dermatol* 2002; **12:** 38–49.
3. Anonymous. Propecia and Rogaine Extra Strength for alopecia. *Med Lett Drugs Ther* 1998; **40:** 25–7.
4. McClellan KJ, Markham A. Finasteride: a review of its use in male pattern hair loss. *Drugs* 1999; **57:** 111–26.
5. Mazzerella F, *et al.* Topical finasteride in the treatment of androgenic alopecia. *J Dermatol Treat* 1997; **8:** 189–92.


**Benign prostatic hyperplasia.** Benign enlargement of the prostate gland is common in men with increasing age: at least 50% of men aged over 60 years have histological evidence of hyperplasia.[1] Men with an enlarged prostate may exhibit overt symptoms of obstruction, such as acute or chronic urinary retention, or irritative symptoms such as frequency, urgency, nocturia, or occasionally urge incontinence, resulting from secondary bladder instability.

In men with mild symptoms, or moderate symptoms that are not bothersome, no treatment may be required, although symptoms need to be monitored ('watchful waiting').[1] In those with more severe symptoms or complications the mainstay of treatment is *transurethral resection of the prostate* (TURP).[1] This is the most effective treatment, but is associated with the greatest risk of complications and morbidity, including potential impotence. In consequence drug therapy may be tried first in men with moderate symptoms but no definite indications for surgery.[1,2]

Therapy with an *alpha₁-adrenoceptor blocker* (such as alfuzosin, doxazosin, prazosin, tamsulosin, or terazosin) can produce rapid symptomatic relief, apparently by an action on smooth muscle in the hyperplastic tissue and in the bladder.[2] However, adverse effects include orthostatic hypotension.[1]

The *5α-reductase inhibitor* finasteride offers an alternative approach.[1-6] Finasteride produces moderate reductions in prostate volume, although this takes a number of months and is not always associated with much symptomatic improvement. Like the alpha blockers, therapy must be continued indefinitely for benefit to be maintained. A 4-year study found that finasteride reduced the probability of surgery and acute urinary retention in men with symptomatic benign prostatic hyperplasia with prostatic enlargement.[7] Although the need for prostatectomy was reduced by 55% it was pointed out[8] that only 6% extra patients would benefit from treatment with finasteride. For every 100 men treated, 7 finasteride and 13 placebo recipients required surgery. A comparative 12-month study[9] found the alpha blocker terazosin to be more effective than finasteride in relieving symptoms and improving peak urine flow rates; the combination of finasteride plus terazosin was no more effective than terazosin alone. Moreover, although finasteride reduced prostatic volume, it was no more effective than placebo, a finding that is at odds with previous placebo-controlled studies. It has been suggested that the smaller median prostate size in this study may explain the negative findings,[10] and that men with larger prostates do benefit from finasteride. Similar results were reported in a 12-month study using doxazosin.[11] A later study[12] found that over a longer period of 4 years the combination of doxazosin and finasteride reduced the risk of clinical progression more than either drug alone. The combination of an alpha blocker and 5α-reductase inhibitor is therefore considered by US guidelines[1] to be a suitable option for patients with urinary symptoms and demonstrable prostatic enlargement, and who are at significant risk of progression. Dutasteride is another 5α-reductase inhibitor that is used similarly.

*Other drug therapies* exist but are largely unproven or unsuitable for general use. Gonadorelin analogues such as leuprorelin or nafarelin can produce a reduction in prostate size, but adverse effects make these drugs unsuitable for indefinite therapy. More recently, gonadorelin antagonists such as cetrorelix have been tried. The antifungal mepartricin has been reported to produce symptomatic improvement, possibly by binding to oestrogen in the intestinal lumen and lowering plasma-oestrogen concentrations. A number of plant extracts such as saw palmetto and *Pygeum africanum* are also in use,[13-16] and the phytosterol sitosterol, which is a constituent of these, is reported to be effective.[17]

Various *surgical alternatives to TURP* use heat to destroy tissue surrounding the urethra. These minimally invasive therapies include transurethral microwave thermotherapy, water-induced thermotherapy, transurethral needle ablation, and interstitial laser treatment.[18]


1. AUA Practice Guidelines Committee. AUA guideline on management of benign prostatic hyperplasia (2003). Chapter 1: diagnosis and treatment recommendations. *J Urol (Baltimore)* 2003; **170:** 530–47. Also available at: http://www.auanet.org/timssnet/products/guidelines/main_reports/bph_management/chapt_1_appendix.pdf (accessed 16/06/04)
2. Lieber MM. Pharmacologic therapy for prostatism. *Mayo Clin Proc* 1998; **73:** 590–6.
3. Gormley GJ, *et al.* The effect of finasteride in men with benign prostatic hyperplasia. *N Engl J Med* 1992; **327:** 1185–91.
4. Finasteride Study Group. Finasteride (MK-906) in the treatment of benign prostatic hyperplasia. *Prostate* 1993; **22:** 291–9.
5. Nickel JC, *et al.* Efficacy and safety of finasteride for benign prostatic hyperplasia: results of a 2-year randomized controlled trial (the PROSPECT study). *Can Med Assoc J* 1996; **155:** 1251–9.
6. Wilde MI, Goa KL. Finasteride: an update of its use in the management of symptomatic benign prostatic hyperplasia. *Drugs* 1999; **57:** 557–81.
7. McConnell JD, *et al.* The effect of finasteride on the risk of acute urinary retention and the need for surgical treatment among men with benign prostate hyperplasia. *N Engl J Med* 1998; **338:** 557–63.
8. Wasson JH. Finasteride to prevent morbidity from benign prostatic hyperplasia. *N Engl J Med* 1998; **338:** 612–13.
9. Lepor H, *et al.* The efficacy of terazosin, finasteride, or both in benign prostatic hyperplasia. *N Engl J Med* 1996; **335:** 533–9.
10. Walsh PC. Treatment of benign prostatic hyperplasia. *N Engl J Med* 1996; **335:** 586–7.
11. Kirby RS, *et al.* Efficacy and tolerability of doxazosin and finasteride, alone or in combination, in treatment of symptomatic benign prostatic hyperplasia: the Prospective European Doxazosin and Combination Therapy (PREDICT) trial. *Urology* 2003; **61:** 119–26.
12. McConnell JD, *et al.* The long-term effect of doxazosin, finasteride, and combination therapy on the clinical progression of benign prostatic hyperplasia. *N Engl J Med* 2003; **349:** 2387–98.
13. Buck AC. Phytotherapy for the prostate. *Br J Urol* 1996; **78:** 325–36.
14. Wilt TJ, *et al.* Saw palmetto extracts for treatment of benign prostatic hyperplasia: a systematic review. *JAMA* 1998; **280:** 1604–9. Correction. *ibid.* 1999; **281:** 515.
15. Lowe FC, Fagelman E. Phytotherapy in the treatment of benign prostatic hyperplasia: an update. *Urology* 1999; **53:** 671–8.
16. Ishani A, *et al.* Pygeum africanum for the treatment of patients with benign prostatic hyperplasia: a systematic review and quantitative meta-analysis. *Am J Med* 2000; **109:** 654–64.
17. Wilt TJ, *et al.* β-Sitosterol for the treatment of benign prostatic hyperplasia: a systematic review. *BJU Int* 1999; **83:** 976–83.
18. Larson TR. Rationale and assessment of minimally invasive approaches to benign prostatic hyperplasia therapy. *Urology* 2002; **59** (suppl 2A): 12–16.


**Hirsutism.** Finasteride is reported to be effective for the treatment of hirsutism (p.1545) in women.[1-3] It should be noted that finasteride should not be used in women who are or may become pregnant (see Precautions, above).


1. Wong IL, *et al.* A prospective randomized trial comparing finasteride to spironolactone in the treatment of hirsute women. *J Clin Endocrinol Metab* 1995; **80:** 233–8.
2. Falsetti L, *et al.* Comparison of finasteride versus flutamide in the treatment of hirsutism. *Eur J Endocrinol* 1999; **141:** 361–7.
3. Moghetti P. *et al.* Comparison of spironolactone, flutamide, and finasteride efficacy in the treatment of hirsutism: a randomized, double blind, placebo-controlled trial. *J Clin Endocrinol Metab* 2000; **85:** 89–94.


**Malignant neoplasms of the prostate.** Finasteride appears to have little effect in men with established prostate cancer,[1,2] but is under investigation for the prevention of prostate cancer (p.521). The results of 1 small study[3] of its effects on the prostate found little evidence to support its use for prevention of malignancy in patients at high risk. In healthy men, a large controlled trial[4] found that seven years of finasteride prophylaxis reduced the incidence of prostate cancer by about 25% compared with placebo, but this benefit was offset by an increased risk of high-grade tumours associated with finasteride.


1. Presti JC, *et al.* Multicenter, randomized, double-blind placebo controlled study to investigate the effect of finasteride (MK-906) on stage D prostate cancer. *J Urol (Baltimore)* 1992; **148:** 1201–4.
2. Rittmaster RS. Finasteride. *N Engl J Med* 1994; **330:** 120–5.
3. Cote RJ, *et al.* The effect of finasteride on the prostate gland in men with elevated serum prostate-specific antigen levels. *Br J Cancer* 1998; **78:** 413–18.
4. Thompson IM, *et al.* The influence of finasteride on the development of prostate cancer. *N Engl J Med* 2003; **349:** 215–24.


## Preparations

***USP 27:*** Finasteride Tablets.

**Proprietary Preparations** (details are given in Part 3)
***Arg.:*** Anatine; Andropel; Avertex; Conef; Eutiz; Finasterin; Finprostat; Flutiamik; HPB; Nasteril; Pelicrep; Propecia; Proscar; Prosmin; Prostanovag; Prostene; Renacidin; Sutrico; Tealep; Tricofarma; Vetiprost; ***Austral.:*** Propecia; Proscar; ***Austria:*** Proscar; ***Belg.:*** Proscar; ***Braz.:*** Alfasin; Finalop; Finastil; Flaxin; Nasterid; Pracap; Prohair; Pronasteron; Propecia; Proscar; Prostide; Reduscar; ***Canad.:*** Propecia; Proscar; ***Chile:*** Apeplus; Prohair; Proscar; Saniprostol; Vastus; ***Denm.:*** Propecia; Proscar; ***Fin.:*** Gefina; Propecia; Proscar; ***Fr.:*** Chibro-Proscar; Propecia; ***Ger.:*** Propecia; Proscar; ***Gr.:*** Proscar; ***Hong Kong:*** Propecia; Proscar; ***India:*** Fincar; ***Irl.:*** Proscar; ***Israel:*** Pro-Cure; Propecia; ***Ital.:*** Finastid; Genaprost; Propecia; Proscar; Prostide; ***Malaysia:*** Propecia; Proscar; ***Mex.:*** Propeshia; Proscar; ***Neth.:*** Proscar; ***Norw.:*** Proscar; ***NZ:*** Propecia; Proscar; ***Port.:*** Propecia; Proscar; ***S.Afr.:*** Propecia; Proscar; ***Singapore:*** Propecia; Proscar; ***Spain:*** Eucoprost; Folitabs†; Propecia; Proscar; ***Swed.:*** Propecia; Proscar; ***Switz.:*** Propecia; Proscar; ***Thai.:*** Propecia; Proscar; ***UK:*** Propecia; Proscar; ***USA:*** Propecia; Proscar.

**Multi-ingredient: *Arg.:*** Tricoplus Conef.

---

## Flugestone Acetate *(BANM)*

Acetato de flugestona; Flurogestone Acetate *(USAN)*; NSC-65411; SC-9880. 9α-Fluoro-11β,17α-dihydroxypregn-4-ene-3,20-dione 17-acetate.

$C_{23}H_{31}FO_5$ = 406.5.
*CAS — 337-03-1 (flugestone); 2529-45-5 (flugestone acetate).*

### Profile

Flugestone acetate is a progestogen (see Progesterone, p.1566) used in veterinary medicine.

---

## Fluoxymesterone *(BAN, rINN)*

Fluximesterona; NSC-12165. 9α-Fluoro-11β,17β-dihydroxy-17α-methylandrost-4-en-3-one.

$C_{20}H_{29}FO_3$ = 336.4.
*CAS — 76-43-7.*
*ATC — G03BA01.*

**Pharmacopoeias.** In *Jpn* and *US*.

**USP 27** (Fluoxymesterone). A white or practically white, odourless, crystalline powder. Practically insoluble in water; sparingly soluble in alcohol; slightly soluble in chloroform. Protect from light.

### Adverse Effects and Precautions

As for androgens and anabolic steroids in general (see Testosterone, p.1570).

As with other 17α-alkylated compounds fluoxymesterone may cause hepatotoxicity, and is probably best avoided in patients with hepatic impairment, and certainly if this is severe. Hepatic function should be monitored during therapy.

### Uses and Administration

Fluoxymesterone has androgenic properties (see Testosterone, p.1571). It is effective when given by mouth and is more potent than methyltestosterone.

In the treatment of male hypogonadism, fluoxymesterone has been given in a dosage of 5 to 20 mg daily. In the treatment of delayed puberty in the male it has been given in usual daily doses of 2.5 to 10 mg, adjusted according to response; care was necessary because of the risk of epiphyseal closure and treatment was generally only given for 4 to 6 months. In the palliation of inoperable neoplasms of the breast in postmenopausal women, it has been given in daily doses of up to 40 mg. Fluoxymesterone has also been used in the treatment of aplastic anaemia.

**Growth retardation.** Fluoxymesterone has been used to try to increase final adult height in boys with constitutional delay of growth associated with delayed puberty (see p.1314).

### Preparations

***USP 27:*** Fluoxymesterone Tablets.

**Proprietary Preparations** (details are given in Part 3)
***Austral.:*** Halotestin†; ***Canad.:*** Halotestin†; ***Fr.:*** Halotestin†; ***Hong Kong:*** Halotestin; ***Israel:*** Halotestin†; ***Ital.:*** Halotestin†; ***Mex.:*** Stenox; ***Neth.:*** Halotestin†; ***Norw.:*** Halotestin†; ***S.Afr.:*** Halotestin†; ***Singapore:*** Halotestin†; ***Thai.:*** Halotestin; ***USA:*** Halotestin†.

**Multi-ingredient: *Arg.:*** Ferona.

---

## Formebolone *(BAN, rINN)*

Formebolona; Formyldienolone. 11α,17β-Dihydroxy-17β-methyl-3-oxoandrosta-1,4-diene-2-carbaldehyde.

$C_{21}H_{28}O_4$ = 344.4.
*CAS — 2454-11-7.*

### Profile

Formebolone has anabolic properties (see Testosterone, p.1569) and has been given by mouth or by intramuscular injection.

---

## Fosfestrol *(BAN, rINN)*

Diethylstilbestrol Diphosphate; Phosphoestrolum; Stilboestrol Diphosphate. (*E*)-αα′-Diethylstilbene-4,4′-diol bis(dihydrogen phosphate); (*E*)-4,4′-(1,2-Diethylvinylene)bis(phenyl dihydrogen orthophosphate).

$C_{18}H_{22}O_8P_2$ = 428.3.
*CAS — 522-40-7.*
*ATC — L02AA04.*

**Pharmacopoeias.** In *Jpn* and *US*.

**USP 27** (Diethylstilbestrol Diphosphate). An off-white, odourless, crystalline powder. Sparingly soluble in water; soluble in alcohol and in dilute alkali. Store in airtight containers at a temperature not exceeding 21°.

## Fosfestrol Sodium *(BANM, rINNM)*

Fosfestrol sódico.

$C_{18}H_{18}Na_4O_8P_2$ = 516.2.
*CAS — 23519-26-8 (fosfestrol tetrasodium $xH_2O$); 4719-75-9 (anhydrous fosfestrol tetrasodium).*
*ATC — L02AA04.*

**Pharmacopoeias.** In *Br.*, which specifies $xH_2O$.

**BP 2003** (Fosfestrol Sodium). A white or almost white powder. Freely soluble in water; practically insoluble in dehydrated alcohol and in ether. A 5% solution in water has a pH of 7.0 to 9.0. Protect from light.

### Adverse Effects and Precautions

As for Diethylstilbestrol, see p.1548.

Following intravenous injection of fosfestrol sodium there may be a temporary burning sensation in the perineal region and pain at the site of bony metastases. Slow infusion is not recommended as cytotoxic concentrations of the drug may not be achieved.

### Uses and Administration

Fosfestrol is a synthetic nonsteroidal oestrogen that requires dephosphorylation to diethylstilbestrol (p.1548) before it is active. It is used in the treatment of malignant neoplasms of the prostate (p.521).

Anhydrous fosfestrol sodium 100 mg is approximately equivalent to 83 mg of fosfestrol. Expressed in terms of fosfestrol sodium, initial therapy for at least the first 5 days may range from 600 to 1200 mg daily by slow intravenous injection. In terms of fosfestrol, these doses are equivalent to 500 to 1000 mg. Injections should be given preferably with the patient lying down. Maintenance intravenous therapy may be with 300 to 600 mg fosfestrol sodium one to four times a week. Fosfestrol sodium may also be given by mouth, in a dose of up to 240 mg three times daily for 7 days then reducing over 14 days to 120 to 360 mg daily in divided doses.

Fosfestrol disodium has also been used.

### Preparations

**BP 2003:** Fosfestrol Injection; Fosfestrol Tablets;
**USP 27:** Diethylstilbestrol Diphosphate Injection.

**Proprietary Preparations** (details are given in Part 3)
**Arg.:** Fosfostilben; Honvan; **Austral.:** Honvan†; **Austria:** Honvan; **Belg.:** Honvan; **Braz.:** Honvan†; Ronvan; **Canad.:** Honvol; **Fr.:** ST-52; **Ger.:** Honvan; **Gr.:** Honvan; **Hong Kong:** Honvan; **India:** Honvan; **Mex.:** Honvan; **Neth.:** Honvan; **Norw.:** Honvan†; **NZ:** Honvan†; **Port.:** Honvan; **Singapore:** Honvan†; **Spain:** Honvan; **Switz.:** Honvan; **UK:** Honvan†; **USA:** Stilphostrol†.

## Gestodene *(BAN, USAN, rINN)*

Gestodeno; SH-B-331. 13β-Ethyl-17β-hydroxy-18,19-dinor-17α-pregna-4,15-dien-20-yn-3-one.
$C_{21}H_{26}O_2$ = 310.4.
*CAS — 60282-87-3.*

### Adverse Effects and Precautions

As for progestogens in general (see Progesterone, p.1566). See also under Hormonal Contraceptives, p.1527. Gestodene is reported to have few androgenic effects, and to have less adverse effect on the serum lipid profile than older 19-nortestosterone derivatives. However, there is some evidence that gestodene-containing combined oral contraceptives are associated with a small increased risk of venous thromboembolism (see p.1531, and for precautions, see p.1533).

### Interactions

As for progestogens in general (see Progesterone, p.1567). See also under Hormonal Contraceptives, p.1534.

**Antiepileptics.** *Felbamate* treatment significantly increased gestodene clearance from a low-dose combined oral contraceptive, and might decrease contraceptive efficacy.[1] See also p.1534.

1. Saano V, *et al.* Effects of felbamate on the pharmacokinetics of a low-dose combination oral contraceptive. *Clin Pharmacol Ther* 1995; **58:** 523–31.

### Pharmacokinetics

Gestodene is well absorbed with a high bioavailability when given by mouth. It is extensively bound to plasma proteins (75 to 87% to sex hormone binding globulin, and 13 to 24% to albumin). Gestodene is metabolised in the liver, less than 1% of a dose being excreted in the urine unchanged.

### Uses and Administration

Gestodene is a progestogen (see Progesterone, p.1566) structurally related to levonorgestrel. It is used as the progestogenic component of combined oral contraceptives (see p.1535); a typical daily dose is 75 micrograms in monophasic preparations, and 50 to 100 micrograms in triphasic preparations.

◊ Reviews.


1. Anonymous. Femodene/Minulet—how different is gestodene? *Drug Ther Bull* 1990; **28:** 41–2.
2. Wilde MI, Balfour JA. Gestodene: a review of its pharmacology, efficacy and tolerability in combined contraceptive preparations. *Drugs* 1995; **50:** 364–95.


### Preparations

**Proprietary Preparations** (details are given in Part 3)
**Multi-ingredient: Arg.:** Femiane; Ginelea; Ginelea T; Gynovin; Harmonet; Minesse; Minulet; Mirelle; Secret 28; **Austral.:** Femoden ED; Minulet; Tri-Minulet; Trioden; **Austria:** Gynovin; Harmonette; Meliane; Minesse; Minulet; Mirelle; Monogestin†; Myvlar†; Tri-Minulet; Triodena; Triogestena†; Triogestin†; **Belg.:** Femodene; Harmonet; Meliane; Minulet; Mirelle; Tri-Minulet; Triodene; **Braz.:** Diminut; Femiane; Gestinol; Ginesse; Gynera; Harmonet; Micropil; Minesse; Minulet; Mirelle; Tamisa; **Chile:** Careza; Ciclomex; Feminol; Gynera; Harmonet; Microgen; Minesse; Minulet; Mirelle; Tri-Ciclomex; **Denm.:** Gynera; Harmonet; Meloden; Milvane; Minulet; Tri-Minulet; **Fin.:** Femoden; Harmonet; Meliane; Minulet; Mirelle; Tri-Femoden; Tri-Minulet; **Fr.:** Avadene; Harmonet; Meliane; Melodia; Minesse; Minulet; Moneva; Phaeva; Successia; Tri-Minulet; **Ger.:** Femovan; Minulet; **Gr.:** Gynera; Harmonette; Meliane; Minulet; Tri-Minulet; Trigynera; **Hong Kong:** Gynera; Harmonet; Meliane; Minulet; **Irl.:** Femodene; Minesse†; Minulet; Tri-Minulet; Triodene; **Israel:** Gynera; Harmonet; Meliane; Minesse; Minulet; **Ital.:** Arianna; Fedra; Ginoden; Harmonet; Milvane; Minesse; Minulet; Tri-Minulet; **Malaysia:** Gynera; Meliane; Minulet; **Mex.:** Gynovin; Minulet; **Neth.:** Femodeen; Harmonet; Meliane; Minulet; Tri-Minulet; Triodeen; **NZ:** Femodene; Melodene; Minulet; **Port.:** Gynera; Harmonet; Microgeste; Minigeste; Minulet; Tri-Gynera; Tri-Minulet; **S.Afr.:** Femodene ED; Melodene; Minesse; Minulette; Mirelle; Tri-Minulet; Triodene; **Singapore:** Gynera; Meliane; Minulet; **Spain:** Gynovin; Harmonet; Meliane; Melodene 15; Minesse; Minulet; Tri-Minulet; Trigynovin; **Switz.:** Gynera; Harmonet; Meloden; Milvane; Minesse; Minulet; Mirelle; Tri-Minulet; **Thai.:** Gynera; Meliane; Minulet; **UK:** Femodene; Femodette; Minulet; Tri-Minulet; Triadene.

## Gestonorone Caproate *(BANM, USAN, rINN)*

Caproato de gestonorona; Gestronol Hexanoate; NSC-84054; SH-582. 17α-Hydroxy-19-norpregn-4-ene-3,20-dione hexanoate.
$C_{26}H_{38}O_4$ = 414.6.
*CAS — 1253-28-7.*
*ATC — G03DA01; L02AB03.*

### Adverse Effects and Precautions

As for progestogens in general (see Progesterone, p.1566).

Local reactions have occurred at the site of injection. Rarely, coughing, dyspnoea, and circulatory disturbances may develop during or immediately after injection but can be avoided by injecting gestonorone very slowly. In males, spermatogenesis is temporarily inhibited.

### Interactions

As for progestogens in general (see Progesterone, p.1567).

### Uses and Administration

Gestonorone caproate is a long-acting potent progestogen structurally related to progesterone (p.1567). It is given in an oily solution by intramuscular injection in doses of 200 to 400 mg every 5 to 7 days for the adjunctive treatment of endometrial carcinoma (p.516). It has also been used in the management of benign prostatic hyperplasia (p.1555) in doses of 200 mg weekly, increased to 300 to 400 mg weekly if necessary.

### Preparations

**Proprietary Preparations** (details are given in Part 3)
**Ger.:** Depostat; **Ital.:** Depostat; **Mex.:** Primostat; **Spain:** Depostat; **Switz.:** Depostat.

## Gestrinone *(BAN, USAN, rINN)*

A-46745; Ethylnorgestrienone; Gestrinona; R-2323; RU-2323. 13β-Ethyl-17β-hydroxy-18,19-dinor-17α-pregna-4,9,11-trien-20-yn-3-one.
$C_{21}H_{24}O_2$ = 308.4.
*CAS — 16320-04-0; 40542-65-2.*
*ATC — G03XA02.*

### Adverse Effects and Precautions

As for Danazol, p.1545.

### Interactions

Antiepileptic drugs and rifampicin may accelerate the metabolism of gestrinone.

### Pharmacokinetics

Gestrinone is well absorbed after oral doses with negligible first-pass hepatic metabolism. Peak plasma concentrations occur about 3 hours after administration. The plasma half-life is about 24 hours. Gestrinone is metabolised in the liver to form conjugated metabolites.

### Uses and Administration

Gestrinone is a synthetic steroidal hormone reported to have androgenic, anti-oestrogenic, and antiprogestogenic properties. It is used in the treatment of endometriosis (p.1546) in doses of 2.5 mg twice weekly by mouth; the first dose is taken on the first day of the menstrual cycle with the second dose taken three days later; thereafter the doses should be taken on the same two days of each week, usually for a period of 6 months. If a dose is missed it should be given as soon as possible and the original dose sequence maintained thereafter; if 2 or more doses are missed gestrinone should be stopped and restarted on the first day of a new cycle after a negative pregnancy test.

Gestrinone has been studied in the management of cyclical mastalgia (p.1546).

◊ References.


1. Thomas EJ, Cooke ID. Impact of gestrinone on the course of asymptomatic endometriosis. *BMJ* 1987; **294:** 272–4.
2. Brosens IA, *et al.* The morphologic effect of short-term medical therapy of endometriosis. *Am J Obstet Gynecol* 1987; **157:** 1215–21.
3. Coutinho EM, Azadian-Boulanger G. Treatment of endometriosis by vaginal administration of gestrinone. *Fertil Steril* 1988; **49:** 418–22.
4. Hornstein MD, *et al.* A randomized double-blind prospective trial of two doses of gestrinone in the treatment of endometriosis. *Fertil Steril* 1990; **53:** 237–41.
5. Peters F. Multicentre study of gestrinone in cyclical breast pain. *Lancet* 1992; **339:** 205–8.
6. Worthington M, *et al.* A randomized comparative study of the metabolic effects of two regimens of gestrinone in the treatment of endometriosis. *Fertil Steril* 1993; **59:** 522–6.
7. Gestrinone Italian Study Group. Gestrinone versus a gonadotropin-releasing hormone agonist for the treatment of pelvic pain associated with endometriosis: a multicenter, randomized, double-blind study. *Fertil Steril* 1996; **66:** 911–19.
8. Dawood MY, *et al.* Clinical, endocrine, and metabolic effects of two doses of gestrinone in treatment of pelvic endometriosis. *Am J Obstet Gynecol* 1997; **176:** 387–94.


### Preparations

**Proprietary Preparations** (details are given in Part 3)
**Arg.:** Nemestran; **Austral.:** Dimetriose; **Belg.:** Dimetrose†; **Braz.:** Dimetrose; **Ital.:** Dimetriose; **Malaysia:** Dimetriose; **Mex.:** Nemestran; **Neth.:** Nemestran; **NZ:** Dimetriose; **Port.:** Dimetriose; **S.Afr.:** Tridomose; **Singapore:** Dimetriose; **Spain:** Nemestran; **Switz.:** Nemestran; **Thai.:** Dimetriose; **UK:** Dimetriose.

## Hexestrol *(rINN)*

Dihydrodiethylstilboestrol; Dihydrostilboestrol; Hexanoestrol; Hexoestrol; NSC-9894; Synestrol; Synoestrol. 4,4′-(1,2-Diethylethylene)diphenol.
$C_{18}H_{22}O_2$ = 270.4.
*CAS — 5635-50-7 (hexestrol); 84-16-2 (meso-hexestrol).*

### Profile

Hexestrol is a synthetic nonsteroidal oestrogen that is used in the treatment of malignant neoplasms and gynaecological disorders.

## Hydroxyestrone Diacetate

Hidroxiestrona, diacetato de; 16α-Hydroxyoestrone Diacetate. 3,16α-Dihydroxyestra-1,3,5(10)-trien-17-one diacetate.
$C_{22}H_{26}O_5$ = 370.4.
*CAS — 566-76-7 (hydroxyestrone); 1247-71-8 (hydroxyestrone diacetate).*

### Profile

Hydroxyestrone diacetate is an oestrogen (see Estradiol, p.1550). It has been given by mouth in vulvovaginal disorders and for female infertility.

### Preparations

**Proprietary Preparations** (details are given in Part 3)
**Braz.:** Hormocervix†.

## Hydroxyprogesterone Caproate *(BANM, rINN)*

17-AHPC; Caproato de hidroxiprogesterona; Hydroxyprogesterone Hexanoate; NSC-17592. 3,20-Dioxopregn-4-en-17α-yl hexanoate; 17α-Hydroxypregn-4-ene-3,20-dione hexanoate.
$C_{27}H_{40}O_4$ = 428.6.
*CAS — 68-96-2 (hydroxyprogesterone); 630-56-8 (hydroxyprogesterone caproate).*
*ATC — G03DA03.*

**Pharmacopoeias.** In *Chin.* and *US.*

**USP 27** (Hydroxyprogesterone Caproate). A white or creamy-white, crystalline powder. Odourless or having a slight odour. Insoluble in water; soluble in ether; slightly soluble in benzene. Protect from light. Store at a temperature of 25°, excursions permitted between 15° and 30°.

### Adverse Effects and Precautions

As for progestogens in general (see Progesterone, p.1566).

There may be local reactions at the site of injection. Rarely, coughing, dyspnoea, and circulatory disturbances may occur during or immediately after injection of hydroxyprogesterone caproate but can be avoided by injecting the drug very slowly.

**Pregnancy.** Abnormalities reported in infants born to mothers who had received hydroxyprogesterone during pregnancy have included tetralogy of Fallot in one infant,[1] genito-urinary abnormalities in 2 infants,[2] and adrenocortical carcinoma in one infant.[3]


1. Heinonen OP, *et al.* Cardiovascular birth defects and antenatal exposure to female sex hormones. *N Engl J Med* 1977; **296:** 67–70.
2. Evans ANW, *et al.* The ingestion by pregnant women of substances toxic to the foetus. *Practitioner* 1980; **224:** 315–19.
3. Mann JR, *et al.* Transplacental carcinogenesis (adrenocortical carcinoma) associated with hydroxyprogesterone hexanoate. *Lancet* 1983; **ii:** 580.


### Interactions

As for progestogens in general (see Progesterone, p.1567).

### Uses and Administration

Hydroxyprogesterone caproate is a progestogen structurally related to progesterone (p.1567) that has been used for recurrent miscarriage and various menstrual disorders. In recurrent miscarriage associated with proven progesterone deficiency, doses of 250 to 500 mg weekly by intramuscular injection have been given during the first half of pregnancy.

The acetate and the enantate have also been used.

**Premature labour.** In women who have a history of spontaneous premature delivery (p.794), there is some evidence to suggest that prophylactic hydroxyprogesterone caproate may reduce the risk for premature delivery in subsequent pregnancies.[1]

1. Meis PJ, *et al.* Prevention of recurrent preterm delivery by 17 alpha-hydroxyprogesterone caproate. *N Engl J Med* 2003; **348:** 2379–85.

### Preparations

*USP 27:* Hydroxyprogesterone Caproate Injection.

**Proprietary Preparations** (details are given in Part 3)

***Arg.:*** Gestageno; Proluton Depot; ***Austria:*** Proluton Depot; ***Chile:*** Primolut Depot; ***Fr.:*** Progesterone-retard Pharlon; ***Ger.:*** Progesteron-Depot; Proluton Depot; ***Gr.:*** Proluton Depot; ***Hong Kong:*** Proluton Depot†; ***India:*** Maintane; Proluton Depot; ***Israel:*** Depolut; Proluton Depot; ***Ital.:*** Lentogest; Proluton Depot; ***Malaysia:*** Proluton Depot; ***Mex.:*** Caposten; Primolut Depot; ***Neth.:*** Proluton Depot; ***S.Afr.:*** Primolut Depot†; ***Singapore:*** Proluton Depot; ***Switz.:*** Proluton Depot†; ***Thai.:*** Proluton Depot; ***UK:*** Proluton Depot†; ***USA:*** Hylutin.

**Multi-ingredient:** ***Arg.:*** Dos Dias N; Primosiston; ***Austria:*** Gravibinon†; ***Braz.:*** Gestadinona; Progest†; Trinestril; ***Chile:*** Gravidinona; ***Ger.:*** Gravibinon; Syngynon; ***Ital.:*** Gravibinan; ***Mex.:*** Gravidinona; Primosiston; ***Mon.:*** Tocogestan†; ***Switz.:*** Primosiston.

## Lynestrenol *(BAN, USAN, rINN)*

Ethinylestrenol; Linestrenol; Lynenol; Lynestrenolum; Lynoestrenol; NSC-37725. 19-Nor-17α-pregn-4-en-20-yn-17β-ol.

$C_{20}H_{28}O$ = 284.4.

*CAS — 52-76-6.*

*ATC — G03AC02; G03DC03.*

**Pharmacopoeias.** In *Eur.* (see p.vi).

**Ph. Eur. 5.0** (Lynestrenol). A white or almost white crystalline powder. Practically insoluble in water; soluble in alcohol and in acetone. Protect from light.

### Profile

Lynestrenol is a progestogen (see Progesterone, p.1566) structurally related to norethisterone that is used alone or as the progestogenic component of oral contraceptives (see p.1527). Typical oral daily doses for contraception are 0.5 mg when used as a progestogen-only preparation, and 0.75 to 2.5 mg when combined with an oestrogen. When used alone for menstrual disorders, doses of 5 to 10 mg daily are given, often as cyclical regimens.

**Porphyria.** Lynestrenol has been associated with acute attacks of porphyria and is considered unsafe in porphyric patients.

### Preparations

**Proprietary Preparations** (details are given in Part 3)

***Arg.:*** Exluton; ***Austria:*** Orgametril; ***Belg.:*** Exluton†; Orgametril; ***Braz.:*** Exluton; ***Chile:*** Exluton; Linosun; Normalac; ***Denm.:*** Exlutona†; Orgametril; ***Fin.:*** Exluton; Orgametril; ***Fr.:*** Exluton†; Orgametril; ***Ger.:*** Exlutona†; Orgametril; ***Gr.:*** Orgametril; ***Mex.:*** Exluton; ***Neth.:*** Exluton†; Orgametril; ***Norw.:*** Exlutona; ***Port.:*** Exluton; Orgametril; ***Spain:*** Orgametril; ***Swed.:*** Exlutena; Orgametril; ***Switz.:*** Exlutona†; ***Thai.:*** Exluton.

**Multi-ingredient:** ***Arg.:*** Lindiol; ***Austria:*** Lyndiol†; Ovanon†; Yermonil; ***Belg.:*** Fysioquens†; Lyndiol†; Ministat†; Ovanon†; Ovostat†; ***Braz.:*** Anacyclin; Ovoresta; ***Chile:*** Anovulatorios; ***Denm.:*** Lyndiol†; ***Fr.:*** Ovanon†; Physiostat†; ***Ger.:*** Anacyclin†; Lyn-ratiopharm-Sequenz; Lyn-ratiopharm†; Lyndiol†; Nuriphasic†; Ovanon†; Ovoresta M; Ovoresta†; Pregnon L†; Yermonil†; ***Hong Kong:*** Lyndiol†; ***Neth.:*** Fysioquens; Mini Pregnon; Ministat; Ovanon; Ovostat; ***S.Afr.:*** Ovostat†; ***Spain:*** Neo Lyndiol†; ***Swed.:*** Lyndiolett†; Restovar; ***Switz.:*** Normophasic†; Ovanon†; Yermonil†; ***Thai.:*** Lyndiol.

## Medrogestone *(BAN, USAN, rINN)*

AY-62022; Medrogestona; Metrogestone; NSC-123018; R-13-615. 6,17α-Dimethylpregna-4,6-diene-3,20-dione.

$C_{23}H_{32}O_2$ = 340.5.

*CAS — 977-79-7.*

*ATC — G03DB03.*

### Profile

Medrogestone is a progestogen structurally related to progesterone (p.1566) that is used in the treatment of menstrual disorders, and as the progestogen in menopausal HRT (see p.1536). It is usually given in daily doses of 5 to 10 mg by mouth, generally in a cyclical regimen. Higher doses were used in the treatment of endometrial carcinoma, prostatic hyperplasia, and breast disorders including carcinoma. It has also been used for threatened or recurrent miscarriage, but such use is not recommended unless there is proven progesterone deficiency.

### Preparations

**Proprietary Preparations** (details are given in Part 3)

***Austria:*** Colpron; ***Belg.:*** Colpro; ***Canad.:*** Colprone†; ***Fr.:*** Colprone; ***Ger.:*** Prothil; ***Hong Kong:*** Colprone; ***Ital.:*** Colprone†; ***Neth.:*** Colpro†; ***S.Afr.:*** Colpro; ***Spain:*** Colpro; ***Switz.:*** Colpro; ***Thai.:*** Colprone†.

**Multi-ingredient:** ***Austria:*** Premarin compositum; Premarin Plus; ***Belg.:*** Premplus; ***Ger.:*** Presomen compositum; ***Hong Kong:*** Prempak; ***Ital.:*** Prempak; ***Malaysia:*** Prempak; ***Mex.:*** Premarin Pak†; ***Neth.:*** Premarin Plus; ***Port.:*** Premarin Plus; ***S.Afr.:*** Prempak N; ***Switz.:*** Premarin Plus; ***Thai.:*** Prempak†.

## Medroxyprogesterone Acetate

*(BANM, rINNM)*

Acetato de medroxiprogesterona; Medroxyprogesteroni Acetas; Methylacetoxyprogesterone; Metipregnone; NSC-26386. 6α-Methyl-3,20-dioxopregn-4-en-17α-yl acetate; 17α-Hydroxy-6α-methylpregn-4-ene-3,20-dione acetate.

$C_{24}H_{34}O_4$ = 386.5.

*CAS — 520-85-4 (medroxyprogesterone); 71-58-9 (medroxyprogesterone acetate).*

*ATC — G03AC06; G03DA02; L02AB02.*

**Pharmacopoeias.** In *Chin., Eur.* (see p.vi), *Int., Pol.,* and *US.*

**Ph. Eur. 5.0** (Medroxyprogesterone Acetate). A white or almost white crystalline powder. Practically insoluble in water; sparingly soluble in alcohol; soluble in acetone and in dioxan; freely soluble in dichloromethane. Protect from light.

**USP 27** (Medroxyprogesterone Acetate). A white to off-white, odourless, crystalline powder. Insoluble in water; sparingly soluble in alcohol and in methyl alcohol; soluble in acetone and in dioxan; freely soluble in chloroform; slightly soluble in ether. Store in airtight containers at a temperature of 25°, excursions permitted between 15° and 30°. Protect from light.

### Adverse Effects and Precautions

As for progestogens in general (see Progesterone, p.1566). See also under Hormonal Contraceptives, p.1527. Medroxyprogesterone acetate may have glucocorticoid effects when given long term at high doses.

**Breast feeding.** Medroxyprogesterone is reported to be distributed into breast milk when given as a depot progestogen-only contraceptive.[1] No adverse effects have been observed in breast-fed infants whose mothers were receiving medroxyprogesterone, and the American Academy of Pediatrics considers[2] that it is therefore usually compatible with breast feeding. Progestogen-only parenteral contraceptives should not be given until 6 weeks after birth if the women is breast feeding (see Breast Feeding under Hormonal Contraceptives, p.1533).

1. Schwallie PC. The effect of depot-medroxyprogesterone acetate on the fetus and nursing infant: a review. *Contraception* 1981; **23:** 375–86.
2. American Academy of Pediatrics. The transfer of drugs and other chemicals into human milk. *Pediatrics* 2001; **108:** 776–89. Correction. *ibid.*; 1029. Also available at: http://aappolicy.aappublications.org/cgi/content/full/pediatrics%3b108/3/776 (accessed 21/06/04)

**Carcinogenicity.** The risk of various cancers associated with the use of depot medroxyprogesterone acetate as a contraceptive has been evaluated by WHO.[1] Overall, there was no increase in risk of breast cancer, although there is some evidence that current or recent use may be associated with a slight increase in risk (see also p.1528). There was no increased risk of cervical cancer (see also p.1528), and a protective effect against endometrial cancer (see p.1529). In contrast to combined oral contraceptives, there was no evidence of a protective effect against ovarian cancer (p.1529).

1. Anonymous. Depot-medroxyprogesterone acetate (DMPA) and cancer: memorandum from a WHO meeting. *Bull WHO* 1993; **71:** 669–76.

**Effects on bone density.** Use of medroxyprogesterone acetate as a parenteral progestogen-only contraceptive has been associated with reductions in bone density (see under Effects on the Musculoskeletal System, p.1532). This effect has also been reported after oral doses for menstrual disorders,[1] and is thought to be due to medroxyprogesterone-induced oestrogen deficiency.

1. Cundy T, *et al.* Short-term effects of high dose oral medroxyprogesterone acetate on bone density in premenopausal women. *J Clin Endocrinol Metab* 1996; **81:** 1014–17.

**Effects on the skin.** Acute local skin necrosis has been reported[1] following the intramuscular injection of medroxyprogesterone acetate as a depot contraceptive.

1. Clark SM, Lanigan SW. Acute necrotic skin reaction to intramuscular Depo-Provera®. *Br J Dermatol* 2000; **143:** 1356–7.

**Glucocorticoid effects.** There have been reports of Cushing's syndrome induced by medroxyprogesterone acetate in patients receiving long-term therapy with high doses for the treatment of malignant neoplasms.[1-5] Cushingoid symptoms regressed when treatment was stopped. Medroxyprogesterone possesses glucocorticoid activity and there is a risk of adrenal insufficiency during periods of stress or after sudden withdrawal of treatment. Some[4] consider that patients should be monitored for glucose intolerance and adrenal insufficiency during treatment.

1. Siminoski K, *et al.* The Cushing syndrome induced by medroxyprogesterone acetate. *Ann Intern Med* 1989; **111:** 758–60.
2. Donckier JE, *et al.* Cushing syndrome and medroxyprogesterone acetate. *Lancet* 1990; **335:** 1094.
3. Grenfell A, *et al.* Cushing's syndrome and medroxyprogesterone acetate. *Lancet* 1990; **336:** 256.
4. Merrin PK, Alexander WD. Cushing's syndrome induced by medroxyprogesterone. *BMJ* 1990; **301:** 345.
5. Shotliff K, Nussey SS. Medroxyprogesterone acetate induced Cushing's syndrome. *Br J Clin Pharmacol* 1997; **44:** 304.

**Porphyria.** Medroxyprogesterone has been associated with acute attacks of porphyria and is considered unsafe in porphyric patients. However, for a reference to the use of medroxyprogesterone acetate with buserelin acetate in the prevention of premenstrual exacerbations of porphyria in 2 women, see p.1320.

### Interactions

As for progestogens in general (see Progesterone, p.1567). Aminoglutethimide markedly reduces plasma concentrations of medroxyprogesterone so that an increase in medroxyprogesterone dosage is likely to be required.

### Pharmacokinetics

Medroxyprogesterone is absorbed from the gastrointestinal tract. In the blood, it is highly protein bound, principally to albumin. It is metabolised in the liver and excreted mainly as glucuronide conjugates in the urine and faeces. It has a half-life of 24 to 30 hours after oral doses; the half-life may be as long as 50 days after intramuscular injection. Medroxyprogesterone is reported to be distributed into breast milk.

### Uses and Administration

Medroxyprogesterone acetate is a progestogen structurally related to progesterone, with actions and uses similar to those of the progestogens in general (see Progesterone, p.1567). It is given by mouth or, for prolonged action, by intramuscular injection as an aqueous suspension.

It is used for the treatment of **menorrhagia** (p.1567) and **secondary amenorrhoea** in doses of 2.5 to 10 mg daily by mouth for 5 to 10 days starting on the assumed or calculated 16th to 21st day of the menstrual cycle, although some sources suggest that treatment may begin on any day in secondary amenorrhoea.

In the treatment of mild to moderate **endometriosis** (p.1546) usual doses are 10 mg three times daily by mouth, or 50 mg weekly or 100 mg every 2 weeks by intramuscular injection. In the UK it is recommended that treatment continue for 90 consecutive days; US sources recommend treatment for at least 6 months.

Medroxyprogesterone acetate is also given by intramuscular injection as a **contraceptive** (see under Hormonal Contraceptives, p.1535). As a progestogen-only contraceptive a dose of 150 mg is given every 12 weeks. A combined contraceptive injection containing medroxyprogesterone acetate 25 mg with estradiol cipionate 5 mg is given monthly.

When used as the progestogen component of **menopausal HRT** (see p.1540), medroxyprogesterone acetate is given orally in a variety of regimens including 1.5, 2.5, or 5 mg daily continuously, 5 or 10 mg daily for 12 to 14 days of a 28-day cycle, and 20 mg daily for 14 days of a 91-day cycle.

Medroxyprogesterone acetate may also be used in the palliative treatment of some hormone-dependent malignant neoplasms. In **breast carcinoma** (see below) doses have ranged from 0.4 to 2 g daily by mouth and from 0.5 g twice weekly to 1 g daily by intramuscular injection. In **endometrial** and **renal carcinoma** (p.516 and p.518, respectively) doses have ranged from 100 to 500 mg daily by mouth and from 0.25 to 1 g weekly by intramuscular injection. Some regimens using intramuscular injections have started with twice-weekly or alternate-day dosing before reducing to a weekly dosage interval, or have started treatment with weekly doses and reduced to a maintenance schedule of as little as 400 mg monthly. In **prostatic carcinoma** (p.521) doses have been 100 to 500 mg daily by mouth and 0.5 g weekly or twice weekly by intramuscular injection.

**Cachexia.** Medroxyprogesterone may improve appetite and food intake, and prevent loss of body-weight in cachexia (p.1558) associated with severe chronic disorders,[1,2] although information is limited.

1. Simons JPFHA, *et al.* Effects of medroxyprogesterone acetate on appetite, weight, and quality of life in advanced-stage non-hormone-sensitive cancer: a placebo-controlled multicenter study. *J Clin Oncol* 1996; **14:** 1077–84.
2. Simons JPFHA, *et al.* Effects of medroxyprogesterone acetate on food intake, body composition, and resting energy expenditure in patients with advanced, nonhormone-sensitive cancer: a randomized, placebo-controlled trial. *Cancer* 1998; **82:** 553–60.

**Contraception.** Medroxyprogesterone acetate has an established use as a parenteral progestogen-only contraceptive (p.1535). It has also been developed as the progestogenic component of a combined injectable contraceptive.

References.
1. Garza-Flores J, *et al.* Introduction of Cyclofem® once-a-month injectable contraceptive in Mexico. *Contraception* 1998; **58:** 7–12.
2. Kaunitz AM, *et al.* Comparative safety, efficacy, and cycle control of Lunelle monthly contraceptive injection (medroxyprogesterone acetate and estradiol cypionate injectable suspension) and Ortho-Novum 7/7/7 oral contraceptive (norethindrone/ethinyl estradiol triphasic). *Contraception* 1999; **60:** 179–87.

**Epilepsy.** Preliminary findings[1] suggested that medroxyprogesterone acetate might be of value in the management of catamenial epilepsy (p.349). In a later review[2] it was suggested that hormonal manipulation with drugs such as medroxyprogesterone should be reserved for highly selected groups under close supervision.

1. Mattson RH, *et al.* Treatment of seizures with medroxyprogesterone acetate: preliminary report. *Neurology* 1984; **34:** 1255–8.
2. Herkes GK. Drug treatment of catamenial epilepsy. *CNS Drugs* 1995; **3:** 260–6.

**Male hypersexuality.** The anti-androgenic action of medroxyprogesterone has been used for suppression of libido in the control of men with deviant or disinhibited sexual behaviour[1-3] (see Disturbed Behaviour, p.665).

1. Kiersch TA. Treatment of sex offenders with Depo-Provera. *Bull Am Acad Psychiatry Law* 1990; **18:** 179–87.
2. Weiner MF, *et al.* Intramuscular medroxyprogesterone acetate for sexual aggression in elderly men. *Lancet* 1992; **339:** 1121–2.
3. Kravitz HM, *et al.* Medroxyprogesterone treatment for paraphiliacs. *Bull Am Acad Psychiatry Law* 1995; **23:** 19–33.

**Malignant neoplasms.** BREAST. Progestogens are used as second- or third-choice drugs in the hormonal therapy of advanced breast cancer (p.514). Some references to the use of medroxyprogesterone acetate in advanced breast cancer are cited below.[1-6] Comparative studies have shown that patients respond equally well to medroxyprogesterone and either mepitiostane,[1] aminoglutethimide,[2] or oophorectomy.[3]

1. Izuo M, *et al.* A phase III trial of oral high-dose medroxyprogesterone acetate (MPA) versus mepitiostane in advanced postmenopausal breast cancer. *Cancer* 1985; **56:** 2576–9.
2. Canney PA, *et al.* Randomized trial comparing aminoglutethimide with high-dose medroxyprogesterone acetate in therapy for advanced breast carcinoma. *J Natl Cancer Inst* 1988; **80:** 1147–51.
3. Martoni A, *et al.* High-dose medroxyprogesterone acetate versus oophorectomy as first-line therapy of advanced breast cancer in premenopausal patients. *Oncology* 1991; **48:** 1–6.
4. Muss HB, *et al.* Tamoxifen versus high-dose oral medroxyprogesterone acetate as initial endocrine therapy for patients with metastatic breast cancer: a Piedmont Oncology Association study. *J Clin Oncol* 1994; **12:** 1630–8.
5. Clinton OP, *et al.* A prospective randomized trial to evaluate different oral dose regimens of medroxyprogesterone acetate in women with advanced breast cancer. *Clin Oncol* 1995; **7:** 251–6.
6. Byrne MJ, *et al.* Medroxyprogesterone acetate addition or substitution for tamoxifen in advanced tamoxifen-resistant breast cancer: a phase III randomized trial. *J Clin Oncol* 1997; **15:** 3141–8.

ENDOMETRIUM. Progestogens are used in the treatment of advanced endometrial carcinoma (p.516) but there are doubts about their value in the earlier stages of disease.[1] Medroxyprogesterone acetate was effective in a rare case of low-grade endometrial stromal sarcoma.[2]

1. Martin-Hirsch PL, *et al.* Progestagens for endometrial cancer. Available in The Cochrane Library; Issue 2. Chichester: John Wiley; 2004.
2. Rand RJ, Lowe JW. Low-grade endometrial stromal sarcoma treated with a progestogen. *Br J Hosp Med* 1990; **43:** 154–6.

**Respiratory disorders.** Reviews of the use of medroxyprogesterone acetate in obstructive sleep apnoea have concluded that it has a limited role.[1,2]

Medroxyprogesterone is commonly used in the treatment of pulmonary lymphangioleiomyomatosis, a rare disease affecting only women.[3,4] Anecdotal evidence suggests some patients improve or stabilise on treatment, possibly those with chylous effusions or chylous ascites.[5]

Medroxyprogesterone acetate was reported to be effective in treating congenital central hypoventilation syndrome in 2 children.[6]

1. Millman RP. Medroxyprogesterone and obstructive sleep apnea. *Chest* 1989; **96:** 225–6.
2. Terra SG, Oberg KC. Medroxyprogesterone acetate in the treatment of obstructive sleep apnea. *Ann Pharmacother* 1997; **31:** 776–8.
3. Johnson S. Lymphangioleiomyomatosis: clinical features, management and basic mechanisms. *Thorax* 1999; **54:** 254–64.
4. Johnson SR, Tattersfield AE. Clinical experience of lymphangioleiomyomatosis in the UK. *Thorax* 2000; **55:** 1052–7.
5. Taylor JR, *et al.* Lymphangioleiomyomatosis: clinical course in 32 patients. *N Engl J Med* 1990; **323:** 1254–60.
6. Milerad J, *et al.* Alveolar hypoventilation treated with medroxyprogesterone. *Arch Dis Child* 1985; **60:** 150–5.

**Sickle-cell disease.** Intramuscular medroxyprogesterone reduced the frequency of painful crises in patients with homozygous sickle-cell disease (p.734),[1] and is considered a suitable contraceptive in women with the condition[2,3] in whom combined oral contraceptives should probably be avoided (see also p.1533).

1. de Ceulaer K, *et al.* Medroxyprogesterone acetate and homozygous sickle-cell disease. *Lancet* 1982; **ii:** 229–31.
2. Guillebaud J. Sickle cell disease and contraception. *BMJ* 1993; **307:** 506–7.
3. Kirkman REJ, Elstein M. Management of sickle cell disease: contraception with medroxyprogesterone may be beneficial. *BMJ* 1998; **316:** 935.

## Preparations

***USP 27:*** Medroxyprogesterone Acetate Injectable Suspension; Medroxyprogesterone Acetate Tablets.

**Proprietary Preparations** (details are given in Part 3)

***Arg.:*** Cycrin; Depo-Provera; Farlutale; Livomedrox; Map An; Medrosterona; Veraplex; ***Austral.:*** Depo-Provera; Depo-Ralovera; Medroxyhexal; Provera; Ralovera; ***Austria:*** Depo-Provera; Depocon; Farlutal; Prodafem; Provera; ***Belg.:*** Depo-Provera; Farlutal; Provera; ***Braz.:*** Acemedrox; Acetoflux; Contracep; Cycrin; Depo-Provera; Farlutal; Medroxitest; Provera; Tricilon; ***Canad.:*** Alti-MPA; Depo-Provera; Gen-Medroxy; Novo-Medrone; Proclim†; Provera; ***Chile:*** Depo-Prodasone; Farlutal; Farlutes; Prodasone; Provera; Sicrit; ***Denm.:*** Depo-Provera; Perlutex; Provera; ***Fin.:*** Cykrina†; Depo-Provera; Farlutal; Gestapuran; Lutopolar; Mepastat; Provera; ***Fr.:*** Depo-Prodasone; Depo-Provera; Farlutal; Gestoral; Prodasone†; ***Ger.:*** Clinofem; Clinovir; Depo-Clinovir; Farlutal; G-Farlutal; GestaPolar†; MPA; MPA Gyn; MPA-beta; MPA-Noury; ***Gr.:*** Depo-Provera; Farlutal; Gestoral; Progevera; Provera; ***Hong Kong:*** Depo-Provera; Farlutal; Provera; ***India:*** Depo-Provera; Meprate; ***Irl.:*** Depo-Provera; Provera; ***Israel:*** Aragest; Depo-Provera; Provera; ***Ital.:*** Depo-Provera; Farlutal; Lutoral†; Provera; ***Malaysia:*** Depo-Provera; Farlutal; Petogen; Provera; Veraplex; ***Mex.:*** Ciclotal; Cycrin; Depo-Provera; Farlutal; Progezzard†; Protarin†; Provera; ***Neth.:*** Depo-Provera; Farlutal; Provera; ***Norw.:*** Depo-Provera; Farlutal; Perlutex; Provera; ***NZ:*** Depo-Provera; Farlutal; Provera; ***Port.:*** Depo-Provera; Provera; ***S.Afr.:*** Depo-Provera; Farlutal†; Petogen†; Provera; ***Singapore:*** Depo-Provera; Farlutal; Provera; ***Spain:*** Depo-Progevera; Farlutal; Progevera; Progevera 250; ***Swed.:*** Cykrina†; Depo-Provera; Farlutal; Gestapuran; Provera; ***Switz.:*** Depo-Provera; Farlutal; Prodafem; ***Thai.:*** Contracep; Depo-Gestin; Depo-Progesno; Depo-Progesta; Depo-Provera; Farlutal; Manodepo; Medeton; Provera; ***UK:*** Adgyn Medro†; Depo-Provera; Farlutal; Provera; ***USA:*** Amen; Cycrin; Depo-Provera; Provera.

**Multi-ingredient:** ***Arg.:*** Dilena; Farludiol; Farludiol Ciclo; Periofem Ciclico; Periofem Continuo; Premelle Ciclico; Premelle Continuo; ***Austral.:*** Divina†; Estrapak†; Menoprem; Premia; Premia Continuous; Premia Low; Provelle; ***Austria:*** Cyclo-Premarin-MPA†; Femipak; Filena; Perennia; Premarin MPA†; Sequennia; Tri-Filena†; ***Belg.:*** Diviplus; Diviva; Premelle; Trivina; ***Braz.:*** Cyclofemina; Dilena; Menosedan Ciclo; Menosedan Fase; Menosedan MPA; Premarin MPA; Premelle; Premelle Ciclo; Prempro Bifasico; Prempro Monofasico; Repogen Ciclo; Repogen Conti; ***Canad.:*** Premplus; ***Chile:*** Climatrol Ht; Climatrol Ht Continuo; Conpremin Pak; Conpremin Pak Plus; Cyclofem; Enadiol CC; Enadiol MP; Estranova 30 Simple; Estranova CC; Farlupost; Farlutal Estrogeno; Kilios; Novafac; Novafac 30; Novafac CC; Novafem; Prempak; Primaquin MP; Primaquin MP Continuo; Profemina CC; Profemina MP; ***Denm.:*** Divina; Divina Plus; Indivina; Klimalet; Klimaxil; Trevina; ***Fin.:*** Divina; Divitren; Indivina; ***Fr.:*** Divina; Diviseq; Duova; Precyclan; ***Ger.:*** Climopax; Climopax Cyclo; Cyclo-Polar†; Estrafemol; Gianda; Indivina; Osmil; Procyclo; Sisare; ***Gr.:*** Divina; Estopause; Premelle; ***Hong Kong:*** Dilena; Premelle; Premelle Cycle; ***Irl.:*** Diviseq; Femplan-MA†; Indivina; Premique; Premique Cycle; Tridestra†; ***Israel:*** Meno-MPA; Premaril MP; Premaril Plus MP; ***Ital.:*** Filena; Premelle C; Premelle S; Premelle Sequenziale; ***Malaysia:*** Plentiva; Plentiva Cycle 5; Premelle; ***Mex.:*** Cyclofemina; Dilena; Premelle; ***Neth.:*** Divina; Premelle; Premelle Cycle; ***Norw.:*** Diviseq; Indivina; ***NZ:*** Menoprem; Premia; Premia Continuous; Provette Continuous†; Provette Sequential†; ***Port.:*** Dilena; Medrivas Antibiotico; Medrivas†; Premelle; Premelle Cycle; ***S.Afr.:*** Divina; Premelle; Trivina; ***Singapore:*** Premelle; Premelle Cycle; ***Spain:*** Medricol†; Medrivas; Medrivas Antib; Perifem; Premelle; Premelle Ciclico; ***Swed.:*** Divina; Divina Plus; Indivina; Premelle; Premelle Sekvens; Trivina; ***Switz.:*** Cyclo-Premella ST; Cyclo-Premella†; Diviseq; Indivina; OestroTabs Plus Cyclic; Premella; Triaval; ***Thai.:*** Indivina; Premelle; Premelle Cycle; ***UK:*** Indivina; Premique; Premique Cycle; Tridestra; ***USA:*** Lunelle; Premphase; Prempro.

# Megestrol Acetate *(BANM, USAN, rINNM)*

Acetato de megestrol; BDH-1298; Compound 5071; Megestroli Acetas; NSC-71423; SC-10363. 6-Methyl-3,20-dioxopregna-4,6-dien-17α-yl acetate; 17α-Hydroxy-6-methylpregna-4,6-diene-3,20-dione acetate.

$C_{24}H_{32}O_4$ = 384.5.

*CAS — 3562-63-8 (megestrol); 595-33-5 (megestrol acetate).*

*ATC — G03AC05; G03DB02; L02AB01.*

**Pharmacopoeias.** In *Chin., Eur.* (see p.vi), and *US.*

**Ph. Eur. 5.0** (Megestrol Acetate). A white or almost white crystalline powder. Practically insoluble in water; sparingly soluble in alcohol; soluble in acetone. Protect from light.

**USP 27** (Megestrol Acetate). A white to creamy-white, essentially odourless, crystalline powder. Insoluble in water; sparingly soluble in alcohol; soluble in acetone; very soluble in chloroform; slightly soluble in ether and in fixed oils. Protect from light.

## Adverse Effects and Precautions

As for progestogens in general (see Progesterone, p.1566). The weight gain that may be observed with megestrol acetate appears to be associated with an increased appetite and food intake rather than with fluid retention. Megestrol acetate may have glucocorticoid effects when given long term.

**Effects on carbohydrate metabolism.** Megestrol therapy has been associated with hyperglycaemia[1,2] or diabetes mellitus[3] in AIDS patients being treated for cachexia. It has been suggested that megestrol produces peripheral insulin resistance due to a glucocorticoid action.[4]

1. Panwalker AP. Hyperglycemia induced by megestrol acetate. *Ann Intern Med* 1992; **116:** 878.
2. Bornemann M, Johnson AC. Endocrine effects of HIV infection. *N Engl J Med* 1993; **328:** 890.
3. Henry K, *et al.* Diabetes mellitus induced by megestrol acetate in a patient with AIDS and cachexia. *Ann Intern Med* 1992; **116:** 53–4.
4. Leinung MC, *et al.* Induction of adrenal suppression by megestrol acetate in patients with AIDS. *Ann Intern Med* 1995; **122:** 843–5.

**Effects on the musculoskeletal system.** Severe pain of the hands reminiscent of carpal tunnel syndrome occurred in 4 women while taking megestrol acetate and melphalan;[1] megestrol appeared to be responsible.

1. DiSaia PJ, Morrow CP. Unusual side effect of megestrol acetate. *Am J Obstet Gynecol* 1977; **129:** 460–1.

**Effects on the respiratory system.** Two cases of hyperpnoea occurred in patients receiving megestrol acetate 80 mg three times daily.[1]

1. Fessel WJ. Megestrol acetate and hyperpnea. *Ann Intern Med* 1989; **110:** 1034–5.

**Glucocorticoid effects.** Megestrol has glucocorticoid-like properties which can result in adrenocortical insufficiency severe enough to require replacement therapy with hydrocortisone.[1-5]

1. Leinung MC, *et al.* Induction of adrenal suppression by megestrol acetate in patients with AIDS. *Ann Intern Med* 1995; **122:** 843–5.
2. Maurer M. Megestrol for AIDS-related anorexia. *Ann Intern Med* 1995; **122:** 880.
3. Stoffer SS, Krakauer JC. Induction of adrenal suppression by megestrol acetate. *Ann Intern Med* 1996; **124:** 613–14.
4. Mann M, *et al.* Glucocorticoidlike activity of megestrol: a summary of Food and Drug Administration experience and a review of the literature. *Arch Intern Med* 1997; **157:** 1651–6.
5. Stockheim JA, *et al.* Adrenal suppression in children with the human immunodeficiency virus treated with megestrol acetate. *J Pediatr* 1999; **134:** 368–70.

**Porphyria.** Megestrol is considered to be unsafe in patients with porphyria because it has been shown to be porphyrinogenic in *animals.*

## Interactions

As for progestogens in general (see Progesterone, p.1567).

## Pharmacokinetics

Absorption of megestrol acetate from the gastrointestinal tract is variable after oral doses; peak drug concentrations in plasma occur 1 to 3 hours after a dose by mouth. Megestrol acetate is highly protein bound in plasma. It undergoes hepatic metabolism, with 57 to 78% of a dose being excreted in the urine and 8 to 30% in the faeces.

## Uses and Administration

Megestrol acetate is a progestogen structurally related to progesterone (p.1567) that is used for the palliative treatment of various cancers.

It is given by mouth in endometrial carcinoma in doses of 40 to 320 mg daily in divided doses, and in doses of 40 mg four times daily or 160 mg once daily in breast cancer.

Megestrol acetate is also used in the treatment of anorexia and cachexia in patients with cancer or AIDS. The usual dose is 800 mg daily, as oral suspension, for one month, followed by a maintenance dose of 400 to 800 mg daily.

**Cachexia.** In some patients with severe chronic disorders or malignant neoplasms, anorexia (loss of appetite) forms part of a syndrome of metabolic abnormalities and progressive physical wasting known as cachexia. Improved nutrition and dietary counselling are usually insufficient to reverse cachexia, and drug therapy has been tried to stimulate appetite and promote weight gain.

In **cancer-related cachexia**, corticosteroids are frequently used for appetite stimulation in patients with advanced malignancies. They appear to be effective in stimulating appetite, although do not appear to promote weight gain.[1-3] High-dose megestrol has produced weight gain in some randomised controlled trials,[4,5] and has been recommended,[1] particularly in slowly progressive disease accompanied by anorexia.[2] Similar properties have been reported with medroxyprogesterone.[3] Anabolic steroids have also been tried, but further evaluation is necessary:[1,2] a comparison of megestrol or dexamethasone with fluoxymesterone found the latter to be less effective than the progestogen or the corticosteroid.[6] Prokinetic drugs such as metoclopramide may be useful in patients whose symptoms are secondary to decreased gastrointestinal motility.[2] Other drugs studied but with little, if any, benefit include cannabinoids, cyproheptadine and hydrazine.[1-3] Megestrol has also been given with ibuprofen.[7]

High-dose megestrol is also effective in adults and children with **HIV-related cachexia**,[8-10] a topic which is discussed further on p.623.

1. Loprinzi CL. Management of cancer anorexia/cachexia. *Support Care Cancer* 1995; **3:** 120–2.
2. Bruera E. Anorexia, cachexia, and nutrition. *BMJ* 1997; **315:** 1219–22.

3. Mantovani G, *et al.* Managing cancer-related anorexia/cachexia. *Drugs* 2001; **61:** 499–514.
4. Loprinzi CL, *et al.* Controlled trial of megestrol acetate for the treatment of cancer anorexia and cachexia. *J Natl Cancer Inst* 1990; **82:** 1127–32.
5. Tchekmedyian NS, *et al.* Megestrol acetate in cancer anorexia and weight loss. *Cancer* 1992; **69:** 1268–74.
6. Loprinzi CL, *et al.* Randomized comparison of megestrol acetate versus dexamethasone versus fluoxymesterone for the treatment of cancer anorexia/cachexia. *J Clin Oncol* 1999; **17:** 3299–3306.
7. McMillan DC, *et al.* A prospective randomized study of megestrol acetate and ibuprofen in gastrointestinal cancer patients with weight loss. *Br J Cancer* 1999; **79:** 495–500.
8. Von Roenn JH, *et al.* Megestrol acetate in patients with AIDS-related cachexia. *Ann Intern Med* 1994; **121:** 393–9.
9. Oster MH, *et al.* Megestrol acetate in patients with AIDS and cachexia. *Ann Intern Med* 1994; **121:** 400–408.
10. Clarick RH, *et al.* Megestrol acetate treatment of growth failure in children infected with human immunodeficiency virus. *Pediatrics* 1997; **99:** 354–7.

**Hot flushes.** Megestrol has been used in female patients with breast cancer who were experiencing hot flushes (to avoid the potentially tumour-stimulating effects of an oestrogen—see Malignant Neoplasms, under Precautions of HRT, p.1539), as well as in men with hot flushes after orchidectomy or anti-androgen therapy for prostate cancer.[1] Therapy, which involved low doses of 20 mg twice daily, was associated with a decrease in frequency of flushes of 50% or more in about three-quarters of all patients.

1. Loprinzi CL, *et al.* Megestrol acetate for the prevention of hot flashes. *N Engl J Med* 1994; **331:** 347–52.

**Malignant neoplasms.** Like some other progestogens megestrol acetate is used in endometrial cancer (p.516), and it has been reported to have similar efficacy to anastrozole[1] and tamoxifen[2] in postmenopausal women with advanced breast cancer (p.514). There was no advantage in terms of response or survival in escalating the standard dose of megestrol (160 mg daily) to 800 or 1600 mg daily in a randomised study in women with breast cancer.[3]

1. Buzdar A, *et al.* Anastrozole, a potent and selective aromatase inhibitor, versus megestrol acetate in postmenopausal women with advanced breast cancer: results of overview analysis of two phase III trials. *J Clin Oncol* 1996; **14:** 2000–11.
2. Stuart NSA, *et al.* A randomised phase III cross-over study of tamoxifen versus megestrol acetate in advanced and recurrent breast cancer. *Eur J Cancer* 1996; **32A:** 1888–92.
3. Abrams J, *et al.* Dose-response trial of megestrol acetate in advanced breast cancer: cancer and Leukemia Group B phase III study 8741. *J Clin Oncol* 1999; **17:** 64–73.

### Preparations

***BP 2003:*** Megestrol Tablets;
***USP 27:*** Megestrol Acetate Oral Suspension; Megestrol Acetate Tablets.

**Proprietary Preparations** (details are given in Part 3)
***Arg.:*** Megace; Meltonar; Varigestrol; ***Austral.:*** Megace; Megostat†; ***Austria:*** Megace; Nia†; ***Belg.:*** Megace; ***Braz.:*** Gynodal; Megastrol†; Megestat; ***Canad.:*** Megace; ***Chile:*** Megace; Mestrel; ***Denm.:*** Megace; Megestin†; ***Fin.:*** Megace; Megestin; ***Fr.:*** Megace; ***Ger.:*** Megestat; ***Gr.:*** Megace; ***Hong Kong:*** Megace; ***India:*** Endace; ***Irl.:*** Megace; ***Israel:*** Megace; ***Ital.:*** Megace; Megestil; Meprogest; ***Malaysia:*** Megace; ***Mex.:*** Megace; Mestrel; Prazoken†; ***Neth.:*** Megace; ***Norw.:*** Megace; ***NZ:*** Megace; Megostat†; ***Port.:*** Acestrol; Megace; ***Singapore:*** Megace; ***Spain:*** Borea; Maygace; Megefren; Megostat; ***Swed.:*** Megace; ***Switz.:*** Megestat; ***Thai.:*** Megace; Mestrel; ***UK:*** Megace; ***USA:*** Megace.

---

## Mepitiostane *(rINN)*

Mepitiostano; S-10364. 17β-(1-Methoxycyclopentyloxy)-2α,3α-epithio-5α-androstane; Cyclopentanone 2α,3α-epithio-5α-androstan-17β-yl methyl acetal.

$C_{25}H_{40}O_2S$ = 404.6.
*CAS — 21362-69-6.*

**Pharmacopoeias.** In *Jpn.*

### Profile

Mepitiostane has androgenic and anabolic properties (see Testosterone, p.1569) and is given by mouth in usual doses of 10 mg twice daily for the management of neoplasms of the breast and anaemia associated with renal failure.

### Preparations

**Proprietary Preparations** (details are given in Part 3)
***Jpn:*** Thioderon.

---

## Mesterolone *(BAN, USAN, rINN)*

Mesterolona; Mesterolonum; NSC-75054; SH-723. 17β-Hydroxy-1α-methyl-5α-androstan-3-one.

$C_{20}H_{32}O_2$ = 304.5.
*CAS — 1424-00-6.*
*ATC — G03BB01.*

**Pharmacopoeias.** In *Eur.* (see p.vi).

**Ph. Eur. 5.0** (Mesterolone). A white or yellowish crystalline powder. Practically insoluble in water; sparingly soluble in acetone, in ethyl acetate, and in methyl alcohol.

### Adverse Effects and Precautions

As for androgens in general (see Testosterone, p.1570).

Mesterolone is reported not to inhibit gonadotrophin secretion or spermatogenesis.

### Uses and Administration

Mesterolone has androgenic properties (see Testosterone, p.1571) but is reported to have less inhibitory effect on intrinsic testicular function than testosterone.

Mesterolone is given by mouth in the treatment of androgen deficiency or male infertility associated with hypogonadism (p.1316) in initial doses of 75 to 100 mg daily followed by doses of 50 to 75 mg daily for maintenance.

### Preparations

**Proprietary Preparations** (details are given in Part 3)
***Austral.:*** Proviron; ***Austria:*** Proviron; ***Belg.:*** Proviron; ***Braz.:*** Proviron; ***Chile:*** Proviron; ***Denm.:*** Mestoranum; ***Fin.:*** Proviron; ***Fr.:*** Proviron†; ***Ger.:*** Proviron; Vistimon; ***Gr.:*** Proviron; ***Hong Kong:*** Proviron; ***India:*** Provironum; ***Israel:*** Proviron; ***Ital.:*** Proviron; ***Malaysia:*** Provironum; Vistimon; ***Mex.:*** Proviron; ***Neth.:*** Proviron; ***Norw.:*** Mestoranum†; ***Port.:*** Proviron; ***S.Afr.:*** Proviron; ***Singapore:*** Provironum; ***Spain:*** Proviron; ***Swed.:*** Mestoranum†; ***Switz.:*** Proviron†; ***Thai.:*** Provironum; ***UK:*** Proviron.

---

## Mestranol *(BAN, USAN, rINN)*

Compound 33355; EE3ME; $EE_3ME$; Ethinyloestradiol-3-methyl Ether; Mestranolum. 3-Methoxy-19-nor-17α-pregna-1,3,5(10)-trien-20-yn-17β-ol.

$C_{21}H_{26}O_2$ = 310.4.
*CAS — 72-33-3.*

**Pharmacopoeias.** In *Eur.* (see p.vi), *Jpn, Pol.,* and *US.*

**Ph. Eur. 5.0** (Mestranol). A white or almost white crystalline powder. Practically insoluble in water; sparingly soluble in alcohol. Protect from light.

**USP 27** (Mestranol). A white to creamy-white, odourless, crystalline powder. Insoluble in water; sparingly soluble in dehydrated alcohol; freely soluble in chloroform; soluble in dioxan; slightly soluble in methyl alcohol. Protect from light.

### Adverse Effects and Precautions

As for oestrogens in general (see Estradiol, p.1550). See also under Hormonal Contraceptives, p.1527.

**Porphyria.** Mestranol is considered to be unsafe in patients with porphyria because it has been shown to be porphyrinogenic in *animals* or *in-vitro* systems.

### Interactions

See under Hormonal Contraceptives, p.1534.

### Pharmacokinetics

Mestranol is readily absorbed from the gastrointestinal tract. About 70% is metabolised in the liver to ethinylestradiol and its glucuronide. Excretion is via the kidneys and bile; metabolites undergo enterohepatic recycling. Compared with many other oestrogens, its metabolism is slow. The biological half-life is about 50 hours.

### Uses and Administration

Mestranol is a synthetic oestrogen prodrug that is rapidly metabolised to ethinylestradiol; it therefore has actions similar to those of estradiol (see p.1551). It is used as the oestrogen component of combined oral contraceptive preparations (see p.1535) in a usual dose of 50 micrograms daily. The progestogen component is often norethisterone. Mestranol has also been used as the oestrogen component of some preparations for menopausal HRT (see p.1536), although natural oestrogens are often preferred. It has usually been given in a sequential regimen with doses ranging from 12.5 to 50 micrograms daily, with a cyclical progestogen.

### Preparations

***USP 27:*** Ethynodiol Diacetate and Mestranol Tablets; Norethindrone and Mestranol Tablets.

**Proprietary Preparations** (details are given in Part 3)
**Multi-ingredient:** ***Austral.:*** Norinyl-1; ***Austria:*** Ortho-Novum; ***Belg.:*** Ortho-Novum 1/50†; ***Braz.:*** Biofim†; Megestran; ***Canad.:*** Norinyl 1/50†; Ortho-Novum 1/50; ***Chile:*** Anovulatorios; ***Ger.:*** Gestamestrol N; Ortho-Novum 1/50†; Ovosiston; ***Hong Kong:*** Norinyl-1; ***Irl.:*** Menophase†; Norinyl-1†; Ortho-Novin†; ***Mex.:*** Lutoral E; Norace; Norinyl; Ortho-Novum; Secuentex-21; ***NZ:*** Norinyl-1; ***S.Afr.:*** Norinyl-1/28; ***Thai.:*** Anamai; ***UK:*** Norinyl-1; ***USA:*** Genora 1/50†; Necon 1/50; Nelova 1/50M†; Norethin 1/50M†; Norinyl 1 + 50; Ortho-Novum 1/50.

---

## Metenolone Acetate *(BANM, rINNM)*

Acetato de metenolona; Methenolone Acetate *(USAN)*; NSC-74226; SH-567; SQ-16496. 17β-Hydroxy-1-methyl-5α-androst-1-en-3-one acetate.

$C_{22}H_{32}O_3$ = 344.5.
*CAS — 153-00-4 (metenolone); 434-05-9 (metenolone acetate).*
*ATC — A14AA04.*

**Pharmacopoeias.** In *Jpn.*

## Metenolone Enantate *(BANM, rINNM)*

Enantato de metenolona; Methenolone Enanthate *(USAN)*; Methenolone Oenanthate; NSC-64967; SH-601; SQ-16374. 17β-Hydroxy-1-methyl-5α-androst-1-en-3-one heptanoate.

$C_{27}H_{42}O_3$ = 414.6.
*CAS — 303-42-4.*
*ATC — A14AA04.*

**Pharmacopoeias.** In *Jpn.*

### Profile

Metenolone is an anabolic steroid (see Testosterone, p.1569) that has been used in treating aplastic anaemia, breast cancer, and postmenopausal osteoporosis. It has been given by mouth as the acetate in usual doses of 10 to 20 mg daily (although higher doses have been given), and intramuscularly as the enantate in doses of 100 mg every 2 to 4 weeks.

### Preparations

**Proprietary Preparations** (details are given in Part 3)
***Austral.:*** Primobolan; ***Austria:*** Primobolan†; ***Ger.:*** Primobolan; ***Gr.:*** Primobolan Depot; ***Ital.:*** Primobolan Depot†; ***Mex.:*** Primobolan; ***Neth.:*** Primobolan S; ***Norw.:*** Primobolan†; ***S.Afr.:*** Primobolan; ***Spain:*** Primobolan Depot.

**Multi-ingredient:** ***Ger.:*** AntiFocal N; NeyChondrin N (Revitorgan-Dilutionen N Nr 68); NeyGeront N (Revitorgan-Dilutionen N Nr 64); Ney-Pulpin N (Revitorgan-Dilutionen N Nr 10); NeyTumorin N (Revitorgan-Dilutionen N Nr 66).

---

## Methandienone *(BAN)*

Metandienone *(pINN)*; Metandienona; Methandrostenolone; NSC-42722. 17β-Hydroxy-17α-methylandrosta-1,4-dien-3-one.

$C_{20}H_{28}O_2$ = 300.4.
*CAS — 72-63-9.*
*ATC — A14AA03; D11AE01.*

**Pharmacopoeias.** In *Pol.*

### Adverse Effects and Precautions

As for androgens and anabolic steroids in general (see Testosterone, p.1570).

As with other 17α-alkylated compounds, methandienone is associated with hepatotoxicity and hepatic function should be monitored during therapy. It should probably be avoided in patients with hepatic impairment, and certainly if this is severe.

**Effects on the liver.** References to carcinoma of the liver in one patient[1] given methandienone and benign liver-cell adenoma in another.[2]

1. Johnson FL, *et al.* Association of androgenic-anabolic steroid therapy with development of hepatocellular carcinoma. *Lancet* 1972; **ii:** 1273–6.
2. Hernandez-Nieto L, *et al.* Benign liver-cell adenoma associated with long-term administration of an androgenic-anabolic steroid (methandienone). *Cancer* 1977; **40:** 1761–4.

### Uses and Administration

Methandienone has anabolic and some androgenic properties (see Testosterone, p.1571). It has little progestogenic activity. Methandienone has been given by mouth as an anabolic drug.

### Preparations

**Proprietary Preparations** (details are given in Part 3)
***Thai.:*** Anabol; Melic.

---

## Methyltestosterone *(BAN, rINN)*

Methyltestosteronum; Metiltestosterona; NSC-9701. 17β-Hydroxy-17α-methylandrost-4-en-3-one.

$C_{20}H_{30}O_2$ = 302.5.
*CAS — 58-18-4.*
*ATC — G03BA02.*

**Pharmacopoeias.** In *Chin., Eur.* (see p.vi), *Int., Jpn, Pol.,* and *US.*

**Ph. Eur. 5.0** (Methyltestosterone). A white or slightly yellowish-white, crystalline powder. Practically insoluble in water; freely soluble in alcohol. Protect from light.

**USP 27** (Methyltestosterone). White or creamy-white, odourless, slightly hygroscopic, crystals or crystalline powder. Practically insoluble in water; soluble in alcohol, in ether, in methyl alcohol, and in other organic solvents; sparingly soluble in vegetable oils. Protect from light.

### Adverse Effects and Precautions

As for androgens and anabolic steroids in general (see Testosterone, p.1570).

As with other 17α-alkylated compounds, methyltestosterone can produce a cholestatic hepatitis with jaundice, and has caused peliosis hepatis and hepatic neoplasms (see below). Methyltestosterone should be used with caution in patients with liver impairment, and is probably best avoided if this is severe. Liver function should be monitored during therapy.

**Effects on the liver.** Reports of peliosis hepatis[1] and liver damage[2-4] associated with methyltestosterone.

See also under Malignant Neoplasms, below.


1. Bagheri SA, *et al.* Peliosis hepatis associated with androgenic-anabolic steroid therapy: a severe form of hepatic injury. *Ann Intern Med* 1974; **81:** 610–18.
2. Westaby D, *et al.* Liver damage from long-term methyltestosterone. *Lancet* 1977; **ii:** 261–3.
3. Lowdell CP, Murray-Lyon IM. Reversal of liver damage due to long term methyltestosterone and safety of non-17 α-alkylated androgens. *BMJ* 1985; **291:** 637.
4. Borhan-Manesh F, Farnum JB. Methyltestosterone-induced cholestasis: the importance of disproportionately low serum alkaline phosphatase level. *Arch Intern Med* 1989; **124:** 2127–9.


MALIGNANT NEOPLASMS. Reports of hepatocellular carcinoma[1-6] and hepatic adenoma[5,7] associated with methyltestosterone.


1. Johnson FL, *et al.* Association of androgenic-anabolic steroid therapy with development of hepatocellular carcinoma. *Lancet* 1972; **ii:** 1273–6.
2. Henderson JT, *et al.* Androgenic-anabolic steroid therapy and hepatocellular carcinoma. *Lancet* 1973; **i:** 934.
3. Farrell GC, *et al.* Androgen-induced hepatoma. *Lancet* 1975; **i:** 430–2.
4. Goodman MA, Laden AMJ. Hepatocellular carcinoma in association with androgen therapy. *Med J Aust* 1977; **1:** 220–1.
5. Boyd PR, Mark GJ. Multiple hepatic adenomas and a hepatocellular carcinoma in a man on oral methyl testosterone for eleven years. *Cancer* 1977; **40:** 1765–70.
6. Gleeson D, *et al.* Androgen associated hepatocellular carcinoma with an aggressive course. *Gut* 1991; **32:** 1084–6.
7. Coombes GB, *et al.* An androgen-associated hepatic adenoma in a trans-sexual. *Br J Surg* 1978; **65:** 869–70.


**Pregnancy.** For reference to virilisation of a female fetus whose mother received methyltestosterone during pregnancy, see p.1571.

## Interactions

As for androgens and anabolic steroids in general (see Testosterone, p.1571).

## Pharmacokinetics

Methyltestosterone is absorbed from the gastrointestinal tract and from the oral mucosa. It undergoes less extensive first-pass hepatic metabolism than testosterone after oral doses, and has a longer half-life.

## Uses and Administration

As for androgens and anabolic steroids in general (see Testosterone, p.1571).

Methyltestosterone is effective when given by mouth; its effect is increased about twofold when given buccally, as this avoids first-pass hepatic metabolism.

Suggested doses of methyltestosterone for androgen replacement therapy in male hypogonadism (p.1316) have been 10 to 50 mg daily by mouth or 5 to 25 mg daily buccally. Doses of 50 to 200 mg daily by mouth or 25 to 100 mg daily buccally have been given for metastatic breast carcinoma (p.514) in postmenopausal women. Doses of 1.25 to 2.5 mg daily by mouth have been given with oestrogens for the short-term treatment of menopausal vasomotor symptoms unresponsive to oestrogens alone.

## Preparations

***USP 27:*** Methyltestosterone Capsules; Methyltestosterone Tablets.

**Proprietary Preparations** (details are given in Part 3)

***Canad.:*** Metandren†; ***Israel:*** Testotonic B†; ***USA:*** Android; Oreton Methyl†; Testred; Virilon.

**Multi-ingredient:** ***Austria:*** Pasuma-Dragees; ***Braz.:*** Ero Test†; Gabecon M; Gabormon†; Gerosenil†; Ioimbina Composta†; Neurofitol†; Sexormom†; Testonus†; ***Chile:*** Delitan; Feminova-T; ***Fin.:*** Potentol; ***Hong Kong:*** Gerivit†; Wari-Procomil; ***India:*** Mixogen; ***Mex.:*** Bigenol; ***Thai.:*** Hormone Multicap; Horon; Men Hormone; Wari-Procomil; ***UK:*** Prowess†; ***USA:*** Estratest; Menogen†; Premarin with Methyltestosterone†.

## Mibolerone *(BAN, USAN, rINN)*

Mibolerona; NSC-72260; U-10997. 17β-Hydroxy-7α,17-dimethylestr-4-en-3-one.

$C_{20}H_{30}O_2$ = 302.5.

*CAS — 3704-09-4.*

**Pharmacopoeias.** In *US* for veterinary use only.

**USP 27** (Mibolerone). A white to off-white powder. Practically insoluble in water; slightly soluble in chloroform, in dioxan, and in dichloromethane.

### Profile

Mibolerone is an androgen that is used in veterinary practice as a contraceptive for female dogs. It also has anabolic properties.

## Mifepristone *(BAN, USAN, rINN)*

Mifepristona; RU-486; RU-38486. 11β-(4-Dimethylaminophenyl)-17β-hydroxy-17α-prop-1-ynylestra-4,9-dien-3-one.

$C_{29}H_{35}NO_2$ = 429.6.

*CAS — 84371-65-3.*

*ATC — G03XB01.*

## Adverse Effects

In a small proportion of patients given mifepristone uterine bleeding may be severe enough to warrant transfusion and curettage. Few patients have experienced pain after use of mifepristone although uterine pain is often experienced after subsequent use of a prostaglandin. Malaise, faintness, dizziness, chills, fever, headache, nausea, vomiting, and skin rashes have been reported. Uterine and urinary-tract infections have occurred in a small number of patients.

**Effects on the cardiovascular system.** A 31-year-old woman died from cardiovascular shock during an abortion induced by mifepristone followed by sulprostone.[1] She was a heavy cigarette smoker.


1. Anonymous. A death associated with mifepristone/sulprostone. *Lancet* 1991; **337:** 969–70.


## Precautions

Mifepristone should not be given to women with a suspected ectopic pregnancy, to those with chronic adrenal failure or severe uncontrolled asthma. Use in those with renal or hepatic impairment is also not recommended. Women over 35 years of age who are smokers should not receive mifepristone with a prostaglandin for pregnancy termination. Mifepristone should be given with care to patients with less severe asthma or with chronic obstructive airways diseases, haemorrhagic or cardiovascular disease or associated risk factors, or anaemia. Therapy may need to be adjusted in patients receiving long-term corticosteroid treatment; a corticosteroid may need to be given if acute adrenal suppression is suspected. Care is also required in patients receiving anticoagulants because of the increased risk of severe bleeding. Patients with prosthetic heart valves or those with a history of infective endocarditis should be given chemoprophylaxis when undergoing pregnancy termination. As with other means of terminating pregnancy, rhesus-negative women who have not been rhesus immunised will require protection with anti-D immunoglobulin.

**Porphyria.** Mifepristone is considered to be unsafe in patients with porphyria although there is conflicting experimental evidence of porphyrinogenicity.

**Pregnancy.** Studies in *rabbits*, but not *rats* or *mice*, suggest mifepristone causes fetal malformation. There have been reports of normal fetal development following the use of mifepristone alone in mothers who subsequently decided to continue their pregnancy.[1,2] However, in one woman, use of mifepristone was possibly related to malformations of the fetus including sirenomelia.[2]


1. Lim BH, *et al.* Normal development after exposure to mifepristone in early pregnancy. *Lancet* 1990; **336:** 257–8.
2. Pons J-C, *et al.* Development after exposure to mifepristone in early pregnancy. *Lancet* 1991; **338:** 763.


## Interactions

Aspirin and NSAIDs should be avoided until complete termination of pregnancy has been confirmed, because of a theoretical risk that prostaglandin synthetase inhibitors may alter the efficacy of mifepristone.

## Pharmacokinetics

After oral doses peak plasma concentrations of mifepristone occur after 1.3 hours; bioavailability is about 70%. Elimination is biphasic; a slow phase is followed by a more rapid terminal phase, with an elimination half-life of about 18 hours. Mifepristone undergoes hepatic metabolism, and metabolites are excreted in the bile and eliminated in the faeces. Only a small fraction is detected in the urine. Mifepristone is about 98% bound to plasma proteins, mainly $\alpha_1$-acid glycoprotein.

## Uses and Administration

Mifepristone is a steroid derived from norethisterone. It has potent antiprogestogenic activity, and is used for the medical termination of pregnancy (p.1512), softening and dilatation of the cervix prior to surgical termination of pregnancy, and for the induction of labour following fetal death *in utero*.

In the UK the licensed regimen for the **termination** of pregnancies of up to 63 days' gestation, is to give a single oral dose of 600 mg of mifepristone followed by the prostaglandin gemeprost 1 mg vaginally 36 to 48 hours later, unless abortion has already been completed. In the USA the licensed regimen for the termination of pregnancies up to 49 days' gestation is a single oral dose of 600 mg of mifepristone followed 2 days later by 400 micrograms of misoprostol by mouth, unless abortion has already been completed. Lower doses of mifepristone have been employed effectively in some studies, as have different prostaglandins. See also Termination of Pregnancy, below. For the termination of pregnancy between 13 and 24 weeks' gestation the licensed dose in the UK is a single oral dose of mifepristone 600 mg; this is given 36 to 48 hours before scheduled prostaglandin termination of pregnancy, thus shortening the duration of the procedure and reducing the dose of prostaglandin required.

For **softening** and **dilatation of the cervix** prior to surgical termination of pregnancy a single 600-mg dose of mifepristone is given 36 to 48 hours before the procedure.

For labour induction following intra-uterine **fetal death**, mifepristone 600 mg is given daily for 2 consecutive days; if labour has not started within 72 hours of the first dose, other methods of induction should be used.

Mifepristone has been tried for **other uses** such as postcoital contraception, endometriosis, uterine fibroids (leiomyomas), and for progestogen-dependent neoplasms such as meningiomas. Mifepristone also has anti-glucocorticoid activity and has been used in the treatment of Cushing's syndrome.

◊ General references.


1. Heikinheimo O. Clinical pharmacokinetics of mifepristone. *Clin Pharmacokinet* 1997; **33:** 7–17.
2. Mahajan DK, London SN. Mifepristone (RU486): a review. *Fertil Steril* 1997; **68:** 967–76.
3. Koide SS. Mifepristone: auxiliary therapeutic use in cancer and related disorders. *J Reprod Med* 1998; **43:** 551–60.
4. DeHart RM, Morehead MS. Mifepristone. *Ann Pharmacother* 2001; **35:** 707–19.


**Contraception.** A single 600-mg dose of mifepristone has been established as an effective emergency contraceptive (p.1536) when given within 72 hours postcoitally (pre-implantation).[1,2] More recently, mifepristone has also been shown to be effective within 120 hours of unprotected coitus; a very low dose of 10 mg appeared to be similar in efficacy to the 600-mg dose and caused less disturbance of the menstrual cycle.[3] Mifepristone has also been used 2 to 3 weeks postcoitally (post-implantation).[4] The development of a mifepristone-based standard contraceptive (p.1535) has been less successful. Regimens based on daily,[5] weekly,[6] or monthly[7] administration of mifepristone have been investigated.


1. Glasier A, *et al.* Mifepristone (RU 486) compared with high-dose estrogen and progestogen for emergency postcoital contraception. *N Engl J Med* 1992; **327:** 1041–4.
2. Webb AMC, *et al.* Comparison of Yuzpe regimen, danazol, and mifepristone (RU 486) in oral postcoital contraception. *BMJ* 1992; **305:** 927–31.
3. Task Force on Postovulatory Methods of Fertility Regulation. Comparison of three single doses of mifepristone as emergency contraception: a randomised trial. *Lancet* 1999; **353:** 697–702.
4. Lähteenmäki P, *et al.* Late postcoital treatment against pregnancy with antiprogesterone RU 486. *Fertil Steril* 1988; **50:** 36–8.
5. Brown A, *et al.* Daily low-dose mifepristone has contraceptive potential by suppressing ovulation and menstruation: a double-blind randomized control trial of 2 and 5 mg per day for 120 days. *J Clin Endocrinol Metab* 2002; **87:** 63–70.
6. Marions L, *et al.* Contraceptive efficacy of low doses of mifepristone. *Fertil Steril* 1998; **70:** 813–16.
7. Swahn ML, *et al.* Contraception with mifepristone. *Lancet* 1991; **338:** 942–3.


**Cushing's syndrome.** Mifepristone may be useful in Cushing's syndrome (p.1313) because of its glucocorticoid antagonist effects.

References.


1. Nieman LK, *et al.* Successful treatment of Cushing's syndrome with the glucocorticoid antagonist RU 486. *J Clin Endocrinol Metab* 1985; **61:** 536–40.
2. van der Lely A-J, *et al.* Rapid reversal of acute psychosis in the Cushing syndrome with the cortisol-receptor antagonist mifepristone (RU 486). *Ann Intern Med* 1991; **114:** 143–4.
3. Sartor O, Cutler GB. Mifepristone: treatment of Cushing's syndrome. *Clin Obstet Gynecol* 1996; **39:** 506–10.
4. Chu JW, *et al.* Successful long-term treatment of refractory Cushing's disease with high-dose mifepristone (RU 486). *J Clin Endocrinol Metab* 2001; **86:** 3568–73.

**Ectopic pregnancy.** Methotrexate with mifepristone may be more effective than methotrexate alone for the medical treatment of ectopic pregnancy (p.572).

References.


1. Gazvani MR, *et al.* Mifepristone in combination with methotrexate for the medical treatment of tubal pregnancy: a randomized, controlled trial. *Hum Reprod* 1998; **13:** 1987–90.
2. Perdu M, *et al.* Treating ectopic pregnancy with the combination of mifepristone and methotrexate: a phase II nonrandomized study. *Am J Obstet Gynecol* 1998; **179:** 640–3.


**Endometriosis.** Some results[1,2] have suggested that mifepristone, which is capable of suppressing ovarian function, may be of benefit in patients with endometriosis (p.1546).


1. Kettel LM, *et al.* Endocrine responses to long-term administration of the antiprogesterone RU486 in patients with pelvic endometriosis. *Fertil Steril* 1991; **56:** 402–7.
2. Kettel LM, *et al.* Preliminary report on the treatment of endometriosis with low-dose mifepristone (RU 486). *Am J Obstet Gynecol* 1998; **178:** 1151–6.


**Fibroids.** Mifepristone has been reported to produce significant decreases in tumour volume when given to patients with uterine leiomyomas,[1,2] and produced comparable results to a gonadorelin analogue (p.1326) as an adjunct to surgery.


1. Murphy AA, *et al.* Regression of uterine leiomyomata in response to the antiprogesterone RU 486. *J Clin Endocrinol Metab* 1993; **76:** 513–17.
2. Murphy AA, *et al.* Regression of uterine leiomyomata to the antiprogesterone RU486: dose-response effect. *Fertil Steril* 1995; **64:** 187–90.


**Induction of labour.** Some references to the use of mifepristone for cervical ripening and labour induction where intra-uterine fetal death has occurred,[1] or at term.[2-5] A systematic review[6] of the latter use considered that mifepristone was better than placebo but that there was still insufficient evidence to support its use. See also p.1511.


1. Cabrol D, *et al.* Induction of labor with mifepristone (RU 486) in intrauterine fetal death. *Am J Obstet Gynecol* 1990; **163:** 540–2.
2. Frydman R, *et al.* Labor induction in women at term with mifepristone (RU486): a double-blind, randomized, placebo-controlled study. *Obstet Gynecol* 1992; **80:** 972–5.
3. Giacalone PL, *et al.* Cervical ripening with mifepristone before labor induction: a randomized study. *Obstet Gynecol* 1998; **92:** 487–92.
4. Elliott CL, *et al.* The effects of mifepristone on cervical ripening and labor induction in primigravidae. *Obstet Gynecol* 1998; **92:** 804–9.
5. Stenlund PM, *et al.* Induction of labor with mifepristone—a randomized, double-blind study versus placebo. *Acta Obstet Gynecol Scand* 1999; **78:** 793–8.
6. Neilson JP. Mifepristone for induction of labour. Available in The Cochrane Library; Issue 2. Chichester: John Wiley; 2004.


**Malignant neoplasms.** Mifepristone has been used successfully in some patients with inoperable meningioma,[1-3] a brain tumour that may be progestogen-receptor positive. Preliminary data on mifepristone in patients with breast cancer (p.514) had been encouraging,[4] but in a later study response rates were low.[5]


1. Haak HR, *et al.* Successful mifepristone treatment of recurrent, inoperable meningioma. *Lancet* 1990; **336:** 124–5.
2. Grunberg SM, *et al.* Treatment of unresectable meningiomas with the antiprogesterone agent mifepristone. *J Neurosurg* 1991; **74:** 861–6.
3. Lamberts SWJ, *et al.* Mifepristone (RU 486) treatment of meningiomas. *J Neurol Neurosurg Psychiatry* 1992; **55:** 486–90.
4. Bakker G, *et al.* Treatment of breast cancer with different antiprogestins: preclinical and clinical studies. *J Steroid Biochem Mol Biol* 1990; **37:** 789–94.
5. Perrault D, *et al.* Phase II study of the progesterone antagonist mifepristone in patients with untreated metastatic breast carcinoma: a National Cancer Institute of Canada Clinical Trials Group study. *J Clin Oncol* 1996; **14:** 2709–12.


**Termination of pregnancy.** For the termination of early pregnancy (prior to 9 weeks' gestation), mifepristone combined with a prostaglandin is an effective alternative to surgical methods.[1,2] Termination success rates are highest prior to 7 weeks' gestation; after this the success rate for mifepristone with oral misoprostol tends to decrease compared with other regimens.[1,2] Mifepristone has been used alone, but it is not sufficiently effective as a single agent.[2] The usual dose of mifepristone is 600 mg, although lower doses of 200 and 400 mg have been studied in various regimens with prostaglandins and found to be as effective. However, the manufacturers have commented that there was no evidence that a lower dose was better tolerated, and that early studies using mifepristone without a prostaglandin had indicated a significantly higher risk of ongoing pregnancy with lower doses.[3] Mifepristone is also used to ripen the cervix prior to surgical termination of pregnancy,[4-8] and in combination with a prostaglandin for second trimester termination (13 to 20 weeks' gestation).[9-13] Similarly to early termination, a study found mifepristone 200 mg to be as effective as 600 mg when combined with misoprostol for second trimester termination.[13] A further review of 500 cases also reported mifepristone 200 mg combined with misoprostol to be effective.[14] Preliminary evidence indicated that mifepristone plus a prostaglandin is also effective for medical termination of pregnancy at 9 to 13 weeks' gestation.[15]

In the UK the Royal College of Obstetricians and Gynaecologists' guidelines[16] for both early and mid-trimester terminations include the following regimens:

- For gestation up to 7 weeks (and as an option for gestation of 7 to 9 weeks), mifepristone 200 mg by mouth followed 36 hours later by gemeprost 500 micrograms vaginally.
- For mid-trimester termination (over 15 weeks), mifepristone 200 mg by mouth followed 36 hours later by gemeprost 1 mg every 6 hours vaginally.

For a discussion of the termination of pregnancy, see p.1512.


1. Kahn JG, *et al.* The efficacy of medical abortion: a meta analysis. *Contraception* 2000; **61:** 29–40.
2. Christin-Maitre S, *et al.* Medical termination of pregnancy. *N Engl J Med* 2000; **342:** 946–56.
3. Ulmann A, Barnard J. Termination of pregnancy with mifepristone. *BMJ* 1993; **307:** 684.
4. Rådestad A, *et al.* Induced cervical ripening with mifepristone in first trimester abortion: a double-blind randomized biomechanical study. *Contraception* 1988; **38:** 301–12.
5. Gupta JK, Johnson N. Effect of mifepristone on dilatation of the pregnant and non-pregnant cervix. *Lancet* 1990; **335:** 1238–40.
6. Lefebvre Y, *et al.* The effects of RU-38486 on cervical ripening. *Am J Obstet Gynecol* 1990; **162:** 61–5.
7. WHO. The use of mifepristone (RU 486) for cervical preparation in first trimester pregnancy termination by vacuum aspiration. *Br J Obstet Gynaecol* 1990; **97:** 260–6.
8. Henshaw RC, Templeton AA. Pre-operative cervical preparation before first trimester vacuum aspiration: a randomized controlled comparison between gemeprost and mifepristone (RU 486). *Br J Obstet Gynaecol* 1991; **98:** 1025–30.
9. Gottlieb C, Bygdeman M. The use of antiprogestin (RU 486) for termination of second trimester pregnancy. *Acta Obstet Gynecol Scand* 1991; **70:** 199–203.
10. Urquhart DR, Templeton AA. The use of mifepristone prior to prostaglandin-induced mid-trimester abortion. *Hum Reprod* 1990; **5:** 883–6.
11. Rodger M, Baird D. Pretreatment with mifepristone (RU486) reduces interval between prostaglandin administration and expulsion in second trimester abortion. *Br J Obstet Gynaecol* 1990; **97:** 41–5.
12. Thong KJ, Baird DT. Induction of second trimester abortion with mifepristone and gemeprost. *Br J Obstet Gynaecol* 1993; **100:** 758–61.
13. Webster D, *et al.* A comparison of 600 and 200 mg mifepristone prior to second trimester abortion with the prostaglandin misoprostol. *Br J Obstet Gynaecol* 1996; **103:** 706–9.
14. Ashok PW, Templeton A. Nonsurgical mid-trimester termination of pregnancy: a review of 500 consecutive cases. *Br J Obstet Gynaecol* 1999; **106:** 706–10.
15. Ashok PW, *et al.* Termination of pregnancy at 9-13 weeks' amenorrhoea with mifepristone and misoprostol. *Lancet* 1998; **352:** 542–3.
16. Royal College of Obstetricians and Gynaecologists. The care of women requesting induced abortion. Available at: http://www.rcog.org.uk/guidelines.asp?PageID=108&GuidelineID=31 (accessed 21/06/04)


## Preparations

**Proprietary Preparations** (details are given in Part 3)
***Austria:*** Mifegyne; ***Denm.:*** Mifegyne; ***Fin.:*** Mifegyne; ***Fr.:*** Mifegyne; ***India:*** Mifegest; ***Israel:*** Mifegyne; ***Norw.:*** Mifegyne; ***Spain:*** Mifegyne; ***Swed.:*** Mifegyne; ***Switz.:*** Mifegyne; ***UK:*** Mifegyne; ***USA:*** Mifeprex.

---

## Nandrolone *(BAN, rINN)*

Nandrolona; 19-Nortestosterone. 17β-Hydroxyestr-4-en-3-one; 3-Oxoestr-4-en-17β-yl.

$C_{18}H_{26}O_2$ = 274.4.
*CAS — 434-22-0.*
*ATC — A14AB01; S01XA11.*

## Nandrolone Cyclohexylpropionate *(BANM, rINNM)*

Ciclohexilpropionato de nandrolona; Nandrolone Cyclohexanepropionate; Nortestosterone Cyclohexylpropionate. 3-Oxoestr-4-en-17β-yl 3-cyclohexylpropionate; 17β-Hydroxyestr-4-en-3-one cyclohexylpropionate.

$C_{27}H_{40}O_3$ = 412.6.
*CAS — 912-57-2.*
*ATC — A14AB01; S01XA11.*

## Nandrolone Decanoate *(BANM, USAN, rINNM)*

Decanoato de nandrolona; Nortestosterone Decanoate; Nortestosterone Decylate. 3-Oxoestr-4-en-17β-yl decanoate; 17β-Hydroxyestr-4-en-3-one decanoate.

$C_{28}H_{44}O_3$ = 428.6.
*CAS — 360-70-3.*
*ATC — A14AB01; S01XA11.*

**Pharmacopoeias.** In *Br.* and *US.*

**BP 2003** (Nandrolone Decanoate). A white to creamy-white crystalline powder with a faint characteristic odour. Practically insoluble in water; freely soluble in alcohol, in chloroform, in ether, in fixed oils, and in esters. Store under nitrogen at 2° to 8°. Protect from light.

**USP 27** (Nandrolone Decanoate). A white to creamy-white fine crystalline powder, odourless or may have a slight odour. Practically insoluble in water; soluble in alcohol, in acetone, in chloroform, and in vegetable oils. Store at 2° to 8° in airtight containers. Protect from light.

## Nandrolone Laurate *(BANM, rINNM)*

Laurato de nandrolona; Nandrolone Dodecanoate; Nortestosterone Laurate. 3-Oxoestr-4-en-17β-yl dodecanoate; 17β-Hydroxyestr-4-en-3-one dodecanoate.

$C_{30}H_{48}O_3$ = 456.7.
*CAS — 26490-31-3.*
*ATC — A14AB01; S01XA11.*

**Pharmacopoeias.** In *BP(Vet).*

**BP(Vet) 2003** (Nandrolone Laurate). A white to creamy-white crystalline powder with a faint characteristic odour. Practically insoluble in water; freely soluble in alcohol, in chloroform, in ether, in fixed oils, and in esters of fatty acids. Store at 2° to 8°. Protect from light.

## Nandrolone Phenylpropionate *(BANM, rINNM)*

Fenilpropionato de nandrolona; Nandrolone Hydrocinnamate; Nandrolone Phenpropionate; 19-Norandrostenolone Phenylpropionate; Nortestosterone Phenylpropionate; NSC-23162. 3-Oxoestr-4-en-17β-yl 3-phenylpropionate; 17β-Hydroxyestr-4-en-3-one 3-phenylpropionate.

$C_{27}H_{34}O_3$ = 406.6.
*CAS — 62-90-8.*
*ATC — A14AB01; S01XA11.*

**Pharmacopoeias.** In *Br., Chin., Pol.,* and *US.*

**BP 2003** (Nandrolone Phenylpropionate). A white to creamy-white crystalline powder with a characteristic odour. Practically insoluble in water; soluble in alcohol. Protect from light.

**USP 27** (Nandrolone Phenpropionate). Store in airtight containers. Protect from light.

## Nandrolone Sodium Sulfate *(rINNM)*

Nandrolone Sodium Sulphate *(BANM)*; Nortestosterone Sodium Sulphate; Sulfato sódico de nandrolona. 3-Oxoestr-4-en-17β-yl sodium sulphate; 17β-Hydroxyestr-4-en-3-one sodium sulphate.

$C_{18}H_{25}O_5SNa$ = 376.4.
*CAS — 60672-82-4.*
*ATC — A14AB01; S01XA11.*

## Nandrolone Undecylate *(rINNM)*

Nandrolone Undecanoate *(BANM)*; Nortestosterone Undecanoate; Undecilato de nandrolona. 3-Oxoestr-4-en-17β-yl undecanoate; 17β-Hydroxyestr-4-en-3-one undecanoate.

$C_{29}H_{46}O_3$ = 442.7.
*CAS — 862-89-5.*
*ATC — A14AB01; S01XA11.*

### Adverse Effects and Precautions

As for androgens and anabolic steroids in general (see Testosterone, p.1570).

**Abuse.** Nandrolone, like other anabolic compounds, has been abused by athletes and bodybuilders. However, controversy has arisen over the methods used to detect abuse in the former group, and there is some evidence that metabolites of nandrolone may be produced endogenously (see under Precautions of Testosterone, p.1570).

**Effects on the liver.** Intrahepatic cholestasis occurred in a patient receiving nandrolone cyclohexylpropionate.[1]


1. Gil VG, *et al.* A non-C17-alkylated steroid and long-term cholestasis. *Ann Intern Med* 1986; **104:** 135–6.


**Porphyria.** Nandrolone has been associated with acute attacks of porphyria and is considered unsafe in porphyric patients.

### Interactions

As for androgens and anabolic steroids in general (see Testosterone, p.1571).

### Uses and Administration

Nandrolone is an anabolic steroid with some androgenic properties (see Testosterone, p.1571). It is usually given as the decanoate ester in the form of oily intramuscular injections. The hexyloxyphenylpropionate, propionate, phenylpropionate, and undecylate esters have also been used.

Doses of nandrolone decanoate 25 to 100 mg once every 3 to 4 weeks have been used as an anabolic after debilitating illness, for postmenopausal osteoporosis, and for postmenopausal metastatic breast carcinoma. Doses of between 50 and 200 mg weekly have been suggested for the treatment of anaemia of chronic renal failure, and doses of 50 to 150 mg weekly for aplastic anaemia.

Nandrolone sodium sulfate has been used topically in the treatment of corneal damage.

Nandrolone cyclohexylpropionate, laurate, and phenylpropionate are used in veterinary medicine.

**Cachexia.** Nandrolone increased body-weight in patients with HIV-associated wasting[1] and in patients with end-stage renal failure undergoing dialysis.[2]


1. Gold J, *et al.* Safety and efficacy of nandrolone decanoate for treatment of wasting in patients with HIV infection. *AIDS* 1996 **10:** 745–52.
2. Johansen KL, *et al.* Anabolic effects of nandrolone decanoate in patients receiving dialysis: a randomized controlled trial. *JAMA* 1999; **281:** 1275–81.


**Male contraception.** Preliminary findings showed that nandrolone suppressed spermatogenesis,[1-3] suggesting potential as a male contraceptive (p.1535), but more recent studies seem to have favoured other androgens.


1. Schürmeyer T, *et al.* Reversible azoospermia induced by the anabolic steroid 19-nortestosterone. *Lancet* 1984; **i:** 417–20.
2. Knuth UA, *et al.* Combination of 19-nortestosterone-hexyloxyphenyl-propionate (Anadur) and depot-medroxyprogesterone-acetate (Clinovir) for male contraception. *Fertil Steril* 1989; **51:** 1011–18.
3. WHO Task Force on Methods for the Regulation of Male Fertility. Comparison of two androgens plus depot-medroxyprogesterone acetate for suppression to azoospermia in Indonesian men. *Fertil Steril* 1993; **60:** 1062–8.

### Preparations

**BP 2003:** Nandrolone Decanoate Injection; Nandrolone Phenylpropionate Injection;
**USP 27:** Nandrolone Decanoate Injection; Nandrolone Phenpropionate Injection.

**Proprietary Preparations** (details are given in Part 3)
***Arg.:*** Deca-Durabolin; Keratyl; ***Austral.:*** Deca-Durabolin; ***Austria:*** Deca-Durabolin; ***Belg.:*** Deca-Durabolin; ***Braz.:*** Deca-Durabolin; Nandrol†; ***Canad.:*** Deca-Durabolin; ***Chile:*** Anaprolina; Deca-Durabolin; Nandrosande; ***Fin.:*** Deca-Durabolin; ***Fr.:*** Keratyl; ***Ger.:*** Deca-Durabolin; Keratyl; ***Gr.:*** Anaboline Depot; Deca-Durabolin; Extraboline; ***Hong Kong:*** Deca-Durabolin; ***India:*** Deca-Durabolin; Decaneurabol; Durabolin; Metabol; Metadec; Neurabol; ***Irl.:*** Deca-Durabolin†; ***Israel:*** Deca-Durabolin†; Deca-Noralone†; Durabolin†; Noralone†; ***Ital.:*** Deca-Durabolin; Dynabolon; ***Malaysia:*** Deca-Durabolin; ***Mex.:*** Deca-Durabolin; ***Neth.:*** Deca-Durabolin; ***Norw.:*** Deca-Durabolin; ***NZ:*** Deca-Durabolin; ***Port.:*** Deca-Durabolin; Nandain; ***S.Afr.:*** Deca-Durabolin; ***Singapore:*** Deca-Durabolin; ***Spain:*** Deca-Durabolin; Nandrol†; ***Swed.:*** Deca-Durabol; ***Switz.:*** Deca-Durabolin; Keratyl; ***Thai.:*** Deca-Durabolin; Keratyl; ***UK:*** Deca-Durabolin; ***USA:*** Androlone-D; Deca-Durabolin; Durabolin; Hybolin; Neo-Durabolic.

**Multi-ingredient:** ***Arg.:*** Dexatopic; ***Fin.:*** Dexatopic†; ***Neth.:*** Dexatopic†.

## Nomegestrol Acetate *(BANM, rINNM)*

Acetato de nomegestrol; Nomegestroli Acetas. 17-Hydroxy-6-methyl-19-norpregna-4,6-diene-3,20-dione acetate.

$C_{23}H_{30}O_4$ = 370.5.
*CAS — 58691-88-6 (nomegestrol); 58652-20-3 (nomegestrol acetate).*
*ATC — G03DB04.*

**Pharmacopoeias.** In *Eur.* (see p.vi).

**Ph. Eur. 5.0** (Nomegestrol Acetate). A white or almost white crystalline powder. Practically insoluble in water; soluble in alcohol; freely soluble in acetone. Protect from light.

### Profile

Nomegestrol acetate is a progestogen structurally related to progesterone (p.1566) that has been used in the treatment of menstrual disorders and as the progestogen component of menopausal HRT (p.1540). Typical doses are 5 mg daily by mouth for 10 to 14 days of a 28-day cycle. A subdermal implant is under investigation as a long-acting progestogen-only contraceptive.

◊ References.

1. Coutinho EM, *et al.* Multicenter clinical trial on the efficacy and acceptability of a single contraceptive implant of nomegestrol acetate, Uniplant. *Contraception* 1996; **53:** 121–5.
2. Devoto L, *et al.* Hormonal profile, endometrial histology and ovarian ultrasound assessment during 1 year of nomegestrol acetate implant (Uniplant). *Hum Reprod* 1997; **12:** 708–13.
3. Barbosa IC, *et al.* Carbohydrate metabolism in sickle cell patients using a subdermal implant containing nomegestrol acetate (Uniplant). *Contraception* 2001; **63:** 263–5.

### Preparations

**Proprietary Preparations** (details are given in Part 3)
***Arg.:*** Lutenyl; ***Belg.:*** Lutenyl; ***Braz.:*** Lutenil; ***Chile:*** Lutenyl; ***Hong Kong:*** Lutenyl; ***Ital.:*** Lutenyl; ***Mon.:*** Lutenyl; ***Port.:*** Lutenyl.

## Norelgestromin *(BAN, USAN, rINN)*

17-Deacylnorgestimate; RWJ-10553. 13-Ethyl-17-hydroxy-18,19-dinor-17α-pregn-4-en-20-yn-3-one oxime.

$C_{21}H_{29}NO_2$ = 327.5.
*CAS — 53016-31-2.*

### Profile

Norelgestromin is a progestogen (see Progesterone, p.1566); it is the primary active metabolite of norgestimate (p.1563). Norelgestromin is used as the progestogenic component of a combined contraceptive transdermal patch. A dose of 150 micrograms norelgestromin is released daily with ethinylestradiol. A new patch is applied each week for 3 weeks of a 4-week cycle.

◊ References.

1. Audet M-C, *et al.* Evaluation of contraceptive efficacy and cycle control of a transdermal contraceptive patch vs an oral contraceptive: a randomized controlled trial. *JAMA* 2001; **285:** 2347–54.
2. Abrams LS, *et al.* Pharmacokinetics of norelgestromin and ethinyl estradiol from two consecutive contraceptive patches. *J Clin Pharmacol* 2001; **41:** 1232–7.
3. Abrams LS, *et al.* Pharmacokinetics of norelgestromin and ethinyl estradiol delivered by a contraceptive patch (Ortho Evra™/Evra™) under conditions of heat, humidity, and exercise. *J Clin Pharmacol* 2001; **41:** 1301–9.
4. Anonymous. Ortho Evra—a contraceptive patch. *Med Lett Drugs Ther* 2002; **44:** 8.
5. Abrams LS, *et al.* Pharmacokinetics of a contraceptive patch (Evra™/Ortho Evra™) containing norelgestromin and ethinyloestradiol at four application sites. *Br J Clin Pharmacol* 2002; **53:** 141–6.

### Preparations

**Proprietary Preparations** (details are given in Part 3)
**Multi-ingredient:** ***Fr.:*** Evra; ***UK:*** Evra; ***USA:*** Ortho Evra.

## Norethandrolone *(BAN, rINN)*

17α-Ethyl-17β-hydroxyestr-4-en-3-one; 17β-Hydroxy-19-nor-17α-pregn-4-en-3-one; Noretandrolona.

$C_{20}H_{30}O_2$ = 302.5.
*CAS — 52-78-8.*
*ATC — A14AA09.*

### Adverse Effects and Precautions

As for androgens and anabolic steroids in general (see Testosterone, p.1570). As with other 17α-alkylated compounds, norethandrolone may produce hepatotoxicity and liver function should be monitored. It should probably be avoided in patients with impaired liver function, and certainly if this is severe.

### Uses and Administration

Norethandrolone is an anabolic steroid (see Testosterone, p.1571). It is given by mouth in the treatment of aplastic anaemia in a dose of 0.25 to 2 mg/kg daily.

### Preparations

**Proprietary Preparations** (details are given in Part 3)
***Fr.:*** Nilevar.

## Norethisterone *(BAN, pINN)*

Ethinylnortestosterone; Norethindrone; Norethisteronum; Noretisterona; Noretisterone; Norpregneninolone; NSC-9564. 17β-Hydroxy-19-nor-17α-pregn-4-en-20-yn-3-one.

$C_{20}H_{26}O_2$ = 298.4.
*CAS — 68-22-4.*
*ATC — G03AC01; G03DC02.*

**Pharmacopoeias.** In *Chin., Eur.* (see p.vi), *Int., Jpn,* and *US.*

**Ph. Eur. 5.0** (Norethisterone). A white or yellowish-white crystalline powder. Practically insoluble in water; slightly soluble in alcohol. Protect from light.

**USP 27** (Norethindrone). A white to creamy-white odourless crystalline powder. Practically insoluble in water; sparingly soluble in alcohol; soluble in chloroform and in dioxan; slightly soluble in ether.

## Norethisterone Acetate *(BANM, pINNM)*

Acetato de noretisterona; Norethindrone Acetate; Norethisteroni Acetas. 17β-Hydroxy-19-nor-17α-pregn-4-en-20-yn-3-one acetate; 3-Oxo-19-nor-17α-pregn-4-en-20-yn-17β-yl acetate.

$C_{22}H_{28}O_3$ = 340.5.
*CAS — 51-98-9.*
*ATC — G03AC01; G03DC02.*

**Pharmacopoeias.** In *Eur.* (see p.vi), *Int.,* and *US.*

**Ph. Eur. 5.0** (Norethisterone Acetate). A white or yellowish-white crystalline powder. It exhibits polymorphism. Practically insoluble in water; soluble in alcohol; freely soluble in dichloromethane. Protect from light.

**USP 27** (Norethindrone Acetate). A white to creamy-white odourless crystalline powder. Practically insoluble in water; soluble 1 in 10 of alcohol, 1 in less than 1 of chloroform, 1 in 2 of dioxan, and 1 in 18 of ether.

## Norethisterone Enantate *(BANM, pINNM)*

Enantato de noretisterona; Norethindrone Enanthate; Norethisterone Enanthate; Norethisterone Heptanoate. 17β-Hydroxy-19-nor-17α-pregn-4-en-20-yn-3-one heptanoate.

$C_{27}H_{38}O_3$ = 410.6.
*CAS — 3836-23-5.*
*ATC — G03AC01; G03DC02.*

**Pharmacopoeias.** In *Int.*

### Adverse Effects and Precautions

As for progestogens in general (see Progesterone, p.1566). See also under Hormonal Contraceptives, p.1527.

**Effects on the liver.** There were 6 cases of jaundice among 107 patients with breast cancer treated with high-dose norethisterone acetate;[1] the jaundice was reversible and of an obstructive type.

1. Langlands AO, Martin WMC. Jaundice associated with norethisterone-acetate treatment of breast cancer. *Lancet* 1975; **i:** 584–5.

**Porphyria.** Norethisterone has been associated with acute attacks of porphyria and is considered unsafe in porphyric patients.

**Pregnancy.** Abnormalities seen in the offspring of women who had received norethisterone during pregnancy (either alone or with ethinylestradiol) included hypospadias,[1] masculinisation of female infants,[2] meningomyelocele or hydrocephalus,[3] and neonatal choreoathetosis associated with oral contraceptive use.[4] For reference to the fact that oral contraceptives have not generally been associated with teratogenicity, even when used inadvertently in pregnancy, see p.1533.

1. Aarskog D. Clinical and cytogenetic studies in hypospadias. *Acta Paediatr Scand* 1970; (suppl 203): 1–62.
2. Wilkins L. Masculinization of female fetus due to use of orally given progestins. *JAMA* 1960; **172:** 1028–32.
3. Gal I, *et al.* Hormonal pregnancy tests and congenital malformation. *Nature* 1967; **216:** 83.
4. Profumo R, *et al.* Neonatal choreoathetosis following prenatal exposure to oral contraceptives. *Pediatrics* 1990; **86:** 648–9.

**Venous thromboembolism.** For mention that combined oral contraceptives containing older progestogens such as norethisterone appear to be associated with a lower incidence of venous thromboembolism than desogestrel- or gestodene-containing preparations, see p.1531.

### Interactions

As for progestogens in general (see Progesterone, p.1567). See also under Hormonal Contraceptives, p.1534.

### Pharmacokinetics

Norethisterone is absorbed from the gastrointestinal tract, undergoing first-pass hepatic metabolism, with peak plasma concentrations occurring 1 to 2 hours after a dose by mouth. It exhibits biphasic pharmacokinetics; an initial distribution phase is followed by a prolonged elimination phase with a half-life of about 8 hours or more. Norethisterone is highly protein bound; about 60% to albumin and 35% to sex hormone binding globulin. Administration with an oestrogen increases the proportion bound to sex hormone binding globulin. It is metabolised in the liver with 50 to 80% of a dose being excreted in the urine and up to 40% in the faeces.

Norethisterone acetate may have a more prolonged elimination than norethisterone after oral use. It is hydrolysed to norethisterone, principally by intestinal tissue.

Following intramuscular injection of norethisterone enantate peak concentrations of norethisterone in plasma are not attained for several days.

### Uses and Administration

Norethisterone and its acetate and enantate esters are progestogens (see Progesterone, p.1567) derived from nortestosterone that have weak oestrogenic and androgenic properties. They are commonly used as **hormonal contraceptives** (see p.1535). Norethisterone and norethisterone acetate are both given by mouth. Typical daily doses are 0.35 mg for norethisterone and 0.6 mg for norethisterone acetate when used alone, or 0.5 to 1 mg for norethisterone and 1 to 1.5 mg for norethisterone acetate when used with an oestrogen. Norethisterone enantate is given by intramuscular injection; a dose of 200 mg provides contraception for 8 weeks.

Norethisterone and norethisterone acetate are used as the progestogen component of **menopausal HRT** (p.1540) to oppose the effects of oestrogens on the endometrium. Typical regimens have included either continuous daily doses of norethisterone 0.7 mg or norethisterone acetate 0.5 to 1 mg, or cyclical regimens of norethisterone or norethisterone acetate 1 mg daily for 10 to 12 days of a 28-day cycle. Norethisterone acetate is also available as transdermal patches supplying 170 or 250 micrograms in 24 hours, that are applied twice weekly for 2 weeks of a 4-week cycle; the lower strength may also be applied twice weekly on a continuous basis.

Norethisterone and norethisterone acetate may be given by mouth for the treatment of conditions such as **menorrhagia** (p.1567) and **endometriosis** (p.1546). In menorrhagia (dysfunctional uterine bleeding), norethisterone is given in usual doses of 10 to 15 mg daily and norethisterone acetate in doses of 2.5 to 10 mg daily, in a cyclical regimen. In endometriosis the dosage of norethisterone is 10 to 25 mg daily and of norethisterone acetate 5 to 15 mg daily. Treatment of endometriosis is usually continuous for 4 to 9 months.

Norethisterone has been used in daily doses of up to 15 mg by mouth in a cyclical regimen in the treatment of **premenstrual syndrome** (p.1551).

In **breast cancer** (p.514) doses of up to 60 mg daily by mouth of norethisterone have been used.

**Menorrhagia.** Although cyclical norethisterone has been widely used for menorrhagia (p.1567), it is of limited efficacy during ovulatory cycles being most effective for anovulatory bleeding, which occurs in a minority of women with menorrhagia.

References.

1. Cameron IT, *et al.* The effects of mefenamic acid and norethisterone on measured menstrual blood loss. *Obstet Gynecol* 1990; **76:** 85–8.
2. Preston JT, *et al.* Comparative study of tranexamic acid and norethisterone in the treatment of ovulatory menorrhagia. *Br J Obstet Gynaecol* 1995; **102:** 401–6.

## Preparations

***BP 2003:*** Norethisterone Tablets;
***USP 27:*** Norethindrone Acetate and Ethinyl Estradiol Tablets; Norethindrone Acetate Tablets; Norethindrone and Ethinyl Estradiol Tablets; Norethindrone and Mestranol Tablets; Norethindrone Tablets.

**Proprietary Preparations** (details are given in Part 3)
***Arg.:*** Primolut-Nor; Selectan; ***Austral.:*** Locilan; Micronor; Noriday; Primolut N; ***Austria:*** Micronovum; Primolut-Nor; ***Belg.:*** Primolut-Nor; ***Braz.:*** Micronor; Norestin; Primolut-Nor; ***Canad.:*** Micronor; Norlutate; ***Chile:*** Primolut-Nor; ***Denm.:*** Mini-Pe; ***Fin.:*** Mini-Pill; Primolut N; Primolut-Nor; ***Fr.:*** Milligynon; Noristerat†; Norluten†; Primolut-Nor; ***Ger.:*** Gestakadin; Micronovum†; Noristerat; Primolut-Nor; Sovel; ***Gr.:*** Fortilut; Primolut-Nor; ***Hong Kong:*** Norcolut; Primolut N; ***India:*** Noristerat; Primolut N; Styptin; ***Irl.:*** Micronor†; Noriday; Primolut N; ***Israel:*** Primolut-Nor; ***Ital.:*** Primolut-Nor; ***Malaysia:*** Norcolut; Noriday; Noristerat; Primolut N; Sunolut; Trisequens; ***Mex.:*** Noristerat; Primolut-Nor; ***Neth.:*** Primolut N; ***Norw.:*** Conludag; Primolut N; ***NZ:*** Noriday; Primolut N; ***Port.:*** Primolut-Nor; ***S.Afr.:*** Micronovum; Nur-Isterate; Primolut N; ***Singapore:*** Norcolut; Noristerat; Primolut N; ***Spain:*** Primolut-Nor; ***Swed.:*** Mini-Pe; Primolut-Nor; ***Switz.:*** Micronovum; Primolut N; Primolut-Nor†; ***Thai.:*** Noristerat; Primolut N; Steron; ***UK:*** Micronor; Micronor HRT; Noriday; Noristerat; Primolut N; Utovlan; ***USA:*** Aygestin; Jolivette; Nor-QD; Ortho Micronor.

**Multi-ingredient:** ***Arg.:*** Activelle; Estracomb; Estragest; Evorel Conti; Evorel Sequi; Kliogest; Mesigyna; Trial Combi; Trial Gest; Trial Pack; Trisequens; ***Austral.:*** Brevinor; Estalis Continuous; Estalis Sequi; Estracombi; Improvil; Kliogest; Kliovance; Norimin; Norinyl-1; Synphasic; Trisequens; ***Austria:*** Activelle; Estalis; Estalis Sequens; Estracomb; Estragest†; Fem-HRT; Kliogest; Mericomb; Merigest; Ortho-Novum; Ovysmen; Perikliman; Primosiston; Trinovum; Trisequens; ***Belg.:*** Activelle; Estracombi; Kliogest; Minestril; Ortho-Novum 1/50†; Ovysmen; Trinovum; Trisequens; ***Braz.:*** Activelle; Biofim†; Ciclovulon; Cliane; Estalis; Estracomb; Estragest; Ginedisc 50 Plus; Kliogest; Megestran; Mericomb; Merigest; Mesigyna; Primosiston; Suprema; Trinovum; Trisequens; ***Canad.:*** Brevicon; Estalis; Estalis Sequi; Estracomb; FemHRT; Loestrin 1.5/30; Minestrin; Norinyl 1/50†; Ortho 0.5/35; Ortho 1/35; Ortho 10/11†; Ortho 7/7/7; Ortho-Novum 1/50; Select 1/35; Synphasic; ***Chile:*** Activelle; Cliane; Estracomb; Estragest; Kliogest; Mesigyna; Primosiston; Trisequens; ***Denm.:*** Activelle; Econ; Estracomb; Evo-Conti; Evo-Sequi; Femanor; Femasekvens; Kliogest; Ostranorm; Trinorm; Trinovum; Trisekvens; ***Fin.:*** Activelle; Estalis; Estalis Sekvens; Estracomb; Evorel Conti; Evorel Sequi; Kliogest; Mericomb; Merigest; Trisekvens; ***Fr.:*** Activelle; Kliogest; Milli Anovlar†; Miniphase; Novofemme; Ortho-Novum 1/35; Triella; Trisequens; ***Ger.:*** Activelle; Conceplan M; Estalis Sequi; Estracomb; Estragest; Eve; Gynamon; Kliogest N; Mericomb; Merigest; Neorlest†; Non-Ovlon; Nora-ratiopharm; Novofem; Ortho-Novum 1/50†; Ostro-Primolut; Ovysmen; Primosiston; Prosiston; Sequostat; Sinovula; Synphasec; Trinovum; Trisequens; ***Gr.:*** Activelle; Estracomb TTS; Kliogest; Trisequens; ***Hong Kong:*** Activelle; Brevinor; Estracomb; Kliogest; Norimin; Norinyl-1; Synphase; Trinovum; Trisequens; ***Irl.:*** Activelle; Binovum†; Brevinor; Estalis; Estalis Sequi; Estracombi; Estrapak; Evorel Conti; Kliogest; Menophase†; Norinyl-1†; Normin†; Novofem; Ortho-Novin†; Ovysmen†; Trinovum†; Trisequens; ***Israel:*** Activelle; Evorel Conti; Evorel Sequi; Kliogest; Meno-Net; Trisequens; ***Ital.:*** Activelle; Estalis Sequi; Estracomb; Kliogest; Tesor-C†; Trinovum†; Trisequens; ***Malaysia:*** Activelle; Kliogest; ***Mex.:*** Cliane; Estracomb; Estrapak†; Evorelconti; Mesigyna; Norace; Norinyl; Ortho-Novum; Ortho-Novum 1/35†; ***Neth.:*** Activelle; Estracomb; Kliogest; Modicon; Neocon; Trinovum; Trisequens; ***Norw.:*** Activelle; Estalis; Estalis Sekvens; Estracomb†; Kliogest; Novofem; Synfase; Trisekvens; ***NZ:*** Brevinor; Cliane; Estrapak; Kliogest; Kliovance; Norimin; Norinyl-1; Synphasic; Trisequens; ***Port.:*** Activelle; Estalis; Estalis Sequi; Estracomb; Kliogest; Trisequens; ***S.Afr.:*** Activelle; Brevinor†; Estracombi; Evorel Conti; Evorel Sequi; Kliogest; Norinyl-1/28; Trinovum; Trisequens; ***Singapore:*** Activelle; Estracomb; Kliogest; Trisequens; ***Spain:*** Absorlent Plus; Activelle; Estalis; Estalis Sequi; Estracomb; Merigest; Merigest Sequi; Primosiston†; Trisequens; ***Swed.:*** Activelle; Estalis; Estalis Sekvens; Estracomb; Evorel Micronor; Femanor; Femasekvens; Kliogest; Orthonett Novum; Synfase; Trinovum; Trisekvens; ***Switz.:*** Activelle; Estalis; Estalis Sequi; Estracomb; Estragest; Kliogest N; Mericomb; Merigest; Ovysmen; Primosiston; Systen Conti; Systen Sequi; Trinovum; Trisequens; ***Thai.:*** Activelle; Anamai; Kliogest†; Trisequens†; ***UK:*** Adgyn Combi†; Binovum; Brevinor; Climagest; Climesse; Elleste Duet Conti; Elleste-Duet; Estracombi; Estrapak†; Evorel Conti; Evorel Pak; Evorel Sequi; FemTab Continuous; Kliofem; Kliovance; Loestrin; Norimin; Norinyl-1; Novofem; Nuvelle Continuous; Ovysmen; Synphase; Trinovum; Trisequens; ***USA:*** Activella; Brevicon; CombiPatch; Estrostep; Estrostep Fe; FemHRT; Genora 0.5/35 and 1/35†; Genora 1/50†; Jenest†; Junel Fe; Loestrin; Loestrin Fe; Modicon; Necon 1/50; Necon 10/11; Necon 0.5/35, 1/35; NEE 1/35; Nelova 0.5/35E and 1/35E†; Nelova 1/50M†; Nelova 10/11†; Norethin 1/35E†; Norethin 1/50M†; Norinyl 1 + 35; Norinyl 1 + 50; Ortho-Novum 1/35; Ortho-Novum 1/50; Ortho-Novum 10/11; Ortho-Novum 7/7/7; Ovcon 35; Ovcon 50; Tri-Norinyl.

---

## Noretynodrel *(BAN, rINN)*

Norethynodrel *(USAN)*; Noretinodrel; NSC-15432; SC-4642. 17β-Hydroxy-19-nor-17α-pregn-5(10)-en-20-yn-3-one.

$C_{20}H_{26}O_2$ = 298.4.
*CAS — 68-23-5.*

**Pharmacopoeias.** In *US.*

**USP 27** (Norethynodrel). A white or practically white, odourless, crystalline powder. Very slightly soluble in water and in petroleum spirit; sparingly soluble in alcohol; soluble in acetone; freely soluble in chloroform.

### Profile

Noretynodrel is a progestogen (see Progesterone, p.1566) structurally related to norethisterone that has been given by mouth with an oestrogen such as mestranol for the treatment of various menstrual disorders and endometriosis.

**Breast feeding.** Approximately 1% of an oral dose of radiolabelled noretynodrel was detected in breast milk in a study of 4 women.[1] No adverse effects have been observed in breast-fed infants whose mothers were receiving noretynodrel, and the American Academy of Pediatrics considers[2] that it is therefore usually compatible with breast feeding.

1. Laumas KR, *et al.* Radioactivity in the breast milk of lactating women after oral administration of $^3$H-norethynodrel. *Am J Obstet Gynecol* 1967; **98:** 411–3.
2. American Academy of Pediatrics. The transfer of drugs and other chemicals into human milk. *Pediatrics* 2001; **108:** 776–89. Correction. *ibid.*; 1029. Also available at: http://aappolicy.aappublications.org/cgi/content/full/pediatrics%3b108/3/776 (accessed 21/06/04)

**Porphyria.** Noretynodrel is considered to be unsafe in patients with porphyria because it has been shown to be porphyrinogenic in *animals* or *in-vitro* systems.

**Pregnancy.** A woman who had received noretynodrel during pregnancy to prevent threatened miscarriage gave birth to a female infant showing evidence of masculinisation.[1]

1. Wilkins L. Masculinization of female fetus due to use of orally given progestins. *JAMA* 1960; **172:** 1028–32.

---

## Norgestimate *(BAN, USAN, rINN)*

D-138; Dexnorgestrel Acetime; Norgestimato; ORF-10131; RWJ-10131. 13β-Ethyl-3-hydroxyimino-18,19-dinor-17α-pregn-4-en-20-yn-17β-yl acetate.

$C_{23}H_{31}NO_3$ = 369.5.
*CAS — 35189-28-7.*

**Pharmacopoeias.** In *US.*

**USP 27** (Norgestimate). A mixture of (*E*)- and (*Z*)-isomers having a ratio of (*E*)- to (*Z*)-isomer between 1.27 and 1.78. A white to pale yellow powder. Insoluble in water; sparingly soluble in acetonitrile; freely to very soluble in dichloromethane.

### Profile

Norgestimate is a progestogen (see Progesterone, p.1566) structurally related to levonorgestrel (to which it is partly metabolised) that is used as the progestogenic component of combined oral contraceptives (see p.1527) and in menopausal HRT (see p.1536). A typical daily dose is 250 micrograms in monophasic contraceptive preparations, and 180 to 250 micrograms in triphasic preparations. For HRT, a regimen of estradiol daily for 3 days followed by estradiol combined with norgestimate 90 micrograms daily for 3 days is used; this 6-day cycle is repeated continuously without interruption.

### Preparations

**Proprietary Preparations** (details are given in Part 3)
**Multi-ingredient:** ***Arg.:*** Cilest; Prefest; Tridette; ***Austria:*** Cileste; Tri-Cilest; Vivelle; ***Belg.:*** Cilest; ***Braz.:*** Prefest; ***Canad.:*** Cyclen; Tri-Cyclen; ***Chile:*** Mactex; Neofam; Orlon; Tri-Mactex; Trifas; ***Denm.:*** Cilest; ***Fin.:*** Cilest; ***Fr.:*** Cilest; Effiprev; ***Ger.:*** Cilest; Pramino; ***Irl.:*** Cilest; ***Israel:*** Ortho Cyclen; ***Mex.:*** Cilest; ***Neth.:*** Cilest; ***S.Afr.:*** Cilest; Prefesta; TriCilest; ***Swed.:*** Cilest; ***Switz.:*** Cilest; ***UK:*** Cilest; ***USA:*** Ortho Cyclen; Ortho Tri-Cyclen; Prefest; Previfem; Sprintec; Tri-Sprintec; TriNessa.

---

## Norgestomet *(BAN, USAN, rINN)*

SC-21009. 11β-Methyl-3,20-dioxo-19-norpregn-4-en-17α-yl acetate.

$C_{23}H_{32}O_4$ = 372.5.
*CAS — 25092-41-5.*

### Profile

Norgestomet is a progestogen (see Progesterone, p.1566) used in veterinary medicine with estradiol.

---

# Norgestrel *(BAN, USAN, rINN)*

*dl*-Norgestrel; DL-Norgestrel; Norgestrelum; Wy-3707. (±)-13-Ethyl-17β-hydroxy-18,19-dinor-17α-pregn-4-en-20-yn-3-one.

$C_{21}H_{28}O_2$ = 312.4.
*CAS — 6533-00-2.*

**Pharmacopoeias.** In *Chin., Eur.* (see p.vi), *Jpn,* and *US.*

**Ph. Eur. 5.0** (Norgestrel). A white or almost white crystalline powder. Practically insoluble in water; slightly soluble in alcohol; sparingly soluble in dichloromethane. Protect from light.

**USP 27** (Norgestrel). A white or practically white, practically odourless crystalline powder. Insoluble in water; sparingly soluble in alcohol; freely soluble in chloroform.

## Levonorgestrel *(BAN, USAN, rINN)*

Levonorgestrelum; D-Norgestrel; Wy-5104. (−)-13β-Ethyl-17β-hydroxy-18,19-dinor-17α-pregn-4-en-20-yn-3-one.

*CAS — 797-63-7.*
*ATC — G03AC03.*

NOTE. The name Dexnorgestrel has also been used.

**Pharmacopoeias.** In *Chin., Eur.* (see p.vi), *Int.,* and *US.*

**Ph. Eur. 5.0** (Levonorgestrel). A white or almost white crystalline powder. Practically insoluble in water; slightly soluble in alcohol; sparingly soluble in dichloromethane. Protect from light.

**USP 27** (Levonorgestrel). A white or practically white, odourless powder. Practically insoluble in water; slightly soluble in alcohol; soluble in chloroform. Protect from light.

### Adverse Effects and Precautions

As for progestogens in general (see Progesterone, p.1566). See also under Hormonal Contraceptives, p.1527.

◊ Following the introduction of levonorgestrel in a subdermal implant formulation in February 1991, the US FDA had received about 5800 reports of adverse effects as of December 1993 (out of an estimated 891 000 implants distributed).[1] Serious adverse effects associated with the implant included 24 cases of infection related to insertion of the implant, 15 cases of stroke and 39 of benign intracranial hypertension, 3 cases of thrombocytopenic purpura and 6 of thrombocytopenia (1 fatal). None of the reporting rates for these disorders exceeded the expected rate in this population. In a 5-year cohort study[2] of more than 16 000 women who received either a levonorgestrel implant or an IUD (not progestogen-releasing), or underwent sterilisation, there was no significant risk of major morbidity associated with the implant, although there were moderately elevated risks of gallbladder disease and raised blood pressure in current users.

1. Wysowski DK, Green L. Serious adverse events in Norplant users reported to the Food and Drug Administration's MedWatch Spontaneous Reporting System. *Obstet Gynecol* 1995; **85:** 538–42.
2. Meirik O, *et al.* Safety and efficacy of levonorgestrel implant, intrauterine device, and sterilization. *Obstet Gynecol* 2001; **97:** 539–47.

**Benign intracranial hypertension.** Intracranial hypertension, presenting as headaches, vomiting, and visual obscuration associated with florid bilateral papilloedema developed in 2 patients four to five months after subdermal implantation of levonorgestrel.[1] Despite a further 56 cases reported to various drug monitoring centres, and 70 cases known to the manufacturers,[2] it remained unclear whether the drug actually caused intracranial hypertension, but removal of implants in patients in whom intracranial pressure increases is recommended.

1. Alder JB, *et al.* Levonorgestrel implants and intracranial hypertension. *N Engl J Med* 1995; **332:** 1720–1.
2. Weber ME, *et al.* Levonorgestrel implants and intracranial hypertension. *N Engl J Med* 1995; **332:** 1721.

**Breast feeding.** Levonorgestrel was detected in breast milk and the circulation of breast-fed infants during the use of either a levonorgestrel IUD, subcutaneous implant, or progestogen-only oral contraceptive.[1] A review[2] of studies of a levonorgestrel implant used during lactation concluded that it was generally shown to have no adverse effect on the duration of lactation, infant growth or development. The American Academy of Pediatrics considers that levonorgestrel is usually compatible with breast feeding.[3] Progestogen-only contraceptives should not be started until several weeks after birth if the woman is breast feeding (see Breast Feeding under Hormonal Contraceptives, p.1533).

1. Shikary ZK, *et al.* Transfer of levonorgestrel (LNG) administered through different drug delivery systems from the maternal circulation into the newborn infant's circulation via breast milk. *Contraception* 1987; **35:** 477–86.
2. Díaz S. Contraceptive implants and lactation. *Contraception* 2002; **65:** 39–46.
3. American Academy of Pediatrics. The transfer of drugs and other chemicals into human milk. *Pediatrics* 2001; **108:** 776–89. Correction. *ibid.*; 1029. Also available at: http://aappolicy.aappublications.org/cgi/content/full/pediatrics%3b108/3/776 (accessed 21/06/04)

**Effects on the blood.** A long-term study of the use of levonorgestrel subdermal implants (Norplant) in 100 Singaporean women indicated that during 12 months of use patients possibly had an increased tendency for thrombosis and an increased potential for hypercoagulation.[1] Some of the haematological changes observed after 1 year persisted throughout the second year of the study whereas others returned to normal.[2]

1. Viegas OAC, *et al.* The effects of Norplant on clinical chemistry in Singaporean acceptors after 1 year of use I: haemostatic changes. *Contraception* 1988; **38:** 313–23.
2. Singh K, *et al.* Two-year follow-up of changes in clinical chemistry in Singaporean Norplant-2 rod acceptors: haemostatic changes. *Contraception* 1989; **39:** 155–64.

**Effects on carbohydrate metabolism.** For a mention that levonorgestrel has been reported to be the most potent progestogen in decreasing glucose tolerance when used as a combined oral contraceptive, see p.1530.

**Glucocorticoid effects.** Reference to the minimal suppressive effect of subdermal levonorgestrel on adrenal function.[1]

1. Toppozada MK, *et al.* Effect of Norplant implants on the pituitary-adrenal axis function and reserve capacity. *Contraception* 1997; **55:** 7–10.

**Myasthenia gravis.** Myasthenia gravis occurring after insertion of a levonorgestrel implant improved on removal of the implant.[1]

1. Brittain J, Lange LS. Myasthenia gravis and levonorgestrel implant. *Lancet* 1995; **346:** 1556.

**Porphyria.** Levonorgestrel has been associated with acute attacks of porphyria and is considered unsafe in porphyric patients.

**Pregnancy.** Adverse effects in infants whose mothers had received oral contraceptives containing norgestrel during early pregnancy have included tracheo-oesophageal fistula in one infant[1] and inoperable hepatoblastoma in another.[2] However, many epidemiological studies have failed to show any association between fetal malformations and oral contraceptives, even when used inadvertently during pregnancy, see p.1533.

1. Frost O. Tracheo-oesophageal fistula associated with hormonal contraception during pregnancy. *BMJ* 1976; **2:** 978.
2. Otten J, *et al.* Hepatoblastoma in an infant after contraceptive intake during pregnancy. *N Engl J Med* 1977; **297:** 222.

**Venous thromboembolism.** For mention that levonorgestrel-containing combined oral contraceptives appeared to be associated with a lower incidence of venous thromboembolism than desogestrel- or gestodene-containing preparations, see p.1531. See also Effects on the Blood, above.

## Interactions

As for progestogens in general (see Progesterone, p.1567). See also under Hormonal Contraceptives, p.1534.

## Pharmacokinetics

Levonorgestrel is rapidly and almost completely absorbed after a dose by mouth, and undergoes little first-pass hepatic metabolism. It is highly bound to plasma proteins; 42 to 68% to sex hormone binding globulin and 30 to 56% to albumin. The proportion bound to sex hormone binding globulin is higher when it is given with an oestrogen. Levonorgestrel and norgestrel are metabolised in the liver to sulfate and glucuronide conjugates, which are excreted in the urine and to a lesser extent in the faeces. Levonorgestrel is distributed into breast milk.

◊ References.

1. Fotherby K. Levonorgestrel: clinical pharmacokinetics. *Clin Pharmacokinet* 1995; **28:** 203–15.

## Uses and Administration

Norgestrel and its active (−)-isomer levonorgestrel are progestogens (see Progesterone, p.1567) derived from nortestosterone. They are more potent inhibitors of ovulation than norethisterone and have androgenic activity. Levonorgestrel is more commonly used than norgestrel and is twice as potent. For example, levonorgestrel 37.5 micrograms is equivalent to norgestrel 75 micrograms.

They are both used as **hormonal contraceptives** (see p.1535). The typical daily dose is the equivalent of:

- 30 or 37.5 micrograms of levonorgestrel as an oral progestogen-only contraceptive
- 150 to 250 micrograms of levonorgestrel in monophasic combined oral contraceptives
- 50 to 125 micrograms of levonorgestrel in triphasic preparations

Levonorgestrel is also used as a long-acting progestogen-only contraceptive by subcutaneous implantation; 6 implants each containing 36 mg of levonorgestrel are inserted under the skin within the first 7 days of the menstrual cycle and are replaced at intervals of up to 5 years. Insertion and removal must be carried out by personnel fully trained in the technique. A 2-implant preparation providing up to 5 years of contraception is also available. Uterine, cervical, and vaginal devices containing levonorgestrel have also been investigated. An intra-uterine device is available for contraception or **menorrhagia**, containing a total of 52 mg of levonorgestrel which is released at an initial rate of 20 micrograms per 24 hours. The device is effective for 5 years.

For **emergency contraception** (p.1536), levonorgestrel may be given alone by mouth in a single dose of 1.5 mg within 72 hours of coitus (preferably as soon as possible). Alternatively, a dose of 750 micrograms is given within 72 hours of coitus (preferably as soon as possible), and repeated after 12 hours. Another regimen uses the equivalent of levonorgestrel 500 micrograms plus ethinylestradiol 100 micrograms, given within 72 hours of coitus and repeated after 12 hours.

Both levonorgestrel and norgestrel are used as the progestogenic component of **menopausal HRT** (see p.1540). Typical regimens are the equivalent of 75 to 250 micrograms of levonorgestrel by mouth for 10 to 12 days of a 28-day cycle. Levonorgestrel may also be given via a combined transdermal patch, releasing 10 micrograms per 24 hours with an oestrogen, which is applied once weekly for 2 weeks of a 4-week cycle. Alternatively, a patch releasing 7 or 15 micrograms per 24 hours with an oestrogen is applied once weekly for continuous HRT. The intra-uterine levonorgestrel device is under investigation for use with oestrogen for this indication.

**Administration.** IMPLANTS. Some references to the use of levonorgestrel by subcutaneous implant for hormonal contraception.[1-5]

1. Shoupe D, Mishell DR. Norplant: subdermal implant system for long-term contraception. *Am J Obstet Gynecol* 1989; **160:** 1286–92.
2. Polaneczky M, *et al.* The use of levonorgestrel implants (Norplant) for contraception in adolescent mothers. *N Engl J Med* 1994; **331:** 1201–6.
3. Anonymous. Long-acting progestogen-only contraception. *Drug Ther Bull* 1996; **34:** 93–6.
4. Coukell AJ, Balfour JA. Levonorgestrel subdermal implants: a review of contraceptive efficacy and acceptability. *Drugs* 1998; **55:** 861–87.
5. Sivin I. Risks and benefits, advantages and disadvantages of levonorgestrel-releasing contraceptive implants. *Drug Safety* 2003; **26:** 303–35.

INTRA-UTERINE DEVICES. Some references to the use of levonorgestrel-releasing intra-uterine devices for contraception[1-3] and menopausal HRT.[4,5]

1. Sturridge F, Guillebaud J. A risk-benefit assessment of the levonorgestrel-releasing intrauterine system. *Drug Safety* 1996; **15:** 430–40.
2. Backman T, *et al.* Length of use and symptoms associated with premature removal of the levonorgestrel intrauterine system: a nation-wide study of 17,360 users. *Br J Obstet Gynaecol* 2000; **107:** 335–9.
3. French RS, *et al.* Levonorgestrel-releasing (20 microgram/day) intrauterine systems (Mirena) compared with other methods of reversible contraceptives. *Br J Obstet Gynaecol* 2000; **107:** 1218–25.
4. Suvanto-Luukkonen E, Kauppila A. The levonorgestrel intrauterine system in menopausal hormone replacement therapy: five-year experience. *Fertil Steril* 1999; **72:** 161–3.
5. Varila E, *et al.* A 5-year follow-up study on the use of a levonorgestrel intrauterine system in women receiving hormone replacement therapy. *Fertil Steril* 2001; **76:** 969–73.

**Menorrhagia.** Although oral cyclical progestogens have limited efficacy in the treatment of menorrhagia (p.1567), the levonorgestrel-containing intra-uterine device appears to be particularly useful in reducing menstrual blood loss. The *British National Formulary* notes that another treatment should be considered if bleeding does not improve within 3 to 6 months of insertion. References[1-4] and a systematic review[5] of the use of levonorgestrel are given below.

1. Andersson JK, Rybo G. Levonorgestrel-releasing intrauterine device in the treatment of menorrhagia. *Br J Obstet Gynaecol* 1990; **97:** 690–4.
2. Milsom I, *et al.* A comparison of flurbiprofen, tranexamic acid, and a levonorgestrel-releasing intrauterine contraceptive device in the treatment of idiopathic menorrhagia. *Am J Obstet Gynecol* 1991; **164:** 879–83.
3. Crosignani PC, *et al.* Levonorgestrel releasing intrauterine device versus hysteroscopic endometrial resection in the treatment of dysfunctional uterine bleeding. *Obstet Gynecol* 1997; **90:** 257–63.
4. Lähteenmäki P, *et al.* Open randomised study of use of levonorgestrel releasing intrauterine system as alternative to hysterectomy. *BMJ* 1998; **316:** 1122–6.
5. Lethaby AE, *et al.* Progesterone/progestogen releasing intrauterine systems for heavy menstrual bleeding. Available in The Cochrane Library; Issue 2. Chichester: John Wiley; 2004.

## Preparations

***BP 2003:*** Levonorgestrel and Ethinylestradiol Tablets; Levonorgestrel Tablets; Norgestrel Tablets;
***USP 27:*** Levonorgestrel and Ethinyl Estradiol Tablets; Norgestrel and Ethinyl Estradiol Tablets; Norgestrel Tablets.

**Proprietary Preparations** (details are given in Part 3)
***Arg.:*** Imediat N; Microlut; Mirena; Norgeal; Norgestrel Max; ***Austral.:*** Microlut; Microval; Mirena; Postinor-2; ***Austria:*** Mirena; Vikela; ***Belg.:*** Microlut; Microval; Mirena; Norlevo; ***Braz.:*** Minipil; Mirena; Norlevo; Nortrel; Pilem; Postinor; Pozato; ***Canad.:*** Mirena; Norplant; Plan B; ***Chile:*** Microlut; Microval; Mirena; Postinor-2; ***Denm.:*** Levonova; Microluton; Microval†; Norlevo; ***Fin.:*** Jadelle; Levonova; Microluton; Norlevo; Postinor; ***Fr.:*** Microval; Mirena; Norlevo; Vikela; ***Ger.:*** 28 mini; Duofem; Microlut; Mikro-30; Mirena; ***Gr.:*** Norlevo; ***Hong Kong:*** Mirena; Postinor-2; ***India:*** Ecee2; ***Irl.:*** Mirena; ***Israel:*** Mirena; Norplant†; Postinor-2; ***Ital.:*** Levonelle; Microlut†; Mirena; Norlevo; ***Malaysia:*** Mirena; Norplant; Postinor; ***Mex.:*** Microlut; Norplant†; ***Neth.:*** Mirena; ***Norw.:*** Levonova; Microluton; Norlevo; ***NZ:*** Levonelle; Microlut; Microval; Mirena; Postinor-2; ***Port.:*** Levonelle; Mirena; Norlevo; ***S.Afr.:*** Microval; Mirena; Norlevo; ***Singapore:*** Mirena; Norplant; Postinor; ***Spain:*** Mirena; Norlevo; Postinor; ***Swed.:*** Follistrel; Levonova; Norlevo; Norplant; ***Switz.:*** Microlut; Mirena; ***Thai.:*** Madonna; Mirena; Norplant; Postinor; ***UK:*** Levonelle; Microval; Mirena; Neogest; Norgeston; Postinor-2; ***USA:*** Mirena; Norplant†; Ovrette; Plan B.

**Multi-ingredient:** ***Arg.:*** April; Ciclocur; Dos Dias N; Evelea; Femexin; Microgynon; Microvlar; Miranova; Neogynon; Nordette; Nordiol; Norgestrel Plus; Ovral; Plenifem; Tridestan N; Trinordiol; Triquilar; ***Austral.:*** Biphasil; Levlen ED; Loette; Logynon ED; Microgynon; Microlevlen ED; Monofeme; Nordette; Nordiol; Sequilar ED; Trifeme; Triphasil; Triquilar; ***Austria:*** Climabelle; Cyclacur; FemSeven Combi; Levlen†; Liogynon†; Loette; Microgynon; Neo-Stediril; Neogynon; Ovranette; Perikursal; Sequilar; Stediril D; Trigynon; Trinordiol; ***Belg.:*** Binordiol; Cyclocur; Feminova Plus; Microgynon; Neo-Stediril; Neogynon; Stediril 30; Stediril D; Trigynon; Trinordiol; ***Braz.:*** Anfertil; Ciclo; Ciclomestril†; Ciclon; Cicloprimogyna; Evanor; Gestrelan; Karin†; Levordiol; Lindisc Duo; Lovelle; Microvlar; Neovlar; Nociclin; Nordette; Normamor; Postoval; Primovlar†; Trinordiol; Triquilar; ***Canad.:*** Alesse; Min-Ovral; Ovral; Triphasil; Triquilar; ***Chile:*** Anovulatorio Micro-Dosis; Anulette; Fem 7 Combi; Innova Cd; Loette; Microfemin; Microgynon; Modutrol; Nordette; Nordiol; Norvetal; Postoval; Progyluton; Trinordiol; Triquilar; Trolit; ***Denm.:*** Cyclo-Progynon; Dystrol†; Fironetta; Gynatrol; Microgyn; Neogentrol; Neogynon; Nuvelle; Tetragynon; Trinordiol; Triquilar; ***Fin.:*** Climara Duo; Cyclabil; Microgynon; Neo-Primovlar; Trikvilar; Trinordiol; ***Fr.:*** Adepal; Daily; Ludeal; Minidril; Stediril; Tetragynon; Trinordiol; ***Ger.:*** Cyclo-Menorette; Cyclo-Progynova; CycloOstrogynal; Fem 7 Combi; Femigoa; Femranette mikro; Gravistat; Klimonorm; Leios; Microgynon; Minisiston; Miranova; MonoStep; Neo-Stediril; Neogynon; NovaStep; Ostronara; Perikursal; Sequilar; Stediril; Stediril 30; Stediril D; Tetragynon; Triette; Trigoa; Trinordiol; Triquilar; Trisiston; TriStep; ***Gr.:*** Cyclacur; Neogynon; Nordette; Nordiol-21; Ovral; Trinordiol; Triquilar; ***Hong Kong:*** Duoluton†; Eugynon; Klimonorm; Microgynon; Neogynon; Nordette; Nordiol†; Ovral†; Rigevidon; Tri-Regol; Trinordiol; Triquilar; ***India:*** Duoluton-L; Ovral; Triquilar; ***Irl.:*** Logynon; Microgynon 30; Microlite; Nuvelle; Ovran; Ovran 30†; Ovranette; Prempak-C; Trinordiol; ***Israel:*** Logynon; Microgynon; Neogynon; Nordette; Progyluton; Trinordiol; ***Ital.:*** Combiseven; Egogyn 30; Eugynon; Evanor-D; Loette; Microgynon; Miranova; Novogyn; Nuvelle; Nuvelle TS; Ovranet; Trigynon; Trinordiol; ***Jpn:*** Ange; ***Malaysia:*** Klimonorm; Loette; Microgynon 30; Nordette; Progyluton; Rigevidon; Tri-Regol; Trinordiol; Triquilar; ***Mex.:*** Microgynon; Neogynon; Nordet; Nordiol; Ovral; Progyluton; Trinordiol; Triquilar; ***Mon.:*** FemseptCombi; ***Neth.:*** Binordiol†; Cyclocur; Fem 7 Sequi; Microgynon; Neo-Stediril†; Neogynon; Prempak-C; Stediril 30, Stediril D; Trigynon; Trinordiol; ***Norw.:*** Cyclabil; Eugynon†; Follimin; Microgynon; Tetragynon; Trinordiol; Trionetta; ***NZ:*** Biphasil†; Levlen ED; Loette; Microgynon; Monofeme; Nordette; Nordiol; Nuvelle; Ovral; Prempak-C; Trifeme; Triphasil; Triquilar; ***Port.:*** Climara Duo; Microginon; Miranova; Neomonovar; Nuvelle; Progyluton; Tetragynon†; Trinordiol; Triquilar; ***S.Afr.:*** Biphasil; E-Gen-C; Loette; Logynon ED; Nordette; Nordiol; Normovlar ED†; Ovral; Postoval; Triphasil; ***Singapore:*** Loette; Microgynon; Nordette; Prempak-C; Progyluton; Trinordiol; Triquilar; ***Spain:*** Auroclim; Loette; Microgynon; Neogynona; Nuvelle; Ovoplex; Progyluton; Triagynon; Triciclor; ***Swed.:*** Cyclabil; Follimin; Follinett; Neovletta; Regunon†; Trinordiol; Trionetta; ***Switz.:*** Binordiol; Cyclacur; Fem 7 Combi; Microgynon; Neo-Stediril†; Neogynon; Ologyn; Sequilar†; Stediril 30; Stediril D; Tetragynon; Trinordiol; Triquilar; ***Thai.:*** Anna; Cyclo-Progynova; Eugynon 250; FMP; Klimonorm†; Microgest; Microgynon; Nordette; Nordiol†; Ovral†; R-Den; Riget; Rigevidon; Trinordiol†; Triquilar; ***UK:*** Cyclo-Progynova 1 mg; Cyclo-Progynova 2 mg; Eugynon 30; FemSeven Conti; FemSeven Sequi; FemTab Sequi; Logynon; Microgynon 30; Nuvelle; Nuvelle TS†; Ovran 30; Ovran†; Ovranette; Prempak-C; Schering PC4†; Trinordiol; ***USA:*** Alesse; Aviane; ClimaraPro; Cryselle; Enpresse; Lessina; Levlen; Levlite; Levora; Lo/Ovral; Nordette; Ovral; Portia; Preven; Seasonale; Tri-Levlen; Triphasil; Trivora.

---

# Norgestrienone *(rINN)*

Norgestrienona. 17β-Hydroxy-19-nor-17α-pregna-4,9,11-trien-20-yn-3-one.

$C_{20}H_{22}O_2$ = 294.4.
*CAS — 848-21-5.*
*ATC — G03AC07.*

## Profile

Norgestrienone is a progestogen (see Progesterone, p.1566) structurally related to norethisterone that is used as an oral contraceptive (see p.1527). Typical doses are 2 mg daily with an oestrogen, and 350 micrograms daily when used alone.

## Preparations

**Proprietary Preparations** (details are given in Part 3)
***Fr.:*** Ogyline†.

**Multi-ingredient:** ***Fr.:*** Planor.

---

# Ormeloxifene *(rINN)*

Centchroman; Ormeloxifeno. *trans*-1-{2-[4-(3,4-Dihydro-7-methoxy-2,2-dimethyl-3-phenyl-2*H*-1-benzopyran-4-yl)phenoxy]ethyl}pyrrolidine.

$C_{30}H_{35}NO_3$ = 457.6.
*CAS — 31477-60-8.*

## Profile

Ormeloxifene is a nonsteroidal benzopyran derivative with anti-oestrogenic and antiprogestogenic actions that has been administered weekly as an oral contraceptive. Ormeloxifene has also been investigated in the management of osteoporosis. The *l*-isomer, levormeloxifene, has also been investigated.

◊ References.

1. Kamboj VP, *et al.* New products: centchroman. *Drugs Today* 1992; **28:** 227–32.
2. Gupta RC, *et al.* Centchroman: a new non-steroidal oral contraceptive in human milk. *Contraception* 1995; **52:** 301–5.
3. Lal J, *et al.* Pharmacokinetics of centchroman in healthy female subjects after oral administration. *Contraception* 1995; **52:** 297–300.
4. Lal J, *et al.* Optimization of contraceptive dosage regimen of centchroman. *Contraception* 2001; **63:** 47–51.
5. Alexandersen P, *et al.* Efficacy of levormeloxifene in the prevention of postmenopausal bone loss and on the lipid profile compared to low dose hormone replacement therapy. *J Clin Endocrinol Metab* 2001; **86:** 755–60.
6. Skrumsager BK, *et al.* Levormeloxifene: safety, pharmacodynamics and pharmacokinetics in healthy postmenopausal women following single and multiple doses of a new selective oestrogen receptor modulator. *Br J Clin Pharmacol* 2002; **53:** 284–95.

## Preparations

**Proprietary Preparations** (details are given in Part 3)
***India:*** Centron.

---

## Ovary Extracts

Extractos de ovario; Ovarian Extracts.

### Profile

Ovary extracts of animal origin (usually porcine or bovine) have been used for a variety of disorders including gynaecological and menopausal disorders. They are often used in preparations containing other mammalian tissue extracts or herbal medicines.

### Preparations

**Proprietary Preparations** (details are given in Part 3)
**Multi-ingredient: Ger.:** Intradermi N†.

## Oxabolone Cipionate *(rINN)*

Cipionato de oxabolona; FI-5852; Oxabolone Cypionate. 4,17β-Dihydroxyestr-4-en-3-one 17-(β-cyclopentylpropionate).

$C_{26}H_{38}O_4$ = 414.6.
*CAS — 1254-35-9.*
*ATC — A14AB03.*

### Profile

Oxabolone cipionate has anabolic properties.

### Preparations

**Proprietary Preparations** (details are given in Part 3)
**Ital.:** Steranabol Ritardo†.

## Oxandrolone *(BAN, USAN, rINN)*

NSC-67068; Oxandrolona; SC-11585. 17β-Hydroxy-17α-methyl-2-oxa-5α-androstan-3-one.

$C_{19}H_{30}O_3$ = 306.4.
*CAS — 53-39-4.*
*ATC — A14AA08.*

**Pharmacopoeias.** In *US.*

**USP 27** (Oxandrolone). A white odourless crystalline powder. Soluble 1 in 5200 of water, 1 in 57 of alcohol, 1 in 69 of acetone, 1 in less than 5 of chloroform, and 1 in 860 of ether. Protect from light.

### Adverse Effects and Precautions

As for androgens and anabolic steroids in general (see Testosterone, p.1570). As with other 17α-alkylated compounds, oxandrolone may cause hepatotoxicity, and liver function should be monitored. It should be avoided if hepatic impairment is severe.

### Pharmacokinetics

Oxandrolone is rapidly absorbed from the gastrointestinal tract. It is excreted mainly in the urine as metabolites and unchanged oxandrolone. A small amount is excreted in the faeces.

### Uses and Administration

Oxandrolone has anabolic and androgenic properties (see Testosterone, p.1571) and is given in doses of 2.5 to 20 mg daily by mouth; the usual dose is 5 to 10 mg daily in divided doses for 2 to 4 weeks. In the promotion of growth in constitutional delayed growth and puberty in boys, usual daily doses of up to 100 micrograms/kg have been given (see also below). Courses of treatment should generally be short to avoid the risk of premature epiphyseal closure.

**Cachexia.** Oxandrolone has been used for its protein anabolic effect in a number of conditions associated with cachexia (p.1558) or wasting, including alcoholic hepatitis,[1] burn injury,[2] HIV-infection,[3,4] and muscular dystrophy[5,6] (p.1083).

1. Mendenhall CL, *et al.* A study of oral nutritional support with oxandrolone in malnourished patients with alcoholic hepatitis: results of a Department of Veterans Affairs Cooperative Study. *Hepatology* 1993; **17:** 564–76.
2. Demling RH. Comparison of the anabolic effects and complications of human growth hormone and the testosterone analog, oxandrolone, after severe burn injury. *Burns* 1999; **25:** 215–21.
3. Berger JR, *et al.* Oxandrolone in AIDS-wasting myopathy. *AIDS* 1996; **10:** 1657–62.
4. Strawford A, *et al.* Resistance exercise and supraphysiologic androgen therapy in eugonadal men with HIV-related weight loss. *JAMA* 1999; **281:** 1282–90.
5. Fenichel G, *et al.* A beneficial effect of oxandrolone in the treatment of Duchenne muscular dystrophy: a pilot study. *Neurology* 1997; **48:** 1225–6.
6. Fenichel GM, *et al.* A randomized efficacy and safety trial of oxandrolone in the treatment of Duchenne dystrophy. *Neurology* 2001; **56:** 1075–9.

**Growth retardation.** A beneficial effect of oxandrolone on growth rate in *boys* with constitutional delay of growth and puberty (p.1314) has been shown in various studies,[1-5] two of which[2,5] were placebo-controlled. Doses used have included 1.25 or 2.5 mg daily[1-3] and 50 or 100 micrograms/kg daily,[4,5] generally for 3 to 12 months. Although a slight advance in bone age has been noted,[1,4,5] final predicted height[5] and actual adult height[3] was not compromised by oxandrolone therapy. Oxandrolone did not affect the rate of pubertal progression and as the aim of such therapy is primarily to relieve psychosocial difficulties associated with short stature and sexual immaturity, it is not clear that it achieves this.[5]

Oxandrolone is also used for the promotion of growth in *girls* with Turner's syndrome (p.1317) in daily doses of 50 to 125 micrograms/kg.

1. Stanhope R, Brook CGD. Oxandrolone in low dose for constitutional delay of growth and puberty in boys. *Arch Dis Child* 1985; **60:** 379–81.
2. Stanhope R, *et al.* Double blind placebo controlled trial of low dose oxandrolone in the treatment of boys with constitutional delay of growth and puberty. *Arch Dis Child* 1988; **63:** 501–5.
3. Tse W-Y, *et al.* Long-term outcome of oxandrolone treatment in boys with constitutional delay of growth and puberty. *J Pediatr* 1990; **117:** 588–91.
4. Papadimitriou A, *et al.* Treatment of constitutional growth delay in prepubertal boys with a prolonged course of low dose oxandrolone. *Arch Dis Child* 1991; **66:** 841–3.
5. Wilson DM, *et al.* Oxandrolone therapy in constitutionally delayed growth and puberty. *Pediatrics* 1995; **96:** 1095–1100.

### Preparations

**USP 27:** Oxandrolone Tablets.

**Proprietary Preparations** (details are given in Part 3)
**Austral.:** Lonavar†; Oxandrin; **Israel:** Lonavar; **USA:** Oxandrin.

## Oxendolone *(USAN, rINN)*

TSAA-291. 16β-Ethyl-17β-hydroxyestr-4-en-3-one.

$C_{20}H_{30}O_2$ = 302.5.
*CAS — 33765-68-3.*

### Profile

Oxendolone is an anti-androgen that has been used in the treatment of benign prostatic hyperplasia.

### Preparations

**Proprietary Preparations** (details are given in Part 3)
**Jpn:** Prostetin†.

## Oxymetholone *(BAN, USAN, rINN)*

CI-406; HMD; Oximetolona. 17β-Hydroxy-2-hydroxymethylene-17α-methyl-5α-androstan-3-one.

$C_{21}H_{32}O_3$ = 332.5.
*CAS — 434-07-1.*
*ATC — A14AA05.*

**Pharmacopoeias.** In *Br., Jpn,* and *US.*

**BP 2003** (Oxymetholone). A white to creamy-white, odourless or almost odourless, crystalline powder. It exhibits polymorphism. Practically insoluble in water; soluble in alcohol; freely soluble in chloroform; slightly soluble in ether. Protect from light. Avoid contact with ferrous metals.

**USP 27** (Oxymetholone). A white to creamy-white, odourless crystalline powder. Practically insoluble in water; soluble 1 in 40 of alcohol, 1 in 5 of chloroform, 1 in 82 of ether, and 1 in 14 of dioxan.

### Adverse Effects and Precautions

As for androgens and anabolic steroids in general (see Testosterone, p.1570).

Liver disturbances and jaundice are common with normal doses and hepatic neoplasms have also been reported (see below). Liver function should be monitored during therapy. As with other 17α-alkylated compounds, oxymetholone should probably be avoided in patients with liver impairment, and certainly if this is severe.

**Effects on the blood.** Although there were some early reports[1,2] of leukaemia developing in patients given oxymetholone for aplastic anaemia, it has also been pointed out that of patients who present with aplastic anaemia, 1 to 5% actually have leukaemia.[3]

1. Delamore IW, Geary CG. Aplastic anaemia, acute myeloblastic leukaemia, and oxymetholone. *BMJ* 1971; **2:** 743–5.
2. Ginsburg AD. Oxymetholone and hematologic disease. *Ann Intern Med* 1973; **79:** 914.
3. Camitta BM, *et al.* Aplastic anemia (first of two parts): pathogenesis, diagnosis, treatment, and prognosis. *N Engl J Med* 1982; **306:** 645–52.

**Effects on carbohydrate metabolism.** Pronounced hyperglucagonaemia developed in 6 patients receiving oxymetholone.[1]

1. Williams G, *et al.* Severe hyperglucagonaemia during treatment with oxymetholone. *BMJ* 1986; **292:** 1637–8.

**Effects on the liver.** Reports of peliosis hepatis[1-4] and various liver tumours[4-8] associated with oxymetholone.

1. Bagheri SA, Boyer JL. Peliosis hepatis associated with androgenic-anabolic steroid therapy: a severe form of hepatic injury. *Ann Intern Med* 1974; **81:** 610–18.
2. McDonald EC, Speicher CE. Peliosis hepatis associated with administration of oxymetholone. *JAMA* 1978; **240:** 243–4.
3. Hirose H, *et al.* Fatal splenic rupture in anabolic steroid-induced peliosis in a patient with myelodysplastic syndrome. *Br J Haematol* 1991; **78:** 128–9.
4. Linares M, *et al.* Hepatocellular carcinoma and squamous cell carcinoma in a patent with Fanconi's anemia. *Ann Hematol* 1991; **63:** 54–5.
5. Lesna M, *et al.* Liver nodules and androgens. *Lancet* 1976; **i:** 1124.
6. Mokrohisky ST, *et al.* Fulminant hepatic neoplasia after androgen therapy. *N Engl J Med* 1977; **296:** 1411–12.
7. Kosaka A, *et al.* Hepatocellular carcinoma associated with anabolic steroid therapy: report of a case and review of the Japanese literature. *J Gastroenterol* 1996; **31:** 450–4.
8. Nakao A, *et al.* Multiple hepatic adenomas caused by long-term administration of androgenic steroids for aplastic anemia in association with familial adenomatous polyposis. *J Gastroenterol* 2000; **35:** 557–62.

**Effects on the nervous system.** Toxic confusional state and choreiform movements developed in an elderly man given oxymetholone 200 to 300 mg daily.[1]

1. Tilzey A, *et al.* Toxic confusional state and choreiform movements after treatment with anabolic steroids. *BMJ* 1981; **283:** 349–50.

### Uses and Administration

Oxymetholone has anabolic and androgenic properties (see Testosterone, p.1571). It has been used mainly in the treatment of anaemias such as aplastic anaemia at a usual dosage by mouth of 1 to 5 mg/kg daily. Treatment for 3 to 6 months has been suggested, with the drug either withdrawn gradually on remission or reduced to an appropriate maintenance dose.

**Aplastic anaemia.** There have been mixed results[1-5] with oxymetholone in the treatment of aplastic anaemia (p.732); generally, the response and survival rates have been disappointing.

1. Davis S, Rubin AD. Treatment and prognosis in aplastic anaemia. *Lancet* 1972; **i:** 871–3.
2. Mir MA, Delamore IW. Oxymetholone in aplastic anaemia. *Postgrad Med J* 1974; **50:** 166–71.
3. Camitta BM, *et al.* A prospective study of androgens and bone marrow transplantation for treatment of severe aplastic anemia. *Blood* 1979; **53:** 504–14.
4. Mir MA, Geary CG. Aplastic anaemia: an analysis of 174 patients. *Postgrad Med J* 1980; **56:** 322–9.
5. Webb DKH, *et al.* Acquired aplastic anaemia: still a serious disease. *Arch Dis Child* 1991; **66:** 858–61.

### Preparations

**BP 2003:** Oxymetholone Tablets;
**USP 27:** Oxymetholone Tablets.

**Proprietary Preparations** (details are given in Part 3)
**Braz.:** Hemogenin; **India:** Adroyd; **Thai.:** Androlic; **UK:** Anapolon†; **USA:** Anadrol.

## Polyestradiol Phosphate *(BAN, rINN)*

Fosfato de poliestradiol; Leo-114; Polyoestradiol Phosphate. A water-soluble polymeric ester of estradiol and phosphoric acid with a molecular weight of about 26 000.

*CAS — 28014-46-2.*
*ATC — L02AA02.*

### Adverse Effects and Precautions

As for oestrogens in general (see Estradiol, p.1550). Pain may occur at the site of injection, and mepivacaine is included in some preparations to minimise this.

### Pharmacokinetics

Following intramuscular injection polyestradiol phosphate is released slowly into the bloodstream where it is slowly metabolised to estradiol.

### Uses and Administration

Polyestradiol phosphate is a polymer of estradiol (see p.1550) which has a prolonged duration of action, and is used in the treatment of metastatic prostatic carcinoma (p.521). It has been given by deep intramuscular injection in initial doses of 80 to 160 mg every 4 weeks for 2 to 3 months, reduced to 40 to 80 mg every 4 weeks for maintenance. Higher doses of 240 mg every 2 weeks for 2 months, followed by a maintenance dose of 240 mg every 4 weeks, have also been used.

### Preparations

**Proprietary Preparations** (details are given in Part 3)
**Austria:** Estradurin; **Belg.:** Estradurine; **Denm.:** Estradurin; **Fin.:** Estradurin; **Ger.:** Estradurin; **Neth.:** Estradurin; **Norw.:** Estradurin; **Spain:** Estradurin†; **Swed.:** Estradurin; **Switz.:** Estradurin.

## Polyestriol Phosphate

Poliestriol, fosfato de; Polyoestriol Phosphate.

*CAS — 37452-43-0.*

### Profile

Polyestriol phosphate is a polymer of estriol (p.1552) with phosphoric acid. It has the properties of oestrogens in general and has been given in the treatment of menopausal disorders.

## Prasterone *(rINN)*

Dehydroandrosterone; Dehydroepiandrosterone; Dehydroisoandrosterone; DHEA; GL-701; Prasterona. 3β-Hydroxyandrost-5-en-17-one.

$C_{19}H_{28}O_2$ = 288.4.
*CAS — 53-43-0.*
*ATC — A14AA07.*

**Pharmacopoeias.** In *Fr.*

## Prasterone Enantate *(rINNM)*

Dehydroepiandrosterone Enanthate; EDHEA; Enantato de prasterona; Prasterone Enanthate. 3β-Hydroxyandrost-5-en-17-one heptanoate.

$C_{26}H_{40}O_3$ = 400.6.
*CAS — 23983-43-9.*
*ATC — A14AA07.*

### Prasterone Sodium Sulfate *(rINNM)*

Dehydroepiandrosterone Sulphate Sodium; DHA-S; DHEAS; PB-005; Prasterone Sodium Sulphate; Sulfato sódico de prasterona. 3β-Hydroxyandrost-5-en-17-one hydrogen sulphate sodium.

$C_{19}H_{27}NaO_5S$ = 390.5.
*CAS — 651-48-9 (prasterone sulfate); 1099-87-2 (prasterone sodium sulfate).*
*ATC — A14AA07.*

**Pharmacopoeias.** In *Jpn. Chin.* includes the dihydrate.

#### Profile

Prasterone is a naturally occurring adrenal androgen that is a precursor of androgens and oestrogens. Prasterone enantate, in a dose of 200 mg every 4 weeks, is given by intramuscular depot injection with estradiol valerate as menopausal HRT (p.1540). Prasterone is also being investigated in adrenal insufficiency and in systemic lupus erythematosus, and the sodium sulfate is under investigation for the treatment of burns and acute asthma.

◊ General reviews.

1. Kroboth PD, *et al.* DHEA and DHEA-S: a review. *J Clin Pharmacol* 1999; **39:** 327–48.
2. Pepping J. DHEA: dehydroepiandrosterone. *Am J Health-Syst Pharm* 2000; **57:** 2048–56.

**HIV infection and AIDS.** Plasma concentrations of prasterone are reported to be abnormally low in patients with AIDS, and it has been suggested that use of prasterone might be of benefit; however, large controlled studies are lacking.[1] One small controlled trial[2] of patients with advanced HIV disease reported that supplementation raised concentrations of prasterone, and improved some quality of life measures.

1. Centurelli MA, *et al.* The role of dehydroepiandrosterone in AIDS. *Ann Pharmacother* 1997; **31:** 639–42.
2. Piketty C, *et al.* Double-blind placebo-controlled trial of oral dehydroepiandrosterone in patients with advanced HIV disease. *Clin Endocrinol (Oxf)* 2001; **55:** 325–30.

**Replacement therapy.** There has been much speculation about the physiological role and importance of prasterone, which is the most abundant steroid hormone in the circulation. It is produced by the adrenal gland and is a precursor of androgens and oestrogens.[1] Serum concentrations of the sulfate conjugate peak at about 20 years then gradually decline with age. Epidemiological studies suggest that certain age-related diseases are linked to this decline, including an increased risk of cardiovascular disease in men, and breast cancer in premenopausal women.[1] It has been suggested, therefore, that replacement therapy with prasterone might alleviate some of the problems of ageing. However, there is insufficient evidence of safety and efficacy to recommend such use. A systematic review[2] of studies in healthy adults taking prasterone supplementation found no support for an improvement in memory or cognitive function. A study of healthy adults who took prasterone or placebo for one year reported improved bone turnover and skin condition, particularly in women over 70 years old.[3] A review[4] of the use of prasterone as a 'food supplement' noted that although it was being taken in the belief that it could reverse some of the effects of ageing there was no good evidence of this. Various androgenic effects, including hirsutism and voice changes, have been reported in women taking prasterone and there is a theoretical possibility that it might promote growth of hormone-sensitive tumours in both sexes.[1,4]

Prasterone has also been studied as replacement therapy for patients with adrenal insufficiency, who have subnormal levels of prasterone. Such therapy has been reported to raise serum levels of prasterone to normal, and improve measures of well-being, mood, and fatigue.[5,6]

1. Weksler ME. Hormone replacement for men. *BMJ* 1996; **312:** 859–60.
2. Huppert FA, Van Niekerk JK. Dehydroepiandrosterone (DHEA) supplementation for cognitive function. Available in The Cochrane Library; Issue 2. Chichester: John Wiley; 2004.
3. Baulieu E-E, *et al.* Dehydroepiandrosterone (DHEA), DHEA sulfate, and aging: contribution of the DHEAge study to a sociobiomedical issue. *Proc Natl Acad Sci U S A* 2000; **97:** 4279–84.
4. Anonymous. Dehydroepiandrosterone (DHEA). *Med Lett Drugs Ther* 1996; **38:** 91–2.
5. Arlt W, *et al.* Dehydroepiandrosterone replacement in women with adrenal insufficiency. *N Engl J Med* 1999; **341:** 1013–20.
6. Hunt PJ, *et al.* Improvement in mood and fatigue after dehydroepiandrosterone replacement in Addison's disease in a randomized, double blind trial. *J Clin Endocrinol Metab* 2000; **85:** 4650–6.

**Systemic lupus erythematosus.** Symptomatic improvement was seen in 8 of 10 women with systemic lupus erythematosus (p.1088) who received prasterone 200 mg daily by mouth for several months.[1] Improvement permitted a reduction in their corticosteroid dosage. Similar findings have been reported by one group in a number of small studies,[2-5] but although they considered that there was clear evidence of benefit,[6] two larger, and thus far unpublished, studies have produced more statistically ambiguous results; as a result, as of July 2001 the FDA had not approved licensing of prasterone for this indication.

1. van Vollenhoven RF, *et al.* An open study of dehydroepiandrosterone in systemic lupus erythematosus. *Arthritis Rheum* 1994; **37:** 1305–10.
2. van Vollenhoven RF, *et al.* Dehydroepiandrosterone in systemic lupus erythematosus. *Arthritis Rheum* 1995; **38:** 1826–31.
3. van Vollenhoven RF, *et al.* Treatment of systemic lupus erythematosus with dehydroepiandrosterone: 50 patients treated up to 12 months. *J Rheumatol* 1998; **25:** 285–9.
4. Barry NN, *et al.* Dehydroepiandrosterone in systemic lupus erythematosus: relationship between dosage, serum levels, and clinical response. *J Rheumatol* 1998; **25:** 2352–6.
5. van Vollenhoven RF, *et al.* A double-blind, placebo-controlled, clinical trial of dehydroepiandrosterone in severe systemic lupus erythematosus. *Lupus* 1999; **8:** 181–7.
6. van Vollenhoven RF. Dehydroepiandrosterone in systemic lupus erythematosus. *Rheum Dis Clin North Am* 2000; **26:** 349–62.

#### Preparations

**Proprietary Preparations** (details are given in Part 3)
***Port.:*** Dinistenile.

**Multi-ingredient: *Arg.:*** Dastonil; Gynodian Depot; ***Austria:*** Gynodian Depot; ***Chile:*** Gynodian Depot; ***Ger.:*** Gynodian Depot; ***Gr.:*** Cyclacur; Divina; ***Ital.:*** Gynodian Depot; Sinsurrene†; ***Mex.:*** Binodian; Sten; ***Spain:*** Gynodian Depot†; ***Switz.:*** Gynodian Depot.

## Progesterone *(BAN, rINN)*

Corpus Luteum Hormone; Luteal Hormone; Luteine; Luteohormone; NSC-9704; Pregnenedione; Progesterona; Progesteronum. Pregn-4-ene-3,20-dione.

$C_{21}H_{30}O_2$ = 314.5.
*CAS — 57-83-0.*
*ATC — G03DA04.*

**Pharmacopoeias.** In *Chin., Eur.* (see p.vi), *Int., Jpn, Pol., US,* and *Viet.*

**Ph. Eur. 5.0** (Progesterone). A white or almost white crystalline powder or colourless crystals. It exhibits polymorphism. Practically insoluble in water; freely soluble in dehydrated alcohol; sparingly soluble in acetone and in fatty oils. Protect from light.

**USP 27** (Progesterone). A white or creamy-white, odourless, crystalline powder. Practically insoluble in water; soluble in alcohol, in acetone, and in dioxan; sparingly soluble in vegetable oils. Store in airtight containers at a temperature of 25°, excursions permitted between 15° and 30°. Protect from light.

### Adverse Effects

Progesterone and the progestogens may cause gastrointestinal disturbances, changes in appetite or weight, fluid retention, oedema, acne, chloasma (melasma), allergic skin rashes, urticaria, mental depression, breast changes including discomfort or occasionally gynaecomastia, changes in libido, hair loss, hirsutism, fatigue, drowsiness or insomnia, fever, headache, premenstrual syndrome-like symptoms, and altered menstrual cycles or irregular menstrual bleeding. Anaphylaxis or anaphylactoid reactions may occur rarely. Alterations in the serum lipid profile may occur, and rarely alterations in liver-function tests and jaundice. Pain, diarrhoea, and flatulence have followed rectal use. Injection-site reactions have followed parenteral use.

Adverse effects vary depending on the dose and type of progestogen. For example, androgenic effects such as acne and hirsutism are more likely to occur with nortestosterone derivatives such as norethisterone and norgestrel. These derivatives may also be more likely to adversely affect serum lipids. Conversely, adverse effects on serum lipids appear less likely with gestodene and desogestrel, but these 2 drugs have been associated with a higher incidence of thromboembolism than norethisterone and norgestrel when used in combined oral contraceptives (see p.1531). High doses of progestogens such as those used in treating cancer have also been associated with thromboembolism. For a discussion of the effect of progestogens on the cardiovascular risk profile of menopausal HRT see p.1538. Breakthrough uterine bleeding is more common with oral progestogen-only contraceptives than when progestogens are used for menstrual irregularities or as part of menopausal HRT.

Some progestogens when given during pregnancy have been reported to cause virilisation of a female fetus. This appears to have been associated with those progestogens with more pronounced androgenic activity such as norethisterone; the natural progestogenic hormone progesterone and its derivatives such as dydrogesterone and medroxyprogesterone do not appear to have been associated with such effects.

For the adverse effects of progestogens when administered either alone or with oestrogens as contraceptives, see p.1527. For those of menopausal HRT, see p.1536.

**Effects on the skin.** A case report and discussion of progesterone-induced urticaria.[1]

1. Wilkinson SM, *et al.* Progesterone-induced urticaria—need it be autoimmune? *Br J Dermatol* 1995; **133:** 792–4.

### Precautions

Progesterone and the progestogens should be used with caution in patients with cardiovascular or renal impairment, diabetes mellitus, asthma, epilepsy, and migraine, or other conditions which may be aggravated by fluid retention. They should also be used with care in persons with a history of depression. High doses should be used with caution in patients susceptible to thromboembolism.

Progesterone and the progestogens should not be given to patients with undiagnosed vaginal bleeding, nor to those with a history or current high risk of arterial disease and should generally be avoided in hepatic impairment, especially if severe. Unless progestogens are being used as part of the management of breast or genital-tract carcinoma they should not be given to patients with these conditions.

Although progestogens have been given as hormonal support during early pregnancy such use is not now generally advised. Some, however, allow the use of a progesterone-type progestogen for women who are progesterone-deficient. Such use may prevent spontaneous evacuation of a dead fetus, therefore careful monitoring of pregnancy is required. Progestogens should not be used diagnostically for pregnancy testing and should not be given in missed or incomplete abortion.

For precautions to be observed when progestogens are used as contraceptives, see p.1532. For those to be observed when progestogens are used in preparations for menopausal HRT, see p.1539.

**Abuse.** A case report of abuse of and dependency on progesterone.[1]

1. Keefe DL, Sarrel P. Dependency on progesterone in woman with self-diagnosed premenstrual syndrome. *Lancet* 1996; **347:** 1182.

**Breast feeding.** A large study[1] compared a contraceptive progesterone-releasing vaginal ring and a copper IUD for 1 year in breast-feeding women. There was little difference in infant weight gain during the study, although at 12 months the infants of mothers using the IUD were breast-fed less frequently, receiving more supplementary feeding, and were heavier. There was no adverse effect of progesterone on lactation or infant growth. The American Academy of Pediatrics has found no reports of adverse effects in breast-fed infants whose mothers were receiving progesterone, and therefore considers it to be usually compatible with breast feeding.[2]

1. Sivin I, *et al.* Contraceptives for lactating women: a comparative trial of a progesterone-releasing vaginal ring and the copper T 380A IUD. *Contraception* 1997; **55:** 225–32.
2. American Academy of Pediatrics. The transfer of drugs and other chemicals into human milk. *Pediatrics* 2001; **108:** 776–89. Correction. *ibid.*; 1029. Also available at: http://aappolicy.aappublications.org/cgi/content/full/pediatrics%3b108/3/776 (accessed 21/06/04)

**Porphyria.** Progesterone and progestogens have been associated with acute attacks of porphyria and are considered unsafe in patients with porphyria (but medroxyprogesterone has been used with buserelin to suppress premenstrual exacerbations of porphyria, see p.1320). Progestogens should generally be avoided by all women with porphyria; however, where non-hormonal contraception is inappropriate, progestogens may be used with extreme caution if the potential benefit outweighs the risk. The risk of an acute attack is greatest in women who have had a previous attack or are under 30 years of age. Long-acting progestogen preparations should never be used in those at risk.

**Pregnancy.** In Hungary where 30% of all pregnant women were given hormonal support therapy with progestogens during the early 1980s, a case-control study suggested that there was a causal relationship between such treatment and hypospadias in their offspring.[1] Reports of abnormalities in infants following exposure *in utero* to progestogens have included hypospadias[2] with norethisterone and hydroxyprogesterone; other genito-urinary anomalies with dydrogesterone[3] and hydroxyprogesterone;[4] tetralogy of Fallot[5] and adrenocortical carcinoma[6] with hydroxyprogesterone; fetal masculinisation[7] with norethisterone, noretynodrel, and ethisterone; and meningomyelocele or hydrocephalus[8] with norethisterone and ethisterone. For further details see under Pregnancy in the individual monographs. For the effects on the fetus when progestogens are used as contraceptives, see p.1533. For the risk of ectopic pregnancy with progestogen-only contraceptives, see p.1529.

1. Czeizel A. Increasing trends in congenital malformations of male external genitalia. *Lancet* 1985; **i:** 462–3.
2. Aarskog D. Clinical and cytogenetic studies in hypospadias. *Acta Paediatr Scand* 1970; (suppl 203): 1–62.

3. Roberts IF, West RJ. Teratogenesis and maternal progesterone. *Lancet* 1977; **ii:** 982.
4. Evans ANW, *et al.* The ingestion by pregnant women of substances toxic to the foetus. *Practitioner* 1980; **224:** 315–19.
5. Heinonen OP, *et al.* Cardiovascular birth defects and antenatal exposure to female sex hormones. *N Engl J Med* 1977; **296:** 67–70.
6. Mann JR, *et al.* Transplacental carcinogenesis (adrenocortical carcinoma) associated with hydroxyprogesterone hexanoate. *Lancet* 1983; **ii:** 580.
7. Wilkins L. Masculinization of female fetus due to use of orally given progestins. *JAMA* 1960; **172:** 1028–32.
8. Gal I, *et al.* Hormonal pregnancy tests and congenital malformation. *Nature* 1967; **216:** 83.

**Veterinary use.** An expert committee of the FAO and WHO considered it unnecessary to establish an acceptable daily intake or acceptable residue level in food for endogenous hormones such as progesterone.[1] Residues resulting from the use of progesterone as a growth promotor in accordance with good animal husbandry practice are unlikely to pose a hazard to human health. However, it should be noted that in the European Union the use of steroidal hormones such as progestogens in veterinary practice is restricted, and their use as growth promotors is banned.

1. FAO/WHO. Evaluation of certain veterinary drug residues in food: thirty-second report of the joint FAO/WHO expert committee on food additives. *WHO Tech Rep Ser 763* 1988.

## Interactions

Enzyme-inducing drugs such as carbamazepine, griseofulvin, phenobarbital, phenytoin, and rifampicin may enhance the clearance of progesterone and the progestogens. These interactions are likely to reduce the efficacy of progestogen-only contraceptives (see p.1534), and additional or alternative contraceptive measures are recommended.

Aminoglutethimide markedly reduces the plasma concentrations of medroxyprogesterone acetate and megestrol, possibly through a hepatic enzyme-inducing effect; an increase in progestogen dose is likely to be required.

Since progesterone and other progestogens can influence diabetic control an adjustment in antidiabetic dosage could be required. Progestogens may inhibit ciclosporin metabolism leading to increased plasma-ciclosporin concentrations and a risk of toxicity (see p.1356).

## Pharmacokinetics

Progesterone has a short elimination half-life and undergoes extensive first-pass hepatic metabolism when given by mouth; oral bioavailability is very low although it may be increased somewhat by an oily vehicle and by micronisation. Progesterone is absorbed when given buccally, rectally, or vaginally, and rapidly absorbed from the site of an oily intramuscular injection.

Various derivatives have been produced to extend the duration of action and to improve oral activity. Esters of progesterone derivatives such as hydroxyprogesterone caproate are used intramuscularly, and megestrol acetate is orally active. The ester medroxyprogesterone acetate is used orally and parenterally. 19-Nortestosterone progestogens have good oral activity because the 17-ethinyl substituent slows hepatic metabolism.

Progesterone and the progestogens are highly protein bound; progesterone is bound to albumin and corticosteroid binding globulin; esters such as medroxyprogesterone acetate are principally bound to albumin; and 19-nortestosterone analogues are bound to sex-steroid binding globulin and albumin. Progesterone is metabolised in the liver to various metabolites including pregnanediol, which are excreted in the urine as sulfate and glucuronide conjugates. Similarly, progestogens undergo hepatic metabolism to various conjugates, which are excreted in the urine. Progesterone is distributed into breast milk.

◊ Reviews.

1. Kuhl H. Comparative pharmacology of newer progestogens. *Drugs* 1996; **51:** 188–215.
2. Stanczyk FZ. Structure-function relationships, metabolism, pharmacokinetics and potency of progestins. *Drugs Today* 1996; **32** (suppl H): 1–14.

## Uses and Administration

Progesterone is a natural hormone whereas progestogens are synthetic compounds, derived from progesterone or 19-nortestosterone, with actions similar to those of progesterone (for further details, see p.1527).

Progestogens derived from 19-nortestosterone are used as **hormonal contraceptives** (see p.1535), either alone or combined with an oestrogen. The progesterone derivative medroxyprogesterone acetate is also used, and progesterone itself has been used.

Progestogens, and sometimes progesterone, are used with oestrogens for **menopausal HRT** (p.1540) to reduce the increased risk of endometrial hyperplasia and carcinoma which occurs when unopposed long-term oestrogen therapy is employed.

Similarly, drugs with progestogenic actions may be used in **menstrual disorders** such as dysmenorrhoea (p.6) and menorrhagia associated with dysfunctional uterine bleeding (below). Progestogens may also be used in the management of endometriosis (p.1546). Although progestogens and progesterone have been used for the management of the premenstrual syndrome, such a practice is of debatable value (p.1551).

Progestogens may be valuable in advanced **endometrial cancer** (p.516) and have been tried in some other malignancies. The progestogens typically used for malignant disease include medroxyprogesterone acetate, megestrol, and norethisterone. Some progestogens such as megestrol and medroxyprogesterone are used for the **cachexia** or wasting associated with severe illness including cancer and AIDS (p.1558).

Progestogens have been widely advocated for either the prevention of **recurrent miscarriage** or the treatment of threatened miscarriage. However, there is little evidence of any benefit from such a practice and the use of progestogens in early pregnancy is not now generally advised, with the exception of the use of progesterone or a progesterone derivative in women who are progesterone deficient (see also under Precautions, above).

USES AND ADMINISTRATION OF PROGESTERONE. Progesterone is usually given as an oily intramuscular injection, a vaginal gel or pessaries, or as suppositories. An oral micronised preparation of progesterone is also available.

In dysfunctional uterine bleeding or amenorrhoea 5 to 10 mg daily of progesterone may be given by intramuscular injection for about 5 to 10 days until 2 days before the anticipated onset of menstruation. Alternatively, progesterone may be given as a vaginal gel at a usual dose of 45 mg on alternate days from day 15 to 25 of the cycle, or orally at a dose of 400 mg daily for 10 days.

In women with a history of recurrent miscarriage and proven progesterone deficiency, twice weekly intramuscular injection (increased to daily if necessary) of 25 to 100 mg of progesterone, from about day 15 of the pregnancy until 8 to 16 weeks, has been used. A similar schedule has been used in *in vitro* fertilisation or gamete intra-fallopian transfer techniques with treatment beginning on the day of transfer of embryo or gametes. The dose may be increased to 200 mg daily if necessary. Alternatively, progesterone may be given as a vaginal gel at a dose of 90 mg daily continued for 30 days after laboratory evidence of pregnancy; 90 mg twice daily has been used in women with ovarian failure.

Progesterone may be given vaginally or rectally in doses of 200 mg daily to 400 mg twice daily for the management of the premenstrual syndrome. Treatment usually starts on day 12 to 14 of the menstrual cycle and continues until the onset of menstruation. Similar vaginal or rectal doses have also been used in the treatment of puerperal (post-natal) depression.

Progesterone gel may be given intravaginally at a dose of 45 mg on alternate days for 12 days of a 28-day cycle as the progestogen component of menopausal HRT.

A progesterone-releasing intra-uterine device has also been used as a hormonal contraceptive; the device contains 38 mg of progesterone and is effective for up to 12 months.

**Menorrhagia.** Menorrhagia, or excessive menstrual bleeding, is usually defined as a blood loss exceeding 80 mL per menstrual period,[1,2] compared with a normal loss of about 30 mL. However, many women consider losses below 80 mL to be excessive particularly if 'flooding' occurs. Although not life-threatening, menorrhagia can lead to iron deficiency anaemia as well as considerably impairing quality of life. Menorrhagia may be associated with pelvic disorders such as fibroids or endometriosis, or the use of copper intra-uterine devices, or some systemic disorders.[1,2] However, most commonly it is associated with dysfunctional uterine bleeding; a term used to denote frequent, prolonged or heavy uterine bleeding for which no specific cause is found (essential, idiopathic, or primary menorrhagia). Both ovulatory (regular) and anovulatory cycles may give rise to dysfunctional uterine bleeding.[2] If the patient has regular ovulatory cycles and does not require contraception or wish to take a hormonal treatment, then an NSAID or tranexamic acid is usually the preferred treatment.[1-3] These have the advantage that they are only taken during menstruation, which increases compliance.[2] Therapy is generally tried for 3 months, and continued if the response is good and there are no adverse effects; nonresponders may be switched to the alternative therapy while awaiting referral to a specialist.[3]

UK summary guidelines for the initial management of menorrhagia recommend the use of mefenamic acid as the *NSAID* of choice[3] but other NSAIDs such as ibuprofen or naproxen have been used and there does not seem to be evidence to suggest that one NSAID is more effective than another. They reduce menstrual blood loss by about 30%,[2,4] and relieve dysmenorrhoea (p.6). Systematic review suggests that NSAIDs are less effective than tranexamic acid or danazol in reducing bleeding,[5] but they may have fewer adverse effects.

Given during menstruation *tranexamic acid* reduces menstrual blood loss by about half;[2,4] the benefits of tranexamic therapy have been confirmed by systematic review.[6] However, gastrointestinal adverse effects are common and it is contra-indicated in women with thromboembolic disorders. *Etamsylate* has been reported to have similar efficacy to an NSAID in 1 study,[7] but to be ineffective in another.[8] An analysis, which included these and 2 earlier studies, concluded that etamsylate reduced menstrual blood loss by about 10 to 15%.[4]

In women who require contraception, a *combined oral contraceptive* appears to be effective,[1,2] although good evidence of this is actually lacking.[9] UK summary guidelines recommend use with mefenamic acid in those women in whom an oral contraceptive alone is inadequate.[3] Traditional therapy with *progestogens* such as norethisterone or medroxyprogesterone given during the luteal phase appears to be ineffective in women with normal ovulatory cycles,[2,10] although cyclical therapy may be of benefit in anovulatory patients as it imposes a cycle.[2] Progestogen therapy for 21 days of the cycle results in a significant reduction in menstrual blood loss,[10] but is associated with adverse effects that may limit its acceptability.

More recently, a *levonorgestrel-containing intra-uterine device* has been shown to be very effective in reducing menstrual blood loss,[11,12] and to be an alternative to hysterectomy in menorrhagia.[13,14] It has been suggested that this may become the preferred long-term medical treatment for menorrhagia,[1] although comparative data are scanty.[15]

*Danazol* is also effective, producing about a 50% reduction in menstrual blood loss,[4] but has significant adverse effects and treatment is usually limited to 3 to 6 months. *Gonadorelin analogues* are effective for menorrhagia associated with fibroids (p.1326), but can only be used short term because of the resultant ovarian suppression.[1] When used pre-operatively for endometrial thinning, gonadorelin analogues produce more consistent results than danazol.[16]

In patients who fail to respond to drug treatment, or in whom such therapy is inappropriate, various *surgical options* exist. Conservative surgical techniques, where the endometrium is ablated or resected, are increasingly being used, and appear to be an effective alternative to hysterectomy.[17] Hysterectomy is the ultimate therapy, but is associated with significant morbidity.

1. Wood CE. Menorrhagia: a clinical update. *Med J Aust* 1996; **165:** 510–14.
2. Prentice A. Medical management of menorrhagia. *BMJ* 1999; **319:** 1343–5.
3. Royal College of Obstetricians and Gynaecologists. The initial management of menorrhagia [summary]. Available at: http://www.rcog.org.uk/guidelines.asp?PageID=108&GuidelineID=28 (accessed 17/05/02)
4. Coulter A, *et al.* Treating menorrhagia in primary care: an overview of drug trials and a survey of prescribing practice. *Int J Technol Assess Health Care* 1995; **11:** 456–71.
5. Lethaby A, *et al.* Nonsteroidal anti-inflammatory drugs for heavy menstrual bleeding. Available in The Cochrane Library; Issue 2. Chichester: John Wiley; 2004.
6. Lethaby A, *et al.* Antifibrinolytics for heavy menstrual bleeding. Available in The Cochrane Library; Issue 2. Chichester: John Wiley; 2004.
7. Chamberlain G, *et al.* A comparative study of ethamsylate and mefenamic acid in dysfunctional uterine bleeding. *Br J Obstet Gynaecol* 1991; **98:** 707–11.
8. Bonnar J, Sheppard BL. Treatment of menorrhagia during menstruation: randomised controlled trial of ethamsylate, mefenamic acid, and tranexamic acid. *BMJ* 1996; **313:** 579–82.
9. Iyer V, *et al.* Oral contraceptive pills for heavy menstrual bleeding. Available in The Cochrane Library; Issue 2. Chichester: John Wiley; 2004.
10. Lethaby A, *et al.* Cyclical progestogens for heavy menstrual bleeding. Available in The Cochrane Library; Issue 2. Chichester: John Wiley; 2004.

11. Andersson JK, Rybo G. Levonorgestrel-releasing intrauterine device in the treatment of menorrhagia. *Br J Obstet Gynaecol* 1990; **97:** 690–4.
12. Milsom I, *et al.* A comparison of flurbiprofen, tranexamic acid, and a levonorgestrel-releasing intrauterine contraceptive device in the treatment of idiopathic menorrhagia. *Am J Obstet Gynecol* 1991; **164:** 879–83.
13. Lähteenmäki P, *et al.* Open randomised study of use of levonorgestrel releasing intrauterine system as alternative to hysterectomy. *BMJ* 1998; **316:** 1122–6.
14. Hurskainen R, *et al.* Quality of life and cost-effectiveness of levonorgestrel-releasing intrauterine system versus hysterectomy for treatment of menorrhagia: a randomised trial. *Lancet* 2001; **357:** 273–77.
15. Lethaby AE, *et al.* Progesterone/progestogen releasing intrauterine systems for heavy menstrual bleeding. Available in The Cochrane Library; Issue 2. Chichester: John Wiley; 2004.
16. Sowter MC, *et al.* Pre-operative endometrial thinning agents before endometrial destruction for heavy menstrual bleeding. Available in The Cochrane Library; Issue 2. Chichester: John Wiley; 2004.
17. Lethaby A, *et al.* Endometrial resection and ablation versus hysterectomy for heavy menstrual bleeding. Available in The Cochrane Library; Issue 2. Chichester: John Wiley; 2004.

**Premenstrual syndrome.** Progestogen therapy was once popular for premenstrual syndrome, but beneficial responses have not been universally achieved and the theory that progesterone was necessary to correct a hormone imbalance is now losing ground (see p.1551). A double-blind, placebo-controlled crossover study[1] involving 168 women showed that progesterone 0.4 or 0.8 g daily by the vaginal route did not significantly improve symptoms of the premenstrual syndrome. However, the view has been expressed[2] that since absorption of progesterone from the vagina or rectum may vary between patients, the dose and frequency of administration needs to be individualised and that if the response to treatment is inadequate the intramuscular route should be tried. A more recent study found oral micronised progesterone, in an initial dose of 1.2 g daily in divided doses, increased as required to 3.6 g daily, to be no better than placebo in the management of severe premenstrual syndrome.[3]

1. Freeman E, *et al.* Ineffectiveness of progesterone suppository treatment for premenstrual syndrome. *JAMA* 1990; **264:** 349–53.
2. Dalton K. Treating the premenstrual syndrome. *BMJ* 1988; **297:** 490.
3. Freeman EW, *et al.* A double-blind trial of oral progesterone, alprazolam, and placebo in treatment of severe premenstrual syndrome. *JAMA* 1995; **274:** 51–7.

## Preparations

***BP 2003:*** Progesterone Injection;
***USP 27:*** Progesterone Injectable Suspension; Progesterone Injection; Progesterone Intrauterine Contraceptive System; Progesterone Vaginal Suppositories.

**Proprietary Preparations** (details are given in Part 3)
***Arg.:*** Crinone; Faselut; Gester; Mafel; Progest; Proluton; Utrogestan; ***Austral.:*** Proluton; ***Austria:*** Utrogestan; ***Belg.:*** Progestogel; Utrogestan; ***Braz.:*** Crinone; Utrogestan; ***Canad.:*** Crinone; Gesterol†; Prometrium; ***Chile:*** Progendo; ***Fin.:*** Crinone; Lugesteron; ***Fr.:*** Estima; Evapause; Progestasert†; Progestogel; Progestosol†; Utrogestan; ***Ger.:*** Crinone; Progestogel; Utrogest; ***Gr.:*** Crinone; ***Hong Kong:*** Crinone; Cyclogest; Progestogel; Utrogestan; ***India:*** Naturogest; Progest; ***Irl.:*** Crinone; Utrogestan; ***Israel:*** Endometrin; Gestone; Utrogestan; ***Ital.:*** Crinone; Esolut; Lutogin; Progeffik; Progestogel; Progestol; Prometrium; Prontogest; ***Malaysia:*** Utrogestan; ***Mex.:*** Crinone; Cuerpo Amarillo Fuerte; Geproml; Geslutin; Prolidon†; Utrogestan; ***Neth.:*** Progestan; ***Norw.:*** Crinone; ***NZ:*** Gestone; ***Port.:*** Crinone; Progenar; Progestogel; Utrogestan; ***S.Afr.:*** Cyclogest; Utrogestan; ***Singapore:*** Crinone†; Cyclogest; Utrogestan; ***Spain:*** Crinone; Cutifitol†; Progeffik; Progestogel; Utrogestan; ***Swed.:*** Crinone; ***Switz.:*** Crinone; Progestogel; Utrogestan; ***Thai.:*** Cyclogest; Gestone; Progestogel; Proluton†; Utrogestan; ***UK:*** Crinone; Cyclogest; Gestone; ***USA:*** Crinone; Prochieve; Progestasert; Prometrium.

**Multi-ingredient:** ***Arg.:*** Cristerona; Hosterona; Lubriderm; Menstrogen; Tropivag Plus; ***Braz.:*** Ginecoside; Hormoginase†; Normomensil; Progest†; ***Fr.:*** Florgynal; Synergon; Trophigil; ***Ger.:*** Jephagynon; ***Ital.:*** Biormon; Duo-Ormogyn†; Menovis; ***Mex.:*** Damax; Lutoginestryl F; Metrigen Fuerte; Ominol; Progediol; Proger-F; ***Mon.:*** Tocogestan†; ***Port.:*** Emmenovis; ***Thai.:*** Duoton.

## Proligestone *(BAN, rINN)*

Proligestona. 14a,17α-Propylidene dioxypregn-4-ene-3,20-dione.
$C_{24}H_{34}O_4$ = 386.5.
*CAS — 23873-85-0.*

### Profile

Proligestone is a progestogen used in veterinary medicine.

## Promegestone *(rINN)*

Promegestona; R-5020. 17α-Methyl-17-propionylestra-4,9-dien-3-one.
$C_{22}H_{30}O_2$ = 326.5.
*CAS — 34184-77-5.*
*ATC — G03DB07.*

### Profile

Promegestone is a progestogen structurally related to progesterone (p.1566). It has been given by mouth on a cyclical basis, in doses of 125 to 500 micrograms daily, in the treatment of menstrual disorders and mastalgia, and as the progestogen component of menopausal HRT.

### Preparations

**Proprietary Preparations** (details are given in Part 3)
***Fr.:*** Surgestone; ***Port.:*** Surgestone.

## Promestriene *(rINN)*

Promestrieno. 17β-Methoxy-3-propoxyestra-1,3,5(10)-triene.
$C_{22}H_{32}O_2$ = 328.5.
*CAS — 39219-28-8.*
*ATC — G03CA09.*

### Profile

Promestriene is a derivative of estradiol (p.1550) that has been used topically in menopausal atrophic vaginitis, and in seborrhoea.

### Preparations

**Proprietary Preparations** (details are given in Part 3)
***Arg.:*** Colpotrophine; ***Braz.:*** Colpotrofine; ***Hong Kong:*** Colpotrophine; ***Ital.:*** Colpotrophine; ***Mon.:*** Colpotrophine; ***Port.:*** Colpotrophine; ***Singapore:*** Colpotrophine; ***Spain:*** Colpotrofin; Delipoderm; ***Switz.:*** Colpotrophine.

**Multi-ingredient:** ***Hong Kong:*** Colposeptine; ***Mon.:*** Colposeptine; ***Port.:*** Trophoseptine†.

## Pygeum Africanum

African Prune; Pruni Africanae; Prunier d'Afrique.
*ATC — G04CX01.*

**Pharmacopoeias.** In *Eur.* (see p.vi).
**Ph. Eur. 5.0** (Pygeum Africanum Bark; Pygeum Bark BP 2003). The whole or cut, dried bark of the stems and branches of *Prunus africana* (*Pygeum africanum*).

### Profile

An extract of the bark of *Pygeum africanum* is used in the treatment of benign prostatic hyperplasia (p.1555). Like some other phytotherapies for this disorder, it appears to contain various sitosterols. A usual dosage is 100 mg daily by mouth.

**Benign prostatic hyperplasia.** Pygeum africanum appears to produce a modest benefit on urological symptoms and measures of urinary flow.

References.

1. Andro M-C, Riffaud J-P. Pygeum africanum extract for the treatment of patients with benign prostatic hyperplasia: a review of 25 years of published experience. *Curr Ther Res* 1995; **56:** 796–817.
2. Buck AC. Phytotherapy for the prostate. *Br J Urol* 1996; **78:** 325–36.
3. Ishani A, *et al.* Pygeum africanum for the treatment of patients with benign prostatic hyperplasia: a systematic review and quantitative meta-analysis. *Am J Med* 2000; **109:** 654–64.

### Preparations

**Proprietary Preparations** (details are given in Part 3)
***Austria:*** Tadenan; ***Braz.:*** Prolitrol†; Prostem; ***Fr.:*** Tadenan; ***Hong Kong:*** Tadenan†; ***Ital.:*** Pigenil; Tadenan; ***Mex.:*** Tadenom; ***Port.:*** Tadenan; ***Spain:*** Acubiron; Bidrolar; Pronitol; Prostamal†; Tuzanil; ***Switz.:*** Tadenan; ***Thai.:*** Tadenan.

**Multi-ingredient:** ***Arg.:*** Catiz Plus; Normoprost Compuesto; Normoprost Plus; Ultracal; ***Austria:*** Prostatonin; ***Braz.:*** Prostem Plus; ***Canad.:*** Prostease; ***Port.:*** Neo Urgenin†; ***Spain:*** Neo Urgenin; Prosturol; Tebetane Compuesto; ***Switz.:*** Prostatonin.

## Quinestradol *(BAN, rINN)*

Oestriol 3-Cyclopentyl Ether; Quinestradiol. 3-Cyclopentyloxyestra-1,3,5(10)-triene-16α,17β-diol.
$C_{23}H_{32}O_3$ = 356.5.
*CAS — 1169-79-5.*

### Profile

Quinestradol is a synthetic oestrogen that has been given by mouth for the treatment of menopausal vaginal symptoms.

### Preparations

**Proprietary Preparations** (details are given in Part 3)
***Ital.:*** Colpovis†.

## Quinestrol *(BAN, USAN, rINN)*

17α-Ethinyloestradiol 3-cyclopentyl Ether; W-3566. 3-Cyclopentyloxy-19-nor-17α-pregna-1,3,5(10)-trien-20-yn-17β-ol.
$C_{25}H_{32}O_2$ = 364.5.
*CAS — 152-43-2.*

**Pharmacopoeias.** In *Chin.*

### Profile

Quinestrol is a synthetic oestrogen that has a prolonged duration of action and is metabolised to ethinylestradiol (p.1553). Quinestrol has been given by mouth for the treatment of menopausal symptoms and other conditions arising from oestrogen deficiency.

### Preparations

**Proprietary Preparations** (details are given in Part 3)
***Arg.:*** Qui-Lea.
**Multi-ingredient:** ***Arg.:*** Soluna.

## Raloxifene Hydrochloride

*(BANM, USAN, rINNM)*

Hidrocloruro de raloxifeno; Keoxifene Hydrochloride; LY-156758; LY-139481 (raloxifene). 6-Hydroxy-2-(*p*-hydroxyphenyl)benzo[*b*]thien-3-yl-*p*-(2-piperidinoethoxy)phenyl ketone hydrochloride.
$C_{28}H_{27}NO_4S,HCl$ = 510.0.
*CAS — 84449-90-1 (raloxifene); 82640-04-8 (raloxifene hydrochloride).*
*ATC — G03XC01.*

### Adverse Effects

The most common adverse effects of raloxifene are hot flushes and leg cramps. Raloxifene is associated with an increased risk of venous thromboembolic events, particularly during the first 4 months of treatment. Peripheral oedema has also been reported. Rashes and gastrointestinal disturbances have occurred rarely.

**Effects on the liver.** Hepatitis, probably associated with the drug, occurred in a woman a month after starting raloxifene.[1]

1. Vilches AR, *et al.* Raloxifene-associated hepatitis. *Lancet* 1998; **352:** 1524–5.

### Precautions

Raloxifene should be avoided in women with active venous thromboembolism, or a history of thromboembolic disorders. It should be stopped at least 72 hours before periods of prolonged immobilisation, such as post-surgical recovery. Raloxifene should be used with caution in women with risk factors for venous thromboembolism including congestive heart failure or active malignancy. It should be avoided in hepatic and severe renal impairment.

Raloxifene had adverse effects in *animal* teratogenicity studies and should not be used in women who are or may become pregnant. It should not be given to women with undiagnosed uterine bleeding. An increase in triglycerides has been reported in some women with a history of hypertriglyceridaemia caused by oestrogen therapy.

### Interactions

Colestyramine reduces the absorption and enterohepatic recycling of raloxifene, and they should not be given together. Raloxifene may decrease the efficacy of warfarin.

### Pharmacokinetics

Raloxifene is absorbed from the gastrointestinal tract and undergoes extensive first-pass hepatic metabolism to the glucuronide conjugates. It is highly bound to plasma proteins, principally albumin and $\alpha_1$-acid glycoprotein. Raloxifene undergoes enterohepatic recycling, and has a half-life of about 27 hours. It is excreted almost entirely in the faeces.

### Uses and Administration

Raloxifene hydrochloride is a selective oestrogen receptor modulator; it is a benzothiophene related to the nonsteroidal anti-oestrogens clomifene and tamoxifen. It is used, in doses of 60 mg daily by mouth, for the prevention and treatment of postmenopausal osteoporosis (p.763).

It is also under investigation for the prophylaxis of breast cancer (p.515).

◊ References.

1. Delmas PD, *et al.* Effects of raloxifene on bone mineral density, serum cholesterol concentrations, and uterine endometrium in postmenopausal women. *N Engl J Med* 1997; **337:** 1641–7.
2. Walsh BW, *et al.* Effects of raloxifene on serum lipids and coagulation factors in healthy postmenopausal women. *JAMA* 1998; **279:** 1445–51.
3. Balfour JA, Goa KL. Raloxifene. *Drugs Aging* 1998; **12:** 335–41.
4. Lufkin EG, *et al.* Treatment of established postmenopausal osteoporosis with raloxifene: a randomized trial. *J Bone Miner Res* 1998; **13:** 1747–54.
5. Khovidhunkit W, Shoback DM. Clinical effects of raloxifene hydrochloride in women. *Ann Intern Med* 1999; **130:** 431–9.
6. Ettinger B, *et al.* Reduction of vertebral fracture risk in postmenopausal women with osteoporosis treated with raloxifene: results from a 3-year randomized clinical trial. *JAMA* 1999; **282:** 637–45.

7. Clemett D, Spencer CM. Raloxifene: a review of its use in postmenopausal osteoporosis. *Drugs* 2000; **60:** 379–411.
8. Johnston CC, *et al.* Long-term effects of raloxifene on bone mineral density, bone turnover, and serum lipid levels in early postmenopausal women: three-year data from 2 double-blind, randomized, placebo-controlled trials. *Arch Intern Med* 2000; **160:** 3444–50.
9. Barrett-Connor E, *et al.* Raloxifene and cardiovascular events in osteoporotic postmenopausal women: four-year results from the MORE (Multiple Outcomes of Raloxifene Evaluation) randomized trial. *JAMA* 2002; **287:** 847–57.
10. Maricic M, *et al.* Early effects of raloxifene on clinical vertebral fractures at 12 months in postmenopausal women with osteoporosis. *Arch Intern Med* 2002; **162:** 1140–3.
11. Delmas PD, *et al.* Efficacy of raloxifene on vertebral fracture risk reduction in postmenopausal women with osteoporosis: four-year results from a randomized clinical trial. *J Clin Endocrinol Metab* 2002; **87:** 3609–17.


**Malignant neoplasms of the breast.** References.


1. Cummings SR, *et al.* The effect of raloxifene on risk of breast cancer in postmenopausal women: results from the MORE randomized trial. *JAMA* 1999; **281:** 2189–97.
2. Chlebowski RT, *et al.* American Society of Clinical Oncology technology assessment of pharmacologic interventions for breast cancer risk reduction including tamoxifen, raloxifene, and aromatase inhibition. *J Clin Oncol* 2002; **20:** 3328–43.


### Preparations

**Proprietary Preparations** (details are given in Part 3)
***Arg.:*** Biofem; Ciclotran; Evista; Ketidin; Loxifen; Raxeto; ***Austral.:*** Evista; ***Austria:*** Evista; Optruma; ***Belg.:*** Evista; ***Braz.:*** Evista; ***Canad.:*** Evista; ***Chile:*** Evista; ***Denm.:*** Evista; ***Fin.:*** Evista; ***Fr.:*** Evista; Optruma; ***Ger.:*** Evista; ***Gr.:*** Evista; ***Hong Kong:*** Evista; ***India:*** Bonmax; ***Irl.:*** Evista; ***Israel:*** Evista; ***Ital.:*** Evista; Optruma; ***Malaysia:*** Evista; ***Mex.:*** Evista; ***Neth.:*** Evista; ***Norw.:*** Evista; ***NZ:*** Evista; ***Port.:*** Evista; Optruma; ***S.Afr.:*** Evista; ***Singapore:*** Evista; ***Spain:*** Evista; Optruma; ***Swed.:*** Evista; ***Switz.:*** Evista; ***Thai.:*** Celvista; ***UK:*** Evista; ***USA:*** Evista.

## Saw Palmetto

American Dwarf Palm; *Brahea serrulata*; PA-109; Sabal; *Sabal serrulata*; Sabalis Serrulatae; *Serenoa repens*; *Serenoa serrulatum*.
*ATC — G04CX02.*

**Pharmacopoeias.** In *Eur.* (see p.vi). Also in *USNF*, which also includes the extract and the powdered form.
**Ph. Eur. 5.0** (Saw Palmetto Fruit). The dried, ripe fruit of *Serenoa repens* (*Sabal serrulata*). It contains not less than 11.0% of total fatty acids, calculated with reference to the dried drug. Protect from light.
**USNF 22** (Saw Palmetto). The partially dried, ripe fruit of *Serenoa repens* (Arecaceae). Store in airtight containers. Protect from light.

### Profile

Saw palmetto is the dried fruit of the American dwarf palm, *Serenoa repens* (Arecaceae). It contains various steroidal compounds with anti-androgenic and oestrogenic activities, one of which is sitosterol (p.982). Saw palmetto is used for the treatment of benign prostatic hyperplasia. Preparations of alcoholic or lipophilic extracts have typically been administered in doses of 160 mg twice daily, or 320 mg once daily, by mouth.

**Adverse effects.** EFFECTS ON THE LIVER. Cholestatic hepatitis occurred in a man who took a herbal preparation containing saw palmetto for 2 weeks to treat nocturia and hesitancy.[1]


1. Hamid S, *et al.* Protracted cholestatic hepatitis after the use of Prostata. *Ann Intern Med* 1997; **127:** 169–70.


**Uses.** BENIGN PROSTATIC HYPERPLASIA. A lipid hexane extract of saw palmetto has been shown to be generally superior to placebo,[1,2] and of similar efficacy to finasteride[3] in the treatment of benign prostatic hyperplasia (p.1555). A systematic review of randomised studies of various saw palmetto extracts concluded that they improve urological symptoms and flow measures.[4]


1. Champault G, *et al.* A double-blind trial of an extract of the plant Serenoa repens in benign prostatic hyperplasia. *Br J Clin Pharmacol* 1984; **18:** 461.
2. Plosker GL, Brogden RN. Serenoa repens (Permixon): a review of its pharmacology and therapeutic efficacy in benign prostatic hyperplasia. *Drugs Aging* 1996; **9:** 379–95.
3. Carraro J-C, *et al.* Comparison of phytotherapy (Permixon) with finasteride in the treatment of benign prostate hyperplasia: a randomized international study of 1,098 patients. *Prostate* 1996; **29:** 231–40.
4. Wilt T, *et al.* Serenoa repens for benign prostatic hyperplasia. Available in The Cochrane Library; Issue 2. Chichester: John Wiley; 2004.


### Preparations

***USNF 22:*** Saw Palmetto Capsules.

**Proprietary Preparations** (details are given in Part 3)
***Arg.:*** Beltrax Uno; Herbaccion Prostatico; Permicaps; Permixon; Sereprostat; ***Austral.:*** Bioglan Pro-Guard†; Prosta†; ***Austria:*** Permixon; Prosta-Urgenin; ***Belg.:*** Prosta-Urgenin; Prostaserene; ***Braz.:*** Permixon; Prostalium; Prostatal; Renopen; ***Chile:*** Prostafort; ***Fr.:*** Capistan†; Permixon; ***Ger.:*** Azuprostat Sabal; Eviprostat-S; Prosta Urgenin Uno; Prosta-Urgenin†; Prostagutt mono; Prostagutt uno; Prostess; Remiprostan uno; Sabacur uno; Sabal; Sabal uno; Sabalvit; Sabonal Uno; Sita; Steiprostat; Strogen; SX Sabal†; Talso; Valverde Sabal†; ***Ital.:*** Biosern; Permixon; Proser†; Prosteren; Rilaprost; Saba; Sere-Mit†; Serpens; ***Mex.:*** Permixon; Prostex; Urogutt; ***Port.:*** Permixon; ***Singapore:*** Permixon; ***Spain:*** Permixon; Sereprostat; ***Switz.:*** Permixon; Prosta-Urgenine; Prostasan; SabCaps; ***Thai.:*** Permixon; Urogutt†; ***UK:*** Sabalin.

**Multi-ingredient:** ***Arg.:*** Anastim con RTH; Catiz Plus; Keracnyl; Normoprost Plus; Sabal; Ultracal; ***Austral.:*** Bioglan Mens Super Soy/Clover†; Extralife Flow-Care†; Lifechange Mens Complex with Saw Palmetto†; Serenoa Complex†; Urapro†; Urgenin†; Urinase†; ***Austria:*** Prostagutt; Spasmo-Urgenin; Urgenin; ***Belg.:*** Urgenin; ***Canad.:*** Damiana-Sarsaparilla Formula; Prostease; ProstGard; ***Fr.:*** Argeal; Keracnyl; Sabal; Salucur†; ***Ger.:*** Cefasabal; Granu Fink Prosta; Nephroselect M; Prosta Fink N†; Prostagutt forte; ***Hong Kong:*** Palmetto Plus; Sawmetto Vivo-Livo; Urgenin; ***Israel:*** Urgenin; ***Ital.:*** Biothymus M Urto; ***Malaysia:*** Prostakan; ***Mex.:*** Prosgutt; ***Port.:*** Efluvium Anti-caspa; Efluvium Anti-seborreico; Neo Urgenin†; Spasmo-Urgenin; ***S.Afr.:*** Spasmo-Urgenin; ***Spain:*** Neo Urgenin; Spasmo-Urgenin; Urgenin; ***Switz.:*** Granu Fink Prosta; Phytomed Prosta; Prosta-Caps Chassot N; Prosta-Caps Fink†; Prostagutt-F; Urgenine†; ***Thai.:*** Spasmo-Urgenin; ***UK:*** Antiglan; Daily Fatigue Relief; Damiana and Kola Tablets; Elixir Damiana and Saw Palmetto; Regina Royal Concorde; Serenoa-C†; Strength.

## Stanozolol *(BAN, USAN, rINN)*

Androstanazole; Estanozolol; Methylstanazole; NSC-43193; Stanozololum; Win-14833. 17α-Methyl-2′H-5α-androst-2-eno[3,2-c]pyrazol-17β-ol.
$C_{21}H_{32}N_2O$ = 328.5.
*CAS — 10418-03-8.*
*ATC — A14AA02.*

**Pharmacopoeias.** In *Chin.*, *Eur.* (see p.vi), and *US*.
**Ph. Eur. 5.0** (Stanozolol). A white or almost white, hygroscopic crystalline powder. It exhibits polymorphism. Practically insoluble in water; slightly soluble in alcohol; very slightly soluble in dichloromethane; soluble in dimethylformamide. Store in airtight containers. Protect from light.
**USP 27** (Stanozolol). An odourless crystalline powder occurring in 2 forms; needles melt at about 155° and prisms at about 235°. Insoluble in water; soluble 1 in 41 of alcohol, 1 in 74 of chloroform, and 1 in 370 of ether; slightly soluble in acetone and in ethyl acetate; soluble in dimethylformamide; very slightly soluble in benzene. Store in airtight containers. Protect from light.

### Adverse Effects and Precautions

As for androgens and anabolic steroids in general (see Testosterone, p.1570). As with other 17α-alkylated compounds stanozolol may produce hepatotoxicity, and liver function should be monitored. It is probably best avoided in patients with hepatic impairment, and certainly if this is severe. Haematocrit and haemoglobin concentrations should also be monitored.

Because of its androgenic effects it has been recommended that stanozolol should not be used to treat hereditary angioedema in premenopausal women except in life-threatening situations.

**Effects on the liver.** Some reports of jaundice associated with stanozolol.[1,2]


1. Slater SD, *et al.* Jaundice induced by stanozolol hypersensitivity. *Postgrad Med J* 1976; **52:** 229–32.
2. Evely RS, *et al.* Severe cholestasis associated with stanozolol. *BMJ* 1987; **294:** 612–13.


**Effects on the nervous system.** Benign intracranial hypertension developed in an elderly woman receiving stanozolol; CSF pressure returned to normal after stanozolol was discontinued.[1]


1. Tully MP, *et al.* Intracranial hypertension associated with stanozolol. *DICP Ann Pharmacother* 1990; **24:** 1234.


**Porphyria.** Stanozolol is considered to be unsafe in patients with porphyria because it has been shown to be porphyrinogenic in *animals*.

### Interactions

As mentioned under Testosterone, p.1571, anabolic steroids may enhance the activity of a number of drugs. For the effect of stanozolol on some anticoagulants, see p.1027.

### Uses and Administration

Stanozolol has anabolic and androgenic properties (see Testosterone, p.1571). It has been used in the treatment of vascular manifestations of Behçet's syndrome in usual doses of 10 mg daily by mouth.

In the management of hereditary angioedema, an initial dose of 2.5 to 10 mg daily by mouth is given to prevent attacks. The dosage may then be reduced, according to the patient's response; maintenance doses of 2 mg daily or on alternate days, or 2.5 mg three times weekly have been used successfully. In the USA doses of 1 mg daily for children under 6 years and up to 2 mg in those aged 6 to 12 years have been suggested. Slightly higher doses have been permitted in children in the UK.

As with other anabolic steroids, stanozolol has been used for breast cancer in postmenopausal women, and for anaemias, osteoporosis, and catabolic disorders. Stanozolol has also been given by intramuscular injection in doses of 50 mg every 2 or 3 weeks.

**Hereditary angioedema.** Stanozolol has been used successfully to prevent attacks of hereditary angioedema (p.761). References.


1. Sheffer AL, *et al.* Hereditary angioedema: a decade of management with stanozolol. *J Allergy Clin Immunol* 1987; **80:** 855–60.


**Vascular disorders.** Stanozolol has been used in the treatment of vascular manifestations of Behçet's syndrome (p.1076). It has also been reported to promote fibrinolysis in vascular disorders, including long-standing liposclerosis of the leg,[1-3] necrobiosis lipoidica,[4] Raynaud's syndrome,[5,6] systemic sclerosis,[6] idiopathic recurrent superficial thrombophlebitis,[7] cryofibrinogenaemia,[8] and venous ulceration.[9-11] Most of these studies were noncomparative and in small numbers of patients, and results have been variable.


1. Browse NL, *et al.* Treatment of liposclerosis of the leg by fibrinolytic enhancement: a preliminary report. *BMJ* 1977; **2:** 434–5.
2. Burnand K, *et al.* Venous lipodermatosclerosis: treatment by fibrinolytic enhancement and elastic compression. *BMJ* 1980; **280:** 7–11.
3. Muston HL. Treatment of liposclerosis. *BMJ* 1980; **280:** 254–5.
4. Rhodes EL. Fibrinolytic agents in the treatment of necrobiosis lipoidica. *Br J Dermatol* 1976; **95:** 673–4.
5. Jarrett PEM, *et al.* Treatment of Raynaud's phenomenon by fibrinolytic enhancement. *BMJ* 1978; **2:** 523–5.
6. Jayson MIV, *et al.* A controlled study of stanozolol in primary Raynaud's phenomenon and systemic sclerosis. *Ann Rheum Dis* 1991; **50:** 41–7.
7. Jarrett PEM, *et al.* Idiopathic recurrent superficial thrombophlebitis: treatment with fibrinolytic enhancement. *BMJ* 1977; **1:** 933–4.
8. Amdo TD, Welker JA. An approach to the diagnosis and treatment of cryofibrinogenemia. *Am J Med* 2004; **116:** 332–7.
9. Anonymous. Does stanozolol prevent venous ulceration? *Drug Ther Bull* 1985; **23:** 91–2.
10. Browse NL, Burnand KG. Getting the balance right. *BMJ* 1986; **292:** 825.
11. Herxheimer A. Getting the balance right. *BMJ* 1986; **292:** 1014.


### Preparations

***BP 2003:*** Stanozolol Tablets;
***USP 27:*** Stanozolol Tablets.

**Proprietary Preparations** (details are given in Part 3)
***Belg.:*** Stromba†; Strombaject†; ***India:*** Menabol; Neurabol; ***Irl.:*** Stromba; ***Neth.:*** Stromba†; ***Spain:*** Winstrol; ***Thai.:*** Stanol; ***UK:*** Stromba†; ***USA:*** Winstrol.

**Multi-ingredient:** ***Thai.:*** Cetabon.

## Testis Extracts

Extractos testiculares; Testicular Extracts.

### Profile

Testis extracts are usually of bovine origin and have been used in a variety of disorders. They have been given to elderly men as androgenic supplements. They have also been used topically, often in preparations containing other mammalian tissue extracts, in the treatment of peripheral circulatory or musculoskeletal disorders.

### Preparations

**Proprietary Preparations** (details are given in Part 3)
***Austria:*** Testiculi†; ***Ger.:*** Orchibion.

**Multi-ingredient:** ***Canad.:*** Heracline; Revitonus C; ***Ger.:*** Intradermi N†; poliomyelan; tactu-nerval; ***Hong Kong:*** Wari-Procomil; ***Thai.:*** Wari-Procomil.

## Testosterone *(BAN, rINN)*

Testosterona; Testosteronum. 17β-Hydroxyandrost-4-en-3-one.
$C_{19}H_{28}O_2$ = 288.4.
*CAS — 58-22-0.*
*ATC — G03BA03.*

**Pharmacopoeias.** In *Eur.* (see p.vi) and *US*.
**Ph. Eur. 5.0** (Testosterone). A white crystalline powder, or colourless or yellowish-white crystals. Practically insoluble in water and in fatty oils; freely soluble in alcohol and in dichloromethane. Protect from light.
**USP 27** (Testosterone). White or slightly creamy-white, odourless, crystals or crystalline powder. Practically insoluble in water; soluble 1 in 6 of dehydrated alcohol, 1 in 2 of chloroform, and 1 in 100 of ether; soluble in dioxan and in vegetable oils. Store at a temperature of 25°, excursions permitted between 15° and 30°.

## Testosterone Cipionate *(BANM, rINNM)*

Cipionato de testosterona; Testosterone Cyclopentylpropionate; Testosterone Cypionate. 3-Oxoandrost-4-en-17β-yl 3-cyclopentylpropionate; 17β-Hydroxyandrost-4-en-3-one cyclopentanepropionate; 17β-(3-Cyclopentyl-1-oxopropoxy)androst-4-en-3-one.
$C_{27}H_{40}O_3$ = 412.6.
*CAS — 58-20-8.*
*ATC — G03BA03.*

**Pharmacopoeias.** In *US*.
**USP 27** (Testosterone Cypionate). A white or creamy-white, crystalline powder, odourless or has a slight odour. Insoluble in water; freely soluble in alcohol, in chloroform, in dioxan, and in ether; soluble in vegetable oils. Protect from light.

### Testosterone Decanoate *(BANM, rINNM)*

Decanoato de testosterona. 3-Oxoandrost-4-en-17β-yl decanoate; 17β-Hydroxyandrost-4-en-3-one decanoate.

$C_{29}H_{46}O_3$ = 442.7.
*CAS — 5721-91-5.*
*ATC — G03BA03.*

**Pharmacopoeias.** In *Br.*

**BP 2003** (Testosterone Decanoate). White to creamy-white crystals or crystalline powder. Practically insoluble in water; very soluble in alcohol and in chloroform. Store at a temperature not exceeding 15°. Protect from light.

### Testosterone Enantate *(BANM, rINNM)*

Enantato de testosterona; NSC-17591; Testosterone Enanthate; Testosterone Heptanoate; Testosteroni Enantas. 3-Oxoandrost-4-en-17β-yl heptanoate; 17β-Hydroxyandrost-4-en-3-one heptanoate.

$C_{26}H_{40}O_3$ = 400.6.
*CAS — 315-37-7.*
*ATC — G03BA03.*

**Pharmacopoeias.** In *Eur.* (see p.vi), *Int., Jpn, Pol.,* and *US.*

**Ph. Eur. 5.0** (Testosterone Enantate). A white or yellowish-white crystalline powder. Practically insoluble in water; very soluble in dehydrated alcohol; freely soluble in fatty oils. Store at a temperature of 2° to 8°. Protect from light.

**USP 27** (Testosterone Enanthate). A white or creamy-white crystalline powder. It is odourless or has a faint odour characteristic of heptanoic acid. Insoluble in water; very soluble in ether; soluble in vegetable oils. Store in a cool place.

### Testosterone Isocaproate *(BANM, rINNM)*

Isocaproato de testosterona; Testosterone Isohexanoate. 3-Oxoandrost-4-en-17β-yl 4-methylpentanoate; 17β-Hydroxyandrost-4-en-3-one 4-methylpentanoate.

$C_{25}H_{38}O_3$ = 386.6.
*CAS — 15262-86-9.*
*ATC — G03BA03.*

**Pharmacopoeias.** In *Br.*

**BP 2003** (Testosterone Isocaproate). White to creamy-white crystals or crystalline powder. Practically insoluble in water; very soluble in alcohol and in chloroform. Store at a temperature not exceeding 15°. Protect from light.

### Testosterone Phenylpropionate *(BANM, rINNM)*

Fenilpropionato de testosterona. 3-Oxoandrost-4-en-17β-yl 3-phenylpropionate; 17β-Hydroxyandrost-4-en-3-one 3-phenylpropionate.

$C_{28}H_{36}O_3$ = 420.6.
*CAS — 1255-49-8.*
*ATC — G03BA03.*

**Pharmacopoeias.** In *BP(Vet).*

**BP(Vet) 2003** (Testosterone Phenylpropionate). A white to almost white crystalline powder with a characteristic odour. Practically insoluble in water; sparingly soluble in alcohol. Protect from light.

### Testosterone Propionate *(BANM, rINNM)*

NSC-9166; Propionato de testosterona; Testosteroni Propionas. 3-Oxoandrost-4-en-17β-yl propionate; 17β-Hydroxyandrost-4-en-3-one propionate.

$C_{22}H_{32}O_3$ = 344.5.
*CAS — 57-85-2.*
*ATC — G03BA03.*

**Pharmacopoeias.** In *Chin., Eur.* (see p.vi), *Int., Jpn, Pol.,* and *US.*

**Ph. Eur. 5.0** (Testosterone Propionate). A white or almost white powder or colourless crystals. Practically insoluble in water; freely soluble in alcohol and in acetone; soluble in fatty oils.

**USP 27** (Testosterone Propionate). White or creamy-white, odourless, crystals or crystalline powder. Insoluble in water; freely soluble in alcohol, in dioxan, in ether, and in other organic solvents; soluble in vegetable oils. Protect from light.

### Testosterone Undecylate *(rINNM)*

Org-538; Testosterone Undecanoate *(BANM, USAN)*; Undecilato de testosterona. 3-Oxoandrost-4-en-17β-yl undecanoate; 17β-Hydroxyandrost-4-en-3-one undecanoate.

$C_{30}H_{48}O_3$ = 456.7.
*CAS — 5949-44-0.*
*ATC — G03BA03.*

**Pharmacopoeias.** In *Chin.*

## Adverse Effects

Testosterone and other **androgens** may give rise to side-effects which can be related to their androgenic or anabolic activities. They include increased retention of nitrogen, sodium, and water, oedema, increased vascularity of the skin, hypercalcaemia, impaired glucose tolerance, and increased bone growth and skeletal weight. Other effects include increased low-density-lipoprotein cholesterol, decreased high-density-lipoprotein cholesterol, increased haematocrit, and increased fibrinolytic activity. Androgens may cause headache, depression, and gastrointestinal bleeding. It has been suggested that androgens may induce sleep apnoea in susceptible patients.

Abnormal liver function tests may occur and there have been reports of liver toxicity including jaundice and cholestatic hepatitis. There have also been reports of peliosis hepatis and hepatic tumours in patients who have received high doses over prolonged periods. These adverse hepatic effects have occurred primarily with the 17α-alkylated derivatives (e.g. methyltestosterone, stanozolol).

In men, large doses suppress spermatogenesis and cause degenerative changes in the seminiferous tubules. Priapism is a sign of excessive dosage and may occur especially in elderly males. Gynaecomastia may occur. Androgens may cause prostatic hyperplasia and accelerate the growth of malignant neoplasms of the prostate.

In women, the inhibitory action of androgens on the activity of the anterior pituitary results in the suppression of ovarian activity and menstruation. Continued use produces symptoms of virilism, such as hirsutism or male-pattern baldness, deepening of the voice, atrophy of the breasts and endometrial tissue, oily skin, acne, and hypertrophy of the clitoris; libido is increased and lactation suppressed. Virilisation may not be reversible, even after stopping therapy.

Large and repeated doses in early puberty may cause closure of the epiphyses and stop linear growth. Children may experience symptoms of virilisation: in boys there may be precocious sexual development with phallic enlargement and increased frequency of erection, and in girls, clitoral enlargement. Gynaecomastia may also occur in boys.

Masculinisation of the external genitalia of the female fetus may occur if androgens are given during pregnancy.

Following transdermal application of testosterone, skin reactions may include irritation, erythema, allergic contact dermatitis, and sometimes burn-like lesions. Skin reactions are more common with patches that contain permeation enhancers.

The **anabolic steroids**, because they generally retain some androgenic activity, share the adverse effects of the androgens described above, but their virilising effects, especially in women, are usually less. There have been reports of adverse psychiatric effects in athletes taking large doses to try and improve performance. For adverse effects following the misuse of anabolic steroids, see Abuse under Precautions, below.

**Carcinogenicity.** Reports of malignant neoplasms associated with testosterone therapy have included prostatic cancer (with testosterone cipionate therapy),[1] and renal cell carcinoma (testosterone ester unspecified).[2] Concern has been expressed[3] about the possibility that long-term use of testosterone esters for male contraception may lead to an increase in the number of cases of prostatic cancer or benign prostatic hyperplasia. For reference to hepatic malignancies associated with androgens and anabolic steroids, see Effects on the Liver, below.

1. Jackson JA, *et al.* Prostatic complications of testosterone replacement therapy. *Arch Intern Med* 1989; **149:** 2365–6.
2. Rosner F, Khan MT. Renal cell carcinoma following prolonged testosterone therapy. *Arch Intern Med* 1992; **152:** 426, 429.
3. Schally AV, Comaru-Schally AM. Male contraception involving testosterone supplementation: possible increased risks of prostate cancer? *Lancet* 1987; **i:** 448–9.

**Effects on the cardiovascular system.** A cerebrovascular accident has been reported in a young man following the overzealous self-administration of testosterone enantate intramuscularly for hypogonadism.[1] It was noted that thromboembolic complications are not generally recognised as side-effects of androgen therapy although there is some experimental evidence that testosterone stimulates thrombus formation.

1. Nagelberg SB, *et al.* Cerebrovascular accident associated with testosterone therapy in a 21-year-old hypogonadal man. *N Engl J Med* 1986; **314:** 649–50.

**Effects on the liver.** As mentioned above, hepatotoxicity, including elevations in liver enzymes, hepatic cholestasis and jaundice, and rarely peliosis hepatis and hepatic tumours, has occurred with androgens and anabolic steroids, particularly the 17α-alkylated derivatives. Prolonged treatment and high doses may be significant contributory factors. Tumours have included hepatocellular carcinomas, benign adenomas, and less commonly angiosarcomas and cholangiocarcinomas. Tumours and peliosis may regress on stopping therapy, but they can also progress to liver failure and death. Some reviews of the hepatic effects of androgens and anabolic steroids are cited below.[1-4] There has been a specific report of benign hepatic adenoma in a patient treated with testosterone enantate for 11 years,[5] and of hepatocellular carcinoma in a patient receiving testosterone enantate and methyltestosterone.[6] Further specific references may be found under individual drug monographs.

1. Bagheri SA, Boyer JL. Peliosis hepatis associated with androgenic-anabolic steroid therapy. *Ann Intern Med* 1974; **81:** 610–18.
2. Ishak KG, Zimmerman HJ. Hepatotoxic effects of the anabolic/androgenic steroids. *Semin Liver Dis* 1987; **7:** 230–6.
3. Søe KL, *et al.* Liver pathology associated with the use of anabolic-androgenic steroids. *Liver* 1992; **12:** 73–9.
4. Touraine RL, *et al.* Hepatic tumours during androgen therapy in Fanconi anaemia. *Eur J Pediatr* 1993; **152:** 691–3.
5. Carrasco D, *et al.* Hepatic adenomata and androgen treatment. *Ann Intern Med* 1984; **100:** 316.
6. Johnson FL. *et al.* Association of androgenic-anabolic steroid therapy with development of hepatocellular carcinoma. *Lancet* 1972; **ii:** 1273–6.

**Effects on sexual function.** Reports of severe priapism following the use of testosterone for the management of delayed puberty.[1,2]

1. Zelissen PMJ, Stricker BHC. Severe priapism as a complication of testosterone substitution therapy. *Am J Med* 1988; **85:** 273–4.
2. Ruch W, Jenny P. Priapism following testosterone administration for delayed male puberty. *Am J Med* 1989; **86:** 256.

## Precautions

Testosterone and other androgens and anabolic steroids should be used cautiously in patients with cardiovascular disorders, renal or hepatic impairment, epilepsy, migraine, diabetes mellitus or other conditions which may be aggravated by the possible fluid retention or oedema caused. They should not be given to patients with hypercalcaemia or hypercalciuria, and should be used cautiously in conditions in which there is a risk of these developing such as skeletal metastases. The use of the 17α-alkylated derivatives, which are associated with an increased risk of hepatotoxicity, is probably best avoided in patients with hepatic impairment, and certainly if this is severe. Hepatic function should be monitored during therapy.

In men, androgens and anabolic steroids should not be given to those with carcinoma of the breast or prostate (although in women they have been used in the treatment of certain breast carcinomas). The prostate should be examined regularly during treatment.

Androgens and anabolic steroids should not be given during pregnancy because of the risk of virilisation of the female fetus.

Androgens and anabolic steroids should be used with extreme care in children because of the masculinising effects and also because premature closure of the epiphyses may occur resulting in inhibited linear growth and small stature. Skeletal maturation should be monitored during therapy.

Androgens and anabolic steroids may interfere with a number of clinical laboratory tests such as those for glucose tolerance and thyroid function.

**Abuse.** The adverse effects arising from the illicit use of androgens and anabolic steroids by athletes, often taken together at doses well in excess of those used therapeutically, have been discussed.[1-6] Effects have included abnormal liver function and hepatic neoplasms (see also Effects on the Liver, above), an atherogenic blood lipid profile[7] and increased risk of cardiovascular disease,[8] and reduced glucose tolerance. Hypogonadal states are commonly induced (azoospermia or oligospermia and testicular atrophy in men, and amenorrhoea or oligomenorrhoea in women). Gynaecomastia is relatively common in men, and virilisation in women. Psychiatric disturbances such as mania, hypomania, depression, aggression, and emotional lability, have been described.[9,10] There is also some evidence that dependence associated with an acute withdrawal syndrome can occur.[11,12] Rare reports include alterations in immune response,[13,14] bleeding oesophageal varices,[15] tendon damage,[16] renal cell carcinoma,[17] and peliosis hepatis.[18]

There has been some dispute about the methods used to detect abuse of certain anabolic steroids in athletes; a study in healthy subjects has apparently confirmed endogenous production of small amounts of nandrolone metabolites.[19]

1. American Medical Association Council on Scientific Affairs. Drug abuse in athletes: anabolic steroids and human growth hormone. *JAMA* 1988; **259:** 1703–5.
2. Hallagan JB, *et al.* Anabolic-androgenic steroid use by athletes. *N Engl J Med* 1989; **321:** 1042–5.
3. Graham S, Kennedy M. Recent developments in the toxicology of anabolic steroids. *Drug Safety* 1990; **5:** 458–76.

4. Kennedy M. Drugs and athletes—an update. *Adverse Drug React Bull* 1994; (Dec): 639–42.
5. O'Sullivan AJ, *et al.* Anabolic-androgenic steroids: medical assessment of present, past and potential users. *Med J Aust* 2000; **173:** 323–7.
6. Pärssinen M, Seppälä T. Steroid use and long-term health risks in former athletes. *Sports Med* 2002; **32:** 83–94.
7. Glazer G. Atherogenic effects of anabolic steroids on serum lipid levels. *Arch Intern Med* 1991; **151:** 1925–33.
8. Madea B, Grellner W. Long-term cardiovascular effects of anabolic steroids. *Lancet* 1998; **352:** 33.
9. Su T-P, *et al.* Neuropsychiatric effects of anabolic steroids in male normal volunteers. *JAMA* 1993; **269:** 2760–4.
10. Pope HG, Katz DL. Psychiatric and medical effects of anabolic-androgenic steroid use: a controlled study of 160 athletes. *Arch Gen Psychiatry* 1994; **51:** 375–82.
11. Kashkin KB, Kleber HD. Hooked on hormones: an anabolic steroid addiction hypothesis. *JAMA* 1989; **262:** 3166–70.
12. Brower KJ, *et al.* Evidence for physical and psychological dependence on anabolic androgenic steroids in eight weight lifters. *Am J Psychiatry* 1990; **147:** 510–12.
13. Widder RA, *et al.* Candida albicans endophthalmitis after anabolic steroid abuse. *Lancet* 1995; **345:** 330–1.
14. Johnson AS, *et al.* Severe chickenpox in an anabolic steroid user. *Lancet* 1995; **345:** 1447–8.
15. Winwood PJ, *et al.* Bleeding oesophageal varices associated with anabolic steroid use in an athlete. *Postgrad Med J* 1990; **66:** 864–5.
16. Laseter JT, Russell JA. Anabolic steroid-induced tendon pathology: a review of the literature. *Med Sci Sports Exerc* 1991; **23:** 1–3.
17. Bryden AAG, *et al.* Anabolic steroid abuse and renal-cell carcinoma. *Lancet* 1995; **346:** 1306–7.
18. Cabasso A. Peliosis hepatis in a young adult bodybuilder. *Med Sci Sports Exerc* 1994; **26:** 2–4.
19. Reznik Y, *et al.* Urinary nandrolone metabolites of endogenous origin in man: a confirmation by output regulation under human chorionic gonadotropin stimulation. *J Clin Endocrinol Metab* 2001; **86:** 146–50.


**Breast feeding.** Testosterone should be avoided in women who are breast feeding because of the theoretical potential androgenic effect on the infant.

**Porphyria.** Androgens are considered to be unsafe in patients with porphyria although there is conflicting experimental evidence of porphyrinogenicity.

A female patient with acute intermittent porphyria (p.1040) who suffered from severe attacks pre-menstrually was successfully managed with subcutaneous implants of testosterone when suppression of the menstrual cycle with buserelin met with limited success.[1]


1. Savage MW, *et al.* Acute intermittent porphyria treated by testosterone implant. *Postgrad Med J* 1992; **68:** 479–81.


**Pregnancy.** Reports of female fetal virilisation following maternal use of testosterone[1] or methyltestosterone[2] during pregnancy.


1. Reschini E, *et al.* Female pseudohermaphroditism due to maternal androgen administration: 25-year follow-up. *Lancet* 1985; **i:** 1226.
2. Dewhurst J, Gordon RR. Fertility following change of sex. *Lancet* 1984; **ii:** 1461.


**Veterinary use.** It was considered unnecessary to establish an acceptable daily intake or acceptable residual level in food for endogenous hormones such as testosterone. Residues resulting from the use of testosterone as a growth promotor in accordance with good animal husbandry practice are unlikely to pose a hazard to human health.[1] However, it should be noted that, in the European Union the use of androgens in veterinary practice is restricted and their use as growth promotors is banned. In addition, the use of anabolic steroids is banned in animals intended for human consumption.


1. FAO/WHO. Evaluation of certain veterinary drug residues in food: thirty-second report of the joint FAO/WHO expert committee on food additives. *WHO Tech Rep Ser 763* 1988.


## Interactions

Testosterone and other androgens and anabolic steroids have been reported to enhance the activity of a number of drugs, with resulting increases in toxicity. Drugs affected include ciclosporin (see p.1356), antidiabetics, levothyroxine (see p.1601), and anticoagulants such as warfarin (see p.1027). Resistance to the effects of neuromuscular blockers (p.1402) has also been reported.

## Pharmacokinetics

Testosterone is absorbed from the gastrointestinal tract, the skin, and the oral mucosa. However, testosterone undergoes extensive first-pass hepatic metabolism when given by mouth and is therefore usually given intramuscularly, subcutaneously, or transdermally. In addition, the basic molecule of testosterone has been modified to produce orally active compounds and to extend the duration of action. Alkylation of the 17$\alpha$ position produces compounds that are more slowly metabolised by the liver, and hence may be administered orally. Esterification of the 17$\beta$ hydroxyl group increases lipid solubility and results in slower systemic absorption following intramuscular injection. The rate of absorption of the esters is related to the size of the ester group. The undecylate ester undergoes less complete inactivation after oral doses because of distribution into the lymphatic system. Testosterone esters are hydrolysed to testosterone following absorption.

Testosterone is about 80% bound to sex-hormone binding globulin. Derivatives of 19-nortestosterone and 17-$\alpha$-methylated compounds have reduced binding to this globulin. The plasma half-life of testosterone is reported to range from about 10 to 100 minutes. It is largely metabolised in the liver via oxidation at the 17-OH group with the formation of androstenedione, which is further metabolised to the weakly androgenic androsterone and inactive etiocholanolone which are excreted in the urine mainly as glucuronides and sulfates. About 6% is excreted unchanged in the faeces after undergoing enterohepatic recirculation. Testosterone is converted to the more active dihydrotestosterone in some target organs by 5$\alpha$-reductase. 19-Nortestosterone derivatives appear to be less susceptible to this enzyme. Small amounts of testosterone are aromatised to form oestrogenic derivatives in the body. Compounds with a saturated A-ring, such as mesterolone, appear to be less likely to be aromatised to oestrogen.

◊ References to the pharmacokinetics of subcutaneous testosterone pellets,[1] scrotal[2,3] and non-scrotal[4-7] transdermal patches, and gel[8] are given below.


1. Handelsman DJ, *et al.* Pharmacokinetics and pharmacodynamics of testosterone pellets in man. *J Clin Endocrinol Metab* 1990; **71:** 216–22.
2. Findlay JC, *et al.* Transdermal delivery of testosterone. *J Clin Endocrinol Metab* 1987; **64:** 266–8.
3. Cunningham GR, *et al.* Testosterone replacement with transdermal therapeutic systems: physiological serum testosterone and elevated dihydrotestosterone levels. *JAMA* 1989; **261:** 2525–30.
4. Meikle AW, *et al.* Pharmacokinetics and metabolism of a permeation-enhanced testosterone transdermal system in hypogonadal men: influence of application site. *J Clin Endocrinol Metab* 1996; **81:** 1832–40.
5. Yu Z, *et al.* Transdermal testosterone administration in hypogonadal men: comparison of pharmacokinetics at different sites of application and at the first and fifth days of application. *J Clin Pharmacol* 1997; **37:** 1129–38.
6. Dobs AS, *et al.* Pharmacokinetics, efficacy, and safety of a permeation-enhanced testosterone transdermal system in comparison with bi-weekly injections of testosterone enanthate for the treatment of hypogonadal men. *J Clin Endocrinol Metab* 1999; **84:** 3469–78.
7. Singh AB, *et al.* Pharmacokinetics of a transdermal testosterone system in men with end stage renal disease receiving maintenance hemodialysis and healthy hypogonadal men. *J Clin Endocrinol Metab* 2001; **86:** 2437–45.
8. Swerdloff RS, *et al.* Long-term pharmacokinetics of transdermal testosterone gel in hypogonadal men. *J Clin Endocrinol Metab* 2000; **85:** 4500–10.


## Uses and Administration

The natural hormone testosterone and its derivatives have anabolic and androgenic properties (for further details, see p.1527).

The primary indication for androgens, such as testosterone or its esters, is as replacement therapy in **male hypogonadal disorders** (p.1316) caused by either pituitary or testicular disorders or in hypogonadism following orchidectomy. Testosterone may be used as a subcutaneous implant in a dose of 100 to 600 mg; plasma concentrations of testosterone are usually maintained within the physiological range for 4 to 5 months with a dose of 600 mg. It may also be given by transdermal delivery systems. The scrotal patch contains 10 or 15 mg of testosterone and supplies approximately 4 or 6 mg of testosterone in 24 hours. Non-scrotal patches are applied to the back, abdomen, thighs or upper arms to supply 2.5 to 10 mg daily. A hydroalcoholic gel containing 1% testosterone, which is applied daily to the shoulders and upper arms and/or abdomen, is also available. About 10% of the applied dose is absorbed across the skin to provide a systemic dose of testosterone 5 to 10 mg (see also Hypogonadism, below). A sustained-release adhesive buccal system that contains testosterone 30 mg is applied twice daily. Testosterone has also been given by intramuscular injection in a dose of up to 50 mg two or three times weekly, but testosterone esters are generally preferred by this route.

The testosterone esters are usually formulated as oily solutions for intramuscular use to give a prolonged duration of action. Suggested doses for the various esters are: 50 to 400 mg every 2 to 4 weeks for the cipionate; 50 to 400 mg every 2 to 4 weeks for the enantate (or an initial dose of 250 mg every 2 to 3 weeks followed by maintenance dosing every 3 to 6 weeks may be employed); and up to 50 mg two or three times weekly for the propionate. The isocaproate, phenylpropionate, and propionate esters may be given as a combined intramuscular preparation, sometimes also containing testosterone decanoate. Testosterone hexahydrobenzoate and testosterone hexahydrobenzylcarbonate have also been used. The undecylate ester is given by mouth in an initial dose of 120 to 160 mg daily for 2 to 3 weeks, followed by a maintenance dose of 40 to 120 mg daily.

Androgens and anabolic steroids have also been used in adolescent males with constitutionally delayed puberty or growth, and anabolic steroids have been used in the treatment of short stature in girls with Turner's syndrome. However, great care is necessary when using androgens for such conditions as bone growth may be inhibited by the early fusion of the epiphyses. This effect has been utilised by the administration of supraphysiological doses of androgens to reduce final height in boys with constitutionally tall stature.

In postmenopausal women androgens, and sometimes anabolic steroids are occasionally used in the hormonal therapy of disseminated breast carcinoma but care should be taken to choose a compound with a lower masculinising effect; the short-acting synthetic compounds are usually preferred for such purposes. Androgens and anabolic steroids have also sometimes been used with oestrogens in the management of certain menopausal disorders, but the use of androgens and anabolic steroids in women with osteoporosis is no longer advocated because their adverse effects essentially outweigh any benefit they may produce.

Anabolic steroids, and sometimes androgens, have been used in the treatment of refractory anaemias characterised by deficient red cell production, such as aplastic anaemia. Anabolic steroids and synthetic androgens with an attenuated action (sometimes known as 'attenuated androgens') such as danazol are also used in the management of hereditary angioedema.

Topical androgens may be used in the treatment of lichen sclerosus. Anabolic steroids may be useful to relieve the itching associated with obstructive jaundice.

Androgens and anabolic steroids have been used for their anabolic properties in various catabolic states.

Some testosterone esters are being investigated as male contraceptives.

Testosterone hemisuccinate is an ingredient of preparations promoted for the management of cataracts.

◊ General reviews of androgens and anabolic steroids.


1. Hickson RC, *et al.* Adverse effects of anabolic steroids. *Med Toxicol Adverse Drug Exp* 1989; **4:** 254–71.
2. Bagatell CJ, Bremner WJ. Androgens in men—uses and abuses. *N Engl J Med* 1996; **334:** 707–14.
3. Conway AJ, *et al.* Use, misuse and abuse of androgens: the Endocrine Society of Australia consensus guidelines for androgen prescribing. *Med J Aust* 2000; **172:** 220–4.


**Anabolic effects.** The androgens generally possess anabolic activity and were formerly used to increase weight in patients suffering from emaciation or debilitating diseases but effectiveness was doubtful. The anabolic steroids were developed in order to enhance the ability to build proteins and diminish the virilising and masculinising effects of the natural androgens, but all anabolics retain some androgenic activity. The anabolic steroids have again, like the androgens, been used in an attempt to produce weight gain in cachexia and wasting diseases (p.1558).

The anabolic steroids and androgens have been the subject of much misuse and abuse by athletes, sports persons, and body builders (see under Precautions, above) in an attempt to increase muscle mass and body-weight but such use cannot be justified.

References to the anabolic effects of testosterone.


1. Bhasin S, *et al.* The effects of supraphysiologic doses of testosterone on muscle size and strength in normal men. *N Engl J Med* 1996; **335:** 1–7.
2. Grinspoon S, *et al.* Effects of androgen administration in men with the AIDS wasting syndrome: a randomized, double-blind, placebo-controlled trial. *Ann Intern Med* 1998; **129:** 18–26.
3. Grinspoon S, *et al.* Effects of testosterone and progressive resistance training in eugonadal men with AIDS wasting: a randomized, controlled trial. *Ann Intern Med* 2000; **133:** 348–55.
4. Basaria S, *et al.* Anabolic-androgenic steroid therapy in the treatment of chronic diseases. *J Clin Endocrinol Metab* 2001; **86:** 5108–17.


**Antineoplastic-induced infertility.** For reference to the use of testosterone to preserve gonadal function during cyclophosphamide therapy, see Effects on Reproductive Potential, p.541.

**Constitutionally delayed puberty.** Testosterone enantate given by intramuscular injection every one to two months for periods ranging from 3 months to several years, produced beneficial effects in boys with constitutionally delayed puberty and growth;[1,2] growth rate increased, sexual and skeletal maturation were stimulated, and full height potential did not appear to be compromised. However, it has been pointed out that repeated intramuscular injections are painful and are disliked by adolescents;[3] oral testosterone undecylate or oxandrolone have been shown to be effective in the treatment of delayed puberty and growth in boys,[4,5] and may be preferred.[3] It should be noted that giving androgens to boys with constitutional delay of growth and puberty is controversial (see p.1314). For reference to the use of testosterone in boys with delayed puberty due to hypogonadism see below.


1. Donaldson MDC, Savage DCL. Testosterone therapy in boys with delayed puberty. *Arch Dis Child* 1987; **62:** 647–8.
2. Richman RA, Kirsch LR. Testosterone treatment in adolescent boys with constitutional delay in growth and development. *N Engl J Med* 1988; **319:** 1563–7.
3. Kelnar CJH. Treatment of the short, sexually immature adolescent boy. *Arch Dis Child* 1994; **71:** 285–7.
4. Albanese A, *et al.* Oral treatment for constitutional delay of growth and puberty in boys: a randomised trial of an anabolic steroid or testosterone undecanoate. *Arch Dis Child* 1994; **71:** 315–17.
5. Brown DC, *et al.* A double blind, placebo controlled study of the effects of low dose testosterone undecanoate on the growth of small for age, prepubertal boys. *Arch Dis Child* 1995; **73:** 131–5.


**Constitutionally tall stature.** Supraphysiological doses of androgens have been used to *reduce* final height in tall adolescent boys. Testosterone esters in monthly doses of up to 1000 mg have been used. Preliminary evidence after a mean of 10 years follow-up suggests that there was no long-term effect on reproductive function.[1] For reference to the use of testosterone to *increase* growth rate, see Constitutionally Delayed Puberty, above.


1. de Waal WJ, *et al.* Long term sequelae of sex steroid treatment in the management of constitutionally tall stature. *Arch Dis Child* 1995; **73:** 311–15.


**Erectile dysfunction.** For reference to the use of a cream containing testosterone, isosorbide dinitrate, and co-dergocrine mesilate in the treatment of erectile dysfunction, see under Glyceryl Trinitrate, p.925.

**Gender reassignment.** Testosterone is used in female-to-male transsexuals to develop and maintain secondary sexual characteristics. Suggested doses of the cipionate and enantate esters are 200 mg intramuscularly every 2 weeks.

**Hypogonadism.** Replacement therapy with testosterone or a testosterone ester is the standard treatment for primary hypogonadism in men (see p.1316). The androgen is often given as an intramuscular depot injection of one of the esters, although subcutaneous implants, oral formulations, transdermal systems, and a topical gel are also used (for doses see above).[1-8] A sublingual testosterone tablet is under investigation. Testosterone is also used to promote masculinisation in hypogonadal adolescent boys,[9,10] and is of value in the treatment of osteoporosis in hypogonadal men.[11] Testosterone has a negative feedback effect on gonadotrophin secretion, therefore any remaining spermatogenesis is generally suppressed; androgens are thus rarely useful in reversing male infertility (p.1316). Recommendations for monitoring therapy have been made.[8]

Transdermal testosterone may possibly be of benefit as an adjunct to oestrogen replacement in women who have undergone hysterectomy and oophorectomy.[12]


1. Bals-Pratch M, *et al.* Transdermal testosterone substitution therapy for male hypogonadism. *Lancet* 1986; **ii:** 943–6.
2. Korenman SG, *et al.* Androgen therapy of hypogonadal men with transscrotal testosterone systems. *Am J Med* 1987; **83:** 471–8.
3. Findlay JC, *et al.* Treatment of primary hypogonadism in men by the transdermal administration of testosterone. *J Clin Endocrinol Metab* 1989; **68:** 369–73.
4. Anonymous. Testosterone patches for hypogonadism. *Med Lett Drugs Ther* 1996; **38:** 49–50.
5. Arver S, *et al.* Improvement of sexual function in testosterone deficient men treated for 1 year with a permeation enhanced testosterone transdermal system. *J Urol (Baltimore)* 1996; **155:** 1604–8.
6. Anonymous. Replacing testosterone in men. *Drug Ther Bull* 1999; **37:** 3–5.
7. Wang C, *et al.* Transdermal testosterone gel improves sexual function, mood, muscle strength, and body composition parameters in hypogonadal men. *J Clin Endocrinol Metab* 2000; **85:** 2839–53.
8. Rhoden EL, Morgentaler A. Risks of testosterone-replacement therapy and recommendations for monitoring. *N Engl J Med* 2004; **350:** 482–92.
9. Moorthy B, *et al.* Depot testosterone in boys with anorchia or gonadotrophin deficiency: effect on growth rate and adult height. *Arch Dis Child* 1991; **66:** 197–9.
10. Zacharin MR, Warne GL. Treatment of hypogonadal adolescent boys with long acting subcutaneous testosterone pellets. *Arch Dis Child* 1997; **76:** 495–9.
11. Finkelstein JS, *et al.* Increases in bone density during treatment of men with idiopathic hypogonadotropic hypogonadism. *J Clin Endocrinol Metab* 1989; **69:** 776–83.
12. Shifren JL, *et al.* Transdermal testosterone treatment in women with impaired sexual function after oophorectomy. *N Engl J Med* 2000; **343:** 682–8.


**Lichen sclerosus.** Topical androgens such as androstanolone and testosterone have been used to treat pruritus associated with vulvar lichen sclerosus (p.1136) in postmenopausal women.[1-4] However, a topical corticosteroid is likely to be preferred.[5]


1. Friedrich EG, Kalra PS. Serum levels of sex hormones in vulvar lichen sclerosus, and the effect of topical testosterone. *N Engl J Med* 1984; **310:** 488–91.
2. Paslin D. Treatment of lichen sclerosus with topical dihydrotestosterone. *Obstet Gynecol* 1991; **78:** 1046–9.
3. Paslin D. Androgens in the topical treatment of lichen sclerosus. *Int J Dermatol* 1996; **35:** 298–301.
4. Bracco GL, *et al.* Clinical and histologic effects of topical treatments of vulval lichen sclerosus: a critical evaluation. *J Reprod Med* 1993; **38:** 37–40.
5. Powell JJ, Wojharowska F. Lichen sclerosus. *Lancet* 1999; **353:** 1777–83.


**Male contraception.** In male contraceptive trials it was found that high-dose testosterone severely reduced sperm production.[1] In those in whom azoospermia was not induced there was oligozoospermia with remaining sperm having a markedly diminished fertilising capacity. In a multicentre study carried out by the WHO[2] involving 271 healthy fertile men, weekly intramuscular injection of testosterone enantate 200 mg produced azoospermia in 157 men within 6 months. In a subsequent 12-month study of these azoospermic men, during which time testosterone enantate was the only contraceptive measure used, there was only 1 pregnancy. Spermatogenesis was re-established on withdrawal of testosterone. These findings have been confirmed in a larger trial of the same regimen, which additionally assessed contraceptive efficacy in men who achieved oligozoospermia (less than $3 \times 10^6$ per mL).[3] No pregnancies occurred in couples where the man was azoospermic. However, the pregnancy rate was 8.1 per 100-person-years in the subgroup of couples where the man was oligozoospermic. This rate is sixfold higher than is generally seen with hormonal contraceptives in women.[4] Both studies found that consistent azoospermia was achieved in a higher percentage of Asian men (95%) than Western men (70%).[4]

An alternative approach being investigated is the suppression of spermatogenesis with a progestogen such as desogestrel combined with low-dose testosterone.[5,6]

For a general discussion on choice of contraceptive method, including mention of male contraception, see p.1535.


1. Matsumoto AM. Is high dosage testosterone an effective male contraceptive agent? *Fertil Steril* 1988; **50:** 324–8.
2. WHO Task Force on Methods for the Regulation of Male Fertility. Contraceptive efficacy of testosterone-induced azoospermia in normal men. *Lancet* 1990; **336:** 955–9.
3. WHO Task Force on Methods for the Regulation of Male Fertility. Contraceptive efficacy of testosterone-induced azoospermia and oligozoospermia in normal men. *Fertil Steril* 1996; **65:** 821–9.
4. Anonymous. An androgen contraceptive for men: preliminary findings. *WHO Drug Inf* 1996; **10:** 50–3.
5. Wu FCW, *et al.* Oral progestogen combined with testosterone as a potential male contraceptive: additive effects between desogestrel and testosterone enanthate in suppression of spermatogenesis, pituitary-testicular axis, and lipid metabolism. *J Clin Endocrinol Metab* 1999; **84:** 112–22.
6. Hair WM, *et al.* A novel male contraceptive pill-patch combination: oral desogestrel and transdermal testosterone in the suppression of spermatogenesis in normal men. *J Clin Endocrinol Metab* 2001; **86:** 5201–9.


**Menopausal hormone replacement therapy.** In the UK menopausal women are sometimes given implants of testosterone (in a dose of 50 to 100 mg every 4 to 8 months) as an adjunct to menopausal HRT (p.1536). In the USA, preparations containing an androgen and an oestrogen are available for the treatment of menopausal vasomotor symptoms, but there is conflicting opinion as to their usefulness, and further data are needed.[1] For mention of the use of transdermal testosterone in women who have undergone oophorectomy see under Hypogonadism, above.


1. Abraham D, Carpenter PC. Issues concerning androgen replacement therapy in postmenopausal women. *Mayo Clin Proc* 1997; **72:** 1051–5.


**Rheumatoid arthritis.** A hypogonadic condition characterised by low serum-testosterone concentrations appears to be associated with at least the active stages of rheumatoid arthritis (p.9) in men.[1] Clinical improvement and reductions in IgM rheumatoid factor concentration, tender joint count, and the daily dosage of NSAIDs required, were observed in men with rheumatoid arthritis given oral testosterone undecylate 40 mg three times daily for 6 months. Improvements in rheumatoid arthritis were also seen in 12 of 36 postmenopausal women treated with intramuscular testosterone 50 mg plus progesterone 2.5 mg once every 2 weeks compared with 2 of 32 women receiving placebo.[2]


1. Cutolo M, *et al.* Androgen replacement therapy in male patients with rheumatoid arthritis. *Arthritis Rheum* 1991; **34:** 1–5.
2. Booji A, *et al.* Androgens as adjuvant treatment in postmenopausal female patients with rheumatoid arthritis. *Ann Rheum Dis* 1996; **55:** 811–15.


## Preparations

***BP 2003:*** Testosterone Implants; Testosterone Propionate Injection;
***USP 27:*** Testosterone Cypionate Injection; Testosterone Enanthate Injection; Testosterone Injectable Suspension; Testosterone Propionate Injection.

**Proprietary Preparations** (details are given in Part 3)
***Arg.:*** Sustanon 250; Testoviron Depot 100; Testoviron Depot 250; Undestor; ***Austral.:*** Andriol; Androderm; Primoteston Depot; Sustanon 100; Sustanon 250; ***Austria:*** Andriol; Testoderm; Testoviron 250; Virormone; ***Belg.:*** Sustanon; Testoderm†; Testoviron Depot†; Undestor; ***Braz.:*** Androxon; Deposteron; Testiormina†; Tesurene†; Virilisterona†; ***Canad.:*** Andriol; Androderm; Delatestryl; Malogen Aqueous†; Malogen in Oil†; Malogex†; Scheinpharm Testone-Cyp†; ***Chile:*** Primoniat Depot; Sustenan; Sustenan 250; ***Denm.:*** Restandol; Testoviron Depot 135; Testoviron Depot 250; ***Fin.:*** Atmos; Panteston; Sustanon 250; ***Fr.:*** Androtardyl; Pantestone; ***Ger.:*** Andriol; Androderm; Testoderm†; Testoviron Depot 250; ***Gr.:*** Restandol; Testoviron; ***Hong Kong:*** Andriol; Sustanon; Testoviron Depot; ***India:*** Aquaviron; Nuvir; Sustanon 100; Sustanon 250; Testanon 25; Testanon 50; Testoviron Depot; ***Irl.:*** Andropatch; Restandol; Sustanon 100; Sustanon 250; ***Israel:*** Androxon; Sustanon 250; Testoviron Depot; ***Ital.:*** Andriol; Androderm; Sustanon; Testo-Enant; Testovis; ***Malaysia:*** Andriol; Jenasteron; ***Mex.:*** Andriol; Primoteston Depot; Sostenon; Testozzard†; ***Neth.:*** Andriol; Sustanon 100; Sustanon 250; Testoderm; Testoviron Depot; ***Norw.:*** Androxon; Atmos; ***NZ:*** Panteston; Primoteston Depot; Sustanon; ***Port.:*** Andriol; Testoviron Depot; ***S.Afr.:*** Androxon; Depotrone; Sustanon 250; ***Singapore:*** Andriol; Sustanon 250; Testoviron Depot†; ***Spain:*** Androderm; Testex; Testoviron Depot 250; ***Swed.:*** Atmos; Testoviron Depot; Undestor; ***Switz.:*** Andriol; Androderm; Testoderm; Testoviron Depot; ***Thai.:*** Andriol; Testoviron 100; Testoviron 250; Virormone; ***UK:*** Andropatch; Primoteston Depot†; Restandol; Striant; Sustanon 100; Sustanon 250; Testoderm†; Testogel; Testosterone Implants; Virormone; ***USA:*** Androderm; AndroGel; Androposityory†; Delatestryl; depAndro†; Depotest†; Durathate†; Everone†; Histerone†; Striant; Tesamone†; Testim; Testoderm; Testopel; Virilon.

**Multi-ingredient:** ***Arg.:*** Supligol; ***Austria:*** Testoviron 100†; ***Braz.:*** Durateston; Estandron P; Trinestril; ***Canad.:*** Climacteron; ***Chile:*** Estandron Prolongado; ***Ger.:*** Androfemon; Tachynerg N†; Testoviron Depot 100; Testoviron Depot 50; ***India:*** Mixogen; ***Ital.:*** Facovit; Rubidiosin Composto†; Testoviron Depot; ***Malaysia:*** Sustanon 250; ***Mex.:*** Despamen; Sten; ***Norw.:*** Primoteston Depot; ***Port.:*** Sustenon 250; ***S.Afr.:*** Mixogen; Primodian Depot; ***Spain:*** Testoviron Depot 100; ***Thai.:*** Metharmon-F; Primodian Depot; ***USA:*** depAndrogyn†; Depo-Testadiol; Depotestogen; Duo-Cyp†; Duratestrin†; Test-Estro†; Valertest†.

---

# Tibolone *(BAN, USAN, rINN)*

7α-Methylnorethynodrel; Org-OD-14; Tibolona. 17β-Hydroxy-7α-methyl-19-nor-17α-pregn-5(10)-en-20-yn-3-one.

$C_{21}H_{28}O_2$ = 312.4.

*CAS — 5630-53-5.*

*ATC — G03DC05.*

## Adverse Effects

Irregular vaginal bleeding or spotting may occur with tibolone, mainly during the first few months of treatment, and particularly in women undergoing a natural menopause who use tibolone within 12 months of their last menstrual period. Unlike cyclical, but similar to continuous, combination HRT (p.1536), tibolone does not produce regular withdrawal bleeding. Other adverse effects have included changes in body-weight, ankle oedema, dizziness, skin reactions, headache, migraine, visual disturbances, gastrointestinal disturbances, increased growth of facial hair, altered liver function, depression, and arthralgia or myalgia.

**Incidence of adverse effects.** In 1994, the UK Committee on Safety of Medicines had received reports of 2796 suspected adverse reactions with tibolone over 3 years, out of about 666 000 prescriptions.[1] The commonest reported effects were headache, dizziness, nausea, rash, itching, and weight gain. Vaginal bleeding appeared to occur in about 8 to 9% of recipients. There had also been 52 reports of migraine, 4 of exacerbation of migraine, and 49 reports of visual disturbances, some suggestive of migraine.


1. Committee on Safety of Medicines/Medicines Control Agency. Tibolone (Livial). *Current Problems* 1994; **20:** 14.


**Effects on the endometrium.** Endometrial hyperplasia and endometrial carcinoma have been rarely reported after investigation of uterine bleeding in women receiving tibolone therapy,[1,2] as has exacerbation of adenomyosis.[3] Some of these women had previously received oestrogens. One report concluded that it was unclear whether tibolone was an aetiological agent or a cofactor in these cases,[1] and emphasised that, although tibolone has progestogenic properties, it cannot be expected to reverse pre-existing endometrial hyperplasia or to protect against the development of endometrial malignancy.[1]


1. von Dadelszen P, *et al.* Endometrial hyperplasia and adenocarcinoma during tibolone (Livial) therapy. *Br J Obstet Gynaecol* 1994; **101:** 158–61.
2. Ginsburg J, Prelevic GM. Cause of vaginal bleeding in postmenopausal women taking tibolone. *Maturitas* 1996; **24:** 107–10.
3. Prys Davies A, Oram D. Exacerbation of adenomyosis in a postmenopausal woman taking tibolone associated with an elevation in serum CA 125. *Br J Obstet Gynaecol* 1994; **101:** 632–3.


## Precautions

Tibolone is contra-indicated in women with hormone-dependent tumours, cardiovascular or cerebrovascular disorders including thrombophlebitis, thromboembolic processes, or a history of these conditions, undiagnosed vaginal bleeding, and severe liver disorders. It should not be given to pregnant women and should not be used prior to the menopause because menstrual regularity may be disturbed. Use of tibolone within 12 months of a natural menopause is also not recommended because irregular vaginal bleeding is likely. In postmenopausal women, vaginal bleeding starting after 3 months or more of treatment, or recurrent or persistent bleeding should be investigated. Care should be taken when giving tibolone to patients with liver disease or disorders that may be exacerbated by fluid retention such as kidney dysfunction, epilepsy, or migraine, or with a history of these conditions. It should also be given with caution to patients with hypercholesterolaemia and impaired glucose tolerance. Tibolone should be stopped if there are signs of thromboembolism or if abnormal liver function tests or cholestatic jaundice occur. Consideration should be given to stopping tibolone 4 weeks before elective surgery when prolonged immobilisation after surgery is likely.

In women transferring from another form of HRT to tibolone it is suggested that a withdrawal bleed be induced with a progestogen prior to starting tibolone treatment since the endometrium may already be stimulated.

**Breast feeding.** The manufacturer recommends that tibolone should be avoided during breast feeding.

## Interactions

On theoretical grounds, it is anticipated that compounds that induce liver enzymes such as phenytoin, carbamazepine, and rifampicin may enhance the metabolism of tibolone and thus reduce its activity.

## Pharmacokinetics

After oral doses, peak-plasma concentrations are attained in 1 to 4 hours. Tibolone is rapidly metabolised into 3 active metabolites, 2 of which have predominantly oestrogenic activity while the third, like the parent compound, has predominantly progestogenic activity. Metabolites are excreted in the bile and eliminated in the faeces. A small amount is excreted in the urine.

## Uses and Administration

Tibolone is a steroid derived from noretynodrel that has oestrogenic, progestogenic, and weak androgenic properties. It is used as menopausal HRT (see p.1540) in the treatment of menopausal vasomotor symptoms and the prevention of postmenopausal osteoporosis. The usual dose is 2.5 mg daily by mouth in a continuous regimen.

**'Add-back' therapy.** Tibolone reduces vasomotor symptoms associated with the use of gonadorelin analogues for endometriosis (p.1546) or fibroids (p.1326).[1]

1. Lindsay PC, *et al.* The effect of add-back treatment with tibolone (Livial) on patients treated with the gonadotropin-releasing hormone agonist triptorelin (Decapetyl). *Fertil Steril* 1996; **65:** 342–8.

**Menopausal disorders.** References and a review[1] of the use of tibolone for menopausal symptoms[2,3] and prevention[4,5] or treatment[6] of postmenopausal bone loss.

1. Modelska K, Cummings S. Tibolone for postmenopausal women: systematic review of randomized trials. *J Clin Endocrinol Metab* 2002; **87:** 16–23.
2. Egarter C, *et al.* Tibolone versus conjugated estrogens and sequential progestogen in the treatment of climacteric complaints. *Maturitas* 1996; **23:** 55–62.
3. Hammar M, *et al.* A double-blind, randomised trial comparing the effects of tibolone and continuous combined hormone replacement therapy in postmenopausal women with menopausal symptoms. *Br J Obstet Gynaecol* 1998; **105:** 904–11.
4. Berning B, *et al.* Effects of two doses of tibolone on trabecular and cortical bone loss in early postmenopausal women: a two-year randomized, placebo-controlled study. *Bone* 1996; **19:** 395–9.
5. Lippuner K, *et al.* Prevention of postmenopausal bone loss using tibolone or conventional peroral or transdermal hormone replacement therapy with 17β-estradiol and dydrogesterone. *J Bone Miner Res* 1997; **12:** 806–12.
6. Studd J, *et al.* A randomized study of tibolone on bone mineral density in osteoporotic postmenopausal women with previous fractures. *Obstet Gynecol* 1998; **92:** 574–9.

## Preparations

**Proprietary Preparations** (details are given in Part 3)

***Arg.:*** Discretal; Paraclim; Tibofem; ***Austral.:*** Livial; ***Austria:*** Liviel; ***Belg.:*** Livial; ***Braz.:*** Donna; Libiam; Livial; Livolon; ***Chile:*** Lifar; Livial; Tinox; Tobe; ***Denm.:*** Livial; ***Fin.:*** Livial; ***Fr.:*** Livial; ***Ger.:*** Liviella; ***Gr.:*** Livial; ***Hong Kong:*** Livial; ***India:*** Livial; ***Irl.:*** Livial; ***Ital.:*** Livial; ***Malaysia:*** Livial; ***Mex.:*** Livial; ***Neth.:*** Livial; ***Norw.:*** Livial; ***NZ:*** Livial; ***Port.:*** Livial; ***S.Afr.:*** Livifem; ***Singapore:*** Livial; ***Spain:*** Boltin; ***Swed.:*** Livial; ***Switz.:*** Livial; ***Thai.:*** Livial; ***UK:*** Livial.

---

## Trenbolone Acetate *(BANM, USAN, rINNM)*

Acetato de trenbolona; RU-1697; Trienbolone Acetate. 17β-Hydroxyestra-4,9,11-trien-3-one acetate.

$C_{20}H_{24}O_3 = 312.4.$

*CAS — 10161-33-8 (trenbolone); 10161-34-9 (trenbolone acetate).*

**Pharmacopoeias.** In *US*, for veterinary use only.

**USP 27** (Trenbolone Acetate). Store in airtight containers at a temperature of 2° to 8°.

### Profile

Trenbolone acetate has been used as an anabolic agent in veterinary practice. The hexahydrobenzylcarbonate has also been used for its anabolic properties.

◊ WHO specifies an acceptable daily intake of trenbolone acetate as a residue in foods, and recommends maximum residue limits in various animal tissues.[1] However, it should be noted that, in the European Union the use of trenbolone acetate and other anabolic steroids is restricted to certain therapeutic indications in non-food producing animals and their use as growth promotors is banned.

1. FAO/WHO. Evaluation of certain veterinary drug residues in food: thirty-fourth report of the joint FAO/WHO expert committee on food additives. *WHO Tech Rep Ser 788* 1989.

---

## Trimegestone *(BAN, USAN, rINN)*

RU-27987; Trimegestona. 17β-(S)-Lactoyl-17-methylestra-4,9-dien-3-one; 17β-[(S)-2-Hydroxypropionyl]-17α-methylestra-4,9-dien-3-one.

$C_{22}H_{30}O_3 = 342.5.$

*CAS — 74513-62-5.*

### Profile

Trimegestone is a progestogen (see Progesterone, p.1566) used in menopausal HRT (see p.1536). It is given in daily doses of 500 micrograms by mouth, in a cyclical regimen. Trimegestone is also under investigation as a component of a combined oral contraceptive.

◊ References.

1. Ross D. Endometrial effects of three doses of trimegestone, a new orally active progestogen, on the postmenopausal endometrium. *Maturitas* 1997; **28:** 83–8.
2. Al-Azzawi F, *et al.* Acceptability and patterns of uterine bleeding in sequential trimegestone-based hormone replacement therapy: a dose-ranging study. *Hum Reprod* 1999; **14:** 636–41.
3. Meuwissen JH, *et al.* A 1-year comparison of the efficacy and clinical tolerance in postmenopausal women of two hormone replacement therapies containing estradiol in combination with either norgestrel or trimegestone. *Gynecol Endocrinol* 2001; **15:** 349–58.
4. Al-Azzawi F, *et al.* Acceptability and patterns of endometrial bleeding in estradiol-based HRT regimens: a comparative study of cyclical sequential combinations of trimegestone or norethisterone acetate. *Climacteric* 2001; **4:** 343–54.

### Preparations

**Proprietary Preparations** (details are given in Part 3)

**Multi-ingredient:** ***Austria:*** Totelle cyclo; ***Belg.:*** Totelle; ***Chile:*** Totelle; ***Denm.:*** Totelle; ***Fin.:*** Totelle Sekvens; ***Ital.:*** Totelle; ***Swed.:*** Totelle Sekvens.

---

## Zeranol *(BAN, USAN, rINN)*

MK-188; P-1496; THFES (HM); Zearalanol. (3S,7R)-3,4,5,6,7,8,9,10,11,12-Decahydro-7,14,16-trihydroxy-3-methyl-1H-2-benzoxacyclotetradecin-1-one.

$C_{18}H_{26}O_5 = 322.4.$

*CAS — 26538-44-3.*

### Profile

Zeranol is a nonsteroidal oestrogen that has been used for the management of menopausal and menstrual disorders. It has also been used as a growth promotor in veterinary practice.

◊ WHO specifies an acceptable daily intake of zeranol as a residue in foods and recommends maximum residue limits in various animal tissues.[1] However, it should be noted that, in the European Union the use of zeranol in veterinary medicine is prohibited. Certain other steroidal hormones are permitted for restricted use but their use as growth promotors is banned.

1. FAO/WHO. Evaluation of certain veterinary drug residues in food: thirty-second report of the joint FAO/WHO expert committee on food additives. *WHO Tech Rep Ser 763* 1988.

# Soaps and Other Anionic Surfactants

Soaps and other anionic surfactants dissociate in aqueous solution to form an anion, which is responsible for the surface activity, and a cation which is devoid of surface-active properties. They are widely used for their emulsifying and cleansing properties. The term detergent is used to describe a surface-active agent that concentrates at oil-water interfaces and possesses emulsifying and cleansing properties. The principal groups of anionic surfactants used in pharmaceutical preparations include:

**Alkali-metal** and **ammonium soaps** (monovalent alkyl carboxylates) which are the sodium, potassium, and ammonium salts of the higher fatty acids.

**Metallic soaps** (polyvalent alkyl carboxylates) are the calcium, zinc, magnesium, and aluminium salts of the higher fatty acids and produce water-in-oil emulsions; the soaps are often made by chemical reaction during the preparation of the emulsion.

**Amine soaps** are salts of amines with fatty acids.

**Alkyl sulfates** or **sulfated fatty alcohols** are salts of the sulfuric acid esters of the higher fatty alcohols.

**Alkyl ether sulfates** or **ethoxylated alkyl sulfates** are formed by sulfating ethoxylated alcohols.

**Sulfated oils** are prepared by treating fixed oils with sulfuric acid and neutralising with sodium hydroxide solution.

Many **sulfonated compounds** have been produced which possess surface-active properties and are used as detergents; they include alkyl sulfonates, alkyl aryl sulfonates, and amide sulfonates. Docusate sodium (p.1262), a sulfonated dibasic acid ester, has medicinal and pharmaceutical uses.

**Ampholytic (or amphoteric) surfactants** possess at least one anionic group and at least one cationic group in the molecule and can therefore have anionic, nonionic, or cationic properties depending on the pH. When the strength of the cationic portion of the molecule is equivalent to that of the anionic portion the isoelectric point occurs at pH 7 and the molecule is said to be balanced. Ampholytic surfactants have the detergent properties of anionic surfactants and the disinfectant properties of cationic surfactants. Their activity depends on the pH of the media in which they are used. Compounds used include aminocarboxylic acids, aminopropionic acid derivatives, imidazoline derivatives, and dodicin. Long-chain betaines are sometimes classed as ampholytic surfactants.

Balanced ampholytic surfactants are reputed to be non-irritant to the eyes and skin and have therefore been used in baby shampoos.

## Aluminium Monostearate

Aluminii Monostearas; Aluminum Monostearate; Monoestearato de aluminio. Dihydroxy(octadecanoato-*O*-)aluminium; Dihydroxy(stearato)aluminium.

*CAS — 7047-84-9.*

**Pharmacopoeias.** In *Jpn* and *Pol.* Also in *USNF.*

**USNF 22** (Aluminum Monostearate). A compound of aluminium with a mixture of solid organic acids obtained from fats and consisting mainly of variable proportions of aluminium monostearate and aluminium monopalmitate. A fine, white to yellowish-white, bulky powder with a faint characteristic odour. Insoluble in water, in alcohol, and in ether.

### Profile

Aluminium monostearate forms gels with fixed or mineral oils when heated to about 60°; such gels are used to suspend medicaments in oily injections.

## Calcium Stearate

Calcii Stearas; Estearato de calcio. Calcium octadecanoate.

*CAS — 542-42-7 (calcium palmitate); 1592-23-0 (calcium stearate).*

**Pharmacopoeias.** In *Eur.* (see p.vi), *Int.*, and *Jpn.* Also in *USNF.*

**Ph. Eur. 5.0** (Calcium Stearate). A mixture of calcium salts of different fatty acids consisting mainly of stearic acid ($C_{36}H_{70}CaO_4$ = 607.0) and palmitic acid ($C_{32}H_{62}CaO_4$ = 550.9) with minor proportions of other fatty acids. The fatty acid fraction contains not less than 40.0% of stearic acid and the sum of stearic acid and palmitic acids is not less than 90.0%. A fine, white or almost white, crystalline powder. Practically insoluble in water and in alcohol.

**USNF 22** (Calcium Stearate). A compound of calcium with a mixture of solid organic acids obtained from fats, consisting mainly of variable proportions of calcium stearate ($C_{36}H_{70}CaO_4$ = 607.0) and calcium palmitate ($C_{32}H_{62}CaO_4$ = 550.9). A fine, white to yellowish-white bulky, unctuous powder, free from grittiness with a slight characteristic odour. Insoluble in water, in alcohol, and in ether.

### Profile

Calcium stearate is added to granules as a lubricant in the manufacture of tablets and capsules.

## Magnesium Stearate

572; Estearato de magnesio; Magnesii Stearas.

*CAS — 1555-53-9 (magnesium oleate); 2601-98-1 (magnesium palmitate); 557-04-0 (magnesium stearate).*

**Pharmacopoeias.** In *Chin.*, *Eur.* (see p.vi), *Int.*, *Jpn*, *Pol.*, and *Viet.* Also in *USNF.*

**Ph. Eur. 5.0** (Magnesium Stearate). A mixture of the magnesium salts of different fatty acids consisting mainly of stearic acid ($C_{36}H_{70}MgO_4$ = 591.2) and palmitic acid ($C_{32}H_{62}MgO_4$ = 535.1) and in minor proportions other fatty acids. The fatty acid fraction contains not less than 40.0% of stearic acid and the sum of stearic acid and palmitic acid is not less than 90.0%. A white, very fine, light powder, greasy to the touch. Practically insoluble in water and in dehydrated alcohol.

**USNF 22** (Magnesium Stearate). A compound of magnesium with a mixture of solid organic acids, and consisting mainly of variable proportions of magnesium stearate ($C_{36}H_{70}MgO_4$ = 591.2) and magnesium palmitate ($C_{32}H_{62}MgO_4$ = 535.1). It is a very fine, light, white powder, slippery to touch. Insoluble in water, in alcohol, and in ether.

### Profile

Magnesium stearate is added as a lubricant to the granules in tablet-making and has been used as a dusting powder and in barrier creams.

## Sodium Cetostearyl Sulfate

Cetoestearilsulfato de sodio; Cetylstearylschwefelsaures Natrium; Natrii Cetylo- et Stearylosulfas; Natrium Cetylosulphuricum; Natrium Cetylstearylosulphuricum; Sodium Cetostearyl Sulphate.

*CAS — 1120-01-0 (sodium cetyl sulfate); 1120-04-3 (sodium stearyl sulfate).*

**Pharmacopoeias.** In *Eur.* (see p.vi) and *Pol.* Also in *USNF.*

**Ph. Eur. 5.0** (Sodium Cetostearyl Sulphate). A mixture of sodium cetyl sulfate ($C_{16}H_{33}NaO_4S$ = 344.5) and sodium stearyl sulfate ($C_{18}H_{37}NaO_4S$ = 372.5). A white or pale yellow, amorphous or crystalline powder. Soluble in hot water giving an opalescent solution; practically insoluble in cold water; partly soluble in alcohol.

**USNF 22** (Sodium Cetostearyl Sulfate). A mixture of sodium cetyl sulfate ($C_{16}H_{33}NaSO_4$ = 344.5) and sodium stearyl sulfate ($C_{18}H_{37}NaSO_4$ = 372.5). It contains not less than 40% of sodium cetyl sulfate and the sum of the sodium cetyl sulfate content and sodium stearyl sulfate content is not less than 90%, both contents calculated on the anhydrous basis. A white or pale yellow, amorphous or crystalline powder. Soluble in hot water giving an opalescent solution; practically insoluble in cold water; partly soluble in alcohol.

### Profile

Sodium cetostearyl sulfate is used for similar purposes to sodium laurilsulfate (see below).

## Sodium Laurilsulfate *(pINNM)*

Laurilsulfato de sodio; Natrii Laurilsulfas; Natrium Lauryl Sulphuricum; Sodium Dodecyl Sulphate; Sodium Lauryl Sulfate; Sodium Lauryl Sulphate.

*CAS — 151-21-3.*

**Pharmacopoeias.** In *Chin.*, *Eur.* (see p.vi), *Jpn*, and *Pol.* Also in *USNF.*

**Ph. Eur. 5.0** (Sodium Laurilsulfate; Sodium Lauryl Sulphate BP 2003). A mixture of sodium alkyl sulfates, consisting mainly of sodium dodecyl sulfate ($C_{12}H_{25}NaO_4S$ = 288.4). It contains not less than 85% of sodium alkyl sulfates and not more than a total of 8% of sodium chloride and sodium sulfate. A white or pale yellow powder or crystals. Freely soluble in water giving an opalescent solution; partly soluble in alcohol.

**USNF 22** (Sodium Lauryl Sulfate). A mixture of sodium alkyl sulfates, consisting mainly of sodium laurilsulfate ($C_{12}H_{25}NaO_4S$ = 288.4). The combined content of sodium chloride and sodium sulfate is not more than 8%. Small, white or light yellow crystals with a slight, characteristic odour. Soluble 1 in 10 of water giving an opalescent solution.

**Incompatibility.** Sodium laurilsulfate interacts with cationic surfactants such as cetrimide, resulting in a loss of activity. It is also incompatible with salts of polyvalent metal ions (e.g. aluminium, lead, tin, or zinc) and with acids of pH below 2.5. It is not affected by hard water due to the solubility of the corresponding calcium and magnesium salts.

### Profile

Sodium laurilsulfate is an anionic emulsifying agent. It is a detergent and wetting agent, effective in both acid and alkaline solution and in hard water. It is used in medicated shampoos and as a skin cleanser and in toothpastes. It is used in the preparation of Emulsifying Wax (p.1481).

Other salts of laurilsulfate have been used for their surfactant properties. These include monoethanolamine, diolamine, and trolamine laurilsulfates, and magnesium and ammonium laurilsulfates. Similar surfactants include sodium lauril ether sulfate and sodium alkyl sulfoacetates such as sodium lauril sulfoacetate.

Sodium laurilsulfate and related surfactants are also included in some combination preparations used rectally for the management of constipation.

### Preparations

*BP 2003:* Emulsifying Wax.

**Proprietary Preparations** (details are given in Part 3)

***Arg.:*** Limectant; ***Braz.:*** Endocris†; ***Canad.:*** Pro-Sope†; ***Chile:*** Solucion Detergente; ***Fr.:*** Gyalme; ***Hong Kong:*** Lowila Cake; ***Mex.:*** Aquanil; ***Spain:*** Anticerumen.

**Multi-ingredient:** ***Arg.:*** Nigalax; Plus & Plus; ***Austral.:*** Fleet Micro-Enema; Microlax; Pinetarsol; ***Austria:*** Microklist; ***Belg.:*** Microlax; Neo-Sabenyl; ***Canad.:*** Aseptone 2†; Microlax; Plax; ***Denm.:*** Microlax; ***Fin.:*** Microlax; ***Fr.:*** Bactident; Microlax; Ysol 206; ***Ger.:*** Dermofug†; Dermowas; Microklist; ***Hong Kong:*** Fleet Micro-Enema; Microlax; ***Irl.:*** Micolette; Microlax; ***Israel:*** Microlet; ***Ital.:*** Eso Zim; Florigien†; Novilax; Si-Cliss†; ***Malaysia:*** Dentinox Cradle Cap; Microlax; ***Mex.:*** Microlax; ***Neth.:*** Microlax; ***Norw.:*** Microlax; ***NZ:*** Fleet Micro-Enema; Microlax; ***Port.:*** Microlax; ***S.Afr.:*** Medigel; Microlax; ***Singapore:*** Dentinox Cradle Cap; Microlax; ***Spain:*** Micralax; Microcasen†; ***Swed.:*** Fleet Micro; Microlax; ***Switz.:*** Microklist; Microlax†; Stellisept†; ***UK:*** Dentinox Cradle Cap; Micolette; Micralax; Relaxit; ***USA:*** Maxilube; Summers Eve Post-Menstrual; Trichotine; Trimo-San.

## Sodium Oleate

Oleato de sodio.

*CAS — 143-19-1.*

### Profile

Sodium oleate is an anionic surfactant used as an ingredient in preparations for the symptomatic relief of haemorrhoids and pruritus ani.

Zinc oleate and potassium oleate have also been used in skin preparations, while the sodium, potassium, and calcium salts have applications as food additives.

### Preparations

**Proprietary Preparations** (details are given in Part 3)

**Multi-ingredient:** ***Belg.:*** Cose-Anal; Neo-Alcos-Anal†; ***Fr.:*** Bilifluine†; ***Ger.:*** Alcos-Anal; Neo-Ballistol; ***Neth.:*** Epianal; ***Norw.:*** Alcos-Anal; ***Swed.:*** Alcos-Anal.

## Sodium Stearate

Estearato de sodio; Natrii Stearas.

*CAS — 408-35-5 (sodium palmitate); 822-16-2 (sodium stearate).*

**Pharmacopoeias.** In *Eur.* (see p.vi) and *Pol.* Also in *USNF.*

**Ph. Eur. 5.0** (Sodium Stearate). A mixture of sodium salts of different fatty acids consisting mainly of stearic acid ($C_{18}H_{35}O_2Na$ = 306.5) and palmitic acid ($C_{16}H_{31}O_2Na$ = 278.4). It contains 7.4 to 8.5% of sodium, calculated with reference to the dried substance. The fatty acid fraction contains not less than 40% of stearic acid and the sum of stearic acid and palmitic acid is not less than 90%. A white or yellowish, fine powder, with a greasy touch. Slightly soluble in water and in alcohol. Store in airtight containers. Protect from light.

**USNF 22** (Sodium Stearate). A mixture containing not less than 90% of sodium stearate ($C_{18}H_{35}NaO_2$ = 306.5) and sodium palmitate ($C_{16}H_{31}NaO_2$ = 278.4); the content of sodium stearate is not less than 40% of the total. It contains small amounts of the sodium salts of other fatty acids. A fine, white powder, soapy to the touch, usually with a slight tallow-like odour. Slowly soluble in cold water and in cold alcohol; readily soluble in hot water and in hot alcohol. Protect from light.

### Profile

Sodium stearate is an emulsifying and stiffening agent used in a variety of topical preparations. It is an ingredient of Glycerin Suppositories (USP 27).

## Sodium Stearyl Fumarate

Estearilfumarato de sodio; Natrii Stearylis Fumaras.

$C_{22}H_{39}NaO_4$ = 390.5.

**Pharmacopoeias.** In *Eur.* (see p.vi). Also in *USNF.*

**Ph. Eur. 5.0** (Sodium Stearyl Fumarate). A fine, white or almost white powder with agglomerates of flat, circular shaped particles. Practically insoluble in water, in alcohol, and in acetone; slightly soluble in methyl alcohol.

**USNF 22** (Sodium Stearyl Fumarate). A fine white powder. Practically insoluble in water; slightly soluble in methyl alcohol.

### Profile

Sodium stearyl fumarate is used as a lubricant in the manufacture of tablets and capsules.

## Sodium Tetradecyl Sulfate *(rINN)*

Sodium Tetradecyl Sulphate; Tetradecilsulfato de sodio. Sodium 4-ethyl-1-isobutyloctyl sulfate.

$C_{14}H_{29}NaO_4S$ = 316.4.

*CAS — 139-88-8.*

*ATC — C05BB04.*

**Pharmacopoeias.** *Br.* includes as a concentrated form.

**BP 2003** (Sodium Tetradecyl Sulphate Concentrate). A clear, colourless gel. Store at a temperature not exceeding 25°. Protect from light.

### Adverse Effects and Precautions

The complications of injection sclerotherapy with sclerosants such as sodium tetradecyl sulfate are discussed under Monoethanolamine Oleate, p.1716.

### Uses and Administration

Sodium tetradecyl sulfate is an anionic surfactant. It has sclerosing properties and is used in the treatment of varicose veins (p.1717). It has also been given in the management of bleeding oesophageal varices (p.1716).

Sclerotherapy for varicose veins is a specialised technique. A solution of sodium tetradecyl sulfate is injected slowly into the lumen of an isolated segment of an emptied superficial vein, followed by compression. Solutions are available in a variety of strengths (0.2 to 3%); doses depend on the site and condition being treated. A test dose is advisable in patients with a history of allergy. Facilities for treating anaphylaxis should be available.

### Preparations

***BP 2003:*** Sodium Tetradecyl Sulphate Injection.

**Proprietary Preparations** (details are given in Part 3)

***Arg.:*** Fibro-Vein; ***Austral.:*** Fibro-Vein; ***Canad.:*** Tromboject; Trombovar; ***Fr.:*** Trombovar; ***Irl.:*** Fibro-Vein; ***Ital.:*** Fibro-Vein; Trombovar; ***Malaysia:*** Trombovar; ***NZ:*** Fibro-Vein; ***S.Afr.:*** Fibrovein†; STD†; ***UK:*** Fibro-Vein; ***USA:*** Sotradecol.

## Soft Soap

Green Soap; Jabón blando; Medicinal Soft Soap; Potassium Soap; Sabão Mole; Sapo Mollis; Soft soap.

**Pharmacopoeias.** In *Br., Chin.,* and *US.*

**BP 2003** (Soft Soap). It is made by the interaction of potassium hydroxide or sodium hydroxide with a suitable vegetable oil or oils or their fatty acids. It may be coloured with chlorophyll or not more than 0.015% of a suitable green soap dye. A yellowish-white to green or brown, unctuous substance. Soluble in water and in alcohol.

**USP 27** (Green Soap). It is made by the saponification of suitable vegetable oils, excluding coconut oil and palm kernel oil, without the removal of glycerol. The method given in the USP 27 involves mixing the oil with oleic acid and to the heated mixture adding potassium hydroxide dissolved in glycerol and water. The homogeneous emulsion is then adjusted to weight with hot water. A yellowish-white to brownish- or greenish-yellow, transparent to translucent, soft unctuous mass with a slight, characteristic odour.

### Adverse Effects and Treatment

Soaps and anionic detergents, in general, may be irritant to the skin by removing natural oils and may produce redness, soreness, cracking and scaling, and papular dermatitis. There may be some irritation of the eyes and mucous membranes and this limits the use of soap enemas. Ingestion of anionic detergents may cause gastrointestinal irritation with nausea, diarrhoea, intestinal distension, and occasionally vomiting. Treatment is symptomatic.

### Uses

Soft soap is used to remove incrustations in chronic scaly skin diseases such as psoriasis (p.1137) and to cleanse the scalp before the application of lotions. A solution in industrial methylated spirit, with the addition of solvent ether, has been used to cleanse the skin. A solution of soft soap in warm water has been used as an enema to soften impacted faeces but should be avoided as it may inflame the colonic mucosa; other measures are now employed to soften impacted faeces (see Constipation, p.1240). Soft soap is an ingredient of Soap Spirit (BP 2003) and Green Soap Tincture (USP 27).

Potash soap (linseed oil soap) has been used in the preparation of liquid soaps. Hard soap (castile soap) and curd soap were formerly used as pill excipients and hard soap was also formerly used in the preparation of plasters.

### Preparations

***BP 2003:*** Soap Spirit;
***USP 27:*** Green Soap; Green Soap Tincture.

**Proprietary Preparations** (details are given in Part 3)

***USA:*** Fleet Bagenema.

***Multi-ingredient:*** ***Austria:*** Abfuhrdragees; Abfuhrdragees mild; ***Spain:*** Linimento Naion; ***USA:*** Therevac Plus; Therevac SB.

## Sulfated Castor Oil

Aceite de ricino sulfatado; Ol. Ricin. Sulphat.; Oleum Ricini Sulphatum; Sulfonated Castor Oil; Sulphated Castor Oil.

*CAS — 8002-33-3.*

### Profile

Sulfated castor oil is a detergent and wetting agent that has been used as a skin cleanser and emulsifying agent.

Sulfated hydrogenated castor oil (hydroxystearin sulfate) has been used in the manufacture of hydrophilic ointment bases and other emulsions.

Sodium ricinoleate has been used for its surfactant properties.

### Preparations

**Proprietary Preparations** (details are given in Part 3)

***Mex.:*** Dermac.

***Multi-ingredient:*** ***Fr.:*** Pyorex.

## Zinc Stearate

Estearato de zinc; Zinci Stearas.

*CAS — 4991-47-3 (zinc palmitate); 557-05-1 (zinc stearate).*

**Pharmacopoeias.** In *Eur.* (see p.vi), *Pol.,* and *US.*

**Ph. Eur. 5.0** (Zinc Stearate). Zinc stearate [$(C_{17}H_{35}CO_2)_2Zn$ = 632.3] may contain varying proportions of zinc palmitate [$(C_{15}H_{31}CO_2)_2Zn$ = 576.2] and zinc oleate [$(C_{17}H_{33}CO_2)2Zn$ = 628.3]. A light, white, amorphous powder, free from gritty particles. Practically insoluble in water and in dehydrated alcohol.

**USP 27** (Zinc Stearate). A compound of zinc with a mixture of solid organic acids obtained from fats and consisting mainly of variable proportions of zinc stearate [$(C_{17}H_{35}CO_2)_2Zn$ = 632.3] and zinc palmitate [$(C_{15}H_{31}CO_2)_2Zn$ = 576.2]. A fine, white, bulky powder, free from grittiness, with a faint characteristic odour. Insoluble in water, in alcohol, and in ether.

### Adverse Effects

Zinc stearate inhalation has caused fatal pneumonitis, particularly in infants.

### Uses

Zinc stearate is used as a soothing and protective application in the treatment of skin inflammation. It is used either alone or with other powders or in the form of a cream.

Zinc stearate is also added as a lubricant to the granules in tablet-making.

### Preparations

***USP 27:*** Compound Clioquinol Topical Powder.

**Proprietary Preparations** (details are given in Part 3)

***Multi-ingredient:*** ***Arg.:*** Prurisedan; ***Belg.:*** Baseler Haussalbe†; Pelsano†; ***Ital.:*** Neo Zeta-Foot†; Steril Zeta; ***Switz.:*** Adrectal†; Hydrocortisone comp; Rocanal Permanent Gangrene†; Rocanal Permanent Vital†; ***Thai.:*** Banocin; ***UK:*** Simpsons.

# Stabilising and Suspending Agents

The stabilising and suspending agents described in this chapter have the property of increasing the viscosity of water when dissolved or dispersed. The rheological properties of the dispersions can vary widely from thin liquids to thick gels.

They have wide applications both in pharmaceutical manufacturing and in the food industry. As well as being used as thickening and suspending agents many are used in emulsions as stabilisers and in some cases as emulsifying agents; some are also used in the manufacture of tablets as disintegrants, binding and granulating agents, and for film or enteric coating.

Some are used in artificial tear and artificial saliva preparations which are employed in the management of dry eye and dry mouth respectively. Those most commonly used are carbomers, cellulose ethers such as carmellose and hypromellose, polyvinyl alcohol, and povidone. Some, such as the alginates and methylcellulose, are also used in gastrointestinal disorders.

## Dry eye

Dry eye is a chronic condition caused by instability of the tear film covering the eye; the tear film breaks up into dry spots rather than being maintained between blinks. Tears consist of a slightly alkaline fluid that is spread across the eye by blinking and is lost via the lachrymal ducts or by evaporation. Mucus secreted by the conjunctiva is also required to maintain tear film stability and dry eye can result from reduced production of either tears or conjunctival mucus. Reduced tear secretion is common in the elderly, but also occurs in some systemic disorders or as an adverse effect of drugs such as those, like tricyclic antidepressants, that have antimuscarinic effects. Tear film instability may also result from increased tear evaporation, for example due to corneal exposure in thyroid disease, or from lid, corneal, or other eye disorders.

The main symptoms of dry eye are discomfort, typically with a chronic gritty sensation, visual disturbances, and sometimes photophobia. If left untreated corneal ulceration and eventual loss of sight may occur. Keratoconjunctivitis sicca (corneal inflammation) may result from severe dry eye in Sjögren's syndrome (see below).

Treatment of dry eye is primarily symptomatic using 'artificial tears' preparations; eye drops containing hypromellose or other cellulose ethers (carmellose, hyetellose, methylcellulose), polyvinyl alcohol, or povidone are used. Carbomer, in liquid gel formulations, and ointments containing soft or liquid paraffins are also employed. Ointments have a longer duration of action than drops, but tend to blur the vision and are most suitable for use at night. Drops should be used as frequently as required, up to hourly or more often if necessary. Frequent use of eye drops may cause sensitivity to the preservative, in which case preservative-free preparations should be considered. An alternative in patients requiring very frequent instillation of drops is a slow-release ophthalmic insert of hyprolose. Punctal occlusion with gelatin rods or collagen implants is used diagnostically to block tear outflow and treatment by permanent occlusion may be considered. Mucus build-up due to reduced tear production may respond to topical mucolytics such as acetylcysteine or bromhexine. Topical immunosuppressants such as ciclosporin may be of benefit in some patients with keratoconjunctivitis sicca.[1]

**Sjögren's syndrome** is an auto-immune inflammatory disease primarily affecting the lachrymal and salivary glands, and manifests as dry eye and dry mouth. It is often secondary to an auto-immune disorder such as rheumatoid arthritis. Treatment is mainly symptomatic[2] using artificial tears and topical mucolytics for dry eye; dry mouth is treated with artificial saliva as outlined below. Oral pilocarpine may be of benefit for both dry eye and dry mouth;[3] systemic treatment with the mucolytic bromhexine has produced conflicting results.[4-6] Corticosteroids and immunosuppressants may have a role in patients with CNS involvement.[7]


1. Anonymous. Ophthalmic cyclosporine (Restasis) for dry eye disease. *Med Lett Drugs Ther* 2003; **45:** 42–3.
2. Oxholm P, *et al.* Rational drug therapy: recommendations for the treatment of patients with Sjögren's syndrome. *Drugs* 1998; **56:** 345–53.
3. Vivino FB, *et al.* Pilocarpine tablets for the treatment of dry mouth and dry eye symptoms in patients with Sjögren syndrome: a randomized, placebo-controlled, fixed-dose, multicenter trial. *Arch Intern Med* 1999; **159:** 174–81.
4. Frost-Larsen K, *et al.* Sjögren's syndrome treated with bromhexine: a randomised clinical study. *BMJ* 1978; **i:** 1579–81.
5. Tapper-Jones LM, *et al.* Sjögren's syndrome treated with bromhexine: a reassessment. *BMJ* 1980; **280:** 1356.
6. Prause JU, *et al.* Lacrimal and salivary secretion in Sjögren's syndrome: the effect of systemic treatment with bromhexine. *Acta Ophthalmol (Copenh)* 1984; **62:** 489–97.
7. Rogers SJ, *et al.* Myelopathy in Sjögren's syndrome: role of nonsteroidal immunosuppressants. *Drugs* 2004; **64:** 123–32.


## Dry mouth

Dryness of the mouth (xerostomia) resulting from decreased salivary secretion is often an adverse effect of therapy with drugs such as antimuscarinics, antihistamines, tricyclic antidepressants, and diuretics. Other causes include dehydration, anxiety, Sjögren's syndrome (see Dry Eye, above), and radiotherapy of the head and neck. Dry mouth can cause eating difficulties and lead to oral disease such as candidiasis, dental caries, and bacterial infections.[1] Where possible any underlying disorder should be treated first.

Frequent sips of fluids help to relieve dry mouth. Artificial saliva products are also important in the symptomatic treatment of dry mouth. They aim to mimic normal saliva and generally contain viscosity-increasing agents, such as mucins or cellulose derivatives such as carmellose,[2,3] as well as electrolytes, including fluoride; they seldom relieve symptoms for more than 1 or 2 hours. It may be possible to stimulate saliva production with sialogogues such as sugarless chewing gum or citrus products but the low pH of the latter can damage the teeth. Malic acid has also been used as a sialogogue.

A number of systemic therapies have also been tried. Pilocarpine is an effective sialogogue, increasing salivary production where some function remains,[4] and is used in dry mouth following radiotherapy; it may also be effective in Sjögren's syndrome or other causes of dry mouth. Adverse effects, particularly increased sweating, may, however, limit its use. Carbachol has been suggested as an alternative to pilocarpine with a study[5] reporting comparable efficacy but less sweating. Anethole trithione and cevimeline have been used similarly. Amifostine is used for the prevention of dry mouth associated with radiotherapy.


1. Fox PC. Management of dry mouth. *Dent Clin North Am* 1997; **41:** 863–75.
2. Vissink A, *et al.* A clinical comparison between commercially available mucin- and CMC-containing saliva substitutes. *Int J Oral Surg* 1983; **12:** 232–8.
3. Duxbury AJ, *et al.* A double-blind cross-over trial of a mucin-containing artificial saliva. *Br Dent J* 1989; **166:** 115–20.
4. Wiseman LR, Faulds D. Oral pilocarpine: a review of its pharmacological properties and clinical potential in xerostomia. *Drugs* 1995; **49:** 143–55.
5. Joensuu H. Treatment for post-irradiation xerostomia. *N Engl J Med* 1994; **330:** 141–2.


---

## Acacia

Acac.; Acaciae Gummi; E414; Goma arábiga; Gomme Arabique; Gomme de Sénégal; Gum Acacia; Gum Arabic; Gummi Africanum; Gummi Arabicum; Gummi Mimosae.

*CAS — 9000-01-5.*

**Pharmacopoeias.** In *Eur.* (see p.vi), *Int.*, *Jpn*, and *Pol.* Also in *USNF.*

**Ph. Eur. 5.0** (Acacia). The air-hardened gummy exudate from the trunk and branches of *Acacia senegal*, other species of *Acacia* of African origin, and *Acacia seyal*. Yellowish-white, yellow, or pale amber tears, sometimes with a pinkish tint. It is friable, opaque, frequently with a cracked surface, easily broken into irregular, whitish or slightly yellowish angular fragments with conchoidal fracture and a glassy and transparent appearance. Very slowly but almost completely soluble, after about 2 hours, in twice its mass of water leaving only a very small residue of vegetable particles; the liquid obtained is colourless or yellowish, dense, viscous, adhesive, translucent, and weakly acid to blue litmus paper. Practically insoluble in alcohol. Protect from light.

**Ph. Eur. 5.0** (Acacia, Spray-dried; Acaciae Gummi Dispersione Desiccatum). It is obtained from a solution of acacia. Dissolves, rapidly and completely, after about 20 minutes, in twice its mass of water. The liquid obtained is colourless or yellowish, dense, viscous, adhesive, translucent, and weakly acid to blue litmus paper. Practically insoluble in alcohol. Protect from light.

**USNF 22** (Acacia). The dried gummy exudate from the stems and branches of *Acacia senegal* (Leguminosae) or of other related African species of *Acacia*. Spheroidal tears or angular fragments of white to yellowish-white colour. It is translucent or somewhat opaque from the presence of numerous minute fissures. It is very brittle, the fractured surface is glassy and occasionally iridescent. It is also available as flakes, powder, granules, or as a spray-dried form. It is practically odourless. Insoluble in alcohol. Store in airtight containers.

**Incompatibility.** Incompatibilities of acacia have been reported with a number of substances including alcohol, aminophenazone, apomorphine, cresol, ferric salts, morphine, phenol, physostigmine, tannins, thymol, and vanillin. Acacia contains an oxidising enzyme that may affect preparations containing easily oxidised substances; the enzyme may be inactivated by heating at 100° for a short time.

### Adverse Effects

Hypersensitivity reactions have occurred rarely after inhalation or ingestion of acacia.

### Uses

Acacia is used in pharmaceutical manufacturing as a suspending and emulsifying agent, as a tablet binder, and in pastilles. It is often used with tragacanth.

It is used as an emulsifier and stabiliser in the food industry.

### Preparations

***USNF 22:*** Acacia Syrup.

---

## Agar

Agar-agar; Colle du Japon; E406; Gelosa; Gélose; Japanese Isinglass; Layor Carang.

*CAS — 9002-18-0.*

**Pharmacopoeias.** In *Chin.*, *Eur.* (see p.vi), and *Jpn.* Also in *USNF.*

**Ph. Eur. 5.0** (Agar). Polysaccharides extracted from various species of Rhodophyceae algae, mainly those belonging to the genus *Gelidium*. It is prepared by treating the algae with boiling water; the extract is filtered while hot, concentrated, and dried. Colourless to pale yellow translucent strips, flakes, or powder; tough when damp but becoming more brittle on drying.

**USNF 22** (Agar). The dried, hydrophilic, colloidal substance extracted from *Gelidium cartilagineum* (Gelidiaceae), *Gracilaria confervoides* (Sphaerococcaceae), and related red algae (Class Rhodophyceae). It usually consists of thin, membranous, agglutinated strips, but may occur in cut, flaked, or granulated forms. May be weak yellowish-orange, yellowish-grey to pale yellow, or colourless. It is tough when damp, brittle when dry. Odourless or has a slight odour. Insoluble in cold water; soluble in boiling water.

### Uses and Administration

Agar is used as a suspending or thickening agent in pharmaceutical manufacturing and as an emulsifying and stabilising agent in the food industry.

It was formerly used similarly to methylcellulose (p.1580) as a bulk laxative. Preparations containing agar with liquid paraffin and phenolphthalein are available to treat constipation, but the relatively small amount of agar in these probably acts solely as an emulsion stabiliser.

### Preparations

**Proprietary Preparations** (details are given in Part 3)

**Multi-ingredient:** ***Arg.:*** Agarol; Usar Fibras; ***Austral.:*** Lexat†; ***Braz.:*** Agarol; Fenogar†; Laxantil†; Manon†; ***Canad.:*** Agarol†; ***Fr.:*** Gelogastrine†; Pseudophage; ***India:*** Agarol; ***Irl.:*** Agarol†; ***Port.:*** Byl; ***S.Afr.:*** Agarol†; ***Switz.:*** Agarol†; Demosvelte N†; Paragar; ***UK:*** Agarol†; ***USA:*** Agoral.

---

## Alginic Acid

Ácido algínico; Acidum Alginicum; E400; Polymannuronic Acid.

*CAS — 9005-32-7.*
*ATC — A02BX13.*

**Pharmacopoeias.** In *Eur.* (see p.vi) and *Int.* Also in *USNF.*

**Ph. Eur. 5.0** (Alginic Acid). A mixture of polyuronic acids composed of residues of D-mannuronic and L-guluronic acids extracted from algae belonging to the Phaeophyceae. A white or pale yellowish-brown, crystalline or amorphous powder. It swells in water. Very slightly soluble or practically insoluble in alcohol; practically insoluble in organic solvents; dissolves in solutions of alkali hydroxides.

**USNF 22** (Alginic Acid). A hydrophilic colloidal carbohydrate extracted with dilute alkali from various species of brown seaweeds (Phaeophyceae). A white to yellowish-white, odourless or practically odourless, fibrous powder. Insoluble in water and in organic solvents; soluble in alkaline solutions. pH of a 3% dispersion in water is between 1.5 and 3.5.

## Propylene Glycol Alginate

Alginato de propilenglicol; E405. Propane-1,2-diol Alginate.

*ATC — A02BX13.*

**Pharmacopoeias.** In *USNF.*

**USNF 22** (Propylene Glycol Alginate). A white to yellowish, practically odourless, fibrous or granular powder. Soluble in water, in solutions of dilute organic acids, and, depending on the degree of esterification, in hydroalcoholic mixtures containing up to 60% by weight of alcohol, to form stable, viscous colloidal solutions at a pH of 3.

## Sodium Alginate

Algin; Alginato sódico; E401; Natrii Alginas; Sodium Polymannuronate.

*CAS — 9005-38-3.*

*ATC — A02BX13.*

**Pharmacopoeias.** In *Eur.* (see p.vi). Also in *USNF.*

**Ph. Eur. 5.0** (Sodium Alginate). It consists chiefly of the sodium salt of alginic acid. A white or pale yellowish-brown powder. Slowly soluble in water, forming a viscous, colloidal solution; practically insoluble in alcohol.

**USNF 22** (Sodium Alginate). A yellowish-white, practically odourless, coarse or fine powder. Soluble in water, forming a viscous, colloidal solution; insoluble in alcohol, in chloroform, and in ether, in hydroalcoholic solutions in which the alcohol content is greater than 30% by weight, and in acids when the pH of the resulting solution becomes lower than about 3. Store in airtight containers.

**Incompatibility.** Incompatibilities of sodium alginate have been observed with acridine derivatives, methylrosanilinium chloride, phenylmercuric acetate and nitrate, calcium salts, alcohol in concentrations greater than 5%, and heavy metals. High concentrations of electrolytes cause an increase in viscosity until salting-out of sodium alginate occurs; salting-out occurs if more than 4% of sodium chloride is present.

### Uses and Administration

Alginic acid and alginates such as propylene glycol alginate and sodium alginate are used in pharmaceutical manufacturing as suspending and thickening agents. They may be used as stabilisers for oil-in-water emulsions and as binding and disintegrating agents in tablets. Various grades are usually available commercially for different applications and yield solutions of varying viscosity. A reduction in viscosity has been said to occur following sterilisation by autoclaving of sodium alginate solutions.

Alginic acid and alginates (ammonium alginate, calcium alginate (p.745), potassium alginate, propylene glycol alginate, and sodium alginate) are also used as emulsifiers and stabilisers in the food industry.

Alginic acid or the alginates, magnesium alginate and sodium alginate, are used with an antacid or a histamine $H_2$-antagonist such as cimetidine in the management of gastro-oesophageal reflux disease (p.1242). Alginic acid or the alginate reacts with gastric acid to form a viscous gel (often termed a raft) that floats on top of the gastric contents. This raft then acts as a mechanical barrier to reduce reflux.

Alginic acid is also used, usually in the form of a mixed calcium-sodium salt, as a haemostatic and wound dressing; it is employed in the form of a fibre made into a dressing or packing material.

### Preparations

**Proprietary Preparations** (details are given in Part 3)
***Austral.:*** Kaltostat; ***Fr.:*** Nu-Gel; ***Ger.:*** Gaviscon; Gaviscon Advance; ***Irl.:*** Kaltostat; ***Israel:*** Nu-Gel; ***Ital.:*** Kaltostat; Nu-Gel; ***NZ:*** Gaviscon; ***S.Afr.:*** Gaviscon; Kaltostat; ***UK:*** Comfeel Seasorb; Heartburn & Indigestion Liquid†.

**Multi-ingredient:** ***Arg.:*** Comfeel Seasorb; Gaviscon; Glicalox; Mylanta Reflux; Redudiet; ***Austral.:*** Algicon†; Gaviscon; Gaviscon Double Strength; Infant Gaviscon; Meracote; Mylanta Heartburn Relief; ***Austria:*** Rennie Duo; ***Belg.:*** Gaviscon; Gaviscon Advance; ***Braz.:*** Algicote†; ***Canad.:*** Gastrifom; Gastrocote†; Gaviscon Heartburn Relief; Heartburn Relief; Maalox HRF; Rafton; ***Chile:*** Algicote; Gaviscon; ***Denm.:*** Gaviscon; ***Fin.:*** Gaviscon; Refluxin†; ***Fr.:*** Comfeel Seasorb; Gaviscon; Hyalogran; Pseudophage; Rennie Refluxine†; Topaal; ***Ger.:*** Nu-Gel; Recatol Algin; ***Hong Kong:*** Gaviscon; ***India:*** Acigon; Gaviscon; Raftace; ***Irl.:*** Acidex; Algitec†; Gaviscon; Gaviscon Advance; Gaviscon Infant; Pyrogastrone; Rennie Duo; ***Israel:*** Gaviscon†; Kaltocarb; Kaltostat; ***Ital.:*** Digerall; Gaviscon; Gaviscon Advance; ***Malaysia:*** Gaviscon; ***Mex.:*** Algicon; ***Neth.:*** Aciflux; Algicon; Gaviscon; ***Norw.:*** Algicon†; Gaviscon; ***NZ:*** Gaviscon; Mylanta Heartburn Relief; ***Port.:*** Carboflex; Gaviscon†; Kaltostat; ***S.Afr.:*** Gaviscon; Gelacid; Infant Gaviscon; ***Singapore:*** Gaviscon; ***Spain:*** Dolcopin; Gaviscon†; ***Swed.:*** Gaviscon; ***Switz.:*** Demosvelte N†; Gaviscon; Refluxine; ***UK:*** Acidex; Algicon; Asilone Heartburn; Bisodol Heartburn Relief; Gastrocote; Gaviscon; Gaviscon Advance; Gaviscon Infant; Peptac; Pyrogastrone; Raft-Eze; Rennie Duo; Setlers Heartburn & Indigestion Liquid; Topal; ***USA:*** Foamicon; Gaviscon; Genaton; Pretts Diet Aid.

---

## Aluminium Magnesium Silicate

Aluminii Magnesii Silicas; Aluminosilicato magnésico; Magnesium Aluminium Silicate; Magnesium Aluminum Silicate; Saponite.

*CAS — 1327-43-1; 12511-31-8.*

**Pharmacopoeias.** In *Eur.* (see p.vi) and *Int.* Also in *USNF. USNF* also includes Magnesium Aluminosilicate and Magnesium Aluminometasilicate.

**Ph. Eur. 5.0** (Aluminium Magnesium Silicate). A mixture of colloidal-size particles of montmorillonite and saponite, free from grit and nonswellable ore. Almost white powder, granules, or plates. Practically insoluble in water and in organic solvents; swells in water to form a colloidal dispersion. A 5% dispersion in water has a pH of 9.0 to 10.0.

**USNF 22** (Magnesium Aluminum Silicate). A blend of colloidal montmorillonite and saponite that has been processed to remove grit and nonswellable ore components. There are several types, differing in viscosity and in ratio of aluminium content to magnesium content. It is an odourless, fine (micronised) powder, small cream to tan granules, or small flakes that are creamy when viewed on their flat surfaces and tan to brown when viewed on their edges. Insoluble in water and in alcohol; swells when added to water or glycerol. pH of a 5% suspension in water is between 9.0 and 10.0. Store in airtight containers.

**USNF 22** (Magnesium Aluminosilicate). A synthetic material that contains 20.5 to 27.7% of magnesium oxide, 27.0 to 34.3% of aluminium oxide, and 14.4 to 21.7% of silicon dioxide, calculated on the dried basis. A white powder or granules having an amorphous structure. Practically insoluble in water and in alcohol; partially soluble in acids and alkalis. A 4% suspension in water has a pH of 8.5 to 10.5. Store at a temperature not exceeding 40° in airtight containers.

**USNF 22** (Magnesium Aluminometasilicate). A synthetic material that contains 29.1 to 35.5% of aluminium oxide, 11.4 to 14.0% of magnesium oxide, and 29.2 to 35.6% of silicon dioxide, calculated on the dried basis. It exists in two forms, Type I-A and Type I-B. A white powder or granules having an amorphous structure. Practically insoluble in water and in alcohol; partially soluble in acids and alkalis. A 4% suspension in water has a pH of 6.5 to 8.5 (Type I-A) and 8.5 to 10.5 (Type I-B). Store at a temperature not exceeding 40° in airtight containers.

### Uses

Aluminium magnesium silicate has a variety of pharmaceutical uses, including use as a suspending and thickening agent, as an emulsion stabiliser, and as a binder and disintegrating agent in tablets.

Other forms of aluminium magnesium silicate include an artificial hydrate known as almasilate (p.1248), which is used as an antacid, and attapulgite (p.1251), a purified native hydrated aluminium magnesium silicate that is highly adsorbent and is used in a wide range of products including fertilisers and pesticides. Activated attapulgite, which is attapulgite that has been carefully heated to increase its adsorptive capacity, is used in preparations for diarrhoea.

### Preparations

**Proprietary Preparations** (details are given in Part 3)
**Multi-ingredient:** ***Denm.:*** Alkasid; ***Ger.:*** Mucal†; ***Hong Kong:*** Gl†; ***Switz.:*** TRI-OM†; ***Thai.:*** Almaxane†; Diasgest; ***UAE:*** Alkasid.

---

## Bentonite

Bentonita; Bentonitum; E558; Mineral Soap; Soap Clay; Wilkinite.

*CAS — 1302-78-9.*

**Pharmacopoeias.** In *Eur.* (see p.vi), *Int., Jpn,* and *Pol.* Also in *USNF,* which also includes a purified form.

**Ph. Eur. 5.0** (Bentonite). A natural clay containing a high proportion of montmorillonite, a native hydrated aluminium silicate in which some aluminium and silicon atoms may be replaced by other atoms such as magnesium and iron. A very fine, homogeneous, greyish-white powder with a more or less yellowish or pinkish tint. Practically insoluble in water and in aqueous solutions, but swells with a little water forming a malleable mass.

**USNF 22** (Bentonite). A native, colloidal, hydrated aluminium silicate. A very fine, odourless, hygroscopic, pale buff or cream-coloured to greyish powder, free from grit. Insoluble in water, but swells to approximately 12 times its volume when added to water; insoluble in, and does not swell in, organic solvents. pH of a 2% suspension in water, mixed vigorously to facilitate wetting, is between 9.5 and 10.5. Store in airtight containers.

**USNF 22** (Purified Bentonite). A colloidal montmorillonite that has been processed to remove grit and nonswellable ore components. An odourless, fine, micronised powder, or small flakes that are creamy when viewed on their flat surfaces and tan to brown when viewed on their edges. Insoluble in water and in alcohol. Swells when added to water or glycerol. pH of a 5% suspension in water is between 9.0 and 10.0. Store in airtight containers.

### Uses

Bentonite absorbs water readily to form sols or gels, depending on its concentration. It is used in pharmaceutical manufacturing as a suspending and stabilising agent and as an adsorbent or clarifying agent. It is also used as an anticaking agent in the food industry.

Bentonite may be used as an oral adsorbent in paraquat poisoning (p.1508).

### Preparations

***USNF 22:*** Bentonite Magma.

**Proprietary Preparations** (details are given in Part 3)
***Gr.:*** Bentonine.

---

## Carbomers

Acrylic Acid Polymers; Carbomera; Carbómeros; Carbopols; Carboxypolymethylene; Carboxyvinyl Polymers; Polyacrylic Acid.

*CAS — 9003-01-4; 54182-57-9.*

NOTE. Carbomer is *BAN, USAN,* and *rINN.*

**Pharmacopoeias.** In *Chin., Eur.* (see p.vi), and *Int. USNF* has separate monographs for a range of carbomers.

*USNF* also includes Carbomer Copolymer and Carbomer Interpolymer.

**Ph. Eur. 5.0** (Carbomers). High-molecular-weight polymers of acrylic acid cross-linked with polyalkenyl ethers of sugars or polyalcohols. They are produced in several grades characterised by the viscosity of a defined solution. White, fluffy, hygroscopic powders. They swell in water and in other polar solvents after dispersion and neutralisation with sodium hydroxide solution. Store in airtight containers.

**USNF 22** (Carbomer 934; Carbomer 934P; Carbomer 940; Carbomer 941; Carbomer 1342). Carbomers are high-molecular-weight polymers of acrylic acid cross-linked with allyl ethers of pentaerythritol. The viscosity of a neutralised aqueous dispersion for each carbomer is:

- Carbomer 934 (0.5%), 30 500 to 39 400 cP
- Carbomer 934P (0.5%), 29 400 to 39 400 cP
- Carbomer 940 (0.5%), 40 000 to 60 000 cP
- Carbomer 941 (0.5%), 4000 to 11 000 cP
- Carbomer 1342 (1.0%), 9500 to 26 500 cP

They are white, fluffy, hygroscopic powders having a slight characteristic odour. pH of a 1% dispersion in water is about 3. When neutralised with alkali hydroxides or with amines, they dissolve in water, in alcohol, and in glycerol. Store in airtight containers.

**USNF 22** (Carbomer Copolymer). A high-molecular-weight copolymer of acrylic acid and a long chain alkyl methacrylate cross-linked with polyalkenyl ethers of polyalcohols. Different types of Carbomer Copolymer are characterised by the viscosity of a defined solution. Store in airtight containers at a temperature not exceeding 45°.

**USNF 22** (Carbomer Interpolymer). A carbomer homopolymer or copolymer that contains a block copolymer of macrogol and a long chain alkyl acid ester. Different types of Carbomer Interpolymer are characterised by the viscosity of a defined solution. Store in airtight containers at a temperature not exceeding 45°.

### Uses and Administration

Carbomers are used in pharmaceutical manufacturing as suspending agents, gel bases, emulsifiers, and binding agents in tablets.

Carbomers, in liquid gel formulations containing typically 0.2 or 0.3%, are used topically as tear substitutes in the management of dry eye (p.1576).

### Preparations

***BP 2003:*** Carbomer Eye Drops.

**Proprietary Preparations** (details are given in Part 3)
***Arg.:*** Acrylarm; Lacryvisc; Liposic; Refresh Gel; Siccafluid; Teargel; Viscotears; ***Austral.:*** GelTears†; Poly Gel; Viscotears; ***Austria:*** AquaTears; Tears Naturale; Vidisic; ***Belg.:*** Alcon Eye Gel; Ocugel; Thilo Tears†; Vidisic; ***Braz.:*** Vidisic; Viscotears; ***Canad.:*** Lacrinorm; Tear-Gel; ***Chile:*** Lacryvisc; Nicotears; Viscotears; ***Denm.:*** Oftagel; Viscotears; ***Fin.:*** Oftagel; Viscotears; ***Fr.:*** Aqualarm; Civigel; Gel-Larmes; Lacrinorm; Lacryvisc; Liposic; Siccafluid; ***Ger.:*** Liposic; Liquigel; Siccapos; Thilo-Tears; Vidisic; Visc-Ophtal; ***Gr.:*** Dacrio Gel; Thilogel; Viscoter; ***Hong Kong:*** Lacryvisc; Viscotears; ***Irl.:*** GelTears; Vidisic; ***Israel:*** Viscotears; ***Ital.:*** Dacriogel; Dropgel; Lacrigel; Lacrinorm; Siccafluid; Viscotirs; ***Malaysia:*** Vidisic; ***Mex.:*** Lubrigel†; Viscotears; ***Mon.:*** Lacrifluid; Lacrigel; ***Neth.:*** Vidisic; ***Norw.:*** Viscotears; ***NZ:*** Viscotears; ***Port.:*** Lacryvisc; Vidisic; ***S.Afr.:*** Teargel; ***Singapore:*** Lacryvisc; Vidisic; ***Spain:*** Lacryvisc; Revic†; Siccafluid; Viscotears; ***Swed.:*** Lacryvisc†; Oftagel; Viscotears; ***Switz.:*** Lacrinorm; Lacryvisc; Thilo-Tears†; Viscotears; ***Thai.:*** Lacryvisc; Vidisic; ***UK:*** GelTears; Liposic; Liquivisc; Viscotears.

**Multi-ingredient:** ***Austral.:*** Genteal Moisturising; ***Chile:*** Gelsolets; ***Hong Kong:*** Hypotears; ***Irl.:*** Liposic; ***Ital.:*** Dropyal; ***Port.:*** Hidratante VG; ***Switz.:*** Lacrycon; ***USA:*** Maxilube.

---

## Carmellose *(rINN)*

Carboxymethylcellulose; Carmelosa; CMC; E466.

**Pharmacopoeias.** In *Jpn.*

## Carmellose Calcium *(rINNM)*

Calcium Carboxymethylcellulose; Carboxymethylcellulose Calcium; Carmellosum Calcicum; Carmelosa cálcica.

*CAS — 9050-04-8.*

**Pharmacopoeias.** In *Eur.* (see p.vi) and *Jpn.* Also in *USNF.*

**Ph. Eur. 5.0** (Carmellose Calcium). A white or yellowish-white, hygroscopic powder. It swells in water to form a suspension; practically insoluble in alcohol, in acetone, and in toluene. Store in airtight containers.

**USNF 22** (Carboxymethylcellulose Calcium). A white to yellowish-white, hygroscopic powder. It swells in water to form a suspension; practically insoluble in alcohol, in acetone, in chloroform, in ether, and in benzene. pH of a 1% suspension in water is between 4.5 and 6.0. Store in airtight containers.

## Carmellose Sodium *(BAN, rINNM)*

Carboxymethylcellulose Sodium; Carboxymethylcellulosum Natricum; Carmellosum Natricum; Carmelosa sódica; Cellulose Gum; E466; SCMC; Sodium Carboxymethylcellulose; Sodium Cellulose Glycollate.

*CAS — 9004-32-4.*

**Pharmacopoeias.** In *Eur.* (see p.vi), *Int., Jpn, Pol.,* and *US. Eur.* and *USNF* also include low-substituted carmellose sodium. *USNF* also includes Carboxymethylcellulose Sodium 12.

**Ph. Eur. 5.0** (Carmellose Sodium). A white or almost white, hygroscopic granular powder. It has a sodium content of 6.5 to 10.8% calculated on the dry substance. Easily dispersed in water forming colloidal solutions; practically insoluble in dehydrated alcohol, in acetone, in ether, and in toluene. A 1% colloidal solution in water has a pH of 6.0 to 8.0.

**Ph. Eur. 5.0** (Carmellose Sodium, Low-substituted; Carmellosum Natricum, Substitutum Humile). It contains not less than 2.0% and not more than 4.5% of sodium, calculated with reference to the dried substance. A white or almost white powder or short fibres. It swells in water to form a gel; practically insoluble in dehydrated alcohol, in acetone, and in toluene. A 1% suspension in water has a pH of 6.0 to 8.5.

**USP 27** (Carboxymethylcellulose Sodium). A white to cream-coloured, hygroscopic powder or granules. It contains not less than 6.5% and not more than 9.5% of sodium, calculated on the dried basis. Easily dispersed in water to form colloidal solutions; insoluble in alcohol, in ether, and in most other organic solvents. pH of a 1% solution in water is between 6.5 and 8.5. Store in airtight containers.

**USNF 22** (Low-Substituted Carboxymethylcellulose Sodium). It has a sodium content of 2.0 to 4.5%, calculated on the dried basis. A white or almost white powder or short fibres. Practically insoluble in alcohol, in acetone, and in toluene. It swells in water to form a gel. pH of a 1% suspension in water is between 6.0 and 8.5.

**USNF 22** (Carboxymethylcellulose Sodium 12). It has a sodium content of 10.4 to 12.0%, calculated on the dry substance. Store in airtight containers.

**Incompatibility.** Incompatibilities of carmellose sodium have been reported with strongly acidic solutions, with soluble salts of iron and some other metals, and with xanthan gum.

## Croscarmellose Sodium *(USAN)*

Carmellosum Natricum Conexum; Croscarmelosa sódica; Crosslinked Carboxymethylcellulose Sodium; E468; Modified Cellulose Gum.

**Pharmacopoeias.** In *Eur.* (see p.vi). Also in *USNF.*

**Ph. Eur. 5.0** (Croscarmellose Sodium). A cross-linked polymer of carmellose sodium. A white or greyish-white powder. Practically insoluble in dehydrated alcohol, in acetone, and in toluene. A 1% suspension in water has a pH of 5.0 to 7.0.

**USNF 22** (Croscarmellose Sodium). A cross-linked polymer of carmellose sodium. A white, free-flowing powder. Partially soluble in water; insoluble in alcohol, in ether, and in other organic solvents. pH of a dispersion containing 1 g mixed with 99 mL of water for 1 hour is between 5.0 and 7.0. Store in airtight containers.

### Uses and Administration

Carmellose calcium and carmellose sodium have a variety of pharmaceutical uses, including use as suspending, thickening, and emulsifying agents, and as disintegrants, binders, and coating agents in tablets. Carmellose sodium is also used as an emulsifier or stabiliser in the food industry. Croscarmellose sodium is used as a tablet disintegrant.

Carmellose sodium is used topically as an ingredient of protective preparations for stoma care, in the management of wounds, and for the mechanical protection of oral and perioral lesions, such as mouth ulceration (p.1245). It is also used, in concentrations of up to 1%, in artificial saliva preparations for the treatment of dry mouth (p.1576), and in eye drops for the management of dry eye (p.1576).

Carmellose sodium given orally absorbs water and acts as a bulk-forming agent; the volume of faeces is increased and peristalsis promoted. It is used in the treatment of constipation (p.1240). Carmellose sodium has been included in preparations to control appetite in the management of obesity (p.1583) but there is little evidence of efficacy. For precautions to be observed with bulk-forming agents, see under Methylcellulose, p.1580.

### Preparations

***USP 27:*** Carboxymethylcellulose Sodium Paste; Carboxymethylcellulose Sodium Tablets.

**Proprietary Preparations** (details are given in Part 3)

***Arg.:*** Aquacel; Cellufresh; Celluvisc; Comfeel; Natura Fresh; Refresh Tears; ***Austral.:*** Aquacel; Cellufresh; Celluvisc; Refresh Liquigel; Refresh Tears Plus; ***Braz.:*** Cellufresh; Fresh Tears; Salivan†; ***Canad.:*** Cellufresh†; Celluvisc; Refresh Plus; Refresh Tears; ***Chile:*** Refresh Tears; ***Denm.:*** Celluvisc; ***Fin.:*** Celluvisc; ***Fr.:*** Aquacel; Askina Biofilm; Celluvisc; Comfeel; Hydrocoll; Physiotulle; Sureskin; Tegasorb†; Urgomed; Urgotul; ***Ger.:*** Algoplaque; Celluvisc; Urgotul; ***Gr.:*** Celluvisc; ***Hong Kong:*** Celluvisc†; Refresh Plus; Refresh Tears; ***Ital.:*** Cellufresh; Celluvisc; ***Mex.:*** Celluvisc; Refresh Tears; Thera Tears; ***NZ:*** Cellufresh; Celluvisc; Refresh Tears Plus; ***Port.:*** Aquacel; Celluvisc; ***S.Afr.:*** Cellufresh; Celluvisc; ***Singapore:*** Cellufresh†; Celluvisc; Refresh Plus; ***Spain:*** Cellufresh; Celluvisc; Optrelam†; Viscofresh; ***Swed.:*** Celluvisc; ***Switz.:*** Celluvisc; Comfeel†; ***Thai.:*** Cellufresh; Celluvisc; ***UK:*** Celluvisc; Comfeel; Intrasite; Physiotulle; Revive†; ***USA:*** Celluvisc; Refresh Plus; Refresh Tears; Tears Again.

**Multi-ingredient:** ***Arg.:*** Comfeel Purilon; Comfeel Seasorb; Humectante Bucal; Razagleda Plus; ***Austral.:*** Aquae; Orabase; Orahesive; Solo-Site; Stomahesive; ***Austria:*** Glandosane; Sialin; ***Braz.:*** Chofranina; ***Canad.:*** Appedrine; Dexatrim†; Moi-Stir; Orabase; Orahesive; Salivart; ***Chile:*** K.C.M.C; Novafix Extra Fuerte; Salivart; ***Fr.:*** Amivia; Artisial; Askina Sorb; Comfeel Seasorb; Intrasite; Melgisorb; Purilon; Urgosorb; ***Ger.:*** Artisial†; Glandosane; Lary-Phary; Nu-Gel; Recatol Algin; ***Hong Kong:*** Aquae; Salivart; ***India:*** Digene; ***Irl.:*** Luborant†; Orabase; ***Israel:*** Glandosane; Orabase; ***Ital.:*** Idrum†; ***NZ:*** Orabase; Stomahesive; ***Port.:*** Carboflex; Combiderm†; Glandosane; Varihesive; ***S.Afr.:*** Granuflex; Granugel; ***Spain:*** Laxvital; ***Switz.:*** Glandosane; Varihesive Hydroactive†; ***Thai.:*** Bisolax; Emulax; Glandosane; ***UK:*** Comfeel Plus; Glandosane; Luborant; Orabase; Orahesive; Salivace†; Seasorb Soft; Seprafilm; Stomahesive; ***USA:*** Dieutrim†; Entertainer's Secret; Glandosane†; Moi-Stir; Pretts Diet Aid; Salivart; Seprafilm; Surgel; Tears Night & Day†.

## Carrageenan

Carrageenin; Carragenina; Carraghénates; Chondrus Extract; E407; Irish Moss Extract.

*CAS — 9000-07-1 (carrageenan); 11114-20-8 (κ-carrageenan); 9064-57-7 (λ-carrageenan).*

**Pharmacopoeias.** In *Fr.* Also in *USNF.*

**USNF 22** (Carrageenan). The hydrocolloid obtained by extraction with water or aqueous alkali from some members of the class Rhodophyceae (red seaweeds). It consists chiefly of a mixture of the ammonium, calcium, magnesium, potassium, and sodium sulfate esters of galactose and 3,6-anhydrogalactose copolymers. The prevalent copolymers in the hydrocolloids are κ-carrageenan, ι-carrageenan, and λ-carrageenan.

A yellowish or tan to white, coarse to fine, practically odourless, powder. Soluble in water at 80° forming a viscous, clear or slightly opalescent solution that flows readily. It disperses more readily in water if first moistened with alcohol, with glycerol, or with a saturated solution of glucose in water. Store in airtight containers at a temperature of 8° to 15°.

### Uses and Administration

Carrageenan is used in pharmaceutical manufacturing and the food industry as a suspending and gelling agent.

It has been used as a bulk-forming laxative to treat constipation; for precautions to be observed with bulk-forming laxatives, see under Methylcellulose, p.1580. Carrageenan is also included in topical preparations for the symptomatic relief of anorectal disorders. A gel containing carrageenan is under investigation as a topical microbicide.

A degraded form of carrageenan was formerly used in gastrointestinal disorders but it was associated with lesions in *animals* and is no longer used.

Irish moss (*Chondrus crispus*), a source of carrageenan, is used in herbal medicine.

◊ Refined non-degraded carrageenan and furcellaran, a similar extract from Rhodophyceae that is included in the specifications for food-grade carrageenan, have generally been considered safe for use as food additives, although this may not be the case with degraded and 'semi-refined' forms.[1] However, in the UK the Food Advisory Committee has recommended that carrageenan should not be permitted as an additive for infant formulas because of the possibility of immunological consequences following absorption from the immature gut.[2] Carrageenans affect the immune system of experimental *animals* after parenteral or oral use, and small amounts of food-grade carrageenan cross the intestinal epithelium in *rats* and are taken up by gut-associated lymphoid tissue.[3]

1. FAO/WHO. Evaluation of certain food additives and contaminants: twenty-eighth report of the joint FAO/WHO expert committee on food additives. *WHO Tech Rep Ser 710* 1984.
2. MAFF. Food Advisory Committee: report on the review of the use of additives in foods specially prepared for infants and young children. FdAC/REP/12. London: HMSO, 1992.
3. MAFF. Food Advisory Committee: report on the review of the emulsifiers and stabilisers in food regulations. FdAC/REP/11. London: HMSO, 1992.

### Preparations

**Proprietary Preparations** (details are given in Part 3)

***Austria:*** Coreine.

**Multi-ingredient:** ***Austral.:*** Bonningtons Irish Moss†; ***Austria:*** Anoreine; Anoreine mit Lidocain; ***Belg.:*** Tisane Pectorale†; ***Fr.:*** Anoreine; Titanoreine; Titanoreine Lidocaine; ***Ital.:*** Resource Gelificata; ***NZ:*** Bonningtons Irish Moss; ***Spain:*** Laxante Bescansa†; Titanorein†; ***Switz.:*** Flogecyl; Titanoreine; ***UK:*** Biobalm†; Fam-Lax Senna; Liminate†.

## Cellacefate *(BAN, rINN)*

CAP; Celacefato; Cellacephate; Cellulose Acetate Phthalate; Cellulosi Acetas Phthalas; Cellulosum Acetylphthalicum; Celophthalum.

*CAS — 9004-38-0.*

**Pharmacopoeias.** In *Chin., Eur.* (see p.vi), *Int., Jpn,* and *Pol.* Also in *USNF.*

**Ph. Eur. 5.0** (Cellulose Acetate Phthalate; Cellacefate BP 2003). Cellulose in which some of the hydroxyl groups are acetylated (21.5 to 26.0%) and some are phthalylated (30.0 to 36.0%), both calculated with reference to the anhydrous, acid-free substance. A hygroscopic, white, free-flowing powder or colourless flakes. Practically insoluble in water, in dehydrated alcohol, and in dichloromethane; freely soluble in acetone; soluble in diethylene glycol; it dissolves in dilute solutions of alkalis. Store in airtight containers.

**USNF 22** (Cellacefate). A reaction product of phthalic anhydride and a partial acetate ester of cellulose. It contains 21.5 to 26.0% of acetyl groups, and 30.0 to 36.0% of phthalyl(*o*-carboxy-benzoyl) groups, calculated on the anhydrous, acid-free basis. A white, free-flowing powder that may have a slight odour of acetic acid. Insoluble in water and in alcohol; soluble in acetone and in dioxan. Store in airtight containers.

### Uses

Cellacefate is unaffected by immersion in acid media in the stomach but softens and swells in intestinal fluid. It is used in pharmaceutical manufacturing as an enteric-coating material for tablets and capsules, usually with a plasticiser. Films of cellacefate are reported to be permeable to some ionic substances such as ammonium chloride and potassium iodide, and such substances require a sealing coat.

## Cellulose

Celulosa.

**Description.** Cellulose is an unbranched polysaccharide polymer consisting of 1,4-β-linked glucopyranose units. It is the chief constituent of fibrous plant material.

## Dispersible Cellulose *(BAN)*

Celulosa dispersable; Microcrystalline Cellulose and Carboxymethylcellulose Sodium.

**Pharmacopoeias.** In *Br.* Also in *USNF.*

**BP 2003** (Dispersible Cellulose). An odourless or almost odourless, white or off-white, coarse or fine powder consisting of a colloid-forming attrited mixture of microcrystalline cellulose and carmellose sodium. Disperses in water to produce a white, opaque dispersion or gel; practically insoluble in organic solvents and in dilute acids. Store at a temperature between 8° and 15°.

**USNF 22**( Microcrystalline Cellulose and Carboxymethylcellulose Sodium). A colloid-forming, attrited mixture of microcrystalline cellulose and carmellose sodium. A white to off-white, odourless, coarse to fine, powder. It swells in water, producing, when dispersed, a white, opaque dispersion or gel; insoluble in organic solvents and in dilute acids. Store in airtight containers in a dry place, and at a temperature not exceeding 40°.

## Microcrystalline Cellulose

Cellulosa Microgranulare; Cellulose Gel; Cellulosum Microcrystallinum; Celulosa microcristalina; Crystalline Cellulose; E460.

*CAS — 9004-34-6.*

**Pharmacopoeias.** In *Chin., Eur.* (see p.vi), *Int., Jpn,* and *Pol.* Also in *USNF.*

**Ph. Eur. 5.0** (Cellulose, Microcrystalline). A purified, partly depolymerised cellulose, prepared by treating alpha-cellulose, obtained as a pulp from fibrous plant materials, with mineral acids. It is a white or almost white, fine or granular powder. Practically insoluble in water, in dehydrated alcohol, in acetone, in toluene, in dilute acids, and in sodium hydroxide solution (1 in 20). The pH of the supernatant liquid obtained from a 12.5% mixture in water after 20 minutes of shaking is 5.0 to 7.5.

**USNF 22** (Microcrystalline Cellulose). A purified, partially depolymerised cellulose, prepared by treating alpha-cellulose, obtained as a pulp from fibrous plant material, with mineral acids. It is a fine, white or almost white powder consisting of free-flowing, nonfibrous particles. Insoluble in water, in dilute acids, and in most organic solvents; practically insoluble in sodium hydroxide solution (1 in 20). The pH of the supernatant liquid obtained from a 12.5% mixture in water after 20 minutes of shaking is between 5.0 and 7.0. Store in airtight containers.

## Powdered Cellulose

Cellulose Powder; Cellulosi Pulvis; Celulosa en polvo; E460.

**Pharmacopoeias.** In *Eur.* (see p.vi) and *Jpn.* Also in *USNF.*

**Ph. Eur. 5.0** (Cellulose, Powdered). A purified mechanically disintegrated cellulose prepared from alpha-cellulose obtained as a pulp from fibrous plant materials. It is a white or almost white, fine or granular powder. Practically insoluble in water, in dehydrated alcohol, in acetone, in toluene, in most organic solvents, and in dilute acids; slightly soluble in sodium hydroxide solution (1 in 20). The pH of the supernatant liquid of a 11.1% mixture in water is between 5.0 and 7.5 one hour after preparation.

**USNF 22** (Powdered Cellulose). A purified, mechanically disintegrated cellulose prepared by processing alpha-cellulose obtained as a pulp from fibrous plant materials. It is a white or almost white powder. Exhibits degrees of fineness ranging from a free-flowing, dense powder to a coarse, fluffy, nonflowing material. Insoluble in water, in nearly all organic solvents, and in dilute acids; slightly soluble in sodium hydroxide solution (1 in 20). The pH of the supernatant liquid of a 11.1% mixture in water is between 5.0 and 7.5 one hour after preparation. Store in airtight containers.

### Uses and Administration

Powdered cellulose and microcrystalline cellulose are used in pharmaceutical manufacturing as tablet binders and disintegrants and as capsule and tablet diluents. These two forms of cellulose are also used in the food industry. Dispersible cellulose (which also contains some carmellose sodium) forms a thixotropic gel with water and is used pharmaceutically as a suspending and thickening agent.

Various forms of cellulose have been included in preparations used in the management of constipation and obesity. Cellulose is also used in adsorbent powder preparations used for skin disorders including hyperhidrosis.

## Preparations

**Proprietary Preparations** (details are given in Part 3)
***Ital.:*** Fibrasan; ***UK:*** Nasaleze; Sterigel; ***USA:*** Unifiber.

**Multi-ingredient:** ***Arg.:*** Usar Fibras; ZeaSorb; ***Austral.:*** ZeaSorb; ***Canad.:*** ZeaSorb; ***Chile:*** ZeaSorb; ***Fr.:*** Gelopectose; Hydroclean; ZeaSorb; ***Ger.:*** ZeaSorb†; ***Irl.:*** ZeaSorb; ***Israel:*** Celluspan; ***Port.:*** Fermetone Composto; ***Thai.:*** ZeaSorb; ***UK:*** ZeaSorb.

# Ceratonia

Carob Bean Gum; Carob Gum; Cerat.; Ceratonia Gum; E410; Goma de garrofín; Gomme de Caroube; Locust Bean Gum.
*CAS — 9000-40-2.*
*ATC — A07XA02.*

## Uses

Ceratonia consists of the endosperms separated from the seeds of the locust bean tree, *Ceratonia siliqua* (Leguminosae). It is used as a thickening agent and stabiliser in the food industry.

## Preparations

**Proprietary Preparations** (details are given in Part 3)
***Austria:*** Arobon; ***Irl.:*** Carobel; ***Ital.:*** Arobon; ***Norw.:*** Arobon†; ***Switz.:*** Nestargel; ***UK:*** Carobel; Nestargel.

**Multi-ingredient:** ***Austria:*** China-Eisenwein; ***Belg.:*** Kestomatine Baby; ***Braz.:*** Enteroftal†; Licor de Tayuya†; ***Fr.:*** Gumilk; Polysilane Joullie†; ***Switz.:*** Gastricure†; Kestomatine Bebe†.

# Dextrates *(USAN)*

Dextratos.
*CAS — 39404-33-6.*

**Pharmacopoeias.** In *USNF.*

**USNF 22** (Dextrates). A purified, anhydrous or hydrated, mixture of saccharides obtained by the controlled enzymatic hydrolysis of starch. Free-flowing, porous, white, odourless, spherical granules consisting of aggregates of microcrystals. Freely soluble in water (heating increases its solubility in water); soluble in dilute acids and alkalis and in basic organic solvents such as pyridine; insoluble in the common organic solvents. pH of a 20% solution in water is between 3.8 and 5.8. Store in a dry place at a temperature of 8° to 15°.

## Uses

Dextrates is used as a capsule and tablet diluent and as a tablet binding agent.

# Ethylcellulose *(rINN)*

Cellulose Ethyl Ether; E462; Ethylcellulosum; Etilcelulosa.
*CAS — 9004-57-3.*

**Pharmacopoeias.** In *Chin., Eur.* (see p.vi), and *Int.* Also in *USNF.*

**Ph. Eur. 5.0** (Ethylcellulose). A partly *O*-ethylated cellulose. It contains 44 to 51% of ethoxy ($-OC_2H_5$) groups, calculated on the dried basis. A white to yellowish-white, odourless or almost odourless, powder or granular powder. Solutions of ethylcellulose may show a slight opalescence. Practically insoluble in water, in glycerol (85%), and in propylene glycol; soluble in dichloromethane and in a mixture of 20 parts alcohol and 80 parts toluene (w/w); slightly soluble in ethyl acetate and methyl alcohol.

**USNF 22** (Ethylcellulose). The ethyl ether of cellulose. When dried at 105° for 2 hours, it contains 44.0 to 51.0% of ethoxy groups. A free-flowing white to light tan powder. Its aqueous suspensions are neutral to litmus. Insoluble in water, in glycerol, and in propylene glycol. Ethylcellulose containing less than 46.5% of ethoxy groups is freely soluble in chloroform, in methyl acetate, in tetrahydrofuran, and in mixtures of aromatic hydrocarbons with alcohol; ethylcellulose containing 46.5% or more of ethoxy groups is freely soluble in alcohol, in chloroform, in ethyl acetate, in methyl alcohol, and in toluene.

## Uses

Ethylcellulose is used as a binder in tablets and as a coating material for tablets, granules, and microcapsules. It is also used as a thickening agent.

## Preparations

***USNF 22:*** Ethylcellulose Aqueous Dispersion.

# Gastric Mucin *(BAN)*

Mucina gástrica.

## Uses and Administration

Gastric mucin is a high-molecular-weight glycoprotein precipitated by alcohol (60%) after digestion of hogs' stomach linings by pepsin and hydrochloric acid. It is used in artificial saliva formulations for dry mouth (p.1576) as an oral spray containing 3.5% or as lozenges.

## Preparations

**Proprietary Preparations** (details are given in Part 3)
***Ger.:*** Saliva medac.

**Multi-ingredient:** ***UK:*** Saliva Orthana.

# Hyetellose *(rINN)*

Hidroxietilcelulosa; Hydroxyethyl Cellulose; Hydroxyethylcellulose; Hydroxyethylcellulosum.
*CAS — 9004-62-0.*

NOTE. HECL is a code approved by the BP 2003 for use on single unit doses of eye drops containing hyetellose and sodium chloride where the individual container may be too small to bear all the appropriate labelling information.

**Pharmacopoeias.** In *Eur.* (see p.vi), *Int.,* and *Pol.* Also in *USNF.*

**Ph. Eur. 5.0** (Hydroxyethylcellulose). A partially substituted 2-hydroxyethyl ether of cellulose. Various grades are available and are distinguished by appending a number indicative of the apparent viscosity in millipascal seconds of a 2% solution measured at 25°. A white, yellowish-white, or greyish-white, powder or granules. Soluble in cold or hot water, forming colloidal solutions; practically insoluble in alcohol, in acetone, and in toluene. A 1% solution in water has a pH of 5.5 to 8.5.

**USNF 22** (Hydroxyethyl Cellulose). A partially substituted poly(hydroxyethyl) ether of cellulose. It is available in several grades, varying in viscosity and degree of substitution, and some grades are modified to improve their dispersion in water. It may contain suitable anticaking agents. A white to light tan, practically odourless, hygroscopic, powder. Soluble in cold or hot water, giving a colloidal solution; practically insoluble in alcohol and in most organic solvents. pH of a 1% solution in water is between 6.0 and 8.5.

## Uses and Administration

Hyetellose is used in pharmaceutical manufacturing as a thickener and stabiliser and as a tablet coating and binding agent. It is present in lubricant preparations for dry eye (p.1576), contact lens care (p.1164), and dry mouth (p.1576).

## Preparations

**Proprietary Preparations** (details are given in Part 3)
***Austral.:*** Rohto Zi Contact; ***Ger.:*** Lacrigel; ***Israel:*** V-Tears; ***USA:*** Comfort Tears; Gonioscopic; TearGard.

**Multi-ingredient:** ***Arg.:*** Hidratagel; ***Austral.:*** Minims Artificial Tears; ***Fr.:*** Premicia; ***Ger.:*** Lubrikano; Nu-Gel; ***Irl.:*** Minims Artificial Tears; ***UK:*** Minims Artificial Tears; ***USA:*** Optimoist.

# Hymetellose *(rINN)*

HEMC; Hidroxietilmetilcelulosa; Hydroxyethyl Methylcellulose; Hydroxyethylmethylcellulose; Methylhydroxyethylcellulose; Methylhydroxyethylcellulosum.
*CAS — 9032-42-2.*

**Pharmacopoeias.** In *Eur.* (see p.vi). Also in *USNF.*

**Ph. Eur. 5.0** (Methylhydroxyethylcellulose; Hydroxyethylmethylcellulose BP 2003). A partially substituted ether of cellulose containing methoxy and 2-hydroxyethyl groups. Various grades are available and are distinguished by appending a number indicative of the apparent viscosity in millipascal seconds of a 2% w/w solution measured at 20°. A white, yellowish-white, or greyish-white powder or granules; hygroscopic after drying. Practically insoluble in hot water, in dehydrated alcohol, in acetone, and in toluene; dissolves in cold water forming a colloidal solution. A 1% w/w solution in water has a pH of 5.5 to 8.0.

**USNF 22** (Hymetellose). A partly *O*-(methylated) and *O*-(2-hydroxyethylated) cellulose. Various grades are available, labelled with the viscosity of a 2% w/w solution measured at 20°. A white, yellowish-white, or greyish-white powder or granules; hygroscopic after drying. Insoluble in hot water, in alcohol, in acetone, in ether, and in toluene; dissolves in cold water forming a colloidal solution. pH of a 1% w/w solution in water is between 5.5 and 8.0.

## Uses

Hymetellose is used similarly to other cellulose ethers, such as methylcellulose (p.1580), as a pharmaceutical excipient.

## Preparations

**Proprietary Preparations** (details are given in Part 3)
**Multi-ingredient:** ***Fr.:*** Pharmatex.

# Hyprolose *(rINN)*

E463; Hidroxipropilcelulosa; Hydroxypropyl Cellulose; Hydroxypropylcellulose; Hydroxypropylcellulosum.
*CAS — 9004-64-2.*

**Pharmacopoeias.** In *Chin., Eur.* (see p.vi), *Int.,* and *Jpn.* Also in *USNF* which has two separate monographs, for Hydroxypropyl Cellulose and for Low-substituted Hydroxypropyl Cellulose.

**Ph. Eur. 5.0** (Hydroxypropylcellulose). A partially substituted 2-hydroxypropyl ether of cellulose. Various grades are available and may be distinguished by appending a number indicative of the apparent viscosity in millipascal seconds of a 2% w/w solution measured at 20°. White or yellowish-white, granules or powder; hygroscopic after drying. Soluble in cold water, in dehydrated alcohol, in glacial acetic acid, in methyl alcohol, in propylene glycol, and in a mixture of 10 parts methyl alcohol and 90 parts dichloromethane, forming colloidal solutions; practically insoluble in hot water, in ethylene glycol, and in toluene; sparingly soluble or slightly soluble in acetone. A 1% w/w solution in water has a pH of 5.0 to 8.5.

**USNF 22** (Hydroxypropyl Cellulose). A partially substituted poly(hydroxypropyl) ether of cellulose. When dried at 105° for 1 hour, it contains not more than 80.5% of hydroxypropoxy groups. It may contain not more than 0.60% of silica or other suitable anticaking agent. A white to cream-coloured, practically odourless, granular solid or powder, hygroscopic after drying. Soluble in cold water, in alcohol, in chloroform, and in propylene glycol, giving a colloidal solution; insoluble in hot water. pH of a 1% solution in water is between 5.0 and 8.0.

**USNF 22** (Low-Substituted Hydroxypropyl Cellulose). It contains not less than 5.0% and not more than 16.0% of hydroxypropoxy groups. A white to yellowish-white, practically odourless, hygroscopic, fibrous or granular powder. Practically insoluble in dehydrated alcohol and in ether; dissolves in a solution of sodium hydroxide (1 in 10) and produces a viscous solution; swells in water, in sodium carbonate, and in 2N hydrochloric acid. pH of the suspension obtained by shaking 1.0 g with 100 mL of water is between 5.0 and 7.5. Store in airtight containers.

## Adverse Effects

Hyprolose used as a solid ocular insert may result in blurred vision and ocular discomfort or irritation including hypersensitivity and oedema of the eyelids.

**Hypersensitivity.** Allergic contact dermatitis was reported in a patient, associated with the hyprolose present in the reservoir layer of a transdermal estradiol patch.[1]

1. Schwartz BK, Clendenning WE. Allergic contact dermatitis from hydroxypropyl cellulose in a transdermal estradiol patch. *Contact Dermatitis* 1988; **18:** 106–7.

## Uses and Administration

Hyprolose is used in pharmaceutical manufacturing in the film coating of tablets, as a tablet excipient, as a thickener, and in microencapsulation. It is used as an emulsifier and stabiliser in the food industry.

Hyprolose is also used as a modified-release solid ophthalmic insert in the management of dry eye (p.1576).

## Preparations

***USP 27:*** Hydroxypropyl Cellulose Ocular System.

**Proprietary Preparations** (details are given in Part 3)
***Austral.:*** Lacrisert; ***Canad.:*** Lacrisert; ***Denm.:*** Lacrisert†; ***Fin.:*** Lacrisert; ***Fr.:*** Lacrisert; ***Ital.:*** Lacrisert†; ***Neth.:*** Lacrisert; ***Norw.:*** Lacrisert; ***S.Afr.:*** Lacrisert†; ***Swed.:*** Lacrisert; ***USA:*** Lacrisert.

# Hypromellose *(BAN, rINN)*

E464; Hipromelosa; Hydroxypropyl Methylcellulose; Hydroxypropylmethylcellulose; Hypromellosum; Methyl Hydroxypropyl Cellulose; Methylcellulose Propylene Glycol Ether; Methylhydroxypropylcellulose; Methylhydroxypropylcellulosum.
*CAS — 8063-82-9; 9004-65-3.*
*ATC — S01KA02.*

NOTE. HPRM is a code approved by the BP 2003 for use on single unit doses of eye drops containing hypromellose where the individual container may be too small to bear all the appropriate labelling information.

**Pharmacopoeias.** In *Chin., Eur.* (see p.vi), *Int., Jpn, Pol.,* and *US.*

**Ph. Eur. 5.0** (Hypromellose). A mixed ether of cellulose containing a variable proportion of methoxy and 2-hydroxypropoxy groups. Various grades are available (see Labelling, below). A white, yellowish-white, or greyish-white powder or granules; hygroscopic after drying. Dissolves in cold water, forming a colloidal solution; practically insoluble in hot water, in dehydrated alcohol, in acetone, and in toluene. A 1% w/w solution in water has a pH of 5.5 to 8.0.

**USP 27** (Hypromellose). A propylene glycol ether of methylcellulose. When dried at 105° for 2 hours, it contains methoxy and hydroxypropoxy groups conforming to the limits for the types 1828, 2208, 2906, and 2910 (see Labelling, below). A white to slightly off-white fibrous or granular powder. Swells in water and produces a clear to opalescent, viscous, colloidal mixture; insoluble in dehydrated alcohol, in chloroform, and in ether.

**Labelling.** In Europe, grades of hypromellose are distinguished by appending a number indicative of the apparent viscosity in millipascal seconds of a 2% w/w solution measured at 20° (e.g. hypromellose 4500). In the USA, they are distinguished by appending a number in which the first 2 digits represent the approximate percentage content of methoxy groups, and the third and fourth digits the approximate percentage content of hydroxypropoxy groups.

# Hypromellose Phthalate *(BANM, rINNM)*

Ftalato de hipromelosa; Hydroxypropyl Methylcellulose Phthalate; Hypromellosi Phthalas; Methylhydroxypropylcellulose Phthalate; Methylhydroxypropylcellulosi Phthalas.

**Pharmacopoeias.** In *Eur.* (see p.vi) and *Jpn.* Also in *USNF.*

**Ph. Eur. 5.0** (Hypromellose Phthalate). A monophthalic acid ester of hypromellose containing methoxy and 2-hydroxypropoxy groups and 21 to 35% of phthalyl groups, calculated with reference to the anhydrous substance. White or slightly off-white, free-flowing flakes or a granular powder. Practically insoluble in water and in dehydrated alcohol; very slightly soluble in acetone and in toluene; soluble in a mixture of equal volumes of acetone and methyl alcohol, and of dichloromethane and methyl alcohol. Store in airtight containers.

**USNF 22** (Hypromellose Phthalate). A monophthalic acid ester of hypromellose. It contains methoxy, hydroxypropoxy, and phthalyl groups. It contains 21.0 to 35.0% of phthalyl groups, calculated on the anhydrous basis. Store in airtight containers. A white, odourless, powder or granules. Practically insoluble in water, in dehydrated alcohol, and in hexane; produces a viscous solution in a mixture of dehydrated alcohol and acetone (1:1), or in a mixture of methyl alcohol and dichloromethane (1:1); dissolves in 1N sodium hydroxide. Store in airtight containers.

**Labelling.** Different grades of hypromellose phthalate in the USA are distinguished by appending a number in which the first 2 digits represent the approximate percentage content of the methoxy groups, the next 2 digits the approximate percentage content of hydroxypropoxy groups, and the last 2 digits the approximate percentage content of the phthalyl groups. Another system of nomenclature involves appending a number which indicates the pH value (×10) at which the polymer dissolves in aqueous buffer solutions; letters such as S or F may also be used to indicate grades of high molecular-weight or small particle size respectively.

## Uses and Administration

Hypromellose has properties similar to those of methylcellulose (below). It is used in pharmaceutical manufacturing for film-coating tablets, as a tablet binder, as a modified-release matrix, and as an emulsifier, suspending agent, and stabiliser in topical gels and ointments. Hypromellose may also be used as an emulsifier and stabiliser in the food industry.

Hypromellose phthalate is used to provide enteric coating for tablets and granules, for the preparation of modified-release granules, and as a coating to mask the unpleasant taste of some tablets.

Hypromellose is widely used clinically in ophthalmic solutions; it is preferred to methylcellulose since mucilages of hypromellose have greater clarity and usually contain fewer undispersed fibres. Hypromellose is used to prolong the action of medicated eye drops and, either alone or with other viscosity-increasing agents, in artificial tears preparations for the management of dry eye (p.1576); solutions containing 0.3 to 1% of hypromellose are commonly used. Solutions for contact lens care (p.1164) and for lubricating artificial eyes contain similar concentrations. Hypromellose is also administered intra-ocularly, usually as a 2% solution, as an adjunct in ophthalmic surgery (below) and concentrations of up to 2.5% may be used topically to protect the cornea during gonioscopy procedures.

Hypromellose has been included in artificial saliva preparations used in the management of dry mouth (p.1576), but other drugs are usually preferred.

**Ophthalmic surgery.** Intra-ocular hypromellose may be used as a visco-elastic agent to protect the eye during surgery. In cataract extraction it is employed to maintain the anterior chamber and to coat the intra-ocular lens to facilitate its implantation. Although intra-ocular hypromellose is generally considered to be well tolerated, some workers[1] reported an increased incidence of pupil abnormalities (non-reactive semi-dilated pupils) following such use; others[2] did not confirm this. There has also been a report[3] of corneal opacities in a number of patients following the use of intra-ocular hypromellose.

1. Tan AKK, Humphry RC. The fixed dilated pupil after cataract surgery—is it related to intraocular use of hypromellose? *Br J Ophthalmol* 1993; **77:** 639–41.
2. Eason J, Seward HC. Pupil size and reactivity following hydroxypropyl methylcellulose and sodium hyaluronate. *Br J Ophthalmol* 1995; **79:** 541–3.
3. Newton JN, *et al.* Corneal opacities after cataract surgery with hypromellose. *Lancet* 2000; **355:** 290.

## Preparations

***BP 2003:*** Hypromellose Eye Drops;
***USP 27:*** Hypromellose Ophthalmic Solution.

**Proprietary Preparations** (details are given in Part 3)
***Arg.:*** Artelac; Genteal; Lacrisifi; Natura Lagrimas; ***Austral.:*** Genteal Lubricant; Isopto Tears; Methopt; ***Austria:*** Artelac; Okuzell; Prosicca; Visacare; ***Belg.:*** Artelac; Isopto Tears†; Ocucoat†; ***Braz.:*** Artelac; Filmcel; Genteal; Lubrik; ***Canad.:*** Eyelube; Genteal; Isopto Tears; Lacril; Visine Contact Lens; ***Chile:*** Genteal; ***Fin.:*** Artelac; Isopto Alkaline; Isopto Plain; ***Fr.:*** Artelac; Contactol†; ***Ger.:*** Artelac; Berberil Dry Eye; Cellugel; Celoftal; Genteal; HPMC-Ophtal; Isopto Fluid†; Methocel; Sic-Ophtal; Sicca-Stulln; ***Gr.:*** Vidilac; ***Hong Kong:*** Genteal; Isopto Tears; Methocel; ***India:*** Hyprosol; Moisol; Nova Vizol; Occu System; ***Irl.:*** Artelac; Isopto Alkaline; Isopto Plain; ***Israel:*** Adato-Cel; Genteal; Ocucoat; ***Ital.:*** Gel 4000; Genteal; Lacrimill; Lacrisifi; Lacrisol; Methocel†; ***Mex.:*** Celulose; Filmexil; Meticel; Naturalag; Oftalmet†; ***Norw.:*** Artelac; ***NZ:*** Genteal; Isopto Tears†; Methopt; ***Port.:*** Artelac; Hidrocil; ***S.Afr.:*** Methocel; Spersatear; Viscotraan; ***Singapore:*** Celoftal†; Eye Mo Moist; Isopto Tears†; Lacrisifi; Methocel; ***Spain:*** Acuolens; ***Swed.:*** Artelac; Isopto Plain; ***Switz.:*** Isopto Tears; Ultra Tears†; ***Thai.:*** Isopto Tears; Lac-Oph; Opsil Tears; Simoph Tears; ***UK:*** Artelac; Brolene Cool Eyes; Isopto Alkaline; Isopto Plain; Moisture Eyes†; Ocucoat†; ***USA:*** Artificial Tears; Genteal; Gonak; Goniosoft; Goniosol; Isopto Plain; Isopto Tears; Lacril; Ocucoat; Tearisol; Tears Again MC; Ultra Tears.

**Multi-ingredient:** ***Arg.:*** Alcon Lagrimas; Irix Lagrimas; ***Austral.:*** Bausch & Lomb Sensitive Eyes Lens Lubricant†; Bion Tears†; Genteal Moisturising; Murine Contact†; Poly-Tears; Tears Naturale; Visine True Tears; ***Belg.:*** Alcon Adequad; Lacrystat; Tears Naturale; ***Braz.:*** Lacrima; Lacrima Plus; Opti-Tears; ***Canad.:*** Bion Tears; Moisture Drops; Ocutears†; Tears Naturale; ***Chile:*** Nicotears; Novo-Tears; Tears Naturale; ***Denm.:*** Dacriosol; ***Ger.:*** Isopto Naturale†; Lacrisic; Oculotect; ***Gr.:*** Tears Natural; ***Hong Kong:*** Bion Tears; Visine for Contacts; ***Irl.:*** Ilube; Tears Naturale; ***Israel:*** Tears Naturale; V-Crima; ***Ital.:*** Dacriosol; Hamamilla; Ipragocce; Tirs; ***Malaysia:*** Dacrolux; Tears Naturale; ***Mex.:*** Naphacel; ***Norw.:*** Tears Naturale; ***NZ:*** Poly-Tears; Tears Naturale; ***Port.:*** Tears Naturale; ***S.Afr.:*** Moisture Drops; Tears Naturale; ***Singapore:*** Bion Tears; Dacrolux; Tears Naturale; ***Spain:*** Dacrolux; Humectante; Tears Humectante; ***Swed.:*** Bion Tears; Tears Naturale†; ***Switz.:*** Tears Naturale; ***Thai.:*** Bion Tears; Tears Naturale; ***UK:*** Ilube; Tears Naturale; ***USA:*** Bion Tears; Clear Eyes CLR; Lacri-Tears; LubriTears; Maximum Strength Allergy Drops; Moisture Drops; Nature's Tears; Ocucoat; Tears Naturale; Tears Renewed.

---

# Magnesium Silicate

E553(a); Silicato de magnesio.
*CAS — 1343-88-0.*
*ATC — A02AA05.*

NOTE. The code E553(a) has also been applied to magnesium trisilicate.

**Pharmacopoeias.** In *Jpn.* Also in *USNF.*

**USNF 22** (Magnesium Silicate). A compound of magnesium oxide and silicon dioxide. It contains not less than 15.0% of magnesium oxide and not less than 67.0% of silicon dioxide, calculated on the ignited basis. It is a fine, white, odourless powder, free from grittiness. Insoluble in water and in alcohol. It is readily decomposed by mineral acids. pH of a well-mixed 10% suspension in water is between 7.0 and 10.8.

## Uses

Magnesium silicate is used in the food industry and in pharmaceutical manufacturing as an anticaking agent.

## Preparations

**Proprietary Preparations** (details are given in Part 3)
***Port.:*** Acnoil Free.

**Multi-ingredient:** ***Belg.:*** Mucal†; ***Braz.:*** Cutisanol; ***Fr.:*** ZeaSorb; ***Ital.:*** Babigoz Crema Protettiva; ***Port.:*** Mucal; ***Switz.:*** Bigasan†.

---

# Methylcellulose *(rINN)*

E461; Methylcellulosum; Metilcelulosa.
*CAS — 9004-67-5.*
*ATC — A06AC06.*

**Pharmacopoeias.** In *Chin., Eur.* (see p.vi), *Int., Jpn, Pol.,* and *US.*

**Ph. Eur. 5.0** (Methylcellulose). A cellulose having some of the hydroxyl groups in the form of the methyl ether. Various grades of methylcellulose are available and are distinguished by appending a number indicating the apparent viscosity in millipascal seconds of a 2% w/w solution at 20°. It is a white, yellowish-white, or greyish-white powder or granules; hygroscopic after drying. Practically insoluble in hot water, in dehydrated alcohol, in acetone, and in toluene; dissolves in cold water, forming a colloidal solution. A 1% w/w solution in water has a pH of 5.5 to 8.0.

**USP 27** (Methylcellulose). A methyl ether of cellulose. When dried at 105° for 2 hours, it contains 27.5 to 31.5% of methoxy groups. It is a white, fibrous powder or granules. It swells in water and produces a clear to opalescent, viscous, colloidal suspension; insoluble in alcohol, in chloroform, and in ether; soluble in glacial acetic acid and in a mixture of equal volumes of alcohol and chloroform. Its aqueous suspensions are neutral to litmus.

**Incompatibility.** Incompatibilities of methylcellulose have been reported with a number of compounds including chlorocresol, hydroxybenzoates, and phenol. Large amounts of electrolytes increase the viscosity of methylcellulose mucilages owing to salting-out of the methylcellulose; in very high concentrations of electrolytes, the methylcellulose may be completely precipitated.

## Adverse Effects

Large quantities of methylcellulose may temporarily increase flatulence and distension and there is a risk of intestinal obstruction. Oesophageal obstruction may occur if compounds such as methylcellulose are swallowed dry.

## Precautions

Methylcellulose and other bulk-forming agents should not be given to patients with intestinal obstruction or conditions likely to lead to intestinal obstruction. They should be taken with sufficient fluid to prevent faecal impaction or oesophageal obstruction, and should not be taken immediately before going to bed. Methylcellulose should not be used in infective bowel disease.

## Interactions

Bulk laxatives such as methylcellulose lower the transit time through the gut and could affect the absorption of other drugs.

## Uses and Administration

The various grades of methylcellulose are widely used in pharmaceutical manufacturing as emulsifying, suspending, and thickening agents and as binding, disintegrating, and coating agents in tablet manufacturing. Low-viscosity grades are preferred for use as emulsifying agents as the surface tension produced is lower than with the higher-viscosity grades. Low-viscosity grades may also be used as suspending or thickening agents for liquid oral dosage forms and solutions of methylcellulose may be used as replacements for sugar-based syrups or other suspension bases. For thickening topically applied products such as gels and creams a high-viscosity grade is usually used. In tablet technology low- or medium-viscosity grades are used as binding agents while high-viscosity grades act as tablet disintegrants by swelling on contact with the disintegration medium. For tablet coating, highly substituted low-viscosity grades are usually used. Methylcellulose may also be included in modified-release tablet formulations.

Methylcellulose is also used as an emulsifier and stabiliser in the food industry.

Methylcellulose is used clinically as a bulk-forming agent. Medium- or high-viscosity grades are used as bulk laxatives in the treatment of constipation (p.1240); by taking up moisture they increase the volume of the faeces and promote peristalsis. Methylcellulose is usually given in a dosage of up to 6 g daily in divided doses, taken with plenty of fluid. It is also given in similar doses but with a minimum amount of water for the control of diarrhoea (p.1241) and for the control of faecal consistency in ostomies. It is also used in the management of diverticular disease (p.1241). Methylcellulose has also been used as an aid to appetite control in the management of obesity (p.1583) but there is little evidence of efficacy.

A 0.5 to 1% solution of a high-viscosity grade of methylcellulose has been used as a vehicle for eye drops, as artificial tears, and in contact lens care, but hypromellose (p.1580) is now generally preferred for this purpose.

## Preparations

***BP 2003:*** Methylcellulose Granules; Methylcellulose Tablets;
***USP 27:*** Methylcellulose Ophthalmic Solution; Methylcellulose Oral Solution; Methylcellulose Tablets.

**Proprietary Preparations** (details are given in Part 3)
***Austral.:*** Cellulone†; ***Austria:*** Bulk; ***Canad.:*** Murocel†; ***Fr.:*** Dacryolarmes; ***Irl.:*** Celevac; ***Ital.:*** Lacrimart; ***Malaysia:*** Methocel; ***Port.:*** Davilose; ***Spain:*** Muciplasma; ***UK:*** Celevac; ***USA:*** Citrucel; Murocel.

**Multi-ingredient:** ***Austral.:*** Bioglan 3B Beer Belly Buster†; Citri Slim+Trim†; Le Trim-BM†; Neo-Trim Fibre†; Parachoc; Pro-Shape†; ***Austria:*** Cellobexon; ***Braz.:*** Kolantyl; Kolantyl DMP; ***Canad.:*** Slim Mint†; ***Ital.:*** Conta-Lens Wetting†; ***S.Afr.:*** Kolantyl; Medigel; Merasyn.

---

# Pectin

E440 (amidated pectin or pectin); Pectina.
*CAS — 9000-69-5.*
*ATC — A07BC01.*

**Pharmacopoeias.** In *US.*

**USP 27** (Pectin). A purified carbohydrate product obtained from the dilute acid extract of the inner portion of the rind of citrus fruits or from apple pomace; it consists mainly of partially methoxylated polygalacturonic acids. A yellowish-white, almost odourless, coarse or fine powder. Almost completely soluble in 1 in 20 of water, forming a viscous, opalescent, colloidal solution which flows readily and is acid to litmus; practically insoluble in alcohol or in diluted alcohol and in other organic solvents. It dissolves more readily in water if first moistened with alcohol, glycerol, or simple syrup, or if mixed with 3 or more parts of sucrose. Store in airtight containers.

## Interactions

Bulk-forming agents such as dietary fibre lower the transit time through the gut and may affect the absorption of other drugs.

**Lipid regulating drugs.** Pectin, employed as a source of fibre, together with a lipid-lowering diet and *lovastatin,* has resulted in a paradoxical increase in low-density lipoprotein (LDL)-cholesterol in patients with hypercholesterolaemia. It was believed the pectin reduced the absorption of lovastatin from the gut.[1]

1. Richter WO, *et al.* Interaction between fibre and lovastatin. *Lancet* 1991; **338:** 706.

## Uses and Administration

Pectins are used as emulsifiers and stabilisers in the food industry. They are non-starch polysaccharide constituents of dietary fibre (see under Dietary Role in Bran, p.1253).

Pectin is an adsorbent and bulk-forming agent and is present in multi-ingredient preparations for the management of diarrhoea, constipation, and obesity. Pectin has also been tried for reducing or slowing carbohydrate absorption in the dumping syndrome (p.1242).

## Preparations

**Proprietary Preparations** (details are given in Part 3)
***Braz.:*** Kaogel; ***Fr.:*** Arhemapectine Antihemorragique; Hydrocoll.

**Multi-ingredient:** ***Arg.:*** Endomicina; Opocler; ***Austral.:*** Betaine Digestive Aid†; Bioglan 3B Beer Belly Buster†; Bioglan Psylli-Mucil Plus†; Bioglan Zellulean with Escin†; Bis-Pectin; Citri Slim+Trim†; Diarcalm†; Diareze; Donnagel; Enterocare†; Kaomagma with Pectin†; Kaopectate†; Natures Own Acidophilus Plus†; Orabase; Orahesive; PC Regulax†; Pro-Shape†; Stomahesive; ***Austria:*** Diarrhoesan; ***Belg.:*** Kaopectate†; Tanalone; ***Braz.:*** Atacoly†; Atalin; Atapec; Diapool†; Enterobion†; Enterocler†; Enterodina†; Enteropen†; Fluocal com Pectina†; Furazolin†; Kal Sept†; Kaomagma; Kaopectate†; Kaopectin†; Kaostase Suspension†; Linadin†; Magnostase†; Parenterin; Pectalin†; Pectimax†; Plasmocolit†; Plexo Enterin†; Sanadiar†; Suspectim†; Tratocoli†; ***Canad.:*** Diarex†; Diban†; Donnagel-PG†; Orabase; Orahesive; ***Chile:*** Enterol; Furazolidona; ***Fr.:*** Gelopectose; ***Ger.:*** Diarrhoesan; Kaoprompt-H; ***Gr.:*** Kaopectate; ***Hong Kong:*** Uni-Kaotin; ***Irl.:*** Kaopectate; Orabase; ***Israel:*** Kaopectin; Kapectin Forte; Orabase; ***Ital.:*** Cruscasohn; Streptomagma; ***Malaysia:*** Beakopectin; Kaopectate; ***Mex.:*** Caopecfar; Colfur; Contefur; Coralzul; Dibapec Compuesto; Facetin-D; Farpectol; Fuzotyl; Hidromagma; Isocar; Kaomycin; Kaopectate; Lactopectin; Neo-Kap; Neoxil; Olam; Optazol; Quimefuran; Tapzol con Neomicina; Tapzol†; Treda; Trilor; Yodozona; ***NZ:*** Orabase; Stomahesive; ***Port.:*** Cloranpectina; Combiderm†; Varihesive; ***S.Afr.:*** Betapect; Bipectinol; Biskapect; Chloropect; Collodyne†; Enterolyte; Gastropect; Granuflex; Granugel; Kantrexil; Kao; Kaopectin; Kaostatex; Pectin-K; Pectrolyte; ***Singapore:*** Kaopectate; ***Spain:*** Dextricea; Estreptoenterol; ***Switz.:*** Demosvelte N†; HEC; Kaopectate†; Varihesive Hydroactive†; ***Thai.:*** Biodan; Carbonpectate; Di-Su-Frone; Difuran; Diolin†; Disento PF; Furasian; Furopectin; Kaopectal; Kaopectal-N†; Kaopectate†; Med-Kafuzone; **UAE:** Kaptin; **UK:** Entrotabs†; Goodypops; KLN; Orabase; Orahesive; Stomahesive; **USA:** K-C; Kao-Paverin; Kao-Spen; Kaodene Non-Narcotic.

## Polyethylene Oxide

Óxido de polietileno.

**Pharmacopoeias.** In *USNF.*

**USNF 22** (Polyethylene Oxide). A nonionic homopolymer of ethylene oxide, represented by the formula $(OCH_2CH_2)_n$, in which *n* represents the average number of oxyethylene groups (about 2000 to over 100 000). It is obtainable in several grades, varying in viscosity profile in an aqueous isopropyl alcohol solution. It may contain not more than 3% of silicon dioxide. A white to off-white powder. Miscible with water; freely soluble in acetonitrile, in dichloromethane, in ethylene dichloride, and in trichloroethylene; insoluble in aliphatic hydrocarbons, in ethylene glycol, in diethylene glycol, and in glycerol. Store in airtight containers. Protect from light.

### Uses

Polyethylene oxide is used as a tablet binder and as a suspending and thickening agent in pharmaceutical preparations. Polyethylene oxide has been used in hydrogel wound dressings.

### Preparations

**Proprietary Preparations** (details are given in Part 3)
**UK:** Vigilon†.

## Polyvinyl Acetate Phthalate

Acetato ftalato de polivinilo.

**Pharmacopoeias.** In *USNF.*

**USNF 22** (Polyvinyl Acetate Phthalate). A reaction product of phthalic anhydride and a partially hydrolysed polyvinyl acetate. It contains 55.0 to 62.0% of phthalyl groups, calculated on an anhydrous acid-free basis. It is a free-flowing white powder that may have a slight odour of acetic acid. Insoluble in water, in chloroform, and in dichloromethane; soluble in alcohol and in methyl alcohol. Store in airtight containers.

### Uses

Polyvinyl acetate phthalate is a viscosity-modifying agent that is used in the manufacture of enteric coating for tablets.

## Polyvinyl Alcohol

Alcohol polivinílico; Poly(alcohol Vinylicus).
*CAS — 9002-89-5.*

**Pharmacopoeias.** In *Eur.* (see p.vi), *Pol.,* and *US.*

**Ph. Eur. 5.0** (Poly(Vinyl Alcohol)). It is obtained by polymerisation of vinyl acetate followed by partial or complete hydrolysis of polyvinyl acetate in the presence of catalytic amounts of alkali or mineral acids. Various grades are available and they differ in their degree of polymerisation and their degree of hydrolysis, which determine the physical properties of the different grades. They are characterised by the viscosity and the ester value of the substance. The mean relative molecular mass lies between 20 000 and 150 000. The viscosity is 3 to 70 millipascal seconds. The ester value, which characterises the degree of hydrolysis, is not greater than 280.

Polyvinyl alcohol occurs as a yellowish-white powder or translucent granules. Soluble in water; slightly soluble in dehydrated alcohol; practically insoluble in acetone. A 4% solution in water has a pH of 4.5 to 6.5.

**USP 27** (Polyvinyl Alcohol). A synthetic resin represented by the formula $(CH_2CHOH)_n$, where the average value of *n* is 500 to 5000. It is prepared by 85 to 89% hydrolysis of polyvinyl acetate. White to cream-coloured, odourless, granules or powder. Freely soluble in water at room temperature; solution may be effected more rapidly at somewhat higher temperatures. pH of a 4% solution in water is between 5.0 and 8.0.

### Uses and Administration

Polyvinyl alcohol is a nonionic surfactant that is used in pharmaceutical manufacturing as a stabilising agent and as a viscosity-increasing agent and lubricant.

Polyvinyl alcohol has also been used in the preparation of jellies that dry rapidly when applied to the skin to form a soluble plastic film.

Polyvinyl alcohols of various grades are used for a wide variety of industrial applications.

Polyvinyl alcohol has been used to increase the viscosity of ophthalmic preparations thus prolonging contact of the active ingredient with the eye. It is included in artificial tears preparations used for dry eye (p.1576) and in contact lens solutions (p.1164). For dry eye it is often used in a concentration of 1.4% with or without povidone.

### Preparations

**Proprietary Preparations** (details are given in Part 3)
**Arg.:** Bio Tears; Lagrima Artificial; Lagrima Humectante; Lentisol; Liquifilm Lagrimas; Natura Wet; **Austral.:** Liquifilm; PVA; **Austria:** Liquifilm†; **Belg.:** Liquifilm; **Braz.:** Duracare; Lacril; Totalens; **Canad.:** Artificial Tears; Cooper Tears†; Duracare†; Hypotears; Liquifilm; Optilube PVA; PMS-Artificial Tears; Revitaleyes†; RO-Dry Eyes†; Scheinpharm Artificial Tears; Total; **Chile:** Lagrimas Artificiales; Liquifilm Lagrimas; Visidic; **Denm.:** Lacril; **Fin.:** Liquifilm; Oftan; **Fr.:** Liquifilm†; **Ger.:** Alltotal†; Contafilm†; Lacrimal; Liquifilm; Vistofilm†; **Gr.:** Liquifilm Tears; **Hong Kong:** Liquifilm; PMS-Artificial Tears; **Irl.:** Liquifilm; Sno Tears; **Israel:** Hypotears; Liquifilm Tears; **Ital.:** Lacrilux; **Malaysia:** Liquifilm; **Mex.:** Acuafil Ofteno; Lubrik; **Norw.:** Ocufri; **NZ:** Liquifilm; **Port.:** Liquifilm; **S.Afr.:** Liquifilm Tears; **Singapore:** Hypotears; Liquifilm Tears; PMS-Artificial Tears†; **Spain:** Hypo Tears; Liquifilm Lagrimas; **Swed.:** Sincon; **Switz.:** Liquifilm; **Thai.:** Liquifilm Tears; **UK:** Liquifilm Tears; Refresh; Sno Tears; **USA:** Akwa Tears; Dry Eyes; Liquifilm; Nu-Tears; Ocu-Tears; Puralube; Tears Again.

**Multi-ingredient: Arg.:** Consil; Refresh Free; Soquette; **Austral.:** Murine Revital Eyes; Murine Tears for Eyes; Refresh; Teardrops†; Tears Plus; **Austria:** Siccaprotect; **Braz.:** Polipred; Refresh; **Canad.:** Murine; PMS-Artificial Tears Extra; Refresh; Scheinpharm Artificial Tears Plus; Teardrops; Tears Plus; **Fr.:** Refresh; **Ger.:** Dispatenol; Duracare†; Lacrimal OK; Liquifilm OK; Siccaprotect; **Gr.:** Refresh; **Hong Kong:** Hypotears; **India:** I-Lube; **Israel:** Hypotears PF†; Refresh; **Ital.:** Collyria; Hypotears; **Malaysia:** Hypotears; Murine NTF; Murine Plus; Refresh; **Mex.:** Lagrifilm Plus; Refresh; Soltrictor con Lagrifilm; **NZ:** Refresh; Teardrops†; Tears Plus; **S.Afr.:** Refresh; Tears Plus; **Singapore:** Refresh; **Spain:** Liquifresh; **Switz.:** Collylarm; Hypotears; Tears Plus; **Thai.:** Refresh; **UK:** Blink; Hypotears; **USA:** Hypotears; Murine; Murine Plus; Nu-Tears II; Refresh; Tears Plus; VasoClear.

## Povidone *(BAN, USAN, rINN)*

E1201; Polyvidone; Polyvidonum; Polyvinylpyrrolidone; Povidona; Povidonum; PVP; Vinylpyrrolidinone Polymer. Poly (2-oxopyrrolidin-1-ylethylene).
$(C_6H_9NO)_n$.
*CAS — 9003-39-8.*
*ATC — A07BC03.*

**Pharmacopoeias.** In *Chin., Eur.* (see p.vi), *Int., Jpn, Pol.,* and *US.*

**Ph. Eur. 5.0** (Povidone). Linear polymers of 1-ethenylpyrrolidin-2-one. The different types of povidone are characterised by their viscosity in solution. A white or yellowish-white, hygroscopic powder or flakes. Freely soluble in water, in alcohol, and in methyl alcohol; slightly soluble in acetone. A 5% solution in water has a pH of 3.0 to 7.0 depending on the viscosity. Store in airtight containers.

**USP 27** (Povidone). A synthetic polymer consisting essentially of linear 1-vinyl-2-pyrrolidinone groups, the degree of polymerisation of which results in polymers of various molecular weights. The different types of povidone are characterised by their viscosity in aqueous solution, relative to that of water, expressed as a K-value. A white to slightly creamy-white, hygroscopic powder. Freely soluble in water, in alcohol, and in methyl alcohol; slightly soluble in acetone; practically insoluble in ether. pH of a 5% solution in water is between 3.0 and 7.0. Store in airtight containers.

## Copovidone

Copolyvidone; Copolyvidonum; Copovidona; Copovidonum.
*ATC — A07BC03.*

**Pharmacopoeias.** In *Eur.* (see p.vi).

**Ph. Eur. 5.0** (Copovidone). A copolymer of 1-vinylpyrrolidin-2-one and vinyl acetate in the mass proportion 3:2. A white or yellowish-white, hygroscopic powder or flakes. Freely soluble in water, in alcohol, and in dichloromethane. Protect from moisture.

## Crospovidone *(rINN)*

Crospovidona; Crospovidonum; Polyplasdone XL.
*CAS — 9003-39-8.*
*ATC — A07BC03.*

**Pharmacopoeias.** In *Eur.* (see p.vi). Also in *USNF.*

**Ph. Eur. 5.0** (Crospovidone). A cross-linked homopolymer of 1-vinylpyrrolidin-2-one. A white or yellowish-white, hygroscopic powder or flakes. Practically insoluble in water, in alcohol, and in dichloromethane. Protect from moisture.

**USNF 22** (Crospovidone). A synthetic cross-linked homopolymer of *N*-vinyl-2-pyrrolidinone. A white to creamy-white, hygroscopic powder having a faint odour. Insoluble in water and in ordinary organic solvents. pH of a 1% suspension in water is between 5.0 and 8.0. Store in airtight containers.

### Adverse Effects

Some products intended for parenteral administration contain povidone as an excipient and injection has led to deposition of povidone in various tissues with consequent lesions and pain. There have been occasional reports of liver involvement.

◊ Reviews of adverse effects associated with pharmaceutical excipients including povidone.

1. Golightly LK, *et al.* Pharmaceutical excipients: adverse effects associated with 'inactive ingredients' in drug products (part II). *Med Toxicol* 1988; **3:** 209–40.

### Uses and Administration

Povidone is used in pharmaceutical manufacturing as a suspending and dispersing agent and as a tablet binding, granulating, and coating agent. It is used as a carrier for iodine (see Povidone-Iodine, p.1190). An insoluble cross-linked form of povidone known as crospovidone is used as a tablet disintegrant. Copovidone, a copolymer with vinyl acetate, is used as a tablet binding and coating agent.

Povidone is included in artificial tears preparations used in the management of dry eye (p.1576) and in solutions for contact lens care (p.1164). For dry eye it is often used in a concentration of 0.6% together with other viscosity-increasing agents (such as polyvinyl alcohol); it may also be used alone in solutions containing 1.5 to 5%.

Povidone has also been used as an adsorbent in gastrointestinal disorders.

Povidone was formerly used as a plasma expander but other compounds are now preferred.

### Preparations

**Proprietary Preparations** (details are given in Part 3)
**Arg.:** Hypotears Plus; Megatears; **Austral.:** Clerz Moisturising Drops†; In A Wink Moisturing†; Rohto Zi Fresh; **Austria:** Oculotect; Protagent; **Belg.:** Protagent†; Siccagent; **Braz.:** Hypotears; **Chile:** Oculotec; **Denm.:** Oculac; **Fin.:** Oculac; **Fr.:** Bolinan; Dulcilarmes; Fluidabak; Larmecran; Nu-Gel; Nutrivisc; Unifluid; **Ger.:** Arufil; Lacophtal; Lacri-Stulln; Oculotect Fluid; Protagent; Vidirakt S; Vidisept; Vidisept EDO; Yxin Tears; **Gr.:** Oculotect; Protagent; **Hong Kong:** Hypotears Plus; Protagent; **Israel:** Hypotears E; Lacrimol; **Ital.:** Clarover; Nu-Gel; Protagent; **Malaysia:** Oculotect; Vidisept N; **Mex.:** Hypotears Plus; Logical; **Neth.:** Oculotect; **Norw.:** Oculac; **NZ:** In A Wink†; **Port.:** Oculotect; **S.Afr.:** Hypotears; **Singapore:** Oculotect; Vidisept N; **Spain:** Oculotect; **Swed.:** Oculac; **Switz.:** Oculac; Protagent; **Thai.:** Hypotears Plus; **UK:** Aloclair; Oculotect.

**Multi-ingredient: Arg.:** Refresh Free; **Austral.:** Bausch & Lomb Sensitive Eyes Lens Lubricant†; Murine Revital Eyes; Murine Tears for Eyes; Refresh; Teardrops†; Tears Plus; Visine Advanced Relief; **Braz.:** Refresh; **Canad.:** Moisture Drops; Murine; PMS-Artificial Tears Extra; Refresh; Scheinpharm Artificial Tears Plus; Teardrops; Tears Plus; **Fr.:** Poly-Karaya; Refresh; **Ger.:** Lacrimal OK; Lacrisic; Liquifilm OK; **Gr.:** Refresh; **India:** I-Lube; **Israel:** Refresh; V-Crima; **Malaysia:** Murine NTF; Murine Plus; Refresh; **Mex.:** Lagrifilm Plus; Refresh; Soyaloid; Soydex; **NZ:** Refresh; Teardrops†; Tears Plus; Visine Advanced Relief; **S.Afr.:** Moisture Drops; Refresh; Tears Plus; **Singapore:** Refresh; **Spain:** Liquifresh; **Switz.:** Collylarm; Poly-Karaya†; Tears Plus; **Thai.:** Refresh; **UK:** Gelclair; **USA:** Advanced Relief Visine; Murine; Murine Plus; Refresh; Tears Night & Day†; Tears Plus.

## Silicas

Sílice.

## Purified Siliceous Earth

Diatomaceous Earth; Diatomite; Purified Infusorial Earth; Purified Kieselguhr; Terra Silicea Purificada; Tierra de diatomeas.
*CAS — 7631-86-9.*

**Pharmacopoeias.** In *USNF.*

**USNF 22** (Purified Siliceous Earth). A form of silicon dioxide consisting of frustules and fragments of diatoms purified by calcining. A very fine, white, light grey, or pale buff mixture of amorphous powder and lesser amounts of crystalline polymorphs, including quartz and cristobalite. It is gritty and readily absorbs moisture, and retains about four times its weight of water before becoming fluid. Insoluble in water, in acids, and in dilute solutions of alkali hydroxides.

## Silicon Dioxide

Colloidal Hydrated Silica; Dióxido de silicio; E551; Precipitated Silica; Silica Colloidalis Hydrica; Silica Gel.
$SiO_2,xH_2O$ = 60.08 (anhydrous).
*CAS — 63231-67-4; 7631-86-9.*

**Pharmacopoeias.** In *Eur.* (see p.vi). Also in *USNF. Eur.* and *USNF* also include dental-type silica.

**Ph. Eur. 5.0** (Silica, Colloidal Hydrated). A light, fine, white or almost white, amorphous powder. Practically insoluble in water, and in mineral acids except hydrofluoric acid; dissolves in hot solutions of alkali hydroxides.

**Ph. Eur. 5.0** (Silica, Dental Type). An amorphous silica (precipitated, gel, or obtained by flame hydrolysis). A white or almost white, light, fine amorphous powder. Practically insoluble in water and in mineral acids; dissolves in hydrofluoric acid and in hot solutions of alkali hydroxides.

**USNF 22** (Silicon Dioxide). It is obtained by insolubilising the dissolved silica in sodium silicate solution. Where obtained by the addition of sodium silicate to a mineral acid, the product is termed silica gel; where obtained by the destabilisation of a solution of sodium silicate in such a manner as to yield very fine particles, the product is termed precipitated silica. A fine, white, odourless, hygroscopic, amorphous powder in which the diameter of the average particles ranges from 2 to 10 micrometres. Insoluble in water, in alcohol, and in other organic solvents; soluble in hot solutions of alkali hydroxides. pH of 5% slurry in water is between 4.0 and 8.0. Store in airtight containers. Protect from moisture.

**USNF 22** (Dental-Type Silica). It is obtained from sodium silicate solution by destabilising with acid in such a way as to yield very fine particles. A fine, white, odourless, hygroscopic, amorphous powder in which the diameter of the average particles ranges from 0.5 to 40 micrometres. Insoluble in water, in alcohol, and in acid (except hydrofluoric acid); soluble in hot solutions of alkali hydroxides. pH of 5% slurry in water is between 4.0 and 8.5. Store in airtight containers.

## Colloidal Silicon Dioxide

Acidum Silicicum Colloidale; Colloidal Anhydrous Silica; Colloidal Silica; Dióxido de silicio coloidal; Hochdisperses Silicumdioxid; Silica Colloidalis Anhydrica.
$SiO_2$ = 60.08.
*CAS — 7631-86-9.*

**Pharmacopoeias.** In *Eur.* (see p.vi) and *Pol.* Also in *USNF.*

**Ph. Eur. 5.0** (Silica, Colloidal Anhydrous). A light, fine, white, amorphous powder. It has a particle size of about 15 nm. Practically insoluble in water and in mineral acids except hydrofluoric acid; dissolves in hot solutions of alkali hydroxides. A 3.3% suspension in water has a pH of 3.5 to 5.5.

**USNF 22** (Colloidal Silicon Dioxide). A submicroscopic fumed silicon dioxide, prepared by the vapour-phase hydrolysis of a silicon compound. A light, white, non-gritty powder of extremely fine particle size (about 15 nm). Insoluble in water and in acid (except hydrofluoric acid); soluble in hot solutions of alkali hydroxides. pH of a 4% dispersion in water is between 3.5 and 5.5.

### Adverse Effects

Prolonged inhalation of some forms of silica dust may be associated with the development of fibrosis of the lung (silicosis). The forms of silica described here and used as pharmaceutical excipients may cause irritation of the respiratory tract if inhaled but do not appear to be associated with silicosis.

### Uses

The different forms of silica have various pharmaceutical uses. Purified siliceous earth is used as a filtering medium and adsorbent. Silicon dioxide is used as a suspending and thickening agent and, as silica gel, as a desiccant. Colloidal silicon dioxide is used as a suspending agent and thickener, as a stabiliser in emulsions, and as an anticaking agent and desiccant. Silicon dioxide is also used as an anticaking agent in the food industry.

Silicon dioxide (Silicea) is used in homoeopathic medicine.

### Preparations

**Proprietary Preparations** (details are given in Part 3)
***Austral.:*** Celloids S 79†; ***Ger.:*** Aktiv-Puder†; Entero-Teknosal; Sklerosol N; ***Mon.:*** Dissolvurol; ***NZ:*** Biosil; ***UK:*** Aerosil.

**Multi-ingredient:** ***Austral.:*** Bio-Disc†; Duo Celloids SCF†; Duo Celloids SPS†; Duo Celloids SSS†; Silicic Complex†; ***Austria:*** $CO_2$ Granulat; Kephalodoron; ***Chile:*** Xeragel; ***Fin.:*** Wicne; ***Fr.:*** Gelopectose; Topaal; ***Ger.:*** Aplona; $CO_2$ Granulat; Equisil N; ***Gr.:*** Gastrovison; ***Hong Kong:*** Biscasil†; Disflatyl; ***Israel:*** Adinol; Kelo-Cote; ***Ital.:*** Gastrovison†; Lacalut; ***NZ:*** Odor Eze; ***Singapore:*** Disflatyl; ***Switz.:*** Acne Creme; Fissan; ***UK:*** New Era Zief†.

## Sodium Starch Glycolate

Carboxymethylamylum Natricum; Glicolato sódico de almidón; Sodium Carboxymethyl Starch; Sodium Starch Glycollate; Starch Sodium Glycolate.

*CAS — 9063-38-1.*

**Pharmacopoeias.** In *Chin.* and *Eur.* (see p.vi). Also in *USNF.*

**Ph. Eur. 5.0** (Sodium Starch Glycolate (Type A); Carboxymethylamylum Natricum A). The sodium salt of a cross-linked partly *O*-carboxymethylated potato starch. It contains 2.8 to 4.2% of sodium, calculated with reference to the substance washed with alcohol (80%) and dried. A fine, white or almost white, very hygroscopic, free-flowing powder. It forms a translucent suspension in water; practically insoluble in dichloromethane. pH of the supernatant of a 3.33% suspension in water is 5.5 to 7.5. Store in airtight containers. Protect from light.

**Ph. Eur. 5.0** (Sodium Starch Glycolate (Type B); Carboxymethylamylum Natricum B). The sodium salt of a cross-linked partly *O*-carboxymethylated potato starch. It contains 2.0 to 3.4% of sodium, calculated with reference to the substance washed with alcohol (80%) and dried. A fine, white or almost white, very hygroscopic, free-flowing powder. It forms a translucent suspension in water; practically insoluble in dichloromethane. pH of the supernatant of a 3.33% suspension in water is 3.0 to 5.0. Store in airtight containers. Protect from light.

**Ph. Eur. 5.0** (Sodium Starch Glycolate (Type C); Carboxymethylamylum Natricum C). The sodium salt of a cross-linked by physical dehydration, partly *O*-carboxymethylated starch. It contains 2.8 to 5.0% of sodium, calculated with reference to the substance washed with alcohol (80%) and dried. A fine, white or almost white, very hygroscopic, free-flowing powder. It forms a translucent gel-like product in water; practically insoluble in dichloromethane. pH of a 3.33% gel in water is 5.5 to 7.5. Store in airtight containers. Protect from light.

**USNF 22** (Sodium Starch Glycolate). The sodium salt of a carboxymethyl ether of starch. It contains not less than 2.8% and not more than 4.2% of sodium on the dried, alcohol-washed basis. A white, odourless, relatively free-flowing powder available in several different viscosity grades. A 2% dispersion in cold water settles, on standing, in the form of a highly hydrated layer. Protect from variations in temperature and humidity which may cause caking. pH of a 1 g in 30 mL suspension in water is either between 3.0 and 5.0 or between 5.5 and 7.5.

### Uses

Sodium starch glycolate is used as a disintegrating agent in tablet manufacture.

## Tragacanth

E413; Goma Alcatira; Goma de tragacanto; Gomme Adragante; Gum Dragon; Gum Tragacanth; Trag.; Tragacantha; Tragacanto; Tragant.

*CAS — 9000-65-1.*

**Pharmacopoeias.** In *Eur.* (see p.vi), *Jpn*, and *Pol.* Also in *USNF.*

**Ph. Eur. 5.0** (Tragacanth). The air-hardened gummy exudation flowing naturally or obtained by incision from the trunk and branches of *Astragalus gummifer* and some other species of *Astragalus* (Leguminosae) from western Asia. It occurs as thin, flattened, ribbon-like, white or pale yellow, translucent, horny strips. When reduced to a powder it forms a mucilaginous gel with about ten times its weight of water. Protect from light.

**USNF 22** (Tragacanth). The dried gummy exudation from *Astragalus gummifer* or other Asiatic species of *Astragalus* (Leguminosae). It occurs as odourless, flattened, lamellated, frequently curved fragments or straight or spirally twisted linear pieces. It is white to weak yellow, translucent, and horny in texture. Powdered tragacanth is white to yellowish-white.

### Adverse Effects

Hypersensitivity reactions, sometimes severe, have occurred rarely after the ingestion of products containing tragacanth. Contact dermatitis has been reported following the external use of tragacanth.

### Uses

Tragacanth forms viscous solutions or gels with water, depending on the concentration. It is used in pharmaceutical manufacturing as a suspending agent and as an emulsifying agent. In dispensing aqueous preparations of tragacanth, the powdered tragacanth is first dispersed in a wetting agent, such as alcohol, to prevent agglomeration on the addition of water.

Tragacanth is also used for similar purposes in the food industry.

## Xanthan Gum

Corn Sugar Gum; E415; Goma de xantana; Polysaccharide B 1459; Xantham Gum; Xanthani Gummi.

*CAS — 11138-66-2.*

**Pharmacopoeias.** In *Eur.* (see p.vi). Also in *USNF.*

**Ph. Eur. 5.0** (Xanthan Gum). A gum produced by fermentation of a carbohydrate with *Xanthomonas campestris* and purified. It is the sodium, potassium, or calcium salt of a high-molecular-weight polysaccharide containing D-glucose, mannose, and glucuronic acid. It also contains not less than 1.5% of pyruvic acid, calculated with reference to the dried substance. A white or yellowish-white, free-flowing powder. Soluble in water giving a highly viscous solution; practically insoluble in organic solvents. A 1% solution in water has a pH of 6.0 to 8.0.

**USNF 22** (Xanthan Gum). A high-molecular-weight polysaccharide gum produced by a pure-culture fermentation of a carbohydrate with *Xanthomonas campestris* and purified. It contains D-glucose, D-mannose, and D-glucuronic acid. It is prepared as the sodium, potassium, or calcium salt. A cream-coloured powder. Soluble in hot or cold water. Its solutions are neutral to litmus.

### Uses

Xanthan gum is used in pharmaceutical manufacturing as a suspending, stabilising, thickening, and emulsifying agent. It is also used similarly in the food industry.

◊ Suspensions of crushed tablets or insoluble powders made with xanthan gum were reported to be preferable to those made with tragacanth.[1]

The stability was generally good and only a small number of drugs had been found to be incompatible (amitriptyline, tamoxifen, and verapamil).[1] For extemporaneous dispensing, a 1% solution of xanthan gum with hydroxybenzoate, prepared in advance, was diluted to 0.5% with water when preparing the suspension.

Xanthan gum was found to be a suitable suspending vehicle for delivering antispasmodics topically along the length of the oesophagus in patients with oesophageal spasm.[2] Coagulation of the gum had been observed when it was used for suspensions of certain film-coated tablets.

1. Anonymous. "Extremely useful" new suspending agent. *Pharm J* 1986; **237:** 665.
2. Evans BK, Fenton-May V. Keltrol. *Pharm J* 1986; **237:** 736–7.

### Preparations

***USNF 22:*** Xanthan Gum Solution.

**Proprietary Preparations** (details are given in Part 3)
***Ger.:*** Ronfnyl; ***Malaysia:*** Ronfnyl; ***Switz.:*** TenderWet.

**Multi-ingredient:** ***Ital.:*** Resource Gelificata.

# Stimulants and Anorectics

Hyperactivity, p.1583
Narcoleptic syndrome, p.1583
Obesity, p.1583
Prader-Willi syndrome, p.1584

This chapter includes compounds used, generally under specialist supervision, for their central stimulant or their anorectic effects. Many are sympathomimetics and are subject to extensive abuse, which has led to strict limitations on their availability.

## Hyperactivity

Attention deficit hyperactivity disorder (ADHD) is a syndrome of developmentally inappropriate and socially disruptive behaviour beginning in childhood and characterised by varying degrees of hyperactivity, inattention, and impulsiveness. Children with ADHD are easily distracted and have difficulty in completing tasks. Associated features may include low frustration tolerance, mood lability, and defiance. Some children continue to have symptoms throughout adolescence and into adulthood. The terms hyperkinesis, hyperkinetic syndrome, minimal brain dysfunction, attention deficit disorder, and attention deficit disorder with hyperactivity have sometimes been used synonymously for ADHD, but patients described as having these disorders do not necessarily satisfy the diagnostic criteria for ADHD.

Both drug and behaviour therapy may be used for the management of ADHD. Drug therapy is useful for the control of symptoms but is not curative. In the USA drug treatment for ADHD is quite common even in mild forms, and in the hands of specialists appears superior to behavioural therapy, but in the UK drugs are generally reserved for the more severely affected child who fails to respond to counselling and behaviour therapy.

Dexamfetamine and methylphenidate are usually the drugs of first choice but there is no consensus on which is the more effective. Pemoline has been used but is associated with hepatotoxicity. Most children who benefit from drug therapy appear to require several years of treatment. Prolonged use of central stimulants can retard growth and some recommend occasional drug holidays to allow catch-up growth and determine whether continued therapy is necessary; many authorities consider that young children should not receive stimulants. Stimulants appear to be of use when the disorder persists into adulthood.

Tricyclic antidepressants such as imipramine and desipramine are also used for ADHD in both children and adults and their effect appears to be independent of their antidepressant action. However, they tend to be reserved for patients who fail to respond to, or are intolerant of, central stimulants. Tricyclic antidepressants may be useful in patients with co-existing Tourette's syndrome or in those with a family history of the disorder, as stimulants are believed to precipitate or exacerbate associated tics (p.664). Tricyclic antidepressants might also be preferred in patients with co-existing anxiety, depression, or enuresis, or in those with a history of drug abuse. Use with central stimulants has been studied but careful monitoring is advised (see also Interactions under Dexamfetamine, p.1586). MAOIs have been used successfully but problems with dietary restriction and potential drug interactions have limited their use. SSRIs such as fluoxetine have produced beneficial results as an adjunct to central stimulants in a small number of patients with associated depression or obsessive-compulsive disorder, but their value in ADHD alone is unclear. Bupropion has shown promising results in controlled studies in children but may exacerbate tics and increase the risk of seizures in predisposed patients. Venlafaxine has been effective in open trials in a small number of adult patients. The selective noradrenaline reuptake inhibitor atomoxetine is also effective.

There is some evidence that carbamazepine may be an effective alternative to central stimulants. Clonidine has been used successfully with stimulants in children with an inadequate response to stimulants alone. However, there have been reports of adverse cardiac events associated with such combinations. Antipsychotics can produce severe adverse effects and are probably only warranted as adjunctive therapy to central stimulants in severe cases or when there is also extremely violent or destructive behaviour. Dopaminergics such as levodopa or pergolide have been tried with beneficial results for the treatment of restless legs syndrome and periodic limb movements in sleep associated with ADHD; some improvements in ADHD symptoms were also noted following resolution of the parasomnias.

Much controversy has surrounded the hypothesis that certain synthetic food additives including preservatives and artificial flavours and colours are aetiological agents in ADHD. Controlled studies have not proved the efficacy of dietary manipulation.

References.

1. Fox AM, Rieder MJ. Risks and benefits of drugs used in the management of the hyperactive child. *Drug Safety* 1993; **9:** 38–50.
2. Barbaresi WJ. Primary-care approach to the diagnosis and management of attention-deficit hyperactivity disorder. *Mayo Clin Proc* 1996; **71:** 463–71.
3. Committee on Children With Disabilities and Committee on Drugs. Medication for children with attention disorders. *Pediatrics* 1996; **98:** 301–4.
4. Cyr M, Brown CS. Current drug therapy recommendations for the treatment of attention deficit hyperactivity disorder. *Drugs* 1998; **56:** 215–23.
5. Goldman LS, *et al.* Diagnosis and treatment of attention-deficit/hyperactivity disorder in children and adolescents. *JAMA* 1998; **279:** 1100–1107.
6. Wender PH. Pharmacotherapy of attention-deficit/hyperactivity disorder in adults. *J Clin Psychiatry* 1998; **59** (suppl 7): 76–9.
7. Swanson JM, *et al.* Attention-deficit hyperactivity disorder and hyperkinetic disorder. *Lancet* 1998; **351:** 429–33.
8. Zametkin AJ, Ernst M. Problems in the management of attention-deficit-hyperactivity disorder. *N Engl J Med* 1999; **340:** 40–6.
9. Elia J, *et al.* Treatment of attention-deficit-hyperactivity disorder. *N Engl J Med* 1999; **340:** 780–8.
10. The MTA Cooperative Group. A 14-month randomized clinical trial of treatment strategies for attention-deficit/hyperactivity disorder. *Arch Gen Psychiatry* 1999; **56:** 1073–86.
11. Overmeyer S, Taylor E. Annotation: principles of treatment for hyperkinetic disorder: practice approaches for the UK. *J Child Psychol Psychiatry* 1999; **40:** 1147–57.
12. Trollor JN. Attention deficit hyperactivity disorder in adults: conceptual and clinical issues. *Med J Aust* 1999; **171:** 421–5.
13. Jadad AR, *et al. Treatment of attention-deficit/hyperactivity disorder.* Rockville, MD: Agency for Healthcare Research and Quality; 1999. Available at: http://www.ahcpr.gov/clinic/epcsums/adhdsum.htm (accessed 15/04/04)
14. Spencer T, *et al.* Pharmacotherapy of attention deficit hyperactivity disorder. *Child Adolesc Psychiatr Clin North Am* 2000; **9:** 77–97.
15. National Institute for Clinical Excellence. Guidance on the use of methylphenidate (Ritalin, Equasym) for attention deficit/hyperactivity disorder (ADHD) in childhood (issued October 2000). Available at: http://www.nice.org.uk/pdf/Methylph-guidance13.pdf (accessed 15/04/04)
16. Anonymous. Stimulant drugs for severe hyperactivity in childhood. *Drug Ther Bull* 2001; **39:** 52–4.
17. Scottish Intercollegiate Guidelines Network. Attention deficit and hyperkinetic disorders in children and young people: a national clinical guideline (issued June 2001). Available at: http://www.sign.ac.uk/pdf/sign52.pdf (accessed 15/04/04)
18. American Academy of Pediatrics, Subcommittee on Attention-Deficit/Hyperactivity Disorder and Committee on Quality Improvement. Clinical practice guideline: treatment of the school-aged child with attention-deficit/hyperactivity disorder. *Pediatrics* 2001; **108:** 1033–44. Also available at http://aappolicy.aappublications.org/cgi/reprint/pediatrics;108/4/1033.pdf (accessed 15/04/04)
19. Maidment ID. Efficacy of stimulants in adult ADHD. *Ann Pharmacother* 2003; **37:** 1884–90.
20. Wilens TE. Drug therapy for adults with attention-deficit hyperactivity disorder. *Drugs* 2003; **63:** 2395–2411.
21. Kutcher S, *et al.* International consensus statement on attention-deficit/hyperactivity disorder (ADHD) and disruptive behaviour disorders (DBDs): clinical implications and treatment practice suggestions. *Eur Neuropsychopharmacol* 2004; **14:** 11–28.

## Narcoleptic syndrome

**Narcolepsy** is characterised by excessive daytime sleepiness and irresistible sleep attacks that last from a few minutes to hours. The narcoleptic syndrome often includes **cataplexy**, a sudden short-lived loss of muscle tone and paralysis of voluntary muscles induced by strong emotions. The severity of the attack can vary and some patients experience complete collapse but there is no loss of consciousness. **Sleep paralysis** consists of transient episodes of complete paralysis while falling asleep or during waking; respiration is unaffected. Some patients also have vivid auditory or visual hallucinations while falling asleep (**hypnagogic hallucinations**) or disturbed sleep.

For the management of narcoleptic syndrome the patient is initially encouraged to take planned regular short periods of sleep during the day and to avoid stressful events that may provoke attacks. If drug treatment is required then central stimulants are the main drugs used for the sleep attacks of narcolepsy. However, most are ineffective against cataplexy. The selection, dose, and timing of administration of these drugs needs to be titrated for each patient and drug holidays have been suggested to reduce the risk of developing tolerance. Amfetamines were the first drugs used. However, methylphenidate is often preferred to dexamfetamine as it has a rapid action and is considered to have fewer adverse effects. Alternative non-amfetamine stimulants used in the treatment of narcolepsy include mazindol, which also appears to be effective in cataplexy, and modafinil. Selegiline has been reported to improve excessive daytime sleepiness and cataplexy. There is a wide range of other drugs for which there is anecdotal or other limited evidence of efficacy in narcolepsy but there appears to be no evidence that they are superior to the central stimulants.

Tricyclic antidepressants are the primary treatment for cataplexy and sleep paralysis. Imipramine appears to be one of the most widely used and has been reported to act more rapidly and to require a lower dose for cataplexy than when used as an antidepressant. The daily dose should be titrated to provide maximal protection for the time of day when symptoms usually occur. Clomipramine and protriptyline are also commonly used.

The use of sodium oxybate at night with stimulants during the day has been reported to improve the symptoms of patients with narcoleptic syndrome.

Patients requiring treatment for both narcolepsy and cataplexy may be given central stimulants and tricyclic antidepressants but require careful monitoring as the combination may produce serious adverse effects such as cardiac arrhythmias or hypertension; see also Interactions of Dexamfetamine, p.1586.

References.

1. Richardson JW, *et al.* Narcolepsy update. *Mayo Clin Proc* 1990; **65:** 991–8.
2. Aldrich MS. Narcolepsy. *N Engl J Med* 1990; **323:** 389–94.
3. Parkes JD. Daytime sleepiness. *BMJ* 1993; **306:** 772–5.
4. Eisen J, *et al.* Psychotropic drugs and sleep. *BMJ* 1993; **306:** 1331–4.
5. Wise MS. Childhood narcolepsy. *Neurology* 1998; **50** (suppl 1): S37–S42.
6. Nishino S, Mignot E. Drug treatment of patients with insomnia and excessive daytime sleepiness. *Clin Pharmacokinet* 1999; **37:** 305–30.
7. Krahn LE, *et al.* Narcolepsy: new understanding of irresistible sleep. *Mayo Clin Proc* 2001; **76:** 185–94.
8. Mitler MM, Hayduk R. Benefits and risks of pharmacotherapy for narcolepsy. *Drug Safety* 2002; **25:** 791–809.

## Obesity

Obesity results from an imbalance between energy intake and energy expenditure and increases the risk of cardiovascular disease, diabetes mellitus, gallstones, respiratory disease, osteoarthritis, and some forms of cancer. The prevalence of obesity is increasing especially in developed countries. Obesity may be defined in terms of the body-mass index (BMI), which is the weight (kg) divided by the square of the height ($m^2$):

- BMI 25.0 to 29.9: overweight
- BMI 30.0 to 34.9: obese, moderate risk of co-morbidity
- BMI 35.0 to 39.9: obese, severe risk of co-morbidity
- BMI 40.0 or more: obese, very severe risk of co-morbidity

Weight loss appears to improve control of diabetes mellitus and hypertension, and to reduce cardiovascular risk factors but long-term benefits are difficult to assess as weight is often regained.

Initial management involves dietary modification and includes calorie restriction and changes in the dietary proportions of fat, protein, and carbohydrates. Physical activity should also be increased and excess alcohol avoided. These measures should be followed for at least 3 months. If there has then been less than 10% reduction in weight and the BMI is still above 30, drug treatment may be considered. For patients with associated risk factors such as diabetes mellitus, ischaemic heart disease, hyperlipidaemias, hypertension, or sleep apnoea, drugs may be considered when the BMI is 27 or 28. Combination drug therapy is not recommended. Drugs should be given initially for 12 weeks. If weight loss is less than 5% then they should be considered a failure and discontinued. If weight loss is more than 5% they may be continued and the patient monitored at monthly intervals. Treatment should be stopped once the BMI falls below 30 (or 27/28 as appropriate, see above), or if weight is regained, or there is any suspicion of toxicity.

Many drugs are capable of reducing appetite and have been used as such in the treatment of obesity. Both centrally acting (appetite suppressant, anorectic) drugs and those with a local action on the gastrointestinal tract have been used. However, toxicity has been a major problem with centrally acting drugs and very few are still in current use.

Appetite suppressants can be divided into two main groups: central stimulants that act on central catecholamine pathways and drugs acting on central serotonin pathways. Stimulants such as the amfetamines and phenmetrazine are no longer recommended because of their addictive potential. Other stimulants that have been used include diethylpropion, phentermine, mazindol, and phenylpropanolamine but they are also no longer recommended. The serotonergic drugs dexfenfluramine and fenfluramine were formerly used in long-term therapy (up to 1 year) but have both been associated with valvular heart defects and have generally been withdrawn worldwide. There have also been reports of valvular heart defects in patients receiving combinations of anorectics. UK and US guidelines therefore emphasise the centrally-acting serotonin and noradrenaline reuptake inhibitor sibutramine, and the gastric lipase inhibitor orlistat, as appropriate choices for the drug treatment of obesity, in combination with diet and exercise.

Other drugs that have been investigated include fluoxetine, which has been tried with some success, and ephedrine with caffeine. Bulk-forming drugs such as methylcellulose and sterculia have been used in an attempt to control appetite by the local effect they might exert when they swell in the gastrointestinal tract, but there is little evidence of efficacy. Nondigestible fat substitutes such as sucrose polyesters have been promoted by the food industry, as part of a strategy to reduce fat and calories in the diet to aid body-weight control.

The control of appetite and the mechanisms of obesity are under investigation. A gene, called the ob-gene, and its protein product, leptin, have been identified and appear to be involved in regulation of food intake.

References.


1. Epstein LH, *et al.* Treatment of pediatric obesity. *Pediatrics* 1998; **101:** 554–70.
2. Kolanowski J. A risk-benefit assessment of anti-obesity drugs. *Drug Safety* 1999; **20:** 119–31.
3. Carek PJ, Dickerson LM. Current concepts in the pharmacological management of obesity. *Drugs* 1999; **57:** 883–904.
4. Collazo-Clavell ML. Safe and effective management of the obese patient. *Mayo Clin Proc* 1999; **74:** 1255–60.
5. Egger G, *et al.* The effectiveness of popular, non-prescription weight loss supplements. *Med J Aust* 1999; **171:** 604–8.
6. WHO. Obesity: preventing and managing the global epidemic. *WHO Tech Rep Ser 894* 2000.
7. National Heart, Lung, and Blood Institute. The practical guide: identification, evaluation, and treatment of overweight and obesity in adults (October 2000). Available at: http://www.nhlbi.nih.gov/guidelines/obesity/practgde.htm (accessed 15/04/04)
8. Glazer G. Long-term pharmacotherapy of obesity 2000: a review of efficacy and safety. *Arch Intern Med* 2001; **161:** 1814–24.
9. Royal College of Physicians of London. *Anti-obesity drugs: guidance on appropriate prescribing and management.* Salisbury: Royal College of Physicians of London, 2003.
10. ASHP Commission on Therapeutics. ASHP therapeutic position statement on the safe use of pharmacotherapy for obesity management in adults (approved April 23, 2001). *Am J Health-Syst Pharm* 2001; **58:** 1645–55.
11. Yanovski SZ, Yanovski JA. Obesity. *N Engl J Med* 2002; **346:** 591–602.
12. Hitchcock Noël P, Pugh JA. Management of overweight and obese adults. *BMJ* 2002; **325:** 757–61.
13. Fernández-López JA, *et al.* Pharmacological approaches for the treatment of obesity. *Drugs* 2002; **62:** 915–44.


### Prader-Willi syndrome

Compulsive eating and a voracious appetite are two of the many clinical features of Prader-Willi syndrome, a congenital disorder characterised by infantile hypotonia, hypogonadism, and facial dysmorphism, with subsequent development of abnormalities of behaviour and intellect.[1,2] Supervision and restricted access to food are the mainstay in preventing obesity, but are commonly not sufficient. Fluoxetine may decrease food intake in some patients. It has also been tried for associated self-mutilatory behaviour (skin picking) with variable results.[3,4] Growth hormone may be of benefit in increasing associated short stature and decreasing percentage body fat,[5-7] but close surveillance of glucose homoeostasis is advisable and there have been reports of fatalities in patients with severe obesity or risk factors for respiratory impairment or obstruction. Anorectics have been ineffective.[2]


1. Donaldson MDC, *et al.* The Prader-Willi syndrome. *Arch Dis Child* 1994; **70:** 58–63.
2. Couper RTL, Couper JJ. Prader-Willi syndrome. *Lancet* 2000; **356:** 673–5.
3. Warnock JK, Kestenbaum T. Pharmacologic treatment of severe skin-picking behaviors in Prader-Willi syndrome. *Arch Dermatol* 1992; **128:** 1623–5.
4. Schepis C, *et al.* Failure of fluoxetine to modify the skin-picking behaviour of Prader-Willi syndrome. *Australas J Dermatol* 1998; **39:** 57–60.
5. Lindgren AC, *et al.* Five years of growth hormone treatment in children with Prader-Willi syndrome. *Acta Paediatr Suppl* 1999; **433:** 109–11.
6. Myers SE, *et al.* Physical effects of growth hormone treatment in children with Prader-Willi syndrome. *Acta Paediatr Suppl* 1999; **433:** 112–14.
7. Paterson WF, Donaldson MDC. Growth hormone therapy in the Prader-Willi syndrome. *Arch Dis Child* 2003; **88:** 283–5.


## Adrafinil *(rINN)*

Adrafinilo; CRL-40048. 2-[(Diphenylmethyl)sulfinyl]acetohydroxamic acid.

$C_{15}H_{15}NO_3S$ = 289.3.

*CAS — 63547-13-7.*

*ATC — N06BX17.*

### Profile

Adrafinil is a central stimulant and alpha$_1$-adrenergic agonist chemically related to modafinil (p.1591). It is given by mouth for mental function impairment in the elderly in doses of 600 mg to 1.2 g daily.

### Preparations

**Proprietary Preparations** (details are given in Part 3)
***Fr.:*** Olmifon.

## Almitrine Dimesilate *(BANM, rINNM)*

Almitrine Bismesylate; Almitrine Dimesylate; Almitrine Mesylate *(USAN)*; Dimesilato de almitrina; S-2620 (almitrine or almitrine dimesilate). *NN*′-Diallyl-6-[4-(4,4′-difluorobenzhydryl)piperazin-1-yl]-1,3,5-triazine-2,4-diyldiamine bis(methanesulphonate).

$C_{26}H_{29}F_2N_7,2CH_4SO_3$ = 669.8.

*CAS — 27469-53-0 (almitrine); 29608-49-9 (almitrine dimesilate).*

*ATC — R07AB07.*

### Profile

Almitrine dimesilate has been used as a respiratory stimulant in acute respiratory failure associated with conditions such as chronic obstructive pulmonary disease. Usual oral doses range from 50 to 100 mg daily and treatment may be intermittent. Up to 3 mg/kg has been given daily by intravenous infusion in 2 or 3 divided doses, each dose being infused over 2 hours. It is also available in a compound preparation with raubasine for mental function impairment in the elderly.

**Mental impairment.** References.


1. Poitrenaud J, *et al.* Almitrine-raubasine and cognitive impairment in the elderly: results of a 6-month controlled multicenter study. *Clin Neuropharmacol* 1990; **13** (suppl 3): S100–S108.
2. Poitrenaud J, *et al.* Time course of age-associated memory impairment in 8037 patients treated with Duxil for 6 months. *Rev Geriatr* 1994; **19:** 531–8.
3. Poitrenaud J, *et al.* Memory disorders in 8037 elderly patients with age-associated memory impairment: multicenter trial with a 6-month follow-up under almitrine-raubasine. *Eur Neurol* 1995; **35** (suppl 1): 43–6.
4. Allain H, Bentue-Ferrer D. Clinical efficacy of almitrine-raubasine: an overview. *Eur Neurol* 1998; **39:** (suppl 1) 39–44.


**Respiratory system disorders.** Respiratory stimulants (such as almitrine) have a limited and short-term role in acute respiratory failure in chronic obstructive pulmonary disease (p.779). Almitrine has been reported[1-3] to improve ventilation and blood oxygenation, and to decrease the number of episodes of dyspnoea and hospital admissions. There are also reports[4,5] of beneficial effects when used with inhaled nitric oxide in patients with severe hypoxaemic acute respiratory distress syndrome (p.1075) as well as in patients with hypoxia caused by focal lung lesions.[6] However, these modest benefits may be outweighed by the adverse effects, which have included peripheral paraesthesia and weight loss,[1] and headache, urticaria, breathlessness, diarrhoea, chest pain, nausea, and vomiting.[3] The peripheral neuropathy that sometimes occurs during long-term use of almitrine[7,8] may be due to an underlying feature of the pulmonary disease being treated,[9-11] although some disagree with this.[12]


1. Watanabe S, *et al.* Long-term effect of almitrine bismesylate in patients with hypoxemic chronic obstructive pulmonary disease. *Am Rev Respir Dis* 1989; **140:** 1269–73.
2. Daskalopoulou E, *et al.* Comparison of almitrine bismesylate and medroxyprogesterone acetate on oxygenation during wakefulness and sleep in patients with chronic obstructive lung disease. *Thorax* 1990; **45:** 666–9.
3. Bakran I, *et al.* Double-blind placebo controlled clinical trial of almitrine bismesylate in patients with chronic respiratory insufficiency. *Eur J Clin Pharmacol* 1990; **38:** 249–53.
4. Jolliet P, *et al.* Additive beneficial effects of the prone position, nitric oxide, and almitrine bismesylate on gas exchange and oxygen transport in acute respiratory distress syndrome. *Crit Care Med* 1997; **25:** 786–94.
5. Gallart L, *et al.* The NO Almitrine Study Group. Intravenous almitrine combined with inhaled nitric oxide for acute respiratory distress syndrome. *Am J Respir Crit Care Med* 1998; **158:** 1770–7.
6. Payen D, *et al.* Inhaled nitric oxide, almitrine infusion, or their coadministration as a treatment of severe hypoxemic focal lung lesions. *Anesthesiology* 1998; **89:** 1157–65.
7. Chedru F, *et al.* Peripheral neuropathy during treatment with almitrine. *BMJ* 1985; **290:** 896.
8. Gherardi R, *et al.* Peripheral neuropathy in patients treated with almitrine dimesylate. *Lancet* 1985; **i:** 1247–50.
9. Suggett AJ, *et al.* Almitrine and peripheral neuropathy. *Lancet* 1985; **ii:** 830–1.
10. Alani SM, *et al.* Almitrine and peripheral neuropathy. *Lancet* 1985; **ii:** 1251.
11. Moore N, *et al.* Peripheral neuropathy in chronic obstructive lung disease. *Lancet* 1985; **ii:** 1311.
12. Louarn F, Gherardi R. Almitrine and peripheral neuropathy. *Lancet* 1985; **ii:** 1068.


### Preparations

**Proprietary Preparations** (details are given in Part 3)
***Belg.:*** Vectarion; ***Braz.:*** Vectarion; ***Denm.:*** Vectarion; ***Fr.:*** Vectarion; ***Ger.:*** Vectarion†; ***Irl.:*** Vectarion; ***Port.:*** Vectarion†; ***Spain:*** Vectarion.

**Multi-ingredient: *Fr.:*** Duxil; ***Hong Kong:*** Duxaril; ***Port.:*** Duxil; Transoxyl; ***Singapore:*** Duxaril; ***Spain:*** Duxor; Salvalion†; ***Thai.:*** Duxaril.

## Amfetamine *(BAN, rINN)*

Amphetamine; Anfetamina; Racemic Desoxynorephedrine. (*R*,*S*)-α-Methylphenethylamine.

$C_9H_{13}N$ = 135.2.

*CAS — 300-62-9 (amfetamine); 139-10-6 (amfetamine phosphate).*

*ATC — N06BA01.*

## Amfetamine Sulfate *(rINNM)*

Amfetamine Sulphate *(BANM)*; Amfetamini Sulfas; Amphetamine Sulfate; Amphetamine Sulphate; Phenaminum; Phenylaminopropanum Racemicum Sulfuricum; Sulfato de anfetamina. (*R*,*S*)-α-Methylphenethylamine sulphate.

$(C_9H_{13}N)_2,H_2SO_4$ = 368.5.

*CAS — 60-13-9.*

*ATC — N06BA01.*

**Pharmacopoeias.** In *Chin., Eur.* (see p.vi), and *US.*

**Ph. Eur. 5.0** (Amfetamine Sulphate). A white powder. Freely soluble in water; slightly soluble in alcohol. Protect from light.

**USP 27** (Amphetamine Sulfate). A white odourless crystalline powder. Freely soluble in water; slightly soluble in alcohol; practically insoluble in ether. Its solutions are acid to litmus, having a pH of 5 to 6.

**Incompatibility.** Amfetamine sulfate is incompatible with alkalis and calcium salts.

### Profile

Amfetamine is an indirect-acting sympathomimetic with actions and uses similar to those of its isomer dexamfetamine (p.1585). Amfetamine, amfetamine sulfate, and amfetamine aspartate are given by mouth in doses similar to those of dexamfetamine sulfate. The laevo-isomer, levamfetamine was formerly used in a similar manner. Amfetamine, being volatile, was formerly employed by inhalation.

**Breast feeding.** Amfetamine is concentrated in breast milk and the American Academy of Pediatrics has stated[1] that it has caused irritability and poor sleep pattern in breast-feeding infants when used as a drug of abuse by mothers.


1. American Academy of Pediatrics. The transfer of drugs and other chemicals into human milk. *Pediatrics* 2001; **108:** 776–89. Correction. *ibid.*; 1029. Also available at: http://aappolicy.aappublications.org/cgi/content/full/pediatrics%3b108/3/776 (accessed 15/04/04)


### Preparations

***USP 27:*** Amphetamine Sulfate Tablets.

**Proprietary Preparations** (details are given in Part 3)
***Spain:*** Centramina†.

**Multi-ingredient: *Belg.:*** Epipropane; ***Fr.:*** Ortenal†; ***USA:*** Adderall.

## Amfetaminil *(rINN)*

Amphetaminil; Anfetaminilo. α-(α-Methylphenethylamino)-α-phenylacetonitrile.

$C_{17}H_{18}N_2$ = 250.3.

*CAS — 17590-01-1.*

### Profile

Amfetaminil is a central stimulant that has been given by mouth in doses of 10 to 30 mg daily in the treatment of narcolepsy (p.1583).

### Preparations

**Proprietary Preparations** (details are given in Part 3)
***Ger.:*** AN 1.

## Amiphenazole Hydrochloride *(BANM, rINNM)*

Amiphenazole Chloride; Hidrocloruro de amifenazol. 5-Phenylthiazole-2,4-diamine hydrochloride.

$C_9H_9N_3S,HCl$ = 227.7.

*CAS — 490-55-1 (amiphenazole); 942-31-4 (amiphenazole hydrochloride).*

### Profile

Amiphenazole hydrochloride has properties similar to those of doxapram hydrochloride (p.1587) and has been used intramuscularly or intravenously as a respiratory stimulant.

Lichenoid reactions have been reported in addition to those reactions expected from its central activity.

## Ammonium Camphocarbonate

Canfocarbonato de amonio.

$C_{11}H_{19}NO_3$ = 213.3.

*CAS — 5972-75-8.*

### Profile

Ammonium camphocarbonate has been used in preparations for the treatment of respiratory-tract disorders.

### Preparations

**Proprietary Preparations** (details are given in Part 3)

**Multi-ingredient:** ***Spain:*** Pulmofasa; Pulmofasa Antihist†.

## Atomoxetine Hydrochloride *(BANM, USAN, rINNM)*

Hidrocloruro de tomoxetina; LY-135252; LY-139602; LY-139603; Tomoxetine Hydrochloride. (−)-*N*-Methyl-γ-(2-methylphenoxy)-benzenepropanamine hydrochloride.

$C_{17}H_{21}NO,HCl$ = 291.8.

*CAS — 83015-26-3 (atomoxetine); 82248-59-7 (atomoxetine hydrochloride).*

*ATC — N06BA09.*

### Adverse Effects and Precautions

Adverse effects reported in patients receiving atomoxetine include dyspepsia and other gastrointestinal disturbances, anorexia and weight loss, fatigue, sleep disturbances, dizziness, irritability and emotional lability, cough, sinusitis or rhinorrhoea, urinary hesitancy or retention, decreased libido and sexual dysfunction, skin rashes, increased sweating, and hot flushes. Hypersensitivity reactions have occurred rarely.

There may be increases in blood pressure and heart rate, and atomoxetine should be given with caution to patients with hypertension, tachycardia or pre-existing cardiovascular disease. Orthostatic hypotension has also been reported.

Use of atomoxetine is contra-indicated in patients with angle-closure glaucoma. The effects of long-term therapy on growth in children and adolescents are uncertain: the manufacturer recommends that growth be monitored and consideration given to interrupting treatment in patients who are not growing or gaining weight satisfactorily.

Poor metabolisers of atomoxetine (see Pharmacokinetics, below) may have an increased risk of adverse reactions.

### Interactions

Atomoxetine should not be taken with an MAOI, or within 2 weeks of stopping MAOI therapy, nor should MAOI therapy be begun for 2 weeks after stopping atomoxetine. Care should be taken if given with other drugs that raise blood pressure, because of a possible additive affect; the actions of salbutamol on the cardiovascular system may be potentiated.

Atomoxetine is metabolised via the cytochrome P450 isoenzyme CYP2D6 and inhibitors of this enzyme such as paroxetine, fluoxetine, and quinidine may increase plasma concentrations of atomoxetine in extensive, but not poor, metabolisers.

**Antidepressants.** *Paroxetine* was found to inhibit atomoxetine's metabolism by cytochrome P450 isoenzyme CYP2D6 in extensive metabolisers resulting in pharmacokinetics for atomoxetine similar to those in poor metabolisers.[1]

1. Belle DJ, *et al.* Effect of potent CYP2D6 inhibition by paroxetine on atomoxetine pharmacokinetics. *J Clin Pharmacol* 2002; **42:** 1219–27.

### Pharmacokinetics

Atomoxetine is well absorbed after oral administration, with peak plasma concentrations 1 to 2 hours after a dose. Bioavailability is about 94% in poor metabolisers but only 63% in extensive metabolisers. Atomoxetine is metabolised primarily via the cytochrome P450 isoenzyme CYP2D6 to the active metabolite 4-hydroxyatomoxetine; a minority of the population are poor metabolisers and experience plasma concentrations about 5 times those in extensive metabolisers. It is excreted in the urine as glucuronide metabolites and a small amount of unchanged drug; less than 17% of a dose is excreted in the faeces. The half-life of atomoxetine is about 5.2 hours in extensive and 21.6 hours in poor metabolisers.

### Uses and Administration

Atomoxetine hydrochloride is a selective noradrenaline reuptake inhibitor used in the treatment of attention deficit hyperactivity disorder (p.1583) in adults and children. It is given as the hydrochloride although doses are expressed in terms of the base; atomoxetine hydrochloride 11.4 mg is approximately equivalent to 10 mg atomoxetine base.

In *adults and children over 70 kg*, the initial dose is the equivalent of 40 mg daily gradually increased after at least 7 days to 80 mg daily. A further increase to a maximum of 100 mg daily may be made after 2 to 4 weeks. In *children and adolescents of 70 kg and under*, the initial dose is the equivalent of about 500 micrograms/kg daily; this may be gradually increased after at least 7 days to about 1.2 mg/kg daily. The total daily dose in this group should not exceed 1.4 mg/kg or 100 mg, whichever is less. Doses may be given as either a single dose in the morning or as equally divided doses in the morning and late afternoon or early evening.

Reduced doses are recommended in patients with hepatic impairment, see below.

◊ References.

1. Spencer T, *et al.* Effectiveness and tolerability of tomoxetine in adults with attention deficit hyperactivity disorder. *Am J Psychiatry* 1998; **155:** 693–5.
2. Michelson D, *et al.* Atomoxetine in the treatment of children and adolescents with attention-deficit/hyperactivity disorder: a randomized, placebo-controlled, dose-response study. *Pediatrics* 2001; **108:** 1197. Full version: http://pediatrics.aappublications.org/cgi/content/full/108/5/e83 (accessed 15/04/04)
3. Simpson D, Plosker GL. Atomoxetine: a review of its use in adults with attention deficit hyperactivity disorder. *Drugs* 2004; **64:** 205–22.

**Administration in hepatic impairment.** In patients with moderate hepatic impairment the dose of atomoxetine (see above) should be reduced by 50%, while in those with severe impairment it should be reduced by 75%.

References.

1. Chalon SA, *et al.* Effect of hepatic impairment on the pharmacokinetics of atomoxetine and its metabolites. *Clin Pharmacol Ther* 2003; **73:** 178–91.

### Preparations

**Proprietary Preparations** (details are given in Part 3)

***Austral.:*** Strattera; ***UK:*** Strattera; ***USA:*** Strattera.

## Bemegride *(BAN, rINN)*

Bemegrida; Bemegridum. 3-Ethyl-3-methylglutarimide; 4-Ethyl-4-methylpiperidine-2,6-dione.

$C_8H_{13}NO_2$ = 155.2.

*CAS — 64-65-3.*

*ATC — R07AB05.*

### Profile

Bemegride has properties similar to those of doxapram (p.1587). It has been given intravenously as a respiratory stimulant.

**Porphyria.** Bemegride has been associated with acute attacks of porphyria and is considered unsafe in porphyric patients.

## Benzfetamine Hydrochloride *(BANM, rINNM)*

Benzphetamine Hydrochloride; Hidrocloruro de benzfetamina. (+)-*N*-Benzyl-*N*,α-dimethylphenethylamine hydrochloride.

$C_{17}H_{21}N,HCl$ = 275.8.

*CAS — 156-08-1 (benzfetamine); 5411-22-3 (benzfetamine hydrochloride).*

### Profile

Benzfetamine hydrochloride is a central stimulant and sympathomimetic with properties similar to those of dexamfetamine (below). It has been used as an anorectic in the treatment of obesity (p.1583), although amfetamines are no longer recommended for this indication. The usual initial dose is 25 to 50 mg given once daily by mouth, subsequently adjusted, according to requirements, to a dose of 25 to 50 mg up to three times daily.

### Preparations

**Proprietary Preparations** (details are given in Part 3)

***USA:*** Didrex.

## Catha

Abyssinian, African, or Arabian Tea; Kat; Kath; Khat; Miraa; Qat.

**Description.** Catha consists of the leaves of *Catha edulis* (Celastraceae), and contains cathine, cathinone, celastrin, choline, tannins, and inorganic salts.

## Cathine *(pINN)*

Catina; (+)-Norpseudoephedrine. *threo*-2-Amino-1-phenylpropan-1-ol.

$C_9H_{13}NO$ = 151.2.

*CAS — 492-39-7; 36393-56-3.*

*ATC — A08AA07.*

## Cathinone *(pINN)*

Catinona. (*S*)-2-Aminopropiophenone.

$C_9H_{11}NO$ = 149.2.

*CAS — 71031-15-7.*

### Profile

Catha is used for its stimulant properties among some cultures of Africa and the Middle East, usually by chewing the leaves. Its effects are reported to resemble those of the amfetamines (see Dexamfetamine Sulfate, below), and are thought to be largely due to the content of cathinone. Dependence and psychotic reactions have been reported. Cathine, another constituent, is used as the hydrochloride as an anorectic.

◊ References to the pharmacology and pharmacokinetics of catha and its constituents[1-8] and reports of adverse effects.[9-14]

1. Brenneisen R, *et al.* Metabolism of cathinone to (−)-norephedrine and (−)-norpseudoephedrine. *J Pharm Pharmacol* 1986; **38:** 298–300.
2. Brenneisen R, *et al.* Amphetamine-like effects in humans of the khat alkaloid cathinone. *Br J Clin Pharmacol* 1990; **30:** 825–8.
3. Kalix P. Pharmacological properties of the stimulant khat. *Pharmacol Ther* 1990; **48:** 397–416.
4. Kalix P. Chewing khat, an old drug habit that is new in Europe. *Int J Risk Safety Med* 1992; **3:** 143–56.
5. Kalix P. Cathinone, a natural amphetamine. *Pharmacol Toxicol* 1992; **70:** 77–86.
6. Widler P, *et al.* Pharmacodynamics and pharmacokinetics of khat: a controlled study. *Clin Pharmacol Ther* 1994; **55:** 556–62.
7. Kalix P. Catha edulis, a plant that has amphetamine effects. *Pharm World Sci* 1996; **18:** 69–73.
8. Toennes SW, *et al.* Pharmacokinetics of cathinone, cathine and norephedrine after the chewing of khat leaves. *Br J Clin Pharmacol* 2003; **56:** 125–30.
9. Rumpf KW, *et al.* Rhabdomyolysis after ingestion of an appetite suppressant. *JAMA* 1983; **250:** 2112.
10. Gough SP, Cookson IB. Khat-induced schizophreniform psychosis in UK. *Lancet* 1984; **i:** 455.
11. Roper JP. The presumed neurotoxic effects of Catha edulis—an exotic plant now available in the United Kingdom. *Br J Ophthalmol* 1986; **70:** 779–81.
12. Zureikat N, *et al.* Chewing khat slows the orocaecal transit time. *Gut* 1992; **33** (suppl): S23.
13. Yousef G, *et al.* Khat chewing as a cause of psychosis. *Br J Hosp Med* 1995; **54:** 322–6.
14. Al-Motarreb A, *et al.* Khat chewing and acute myocardial infarction. *Heart* 2002; **87:** 279–280.

### Preparations

**Proprietary Preparations** (details are given in Part 3)

***Ger.:*** Antiadipositum X-112 S†; Mirapront N†; Vita-Schlanktropfen†; ***Hong Kong:*** Mirapront N†; ***Mex.:*** Insacial†; ***S.Afr.:*** Appetrol†; Dietene; Eetless; Leanor; Nobese No. 1; Slim 'n Trim; Thinz; ***Singapore:*** Mirapront N†; ***Switz.:*** Adistop†; Antiadipositum X-112; Belloform nouvelle formule; Limit-X; Miniscap; ***Thai.:*** Mirapront N.

## Clobenzorex Hydrochloride *(rINNM)*

Hidrocloruro de clobenzorex; SD-271-12. (+)-*N*-(2-Chlorobenzyl)-α-methylphenethylamine hydrochloride.

$C_{16}H_{18}ClN,HCl$ = 296.2.

*CAS — 13364-32-4 (clobenzorex); 5843-53-8 (clobenzorex hydrochloride).*

*ATC — A08AA08.*

### Profile

Clobenzorex hydrochloride is a central stimulant and sympathomimetic with properties similar to those of dexamfetamine (below). It has been used as an anorectic in the treatment of obesity (p.1583) but regulatory authorities in the European Union have called for the withdrawal of all anorectics from the market (see under Effects on the Cardiovascular System in Fenfluramine, p.1588).

### Preparations

**Proprietary Preparations** (details are given in Part 3)

***Mex.:*** Asenlix; Itravil; ***Port.:*** Dinintel†; ***Singapore:*** Dinintel†; ***Spain:*** Finedal†.

## Deanol *(BAN)*

Démanol. 2-Dimethylaminoethanol.

$C_4H_{11}NO$ = 89.14.

*CAS — 108-01-0 (deanol); 3342-61-8 (deanol aceglumate); 968-46-7 (deanol benzilate); 71-79-4 (deanol benzilate hydrochloride).*

*ATC — N06BX04.*

NOTE. Deanol Aceglumate is *pINN.*

### Profile

Deanol, a precursor of choline, may enhance central acetylcholine formation. It has been used as a central stimulant in the treatment of hyperactivity in children but its efficacy is not proven. It has been included in preparations used as tonics and for the management of impaired mental function.

It has been used as a variety of salts and esters including deanol aceglumate, deanol acetamidobenzoate, deanol bisorcate, deanol cyclohexylpropionate (cyprodenate; cyprodemanol), deanol hemisuccinate, deanol pidolate, and deanol tartrate. Deanol benzilate (deanol diphenylglycolate; benzacine) has been used as the hydrochloride in antispasmodic preparations.

### Preparations

**Proprietary Preparations** (details are given in Part 3)

***Belg.:*** Actebral; ***Fr.:*** Astyl; Cleregil†; Tonibral Adulte†; ***Ger.:*** Medacaps N†; Risatarun; ***Ital.:*** Rischiaril; ***Port.:*** Tonibral.

**Multi-ingredient:** ***Fr.:*** Acti 5; Debrumyl; ***Ger.:*** Rowachol comp; ***Port.:*** Actilam; Debrumyl; Forticol; Projuvex†; Tonice; ***Spain:*** Acticinco†; Anti Anorex Triple; Denubil; ***Switz.:*** Vigoran.

## Dexamfetamine Sulfate *(pINNM)*

Dexamfetamine Sulphate *(BANM)*; Dexamphetamine Sulphate; Dexamphetamini Sulfas; Dextro Amphetamine Sulphate; Dextroamphetamine Sulfate; NSC-73713 (dexamfetamine); Sulfato de dexanfetamina. (*S*)-α-Methylphenethylammonium sulphate; (+)-α-Methylphenethylamine sulphate.

$(C_9H_{13}N)_2,H_2SO_4$ = 368.5.

*CAS — 51-64-9 (dexamfetamine); 7528-00-9 (dexamfetamine phosphate); 51-63-8 (dexamfetamine sulfate).*

*ATC — N06BA02.*

**Pharmacopoeias.** In *Br., Swiss,* and *US.*

**BP 2003** (Dexamfetamine Sulphate). A white or almost white, odourless or almost odourless, crystalline powder. Freely soluble in water; slightly soluble in alcohol; practically insoluble in ether.

**USP 27** (Dextroamphetamine Sulfate). A white, odourless, crystalline powder. Soluble 1 in 10 of water and 1 in 800 of alcohol; insoluble in ether. pH of a 5% solution in water is between 5.0 and 6.0.

## Adverse Effects

The adverse effects of dexamfetamine are commonly symptoms of overstimulation of the CNS and include insomnia, night terrors, nervousness, restlessness, irritability, and euphoria that may be followed by fatigue and depression. There may be dryness of the mouth, anorexia, abdominal cramps and other gastrointestinal disturbances, headache, dizziness, tremor, sweating, tachycardia, palpitations, increased or sometimes decreased blood pressure, altered libido, and impotence. Psychotic reactions have occurred, as has muscle damage with associated rhabdomyolysis and renal complications. Rarely, cardiomyopathy has occurred with chronic use. In children, growth retardation may occur during prolonged treatment.

In *acute overdosage*, the adverse effects are accentuated and may be accompanied by hyperpyrexia, mydriasis, hyperreflexia, chest pain, cardiac arrhythmias, confusion, panic states, aggressive behaviour, hallucinations, delirium, convulsions, respiratory depression, coma, circulatory collapse, and death. Individual patient response may vary widely and toxic manifestations may occur with quite small overdoses.

*Tolerance* can develop to some of dexamfetamine's central effects leading to increased doses and habituation. Abrupt cessation after prolonged treatment or abuse of amfetamines has been associated with extreme fatigue, hyperphagia, and depression. However, it is generally accepted that the amfetamines, although widely abused, are not associated with substantial physical dependence.

*Abuse* of amfetamines for their euphoriant effects has resulted in personality changes, compulsive and stereotyped behaviour, and may induce a toxic psychosis with auditory and visual hallucinations and paranoid delusions.

**Abuse.** Abuse of amfetamines can lead to toxicity affecting many organs or body systems. There have been reports of *intracerebral haemorrhage*[1-3] and of *cardiomyopathy*.[4-6] *Acute myocardial infarction* has also occurred.[7]

A syndrome characterised by *circulatory collapse, fever, leukaemoid reaction, disseminated intravascular coagulation*, and *rhabdomyolysis* with *diffuse myalgias* and *muscle tenderness* has been described[8] in 5 drug abusers who had used amfetamines or phenmetrazine intravenously. In an earlier study,[9] *necrotising angiitis* was associated with intravenous metamfetamine abuse. A 30-year-old man who had ingested 50 amfetamine sulfate tablets developed *rhabdomyolysis* and *myoglobinuric renal failure*, possibly secondary to a crush syndrome, but in the absence of prolonged coma or other major myotoxic factors.[10] However, *acute interstitial nephritis* and *acute renal failure* have followed oral amfetamine abuse without the associated factors of rhabdomyolysis, hyperpyrexia, or necrotising angiitis.[11]

Chronic use may result in adverse effects such as *hallucinations*, a *delusional disorder* resembling *paranoid schizophrenia, stereotyped behaviour*, and *movement disorders*.[12] Although chronic intoxication is the most common precondition for psychosis, individual sensitivities are an important aspect of the drug reaction.

Increased serum concentrations of *thyroxine* have been associated with heavy amfetamine abuse in 4 psychiatric patients.[13]

Abrupt cessation after prolonged treatment or abuse of amfetamines may cause *extreme fatigue, hyperphagia*, and *depression*. *Depressive stupor* has been reported in 3 long-term abusers of amfetamine after sudden withdrawal.[14]

1. Delaney P, Estes M. Intracranial hemorrhage with amphetamine abuse. *Neurology* 1980; **30:** 1125–8.
2. Harrington H, *et al.* Intracerebral hemorrhage and oral amphetamine. *Arch Neurol* 1983; **40:** 503–7.
3. Salanova V, Taubner R. Intracerebral haemorrhage and vasculitis secondary to amphetamine use. *Postgrad Med J* 1984; **60:** 429–30.
4. Smith HJ, *et al.* Cardiomyopathy associated with amphetamine administration. *Am Heart J* 1976; **91:** 792–7.
5. Call TD, *et al.* Acute cardiomyopathy secondary to intravenous amphetamine abuse. *Ann Intern Med* 1982; **97:** 559–60.
6. Hong R, *et al.* Cardiomyopathy associated with the smoking of crystal methamphetamine. *JAMA* 1991; **265:** 1152–4.
7. Waksman J, *et al.* Acute myocardial infarction associated with amphetamine use. *Mayo Clin Proc* 2001; **76:** 323–6.
8. Kendrick WC, *et al.* Rhabdomyolysis and shock after intravenous amphetamine administration. *Ann Intern Med* 1977; **86:** 381–7.
9. Citron BP, *et al.* Necrotizing angiitis associated with drug abuse. *N Engl J Med* 1970; **283:** 1003–11.
10. Scandling J, Spital A. Amphetamine-associated myoglobinuric renal failure. *South Med J* 1982; **75:** 237–40.
11. Foley RJ, *et al.* Amphetamine-induced acute renal failure. *South Med J* 1984; **77:** 258–60.
12. Ellinwood EH, Kilbey MM. Fundamental mechanisms underlying altered behavior following chronic administration of psychomotor stimulants. *Biol Psychiatry* 1980; **15:** 749–57.
13. Morley JE, *et al.* Amphetamine-induced hyperthyroxinemia. *Ann Intern Med* 1980; **93:** 707–9.
14. Tuma TA. Depressive stupor following amphetamine withdrawal. *Br J Hosp Med* 1993; **49:** 361–3.

**Effects on growth.** The Pediatric Subcommittee of the FDA Psychopharmacologic Drugs Advisory Committee reviewed the growth-suppressing effects of stimulant medication in hyperkinetic children.[1] There was reasonable evidence that stimulant drugs, particularly in higher doses, moderately suppressed growth in weight and might have a minor suppressing effect on growth in stature. There were indications that some growth caught up during drug holidays, and that early growth suppression was not evident in adulthood. Careful monitoring during treatment was recommended.

See also under Methylphenidate Hydrochloride, p.1590.

1. Roche AF, *et al.* The effects of stimulant medication on the growth of hyperkinetic children. *Pediatrics* 1979; **63:** 847–50.

## Treatment of Adverse Effects

Activated charcoal may be given to delay absorption if the patient presents within 1 hour; gastric lavage may be considered in recent large ingestions. In general the management of overdosage with amfetamines involves supportive and symptomatic therapy. Sedation is usually sufficient. Forced acid diuresis has been advocated to increase amfetamine excretion but is seldom necessary and should only be considered in severely poisoned patients; it requires close supervision and monitoring.

## Precautions

Dexamfetamine is contra-indicated in patients with cardiovascular disease including moderate to severe hypertension, and in patients with hyperthyroidism, glaucoma, hyperexcitability, or agitated states. It should not be given to patients with a history of drug or alcohol abuse and it should be avoided in pregnant or breast-feeding women. It should be given with caution to patients with mild hypertension, renal impairment or unstable personality.

Height and weight in children should be monitored as growth retardation may occur. Behavioural disturbances and thought disorders may be exacerbated in psychotic children.

Prolonged high doses may need gradual withdrawal as abrupt cessation may produce fatigue and mental depression.

Care may be needed in certain patients predisposed to tics or Tourette's syndrome as symptoms may be provoked. Dexamfetamine is likely to reduce the convulsive threshold; caution is therefore advised in patients with epilepsy. However, it appears that in some countries amfetamines have been included in antiepileptic preparations containing phenytoin or phenobarbital in an attempt to increase their antiepileptic action. Amfetamines may impair patients' ability to drive or to operate machinery.

Diabetic control should be monitored when central stimulants are used for the control of obesity.

**Abuse.** Dexamfetamine is subject to extensive abuse and for this reason its availability is severely curtailed. For adverse effects associated with abuse, see above.

**Porphyria.** Amfetamines are considered to be unsafe in patients with porphyria although there is conflicting experimental evidence of porphyrinogenicity. Metamfetamine has been associated with acute attacks of porphyria.

**Pregnancy.** No difference was found in the incidence of severe congenital anomalies between 1824 children of mothers prescribed amfetamines or phenmetrazine during pregnancy and 8989 children of mothers who had not received these drugs.[1] Though an excess of oral clefts was noted in the offspring of mothers prescribed amfetamines, there was no excess of congenital heart disease.[1] This was contrary to a previous suggestion[2] in which congenital heart disease in 184 infants had been studied and a link to maternal dexamfetamine exposure postulated. There has been a report of a bradycardia followed by death in a fetus due to maternal intravenous self-administration of 500 mg of amfetamine.[3]

1. Milkovich L, van den Berg BJ. Effects of antenatal exposure to anorectic drugs. *Am J Obstet Gynecol* 1977; **129:** 637–42.
2. Nora JJ, *et al.* Dexamphetamine: a possible environmental trigger in cardiovascular malformations. *Lancet* 1970; **i:** 1290–1.
3. Dearlove JC, Betteridge TJ. Stillbirth due to intravenous amphetamine. *BMJ* 1992; **304:** 548.

**Tourette's syndrome.** A review[1] of clinical reports concluded that there was virtually no evidence that central stimulants caused or provoked Tourette's syndrome and weak or inadequate evidence that clinically appropriate doses of central stimulants caused tics in previously asymptomatic patients or exacerbated pre-existing symptoms. However, the authors suggested that there was evidence that high or toxic doses might exacerbate or provoke tics in predisposed patients. Long-term methylphenidate therapy did not appear to exacerbate motor or vocal tics in a study[2] of 34 children with ADHD and chronic multiple tic disorder who were followed up for 2 years. However, the authors did point out that careful clinical monitoring is essential to eliminate the possibility of drug-induced exacerbation in individual patients. In contrast, a report[3] on 15 children who developed Tourette's syndrome while receiving stimulant medication for hyperactivity considered that such therapy was contra-indicated in children with motor tics or diagnosed Tourette's syndrome and should be used with caution in children with a family history of these symptoms. In addition, it suggested that the development of motor tic symptoms in any child receiving stimulants should be a clear indication for immediate discontinuation to minimise the possibility of eliciting a full-blown Tourette's syndrome.

1. Shapiro AK, Shapiro E. Do stimulants provoke, cause, or exacerbate tics and Tourette syndrome? *Compr Psychiatry* 1981; **22:** 265–73.
2. Gadow KD, *et al.* Long-term methylphenidate therapy in children with comorbid attention-deficit hyperactivity disorder and chronic multiple tic disorder. *Arch Gen Psychiatry* 1999; **56:** 330–6.
3. Lowe TL, *et al.* Stimulant medications precipitate Tourette's syndrome. *JAMA* 1982; **247:** 1729–31.

## Interactions

Dexamfetamine is an indirect-acting sympathomimetic and may interact with a number of other drugs. To avoid precipitating a hypertensive crisis, it should not be given to patients being treated with an MAOI or within 14 days of stopping such treatment. Use of beta blockers with amfetamines may produce severe hypertension. Dexamfetamine may also diminish the effects of other antihypertensives, including guanethidine and similar drugs, and concurrent use should be avoided. Patients receiving amfetamines and tricyclic antidepressants require careful monitoring as the risk of cardiovascular effects including arrhythmias may be increased. The urinary excretion of amfetamines is reduced by urinary alkalinisers, which may enhance or prolong their effects; excretion is increased by urinary acidifiers.

Amfetamines may delay the absorption of ethosuximide, phenobarbital, and phenytoin. The stimulant effects of amfetamines are inhibited by chlorpromazine, haloperidol, and lithium. Disulfiram may inhibit the metabolism and excretion of amfetamines.

Use of sympathomimetics with volatile liquid anaesthetics such as halothane is associated with an increased risk of cardiac arrhythmias.

## Pharmacokinetics

Amfetamines are readily absorbed from the gastrointestinal tract and are distributed into most body tissues with high concentrations in the brain and CSF. They are partially metabolised in the liver but a considerable fraction may be excreted in the urine unchanged. Urinary elimination is pH-dependent and enhanced in acid urine. Amfetamines are distributed into breast milk.

◊ References.

1. Steiner E, *et al.* Amphetamine secretion in breast milk. *Eur J Clin Pharmacol* 1984; **27:** 123–4.

## Uses and Administration

Dexamfetamine, the dextrorotatory isomer of amfetamine, is an indirect-acting sympathomimetic with alpha- and beta-adrenergic agonist activity. It has a marked stimulant effect on the CNS, particularly the cerebral cortex.

Dexamfetamine is used in the treatment of narcolepsy (p.1583) and as an adjunct in the management of refractory hyperactivity disorders in children (p.1583). Dexamfetamine has been given in the treatment of obesity (p.1583), although amfetamines are no longer recommended for this indication. Amfetamines have also been used to overcome fatigue but, again, such use is considered undesirable.

Dexamfetamine is used as the sulfate and is given by mouth.

In the treatment of **narcolepsy**, the usual starting dose is 5 to 10 mg daily in divided doses, increased if necessary by 5 to 10 mg at weekly intervals to a maximum of 60 mg daily. The lower initial dose of 5 mg daily is recommended for the elderly and any weekly increments should also be restricted to 5 mg in such patients.

In children with **hyperactivity** individualisation of treatment is especially important. In the UK, children aged 6 years and over usually start with a dose of 5 mg once or twice daily; the daily dose may be increased if necessary by 5 mg at weekly intervals to an upper limit of 20 mg daily, although older children might require up to 40 mg or more daily. Although dexamfetamine is licensed for the treatment of children younger than 6 years of age in some countries, including the UK, WHO has recommended against the use of stimulants in children under 5 years of age and the *British National Formulary* considers such use inappropriate below 6 years of age.

Dexamfetamine has also been given as the saccharate.

## Preparations

***BP 2003:*** Dexamfetamine Tablets;
***USP 27:*** Dextroamphetamine Sulfate Capsules; Dextroamphetamine Sulfate Elixir; Dextroamphetamine Sulfate Tablets.

**Proprietary Preparations** (details are given in Part 3)
***Canad.:*** Dexedrine; ***Switz.:*** Dexamin; ***UK:*** Dexedrine; ***USA:*** Dexedrine; Dextrostat.

**Multi-ingredient:** ***USA:*** Adderall.

---

# Dexfenfluramine Hydrochloride *(BANM, USAN, rINNM)*

Hidrocloruro de dexfenfluramina; S-5614 (dexfenfluramine). (*S*)-*N*-Ethyl-α-methyl-3-trifluoromethylphenethylamine hydrochloride.

$C_{12}H_{16}F_3N,HCl = 267.7.$
*CAS — 3239-44-9 (dexfenfluramine); 3239-45-0 (dexfenfluramine hydrochloride).*
*ATC — A08AA04.*

## Profile

Dexfenfluramine is the *S*-isomer of fenfluramine (p.1588). It stimulates the release of serotonin and selectively inhibits its reuptake, but differs from fenfluramine in not possessing any catecholamine agonist activity.

Dexfenfluramine was formerly given by mouth as the hydrochloride in the treatment of obesity but, like fenfluramine, was withdrawn worldwide following reports of valvular heart defects.

**Porphyria.** Dexfenfluramine is considered to be unsafe in patients with porphyria because it has been shown to be porphyrinogenic in *in-vitro* systems.

## Dexmethylphenidate Hydrochloride *(USAN, rINNM)*

d-Methylphenidate Hydrochloride; d-MPH; *d-threo*-Methylphenidate. Methyl (2*R*)-phenyl[(2*R*)-piperidin-2-yl]acetate hydrochloride.

$C_{14}H_{19}NO_2$,HCl = 269.8.

*CAS — 40431-64-9 (dexmethylphenidate); 19262-68-1 (dexmethylphenidate hydrochloride).*

### Profile

Dexmethylphenidate hydrochloride is the *d-threo*-enantiomer of racemic methylphenidate hydrochloride (p.1590). It is used as a central stimulant in the treatment of hyperactivity disorders in children.

For patients new to methylphenidate the starting dose of dexmethylphenidate hydrochloride is 2.5 mg twice daily. Each dose should be given at least four hours apart. Dosage may be adjusted in 2.5 to 5 mg increments weekly to a maximum of 10 mg twice daily.

For patients currently using methylphenidate the starting dose of dexmethylphenidate hydrochloride is half the dose of the racemic substance. The maximum recommended dose is 10 mg twice daily. Dexmethylphenidate should be discontinued if there is no improvement in symptoms after appropriate adjustments in dosage over one month. It also needs to be discontinued from time to time in those who do respond to assess the patient's condition.

### Preparations

**Proprietary Preparations** (details are given in Part 3)
***USA:*** Focalin.

---

## Diethylaminoethanol

Dietilaminoetanol. 2-Diethylaminoethanol.

$C_6H_{15}NO$ = 117.2.

*CAS — 100-37-8.*

### Profile

Diethylaminoethanol is an analogue of deanol (p.1585) and has been used similarly as the malate. The hydrochloride has also been used.

### Preparations

**Proprietary Preparations** (details are given in Part 3)
***Fr.:*** Cerebrol†.

**Multi-ingredient:** ***Austria:*** Barokaton.

---

## Diethylpropion Hydrochloride *(BANM)*

Amfepramone Hydrochloride *(pINNM)*; Hidrocloruro de anfepramona. *N*-(1-Benzoylethyl)-*NN*-diethylammonium chloride; 2-Diethylaminopropiophenone hydrochloride; (*RS*)-α-Diethylaminopropiophenone hydrochloride.

$C_{13}H_{19}NO$,HCl = 241.8.

*CAS — 90-84-6 (diethylpropion); 134-80-5 (diethylpropion hydrochloride).*

*ATC — A08AA03.*

**Pharmacopoeias.** In *US.*

**USP 27** (Diethylpropion Hydrochloride). A white to off-white, fine crystalline powder. Is odourless or has a slight characteristic odour. It may contain tartaric acid as a stabilising agent. Soluble 1 in 0.5 of water, 1 in 3 of alcohol, and 1 in 3 of chloroform; practically insoluble in ether. Protect from light.

### Adverse Effects, Treatment, and Precautions

As for Dexamfetamine Sulfate, p.1586. In addition gynaecomastia has been reported rarely. The incidence of central adverse effects may be lower with diethylpropion than with dexamfetamine. Diethylpropion should not be given to patients with emotional instability or a history of psychiatric illness. It should be avoided in children and the elderly. Diethylpropion hydrochloride is subject to abuse.

**Porphyria.** Diethylpropion is considered to be unsafe in patients with porphyria because it has been shown to be porphyrinogenic in *animals*.

### Interactions

Diethylpropion is an indirect-acting sympathomimetic and, similarly to dexamfetamine (p.1586), may interact with a number of other drugs.

### Pharmacokinetics

Diethylpropion is readily absorbed from the gastrointestinal tract. It is extensively metabolised in the liver and possibly the gastrointestinal tract and is excreted in the urine. Diethylpropion crosses the blood-brain barrier and the placenta. Diethylpropion and its metabolites are distributed into breast milk.

### Uses and Administration

Diethylpropion hydrochloride is a central stimulant and indirect-acting sympathomimetic with the actions of dexamfetamine (p.1586). It is used as an anorectic administered by mouth in the short term treatment of obesity (p.1583), although stimulants are not generally recommended for this indication.

Doses of 25 mg three times daily 1 hour before meals or 75 mg once daily in mid-morning as a modified-release preparation, are given. To reduce the risk of dependence, diethylpropion should not be given for more than a few weeks at a time.

Regulatory authorities in the European Union have called for the withdrawal of diethylpropion from the market (see under Effects on the Cardiovascular System in Fenfluramine, p.1588)

### Preparations

***USP 27:*** Diethylpropion Hydrochloride Tablets.

**Proprietary Preparations** (details are given in Part 3)
***Austral.:*** Tenuate; ***Austria:*** Regenon†; ***Belg.:*** Atractil†; Dietil†; Menutil†; Prefamone†; Regenon†; Tenuate Dospan†; ***Braz.:*** Dualid S; Hipofagin S; Inibex S; ***Canad.:*** Tenuate; ***Chile:*** Sacin; ***Denm.:*** Dobesin†; Regenon†; ***Ger.:*** Regenon†; Tenuate Retard†; ***Ital.:*** Linea†; Tenuate Dospan†; ***Mex.:*** Ifa Norex; Neobes; Tenuate Dospan†; ***NZ:*** Tenuate Dospan; ***S.Afr.:*** Tenuate Dospan; ***Spain:*** Delgamer†; ***Switz.:*** Prefamone; Regenon; Tenuate Retard†; ***Thai.:*** Atractil; Dietil; Prefamone†; Regenon; ***USA:*** Tenuate.

**Multi-ingredient:** ***Arg.:*** Tratobes; ***Braz.:*** Fastium†.

---

## Dimefline Hydrochloride *(BANM, USAN, rINNM)*

DW-62; Hidrocloruro de dimeflina; NSC-114650; Rec-7/0267. 8-Dimethylaminomethyl-7-methoxy-3-methyl-2-phenylchromen-4-one hydrochloride.

$C_{20}H_{21}NO_3$,HCl = 359.8.

*CAS — 1165-48-6 (dimefline); 2740-04-7 (dimefline hydrochloride).*

*ATC — R07AB08.*

### Profile

Dimefline has actions similar to those of doxapram (below) and has been used as the hydrochloride by mouth and parenterally as a respiratory stimulant.

### Preparations

**Proprietary Preparations** (details are given in Part 3)
***Ital.:*** Remeflin.

---

## Doxapram Hydrochloride *(BANM, USAN, rINNM)*

AHR-619; Doxaprami Hydrochloridum; Hidrocloruro de doxapram. 1-Ethyl-4-(2-morpholinoethyl)-3,3-diphenyl-2-pyrrolidinone hydrochloride monohydrate.

$C_{24}H_{30}N_2O_2$,HCl,$H_2O$ = 433.0.

*CAS — 309-29-5 (doxapram); 113-07-5 (anhydrous doxapram hydrochloride); 7081-53-0 (doxapram hydrochloride monohydrate).*

*ATC — R07AB01.*

**Pharmacopoeias.** In *Chin., Eur.* (see p.vi), *Jpn,* and *US.*

**Ph. Eur. 5.0** (Doxapram Hydrochloride). A white or almost white crystalline powder. Sparingly soluble in water, in alcohol and in dichloromethane. A 1% solution in water has a pH of 3.5 to 5.0.

**USP 27** (Doxapram Hydrochloride). A white to off-white, odourless, crystalline powder. Soluble 1 in 50 of water; soluble in chloroform; sparingly soluble in alcohol; practically insoluble in ether. pH of a 1% solution in water is between 3.5 and 5.0. Store in airtight containers.

**Incompatibility.** The commercial injection of doxapram hydrochloride is reported to be incompatible with alkaline solutions such as aminophylline, furosemide, or thiopental sodium.

### Adverse Effects

As with other respiratory stimulants, there is a risk that doxapram will produce adverse effects due to general stimulation of the CNS.

Doxapram may produce dyspnoea and other respiratory problems such as coughing, bronchospasm, laryngospasm, hiccup, hyperventilation, and rebound hypoventilation. Muscle involvement may range from fasciculations to spasticity. Convulsions, headache, dizziness, hyperactivity, and confusion can occur as can sweating, flushing, fever or a sensation of warmth, particularly in the genital or perineal regions. Hallucinations may occur rarely. There may be nausea, vomiting, diarrhoea, and problems with urination. Cardiovascular effects include hypertension and various arrhythmias although sudden hypotension may also occur.

Thrombophlebitis may follow extravasation of doxapram during injection.

**Effects on the heart.** Second-degree atrioventricular block caused by prolongation of the QT interval has been associated with doxapram use in 3 neonates.[1] Although the preparation used contained benzyl alcohol this was not considered to play a role in the adverse effect. A prospective study[2] involving 40 premature infants given doxapram for apnoea of prematurity also found QT interval lengthening at 48 and 72 hours of treatment, even when the drug plasma concentrations were kept within therapeutic ranges. In 6 infants, the QT interval lengthened to a degree considered to be life-threatening. There was also a trend towards moderate increases in blood pressure. The authors recommended heart monitoring when doxapram was given to premature infants.

1. De Villiers GS, *et al.* Second-degree atrioventricular heart block after doxapram administration. *J Pediatr* 1998; **133:** 149–50.
2. Maillard C, *et al.* QT interval lengthening in premature infants treated with doxapram. *Clin Pharmacol Ther* 2001; **70:** 540–5.

**Effects on the liver.** Acute hepatic necrosis in a patient was attributed to a 24-hour infusion of doxapram.[1] Liver function tests returned to normal over 3 weeks.

1. Fancourt GJ, *et al.* Hepatic necrosis with doxapram hydrochloride. *Postgrad Med J* 1985; **61:** 833–5.

### Precautions

Doxapram should not be given to patients with epilepsy or other convulsive disorders, cerebral oedema, cerebrovascular accident, head injury, acute severe asthma, physical obstruction of the airway, severe hypertension, ischaemic heart disease, hyperthyroidism, or phaeochromocytoma. Caution is also advisable if doxapram is used in patients with less severe degrees of hypertension or impaired cardiac reserve. It should be given with care to patients with significantly hepatic or renal impairment.

Patients should be carefully supervised during administration of doxapram; special attention should be paid to changes in blood gas measurements. Doxapram should be given with oxygen in severe irreversible airways obstruction or severely decreased lung compliance because of the increased work of breathing. A $beta_2$ agonist should be given concomitantly in patients with bronchoconstriction.

### Interactions

Additive pressor effects may occur when doxapram is used with sympathomimetics or MAOIs. Cardiac arrhythmias may occur when doxapram is given with anaesthetics known to sensitise the myocardium, such as halothane, enflurane, and isoflurane; it has been recommended that doxapram should not be given for at least 10 minutes after discontinuation of these anaesthetics. Doxapram may temporarily mask the residual effects of neuromuscular blockers. The manufacturers have reported that there may be an interaction between doxapram and aminophylline manifested by agitation and increased skeletal muscle activity.

### Pharmacokinetics

After intravenous administration doxapram is rapidly distributed into the tissues. Onset of respiratory stimulation usually occurs in 20 to 40 seconds, with a peak effect achieved in 1 to 2 minutes. Duration of effect following a single dose varies from 5 to 12 minutes. Doxapram is extensively metabolised in the liver. The major route of excretion of metabolites and a small amount of unchanged drug is thought to be via bile to the faeces. It is also excreted in the urine.

Some absorption occurs when doxapram is given orally.

◊ References.

1. Robson RH, Prescott LF. A pharmacokinetic study of doxapram in patients and volunteers. *Br J Clin Pharmacol* 1978; **7:** 81–7.
2. Baker JR, *et al.* Normal pharmacokinetics of doxapram in a patient with renal failure and hypothyroidism. *Br J Clin Pharmacol* 1981; **11:** 305–6.

### Uses and Administration

Doxapram hydrochloride is a central and respiratory stimulant with a brief duration of action. It acts by stimulation of peripheral chemoreceptors and central respiratory centres; at higher doses, it stimulates other parts of the brain and spinal cord. Doxapram has a pressor action and may also increase catecholamine release.

Doxapram has limited uses in the treatment of acute respiratory failure (for example where this is superimposed on chronic obstructive pulmonary disease), and of postoperative respiratory depression (see Respiratory Failure under Oxygen, p.1237).

Doxapram hydrochloride may be infused at a rate of 1.5 to 4 mg/minute in the treatment of acute respiratory failure.

For postoperative respiratory depression it has been given in a dose of 0.5 to 1.5 mg/kg by intravenous injection over a period of at least 30 seconds. This dose may be repeated at hourly intervals. It may also be given by intravenous infusion, initially administered at a rate of 2 to 5 mg/minute and then reduced, according to the patient's response, to 1 to 3 mg/minute; a recommended maximum total dosage is 4 mg/kg.

Doxapram hydrochloride has also been used to treat respiratory and CNS depression following drug overdose but its use for this indication is no longer recommended.

**Chronic obstructive pulmonary disease.** Respiratory stimulants such as doxapram have a limited and short-term role in hypercapnic respiratory failure in patients with chronic obstructive pulmonary disease (p.779). Benefit has been reported in such patients in whom doxapram was used as an alternative to intubation.[1,2] However, a systematic review suggested that despite short-term improvements in blood-gas exchange with doxapram, techniques such as non-invasive ventilation might be more effective.[3]

1. Hirshberg AJ, *et al.* Use of doxapram hydrochloride injection as an alternative to intubation to treat chronic obstructive pulmonary disease patients with hypercapnia. *Ann Emerg Med* 1994; **24:** 701–3.
2. Kerr HD. Doxapram in hypercapric chronic obstructive pulmonary disease with respiratory failure. *J Emerg Med* 1997; **15:** 513–15.
3. Greenstone M, Lasserson TJ. Doxapram for ventilatory failure due to exacerbations of chronic obstructive pulmonary disease. Available in The Cochrane Library; Issue 1. Chichester: John Wiley; 2004.

**Neonatal apnoea.** Doxapram is effective in neonatal apnoea (p.806) and may be considered as an alternative, or in addition, to xanthines in infants with apnoea that does not respond to xanthine therapy alone. However, it is less convenient to use as it must be given by continuous intravenous infusion and blood pressure must be monitored. Additionally, some preparations may contain benzyl alcohol as a preservative making them unsuitable for use in neonates. It has been used in doses of 2.5 mg/kg per hour.[1-3] Adverse CNS effects have been reported.[3] Lower doses of 0.25 or 1.5 mg/kg per hour have been shown to be effective.[4,5] However, use of low doses of 500 micrograms/kg per hour in very low birth-weight premature infants produced higher than expected plasma-doxapram concentrations and a greater increase in systolic blood pressure compared with controls.[6]


1. Sagi E, *et al.* Idiopathic apnoea of prematurity treated with doxapram and aminophylline. *Arch Dis Child* 1984; **59:** 281–3.
2. Eyal F, *et al.* Aminophylline versus doxapram in idiopathic apnea of prematurity: a double-blind controlled study. *Pediatrics* 1985; **75:** 709–13.
3. Dear PRF, Wheeler D. Doxapram and neonatal apnoea. *Arch Dis Child* 1984; **59:** 903–4.
4. Bairam A, Vert P. Low-dose doxapram for apnoea of prematurity. *Lancet* 1986; **i:** 793–4.
5. Peliowski A, Finer NN. A blinded, randomized, placebo-controlled trial to compare theophylline and doxapram for the treatment of apnea of prematurity. *J Pediatr* 1990; **116:** 648–53.
6. Huon C, *et al.* Low-dose doxapram for treatment of apnoea following early weaning in very low birthweight infants: a randomized, double-blind study. *Acta Paediatr* 1998; **87:** 1180–4.


**Respiratory depression.** References to the use of doxapram in postoperative respiratory depression.


1. Jansen JE, *et al.* Effect of doxapram on postoperative pulmonary complications after upper abdominal surgery in high-risk patients. *Lancet* 1990; **335:** 936–8.
2. Thangathurai D, *et al.* Doxapram for respiratory depression after epidural morphine. *Anaesthesia* 1990; **45:** 64–5.
3. Sajjad T. Comparison of the effects of doxapram or carbon dioxide on ventilatory frequency and tidal volume during induction of anaesthesia with propofol, *Br J Anaesth* 1994; **73:** 266P.
4. Alexander-Williams M, *et al.* Doxapram and the prevention of postoperative hypoxaemia. *Br J Anaesth* 1995; **75:** 233P.


**Shivering.** Doxapram is one of a number of drugs that have been used in postoperative shivering, see p.1295.

References.


1. Sarma V, Fry ENS. Doxapram after general anaesthesia: its role in stopping shivering during recovery. *Anaesthesia* 1991; **46:** 460–1.
2. Singh P, *et al.* Double-blind comparison between doxapram and pethidine in the treatment of postanaesthetic shivering. *Br J Anaesth* 1993; **71:** 685–8.
3. Wrench IJ, *et al.* The minimum effective doses of pethidine and doxapram in the treatment of post-anaesthetic shivering. *Anaesthesia* 1997; **52:** 32–6.


### Preparations

***BP 2003:*** Doxapram Injection;
***USP 27:*** Doxapram Hydrochloride Injection.

**Proprietary Preparations** (details are given in Part 3)
***Austral.:*** Dopram; ***Austria:*** Dopram; ***Belg.:*** Dopram; ***Canad.:*** Dopram†; ***Denm.:*** Dopram; ***Fin.:*** Dopram; ***Ger.:*** Dopram; ***Gr.:*** Dopram; ***Hong Kong:*** Dopram; ***Irl.:*** Dopram; ***Neth.:*** Dopram; ***Norw.:*** Dopram; ***NZ:*** Dopram; ***S.Afr.:*** Dopram; ***Spain:*** Docatone; ***Switz.:*** Dopram; ***UK:*** Dopram; ***USA:*** Dopram.

## Etamivan *(BAN, rINN)*

Etamiván; Ethamivan *(USAN)*; NSC-406087; Vanillic Acid Diethylamide; Vanillic Diethylamide. *N,N*-Diethylvanillamide.

$C_{12}H_{17}NO_3$ = 223.3.
*CAS — 304-84-7.*
*ATC — R07AB04.*

### Profile

Etamivan has actions similar to those of doxapram (above). It was formerly used as a respiratory stimulant, but the risk of toxicity associated with effective doses is now considered to be unacceptable.

Etamivan is available in compound preparations for administration by mouth in cerebrovascular and circulatory disorders and hypotension, but such use is not recommended.

### Preparations

**Proprietary Preparations** (details are given in Part 3)
***Multi-ingredient: Arg.:*** Dosulfin Bronquial; ***Austria:*** Cinnarplus; Instenon; ***Ger.:*** Normotin-R; ***Hong Kong:*** Instenon; ***Spain:*** Vasperdil†; ***Thai.:*** Instenon.

## Etilamfetamine Hydrochloride *(rINN)*

Ethylamphetamine Hydrochloride. *N*-Ethyl-α-methylphenethylamine hydrochloride.

$C_{11}H_{17}N,HCl$ = 199.7.
*CAS — 457-87-4 (etilamfetamine); 1858-47-5 (etilamfetamine hydrochloride).*
*ATC — A08AA06.*

### Profile

Etilamfetamine hydrochloride is a central stimulant with properties similar to those of dexamfetamine (p.1585). It has been used as an anorectic in the treatment of obesity.

### Preparations

**Proprietary Preparations** (details are given in Part 3)
***Switz.:*** Apetinil-Depot†.

## Fencamfamin Hydrochloride *(BANM, rINNM)*

H-610; Hidrocloruro de fencanfamina. *N*-Ethyl-3-phenylbicyclo[2.2.1]hept-2-ylamine hydrochloride.

$C_{15}H_{21}N,HCl$ = 251.8.
*CAS — 1209-98-9 (fencamfamin); 2240-14-4 (fencamfamin hydrochloride).*
*ATC — N06BA06.*

### Profile

Fencamfamin hydrochloride has been given by mouth as a central stimulant.

### Preparations

**Proprietary Preparations** (details are given in Part 3)
***Multi-ingredient: S.Afr.:*** Reactivan.

## Fenetylline Hydrochloride *(BANM, rINNM)*

Amfetyline Hydrochloride; 7-Ethyltheophylline Amphetamine Hydrochloride; Fenethylline Hydrochloride *(USAN)*; H-814; Hidrocloruro de fenetilina; R-720-11. 7-[2-(α-Methylphenethylamino)ethyl]theophylline hydrochloride.

$C_{18}H_{23}N_5O_2,HCl$ = 377.9.
*CAS — 3736-08-1 (fenetylline); 1892-80-4 (fenetylline hydrochloride).*

### Profile

Fenetylline is a theophylline derivative of amfetamine with properties similar to those of dexamfetamine (p.1585). It has been given by mouth in usual doses of 25 to 50 mg once or twice daily, in the management of hyperactivity disorders. Fenetylline is subject to abuse.

### Preparations

**Proprietary Preparations** (details are given in Part 3)
***Belg.:*** Captagon; ***Ger.:*** Captagon; ***Israel:*** Fitton†.

## Fenfluramine Hydrochloride *(BANM, USAN, rINNM)*

AHR-3002; Hidrocloruro de fenfluramina; S-768. *N*-Ethyl-α-methyl-3-trifluoromethylphenethylamine hydrochloride.

$C_{12}H_{16}F_3N,HCl$ = 267.7.
*CAS — 458-24-2 (fenfluramine); 404-82-0 (fenfluramine hydrochloride).*
*ATC — A08AA02.*

### Adverse Effects and Precautions

As for Dexamfetamine, p.1586, but fenfluramine usually depresses rather than stimulates the CNS. Fenfluramine has been associated with serious cardiovascular toxicity. Pulmonary hypertension led to certain precautions being imposed upon its use and subsequent reports of valvular heart defects led to its general withdrawal worldwide.

**Effects on the cardiovascular system.** The association of primary *pulmonary hypertension* with the use of anorectics including fenfluramine, dexfenfluramine, and phentermine is well recognised.[1-3] Both reversible and irreversible cases have been reported and in some cases it has proved fatal.[1,4-9] The condition appears to be linked to prolonged or repeated therapy.[1,10] In 1992 the UK Committee on Safety of Medicines (CSM) advised that treatment should not exceed 3 months[1] but later in 1997 it revised its recommendations for fenfluramine and dexfenfluramine allowing treatment for up to 12 months under certain conditions.[2] The CSM stated that treatment could be continued beyond 3 months only if there had been a satisfactory response (more than 10% weight loss) and that this loss was maintained. Patients should also be monitored for symptoms of pulmonary hypertension. For other anorectics such as phentermine the maximum duration of treatment remained 3 months.

However, shortly after this, a report was published[11] that outlined an association between the use of a fenfluramine-phentermine combination and the development of *valvular heart disease* in 24 patients. Initially, the response by the CSM was to advise against the use of combinations of anorectics[12] although subsequently fenfluramine, along with dexfenfluramine, was withdrawn from the world market after more cases became known.[13,14] By September 1997 the FDA in the USA[14] had received 144 reports of valvulopathy, including the original 24, associated with fenfluramine or dexfenfluramine, with or without phentermine; none were associated with phentermine treatment alone. As a consequence the US authorities made recommendations[14] for the screening of all patients who had previously received fenfluramine or dexfenfluramine in order to detect heart valve lesions and to provide optimal care. Further studies[15-20] have supported the association with valvular abnormalities, and suggested that prolonged exposure or exposure to high doses of dexfenfluramine or fenfluramine increased the risk; clinically important disease would probably not develop in most patients with only short-term exposure.[21]

In 2000, the European Commission called for the withdrawal of all anorectics from the European market. Those anorectics involved in the decision included clobenzorex, diethylpropion, fenproporex, mazindol, mefenorex, phendimetrazine, phentrazine, and phentermine. However in 2002, following an appeal by some manufacturers, the European Court ruled that the Commission did not have the authority to withdraw marketing authorisations.


1. Committee on Safety of Medicines. Fenfluramine (Ponderax Pacaps), dexfenfluramine (Adifax) and pulmonary hypertension. *Current Problems 34* 1992.
2. Committee on Safety of Medicines/Medicines Control Agency. Anorectic agents: risks and benefits. *Current Problems* 1997; **23:** 1–2. Also available at: http://www.mca.gov.uk/ourwork/monitorsafequalmed/currentproblems/volume23.htm (accessed 15/04/04)
3. Abenhaim L, *et al.* Appetite-suppressant drugs and the risk of primary pulmonary hypertension. *N Engl J Med* 1996; **335:** 609–16.
4. Douglas JG, *et al.* Pulmonary hypertension and fenfluramine. *BMJ* 1981; **283:** 881–3.
5. McMurray J, *et al.* Irreversible pulmonary hypertension after treatment with fenfluramine. *BMJ* 1986; **292:** 239–40.
6. Fotiadis I, *et al.* Fenfluramine-induced irreversible pulmonary hypertension. *Postgrad Med J* 1991; **67:** 776–7.
7. Atanassoff PG, *et al.* Pulmonary hypertension and dexfenfluramine. *Lancet* 1992; **339:** 436.
8. Cacoub P, *et al.* Pulmonary hypertension and dexfenfluramine. *Eur J Clin Pharmacol* 1995; **48:** 81–3.
9. Roche N, *et al.* Pulmonary hypertension and dexfenfluramine. *Lancet* 1992; **339:** 436–7.
10. Thomas SHL, *et al.* Appetite suppressants and primary pulmonary hypertension in the United Kingdom. *Br Heart J* 1995; **74:** 600–63.
11. Connolly HM, *et al.* Valvular heart disease associated with fenfluramine-phentermine. *N Engl J Med* 1997; **337:** 581–8. Correction. *ibid.*; 1783.
12. Committee on Safety of Medicines/Medicines Control Agency. Anorectic agents and valvular heart disease. *Current Problems* 1997; **23:** 12. Also available at: http://www.mca.gov.uk/ourwork/monitorsafequalmed/currentproblems/page4.htm (accessed 15/04/04)
13. Committee on Safety of Medicines/Medicines Control Agency. Fenfluramine and dexfenfluramine withdrawn. *Current Problems* 1997; **23:** 13–14. Also available at: http://www.mca.gov.uk/ourwork/monitorsafequalmed/currentproblems/first.htm (accessed 15/04/04)
14. Anonymous. Cardiac valvulopathy associated with exposure to fenfluramine or dexfenfluramine: US Department of Health and Human Services interim public health recommendations, November 1997. *MMWR* 1997; **46:** 1061–6.
15. Khan MA, *et al.* The prevalence of cardiac valvular insufficiency assessed by transthoracic echocardiography in obese patients treated with appetite-suppressant drugs. *N Engl J Med* 1998; **339:** 713–18.
16. Jick H, *et al.* A population-based study of appetite-suppressant drugs and the risk of cardiac-valve regurgitation. *N Engl J Med* 1998; **339:** 719–24.
17. Weissman NJ, *et al.* An assessment of heart-valve abnormalities in obese patients taking dexfenfluramine, sustained-release dexfenfluramine, or placebo. *N Engl J Med* 1998; **339:** 725–32.
18. Gardin JM, *et al.* Valvular abnormalities and cardiovascular status following exposure to dexfenfluramine or phentermine/fenfluramine. *JAMA* 2000; **283:** 1703–9.
19. Lepor NE, *et al.* Dose and duration of fenfluramine-phentermine therapy impacts the risk of significant valvular heart disease. *Am J Cardiol* 2000; **86:** 107–10.
20. Jollis JG, *et al.* Fenfluramine and phentermine and cardiovascular findings: effect of treatment duration on prevalence of valve abnormalities. *Circulation* 2000; **101:** 2071–7.
21. Devereux RB. Appetite suppressants and valvular heart disease. *N Engl J Med* 1998; **339:** 765–6.


**Effects on the liver.** The UK Medicines and Healthcare products Regulatory Agency had warned[1] that there had been cases of hepatotoxicity associated with adulteration of traditional Chinese slimming medicines with fenfluramine and/or nitrosofenfluramine. Nitrosofenfluramine was known to be hepatotoxic.


1. Medicines and Healthcare products Regulatory Agency (MHRA). Shubao slimming capsules containing fenfluramine and nitrosofenfluramine (issued 28 April 2004). Available at: http://medicines.mhra.gov.uk/ourwork/licensingmeds/herbalmeds/shubaoletter_april2004.pdf (accessed 10/05/04)


**Porphyria.** Fenfluramine is considered to be unsafe in patients with porphyria because it has been shown to be porphyrinogenic in *animals*.

### Uses and Administration

Fenfluramine is an indirect-acting sympathomimetic related to amfetamine, but at standard doses it usually depresses rather than stimulates the CNS. It appears to stimulate the release of serotonin and selectively inhibits its reuptake resulting in increased CNS serotonin concentrations. It may also increase glucose utilisation and lower blood-glucose concentrations.

Fenfluramine was formerly given by mouth as the hydrochloride in the treatment of obesity (p.1583) but was generally withdrawn worldwide following reports of valvular heart defects.

### Preparations

**Proprietary Preparations** (details are given in Part 3)
***Chile:*** Megaval.

## Fenproporex Hydrochloride *(rINNM)*

*N*-2-Cyanoethylamphetamine Hydrochloride; Hidrocloruro de fenproporex. (±)-3-(α-Methylphenethylamino)propionitrile hydrochloride.

$C_{12}H_{16}N_2,HCl$ = 224.7.
*CAS — 15686-61-0 (fenproporex); 18305-29-8 (fenproporex hydrochloride).*

### Profile

Fenproporex is a central stimulant and indirect-acting sympathomimetic with actions similar to those of dexamfetamine (p.1585). Following administration by mouth it is reported to be metabolised to amfetamine. Fenproporex has been given as the hydrochloride, the diphenylacetate, and as a resinate.

Fenproporex hydrochloride has been used as an anorectic in the treatment of obesity (p.1583) although the use of stimulants in this way is no longer recommended. Regulatory authorities in the European Union have called for the withdrawal of all anorectics from the market (see under Effects on the Cardiovascular System in Fenfluramine, p.1588)

### Preparations

**Proprietary Preparations** (details are given in Part 3)
***Braz.:*** Desobesi-M; Inobesin†; Lipomax†; Nobese†; ***Chile:*** Salcal; Sinapet; ***Mex.:*** Delgafen†; Fenisec†; Ifa Dex†; Ifa Diety; Obisin†; ***Port.:*** Drenur†; Pesex-R†; Tegisec†; ***Spain:*** Antiobes†; Grasmin†; Tegisec†.

**Multi-ingredient:** ***Arg.:*** Tratobes; ***Mex.:*** Esbelcaps.

## Lobelia

Indian Tobacco.

**Description.** Lobelia consists of the dried aerial parts of *Lobelia inflata* (Lobeliaceae). Lobeline is the main alkaloidal constituent.

## Lobeline Hydrochloride *(BANM, rINNM)*

Alpha-lobeline Hydrochloride; Hidrocloruro de lobelina; Lobelini Hydrochloridum. 2-[6-(β-Hydroxyphenethyl)-1-methyl-2-piperidyl]acetophenone hydrochloride.

$C_{22}H_{27}NO_2,HCl = 373.9.$

*CAS — 90-69-7 (lobeline); 134-63-4 (lobeline hydrochloride).*

**Pharmacopoeias.** In *Chin.* and *Eur.* (see p.vi).

**Ph. Eur. 5.0** (Lobeline Hydrochloride). A white or almost white microcrystalline powder. Sparingly soluble in water; freely soluble in alcohol; soluble in dichloromethane. A 1% solution in water has a pH of 4.6 to 6.4. Protect from light.

## Lobeline Sulfate *(rINNM)*

Lobeline Sulphate *(BANM)*; Sulfato de Lobelina.

$(C_{22}H_{27}NO_2)_2,H_2SO_4 = 773.0.$

*CAS — 134-64-5.*

### Adverse Effects

Side-effects of lobelia and lobeline include nausea and vomiting, coughing, tremor, and dizziness. Symptoms of overdosage include profuse diaphoresis, paresis, tachycardia, hypothermia, hypotension, and coma; fatalities have occurred.

### Uses and Administration

Lobeline, which chiefly accounts for the activity of lobelia, has peripheral and central effects similar to those of nicotine (p.1720).

Lobelia has been used mainly in preparations aimed at relieving respiratory-tract disorders. Lobeline has been given by mouth as the hydrochloride or sulfate as a smoking deterrent (see Smoking Cessation, p.1721). Lobelia has been used similarly given either by mouth or incorporated into herbal cigarettes.

**Smoking cessation.** Reviews of anti-smoking therapy generally consider lobeline to have little benefit compared with placebo.[1-3]


1. Nunn-Thompson CL, Simon PA. Pharmacotherapy for smoking cessation. *Clin Pharm* 1989; **8:** 710–20.
2. Gourlay SG, McNeil JJ. Antismoking products. *Med J Aust* 1990; **153:** 699–707.
3. Stead LF, Hughes JR. Lobeline for smoking cessation. Available in The Cochrane Library; Issue 1. Chichester: John Wiley; 2004.


### Preparations

**Proprietary Preparations** (details are given in Part 3)
***Austral.:*** Cig-Ridettes†; ***Canad.:*** Butt-Out; ***Spain:*** Smokeless; ***UK:*** Anti-Smoking Tablets†.

**Multi-ingredient:** ***Austral.:*** Potassium Iodide and Stramonium Compound†; ***Belg.:*** Kamfeine; Sirop Toux du Larynx†; ***Braz.:*** Asmatiron†; Broncofenil; Broncotussan†; Bronquidex; Brontoss; Efedronal†; Expectobron; Expectol; Expectolu†; Iodeto de Potassio; Iol; Iolin; Lobelia Composta†; MM Expectorante; Pinosil†; Pulmoformil†; Pulmoforte†; Sedatux; Subitan†; Tosseina†; Xarope de Eucalipto†; Xarope de Iodeto de Potassio Composto†; Xarope de Lobelia Composto†; Xarope Peitoral de Ameixa Composto; ***Chile:*** Paltomiel Plus; Pulmagol; Ramistos; ***Port.:*** Lactucol†; ***Spain:*** Pazbronquial; ***UK:*** Antibron; Asthma & Catarrh Relief; Balm of Gilead; Chest Mixture; Herbelix; Horehound and Aniseed Cough Mixture; Lobelia Compound†; Modern Herbals Cold & Congestion; Vegetable Cough Remover.

## Mazindol *(BAN, USAN, rINN)*

42-548; AN-448; SaH-42548. 5-(4-Chlorophenyl)-2,5-dihydro-3*H*-imidazo[2,1-*a*]isoindol-5-ol.

$C_{16}H_{13}ClN_2O = 284.7.$

*CAS — 22232-71-9.*

*ATC — A08AA05.*

**Pharmacopoeias.** In *US.*

**USP 27** (Mazindol). A white to off-white crystalline powder, having not more than a faint odour. Insoluble in water; slightly soluble in chloroform and in methyl alcohol. Store in airtight containers.

### Adverse Effects, Treatment, and Precautions

As for Dexamfetamine Sulfate, p.1586.

**Effects on the testes.** A report of 8 men who developed testicular pain after taking mazindol.[1]


1. McEwen J, Meyboom RHB. Testicular pain caused by mazindol. *BMJ* 1983; **287:** 1763–4.


### Interactions

As for Dexamfetamine Sulfate, p.1586.

**Lithium.** For a report of mazindol interacting with lithium to cause lithium toxicity, see p.304.

### Pharmacokinetics

Mazindol is readily absorbed from the gastrointestinal tract and is excreted in the urine, partly unchanged and partly as metabolites.

### Uses and Administration

Mazindol is a central stimulant with actions similar to those of dexamfetamine (p.1586), although structurally the two compounds are unrelated. It appears to inhibit reuptake of dopamine and noradrenaline. It has been used as an anorectic, given by mouth in the treatment of obesity (p.1583), although stimulants are no longer recommended for this indication. Regulatory authorities in the European Union have called for the withdrawal of all anorectics from the market (see under Effects on the Cardiovascular System in Fenfluramine, p.1588).

Mazindol has been investigated in the treatment of Duchenne muscular dystrophy.

**Narcolepsy.** Mazindol has been reported[1-4] to be beneficial in patients with narcolepsy and associated cataplexy (p.1583). A wide range of doses has been used: 3 to 8 mg daily in one study,[1] 1 mg weekly to 16 mg daily in another;[3] children have been given 1 to 2 mg daily.[4]


1. Parkes JD, Schachter M. Mazindol in the treatment of narcolepsy. *Acta Neurol Scand* 1979; **60:** 250–4.
2. Shindler J, *et al.* Amphetamine, mazindol, and fencamfamin in narcolepsy. *BMJ* 1985; **290:** 1167–70.
3. Alvarez B, *et al.* Mazindol in long-term treatment of narcolepsy. *Lancet* 1991; **337:** 1293–4.
4. Allsopp MR, Zaiwalla Z. Narcolepsy. *Arch Dis Child* 1992; **67:** 302–6.


### Preparations

***USP 27:*** Mazindol Tablets.

**Proprietary Preparations** (details are given in Part 3)
***Arg.:*** Afilan; Samonter; ***Braz.:*** Absten S; Dasten†; Fagolipo; Magrinex†; ***Canad.:*** Sanorex; ***Israel:*** Teronac; ***Mex.:*** Diestet; Liofindol†; Sanorex; Solucaps; ***Neth.:*** Teronac†; ***Singapore:*** Teronac; ***Switz.:*** Teronac; ***USA:*** Mazanor†; Sanorex†.

**Multi-ingredient:** ***Arg.:*** Dimagrir Triac; Maxitratobes; ***Braz.:*** Dobesix†; Moderine; Nofagus†.

## Mefenorex Hydrochloride *(USAN, pINNM)*

Hidrocloruro de mefenorex; Ro-4-5282. *N*-(3-Chloropropyl)-α-methylphenethylamine hydrochloride.

$C_{12}H_{18}ClN,HCl = 248.2.$

*CAS — 17243-57-1 (mefenorex); 5586-87-8 (mefenorex hydrochloride).*

*ATC — A08AA09.*

### Profile

Mefenorex hydrochloride is a central stimulant and indirect-acting sympathomimetic with actions similar to those of dexamfetamine (p.1585). It has been used as an anorectic in the treatment of obesity although stimulants are no longer recommended for this indication. Regulatory authorities in the European Union have called for the withdrawal of all anorectics from the market (see under Effects on the Cardiovascular System in Fenfluramine, p.1588).

### Preparations

**Proprietary Preparations** (details are given in Part 3)
***Ger.:*** Rondimen†.

## Mesocarb *(rINN)*

3-(α-Methylphenethyl)-*N*-(phenylcarbamoyl)syndnone imine.

$C_{18}H_{18}N_4O_2 = 322.4.$

*CAS — 34262-84-5.*

### Profile

Mesocarb is reported to be a central stimulant.

## Metamfetamine Hydrochloride *(rINNM)*

*d*-Deoxyephedrine Hydrochloride; *d*-Desoxyephedrine Hydrochloride; Hidrocloruro de metanfetamina; Methamphetamine Hydrochloride; Methamphetamini Hydrochloridum; Methylamphetamine Hydrochloride; Phenylmethylaminopropane Hydrochloride. (+)-*N*,α-Dimethylphenethylamine hydrochloride.

$C_{10}H_{15}N,HCl = 185.7.$

*CAS — 537-46-2 (metamfetamine); 51-57-0 (metamfetamine hydrochloride).*

*ATC — N06BA03.*

NOTE. Metamfetamine abused in a smokeable form has been known as Crank, Crystal, Crystal Meth, Ice, Meth, and Speed.

**Pharmacopoeias.** In *Jpn, Swiss,* and *US.*

**USP 27** (Methamphetamine Hydrochloride). White, odourless or practically odourless, crystals or crystalline powder. Freely soluble in water, in alcohol, and in chloroform; very slightly soluble in ether. Its solutions in water have a pH of about 6. Store in airtight containers. Protect from light.

### Adverse Effects, Treatment, and Precautions

As for Dexamfetamine Sulfate, p.1586.

Metamfetamine has been subject to extensive abuse.

**Abuse.** Pulmonary oedema,[1,2] cardiomyopathy,[2] and choreoathetosis and rhabdomyolysis[3] have occurred following smoking of metamfetamine crystals. It is also abused by mouth and intravenously, and has been associated with fatalities.[4]

A study of former users suggests that metamfetamine abuse may cause long-term neuronal damage.[5]


1. Nestor TA, *et al.* Acute pulmonary oedema caused by crystalline methamphetamine. *Lancet* 1989; **ii:** 1277–8.
2. Hong R, *et al.* Cardiomyopathy associated with the smoking of crystal methamphetamine. *JAMA* 1991; **265:** 1152–4.
3. Sperling LS, Horowitz JL. Methamphetamine-induced choreoathetosis and rhabdomyolysis. *Ann Intern Med* 1994; **121:** 986.
4. Albertson TE, *et al.* Methamphetamine and the expanding complications of amphetamines. *West J Med* 1999; **170:** 214–19.
5. Ernst T, *et al.* Evidence for long-term neurotoxicity associated with methamphetamine abuse: a $^1$H MRS study. *Neurology* 2000; **54:** 1344–9.


**Porphyria.** Metamfetamine has been associated with acute attacks of porphyria and is considered unsafe in porphyric patients.

### Interactions

As for Dexamfetamine Sulfate, p.1586.

### Pharmacokinetics

Like most amfetamines (see Dexamfetamine Sulfate, p.1586) metamfetamine is readily absorbed from the gastrointestinal tract and is distributed into most body tissues. It is partially metabolised in the liver and excreted in the urine.

◊ References.


1. Shappell SA, *et al.* Chronopharmacokinetics and chronopharmacodynamics of dextromethamphetamine in man. *J Clin Pharmacol* 1996; **36:** 1051–63.


### Uses and Administration

Metamfetamine hydrochloride is a central stimulant and indirect-acting sympathomimetic with actions and uses similar to those of dexamfetamine (p.1586).

It has been given by mouth in the treatment of hyperactivity disorders in children aged 6 years and over, although dexamfetamine and methylphenidate are the main stimulants used (p.1583). Initial doses are 5 mg once or twice daily, increased if necessary by 5 mg at weekly intervals to the optimum effective dose, usually 20 to 25 mg daily.

Metamfetamine hydrochloride has also been used as an anorectic in the management of obesity (p.1583), although amfetamines are no longer recommended for this indication. A dose of 5 mg before each meal has been given by mouth. Treatment should be for no longer than a few weeks.

Metamfetamine hydrochloride has also been used parenterally as a pressor agent.

The laevorotatory form, levmetamfetamine (p.1124) is used as a nasal decongestant.

### Preparations

***USP 27:*** Methamphetamine Hydrochloride Tablets.

**Proprietary Preparations** (details are given in Part 3)
***Chile:*** Cidrin; Escancil; ***USA:*** Desoxyn.

**Multi-ingredient:** ***Port.:*** Davicaina†.

## Methylenedioxymethamfetamine

MDMA; Methylenedioxymethamphetamine; 3,4-Methylenedioxymethamphetamine; Metilendioximetanfetamina. *N*,α-Dimethyl-1,3-benzodioxole-5-ethanamine.

$C_{11}H_{15}NO_2 = 193.2.$

*CAS — 42542-10-9.*

NOTE. Methylenedioxymethamfetamine has also been known as Adam, Disco Biscuits, Doves, E, Ecstasy, M&M, MDM, and XTC.

### Profile

Methylenedioxymethamfetamine is a phenylethylamine compound structurally related to amfetamine and mescaline and is an analogue of tenamfetamine (p.1593). It is subject to abuse. Its toxicity is similar to that of dexamfetamine (see Abuse, below and under Dexamfetamine, p.1586) and may be treated similarly.

**Abuse.** Methylenedioxymethamfetamine may be ingested as tablets, capsules, or inhaled as a powder. It is often mixed with a combination of adulterants such as amfetamines, caffeine, ephedrine, and pseudoephedrine.[1]

The toxicity associated with abuse of methylenedioxymethamfetamine has been the subject of a number of discussions.[2-7] Acute effects can be severe and symptoms have included cardiac arrhythmias, fulminant hyperthermia, convulsions, disseminated intravascular coagulation, rhabdomyolysis, and acute renal failure; fatalities may occur. Repeated use may cause hepatic damage. Psychiatric effects reported include psychosis[8-10] and depression.[9-11] Damage to central serotonergic nerves has been implicated[8-12] and hence there is some concern regarding the long-term effects of methylenedioxymethamfetamine abuse.[13,14] Hyponatraemia, inappropriate antidiuretic hormone secretion, and cerebral oedema have also been reported;[15-20] the severity may be increased by excessive fluid intake that is frequently advocated to prevent dehydration and hyperthermia.[18-22] Urinary retention has also been reported.[23]

Concern has been expressed regarding abuse during *pregnancy*. Twelve congenital malformations, including 2 cases of congenital heart disease, have been noted among 78 liveborn infants whose mothers had taken methylenedioxymethamfetamine, often with other drugs of abuse, during their pregnancies.[24]

For reviews of the properties of other phenylethylamine compounds, see under Tenamfetamine, p.1593.


1. Smith KM, *et al.* Club drugs: methylenedioxymethamphetamine, flunitrazepam, ketamine hydrochloride, and γ-hydroxybutyrate. *Am J Health-Syst Pharm* 2002; **59:** 1067–76.
2. Henry JA. Ecstasy and the dance of death. *BMJ* 1992; **305:** 5–6.
3. Henry JA, *et al.* Toxicity and deaths from 3,4-methylenedioxymethamphetamine ("ecstasy"). *Lancet* 1992; **340:** 384–7.
4. O'Connor B. Hazards associated with the recreational drug 'ecstasy'. *Br J Hosp Med* 1994; **52:** 507–14.
5. McCann UD, *et al.* Adverse reactions with 3,4-methylenedioxymethamphetamine (MDMA; 'Ecstasy'). *Drug Safety* 1996; **15:** 107–115.
6. Hall AP. Ecstasy and the anaesthetist. *Br J Anaesth* 1997; **79:** 697–8.
7. Schwartz RH, Miller NS. MDMA (ecstasy) and the rave: a review. *Pediatrics* 1997; **100:** 705–8.
8. McGuire P, Fahy T. Chronic paranoid psychosis after misuse of MDMA ("ecstasy"). *BMJ* 1991; **302:** 697.
9. Winstock AR. Chronic paranoid psychosis after misuse of MDMA. *BMJ* 1991; **302:** 1150–1.
10. Schifano F. Chronic atypical psychosis associated with MDMA ("ecstasy") abuse. *Lancet* 1991; **338:** 1335.
11. Benazzi F, Mazzoli M. Psychiatric illness associated with "ecstasy". *Lancet* 1991; **338:** 1520.
12. McCann UD, *et al.* Positron emission tomographic evidence of toxic effect of MDMA ("Ecstasy") on brain serotonin neurons in human beings. *Lancet* 1998; **352:** 1433–7.
13. Green AR, Goodwin GM. Ecstasy and neurodegeneration. *BMJ* 1996; **312:** 1493–4.
14. Bolla KI, *et al.* Memory impairment in abstinent MDMA ("Ecstasy") users. *Neurology* 1998; **51:** 1532–7.
15. Maxwell DL, *et al.* Hyponatraemia and catatonic stupor after taking "ecstasy". *BMJ* 1993; **307:** 1399.
16. Kessel B. Hyponatraemia after ingestion of "ecstasy". *BMJ* 1994; **308:** 414.
17. Satchell SC, Connaughton M. Inappropriate antidiuretic hormone secretion and extreme rises in serum creatinine kinase following MDMA ingestion. *Br J Hosp Med* 1994; **51:** 495.
18. Holden R, Jackson MA. Near-fatal hyponatraemic coma due to vasopressin over-secretion after ecstasy (3,4-MDMA). *Lancet* 1996; **347:** 1052.
19. Matthai SM, *et al.* Cerebral oedema after ingestion of MDMA (ecstasy) and unrestricted intake of water. *BMJ* 1996; **312:** 1359.
20. Parr MJA, *et al.* Hyponatraemia and death after ecstasy ingestion. *Med J Aust* 1997; **166:** 136–7.
21. Cook TM. Cerebral oedema after MDMA ('ecstasy') and unrestricted water intake. *BMJ* 1996; **313:** 689.
22. Henry JA, *et al.* Low-dose MDMA ("ecstasy") induces vasopressin secretion. *Lancet* 1998; **351:** 1784.
23. Bryden AA, *et al.* Urinary retention with misuse of 'ecstasy'. *BMJ* 1995; **310:** 504.
24. McElhatton PR, *et al.* Congenital anomalies after prenatal ecstasy exposure. *Lancet* 1999; **354:** 1441–2.


**Interactions.** A psychotic reaction has been reported in a patient who took methylenedioxymethamfetamine while receiving therapy with *citalopram*.[1]

A patient receiving *phenelzine* and lithium therapy experienced a serotonin syndrome (p.313) after ingesting methylenedioxymethamfetamine.[2] Symptoms included markedly increased muscle tension, tremulousness, abnormal posturing, limited pain response, tachycardia, hypertension, hyperthermia, increased white blood cell count, increased creatine phosphokinase concentration, respiratory acidosis, metabolic acidosis, delirium, and agitation. Within 15 minutes of methylenedioxymethamfetamine ingestion the patient was comatose; within 5 hours the patient was alert with a normal muscle tone. An interaction between phenelzine and methylenedioxymethamfetamine was suggested as the cause of the serotonin syndrome.

A fatal serotonergic reaction to methylenedioxymethamfetamine possibly due to an interaction with *ritonavir* has been described.[3] A prolonged and exaggerated effect from a small dose of methylenedioxymethamfetamine has been reported[4] in another patient also receiving ritonavir. Although this patient was also receiving saquinavir, the authors postulated that the mechanism may be ritonavir-induced inhibition of the cytochrome P450 isoenzyme CYP2D6.


1. Lauerma H, *et al.* Interaction of serotonin reuptake inhibitor and 3,4-methylenedioxymethamphetamine? *Biol Psychiatry* 1998; **43:** 923–8.
2. Kaskey GB. Possible interaction between an MAOI and "ecstasy". *Am J Psychiatry* 1992; **149:** 411–12.
3. Henry JA, Hill IR. Fatal interaction between ritonavir and MDMA. *Lancet* 1998; **352:** 1751–2.
4. Harrington RD, *et al.* Life-threatening interactions between HIV-1 protease inhibitors and the illicit drugs MDMA and γ-hydroxybutyrate. *Arch Intern Med* 1999; **159:** 2221–4.


## Methylphenidate Hydrochloride *(BANM, rINNM)*

Hidrocloruro de metilfenidato; Methyl Phenidate Hydrochloride. Methyl α-phenyl-2-piperidylacetate hydrochloride.

$C_{14}H_{19}NO_2,HCl = 269.8.$

*CAS — 113-45-1 (methylphenidate); 298-59-9 (methylphenidate hydrochloride).*

*ATC — N06BA04.*

**Pharmacopoeias.** In *Chin., Swiss,* and *US.*

**USP 27** (Methylphenidate Hydrochloride). A white, odourless, fine crystalline powder. Freely soluble in water and in methyl alcohol; soluble in alcohol; slightly soluble in acetone and in chloroform. Solutions are acid to litmus.

### Adverse Effects, Treatment, and Precautions

As for Dexamfetamine Sulfate, p.1586. Hypersensitivity reactions have been reported. Skin reactions have included exfoliative dermatitis and erythema multiforme. Purpura, thrombocytopenia, and leucopenia have occurred. Blood counts should be monitored periodically during prolonged therapy.

◊ References.


1. Ahmann PA, *et al.* Placebo-controlled evaluation of Ritalin side effects. *Pediatrics* 1993; **91:** 1101–6.
2. Efron D, *et al.* Side effects of methylphenidate and dexamphetamine in children with attention deficit hyperactivity disorder: a double-blind, crossover trial. *Pediatrics* 1997; **100:** 662–6.
3. Rappley MD. Safety issues in the use of methylphenidate: an American perspective. *Drug Safety* 1997; **17:** 143–8.


**Abuse.** Reports of adverse effects following the abuse of methylphenidate by injecting solutions of crushed tablets.[1-3] Intravenous abuse of methylphenidate with pentazocine has also been reported.[4,5] In addition, there are also reports of intranasal methylphenidate abuse,[6-8] including fatalities.[8]

See also under Effects on the Liver, below.


1. Wolf J, *et al.* Eosinophilic syndrome with methylphenidate abuse. *Ann Intern Med* 1978; **89:** 224–5.
2. Gunby P. Methylphenidate abuse produces retinopathy. *JAMA* 1979; **241:** 546.
3. Parran TV, Jasinski DR. Intravenous methylphenidate abuse: prototype for prescription drug abuse. *Arch Intern Med* 1991; **151:** 781–3.
4. Debooy VD, *et al.* Intravenous pentazocine and methylphenidate abuse during pregnancy: maternal lifestyle and infant outcome. *Am J Dis Child* 1993; **147:** 1062–5.
5. Carter HS, Watson WA. IV pentazocine/methylphenidate abuse—the clinical toxicity of another Ts and blues combination. *J Toxicol Clin Toxicol* 1994; **32:** 541–7.
6. Jaffe SL. Intranasal abuse of prescribed methylphenidate by an alcohol and drug abusing adolescent with ADHD. *J Am Acad Child Adolesc Psychiatry* 1991; **30:** 773–5.
7. Garland EJ. Intranasal abuse of prescribed methylphenidate. *J Am Acad Child Adolesc Psychiatry* 1998; **37:** 573–4.
8. Massello W, Carpenter DA. A fatality due to the intranasal abuse of methylphenidate (Ritalin®). *J Forensic Sci* 1999; **44:** 220–1.


**Effects on growth.** Concern has been expressed about the effects of central stimulants such as methylphenidate on growth rate when used to treat hyperactivity in children. One study showed that methylphenidate produced decreases in weight percentiles after 1 year of therapy and progressive decrement in height percentiles that became significant after 2 years of use.[1] However, another suggested that moderate doses might have a lower risk for long-term height suppression than dexamfetamine.[2] There has also been a study which showed that, even when methylphenidate had an adverse effect on growth rate during active treatment, final height was not compromised and that a compensatory rebound of growth appeared to occur following discontinuation of the stimulant treatment.[3]

See also under Dexamfetamine Sulfate, p.1586.


1. Mattes JA, Gittelman R. Growth of hyperactive children on maintenance regimen of methylphenidate. *Arch Gen Psychiatry* 1983; **40:** 317–21.
2. Greenhill LL, *et al.* Prolactin, growth hormone and growth responses in boys with attention deficit disorder and hyperactivity treated with methylphenidate. *J Am Acad Child Psychiatry* 1984; **23:** 58–67.
3. Klein RG, Mannuzza S. Hyperactive boys almost grown up III: methylphenidate effects on ultimate height. *Arch Gen Psychiatry* 1988; **45:** 1131–4.


**Effects on the liver.** Hepatotoxicity with raised liver enzyme values in a 67-year-old woman was associated with the administration of methylphenidate hydrochloride 30 mg daily by mouth.[1] Methylphenidate-induced hepatocellular injury was reported in a 19-year old woman who developed jaundice, fever, and malaise after intravenous abuse of methylphenidate hydrochloride tablets.[2]


1. Goodman CR. Hepatotoxicity due to methylphenidate hydrochloride. *N Y State J Med* 1972; **72:** 2339–40.
2. Mehta H, *et al.* Hepatic dysfunction due to intravenous abuse of methylphenidate hydrochloride. *J Clin Gastroenterol* 1984; **6:** 149–51.


**Effects on the skin.** A fixed drug eruption of the scrotum has been reported in 2 children treated with methylphenidate for attention deficit disorder.[1]


1. Cohen HA, *et al.* Fixed drug eruption of the scrotum due to methylphenidate. *Ann Pharmacother* 1992; **26:** 1378–9.


**Tourette's syndrome.** For a discussion on whether central stimulants provoke Tourette's syndrome, see Dexamfetamine Sulfate, p.1586.

### Interactions

As for Dexamfetamine Sulfate, p.1586.

**Anticoagulants.** For the effect of methylphenidate on ethyl biscoumacetate, see Central Stimulants under the Interactions of Warfarin, p.1026.

**Antidepressants.** For the effect of methylphenidate on tricyclic antidepressants, see under Amitriptyline, p.284.

**Antiepileptics.** Methylphenidate blood concentrations decreased, and symptoms of attention deficit hyperactivity disorder worsened, in a 13-year-old girl after starting therapy with *carbamazepine*.[1]

For the effect of methylphenidate on antiepileptics, see under Phenytoin, p.374.


1. Schaller JL, *et al.* Carbamazepine and methylphenidate in ADHD. *J Am Acad Child Adolesc Psychiatry* 1999; **38:** 112–13.


**NSAIDs.** For the effect of methylphenidate on phenylbutazone, see p.83.

### Pharmacokinetics

Methylphenidate is readily absorbed from the gastrointestinal tract. The presence of food in the stomach accelerates the rate of absorption but not the total amount absorbed. Peak plasma concentrations are reached about 2 hours after oral administration; methylphenidate undergoes extensive first-pass metabolism. Protein binding is low. It is excreted as metabolites mainly in the urine with small amounts appearing in the faeces; less than 1% appears in the urine as unchanged methylphenidate. The major metabolite is ritalinic acid (2-phenyl-2-piperidyl acetic acid). The plasma elimination half-life is about 2 hours.

◊ References.


1. Aoyama T, *et al.* Nonlinear kinetics of threo-methylphenidate enantiomers in a patient with narcolepsy and in healthy volunteers. *Eur J Clin Pharmacol* 1993; **44;** 79–84.
2. Aoyama T, *et al.* Pharmacokinetics and pharmacodynamics of (+)-threo-methylphenidate enantiomer in patients with hypersomnia. *Clin Pharmacol Ther* 1994; **55:** 270–6.
3. Shader RI, *et al.* Population pharmacokinetics of methylphenidate in children with attention-deficit hyperactivity disorder. *J Clin Pharmacol* 1999; **39:** 775–785.
4. Kimko HC, *et al.* Pharmacokinetics and clinical effectiveness of methylphenidate. *Clin Pharmacokinet* 1999; **37:** 457–70.
5. Modi NB, *et al.* Single- and multiple-dose pharmacokinetics of an oral once-a-day osmotic controlled-release OROS® (methylphenidate HCl) formulation. *J Clin Pharmacol* 2000; **40:** 379–88.


### Uses and Administration

Methylphenidate hydrochloride is a central stimulant and indirect-acting sympathomimetic with actions and uses similar to those of dexamfetamine (p.1586). It is used in the treatment of narcolepsy (p.1583) and as an adjunct to psychological, educational, and social measures in the treatment of hyperactivity disorders in children.

In the treatment of **narcolepsy** the usual dose is 20 to 30 mg daily by mouth in divided doses, normally 30 to 45 minutes before meals, but the effective dose may range from 10 to 60 mg daily.

In **hyperactivity disorders** in children aged 6 years and over, the usual initial dose is 5 mg once or twice daily by mouth, increased if necessary by 5 to 10 mg at weekly intervals to a maximum of 60 mg daily in divided doses. Methylphenidate may be given before breakfast and lunch. A bedtime dose may be considered if the effect wears off in the evening causing rebound hyperactivity. Methylphenidate should be discontinued if there is no improvement in symptoms after appropriate adjustments in dosage over one month. It also needs to be discontinued from time to time in those who do respond, to assess the patient's condition. Treatment is not usually continued beyond puberty, however, in some patients drug therapy may be required into adulthood. In such cases doses are similar to those used in the treatment of narcolepsy.

Methylphenidate hydrochloride is also given as a modified-release preparation.

A single isomer form of methylphenidate, dexmethylphenidate (p.1587) is also used for hyperactivity disorders.

◊ References.


1. Challman TD, Lipsky JJ. Methylphenidate: its pharmacology and uses. *Mayo Clin Proc* 2000; **75:** 711–21.


**Depression.** Stimulants are no longer recommended as sole treatment for depression (p.279), although they have been tried in augmenting the effect of standard antidepressants such as the SSRIs[1] in patients with refractory depressive disorders.


1. Stoll AL, *et al.* Methylphenidate augmentation of serotonin selective reuptake inhibitors: a case series. *J Clin Psychiatry* 1996; **57:** 72–6.


**Disturbed behaviour.** Disturbed behaviour can have a number of causes and is usually treated with an antipsychotic or benzodiazepine (see p.665). However, a study of methylphenidate in patients who had sustained serious brain injury found that methylphenidate 30 mg daily reduced anger and temper outbursts and improved memory and general measure of psychopathological outcome.[1]


1. Mooney GF, Haas LJ. Effect of methylphenidate on brain injury-related anger. *Arch Phys Med Rehabil* 1993; **74:** 153–60.


**Hyperactivity.** Methylphenidate is one of the main drugs used in hyperactivity, including attention deficit hyperactivity disorder (ADHD) (p.1583).

Small studies have indicated that different aspects of attention deficit disorders in children might respond to different doses of methylphenidate.[1-4] In addition to the morning and noon doses commonly used in hyperactivity disorders, studies[5,6] have shown improved clinical outcome with little adverse effect on sleep patterns if a third late afternoon dose is given. Although modified-release preparations with a slow onset of action have been developed to overcome the short duration of action of methylphenidate they are considered to be less effective than immediate-release preparations. A study,[7] using a regimen to simulate the prolonged steady plasma concentration profile obtained with the slow-onset, modified-release preparations, has suggested that unlike twice daily treatment acute tolerance might develop with the use of modified-release preparations. However, a newer modified-release preparation has been reported to be as effective as an immediate release preparation in short-term studies.[8,9]

UK guidelines for the use of methylphenidate in children and adolescents with ADHD are available.[10]


1. Sprague RL, Sleator EK. Methylphenidate in hyperkinetic children: differences in dose effects on learning and social behavior. *Science* 1977; **198:** 1274–6.
2. Tannock R, *et al.* Dose-response effects of methylphenidate on academic performance and overt behavior in hyperactive children. *Pediatrics* 1989; **84:** 648–57.
3. Sebrechts MM, *et al.* Components of attention, methylphenidate dosage, and blood levels in children with attention deficit disorder. *Pediatrics* 1986; **77:** 222–8.
4. Barkley RA, *et al.* Attention deficit disorder with and without hyperactivity: clinical response to three dose levels of methylphenidate. *Pediatrics* 1991; **87:** 519–31.
5. Kent JD, *et al.* Effects of late-afternoon methylphenidate administration on behavior and sleep in attention-deficit hyperactivity disorders. *Pediatrics* 1995; **96:** 320–5.
6. Stein MA, *et al.* Methylphenidate dosing: twice daily versus three times daily. *Pediatrics* 1996; **98:** 748–56.
7. Swanson J, *et al.* Acute tolerance to methylphenidate in the treatment of attention deficit hyperactivity disorder in children. *Clin Pharmacol Ther* 1999; **66:** 295–305.
8. Pelham WE, *et al.* Once-a-day Concerta methylphenidate versus three-times-daily methylphenidate in laboratory and natural settings. *Pediatrics* 2001; **107:** 1417. Full version available at: http://pediatrics.aappublications.org/cgi/content/full/107/6/e105 (accessed 15/04/04)
9. Wolraich ML, *et al.* Randomized, controlled trial of OROS methylphenidate once a day in children with attention-deficit/hyperactivity disorder. *Pediatrics* 2001; **108:** 883–92.
10. National Institute for Clinical Excellence. Guidance on the use of methylphenidate (Ritalin, Equasym) for attention deficit/hyperactivity disorder (ADHD) in childhood (issued October 2000). Available at: http://www.nice.org.uk/pdf/Methylph-guidance13.pdf (accessed 15/04/04)


## Preparations

***USP 27:*** Methylphenidate Hydrochloride Extended-release Tablets; Methylphenidate Hydrochloride Tablets.

**Proprietary Preparations** (details are given in Part 3)

***Arg.:*** Methylin; Ritalina; Rubifen; ***Austral.:*** Attenta; Concerta; Lorentin; Ritalin; ***Austria:*** Ritalin; ***Belg.:*** Rilatine; ***Braz.:*** Ritalina; ***Canad.:*** Riphenidate; Ritalin; ***Chile:*** Aradix; Elem; Nebapul; Ritalin; Ritrocel; ***Denm.:*** Ritalin; ***Fr.:*** Ritaline; ***Ger.:*** Ritalin; ***Hong Kong:*** Ritalin; ***Irl.:*** Ritalin; ***Israel:*** Metadate; Ritalin; ***Malaysia:*** Ritalin; ***Mex.:*** Ritalin; ***Neth.:*** Ritalin; ***Norw.:*** Ritalin; ***NZ:*** Ritalin; Rubifen; ***S.Afr.:*** Ritalin; Ritaphen; ***Singapore:*** Ritalin; Rubifen; ***Spain:*** Rubifen; ***Swed.:*** Concerta; ***Switz.:*** Ritaline; ***Thai.:*** Rubifen; ***UK:*** Concerta; Equasym; Ritalin; Tranquilyn†; ***USA:*** Concerta; Metadate; Methylin; Ritalin.

## Modafinil *(BAN, USAN, rINN)*

CEP-1538; CRL-40476; Modafinilo. 2-[(Diphenylmethyl)sulfinyl]acetamide.

$C_{15}H_{15}NO_2S = 273.4.$

*CAS — 68693-11-8.*

*ATC — N06BA07.*

### Adverse Effects, Treatment, and Precautions

Adverse effects of modafinil may be a result of CNS stimulation and effects such as nervousness, insomnia, excitation, aggressive tendencies, personality disorder, tremor, and euphoria have been noted. There may also be gastrointestinal disturbances, including nausea and abdominal pain, dry mouth, headache, anorexia, and cardiovascular effects such as hypertension, palpitations, and tachycardia. Pruritic skin rashes, dose-related increases in alkaline phosphatase and, very rarely, bucco-facial dyskinesia have been observed.

Modafinil is contra-indicated in patients with moderate to severe hypertension or cardiac arrhythmias. It is not recommended in patients with a history of left ventricular hypertrophy or ischaemic ECG changes, chest pain, or other signs of mitral valve prolapse.

As with other stimulants, there is the possibility of dependence with long-term use.

### Interactions

Modafinil has enzyme-inducing activity and may impair the efficacy of drugs such as oral contraceptives and antiepileptics.

### Pharmacokinetics

Modafinil is well absorbed from the gastrointestinal tract following oral administration with peak plasma concentrations occurring after 2 to 4 hours. Plasma protein binding is about 60%. Modafinil is metabolised in the liver, the major metabolite being acid modafinil, which is inactive. Excretion is mainly through the kidneys with less than 10% of the dose being eliminated unchanged. The elimination half-life after multiple doses is 15 hours.

◊ References.


1. Wong YN, *et al.* A double-blind, placebo-controlled, ascending-dose evaluation of the pharmacokinetics and tolerability of modafinil tablets in healthy male volunteers. *J Clin Pharmacol* 1999; **39:** 30–40.
2. Wong YN, *et al.* Open-label, single-dose pharmacokinetic study of modafinil tablets: influence of age and gender in normal subjects. *J Clin Pharmacol* 1999; **39:** 281–8.


### Uses and Administration

Modafinil is a central stimulant chemically related to adrafinil (p.1584). It is used in the treatment of excessive daytime sleepiness associated with the narcoleptic syndrome (p.1583), obstructive sleep apnoea, and shift-work sleep disorder. In the treatment of the narcoleptic syndrome or obstructive sleep apnoea, modafinil is given orally in a dose of 200 to 400 mg daily, in two divided doses, in the morning and at midday, or as a single dose in the morning. For the treatment of shift-work sleep disorder, the daily dose is 200 mg taken as a single dose 1 hour before starting work. An initial dose of 100 mg daily should be used in the elderly and adjusted as necessary. For doses in hepatic and renal impairment, see below.

Modafinil has also been investigated for the treatment of fatigue associated with multiple sclerosis.

◊ References.


1. Broughton RJ, *et al.* Randomized, double-blind, placebo-controlled crossover trial of modafinil in the treatment of excessive daytime sleepiness in narcolepsy. *Neurology* 1997; **49:** 444–51.
2. US Modafinil in Narcolepsy Multicenter Study Group. Randomized trial of modafinil for the treatment of pathological somnolence in narcolepsy. *Ann Neurol* 1998; **43:** 88–97.
3. McClellan KJ, Spencer CM. Modafinil: a review of its pharmacology and clinical efficacy in the management of narcolepsy. *CNS Drugs* 1998; **9:** 311–24.
4. Fry JM. Treatment modalities for narcolepsy. *Neurology* 1998; **50:** S43–S48.
5. Anonymous. Modafinil for narcolepsy. *Med Lett Drugs Ther* 1999; **41:** 30–1.
6. US Modafinil in Narcolepsy Multicenter Study Group. Randomized trial of modafinil as a treatment for the excessive daytime somnolence of narcolepsy. *Neurology* 2000; **54:** 1166–75.
7. Kingshott RN, *et al.* Randomized, double-blind, placebo-controlled crossover trial of modafinil in the treatment of residual excessive daytime sleepiness in the sleep apnea/hypopnea syndrome. *Am J Respir Crit Care Med* 2001; **163:** 918–23.


**Administration in hepatic or renal impairment.** The total daily dose of modafinil should be reduced to 100 to 200 mg in any patient with severe hepatic or renal impairment.

### Preparations

**Proprietary Preparations** (details are given in Part 3)

***Arg.:*** Vigicer; ***Austral.:*** Modavigil; ***Austria:*** Modasomil; ***Belg.:*** Provigil; ***Canad.:*** Alertec; ***Denm.:*** Modiodal; ***Fr.:*** Modiodal; ***Ger.:*** Vigil; ***Gr.:*** Modiodal; ***Irl.:*** Provigil; ***Israel:*** Provigil; ***Ital.:*** Provigil; ***Neth.:*** Modiodal; ***NZ:*** Modavigil; ***Port.:*** Modiodal; ***Spain:*** Modiodal; ***Swed.:*** Modiodal; ***Switz.:*** Modasomil; ***UK:*** Provigil; ***USA:*** Provigil.

## Nikethamide *(BAN, rINN)*

Cordiaminum; Nicethamidum; Nicotinic Acid Diethylamide; Nicotinoyldiaethylamidum; Nikethylamide; Niquetamida. *N,N*-Diethylnicotinamide; *N,N*-Diethylpyridine-3-carboxamide.

$C_{10}H_{14}N_2O = 178.2.$

*CAS — 59-26-7.*

*ATC — R07AB02.*

**Pharmacopoeias.** In *Chin., Eur.* (see p.vi), *Pol.,* and *Viet.*

**Ph. Eur. 5.0** (Nikethamide). A colourless or slightly yellow oily liquid or crystalline mass. Miscible with water and with alcohol. A 25% solution in water has a pH of 6.0 to 7.8.

### Profile

Nikethamide has actions similar to those of doxapram (p.1587). It was formerly used as a respiratory stimulant but this has largely been abandoned because of toxicity. Nikethamide and its calcium thiocyanate salt have also been used in some countries as central stimulants and for hypotensive disorders.

**Porphyria.** Nikethamide has been associated with acute attacks of porphyria and is considered unsafe in porphyric patients.

### Preparations

***BP 2003:*** Nikethamide Injection.

**Proprietary Preparations** (details are given in Part 3)

***Braz.:*** Cinclamina†.

**Multi-ingredient:** ***Braz.:*** Cardioregis†; ***Fr.:*** Coramine Glucose; ***Ger.:*** Felsol Neo†; Zellaforte N Plus; ***Switz.:*** Gly-Coramin.

## Pemoline *(BAN, USAN, rINN)*

LA-956; NSC-25159; Pemolina; Phenoxazole; Phenylisohydantoin; Phenylpseudohydantoin. 2-Imino-5-phenyl-4-oxazolidinone.

$C_9H_8N_2O_2 = 176.2.$

*CAS — 2152-34-3 (pemoline); 68942-31-4 (pemoline hydrochloride); 18968-99-5 (magnesium pemoline).*

*ATC — N06BA05.*

### Adverse Effects, Treatment, and Precautions

As for Dexamfetamine Sulfate, p.1586; however, the effects of over-stimulation and sympathomimetic activity are considered to be less with pemoline.

Reports of liver toxicity in patients taking pemoline (see Effects on the Liver, below) have limited its use; it is contra-indicated in patients with liver disorders and there are stringent precautions to be observed with its use. Treatment should be initiated only in patients with normal baseline liver function tests and liver function should be monitored every 2 weeks. Pemoline should be discontinued if serum alanine aminotransferase is increased to a clinically significant level or there is any increase greater than or equal to twice the upper limit of normal, or if any clinical signs or symptoms suggestive of liver failure develop. Pemoline should also be withdrawn from patients who have failed to show a substantial clinical response within 3 weeks of completing dose titration. There have also been rare or isolated reports of chorea, tics, mania, and neutropenia.

**Abuse.** Paranoid psychosis was observed in a 38-year-old man taking pemoline 75 to 225 mg daily.[1] His compulsive use of the drug, development of tolerance, depressive withdrawal syndrome, and inability to abstain indicated dependence and it was evident that the patient was addicted to pemoline.

Choreoathetosis and rhabdomyolysis developed in a patient following a marked increase in intake of pemoline.[2] Abnormal movements responded to diazepam.


1. Polchert SE, Morse RM. Pemoline abuse. *JAMA* 1985; **254:** 946–7.
2. Briscoe JG, *et al.* Pemoline-induced choreoathetosis and rhabdomyolysis. *Med Toxicol* 1988; **3:** 72–6.


**Effects on growth.** Results of a study in 24 hyperkinetic children suggested that growth suppression was a potential side-effect of prolonged treatment with clinically effective doses of pemoline and that this effect might be dose-related.[1]

See also under Dexamfetamine Sulfate, p.1586.


1. Dickinson LC, *et al.* Impaired growth in hyperkinetic children receiving pemoline. *J Pediatr* 1979; **94:** 538–41.


**Effects on the liver.** Pemoline has been associated with hepatotoxicity.

Elevated concentrations of serum aspartate aminotransferase and serum alanine aminotransferase have been noted in 2% of children taking pemoline for hyperactivity; the effect was stated to be transient and reversible.[1]

However, more serious reactions have also occurred. Acute hepatitis was associated with pemoline in a 10-year-old boy[2] and the drug was believed to be the cause of fatal fulminant liver failure in a 14-year-old boy and in 2 previously published cases.[3] The UK Committee on Safety of Medicines[4] subsequently became aware of 33 reports of serious hepatic reactions in the USA, including a total of 6 fatalities and the need for liver transplantation in 2 cases. This prompted the withdrawal of pemoline for the treatment of hyperactivity in the UK.


1. Anonymous. 'Hyperkinesis' can have many causes, symptoms. *JAMA* 1975; **232:** 1204–16.
2. Patterson JF. Hepatitis associated with pemoline. *South Med J* 1984; **77:** 938.
3. Berkovitch M, *et al.* Pemoline-associated fulminant liver failure: testing the evidence for causation. *Clin Pharmacol Ther* 1995; **57:** 696–8.
4. Committee on Safety of Medicines/Medicines Control Agency. Volital (pemoline) has been withdrawn. *Current Problems* 1997; **23:** 10. Also available at: http://www.mca.gov.uk/ourwork/monitorsafequalmed/currentproblems/page2.htm (accessed 15/04/04)


**Effects on the prostate.** Experience in one patient suggested that pemoline might adversely affect the prostate gland or interfere with tests for prostatic acid phosphatase used in the diagnosis of prostatic carcinoma.[1]


1. Lindau W, de Girolami E. Pemoline and the prostate. *Lancet* 1986; **i:** 738.


### Interactions

Hypertensive crisis may possibly occur if pemoline is given with MAOIs. Reduced seizure threshold has been reported in epileptic patients taking pemoline and antiepileptics.

### Pharmacokinetics

Pemoline is readily absorbed from the gastrointestinal tract. About 50% is bound to plasma protein. It is metabolised in the liver and excreted in the urine as unchanged pemoline and metabolites.

◊ References.


1. Vermeulen NPE, *et al.* Pharmacokinetics of pemoline in plasma, saliva and urine following oral administration. *Br J Clin Pharmacol* 1979; **8:** 459–63.
2. Sallee F, *et al.* Oral pemoline kinetics in hyperactive children. *Clin Pharmacol Ther* 1985; **37:** 606–9.
3. Collier CP, *et al.* Pemoline pharmacokinetics and long term therapy in children with attention deficit disorder and hyperactivity. *Clin Pharmacokinet* 1985; **10:** 269–78.


### Uses and Administration

Pemoline is a central stimulant with actions similar to those of dexamfetamine (p.1586).

It has been used in the management of hyperactivity disorders in children (p.1583). In the USA 37.5 mg is given by mouth each morning initially, increased gradually at weekly intervals by 18.75 mg; the usual range is 56.25 to 75 mg daily and the maximum recommended daily dose is 112.5 mg. In the UK, pemoline was withdrawn from use for hyperactivity in children after reports of serious hepatotoxicity in the USA.

Pemoline has been included in preparations also containing yohimbine hydrochloride and methyltestosterone that are claimed to combat failure of sexual desire and functioning in males and females; such preparations are not recommended.

Pemoline has been given with magnesium hydroxide (magnesium pemoline) in an attempt to increase its absorption.

### Preparations

**Proprietary Preparations** (details are given in Part 3)

***Arg.:*** Tamilan; ***Belg.:*** Stimul†; ***Canad.:*** Cylert†; ***Chile:*** Bimolin; Ceractiv; Cylert; ***Ger.:*** Hyperilex†; Senior†; Tradon; ***Israel:*** Cylert; Nitan; ***S.Afr.:*** Dynalert†; ***USA:*** Cylert; PemADD.

**Multi-ingredient:** ***S.Afr.:*** Lentogesic; ***UK:*** Prowess†.

## Pentetrazol *(BAN, rINN)*

Corazol; Leptazol; Pentamethazol; 1,5-Pentamethylenetetrazole; Pentazol; Pentetrazolum; Pentylenetetrazol. 6,7,8,9-Tetrahydro-5*H*-tetrazoloazepine.

$C_6H_{10}N_4$ = 138.2.

*CAS — 54-95-5.*

*ATC — R07AB03.*

**Pharmacopoeias.** In *It.*

### Profile

Pentetrazol is a central and respiratory stimulant similar to doxapram (p.1587). It has been used in respiratory depression and in multi-ingredient preparations intended for the treatment of respiratory-tract disorders including cough, cardiovascular disorders including hypotension, and for the treatment of pruritus. Administration has been by mouth and by injection.

**Porphyria.** Pentetrazol has been associated with acute attacks of porphyria and is considered unsafe in porphyric patients.

### Preparations

**Proprietary Preparations** (details are given in Part 3)

**Multi-ingredient:** ***Braz.:*** Belacodid; Piritosse†; Revulsan; Suprasten; ***India:*** Cardiazol-Dicodid; ***Ital.:*** Cardiazol-Paracodina; ***Port.:*** Broncodiazina.

## Phendimetrazine Tartrate *(BANM, rINNM)*

Phendimetrazine Acid Tartrate; Phendimetrazine Bitartrate; Tartrato de fendimetrazina. (+)-3,4-Dimethyl-2-phenylmorpholine hydrogen tartrate.

$C_{12}H_{17}NO,C_4H_6O_6$ = 341.4.

*CAS — 634-03-7 (phendimetrazine); 7635-51-0 (phendimetrazine hydrochloride); 50-58-8 (phendimetrazine tartrate).*

**Pharmacopoeias.** In *US.*

**USP 27** (Phendimetrazine Tartrate). A white odourless crystalline powder. Freely soluble in water; sparingly soluble in warm alcohol; insoluble in acetone, in chloroform, in ether, and in benzene. pH of a 2.5% solution in water is between 3.0 and 4.0. Store in airtight containers.

### Adverse Effects, Treatment, and Precautions

As for Dexamfetamine Sulfate, p.1586.

Pulmonary hypertension and valvular heart defects have been reported in patients receiving phendimetrazine with other anorectics; these adverse effects, with the relevant precautions to be observed, are discussed under Fenfluramine Hydrochloride, p.1588. Phendimetrazine should not be used with other anorectics nor within a year of their use.

### Interactions

Phendimetrazine is an indirect-acting sympathomimetic and may interact with other drugs similarly to dexamfetamine (p.1586).

### Pharmacokinetics

Phendimetrazine tartrate is readily absorbed from the gastrointestinal tract and is excreted in the urine, partly unchanged and partly as phenmetrazine and other metabolites.

### Uses and Administration

Phendimetrazine tartrate is a central stimulant and indirect-acting sympathomimetic with actions similar to those of dexamfetamine (p.1586). It has been used as an anorectic in the short-term treatment of obesity (p.1583), although stimulants are no longer recommended for this indication. The usual dose is 35 mg two or three times daily by mouth before food. An alternative dose is 105 mg once daily in the morning as a modified-release preparation.

Phendimetrazine hydrochloride has been used similarly.

Regulatory authorities in the European Union have called for the withdrawal of all anorectics from the market. (see under Effects on the Cardiovascular System in Fenfluramine, p.1588)

### Preparations

***USP 27:*** Phendimetrazine Tartrate Capsules; Phendimetrazine Tartrate Tablets.

**Proprietary Preparations** (details are given in Part 3)

***Belg.:*** Anoran†; ***Ital.:*** Plegine†; ***S.Afr.:*** Obesan-X; Obex-LA; ***USA:*** Adipost†; Bontril; Dyrexan-OD†; Melfiat; Plegine†; Prelu-2; Rexigen Forte†.

## Phenmetrazine Hydrochloride *(BANM, rINNM)*

Hidrocloruro de fenmetrazina; Oxazimédrine. (±)-*trans*-3-Methyl-2-phenylmorpholine hydrochloride.

$C_{11}H_{15}NO,HCl$ = 213.7.

*CAS — 134-49-6 (phenmetrazine); 1707-14-8 (phenmetrazine hydrochloride); 13931-75-4 (phenmetrazine teoclate).*

**Pharmacopoeias.** In *US.*

**USP 27** (Phenmetrazine Hydrochloride). A white to off-white crystalline powder. Soluble 1 in 0.4 of water, 1 in 2 of alcohol, and 1 in 2 of chloroform. pH of a 2.5% solution in water is between 4.5 and 5.5. Store in airtight containers.

### Profile

Phenmetrazine hydrochloride is a central stimulant and indirect-acting sympathomimetic with actions similar to those of dexamfetamine (p.1585). It has been used as an anorectic in the treatment of obesity. Regulatory authorities in the European Union have called for the withdrawal of all anorectics from the market (see under Effects on the Cardiovascular System in Fenfluramine, p.1588). It has been subject to extensive abuse.

**Abuse.** For reference to a serious syndrome involving rhabdomyolysis following intravenous abuse of phenmetrazine, see Dexamfetamine Sulfate, p.1586.

### Preparations

***USP 27:*** Phenmetrazine Hydrochloride Tablets.

## Phentermine *(BAN, USAN, rINN)*

Fentermina. α,α-Dimethylphenethylamine.

$C_{10}H_{15}N$ = 149.2.

*CAS — 122-09-8.*

*ATC — A08AA01.*

## Phentermine Hydrochloride *(BANM, rINNM)*

Hidrocloruro de fentermina.

$C_{10}H_{15}N,HCl$ = 185.7.

*CAS — 1197-21-3.*

*ATC — A08AA01.*

**Pharmacopoeias.** In *US.*

**USP 27** (Phentermine Hydrochloride). A white, odourless, hygroscopic, crystalline powder. Soluble in water and in the lower alcohols; slightly soluble in chloroform; insoluble in ether. pH of a 2% solution in water is between 5.0 and 6.0. Store in airtight containers.

### Adverse Effects, Treatment, and Precautions

As for Dexamfetamine Sulfate, p.1586. Urticaria may occur with use of phentermine.

Pulmonary hypertension has been reported in patients receiving phentermine and valvular heart defects in patients receiving the drug with other anorectics such as fenfluramine or dexfenfluramine; these adverse effects, with the relevant precautions to be observed, are discussed under Fenfluramine Hydrochloride, p.1588.

### Interactions

Phentermine is an indirect-acting sympathomimetic and may interact with other drugs, similarly to dexamfetamine (p.1586).

### Pharmacokinetics

Phentermine is readily absorbed from the gastrointestinal tract and is excreted in the urine, partly unchanged and partly as metabolites.

### Uses and Administration

Phentermine is a central stimulant and indirect-acting sympathomimetic with actions similar to those of dexamfetamine (p.1586). It has been given by mouth as the base or hydrochloride as an anorectic in the short-term treatment of moderate to severe obesity (p.1583), although stimulants are no longer recommended for this indication.

The usual dose of phentermine is 15 to 30 mg once daily before breakfast given as an ion-exchange resin complex that provides modified release. A suggested dose for phentermine hydrochloride is 8 mg three times daily before meals or 15 to 37.5 mg once daily in the morning. It should not be given for longer than a few weeks.

Regulatory authorities in the European Union have called for the withdrawal of phentermine from the market (see under Effects on the Cardiovascular System in Fenfluramine, p.1588).

### Preparations

***USP 27:*** Phentermine Hydrochloride Capsules; Phentermine Hydrochloride Tablets.

**Proprietary Preparations** (details are given in Part 3)

***Austral.:*** Duromine; ***Austria:*** Adipex†; ***Belg.:*** Ionamin†; ***Canad.:*** Fastin†; Ionamin; ***Hong Kong:*** Duromine; Panbesy; Redusa; ***Israel:*** Novirasin; ***Malaysia:*** Adipex; Duromine; Ionamin; ***Mex.:*** Diminex†; Ifa Reduccing S; Ionamin†; Reducap†; Sinpet; ***NZ:*** Duromine; Umine; ***S.Afr.:*** Duromine; Minobese†; ***Singapore:*** Duromine; Ionamin; Panbesy; Umine; ***Switz.:*** Adipex; Ionamine; Normaform†; ***Thai.:*** Duromine; Panbesy; ***UK:*** Duromine†; Ionamin†; ***USA:*** Adipex-P; Fastin†; Ionamin; Obe-Nix†; Zantryl†.

## Pipradrol Hydrochloride *(BANM, rINNM)*

Hidrocloruro de pipradrol. α-2-Piperidylbenzhydrol hydrochloride; α,α-Diphenyl-2-piperidinemethanol hydrochloride.

$C_{18}H_{21}NO,HCl$ = 303.8.

*CAS — 467-60-7 (pipradrol); 71-78-3 (pipradrol hydrochloride).*

*ATC — N06BX15.*

### Profile

Pipradrol hydrochloride has been given by mouth in tonic preparations as a CNS stimulant.

### Preparations

**Proprietary Preparations** (details are given in Part 3)

**Multi-ingredient:** ***Austral.:*** Alertonic; ***Canad.:*** Alertonic; ***S.Afr.:*** Alertonic.

## Prethcamide

G-5668; Pretcamida. *N,N*-Dimethyl-2-(*N*-propylcrotonamido)butyramide (cropropamide, $C_{13}H_{24}N_2O_2$ = 240.3); 2-(*N*-Ethylcrotonamido)-*N,N*-dimethylbutyramide (crotetamide, $C_{12}H_{22}N_2O_2$ = 226.3).

*CAS — 8015-51-8 (prethcamide); 633-47-6 (cropropamide); 6168-76-9 (crotetamide).*

*ATC — R07AB06.*

**Description.** Prethcamide is a mixture of equal parts by weight of cropropamide (*pINN*) and crotetamide (*BAN, rINN*)(crotethamide).

### Profile

Prethcamide has actions similar to those of doxapram (p.1587) and has been used as a respiratory stimulant. Doses of 100 mg have been given three times daily by mouth.

### Preparations

**Proprietary Preparations** (details are given in Part 3)

***Ital.:*** Micoren.

## Prolintane Hydrochloride *(BANM, USAN, rINNM)*

Hidrocloruro de prolintano; SP-732. 1-(α-Propylphenethyl)pyrrolidine hydrochloride.

$C_{15}H_{23}N,HCl$ = 253.8.

*CAS — 493-92-5 (prolintane); 1211-28-5 (prolintane hydrochloride).*

*ATC — N06BX14.*

### Profile

Prolintane hydrochloride is a mild central stimulant and has properties similar to those of dexamfetamine (p.1585). It has been available mainly in tonic preparations that also contained vitamin supplements. It has also been used in narcolepsy.

### Preparations

**Proprietary Preparations** (details are given in Part 3)

***Belg.:*** Catorid†; ***S.Afr.:*** Catovit N†.

**Multi-ingredient:** ***S.Afr.:*** Catovit†; ***Spain:*** Katovit†.

## Propylhexedrine *(BAN, rINN)*

Hexahydrodesoxyephedrine; Propilhexedrina; Propylhexed. 2-Cyclohexyl-1-methylethyl-(methyl)amine; (±)-*N*-α-Dimethylcyclo-hexaneethylamine.

$C_{10}H_{21}N$ = 155.3.

*CAS — 101-40-6; 3595-11-7 ((±)-propylhexedrine).*

**Pharmacopoeias.** In *US.*

**USP 27** (Propylhexedrine). A clear colourless liquid having a characteristic amine-like odour. It slowly volatilises at room temperature and absorbs carbon dioxide from the air. Very slightly soluble in water; soluble 1 in 0.4 of alcohol, 1 in 0.2 of chloroform, and 1 in 0.1 of ether. Its solutions are alkaline to litmus. Store in airtight containers.

## Propylhexedrine Hydrochloride *(BANM, rINNM)*

Hidrocloruro de propilhexedrina.

$C_{10}H_{21}N,HCl$ = 191.7.

*CAS — 1007-33-6; 6192-95-6 ((±)-propylhexedrine hydrochloride).*

### Adverse Effects, Treatment and Precautions

As for Dexamfetamine Sulfate, p.1586.

Nasal inhalation may cause transient burning, stinging, mucosal dryness, and sneezing. Prolonged use can cause rebound congestion, redness, swelling, and rhinitis. Systemic effects such as headache, hypertension, nervousness, and increased heart rate may occur.

Propylhexedrine is subject to abuse by mouth or intravenously; fatalities due to myocardial infarction, heart failure, or pulmonary hypertension have been reported. Psychosis may occur.

**Abuse.** References.

1. White L, DiMaio VJM. Intravenous propylhexedrine and sudden death. *N Engl J Med* 1977; **297:** 1071.
2. Anderson RJ, *et al.* Intravenous propylhexedrine (Benzedrex®) abuse and sudden death. *Am J Med* 1979; **67:** 15–20.
3. Cameron J, *et al.* Possible association of pulmonary hypertension with an anorectic drug. *Med J Aust* 1984; **140:** 595–7.

## Uses and Administration

Propylhexedrine is a central stimulant and indirect-acting sympathomimetic with actions similar to those of dexamfetamine (p.1586). It has been used as an inhalant for nasal decongestion (p.1112).

Propylhexedrine hydrochloride has been given by mouth as an anorectic in the treatment of obesity (p.1583) but stimulants are no longer recommended for this indication. The (−)-isomer, levopropylhexedrine hydrochloride, has been used similarly.

## Preparations

*USP 27:* Propylhexedrine inhalant.

**Proprietary Preparations** (details are given in Part 3)
***Mex.:*** Colloidine†; ***USA:*** Benzedrex.
**Multi-ingredient:** ***S.Afr.:*** Reducealin.

# Sibutramine Hydrochloride *(BANM, USAN, rINNM)*

BTS-54524; Hidrocloruro de sibutramina. (±)-1-(*p*-Chlorophenyl)-α-isobutyl-*N*,*N*-dimethylcyclobutanemethylamine hydrochloride monohydrate.

$C_{17}H_{26}ClN,HCl,H_2O$ = 334.3.
*CAS — 106650-56-0 (sibutramine); 84485-00-7 (anhydrous sibutramine hydrochloride); 125494-59-9 (sibutramine hydrochloride monohydrate).*
*ATC — A08AA10.*

## Adverse Effects

Commonly reported side-effects of sibutramine are dry mouth, headache, insomnia, and constipation. Diarrhoea, back pain, increased appetite, dizziness, flu-like symptoms, and rhinitis have also occurred. Less frequently reported side-effects include dyspepsia, nausea, dysmenorrhoea, increased sweating and thirst, oedema, paraesthesia, skin rashes, taste perversion, palpitations, vasodilatation, anxiety, nervousness, drowsiness, and depression. Abnormal bleeding including Henoch-Schönlein purpura and thrombocytopenia, acute interstitial nephritis, glomerulonephritis, emotional lability, seizures, and blurred vision have been reported rarely. Clinically significant increases in heart rate and blood pressure may occur. Sibutramine may decrease salivary flow and therefore increase the risk of dental caries, periodontal disease, or other oral disorders. It may also produce mydriasis. Reversible increases in liver enzymes have been reported.

## Precautions

Sibutramine should be avoided in patients with a history of eating disorders such as anorexia nervosa and bulimia nervosa. It is also contra-indicated in patients with uncontrolled or poorly controlled hypertension and should be used with caution in patients with a history of, or with, well-controlled hypertension. Blood pressure and heart rate should be monitored (see below for details). In the event of sustained elevations, the dose should be reduced or treatment discontinued.

Sibutramine should not be used in patients with a history of cerebrovascular disease or cardiovascular disorders such as cardiac arrhythmias, heart failure, peripheral arterial occlusive disease, and coronary artery disease; it should be avoided in patients with severe hepatic or renal impairment. Sibutramine should also not be used in patients with bipolar disorder, Tourette's syndrome, hyperthyroidism, phaeochromocytoma, benign prostatic hyperplasia, or a history of drug or alcohol abuse. It should be used with caution, if at all, in patients with glaucoma. Sibutramine should also be used with caution in patients with a history of depression, seizures or gallstones (which may be precipitated or exacerbated by weight loss), or a family history of motor or verbal tics.

Any centrally-acting drug such as sibutramine may impair the ability to perform tasks requiring judgement or motor or cognitive skills; if affected, patients should not drive or operate machinery.

**Bleeding disorders.** Because other drugs that inhibit reuptake of serotonin have occasionally been associated with bleeding disorders and other effects on the blood (see under Fluoxetine, p.292) the UK manufacturers of sibutramine recommend that it should be used with caution in patients predisposed to bleeding disorders and in those taking other drugs known to affect haemostasis or platelet function.

**Cardiovascular monitoring.** Sibutramine may cause clinically significant increases in blood pressure and heart rate and monitoring is recommended in all patients during treatment. In the first 3 months, blood pressure and heart rate should be checked every 2 weeks; this may be reduced to every month for the next 3 months, and at least every 3 months thereafter. Treatment should be discontinued if resting heart rate increases by 10 beats/minute or more, or blood pressure by 10 mmHg or more, at two consecutive visits. In patients with previously well-controlled hypertension, treatment should be discontinued if their blood pressure exceeds 145/90 mmHg at two consecutive visits.

## Interactions

Sibutramine should not be given with, or within at least 2 weeks of stopping an MAOI; at least 2 weeks should elapse between discontinuation of sibutramine and starting therapy with an MAOI. There is a risk of the serotonin syndrome (p.313) developing if sibutramine is used with other serotonergic drugs such as SSRIs, sumatriptan, lithium, pethidine, fentanyl, dextromethorphan, and pentazocine. Caution is advised when sibutramine is given with other drugs that may increase heart rate or blood pressure such as ephedrine, phenylpropanolamine, and pseudoephedrine. It should not be used with other centrally acting anorectics. Alcohol should be avoided.

Inhibitors of the cytochrome P450 isoenzyme CYP3A4, such as ketoconazole and erythromycin, may increase plasma concentrations of sibutramine. Conversely, inducers of this isoenzyme, such as rifampicin, phenytoin, carbamazepine, and phenobarbital, may reduce plasma concentrations of sibutramine.

**Antibacterials.** A study in 12 obese subjects indicated that addition of *erythromycin* to sibutramine therapy resulted in little significant alteration in sibutramine pharmacokinetics beyond a modest increase in maximum plasma concentration of one of the active metabolites.[1] A small increase in the QT interval was not considered clinically meaningful.

1. Hinson JL, *et al.* Steady-state interaction study of sibutramine (Meridia™) and erythromycin in uncomplicated obese subjects. *Pharm Res* 1996; **13** (suppl): S116.

**Antifungals.** A study in 12 obese subjects given sibutramine found that *ketoconazole* moderately increased steady-state plasma concentrations of sibutramine and its active metabolites.[1] There was a significant increase in heart rate but no clinically relevant change in the QT interval.

1. Hinson JL, *et al.* Steady-state interaction study of sibutramine (Meridia™) and ketoconazole in uncomplicated obese subjects. *Pharm Res* 1996; **13** (suppl): S116.

## Pharmacokinetics

Sibutramine is well-absorbed from the gastrointestinal tract; peak plasma concentrations appear after 1.2 hours (parent drug) and 3 to 4 hours (metabolites). It undergoes extensive first-pass hepatic metabolism, mediated mainly by the cytochrome P450 isoenzyme CYP3A4. Demethylation produces mono- and di-desmethylsibutramine (both of which are pharmacologically active) and is followed by hydroxylation and conjugation to inactive metabolites. Protein binding is 97%. Plasma-elimination half-life is 14 to 16 hours. Elimination is mainly in the urine as inactive metabolites, and partly in the faeces.

◊ References.

1. Hind ID, *et al.* Sibutramine pharmacokinetics in young and elderly healthy subjects. *Eur J Clin Pharmacol* 1999; **54:** 847–9.

## Uses and Administration

Sibutramine, which is structurally related to amfetamine (p.1584), is a serotonin and noradrenaline reuptake inhibitor; it also inhibits dopamine reuptake but to a lesser extent. Sibutramine is used in the management of obesity (p.1583). It may also be used in overweight patients (body-mass index of 27 kg/m² or more) if other risk factors such as hypertension (but see Precautions, above), diabetes mellitus, or hyperlipidaemias are present.

Sibutramine hydrochloride is given by mouth in an initial daily dose of 10 mg, usually taken in the morning. Patients who cannot tolerate 10 mg daily may benefit from a dose of 5 mg daily. Treatment with sibutramine should be re-evaluated if weight loss is less than 2 kg in the first 4 weeks of therapy. At this stage, the dose may be increased to a maximum of 15 mg daily, taking into consideration effects on heart rate and blood pressure, or treatment may need to be discontinued. It should be re-assessed again after a further 4 weeks at maximum dose, and discontinued if weight loss is less than 2 kg. Treatment should also be stopped if:

- weight loss stabilises at less than 5% of the initial body-weight
- weight loss after 3 months is less than 5% of the initial body-weight
- weight gain of 3 kg or more occurs after previous weight loss.

Treatment should not be given for longer than 1 year.

In patients with other risk factors (see Precautions, above), it is recommended that sibutramine is continued only if weight loss is associated with other clinical benefits.

◊ References.

1. McNeely W, Goa KL. Sibutramine: a review of its contribution to the management of obesity. *Drugs* 1998; **56:** 1093–1124.
2. Luque CA, Rey JA. Sibutramine: a serotonin-norepinephrine reuptake-inhibitor for the treatment of obesity. *Ann Pharmacother* 1999; **33:** 968–78.
3. James WPT, *et al.* Effect of sibutramine on weight maintenance after weight loss: a randomised trial. *Lancet* 2000; **356:** 2119–25.
4. McMahon FG, *et al.* Efficacy and safety of sibutramine in obese white and African American patients with hypertension: a 1-year, double-blind, placebo-controlled, multicenter trial. *Arch Intern Med* 2000; **160:** 2185–91.
5. National Institute for Clinical Excellence. Guidance on the use of sibutramine for the treatment of obesity in adults (issued October 2001). Available at: http://www.nice.org.uk/pdf/SIBUTRAME%2031%20GUIDANCE.pdf (accessed 15/04/04)
6. Nisoli E, Carruba MO. A benefit-risk assessment of sibutramine in the management of obesity. *Drug Safety* 2003; **26:** 1027–48.

## Preparations

**Proprietary Preparations** (details are given in Part 3)
***Arg.:*** Aderan; Ipomex; Raductil; Societyl; Sibu-Estirol; ***Austral.:*** Reductil; ***Austria:*** Meridia; Reductil; ***Belg.:*** Reductil; ***Braz.:*** Plenty; Reductil; ***Canad.:*** Meridia; ***Chile:*** Adisar; Atenix; Ipogras; Medixil; Mesura; Milical; Noducil; Reductil; Reduten; Saton; ***Denm.:*** Reductil; ***Fin.:*** Reductil; ***Fr.:*** Sibutral; ***Ger.:*** Reductil; ***Hong Kong:*** Reductil; ***India:*** Obestat; ***Irl.:*** Reductil; ***Israel:*** Reductil; ***Ital.:*** Ectiva; Reductil; Reduxade; ***Mex.:*** Ectiva; Raductil; ***Neth.:*** Reductil; ***NZ:*** Reductil; ***Port.:*** Reductil; ***S.Afr.:*** Reductil; ***Singapore:*** Reductil; ***Spain:*** Reductil; ***Swed.:*** Reductil; ***Switz.:*** Reductil; ***Thai.:*** Reductil; ***UK:*** Reductil; ***USA:*** Meridia.

# Tenamfetamine *(rINN)*

MDA; Methylenedioxyamphetamine; 3,4-Methylenedioxyamphetamine; SKF-5; Tenanfetamina. α-Methyl-3,4-methylenedioxyphenethylamine.

$C_{10}H_{13}NO_2$ = 179.2.
*CAS — 4764-17-4; 51497-09-7.*

NOTE. Tenamfetamine has also been known as Love Drug, Love Pill, and Mellow Drug of America.

## Profile

Tenamfetamine is a phenylethylamine compound, structurally related to amfetamine and mescaline, with hallucinogenic effects. It has been subject to abuse and dependence. A number of similar compounds are known because of their abuse and include:

- brolamfetamine (4-bromo-2,5-dimethoxyamfetamine; bromo-DMA; bromo-DOM; 2,5-dimethoxy-4-bromoamfetamine; DOB);
- 4-bromo-2,5-methoxyphenylethylamine (afterburner; 2-CB; MFT);
- 2,5-dimethoxy-4-metamfetamine (DOM; methyl-2,5-dimethoxyamfetamine; Serenity, Tranquillity and Peace; STP);
- *N*-ethyltenamfetamine (Eve; MDE; MDEA; 3,4-methylenedioxyethamfetamine);
- *N*-hydroxytenamfetamine (*N*-hydroxy MDA; 3,4-methylenedioxy-*N*-hydroxyamfetamine);
- methoxyamfetamine (4-methoxyamfetamine; *p*-methoxyamfetamine; PMA);
- methylenedioxymethamfetamine (Ecstasy) (see p.1589);
- 2,4,5-trimethoxyamfetamine (TMA; TMA-2).

In large doses the side-effects of tenamfetamine and related compounds are similar to those of dexamfetamine and may be treated similarly (see p.1586). Fatalities have been associated with the abuse of some of these compounds.

◊ Reviews of the properties of some designer drugs, including phenylethylamine compounds.

1. Buchanan JF, Brown CR. 'Designer drugs': a problem in clinical toxicology. *Med Toxicol* 1988; **3:** 1–17.
2. Chesher G. Designer drugs—the "whats" and the "whys". *Med J Aust* 1990; **153:** 157–61.
3. Christophersen AS. Amphetamine designer drugs–an overview and epidemiology. *Toxicol Lett* 2000; **112-113:** 127–31.
4. Kraemer T, *et al.* Toxicokinetics of amphetamines: metabolism and toxicokinetic data of designer drugs, amphetamine, methamphetamine, and their N-alkyl derivatives. *Ther Drug Monit* 2002; **24:** 277–89.
5. Reneman L. Designer drugs: how dangerous are they? *J Neural Transm* 2003; **66** (suppl): 61–83.

# Thyroid and Antithyroid Drugs

The principal role of the thyroid gland is to regulate tissue metabolism through production of the **thyroid hormones** 3,5,3′,5′-tetra-iodo-L-thyronine (L-thyroxine, levothyroxine; $T_4$) and, in smaller amounts, 3,5,3′-tri-iodo-L-thyronine (liothyronine, or triiodothyronine; $T_3$). In infants and children thyroid hormones are also necessary for the development of the CNS and for normal growth and bone maturation.

The production of thyroid hormones is dependent on an adequate supply of dietary iodine. Iodine is reduced to iodide in the gastrointestinal tract and is then readily absorbed and actively transported into the thyroid, where it undergoes oxidation, catalysed by thyroid peroxidase. Oxidised iodide is incorporated into the glycoprotein thyroglobulin to form L-mono-iodotyrosine (MIT) and L-di-iodotyrosine (DIT), which are inactive. A coupling reaction, also catalysed by thyroid peroxidase, yields the hormonally active iodothyronines, $T_3$ and $T_4$, joined by a peptide bond to thyroglobulin for storage in the follicular colloid. The release of proteolytic enzymes from lysosomes degrades the thyroglobulin into its constituent amino acids to release $T_3$ and $T_4$ into the circulation; iodide resulting from this reaction is recycled.

Whereas $T_4$ enters the circulation only by direct glandular secretion, most of the $T_3$ in the body is produced by the mono-deiodination of $T_4$ in the peripheral tissues. About 35% of secreted $T_4$ is converted to $T_3$ and about 40% is converted to inactive reverse tri-iodothyronine (reverse $T_3$; $rT_3$). The metabolic activity of $T_3$ is about 3 to 5 times that of $T_4$ and it has been suggested that $T_3$ is the active thyroid hormone with $T_4$ acting primarily as a prohormone.

Thyroid hormones are extensively protein bound in plasma, principally to thyroxine-binding globulin (TBG) but also to a lesser extent to thyroxine-binding pre-albumin (TBPA) or to albumin.

**Thyroid hormone homoeostasis** is maintained by autoregulatory mechanisms within the gland, and by the hypothalamic-pituitary-thyroid axis. In response to falling plasma concentrations of unbound $T_3$ and $T_4$, the hypothalamus secretes thyrotropin releasing hormone (protirelin; TRH—see p.1337), which in turn stimulates the synthesis and release of thyroid stimulating hormone (thyrotropin; TSH—see p.1341) by the anterior pituitary gland. TSH acts on its receptor in the thyroid gland to increase production of $T_3$ and $T_4$, and also to release hormone stored in the gland. As thyroid hormone concentrations in blood increase the secretion of TSH and possibly TRH will be suppressed. The term euthyroidism is used when the thyroid gland is functioning normally and there are normal amounts of thyroid hormone in the blood.

◊ References.


1. Ladenson PW, *et al.* American Thyroid Association guidelines for detection of thyroid dysfunction. *Arch Intern Med* 2000; **160:** 1573–5.
2. Dayan CM. Interpretation of thyroid function tests. *Lancet* 2001; **357:** 619–24.


## Goitre and thyroid nodules

Goitre is the enlargement of the thyroid gland. The swelling may be focal (caused by a solitary thyroid nodule, adenoma, or cyst) or generalised, in which case it is usually diffuse at first, later becoming multinodular. Non-toxic goitres may be associated with hypothyroidism (see below) or euthyroidism. The management of toxic goitres is discussed under Hyperthyroidism, below.

Non-toxic goitres may be associated with intrinsic defects in hormone production, or extrinsic factors such as dietary-iodine deficiency in endemic goitre (see Iodine Deficiency Disorders, p.1599). Decreased secretion of thyroid hormone results in an excessive output of thyroid-stimulating hormone (TSH) from the pituitary. This stimulates thyroid-hormone production but also leads to hypertrophy and hyperplasia of the thyroid gland. If the response to TSH overcomes the deficiency in thyroid-hormone synthesis then the patient is goitrous and euthyroid but if the compensatory response to TSH is inadequate then goitre with hypothyroidism is observed. Other factors such as autoantibodies might stimulate thyroid growth, and thyroid autonomy, in which the gland functions independently of TSH control, can also occur.

The general aims in the management of thyroid masses are:

- the detection and treatment of malignancy
- the reduction of goitre or prevention of further enlargement, and the relief of obstructive symptoms
- the maintenance of a euthyroid state.

Ultrasound or radionuclide imaging may be used to determine the number and size of any nodules present but cannot distinguish a benign from a malignant nodule. Levothyroxine has been given short-term in an attempt to do so, with failure of the nodule to shrink being regarded as an indication of malignancy, but it is much less reliable than cytological analysis, which is the most reliable means of diagnosing malignancy.[1-3]

In established **malignancy**, surgery, followed by levothyroxine replacement therapy, is the usual course (for further discussion of the treatment of thyroid cancer, see p.523).

The treatment of non-toxic **benign solitary nodules** is a matter of dispute. Many prefer simply to observe patients with benign solitary nodules.[1,2] Suppressive therapy with doses of levothyroxine (or, less often, liothyronine) sufficient to suppress TSH production and reduce the size of the nodule has been widely practised, but results conflict as to whether such therapy is effective.[2-4] A meta-analysis of 7 studies[5] suggested that although levothyroxine treatment produced some benefit, the number of patients who responded was quite small. Another meta-analysis[6] (which included 5 of the same studies and a later one) found an overall non-significant treatment response; the authors concluded that routine suppressive levothyroxine for single benign thyroid nodules could not be recommended, but that a subgroup of patients with small, solid nodules might benefit from therapy. There has been some concern about the possible risk of osteoporosis[1,2,7] with levothyroxine (see Effects on the Bones, p.1600). An alternative to levothyroxine is treatment with potassium iodide, although it is somewhat less effective,[8] and has adverse effects of its own.[7] Sclerotherapy by alcohol injection has been investigated.[9,10]

Levothyroxine suppression therapy is effective in patients with **diffuse** non-toxic goitre, and may be of benefit in some patients with **multinodular** disease.[3] However, many patients with large multinodular goitres have autonomous thyroid hormone production, and in such patients levothyroxine is of no benefit and may cause overt hyperthyroidism. Radio-iodine ($^{131}I$) treatment appears to be more effective and better tolerated than levothyroxine,[11] and has been a useful alternative to surgery in selected cases of multinodular non-toxic goitre.[3,12]


1. Mazzaferri EL. Management of a solitary thyroid nodule. *N Engl J Med* 1993; **328:** 553–9.
2. Giuffrida D, Gharib H. Controversies in the management of cold, hot, and occult thyroid nodules. *Am J Med* 1995; **99:** 642–50.
3. Hermus AR, Huysmans DA. Treatment of benign nodular thyroid disease. *N Engl J Med* 1998; **338:** 1438–47.
4. Gharib H, Mazzaferri EL. Thyroxine suppressive therapy in patients with nodular thyroid disease. *Ann Intern Med* 1998; **128:** 386–94.
5. Zelmanovitz F, *et al.* Suppressive therapy with levothyroxine for solitary thyroid nodules: a double-blind controlled clinical study and cumulative meta-analyses. *J Clin Endocrinol Metab* 1998; **83:** 3881–5.
6. Castro MR, *et al.* Effectiveness of thyroid hormone suppressive therapy in benign solitary thyroid nodules: a meta-analysis. *J Clin Endocrinol Metab* 2002; **87:** 4154–9.
7. Blum M. Why do clinicians continue to debate the use of levothyroxine in the diagnosis and management of thyroid nodules? *Ann Intern Med* 1995; **122:** 63–4.
8. La Rosa GL, *et al.* Levothyroxine and potassium iodide are both effective in treating benign solitary cold nodules of the thyroid. *Ann Intern Med* 1995; **122:** 1–8.
9. Bennedbaek FN *et al.*. Effect of percutaneous ethanol injection therapy versus suppressive doses of L-thyroxine on benign solitary cold thyroid nodules: a randomized trial. *J Clin Endocrinol Metab* 1998; **83:** 830–5.
10. Bennedbaek FN, Hegedüs L. Percutaneous ethanol injection therapy in benign solitary solid cold thyroid nodules: a randomized trial comparing one injection with three injections. *Thyroid* 1999; **9:** 225–33.
11. Wesche MFT, *et al.* A randomized trial comparing levothyroxine with radioactive iodine in the treatment of sporadic nontoxic goiter. *J Clin Endocrinol Metab* 2001; **86:** 998–1005.
12. Nygaard B, *et al.* Radio iodine treatment of multinodular nontoxic goitre. *BMJ* 1993; **307:** 828–32.


## Hyperthyroidism

Hyperthyroidism is overactivity of the thyroid gland, with consequent excess secretion of hormones. The terms thyrotoxicosis and hyperthyroidism are used interchangeably, although some apply 'thyrotoxicosis' to the *effects* of excessive thyroid hormone. The most common causes of hyperthyroidism are Graves' disease (diffuse toxic goitre) and hyperactivity arising from single or multiple thyroid nodules (toxic nodular goitre). Graves' disease (or Basedow's disease) is an auto-immune condition in which thyroid-stimulating antibodies in the plasma are directed against the thyroid-stimulating hormone (TSH) receptor or a closely associated protein on the thyroid cell. Graves' disease, which is more prevalent in females, frequently occurs in association with other diseases such as Addison's disease, type 1 diabetes mellitus, and pernicious anaemia, and there may be a genetic predisposition. Iodine and its salts, or iodine-containing drugs such as amiodarone, can also be a cause of both hyperthyroidism and hypothyroidism.

The major clinical manifestations associated with clinical hyperthyroidism include goitre, nervousness, agitation, tremor, tachycardia or atrial fibrillation, weight loss (often despite increased appetite), emotional lability, muscle weakness, fatigue, heat intolerance and excessive perspiration, and increased bowel frequency. Exaggerated growth may occur in children. Females may occasionally experience amenorrhoea or oligomenorrhoea and males may develop gynaecomastia. Occasionally there is subcutaneous deposition of mucopolysaccharides around the shins, causing a non-pitting oedema (pretibial myxoedema).

A **diagnosis** of primary hyperthyroidism may be confirmed by demonstration of a low TSH value and a high concentration of free $T_4$ or $T_3$ in the circulation. Determination of TSH, which is low in hyperthyroidism due to negative feedback, allows differential diagnosis of hyperthyroidism from a TSH-secreting pituitary tumour.

**Subclinical hyperthyroidism** is characterised by normal thyroid hormone concentrations, decreased TSH concentrations, but no clinical symptoms. It has been reported to occur less frequently than subclinical hypothyroidism. Consensus on management has been lacking;[1-3] while treatment is not routinely recommended for mild subclinical hyperthyroidism, certain subgroups of patients, such as those at risk of atrial fibrillation or osteoporosis, may benefit from therapy.[4]

There are three forms of **treatment** for hyperthyroidism: drug therapy, use of radio-iodine, or surgery.

*Drug therapy.* The main **antithyroid drugs** are all thiourea derivatives that block the production of thyroid hormones through inhibition of thyroid peroxidase. Carbimazole (in the UK) or thiamazole (in the USA), or propylthiouracil, are the mainstays of treatment. Antithyroid drugs do not block the release of stored thyroid hormones and it is only when the preformed hormones are depleted and concentrations of circulating hormones decline that clinical effects become apparent. An additional action of propylthiouracil is inhibition of the peripheral deiodination of thyroxine to tri-iodothyronine. The place of immunosuppression in the antithyroid activity of these drugs is subject to debate.

Many patients begin treatment with an antithyroid drug; they receive high doses initially until they become euthyroid, generally within 1 to 2 months. Once a response to the antithyroid drug has been obtained, patients with more severe or recurrent disease may require ablative treatment with either radio-iodine or surgery (see below), while those with mild to moderate disease may be best managed with lower maintenance doses of antithyroid drugs. These are either given indefinitely, or more usually for at least a year (often 18 months), followed by observation to see if remission is maintained in the absence of therapy.[1,5-7] Relapse at some stage following cessation of therapy is fairly common but unpredictable. Addition of levothyroxine to the maintenance dose of thiamazole has been reported to reduce the rate of relapse in patients with Graves' disease when therapy is subsequently withdrawn,[8] but later studies have not shown benefit.[9-12]

An alternative maintenance regimen is to add the thyroid hormone while maintaining the high initial doses of antithyroid drug. This '*blocking-replacement therapy*' has been suggested to help to prevent hypothyroidism which may be induced when antithyroid drugs are used alone. Because of the high doses of thioureas required and the insufficient placental transfer of levothyroxine,[13,14] the blocking-replacement regimen should not be used in pregnancy.

More rapid relief of the symptoms of hyperthyroidism can be achieved with beta blockers or iodide.[5,7] Beta blockers usually achieve a response within 48 hours, and are given as short-term adjuncts to antithyroid drugs to control severe sympathetic overactivity in patients such as those with thyroid storm (see below), but their use in heart failure associated with thyrotoxicosis is controversial because of the risk of cardiac deterioration.[15] The use of beta blockers in patients with mild to moderate hyperthyroidism is usually unnecessary.

Iodine and iodides are given with antithyroid drugs for 7 to 14 days as pre-operative preparation for patients who are to undergo thyroidectomy (but see also under Surgical Therapy, below); a combination of iodide and a beta blocker has also been used. Iodide has been used with antithyroid drugs, for control of thyroid storm. It is suggested that the antithyroid drugs should always be given first to prevent incorporation of iodide into new hormone stores.[5]

Other drugs tried in hyperthyroidism have included lithium, though its practical value is a matter of debate.[5] Potassium and sodium perchlorate have been used; they increase responsiveness to conventional antithyroid drugs and may be useful in patients with iodine-induced hyperthyroidism.[16]

In those patients in whom drug therapy fails to achieve long-term remission, ablative therapy may be considered in the form of radio-iodine therapy or surgery.

*Radio-iodine therapy* with $^{131}$I as oral $^{131}$I-sodium iodide cures hyperthyroidism by destroying the functioning cells of the thyroid gland. It is increasingly used as initial therapy,[5,13,17,18] especially in the USA.[19] It is also useful for patients who have not responded to antithyroid drug therapy or who have relapsed following it.[1,6]

Pretreatment of patients with an antithyroid drug for 2 to 8 weeks before radio-iodine therapy has been advocated, to avoid the risk of precipitating thyroid storm. However, many no longer consider this to be necessary for all patients,[5,13,17] although it is generally agreed that the elderly or those with severe disease or increased risk of cardiac symptoms should receive some form of pretreatment. In younger patients, a study has suggested that antithyroid pretreatment may exacerbate the risks when the drugs are withdrawn.[20] Such withdrawal, 2 to 4 days before radio-iodine is given, is standard practice to maximise the latter's effect, although some consider it unnecessary.[5] There is also some evidence that pretreated patients respond less well, and an increased dose of radio-iodine has been advocated in such patients.[17] Pretreatment or ancillary treatment with a beta blocker is a possible alternative to antithyroid drugs in patients receiving radio-iodine.[5,7,13,17]

The dose of radio-iodine required to achieve euthyroidism is difficult to predict and there is little agreement on the most appropriate dosage schedule.[1,7,17] Radio-iodine therapy may take up to 10 weeks to achieve a clinical response, and cover with an antithyroid drug may be required during this period. Radio-iodine is not generally considered to increase the risk of malignancy,[5,17,21] or teratogenicity[13] but it is contra-indicated in pregnancy and while breast feeding. The commonest unwanted effect of radio-iodine therapy is hypothyroidism and all patients require long-term follow-up and possible levothyroxine replacement therapy. Iodide may be given after radio-iodine therapy to help the return of normal thyroid function.[5] Controversy exists as to whether radio-iodine therapy exacerbates Graves' ophthalmopathy[5,22,23] although it is considered to worsen disease in smokers.[13,18]

*Surgical treatment* is usually reserved for patients with severe hyperthyroidism or for those with extreme thyroid enlargement or a single nodule. Euthyroidism is first established using antithyroid drugs and then iodide is given for 7 to 14 days before surgery to reduce the vasculature of the gland. Alternatively, a beta blocker and iodide may be used together for pre-operative preparation. However, a consensus view[2] suggested that pre-operative iodine probably has no beneficial effect. Levothyroxine replacement therapy may be required following surgical treatment.

If untreated or inadequately controlled, hyperthyroidism can complicate **pregnancy** and have adverse perinatal effects.[13,14,18,24] Hyperthyroidism is generally treated throughout pregnancy with an antithyroid drug, usually propylthiouracil[13,14,18,24] at the minimum dose needed to maintain a borderline euthyroid state. Occasionally, the antithyroid drug can be withdrawn in the third trimester.[13,18,19] Drug therapy during pregnancy may cause fetal or neonatal hypothyroidism, with or without goitre. This risk appears unrelated to the dose of the drug,[14,24] and the condition may mask neonatal hyperthyroidism[24] (see below).

Failure to control symptoms of hyperthyroidism with antithyroid drugs during pregnancy may indicate the need for surgery which is often delayed where possible until after the first trimester.[14,18,24,25] Iodide and radio-iodine are contra-indicated during pregnancy,[7,13,14,18,24,25] as is the blocking-replacement regimen.[13,14,19,24]

**Neonatal hyperthyroidism** may occur rarely due to transfer of thyroid-stimulating immunoglobulins across the placenta, and should be treated with antithyroid drugs, iodide, and appropriate therapy for cardiovascular complications.[26]

**Thyroid storm** (also known as thyroid crisis or thyrotoxic crisis) is an extreme accentuation of the hyperthyroid state and should be treated as a medical emergency. It is usually abrupt in onset and is often related to some precipitating factor such as inadequate preparation for thyroidectomy or radio-iodine therapy, or infection in previously unrecognised hyperthyroid subjects. The most common clinical manifestations are hyperpyrexia and extreme tachycardia; others may include arrhythmia, heart failure, shock, agitation, tremor, mania, delirium, stupor, coma, abdominal pain, diarrhoea, vomiting, jaundice, and hepatomegaly. Treatment consists of high-dose antithyroid drugs, gradually reduced as the condition improves, along with a beta blocker and iodide to control cardiovascular symptoms and prevent thyroid hormone release from the thyroid gland. Additional symptomatic treatment may also be required.

The clinical manifestations of **Graves' ophthalmopathy** may not occur in conjunction with those of systemic hyperthyroidism, and it has been characterised as an independent manifestation of the immunological abnormality in Graves' disease.[27]

In Graves' ophthalmopathy, oedema and inflammation of the muscles around the eyes produces exophthalmos or proptosis and diplopia. On rare occasions patients may develop papilloedema and loss of vision. Treatment is generally unsatisfactory and signs of disease may persist indefinitely.[28] Opinions differ as to whether controlling associated hyperthyroidism improves ocular symptoms.[27] Reports that radio-iodine therapy may exacerbate Graves' ophthalmopathy are disputed,[5,13,17,22,23] but some prefer to avoid its use in active ocular disease.[1] Most patients with mild ocular involvement in hyperthyroidism require no specific therapy; dry eye should be managed appropriately (see p.1576). Patients with moderate to severe ophthalmopathy may be treated with high-dose systemic corticosteroids, or with orbital radiotherapy, which appears to be equally effective,[29] or a combination of both.[30] High dose intravenous methylprednisolone has been found to be more effective and better tolerated than oral prednisone.[30,31] Other immunosuppressants, particularly ciclosporin, have also been used but have produced equivocal results.[27] Surgical decompression may be required if patients do not respond to such therapy or cannot tolerate its adverse effects, or if vision is threatened by severe optic nerve compression.


1. Gittoes NJL, Franklyn JA. Hyperthyroidism: current treatment guidelines. *Drugs* 1998; **55:** 543–53.
2. Vanderpump MPJ, *et al.* Consensus statement for good practice and audit measures in the management of hypothyroidism and hyperthyroidism *BMJ* 1996; **313:** 539–44.
3. Helfand M, Redfern CC. Screening for thyroid disease: an update. *Ann Intern Med* 1998; **129:** 144–58. Correction. *ibid.*; **130:** 246.
4. Surks MI, *et al.* Subclinical thyroid disease: scientific review and guidelines for diagnosis and management. *JAMA* 2004; **291:** 228–38.
5. Klein I, *et al.* Treatment of hyperthyroid disease. *Ann Intern Med* 1994; **121:** 281–8.
6. Cheetham TD, *et al.* Treatment of hyperthyroidism in young people. *Arch Dis Child* 1998; **78:** 207–9.
7. Franklyn J. Thyrotoxicosis. *Prescribers' J* 1999; **39:** 1–8.
8. Hashizume K, *et al.* Administration of thyroxine in treated Graves' disease: effects on the level of antibodies to thyroid-stimulating hormone receptors and on the risk of recurrence of hyperthyroidism. *N Engl J Med* 1991; **324:** 947–53.
9. Tamai H, *et al.* Lack of effect of thyroxine administration on elevated thyroid stimulating hormone receptor antibody levels in treated Graves' disease patients. *J Clin Endocrinol Metab* 1995; **80:** 1481–4.
10. Hershman JM. Does thyroxine therapy prevent recurrence of Graves' hyperthyroidism? *J Clin Endocrinol Metab* 1995; **80:** 1479–80.
11. McIver B, *et al.* Lack of effect of thyroxine in patients with Graves' hyperthyroidism who are treated with an antithyroid drug. *N Engl J Med* 1996; **334:** 220–4.
12. Rittmaster RS, *et al.* Effect of methimazole, with or without L-thyroxine, on remission rates in Graves' disease. *J Clin Endocrinol Metab* 1998; **83:** 814–18.
13. Weetman AP. Graves' disease. *N Engl J Med* 2000; **343:** 1236–48.
14. Atkins P, *et al.* Drug therapy for hyperthyroidism in pregnancy: safety issues for mother and fetus. *Drug Safety* 2000; **23:** 229–244.
15. Ko GTC, *et al.* Should β-blocking agents be used in thyrotoxic heart disease? *Med J Aust* 1995; **162:** 426–7.
16. Wolff J. Perchlorate and the thyroid gland. *Pharmacol Rev* 1998; **50:** 89–105.
17. Kaplan MM, *et al.* Treatment of hyperthyroidism with radioactive iodine. *Endocrinol Metab Clin North Am* 1998; **27:** 205–23.
18. Woeber KA. Update on the management of hyperthyroidism and hypothyroidism. *Arch Intern Med* 2000; **160:** 1067–71.
19. Cooper DS. Hyperthyroidism. *Lancet* 2003; **362:** 459–68.
20. Burch HB, *et al.* Discontinuing antithyroid drug therapy before ablation with radioiodine in Graves disease. *Ann Intern Med* 1994; **121:** 553–9.
21. Ron E, *et al.* Cancer mortality following treatment for adult hyperthyroidism. *JAMA* 1998; **280:** 347–55.
22. Tallstedt L, *et al.* Occurrence of ophthalmopathy after treatment for Graves' hyperthyroidism. *N Engl J Med* 1992; **326:** 1733–8.
23. Bartalena L, *et al.* Relation between therapy for hyperthyroidism and the course of Graves' ophthalmopathy. *N Engl J Med* 1998; **338:** 73–8.
24. Girling JC. Thyroid disease in pregnancy. *Hosp Med* 2000; **61:** 834–40.
25. Masiukiewicz US, Burrow GN. Hyperthyroidism in pregnancy: diagnosis and treatment. *Thyroid* 1999; **9:** 647–52.
26. Ogilvy-Stuart AL. Neonatal thyroid disorders. *Arch Dis Child Fetal Neonatal Ed* 2002; **87:** F165–F171.
27. Char DH. Thyroid eye disease. *Br J Ophthalmol* 1996; **80:** 922–6.
28. Fleck BW, Toft AD. Graves' ophthalmopathy. *BMJ* 1990; **300:** 1352–3.
29. Prummel MF, *et al.* Randomised double-blind trial of prednisone versus radiotherapy in Graves' ophthalmopathy. *Lancet* 1993; **342:** 949–54.
30. Marcocci C, *et al.* Comparison of the effectiveness and tolerability of intravenous or oral glucocorticoids associated with orbital radiotherapy in the management of severe Graves' ophthalmopathy: results of a prospective, single-blind, randomized study. *J Clin Endocrinol Metab* 2001; **86:** 3562–7.
31. Macchia PE, *et al.* High-dose intravenous corticosteroid therapy for Graves' ophthalmopathy. *J Endocrinol Invest* 2001; **24:** 152–8.


## Hypothyroidism

Hypothyroidism is the clinical syndrome resulting from deficiency of thyroid hormones. It predominantly affects women and is more prevalent in the middle-aged and elderly. The symptoms of hypothyroidism may be due to general deceleration of metabolism or to accumulation of mucopolysaccharide in the subcutaneous tissues and vocal cords. Common clinical manifestations include weakness, fatigue, lethargy, physical and mental slowness, and weight gain; puffy, nonpitted swelling of subcutaneous tissue often develops, particularly around the eyes. Menstrual disorders, hyperlipidaemia, and constipation can occur and goitre may develop despite associated cell destruction.

The term **myxoedema** is often reserved for severe or advanced hypothyroidism. In the most severely affected patients, progressive somnolence and torpor combine with cold intolerance and bradycardia to induce a state of coma often known as 'hypothyroid' or 'myxoedema coma' (see below).

In children, untreated hypothyroidism results in retardation of growth and mental development. Endemic cretinism is a result of maternal, and hence fetal, iodine deficiency and consequent lack of thyroid hormone production (see Iodine Deficiency Disorders, p.1599).

Hypothyroidism is usually primary, resulting from malfunction of the thyroid gland. In areas where iodine intake is sufficient the commonest cause of hypothyroidism is auto-immune lymphocytic thyroiditis of which there are two major variants. In **Hashimoto's thyroiditis** there is also goitre whereas in **idiopathic** or **primary myxoedema** (**atrophic thyroiditis**) there is no thyroid enlargement. Hypothyroidism can also be caused by either an excess or a deficiency of iodine. An excess may result from intake of iodine or its salts or iodine-containing drugs such as amiodarone. Drugs that decrease thyroid hormone synthesis such as lithium can also be a cause of hypothyroidism. In some patients hypothyroidism may be secondary to disorders of the hypothalamus or pituitary gland.

The **diagnosis** of hypothyroidism is essentially clinical but, given the non-specific nature of many of the symptoms, biochemical tests are performed for confirmation.[1-3] A raised thyroid stimulating hormone (TSH) value and a low free $T_4$ or $T_3$ concentration indicates primary hypothyroidism. Protirelin and thyrotrophin have also been used for the differential diagnosis of hypothyroidism.

**Subclinical hypothyroidism** is a condition in which there are normal concentrations of thyroid hormones, raised concentrations of TSH, but no clinical symptoms. Patients with subclinical hypothyroidism are at a greater risk of developing clinical hypothyroidism if they also have thyroid antibodies against thyroid peroxidase/microsomal antigen although the best strategy for identifying those at risk is not yet known.[2]

Hypothyroidism is readily **treated** by lifelong replacement therapy with levothyroxine.[1,2,4,5] Although the thyroid gland produces $T_3$ (liothyronine) and $T_4$ (thyroxine), $T_3$ is mainly produced by peripheral monodeiodination of circulating $T_4$ and it is therefore sufficient to give levothyroxine alone. There is no rationale for the use of combined preparations containing liothyronine and levothyroxine, or of dried thyroid hormone extracts, which may lead to elevated serum concentrations of $T_3$ and thyrotoxic symptoms. Liothyronine may, however, be used initially for its rapid onset of action in severe hypothyroid states such as myxoedema coma (see below). Initial checks should be made to ensure that thyroid replacement treatment is restoring deficiencies in thyroid hormone but not providing an excess. This is best done by monitoring hormone concentrations and the goal of replacement therapy has been advocated as a normal TSH value, which is generally associated with a normal or slightly elevated $T_4$ value.[2,5]

In subclinical hypothyroidism, treatment with levothyroxine is controversial. It has been recommended[2-4,6] if thyroid peroxidase antibodies are present or if TSH levels are above 10 milliunits/litre.

Although titres of antithyroid antibodies may fall during **pregnancy**, some patients may require progressive increases in levothyroxine dosage,[7] and therefore thyroid function tests should be performed in each trimester.[1,2,4,8]

The diagnosis of **congenital hypothyroidism** (neonatal hypothyroidism) is now most commonly made on the basis of screening programmes.[9] Early treatment with adequate doses of levothyroxine is required to minimise the effects of hypothyroidism on mental and physical development. Administration should be started as soon as possible after birth and should be reviewed regularly.[9,10] However, it is generally accepted that in those with more severe hypothyroidism at diagnosis some small degree of deficit and incoordination remains, although they should be mild enough to permit a normal life.[11]

**Hypothyroid (myxoedema) coma** is a medical emergency requiring prompt treatment usually with liothyronine given by intravenous injection because of its rapid action, although some centres use intravenous levothyroxine. Alternatively, the nasogastric route may be employed. In some patients, liothyronine given intravenously is followed by oral levothyroxine. Other treatment includes intravenous hydrocortisone (because of the likelihood of adrenocortical insufficiency) and intravenous fluids (to maintain plasma-glucose and electrolyte concentrations). Respiratory function should be supported by assisted ventilation and oxygen administration.


1. Singer PA, *et al.* Treatment guidelines for patients with hyperthyroidism and hypothyroidism. *JAMA* 1995; **273:** 808–12.
2. Lindsay RS, Toft AD. Hypothyroidism. *Lancet* 1997; **349:** 413–17. Correction. *ibid.*; 1023.
3. Woeber KA. Update on the management of hyperthyroidism and hypothyroidism. *Arch Intern Med* 2000; **160:** 1067–71.
4. Vanderpump MPJ, *et al.* Consensus statement for good practice and audit measures in the management of hypothyroidism and hyperthyroidism. *BMJ* 1996; **313:** 539–44.
5. Toft AD. Thyroxine therapy. *N Engl J Med* 1994; **331:** 174–80.
6. Surks MI, *et al.* Subclinical thyroid disease: scientific review and guidelines for diagnosis and management. *JAMA* 2004; **291:** 228–38.
7. Drake WM, Wood DF. Thyroid disease in pregnancy. *Postgrad Med J* 1998; **74:** 583–6.
8. Girling JC. Thyroid disease in pregnancy. *Hosp Med* 2000; **61:** 834–40.
9. LaFranchi S. Congenital hypothyroidism: etiologies, diagnosis, and management. *Thyroid* 1999; **9:** 735–40.
10. Hopwood NJ. Treatment of the infant with congenital hypothyroidism. *J Pediatr* 2002; **141:** 752–4.
11. Rovet JF. Congenital hypothyroidism: long term outcome. *Thyroid* 1999; **9:** 741–8.


## Benzylthiouracil

Benciltiouracilo. 6-Benzyl-2,3-dihydro-2-thioxopyrimidin-4(1*H*)-one; 6-Benzyl-2-mercaptopyrimidin-4-ol; 6-Benzyl-2-thiouracil.

$C_{11}H_{10}N_2OS$ = 218.3.

*CAS — 33086-27-0; 6336-50-1.*

*ATC — H03BA03.*

### Profile

Benzylthiouracil is a thiourea antithyroid drug. It is given by mouth in the treatment of hyperthyroidism (p.1594) in an initial dose of 150 to 200 mg daily, reducing to a maintenance dose of 100 mg daily after several months.

**Porphyria.** Benzylthiouracil is considered to be unsafe in patients with porphyria although there is conflicting experimental evidence of porphyrinogenicity.

### Preparations

**Proprietary Preparations** (details are given in Part 3)

**Fr.:** Basdene.

## Carbimazole *(BAN, rINN)*

Carbimazol; Carbimazolum. Ethyl 3-methyl-2-thioxo-4-imidazoline-1-carboxylate.

$C_7H_{10}N_2O_2S$ = 186.2.

*CAS — 22232-54-8.*

*ATC — H03BB01.*

**Pharmacopoeias.** In *Chin.* and *Eur.* (see p.vi).

**Ph. Eur. 5.0** (Carbimazole). A white or yellowish-white crystalline powder. Slightly soluble in water; soluble in alcohol and in acetone.

### Adverse Effects and Precautions

Adverse effects from carbimazole and other thiourea antithyroid drugs occur most frequently during the first 8 weeks of treatment. The most common minor adverse effects are nausea and vomiting, gastric discomfort, headache, arthralgia, skin rashes, and pruritus. Hair loss has also been reported.

Bone-marrow depression may occur and mild leucopenia is common. Rarely, agranulocytosis can develop and this is the most serious adverse reaction associated with this class of drugs. Patients or their carers should be told how to recognise such toxicity and should be advised to seek immediate medical attention if mouth ulcers or sore throat, fever, bruising, malaise, or non-specific illness develop. Full blood counts should be performed, and treatment should be discontinued immediately if there is any clinical or laboratory evidence of neutropenia. Aplastic anaemia or isolated thrombocytopenia have been reported rarely, as has hypoprothrombinaemia.

There have been several reports of liver damage, most commonly jaundice, in patients taking thiourea antithyroid drugs; the drug should be withdrawn if hepatic effects occur.

Other adverse effects sometimes observed with the thiourea antithyroid compounds include fever, a lupus-like syndrome, myopathy, vasculitis and nephritis, and taste disturbances. Creatine phosphokinase values should be measured if patients experience myalgia.

Excessive doses of antithyroid drugs may cause hypothyroidism and goitre. High doses in pregnancy may result in fetal hypothyroidism and goitre (see Pregnancy, below).

An immune mechanism has been implicated in many of these reactions and cross-sensitivity between the thiourea antithyroid drugs may occur.

**Breast feeding.** The safety of breast feeding during maternal treatment depends partly on how much drug is distributed into the breast milk. Thiourea antithyroid drugs may be used with care in breast-feeding mothers; neonatal development and thyroid function of the infant should be closely monitored and the lowest effective dose used.

Propylthiouracil has been preferred to carbimazole or thiamazole since it enters breast milk less readily.[1-3] In a small study[4] of breast-feeding mothers taking doses of propylthiouracil as high as 750 mg daily for Graves' disease, no adverse effects were observed on the thyroid status of their infants.

Thiamazole enters breast milk freely, with plasma to milk ratios almost one.[3,5] The infant's intake of thiamazole following administration of carbimazole (or thiamazole) might be greatly reduced by discarding the breast milk produced 2 to 4 hours after a dose,[6] since the highest concentration was found at this time. Two studies found no adverse effects on thyroid function,[7,8] thyroid hormone levels,[7] or physical and intellectual development, in breast-fed infants during up to 6 months[7] to 1 year[8] of maternal treatment with thiamazole. Maximum maternal daily doses of 10 mg of thiamazole,[3] 15 mg of carbimazole, and 150 mg of propylthiouracil[9] have been recommended, although thiamazole 20 to 30 mg has been administered to thyrotoxic lactating women for the first month of a year of therapy with no observable adverse effects on the thyroid function of their breast-fed infants.[10] Despite stating that goitre has been associated with the use of carbimazole, the American Academy of Pediatrics considers the use of all three drugs to be compatible with breast feeding.[11]


1. Kampmann JP, *et al.* Propylthiouracil in human milk: revision of a dogma. *Lancet* 1980; **i:** 736–8.
2. Johansen K, *et al.* Excretion of methimazole in human milk. *Eur J Clin Pharmacol* 1982; **23:** 339–41.
3. Cooper DS. Antithyroid drugs: to breast-feed or not to breast-feed. *Am J Obstet Gynecol* 1987; **157:** 234–5.
4. Momotani N, *et al.* Thyroid function in wholly breast-feeding infants whose mothers take high doses of propylthiouracil. *Clin Endocrinol (Oxf)* 2000; **53:** 177–81.
5. Cooper DS, *et al.* Methimazole pharmacology in man: studies using a newly developed radioimmunoassay for methimazole. *J Clin Endocrinol Metab* 1984; **58:** 473–9.
6. Rylance GW, *et al.* Carbimazole and breastfeeding. *Lancet* 1987; **i:** 928.
7. Azizi F. Effect of methimazole treatment of maternal thyrotoxicosis on thyroid function in breast-feeding infants. *J Pediatr* 1996; **128:** 855–8.
8. Azizi F, *et al.* Thyroid function and intellectual development of infants nursed by mothers taking methimazole. *J Clin Endocrinol Metab* 2000; **85:** 3233–8.
9. Lamberg B-A, *et al.* Antithyroid treatment of maternal hyperthyroidism during lactation. *Clin Endocrinol (Oxf)* 1984; **21:** 81–7.
10. Azizi F, Hedayati M. Thyroid function in breast-fed infants whose mothers take high doses of methimazole. *J Endocrinol Invest* 2002; **25:** 493–6.
11. American Academy of Pediatrics. The transfer of drugs and other chemicals into human milk. *Pediatrics* 2001; **108:** 776–89. Correction. *ibid.*; 1029. Also available at: http://aappolicy.aappublications.org/cgi/content/full/pediatrics%3b108/3/776 (accessed 17/5/04)


**Effects on the blood.** While **leucopenia** is considered to be a common adverse effect of the thiourea antithyroid drugs, occurring in up to a quarter of patients, it is usually mild and improves as treatment continues.[1]

**Agranulocytosis**, a more serious hazard, is usually reported to affect 0.03% of patients in Europe,[2] who are mostly treated with carbimazole. However the incidence has been reported to be higher (0.4%) in areas where thiamazole is used.[3,4] Fatalities have been reported.[1,2,4,5] Although a direct toxic effect had been suggested, the agranulocytosis associated with the thiourea drugs is now generally considered to be immunologically mediated.[1,6] The onset of agranulocytosis is usually rapid and monitoring of the blood count is not always of predictive value;[3] routine monitoring is not indicated.[2] Agranulocytosis has occurred in patients receiving propylthiouracil for a second time who had no such complications in their first course of therapy.[7] There is limited evidence that agranulocytosis is more common at higher doses, and in older patients. However this has not been proved conclusively.[1]

There have been some case reports of **aplastic anaemia** being produced by antithyroid drugs, but the excess risk associated with their use is considered to be very low[6,8] and complete recovery has been reported following withdrawal of the antithyroid drug. An immune mechanism has been implicated.

Carbimazole has produced **haemolytic anaemia**.[9] In this case the immune reaction was specific to carbimazole and could not be demonstrated with thiamazole.

On very rare occasions patients taking propylthiouracil have experienced a reduction in prothrombin values and bleeding.[10-12] In one patient bleeding was linked to propylthiouracil-induced **thrombocytopenia**.[13]


1. Bartalena L *et al.* Adverse effects of thyroid hormone preparations and antithyroid drugs. *Drug Safety* 1996; **15:** 53–63.
2. Committee on Safety of Medicines/Medicines Control Agency. Reminder: agranulocytosis with antithyroid drugs. *Current Problems* 1999; **25:** 3. Also available at: http://www.mca.gov.uk/ourwork/monitorsafequalmed/currentproblems/volume25feb.htm (accessed 17/05/04)
3. Tajiri J, *et al.* Antithyroid drug-induced agranulocytosis: the usefulness of routine white blood cell count monitoring. *Arch Intern Med* 1990; **150:** 621–4.
4. Anonymous. Elaboration: drug-induced agranulocytosis–monitoring antithyroid treatment. *Drug Ther Bull* 1997; **35:** 88.
5. Anonymous. Drug-induced agranulocytosis. *Drug Ther Bull* 1997; **35:** 49–52.
6. International Agranulocytosis and Aplastic Anaemia Study. Risk of agranulocytosis and aplastic anaemia in relation to use of antithyroid drugs. *BMJ* 1988; **297:** 262–5.
7. Shiran A, *et al.* Propylthiouracil-induced agranulocytosis in four patients previously treated with the drug. *JAMA* 1991; **266:** 3129–30.
8. Bishara J. Methimazole-induced aplastic anemia. *Ann Pharmacother* 1996; **30:** 684.
9. Salama A, *et al.* Carbimazole-induced immune haemolytic anaemia: role of drug-red blood cell complexes for immunization. *Br J Haematol* 1988; **68:** 479–82.
10. D'Angelo G, Le Gresley LP. Severe hypoprothrombinaemia after propylthiouracil therapy. *Can Med Assoc J* 1959; **81:** 479–81.
11. Naeye RL, Terrien CM. Hemorrhagic state after therapy with propylthiouracil. *Am J Clin Pathol* 1960; **34:** 254–7.
12. Gotta AW, *et al.* Prolonged intraoperative bleeding caused by propylthiouracil-induced hypoprothrombinemia. *Anesthesiology* 1972; **37:** 562–3.
13. Ikeda S, Schweiss JF. Excessive blood loss during operation in the patient treated with propylthiouracil. *Can Anaesth Soc J* 1982; **29:** 477–80.


**Effects on the ears.** Earache, high-frequency hearing loss, and tinnitus in a patient with Graves' disease were considered to be associated with hypersensitivity to carbimazole therapy;[1] hearing loss, but not the tinnitus, resolved when carbimazole was replaced with propylthiouracil.


1. Hill D, *et al.* Hearing loss and tinnitus with carbimazole *BMJ* 1994; **309:** 929.


**Effects on the kidneys.** There have been reports of glomerulonephritis associated with the development of antineutrophil cytoplasmic antibodies in patients receiving thiourea antithyroid drugs.[1-5]


1. Vogt BA, *et al.* Antineutrophil cytoplasmic autoantibody-positive crescentic glomerulonephritis as a complication of treatment with propylthiouracil in children. *J Pediatr* 1994; **124:** 986–8.
2. D'Cruz D, *et al.* Antineutrophil cytoplasmic antibody-positive crescentic glomerulonephritis associated with anti-thyroid drug treatment. *Br J Rheumatol* 1995; **34:** 1090–1.
3. Yuasa S, *et al.* Antineutrophil cytoplasmic antibodies (ANCA)-associated crescentic glomerulonephritis and propylthiouracil therapy. *Nephron* 1996; **73:** 701–3.

4. Kudoh Y, *et al.* Propylthiouracil-induced rapidly progressive glomerulonephritis associated with antineutrophil cytoplasmic autoantibodies. *Clin Nephrol* 1997; **48:** 41–3.
5. Prasad GVR, *et al.* Propylthiouracil-induced diffuse proliferative lupus nephritis: review of immunological complications. *J Am Soc Nephrol* 1997; **8:** 1205–10.

**Effects on the liver.** Jaundice, usually cholestatic, has been reported with thiamazole and carbimazole.[1-5] An immune-mediated mechanism rather than a toxic reaction has been proposed. Hepatitis (sometimes progressing to cirrhosis[6]) and hepatic necrosis have been associated with propylthiouracil,[6-9] sometimes with fatal consequences.[7,8] However, in one study[10] almost 30% of patients being treated with propylthiouracil developed asymptomatic liver changes (increased alanine aminotransferase values) that were mostly reversible as treatment continued at a reduced dose.

Despite reports of liver damage, propylthiouracil has been investigated in the treatment of patients with alcoholic liver disease (see p.1603).

1. Becker CE, *et al.* Hepatitis from methimazole during adrenal steroid therapy for malignant exophthalmos. *JAMA* 1968; **206:** 1787–9.
2. Fischer MG, *et al.* Methimazole-induced jaundice. *JAMA* 1973; **223:** 1028–9.
3. Blom H, *et al.* A case of carbimazole-induced intrahepatic cholestasis. *Arch Intern Med* 1985; **145:** 1513–15.
4. Schmidt G, *et al.* Methimazole-associated cholestatic liver injury: case report and brief literature review. *Hepatogastroenterology* 1986; **33:** 244–6.
5. Arab DM, *et al.* Severe cholestatic jaundice in uncomplicated hyperthyroidism treated with methimazole. *J Clin Endocrinol Metab* 1995; **80:** 1083–5.
6. Özenírler S, *et al.* Propylthiouracil-induced hepatic damage. *Ann Pharmacother* 1996; **30:** 960–3.
7. Hanson JS. Propylthiouracil and hepatitis. Two cases and a review of the literature. *Arch Intern Med* 1984; **144:** 994–6.
8. Limaye A, Ruffolo PR. Propylthiouracil-induced fatal hepatic necrosis. *Am J Gastroenterol* 1987; **82:** 152–4.
9. Ichiki Y, *et al.* Propylthiouracil-induced severe hepatitis: a case report and review of the literature. *J Gastroenterol* 1998; **33:** 747–50.
10. Liaw Y-F, *et al.* Hepatic injury during propylthiouracil therapy in patients with hyperthyroidism. *Ann Intern Med* 1993; **118:** 424–8.

**Effects on the lungs.** A report of a diffuse interstitial pneumonitis in 2 patients given propylthiouracil.[1] A hypersensitivity reaction to propylthiouracil was suggested. Propylthiouracil was also implicated in 2 cases of alveolar haemorrhage, associated with antineutrophil cytoplasmic antibody.[2,3]

1. Miyazono K, *et al.* Propylthiouracil-induced diffuse interstitial pneumonitis. *Arch Intern Med* 1984; **144:** 1764–5.
2. Ohtsuka M, *et al.* Propylthiouracil-induced alveolar haemorrhage associated with antineutrophil cytoplasmic antibody. *Eur Respir J* 1997; **10:** 1405–7.
3. Dhillon SS, *et al.* Diffuse alveolar hemorrhage and pulmonary capillaritis due to propylthiouracil. *Chest* 1999; **116:** 1485–8.

**Effects on the muscles.** Myositis with pain, weakness, and increased creatine kinase concentrations has been reported with carbimazole.[1,2] This effect might be explained by 'tissue hypothyroidism', and might respond to dosage reduction.[3]

1. Page SR, Nussey SS. Myositis in association with carbimazole therapy. *Lancet* 1989; **i:** 964.
2. Pasquier E, *et al.* Biopsy-proven myositis with microvasculitis in association with carbimazole. *Lancet* 1991; **338:** 1082–3.
3. O'Malley B. Carbimazole-induced cramps. *Lancet* 1989; **i:** 1456.

**Hypersensitivity.** Many of the adverse effects associated with the thiourea antithyroid drugs appear to have an immune basis. These effects may be associated with polyarthritis[1] or hypersensitivity vasculitis.[2-7] The latter is sometimes severe and multisystemic, and fatalities have occurred.

Hypersensitivity reactions may also be associated with the development of antineutrophil cytoplasmic antibodies (ANCA), or sometimes with a lupus-like syndrome with or without the presence of antinuclear antibodies.[2,5]

Serum sickness with arthralgias and raised immunoglobulin M (IgM) concentrations has been reported with thiamazole,[8] and the production of antibodies to insulin, resulting in episodes of hypoglycaemia, has been associated with thiamazole[9] and carbimazole.[10]

The thiourea antithyroid drugs all contain a thioamide group and cross-sensitivity between them might be expected; in particular, complete cross-reactivity may be expected between thiamazole and carbimazole since the latter is converted *in vivo* to thiamazole. Cross-sensitivity between propylthiouracil and carbimazole[11] or thiamazole[12] has been reported but the incidence and clinical importance is not clear. Although it has been suggested that carbimazole or thiamazole may be substituted for propylthiouracil in hypersensitive patients, it is safer to discontinue antithyroid drugs in such patients.[11]

1. Bajaj S, *et al.* Antithyroid arthritis syndrome. *J Rheumatol* 1998; **25:** 1235–9.
2. Kawachi Y, *et al.* ANCA-associated vasculitis and lupus-like syndrome caused by methimazole. *Clin Exp Dermatol* 1995; **20:** 345–7.
3. Chastain MA, *et al.* Propylthiouracil hypersensitivity: report of two patients with vasculitis and review of the literature. *J Am Acad Dermatol* 1999; **41:** 757–64.
4. Gunton JE, *et al.* Clinical case seminar: antithyroid drugs and antineutrophil cytoplasmic antibody positive vasculitis. A case report and review of the literature. *J Clin Endocrinol Metab* 1999; **84:** 13–16.
5. Mathieu E, *et al.* Systemic adverse effect of antithyroid drugs. *Clin Rheumatol* 1999; **18:** 66–8.
6. Dolman KM, *et al.* Vasculitis and antineutrophil cytoplasmic autoantibodies associated with propylthiouracil therapy. *Lancet* 1993; **342:** 651–2.
7. ten Holder SM, *et al.* Cutaneous and systemic manifestations of drug-induced vasculitis. *Ann Pharmacother* 2002; **36:** 130–47.
8. Van Kuyk M, *et al.* Methimazole-induced serum sickness. *Acta Clin Belg* 1983; **38:** 68–9.
9. Hakamata M, *et al.* Insulin autoimmune syndrome after the third therapy with methimazole. *Intern Med* 1995; **34:** 410–12.
10. Burden AC, Rosenthal FD. Methimazole and insulin autoimmune syndrome. *Lancet* 1983; **ii:** 1311.
11. Smith A, *et al.* Cross sensitivity to antithyroid drugs. *BMJ* 1989; **298:** 1253.
12. De Weweire A, *et al.* Failure to control hyperthyroidism with a thionamide after potassium perchlorate withdrawal in a patient with amiodarone associated thyrotoxicosis. *J Endocrinol Invest* 1987; **10:** 529.

**Pregnancy.** Thiourea antithyroid drugs have been used successfully in pregnancy (see Hyperthyroidism, p.1594).

Thiamazole (the metabolite of carbimazole) has been the antithyroid drug most frequently involved in the few reports of **congenital defects** following maternal use of such compounds. Several infants exposed to thiamazole *in utero* have been born with scalp defects (aplasia cutis congenita—a localised absence of skin at birth)[1,2] although hyperthyroidism itself may give rise to such defects.[3] Individual case reports of other congenital defects associated with thiamazole have included choanal atresia (an upper respiratory-tract defect), oesophageal atresia, and tracheo-oesophageal fistula[3] but the incidence of congenital abnormalities is not increased compared with the general population.[4] Gastroschisis (an abdominal wall defect) has been reported in an infant after maternal exposure to carbimazole.[5] There have been some reports of neonates exposed to thiourea antithyroid drugs *in utero* displaying signs of **hypothyroidism** including goitre.[6,7]

1. Milham S. Scalp defects in infants of mothers treated for hyperthyroidism with methimazole or carbimazole during pregnancy. *Teratology* 1985; **32:** 321.
2. Vogt T, *et al.* Aplasia cutis congenita after exposure to methimazole: a causal relationship? *Br J Dermatol* 1995; **133:** 994–6.
3. Johnsson E, *et al.* Severe malformations in infant born to hyperthyroid woman on methimazole. *Lancet* 1997; **350:** 1520.
4. Wing DA, *et al.* A comparison of propylthiouracil versus methimazole in the treatment of hyperthyroidism in pregnancy. *Am J Obstet Gynecol* 1994; **170:** 90–5.
5. Guignon A-M, *et al.* Carbimazole-related gastroschisis. *Ann Pharmacother* 2003; **37:** 829–31.
6. O'Doherty MJ, *et al.* Treating thyrotoxicosis in pregnant or potentially pregnant women. *BMJ* 1999; **318:** 5–6.
7. Masiukiewicz US, Barrow GN. Hyperthyroidism in pregnancy: diagnosis and treatment. *Thyroid* 1999; **9:** 647–52.

## Pharmacokinetics

The pharmacokinetics of carbimazole and thiamazole can be considered together since carbimazole is rapidly and completely metabolised to thiamazole in the body. The antithyroid activity of carbimazole is dependent upon this conversion to thiamazole.

Carbimazole and other thiourea antithyroid drugs are rapidly absorbed from the gastrointestinal tract with peak plasma concentrations occurring about 1 to 2 hours following doses by mouth.

They are concentrated in the thyroid gland; since their duration of action is more closely related to the intrathyroidal drug concentration than their plasma half-life, prolonged antithyroid activity results from single daily doses. Thiamazole is not bound to plasma proteins.

Thiamazole has an elimination half-life from plasma of about 3 to 6 hours and is metabolised, probably by the liver, and excreted in the urine. Less than 12% of a dose of thiamazole may be excreted as unchanged drug. 3-Methyl-2-thiohydantoin has been identified as a metabolite of thiamazole. The elimination half-life may be increased in hepatic and renal impairment.

Thiamazole crosses the placenta and is distributed into breast milk.

◊ References to the pharmacokinetics of carbimazole and thiamazole.

1. Skellern GG, *et al.* The pharmacokinetics of methimazole after oral administration of carbimazole and methimazole, in hyperthyroid patients. *Br J Clin Pharmacol* 1980; **9:** 137–43.
2. Kampmann JP, Hansen JM. Clinical pharmacokinetics of antithyroid drugs. *Clin Pharmacokinet* 1981; **6:** 401–28.
3. Jansson R, *et al.* Intrathyroidal concentrations of methimazole in patients with Graves' disease. *J Clin Endocrinol Metab* 1983; **57:** 129–32.
4. Cooper DS, *et al.* Methimazole pharmacology in man: studies using a newly developed radioimmunoassay for methimazole. *J Clin Endocrinol Metab* 1984; **58:** 473–9.
5. Jansson R, *et al.* Pharmacokinetic properties and bioavailability of methimazole. *Clin Pharmacokinet* 1985; **10:** 443–50.

## Uses and Administration

Carbimazole is a thiourea antithyroid drug that acts by blocking the production of thyroid hormones (see p.1594). It is used in the management of hyperthyroidism (p.1594), including the treatment of Graves' disease, the preparation of hyperthyroid patients for thyroidectomy, use as an adjunct to radio-iodine therapy, and the treatment of thyroid storm.

Carbimazole is completely metabolised to thiamazole and it is this metabolite that is responsible for the clinical antithyroid activity of carbimazole.

Carbimazole is given by mouth typically in an initial dosage of 15 to 40 mg daily. It has often been given in divided daily doses but once daily administration is also possible. Improvement is usually seen in 1 to 3 weeks and control of symptoms is achieved in 1 to 2 months. When the patient is euthyroid the dose is gradually reduced to the smallest amount that will maintain the euthyroid state. Typical maintenance doses are 5 to 15 mg daily.

Children may be given an initial dose of 250 micrograms/kg three times daily, adjusted according to response; treatment in children should be undertaken by a specialist.

Carbimazole is also given in an initial dose of 20 to 60 mg with supplemental levothyroxine as a *blocking-replacement regimen*. Either form of maintenance treatment is usually continued for at least a year, and often for 18 months.

**Action.** There is evidence to suggest that thiourea antithyroid drugs suppress the immune response. However, it is not clear whether this immunosuppressive effect contributes to their antithyroid action or has any clinical significance in the treatment of auto-immune thyroid disorders.[1-5] Increasing the daily dose of thiamazole with the aim of immunosuppression was of no benefit in a large study of patients with Graves' disease.[6]

A number of the adverse effects of the thiourea drugs are considered to have an immune basis (see under Hypersensitivity, above).

1. Kendall-Taylor P. Are antithyroid drugs immunosuppressive? *BMJ* 1984; **288:** 509–11.
2. Ludgate ME, *et al.* Analysis of T cell subsets in Graves' disease: alterations associated with carbimazole. *BMJ* 1984; **288:** 526–30.
3. Jansson R, *et al.* Thyroxine, methimazole, and thyroid microsomal autoantibody titres in hypothyroid Hashimoto's thyroiditis. *BMJ* 1985; **290:** 11–12.
4. Tötterman TH, *et al.* Induction of circulating activated suppressor-like T cells by methimazole therapy for Graves' disease. *N Engl J Med* 1987; **316:** 15–22.
5. Volpé R. Immunoregulation in autoimmune thyroid disease. *N Engl J Med* 1987; **316:** 44–6.
6. Reinwein D, *et al.* A prospective randomised trial of antithyroid drug dose in Graves' disease therapy. *J Clin Endocrinol Metab* 1993; **76:** 1516–21.

## Preparations

***BP 2003:*** Carbimazole Tablets.

**Proprietary Preparations** (details are given in Part 3)
***Austral.:*** Neo-Mercazole; ***Austria:*** Carbistad; ***Denm.:*** Neo-Mercazole; ***Fin.:*** Tyrazol; ***Fr.:*** Neo-Mercazole; ***Ger.:*** Neo-Thyreostat; ***Gr.:*** Thyrostat; ***Hong Kong:*** Cazole; Neo-Mercazole†; ***India:*** Neo-Mercazole; ***Irl.:*** Neo-Mercazole; ***Malaysia:*** Camazol; ***Norw.:*** Neo-Mercazole; ***NZ:*** Neo-Mercazole; ***S.Afr.:*** Neo-Mercazole; ***Singapore:*** Camazol; Cazole; Neo-Mercazole†; ***Spain:*** Neo Tomizol; ***Switz.:*** Neo-Mercazole; ***UK:*** Neo-Mercazole.

---

## Dibromotyrosine

Dibromotirosina. 3,5-Dibromo-L-tyrosine.

$C_9H_9Br_2NO_3 = 339.0.$
*CAS — 300-38-9.*
*ATC — H03BX02.*

### Profile

Dibromotyrosine is an antithyroid drug used in the treatment of hyperthyroidism (p.1594) in doses of 300 to 900 mg daily by mouth.

### Preparations

**Proprietary Preparations** (details are given in Part 3)
***Ital.:*** Bromotiren.
**Multi-ingredient:** ***Ital.:*** Bromazolo.

---

## Diiodotyrosine

Diiodotirosina; Diotyrosine; Iodogorgoic Acid. 3,5-Di-iodo-L-tyrosine dihydrate.

$C_9H_9I_2NO_3,2H_2O = 469.0.$
*CAS — 66-02-4 (anhydrous diiodotyrosine); 300-39-0 (anhydrous L-diiodotyrosine).*
*ATC — H03BX01.*

### Profile

Diiodotyrosine is an antithyroid drug. It is given by mouth in usual doses of 177.5 to 355 micrograms daily for the treatment of hyperthyroidism and iodine deficiency disorders.

### Preparations

**Proprietary Preparations** (details are given in Part 3)
***Ger.:*** Strumedical 400†.

---

### Fluorotyrosine

Fluorotirosina; Fluorotyrosinum; Fluortyrosine. 3-Fluorotyrosine.

$C_9H_{10}FNO_3$ = 199.2.

*CAS — 139-26-4.*

#### Profile

Fluorotyrosine is an antithyroid drug that has been used in the treatment of hyperthyroidism.

#### Preparations

**Proprietary Preparations** (details are given in Part 3)

***Austria:*** Fluorthyrin.

## Iodine

Iode; Iodo; Iodum; Jodum; Yodo.

$I_2$ = 253.80894.

*CAS — 7553-56-2.*

*ATC — D08AG03.*

**Pharmacopoeias.** In *Chin., Eur.* (see p.vi), *Int., Jpn, Pol., US,* and *Viet.*

**Ph. Eur. 5.0** (Iodine). Greyish-violet, brittle plates or fine crystals, with a metallic sheen. It is slowly volatile at room temperature. Very slightly soluble in water; soluble in alcohol; slightly soluble in glycerol; very soluble in concentrated solutions of iodides.

**USP 27** (Iodine). Heavy, greyish-black plates or granules with a metallic sheen and a characteristic odour. Soluble 1 in 3000 of water, 1 in 13 of alcohol, 1 in 4 of carbon disulfide, and 1 in 80 of glycerol; freely soluble in chloroform, in ether, and in carbon tetrachloride; soluble in solutions of iodides. Store in airtight containers.

**Incompatibility.** With acetone, iodine forms a pungent irritating compound.

### Potassium Iodate

Iodato potásico.

$KIO_3$ = 214.0.

*CAS — 7758-05-6.*

**Pharmacopoeias.** In *Br., Chin.,* and *It.*

**BP 2003** (Potassium Iodate). A white crystalline powder with a slight odour. Slowly soluble in water; insoluble in alcohol. A 5% solution in water has a pH of 5.0 to 8.0.

### Potassium Iodide

Iodeto de Potássio; Ioduro potásico; Kalii Iodetum; Kalii Iodidum; Kalii Jodidum; Kalium Iodatum; Kalium Jodatum; Pot. Iod.; Potassii Iodidum; Potassium (Iodure de).

KI = 166.0.

*CAS — 7681-11-0.*

*ATC — R05CA02; S01XA04; V03AB21.*

**Pharmacopoeias.** In *Chin., Eur.* (see p.vi), *Int., Jpn, Pol., US,* and *Viet.*

**Ph. Eur. 5.0** (Potassium Iodide). A white powder or colourless crystals. Very soluble in water; soluble in alcohol; freely soluble in glycerol. Protect from light.

**USP 27** (Potassium Iodide). Hexahedral crystals, either transparent and colourless or somewhat opaque and white, or a white, granular powder. It is slightly hygroscopic. Soluble 1 in 0.7 of water and 1 in 0.5 of boiling water, 1 in 22 of alcohol, and 1 in 2 of glycerol. Its solutions are neutral or alkaline to litmus.

### Sodium Iodide

Iodeto de Sódio; Ioduro sódico; Natrii Iodetum; Natrii Iodidum; Natrii Jodidum; Natrium Iodatum; Sod. Iod.; Sodii Iodidum; Sodium (Iodure de).

NaI = 149.9.

*CAS — 7681-82-5.*

**Pharmacopoeias.** In *Chin., Eur.* (see p.vi), *Jpn, Pol.,* and *US.*

**Ph. Eur. 5.0** (Sodium Iodide). Colourless crystals or white crystalline powder. It is hygroscopic. Very soluble in water; freely soluble in alcohol. Protect from light.

**USP 27** (Sodium Iodide). Colourless, odourless crystals, or white crystalline powder. It is deliquescent in moist air and develops a brown tint upon decomposition. Soluble 1 in 0.6 of water, 1 in 2 of alcohol, and 1 in 1 of glycerol. Store in airtight containers.

### Adverse Effects and Treatment

Iodine and iodides, whether applied topically or administered systemically, can give rise to hypersensitivity reactions which may include urticaria, angioedema, cutaneous haemorrhage or purpuras, fever, arthralgia, lymphadenopathy, and eosinophilia.

Inhalation of iodine vapour is very irritating to mucous membranes.

Iodine and iodides have variable effects on the thyroid (see below) and can produce goitre and hypothyroidism as well as hyperthyroidism (the Iod-Basedow or Jod-Basedow phenomenon). Goitre and hypothyroidism have also occurred in infants born to mothers who had taken iodides during pregnancy.

Prolonged administration may lead to a range of adverse effects, often called 'iodism', some of which may again be due to hypersensitivity. Adverse effects include metallic taste, increased salivation, burning or painful mouth; there may be acute rhinitis, coryza-like symptoms, and swelling and inflammation of the throat. Eyes may be irritated and swollen and there may be increased lachrymation. Pulmonary oedema, dyspnoea, and bronchitis may develop. Skin reactions include acneform or, more rarely, severe eruptions (iododerma). Other reported effects include depression, insomnia, impotence, headache, and gastrointestinal disturbances, notably nausea, vomiting, and diarrhoea.

The symptoms of acute poisoning from ingestion of iodine are mainly due to its corrosive effects on the gastrointestinal tract; a disagreeable metallic taste, vomiting, abdominal pain, and bloody diarrhoea occur. Thirst and headache have been reported. Systemic toxicity may lead to shock, tachycardia, fever, metabolic acidosis and renal impairment. Death may be due to circulatory failure, oedema of the epiglottis resulting in asphyxia, aspiration pneumonia, or pulmonary oedema. Oesophageal stricture may occur if the patient survives the acute stage.

Victims of acute poisoning have been given copious draughts of milk or starch mucilage; lavage should probably not be attempted, and certainly not unless the ingested iodine was in sufficiently dilute form not to produce gastrointestinal corrosion. Other treatments include activated charcoal or sodium thiosulfate solution (usually as a 1% solution) to reduce iodine to the less toxic iodides.

**Effects on the thyroid.** Iodide may be isolated by the body from a variety of sources, including an iodine-rich diet, or some disinfectants and drugs containing iodine (see also under Amiodarone, p.860). Although iodine is required for the production of thyroid hormones, excessive quantities can cause hyperthyroidism, or even paradoxical goitre and hypothyroidism.

The normal daily requirement ranges from 100 to 300 micrograms.[1,2] Quantities of 500 micrograms to 1 mg daily probably have no untoward effects on thyroid function in most cases.[2] When progressively larger doses are given there is an initial rise in thyroid hormone production, but at still higher doses, production decreases (the Wolff-Chaikoff effect). This effect is usually seen with doses of more than about 2 mg daily, but is normally transient, adaptation occurring on repeated administration. In certain individuals a lack of adaptation produces a chronic inhibition of thyroid hormone synthesis leading to goitre and **hypothyroidism**.[1,2]

Excess iodine may also induce **hyperthyroidism** (the Iod-Basedow or Jod-Basedow phenomenon). Iodine-induced hyperthyroidism has been associated with iodine prophylaxis programmes in developing countries.[3] The highest incidence of hyperthyroidism has been reported to occur 1 to 3 years after supplementation commences, with the incidence returning to normal within 3 to 10 years despite continued iodine exposure.[4] Elderly subjects and those with nodular goitres have been found to be at greatest risk.

To overcome any adverse effects on thyroid function as a result of iodine prophylaxis during **pregnancy**, WHO has issued guidelines on the safe use of iodised oil during gestation.[5,6] There is some evidence that the use of iodine-containing antiseptics on pregnant women and neonates may cause disturbances in thyroid function.[7,8]


1. Arthur JR, Beckett GJ. Thyroid function. *Br Med Bull* 1999; **55:** 658–68.
2. WHO. Iodine. In *Trace elements in human nutrition and health.* Geneva: WHO, 1996: 49–71.
3. Delange F, *et al.* Risks of iodine-induced hyperthyroidism after correction of iodine deficiency by iodized salt. *Thyroid* 1999; **9:** 545–56.
4. Fradkin JE, Wolff J. Iodide-induced thyrotoxicosis. *Medicine (Baltimore)* 1983; **62:** 1–20.
5. WHO. Safe use of iodized oil to prevent iodine deficiency in pregnant women. *Bull WHO* 1996; **74:** 1–3.
6. Delange F. Administration of iodized oil during pregnancy: a summary of the published evidence. *Bull WHO* 1996; **74:** 101–8.
7. Linder N *et al.* Topical iodine-containing antiseptics and subclinical hypothyroidism in preterm infants. *J Pediatr* 1997; **131:** 434–9.
8. Weber G *et al.* Neonatal transient hypothyroidism: aetiological study. *Arch Dis Child Fetal Neonatal Ed* 1998; **79:** F70–2.


### Precautions

Caution is necessary if preparations containing iodine or iodides are taken for prolonged periods, and such preparations should not be taken regularly during pregnancy except when iodine supplementation is required. Caution is also required when giving iodine or iodides to children. Patients over the age of 45 years or with nodular goitres are especially susceptible to hyperthyroidism when given iodine supplementation. Reduced doses should therefore be used and supplementation with iodised oil may not be appropriate.

Solutions of iodine applied to the skin should not be covered with occlusive dressings. The disinfectant activity of iodine is reduced by alkalis as well as by protein.

As iodine and iodides can affect the thyroid gland the administration of such preparations may interfere with tests of thyroid function.

**Breast feeding.** Iodine is concentrated by the mammary gland into breast milk to ensure an adequate supply to the breast-fed infant. Since this is dependent on the maternal dietary intake,[1] the WHO recommends a daily iodine intake of 200 micrograms for lactating women, see Iodine Deficiency Disorders, below.

The *British National Formulary* considers treatment with iodine or iodides to be a contra-indication to breast feeding. However, the American Academy of Pediatrics[2] considers that such treatment is usually compatible with breast feeding although it is noted that goitre or effects on thyroid function have been reported.


1. Semba RD, Delange F. Iodine in human milk: perspectives for infant health. *Nutr Rev* 2001; **59:** 269–78.
2. American Academy of Pediatrics. The transfer of drugs and other chemicals into human milk. *Pediatrics* 2001; **108:** 776–89. Correction. *ibid.*; 1029. Also available at: http://aappolicy.aappublications.org/cgi/content/full/pediatrics%3b108/3/776 (accessed 17/05/04)


### Interactions

The effects of iodine and iodides on the thyroid may be altered by other compounds including amiodarone and lithium.

### Pharmacokinetics

Iodine is slightly absorbed when applied to the skin. When taken by mouth iodine preparations (which are converted to iodide) and iodides are transported to and concentrated in the thyroid gland (see p.1594). Iodides not taken up by the thyroid are excreted mainly in the urine, with smaller amounts appearing in the faeces, saliva, and sweat. They cross the placenta and are distributed into breast milk.

### Uses and Administration

Iodine is an essential trace element in the human diet, necessary for the formation of thyroid hormones (see p.1594), and consequently it is used in iodine deficiency and thyroid disorders. It also has antimicrobial activity.

For the prophylaxis and treatment of **iodine deficiency disorders** (below) it may be given as potassium or sodium iodide, iodised oil, or potassium iodate.

In the pre-operative management of **hyperthyroidism** (p.1594) iodine and iodides are used with antithyroid drugs such as carbimazole, thiamazole, or propylthiouracil. Administration has been thought to render the thyroid firm and avoid the increased vascularity and friability with increased risk of haemorrhage that may result from the use of an antithyroid drug alone. However, there is little evidence of a beneficial effect. Iodine may be given as a solution with potassium iodide (Aqueous Iodine Oral Solution BP 2003; Lugol's Solution or Strong Iodine Solution USP 27) which contains in each mL 130 mg of free and combined iodine; a dose of 0.1 to 0.3 mL in milk or water is given three times daily for 10 to 14 days. Alternatively, potassium iodide has been given in doses of up to 250 mg three times daily with food. Solutions of potassium iodide intended for oral administration should be given well diluted to avoid gastric irritation. Potassium iodide may also be given as part of the management of thyroid storm 1 hour after administration of an antithyroid drug; doses as high as 500 mg every 4 hours have been suggested. Each g of potassium iodide represents 6 mmol of potassium and of iodide. Sodium iodide has been given by intravenous injection as part of the management of thyroid storm.

Potassium iodide has been tried in the treatment of benign **thyroid nodules** (p.1594).

Potassium iodide or potassium iodate are taken by mouth for **radiation protection** (below) to saturate the thyroid when uptake of radio-iodine by the gland is not desired.

Iodine has a powerful bactericidal action. It is also active against fungi, viruses, protozoa, cysts, and spores. Potassium iodide has been used in the treatment of fungal infections such as sporotrichosis (below). Iodine is used as an **antiseptic** and **disinfectant** generally as a 2% or 2.5% solution. Its activity is reduced in the presence of organic matter, though not to the same extent as with the other halogen disinfectants. If industrial methylated spirit is used for the solution, it should be free from acetone with which iodine forms an irritant and lachrymatory compound. Iodine solutions may be applied to small wounds or abrasions as well as to unbroken skin, but an iodophore such as povidone-iodine (p.1190) may be preferred.

Iodine may also be used to sterilise drinking water; 5 drops of a 2% alcoholic solution added to about one litre (one US quart) of water is reported to kill amoebae and bacteria within 15 minutes. Water contaminated with *Giardia* requires 12 drops of a 2% alcoholic solution for each litre which may take one hour to achieve its effect.

When iodine combines chemically it is decolorised and so-called colourless iodine preparations do not have the disinfectant properties of iodine.

Iodine stains the skin a deep reddish-brown; the stain can be readily removed by dilute solutions of alkalis or sodium thiosulfate. A dilute solution of iodine (Schiller's Iodine) has been used as a **diagnostic** stain in colposcopy.

There have been numerous other uses of iodine and iodides. Iodides have long been used as ingredients of expectorant mixtures (see Cough, p.1112) but there is little evidence of their effectiveness. A diatomic iodine formulation is under investigation for the treatment of fibrocystic breast disease. Iodinated organic compounds including iodised oil are used as X-ray contrast media (p.1059). Iodine radionuclides are often administered as preparations of sodium iodide. Potassium iodide has been given in the treatment of Sweet's syndrome (acute febrile neutrophilic dermatosis). A mixture of iodine and sodium iodide is used as sclerotherapy for varicose veins (p.1717).

**Fungal infections.** Potassium iodide is used in the treatment of cutaneous sporotrichosis (p.391), although how it acts is unclear since antifungal activity was not demonstrated *in vitro* against *Sporothrix schenkii*.[1] It is usually given by mouth in a gradually increasing dosage up to the limit of tolerance. The WHO recommended initial dose is 5 drops [about 250 mg] of a saturated solution of potassium iodide (1 g/mL) given three times daily; treatment should be continued for at least 1 month after the disappearance or stabilisation of the lesions.

Potassium iodide has also been found to be effective in the treatment of phycomycosis caused by *Basidiobolus haptosporus*;[2,3] once again the mode of action is unclear.[4]

Potassium iodide and sodium iodide have been tried by local intracavitary instillation for the treatment of life-threatening haemoptysis from pulmonary aspergillomas.[5] Mechanical factors may have accounted for a beneficial effect rather than any antifungal action. Aspergillomas are usually managed conservatively or, in more severe disease, with antifungals or surgery (see p.386).

1. WHO. *WHO model prescribing information: drugs used in skin diseases*. Geneva: WHO, 1997.
2. Kelly S, *et al.* Subcutaneous phycomycosis in Sierra Leone. *Trans R Soc Trop Med Hyg* 1980; **74:** 396–7.
3. Kamalam A, Thambiah AS. Muscle invasion by Basidiobolus haptosporus. *Sabouraudia* 1984; **22:** 273–7.
4. Yangco BG, *et al.* In vitro susceptibilities of human and wild-type isolates of Basidiobolus and Conidiobolus species. *Antimicrob Agents Chemother* 1984; **25:** 413–16.
5. Rumbak M, *et al.* Topical treatment of life threatening haemoptysis from aspergillomas. *Thorax* 1996; **51:** 253–5.

**Iodine deficiency disorders.** Iodine is an essential trace element required for thyroid hormone production. In the UK the reference nutrient intake (RNI) for adults is 140 micrograms (1.1 micromoles) of iodine daily[1] and in the USA the recommended dietary allowance (RDA) is 150 micrograms daily.[2] A full explanation of the terms RNI and RDA can be found under Human Requirements of Vitamins, p.1419. In 1996, WHO[3] recommended the following daily iodine intakes:

- 50 micrograms up to 12 months of age
- 90 micrograms from 1 to 6 years
- 120 micrograms from 7 to 12 years
- 150 micrograms from 12 years of age
- 200 micrograms during pregnancy and lactation.

A subsequent document from the International Council for Control of Iodine Deficiency Disorders recommended 90 micrograms daily for all infants and children under 7 years of age.[4]

When iodine requirements are not met, a range of disorders can develop. These iodine deficiency disorders include endemic goitre (enlargement of the thyroid), endemic cretinism (a syndrome characterised by deaf-mutism, intellectual deficit, spasticity, and sometimes hypothyroidism), impaired mental function in children and adults, and an increased incidence of still-births as well as perinatal and infant mortality.[3]

Iodine deficiency disorders can be prevented by iodine supplementation. The incidence of endemic goitre, endemic cretinism, and mental retardation can be reduced and some of the effects of established iodine deficiency ameliorated, with only modest risks.[5]

Although various methods of iodine supplementation, including iodination of sugar, water, and bread, as well as the administration of potassium iodide, have been investigated, the two methods generally used are iodination of culinary salt and the administration of iodised oil.[3]

*Salt* may be iodinated by the addition of potassium iodide. However, in countries where impurities or environmental factors such as moisture and temperature are likely to cause a reduction in the iodine content of the salt, potassium iodate is the preferred compound since it is more stable than iodide under varying climatic conditions. The concentration used in different countries varies over a wide range from 10 to about 80 ppm of elemental iodine.[4]

The chief alternative to supplementation with iodinated salt is *iodised oil*, usually by intramuscular injection; it is useful where salt consumption is unreliable or inadequate or where immediate action is necessary to correct severe iodine deficiency.[3] A commonly used type of iodised oil has been a poppyseed oil containing about 38% w/w or 480 mg/mL of iodine (see Iodised Oil, p.1063). Some countries have produced iodised oil based on alternatives such as peanut or rapeseed oil.[6,7] Single intramuscular doses can provide adequate protection from iodine deficiency for up to 3 years. WHO has recommended[8] that infants up to 1 year receive 190 mg iodine, as iodised oil (480 mg/mL iodine), by intramuscular injection; children and adults up to age 45 are given 380 mg. Subjects over the age of 45 years and those with nodular goitre are susceptible to hyperthyroidism when given iodine, and iodised oil may not be a suitable means of supplementation. If it is used, doses of 76 mg are given.[8]

Iodised oil may also be given by mouth once yearly. WHO recommends[8] that infants up to 1 year be given a single dose of 100 mg iodine, children from 1 to 5 years 200 mg, and those over 6 years 400 mg. The evidence suggests that oral administration of iodised oil is as effective as intramuscular for preventing iodine deficiency disorders in children.[9] Adults are also given 400 mg, except during pregnancy, when a single dose of 200 mg is recommended.

Iodine or iodides may suppress neonatal thyroid function and it is generally recommended that iodine compounds should be avoided during **pregnancy**. However, where it is essential to prevent neonatal goitre and cretinism, iodine supplementation should not be withheld from pregnant women.[10,11] Iodine supplementation has been found to be effective in preventing brain-damage in the fetus provided it is given to the mother in the first or second trimester;[10] treatment later in pregnancy was not effective in improving neurological status, although some developmental improvement was seen and hypothyroidism will be corrected. WHO has stated that in areas where iodine deficiency disorders are moderate to severe, iodised oil given either before or at any stage of gestation is beneficial.[8,11] A dose of 480 mg iodine intramuscularly each year, or 300 to 480 mg iodine by mouth each year, or 100 to 300 mg iodine by mouth every 6 months, is recommended for pregnant women and for at least one year postpartum. Similar intramuscular doses are recommended for non-pregnant fertile women with oral doses being 400 to 960 mg iodine every year, or 200 to 480 mg every 6 months.

*Indirect iodine supplementation*, by addition of potassium iodate to the water used to irrigate crops, has been tried in areas of iodine deficiency where other methods had proved difficult to implement.[12]

1. DoH. Dietary reference values for food energy and nutrients for the United Kingdom: report of the panel on dietary reference values of the Committee on Medical Aspects of Food Policy. *Report on health and social subjects 41*. London: HMSO, 1991.
2. Standing Committee on the Scientific Evaluation of Dietary Reference Intakes of the Food and Nutrition Board. *Dietary Reference Intakes for Vitamin A, Vitamin K, Arsenic, Boron, Chromium, Copper, Iodine, Iron, Manganese, Molybdenum, Nickel, Silicon, Vanadium, and Zinc*. Washington DC: National Academy Press, 2001.
3. WHO. Iodine. In *Trace elements in human nutrition and health*. Geneva: WHO, 1996: 49–71.
4. International Council for Control of Iodine Deficiency Disorders. Iodine deficiency disorder. Available at: http://www.people.virginia.edu/~jtd/iccidd/aboutidd.htm (accessed 17/05/04)
5. Delange F, Lecomte P. Iodine supplementation: benefits outweigh risks. *Drug Safety* 2000; **22:** 89–95.
6. Ingenbleek Y, *et al.* Iodised rapeseed oil for eradication of severe endemic goitre. *Lancet* 1997; **350:** 1542–5.
7. Untoro J, *et al.* Efficacy of different types of iodised oil. *Lancet* 1998; **351:** 752–3.
8. WHO. *WHO model formulary*. Geneva: WHO, 2004.
9. Angermayr L, Clar C. Iodine supplementation for preventing iodine deficiency disorders in children. Available in The Cochrane Library; Issue 2. Chichester: John Wiley; 2004.
10. Delange F. Administration of iodized oil during pregnancy: a summary of the published evidence. *Bull WHO* 1996; **74:** 101–8.
11. WHO. Safe use of iodized oil to prevent iodine deficiency in pregnant women. *Bull WHO* 1996; **74:** 1–3.
12. Cao X-Y, *et al.* Iodination of irrigation water as a method of supplying iodine to a severely iodine-deficient population in Xinjiang, China. *Lancet* 1994; **344:** 107–10.

**Radiation protection.** The administration of a radiologically stable form of iodine to saturate the thyroid gland confers thyroid protection from iodine radionuclides.[1,2] When thyroid protection from a *medical procedure* involving radio-iodine is needed 100 to 150 mg of iodide as potassium iodide may be given by mouth 24 hours before the procedure and daily for up to 10 days following it.

In the event of a *nuclear accident* authorities in the USA recommend[1,3] a dose of 130 mg of potassium iodide by mouth daily in adults (including pregnant and lactating women). Daily administration should continue until risk of exposure has passed and adjunctive measures have been implemented. Recommended daily doses of potassium iodide for children are: up to 1 month of age, 16 mg; 1 month to 3 years, 32 mg; 3 to 12 years (up to 18 years if body-weight is less than 70 kg), 65 mg. In the UK the Department of Health[4] recommends a single oral dose of 100 mg of stable iodine (as 170 mg of potassium iodate) for adults (including pregnant women and women who are breast feeding) as soon as possible after exposure and before evacuation. Dosages for children are: 3 to 12 years, 50 mg of stable iodine (85 mg of potassium iodate); 1 month to 3 years, 25 mg of stable iodine (42.5 mg of potassium iodate); and for neonates, 12.5 mg of stable iodine (21.25 mg of potassium iodate) given as a single dose. When evacuation is delayed, repeated daily administration is recommended.

1. Halperin JA. Potassium iodide as a thyroid blocker— Three Mile Island today. *Drug Intell Clin Pharm* 1989; **23:** 422–7.
2. Nauman J, Wolff J. Iodide prophylaxis in Poland after the Chernobyl reactor accident: benefits and risks. *Am J Med* 1993; **94:** 524–32.
3. FDA Center for Drug Evaluation and Research. Guidance: potassium iodide as a thyroid blocking agent in radiation emergencies (issued December 2001). Available at: http://www.fda.gov/cder/guidance/4825fnl.htm (accessed 17/05/04)
4. DoH. Practical guidance on planning for incidents involving radioactivity: potassium iodate (stable iodine) prophylaxis in the event of a nuclear accident. PL/CMO(93)1 (issued 15 February 1993).

## Preparations

***BP 2003:*** Alcoholic Iodine Solution; Aqueous Iodine Oral Solution; Potassium Iodate Tablets; Sodium Iodide Injection;
***BPC 1968:*** Compound Iodine Paint;
***USP 27:*** Iodine Tincture; Iodine Topical Solution; Potassium Iodide Delayed-release Tablets; Potassium Iodide Oral Solution; Potassium Iodide Tablets; Strong Iodine Solution; Strong Iodine Tincture.

**Proprietary Preparations** (details are given in Part 3)

***Austria:*** Jodid; Jodonorm; Leukona-Jod-Bad; ***Braz.:*** Elixir Americano†; Iodetal†; Iodeton; Iodetoss; Iodex; Xarope Neo; ***Canad.:*** Micro I†; Sclerodine; Thyro-Block; ***Chile:*** Solucion De Lugol; ***Fin.:*** Jodix; ***Fr.:*** Axyol†; ***Ger.:*** Jodetten; Jodgamma; Jodid; jodminerase†; Kaliklora Jod med†; Leukona-Jod-Bad; Mono-Jod; Strumex; Varigloban; ***India:*** Collosol; ***Ital.:*** Chitodine; Goccemed; Iodosan Collutorio†; Sol-Jod; ***Mex.:*** Yodolactina; ***Norw.:*** Jodosan; ***Port.:*** Iodisis; ***UK:*** Bioiodine; ***USA:*** Iodopen; Pima; SSKI; Thyro-Block.

**Multi-ingredient:** ***Arg.:*** Azufracid; Iodotiazol; Yodofrixon Salicilado; ***Austral.:*** Asa Tones†; Potassium Iodide and Stramonium Compound†; ***Austria:*** Jodthyrox; Jopinol; ***Belg.:*** Aperop†; ITC†; ***Braz.:*** Antimic†; Antiphlogistine; Atatosse Balsamico†; Axol†; Becantosse†; Bontoss; Boralina†; Broncofisin; Bronquidex; Brontoss; CAM†; Dermicon; Dermofytol†; Dermol; Dermycose; Elixir 914; Elixir de Marinheiro†; Endotussin; Etercilina†; Expec; Expectobron; Expectolu†; Formitonicum†; Frenotossil†; Fungodermol†; Fungol†; Glicodin†; Glycon; Glyteol Balsamico†; Hebrin; Ikaflux†; Iodepol; Iodermol†; Iodesin; Iodetal; Iodeto de Potassio; Iodeto de Potassio Composto; Iodeto de Potassium Composto; Iodex com Salicilato de Metila; Iodobec†; Iodopulmin†; Iol; Iolin; KI-Expectorante; Locao Mancha Branca†; Micocid†; Micotiazol; Micotissim†; MM Expectorante; Pulmoforte†; Pulmonix; Salutina†; Sanoclorofila†; Sedatux; Solucao ABC†; Subitan†; Sudonol†; Tetrabronco†; Teutoss; Thiodeol†; Tolusil†; Tossivitan; Tussin-Pinho†; Tussivit; Tussol†; Tuzo†; Um Segundo†; Xarope de Iodeto de Potassio Composto†; Xarope de Iodeto de Potassio†; Xarope Iodo-Suma; ***Canad.:*** Diodine†; IDM Solution†; Iode; Mathieu Cough Syrup†; Theo-Bronc; Vito Bronches; ***Fr.:*** Marinol; Nitrol; ***Ger.:*** Adelheid-Jodquelle, Tolzer; Jodthyrox; Krophan N; Thyreocomb N; Thyronajod; ***Hong Kong:*** Colircusi Iodine-Thio-Calcic†; Vitreolent; ***India:*** Cato-Bell; ***Israel:*** Iodax; ***Ital.:*** Antiadiposo; Esoform Jod 20 and 50; Facovit; Fertomcidina-U; Jodo Calcio Vitaminico; Polijodurato; Rubidiosin Composto†; Rubistenol†; Rubjovit; ***Malaysia:*** Vitreolent; ***Mex.:*** Iodarsolo B12; ***Port.:*** Fluidin Adulto†; Fluidin Antiasmatico†; Prelus; ***Singapore:*** Vitreolent; ***Spain:*** Adiod; Audione; Callicida Rojo; Depurativo Richelet; Encialina; Lasa Antiasmatico†; Nitroina; Yodo Tio Calci†; ***Switz.:*** Dental-Phenjoca†; Perpector; Variglobin; Vitreolent; ***UK:*** Nasciodine; TCP; ***USA:*** Elixophyllin-KI; Iodex with Methyl Salicylate; KIE; Mudrane†; ORA5; Pediacof; Producing Pedituss Cough; Phylorinol; Quadrinal.

## Levothyroxine Sodium *(BANM, rINN)*

Levothyroxinnatrium; Levothyroxinum Natricum; Levotiroxina sódica; 3,5,3′,5′-Tetra-iodo-L-thyronine Sodium; Thyroxine Sodium; L-Thyroxine Sodium; Thyroxinum Natricum; Tirossina; Tiroxina Sodica. Sodium 4-O-(4-hydroxy-3,5-di-iodophenyl)-3,5-di-iodo-L-tyrosine hydrate.

$C_{15}H_{10}I_4NNaO_4,xH_2O$ = 798.9 (anhydrous).

*CAS — 51-48-9 (levothyroxine); 55-03-8 (anhydrous levothyroxine sodium); 25416-65-3 (levothyroxine sodium, hydrate); 8065-29-0 (liotrix).*

*ATC — H03AA01.*

NOTE. The abbreviation $T_4$ is often used for endogenous thyroxine in medical and biochemical reports. Liotrix is *USAN* for a mixture of liothyronine sodium with levothyroxine sodium.

**Pharmacopoeias.** In *Eur.* (see p.vi), *Int., Jpn, US,* and *Viet. Int.* includes the anhydrous form.

**Ph. Eur. 5.0** (Levothyroxine Sodium). An almost white or slightly brownish-yellow powder or a fine, crystalline powder. Very slightly soluble in water; slightly soluble in alcohol. It dissolves in dilute solutions of alkali hydroxides. Store at 2° to 8° in airtight containers. Protect from light.

**USP 27** (Levothyroxine Sodium). The sodium salt of the laevo-isomer of levothyroxine, obtained from the thyroid gland of domesticated animals used for food by man or prepared synthetically. A light yellow to buff-coloured, odourless, hygroscopic, powder. It may assume a slight pink colour on exposure to light. Soluble 1 in 700 of water and 1 in 300 of alcohol; insoluble in acetone, in chloroform, and in ether; soluble in solutions of alkali hydroxides and in hot solutions of alkali carbonates. pH of a saturated solution in water is about 8.9. Store in airtight containers. Protect from light.

### Adverse Effects and Treatment

The adverse effects of levothyroxine are generally associated with excessive dosage and correspond to symptoms of hyperthyroidism. They may include tachycardia, palpitations, cardiac arrhythmias, anginal pain, headache, restlessness, excitability, insomnia, tremors, muscle weakness and cramps, heat intolerance, sweating, flushing, fever, weight loss, menstrual irregularities, diarrhoea, and vomiting. These adverse reactions usually disappear after dosage reduction or temporary withdrawal of treatment. Thyroid storm has occasionally been reported following massive or chronic intoxication and convulsions, cardiac arrhythmias, heart failure, coma, and death have occurred.

In acute overdosage, gastrointestinal absorption may be reduced by activated charcoal. Treatment is usually symptomatic and supportive; propranolol may be useful in controlling the symptoms of sympathetic overactivity. Levothyroxine overdosage requires an extended follow-up period as symptoms may be delayed for up to 6 days due to the gradual peripheral conversion of levothyroxine to tri-iodothyronine.

**Carcinogenicity.** An association between the use of thyroid hormones and an increased risk of breast cancer in women has been proposed,[1] but a further analysis of the data did not confirm such an association,[2] and nor did later studies.[3-5]


1. Kapdi CC, Wolfe JN. Breast cancer. Relationship to thyroid supplements for hypothyroidism. *JAMA* 1976; **236:** 1124–7.
2. Mustacchi P, Greenspan F. Thyroid supplementation for hypothyroidism. An iatrogenic cause of breast cancer? *JAMA* 1977; **237:** 1446–7.
3. Wallace RB, *et al.* Thyroid hormone use in patients with breast cancer. Absence of an association. *JAMA* 1978; **239:** 958.
4. Shapiro S, *et al.* Use of thyroid supplements in relation to the risk of breast cancer. *JAMA* 1980; **244:** 1685–7.
5. Hoffman DA, *et al.* Breast cancer in hypothyroid women using thyroid supplements. *JAMA* 1984; **251:** 616–19.


**Effects on the bones.** Hyperthyroidism is a known risk factor for osteoporosis and some studies have indicated that women receiving long-term levothyroxine therapy may have decreased bone density or accelerated bone mineralisation and thus be at greater risk of developing osteoporosis.[1-5] The bone changes were greatest in those who had some degree of overtreatment resulting in subclinical hyperthyroidism (usually indicated by low TSH concentrations). Strict attention to monitoring of therapy by using sensitive TSH assays, and possibly the use of bone studies, has been advised.[1-6] A meta-analysis of the effects of thyroid hormones on bone density also suggested that prolonged therapy (some 10 years) reduced bone density.[7] Conversely, other studies have not found levothyroxine treatment to affect bone density,[8,9] and even in postmenopausal women receiving relatively high doses of levothyroxine there is evidence that any deleterious effect on the bones may be prevented by oestrogen replacement therapy.[10]


1. Paul TL, *et al.* Long-term L-thyroxine therapy is associated with decreased hip bone density in premenopausal women. *JAMA* 1988; **259:** 3137–41.
2. Stall GM, *et al.* Accelerated bone loss in hypothyroid patients overtreated with L-thyroxine. *Ann Intern Med* 1990; **113:** 265–9.
3. Adlin EV, *et al.* Bone mineral density in postmenopausal women treated with L-thyroxine. *Am J Med* 1991; **90:** 360–6.
4. Kung AWC, Pun KK. Bone mineral density in premenopausal women receiving long-term physiological doses of levothyroxine. *JAMA* 1991; **265:** 2688–91.
5. Greenspan SL, *et al.* Skeletal integrity in premenopausal and postmenopausal women receiving long-term L-thyroxine therapy. *Am J Med* 1991; **91:** 5–14.
6. Greenspan SL, Greenspan FS. The effect of thyroid hormone on skeletal integrity. *Ann Intern Med* 1999; **130:** 750–8.
7. Uzzan B, *et al.* Effects on bone mass of long-term treatment with thyroid hormones: a meta-analysis. *J Clin Endocrinol Metab* 1996; **81:** 4278–89.
8. Franklyn JA, *et al.* Long-term thyroxine treatment and bone mineral density. *Lancet* 1992; **340:** 9–13.
9. Ross DS. Bone density is not reduced during the short-term administration of levothyroxine to postmenopausal women with subclinical hypothyroidism: a randomized prospective study. *Am J Med* 1993; **95:** 385–8.
10. Schneider DL, *et al.* Thyroid hormone use and bone mineral density in elderly women: effects of estrogen. *JAMA* 1994; **271:** 1245–9.


**Effects on the nervous system.** Two children aged 8 and 11 years developed pseudotumor cerebri (benign intracranial hypertension) shortly after the initiation of levothyroxine therapy for hypothyroidism.[1] There have been further reports on individual children[2,3] and infants.[4]

Partial complex status epilepticus, with confusion, agitation, and continuous myoclonic jerks in the left side of the face and left hand, was seen in a hypothyroid patient with Turner's syndrome who was receiving treatment with levothyroxine for myxoedema coma.[5] The condition responded to anticonvulsant therapy; the patient subsequently remained seizure-free on a reduced dose of levothyroxine and concomitant phenytoin.


1. Van Dop C, *et al.* Pseudotumor cerebri associated with initiation of levothyroxine therapy for juvenile hypothyroidism. *N Engl J Med* 1983; **308:** 1076–80.
2. McVie R. Pseudotumor cerebri and thyroid-replacement therapy. *N Engl J Med* 1983; **309:** 731.
3. Hymes LC, *et al.* Pseudotumor cerebri and thyroid-replacement therapy. *N Engl J Med* 1983; **309:** 732.
4. Raghavan S, *et al.* Pseudotumor cerebri in an infant after L-thyroxine therapy for transient neonatal hypothyroidism. *J Pediatr* 1997; **130:** 478–80.
5. Duarte J, *et al.* Thyroxine-induced partial complex status epilepticus. *Ann Pharmacother* 1993; **27:** 1139.


**Hypersensitivity.** A hypersensitivity reaction to synthetic thyroid hormones was reported in a 63-year-old hypothyroid woman with Hashimoto's thyroiditis.[1] Fever, eosinophilia, and liver dysfunction developed after replacement treatment with liothyronine or levothyroxine, but disappeared when therapy was discontinued. After an interval of 4 months liothyronine was gradually reintroduced without adverse effect.

Urticaria and angioedema have been described in a patient who received thyroid and levothyroxine.[2] In a further case similar reactions were attributed to the presence of sunset yellow as colouring agent in the proprietary levothyroxine preparation.[3]


1. Shibata H, *et al.* Hypersensitivity caused by synthetic thyroid hormones in a hypothyroid patient with Hashimoto's thyroiditis. *Arch Intern Med* 1986; **146:** 1624–5.
2. Pandya AG, *et al.* Chronic urticaria associated with exogenous thyroid use. *Arch Dermatol* 1990; **126:** 1238–9.
3. Lévesque H, *et al.* Reporting adverse drug reactions by proprietary name. *Lancet* 1991; **338:** 393.


**Overdosage.** The clinical features and management of overdosage with thyroid drugs have been reviewed.[1] Although aggressive therapy is not normally justified in asymptomatic patients, various regimens have been tried.

Massive overdoses of levothyroxine ranging from 70 to 1200 mg over 2 to 12 days have been described in 6 patients.[2] All the patients developed symptoms of thyrotoxicosis within 3 days of taking the first dose. Treatment was tried using propranolol 120 to 140 mg daily, with hydrocortisone 400 mg daily, and in 3 patients, propylthiouracil 400 to 1200 mg daily, but the benefits of such therapy were considered doubtful. Seven to 10 days after the first dose of levothyroxine, all 6 patients developed neurological complications and 5 went into coma. Cardiac disturbances were also noted; 2 had left ventricular failure and 3 developed severe arrhythmias. Plasmapheresis and charcoal haemoperfusion were both found to increase the elimination of levothyroxine from serum. Plasmapheresis appeared to be the more effective procedure, though the magnitude of the extraction of levothyroxine depended on the serum concentration. One patient died of septic shock and acute renal failure; the other 5 recovered after troubled courses.

In another report,[3] fever, confusion, agitation, and tachycardia developed 5 days after ingestion of approximately 720 mg of levothyroxine, despite treatment with activated charcoal and a cathartic at the time of ingestion (at which point the patient was asymptomatic). Despite treatment with diazepam 380 mg and phenobarbital 1 g intravenously complete sedation could not be achieved; the patient remained tachycardic and febrile for a further 7 days, during which propranolol 10 mg was given intravenously about every 6 hours, along with further diazepam as required. Symptoms subsequently resolved over about 2 weeks.

Symptoms of hyperthyroidism developed in 11 of 41 children, aged 1 to 5 years, who had accidentally ingested levothyroxine sodium in estimated amounts ranging from 0.05 to 13 mg. Symptoms occurred between 12 hours and 11 days after ingestion. Treatment was limited to initial measures to decrease absorption; no adverse effect was considered severe enough to warrant specific symptomatic treatment and all symptoms fully resolved within 14 days. These findings appeared to be consistent with previous reports, although there has been a report[4] of a 2-year-old boy who developed clinical signs of hyperthyroidism and suffered 2 episodes of tonic-clonic seizures 7 days after the ingestion of up to 18 mg of levothyroxine sodium. However, since serious complications appeared to be uncommon and most symptoms remitted without treatment, a conservative approach to the management of acute levothyroxine overdosage in children was recommended.[5]


1. Lin T-H, *et al.* Clinical features and management of overdosage with thyroid drugs. *Med Toxicol* 1988; **3:** 264–72.
2. Binimelis J, *et al.* Massive thyroxine intoxication: evaluation of plasma extraction. *Intensive Care Med* 1987; **13:** 33–8.
3. Hack JB, *et al.* Severe symptoms following a massive intentional L-thyroxine ingestion. *Vet Hum Toxicol* 1999; **41:** 323–6.
4. Kulig K, *et al.* Levothyroxine overdose associated with seizures in a young child. *JAMA* 1985; **254:** 2109–10.
5. Golightly LK, *et al.* Clinical effects of accidental levothyroxine ingestion in children. *Am J Dis Child* 1987; **141:** 1025–7.


### Precautions

Levothyroxine is contra-indicated in untreated hyperthyroidism. It should be used with extreme caution in patients with cardiovascular disorders including angina, heart failure, myocardial infarction, and hypertension; lower initial doses, smaller increments, and longer intervals between increases should be used as necessary. An ECG performed before starting treatment with levothyroxine may help to distinguish underlying myocardial ischaemia from changes induced by hypothyroidism. Levothyroxine should also be introduced very gradually in elderly patients and those with long-standing hypothyroidism to avoid any sudden increase in metabolic demands. It should not be given to patients with adrenal insufficiency without adequate corticosteroid cover otherwise the thyroid replacement therapy might precipitate an acute adrenal crisis. Care is also required when levothyroxine is given to patients with diabetes mellitus or diabetes insipidus.

Tests of thyroid function are subject to alteration by a number of nonthyroidal clinical conditions and by a wide variety of drugs, some of which are mentioned under Interactions, below.

**Abuse.** For mention of abuse of levothyroxine by athletes for weight loss see Obesity, under Uses and Administration, below.

**Adrenocortical insufficiency.** Thyroid-hormone replacement without concomitant treatment with corticosteroids may precipitate acute adrenocortical insufficiency in patients with impaired adrenocortical function, including those with subclinical or unrecognised adrenocortical disease.[1] Prompt diagnosis and replacement of corticosteroids can prevent the development of a potentially fatal crisis. It has been pointed out that a raised concentration of thyroid-stimulating-hormone alone may not necessarily imply hypothyroidism in patients with chronic adrenocortical insufficiency.[2] Even confirmed hypothyroidism in these patients may not be permanent.


1. Fonseca V, *et al.* Acute adrenal crisis precipitated by thyroxine. *BMJ* 1986; **292:** 1185–6.
2. Davis J, Sheppard M. Acute adrenal crisis precipitated by thyroxine. *BMJ* 1986; **292:** 1595.


**Anaemia.** Four patients with iron deficiency anaemia and primary hypothyroidism developed palpitations and restlessness upon treatment with levothyroxine sodium, necessitating discontinuation of the drug. Upon correction of the anaemia with ferrous sulfate, all were able to tolerate levothyroxine therapy.[1] (For a warning that ferrous sulfate reduces absorption of levothyroxine from the gastrointestinal tract, see under Interactions, below.)


1. Shakir KMM, *et al.* Anemia: a cause of intolerance to thyroxine sodium. *Mayo Clin Proc* 2000; **75:** 189–92.


**Breast feeding.** Minimal amounts of thyroid hormones are distributed into breast milk.[1] There is insufficient thyroid hormone to meet the biological needs of a suckling infant with a nonfunctioning thyroid gland but it has been suggested that levothyroxine in breast milk might mask any hypothyroidism in the suckling newborn.[2] However, the *British National Formulary* considers that the amounts involved are too small to affect tests for neonatal hypothyroidism. The American Academy of Pediatrics noted that there have been no observable effects in breast-fed infants whose mothers were taking levothyroxine and as such considers its use to be usually compatible with breast feeding.[3]


1. Bennett PN, ed. *Drugs and human lactation.* Amsterdam: Elsevier, 1988.
2. Anonymous. Can a woman on thyroxine safely breast-feed her baby? *BMJ* 1977; **2:** 1589.
3. American Academy of Pediatrics. The transfer of drugs and other chemicals into human milk. *Pediatrics* 2001; **108:** 776–89. Correction. *ibid.*; 1029. Also available at: http://aappolicy.aappublications.org/cgi/content/full/pediatrics%3b108/3/776 (accessed 17/05/04)

**Cardiovascular disorders.** There is a complex relationship between the heart and thyroid.[1] Cardiovascular abnormalities may be associated with hypothyroidism as well as with levothyroxine replacement therapy, hence the need for caution.

1. Gammage M, Franklyn J. Hypothyroidism, thyroxine treatment, and the heart. *Heart* 1997; **77:** 189–90.

**Myasthenia.** Thyroid hormones may occasionally precipitate or exacerbate a pre-existing myasthenic syndrome.[1,2]

1. Mastaglia FL. Adverse effects of drugs on muscle. *Drugs* 1982; **24:** 304–21.
2. Lane RJM, Routledge PA. Drug-induced neurological disorders. *Drugs* 1983; **26:** 124–47.

**Pregnancy.** Most authorities consider that thyroid hormones do not readily cross the placenta. Placental transfer has been reported,[1] but in amounts so limited that a mother with physiological concentrations of thyroxine and tri-iodothyronine would not provide normal thyroid hormone concentrations to a fetus with congenital hypothyroidism.[2-4]

1. Vulsma T, *et al.* Maternal-fetal transfer of thyroxine in congenital hypothyroidism due to a total organification defect or thyroid agenesis. *N Engl J Med* 1989; **321:** 13–16.
2. Sack J, *et al.* Maternal-fetal transfer of thyroxine. *N Engl J Med* 1989; **321:** 1549–50.
3. Bachrach LK, Burrow GN. Maternal-fetal transfer of thyroxine. *N Engl J Med* 1989; **321:** 1549.
4. Vulsma T, *et al.* Maternal-fetal transfer of thyroxine. *N Engl J Med* 1989; **321:** 1550.

## Interactions

**Antiarrhythmics.** *Amiodarone*[1] may inhibit the de-iodination of thyroxine to tri-iodothyronine resulting in a decreased concentration of tri-iodothyronine with a concomitant rise in the concentration of inactive reverse tri-iodothyronine.

1. Hershman JM, *et al.* Thyroxine and triiodothyronine kinetics in cardiac patients taking amiodarone. *Acta Endocrinol (Copenh)* 1986; **111:** 193–9.

**Antibacterials.** Enzyme induction by *rifampicin*[1] enhances thyroid hormone metabolism resulting in reduced serum concentrations of thyroid hormones.

1. Ohnhaus EE, Studer H. A link between liver microsomal enzyme activity and thyroid hormone metabolism in man. *Br J Clin Pharmacol* 1983; **15:** 71–6.

**Anticoagulants.** Thyroid hormones enhance the effects of *oral anticoagulants* (see under the interactions of Warfarin, p.1027). Patients on anticoagulant therapy therefore require careful monitoring when treatment with thyroid drugs is initiated or altered as the oral anticoagulant dose may need to be adjusted.

**Antidepressants.** Some drugs such as *lithium* act directly on the thyroid gland and inhibit the release of thyroid hormones leading to clinical hypothyroidism.[1]

The effects of levothyroxine in hypothyroid patients may be decreased by concomitant use of *sertraline*, and the dose of levothyroxine may need to be increased.[2]

For the effects of thyroid hormones on *tricyclic antidepressants* see under Amitriptyline, p.285.

1. Ramsay I. Drugs and non-thyroid induced changes in thyroid function tests. *Postgrad Med J* 1985; **61:** 375–7.
2. McCowen KC, *et al.* Elevated serum thyrotropin in thyroxine-treated patients with hypothyroidism given sertraline. *N Engl J Med* 1997; **337:** 1010–11.

**Antidiabetics.** As thyroid status influences metabolic activity and most body systems, correction of hypothyroidism may affect other disease states and dosage of any drug treatment. In hypothyroid diabetics for instance, the initiation of thyroid replacement therapy may increase their *insulin* or *oral hypoglycaemic* requirements.[1]

1. Refetoff S. Thyroid hormone therapy. *Med Clin North Am* 1975; **59:** 1147–62.

**Antiepileptics.** Enzyme induction by drugs such as *carbamazepine*,[1,2] *phenytoin*,[2,3] or *barbiturates*[4] enhances thyroid hormone metabolism resulting in reduced serum concentrations of thyroid hormones. Therefore, patients on thyroid replacement therapy may require an increase in their dose of thyroid hormone if these drugs are given concurrently[5] and a decrease if the enzyme-inducing drug is withdrawn.[6] *Phenytoin*,[3] and *carbamazepine* may reduce protein binding by displacing the thyroid hormones from their plasma-binding sites. As thyroid hormones are highly protein bound, changes in binding might be expected to influence requirements in thyroid replacement therapy, but in practice there is little clinical evidence of any problems except with thyroid-function testing.

1. Connell JMC, *et al.* Changes in circulating thyroid hormones during short-term hepatic enzyme induction with carbamazepine. *Eur J Clin Pharmacol* 1984; **26:** 453–6.
2. Larkin JG, *et al.* Thyroid hormone concentrations in epileptic patients. *Eur J Clin Pharmacol* 1989; **36:** 213–6.
3. Franklyn JA, *et al.* Measurement of free thyroid hormones in patients on long-term phenytoin therapy. *Eur J Clin Pharmacol* 1984; **26:** 633–4.
4. Ohnhaus EE, Studer H. A link between liver microsomal enzyme activity and thyroid hormone metabolism in man. *Br J Clin Pharmacol* 1983; **15:** 71–6.
5. Blackshear JL, *et al.* Thyroxine replacement requirements in hypothyroid patients receiving phenytoin. *Ann Intern Med* 1983; **99:** 341–2.
6. Hoffbrand BI. Barbiturate/thyroid-hormone interaction. *Lancet* 1979; **ii:** 903–4.

**Antimalarials.** Increased thyroid-stimulating hormone concentration has been noted following the use of combined *chloroquine* and *proguanil* chemoprophylaxis for malaria in a patient stabilised on levothyroxine.[1] Induction of liver enzymes by chloroquine resulting in increased metabolism of levothyroxine was suggested as the mechanism.

1. Munera Y, *et al.* Interaction of thyroxine sodium with antimalarial drugs. *BMJ* 1997; **314:** 1593.

**Antivirals.** There has been an isolated report of an interaction between *ritonavir* and levothyroxine, resulting in an increased requirement for levothyroxine supplementation.[1]

1. Tseng A, Fletcher D. Interaction between ritonavir and levothyroxine. *AIDS* 1998; **12:** 2235–6.

**Beta blockers.** Studies have indicated that plasma concentrations of *propranolol* are reduced in hyperthyroidism compared with the euthyroid state, probably due to increased clearance[1-4] and hypothyroid patients receiving chronic propranolol therapy have had a reduction in plasma-propranolol concentrations when given levothyroxine treatment.[2]

*Propranolol*[5,6] may inhibit the de-iodination of thyroxine to tri-iodothyronine resulting in a decreased concentration of tri-iodothyronine with a concomitant rise in the concentration of inactive reverse tri-iodothyronine.

1. Feely J, *et al.* Increased clearance of propranolol in thyrotoxicosis. *Ann Intern Med* 1981; **94:** 472–4.
2. Feely J, *et al.* Plasma propranolol steady state concentrations in thyroid disorders. *Eur J Clin Pharmacol* 1981; **19:** 329–33.
3. Aro A, *et al.* Pharmacokinetics of propranolol and sotalol in hyperthyroidism. *Eur J Clin Pharmacol* 1982; **21:** 373–7.
4. Hallengren B, *et al.* Influence of hyperthyroidism on the kinetics of methimazole, propranolol, metoprolol, and atenolol. *Eur J Clin Pharmacol* 1982; **21:** 379–84.
5. Chambers JB, *et al.* The effects of propranolol on thyroxine metabolism and triiodothyronines production in man. *J Clin Pharmacol* 1982; **22:** 110–16.
6. Wilkins MR, *et al.* Effect of propranolol on thyroid homeostasis of healthy volunteers. *Postgrad Med J* 1985; **61:** 391–4.

**Cardiac glycosides.** Serum-digoxin concentrations appear to be lower in hyperthyroidism and higher in hypothyroidism[1] which may contribute in part to the observed insensitivity of hyperthyroid patients to *digoxin* therapy[2] although other mechanisms have been proposed.[3]

1. Croxson MS, Ibbertson HK. Serum digoxin in patients with thyroid disease. *BMJ* 1975; **3:** 566–8.
2. Huffman DH, *et al.* Digoxin in hyperthyroidism. *Clin Pharmacol Ther* 1977; **22:** 533–8.
3. Lawrence JR, *et al.* Digoxin kinetics in patients with thyroid dysfunction. *Clin Pharmacol Ther* 1977; **22:** 7–13.

**Gastrointestinal drugs.** *Sucralfate* reduces absorption of levothyroxine from the gastrointestinal tract[1,2] as does *aluminium hydroxide*,[3] and *calcium carbonate*.[4,5]

1. Sherman SI, *et al.* Sucralfate causes malabsorption of L-thyroxine. *Am J Med* 1994; **96:** 531–5.
2. Campbell JA, *et al.* Sucralfate and the absorption of L-thyroxine. *Ann Intern Med* 1994; **121:** 152.
3. Liel Y, *et al.* Nonspecific intestinal adsorption of levothyroxine by aluminium hydroxide. *Am J Med* 1994; **97:** 363–5.
4. Schneyer CR. Calcium carbonate and reduction of levothyroxine efficacy. *JAMA* 1998; **279:** 750.
5. Singh N, *et al.* Effect of calcium carbonate on the absorption of levothyroxine. *JAMA* 2000; **283:** 2822–5.

**General anaesthetics.** Severe hypertension and tachycardia have been reported[1] when *ketamine* was used in patients taking levothyroxine.

1. Kaplan JA, Cooperman LH. Alarming reactions to ketamine in patients taking thyroid medication-treatment with propranolol. *Anesthesiology* 1971; **35:** 229–30.

**Ion-exchange resins.** *Colestyramine* significantly reduces the absorption of ingested levothyroxine by binding with thyroid hormones in the gastrointestinal tract. The malabsorption of levothyroxine is minimised by allowing an interval of 4 to 5 hours to elapse between the ingestion of the two drugs.[1] A similar effect has been observed with *sodium polystyrene sulfonate*.[2]

1. Northcutt RC, *et al.* The influence of cholestyramine on thyroxine absorption. *JAMA* 1969; **208:** 1857–61.
2. McLean M, *et al.* Cation-exchange resin and inhibition of intestinal absorption of thyroxine. *Lancet* 1993; **341:** 1286.

**Iron salts.** *Ferrous sulfate* reduces absorption of levothyroxine from the gastrointestinal tract.[1]

1. Campbell NRC, *et al.* Ferrous sulfate reduces thyroxine efficacy in patients with hypothyroidism. *Ann Intern Med* 1992; **117:** 1010–13.

**Lipid regulating drugs.** Both decreased efficacy[1] and increased efficacy[2] of levothyroxine have been reported in individual patients given *lovastatin*.

1. Demke DM. Drug interaction between thyroxine and lovastatin. *N Engl J Med* 1989; **321:** 1341–2.
2. Gormley GJ, Tobert JA. Drug interaction between thyroxine and lovastatin. *N Engl J Med* 1989; **321:** 1342.

**NSAIDs.** Falsely low total plasma concentrations of levothyroxine have reportedly been observed during concurrent treatment with some anti-inflammatory drugs.

**Sex hormones.** *Oestrogen* therapy increases serum concentrations of thyroxine-binding globulin, thus increasing the amount of bound thyroxine. Normal thyroid function stimulates thyroxine synthesis to compensate for this effect and maintain normal free-thyroxine serum concentrations. In hypothyroidism, however, patients treated with exogenous levothyroxine who receive oestrogens, as in oral contraceptives or HRT,[1] may require an increase in levothyroxine dose. In contrast, *androgens* reduce the concentration of the binding globulin, which has resulted in clinical hyperthyroidism when given to postmenopausal women maintained on levothyroxine replacement therapy.[2]

1. Arafah BM. Increased need for thyroxine in women with hypothyroidism during estrogen therapy. *N Engl J Med* 2001; **344:** 1743–9.
2. Arafah BM. Decreased levothyroxine requirement in women with hypothyroidism during androgen therapy for breast cancer. *Ann Intern Med* 1994; **121:** 247–51.

**Sympathomimetics.** Thyroid drugs increase metabolic demands and should therefore be used with caution with other drugs known to influence cardiac function, such as the *sympathomimetics*, as they may enhance this effect. In addition, thyroid hormones may increase receptor sensitivity to catecholamines.

## Pharmacokinetics

Levothyroxine is variably absorbed from the gastrointestinal tract after oral doses. Fasting increases absorption. Once in the circulation, levothyroxine is extensively protein bound, principally to thyroxine-binding globulin (TBG) but also to a lesser extent to thyroxine-binding pre-albumin (TBPA) or to albumin. Levothyroxine has a plasma half-life of about 6 to 7 days in euthyroid subjects; the half-life is prolonged in hypothyroidism and reduced in hyperthyroidism.

Levothyroxine is primarily metabolised in the liver and kidney to tri-iodothyronine (liothyronine) and, about 40%, to inactive reverse triiodothyronine (reverse $T_3$) both of which undergo further deiodination to inactive metabolites. Further metabolites result from the deamination and decarboxylation of levothyroxine to tetrac.

Levothyroxine is reported to undergo enterohepatic recycling and excretion in the faeces.

The distribution of thyroid hormones into breast milk and across the placenta is discussed under Breast Feeding and Pregnancy (above).

## Uses and Administration

Levothyroxine is a thyroid hormone (see p.1594 for a description of the endogenous hormones) used as replacement therapy in the treatment of hypothyroidism (p.1595). It is given in conditions such as diffuse non-toxic goitre (see Goitre and Thyroid Nodules, p.1594) and Hashimoto's thyroiditis (see Hypothyroidism, p.1595) to suppress the secretion of thyroid-stimulating hormone (TSH) and hence prevent or reverse enlargement of the thyroid gland. Levothyroxine is also used to suppress TSH production in the treatment of thyroid carcinoma (p.523) and as a diagnostic agent for the differential diagnosis of hyperthyroidism. It is given with antithyroid drugs in the blocking-replacement regimen for the management of hyperthyroidism (p.1594).

The peak therapeutic effect of regular oral levothyroxine may not be achieved for several weeks and there is a slow response to changes in dosage. Similarly, effects may persist for several weeks after withdrawal. Levothyroxine is given as the sodium salt in a single daily dose. Its absorption can be irregular and it is probably best taken on an empty stomach, usually before breakfast.

The dose of levothyroxine sodium for the treatment of any thyroid disorder should be individualised on the basis of clinical response and biochemical tests and should be monitored regularly.

In hypothyroidism an initial adult dose of 50 to 100 micrograms of levothyroxine sodium daily by mouth may be increased by 25 to 50 micrograms at intervals of about 4 weeks until the thyroid deficiency is corrected and a maintenance dose is established. The adult maintenance dose is usually between 100 and 200 micrograms daily. In elderly patients, in those with cardiovascular disorders, or in those with severe hypothyroidism of long standing, treatment should be introduced more gradually: an initial dose of 12.5 to 50 micrograms daily increased by increments of 12.5 to 25 micrograms at intervals of about 4 weeks may be appropriate.

In children, individualisation of dosage and monitoring of treatment is especially important. One recommended regimen for the treatment of congenital hypothyroidism is 10 to 15 micrograms/kg daily in neonates, adjusted as necessary. Another regimen suggests an initial dose of 5 to 10 micrograms/kg daily in children up to 1 month of age (or 5 micrograms/kg in children over 1 month), adjusted in steps of 25 micrograms every 2 to 4 weeks until mild toxic symptoms appear, at which time the dosage is slightly reduced. For juvenile myxoedema, children over 1 year of age may be given 2.5 to 5 micrograms/kg daily initially.

Levothyroxine sodium may be given by intravenous injection. It has also been given intramuscularly. In myxoedema (hypothyroid) coma doses of 200 to 500 micrograms by intravenous injection may be given initially. A further dose of 100 to 300 micrograms is given on the second day if no improvement is evident, and followed by daily supplements of about 100 to 200 micrograms until the patient is euthyroid and can tolerate administration by mouth.

◊ General references.

1. Mandel SJ, *et al.* Levothyroxine therapy in patients with thyroid disease. *Ann Intern Med* 1993; **119:** 492–502.
2. Toft AD. Thyroxine therapy. *N Engl J Med* 1994; **331:** 174–80. Correction. *ibid.*; 1035.

**Administration.** There has been controversy over the bioequivalence or otherwise of different brands of levothyroxine. Most studies and reports have come from the USA and results may have depended to some extent on the particular brands compared. Formulations may also have changed which makes comparison of results difficult. One study[1] concluded that 2 generic levothyroxine products were bioequivalent and interchangeable with 2 branded products.

1. Dong BJ, *et al.* Bioequivalence of generic and brand-name levothyroxine products in the treatment of hypothyroidism. *JAMA* 1997; **277:** 1205–13.

**Cardiomyopathies.** Management of dilated cardiomyopathy (p.818) usually involves conventional therapy for heart failure, but a small study has reported benefit from short-term administration of levothyroxine.[1] Levothyroxine administration was well tolerated but thyroid-stimulating hormone levels were reduced and this might limit long-term therapy with levothyroxine.

1. Moruzzi P, *et al.* Medium-term effectiveness of L-thyroxine treatment in idiopathic dilated cardiomyopathy. *Am J Med* 1996; **101:** 461–7.

**Depression.** While thyroid hormones may increase the activity of tricyclic antidepressants (see Thyroid Hormones, under Interactions of Amitriptyline, p.285), the benefits in the augmentation treatment of refractory depression (p.279) are debatable. A meta-analysis[1] of 8 studies involving 292 patients treated with liothyronine in addition to tricyclic antidepressants indicated that such therapy was effective in a subgroup of cases but that the small number of patients studied made additional placebo-controlled data desirable. It was also noted that trends in the treatment of depression favoured drugs other than tricyclics, so that future trials with liothyronine may need to investigate combination treatment with SSRIs.

1. Aronson R, *et al.* Triiodothyronine augmentation in the treatment of refractory depression: a meta-analysis. *Arch Gen Psychiatry* 1996; **53:** 842–8.

**Obesity.** Thyroid drugs have been tried in the treatment of obesity (p.1583) in euthyroid patients, but they produce only temporary weight loss, mainly of lean body-mass, and can produce serious adverse effects, especially cardiac complications.[1] Hypothyroidism has also been reported[2] when these drugs were withdrawn from previously euthyroid patients being treated for simple obesity. Levothyroxine appears to have been abused by some athletes to promote weight loss.[3]

1. Rivlin RS. Therapy of obesity with hormones. *N Engl J Med* 1975; **292:** 26–9.
2. Dornhorst A, *et al.* Possible iatrogenic hypothyroidism. *Lancet* 1981; **i:** 52.
3. MacAuley D. Drugs in sport. *BMJ* 1996; **313:** 211–15.

**Urticaria.** There is some suggestion that chronic urticaria (p.1138) may be associated with thyroid autoimmunity and that treatment with thyroid hormones may result in clinical remission.[1] In one study, a nine-year-old boy was successfully treated for chronic urticaria with levothyroxine therapy at doses of 50 to 100 micrograms daily.[2] The authors advised screening for thyroid function and anti-thyroid microsomal antibodies in cases of chronic urticaria as these patients may benefit from thyroid hormone therapy.

1. Rumbyrt JS, *et al.* Resolution of chronic urticaria in patients with thyroid autoimmunity. *J Allergy Clin Immunol* 1995; **96:** 901–5.
2. Dreyfus DH, *et al.* Steroid-resistant chronic urticaria associated with anti-thyroid microsomal antibodies in a nine-year-old boy. *J Pediatr* 1996; **128:** 576–8.

## Preparations

***BP 2003:*** Levothyroxine Tablets;
***USP 27:*** Levothyroxine Sodium Tablets; Liotrix Tablets.

**Proprietary Preparations** (details are given in Part 3)
***Arg.:*** Euthyrox; T4; ***Austral.:*** Eutroxsig; Oroxine; ***Austria:*** Euthyrox†; Thyrex; ***Belg.:*** Elthyrone; Euthyrox; Thyrax; ***Braz.:*** Euthyrox; Puran T4; Synthroid; Tetroid; ***Canad.:*** Eltroxin; Levo-T†; Levotec†; Synthroid; ***Chile:*** Eutirox; ***Denm.:*** Eltroxin; ***Fr.:*** Levothyrox; ***Ger.:*** Berlthyrox; Eferox; Euthyrox; Thevier; ***Gr.:*** T4; Thyro-4; Thyrohormone; ***Hong Kong:*** Eltroxin; ***India:*** Eltroxin; ***Irl.:*** Eltroxin; ***Israel:*** Eltroxin; ***Ital.:*** Eutirox; Tiracrin; Tirosint; ***Jpn:*** Thyradin-S; ***Malaysia:*** Oroxine; ***Mex.:*** Abutiroi; Dal-troid; Eutirox; Sintrocid; Tiroidine; ***Neth.:*** Eltroxin; Euthyrox; Thyrax; ***Norw.:*** Levaxin; ***NZ:*** Eltroxin; ***Port.:*** Letequatro; Letter; Thyrax; ***S.Afr.:*** Eltroxin; ***Singapore:*** Eltroxin; Euthyrox; Oroxine; ***Spain:*** Dexnon; Levothroid; Thyrax†; ***Swed.:*** Levaxin; ***Switz.:*** Eltroxine; Euthyrox; ***Thai.:*** Eltroxin; Pondtroxin; Thyrosit; ***UK:*** Eltroxin; ***USA:*** Eltroxin†; Levo-T†; Levothroid; Levoxyl; Novothyrox; Synthroid; Unithroid.

**Multi-ingredient:** ***Arg.:*** Eutroid; Levotrin; ***Austria:*** Combithyrex; Jodthyrox; Novothyral; Prothyrid; ***Belg.:*** Novothyral; ***Braz.:*** Levotiroxina†; Tyroplus; ***Chile:*** Novothyral; ***Fr.:*** Euthyral; ***Ger.:*** Jodthyrox; Novothyral; Prothyrid; Thyreocomb N; Thyreotom; Thyronajod; ***Ital.:*** Dermocinetic; Somatoline; Tiroide Amsa; ***Mex.:*** Cynoplus; Novotiral; Proloid S; ***S.Afr.:*** Diotroxin; ***Switz.:*** Novothyral; ***USA:*** Thyrolar.

---

# Liothyronine Sodium *(BANM, rINNM)*

Liothyroninum Natricum; Liotironina sódica; Sodium Liothyronine; L-Tri-iodothyronine Sodium; 3,5,3′-Tri-iodo-L-thyronine Sodium. Sodium 4-*O*-(4-hydroxy-3-iodophenyl)-3,5-di-iodo-L-tyrosine.

$C_{15}H_{11}I_3NNaO_4$ = 673.0.
*CAS — 6893-02-3 (liothyronine); 55-06-1 (liothyronine sodium); 8065-29-0 (liotrix).*
*ATC — H03AA02.*

NOTE. The abbreviation $T_3$ is often used for endogenous tri-iodothyronine in medical and biochemical reports. Liotrix is *USAN* for a mixture of liothyronine sodium with levothyroxine sodium.

**Pharmacopoeias.** In *Eur.* (see p.vi), *Jpn, Pol.,* and *US.*
**Ph. Eur. 5.0** (Liothyronine Sodium). A white or slightly coloured powder. Practically insoluble in water; slightly soluble in alcohol. It dissolves in dilute solutions of alkali hydroxides. Store at 2° to 8° in airtight containers. Protect from light.
**USP 27** (Liothyronine Sodium). A light tan, odourless, crystalline powder. Very slightly soluble in water; slightly soluble in alcohol; practically insoluble in most other organic solvents. Store in airtight containers.

## Adverse Effects, Treatment, and Precautions

As for Levothyroxine Sodium, p.1600.

## Interactions

As for Levothyroxine Sodium, p.1601.

## Pharmacokinetics

Liothyronine is readily and almost completely absorbed from the gastrointestinal tract following oral administration. Once in the circulation, liothyronine binds principally to thyroxine-binding globulin (TBG), although less strongly than levothyroxine; some is also bound to thyroxine-binding pre-albumin (TBPA) or to albumin. Liothyronine has a plasma half-life in euthyroidism of about 1 to 2 days; the half-life is prolonged in hypothyroidism and reduced in hyperthyroidism.

Liothyronine is metabolised by deiodination to inactive di-iodothyronine and mono-iodothyronine. Iodine released by deiodination is largely reused within the thyroid cells. Further metabolites result from deamination and decarboxylation to tiratricol (triac).

## Uses and Administration

Liothyronine is a thyroid hormone (see p.1594). It is used in the treatment of hypothyroidism (p.1595), and is believed to be more active than levothyroxine (p.1601). The onset of action of liothyronine is rapid, developing within a few hours of administration, and therefore it tends to be used in circumstances where this, and its short duration of action, are useful, particularly in hypothyroid (myxoedema) coma.

With regular dosing the peak therapeutic effect is usually achieved by 3 days; on withdrawal its effects may persist for 1 to 3 days.

The dose of liothyronine should be individualised on the basis of clinical response and biochemical tests and should be monitored regularly. Although liothyronine is administered as the sodium salt, doses can be expressed in terms of liothyronine sodium or liothyronine; the doses below are in terms of liothyronine sodium. Liothyronine sodium 10.3 micrograms is approximately equivalent to 10 micrograms of liothyronine. Liothyronine sodium 20 to 25 micrograms is generally considered to be approximately equivalent in activity to levothyroxine sodium 100 micrograms.

In **hypothyroidism** a usual initial adult dose is 5 to 25 micrograms daily by mouth increased gradually to a maintenance dose of 60 to 75 micrograms daily in 2 to 3 divided doses, although up to 100 micrograms daily may be required in some patients. In elderly patients, in those with cardiovascular disorders, or in those with severe long-standing hypothyroidism, treatment should be introduced with doses at the low end of the range, with smaller increments, and longer intervals between increases, as necessary.

In **myxoedema coma** liothyronine sodium may be given intravenously in a dose of 5 to 20 micrograms by slow intravenous injection, repeated as necessary, usually at intervals of 12 hours; the minimum interval between doses is 4 hours. An alternative regimen advocates an initial dose of 50 micrograms intravenously followed by further injections of 25 micrograms every 8 hours until improvement occurs; the dosage may then be reduced to 25 micrograms intravenously twice daily.

Liothyronine has also been given in the **diagnosis** of hyperthyroidism in adults. Failure to suppress the uptake of radio-iodine after several days of receiving liothyronine sodium suggests a diagnosis of hyperthyroidism.

Liothyronine hydrochloride has also been used.

## Preparations

***BP 2003:*** Liothyronine Tablets;
***USP 27:*** Liothyronine Sodium Tablets; Liotrix Tablets.

**Proprietary Preparations** (details are given in Part 3)
***Austral.:*** Tertroxin; ***Belg.:*** Cytomel†; ***Braz.:*** Cynomel; ***Canad.:*** Cytomel; ***Fr.:*** Cynomel; ***Ger.:*** Thybon; Thyrotardin N; ***Gr.:*** T3; ***Ital.:*** Dispon; Ti-Tre; ***Mex.:*** Cynomel; Triyodisan†; Triyotex; ***Neth.:*** Cytomel; ***NZ:*** Tertroxin; ***Port.:*** Neo-Tiroimade; ***S.Afr.:*** Tertroxin; ***Thai.:*** Tertroxin; ***UK:*** Tertroxin; Triiodothyronine Injection; ***USA:*** Cytomel; Triostat.

**Multi-ingredient:** ***Arg.:*** Eutroid; Levotrin; Tresite F; ***Austria:*** Combithyrex; Novothyral; Prothyrid; ***Belg.:*** Novothyral; ***Braz.:*** Levotiroxina†; Tyroplus; ***Chile:*** Novothyral; ***Fr.:*** Euthyral; ***Ger.:*** AntiFocal N; NeyNormin N (Revitorgan-Dilutionen N Nr 65); NeyTumorin N (Revitorgan-Dilutionen N Nr 66); Novothyral; Prothyrid; Thyreotom; ***Ital.:*** Tiroide Amsa; ***Mex.:*** Cynoplus; Novotiral; Proloid S; ***S.Afr.:*** Diotroxin; ***Switz.:*** Novothyral; ***USA:*** Thyrolar.

---

# Methylthiouracil *(rINN)*

Metiltiouracilo. 2,3-Dihydro-2-thioxo-6-methylpyrimidin-4(1*H*)-one; 2-Mercapto-6-methylpyrimidin-4-ol; 6-Methyl-2-thiouracil.

$C_5H_6N_2OS$ = 142.2.
*CAS — 56-04-2.*
*ATC — H03BA01.*

## Profile

Methylthiouracil is a thiourea antithyroid drug that has been used in the treatment of hyperthyroidism.

---

# Potassium Perchlorate

Kalii Perchloras; Perclorato potásico.

$KClO_4$ = 138.5.
*CAS — 7778-74-7.*
*ATC — H03BC01.*

**Pharmacopoeias.** In *Eur.* (see p.vi) and *US.*
**Ph. Eur. 5.0** (Potassium Perchlorate). A white crystalline powder or colourless crystals. Sparingly soluble in water; practically insoluble in alcohol.
**USP 27** (Potassium Perchlorate). pH of a 0.1M solution in water is between 5.0 and 6.5.

**Handling.** Potassium perchlorate has been used for the illicit preparation of explosives or fireworks; care is required with its supply. Great caution should be taken in handling potassium perchlorate in solution or in the dry state as explosions may occur if it is brought into contact with organic or other readily oxidisable substances.

## Adverse Effects

Fever and rashes have occurred after use of potassium perchlorate. Some patients may experience nausea and vomiting. Potassium perchlorate seldom produces adverse effects when given as a single dose for diagnostic purposes. Prolonged use as an antithyroid drug has been associated with serious dose-related adverse effects. Aplastic anaemia (with some fatalities), agranulocytosis, leucopenia, pancytopenia, and the nephrotic syndrome have been reported. Excessive doses may cause hypothyroidism and goitre.

**Effects on the blood.** There have been reports of fatal aplastic anaemia[1,2] and of leucopenia and agranulocytosis[1] associated with the use of potassium perchlorate for the treatment of hyperthyroidism. A review[3] in 1998 noted that despite an increase in perchlorate use in recent years there did not appear to have been any further cases of aplastic anaemia since the 1960s.


1. Anonymous. Potassium perchlorate and aplastic anaemia. *BMJ* 1961; **i:** 1520–1.
2. Krevans JR, *et al.* Fatal aplastic anemia following use of potassium perchlorate in thyrotoxicosis. *JAMA* 1962; **181:** 182–4.
3. Wolff J. Perchlorate and the thyroid gland. *Pharmacol Rev* 1998; **50:** 89–105.


## Uses and Administration

Potassium perchlorate reduces the uptake and concentration of iodide, pertechnetate, and other anions by the thyroid, choroid plexus, gastric mucosa, and salivary glands, probably by competitive inhibition of active transport mechanisms.

It is used **diagnostically** as an adjunct to pertechnetate ($^{99m}$Tc) to enhance visualisation of the brain, Meckel's diverticulum, or the placenta by reducing unwanted images of other organs. The usual adult dose is 200 to 400 mg by mouth given 30 to 60 minutes before the administration of sodium pertechnetate ($^{99m}$Tc). For children aged 2 to 12 years, a dose of 200 mg by mouth has been suggested; for children younger than 2 years of age, 100 mg has been given by mouth.

Potassium perchlorate is also used with sodium iodide ($^{131}$I) in the perchlorate discharge test of thyroid function. The release of radio-iodine from the gland following an oral dose of potassium perchlorate indicates a defect in the binding of iodide by the thyroid and thus a defect in thyroid hormone synthesis. The test has also been used to investigate the action of antithyroid drugs.

Potassium perchlorate has been used in the treatment of **hyperthyroidism** (p.1594), but because of its toxicity it has been largely replaced by alternative treatments. However, it may be useful in patients with iodine-induced hyperthyroidism such as that associated with amiodarone therapy, by increasing responsiveness to conventional antithyroid drugs. An adult dose of 600 mg to 1 g daily by mouth in 3 or 4 divided doses is used as initial therapy with maintenance doses of 200 to 500 mg daily in divided doses. The total daily dose should not exceed 1 g.

◊ References.


1. Bartalena L, *et al.* Treatment of amiodarone-induced thyrotoxicosis, a difficult challenge: results of a prospective study. *J Clin Endocrinol Metab* 1996; **81:** 2930–3.
2. Wolff J. Perchlorate and the thyroid gland. *Pharmacol Rev* 1998; **50:** 89–105.
3. Soldin OP, *et al.* Perchlorate clinical pharmacology and human health: a review. *Ther Drug Monit* 2001; **23:** 316–31.


### Preparations

***USP 27:*** Potassium Perchlorate Capsules.

**Proprietary Preparations** (details are given in Part 3)
***Ital.:*** Pertiroid; ***USA:*** Perchloracap.

---

## Prolonium Iodide *(rINN)*

Ioduro de prolonio. *NN*-(2-Hydroxytrimethylene)bis(trimethylammonium) di-iodide.

$C_9H_{24}I_2N_2O$ = 430.1.

*CAS — 123-47-7.*

**Pharmacopoeias.** In *Chin.*

### Profile

Prolonium iodide has been given by injection as a source of iodine (p.1598) as part of the treatment of thyroid storm and for the pre-operative management of hyperthyroidism.

---

# Propylthiouracil *(BAN, rINN)*

Propiltiouracilo; Propylthiouracilum. 2,3-Dihydro-6-propyl-2-thioxopyrimidin-4(1*H*)-one; 2-Mercapto-6-propylpyrimidin-4-ol; 6-Propyl-2-thiouracil.

$C_7H_{10}N_2OS$ = 170.2.

*CAS — 51-52-5.*

*ATC — H03BA02.*

**Pharmacopoeias.** In *Chin., Eur.* (see p.vi), *Int., Jpn,* and *US.*

**Ph. Eur. 5.0** (Propylthiouracil). White or almost white crystals or crystalline powder. Very slightly soluble in water; sparingly soluble in alcohol; dissolves in solutions of alkali hydroxides. Protect from light.

**USP 27** (Propylthiouracil). A white, powdery, crystalline substance. It is starch-like in appearance and to the touch. Slightly soluble in water, in chloroform, and in ether; sparingly soluble in alcohol; soluble in ammonium hydroxide and in alkali hydroxides. Protect from light.

## Adverse Effects and Precautions

As for Carbimazole, p.1596.

Propylthiouracil has been associated with greater hepatotoxicity than other thiourea antithyroid drugs (such as carbimazole or thiamazole). Rarely hepatitis, hepatic necrosis, encephalopathy, and death have occurred; asymptomatic liver damage is more common (see Effects on the Liver, under Carbimazole, p.1597).

Propylthiouracil should be given with care, and in reduced doses, to patients with renal impairment.

**Breast feeding.** Propylthiouracil has been preferred to carbimazole or thiamazole since it enters breast milk less readily, see Breast Feeding, under Carbimazole, p.1596.

## Pharmacokinetics

Propylthiouracil is rapidly absorbed from the gastrointestinal tract with peak plasma concentrations occurring about 1 to 2 hours after oral doses. It is concentrated in the thyroid gland; since its duration of action is more closely related to the intrathyroidal drug concentration than its plasma half-life, prolonged antithyroid activity results from single daily doses. Propylthiouracil is 75 to 80% bound to plasma proteins.

Propylthiouracil has an elimination half-life of about 1 to 2 hours and is metabolised, probably by the liver, and excreted in the urine as unchanged drug (less than 2% of a dose) and metabolites; more than 50% of a dose is excreted as the glucuronic acid conjugate. The elimination half-life may be increased in renal or hepatic impairment.

Propylthiouracil crosses the placenta and is distributed into breast milk.

◊ References.


1. Kampmann JP, Hansen JM. Clinical pharmacokinetics of antithyroid drugs. *Clin Pharmacokinet* 1981; **6:** 401–28.
2. Giles HG, *et al.* Disposition of intravenous propylthiouracil. *J Clin Pharmacol* 1981; **21:** 466–71.
3. Kampmann JP, Hansen JEM. Serum protein binding of propylthiouracil. *Br J Clin Pharmacol* 1983; **16:** 549–52.


## Uses and Administration

Propylthiouracil is a thiourea antithyroid drug that acts by blocking the production of thyroid hormones (see p.1594); it also inhibits the peripheral deiodination of thyroxine to tri-iodothyronine. It is used in the management of hyperthyroidism (p.1594), including the treatment of Graves' disease, preparation of hyperthyroid patients for thyroidectomy, use as an adjunct to radio-iodine therapy, and the treatment of thyroid storm.

Propylthiouracil is given by mouth. Usual initial doses range from 150 to 450 mg daily (the *British National Formulary* recommends 200 to 400 mg daily), although in severe cases initial doses of 600 mg to 1.2 g daily have been used. It has often been given in divided daily doses but once daily administration is also possible. Improvement is usually seen in 1 to 3 weeks and control of symptoms is achieved in 1 to 2 months. When the patient is euthyroid the dose is gradually reduced to a maintenance dose, usually 50 to 150 mg daily. Treatment is usually continued for at least a year, and often for 18 months. A suggested initial dose for children aged 6 to 10 years is 50 to 150 mg daily, and for children over 10 years 150 to 300 mg daily.

Doses should be reduced in renal impairment (below). Doses may also need to be reduced in hepatic impairment.

**Administration in renal impairment.** Dosage of propylthiouracil should be reduced by 25% in mild to moderate renal impairment and by 50% in severe renal impairment.

**Alcoholic liver disease.** Propylthiouracil has been said to reduce hyperoxic liver injury in hypermetabolic *animals* and despite reports of hepatotoxicity, including some fatalities, associated with propylthiouracil (see Effects on the Liver, under Carbimazole, p.1597), it has been investigated in the treatment of patients with alcoholic liver disease. In a 2-year double-blind study[1] the 13% mortality rate in patients receiving propylthiouracil 300 mg daily was significantly lower than the 25% mortality rate in patients receiving placebo. The main effect of propylthiouracil appeared to be on acute alcoholic hepatitis as the difference in mortality rate was greatest during the first 12 weeks. However, Sherlock commented[2] that propylthiouracil had never gained general acceptance for the treatment of alcoholic liver disease.


1. Orrego H, *et al.* Long-term treatment of alcoholic liver disease with propylthiouracil. *N Engl J Med* 1987; **317:** 1421–7.
2. Sherlock S. Alcoholic liver disease. *Lancet* 1995; **345:** 227–9.


**Psoriasis.** Propylthiouracil has been tried orally[1] and topically[2] in a few patients with psoriasis (p.1137). The beneficial effects may be due to its immunomodulatory properties.[3]


1. Elias AN, *et al.* Propylthiouracil in psoriasis: results of an open trial. *J Am Acad Dermatol* 1993; **29:** 78–81.
2. Elias AN, *et al.* A controlled trial of topical propylthiouracil in the treatment of patients with psoriasis. *J Am Acad Dermatol* 1994; **31:** 455–8.
3. Köse K, *et al.* Effect of propylthiouracil on adenosine deaminase activity and thyroid function in patients with psoriasis. *Br J Dermatol* 2001; **144:** 1121–6.


## Preparations

***BP 2003:*** Propylthiouracil Tablets;
***USP 27:*** Propylthiouracil Tablets.

**Proprietary Preparations** (details are given in Part 3)
***Austria:*** Prothiucil; ***Braz.:*** Propil; Propilracil; ***Canad.:*** Propyl-Thyracil; ***Ger.:*** Propycil; Thyreostat II; ***Gr.:*** Prothuril; ***Israel:*** Propylthiocil; ***Port.:*** Propycil; ***Swed.:*** Tiotil; ***Thai.:*** Propacil†; Propyl; Uracil.

---

## Sodium Perchlorate

Perclorato sódico.

$NaClO_4$ = 122.4.

*CAS — 7601-89-0 (anhydrous sodium perchlorate); 7791-07-3 (sodium perchlorate monohydrate).*

**Handling.** Sodium perchlorate has been used for the illicit preparation of explosives or fireworks; care is required with its supply.

### Profile

Sodium perchlorate has actions and uses similar to those of potassium perchlorate (p.1602). A dose of 200 to 400 mg by mouth has been given 30 to 60 minutes before radionuclide brain scanning.

Sodium perchlorate has been used to treat hyperthyroidism (p.1594) in an initial dose of 800 mg to 1 g daily by mouth in divided doses (some countries permit an initial dose of 1.2 to 2 g daily), reduced as required to a maintenance dose of 100 to 400 mg daily. Because of their toxicity the perchlorates have largely been replaced by other antithyroid drugs.

### Preparations

**Proprietary Preparations** (details are given in Part 3)
***Austria:*** Irenat; ***Ger.:*** Irenat.

---

# Thiamazole *(BAN, rINN)*

Mercazolylum; Methimazole; Methylmercaptoimidazole; Thiamazolum; Tiamazol. 1-Methylimidazole-2-thiol.

$C_4H_6N_2S$ = 114.2.

*CAS — 60-56-0.*

*ATC — H03BB02.*

**Pharmacopoeias.** In *Chin., Eur.* (see p.vi), *Jpn, Pol.,* and *US.*

**Ph. Eur. 5.0** (Thiamazole). A white or pale brown, crystalline powder. Freely soluble in water and in dichloromethane; freely soluble or soluble in alcohol.

**USP 27** (Methimazole). A white to pale buff crystalline powder having a faint characteristic odour. Soluble 1 in 5 of water, 1 in 5 of alcohol, 1 in 4.5 of chloroform, and 1 in 125 of ether. Its solutions are practically neutral to litmus. Protect from light.

## Adverse Effects and Precautions

As for Carbimazole, p.1596.

**Breast feeding.** The administration of thiamazole during breast feeding is discussed under Carbimazole, p.1596.

## Pharmacokinetics

The pharmacokinetics of thiamazole can be considered together with those of carbimazole (p.1597) since the latter is rapidly and completely metabolised to thiamazole in the body.

## Uses and Administration

Thiamazole is a thiourea antithyroid drug that acts by blocking the production of thyroid hormones (see p.1594). It is used in the management of hyperthyroidism (p.1594), including the treatment of Graves' disease, the preparation of hyperthyroid patients for thyroidectomy, use as an adjunct to radio-iodine therapy, and the treatment of thyroid storm.

Thiamazole is given by mouth usually in an initial dosage of 15 to 60 mg daily. It has often been given in divided doses but once daily administration is also possible. Improvement is usually seen in 1 to 3 weeks and control of symptoms in 1 to 2 months. When the patient is euthyroid the dose is gradually reduced to a maintenance dose, usually 5 to 15 mg daily. Alternatively, the dose may be continued at the initial level together with supplemental levothyroxine as a blocking-replacement regimen. Either form of maintenance treatment is usually continued for at least a year, and often for 18 months. A recommended initial dose for children is 400 micrograms/kg daily in 3 divided doses; for maintenance this dose may be halved.

**Action.** For reference to the possible immunosuppressant effects of thiourea antithyroid drugs, see under Uses and Administration of Carbimazole, p.1597.

## Preparations

***USP 27:*** Methimazole Tablets.

**Proprietary Preparations** (details are given in Part 3)
***Arg.:*** Danantizol; ***Austria:*** Favistan; ***Belg.:*** Strumazol; ***Braz.:*** Tapazol; ***Canad.:*** Tapazole; ***Chile:*** Tirozol 5/10; ***Denm.:*** Thycapzol; ***Ger.:*** Favistan; Thyrozol; ***Gr.:*** Unimazole; ***Hong Kong:*** Tapazole†; ***Israel:*** Mercaptizol; Tapazole; ***Ital.:*** Tapazole; ***Mex.:*** Tapazol; ***Neth.:*** Strumazol; ***Port.:*** Metibasol; ***Singapore:*** Thyrozol; ***Spain:*** Tirodril; ***Swed.:*** Thacapzol; ***Switz.:*** Tapazole; ***Thai.:*** Tapazole; ***USA:*** Tapazole.

**Multi-ingredient:** ***Ital.:*** Bromazolo.

## Thyroglobulin *(USAN, rINN)*

Tiroglobulina.

*CAS — 9010-34-8.*

### Profile

Thyroglobulin is an extract obtained by the fractionation of porcine thyroid glands, that yields levothyroxine and liothyronine on hydrolysis. It has been used in the treatment of hypothyroidism, but such treatment with mixtures of thyroid hormones or preparations of animal extracts is not recommended.

### Preparations

**Proprietary Preparations** (details are given in Part 3)
***Ital.:*** Tiroide Vister.

## Thyroid

Dry Thyroid; Getrocknete Schilddrüse; NSC-26492; Thyreoidin; Thyroid Extract; Thyroid Gland; Thyroidea; Thyroideum Siccum; Tiroide Secca; Tiroides.

*ATC — H03AA05.*

**Pharmacopoeias.** In *Chin.*, *Jpn*, and *US*.

**USP 27** (Thyroid). It is the cleaned, dried, and powdered thyroid gland, previously deprived of connective tissue and fat, obtained from domesticated animals used for food by humans. On hydrolysis it yields not less than 90% and not more than 110% each of the labelled amounts of levothyroxine and liothyronine calculated on the dried basis. It is free from iodine in inorganic or any form of combination other than that peculiar to the thyroid gland. It may contain a suitable diluent such as glucose, lactose, sodium chloride, starch, or sucrose. A yellowish to buff-coloured amorphous powder, having a slight, characteristic, meat-like odour. Store in airtight containers.

### Profile

Thyroid has been used in the treatment of hypothyroidism, but treatment with mixtures of thyroid hormones or preparations of animal extracts is not recommended.

### Preparations

***USP 27:*** Thyroid Tablets.

**Proprietary Preparations** (details are given in Part 3)
***Ital.:*** Cinetic; ***USA:*** Nature Throid; Thyrar†.

**Multi-ingredient:** ***Braz.:*** Emagrex†; Esbelt†; Esbeltrat†; Macroten†; Magroton†; Normagrin†; Obesidex; Obesifran; ***Ger.:*** AntiFocal; ***India:*** Ebexid; ***Thai.:*** Metharmon-F.

## Tiratricol *(rINN)*

Triac; Triiodothyroacetic Acid. [4-(4-Hydroxy-3-iodophenoxy)-3,5-di-iodophenyl]acetic acid.

$C_{14}H_9I_3O_4$ = 621.9.

*CAS — 51-24-1.*

*ATC — D11AX08; H03AA04.*

NOTE. Tri-ac has also been used as a name for proprietary preparations containing other drugs.

### Profile

Tiratricol, a metabolite of tri-iodothyronine, is reported to be less active than the thyroid hormones but is given by mouth to suppress the secretion of thyroid-stimulating hormone.

**Obesity.** Abnormal thyroid function tests, severe diarrhoea, fatigue, lethargy, and profound weight loss have occurred in patients taking dietary supplements containing tiratricol.[1] The FDA has warned that tiratricol may cause heart attacks and strokes, and has advised consumers not to take these products.[1]

1. Anonymous. Triax®: a harmful product sold on the internet. *WHO Drug Inf* 2000; **14:** 30.

### Preparations

**Proprietary Preparations** (details are given in Part 3)

***Arg.:*** Nulobes; Triacana; ***Braz.:*** Dimagress†; Obelin†; Redulip; Triac; Trimag; ***Chile:*** Triacana; ***Fr.:*** Teatrois; Triacana.

**Multi-ingredient:** ***Arg.:*** Dimagrir Triac.

# Vaccines Immunoglobulins and Antisera

The agents described in this section are immunological agents used for both active immunisation and passive immunisation.

*Active immunisation* is a process of increasing resistance to infection whereby micro-organisms or products of their activity act as antigens and stimulate certain body cells to produce antibodies with a specific protective capacity. It may be a natural process following recovery from an infection, or an artificial process induced by the administration of *vaccines*. It is inevitably a slow process dependent upon the rate at which the antibodies can be produced. Although the terms vaccination and immunisation are often used synonymously and interchangeably, *vaccination* simply refers to the administration of a vaccine whereas *immunisation* implies the development of protective levels of antibodies confirmed usually by serological testing.

*Passive immunisation*, which results in immediate short-term protection, may be achieved by giving the antibodies themselves usually in the form of *antisera* (of animal origin) or *immunoglobulins*.

## Antisera

Antisueros.

### Description

Antisera (immunosera) are sterile preparations containing immunoglobulins obtained from the serum of immunised animals by purification. The term antisera includes antitoxins, which are antibodies that combine with and neutralise specific toxins, and antivenins (antivenoms), which are antitoxins directed against the toxic principle of the venoms of poisonous animals such as certain snakes and arthropods.

Antisera are obtained from healthy animals immunised by injections of the appropriate toxins or toxoids, venins, or suspensions of micro-organisms or other antigens. The specific immunoglobulins may be obtained from the serum by fractional precipitation and enzyme treatment or by other chemical or physical means. A suitable antimicrobial preservative may be added, and is invariably added if the product is issued in multidose containers. The Ph. Eur. 5.0 directs that when antisera contain phenol, the concentration is not more than 0.25%. The antiserum is distributed aseptically into sterile containers, which are sealed so as to exclude micro-organisms. Alternatively they may be supplied as freeze-dried preparations for reconstitution immediately before use.

### Adverse Effects and Precautions

Reactions are liable to occur after the injection of any serum of animal origin. Anaphylaxis (type I hypersensitivity reaction, p.419) may occur, with hypotension, dyspnoea, urticaria, and shock, which requires management as a medical emergency (see p.855).

Serum sickness (type III hypersensitivity reaction, p.419) may occur, frequently 7 to 10 days after the injection of serum of animal origin.

Before injecting serum, information should be obtained whenever possible as to whether previous injections of serum have been received and whether the patient is subject to hypersensitivity disorders. Sensitivity testing should be performed before giving antisera. The patient must be kept under observation after the administration of full doses of antisera. Adrenaline injection and resuscitation facilities should be available.

### Uses and Administration

Antisera have the specific power of neutralising venins or bacterial toxins, or combining with the bacterium, virus, or other antigen used for their preparation. Most antisera in current use are antitoxins or antivenins. The use of antisera to induce passive immunity has declined; immunoglobulins are preferred. Although antisera are defined as being of animal origin (see above), the term antisera has been used in some countries to describe antitoxins of human origin (immunoglobulins).

## Immunoglobulins

Inmunoglobulinas.

### Description

Immunoglobulins are produced by B lymphocytes as part of the humoral response to foreign antigens. Immunoglobulins used in clinical practice are preparations containing antibodies, usually prepared from human plasma or serum, and mainly comprise IgG. Normal immunoglobulin, prepared from material from blood donors, contains several antibodies against infectious diseases prevalent in the general population, whereas specific immunoglobulins contain minimum specified levels of one antibody. Antibodies may also be prepared by genetic engineering techniques.

### Adverse Effects

Local reactions with pain and tenderness at the site of intramuscular injection may follow the administration of immunoglobulins. Hypersensitivity reactions, including, rarely, anaphylactic reactions, have also been reported; such reactions, though, are far less frequent than following the use of antisera of animal origin.

Some immunoglobulins are available as intravenous preparations. Systemic reactions with fever, chills, facial flushing, headache, and nausea may occur after their administration, particularly at high rates of infusion.

### Precautions

Strenuous efforts are made to screen human donor material used in the preparation of immunoglobulins; the transmission of infections, including hepatitis B and HIV, which has been associated with the use of certain blood products (see p.744), does not appear to be a problem with the immunoglobulins currently in use.

IgA, present in some immunoglobulin preparations, may give rise to the production of anti-IgA antibodies in patients with IgA deficiencies, with the consequent risk of anaphylactic reactions. For precautions in such patients, see Hypersensitivity under Adverse Effects and Precautions in Normal Immunoglobulins, p.1628.

### Interactions

Immunoglobulins may interfere with the ability of live vaccines to induce an immune response and a suitable interval should separate their administration (see Vaccines, Interactions, p.1606).

◊ Reviews of possible interactions between immunoglobulins and other drugs.

1. Grabenstein JD. Drug interactions involving immunologic agents. Part I. Vaccine-vaccine, vaccine-immunoglobulin, and vaccine-drug interactions. *DICP Ann Pharmacother* 1990; **24:** 67–81.
2. Grabenstein JD. Drug interactions involving immunologic agents. Part II. Immunodiagnostic and other immunologic drug interactions. *DICP Ann Pharmacother* 1990; **24:** 186–93.

### Uses and Administration

Immunoglobulins are used for passive immunisation, thus conferring immediate protection against some infectious diseases. They are preferred to antisera of animal origin as the incidence of adverse reactions is less.

It is generally important to follow the conferment of passive immunity, which is largely an emergency procedure, by the injection of suitable antigens to produce active immunity.

## Vaccines

Vacunas.

### Description

Vaccines are traditionally preparations of antigenic materials that are given with the object of inducing in the recipient active immunity to specific infecting agents or toxins or antigens produced by them. They may contain living or killed micro-organisms, bacterial toxoids, or antigenic material from particular parts of the infecting organism, which may be derived from the organism or produced by recombinant DNA technology. Vaccines may be single-component vaccines or mixed combined vaccines. Vaccines against some non-infectious diseases are being developed.

**Storage.** Advice concerning the effects of temperature on vaccines.

1. Miller LG, Loomis JH. Advice of manufacturers about effects of temperature on biologicals. *Am J Hosp Pharm* 1985; **42:** 843–8.
2. Longland PW, Rowbotham PC. Stability at room temperature of medicines normally recommended for cold storage. *Pharm J* 1987; **238:** 147–51. Correction. *ibid.*; 220.
3. Anonymous. Stability of vaccines. *Bull WHO* 1990; **68:** 118–20.
4. Casto DT, Brunell PA. Safe handling of vaccines. *Pediatrics* 1991; **87:** 108–12.
5. André FE. Stability of vaccines. *BMJ* 1993; **307:** 939.
6. CDC. Notice to readers: guidelines for maintaining and managing the vaccine cold chain. *MMWR* 2003; **52:** 1023–5.

### Adverse Effects

Injection of a vaccine may be followed by a local reaction, possibly with inflammation and lymphangitis. An induration or sterile abscess may develop at the site of injected vaccine. Fever, headache, and malaise may start a few hours after injection and last for 1 or 2 days. Hypersensitivity reactions may occur and anaphylaxis has been reported rarely.

Further details, if appropriate, of adverse effects of vaccines may be found in the respective individual monographs.

**Long-term effects.** The introduction of routine childhood vaccination has been accompanied by concerns over the safety and possible long term sequelae of some commonly used vaccines. Difficulties have arisen in distinguishing temporal and causal associations and in some cases the perceived dangers of vaccination have impeded uptake. Among the disorders that have been temporally associated with childhood vaccination are neurological disorders, sudden infant death syndrome, type 1 diabetes mellitus, and demyelinating disorders. Information on adverse effects associated with specific vaccines can be found under individual monographs.

Additives or excipients such as the preservative thiomersal (p.1194) have sometimes been alleged to be the cause of adverse reactions.

References.

1. Stratton KR, *et al.* Adverse events associated with childhood vaccines other than pertussis and rubella: summary of a report from the Institute of Medicine. *JAMA* 1994; **271:** 1602–5.
2. Mitchell EA, *et al.* Immunisation and the sudden infant death syndrome. *Arch Dis Child* 1995; **73:** 498–501.
3. Freed GL, *et al.* Safety of vaccinations: Miss America, the media, and public health. *JAMA* 1996; **276:** 1869–72.
4. Centers for Disease Control. Update: vaccine side effects, adverse reactions, contraindications, and precautions: recommendations of the Advisory Committee on Immunization Practices (ACIP). *MMWR* 1996; **45** (RR-12): 1–45.
5. Braun MM, Ellenberg SS. Descriptive epidemiology of adverse events after immunization: reports to the vaccine adverse event reporting system (VAERS), 1991-1994. *J Pediatr* 1997; **131:** 529–35.
6. Jefferson T. Vaccination and its adverse effects: real or perceived. *BMJ* 1998; **317:** 159–60.
7. Ball LK, *et al.* Risky business: challenges in vaccine risk communication. *Pediatrics* 1998; **101:** 453–8.
8. Hiltunen M, *et al.* Immunisation and type 1 diabetes mellitus: is there a link? *Drug Safety* 1999; **20:** 207–12.
9. Institute for Vaccine Safety Diabetes Workshop Panel. Childhood immunizations and type 1 diabetes: summary of an Institute for Vaccine Safety workshop. *Pediatr Infect Dis J* 1999; **18:** 217–22.
10. Hviid A, *et al.* Childhood vaccination and type 1 diabetes. *N Engl J Med* 2004; **350:** 1398–1404.

**Effects on the nervous system.** GUILLAIN-BARRÉ SYNDROME. Guillain-Barré syndrome (see p.1630) has occasionally been associated with vaccination, although causal relationships have been difficult to evaluate. Vaccines implicated include a swine influenza vaccine, diphtheria and tetanus vaccines, some rabies vaccines, and oral poliomyelitis vaccines.[1] A summary[2] of a report by the Institute of Medicine in the USA concluded that there was evidence favouring a causal relation with tetanus or diphtheria and tetanus vaccines (mainly in immunocompromised patients), and with oral poliomyelitis vaccines, but that the evidence was inadequate for measles vaccines, inactivated poliomyelitis vaccines, hepatitis B vaccines, or Haemophilus influenzae vaccines. See individual monographs for further details.

1. Awong IE, *et al.* Drug-associated Guillain-Barré syndrome: a literature review. *Ann Pharmacother* 1996; **30:** 173–80.
2. Stratton KR, *et al.* Adverse events associated with childhood vaccines other than pertussis and rubella: summary of a report from the Institute of Medicine. *JAMA* 1994; **271:** 1602–5.

**Effects on the skin.** Granuloma at the injection site of adsorbed vaccines was reported in 3 patients.[1] Biopsy and microscopy suggested that the granuloma was due to aluminium used as the adsorbent in the vaccines.

1. Fawcett HA, Smith NP. Injection-site granuloma due to aluminum. *Arch Dermatol* 1984; **120:** 1318–22.

## Precautions

Vaccination should be postponed in patients suffering from any acute illness although minor infections without fever or systemic upset are not regarded as contra-indications.

Any history of hypersensitivity, either local or generalised, should be determined before giving a vaccine and measures to treat hypersensitivity reactions up to and including anaphylactic shock (p.855) should be immediately available. Immunisation should not be carried out in individuals who have previously had a severe local or generalised reaction to the vaccine. Reactions which should be regarded as severe include extensive redness and swelling with induration involving large areas of the vaccinated limb, fever of 39.5° or more within 48 hours of vaccination, anaphylaxis, bronchospasm, laryngeal oedema, generalised collapse, prolonged unresponsiveness, prolonged inconsolable or high-pitched screaming (more than 4 hours), convulsions, or encephalopathy within 72 hours. Some vaccines contain small amounts of antibacterials and should not be given to patients with a history of anaphylaxis to them. Caution should be observed in patients with less severe manifestations of antibacterial hypersensitivity. Additionally some vaccines are prepared using hens' eggs and a history of anaphylaxis to the ingestion of eggs is a contra-indication to the use of such vaccines. Similarly, caution should be observed in patients with less severe manifestations of egg hypersensitivity. Asthma, eczema, hay fever, or a history of other allergies, should not be regarded as contra-indications to vaccination.

Before injection of a vaccine any alcohol or disinfectant used for cleansing the skin should be allowed to evaporate otherwise inactivation of live vaccines may occur.

It is recommended that immunisation of infants should not be postponed because of prematurity and that the normal schedules and timings based on the actual birth date should be adhered to.

Certain precautions and contra-indications apply specifically to vaccines containing live attenuated micro-organisms.

Live vaccines should not be given to patients receiving immunosuppressive therapy (see under Interactions, below); to patients suffering from certain malignant conditions such as lymphoma, leukaemia, Hodgkin's disease, or other tumours of the reticuloendothelial system; to patients who have received bone marrow transplants within the previous 6 months (after which time they should have their immune status checked and be immunised appropriately); or to patients with other types of impaired immunological responses, such as hypogammaglobulinaemia.

Live vaccines should not be given during pregnancy because of a theoretical risk to the fetus, unless it is considered there is a significant risk of exposure to infection.

It should be remembered that the immune response to all vaccines (live or inactivated) may be diminished in immunocompromised patients.

**HIV-infected patients.** A review[1] of experience of the safety and efficacy of vaccines in patients infected with HIV found that the theoretical risk of accelerating HIV infection by immunisation was not supported by the limited clinical information available, and the risks may be trivial compared with other natural sources of antigenic stimulation, especially in areas of the world with high levels of endemic infectious diseases. Recommendations for immunisation of HIV-positive individuals vary, particularly with regard to the use of live vaccines[2] (see Immunisation of Immunocompromised Patients, below for UK recommendations). Where an alternative is available an inactivated vaccine may be preferred to a live one (for example, poliomyelitis vaccines), but in general, vaccines recommended for routine immunisation in childhood may be given to HIV-positive individuals. For asymptomatic HIV-positive persons, WHO and UNICEF[3] recommend that routine immunisation should be carried out according to their usual Expanded Programme on Immunization (see below). In addition, an extra dose of measles vaccine should be given at 6 months of age with the standard dose given as soon after 9 months of age as possible. BCG vaccines and yellow fever vaccines (pending further studies) should not be given to those with symptomatic disease. See individual monographs for further information.

1. von Reyn CF, *et al.* Human immunodeficiency virus infection and routine childhood immunisation. *Lancet* 1987; **ii:** 669–72.
2. Centers for Disease Control. Recommendations of the Advisory Committee on Immunization Practices (ACIP): use of vaccines and immune globulins for persons with altered immunocompetence. *Clin Pharm* 1993; **12:** 675–84. Also available at: http://www.cdc.gov/mmwr/PDF/rr/rr4204.pdf (accessed 22/06/04)
3. WHO. *EPI vaccines in HIV-infected individuals: 5 October 2001.* Available at: http://www.who.int/vaccines-diseases/diseases/HIV.shtml (accessed 22/06/04)

**Premature infants.** References.

1. Anonymous. Routine immunisation of preterm infants. *Lancet* 1990; **335:** 23–4.
2. Khalak R, *et al.* Three-year follow-up of vaccine response in extremely preterm infants. *Pediatrics* 1998; **101:** 597–603.
3. Kirmani KI, *et al.* Seven-year follow-up of vaccine response in extremely premature infants. *Pediatrics* 2002; **109:** 498–504.
4. Saari TN, American Academy of Pediatrics Committee on Infectious Diseases. Immunization of preterm and low birth weight infants. *Pediatrics* 2003; **112:** 193–8.

## Interactions

The ability of vaccines to induce an immune response can be influenced by the recent administration of other vaccines or immunoglobulins. Live vaccines should either be given simultaneously (but at different sites) or an interval of at least 3 weeks allowed between administration. Live vaccines should normally be given at least 2 to 3 weeks before or at least 3 months after the administration of immunoglobulin. However, travellers should receive appropriate vaccines regardless of these limitations if time is short.

Patients receiving immunosuppressant therapy, including antineoplastics or therapeutic doses of corticosteroids, may also display a reduced response to vaccines, and there is a possibility of generalised infections with live viral vaccines. In the UK, the Department of Health suggests that immunosuppression may be expected in children receiving the equivalent of 2 mg prednisolone per kg daily for at least 1 week or 1 mg/kg daily for 1 month, and in adults receiving the equivalent of 40 mg daily for more than 1 week. Vaccination should also be postponed for at least 6 months after the end of antineoplastic chemotherapy and for at least 3 months after systemic corticosteroid therapy.

Any agent that is active against the bacterial or viral strain present in the vaccine may interfere with development of a protective immune response but treatment with antibacterials should not be considered to be a contra-indication to immunisation.

◊ References.

1. Grabenstein JD. Drug interactions involving immunologic agents. Part I. Vaccine-vaccine, vaccine-immunoglobulin, and vaccine-drug interactions. *DICP Ann Pharmacother* 1990; **24:** 67–81.
2. Grabenstein JD. Drug interactions involving immunologic agents. Part II. Immunodiagnostic and other immunologic drug interactions. *DICP Ann Pharmacother* 1990; **24:** 186–93.

## Uses and Administration

Vaccines are used for active immunisation as a prophylactic measure against some infectious diseases. They provide partial or complete protection for months or years. For inactivated vaccines, a slight and rather slow antibody response of primarily immunoglobulin M (IgM) (the primary response) is produced after the first or second dose but, when a further dose is given after a suitable interval, a prompt antibody response follows and high concentrations of IgG occur in the blood (the secondary response). Though the antibody concentration may later fall, a further dose of vaccine promptly restores it. For most live vaccines only one dose is required, although 3 doses of live (oral) poliomyelitis vaccines are needed to achieve complete immunisation. Some inactivated vaccines contain an adjuvant such as aluminium hydroxide or aluminium phosphate to enhance the immune response.

Protection against several infectious diseases may be provided in early life by active immunisation and national schedules for childhood immunisation are regularly reviewed and updated. Schedules for routine immunisation of infants and children are generally designed to fit in with routine health checks and landmark events such as school starting and leaving ages. National immunisation schedules should be consulted for full details of local recommendations.

In the **UK**, the following schedule of vaccination and immunisation is recommended:

- at 2, 3, and 4 months of age, doses of a combined diphtheria, tetanus, pertussis (acellular component), poliomyelitis (inactivated), and *Haemophilus influenzae* vaccine (p.1615), together with a meningococcal C conjugate vaccine (p.1626)
- at about 13 months, measles, mumps, and rubella vaccine (p.1625)
- at 3 years 4 months to 5 years, reinforcing doses of a combined diphtheria, tetanus, pertussis (acellular component), and poliomyelitis (inactivated) vaccine (p.1615) and a second dose of measles, mumps, and rubella vaccine
- between 10 and 14 years, BCG vaccine (p.1609) may be given to tuberculin-negative children if it has not been given in infancy
- before leaving school (age 13 to 18 years), reinforcing doses of a low-dose diphtheria, tetanus, and poliomyelitis (inactivated) vaccine (p.1613)
- a further reinforcing dose of an appropriate vaccine containing a tetanus component may be given after 10 years.

The following schedule is recommended in the **USA**:

- at birth or up to 2 months of age, the first dose of hepatitis B vaccine (p.1618)
- at age 1 to 4 months, a second dose of hepatitis B vaccine, not less than 1 month after the first
- at 2 months and 4 months, diphtheria, tetanus, and pertussis vaccine, together with a *Haemophilus influenzae* vaccine, a pneumococcal conjugate vaccine (p.1633), and a poliomyelitis vaccine
- at 6 months, the third dose of *Haemophilus influenzae* vaccine if necessary (depending on the type of vaccine used), a third dose of diphtheria, tetanus, and pertussis vaccine, and a third dose of pneumococcal conjugate vaccine
- at 6 to 18 months, the third doses of hepatitis B and poliomyelitis vaccines; alternatively, hepatitis B vaccine may be given at any time between the ages of 2 to 18 years if any previous doses have not been given
- from 6 months to 18 years, annual influenza vaccine in high-risk patients, although influenza vaccine is also recommended in healthy infants aged 6 months to 2 years
- at 12 to 15 months, a reinforcing dose of *Haemophilus influenzae* vaccine, the first dose of measles, mumps, and rubella vaccine, and the fourth dose of pneumococcal conjugate vaccine; pneumococcal conjugate vaccine may alternatively be given between the ages of 2 and 5 years if any dose has not been given previously
- at 12 to 18 months (or at any subsequent time between the ages of 2 to 18 years if not given previously), a varicella-zoster vaccine (p.1643)
- at 15 to 18 months, the fourth dose of diphtheria, tetanus, and pertussis vaccine
- at 2 to 18 years, pneumococcal polysaccharide vaccine (in addition to previously administered pneumococcal conjugate vaccine) in certain high-risk groups
- at 2 to 18 years, hepatitis A vaccine in selected geographical areas and for certain high-risk groups

- at 4 to 6 years, the fifth dose of diphtheria, tetanus, and pertussis vaccine and the fourth dose of poliomyelitis vaccine; the second dose of measles, mumps, and rubella vaccine may be given at this age (or at age 11 to 18 years if not previously given)
- at age 11 to 12 years, tetanus and low-dose diphtheria toxoids (or at any time between 13 and 18 years if not previously given)
- susceptible children 13 years of age and older should receive 2 doses of varicella vaccine, at least 1 month apart
- subsequently routine booster doses of tetanus and low-dose diphtheria toxoids are recommended every 10 years.

Immunisation schedules for older children and adults are also produced, along with recommendations for vaccination of high-risk groups, including the immunocompromised and the elderly, and of travellers.

In addition to vaccines directed against bacteria and viruses, advances are being made in producing vaccines against fungi, protozoa, and helminths, and for non-infective diseases including cancer and auto-immune disorders.

Development of novel vaccine formulations and delivery methods is continuing, including transdermal and transmucosal systems. Genetic manipulations of foodstuffs is being investigated with the aim of producing edible vaccines.

**Immunisation schedules.** References to routine immunisation schedules in the UK[1] and USA.[2]


1. Department of Health. *Immunisation against infectious disease 1996: "The Green Book"*. Available at: http://www.dh.gov.uk/PublicationsAndStatistics/Publications/PublicationsPolicyAndGuidance/PublicationsPolicyAndGuidanceArticle/fs/en?CONTENT_ID=4072977&chk=87uz6M (accessed 12/08/04)
2. American Academy of Pediatrics Advisory Committee on Immunization Practices. Recommended childhood and adolescent immunization schedule—United States, January-June 2004. *Pediatrics* 2004; **113:** 142–3. Also available at: http://www.cdc.gov/nip/recs/child-schedule.PDF (accessed 22/06/04)


EXPANDED PROGRAMME ON IMMUNIZATION. In 1974 the World Health Assembly adopted a resolution creating the Expanded Programme on Immunization (EPI), the aim of which was to provide immunisation against six target diseases (diphtheria, measles, pertussis, poliomyelitis, tetanus, and tuberculosis) for all children throughout the world by 1990. More recently, EPI has added hepatitis B and yellow fever to the list of target diseases. Although the attention of WHO had been focussed primarily on the developing countries, it was emphasised that the programme was not created exclusively for these countries. Besides WHO, many other organisations, including UNICEF, were involved.

Vaccine uptake was around 70% in 1990 compared with less than 5% in 1974. Although many cases of the target diseases and many deaths have been prevented, vaccine coverage, especially for measles and neonatal tetanus is still low. It is particularly important to immunise children as early in life as possible and not to withhold vaccines from those suffering from minor illness or malnutrition.

A schedule designed to provide protection at the earliest possible age consists of: trivalent oral poliomyelitis vaccine together with BCG vaccine at birth; hepatitis B vaccine at birth, 6 weeks, and 14 weeks (where transmission at birth is likely), or at 6, 10, and 14 weeks (where transmission at birth is less likely); trivalent oral poliomyelitis vaccine together with diphtheria, tetanus, and pertussis vaccine at 6, 10, and 14 weeks of age; and measles vaccine and yellow fever vaccine at 9 months of age. Tetanus vaccine is also administered to all women of child-bearing age. Also included in the programme in parts of the Far East is Japanese encephalitis vaccine.

Some references to the Expanded Programme on Immunization.


1. WHO Global Programme for Vaccines and Immunization: Expanded Programme on Immunization: Module 1: EPI target diseases. Geneva: WHO, 1998. Available at: http://www.who.int/vaccines-documents/DaxTrng/IIP-E/www9556-01.pdf (accessed 22/06/04)
2. WHO. Department of Vaccines and Biologicals: Module 2: EPI vaccines. Geneva: WHO, 2001. Available at: http://www.who.int/vaccines-documents/DaxTrng/IIP-E/www9556-02.pdf (accessed 22/06/04)


**Immunisation of immunocompromised patients.** Immunocompromised and asplenic patients and recipients of bone marrow transplants may require immunisation against opportunistic infections. As discussed under Precautions, above, immune response to vaccination may be impaired, and there is a risk of disseminated infection with live vaccines.

In the UK, the Department of Health recommends that HIV-positive individuals (whether symptomatic or asymptomatic) may receive, where appropriate, live vaccines against measles, mumps, poliomyelitis, and rubella and inactivated vaccines against cholera, diphtheria, *Haemophilus influenzae* type b infections, hepatitis B, pertussis, poliomyelitis, tetanus, and typhoid. Hepatitis A, meningococcal, pneumococcal, and rabies vaccines may also be given. In the UK it is recommended that BCG vaccine should not be given to HIV-positive individuals; WHO have, however, advised immunisation of asymptomatic infants when the risk of tuberculosis is high, but state that BCG vaccine should not be given to symptomatic individuals. There is as yet insufficient data on the safety of yellow fever vaccine in HIV-positive individuals. In the UK administration of yellow fever vaccine to all HIV-positive individuals, whether asymptomatic or not, is not recommended. WHO advise that the vaccine may be administered to asymptomatic persons, but that it should not be given to those with symptomatic infection.

As with other causes of immunosuppression, the efficacy of vaccines may be reduced in HIV-positive individuals. Administration of normal immunoglobulins is suggested for HIV-positive individuals exposed to measles.

For references to the use of vaccines in HIV-infected patients, see under Precautions, above.

**Immunisation for travellers.** A booklet entitled *International Travel and Health* is published annually by WHO. In the 2003 edition the following information regarding certification of vaccination was given.

A *yellow fever* vaccination certificate is now the only one that may be required in international travel. The vaccine used must be approved by WHO and administered at a designated vaccinating centre. Vaccination is strongly recommended for travel outside the urban areas of countries in the yellow fever endemic zone even if these countries have not officially reported the disease and do not require evidence of vaccination on entry. Many countries require a certificate from travellers arriving from infected areas or from countries with infected areas, or who have been in transit through those areas. Some countries require a certificate from all entering travellers including those in transit; although there is no epidemiological justification for this requirement, and it is clearly in excess of the International Health Regulations (WHO recommendations for prevention of the international spread of diseases), travellers may find that it is strictly enforced, particularly for persons going to Asia from Africa or South America. The validity period of international certificates of vaccination against yellow fever is 10 years, beginning 10 days after vaccination.

No country or territory any longer requires a certificate of *cholera* immunisation as the introduction of cholera into any country cannot be prevented by cholera vaccination.

Now that *smallpox* has been eradicated, smallpox vaccination is no longer required by any country.

Apart from vaccinations required by countries for entry to their territory, other vaccinations are either recommended by WHO for general protection against certain diseases or advised in certain circumstances. A vaccination plan should be established, taking into account the traveller's destination, overall state of health and current immune status, the duration and type of travel, and the time available.

Further information for international travellers is also often provided by national authorities. In the UK, the Department of Health issues *Health Advice for Travellers* for the public and *Health Information for Overseas Travel* for the medical profession. In the USA, guidelines are produced by the Centers for Disease Control.

**Infection eradication.** Eradication of infectious diseases has proved more difficult than was hoped, and smallpox is the only disease to have been recognised officially as having been eradicated so far. Eradication is defined as the extinction of the pathogen that causes the infectious disease in question, whereas in elimination the disease disappears but the causative agent remains. Of the target diseases of WHO's Expanded Programme on Immunization (see above), many of the factors necessary for elimination are present for each of the diseases, but some are not. *Measles* is so highly communicable a disease that a vaccine efficacy rate of about 95% is probably not high enough even to eliminate, much less eradicate, the disease. However, immunisation campaigns have produced substantial reductions of infection rate in some countries, although repeated vaccination may be necessary. *Pertussis* is also highly infectious and the vaccine is almost certainly not effective enough. *Tetanus* is not eradicable as the causative organism is ubiquitous. However, elimination of neonatal tetanus may be possible although it depends on protection of more than 80% of infants at birth. This depends not only on maternal vaccination but also on delivery practices. For *poliomyelitis*, countries that are efficient at giving vaccines have proved remarkably successful not only in practically eliminating the disease but also in virtually eradicating the organism. *Tuberculosis* is clearly not eradicable at present and *diphtheria* has many features that suggest it cannot be easily eradicated. Prospects for eradicating *congenital rubella syndrome* are more encouraging and the prospects for elimination or eradication of *mumps* are probably similar to those of rubella.

Other factors that may contribute to the failure of vaccination policies in eradicating disease include: concern, often unfounded, over the safety of vaccines and the perpetuation of invalid contra-indications, the use of inappropriate indicators for the effectiveness of vaccines, the suitability of different types of vaccine and of vaccination schedules, difficulties in vaccine supply, and social and behavioural pressures which reduce compliance with vaccination schedules.

**Vaccine development.** References to vaccine development and research.


1. Gilligan CA, Li Wan Po A. Oral vaccines: design and delivery. *Int J Pharmaceutics* 1991; **75:** 1–24.
2. O'Hagan DT. Oral delivery of vaccines: formulation and clinical pharmacokinetic considerations. *Clin Pharmacokinet* 1992; **22:** 1–10.
3. McDonnell WM, Askari FK. Molecular medicine: DNA vaccines. *N Engl J Med* 1996; **334:** 42–5.
4. McCarthy M. DNA vaccination: a direct line to the immune system. *Lancet* 1996; **348:** 1232.
5. Seder RA, Gurunathan S. DNA vaccines—designer vaccines for the 21st century. *N Engl J Med* 1999; **341:** 277–8.
6. Ellis RW. New technologies for making vaccines. *Vaccine* 1999; **17:** 1596–1604.
7. Lewis PJ, Babiuk LA. DNA vaccines: a review. *Adv Virus Res* 1999; **54:** 129–88.
8. Leitner WW, *et al.* DNA and RNA-based vaccines: principles, progress and prospects. *Vaccine* 2000; **18:** 765–77.
9. Restifo NP, *et al.* The promise of nucleic acid vaccines. *Gene Ther* 2000; **7:** 89–92.
10. Srivastava IK, Liu MA. Gene vaccines. *Ann Intern Med* 2003; **138:** 550–9.


## AIDS Immunoglobulins

HIV Immunoglobulins; Inmunoglobulinas contra el SIDA.

### Profile

AIDS immunoglobulin preparations containing HIV-neutralising antibodies have been prepared from the plasma of asymptomatic HIV-positive subjects. They have been tried for passive immunisation in patients with AIDS or AIDS-related complex.

◊ References.


1. Lambert JS, *et al.* Pediatric AIDS Clinical Trials Group Protocol 185 Pharmacokinetic Study Group. Safety and pharmacokinetics of hyperimmune anti-human immunodeficiency virus (HIV) immunoglobulin administered to HIV-infected pregnant women and their newborns. *J Infect Dis* 1997; **175:** 283–91.
2. Stiehm ER, *et al.* Efficacy of zidovudine and human immunodeficiency virus (HIV) hyperimmune immunoglobulin for reducing perinatal HIV transmission from HIV-infected women with advanced disease: results of Pediatric AIDS Clinical Trials Group protocol 185. *J Infect Dis* 1999; **179:** 567–75.
3. Stiehm ER, *et al.* Use of human immunodeficiency virus (HIV) human hyperimmune immunoglobulin in HIV type 1-infected children (Pediatric AIDS Clinical Trials Group protocol 273). *J Infect Dis* 2000; **181:** 548–54.


## AIDS Vaccines

HIV Vaccines; Vacunas del SIDA.

### Profile

Many prototype vaccines against the acquired immunodeficiency syndrome have been or are being developed but the results of clinical studies have generally been disappointing.

◊ Research into AIDS vaccines has continued into both therapeutic vaccines, aimed at reducing the rate of disease progression in HIV-infected individuals, and prophylactic vaccines, aimed at preventing primary infection. It is now appreciated that both humoral and cell-mediated immune mechanisms play a vital role in controlling HIV infection. Among a number of possible approaches, subunit recombinant viral envelope proteins (gp120 or gp160) have been candidates for both therapeutic and prophylactic vaccines, either as monovalent or polyvalent formulations. They mainly produce a humoral (antibody) response although cell-mediated responses, possibly to other components of the vaccine, have been detected. Clinical studies have not demonstrated a delay in disease progression. Attenuated live viral vaccines are potentially useful for prophylaxis but were initially dismissed because the risk of reversion to virulent strains was felt to be too great. However, they are now being re-examined since they are capable of producing both cell-mediated and humoral immune responses, although the problem of safety remains to be resolved. Another recent development is investigation of nucleic acid vaccines. Free DNA encoding for viral antigens injected into the muscle results in expression of the encoded antigens promoting a humoral and cell-mediated response. Although these vaccines are still at an early stage of development, they may represent a safer alternative to live viral vaccines.

Reviews.


1. Bangham CRM, Phillips RE. What is required of an HIV vaccine? *Lancet* 1997; **350:** 1617–21.
2. Frey SE. HIV vaccines. *Infect Dis Clin North Am* 1999; **13:** 95–112.
3. Rousseau MC, *et al.* Vaccination and HIV: a review of the literature. *Vaccine* 1999; **18:** 825–31.
4. Esparza J, Bhamarapravati N. Accelerating the development and future availability of HIV-1 vaccines: why, when, where, and how? *Lancet* 2000; **355:** 2061–6.
5. Hanke T. Prospect of a prophylactic vaccine for HIV. *Br Med Bull* 2001; **58:** 205–18.
6. Makgoba MW, *et al.* The search for an HIV vaccine. *BMJ* 2002; **324:** 211–13.

7. Weidle PJ, *et al.* HIV/AIDS treatment and HIV vaccines for Africa. *Lancet* 2002; **359:** 2261–7.
8. Tramont EC, Johnston MI. Progress in the development of an HIV vaccine. *Expert Opin Emerg Drugs* 2003; **8:** 37–45.
9. Stevceva L, Strober W. Mucosal HIV vaccines: where are we now? *Curr HIV Res* 2004; **2:** 1–10.

## Anthrax Vaccines

Vacunas del carbunco.

*ATC — J07AC01.*

### Adverse Effects and Precautions

As for vaccines in general, p.1605.

### Interactions

As for vaccines in general, p.1606.

### Uses and Administration

An anthrax vaccine that is an alum precipitate of the antigen found in the sterile filtrate of suitable cultures of the Sterne strain of *Bacillus anthracis* is available in the UK for human use. It is used for active immunisation against anthrax and is recommended for persons working with potentially infected animals or animal products. It is given in 4 doses, each of 0.5 mL by intramuscular injection. The first 3 doses are separated by intervals of 3 weeks and the fourth dose follows after an interval of 6 months. In the USA, where an anthrax vaccine is also available, 6 doses, each of 0.5 mL, are given subcutaneously, the first 3 at intervals of 2 weeks and the last 3 at intervals of 6 months. Reinforcing doses of 0.5 mL are required each year.

◊ References.

1. Centers for Disease Control. Use of anthrax vaccine in the United States: recommendations of the Advisory Committee on Immunization Practices (ACIP). *MMWR* 2000; **49** (RR-15): 1–20.
2. Centers for Disease Control. Use of anthrax vaccine in response to terrorism: supplemental recommendations of the Advisory Committee on Immunization Practices. *MMWR* 2002; **51:** 1024–6.
3. Health Protection Agency. Interim guidelines for action in the event of a deliberate release: anthrax. Available at: http://www.hpa.org.uk/infections/topics_az/deliberate_release_static/anthrax/PDFs/anthrax_guidelines.pdf (accessed 22/06/04)

### Preparations

***USP 27:*** Anthrax Vaccine Adsorbed.

## Anti-D Immunoglobulins

Inmunoglobulinas anti-D.

*ATC — J06BB01.*

**Pharmacopoeias.** Many pharmacopoeias have monographs including *Eur.* (see p.vi) and *US.*

**Ph. Eur. 5.0** (Human Anti-D Immunoglobulin; Immunoglobulinum Humanum Anti-D; Anti-D ($Rh_o$) Immunoglobulin BP 2003). A liquid or freeze-dried preparation containing immunoglobulins, mainly immunoglobulin G (IgG). It is intended for intramuscular administration. It is obtained from plasma from D-negative donors who have been immunised against the D-antigen. It contains specific antibodies against the erythrocyte D-antigen and may also contain small quantities of other blood group antibodies, such as anti-C, anti-E, anti-A, and anti-B. Normal immunoglobulin may be added. The liquid and freeze-dried preparations should be stored, protected from light, in a colourless, glass container. The freeze-dried preparation should be stored in an airtight container.

**Ph. Eur. 5.0** (Human Anti-D Immunoglobulin for Intravenous Administration; Immunoglobulinum Humanum Anti-D ad Usum Intravenosum; Anti-D Immunoglobulin for Intravenous Use BP 2003). A liquid or freeze-dried preparation containing immunoglobulins, mainly immunoglobulin G (IgG). It is obtained from plasma from D-negative donors who have been immunised against the D-antigen. It contains specific antibodies against the erythrocyte D-antigen and may also contain small quantities of other blood group antibodies. Human normal immunoglobulin for intravenous administration may be added. Storage requirements are similar to those for Human Anti-D Immunoglobulin, except that the freeze-dried preparation is stored at a temperature not exceeding 25°.

**USP 27** ($Rh_o$ (D) Immune Globulin). A sterile solution of globulins derived from human plasma containing antibody to the erythrocyte factor $Rh_o$ (D). It contains 10 to 18% of protein, of which not less than 90% is gamma globulin. It contains glycine as a stabilising agent, and a suitable preservative. It should be stored at 2° to 8°.

### Adverse Effects and Precautions

As for immunoglobulins in general, p.1605.

Anti-D immunoglobulin should be administered with caution to rhesus-positive persons for the treatment of blood disorders; the resultant haemolysis may exacerbate pre-existing anaemia.

### Interactions

As for immunoglobulins in general, p.1605.

### Uses and Administration

Anti-D immunoglobulin is used to prevent a rhesus-negative mother actively forming antibodies to fetal rhesus-positive red blood cells that may pass into the maternal circulation during childbirth, abortion, or certain other sensitising events. In subsequent rhesus-positive pregnancies these antibodies could produce haemolytic disease of the newborn (erythroblastosis foetalis). The injection of anti-D immunoglobulin is not effective once the mother has formed anti-D antibodies. Anti-D immunoglobulin is also used in the management of some blood disorders, primarily idiopathic thrombocytopenic purpura.

Anti-D immunoglobulin should always be given to rhesus-negative mothers with no anti-D antibodies in their serum and who have just delivered rhesus-positive infants. It should be given as soon as possible after delivery but may give some protection even if administration is delayed beyond 72 hours. In the UK, the Blood Transfusion Services recommend a dose of 500 units (100 micrograms) by intramuscular injection and this will clear up to 4 mL of fetal red cells. An additional dose may be required depending on the amount of transplacental bleeding as assessed by the Kleihauer test; for bleeds exceeding 4 mL an additional 125 units for each mL of red cells will be required.

For routine antenatal prophylaxis, two doses of at least 500 units of anti-D immunoglobulin should be given at 28 and 34 weeks' gestation. Postnatal prophylaxis is still necessary.

There is also a risk of sensitisation during pregnancy from spontaneous, induced, or threatened abortion, amniocentesis, or external version. Any rhesus-negative woman at risk of transplacental haemorrhage during pregnancy and not known to be sensitised should be given 250 units at up to 20 weeks' gestation and 500 units of anti-D immunoglobulin after 20 weeks' gestation.

Anti-D immunoglobulin is also given to rhesus-negative women of child-bearing potential after the inadvertent transfusion of Rh-incompatible blood, or after receiving blood components containing rhesus-positive red cells or organ donations from rhesus-positive donors. The dose is based on the amount of red blood cells transfused; up to 125 units/mL of transfused cells may be used.

In the USA, doses of anti-D immunoglobulins have traditionally been higher than in the UK; dosage recommendations are based on a standard dose that is capable of suppressing the immune response to 15 mL of incompatible red blood cells. One-sixth of this dose may be used up to 12 weeks of gestation for sensitising episodes.

For idiopathic thrombocytopenic purpura, an initial dose of 250 units/kg (50 micrograms/kg) of anti-D immunoglobulin by intravenous injection is given. Maintenance doses will depend on the clinical response.

**Haemolytic disease of the newborn.** Rhesus (Rh) incompatibility, in particular Rh(D) incompatibility, is a major cause of potentially severe haemolytic disease of the newborn, although other blood group antibodies may also cause the disease.[1] The use of anti-D immunoglobulin to suppress the production of anti-D antibodies in a Rh(D)-negative mother in response to leakage of red blood cells across the placenta from a Rh(D)-positive fetus has produced a major reduction in the incidence of this disorder.[1]

**Prophylaxis.** Postnatal prophylaxis of Rh(D)-negative mothers following the birth of a Rh(D)-positive infant is well established. In 1971, WHO[2] suggested a standard dose of 200 to 300 micrograms but stated that a 100-microgram dose was likely to have a success rate only slightly inferior to that of a 200-microgram dose, thus allowing optimum use to be made of a limited resource. Clinical experience in the UK has confirmed the efficacy of the 100-microgram (500 units) dose and this is the amount officially recommended in the UK in such situations.[3]

Despite the success of anti-D immunoglobulin prophylaxis, sensitisations have continued to occur.[4] There are several possible reasons for this. Failures may occur when an inadequate dose has been administered or when anti-D immunoglobulin prophylaxis is omitted following a sensitising event.[5,6] Postpartum doses may be omitted due to oversight or loss to follow-up. Sensitisation may occur spontaneously during the first pregnancy without any identifiable event causing feto-maternal haemorrhage. Inadequate dosing can be avoided by application of the Kleihauer test to estimate the size of any transplacental haemorrhage.[1]

Significant feto-maternal transfusion may also occur following still-birth, abortion (both therapeutic and spontaneous), threatened abortion, external fetal version, abdominal injury, or amniocentesis.

The efficacy of postpartum prophylaxis is not in question but opinions differ on the need for prophylaxis during pregnancy. It is generally agreed that prophylaxis is necessary following therapeutic terminations at any stage of pregnancy,[7,8] including medical termination utilising mifepristone,[9] but there is no generally accepted policy for other possibly sensitising events. A study of 655 Rh(D)-negative women in Denmark,[10] where antepartum prophylaxis is not common practice, suggested that the sensitisation rate following amniocentesis was no higher than the spontaneous sensitisation rate. Surveys of general medical practitioners and consultant obstetricians and haematologists in the UK[11,12] have suggested that many do not recommend routine prophylaxis following early complete or threatened miscarriages; 74% of general practitioners in one survey[12] never gave anti-D immunoglobulin after threatened miscarriages. Spontaneous miscarriages during early pregnancy might not cause sensitisation so long as there is no surgical intervention.[7,8,13] Nonetheless, the Royal College of Obstetricians and Gynaecologists and other authorities in the UK urge routine antenatal prophylaxis for all Rh(D)-negative women. Others[14,15] represent the alternative opinion that, with the shortage of anti-D immunoglobulin, indiscriminate use should be avoided[14] and attention should be focussed upon administration of adequate doses following term deliveries and terminations of pregnancy in Rh(D)-negative women.[5,15]

Further debate arises over the significance of spontaneous sensitisation during the first pregnancy. In one study,[16] administration of anti-D immunoglobulin to 2069 Rh(D)-negative primigravidas at 28 and 34 weeks as well as standard postpartum administration was more effective at preventing immunisation than standard postpartum prophylaxis in 2000 primigravidas. In a subsequent analysis of women from this study[17] following further pregnancies, comparison with a group of Rh(D)-positive mothers showed no detrimental effects to mothers or infants. In addition, antenatal prophylaxis may not need to be given beyond the first pregnancy. Nevertheless, concerns have been expressed[18] over the consequent unnecessary administration of anti-D immunoglobulin to women who are carrying Rh(D)-negative fetuses and the possible long-term effects, although anti-D immunoglobulin has had a good safety record.[19] Both factions agree[18,20] on the desirability of identifying high-risk women to reduce the indiscriminate use of anti-D immunoglobulin. A remaining major stumbling block, in the UK at least, is the continuing expense and scarcity of anti-D immunoglobulin. Supplies are derived from plasma collected from Rh-negative donors who have to undergo potentially hazardous sensitisation with Rh-positive red blood cells. The development of genetically-engineered anti-D immunoglobulin should help to improve availability. The UK[3] and WHO[2] guidelines may represent a counsel of perfection, but until difficulties with supply are overcome, prophylaxis during the first pregnancy for Rh(D)-negative women, thus ensuring the possibility of two unaffected infants, would seem a reasonable priority.

**Treatment.** In mild cases, the resultant hyperbilirubinaemia can be managed with phototherapy. In severe cases, exchange transfusions may be necessary and intra-uterine transfusions may be considered in pregnancies of less than about 34 weeks' gestation; beyond this, premature delivery is often preferable.[21] Some clinicians[22] have reported treatment failures with intra-uterine transfusions but have found the intravenous administration of normal immunoglobulin 400 mg/kg daily for 5 days every 2 to 3 weeks to the mother to be effective. There are several case reports[23,24] of beneficial responses using similar doses, but no benefit was seen in 4 patients receiving 1000 mg/kg once a week.[25] This dose, however, appeared to reduce the severity of the disease in a patient with Kell sensitisation.[25] Reductions in bilirubin concentrations have been reported following intravenous administration of normal immunoglobulin 500 mg/kg as a single dose to newborn infants.[26] Preliminary studies in small numbers of infants[27,28] suggest that epoetins may be of value in controlling anaemia which develops 2 to 8 weeks after birth.

1. Tovey LAD. Haemolytic disease of the newborn and its prevention. *BMJ* 1990; **300:** 313–16.
2. WHO. Prevention of Rh sensitization: report of a WHO scientific group. *WHO Tech Rep Ser 468* 1971.
3. McClelland DBL, ed. *Handbook of transfusion medicine: Blood Transfusion Services of the United Kingdom.* 3rd ed. London: The Stationery Office, 2001.
4. Robson SC, *et al.* Anti-D immunoglobulin in RhD prophylaxis. *Br J Obstet Gynaecol* 1998; **105:** 129–34.
5. James D. Anti-D prophylaxis in 1997: the Edinburgh consensus statement. *Arch Dis Child* 1998; **78:** F161–F165.
6. Howard HL, *et al.* Preventing rhesus D haemolytic disease of the newborn by giving anti-D immunoglobulin: are the guidelines being adequately followed? *Br J Obstet Gynaecol* 1997; **104:** 37–41.
7. Contreras M. Is anti-D immunoglobulin unnecessary in the domiciliary treatment of miscarriages? *BMJ* 1988; **297:** 733.
8. Tovey LAD. Anti-D and miscarriages. *BMJ* 1988; **297:** 977–8.
9. Lee D. Recommendations for the use of anti-D immunoglobulin. *Prescribers' J* 1991; **31:** 262–3.
10. Tabor A, *et al.* Incidence of rhesus immunisation after genetic amniocentesis. *BMJ* 1986; **293:** 533–6.
11. Contreras M, *et al.* Why women are not receiving anti-Rh prophylaxis. *BMJ* 1986; **293:** 1373.
12. Everett C, *et al.* Reported management of threatened miscarriage by general practitioners in Wessex. *BMJ* 1987; **295:** 583–6.

13. Everett CB. Is anti-D immunoglobulin unnecessary in the domiciliary treatment of miscarriages? *BMJ* 1988; **297:** 732.
14. Everett CB. Anti-D immunoglobulin for bleeding in early pregnancy. *BMJ* 1990; **301:** 1329.
15. Hussey RM. Why women are not receiving anti-Rh prophylaxis. *BMJ* 1987; **294:** 119.
16. Tovey LAD, *et al.* The Yorkshire antenatal anti-D immunoglobulin trial in primigravidae. *Lancet* 1983; **ii:** 244–6.
17. Thornton JG, *et al.* Efficacy and long term effects of antenatal prophylaxis with anti-D immunoglobulin. *BMJ* 1989; **298:** 1671–3.
18. Hussey R. Antenatal prophylaxis with anti-D immunoglobulin. *BMJ* 1989; **299:** 568.
19. Lee D. Antenatal prophylaxis with anti-D immunoglobulin. *BMJ* 1989; **299:** 920.
20. Thornton JG, Tovey LAD. Antenatal prophylaxis with anti-D immunoglobulin. *BMJ* 1989; **299:** 919–20.
21. Whittle MJ. Rhesus haemolytic disease. *Arch Dis Child* 1992; **67:** 65–8.
22. Margulies M, Voto LS. High-dose intravenous gamma globulin: does it have a role in the treatment of severe erythroblastosis fetalis? *Obstet Gynecol* 1991; **77:** 804–5.
23. Berlin G, *et al.* Rhesus haemolytic disease treated with high-dose intravenous immunoglobulin. *Lancet* 1985; **i:** 1153.
24. de la Cámara C, *et al.* High-dose intravenous immunoglobulin as the sole prenatal treatment for severe Rh immunization. *N Engl J Med* 1988; **318:** 519–20.
25. Chitkara U, *et al.* High-dose intravenous gamma globulin: does it have a role in the treatment of severe erythroblastosis fetalis? *Obstet Gynecol* 1990; **76:** 703–8.
26. Rübo J, *et al.* High-dose intravenous immune globulin therapy for hyperbilirubinemia caused by Rh hemolytic disease. *J Pediatr* 1992; **121:** 93–7.
27. Ohls RK, *et al.* Recombinant erythropoietin as treatment for the late hyporegenerative anemia of Rh hemolytic disease. *Pediatrics* 1992; **90:** 678–80.
28. Scaradavou A, *et al.* Suppression of erythropoiesis by intrauterine transfusions in hemolytic disease of the newborn: use of erythropoietin to treat the late anemia. *J Pediatr* 1993; **123:** 279–84.

**Idiopathic thrombocytopenic purpura.** Normal immunoglobulin is used for chronic idiopathic thrombocytopenic purpura (p.1082), and anti-D immunoglobulin has been found to have similar properties.[1] Treatment of an Rh(D)-positive patient with a long history of severe immune thrombocytopenic purpura with a single dose of 500 units (100 micrograms) of anti-D immunoglobulin intravenously was reported to result in a steady rise in platelet count and rapid resolution of a cephalic haematoma.[2] Responses to anti-D immunoglobulin were reported in 23 of 25 children with chronic idiopathic thrombocytopenia[3] following treatment with 25 micrograms/kg on each of two consecutive days. It has been stated[4] that children with *acute* disease usually recover regardless of therapy but the small risk of intracranial haemorrhage leads many to recommend treatment. In one study[4] involving children with acute disease, a similar dose of anti-D immunoglobulin was less effective in restoring platelet count and produced a greater fall in haemoglobin than either normal immunoglobulin or corticosteroids.

Beneficial results in both rhesus-positive and rhesus-negative patients with HIV-related thrombocytopenia were reported[5-8] with doses in the order of 1 to 3 mg daily, given intravenously.

1. Anonymous. Rho(D) immunoglobulin iv for prevention of Rh isoimmunization and for treatment of ITP. *Med Lett Drugs Ther* 1996; **38:** 6–8.
2. Baglin TP, *et al.* Rapid and complete response of immune thrombocytopenic purpura to a single injection of rhesus anti-D immunoglobulin. *Lancet* 1986; **i:** 1329–30.
3. Andrew M, *et al.* A multicenter study of the treatment of childhood chronic idiopathic thrombocytopenic purpura with anti-D. *J Pediatr* 1992; **120:** 522–7.
4. Blanchette V, *et al.* Randomised trial of intravenous immunoglobulin G, intravenous anti-D, and oral prednisone in childhood acute immune thrombocytopenic purpura. *Lancet* 1994; **344:** 703–7.
5. Durand JM, *et al.* Anti-Rh(D) immunoglobulin for immune thrombocytopenic purpura. *Lancet* 1986; **ii:** 49–50.
6. Biniek R, *et al.* Anti-Rh(D) immunoglobulin for AIDS-related thrombocytopenia. *Lancet* 1986; **ii:** 627.
7. Bierling P, *et al.* Anti-rhesus antibodies, immune thrombocytopenia, and human immunodeficiency virus infection. *Ann Intern Med* 1987; **106:** 773–4.
8. Landonio G, *et al.* HIV-related severe thrombocytopenia in intravenous drug users: prevalence, response to therapy in a medium-term follow-up, and pathogenic evaluation. *AIDS* 1990; **4:** 29–34.

## Preparations

***Ph. Eur.:*** Human Anti-D Immunoglobulin; Human Anti-D Immunoglobulin for Intravenous Administration;
***USP 27:*** $Rh_0$ (D) Immune Globulin.

**Proprietary Preparations** (details are given in Part 3)
***Arg.:*** BayRho-D; Kam Rho-D; Partoben; Partogamma-T; ***Austral.:*** WinRho; ***Austria:*** Partobulin; Rhesogam; ***Belg.:*** Rhesuman†; ***Braz.:*** BayRho-D†; Matergam; Partogamma†; Rhesonativ†; ***Canad.:*** BayRho-D; HypRho-D†; WinRho; ***Chile:*** BayRho-D; Igamad; Rhesogamma P; ***Denm.:*** Rhesogamma P; ***Fr.:*** Natead; ***Ger.:*** Partobulin; Rhesogam; ***Gr.:*** Rhesogamma P; ***Hong Kong:*** BayRho-D; Partobulin; Rhesuman†; RhoGAM; ***India:*** Matergam-P; ***Irl.:*** Rhesonativ; ***Israel:*** BayRho-D; IgRho†; Kam-Rho-D; WinRho; ***Ital.:*** Gamma-Men†; Haima-D; Igamad; Immunorho; Parto-Gamma; Partobulin; Rhesuman†; Venogamma Anti-Rho (D)†; ***Malaysia:*** Rhesonativ; ***Mex.:*** BayRho-D; Probi-Rho D; Rhesogamma†; ***Norw.:*** Rhesogamma; Rhesonativ†; ***NZ:*** WinRho; ***Port.:*** Igantid; Rhesuman; ***S.Afr.:*** Rhesugam; ***Singapore:*** BayRho-D; ***Spain:*** Berigobina Anti D-P†; Gamma Anti D; Gammaglob Anti D†; Globulina Lloren Anti RH†; Rhesogamma; Rhesuman†; ***Swed.:*** Rhesogamma; Rhesonativ; ***Switz.:*** Rhesuman†; Rhophylac; ***Thai.:*** Rhesuman†; ***UK:*** D-Gam; Partobulin; Rhophylac; WinRho; ***USA:*** BayRho-D; Gamulin Rh†; MICRhoGAM; Mini-Gamulin Rh†; RhoGAM; WinRho.



## Argentine Haemorrhagic Fever Vaccines

Junin Haemorrhagic Fever Vaccines; Vacunas de la fiebre hemorrágica argentina.

### Profile

A live attenuated vaccine has been investigated for active immunisation against Argentine haemorrhagic fever.

◊ References.

1. Maiztegui JI, *et al.* Protective efficacy of a live attenuated vaccine against Argentine hemorrhagic fever. *J Infect Dis* 1998; **177:** 277–83.

## BCG Vaccines

Bacillus Calmette-Guérin Vaccines; Vacunas BCG.

*ATC — J07AN01; L03AX03.*

**Pharmacopoeias.** Many pharmacopoeias have monographs including *Br., Eur.* (see p.vi), and *US.*

**Ph. Eur. 5.0** (BCG Vaccine, Freeze-dried; Vaccinum Tuberculosis (BCG) Cryodesiccatum; Bacillus Calmette-Guérin Vaccine BP 2003). A freeze-dried preparation containing live bacteria obtained from a strain derived from the bacillus of Calmette and Guérin (*Mycobacterium bovis* BCG) whose capacity to protect against tuberculosis has been established. It may contain a stabiliser. The dried vaccine should be stored at 2° to 8° and be protected from direct sunlight.

The BP 2003 states that Dried/Tub/Vac/BCG may be used on the label.

The BP 2003 gives BCG Vaccine as an approved synonym.

**BP 2003** (Percutaneous Bacillus Calmette-Guérin Vaccine). A suspension of living cells of an authentic strain of the bacillus of Calmette and Guérin with a higher viable bacterial count than Bacillus Calmette-Guérin Vaccine. It is supplied as a dried vaccine and is reconstituted immediately before use by the addition of a suitable sterile liquid. The dried vaccine should be stored at a temperature below −20° and be protected from light.

The BP 2003 states that Tub/Vac/BCG (Perc) may be used on the label.

The BP 2003 gives Percut. BCG Vaccine as an approved synonym.

**USP 27** (BCG Vaccine). A dried living culture of the bacillus Calmette-Guérin strain of *Mycobacterium tuberculosis* var. *bovis*; it is grown from a strain that has been maintained to preserve its capacity for conferring immunity. It contains an amount of viable bacteria such that inoculation, in the recommended dose, of tuberculin-negative persons results in an acceptable tuberculin conversion rate. It contains a suitable stabiliser and no antimicrobial agent. The dried vaccine should be stored in hermetically sealed containers at 2° to 8°. The reconstituted vaccine should be used immediately after preparation and any portion not used within 2 hours should be discarded.

**Ph. Eur. 5.0** (BCG for Immunotherapy; BCG ad Immunocurationem). A freeze-dried preparation of live bacteria derived from a culture of the bacillus of Calmette and Guérin (*Mycobacterium bovis* BCG) whose capacity for treatment has been established. It may contain a stabiliser. It is for intravesical use only. The product should be stored at 2° to 8° and be protected from direct sunlight.

### Adverse Effects

As for vaccines in general, p.1605.

Side-effects occur rarely with BCG vaccines. They include ulceration of the inoculation site, lymphadenitis, and keloid formation. Serious local reactions are usually due to faulty injection techniques. Very rarely, a lupoid type of reaction has occurred. Generalised reactions, possibly due to hypersensitivity, have been reported with a few fatalities. Disseminated BCG infection may occur. Osteitis has been reported with some BCG vaccines.

◊ Reviews and studies of the adverse effects of BCG vaccines.[1-3] An increased incidence of local effects has followed intradermal injection of high doses of BCG vaccines.[4,5]

1. Lotte A, *et al.* Second IUATLD study on complications induced by intradermal BCG-vaccination. *Bull Int Union Tuberc Lung Dis* 1988; **63:** 47–59.
2. Milstien JB, Gibson JJ. Quality control of BCG vaccine by WHO: a review of factors that may influence vaccine effectiveness and safety. *Bull WHO* 1990; **68:** 93–108.
3. Grange JM. Complications of bacille Calmette-Guérin (BCG) vaccination and immunotherapy and their management. *Commun Dis Public Health* 1998; **1:** 84–8.
4. Miles MM, Shaw RJ. Effect of inadvertent intradermal administration of high dose percutaneous BCG vaccine. *BMJ* 1996; **312:** 1014.
5. Puliyel JM, *et al.* Adverse local reactions from accidental BCG overdose in infants. *BMJ* 1996; **313:** 528–9.

**Effects on the bones and joints.** The risk of osteitis following BCG vaccination varies from country to country and appears to be linked to the strain of bacillus used.[1]

Osteitis or arthritis has also been reported following intravesicular administration of BCG (see below).

1. Milstien JB, Gibson JJ. Quality control of BCG vaccine by WHO: a review of factors that may influence vaccine effectiveness and safety. *Bull WHO* 1990; **68:** 93–108.

**Effects on the eyes.** Follicular conjunctivitis occurred following accidental contamination of the eye with BCG vaccine.[1] The conjunctivitis responded to topical corticosteroid therapy, but a course of isoniazid was given as a precautionary measure.

1. Pollard AJ, George RH. Ocular contamination with BCG vaccine. *Arch Dis Child* 1994; **70:** 71.

**Effects on the lymphatic system.** Increases in the incidence and severity of lymphadenitis have been reported following changes in BCG vaccine to one containing more virulent strains or with different dosage recommendations.[1,2]

1. Hengster P, *et al.* Occurrence of suppurative lymphadenitis after a change of BCG vaccine. *Arch Dis Child* 1992; **67:** 952–5.
2. Kabra SK, *et al.* BCG-associated adenitis. *Lancet* 1993; **341:** 970.

**Intravesicular administration.** Intravesicular instillation of BCG can give rise to both localised and systemic adverse effects.[1] Local effects include bladder irritation and urinary-tract infections. A case of local infection with vaccine-derived *Mycobacterium bovis* has been reported.[2] Symptoms of hypersensitivity reactions include malaise, fever, and chills. The most serious reactions are severe sepsis with cardiorespiratory manifestations and a disseminated mycobacterial infection with lung granulomas and impaired liver function; both require prompt treatment with antimycobacterials.[1] There have been case reports of systemic granulomatous disease[3] and of arthritis and osteitis[4-6] following intravesicular administration of BCG.

1. Lamm DL, *et al.* Incidence and treatment of complications of bacillus Calmette-Guerin intravesical therapy in superficial bladder cancer. *J Urol (Baltimore)* 1992; **147:** 596–600.
2. Ribera M, *et al.* Mycobacterium bovis-BCG infection of the glans penis: a complication of intravesical administration of bacillus Calmette-Guerin. *Br J Dermatol* 1995; **132:** 309–10.
3. Mooren FC, *et al.* Systemic granulomatous disease after intravesical BCG instillation. *BMJ* 2000; **320:** 219.
4. Puett DW, Fuchs HA. Arthritis after bacillus Calmette-Guerin therapy. *Ann Intern Med* 1992; **117:** 537.
5. Devlin M, *et al.* Arthritis as a complication of intravesical BCG vaccine. *BMJ* 1994; **308:** 1638.
6. Morgan MB, Iseman MD. Mycobacterium bovis vertebral osteomyelitis as a complication of intravesical administration of Bacille Calmette-Guérin. *Am J Med* 1996; **100:** 372–3.

### Precautions

As for vaccines in general, p.1606. BCG vaccines may be given concomitantly with other live vaccines, but if they are not given at the same time it is preferable to allow an interval of 4 weeks between administration although the period may be reduced to 10 days if absolutely necessary. However, routine immunisation with live poliomyelitis vaccine need not be delayed. No further vaccination should be given in the arm used for BCG vaccination for at least 3 months because of the risk of lymphadenitis. Because of the possible risk of disseminated infections, it is recommended in the UK that BCG vaccines should not be given to immunocompromised patients including those with HIV infection. WHO has, however, advised immunisation of asymptomatic HIV-positive children when the risk of tuberculosis is high. In patients with eczema, BCG vaccines should be given at a site free from lesions. They should not be given to patients receiving antimycobacterial therapy.

**Immunocompromised patients.** Like other live vaccines, BCG vaccine should not be given to immunocompromised patients including those with symptomatic HIV infections and AIDS. However, the risk of possible adverse effects in patients with asymptomatic HIV infections may be outweighed by the possible advantages of vaccination (see Tuberculosis, HIV-infected Patients, below). Disseminated BCG infections have been reported in children with HIV infections,[1] but large studies have shown that infants born to HIV-positive mothers had only a slightly increased risk of adverse reactions, and many of these were generally mild.[2,3]

1. Ryder RW, *et al.* Safety and immunogenicity of bacille Calmette-Guérin, diphtheria-tetanus-pertussis, and oral polio vaccines in newborn children in Zaire infected with human immunodeficiency virus type 1. *J Pediatr* 1993; **122:** 697–702.
2. Besnard M, *et al.* Bacillus Calmette-Guérin infection after vaccination of human immunodeficiency virus-infected children. *Pediatr Infect Dis J* 1993; **12:** 993–7.
3. O'Brien KL, *et al.* Bacillus Calmette-Guérin complications in children born to HIV-1-infected women with a review of the literature. *Pediatrics* 1995; **95:** 414–18.

### Interactions

As for vaccines in general, p.1606.

**Theophylline.** For a report of increased theophylline half-life and serum concentrations after BCG vaccination, see under Theophylline Hydrate, p.803.

## Uses and Administration

BCG vaccines are used for active immunisation against tuberculosis, principally for the vaccination of selected groups of the population and of persons likely to be exposed to infection. In some countries it is administered only to persons who give a negative tuberculin reaction, but in countries with a high prevalence of tuberculosis, routine vaccination in infancy is recommended (see under Tuberculosis, below for further details). A form suitable for immunotherapy is also used locally in the treatment of bladder cancers (see under Malignant Neoplasms, Bladder, below for further details).

In the UK, vaccination is recommended in the following groups of persons, if there is *no evidence of previous immunisation* and they are found to be *tuberculin-negative* (see under Tuberculins, p.1759):

- children aged 10 to 14 years (as part of the standard schedule for immunisation—see p.1606)
- contacts of persons suffering from active respiratory tuberculosis
- immigrants in whose communities there is known to be a high incidence of tuberculosis and all their children wherever born
- health service staff at high risk of infection
- veterinary and other staff who handle animals known to be susceptible to tuberculosis
- staff in any institution where the incidence of tuberculosis is high
- persons intending to stay in countries with a high incidence of tuberculosis for more than a month
- any other individual upon request.

Sensitivity testing to tuberculin need not be performed for infants less than 3 months old.

The BCG vaccine is given intradermally (intracutaneously) at the insertion of the deltoid muscle in a dose of 0.1 mL; infants under 12 months of age are given 0.05 mL. For cosmetic reasons, the injection may be given into the upper and lateral surface of the thigh, except in neonates when the upper arm must be used.

A BCG vaccine approximately 10 times the strength of the intradermal vaccine has been given percutaneously using a multiple-puncture device, but such administration is only recommended in infants and young children (up to 5 years of age).

Contacts of patients with active pulmonary tuberculosis may require chemoprophylaxis despite previous vaccination (see under Tuberculosis, p.150). Neonates and children under 2 years of age should be given chemoprophylaxis and immunised, if appropriate, once the course is completed. An isoniazid-resistant form of the vaccine has been produced for use in patients who have received isoniazid, but its use is not recommended.

◊ General references and reviews.


1. Lugosi L. Theoretical and methodological aspects of BCG vaccine from the discovery of Calmette and Guérin to molecular biology: a review. *Tubercle Lung Dis* 1992; **73:** 252–61.


**Leishmaniasis.** For reference to the use of BCG vaccines in leishmaniasis, see Leishmaniasis Vaccines, p.1622.

**Leprosy.** BCG vaccination has been shown to protect recipients against leprosy[1] and is considered to be one of the factors responsible for the decrease in the incidence of leprosy. As in tuberculosis considerable variation has been noted in the efficacy of BCG in leprosy, and it appears to be more effective in Africa[2-4] and South America than in Asia.[5,6] Protection appears to be afforded against both multibacillary and paucibacillary leprosy[7,8] and a second dose may provide additional protection.[9] Adding killed *Mycobacterium leprae* has not improved the response further.[9] BCG is considered to be an important addition to multidrug treatment in long-term eradication programmes.[1] Specific vaccines against leprosy are under development (see p.1622).


1. Lienhardt C, Fine PEM. Controlling leprosy. *BMJ* 1992; **305:** 206–7.
2. Stanley SJ, *et al.* BCG vaccination of children against leprosy in Uganda: final results. *J Hyg (Camb)* 1981; **87:** 233–48.
3. Fine PEM, *et al.* Protective efficacy of BCG against leprosy in northern Malawi. *Lancet* 1986; **ii:** 499–502.
4. Baker DM, Nguyen-Van-Tam JS. BCG vaccine and leprosy. *Lancet* 1992; **339:** 1236.
5. Lwin KW, *et al.* BCG vaccination of children against leprosy: fourteen-year findings of the trial in Burma. *Bull WHO* 1985; **63:** 1069–78.
6. Tripathy SP. The case for BCG. *Ann Natl Med Sci (India)* 1983; **19:** 11–21.
7. Pönnighaus JM, *et al.* Efficacy of BCG vaccine against leprosy and tuberculosis in northern Malawi. *Lancet* 1992; **339:** 636–9.
8. Muliyil J, *et al.* Effect of BCG on the risk of leprosy in an endemic area: case control study. *Int J Lepr* 1991; **59:** 229–36.
9. Karonga Prevention Trial Group. Randomised controlled trial of single BCG, repeated BCG, or combined BCG and killed mycobacterium leprae vaccine for prevention of leprosy and tuberculosis in Malawi. *Lancet* 1996; **348:** 17–24.


**Malignant neoplasms.** Immunotherapy with BCG vaccines has been tried in various malignant disorders and is most successful when administered locally. The possibility that BCG vaccination might protect children against malignancies has been discussed.[1]


1. Grange JM, Stanford JL. BCG vaccination and cancer. *Tubercle* 1990; **71:** 61–4.


BLADDER. Immunotherapy with adjuvant intravesicular BCG is used in the management of bladder cancers and is the treatment of choice for carcinoma *in situ* (p.512). Local and systemic adverse effects, although rarely severe, are relatively common. Treatment is not started until 10 to 14 days after bladder biopsy or transurethral resection. A number of regimens have been tried, but one manufacturer (Cambridge, UK) recommends that BCG is instilled into the bladder once weekly for 6 weeks, followed after a 6-week pause by further instillations once weekly for 1 to 3 weeks. Maintenance therapy is recommended and consists of instillations every 1 to 3 weeks at 6 months after initiation of treatment and then every 6 months thereafter until 36 months. Another manufacturer (Organon, UK) recommends that the initial 6-week course may be followed by a 2-week pause and then monthly instillations for at least 6 months; maintenance may be required for up to 24 months in this regimen.

Urine voided for 6 hours after instillation of BCG vaccines should be disinfected with sodium hypochlorite solution.

Reviews.


1. Alexandroff AB, *et al.* BCG immunotherapy of bladder cancer: 20 years on. *Lancet* 1999; **353:** 1689–94.
2. Böhle A, *et al.* Intravesical bacillus Calmette-Guerin versus mitomycin C for superficial bladder cancer: a formal meta-analysis of comparative studies on recurrence and toxicity. *J Urol (Baltimore)* 2003; **169:** 90–5.
3. Shelley MD, *et al.* Intravesical bacillus Calmette-Guerin in Ta and T1 bladder cancer. Available in The Cochrane Library; Issue 2. Chichester: John Wiley; 2004.
4. Shelley MD, *et al.* Intravesical bacillus Calmette-Guerin versus mitomycin C for Ta and T1 bladder cancer. Available in The Cochrane Library; Issue 2. Chichester: John Wiley; 2004.


SKIN. Several studies have reported that BCG vaccine injected into intradermal metastases of melanoma can result in regression of the injected, and sometimes also the uninjected nodules. BCG therapy has been disappointing for visceral metastases. Many anecdotal reports and nonrandomised studies have shown benefit from BCG vaccine as adjuvant therapy, but these results have not been confirmed in large randomised, controlled studies.[1,2] More specific immunological interventions such as therapeutic vaccines are now being investigated in the treatment of melanomas (p.522).


1. Ho VC, Sober AJ. Therapy for cutaneous melanoma: an update. *J Am Acad Dermatol* 1990; **22:** 159–76.
2. Agarwala SS, *et al.* Mature results of a phase III randomized trial of bacillus Calmette-Guerin (BCG) versus observation and BCG plus dacarbazine versus BCG in the adjuvant therapy of American Joint Committee on Cancer stage I-III melanoma (E1673): a trial of the Eastern Oncology Group. *Cancer* 2004; **100:** 1692–8.


**Tuberculosis.** Studies from many parts of the world have evaluated the efficacy of BCG vaccine to protect against tuberculosis. Levels of protection have varied from 0 to over 80%.[1] Many explanations for such variability have been proposed: interaction with the immune response to other mycobacterial infections; antigenic, microbiological, or formulation differences between BCG vaccines; differences in the natural history of infection and disease; variations in host genetics or nutrition; methodological differences between studies.[1,2] It has been noted that in general the efficacy of BCG vaccine in any region is proportional to its distance from the equator and this possibly reflects differences in exposure to environmental mycobacteria.[3] This could be the strongest influence on efficacy,[3] with the implication that BCG may be least effective in areas of the world where the risk of tuberculosis is greatest. BCG also appears to be more effective against systemic (miliary and meningitic tuberculosis) than against pulmonary tuberculosis. It is likely that BCG cannot produce complete protection against infection, and the development of new vaccines is underway.

National policies of BCG vaccination vary widely. In the USA, vaccination is recommended only for tuberculin-negative infants and children at high risk of tuberculosis.[4] Most other countries recommend routine vaccination (the UK recommendations are described under Uses and Administration, above).[1] Schedules vary from single vaccination at birth (as recommended by WHO),[5] to single vaccination at age 10 to 14 (as in the UK), to repeated vaccination every few years (particularly in eastern Europe). These policy differences appear to be related as much to differences of opinion about the mechanism of action and effectiveness of vaccines as to local differences in the epidemiology of tuberculosis.[1] WHO considers BCG vaccination to be an adjunct to case detection and treatment in the control of tuberculosis,[5] and recommends that neither tuberculin skin testing nor repeat vaccination should be used.


1. Fine PEM, Rodrigues LC. Modern vaccines: mycobacterial diseases. *Lancet* 1990; **335:** 1016–20.
2. Fine PEM. BCG vaccination against tuberculosis and leprosy. *Br Med Bull* 1988; **44:** 691–703.
3. Fine PEM. Variation in protection by BCG: implications of and for heterologous immunity. *Lancet* 1995; **346:** 1339–45. Correction. *ibid.*; **347:** 340.
4. Centers for Disease Control. The role of BCG vaccine in the prevention and control of tuberculosis in the United States: a joint statement by the Advisory Council for the Elimination of Tuberculosis and the Advisory Committee on Immunization Practices. *MMWR* 1996; **45** (RR-4): 1–18.
5. Anonymous. WHO statement on BCG revaccination for the prevention of tuberculosis. *Bull WHO* 1995; **73:** 805–6.


HIV-INFECTED PATIENTS. Like other live vaccines, BCG vaccine should not be given to immunocompromised patients, including patients with symptomatic HIV infection or AIDS. Doubts about the safety (see under Precautions, above) and efficacy of BCG vaccines in patients with asymptomatic HIV infection have resulted in differing national policies. WHO recommends that the national policy should depend on the local prevalence of tuberculosis.[1] In countries where prevalence is high, the possible benefits of immunisation outweigh the possible disadvantages, and routine BCG vaccination should be given to all children except those with symptomatic HIV infection or AIDS. In countries with low tuberculosis prevalence, BCG vaccination should not be given to children with HIV infection. In the UK[2] and USA,[3] BCG vaccination is not recommended for HIV-positive patients. Similar policies apply to infants born to HIV-positive mothers, although it is not necessary to screen mothers for HIV infection before giving routine BCG vaccination.[2]


1. WHO. *TB/HIV: a clinical manual.* Geneva: WHO, 1996.
2. Department of Health. *Immunisation against infectious disease* 1996: "The Green Book". Available at: http://www.dh.gov.uk/PublicationsAndStatistics/Publications/PublicationsPolicyAndGuidance/PublicationsPolicyAndGuidanceArticle/fs/en?CONTENT_ID=4072977&chk=87uz6M (accessed 22/06/04) See also http://www.hpa.org.uk/infections/topics_az/vaccination/vac_sced.htm (accessed 22/06/04)
3. Centers for Disease Control. The role of BCG vaccine in the prevention and control of tuberculosis in the United States: a joint statement by the Advisory Council for the Elimination of Tuberculosis and the Advisory Committee on Immunization Practices. *MMWR* 1996; **45** (RR-4) 1–18.


## Preparations

***BP 2003:*** Percutaneous Bacillus Calmette-Guérin Vaccine;
***Ph. Eur.:*** BCG for Immunotherapy; Freeze-dried BCG Vaccine;
***USP 27:*** BCG Vaccine.

**Proprietary Preparations** (details are given in Part 3)
***Arg.:*** ImmuCyst; Pacis; ***Austral.:*** ImmuCyst; OncoTICE; ***Austria:*** ImmuCyst; OncoTICE; ***Belg.:*** ImmuCyst; Pastimmun†; ***Braz.:*** ImmuCyst; OncoTICE†; ***Canad.:*** ImmuCyst; OncoTICE; Pacis; ***Chile:*** ImmuCyst; ***Denm.:*** OncoTICE; ***Fin.:*** OncoTICE; ***Fr.:*** ImmuCyst; Monovax; ***Ger.:*** ImmuCyst; OncoTICE; ***Gr.:*** OncoTICE; ***Hong Kong:*** ImmuCyst; OncoTICE; ***Israel:*** ImmuCyst; OncoTICE; ***Ital.:*** ImmuCyst; Imovax BCG; OncoTICE; ***Malaysia:*** ImmuCyst; ***Mex.:*** Cultivo BCG; ***Neth.:*** OncoTICE; ***Norw.:*** OncoTICE; ***NZ:*** ImmuCyst; OncoTICE; ***Port.:*** ImmuCyst; OncoTICE; ***Singapore:*** ImmuCyst; ***Spain:*** ImmuCyst; OncoTICE; ***Swed.:*** OncoTICE; ***Switz.:*** ImmuCyst†; OncoTICE; ***Thai.:*** ImmuCyst; ***UK:*** ImmuCyst; OncoTICE; ***USA:*** Pacis; TheraCys; Tice.

---

## Botulism Antitoxins

Antitoxinas botulínicas.

*ATC — J06AA04.*

**Pharmacopoeias.** Many pharmacopoeias have monographs including *Eur.* (see p.vi) and *US.*

**Ph. Eur. 5.0** (Botulinum Antitoxin; Immunoserum Botulinicum). A sterile preparation containing the specific antitoxic globulins that have the power of neutralising the toxins formed by type A, type B, type E, or any mixture of types A, B, and E, of *Clostridium botulinum*. It contains not less than 500 international units of each of type A and type B and not less than 50 units of type E per mL. It should be stored at 2° to 8°, and not be allowed to freeze.

The BP 2003 states that Bot/Ser may be used on the label.

The BP 2003 states that when Mixed Botulinum Antitoxin or Botulinum Antitoxin is prescribed or demanded and the types to be present are not stated, Botulinum Antitoxin prepared from types A, B, and E shall be dispensed or supplied.

**USP 27** (Botulism Antitoxin). A sterile solution of the refined and concentrated antitoxic antibodies, chiefly globulins, obtained from the blood of healthy horses that have been immunised against the toxins produced by type A and type B and/or E strains of *Clostridium botulinum*. It contains a suitable antimicrobial agent. It should be stored at 2° to 8° in single-use containers.

◊ NOTE. Some antitoxins available in the UK have not conformed to the requirements of the BP 2003 and Ph. Eur. 5.0 (having a higher phenol content than the pharmacopoeias allow), and thus have been referred to as **botulism antitoxin** rather than botulinum antitoxin.

## Adverse Effects and Precautions

As for antisera in general, p.1605.

## Uses and Administration

Botulism antitoxins are used in the postexposure prophylaxis and treatment of botulism. Treatment should be given as early as possible in the course of the disease. Botulism antitoxins are generally not effective for infant botulism.

Since the type of botulism toxin is seldom known the polyvalent antitoxin is usually given. Sensitivity testing should always be performed before administration of the antitoxin.

In the UK, a trivalent antitoxin containing antitoxin types A, B, and E is employed. For the treatment of botulism, 20 mL of this antitoxin should be diluted to 100 mL with sodium chloride 0.9% and given by slow intravenous infusion over at least 30 minutes; another 10 mL may be given 2 to 4 hours later if necessary, and further doses at 12- to 24-hour intervals if indicated. Persons who have been exposed to the toxin and in whom symptoms have not developed should be given 20 mL intramuscularly as a prophylactic measure.

In some countries the mixed antitoxin contains differing amounts of types A, B, and E antitoxin.

**Botulism.** Botulism is caused by the exotoxin of *Clostridium botulinum*, a spore-forming, Gram-positive anaerobe which occurs in soil and mud. The disease usually follows ingestion of contaminated preserved foodstuffs, but may develop from infected wounds or following gastrointestinal colonisation in infants. The toxin is heat labile, but the spores can survive temperatures of up to 120°. Eight types of *C. botulinum* can be distinguished, each producing a different exotoxin; human disease is usually caused by types A, B, and E.

Symptoms arise from inhibition of acetylcholine-mediated neurotransmission and include descending weakness or paralysis, gastrointestinal symptoms, orthostatic hypotension, dry mouth, and dilated pupils. Death is usually from respiratory arrest.

Treatment of botulism is with antitoxins and intensive respiratory and supportive therapy. Antitoxins should be given as early as possible but may still be beneficial if treatment is delayed.

Drug therapy aimed at reversing the neuromuscular blockade has included fampridine and guanidine and some patients may benefit from this treatment.

Infant botulism is of increasing importance, especially in the USA where it is reported to be the most commonly occurring form of botulism, with honey (see p.1434) reputed to be the most frequent source of infection. Treatment is with intensive supportive care; antitoxins are not generally considered to be effective although some products specifically designed for infants are becoming available.

References.


1. Shapiro RL, *et al.* Botulism in the United States: a clinical and epidemiologic review. *Ann Intern Med* 1998; **129:** 221–8.
2. Robinson RF, Nahata MC. Management of botulism. *Ann Pharmacother* 2003; **37:** 127–31.
3. Health Protection Agency. Interim guidelines for action in the event of a deliberate release: botulism. Available at: http://www.hpa.org.uk/infections/topics_az/deliberate_release_static/botulism/PDFs/botulism_guidelines.pdf (accessed 04/06/04)


### Preparations

***Ph. Eur.:*** Botulinum Antitoxin;
***USP 27:*** Botulism Antitoxin.

**Proprietary Preparations** (details are given in Part 3)
***Ital.:*** Liosiero†; ***USA:*** BabyBIG.

## Bovine Colostrum

Calostro bovino.

### Profile

Bovine colostrum has been used similarly to antisera and human immunoglobulin preparations to provide passive immunity against infectious diseases. Hyperimmune bovine colostra have been prepared from cows previously immunised with specific antigens. In particular, these specific hyperimmune bovine colostra have been tried in cryptosporidiosis and in the prevention of rotavirus diarrhoea in infants.

### Preparations

**Proprietary Preparations** (details are given in Part 3)
***Austral.:*** Gastrogard-R†.
**Multi-ingredient: *Ital.:*** Colostrum; ***UK:*** BioXtra.

## Brucellosis Vaccines

Vacunas de la brucelosis.

*ATC — J07AD01.*

### Profile

A brucellosis vaccine prepared from an antigenic extract of *Brucella abortus* has been used for active immunisation against brucellosis in persons at high risk of contracting the disease.

### Preparations

**Proprietary Preparations** (details are given in Part 3)
***Braz.:*** Bruvac†.

## Campylobacter Jejuni Vaccines

Vacunas contra el Campylobacter jejuni.

### Profile

An oral vaccine is under development to provide active immunisation against *Campylobacter jejuni* infection.

## Cancer Vaccines

Vacunas contra el cáncer.

### Profile

Vaccines are under investigation for a variety of neoplastic diseases including breast, cervical, colorectal, head and neck, lung, ovarian, pancreatic, prostate, and renal cancers, lymphomas, and melanoma. BCG vaccine (p.1610) is used locally in the treatment of bladder cancer and has been tried in other neoplastic diseases. Human papilloma virus vaccines (p.1620) are under investigation for the treatment of some cancers.

◊ General reviews of cancer vaccines under development.


1. Herlyn D, Birebent B. Advances in cancer vaccine development. *Ann Med* 1999; **31:** 66–78.
2. Minev BR, *et al.* Cancer vaccines: novel approaches and new promise. *Pharmacol Ther* 1999; **81:** 121–39.
3. Greten TF, Jaffee EM. Cancer vaccines. *J Clin Oncol* 1999; **17:** 1047–60.
4. Chamberlain RS. Prospects for the therapeutic use of anticancer vaccines. *Drugs* 1999; **57:** 309–25.
5. Jaffee EM. Immunotherapy of cancer. *Ann N Y Acad Sci* 1999; **886:** 67–72.
6. Sinkovics JF, Horvath JC. Vaccination against human cancers (review). *Int J Oncol* 2000; **16:** 81–96.
7. Moingeon P. Cancer vaccines. *Vaccine* 2001; **19:** 1305–26.
8. Dermime S, *et al.* Cancer vaccines and immunotherapy. *Br Med Bull* 2002; **62:** 149–62.


**Melanoma.** Reviews.


1. Bonn D. Getting under the skin with melanoma vaccines. *Lancet* 1996; **348:** 396.
2. Haigh PI, *et al.* Vaccine therapy for patients with melanoma. *Oncology (Huntingt)* 1999; **13:** 1561–74.
3. Brinckerhoff LH, *et al.* Melanoma vaccines. *Curr Opin Oncol* 2000; **12:** 163–73.


## Cholera Vaccines

Vacunas del cólera.

*ATC — J07AE01; J07AE02.*

**Pharmacopoeias.** Many pharmacopoeias have monographs including *Br.* and *Eur.* (see p.vi).

**Ph. Eur. 5.0** (Cholera Vaccine; Vaccinum Cholerae). A sterile homogeneous suspension of a suitable killed strain or strains of *Vibrio cholerae*. It consists of a mixture of equal parts of vaccines prepared from smooth strains of 2 main serological types, Inaba and Ogawa of the classical biotype with or without the El Tor biotype. A single strain or several strains of each type may be included. All strains must contain, in addition to their type O antigens, the heat-stable O antigen common to the Inaba and Ogawa types. If more than one strain each of Inaba and Ogawa are used they may be selected to contain other O antigens. It contains not less than 8000 million *V. cholerae* per dose, which does not exceed 1 mL. It contains not more than 0.5% of phenol. It should be stored at 2° to 8° and protected from light.

**Ph. Eur. 5.0** (Cholera Vaccine, Freeze-dried; Vaccinum Cholerae Cryodesiccatum). Cholera vaccine that is freeze-dried and reconstituted immediately before use by the addition of a suitable sterile liquid. Phenol may not be used in the preparation of the dried vaccine. It should be stored at 2° to 8° and be protected from light.

**BP 2003** (Cholera Vaccine). When Cholera Vaccine is issued as a liquid, it complies with the requirements of Cholera Vaccine (Ph. Eur. 5.0). When Cholera Vaccine is prepared immediately before use by reconstitution from the dried vaccine, the dried vaccine complies with the requirements of Cholera Vaccine, Freeze-dried (Ph. Eur. 5.0).

The BP 2003 states that Cho/Vac or Dried/Cho/Vac may be used on the label as appropriate.

### Adverse Effects and Precautions

As for vaccines in general, p.1605.

Slight swelling, erythema, and tenderness occasionally occur at the injection site. Fever and malaise have been reported and general reactions, including anaphylaxis and hypersensitivity reactions, have occurred. Neurological and psychiatric reactions have occasionally occurred.

### Interactions

As for vaccines in general, p.1606.

◊ For reference to the effect of cholera vaccination on the response to *yellow fever vaccines*, see under Yellow Fever Vaccines, p.1644.

### Uses and Administration

Injectable inactivated whole-cell cholera vaccines have been used for active immunisation against cholera but are not considered to be very effective and the immunity conferred is short-lived. They have no role in the management of contacts of cases or in controlling the spread of infection. The WHO International Health Regulations do not require cholera vaccination for travellers as the introduction of cholera into any country cannot be prevented by cholera vaccination. However, travellers may still be asked for evidence of immunisation at some borders.

Oral vaccines containing either live attenuated or inactivated strains are available in some countries and appear to be more effective than parenteral vaccines (see below).

**Oral cholera vaccines.** Since parenteral cholera vaccines are not considered to be very effective, providing at best 50% protection and confer immunity lasting only 3 to 6 months, attention has turned towards oral vaccines that stimulate intestinal immunity. Both killed and living oral vaccines have been developed, and both types have been shown to be non-toxic and immunogenic.

Killed vaccines contain inactivated whole *V. cholerae* O1 either alone or with B subunit component of cholera toxin.[1-6] These vaccines produce a protective efficacy of about 60 to 70%[1,2,6] and both modify established infections and prevent new ones. Although the vaccines are effective in areas where the El Tor biotype predominates,[5,6] they are more effective against classical strains.[1] Immunity particularly against El Tor may be less sustained in children under 5 years of age than in older children and adults.[1,2,7] The main drawback is the need to administer two or more doses at 1- to 2-week intervals to achieve a protective effect.[4,5,8] The protective effect is rapidly established[5] but wanes over time[1,7] and booster doses after 1 year may be necessary to maintain a high level of immunity.[9]

The most widely investigated live attenuated vaccine is CVD 103-HgR in which the genes encoding the toxic A subunit are deleted by recombinant techniques.[10-14] This vaccine is effective 8 days after a single dose but less so against El Tor than against classical strains. Live oral vaccines effective against El Tor are now being developed,[15,16] and promising responses have also been reported with a live attenuated O139 vaccine.[17]

The efficacy and cost-effectiveness of oral vaccines to control cholera outbreaks in refugee populations remains uncertain.[18,19]


1. Clemens JD, *et al.* Field trial of oral cholera vaccines in Bangladesh: results from three-year follow-up. *Lancet* 1990; **335:** 270–3.
2. Clemens JD, *et al.* Evidence that inactivated oral cholera vaccines both prevent and mitigate Vibrio cholerae O1 infections in a cholera-endemic area. *J Infect Dis* 1992; **166:** 1029–34.
3. Jertborn M, *et al.* Evaluation of different immunization schedules for oral cholera B subunit-whole cell vaccine in Swedish volunteers. *Vaccine* 1993; **11:** 1007–12.
4. Sanchez JL, *et al.* Safety and immunogenicity of the oral, whole cell/recombinant B subunit cholera vaccine in North American volunteers. *J Infect Dis* 1993; **167:** 1446–9.
5. Sanchez JL, *et al.* Protective efficacy of oral whole-cell/recombinant-B-subunit cholera vaccine in Peruvian military recruits. *Lancet* 1994; **344:** 1273–6.
6. Trach DD, *et al.* Field trial of a locally produced, killed, oral cholera vaccine in Vietnam. *Lancet* 1997; **349:** 231–5.
7. van Loon FPL, *et al.* Field trial of inactivated oral cholera vaccines in Bangladesh: results from 5 years of follow-up. *Vaccine* 1996; **14:** 162–6.
8. Sanchez JL, *et al.* Immunological response to Vibrio cholerae O1 infection and an oral cholera vaccine among Peruvians. *Trans R Soc Trop Med Hyg* 1995; **89:** 542–5.
9. Begue RE, *et al.* Immunogenicity in Peruvian volunteers of a booster dose of oral cholera vaccine consisting of whole cells plus recombinant B subunit. *Infect Immun* 1995; **63:** 3726–8.
10. Levine MM, *et al.* Safety, immunogenicity, and efficacy of recombinant live oral cholera vaccines, CVD 103 and CVD 103-HgR. *Lancet* 1988; **ii:** 467–70.
11. Suharyono, *et al.* Safety and immunogenicity of single-dose live oral cholera vaccine CVD 103-HgR in 5-9-year-old Indonesian children. *Lancet* 1992; **340:** 689–94.
12. Su-Arehawaratana P, *et al.* Safety and immunogenicity of different immunization regimens of CVD 103-HgR live oral cholera vaccine in soldiers and civilians in Thailand. *J Infect Dis* 1992; **165:** 1042–8.
13. Barrett P, *et al.* Oral cholera vaccine well tolerated. *BMJ* 1993; **307:** 1425.
14. Tacket CO, *et al.* Onset and duration of protective immunity in challenged volunteers after vaccination with live oral cholera vaccine CVD 103-HgR. *J Infect Dis* 1992; **166:** 837–41.
15. Tacket CO, *et al.* Volunteer studies investigating the safety and efficacy of live El Tor Vibrio cholerae O1 vaccine strain CVD 111. *Am J Trop Med Hyg* 1997; **56:** 533–7.
16. Sack DA, *et al.* Evaluation of Peru-15, a new live oral vaccine for cholera, in volunteers. *J Infect Dis* 1997; **176:** 201–5.
17. Coster TS, *et al.* Safety, immunogenicity, and efficacy of live attenuated Vibrio cholerae O139 vaccine prototype. *Lancet* 1995; **345:** 949–52.
18. Naficy A, *et al.* Treatment and vaccination strategies to control cholera in sub-Saharan refugee settings: a cost-effectiveness analysis. *JAMA* 1998; **279:** 521–5.
19. Waldman RJ. Cholera vaccination in refugee settings. *JAMA* 1998; **279:** 552–3.


### Preparations

***Ph. Eur.:*** Cholera Vaccine; Freeze-dried Cholera Vaccine.

**Proprietary Preparations** (details are given in Part 3)
***Arg.:*** Orochol; ***Austral.:*** Orochol; ***Canad.:*** Mutacol; ***Denm.:*** Dukoral; ***Norw.:*** Dukoral; ***NZ:*** Dukoral; Orochol†; ***Swed.:*** Dukoral; ***Switz.:*** Orochol; ***UK:*** Dukoral.

## Contraceptive Vaccines

Vacunas anticonceptivas.

### Profile

Various approaches to development of a contraceptive vaccine are under investigation. A synthetic contraceptive vaccine that stimulates the production of an antibody against human chorionic gonadotrophin has been studied in human trials.

◊ Reviews.

1. Delves PJ. The development of contraceptive vaccines. *Expert Opin Invest Drugs* 2002; **11:** 1225–37.
2. Aitken RJ. Immunocontraceptive vaccines for human use. *J Reprod Immunol* 2002; **57:** 273–87.

## Crimean-Congo Haemorrhagic Fever Immunoglobulins

Inmunoglobulinas contra la fiebre hemorrágica de Congo-Crimea.

### Profile

Preparations containing antibodies against Crimean-Congo haemorrhagic fever are available in some countries for passive immunisation against the disease.

◊ References.

1. Vassilenko SM, *et al.* Specific intravenous immunoglobulin for Crimean-Congo haemorrhagic fever. *Lancet* 1990; **335:** 791–2.

## Cytomegalovirus Immunoglobulins

Inmunoglobulinas contra el citomegalovirus.

*ATC — J06BB09.*

**Description.** Cytomegalovirus immunoglobulins containing high levels of specific antibody against cytomegalovirus have been prepared from human plasma.

### Adverse Effects and Precautions

As for immunoglobulins in general, p.1605.

### Interactions

As for immunoglobulins in general, p.1605.

### Uses and Administration

Cytomegalovirus immunoglobulins are used for passive immunisation against cytomegalovirus infection. They may be used prophylactically, especially in patients undergoing certain transplant procedures, or therapeutically for the treatment of established cytomegalovirus infections. For therapeutic and some prophylactic uses, they are commonly given with ganciclovir.

In the USA a cytomegalovirus immunoglobulin G is available for use in recipients of heart, kidney, liver, lung, and pancreas transplants from cytomegalovirus seropositive donors. The dosage schedule for kidney transplant recipients is 150 mg/kg by intravenous infusion within 72 hours of transplantation, then 100 mg/kg once every 2 weeks for 4 doses, then 50 mg/kg every 4 weeks for 2 doses. The rate of infusion should start at 15 mg/kg per hour increasing to a maximum rate of 60 mg/kg per hour. For recipients of transplants other than kidney, the recommended dosage schedule is 150 mg/kg within 72 hours of transplantation and then once every 2 weeks for 4 further doses, then 100 mg/kg every 4 weeks for 2 doses. Ganciclovir should be given concomitantly.

The name sevirumab is applied to a $\chi$-chain human monoclonal cytomegalovirus immunoglobulin G1.

### Preparations

**Proprietary Preparations** (details are given in Part 3)

***Arg.:*** CytoGam; Megalotect; ***Austral.:*** CMV Immunoglobulin; ***Austria:*** Cytoglobin; Cytotect; ***Canad.:*** CMV Iveegam†; ***Chile:*** Cytotect; ***Fin.:*** Megalotect†; ***Ger.:*** Cytoglobin; Cytotect; ***Gr.:*** Megalotect; ***Hong Kong:*** Cytotect; ***Irl.:*** Megalotect; ***Israel:*** Megalotect; ***Ital.:*** Cytotect; Haimacig†; Immunoendocig; Uman-Cig; ***Port.:*** Megalotect; ***S.Afr.:*** Megalotect; ***Swed.:*** Megalotect†; ***Switz.:*** Cytotect; Globuman iv CMV†; ***Thai.:*** Megalotect; ***USA:*** CytoGam.

## Cytomegalovirus Vaccines

Vacunas contra el citomegalovirus.

### Profile

A live attenuated cytomegalovirus vaccine containing human cytomegalovirus Towne strain has been investigated in humans since the late 1970s, particularly for the prevention of cytomegalovirus infection in renal transplant recipients. However, there are doubts over its safety. Vaccines produced by recombinant technology are also being studied.

◊ In a placebo-controlled study involving 237 renal transplant patients[1] cytomegalovirus vaccine (Towne strain) given subcutaneously had no effect on the overall incidence of cytomegalovirus infection or disease, but there was less severe disease in seronegative recipients who received kidneys from seropositive donors. The vaccine also appeared to prolong graft survival in this subset of patients. However, the Towne vaccine failed to prevent infection in immunocompetent women exposed to infectious young children.[2]

Studies of subunit vaccines have produced some promising results.[3-5]

1. Plotkin SA, *et al.* Effect of Towne live virus vaccine on cytomegalovirus disease after renal transplant. *Ann Intern Med* 1991; **114:** 525–31.
2. Adler SP, *et al.* Immunity induced by primary human cytomegalovirus infection protects against secondary infection among women of childbearing age. *J Infect Dis* 1995; **171:** 26–32.
3. Britt WJ. Vaccines against human cytomegalovirus: time to test. *Trends Microbiol* 1996; **4:** 34–8.
4. Pass RF, *et al.* A subunit cytomegalovirus vaccine based on recombinant envelope glycoprotein B and a new adjuvant. *J Infect Dis* 1999; **180:** 970–5.
5. Frey SE, *et al.* Effects of antigen dose and immunization regimens on antibody responses to a cytomegalovirus glycoprotein B subunit vaccine. *J Infect Dis* 1999; **180:** 1700–3.

## Dengue Fever Vaccines

Vacunas del dengue.

### Profile

Live attenuated vaccines under study for active immunisation against dengue fever contain dengue virus types 1, 2, 3, and 4 alone or in various combinations. The ultimate aim is to produce a vaccine active against all types of dengue virus.

Recombinant vaccines are also under investigation.

◊ References.

1. Velzing J, *et al.* Induction of protective immunity against dengue virus type 2: comparison of candidate live attenuated and recombinant vaccines. *Vaccine* 1999; **17:** 1312–30.
2. Kanesa-Thasan N, *et al.* Safety and immunogenicity of attenuated dengue virus vaccines (Aventis Pasteur) in human volunteers. *Vaccine* 2001; **19:** 3179–88.
3. Rothman AL, *et al.* Induction of T lymphocyte responses to dengue virus by a candidate tetravalent live attenuated dengue virus vaccine. *Vaccine* 2001; **19:** 4694–99.

## Dental Caries Vaccines

Vacunas de la caries dental.

### Profile

Dental caries vaccines consisting of purified proteins from *Streptococcus mutans* are under investigation. Monoclonal antibodies are also being studied for local passive immunisation.

◊ References.

1. Russell MW. Immunization against dental caries. *Curr Opin Dent* 1992; **2:** 72–80.
2. Hajishengallis G, Michalek SM. Current status of a mucosal vaccine against dental caries. *Oral Microbiol Immunol* 1999; **14:** 1–20.
3. Ma JK-C. The caries vaccine: a growing prospect. *Dent Update* 1999; **26:** 374–80.
4. Koga T, *et al.* Immunization against dental caries. *Vaccine* 2002; **20:** 2027–44.

## Diphtheria Antitoxins

Antitoxinas diftéricas.

*ATC — J06AA01.*

**Pharmacopoeias.** Many pharmacopoeias have monographs including *Eur.* (see p.vi).

**Ph. Eur. 5.0** (Diphtheria Antitoxin; Immunoserum Diphthericum). A sterile preparation containing the specific antitoxic globulins that have the power of neutralising the toxin formed by *Corynebacterium diphtheriae*. It has a potency of not less than 1000 international units per mL when obtained from horse serum and not less than 500 international units/mL when obtained from other mammals. It should be stored at 2° to 8°, and not be allowed to freeze.

The BP 2003 states that Dip/Ser may be used on the label.

### Adverse Effects and Precautions

As for antisera in general, p.1605.

### Uses and Administration

Diphtheria antitoxins neutralise the toxin produced by *Corynebacterium diphtheriae* locally at the site of infection and in the circulation.

Diphtheria antitoxin is used for passive immunisation in suspected cases of diphtheria and should be given without waiting for bacteriological confirmation of the infection. An antibacterial is usually given concomitantly (see p.125). Diphtheria antitoxin is generally not used for the prophylaxis of diphtheria because of the risk of provoking a hypersensitivity reaction. Contacts of a diphtheria case should be promptly investigated, given antibacterial prophylaxis and active immunisation with a suitable diphtheria-containing vaccine as appropriate (see p.1612), and kept under observation.

A test dose of diphtheria antitoxin should always be given to exclude hypersensitivity. For the treatment of diphtheria of mild or moderate severity doses of 10 000 to 40 000 units of diphtheria antitoxin may be given intramuscularly; doses of 40 000 to 100 000 units may be given in severe cases. Higher doses have been used in some countries. For doses of more than 40 000 units a portion of the dose is given intramuscularly followed by the bulk of the dose intravenously after about 0.5 to 2 hours.

### Preparations

***Ph. Eur.:*** Diphtheria Antitoxin.

## Diphtheria Vaccines

Vacunas de la difteria.

*ATC — J07AF01.*

**Pharmacopoeias.** Many pharmacopoeias have monographs including *Eur.* (see p.vi).

**Ph. Eur. 5.0** (Diphtheria Vaccine (Adsorbed); Vaccinum Diphtheriae Adsorbatum). A preparation of diphtheria formol toxoid adsorbed on a mineral carrier. The formol toxoid is prepared from the toxin produced by the growth of *Corynebacterium diphtheriae*. The mineral carrier may be hydrated aluminium phosphate or aluminium hydroxide and the resulting mixture is approximately isotonic with blood. The antigenic properties are adversely affected by certain antimicrobial preservatives, particularly those of the phenolic type. It contains not less than 30 international units per dose. It should be stored at 2° to 8°, not be allowed to freeze, and be protected from light.

The BP 2003 states that Dip/Vac/Ads(Child) may be used on the label.

The BP 2003 gives Adsorbed Diphtheria Prophylactic as an approved synonym.

**Ph. Eur. 5.0** (Diphtheria Vaccine (Adsorbed) for Adults and Adolescents; Vaccinum Diphtheriae Adulti et Adulescentis Adsorbatum). It is an adsorbed diphtheria vaccine containing not less than 2 international units per dose.

The BP 2003 states that for a vaccine for use in the UK, the amount of toxoid used is adjusted so that the final vaccine contains not more than 2.0 Limes flocculationis (Lf) per dose.

The BP 2003 states that Dip/Vac/Ads(Adults) may be used on the label.

### Adverse Effects and Precautions

As for vaccines in general, p.1605.

Local reactions may occur but are generally not severe in young children; the frequency and severity of reactions is reported to be less in children under 2 years of age than in older children and adults.

If diphtheria vaccines or vaccines containing a diphtheria component need to be given to children over the age of 10 years or to adults, vaccines with a reduced content of diphtheria toxoid and intended for adults and adolescents should be used. For further details see under Uses and Administration, below.

### Uses and Administration

Diphtheria vaccines are used for active immunisation against diphtheria. The non-adsorbed vaccine has poor immunogenic properties and its effects are enhanced by administration as an adsorbed preparation. For primary immunisation combined diphtheria vaccines are usually used. A single-component diphtheria vaccine has sometimes been used, for example in the event of contact with an infected patient or a carrier. For discussion of immunisation schedules, see under Vaccines, p.1606.

For primary immunisation, three doses of a combined vaccine are given at intervals of one month. For children who receive primary immunisation during infancy reinforcing doses should be given at school entry (preferably at least 3 years after primary immunisation) and again on leaving school.

Individuals coming into contact with a case of diphtheria or carriers of a toxigenic strain, or those travelling to an endemic or epidemic area should receive a complete primary course or a reinforcing dose according to age and immunisation history; those not previously immunised should receive a 3-dose primary course using the appropriate vaccine as outlined above, those previously immunised should receive a single 0.5 mL dose. Unimmunised contacts of a case of diphtheria should in addition receive a prophylactic course of a suitable antibacterial (see p.125). Individuals at repeated risk of exposure to infection may be offered booster doses every 10 years.

Schick testing (p.1742) to ascertain immune status is no longer considered necessary before administering diphtheria vaccine to adults provided that a low dose is given; antibody testing is used to check immunity in those regularly exposed to diphtheria.

In some countries, booster doses of diphtheria in combination with tetanus vaccine are recommended every 10 years (see under Diphtheria and Tetanus Vaccines, p.1613).

Conjugation to diphtheria toxoid has been used to increase the immunogenicity of other vaccines (see Haemophilus Influenzae Vaccines, p.1616).

### Preparations

***Ph. Eur.:*** Diphtheria Vaccine (Adsorbed); Diphtheria Vaccine (Adsorbed) for Adults and Adolescents.

**Proprietary Preparations** (details are given in Part 3)

***Ital.:*** H-Adiftal†; ***NZ:*** Di Anatoxal; ***Switz.:*** Anatoxal Di†.

## Diphtheria and Tetanus Vaccines

Vacunas de la difteria y el tétanos.

*ATC — J07AM51.*

**Pharmacopoeias.** Many pharmacopoeias have monographs including *Eur.* (see p.vi) and *US*.

**Ph. Eur. 5.0** (Diphtheria and Tetanus Vaccine (Adsorbed); Vaccinum Diphtheriae et Tetani Adsorbatum). A preparation of diphtheria formol toxoid and tetanus formol toxoid adsorbed on a mineral carrier. The mineral carrier may be hydrated aluminium phosphate or aluminium hydroxide and the resulting mixture is approximately isotonic with blood. The antigenic properties are adversely affected by certain antimicrobial preservatives particularly those of the phenolic type. It contains not less than 30 international units of diphtheria toxoid and not less than 40 international units of tetanus toxoid per dose. It should be stored at 2° to 8°, not be allowed to freeze, and be protected from light.

The BP 2003 states that DT/Vac/Ads(Child) may be used on the label.

The BP 2003 gives Adsorbed Diphtheria-Tetanus Prophylactic as an approved synonym.

**Ph. Eur. 5.0** (Diphtheria and Tetanus Vaccine (Adsorbed) for Adults and Adolescents; Vaccinum Diphtheriae et Tetani Adulti et Adulescentis Adsorbatum). It is diphtheria and tetanus vaccine (adsorbed) containing not less than 2 units of diphtheria toxoid and not less than 20 units of tetanus toxoid per dose.

The BP 2003 states that for a vaccine for use in the UK, the amount of diphtheria toxoid used is adjusted so that the final vaccine contains not more than 2.0 Limes flocculationis (Lf) of diphtheria toxoid per dose.

The BP 2003 states that DT/Vac/Ads(Adult) may be used on the label.

**USP 27** (Diphtheria and Tetanus Toxoids Adsorbed). A sterile suspension prepared by mixing suitable quantities of plain or adsorbed diphtheria toxoid and plain or adsorbed tetanus toxoid and, if plain toxoids are used, an aluminium adsorbing agent. The antigenicity or potency and the proportions of the toxoids are such as to provide an immunising dose of each toxoid in the labelled dose. It should be stored at 2° to 8° and not be allowed to freeze.

**USP 27** (Tetanus and Diphtheria Toxoids Adsorbed for Adult Use). A sterile suspension prepared by mixing suitable quantities of adsorbed diphtheria toxoid and adsorbed tetanus toxoid using the same precipitating or adsorbing agent for both toxoids. The antigenicity or potency and the proportions of the toxoids are such as to provide, in the labelled dose, an immunising dose of adsorbed tetanus toxoid and one-tenth of the immunising dose of adsorbed diphtheria toxoid specified for children and not more than 2 Lf of diphtheria toxoid. It should be stored at 2° to 8° and not be allowed to freeze.

### Adverse Effects and Precautions

As for vaccines in general, p.1605. See also under Diphtheria Vaccines, p.1612, and Tetanus Vaccines, p.1640. Diphtheria and tetanus vaccines are reported to produce fewer adverse effects than diphtheria, tetanus, and pertussis vaccines (see under Adverse Effects, p.1614).

**Dose-related effects.** A high incidence of adverse effects was reported in teenagers inadvertently given a high-dose diphtheria and tetanus vaccine intended for use in infants.[1] Most reactions were classified as mild or moderately severe, but severe local or systemic reactions occurred in a third of those reporting reactions.

1. Sidebotham PD, Lenton SW. Incidence of adverse reactions after administration of high dose diphtheria with tetanus vaccine to school leavers: retrospective questionnaire study. *BMJ* 1996; **313:** 533–4.

**Effects on the nervous system.** Encephalopathy more commonly follows vaccination with diphtheria, tetanus, and pertussis vaccine than with diphtheria and tetanus vaccine (p.1614). Several cases of encephalopathy occurred in a small region in Italy in children following immunisation against diphtheria and tetanus,[1] although it was not possible to infer a causal relationship. A case of polyradiculoneuritis has been reported in a patient following the use of a diphtheria-tetanus vaccine and was considered most likely to have been due to the tetanus component.[2]

1. Greco D. Case-control study on encephalopathy associated with diphtheria-tetanus immunization in Campania, Italy. *Bull WHO* 1985; **63:** 919–25.
2. Holliday PL, Bauer RB. Polyradiculoneuritis secondary to immunization with tetanus and diphtheria toxoids. *Arch Neurol* 1983; **40:** 56–7.

GUILLAIN-BARRÉ SYNDROME. Evidence mainly from case reports and uncontrolled studies favoured a causal relationship between vaccination with diphtheria and tetanus vaccines or single-antigen tetanus vaccines and Guillain-Barré syndrome. The data came primarily from immunocompromised patients.[1]

1. Stratton KR, *et al.* Adverse events associated with childhood vaccines other than pertussis and rubella: summary of a report from the Institute of Medicine. *JAMA* 1994; **271:** 1602–5.

### Uses and Administration

Combined adsorbed diphtheria and tetanus vaccines are used for active immunisation against diphtheria and tetanus; they are used in some countries for reinforcing doses following primary immunisation. For discussion of immunisation schedules, see under Vaccines, p.1606.

The non-adsorbed combined diphtheria and tetanus vaccines have weaker immunogenic properties than adsorbed vaccines and are no longer recommended.

**Booster doses.** In some countries, booster doses of combined diphtheria and tetanus vaccines are recommended every 10 years, and studies have been conducted to assess whether this is necessary. Since the incidence of clinical diphtheria in many countries in western Europe and North America approaches zero, it had been considered that there was no need for booster doses in adults, despite low antibody titres, so long as the policy of immunisation during infancy was maintained.[1,2] However, following a report[3] of an outbreak of clinical diphtheria in Sweden after a period of many years during which no indigenous cases of diphtheria had occurred and the disease was regarded as being eliminated from the country, the question of immunity in adults and the need for revaccination again arose. In the USA, it was considered[4] that re-immunisation every 10 years with a diphtheria and tetanus combined vaccine was mandatory and that this combined vaccine should be used whenever a tetanus vaccine was indicated as in treating emergency wounds. Outbreaks of diphtheria in Russia and neighbouring countries[5] have prompted recommendations for booster doses in travellers to these countries.

A study has shown that an intranasal formulation could produce an adequate booster response and may be advantageous in some patients.[6]

1. Mathias RG, Schechter MT. Booster immunisation for diphtheria and tetanus: no evidence of need in adults. *Lancet* 1985; **i:** 1089–91.
2. Anonymous. Diphtheria and tetanus boosters. *Lancet* 1985; **i:** 1081–2.
3. Rappuoli R, *et al.* Molecular epidemiology of the 1984–1986 outbreak of diphtheria in Sweden. *N Engl J Med* 1988; **318:** 12–14.
4. Karzon DT, Edwards KM. Diphtheria outbreaks in immunized populations. *N Engl J Med* 1988; **318:** 41–3.
5. Anonymous. Diphtheria immunisation—advice from the Chief Medical Officer. *Commun Dis Rep* 1993; **3:** 27.
6. Aggerbeck H, *et al.* Intranasal booster vaccination against diphtheria and tetanus in man. *Vaccine* 1997; **15:** 307–16.

### Preparations

***Ph. Eur.:*** Diphtheria and Tetanus Vaccine (Adsorbed); Diphtheria and Tetanus Vaccine (Adsorbed) for Adults and Adolescents;
***USP 27:*** Diphtheria and Tetanus Toxoids Adsorbed; Tetanus and Diphtheria Toxoids Adsorbed for Adult Use.

**Proprietary Preparations** (details are given in Part 3)

***Arg.:*** Diftavax; DT Vax; Vacuna Doble; ***Austral.:*** ADT; CDT; ***Austria:*** Anatoxal Di Te; Ditanrix†; DT-reduct; Td-pur; ***Belg.:*** Anatoxal Di Te†; Ditemer; Tedivax; ***Braz.:*** DT Vax; Refortrix; Vacina Dupla DT†; ***Denm.:*** DiTe Booster; ***Fin.:*** DiTe Booster; ***Fr.:*** Diftavax†; DT Bis†; ***Ger.:*** DT-Impfstoff; DT-Rix†; DT-Vaccinol†; Td-Impfstoff; Td-pur; Td-Rix; Td-Vaccinol†; ***Gr.:*** Anatoxal Di Te Berna; D.T.Vax Adsorbe; ***Hong Kong:*** Adsorbed DT Vax†; DiTe Anatoxal; ***India:*** Dual Antigen; ***Irl.:*** Diftavax; ***Ital.:*** Anatoxal Di Te; Dif-Tet-All; Diftavax; Ditanrix; H-Adiftetal†; Imovax DT†; Vaccino Difto Tetano†; ***NZ:*** ADT†; CDT†; DiTe Anatoxal; ***Port.:*** Anatoxal Di Te†; ***S.Afr.:*** DT Vax; ***Singapore:*** Di Te Anatoxal†; ***Spain:*** Anatoxal Di Te; Anatoxal Te Di; Diftavax; Ditanrix; Divacuna DT†; TD; ***Swed.:*** DiTe Booster; Duplex†; ***Switz.:*** Anatoxal Di Te; Ditanrix; ***Thai.:*** Di Te Anatoxal; Dif-Tet-All; DT Vax; ***UK:*** Diftavax.

## Diphtheria, Tetanus, and Haemophilus Influenzae Vaccines

Vacunas de la difteria, el tétanos y Haemophilus influenzae.

### Profile

Combined adsorbed diphtheria, tetanus, and *Haemophilus influenzae* type b vaccines have been used in some countries for active immunisation of infants. For discussion of immunisation schedules see under Vaccines, p.1606. For concern over the antigenicity of *Haemophilus influenzae* type b vaccine in combined vaccines, see under Haemophilus Influenzae Vaccines, Interactions, p.1616.

### Preparations

**Proprietary Preparations** (details are given in Part 3)
***Ger.:*** HIB-DT†.

## Diphtheria, Tetanus, and Hepatitis B Vaccines

*ATC — J07CA07.*

**Pharmacopoeias.** Many pharmacopoeias have monographs including *Eur.* (see p.vi).

**Ph. Eur. 5.0** ( Diphtheria, Tetanus, and Hepatitis B (rDNA) Vaccine (Adsorbed); Vaccinum Diphtheriae, Tetani et Hepatitidis B (ADNr) Adsorbatum). A combined vaccine composed of diphtheria formol toxoid, tetanus formol toxoid, hepatitis B surface antigen, and a mineral carrier such as aluminium hydroxide or hydrated aluminium phosphate. It should be stored at 2° to 8°, not be allowed to freeze, and be protected from light.

### Profile

Combined diphtheria, tetanus, and hepatitis B vaccines have been used in some countries for active immunisation.

### Preparations

***Ph. Eur.:*** Diphtheria, Tetanus and Hepatitis B (rDNA) Vaccine (Adsorbed).

**Proprietary Preparations** (details are given in Part 3)
***Ital.:*** Primavax†.

## Diphtheria, Tetanus, and Pertussis Vaccines

Vacunas de la difteria, el tétanos y la tos ferina.

**Pharmacopoeias.** Many pharmacopoeias have monographs including *Eur.* (see p.vi).

**Ph. Eur. 5.0** (Diphtheria, Tetanus and Pertussis Vaccine (Adsorbed); Vaccinum Diphtheriae, Tetani et Pertussis Adsorbatum). A preparation of diphtheria formol toxoid and tetanus formol toxoid on a mineral carrier to which a suspension of killed *Bordetella pertussis* has been added. The mineral carrier may be hydrated aluminium phosphate or aluminium hydroxide and the resulting mixture is approximately isotonic with blood. The antigenic properties are adversely affected by certain antimicrobial preservatives particularly those of the phenolic type. It contains not less than 30 international units of diphtheria toxoid, not less than 40 international units if the test is performed in *guinea-pigs*, or 60 international units if the test is performed in *mice*, of tetanus toxoid, and not less than 4 international units of the pertussis component per dose. It should be stored at 2° to 8°, not be allowed to freeze, and be protected from light.

The BP 2003 states that DTPer/Vac/Ads may be used on the label.

The BP 2003 gives Adsorbed Diphtheria–Tetanus–Whooping-cough Prophylactic as an approved synonym.

**Ph. Eur. 5.0** (Diphtheria, Tetanus and Pertussis (Acellular, Component) Vaccine (Adsorbed); Vaccinum Diphtheriae, Tetani et Pertussis Sine Cellulis ex Elementis Praeparatum Adsorbatum). A combined vaccine composed of diphtheria formol toxoid, tetanus formol toxoid, individually purified antigenic components of *Bordetella pertussis*, and a mineral carrier such as aluminium hydroxide or hydrated aluminium phosphate. It should be stored at 2° to 8°, not be allowed to freeze, and be protected from light.

### Adverse Effects and Precautions

As for vaccines in general, p.1605. See also under Diphtheria Vaccines, p.1612, Pertussis Vaccines, p.1631, and Tetanus Vaccines, p.1640.

The incidence of local reactions and fever is reported to be lower with accelerated immunisation schedules than schedules spreading primary immunisation over 6 months. Local reactions and pyrexia occur less commonly after acellular pertussis vaccines, especially in children older than 6 months.

In infants with a personal or close family history of seizures, precautions should be taken to avoid pyrexia. See under Pertussis Vaccines for further details of precautions and contra-indications in individuals with a history of neurological problems.

As with other vaccines, immunisation should not be carried out in individuals with a definite history of severe reactions. However, in individuals with a history of a less severe general reaction to a preceding dose, immunisation should be completed using diphtheria and tetanus vaccine; acellular pertussis vaccine can be used if the previous reaction was a local one.

◊ Local and systemic reactions are more common following diphtheria, tetanus, and pertussis (DTP) vaccines than diphtheria and tetanus (DT) vaccines. However, they are generally mild and self-limiting.[1] Infrequently, high fever, persistent or inconsolable crying (possibly as a reaction to pain), hypotonic-hyporesponsive collapse, or short-lived convulsions (frequently febrile convulsions) may occur, and have been reported after both DT and DTP vaccines.[2] These reactions do not appear to have any long-term consequences.[1] Rare but serious acute neurological complications including encephalopathy and prolonged seizures have been reported after DTP and have been attributed to the whole-cell pertussis component (see Effects on the Nervous System, p.1631) but the association could be coincidental. Epidemiological studies have shown that such events are exceedingly rare and only occasionally followed by long-term neurological damage. Analysis of these studies has been difficult but the National Vaccine Advisory Committee and the Advisory Committee on Immunization Practices[1] concluded that the evidence was insufficient for a link, and this was also the view of the Department of Health Joint Committee on Vaccination and Immunisation in the UK.[2]

The risk of febrile convulsions following DTP vaccination is reported not to be increased in children immunised before 6 months of age,[2] but there appears to be an increased risk beyond this. Children with a personal or close family history of epilepsy may also be at increased risk of seizures after DTP vaccination. Current recommendations are that immunisation should be given to children with stable neurological conditions, using precautions (such as paracetamol administration and tepid sponging) to prevent pyrexia.

Children experiencing a seizure during the course of immunisation should be carefully assessed before deciding whether to continue immunisation with DTP or DT vaccine. A causal relationship between DTP vaccination and sudden infant death syndrome (SIDS) has not been established and any temporal relationship is likely to be due to chance.[3,4] There is evidence that the risk of SIDS is lower in infants who have been vaccinated.[5]

Immediate anaphylactic reactions have been reported and are regarded as a contra-indication to further use of DTP vaccine. However, the appearance of a rash is not generally regarded as a contra-indication to further doses.

1. Centers for Disease Control. Update: vaccine side effects, adverse reactions, contraindications, and precautions: recommendations of the Advisory Committee on Immunization Practices (ACIP). *MMWR* 1996; **45** (RR-12): 1–45.
2. Department of Health. *Immunisation against infectious disease* 1996: "The Green Book". Available at: http://www.dh.gov.uk/PublicationsAndStatistics/Publications/PublicationsPolicyAndGuidance/PublicationsPolicyAndGuidanceArticle/fs/en?CONTENT_ID=4072977&chk=87uz6M (accessed 12/08/04)
3. Hoffman HJ, *et al.* Diphtheria-tetanus-pertussis immunization and sudden infant death: results of the National Institute of Child Health and Human Development Cooperative Epidemiological Study of Sudden Infant Death Syndrome Risk Factors. *Pediatrics* 1987; **79:** 598–611.
4. Griffin MR, *et al.* Risk of sudden infant death syndrome after immunization with the diphtheria-tetanus-pertussis vaccine. *N Engl J Med* 1988; **319:** 618–23.
5. Mitchell EA, *et al.* Immunisation and the sudden infant death syndrome. *Arch Dis Child* 1995; **73:** 498–501.

## Interactions

As for vaccines in general, p.1606.

For a report of a diminished immune response to the pertussis component of diphtheria, tetanus, and pertussis vaccine when mixed with inactivated poliomyelitis vaccine, see Pertussis Vaccines, p.1632.

For a report of a diminished immune response to *Haemophilus influenzae* conjugated vaccine when mixed with diphtheria, tetanus, and acellular pertussis vaccine, see Haemophilus Influenzae Vaccines, p.1616.

## Uses and Administration

Combined diphtheria, tetanus, and pertussis vaccines are used for active immunisation of children against diphtheria, tetanus, and pertussis (whooping cough). For discussion of immunisation schedules see below.

Combined adsorbed vaccines may be given by deep subcutaneous or intramuscular injection (vaccines with acellular pertussis components are for intramuscular injection only) in usual doses of 0.5 mL. In the USA a vaccine with an acellular pertussis component is used and three doses are given at intervals of 2 months, a fourth dose at least 6 months after the third, and a fifth dose at school entry.

For a discussion of vaccines containing an acellular pertussis component rather than the standard whole-cell component, which are now preferred in some countries, see under Uses and Administration of Pertussis Vaccines, p.1632. The non-adsorbed type of combined diphtheria, tetanus, and pertussis vaccines have weaker immunogenic properties than adsorbed vaccines and are no longer recommended.

## Preparations

**Ph. Eur.:** Diphtheria, Tetanus and Pertussis (Acellular, Component) Vaccine (Adsorbed); Diphtheria, Tetanus and Pertussis Vaccine (Adsorbed).

**Proprietary Preparations** (details are given in Part 3)

***Arg.:*** Bustrix; Triacel; Vacuna Triple; ***Austral.:*** Boostrix; Infanrix; Tripacel; Triple Antigen†; ***Austria:*** Anatoxal Di Te Per; Boostrix; Infanrix; ***Belg.:*** Boostrix; Combivax†; Infanrix; Triamer; ***Braz.:*** DTCoq/DTP; DTP†; Infanrix; Pertacel; Vacina Triplice DPT†; ***Canad.:*** Adacel; Tri-Immunol†; Tripacel†; ***Fin.:*** Boostrix; Di-Te-Kik; Infanrix; ***Fr.:*** DT Coq†; ***Ger.:*** Boostrix; Covaxis; DPT Merieux†; DPT-Impfstoff†; DPT-Vaccinol†; DTP-Rix†; Infanrix; ***Gr.:*** Di-Te-Per Anatoxal; Infanrix; ***Hong Kong:*** Adsorbed DT Coq; Di Te Per Anatoxal†; Infanrix; Tripacel; Triple Antigen; ***India:*** Tripvac; ***Irl.:*** Infanrix; Trivax-AD†; Trivax†; ***Israel:*** Acelluvax DTP; Boostrix; DTCoq/DTP; Infanrix; ***Ital.:*** Adifteper†; Anatoxal Di Te Per†; Boostrix; Dif-Per-Tet-All†; Imovax DTP†; Infanrix; Triacelluvax†; Tritanrix†; Vaccino DPT†; ***Malaysia:*** Infanrix; Tripacel; ***Mex.:*** Infanrix; ***Norw.:*** Boostrix; Infanrix†; ***NZ:*** Boostrix; DiTePer Anatoxal†; Infanrix†; Tripacel; ***Port.:*** Anatoxal Di Te Per†; Infanrix; ***S.Afr.:*** DTP-Merieux; ***Singapore:*** Di Te Per Anatoxal†; Infanrix; Tripacel; ***Spain:*** Anatoxal Di Te Per; Boostrix; DTP-Merieux; Infanrix; Trivacuna†; ***Swed.:*** Di-Te-Kik; Infanrix; ***Switz.:*** Acel-Imune†; Anatoxal Di Te Per†; Boostrix; Infanrix DTPa; ***Thai.:*** Acelluvax DTP†; Di Te Per Anatoxal†; Dif-Per-Tet-All†; DTCoq/DTP; Infanrix; Tripacel; ***UK:*** Infanrix; Trivax-AD; ***USA:*** Acel-Imune†; Certiva†; Daptacel; Infanrix; Tri-Immunol†; Tripedia.

# Diphtheria, Tetanus, Pertussis, and Haemophilus Influenzae Vaccines

Vacunas de la difteria, el tétanos, la tos ferina y Haemophilus influenzae.

**Pharmacopoeias.** Many pharmacopoeias have monographs including *Eur.* (see p.vi).

**Ph. Eur. 5.0** (Diphtheria, Tetanus, Pertussis (Acellular, Component) and Haemophilus type b Conjugate Vaccine (Adsorbed); Vaccinum Diphtheriae, Tetani, Pertussis Sine Cellulis ex Elementis Praeparatum et Haemophili Stirpe b Conjugatum Adsorbatum). A combined vaccine composed of diphtheria formol toxoid, tetanus formol toxoid, individually purified antigenic components of *Bordetella pertussis*, polyribosylribitol phosphate derived from a suitable strain of *Haemophilus influenzae* type b and covalently bound to a carrier protein, and a mineral carrier such as aluminium hydroxide or hydrated aluminium phosphate. The product may be presented with the Haemophilus type b component in a separate container, the contents of which are mixed with the other components immediately before use. It should be stored at 2° to 8°, not be allowed to freeze, and be protected from light.

## Adverse Effects and Precautions

As for vaccines in general, p.1605.

## Interactions

As for vaccines in general, p.1606.

## Uses and Administration

Combined adsorbed diphtheria, tetanus, whole-cell or acellular pertussis, and *Haemophilus influenzae* type b vaccines are available in some countries for active immunisation of infants. For discussion of immunisation schedules, see under Vaccines, p.1606.

Some combined vaccines are not licensed for use in primary immunisation regimens because of concerns over the response to the *Haemophilus influenzae* type b component (see under Interactions of Haemophilus Influenzae Vaccines, p.1616).

## Preparations

**Ph. Eur.:** Diphtheria, Tetanus, Pertussis (Acellular, Component) and Haemophilus Type b Conjugate Vaccine (Adsorbed); Diphtheria, Tetanus, Pertussis (Acellular, Component), Poliomyelitis (Inactivated) and Haemophilus Type b Conjugate Vaccine (Adsorbed); Diphtheria, Tetanus, Pertussis, Poliomyelitis (Inactivated) and Haemophilus Type b Conjugate Vaccine (Adsorbed).

**Proprietary Preparations** (details are given in Part 3)

***Arg.:*** Actacel; ***Austral.:*** Infanrix Hib; ***Austria:*** Act-HIB plus DPT; Infanrix + Hib; ***Belg.:*** Infanrix + Hib; Tetract-HIB†; ***Braz.:*** Tetract-HIB; ***Canad.:*** Tetramune†; ***Chile:*** Actacel; Tetract-HIB; ***Ger.:*** HIB-DPT†; Infanrix + Hib; ***Hong Kong:*** Tetramune†; ***Israel:*** Infanrix Hib; Tetract-HIB; ***Ital.:*** Tetract-HIB†; ***Malaysia:*** Tetract-HIB; ***Mex.:*** Tetramune†; ***NZ:*** Infanrix Hib; Tetramune†; ***S.Afr.:*** Combact-HIB; TetraTITER†; ***Singapore:*** Actacel; Infanrix Hib; Tetract-HIB; Tetramune†; ***Spain:*** Infanrix Hib; Tetract-HIB; ***Switz.:*** Infanrix DTPa-Hib; Tetramune†; ***Thai.:*** Actacel; Tetract-HIB; ***UK:*** Act-HIB DTP; Infanrix Hib; Trivax-Hib†; ***USA:*** Tetramune†; TriHIBit.

# Diphtheria, Tetanus, Pertussis, Haemophilus Influenzae, and Hepatitis B Vaccines

## Profile

Combined diphtheria, tetanus, pertussis, Haemophilus influenzae, and hepatitis B vaccines are available in some countries for active immunisation.

## Preparations

**Proprietary Preparations** (details are given in Part 3)

***Arg.:*** Tritanrix HB-HIB; ***Mex.:*** Tritanrix HB/Hiberix.

# Diphtheria, Tetanus, Pertussis, and Hepatitis B Vaccines

Vacunas de la difteria, el tétanos, la tos ferina y la hepatitis B.

*ATC — J07CA05.*

**Pharmacopoeias.** Many pharmacopoeias have monographs including *Eur.* (see p.vi).

**Ph. Eur. 5.0** (Diphtheria, Tetanus, Pertussis (Acellular, Component) and Hepatitis B (rDNA) Vaccine (Adsorbed); Vaccinum Diphtheriae, Tetani, Pertussis Sine Cellulis ex Elementis Praeparatum et Hepatitidis B (ADNr) Adsorbatum). A combined vaccine composed of diphtheria formol toxoid, tetanus formol toxoid, individually purified antigenic components of *Bordetella pertussis*, hepatitis B surface antigen, and a mineral carrier such as aluminium hydroxide or hydrated aluminium phosphate. It should be stored at 2° to 8°, not be allowed to freeze, and be protected from light.

## Profile

Combined diphtheria, tetanus, pertussis, and hepatitis B vaccines are available in some countries for active immunisation.

## Preparations

**Ph. Eur.:** Diphtheria, Tetanus, Pertussis (Acellular, Component) and Hepatitis B (rDNA) Vaccine (Adsorbed).

**Proprietary Preparations** (details are given in Part 3)

***Austral.:*** Infanrix HepB; ***Braz.:*** Infanrix DTPa HB†; ***Fin.:*** Infanrix HepB; ***Gr.:*** Infanrix HepB; ***India:*** Tritanrix HB; ***Ital.:*** Infanrix HepB; ***Malaysia:*** Tritanrix HB; ***NZ:*** Infanrix HepB; ***S.Afr.:*** Infanrix HB; ***Spain:*** Infanrix HepB; Tritanrix HB; ***Swed.:*** Infanrix HepB; ***Switz.:*** Infanrix DTPa-HepB†; ***Thai.:*** Tritanrix HB.

# Diphtheria, Tetanus, Pertussis, Hepatitis B, Poliomyelitis, and Haemophilus Influenzae Vaccines

*ATC — J07CA09.*

**Pharmacopoeias.** Many pharmacopoeias have monographs including *Eur.* (see p.vi).

**Ph. Eur. 5.0** ( Diphtheria, Tetanus, Pertussis (Acellular, Component), Hepatitis B (rDNA), Poliomyelitis (Inactivated) and Haemophilus type b Conjugate Vaccine (Adsorbed); Vaccinum Diphtheriae, Tetani, Pertussis Sine Cellulis ex Elementis Praeparatum, Hepatitidis B (ADNr), Poliomyelitidis Inactivatum et Haemophili Stirpe b Coniugatum Adsorbatum). A combined vaccine composed of diphtheria formol toxoid, tetanus formol toxoid, individually purified antigenic components of *Bordetella pertussis*, hepatitis B surface antigen, suitable strains of human polioviruses type 1, 2, and 3 grown in suitable cell cultures and inactivated by a validated method, polyribosylribitol phosphate derived from a suitable strain of *Haemophilus influenzae* type b and covalently bound to a carrier protein, and a mineral carrier such as aluminium hydroxide or hydrated aluminium phosphate. The product may be presented with the Haemophilus type b component in a separate container, the contents of which are mixed with the other components immediately before or during use. It should be stored at 2° to 8°, not be allowed to freeze, and be protected from light.

## Profile

A combined diphtheria, tetanus, pertussis, hepatitis B, poliomyelitis, and Haemophilus influenzae vaccine is available in some countries for active immunisation.

◊ References.

1. Curran MP, Goa KL. DTPa-HBV-IPV/Hib vaccine (Infanrix hexa™) *Drugs* 2003; **63:** 673–82.

## Preparations

**Ph. Eur.:** Diphtheria, Tetanus, Pertussis (Acellular, Component), Hepatitis B (rDNA), Poliomyelitis (Inactivated) and Haemophilus Type b Conjugate Vaccine (Adsorbed).

**Proprietary Preparations** (details are given in Part 3)

***Arg.:*** Hexavac; Infanrix Hexa; ***Belg.:*** Infanrix Hexa; ***Chile:*** Infanrix Hexa; ***Fin.:*** Infanrix Hexa; ***Fr.:*** Hexavac; Infanrix Hexa; Infanrixhexa; ***Ger.:*** Hexavac; Infanrix Hexa; ***Gr.:*** Hexavac; Infanrix Hexa; ***Ital.:*** Hexavac; Infanrix Hexa; ***Spain:*** Hexavac; Infanrix Hexa; ***Swed.:*** Infanrix Hexa; ***Switz.:*** Hexavac; Infanrix Hexa.

## Diphtheria, Tetanus, Pertussis, and Poliomyelitis Vaccines

Vacunas de la difteria, el tétanos, la tos ferina y la poliomielitis.

*ATC — J07CA02.*

**Pharmacopoeias.** Many pharmacopoeias have monographs including *Eur.* (see p.vi).

**Ph. Eur. 5.0** (Diphtheria, Tetanus, Pertussis (Acellular, Component) and Poliomyelitis (Inactivated) Vaccine (Adsorbed); Vaccinum Diphtheriae, Tetani, Pertussis Sine Cellulis ex Elementis Praeparatum et Poliomyelitidis Inactivatum Adsorbatum). A combined vaccine containing diphtheria formol toxoid, tetanus formol toxoid, individually purified antigenic components of *Bordetella pertussis*, suitable strains of human polioviruses type 1, 2, and 3 grown in suitable cell cultures and inactivated by a validated method, and a mineral carrier such as aluminium hydroxide or hydrated aluminium phosphate. It should be stored at 2° to 8°, not be allowed to freeze, and be protected from light.

**Ph. Eur. 5.0** (Diphtheria, Tetanus, Pertussis and Poliomyelitis (Inactivated) Vaccine (Adsorbed); Vaccinum Diphtheriae, Tetani, Pertussis et Poliomyelitidis Inactivatum Adsorbatum). A combined vaccine containing diphtheria formol toxoid, tetanus formol toxoid, an inactivated suspension of *Bordetella pertussis*, suitable strains of human polioviruses type 1, 2, and 3 grown in suitable cell cultures and inactivated by a validated method, and a mineral carrier such as aluminium hydroxide or hydrated aluminium phosphate. It should be stored at 2° to 8°, not be allowed to freeze, and be protected from light.

### Adverse Effects and Precautions

As for vaccines in general, p.1605.

See also under Diphtheria Vaccines, p.1612, Diphtheria, Tetanus, and Pertussis Vaccines, p.1613, Pertussis Vaccines, p.1631, and Tetanus Vaccines, p.1641.

### Uses and Administration

A combined diphtheria, tetanus, pertussis (acellular component), and poliomyelitis (inactivated) vaccine is used for active immunisation. For discussion of immunisation schedules see under Vaccines, p.1606.

In the UK it is given by intramuscular injection in a single dose (usually 0.5 mL) as a booster at pre-school age (3 years 4 months to 5 years).

### Preparations

***Ph. Eur.:*** Diphtheria, Tetanus, Pertussis (Acellular, Component) and Poliomyelitis (Inactivated) Vaccine (Adsorbed); Diphtheria, Tetanus, Pertussis and Poliomyelitis (Inactivated) Vaccine (Adsorbed).

**Proprietary Preparations** (details are given in Part 3)
***Belg.:*** Infanrix IPV; Tetracoq; Tetravac; ***Braz.:*** Tetracoq; ***Canad.:*** Quadracel; ***Denm.:*** Di-Te-Ki-Pol; ***Fin.:*** Di-Te-Ki-Pol; ***Fr.:*** Infanrixtetra; Tetracoq†; Tetravac; Vaccin DTCP†; ***Ger.:*** Quatro-Virelon; Repevax; Tetravac; ***Gr.:*** Tetravac; ***Hong Kong:*** Tetracoq†; ***Irl.:*** Tetravac; ***Israel:*** Tetracoq; ***Ital.:*** Tetravac; ***Malaysia:*** Tetracoq; ***NZ:*** Infanrix IPV; ***Swed.:*** Di-Te-Ki-Pol; DTap-IPV†; ***Switz.:*** DiTePerPol Vaccin†; Infanrix DTPa-IPV; Tetravac; ***Thai.:*** Tetracoq; ***UK:*** Repevax.

## Diphtheria, Tetanus, Pertussis, Poliomyelitis, and Haemophilus Influenzae Vaccines

Vacunas de la difteria, el tétanos, la tos ferina, la poliomielitis y Haemophilus influenzae.

*ATC — J07CA06.*

**Pharmacopoeias.** Many pharmacopoeias have monographs including *Eur.* (see p.vi).

**Ph. Eur. 5.0** (Diphtheria, Tetanus, Pertussis (Acellular, Component), Poliomyelitis (Inactivated) and Haemophilus type b Conjugate Vaccine (Adsorbed); Vaccinum Diphtheriae, Tetani, Pertussis Sine Cellulis ex Elementis Praeparatum Poliomyelitidis Inactivatum et Haemophili Stirpe b Conjugatum Adsorbatum). A combined vaccine composed of diphtheria formol toxoid, tetanus formol toxoid, individually purified antigenic components of *Bordetella pertussis*, suitable strains of human polioviruses type 1, 2, and 3 grown in suitable cell cultures and inactivated by a validated method, polyribosylribitol phosphate derived from a suitable strain of *Haemophilus influenzae* type b and covalently bound to a carrier protein, and a mineral carrier such as aluminium hydroxide or hydrated aluminium phosphate. The product is presented with the Haemophilus type b component in a separate container, the contents of which are mixed with the other components immediately before use. It should be stored at 2° to 8°, not be allowed to freeze, and be protected from light.

**Ph. Eur. 5.0** (Diphtheria, Tetanus, Pertussis, Poliomyelitis (Inactivated) and Haemophilus type b Conjugate Vaccine (Adsorbed); Vaccinum Diphtheriae, Tetani, Pertussis, Poliomyelitidis Inactivatum et Haemophili Stirpe b Conjugatum Adsorbatum). A combined vaccine composed of diphtheria formol toxoid, tetanus formol toxoid, an inactivated suspension of *Bordetella pertussis*, suitable strains of human polioviruses type 1, 2, and 3 grown in suitable cell cultures and inactivated by a validated method, polyribosylribitol phosphate derived from a suitable strain of *Haemophilus influenzae* type b and covalently bound to a carrier protein, and a mineral carrier such as aluminium hydroxide or hydrated aluminium phosphate. The product is presented with the Haemophilus type b component in a separate container, the contents of which are mixed with the other components immediately before use. It should be stored at 2° to 8°, not be allowed to freeze, and be protected from light.

### Adverse Effects and Precautions

As for vaccines in general, p.1605.

See also under Diphtheria Vaccines, p.1612, Diphtheria, Tetanus, and Pertussis Vaccines, p.1613, Haemophilus Influenzae Vaccines, p.1616, Pertussis Vaccines, p.1631, and Tetanus Vaccines, p.1641.

### Uses and Administration

A combined diphtheria, tetanus, pertussis (acellular component), poliomyelitis (inactivated), and Haemophilus influenzae vaccine is used for active immunisation. For discussion of immunisation schedules see under Vaccines, p.1606.

In the UK it is used for primary immunisation of infants over 2 months of age and children under 10 years. It is given by intramuscular injection in usual doses of 0.5 mL; three doses are given at intervals of one month.

### Preparations

**Proprietary Preparations** (details are given in Part 3)
***Arg.:*** Poliacel; ***Austria:*** Infanrix IPV + Hib; ***Belg.:*** Infanrix IPV + Hib; ***Braz.:*** Infanrix IPV + Hib; Pentact; Poliacel; ***Canad.:*** Pentacel; ***Chile:*** Pentact-HIB; ***Fin.:*** Infanrix Polio + Hib; ***Fr.:*** Infanrixquinta; Pentacoq; Pentavac; Pent-HIBest†; ***Ger.:*** Infanrix IPV + Hib; Pentavac; ***Gr.:*** Infanrix IPV + Hib; ***Hong Kong:*** Infanrix IPV + Hib; Pentact-HIB; ***Irl.:*** Pentavac.; ***Israel:*** Infanrix Polio + Hib; Pentact-HIB; Poliacel-Act-Hib; ***Ital.:*** Cinquerix; Pentavac; Quinivax-in; ***Norw.:*** Infanrix Polio + Hib; ***Singapore:*** Infanrix IPV + Hib; ***Spain:*** Pentavac; ***Swed.:*** Infanrix Polio + Hib; Pentavac; ***Switz.:*** Infanrix DTPa-IPV+Hib; Pentavac; ***Thai.:*** Infanrix IPV + Hib; Pentact-HIB; ***UK:*** Pediacel.

## Diphtheria, Tetanus, Pertussis, Poliomyelitis, and Hepatitis B Vaccines

### Adverse Effects and Precautions

As for vaccines in general, p.1605.

### Interactions

As for vaccines in general, p.1606.

### Uses and Administration

A combined diphtheria, tetanus, pertussis, poliomyelitis, and hepatitis B vaccine is available in some countries for active immunisation as part of the primary immunisation of infants. In the USA, it is given in a schedule of three doses of 0.5 mL intramuscularly at 6- to 8-week intervals, usually starting at 2 months of age.

### Preparations

**Proprietary Preparations** (details are given in Part 3)
***Gr.:*** Infanrix Penta; ***Ital.:*** Infanrix Penta; ***USA:*** Pediarix.

## Diphtheria, Tetanus, and Poliomyelitis Vaccines

Vacunas de la difteria, el tétanos y la poliomielitis.

*ATC — J07CA01.*

### Adverse Effects and Precautions

As for vaccines in general, p.1605.

See also under Diphtheria Vaccines, p.1612, Diphtheria, Tetanus, and Pertussis Vaccines, p.1613, and Tetanus Vaccines, p.1641.

### Uses and Administration

A combined diphtheria, tetanus, and poliomyelitis (inactivated) vaccine is used for active immunisation. For discussion of immunisation schedules see under Vaccines, p.1606.

In the UK it is given by intramuscular injection in a single dose (usually 0.5 mL) as a booster at the ages of 13 to 18 years.

### Preparations

**Proprietary Preparations** (details are given in Part 3)
***Belg.:*** Revaxis; ***Canad.:*** Td-Polio; ***Denm.:*** Di-Te-Pol†; ***Fr.:*** DT Polio; Revaxis; Vaccin DTP; ***Ger.:*** Revaxis; Td-Virelon; ***Gr.:*** Revaxis; ***Irl.:*** Revaxis; ***Ital.:*** Revaxis; ***Switz.:*** Revaxis; ***UK:*** Revaxis.

## Diphtheria, Tetanus, and Rubella Vaccines

Vacunas de la difteria, el tétanos y la rubéola.

*ATC — J07CA03.*

### Profile

Diphtheria, tetanus, and rubella vaccines have been used in some countries for active immunisation against diphtheria, tetanus, and rubella.

## Endotoxin Antibodies

Anticuerpos antiendotoxinas.

### Profile

Antibodies against the endotoxin of Gram-negative bacteria have been tried as adjunctive therapy for the treatment and prevention of Gram-negative bacteraemia and shock.

Early preparations consisted of antisera prepared from the sera of donors immunised with *Escherichia coli* J5; these were superseded by human and murine IgM monoclonal antibodies. Nebacumab (HA-1A) is a human monoclonal IgM antibody that binds specifically to the lipid A domain of endotoxin. Lipid A in the circulation releases tumour necrosis factor and other cytokines from macrophages and endothelial cells which may ultimately culminate in physiological effects such as multiple organ failure. Despite early promising results of clinical studies the safety of nebacumab in patients without Gram-negative septicaemia was questioned and the product was withdrawn.

A murine monoclonal IgM antibody (edobacomab; E5) has also undergone clinical trials although results have been disappointing.

◊ References.


1. Ziegler EJ, *et al.* Treatment of Gram-negative bacteremia and septic shock with HA-1A human monoclonal antibody against endotoxin. *N Engl J Med* 1991; **324:** 429–36.
2. McCloskey RV, *et al.* Treatment of septic shock with human monoclonal antibody HA-1A: a randomized, double-blind, placebo-controlled trial. *Ann Intern Med* 1994; **121:** 1–5.
3. Horton R. Voluntary suspension of Centoxin. *Lancet* 1993; **341:** 298.
4. Greenman RL, *et al.* A controlled clinical trial of E5 murine monoclonal IgM antibody to endotoxin in the treatment of Gram-negative sepsis. *JAMA* 1991; **266:** 1097–1102.
5. Bone RC, *et al.* A second large controlled clinical study of E5, a monoclonal antibody to endotoxin: results of a prospective, multicenter, randomized controlled trial. *Crit Care Med* 1995; **23:** 994–1005.
6. Angus DC, *et al.* E5 murine monoclonal antiendotoxin antibody in Gram-negative sepsis: a randomized controlled trial. *JAMA* 2000; **283:** 1723–30.


## Epstein-Barr Virus Vaccines

Vacunas del virus de Epstein-Barr.

### Profile

Several Epstein-Barr virus vaccines are under investigation for active immunisation against infectious mononucleosis and post-transplant lymphoproliferative disorders.

◊ References.


1. Moss DJ, *et al.* Candidate vaccines for Epstein-Barr virus. *BMJ* 1998; **317:** 423–4.
2. Macsween KF, Crawford DH. Epstein-Barr virus — recent advances. *Lancet Infect Dis* 2003; **3:** 131–40.


## Escherichia Coli Vaccines

Vacunas de Escherichia coli.

### Profile

Vaccines against enterotoxigenic strains of *Escherichia coli* are under investigation. Vaccine candidates include toxoids, inactivated whole bacteria, purified surface antigens, and live oral vaccines.

◊ References.


1. Konadu EY, *et al.* Investigational vaccine for Escherichia coli O157: phase 1 study of O157 O-specific polysaccharide-Pseudomonas aeruginosa recombinant exoprotein A conjugates in adults. *J Infect Dis* 1998; **177:** 383–7.
2. Savarino SJ, *et al.* Safety and immunogenicity of an oral, killed enterotoxigenic Escherichia coli-cholera toxin B subunit vaccine in Egyptian adults. *J Infect Dis* 1998; **177:** 796–9.
3. Jertborn M, *et al.* Safety and immunogenicity of an oral inactivated enterotoxigenic Escherichia coli vaccine. *Vaccine* 1998; **16:** 255–60.
4. Cohen D, *et al.* Safety and immunogenicity of two different lots of the oral, killed enterotoxigenic escherichia coli-cholera toxin B subunit vaccine in Israeli young adults. *Infect Immun* 2000; **68:** 4492–7.
5. Guerena-Burgueno F, *et al.* Safety and immunogenicity of a prototype enterotoxigenic Escherichia coli vaccine administered transcutaneously. *Infect Immun* 2002; **70:** 1874–80.
6. Katz DE, *et al.* Oral immunization of adult volunteers with microencapsulated enterotoxigenic Escherichia coli (ETEC) CS6 antigen. *Vaccine* 2003; **21:** 341–6.


## Gas-gangrene Antitoxins

Antitoxinas de la gangrena gaseosa.

*ATC — J06AA05.*

**Pharmacopoeias.** Many pharmacopoeias have monographs including *Eur.* (see p.vi).

**Ph. Eur. 5.0** (Gas-gangrene Antitoxin (Novyi); Immunoserum Gangraenicum (Clostridium Novyi)). A sterile preparation containing the specific antitoxic globulins that have the power of neutralising the alpha toxin formed by *Clostridium novyi*. It has a potency of not less than 3750 international units/mL. It should be stored at 2° to 8°, and not be allowed to freeze.

The BP 2003 states that Nov/Ser may be used on the label.

The BP 2003 gives Gas-gangrene Antitoxin (Oedematiens) as an approved synonym.

**Ph. Eur. 5.0** (Gas-gangrene Antitoxin (Perfringens); Immunoserum Gangraenicum (Clostridium Perfringens)). A sterile preparation containing the specific antitoxic globulins that have the power of neutralising the alpha toxin formed by *Clostridium perfringens*. It has a potency of not less than 1500 international units/mL. It should be stored at 2° to 8°, and not be allowed to freeze.

The BP 2003 states that Perf/Ser may be used on the label.

**Ph. Eur. 5.0** (Gas-gangrene Antitoxin (Septicum); Immunoserum Gangraenicum (Clostridium Septicum)). A sterile preparation containing the specific antitoxic globulins that have the power of neutralising the alpha toxin formed by *Clostridium septicum*. It has a potency of not less than 1500 international units/mL. It should be stored at 2° to 8°, and not be allowed to freeze.

The BP 2003 states that Sep/Ser may be used on the label.

**Ph. Eur. 5.0** (Gas-gangrene Antitoxin, Mixed; Immunoserum Gangraenicum Mixtum). It is prepared by mixing Gas-gangrene Antitoxin (Novyi), Gas-gangrene Antitoxin (Perfringens), and Gas-gangrene Antitoxin (Septicum) in appropriate quantities. It has a potency of not less than 1000 international units/mL of Gas-gangrene Antitoxin (Novyi), not less than 1000 international units/mL of Gas-gangrene Antitoxin (Perfringens), and not less than 500 international units/mL of Gas-gangrene Antitoxin (Septicum). It should be stored at 2° to 8°, and not be allowed to freeze.

The BP 2003 states that Gas/Ser may be used on the label.

### Profile

Gas-gangrene antitoxins have been used for the treatment of gas gangrene and for prophylaxis in patients at risk following injury. They are now seldom used and have been superseded by antibacterials. Monovalent gas-gangrene antitoxins have been little used in practice owing to the difficulty of rapidly identifying the infecting organism.

### Preparations

**Ph. Eur.:** Gas-gangrene Antitoxin (Novyi); Gas-gangrene Antitoxin (Perfringens); Gas-gangrene Antitoxin (Septicum); Mixed Gas-gangrene Antitoxin.

**Proprietary Preparations** (details are given in Part 3)
**Ger.:** Gasbrand-Antitoxin†.

---

## Gonococcal Vaccines

Gonorrhoea Vaccines; Vacunas de la gonorrea.

### Profile

Several experimental gonococcal vaccines, produced usually from the surface antigens of *Neisseria gonorrhoeae*, are under investigation.

---

## Haemophilus Influenzae Vaccines

Vacunas de Haemophilus influenzae.

*ATC — J07AG01 (B, purified antig. conjugate).*

**Pharmacopoeias.** Many pharmacopoeias have monographs including *Eur.* (see p.vi).

**Ph. Eur. 5.0** (Haemophilus type b Conjugate Vaccine; Vaccinum Haemophili Stirpe B Conjugatum). A liquid or freeze-dried preparation of a polysaccharide, polyribosylribitol phosphate (PRP), derived from a suitable strain of *Haemophilus influenzae* type b, covalently bound to a carrier protein. The carrier protein, when conjugated to PRP, is capable of inducing a T-cell-dependent B-cell immune response to the polysaccharide. Carrier proteins currently approved are diphtheria toxoid, tetanus toxoid, CRM 197 diphtheria protein, and meningococcal group B outer membrane protein (OMP). It should be stored at 2° to 8° and protected from light.

The BP 2003 states that Hib/Vac may be used on the label.

### Adverse Effects and Precautions

As for vaccines in general, p.1605.

Erythema multiforme, convulsions, and transient cyanosis of the lower limbs have been reported rarely in children receiving haemophilus influenzae vaccines.

**Effects on the nervous system.** Guillain-Barré syndrome has been reported[1] in 3 infants, with onset of symptoms within 1 week of vaccination with an haemophilus influenzae conjugate vaccine (diphtheria toxoid conjugate).

1. D'Cruz OF, *et al.* Acute inflammatory demyelinating polyradiculoneuropathy (Guillain-Barré syndrome) after immunization with Haemophilus influenzae type b conjugate vaccine. *J Pediatr* 1989; **115:** 743–6.

### Interactions

As for vaccines in general, p.1606.

**Antineoplastics.** Haemophilus influenzae infection occurred in a child who had received antineoplastic therapy despite having completed a primary course of immunisation before the neoplasia was diagnosed.[1] A subsequent booster dose produced an adequate antibody response. Antineoplastic therapy may have impaired the T-cell response to infection.

1. Jenkins DR, *et al.* Childhood neoplasia and Haemophilus influenzae type b vaccine failure. *Lancet* 1996; **348:** 131.

**Diphtheria, tetanus, and pertussis vaccines.** Some haemophilus influenzae conjugated vaccines may be mixed with diphtheria, tetanus, and pertussis vaccines before administration without adversely affecting the immunogenicity of the components.[1,2] However the immunogenicity of a haemophilus influenzae conjugated vaccine was reduced when mixed with a diphtheria, tetanus, and acellular pertussis vaccine.[3]

1. Miller MA, *et al.* Safety and immunogenicity of PRP-T combined with DTP: excretion of capsular polysaccharide and antibody response in the immediate post-vaccination period. *Pediatrics* 1995; **95:** 522–7.
2. Mulholland EK, *et al.* The use of Haemophilus influenzae type b-tetanus toxoid conjugate vaccine mixed with diphtheria-tetanus-pertussis vaccine in Gambian infants. *Vaccine* 1996; **14:** 905–9.
3. Eskola J, *et al.* Randomised trial of the effect of co-administration with acellular pertussis DTP vaccine on immunogenicity of Haemophilus influenzae type b conjugated vaccine. *Lancet* 1996; **348:** 1688–92.

### Uses and Administration

Haemophilus influenzae (Hib) vaccines are used for active immunisation against *Haemophilus influenzae* type b infections. Vaccines are prepared from the capsular polysaccharide of *H. influenzae* type b and immunogenicity, especially in young children, is improved by linking the polysaccharide to a protein carrier to form a conjugate vaccine. For discussion of immunisation schedules see below.

Different proprietary vaccines may be conjugated to differing proteins but are generally regarded as interchangeable.

Haemophilus Influenzae Conjugate Vaccine (Diphtheria Toxoid Conjugate) (PRP-D) consists of the purified capsular polysaccharide of *Haemophilus influenzae* type b covalently linked to diphtheria toxoid.

Haemophilus Influenzae Conjugate Vaccine (Diphtheria $CRM_{197}$ Protein Conjugate) (HbOC) consists of oligosaccharides derived from the purified capsular polysaccharide of *Haemophilus influenzae* type b covalently linked to a non-toxic variant of diphtheria toxin isolated from *Corynebacterium diphtheriae.*

Haemophilus Influenzae Conjugate Vaccine (Meningococcal Protein Conjugate) (PRP-OMP or PRP-OMPC) consists of the purified capsular polysaccharide of *Haemophilus influenzae* type b covalently linked to an outer membrane protein complex of *Neisseria meningitidis* group B.

Haemophilus Influenzae Conjugate Vaccine (Tetanus Toxoid Conjugate) (PRP-T) consists of the purified capsular polysaccharide of *Haemophilus influenzae* type b covalently linked to tetanus toxoid.

In the UK, a combined diphtheria, tetanus, pertussis (acellular component), poliomyelitis (inactivated), and Haemophilus influenzae vaccine is given by intramuscular injection in doses of 0.5 mL. For primary immunisation of infants from 2 months of age, three doses are given at intervals of one month. Children aged under one year who have already completed the rest of a non-UK primary immunisation schedule should receive three doses of a single-component Hib vaccine at intervals of one month. Children aged 1 to 10 years should be given a single dose of a single-component Hib vaccine. Routine use in older children or adults is not recommended in the UK. Asplenic children (over 10 years of age) and adults should receive a single dose of Hib vaccine, or three doses for children under 1 year of age.

In the USA, primary immunisation is also carried out in conjunction with diphtheria, tetanus, and pertussis vaccination. If a meningococcal protein conjugate vaccine is used, only 2 doses are given for the primary course. A reinforcing dose using any of the available vaccines is given at 12 to 15 months of age.

Where compatibility has been demonstrated, Hib vaccines may be given as mixtures with diphtheria, tetanus, and pertussis vaccines (but see Interactions, above).

**Immunisation schedules.** Various regimens for vaccination against *Haemophilus influenzae* type b infection (Hib) have been tried. In the USA a reinforcing dose is given at 12 to 15 months of age to children who have received a primary course and studies in other countries have shown that a booster dose substantially reduces the risk of infection.[1] In the UK this is considered unnecessary[2,3] and a reinforcing dose is not included in the routine schedule (see under Vaccines, p.1606). Follow-up of children using a schedule without such reinforcing doses has shown that satisfactory serum-antibody concentrations persist at 4.5 years of age.[4] This difference in recommendations may reflect the high vaccine uptake, the use of a three-dose primary schedule, and the use of a highly immunogenic vaccine in the UK.[1] Studies have shown that two-dose schedules[5,6] or giving one-half or one-third of the full dose at 2, 4, and 6 months of age[7] can produce an adequate immune response although the usual three-dose schedule produces higher antibody concentrations.[6]

Differing immunogenicity of conjugate vaccines led to concern over the interchangeability of vaccines during primary immunisation.[8] In general, studies have shown that, despite some differences in antibody concentrations when different vaccines are used for doses during the primary course, the immune response was usually adequate.[9-12]

Response to some Hib vaccines may be inadequate in premature infants,[13,14] although adequate responses even in very premature infants have been reported.[15] Raised antibody titres have been reported in infants following maternal immunisation during the third trimester of pregnancy.[16]

1. Böhm O, von Kries R. Are Hib booster vaccinations redundant? *Lancet* 1997; **350:** 68.
2. Booy R, *et al.* Vaccine failures after primary immunisation with Haemophilus influenzae type-b conjugate vaccine without booster. *Lancet* 1997; **349:** 1197–1202.
3. Goldblatt D, *et al.* Immunological response to conjugate vaccines in infants: follow up study. *BMJ* 1998; **316:** 1570–1.
4. Heath PT, *et al.* Antibody persistence and Haemophilus influenzae type b carriage after infant immunisation with PRP-T. *Arch Dis Child* 1997; **77:** 488–92.
5. Kurikka S, *et al.* Immunologic priming by one dose of Haemophilus influenzae type b conjugate vaccine in infancy. *J Infect Dis* 1995; **172:** 1268–72.
6. Kurikka S, *et al.* Comparison of five different vaccination schedules with Haemophilus influenzae type b-tetanus toxoid conjugate vaccine. *J Pediatr* 1996; **128:** 524–30.
7. Lagos R, *et al.* Economisation of vaccination against Haemophilus influenzae type b: a randomised trial of immunogenicity of fractional-dose and two-dose regimens. *Lancet* 1998; **351:** 1472–6.
8. Granoff DM, *et al.* Differences in the immunogenicity of three Haemophilus influenzae type b vaccines in infants. *J Pediatr* 1992; **121:** 187–94.
9. Anderson EL, *et al.* Interchangeability of conjugated Haemophilus influenzae type b vaccines in infants. *JAMA* 1995; **273:** 849–53.
10. Greenberg DP, *et al.* Enhanced antibody responses in infants given different sequences of Haemophilus influenzae type b conjugate vaccines. *J Pediatr* 1995; **126:** 206–11.
11. Goldblatt D, *et al.* Interchangeability of conjugated Haemophilus influenzae type b vaccines during primary immunisation of infants. *BMJ* 1996; **312:** 817–18.
12. Bewley KM, *et al.* Interchangeability of Haemophilus influenzae type b vaccines in the primary series: evaluation of a two-dose mixed regimen. *Pediatrics* 1996; **98:** 898–904.
13. Munoz A, *et al.* Antibody response of low birth weight infants to Haemophilus influenzae type b polyribosylribitol phosphate-outer membrane protein conjugate vaccine. *Pediatrics* 1995; **96:** 216–19.
14. Kristensen K, *et al.* Antibody response to Haemophilus influenzae type b capsular polysaccharide conjugated to tetanus toxoid in preterm infants. *Pediatr Infect Dis J* 1996; **15:** 525–9.
15. D'Angio CT, *et al.* Immunologic response of extremely premature infants to tetanus, Haemophilus influenzae, and polio immunizations. *Pediatrics* 1995; **96:** 18–22.
16. Englund JA, *et al.* Haemophilus influenzae type b-specific antibody in infants after maternal immunization. *Pediatr Infect Dis J* 1997; **16:** 1122–30.

### Preparations

**Ph. Eur.:** Haemophilus Type b Conjugate Vaccine.

**Proprietary Preparations** (details are given in Part 3)
**Arg.:** PedvaxHIB; **Austral.:** Hiberix; HibTITER; PedvaxHIB; **Austria:** Act-HIB; Hiberix; HibTITER; ProHIBiT; **Belg.:** Act-HIB; Hiberix; HibTITER; **Braz.:** Act-HIB; Hiberix; HibTITER†; PedvaxHIB; **Canad.:** Act-HIB; HibTITER†; PedvaxHIB; **Chile:** Act-Hib; **Denm.:** Act-HIB; HibTITER; **Fin.:** Hiberix; HibTITER; **Fr.:** Act-HIB; HIBest†; **Ger.:** Act-HIB; HIB Merieux†; HIB-Vaccinol†; HibTITER; PedvaxHIB; **Gr.:** ACT-HIB; Hiberix; HibTITER; **Hong Kong:** Act-HIB; Hiberix; PedvaxHIB; **India:** Hiberix; Vaxim HIB; **Irl.:** Act-HIB; Hiberix; HibTITER; **Israel:** Act-HIB; HibTITER; PedvaxHIB; **Ital.:** Act-HIB; Hiberix; HibTITER; Vaxem Hib; **Malaysia:** Act-HIB; Hiberix; PedvaxHIB; **Mex.:** HibTITER; PedvaxHIB; Vaxem Hib; **Neth.:** Act-HIB; **Norw.:** Act-HIB; **NZ:** Hiberix; HibTITER; **Port.:** HibTITER; **S.Afr.:** Act-HIB; Hiberix; HibTITER†; **Singapore:** Act-HIB; Hiberix; HibTITER†; PedvaxHIB; **Spain:** Act-HIB; Hiberix; HibTITER; **Swed.:** Act-HIB; HibTITER; PedvaxHIB†; **Switz.:** Act-HIB†; Hiberix; HibTITER†; **Thai.:** Act-HIB; Hiberix; PedvaxHIB; Vaxem Hib; **UK:** Act-HIB†; Hiberix; HibTITER†; **USA:** Act-HIB; HibTITER; OmniHIB; PedvaxHIB; ProHIBiT.

---

## Haemophilus Influenzae and Hepatitis B Vaccines

Vacunas de Haemophilus influenzae y la hepatitis B.

*ATC — J07CA08.*

### Adverse Effects and Precautions

As for vaccines in general, p.1605.

### Interactions

As for vaccines in general, p.1606.

### Uses and Administration

Haemophilus influenzae type b (Hib) conjugate and hepatitis B vaccines are available in some countries for active immunisation as part of the primary immunisation of infants. In the USA, an Haemophilus influenzae type b conjugate (meningococcal protein conjugate) and hepatitis B (recombinant) vaccine is used. It is given in a schedule of 3 doses, 0.5 mL being administered intramuscularly at 2 months, 4 months, and 12 to 15 months of age. Administration to infants less than 6 weeks old is not recommended.

### Preparations

**Proprietary Preparations** (details are given in Part 3)
**Austral.:** Comvax; **Ger.:** Procomvax; **Gr.:** Procomvax; **Ital.:** Procomvax; **Mex.:** Comvax; **USA:** Comvax.

---

## Haemophilus Influenzae and Poliomyelitis Vaccines

*ATC — J07CA04.*

### Profile

Combined haemophilus influenzae type b conjugate and inactivated poliomyelitis vaccines are available in some countries for active immunisation of infants.

### Preparations

**Proprietary Preparations** (details are given in Part 3)
**Norw.:** Act-HIB Polio; **Swed.:** Act-HIB Polio†; PolioHib.

## Haemorrhagic Fever with Renal Syndrome Vaccines

HFRS Vaccine; Vaccinum Haemorrhagia Febris cum Renis Sindronum; Vacunas de la fiebre renal epidémica.

**Description.** A fluid or freeze-dried preparation of a suitable hantavirus grown in the neural tissue of suckling rodents or in cell cultures and inactivated. The fluid vaccine should be stored at 2° to 8° and not allowed to freeze. The freeze-dried form should be stored below 10°.

### Profile

Inactivated viral vaccines against haemorrhagic fever with renal syndrome have been investigated in several countries.

◊ References.


1. Lee HW, *et al.* Field trial of an inactivated vaccine against hemorrhagic fever with renal syndrome in humans. *Arch Virol* 1990; (suppl 1): 35–47.
2. Song G, *et al.* Preliminary trials of inactivated vaccine against haemorrhagic fever with renal syndrome. *Lancet* 1991; **337:** 801.
3. Zhu Z-Y, *et al.* Investigation on inactivated epidemic hemorrhagic fever tissue culture vaccine in humans. *Chin Med J* 1994; **107:** 167–70.


## Helicobacter Pylori Vaccines

Vacunas de Helicobacter pylori.

### Profile

Vaccines against *Helicobacter pylori* are being developed for prophylaxis of peptic ulcer disease and gastric cancer.

◊ Reviews.


1. Sutton P, Doidge C. Helicobacter pylori vaccines spiral into the new millennium. *Dig Liver Dis* 2003; **35:** 675–87.


## Hepatitis A Immunoglobulins

Inmunoglobulinas contra la hepatitis A.

*ATC — J06BB11.*

**Pharmacopoeias.** Many pharmacopoeias have monographs including *Eur.* (see p.vi).

**Ph. Eur. 5.0** (Human Hepatitis A Immunoglobulin; Immunoglobulinum Humanum Hepatitidis A). A liquid or freeze-dried preparation containing human immunoglobulins, mainly immunoglobulin G (IgG). It is obtained from plasma from selected donors having specific antibodies against the hepatitis A virus. Normal immunoglobulin may be added. It contains not less than 600 international units/mL. The liquid preparation should be stored, protected from light, in a sealed, colourless, glass container. The freeze-dried preparation should be stored, protected from light, in a colourless, glass container under vacuum or under an inert gas.

### Profile

Immunoglobulins containing high levels of specific antibodies against hepatitis A have been used in some countries for passive immunisation against hepatitis A infection; in the UK, normal immunoglobulin is usually given.

### Preparations

***Ph. Eur.:*** Human Hepatitis A Immunoglobulin.

**Proprietary Preparations** (details are given in Part 3)

***Belg.:*** Globuman Hepatite A†; ***Ger.:*** Gammabulin A†; ***Hong Kong:*** Globuman Hepatitis A†; ***Port.:*** Globuman Hepatite A; ***S.Afr.:*** Globuman Hepatitis A†; ***Switz.:*** Globuman Hepatite A†; ***Thai.:*** Globuman Hepatitis A†.

# Hepatitis A Vaccines

Vacunas de la hepatitis A.

*ATC — J07BC02.*

**Pharmacopoeias.** Many pharmacopoeias have monographs including *Eur.* (see p.vi).

**Ph. Eur. 5.0** (Hepatitis A Vaccine (Inactivated, Adsorbed); Vaccinum Hepatitidis A Inactivatum Adsorbatum; Inactivated Hepatitis A Vaccine BP 2003). A liquid preparation of a suitable strain of hepatitis A virus grown in cell cultures, inactivated by a validated method, and adsorbed on a mineral carrier. It should be stored at 2° to 8°, not be allowed to freeze, and be protected from light.

The BP 2003 states that Hep A/Vac may be used on the label.

**Ph. Eur. 5.0** (Hepatitis A Vaccine (Inactivated, Virosome); Vaccinum Hepatitidis A Inactivatum Virosomale). A liquid preparation of a suitable strain of hepatitis A virus grown in cell cultures and inactivated by a validated method. Virosomes composed of influenza proteins and phospholipids are used as adjuvants. It should be stored at 2° to 8°, not be allowed to freeze, and be protected from light.

## Adverse Effects and Precautions

As for vaccines in general, p.1605.

◊ General references.


1. Niu MT, *et al.* Two-year review of hepatitis A vaccine safety: data from the Vaccine Adverse Event Reporting System (VAERS). *Clin Infect Dis* 1998; **26:** 1475–6.


**Effects on the blood.** WHO has received reports of 5 cases of thrombocytopenia, 3 with purpura, associated with hepatitis A vaccine.[1]


1. Meyboom RHB, *et al.* Thrombocytopenia reported in association with hepatitis B and A vaccines. *Lancet* 1995; **345:** 1638.


**Effects on the nervous system.** Neurological symptoms resembling encephalitis have followed a third dose of hepatitis A vaccine.[1] Other serious neurological reactions reported in patients receiving inactivated hepatitis A vaccine include transverse myelitis, Guillain-Barré syndrome, and neuralgic amyotrophy.[2] Such reactions appear to be very rare, and, since other vaccines have often been given simultaneously, may not be directly attributable to hepatitis A vaccine.


1. Hughes PJ, *et al.* Probable post-hepatitis A vaccination encephalopathy. *Lancet* 1993; **342:** 302.
2. Committee on Safety of Medicines/Medicines Control Agency. Hepatitis A vaccination (Havrix). *Current Problems* 1994; **20:** 16.


## Interactions

As for vaccines in general, p.1606.

## Uses and Administration

Hepatitis A vaccines are used for active immunisation against hepatitis A infection.

In the UK, the use of an inactivated vaccine is recommended as an alternative to normal immunoglobulin for frequent travellers to areas of high or moderate hepatitis A endemicity or for those staying for more than 3 months in such areas; in some countries a hepatitis A immunoglobulin (p.1617) is available for those making shorter or less frequent journeys. Immunisation is also recommended in haemophiliacs and in those at risk of exposure to hepatitis A by virtue of their occupation, and should be considered in persons whose lifestyle is likely to place them at risk. The vaccine is given intramuscularly in the deltoid region, except in haemophiliacs in whom it should be given subcutaneously. In the UK, vaccines containing 1440 ELISA units/mL (derived from the HM175 strain of virus), or 320 antigen units/mL (GBM strain) may be used: adult doses are 1 mL of the former, or 0.5 mL of the latter. The dose is repeated 6 to 12 months later. Children under the age of 15 years may be given a dose of 0.5 mL containing 720 ELISA units with a booster dose of 0.5 mL 6 to 12 months later. Alternatively 0.5 mL of a preparation containing 50 antigen units/mL may be given to adolescents or children over 2 years of age, and repeated after 6 to 18 months.

Immunity is provided for up to 10 years following these doses.

◊ Commercially available hepatitis A vaccines are usually produced from inactivated hepatitis A virus strains propagated in cell culture, commonly of human diploid fibroblast cells. Live attenuated hepatitis A vaccines have also been developed, although an oral live vaccine does not appear to have yet been produced. 'Virosome' hepatitis A vaccines consisting of inactivated hepatitis A virus epitopes formulated into liposomes are under investigation.

### Preparations

***Ph. Eur.:*** Hepatitis A Vaccine (Inactivated, Adsorbed).

**Proprietary Preparations** (details are given in Part 3)

***Arg.:*** Avaxim; Havrix; VAQTA; Virohep-A; ***Austral.:*** Avaxim; Havrix; VAQTA; ***Austria:*** Avaxim†; Havrix; ***Belg.:*** Epaxal†; Havrix; VAQTA; ***Braz.:*** Avaxim; Havrix; VAQTA; ***Canad.:*** Avaxim; Epaxal; Havrix; VAQTA; ***Chile:*** Avaxim; Havrix; ***Denm.:*** Avaxim†; Epaxal; Havrix; ***Fin.:*** Epaxal; Havrix; VAQTA; ***Fr.:*** Avaxim; Havrix; VAQTA; ***Ger.:*** Epaxal; Havpur; Havrix; VAQTA; ***Gr.:*** Havrix; VAQTA; ***Hong Kong:*** Avaxim; Epaxal; Havrix; VAQTA; ***India:*** Havrix; ***Irl.:*** Avaxim; Havrix; VAQTA; ***Israel:*** Avaxim; Havrix; VAQTA; ***Ital.:*** Avaxim†; Epaxal; Havrix; Nothav; VAQTA; ***Malaysia:*** Avaxim; Havrix; VAQTA; ***Mex.:*** Havrix; VAQTA; ***Neth.:*** Avaxim; Havrix; ***Norw.:*** Epaxal; Havrix; ***NZ:*** Avaxim; Epaxal; Havrix; VAQTA; ***Port.:*** Havrix; ***S.Afr.:*** Avaxim; Havrix; ***Singapore:*** Avaxim; Havrix; VAQTA; ***Spain:*** Avaxim; Havrix; VAQTA; ***Swed.:*** Avaxim†; Epaxal; Havrix; VAQTA; ***Switz.:*** Epaxal; Havrix; VAQTA; ***Thai.:*** Avaxim; Havrix; VAQTA; ***UK:*** Avaxim; Epaxal; Havrix; VAQTA; ***USA:*** Havrix; VAQTA.

# Hepatitis B Immunoglobulins

Inmunoglobulinas contra la hepatitis B.

*ATC — J06BB04.*

**Pharmacopoeias.** Many pharmacopoeias have monographs including *Eur.* (see p.vi) and *US.*

**Ph. Eur. 5.0** (Human Hepatitis B Immunoglobulin; Immunoglobulinum Humanum Hepatitidis B). A liquid or freeze-dried preparation containing immunoglobulins, mainly immunoglobulin G (IgG). It is obtained from plasma from selected and/or immunised donors having antibodies against hepatitis B surface antigen. Normal immunoglobulin may be added. It contains not less than 100 international units/mL. The liquid preparation should be stored, protected from light, in a sealed, colourless, glass container. The freeze-dried preparation should be stored, protected from light, in a colourless, glass container, under vacuum or under an inert gas.

**Ph. Eur. 5.0** (Human Hepatitis B Immunoglobulin for Intravenous Administration; Immunoglobulinum Humanum Hepatitidis B ad Usum Intravenosum). A liquid or freeze-dried preparation containing immunoglobulins, mainly immunoglobulin G (IgG). It is obtained from plasma from selected and/or immunised donors having antibodies against hepatitis B surface antigen. Human normal immunoglobulin for intravenous administration may be added. It contains not less than 50 international units/mL. Storage requirements are similar to those for Human Hepatitis B Immunoglobulin, except that the freeze-dried preparation is stored at a temperature not exceeding 25°.

**USP 27** (Hepatitis B Immune Globulin). A is a sterile solution consisting of globulins derived from the plasma of human donors who have high titres of antibodies against hepatitis B surface antigen. It contains 10 to 18% of protein, of which not less than 80% is monomeric immunoglobulin G. It contains glycine as a stabilising agent, and a suitable preservative. It should be stored at 2° to 8°.

## Adverse Effects and Precautions

As for immunoglobulins in general, p.1605.

**Preparation strength.** For a warning concerning possible lack of equivalence between different preparations of hepatitis B immunoglobulins, see under Uses and Administration, below.

## Uses and Administration

Hepatitis B immunoglobulins are used for passive immunisation of persons exposed or possibly exposed to hepatitis B virus, including by sexual contact. They are not appropriate for treatment. Active immunisation with hepatitis B vaccine should always be started in conjunction with administration of hepatitis B immunoglobulins in patients exposed to hepatitis B virus.

In the UK, a hepatitis B immunoglobulin containing 100 international units/mL is available for intramuscular use. The dose in adults and children over 10 years of age is a single dose of 500 international units by intramuscular injection given preferably within 48 hours of exposure and not more than 1 week after exposure. Children aged 5 to 9 years may be given 300 international units, and children under 5 years 200 international units. Hepatitis B immunoglobulin should also be given to newborn infants at risk whose mothers are persistent carriers of hepatitis B surface antigen or whose mothers are HBsAg-positive as a result of recent infection. The dose is 200 international units by intramuscular injection preferably at birth, and certainly within 48 hours of birth.

There is now a UK and European standard for a preparation for intravenous use containing not less than 50 international units/mL.

In the USA, a hepatitis B immunoglobulin containing 15 to 18% of protein is available for intramuscular use. The dose for adults is 0.06 mL/kg. A dose of 0.5 mL is given to infants perinatally exposed to hepatitis B; this appears to be a significantly lower dose than that employed in the UK.

**Preparation strength.** The US Immunization Practices Advisory Committee has issued recommendations on the use of hepatitis B vaccines and hepatitis B immunoglobulins.[1] *The content of hepatitis B immunoglobulin may vary between countries and between manufacturers. Care should be taken in interpreting dosage recommendations which are not given in terms of international units.*[2] Products available in the USA have their strength expressed with reference to an FDA standard but are considered to contain[3] the equivalent of at least 200 international units/mL.


1. Immunization Practices Advisory Committee. Hepatitis B virus: a comprehensive strategy for eliminating transmission in the United States through universal childhood vaccination. *MMWR* 1991; **40** (RR-13).
2. Vegnente A, *et al.* Universal hepatitis B immunization: the dose of HBIg that should be administered at birth. *Pediatrics* 1994; **94:** 242.
3. Halsey NA, Hall CB. Universal hepatitis B immunization: the dose of HBIg that should be administered at birth. *Pediatrics* 1994; **94:** 242–3.


**Monoclonal antibodies.** The name tuvirumab is applied to a human hepatitis B monoclonal antibody. A murine monoclonal antibody has been tried in a few patients with primary antibody deficiency.[1]


1. Lever AML, *et al.* Monoclonal antibody to HBsAg for chronic hepatitis B virus infection with hypogammaglobulinaemia. *Lancet* 1990; **335:** 1529.


**Organ and tissue transplantation.** Studies[1-5] in patients positive for hepatitis B surface antigen undergoing liver transplantation (p.1346) suggest that long-term passive immunisation with hepatitis B immunoglobulin could reduce hepatitis B re-infection and improve survival in these patients.


1. Samuel D, *et al.* Passive immunoprophylaxis after liver transplantation in HBsAg-positive patients. *Lancet* 1991; **337:** 813–15.
2. Nymann T, *et al.* Prevention of hepatitis B recurrence with indefinite hepatitis B immune globulin (HBIG) prophylaxis after liver transplantation. *Clin Transplant* 1996; **10:** 663–7.
3. McGory RW, *et al.* Improved outcome of orthotopic liver transplantation for chronic hepatitis B cirrhosis with aggressive passive immunization. *Transplantation* 1996; **61:** 1358–64.
4. Terrault NA, *et al.* Prophylaxis in liver transplant recipients using a fixed dosing schedule of hepatitis B immunoglobulin. *Hepatology* 1996; **24:** 1327–33.
5. Sanchez-Fueyo A, *et al.* Hepatitis B immunoglobulin discontinuation followed by hepatitis B virus vaccination: a new strategy in the prophylaxis of hepatitis B virus recurrence after liver transplantation. *Hepatology* 2000; **31:** 496–501.


**Postexposure prophylaxis.** For discussion of the use of hepatitis B immunoglobulins in patients exposed to hepatitis B virus, see Postexposure Prophylaxis under Uses and Administration of Hepatitis B Vaccines, below.

## Preparations

**Ph. Eur.:** Human Hepatitis B Immunoglobulin; Human Hepatitis B Immunoglobulin for Intravenous Administration;
**USP 27:** Hepatitis B Immune Globulin.

**Proprietary Preparations** (details are given in Part 3)
***Arg.:*** Anti B; ***Austria:*** Aunativ; Hepatect; ***Belg.:*** Hepuman†; ***Canad.:*** Bay-Hep B; HyperHep†; ***Chile:*** Igantibe; ***Denm.:*** Aunativ; ***Fr.:*** Ivhebex; ***Ger.:*** Aunativ†; Hepatect; ***Gr.:*** Aunativ S.D.; ***Hong Kong:*** BayHep B; Hepatect; Hepuman; ***Irl.:*** Hepatect; ***Israel:*** BayHep; Hepatect; Omri-Hep-B; ***Ital.:*** Haimabig; Hepatect†; Hepuman B; ImmunoHBs; Uman-Big; Venbig; ***Jpn:*** Hebsbulin-IH; ***Malaysia:*** Hepabig; ***Norw.:*** Aunativ; ***Port.:*** Hepatect; ***S.Afr.:*** Hebagam IM; ***Singapore:*** BayHep B; ***Spain:*** Gamma Antihep B; Gamma Glob Antihepa B†; Gammaglob Antihep B P BE; Glogama Antihepatitis B†; Hepuman; ***Swed.:*** Aunativ; ***Switz.:*** Hepatect; Hepuman; ***Thai.:*** Hepuman†; ***USA:*** BayHep B; H-BIG†; Nabi-HB.

# Hepatitis B Vaccines

Vacunas de la hepatitis B.
*ATC — J07BC01.*

**Pharmacopoeias.** Many pharmacopoeias have monographs including *Eur.* (see p.vi) and *US.*

**Ph. Eur. 5.0** (Hepatitis B Vaccine (rDNA); Vaccinum Hepatitidis B (ADNr)). A preparation of hepatitis B surface antigen, that is obtained by recombinant DNA technology. It should be stored at a temperature of 2° to 8°, not be allowed to freeze, and be protected from light. Under these storage conditions it may be expected to retain its potency for 24 months.

The BP 2003 states that Hep B/Vac may be used on the label.

**USP 27** (Hepatitis B Virus Vaccine Inactivated). A sterile preparation consisting of a suspension of particles of hepatitis B surface antigen (HBsAg) isolated from the plasma of HBsAg carriers; it is treated so as to inactivate any hepatitis B virus and other viruses. It is adsorbed onto aluminium hydroxide and contains thiomersal as a preservative. It should be stored at 2° to 8° and not be allowed to freeze.

## Adverse Effects

As for vaccines in general, p.1605.

In addition, hepatitis B vaccines have been reported to cause abdominal pain and gastrointestinal disturbance, and musculoskeletal and joint pain and inflammation. There may also be dizziness and sleep disturbance. Cardiovascular effects include occasional hypotension and, rarely, tachycardia. Other rare adverse effects include dysuria, visual disturbances, and earache.

◊ General references.


1. McMahon BJ, *et al.* Frequency of adverse reactions to hepatitis B vaccine in 43,618 persons. *Am J Med* 1992; **92:** 254–6.
2. Anonymous. Adverse events after hepatitis B vaccination. *Can Med Assoc J* 1992; **147:** 1023–6.


**Effects on the blood.** Rare cases of thrombocytopenia associated with hepatitis B vaccination have been reported.[1-3]


1. Poullin P, Gabriel B. Thrombocytopenic purpura after recombinant hepatitis B vaccine. *Lancet* 1994; **344:** 1293.
2. Meyboom RHB, *et al.* Thrombocytopenia reported in association with hepatitis B and A vaccines. *Lancet* 1995; **345:** 1638.
3. Ronchi F, *et al.* Thrombocytopenic purpura as adverse reaction to recombinant hepatitis B vaccine. *Arch Dis Child* 1998; **78:** 273–4.


**Effects on bones and joints.** Reactive arthritis[1,2] and Reiter's syndrome[2] have been reported after hepatitis B vaccination. A number of reports of arthralgia have been received by the UK Committee on Safety of Medicines and by the manufacturers of Engerix B.[2]


1. Rogerson SJ, Nye FJ. Hepatitis B vaccine associated with erythema nodosum and polyarthritis. *BMJ* 1990; **301:** 345.
2. Hassan W, Oldham R. Reiter's syndrome and reactive arthritis in health care workers after vaccination. *BMJ* 1994; **309:** 94–5.


**Effects on the eyes.** There have been isolated case reports of acute posterior uveitis,[1] visual loss associated with eosinophilia,[2] acute posterior multifocal placoid pigment epitheliopathy,[3] and central retinal vein occlusion[4] following vaccination against hepatitis B.

For mention of optic neuritis in patients receiving hepatitis B vaccine, see under Effects on the Nervous System, below.


1. Fried M, *et al.* Uveitis after hepatitis B vaccination. *Lancet* 1987; **ii:** 631–2.
2. Brézin AP, *et al.* Visual loss and eosinophilia after recombinant hepatitis B vaccine. *Lancet* 1993; **342:** 563–4.
3. Brézin AP, *et al.* Acute posterior multifocal placoid pigment epitheliopathy after hepatitis B vaccine. *Arch Ophthalmol* 1995; **113:** 297–300.
4. Devin F, *et al.* Occlusion of central retinal vein after hepatitis B vaccination. *Lancet* 1996; **347:** 1626.


**Effects on the kidneys.** Acute glomerulonephritis was reported in a patient after the third injection of hepatitis B vaccine.[1]


1. Carmeli Y, Oren R. Hepatitis B vaccine side-effect. *Lancet* 1993; **341:** 250–1.


**Effects on the liver.** There have been occasional reports of transient abnormalities in liver function associated with hepatitis B vaccine.[1-3] The appearance of autoantibodies has been reported in a patient,[2] and severe cytolysis consistent with an allergic mechanism in another.[3]


1. Rajendran V, Brooks AP. Symptomatic reaction to hepatitis B vaccine with abnormal liver function values. *BMJ* 1985; **290:** 1476.
2. Lilic D, Ghosh SK. Liver Dysfunction and DNA antibodies after hepatitis B vaccination. *Lancet* 1994; **344:** 1292–3.
3. Germanaud J, *et al.* A case of severe cytolysis after hepatitis B vaccination. *Am J Med* 1995; **98:** 595.


**Effects on the nervous system.** In the years 1982 to 1985 the Centers for Disease Control, the FDA, and the manufacturer of plasma-derived hepatitis B vaccine received 41 reports of adverse neurological effects.[1] It was estimated that about 850 000 persons had received the vaccine in this time. Neurological events were convulsions (5 cases), Bell's palsy (10), Guillain-Barré syndrome (9), lumbar radiculopathy (5), brachial plexus neuropathy (3), optic neuritis (5), and transverse myelitis (4). In some analyses Guillain-Barré syndrome was reported significantly more often than expected. However, no conclusive epidemiological association could be made between any neurological adverse effect and the vaccine.

In France, spontaneous reports of multiple sclerosis and central demyelinating disease in patients who had received hepatitis B vaccine led to the suspension by the French authorities of hepatitis B vaccination in schools in 1998. This decision has been widely condemned by many authorities including WHO, the US National Multiple Sclerosis Society, and the Viral Hepatitis Prevention Board, and there is a fear that reduced confidence in the vaccine could have a profound effect on uptake. Arguments[2] against a link between hepatitis B vaccine and multiple sclerosis include the lack of correlation between the incidence of hepatitis B infection and demyelinating diseases, data from clinical studies including extensive postmarketing surveillance, and analysis of the French cases which concluded that the incidence of multiple sclerosis amongst vaccine recipients was not higher than would be expected in the population as a whole. A consultative group concluded[3] that, in the light of the evidence, the benefits of hepatitis B vaccination supported current WHO recommendations that all countries should have universal infant and/or adolescent hepatitis B immunisation programmes and that adults at increased risk of infection should also be immunised. More recent studies[4] have also indicated no association between hepatitis B vaccine and multiple sclerosis.


1. Shaw FE, *et al.* Postmarketing surveillance for neurologic adverse events reported after hepatitis B vaccination: experience of the first three years. *Am J Epidemiol* 1988; **127:** 337–52.
2. Anonymous. Expanded Programme on Immunization (EPI): lack of evidence that hepatitis B vaccine causes multiple sclerosis. *Wkly Epidem Rec* 1997; **72:** 149–52.
3. Halsey NA, *et al.* Hepatitis B vaccine and central nervous system demyelinating diseases. *Pediatr Infect Dis J* 1999; **18:** 23–4.
4. Ascherio A, *et al.* Hepatitis B vaccination and the risk of multiple sclerosis. *N Engl J Med* 2001; **344:** 327–32.


**Effects on the skin.** Skin reactions which have been reported in a few individuals after hepatitis B vaccination include erythema multiforme,[1,2] erythema nodosum,[3-5] lichen planus,[6,7] and vasculitis.[8,9]


1. Feldshon SD, Sampliner RE. Reaction to hepatitis B virus vaccine. *Ann Intern Med* 1984; **100:** 156–7.
2. Wakeel RA, White MI. Erythema multiforme associated with hepatitis B vaccine. *Br J Dermatol* 1992; **126:** 94–5.
3. Di Giusto CA, Bernhard JD. Erythema nodosum provoked by hepatitis B vaccine. *Lancet* 1986; **ii:** 1042.
4. Goolsby PL. Erythema nodosum after Recombivax HB hepatitis B vaccine. *N Engl J Med* 1989; **321:** 1198–9.
5. Rogerson SJ, Nye FJ. Hepatitis B vaccine associated with erythema nodosum and polyarthritis. *BMJ* 1990; **301:** 345.
6. Ciaccio M, Rebora A. Lichen planus following HBV vaccination: a coincidence? *Br J Dermatol* 1990; **122:** 424.
7. Ferrnado MF, *et al.* Lichen planus following hepatitis B vaccination. *Br J Dermatol* 1998; **139:** 350.
8. Cockwell P, *et al.* Vasculitis related to hepatitis B vaccine. *BMJ* 1990; **301:** 1281.
9. Le Helto C, *et al.* Suspected hepatitis B vaccination related vasculitis. *J Rheumatol* 1999; **26:** 191–4.


**Hypersensitivity.** Acute exacerbation of eczema[1] occurred in a patient on the day after vaccination against hepatitis B; the pruritus experienced and the exacerbation of the eczema was probably due to the formaldehyde in the vaccine. Hypersensitivity to thiomersal included in recombinant hepatitis B vaccine has also been reported.[2]

There has also been a report of a hypersensitivity reaction after administration of a yeast-derived recombinant DNA hepatitis B vaccine to a patient with a history of reactions to mouldy foods.[3] The clinical history and skin-prick testing suggested a type I hypersensitivity reaction to small quantities of *Saccharomyces cerevisiae* remaining in the vaccine.


1. Ring J. Exacerbation of eczema by formalin-containing hepatitis B vaccine in formaldehyde-allergic patient. *Lancet* 1986; **ii:** 522–3.
2. Noel I, *et al.* Hypersensitivity to thiomersal in hepatitis B vaccine. *Lancet* 1991; **338:** 705.
3. Brightman CAJ, *et al.* Yeast-derived hepatitis B vaccine and yeast sensitivity. *Lancet* 1989; **i:** 903.


## Precautions

As for vaccines in general, p.1606.

**Reduced immune response.** The immune response to hepatitis B vaccine is dependent on both host- and immunisation-related factors.[1] Host-related factors that appear to diminish the response include increasing age, increasing body-weight, smoking,[1,2] and male sex;[3] particular HLA haplotypes may also be associated with poor response.[4] Failure of hepatitis B immunisation in infants could be related to high perinatal maternal viraemia[5] rather than to inherent resistance to the vaccine.

Some studies have observed a defective response in chronic alcoholics[6,7] whereas others have not;[8] the degree of liver impairment may be a significant factor. It has been suggested that an increased dose of hepatitis B vaccine may be appropriate in those with a history of alcoholism.[9] Active infection with *Schistosoma mansoni* also appears to decrease the response to hepatitis B vaccination.[10] A diminished response occurs in HIV-positive patients[11-13] and in patients on haemodialysis;[1] an increased dose of hepatitis B vaccine is recommended in these patients. In patients with haemophilia who are not HIV-positive[14] immunity is reported to wane rapidly after vaccination and frequent booster doses may be required. Biological response modifiers such as thymopentin[15] and interferon,[16] have been used successfully in some patients on haemodialysis to overcome the immune deficit. Administration of interleukin-2 has met with variable success.

The immune response to hepatitis B vaccine is affected by the site of intramuscular injection. The deltoid region is recommended for adults and the anterolateral thigh for infants. A diminished response has been associated with administration in the gluteal region (buttock).[1]

A related problem is posed by subjects who become infected with hepatitis B despite mounting an adequate response to immunisation. Evidence of viral replication was detected in 44 of 1590 hepatitis B vaccinees despite development of protective titres of antibody.[17] Acute hepatitis occurred in one patient. Although the infection may have been incubating at the time of vaccination, the virus isolated from the child with acute disease was an escape mutant with a different DNA sequence from that isolated from the mother.


1. Hollinger FB. Factors influencing the immune response to hepatitis b vaccine, booster dose guidelines, and vaccine protocol recommendations. *Am J Med* 1989; **87** (suppl 3A): 36S–40S.
2. Horowitz MM, *et al.* Duration of immunity after hepatitis B vaccination: efficacy of low-dose booster vaccine. *Ann Intern Med* 1988; **108:** 185–9.
3. Morris CA, *et al.* Intradermal hepatitis B immunization with yeast-derived vaccine: serological response by sex and age. *Epidemiol Infect* 1989; **103:** 387–94.
4. Alper CA, *et al.* Genetic prediction of nonresponse to hepatitis B vaccine. *N Engl J Med* 1989; **321:** 708–12.
5. del Canho R, *et al.* Failure of neonatal hepatitis B vaccination: the role of HBV-DNA levels in hepatitis B carrier mothers and HLA antigens in neonates. *J Hepatol* 1994; **20:** 483–6.
6. Degos F, *et al.* Hepatitis B vaccination and alcoholic cirrhosis. *Lancet* 1983; **ii:** 1498.
7. Mendenhall C, *et al.* Hepatitis B vaccination: response of alcoholic with and without liver injury. *Dig Dis Sci* 1988; **33:** 263–9.
8. McMahon BJ, *et al.* Response to hepatitis B vaccine in Alaska Natives with chronic alcoholism compared with non-alcoholic control subjects. *Am J Med* 1990; **88:** 460–4.
9. Rosman AS, *et al.* Efficacy of a high and accelerated dose of hepatitis B vaccine in alcoholic patients: a randomized clinical trial. *Am J Med* 1997; **103:** 217–22.
10. Ghaffar YA, *et al.* Response to hepatitis B vaccine in infants born to mothers with schistosomiasis. *Lancet* 1989; **ii:** 272.
11. Carne CA, *et al.* Impaired responsiveness of homosexual men with HIV antibodies to plasma derived hepatitis B vaccine. *BMJ* 1987; **294:** 866–8.
12. Collier AC, *et al.* Antibody to human immunodeficiency virus (HIV) and suboptimal response to hepatitis B vaccination. *Ann Intern Med* 1988; **109:** 101–5.
13. Chan W, *et al.* Response to hepatitis B immunization in children with hemophilia: relationship to infection with human immunodeficiency virus type 1. *J Pediatr* 1990; **117:** 427–30.
14. Maris JM, *et al.* Loss of detectable antibody to hepatitis B surface antigen in immunized patients with hemophilia but without human immunodeficiency virus infection. *J Pediatr* 1995; **126:** 269–71.
15. Donati D, Gastaldi L. Controlled trial of thymopentin in hemodialysis patients who fail to respond to hepatitis B vaccination. *Nephron* 1988; **50:** 133–6.
16. Quiroga JA, Carreño V. Interferon and hepatitis B vaccine in haemodialysis patients. *Lancet* 1989; **i:** 1264.
17. Carman WF, *et al.* Vaccine-induced escape mutant of hepatitis B virus. *Lancet* 1990; **336:** 325–9.


## Uses and Administration

Hepatitis B vaccines are used for active immunisation against hepatitis B infection. Two types of vaccine have been available each containing hepatitis B surface antigen (HBsAg) adsorbed onto aluminium hydroxide or a similar adsorbent. The type of vaccine in which the surface antigen is produced in yeast cells using recombinant DNA techniques is now widely used and there has been considerable interest in further developments to improve immunogenicity. The second type of vaccine, in which the surface antigen is obtained from plasma after purification and inactivation processes is now not generally available.

WHO had recommended that national immunisation policies should include routine hepatitis B immunisation for the whole population by 1997 and this has been implemented in some countries including the USA (see Administration, below). The current recommendations in the UK are for immunisation of persons at high risk of contracting hepatitis B. High-risk groups include: health care personnel, laboratory workers, or any other personnel who have direct contact with patients or their body fluids or tissues; staff and residents of accommodation for those with severe learning difficulties; patients with chronic renal failure including those requiring haemodialysis; haemophiliacs and those receiving regular blood transfusions or blood products; close family contacts or sexual partners of cases or carriers of hepatitis B; families adopting children from countries with a high prevalence of hepatitis B; individuals who frequently change sexual partners; parenteral drug abusers; inmates of custodial institutions; and some travellers to areas where hepatitis B is endemic. Immunisation should also be performed in infants born to women who are persistent carriers of hepatitis B surface antigen or infants born to women who are HBsAg-positive as a result of recent infection. Hepatitis C carriers who are not immunised against hepatitis B should also receive immunisation.

The basic immunisation schedule consists of 3 doses of a hepatitis B vaccine, with the second and third doses 1 and 6 months, respectively, after the first. In the USA, some products may be given in an alternative 2-dose regimen to adolescents with doses given 4 to 6 months apart. Doses should be given intramuscularly, with the deltoid region being the preferred site in adults and older children and the anterolateral thigh the preferred site in neonates, infants, and younger children; the gluteal region (buttock) should not be used as efficacy may be reduced. The dose of the recombinant vaccine depends on the product used. Typical doses for adults are 10 or 20 micrograms and for children 5 or 10 micrograms. Products containing 40 micrograms are available for patients on haemodialysis who have a reduced immune response to the vaccine. However, *the dose of one recombinant preparation should not be seen as equivalent to the dose of another.*

The recombinant vaccine has also been used where more rapid immunisation, for instance with travellers, is required. This schedule has involved giving the third dose 2 months after the initial dose with a further booster at 1 year. In exceptional circumstances in adults travelling to an endemic area who commence their vaccination course within a month of departure, an even more rapid schedule involving injections at 0, 7, and 21 days has been used; when this schedule is used, a booster dose is recommended after 1 year.

For newborn infants at risk combined active and passive immunisation against hepatitis B is recommended. The first dose of vaccine should preferably be given at birth, and certainly within 48 hours of birth. A single dose of hepatitis B immunoglobulin (200 international units) should be administered at the same time into a different site. Additionally, in any patient in whom immediate protection is required, combined active and passive immunisation may be considered with a single dose of 500 international units of hepatitis B immunoglobulin being the dose for adults. See under Hepatitis B Immunoglobulins, p.1617, for children's doses.

The subcutaneous route should be used in patients with haemophilia. Some authorities have suggested that intradermal administration, in a dose of about 2 micrograms, may be considered for haemophiliacs, but the likelihood of effective antibody response is reduced and the risk of local adverse effects may be increased.

◊ General references.


1. Buynak EB, *et al.* Vaccine against human hepatitis B. *JAMA* 1976; **235:** 2832–4.
2. Douglas RG. The heritage of hepatitis B vaccine. *JAMA* 1996; **276:** 1796–8.
3. Lemon SM, Thomas DL. Vaccines to prevent viral hepatitis. *N Engl J Med* 1997; **336:** 196–204.
4. Keating GM, Noble S. Recombinant hepatitis B vaccine (Engerix-B): a review of its immunogenicity and protective efficacy against hepatitis B. *Drugs* 2003; **63:** 1021–51.


**Administration.** The major public health burden of hepatitis B infection in the developing world is due to the consequences of chronic carriage of hepatitis B virus (hepatocellular carcinoma and chronic cirrhosis) rather than acute infection. WHO[1] considered that the most important means of controlling hepatitis B on a global scale and of reducing mortality from its sequelae was mass immunisation of infants. It stated that hepatitis B vaccine should be incorporated into the Expanded Programme on Immunization (EPI) and many countries have since done so. WHO later reiterated this aim[2] stating that hepatitis B vaccine should be integrated into national immunisation programmes in all countries with a hepatitis B carrier prevalence (HBsAg) of 8% or greater by 1995 and in all countries by 1997. WHO's aim was to reduce the incidence of new child carriers of hepatitis B by 80% by 2001. Results from Taiwan, where mass immunisation of infants has been in place since the mid-1980s have shown a marked decline in the number of child carriers under 10 years of age.[3,4] The incidence of hepatocellular carcinoma in children has also been reduced.[5,6]

Opinion has been divided in the UK regarding implementation of universal hepatitis B immunisation,[7-9] with some advising increased emphasis on alternative strategies already in place such as antenatal screening.[7,8]

The optimum vaccination strategy depends on the pattern of hepatitis B viral transmission in a particular country. In hyperendemic regions where most infections are acquired early in life, the vaccine should be administered shortly after birth and hepatitis B immunisation integrated into the EPI. Immunisation of all infants should be considered for population groups with chronic hepatitis B virus carrier rates greater than 2% and should be a public health priority where carrier rates are greater than 10%. Countries with a lower carrier rate might opt to immunise all adolescents as an alternative to infant immunisation. Immunisation of individuals at high risk of infection should be continued in addition to routine vaccination schedules[2] and, if hepatitis B is not integrated into infant vaccination schedules, screening pregnant women for HBsAg and immunising the infants of HBsAg-positive mothers should continue.[1]

If use of hepatitis B vaccine is integrated into the EPI, three doses should be given intramuscularly, the first dose being given as soon as possible after birth with the first EPI immunisation. The exact timing of these doses will depend on the EPI schedule in operation. In the USA, these recommendations have been implemented by immunisation of all infants and of children at any age between 2 and 18 years who have not previously received three doses of vaccine. The recommended schedule[10] is: infants of HBsAg-negative mothers, the initial dose is given at birth or at up to 2 months of age, a second dose at 1 to 4 months of age but at least 1 month after the first dose and the third dose at 6 to 18 months of age; infants of HBsAg-positive mothers, hepatitis B vaccine plus hepatitis B immunoglobulin at birth, then additional doses of vaccine at age 1 to 2 months and at 6 months; infants of mothers whose HBsAg status is unknown, hepatitis B vaccine at birth, with maternal blood checked at delivery and, if positive for HBsAg, hepatitis B immunoglobulin as soon as possible (no later than 1 week of age). Children aged 2 to 18 years who have not received immunisation as an infant should be given three doses with the second dose given at least one month after the first and the third given at least 4 months after the first and 2 months after the second. Alternatively, some products may be administered in a two-dose regimen, with doses given 4 to 6 months apart. For further details, see p.1606. For premature infants of HBsAg-negative mothers, it has been suggested that the initial dose of vaccine could be delayed until the infant weighs at least 2000 g or until about 2 months of age.[11]


1. WHO. Progress in the control of viral hepatitis: memorandum from a WHO meeting. *Bull WHO* 1988; **66:** 443–55.
2. Anonymous. Hepatitis B vaccine. *WHO Drug Inf* 1993; **7:** 130–1.
3. Chen H-L, *et al.* Seroepidemiology of hepatitis B virus infection in children: ten years of mass vaccination in Taiwan. *JAMA* 1996; **276:** 906–8.
4. Hsu H-M, *et al.* Seroepidemiologic survey for hepatitis B virus infection in Taiwan: the effect of hepatitis B mass immunization. *J Infect Dis* 1999; **179:** 367–70.
5. Lee C-L, Ko Y-C. Hepatitis B vaccination and hepatocellular carcinoma in Taiwan. *Pediatrics* 1997; **99:** 351–3.
6. Chang M-H, *et al.* Universal hepatitis B vaccination in Taiwan and the incidence of hepatocellular carcinoma in children. *N Engl J Med* 1997; **336:** 1855–9.
7. Mortimer PP, Miller E. Commentary: antenatal screening and targeting should be sufficient in some countries. *BMJ* 1997; **314:** 1036–7.
8. Dunn J, *et al.* Integration of hepatitis B vaccination into national immunisation programmes: alternative strategies must be considered before universal vaccination is adopted. *BMJ* 1997; **315:** 121–2.
9. Goldberg D, McMenamin J. The United Kingdom's hepatitis B immunisation strategy—where now? *Commun Dis Public Health* 1998; **1:** 79–83.
10. American Academy of Pediatrics Advisory Committee on Immunization Practices. Recommended childhood and adolescent immunization schedule—United States, January-June 2004. *Pediatrics* 2004; **113:** 142–3.
11. Committee on Infectious Diseases. Update on timing of hepatitis B vaccination for premature infants and for children with lapsed immunization. *Pediatrics* 1994; **94:** 403–4.


BOOSTER DOSES. There has been considerable interest in the duration of immunity conferred by hepatitis B vaccination and the possible need for booster doses. However there are no official guidelines yet on administering booster doses after the recommended schedules, apart from recommendations that health care workers who have already been successfully vaccinated should be given a booster dose of vaccine after contamination of skin or eyes with blood from a HBsAg-positive person, unless they are known to have protective concentrations of antibody. A booster dose is also recommended for adults who receive a rapid immunisation schedule.

References.


1. Hollinger FB. Factors influencing the immune response to hepatitis B vaccine, booster dose guidelines, and vaccine protocol recommendations. *Am J Med* 1989; **87** (suppl 3A): 36S–40S.
2. Hadler SC. Are booster doses of hepatitis B vaccine necessary? *Ann Intern Med* 1988; **108:** 457–8.
3. Nommensen FE, *et al.* Half-life of HBs antibody after hepatitis B vaccination: an aid to timing of booster vaccination. *Lancet* 1989; **ii:** 847–9.
4. Gilks WR, *et al.* Timing of booster doses of hepatitis B vaccine. *Lancet* 1989; **ii:** 1273–4.
5. Coursaget P, *et al.* Scheduling of revaccination against hepatitis B virus. *Lancet* 1991; **337:** 1180–3.
6. Prince AM. Revaccination against hepatitis B. *Lancet* 1991; **338:** 61.
7. Hall AJ. Hepatitis B vaccination: protection for how long and against what? *BMJ* 1993; **307:** 276–7.
8. Tilzey AJ. Hepatitis B vaccine boosting: the debate continues. *Lancet* 1995; **345:** 1000–1.
9. Simó Miñana J, *et al.* Hepatitis B vaccine immunoresponsiveness in adolescents: a revaccination proposal after primary vaccination. *Vaccine* 1996; **14:** 103–6.
10. Edmunds WJ, *et al.* Vaccination against hepatitis B virus in highly endemic areas: waning vaccine-induced immunity and the need for booster doses. *Trans R Soc Trop Med Hyg* 1996; **90:** 436–40.
11. European Consensus Group on Hepatitis B Immunity. Are booster immunisations needed for lifelong hepatitis B immunity? *Lancet* 2000; **355:** 561–5.


**Postexposure prophylaxis.** A combination of passive immunisation with a hepatitis B immunoglobulin and active immunisation with a hepatitis B vaccine is generally recommended for postexposure prophylaxis against hepatitis B.

One group of patients who should be considered for postexposure prophylaxis are infants born to mothers who are persistent carriers of hepatitis B surface antigen (HBsAg). The risk is particularly high if the mother has detectable hepatitis B e antigen (HBeAg) or hepatitis B virus DNA or absence of detectable antibody to hepatitis e antigen (anti-HBe). Postexposure prophylaxis is also recommended in the UK for persons accidentally inoculated, or who contaminate the eye or mouth or breaks to the skin with blood from a known HBsAg-positive person, as well as in sexual contacts (and sometimes close family contacts) of sufferers from acute hepatitis B and who are seen within a week of the onset of jaundice in the contact.

In the UK, the recommended schedule for postexposure prophylaxis is the first dose of vaccine given preferably within 48 hours of exposure and no later than one week after exposure, or, for babies exposed to hepatitis B at birth, no later than 48 hours after birth, in conjunction with a single dose of hepatitis B immunoglobulin given at a separate site. The second and third doses of vaccine are given 1 and 2 months after the first dose, with a booster dose at 12 months. Health care workers who have been successfully immunised should be given a booster dose after subsequent contamination with blood from an infected person, unless they are known to have adequate antibody concentration.

## Preparations

***Ph. Eur.:*** Hepatitis B Vaccine (rDNA);
***USP 27:*** Hepatitis B Virus Vaccine Inactivated.

**Proprietary Preparations** (details are given in Part 3)

***Arg.:*** AGB; Biovac HB; Engerix-B; H-B-Vax II; Hepativax; ***Austral.:*** Engerix-B; H-B-Vax II; ***Austria:*** Engerix-B; Gen H-B-Vax; ***Belg.:*** Engerix-B; H-B-Vax II†; HBVaxPro; ***Braz.:*** Engerix-B; Heberbiovac HB; Hevac B†; Recombivax HB; ***Canad.:*** Engerix-B; Recombivax HB; ***Chile:*** Engerix-B; Heberbiovac HB; Recomvax B; ***Denm.:*** Engerix-B; H-B-Vax; ***Fin.:*** Engerix-B; HBVaxPro; ***Fr.:*** Engerix-B; GenHevac B; HB-Vax-DNA; HBVaxPro; ***Ger.:*** Engerix-B; Gen H-B-Vax; HBVaxPro; ***Gr.:*** Engerix; HbVaxPro; ***Hong Kong:*** Engerix-B; H-B-Vax II; HBVaxPro; ***India:*** Engerix-B; HB Vac; Shanvac-B; ***Irl.:*** Engerix-B; H-B-Vax II; ***Israel:*** Bio-Hep-B; Engerix-B; Recombinant H-B Vax II; ***Ital.:*** Engerix-B; HBVaxPro; Recombivax HB; ***Malaysia:*** Engerix-B; Euvax-B; H-B-Vax II; Hepavax-Gene; ***Mex.:*** Engerix-B; H-B-Vax II; Heberbiovac HB; ***Neth.:*** Engerix-B; HB-Vax-DNA; ***Norw.:*** Engerix-B; ***NZ:*** Engerix-B; H-B-Vax II; ***Port.:*** Engerix-B; Recombivax HB; ***S.Afr.:*** Engerix-B; H-B-Vax II; Hepaccine-B; ***Singapore:*** Engerix-B; H-B-Vax II; ***Spain:*** Engerix-B; Recombivax HB; ***Swed.:*** Engerix-B; HBVaxPro; ***Switz.:*** Engerix-B; Gen H-B-Vax; Heprecomb; ***Thai.:*** Engerix-B; Euvax-B; H-B-Vax II; Heberbiovac HB; Hepavax-Gene; ***UK:*** Engerix-B; H-B-Vax II†; HBVaxPro; ***USA:*** Engerix-B; Recombivax HB.

## Hepatitis A and B Vaccines

Vacunas de las hepatitis A y B.

**Pharmacopoeias.** Many pharmacopoeias have monographs including *Eur.* (see p.vi).

**Ph. Eur. 5.0** (Hepatitis A (Inactivated) and Hepatitis B (rDNA) Vaccine (Adsorbed); Vaccinum Hepatitidis A Inactivatum et Hepatitidis B (ADNr) Adsorbatum). A suspension consisting of a suitable strain of hepatitis A virus, grown in cell cultures and inactivated by a validated method, and of hepatitis B surface antigen obtained by recombinant DNA technology; the antigens are adsorbed on a mineral carrier, such as aluminium hydroxide or hydrated aluminium phosphate. It should be stored at 2° to 8°, not be allowed to freeze, and be protected from light.

### Adverse Effects and Precautions

As for vaccines in general, p.1605.

See also under Hepatitis A Vaccines, p.1617, and Hepatitis B Vaccines, p.1618.

### Uses and Administration

Combined hepatitis A and B vaccines are used for active immunisation against hepatitis A and hepatitis B.

In the UK, a hepatitis A and B vaccine is available containing not less than 720 ELISA units of inactivated hepatitis A virus and not less than 20 micrograms of recombinant hepatitis B surface antigen (HBsAg) protein in 1 mL. For primary immunisation, three doses of 1 mL are given by intramuscular injection, with the second and third doses 1 and 6 months after the first. For children up to the age of 16 years a 0.5-mL dose is given.

Alternatively, in exceptional circumstances when travel is anticipated within one month or more after the first dose but when insufficient time is available for the standard course, an accelerated schedule may be given to adults consisting of three doses at 0, 7 and 21 days.

Booster doses may be given as appropriate with the monovalent component vaccines since protection against hepatitis A and B declines at different rates, or a booster dose of the combined vaccine may be given after 5 years in adults or 4 years in children. A booster is recommended 1 year after the accelerated schedule.

◊ References.

1. Murdoch DL, *et al.* Combined hepatitis A and B vaccines: a review of their immunogenicity and tolerability. *Drugs* 2003; **63:** 2625–49.

### Preparations

***Ph. Eur.:*** Hepatitis A (Inactivated) and Hepatitis B (rDNA) Vaccine (Adsorbed).

**Proprietary Preparations** (details are given in Part 3)
***Arg.:*** Twinrix; ***Austral.:*** Twinrix; ***Austria:*** Twinrix; ***Belg.:*** Twinrix; ***Braz.:*** Twinrix; ***Canad.:*** Twinrix; ***Chile:*** Twinrix; ***Denm.:*** Twinrix; ***Fin.:*** Twinrix; ***Fr.:*** Twinrix; ***Ger.:*** Twinrix; ***Hong Kong:*** Twinrix; ***Irl.:*** Twinrix; ***Israel:*** Twinrix; ***Ital.:*** Twinrix; ***Malaysia:*** Twinrix; ***Mex.:*** Twinrix; ***Neth.:*** Twinrix; ***Norw.:*** Twinrix; ***NZ:*** Twinrix; ***Port.:*** Twinrix; ***S.Afr.:*** Twinrix; ***Singapore:*** Twinrix; ***Spain:*** Twinrix; ***Swed.:*** Ambirix; Twinrix; ***Switz.:*** Twinrix; ***UK:*** Twinrix; ***USA:*** Twinrix.

## Hepatitis A and Typhoid Vaccines

Vacunas de la hepatitis A y fiebre tifoidea.

### Adverse Effects and Precautions

As for vaccines in general, p.1605.

### Uses and Administration

Combined hepatitis A and typhoid vaccines are used for active immunisation. One consists of inactivated HM175 hepatitis A virus strain together with the Vi capsular polysaccharide from *Salmonella typhi* Ty 2 strain, and is given to adults and adolescents over 15 years of age by intramuscular injection in a dose of 1 mL, containing not less than 1440 ELISA units of inactivated hepatitis A antigen and 25 micrograms of Vi polysaccharide antigen, at least 2 weeks prior to risk of exposure to typhoid and hepatitis A. A booster dose may be given after 6 to 12 months to provide long-term protection. An alternative vaccine, containing 160 antigen units of inactivated hepatitis A virus (expressed according to the manufacturers' standard) and 25 micrograms of Vi polysaccharide antigen, is given in the same dose.

### Preparations

**Proprietary Preparations** (details are given in Part 3)
***UK:*** Hepatyrix; ViATIM.

## Herpes Simplex Vaccines

Vacunas del herpes simple.

### Profile

Several types of vaccines against herpes simplex virus types 1 and 2 have been developed. They have been tried in patients with both oral and genital herpes infections. They are also being studied for the prevention of infection in sexual partners of patients with genital herpes.

◊ References.

1. Stanberry LR, *et al.* Prospects for control of herpes simplex virus disease through immunization. *Clin Infect Dis* 2000; **30:** 549–66.
2. Morrison LA. Vaccines against genital herpes: progress and limitations. *Drugs* 2002; **62:** 1119–29.
3. Stanberry LR, *et al.* Glycoprotein-D-adjuvant vaccine to prevent genital herpes. *N Engl J Med* 2002; **347:** 1652–61.

### Preparations

**Proprietary Preparations** (details are given in Part 3)
***Hong Kong:*** Lupidon G†; ***Ital.:*** Lupidon G†; Lupidon H†; ***Switz.:*** Lupidon H+G†.

## Human Papilloma Virus Vaccines

Vacunas del virus del papiloma humano.

### Profile

Vaccines against human papilloma virus are under investigation for the treatment of genital warts and several malignant neoplasms including cervical and laryngeal cancers.

## Influenza Vaccines

Vacunas de la gripe.
*ATC — J07BB01; J07BB02.*

**Pharmacopoeias.** Many pharmacopoeias have monographs including *Eur.* (see p.vi) and *US.*

**Ph. Eur. 5.0** (Influenza Vaccine (Whole Virion, Inactivated); Vaccinum Influenzae Inactivatum ex Viris Integris Praeparatum). A sterile aqueous suspension of a suitable strain or strains of influenza virus types A and B, either individually or mixed, grown individually in embryonated hen eggs and inactivated so that they retain their antigenic properties. The stated amount of haemagglutinin antigen for each strain present is usually 15 micrograms per dose. Suitable strains of influenza virus are those recommended by WHO. An antimicrobial preservative may be added. The vaccine should be stored at 2° to 8°, not be allowed to freeze, and be protected from light. Under these conditions it may be expected to be suitable for use for 1 year, provided that the strains of virus continue to be appropriate.

The BP 2003 states that Flu/Vac may be used on the label.

The BP 2003 directs that when Inactivated Influenza Vaccine or Influenza Vaccine is prescribed or demanded and the form is not stated, Influenza Vaccine (Whole Virion, Inactivated), Influenza Vaccine (Split Virion, Inactivated), or Influenza Vaccine (Surface Antigen, Inactivated) may be dispensed or supplied.

**Ph. Eur. 5.0** (Influenza Vaccine (Split Virion, Inactivated); Vaccinum Influenzae Inactivatum ex Virorum Fragmentis Praeparatum). A sterile aqueous suspension of a suitable strain or strains of influenza virus types A and B, either individually or mixed, grown individually in embryonated hen eggs and inactivated so that the integrity of the virus particles has been disrupted without diminishing their antigenic properties. The stated amount of haemagglutinin antigen for each strain present is usually 15 micrograms per dose. Suitable strains of influenza virus are those recommended by WHO. An antimicrobial preservative may be added. The vaccine should be stored at 2° to 8°, not be allowed to freeze, and be protected from light. Under these conditions it may be expected to be suitable for use for 1 year, provided that the strains of virus continue to be appropriate.

The BP 2003 states that Flu/Vac/Split may be used on the label.

The BP 2003 directs that when Inactivated Influenza Vaccine or Influenza Vaccine is prescribed or demanded and the form is not stated, Influenza Vaccine (Whole Virion, Inactivated), Influenza Vaccine (Split Virion, Inactivated), or Influenza Vaccine (Surface Antigen, Inactivated) may be dispensed or supplied.

**Ph. Eur. 5.0** (Influenza Vaccine (Surface Antigen, Inactivated); Vaccinum Influenzae Inactivatum ex Corticis Antigeniis Praeparatum). A sterile suspension consisting predominantly of haemagglutinin and neuraminidase antigens of a suitable strain or strains of influenza virus types A and B either individually or mixed, grown individually in embryonated hen eggs and inactivated so that they retain their antigenic properties. The stated amount of haemagglutinin antigen for each strain is usually 15 micrograms per dose. It may contain an adjuvant. Suitable strains of influenza virus are those recommended by WHO. An antimicrobial preservative may be added. The vaccine should be stored at 2° to 8°, not be allowed to freeze, and be protected from light. Under these conditions it may be expected to be suitable for use for 1 year, provided that the strains of virus continue to be appropriate.

The BP 2003 states that Flu/Vac/SA may be used on the label.

The BP 2003 directs that when Inactivated Influenza Vaccine or Influenza Vaccine is prescribed or demanded and the form is not stated, Influenza Vaccine (Whole Virion, Inactivated), Influenza Vaccine (Split Virion, Inactivated), or Influenza Vaccine (Surface Antigen, Inactivated) may be dispensed or supplied.

**Ph. Eur. 5.0** (Influenza Vaccine (Surface Antigen, Inactivated, Virosome); Vaccinum Influenzae Inactivatum ex Corticis Antigeniis Praeparatum Virosomale). A sterile aqueous suspension consisting predominantly of haemagglutinin and neuraminidase antigens of a suitable strain or strains of influenza virus types A and B either individually or mixed, grown individually in embryonated hen eggs and inactivated so that they retain their antigenic properties and reconstituted to virosomes with phospholipids and without diminishing the antigenic properties of the antigens. The stated amount of haemagglutinin antigen for each strain is 15 micrograms per dose. Suitable strains of influenza virus are those recommended by WHO. An antimicrobial preservative may be added. The vaccine should be stored at 2° to 8°, not be allowed to freeze, and be protected from light. Under these conditions it may be expected to be suitable for use for 1 year, provided that the strains of virus continue to be appropriate.

**USP 27** (Influenza Virus Vaccine). A sterile aqueous suspension of suitably inactivated influenza virus types A and B, either individually or combined, or virus subunits prepared from the extra-embryonic fluid of virus-infected chick embryos. Suitable strains of influenza virus are those designated by the US Government's Expert Committee on Influenza and recommended by the Surgeon General of the US Public Health Service. It may contain a suitable antimicrobial agent. It should be stored at 2° to 8° and not be allowed to freeze.

**Nomenclature of strains.** The strain designation for influenza virus types A, B, and C contains: a description of the antigenic specificity of the nucleoprotein antigen (types A, B, or C) (an internal antigen, the matrix antigen, has also been described); the host of origin (if not man, including, if appropriate, the inanimate source); the geographical origin; the strain number; and the year of isolation; e.g. A/lake water/Wisconsin/1/79. For type A viruses the antigenic description follows (in parentheses) including the antigenic character of the haemagglutinin (e.g. H1) and the antigenic character of the neuraminidase (e.g. N1). There is no provision for describing subtypes of B and C viruses. Recombination between viruses within a type is readily accomplished; the letter R should be added after the strain description to indicate the recombinant nature of the virus, e.g. A/Hong Kong/1/68(H3N2)R. In addition the strain of origin of the H and N antigens of antigenic hybrid recombinant A and B viruses should be given, e.g. A/BEL/42(H1)—Singapore/1/57(N2)R.[1]

1. Assaad FA, *et al.* Revision of the system of nomenclature for influenza viruses: a WHO Memorandum. *Bull WHO* 1980; **58:** 585–91.

### Adverse Effects

As for vaccines in general, p.1605.

Local and systemic reactions may occur but are usually mild. Fever and malaise sometimes occur and severe febrile reactions have been reported particularly after administration of whole-virion vaccine to children.

Various neurological syndromes have been temporally associated with administration of influenza vaccine, the most notable report being of the Guillain-Barré syndrome occurring after vaccination with inactivated swine influenza vaccine in 1976 (see below).

**Effects on the nervous system.** GUILLAIN-BARRÉ SYNDROME. In 1976 a limited outbreak of influenza in the USA caused by a virus closely resembling the swine influenza virus led to the use of a killed swine influenza virus vaccine.[1] After about 45 million doses of the vaccine had been administered the vaccination programme ceased because there was some evidence of a temporal association between vaccination and the onset of a paralytic polyneuropathy of the Guillain-Barré type. An epidemiologic and clinical evaluation of these cases suggested a definite link between vaccination and the onset of the syndrome with extensive paralysis but no association with the onset of limited motor lesions. Influenza virus vaccines which lack a swine influenza virus component seem not to raise the risk of paralysis above background levels.

An increased number of reports of Guillain-Barré syndrome following vaccination with the 1993-94 influenza vaccine in the USA was not found to be associated with an increased risk from the vaccine itself, but was considered to be probably due to increases in vaccine coverage and in the baseline incidence of the syndrome.[2]

1. Anonymous. Influenza and the Guillain-Barré syndrome. *Lancet* 1984; **ii:** 850–1.
2. Lasky T, *et al.* The Guillain-Barré syndrome and the 1992-1993 and 1993-1994 influenza vaccines. *N Engl J Med* 1998; **339:** 1797–1802.

MULTIPLE SCLEROSIS. Analysis[1] indicated that there was no association between the use in the USA during 1976 of influenza vaccines containing a swine virus component and the development of multiple sclerosis.

1. Kurland LT, *et al.* Swine flu vaccine and multiple sclerosis. *JAMA* 1984; **251:** 2672–5.

**Henoch-Schönlein purpura.** Influenza vaccination has been associated with both development[1] and exacerbation[2] of Henoch-Schönlein purpura.

1. Patel U, *et al.* Henoch-Schönlein purpura after influenza vaccination. *BMJ* 1988; **296:** 1800.
2. Damjanov I, Amato JA. Progression of renal disease in Henoch-Schönlein purpura after influenza vaccination. *JAMA* 1979; **242:** 2555–6.

## Precautions

As for vaccines in general, p.1606.

Whole-virion influenza vaccine is not recommended for use in children because of the increased risk of febrile reactions.

Influenza vaccines should not be given to individuals with a known hypersensitivity to egg products.

Vaccination should be postponed in patients with active infection or acute febrile illness.

**Asthma.** There have been reports of exacerbations of asthma following influenza vaccination,[1,2] but reviews[3,4] have concluded that evidence of a causal relationship is lacking and that any risk of exacerbation which might exist is outweighed by the risk of influenza itself. Chronic respiratory disease, including asthma, is an indication for influenza vaccination in both the UK and USA. However, systematic reviews, while supporting the use of inactivated vaccines for patients with chronic obstructive pulmonary disease,[5] have concluded that there is not enough evidence to assess the risks and benefits for people with asthma.[6]

1. Hassan WU, *et al.* Influenza vaccination in asthma. *Lancet* 1992; **339:** 194.
2. Nicholson KG, *et al.* Randomised placebo-controlled crossover trial on effect of inactivated influenza vaccine on pulmonary function in asthma. *Lancet* 1998; **351:** 326–31.
3. Watson JM, *et al.* Does influenza immunisation cause exacerbations of chronic airflow obstruction or asthma? *Thorax* 1997; **52:** 190–4.
4. Park CL, Frank A. Does influenza vaccination exacerbate asthma? *Drug Safety* 1998; **19:** 83–8.
5. Poole PJ, *et al.* Influenza vaccine for patients with chronic obstructive pulmonary disease. Available in The Cochrane Library; Issue 2. Chichester: John Wiley; 2004.
6. Cates CJ, *et al.* Vaccines for preventing influenza in people with asthma. Available in The Cochrane Library; Issue 2. Chichester: John Wiley; 2004.

**Diagnostic tests.** False-positive screening enzyme-linked immunosorbent assays (ELISAs) for antibodies to HIV-1, HTLV-1 and hepatitis C virus were reported in blood donors who had recently received influenza vaccine.[1] The reaction was attributed to cross-reactivity of the test kit in use at the time with non-specific IgM.

1. Anonymous. False-positive serologic tests for human T-cell lymphotropic virus type 1 among blood donors following influenza vaccination, 1992. *JAMA* 1993; **269:** 2076 and 2078.

## Interactions

◊ For the effect of influenza vaccination on some other drugs see under Phenobarbital Sodium, p.369, Phenytoin Sodium, p.374, Theophylline Hydrate, p.803, and Warfarin Sodium, p.1027.

## Uses and Administration

Influenza vaccines are used for active immunisation against influenza.

Three types of the influenza virus occur, namely types A, B, and C, and the formulation and composition of influenza vaccines is constantly reviewed with changes made to accommodate the antigenic shifts and drifts of the influenza virus. Recommendations concerning the antigenic nature of influenza vaccines are made annually by WHO. Currently, influenza vaccines are of the inactivated type and may be available in three forms, as a whole-virion vaccine, as a split-virion vaccine, or as a surface-antigen vaccine.

Influenza vaccination is recommended for persons considered to be at special risk, particularly the elderly, those with chronic heart disease, chronic respiratory disease including asthma (see above), chronic renal disease, diabetes mellitus, and patients who are immunosuppressed. Vaccination should also be considered for residents, particularly elderly persons and children, in closed institutions. Medical personnel and other persons at risk from infection through contact with infected patients should also receive vaccination. Vaccination usually produces immunity after about 14 days, lasting for about 6 months to 1 year. Injections are therefore scheduled annually so that the period of maximum immunity coincides with the usual period of influenza infection. In the UK and USA, they are generally given in October or November.

Influenza vaccines are administered in the UK by deep subcutaneous injection or intramuscular injection. The preferred site for injection is the deltoid muscle in adults and older children and, in infants and young children, the anterolateral aspect of the thigh. The recommended dose is 0.5 mL for adults and children aged over 3 years. In children aged 6 months to 3 years, doses of 0.25 or 0.5 mL have been used. Children should be given a second dose at least 4 weeks after the first if receiving the vaccine for the first time. A live influenza vaccine is given in the USA by intranasal administration in a dose of 0.5 mL in adults and children aged over 9 years and in children aged 5 to 8 years who have received it previously. Children aged 5 to 8 years who have not previously received the vaccine are given a repeat dose after about 60 days.

◊ Reviews.

1. Palache AM. Influenza vaccines: a reappraisal of their use. *Drugs* 1997; **54:** 841–56.
2. Demicheli V, *et al.* Vaccines for preventing influenza in healthy adults. Available in The Cochrane Library; Issue 2. Chichester: John Wiley; 2004.

**Administration.** Haemagglutinin on the surface of the influenza virus allows the virus to attach to the host cells, and antibody against it is the main form of immunity to influenza. Antibody to neuraminidase on the virus surface and cell-mediated immunity may be important as well. Adults with previous exposure to the relevant subtype usually get a fourfold or greater increase in haemagglutinin antibody after vaccination with 20 to 30 micrograms of haemagglutinin [approximately equivalent to one 0.5-mL dose], but in some cases most of the new antibody is against the original strain rather than the variant in the vaccine. Children and unprimed adults need two injections of a much larger dose of haemagglutinin (60 micrograms or more) for an adequate antibody response. The level of antibody falls by about 75% over 8 months after split-virus vaccine and by 50% over 6 months after whole-virus vaccine. Because of this decrease in antibody level, and antigenic drift, immunisation against influenza is required each year. After one or two doses of killed vaccine, clinical infection rates are reduced by 60 to 80% in children and young adults. Vaccination reduces clinical infection by only about 30% in elderly patients in institutions, but serious illness and death are probably cut by about 70%. The effectiveness of vaccination has varied widely in different studies, probably because of differences in previous exposure to the influenza subtype, vaccine dose, interval between vaccination and challenge, and matching of vaccine and challenge antigens.

## Preparations

***Ph. Eur.:*** Inactivated Influenza Vaccine (Split Virion, Inactivated); Influenza Vaccine (Surface Antigen, Inactivated); Influenza Vaccine (Surface Antigen, Inactivated, Virosome); Influenza Vaccine (Whole Virion, Inactivated); ***USP 27:*** Influenza Virus Vaccine.

**Proprietary Preparations** (details are given in Part 3)
***Arg.:*** Berigripina; Evagrip; Fluarix; Fluzone; Imovax Gripe; Influvac; Isiflu Zonale; Istivac; Nilgrip; Vaxigrip; ***Austral.:*** Fluarix; Fluvax; Fluvirin†; Influvac; Vaxigrip; Xflu†; ***Austria:*** Addigrip; Begrivac; Fluad; Fluarix; Inflexal; Influvac; Sandovac; Vaxigrip; ***Belg.:*** α-Rix; Addigrip; Fluvirin; Influvac S; Mutagrip; Vaxigrip; ***Braz.:*** Fluarix; Fluzone†; Vaxigrip; ***Canad.:*** Fluviral; Fluzone; Vaxigrip; ***Chile:*** Fluarix; Vaxigrip; ***Denm.:*** Begrivac†; Fluarix; Influvac; Vaxigrip; ***Fin.:*** Begrivac; Fluarix; Flupar; Fluvirin; Influvac; Vaxigrip; ***Fr.:*** Agrippal; Fluarix; Fluvirine; Immugrip; Influvac; Mutagrip; Previgrip; Vaxigrip; ***Ger.:*** Addigrip; Begrivac; Inflexal S; Influsplit SSW; Influvac; Mutagrip; ***Gr.:*** Agrippal; Fluarix; Influvac Sub-Unit; Vaxigrip; ***Hong Kong:*** Fluarix; Fluvax; Inflexal†; Vaxigrip; ***Irl.:*** Begrivac; Fluarix; Fluvirin; Fluzone†; Influvac; ***Israel:*** Fluvirin; Influvac; Vaxigrip; ***Ital.:*** Adiugrip; Agrippal; Begrivac; Biaflu-Zonale SU†; Biaflu†; Fluad; Fluarix; Fluvirin†; Inflexal; Influpozzi; Influsplit; Influvac S; Influvirus; Isiflu V; Isigrip Zonale; Mutagrip; Vaxigrip; ***Malaysia:*** Vaxigrip; ***Mex.:*** Agrippal; Fluarix; Flushield†; ***Neth.:*** Fluarix; Influvac; Vaxigrip; ***Norw.:*** Begrivac; Fluarix; Fluvirin; Fluzone†; Influvac; Vaxigrip; ***NZ:*** Begrivac; Fluarix; Fluvax; Vaxigrip; ***Port.:*** Chiroflu; Fluarix; Fluvirin; Inflexal; Influvac; Istivac; Vaxigrip; ***S.Afr.:*** Agrippal; Fluarix; Fluvirin; Inflexal†; Influvac; Vaxigrip; Xflu; ***Singapore:*** Aggripal S1; Fluad; Fluarix; Inflexal†; Vaxigrip; ***Spain:*** Chiroflu; Chiromas; Evagrip; Fluarix; Gripavac; Imuvac; Inflexal†; Mutagrip; Procigrip; Vac Antigrip Frac; Vacuna Antigripal; Vitagripe; ***Swed.:*** Agrippal; Batrevac; Begrivac; Fluad; Fluarix; Fluvirin; Influvac; Vaxigrip; ***Switz.:*** Fluarix; Inflexal; Influvac; Mutagrip; Nasalflu; ***Thai.:*** Agrippal; Fluarix; Vaxigrip; ***UK:*** Agrippal; Begrivac; Fluarix; Fluvirin; Fluzone†; Inflexal; Influvac; Mastaflu; MFV-Ject†; ***USA:*** FluMist; Fluogen†; Flushield†; Fluvirin; Fluzone.

# Japanese Encephalitis Vaccines

Vacunas de la encefalitis japonesa.

*ATC — J07BA02.*

## Adverse Effects and Precautions

As for vaccines in general, p.1605.

Hypersensitivity reactions including urticaria, angioedema, hypotension, and dyspnoea have been reported mainly in travellers from non-endemic areas.

◊ References.

1. Andersen MM, Rønne T. Side-effects with Japanese encephalitis vaccine. *Lancet* 1991; **337:** 1044.
2. Ruff TA, *et al.* Adverse reactions to Japanese encephalitis vaccine. *Lancet* 1991; **338:** 881–2.
3. Plesner A-M, *et al.* Neurological complications and Japanese encephalitis vaccination. *Lancet* 1996; **348:** 202–3.
4. Nothdurft HD, *et al.* Adverse reactions to Japanese encephalitis vaccine in travellers. *J Infect* 1996; **32:** 119–22.
5. Jelinek T, Nothdurft HD. Japanese encephalitis vaccine in travellers: is wider use prudent? *Drug Safety* 1997; **16:** 153–6.
6. Berg SW, *et al.* Systemic reactions in US Marine Corps personnel who received Japanese encephalitis vaccine. *Clin Infect Dis* 1997; **24:** 265–6.
7. Liu ZL, *et al.* Short-term safety of live attenuated Japanese encephalitis vaccine (SA14-14-2): results of a randomized trial with 26,239 subjects. *J Infect Dis* 1997; **176:** 1366–9.
8. Plesner A, *et al.* Case-control study of allergic reactions to Japanese encephalitis vaccine. *Vaccine* 2000; **18:** 1830–6.

## Interactions

As for vaccines in general, p.1606.

## Uses and Administration

Two types of inactivated Japanese encephalitis vaccine are used for active immunisation against encephalitis due to Japanese encephalitis virus, an infection against which there is currently no specific treatment. One type of vaccine is derived from mouse brain and the other from primary hamster kidney cells. The vaccines are widely used in Japan and other parts of Asia and may form part of the WHO Expanded Programme on Immunization.

Vaccination is recommended for visitors to rural areas of South East Asia and the Far East where infection is endemic and where the visit is to be for more than one month; it is also recommended for shorter visits in individuals likely to be at exceptional risk. Adults are usually given 3 doses each of 1 mL of the inactivated vaccine subcutaneously at 0, 7 to 14, and 28 to 30 days; full immunity will take up to one month to develop. A two-dose schedule with doses given 7 to 14 days apart is suggested to provide short-term immunity but is effective in only 80% of recipients; in the USA, an abbreviated dosage schedule with administration at 0, 7, and 14 days is suggested if time is not available for the standard schedule. Children under 3 years of age may be given 3 doses of 0.5 mL; in the USA, the vaccine is not recommended for children under 1 year. A reinforcing dose may be given after 2 years.

Live attenuated Japanese encephalitis vaccines are used in some countries.

◊ Inactivated Japanese encephalitis vaccines have been widely used in Asia for some years. In Japan, the incidence of the disease has decreased since the introduction of nationwide vaccination in the mid-1960s.[1] A study in Thailand in 1984–5 compared a monovalent Nakayama strain vaccine (21 628 subjects), a bivalent Nakayama-Beijing 1 strain vaccine (22 080 subjects), and a tetanus toxoid placebo (21 516 subjects) in children aged 1 to 14 years.[2] Two subcutaneous 1-mL doses (0.5 mL for children under 3 years of age) were given 7 days apart. The attack rate for encephalitis caused by Japanese encephalitis virus was 51 per 100 000 in the placebo group and 5 per 100 000 in both vaccine groups. Vaccine efficacy in both groups combined was calculated to be 91%. Results suggested that Japanese encephalitis vaccine does not prevent virus infection but protects against symptomatic Japanese encephalitis. Immunisation had no significant effect on the incidence of dengue haemorrhagic fever although the severity of episodes may be decreased. The vaccines were associated with minimal short-term side-effects. Findings suggested that post-vaccine encephalomyelitis does not occur or is very rare with these vaccines.

A case-control study of a live attenuated vaccine (SA14-14-2) indicated that 2 doses given a year apart were 97% effective in an endemic region of rural China.[3] Similar results were obtained when the interval between doses was reduced to 1 to 3 months.[4] A further case-control study[5] in Nepal found that single-dose administration was more than 99% effective.

Other vaccines are under development.[6]

1. Denning DW, Kaneko Y. Should travellers to Asia be vaccinated against Japanese encephalitis? *Lancet* 1987; **i:** 853–4.
2. Hoke CH, *et al.* Protection against Japanese encephalitis by inactivated vaccines. *N Engl J Med* 1988; **319:** 608–14.
3. Hennessy S, *et al.* Effectiveness of live-attenuated Japanese encephalitis vaccine (SA14-14-2): a case-control study. *Lancet* 1996; **347:** 1583–6.
4. Tsai TF, *et al.* Immunogenicity of live attenuated SA14-14-2 Japanese encephalitis vaccine—a comparison of 1- and 3-month immunization schedules. *J Infect Dis* 1998; **177:** 221–3.
5. Bista MB, *et al.* Efficacy of single-dose SA 14-14-2 vaccine against Japanese encephalitis: a case control study. *Lancet* 2001; **358:** 791–5.
6. Barrett ADT. Japanese encephalitis and dengue vaccines. *Biologicals* 1997; **25:** 27–34.

## Preparations

**Proprietary Preparations** (details are given in Part 3)
***Austral.:*** JE-Vax; ***Canad.:*** JE-Vax; ***Thai.:*** JE-Vaccine; ***USA:*** JE-Vax.

# Jellyfish Venom Antisera

Antisuero contra el veneno de la medusa; Jellyfish Antivenins; Jellyfish Antivenoms.

## Adverse Effects and Precautions

As for antisera in general, p.1605.

## Uses and Administration

An antiserum for use in the management of severe stings by the box jellyfish or sea wasp (*Chironex fleckeri*) is available in Australia. The preparation contains the specific antitoxic globulins that have the power of neutralising the venom of *Chironex fleckeri*. The globulins are obtained from the serum of sheep that have been immunised with the venom of the box jellyfish.

Box jellyfish antivenom is usually given by the intravenous route in a dose of 20 000 units. Alternatively, 60 000 units may be injected intramuscularly.

**Box jellyfish sting.** The sting of the box jellyfish (*Chironex fleckeri*) can be rapidly fatal so immediate first aid is vital. Fragments of tentacle adhering to the skin should be inactivated by the application of vinegar or 3 to 10% acetic acid solution. Artificial respiration and external cardiac massage may be necessary. The antiserum can be effective if administered quickly and in adequate dosage.[1-3] Studies in *rodents*[4] suggest that verapamil may be useful for treatment of the cardiotoxic effects of the venom and allow more time for the antiserum to exert its action.

Some have suggested that the box jellyfish antiserum may be effective for severe envenomation by related species.[5]


1. Lumley J, *et al.* Fatal envenomation by Chironex fleckeri, the north Australian box jellyfish: the continuing search for lethal mechanisms. *Med J Aust* 1988; **148:** 527–34.
2. Horne TW. Box-jellyfish envenomation. *Med J Aust* 1988; **148:** 540.
3. Fenner PJ, *et al.* Successful use of chironex antivenom by members of the Queensland Ambulance Transport Brigade. *Med J Aust* 1989; **151:** 708–10.
4. Burnett JW. The use of verapamil to treat box-jellyfish stings. *Med J Aust* 1990; **153:** 363.
5. Fenner PJ, Williamson JA. Worldwide deaths and severe envenomation from jellyfish stings. *Med J Aust* 1996; **165:** 658–61.


## Leishmaniasis Vaccines

Vacunas de la leishmaniasis.

### Profile

Vaccines containing *Leishmania* spp. are under investigation in an attempt to prevent cutaneous leishmaniasis.

◊ The inoculation of an infective strain of a *Leishmania* sp. into the skin, a technique known as leishmanisation, has been used to protect against cutaneous leishmaniasis. Although the technique has been standardised it is not generally recommended since large, slow-healing lesions have occurred in some patients.

Vaccines containing strains of killed leishmanial promastigotes have been developed and have conferred some protection against cutaneous leishmaniasis although this has waned relatively quickly in some cases. The safety and efficacy of killed *Leishmania* vaccines is under clinical investigation. Killed vaccines combined with BCG as an adjuvant have also been tried.[1-4] A killed vaccine with BCG has also been tried for visceral leishmaniasis but with disappointing results. Also under development are live vaccines containing stable mutants of *Leishmania* or recombinant subunit and synthetic vaccines.

Immunotherapy with a mixture of heat-killed promastigotes of *Leishmania mexicana amazonensis* and live BCG has compared favourably with meglumine antimonate treatment in patients with cutaneous leishmaniasis.[5] Immunotherapy resulted in fewer side-effects than chemotherapy. For a discussion of the difficulties in treating cutaneous leishmaniasis, see p.597.


1. Armijos RX, *et al.* Field trial of a vaccine against New World cutaneous leishmaniasis in an at-risk child population: safety, immunogenicity, and efficacy during the first 12 months of follow-up. *J Infect Dis* 1998; **177:** 1352–7.
2. Momeni AZ, *et al.* A randomised, double-blind, controlled trial of a killed L. major vaccine plus BCG against zoonotic cutaneous leishmaniasis in Iran. *Vaccine* 1999; **17:** 466–72.
3. Vélez ID, *et al.* Safety and immunogenicity of a killed Leishmania (L.) amazonensis vaccine against cutaneous leishmaniasis in Colombia: a randomized controlled trial. *Trans R Soc Trop Med Hyg* 2000; **94:** 698–703.
4. Satti IN, *et al.* Immunogenicity and safety of autoclaved Leishmania major plus BCG vaccine in healthy Sudanese volunteers. *Vaccine* 2001; **19:** 2100–6.
5. Convit J, *et al.* Immunotherapy of localized, intermediate, and diffuse forms of American cutaneous leishmaniasis. *J Infect Dis* 1989; **160:** 104–15.


## Leprosy Vaccines

Vacunas de la lepra.

### Profile

Vaccines against leprosy including those using *Mycobacterium leprae*, as well as other mycobacteria, are under investigation. A killed vaccine has been developed in India for use as an adjunct to standard multidrug therapy in the treatment of leprosy. Although studies of new vaccines are continuing, BCG vaccine (p.1610) also appears to be effective.

◊ Attempts to develop a vaccine against leprosy are based on the assumption that induction of a cell-mediated immune response to *Mycobacterium leprae* will lead to protection against the bacillus.[1-4] Considerable protection against leprosy is afforded by BCG vaccination (see p.1610), and a study in Malawi showed that repeated vaccination provided additional protection.[5] However, the addition of killed *M. leprae* did not produce any further improvement, confirming preliminary results of a study in Venezuela.[6] The fortuitous finding that BCG vaccine, which is inexpensive and widely available, is effective against leprosy has important implications for leprosy control programmes.[7] Vaccines from non-pathogenic species of mycobacteria, *Mycobacterium w*, have been developed in India.

Leprosy vaccines are being studied both to prevent infection with *M. leprae* (immunoprophylaxis) and to prevent disease in infected individuals (immunotherapeutic). Beneficial responses have been reported[8-12] from the immunotherapeutic use of *Mycobacterium w* vaccine in combination with standard multidrug therapy (p.133) although a small increase in Type 1 lepra reactions has been observed.[13] A similar, and possibly identical, vaccine based on the ICRC bacillus is also being evaluated.[14,15] Immunotherapy with BCG and heat killed *M.leprae* has produced beneficial responses when given as an adjunct to chemotherapy.[16] WHO has suggested that the immunotherapeutic use of vaccines may ultimately prove to be more clinically relevant than the immunoprophylactic use,[14] and high compliance with immunotherapy appears to be attainable.[17]


1. Anonymous. Vaccines against leprosy. *Lancet* 1987; **i:** 1183–4.
2. WHO. WHO expert committee on leprosy: sixth report. *WHO Tech Rep Ser 768* 1988.
3. Fine PEM, Ponnighaus JM. Leprosy in Malawi 2: background, design and prospects of the Karonga Prevention Trial, a leprosy vaccine trial in northern Malawi. *Trans R Soc Trop Med Hyg* 1988; **82:** 810–17.
4. Anonymous. Bettering BCG. *Lancet* 1992; **339:** 462–3.
5. Karonga Prevention Trial Group. Randomised controlled trial of single BCG, repeated BCG, or combined BCG and killed Mycobacterium leprae vaccine for prevention of leprosy and tuberculosis in Malawi. *Lancet* 1996; **348:** 17–24.
6. Convit J, *et al.* Immunoprophylactic trial with combined Mycobacterium leprae/BCG vaccine against leprosy: preliminary results. *Lancet* 1992; **339:** 446–50.
7. Fine PEM, Smith PG. Vaccination against leprosy—the view from 1996. *Lepr Rev* 1996; **67:** 249–52.
8. Zaheer SA, *et al.* Combined multidrug and Mycobacterium w vaccine therapy in patients with multibacillary leprosy. *J Infect Dis* 1993; **167:** 401–10.
9. Zaheer SA, *et al.* Immunotherapy with Mycobacterium w vaccine decreases the incidence and severity of type 2 (ENL) reactions. *Lepr Rev* 1993; **64:** 7–14.
10. Zaheer SA, *et al.* Addition of immunotherapy with Mycobacterium w vaccine to multi-drug therapy benefits multibacillary leprosy patients. *Vaccine* 1995; **13:** 1102–10.
11. Katoch K, *et al.* Treatment of bacilliferous BL/LL cases with combined chemotherapy and immunotherapy. *Int J Lepr* 1995; **63:** 202–12.
12. Talwar GP. An immunotherapeutic vaccine for multibacillary leprosy. *Int Rev Immunol* 1999; **18:** 229–49.
13. Kar HK, *et al.* Reversal reaction in multibacillary leprosy patients following MDT with and without immunotherapy with a candidate for an antileprosy vaccine, Mycobacterium w. *Lepr Rev* 1993; **64:** 219–26.
14. Mangla B. Leprosy vaccine debate in India re-ignited. *Lancet* 1993; **342:** 233.
15. Jayaraman KS. Charges fly over rival leprosy vaccines. *Nature* 1994; **367:** 403.
16. Rada E, *et al.* A follow-up study of multibacillary Hansen's disease patients treated with multidrug therapy (MDT) or MDT + immunotherapy (IMT). *Int J Lepr* 1997; **65:** 320–7.
17. Walia R, *et al.* Field trials on the use of Mycobacterium w vaccine in conjunction with multidrug therapy in leprosy patients for immunotherapeutic and immunoprophylactic purposes. *Lepr Rev* 1993; **64:** 302–11.


## Leptospirosis Vaccines

Leptospira Vaccines; Vacunas de la leptospirosis.

### Profile

Leptospirosis vaccines prepared from killed *Leptospira interrogans* are available in some countries. They are used for active immunisation against leptospirosis icterohaemorrhagica (spirochaetal jaundice; Weil's disease) in persons at high risk of contracting the disease.

### Preparations

**Proprietary Preparations** (details are given in Part 3)
***Fr.:*** Spirolept.

## Lyme Disease Vaccines

Vacunas de la enfermedad de Lyme.

### Adverse Effects and Precautions

As for vaccines in general, p.1605.

Lyme arthritis refractory to treatment with antibacterials has occurred rarely as an immune reaction to vaccine-derived outer surface proteins of *Borrelia burgdorferi*.

### Uses and Administration

Vaccines based on recombinant outer surface proteins of *Borrelia burgdorferi* have been developed and used in some countries for active immunisation against Lyme disease in persons at risk of contracting the disease.

### Preparations

**Proprietary Preparations** (details are given in Part 3)
***Canad.:*** LYMErix†; ***USA:*** LYMErix†.

## Malaria Vaccines

Vacunas del paludismo.

### Profile

Malaria vaccines acting against the sporozoite, asexual, and sexual stages of the *Plasmodium falciparum* life cycle are under investigation, as well as multicomponent vaccines consisting of combined antigens from various stages.

**Vaccine development.** Chemoprophylaxis of malaria is becoming increasingly problematical (see p.444), resulting in the increased desirability of effective malaria vaccines, several of which have been, or are being, studied clinically. The various approaches to malaria vaccine development have been reviewed.[1-3] Malaria vaccines can be categorised into 3 main groups:

- vaccines against pre-erythrocytic forms of the parasite or specifically sporozoites would prevent development of clinical disease and interrupt transmission by insect vectors. However, infection acquired by blood transfusion would not be prevented. RTS,S, a recombinant circumsporozoite protein fused with the more immunogenic adjuvant hepatis B surface antigen, produced encouraging results in a preliminary study[4] although results in a follow-up study[5] were disappointing and it was considered that further development of vaccine composition was needed. Subsequent combination with an adjuvant, AS02, led to more promising protection rates with RTS,S/AS02.[6] Other pre-erythrocytic vaccines under investigation include ICC-1132 and NYU-CS.[2]
- vaccines against asexual stages of the parasite would inhibit development of clinical disease but would not interrupt transmission. Infection of the liver would not be impeded. Candidates include AMA-1, MSP-1, MSP-2, MSP-3, MSP/RESA, FMP-1, and GLURP.[2]
- vaccines against the sexual stages of the life cycle (so called 'altruistic' vaccines) would interrupt malaria transmission but would not prevent infection with sporozoites or development of asexual forms in the blood or liver.

A further approach that has been studied involves the development of vaccines to induce production of cytotoxic T-lymphocytes which confer immunity from malaria via destruction of parasite-infected hepatocytes.[7]

WHO envisages that different types of vaccine could be used in combination. Various malarial antigens have been identified and studied in the hope of developing a multicomponent vaccine. One such vaccine, SPf66, was developed in Colombia where it was shown to be effective in semi-immune populations in endemic areas.[8,9] The vaccine consists of a synthetic preparation of three antigens from the asexual phase of the parasite in the blood linked by a sporozoite antigen. Subsequent studies in Ecuador[10] and Venezuela[11] demonstrated efficacy of 67 and 55% respectively. However, the reproducibility of the results and the efficacy of this vaccine in highly endemic regions was the cause of considerable controversy[12-14] which, it was hoped, had been resolved by the results of a clinical study from Tanzania[15,16] where vaccine efficacy was reported to be 31%. Although low, it was thought that this degree of efficacy could substantially reduce mortality.[17] Unfortunately, however, SPf66 did not protect against clinical falciparum malaria in studies from The Gambia[18] and Thailand.[19]

Another multicomponent vaccine, NYVAC-Pf7, using a recombinant vaccinia viral vector that expresses 7 proteins from different stages of malarial infection, has also been studied,[20] but results have been disappointing. A further multicomponent vaccine, CDC/NIIMALVAC-1 has provided encouraging preliminary results in *animals* and *in vitro*.[21]

DNA vaccines against malaria are also under investigation.[22]


1. Webster D, Hill AVS. Progress with new malaria vaccines. *Bull WHO* 2003; **81:** 902–9.
2. Moorthy VS, *et al.* Malaria vaccine developments. *Lancet* 2004; **363:** 150–6.
3. Graves P, Gelbrand H. Vaccines for preventing malaria. Available in The Cochrane Library; Issue 1. Chichester: John Wiley; 2004.
4. Stoute JA, *et al.* A preliminary evaluation of a recombinant circumsporozoite protein vaccine against Plasmodium falciparum malaria. *N Engl J Med* 1997; **336:** 86–91.
5. Stoute JA, *et al.* Long-term efficacy and immune responses following immunization with the RTS,S malaria vaccine. *J Infect Dis* 1998; **178:** 1139–44.
6. Bojang KA, *et al.* Efficacy of RTS,S/AS02 malaria vaccine against Plasmodium falciparum infection in semi-immune adult men in The Gambia: a randomised trial. *Lancet* 2001; **358:** 1927–34.
7. Aidoo M, *et al.* Identification of conserved antigenic components for a cytotoxic T lymphocyte-inducing vaccine against malaria. *Lancet* 1995; **345:** 1003–7.
8. Valero MV, *et al.* Vaccination with SPf66, a chemically synthesised vaccine, against Plasmodium falciparum malaria in Colombia. *Lancet* 1993; **341:** 705–10.
9. Amador R, *et al.* The first field trials of the chemically synthesized malaria vaccine SPf66: safety, immunogenicity and protectivity. *Vaccine* 1992; **10:** 179–84.
10. Sempertegui F, *et al.* Safety, immunogenicity and protective effect of the SPf66 malaria synthetic vaccine against Plasmodium falciparum infection in a randomised double-blind placebo-controlled field trial in an endemic area of Ecuador. *Vaccine* 1994; **12:** 337–42.
11. Noya O, *et al.* A population based clinical trial with the SPf66 synthetic Plasmodium falciparum malaria vaccine in Venezuela. *J Infect Dis* 1994; **170:** 396–402.
12. Anonymous. Towards a malarial vaccine. *Lancet* 1992; **339:** 586–7.
13. Marsh K. Patarroyo's vaccine. *Lancet* 1993; **341:** 729–30.
14. Anonymous. Malaria: a first stride towards effective vaccination? *WHO Drug Inf* 1993; **7:** 45–7.
15. Teuscher T, *et al.* SPf66, a chemically synthesized subunit malaria vaccine, is safe and immunogenic in Tanzanians exposed to intense malaria transmission. *Vaccine* 1994; **12:** 328–36.
16. Alonso PL, *et al.* Randomised trial of efficacy of SPf66 vaccine against Plasmodium falciparum malaria in children in southern Tanzania. *Lancet* 1994; **344:** 1175–81.
17. White NJ. Tough test for malaria vaccine. *Lancet* 1994; **344:** 1172–3.
18. D'Alessandro U, *et al.* Efficacy trial of malaria vaccine SPf66 in Gambian infants. *Lancet* 1995; **346:** 462–7.
19. Nosten F, *et al.* Randomised double-blind placebo-controlled trial of SPf66 malaria vaccine in children in northwestern Thailand. *Lancet* 1996; **348:** 701–7.
20. Ockenhouse CF, *et al.* Phase I/IIa safety, immunogenicity, and efficacy trial of NYVAC-Pf7, a pox-vectored, multiantigen, multistage vaccine candidate for Plasmodium falciparum malaria. *J Infect Dis* 1998; **177:** 1664–73.
21. Shi YP, *et al.* Immunogenicity and in vitro protective efficacy of a recombinant multistage Plasmodium falciparum candidate vaccine. *Proc Natl Acad Sci U S A* 1999; **96:** 1615–20.
22. Moorthy VS, *et al.* Safety and immunogenicity of DNA/modified vaccinia virus ankara malaria vaccination in African adults. *J Infect Dis* 2003; **188:** 1239–44.

## Measles Immunoglobulins

Inmunoglobulinas contra el sarampión.

*ATC — J06BB14.*

**Pharmacopoeias.** Many pharmacopoeias have monographs including *Eur.* (see p.vi).

**Ph. Eur. 5.0** (Human Measles Immunoglobulin; Immunoglobulinum Humanum Morbillicum). A liquid or freeze-dried preparation containing immunoglobulins, mainly immunoglobulin G (IgG). It is obtained from plasma containing specific antibodies against the measles virus. Normal immunoglobulin may be added. It contains not less than 50 international units/mL. Both the liquid and freeze-dried preparations should be stored, protected from light, in a colourless, glass container. The freeze-dried preparation should be stored under vacuum or under an inert gas.

### Adverse Effects and Precautions

As for immunoglobulins in general, p.1605.

### Interactions

As for immunoglobulins in general, p.1605.

### Uses and Administration

Measles immunoglobulins may be used for passive immunisation against measles. They have been used to prevent or modify measles in susceptible persons who have been exposed to infection; in the UK, normal immunoglobulin is usually given.

### Preparations

***Ph. Eur.:*** Human Measles Immunoglobulin.

**Proprietary Preparations** (details are given in Part 3)
***Ital.:*** Immunomorb†; Morbil†; Moruman†; ***S.Afr.:*** Measlegam†.

## Measles Vaccines

Vacunas del sarampión.

*ATC — J07BD01.*

**Pharmacopoeias.** Many pharmacopoeias have monographs including *Eur.* (see p.vi) and *US.*

**Ph. Eur. 5.0** (Measles Vaccine (Live); Vaccinum Morbillorum Vivum). A freeze-dried preparation of a suitable live attenuated strain of measles virus grown in cultures of chick-embryo cells or human diploid cells. It is prepared immediately before use by reconstitution from the dried vaccine. The virus titre is not less than $1 \times 10^3$ $CCID_{50}$ per dose. The dried vaccine should be stored at 2° to 8° and be protected from light.

The BP 2003 states that Meas/Vac(Live) may be used on the label.

**USP 27** (Measles Virus Vaccine Live). A bacterially sterile preparation of a suitable live strain of measles virus grown in cultures of chick-embryo cells. It contains not less than the equivalent of $1 \times 10^3$ $TCID_{50}$ in each immunising dose, and may contain suitable antimicrobial agents. It should be stored at 2° to 8° and be protected from light.

### Adverse Effects

As for vaccines in general, p.1605.

Fever and skin rashes may occur following the administration of measles vaccines. The fever generally starts 5 to 10 days after the injection, lasts for about 1 or 2 days, and has sometimes been accompanied by convulsions. More serious effects reported rarely include encephalitis and thrombocytopenia.

◊ Reviews.

1. Duclos P, Ward BJ. Measles vaccines: a review of adverse events. *Drug Safety* 1998; **19:** 435–54.

**Incidence of adverse effects.** Some brief comments made by the Advisory Committee on Immunization Practices in the USA on adverse effects of standard measles vaccines.[1] An excellent safety record of measles vaccines has been indicated by the experience gained through the use of more than 160 million doses up to 1986. Fever with a temperature of 39.4° or more may develop in 5 to 15% of vaccinees beginning about the fifth day after vaccination and usually lasts several days. Transient rashes have been reported in about 5% of vaccinees. CNS disorders, including encephalitis and encephalopathy, have been reported with a frequency of less than one case per million doses given. The incidence of encephalitis or encephalopathy after vaccination is lower than the incidence rate of encephalitis of unknown origin suggesting that such events after vaccination may be only temporally related to, rather than due to, vaccination.

1. Immunization Practices Advisory Committee. Measles prevention. *JAMA* 1987; **258:** 890–5.

**Atypical measles.** The atypical-measles syndrome has occurred in persons vaccinated against measles and later exposed to the natural infection. The syndrome has been characterised by high fever and atypical rash; abdominal pain has been common and pneumonia almost universal.[1] Although atypical measles has occurred particularly in patients given killed vaccine[1] (no longer used) it has been reported in recipients of live measles vaccines.[2-4]

Measles occurring in patients previously vaccinated with live measles vaccines may be mild and go unrecognised. However, secondary vaccine failure does not appear to be a major problem (see Immunisation Schedules under Uses, below).

1. Anonymous. The atypical-measles syndrome. *Lancet* 1979; **i:** 962–3.
2. Chatterji M, Mankad V. Failure of attenuated viral vaccine in prevention of atypical measles. *JAMA* 1977; **238:** 2635.
3. Henderson JAM, Hammond DI. Delayed diagnosis in atypical measles syndrome. *Can Med Assoc J* 1985; **133:** 211–13.
4. Hirose M, *et al.* Five cases of measles secondary vaccine failure with confirmed seroconversion after live measles vaccination. *Scand J Infect Dis* 1997; **29:** 187–90.

**Effects on hearing.** There have been individual case reports of sensorineural hearing loss after measles vaccination.[1,2] Similar reports have been made after vaccination with measles and rubella vaccines (p.1624) and measles, mumps, and rubella vaccines (p.1625).

1. Watson JG. Bilateral hearing loss in a 3-year-old girl following measles immunisation at the age of 15 months. *Int J Pediatr Otorhinolaryngol* 1990; **19:** 189–90.
2. Jayarajan V, Sedler PA. Hearing loss following measles vaccination. *J Infect* 1995; **30:** 184–5.

**Effects on the nervous system.** Subacute sclerosing panencephalitis (SSPE) is a rare complication of measles infection (p.624) and has been reported in children who have received measles vaccine but have no history of clinical disease. Nevertheless mass measles vaccination has been effective in reducing the incidence of SSPE in both developing and industrialised countries,[1] and the risks of remaining unimmunised are considered to be greater than those arising from immunisation.

1. Anonymous. SSPE in the developing world. *Lancet* 1990; **336:** 600.

GUILLAIN-BARRÉ SYNDROME. No association was found between measles vaccination and Guillain-Barré syndrome in an analysis of 2296 cases.[1]

1. da Silveira CM, *et al.* Measles vaccination and Guillain-Barré syndrome. *Lancet* 1997; **349:** 14–16.

OPTIC NEURITIS. For a report of optic neuritis in 2 children following administration of measles and rubella vaccine, see under Adverse Effects of Measles and Rubella Vaccines, p.1625.

**Effects on the skin.** Stevens-Johnson syndrome was associated with measles vaccination in a 10-month-old infant.[1]

1. Hazir T, *et al.* Stevens-Johnson syndrome following measles vaccination. *J Pakistan Med Assoc* 1997; **47:** 264–5.

**High-titre vaccines and mortality.** Following reports of excess mortality in children, especially among girls, who received high-titre Edmonston-Zagreb (EZ) measles vaccine,[1] WHO reversed its recommendation for the use of this vaccine in its Expanded Programme on Immunization in developing countries.[2,3] Subsequent study[4] of children who had received high-titre EZ vaccine showed adverse effects on the nutritional status in either sex, confirming a generally deleterious effect of the vaccine. Others, however, have argued that the problems associated with the use of EZ vaccine have been exaggerated.[5]

1. Knudsen KM, *et al.* Child mortality following standard, medium or high titre measles immunization in West Africa. *Int J Epidemiol* 1996; **25:** 665–73.
2. Anonymous. High-titre measles vaccines dropped. *Lancet* 1992; **340:** 232.
3. WHO. Expanded Programme on Immunization; safety of high-titre measles vaccines. *Wkly Epidem Rec* 1992; **67:** 357–61.
4. Garenne M. Effect of Edmonston-Zagreb high-titre vaccine on nutritional status. *Lancet* 1994; **344:** 261–2.
5. Bennett JV, *et al.* Edmonston-Zagreb measles vaccine: a good vaccine with an image problem. *Pediatrics* 1999; **104:** 1123–4.

### Precautions

As for vaccines in general, p.1606.

In the UK it was formerly recommended that children with a personal history of convulsions or those whose parents or siblings have a history of idiopathic epilepsy should receive measles vaccine but simultaneously with a specially diluted human normal immunoglobulin; it is now, however, recommended that such children be vaccinated with combined measles, mumps, and rubella vaccine in the same manner as normal healthy children. Carers should understand that a febrile reaction is possible and that suitable prophylactic treatment against febrile convulsions be undertaken (see Fever and Hyperthermia, p.8, for comments on the prevention of fever following immunisation). Immunoglobulin should not be given with the combined vaccine.

Measles vaccines are not generally recommended for children below the age of 1 year in whom maternal antibodies might prevent a response, but they have been given to younger infants when the risk of measles is particularly high (see Immunisation Schedules, under Uses, below, for further discussion).

**Hypersensitivity.** For discussion of precautions to be taken on administration of measles vaccines to children allergic to egg, see Measles, Mumps, and Rubella Vaccines, p.1625.

**Immunocompromised patients.** For a discussion of the use of live vaccines in immunocompromised patients including those with HIV infections, see under Uses on p.1607.

As with other live vaccines, measles vaccine is generally not recommended for use in patients with impaired immunity, although combined measles, mumps, and rubella vaccine may be given to HIV-positive individuals in the absence of other contra-indications. The WHO and UNICEF[1] recommend that children with suspected or confirmed HIV infection should receive a dose of measles vaccine at 6 months of age in addition to the scheduled dose at 9 months. The immunogenicity of measles vaccine in children with HIV infections has been shown to be low[2,3] although immunisation at 6 months of age was more effective than at 12 months of age.[3] Immunocompromised patients who come into contact with measles should be given normal immunoglobulin. Specific measles immunoglobulins are available in some countries. Although measles vaccines have been given to immunocompromised patients without causing adverse effects[2] there have been some reports of severe reactions; disseminated measles infection was reported in a child with severe congenital immunodeficiency,[4] and fatal giant-cell pneumonitis was reported in an adult with AIDS.[5] The American Academy of Pediatrics has recommended[6] that *severely* immunosuppressed HIV-infected children and young adults should not receive any measles-containing vaccines, whereas those with HIV infection but without evidence of severe immunosuppression should receive measles, mumps, and rubella vaccine. They also recommend that if HIV-infected children or adolescents are exposed to wild type measles, they should receive normal immunoglobulin regardless of their degree of immunosuppression or measles immunisation status.[6]

1. WHO. *EPI vaccines in HIV-infected individuals: 5 October 2001.* Available at: http://www.who.int/vaccines-diseases/diseases/HIV.shtml (accessed 22/06/04)
2. Krasinski K, Borkowsky W. Measles and measles immunity in children infected with human immunodeficiency virus. *JAMA* 1989; **261:** 2512–16.
3. Rudy BJ, *et al.* Responses to measles immunization in children infected with human immunodeficiency virus. *J Pediatr* 1994; **125:** 72–4.
4. Monafo WJ, *et al.* Disseminated measles infection after vaccination in a child with a congenital immunodeficiency. *J Pediatr* 1994; **124:** 273–6.
5. Angel JB, *et al.* Vaccine-associated measles pneumonitis in an adult with AIDS. *Ann Intern Med* 1998; **129:** 104–6.
6. American Academy of Pediatrics Committee on Infectious Diseases and Committee on Pediatric AIDS. Measles immunization in HIV-infected children. *Pediatrics* 1999; **103:** 1057–60.

**Inflammatory bowel disease.** Measles vaccination has been suggested as a possible factor in the development of inflammatory bowel disease.[1] However a case-control study involving 140 patients with inflammatory bowel disease provided no support for this hypothesis,[2] and measles virus has not been detected in biopsy specimens from patients with inflammatory bowel disease.[3] A suggested link between measles vaccine-associated inflammatory bowel disease and autism has proved controversial (see p.1625).

1. Thompson NP, *et al.* Is measles vaccination a risk factor for inflammatory bowel disease? *Lancet* 1995; **345:** 1071–4.
2. Feeney M, *et al.* A case-control study of measles vaccination and inflammatory bowel disease. *Lancet* 1997; **350:** 764–6.
3. Afzal MA, *et al.* Absence of measles-virus genome in inflammatory bowel disease. *Lancet* 1998; **351:** 646–7.

### Interactions

As for vaccines in general, p.1606

**Vitamin A.** Supplementation with vitamin A (p.1453) is now included as part of WHO's Expanded Programme on Immunization. There is conflicting evidence of the effects of such supplementation on the response to measles vaccination. One study[1] reported a reduced response if vaccination occurs at 6 months while another[2] found the response to be unaffected in children vaccinated at 9 months. This difference, if confirmed, could be due to the influence of maternal antibodies, which would still be present at 6 months but not at 9 months of age.[3]

1. Semba RD, *et al.* Reduced seroconversion to measles in infants given vitamin A with measles vaccination. *Lancet* 1995; **345:** 1330–2.
2. Benn CS, *et al.* Randomised trial of effect of vitamin A supplementation on antibody response to measles vaccine in Guinea-Bissau, West Africa. *Lancet* 1997; **350:** 101–5.
3. Semba RD. Vitamin A supplementation. *Lancet* 1997; **350:** 1031–2.

### Uses and Administration

Measles vaccines are used for active immunisation against measles.

For primary immunisation a combined measles, mumps, and rubella vaccine (p.1625) is usually used. For discussion of immunisation schedules, see below.

In the UK, single-antigen measles vaccine prepared from the Schwarz strain of the measles virus was formerly used. It was given in a dose of 0.5 mL by deep subcutaneous or intramuscular injection.

Measles vaccines are not generally recommended for children below the age of 1 year in whom maternal antibodies might prevent a response. However, they have been given to infants at 6 to 9 months of age in developing countries and in the USA in certain circumstances (see also Immunisation Schedules, below). A high-potency measles vaccine prepared from the Edmonston-Zagreb strain of measles virus was formerly used but was discontinued following evidence of increased mortality (see High-titre Vaccines and Mortality, under Adverse Effects, above).

Single-antigen measles vaccines have also been used for prophylaxis after exposure to measles provided they are given within 72 hours of contact.

**Administration.** Several alternative routes of administration of measles vaccines have been investigated in an attempt to overcome some of the disadvantages of subcutaneous or intramuscular injection.[1] Intradermal injection is effective if a needle is to be used but carries the same risk of secondary infection as subcutaneous administration; the use of a jet injector has produced less reliable immunisation. The conjunctival and oral routes are not sufficiently effective, and the intranasal route produced variable responses and could be influenced by concurrent upper respiratory-tract infections. A review of clinical studies[1] has shown that aerosol administration has produced good responses in children over 9 months of age, although this route was not so effective in younger children. The Edmonston-Zagreb strain generally produced higher rates of seroconversion than the Schwarz strain. Aerosol administration could be potentially useful for mass immunisation campaigns and this suggestion was confirmed in a randomised study.[2]

1. Cutts FT, *et al.* Alternative routes of measles immunization: a review. *Biologicals* 1997; **25:** 323–38.
2. Dilraj A, *et al.* Response to different measles vaccine strains given by aerosol and subcutaneous routes to schoolchildren: a randomised trial. *Lancet* 2000; **355:** 798–803.

**Immunisation schedules.** In the developed world measles vaccine (usually as measles, mumps, and rubella vaccine) is usually given in the second year of life.[1] As a result of concern that measles vaccine would not elicit an appropriate immune response in young infants due to the persistence of maternal antibodies in circulation, vaccination has generally not been attempted in children under 12 months old. Studies have shown that seroconversion rates are similar following vaccination at 12, 13, 14, and 15 to 18 months.[2] However, infants born to vaccinated mothers tend to have lower levels of maternal antibodies and are susceptible to measles infection at under 12 months of age; vaccination has been shown to be effective at 6 to 9 months of age in such children,[3-5] although antibody titres were lower in infants vaccinated at 6 months of age than in those vaccinated later.[3,6]

In the UK and USA, routine vaccination is given at 12 to 15 months, with a second dose given at 3 to 6 years or 11 to 18 years of age (see the immunisation schedules summarised under Vaccines, p.1606). Similar schedules are used in other countries. There is evidence that these 2-dose strategies will produce high levels of immunity in the community.[7] During an outbreak of measles, vaccination may be given as early as 6 months of age;[8] revaccination is recommended in any child who is vaccinated before their first birthday. Vaccine may be given to non-immune persons of any age considered to be at risk of infection even if their immune status is uncertain.

Immunisation strategies involving a single dose of measles vaccine have not been successful in eradicating or eliminating the disease in developed countries.[9,10] Immunisation has changed the epidemiology of measles and several isolated outbreaks have occurred among both unvaccinated and vaccinated persons.[9] Primary vaccine failure (approximately 2 to 10% of vaccinees fail to seroconvert after measles vaccination) has played a substantial role in transmission of measles.[9] Furthermore, waning of immunity in the vaccinated cohort coupled with a reduction in the prevalence of the natural infection has resulted in increasing numbers of young adults with low concentrations of antibodies.[11,12] As these young adults reach child-bearing age, their children in turn have lower, faster-waning immunity and are susceptible to infection before the usual age of immunisation.[13] Immunisation schedules which include a second dose of measles vaccine in adolescence would boost immunity in young adults and hence in their offspring, but there is evidence that revaccination is ineffective in a proportion of recipients.[14,15] The alternative is to give the first dose of vaccine earlier, for example at 6 months of age, and a second dose in early childhood. However this too would not overcome the problem of secondary vaccine failures in young adults. This dilemma over the most appropriate schedule is most pressing in developing countries where transmission rates are usually high. For discussion of immunisation schedules in the developing world, see under Expanded Programme on Immunization, below.

1. Isaacs D, Menser M. Modern vaccines: measles, mumps, rubella, and varicella. *Lancet* 1990; **335:** 1384–7.
2. Kakakios AM, *et al.* Optimal age for measles and mumps vaccination in Australia. *Med J Aust* 1990; **152:** 472–4.
3. Johnson CE, *et al.* Measles vaccine immunogenicity in 6- versus 15-month-old infants born to mothers in the measles vaccine era. *Pediatrics* 1994; **93:** 939–44.
4. Carson MM, *et al.* Measles vaccination of infants in a well-vaccinated population. *Pediatr Infect Dis J* 1995; **14:** 17–22.
5. Markowitz LE, *et al.* Changing levels of measles antibody titers in women and children in the United States: impact on response to vaccination. *Pediatrics* 1996; **97:** 53–8.
6. Gans HA, *et al.* Deficiency of the humoral immune response to measles vaccine in infants immunized at age 6 months. *JAMA* 1998; **280:** 527–32.
7. Poland GA, *et al.* Measles reimmunization in children seronegative after initial immunization. *JAMA* 1997; **277:** 1156–8.
8. De Serres G, *et al.* Effectiveness of vaccination at 6 to 11 months of age during an outbreak of measles. *Pediatrics* 1996; **97:** 232–5.
9. Immunization Practices Advisory Committee. Measles prevention: supplementary statement. *JAMA* 1989; **261:** 827 and 831.
10. Levy MH, Bridges-Webb C. "Just one shot" is not enough — measles control and eradication. *Med J Aust* 1990; **152:** 489–91.
11. Mulholland K. Measles and pertussis in developing countries with good vaccine coverage. *Lancet* 1995; **345:** 305–7.
12. McLean AR. After the honeymoon in measles control. *Lancet* 1995; **345:** 272.
13. Maldonado YA, *et al.* Early loss of passive measles antibody in infants of mothers with vaccine-induced immunity. *Pediatrics* 1995; **96:** 447–50.
14. Markowitz LE, *et al.* Persistence of measles antibody after revaccination. *J Infect Dis* 1992; **166:** 205–8.
15. Cohn ML, *et al.* Measles vaccine failures: lack of sustained measles-specific immunoglobulin G responses in revaccinated adolescents and young adults. *Pediatr Infect Dis J* 1994; **13:** 34–8.

EXPANDED PROGRAMME ON IMMUNIZATION. In the developed world measles vaccine (usually as measles, mumps, and rubella vaccine) is usually given in the second year of life. If given earlier, passively-acquired maternal antibodies against measles may interfere with development of protective immunity although this situation is changing as vaccinated women reach child-bearing age (see Immunisation Schedules, above). In the developing world, protection given by maternal antibodies is often rapidly lost.[1] Thus in hyperendemic areas, such as urban and peri-urban areas, clinical measles may occur in children as young as 5 to 6 months of age. Immunisation against measles is part of WHO's Expanded Programme on Immunization.[2] It is given as a single-antigen vaccine generally at 9 months of age. However control of measles in children less than 9 months of age is a major concern in some countries, in particular in areas of high population density.[3] WHO no longer recommends the use of high-titre Edmonston-Zagreb measles vaccine. Unlike conventional vaccines, this vaccine was shown to be effective at 6 months of age but, despite the resulting increase in immunity, increased mortality has been observed (see High-titre Vaccines and Mortality, under Adverse Effects, above). For comments on the possibility of a resurgence of measles infection in young adults and infants in countries with good vaccine coverage, see under Immunisation Schedules, above. WHO recognises that vaccination strategies will need to be formulated to cope with local disease patterns and available resources.[3]

In some situations high coverage with a single dose of vaccine can produce a high degree of immunity[3] and standard titre vaccines have been shown to be as effective as high-titre vaccines.[4,5] Mass immunisation campaigns can also be very effective[6] but can be expensive when a large proportion of the community is already immune.[7,8]

Early 2-dose schedules[3] may be more applicable in areas with high transmission rates among young infants. The first dose is typically given at 9 months of age and the second dose 3 to 6 months later. In very high-risk situations, such as refugee camps and following disasters, the first dose may be given at 6 months of age and the second dose as soon as possible after the child reaches 9 months of age.

Late 2-dose schedules[3] may be more appropriate in industrialised countries in which measles transmission among young infants is limited. The schedule is aimed at preventing infection in older children following primary or secondary vaccine failure. The first dose is typically given at 9 to 12 months of age, and the second dose at school entry.

Several studies have examined the effect of measles immunisation on mortality and morbidity in developing countries.[9] Data suggest that the reduction in mortality following immunisation is greater than that expected simply from a reduction in death from acute measles. Measles immunisation may protect children dying not only from an acute measles attack but also from late causes which may be attributable to measles. It is also possible that measles vaccine has an immunostimulant effect.

For discussion of the link between vitamin A status and measles see Measles, under Uses and Administration of Vitamin A Substances, p.1453.

1. Toole MJ, *et al.* Measles prevention and control in emergency settings. *Bull WHO* 1989; **67:** 381–8.
2. Hall AJ, *et al.* Modern vaccines: practice in developing countries. *Lancet* 1990; **335:** 774–7.
3. Rosenthal SR, Clements CJ. Two-dose measles vaccination schedules. *Bull WHO* 1993; **71:** 421–8.
4. Garenne M, *et al.* Efficacy of measles vaccines after controlling for exposure. *Am J Epidemiol* 1993; **138:** 182–95.
5. Diaz-Ortega J-L, *et al.* The relationship between dose and response of standard measles vaccines. *Biologicals* 1994; **22:** 35–44.
6. de Quadros CA, *et al.* Measles elimination in the Americas: evolving strategies. *JAMA* 1996; **275:** 224–9.
7. Cutts FT. Measles control in young infants: where do we go from here? *Lancet* 1993; **341:** 290–1.
8. Global Programme for Vaccines of the World Health Organization. Role of mass campaigns in global measles control. *Lancet* 1994; **344:** 174–5.
9. Aaby P, Clements CJ. Measles immunization research: a review. *Bull WHO* 1989; **67:** 443–8.

**Immunisation for travellers.** The Advisory Committee on Immunization Practices in the USA has recommended that administration of measles vaccine be considered for all persons travelling abroad who were born after 1956, regardless of their vaccination status.[1] Travellers who have had measles or were born before 1957 are considered immune secondary to natural infection.[2] Single-antigen measles vaccine or measles, mumps, and rubella vaccine may be used.[1] Children aged 6 to 11 months should receive a dose of single-antigen vaccine if travelling to areas where measles is endemic or epidemic.[1] A dose of measles, mumps, and rubella vaccine is given at 15 months, or 12 months if the child remains in a high-risk area.

1. Immunization Practices Advisory Committee. Measles prevention. *JAMA* 1987; **258:** 890–5.
2. Hill DR, Pearson RD. Measles prophylaxis for international travel. *Ann Intern Med* 1989; **111:** 699–701.

## Preparations

***Ph. Eur.:*** Measles Vaccine (Live);
***USP 27:*** Measles Virus Vaccine Live.

**Proprietary Preparations** (details are given in Part 3)
***Arg.:*** Lirugen; ***Austral.:*** Rimevax; ***Belg.:*** Rimevax†; ***Braz.:*** Attenuvax†; Rouvax; ***Denm.:*** Attenuvax; ***Fr.:*** Rouvax; ***Ger.:*** Masern-Impfstoff Merieux; Masern-Lebend-Impfstoff†; Masern-Vaccinol†; Masern-Virus-Impfstoff†; ***Gr.:*** Rouvax Merieux; ***Hong Kong:*** Moraten†; Rouvax†; ***India:*** M-Vac; ***Israel:*** Mevilin-L†; Rimevax; Rouvax; ***Ital.:*** Attenuvax†; Lio-Morbilo†; Moraten†; Morbilvax; Rimevax†; Rouvax; ***Malaysia:*** Rimevax; ***Mex.:*** Rimevax; ***NZ:*** Moraten†; Rimevax†; ***Port.:*** Moraten†; ***S.Afr.:*** Diplovax; Moraten†; Morbilvax; Rimevax; Rouvax; ***Singapore:*** Moraten†; ***Spain:*** Amunovax; Rimevax; ***Switz.:*** Attenuvax; Moraten; Rimevax; ***Thai.:*** Moraten†; Morbilvax; Rimevax†; Rouvax; ***UK:*** Mevilin-L†; ***USA:*** Attenuvax.

## Measles and Mumps Vaccines

Vacunas del sarampión y la parotiditis.

*ATC — J07BD51.*

### Adverse Effects and Precautions

As for vaccines in general, p.1605.

See also under Measles Vaccines, p.1623, and Mumps Vaccines, p.1626.

**Effects on the bones and joints.** For a reference to arthritis occurring after administration of measles and mumps vaccine, see under Adverse Effects and Precautions of Measles, Mumps, and Rubella Vaccines, p.1625.

### Interactions

As for vaccines in general, p.1606.

See also under Measles Vaccines, p.1623.

### Uses and Administration

Measles and mumps vaccines may be used for active immunisation against measles and mumps. Vaccination against measles and mumps is normally performed using a combined measles, mumps, and rubella vaccine (p.1625) but bivalent measles and mumps vaccines have been employed when vaccination against rubella is not indicated. For discussion of immunisation schedules, see under Vaccines, p.1606.

Two types of vaccine have been used. The first has been prepared from a more attenuated line of measles virus derived from Enders' attenuated Edmonston strain and the Jeryl Lynn (B level) strain of mumps virus, and the second from the attenuated Schwarz strain of measles virus and the attenuated Urabe Am 9 strain of mumps virus. For both types, a 0.5-mL dose has been given by intramuscular or subcutaneous injection.

Measles and mumps vaccines may also be used for prophylaxis after exposure to measles provided it is given within 72 hours of contact.

### Preparations

**Proprietary Preparations** (details are given in Part 3)
***Belg.:*** Duovax†; ***Ger.:*** M-M Vax; MM Diplovax†; ***S.Afr.:*** Biviraten†; ***Switz.:*** Biviraten†; M-M Vax†.

## Measles and Rubella Vaccines

Vacunas del sarampión y la rubéola.

*ATC — J07BD53.*

**Pharmacopoeias.** Many pharmacopoeias have monographs including *US.*

**USP 27** (Measles and Rubella Virus Vaccine Live). Bacterially sterile preparation of suitable live strains of measles virus and live rubella virus. It may contain suitable antimicrobial agents. Each labelled dose provides an immunising dose of each component. It should be stored at 2° to 8° and be protected from light.

### Adverse Effects and Precautions

As for vaccines in general, p.1605.

See also under Measles Vaccines, p.1623, and Rubella Vaccines, p.1637.

**Incidence of adverse effects.** Eight million children aged between 5 and 16 years were immunised with a measles and rubella vaccine in 1994 in the UK. By October 1995 the UK Committee on Safety of Medicines had received reports on 2735 suspected adverse reactions most of which were minor and self-limiting.[1] Serious suspected reactions were rare and generally the number of reported cases was consistent with the background frequency of the particular disorder.

1. Committee on Safety of Medicines/Medicines Control Agency. Adverse reactions to measles rubella vaccine. *Current Problems* 1995; **21:** 9–10.

**Effects on hearing.** Profound, irreversible sensorineural deafness was reported in a 27-year-old woman after administration of a measles and rubella vaccine.[1] Sensorineural deafness has also been reported after administration of measles, mumps, and rubella vaccine (p.1625), and monovalent measles vaccine (p.1623).

1. Hulbert TV, *et al.* Bilateral hearing loss after measles and rubella vaccination in an adult. *N Engl J Med* 1991; **325:** 134.

**Effects on the nervous system.** Optic neuritis was reported in 2 children who had received measles and rubella vaccine 2 to 3 weeks previously.[1]

1. Stevenson VL, *et al.* Optic neuritis following measles/rubella vaccination in two 13-year-old children. *Br J Ophthalmol* 1996; **80:** 1110–11.

### Interactions

As for vaccines in general, p.1606.

See also under Measles Vaccines, p.1623.

### Uses and Administration

Measles and rubella vaccines may be used for active immunisation against measles and rubella. For primary immunisation a combined measles, mumps, and rubella vaccine (p.1625) is usually used but bivalent measles and rubella vaccines have been employed when vaccination against mumps is not indicated. For discussion of immunisation schedules, see under Vaccines, p.1606.

Vaccines have been prepared from either a more attenuated line of measles virus derived from Enders' attenuated Edmonston strain or attenuated Schwarz strain, and the Wistar RA 27/3 strain of rubella virus. They are generally given in a dose of 0.5 mL by subcutaneous or intramuscular injection to infants or to other susceptible children or adults considered to be at risk.

### Preparations

***USP 27:*** Measles and Rubella Virus Vaccine Live.

**Proprietary Preparations** (details are given in Part 3)
***Braz.:*** Rudi-Rouvax; ***Canad.:*** MoRu-Viraten†; ***Ital.:*** Morubel†; ***Switz.:*** MoRu-Viraten†; ***Thai.:*** Rudi-Rouvax; ***USA:*** M-R-Vax II†.

## Measles, Mumps, and Rubella Vaccines

Vacunas del sarampión, la parotiditis y la rubéola.

*ATC — J07BD52.*

**Pharmacopoeias.** Many pharmacopoeias have monographs including *Eur.* (see p.vi) and *US.*

**Ph. Eur. 5.0** (Measles, Mumps and Rubella Vaccine (Live); Vaccinum Morbillorum, Parotitidis et Rubellae Vivum). A freeze-dried preparation containing suitable live attenuated strains of measles virus, mumps virus (*Paramyxovirus parotitidis*), and rubella virus. The vaccine is prepared immediately before use by reconstitution from the dried vaccine. It contains in each dose not less than $1 \times 10^3$ $CCID_{50}$ of infective measles virus, not less than $5 \times 10^3$ $CCID_{50}$ of infective mumps virus, and not less than $1 \times 10^3$ $CCID_{50}$ of infective rubella virus. The dried vaccine should be stored at 2° to 8° and be protected from light.

The BP 2003 states that MMR/Vac(Live) may be used on the label.

**USP 27** (Measles, Mumps, and Rubella Virus Vaccine Live). A bacterially sterile preparation of suitable live strains of measles virus, mumps virus, and rubella virus. It may contain suitable antimicrobial agents. Each labelled dose provides an immunising dose of each component. It should be stored at 2° to 8° and be protected from light.

### Adverse Effects and Precautions

As for vaccines in general, p.1605.

See also under Measles Vaccines, p.1623, Mumps Vaccines, p.1626, and Rubella Vaccines, p.1637.

Adverse effects tend to be less frequent after the second dose of vaccine than after the first dose.

Measles, mumps, and rubella vaccines should not be given to individuals hypersensitive to any antibacterial such as neomycin or kanamycin, that may be used in the manufacturing process.

Recommendations on vaccination in persons with egg allergy have been modified (see Hypersensitivity, below). A history of mild reactions to egg is not regarded as a contra-indication.

Children with a history of convulsions should receive measles, mumps, and rubella vaccination, but advice should be given on controlling fever.

**Incidence of adverse effects.** A double-blind placebo-controlled crossover study[1] in 581 pairs of twins showed that the true frequency of side-effects was between 0.5 and 4.0%, indicating that adverse reactions are much less common than was previously thought.

A study in the USA[2] showed that children receiving the vaccine at age 4 to 6 years had fewer adverse effects than those receiving it at 10 to 12 years.

A study[3] that assessed the effect of almost 3 million doses of vaccines in 1.8 million individuals revealed that 173 potentially serious reactions were claimed to have been caused by vaccination. There were 77 neurologic, 73 allergic, and 22 miscellaneous reactions recorded, and 1 death reported. However, 45% of the reactions were probably caused by some other factor. It was therefore concluded that serious events caused by measles, mumps, and rubella vaccine are rare and are greatly outweighed by the risks of the natural diseases.

1. Peltola H, Heinonen OP. Frequency of true adverse reactions to measles-mumps-rubella vaccine: a double-blind placebo-controlled trial in twins. *Lancet* 1986; **i:** 939–42.
2. Davis RL, *et al.* MMR2 immunization at 4 to 5 years and 10 to 12 years of age: a comparison of adverse clinical events after immunization in the vaccine safety datalink project. *Pediatrics* 1997; **100:** 767–71.
3. Patja A, *et al.* Serious adverse events after measles-mumps-rubella vaccination during a fourteen-year prospective follow-up. *Pediatr Infect Dis J* 2000; **19:** 1127–34.

**Effects on the blood.** Thrombocytopenia occurs rarely in children receiving measles, mumps, and rubella vaccine and usually resolves spontaneously. An increased incidence of thrombocytopenia following the second dose of the vaccine has been reported in children who developed thrombocytopenia after the first dose.[1] A study[2] by the Public Health Laboratory Service in the UK has suggested a link between measles, mumps, and rubella vaccine and the occurrence of idiopathic thrombocytopenic purpura, with an absolute risk of 1 in 22 300 of occurrence within 6 weeks of the first dose of the vaccine, and 2 out of every 3 cases attributable to it. Children with idiopathic thrombocytopenic purpura before receiving measles, mumps, and rubella vaccine experienced no vaccine-associated recurrences. As a consequence of these findings, the UK Committee on Safety of Medicines has recommended[3] that children developing idiopathic thrombocytopenic purpura within 6 weeks of vaccination with measles, mumps, and rubella vaccine, or any of its components, should have serological testing before their second dose is due; if this suggests that full immunity is not established, then a second dose should be given.

1. Vlacha V, *et al.* Recurrent thrombocytopenic purpura after repeated measles-mumps-rubella vaccination. *Pediatrics* 1996; **97:** 738–9.
2. Miller E, *et al.* Idiopathic thrombocytopenic purpura and MMR vaccine. *Arch Dis Child* 2001; **84:** 227–9.
3. Committee on Safety of Medicines/Medicines Control Agency. MMR vaccine and idiopathic thrombocytopenic purpura. *Current Problems* 2001; **27:** 15. Also available at: http://www.mca.gov.uk/ourwork/monitorsafequalmed/currentproblems/cpaug2001.pdf (accessed 22/06/04)

**Effects on the bones and joints.** Arthralgia and arthritis occurring in patients receiving mumps, measles, and rubella vaccines have generally been attributed to the rubella component.[1] However, arthritis has been reported in an infant following vaccination with measles and mumps vaccine.[2]

1. Benjamin CM, *et al.* Joint and limb symptoms in children after immunisation with measles, mumps, and rubella vaccine. *BMJ* 1992; **304:** 1075–8.
2. Nussinovitch M, *et al.* Arthritis after mumps and measles vaccination. *Arch Dis Child* 1995; **72:** 348–9.

**Effects on hearing.** Nine cases of sensorineural hearing loss following measles, mumps, and rubella vaccine administration were reported to the UK Committee on Safety of Medicines between 1988 and 1993.[1] Of these, 3 cases were judged not to have been associated with the vaccine. In the remaining 6, the mumps virus component was considered to be the most likely cause of deafness if the vaccine was to blame, but the risk was considered to be small compared with the risks of natural infection. However, sensorineural deafness has also been reported following administration of measles and rubella vaccine (see p.1624), and monovalent measles vaccine (see p.1623).

1. Stewart BJA, Prabhu PU. Reports of sensorineural deafness after measles, mumps, and rubella immunisation. *Arch Dis Child* 1993; **69:** 153–4.

**Effects on the nervous system.** Although there have been case reports[1] linking Guillain-Barré syndrome with measles, mumps, and rubella vaccine, a retrospective study[2] that involved 189 patients with the syndrome and about 630 000 recipients of could not find a causal association.

Prolonged tonic-clonic seizures were associated with prolonged hemiparesis in a 16-month-old girl 6 days after measles, mumps, and rubella vaccination.[3] There was evidence of transient encephalopathy. However, a causal relationship between measles-containing vaccines and encephalitis is generally considered to be unlikely. Other reported neurological effects following vaccination include gait disturbances[4] and transverse myelitis.[5]

For discussion of meningitis and encephalitis occurring after measles, mumps, and rubella vaccination, see under Adverse Effects of Mumps Vaccines, p.1627.

1. Morris K, Rylance G. Guillain-Barré syndrome after measles, mumps, and rubella vaccine. *Lancet* 1994; **343:** 60.
2. Patja A, *et al.* Risk of Guillain-Barré syndrome after measles-mumps-rubella vaccination. *J Pediatr* 2001; **138:** 250–4.
3. Sackey AH, Broadhead RL. Hemiplegia after measles, mumps, and rubella vaccination. *BMJ* 1993; **306:** 1169.
4. Plesner A-M. Gait disturbances after measles, mumps, and rubella vaccine. *Lancet* 1995; **345:** 316.
5. Joyce KA, Rees JE. Transverse myelitis after measles, mumps, and rubella vaccine. *BMJ* 1995; **311:** 422.

**Hypersensitivity.** Since the measles and mumps components of measles, mumps, and rubella vaccines are grown in cell cultures of chick embryos the vaccine has in the past been contra-indicated in individuals with a history of anaphylactic reactions to egg. It is generally agreed that the vaccine can be given safely to children with less severe reactions to eggs. In both the UK and USA, even serious reactions to egg including anaphylaxis are no longer regarded as absolute contra-indications to vaccination,[1-4] and skin testing and desensitisation are considered to be of questionable value.[3,4] Nevertheless, a history of severe hypersensitivity to gelatin, kanamycin, or neomycin is regarded as a contra-indication to measles, mumps, and rubella vaccines.[1,4]

1. Centers for Disease Control. Update: vaccine side effects, adverse reactions, contraindications, and precautions: recommendations of the Advisory Committee on Immunization Practices (ACIP). *MMWR* 1996; **45:** (RR-12): 1–45.
2. Department of Health. *Immunisation against infectious disease* 1996: "The Green Book". Available at: http://www.dh.gov.uk/PublicationsAndStatistics/Publications/PublicationsPolicyAndGuidance/PublicationsPolicyAndGuidanceArticle/fs/en?CONTENT_ID=4072977&chk=87uz6M (accessed 22/06/04) See also http://www.hpa.org.uk/infections/topics_az/vaccination/vac_sced.htm (accessed 22/06/04)
3. Khakoo GA, Lack G. Recommendations for using MMR vaccine in children allergic to eggs. *BMJ* 2000; **320:** 929–32.
4. Centers for Disease Control. Measles, mumps, and rubella—vaccine use and strategies for elimination of measles, rubella, and congenital rubella syndrome and control of mumps: recommendations of the Advisory Committee on Immunization Practices (ACIP). *MMWR* 1998; **47** (RR-8): 1–57.

**Inflammatory bowel disease and autism.** A controversial report[1] in 1998 by Wakefield and coworkers linking measles, mumps, and rubella vaccination with the development of inflammatory bowel disease and behavioural abnormalities including autism was not supported by epidemiological evidence[2-4] and prompted the UK Committee on Safety of Medicines (CSM) to issue in 1999 a statement to this effect.[5] However, Wakefield, with another co-author,[6] in 2000 again raised issues concerning the safety of vaccination and alleged that the licensing procedures had not been properly carried out. The response by the UK Medicines Control Agency and Department of Health, reflecting additionally the view of the CSM and the Joint Committee on Vaccination and Immunisation,[7] was that the evidence did not support an association between measles, mumps, and rubella vaccine and inflammation of the bowel and autism. Moreover, it was re-iterated that this view was based not on a lack of evidence but, rather, that it was based on evidence that did not show an association. Other retrospective analyses[8-10] followed assessing the possible relationship of autism to measles, mumps, and rubella vaccine but again failed to document any association. Other suggestions of links between measles vaccines and inflammatory bowel disease have not been substantiated (see under Precautions for Measles Vaccines, p.1623).

1. Wakefield AJ, *et al.* Ileal-lymphoid-nodular hyperplasia, non-specific colitis, and pervasive developmental disorder in children. *Lancet* 1998; **351:** 637–41.
2. Peltola H, *et al.* No evidence for measles, mumps, and rubella vaccine-associated inflammatory bowel disease or autism in a 14-year prospective study. *Lancet* 1998; **351:** 1327–8.
3. Roberts R. There is no causal link between MMR vaccine and autism. *BMJ* 1998; **316:** 1824.
4. Taylor B, *et al.* Autism and measles, mumps, and rubella vaccine: no epidemiological evidence for a causal association. *Lancet* 1999; **353:** 2026–9.
5. Committee on Safety of Medicines. The safety of MMR Vaccine. *Current Problems* 1999; **25:** 9–10. Also available at: http://www.mca.gov.uk/ourwork/monitorsafequalmed/currentproblems/volume25jun.htm (accessed 08/07/04)
6. Wakefield AJ, Montgomery SM. Measles, mumps, rubella vaccine: through a glass, darkly. *Adverse Drug React Toxicol Rev* 2000; **19:** 265–83.
7. Arlett P, *et al.* A response to 'Measles, mumps, rubella vaccine: through a glass, darkly' by Drs AJ Wakefield and SM Montgomery and published reviewers' comments. *Adverse Drug React Toxicol Rev* 2001; **20:** 37–45. Also available at: http://www.dh.gov.uk/assetRoot/04/06/88/93/04068893.pdf (accessed 22/06/04)
8. Kaye JA, *et al.* Mumps, measles, and rubella vaccine and the incidence of autism recorded by general practitioners: a time trend analysis. *BMJ* 2001; **322:** 460–3. Correction. *ibid.*; 720.
9. Dales L, *et al.* Time trends in autism and in MMR immunization coverage in California. *JAMA* 2001; **285:** 1183–5.
10. Halsey NA, *et al.* Measles-mumps-rubella vaccine and autistic spectrum disorder: report from the new challenges in childhood immunizations conference convened in Oak Brook, Illinois, June 12-13, 2000. Abstract: *Pediatrics* 2001; **107:** 1174. Full version: http://pediatrics.aappublications.org/cgi/content/full/107/5/e84 (accessed 22/06/04)

### Interactions

As for vaccines in general, p.1606.

See also under Measles Vaccines, p.1623.

### Uses and Administration

Measles, mumps, and rubella vaccines are used for active immunisation against measles, mumps, and rubella. They are used for primary immunisation in children 12 months of age or older and to protect susceptible contacts during an outbreak of measles. For discussion of immunisation schedules, see under Vaccines, p.1606.

In the UK and USA, the vaccine is prepared from an attenuated line of measles virus derived from Enders' attenuated Edmonston strain, the Jeryl Lynn (B level) strain of mumps virus, and the Wistar RA 27/3 strain of rubella virus. An alternative in the UK contains measles virus prepared from the Schwarz strain. Another type, no longer used in several countries because of an increased risk of meningoencephalitis (see Effects on the Nervous System under Mumps Vaccines, p.1627), has been prepared from the Schwarz strain of measles virus, the Urabe Am 9 strain of mumps virus, and the Wistar RA 27/3 strain of rubella virus.

In the UK, it is recommended that all children receive two doses of 0.5 mL of a measles, mumps, and rubella vaccine by deep subcutaneous or intramuscular injection. These are usually given shortly after the first birthday and before school entry, but may be given at any age if routine administration has been omitted, allowing 3 months between doses. The combined vaccine may also be used for prophylaxis after exposure to measles provided it is given within 72 hours of contact. However, it is not considered to be effective for postexposure prophylaxis against either mumps or rubella. If the vaccine is given before 12 months of age, re-immunisation will be necessary starting at between 12 and 15 months with a further dose according to national schedules.

In the USA, the second dose is recommended at age 4 to 6 years. Children who have not previously received the second dose should complete the vaccination schedule between the ages of 11 to 18 years.

## Preparations

**Ph. Eur.:** Measles, Mumps, and Rubella Vaccine (Live);
**USP 27:** Measles, Mumps, and Rubella Virus Vaccine Live.

**Proprietary Preparations** (details are given in Part 3)
**Arg.:** MMR II; Trimovax; Triviraten; **Austral.:** MMR II; Priorix; **Austria:** MMR Vax; Priorix; **Belg.:** MMR Vax; Priorix; **Braz.:** MMR II; Priorix; Trimovax; **Canad.:** MMR II; Priorix; **Denm.:** MMR; Virivac†; **Fin.:** MMR II; Priorix; **Fr.:** Priorix; R.O.R.; **Ger.:** MMR Triplovax; MMR Vax; Priorix; **Gr.:** MMR II; Priorix; **Hong Kong:** MMR II; Priorix; Trimovax; Triviraten; **India:** Tresivac; **Irl.:** MMR II; Priorix; **Israel:** MMR II; Priorix; **Ital.:** MMR II; Morupar; Priorix; Trimovax†; Triviraten†; **Malaysia:** MMR II; Priorix; Triviraten; **Mex.:** MMR II; Morupar; Priorix; **NZ:** Triviraten; **Port.:** Priorix†; Triviraten†; **S.Afr.:** MMR II†; Morupar; Priorix; Trimovax; Triviraten†; **Singapore:** MMR II; Priorix; **Spain:** Priorix; Triviraten; Vac Triple MSD; **Swed.:** MMR II; Priorix; Virivac†; **Switz.:** MMR II; Priorix; Triviraten; **Thai.:** MMR II; Priorix; Trimovax; Triviraten; **UK:** MMR II; Priorix; **USA:** MMR II.

**Multi-ingredient: NZ:** MMR II.

## Measles, Mumps, Rubella, and Varicella-Zoster Vaccines

### Profile

A live, attenuated measles, mumps, rubella, and varicella-zoster vaccine is under investigation for active immunisation against measles, mumps, rubella and varicella (chickenpox).

# Meningococcal Vaccines

Vacunas de polisacáridos meningocócicos.

*ATC — J07AH01; J07AH02; J07AH03; J07AH04; J07AH05; J07AH06; J07AH07.*

**Pharmacopoeias.** Many pharmacopoeias have monographs including *Eur.* (see p.vi).

**Ph. Eur. 5.0** (Meningococcal Polysaccharide Vaccine; Vaccinum Meningitidis Cerebrospinalis). It consists of one or more purified capsular polysaccharides obtained from one or more suitable strains of *Neisseria meningitidis* group A, group C, group Y, and group W135; it may contain a single type of polysaccharide or any mixture of the types. It is prepared immediately before use by reconstitution from the stabilised freeze-dried vaccine with a suitable sterile liquid. The freeze-dried vaccine should be stored at 2° to 8° and be protected from light.

The BP 2003 states that Neimen/Vac may be used on the label.

**Ph. Eur. 5.0** (Meningococcal Group C Conjugate Vaccine; Vaccinum Meningococcale Classis C Coniugatum). A liquid or freeze-dried preparation of purified capsular polysaccharide derived from a suitable strain of *Neisseria meningitidis* group C covalently linked to a carrier protein. The vaccine may contain an adjuvant. The freeze-dried vaccine should be stored at 2° to 8° and be protected from light.

## Adverse Effects and Precautions

As for vaccines in general, p.1605.

Immunity to some meningococcal vaccines may be insufficient to confer adequate protection against infection in infants under about 2 years of age (for further discussion see Immunisation, below).

**Pregnancy and the neonate.** A mixed meningococcal vaccine (A and C) was evaluated in pregnant women and infants during an epidemic of meningitis in Brazil.[1] Antibodies were detected in the women and there was some placental transfer of antibody although this was irregular. Vaccination of children in the first 6 months of life was unsuccessful. These results were supported by a subsequent study in the Gambia.[2] Maternal antibodies were high in all women at the time of delivery, but only a proportion of the antibody crossed the placenta. There was considerable individual variation in the cord blood:maternal blood antibody ratios. Antibody concentrations declined rapidly in the infants and had effectively disappeared by 3 to 4 months of age.

1. Carvalho A de A, *et al.* Maternal and infant antibody response to meningococcal vaccination in pregnancy. *Lancet* 1977; **ii:** 809–11.
2. O'Dempsey TJD, *et al.* Meningococcal antibody titres in infants of women immunised with meningococcal polysaccharide vaccine during pregnancy. *Arch Dis Child* 1996; **74:** F43–6.

## Interactions

As for vaccines in general, p.1606.

## Uses and Administration

Meningococcal vaccines are used for active immunisation against *Neisseria meningitidis* infections, which include meningitis and septicaemia. They are preparations of purified polysaccharide antigens from *N. meningitidis* and may be monovalent, containing the antigen of only one serotype of *N. meningitidis* or polyvalent, containing antigens of two or more serotypes. Vaccines available in the UK are a bivalent vaccine from groups A and C, a tetravalent vaccine from groups A, C, Y, and W135, and meningococcal group C conjugate vaccines conjugated to diphtheria $CRM_{197}$ protein conjugate or to tetanus toxoid protein. In the USA, a tetravalent vaccine from groups A, C, Y, and W135 is used. Both the bivalent and the tetravalent vaccines are given in a single dose of 0.5 mL; the bivalent vaccine is given by deep subcutaneous or intramuscular injection and the tetravalent vaccine by deep subcutaneous injection. The meningococcal C conjugate vaccines in the UK are generally given by intramuscular injection with the subcutaneous route reserved for patients with haemophilia or thrombocytopenia. Infants aged 2 to 4 months are given 3 doses of 0.5 mL at monthly intervals for primary immunisation. Children who have not received primary immunisation should receive 3 doses similarly up to the age of 1 year; a single dose of 0.5 mL is given to adults and children over 1 year of age. For discussion of immunisation schedules see under Vaccines, p.1606.

Meningococcal vaccines are indicated in persons at risk, in epidemic or endemic areas, of meningococcal disease caused by the specific serotypes contained in the vaccines. They are given as an adjunct to chemoprophylaxis in close contacts of persons with the disease. Persons travelling to countries where the risk of infection is high should receive tetravalent meningococcal polysaccharide vaccine rather than the group C conjugate vaccine, and should be immunised even if they have already received the latter. Vaccination is indicated particularly for visits of 1 month or more and for those backpacking or living or working with local residents. Asplenic persons or those who have terminal complement component deficiencies are at higher than normal risk of acquiring meningococcal infection. The polyvalent vaccine may also be considered in college students living in dormitories or halls of residence.

The minimum recommended age for administration of meningococcal vaccines has varied from 2 months to 2 years because of reports of poor immune response to the unconjugated polysaccharide vaccines in younger infants although the immunogenicity of the conjugate group C vaccine in these patients appears to be greater (see below).

**Immunisation.** *Neisseria meningitidis* is an important cause of meningitis. Polysaccharide vaccines of meningococci of groups A, C, W135, and Y are successful in producing short-term immunity (up to about 5 years) and controlling epidemics and outbreaks. Conjugate vaccines against group A and C meningococci have been developed in order to improve immunogenicity and their use is now established. About 60% of meningococcal infections (p.135) in the UK and the USA, however, are caused by *Neisseria meningitidis* of group B serotype. Unfortunately there is no available vaccine against these organisms because the purified group B polysaccharide is only poorly immunogenic, even after conjugation with proteins.[1] Several avenues of research are being followed in the development of an effective vaccine against the group B serotype.[2-4] A number of candidate vaccines based on class 1 outer membrane proteins have been field-tested but efficacy has been variable. Favourable results with a fairly crude vaccine in Cuba were not confirmed by a study in Brazil using the same vaccine,[5] and the response in young children was especially disappointing. Similarly, a vaccine produced in Norway gave a protection rate of about 60%, judged to be too low for use in a general immunisation programme.[6] A direct comparison of the two vaccines[7] found that the Norwegian vaccine produced greater immunity in adolescents than the Cuban vaccine. A subsequent study,[8] however, has reiterated that neither vaccine would confer adequate protection during an epidemic with non-vaccine type strains of meningococcus. Other strategies have included vaccines based on other outer membrane proteins and lipopolysaccharide derivatives.[2-4]

1. Anonymous. Preventing meningococcal infection. *Drug Ther Bull* 1990; **28:** 34–6.
2. Zollinger WD, Moran E. Meningococcal vaccines—present and future. *Trans R Soc Trop Med Hyg* 1991; **85** (suppl 1): 37–43.
3. Herbert MA, *et al.* Meningococcal vaccines for the United Kingdom. *Commun Dis Rep* 1995; **5** (review 9): R130–5.
4. Ala'Aldeen DAA, Cartwright KAV. Neisseria meningitidis: vaccines and vaccine candidates. *J Infect* 1996; **33:** 153–7.
5. de Morales JC, *et al.* Protective efficacy of a serogroup B meningococcal vaccine in Sao Paulo, Brazil. *Lancet* 1992; **340:** 1074–8.
6. Bjune G, *et al.* Effect of outer membrane vesicle vaccine against group B meningococcal disease in Norway. *Lancet* 1991; **338:** 1093–6.
7. Perkins BA, *et al.* Immunogenicity of two efficacious outer membrane protein-based serogroup B meningococcal vaccines among young adults in Iceland. *J Infect Dis* 1998; **177:** 683–91.
8. Tappero JW, *et al.* Immunogenicity of 2 serogroup B outer-membrane protein meningococcal vaccines: a randomized controlled trial in Chile. *JAMA* 1999; **281:** 1520–7.

## Preparations

**Ph. Eur.:** Meningococcal Group C Conjugate Vaccine; Meningococcal Polysaccharide Vaccine.

**Proprietary Preparations** (details are given in Part 3)
**Arg.:** Meningitec; Va-Mengoc-BC; **Austral.:** Mencevax ACWY; Meningitec; Menjugate; Menomune; NeisVac-C; **Austria:** Mencevax ACWY; Menomune ACYW; **Belg.:** Mencevax ACWY; Meningitec; Meningovax A+C; Menjugate; **Braz.:** Meningo A+C†; Va-Mengoc-BC; Vacina Meningococica A+C; Vacina Meningococica Conjugada Grupo C; **Canad.:** Menomune; **Denm.:** Meningovax A+C; NeisVac-C; **Fin.:** Mencevax ACWY; Meningovax A+C; NeisVac-C; **Fr.:** Meningitec; Meninvact; Menjugate; Menomune; NeisVac; **Ger.:** Mencevax ACWY; Meningitec; Meningokokken-Impfstoff A + C; NeisVac-C; **Gr.:** Meningitec; Menomune; NeisVac-C; Vaccin Meningococcique Merieux; **Hong Kong:** Mencevax ACWY; Meningococcal A+C; **Irl.:** Mengivac (A+C); Meningitec; Menjugate; **Israel:** Mencevax AC; **Ital.:** Mencevax ACWY; Meningitec; Menjugate; Menomune; Menpovax 4†; Menpovax A+C†; NeisVac-C; **Malaysia:** Menomune; **Neth.:** Meningovax A+C; **Norw.:** Mencevax AC; Meningovax A+C; **NZ:** Mencevax ACWY; Menomune; **Port.:** Meningitec; Menjugate; **S.Afr.:** Imovax Meningo A & C; Mencevax; **Singapore:** Mencevax AC†; Mencevax ACWY; Menomune; **Spain:** Mencevax AC; Meningitec; Meninvact; Menjugate; NeisVac-C; Vac Antimeningococic A+C; **Swed.:** Meningovax A+C; NeisVac-C; **Switz.:** Meningitec; **Thai.:** Meningococcal A+C; Menpovax 4†; Menpovax A+C†; **UK:** ACWY Vax; Mengivac (A+C)†; Meningitec; Menjugate; NeisVac-C; **USA:** Menomune.

## Multiple Sclerosis Vaccines

Vacunas de la esclerosis múltiple.

### Profile

Vaccines based on T cells have been investigated for the management of multiple sclerosis.

◊ References.

1. Medaer R, *et al.* Depletion of myelin-basic-protein autoreactive T cells by T-cell vaccination: pilot trial in multiple sclerosis. *Lancet* 1995; **346:** 807–8.
2. Vandenbark AA, *et al.* Treatment of multiple sclerosis with T-cell receptor peptides: results of a double-blind pilot trial. *Nat Med* 1996; **2:** 1109–15. Correction. *ibid.* 1997; **3:** 240.
3. Goodkin DE, *et al.* A phase I trial of solubilized DR2:$MBP^{84-102}$ (AG284) in multiple sclerosis. *Neurology* 2000; **54:** 1414–20.

## Mumps Immunoglobulins

Inmunoglobulinas contra la parotiditis.

*ATC — J06BB15.*

### Profile

Preparations containing antibodies against mumps virus have been used in some countries for passive immunisation against mumps.

### Preparations

**Proprietary Preparations** (details are given in Part 3)
**Ital.:** Haima-Parot†; Immunoparot†; Par-Gamma†; Paruman†.

# Mumps Vaccines

Vacunas de la parotiditis.

*ATC — J07BE01.*

**Pharmacopoeias.** Many pharmacopoeias have monographs including *Eur.* (see p.vi) and *US.*

**Ph. Eur. 5.0** (Mumps Vaccine (Live); Vaccinum Parotitidis Vivum). A freeze-dried preparation containing a suitable live attenuated strain of mumps virus (*Paramyxovirus parotitidis*) grown in cultures of human diploid cells or chick-embryo cells or the amniotic cavity of chick embryos. It is prepared immediately before use by reconstitution from the dried vaccine. The cell-culture medium may contain the lowest effective concentration of a suitable antibacterial. The virus titre is not less than $5 \times 10^3$ $CCID_{50}$ per dose. The dried vaccine should be stored at 2° to 8° and be protected from light.

The BP 2003 states that Mump/Vac(Live) may be used on the label.

**USP 27** (Mumps Virus Vaccine Live). A bacterially sterile preparation of a suitable strain of mumps virus grown in cultures of chick-embryo cells. It contains not less than the equivalent of $5 \times 10^3$ $TCID_{50}$ in each immunising dose. It may contain suitable antimicrobial agents. It should be stored at 2° to 8° and be protected from light.

## Adverse Effects and Precautions

As for vaccines in general, p.1605.

Parotid swelling may occur. Unilateral nerve deafness, meningitis, and encephalitis have occurred rarely (see below for further discussion).

Mumps vaccines are not generally recommended for children below the age of 1 year in whom maternal antibodies might prevent a response.

**Effects on hearing.** For a report of sensorineural hearing loss following measles, mumps, and rubella vaccination, see p.1625.

**Effects on the nervous system.** There have been a few reports of neurological reactions including meningitis and encephalitis after vaccination with measles, mumps, and rubella vaccines. These reactions have been attributed to the mumps component. However, it has not been possible to isolate the virus from the CSF in every case and identify it as either the vaccine strain or a wild-type strain. Meningitis develops up to 35 days after immunisation, is mild, and sequelae are rare.[1,2] One study[3] found the incidence of virus-positive post-immunisation meningitis from the Urabe strain of mumps vaccine to be approximately 1 in 11 000 immunised children, with the incidence following Jeryl Lynn mumps vaccine being much lower. This result was supported by the incidence of 1 in about 4000 in another study,[4] making it less likely that this was a chance result, and much higher than the estimates of up to 1 in 1 million reported previously.[5] Subsequent research[6] identified the Urabe vaccine strain in CSF samples from all of 20 children with post-vaccination meningitis in the UK, and no isolates of the Jeryl Lynn strain in patients with meningitis among 80 samples tested. Thus, vaccines containing the Urabe strain, including combined measles, mumps, and rubella vaccines are no longer used in the UK and some other countries.[7] A relatively high incidence of meningitis of about 1 in 1000 has also been observed after use of a measles and mumps vaccine prepared from the Leningrad-3 strain of mumps virus.[8,9]

Encephalitis has been associated with mumps vaccination less frequently than meningitis, but may be more serious.[1] The Advisory Committee on Immunization Practices in the USA has reported that the incidence of encephalitis within 30 days of receiving a mumps-containing vaccine is 0.4 per one million doses.[10] This is no higher than the observed background incidence for CNS dysfunction in the general population.

In considering the above data it should be remembered that mumps is the most common cause of meningoencephalitis in children under 15 years of age in the UK and an important cause of permanent sensorineural deafness in childhood.[1] Meningitis after natural mumps infection is estimated to occur in 1 in 400 cases, an incidence that is very considerably above any reported with vaccination.


1. Anonymous. Mumps meningitis and MMR vaccination. *Lancet* 1989; **ii:** 1015–16.
2. Maguire HC, *et al.* Meningoencephalitis associated with MMR vaccine. *Commun Dis Rep* 1991; **1** (review 6): R60–R61.
3. Miller E, *et al.* Risk of aseptic meningitis after measles, mumps, and rubella vaccine in UK children. *Lancet* 1993; **341:** 979–82.
4. Colville A, Pugh S. Mumps meningitis and measles, mumps, and rubella vaccine. *Lancet* 1992; **340:** 786. Correction. *ibid.*: 986.
5. McDonald JC, *et al.* Clinical and epidemiologic features of mumps meningoencephalitis and possible vaccine-related disease. *Pediatr Infect Dis J* 1989; **8:** 751–5.
6. Forsey T, *et al.* Mumps vaccine and meningitis. *Lancet* 1992; **340:** 980.
7. Anonymous. Two MMR vaccines withdrawn. *Lancet* 1992; **340:** 722.
8. Čižman M, *et al.* Aseptic meningitis after vaccination against measles and mumps. *Pediatr Infect Dis J* 1989; **8:** 302–8.
9. Tešović G, *et al.* Aseptic meningitis after measles, mumps, and rubella vaccine. *Lancet* 1993; **341:** 1541.
10. Immunization Practices Advisory Committee. Mumps prevention. *MMWR* 1989; **38:** 388–400.


## Interactions

As for vaccines in general, p.1606.

## Uses and Administration

Mumps vaccines are used for active immunisation against mumps.

For primary immunisation a combined measles, mumps, and rubella vaccine (p.1625) is usually used. For discussion of immunisation schedules, see under Vaccines, p.1606.

In the UK, a vaccine prepared from the Jeryl Lynn (B level) strain of mumps virus was formerly available. The vaccine is, however, available in the USA, and may be given in a dose of 0.5 mL by subcutaneous injection.

## Preparations

***Ph. Eur.:*** Mumps Vaccine (Live);
***USP 27:*** Mumps Virus Vaccine Live.

**Proprietary Preparations** (details are given in Part 3)
***Arg.:*** Imovax Parotiditis; ***Braz.:*** Imovax Mumps; Mumpsvax†; ***Canad.:*** Mumpsvax; ***Denm.:*** Mumpsvax; ***Fr.:*** Imovax†; ***Ger.:*** Mumpsvax; ***Hong Kong:*** Imovax Mumps†; Mumaten†; ***Irl.:*** Mumpsvax†; ***Ital.:*** Mumaten†; Mumpsvax†; Vaxipar; ***S.Afr.:*** Mumaten†; ***Spain:*** Vac Antiparotiditis; ***Switz.:*** Mumaten†; Mumpsvax; ***Thai.:*** Mumaten†; ***UK:*** Mumpsvax†; ***USA:*** Mumpsvax.

## Mycobacterium Vaccae Vaccines

Vacunas de Mycobacterium vaccae.

### Profile

Vaccines containing *Mycobacterium vaccae* are under investigation for the prevention and immunotherapy of tuberculosis and other mycobacterial infections. They are also being studied for therapeutic use in psoriasis and some neoplastic diseases.

**Malignant neoplasms.** References.


1. O'Brien ME, *et al.* A randomized phase II study of SRL172 (Mycobacterium vaccae) combined with chemotherapy in patients with advanced inoperable non-small-cell lung cancer and mesothelioma. *Br J Cancer* 2000; **83:** 853–7.


**Psoriasis.** References.


1. Balagon MV, *et al.* Improvement in psoriasis after intradermal administration of heat-killed Mycobacterium vaccae. *Int J Dermatol* 2000; **39:** 51–8.


**Tuberculosis.** IMMUNISATION. References.


1. von Reyn CF, *et al.* Cellular immune responses to mycobacteria in healthy and human immunodeficiency virus-positive subjects in the United States after a five-dose schedule of Mycobacterium vaccae vaccine. *Clin Infect Dis* 1998; **27:** 1517–20.
2. Waddell RD, *et al.* Safety and immunogenicity of a five-dose series of inactivated Mycobacterium vaccae vaccination for the prevention of HIV-associated tuberculosis. *Clin Infect Dis* 2000; **30** (suppl 3): S309–S315.


IMMUNOTHERAPY. A systematic review[1] found that immunotherapy with *Mycobacterium vaccae* produced no beneficial effects in patients with tuberculosis.


1. de Bruyn G, Garner P. Mycobacterium vaccae immunotherapy for treating tuberculosis. Available in The Cochrane Library; Issue 2. Chichester: John Wiley; 2004.


# Normal Immunoglobulins

Inmunoglobulinas inespecíficas.

*ATC — J06BA01; J06BA02.*

**Pharmacopoeias.** Many pharmacopoeias have monographs including *Eur.* (see p.vi) and *US.*

**Ph. Eur. 5.0** (Human Normal Immunoglobulin; Immunoglobulinum Humanum Normale). A liquid or freeze-dried preparation containing immunoglobulins, mainly immunoglobulin G (IgG) antibodies, of normal subjects. Other proteins may be present; it contains not less than 10% and not more than 18% of total protein. It is intended for intramuscular injection. It is obtained from the pooled plasma collected from at least 1000 donors who must be healthy, must not have been treated with substances of human pituitary origin, and as far as can be ascertained be free from detectable agents of infection transmissible by transfusion of blood or blood components. No antibacterial is added to the plasma used. It is prepared as a stabilised solution and passed through a bacteria-retentive filter. Multidose, but not single dose, preparations contain an antimicrobial preservative. The pH of a solution in sodium chloride 0.9% containing 1% of protein is 5.0 to 7.2. The liquid preparation should be stored, protected from light, in a sealed, colourless, glass container. The freeze-dried preparation should be stored, protected from light, in an airtight, colourless, glass container.

**Ph. Eur. 5.0** (Human Normal Immunoglobulin for Intravenous Administration; Immunoglobulinum Humanum Normale ad Usum Intravenosum). A liquid or freeze-dried preparation containing immunoglobulins, mainly immunoglobulin G (IgG); other proteins may be present and the total protein content is not less than 3%. It contains IgG antibodies of normal subjects; the standard does not apply to products intentionally prepared to contain fragments or chemically modified IgG. It is prepared as a stabilised solution and passed through a bacteria-retentive filter. It does not contain an antimicrobial preservative. The pH of a solution in sodium chloride 0.9% containing 1% of protein is 4.0 to 7.4. Storage requirements are similar to those for Human Normal Immunoglobulin, except that the freeze-dried preparation is stored in an airtight container at a temperature not exceeding 25°.

**USP 27** (Immune Globulin). A sterile solution of globulins that contains many antibodies normally present in human adult blood. It is prepared from pooled material (approximately equal quantities of blood, plasma, serum, or placentas) from not fewer than 1000 donors. It contains 15 to 18% of protein, of which not less than 90% is gamma globulin. It is intended for intramuscular injection. It contains glycine as a stabiliser, and a suitable preservative. It contains antibodies against diphtheria, measles, and poliomyelitis. It should be stored at 2° to 8°.

## Adverse Effects and Precautions

As for immunoglobulins in general, p.1605. Intravenous immunoglobulin preparations should be used with caution in patients with renal impairment. Immunoglobulin products containing sucrose may be associated with an increased risk of inducing acute renal failure (see Effects on the Kidneys, below).

Antibody titres for some common pathogens can vary widely not only between products from different manufacturers, but also from lot to lot. Formulations of intravenous immunoglobulins should therefore not be regarded as equivalent.

◊ Reviews.


1. Nydegger UE, Sturzenegger M. Adverse effects of intravenous immunoglobulin therapy. *Drug Safety* 1999; **21:** 171–85.


**Effects on the blood.** Adverse effects on the blood have occasionally been reported following intravenous administration of normal immunoglobulin to increase the platelet count in patients with idiopathic thrombocytopenic purpura. Reduced platelet adhesiveness with multiple subcutaneous haematomas occurred in one patient.[1] Thrombotic events have occurred after intravenous administration,[2,3] particularly in elderly subjects (sometimes fatal) suggesting that a rising platelet count during normal immunoglobulin treatment may represent a risk in patients with severe atherosclerotic disease.[2] A review in Scotland of 34 patients over 60 years of age treated with normal immunoglobulin could not, however, confirm the association.[4]

Passive transfer of anti-A, anti-B, or anti-D antibodies or active immunisation by blood group substances from normal immunoglobulin preparations has been implicated in the production of haemolytic reactions including a case of haemolytic disease of the newborn.[5,6] It has been suggested[6] that blood phenotyping be carried out before treatment with normal immunoglobulin is started.

Transient neutropenia has occurred after use of normal immunoglobulin in patients with thrombocytopenic purpura, but the clinical significance of this effect has been disputed.[7-9]


1. Ljung R, Nilsson IM. High-dose intravenous gammaglobulin: a cautionary note. *Lancet* 1985; **i:** 467.
2. Woodruff RK, *et al.* Fatal thrombotic events during treatment of autoimmune thrombocytopenia with intravenous immunoglobulin in elderly patients. *Lancet* 1986; **ii:** 217–18.
3. Go RS, Call TG. Deep venous thrombosis of the arm after intravenous immunoglobulin infusion: case report and literature review of intravenous immunoglobulin-related thrombotic complications. *Mayo Clin Proc* 2000; **75:** 83–5.
4. Frame WD, Crawford RJ. Thrombotic events after intravenous immunoglobulin. *Lancet* 1986; **ii:** 468.
5. Potter M, *et al.* ABO alloimmunisation after intravenous immunoglobulin infusion. *Lancet* 1988; **i:** 932–3.
6. Nicholls MD, *et al.* Haemolysis induced by intravenously-administered immunoglobulin. *Med J Aust* 1989; **150:** 404–6.
7. Majer RV, Green PJ. Neutropenia caused by intravenous immunoglobulin. *BMJ* 1988; **296:** 1262.
8. Veys PA, *et al.* Neutropenia following intravenous immunoglobulin. *BMJ* 1988; **296:** 1800.
9. Ben-Chetrit E, Putterman C. Transient neutropenia induced by intravenous immune globulin. *N Engl J Med* 1992; **326:** 270–1.


**Effects on the kidneys.** Acute renal failure was reported after intravenous administration of normal immunoglobulin to a patient who had serum rheumatoid factor associated with lymphoma.[1] A symptomless, transient rise in plasma-creatinine concentrations was also noted in 6 patients with nephrotic syndrome after administration of intravenous normal immunoglobulin.[2] A similar rise in plasma creatinine was seen in 2 other patients with pre-existing renal impairment but no nephrotic syndrome. An elderly patient with lymphoproliferative disorder and idiopathic thrombocytopenic purpura received normal immunoglobulin and developed acute renal failure within 48 hours, with subsequently fatal heart failure and pulmonary oedema.[3] The incidence of renal failure appears to be greatest with immunoglobulin products containing sucrose. As a consequence, the FDA in the USA has issued a warning alerting physicians to the potential risks of acute renal failure associated with intravenous administration of normal immunoglobulin products, particularly those containing sucrose.


1. Barton JC, *et al.* Acute cryoglobulinemic renal failure after intravenous infusion of gamma globulin. *Am J Med* 1987; **82:** 624–9.
2. Schifferli J, *et al.* High-dose intravenous IgG treatment and renal function. *Lancet* 1991; **337:** 457–8.
3. Winward DB, Brophy MT. Acute renal failure after administration of intravenous immunoglobulin: review of the literature and case report. *Pharmacotherapy* 1995; **15:** 765–72.


**Effects on the nervous system.** Aseptic meningitis has been reported after intravenous administration of normal immunoglobulin.[1-5]

Migraine was associated with intravenous immunoglobulin therapy in a patient on two occasions.[6] Migraine did not recur after prophylaxis with propranolol was instituted.

Hemiplegia has been reported in a 4-year-old child receiving intravenous immunoglobulin for immune thrombocytopenic purpura.[7]


1. Kato E, *et al.* Administration of immune globulin associated with aseptic meningitis. *JAMA* 1988; **259:** 3269–71.
2. Casteels-Van Daele M, *et al.* Intravenous immune globulin and acute aseptic meningitis. *N Engl J Med* 1990; **323:** 614–15.
3. Sekul EA, *et al.* Aseptic meningitis associated with high-dose intravenous immunoglobulin therapy: frequency and risk factors. *Ann Intern Med* 1994; **121:** 259–62.
4. Picton P, Chisholm M. Aseptic meningitis associated with high dose immunoglobulin: case report. *BMJ* 1997; **315:** 1203–4.
5. Boyce TG, Spearman P. Acute aseptic meningitis secondary to intravenous immunoglobulin in a patient with Kawasaki syndrome. *Pediatr Infect Dis J* 1998; **17:** 1054–6.
6. Constantinescu CS, *et al.* Recurrent migraine and intravenous immune globulin therapy. *N Engl J Med* 1993; **329:** 583–4.
7. Tsiouris J, Tsiouris N. Hemiplegia as a complication of treatment of childhood immune thrombocytopenic purpura with intravenously administered immunoglobulin. *J Pediatr* 1998; **133:** 717.


**Effects on the skin.** Diffuse alopecia has been reported[1] in 3 women within 1 to 4 weeks of treatment with intravenous normal immunoglobulin. There have been reports[2,3] of severe and extensive eczema in elderly patients up to 3 weeks after receiving normal immunoglobulin intravenously. There has also been a report of cutaneous vasculitic rash on the face of a woman receiving intravenous normal immunoglobulin.[4]

For mention of a patient with AIDS who developed erythema characteristic of fifth disease following intravenous normal immunoglobulin, see Infection, below.


1. Chan-Lam D, *et al.* Alopecia after immunoglobulin infusion. *Lancet* 1987; **i:** 1436.
2. Barucha C, McMillan JC. Eczema after intravenous infusion of immunoglobulin. *BMJ* 1987; **295:** 1141.
3. Whittam LR, *et al.* Eczematous reactions to human immune globulin. *Br J Dermatol* 1997; **137:** 481–2.
4. Howse M, *et al.* Facial vasculitic rash associated with intravenous immunoglobulin. *BMJ* 1998; **317:** 1291.


**Hypersensitivity.** Hypersensitivity reactions may occasionally occur after intramuscular or intravenous administration of normal immunoglobulins particularly in hypogammaglobulinaemic or agammaglobulinaemic patients. Both immediate and late[1] reactions have occurred.

The IgA content of normal immunoglobulins can result in the development of IgE and IgG anti-IgA antibodies in immunodeficient patients with IgA deficiency. It has been suggested by some[2] that the IgE anti-IgA antibodies are responsible for anaphylaxis although others have disagreed.[3] Two patients who had reactions to conventional normal immunoglobulin preparations tolerated preparations with a low content of IgA.[2] Some manufacturers of normal immunoglobulin preparations recommend that they should not be used in patients with selective IgA deficiencies who have known antibody against IgA.

The IgE content of some preparations has also been suggested as a cause of hypersensitivity reactions[4] although this has been disputed.[5] Complement-activating IgG aggregates may also be involved although the anticomplementary activity of the products does not appear to be related to the incidence of side-effects.[5]


1. Hachimi-Idrissi S, *et al.* Type III allergic reaction after infusion of immunoglobulins. *Lancet* 1990; **336:** 55.
2. Burks AW, *et al.* Anaphylactic reactions after gamma globulin administration in patients with hypogammaglobulinemia. *N Engl J Med* 1986; **314:** 560–4.
3. Hammarström L, Smith CIE. Anaphylaxis after administration of gamma globulin for hypogammaglobulinemia. *N Engl J Med* 1986; **315:** 519.
4. Tovo P-A, *et al.* IgE content of commercial intravenous IgG preparations. *Lancet* 1984; **i:** 458.
5. Newland AC, *et al.* IgE in intravenous IgG. *Lancet* 1984; **i:** 1406–7.


**Infection.** An association between administration of certain intravenous immunoglobulin preparations and hepatitis C infections led to changes in manufacturing procedures and withdrawal of the affected products from the market.[1-3]

In addition, there has been a report[4] of a patient with AIDS who developed fifth disease (erythema infectiosum) following intravenous normal immunoglobulin treatment for infection with parvovirus.


1. Quinti I, *et al.* Intravenous gammaglobulin may still infect patients. *BMJ* 1994; **308:** 856.
2. Bader J-M. HCV and Gammagard in France. *Lancet* 1994; **343:** 1628. Corrections. *ibid.*; **344:** 201 and 206.
3. Anonymous. Outbreak of hepatitis C associated with intravenous immunoglobulin administration—United States, October 1993–June 1994. *JAMA* 1994; **272:** 424–5.
4. French AL, *et al.* Fifth disease after immunoglobulin administration in an AIDS patient with parvovirus-induced red cell aplasia. *Am J Med* 1996; **101:** 108–9.


## Interactions

Normal immunoglobulin may interfere with the immune response to live viral vaccines. Such vaccines should therefore be given at least 3 weeks before, or 3 months after, normal immunoglobulins. This does not apply to yellow fever vaccine for immunoglobulins prepared in the UK, nor for booster doses of oral poliomyelitis vaccines. Where such an interval is impractical for immunisation preceding foreign travel it may have to be ignored.

**Poliomyelitis vaccine.** For a study indicating that normal immunoglobulin has no effect on the antibody response to oral poliomyelitis vaccine, see p.1634.

## Uses and Administration

Normal immunoglobulin is available as two distinct preparations and formulations. One type of injection generally containing 16% of protein is used for passive immunisation, and sometimes also for primary antibody deficiencies, and should only be given intramuscularly; Human Normal Immunoglobulin (Ph. Eur. 5.0) and Immune Globulin (USP 27) are intended for intramuscular use only. The second type of preparation is formulated for intravenous administration (Human Normal Immunoglobulin for Intravenous Administration (Ph. Eur. 5.0)) and is used in disorders such as primary antibody deficiencies and idiopathic thrombocytopenic purpura; solutions generally contain about 3 to 6% of protein, although some may contain up to 12%. Doses of normal immunoglobulin often appear confusing, being expressed variously in terms of weight (protein or immunoglobulin G content) or in terms of volume to be given, and the two do not always appear to correspond. It should be remembered that there may be differences between intravenous preparations of normal immunoglobulin including differing IgA content and IgG subclass distribution.

Normal immunoglobulin, being derived from the pooled plasma of blood donors, contains antibodies to bacteria and viruses currently prevalent in the general population; in the UK, and also in some other countries, typical antibodies present include those against hepatitis A, measles, mumps, rubella, and varicella. Normal immunoglobulin, therefore, may be used to provide passive immunisation against such diseases.

Normal immunoglobulin may be used to control outbreaks of **hepatitis A**, the recommended dose for close contacts being 250 mg in those under 10 years of age and 500 mg in older children and adults. It may also be used for prophylaxis against hepatitis A in immunocompromised patients if their response to hepatitis A vaccine is unlikely to be adequate.

Normal immunoglobulin may be used to prevent or possibly modify an attack of **measles** in children and adults at special risk (such as those who are immunocompromised) but should be given as soon as possible after contact with measles. In the UK recommended doses, given intramuscularly, for the prevention of an attack are 250 mg for those under 1 year of age, 500 mg for those aged 1 to 2 years, and 750 mg for those aged 3 years and over; to modify an attack, recommended doses are 100 mg for those under 1 year of age and 250 mg for older children.

Normal immunoglobulin does not prevent **rubella** infection but may reduce the likelihood of clinical symptoms in pregnant women exposed to rubella thereby lessening the risk to the fetus; it should be given as soon as possible after exposure. The recommended dose is 750 mg by intramuscular injection.

Normal immunoglobulin may be used in the management of patients with **primary antibody deficiencies** such as congenital agammaglobulinaemia, hypogammaglobulinaemia, or **immunocompromised patients** including those with immunodeficiency syndromes; the immunoglobulin is given to provide protection against infectious diseases that such patients may suffer. The intramuscular preparation has been used but the intravenous route is usually preferred since administration is less painful for the doses required. For intravenous infusion the dose, expressed in terms of weight (protein or immunoglobulin G content), is usually 400 to 800 mg/kg initially, then 200 mg/kg every 3 weeks adjusted as necessary according to trough-immunoglobulin concentrations; the maintenance dose is usually 200 to 800 mg/kg per month. In patients with secondary immunodeficiency syndromes, doses of 200 to 400 mg/kg every 3 to 4 weeks have been recommended. Other dosage regimens have been used. When infused intravenously, normal immunoglobulin should always be given very carefully and slowly with gradual increases in the rate of administration.

For prophylaxis of infection after **bone marrow transplantation**, normal immunoglobulin is given intravenously in a dose of 500 mg/kg weekly, adjusted according to response.

Intravenous infusion of normal immunoglobulin is also employed to raise the platelet count in patients with **idiopathic thrombocytopenic purpura**. Doses of 400 mg/kg are given daily for 2 to 5 consecutive days. Alternatively, doses of 800 to 1000 mg/kg may be given on day 1 and repeated on day 3 if necessary. Further doses may be given as necessary.

For **Kawasaki disease**, normal immunoglobulin (in conjunction with aspirin) is given intravenously in a dose of 1.6 to 2 g/kg in divided doses over 2 to 5 days, or 2 g/kg given as a single dose. Similar doses of intravenous normal immunoglobulin have been tried in a range of disorders believed to have an auto-immune origin. The precise mode of action of normal immunoglobulin in such disorders is unknown.

For the treatment of **Guillain-Barré syndrome**, normal immunoglobulin is given intravenously in a dose of 400 mg/kg for 5 consecutive days, repeated every 4 weeks if required.

◊ Reviews and discussions of the actions and uses of intravenous normal immunoglobulins.


1. National Institutes of Health Consensus Conference. Intravenous immunoglobulin: prevention and treatment of disease. *JAMA* 1990; **264:** 3189–93.
2. Anonymous. Consensus on IVIG. *Lancet* 1990; **336:** 470–2.
3. ASHP Commission on Therapeutics. ASHP therapeutic guidelines for intravenous immune globulin. *Clin Pharm* 1992; **11:** 117–36.
4. Dwyer JM. Manipulating the immune system with immune globulin. *N Engl J Med* 1992; **326:** 107–16.
5. Pirofsky B, Kinzey DM. Intravenous immune globulins: a review of their uses in selected immunodeficiency and autoimmune diseases. *Drugs* 1992; **43:** 6–14.
6. Keller T, *et al.* Indications for the use of intravenous immunoglobulin: recommendations of the Australasian Society of Blood Transfusion consensus symposium. *Med J Aust* 1993; **159:** 204–6.
7. Ratko TA, *et al.* Recommendations for off-label use of intravenously administered immunoglobulin preparations. *JAMA* 1995; **273:** 1865–70.
8. Stiehm ER. Appropriate therapeutic use of immunoglobulin. *Transfus Med Rev* 1996; **10:** 203–21.
9. Kazatchkine MD, Kaveri SV. Immunomodulation of autoimmune and inflammatory diseases with intravenous immune globulin. *N Engl J Med* 2001; **345:** 747–55.
10. Ahmed AR, Dahl MV. Consensus statement on the use of intravenous immunoglobulin therapy in the treatment of autoimmune mucocutaneous blistering diseases. *Arch Dermatol* 2003; **139:** 1051–9.


**Administration.** In order to overcome some of the problems associated with ensuring regular venous access necessary for long-term intravenous immunoglobulin therapy, administration by rapid subcutaneous infusion has been evaluated. Subcutaneous infusion of approximately 16% preservative-free solutions or solutions not containing a mercurial preservative were administered to adults[1] through 2 pumps at a rate of 17 to 20 mL/hour at each pump and to children[2,3] at a rate of 10 to 20 mL/hour. Adequate immunoglobulin concentrations were achieved and this route of administration was generally well tolerated. A subsequent review[4] of subcutaneous infusion therapy in 165 patients receiving doses of between 80 and 800 mg/kg per month in divided doses supported these results.

Oral administration of normal immunoglobulins has been proposed to reduce the incidence and severity of gastrointestinal infections, particularly in patients with defective immune systems including neonates. Although the predominant immunoglobulin secreted into the gastrointestinal tract in subjects with a normal immune system is IgA, a species not present in large quantities in commercial normal immunoglobulins, beneficial responses, especially in viral infections, have been reported following oral administration. Systematic reviews have not, however, supported routine use of oral immunoglobulin for the prevention or treatment of gastrointestinal infections.[5-7] Preparations of immunoglobulin A are available in some countries and have been tried, mainly in bacterial gastrointestinal infections.[8,9]


1. Gardulf A, *et al.* Home treatment of hypogammaglobulinaemia with subcutaneous gammaglobulin by rapid infusion. *Lancet* 1991; **338:** 162–6.
2. Thomas MJ, *et al.* Rapid subcutaneous immunoglobulin infusions in children. *Lancet* 1993; **342:** 1432–3.
3. Gaspar J, *et al.* Immunoglobulin replacement treatment by rapid subcutaneous infusion. *Arch Dis Child* 1998; **79:** 48–51.
4. Gardulf A, *et al.* Subcutaneous immunoglobulin replacement in patients with primary antibody deficiencies: safety and costs. *Lancet* 1995; **345:** 365–9.
5. Foster J, Cole M. Oral immunoglobulin for preventing necrotizing enterocolitis in preterm and low birth-weight neonates. Available in The Cochrane Library; Issue 2. Chichester: John Wiley; 2004.
6. Mohan P, Haque K. Oral immunoglobulin for the prevention of rotavirus infection in low birth weight infants. Available in The Cochrane Library; Issue 2. Chichester: John Wiley; 2004.

7. Mohan P, Haque K. Oral immunoglobulin for the treatment of rotavirus diarrhoea in low birth weight infants. Available in The Cochrane Library; Issue 2. Chichester: John Wiley; 2004.
8. Tjellström B, *et al.* Oral immunoglobulin A supplement in treatment of Clostridium difficile enteritis. *Lancet* 1993; **341:** 701–2.
9. Hammarström V, *et al.* Oral immunoglobulin treatment in Campylobacter jejuni enteritis. *Lancet* 1993; **341:** 1036.


**Blood disorders.** Intravenous normal immunoglobulins are used in the treatment of symptomatic severe acute and chronic idiopathic thrombocytopenic purpura (p.1082). Other blood disorders in which normal immunoglobulins have been tried include agranulocytosis[1] and haemolytic disease of the newborn (p.1608), aplastic and haemolytic anaemias (p.732), red cell aplasia caused by parvovirus B19 infections (see under Passive Immunisation, below), thrombotic thrombocytopenic purpura and haemolytic-uraemic syndrome (see Thrombotic Microangiopathies p.758), and thrombocytopenia with a variety of causes.[2-10]


1. Fasth A. Immunoglobulin for neonatal agranulocytosis. *Arch Dis Child* 1986; **61:** 86–7.
2. Hoffman DM, *et al.* Human immunodeficiency virus-associated thrombocytopenia. *DICP Ann Pharmacother* 1989; **23:** 157–160.
3. Frame JN, *et al.* Correction of severe heparin-associated thrombocytopenia with intravenous immunoglobulin. *Ann Intern Med* 1989; **111:** 946–7.
4. Howrie DL, *et al.* Use of iv immune globulin for treatment of phenytoin-induced thrombocytopenia. *Clin Pharm* 1989; **8:** 734–7.
5. Landonio G, *et al.* HIV-related severe thrombocytopenia in intravenous drug users: prevalence, response to therapy in a medium-term follow-up, and pathogenic evaluation. *AIDS* 1990; **4:** 29–34.
6. Goulder P, *et al.* Intravenous immunoglobulin in virus associated haemophagocytic syndrome. *Arch Dis Child* 1990; **65:** 1275–7.
7. Larner AJ, *et al.* Life threatening thrombocytopenia in sarcoidosis: response to vincristine, human immunoglobulin, and corticosteroids. *BMJ* 1990; **300:** 317–19.
8. Ray JB, *et al.* Intravenous immune globulin for the treatment of presumed quinidine-induced thrombocytopenia. *DICP Ann Pharmacother* 1990; **24:** 693–5.
9. Salzman MB, Smith EM. Phenytoin-induced thrombocytopenia treated with intravenous immune globulin. *J Pediatr Hematol Oncol* 1998; **20:** 152–3.
10. Majluf-Cruz A, *et al.* Usefulness of a low-dose intravenous immunoglobulin regimen for the treatment of thrombocytopenia associated with AIDS. *Am J Hematol* 1998; **59:** 127–32.


**Epilepsy.** Normal immunoglobulins have sometimes been of benefit[1-3] in the treatment of children with intractable epilepsy, including Lennox-Gastaut syndrome or West's syndrome, but a review of the literature found that few well controlled studies had been conducted.[4] Although a positive trend in favour of intravenous immunoglobulin therapy for refractory epilepsy was noted in one double-blind controlled study[5] involving 61 patients, the results were not considered to be statistically significant.


1. Ariizumi M, *et al.* High dose gammaglobulin for intractable childhood epilepsy. *Lancet* 1983; **ii:** 162–3.
2. Sandstedt P, *et al.* Intravenous gammaglobulin for post-encephalitic epilepsy. *Lancet* 1984; **ii:** 1154–5.
3. van Engelen BGH, *et al.* High-dose intravenous immunoglobulin treatment in cryptogenic West and Lennox-Gastaut syndrome: an add-on study. *Eur J Pediatr* 1994; **153:** 762–9.
4. Duse M, *et al.* Intravenous immune globulin in the treatment of intractable childhood epilepsy. *Clin Exp Immunol* 1996; **104** (suppl 1): 71–6.
5. van Rijckevorsel-Harmant K, *et al.* Treatment of refractory epilepsy with intravenous immunoglobulins: results of the first double-blind/dose finding clinical study. *Int J Clin Lab Res* 1994; **24:** 162–6.


**Hypogammaglobulinaemia.** See under Primary Antibody Deficiency, below.

**Immunocompromised patients.** Immunodeficiency states may arise from primary disorders of the immune system, or, more commonly, they are secondary to immunosuppressive therapy, HIV infection, or haematological malignancies. Premature neonates may have deficits in their immune systems due to their immaturity; placental transfer of maternal antibodies usually occurs after about 32 weeks of gestation. Such patients and neonates may be deficient in gammaglobulins and they could potentially benefit from the administration of normal immunoglobulins to address their increased susceptibility to infection. For information on the use of immunoglobulins in specific conditions, see the following sections and under Neonatal Sepsis, below.

BONE MARROW TRANSPLANTATION. In patients undergoing allogeneic bone marrow transplantation (see Haematopoietic Stem Cell Transplantation, p.1344), intravenous normal immunoglobulin has decreased the incidence of both bacterial infections[1] and of symptomatic cytomegalovirus infection, particularly interstitial pneumonia.[1,2] Overall survival[1] or overall incidence of cytomegalovirus infection[1,2] was not decreased. A combination of normal immunoglobulin and ganciclovir appears to improve the outcome of cytomegalovirus pneumonia subsequent to bone marrow transplantation.[3] No patients treated with normal immunoglobulin alone survived. Cytomegalovirus immunoglobulins (p.1612) may be more appropriate for the specific prophylaxis and treatment of cytomegalovirus infections.

Intravenous immunoglobulin therapy has been found to be ineffective in preventing infections in patients receiving autologous bone marrow transplants[4] and may have contributed to an increased incidence of fatal hepatic veno-occlusive disease.

Normal immunoglobulin administration has been associated with a reduced frequency of acute graft-versus-host disease, possibly as a result of a direct immunomodulatory effect.


1. Sullivan KM, *et al.* Immunomodulatory and antimicrobial efficacy of intravenous immunoglobulin in bone marrow transplantation. *N Engl J Med* 1990; **323:** 705–12.
2. Winston DJ, *et al.* Intravenous immune globulin for prevention of cytomegalovirus infection and interstitial pneumonia after bone marrow transplantation. *Ann Intern Med* 1987; **106:** 12–18.
3. Emanuel D, *et al.* Cytomegalovirus pneumonia after bone marrow transplantation successfully treated with the combination of ganciclovir and high-dose intravenous immune globulin. *Ann Intern Med* 1988; **109:** 777–82.
4. Wolff SN, *et al.* High-dose weekly intravenous immunoglobulin to prevent infections in patients undergoing autologous bone marrow transplantation or severe myelosuppressive therapy: a study of the American Bone Marrow Transplant Group. *Ann Intern Med* 1993; **118:** 937–42.


HIV INFECTION AND AIDS. Immunoglobulin levels are typically raised in patients with AIDS, but hypogammaglobulinaemia has been observed and, even in the presence of hypergammaglobulinaemia, patients exhibit signs of being hypogammaglobulinaemic. Normal immunoglobulin has therefore been administered to some symptomatic HIV-positive children. A significant improvement was noted[1] in 8 children given intravenous normal immunoglobulin, in terms of weight gain, number of infectious episodes, and diarrhoea. HIV core antigen was detected in 4 children before treatment. All became core-antigen negative after treatment was commenced although the effect was only maintained in 3. The validity of these results was questioned.[2] Larger studies have reported improvements in the rate of decline of the CD4+ T lymphocyte count[3] and the incidence of serious bacterial infections[4,5] but could not demonstrate improved survival. However, a further controlled study[6] in adult patients with AIDS given intravenous normal immunoglobulin demonstrated both an increase in the time free from bacterial or viral infection and also an improvement in survival rate after 31 weeks, and a small study in 24 patients[7] has reported improved survival at up to 12 months in patients who received normal immunoglobulin.


1. Hague RA, *et al.* Intravenous immunoglobulin in HIV infection: evidence for the efficacy of treatment. *Arch Dis Child* 1989; **64:** 1146–50.
2. Gibb D, Levin M. Intravenous immunoglobulin in HIV infection. *Arch Dis Child* 1990; **65:** 247–8.
3. Mofenson LM, *et al.* Effect of intravenous immunoglobulin (IVIG) on CD4+ lymphocyte decline in HIV-infected children in a clinical trial of IVIG infection prophylaxis. *J Acquir Immune Defic Syndr* 1993; **6:** 1103–13.
4. The National Institute of Child Health and Human Development Intravenous Immunoglobulin Study Group. Intravenous immune globulin for the prevention of bacterial infections in children with symptomatic human immunodeficiency virus infection. *N Engl J Med* 1991; **325:** 73–80.
5. Spector SA, *et al.* A controlled trial of intravenous immune globulin for the prevention of serious bacterial infections in children receiving zidovudine for advanced human immunodeficiency virus infection. *N Engl J Med* 1994; **331:** 1181–7.
6. Kiehl MG, *et al.* A controlled trial of intravenous immune globulin for the prevention of serious infections in adults with advanced human immunodeficiency virus infection. *Arch Intern Med* 1996; **156:** 2545–50.
7. Saint-Marc T, *et al.* Beneficial effects of intravenous immunoglobulins in AIDS. *Lancet* 1992; **340:** 1347.


MALIGNANCIES. Hypogammaglobulinaemia and the effects of treatment may increase the susceptibility to infection of patients with *chronic lymphocytic leukaemia*.[1] In a study of 81 patients with chronic lymphocytic leukaemia considered to be at an increased risk of infection, intravenous normal immunoglobulin 400 mg/kg given every 3 weeks for one year reduced the incidence of bacterial infection compared with saline placebo. The incidence of viral and fungal infections was not affected. A study in 34 patients[2] suggested that a dose of normal immunoglobulin 250 mg/kg per month was adequate for routine prophylaxis in most patients. Beneficial effects on infection rates have been reported in patients with *multiple myeloma* receiving normal immunoglobulins.[3]


1. Cooperative Group for the Study of Immunoglobulin in Chronic Lymphocytic Leukemia. Intravenous immunoglobulin for *N Engl J Med* 1988; **319:** 902–7.
2. Chapel H, *et al.* Immunoglobulin replacement in patients with chronic lymphocytic leukaemia: a comparison of two dose regimes. *Br J Haematol* 1994; **88:** 209–12.
3. Chapel HM, *et al.* Randomised trial of intravenous immunoglobulin as prophylaxis against infection in plateau-phase multiple myeloma. *Lancet* 1994; **343:** 1059–63.


PRIMARY ANTIBODY DEFICIENCY. There are three major forms of primary antibody deficiency: X-linked agammaglobulinaemia (XLA, Bruton's agammaglobulinaemia), common variable immunodeficiency (CVID) which includes IgG subclass and specific antibody deficiencies, and selective IgA deficiency. The disease is characterised by a wide range of infective complications as well as auto-immune disorders. Management is by replacement therapy with normal immunoglobulin accompanied by appropriate antimicrobial therapy for breakthrough infections. Immunisation against infection is of no value and is contra-indicated for live viral vaccines.

Normal immunoglobulin was traditionally administered by the intramuscular route. However, the maximum dose that could be reasonably given by this route was 25 mg/kg weekly, and it was therefore only satisfactory for patients with mild disease.[1] The introduction of intravenous preparations of normal immunoglobulin allowed high doses to be given to those with severe disease. This route should therefore be used for all patients with XLA and for patients with CVID who have more than mild disease.[2] The use of intravenous normal immunoglobulin in IgG subclass deficiency, with or without IgA deficiency, or in specific antibody deficiency is successful, though less well established. The dose and frequency of administration of intravenous normal immunoglobulin is variable and should be adjusted to prevent breakthrough infection. Most patients require 200 to 600 mg/kg every 2 or 3 weeks to maintain optimum protection.[1] In one study,[3] doses of between 260 and 1120 mg/kg every 3 weeks were necessary to maintain residual serum IgG concentrations above 500 mg/dL. These doses were found to be effective in reducing the incidence of severe acute bacterial infections and pulmonary insufficiency in children with XLA. Surgical procedures should be covered with additional normal immunoglobulin and appropriate prophylactic antibacterials. Home treatment with intravenous normal immunoglobulin has been used successfully in several countries in both adults and children.[1,4-7] Adverse reactions have been few and generally mild.[1,5,6] They are most likely to occur during the first infusion and during intercurrent illness, and may be precipitated by a high infusion rate.[7] Long-term treatment of children with antibody deficiencies with intravenous normal immunoglobulin has been shown to lead to normal growth and similar rates of infection to those found in non-immunodeficient children.[8]

Some patients have been successfully treated with subcutaneous infusion of normal immunoglobulin (see Administration, above) and the intraventricular route has been of benefit in some patients with echovirus encephalitis.[1,9]

In a pilot study, normal immunoglobulin given subcutaneously to 10 patients with selective IgA deficiency was safe and reduced the rate of respiratory-tract infections.[10]


1. Spickett GP, *et al.* Primary antibody deficiency in adults. *Lancet* 1991; **337:** 281–4.
2. Carrock Sewell WA, *et al.* Therapeutic strategies in common variable immunodeficiency. *Drugs* 2003; **63:** 1359–71.
3. Quartier P, *et al.* Early and prolonged intravenous immunoglobulin replacement therapy in childhood agammaglobulinemia: a retrospective survey of 31 patients. *J Pediatr* 1999; **134:** 589–96.
4. Ochs HD, *et al.* Intravenous immunoglobulin home treatment for patients with primary immunodeficiency diseases. *Lancet* 1986; **i:** 610–11.
5. Ryan A, *et al.* Home intravenous immunoglobulin therapy for patients with primary hypogammaglobulinaemia. *Lancet* 1988; **ii:** 793.
6. Kobayashi RH, *et al.* Home self-administration of intravenous immunoglobulin therapy in children. *Pediatrics* 1990; **85:** 705–9.
7. Chapel HM. Consensus on diagnosis and management of primary antibody deficiencies. *BMJ* 1994; **308:** 581–5.
8. Skull S, Kemp A. Treatment of hypogammaglobulinaemia with intravenous immunoglobulin, 1973-93. *Arch Dis Child* 1996; **74:** 527–30.
9. Erlendsson K, *et al.* Successful reversal of echovirus encephalitis in x-linked hypogammaglobulinemia by intraventricular administration of immunoglobulin. *N Engl J Med* 1985; **312:** 351–30.
10. Gustafson R, *et al.* Prophylactic therapy for selective IgA deficiency. *Lancet* 1997; **350:** 865.


**Inflammatory bowel diseases.** Intravenous normal immunoglobulin may be beneficial[1-3] in inducing remission of Crohn's disease and ulcerative colitis and has been tried[4] in antibiotic-associated colitis.


1. Rohr G, *et al.* Treatment of Crohn's disease and ulcerative colitis with 7S-immunoglobulin. *Lancet* 1987; **i:** 170.
2. Knoflach P, *et al.* Crohn disease and intravenous immunoglobulin G. *Ann Intern Med* 1990; **112:** 385–6.
3. Körber J, *et al.* A case of Crohn's disease with increased CD8 T-cell activation and remission during therapy with intravenous immunoglobulins. *Scand J Gastroenterol* 1998; **33:** 1113–17.
4. Leung DYM, *et al.* Treatment with intravenously administered gamma globulin of chronic relapsing colitis induced by Clostridium difficile toxin. *J Pediatr* 1991; **118:** 633–7.


**Kawasaki disease.** Kawasaki disease, also known as mucocutaneous lymph node syndrome of childhood, occurs mainly in children under 5 years of age. It is epidemic and endemic worldwide but is a particular problem in Japan. Kawasaki disease presents with high fever which persists for at least 5 days and may be followed by bilateral conjunctivitis, changes in the oropharyngeal mucosa, signs of vasculitis in the extremities, rash, and cervical lymphadenopathy. The major complications of Kawasaki disease are cardiac effects including coronary artery aneurysm, aortic or mitral incompetence, myocarditis, and pericarditis with effusion. The cause of the disease is unknown, although an infective aetiology has been suggested. Early diagnosis, expert cardiac assessment, and immediate treatment are essential for improved outcome.

Treatment aims to reduce inflammation, particularly in the coronary arterial wall and myocardium, and therefore prevent the development of cardiac complications. Long-term antiplatelet treatment is given as necessary to prevent coronary thrombosis.

**Initial treatment** is with aspirin and normal immunoglobulin.[1-3] A decreased incidence of coronary-artery abnormalities has been demonstrated after such a combination as compared with aspirin alone.[4] Normal immunoglobulin has generally been given by intravenous infusion in divided doses over 2 to 5 days, although high-dose administration as a single dose is recommended as an alternative,[5] and a meta-analysis[6] and a systematic review[7] have concluded that single-dose administration is associated with a lower incidence of coronary abnormalities after 30 days than multiple-dose treatment. The optimum dosage and duration of treatment with aspirin is not yet established, but the usual practice is to use an anti-inflammatory regimen until the fever has settled and then to convert to an antithrombotic regimen. A few patients fail to respond to treatment with aspirin and normal immunoglobulin. A small study[8] suggested that re-treatment with normal immunoglobulin may be considered for those with persistent or recurring fever. The use of corticosteroids remains controversial.[1] They have been given in some centres[9] but since the introduction of immunoglobulin therapy they have not been routinely used as there is a risk that they may exacerbate coronary artery aneurysms. Nevertheless, their use has received renewed attention; randomised studies comparing the adjunctive use of corticosteroids with standard therapy alone have suggested they may be of benefit.[10,11]

**Long-term management.** Aspirin should be continued for 6 to 8 weeks after the onset of illness and then discontinued if there are no coronary abnormalities. Some practitioners use aspirin and dipyridamole as antithrombotic therapy although it is not known whether this combination provides benefit over aspirin alone. Dipyridamole may be used as an alternative antithrombotic agent for patients who cannot tolerate aspirin. Aspirin is usually continued for at least one year if coronary abnormalities are present and should be continued indefinitely if coronary aneurysms persist. Anticoagulation with warfarin or heparin in addition to aspirin may be necessary in some patients such as those with giant or multiple aneurysms.


1. Onouchi Z, Kawasaki T. Overview of pharmacological treatment of Kawasaki disease. *Drugs* 1999; **58:** 813–22.
2. Williams RV, *et al.* Pharmacological therapy for patients with Kawasaki disease. *Paediatr Drugs* 2001; **3:** 649–60.
3. Brogan PA, *et al.* Kawasaki disease: an evidence based approach to diagnosis, treatment, and proposals for future research. *Arch Dis Child* 2002; **86:** 286–90.
4. Newburger JW, *et al.* The treatment of Kawasaki syndrome with intravenous gamma globulin. *N Engl J Med* 1986; **315:** 341–7.
5. Newburger JW, *et al.* A single intravenous infusion of gamma globulin as compared with four infusions in the treatment of acute Kawasaki syndrome. *N Engl J Med* 1991; **324:** 1633–9.
6. Durongpisitkul K, *et al.* The prevention of coronary artery aneurysm in Kawasaki disease: a meta-analysis on the efficacy of aspirin and immunoglobulin treatment. *Pediatrics* 1995; **96:** 1057–61.
7. Oates-Whitehead RM, *et al.* Intravenous immunoglobulin for the treatment of Kawasaki disease in children. Available in The Cochrane Library; Issue 2. Chichester: John Wiley; 2004.
8. Sundel RP, *et al.* Gamma globulin re-treatment in Kawasaki disease. *J Pediatr* 1993; **123:** 657–9.
9. Shinohara M, *et al.* Corticosteroids in the treatment of the acute phase of Kawasaki disease. *J Pediatr* 1999; **135:** 465–9.
10. Sundel RP, *et al.* Corticosteroids in the initial treatment of Kawasaki disease: report of a randomized trial. *J Pediatr* 2003; **142:** 611–16.
11. Okada Y, *et al.* Effect of corticosteroids in addition to intravenous gamma globulin therapy on serum cytokine levels in the acute phase of Kawasaki disease in children. *J Pediatr* 2003; **143:** 363–7.


**Kidney disorders.** Treatment with normal immunoglobulin has been of benefit in some patients with haemolytic-uraemic syndrome and in those with lupus nephritis (see under Musculoskeletal and Nerve Disorders, below). For mention of the use of normal immunoglobulin in IgA nephropathy, see Glomerular Kidney Disease, p.1080.

**Musculoskeletal and nerve disorders.** High-dose intravenous normal immunoglobulin has been tried with some benefit in various disorders of the nerves, muscles, joints, and connective tissues which may have an auto-immune basis. These include multiple sclerosis,[1] chronic inflammatory demyelinating polyneuropathy,[2-4] polymyositis and dermatomyositis,[5-10] myasthenia gravis,[11-14] stiff-man syndrome,[15-19] chronic systemic juvenile arthritis,[20-22] systemic lupus erythematosus[23] including lupus nephritis,[24] Guillain-Barré syndrome (see below), and motor neurone disease (see also below).


1. Fazekas F, *et al.* Randomised placebo-controlled trial of monthly intravenous immunoglobulin therapy in relapsing-remitting multiple sclerosis. *Lancet* 1997; **349:** 589–93.
2. van Doorn PA, *et al.* High-dose intravenous immunoglobulin treatment in chronic inflammatory demyelinating polyneuropathy: a double-blind, placebo-controlled, crossover study. *Neurology* 1990; **40:** 209–12.
3. Mendell JR, *et al.* Randomized controlled trial of IVIg in untreated chronic inflammatory demyelinating polyradiculoneuropathy. *Neurology* 2001; **56:** 445–9.
4. Sharma KR, *et al.* Diabetic demyelinating polyneuropathy responsive to intravenous immunoglobulin therapy. *Arch Neurol* 2002; **59:** 751–7.
5. Cherin P, *et al.* Efficacy of intravenous gammaglobulin therapy in chronic refractory polymyositis and dermatomyositis: an open study with 20 adult patients. *Am J Med* 1991; **91:** 162–8.
6. Lang BA, *et al.* Treatment of dermatomyositis with intravenous gammaglobulin. *Am J Med* 1991; **91:** 169–72.
7. Dalakas MC, *et al.* A controlled trial of high-dose intravenous immune globulin infusions as treatment for dermatomyositis. *N Engl J Med* 1993; **329:** 1993–2000.
8. Brownell AKW. Intravenous immune globulin for dermatomyositis. *N Engl J Med* 1994; **330:** 1392.
9. Collet E, *et al.* Juvenile dermatomyositis: treatment with intravenous gammaglobulin. *Br J Dermatol* 1994; **130:** 231–4.
10. Cherin P, *et al.* Results and long-term followup of intravenous immunoglobulin infusions in chronic, refractory polymyositis: an open study with thirty-five adult patients. *Arthritis Rheum* 2002; **46:** 467–74.
11. Bassan H, *et al.* High-dose intravenous immunoglobulin in transient neonatal myasthenia gravis. *Pediatr Neurol* 1998; **18:** 181–3.
12. Jongen JLM, *et al.* High-dose intravenous immunoglobulin therapy for myasthenia gravis. *J Neurol* 1998; **245:** 26–31.
13. Howard JF. Intravenous immunoglobulin for the treatment of acquired myasthenia gravis. *Neurology* 1998; **51** (suppl 5): S30–S36.
14. Selcen D, *et al.* High-dose intravenous immunoglobulin therapy in juvenile myasthenia gravis. *Pediatr Neurol* 2000; **22:** 40–3.
15. Karlson EW, *et al.* Treatment of stiff-man syndrome with intravenous immune globulin. *Arthritis Rheum* 1994; **37:** 915–18.
16. Amato AA, *et al.* Treatment of stiff-man syndrome with intravenous immunoglobulin. *Neurology* 1994; **44:** 1652–4.
17. Barker RA, Marsden CD. Successful treatment of stiff man syndrome with intravenous immunoglobulin. *J Neurol Neurosurg Psychiatry* 1997; **62:** 426–7.
18. Khanlou H, Eiger G. Long-term remission of refractory stiff-man syndrome after treatment with intravenous immunoglobulin. *Mayo Clin Proc* 1999; **74:** 1231–2.
19. Dalakas MC, *et al.* High-dose intravenous immune globulin for stiff-person syndrome. *N Engl J Med* 2001; **345:** 1870–6.
20. Groothoff JW, van Leeuwen EF. High dose intravenous gammaglobulin in chronic systemic juvenile arthritis. *BMJ* 1988; **296:** 1362–3.
21. Giannini EH, *et al.* Intravenous immunoglobulin in the treatment of polyarticular juvenile rheumatoid arthritis: a phase I/II study. *J Rheumatol* 1996; **23:** 919–24.
22. Uziel Y, *et al.* Intravenous immunoglobulin therapy in systemic onset juvenile rheumatoid arthritis: a followup study. *J Rheumatol* 1996; **23:** 910–18.
23. Francioni C, *et al.* Long term IV Ig treatment in systemic lupus erythematosus. *Clin Exp Rheumatol* 1994; **12:** 163–8.
24. Lin C-Y, *et al.* Improvement of histological and immunological change in steroid and immunosuppressive drug-resistant lupus nephritis by high-dose intravenous gamma globulin. *Nephron* 1989; **53:** 303–10.


GUILLAIN-BARRÉ SYNDROME. Guillain-Barré syndrome (acute idiopathic inflammatory polyneuropathy; acute idiopathic demyelinating neuropathy; acute infectious polyneuropathy) may follow an infection or, more rarely, immunisation, but very often no predisposing factor can be identified. There may be an association with infection with *Campylobacter jejuni*.[1] Reversible demyelination results in pain and progressive flaccid paralysis. An auto-immune aetiology seems likely. Severely affected patients require cardiovascular monitoring and respiratory support if respiratory muscles are affected or autonomic instability is present. Corticosteroids have been given but are generally considered to be of little value[2] (see Polyneuropathies, p.1086). Plasma exchange (see p.758) is effective if given early,[3] but is not universally available and is not suitable for all patients. A systematic review[4] has concluded that administration of normal immunoglobulins is at least as effective as plasma exchange, but that there is no advantage from combining the two forms of treatment. Deterioration has also been noted in some patients following immunoglobulin therapy.[5,6]


1. Rees JH, *et al.* Campylobacter jejuni infection and Guillain-Barré syndrome. *N Engl J Med* 1995; **333:** 1374–9.
2. Hughes RAC, van der Meché FGA. Corticosteroids for Guillain-Barré syndrome. Available in The Cochrane Library; Issue 2. Chichester: John Wiley; 2004.
3. Raphaël JC, *et al.* Plasma exchange for Guillain-Barré syndrome. Available in The Cochrane Library; Issue 2. Chichester: John Wiley; 2004.
4. Hughes RAC, *et al.* Intravenous immunoglobulin for Guillain-Barré syndrome. Available in The Cochrane Library; Issue 2. Chichester: John Wiley; 2004.
5. Irani DN, *et al.* Relapse in Guillain-Barré syndrome after treatment with human immune globulin. *Neurology* 1993; **43:** 872–5.
6. Castro LHM, Ropper AH. Human immune globulin infusion in Guillain-Barré syndrome: worsening during and after treatment. *Neurology* 1993; **43:** 1034–6.


MOTOR NEURONE DISEASE. Normal immunoglobulins have been tried in the treatment of multifocal motor neuropathy, a form of motor neurone disease (p.1739) associated with anti-$GM_1$ antibody formation.[1-5]


1. Van den Berg LH, *et al.* Treatment of multifocal motor neuropathy with high dose intravenous immunoglobulins: a double blind, placebo controlled study. *J Neurol Neurosurg Psychiatry* 1995; **59:** 248–52.
2. Azulay J-P, *et al.* Long term follow up of multifocal motor neuropathy with conduction block under treatment. *J Neurol Neurosurg Psychiatry* 1997; **62:** 391–4.
3. Meucci N, *et al.* Long term effect of intravenous immunoglobulins and oral cyclophosphamide in multifocal motor neuropathy. *J Neurol Neurosurg Psychiatry* 1997; **63:** 765–9.
4. Van den Berg LH, *et al.* The long-term effect of intravenous immunoglobulin treatment in multifocal motor neuropathy. *Brain* 1998; **121:** 421–8.
5. Ellis CM, *et al.* Use of human intravenous immunoglobulin in lower motor neuron syndromes. *J Neurol Neurosurg Psychiatry* 1999; **67:** 15–19.


**Neonatal disorders.** HAEMOLYTIC DISEASE OF THE NEWBORN. For a discussion of haemolytic disease of the newborn and its management, including the use of intravenous immunoglobulin as an alternative to exchange transfusions in affected pregnancies, see p.1608.

NEONATAL SEPSIS. Sepsis is a serious problem in premature infants despite appropriate antimicrobial therapy. Preterm infants are born with low serum-immunoglobulin concentrations which decrease over the next several weeks of life. There is also a deficiency of antibodies to specific organisms such as group B streptococci, *Staphylococcus epidermidis*, and *Escherichia coli*.

Some, but not all, studies suggest that prophylactic use of intravenous normal immunoglobulin in premature infants shortly after birth can decrease the incidence of septicaemia.[1] Aspects of the methodology of these studies have, however, been criticised[2] and a systematic review[3] concluded that prophylactic use of intravenous immunoglobulin for prevention of sepsis in preterm or low birth-weight neonates was of marginal benefit only and did not recommend routine use. Some benefit has been seen after use of intravenous immunoglobulin to treat infants with suspected sepsis,[1] and it may improve the response to antibacterials[4] although a further systematic review[5] found insufficient evidence to support routine treatment in infants with suspected, or subsequently proved, neonatal infection.

The optimum effective dosage of intravenous immunoglobulin is not established. A prophylactic dose of 500 mg/kg on admission repeated every 1 to 2 weeks has been suggested for units where infection is common in very low birth-weight infants.[1] Others have suggested adjusting the dose to maintain a specified serum-immunoglobulin concentration.[6,7] Alternatively, normal immunoglobulin could be given only to infants with immunoglobulin concentrations below a certain level, or be reserved for immediate use in those who become ill with suspected sepsis.[1]

Normal immunoglobulin cannot protect against all types of infection. Normal immunoglobulin preparations from different manufacturers may demonstrate, for a specific pathogen (group B streptococcus), differing levels of specific antibody and differing levels of functional activity both *in vitro* and in *animals*.[8] Lot-to-lot variability in functional activity was also observed for normal immunoglobulin from a specific manufacturer. Such variability, resulting in low concentrations of functional antibodies in the 4 batches of immunoglobulins used in the National Institute of Child Health Study,[9] was held responsible for the lack of demonstrable effectiveness of immunoglobulins in that study, one of the largest to date. It has been suggested[10] that normal immunoglobulin would probably not be effective for the prevention of serious *Herpes simplex* virus infection in neonates at risk.

The use of fresh frozen plasma as an alternative to normal immunoglobulin could not be recommended following a study[11] that showed that it did not produce the beneficial effects on humoral immune markers seen with normal immunoglobulin.


1. Whitelaw A. Treatment of sepsis with IgG in very low birth-weight infants. *Arch Dis Child* 1990; **65:** 347–8.
2. Noya FJD, Baker CJ. Intravenously administered immune globulin for premature infants: a time to wait. *J Pediatr* 1989; **115:** 969–71.
3. Ohlsson A, Lacy JB. Intravenous immunoglobulin for preventing infection in preterm and/or low-birth-weight infants. Available in The Cochrane Library; Issue 2. Chichester: John Wiley; 2004.
4. Christensen RD, *et al.* Effect on neutrophil kinetics and serum opsonic capacity of intravenous administration of immune globulin to neonates with clinical signs of early-onset sepsis. *J Pediatr* 1991; **118:** 606–14.
5. Ohlsson A, Lacy JB. Intravenous immunoglobulin for suspected or subsequently proven infection in neonates. Available in The Cochrane Library; Issue 2. Chichester: John Wiley; 2004.
6. Clapp DW, *et al.* Use of intravenously administered immune globulin to prevent nosocomial sepsis in low birth weight infants: report of a pilot study. *J Pediatr* 1989; **115:** 973–8.
7. Kyllonen KS, *et al.* Dosage of intravenously administered immune globulin and dosing interval required to maintain target levels of immunoglobulin G in low birth weight infants. *J Pediatr* 1989; **115:** 1013–16.
8. Givner LB. Human immunoglobulins for intravenous use: comparison of available preparations for group B streptococcal antibody levels, opsonic activity, and efficacy in animal models. *Pediatrics* 1990; **86:** 955–62.
9. Fanaroff AA, *et al.* A controlled trial of intravenous immune globulin to reduce nosocomial infections in very-low-birth-weight infants. *N Engl J Med* 1994; **330:** 1107–13.
10. Kohl S, *et al.* Effect of intravenously administered immune globulin on functional antibody to herpes simplex virus in low birth weight neonates. *J Pediatr* 1989; **115:** 135–9.
11. Acunas BA, *et al.* Effect of fresh frozen plasma and gammaglobulin on humoral immunity in neonatal sepsis. *Arch Dis Child* 1994; **70:** F182–7.


**Obsessive-compulsive disorder.** Benefit has been demonstrated from plasma exchange and administration of intravenous immunoglobulin in children with exacerbations of obsessive-compulsive disorder or tic disorders including Tourette's syndrome associated with streptococcal infection.[1] These results suggest that these disorders may respond to immunomodulatory therapy in a subgroup of patients with paediatric auto-immune neuropsychiatric disorders associated with streptococcal infections (PANDAS), believed to be due to cross-reaction of antistreptococcal antibodies with neural tissue.


1. Perlmutter SJ, *et al.* Therapeutic plasma exchange and intravenous immunoglobulin for obsessive-compulsive disorder and tic disorders in childhood. *Lancet* 1999; **354:** 1153–8.


**Passive immunisation.** CYTOMEGALOVIRUS INFECTION. See Bone Marrow Transplantation, under Immunocompromised Patients, above.

HEPATITIS C. In a randomised, placebo-controlled study[1] in seronegative sexual partners of patients positive for antibody to hepatitis C, normal immunoglobulin administered intramuscularly every 2 months was found to significantly reduce the incidence of subsequent seroconversion. One of 450 subjects who received normal immunoglobulin became seropositive during follow-up compared with 6 of 449 who had received placebo.


1. Piazza M, *et al.* Sexual transmission of the hepatitis C virus and efficacy of prophylaxis with intramuscular immune serum globulin: a randomized controlled trial. *Arch Intern Med* 1997; **157:** 1537–44.


PARVOVIRUS B19 INFECTION. Persistent infection with human parvovirus B19 can cause red-cell aplasia with resultant anaemia, particularly in immunocompromised patients. Resolution of anaemia and clearance of parvovirus B19 from the circulation have been reported after administration of normal immunoglobulin to a patient who had had red-cell aplasia for 10 years.[1] Normal immunoglobulin was given by intravenous infusion in a dose of 400 mg/kg daily for 10 days and then periodically for several months. Successful treatment of anaemia due to parvovirus B19-induced red-cell aplasia with plasmapheresis and intravenous immunoglobulin has been described in a liver transplant recipient.[2] Clearance of parvovirus B19 from the circulation has been reported in patients who also have AIDS, but the presence of concomitant opportunistic infections may prevent resolution of the anaemia.[3,4]

Beneficial responses to intravenous immunoglobulin have also been reported in a few patients with parvovirus B19 infections associated with vasculitic syndromes.[5,6]

1. Kurtzman G, *et al.* Pure red-cell aplasia of 10 years' duration due to persistent parvovirus B19 infection and its cure with immunoglobulin therapy. *N Engl J Med* 1989; **321:** 519–23.
2. Ramage JK, *et al.* Parvovirus B19-induced red cell aplasia treated with plasmapheresis and immunoglobulin. *Lancet* 1994; **343:** 667–8.
3. Frickhofen N, *et al.* Persistent B19 parvovirus infection in patients infected with human immunodeficiency virus type 1 (HIV-1): a treatable cause of anemia in AIDS. *Ann Intern Med* 1990; **113:** 926–33.
4. Bowman CA, *et al.* Red cell aplasia associated with human parvovirus B19 and HIV infection: failure to respond clinically to intravenous immunoglobulin. *AIDS* 1990; **4:** 1038–9.
5. Finkel TH, *et al.* Chronic parvovirus B19 infection and systemic necrotising vasculitis: opportunistic infection or aetiological agent? *Lancet* 1994; **343:** 1255–8.
6. Viguier M, *et al.* Treatment of parvovirus B19-associated polyarteritis nodosa with intravenous immune globulin. *N Engl J Med* 2001; **344:** 1481–2.

RUBELLA. Normal immunoglobulin does not prevent rubella infection but may reduce the likelihood of clinical symptoms in pregnant women exposed to rubella thereby lessening the risk to the fetus; it should be given as soon as possible after exposure.

TOXIC SHOCK SYNDROME. For a discussion of toxic shock syndrome and its treatment, including reference to clinical improvement after administration of intravenous normal immunoglobulins, see p.149.

**Skin disorders.** Normal immunoglobulins have been tried in a few patients with blistering skin diseases.[1,2] The usual treatment for pemphigus and pemphigoid is with systemic corticosteroids; normal immunoglobulins in high doses have produced generally transient improvement when used alone,[3] although steroid-sparing effects have been reported.[4] A patient with severe epidermolysis bullosa responded to therapy with high-dose intravenous immunoglobulins.[5] Clinical benefit was noted in 9 of 10 patients with auto-immune chronic urticaria who were given a 5-day course of intravenous immunoglobulins, 2 of whom experienced prolonged remission over 3 years of follow-up.[6] Benefit has also occurred after intravenous immunoglobulin therapy for atopic dermatitis,[7] psoriasis,[8] and pyoderma gangrenosum.[9]

1. Harman KE, Black MM. High-dose intravenous immune globulin for the treatment of autoimmune blistering diseases: an evaluation of its use in 14 cases. *Br J Dermatol* 1999; **140:** 865–74.
2. Ahmed AR, Dahl MV. Consensus statement on the use of intravenous immunoglobulin therapy in the treatment of autoimmune mucocutaneous blistering diseases. *Arch Dermatol* 2003; **139:** 1051–9.
3. Godard W, *et al.* Bullous pemphigoid and intravenous gammaglobulin. *Ann Intern Med* 1985; **103:** 965.
4. Beckers RCY, *et al.* Adjuvant high-dose intravenous gammaglobulin in the treatment of pemphigus and bullous pemphigoid: experience in six patients. *Br J Dermatol* 1995; **133:** 289–93.
5. Mohr C, *et al.* Successful treatment of epidermolysis bullosa acquisita using intravenous immunoglobulins. *Br J Dermatol* 1995; **132:** 824–6.
6. O'Donnell BF, *et al.* Intravenous immunoglobulin in autoimmune chronic urticaria. *Br J Dermatol* 1998; **138:** 101–6.
7. Jolles S, *et al.* The treatment of atopic dermatitis with adjunctive high-dose intravenous immunoglobulin: a report of three patients and review of the literature. *Br J Dermatol* 2000; **142:** 551–4.
8. Gurmin V, *et al.* Psoriasis: response to high-dose intravenous immunoglobulin in three patients. *Br J Dermatol* 2002; **147:** 554–7.
9. Dirschka T, *et al.* Successful treatment of pyoderma gangrenosum with intravenous human immunoglobulin. *J Am Acad Dermatol* 1998; **39:** 789–90.

**Spontaneous abortion.** Fetal loss has been attributed in some cases to the presence of antiphospholipid antibodies (lupus anticoagulant and anticardiolipin) in the mother. Successful pregnancy outcome has been reported after administration of intravenous normal immunoglobulin during pregnancy to a few such women.[1-5]

1. Carreras LO, *et al.* Lupus anticoagulant and recurrent fetal loss: successful treatment with gammaglobulin. *Lancet* 1988; **ii:** 393–4.
2. Francois A, *et al.* Repeated fetal losses and the lupus anticoagulant. *Ann Intern Med* 1988; **109:** 993–4.
3. Parke A, *et al.* Intravenous gamma-globulin, antiphospholipid antibodies, and pregnancy. *Ann Intern Med* 1989; **110:** 495–6.
4. Katz VL, *et al.* Human immunoglobulin therapy for preeclampsia associated with lupus anticoagulant and anticardiolipin antibody. *Obstet Gynecol* 1990; **76:** 986–8.
5. Mueller-Eckhardt G, *et al.* IVIG to prevent recurrent spontaneous abortion. *Lancet* 1991; **337:** 424–5.

## Preparations

***Ph. Eur.:*** Human Normal Immunoglobulin; Human Normal Immunoglobulin for Intravenous Administration;
***USP 27:*** Immune Globulin.

**Proprietary Preparations** (details are given in Part 3)

***Arg.:*** Citax F; Endobulin; Flebogamma; Gamimune; Gammaglobulina; IgG; Isiven; Pentaglobin; Sandoglobulina; Seroglubin; ***Austral.:*** Intragam; Intraglobin; Sandoglobulin; ***Austria:*** Beriglobin; Endobulin; Gamma-Venin; Gammagard; Intragam†; Intraglobin; Octagam; Pentaglobin; Sandoglobulin; Venimmun N; ***Belg.:*** Gammagard†; Globuman†; Sandoglobuline; ***Braz.:*** Armoglobulina; Beriglobina; Gama Venina; Gamimune; Intraglobin F†; Isiven†; Pentaglobin†; Sandoglobulina; Veinoglobuline†; Venimmuna; Vigam; ***Canad.:*** Baygam; Gamimune N; Gammagard; Iveegam; ***Chile:*** Beriglobina P; Flebogamma; Gamimune N; Octagam; Sandoglobulina; ***Denm.:*** Beriglobin; Endobulin; Gammagard; Gammaglobulin†; Gammanorm; Gammonativ; Nordimmun†; ***Fin.:*** Endobulin; Gammagard; Gammaglobulin SPR; Sandoglobulin†; Venogamma; ***Fr.:*** Endobuline; Gammagard; Octagam; Sandoglobuline†; Tegeline; ***Ger.:*** Alphaglobin†; Beriglobin; Endobulin; Flebogamma; Gamma-Venin; Gammabulin†; Gammagard; Gammonativ; Intraglobin; Intrimun†; Octagam; Pentaglobin; Polyglobin; Sandoglobulin; Venimmun; ***Gr.:*** Flebogamma; Gamma-Venin P; Gammagard SD; Intraglobin F; Sandoglobulin; ***Hong Kong:*** Gamimune N†; Gammabulin†; Gammagard; Globuman; Intraglobin F; Octagam†; Pentaglobin; Venoglobulin-S; ***India:*** Gamafine; ***Irl.:*** Gammabulin†; Intraglobin; Sandoglobulin†; ***Israel:*** Beriglobin P; Endobulin; Gamimune N; Gamma-Venin†; Gammagard; Ig Gamma†; Intraglobin F; Omr-IgG; Sandoglobulin; Venoglobulin; Vigam; ***Ital.:*** Alphaglobin†; Biaven; Endobulin; Flebogamma; Gamma-Venin P; Gammabulin†; Gammagard; Globuman; Haimaven; Ig Gamma; Ig Vena N; Intraglobin F; Isiven; Normogamma†; Pentaglobin; Sandoglobulina; Uman-Gamma; Venimmun; Venogamma Polivalente†; ***Jpn:*** Venoglobulin-H; ***Malaysia:*** Gammagard; Globuman; Intraglobin F; Pentaglobin; Venoglobulin-S; Vigam; ***Mex.:*** Beriglobina P†; Intacglobin†; Isiven; Pentaglobin†; Sandoglobulina; Seroglubin; ***Norw.:*** Gammaglobulin; Gammanorm; Gammonativ†; Octagam; ***NZ:*** Intragam; Sandoglobulin; ***Port.:*** Flebogamma; Globuman; Sandoglobulina; ***S.Afr.:*** Beriglobin; Endobulin; Globuman†; Intragam; Intraglobin F; Pentaglobin; Polygam; ***Singapore:*** Flebogamma; Gammagard†; Intraglobin F; Pentaglobin; Venoglobulin; Vigam; ***Spain:*** Beriglobina P; Endobulin; Flebogamma; Gamma-Venin†; Gammagard; Gammaglob; Globuman; Polyglobin†; ***Swed.:*** Beriglobin; Endobulin; Gammagard; Gammanorm; Gammonativ; Nordimmun†; Octagam; Polyglobin; Sandoglobulin†; ***Switz.:*** Endobulin†; Gammagard; Globuman; Intraglobin F; Octagam; Pentaglobin; Redimune; Sandoglobuline†; ***Thai.:*** Globuman†; Intraglobin; Pentaglobin; Venoglobulin-S; Vigam-S; ***UK:*** Flebogamma; Gammabulin†; Gammagard; Kabiglobulin†; Octagam; Sandoglobulin; Subcuvia; Vigam; ***USA:*** Flebogamma; Gamimune N; Gammagard; Gammar-P; Gamunex; Iveegam; Panglobulin; Polygam; Sandoglobulin†; Venoglobulin.

**Multi-ingredient:** ***Arg.:*** Biotaer Gamma; Histaglobin; ***Austria:*** Histaglobin; ***Chile:*** Pentaglobin; ***Ger.:*** Histadestal; ***India:*** Histaglobulin; ***S.Afr.:*** Histaglobin; ***Thai.:*** Histaglobin†.

## Pertussis Immunoglobulins

Inmunoglobulinas contra la tos ferina.

*ATC — J06BB13.*

**Pharmacopoeias.** Many pharmacopoeias have monographs including *US.*

**USP 27** (Pertussis Immune Globulin). A sterile solution of globulins derived from the plasma of adult human donors who have been immunised with pertussis vaccine. It may contain glycine as a stabilising agent, and a suitable preservative. It should be stored at 2° to 8°.

### Adverse Effects and Precautions

As for immunoglobulins in general, p.1605.

### Interactions

As for immunoglobulins in general, p.1605.

### Uses and Administration

Pertussis immunoglobulins may be used for passive immunisation against pertussis (whooping cough). They have been used to prevent or modify pertussis in susceptible persons who have been exposed to infection.

### Preparations

***USP 27:*** Pertussis Immune Globulin.

**Proprietary Preparations** (details are given in Part 3)

***Ital.:*** Haimapertus†; Immunopertox†; Pertoglobulin†; Pertus-Gamma†; Tosuman†.

# Pertussis Vaccines

Vacunas de la tos ferina.

*ATC — J07AJ01; J07AJ02.*

**Pharmacopoeias.** Many pharmacopoeias have monographs including *Br.* and *Eur.* (see p.vi).

**Ph. Eur. 5.0** (Pertussis Vaccine; Vaccinum Pertussis). A sterile suspension of inactivated whole cells of one or more strains of *Bordetella pertussis* in saline. The estimated potency is not less than 4 international units per dose. It may contain a suitable antimicrobial preservative. It should be stored at 2° to 8°, not be allowed to freeze, and be protected from light.

**Ph. Eur. 5.0** (Pertussis Vaccine (Adsorbed); Vaccinum Pertussis Adsorbatum). A sterile suspension of inactivated whole cells of one or more strains of *Bordetella pertussis* in saline to which hydrated aluminium phosphate or aluminium hydroxide has been added. It may contain a suitable antimicrobial preservative. The estimated potency is not less than 4 units per dose. It should be stored at 2° to 8°, not be allowed to freeze, and be protected from light.

**BP 2003** (Pertussis Vaccine). When Pertussis Vaccine is issued as a plain vaccine, it complies with the requirements of Pertussis Vaccine (Ph. Eur. 5.0). When Pertussis Vaccine is issued as an adsorbed vaccine, it complies with the requirements of Pertussis Vaccine (Adsorbed) (Ph. Eur. 5.0).

The BP 2003 states that Per/Vac or Per/Vac/Ads may be used on the label as appropriate.

The BP 2003 gives Whooping-cough Vaccine as an approved synonym.

The BP 2003 directs that when Pertussis Vaccine is prescribed or demanded and the form is not stated, either the plain or the adsorbed vaccine may be dispensed or supplied.

**Ph. Eur. 5.0** (Pertussis Vaccine (Acellular, Component, Adsorbed); Vaccinum Pertussis sine Cellulis ex Elementis Praeparatum Adsorbatum). A preparation of individually prepared and purified antigenic components of *Bordetella pertussis* adsorbed on a mineral carrier such as aluminium hydroxide or hydrated aluminium phosphate. It contains either a suitably prepared pertussis toxoid or a pertussis toxin-like protein free from toxic properties produced by expression of a genetically modified form of the corresponding gene. It may also contain filamentous haemagglutinin, pertactin, and other defined antigens such as fimbrial-2 and fimbrial-3 antigens. The final vaccine contains not more than 100 units of bacterial endotoxin per dose. It may contain a suitable antimicrobial preservative. It should be stored at 2° to 8°, not be allowed to freeze, and be protected from light.

**Ph. Eur. 5.0** (Pertussis Vaccine (Acellular, Co-purified, Adsorbed); Vaccinum Pertussis Sine Cellulis Copurificatum Adsorbatum). A preparation of antigenic components of *Bordetella pertussis* adsorbed on a mineral carrier such as aluminium hydroxide or hydrated aluminium phosphate. It should be stored at 2° to 8°, not be allowed to freeze, and be protected from light.

## Adverse Effects

As for vaccines in general, p.1605.

Local reactions may occur at the site of injection of pertussis vaccines or pertussis-containing vaccines and administration may be followed by fever and irritability. Local reactions and fever occur less frequently following use of the acellular vaccine than after whole-cell vaccine, especially in children over 6 months of age and adults.

Severe reactions which have been reported include persistent screaming and generalised collapse but these effects were generally associated with an earlier type of vaccine and the reactions are stated to be rarely observed with the currently available vaccines.

Rare neurological adverse reactions have included convulsions and encephalopathy. There has been much debate, however, on the causal role of pertussis vaccine in such reactions (see below for detailed discussion). It should be remembered that neurological complications occur more frequently as a consequence of pertussis infection than in association with vaccination.

**Asthma.** A higher incidence of asthma was reported in 243 children who had received pertussis vaccine than in 203 children who had not.[1] However, follow-up of a large Swedish study[2] showed no difference in the incidence of wheezing or allergic reactions between children who had received diphtheria, tetanus, and pertussis vaccines and those who had not. A later prospective study[3] also found no evidence that pertussis vaccination increased the risk of wheezing illness in young children.

1. Odent MR, *et al.* Pertussis vaccination and asthma: is there a link? *JAMA* 1994; **272:** 592–3.
2. Nilsson L, *et al.* Lack of association between pertussis vaccination and symptoms of asthma and allergy. *JAMA* 1996; **275:** 760.
3. Henderson J, *et al.* Pertussis vaccination and wheezing illnesses in young children: prospective cohort study. *BMJ* 1999; **318:** 1173–6.

**Effects on the nervous system.** There has been continuing debate over several decades concerning the perceived link between pertussis vaccination and brain damage. Anxiety among both the public and health care professionals in the UK in the mid-1970s over the safety of pertussis vaccines led to a fall in the acceptance rates for infant vaccination and major epidemics of pertussis in 1977/79 and 1981/83. Since that time confidence has been restored, and, by 1995, 94% of infants were receiving the vaccine before their second birthday.

The consensus of opinion now seems to be that there is a temporal, but not necessarily causal, relationship between pertussis vaccine and acute neurological illness that may occasionally lead to long-term dysfunction, and that risks of not immunising are greater than the potential risks associated with the vaccine.

The difficulty in ascertaining whether a causal relationship exists between pertussis vaccine (usually given as diphtheria, tetanus, and pertussis (DTP) vaccine) and acute neurological reactions arises partly because primary vaccination is given at an age when neurological dysfunction with other causes is often first manifested. The observed temporal relationship may be entirely coincidental, may result from indirect factors such as pyrexia following vaccination, or may represent a direct effect of DTP vaccine. Much of the evidence is based on large epidemiological studies,[1-6] in particular the National Childhood Encephalopathy Study (NCES)[7] from the UK and its 10-year follow-up.[8] Serious acute neurological illnesses reported to the NCES[7] were found to be more common in infants immunised within 7 days (relative risk 2.4), and especially within 72 hours of onset, than in unimmunised children. For previously normal children, irrespective of outcome, the risk was estimated as 1 in 110 000 injections. In a subset of cases diagnosed as infantile spasms,[9] no link with vaccination was found overall, but there was a small excess of cases of infantile spasm in previously normal children who had received either DTP or diphtheria and tetanus vaccines during the previous 7 days (relative risk 2.0-2.5) followed by a corresponding deficit during the next 3 weeks. This suggested that vaccination may trigger the onset of spasms in a child with an underlying predisposition.

In 1991, the Institute of Medicine in the USA reviewed the available data, including the NCES results, and concluded that a causal relationship between DTP vaccine and acute encephalopathy probably existed, with an estimated excess risk of 0 to 10.5 per million vaccinations.[10] They concurred with the conclusion that a causal relationship between vaccination and infantile spasm was unlikely.

The NCES 10-year follow-up found that children who had had a serious acute neurological illness (excluding infantile spasms) had an increased risk of death or long-term dysfunction, but the risk was no greater in children who had received DTP vaccine in the 7 days before the original acute illness.[8] The National Vaccines Advisory Committee concluded that the results were insufficient to determine whether DTP vaccine influenced the development of chronic neurological dysfunction, and this conclusion has been accepted by both the Advisory Committee on Immunization Practices[11] and the American Academy of Pediatrics.[12]

1. Pollock TM, Morris J. A 7-year survey of disorders attributed to vaccination in North West Thames Region. *Lancet* 1983; **i:** 753–7.
2. Pollock TM, *et al.* Symptoms after primary immunisation with DTP and with DT vaccine. *Lancet* 1984; **ii:** 146–9.
3. Walker AM, *et al.* Neurologic events following diphtheria-tetanus-pertussis immunization. *Pediatrics* 1988; **81:** 345–9.
4. Shields WD, *et al.* Relationship of pertussis immunization to the onset of neurologic disorders: a retrospective epidemiologic study. *J Pediatr* 1988; **113:** 801–5.
5. Griffin MR, *et al.* Risk of seizures and encephalopathy after immunization with the diphtheria-tetanus-pertussis vaccine. *JAMA* 1990; **263:** 1641–5.
6. Gale JL, *et al.* Risk of serious acute neurological illness after immunization with diphtheria-tetanus-pertussis vaccine: a population-based case-control study. *JAMA* 1994; **271:** 37–41.
7. Miller DL, *et al.* Pertussis immunisation and serious acute neurological illness in children. *BMJ* 1981; **282:** 1595–9.
8. Miller D, *et al.* Pertussis immunisation and serious acute neurological illnesses in children. *BMJ* 1993; **307:** 1171–6.
9. Bellman MH, *et al.* Infantile spasms and pertussis immunisation. *Lancet* 1983; **i:** 1031–4.
10. Howson CP, Fineberg HV. Adverse events following pertussis and rubella vaccines: summary of a report of the Institute of Medicine. *JAMA* 1992; **267:** 392–6.
11. Centers for Disease Control. Update: vaccine side effects, adverse reactions, contraindications, and precautions: recommendations of the Advisory Committee on Immunization Practices (ACIP). *MMWR* 1996; **45** (RR-12): 1–45.
12. Committee on Infectious Disease, American Academy of Pediatrics. The relationship between pertussis vaccine and central nervous system sequelae: continuing assessment. *Pediatrics* 1996; **97:** 279–81.

## Precautions

As for vaccines in general, p.1606. The precautions and contra-indications to the use of pertussis vaccines have sometimes been more stringent than is now considered necessary because of the controversy concerning their potential adverse effects, especially neurotoxicity (see under Adverse Effects, above). As with other vaccines, immunisation should not be carried out in individuals with a definite history of a severe local or general reaction to a preceding dose. In children who have a history of less severe general reactions, immunisation may be completed omitting the pertussis component, or, in the case of local reactions or pyrexia, substituting an acellular pertussis vaccine.

Whether or not children with a personal or family history of convulsions or epilepsy or who have suffered cerebral damage in the neonatal period should receive pertussis vaccines appears to have been the most difficult question to resolve in the past. In the UK, the Department of Health now recommends that children with a personal or family history of febrile convulsions and children with a close family history of idiopathic epilepsy should be immunised and children whose epilepsy is well controlled may receive pertussis vaccine; advice on the prevention of fever should be given at the time of immunisation (see Fever and Hyperthermia, p.8 for comments on the prevention of fever after immunisation). Immunisation should also be carried out in children with a history of cerebral damage in the neonatal period unless there is evidence of an evolving neurological abnormality. In children with a neurological problem that is still evolving it is recommended that immunisation should be deferred until the condition is stable.

A personal or family history of hypersensitivity reactions is not generally considered to be a contra-indication to the use of pertussis vaccines, nor are stable neurological conditions such as cerebral palsy or spina bifida.

◊ Although collapse (hypotonic-hyporesponsive episode) after pertussis vaccination remains a contra-indication to further doses of the whole-cell vaccine in the UK, a follow-up study of infants who had experienced such an episode in the Netherlands showed a very low incidence of recurrence on second and subsequent doses[1] and a review[2] from Australia concluded that there were no long-term sequelae and that children who have experienced such an episode may be revaccinated.

1. Vermeer-de Bondt PE, *et al.* Rate of recurrent collapse after vaccination with whole cell pertussis vaccine: follow up study. *BMJ* 1998; **316:** 902–3.
2. Gold MS. Hypotonic-hyporesponsive episodes following pertussis vaccination: a cause for concern? *Drug Safety* 2002; **25:** 85–90.

## Interactions

As for vaccines in general, p.1606.

**Poliomyelitis vaccines.** A diminished immune response to pertussis vaccine was reported in infants given inactivated poliomyelitis vaccine mixed with diphtheria, tetanus, and pertussis vaccine compared with infants given the two vaccines as separate injections on the same visit.[1]

1. Halperin SA, *et al.* Effect of inactivated poliovirus vaccine on the antibody response to Bordetella pertussis antigens when combined with diphtheria-pertussis-tetanus vaccine. *Clin Infect Dis* 1996; **22:** 59–62.

## Uses and Administration

Pertussis vaccines are used for active immunisation against pertussis (whooping cough) (p.140).

For primary immunisation combined diphtheria, tetanus, and whole-cell pertussis vaccines (p.1613) have usually been used. For discussion of immunisation schedules, see below. Acellular pertussis vaccines are taking the place of whole-cell vaccines in several countries including the UK and the USA and are being incorporated into primary immunisation schedules for infants and children and for reinforcing doses in older children and adults.

◊ Reviews.

1. Tinnion ON, Hanlon M. Acellular vaccines for preventing whooping cough in children. Available in The Cochrane Library; Issue 2. Chichester: John Wiley; 2004.

**Acellular vaccines.** Vaccination using whole-cell pertussis vaccines has been effective but adverse reactions are common. The immunogenicity of the UK whole-cell vaccine is estimated at about 90% using the current accelerated three-dose schedule.[1] Dissatisfaction with whole-cell vaccines in the 1970s led to reduced uptake and a resurgence of pertussis in several countries. In Japan, research into less reactogenic pertussis vaccines resulted in the introduction of acellular vaccines for routine vaccination in the early 1980s.

The antigenic components of acellular pertussis vaccines are pertussis toxin (PT; also formerly known as lymphocytosis-promoting factor, LPF) either alone or more usually in combination with filamentous haemagglutinin (FHA), the 69 kilodalton outer membrane protein pertactin, and/or fimbrial agglutinogens (with 3 major serotypes; also referred to as fimbrial antigens). Adverse reactions to acellular vaccines are less frequent and less severe than those associated with whole-cell vaccines.[2] The acellular vaccines have successfully controlled pertussis infections but formal comparisons of efficacy with whole-cell vaccines have only been reported more recently. For studies of primary immunisation pertussis vaccine is used in combination with diphtheria and tetanus toxoids, and diphtheria and tetanus vaccines are used in the placebo groups.

As with whole-cell vaccines,[3,4] acellular vaccines varied in their efficacy. Multivalent vaccines were generally more effective than monovalent vaccines.[5] It has been argued that a monovalent pertussis toxoid, while providing incomplete protection for the individual, may nevertheless produce adequate herd immunity to inhibit disease transmission.[6] However, the use of multivalent vaccines seems preferable.[7,8]

In general, acellular vaccines approached the efficacy of, and were better tolerated than, whole-cell vaccines.[5,9-12] A surprising result of large studies in Sweden[5] and Italy,[10] in which the acellular vaccines were considerably more effective than the whole-cell vaccines, was the low efficacy of the US whole-cell vaccine (less than 50%). This was attributed to a rapidly waning effect after 3 doses given at 2, 4, and 6 months of age, suggesting that the booster doses at age 15 to 18 months and at school entry are essential to the US schedule. The UK whole-cell vaccine was found to be as effective as a pentavalent acellular vaccine and both were more effective than a trivalent vaccine in a large study in Sweden.[13]

In the UK, confidence in the whole-cell vaccine was largely restored, and uptake of primary immunisation in infants approached 90%.[1] However, there has been some concern over the incidence of pertussis infection in adults[15] and it is possible that acellular vaccines, which are better tolerated in older recipients than whole-cell vaccines, would be more acceptable if booster doses are added at school entry and in school leavers. In both the UK and the USA, acellular pertussis vaccines are now recommended for both primary immunisation in infants and for the booster doses in young children and before school entry.

1. White JM, *et al.* The effect of an accelerated immunisation schedule on pertussis in England and Wales. *Commun Dis Rep* 1996; **6** (review 6): R86–R91.
2. Decker MD, *et al.* Comparison of 13 acellular pertussis vaccines: adverse reactions. *Pediatrics* 1995; **96** (suppl): 557–66.
3. Edwards KM, *et al.* Differences in antibody response to whole-cell pertussis vaccines. *Pediatrics* 1991; **88:** 1019–23.
4. Baker JD, *et al.* Antibody response to Bordetella pertussis antigens after immunization with American and Canadian whole-cell vaccines. *J Pediatr* 1992; **121:** 523–7.
5. Gustafsson L, *et al.* A controlled trial of a two-component acellular, five-component acellular, and a whole-cell pertussis vaccine. *N Engl J Med* 1996; **334:** 349–55. Correction. *ibid.;* 1207.
6. Schneerson R, *et al.* A toxoid vaccine for pertussis as well as diphtheria? Lessons to be relearned. *Lancet* 1996; **348:** 1289–92.
7. Wirsing von König CH, Schmitt HJ. Toxoid vaccine for pertussis. *Lancet* 1997; **349:** 136.
8. He Q, *et al.* Toxoid vaccine for pertussis. *Lancet* 1997; **349:** 136–7.
9. Schmitt H-J, *et al.* Efficacy of acellular pertussis vaccine in early childhood after household exposure. *JAMA* 1996; **275:** 37–41.
10. Greco D, *et al.* A controlled trial of two acellular vaccines and one whole-cell vaccine against pertussis. *N Engl J Med* 1996; **334:** 341–8.
11. Stehr K, *et al.* A comparative efficacy trial in Germany in infants who received either the Lederle/Takeda acellular pertussis component DTP (DTaP) vaccine, the Lederle whole-cell component DTP vaccine, or DT vaccine. *Pediatrics* 1998; **101:** 1–11.
12. Giuliano M, *et al.* Antibody responses and persistence in the two years after immunization with two acellular vaccines and one whole-cell vaccine against pertussis. *J Pediatr* 1998; **132:** 983–8.
13. Olin P, *et al.* Randomised controlled trial of two-component, three-component, and five-component acellular pertussis vaccines compared with whole-cell pertussis vaccine. *Lancet* 1997; **350:** 1569–77. Correction. *ibid.;* **351:** 454.
14. Miller E. Acellular pertussis vaccines. *Arch Dis Child* 1995; **73:** 390–1.
15. Nenning ME. Prevalence and incidence of adult pertussis in an urban population. *JAMA* 1996; **275:** 1672–4.

**Immunisation schedules.** A review of the epidemiology and control of pertussis.[1] Pertussis is a common, highly infectious, respiratory disease, predominantly affecting children, and for which there is no effective treatment. WHO has estimated that 60 million cases of pertussis occur annually and that the disease is responsible for half a million to one million deaths each year. The highest incidence of pertussis is observed in developing countries where immunisation is low.

A combined adsorbed diphtheria, tetanus, and pertussis vaccine is now used in most countries but both the strength of the pertussis component and production methods vary, leading to vaccines of different potencies. In some countries a combined vaccine with additional poliomyelitis and Haemophilus influenzae components is used.

Depending upon the country, the age at which a child is given the first dose of the combined vaccine varies from 5 weeks to 6 months. (For summaries of immunisation schedules in the UK and USA, see under Vaccines, p.1606.) In countries with a high incidence of pertussis, WHO recommends that immunisation should start at 6 weeks of age and that the schedule involve three doses at monthly intervals followed by a booster dose at 3 to 4 years of age. In the UK and USA, booster doses should be given after the end of the primary series of 3 injections and before entry to school. Several reports have described the use of a two-dose widely-spaced primary immunisation schedule and this would indeed simplify procedures in developing countries; however, the limitation of such a schedule is the long period of risk between doses without adequate protection and unless the interval can be shortened to 4 weeks, the wide use of such a schedule is not advisable in endemic areas.

1. Muller AS, *et al.* Pertussis: epidemiology and control. *Bull WHO* 1986; **64:** 321–31.

## Preparations

***Ph. Eur.:*** Pertussis Vaccine; Pertussis Vaccine (Acellular Component, Adsorbed); Pertussis Vaccine (Acellular, Co-purified, Adsorbed); Pertussis Vaccine (Adsorbed).

**Proprietary Preparations** (details are given in Part 3)
***Canad.:*** Acel-P†; ***Fr.:*** Vaxicoq†; ***Ger.:*** Acel-P†; Pa-Vaccinol†; Pac Merieux; Pertuvac†; ***Ital.:*** Acelluvax†; ***Switz.:*** Acel-P†; ***Thai.:*** Acelluvax†.

# Pigbel Vaccines

Vacunas de la enteritis necrotizante.

## Profile

A vaccine against pigbel (necrotising enteritis), a disease occurring predominantly in children in the highlands of Papua New Guinea, is used for active immunisation against the disease. The vaccine consists of an adsorbed *Clostridium perfringens* type C toxoid.

◊ An immunisation programme, in which pigbel vaccine was given to children at 2, 4, and 6 months of age and, initially, to older children, was introduced in Papua New Guinea in 1980.[1] A survey found a sustained overall fall in the incidence of severe pigbel in children coincident with the increased induced immunity. However, protection may be relatively short-lived and boosters may be necessary for full protection of young children.

1. Lawrence GW, *et al.* Impact of active immunisation against enteritis necroticans in Papua New Guinea. *Lancet* 1990; **336:** 1165–7.

## Plague Vaccines

Vacunas de la peste.

*ATC — J07AK01.*

### Adverse Effects and Precautions

As for vaccines in general, p.1605.

### Interactions

As for vaccines in general, p.1606.

### Uses and Administration

Plague vaccines have been used for active immunisation against plague in those occupationally exposed to the organism and in some field workers in infected areas. They may reduce morbidity and mortality in bubonic plague but their activity against pneumonic plague is unknown.

## Pneumococcal Vaccines

Vacunas neumocócicas.

*ATC — J07AL01; J07AL02.*

**Pharmacopoeias.** Many pharmacopoeias have monographs including *Eur.* (see p.vi).

**Ph. Eur. 5.0** (Pneumococcal Polysaccharide Vaccine; Vaccinum Pneumococcale Polysaccharidum). A mixture of purified polysaccharide capsular antigens from 23 differing serotypes of *Streptococcus pneumoniae*. Each 0.5-mL dose contains 25 micrograms of each of the 23 polysaccharide types. An antimicrobial preservative may be added. The vaccine has a pH of 4.5 to 7.4. It should be stored at 2° to 8°, not be allowed to freeze, and be protected from light.

The BP 2003 states that Pneumo/Vac may be used on the label.

### Adverse Effects and Precautions

As for vaccines in general, p.1605. Unless otherwise stated, the information below refers to the unconjugated polyvalent vaccine.

Revaccination of adults is not generally recommended because of the increased incidence and severity of adverse reactions. For details of patient groups in whom revaccination may be considered and timings, see under Uses and Administration, below.

Pneumococcal vaccination is relatively ineffective in patients with multiple myeloma, Hodgkin's and non-Hodgkin's lymphoma, especially during treatment, and in chronic alcoholism. In patients with Hodgkin's disease the use of pneumococcal vaccines is not recommended in those who have received extensive chemotherapy or nodal irradiation. Pneumococcal vaccines should be given at least 10 days before starting immunosuppressive therapy or be delayed until at least 6 months after completion of therapy.

A satisfactory response to the unconjugated polyvalent pneumococcal vaccines is not obtained in children less than 2 years of age and therefore immunisation of this age group with this vaccine is not recommended. However, a pneumococcal conjugate vaccine is available that may be given to infants from 6 weeks of age.

**Effects on the blood.** The manufacturer reports that on rare occasions, relapses have occurred in patients with stabilised idiopathic thrombocytopenic purpura at 2 to 14 days after vaccination against pneumococcal infections, lasting for up to 2 weeks. One such case was reported[1] following revaccination less than 2.5 years after an uneventful primary vaccination with pneumococcal vaccine.

1. Neil VS. Long term management after splenectomy: revaccination may cause relapse. *BMJ* 1994; **308:** 339.

**Effects on the kidneys.** Glomerulonephritis was described[1] in a splenectomised patient following administration of pneumococcal vaccine. It was postulated that high antibody titres from a recent pneumococcal infection could have contributed.

1. Tan SY, Cumming AD. Vaccine related glomerulonephritis. *BMJ* 1993; **306:** 248.

**Effect of nutritional status.** An impaired antibody response to pneumococcal vaccine was reported[1] in elderly patients with low serum concentrations of vitamin $B_{12}$.

1. Fata FT, *et al.* Impaired antibody responses to pneumococcal polysaccharide in elderly patients with low serum vitamin B12 levels. *Ann Intern Med* 1996; **124:** 299–304.

### Interactions

As for vaccines in general, p.1606.

### Uses and Administration

Of the many serotypes of *Streptococcus pneumoniae* the 23 from which antigens are obtained for the most commonly available pneumococcal vaccine are considered to cause about 90% of pneumococcal disease.

Pneumococcal vaccines are used for active immunisation in those at increased risk from infection with the types of *Streptococcus pneumoniae* contained in the vaccine. Pneumococcal vaccines may be in the form of a 23-valent polysaccharide vaccine (suitable only for patients over 2 years of age) or as a conjugate vaccine containing 7 serotypes (suitable for infants aged 2 months to 2 years). In the UK, it is recommended that immunisation should be considered in all persons aged 65 and over; persons who have undergone splenectomy and those with splenic dysfunction, including that due to sickle-cell anaemia and coeliac disease; patients with immunodeficiency or immunosuppression due to disease or treatment, including HIV infection at all stages; persons with chronic cardiac, pulmonary, hepatic, or renal impairment, including nephrotic syndrome, or diabetes mellitus; and persons with cochlear implants.

An antibody response develops by the third week, and usually lasts about 5 years. The antibody response is less reliable and declines more rapidly in young children and persons with impaired immune function.

A single dose of 0.5 mL of the 23-valent vaccine, containing 25 micrograms of each of the 23 polysaccharide types, is given by subcutaneous or intramuscular injection. The vaccine should be given at least 2 weeks before elective splenectomy, chemotherapy, or other immunosuppressive treatment. Revaccination is not generally recommended except, after 5 years, in patients likely to have rapidly declining antibody concentrations; see below for further discussion.

The pneumococcal conjugate vaccine is given by intramuscular injection. In the UK, the Department of Health recommends that infants under 6 months should be given three single doses of 0.5 mL at intervals of 1 month, starting at 2 months of age, with a fourth dose given in the second year of life; those aged 7 to 11 months should receive 2 doses at least one month apart with a third dose given in the second year of life; and those aged 12 to 23 months should receive 2 doses at least two months apart.

In the USA, three doses of the pneumococcal conjugate vaccine are recommended at 2, 4, and 6 months of age, followed by a fourth dose at 12 to 15 months; it is stated that at least 2 months must elapse before the fourth dose is given. Previously unvaccinated infants aged 7 to 11 months are given two doses of 0.5 mL with an interval of at least 1 month between doses; a third dose is recommended in the second year of life with a time interval of 2 months recommended before this third dose. Previously unvaccinated children aged 12 to 23 months are given two doses of 0.5 mL, separated by an interval of at least 2 months. In the USA, a single dose is used for children aged 2 to 9 years. Pneumococcal conjugate vaccine may alternatively be given in the USA between the ages of 2 and 5 years if any dose has not been given previously. Pneumococcal polysaccharide vaccine should be given to certain high-risk groups between the ages of 2 and 18 years in addition to previously administered pneumococcal conjugate vaccine.

◊ Reviews.

1. Dear K, *et al.* Vaccines for preventing pneumococcal infection in adults. Available in The Cochrane Library; Issue 1. Chichester: John Wiley; 2004.
2. Sheikh A, *et al.* Pneumococcal vaccine for asthma. Available in The Cochrane Library; Issue 1. Chichester: John Wiley; 2004.
3. Davies EG, *et al.* Pneumococcal vaccines for sickle cell disease. Available in The Cochrane Library; Issue 1. Chichester: John Wiley; 2004.
4. Straetemans M, *et al.* Pneumococcal vaccines for preventing otitis media. Available in The Cochrane Library; Issue 1. Chichester: John Wiley; 2004.

◊ Although pneumococcal vaccines are effective in protecting against *Streptococcus pneumoniae* infection in healthy subjects there has been much debate over their **efficacy** in patients at increased risk of infection. There have been several studies demonstrating either adequate or inadequate protection in high-risk groups of patients, but most used the now discontinued 14-valent pneumococcal vaccine. Most,[1-4] but not all,[5] studies using the current 23-valent pneumococcal vaccines have demonstrated a useful degree of protection against pneumococcal infections in high-risk groups including the elderly.

One major consequence of the doubts over the efficacy and safety of pneumococcal vaccines has been a low **uptake** of vaccination in persons at risk of infection. It has been estimated that as few as 10% of subjects for whom vaccination is recommended have received it.[6] Doubts have been expressed[7] over the necessity to vaccinate any but those at highest risk, despite evidence of efficacy of the 23-valent vaccine in those patient groups covered by existing recommendations.[8]

The **recommendations** of the Department of Health in the UK are outlined under Uses and Administration, above. Similar recommendations have been made elsewhere. Pneumococcal vaccine is also recommended for persons living in environments or social settings with an identified increased risk of pneumococcal disease. Pneumococcal vaccine is not indicated for children with recurrent upper respiratory tract disease including otitis media and sinusitis.

Routine **revaccination** of adults with pneumococcal vaccines is not recommended, although in the UK the Department of Health recommend it every 5 years in individuals likely to have a rapid decline in antibody titre such as asplenic patients, those with dysfunction of the spleen, or those with nephrotic syndrome. In the USA, the CDC has stated that revaccination may be considered after 3 to 5 years for children at highest risk of pneumococcal infection who would be aged 10 years or under at revaccination.[9]

A **combined schedule** of 7-valent pneumococcal conjugate vaccine followed by 23-valent unconjugated vaccine has been shown to elicit an improved immune response in children and young adults with sickle- cell disease[10] and, in the USA, such combined vaccination is recommended for children aged 24 to 59 months who are at increased risk of pneumococcal infection (such as those with sickle-cell haemoglobinopathies, HIV infection, or other immunocompromising or chronic medical conditions). These children should be given two doses of the 7-valent pneumococcal conjugate vaccine, 2 months apart, followed by one dose of a 23-valent pneumococcal polysaccharide vaccine given at least 2 months after the second dose of pneumococcal conjugate vaccine.

1. Lee H, *et al.* Immunogenicity and safety of a 23-valent pneumococcal polysaccharide vaccine in healthy children and in children at increased risk of pneumococcal infection. *Vaccine* 1995; **13:** 1533–8.
2. Farr BM, *et al.* Preventing pneumococcal bacteremia in patients at risk. *Arch Intern Med* 1995; **155:** 2336–8.
3. Sankilampi U, *et al.* Antibody response to pneumococcal capsular polysaccharide vaccine in the elderly. *J Infect Dis* 1996; **173:** 387–93.
4. Furth SL, *et al.* Pneumococcal polysaccharide vaccine in children with chronic renal disease: a prospective study of antibody response and duration. *J Pediatr* 1996; **128:** 99–101.
5. Örtqvist Å, *et al.* Randomised trial of 23-valent pneumococcal capsular polysaccharide vaccine in prevention of pneumonia in middle-aged and elderly people. *Lancet* 1998; **351:** 399–403.
6. Williams WW, *et al.* Immunization policies and vaccine coverage among adults: the risk for missed opportunities. *Ann Intern Med* 1988; **108:** 616–25.
7. Hirschman JV, Lipsky BA. The pneumococcal vaccine after 15 years of use. *Arch Intern Med* 1994; **154:** 373–7.
8. Butler JC, *et al.* Pneumococcal polysaccharide vaccine efficacy: an evaluation of current recommendations. *JAMA* 1993; **270:** 1826–31.
9. Centers for Disease Control. Prevention of pneumococcal disease: recommendations of the Advisory Committee on Immunization Practices (ACIP). *MMWR* 1997; **46** (RR-8): 1–24.
10. Vernacchio L, *et al.* Combined schedule of 7-valent pneumococcal conjugate vaccine followed by 23-valent pneumococcal vaccine in children and young adults with sickle cell disease. *J Pediatr* 1998; **133:** 275–8.

### Preparations

***Ph. Eur.:*** Pneumococcal Polysaccharide Vaccine.

**Proprietary Preparations** (details are given in Part 3)

***Arg.:*** Imovax Pneumo; Neumak; Pneumo 23; Pneumovax 23; Prevenar; ***Austral.:*** Pneumovax 23; Prevenar; ***Austria:*** Pneumo 23; Pnu-Imune; Prevenar; ***Belg.:*** Pneumovax 23; Pneumune; ***Braz.:*** Pneumo 23; Pneumovax 23; Vacina Pneumococica Conjugada 7-valate; ***Canad.:*** Pneumo 23; Pneumovax 23; Pnu-Imune 23†; Prevnar; ***Chile:*** Pneumo 23; Prevenar; ***Denm.:*** Pneumovax; Prevenar; ***Fin.:*** Pneumovax; Pnu-Imune 23†; Prevenar; ***Fr.:*** Pneumo 23; Prevenar; ***Ger.:*** Pneumopur; Pneumovax 23; Prevenar; ***Gr.:*** Pneumo 23; Pnu-Imune 23; ***Hong Kong:*** Pneumo 23; Pneumovax 23; ***Irl.:*** Pneumovax II; Pnu-Imune; Prevenar; ***Israel:*** Pneumo 23 Imovax; Pneumovax 23; ***Ital.:*** Pneumo 23; Pneumovax; Pnu-Imune 23; Prevenar; ***Malaysia:*** Pneumo 23; Pneumovax 23; ***Mex.:*** Pnu-Imune 23; Pulmovax; ***Neth.:*** Pneumovax 23; Pneumune†; ***Norw.:*** Pneumovax; Pnu-Imune; Prevenar; ***NZ:*** Pneumo 23; Pneumovax 23; ***Port.:*** Pneumo 23; Pnu-Imune; Prevenar; ***S.Afr.:*** Imovax Pneumo 23; Pneumovax 23; ***Singapore:*** Pneumo 23; Pneumovax 23; ***Spain:*** Pneumo 23; Pnu-Inmune; Prevenar; ***Swed.:*** Pneumovax; Pnu-Imune; Prevenar; ***Switz.:*** Pneumovax 23; Pnu-Imune 23; Prevenar; ***Thai.:*** Pneumo 23; Pneumovax 23; ***UK:*** Pneumovax II; Pnu-Imune†; Prevenar; ***USA:*** Pneumovax 23; Pnu-Imune 23†; Prevnar.

## Poliomyelitis Vaccines

Polio Vaccines; Poliovirus Vaccines; Vacunas de la poliomielitis.

*ATC — J07BF01; J07BF02; J07BF03.*

NOTE. Inactivated poliomyelitis vaccines are sometimes termed Salk Vaccine and live (oral) poliomyelitis vaccines are sometimes termed Sabin Vaccine.

**Pharmacopoeias.** Many pharmacopoeias have monographs including *Eur.* (see p.vi) and *US.*

**Ph. Eur. 5.0** (Poliomyelitis Vaccine (Inactivated); Vaccinum Poliomyelitidis Inactivatum). A liquid preparation of suitable strains of poliomyelitis virus, types 1, 2, and 3, grown in suitable cell cultures and inactivated by a suitable method. Permitted antibacterials may be used in its production and it may contain preservatives. It should be stored at 2° to 8° and be protected from light.

The BP 2003 states that Pol/Vac(Inact) may be used on the label

**Ph. Eur. 5.0** (Poliomyelitis Vaccine (Oral); Vaccinum Poliomyelitidis Perorale; Poliomyelitis Vaccine, Live (Oral) BP 2003). A liquid preparation of suitable live attenuated strains of poliomyelitis virus, types 1, 2, or 3, grown in suitable, approved cell cultures; it may contain any one of the 3 virus types or combinations of them. The trivalent vaccine is standardised for virus titre which is not less than $1 \times 10^6$ $CCID_{50}$ for type 1, not less than $1 \times 10^5$ $CCID_{50}$ for type 2, and not less than $1 \times 10^{5.5}$ $CCID_{50}$ for type 3 per dose. Permitted antibacterials may be used in its production. It should be stored at 2° to 8°, not be allowed to freeze, and be protected from light.

The BP 2003 states that Pol/Vac(Oral) may be used on the label. For vaccine presented in single doses where the individual container is too small to accommodate the abbreviation Pol/Vac(Oral), the code OPV may be stated on the label on the container provided that the code OPV is also stated on the label on the package.

**USP 27** (Poliovirus Vaccine Inactivated). A sterile aqueous suspension of poliomyelitis virus, types 1, 2, and 3, grown separately in cultures of monkey kidney tissue and inactivated. Suitable antimicrobial agents may be used during production. It should be stored at 2° to 8°.

## Adverse Effects

As for vaccines in general, p.1605.

Vaccine-associated poliomyelitis has been reported in a small number of recipients of oral poliomyelitis vaccines and in contacts of recipients.

**Effects on the nervous system.** Case reports of the isolation of poliovaccine virus from the CSF after administration of oral poliomyelitis vaccine.

1. Rantala H, *et al.* Poliovaccine virus in the cerebrospinal fluid after oral polio vaccination. *J Infect* 1989; **19:** 173–6.
2. Gutierrez K, Abzug MJ. Vaccine-associated poliovirus meningitis in children with ventriculoperitoneal shunts. *J Pediatr* 1990; **117:** 424–7.

GUILLAIN-BARRÉ SYNDROME. A small cluster of cases of Guillain-Barré syndrome was observed[1] in children after a mass poliomyelitis vaccination campaign in Finland in 1985. An increased frequency of Guillain-Barré syndrome was also seen in adults. However, a direct link with poliovaccine virus infection could not be established and no link between Guillain-Barré syndrome and oral polio vaccine was revealed by a subsequent, epidemiological study in California.[2]

1. Uhari M, *et al.* Cluster of childhood Guillain-Barré cases after an oral poliovaccine campaign. *Lancet* 1989; **ii:** 440–1.
2. Rantala H, *et al.* Epidemiology of Guillain-Barré syndrome in children: relationship of oral polio vaccine administration to occurrence. *J Pediatr* 1994; **124:** 220–3.

PARALYTIC POLIOMYELITIS. A survey of the incidence of paralytic poliomyelitis after vaccination conducted by WHO[1] reported that, in all but one of the 13 participating countries, the risk was 0.03 per million vaccine recipients. The incidence was least with the use of type 1 strains and greatest with type 3 strains. Paralytic poliomyelitis in contacts of vaccine recipients could be further reduced by ensuring that parents without evidence of previous immunisation receive the vaccine at the same time as their children. The risk of vaccine-associated paralytic poliomyelitis may be increased in immunocompromised patients.

Until recently there has been no satisfactory explanation of the high risk of paralytic poliomyelitis found in Romania by the WHO survey.[1] A case-control study[2] identified intramuscular injections given within 30 days of polio vaccination as a risk factor in the development of paralytic poliomyelitis. This phenomenon, known as provocation paralysis or provocation poliomyelitis has been described with the wild virus[3] and more recently has been recognised as a factor in vaccine-associated paralysis in the UK and USA.[4] Romanian children may be further predisposed to vaccine-associated paralysis because the first dose of polio vaccine is delayed until 2 to 7 months of age, by which time they possess little or no residual maternal antibody.[5]

In the USA, where the majority of cases of clinical poliomyelitis are associated with vaccination, there is evidence that the incidence of paralytic poliomyelitis is still falling.[6-8]

1. Esteves K. Safety of oral poliomyelitis vaccine: results of a WHO enquiry. *Bull WHO* 1988; **66:** 739–46.
2. Strebel PM, *et al.* Intramuscular injections within 30 days of immunization with oral poliovirus vaccine—a risk factor for vaccine-associated paralytic poliomyelitis. *N Engl J Med* 1995; **332:** 500–6.
3. Anonymous. Provocation paralysis. *Lancet* 1992; **340:** 1005–6.
4. Wyatt HV. Vaccine-associated poliomyelitis. *Lancet* 1994; **343:** 610.
5. Wright PF, Karzon DT. Minimizing the risks associated with the prevention of poliomyelitis. *N Engl J Med* 1995; **332:** 529–30.
6. Nkowane BM, *et al.* Vaccine-associated paralytic poliomyelitis. United States: 1973 through 1984. *JAMA* 1987; **257:** 1335–40.
7. Centers for Disease Control. Paralytic poliomyelitis—United States, 1980-1994. *MMWR* 1997; **46:** 79–83.
8. Sepkowitz S. Vaccine-associated paralytic poliomyelitis. *Pediatrics* 1997; **99:** 145.

## Precautions

As for vaccines in general, p.1606.

Oral poliomyelitis vaccine may contain trace amounts of penicillin, neomycin, polymyxin, and streptomycin and the inactivated vaccine may contain trace amounts of neomycin and polymyxin: both should be used with caution in patients with severe hypersensitivity to these antibacterials.

Oral poliomyelitis vaccines should not be given to patients with diarrhoea or vomiting.

Because the vaccine virus of oral poliomyelitis vaccines is excreted in the faeces for up to 6 weeks, the contacts of recently vaccinated babies and infants should be advised of the need for strict personal hygiene, particularly hand washing after napkin changing, in order to reduce the possibility of infection in unimmunised contacts. Unimmunised adults can be immunised at the same time as their children.

Immunocompromised patients are at increased risk of developing vaccine-associated paralytic poliomyelitis. Oral poliomyelitis vaccines should not be given to immunocompromised patients or their household contacts and in these persons an inactivated vaccine should be used (see Uses and Administration, below). Asymptomatic HIV-positive persons may receive oral poliomyelitis vaccines but faecal excretion of the vaccine virus may continue for longer than in uninfected individuals. For symptomatic HIV-positive persons the use of inactivated poliomyelitis vaccine may be considered.

Intramuscular injections given after the oral vaccine may also increase the risk of vaccine-associated paralytic poliomyelitis (see above).

**Pregnancy.** Live vaccines such as *oral poliomyelitis vaccines* are generally contra-indicated in pregnancy because of a theoretical risk to the fetus. Population-wide mass vaccination programmes become impossible, however, if pregnant mothers and women of child-bearing age are to be excluded.[1] In February 1985, mass vaccination with live oral poliomyelitis vaccine was started during a poliomyelitis outbreak in Finland.[1] Pregnant women were advised to take the vaccine. An analysis of all reported congenital malformations in the years 1982 to 1986 suggested that oral poliomyelitis vaccine had no harmful effects on fetal development as measured by overall prevalence of malformations or by the incidence of either CNS or orofacial defects. The results did not, however, exclude an effect measurable by other criteria of fetal development.

The incidence of spontaneous abortions was measured during a mass poliomyelitis vaccination campaign in Israel.[2] The number of spontaneous abortions did not differ between controls and women vaccinated during the first trimester of pregnancy; the percentage of spontaneous abortions in relation to live births was also similar. Microscopic examination of placentas from spontaneous abortions indicated no effect of oral poliomyelitis vaccine on the frequency or type of pathological changes. In addition, subsequent epidemiological study[3] found no increases in congenital malformations or in premature births during the period of and immediately following the vaccination campaign compared with those born before the campaign.

The Collaborative Perinatal Project in the USA[4] followed up 50 897 pregnancies to examine risk factors for the development of malignancies in offspring born between 1959 and 1966. In 18 342 children whose mothers were vaccinated during pregnancy with *inactivated poliomyelitis vaccines*, there were 14 malignancies (7.6 per 10 000), while in 32 555 non-exposed children there were 10 malignancies (3.1 per 10 000). There were 7 tumours derived from neural tissue in the exposed children (3.8 per 10 000) and one in non-exposed children (0.3 per 10 000). Thus there was an excess of neural tumours but not of leukaemias or other malignancies in children exposed *in utero* to inactivated poliomyelitis vaccine. No malignancies occurred among the children born to 3056 women who received oral poliomyelitis vaccine. Serum samples collected from mothers on entry into the Collaborative Perinatal Project and at delivery have subsequently been analysed[5] for the presence of antibodies to Simian virus 40 (SV40). None of the serum samples from 8 mothers of infants with neural tumours had antibodies to SV40. Two of the 7 mothers of infants with leukaemia had SV40 antibodies, but only one had conversion during pregnancy. None of the samples from the 7 mothers of children with other types of cancer had antibodies. Three of 36 controls had antibodies, but in both the first and second samples. The association between administration of inactivated poliomyelitis vaccine to mothers and neural tumours in their offspring could not be attributed to contamination of vaccine with SV40.

1. Harjulehto T, *et al.* Congenital malformations and oral poliovirus vaccination during pregnancy. *Lancet* 1989; **i:** 771–2.
2. Ornoy A, *et al.* Spontaneous abortions following oral poliovirus vaccination in first trimester. *Lancet* 1990; **i:** 800.
3. Ornoy A, Ben Ishai P. Congenital anomalies after oral poliovirus vaccination during pregnancy. *Lancet* 1993; **341:** 1162.
4. Heinonen OP, *et al.* Immunization during pregnancy against poliomyelitis and influenza in relation to childhood malignancy. *Int J Epidemiol* 1973; **2:** 229–35.
5. Rosa FW, *et al.* Absence of antibody response to simian virus 40 after inoculation with killed-poliovirus vaccine of mothers of offspring with neurologic tumors. *N Engl J Med* 1988; **318:** 1469.

## Interactions

As for vaccines in general, p.1606.

**Normal immunoglobulins.** Although the concurrent administration of live vaccines and immunoglobulins is generally not recommended, normal immunoglobulin had no effect on the antibody response to oral poliomyelitis vaccine when the 2 preparations were given simultaneously to 50 subjects.[1]

1. Green MS, *et al.* Response to trivalent oral poliovirus vaccine with and without immune serum globulin in young adults in Israel in 1988. *J Infect Dis* 1990; **162:** 971–4.

**Pertussis vaccines.** For a report of a diminished immune response to the pertussis component of diphtheria, tetanus, and pertussis vaccine when mixed with inactivated poliomyelitis vaccine, see Pertussis Vaccines, p.1632.

## Uses and Administration

Poliomyelitis vaccines are used for active immunisation against poliomyelitis. For discussion of immunisation schedules, see under Vaccines, p.1606. Both live (oral) poliomyelitis vaccines and inactivated poliomyelitis vaccines are available. The oral vaccine stimulates the formation of antibodies both in the blood and in the mucosal tissues of the gastrointestinal tract.

In the UK, an inactivated poliomyelitis vaccine containing the three types of poliovirus (trivalent) is recommended for the primary immunisation of all age groups, given as a course of 3 doses at intervals of 4 weeks. It is given intramuscularly as a combined diphtheria, tetanus, pertussis (acellular component), poliomyelitis (inactivated), and Haemophilus influenzae vaccine. For children who received primary immunisation during infancy, reinforcing doses are recommended at school entry (diphtheria, tetanus, pertussis, and poliomyelitis) and before leaving school (diphtheria, tetanus, and poliomyelitis). Further reinforcing doses are necessary only in adults exposed to infection including travellers to countries where poliomyelitis is epidemic or endemic and health care workers in contact with poliomyelitis cases. A single dose is given, repeated every 10 years if necessary.

In the USA, both the oral and the inactivated vaccine have been used for primary immunisation. In 1997, the controversial decision was made to recommend the use of inactivated vaccine for the first two doses given at 2 and 4 months of age, completing immunisation with two doses of oral vaccine given at between 12 and 18 months, and at 4 to 6 years of age. Subsequently, the recommended schedule has been further changed and now consists of four doses of inactivated vaccine given at 2 months, 4 months, 6 to 18 months, and 4 to 6 years of age. See Choice of Vaccine, below for further discussion.

On the occurrence of a single case of paralytic poliomyelitis from wild virus, a single dose of the oral vaccine is recommended for all persons in the neighbourhood, regardless of whether they have previously been immunised. A primary course should be completed in previously unimmunised individuals. Immunisation of contacts is unnecessary in the case of vaccine-associated infections.

**Choice of vaccine.** In the USA, both oral and inactivated poliomyelitis vaccines (OPV and IPV respectively) have previously been used for primary immunisation. Three schedule options, each involving a total of four doses of vaccine at or before school entry, were available to physicians:[1]

- sequential IPV and OPV (2 doses of IPV at 2 and 4 months of age, followed by 2 doses of OPV at 12 to 18 months and 4 to 6 years), intended to minimise the risk of vaccine associated paralytic poliomyelitis (VAPP) while producing adequate intestinal immunity
- IPV only (dose intervals as above), recommended when OPV was contra-indicated and to reduce the risk of VAPP in unimmunised household contacts of the vaccine recipient
- OPV only (with the third dose given 2 months after the second dose), recommended when rapid immunisation was necessary, for example in older children, or in areas of low vaccine uptake. It also had the advantage of requiring no injections.

However, in 1997, the Advisory Committee on Immunization Practices (ACIP) of the Centers for Disease Control and Prevention recommended that the sequential IPV and OPV schedule should be preferred on the basis that, while there had been no cases of poliomyelitis from wild poliovirus in the USA since 1979, 8 to 10 cases of VAPP continued to occur each year. This decision was criticised by commentators both in the USA and elsewhere. Objections raised included the lack of experience with the recommended combined schedule, the lack of evidence that it would reduce the incidence of VAPP, and a possible reduction in compliance because of the increased number of injections needed.[2] Added to this was the greater cost of IPV than OPV which may have further reduced compliance and raised doubts over the cost-effectiveness of the strategy.[3,4] Subsequently, in 1999 both the ACIP and the American Academy of Pediatrics (AAP) issued revised recommendations[5,6] in which they advocated the use of IPV only and recommended that OPV no longer be given for routine immunisation: they recommended that use of OPV be limited to special situations such as mass vaccination campaigns to control outbreaks.

Commentators for WHO[7] stressed the necessity of the continued use of OPV for global eradication of poliomyelitis (see below). WHO was concerned that the change in US policy could be interpreted as implying that OPV alone is ineffective or unsafe, and might lead to the adoption of inappropriate vaccine policies in countries where wild polio still exists. The continued use of OPV for the global eradication strategy was again endorsed by both the ACIP[6] and the AAP.[5]

1. Committee on Infectious Diseases, American Academy of Pediatrics. Poliomyelitis prevention: recommendations for use of inactivated poliovirus vaccine and live oral poliovirus vaccine. *Pediatrics* 1997; **99:** 300–305.
2. Judelsohn R. Changing the US polio immunization schedule would be bad public health policy. *Pediatrics* 1996; **98:** 115–16.
3. Miller MA, *et al.* Cost-effectiveness of incorporating inactivated poliovirus vaccine into the routine childhood immunization schedule. *JAMA* 1996; **276:** 967–71.
4. Schneider S. The new immunization debate. *Pediatrics* 1996; **98:** 795.
5. Committee on Infectious Diseases, American Academy of Pediatrics. Prevention of poliomyelitis: recommendations for use of only inactivated poliovirus vaccine for routine immunization. *Pediatrics* 1999; **104:** 1404–6.
6. Centers for Disease Control. Recommendations of the Advisory Committee on Immunization Practices: revised recommendations for routine poliomyelitis vaccination. *MMWR* 1999; **48:** 590.
7. Hull HF, Lee JW. Sabine, Salk, or sequential? *Lancet* 1996; **347:** 630.

**Eradication of infection.** In 1988, WHO announced[1] their goal of eradicating poliomyelitis by the year 2000 and, while considerable progress was made towards achieving it, sporadic outbreaks of disease do still occur in unimmunised or inadequately immunised populations[2,3] and are reminders of the importance of maintaining the momentum of the WHO campaign. The campaign continues, with the renewed goal of global polio eradication by the year 2005.

The WHO campaign[1] depended on four strategies:

- routine immunisation—although routine immunisation alone cannot eliminate polio, it remains the foundation of eradication policy
- national immunisation days—regular (usually annual) nationwide immunisation of all children under 5 years of age regardless of immunisation history
- immunisation after an outbreak—all children under 5 years of age living in the vicinity of a suspected case receive one dose of oral vaccine
- mopping-up immunisation—house-to-house immunisation of children in high-risk areas to reach children missed during routine immunisation or national immunisation days.

WHO has consistently argued for the continued use of oral poliomyelitis vaccine (OPV) rather than inactivated vaccine (IPV) in immunisation schedules. The main argument has been the proven efficacy of repeated doses of OPV to abort outbreaks[4] and eliminate wild virus entirely, notably in South America.[1] Other advantages include the rapid induction of both humoral and intestinal immunity which is necessary to interrupt wild virus transmission; passive transfer of vaccine virus to non-immunised individuals improving population immunity; ease of administration by non-medical personnel; and the low cost of OPV.[5]

OPV produces a lower rate of seroconversion in developing countries than in developed countries, typically needing at least 5 doses to produce an adequate response.[1] There have been reports of poliomyelitis occurring in children who have completed a three-dose course of OPV.[6-8] Possible reasons for this suboptimal response include high levels of maternal antibodies, inhibition of types 1 and 3 viruses by type 2, interference from competing enteroviruses, and diarrhoea.[1,9] Mass immunisation campaigns are reported to produce a higher immune response than equivalent doses given in the routine schedule, and are seen as an essential adjunct to routine immunisation.[10] Seroconversion rates are highest when the vaccine is administered during mass campaigns in the cool and dry season.[1]

There have been several advocates of IPV either as an alternative or in addition to OPV. Most cite the higher immunogenicity of IPV and its successful use in some, albeit mainly industrialised, countries.[11,12] Combined IPV and OPV schedules have been shown to produce high levels of humoral immunity, with intestinal immunity equivalent to that produced by OPV alone.[13] The use of combined IPV and OPV schedules in countries which have not eliminated the wild virus could improve the effectiveness of routine vaccination schedules.[11,14] In the USA, a combined schedule was previously advocated to reduce vaccine associated paralytic poliomyelitis while still providing protection against transmission of imported wild virus, although use of OPV is now no longer recommended for routine immunisation (see Choice of Vaccine, above).

However, most cases of poliomyelitis in endemic countries occur among unimmunised children and the main priority remains to improve vaccine uptake rather than to alter immunisation schedules.[1,15] There is concern that uncertainty fostered by a change in vaccination policy could be interpreted as implying that OPV alone is ineffective or unsafe, and the central message that high uptake of vaccine is essential could be lost.[5]

1. Hull HF, *et al.* Paralytic poliomyelitis: seasoned strategies, disappearing disease. *Lancet* 1994; **343:** 1331–7.
2. van Niekerk ABW, *et al.* Outbreak of paralytic poliomyelitis in Namibia. *Lancet* 1994; **344:** 661–4.
3. Oostvogel PM, *et al.* Poliomyelitis outbreak in an unvaccinated community in the Netherlands, 1992-93. *Lancet* 1994; **344:** 665–70.
4. Greco D, *et al.* Poliomyelitis vaccination strategies for Europe. *Lancet* 1997; **349:** 437.
5. Hull HF, Lee JW. Sabine, Salk, or sequential? *Lancet* 1996; **347:** 630.
6. Sutter RW, *et al.* Outbreak of paralytic poliomyelitis in Oman: evidence for widespread transmission among fully vaccinated children. *Lancet* 1991; **338:** 715–20.
7. Samuel R, *et al.* Persisting poliomyelitis after high coverage with oral poliovaccine. *Lancet* 1993; **341:** 903.
8. Mudur G. Flawed immunisation policies in India led to polio paralysis. *BMJ* 1998; **316:** 1264.
9. WHO Collaborative Study Group on Oral Poliovirus Vaccine. Factors affecting the immunogenicity of oral poliovirus vaccine: a prospective evaluation in Brazil and the Gambia. *J Infect Dis* 1995; **171:** 1097–1106.
10. Richardson G, *et al.* Immunogenicity of oral poliovirus vaccine administered in mass campaigns versus routine immunization programmes. *Bull WHO* 1995; **73:** 769–77.
11. Patriarca PA, *et al.* Progress in polio eradication. *Lancet* 1993; **342:** 1461–4.
12. Preston NW. Polio eradication. *Lancet* 1994; **344:** 1163.
13. WHO Collaborative Study Group on Oral and Inactivated Poliovirus Vaccines. Combined immunization of infants with oral and inactivated poliovirus vaccines: results of a randomized trial in the Gambia, Oman, and Thailand. *Bull WHO* 1996; **75:** 253–68.
14. Moriniere BJ, *et al.* Immunogenicity of a supplemental dose of oral versus inactivated poliomyelitis vaccine. *Lancet* 1993; **341:** 1545–50.
15. Chander J, Subrahmanyan S. Mass polio vaccination. *BMJ* 1996; **312:** 1178–9.

## Preparations

***Ph. Eur.:*** Poliomyelitis Vaccine (Inactivated); Poliomyelitis Vaccine (Oral); ***USP 27:*** Poliovirus Vaccine Inactivated.

**Proprietary Preparations** (details are given in Part 3)

***Arg.:*** Imovax Polio; Sabin; ***Austral.:*** Enpovax HDC; Ipol; ***Belg.:*** Imovax Polio; Sabin; ***Braz.:*** Imovax Polio; IPV†; Vacina Poliomielitica; ***Fin.:*** Imovax Polio; ***Fr.:*** Imovax Polio; ***Ger.:*** IPV Merieux; IPV-Virelon; Oral-Virelon†; Polio-Vaccinol†; Virelon C†; ***Gr.:*** Imovax Polio; Vaccine Antipoliomyelitique/Merieux; ***Hong Kong:*** Buccapol†; Imovax Polio; ***Israel:*** Imovax Polio; Polioral; ***Ital.:*** Imovax Polio; Polio Sabin; Polioral; Poliovax-IN; ***Malaysia:*** Polioral; ***Mex.:*** Polio Sabin; Polioral; ***Norw.:*** Imovax Polio; ***NZ:*** Ipol; ***S.Afr.:*** OPV-Merieux; Polioral; ***Singapore:*** Buccapol†; Imovax Polio†; ***Spain:*** Vac Antipolio Or; Vac Antipolio Oral†; Vac Polio Sabin; Vac Poliomielitica; ***Swed.:*** Imovax Polio; ***Switz.:*** Poloral†; ***Thai.:*** Polio Sabin; Polioral; ***USA:*** Ipol; Orimune†.

## Pseudomonas Immunoglobulins

Inmunoglobulinas contra pseudomonas.

### Profile

Preparations containing antibodies against *Pseudomonas aeruginosa* have been used in some countries for passive immunisation against severe pseudomonal infections.

## Pseudomonas Vaccines

Vacunas de pseudomonas.

### Profile

A number of polyvalent *Pseudomonas aeruginosa* conjugate vaccines are under investigation for the prevention of pseudomonal infections in a variety of disease states.

◊ Reviews.

1. Keogan MT, Johansen HK. Vaccines for preventing infection with Pseudomonas aeruginosa in people with cystic fibrosis. Available in The Cochrane Library; Issue 2. Chichester: John Wiley; 2004.

## Q Fever Vaccines

Vacunas de la fiebre Q.

### Profile

A Q fever vaccine consisting of a purified killed suspension of *Coxiella burnetii* is available in Australia. It is prepared from Phase I Henzerling strain of *C. burnetii* grown in the yolk sacs of embryonated eggs. A single 0.5-mL subcutaneous dose is given for active immunisation in individuals at high risk of Q fever. These include abattoir workers, veterinarians, farmers and others exposed to farm animals, and laboratory workers handling potentially infected tissue.

### Preparations

**Proprietary Preparations** (details are given in Part 3)
***Austral.:*** Q-Vax.

## Rabies Antisera

Antisuero de la rabia.
*ATC — J06AA06.*

### Profile

Rabies antisera have been used to provide passive immunisation against rabies but the use of rabies immunoglobulins (see below) is preferred.

## Rabies Immunoglobulins

Inmunoglobulinas contra la rabia.
*ATC — J06BB05.*

**Pharmacopoeias.** Many pharmacopoeias have monographs including *Eur.* (see p.vi) and *US.*

**Ph. Eur. 5.0** (Human Rabies Immunoglobulin; Immunoglobulinum Humanum Rabicum). A liquid or freeze-dried preparation containing human immunoglobulins, mainly immunoglobulin G (IgG). It is obtained from plasma from donors immunised against rabies and contains specific antibodies that neutralise the rabies virus. Normal immunoglobulin may be added. It contains not less than 150 international units/mL. The liquid preparation should be stored, protected from light, in a colourless, glass container. The freeze-dried preparation should be stored, protected from light, in a colourless, glass container, under vacuum or under an inert gas.

**USP 27** (Rabies Immune Globulin). A sterile solution of globulins derived from plasma or serum from selected adult human donors who have been immunised with rabies vaccine and have developed high titres of rabies antibody. It contains 10 to 18% of protein of which not less than 80% is monomeric immunoglobulin G. It has a potency of 150 international units/mL. It contains glycine as a stabilising agent, and a suitable preservative. A solution diluted to contain 1% of protein has a pH of 6.4 to 7.2. It should be stored at 2° to 8°.

### Adverse Effects and Precautions

As for immunoglobulins in general, p.1605.

### Uses and Administration

Rabies immunoglobulins are used for passive immunisation against rabies. They are used in conjunction with active immunisation with rabies vaccines (see below) as part of the postexposure treatment for the prevention of rabies in previously unimmunised persons who have been bitten by rabid animals or animals suspected of being rabid. The recommended dose of rabies immunoglobulin is 20 international units/kg, half of which should be infiltrated around the wound and half given intramuscularly at a different site to that at which the vaccine was administered.

### Preparations

***Ph. Eur.:*** Human Rabies Immunoglobulin;
***USP 27:*** Rabies Immune Globulin.

**Proprietary Preparations** (details are given in Part 3)
***Arg.:*** Imogam Rabia; ***Austral.:*** Imogam; ***Austria:*** Berirab; ***Canad.:*** BayRab; Hyperab†; Imogam; ***Fr.:*** Imogam Rage; ***Ger.:*** Berirab; Tollwutglobulin†; ***Hong Kong:*** BayRab; Rabuman; ***India:*** Berirab-P; ***Israel:*** Berirab; Hyperab†; Imogam Rabies; ***Ital.:*** Haimarab†; Rabies Gamma†; Rabuman†; ***Mex.:*** BayRab; ***S.Afr.:*** Rabigam; ***Singapore:*** BayRab; ***Spain:*** Imogam Rabia; Lyssuman†; ***Switz.:*** Rabuman; ***Thai.:*** Rabuman†; ***USA:*** BayRab; Imogam Rabies.

# Rabies Vaccines

Vacunas de la rabia.
*ATC — J07BG01.*

**Pharmacopoeias.** Many pharmacopoeias have monographs including *Eur.* (see p.vi) and *US.*

**Ph. Eur. 5.0** (Rabies Vaccine for Human Use Prepared in Cell Cultures; Vaccinum Rabiei ex Cellulis ad Usum Humanum; Rabies Vaccine BP 2003). A sterile freeze-dried suspension of inactivated rabies virus; a suitable strain is grown in an approved cell culture. The cell-culture medium may contain suitable antibacterials at the smallest effective concentration. The vaccine is prepared immediately before use by the addition of a suitable sterile liquid. The estimated potency is not less than 2.5 international units per dose. The dried vaccine should be stored at 2° to 8° and be protected from light.

The BP 2003 states that Rab/Vac may be used on the label.

**USP 27** (Rabies Vaccine). A sterile preparation, in dried or liquid form, of inactivated rabies virus obtained from inoculated diploid cell cultures. It has a potency of not less than 2.5 international units per dose. It should be stored at 2° to 8°.

## Adverse Effects and Precautions

As for vaccines in general, p.1605.

Patients may experience pain, erythema, and induration at the injection site after the use of any type of rabies vaccine; nausea, headache, fever, malaise, or myalgia may also occur. Hypersensitivity reactions including anaphylaxis occur more commonly with vaccines prepared from non-human sources than with human diploid-cell vaccine.

Neuroparalytic reactions (transverse myelitis, neuropathy, or encephalopathy) have been associated with the use of animal brain-tissue vaccines and, to a lesser extent with duck-embryo vaccines.

There are only isolated reports of neurological reactions after use of human diploid-cell vaccines.

**Effects on the nervous system.** The incidence of neuroparalytic accidents following a course of nerve-tissue vaccines is known to vary from country to country.[1] The risk of CNS damage associated with the use of rabies vaccines prepared in the brains of adult *animals* has been stated to be about 1 in 2000 doses administered.[2] Paralytic accidents have occurred much less frequently with vaccines produced from brain tissue of mice younger than 9 days of age compared with older animals[1] and a particularly high risk of neurological complications has been observed with a sheep-brain vaccine.[3]

Neuroparalytic reactions occur less frequently with duck-embryo than nerve-tissue vaccines.[1] In an estimated 424 000 patients receiving duck-embryo rabies vaccine in the USA from 1958 to 1971 there were 137 reports of minor transient neurological reactions, 4 of transverse myelitis, 5 of neuropathy, and 4 of encephalopathy (2 fatal).[4]

There are only isolated reports of neuroparalytic reactions associated with human diploid-cell vaccines.[5,6]


1. WHO. WHO expert committee on rabies: seventh report. *WHO Tech Rep Ser 709* 1984.
2. WHO. WHO expert committee on biological standardization: thirty-seventh report. *WHO Tech Rep Ser 760* 1987.
3. Swaddiwuthipong W, *et al.* A high rate of neurological complications following Semple anti-rabies vaccine. *Trans R Soc Trop Med Hyg* 1988; **82:** 472–5.
4. Rubin RH, *et al.* Adverse reactions to duck embryo rabies vaccine: range and incidence. *Ann Intern Med* 1973; **78:** 643–9.
5. Knittel T, *et al.* Guillain-Barré syndrome and human diploid cell rabies vaccine. *Lancet* 1989; **i:** 1334–5.
6. Tornatore CS, Richert JR. CNS demyelination associated with diploid cell rabies vaccine. *Lancet* 1990; **335:** 1346–7.


**Hypersensitivity.** An analysis[1] based on clinical observation of 108 cases of systemic hypersensitivity reactions following immunisation with human diploid-cell rabies vaccine, reported to the Centers for Disease Control in the USA over the period June 1980 to March 1984, revealed 9 cases of presumed type I immediate hypersensitivity (incidence of 1 in 10 000 vaccinees), 87 cases of presumed type III hypersensitivity (9 in 10 000 vaccinees), and 12 cases of indeterminate type. All the reactions presumed to be type I occurred during either primary pre- or postexposure immunisation, whereas 93% of the presumed type III reactions were observed following booster immunisations. Presenting features of the type III reaction included generalised or pruritic rash or urticaria, angioedema, arthralgias, fever, nausea, vomiting, and malaise.


1. Centers for Disease Control. Systemic allergic reactions following immunization with HDCV. *JAMA* 1984; **251:** 2194–5.


**Spongiform encephalopathies.** Possible transmission of Creutzfeldt-Jakob disease associated with sheep-brain rabies vaccine has been reported from India.[1] It was suggested that transmission of the abnormal prion protein from sheep with scrapie might be implicated.


1. Arya SC. Acquisition of spongiform encephalopathies in India through sheep-brain rabies vaccination. *Natl Med J India* 1992; **4:** 311–12.


## Interactions

As for vaccines in general, p.1606.

**Antimalarials.** Studies have suggested that continuous antimalarial chemoprophylaxis with *chloroquine* during primary immunisation with human diploid-cell rabies vaccine, given intradermally for pre-exposure prophylaxis, may be associated with a poor antibody response.[1,2]


1. Taylor DN, *et al.* Chloroquine prophylaxis associated with a poor antibody response to human diploid cell rabies vaccine. *Lancet* 1984; **i:** 1405.
2. Pappaioanou M, *et al.* Antibody response to preexposure human diploid-cell rabies vaccine given concurrently with chloroquine. *N Engl J Med* 1986; **314:** 280–4.


## Uses and Administration

Rabies vaccines are used for active immunisation against rabies. They are used as part of postexposure treatment to prevent rabies in patients who have been bitten by rabid animals or animals suspected of being rabid. Infection does not take place through unbroken skin but is possible through uninjured mucous membranes and has been reported after the inhalation of virus in the laboratory. Rabies vaccines are also used for pre-exposure prophylaxis against rabies in persons exposed to a high risk of being bitten by rabid or potentially rabid animals.

Schedules for prophylaxis and treatment of rabies are recommended by WHO (see Pre-exposure Immunisation, below) and many countries have immunisation schedules based on these.

In the UK, a rabies vaccine prepared from inactivated Wistar rabies virus strain PM/WI38 1503-3M cultured on human diploid cells is used. It contains not less than 2.5 international units/mL. The vaccine should be given by deep subcutaneous or intramuscular injection into the deltoid region, or in a child, the anterolateral aspect of the thigh.

For **pre-exposure prophylaxis** against rabies, the recommended schedule in the UK for the human diploid-cell vaccine is 3 doses, each of 1 mL, by deep subcutaneous or intramuscular injection on days 0, 7, and 28; alternatively a dose of 0.1 mL has been given intradermally on the same days. Booster doses may be given every 2 to 3 years depending upon the risk of exposure, but where postexposure treatment is readily available booster doses are not normally required in individuals who have received three doses of vaccine.

A two-dose schedule has also been employed for travellers to enzootic areas who are not animal handlers: doses of 1 mL by deep subcutaneous or intramuscular injection, or 0.1 mL intradermally, are given 4 weeks apart. This schedule is somewhat less effective than the 3-dose schedule and should only be used where postexposure treatment will be readily available.

It has been suggested that rapid immunisation of personnel engaged in the care of a patient with rabies may be achieved by the intradermal administration of 0.1 mL into each limb (total of 0.4 mL) on the first day of exposure to the patient.

For **postexposure treatment**, thorough cleansing of the wound with soap and water is imperative. The recommended schedule in the UK for the human diploid-cell vaccine is 5 doses, each of 1 mL, by deep subcutaneous or intramuscular injection on days 0, 3, 7, 14, and 30. The UK manufacturers also recommend a further dose on day 90. Vaccination should be started as soon as possible after exposure, and may be discontinued if it is proved that the patient was not at risk. In previously unimmunised patients at high risk, rabies immunoglobulin (see above) should also be given at the same time as the first dose of vaccine. A modified course of vaccine administration may be employed in previously immunised persons consisting of two doses on day 0 and between days 3 to 7; rabies immunoglobulin is not required in these patients.

**Rabies.** Rabies is caused by infection with a rhabdovirus of the genus Lyssavirus, which also contains a number of related viruses some of which have caused disease in man. The rabies virus is usually transmitted by the bite of an infected animal or contamination of broken skin by saliva. Infection is possible via intact mucous membranes and by aerosol transmission, but infection is unlikely following contamination of intact skin. Other body fluids such as urine and tears should be regarded as potentially infectious.

Human rabies is almost always fatal once symptoms have appeared. After an incubation period of about 30 to 90 days there is a prodrome lasting up to about 10 days of generally non-specific symptoms. This prodrome is followed by the onset of acute neurological symptoms. Periods of hyperexcitability accompanied by severe agitation and bizarre behaviour alternate with periods of lucidity. Severe spasms of the larynx and pharynx may be provoked by attempts at swallowing leading to hydrophobia or by air blown at the face (aerophobia). Other symptoms include hypersalivation, fever, and convulsions. An alternative presentation of nervous system involvement is a progressive flaccid paralysis. Patients not dying through respiratory or cardiac arrest during the acute phase may develop any of a number of complications culminating in coma and death or (very rarely) recovery; only a few patients are documented as having survived after the onset of coma, and all had received either pre- or postexposure immunisation.

Rabies has a worldwide distribution, primarily in domesticated and wild dogs but also in bats and other warm-blooded animals, although some countries, including the UK, most of Australasia, and Antarctica are designated as rabies-free areas. National control programmes involve epidemiological surveillance, mass canine immunisation campaigns, and dog population management. The recent development of oral animal vaccines delivered on baited food has met with considerable success in a number of areas and has become an essential tool for eliminating rabies in wild animals. Rigorously applied controls of international transfer of animals including certification of vaccination and quarantine for animals entering rabies-free areas are necessary to prevent re-introduction of rabies.

Although a number of treatments have been tried including various antivirals including interferons, high doses of rabies immunoglobulin, and corticosteroids, none has shown evidence of effectiveness. Avoidance of rabies after contact with a suspected or confirmed rabid animal depends upon prompt and thorough cleansing of the contaminated site and administration of rabies vaccine with or without rabies immunoglobulins immediately. For a brief outline of postexposure treatment, see below; however, readers are strongly advised to consult the complete guidelines published by WHO if they are likely to be involved with the management of patients exposed to rabies.

Prophylaxis is recommended in persons at high risk of exposure, either due to their occupation or those travelling in enzootic areas. The main obstacle to mass pre-exposure vaccination appears to be the high cost of cell culture vaccines. See under Pre-exposure Immunisation (below) for outlines of recommended vaccination schedules.

CHOICE OF VACCINES. Many different rabies vaccines are available for human use: those derived from nerve tissue of animals; those derived from avian tissues (duck embryos); and those prepared in cell cultures. Originally the only source of rabies virus available for vaccine production was infected brain tissue from adult animals; such vaccines contain neuroparalytic and encephalitogenic substances and WHO supports the trend to limit, or abandon completely, their production.[1] Vaccines prepared from virus grown in duck embryos have been developed and a purified duck-embryo vaccine (PDEV) may provide similar efficacy and safety to vaccines produced from cell cultures.[1] Improvements in biotechnology may reduce the costs of cell-culture production. Among the vaccines prepared in this way is one developed from an adapted Pasteur strain of virus grown in a human diploid cell strain (HDCV), a purified chick embryo-cell vaccine (PCECV), and a purified Vero-cell vaccine (PVRV).[2] There appears to be little difference in terms of safety and antigenicity between HDCV, PCECV, PVRV, and PDEV in recommended regimens.[2] The incidence of severe hypersensitivity reactions should, however, be lower with PVRV and PCECV than with HDCV since the purification process removes most human serum albumin in the cell-growth medium before virus inactivation.[2]

There is little data concerning the efficacy of rabies vaccines.[2] It appears that nerve-tissue vaccines afford limited protection after minor exposures to rabies virus, are less effective after head bites, and are of little use after very severe exposures. Failure rates for HDCV, PCECV, and PVRV (including cases with less than the recommended therapy) has been estimated as less than 1 in 80 000 treatments in the USA, Canada, and Europe, 1 in 12 000 to 20 000 in Thailand, and 1 in 30 000 in the remaining tropical countries. Reported failures of these vaccines are often accounted for by deviation from recommendations, incorrect site of vaccine administration, or delay in treatment.

The cost of cell-culture rabies vaccines is prohibitively high in the developing world. Although the adverse effects of nerve-tissue vaccines preclude their use for pre-exposure prophylaxis, they are still used for postexposure prophylaxis.[2] WHO is anxious that nerve-tissue vaccines should be replaced with affordable cell-culture vaccines as soon as possible. In the meantime, cost-cutting regimens have been devised for use of cell-culture rabies vaccines by the intradermal route. Rapid immunisation is achieved by the use of several sites of injection; fewer injections are required than with traditional intramuscular regimens.[2]


1. WHO. WHO expert committee on rabies: eighth report. *WHO Tech Rep Ser 824* 1992.
2. Nicholson KG. Modern vaccines: rabies. *Lancet* 1990; **335:** 1201–5. Correction. *ibid.*; 1540.


PRE-EXPOSURE IMMUNISATION. Pre-exposure prophylaxis with rabies vaccine is generally recommended for use in persons at high risk of infection with rabies virus. Where available, the vaccines produced in cell culture are preferred over the vaccines produced in animal tissues (see under Choice of Vaccine, above). WHO recommends[1] pre-exposure prophylaxis for persons regularly at high risk of exposure, such as certain laboratory workers, veterinarians, animal handlers, and wildlife officers, and those living in or travelling to areas where rabies is endemic. The immunisation schedule should preferably consist of 3 injections of a tissue-culture rabies vaccine of potency at least 2.5 international units given on days 0, 7, and 28, but a few days' variation is unimportant. Administration should be into the deltoid area of the arm or for young children into the anterolateral area of the thigh. Titres of virus-neutralising antibodies can be checked in serum samples collected 1 to 3 weeks after the last dose. Those who work with the live virus should have their antibody titres checked every 6 months and if the figure falls below 0.5 international units/mL they should receive a booster. Other individuals at continuing risk should have their titres checked every 12 months and a booster given if the titre is below 0.5 international units/mL.

The intradermal administration of rabies vaccine in doses of 0.1 mL on days 0, 7, and 28 has also been shown to induce seroconversion.

National policies vary somewhat from that of WHO, depending on the local risk of contracting rabies and the vaccines available.

In the UK, the schedule for immunisation (see Uses and Administration, above) is similar to that recommended by WHO.

In the USA, immunisation with a human diploid cell vaccine, a vaccine adsorbed onto an aluminium salt, or a purified chick embryo cell vaccine is carried out similarly to the WHO schedule, with serum-antibody titres determined every 6 months to 2 years, depending upon the level of exposure, and booster doses given as necessary.[2]


1. WHO. WHO expert committee on rabies: eighth report. *WHO Tech Rep Ser 824* 1992.
2. Centers for Disease Control. Human rabies prevention—United States, 1999: recommendations of the Advisory Committee on Immunization Practices (ACIP). *MMWR* 1999; **48** (RR-1): 1–21.


POSTEXPOSURE TREATMENT. WHO[1] emphasises the importance of prompt local treatment for all bite wounds and scratches that may be contaminated with rabies virus and that, depending on the category of animal contact, rabies vaccine on its own or with rabies immunoglobulin should be given. The combination of these measures immediately after exposure is considered to almost guarantee complete protection. Pregnancy and infancy are not contra-indications to postexposure vaccination. Also these measures should be instituted in patients who present even months after having been bitten.

First aid or local treatment consists of immediate thorough flushing and washing of the wound with water, or soap and water, or detergent followed by the application of alcohol 70% or tincture or aqueous solution of iodine. Medical care may then consist of the instillation of rabies immunoglobulin into the depth of the wound and infiltration around the wound. Ideally the wound should not be sutured, but if suturing is necessary then it is essential that it be preceded by the administration of rabies immunoglobulin as above.

The administration of rabies vaccine and of rabies immunoglobulin depends on the category of animal contact. WHO classifies the type of contact with a suspect or rabid animal into 3 categories:

- category I covers touching or feeding of animals and licks on intact skin
- category II covers nibbling of uncovered skin, minor scratches or abrasions without bleeding, and licks on broken skin
- category III covers single or multiple transdermal bites or scratches and contamination of mucous membranes with the animal's saliva

Generally no treatment is required for category I contact. Patients who have experienced category II contact should be given rabies vaccine but the course may be stopped if the contact has been with a cat or dog that remains healthy throughout an observation period of 10 days or if postmortem study of the contact animal shows it to be negative for rabies. Patients who have experienced category III contact should be given rabies vaccine preceded by rabies immunoglobulin infiltrated around the wound and instilled into it as described above.

The dose for rabies immunoglobulin is 20 international units/kg; as much as possible of the dose should be infiltrated into and around the wound with the remainder being injected intramuscularly into the gluteal region.

The potency of rabies vaccines should be at least 2.5 international units per single human dose. For intramuscular vaccination schedules one dose should be administered on days 0, 3, 7, 14, and 30 into the deltoid region or, for small children, into the anterolateral area of the thigh. An abbreviated multisite schedule (the 2-1-1 regimen) induces an early antibody response and may be particularly effective when postexposure treatment has not included a rabies immunoglobulin. This schedule consists of one dose given in the right arm and one in the left arm on day 0, and one dose intramuscularly into the deltoid region on days 7 and 21. For intradermal vaccination one dose (0.1 mL) should be given at each of two sites, either the forearm or the upper arm, on days 0, 3, and 7, and one dose at one site on days 30 and 90.

In the UK, rabies immunoglobulin is given if the patient is previously unimmunised and at high risk. Human diploid cell vaccine is given on days 0, 3, 7, 14, and 30 (five doses) in unimmunised persons (although the UK manufacturers also recommend a sixth dose on day 90), and on days 0 and 3 to 7 (two doses) in previously fully immunised persons.

In the USA, a human diploid cell vaccine, an adsorbed rabies vaccine, or a purified chick embryo cell vaccine may be used for postexposure treatment.[2] In previously unimmunised individuals, a 1 mL dose of either vaccine is given intramuscularly on days 0, 3, 7, 14, and 28, together with rabies immunoglobulin as in the WHO schedule. In previously immunised individuals, two doses of vaccine are given on days 0 and 3, and rabies immunoglobulin is not required.


1. WHO. WHO expert committee on rabies: eighth report. *WHO Tech Rep Ser 824* 1992.
2. Centers for Disease Control. Human rabies prevention—United States, 1999: recommendations of the Advisory Committee on Immunization Practices (ACIP). *MMWR* 1999; **48** (RR-1): 1–21.


### Preparations

***Ph. Eur.:*** Rabies Vaccine for Human Use Prepared in Cell Cultures;
***USP 27:*** Rabies Vaccine.

**Proprietary Preparations** (details are given in Part 3)
***Arg.:*** Verorab; ***Austria:*** Rabipur; ***Braz.:*** HDCV†; Verorab; ***Canad.:*** Imovax Rabies; ***Chile:*** Verorab; ***Denm.:*** Rabies-Imovax; ***Fin.:*** Rabies-Imovax; ***Ger.:*** Rabipur; Rabivac; Tollwut-Impfstoff (HDC); ***Hong Kong:*** Lyssavac N†; ***India:*** Rabipur; ***Ital.:*** Imovax Rabbia; Lyssavac N; Rasilvax; ***Norw.:*** Rabies-Imovax; ***S.Afr.:*** Rabipor; Verorab; ***Spain:*** Vac Antirrabica; ***Swed.:*** Rabies-Imovax; ***Switz.:*** Lyssavac N; ***Thai.:*** Lyssavac N†; Rabipur; TRCS-Verorab; ***UK:*** Rabipur; ***USA:*** Imovax Rabies; RabAvert.

## Respiratory Syncytial Virus Immunoglobulins

Inmunoglobulinas contra el virus sincitial respiratorio.

### Palivizumab *(BAN, rINN)*

*CAS — 188039-54-5.*
*ATC — J06BB16.*

### Adverse Effects and Precautions

As for immunoglobulins in general, p.1605.

### Uses and Administration

Respiratory syncytial virus immunoglobulin is available in some countries for the passive immunisation of infants against lower respiratory-tract infections caused by respiratory syncytial virus. It is prepared from the pooled plasma of adults selected for high titres of antibodies that neutralise the virus. Each mL of respiratory syncytial virus immunoglobulin contains approximately 50 mg of protein.

In the USA, children under 2 years of age with bronchopulmonary dysplasia or a history of premature birth may receive a prophylactic intravenous infusion once a month during the respiratory syncytial virus season (typically November to April or early May). The drug is given in a dose of up to 750 mg/kg at an initial rate of 75 mg/kg per hour for 15 minutes, followed by 150 mg/kg per hour for a further 15 minutes, and then 300 mg/kg per hour until the end of the infusion.

Palivizumab, a human monoclonal antibody to respiratory syncytial virus, is available in some countries and is used intramuscularly for similar purposes, in a dose of 15 mg/kg monthly. Palivizumab is also recommended in children under 2 years of age with haemodynamically significant congenital heart disease.

### Preparations

**Proprietary Preparations** (details are given in Part 3)
***Arg.:*** Synagis; ***Austral.:*** Synagis; ***Belg.:*** Synagis; ***Braz.:*** Synagis; ***Denm.:*** Synagis; ***Fin.:*** Synagis; ***Fr.:*** Synagis; ***Ger.:*** Synagis; ***Gr.:*** Synagis; ***Hong Kong:*** Synagis; ***Irl.:*** Synagis; ***Israel:*** Abbosynagis; ***Ital.:*** Synagis; ***Mex.:*** Synagis; ***Neth.:*** Synagis; ***Norw.:*** Synagis; ***NZ:*** Synagis; ***S.Afr.:*** Synagis; ***Singapore:*** Synagis; ***Spain:*** Synagis; ***Swed.:*** Synagis; ***Switz.:*** Synagis; ***UK:*** Synagis; ***USA:*** RespiGam; Synagis.

## Respiratory Syncytial Virus Vaccines

Vacunas del virus sincitial respiratorio.

### Profile

Vaccines containing respiratory syncytial virus protein subunit are being studied for active immunisation.

◊ References.


1. Karron RA, Ambrosino DM. Respiratory syncytial virus vaccines. *Pediatr Infect Dis J* 1998; **17:** 919–20.
2. Gonzalez IM, *et al.* Evaluation of the live attenuated cpts 248/404 RSV vaccine in combination with a subunit RSV vaccine (PFP-2) in healthy young and older adults. *Vaccine* 2000; **18:** 1763–72.
3. Wright PF, *et al.* Evaluation of a live, cold-passaged, temperature-sensitive, respiratory syncytial virus vaccine candidate in infancy. *J Infect Dis* 2000; **182:** 1331–42.
4. Power UF, *et al.* Safety and immunogenicity of a novel recombinant subunit respiratory syncytial virus vaccine (BBG2Na) in healthy young adults. *J Infect Dis* 2001; **184:** 1456–60.


## Rift Valley Fever Vaccines

Vacunas de la fiebre del valle del Rift.

### Profile

An inactivated rift valley fever vaccine has been developed for the active immunisation of persons at high risk of contracting the disease.

## Rotavirus Vaccines

Vacunas de rotavirus.
*ATC — J07BH01.*

### Profile

Several live oral rotavirus vaccines for use in the prevention of childhood diarrhoea have been developed. A live oral tetravalent rotavirus vaccine (RRV-TV) was formerly available in the USA but was withdrawn by the manufacturer in October 1999 following reports of intussusception associated with its use.

◊ Rotaviruses are an important cause of severe diarrhoea in both developed and developing countries (see Gastro-enteritis, p.618), being most prevalent among children 6 to 24 months of age.[1] Human rotavirus diarrhoea is caused by group A, B, or C rotaviruses.[2] Development of a suitable vaccine has been made difficult by the diversity of rotaviruses.[2] Initial attempts at vaccine development used single bovine or rhesus monkey strains but these were associated with variable efficacy and adverse effects.[1,3-5]

To overcome these problems reassortant rotavirus (RRV) strains were constructed. These combined animal rotavirus strains with human rotavirus genes coding for serotype-specific antigens, enabling polyvalent vaccines to be produced against the major rotavirus serotypes causing disease. One of these, a live oral tetravalent vaccine (RRV-TV) became available in the USA in August 1998 but was withdrawn from the market by the manufacturer in October 1999 following reports of intussusception (a condition when part of the intestine prolapses into the lumen of an adjacent part causing an obstruction). From September 1998 until July 1999, 15 patients with intussusception had been reported to the Vaccine Adverse Event Reporting System (VAERS), 12 of whom developed symptoms within a week of vaccination.[6] While this evidence was considered inconclusive, further studies were expected to clarify the risks associated with routine use of this vaccine. One such study,[7] in which 429 infants with intussusception were retrospectively analysed, found that 74 (17.2%) had received RRV-TV compared with 226 of 1763 controls (12.8%) and concluded that there was evidence of a causal relationship with the vaccine. Another retrospective study,[8] however, found that there was no evidence of an increase in hospital admissions due to intussusception during the period of RRV-TV availability and recommended that a large, randomised, double-blind vaccine trial be performed to determine the absolute risk.

A live attenuated rotavirus known as 89-12 is currently under investigation.[9]


1. Anonymous. Rotavirus vaccines. *Bull WHO* 1989; **67:** 583–4.
2. Anonymous. Puzzling diversity of rotaviruses. *Lancet* 1990; **335:** 573–5.
3. Levine MM. Modern vaccines: enteric infections. *Lancet* 1990; **335:** 958–61.
4. Bernstein DI, *et al.* Evaluation of WC3 rotavirus vaccine and correlates of protection in healthy infants. *J Infect Dis* 1990; **162:** 1055–62.
5. Flores J, *et al.* Protection against severe rotavirus diarrhoea by rhesus rotavirus vaccine in Venezuelan infants. *Lancet* 1987; **i:** 882–4.
6. Centers for Disease Control. Intussusception among recipients of rotavirus vaccine—United States, 1998-1999. *MMWR* 1999; **48:** 577–81.
7. Murphy TV, *et al.* Intussusception among infants given an oral rotavirus vaccine. *N Engl J Med* 2001; **344:** 564–72. Correction. *ibid.*; 1564.
8. Simonsen L, *et al.* Effect of rotavirus vaccination programme on trends in admission of infants to hospital for intussusception. *Lancet* 2001; **358:** 1224–9.
9. Bernstein DI, *et al.* Second-year follow-up evaluation of live, attenuated human rotavirus vaccine 89-12 in healthy infants. *J Infect Dis* 2002; **186:** 1487–9.


## Rubella Immunoglobulins

Inmunoglobulinas contra la rubéola.
*ATC — J06BB06.*

**Pharmacopoeias.** Many pharmacopoeias have monographs including *Eur.* (see p.vi).

**Ph. Eur. 5.0** (Human Rubella Immunoglobulin; Immunoglobulinum Humanum Rubellae). A liquid or freeze-dried preparation containing immunoglobulins, mainly immunoglobulin G (IgG). It is obtained from plasma containing specific antibodies against the rubella virus. Normal immunoglobulin may be added. It contains not less than 4500 international units/mL. Both the liquid and freeze-dried preparations should be stored, protected from light, in a colourless, glass container. The freeze-dried preparation should be stored under vacuum or under an inert gas.

### Adverse Effects and Precautions

As for immunoglobulins in general, p.1605.

### Interactions

As for immunoglobulins in general, p.1605.

### Uses and Administration

Rubella immunoglobulins may be used for passive immunisation against rubella (German measles). They have been used to prevent or modify rubella in susceptible persons, although if such a measure is used then normal immunoglobulin is often employed instead.

### Preparations

***Ph. Eur.:*** Human Rubella Immunoglobulin.

**Proprietary Preparations** (details are given in Part 3)
***Ital.:*** Immunoros†; Rosol-Gamma†; Rubeuman†.

# Rubella Vaccines

Vacunas de la rubéola.
*ATC — J07BJ01.*

**Pharmacopoeias.** Many pharmacopoeias have monographs including *Eur.* (see p.vi) and *US.*

**Ph. Eur. 5.0** (Rubella Vaccine (Live); Vaccinum Rubellae Vivum). A freeze-dried preparation of a suitable live attenuated strain of rubella virus grown in human diploid cell cultures. It is reconstituted immediately before use. The cell-culture medium may contain a permitted antibacterial at the smallest effective concentration, and a suitable stabiliser may be added to the bulk vaccine.

The final vaccine contains not less than $1 \times 10^3$ $CCID_{50}$ per dose. The dried vaccine should be stored at 2° to 8° and be protected from light.

The BP 2003 states that Rub/Vac(Live) may be used on the label.

**USP 27** (Rubella Virus Vaccine Live). A bacterially sterile preparation of a suitable live strain of rubella virus grown in cultures of duck-embryo tissue or human tissue. It contains the equivalent of not less than $1 \times 10^3$ $TCID_{50}$ in each immunising dose. It should be stored at 2° to 8° and be protected from light.

## Adverse Effects

As for vaccines in general, p.1605.

Generally, side-effects have not been severe. Those occurring most commonly are skin rashes, pharyngitis, fever, and lymphadenopathy; arthralgia and arthritis may also occur and are reported to be more common in women than young girls. Thrombocytopenia and neurological symptoms including neuropathy and paraesthesia have been reported rarely.

**Effects on bones and joints.** Although acute arthralgia or arthritis occurs in up to 30% of women following rubella vaccination,[1] a retrospective analysis found no evidence of an increased risk of chronic arthropathies.[2]

1. Tingle AJ, *et al.* Randomised double-blind placebo-controlled study on adverse effects of rubella immunisation in seronegative women. *Lancet* 1997; **349:** 1277–81.
2. Ray P, *et al.* Risk of chronic arthropathy among women after rubella vaccination. *JAMA* 1997; **278:** 551–6.

**Effects on the nervous system.** For a report of optic neuritis in 2 children after use of measles and rubella vaccine, see under Adverse Effects of Measles and Rubella Vaccines, p.1625.

## Precautions

As for vaccines in general, p.1606.

Rubella vaccines should not be given during pregnancy and in the UK it is recommended that patients should be advised not to become pregnant within one month of vaccination. However, no case of congenital rubella syndrome has been reported following the inadvertent administration of rubella vaccines shortly before or during pregnancy and there is no evidence that the vaccines are teratogenic. Inadvertent administration of rubella vaccines during pregnancy should not therefore result in a routine recommendation to terminate the pregnancy. There is no risk to a pregnant woman from contact with recently vaccinated persons as the vaccine virus is not transmitted.

Rubella vaccines are not generally recommended for children below the age of 1 year in whom maternal antibodies might prevent a response.

The vaccine available in the UK contains traces of neomycin and/or polymyxin and should therefore not be given to individuals with a history of anaphylaxis to these antibacterials.

**Pregnancy.** Since 1971 the Centers for Disease Control in the USA has followed up women who received rubella vaccines within 3 months before or after conception.[1] Up to 1979 vaccines containing either the Cendehill or HPV-77 strains of rubella virus were available. None of the 290 infants born to the 538 women who had received these vaccines had defects indicative of congenital rubella syndrome; this included 94 live-born infants of women who were known to be susceptible to rubella before receiving the vaccine. In 1979 a rubella vaccine containing the Wistar RA 27/3 strain was introduced. None of 212 infants born live to 254 women known to be susceptible to rubella and who had received the RA 27/3 rubella vaccine from 1979 to 1988 had defects indicative of congenital rubella syndrome. These results are consistent with experiences in Germany[2] and the UK.[3,4] However, because of evidence that rubella vaccine viruses can cross the placenta and infect the fetus a theoretical risk to the fetus cannot be completely ruled out.[1] Thus in both the UK and USA pregnancy is considered a contra-indication to rubella vaccination, and patients are also advised not to become pregnant within one month of vaccination. However, in neither country is termination of pregnancy routinely recommended if the vaccine is inadvertently administered during pregnancy.

1. Anonymous. Rubella vaccination during pregnancy—United States, 1971–1988. *JAMA* 1989; **261:** 3374–83.
2. Enders G. Rubella antibody titers in vaccinated and nonvaccinated women and results of vaccination during pregnancy. *Rev Infect Dis* 1985; **7** (suppl 1): S103–S107.
3. Sheppard S, *et al.* Rubella vaccination and pregnancy: preliminary report of a national survey. *BMJ* 1986; **292:** 727.
4. Tookey PA, *et al.* Rubella vaccination in pregnancy. *Commun Dis Rep* 1991; **1** (review 7): R86–R88.

## Interactions

As for vaccines in general, p.1606.

## Uses and Administration

Rubella vaccines are used for active immunisation against rubella (German measles). The symptoms of rubella infection are generally mild except in the early stages of pregnancy when it leads to fetal damage in most infants.

For primary immunisation combined measles, mumps, and rubella vaccine (p.1625) is usually given. For discussion of immunisation schedules, see under Vaccines, p.1606.

In the UK, administration of a single-antigen rubella vaccine to girls aged 10 to 14 years has been discontinued following the mass immunisation campaign in 1994 and the introduction of a two-dose immunisation schedule in all children. A combined measles, mumps, and rubella vaccine (containing the Wistar RA 27/3 strain of rubella) is now used. Women of child-bearing age should also be vaccinated with the combined vaccine if they are seronegative; women who are found to be seronegative during pregnancy should be vaccinated in the early postpartum period. Effective precautions against pregnancy must be observed for at least one month after vaccination. To avoid the risk of transmitting rubella to pregnant patients, all health service staff, both male and female, should be screened and those found to be seronegative should be vaccinated.

In the USA, a single-antigen rubella vaccine is used. Vaccines containing other strains of rubella virus, such as the Cendehill strain, are available in other countries.

## Preparations

***Ph. Eur.:*** Rubella Vaccine (Live);
***USP 27:*** Rubella Virus Vaccine Live.

**Proprietary Preparations** (details are given in Part 3)
***Arg.:*** Imovax Rubeola; ***Austral.:*** Ervevax; Meruvax II; ***Austria:*** Ervevax; Rubeaten; ***Belg.:*** Ervevax†; ***Braz.:*** Meruvax II†; Rudivax; ***Denm.:*** Meruvax; ***Fr.:*** Rudivax; ***Ger.:*** Ervevax†; Rubellovac; ***Gr.:*** Vaccin Rubeole Merieux; ***Hong Kong:*** Meruvax II†; Rubeaten†; Rudivax; ***India:*** R-Vac; ***Irl.:*** Almevax†; Ervevax; ***Israel:*** Rudivax; ***Ital.:*** Ervevax; Gunevax; Rosovax†; Rubeaten†; Rudivax; ***Malaysia:*** Ervevax; Gunevax; ***Mex.:*** Ervevax; Gunevax; ***NZ:*** Ervevax†; ***Port.:*** Rubeaten; ***S.Afr.:*** Rubeaten†; Rudivax; ***Singapore:*** Rubeaten†; Rudivax†; ***Spain:*** Rubeaten†; Vac Antirrubeola; ***Swed.:*** Meruvax; ***Switz.:*** Ervevax; Meruvax II; Rubeaten; ***Thai.:*** Ervevax†; Gunevax; Rubeaten†; Rudivax; ***UK:*** Almevax; Ervevax†; Rubilin†; ***USA:*** Meruvax II.

---

# Rubella and Mumps Vaccines

Vacunas de la rubéola y la parotiditis.

*ATC — J07BJ51.*

**Pharmacopoeias.** Many pharmacopoeias have monographs including *US.*

**USP 27** (Rubella and Mumps Virus Vaccine Live). A bacterially sterile preparation of a suitable live strain of rubella virus and a suitable live strain of mumps virus. It may contain suitable antimicrobial agents. It should be stored at 2° to 8° and be protected from light.

## Adverse Effects and Precautions

As for vaccines in general, p.1605.

See also under mumps vaccines, p.1626, and rubella vaccines, p.1637.

## Interactions

As for vaccines in general, p.1606.

## Uses and Administration

Rubella and mumps vaccines may be used for active immunisation against mumps and rubella. Vaccination against mumps and rubella is normally performed using a combined measles, mumps, and rubella vaccine (p.1625) but the bivalent rubella and mumps vaccine may be employed when vaccination against measles is not indicated. For discussion of immunisation schedules, see under Vaccines, p.1606.

A vaccine used in the USA is prepared from the Wistar RA 27/3 strain of rubella virus and the Jeryl Lynn (B level) strain of mumps virus. It is generally given in a dose of 0.5 mL by subcutaneous injection to infants during the second year of life or to other children or adults considered to be at risk.

## Preparations

***USP 27:*** Rubella and Mumps Virus Vaccine Live.

**Proprietary Preparations** (details are given in Part 3)
***USA:*** Biavax II.

---

# Schistosomiasis Vaccines

Bilharzia Vaccines; Vacunas de la esquistosomiasis.

## Profile

Vaccines against schistosomiasis are under development.

◊ Reviews.

1. Capron A, *et al.* Vaccine development against schistosomiasis: from concepts to clinical trials. *Br Med Bull* 2002; **62:** 139–48.
2. Pearce EJ. Progress towards a vaccine for schistosomiasis. *Acta Trop* 2003; **86:** 309–13.

---

# Scorpion Venom Antisera

Antisuero contra el veneno de escorpión; Scorpion Antivenins; Scorpion Antivenoms.

## Adverse Effects and Precautions

As for antisera in general, p.1605.

## Uses and Administration

Some scorpion stings are dangerous and even fatal. The use of a scorpion venom antiserum suitable for the species of scorpion can prevent symptoms, provided that it is given with the least possible delay; other general supportive measures and symptomatic treatment are also needed. The effectiveness of scorpion venom antisera is disputed by some clinicians.

**Scorpion stings.** Scorpion stings are common throughout the tropics, but the most dangerous and potentially fatal species are found in India, North Africa and the Middle East, the southern states of North America and Mexico, Latin America and the Caribbean, and southern Africa. Local symptoms following scorpion stings include intense pain and swelling. Systemic symptoms result from excitation of nerve and muscle cells by the venom; the pattern of symptoms depends upon the species of scorpion. Symptoms of parasympathetic stimulation such as dilatation of pupils, hypersalivation, vomiting, and diarrhoea are generally followed by adrenergic features, with release of catecholamines producing hypertension, toxic myocarditis, arrhythmias, heart failure, and pulmonary oedema. The cardiotoxic effects are prominent features of stings in India, North Africa, and the Middle East. Neurotoxic effects such as fasciculations, spasms, and respiratory paralysis are seen with stings from North American species. Stings by the black scorpion of Trinidad may also produce pancreatitis.

Pain is treated with local infiltration or peripheral nerve block with local anaesthetics; opioid analgesics may be necessary, but are regarded as dangerous following stings by some North American species. An appropriate antiserum should be administered as soon as possible after envenomation, although the effectiveness of some antisera has been questioned. Supportive treatment for cardiotoxic effects includes alpha blockers, calcium-channel blockers, and ACE inhibitors. The use of cardiac glycosides, beta blockers, and atropine is controversial. Phenobarbital has been suggested for neurotoxic effects.

References.

1. el Amin EO, *et al.* Scorpion sting: a management problem. *Ann Trop Paediatr* 1991; **11:** 143–8.
2. Bond GR. Antivenin administration for Centruroides scorpion sting: risks and benefits. *Ann Emerg Med* 1992; **21:** 788–91.
3. Warrell DA, Fenner PJ. Venomous bites and stings. *Br Med Bull* 1993; **49:** 423–39.
4. Müller GJ. Scorpionism in South Africa: a report of 42 serious scorpion envenomations. *S Afr Med J* 1993; **83:** 405–11.
5. Gateau T, *et al.* Response to specific centruroides sculpturatus antivenom in 151 cases of scorpion stings. *Clin Toxicol* 1994; **32:** 165–71.
6. Sofer S, *et al.* Scorpion envenomation and antivenom therapy. *J Pediatr* 1994; **124:** 973–8.
7. Karalliedde L. Animal toxins. *Br J Anaesth* 1995; **74:** 319–27.
8. Abroug F, *et al.* Serotherapy in scorpion envenomation: a randomised controlled trial. *Lancet* 1999; **354:** 906–9.
9. Ghalim N, *et al.* Scorpion envenomation and serotherapy in Morocco. *Am J Trop Med Hyg* 2000; **62:** 277–83.

## Preparations

**Proprietary Preparations** (details are given in Part 3)
***Mex.:*** Alacramyn.

---

# Shigella Vaccines

Dysentery Vaccines; Shigellosis Vaccines; Vacunas contra Shigella.

## Profile

Live attenuated shigella vaccines have been under investigation since the 1960s but early prototypes were unsatisfactory. Live oral vaccines and conjugated vaccines are now also under development.

◊ References.

1. Cohen D, *et al.* Double-blind vaccine-controlled randomised efficacy trial of an investigational Shigella sonnei conjugate vaccine in young adults. *Lancet* 1997; **349:** 155–9.
2. Coster TS, *et al.* Vaccination against shigellosis with attenuated Shigella flexneri 2a strain SC602. *Infect Immun* 1999; **67:** 3437–43.
3. Ashkenazi S, *et al.* Safety and immunogenicity of Shigella sonnei and Shigella flexneri 2a O-specific polysaccharide conjugates in children. *J Infect Dis* 1999; **179:** 1565–8.
4. Passwell JH, *et al.* Safety and immunogenicity of Shigella sonnei-CRM9 and Shigella flexneri type 2a-rEPAsucc conjugate vaccines in one- to four-year-old children. *Pediatr Infect Dis J* 2003; **22:** 701–6.
5. Katz DE, *et al.* Two studies evaluating the safety and immunogenicity of a live, attenuated Shigella flexneri 2a vaccine (SC602) and excretion of vaccine organisms in North American volunteers. *Infect Immun* 2004; **72:** 923–30.

### Smallpox Vaccines

Vacunas de la viruela.

**Pharmacopoeias.** Many pharmacopoeias have monographs including *US.*

**USP 27** (Smallpox Vaccine). A suspension or solid containing a suitable strain of the living virus of vaccinia grown in the skin of bovine calves; it may contain a suitable preservative. The liquid vaccine should be stored below 0° and the dried vaccine at 2° to 8°.

### Uses and Administration

Following the global eradication of smallpox, vaccination against smallpox (using vaccinia virus) has been indicated only for investigators at special risk such as laboratory workers handling certain orthopoxviruses.

WHO considers that mass vaccination against smallpox is not appropriate, although individuals who may be at risk of exposure to smallpox or those with confirmed infection may be vaccinated.

Recombinant vaccinia viruses are being investigated as vectors of foreign antigens, for example in a candidate AIDS vaccine (p.1607).

◊ References.


1. Barquet N, Domingo P. Smallpox: the triumph over the most terrible of the ministers of death. *Ann Intern Med* 1997; **127:** 635–42.
2. Centers for Disease Control. Vaccinia (smallpox) vaccine: recommendations of the Advisory Committee on Immunization Practices (ACIP), 2001. *MMWR* 2001; **50** (RR-10): 1–25.
3. Centers for Disease Control. Recommendations for using smallpox vaccine in a pre-event vaccination program: supplemental recommendations of the Advisory Committee on Immunization Practices (ACIP) and the Healthcare Infection Control Practices Advisory Committee (HICPAC). *MMWR* 2003; **52** (RR-7): 1–16.
4. Health Protection Agency. Interim guidelines for action in the event of a deliberate release: smallpox. Available at: http://www.hpa.org.uk/infections/topics_az/deliberate_release_static/smallpox/PDFs/smallpox_guidelines.pdf (accessed 22/06/04)
5. Department of Health. Guidelines for smallpox response and management in the post-eradication era (smallpox plan). Available at: http://www.dh.gov.uk/PublicationsAndStatistics/Publications/PublicationsPolicyAndGuidance/PublicationsPolicyAndGuidanceArticle/fs/en?CONTENT_ID=4070830&chk=XRWF7m (accessed 22/06/04)


### Preparations

***USP 27:*** Smallpox Vaccine.

**Proprietary Preparations** (details are given in Part 3)
***USA:*** Dryvax.

## Snake Venom Antisera

Antisuero contra el veneno de serpiente; Snake Antivenins; Snake Antivenoms.

*ATC — J06AA03.*

**Pharmacopoeias.** Many pharmacopoeias have monographs including *Eur.* (see p.vi) and *US.*

**Ph. Eur. 5.0** (Viper Venom Antiserum, European; Immunoserum Contra Venena Viperarum Europaearum). A preparation containing the specific antitoxic globulins that have the power of neutralising the venom of one or more species of viper (*Vipera ammodytes, V. aspis, V. berus,* or *V. ursinii*). The globulins are obtained by fractionation of the serum of animals that have been immunised against the venom or venoms. Each mL neutralises the venoms in not less than 100 mouse $LD_{50}$ of *V. ammodytes,* 100 of *V. aspis,* 50 of *V. berus,* or 50 of *V. ursinii.* It should be stored at 2° to 8°, and not be allowed to freeze.

The BP 2003 states that the only poisonous snake native to the British Isles is the adder or common viper, *Vipera berus.* In a geographical region where other species of snake (including elapids) are found, antisera able to neutralise the venoms of the species of snake indigenous to the region should be used. When the preparation is intended to neutralise the venom or venoms of one or more snakes other than vipers, the title Snake Venom Antiserum is used.

**USP 27** (Antivenin (Crotalidae) Polyvalent). A sterile freeze-dried preparation of specific venom-neutralising globulins obtained from the serum of healthy horses immunised against 4 species of pit vipers, *Crotalus atrox* (western diamondback), *Crotalus adamanteus, Crotalus durissus terrificus* (South American rattlesnake), and *Bothrops atrox* (South American fer de lance). One dose neutralises the venoms in not less than 180 mouse $LD_{50}$ of *C. atrox,* 1320 of *C. durissus terrificus,* and 780 of *B. atrox.* It may contain a suitable preservative. It should be preserved in single-dose containers and stored at a temperature not exceeding 40°.

**USP 27** (Antivenin (Micrurus Fulvius)). A sterile freeze-dried preparation of specific venom-neutralising globulins obtained from the serum of healthy horses immunised against venom of *Micrurus fulvius* (eastern coral snake). One dose neutralises the venom in not less than 250 mouse $LD_{50}$ of *M. fulvius.* It may contain a suitable preservative. It should be preserved in single-dose containers and stored at a temperature not exceeding 40°.

### Adverse Effects and Precautions

As for antisera in general, p.1605. Serum sickness is not uncommon and anaphylactic reactions may occur.

**Anaphylaxis.** Conjunctival or cutaneous hypersensitivity testing failed to predict early (anaphylactic) reactions to the antivenom given in a study of patients in Nigeria with systemic envenoming by the saw-scaled or carpet viper (*Echis carinatus*) and in Thailand with local or systemic envenoming by green pit vipers (*Trimeresurus albolabris* and *T. macrops*), the monocellate Thai cobra (*Naja kaouthia*), or the Malayan pit viper (*Calloselasma rhodostoma*). It was considered that conventional hypersensitivity testing has no predictive value for the occurrence of allergic reactions to antivenom and that it is not justifiable to delay treatment for 20 or 30 minutes to read the results of these tests. Although the rate of administration of the antiserum can be more easily controlled by intravenous infusion, this method has serious practical disadvantages in the rural tropics where most cases of snake bite occur and an advantage of the intravenous push injection is that the person giving the antiserum must remain with the patient during the period when most severe anaphylactic reactions develop.

There is some evidence that pretreatment with low-dose subcutaneous adrenaline may reduce the incidence of anaphylaxis and other acute adverse reactions to the administration of antiserum.[1] However, the use of premedication with adrenaline, antihistamines, and corticosteroids, although widely practiced, is controversial. In one study,[2] prophylaxis with promethazine was ineffective in preventing anaphylaxis from antiserum against *Bothrops* envenomation.


1. Premawardhena AP, *et al.* Low dose subcutaneous adrenaline to prevent acute adverse reactions to antivenom serum in people bitten by snakes: randomised, placebo controlled trial. *BMJ* 1999; **318:** 1041–3.
2. Fan HW, *et al.* Sequential randomised and double blind trial of promethazine prophylaxis against early anaphylactic reactions to antivenom for bothrops snake bites. *BMJ* 1999; **318:** 1451–2.


### Uses and Administration

Venomous snakes comprise the Viperidae (vipers), Elapidae (cobras, kraits, and mambas), and the Hydrophiidae (sea snakes).

The venom of snakes is a complex mixture chiefly of proteins, many of which have enzymatic activity, and may provoke local inflammatory reactions. The venom may have profound effects on tissue, blood vessels and other organs, blood cells, coagulation, and myotoxic or neurotoxic effects with sensory, motor, cardiac, renal, and respiratory involvement.

Snake venom antisera are the only specific treatment available for venomous snake bites, but can produce severe adverse reactions. They are generally only used if there are clear indications of systemic involvement, severe local involvement, or, in regions where supplies are not limited, in patients at high risk of systemic or severe local involvement. Adrenaline should be available in case of anaphylactic reactions to the antiserum; premedication with adrenaline, corticosteroids, and/or antihistamines is widely practiced but is regarded as controversial.

In Great Britain, the only indigenous poisonous snake is the adder, *Vipera berus*, and European Viper Venom Antiserum (or Zagreb antivenom) may sometimes be indicated as part of the overall treatment. The usual dose for adults and children is 10 mL by intravenous injection over 10 to 15 minutes or by intravenous infusion over 30 minutes after diluting in 5 mL/kg body-weight of sodium chloride 0.9%; the dose may be repeated after about 1 to 2 hours if symptoms of systemic envenoming persist.

In the USA, a polyvalent crotalidae antiserum against *Bothrops atrox, Crotalus adamanteus, C. atrox,* and *C. durissus terrificus,* and an antiserum against the North American coral snake, *Micrurus fulvius,* are available. In Australia, polyvalent antisera against the brown snake, death adder, taipan, and tiger snake, together with either the king brown snake or black snake, are available. A variety of polyvalent and monovalent antisera are also available as appropriate to the indigenous species of snakes in many other countries.

**Snake bites.** Most snake species are non-venomous and belong to the colubrid family although a few colubrids are technically venomous. The three families of venomous front-fanged snakes are the elapids, vipers, and sea snakes. Elapids include cobras, mambas, kraits, coral snakes, and the Australasian venomous land snakes. Vipers are subdivided into crotalids (pit vipers) and viperids. Viper bites are much more common than elapid bites, except in Australasia, where vipers do not occur naturally. Sea snake bites occur among fishermen of the Asian and western Pacific coastal areas. Although there are some notable exceptions, viper bites tend to cause vasculotoxicity, elapids cause neurotoxicity, and sea snakes cause myotoxicity.

Only a few snakes are known to be of medical importance. Of the vipers these include *Bothrops atrox* (Central and South America), *Bitis arietans* (Africa), *Echis carinatus* (Africa and Asia), *Vipera russelli* (Asia), and *Agkistrodon rhodostoma* (south-east Asia). In a few restricted areas of Africa and Asia, cobra bites are common; bites by mambas (Africa) and kraits (Asia) are rare. The carpet viper, *Echis pyramidum,* and saw-scaled viper, *Echis carinatus,* can justifiably be labelled the most dangerous snakes in the world and they cause more deaths and serious poisoning than any other snake.

Management of snake bite involves general supportive care and monitoring of vital functions but in a systemic snake-bite poisoning, specific snake venom antiserum is the most effective therapeutic agent available. If used correctly, it can reverse systemic poisoning when given hours or even days after the bite. It is highly desirable to wait for clear clinical evidence of systemic poisoning before giving an antiserum and therefore it should not be given routinely in all cases of snake bite. Monospecific antisera are more effective, and less likely to cause reactions, than polyvalent antisera. The dosage of antiserum to be used is dependent on the species of snake and the consequent potency of the requisite antiserum. The antiserum should be given intravenously diluted in isotonic saline, either by infusion or bolus injection (see under Adverse Effects and Precautions, above). First aid measures including incisions and suction to remove the venom and application of tourniquets are generally to be discouraged. In most cases, the bitten limb should be immobilised and the victim transferred to a medical facility, together with the snake if possible. For bites by elapids, when respiratory failure may occur before the patient reaches hospital, a tourniquet may be justified to delay the onset of neurotoxicity. Supportive treatment is necessary even in patients who have received an adequate dose of antiserum. Local pain may be treated with a suitable analgesic. Artificial respiration may be required in patients with symptoms of neurotoxicity. Anticholinesterases may be of benefit against the neurotoxic effects of some snake venoms and it has been recommended that an intravenous test dose of edrophonium preceded by atropine should be tried in patients with severe symptoms of neurotoxicity. For those patients who respond, treatment with neostigmine should be started but anticholinesterases are unlikely to affect outcome in patients who already require assisted respiration. Hypovolaemia should be corrected cautiously with parenteral fluids. Hypotension may be treated with subcutaneous adrenaline or, in patients bitten by Russell's viper, a response to dopamine has been noted. Patients with renal impairment may require dialysis if they do not respond to rehydration, diuretics, and dopamine. Broad spectrum antibacterials and tetanus toxoid should be given as prophylactic measures. Surgical decompression and debridement of necrotic tissue may be necessary once normal haemostasis has been restored.

References.


1. Reid HA, Theakston RDG. The management of snake bite. *Bull WHO* 1983; **61:** 885–95.
2. Nelson BK. Snake envenomation: incidence, clinical presentation and management. *Med Toxicol* 1989; **4:** 17–31.
3. Warrell DA. Snake venoms in science and clinical medicine: 1. Russell's viper: biology, venom and treatment of bites. *Trans R Soc Trop Med Hyg* 1989; **83:** 732–40.
4. Theakston RDG. Snakes venoms in science and clinical medicine: 2. applied immunology in snake venom research. *Trans R Soc Trop Med Hyg* 1989; **83:** 741–4.
5. Hulton RA, *et al.* Arboreal green pit vipers (genus Trimeresurus) of South-east Asia: bites by T. albolabris and T. macrops in Thailand and a review of the literature. *Trans R Soc Trop Med Hyg* 1990; **84:** 866–74.
6. Smith TA, Figge HL. Treatment of snakebite poisoning. *Am J Hosp Pharm* 1991; **48:** 2190–6.
7. Warrell DA, Fenner PJ. Venomous bites and stings. *Br Med Bull* 1993; **49:** 423–39.
8. Tibballs J. Premedication for snake antivenom. *Med J Aust* 1994; **160:** 4–7.
9. Caiaffa WT, *et al.* Snake bite and antivenom complications in Belo Horizonate, Brazil. *Trans R Soc Trop Med Hyg* 1994; **88:** 81–5.
10. Trevett AJ, *et al.* The efficacy of antivenom in the treatment of bites by the Papuan taipan (Oxyuranus scutellatus canni). *Trans R Soc Trop Med Hyg* 1995; **89:** 322–5.
11. Jorge MT, *et al.* A randomized 'blinded' comparison of two doses of antivenom in the treatment of Bothrops envenoming in Sao Paulo, Brazil. *Trans R Soc Trop Med Hyg* 1995; **89:** 111–14.
12. Otero R, *et al.* A randomized double-blind clinical trial of two antivenoms in patients bitten by Bothrops atrox in Colombia. *Trans R Soc Trop Med Hyg* 1996; **90:** 696–700.
13. Mead HJ, Jelinek GA. Suspected snakebite in children: a study of 156 patients over 10 years. *Med J Aust* 1996; **164:** 467–70.
14. Paret G, *et al.* Vipera palaestinae snake envenomations: experience in children. *Hum Exp Toxicol* 1997; **16:** 683–7.
15. Ariaratnam CA, *et al.* An open, randomized comparative trial of two antivenoms for the treatment of envenoming by Sri Lankan Russell's viper (Daboia russelii russelii). *Trans R Soc Trop Med Hyg* 2001; **95:** 74–80.
16. Dart RC, *et al.* A randomized multicenter trial of crotalinae polyvalent immune Fab (ovine) antivenom for the treatment for crotaline snakebite in the United States. *Arch Intern Med* 2001; **161:** 2030–6.
17. Offerman SR, *et al.* Crotaline Fab antivenom for the treatment of children with rattlesnake envenomation. *Pediatrics* 2002; **110:** 968–71.
18. Pardal PPO, *et al.* Clinical trial of two antivenoms for the treatment of Bothrops and Lachesis bites in the north eastern Amazon region of Brazil. *Trans R Soc Trop Med Hyg* 2004; **98:** 28–42.

## Preparations

**Ph. Eur.:** European Viper Venom Antiserum;
**USP 27:** Antivenin (Crotalidae) Polyvalent; Antivenin (Micrurus Fulvius).

**Proprietary Preparations** (details are given in Part 3)
**Arg.:** Suero Antiofidico Polivalente; **Austral.:** Polyvalent Snake Antivenom; Snake Bite†; **Canad.:** Antivenin†; **Fr.:** Ipser Europe†; Viperfav; **Hong Kong:** Tiger Snake; **Ital.:** Siero Antiofidico†; **Mex.:** Antivipmyn; Coralmyn; **USA:** CroFab.

## Spider Venom Antisera

Antisuero contra el veneno de arañas; Spider Antivenins; Spider Antivenoms.

**Pharmacopoeias.** Many pharmacopoeias have monographs including *US*.

**USP 27** (Antivenin (Latrodectus Mactans)). A sterile freeze-dried preparation of specific venom-neutralising globulins obtained from the serum of healthy horses immunised against venom of black widow spiders (*Latrodectus mactans*). One dose neutralises the venom in not less than 6000 mouse $LD_{50}$ of *L. mactans*. It contains thiomersal as preservative. It should be preserved in single-dose containers and stored at a temperature not exceeding 40°.

### Adverse Effects and Precautions

As for antisera in general, p.1605.

### Uses and Administration

The use of a spider venom antiserum suitable for the species of spider can prevent symptoms, provided that it is done with the least possible delay; other general supportive measures and symptomatic treatment may also be needed.

An antiserum against the black widow spider (*Latrodectus mactans*) is available in the USA and the contents of a vial containing at least 6000 antivenin units is the usual dose for adults and children. In severe cases and in children under 12 years of age it is given by intravenous infusion in sodium chloride 0.9% over 15 minutes; in less severe cases, it may be given by intramuscular injection.

An antiserum against the funnel-web spider (*Atrax robustus*) is available in Australia.

**Spider bites.** Although many species of spider are venomous, relatively few pose a danger to man. Two main clinical syndromes are recognised; necrotic araneism, produced mainly by members of the genus *Loxosceles* which includes the brown recluse spider *L. reclusa*, and neurotoxic araneism produced by members of the genera *Latrodectus* (including the black widow and red-back spiders), *Phoneutria* (South American banana spiders), and *Atrax* (funnel-web spiders).

Necrotic araneism presents as local pain and erythema at the site of the bite, commonly developing into a necrotic lesion with a black eschar that sloughs after a few weeks, sometimes leaving an ulcer that heals gradually. The area affected can be extensive. Rarely, systemic symptoms including intravascular coagulation, haemolytic anaemia, respiratory distress, and renal failure, occur and may be life-threatening. A number of therapies have been suggested, but conservative management is usually adequate with surgical repair of any persistent defects if necessary. Dapsone is reported to produce beneficial effects on healing. Treatment for systemic manifestations is supportive. Antisera are available in some countries.

Neurotoxic araneism may involve severe pain, headache, vomiting, tachycardia, hypertension, muscle spasms, and occasionally pulmonary oedema, and coma, depending upon the species. Antisera are available and reported to be more effective than those for necrotic araneism, but should be reserved for serious envenomation. Intravenous injection of calcium gluconate 10% has been suggested to relieve muscle spasm as an alternative to conventional muscle relaxants.

References.


1. King LE, Rees RS. Dapsone treatment of a brown recluse bite. *JAMA* 1983; **250:** 648.
2. Hartman LJ, Sutherland SK. Funnel-web spider (Atrax robustus) antivenom in the treatment of human envenomation. *Med J Aust* 1984; **141:** 796–9.
3. Rees RS, *et al.* Brown recluse spider bites: a comparison of early surgical excision versus dapsone and delayed surgical excision. *Ann Surg* 1985; **202:** 659–63.
4. Dieckmann J, *et al.* Efficacy of funnel-web spider antivenom in human envenomation by Hadronyche species. *Med J Aust* 1989; **151:** 706–7.
5. Binder LS. Acute arthropod envenomation: incidence, clinical features and management. *Med Toxicol Adverse Drug Exp* 1989; **4:** 163–73.
6. Clark RF, *et al.* Clinical presentation and treatment of black widow spider envenomation: a review of 163 cases. *Ann Emerg Med* 1992; **21:** 782–7.
7. Warrell DA, Fenner PJ. Venomous bites and stings. *Br Med Bull* 1993; **49:** 423–39.


## Preparations

**USP 27:** Antivenin (Latrodectus Mactans).

**Proprietary Preparations** (details are given in Part 3)
**Canad.:** Antivenin (Latrodectus Mactans); **Mex.:** Aracmyn Plus.

## Staphylococcal Vaccines

Vacunas estafilocócicas.

### Profile

Staphylococcal vaccines, prepared from inactivated *Staphylococcus* spp. have been used for the prophylaxis and treatment of staphylococcal infections. They have been administered orally, topically, and by injection.

◊ References.


1. Shinefield H, *et al.* Use of a Staphylococcus aureus conjugate vaccine in patients receiving hemodialysis. *N Engl J Med* 2002; **346:** 491–6.


### Preparations

**Proprietary Preparations** (details are given in Part 3)
**Braz.:** Anatoxina Estafilococica†; Estafiloide; **USA:** SPL.

## Stone Fish Venom Antisera

Antisuero contra el veneno del pez piedra estuarino; Stone Fish Antivenins; Stone Fish Antivenoms.

### Adverse Effects and Precautions

As for antisera in general, p.1605.

### Uses and Administration

An antiserum for use in the management of stings by the stone fish (*Synanceja trachynis*) is available in Australia. The antiserum is prepared from the serum of horses that have been immunised with the venom of the stone fish. Other symptomatic and supportive treatments are given in addition.

Stone fish venom antiserum may be given by intramuscular injection or, in more severe cases, by intravenous infusion.

◊ References.


1. Sutherland SK. Stone fish bite. *BMJ* 1990; **300:** 679–80.
2. Lehmann DF, Hardy JC. Stonefish envenomation. *N Engl J Med* 1993; **329:** 510–11.


## Streptococcus Group B Vaccines

Vacunas contra estreptococos del grupo B.

### Profile

Vaccines for active immunisation against group B streptococcal infections are being developed. Administration of a vaccine to pregnant women to prevent neonatal infection has been proposed.

◊ References.


1. Baker CJ, *et al.* Immunization of pregnant women with a polysaccharide vaccine of group B streptococcus. *N Engl J Med* 1988; **319:** 1180–5.
2. Coleman RT, *et al.* Prevention of neonatal group B streptococcal infections: advances in maternal vaccine development. *Obstet Gynecol* 1992; **80:** 301–9.
3. Kasper DL, *et al.* Immune response to type III group B streptococcal polysaccharide-tetanus toxoid conjugate vaccine. *J Clin Invest* 1996; **98:** 2308–14.
4. Kotloff KL, *et al.* Safety and immunogenicity of a tetravalent group B streptococcal polysaccharide vaccine in healthy adults. *Vaccine* 1996; **14:** 446–50.
5. Baker CJ, *et al.* Use of capsular polysaccharide-tetanus toxoid conjugate vaccine for type II group B streptococcus in healthy women. *J Infect Dis* 2000; **182:** 1129–38.
6. Baker CJ, Edwards MS. Group B streptococcal conjugate vaccines. *Arch Dis Child* 2003; **88:** 375–8.
7. Baker CJ, *et al.* Safety and immunogenicity of a bivalent group B streptococcal conjugate vaccine for serotypes II and III. *J Infect Dis* 2003; **188:** 66–73.


## Tetanus Antitoxins

Antitoxinas tetánicas.

*ATC — J06AA02.*

**Pharmacopoeias.** Many pharmacopoeias have monographs including *Eur.* (see p.vi).

**Ph. Eur. 5.0** (Tetanus Antitoxin for Human Use; Immunoserum Tetanicum ad Usum Humanum). A sterile preparation containing the specific antitoxic globulins that have the power of neutralising the toxin formed by *Clostridium tetani*. It is obtained by fractionation from the serum of horses, or other mammals, that have been immunised against tetanus toxin. For prophylactic use, it has a potency of not less than 1000 international units/mL, and for therapeutic use not less than 3000 international units/mL. It should be stored at 2° to 8°, and not be allowed to freeze.

The BP 2003 states that Tet/Ser may be used on the label.

### Profile

Tetanus antitoxins neutralise the toxin produced by *Clostridium tetani* and have been used to provide temporary passive immunity against tetanus, but tetanus immunoglobulins (below) are preferred. A test dose of tetanus antitoxin should always be given to identify those who might suffer hypersensitivity reactions.

Whenever a non-immune patient is seen because of injury, a course of active immunisation should be instituted (see Tetanus Vaccines, p.1640).

### Preparations

**Ph. Eur.:** Tetanus Antitoxin for Human Use.

# Tetanus Immunoglobulins

Inmunoglobulinas contra el tétanos.

*ATC — J06BB02.*

**Pharmacopoeias.** Many pharmacopoeias have monographs including *Eur.* (see p.vi) and *US*.

**Ph. Eur. 5.0** (Human Tetanus Immunoglobulin; Immunoglobulinum Humanum Tetanicum). A liquid or freeze-dried preparation containing immunoglobulins, mainly immunoglobulin G (IgG). It is obtained from plasma containing specific antibodies against the toxin of *Clostridium tetani*. Normal immunoglobulin may be added. It contains not less than 100 international units/mL. Both the liquid and freeze-dried preparations should be stored, protected from light, in a colourless, glass container. The freeze-dried preparation should be stored under vacuum or under an inert gas.

**USP 27** (Tetanus Immune Globulin). A sterile solution of globulins derived from the plasma of adult human donors who have been immunised with tetanus vaccine. It contains not less than 50 units of tetanus antitoxin/mL. It contains 10 to 18% of protein of which not less than 90% is gamma globulin. It contains glycine as a stabilising agent, and a suitable preservative. It should be stored at 2° to 8°.

## Adverse Effects and Precautions

As for immunoglobulins in general, p.1605.

## Interactions

As for immunoglobulins in general, p.1605.

Tetanus immunoglobulins will neutralise tetanus toxoid and should not be injected into the same site or in the same syringe as a tetanus vaccine.

## Uses and Administration

Tetanus immunoglobulins are used for passive immunisation against tetanus.

The use of tetanus immunoglobulins is recommended in the UK and the USA as part of the management of tetanus-prone wounds in persons unimmunised or incompletely immunised against tetanus, in persons whose immunisation history is unknown, in persons who received the last dose of tetanus vaccine more than 10 years previously, and in patients with impaired immunity. Active immunisation with a tetanus vaccine (p.1640) should also be started simultaneously, and antibacterials and symptomatic therapy given as appropriate (see p.149 and p.1398). The usual dose of tetanus immunoglobulin is 250 units by intramuscular injection but, if more than 24 hours have elapsed since the wound was sustained, or if there is a risk of heavy contamination, or following burns, 500 units should be given irrespective of the immunisation history.

Tetanus immunoglobulin is also used in the treatment of tetanus, a recommended dose being 150 units/kg in total, given intramuscularly into multiple sites. Doses in the range 30 to 300 units/kg are suggested by the manufacturer in the UK.

A preparation suitable for intravenous use is available in some countries. It is given for the treatment of tetanus in a dose of 5000 to 10 000 units by intravenous infusion.

## Preparations

**Ph. Eur.:** Human Tetanus Immunoglobulin;
**USP 27:** Tetanus Immune Globulin.

**Proprietary Preparations** (details are given in Part 3)
**Arg.:** Gammatet; IT SD-T; Tetabulin; **Austria:** Tetabulin; Tetagam; Tetanosimultan†; Tetavenin; **Belg.:** Tetabuline†; Tetuman†; **Braz.:** Tetaglobulina†; Tetanobulin†; Tetanogamma; **Canad.:** BayTet; Hyper-Tet†; **Chile:** Igantet; **Fr.:** Gammatetanos; **Ger.:** Tetagam N; Tetanobulin; **Gr.:** Tetagam-P; **Hong Kong:** BayTet; Tetabulin; Tetuman; **India:** Tetagam-P; **Irl.:** Tetabulin; **Israel:** BayTet; Ig Tetano†; Tetaglobuline; **Ital.:** Gamma-Tet P; Haima-Tetanus†; Ig Tetano; Igantet; Immunotetan; Imogam Tetano†; Tetabulin; Tetagamma; Tetanus-Gamma; Tetaven; Tetuman†; **Malaysia:** Sero-Tet; Tetuman; **Mex.:** BayTet; Probi-Tet; Tetanogamma†; **Port.:** Tetuman; **S.Afr.:** Tetagam; Tetuman†; **Singapore:** BayTet; **Spain:** Gamma Antitenos†; Gamma Antitetanos; Gammaglob Antite†; Tetagamma P; Tetuman; Torlanbulina Antitenani†; **Switz.:** Tetabuline†; Tetuman; **Thai.:** Tetuman†; **UK:** Liberim T; Tetabulin; **USA:** BayTet.

# Tetanus Vaccines

Vacunas del tétanos.

*ATC — J07AM01.*

**Pharmacopoeias.** Many pharmacopoeias have monographs including *Eur.* (see p.vi) and *US*.

**Ph. Eur. 5.0** (Tetanus Vaccine (Adsorbed); Vaccinum Tetani Adsorbatum). It is prepared from tetanus formol toxoid adsorbed on a mineral carrier which may be hydrated aluminium phosphate or aluminium hydroxide. The resulting mixture is isotonic with blood. Suitable antimicrobial preservatives may be added. The antigenic properties are adversely affected by certain antimicrobial preservatives particularly those of the phenolic type and these should not be added to the vaccine. It contains not less than 40 units per dose. It should be stored at 2° to 8°, not be allowed to freeze, and be protected from light.

The BP 2003 states that Tet/Vac/Ads may be used on the label.

The BP 2003 directs that when Tetanus Vaccine is prescribed or demanded and the form is not stated, Tetanus Vaccine (Adsorbed) may be dispensed or supplied.

**BP 2003** (Tetanus Vaccine). It is prepared from tetanus toxin produced by the growth of *Clostridium tetani*. The toxin is converted to tetanus formol toxoid by treatment with formaldehyde solution. It contains suitable non-phenolic antimicrobial preservatives. It should be stored at 2° to 8° and be protected from light.

The BP 2003 states that Tet/Vac/FT may be used on the label.

The BP 2003 directs that when Tetanus Vaccine is prescribed or demanded and the form is not stated, Tetanus Vaccine (Adsorbed) may be dispensed or supplied.

**USP 27** (Tetanus Toxoid). A sterile solution of the formaldehyde-treated products of growth of *Clostridium tetani*. It contains a non-phenolic preservative. It should be stored at 2° to 8° and not be allowed to freeze.

**USP 27** (Tetanus Toxoid Adsorbed). A sterile preparation of plain tetanus toxoid precipitated or adsorbed by alum, aluminium hydroxide, or aluminium phosphate adjuvants. It should be stored at 2° to 8° and not be allowed to freeze.

## Adverse Effects and Precautions

As for vaccines in general, p.1605.

Local reactions, usually following the use of adsorbed vaccines, and mild systemic reactions may occur. The incidence and severity of reactions increases with the number of doses given.

Anaphylaxis and neurological reactions have occasionally been reported.

Although vaccination is usually postponed in patients suffering from an acute febrile illness, tetanus vaccine should be given to such patients in the presence of a tetanus-prone wound.

Booster doses of tetanus vaccine should not generally be given at intervals of less than 10 years because of an increased risk of severe local reactions.

**Effects of purification.** In a double-blind comparative study[1] involving 205 healthy subjects there was no difference in side-effects in those given a standard (commercial) tetanus vaccine and those given an antibody-affinity-purified vaccine. The results confirmed that side-effects to tetanus vaccines are not eliminated by purification.

1. Leen CLS, *et al.* Double-blind comparative trial of standard (commercial) and antibody-affinity-purified tetanus toxoid vaccines. *J Infect* 1987; **14:** 119–24.

**Effects on the nervous system.** Neuropathies have been reported rarely following tetanus vaccination. Optic neuritis and myelitis occurred[1] in an 11-year-old girl following a routine booster dose. Corticosteroids and immunoglobulin were given, and both vision and muscle power were restored after 11 months. Acute transverse myelitis was reported[2] in a 50-year-old man who received tetanus toxoid and immunoglobulin following an injury. Neurological deficits were unchanged after 1 month despite treatment with corticosteroids. Other causes could not be ruled out in either case. Brachial neuritis which developed in 2 infants following immunisation with diphtheria, tetanus, and pertussis vaccine was attributed to the tetanus component.[3]

1. Topaloglu H, *et al.* Optic neuritis and myelitis after booster tetanus toxoid vaccination. *Lancet* 1992; **339:** 178–9.
2. Read SJ, *et al.* Acute transverse myelitis after tetanus toxoid vaccination. *Lancet* 1992; **339:** 1111–12.
3. Hamati-Haddad A, Fenichel GM. Brachial neuritis following routine childhood immunization for diphtheria, tetanus, and pertussis (DTP): report of two cases and review of the literature. *Pediatrics* 1997; **99:** 602–3.

GUILLAIN-BARRÉ SYNDROME. A possible causal relationship between tetanus-containing vaccines and Guillain-Barré syndrome has been proposed (see Diphtheria and Tetanus Vaccines, p.1613).

**Pregnancy.** No connection has been found between administration of tetanus toxoid during pregnancy and either congenital malformations[1] or spontaneous abortion.[2]

1. Silveira CM, *et al.* Safety of tetanus toxoid in pregnant women: a hospital-based case-control study of congenital anomalies. *Bull WHO* 1995; **73:** 605–8.
2. Catindig N, *et al.* Tetanus toxoid and spontaneous abortions: is there epidemiological evidence of an association? *Lancet* 1996; **348:** 1098–9.

## Interactions

As for vaccines in general, p.1606.

Tetanus immunoglobulins will neutralise tetanus toxoid and should not be injected into the same site or in the same syringe as a tetanus vaccine.

## Uses and Administration

Tetanus vaccines are used for active immunisation against tetanus.

For primary immunisation of infants and children up to 10 years of age a combined diphtheria, tetanus, pertussis (acellular component), poliomyelitis (inactivated), and Haemophilus influenzae vaccine (p.1615) is used in the UK and a combined diphtheria, tetanus, and pertussis vaccine (p.1613) is used in the USA. For discussion of immunisation schedules, see under Vaccines, p.1606. In adults requiring primary immunisation a combined diphtheria, tetanus, and poliomyelitis (inactivated) vaccine is recommended. The primary immunisation course in the UK consists of 3 doses, each of 0.5 mL, administered at intervals of one month by intramuscular injection. In children who complete the primary course in infancy, reinforcing doses are given at school entry and on leaving school using the recommended appropriate combined vaccines. In adults, a reinforcing dose is desirable 10 years later with a further dose after a further 10 years.

The need for tetanus vaccines in wound management depends on both the condition of the wound and the patient's immunisation history. If primary immunisation or a reinforcing dose has been given within the last 10 years, tetanus vaccine should not be given but the patient should receive tetanus immunoglobulin if the risk of infection is considered especially high. If more than 10 years has elapsed, a reinforcing dose of a vaccine should be given. For tetanus-prone wounds, tetanus immunoglobulin (see above) may also be required. Tetanus vaccine and tetanus immunoglobulin may be given concomitantly, but not at the same site. In the event of injury in non-immunised persons or if immunisation status is uncertain, the opportunity is usually taken to initiate a course of primary immunisation. Since this provides no immediate protection, prophylactic treatment with tetanus immunoglobulin is recommended for tetanus-prone wounds. Suitable antibacterial therapy may also be given (see p.149).

**Anergy testing.** For reference to the use of tetanus vaccines for anergy testing in HIV-positive patients, see Tuberculins, p.1759.

**Bone marrow transplant recipients.** In a study[1] of 48 recipients of bone marrow transplants immunity to tetanus was not transferred from seropositive donors to seronegative patients. An unexpected finding was that pre-transplant antibody level of the patient, and not the donor, strongly influenced the antibody level one year after transplantation. Immunity quickly waned, however, after transplantation. Reimmunisation with tetanus vaccine is therefore required in long-term survivors of bone marrow transplants. The study suggested that 3 doses are needed to obtain adequate protection. The necessity for further doses requires study.

1. Ljungman P, *et al.* Response to tetanus toxoid immunization after allogeneic bone marrow transplantation. *J Infect Dis* 1990; **162:** 496–500.

**Neonatal tetanus.** In 1989 WHO adopted a resolution to eliminate neonatal tetanus after estimates revealed that worldwide (but excluding China) it was the cause of 800 000 neonatal deaths each year, a figure representing about 50% of all neonatal deaths in developing countries. Control of neonatal tetanus may be achieved by ensuring adequate hygiene during delivery and by ensuring protective immunity of the mother in late pregnancy. However, by mid-2000 there were 57 countries that had still not eliminated maternal and neonatal tetanus and WHO, UNICEF, and UNFPA agreed to set a target date of 2005 for elimination (defined as a rate of neonatal tetanus below 1 in 1000 live births at district level).

Tetanus vaccine is given to all women of child-bearing age as part of WHO's Expanded Programme on Immunization. For pregnant women, two doses of vaccine should be given, the second dose at least 4 weeks after the first and at least 2 weeks before delivery; this may provide the newborn infant with about 80% protection against tetanus. For all women of child-bearing age, three doses of vaccine, with at least 4 weeks between the first two doses and 6 to 12 months between the second and third doses, provide 95 to 98% protection for at least 5 years. Fourth and fifth doses, each at least one year after the previous dose, prolong the immunity for 10 and 20 years respectively.

**Reinforcing doses in adults.** Although the current recommendation in the UK is that 5 doses of tetanus vaccine (as a 3-dose primary course and 2 reinforcing doses at 10-year intervals) is sufficient to produce life-long immunity to tetanus, there has been concern about immunity in the elderly, and in particular women. Routine primary immunisation against tetanus was introduced in the UK in 1961, so individuals born before that year would not have been immunised in infancy, and unless they had been in the armed forces, may never have received a full primary course.[1] Unless there is a clear immunisation history immunity to tetanus may be difficult to assess.

Studies in the USA,[2] Australia,[3] and Austria[4] have shown that at least half of healthy people over 50 years of age did not have adequate circulating tetanus antibodies. However, the level of circulating antibodies in the absence of an antigen challenge may not be an appropriate measure of the immune status. The low incidence of clinical tetanus in adults provides circumstantial evidence of an adequate inducible antibody response on exposure to tetanus despite a decline in antibody concentrations with increasing age.[5,6] Conversely, there have been reports of tetanus occurring despite high antibody concentrations.[7,8] There have been calls for the introduction of regular booster injections in adults,[4,8-10] as is standard practice in the USA or alternatively a single booster in late middle age[11,12] or administering a primary course to elderly persons who have never received one.[2]

1. Department of Health. *Immunisation against infectious disease* 1996: "The Green Book". Available at: http://www.dh.gov.uk/PublicationsAndStatistics/Publications/PublicationsPolicyAndGuidance/PublicationsPolicyAndGuidanceArticle/fs/en?CONTENT_ID=4072977&chk=87uz6M (accessed 12/08/04)
2. Gergen PJ, *et al.* A population-based serologic survey of immunity to tetanus in the United States. *N Engl J Med* 1995; **332:** 761–6.
3. Heath TC, *et al.* Tetanus immunity in an older Australian population. *Med J Aust* 1996; **164:** 593–6.
4. Steger MM, *et al.* Vaccination against tetanus in the elderly: do recommended vaccination strategies give sufficient protection? *Lancet* 1996; **348:** 762.
5. Bowie C. Tetanus toxoid for adults—too much of a good thing. *Lancet* 1996; **348:** 1185–6.
6. Baily G. Are the elderly inadequately protected against tetanus? *Lancet* 1996; **348:** 1389–90.
7. Passen EL, Andersen BR. Clinical tetanus despite a 'protective' level of toxin-neutralising antibody. *JAMA* 1986; **255:** 1171–3.
8. Bowman C, *et al.* Tetanus toxoid for adults. *Lancet* 1996; **348:** 1664.
9. Rethy LA, Rethy L. Can tetanus boosting be rejected? *Lancet* 1997; **349:** 359–60.
10. Sehgal R. Tetanus toxoid for adults. *Lancet* 1997; **349:** 573.
11. Balestra DJ, Littenberg B. Tetanus immunization in adults. *JAMA* 1994; **272:** 1900.
12. Gardner P, LaForce FM. Protection against tetanus. *N Engl J Med* 1995; **333:** 599.

## Preparations

***BP 2003:*** Tetanus Vaccine;
***Ph. Eur.:*** Tetanus Vaccine (Adsorbed);
***USP 27:*** Tetanus Toxoid; Tetanus Toxoid Adsorbed.

**Proprietary Preparations** (details are given in Part 3)
***Arg.:*** Tetanol; Tetavax; ***Austral.:*** Tet-Tox; ***Austria:*** T-Immun†; Te Anatoxal; Tetanol; ***Belg.:*** Anatoxal Te†; Tetamer†; Tevax; ***Braz.:*** Tetavax; ***Chile:*** Tetavax; ***Ger.:*** T-Immun†; T-Medevax†; Tetamun SSW; Tetanol; Tetasorbat SSW†; Tetavax†; ***Gr.:*** Anatoxal-TE-Berna; ***Hong Kong:*** Te Anatoxal; Tetavax; ***Ital.:*** Anatetall; H-Atetal†; Imovax Tetano; Tanrix; Tetatox; ***Malaysia:*** Te Anatoxal; Tetavax; ***Mex.:*** Tetamyn; Tetanol; Tetinox; Toxanal†; ***Neth.:*** Tetavax; ***Norw.:*** Tetavax; ***NZ:*** Te Anatoxal; Tet-Tox; ***Port.:*** Anatoxal Te†; ***S.Afr.:*** Tetavax; ***Singapore:*** Te Anatoxal; ***Spain:*** Anatoxal Te; Vac Antitetanica†; ***Switz.:*** Anatoxal Te; ***Thai.:*** Anatetall; Te Anatoxal; Tetavax; ***UK:*** Clostet; Tetavax†; ***USA:*** Te Anatoxal.

# Tetanus and Influenza Vaccines

Vacunas del tétanos y la gripe.

## Profile

Tetanus and influenza vaccines are available in some countries for active immunisation against tetanus and influenza.

## Preparations

**Proprietary Preparations** (details are given in Part 3)
***Fr.:*** Tetagrip.

# Tetanus and Poliomyelitis Vaccines

Vacunas del tétanos y la poliomielitis.

## Profile

Tetanus and poliomyelitis (inactivated) vaccines are available in some countries for active immunisation against tetanus and poliomyelitis.

## Preparations

**Proprietary Preparations** (details are given in Part 3)
***Fr.:*** T. Polio; Vaccin TP.

# Tick Venom Antisera

Antisuero contra el veneno de garrapata; Tick Antivenins; Tick Antivenoms.

## Profile

An antiserum is available in Australia for treatment of the neurotoxic effects of envenomation by the tick *Ixodes holocyclus*.

The antiserum is prepared from the serum of dogs that have been immunised with tick venom.

Tick venom antiserum is given by slow intravenous infusion.

## Tick-borne Encephalitis Immunoglobulins

Inmunoglobulinas de la encefalitis transmitida por garrapatas.

*ATC — J06BB12.*

### Profile

Preparations containing antibodies against tick-borne encephalitis are available in some countries for passive immunisation against the disease.

### Preparations

**Proprietary Preparations** (details are given in Part 3)
***Austria:*** FSME-Bulin; ***Ger.:*** Encegam†; FSME-Bulin; ***Switz.:*** FSME-Bulin†.

## Tick-borne Encephalitis Vaccines

Vacunas de la encefalitis transmitida por garrapatas.

*ATC — J07BA01.*

**Pharmacopoeias.** Many pharmacopoeias have monographs including *Eur.* (see p.vi).

**Ph. Eur. 5.0** (Tick-borne Encephalitis Vaccine (Inactivated); Vaccinum Encephalitidis Ixodibus Advectae Inactivatum). A liquid preparation of a suitable strain of tick-borne encephalitis virus grown in cultures of chick-embryo cells or other suitable cell cultures and inactivated by a suitable method. It should be stored at 2° to 8°, not be allowed to freeze, and be protected from light.

### Adverse Effects and Precautions

As for vaccines in general, p.1605.

**Effects on the nervous system.** Severe progressive sensorimotor spastic paralysis occurred in a 54-year-old man after a second booster dose of tick-borne encephalitis vaccine.[1] Partial recovery was noted after about 6 months.

1. Bohus M, *et al.* Myelitis after immunisation against tick-borne encephalitis. *Lancet* 1993; **342:** 239–40.

### Interactions

As for vaccines in general, p.1606.

### Uses and Administration

A vaccine is available in some countries for active immunisation against tick-borne viral encephalitis.

In the UK, vaccination against tick-borne encephalitis is recommended for those who anticipate prolonged exposure to the infective agent, for example persons visiting or working in the warm forested parts of Europe and Scandinavia. The vaccine is given by intramuscular injection in a dose of 0.5 mL. A two-dose regimen with an interval of 3 to 12 weeks will provide protection for 1 year. A third dose 9 to 12 months after the second will give protection for 3 years. A further reinforcing dose may be given up to 6 years later if required. Reinforcing doses every 3 years are recommended for those at continued risk of exposure.

### Preparations

***Ph. Eur.:*** Tick-borne Encephalitis Vaccine (Inactivated).

**Proprietary Preparations** (details are given in Part 3)
***Austria:*** Encepur; FSME-Immun; ***Belg.:*** FSME-Immun†; ***Fin.:*** Encepur; ***Fr.:*** Ticovac†; ***Ger.:*** Encepur; ***Swed.:*** Encepur; ***Switz.:*** Encepur; FSME-Immun; ***UK:*** FSME-Immun.

## Trichomoniasis Vaccines

Vacunas de la tricomoniasis.

### Profile

A trichomoniasis vaccine containing inactivated *Lactobacillus acidophilus* is available in some countries for the prophylaxis of recurrent vaginal trichomoniasis. The vaccine is reported to stimulate production of antibodies against the aberrant coccoid forms of the lactobacilli associated with trichomoniasis and also, by cross-reaction, against the trichomonads themselves.

### Preparations

**Proprietary Preparations** (details are given in Part 3)
***Ger.:*** Gynatren; ***Ital.:*** Ginatren†.

## Tularaemia Vaccines

Vacunas de la tularemia.

### Profile

A tularaemia vaccine prepared from a live attenuated strain of *Francisella tularensis* has been used for active immunisation against tularaemia in persons at high risk of contracting the disease.

◊ References.

1. Titball R, Oyston P. A vaccine for tularaemia. *Expert Opin Biol Ther* 2003; **3:** 645–53.

## Typhoid Vaccines

Vacunas de la fiebre tifoidea.

*ATC — J07AP01; J07AP02; J07AP03.*

**Pharmacopoeias.** Many pharmacopoeias have monographs including *Br.* and *Eur.* (see p.vi).

**Ph. Eur. 5.0** (Typhoid Vaccine; Vaccinum Febris Typhoidi). A sterile suspension of inactivated *Salmonella typhi* containing not less than 500 million and not more than 1000 million bacteria per dose which does not exceed 1 mL. It is prepared from a suitable strain of *S. typhi* such as Ty 2. The bacteria are inactivated by heat, or by treatment with acetone, formaldehyde, or phenol, or by phenol and heat. The vaccine should be stored at 2° to 8°, and be protected from light.

**Ph. Eur. 5.0** (Typhoid Vaccine, Freeze-dried; Vaccinum Febris Typhoidi Cryodesiccatum). A freeze-dried preparation of inactivated *Salmonella typhi* containing not less than 500 million and not more than 1000 million bacteria per dose which does not exceed 1 mL. It is prepared from a suitable strain of *S. typhi* such as Ty 2. The bacteria are inactivated by heat, or by treatment with acetone or formaldehyde. Phenol may not be used in the preparation. The vaccine should be stored at 2° to 8°, and be protected from light. It is reconstituted by the addition of suitable sterile liquid and should be used within 8 hours.

**BP 2003** (Typhoid Vaccine). When Typhoid Vaccine is issued as a liquid, it complies with the requirements of Typhoid Vaccine (Ph. Eur. 5.0). When Typhoid Vaccine is prepared immediately before use by reconstitution from the dried vaccine, the dried vaccine complies with the requirements of Typhoid Vaccine, Freeze-dried (Ph. Eur. 5.0).

The BP 2003 states that Typhoid/Vac or Dried/Typhoid/Vac may be used on the label as appropriate.

**Ph. Eur. 5.0** (Typhoid Vaccine (Live, Oral, Strain Ty 21a); Vaccinum Febris Typhoidis Vivum Perorale (Stirpe Ty 21a)). A freeze-dried preparation of live *S. typhi* strain Ty 21a grown in a suitable medium. It contains not less than $2 \times 10^9$ bacteria per dose. It should be stored at 2° to 8°, and be protected from light.

The BP 2003 states that Typhoid/Vac(Oral) may be used on the label.

**Ph. Eur. 5.0** (Typhoid Polysaccharide Vaccine; Vaccinum Febris Typhoidis Polysaccharidicum). A preparation of purified Vi capsular polysaccharide obtained from *S. typhi* Ty2 strain or some other suitable strain that has the capacity to produce Vi polysaccharide. It contains 25 micrograms of polysaccharide per dose. It should be stored at 2° to 8° and be protected from light.

The BP 2003 states that Typhoid/Vi/Vac may be used on the label.

### Adverse Effects and Precautions

As for vaccines in general, p.1605.

Oral live typhoid and parenteral polysaccharide vaccines have been associated with fewer adverse effects than parenteral killed typhoid vaccines.

### Interactions

As for vaccines in general, p.1606. Oral typhoid vaccine should not be given to individuals receiving antibacterials since the development of immunity may be impaired. Individuals receiving mefloquine for malaria prophylaxis should not take oral typhoid vaccine on the same day or, if this is unavoidable, within 12 hours of the mefloquine dose.

### Uses and Administration

Typhoid vaccines are used for active immunisation against typhoid fever. As with many vaccines, the efficacy of typhoid vaccine is not complete and the importance of maintaining attention to hygiene should be emphasised to those travelling to endemic areas.

Typhoid vaccination is advised for laboratory workers handling specimens which may contain typhoid organisms and for persons travelling to areas where typhoid fever is endemic. In the UK, vaccination of contacts of a known typhoid carrier is not recommended; in the USA such persons are advised to receive the vaccine. Typhoid vaccine is not useful in controlling outbreaks of the disease.

In the UK, two vaccines have been used: a capsular polysaccharide vaccine for parenteral use, and a live oral vaccine that is no longer available.

The capsular polysaccharide typhoid vaccine contains 25 micrograms of the Vi polysaccharide antigen per dose. A single dose of 0.5 mL is given by deep subcutaneous or intramuscular injection. Booster doses may be given every 3 years to those who remain at risk. The response in children under 18 months of age may be suboptimal, and the decision to vaccinate will be governed by the risk of exposure to infection.

The live oral typhoid vaccine contained an attenuated strain of *Salmonella typhi*, Ty 21a, and was administered as enteric-coated capsules containing not less than $2 \times 10^9$ bacteria per dose. A primary immunisation schedule of one capsule every other day for 3 doses was given.

A monovalent whole-cell killed vaccine was also formerly available, and was given parenterally in two doses at an interval of 4 to 6 weeks. The first dose was given by intramuscular or deep subcutaneous injection, although subsequent doses could be given intradermally to reduce adverse reactions.

In the USA, whole-cell parenteral, capsular polysaccharide, and live oral vaccines are available. The former is given in a primary course of two injections of 0.5 mL, given subcutaneously at an interval of 4 or more weeks to adults and children over 10 years of age; children from 6 months to 10 years may be given two doses of 0.25 mL. An additional alternative accelerated schedule of three doses at weekly intervals may be employed, although this may be less effective than the standard two-dose schedule. Booster doses should be given every 3 years. The capsular polysaccharide vaccine is given intramuscularly similarly to that in the UK, with a booster dose suggested every 2 years. For the oral vaccine, 4 doses on alternate days is recommended for both primary immunisation and boosters, which are given every 5 years if exposure continues.

**Immunisation for travellers.** In most developed countries where typhoid is not endemic, the major use for typhoid vaccine is for non-immune travellers visiting endemic areas. Doubts have been raised over the necessity for typhoid vaccination for the majority of travellers because of the rarity of the disease in travellers and the unproven efficacy of the available vaccines in this population.[1] The highest incidence of the disease is associated with travel to the Indian subcontinent and parts of tropical South America, although immunisation is also recommended for travellers to lower risk areas of Africa, Asia, and south-east Europe.[1,2] By far the most important form of protection against gastrointestinal infection is strict attention to personal, food, and water hygiene, although in practice this advice is often difficult to follow.

None of the vaccines used has been 100% effective in preventing disease. The effectiveness of the vaccines has generally been assessed in field trials in the populations of endemic areas. Such populations acquire a degree of natural immunity due to continued exposure and it may not be possible to equate protection rates in these populations to non-immune travellers.[1] The whole-cell vaccine has been evaluated in non-immune subjects[3] and was shown to confer partial protection against a relatively low inoculum compared with that likely to be encountered from foodborne transmission.[1] The live oral vaccine has been shown to confer a useful degree of immunity in field trials[4,5] but the dose used may have been insufficient to protect non-immune individuals. The degree of immunity induced may be increased by the use of higher inocula[6] or liquid preparations.[5,7] In addition, compliance with dosing and storage requirements may further limit the effectiveness of this dosage form.[8]

Two large field studies[9,10] have verified the effectiveness of the capsular polysaccharide vaccine but its efficacy has not been assessed in non-immune populations. However, it does have the advantage of being administered as a single dose.

A meta-analysis[11] of randomised studies concluded that whole-cell vaccines are more efficacious than the capsular polysaccharide and oral vaccines, but are more frequently associated with adverse effects.

For individuals who have previously received the whole-cell vaccine without difficulty, there is no need to change to the newer vaccines, especially since booster doses can be given intradermally to reduce adverse reactions. The single dose required for the capsular polysaccharide vaccine may recommend it for primary immunisation. The oral vaccine may have obvious advantages in patient acceptability but it is expensive and the importance of correct storage and dosing should be stressed.[2]

1. Anonymous. Typhoid vaccination: weighing the options. *Lancet* 1992; **340:** 341–2.
2. Anonymous. Typhoid vaccines—which one to choose? *Drug Ther Bull* 1993; **31:** 9–10.
3. Hornick RB, *et al.* Typhoid fever: pathogenesis and immunologic control, part 2. *N Engl J Med* 1970; **283:** 739–46.
4. Levine MM, *et al.* Large-scale field trial of Ty21a live oral typhoid vaccine in enteric-coated capsule formulation. *Lancet* 1987; **i:** 1049–52.
5. Simanjuntak CH, *et al.* Oral immunisation against typhoid fever in Indonesia with Ty21a vaccine. *Lancet* 1991; **338:** 1055–9.

6. Ferreccio C, *et al.* Comparative efficacy of two, three, or four doses of Ty21a live oral typhoid vaccine in enteric-coated capsules: a field trial in an endemic area. *J Infect Dis* 1989; **159:** 766–9.
7. Levine MM, *et al.* Comparison of enteric-coated capsules and liquid formulation of Ty21a typhoid vaccine in randomised controlled field trial. *Lancet* 1990; **336:** 891–4.
8. Kaplan DT, *et al.* Compliance with live, oral Ty21a typhoid vaccine. *JAMA* 1992; **267:** 1074.
9. Acharya IL, *et al.* Prevention of typhoid fever in Nepal with the Vi capsular polysaccharide of Salmonella typhi: a preliminary report. *N Engl J Med* 1987; **317:** 1101–4.
10. Klugman KP, *et al.* Protective activity of Vi capsular polysaccharide vaccine against typhoid fever. *Lancet* 1987; **ii:** 1165–9.
11. Engels EA, *et al.* Typhoid fever vaccines: a meta-analysis of studies on efficacy and toxicity. *BMJ* 1998; **316:** 110–16.

### Preparations

***Ph. Eur.:*** Freeze-dried Typhoid Vaccine; Typhoid Polysaccharide Vaccine; Typhoid Vaccine; Typhoid Vaccine (Live, Oral, Strain Ty 21a).

**Proprietary Preparations** (details are given in Part 3)

***Arg.:*** Typhim Vi; Vivotif; ***Austral.:*** Typh-Vax; Typherix; Typhim Vi; Vivaxim; ***Austria:*** Typherix; Typhim Vi; Vivotif; ***Belg.:*** Typherix; Typhim Vi; Vivotif; ***Canad.:*** Typherix; Typhim Vi; Vivotif; ***Chile:*** Typhim Vi; ***Denm.:*** Typhim Vi; Vivotif; ***Fin.:*** Typherix; Typhim Vi; Vivotif; ***Fr.:*** Typherix; Typhim Vi; ***Ger.:*** Typherix; Typhim Vi; Typhoral L; Vivotif; ***Hong Kong:*** Typhim Vi; Vivotif; ***India:*** Typhoral; Vactyph; ***Irl.:*** Typherix; Typhim Vi; Vivotif; ***Israel:*** Typherix; Typhim Vi; Vivotif; ***Ital.:*** Enterovaccino ISI (Antitifico)†; Enterovaccino Nuovo ISM†; Neotyf†; Typherix; Typhim Vi; Vivotif; ***Malaysia:*** Typhim Vi; Typhovax; Vivotif; ***Neth.:*** Typherix; Typhim Vi; ***Norw.:*** Typherix; Typhim Vi; Vivotif; ***NZ:*** Typh-Vax; Typherix; Typhim Vi; ***Port.:*** Vivotif; ***S.Afr.:*** Typhim Vi; Vivotif; ***Singapore:*** Typherix; Typhim Vi; Vivotif; ***Spain:*** Typhim Vi; Vac Antitifica Or†; Vivotif; ***Swed.:*** Typherix; Typhim Vi; Vivotif; ***Switz.:*** Vaccin Tab†; Vivotif; ***Thai.:*** Typhim Vi; Vivotif; ***UK:*** Typherix; Typhim Vi; Vivotif†; ***USA:*** Typhim Vi; Vivotif.

## Typhoid and Tetanus Vaccines

Vacunas de la fiebre tifoidea y del tétanos.

### Profile

A combined typhoid and tetanus vaccine has been used by subcutaneous injection for primary immunisation against typhoid fever and tetanus and by intramuscular injection to reinforce immunity.

## Typhus Vaccines

Vacunas de la rickettsiosis típica.

### Profile

Typhus vaccines may be used for active immunisation against louse-borne typhus. Their use may be considered for those living in or visiting the few endemic areas who are likely to have close contact with the indigenous population, including health care workers, and for laboratory workers. They do not provide protection against scrub typhus.

## Vaccinia Immunoglobulins

Inmunoglobulinas contra el virus de la vacuna.

*ATC — J06BB07.*

**Pharmacopoeias.** Many pharmacopoeias have monographs including *US.*

**USP 27** (Vaccinia Immune Globulin). A sterile solution of globulins derived from the plasma of adult human donors who have been immunised with vaccinia virus (smallpox vaccine). It contains 15 to 18% of protein, of which not less than 90% is gamma globulin. It contains glycine as a stabilising agent, and a suitable antimicrobial agent. It should be stored at 2° to 8°.

### Profile

Vaccinia immunoglobulins have been used for the treatment of clinical complications of smallpox vaccination. They are not effective for postviral encephalitis.

### Preparations

***USP 27:*** Vaccinia Immune Globulin.

# Varicella-Zoster Immunoglobulins

Inmunoglobulinas contra el virus de la varicela zóster.

*ATC — J06BB03.*

**Pharmacopoeias.** Many pharmacopoeias have monographs including *Eur.* (see p.vi) and *US.*

**Ph. Eur. 5.0** (Human Varicella Immunoglobulin; Immunoglobulinum Humanum Varicellae). A liquid or freeze-dried preparation containing immunoglobulins, mainly immunoglobulin G (IgG). It is obtained from plasma from selected donors having specific antibodies against *Herpesvirus varicellae*. Normal immunoglobulin may be added. It contains not less than 100 international units/mL. The liquid and freeze-dried preparations should be stored, protected from light, in a colourless, glass container. The freeze-dried preparation should be stored under vacuum or under inert gas.

**Ph. Eur. 5.0** (Human Varicella Immunoglobulin for Intravenous Administration; Immunoglobulinum Humanum Varicellae ad Usum Intravenosum). A liquid or freeze-dried preparation containing immunoglobulins, mainly immunoglobulin G (IgG). It is obtained from plasma from selected donors having antibodies against human herpesvirus 3 (varicella-zoster virus 1). Human normal immunoglobulin for intravenous administration may be added. It contains not less than 25 international units/mL. Storage requirements are similar to those for Human Varicella Immunoglobulin, except that the freeze-dried preparation is stored at a temperature not exceeding 25°.

**USP 27** (Varicella-Zoster Immune Globulin). A sterile solution of globulins derived from the plasma of adult donors selected for high titres of varicella-zoster antibodies. It contains 15 to 18% of globulins, of which not less than 99% is immunoglobulin G with traces of immunoglobulin A and immunoglobulin M. It contains glycine as a stabilising agent and thiomersal as a preservative. It contains not less than 125 units of specific antibody in not more than 2.5 mL of solution. It should be stored at 2° to 8°.

### Adverse Effects and Precautions

As for immunoglobulins in general, p.1605.

### Interactions

As for immunoglobulins in general, p.1605.

### Uses and Administration

Varicella-zoster immunoglobulins are used for passive immunisation against varicella (chickenpox) in susceptible persons considered to be at high risk of developing varicella-associated complications after exposure to varicella or herpes zoster (shingles).

In the UK, varicella-zoster immunoglobulins are recommended for individuals who are at high risk of severe varicella and who have no antibodies to varicella-zoster virus and who have significant exposure to chickenpox or herpes zoster. Those at increased risk include immunosuppressed patients, neonates including those whose mothers develop chickenpox (but not herpes zoster) in the period 7 days before to 7 days after delivery, and pregnant women. Varicella-zoster immunoglobulin does not prevent infection when given after exposure but may modify the course of disease. Treatment with antivirals may be necessary in severe disease (see p.621).

The doses, given by deep intramuscular injection, of the varicella-zoster immunoglobulin available in the UK are: 250 mg for children up to 5 years of age; 500 mg for those aged 6 to 10 years; 750 mg for those aged 11 to 14 years; and 1 g for all those 15 years of age or older. A further dose is required if a second exposure occurs more than 3 weeks later. Varicella-zoster immunoglobulin should be given as soon as possible and not later than 10 days after exposure. Preparations of normal immunoglobulin for intravenous use may be used to provide an immediate source of antibody.

Recommendations in the USA are similar to those in the UK. Doses are 125 units per 10 kg body-weight by intramuscular injection up to a maximum of 625 units. Adults may be given 625 units but higher doses may be required in immunocompromised patients. Administration should start within 96 hours of exposure.

### Preparations

***Ph. Eur.:*** Human Varicella Immunoglobulin; Human Varicella Immunoglobulin for Intravenous Administration;
***USP 27:*** Varicella-Zoster Immune Globulin.

**Proprietary Preparations** (details are given in Part 3)

***Austria:*** Varitect; ***Ger.:*** Varicellon; Varitect; ***Gr.:*** Varitect; ***Hong Kong:*** Varitect; ***Irl.:*** Varitect; ***Israel:*** Varitect; ***Ital.:*** Haimazig†; Immunoendozig†; Immunozig†; Intrazig†; Uman-Vzig; Var-Zeta†; Varitect; ***Port.:*** Varitect; ***S.Afr.:*** Vazigam; ***Singapore:*** Varitect; ***Switz.:*** Varitect; ***Thai.:*** Varitect.

# Varicella-Zoster Vaccines

Vacunas de la varicela zóster.

*ATC — J07BK01.*

**Pharmacopoeias.** Many pharmacopoeias have monographs including *Eur.* (see p.vi).

**Ph. Eur. 5.0** (Varicella Vaccine (Live); Vaccinum Varicellae Vivum). A freeze-dried preparation of a suitable attenuated strain of *Herpesvirus varicellae* grown in cultures of human diploid cells. The culture medium may contain suitable antibiotics at the smallest effective concentration. It is prepared immediately before use by reconstitution from the dried vaccine; it may contain a stabiliser. The vaccine contains not less than 2000 plaque-forming units per dose. The dried vaccine should be stored at 2° to 8°. Protect from light.

The BP 2003 states that Var/Vac(Live) may be used on the label.

### Adverse Effects and Precautions

As for vaccines in general, p.1605.

Rashes at the injection site and varicella-like rashes elsewhere have been reported. It is not known whether the virus becomes latent, which could result in late development of zoster infections, although there are early indications that the incidence of herpes zoster is lower after vaccination than in an unvaccinated population.

◊ General references.

1. Black S, *et al.* Postmarketing evaluation of the safety and effectiveness of varicella vaccine. *Pediatr Infect Dis J* 1999; **18:** 1041–6.

**Pregnancy.** Transmission of the vaccine strain of varicella virus has been reported from a young child to his pregnant mother.[1] After elective termination of the pregnancy, no virus was detected in the fetus.

1. Salzman MB, *et al.* Transmission of varicella-vaccine virus from a healthy 12-month-old child to his pregnant mother. *J Pediatr* 1997; **131:** 151–4.

### Interactions

As for vaccines in general, p.1606.

### Uses and Administration

Varicella-zoster vaccines may be used for active immunisation against varicella (chickenpox) in persons considered to be at high risk of either contracting the infection or to be highly susceptible to any complications it may cause; such patients include susceptible health-care workers, and healthy contacts of immunocompromised patients when continuing close contact is unavoidable.

In the USA, vaccination against varicella is recommended as part of the primary immunisation schedule (see under Vaccines, p.1606). A single dose of 0.5 mL is given subcutaneously at 12 to 18 months of age to healthy children unless there is a reliable history of varicella, although children may receive the vaccine at any subsequent time between the ages of 2 to 18 years if not previously received. Persons over the age of 13 years at increased risk of exposure or complications should receive two doses at an interval of 4 to 8 weeks.

◊ Although the results of studies of varicella-zoster vaccines in healthy and leukaemic children have been largely favourable, until recently these vaccines had not been recommended for routine use in the UK or USA. Protective **efficacy** in healthy children appears to be over 90%. In healthy adolescents and adults, adding a second dose 4 or 8 weeks after the first increased seroconversion rates from about 70 to 80% to 97% or better.[1] A protective efficacy of about 85% has been reported in leukaemic children given one dose of varicella-zoster vaccine.[2,3] A two-dose regimen (doses separated by 3 months) has been tried. Although a second dose is probably of benefit to those who do not seroconvert after one dose, its additional benefit to those who do seroconvert is doubtful.[3] Interruption of chemotherapy for vaccination does not appear necessary in terms of immunogenicity of the vaccine.[2,4] A higher rate of vaccine-associated rashes has, however, been observed in leukaemic children when chemotherapy was suspended for 2 weeks compared with those whose chemotherapy had previously been terminated; this only occurred with certain lots of vaccine.[2]

The **duration of immunity** after varicella-zoster vaccination is also under debate. Studies indicate that the immunity induced by natural infection with wild type virus is superior to that induced by the vaccine. In one study,[3] about one-quarter of all vaccinees (both leukaemic children and healthy adults) were seronegative one year after a second dose of vaccine, but none were seronegative after up to 6 years after breakthrough varicella infection. However, immunity to varicella-zoster is complex, depending not only on circulating antibody but also on cellular immunity and secretory antibody. Thus, although a person may become seronegative after vaccination, protection from varicella may remain, albeit partial.[2] Both humoral and cell mediated immunity have been shown to persist for up to 20 years after vaccination.[5] Leukaemic children observed up to 6 years after immunisation have continued to be well protected[2] and varicella in previously-vaccinated persons is usually mild.[2,3]

There is some controversy over vaccinating healthy children, mainly due to uncertainties over long-term consequences and the impact vaccination may have on unimmunised members of the population. Two studies[6,7] in the USA suggested that inclusion of varicella vaccines into routine **immunisation schedules** in infants could be cost effective, particularly if work time lost by parents caring for sick children is included in the calculation. This view was rigorously opposed by clinicians who considered that such a step would be premature.[8-10] Nevertheless, the American Academy of Pediatrics Committee on Infectious Diseases does recommend universal vaccination of healthy children at age 12 to 18 months, and in susceptible older children and adolescents.[11] Similar recommendations apply to persons with impaired humoral (but not cellular) immunity and some HIV-infected children.[12,13] The US Advisory Committee on Immunization Practices recommends[12] that, in addition, varicella-zoster vaccine be given to all susceptible persons over age 13 who live or work in environments where transmission can or is likely to occur to non-pregnant women of child-bearing age, to those who live in households with children, and to those travelling abroad.

Varicella-zoster vaccine may prevent or modify varicella if given within 3 days of exposure to the infection. In the USA, vaccination is now recommended in all susceptible persons following exposure to varicella.[12,13] It may be useful as an **adjunct** to varicella-zoster immunoglobulin. The treatment of varicella-zoster infections with antivirals is discussed on p.621.

One concern of varicella-zoster vaccination has been the possibility of an **increased risk of herpes zoster** (shingles) in immunised children. Although herpes zoster has been reported in vaccinated persons, a study involving 346 leukaemic children and 84 matched controls concluded that the incidence of herpes zoster following varicella-zoster vaccine was no greater than that following natural varicella infection.[14] The study did suggest that the risk of herpes zoster may be lowered by vaccination but this must be confirmed by long-term follow-up. Postmarketing surveys[12,15] of almost 90 000 vaccine recipients also showed a low incidence of herpes zoster. The vaccine strain of varicella-zoster virus is transmissible, particularly from vaccinees who develop a rash (see also Pregnancy under Adverse Effects, above). There is no evidence of reversion to virulence of the vaccine strain with secondary transmission.

Another concern is that vaccination of children could result in more severe infections in later life after immunity has waned. However, studies have shown that in general varicella is less severe in previously immunised than in non-immunised patients.[16,17]


1. Kuter BJ, *et al.* Safety, tolerability, and immunogenicity of two regimens of Oka/Merck varicella vaccine (Varivax) in healthy adolescents and adults. *Vaccine* 1995; **13:** 967 72.
2. Gershon AA, *et al.* Persistence of immunity to varicella in children with leukemia immunized with live attenuated varicella vaccine. *N Engl J Med* 1989; **320:** 892–7.
3. Gershon AA, *et al.* Live attenuated varicella vaccine: protection in healthy adults compared with leukemic children. *J Infect Dis* 1990; **161:** 661–6.
4. Arbeter AM, *et al.* Immunization of children with acute lymphoblastic leukemia with live attenuated varicella vaccine without complete suspension of chemotherapy. *Pediatrics* 1990; **85:** 338–44.
5. Asano Y, *et al.* Experience and reason: twenty-year follow-up of protective immunity of the Oka strain live varicella vaccine. *Pediatrics* 1994; **94:** 524–6.
6. Huse DM, *et al.* Childhood vaccination against chickenpox: an analysis of benefits and costs. *J Pediatr* 1994; **124:** 869–74.
7. Lieu TA, *et al.* Cost-effectiveness of a routine varicella vaccination program for US children. *JAMA* 1994; **271:** 375–81.
8. Bader M, Oswego L. Varicella vaccine. *JAMA* 1994; **271:** 1744–5.
9. Smukler M. Routine childhood varicella vaccination. *JAMA* 1994; **271:** 1906.
10. Ross LF, Lantos JD. Immunisation against chickenpox. *BMJ* 1995; **310:** 2–3.
11. Committee on Infectious Diseases. Recommendations for the use of live attenuated varicella vaccine. *Pediatrics* 1995; **95:** 791–6. Correction. *ibid.*; **96** (1).
12. Centers for Disease Control. Prevention of varicella: updated recommendations of the Advisory Committee on Immunization Practices (ACIP). *MMWR* 1999; **48** (RR-6): 1–5.
13. Committee on Infectious Diseases, American Academy of Pediatrics. Varicella vaccine update. *Pediatrics* 2000; **105:** 136–41.
14. Lawrence R, *et al.* The risk of zoster after varicella vaccination in children with leukemia. *N Engl J Med* 1988; **318:** 543–8.
15. Black S, *et al.* Postmarketing evaluation of the safety and effectiveness of varicella vaccine. *Pediatr Infect Dis J* 1999; **18:** 1041–6.
16. Watson BM, *et al.* Modified chickenpox in children immunized with the Oka/Merck varicella vaccine. *Pediatrics* 1993; **91:** 17–22.
17. Bernstein HH, *et al.* Clinical survey of natural varicella compared with breakthrough varicella after immunization with live attenuated Oka/Merck varicella vaccine. *Pediatrics* 1993; **92:** 833–7.


## Preparations

***Ph. Eur.:*** Varicella Vaccine (Live).

**Proprietary Preparations** (details are given in Part 3)
***Arg.:*** Varicela Biken; Varilrix; ***Austral.:*** Varilrix; Varivax; ***Austria:*** Varicella†; Varilrix; ***Belg.:*** Varilrix; ***Braz.:*** Varilrix; Varivax; ***Canad.:*** Varivax; ***Chile:*** Varicela Biken; Varilrix; ***Denm.:*** Varilrix; ***Fin.:*** Varilrix; ***Ger.:*** Varilrix; ***Hong Kong:*** Varilrix; Varivax; ***India:*** Varilrix; ***Irl.:*** Varivax; ***Ital.:*** Varilrix; Varivax; ***Malaysia:*** Okavax; Varilrix; Varivax; ***Mex.:*** Varilrix; Varivax; ***Norw.:*** Varilrix; ***NZ:*** Varilrix; ***S.Afr.:*** Varilrix; ***Singapore:*** Varilrix; Varivax; ***Spain:*** Varilrix; ***Swed.:*** Varilrix; ***Switz.:*** Varilrix; ***Thai.:*** Okavax; Varilrix; ***UK:*** Varilrix; Varivax; ***USA:*** Varivax.

# Yellow Fever Vaccines

Vacunas de la fiebre amarilla.
*ATC — J07BL01.*

**Pharmacopoeias.** Many pharmacopoeias have monographs including *Eur.* (see p.vi) and *US.*

**Ph. Eur. 5.0** (Yellow Fever Vaccine (Live); Vaccinum Febris Flavae Vivum). A freeze-dried preparation of the 17D strain of yellow fever virus grown in fertilised hen eggs. It is reconstituted immediately before use. It should be stored at 2° to 8° and be protected from light.

The BP 2003 states that Yel/Vac may be used on the label.

**USP 27** (Yellow Fever Vaccine). A freeze-dried preparation of a selected attenuated strain of live yellow fever virus cultured in chick embryos. It is reconstituted, just prior to use, by the addition of sodium chloride containing no antimicrobial agent. It should be stored under nitrogen preferably below 0° but not above 5°.

## Adverse Effects and Precautions

As for vaccines in general, p.1605.

Local and general reactions are not common after vaccination for yellow fever. Very rarely encephalitis has occurred, generally in infants under 9 months of age. Therefore, yellow fever vaccine is not usually given to infants under 9 months (but see below).

There is as yet insufficient data on the safety of yellow fever vaccine in HIV-positive individuals. In the UK, use of yellow fever vaccine in such individuals is not recommended. WHO advises that the vaccine should be given to HIV-positive individuals who are asymptomatic if the risk of infection is high.

**Fatalities.** There have been a few case reports of fatalities resulting from haemorrhagic fever,[1] hepatitis,[2] and multisystem organ failure[3] associated with the use of yellow fever vaccines.


1. Vasconcelos PFC, *et al.* Serious adverse events associated with yellow fever 17DD vaccine in Brazil: a report of two cases. *Lancet* 2001; **358:** 91–7. Corrections. *ibid.*; 336. *ibid.*; 1018.
2. Chan RC, *et al.* Hepatitis and death following vaccination with 17D-204 yellow fever vaccine. *Lancet* 2001; **358:** 121–2.
3. Martin M, *et al.* Fever and multisystem organ failure associated with 17D-204 yellow fever vaccination: a report of four cases. *Lancet* 2001; **358:** 98–104.


**Effects on the nervous system.** Encephalitis may occur very rarely following vaccination against yellow fever, but WHO in 1986 stated[1] that not more than 17 cases of encephalitis had been recorded over a period of 40 years and all occurred in children; although it was possible that some cases may have gone unrecorded, the number would be very small in proportion to the tens of millions of immunisations performed without known encephalitic complications. As a precaution against possible encephalitic complications, infants under 9 months of age are not generally immunised but it may be advisable to immunise children at 6 months of age if they live in rural areas with a history of yellow fever epidemics, and even at 4 months in an active epidemic focus; no child less than 4 months old should receive yellow fever vaccine.


1. WHO. *Prevention and control of yellow fever in Africa.* Geneva: WHO, 1986.


**Pregnancy.** Although yellow fever vaccine has been given to women during pregnancy without producing adverse effects in the infants,[1] fetal infection has been reported.[2]


1. Nasidi A, *et al.* Yellow fever vaccination and pregnancy: a four-year prospective study. *Trans R Soc Trop Med Hyg* 1993; **87:** 337–9.
2. Tsai TF, *et al.* Congenital yellow fever virus infection after immunization in pregnancy. *J Infect Dis* 1993; **168:** 1520–3.


## Interactions

As for vaccines in general, p.1606.

◊ There have been several studies on the combined use of yellow fever vaccine and other vaccines.[1] The administration of measles vaccine and yellow fever vaccine at the same site has resulted in a decrease in the rate of seroconversions to yellow fever but the injection was made intradermally. When given at different sites, and when diphtheria, tetanus, and pertussis vaccine was also added, no interference was shown. Cholera vaccines should not be given together with yellow fever vaccine, or in the preceding 3 weeks, since the yellow fever neutralising antibody response is reduced at least temporarily. Pooled human immunoglobulin given before, at the same time as, or after yellow fever vaccine does not impair the rate of serological conversion.


1. WHO. *Prevention and control of yellow fever in Africa.* Geneva: WHO, 1986.


## Uses and Administration

Yellow fever vaccines are used for active immunisation against yellow fever. Immunity is usually established within about 10 days of administration and persists for many years. Only one dose is required for immunisation and is given by deep subcutaneous injection; the dose (0.5 mL) is the volume containing at least 1000 mouse $LD_{50}$ units.

In the UK, immunisation against yellow fever is recommended for laboratory workers handling infected material, for persons travelling through or living in areas of infection, and for travellers entering countries which require an International Certificate of Vaccination. The immunity produced may last for life although officially an International Certificate of Vaccination against yellow fever is valid only for 10 years starting 10 days after the primary immunisation and only if the vaccine used has been approved by WHO and administered at a designated vaccinating centre.

Vaccination under 9 months of age is not generally recommended (see under Adverse Effects and Precautions, above).

◊ General references.


1. Barrett ADT. Yellow fever vaccines. *Biologicals* 1997; **25:** 17–25.


◊ Recommendations of the Advisory Committee on Immunization Practices for the prevention of yellow fever in the USA.[1]


1. Centers for Disease Control. Yellow fever vaccine: recommendations of the Advisory Committee on Immunization Practices (ACIP), 2002. *MMWR* 2002; **51** (RR-17): 1–11.


**Immunisation schedules.** The 17D (Rockefeller) yellow fever vaccine is now the only yellow fever vaccine produced.[1] The quantity available in the world has been limited and its relatively short half-life does not permit the accumulation of large stocks. The demand for the vaccine is also somewhat irregular, being suddenly high during epidemics and low during inter-epidemic periods.

In Africa two different strategies for yellow fever immunisation have been followed.[1] Firstly, an emergency immunisation programme takes place once an outbreak has begun, in an attempt to limit the spread of infection by immunising all persons in the focus, regardless of their former immune status. One disadvantage is that immunity does not appear until 7 days after immunisation and deaths may be expected to occur in the interim period. Secondly, a routine mass immunisation programme for yellow fever is aimed at immunising in advance all populations considered to be at risk. Yellow fever vaccine may be considered for inclusion in a national Expanded Programme on Immunization; there are obvious logistic advantages in administering it at the age of 9 months at the same time as measles vaccine. In rural areas of the endemic zone that are considered at high risk, the minimum age for routine immunisation may be lowered to 6 months (see under Adverse Effects and Precautions, above).


1. WHO. *Prevention and control of yellow fever in Africa.* Geneva: WHO, 1986.


**Immunisation for travellers.** A booklet entitled *International Travel and Health* is published annually by WHO. Information is provided concerning the countries in Africa and South America where yellow fever is endemic and also countries requiring a traveller to hold a valid vaccination certificate. For some further details, see p.1607.

## Preparations

***Ph. Eur.:*** Yellow Fever Vaccine (Live);
***USP 27:*** Yellow Fever Vaccine.

**Proprietary Preparations** (details are given in Part 3)
***Arg.:*** Stamaril; ***Austral.:*** Stamaril; ***Belg.:*** Stamaril; ***Canad.:*** YF-Vax; ***Chile:*** Stamaril; ***Denm.:*** Stamaril; ***Fin.:*** Arilvax; Stamaril; ***Fr.:*** Stamaril; ***Ger.:*** Stamaril; ***Irl.:*** Arilvax; Stamaril; ***Israel:*** Arilvax; ***Ital.:*** Stamaril; ***Malaysia:*** Stamaril; ***Neth.:*** Arilvax; Stamaril; ***Norw.:*** Stamaril; ***S.Afr.:*** Arilvax; Stamaril; ***Singapore:*** Arilvax; Stamaril; ***Swed.:*** Arilvax; Stamaril; ***Switz.:*** Arilvax; Stamaril; ***UK:*** Arilvax; Stamaril; ***USA:*** YF-Vax.

# Part 2

# Supplementary Drugs and Other Substances

This chapter includes some drugs not easily classified, herbal medicines, new drugs whose place in therapy is not yet clear, and drugs no longer used clinically but still of interest. There are also monographs on toxic substances, the effects of which may require drug therapy.

## Abrus

Abrus Seed; Indian Liquorice; Jequirity Bean; Jumble Beads; Prayer Beads; Regaliz americano; Rosary Beans.

### Profile

Abrus consists of the seeds of *Abrus precatorius* (Leguminosae), one of whose constituents is abrin. Abrin is considered responsible for the toxic effects of abrus seeds. It is closely related to ricin. Deaths of children have occurred from eating one or more seeds. Toxicity may be less likely to occur if the seeds are swallowed whole, than if they are chewed, because of the hard seed coat. Toxic effects may occur within a few hours or may be delayed for several days following ingestion. Signs and symptoms of abrin poisoning are similar to those described for ricin, p.1738.

Abrus has been used in homoeopathic medicine and as an oral contraceptive in herbal medicine.

◊ References.


1. Aslam M, Shaw JMH. Abrus in Asian medicine. *Pharm J* 1998; **261:** 822–4.
2. Fernando C. Poisoning due to Abrus precatorius (jequirity bean). *Anaesthesia* 2001; **56:** 1178–80.


## Absinthium

Absinthii Herba; Ajenjo; Assenzio; Losna; Pelin; Wermutkraut; Wormwood.

*CAS — 546-80-5 (α-thujone); 471-15-8 (β-thujone).*

**Pharmacopoeias.** In *Eur.* (see p.vi) and *Pol.*

**Ph. Eur. 5.0** (Wormwood). The leaves or flowering tops, or a mixture of these dried, whole or cut organs of wormwood, *Artemisia absinthium*. It contains not less than 2 mL/kg of essential oil, calculated with reference to the dried drug. Protect from light.

### Profile

Absinthium has been used as a bitter. It is also used in small quantities as a flavour in alcoholic beverages, although it is considered in some countries not to be safe for use in foods, beverages, or drugs. Habitual use or large doses cause absinthism, which is characterised by restlessness, vomiting, vertigo, tremors, and convulsions. Absinthium has been used in homoeopathic medicine. Thujone, related to camphor, is the major constituent of the essential oil derived from absinthium.

◊ References.


1. Weisbord SD, *et al.* Poison on line—acute renal failure caused by oil of wormwood purchased through the Internet. *N Engl J Med* 1997; **337:** 825–7.


### Preparations

**Proprietary Preparations** (details are given in Part 3)

**Multi-ingredient:** ***Austria:*** Abdomilon N; Amara; Amylatin; Aponatura Erkaltungs; Aponatura Galle; Aponatura Leber; Aponatura Verdauungs; Bio-Garten Tee fur Leber und Galle; Bio-Garten Tropfen fur Galle und Leber; Bioreform-Leber- und Galletee; Eryval; Felidon neu; Gallogran; Krauterdoktor Gallentreibende Tropfen; Krauterdoktor Verdauungsfordernde Tropfen; Krauterhaus Mag Kottas Tee fur die Verdauung; Magentee EF-EM-ES; Mariazeller; Neuners Krautertee Nr 17 - Lebertee; Neuners Krautertee Nr 28 - zur Unterstutzung der Tatigkeit der Galle; Neuners Krautertee Nr 30 - Stoffwechseltee stark; Pepsiton; Sigman-Haustropfen; St Radegunder Verdauungstee; Vinopepsin; Virgilocard; ***Braz.:*** Camomila†; ***Fr.:*** Tisane Hepatique de Hoerdt; ***Ger.:*** Abdomilon N; Agrimonas N†; Amara-Tropfen; Amara-Tropfen-Pascoe; Anore X N; Aristochol N; Cefagastrin†; Chol-Truw S†; Doppelherz Magenstarkung†; Floradix Multipretten N; Gallemolan forte; Gallemolan G; Gallexier; Gastralon N; Gastritol; Gastrol S; Hepaticum novo; Hepatofalk Neu†; Hevert-Magen-Galle-Leber-Tee†; Leber-Galle-Tropfen 83; Lomatol; Majocarmin forte; Majocarmin mite; Marianon; Nervosana; Neurochol C; Novo Mandrogallan N†; Pascopankreat; Phonix Gastriphon†; Presselin Blahungs K 4 N; Presselin Dyspeptikum; rohasal; Stomachysat N; Stovalid N; Stullmaton; Unex Amarum; ventri-loges N; Ventrimarin novo†; ***India:*** Toniazol; ***Ital.:*** Assenzio (Specie Composta); Genziana (Specie Composta); ***Switz.:*** Baume; Kernosan Heidelberger Poudre; Phytomed Hepato.

## Acedoben *(pINN)*

Acedobén. *p*-Acetamidobenzoic acid.

$C_9H_9NO_3$ = 179.2.

*CAS — 556-08-1.*

### Profile

Acedoben is a component of inosine pranobex (p.640), and has been given by mouth as the potassium salt in the treatment of skin disorders. Acedoben and its sodium salt have been applied topically.

### Preparations

**Proprietary Preparations** (details are given in Part 3)

***Spain:*** Fibroderm†.

**Multi-ingredient:** ***Spain:*** Amplidermis; Hongosan; Perlinsol Cutaneo†.

## Aceglutamide *(rINN)*

Aceglutamida. $N^2$-Acetyl-L-glutamine; 2-Acetylamino-L-glutaramic acid.

$C_7H_{12}N_2O_4$ = 188.2.

*CAS — 2490-97-3.*

### Profile

Aceglutamide has been given in an attempt to improve memory and concentration. Aceglutamide aluminium (p.1248) is used as an antacid.

### Preparations

**Proprietary Preparations** (details are given in Part 3)

**Multi-ingredient:** ***Ital.:*** Acutil Fosforo; Memovisus; Tonoplus; ***Spain:*** Levaliver†; Teovit†.

## Acemannan *(USAN, rINN)*

Acemanán; Polymanoacetate.

*CAS — 110042-95-0.*

### Profile

Acemannan is a highly acetylated, polydispersed, linear mannan obtained from the mucilage of *Aloe vera* (*A. barbadensis*). It has immunomodulating properties and is an ingredient of topical wound dressing products including those formulated for the oral mucosa.

### Preparations

**Proprietary Preparations** (details are given in Part 3)

***USA:*** Carrasyn; DiaB Gel; RadiaGel; SaliCept; Ultrex.

## Acetic Acid

Ácido acético; E260; Eisessig (glacial acetic acid); Essigsäure; Etanoico; Ethanoic Acid.

$C_2H_4O_2$ = 60.05.

*CAS — 64-19-7.*

*ATC — G01AD02; S02AA10.*

NOTE. The nomenclature of acetic acid often leads to confusion over whether concentrations are expressed as percentages of glacial acetic acid ($C_2H_4O_2$) or of a diluted form. In *Martindale*, the percentage figures given against acetic acid represent the amount of $C_2H_4O_2$.

**Pharmacopoeias.** Glacial acetic acid is included in *Chin., Eur.* (see p.vi), *Jpn, Pol.,* and *US.*

Solutions containing about 30 to 37% are included in *Br.* (33%), *Chin.* (36 to 37%), *Jpn* (30 to 32%), *Pol.* (30%), and *Swiss* (30%). Also in *USNF* (36 to 37%).

Dilute acetic acid (6%) is included in *Br.* Also in *USNF.*

**Ph. Eur. 5.0** (Acetic Acid, Glacial; Acidum Aceticum Glaciale). A crystalline mass or a clear colourless volatile liquid. F.p. not lower than 14.8°. Miscible with water, with alcohol, and with dichloromethane. Store in airtight containers.

**BP 2003** (Acetic Acid (33 per cent)). It contains 32.5 to 33.5% w/w of $C_2H_4O_2$. It is a clear colourless liquid with a pungent odour. Miscible with water, with alcohol, and with glycerol.

**BP 2003** (Acetic Acid (6 per cent)). It contains 5.7 to 6.3% w/w of $C_2H_4O_2$. It is prepared by diluting Acetic Acid (33 per cent).

**USP 27** (Glacial Acetic Acid). A clear colourless liquid with a pungent characteristic odour. B.p. about 118°. Miscible with water, with alcohol, and with glycerol. Store in airtight containers.

**USNF 22** (Acetic Acid). It contains 36 to 37% w/v of $C_2H_4O_2$. It is a clear colourless liquid with a strong characteristic odour. Miscible with water, with alcohol, and with glycerol. Store in airtight containers.

**USNF 22** (Diluted Acetic Acid). It contains 5.7 to 6.3% w/v of $C_2H_4O_2$. It is prepared by diluting Acetic Acid. Store in airtight containers.

### Adverse Effects and Treatment

Local or topical application of acetic acid preparations may produce stinging or burning. Ingestion of glacial acetic acid can produce similar adverse effects to those of hydrochloric acid (p.1699), which may be treated similarly.

### Uses and Administration

Glacial acetic acid has been used as an escharotic. Diluted forms have been used as an antibacterial (it is reported to be effective against *Haemophilus* and *Pseudomonas* spp.), antifungal, and antiprotozoal in vaginal gels and douches, irrigations, topical preparations for the skin and nails, and in ear drops. Diluted forms have also been used as an expectorant, an astringent lotion, and as treatments for warts (p.1139), callosities, and for certain jellyfish stings (see below).

A solution containing 4% w/v $C_2H_4O_2$ is known as artificial vinegar or non-brewed condiment. Vinegar is a product of fermentation.

**Jellyfish sting.** Vinegar or acetic acid 3 to 10% is applied to box jellyfish stings to inactivate any fragments of adherent tentacle[1,2] (see p.1621). Acetic acid solutions have been reported to be useful in stings by related species[3] although they may produce further discharge of venom in some jellyfish.[4]


1. Hartwick RJ, *et al.* Disarming the box jellyfish. *Med J Aust* 1980; **1:** 15–20.
2. Fenner PJ, Williamson JA. Worldwide deaths and severe envenomation from jellyfish stings. *Med J Aust* 1996; **165:** 658–61.
3. Fenner PJ, *et al.* "Morbakka", another cubomedusan. *Med J Aust* 1985; **143:** 550–5.
4. Fenner PJ, Fitzpatrick PF. Experiments with the nematocysts of Cyanea capillata. *Med J Aust* 1986; **145:** 174.


**Wounds and burns.** Infection of wounds (p.1139) and burns (p.1134) with *Pseudomonas aeruginosa* may delay healing. Acetic acid has been used, in concentrations of up to 5%, to eradicate these infections.[1]


1. Milner SM. Acetic acid to treat Pseudomonas aeruginosa in superficial wounds and burns. *Lancet* 1992; **340:** 61.


### Preparations

***BP 2003:*** Strong Ammonium Acetate Solution;
***USP 27:*** Acetic Acid Irrigation; Acetic Acid Otic Solution; Hydrocortisone and Acetic Acid Otic Solution.

**Proprietary Preparations** (details are given in Part 3)

***Arg.:*** Ecoshampoo; Pelo Libre; Pil-G Uso; ***Austral.:*** Summers Eve Disposable†; ***Canad.:*** Midol Douche†; ***Chile:*** Soft Kilnits; ***Fr.:*** Para Lentes; ***Gr.:*** Instaret; ***Irl.:*** Aci-Jel; ***Mex.:*** Amigdobis; ***UK:*** Aci-Jel; EarCalm; Meltus Baby; ***USA:*** Feminique; Massengill Disposable; Summers Eve Disposable.

**Multi-ingredient:** ***Arg.:*** Callicida; Microsona Otica; ***Austral.:*** Aci-Jel; Aquaear†; Ear Clear for Swimmer's Ear†; ***Austria:*** Onycho Phytex†; Phytex†; ***Belg.:*** Aporil; ***Braz.:*** A Curitybina; Kalostop; Lacto Vagin; Lacto-Gin†; ***Canad.:*** SH-206; Viron Wart Lotion; VoSoL; VoSoL HC; ***Chile:*** Summer's Eve Vinagre y Agua; ***Fr.:*** Nitrol; Ysol 206; ***Ger.:*** Chol-Truw S†; Gehwol Huhneraugen Tinktur; Solco-Derman; ***Hong Kong:*** Baby Cough with Antihistamine; Solcoderm; ***India:*** Otek-AC; Perfocyn; ***Irl.:*** Phytex; ***Ital.:*** Oleo Calcarea; Silvana†; ***Malaysia:*** Solcoderm; ***Neth.:*** Hexoll†; ***NZ:*** Aci-Jel; Aqua Ear; VoSoL; ***Port.:*** Calicida Indiano; ***Spain:*** Callicida Cor Pik; Callicida Durcall†; Callicida Rojo; Nitroina; Quocin; ***Switz.:*** Coruzol; Solcoderm; Solcogyn; Waruzol; ***Thai.:*** Baby Cough Syrup; Baby Cough with Antihistamine; ***UK:*** Ellimans; Goddards Embrocation; Phytex; Potters Gees Linctus; Sanderson's Throat Specific; ***USA:*** AA-HC Otic†; Acetasol; Acetasol HC; Aci-Jel†; Borofair Otic; Burow's; Fem pH; Otic Domeboro; Star-Otic; Tridesilon; VoSoL; VoSoL HC.

## Acetohydroxamic Acid *(USAN, rINN)*

*N*-Acetyl Hydroxyacetamide; Ácido acetohidroxámico; AHA.

$C_2H_5NO_2$ = 75.07.

*CAS — 546-88-3.*

*ATC — G04BX03.*

**Pharmacopoeias.** In *US.*

**USP 27** (Acetohydroxamic Acid). White, slightly hygroscopic, crystalline powder. Freely soluble in water and in alcohol; very slightly soluble in chloroform. Store in airtight containers at a temperature between 8° and 15°.

### Adverse Effects and Precautions

Phlebitis, thromboembolism, haemolytic anaemia, and iron-deficiency anaemia have occurred. Bone-marrow depression has been reported in *animal* studies. Other adverse effects include headache, gastrointestinal disturbances, alopecia, rash (particularly following ingestion of alcohol), trembling, and mental symptoms including anxiety and depression. Blood counts and renal function should be monitored regularly during treatment. Patients with acute renal failure should not be given acetohydroxamic acid.

**Pregnancy.** Studies in *animals* indicate that acetohydroxamic acid is teratogenic.

### Interactions

Acetohydroxamic acid chelates iron administered orally, resulting in reduced absorption of both. Concomitant consumption of alcohol may precipitate skin rash.

### Pharmacokinetics

Acetohydroxamic acid is rapidly absorbed from the gastrointestinal tract with peak serum concentrations being reached within 1 hour. The plasma half-life is reported to be up to 10 hours, but may be longer in patients with impaired renal function. Acetohydroxamic acid is partially metabolised in the liver to acetamide, which is inactive; up to about two-thirds of a dose may be excreted unchanged in the urine.

### Uses and Administration

Acetohydroxamic acid acts by inhibiting bacterial urease, thus decreasing urinary ammonia concentration and alkalinity. It is used in the prophylaxis of renal calculi (p.936) and as an adjunct in the treatment of chronic urinary-tract infections (p.153).

Acetohydroxamic acid is given by mouth in a usual dose of 250 mg three or four times daily. The total dose should not exceed 1.5 g daily. Children aged over 8 years have been given 10 mg/kg daily in 2 or 3 divided doses. Dosage should be adjusted in patients with renal impairment (see below).

◊ References.

1. Martelli A, *et al.* Acetohydroxamic acid therapy in infected renal stones. *Urology* 1981; **17:** 320–2.
2. Griffith DP. Infection-induced renal calculi. *Kidney Int* 1982; **21:** 422–30.
3. Rodman JS, *et al.* Partial dissolution of struvite calculus with oral acetohydroxamic acid. *Urology* 1983; **22:** 410–12.
4. Burr RG, Nuseibeh I. The effect of oral acetohydroxamic acid on urinary saturation in stone-forming spinal cord patients. *Br J Urol* 1983; **55:** 162–5.
5. Williams JJ, *et al.* A randomized double-blind study of acetohydroxamic acid in struvite nephrolithiasis. *N Engl J Med* 1984; **311:** 760–4.
6. Smith LH. New treatment for struvite urinary stones. *N Engl J Med* 1984; **311:** 792–4.
7. El Nujumi AM, *et al.* Effect of inhibition of Helicobacter pylori urease activity by acetohydroxamic acid on serum gastrin in duodenal ulcer subjects. *Gut* 1991; **32:** 866–70.
8. Zullo A, *et al.* Helicobacter pylori and plasma ammonia levels in cirrhosis: role of urease inhibition by acetohydroxamic acid. *Ital J Gastroenterol Hepatol* 1998; **30:** 405–9.

**Administration in renal impairment.** Acetohydroxamic acid should not be given to patients with serum-creatinine concentrations in excess of about 220 micromoles/litre. If the concentration is between 160 and 220 micromoles/litre, the maximum daily dose should be 1 g and the dosing interval should be extended to every 12 hours.

### Preparations

***USP 27:*** Acetohydroxamic Acid Tablets.

**Proprietary Preparations** (details are given in Part 3)
***Belg.:*** Uronefrex†; ***Fr.:*** Uronefrex†; ***Spain:*** Uronefrex; ***USA:*** Lithostat.

## Acetylcarnitine Hydrochloride

Acetilcarnitina, hidrocloruro de; Acetyl-L-carnitine Chloride; Levacecarnine Hydrochloride; ST-200; ST-200. (3-Carboxy-2-hydroxypropyl)trimethylammonium acetate (ester) chloride.

$C_9H_{17}NO_4,HCl$ = 239.7.

*CAS — 5080-50-2.*

*ATC — N06BX12.*

### Profile

Acetylcarnitine hydrochloride has been given by mouth and by injection in the treatment of cerebrovascular insufficiency and peripheral neuropathies. It is under investigation in Alzheimer's disease and Peyronie's disease.

◊ References.

1. Thal LJ, *et al.* A 1-year multicenter placebo-controlled study of acetyl-L-carnitine in patients with Alzheimer's disease. *Neurology* 1996; **47:** 705–11.
2. Thal LJ, *et al.* A 1-year controlled trial of acetyl-l-carnitine in early-onset AD. *Neurology* 2000; **26:** 805–10.
3. Biagiotti G, Cavallini G. Acetyl-L-carnitine vs tamoxifen in the oral therapy of Peyronie's disease: a preliminary report. *BJU Int* 2001; **88:** 63–7.

### Preparations

**Proprietary Preparations** (details are given in Part 3)
***Arg.:*** Neurex; Neuroactil; ***Chile:*** Actigeron; ***Ital.:*** Acilen†; Branigen; Branitil; Nicetile; Normobren; Zibren.

## Acetylleucine *(rINN)*

Acetileucina; RP-7542. *N*-Acetyl-DL-leucine.

$C_8H_{15}NO_3$ = 173.2.

*CAS — 99-15-0.*

*ATC — N07CA04.*

### Profile

Acetylleucine has been used in the treatment of vertigo (p.423) in usual doses of up to 2 g daily by mouth, in divided doses, or 1 g daily by slow intravenous injection. Higher doses have occasionally been employed.

### Preparations

**Proprietary Preparations** (details are given in Part 3)
***Fr.:*** Tanganil.

## Acexamic Acid *(BAN, rINN)*

Ácido acexámico; CY-153; Epsilon Acetamidocaproic Acid. 6-Acetamidohexanoic acid.

$C_8H_{15}NO_3$ = 173.2.

*CAS — 57-08-9 (acexamic acid); 70020-71-2 (zinc acexamate).*

**Pharmacopoeias.** *Eur.* (see p.vi) includes Zinc Acexamate.

### Profile

Acexamic acid is related structurally to the antifibrinolytic agent aminocaproic acid (p.741). Acexamic acid, usually as the calcium or sodium salt, has been administered topically or systemically to promote the healing of ulcers and various other skin lesions. Zinc acexamate has been given for peptic ulcer disease.

### Preparations

**Proprietary Preparations** (details are given in Part 3)
***Arg.:*** Plastenan; ***Belg.:*** Plastenan†; ***Braz.:*** Plastenan†; ***Fr.:*** Plastenan; ***Mex.:*** Recoveron; ***Port.:*** Plastesol; ***Spain:*** Copinal.

**Multi-ingredient:** ***Arg.:*** Bagoderm; Lisoderma; Plastenan con Neomicina; Restaurene; ***Fr.:*** Trofoseptine; ***Mex.:*** Recoveron N; Recoveron NC; ***Port.:*** Plastenan Neomicina; ***Spain:*** Linitul Antibiotico†; Plaskine Neomicina; Unitul Complex.

## Achillea

Achillée Millefeuille; Aquilea; Milfoil; Millefolii Herba; Schafgarbe; Yarrow.

**Pharmacopoeias.** In *Eur.* (see p.vi) and *Pol.*

**Ph. Eur. 5.0** (Yarrow). The whole or cut, dried flowering tops of yarrow, *Achillea millefolium*. It contains not less than 2 mL/kg of essential oil and not less than 0.02% of proazulenes, expressed as chamazulene ($C_{14}H_{16}$ = 184.3), both calculated with reference to the dried drug. Protect from light.

### Profile

Achillea has been used mainly in herbal and homoeopathic medicine for a great variety of purposes. It has been stated to have diaphoretic, anti-inflammatory, and other miscellaneous properties. It has been reported to cause contact dermatitis.

◊ References.

1. Phillipson JD, Anderson LA. Herbal remedies used in sedative and antirheumatic preparations: part 2. *Pharm J* 1984; **233:** 111–15.
2. Chandler RF. Yarrow. *Can Pharm J* 1989; **122:** 41–3.
3. Anonymous. Final report on the safety assessment of yarrow (Achillea millefolium) extract. *Int J Toxicol* 2001; **20** (suppl 2): 79–84.

### Preparations

**Proprietary Preparations** (details are given in Part 3)
***Ger.:*** Kneipp Schafgarbe-Pflanzensaft Frauentost N†; Schamill†; ***Mex.:*** Blancaler.

**Multi-ingredient:** ***Austral.:*** Crataegus Complex†; Flavons†; ***Austria:*** Abfuhrtee EF-EM-ES; Aktiv Leber- und Gallentee; Aktiv milder Magen- und Darmtee; Amersan; Aurita-Leber-Galletee; Bio-Garten Tee gegen Blahungen; Bio-Garten Tee zur Starkung und Kraftigung; Bio-Garten Tropfen fur Galle und Leber; Bioreform-Windtreibender Tee; Chol-Grandelat; Citochol; Felidon neu; Gallen- und Lebertee EF-EM-ES; Gallogran; Gewusst wie Darmtee; Krauterdoktor Gallentreibende Tropfen; Krauterhaus Mag Kottas Fruhjahrs- und Herbstkurtee; Krauterhaus Mag Kottas Magen- und Darmtee; Krauterhaus Mag Kottas Tee gegen Blahungen; Krauterhaus Mag Kottas Wechseltee; Krauterpfarrer Weidinger Tee bei Sodbrennen; Krauterpfarrer Weidinger Tee fur Leber und Galle; Mag Kottas Krauterexpress-Wechseltee; Mageentee†; Mariazeller; Menodoron; Neuners Krautertee Nr 124 - zur Entspannung vor der Geburt; Neuners Krautertee Nr 16 - Beruhigungstee bei Wechselbeschwerden; Neuners Krautertee Nr 44 - Kreislaufanregender Tee; Sidroga Leber-Galle-Tee; Sidroga Magen-Darm-Tee; ***Fr.:*** Cicadermа†; Gonaxine; Tisane Digestive Weleda†; Tisane Hepatique de Hoerdt; Tisanes de l'Abbe Hamon no 14†; ***Ger.:*** Alasenn; Amara-Tropfen; Aristochol N; Befelka-Tinktur†; Cheiranthol; Dr. Hotz Vollbad†; Floradix Multipretten N; Gallexier; Hevert-Gicht-Rheuma-Tee comp†; Hevert-Magen-Galle-Leber-Tee†; Kamillan plus; Magen-Tee Stada N†; Marianon; Nervosana; Salus Leber-Galle-Tee Nr.18†; Salus Rheuma-Tee Krautertee Nr. 12†; Sedovent; Stomachysat N; Tonsilgon; ***Ital.:*** Fluiven†; Forticrin; Lozione Same Urto; ***Port.:*** Cicaderma; Fade Cream; ***Spain:*** Jaquesor; Menstrunat; Natusor Circusil; Natusor Gastrolen; Natusor Jaquesan; ***Switz.:*** Baume; Enveloppements ECR†; Gastrosan; Kernosan Heidelberger Poudre; Tisane hepatique et biliaire; Tisane pour l'estomac; ***UK:*** Carminative Tea†; Catarrh-eeze; Catarrh†; Rheumatic Pain Remedy; Tabritis; Wellwoman.

## Acid Alpha Glucosidase

Acid Maltase; α-Glucosidasa; Glucosidase, Acid Alpha; Lysosomal α-glucosidase.

### Profile

Recombinant human acid alpha-glucosidase is under investigation as enzyme replacement therapy for the lysosomal storage disease Pompe disease (glycogen storage disease type II). This is a rare fatal autosomal recessive disorder caused by a deficiency of acid α-glucosidase, which cleaves α-1,4- and α-1,6-glucosidic linkages in lysosomal glycogen to liberate glucose. Glycogen accumulation results in progressive myopathy, especially of the skeletal muscles and heart.

◊ References.

1. Amalfitano A, *et al.* Recombinant human acid alpha-glucosidase enzyme therapy for infantile glycogen storage disease type II: results of a phase I/II clinical trial. *Genet Med* 2001; **3:** 132–8.
2. Van den Hout JM, *et al.* Enzyme therapy for Pompe disease with recombinant human alpha-glucosidase from rabbit milk. *J Inherit Metab Dis* 2001; **24:** 266–74.

### Preparations

**Proprietary Preparations** (details are given in Part 3)
**Multi-ingredient:** ***Austral.:*** Digestaid†; Zinc Zenith†.

## Acid Fuchsine

Acid Magenta; Acid Roseine; Acid Rubine; CI Acid Violet 19; Colour Index No. 42685; Fucsina ácida.

### Profile

Acid fuchsine is the disodium or diammonium salt of the trisulfonic acid of magenta. It is used as a microscopic stain and a pH indicator.

## Aconite

Acetylbenzoylaconine (aconitine); Aconit.; Aconit Napel; Aconite Root; Aconiti Tuber; Acónito; Monkshood Root; Radix Aconiti; Wolfsbane Root. 8-Acetoxy-3,11,18-trihydroxy-16-ethyl-1,6,19-trimethoxy-4-methoxymethylaconitan-10-yl benzoate (aconitine).

$C_{34}H_{47}NO_{11}$ = 645.7 (aconitine).

*CAS — 8063-12-5 (aconite); 302-27-2 (aconitine).*

NOTE. Wolfsbane is also used as a common name for arnica flower (p.1656).

**Description.** Aconite consists of the dried tuberous root of *Aconitum napellus* agg. (Ranunculaceae). It contains a number of alkaloids, the main pharmacologically active one being aconitine.

**Pharmacopoeias.** In *Chin.*

### Adverse Effects and Treatment

Aconite has variable effects on the heart leading to heart failure. It also affects the CNS.

Symptoms of aconite poisoning may appear within minutes or up to 2 hours after oral ingestion; in fatal poisoning death usually occurs within 12 hours, although with larger doses it may be instantaneous.

Initial symptoms (and an important diagnostic feature) are tingling sensations of the tongue, mouth, fingers, and toes followed by generalised paraesthesia. Other symptoms include nausea, vomiting, diarrhoea, muscle weakness, skeletal muscle paralysis, and difficult respiration; also sweats, chills and a feeling of intense cold may occur. Respiratory paralysis, hypotension, and cardiac arrhythmias may develop in severe cases.

Although the benefits of gastric decontamination are uncertain, gastric lavage may be tried in patients within one hour of life-threatening oral poisoning; activated charcoal may also be considered. Patients should be observed and monitored, and corrective and supportive treatment administered as necessary. Arrhythmias are relatively resistant to treatment, although atropine has been tried for bradycardia.

**Poisoning.** Reports of poisoning with aconite.

1. Kelly SP. Aconite poisoning. *Med J Aust* 1990; **153:** 499.
2. Tai Y-T, *et al.* Cardiotoxicity after accidental herb-induced aconite poisoning. *Lancet* 1992; **340:** 1254–6.
3. Kolev ST, *et al.* Toxicity following accidental ingestion of Aconitum containing Chinese remedy. *Hum Exp Toxicol* 1996; **15:** 839–42.
4. Mak W, Lau CP. A woman with tetraparesis and missed beats. *Hosp Med* 2000; **61:** 438.
5. Imazio M, *et al.* Malignant ventricular arrhythmias due to Aconitum napellus seeds. *Circulation* 2000; **102:** 2907–8.

### Uses and Administration

Aconite liniments have been used in the treatment of neuralgia, sciatica, and rheumatism. Sufficient aconitine may be absorbed through the skin to cause poisoning; liniments should never be applied to wounds or abraded surfaces. Aconite should not be used internally because of its low therapeutic index and variable potency; however it is reported to be a common ingredient in traditional Chinese remedies and is also an ingredient of some cough mixtures.

A preparation of aconite is used in homoeopathic medicine.

### Preparations

**Proprietary Preparations** (details are given in Part 3)
**Multi-ingredient:** ***Arg.:*** No-Tos Adultos; ***Austria:*** Rheuma; ***Belg.:*** Colimax; Eucalyptine Pholcodine Le Brun; Euphon; Folcodex†; Sirop Toux du Larynx†; Solucamphre†; ***Braz.:*** Agrimel†; Axol†; Broncofenil; Broncotussan†; Expectomel; Gotas Nican; Limao Bravo†; Melagriao†; Pectal; Pinosil†; Xarope Comp Mel e Agriao†; Xarope de Caraguata; Xarope Peitoral de Ameixa Composto; Xarope Sao Joao; ***Chile:*** Gotas Nican; ***Fr.:*** Bronpax†; Euphon†; Gaiarsol†; Peter's Sirop†; Pulmonase†; Sedophon†; Sirop Boin†; Sirop Pectoral adulte†; ***Ital.:*** Lactocol; ***Port.:*** Anti-Gripe; Calmarum; Codoforme†; Lactocol†; ***Spain:*** Encialina; Etermol†; Pectoral Brum†.

## Acridine Orange

Naranja de acridina. 3,6-Bis(dimethylamino)acridine.

$C_{17}H_{19}N_3$ = 265.4.

*CAS — 494-38-2.*

### Profile

Acridine orange is a dye with antiseptic properties. It has been used as a diagnostic stain in microbiology.

For details of the antiseptic properties of acridine derivatives, see p.1165.

**Diagnostic use.** Acridine orange has been used for the diagnostic staining of malarial parasites.[1] For the quantitative buffy coat method, acridine orange is used to stain the parasites in a blood sample that is then centrifuged, and the area just below the buffy coat is examined under a fluorescence microscope. It has been described as easier and quicker to use than the standard examination of stained blood films. However, this method is not specific for diagnosis of malarial type, gives only a rough indication of infection intensity, and can give false-positive results. Acridine orange has also been tried for the staining of blood slides.[2-5]

1. Warhurst DC, Williams JE. ACP Broadsheet no 148, July 1996. Laboratory diagnosis of malaria. *J Clin Pathol* 1996; **49:** 533–8.
2. Gay F, *et al.* Direct acridine orange fluorescence examination of blood slides compared to current techniques for malaria diagnosis. *Trans R Soc Trop Med Hyg* 1996; **90:** 576–18.
3. Craig MH, Sharp BL. Comparative evaluation of four techniques for the diagnosis of Plasmodium falciparum infections. *Trans R Soc Trop Med Hyg* 1997; **91:** 279–82.
4. Tarimo DS, *et al.* Appraisal of the acridine orange method for rapid malaria diagnosis at three Tanzanian district hospitals. *East Afr Med J* 1998; **75:** 504–7.
5. Lema OE, *et al.* Comparison of five methods of malaria detection in the outpatient setting. *Am J Trop Med Hyg* 1999; **60:** 177–82.

## Acrolein

Acraldehyde; Acroleína; Acrylaldehyde; Acrylic Aldehyde. Prop-2-enal.

$C_3H_4O$ = 56.06.

*CAS — 107-02-8.*

### Profile

Acrolein is a volatile, highly flammable liquid at ordinary temperature and pressure. It has various industrial uses, but is also a toxic byproduct of combustion and may be present in exhaust gases, tobacco smoke, and smoke from fires. It is irritant to the skin and may cause skin burns. Ingestion of acrolein produces severe gastrointestinal distress. The vapour causes lachrymation and pulmonary irritation. Inhalation may cause pulmonary oedema and permanent lung damage.

Acrolein is a metabolite of cyclophosphamide (p.540) and may be responsible for the latter's bladder toxicity.

◊ References.

1. Acrolein. *IPCS Health and Safety Guide 67.* Geneva: WHO, 1991.
2. Acrolein. *Environmental Health Criteria 127.* Geneva: WHO, 1992.
3. Kehrer JP, Biswal SS. The molecular effects of acrolein. *Toxicol Sci* 2000; **57:** 6–15.

## Acrylamide

Acrilamida. Propenamide.

$C_3H_5NO$ = 71.08.

*CAS — 79-06-1.*

### Profile

Acrylamide is highly toxic and irritant; it can be absorbed through unbroken skin. Symptoms of poisoning include burning and ulceration of the mouth and throat following ingestion. Excessive sweating is common and other symptoms may include numbness of limbs, paraesthesias, and muscle weakness. CNS effects such as somnolence, confusion, hallucinations, ataxia, tremors, dysarthria, and nystagmus may occur depending on the severity of exposure. Peripheral neuropathies may appear several weeks after severe acute exposure or as a result of chronic exposure. Gastric lavage may be tried in patients within one hour of ingestion; activated charcoal may also be considered. Contamination of eyes and skin should be irrigated and treated as for burns. Patients should be observed and monitored, and corrective and supportive treatment administered as necessary.

Acrylamide has various industrial applications, including use as a plasticiser and a waterproof 'chemical grout'.

◊ References.

1. Kesson CM, *et al.* Acrylamide poisoning. *Postgrad Med J* 1977; **53:** 16–17.
2. Acrylamide health and safety guide. *IPCS Health and Safety Guide 45.* Geneva: WHO, 1991.

**Food toxicity.** Concerns have been expressed by the Swedish National Food Administration about the level of acrylamide they found in certain cooked foods, particularly those exposed to very high temperatures such as fried foods, and the potential carcinogenic risk. However, it has been acknowledged that, although the results have been replicated in other international laboratories, the total sample size is small and none of the methods being used have so far been validated.[1] The WHO has called for further urgent research into the health risks from acrylamide. One subsequent population-based study failed to find any excess risk or convincing trend of cancer of the bowel, bladder, or kidney in high consumers of foods with a high or moderate acrylamide content.[2]

1. Kapp C. WHO urges more research into acrylamide in food. *Lancet* 2002; **360:** 64.
2. Mucci LA, *et al.* Dietary acrylamide and cancer of the large bowel, kidney, and bladder: absence of an association in a population-based study in Sweden. *Br J Cancer* 2003 **88:** 84–9.

## Actinoquinol Sodium *(USAN, rINNM)*

Sodium Etoquinol; Sodium Tequinol. Sodium 8-ethoxy-5-quinolinesulfonate.

$C_{11}H_{10}NNaO_4S$ = 275.3.

*CAS — 15301-40-3 (actinoquinol); 7246-07-3 (actinoquinol sodium).*

### Profile

Actinoquinol and actinoquinol sodium are ingredients of eye drop preparations intended to protect the eyes from the effects of light.

### Preparations

**Proprietary Preparations** (details are given in Part 3)
***Austria:*** Ultra Augenschutz.

**Multi-ingredient:** ***Fr.:*** Uvicol†; ***Ger.:*** duraultra; ***Ital.:*** Fotofil.

## Ademetionine *(rINN)*

Ademethionine; Ademetionina; S-Adenosyl-L-methionine; Methioninyl adenylate; SAMe. (S)-5′-[(3-Amino-3-carboxypropyl)methylsulphonio]-5′-deoxyadenosine hydroxide, inner salt.

$C_{15}H_{22}N_6O_5S$ = 398.4.

*CAS — 29908-03-0; 485-80-3; 17176-17-9.*

*ATC — A16AA02.*

### Profile

Ademetionine is a naturally occurring molecule found in virtually all body tissues and fluids. It acts as a methyl group donor in many transmethylation reactions and therefore is involved in the synthesis or metabolism of a wide range of compounds that maintain normal cell function. Ademetionine sulfate tosilate and ademetionine butanedisulfonate are stable forms of ademetionine that have been used for the treatment of depression (see below), liver disorders, and osteoarthritis.

◊ Reviews.

1. Friedel HA, *et al.* S-Adenosyl-L-methionine: a review of its pharmacological properties and therapeutic potential in liver dysfunction and affective disorders in relation to its physiological role in cell metabolism. *Drugs* 1989; **38:** 389–416.
2. Bottiglieri T, *et al.* The clinical potential of ademetionine (S-adenosylmethionine) in neurological disorders. *Drugs* 1994; **48:** 137–52.
3. Chavez M. SAMe: S-adenosylmethionine. *Am J Health-Syst Pharm* 2000; **57:** 119–23.
4. Fetrow CW, Avila JR. Efficacy of the dietary supplement S-adenosyl-L-methionine. *Ann Pharmacother* 2001; **35:** 1414–25.

**Depression.** Ademetionine has been given by mouth or parenterally in the management of depression (p.279). It appears to be of similar efficacy to the tricyclic antidepressants but evidence is limited to small, heterogeneous groups of patients studied over short periods of time.

References.

1. Bressa GM. S-adenosyl-l-methionine (SAMe) as antidepressant: meta-analysis of clinical studies. *Acta Neurol Scand* 1994; **154** (suppl): 7–14.
2. Anonymous. SAMe for depression. *Med Lett Drugs Ther* 1999; **41:** 107–8.

**Liver disorders.** Some workers have found that administration of ademetionine in doses of 800 mg daily intravenously or 800 mg twice daily by mouth has produced clinical improvement in patients with **intrahepatic cholestasis**,[1,2] including that associated with pregnancy.[3,4] Pruritus associated with the condition has also been relieved. Other studies,[5,6] however, have not found any benefit.

Ademetionine given by intramuscular injection in a dose of 100 mg daily for one month, followed by 100 mg every other day for a further month, produced a good or excellent clinical response in 21 of 28 patients with **hepatic steatosis**,[7] while in a study[8] of patients with **alcoholic liver cirrhosis**, treated with ademetionine 400 mg three times daily by mouth for 2 years, there was a trend towards reduced overall mortality or need for liver transplantation, but only in patients with less severe hepatic dysfunction. However, a systematic review[9] of 8 randomised placebo-controlled trials, which included the latter study, could not demonstrate any significant beneficial effect of ademetionine in patients with alcoholic liver disease, and recommended that it should not be used in such patients outside randomised clinical trials.

1. Frezza M, *et al.* Oral S-adenosylmethionine in the symptomatic treatment of intrahepatic cholestasis: a double-blind, placebo-controlled study. *Gastroenterology* 1990; **99:** 211–15.
2. Almasio P, *et al.* Role of S-adenosyl-L-methionine in the treatment of intrahepatic cholestasis. *Drugs* 1990; **40** (suppl 3): 111–23.
3. Bonfirraro G, *et al.* S-Adenosyl-L-methionine (SAMe)-induced amelioration of intrahepatic cholestasis of pregnancy: results of an open study. *Drug Invest* 1990; **2:** 125–8.
4. Frezza M, *et al.* S-Adenosylmethionine for the treatment of intrahepatic cholestasis of pregnancy: results of a controlled clinical trial. *Hepatogastroenterology* 1990; **37** (suppl 2): 122–5.
5. Ribalta J, *et al.* S-Adenosyl-L-methionine in the treatment of patients with intrahepatic cholestasis of pregnancy: a randomized, double-blind, placebo-controlled study with negative results. *Hepatology* 1991; **13:** 1084–9.
6. Floreani A, *et al.* S-adenosylmethionine versus ursodeoxycholic acid in the treatment of intrahepatic cholestasis of pregnancy: preliminary results of a controlled trial. *Eur J Obstet Gynecol Reprod Biol* 1996; **67:** 109–13.
7. Caballeria E, Moreno J. Therapeutic effects of S-adenosylmethionine (SAMe) in hepatic steatosis. *Acta Ther* 1990; **16:** 253–64.
8. Mato JM, *et al.* S-Adenosylmethionine in alcoholic liver cirrhosis: a randomized, placebo-controlled, double-blind, multicenter clinical trial. *J Hepatol* 1999; **30:** 1081–9.
9. Rambaldi A, Gluud C. S-adenosyl-L-methionine for alcoholic liver diseases. Available in the Cochrane Library; Issue 2. Chichester: John Wiley; 2004.

**Osteoarthritis.** Ademetionine has been reported to possess therapeutic efficacy in the treatment of osteoarthritis (p.9) and similar conditions, possibly due to an effect on cartilage metabolism and formation of anti-inflammatory mediators within the cell; it may also inhibit leukotrienes but does not appear markedly to interfere with prostaglandin synthesis.

References.

1. Domljan Z, *et al.* A double-blind trial of ademetionine vs naproxen in activated gonarthrosis. *Int J Clin Pharmacol Ther Toxicol* 1989; **27:** 329–33.
2. Bradley JD, *et al.* A randomized, double blind, placebo controlled trial of intravenous loading with S-adenosylmethionine (SAM) followed by oral SAM therapy in patients with knee osteoarthritis. *J Rheumatol* 1994; **21:** 905–11.
3. Soeken KL, *et al.* Safety and efficacy of S-adenosylmethionine (SAMe) for osteoarthritis. *J Fam Pract* 2002; **51:** 425–30.

### Preparations

**Proprietary Preparations** (details are given in Part 3)
***Arg.:*** Transmetil; Tunik; ***Austral.:*** MoodLift; ***Ger.:*** Gumbaral; ***Ital.:*** Donamet; Isimet; Samyr; Transmetil; ***Mex.:*** Samyr; ***Spain:*** S Amet.

**Multi-ingredient:** ***Arg.:*** Tunik B12.

## Adenine

Adenina; Adeninum; Vitamin $B_4$. 6-Aminopurine; 1,6-Dihydro-6-iminopurine.

$C_5H_5N_5$ = 135.1.

*CAS — 73-24-5.*

**Pharmacopoeias.** In *Eur.* (see p.vi) and *US.*

**Ph. Eur. 5.0** (Adenine). A white powder. Very slightly soluble in water and in alcohol; dissolves in dilute mineral acids and in dilute solutions of alkali hydroxides.

**USP 27** (Adenine). Odourless white crystals or crystalline powder. Very slightly soluble in water; sparingly soluble in boiling water; slightly soluble in alcohol; practically insoluble in chloroform and in ether.

### Profile

Adenine is a constituent of coenzymes and nucleic acids and has been used to extend the storage life of whole blood (p.743). It has also been given for the management of white blood cell disorders. Adenine hydrochloride has also been used.

### Preparations

***USP 27:*** Anticoagulant Citrate Phosphate Dextrose Adenine Solution.

**Proprietary Preparations** (details are given in Part 3)
***Fr.:*** Leuco-4.

**Multi-ingredient:** ***Fr.:*** TTD-$B_3$-$B_4$; ***Spain:*** Hepadif.

## Adenosine Phosphate *(BAN, USAN, rINN)*

Adenosine 5′-Monophosphate; Adenosine-5′-(dihydrogen phosphate); Adenosine-5′-phosphoric Acid; 5′-Adenylic Acid; AMP; A-5MP; Fosfato de adenosina; Monophosadénine; Muscle Adenylic Acid; NSC-20264. 6-Amino-9-β-D-ribofuranosylpurine 5′-(dihydrogen phosphate).

$C_{10}H_{14}N_5O_7P$ = 347.2.

*CAS — 61-19-8.*

*ATC — C01EB10.*

**Pharmacopoeias.** *Ger.* includes the disodium salt ($C_{10}H_{12}N_5Na_2O_7P,xH_2O$).

### Profile

Adenosine is an endogenous nucleoside involved in many biological processes. As well as the base it is present as various phosphates. The monophosphate, adenosine phosphate, is a vasodilator and has been tried in a variety of disorders including venous insufficiency, haemorrhoids, and varicose veins.

Unlike adenosine (p.851) and adenosine triphosphate (below), adenosine phosphate is not used in supraventricular tachycardias.

### Preparations

**Proprietary Preparations** (details are given in Part 3)
***Fr.:*** Adenyl; ***Ger.:*** Bio-Regenerat S 3†.

**Multi-ingredient:** ***Austria:*** Laevadosin†; ***S.Afr.:*** Lipostabil; ***Spain:*** Artri; Taurobetina.

## Adenosine Triphosphate

Adenosina, trifosfato de; Adenosine 5′-Triphosphate; 5′-Adenyldiphosphoric Acid; Adenylpyrophosphoric Acid; ATP; Triphosadénine. Adenosine 5′-(tetrahydrogen triphosphate).

$C_{10}H_{16}N_5O_{13}P_3$ = 507.2.

*CAS — 56-65-5.*

*ATC — C01EB10.*

**Pharmacopoeias.** *Ger.* includes the disodium salt ($C_{10}H_{14}N_5Na_2O_{13}P_3$ = 551.1).

### Profile

Adenosine triphosphate is a nucleotide constituent of animal cells with a fundamental role in biological energy transformations, being concerned with the storage and release of energy; it is converted to adenosine diphosphate, release of energy occurring during the process.

Adenosine triphosphate and its sodium salt are used as a source of nucleotides. The disodium salt has been given in the treatment of supraventricular tachycardia, but adenosine base (p.851) is the form generally used as an antiarrhythmic. The triphosphate is being investigated for use in cachexia in patients with cancer.

◊ Reviews.

1. Agteresch HJ, *et al.* Adenosine triphosphate: established and potential clinical applications. *Drugs* 1999; **58:** 211–32.

### Preparations

**Proprietary Preparations** (details are given in Part 3)

***Arg.:*** Atepadene; ***Fr.:*** Atepadene; Myoviton†; ***Hong Kong:*** Adesinon-P†; ***Spain:*** Atepodin.

**Multi-ingredient:** ***Austria:*** Laevadosin†; ***Fr.:*** Betriphos-C†; RhinATP†; ***Spain:*** Refulgin†.

---

## Adiphenine *(rINN)*

2-Diethylaminoethyl diphenylacetate.

$C_{20}H_{25}NO_2$ = 311.4.

*CAS — 64-95-9.*

## Adiphenine Hydrochloride *(USAN, rINNM)*

Adiphenini Hydrochloridum; Cloridrato de Adifenina; NSC-129224; Spasmolytine.

$C_{20}H_{25}NO_2,HCl$ = 347.9.

*CAS — 50-42-0.*

### Profile

Adiphenine and adiphenine hydrochloride have been used as antispasmodics.

### Preparations

**Proprietary Preparations** (details are given in Part 3)

**Multi-ingredient:** ***Braz.:*** Analgosedan†; Dipirol; Espasmobel†; Lisador; Sedalene; Somasedin†; ***Chile:*** Abalgin; Andil; Immediat; SAE; ***Switz.:*** Spasmo-Barbamin; Spasmo-Barbamine compositum.

---

## Adipic Acid

Acidum Adipicum; Adípico, ácido; Adipinsäure; Hexanedioic Acid.

$C_6H_{10}O_4$ = 146.1.

*CAS — 124-04-9.*

**Pharmacopoeias.** In *Eur.* (see p.vi).

**Ph. Eur. 5.0** (Adipic Acid). A white crystalline powder. Sparingly soluble in water; soluble in boiling water; freely soluble in alcohol and in methyl alcohol; soluble in acetone.

### Profile

Adipic acid is an acidifier that is used in foods and has been included in preparations for the treatment of urinary-tract infections.

---

## Adonis Vernalis

Adonide; Adonis; Adonis vernal; Adoniskraut; False Hellebore; Herba Adonidis; Vernal Pheasant's Eye.

**Pharmacopoeias.** In *Ger.* and *Pol.*

### Profile

Adonis vernalis, the dried aerial parts of *Adonis vernalis* (Ranunculaceae), contains cardiac glycosides which have actions similar to those of digoxin (p.895). Adonis vernalis is used in herbal and homoeopathic medicine.

### Preparations

**Proprietary Preparations** (details are given in Part 3)

**Multi-ingredient:** ***Braz.:*** Calmazin†; Ritmoneuran†; Serenus; ***Ger.:*** Corguttin N plus†; Miroton; Miroton N; Oxacant N; Oxacant-forte N; Oxacant-Khella N; Raufuncton N†.

---

## Adrenalone *(USAN)*

3′,4′-Dihydroxy-2-(methylamino)acetophenone.

$C_9H_{11}NO_3$ = 181.2.

*CAS — 99-45-6.*

*ATC — A01AD06; B02BC05.*

## Adrenalone Hydrochloride *(pINNM)*

Hidrocloruro de adrenalona.

$C_9H_{11}NO_3,HCl$ = 217.6.

*CAS — 62-13-5.*

*ATC — A01AD06; B02BC05.*

### Profile

Adrenalone hydrochloride is used as a local haemostatic and vasoconstrictor. It has also been used in combination with adrenaline as eye drops for glaucoma.

### Preparations

**Proprietary Preparations** (details are given in Part 3)

***Denm.:*** Stryphnon; ***Ger.:*** Stryphnasal.

**Multi-ingredient:** ***Ger.:*** Links-Glaukosan.

---

## Aesculus

Aesculus hippocastanum; Castaño de indias; Horse-chestnut; Marron d'Inde; Rosskastaniensamen.

*CAS — 6805-41-0 (aescin); 11072-93-8 (β-aescin); 531-75-9 (anhydrous esculoside).*

**Pharmacopoeias.** In *Fr., Ger.,* and *It.* Also in *USNF,* which also includes the powdered form and powdered extract.

*Ger.* also includes esculoside in the sesquihydrate form.

**USNF 22** (Horse Chestnut). The dried seeds of *Aesculus hippocastanum* (Hippocastanaceae), harvested in the autumn. It contains not less than 3.0% of triterpene glycosides, calculated on the dried basis as aescin. Protect from light and moisture.

### Profile

The horse-chestnut, *Aesculus hippocastanum* (conkers), contains several active principles including esculoside (aesculin or esculin; 6-β-D-glucopyranosyloxy-7-hydroxycoumarin, $C_{15}H_{16}O_9$ = 340.3) and aescin (escin), which is a mixture of saponins.

Ingestion of aesculus may cause nausea, vomiting, diarrhoea, abdominal colic, delirium, and with large doses respiratory arrest.

Aescin and esculoside, the major active principles of aesculus, have been used in the prevention and treatment of various peripheral vascular disorders, including haemorrhoids (p.1243). They have been given by mouth, by intravenous injection (in the form of sodium aescinate), by rectal suppository, and applied topically. Aescin has also been given intravenously in the prevention and treatment of postoperative oedema. The maximum intravenous dose in adults for such conditions has been stated to be 20 mg daily; acute renal failure has been reported in patients given higher doses, sometimes with other nephrotoxic drugs.

Other derivatives such as sodium aescin polysulfate have also been used.

*Aesculus hippocastanum* has been used in homoeopathic medicine.

◊ The use of aesculus has been reviewed;[1,2] although there is some evidence suggesting benefit in chronic venous insufficiency, more rigorous studies are needed.[2]

1. Sirtori CR. Aescin: pharmacology, pharmacokinetics and therapeutic profile. *Pharmacol Res* 2001; **44:** 183–93.
2. Pittler MH, Ernst E. Horse chestnut seed extract for chronic venous insufficiency. Available in the Cochrane Library; Issue 2. Chichester: John Wiley; 2004.

**Effects on the kidneys.** A report of the incidence of acute renal failure in patients after cardiac surgery and implicating high-dose intravenous aescin therapy.[1] In 70 patients receiving a mean maximum daily dose of 340 micrograms/kg, no alteration of renal function was observed; in 16 receiving 360 micrograms/kg, mild renal impairment was observed; and in 40 given 510 micrograms/kg, acute renal failure developed.

1. Hellberg K, *et al.* Drug induced acute renal failure after heart surgery. *Thoraxchirurgie* 1975; **23:** 396–400.

**Effects on the skin.** Contact dermatitis[1] to aesculin and contact urticaria[2] to aescin have been reported following the use of topical preparations that contained these extracts. Both reactions were confirmed by positive skin tests.

1. Comaish JS, Kersey PJ. Contact dermatitis to extract of horse chestnut (esculin). *Contact Dermatitis* 1980; **6:** 150–1.
2. Escribano MM, *et al.* Contact urticaria due to aescin. *Contact Dermatitis* 1997; **37:** 233.

**Poisoning.** There have been reports of poisoning in children from eating the seeds, or drinking infusions made from the leaves and twigs of horse-chestnut trees.[1] The toxic substance is considered to be esculoside. Symptoms of poisoning were muscle twitching, weakness, lack of coordination, dilated pupils, vomiting, diarrhoea, paralysis, and stupor.

1. Nagy M. Human poisoning from horse chestnuts. *JAMA* 1973; **226:** 213.

### Preparations

**Proprietary Preparations** (details are given in Part 3)

***Arg.:*** Herbaccion Venotonico; Nadem; Venastat; Venostasin; ***Austria:*** Aesculaforce; Provenen; Reparil; Traumaparil; Venosin; Venostasin; ***Belg.:*** Reparil; ***Braz.:*** Reparil; Varilise; Venostasin; ***Chile:*** Venastat; ***Fr.:*** Flogencyl; Hemorrogel†; ***Ger.:*** Aescorin Forte; Aescusan; Aescuven; Concentrin; Essaven Mono†; Hamos-Tropfen-S; Heweven Phyto; Hoevenol; Noricaven novo; Opino; opino N; Perivar Rosskaven; Plissamur; Proveno N; Reparil; Rexiluven S; Sanaven Venentabletten†; Sklerovenol N; Vasoforte N; Vasotonin; Venalot novo; Venen-Dragees; Venen-Fluid; Venen-Tabletten; Venen-Tropfen N; Venen-Tropfen†; Venentabs; veno-biomo; Venodura; Venogal†; Venoplant; Venopyronum; Venopyronum N; Venostasin; Venotrulan N†; ***Hong Kong:*** Reparil; ***Ital.:*** Curaven; Edeven; Flebostasin; Ginoven†; Reparil; ***Mex.:*** Fluxine†; Venastat; Verisan; ***Neth.:*** Venoplant†; ***Port.:*** Venoparil; ***Spain:*** Fepalitan†; Feparil†; Flebostasin; Provenen; ***Switz.:*** Aesculaforce; AesculaMed; Phlebostasin; Reparil; Sanhelios Venen†; Venastat†; ***Thai.:*** Reparil.

**Multi-ingredient:** ***Arg.:*** Escina Forte; Escina Omega; Feparil; Flaval; Ixana; Nadem Forte; Troxeven; Venoful; Venostasin; ***Austral.:*** Bioglan Cirflo†; Bioglan Fingers & Toes†; Bioglan Zellulean with Escin†; Extralife LegCare†; Herbal Capillary Care†; Proflo†; ***Austria:*** Aesrutan†; Amphodyn; Apoplectal†; Augentropfen Stulln; Dilaescol; Opino; Reparil; Sandoven†; Urelium Neu; Venosin; ***Belg.:*** Rectovasol; Reparil; ***Braz.:*** Castanha de India Composta†; Digestron; Geloril†; Hemoaenus†; Hemorroidex; Hemorrol†; Hemosan†; Hemovirtu's†; Mirorroidin; Novaboin†; Novarrutina; Proctosan†; Reparil; Supositorio Hamamelis Composto; Traumed; Varizin†; Varizol; Venocur Triplex; Venofortan; Venostasin Composto†; ***Canad.:*** Pommade Midy†; Proctomyxin; Proctosedyl; Proctosone; ***Chile:*** Hemorrol; Proctoplex; Repariven; Varicare; ***Denm.:*** Proctosedyl; ***Fin.:*** Proctosedyl; ***Fr.:*** Actisane Hemorroides, Jambes Lourdes†; Anti-Hemorroidaires†; Aphloine P; Arterase; Cepevit†; Circularine†; Climaxol; Creme Rap; Curoveinyl†; Escinogel; Evarose; Fluon; Fragonal†; Hemoluol†; Hemorrogel; Histo-Fluine P; Intrait de Marron D'Inde P; Mediflor Tisane Circulation du Sang No 12; Opo-Veinogene; P. Veinos†; Phlebocreme†; Phlebogel; Phlebosedol; Phlebosup†; Phytomelis; Preparation H; Reparil; Sedorrhoide†; Veinophytum; Veinostase; Veinotonyl; Vivene; ***Ger.:*** Aescorin N; Aescusan; Amphodyn; Apoplectal N; Arnika plus†; Augentropfen Stulln Mono; Cefadysbasin†; Cefasabal; Cycloven Forte N; Diu Venostasin; Essaven; Essaven N; Essaven ultra; Fagorutin Rosskastanien-Balsam N; Hametum-N; Hamos N; Heparin Comp; Heparin Kombi-Gel; Heusin; Heweven P 3†; Heweven P 7†; Hoevenol A†; Hoevenol†; Intradermi; Intradermi Fluid N†; JuPhlebon S†; Lindigoa S; opino N spezial; Pascovenol novo†; PC 30 V; Pe-Ce Ven N†; Posti N; Rectosellan†; Reparil-Gel N; Revicain comp; Revicain comp plus; Salhumin Teilbad N; Salus Venen Krauter Dragees N; Sportupac M; Trauma-cyl; Varicylum-S; Vasesana-Vasoregulans†; Vasotonin forte†; Venacton; Venen-Salbe N; Venen-Salbe†; Venengel; Veno-Kattwiga N; Venoplant AHS; Venostasin; Weleda Hamorrhoidalzapfchen; ***Hong Kong:*** Essaven†; Proctosedyl; Proctosone; Protozone†; Reparil; Roidhemo†; ***India:*** Proctosedyl; ***Irl.:*** Proctosedyl; ***Ital.:*** Bres; Capill; Castindia†; Centella Complex; Centeril H; Dermocinetic; Dermoprolyn; Edeven; Elisir Depurativo Ambrosiano†; Essaven; Flavion; Flogovis IdroGel; Ginkgo Plus†; Hirudex; Inflamase IdroGel; Nitesco Smagliature†; Osmogel; Pomata Midy HC†; Proctonet; Proctopure; Proctosedyl; Recto-Reparil; Reparil; RepaVen; Sedalen Cort; Sedilene Procto; Somatoline; Tioscina†; Varicogel; Venactive; Venoplus; Venotrauma; Venovit†; ***Malaysia:*** Proctosedyl; ***Norw.:*** Proctosedyl; ***Port.:*** Bio-Strath No 1†; Emopads†; Relmus Compositum; Synchrocell; Venoparil; ***S.Afr.:*** Essaven; Proctosedyl; Reparil; ***Singapore:*** Proctosedyl; ***Spain:*** Caprofides Hemostatico; Circovenil Fuerte†; Circovenil†; Contusin; Essavenon; Feparil; Flebo Stop†; Hemodren Compuesto; Killpan†; Liviane Compuesto†; Roidhemo; Ruscimel; Urgenin; Venacol; Venoplant†; ***Swed.:*** Proctosedyl; ***Switz.:*** Augentonicum; Demoven N; Dolo-Veniten; Flavovenyl; Flogecyl; Optazine†; Phlebostasin compositum; Reparil; Reparil N†; Veino-Gouttes-N; Venoplant comp; Venoplant N; ***Thai.:*** Essaven; Proctosedyl; Reparil.

---

## Afelimomab *(rINN)*

*CAS — 156227-98-4.*

### Profile

Afelimomab is a monoclonal tumour necrosis factor antibody that has been investigated for the treatment of sepsis.

◊ References.

1. Vincent JL. Afelimomab. *Int J Clin Pract* 2000; **54:** 190–3.
2. Reinhart K, *et al.* Randomized, placebo-controlled trial of the anti-tumor necrosis factor antibody fragment afelimomab in hyperinflammatory response during severe sepsis: the RAMSES study. *Crit Care Med* 2001; **29:** 765–9.
3. Gallagher J, *et al.* A multicenter, open-label, prospective, randomized, dose-ranging pharmacokinetic study of the anti-TNF-alpha antibody afelimomab in patients with sepsis syndrome. *Intensive Care Med.* 2001; **27:** 1169–78.

---

## Aflatoxins

Aflatoxinas.

*CAS — 1162-65-8 (aflatoxin $B_1$); 7220-81-7 (aflatoxin $B_2$); 1165-39-5 (aflatoxin $G_1$); 7241-98-7 (aflatoxin $G_2$); 6795-23-9 (aflatoxin $M_1$); 6885-57-0 (aflatoxin $M_2$).*

### Profile

Aflatoxins are toxic metabolites produced by many strains of *Aspergillus flavus* and *A. parasiticus,* growing on many vegetable foods, notably maize and peanuts. A number of forms, including aflatoxins $B_1$, $B_2$, $G_1$, and $G_2$ have been identified. Aflatoxins $M_1$ and $M_2$ are metabolites produced by animals following ingestion of aflatoxins $B_1$ and $B_2$; they may be detected in cows' milk.

Aflatoxins can cause hepatitis and cirrhosis. They have been implicated in liver cancer, and may act as co-carcinogens with hepatitis B virus. Aflatoxin $B_1$ is reported to be one of the most potent carcinogens known in *animals.* It has been reported that aflatoxins have been developed in some countries as biological weapons.

◊ References.

1. Ross RK, *et al.* Urinary aflatoxin biomarkers and risk of hepatocellular carcinoma. *Lancet* 1992; **339:** 943–6.
2. Jackson PE, Groopman JD. Aflatoxin and liver cancer. *Baillieres Best Pract Res Clin Gastroenterol* 1999; **13:** 545–55.
3. Peraica M, *et al.* Toxic effects of mycotoxins in humans. *Bull WHO* 1999; **77:** 754–66.
4. Pitt JI. Toxigenic fungi and mycotoxins. *Br Med Bull* 2000; **56:** 184–92.

## Agnus Castus

Agnocasto; Chaste Tree Fruit; Fructus Agni Casti; Gattilier, Fruit de; Keuschlamm; Mönchspfeffer.

**Pharmacopoeias.** In *Swiss.* Also in *USNF.*

**USNF 22** (Chaste Tree). The dried ripe fruits of *Vitex agnus-castus* (Verbenaceae). It contains not less than 0.05% of agnuside and not less than 0.08% of casticin, calculated on the dried basis.

### Profile

Agnus castus is reported to affect the secretion of luteinising hormone, follicle stimulating hormone, and prolactin by the pituitary. Both inhibition and stimulation of prolactin secretion have been reported, and may be dose-dependent. Agnus castus is included in herbal preparations for menstrual or menopausal disorders, but should be avoided in patients receiving exogenous sex hormones, including oral contraceptives.

It is also used in homoeopathic medicine.

◊ References.


1. Houghton P. Agnus castus. *Pharm J* 1994; **253:** 720–1.
2. Christie S, Walker AF. Vitex agnus-castus L.: (1) a review of its traditional and modern therapeutic use; (2) current use from a survey of practitioners. *Eur J Herbal Med* 1997; **3:** 29–45.
3. Schellenberg R. Treatment for the premenstrual syndrome with agnus castus fruit extract: prospective, randomised, placebo controlled study. *BMJ* 2001; **322:** 134–7.
4. Chrubasik S, Roufogalis BD. Chaste tree fruit for female disorders. *Aust J Pharm* 2001; **82:** 156–7.


### Preparations

**Proprietary Preparations** (details are given in Part 3)

***Austral.:*** Premular; ***Austria:*** Agnofem; Agnumens; ***Braz.:*** Lutene; Tenag; Vitex; ***Ger.:*** Agno-Sabona; Agnolyt; Agnucaston; Agnufemil; Biofem; Castufemin; Cefanorm; Femicur N; Feminon A; Gynocastus; Hevertogyn; Kytta-Femin; Strotan; ***Hong Kong:*** Agnucaston†; ***Mex.:*** Cicloplant; ***Switz.:*** Agnolyt; Emoton†; Evana†; Prefemine; PreMens; ***Thai.:*** Agnucaston; ***UK:*** Agnolyt†; Herbal Premens.

**Multi-ingredient:** ***Austral.:*** Dong Quai Complex†; Feminine Herbal Complex†; Lifesystem Herbal Formula 4 Women's Formula†; PMT Complex†; Women's Formula Herbal Formula 3†; ***Ger.:*** Femisana; Presselin Dysmen Olin 3 N†; ***Hong Kong:*** Phytoestrin.

## Agrimony

Agrimonia; Agrimoniae Herba; Aigremoine; Odermennigkraut.

**Pharmacopoeias.** In *Eur.* (see p.vi).

**Ph. Eur. 5.0** (Agrimony). The dried flowering tops of *Agrimonia eupatoria* containing a minimum of 2.0% of tannins expressed as pyrogallol, calculated with reference to the dried drug.

### Profile

Agrimony, the aerial parts of *Agrimonia eupatoria* (Rosaceae) or more rarely *A. procera* (*A. odorata*; fragrant agrimony), has astringent and diuretic properties. It is used internally for diarrhoea, biliary and other gastrointestinal disorders, and urinary-tract disorders; it has also been used for inflammatory mouth and throat disorders. It has been used externally for wound healing and skin disorders.

Agrimony is also used in homoeopathic medicine.

### Preparations

**Proprietary Preparations** (details are given in Part 3)

**Multi-ingredient:** ***Austria:*** Amersan; Gallen- und Lebertee EF-EM-ES; Krauterhaus Mag Kottas Gallen- und Lebertee; Krauterpfarrer Weidinger Tee bei Schlafstorungen; Krauterpfarrer Weidinger Tee fur Leber und Galle; Naturland Heilkrautermundwasser; Neuners Krautertee Nr 28 - zur Unterstutzung der Tatigkeit der Galle; Novocholin; ***Fr.:*** Tisane Hepatique de Hoerdt; ***Ger.:*** Rhoival; Stomasal Med; ***Ital.:*** Allergenid†; ***Spain:*** Natusor Astringel; Natusor Farinol; ***Switz.:*** The Brioni†; ***UK:*** Piletabs.

## Alfalfa

Lucerne; Purple medick.

### Profile

Alfalfa is the plant *Medicago sativa* (Leguminosae) which is cultivated as an animal feedstuff. The seeds and sprouts of alfalfa contain canavanine (2-amino-4-(guanidinooxy)butyric acid), a toxic amino acid structurally related to arginine; content is reported to represent about 1.5% of the dry weight. A syndrome resembling systemic lupus erythematosus has been recorded in *monkeys* fed alfalfa.

Alfalfa is used in herbal preparations for a variety of disorders and in homoeopathic medicine.

### Preparations

**Proprietary Preparations** (details are given in Part 3)

**Multi-ingredient:** ***Austral.:*** Neo-Cleanse†; Panax Complex†; Plantiodine Plus†; Zinc Zenith†; ***Chile:*** Calcio 520; Fucus Compuesto; ***Fr.:*** Gonaxine; Gynosoja; ***Ger.:*** Schneckensirup†; ***UK:*** Fat-Solv†.

## Alglucerase *(BAN, USAN, rINN)*

Alglucerasa; Glucosylceramidase; Macrophage-targeted β-Glucocerebrosidase.

*CAS — 143003-46-7.*

*ATC — A16AB01.*

**Description.** Alglucerase is a modified form of human placental β-glucocerebrosidase (ceramide glucosidase; β-D-glucosyl-*N*-acylsphingosine glucohydrolase). It is a monomeric glycoprotein of 497 amino acids with glycosylation making up about 6% of the molecule.

## Imiglucerase *(BAN, USAN, rINN)*

Imiglucerasa; Recombinant Macrophage-targeted β-Glucocerebrosidase; r-GCR.

*CAS — 154248-97-2.*

*ATC — A16AB02.*

**Description.** Imiglucerase is a recombinant human-derived β-glucocerebrosidase. It is a monomeric glycoprotein of 497 amino acids glycosylated at 4 asparagine residues.

### Adverse Effects and Precautions

Fever, chills, pruritus, flushing, and gastrointestinal symptoms, including cramps, diarrhoea, nausea, and vomiting have been reported following administration of alglucerase or imiglucerase. Some of these may be hypersensitivity reactions; other hypersensitivity reactions, including urticaria and angioedema, respiratory symptoms, and hypotension have also occurred. Anaphylactoid reactions have occurred rarely with imiglucerase. Caution is required in patients who have exhibited signs of hypersensitivity; reduction of the rate of infusion, and pretreatment with antihistamines and/or corticosteroids may permit further treatment. Antibodies have developed in about 15% of patients receiving a glucocerebrosidase enzyme during the first year of therapy. Patients who develop antibodies are at increased risk of hypersensitivity reactions and periodic assessment for antibody formation is recommended.

Pain and irritation at the injection site may occur. Other adverse effects reported include fatigue, dizziness, headache, backache, peripheral oedema, mouth ulcers, and disturbances in sense of smell.

Alglucerase is prepared from human placentas and its infusion therefore carries a risk of transmission of infections although this is minimised by the manufacturing process. Chorionic gonadotrophin, a naturally occurring hormone in human placentas, has been detected in alglucerase. The presence of this hormone may produce early virilisation in young boys if sufficient is given, and has the potential to produce false positive results in pregnancy tests that rely on the detection of this hormone. Alglucerase should be used with caution, if at all, in patients with androgen-sensitive malignancies.

**Effects on the lungs.** Pulmonary hypertension developed in two patients with Gaucher disease after initiation of treatment with alglucerase.[1] Neither patient had evidence of parenchymal lung infiltration with Gaucher cells.


1. Dawson A, *et al.* Pulmonary hypertension developing after alglucerase therapy in two patients with type 1 Gaucher disease complicated by the hepatopulmonary syndrome. *Ann Intern Med* 1996; **125:** 901–4.


### Pharmacokinetics

Following intravenous infusion, plasma enzymatic activities of alglucerase and imiglucerase decline rapidly from steady state, with an elimination half-life of between 3.6 and 10.4 minutes.

### Uses and Administration

Alglucerase and imiglucerase are forms of β-glucocerebrosidase given as long-term enzyme replacement therapy to patients with type 1 or type 3 Gaucher disease (see below) clinically significant non-neurological symptoms. The oligosaccharide chains of the enzyme are modified to terminate with mannose residues to ensure uptake into macrophages.

Alglucerase and imiglucerase are administered by intravenous infusion over 1 to 2 hours. Up to 60 units of alglucerase or imiglucerase per kg may be given as a single infusion. The frequency of administration depends on the severity of symptoms, and initial doses can vary from 2.5 units/kg three times weekly to 60 units/kg once weekly for alglucerase, or once every two weeks for imiglucerase. Once the patient's condition is stabilised the dose should be reduced at intervals of 3 to 12 months to a maintenance dose.

**Gaucher disease.** Gaucher disease[1-4] (glucocerebrosidosis) is a rare, autosomal recessive disorder, although it is the commonest lysosomal storage disease. It is caused by a deficiency of the lysosomal enzyme β-glucocerebrosidase (acid β-glucosidase, ceramide glucosidase, β-D-glucosyl-*N*-acylsphingosine glucohydrolase, or glucosylceramidase) which catalyses the hydrolysis of glucocerebroside, a lipid component of cell membranes, to glucose and ceramide. Deficiency of β-glucocerebrosidase results in accumulation of glucocerebroside in the lysosomes of reticuloendothelial cells, particularly macrophages.

Gaucher disease is classified into three main forms based on clinical signs and symptoms. Hepatosplenomegaly occurs in all forms. Type 1 Gaucher disease (chronic adult non-neuronopathic disease) accounts for 90% or more of cases and occurs especially in Ashkenazi Jews. The disease follows a chronic course of variable severity and onset, with hepatosplenomegaly and blood and bone disorders being the main features; there is no neurological involvement. In type 2 Gaucher disease (acute infantile neuronopathic disease), neurological involvement predominates. Patients show developmental delay by the age of 6 months, suffer seizures, pulmonary infections, and usually die in early childhood. Type 3 Gaucher disease is a subacute neuronopathic form and is slowly progressive.[4] There are 3 subtypes varying in severity and prognosis: in type 3a, there is slow progressive neurological deterioration with death usually occurring during childhood; in type 3b (Norrbotten disease) there is slow cognitive deterioration and patients may survive to adulthood; type 3c typically affects patients of Palestinian, Arab, or Japanese descent, with possible survival to the teenage years.

Treatment of Gaucher disease was previously limited to symptomatic management. Preparations of β-glucocerebrosidase, the deficient enzyme, are now available. Due to the rarity of Gaucher disease, clinical studies have been limited mainly to small case series of patients with type 1 disease. Use of alglucerase or imiglucerase has been shown to reverse hepatosplenomegaly and the haematological abnormalities;[5,6] effects may be seen within a few months, although in many the response is poor during the first 6 to 9 months and then improves rapidly.[2] Return to normal haemoglobin values within 6 to 12 months has been reported, as has reduction in liver size by 20 to 30% within 2 years and 30 to 40% by 5 years; a 50% reduction in spleen size also occurred.[7] Bone symptoms respond more slowly. Decreases in bone pain during the first year of treatment have been reported although there was no radiological improvement.[6] Normalised growth velocity has been reported in children[8] and radiographical assessments have shown improvements in bone density and mineralisation.[9] There is evidence that long-term enzyme replacement therapy for up to 5 years completely or partially ameliorates anaemia, thrombocytopenia, organomegaly, and bone pain in patients with type 1 Gaucher disease, as well as preventing further deterioration.[7] However, successful symptom control is dependent on the degree of damage that has already occurred, and early initiation of therapy is recommended for a more favourable prognosis. Alglucerase has also been tried in rare cases of Gaucher disease affecting the heart[10] or the eye.[11] It is not yet known whether enzyme replacement is able to prevent the development of symptoms in asymptomatic patients.

The efficacy of enzyme replacement therapy in managing neurological symptoms in patients with type 2 or type 3 disease[12] remains to be established. Most of the patients with type 3 Gaucher disease in a small study[13] did not deteriorate neurologically when treated with doses that reversed almost all the systemic manifestations. However, it was pointed out that the amount of enzyme that crosses the blood-brain barrier is unlikely to be significant, and other forms of treatment specifically for neuronopathic Gaucher disease need to be developed.

For those patients in whom enzyme replacement therapy may be unsuitable miglustat may be used. It reduces the synthesis of glucocerebroside by inhibiting glucosyltransferase, one of the early enzymes in the sphingolipid biosynthetic pathway.

Possible future therapies under investigation for Gaucher disease include gene therapy. Other modified forms of β-glucocerebrosidase are also under investigation to improve uptake into the affected macrophages.


1. NIH Technology Assessment Panel on Gaucher Disease. Gaucher disease: current issues in diagnosis and treatment. *JAMA* 1996; **275:** 548–53.
2. Grabowski GA. Current issues in enzyme therapy for Gaucher disease. *Drugs* 1996; **52:** 159–67.
3. Morales LE. Gaucher's disease: a review. *Ann Pharmacother* 1996; **30:** 381–8.
4. Elstein D, *et al.* Gaucher's disease. *Lancet* 2001; **358:** 324–7.
5. Grabowski GA, *et al.* Enzyme therapy in type 1 Gaucher disease: comparative efficacy of mannose-terminated glucocerebrosidase from natural and recombinant sources. *Ann Intern Med* 1995; **122:** 33–9.
6. Pastores GM, *et al.* Enzyme therapy in Gaucher disease type 1: dosage efficacy and adverse effects in 33 patients treated for 6 to 24 months. *Blood* 1993; **82:** 408–16.
7. Weinreb NJ, *et al.* Effectiveness of enzyme replacement therapy in 1028 patients with type 1 Gaucher disease after 2 to 5 years of treatment: a report from the Gaucher Registry. *Am J Med* 2002; **113:** 112–19.
8. Kaplan P, *et al.* Acceleration of retarded growth in children with Gaucher disease after treatment with alglucerase. *J Pediatr* 1996; **129:** 149–53.
9. Rosenthal DI, *et al.* Enzyme replacement therapy for Gaucher disease: skeletal responses to macrophage-targeted glucocerebrosidase. *Pediatrics* 1995; **96:** 629–37.
10. Spada M, *et al.* Cardiac response to enzyme-replacement therapy in Gaucher's disease. *N Engl J Med* 1998; **339:** 1165–6.
11. vom Dahl S, *et al.* Loss of vision in Gaucher's disease and its reversal by enzyme-replacement therapy. *N Engl J Med* 1998; **338:** 1471–2.
12. Bembi B, *et al.* Enzyme replacement treatment in type 1 and type 3 Gaucher's disease. *Lancet* 1994; **344:** 1679–82.
13. Altarescu G, *et al.* The efficacy of enzyme replacement therapy in patients with chronic neuronopathic Gaucher's disease. *J Pediatr* 2001; **138:** 539–47.


### Preparations

**Proprietary Preparations** (details are given in Part 3)

***Austral.:*** Cerezyme; ***Austria:*** Cerezyme; ***Denm.:*** Cerezyme; ***Fr.:*** Cerezyme†; ***Ger.:*** Ceredase†; Cerezyme; ***Hong Kong:*** Cerezyme; ***Israel:*** Ceredase; Cerezyme; ***Ital.:*** Cerezyme; ***Jpn:*** Ceredase; Cerezyme; ***NZ:*** Cerezyme; ***Port.:*** Cerezyme; ***Spain:*** Ceredase†; Cerezyme; ***Switz.:*** Cerezyme; ***UK:*** Cerezyme; ***USA:*** Ceredase; Cerezyme.

## Alibendol *(rINN)*

5-Allyl-*N*-(2-hydroxyethyl)-3-methoxysalicylamide.

$C_{13}H_{17}NO_4$ = 251.3.

*CAS — 26750-81-2.*

### Profile

Alibendol is a choleretic used in the treatment of gastrointestinal disorders.

## Preparations

**Proprietary Preparations** (details are given in Part 3)
*Fr.:* Cebera.

## Allergen Products

Alergenos.

### Adverse Effects and Treatment

Adverse effects to prepared allergens can range from mild local reactions to severe generalised reactions which may be fatal. Severe reactions may be seen after skin tests in sensitive individuals as well as at any time during allergen immunotherapy. Aqueous solutions are more likely to provoke systemic reactions than preparations designed to give slower release rates. Severe reactions have been associated with tyrosine-adsorbed vaccines which have a relatively short half-life.

Hypersensitivity reactions may be immediate or delayed. Local reactions are normally limited to swelling and irritation. Systemic reactions include rhinitis, conjunctivitis, urticaria, bronchospasm, laryngeal oedema, generalised anaphylaxis, and shock. Severe reactions normally occur within 30 minutes and should be treated promptly with intramuscular adrenaline injection 1 in 1000, which should be immediately available when hyposensitising injections are being administered. Full supportive measures should be implemented and treatment with antihistamines and corticosteroids may be required (for a discussion of the treatment of anaphylactic shock, see p.855). Further allergen immunotherapy should be stopped or continued at reduced dosage depending on the severity of the reaction and in accordance with the manufacturer's recommendations.

◊ Reviews.

1. Lockey RF, *et al.* Systemic reactions and fatalities associated with allergen immunotherapy. *Ann Allergy Asthma Immunol* 2001; **87** (suppl 1): 47–55.

◊ In 1986 the UK Committee on Safety of Medicines reported[1] that hyposensitising vaccines have the potential to induce severe bronchospasm and anaphylaxis, and that these reactions had caused 26 deaths in the UK since 1957. The majority of patients had no reaction to previous hyposensitising injections. In 1989 the FDA reported that since 1980, the American Academy of Allergy and Immunology and the FDA had received 14 reports of death following allergen immunotherapy, and 4 deaths following skin testing for allergies.[2] The most common clinical factor in these patients was a history of asthma.

In view of these and other reports, recommendations have been made to minimise the risks of systemic reactions.[3-5] Allergen immunotherapy should only be used for seasonal allergic rhinoconjunctivitis not responding to anti-allergic drugs, and for severe hypersensitivity to Hymenoptera stings. In the UK[4] such treatment is usually avoided in patients with asthma (although asthma is not an absolute contra-indication to Hymenoptera allergen immunotherapy), but elsewhere[3,5] asthmatic patients whose asthma is stable and not severe may be treated. Hyposensitising agents should be used only where facilities for full cardiopulmonary resuscitation are immediately available. The recommended length of time after injection that patients should be kept under medical observation varies from 30 minutes[3] to 1 hour.[4] If the patient develops even mild symptoms of a general reaction observation should be extended until they are completely resolved. The observation period should also be extended for patients at high risk of reactions.

Of twelve samples of *Aspergillus* extract used for allergen immunotherapy, 4 were found to contain aflatoxin (p.1648), one being highly mutagenic as determined by the Ames' test. The results suggested that careful screening of commercially available mould extracts was warranted.[6]

1. Committee on Safety of Medicines. Desensitising vaccines. *BMJ* 1986; **293:** 948.
2. Food and Drug Administration. Fatality risk with allergenic extract use. *JAMA* 1989; **261:** 3368.
3. Malling H-J, Weeke B, eds. Position paper: Immunotherapy. (EAACI) The European Academy of Allergology and Clinical Immunology. *Allergy* 1993; **48** (suppl 14): 9–35.
4. Committee on Safety of Medicines/Medicines Control Agency. Desensitising vaccines: new advice. *Current Problems* 1994; **20:** 5.
5. Bousquet J, *et al.* WHO Position Paper: Allergen immunotherapy: therapeutic vaccines for allergic diseases. *Allergy* 1998; **53** (suppl 44): 1–42.
6. Legator MS, *et al.* Aflatoxin $B_1$ in mould extracts used for desensitisation. *Lancet* 1983; **ii:** 915.

### Precautions

Allergen immunotherapy should not be used in patients with febrile conditions, serious immunological illness, or acute asthma. Allergen preparations should be avoided during pregnancy because of the risk to the fetus of any systemic reactions. Hyposensitising injections should only be administered where facilities for full cardiopulmonary resuscitation are immediately available. It has been recommended that patients should be observed for at least 1 hour after each injection (see under Adverse Effects, above). Patients with asthma may be more susceptible to hypersensitivity reactions with allergen extracts and, in the UK, it is considered that hyposensitising injections should be avoided in patients with asthma, with the possible exception of those at risk of severe hypersensitivity reactions to Hymenoptera stings. Hyposensitising injections should also be avoided in children under 5 years of age.

Whenever possible, the same batch of allergen should be used throughout the treatment course. Injections should be given subcutaneously and not intravenously or intramuscularly.

Hyposensitising injections should be avoided in patients taking beta blockers since adrenaline will be ineffective if hypersensitivity reactions occur in these patients. Severe anaphylactoid reactions have been reported in patients undergoing allergen immunotherapy who are also receiving ACE inhibitors (p.844). Some manufacturers suggest that the reaction could be avoided by temporarily withholding ACE inhibitor therapy during each desensitisation.

Vaccination against infectious diseases should be separated from hyposensitising vaccines by at least 1 week.

Antihistamines should be avoided for at least 48 hours before sensitivity testing is carried out since they may mask skin reactivity; they have been given, during allergen immunotherapy, to very sensitive patients. Systemic or long-term topical use of potent corticosteroids may also mask skin reactivity.

### Uses

Allergen products are used diagnostically in skin tests and provocation tests to confirm the cause of a suspected hypersensitivity reaction. They are also used for allergen immunotherapy in certain patients with hypersensitivity reactions, particularly to insect venoms, pollens, or house-dust mite.

**Allergen immunotherapy.** Allergen immunotherapy (desensitisation or hyposensitisation) is the administration of gradually increasing quantities of allergen extract in a vaccine to ameliorate the effects of subsequent exposure to the allergen. Such therapy has become less popular following reports of severe and fatal anaphylactic reactions during therapy and should only be carried out in specialist centres. Allergen immunotherapy with a specific allergen has been found to be useful in hypersensitivities to pollens and insect venom, particularly that of Hymenoptera.

**Administration.** Allergen vaccines are given as aqueous extracts or as depot preparations bound to aluminium or calcium salts or to tyrosine; allergens modified with glutaral to reduce side-effects while retaining immunogenicity have also been used. Whenever possible, the same batch of allergen should be used during a course of treatment because of possible differences in potency between batches. Allergen extracts are given by subcutaneous injection in dosage regimens as recommended by the manufacturers and depending on the sensitivity of the patient. Skin test titration has been used to determine a safe starting dose. In conventional regimens, increasing doses are given once or twice weekly for aqueous extracts, or every one to two weeks for depot preparations until a maintenance dose is reached. Maintenance doses are given every 4 to 6 weeks. Modified dosage schedules have been used where maintenance needs to be achieved more quickly; such regimens may, however, be associated with an increased risk of adverse reactions. Aqueous extracts should be used for modified schedules until the maintenance dose is reached. In rush schedules, several injections are given once daily on consecutive days. Semi-rush, modified rush, or cluster regimens involve the administration of several injections on a single day, separated by an interval of several days.

The optimal duration of allergen immunotherapy is unknown, but a period of 3 to 5 years is usually recommended.

Oral, nasal, sublingual, and bronchial routes of administration have sometimes been used for allergen immunotherapy.

**Uses.** The use of allergen immunotherapy has been reviewed[1-3] and various authorities have published recommendations.[4-7] Allergen immunotherapy is indicated exclusively for Type I (immediate) hypersensitivity reactions mediated by IgE antibodies. It may be used for the treatment of insect sting hypersensitivity, allergic rhinitis and conjunctivitis, and allergic asthma. Reports of severe and sometimes fatal hypersensitivity reactions to allergen preparations have prompted recommendations to reduce the risk of systemic reactions (see under Adverse Effects, above).

Allergen immunotherapy is used in children[7] and is thought to be more effective than in adults. It has been suggested that its use in children with allergic rhinoconjunctivitis may also prevent the development of asthma. A significant clinical benefit was demonstrated[8] in children 6 years after discontinuation of preseasonal grass pollen immunotherapy. Therapy is generally not recommended for children younger than 5 years of age[4,7] because it is less well tolerated, and in this age group the differential diagnosis between allergic rhinitis and viral infection of the respiratory tract may not be clear.[7]

Allergen immunotherapy is indicated for patients with specific IgE antibodies who have experienced severe anaphylaxis following insect stings, particularly those of Hymenoptera (bees, wasps, and stinging ants).[4,5,7] Vaccines containing purified venom are available for most Hymenoptera and have replaced whole body extract preparations, which were generally found to be ineffective. Venom vaccines are not available for stinging ants but whole body extract vaccines may contain sufficient venom antigens to be effective.[2,7]

Allergen immunotherapy for seasonal allergic rhinitis and conjunctivitis triggered by pollen has generally been reserved for severely affected patients when anti-allergic drugs have failed.[4,7] However, there is some evidence that its use for allergies such as rhinitis may prevent the development of asthma[3] and thus earlier use of allergen immunotherapy may be warranted.[5] Recommendations for the use of allergen immunotherapy in patients with asthma vary. Guidelines in the UK[4] recommend that asthmatic patients should not be treated with allergen immunotherapy because they are more likely to develop severe adverse effects (although asthma is not considered a contra-indication to allergen immunotherapy for anaphylaxis caused by Hymenoptera). Others, including WHO,[5-7] consider that allergen immunotherapy for allergic rhinoconjunctivitis can be given to patients whose asthma is stable and not severe ($FEV_1$ is not less than 70% of predicted value), when avoidance of allergens has not been sufficient or is not possible, and drug treatment has failed. Allergen immunotherapy for rhinoconjunctivitis and asthma due to house-dust mite or animal danders can be considered when the allergen is unavoidable.[5-7,9] However, in the UK the *British National Formulary* considers evidence of benefit from desensitisation to these latter allergens to be inadequate, and it is not recommended.

Allergen immunotherapy to a drug may be warranted on the rare occasions when hypersensitivity has developed and continued use is considered essential, possibly with penicillins or insulin.[4,10] Such regimens produce clinical tolerance, lost on cessation of therapy, without immunological change.[5]

Allergen immunotherapy has also been tried in other disorders such as atopic dermatitis, urticaria, and food allergies, but there is insufficient evidence to support such use.[2,4]

Rush allergen immunotherapy has been successful in a woman hypersensitive to seminal plasma.[11]

Allergen immunotherapy with a single intradermal injection of an enzyme-potentiated allergen extract has been tried.[12]

1. Loblay RH. Allergen immunotherapy: when is it useful? *Drugs* 1990; **40:** 493–7.
2. Weber RW. Immunotherapy with allergens. *JAMA* 1997; **278:** 1881–7.
3. Yang X. Does allergen immunotherapy alter the natural course of allergic disorders? *Drugs* 2001; **61:** 365–74.
4. Frew AJ, British Society for Allergy and Clinical Immunology Working Party. Injection Immunotherapy. *BMJ* 1993; **307:** 919–23.
5. Malling H-J, Weeke B, eds. Position paper: Immunotherapy. (EAACI) The European Academy of Allergology and Clinical Immunology. *Allergy* 1993; **48** (suppl 14): 9–35.
6. Thoracic Society of Australia and New Zealand and Australasian Society of Clinical Immunology and Allergy. Specific allergen immunotherapy for asthma. *Med J Aust* 1997; **167:** 540–44.
7. Bousquet J, *et al.* WHO Position Paper: Allergen immunotherapy: therapeutic vaccines for allergic diseases. *Allergy* 1998; **53** (suppl 44): 1–42.
8. Eng PA, *et al.* Long-term efficacy of preseasonal grass pollen immunotherapy in children. *Allergy* 2002; **57:** 306–12.
9. Abramson MJ, *et al.* Is allergen immunotherapy effective in asthma? A meta-analysis of randomized controlled trials. *Am J Respir Crit Care Med* 1995; **151:** 969–74.
10. Anderson JA, Adkinson NF. Allergic reactions to drugs and biologic agents. *JAMA* 1987; **258:** 2891–9.
11. Frisch C, *et al.* Rush hyposensitisation for allergy to seminal plasma. *Lancet* 1984; **i:** 1073.
12. Fell P, Brostoff J. A single dose desensitization for summer hay fever. *Eur J Clin Pharmacol* 1990; **38:** 77–9.

DIAGNOSTIC USE. Sensitivity testing can be used to confirm that suspected allergens are predominantly responsible for the symptoms of a suspected hypersensitivity reaction. However, sensitivity testing should not form the sole basis of the treatment of hypersensitivity reactions.

Type IV (delayed) hypersensitivity reactions such as contact dermatitis are normally diagnosed using patch tests. A number of standard techniques are available, but in general they all involve maintaining a standard amount of the test substance in contact with the skin for 48 to 72 hours. A positive response is shown by erythema, swelling, or vesiculation. The sensitivity of different parts of the body varies, and this should be accounted for in applying test substances and controls. The test results are normally read half to one hour after removal of the patches to allow any pressure effects of the patches to subside. Patch testing with mixtures of allergens may be necessary to diagnose contact dermatitis in patients hypersensitive to multiple allergens.

Type I (immediate) hypersensitivity reactions such as allergic rhinitis, allergic asthma, and insect-sting hypersensitivity are tested using prick or intradermal tests. Since the allergen is introduced through the skin in these tests the risk of systemic reactions is greater, and adrenaline injection should be kept available. The test involves pricking the skin through a drop of allergen in solution, and comparing the result after 15 to 20 minutes with positive and negative controls. The intradermal test is used if the prick test result does not agree with a strong clinical suspicion. Skin testing is unreliable for evaluating hypersensitivity to drugs, except for penicillins and for certain macromolecules. Skin test titration, that is testing with a series of dilutions, has been used to determine a safe starting dose for allergen immunotherapy.

Provocation tests are designed to reproduce symptoms of hypersensitivity by controlled exposure to a suspected allergen. Provocation may be by the bronchial, oral, nasal, or ocular routes. Facilities for full cardiopulmonary resuscitation should be immediately available.

*In-vitro* methods for measuring antigen-specific IgE include the radioallergosorbent test (RAST).

References.

1. VanArsdel PP, Larson EB. Diagnostic tests for patients with suspected allergic disease: utility and limitations. *Ann Intern Med* 1989; **110:** 304–12.
2. VanArsdel PP, Larson EB. Allergy testing. *Ann Intern Med* 1989; **110:** 317–20.
3. McLelland J, Shuster S. Contact dermatitis with negative patch tests: the additive effects of allergens in combination. *Br J Dermatol* 1990; **122:** 623–30.
4. Anonymous. Allergen testing in patients with type I hypersensitivity. *Drug Ther Bull* 1995; **33:** 45–7. Correction. *ibid.*: 55.

### Preparations

**Proprietary Preparations** (details are given in Part 3)
***Austral.:*** Albay; Allpyral; ***Belg.:*** Pharmalgen†; Pollinex; ***Braz.:*** Nikkho Vac; ***Canad.:*** Pollinex-R; ***Denm.:*** Alutard SQ; Aquagen SQ; Pharmalgen; Sensitiner; Soluprick SQ; True Test; ***Fr.:*** Albey; Allpyral†; Alpha Fraction†; Alyostal; ASAD; Candidine†; ***Ger.:*** ADL†; ALK; Allergovit; Allerset†; Depot-Hal; Hal-oral†; Novo-Helisen; Oralvac; Pollinex Quattro; Purethal; Reless; SDL†; TA Baume; TA Graser; TA MIX; True Test†; Tyrosin TU; Venomenhal; Venomil; ***Ital.:*** Alhydrox†; Alpare†; Conjuvac†; Phostal; Staloral; ***Mex.:*** True Test; ***Neth.:*** Alavac-S†; Allergoid-HAL†; Allerset†; Artoid†; Depot-Hal; Haloral†; Immunovac; Oralgen; Pollinex; Purethal; Sublivac B.E.S.T.; ***Norw.:*** Alutard; ***NZ:*** Albay; Allpyral; True Test; ***Port.:*** Polagen; ***S.Afr.:*** Albay†; Albey; Allpyral Pure Mite; Allpyral Special Grass; Diagnostic Skin Testing Kit†; EH Retard; Tol; ***Swed.:*** Alutard SQ; Aquagen SQ; Pharmalgen†; Soluprick SQ; ***Switz.:*** Alavac-S; ALK; Allergovit; Alutard SQ; Alyostal; ASAD; Novo-Helisen; Pharmalgen; Phostal; Polvac; SDV†; Staloral; ***UK:*** Bencard Skin Testing Solutions†; Pharmalgen; Pollinex; ***USA:*** Albay; Allpyral; Center-Al; Pharmalgen; True Test; Venomil.

**Multi-ingredient:** ***Arg.:*** Summavac; ***Braz.:*** Alergomed†; Alergoral; Aminovac; Insuvac†; Multigen AL; Multivac VR; Munolan†; Rhinovac; Urtivac; Vag Oral; ***Fin.:*** Alutard SQ; Aquagen SQ; Soluprick SQ; ***Ger.:*** BU Pangramin SLIT; Sublivac; ***Neth.:*** Venomhal.

## Almond Oil

Aceite de Almendra; Almendras dulces, aceite de; Bitter Almond Oil; Expressed Almond Oil; Huile d'Amande; Mandelöl; Ol. Amygdal.; Oleo de Amêndoas; Olio di Mandorla; Sweet Almond Oil.
*CAS — 8007-69-0.*

**Pharmacopoeias.** In *USNF.*
*Eur* (see p.vi) includes the virgin oil and a refined oil.
*Fr.* also specifies Huile de Noyaux, an oil obtained from various species of *Prunus.*

**Ph. Eur. 5.0** (Almond Oil, Virgin; Amygdalae Oleum Virginale). A yellow, clear, liquid. It is the fatty oil obtained by cold expression from the ripe seeds of *Prunus dulcis* var. *amara* or *P. dulcis* var. *dulcis* or a mixture of both varieties. Slightly soluble in alcohol; miscible with petroleum spirit. Store in well-filled containers. Protect from light.

**Ph. Eur. 5.0** (Almond Oil, Refined; Amygdalae Oleum Raffinatum). The fatty oil obtained by refining and deodorisation of Almond Oil. It may contain a suitable antioxidant. A pale yellow, clear, transparent liquid. Slightly soluble in alcohol; miscible with petroleum spirit. Store in well-filled containers. Protect from light.

**USNF 22** (Almond Oil). The fixed oil expressed from the kernels of varieties of *Prunus amygdalus* [*Prunus dulcis*] (Rosaceae). A clear, colourless or pale straw-coloured, oily liquid with a bland taste. Slightly soluble in alcohol; miscible with chloroform, with ether, with petroleum spirit, and with benzene. Store in airtight containers.

### Profile

Almond oil, which consists mainly of glycerides of oleic acid with smaller amounts of linoleic and palmitic acid, has nutritive and demulcent properties. It is used as an emollient and to soften ear wax. It is also used as a vehicle in some injections.

### Preparations

***BP 2003:*** Almond Oil Ear Drops;
***USP 27:*** Rose Water Ointment.

**Proprietary Preparations** (details are given in Part 3)
***Fr.:*** Karelyne†; ***Mex.:*** Dermoskin.

**Multi-ingredient:** ***Austral.:*** Curash Babycare; ***Chile:*** Akerat; ***Ital.:*** Babysteril; Otosan Natural Ear Drops; Proctonet; Stilomagic; ***Mex.:*** Caliderm; Liniderm; ***NZ:*** Am-O-Lin; Snorenz; ***Port.:*** Cuidaderma; Olidermil; ***Spain:*** Pasta Lassar Imba; ***Switz.:*** Antidry; Balmandol; Premandol; Viola; Woloderma; ***UK:*** Calendula Nappy Change Cream; Earex; Imuderm; Infaderm; Snor-Away; Snorenz†.

## Alpha Galactosidase A

α-D-Galactosidase; α-Galactosidase A; α-D-Galactoside Galactohydrolase.

## Agalsidase Alfa *(BAN, USAN, rINN)*

*CAS — 104138-64-9 (protein moiety).*
*ATC — A16AB03.*

## Agalsidase Beta *(rINN)*

Alfasidasa β.
*CAS — 104138-64-9 (protein moiety).*
*ATC — A16AB04.*

### Adverse Effects, Treatment, and Precautions

IgG antibodies to agalsidase alfa and beta develop in the majority of patients, who are consequently at increased risk of hypersensitivity reactions. Infusion reactions have been reported in 10% of patients given agalsidase alfa. Onset usually occurs 2 to 4 months after initiation of treatment and common symptoms include chills, dyspnoea, and facial flushing, developing during, or within 1 hour of, infusion. The infusion may be interrupted for about 5 to 10 minutes and restarted once symptoms have subsided. Pre-treatment with oral antihistamines and corticosteroids 1 to 3 hours before infusion has been used to prevent subsequent reactions. Similar infusion reactions have been reported in about 50% of patients treated with agalsidase beta; the frequency of these reactions decreased with continued use.

### Interactions

Agalsidase alfa or beta should not be used with amiodarone, chloroquine, monobenzone, or gentamicin, which all have the potential to inhibit intracellular α-galactosidase activity.

### Pharmacokinetics

The pharmacokinetic properties of agalsidase alfa appear to be unaffected by dose; the elimination half-life from blood following a single dose has been reported to be about 100 minutes. The pharmacokinetics of agalsidase beta indicate a saturated clearance; the elimination half-life following a single dose has been reported to range from 45 to 100 minutes.

### Uses and Administration

Alpha galactosidase A is an endogenous enzyme that hydrolyses terminal α-D-galactose residues in oligosaccharides and galactolipids into more easily digestible mono- and disaccharides. A form derived from a fungal source is used to prevent intestinal gas.

Agalsidase alfa and beta are recombinant forms of alpha galactosidase A used for the long-term enzyme replacement therapy of Fabry disease (see below).

Agalsidase alfa is given by intravenous infusion in a dose of 200 micrograms/kg over 40 minutes, repeated every alternate week.

Agalsidase beta is given by intravenous infusion in a dose of 1 mg/kg at an initial rate of 250 micrograms/minute; the rate may be gradually increased once tolerance has been established, but the total infusion time should not be less than 2 hours. The dose should be repeated every alternate week.

**Fabry disease.** Fabry disease (Anderson-Fabry disease) is a rare X-linked recessive lysosomal storage disorder.[1-3] It is characterised by a deficiency of the enzyme alpha galactosidase A resulting in the intracellular accumulation of globotriaosylceramide ($Gb_3$) and other glycosphingolipids, especially in vascular endothelium and smooth muscle. Symptoms include severe neuropathies, fevers, skin blemishes (angiokeratomas), corneal and lenticular opacities, and gastrointestinal disturbances. Cardiac, cerebrovascular, and renal deterioration is progressive placing patients at increased risk for early-onset myocardial infarction, stroke, and renal failure.

Symptomatic treatment was the only option until the development of enzyme replacement therapy with agalsidase alfa and beta. Results from controlled studies[4-7] show this form of therapy to be effective in clearing deposits from the kidneys, heart, and skin. However, long-term studies are necessary to evaluate the true potential. Gene therapy[8] is also under investigation.


1. Brady RO, Schiffmann R. Clinical features of and recent advances in therapy for Fabry disease. *JAMA* 2000; **284:** 2771–5.
2. Schiffmann R, Brady RO. New prospects for the treatment of lysosomal storage diseases. *Drugs* 2002; **62:** 733–42.
3. Mehta A. Agalsidase alfa: specific treatment for Fabry disease. *Hosp Med* 2002; **63:** 347–50.
4. Moore DF, *et al.* Regional cerebral hyperperfusion and nitric oxide pathway dysregulation in Fabry disease: reversal by enzyme replacement therapy. *Circulation* 2001; **104:** 1506–12.
5. Schiffmann R, *et al.* Enzyme replacement therapy in Fabry disease: a randomized controlled trial. *JAMA* 2001; **285:** 2743–9.
6. Eng CM, *et al.* Safety and efficacy of recombinant human α-galactosidase A replacement therapy in Fabry's disease. *N Engl J Med* 2001; **345:** 9–16.
7. Moore DF, *et al.* Elevated cerebral blood flow velocities in Fabry disease with reversal after enzyme replacement. *Stroke* 2002; **33:** 525–31.
8. Siatskas C, Medin JA. Gene therapy for Fabry disease. *J Inherit Metab Dis* 2001; **24** (suppl 2): 25–41.


### Preparations

**Proprietary Preparations** (details are given in Part 3)
***Canad.:*** Beano; Gaz Away; ***Denm.:*** Fabrazyme; Replagal; ***Fr.:*** Fabrazyme; Replagal; ***Ger.:*** Fabrazyme; Replagal; ***Israel:*** Fabrazyme; Replagal; ***Ital.:*** Fabrazyme; ***Spain:*** Fabrazyme; Replagal; ***UK:*** Beano; Fabrazyme; ***USA:*** Beano; Fabrazyme.

## Alpha$_1$-proteinase Inhibitor

Alpha$_1$ Antitrypsin; Inhibidor de la $\alpha_1$- proteinasa.
*ATC — B02AB02.*

### Adverse Effects and Precautions

Intravenous administration of alpha$_1$-proteinase inhibitor may produce flu-like symptoms, chills, dyspnoea, hypotension, tachycardia, or rashes. Allergic-type reactions have been reported. Preparations derived from pooled human plasma carry a risk of transmission of infection (see Blood, p.744). Vaccination against hepatitis B is recommended before starting treatment with alpha$_1$-proteinase inhibitor.

### Uses and Administration

Endogenous alpha$_1$-proteinase inhibitor is a serum glycoprotein synthesised in the liver that acts as an elastase inhibitor, primarily inhibiting neutrophil elastase. Alpha$_1$-proteinase inhibitor, prepared from pooled human plasma, is used as replacement therapy in patients with emphysema who have congenital alpha$_1$ antitrypsin deficiency (see below). It is given in a dose of 60 mg/kg once a week by intravenous infusion over about 30 minutes.

A recombinant form of alpha$_1$-proteinase inhibitor is under investigation for nebulised delivery in congenital alpha$_1$ antitrypsin deficiency and cystic fibrosis (see below).

Alpha$_1$-proteinase inhibitor is also under investigation for the prevention of bronchopulmonary dysplasia (p.1077) in preterm neonates.

**Alpha$_1$ antitrypsin deficiency.** Alpha$_1$ antitrypsin deficiency is a rare genetic disorder characterised by the development of emphysema usually in the third or fourth decade of life. Patients with this disorder lack alpha$_1$-proteinase inhibitor, which acts in the lungs as an inhibitor of neutrophil elastase, an enzyme released in response to inflammation. A deficiency of this inhibitor thus leaves the lungs vulnerable to destruction by elastase leading to the development of emphysema (p.779).

Management of alpha$_1$ antitrypsin deficiency involves avoidance of factors (mainly cigarette smoking) that cause pulmonary inflammation, and supportive treatment with bronchodilators and oxygen as appropriate. Replacement therapy with alpha$_1$-proteinase inhibitor by intravenous infusion has been shown to correct the biochemical abnormality[1] and has been recommended in those patients with some deterioration of lung function.[2,3] In a short-term study[4] serum and secretion concentrations of alpha$_1$ antitrypsin as well as markers of neutrophilic inflammation were monitored in 12 patients receiving replacement therapy over 4 weeks. Results demonstrated a rise in serum levels of alpha$_1$ antitrypsin to above the protective threshold, and reduction in elastase activity and levels of leukotriene $B_4$ levels (thought to be important in producing airway inflammation in alpha$_1$ antitrypsin deficiency). A small placebo-controlled study[5] found that the rate of decline of $FEV_1$ was not affected in patients treated for at least 3 years. Data[6] from a large registry of patients also suggested that, overall, treatment did not affect the rate of decline of $FEV_1$, but that it decreased mortality, although this may be influenced by other factors. Evaluation[3] of 2 of these studies[5,6] and one other concluded that replacement therapy might reduce the progression of disease in selected patients, but that further randomised placebo-controlled studies are required to provide conclusive evidence for overall clinical efficacy. The authors recommended that replacement therapy should be reserved for patients with an $FEV_1$ between 35 and 50% predicted who are no longer smoking and on optimal medical therapy but continuing to show a rapid decline in $FEV_1$. In a retrospective cohort study[7] in 96 patients followed up for a minimum of 12 months, results indicated that the rate of progression of pulmonary emphysema was reduced during the time that the patients received replacement therapy, and patients with well-maintained lung function and a rapid decline in $FEV_1$ benefited most from therapy. These authors recommended early diagnosis to identify patients at risk and to start augmentation even if lung function is greater than 65% predicted.

Recombinant forms of alpha$_1$-proteinase inhibitor and administration by aerosol are also being investigated, as is gene therapy.[1,2]

Patients with alpha$_1$ antitrypsin deficiency may also have some liver involvement. This may present as neonatal jaundice or in adults as cirrhosis. The liver disease is managed symptomatically; it does not respond to treatment with alpha$_1$-proteinase inhibitor.[2]


1. Coakley RJ, *et al.* α1-Antitrypsin deficiency: biological answers to clinical questions. *Am J Med Sci* 2001; **321:** 33–41.
2. American Thoracic Society/European Respiratory Society. Standards for the diagnosis and management of individuals with alpha-1 antitrypsin deficiency. *Am J Respir Crit Care Med* 2003; **168:** 818–900. Also available at: http://www.thoracic.org/adobe/statements/alpha1.pdf (accessed 02/07/04)
3. Abboud RT, *et al.* Alpha$_1$-antitrypsin deficiency: a position statement of the Canadian Thoracic Society. *Can Respir J* 2001; **8:** 81–8.
4. Stockley RA, *et al.* The effect of augmentation therapy on bronchial inflammation in α1-antitrypsin deficiency. *Am J Respir Crit Care Med* 2002; **165:** 1494–8.
5. Dirksen A, *et al.* A randomized clinical trial of $\alpha_1$-antitrypsin augmentation therapy. *Am J Respir Crit Care Med* 1999; **160:** 1468–72.
6. The Alpha-1-Antitrypsin Deficiency Registry Study Group. Survival and $FEV_1$ decline in individuals with severe deficiency of $\alpha_1$-antitrypsin. *Am J Respir Crit Care Med* 1998; **158:** 49–59.
7. Wencker M, *et al.* Longitudinal follow-up of patients with $\alpha_1$-protease inhibitor deficiency before and during therapy with IV $\alpha_1$-protease inhibitor. *Chest* 2001; **119:** 737–44.


**Cystic fibrosis.** Some of the inflammatory damage that occurs in the lungs of patients with cystic fibrosis is thought to be caused by excessive amounts of elastase released locally. Alpha$_1$-proteinase inhibitor given by nebuliser is therefore under investigation[1,2] in patients with cystic fibrosis (p.123).


1. McElvaney NG, *et al.* Aerosol α1-antitrypsin treatment for cystic fibrosis. *Lancet* 1991; **337:** 392–4.
2. Balfour-Lynn IM. The protease-antiprotease battle in the cystic fibrosis lung. *J R Soc Med* 1999; **92** (suppl 37): 23–30.


### Preparations

**Proprietary Preparations** (details are given in Part 3)
***Canad.:*** Prolastin; ***Ger.:*** Prolastin; ***Hong Kong:*** Prolastin†; ***Ital.:*** Prolastina; ***Spain:*** Prolastina; ***USA:*** Aralast; Prolastin; Zemaira.

## Althaea

Altea; Alteia; Alth.; Eibisch; Guimauve; Malvavisco; Marshmallow.

**Pharmacopoeias.** *Eur.* (see p.vi) and *Pol.* include the root and the leaf. *Fr.* also includes the flower.

**Ph. Eur. 5.0** (Marshmallow Root; Althaeae Radix). The peeled or unpeeled, whole or cut, dried root of marshmallow, *Althaea officinalis*. Protect from light.

**Ph. Eur. 5.0** (Marshmallow Leaf; Althaea Folium). The whole or cut dried leaf of *Althaea officinalis*. Protect from light.

## Profile

Althaea is demulcent and emollient and has been used for irritation and inflammation of the mucous membranes of the mouth and pharynx, and relief of associated dry cough. It has also been used in traditional remedies for a variety of disorders including gastrointestinal disturbances.

## Preparations

**Proprietary Preparations** (details are given in Part 3)

***Austria:*** Risinetten; ***Ger.:*** Phytohustil.

**Multi-ingredient:** ***Austral.:*** Althaea Complex†; Cough Relief†; Garlic and Horseradish + C Complex†; Hydrastis Complex†; Respatona Decongestant Formula†; Respatona Plus Bronchial Cough Relief†; ***Austria:*** Aktiv Husten- und Bronchialtee; Anifer Hustentee; Aponatura Hustenlosende; Aurita-Bronchialtee; Aurita-Erkaltungstee; Bio-Garten Tee gegen Erkaltung; Bioreform-Erkaltungstee; Bronchostop; Bronchostop sine; Erkaltungstee; Gewusst wie Husten-Bronchialtee; Heumann's Bronchialtee; Krauterhaus Mag Kottas Husten- und Bronchialtee; Krauterpfarrer Weidinger Tee bei Darmtragheit; Luuf-Halspastillen fur Kinder; Mag Kottas Husten-Bronchialtee; Mag Kottas Krauterexpress-Husten-Bronchialtee; Mediplant Krauter; Neuners Krautertee Nr 11 - zur Unterstutzung der Tatigkeit der Bronchien und Atemwege; Neuners Krautertee Nr 7 - Bronchial- und Lungentee; Paracodin; Sidroga Brust-Husten-Tee; St Radegunder Hustentee; Synpharma Instant-Brust- und Hustentee; The Chambard-Tee; Tuscalman; Tussimont; ***Belg.:*** Eugiron†; Paracodine; Tisane Antibiliaire et Stomachique†; Tisane Pectorale†; Tisane Purgative†; ***Braz.:*** Limao Bravo†; Peitoral Angico Pelotense; ***Canad.:*** Swiss Herb Cough Drops; ***Fr.:*** Apilaxe; Elixir Contre La Toux Weleda†; Mediflor Tisane No 4 Diuretique; Mediflor Tisane Pectorale d'Alsace†; Tisane des Familles†; Tisane Grande Chartreuse†; ***Ger.:*** Em-eukal Husten- und Brusttee; Heumann Bronchialtee Solubifix; Infantussin N†; Junisana; Tonsilgon; ***Ital.:*** Altea (Specie Composta); Cura†; ***Spain:*** Bronpul; Llantusil; Malvaliz; Natusor Broncopul; Natusor Farinol; Natusor Gastrolen; Natusor Malvasen; Senalsor; ***Switz.:*** Malveol; Neo-DP; Sirop antitussif Wyss a base de codeine†; Sirop pectoral DP1†; Sirop pectoral DP2, DP3†; Sirop Wyss contre la toux†; Tisane pectorale et antitussive; Tisane pectorale pour les enfants; Tisane Provencale No1; Tuscalman; ***UK:*** Biobalm†; Digest†; Garlodex†; Gerard House Golden Seal Compound†; Herb and Honey Cough Elixir; Herbheal Ointment; Modern Herbals Cold & Catarrh; Potter's Catarrh Pastilles; Sinotar.

---

# Alum

Alaun; Allume; Aluin; Alumbre; Alumen; Aluminium Kalium Sulfuricum; Aluminium Potassium Sulphate; Alun; E522; Potash Alum; Potassium Alum. Potassium aluminium sulphate dodecahydrate.

$AlK(SO_4)_2,12H_2O$ = 474.4.

*CAS — 7784-24-9 (alum dodecahydrate); 10043-67-1 (anhydrous alum).*

*ATC — S01XA07.*

**Pharmacopoeias.** In *Chin., Eur.* (see p.vi), *Jpn, Pol.,* and *US.* *US* also includes dodecahydrated ammonia alum (Ammonium Alum). *Jpn* also includes dried alum.

**Ph. Eur. 5.0** (Alum). Colourless, transparent, crystalline masses or a granular powder. Freely soluble in water; very soluble in boiling water; practically insoluble in alcohol; soluble in glycerol. A 10% solution in water has a pH of 3.0 to 3.5.

**USP 27** (Potassium Alum). A white powder or large, colourless crystals or crystalline fragments. It is odourless. Soluble 1 in 7 of water and 1 in 0.3 of boiling water; insoluble in alcohol; freely but slowly soluble in glycerol. Its solutions are acid to litmus. Store in airtight containers.

## Adverse Effects

Large doses of alum are irritant and may be corrosive; gum necrosis and gastrointestinal haemorrhage have occurred. Systemic absorption from bladder irrigation solutions can cause acute aluminium toxicity (see under Aluminium below) including encephalopathy.

◇ Acute encephalopathy has been reported[1,2] following bladder irrigation with alum solutions in the treatment of bladder haemorrhage. Anecdotal evidence would suggest that this practice should be avoided in patients with renal insufficiency.[1]

1. Phelps KR, *et al.* Encephalopathy after bladder irrigation with alum: case report and literature review. *Am J Med Sci* 1999; **318:** 181–5.
2. Nakamura H, *et al.* Acute encephalopathy due to aluminium toxicity successfully treated by combined intravenous deferoxamine and hemodialysis. *J Clin Pharmacol* 2000; **40:** 296–300.

## Uses and Administration

Alum precipitates proteins and is a powerful astringent. It is often included in preparations used as mouthwashes or gargles and in dermatological preparations.

Alum, either as a solid or as a solution, may be used as a haemostatic. Intravesical administration of alum, typically as a 1% solution, has been used as a treatment for bladder haemorrhage.

Alum is also used as a mordant in the dyeing industry.

## Preparations

**Proprietary Preparations** (details are given in Part 3)

**Multi-ingredient:** ***Austral.:*** BFI†; ***Austria:*** EST; ***Braz.:*** Higienex†; Lucretin; ***Canad.:*** Fletchers Sore Mouth Medicine; ***Fr.:*** Denisoline†; ***Ger.:*** Dr. Hotz Vollbad†; Retterspitz Ausserlich†; Retterspitz Gelee†; Retterspitz Innerlich†; Trachitol†; ***Ital.:*** Lavanda Sofar; ***Mex.:*** Forcremol; ***NZ:*** Grans Remedy; ***Spain:*** Cloroboral†; Co Bucal; Lindemil; ***USA:*** BFI; Massengill; Mycinette.

---

# Aluminium

Aluminio; Aluminum; E173.

Al = 26.981538.

*CAS — 7429-90-5.*

**Description.** Aluminium is a malleable and ductile soft silvery-white metal, becoming coated with a thin layer of oxide.

**Pharmacopoeias.** *Br.* includes Aluminium Powder.

**BP 2003** (Aluminium Powder). An odourless or almost odourless, silvery-grey powder. It consists mainly of metallic aluminium in very small flakes, usually with an appreciable quantity of aluminium oxide. It is lubricated with stearic acid to protect the metal from oxidation. Practically insoluble in water and in alcohol; it dissolves in dilute acids and in aqueous solutions of alkali hydroxides, with the evolution of hydrogen.

**Handling.** Aluminium powder has been used for the illicit preparation of explosives or fireworks; care is required with its supply.

**Incompatibility.** Incompatibilities have been reported between aluminium in injection equipment and metronidazole[1,2] and between aluminium and various antineoplastics including cisplatin, daunorubicin, and doxorubicin.[3-6] The suitability of aluminium caps for sugar-containing liquids has also been questioned. Abrasion of the aluminium cap by sugar from Ceporex Syrup [cefalexin] has resulted in the formation of a black slime.[7]

1. Schell KH, Copeland JR. Metronidazole hydrochloride-aluminum interaction. *Am J Hosp Pharm* 1985; **42:** 1040, 1042.
2. Struthers BJ, Parr RJ. Clarifying the metronidazole hydrochloride-aluminum interaction. *Am J Hosp Pharm* 1985; **42:** 2660.
3. Bohart RD, Ogawa G. An observation on the stability of cis-dichlorodiammineplatinum (II): a caution regarding its administration. *Cancer Treat Rep* 1979; **63:** 2117–18.
4. Gardiner WA. Possible incompatibility of doxorubicin hydrochloride with aluminum. *Am J Hosp Pharm* 1981; **38:** 1276.
5. Williamson MJ, *et al.* Doxorubicin hydrochloride-aluminum interaction. *Am J Hosp Pharm* 1983; **40:** 214.
6. Ogawa GS, *et al.* Dispensing-pin problems. *Am J Hosp Pharm* 1985; **42:** 1042.
7. Tressler LJ. Medicine bottle caps. *Pharm J* 1985; **235:** 99.

## Adverse Effects, Treatment, and Precautions

Aluminium toxicity is well recognised in patients with renal impairment. Patients undergoing dialysis have experienced encephalopathy, osteodystrophy, and anaemia associated with an aluminium salt taken as a phosphate binder or with aluminium present in the water supply. For this reason, aluminium-free phosphate binders are often used in dialysis patients and the concentration of aluminium in dialysis fluid has been limited to not more than 10 micrograms/litre (see Aluminium Overload under Dialysis Solutions, p.1221). Serum-aluminium concentrations should be monitored regularly in patients undergoing dialysis.

Aluminium toxicity has followed the use of parenteral fluids and infant feeds with a high concentration of aluminium.

Aluminium toxicity may be treated by removal of the aluminium with desferrioxamine (p.1034).

The adverse effects of aluminium salts and precautions to be observed are described under Aluminium Hydroxide, p.1249.

◇ A review of aluminium toxicity[1] lists possible sources of aluminium including water, antacids, phosphate-binding gels, total parenteral nutrition solutions, processed human serum albumin, fluids used in infants, and environmental pollution; cooking utensils and beverages such as tea have also been suggested as possible sources of aluminium. Toxicity tends to occur when the gastrointestinal barrier to aluminium absorption is circumvented, as in intravenous fluid administration or dialysis, or if the excretion of aluminium is reduced, as in renal impairment. Infants, especially preterm infants, form a special risk group.[2-5]

Accidental deposition of a large amount of aluminium sulfate in a reservoir in Cornwall, UK in 1988 led to contamination of a nearby town's water supply.[6] Symptoms reported included diarrhoea, mouth ulcers or blisters, malaise, joint symptoms (mainly deterioration of existing symptoms), and memory defects (usually beginning 2 to 3 months after the incident). Although some medical experts considered that no long-term toxic effects were to be expected,[6] aluminium deposits were found in the bones of 2 individuals 6 to 7 months later.[7] In a study[8] undertaken 3 years after the incident, 55 adults who claimed to have suffered cerebral damage performed poorly in psychomotor testing. The authors attributed this to aluminium exposure, but the study's design and conclusions have been criticised.[9-11]

1. Monteagudo FSE, *et al.* Recent developments in aluminium toxicology. *Med Toxicol* 1989; **4:** 1–16.
2. Bishop N, *et al.* Aluminium in infant formulas. *Lancet* 1989; **i:** 490.
3. Lawson M, *et al.* Aluminium and infant formulae. *Lancet* 1989; **i:** 614–15.
4. Anonymous. Aluminium content of parenteral drug products. *WHO Drug Inf* 1990; **4:** 70.
5. American Academy of Pediatrics Committee on Nutrition. Aluminum toxicity in infants and children. *Pediatrics* 1996; **97:** 413–16.
6. Anonymous. Camelford two years on. *Lancet* 1990; **336:** 366.
7. Eastwood JB, *et al.* Aluminium deposition in bone after contamination of drinking water supply. *Lancet* 1990; **336:** 462–4.
8. Altmann P, *et al.* Disturbance of cerebral function in people exposed to drinking water contaminated with aluminium sulphate: retrospective study of the Camelford water incident. *BMJ* 1999; **319:** 807–11.
9. David A. Cerebral dysfunction after water pollution incident in Camelford: results were biased by self selection of cases. *BMJ* 2000; **320:** 1337.
10. Esmonde TFG. Cerebral dysfunction after water pollution incident in Camelford: study has several methodological errors. *BMJ* 2000; **320:** 1337–8.
11. McMillan TM. Cerebral dysfunction after water pollution incident in Camelford: study may prolong the agony. *BMJ* 2000; **320:** 1338.

**Effects on mental function.** Encephalopathy with seizures has been associated with the use of aluminium-containing materials used for bone reconstruction.[1,2] In each case, reconstruction of areas of the skull resulted in high concentrations of aluminium in the CSF.

1. Renard JL, *et al.* Post-otoneurosurgery aluminium encephalopathy. *Lancet* 1994; **344:** 63–4.
2. Hantson P, *et al.* Encephalopathy with seizures after use of aluminium-containing bone cement. *Lancet* 1994; **344:** 1647.

ALZHEIMER'S DISEASE. The role of aluminium in the aetiology of Alzheimer's disease (see Dementia, p.1484) is, at best, unclear.[1-4] Circumstantial evidence of a positive association arises from *animal* and *in-vitro* data, together with clinical observations that aluminium is present in senile plaques and neurofibrillary tangles occurring in Alzheimer's disease, that the administration of aluminium chelators to Alzheimer patients may slow the progression of the disease, and that the risk of brain changes is increased in people living in areas with a high aluminium content in the drinking water supply. Some of these findings have been criticised, disproved, or not confirmed by other workers. Listed below are some of the studies which point to an association between aluminium intake and Alzheimer's disease,[5-8] some criticisms,[9-13] and some negative findings.[14,15]

There does not appear to be a risk of aluminium accumulation from normal use of aluminium-containing antacids by patients with normal renal function; consequently use of these antacids by such patients should not be considered to put them at risk of Alzheimer's disease.[16,17]

1. Crapper McLachlan DR, *et al.* Would decreased aluminum ingestion reduce the incidence of Alzheimer's disease? *Can Med Assoc J* 1991; **145:** 793–804.
2. Anonymous. Is aluminium a dementing ion? *Lancet* 1992; **339:** 713–14.
3. Munoz DG. Is exposure to aluminium a risk factor for the development of Alzheimer disease?—No. *Arch Neurol* 1998; **55:** 737–9.
4. Forbes WF, Hill GB. Is exposure to aluminium a risk factor for the development of Alzheimer disease?—Yes. *Arch Neurol* 1998; **55:** 740–1.
5. Martyn CN, *et al.* Geographical relation between Alzheimer's disease and aluminium in drinking water. *Lancet* 1989; **i:** 59–62.
6. Crapper McLachlan DR, *et al.* Intramuscular desferrioxamine in patients with Alzheimer's disease. *Lancet* 1991; **337:** 1304–8.
7. Good PF, *et al.* Selective accumulation of aluminum and iron in the neurofibrillary tangles of Alzheimer's disease: a laser microprobe (LAMMA) study. *Ann Neurol* 1992; **31:** 286–92.
8. Harrington CR, *et al.* Alzheimer's-disease-like changes in tau protein processing: association with aluminium accumulation in brains of renal dialysis patients. *Lancet* 1994; **343:** 993–7.
9. Ebrahim S. Aluminium and Alzheimer's disease. *Lancet* 1989; **i:** 267.
10. Schupf N, *et al.* Aluminium and Alzheimer's disease. *Lancet* 1989; **i:** 267.
11. Lindesay J. Aluminium and Alzheimer's disease. *Lancet* 1989; **i:** 268.
12. Birchall JD, Chappell JS. Aluminium, water chemistry, and Alzheimer's disease. *Lancet* 1989; **i:** 953.
13. Whalley LJ, *et al.* Aluminium and dementia. *Lancet* 1992; **339:** 1235–6.
14. Markesbery WR, *et al.* Instrumental neutron activation analysis of brain aluminum in Alzheimer's disease and aging. *Ann Neurol* 1981; **10:** 511–16.
15. Wettstein A, *et al.* Failure to find a relationship between mnestic skills of octogenarians and aluminum in drinking water. *Int Arch Occup Environ Health* 1991; **63:** 97–103.
16. Anonymous. Aluminium salts and Alzheimer's disease. *Pharm J* 1991; **246:** 809.
17. Flaten TP, *et al.* Mortality from dementia among gastroduodenal ulcer patients. *J Epidemiol Community Health* 1991; **45:** 203–6.

## Uses and Administration

Aluminium is used in packaging and in injection equipment. The foil is also used as a dressing and for insulation. Aluminium may also be employed as a colouring agent for some foodstuffs. It is used as Aluminium Metallicum in homoeopathic medicine. Aluminium powder alone and in paste form with zinc oxide has been used as a dressing. Astringent aluminium salts are used as antiperspirants. Aluminium hydroxide (p.1249) is used as an antacid.

Aluminium oxide (p.1140) has been used as an abrasive agent; it is also used in homoeopathic medicine.

## Preparations

***BP 2003:*** Compound Aluminium Paste.

**Proprietary Preparations** (details are given in Part 3)

**Multi-ingredient:** ***Arg.:*** Effidrate; ***Braz.:*** Belagin; ***Mex.:*** Cidetox; Dicentril; Gavicid; Wingel.

---

# Aluminium Acetate

Aluminio, acetato de; Aluminum Acetate.

$C_6H_9AlO_6$ = 204.1.

*CAS — 139-12-8.*

## Profile

Aluminium acetate is prepared from aluminium sulfate and acetic acid.

Solutions containing aluminium acetate are astringent. Ear drops, which correspond to a solution of aluminium acetotartrate in that they are prepared from aluminium sulfate with the aid of acetic acid and tartaric acid, reduce oedema and inflammation of the ear by producing an acidic environment hostile to pathogenic bacteria; they are also hygroscopic. Solutions, usually prepared from glacial acetic acid and an aluminum subacetate topical solution (which is itself prepared from aluminium sulfate and acetic acid), are also used in dermatology as astringent lotions for irritating skin conditions.

Various preparations containing aluminium acetate have been known as Burow's creams, emulsions, lotions, or solutions.

Aluminium acetotartrate and aluminium subacetate (basic aluminium acetate) are also used as topical astringents.

### Preparations

***BP 2003:*** Aluminium Acetate Ear Drops;
***USP 27:*** Aluminum Subacetate Topical Solution.

**Proprietary Preparations** (details are given in Part 3)
***Canad.:*** Buro-Sol; ***Ger.:*** Alsol; Alsol N; Essigsaure Tonerde-Salbe; Essitol; ***Ital.:*** Euceta†; ***Switz.:*** Euceta; ***USA:*** Bite Rx; Buro-Sol.

**Multi-ingredient:** ***Arg.:*** Aseptalum; Epiprocto; ***Austral.:*** Xyloproct; ***Austria:*** Acetonal; Euceta mit Kamille; Methyment; Nasanal; Neo-Phlogicid†; ***Belg.:*** Xyloproct†; ***Braz.:*** Xyloproct; ***Canad.:*** Buro Derm†; ***Fin.:*** Xyloproct; ***Fr.:*** Gel a l'Acetotartrate d'Alumine Defresne; ***Ger.:*** Anisan; ***Irl.:*** Xyloproct; ***Israel:*** Contra Combustiones†; Proctozorin-N; ***Ital.:*** Betaderm; Micofoot; Neo Zeta-Foot†; Oleo Calcarea; Vegetallumina; Xyloproct†; ***Malaysia:*** Xyloproct; ***Mex.:*** Xyloproct; ***Neth.:*** Xyloproct†; ***Norw.:*** Xyloproct; ***NZ:*** Xyloproct; ***Port.:*** Proctonostrum; ***Singapore:*** Xyloproct†; ***Spain:*** Avril; ***Swed.:*** Xyloproct; ***Switz.:*** Anginesin; Cetona Plus†; Euceta avec camomille et arnica; Euceta Pic; Fortacet; Frigoplasma; Fungex; Mikutan N; Realderm; ***Thai.:*** Xyloproct†; ***UK:*** Xyloproct; ***USA:*** Borofair Otic; Burow's; Otic Domeboro; Star-Otic.

## Aluminium Lactate

Aluminio, lactato de. Tris(lactato)aluminium.

$C_9H_{15}AlO_9$ = 294.2.

*CAS — 537-02-0; 18917-91-4.*

### Profile

Aluminium lactate is used in the local treatment of various disorders of the mouth.

### Preparations

**Proprietary Preparations** (details are given in Part 3)
***Fr.:*** Aluctyl†; ***Ital.:*** Aluctyl.

**Multi-ingredient:** ***Israel:*** Aronal Forte; ***Ital.:*** Lacalut; ***Switz.:*** Deaftol avec lidocaine; Gynasol†.

## Aluminium Sulfate

Aluminii Sulfas; Aluminio, sulfato de; Aluminium Sulfuricum; Aluminium Sulphate; Aluminium Trisulphate; Aluminum Sulfate; E520.

$Al_2(SO_4)_3,xH_2O$ = 342.2 (anhydrous).

*CAS — 10043-01-3 (anhydrous aluminium sulfate); 17927-65-0 (aluminium sulfate hydrate).*

**Pharmacopoeias.** In *Eur.* (see p.vi), *Int., Pol.,* and *US.*

**Ph. Eur. 5.0** (Aluminium Sulphate). Colourless lustrous crystals or crystalline masses. It contains 51 to 59% of $Al_2(SO_4)_3$. Soluble in cold water; freely soluble in hot water; practically insoluble in alcohol. Store in airtight containers.

**USP 27** (Aluminum Sulfate). Contains 54 to 59% of $Al_2(SO_4)_3$. An odourless, white, crystalline powder, shining plates, or crystalline fragments. Soluble 1 in 1 of water; insoluble in alcohol. The pH of a 5% solution in water is not less than 2.9.

### Profile

Aluminium sulfate has an action similar to that of alum (p.1652) but is more astringent. A 20% solution is used for the treatment of envenomation by certain insects and marine organisms. The aluminium may cause precipitation of the proteins contained within the venoms thus reducing local toxicity. Aluminium sulfate is also included in astringent preparations intended to soothe irritating skin conditions.

Aluminium sulfate is also used in the preparation of aluminium acetate solutions.

**Adverse effects.** Possible adverse effects or toxicity associated with aluminium, or aluminium salts such as aluminium sulfate, in the public water supply are discussed under Aluminium, p.1652.

### Preparations

***USP 27:*** Aluminum Subacetate Topical Solution; Aluminum Sulfate and Calcium Acetate Tablets for Topical Solution.

**Proprietary Preparations** (details are given in Part 3)
***Austral.:*** Stingose; ***Hong Kong:*** Stingose; ***Israel:*** Stingose†; ***NZ:*** Stingose; ***S.Afr.:*** Stingose; ***UK:*** Stingose.

**Multi-ingredient:** ***Arg.:*** Gineseptina; ***Austria:*** Citoburol; ***Ger.:*** Schupps Kohlensaurebad†; Tannolil; ***Ital.:*** Cepral†; ***Mex.:*** Domeboro; ***Switz.:*** Gynasol†; ***USA:*** Bluboro; Boropak; Domeboro; Ostiderm; Pedi-Boro Soak Paks.

## Ambucetamide *(BAN, rINN)*

A-16; Ambucetamida; Dibutamide. 2-Dibutylamino-2-(4-methoxyphenyl)acetamide.

$C_{17}H_{28}N_2O_2$ = 292.4.

*CAS — 519-88-0.*

### Profile

Ambucetamide is an antispasmodic and has been given for the relief of dysmenorrhoea. The hydrochloride has also been used.

### Preparations

**Proprietary Preparations** (details are given in Part 3)
**Multi-ingredient:** ***Belg.:*** Neomeritine†; ***Neth.:*** Femerital†.

## Ambutonium Bromide *(BAN)*

BL-700B; R-100. (3-Carbamoyl-3,3-diphenylpropyl)ethyldimethylammonium bromide.

$C_{20}H_{27}BrN_2O$ = 391.3.

*CAS — 14007-49-9 (ambutonium); 115-51-5 (ambutonium bromide).*

### Profile

Ambutonium bromide is a quaternary ammonium antimuscarinic that has been used in gastrointestinal disorders with smooth muscle spasm.

### Preparations

**Proprietary Preparations** (details are given in Part 3)
**Multi-ingredient:** ***Fin.:*** Spasmo-Oxepam†; ***Port.:*** Sedioton.

## Amikhelline Hydrochloride *(rINNM)*

Hidrocloruro de amikelina. 9-(2-Diethylaminoethoxy)-4-hydroxy-7-methyl-5*H*-furo[3,2-*g*][1]benzopyran-5-one hydrochloride.

$C_{18}H_{21}NO_5,HCl$ = 367.8.

*CAS — 4439-67-2 (amikhelline); 40709-23-7 (amikhelline hydrochloride).*

### Profile

Amikhelline hydrochloride has been used as an antispasmodic.

## Amilomer *(rINN)*

*CAS — 42615-49-6.*

### Profile

Amilomer consists of microspheres produced by reaction of partially hydrolysed starch with epichlorohydrin, quickly degradable by amylase (with a half-life of less than 120 minutes); the name is followed by a hyphenated numerical code in which the number preceding the hyphen indicates the half-life in minutes and that following the hyphen indicates the mean diameter of the microspheres in μm.

Amilomer is used in transarterial chemoembolisation procedures in the management of hepatic malignancies.

### Preparations

**Proprietary Preparations** (details are given in Part 3)
***Ger.:*** Spherex.

## Aminohippuric Acid

*p*-Aminobenzoylglycine; *p*-Aminohippuric Acid; Aminohipúrico, ácido; PAHA; Para-aminohippuric Acid. *N*-4-Aminobenzoylaminoacetic acid.

$C_9H_{10}N_2O_3$ = 194.2.

*CAS — 61-78-9 (aminohippuric acid); 94-16-6 (sodium aminohippurate).*

*ATC — V04CH30.*

**Pharmacopoeias.** In *US.*

**USP 27** (Aminohippuric Acid). A white crystalline powder which discolours on exposure to light. Soluble 1 in 45 of water, 1 in 50 of alcohol, and 1 in 5 of 3N hydrochloric acid; very slightly soluble in carbon tetrachloride, in chloroform, in ether, and in benzene; freely soluble in alkaline solutions with some decomposition, and in diluted hydrochloric acid. Store in airtight containers. Protect from light.

### Adverse Effects

Sodium aminohippurate may cause nausea and vomiting, hypersensitivity reactions, vasomotor disturbances, flushing, tingling, cramps, and a feeling of warmth. Patients may develop an urge to urinate or defaecate after infusion.

### Interactions

The estimation of sodium aminohippurate may be affected in patients taking procaine, sulfonamides, or thiazosulfone. Probenecid diminishes the excretion of aminohippuric acid. Clearance is also affected by penicillins, salicylates, and other drugs that compete for the same excretory pathways.

### Uses and Administration

Aminohippuric acid is excreted mainly by proximal tubular secretion, with some glomerular filtration. It is given by intravenous infusion, as sodium aminohippurate (aminohippurate sodium; $C_9H_9N_2NaO_3$ = 216.2), for the estimation of effective renal plasma flow. Doses are aimed at producing a plasma concentration of 20 micrograms/mL; at these concentrations approximately 90% of aminohippurate is cleared from the renal blood stream in a single circuit in patients with normal renal function. Sodium aminohippurate has also been used for the assessment of the renal tubular secretory mechanism. Doses for this purpose are infused slowly to achieve a plasma concentration of 400 to 600 micrograms/mL to saturate the tubular secretion. These tests are used mainly in research procedures.

### Preparations

***USP 27:*** Aminohippurate Sodium Injection.

## Ammi Visnaga Fruit

Biznaga, fruto de la; Khella; Khellah; Picktooth Fruit; Visnaga.

## Khellin *(rINN)*

Kelina; Khelline; Khellinum; Visammin. 4,9-Dimethoxy-7-methyl-5*H*-furo[3,2-*g*]chromen-5-one.

$C_{14}H_{12}O_5$ = 260.2.

*CAS — 82-02-0.*

## Visnadine *(BAN, rINN)*

Visnadina. 10-Acetoxy-9,10-dihydro-8,8-dimethyl-2-oxo-2*H*,8*H*-pyrano[2,3-*f*]chromen-9-yl 2-methylbutyrate.

$C_{21}H_{24}O_7$ = 388.4.

*CAS — 477-32-7.*

*ATC — C04AX24.*

### Profile

*Ammi visnaga* fruit is used in herbal and homoeopathic preparations.

Khellin and visnadine are vasodilators obtained from *Ammi visnaga* fruit or by synthesis. Khellin also has a bronchodilatory action and has been used in angina pectoris and asthma. Khellin has also been tried in conjunction with ultraviolet light to treat vitiligo (see Pigmentation Disorders, p.1137). Visnadine has been used in coronary, cerebral, and peripheral vascular disorders.

◊ References.

1. Hofer A, *et al.* Long-term results in the treatment of vitiligo with oral khellin plus UVA. *Eur J Dermatol* 2001 **11:** 225–9.

### Preparations

**Proprietary Preparations** (details are given in Part 3)
***Ger.:*** Carduben†; Khellangan N; steno-loges N†.

**Multi-ingredient:** ***Austria:*** Urelium Neu; ***Ger.:*** Aesrutal S†; Cefadrin; Hepatofalk Neu†; Oxacant-Khella N; Salusant†; Stenocrat.

## Ammonia

Amoníaco, solución diluida de.

*CAS — 7664-41-7.*

NOTE. The food additive number E527 is used for ammonium hydroxide. Solutions of ammonia in water have been referred to as ammonium hydroxide solutions. Strong solutions of ammonia have also been described by the synonyms Ammoniaca, Ammoniacum, Ammoniaque Officinale, and Liquor Ammoniae Fortis. Dilute solutions of ammonia have also been referred to as Ammonia Water, Ammonium Hydricum Solutum, Liquor Ammoniae, and Liquor Ammoniae Dilutus.

**Pharmacopoeias.** Strong ammonia solutions are included in *Chin.* (25 to 28%), *Eur.* (see p.vi) (25 to 30%), and *USNF* (27 to 31%). Dilute ammonia solutions are included in *Br., Chin., Ger., Jpn, Pol.,* and *Swiss* (all about 10%).

**Ph. Eur. 5.0** (Ammonia Solution, Concentrated; Ammoniae Solutio Concentrata; Strong Ammonia Solution BP 2003). It contains between 25% and 30% (w/w) of ammonia, $NH_3$. A clear colourless liquid. Very caustic. Miscible with water and with alcohol. Store at a temperature not exceeding 20° in airtight containers.

**BP 2003** (Dilute Ammonia Solution). It is prepared by diluting Strong Ammonia Solution with freshly boiled and cooled purified water. It contains 9.5 to 10.5% w/w of $NH_3$.

NOTE. The BP directs that when Ammonia Solution is prescribed or demanded, Dilute Ammonia Solution shall be dispensed or supplied.

**USNF 22** (Strong Ammonia Solution). It contains between 27% and 31% (w/w) of $NH_3$. On exposure to air, it loses ammonia rapidly. A clear colourless liquid with an exceedingly pungent characteristic odour. Store at a temperature not exceeding 25° in airtight containers.

**Handling.** Strong ammonia solutions should be handled with great care because of the caustic nature of the solutions and the irritating properties of the vapour. Cool the container well before opening and avoid inhalation of the vapour.

### Adverse Effects

Ingestion of strong solutions of ammonia causes severe pain in the mouth, throat, and gastrointestinal tract, as well as severe local oedema and salivation, with cough, vomiting, and shock. Burns to the oesophagus and stomach may result in perforation. Stricture formation, usually in the oesophagus, can occur weeks or months later. Ingestion may also cause oedema of the respiratory tract and pneumonitis, though this may not develop for a few hours.

Inhalation of ammonia vapour causes sneezing and coughing and in high concentration causes pulmonary oedema. Asphyxia has been reported following oedema or spasm of the glottis.

Ammonia vapour is irritant to the eyes and causes weeping; there may be conjunctival swelling and temporary blindness.

Ammonia solution in contact with skin and eyes produces blistering and vesiculation; ammonia burns feel 'soapy' because of saponification of the tissues. Strong solutions on the conjunctiva cause a severe reaction with conjunctival oedema, corneal damage, and acute glaucoma. Late complications include angle-closure glaucoma, opaque corneal scars, atrophy of the iris, and formation of cataracts. Ammonia burns have resulted from treating insect bites and stings with the strong solution, and even with the dilute solution, especially if a dressing is subsequently applied.

◊ References.


1. Beare JDL, *et al.* Ammonia burns of the eye: an old weapon in new hands. *BMJ* 1988; **296:** 590.
2. Payne MP, Delic JI. Ammonia. In: *Toxicity Review 24.* London: HMSO, 1991: 1–12.
3. Payne MP, *et al. Toxicology of substances in relation to major hazards: ammonia.* London: HMSO, 1991.
4. Leduc D, *et al.* Acute and long term respiratory damage following inhalation of ammonia. *Thorax* 1992; **47:** 755–7.
5. Michaels RA. Emergency planning and the acute toxic potency of inhaled ammonia. *Environ Health Perspect* 1999; **107:** 617–27.
6. Amshel CE, *et al.* Anhydrous ammonia burns case report and review of the literature. *Burns* 2000; **26:** 493–7.
7. Kerstein MD, *et al.* Acute management of exposure to liquid ammonia. *Mil Med* 2001; **166:** 913–14.


### Treatment of Adverse Effects

Ingestion should not be treated by lavage or emesis. Milk or water have been given as diluents, but small volumes should be used to reduce the risk of inducing emesis. Appropriate measures should be taken to alleviate pain, shock, and pulmonary oedema, and maintain an airway.

Contaminated skin and eyes should be flooded immediately with water and the washing continued for at least 15 minutes. Any affected clothing should be removed while flooding is being carried out.

### Uses and Administration

Dilute solutions of ammonia have been used as reflex stimulants either as smelling salts or solutions for oral administration. They have also been used as rubefacients and counter-irritants (see p.4) and to neutralise insect stings. Users should always be aware of the irritant properties of ammonia.

Hartshorn and Oil was sometimes used as a name for an ammonia liniment. Household ammonia and cloudy ammonia have been used as names for cleaning preparations of ammonia with oleic acid or soap respectively. A saturated solution containing about 35% w/w and known as '0.880 ammonia' has been used in many chemical and industrial applications.

**Stings.** Bathers who were stung by Portuguese men-of-war (*Physalia physalis*) were rapidly and effectively relieved of discomfort, paresis, irritation, and other symptoms by the application of aromatic ammonia spirit compresses.[1]


1. Frohman IG. Treatment of physalia stings. *JAMA* 1966; **197:** 733.


### Preparations

***BP 2003:*** Aromatic Ammonia Solution; Aromatic Ammonia Spirit; Strong Ammonium Acetate Solution; White Liniment.

**Proprietary Preparations** (details are given in Part 3)
***Canad.:*** After Bite; ***Israel:*** After Bite†; ***Spain:*** After Bite; Calmapica; ***UK:*** After Bite.

**Multi-ingredient:** ***Austral.:*** Senega and Ammonia†; ***Austria:*** Apotheker Bauer's Franzbranntwein-Gel; Rowalind; ***Braz.:*** Lactrex; ***Canad.:*** Bronchex; Bronchisaft†; SJ Liniment; ***Chile:*** Rhus Opodeldoc; ***Irl.:*** Rowalind†; ***Ital.:*** Stilomagic; ***Port.:*** Broncodiazina; ***S.Afr.:*** Enterodyne; Famstim†; ***Spain:*** Analgesico Ut Asens Fn†; Licor Amoniacal†; Linimento Sloan†; Masagil; ***UK:*** Blistex Relief Cream; BN†; Goddards Embrocation; Mackenzies Smelling Salts; Pickles Smelling Salts; ***USA:*** Emergent-Ez.

## Ammonium Citrate

Ammon. Cit.; E380; Triammonium Citrate.

$C_6H_5O_7(NH_4)_3$ = 243.2.

*CAS — 3458-72-8.*

### Profile

Ammonium citrate is used as a food additive and has been used in respiratory-tract disorders.

### Preparations

**Proprietary Preparations** (details are given in Part 3)
**Multi-ingredient:** ***Chile:*** Ambrotos; Mucobrol.

## Ammonium Phosphate

545 (ammonium polyphosphates); Diammonium Hydrogen Phosphate; Dibasic Ammonium Phosphate; Fosfato de amonio. Diammonium hydrogen orthophosphate.

$(NH_4)_2HPO_4$ = 132.1.

*CAS — 7783-28-0.*

**Pharmacopoeias.** In *USNF.*

**USNF 22** (Ammonium Phosphate). Colourless or white granules or powder. Freely soluble in water; practically insoluble in alcohol and in acetone. A 1% solution in water has a pH of 7.6 to 8.2. Store in airtight containers.

### Profile

Ammonium phosphate was formerly used as a diuretic. It may be used as a buffering agent in pharmaceutical preparations.

Ammonium biphosphate (monobasic ammonium phosphate; $NH_4H_2PO_4$ = 115.0) has been used to acidify urine and as a phosphate supplement.

### Preparations

**Proprietary Preparations** (details are given in Part 3)
**Multi-ingredient:** ***Fr.:*** Phosphore-Medifa.

## Amnion

Amnios.

### Profile

Human extra-embryonic fetal membranes comprise an inner amniotic membrane, the amnion, and an outer membrane, the chorion. Amnion is used in ocular surgery for a range of conditions. Both amnion and combined membranes have been used as a dressing for raw wounds including chronic ulcers and burns.

### Preparations

**Proprietary Preparations** (details are given in Part 3)
***Ital.:*** Amniex†.

## Amylase

Amilasa; Diastase; Glucogenase; Ptyalin.

*CAS — 9000-92-4 (amylase); 9000-85-5 (bacterial α-amylase); 9000-90-2 (porcine α-amylase, pancreatic).*

*ATC — A09AA01.*

**Pharmacopoeias.** In *Fr.* and *Jpn.*

### Adverse Effects

Hypersensitivity reactions have been reported.

**Hypersensitivity.** References to asthma developing following occupational exposure to amylases used in the flour milling[1-3] and detergent[4,5] manufacturing industries, and studies[6-8] to assess the likelihood of developing amylase hypersensitivity after ingesting wheat products including bread.


1. Smith TA, *et al.* Respiratory symptoms and wheat flour exposure: a study of flour millers. *Occup Med (Lond)* 2000; **50:** 25–9.
2. Cullinan P, *et al.* Allergen and dust exposure as determinants of work-related symptoms and sensitization in a cohort of flour-exposed workers; a case-control analysis. *Ann Occup Hyg* 2001; **45:** 97–103.
3. Quirce S, *et al.* Glucoamylase: another fungal enzyme associated with baker's asthma. *Ann Allergy Asthma Immunol* 2002; **89:** 197–202.
4. Hole AM, *et al.* Occupational asthma caused by bacillary amylase used in the detergent industry. *Occup Environ Med* 2000; **57:** 840–2.
5. Cullinan P, *et al.* An outbreak of asthma in a modern detergent factory. *Lancet* 2000; **356:** 1899–1900.
6. Cullinan P, *et al.* Clinical responses to ingested fungal alpha-amylase and hemicellulase in persons sensitized to Aspergillus fumigatus? *Allergy* 1997; **52:** 346–9.
7. Sander I, *et al.* Is fungal alpha-amylase in bread an allergen? *Clin Exp Allergy* 2000; **30:** 560–5.
8. Simonato B, *et al.* IgE binding to soluble and insoluble wheat flour proteins in atopic and non-atopic patients suffering from gastrointestinal symptoms after wheat ingestion. *Clin Exp Allergy* 2001; **31:** 1771–8.


### Uses and Administration

The term amylase refers to an enzyme catalysing the hydrolysis of α-1,4-glucosidic linkages of polysaccharides such as starch, glycogen, or their degradation products. Amylases may be classified according to the manner in which the glucosidic bond is attacked. Endoamylases attack the α-1,4-glucosidic linkage at random. Alpha-amylases are the only types of endoamylases known and yield dextrins, oligosaccharides, and monosaccharides. The more common alpha-amylases include those isolated from human saliva, mammalian pancreas, *Bacillus subtilis*, *Aspergillus oryzae*, and barley malt. Exoamylases attack the α-1,4-glucosidic linkage only from the non-reducing outer polysaccharide chain ends. They include beta-amylases and glucoamylases (amyloglucosidases or gamma-amylases) and are of vegetable or microbial origin. Beta-amylases yield beta-limit dextrins and maltose, and glucoamylases yield glucose.

Amylase is used in the production of predigested starchy foods and for the conversion of starch to fermentable sugars in the baking, brewing, and fermentation industries.

Amylase from various sources has been used as an ingredient of preparations of digestive enzymes, and has been given by mouth for its supposed activity in reducing respiratory-tract inflammation and local swelling and oedema.

### Preparations

**Proprietary Preparations** (details are given in Part 3)
***Fr.:*** Maxilase; Megamylase; ***Mon.:*** Amylodiastase; ***Port.:*** Maxilase.

**Multi-ingredient:** ***Arg.:*** Dom-Polienzim; Gastridin-E; Homocisteon Compuesto; Pakinase; Polienzim; ***Austral.:*** Enzyme†; ***Austria:*** Wobenzym; ***Belg.:*** Digestomen; ***Braz.:*** Bromelin; Digesnorma†; Enziprid†; Essen; Filogaster; Normopride Enzimatico†; Pantopept; Primeral; Thiomucase; ***Chile:*** Flapex E; ***Fr.:*** Hepatoum†; Maxilase-Bacitracine†; ***Ger.:*** Enzym-Wied; ***Hong Kong:*** Enzyplex; GI†; Magesto; ***India:*** Bestozyme; Catazyme-P; Digeplex; Digeplex-T; Dipep; Farizym; Lupizyme; Molzyme; Neopeptine; Papytazyme; Sanzyme-DS; Unienzyme c MPS; Vitazyme; ***Ital.:*** Digestopan; Essen Enzimatico; Luizym†; ***Malaysia:*** Biotase; Enzyplex; ***Mex.:*** Ochozim; Wobenzym; ***Port.:*** Luizym†; Modulanzime; ***Singapore:*** Enzyplex; Weisen-U; ***Spain:*** Demusin; Digestomen Complex; Espasmo Digestomen†; Paidozim; Polidasa†; ***Switz.:*** Zymoplex; ***Thai.:*** Diasgest; Digestin; Endogest; Enzyplex; Flatulence Gastulence; Magesto; Mesto-Of; Papytazyme; Pepsitase; Polyenzyme-I; ***UK:*** Enzyme Digest; Enzyme Plus; ***USA:*** Arco-Lase Plus†; Arco-Lase†; Enzyme; Gustase Plus†; Gustase†; Ku-Zyme; Kutrase; Papaya Enzyme.

## Anagrelide Hydrochloride *(BANM, USAN, rINNM)*

BL-4162A; BL-4162a; BMY-26538-01; Hidrocloruro de anagrelida. 6,7-Dichloro-1,5-dihydroimidazo[2,1-*b*]quinazolin-2(3*H*)-one hydrochloride.

$C_{10}H_7Cl_2N_3O,HCl$ = 292.5.

*CAS — 68475-42-3 (anagrelide); 58579-51-4 (anagrelide hydrochloride).*

*ATC — B01AC14.*

### Adverse Effects

Anagrelide may cause headache, diarrhoea, abdominal pain, nausea, and oedema. Cardiovascular effects include vasodilatation, positive inotropic effects, and palpitations; myocardial infarction and heart failure have also been reported. Anagrelide has been shown to be embryotoxic and fetotoxic in *animal* studies.

**Erectile dysfunction.** Erectile dysfunction associated with anagrelide therapy has been reported in a patient.[1]


1. Braester A, Laver B. Anagrelide-induced erectile dysfunction. *Ann Pharmacother* 2002; **36:** 1291.


### Precautions

Anagrelide should not be used during pregnancy. It should be used with caution in patients with cardiovascular disease. Platelet counts should be monitored closely, especially during the initial stages of treatment (see below). Hepatic and renal function should also be monitored while the platelet count is being lowered.

### Pharmacokinetics

Anagrelide is rapidly absorbed from the gastrointestinal tract. It is extensively metabolised before elimination in the urine; less than 1% of a dose is excreted unchanged. The plasma half-life is 1.3 hours, and the terminal elimination half-life has been reported to be about 3 days.

### Uses and Administration

Anagrelide reduces platelet production and at higher doses inhibits platelet aggregation. It is used to reduce platelet production in patients with primary (essential) thrombocythaemia (p.509) and thrombocythaemia secondary to other myeloproliferative disorders.

Anagrelide is given by mouth as the hydrochloride but doses are expressed in terms of the base. The initial dose is the equivalent of anagrelide 2 mg daily divided into 2 or 4 doses. After at least a week, the dose is adjusted, by increasing the daily dose by not more than 500 micrograms in any one week, until the platelet count is maintained within the normal range. The usual maintenance dose is 1.5 to 3 mg daily. The dose should not exceed 10 mg daily or 2.5 mg as a single dose.

Platelet counts should be measured every 2 days during the first week of treatment and then at least weekly until the maintenance dose is reached.

◊ References.


1. Anagrelide Study Group. Anagrelide, a therapy for thrombocythemic states: experience in 577 patients. *Am J Med* 1992; **92:** 69–76.
2. Spencer CM, Brogden RN. Anagrelide: a review of its pharmacodynamic and pharmacokinetic properties, and therapeutic potential in the treatment of thrombocythaemia. *Drugs* 1994; **47:** 809–22.
3. Chintagumpala MM, *et al.* Treatment of essential thrombocythemia with anagrelide. *J Pediatr* 1995; **127:** 495–8.
4. Anonymous. Anagrelide for essential thrombocythemia. *Med Lett Drugs Ther* 1997; **39:** 120.
5. Petitt RM, *et al.* Anagrelide for control of thrombocythemia in polycythemia and other myeloproliferative disorders. *Semin Hematol* 1997; **34:** 51–4.
6. Oertel MD. Anagrelide, a selective thrombocytopenic agent. *Am J Health-Syst Pharm* 1998; **55:** 1979–86.
7. Lackner H, *et al.* Treatment of children with anagrelide for thrombocythemia. *J Pediatr Hematol Oncol* 1998; **20:** 469–73.
8. Bellucci S, *et al.* Studies of platelet volume, chemistry and function in patients with essential thrombocythaemia treated with anagrelide. *Br J Haematol* 1999; **104:** 886–92.
9. Pescatore SL, Lindley C. Anagrelide: a novel agent for the treatment of myeloproliferative disorders. *Expert Opin Pharmacother* 2000; **1:** 537–46.


### Preparations

**Proprietary Preparations** (details are given in Part 3)
***Austral.:*** Agrylin; ***Canad.:*** Agrylin; ***Israel:*** Agrylin; ***S.Afr.:*** Agrylin; ***Switz.:*** Xagrid; ***USA:*** Agrylin.

## Anethole

Anethol; Anetol; *p*-Propenylanisole. (*E*)-1-Methoxy-4-(prop-1-enyl)benzene.

$C_{10}H_{12}O$ = 148.2.

*CAS — 104-46-1; 4180-23-8 (E isomer).*

NOTE. Distinguish from Anethole Trithione (below).

**Pharmacopoeias.** In *Ger.* Also in *USNF.*

**USNF 22** (Anethole). Obtained from anise oil or other sources or prepared synthetically. At or above 23° anethole is a colourless or faintly yellow liquid with a sweet taste and the aromatic odour of aniseed. Very slightly soluble in water; soluble 1 in 2 by volume of alcohol; readily miscible with chloroform and with ether. Store in airtight containers. Protect from light.

### Profile

Anethole has similar properties to those of anise oil (below). It is also included in mixed terpene preparations used in urinary-tract disorders.

### Preparations

**Proprietary Preparations** (details are given in Part 3)

**Multi-ingredient:** ***Austria:*** Rowatinex; ***Belg.:*** Calmant Martou†; ***Canad.:*** Beech Nut Cough Drops; Bentasil; Bentasil Licorice with Echinacea; Bentasil†; Bronco Asmol; ***Chile:*** Rowatinex; ***Ger.:*** Pinimenthol Oral N†; Rowatinex; ***Hong Kong:*** Neo-Rowatinex; Rowatinex; ***Irl.:*** Rowatinex; ***Israel:*** Rowatinex; ***Malaysia:*** Rowatinex; ***Spain:*** Pulmofasa; Pulmofasa Antihist†; Rowanefrin; Vicks Formula 44; ***Switz.:*** Dental-Phenjoca†; Neo-Angin exempt de sucre; Pectocalmine Junior N; Spirogel†; ***Thai.:*** Rowatinex; ***UK:*** Rowatinex†.

## Anethole Trithione

Anethole Dithiolthione; Anetol tritiona; SKF-1717; Trithioparamethoxyphenylpropene. 5-(4-Methoxyphenyl)-3*H*-1,2-dithiole-3-thione.

$C_{10}H_8OS_3$ = 240.4.

*CAS — 532-11-6.*

*ATC — A16AX02.*

NOTE. Distinguish from Anethole (above).

### Profile

Anethole trithione has been given orally in the management of dry mouth (p.1576) and as a choleretic. The usual daily dose is 37.5 to 75 mg, generally in divided doses before meals; doses of up to 150 mg daily have sometimes been used. Anethole trithione may cause discoloration of the urine.

### Preparations

**Proprietary Preparations** (details are given in Part 3)

***Belg.:*** Sulfarlem S 25; Sulfarlem†; ***Canad.:*** Sialor; Sulfarlem†; ***Fr.:*** Sulfarlem; ***Ger.:*** Mucinol; ***Hong Kong:*** Sulfarlem†; ***India:*** Hepasulfol; ***Port.:*** Sufralem; ***S.Afr.:*** Sulfarlem†; ***Spain:*** Sonicur; ***Switz.:*** Sulfarlem.

**Multi-ingredient:** ***Belg.:*** Sulfarlem Choline†; ***India:*** Hepasulfol-AA.

## Angelica

Angélica; Angelicae Radix; Archangelica.

**Pharmacopoeias.** In *Eur.* (see p.vi) and *Pol.*

*Jpn* has separate monographs for *Angelica acutiloba* (Japanese Angelica) and *A. dahurica. Chin.* specifies *A. dahurica*, *A. dahurica* var. *formosana*, *A. pubescens*, and *A. sinensis*.

**Ph. Eur. 5.0** (Angelica Root). The whole or cut, carefully dried rhizome and root of *Angelica archangelica* (*Archangelica officinalis*) containing a minimum of 0.2% v/w of essential oil, calculated with reference to the dried drug.

### Profile

Angelica is widely used in herbal and homoeopathic medicine. The root is used as a bitter to stimulate the appetite. Angelica also has diaphoretic and expectorant properties and has been used for circulatory and respiratory disorders. The stems are candied for use in cooking.

Angelica contains furanocoumarins and may cause photosensitivity reactions or interfere with anticoagulant therapy.

Other *Angelica* spp. that are employed in herbal medicine include *A. acutiloba* (Japanese angelica), *A. dahurica*, *A. pubescens*, and *A. sinensis* (*A. polymorpha* var *sinensis*, Chinese angelica, dong quai).

### Preparations

**Proprietary Preparations** (details are given in Part 3)

***Ger.:*** Pascovegeton.

**Multi-ingredient:** ***Austral.:*** Dong Quai Complex†; Extralife Meno-Care†; Feminine Herbal Complex†; Infant Tonic†; Irontona†; Lifesystem Herbal Formula 4 Women's Formula†; Medinat Esten†; Viburnum Complex†; Vitatona†; Women's Formula Herbal Formula 3†; ***Austria:*** Abdomilon N; Amylatin; Aponatura Verdauungs; Apotheker Bauer's Blahungstee; Apotheker Bauer's Magentee; Bio-Garten Tee fur Leber und Galle; Bioreform-Leber- und Galletee; Krauterdoktor Verdauungsfordernde Tropfen; Krauterpfarrer Weidinger Tee bei Darmtragheit; Krauterpfarrer Weidinger Tee bei Vollegefuhl und Blahungen; Krauterpfarrer Weidinger Tee fur das Altersherz; Magentee†; Naturland Magentonikum; Neuners Krautertee Nr 107 - Blahungstee; Neuners Krautertee Nr 28 - zur Unterstutzung der Tatigkeit der Galle; Neuners Krautertee Nr 44 - Kreislaufanregender Tee; ***Belg.:*** Tisane Depurative "les 12 Plantes"†; Tisane Diuretique†; Tisane Pectorale†; Tisane Purgative†; ***Fr.:*** Dystolise; Mediflor Tisane Digestive No 3; ***Ger.:*** Abdomilon N; Anore X N; Carvomin; Doppelherz Melissengeist; Euvitan†; Gastritol; Iberogast; Infi-tract; Melissengeist; Schwedentrunk Elixier; Schwedentrunk mit Ginseng†; Schwedentrunk†; Stovalid N; Ventrimarin novo†; ***Hong Kong:*** Phytoestrin; ***Ital.:*** Bitteridina†; Florelax; Tisana Arnaldi†; Tonactiv†; ***Spain:*** Agua del Carmen; Himelan; ***Switz.:*** Gastrosan; Iberogast; Phytomed Gastro†; ***UK:*** Melissa Comp..

## Aniracetam *(USAN, rINN)*

Ro-13-5057. 1-(4-Methoxybenzoyl)-2-pyrrolidinone.

$C_{12}H_{13}NO_3$ = 219.2.

*CAS — 72432-10-1.*

*ATC — N06BX11.*

### Profile

Aniracetam is a nootropic drug which has been tried in senile dementia (p.1484). It is given by mouth in usual doses of 1.5 g daily.

◊ References.


1. Lee CR, Benfield P. Aniracetam: an overview of its pharmacodynamic and pharmacokinetic properties, and a review of its therapeutic potential in senile cognitive disorders. *Drugs Aging* 1994; **4:** 257–73.
2. Nakamura K. Aniracetam: its novel therapeutic potential in cerebral dysfunctional disorders based on recent pharmacological discoveries. *CNS Drug Rev* 2002; **8:** 70–89.


### Preparations

**Proprietary Preparations** (details are given in Part 3)

***Arg.:*** Conectol; Pergamid; ***Ital.:*** Ampamet; Draganon; Reset†; ***Jpn:*** Sarpul.

## Aniseed

Anice; Anís, semilla de; Anis Verde; Anis Vert; Anise; Anise Fruit; Anisi Fructus; Fructus Anisi Vulgaris.

NOTE. The names Anís Estrellado, Anis Étoilé, Anisum Badium, Anisum Stellatum, Badiana, Badiane de Chine, Star Anise Fruit, and Sternanis are synonyms for Star Anise.

**Pharmacopoeias.** In *Eur.* (see p.vi) and *Pol.*

*Chin.* and *Eur.* also include Star Anise.

**Ph. Eur. 5.0** (Aniseed). The whole dried fruit of *Pimpinella anisum*, containing not less than 2% v/w of essential oil. It has an odour reminiscent of anethole. Protect from light.

**Ph. Eur. 5.0** (Star Anise; Anisi Stellati Fructus). The dried composite fruit of *Illicium verum*, containing not less than 7% v/w of essential oil with reference to the anhydrous drug. The fruit carpels are brown and have an odour of anethole. Protect from light.

### Profile

Aniseed is carminative and mildly expectorant; it is used mainly as anise oil or as preparations of the oil. It may cause contact dermatitis, probably due to its anethole content.

Aniseed and star anise are the source of anise oil (below).

◊ References.


1. Chandler RF, Hawkes D. Aniseed—a spice, a flavor, a drug. *Can Pharm J* 1984; **117:** 28–9.
2. Fraj J, *et al.* Occupational asthma induced by aniseed. *Allergy* 1996; **51:** 337–9.
3. Garcia-Gonzalez JJ, *et al.* Occupational rhinoconjunctivitis and food allergy because of aniseed sensitization. *Ann Allergy Asthma Immunol* 2002; **88:** 518–22.


### Preparations

**Proprietary Preparations** (details are given in Part 3)

**Multi-ingredient:** ***Austral.:*** Neo-Cleanse†; ***Austria:*** Aktiv Husten- und Bronchialtee; Aktiv milder Magen- und Darmtee; Anifer Hustentee; Aponatura Wind; Asthmatee EF-EM-ES; Aurita-Bronchialtee; Brady's-Magentropfen; Euka; Gewusst wie Husten-Bronchialtee; Krauterdoktor Krampf- und Reizhustensirup; Krauterhaus Mag Kottas Tee gegen Durchfall; Mag Kottas Husten-Bronchialtee; Mag Kottas Krauterexpress-Husten-Bronchialtee; Nesthakchen; Neuners Krautertee Nr 10 - Grippetee; Neuners Krautertee Nr 107 - Blahungstee; Neuners Krautertee Nr 11 - zur Unterstutzung der Tatigkeit der Bronchien und Atemwege; Neuners Krautertee Nr 126 - Starkungstee fur stillende Mutter; Neuners Krautertee Nr 211 - Krauterhexlein Kinder-Hustentee; Neuners Krautertee Nr 7 - Bronchial- und Lungentee; Sidroga Brust-Husten-Tee; Spasmo-Granobil-Krampf- und Reizhusten; Species Carvi comp; Teekanne Husten- und Brusttee; Tussimont; ***Belg.:*** Eugiron†; Tisane Antibiliaire et Stomachique†; Tisane pour le Foie†; Tisane Purgative†; ***Braz.:*** Balsamo Branco†; Broncmel†; Camomila†; Fargestium†; Funchicorea†; ***Canad.:*** Pectothymin†; ***Chile:*** Paltomiel; ***Fr.:*** Elixir Bonjean; Elixir Contre La Toux Weleda†; Herbesan; Mediflor Tisane Digestive No 3; Mucinum a l'Extrait de Cascara; Mucinum†; Peter's Sirop†; Santane D₅†; Tisane Clairo†; Tisane des Familles†; Tisane Digestive Weleda†; ***Ger.:*** Echtroferment-N†; Em-eukal; Em-eukal Husten- und Brusttee; Floradix Multipretten N; Grunlicht Hingfong Essenz†; Hevert-Carmin symbio†; Kneipp Magen-Tee†; Majocarmin-Tee; Ramend Krauter; rohasal; Stovalid N; ***Hong Kong:*** Mucinum Cascara; ***Israel:*** Jungborn; ***Ital.:*** Anice (Specie Composta); Cadifen; Cadimint; Dicalmir; Florerbe Lassativa†; Lassatina; Tisana Kelemata; Tonactiv†; ***Spain:*** Broncomicin Bals†; Crislaxo; Digestol Sanatorium†; Digestovital; Laxante Sanatorium; Laxomax; ***Switz.:*** Kernosan Elixir; Kernosan Heidelberger Poudre; The Franklin†; Tisane favorisant l'allaitement; Tisane laxative Natterman no 13†; ***UK:*** Carminative Tea†; Clairo Tea†; Revitonil.

## Anise Oil

Anís, aceite esencial de; Aniseed Oil; Esencia de Anís; Essence d'Anis; Oleum Anisi.

**Pharmacopoeias.** In *Chin., Eur.* (see p.vi), and *Pol.* Also in *USNF.*

**Ph. Eur. 5.0** (Anise Oil; Anisi Aetheroleum). An essential oil obtained by steam distillation from the dry ripe fruits of *Pimpinella anisum*. It contains less than 1.5% linalol, 0.5 to 5.0% estragole, less than 1.2% α-terpineol, 0.1 to 0.4% *cis*-anethole, 87 to 94% *trans*-anethole, 0.1 to 1.4% anisaldehyde, and 0.3 to 2.0% pseudoisoeugenyl 2-methylbutyrate. A clear, colourless or pale yellow liquid. Relative density 0.980 to 0.990. F.p. 15° to 19°. Store in well-filled, airtight containers at a temperature not exceeding 25°. Protect from light.

**Ph. Eur. 5.0** (Star Anise Oil; Anisi Stellati Aetheroleum). An essential oil obtained by steam distillation from the dry ripe fruits of *Illicium verum*. It contains 0.2 to 2.5% linalol, 0.5 to 6.0% estragole, less than 0.3% α-terpineol, 0.1 to 0.5% *cis*-anethole, 86 to 93% *trans*-anethole, 0.1 to 0.5% anisaldehyde, and 0.1 to 3.0% foeniculin. A clear, colourless or pale yellow liquid. Relative density 0.979 to 0.985. F.p. 15° to 19°. Store in well-filled, airtight containers at a temperature not exceeding 25°. Protect from light.

**USNF 22** (Anise Oil). The volatile oil distilled with steam from the dried, ripe fruit of *Pimpinella anisum* (Apiaceae) or from the dried ripe fruit of *Illicium verum* (Illiaceae). Congealing temperature not lower than 15°. Soluble 1 in 3 of alcohol (90%). Store in well-filled airtight containers. If solid material has separated, carefully warm the oil until it is completely liquefied, and mix before using.

**Incompatibility.** PVC bottles softened and distorted fairly rapidly in the presence of anise oil, which should not be stored or dispensed in such bottles.[1]


1. Department of Pharmaceutical Sciences of the Pharmaceutical Society of Great Britain. Plastics medicine bottles of rigid PVC. *Pharm J* 1973; **210:** 100.


### Profile

Anise oil is carminative and mildly expectorant and is a common ingredient of cough preparations. It is also a flavour.

It may cause contact dermatitis, probably due to its anethole content.

◊ For references to aniseed and anise oil, see Aniseed, above.

### Preparations

***BP 2003:*** Camphorated Opium Tincture; Compound Orange Spirit; Concentrated Anise Water; Concentrated Camphorated Opium Tincture;

***USNF 22:*** Compound Orange Spirit.

**Proprietary Preparations** (details are given in Part 3)

**Multi-ingredient:** ***Austral.:*** Cough Relief†; Digestive Aid†; Gartech†; Respatona Decongestant Formula†; Respatona Plus Bronchial Cough Relief†; ***Austria:*** Anitos; Benium; Biokosma Embrocation; Biokosma Medizinalbad; Biokosma Red Point-Massagecreme; Bradosol; Breston; Bronchostop; Expectal-Tropfen; Expigen; Heumann's Bronchialtee; Kamillosan; Luuf-Hustentee; Neo-Angin; Nesthakchen; Synpharma Bronchial; ***Braz.:*** Ovariusedan†; ***Canad.:*** Babys Own Gripe Water†; Beech Nut Cough Drops; Herbal Cough Expectorant†; ***Fr.:*** Paregorique; ***Ger.:*** Aspasmon N; Benium†; Bronchicum Hustentee†; Bronchocedin N†; Bronchoforton; Em-eukal; Em-eukal Husten- und Brusttee; Ephepect-Pastillen N; Ephepect†; Floradix Multipretten N; Grunlicht Hingfong Essenz†; Grunlicht Magenbalsam Tropfen†; Heumann Bronchialtee Solubifix; Hevert-Carmin symbio†; Hevertopect N; Hingfong-Essenz Hofmanns; Infantussin N†; Kamillosan Mundspray; Leber-Galle-Tropfen 83; Neo-Ballistol; Pulmocordio mite SL; Pulmotin; ratioGast; Repha-Os; Salmiak; Salviathymol N; Sinuforton; ***India:*** Bestozyme; Kamillosan-N; Neopeptine; ***Neth.:*** Bronchicum; ***Spain:*** Carminativo Ibys; Carminativo Juventus; H Tussan; Odontocromil c Sulfamida; ***Switz.:*** Bronchofluid N; Bronchol N†; Capsules laxatives Nattermann Nr. 13†; Demo pates pectorales†; Endomethasone†; Kamillosan; Liberol Baby N; Makatussin forte†; Makatussin†; Neo-Bronchol; Pastilles pectorales Demo N; ***Thai.:*** Gas-Nep; Mesto-Of; ***UK:*** Hactos; Honey & Molasses; Lightning Cough Remedy; Potters Strong Bronchial Catarrh Pastilles; Potters Sugar Free Cough Pastilles; Slippery Elm Stomach Tablets; Vegetable Cough Remover; Zubes; Zubes Blackcurrant.

## Apis mellifera

The honey bee.

**Pharmacopoeias.** *Eur.* (see p.vi) includes the live worker honey bee for homoeopathic preparations.

**Ph. Eur. 5.0** (Honey Bee for Homoeopathic Preparations; Apis Mellifera ad Praeparationes Homoeopathicas). Live worker honey bee, *Apis mellifera*.

### Profile

A preparation containing the venom of *Apis mellifera*, the honey bee, is used in homoeopathic medicine where it is known as Apis mellifica or Apis mel. The honey bee is a source of purified honey (p.1434) and royal jelly (p.1740).

**Arthritis.** Bee venom has traditionally been used in the treatment of arthritis.[1,2] Studies *in vitro* have shown that bee venom has anti-inflammatory activity similar to that of cyclophosphamide. Melittin appears to be the active constituent, and seems to act by interfering with superoxide radical production from human leucocytes.[1]


1. Somerfield SD. Bee venom and arthritis: magic, myth or medicine? *N Z Med J* 1986; **99:** 281–3.
2. Caldwell JR. Venoms, copper and zinc in the treatment of arthritis. *Rheum Dis Clin North Am* 1999, **25:** 919–28.


**Hypersensitivity.** For reference to the use of whole body extracts or venom from Hymenoptera spp. for allergen immunotherapy in allergic subjects, see p.1650.

### Preparations

**Proprietary Preparations** (details are given in Part 3)

**Multi-ingredient:** ***Belg.:*** Forapin†; ***Ger.:*** Forapin E; ***Switz.:*** Forapin.

## Aptiganel *(pINN)*

1-(*m*-Ethylphenyl)-1-methyl-3-(1-naphthyl)guanidine.

$C_{20}H_{21}N_3$ = 303.4.

*CAS — 137159-92-3.*

## Aptiganel Hydrochloride *(USAN)*

CNS-1102 (aptiganel hydrochloride).

$C_{20}H_{21}N_3$,HCl = 339.9.

*CAS — 137160-11-3.*

### Profile

Aptiganel is a guanidine derivative that antagonises the effects of the excitatory amino-acid neurotransmitter glutamate at NMDA-receptors. It has been investigated for the prevention of ischaemic brain damage in patients with traumatic head injury or stroke.

◊ Following dose-ranging studies of aptiganel in volunteers[1] and in patients,[2] adverse effects reported[3] in patients with acute ischaemic stroke, at doses that had been neuroprotective in *animals*, included an increase in systolic blood pressure and an excess of CNS effects. A randomised controlled trial[4] in patients with acute ischaemic stroke was suspended because of a lack of efficacy and a potential imbalance in mortality compared with placebo.


1. Muir KW, *et al.* Pharmacological effects of the non-competitive NMDA antagonist CNS 1102 in normal volunteers. *Br J Clin Pharmacol* 1994; **38:** 33–8.
2. Block GA, *et al.* Final results from a dose-escalating safety and tolerance study of the non-competitive NMDA antagonist CNS1102 in patients with acute cerebral ischaemia. *Stroke* 1995; **26:** 185.
3. Dyker AG, *et al.* Safety and tolerability study of aptiganel hydrochloride in patients with an acute ischemic stroke. *Stroke* 1999; **30:** 2038–42.
4. Albers GW, *et al.* Aptiganel hydrochloride in acute ischemic stroke: a randomized controlled trial. *JAMA* 2001; **286:** 2673–82.


## Arachis Oil

Arachidis Oleum Raffinatum; Cacahuete, aceite de; Earth-nut Oil; Erdnussöl; Ground-nut Oil; Huile d'Arachide; Nut Oil; Ol. Arach.; Óleo de Amendoim; Oleum Arachis; Peanut Oil; Refined Arachis Oil.

**Pharmacopoeias.** In *Eur.* (see p.vi) and *Int.* Also in *USNF.*
*Eur.* also includes hydrogenated arachis oil.

**Ph. Eur. 5.0** (Arachis Oil, Refined; Arachis Oil BP 2003). The refined fatty oil obtained from the shelled seeds of *Arachis hypogaea.* A suitable antioxidant may be added. It is a clear, yellowish viscous liquid consisting of glycerides, chiefly of oleic and linoleic acids, with smaller amounts of other acids. It solidifies at about 2°. Very slightly soluble in alcohol; miscible with petroleum spirit. Store in well-filled containers. Protect from light.

The BP 2003 gives Ground-nut Oil and Peanut Oil as approved synonyms.

**Ph. Eur. 5.0** (Arachis Oil, Hydrogenated; Arachidis Oleum Hydrogenatum). Arachis oil that has been refined, bleached, hydrogenated, and deodorised. It is a white or faintly yellowish soft mass that melts to a clear pale yellow liquid when heated. Practically insoluble in water; very slightly soluble in alcohol; freely soluble in dichloromethane and in petroleum spirit (b.p. 65° to 70°). Protect from light.

**USNF 22** (Peanut Oil). The fully-refined (alkali-refined, bleached, and deodorised at 230° to 260°) oil obtained from the seed kernels of one or more of the cultivated varieties of *Arachis hypogaea* (Leguminosae). It is a colourless or pale yellow, oily liquid with a bland taste; it may have a characteristic nutty odour. Very slightly soluble in alcohol; miscible with carbon disulfide, with chloroform, and with ether. Store at a temperature not exceeding 40° in airtight containers. Protect from light.

### Profile

Emulsions containing arachis oil are used in nutrition. Arachis oil is given as an enema for softening impacted faeces. It is used in drops for softening ear wax and in emollient creams. Arachis oil is given by mouth, usually with sorbitol, as a gallbladder evacuant prior to cholecystography.

**Precautions.** It has been suggested that the use during infancy of preparations containing arachis oil, including infant formulae and topical preparations, may be responsible for sensitisation to peanut, with a subsequent risk of hypersensitivity reactions.[1-3] The arachis oil used in such preparations is refined oil and it has been pointed out that such oil should not contain the proteins that produce allergic reactions in susceptible people.[4,5] In the USA, heating of arachis oil during preparation, to further reduce protein content, has been proposed.[6] Nonetheless, some consider that sufficient protein may be present in refined oil to cause sensitisation.[7] In the UK, the Committee on Safety of Medicines considered that there was not enough evidence to conclude that medicinal products containing arachis oil could lead to sensitisation.[8] However, although they considered the risk of a reaction to be low, they recommended that patients known to be allergic to peanuts should not use medicines containing arachis oil (nor, because of the possibility of cross-sensitivity, should patients allergic to soya), and that such medicines should include an appropriate warning in the labelling.


1. de Montis G, *et al.* Sensitisation to peanut and vitamin D oily preparations. *Lancet* 1993; **341:** 1411.
2. Lever LR. Peanut and nut allergy: creams and ointments containing peanut oil may lead to sensitisation. *BMJ* 1996; **313:** 299.
3. Lack G, *et al.* Factors associated with the development of peanut allergy in childhood. *N Engl J Med* 2003; **348:** 977–85.
4. Hourihane J O'B, *et al.* Randomised, double blind, crossover challenge study of allergenicity of peanut oil in subjects allergic to peanuts. *BMJ* 1997; **314:** 1084–8.
5. Committee on Toxicity of chemicals in Food, Consumer Products and the Environment. *Peanut allergy.* London: Department of Health, 1998.
6. Wilkin JK, *et al.* Peanut allergy. *N Engl J Med* 2003; **349:** 302.
7. Lack G, *et al.* Peanut allergy. *N Engl J Med* 2003; **349:** 302–3.
8. Committee on Safety of Medicines/Medicines and Healthcare Regulatory Agency. Medicines containing peanut (arachis) oil. *Current Problems* 2003; **29:** 5. Also available at: http://medicines.mhra.gov.uk/ourwork/monitorsafequalmed/currentproblems/cpsept2003.pdf (accessed 23/07/04)


### Preparations

***BP 2003:*** Arachis Oil Enema.

**Proprietary Preparations** (details are given in Part 3)
***Austral.:*** Calogen; ***Chile:*** Oilatum; ***Fin.:*** Calogen; ***Fr.:*** Matiga†; ***Ger.:*** Olbad Cordes F; ***Irl.:*** Calogen; Oilatum Cream†; ***Ital.:*** Calogen; ***Mex.:*** Oilatum; ***NZ:*** Calogen; ***Singapore:*** Oilatum Cream; ***UK:*** Calogen; Fletchers Arachis Oil Retention Enema.

**Multi-ingredient:** ***Austral.:*** Cerumol; Gold Cross Skin Basics Zinc Cream; Medevac; ***Austria:*** Balneum F; ***Chile:*** Tarytar; ***Fr.:*** Balneum surgras†; ***Ger.:*** Balneum F; Dr. Hotz Vollbad†; Hoecutin Olbad F†; Parfenac Basisbad; ***Hong Kong:*** Cerumol†; ***Irl.:*** Hydromol; ***Israel:*** Balneum F; Cerumol; ***Ital.:*** Balneum Hermal Forte; ***NZ:*** Medevac; ***S.Afr.:*** Cerumol; ***Singapore:*** Cerumol; ***Spain:*** Emolytar; ***Switz.:*** Balneum Hermal F; ***UK:*** Cerumol; Earex; Hewletts; Nowax; Red Oil; Soothol.

## Areca

Areca Nuts; Arecae Semen; Arekasame; Betel; Betel Nuts; Noix d'Arec.

**Pharmacopoeias.** In *Chin.* and *Jpn.*

### Profile

Areca consists of the dried ripe seeds of *Areca catechu* (Palmae) containing the alkaloid arecoline.

Areca is used in Asian countries as a masticatory. It has sialogogue properties and is chewed for its mild intoxicant and euphoriant effects. The usual custom is to chew pieces of areca seed (areca nut; betel nut) wrapped with lime (calcium hydroxide) in the leaf of the betel pepper (betelvine) (*Piper betle*, which is unrelated to areca). This preparation is known as 'betel quid' (betel) or 'paan' (pan-masala), and produces a red juice when chewed, which stains the saliva, teeth and mucosa. Other ingredients that might be added include catechu gum, spices, or tobacco.

Arecoline and arecaidine (produced by the hydrolysis of arecoline when chewed with lime) have cholinergic activity, and adverse effects that may occur with initial or heavy use of areca include excessive salivation, sweating, lachrymation, urinary incontinence, or diarrhoea. An increased incidence of oral submucosal fibrosis, oral leucoplakia, and oral squamous cell carcinoma has been reported following habitual use.

Areca was formerly used in the treatment of tapeworm infection, and arecoline has been used in veterinary medicine as a purgative and taenifuge.

◊ Discussions of the health risks associated with the chewing of preparations containing areca nut by indigenous populations in Asia[1-3] and immigrant groups in the UK,[4] USA,[5] and New Zealand,[6] including acute effects.[2,3,5]


1. Mack TM. The new pan-Asian paan problem. *Lancet* 2001; **357:** 1638–9.
2. Deng JF, *et al.* Acute toxicities of betel nut: rare but probably overlooked events. *J Toxicol Clin Toxicol* 2001; **39:** 355–60.
3. Chu NS. Effects of Betel chewing on the central and autonomic nervous systems. *J Biomed Sci* 2001; **8:** 229–36.
4. Warnakulasuriya S, *et al.* Areca nut use: an independent risk factor for oral cancer. *BMJ* 2002; **324:** 799–800.
5. Nelson BS, Heischober B. Betel nut: a common drug used by naturalized citizens from India, Far East Asia, and the South Pacific Islands. *Ann Emerg Med* 1999; **34:** 238–43.
6. Yoganathan P. Betel chewing creeps into the New World. *N Z Dent J* 2002; **98:** 40–5.


**Carcinogenicity.** Precancerous and cancerous conditions of the oral cavity have been attributed to the chewing of preparations containing areca (see above). In betel-chewer's mucosa, the oral mucosa is discoloured and there is desquamation or peeling of the oral epithelium from the traumatic effect of chewing and possibly a chemical action of the constituents. This condition may be a precursor of oral submucosal fibrosis, which is considered to be precancerous.[1] Oral leucoplakia is another precancerous condition that is reported. The role of areca in the development of these conditions and oral squamous cell carcinoma has been debated. The effects may be due to the arecaidine content of areca, the alkalinity of the lime, presence of tobacco, or a combination of these.[2,3] Results from a case-controlled study[4] point to an independent association between oral squamous cell carcinoma and chewing areca seeds in preparations without tobacco compared with non-users of areca.


1. Reichart PA, Philipsen HP. Betel chewer's mucosa—a review. *J Oral Pathol Med* 1998; **27:** 239–42.
2. Norton SA. Betel: consumption and consequences. *J Am Acad Dermatol* 1998; **38:** 81–8.
3. Nelson BS, Heischober B. Betel nut: a common drug used by naturalized citizens from India, Far East Asia, and the South Pacific Islands. *Ann Emerg Med* 1999; **34:** 238–43.
4. Merchant A, *et al.* Paan without tobacco: an independent risk factor for oral cancer. *Int J Cancer* 2000; **86:** 128–31.


**Effects on the lungs.** Evidence suggesting that there is an association between betel-nut chewing and bronchoconstriction in asthmatic patients.[1,2]


1. Taylor RFH, *et al.* Betel-nut chewing and asthma. *Lancet* 1992; **339:** 1134–6.
2. Kiyingi KS. Betel nut chewing and asthma. *Lancet* 1992; **340:** 59–60.


**Effects on the nervous system.** Areca-nut (betel-nut) chewing is associated with habituation, addiction, and dependence,[1] and CNS symptoms of withdrawal have been described in 2 patients.[2] Psychosis has also been reported.[1]

It has been suggested that the muscarinic action of areca alkaloids may have a beneficial effect on symptoms of schizophrenia, and a study of such patients in a Micronesian population provides some support for this idea.[3] However, severe extrapyramidal symptoms followed betel-nut chewing in 2 patients with chronic schizophrenia who were also receiving antipsychotic therapy.[4]


1. Nelson BS, Heischober B. Betel nut: a common drug used by naturalized citizens from India, Far East Asia, and the South Pacific Islands. *Ann Emerg Med* 1999; **34:** 238–43.
2. Wiesner DM. Betel-nut withdrawal. *Med J Aust* 1987; **146:** 453.
3. Sullivan RJ, *et al.* Effects of chewing betel nut (Areca catechu) on the symptoms of people with schizophrenia in Palau, Micronesia. *Br J Psychiatry* 2000; **177:** 174–8.
4. Deahl MP. Psychostimulant properties of betel nuts. *BMJ* 1987; **294:** 841.


## Aristolochia

Serpentaria.

NOTE. *Aristolochia clematitis* has also been known as asarabacca (p.1658).

**Pharmacopoeias.** *Chin.* allows various species of *Aristolochia.*

### Profile

*Aristolochia* spp. including *A. clematitis* and *A. ringens (A. brasiliensis)* have been used in herbal medicine.

Serpentary (serpentaria) is the dried rhizome and roots of *Aristolochia serpentaria* (Virginian snakeroot) and of *A. reticulata* (Texan snakeroot) (Aristolochiaceae). Snakeroot is also used as a common name to describe poisonous *Eupatorium* spp. Preparations of serpentary have been used as bitters. The active ingredient is aristolochic acid, which has been tried in a number of inflammatory disorders, mainly in folk medicine; the sodium salt of aristolochic acid has also been used. However, there is concern over such use since aristolochic acid has been reported to be carcinogenic and nephrotoxic.

Chinese medicine has employed various species of Aristolochia including *A. contorta*, *A. debilis*, and *A. manshuriensis.* The terms Mu Tong and Fangji have been used for Aristolochia spp. in traditional medicine.

**Adverse effects.** Progressive interstitial fibrosis of the kidney related to a slimming regimen containing Chinese herbs had been reported in 70 patients in Belgium by 1993; 30 of these patients had terminal renal failure.[1] Renal failure has also been reported[2] in 2 patients in the UK following ingestion of Chinese herbal medicines that were subsequently found to contain aristolochic acid, a known nephrotoxin;[3] one of these patients subsequently developed invasive urothelial carcinoma.[4] Inadvertent ingestion of aristolochic acid can originate as a result of the substitution of *Aristolochia* spp. (probably *A. manshuriensis*) for other innocuous herbal substances;[2,5] the Belgian cases were probably as a result of substitution of *A. fangchi* extracts for *Stephania tetrandra.*[1] As a result of these cases, the UK Medicines Control Agency has issued a permanent ban on *Aristolochia* preparations. Similar bans have been made in several other countries.[3] Examination of 39 patients in Belgium with nephropathy associated with *A. fangchi* ingestion had revealed 18 cases of urothelial carcinoma and evidence of mild to moderate dysplasia in 19 patients.[6] There had appeared to be a higher risk of carcinoma with total doses of *A. fangchi* in excess of 200 g.


1. Vanhaelen M, *et al.* Identification of aristolochic acid in Chinese herbs. *Lancet* 1994; **343:** 174.
2. Lord GM, *et al.* Nephropathy caused by Chinese herbs in the UK. *Lancet* 1999; **354:** 481–2.
3. Cosyns JP. Aristolochic acid and 'Chinese herbs nephropathy': a review of the evidence to date. *Drug Safety* 2003; **26:** 33–48.
4. Lord GM, *et al.* Urothelial malignant disease and Chinese herbal nephropathy. *Lancet* 2001; **358:** 1515–6.
5. But PP, Ma S-c. Chinese-herb nephropathy. *Lancet* 1999; **354:** 1731–2.
6. Nortier JL, *et al.* Urothelial carcinoma associated with the use of a chinese herb (Aristolochia fangchi). *N Engl J Med* 2000; **342:** 1686–92.


### Preparations

**Proprietary Preparations** (details are given in Part 3)
***Ital.:*** Euserpina Cellulite.

## Arnica

Árnica; Leopard's Bane; Mountain Tobacco; Wolf's Bane; Wolfsbane.

NOTE. Wolfsbane is also used as a common name for aconite (p.1646).

**Pharmacopoeias.** In *Eur.* (see p.vi).
*Ger.* allows *Arnica montana* or *A. chamissonis* subsp. *foliosa*, or a mixture of both.
*Pol.* allows *A. montana* or *A. chamissonis*.

**Ph. Eur. 5.0** (Arnica Flower; Arnica Flos). It consists of the whole or partially broken, dried flowerheads of *Arnica montana.* It contains not less than 0.4% w/w of total sesquiterpene lactones expressed as dihydrohelenalin tiglate, calculated with reference to the dried drug. It has an aromatic odour. Protect from light.

## Profile

Arnica is generally used in the form of the flowerheads of *Arnica montana* (Compositae).

Arnica flower is irritant to mucous membranes and when ingested has produced severe symptoms including gastrointestinal and nervous system disturbances, both tachycardia and bradycardia, and collapse. Tincture of arnica may cause dermatitis when applied to the skin of sensitive persons.

Preparations of arnica flower and arnica root are used as astringents for topical application to unbroken skin in conditions such as sprains and bruises; such preparations are not considered suitable for internal use.

Herbal and homoeopathic preparations containing arnica are available for oral use.

## Preparations

**Proprietary Preparations** (details are given in Part 3)
***Arg.:*** Herbaccion Desinflamante; ***Austral.:*** Sports Eze Bruising Relief†; ***Chile:*** Arnikaderm; ***Fr.:*** Arnican; Pharmadose teinture d'arnica; ***Ger.:*** Arnica-loges†; Arniflor-N†; Arnikatinktur; Arthrosenex AR; Doc; Hoevenol A†; Hyzum N; Vasotonin; ***Ital.:*** Venustas Lozione Caduta†; ***Neth.:*** Arniflor†; ***Port.:*** Arnigel; ***UK:*** Savlon Natural First Aid for Bruises.

**Multi-ingredient:** ***Austral.:*** Anti-Flamme†; Joint & Muscle Relief Cream†; ***Austria:*** Arnicet; Asthmatee EF-EM-ES; Berggeist; Biokosma Embrocation; Biokosma Red Point-Massagecreme; Cional; Dynexan; Rheuma; Sportino Akut; Varicylum; ***Braz.:*** Dermol; Traumed; ***Chile:*** Lefkaflam; Matikomp; ***Fr.:*** Arnicadol; Carli†; Creme Rap; Dermocica; Evarose; Lelong Contusions; ***Ger.:*** Arnica Kneipp Salbe†; Arnika plus†; Arnikamill; Befelka-Tinktur†; Cefagastrin†; Cefawell; Ceprovit†; Combudoron; derma-loges N†; Dolo-cyl; Essaven Sport; Gothaplast Rheumamed AC; Grunlicht Hingfong Essenz†; Heparin Comp; Heparin Kombi-Gel; Heusin; Hoevenol A†; Lindofluid N; Rhoival; Sportino Akut; Stullmaton; Trauma-cyl; Varicylum-S; Vasesana-Vasoregulans†; Venen-Salbe†; Venengel; Vitosal; ***Hong Kong:*** New Patecs A; ***Ital.:*** Elisir Depurativo Ambrosiano†; Herbavit†; ***Malaysia:*** Arnica Comp; ***S.Afr.:*** Dynexan; ***Spain:*** Arnicon; Encialina; Killpan†; Uralyt†; ***Switz.:*** Alpina Gel a l'arnica avec spilanthes†; Cetona Plus†; Dynexan†; Eubucal; Euceta avec camomille et arnica; Fortacet; ***UK:*** Arnileve; Hansaplast Herbal Heat Plaster; Savlon Natural First Aid for Insect Bites & Stings.

---

# Arsenic Trioxide *(USAN)*

Acidum Arsenicosum Anhydricum; Arseni Trioxydum; Arsenic; Arsenic Oxide; Arsénico, trióxido de; Arsenicum Album; Arsenious Acid; Arsenous Oxide; White Arsenic. Diarsenic trioxide.

$As_2O_3$ = 197.8.

*CAS — 1327-53-3 (arsenic trioxide); 7784-45-4 (arsenic triiodide).*

*ATC — L01XX27.*

**Pharmacopoeias.** In *Jpn.*

*Eur.* (see p.vi) includes a form for homoeopathic preparations.

**Ph. Eur. 5.0** (Arsenious Trioxide for Homoeopathic Preparations; Arsenii Trioxidum ad Praeparationes Homoeopathicae). A white or almost white powder. Practically insoluble to sparingly soluble in water; it dissolves in solutions of alkali hydroxides and carbonates.

## Adverse Effects

The toxicity of inorganic arsenic increases with increasing solubility, and trivalent compounds are considered to be more toxic than pentavalent compounds.

**Acute poisoning.** Symptoms of acute poisoning usually occur within an hour of ingestion but may be delayed for up to 12 hours, especially in the presence of food. Ingested arsenic salts cause oral irritation and a sensation of burning in the mouth and throat. The breath and faeces may have an odour of garlic. In severe poisoning, the principal toxic effect is haemorrhagic gastroenteritis, with acute abdominal pain, severe nausea, vomiting, and diarrhoea, and this can result in profound dehydration, collapse, shock, and death. Cardiac arrhythmias, convulsions, or muscle cramps may also occur. From 70 to 300 mg of arsenic trioxide may be fatal depending on the physical form and the rate of absorption. In the absence of adequate treatment death can occur within one hour but a period of 12 to 48 hours is more usual. Patients who survive the initial effects of arsenic trioxide may develop severe peripheral neuropathies and encephalopathy. Other effects following acute poisoning resemble those seen in chronic poisoning. Acute systemic effects may also be seen following inhalation or contact with the skin; pulmonary irritation may follow inhalation.

**Chronic poisoning.** Chronic poisoning or occupational exposure typically produces varied skin disorders, particularly hyperkeratosis, especially affecting the palms and soles, skin pigmentation, eczematous or follicular dermatitis, oedema especially affecting the eyelids, and alopecia. Muscle aching and weakness, and stomatitis may also occur. Gastrointestinal disturbances are generally mild. Patients may also experience excessive salivation, lachrymation, and inflammation of the conjunctiva and nasal mucosa resembling coryza. Chronic inhalation of arsenic salts may result in perforation of the nasal septum. Characteristic deposits of arsenic may appear in the nails 6 weeks after absorption. Obstructive jaundice may occur as a result of hepatomegaly and portal hypertension may eventually develop. Cirrhosis has been reported rarely. Proteinuria, haematuria, and anuria may occur secondary to renal damage. In advanced poisoning neurological effects are prominent. Encephalopathy has been reported but peripheral neuropathies are more common. There is both sensory and motor involvement and patients may at first experience paraesthesia, and numbness and burning in the extremities, but eventually muscular atrophy and paralysis occur. The legs are usually more affected than the arms. Arsenic is toxic to the bone marrow and produces a wide range of blood disorders including leucopenia, thrombocytopenia, and various anaemias.

Chronic exposure to arsenic has been associated with neoplasms of the skin, lungs, and liver and possibly other organs.

**Adverse effects of therapeutic use.** Reported adverse effects of arsenic trioxide therapy in patients with acute promyelocytic leukaemia (APL) include leucocytosis, neutropenia, raised liver enzyme values, gastrointestinal disturbances, fatigue, oedema, hyperglycaemia, hypokalaemia, dyspnoea, cough, skin rashes, pruritus, pyrexia, headaches, paraesthesia, and dizziness. Prolongation of the QT interval and other cardiac arrhythmias have occurred. The so-called 'leukocyte activation syndrome' ('APL differentiation syndrome') similar to one that develops with tretinoin therapy (see Retinoic Acid Syndrome, p.1161) has occurred in some patients. Sudden death has been reported in a few patients.

◊ Reviews,[1-5] including discussion of epidemic toxicity due to arsenic-contaminated drinking water.[4,5]


1. Arsenic. *Environmental Health Criteria 18.* Geneva: WHO, 1981.
2. Health and Safety Executive. Inorganic arsenic compounds. *Toxicity Review 16.* London: HMSO, 1986.
3. Shannon RL, Strayer DS. Arsenic-induced skin toxicity. *Hum Toxicol* 1989; **8:** 99–104.
4. Gebel T. Confounding variables in the environmental toxicology of arsenic. *Toxicology* 2000; **144:** 155–62.
5. Rahman MM, *et al.* Chronic arsenic toxicity in Bangladesh and West Bengal, India—a review and commentary. *J Toxicol Clin Toxicol* 2001; **39:** 683–700.


**Adulteration.** Arsenical compounds have reportedly been used to "cut" cocaine and symptoms of arsenic poisoning may occur in cocaine abusers.[1] Toxicity due to the presence of arsenic in various ethnic remedies has also been reported.[2-4]


1. Lombard J, *et al.* Arsenic intoxication in a cocaine abuser. *N Engl J Med* 1989; **320:** 869.
2. Kew J, *et al.* Arsenic and mercury intoxication due to Indian ethnic remedies. *BMJ* 1993; **306:** 506–7.
3. Ernst E, Thompson Coon J. Heavy metals in traditional Chinese medicines: a systematic review. *Clin Pharmacol Ther* 2001; **70:** 497–504.
4. Ernst E. Heavy metals in traditional Indian remedies. *Eur J Clin Pharmacol* 2002; **57:** 891–6.


**Treatment of leukaemia.** References[1-5] and a review[6] to adverse effects in patients receiving arsenic trioxide for the treatment of acute promyelocytic leukaemia, including a report of sudden death occurring in 3 patients in a dose-finding study.[5]


1. Huang SY, *et al.* Acute and chronic arsenic poisoning associated with treatment of acute promyelocytic leukaemia. *Br J Haematol* 1998; **103:** 1092–5.
2. Huang CH, *et al.* Complete atrioventricular block after arsenic trioxide treatment in an acute promyelocytic leukemic patient. *Pacing Clin Electrophysiol* 1999; **22:** 965–7.
3. Camacho LH, *et al.* Leukocytosis and the retinoic acid syndrome in patients with acute promyelocytic leukemia treated with arsenic trioxide. *J Clin Oncol* 2000; **18:** 2620–5.
4. Ohnishi K, *et al.* Prolongation of the QT interval and ventricular tachycardia in patients treated with arsenic trioxide for acute promyelocytic leukemia. *Ann Intern Med* 2000; **133:** 881–5.
5. Westervelt P, *et al.* Sudden death among patients with acute promyelocytic leukemia treated with arsenic trioxide. *Blood* 2001; **98:** 266–71.
6. Rust DM, Soignet SL. Risk/benefit profile of arsenic trioxide. *Oncologist* 2001; **6** (suppl 2): 29–32.


## Treatment of Adverse Effects

Acute poisoning due to the ingestion of arsenic compounds should be treated by immediate gastric lavage if the patient presents within 1 hour and has not already vomited. Activated charcoal may be of use to reduce absorption. Intravenous replacement of fluids and electrolytes should be undertaken as necessary to correct dehydration and electrolyte imbalance and to prevent shock; pressor agents and oxygen may be required. Morphine may be given for severe abdominal pain but care should be taken that this does not lead to colonic retention of arsenic compounds.

Chelation therapy with intramuscular dimercaprol (p.1037) should be started immediately the cause of poisoning is suspected. Prompt treatment is necessary to prevent or reduce the severity of neuropathy. It has been suggested that administration of dimercaprol should continue until abdominal symptoms subside and the gut is clear of ingested arsenic. Unithiol (p.1055) given intravenously may be used as an alternative. Oral treatment with succimer (p.1054) or penicillamine (p.1049) may then be substituted. A second course of treatment with penicillamine may be required if symptoms recur.

If renal failure occurs haemodialysis may be required to remove any absorbed or chelated arsenic. Exchange blood transfusion may be required for severe liver damage.

Dimercaprol may also be used in the treatment of chronic poisoning, but penicillamine, succimer, or unithiol (all given orally) may be preferred.

## Precautions

Arsenic trioxide should be used with caution in renal impairment since renal excretion is the main route of elimination. Patients receiving arsenic trioxide for acute promyelocytic leukaemia should have their ECG, blood sugar, electrolytes, blood count, and coagulation monitored at least twice weekly during induction and at least weekly during consolidation. More frequent monitoring may be needed in clinically unstable patients.

## Pharmacokinetics

Water-soluble arsenic acids and their salts are more rapidly absorbed from the gastrointestinal tract than poorly soluble arsenicals such as arsenic trioxide. The absorption of arsenic trioxide is dependent upon the physical form of the compound and coarsely powdered material may be eliminated in the faeces before significant dissolution and absorption can occur. Soluble arsenic salts may also be absorbed following inhalation and through skin.

Once absorbed, arsenic is stored mainly in the liver, kidneys, heart, and lungs, with smaller amounts in the muscles and nervous tissue. About 2 weeks after ingestion, arsenic is deposited in the hair and nails and remains fixed to the keratin for years. It is also deposited in the bones and teeth.

Although pentavalent arsenic is reduced to some degree *in vivo* to the more toxic trivalent form, trivalent arsenic is slowly and extensively oxidised to pentavalent arsenic. Both forms are methylated to relatively non-toxic derivatives and excreted in the urine, mainly as dimethylarsinic acid, with smaller amounts appearing as monomethylarsonic acid and inorganic arsenic compounds. Although 50% of a dose may be eliminated in the urine within 3 to 5 days, small amounts may continue to be excreted for several weeks after a single dose. Less significant amounts of arsenic are excreted in the faeces and sweat and via the lungs and skin. It is also distributed into breast milk and readily crosses the placenta.

## Uses and Administration

Arsenic trioxide is used for induction of remission and consolidation in acute promyelocytic leukaemia (see below). It is given to patients who are refractory to, or who have relapsed from, conventional therapy with retinoids and antineoplastics, as an intravenous infusion over 1 to 2 hours; if acute vasomotor reactions occur, the rate of infusion may be slowed and up to 4 hours may be taken. For induction, a dose of 150 micrograms/kg is given once daily until remission occurs; no more than 50 doses should be given (in the USA, the maximum number of induction doses should not exceed 60). Treatment for consolidation must begin 3 to 4 weeks after completion of induction (or 3 to 6 weeks in the USA). The dose for consolidation is 150 micrograms/kg once daily given for 25 doses spread over a period of up to 5 weeks; the regimen suggested in the UK is to give the daily dose for 5 consecutive days of each week.

Arsenic trioxide is used in homoeopathic medicine and in certain Asian herbal remedies. Arsenic anhydride has also been used.

Arsenic trioxide has been widely used as a constituent of weedkillers and sheepdips and as a rodenticide.

Arsenic trioxide and arsenic triiodide were formerly used internally as solutions or externally as ointments in the treatment of various skin diseases, but such use is generally no longer recommended. Externally, arsenic trioxide has a caustic action.

**Acute myeloid leukaemias.** The use of arsenic trioxide in the management of patients with acute promyelocytic leukaemia (p.506) has been reviewed.[1-3] Remission was achieved in patients who had relapsed despite conventional therapy with retinoids and antineoplastics.[4,5] Treatment was also successful in newly-diagnosed patients but severe liver toxicity occurred in some cases.[4]

For references to adverse effects occurring in patients receiving arsenic trioxide for acute promyelocytic leukaemia, see under Adverse Effects, above.


1. Soignet SL. Clinical experience of arsenic trioxide in relapsed acute promyelocytic leukemia. *Oncologist* 2001; **6** (suppl 2): 11–6.
2. Murgo AJ. Clinical trials of arsenic trioxide in hematologic and solid tumors: overview of the National Cancer Institute Cooperative Research and Development Studies. *Oncologist* 2001; **6** (suppl 2): 22–8.
3. Slack JL, *et al.* Advances in the management of acute promyelocytic leukemia and other hematologic malignancies with arsenic trioxide. *Oncologist* 2002; **7** (suppl 1): 1–13.
4. Niu C, *et al.* Studies on treatment of acute promyelocytic leukemia with arsenic trioxide: remission induction, follow-up, and molecular monitoring in 11 newly diagnosed and 47 relapsed acute promyelocytic leukemia patients. *Blood* 1999; **94:** 3315–24.
5. Soignet SL, *et al.* United States multicenter study of arsenic trioxide in relapsed acute promyelocytic leukemia. *J Clin Oncol* 2001; **19:** 3852–60.


**Multiple myeloma.** Arsenic trioxide is under investigation for the treatment of relapsed or refractory multiple myeloma (p.511).

References.


1. Munshi NC. Arsenic trioxide: an emerging therapy for multiple myeloma. *Oncologist* 2001; **6** (suppl 2): 17–21.
2. Munshi NC, *et al.* Clinical activity of arsenic trioxide for the treatment of multiple myeloma. *Leukemia* 2002; **16:** 1835–7.
3. Bahlis NJ, *et al.* Feasibility and correlates of arsenic trioxide combined with ascorbic acid-mediated depletion of intracellular glutathione for the treatment of relapsed/refractory multiple myeloma. *Clin Cancer Res* 2002; **8:** 3658–68.

**Myelodysplastic syndromes.** The use of arsenic trioxide for the treatment of myelodysplastic syndromes (p.508) is also under investigation and has been reviewed.[1,2]

1. List A, *et al.* Opportunities for Trisenox (arsenic trioxide) in the treatment of myelodysplastic syndromes. *Leukemia* 2003; **17:** 1499–1507.
2. Vey N. Arsenic trioxide for the treatment of myelodysplastic syndromes. *Expert Opin Pharmacother* 2004; **5:** 613–21.

### Preparations

**Proprietary Preparations** (details are given in Part 3)
***UK:*** Trisenox; ***USA:*** Trisenox.
**Multi-ingredient:** ***Ital.:*** Pasta Arsenicale.

## Arsine

Arsenic Trihydride; Arsina; Hydrogen Arsenide.
$AsH_3$ = 77.95.
*CAS — 7784-42-1.*

### Profile

Arsine is a heavy colourless gas with a garlic-like odour, which has no clinical uses but is an environmental or occupational hazard. It is highly toxic and causes severe haemolysis which may result in acute renal failure. It is potentially toxic below the odour threshold of 0.5 ppm and dangerously toxic following exposure to as little as 3 ppm; there may be a latent period of up to 24 hours following exposure before symptoms develop. Symptoms of arsine gas poisoning include generalised weakness, muscle cramps, thirst, headache, abdominal pain, nausea, vomiting, anorexia, jaundice, bronze skin coloration, haemolytic anaemia, haematuria, oliguria, and anuria. Pulmonary oedema, ECG abnormalities, and neurological disorders have also been reported. Treatment involves exchange transfusions and haemodialysis; dimercaprol and other chelating agents have been used but are of no value in the acute stage and do not prevent haemolysis.

◊ References.

1. Fowler BA, Weissberg JB. Arsine poisoning. *N Engl J Med* 1974; **291:** 1171–4.
2. Hesdorffer CS, *et al.* Arsine gas poisoning: the importance of exchange transfusions in severe cases. *Br J Ind Med* 1986; **43:** 353–5.
3. Rael LT, *et al.* The effects of sulfur, thiol, and thiol inhibitor compounds on arsine-induced toxicity in the human erythrocyte membrane. *Toxicol Sci* 2000; **55:** 468–77.

## Asafetida

Asafétida; Asafoetida; Asant; Devil's Dung; Gum Asafetida.
**Pharmacopoeias.** In *Chin.*

### Profile

Asafetida is an oleo-gum resin obtained from various species of *Ferula* (Umbelliferae). It has been used as a carminative and antispasmodic. It was also formerly used as an expectorant. It is used in cooking and is an ingredient of certain foods.

◊ References.

1. Kelly KJ, *et al.* Methemoglobinemia in an infant treated with the folk remedy glycerited asafoetida. *Pediatrics* 1984; **73:** 717–19.

### Preparations

**Proprietary Preparations** (details are given in Part 3)
**Multi-ingredient:** ***Thai.:*** Flatulence Gastulence; ***UK:*** Daily Tension & Strain Relief.

## Asarabacca

Ásaro europeo; Hazelwort; Rhizoma Asari; Wild Nard.

NOTE. Asarabacca has also been used as a common name for *Aristolochia clematitis* (see Aristolochia, p.1656).

### Profile

Asarabacca is the dried rhizome, roots, and leaves of *Asarum europaeum* (Aristolochiaceae), which is an ingredient of snuffs. It is also an irritant emetic and has been used in rodent poisons. Asarabacca has been used in homoeopathic medicine and is an ingredient of preparations given for respiratory disorders.

### Preparations

**Proprietary Preparations** (details are given in Part 3)
***Ger.:*** Escarol.

## Asbestos

Asbesto.

### Profile

The name asbestos is applied to several naturally occurring and widely distributed fibrous mineral silicates of the serpentine and amphibole groups. They include amosite (brown asbestos), anthophyllite, chrysotile (white asbestos), and crocidolite (blue asbestos).

Asbestos has properties of heat resistance, insulation, and reinforcement and has been used extensively for heat or electrical insulation, fire protection, in friction materials, and in the construction industry in a wide variety of materials including cement, pipes, and tiles.

When inhaled, asbestos fibres can cause asbestosis (pulmonary fibrosis), lung cancer, and mesothelioma of the pleura and peritoneum. Mesothelioma has been reported in persons exposed to relatively small amounts of asbestos after an average latent period of 30 to 40 years. An association between occupational exposure and an increased incidence of gastrointestinal, laryngeal, and other cancers has also been reported. Some types of asbestos are more hazardous than others; crocidolite (a member of the amphibole group) is considered to be the most dangerous.

◊ References.

1. Wagner GR. Asbestosis and silicosis. *Lancet* 1997; **349:** 1311–15.
2. Landrigan PJ, *et al.* The hazards of chrysotile asbestos: a critical review. *Ind Health* 1999; **37:** 271–80.
3. Browne K, Gee JB. Asbestos exposure and laryngeal cancer. *Ann Occup Hyg* 2000; **44:** 239–50.
4. Bourdes V, *et al.* Environmental exposure to asbestos and risk of pleural mesothelioma: review and meta-analysis. *Eur J Epidemiol* 2000; **16:** 411–7.
5. British Thoracic Society Standards of Care Committee. Statement on malignant mesothelioma in the United Kingdom. *Thorax* 2001; **56:** 250–65. Correction. *ibid.* 2001; **56:** 820. Also available at: http://www.brit-thoracic.org.uk/docs/mesothelioma.pdf (accessed 11/09/03)
6. Bolton C, *et al.* Asbestos-related disease. *Hosp Med* 2002; **63:** 148–51.

## Avena

Aven; Cultivated White Oats; Oatmeal; Oats.
**Pharmacopoeias.** *US* includes colloidal oatmeal.
**USP 27** (Colloidal Oatmeal). The powder resulting from the grinding and further processing of whole oat grain. When dried at 120° for 4 hours it loses not more than 10% of its weight.

### Profile

Avena is the grain of *Avena sativa* (Gramineae). It is used in herbal and in homoeopathic medicine and is reputed to have sedative activity.

A colloidal fraction extracted from avena is used in the preparation of emollient dermatological preparations.

Whether avenin, a protein present in oats, is harmful to patients with coeliac disease is controversial.

### Preparations

**Proprietary Preparations** (details are given in Part 3)
***Arg.:*** Dermopan; ***Austral.:*** DermaVeen Bath†; DermaVeen Dry Skin†; ***Canad.:*** Aveeno Preparations; ***Fr.:*** Aveeno Preparations†; Emulave†; Sensifluid; ***Hong Kong:*** Sensifluid†; Ultra-Rich†; ***Irl.:*** Aveeno†; ***Israel:*** Nutrasoothe; ***Ital.:*** Avalon; Aveeno Preparations; Emulave; Micaveen; ***Mex.:*** Suavene; ***NZ:*** Dermaveen; ***Port.:*** Aveeno Preparations†; Emulave†; ***Singapore:*** DermaVeen Bath; DermaVeen Dry Skin; DermaVeen Moisturising; DermaVeen Oatmeal Shampoo; DermaVeen Soap Free; ***Switz.:*** Avenaforce; ***UK:*** Aveeno Preparations; ***USA:*** ActiBath.
**Multi-ingredient:** ***Arg.:*** Aveno; Cholesterol Reducing Plan; Dermalibour; Epithelial; Exomega; Valeriana Oligoplex; ***Austral.:*** Avena Complex†; Bioglan The Blue One†; Calmo†; DermaVeen Moisturising†; DermaVeen Shower & Bath†; Dong Quai Complex†; Glycyrrhiza Complex†; Pacifenity†; Panax Complex†; ***Canad.:*** Aveeno Acne Treatment; ***Chile:*** Fucus Compuesto; Homeofortin III; ***Fr.:*** A-Derma Lait Ecran; Acnaveen†; Aveenoderm†; Biocarde; Cytelium; Dermalibour; Epitheliale; Eryase; Exomega; Gonaxine; Micaveen†; Septalibour; ***Ger.:*** Requiesan; Vollmers praparierter gruner N; ***Hong Kong:*** Aderma Dermalibour; Aderma Epitheliale; Aderma Exomega; Aderma Ultra High Protection; Oat Milk Treatment Cream†; ***Ital.:*** Acnaveen; Sebaveen†; ***Mex.:*** Aveendix; ***Port.:*** Acnaveen†; Aveenocream†; Aveenoderm†; D'Aveia; Micaveen†; Sebaveen†; ***Singapore:*** DermaVeen Acne; DermaVeen Shower & Bath; ***Switz.:*** Mucilar Avena; ***UK:*** Avena Sativa Comp; Daily Overwork & Mental Fatigue Relief; Daily Tension & Strain Relief; ***USA:*** Aveeno Cleansing Bar.

## Azadirachta

Margosa; Neem.

### Profile

Azadirachta is the dried stem bark, root bark, and leaves of *Azadirachta indica* (*Melia azadirachta*) (Meliaceae), which has been used as a bitter. It is widely used in South Asia and has been reported to have insecticidal, antimalarial, and spermicidal properties. Neem oil (margosa oil) expressed from the seeds has also been used.

**Insect repellent.** References.

1. Prakash A, *et al.* A preliminary field study on repellency of neem oil against Anopheles dirus (Diptera:Culicidae) in Assam. *J Commun Dis* 2000; **32:** 145–7.

**Poisoning.** Severe poisoning in Indian children given neem oil (margosa oil) as a remedy for minor ailments.[1]

1. Sinniah D, Baskaran G. Margosa oil poisoning as a cause of Reye's syndrome. *Lancet* 1981; **i:** 487–9.

### Preparations

**Proprietary Preparations** (details are given in Part 3)
**Multi-ingredient:** ***NZ:*** Mr Nits.

## Azintamide *(rINN)*

Azintamida; Azinthiamide; ST-9067. 2-[(6-Chloro-3-pyridazinyl)thio]-*N*,*N*-diethylacetamide.
$C_{10}H_{14}ClN_3OS$ = 259.8.
*CAS — 1830-32-6.*

### Profile

Azintamide has been used as a choleretic.

### Preparations

**Proprietary Preparations** (details are given in Part 3)
***Austria:*** Ora-Gallin purum; ***Port.:*** Colerin.
**Multi-ingredient:** ***Arg.:*** Biliuen Enzimatico; ***Austria:*** Ora-Gallin; Ora-Gallin compositum; ***Ger.:*** Oragallin S†; ***Port.:*** Colerin-F; ***Spain:*** Oragallin Espasmolitico.

## Azovan Blue *(BAN)*

Azovanum Caeruleum; Azul de Evans; CI Direct Blue 53; Colour Index No. 23860; Evans Blue; T-1824. Tetrasodium 1,1′-diamino-8,8′-dihydroxy-7,7′-(2,2′-dimethylbiphenyl-4,4′-diylbisdiazo)di-(naphthalene-2,4-disulphonate); Tetrasodium 6,6′-[3,3′-dimethylbiphenyl-4,4′-diylbis(azo)]bis[4-amino-5-hydroxynaphthalene-1,3-disulphonate].
$C_{34}H_{24}N_6Na_4O_{14}S_4$ = 960.8.
*CAS — 314-13-6.*

### Profile

Azovan blue is a dye that has been given intravenously for the determination of blood volume; it is firmly bound to plasma proteins and is slow to leave the circulation. Some patients may experience staining of the skin.

## Azulene

Azuleno; Cyclopentacycloheptene.
$C_{10}H_8$ = 128.2.
*CAS — 275-51-4.*

NOTE. The name 'Azulene' has also been used for a number of derivatives of azulene including azulene sodium sulfonate, chamazulene, guaiazulene, and sodium gualenate.

### Profile

Azulene has been used in preparations for anorectal and skin disorders, and for oral hygiene. The sodium sulfonate salt has been used in preparations for mouth and throat disorders and for dyspepsia; sodium gualenate has also been used in gastrointestinal disorders.

**Hypersensitivity.** Allergic cheilitis occurred in a patient following long-term use of a toothpaste containing azulene.[1]

1. Balato N, *et al.* Allergic cheilitis to azulene. *Contact Dermatitis* 1985; **13:** 39–40.

### Preparations

**Proprietary Preparations** (details are given in Part 3)
***Hong Kong:*** Azunol; ***Israel:*** Kamil Blue.
**Multi-ingredient:** ***Arg.:*** Ninderm; ***Austria:*** Emser Nasensalbe; ***Braz.:*** Eritrex A; Proctosan†; ***Ger.:*** Emser Nasensalbe N; ***Israel:*** Kamil Blue; ***Ital.:*** AZ 15.

## Bactericidal Permeability Increasing Protein

Proteína bactericida incrementadora de la permeabilidad.

## Opebacan *(BAN, USAN, rINN)*

rBPI-21. 132-L-Alanine-1-193-bactericidal/permeability-increasing protein (human).
*CAS — 206254-79-7.*

### Profile

Bactericidal permeability increasing protein is produced by human leucocytes and possesses both gram-negative bactericidal and endotoxin-neutralising properties. It also inhibits angiogenesis. Several derivatives have been developed and are under investigation. Opebacan (rBPI-21) is a modified recombinant fragment of bactericidal permeability increasing protein that is under investigation for the treatment of Crohn's disease and meningococcal septicaemia. Other derivatives of bactericidal permeability increasing protein are under investigation for retinopathies and acne.

Bactericidal permeability increasing protein also possesses antifungal activity.

◊ References.

1. Giroir BP, *et al.* Preliminary evaluation of recombinant amino-terminal fragment of human bactericidal/permeability-increasing protein in children with severe meningococcal sepsis. *Lancet* 1997; **350:** 1439–43.
2. Levin M, *et al.* Recombinant bactericidal/permeability-increasing protein ($rBPI_{21}$) as adjunctive treatment for children with severe meningococcal sepsis: a randomised trial. *Lancet* 2000; **356:** 961–7.

3. Levy O. A neutrophil-derived anti-infective molecule: bactericidal/permeability-increasing protein. *Antimicrob Agents Chemother* 2000; **44:** 2925–31.
4. van der Schaft DW, *et al.* The antiangiogenic properties of bactericidal/permeability-increasing protein (BPI). *Ann Med* 2002; **34:** 19–27.

## Barium

Bario.

Ba = 137.327.

*CAS — 7440-39-3.*

**Description.** Barium is a soft, highly reactive, silvery-white metal.

### Adverse Effects and Treatment

All barium salts that are water- or acid-soluble are very toxic. The symptoms of barium poisoning arise from stimulation of all forms of muscle and include vomiting, excess salivation, colic, diarrhoea, slow or irregular pulse, hypertension, dysarthria, confusion, dizziness, paraesthesias, vertigo, muscle tremors, seizures, muscular paralysis, and respiratory or metabolic acidosis. Hypokalaemia is common. Renal impairment due to barium poisoning has been reported. Death from cardiac or respiratory failure may occur.

In acute poisoning, emptying the stomach by lavage is recommended if possible. Magnesium or sodium sulfate may be given to convert barium to insoluble barium sulfate. Hypokalaemia and metabolic acidosis should be corrected and ventilation assisted if necessary. Excretion may be increased by diuresis. Haemodialysis may be used in severe poisoning.

◊ Reports of barium intoxication.

1. Lewi Z, Bar-Khayim Y. Food poisoning from barium carbonate. *Lancet* 1964; **ii:** 342–3.
2. Diengott D, *et al.* Hypokalaemia in barium poisoning. *Lancet* 1964; **ii:** 343–4.
3. Gould DB, *et al.* Barium sulfide poisoning: some factors contributing to survival. *Arch Intern Med* 1973; **132:** 891–4.
4. Berning J. Hypokalaemia of barium poisoning. *Lancet* 1975; **i:** 110.
5. Wetherill SF, *et al.* Acute renal failure associated with barium chloride poisoning. *Ann Intern Med* 1981; **95:** 187–8.
6. Phelan DM, *et al.* Is hypokalaemia the cause of paralysis in barium poisoning? *BMJ* 1984; **289:** 882.
7. Barium. *Environmental Health Criteria 107.* Geneva: WHO, 1990.
8. Sigue G, *et al.* From profound hypokalemia to life-threatening hyperkalemia: a case of barium sulfide poisoning. *Arch Intern Med* 2000; **160:** 548–51.
9. Wells JA, Wood KE. Acute barium poisoning treated with hemodialysis. *Am J Emerg Med* 2001; **19:** 175–7.
10. Jacobs IA, *et al.* Poisoning as a result of barium styphnate explosion. *Am J Ind Med* 2002; **41:** 285–8.

### Uses and Administration

The soluble barium salts are not used in therapeutics but are widely used in industry. Barium sulfide has been used as a depilatory and barium carbonate was used as a rodenticide. The insoluble barium sulfate (p.1061) is used as a contrast medium.

## Barium Hydroxide Lime

Bario, cal con hidróxido de.

*CAS — 17194-00-2 (anhydrous barium hydroxide); 12230-71-6 (barium hydroxide octahydrate).*

**Pharmacopoeias.** In *US.*

**USP 27** (Barium Hydroxide Lime). A mixture of barium hydroxide octahydrate and calcium hydroxide; it may also contain potassium hydroxide. White or greyish-white granules, or coloured with an indicator to show when absorptive power is exhausted. It absorbs not less than 19% of its weight of carbon dioxide. Store in airtight containers.

### Profile

Barium hydroxide lime is used similarly to soda lime to absorb carbon dioxide in closed-circuit anaesthetic apparatus. Barium hydroxide lime contains a soluble form of barium and is toxic if swallowed.

**Precautions.** Excessive drying out of barium hydroxide lime in anaesthetic apparatus, which may occur if oxygen flow through the equipment is left on for prolonged periods, can lead to the production of carbon monoxide and the risk of inducing carboxyhaemoglobinaemia in patients undergoing anaesthesia using the apparatus.[1]

1. Committee on Safety of Medicines/Medicines Control Agency. Safety issues in anaesthesia: volatile anesthetic agents and carboxyhaemoglobinaemia. *Current Problems* 1997; **23:** 7. Also available at: http://medicines.mhra.gov.uk/ourwork/monitorsafequalmed/currentproblems/volume24.htm (accessed 02/09/03)

## Bay Oil

Laurel dulce, aceite esencial de; Myrcia Oil; Oleum Myrciae.

NOTE. Distinguish from Laurel Leaf Oil (Bay Leaf Oil) which is obtained from the leaves of *Laurus nobilis* (Lauraceae).

### Profile

Bay oil is a yellow volatile oil that darkens rapidly on exposure to air and has a pleasant odour and spicy taste. It is obtained by distillation from the leaves of *Pimenta racemosa* (Myrtaceae) and probably other allied species. The principal use of bay oil is in the preparation of bay rum, which is used as a hair lotion and as an astringent application.

### Preparations

**Proprietary Preparations** (details are given in Part 3)

**Multi-ingredient:** ***UK:*** Adiantine; Medicated Extract of Rosemary.

## Bayberry

Árbol de la cera; Bayberry Bark; Candle Berry Bark; Myrica; Wax Myrtle Bark.

NOTE. Bayberry has also been used as a synonym for bog myrtle (see p.1661).

### Profile

Bayberry, the root bark of *Myrica cerifera* (Myricaceae), is used in upper respiratory-tract disorders and as a gargle for sore throat. It has also been used in gastrointestinal disorders, to treat vaginal discharge, and topically on ulcers and sores.

It is also used in homoeopathic medicine.

### Preparations

**Proprietary Preparations** (details are given in Part 3)

**Multi-ingredient:** ***UK:*** EP&C Essence; Peerless Composition Essence.

## Bearberry

Bärentraubenblätter; Bearberry Leaves; Busserole; Gayuba; Ptarmiganberry Leaves; Uva-Ursi; Uvae Ursi Folium.

**Pharmacopoeias.** In *Eur.* (see p.vi), *Jpn*, and *Pol.*

**Ph. Eur. 5.0** (Bearberry Leaf). The whole or cut dried leaves of the bearberry, *Arctostaphylos uva-ursi*. It contains not less than 7.0% of anhydrous arbutin, calculated with reference to the dried drug. Protect from light.

### Profile

Bearberry has been reported to be a diuretic, bacteriostatic, and astringent and has been used in the treatment of urinary-tract disorders. It has also been used in homoeopathic medicine.

### Preparations

**Proprietary Preparations** (details are given in Part 3)
***Ger.:*** Arctuvan; Cystinol Akut; Uvalysat; ***Ital.:*** Ginocap†.

**Multi-ingredient:** ***Arg.:*** Ajolip; KLB6 Fruit Diet; Water Pill c Potasio; ***Austral.:*** Althaea Complex†; Bioglan Cranbiotic Super†; Cranberry Complex†; De Witts New Pills†; Extralife Fluid-Care†; Extralife PMS-Care†; Extralife Uri-Care†; Fluid Loss†; Herbal Diuretic Formula†; Medinat PMT-Eze†; Profluid†; Protemp†; Urinase†; Uva-Ursi Complex†; Uva-Ursi Plus†; ***Austria:*** Aktiv Blasen- und Nierentee; Apotheker Bauer's Nieren- und Blasentee; Bio-Garten Tee fur Niere und Blase; Bio-Strath Nieren-Blasen; Bioreform-Blasen- und Nierentee; Blasen- und Nierentee; Blasen-Tee†; Mag Kottas Nieren-Blasentee; Neuners Krautertee Nr 204 - Krauterhexlein Kinder Nieren- und Blasentee; Neuners Krautertee Nr 3 - Blasentee; Neuners Krautertee Nr 31 - Harnwegstee; Sidroga Nieren- und Blasentee; St Radegunder Nierentee; Uropurat; ***Belg.:*** Tisane Contre la Tension†; Tisane Diuretique†; ***Braz.:*** Composto Anticelulitico†; Emagrevit; Pilulas De Witt's; ***Chile:*** Primacy Phyto +; ***Fr.:*** Mediflor Tisane Antirhumatismale No 2; Mediflor Tisane No 4 Diuretique; Santane $O_1$†; Santane $R_8$†; Tisane Orientale Soker†; Uromil; Urophytum; ***Ger.:*** Cefanephrin†; Cystinol; Cysto Fink†; Harntee 400; Harntee STADA; Hernia-Tee†; Herniol†; Presselin Nieren-Blasen K 3; Prostatin F; Salusan†; Uro Fink†; ***Israel:*** Jungborn; ***NZ:*** De Witts Pills; ***Port.:*** Asic†; Rilastil Dermo Solar; ***Spain:*** Genurat; Urisor; Vegetalin†; ***Switz.:*** Cysto-Caps Chassot†; Demonatur Dragees pour les reins et la vessie; Dragees pour reins et vessie S†; Tisane pour les reins et la vessie; Urinex; ***UK:*** Antitis; Backache; Backache Relief; Boldo†; Cascade; De Witt's K & B Pills; Diuretabs; Gerard House Buchu Compound†; Gerard House Waterlex†; HealthAid Boldo-Plus; Hofels White Willow and Burdock†; HRI Water Balance; Kas-Bah; Modern Herbals Water Retention; Prementaid; Sciargo; Tabritis; Uvacin; Watershed; Wellwoman†.

## Bendazol Hydrochloride *(rINNM)*

Dibazol. 2-Benzylbenzimidazole hydrochloride.

$C_{14}H_{12}N_2,HCl$ = 244.7.

*CAS — 621-72-7 (bendazol); 1212-48-2 (bendazol hydrochloride).*

### Profile

Bendazol hydrochloride is used as an antispasmodic.

## Bentiromide *(BAN, USAN, rINN)*

Bentiromida; BTPABA; BT-PABA; E-2663; PFT; Ro-11-7891. 4-(*N*-Benzoyl-L-tyrosylamino)benzoic acid.

$C_{23}H_{20}N_2O_5$ = 404.4.

*CAS — 37106-97-1.*

*ATC — V04CK03.*

### Profile

Bentiromide has been given by mouth as a noninvasive test of exocrine pancreatic function, the amount of *p*-aminobenzoic acid and its metabolites excreted in the urine being taken as a measure of the chymotrypsin-secreting activity of the pancreas. Headache and gastrointestinal disturbances have been reported in patients receiving bentiromide. The bentiromide test has given misleading results in patients with gastrointestinal, liver, or kidney disorders, or in patients receiving certain foods or drugs that are excreted as arylamines. Some of these drugs included benzocaine, chloramphenicol, lidocaine, paracetamol, procaine, procainamide, sulfonamides, and some diuretics.

◊ References.

1. Hoek FJ, *et al.* Improved specificity of the PABA test with p-aminosalicylic acid (PAS). *Gut* 1987; **28:** 468–73.
2. Puntis JWL, *et al.* Simplified oral pancreatic function test. *Arch Dis Child* 1988; **63:** 780–4.

### Preparations

**Proprietary Preparations** (details are given in Part 3)
***USA:*** Chymex†.

## Benzaldehyde

Benzaldehído.

$C_7H_6O$ = 106.1.

*CAS — 100-52-7.*

**Pharmacopoeias.** In *Br.* Also in *USNF.*

**BP 2003** (Benzaldehyde). A clear colourless liquid with a characteristic odour of bitter almonds. Slightly soluble in water; miscible with alcohol and with ether. Store at a temperature not exceeding 15° in well-filled containers. Protect from light.

**USNF 22** (Benzaldehyde). A colourless strongly refractive liquid with an odour resembling that of bitter almond oil and a burning aromatic taste. Slightly soluble in water; miscible with alcohol, with ether, and with fixed and volatile oils. Store in well-filled, airtight containers. Protect from light.

### Profile

Benzaldehyde is used as a flavour as an alternative to volatile bitter almond oil. It may cause contact dermatitis.

### Preparations

***USNF 22:*** Compound Benzaldehyde Elixir.

## Benzyl Isothiocyanate

Bencilo, isotiocinato de; Benzyl Mustard Oil; Benzylsenföl; Oleum Tropaeoli.

$C_8H_7NS$ = 149.2.

*CAS — 622-78-6.*

**Pharmacopoeias.** *Fr.* includes Capucine (*Tropaeolum majus*).

### Profile

Benzyl isothiocyanate is an oil obtained from *Tropaeolum majus* (Capuchin cress; common nasturtium) (Tropaeolaceae) that has been given as an antibacterial.

*Tropaeolum majus* has been used in herbal and in homoeopathic medicine.

### Preparations

**Proprietary Preparations** (details are given in Part 3)

**Multi-ingredient:** ***Ger.:*** Angocin Anti-Infekt N; Nephroselect M.

## Berberine

Berberina. 5,6-Dihydro-9,10-dimethoxybenzo[*g*]-1,3-benzodioxolo[5,6-*a*]quinolizinium.

$C_{20}H_{18}NO_4$ = 336.4.

*CAS — 2086-83-1 (berberine); 633-65-8 (berberine chloride); 633-66-9 (berberine sulfate).*

**Pharmacopoeias.** *Chin.* includes berberine chloride. *Jpn* includes berberine chloride and berberine tannate. *Viet.* includes berberine chloride dihydrate.

### Profile

Berberine is a quaternary alkaloid present in hydrastis, in various species of *Berberis*, and in many other plants. It has been used as a bitter and as a flavour in food and alcoholic drinks. It possesses antimicrobial activity and has also been tried as various salts in a number of infections.

◊ References.

1. Khin-Maung-U, *et al.* Clinical trial of berberine in acute watery diarrhoea. *BMJ* 1985; **291:** 1601–5.
2. Rabbani GH, *et al.* Randomized controlled trial of berberine sulfate therapy for diarrhea due to enterotoxigenic Escherichia coli and Vibrio cholerae. *J Infect Dis* 1987; **155:** 979–84.
3. Vennerstrom JL, *et al.* Berberine derivatives as antileishmanial drugs. *Antimicrob Agents Chemother* 1990; **34:** 918–21.
4. Phillipson JD, Wright CW. Medicinal plants in tropical medicine: 1 Medicinal plants against protozoal diseases. *Trans R Soc Trop Med Hyg* 1991; **85:** 18–21.

### Preparations

**Proprietary Preparations** (details are given in Part 3)
***Austral.:*** Murine†; ***NZ:*** Murine†.

**Multi-ingredient:** ***Braz.:*** Lerin; Neo Quimica Colirio; Visolon†; ***Fr.:*** Sedacollyre; ***India:*** Emantid.

## Bergamot Oil

Bergamot Essence; Bergamota, aceite esencial de; Oleum Bergamottae.

**Pharmacopoeias.** In *Fr.* and *It.*

### Profile

Bergamot oil is a greenish or brownish-yellow volatile oil with a characteristic fragrant odour and a bitter aromatic taste, obtained by expression from the fresh peel of fruit of *Citrus bergamia* (Rutaceae). Constituents include linalyl acetate and 5-methoxypsoralen (p.1154) and photosensitivity reactions have occurred following the topical use of preparations containing bergamot oil.

Bergamot oil is used in perfumery and as a flavour in Earl Grey tea. It has been included in some preparations for upper respiratory-tract disorders and hyperhidrosis.

◊ Muscle cramps have been reported[1] in a patient following the ingestion of up to 4 litres of 'Earl Grey' tea daily.

1. Finsterer J. Earl Grey tea intoxication. *Lancet* 2002; **359:** 1484.

### Preparations

**Proprietary Preparations** (details are given in Part 3)
**Multi-ingredient:** ***Fr.:*** Ephydrol; ***Ital.:*** Cura†; Sanaderm†.

## Betahistine *(BAN, rINN)*

*N*-Methyl-2-(2-pyridyl)ethylamine.
$C_8H_{12}N_2$ = 136.2.
*CAS — 5638-76-6.*
*ATC — N07CA01.*

## Betahistine Hydrochloride *(USAN, rINNM)*

Betahistine Dihydrochloride *(BANM)*; Hidrocloruro de betahistina; PT-9. *N*-Methyl-2-(2-pyridyl)ethylamine dihydrochloride.
$C_8H_{12}N_2,2HCl$ = 209.1.
*CAS — 5579-84-0.*
*ATC — N07CA01.*

**Pharmacopoeias.** In *Chin.*

## Betahistine Mesilate *(BANM, rINNM)*

Betahistine Mesylate; Betahistini Mesilas; Mesilato de betahistina. *N*-Methyl-2-(2-pyridyl)ethylamine bismethanesulphonate.
$C_8H_{12}N_2.(CH_4O_3S)_2$ = 328.4.
*CAS — 54856-23-4.*
*ATC — N07CA01.*

**Pharmacopoeias.** In *Eur.* (see p.vi) and *Jpn.*

**Ph. Eur. 5.0** (Betahistine Mesilate). A white, crystalline, very hygroscopic powder. Very soluble in water; freely soluble in alcohol; very slightly soluble in isopropyl alcohol. A 10% solution in water has a pH of 2.0 to 3.0. Store in airtight containers.

### Adverse Effects

Gastrointestinal disturbances, headache, skin rashes, and pruritus have been reported.

### Precautions

Betahistine should not be given to patients with phaeochromocytoma. It should be given with care to patients with asthma, peptic ulcer disease, or a history of peptic ulcer disease.

**Porphyria.** Betahistine hydrochloride is considered to be unsafe in patients with porphyria because it has been shown to be porphyrinogenic in *in-vitro* systems.

### Uses and Administration

Betahistine is an analogue of histamine and is claimed to improve the microcirculation of the labyrinth resulting in reduced endolymphatic pressure. It is used to reduce the symptoms of vertigo (p.423), tinnitus (p.1381), and hearing loss associated with Ménière's disease (p.422).

Betahistine is given by mouth as the hydrochloride or mesilate. The usual initial dose (of the hydrochloride) is 16 mg three times daily taken preferably with meals; maintenance doses are generally in the range of 24 to 48 mg daily. Betahistine mesilate is used in similar doses.

◊ Reviews

1. Lacour M, Sterkers O. Histamine and betahistine in the treatment of vertigo: elucidation of mechanisms of action. *CNS Drugs* 2001; **15:** 853–70.
2. James AL, Burton MJ. Betahistine for Menière's disease or syndrome. Available in The Cochrane Library; Issue 2. Chichester: John Wiley; 2004.

### Preparations

**Proprietary Preparations** (details are given in Part 3)
***Arg.:*** Meniex; Microser; ***Austral.:*** Serc; ***Austria:*** Betaserc; ***Belg.:*** Betaserc; Lobione†; ***Braz.:*** Betaserc; Labirin; ***Canad.:*** Serc; ***Chile:*** Microser; ***Denm.:*** Betaserc; ***Fin.:*** Betaserc; ***Fr.:*** Betaserc; Evolis; Extovyl; Lectil; Serc; Vertigirex†; ***Ger.:*** Aequamen; Betavert; Melopat; Ribrain†; Vasomotal; ***Gr.:*** Antivom; Betaserc; Ribrain; ***Hong Kong:*** Betaserc; Bymeniere; Meniero; Merislon; ***India:*** Vertin; ***Irl.:*** By-Vertin; Serc; Vertigon; ***Israel:*** Agiserc; Betistine; ***Ital.:*** Microser; Vertiserc; ***Jpn:*** Merislon; ***Malaysia:*** Betaserc; ***Mex.:*** Serc; ***Neth.:*** Betaserc; ***NZ:*** Serc; Vergo; ***Port.:*** Betaserc; ***S.Afr.:*** Serc; ***Singapore:*** Betaserc; Merislon; ***Spain:*** Fidium; Serc; ***Switz.:*** Betaserc; ***Thai.:*** Merislon; Merlin; Serc; ***UK:*** Serc.

## Betaine

Betaína; Glycine Betaine; Glycocoll Betaine; Lycine; Trimethylglycine. (Carboxymethyl)trimethylammonium hydroxide inner salt.
$C_5H_{11}NO_2$ = 117.1.
*CAS — 107-43-7.*
*ATC — A16AA06.*

## Betaine Hydrochloride

Betaína, hidrocloruro de; Trimethylglycine Hydrochloride. (Carboxymethyl)trimethylammonium hydroxide inner salt hydrochloride.
$C_5H_{11}NO_2,HCl$ = 153.6.
*CAS — 590-46-5.*
*ATC — A09AB02.*

**Pharmacopoeias.** In *US.*

**USP 27** (Betaine Hydrochloride). A 25% solution in water has a pH of 0.8 to 1.2.

### Profile

Betaine is used as a methyl donor to remethylate homocysteine to methionine in the treatment of patients with homocystinuria (p.1417). It is given by mouth in a usual dose of 3 g twice daily. Doses are adjusted according to plasma-homocysteine concentrations; up to 20 g daily has been required in some patients. In children under 3 years old, an initial dose of 100 mg/kg daily may be used.

Betaine has also been used as a variety of salts in preparations for liver and gastrointestinal disorders. The hydrochloride has been given as a source of hydrochloric acid in the treatment of hypochlorhydria.

**Homocystinuria.** References.

1. Smolin LA, *et al.* The use of betaine for the treatment of homocystinuria. *J Pediatr* 1981; **99:** 467–72.
2. Wilcken DEL, *et al.* Homocystinuria—the effects of betaine in the treatment of patients not responsive to pyridoxine. *N Engl J Med* 1983; **309:** 448–53.
3. Holme E, *et al.* Betaine for treatment of homocystinuria caused by methylenetetrahydrofolate reductase deficiency. *Arch Dis Child* 1989; **64:** 1061–4.
4. Anonymous. Betaine for homocystinuria. *Med Lett Drugs Ther* 1997; **39:** 12.
5. Schwahn BC, *et al.* Pharmacokinetics of oral betaine in healthy subjects and patients with homocystinuria. *Br J Clin Pharmacol* 2003; **55:** 6–13.

**Liver disorders.** Betaine has also been investigated for the treatment of nonalcoholic steatohepatitis.

References.

1. Miglio F, *et al.* Efficacy and safety of oral betaine glucuronate in non-alcoholic steatohepatitis: a double-blind, randomized, parallel-group, placebo-controlled prospective clinical study. *Arzneimittelforschung* 2000; **50:** 722–7.
2. Abdelmalek MF, *et al.* Betaine, a promising new agent for patients with nonalcoholic steatohepatitis: results of a pilot study. *Am J Gastroenterol* 2001; **96:** 2711–7.

### Preparations

**Proprietary Preparations** (details are given in Part 3)
***Austral.:*** Cystadane; ***Canad.:*** Cystadane; ***Israel:*** Cystadan; ***Ital.:*** Somatyl; ***USA:*** Cystadane.

**Multi-ingredient:** ***Austral.:*** Bepep†; Betaine Digestive Aid†; Bioglan Digestive Zyme†; Digestaid†; ***Austria:*** $CO_2$ Granulat; Oroacid; ***Belg.:*** Digestomen; Gastrobul†; ***Braz.:*** Aminotox; Anekron; Betaliver; Biofigado†; Biohepax; Colachofra; Colinvintol†; Cynatrop†; Enterofigon†; Eparex†; Epocler; Eviepar†; Figadobil†; Hepacitron†; Hepalin†; Hepasedan†; Hepatobe†; Hepatocler†; Hepofilina†; Hormo Hepatico; Jecohepat†; Mesitol†; Metiocolin Composto; Necro B-6; Necrohepat†; Xantinon Complex; ***Fr.:*** Citrarginine; Gastrobul; Hepagrume; Nivabetol; Ornitaine; ***Ger.:*** $CO_2$ Granulat; Flacar; Unexym MD S; ***Gr.:*** Kloref; ***Hong Kong:*** Jetepar; ***Israel:*** Betazim; ***Ital.:*** Betascor B12†; Citroepatina; Epabetina; Ietepar; ***Malaysia:*** Jetepar; ***S.Afr.:*** Kloref; ***Singapore:*** Jetepar; ***Spain:*** Espasmo Digestomen†; Levaliver†; ***UK:*** Digezyme†; Enzyme Digest; Enzyme Plus; FatSolv†; Kloref.

## Bibrocathol *(rINN)*

Bibrocathin; Bibrocatol; Bibrokatol; Bismuth Tetrabrompyrocatechinate; Tetrabromopyrocatechol Bismuth. 4,5,6,7-Tetrabromo-2-hydroxy-1,3,2-benzodioxabismole.
$C_6HBiBr_4O_3$ = 649.7.
*CAS — 6915-57-7.*
*ATC — S01AX05.*

### Profile

Bibrocathol is a bismuth-containing compound that has been applied topically in the treatment of eye disorders, wounds, and burns.

### Preparations

**Proprietary Preparations** (details are given in Part 3)
***Ger.:*** Noviform; Posiformin; ***Swed.:*** Noviform; ***Switz.:*** Noviform; Noviforme-Blache†.

**Multi-ingredient:** ***Ger.:*** Novifort.

## Bifemelane *(rINN)*

Bifemelano; MCI-2016 (bifemelane hydrochloride). *N*-Methyl-4-[(α-phenyl-*o*-tolyl)oxy]butylamine.
$C_{18}H_{23}NO$ = 269.4.
*CAS — 90293-01-9 (bifemelane); 62232-46-6 (bifemelane hydrochloride).*
*ATC — N06AX08.*

### Profile

Bifemelane is a nootropic that has been used as the hydrochloride in the treatment of cerebrovascular disorders.

### Preparations

**Proprietary Preparations** (details are given in Part 3)
***Arg.:*** Alemelano; Cordinal; Neurocine; Neurolea.

## Bile Acids and Salts

Biliares, ácidos y sales.
*CAS — 81-25-4 (cholic acid); 11006-55-6 (sodium taurоglycocholate).*

**Pharmacopoeias.** *Jpn* includes bear bile.

### Profile

The principal primary bile acids, cholic acid and chenodeoxycholic acid (p.1670), are produced in the liver from cholesterol and are conjugated with glycine or taurine to give glycocholic acid, taurocholic acid, glycochenodeoxycholic acid, and taurochenodeoxycholic acid, before being secreted into the bile where they are present as the sodium or potassium salts (bile salts). Secondary bile acids are formed in the colon by bacterial deconjugation and 7α-dehydroxylation of cholic acid and chenodeoxycholic acid, producing deoxycholic acid and lithocholic acid, respectively. Ursodeoxycholic acid (p.1760) is a minor bile acid in man although it is the principal bile acid in *bears.* Dehydrocholic acid (p.1679) is a semisynthetic bile acid.

The total body pool of bile salts is about 3 g, and most of the secreted bile salts are reabsorbed in a process of enterohepatic recycling, so that only a small fraction of this amount must be synthesised *de novo* each day.

Bile salts are strongly amphiphilic; with the aid of phospholipids they form micelles and emulsify cholesterol and other lipids in bile. Oral administration of chenodeoxycholic acid also reduces the synthesis of cholesterol in the liver, while ursodeoxycholic acid reduces biliary cholesterol secretion apparently by increasing conversion of cholesterol to other bile acids. The bile acids (but not the bile salts) also have a choleretic action, increasing the secretion of bile, when given by mouth.

Chenodeoxycholic acid and ursodeoxycholic acid are given by mouth in the management of cholesterol-rich gallstones (p.1761) in patients unsuited to, or unwilling to undergo, surgery. Ursodeoxycholic acid is also being studied in some liver disorders.

Preparations containing bile salts have been used to assist the emulsification of fats and absorption of fat-soluble vitamins in conditions in which there is a deficiency of bile in the gastrointestinal tract. Ox bile has also been used in the treatment of chronic constipation. Cholic acid is used for the treatment of inborn errors in primary bile synthesis.

◊ References.

1. Hofmann AF. The continuing importance of bile acids in liver and intestinal disease. *Arch Intern Med* 1999; **159:** 2647–58.

### Preparations

**Proprietary Preparations** (details are given in Part 3)
***Austral.:*** Proslim-Lipid†; ***Ger.:*** Cholecysmon; ***S.Afr.:*** Bilron.

**Multi-ingredient:** ***Arg.:*** Bibol Leloup; Bil 13; Bilagol; Bilidren; Biliosan Compuesto; Carbogasol Digestivo; Cascara Sagrada Sanaplex; Digesplen; Gastron Fuerte; Hepatalgina; Nilflux; Opobyl; Pankreon Compuesto; Veracolate; ***Austral.:*** Digestaid†; Enzyme†; Lexat†; ***Austria:*** Arca-Enzym; Buccalin; Combizym Compositum; Dragees Neunzehn; Helopanzym; Hylakombun†; Nutrizym†; Pankreon compositum†; Peribilan†; Silberne; ***Belg.:*** Buccaline; Grains de Vals; ***Braz.:*** B-Vesil; Colagolen†; Combizym†; Dasc; Digestal†; Emagrex†; Esbelt†; Figatil†; Hepatobyl†; Jurubileno†; Macroten†; Magroton†; Normagrin†; Nutrizim; ***Canad.:*** Aid-Lax†; Alsiline†; Bicholate; Caroid†; Cholasyn II; Herbalax; Herbalax Forte†; Laxat†; Laxative; Phytolax†; Regubil†; Triolax†; Vesilax†; ***Chile:*** Combizym; Combizym Compositum; Flapex E; Hepabil; K.C.M.C; Katin; Onoton; ***Fin.:*** Combizym Compositum; Fellesan†; ***Fr.:*** Bilifluine†; Bilkaby†; Mucinum†; Rectopanbiline; ***Ger.:*** Combizym Compositum; Hepatofalk Neu†; ***Hong Kong:*** Bilsan; Buccaline; Enzyplex; Hepatofalk; Topase; ***India:*** Digeplex-T; Dispeptal; Farizym; Merckenzyme; Panolase; Papytazyme; ***Israel:*** Encypalmed; ***Ital.:*** Pancreon Compositum†; ***Malaysia:*** Enzyplex; ***Mex.:*** Difarben; Dirfaben; Dixiflen; Espaven Enzimatico; Ochozim; Onoton; ***Neth.:*** Combizym Compositum†; ***NZ:*** Combizym Compositum†; ***Port.:*** Byl; Caroid; Combizym Compositum; Fermetone Composto; Nutrizym†; ***Singapore:*** Enzyplex; ***Spain:*** Espasmo Digestomen†; Menabil Complex; ***Swed.:*** Combizym Compositum; Fellesan†; ***Switz.:*** Buccaline; Combizym Compositum†; Opobyl†; ***Thai.:*** Buccaline; Combizym Compositum; Enzyplex; Papytazyme; Veracolate; ***UK:*** Digezyme†; ***USA:*** Digepepsin.

## Birch Leaf

Abedul, hojas de; Betulae Folium; Birkenblätter; Bouleau; Silver Birch Leaf.

**Pharmacopoeias.** In *Eur.* (see p.vi) and *Pol.*

**Ph. Eur. 5.0** (Birch Leaf). The whole or fragmented dried leaves of *Betula pendula* and/or *B. pubescens* as well as hybrids of both species. It contains not less than 1.5% of flavonoids, calculated as hyperoside ($C_{21}H_{20}O_{12}$ = 464.4), with reference to the dried drug. Protect from light.

### Profile

Birch leaf is used in herbal medicine, particularly for urinary-tract disorders.

### Preparations

**Proprietary Preparations** (details are given in Part 3)
***Austria:*** Bakanasan Entwasserungs; Bornosan-Entwasserungsdragees; Entwasserungs-Tabletten; Galama Entschlackungselixier; Sanhelios-Ent-

wasserungsdragees; ***Ger.:*** Kneipp Birkenblatter Pflanzensaft†; Uroflan†; Urorenal.

**Multi-ingredient: *Arg.:*** Sequals G; ***Austria:*** Aktiv Blasen- und Nierentee; Apotheker Bauer's Nieren- und Blasentee; Apotheker Hoyers Brennesseltonikum; Bio-Garten Entschlackungstee; Bio-Garten Tee fur Niere und Blase; Bio-Garten Tee zur Erhohung der Harnmenge; Bio-Garten Tropfen fur Niere und Blase; Bioreform-Blasen- und Nierentee; Bioreform-Entschlackungstee; Bioreform-Harntreibender Tee; Blasen- und Nierentee; Blasentee EF-EM-ES; Brennesseltonikum; Drogimed; Ehrmann's Entschlackungstee; Fruhjahrs-Elixier ohne Alkohol; Kneipp Entwasserungstee; Kneipp Nieren- und Blasen-Tee; Krauterdoktor Entwasserungs-Elixier; Krauterhaus Mag Kottas Blasentee; Krauterhaus Mag Kottas Entschlackungstee; Krauterpfarrer Weidinger Rheumatee; Krauterpfarrer Weidinger Tee zur Entwasserung; Mag Doskar's Nieren- und Blasentonikum; Mag Kottas Entschlackungstee; Mag Kottas Krauterexpress-Entschlackungstee; Naturland Entschlackungstonikum; Neuners Krautertee Nr 19 - Harntreibender Stoffwechseltee; Neuners Krautertee Nr 2 - Fruhjahrskurtee; Neuners Krautertee Nr 204 - Krauterhexlein Kinder Nieren- und Blasentee; Neuners Krautertee Nr 25 - Entschlackungstee; Neuners Krautertee Nr 29 - Stoffwechseltee mild; Neuners Krautertee Nr 30 - Stoffwechseltee stark; Rheuma; Sidroga Nieren- und Blasentee; Solubitrat; St Radegunder Entwasserungs-Elixier; St Radegunder Entwasserungstee; Synpharma Instant-Blasen- und Nierentee; Teekanne Blasen- und Nierentee; ***Fr.:*** B.O.P.; Depuratum; Drainactil; Mediflor no 11 Draineur Renal et Digestif; Mediflor Tisane Antirhumatismale No 2; ***Ger.:*** Agamadon†; Antihypertonicum S; Befelka-Tinktur†; BioCyst; Blasen-Nieren-Tee Stada†; Canephron novo; Cystinol; Cysto Fink†; Discmigon†; Dr Wiemanns Rheumatonikum; Etmoren†; Harntee 400; Harntee 450†; Harntee STADA; Harntee-Steiner; Heumann Blasen- und Nierentee Solubitrat S; Hevert-Blasen-Nieren-Tee N; Hevert-Entwasserungs-Tee†; Hevert-Gicht-Rheuma-Tee comp†; Heweberberol-Tee; Kneipp Blasen- und Nieren-Tee†; Kneipp Entschlackungs-Tee†; Nephro-Pasc; Nephronorm med; Nephropur tri; Nephroselect M; Nephrubin-N; Nierentee 2000; Nieron Blasen- und Nieren-Tee VI; Nieron-Tee N; Presselin Nieren-Blasen K 3; Reducelle†; Renob Blasen- und Nierentee; Salus Rheuma-Tee Krautertee Nr. 12†; Ullus Blasen-Nieren-Tee N†; Uro Fink†; Urodil Blasen-Nieren Arzneitee†; Urodil phyto; Urostei†; ***Ital.:*** Artoxan†; Betulla (Specie Composta); Depurfat†; Fluend†; Ginoday†; Gramigna (Specie Composta); Prexene†; SlimLinea†; ***Spain:*** Diurinat; Genurat; Natusor Artilane; Natusor High Blood Pressure; Natusor Renal; Renusor; Tensiben; ***Switz.:*** Nephrosolid; Phytomed Nephro; Tisane Diuretique; Tisane pour le coeur et la circulation; Tisane pour les reins et la vessie; Urinex; ***UK:*** Massage Balm with Calendula.

## Black Catechu

Cutch.

*CAS — 8001-76-1.*

NOTE. Distinguish from Catechu (p.1668).

**Pharmacopoeias.** In *Chin.*

### Profile

Black catechu is an extract from *Acacia catechu* (Leguminosae) that is used as an astringent.

## Black Currant

Cassis; Grosella negra (casis); Rib. Nig.; Ribes Nigrum.

**Pharmacopoeias.** *Br.* includes the fruit.
*Fr.* includes the leaf.

**BP 2003** (Black Currant). The fresh ripe fruits of *Ribes nigrum* together with their pedicels and rachides. It has a strong, characteristic odour and a pleasantly acidic taste.

### Profile

Black currant fruit is a source of vitamin C (p.1460). It is used to prepare black currant syrup, which is used as a nutritional supplement and as a flavour.

Black currant leaf is included in herbal preparations for urinary, musculoskeletal, and gastrointestinal disorders. Black currant is reported to contain bioflavonoids and is also included in preparations for vascular disorders. It has also been used as a diuretic in folk medicine.

Black currant seed oil (below) is used as a source of gamolenic acid (see p.1690).

### Preparations

***BP 2003:*** Black Currant Syrup.

**Proprietary Preparations** (details are given in Part 3)

**Multi-ingredient: *Austral.:*** Enterocare†; ***Austria:*** Amersan; ***Fr.:*** Arkophytum; Drainactil; IgE; Maxidraine; Mediflor no 11 Draineur Renal et Digestif; Mediflor Tisane Antirhumatismale No 2; Mincifit; Nigrantyl†; Santane $A_4$†; Santane $R_8$†; Veinobiase; ***Ger.:*** Cysto Fink†; Uro Fink†; Venobiase; ***Ital.:*** Allergenid†; Ribovir; ***Spain:*** Fitosvelt; Veinobiase†.

## Black Currant Seed Oil

NOTE. Black currant seed oil is derived from the seeds of *Ribes nigrum* (Grossulariaceae).

### Profile

Black currant seed oil contains gamolenic acid (p.1690) and is used similarly to evening primrose oil (p.1686).

### Preparations

**Proprietary Preparations** (details are given in Part 3)
***Austral.:*** Proglan†.

## Black Nightshade

Hierba mora; Morelle Noire.

### Profile

Black nightshade is the leaves and flowering tops of the black or garden nightshade, *Solanum nigrum* (Solanaceae). It contains solanine and its allied alkaloids. Black nightshade is distributed throughout most of the world as a weed of cultivation. It appears to have little medicinal value but was used in liniments, poultices, and decoctions for external application. Ingestion can cause typical antimuscarinic effects that may require treatment as described under Atropine, p.477.

## Blue Cohosh

Caulófilo; Caulophyllum; Papoose Root; Squaw Root.

NOTE. Distinguish from Black Cohosh, which is Cimicifuga, p.1671.

### Profile

Blue cohosh, the rhizome and roots of *Caulophyllum thalictroides* (Berberidaceae), has uterotonic and antirheumatic properties. It is used for menstrual and other gynaecological disorders.

It is also used in homoeopathic medicine.

**Adverse effects.** Acute myocardial infarction associated with profound congestive heart failure and shock has been reported in a newborn infant whose mother ingested blue cohosh to promote uterine contractions.[1]

1. Jones TK, Lawson BM. Profound neonatal congestive heart failure caused by maternal consumption of blue cohosh herbal medication. *J Pediatr* 1998; **132:** 550–2.

### Preparations

**Proprietary Preparations** (details are given in Part 3)

**Multi-ingredient: *Austral.:*** Lifesystem Herbal Formula 4 Women's Formula†; Women's Formula Herbal Formula 3†.

## Bog Myrtle

Sweet Gale.

NOTE. Bog myrtle has also been used as a common name for *Menyanthes trifoliata* (see Menyanthes, p.1712). Bayberry (see p.1659) has also been used as a synonym for bog myrtle.

### Profile

The essential oil obtained from bog myrtle, *Myrica gale* (Myricaceae), has been used as an insect repellent.

## Boldo

Boldi Folium; Boldo Leaves; Peumus.

*CAS — 476-70-0 (boldine); 1398-22-7 (boldoglucin).*

**Pharmacopoeias.** In *Eur.* (see p.vi).
*Fr.* also includes Boldine.

**Ph. Eur. 5.0** (Boldo Leaf). The whole or fragmented dried leaf of *Peumus boldus.* The whole drug contains not more than 2% v/w, and the fragmented drug not more than 1.5% v/w, of essential oil. It contains not less than 0.1% of total alkaloids, expressed as boldine ($C_{19}H_{21}NO_4$ = 327.4), calculated with reference to the anhydrous drug. It has an aromatic odour especially when rubbed. Protect from light.

### Profile

Boldo is employed in herbal medicine as a diuretic, for hepatobiliary disorders and for gastrointestinal disorders such as constipation. The alkaloid boldine is also used.

Boldo is used in homoeopathic medicine.

### Preparations

**Proprietary Preparations** (details are given in Part 3)
***Ger.:*** Cefabol†; ***Mex.:*** Bliz.

**Multi-ingredient: *Arg.:*** Bil 13; Biliosan Compuesto; Dioxicolagol; Drenocol; Hepacur; Hepatalgina; Hepatodirectol; Hepatotal Family; Herbaccion Dig Fresh; Herbaccion Digestivo; Opobyl; Palatrobil; Radicura; Trixol; ***Austral.:*** Berberis Complex†; Lexat†; ***Austria:*** St Bonifatius-Tee; ***Belg.:*** Tisane pour le Foie†; ***Braz.:*** Alcafelol; Atroveran†; Atrovex†; Bilifel†; Boldigan†; Boldo Jurubeba†; Boldobeba†; Boldopeptan; Boljuprima; Colachofra; Colinex†; Cynarobil†; Dorveran; Ductoveran; Emagrevit; Epagogo†; Eparema; Epatovis†; Espasmolex†; Figadosan†; Figatil†; Gotas Digestivas; Gotas Hepaticas†; Gotas Preciosas†; Hepatilon†; Hepato-Flux†; Hepatobyl†; Hepatophil†; Hepatoregius; Hepavirmo†; Jurubileno†; Kop Hepar†; Litrison†; Metionina Composta†; Prinachol; Solvobil; Transbil†; ***Canad.:*** Alsilax†; ***Chile:*** Hepabil; ***Fr.:*** Actisane Digestion†; Aromabyl†; Bolcitol; Boldoflorine†; Drainactil; Elixir Spark; Gastralsan†; Grains de Vals; Hepaclem; Hepax; Jecopeptol; Mediflor no 11 Draineur Renal et Digestif; Mediflor Tisane Hepatique No 5; Mucinum a l'Extrait de Cascara; Mucinum†; Neo-Boldolaxine†; Opobyl; Oxyboldine; Petites Pilules Carters; Romarinex-Choline†; Santane $C_6$†; Santane $F_{10}$†; Solution Stago Diluee; Tisane des Familles†; Tisane Hepatique de Hoerdt; Tisane Mexicaine†; Vegelax; ***Ger.:*** Cholapret†; Cynarzym N; Gallemolan G; Hepatofalk Neu†; Heumann Leber- und Gallentee Solu-Hepar S; Hevert-Gall S†; ***Hong Kong:*** Mucinum Cascara; ***Ital.:*** Amaro Medicinale; Boldina He; Caramelle alle Erbe Digestive; Certobil†; Coladren; Colax; Confetti Lassativi CM; Critichol; Digelax; Dis-Cinil Complex; Eparema; Eparema-Levul; Eupatol; Fitodorf Rabarbaro†; Florerbe Lassativa†; Frangulina; Hepasil Composto†; Hepatos; Hepatos B12; Magisbile; Mepalax; Raboldo†; Schias-Amaro Medicinale; Sintobil†; Solvobil; Tisana Arnaldi†; Vegebyl†; ***Mex.:*** Chofabol; Ifuchol; ***Port.:*** Solucao Stago†; ***Spain:*** Boldolaxin; Boldosal†; Menabil Complex; Natusor Hepavesical; Nico Hepatocyn; Odisor; Opobyl; Resolutivo Regium; Sambil†; Solucion Schoum; ***Switz.:*** Boldocynara; Boldoflorine†; Dragees pour reins et vessie S†; Grains de Vals†; Laxativum Nouvelle Formule†; Opobyl†; Stago†; The Franklin†; Tisane hepatique et biliaire; ***UK:*** Adios; Boldex; Boldo†; HealthAid Boldo-Plus; Weight Loss Aid.

## Boneset

Eupatorium perfoliatum; Feverwort; Thoroughwort.

NOTE. Boneset has also been used as a common name for *Symphytum officinale* (see Comfrey, p.1675).

### Profile

Boneset, the aerial parts of *Eupatorium perfoliatum* (Compositae), has diaphoretic and immunostimulant properties and has been used in the treatment of fever, influenza, the common cold, and other upper respiratory-tract disorders.

It is also used in homoeopathic medicine.

◊ References.

1. Habtemariam S, Macpherson AM. Cytotoxicity and antibacterial activity of ethanol extract from leaves of a herbal drug, boneset (Eupatorium perfoliatum). *Phytother Res* 2000; **14:** 575–7.

### Preparations

**Proprietary Preparations** (details are given in Part 3)

**Multi-ingredient: *Austral.:*** Flavons†; ***UK:*** Catarrh Mixture.

## Borage

Borraja; Bourrache.

**Pharmacopoeias.** *Fr.* includes monographs for flowers and flowering tops.

### Profile

The aerial parts of borage *Borago officinalis* (Boraginaceae), have been used in herbal medicine as a demulcent and emollient. However, it contains pyrrolizidine alkaloids that may be toxic and internal use is not recommended.

Borage seeds are the source of borage oil (below), which is used as a source of gamolenic acid.

### Preparations

**Proprietary Preparations** (details are given in Part 3)
***Chile:*** Dexol.

**Multi-ingredient: *Fr.:*** Tisanes de l'Abbe Hamon no 15†; ***Mex.:*** Aveendix; ***NZ:*** Mr Nits.

## Borage Oil

Borraja, aceite de; Starflower Oil.

**Description.** Borage oil is derived from the seeds of borage (*Borago officinalis,* Boraginaceae).

### Profile

Borage oil is a source of essential fatty acids, principally gamolenic acid (p.1690). It is included in dietary supplements, often in combination with fish oils or other sources of omega-3 triglycerides (see p.976).

**Eczema.** For the effects of borage oil on eczema, see under Gamolenic Acid, p.1690.

**Rheumatoid arthritis.** For the use of borage oil as a source of gamolenic acid for the management of rheumatoid arthritis, see p.1690.

### Preparations

**Proprietary Preparations** (details are given in Part 3)
***Canad.:*** Boracelle†; ***Fr.:*** Gamatol; Omegaline; ***Ital.:*** Gammavit†; ***Switz.:*** Glandol†; ***UK:*** Boracelle†; Floresse; Super Galanol†.

**Multi-ingredient: *Braz.:*** Emoderm†; ***Canad.:*** GLA-130†; Primanol-Borage; ***Fr.:*** Elteans; Phytophanere; Pruriced; Topialyse; ***Ital.:*** Topialyse; ***Port.:*** Antiestrias; Bioclin Sebo Care; Hidratante VV; Nutraisdin; Rilastil Dermo Solar; Ureadin Facial; ***UK:*** Epopa†; Galanol Gold†; Galmarin†; Gamma Marine†; Naudicelle Forte†; Super GammaOil Marine†.

## Borax

Bórax; Disodium Tetraborate; E285; Natrii Tetraboras; Natrium Boricum; Purified Borax; Sodium Biborate; Sodium Borate; Sodium Pyroborate; Sodium Tetraborate.

$Na_2B_4O_7,10H_2O$ = 381.4.

*CAS — 1330-43-4 (anhydrous borax); 61028-24-8 (anhydrous borax); 1303-96-4 (borax decahydrate).*
*ATC — S01AX07.*

**Pharmacopoeias.** In *Chin., Eur.* (see p.vi), *Jpn,* and *Pol.* Also in *USNF.*

**Ph. Eur. 5.0** (Borax). Colourless crystals or crystalline masses, or white crystalline powder. It effloresces. Soluble in water; very soluble in boiling water; freely soluble in glycerol. A 4% solution in water has a pH of 9.0 to 9.6.

The BP 2003 gives Sodium Borate and Sodium Tetraborate as official synonyms.

**USNF 22** (Sodium Borate). Odourless transparent colourless crystals or white crystalline powder. Its solutions are alkaline to phenolphthalein. It effloresces in warm dry air. Soluble 1 in 16 of water, 1 in 1 of boiling water, and 1 in 1 of glycerol; insoluble in alcohol. Store in airtight containers.

## Boric Acid

Ácido bórico; Acidum Boricum; Boracic Acid; Borsäure; E284; Orthoboric Acid; Sal Sedativa de Homberg.

$H_3BO_3$ = 61.83.

*CAS — 10043-35-3.*

*ATC — S02AA03.*

**Pharmacopoeias.** In *Chin., Eur.* (see p.vi), *Jpn, Pol.,* and *Viet.* Also in *USNF.*

**Ph. Eur. 5.0** (Boric Acid). Colourless shiny plates greasy to the touch, or white crystals, or white crystalline powder. Soluble in water and in alcohol; freely soluble in boiling water and in glycerol (85%). A 3.3% solution in water has a pH of 3.8 to 4.8.

**USNF 22** (Boric Acid). Odourless, colourless, somewhat pearly lustrous scales, or crystals, or white powder, slightly unctuous to the touch. Soluble 1 in 18 of water, 1 in 4 of boiling water, 1 in 18 of alcohol, 1 in 6 of boiling alcohol, and 1 in 4 of glycerol.

**Stability.** Boric acid volatilises in steam. It forms a complex with glycerol which is a stronger acid than boric acid.

### Adverse Effects, Treatment, and Precautions

The main symptoms of acute boric acid poisoning are vomiting and diarrhoea, abdominal pain, an erythematous rash involving both skin and mucous membranes, followed by desquamation, and stimulation or depression of the CNS. There may be convulsions and hyperpyrexia. There may also be renal tubular damage. Abnormal liver function and jaundice have been reported rarely. Death, resulting from circulatory collapse and shock, may occur within several days.

The slow excretion of boric acid can lead to cumulative toxicity during repeated use. Symptoms of chronic intoxication include anorexia, gastrointestinal disturbances, debility, confusion, dermatitis, menstrual disorders, anaemia, convulsions, and alopecia.

Fatalities have occurred most frequently in young children after the accidental ingestion of solutions of boric acid or after the application of boric acid powder to abraded skin. In the UK, the concentration of boric acid is limited to 5% in talcs, to 0.1% in products for oral hygiene, and to 3% in other cosmetic products. Boric-acid containing products should not be used in children under 3 years of age; preparations used for oral hygiene should not be swallowed; and topical preparations containing greater than the equivalent of 1.5% of boric acid should not be applied to peeling or irritated skin.

Deaths have resulted from absorption following lavage of body cavities with solutions of boric acid, and this practice is no longer recommended.

Inhaled boric acid and borax are pulmonary irritants.

Treatment of poisoning is symptomatic. The stomach should be emptied if the patient presents within 1 hour of ingesting a large amount of boric acid; activated charcoal is not effective. Haemodialysis may be of value in severe cases.

◊ In Great Britain pharmacists have been advised not to sell boric acid as such for use as a dusting powder (see also above). Pharmacists have also been advised not to supply Borax Glycerin or Honey of Borax, even with an appropriate warning, because of the hazards associated with the use of these preparations in infants.

### Pharmacokinetics

Boric acid is absorbed from the gastrointestinal tract, from damaged skin, from wounds, and from mucous membranes. It does not readily penetrate intact skin. About 50% of the amount absorbed is excreted in the urine within 24 hours and most of the remainder is excreted within 96 hours of ingestion.

### Uses and Administration

Boric acid possesses weak bacteriostatic and fungistatic properties; it has generally been superseded by more effective and less toxic disinfectants. It is used as a pesticide against ants and cockroaches.

Boric acid is used, usually with borax, as a buffer and antimicrobial in eye drops, and was formerly used as a soluble lubricant in solution-tablets. It is also used as a preservative for urine samples. Boric acid and borax are not used internally.

In the UK, the use of boric acid in cosmetics and toiletries is restricted (see above).

Borax is used similarly to boric acid and has also been used externally as a mild astringent and as an emulsifier in creams. Preparations of borax in glycerol or in honey (Borax Glycerin; Honey of Borax) were formerly used as paints for the throat, tongue, and mouth, but should not be used because of the risk of toxicity.

Other salts of boric acid, including potassium and zinc salts, have been used.

A preparation of borax is used in homoeopathic medicine.

**Antimicrobial activity.** Evaluation of the antimicrobial activity of 1.22% borate buffer.[1]

1. Houlsby RD, *et al.* Antimicrobial activity of borate-buffered solutions. *Antimicrob Agents Chemother* 1986; **29:** 803–6.

**Urine preservation.** Boric acid in concentrations of about 2% may be a suitable preservative for urine samples in transit requiring bacteriological examination.[1,2] However, overnight storage of specimens preserved with boric acid may significantly alter culture results.[3]

1. Porter IA, Brodie J. Boric acid preservation of urine samples. *BMJ* 1969; **2:** 353–5.
2. Lum KT, Meers PD. Boric acid converts urine into an effective bacteriostatic transport medium. *J Infect* 1989; **18:** 51–8.
3. Gillespie T, *et al.* The effect of specimen processing delay on borate urine preservation. *J Clin Pathol* 1999; **52:** 95–8.

**Vaginitis.** Vaginal candidiasis (p.386) caused by *Candida glabrata* and other non-*albicans* species frequently responds to topical boric acid.[1,2] Satisfactory clinical and mycological responses to topical boric acid were reported in 2 patients with *Candida glabrata* vaginitis who had not responded to repeated courses of azole antifungals.[3] Treatment with boric acid effected clinical and mycological cure in 4 of 6 patients with refractory vaginitis caused by *C. krusei.*[4] Long-term boric acid treatment showed promise in the treatment and prevention of relapses of vulvovaginal candidiasis, but its efficacy ended when treatment was stopped.[5]

1. Sobel JD, Chaim W. Treatment of Torulopsis glabrata vaginitis: retrospective review of boric acid therapy. *Clin Infect Dis* 1997; **24:** 649–52.
2. Rex JH, *et al.* Infectious Diseases Society of America. Practice guidelines for the treatment of candidiasis. *Clin Infect Dis* 2000; **30:** 662–78.
3. Redondo-Lopez V, *et al.* Torulopsis glabrata vaginitis: clinical aspects and susceptibility of antifungal agents. *Obstet Gynecol* 1990; **76:** 651–5.
4. Singh S, *et al.* Vaginitis due to Candida krusei: epidemiology, clinical aspects, and therapy. *Clin Infect Dis* 2002; **35:** 1066–70.
5. Guaschino S, *et al.* Efficacy of maintenance therapy with topical boric acid in comparison with oral itraconazole in the treatment of recurrent vulvovaginal candidiasis. *Am J Obstet Gynecol* 2001; **184:** 598–602.

### Preparations

***BP 2003:*** Kaolin Poultice;
***BPC 1973:*** Magenta Paint; Surgical Chlorinated Soda Solution;
***USP 27:*** Rose Water Ointment.

**Proprietary Preparations** (details are given in Part 3)
***Canad.:*** Eye Wash†; RO-Eyewash†; ***Fr.:*** Hydralin; ***Port.:*** Onycho Phytex†.

**Multi-ingredient:** ***Arg.:*** Banoftal; Fungocop; Gineseptina; Griseoplus; Hipoglos Cicatrizante; Hipoglos con Hidrocortisona; Histidanol; Irigal; Lagrimas de Santa Lucia; Parencias; Perfungol; Phylarm; Plusderm; Prurisedan; ***Austral.:*** Floraquin†; Gold Cross BOZ Ointment; ***Austria:*** Coldophthal; Ophtaguttal; Polyrinse-Augenelement†; ***Belg.:*** Alcasol; Amazyl†; Baseler Haussalbe†; Boradrine†; Borostyrol†; Osmoleine†; ***Braz.:*** Adeglos†; Albicon; Antimic†; Antiphlogistine; Bluderm; Boralina†; Borato de Sodio†; Cloraseptic; Colpagex N; Dermobion†; Dermosed†; Dinill; Efederm†; Forsalil†; Fungol†; Gynaseptol†; Gynax-N; Gyrol†; Hipodermon; Lavolho†; Leucocida; Lisofenicol†; Lisoquinol†; Lucretin; Malvona; Novaboin†; Oto-Biotic; Oturga; Po Antisseptico; Polvilho Antisseptico; Pomada Blumen†; Pomaderme; Pomaglos Pomada†; Senophile; Talco Alivio; Topo Worth†; Vagitrin-N; Verlin†; Visiplex; Visogenol†; Visual; Vitacolor†; ***Canad.:*** British Army Foot Powder; Eye Eze†; Ingrown Toe Nail Salve†; Thunas Eye Drops; ***Chile:*** Frescansol; Hipoglos; Homeoplasmina; Perfungol; ***Fin.:*** Otiborin; ***Fr.:*** Antiseptique-Calmante†; Boroclarine; Borostyrol; Dacryoboraline; Dacryoserum; Dacudoses; Dragee Vauban†; Eau Precieuse; Genola†; Gynescal†; Homeoplasmine; Hydralin; Ophtalmine; Paps; Pate a l'Eau Roche-Posay; Phylarm; Sophtal; ***Ger.:*** Ensinger Schiller-Quelle Heilwasser; Ophtopur-N†; ***Gr.:*** Septobore; ***Hong Kong:*** Eye Mo 36†; Eye Mo†; Hydralin; ***India:*** Andre; New Eye Lotion; Proto-Boric; ***Irl.:*** Phytex; ***Israel:*** Gargol; ***Ital.:*** Aquasalina; Bagno Oculare; Boma; Borossigeno Plus Stomatologico†; Fotofil; Fucsina Fenica; ***Mex.:*** Forcremol; Hipoglos Plus; ***Mon.:*** Glyco-Thymoline; ***S.Afr.:*** Anugesic; Anusol-HC†; Universal Eye Drops†; Vagarsol; ***Singapore:*** Buffelin†; Eye Mo; New Daigaku; ***Spain:*** Acnosan†; Banoftal; Boradren†; Cloram Hemidexa; Cloroboral†; Coliriocilina Adren Astr; Dermomycose Liquido; Euboral; Fungusol; Lamnotyl; Milrosina; Natusan; Oftalmol Dexa†; Oftalmol Ocular; Pomada Infantil Vera; Talquissar†; Topico Denticion Vera; Vaselina Boricada; Zolina; ***Swed.:*** Antasten-Privin; ***Switz.:*** Chibro-Boraline†; ***Thai.:*** Eye Mo; Eye-Gene; Eye-Gene Soft; Floraquin†; Mano; Opplin; Opsil; Optal; Quinradon-N; Quinradon†; Visotone; ***UK:*** Oxy Clean Facial Scrub; Phytex; ***USA:*** BFI; Castaderm; Collyrium for Fresh Eyes; Columbia Antiseptic Powder; Dri/Ear; Ear-Dry; Phylorinol; RA Lotion; Saratoga; Seale's Lotion; Star-Otic; Succus Cineraria Maritima; Trimo-San.

---

## Bornyl Acetate *(USAN)*

Borneol Acetate; Bornilo, acetato de. 1,7,7-Trimethylbicyclo[2.2.1]heptan-2-ol acetate.

$C_{12}H_{20}O_2$ = 196.3.

*CAS — 76-49-3.*

### Profile

Bornyl acetate is a constituent of some essential oils. It has been used in aromatic preparations in the treatment of coughs, other respiratory-tract disorders, and musculoskeletal and joint disorders.

### Preparations

**Proprietary Preparations** (details are given in Part 3)

**Multi-ingredient:** ***Arg.:*** Jabonacid; ***Chile:*** Expanden; ***Ger.:*** Lindofluid N; ***Hong Kong:*** Vapex†; ***Singapore:*** Vapex†.

---

## Bromelains *(BAN, USAN, rINN)*

Bromelaína; Bromelins; Plant Protease Concentrate.

*CAS — 9001-00-7.*

*ATC — B06AA11.*

### Units

One Rorer unit of protease activity has been defined as that amount of enzyme which hydrolyses a standardised casein substrate at pH 7 and 25° so as to cause an increase in absorbance of 0.00001 per minute at 280 nm. FIP units are also defined in terms of rate of hydrolysis of bromelain activity of a casein preparation under standard conditions.

Activity has also been described in terms of milk-clotting units.

### Adverse Effects

Bromelains may cause nausea, vomiting, and diarrhoea. Metrorrhagia and menorrhagia have occasionally occurred. Hypersensitivity reactions have been reported and have included skin reactions and asthma.

**Effects on the respiratory system.** Bronchial asthma was experienced by 2 patients after exposure to bromelains.[1] Of 6 workers sensitised to papain, 5 showed positive skin tests to bromelains and 2 of them also showed immediate asthmatic reactions after bronchial challenge with bromelains.[2]

1. Galleguillos F, Rodriguez JC. Asthma caused by bromelin inhalation. *Clin Allergy* 1978; **8:** 21–4.
2. Baur X, Fruhmann G. Allergic reactions, including asthma, to the pineapple protease bromelain following occupational exposure. *Clin Allergy* 1979; **9:** 443–50.

### Precautions

Bromelains should be given with care to patients with coagulation disorders or with severe hepatic or renal impairment.

### Uses and Administration

Bromelains are a concentrate of proteolytic enzymes derived from the pineapple plant, *Ananas comosus* (=*A. sativus*) (Bromeliaceae). They are used as an adjunct in the treatment of soft-tissue inflammation and oedema associated with trauma and surgery. Bromelains have also been given as an aid to digestion, and used in the treatment of partial deep dermal and full thickness burns.

◊ References.

1. Kane S, Goldberg MJ. Use of bromelain for mild ulcerative colitis. *Ann Intern Med* 2000; **132:** 680.
2. Maurer HR. Bromelain: biochemistry, pharmacology and medical use. *Cell Mol Life Sci* 2001; **58:** 1234–45.

### Preparations

**Proprietary Preparations** (details are given in Part 3)
***Chile:*** Ananase Forte; ***Fr.:*** Extranase; ***Ger.:*** Mucozym; Proteozym; Traumanase; ***Hong Kong:*** Ananase†; ***Ital.:*** Ananase; ***Port.:*** Ananase; ***S.Afr.:*** Ananase†; ***Switz.:*** Traumanase.

**Multi-ingredient:** ***Arg.:*** Phlogenzym; ***Austral.:*** Bio-Disc†; Bioglan Discone†; Digestaid†; Digestive Aid†; Natures Own Digestive Enzymes†; Prost-1†; Prozyme†; ***Austria:*** Arca-Enzym; Nutrizym†; Phlogenzym; Wobenzym; ***Braz.:*** Bromelin; Expectoral; Labfcilina†; Monocetin†; Nutrizim; Phlogenzym†; Plasil Enzimatico; Reumat†; Sintozima; Vonil Enzimatico†; ***Ger.:*** Enzym-Wied; Mulsal N; Phlogenzym; Wobenzym N; ***India:*** Merckenzyme; ***Ital.:*** Bres; Derinase Plus†; Flogovis IdroGel; Inflamase IdroGel; ***Mex.:*** Phlogenzym; Plasil Enzimatico; Wobenzym; ***Port.:*** Bioregime SlimKit; Nutrizym†; ***Spain:*** Bequipecto†; Flebo Stop†; ***UK:*** BackOsamine; Cardeymin†; Digezyme†; Enzyme Digest.

---

## Bromides

Bromuros.

*ATC — N05CM11.*

**Pharmacopoeias.** *Eur.* (see p.vi), *Jpn, Pol.,* and *Viet.* include standards for Potassium Bromide and Sodium Bromide. Ammonium Bromide is in *Eur.* and *Pol.*

### Adverse Effects and Precautions

During prolonged exposure bromide accumulation may occur giving rise to bromide intoxication or bromism. Symptoms include nausea and vomiting, slurred speech, memory impairment, drowsiness, irritability, ataxia, tremors, hallucinations, mania, delirium, psychoses, stupor, coma, and other manifestations of CNS depression. Skin rashes of various types may occur and toxic epidermal necrolysis has been reported. Death after acute poisoning appears to be rare as vomiting follows the ingestion of large doses.

There have been reports of neonatal bromide intoxication and growth defects associated with maternal bromide ingestion during pregnancy.

**Breast feeding.** The American Academy of Pediatrics[1] considers that intake of bromides is usually compatible with breast feeding, although rashes, weakness, and absence of crying have been reported in the infant following maternal intake. Exposure to bromides in photographic laboratories may also result in potential absorption and transfer into breast milk.

1. American Academy of Pediatrics. The transfer of drugs and other chemicals into human milk. *Pediatrics* 2001; **108:** 776–89. Correction. *ibid.*; 1029. Also available at: http://aappolicy.aappublications.org/cgi/content/full/pediatrics%3b108/3/776 (accessed 05/07/04)

### Treatment of Adverse Effects

In acute poisoning, the stomach should be emptied (if emesis has not already occurred), and sodium chloride should be given by intravenous infusion. Glucose may also be administered and furosemide may be given to aid diuresis.

In chronic poisoning, bromide administration is stopped and sodium chloride is given intravenously or by mouth with adequate amounts of fluid. Ammonium chloride has been given but is no longer recommended as it may precipitate metabolic acidosis. Diuretics are of value. In severe cases of bromide intoxication or when the usual treatments cannot be used, haemodialysis may be of benefit.

### Pharmacokinetics

Bromides are readily absorbed from the gastrointestinal tract. They displace chloride in extracellular body fluids and have a half-life in the body of about 12 days. They may be detected in the milk of nursing mothers and in the fetus.

### Uses and Administration

Bromides depress the CNS. Calcium, potassium, and sodium bromide have been used as sedatives and anticonvulsants, but have generally been replaced by more effective, less toxic drugs. Ammonium and strontium bromide have been used similarly, as have bromoform and dilute hydrobromic acid. Bromides have also been used in multi-ingredient preparations for the treatment of coughs.

Bromides have been used in homoeopathic medicine.

### Preparations

**Proprietary Preparations** (details are given in Part 3)
***Ger.:*** Dibro-Be Mono.

**Multi-ingredient:** ***Belg.:*** Babygencal†; Normogastryl†; ***Braz.:*** Alergitrat†; Bromidrastina†; Bromosedan†; Broncotussan†; Frenotosse; Gotas Nican; Limao Bravo†; Naquinto†; Tossefedrin†; Uterovarol†; Xarope de Caraguata; Xarope Peitoral de Ameixa Composto; Xarope Sao Joao; Xpe SPC; ***Chile:*** Gotas Nican; Gruben; Ramistos; ***Fr.:*** Dinacode; Galirene; Neurocalcium†; Pectosan†; Sedatif Tiber; Sirop Pectoral adulte†; Sirop Pectoral enfant†; Sirop Teyssedre†; ***Ital.:*** Fertomcidina-U; Neo Soluzione Sulfo Balsamica†; ***Port.:*** Lactucol†; ***S.Afr.:*** Bronchicum; ***Spain:*** Medecitral†; Stomosan†; Topico Denticion Vera.

## Bromine

Bromo; Bromum.

$Br_2$ = 159.808.
*CAS — 7726-95-6.*

**Description.** Bromine is a dark reddish-brown, heavy, mobile liquid which gives off intensely irritating brown fumes.

### Adverse Effects

Bromine is intensely irritating and corrosive to eyes and mucous membranes; it may cause severe gastro-enteritis if swallowed. Contact with the skin can produce severe burns, and inhalation of the vapour causes violent irritation of the respiratory tract and pulmonary oedema.

### Treatment of Adverse Effects

Milk or antacids should be given as soon as possible following ingestion of bromine. Gastric lavage is not recommended. If bromine vapour has been inhaled, oxygen should be administered and assisted ventilation may be necessary. The use of prophylactic corticosteroids for laryngeal and pulmonary oedema is controversial. Splashes on the skin and eyes should be immediately washed off; washing under running water should continue for at least 15 minutes.

### Uses and Administration

Bromine is widely used in industry. It was formerly used, in the form of an adduct with a quaternary ammonium compound, in the treatment of plantar warts.

## Bryonia

Bryony; Nueza.

### Profile

Bryonia, root of *Bryonia alba* or *B. dioica* (Cucurbitaceae), is an ingredient of preparations that have been used in respiratory-tract infections and inflammatory disorders. Toxic symptoms and fatalities have been reported following ingestion of the berries.

Bryonia is also used in homoeopathic medicine.

### Preparations

**Proprietary Preparations** (details are given in Part 3)

**Multi-ingredient:** ***Austral.:*** Cough Relief†; Harpagophytum Complex†; Joint & Muscle Relief Cream†; Respatona Decongestant Formula†; Respatona Plus Bronchial Cough Relief†; ***Fr.:*** Homeoplasmine.

## Buchu

Bucco; Buchú; Buchu Leaves; Diosma; Folia Bucco.

**Pharmacopoeias.** In *Fr.*

### Profile

Buchu, the dried leaves of 'short' or 'round' buchu, *Agathosma betulina* (*Barosma betulina*) (Rutaceae), is a weak diuretic and urinary antiseptic that has been used in multi-ingredient preparations for the treatment of urinary-tract disorders. Oval or long buchu, the leaves of *Agathosma crenulata* (*B.crenulata*), has also been used.

Buchu has been used in homoeopathic medicine.

### Preparations

**Proprietary Preparations** (details are given in Part 3)

**Multi-ingredient:** ***Arg.:*** Water Pill c Potasio; ***Austral.:*** Althaea Complex†; Bioglan Cranbiotic Super†; Cranberry Complex†; De Witts New Pills†; Extralife Uri-Care†; Fluid Loss†; Medinat PMT-Eze†; PMS Support†; Serenoa Complex†; Urinase†; Uva-Ursi Complex†; ***Canad.:*** Herbal Laxative; ***Fr.:*** Urophytum; ***Ger.:*** Hevert-Entwasserungs-Tee†; ***NZ:*** De Witts Pills; ***Port.:*** Solucao Stago†; ***S.Afr.:*** Docrub; ***Switz.:*** Urinex; ***UK:*** Antitis; Backache; Backache Relief; De Witt's K & B Pills; Diuretabs; Gerard House Buchu Compound†; HRI Water Balance; Kas-Bah; Skin Eruptions Mixture; Watershed.

## Bucillamine *(rINN)*

Bucilamina; DE-019; SA-96; Tiobutarit. *N*-(2-Mercapto-2-methylpropionyl)-L-cysteine.

$C_7H_{13}NO_3S_2$ = 223.3.
*CAS — 65002-17-7.*
*ATC — M01CC02.*

### Profile

Bucillamine is structurally related to penicillamine (p.1046) and is reported to be an immunomodulator.

◊ Bucillamine has been used in rheumatoid arthritis.[1] It has been implicated in the development of skin[2] and kidney[3] disorders.


1. Kim HA, Song YW. A comparison between bucillamine and D-penicillamine in the treatment of rheumatoid arthritis. *Rheumatol Int* 1997; **17:** 5–9.
2. Ogata K, *et al.* Drug-induced pemphigus foliaceus with features of pemphigus vulgaris. *Br J Dermatol* 2001; **144:** 421–2.
3. Nagahama K, *et al.* Bucillamine induces membranous glomerulonephritis. *Am J Kidney Dis* 2002; **39:** 706–12.


## Bucladesine Sodium *(rINNM)*

Bucladesina sódica; DBcAMP (bucladesine); Dibutyryl Cyclic AMP Sodium; DT-5621 (bucladesine). *N*-(9-β-D-Ribofuranosyl-9*H*-purin-6-yl)butyramide cyclic 3′,5′-(hydrogen phosphate) 2′-butyrate sodium.

$C_{18}H_{24}N_5O_8PNa$ = 492.4.
*CAS — 362-74-3 (bucladesine); 16980-89-5 (bucladesine sodium).*
*ATC — C01CE04.*

### Profile

Bucladesine sodium has been reported to have cardiotonic properties when given intravenously. It has been applied topically for the treatment of bedsores.

## Bufotenine

Bufotenina; *NN*-Dimethylserotonin; 5-Hydroxy-*NN*-dimethyltryptamine; Mappine. 3-(2-Dimethylaminoethyl)indol-5-ol.

$C_{12}H_{16}N_2O$ = 204.3.
*CAS — 487-93-4.*

### Profile

Bufotenine is an indole alkaloid obtained from the seeds and leaves of *Piptadenia peregrina*, from which the hallucinogenic snuff cohoba is prepared, and *P. macrocarpa* (Mimosaceae). It was first isolated from the skin glands of toads (*Bufo* spp.) and has also been isolated from species of *Amanita* (Agaricaceae). Bufotenine has serotonergic activity and is reported to have hallucinogenic properties. It has no therapeutic use.

## Buphenine Hydrochloride *(BANM)*

Hidrocloruro de bufenina; Nylidrin Hydrochloride; Nylidrinium Chloride. 1-(4-Hydroxyphenyl)-2-(1-methyl-3-phenylpropylamino)propan-1-ol hydrochloride.

$C_{19}H_{25}NO_2,HCl$ = 335.9.
*CAS — 447-41-6 (buphenine); 849-55-8 (buphenine hydrochloride).*
*ATC — C04AA02; G02CA02.*

### Adverse Effects and Precautions

For the adverse effects of sympathomimetics in general and precautions for their use, see under Adrenaline, p.852.

### Uses and Administration

Buphenine produces peripheral vasodilatation through beta-adrenoceptor stimulation and a direct action on the arteries and arterioles of the skeletal muscles.

Buphenine has been used in the treatment of peripheral vascular and cerebrovascular disease. It has also been used in preparations for rhinitis and nasal congestion. Doses of buphenine hydrochloride in the range of 3 to 12 mg by mouth three or four times daily have been given, although total daily doses of up to 90 mg have been used.

An intravenous infusion of buphenine hydrochloride has been used to arrest premature labour. It has also been given orally as a prophylactic tocolytic agent.

### Preparations

**Proprietary Preparations** (details are given in Part 3)
***Austria:*** Dilatol; Dilydrin†; ***Canad.:*** Arlidin; ***India:*** Arlidin; ***Mex.:*** Arlidin; Flumil; Nilken†; ***Spain:*** Diatolil†; ***Switz.:*** Dilydrine Retard†; Tocodrine.

**Multi-ingredient:** ***Austria:*** Apoplectal†; Arbid; Dilaescol; Dilatol-Chinin; Opino; Tropoderm; ***Fr.:*** Ophtadil; Phlebogel; ***Ger.:*** Apoplectal N; opino N spezial; ***Spain:*** Circovenil Fuerte†; Circovenil†; ***Switz.:*** Arbid; Visaline.

## Burnet

Garden Burnet; Greater Burnet; Pimpinela mayor; Sanguisorba.

**Pharmacopoeias.** In *Chin.*

### Profile

Burnet, the aerial parts and roots of *Sanguisorba officinalis* (*Poterium officinalis*) (Rosaceae), has antihaemorrhagic and astringent properties. It has been used internally to treat menorrhagia and gastrointestinal disorders and is also used topically for eczema, burns, and other skin disorders.

It is also used in homoeopathic medicine.

Burnet is also used as an animal fodder and salad vegetable, and as an ingredient in beer making.

### Preparations

**Proprietary Preparations** (details are given in Part 3)
**Multi-ingredient:** ***Canad.:*** Swiss Herb Cough Drops.

## Butinoline Phosphate *(rINNM)*

Fosfato de butinolina. 1,1-Diphenyl-4-pyrrolidino-1′-yl but-2-yn-1-ol phosphate.

$C_{20}H_{21}NO,H_3PO_4$ = 389.4.
*CAS — 968-63-8 (butinoline); 54118-66-0 (butinoline phosphate).*

### Profile

Butinoline phosphate is used as an antispasmodic in preparations for gastrointestinal disorders.

### Preparations

**Proprietary Preparations** (details are given in Part 3)

**Multi-ingredient:** ***Austria:*** Spasmo-Solugastril; ***Ger.:*** Jasicholin N†; Spasmo-Nervogastrol; Spasmo-Solugastril.

## Butterbur

### Profile

The leaves and roots of butterbur, *Petasites hybridus* (*P. officinalis*) (Asteraceae), have antispasmodic and anti-inflammatory properties and have been used in herbal preparations for a variety of disorders, including gastrointestinal and respiratory-tract disorders, and migraine.

◊ References.


1. Schapowal A. Randomised controlled trial of butterbur and cetirizine for treating seasonal allergic rhinitis. *BMJ* 2002; **324:** 144–6.
2. Lee DK, *et al.* Butterbur, a herbal remedy, attenuates adenosine monophosphate induced nasal responsiveness in seasonal allergic rhinitis. *Clin Exp Allergy* 2003; **33:** 882–6.
3. Diener HC, *et al.* The first placebo-controlled trial of a special butterbur root extract for the prevention of migraine: reanalysis of efficacy criteria. *Eur Neurol* 2004; **51:** 89–97.
4. Jackson CM, *et al.* The effects of butterbur on the histamine and allergen cutaneous response. *Ann Allergy Asthma Immunol* 2004; **92:** 250–4.


### Preparations

**Proprietary Preparations** (details are given in Part 3)
***Ger.:*** Petadolex; Petaforce V; ***Switz.:*** Petadolor.

**Multi-ingredient:** ***Ger.:*** Pulmonium N†; ***Switz.:*** Dragees aux figues avec du sene; Dragees pour la detente nerveuse; Relax; Valverde Dragees laxatives; Valverde Dragees pour la detente.

## Butyl Nitrite

Nitrito de butilo.

$C_4H_9NO_2$ = 103.1.

### Profile

Butyl nitrite is not used medicinally but, as with other volatile nitrites, is abused for its vasodilating and related effects following inhalation (see Abuse, under Amyl Nitrite, p.1032).

## Cadmium

Cadmio.

Cd = 112.411.
*CAS — 7440-43-9.*

### Profile

Cadmium is used in a wide range of manufacturing processes and cadmium poisoning presents a recognised industrial hazard. Inhalation of cadmium fumes during welding procedures may not produce symptoms until 12 to 36 hours have passed and these symptoms include respiratory distress leading to pulmonary oedema; kidney toxicity is also a feature of acute cadmium poisoning. Ingestion of cadmium or its salts has the additional hazard of severe gastrointestinal effects. Cadmium has a long biological half-life and accumulates in body tissues, particularly the liver and kidneys. Chelation therapy is not generally recommended for cadmium poisoning, although sodium calcium edetate has been used following acute ingestion. However, chelators do not increase cadmium elimination in chronic poisoning and use of dimercaprol may increase cadmium toxicity and should be avoided. Chronic exposure to cadmium results in progressive renal impairment and other effects (see below).

Cadmium sulfide has been used topically in some countries for the treatment of skin and scalp conditions. Cadmium sulfate has been included in some preparations for the treatment of eye irritation.

**Adverse effects.** The toxicity of cadmium has been reviewed.[1] Environmental or occupational exposure to cadmium has been associated with renal dysfunction,[2-5] although this may be reversible if exposure is reduced.[6] A reduction in bone density may also occur.[7] Fatalities due to industrial exposure or self-poisoning have also been reported.[8,9] No effect on testicular endocrine function was observed in 77 industrial workers exposed to cadmium.[3]

An increased incidence of cancer of the prostate has been reported in subjects exposed to high levels of cadmium but the evidence is not conclusive.[10] There may be an association between cadmium exposure and lung cancer, although observations on this type of cancer are difficult to interpret because of exposure to other hazards such as smoking.


1. Fielder RJ, Dale EA. Cadmium and its compounds. *Toxicity Review 7*. London: HMSO, 1983.
2. Buchet JP, *et al.* Renal effects of cadmium body burden of the general population. *Lancet* 1990; **336:** 699–702. Correction. *ibid.* 1991; **337:** 1554.
3. Mason HJ. Occupational cadmium exposure and testicular endocrine function. *Hum Exp Toxicol* 1990; **9:** 91–4.
4. Cai S, *et al.* Renal dysfunction from cadmium contamination of irrigation water: dose-response analysis in a Chinese population. *Bull WHO* 1998; **76:** 153–9.
5. Satarug S, *et al.* Safe levels of cadmium intake to prevent renal toxicity in human subjects. *Br J Nutr* 2000; **84:** 791–802.
6. Hotz P, *et al.* Renal effects of low-level environmental cadmium exposure: 5-year follow-up of a subcohort from the Cadmibel study. *Lancet* 1999; **354:** 1508–13.
7. Staessen JA, *et al.* Environmental exposure to cadmium, forearm bone density, and risk of fractures: prospective population study. *Lancet* 1999; **353:** 1140–44.
8. Taylor A, *et al.* Poisoning with cadmium fumes after smelting lead. *BMJ* 1984; **288:** 1270–1.
9. Buckler HM, *et al.* Self poisoning with oral cadmium chloride. *BMJ* 1986; **292:** 1559–60. Correction. *ibid.*; **293:** 236.
10. Bell GM. Carcinogenicity of cadmium and its compounds. *Toxicity Review 24*. London: HMSO, 1991.


### Preparations

**Proprietary Preparations** (details are given in Part 3)
***Spain:*** Biocadmio.

**Multi-ingredient:** ***Austria:*** Ichtho-Cadmin†; ***Fr.:*** Visiolyre†.

## Cajuput Oil

Cajeput Oil; Cajuput Essence; Cayeput, aceite esencial de; Oleum Cajuputi.

### Profile

Cajuput oil is a volatile oil obtained by distillation from the fresh leaves and twigs of *Melaleuca cajuputi* (*M. leucadendron*) (Myrtaceae). It contains cineole. Cajuput oil has been applied externally as a stimulant and mild rubefacient in rheumatism. It is also used with other volatile agents in preparations for the relief of respiratory-tract disorders and nasal congestion.

### Preparations

**Proprietary Preparations** (details are given in Part 3)

**Multi-ingredient:** ***Austral.:*** Breathe Eazy Chest Rub†; Capsolin†; Goanna Heat Cream†; Methyl Salicylate Ointment Compound†; Relief Rub†; Silver Clove Medicated Balm†; ***Austria:*** Babix; Luuf-Heilpflanzenol; Tiger Balsam Rot; ***Canad.:*** Broncho Rub†; Penetrating Rub†; Tiger Balm Red; Tiger Balm White; Youngflex Massage 168; ***Fr.:*** Phytolithe; Vegebom; ***Ger.:*** Liniplant; Olbas; Palatol; Palatol N†; ***Hong Kong:*** Vida Salirub; ***Ital.:*** Otosan Natural Ear Drops; ***Singapore:*** Begesic; ***Switz.:*** Frigoplasma; Novital; Olbas†; ***Thai.:*** Dexalin; Olympic Balm; ***UK:*** Bells Muscle Rub; Olbas; Olbas for Children; Soothol; Tiger Balm; Tiger Balm Liquid†; Vadarex.

## Calamus

Acore Vrai; Cálamo aromático; Calamus Rhizome; Kalmus; Sweet Flag Root.

*CAS — 8015-79-0 (calamus oil).*

**Pharmacopoeias.** In *Chin.* and *Swiss.*

### Profile

Calamus, the dried rhizome of the sweet flag, *Acorus calamus* (Araceae), has been used as a bitter and carminative; it is also used as a source of calamus oil which is employed in perfumery. The FDA in the USA has prohibited marketing calamus as a food or food additive; the oil (Jammu variety) is reported to be a carcinogen.

It is also used in homoeopathic preparations.

### Preparations

**Proprietary Preparations** (details are given in Part 3)

**Multi-ingredient:** ***Austria:*** Abdomilon N; Aponatura Starkungs; Aurita-Verdauungstee; Bio-Garten Tee fur Leber und Galle; Bioreform-Leber-und Galletee; Krauterpfarrer Weidinger Tee bei Vollegefuhl und Blahungen; Mag Kottas Krauterexpress-Magen-Darm-Tee; Mag Kottas Magen-und Darmtee; Sidroga Magen-Darm-Tee; ***Fr.:*** Jouvence de l'Abbe Soury; ***Ger.:*** Abdomilon N; Gastrol S; Grunlicht Hingfong Essenz†; Hevert-Gall S†; Hevert-Magen-Galle-Leber-Tee†; Majocarmin mite; Presselin Blahungs K 4 N; Stomasal Med; Stovalid N; ventri-loges N; ***Israel:*** Rekiv; ***Ital.:*** Frerichs Maldifassi; ***Port.:*** Cholagutt; ***Spain:*** Caved-S†; Roter Complex†; ***Switz.:*** Caved-S†; Kernosan Elixir; Tisane pour l'estomac; Urinex; ***UK:*** Pegina.

## Calcium Carbimide *(rINN)*

Calcium Cyanamide; Carbimida cálcica; Cyanamide.

$CCaN_2$ = 80.1.

*CAS — 156-62-7 (calcium carbimide); 8013-88-5 (citrated calcium carbimide).*

*ATC — N07BB02.*

NOTE. The name cyanamide is also used to designate carbimide, which is used in veterinary medicine.

### Adverse Effects and Precautions

Calcium carbimide may cause drowsiness, dizziness, fatigue, skin rash, tinnitus, depression, impotence, and urinary frequency. There may be a reversible increase in the white cell count. It should be used with caution in patients with asthma, coronary artery disease, or myocardial disease. Calcium carbimide causes a reaction in patients who have consumed alcohol similar to that seen with disulfiram (see p.1681).

**Effects on the heart.** Hypotension and tachycardia were reported during the carbimide-alcohol reaction.[1]


1. Peachey JE, *et al.* Cardiovascular changes during the calcium carbimide-ethanol interaction. *Clin Pharmacol Ther* 1981; **29:** 40–6.


**Effects on the liver.** Reports[1,2] of hepatic lesions in patients receiving calcium carbimide.


1. Vázquez JJ, Cervera S. Cyanamide-induced liver injury in alcoholics. *Lancet* 1980; **i:** 361–2.
2. Moreno A, *et al.* Structural hepatic changes associated with cyanamide treatment: cholangiolar proliferation, fibrosis and cirrhosis. *Liver* 1984; **4:** 15–21.


### Uses and Administration

Calcium carbimide has actions and uses similar to those of disulfiram (p.1682). It is an aversive agent used as an adjunct in the treatment of chronic alcoholism (see Alcohol Withdrawal and Abstinence, p.1166). It is given in a dose of up to 60 mg twice daily by mouth. Citrated calcium carbimide has been used similarly.

◊ References.


1. Peachey JE, *et al.* A comparative review of the pharmacological and toxicological properties of disulfiram and calcium carbimide. *J Clin Psychopharmacol* 1981; **1:** 21–6.


### Preparations

**Proprietary Preparations** (details are given in Part 3)
***Austria:*** Colme; ***Canad.:*** Temposil†; ***Irl.:*** Abstem†; ***Spain:*** Colme.

## Calcium Dihydrogen Phosphate

Acid Calcium Phosphate; Calcium Dihydrogenphosphoricum; E341; Fosfato monocálcico; Monobasic Calcium Phosphate; Monocalcium Phosphate. Calcium tetrahydrogen diorthophosphate monohydrate.

$Ca(H_2PO_4)_2,H_2O$ = 252.1.

*CAS — 7758-23-8 (anhydrous calcium dihydrogen phosphate).*

**Pharmacopoeias.** In *Jpn* and *Swiss.*

### Profile

Calcium dihydrogen phosphate is used in fertilisers. It is also used as an antoxidant in baking powders and flours and as a source of calcium in some mineral supplement preparations.

### Preparations

**Proprietary Preparations** (details are given in Part 3)

**Multi-ingredient:** ***Braz.:*** Salutina†; ***Fr.:*** Marinol; Phosphoneuros.

## Calcium Dobesilate *(rINN)*

Calcii Dobesilas; Calcium Doxybenzylate; CLS-2210; Dobesilato de calcio; 205E. Calcium 2,5-dihydroxybenzenesulphonate.

$C_{12}H_{10}CaO_{10}S_2$ = 418.4.

*CAS — 88-46-0 (dobesilic acid); 20123-80-2 (calcium dobesilate).*

*ATC — C05BX01.*

**Pharmacopoeias.** In *Eur.* (see p.vi) which specifies the monohydrate.

**Ph. Eur. 5.0** (Calcium Dobesilate Monohydrate). A white or almost white hygroscopic powder. Very soluble in water; freely soluble in dehydrated alcohol; practically insoluble in dichloromethane; very slightly soluble in isopropyl alcohol. A 10% solution in water has a pH of 4.5 to 6.0. Store in airtight containers. Protect from light.

### Profile

Calcium dobesilate is claimed to reduce capillary permeability and has been used in various peripheral circulatory disorders including diabetic retinopathy and haemorrhoids (p.1243). Gastrointestinal disturbances have occurred with its use, and there are also reports of hypersensitivity reactions.

Calcium dobesilate is given by mouth in usual doses of 0.5 to 1.5 g daily in divided doses. It is also given rectally for haemorrhoids and is an ingredient of some preparations given for various skin disorders.

◊ Reviews.


1. Tejerina T, Ruiz E. Calcium dobesilate: pharmacology and future approaches. *Gen Pharmacol* 1998; **31:** 357–60.
2. Berthet P, *et al.* Calcium dobesilate: pharmacological profile related to its use in diabetic retinopathy. *Int J Clin Pract* 1999; **53:** 631–6.


**Effects on the blood.** Agranulocytosis has been reported[1-3] in a few patients following treatment with calcium dobesilate, and in 2 cases recurred on rechallenge.[1,2]


1. Kulessa W, *et al.* Wiederholte Agranulozytose nach Einnahme von Calciumdobesilat. *Dtsch Med Wochenschr* 1992; **117:** 372–4.
2. Cladera Serra A, *et al.* Agranulocitosis inducida por dobesilato calcico. *Med Clin (Barc)* 1995; **105:** 558–9.
3. García Benayas E, *et al.* Calcium dobesilate-induced agranulocytosis. *Pharm World Sci* 1997; **19:** 251–2.


### Preparations

**Proprietary Preparations** (details are given in Part 3)
***Arg.:*** Doxium; Duflemina; Eflevar; ***Austria:*** Doxium; Vasactin; ***Belg.:*** Doxium†; ***Braz.:*** Doxium†; ***Chile:*** Doxium; ***Ger.:*** Dexium; Dobica; ***Hong Kong:*** Dobesifar; Doxium; ***Ital.:*** Doxium; ***Malaysia:*** Doxium; ***Mex.:*** Doxium; ***Mon.:*** Doxium; ***Port.:*** Doxi-Om; ***Spain:*** Doxium; ***Switz.:*** Doxium.

**Multi-ingredient:** ***Arg.:*** Vasodual; ***Austria:*** Doxiproct; Doxiproct mit Dexamethason; ***Braz.:*** Proctium†; ***Ital.:*** Doxiproct; ***Port.:*** Doxiproct; Doxivenil; ***Spain:*** Acnisdin; Acnisdin Retinoico; Ederal†; Proctium; ***Switz.:*** Doxiproct; Doxiproct Plus; Doxivenil.

## Calcium Hopantenate *(rINNM)*

Calcium Homopantothenate; Hopantenato cálcico. Calcium D-(+)-4-(2,4-dihydroxy-3,3-dimethylbutyramido)butyrate hemihydrate.

$Ca(C_{10}H_{18}NO_5)_2,\frac{1}{2}H_2O$ = 513.6.

*CAS — 18679-90-8 (hopantenic acid); 17097-76-6 (anhydrous calcium hopantenate); 1990-07-4 (calcium hopantenate hemihydrate).*

### Profile

Calcium hopantenate is a homologue of pantothenic acid (p.1442) and has been tried in the treatment of various behavioural and extrapyramidal disorders. Its use is limited by severe metabolic side-effects and fatalities have been reported.

## Calcium Hydroxide

Calcii Hydroxidum; Calcium Hydrate; E526; Hidróxido cálcico; Slaked Lime.

$Ca(OH)_2$ = 74.09.

*CAS — 1305-62-0.*

**Pharmacopoeias.** In *Eur.* (see p.vi), *Jpn, US,* and *Viet.*

**Ph. Eur. 5.0** (Calcium Hydroxide). A fine white or almost white powder. Practically insoluble in water.

**USP 27** (Calcium Hydroxide). A white powder with a slightly bitter alkaline taste. Soluble 1 in 630 of water and 1 in 1300 of boiling water; insoluble in alcohol; soluble in glycerol and in syrup. Store in airtight containers.

### Profile

Calcium hydroxide is a weak alkali. It is used in the form of Calcium Hydroxide Solution (lime water) in some skin lotions and oily preparations to form calcium soaps of fatty acids which produce water-in-oil emulsions.

Calcium hydroxide pastes are used in dentistry. A paste made from a mixture of calcium hydroxide and potassium hydroxide and known as Vienna paste was used as an escharotic. Soda lime (p.1747) is a mixture of calcium hydroxide and potassium hydroxide and/or sodium hydroxide. With sulfur, calcium hydroxide forms sulfurated lime solution (p.1158).

**Adverse effects.** A report of ocular alkali burns in children, leading to severe visual loss, caused by packets of calcium hydroxide ('Chuna') popularly consumed in India as an additive to chewing tobacco.[1]

For the use of disodium edetate in the treatment of calcium hydroxide burns of the eye, see p.1038.


1. Agarwal T, Vajpayee RB. A warning about the dangers of chuna packets. *Lancet* 2003; **361:** 2247.


### Preparations

***BP 2003:*** Calcium Hydroxide Solution;
***USP 27:*** Calcium Hydroxide Topical Solution.

**Proprietary Preparations** (details are given in Part 3)
***Austria:*** Dermi-cyl Allerg; ***Ger.:*** Dermi-cyl; ***Ital.:*** Stomidros†; ***Mex.:*** Lipocal†; Oleocal†; Oleoderm.

**Multi-ingredient:** ***Belg.:*** Oxyplastine†; ***Mex.:*** Caliderm; Liniderm; Oleoderm Plus; ***Spain:*** Cremsol; ***Switz.:*** Calcipulpe†.

## Calcium Oxide

Calcium Oxydatum; Calx; Calx Usta; Chaux Vive; E529; Gebrannter Kalk; Lime; Óxido de calcio; Quicklime.

CaO = 56.08.

*CAS — 1305-78-8.*

**Pharmacopoeias.** In *Jpn, Pol., Swiss,* and *US.*

**USP 27** (Lime). Hard, odourless, white or greyish-white masses, granules, or powder. When it is moistened with water a reaction occurs, heat being evolved and calcium hydroxide formed. Slightly soluble in water; very slightly soluble in boiling water. Store in airtight containers.

### Adverse Effects and Treatment

Calcium oxide may cause burns on contact with moist skin and mucous membranes; it is particularly irritant to the eyes. Washing or flooding of affected areas may need to be prolonged. Pneumonitis may follow inhalation.

◊ For the use of disodium edetate in the treatment of calcium oxide burns of the eye, see p.1038.

### Uses and Administration

Calcium oxide has been used in various dermatological preparations. A paste made from a mixture of calcium oxide and sodium hydroxide and known as London paste was used as an escharotic.

### Preparations

**Proprietary Preparations** (details are given in Part 3)
**Multi-ingredient:** ***Ital.:*** Oleo Calcarea.

## Calcium Saccharate *(rINN)*

Calcii Saccharas; Calcium D-Saccharate; Sacarato cálcico. Calcium D-glucarate tetrahydrate.

$C_6H_8CaO_8,4H_2O$ = 320.3.

*CAS — 5793-88-4 (anhydrous calcium saccharate); 5793-89-5 (calcium saccharate tetrahydrate).*

NOTE. The name calcium saccharate has also been used to describe saccharated lime.

**Pharmacopoeias.** In *US.*

**USP 27** (Calcium Saccharate). A white, odourless, crystalline powder. Very slightly soluble in cold water and in alcohol; slightly soluble in boiling water; practically insoluble in chloroform and in ether; soluble in dilute mineral acids and in solutions of calcium gluconate.

### Profile

Calcium saccharate is used as a stabilising agent in solutions of calcium gluconate for injection. Each g of calcium saccharate contains approximately 3.1 mmol of calcium. Calcium saccharate 8 g is approximately equivalent to 1 g of calcium.

### Preparations

**Proprietary Preparations** (details are given in Part 3)
***Austria:*** Calcium Fresenius; ***Ger.:*** Calcium Fresenius.

**Multi-ingredient:** ***Ger.:*** Calcitrans†; Calcium Braun; Calcium Truw†; Calcium Verla†; ***Switz.:*** C-Calcium.

## Calcium Sulfate

Calcii Sulfas; Calcium Sulphate; E516; Gypsum (calcium sulfate dihydrate); Sulfato cálcico.

$CaSO_4$ = 136.1.

*CAS — 7778-18-9 (anhydrous calcium sulfate); 10101-41-4 (calcium sulfate dihydrate).*

**Pharmacopoeias.** In *Chin., Eur.* (see p.vi), *Int.*, and *Jpn* which specify the dihydrate. Also in *USNF* which specifies the dihydrate or the anhydrous material.

**Ph. Eur. 5.0** (Calcium Sulfate Dihydrate). A white fine powder. Very slightly soluble in water; practically insoluble in alcohol.

**USNF 22** (Calcium Sulfate). It is anhydrous or contains two molecules of water of hydration. A white to slightly yellow-white odourless fine powder. Soluble 1 in 375 of water and 1 in 485 of boiling water; soluble in 3N hydrochloric acid.

### Profile

Calcium sulfate dihydrate is used as an excipient for the preparation of tablets or capsules.

### Preparations

**Proprietary Preparations** (details are given in Part 3)
***Austral.:*** Celloids CS 36†.

## Dried Calcium Sulfate

Calcii Sulfas Hemihydricus; Calcined Gypsum; Calcium Sulfuricum ad Usum Chirurgicum; Calcium Sulphuricum Ustum; Dried Calcium Sulphate; Exsiccated Calcium Sulphate; Gebrannter Gips; Gêsso; Gypsum Siccatum; Plaster of Paris; Plâtre Cuit; Sulfato cálcico anhidro; Sulphate of Lime; Yeso Blanco.

$CaSO_4,\frac{1}{2}H_2O$ = 145.1.

*CAS — 10034-76-1 (calcium sulfate hemihydrate); 26499-65-0 (calcium sulfate hemihydrate).*

**Pharmacopoeias.** In *Br., Chin., Ger., Jpn, Pol.,* and *Viet.*

**BP 2003** (Dried Calcium Sulphate). A white or almost white, odourless or almost odourless hygroscopic powder. It may contain suitable setting accelerators or decelerators. Slightly soluble in water; more soluble in dilute mineral acids; practically insoluble in alcohol.

The BP gives Exsiccated Calcium Sulphate and Plaster of Paris as approved synonyms.

### Profile

Dried calcium sulfate is used for the preparation of Plaster of Paris Bandage, which is used for the immobilisation of limbs and fractures. It is also employed for making dental casts and has been used as a bone graft substitute.

### Preparations

**Proprietary Preparations** (details are given in Part 3)
***Fr.:*** Biplatrix.

## Calendula

Caléndula; Calendulae Flos; Gold-bloom; Marigold; Marybud; Pot Marigold; Souci.

**Pharmacopoeias.** In *Eur.* (see p.vi) and *Pol.*

**Ph. Eur. 5.0** (Calendula Flower). It consists of the whole or cut, dried, and fully opened flowers which have been detached from the receptacle of the cultivated, double-flowered varieties of *Calendula officinalis*. It contains not less than 0.4% of flavonoids, calculated as hyperoside ($C_{21}H_{20}O_{12}$ = 464.4) calculated with reference to the dried drug. Protect from light.

### Profile

Calendula has antiseptic, anti-inflammatory, and astringent properties. It is used in external preparations for minor skin disorders, and also internally for gastrointestinal and menstrual disorders. Calendula is also included in numerous herbal preparations to improve their appearance.

It is also used in homoeopathic medicine.

Calendula oil is also used.

### Preparations

**Proprietary Preparations** (details are given in Part 3)
***Fr.:*** Calendulene; ***UK:*** Calendolon.

**Multi-ingredient:** ***Arg.:*** Acnetrol; Banoftal; Brunavera; Bushi; Eurocolor Post Solar; Europrotec Post Solar; ***Austral.:*** Anti-Flamme†; Galium Complex†; Nappy Rash Relief Cream†; Skin Healing Cream†; ***Austria:*** Apotheker Bauer's Magentee; Bio-Garten Entschlackungstee; Dr. Ernst Richter's Abfuhrtee-Filterbeutel†; Gewusst wie Darmtee; Gewusst wie Leber-Gallentee; Gewusst wie Magentee mild; Kneipp Nieren- und Blasen-Tee; Krauterhaus Mag Kottas Entwasserungstee; Krauterhaus Mag Kottas Fruhjahrs- und Herbstkurtee; Krauterhaus Mag Kottas Gallen- und Lebertee; Krauterhaus Mag Kottas Magen- und Darmtee; Krauterhaus Mag Kottas Nerven- und Schlaftee; Krauterhaus Mag Kottas Tee fur die Verdauung; Krauterhaus Mag Kottas Tee gegen Blahungen; Krauterhaus Mag Kottas Wechseltee; Mag Kottas Blahungs-Verdauungstee; Mag Kottas Entschlackungstee; Mag Kottas Entwasserungstee; Mag Kottas Leber-Gallentee; Mag Kottas Magen- und Darmtee; Mag Kottas Nerven-Beruhigungstee; Mag Kottas Nieren-Blasentee; Mag Kottas Tee fur stillende Mutter; Naturland Heilkrautermundwasser; Neuners Krautertee Nr 16 - Beruhigungstee bei Wechselbeschwerden; Neuners Krautertee Nr 2 - Fruhjahrskurtee; Neuners Krautertee Nr 207 - Krauterhexlein Kinder-Brusttee; Neuners Krautertee Nr 44 - Kreislaufanregender Tee; The Chambard-Tee; ***Belg.:*** Tisane Antibiliaire et Stomachique†; Tisane Depurative "les 12 Plantes"†; Tisane Diuretique†; Tisane Pectorale†; Tisane pour le Foie†; Tisane Purgative†; ***Braz.:*** Calendula Concreta; ***Chile:*** Homeoplasmina; Matikomp; ***Fr.:*** Cicaderma†; Dioptec; Hemorrogel; Homeoplasmine; Mediflor Tisane Pectorale d'Alsace†; Santane $F_{10}$†; Santane $H_7$†; Tisanes de l'Abbe Hamon no 14†; Tisanes de l'Abbe Hamon no 6†; ***Ger.:*** Befelka-Oel; bioplant-Kamillenfluid; Cefagastrin†; Cefaktivon†; Cefawell; Harntee 400; Hevert-Entwasserungs-Tee†; Hevert-Magen-Galle-Leber-Tee†; JuGrippan†; Nephronorm med; Salus Abfuhr-Tee Nr. 2†; Salus Bronchial-Tee Nr.8†; Salus Leber-Galle-Tee Nr.18†; Salus Rheuma-Tee Krautertee Nr. 12†; Unguentum lymphaticum; Urodil Blasen-Nieren Arzneitee†; ***Ital.:*** Alkagin; Babygella; Fluxoten†; Lenirose; Nevril; Proctopure; Sanaderm†; ***Malaysia:*** Arnica Comp; ***Mon.:*** Akipic; ***Port.:*** Alkagin; Cicaderma; ***Spain:*** Banoftal; Menstrunat; ***Switz.:*** Alpina Gel a la consoude†; Alpina Pommade au souci†; Gel a la consoude; Keppur; Pommade Po-Ho N A Vogel†; Urinex; ***UK:*** Calendula Nappy Change Cream; Eucanol; Massage Balm with Calendula; Savlon Natural First Aid for Burns; Savlon Natural First Aid for Cuts & Sores; Savlon Natural First Aid for Insect Bites & Stings; ***USA:*** Nasal-Ease.

## Calumba

Calumba Root; Colombo.

**Pharmacopoeias.** In *Jpn.*

### Profile

Calumba, the dried root of *Jateorhiza palmata* (*J. columba*) (Menispermaceae), has been used as a bitter and as a flavour.

### Preparations

**Proprietary Preparations** (details are given in Part 3)
**Multi-ingredient:** ***Ital.:*** Bitteridina†; ***Switz.:*** Padma-Lax; ***UK:*** Appetiser Mixture; Pegina; Travel-Caps†.

## Camostat Mesilate *(pINNM)*

Camostat Mesylate; FOY-305; Mesilato de camostat. *N,N*-Dimethylcarbamoylmethyl 4-(4-guanidinobenzoyloxy)phenylacetate methanesulphonate.

$C_{20}H_{22}N_4O_5,CH_4O_3S$ = 494.5.

*CAS — 59721-28-7 (camostat); 59721-29-8 (camostat mesilate).*

*ATC — B02AB04.*

**Pharmacopoeias.** In *Jpn.*

### Profile

Camostat mesilate is a protease inhibitor that has been used in the treatment of pancreatitis (p.1726) and postoperative reflux oesophagitis (p.1242). The usual dose is 100 to 200 mg three times daily by mouth.

### Preparations

**Proprietary Preparations** (details are given in Part 3)
***Jpn:*** Foipan.

## Camphor

Alcanfor; 2-Camphanone; D-Camphor (natural); Camphora; Camphre Droit (natural); Camphre du Japon (natural); Cânfora; Kamfer. Bornan-2-one; 1,7,7-Trimethylbicyclo[2.2.1]heptan-2-one.

$C_{10}H_{16}O$ = 152.2.

*CAS — 76-22-2 (± camphor); 21368-68-3 (± camphor); 464-49-3 (+ camphor); 464-48-2 (– camphor).*

*ATC — C01EB02.*

**Pharmacopoeias.** In *Chin., Eur.* (see p.vi), *Jpn, Pol., US,* and *Viet.*; some only describe natural camphor and some only synthetic camphor; *Eur.* and *Jpn* have separate monographs for natural and racemic or synthetic camphor.

**Ph. Eur. 5.0** (Camphor, Racemic). A white crystalline powder or friable crystalline masses, highly volatile even at room temperature. Slightly soluble in water; very soluble in alcohol and in petroleum spirit; very slightly soluble in glycerol; freely soluble in fatty oils.

**Ph. Eur. 5.0** (D-Camphor; Natural Camphor BP 2003). A white crystalline powder or friable crystalline masses, highly volatile even at room temperature. Slightly soluble in water; very soluble in alcohol and in petroleum spirit; very slightly soluble in glycerol; freely soluble in fatty oils.

**USP 27** (Camphor). A ketone obtained from *Cinnamomum camphora* (Lauraceae) or produced synthetically. The natural product is dextrorotatory and the synthetic product is optically inactive.

Colourless or white crystals, granules, or crystalline masses, or colourless to white, translucent, tough masses with a penetrating characteristic odour. It slowly volatilises at ordinary temperatures.

Soluble 1 in 800 of water, 1 in 1 of alcohol, 1 in 0.5 of chloroform, and 1 in 1 of ether; freely soluble in carbon disulfide, in petroleum spirit, and in fixed and volatile oils. Store at a temperature not exceeding 40° in airtight containers.

**Compounding.** A liquid or soft mass is formed when camphor is triturated with cloral hydrate, menthol, phenol, and many other substances. Camphor is readily powdered by triturating with a few drops of alcohol, ether, or chloroform.

### Adverse Effects

In addition to accidental ingestion of preparations containing camphor, poisoning has also occurred after giving camphorated oil (camphor liniment) to children in mistake for castor oil. The symptoms include nausea, vomiting, epigastric pain, headache, dizziness, oropharyngeal burning, delirium, muscle twitching, epileptiform convulsions, depression of the CNS, and coma. Breathing is difficult and the breath has a characteristic odour; anuria may occur. Death from respiratory failure or status epilepticus may occur; fatalities in children have been recorded from 1 g. There have been reports of instant collapse in infants following the local application of camphor to their nostrils.

### Treatment of Adverse Effects

Supportive care, including antiepileptic therapy, is the mainstay of treatment of camphor intoxication. Gastric lavage may be considered if the patient presents within 1 hour of ingestion; any convulsions must be controlled first. Activated charcoal may be given by mouth. Haemodialysis with a lipid dialysate or haemoperfusion have been tried but are of doubtful value.

### Precautions

Camphor should not be applied to the nostrils of infants even in small quantities, as this may cause immediate collapse.

◊ The UK Committee on the Review of Medicines[1] recommended that camphor should not be included in products intended for the treatment of hepatic and biliary disorders, gallstones, colic, renal disorders, urinary-tract infections, or ureteral stones. The administration of camphor parenterally or as irrigants was undesirable due to the associated safety hazard.

1. Anonymous. Camphorated oil: licensing authority takes action on camphor products. *Pharm J* 1984; **232:** 792.

### Pharmacokinetics

Camphor is readily absorbed from all administration sites. It is hydroxylated in the liver to yield hydroxycamphor metabolites which are then conjugated with glucuronic acid and excreted in the urine. Camphor crosses the placenta.

### Uses and Administration

Applied externally, camphor acts as a rubefacient and mild analgesic (see p.4) and is used in liniments as a counter-irritant in fibrositis, neuralgia, and similar conditions. It is also an ingredient of many inhaled nasal decongestant preparations but it is of doubtful efficacy. The use of camphor liniment (camphorated oil) is discouraged because of its potential toxicity. It has been withdrawn from the market in both the UK and the USA. In the USA the concentration of camphor in preparations for external use may not exceed 11%.

Taken internally camphor has irritant and carminative properties and has been used as a mild expectorant. It has also been used in mixed preparations for cardiovascular disorders.

### Preparations

***BP 2003:*** Camphorated Opium Tincture; Concentrated Camphor Water; Concentrated Camphorated Opium Tincture;

***USP 27:*** Camphor Spirit; Camphorated Phenol Topical Gel; Flexible Collodion.

**Proprietary Preparations** (details are given in Part 3)
***Fr.:*** Camphrice Du Canada; ***Ger.:*** Camphoderm N; Mulmicor; Pectocor N; Rheunervol N; Vaopin N; ***UK:*** Rohto Zi.

**Multi-ingredient:** numerous preparations are listed in Part 3.

## Camylofin Hydrochloride *(rINNM)*

Acamylophenine Hydrochloride; Camylofin Dihydrochloride; Hidrocloruro de camilofina. Isopentyl 2-(2-diethylaminoethylamino)-2-phenylacetate dihydrochloride.

$C_{19}H_{32}N_2O_2,2HCl = 393.4.$

*CAS — 54-30-8 (camylofin); 5892-41-1 (camylofin hydrochloride).*

*ATC — A03AA03.*

### Profile

Camylofin is used as an antispasmodic, usually in combination preparations. It is usually used as the hydrochloride; the noramidopyrine mesilate and the sodium salts have also been used.

**Overdosage.** Ingestion of large doses of camylofin by 2 infants produced symptoms similar to those of opioid intoxication.[1] Both infants responded to treatment with naloxone.

1. Schvartsman S, *et al.* Camylofin intoxication reversed by naloxone. *Lancet* 1988; **ii:** 1246.

### Preparations

**Proprietary Preparations** (details are given in Part 3)
***India:*** Anafortan.

**Multi-ingredient:** ***Arg.:*** Apasmo; ***Austria:*** Avamigran; ***Braz.:*** Espasmo Silidron; ***Fr.:*** Avafortan; ***India:*** Anafortan.

## Cannabis

Cáñamo Indiano; Cannab.; Cannabis Indica; Chanvre; Hanfkraut; Indian Hemp.

*CAS — 8063-14-7.*

**Description.** Cannabis consists of the dried flowering or fruiting tops of the pistillate plant of *Cannabis sativa* (Cannabinaceae). In the UK cannabis is defined by law as any part of any plant of the genus *Cannabis*. *Marihuana* usually refers to a mixture of the leaves and flowering tops. *Bhang, dagga, ganja, kif,* and *maconha* are commonly used in various countries to describe similar preparations. *Hashish* and *charas* are names often applied to the resin, although in some countries *hashish* is applied to any cannabis preparation.

A series of cannabinoids has been extracted from the plant, the most important being $\Delta^9$-tetrahydrocannabinol (dronabinol), $\Delta^8$-tetrahydrocannabinol, $\Delta^9$-tetrahydrocannabinolic acid, cannabinol, and cannabidiol. Cannabinol and cannabidiol may be present in large amounts but have little activity.

Cannabis has also been known as: Ait makhlif, Aliamba, Anassa, Anhascha, Assyuni, Bambalacha, Bambia, Bangi-Aku, Bango, Bangue, Bhang, Bhangaku, Canapa, Cangonha, Canhama, Cannacoro, Can-Yac, Caroçuda, Chur ganja, Chutras, Chutsao, Daboa, Dacha, Dagga, Darakte-Bang, Diamba, Dirijo, Djamba, Djoma, Dokka, Donajuanita, Dormilona, Durijo, Elva, Erva maligna, Erva do norte, Esrar, Fêmea, Fininha, Finote, Fokkra, Fumo brabo, Fumo de caboclo, Gandia, Ganga, Ganja, Ganjila, Gnaoui, Gongo, Gozah, Grahni Sherdool, Greefe, Grifa, Guabza, Guaza, Gunjah, Gunza, Hamp, Haouzi, Hen-Nab, Hursini, Hashish, Igbo, Indische-hennepkruid, Indisk hampa, Intianhamppu, Intsangu, Isangu, Janjah, Jatiphaladya churna, Jea, Juana, Kanab, Karpura rasa, Khanh-Chha, Khanje, Kif, Kif Ktami, Kinnab, Liamba, Lianda, Maconha, Maconia, Madi, Magiyam, Makhlif, Malva, Maraguango, Marajuana, Marigongo, Marihuana, Marijuana, Mariquita, Maruamba, Matekwane, Mbanje, Meconha, Misari, Mnoana, Momea, Mota, Mulatinha, Mundyadi vatika, Namba, Ntsangu, Nwonkaka, Peinka, Penek, Penka, Pito, Pot, Pretinha, Rafe, Rafi, Rafo, Riamba, Rongony, Rora, Rosa Maria, Sabsi, Sadda, Siddhi, Soñadora, Soussi, Subji, Summitates cannabis, Suruma, Tahgalim, Takrouri, Tedrika, Teloeut, Teriaki, Tronadora, Umya, Urumogi, Wee, Wewe, Yamba, Yoruba, Zacate chino, Zerouali, and Ziele konopi indyjskich.

Synonyms and approximate synonyms for cannabis resin included: Bheng, Charas, Charris, Chira, Churrus, Chus, Garaouich, Garawiche, Garoarsch, Gauja, Hachiche, Hascisc, Hashish, Hasis, Hasji's, Hasjisj, Haszysz, Haxixe, Heloua, Kamonga, Malak, Manzul, Momeka, N'rama, and Sighirma.

**Pharmacopoeias.** In *Chin.* and *Jpn.*

### Dependence

Prolonged heavy use of cannabis may lead to tolerance and psychological dependence but the existence of physical dependence remains somewhat controversial. Reported withdrawal symptoms have included anorexia, anxiety, insomnia, irritability, restlessness, sweating, headache, and mild gastrointestinal upsets.

◊ References.

1. Smith NT. A review of the published literature into cannabis withdrawal symptoms in human users. *Addiction* 2002; **97:** 621–32.
2. Budney AJ, Moore BA. Development and consequences of cannabis dependence. *J Clin Pharmacol* 2002; **42** (11 suppl): 28S–33S.
3. Haney M. Effects of smoked marijuana in healthy and HIV+ marijuana smokers. *J Clin Pharmacol* 2002; **42** (11 suppl): 34S–40S.

### Adverse Effects, Treatment, and Precautions

Nausea and vomiting may be the first effects of cannabis taken by mouth. The most frequent physical effects of cannabis intoxication are an increase in heart rate with alterations in blood pressure, conjunctival congestion, dry mouth, and increased appetite. Deterioration in motor coordination is common and cannabis has been reported to affect driving. The psychological effects include elation, distortion of time and space perception, irritability, and disturbances of memory and judgement. Anxiety or panic reactions may occur, particularly in inexperienced users. These reactions do not usually require specific therapy; diazepam may be necessary for severe reactions. Psychotic episodes of a paranoid or schizophrenic nature, and usually acute, have occurred in subjects taking cannabis, especially in large doses or after the use of varieties bred for a high yield of cannabinoids (so-called skunk).

◊ Reviews.

1. Johnson BA. Psychopharmacological effects of cannabis. *Br J Hosp Med* 1990; **43:** 114–22.
2. American Academy of Pediatrics. Marijuana: a continuing concern for pediatricians. *Pediatrics* 1991; **88:** 1070–2.
3. Wills S. Cannabis and cocaine. *Pharm J* 1993; **251:** 483–5.
4. Hall W, Solowij N. Adverse effects of cannabis. *Lancet* 1998; **352:** 1611–16.
5. Ashton CH. Adverse effects of cannabis and cannabinoids. *Br J Anaesth* 1999; **83:** 637–49.
6. Ashton CH. Pharmacology and effects of cannabis: a brief review. *Br J Psychiatry* 2001; **178:** 101–6.

**Breast feeding.** The American Academy of Pediatrics deprecates[1] the use of cannabis as a drug of abuse by breast-feeding mothers; a published report[2] indicated that cannabinoids were secreted into breast milk and absorbed by nursing infants, and while no adverse effect was reported to have occurred, some components do have a very long half-life.

1. American Academy of Pediatrics. The transfer of drugs and other chemicals into human milk. *Pediatrics* 2001; **108:** 776–89. Correction. *ibid.*; 1029. Also available at: http://aappolicy.aappublications.org/cgi/content/full/pediatrics%3b108/3/776 (accessed 06/07/04)
2. Perez-Reyes M, Wall ME. Presence of delta9-tetrahydrocannabinol in human milk. *N Engl J Med* 1982; **307:** 819–20.

**Coma.** Coma, reversed by flumazenil, has been reported in 2 children who had ingested cannabis.[1]

1. Rubio F, *et al.* Flumazenil for coma reversal in children after cannabis. *Lancet* 1993; **341:** 1028–9.

**Effects on the cardiovascular system.** References.

1. Jones RT. Cardiovascular system effects of marijuana. *J Clin Pharmacol* 2002; **42** (11 suppl): 58S–63S.
2. Sidney S. Cardiovascular consequences of marijuana use. *J Clin Pharmacol* 2002; **42** (11 suppl): 64S–70S.

**Effects on the CNS.** References to, and reviews of, the CNS effects of cannabis, including effects on cognition,[1-4] anxiety and depression,[5] and psychosis,[6,7] including schizophrenia.[8,9]

1. Pope HG Jr, *et al.* Neuropsychological performance in long-term cannabis users. *Arch Gen Psychiatry* 2001; **58:** 909–15.
2. Solowij N, *et al.* Cognitive functioning of long-term heavy cannabis users seeking treatment. *JAMA* 2002; **287:** 1123–31. Correction: *ibid.*: 1651.
3. Harrison GP Jr, *et al.* Cognitive measures in long-term cannabis users. *J Clin Pharmacol* 2002; **42** (11 suppl): 41S–47S.
4. Gonzalez R, *et al.* Nonacute (residual) neuropsychological effects of cannabis use: a qualitative analysis and systematic review. *J Clin Pharmacol* 2002; **42** (11 suppl): 48S–57S.
5. Patton GC, *et al.* Cannabis use and mental health in young people: cohort study. *BMJ* 2002; **325:** 1195–8.
6. McKay DR, Tennant CC. Is the grass greener? The link between cannabis and psychosis. *Med J Aust* 2000; **172:** 284–6.
7. Johns A. Psychiatric effects of cannabis. *Br J Psychiatry* 2001; **178:** 116–22.
8. Zammit S, *et al.* Self reported cannabis use as a risk factor for schizophrenia in Swedish conscripts of 1969: historical cohort study. *BMJ* 2002; **325:** 1199.
9. Arseneault L, *et al.* Cannabis use in adolescence and risk for adult psychosis: longitudinal prospective study. *BMJ* 2002; **325:** 1212–3.

**Effects on the eyes.** A report of persistent visual abnormalities in a patient following discontinuation of heavy abuse of hashish.[1] No organic cause for the effects, which were accompanied by less persistent mental changes, could be found.

1. Laffi GL, Safran AB. Persistent visual changes following hashish consumption. *Br J Ophthalmol* 1993; **77:** 601–2.

**Effects on the lungs.** References.

1. Tashkin DR, *et al.* Respiratory and immunologic consequences of marijuana smoking. *J Clin Pharmacol* 2002; **42** (11 suppl): 71S–81S.

**Hyperthermia.** Life-threatening hyperthermia was reported[1] in a 24-year-old man who went jogging after smoking cannabis.

1. Walter FG, *et al.* Marijuana and hyperthermia. *J Toxicol Clin Toxicol* 1996; **34:** 217–21.

**Pregnancy.** Cannabis has effects on sperm and can alter reproductive hormonal systems. Infants born to mothers exposed to cannabis during pregnancy tend to have a lower birth-weight[1,2] and may suffer from increased excitation in the postnatal period.[3]

1. Zuckerman B, *et al.* Effects of maternal marijuana and cocaine use on fetal growth. *N Engl J Med* 1989; **320:** 762–8.
2. Frank DA, *et al.* Neonatal body proportionality and body composition after in utero exposure to cocaine and marijuana. *J Pediatr* 1990; **117:** 622–6.
3. Silverman S. Interaction of drug-abusing mother, fetus, types of drugs examined in numerous studies. *JAMA* 1989; **261:** 1689, 1693.

### Interactions

Cannabis and alcohol have additive effects. The sedative effects of cannabis may be potentiated by other CNS depressants. Additive antimuscarinic effects, for example tachycardia, may occur with concomitant use of drugs such as tricyclic antidepressants. Cannabis induces microsomal enzymes and therefore interactions with a wide range of drugs that are metabolised by these enzymes might be expected (see, for example, Theophylline, p.802).

**Disulfiram.** Limited evidence indicates that use of disulfiram with cannabis may produce a hypomanic state.[1]

1. Lacoursiere RB, Swatek R. Adverse interaction between disulfiram and marijuana: a case report. *Am J Psychiatry* 1983; **140:** 243–4.

### Pharmacokinetics

The active principles of cannabis are readily absorbed from the lungs when smoked. Systemic bioavailability of the $\Delta^9$-tetrahydrocannabinol from smoked cannabis generally ranges between about 10 and 35%, with regular users achieving a higher efficiency. This produces an effect almost immediately, reaches a peak in up to 30 minutes, and is dissipated in about 3 to 4 hours.

$\Delta^9$-Tetrahydrocannabinol absorption may be slow and erratic from the gastrointestinal tract. Although highly absorbed (90 to 95%), extensive first-pass liver metabolism reduces the systemic bioavailability to approximately 2 to 14% with high interindividual variation. Effects are not seen for 30 to 90 minutes and persist for about 8 hours when taken by mouth.

Tetrahydrocannabinol is lipophilic and becomes widely distributed in the body. It crosses the placenta and is distributed into breast milk. It is extensively metabolised, primarily in the liver, to the active 11-hydroxy derivative; both are extensively bound to plasma proteins. It is excreted in the urine and faeces, sometimes over prolonged periods.

Duration of detectability of urinary metabolites varies greatly, 3 days for a single use to 27 days for heavy chronic users.

◊ Review.

1. Grotenhermen F. Pharmacokinetics and pharmacodynamics of cannabinoids. *Clin Pharmacokinet* 2003; **42:** 327–60.

### Uses and Administration

Cannabis was formerly employed as a sedative or narcotic. Its main active constituent $\Delta^9$-tetrahydrocannabinol (dronabinol, p.1264) and a synthetic cannabinol (nabilone, p.1277) are used as antiemetics in patients receiving cancer chemotherapy; they are also being investigated for a number of other potential therapeutic uses. Cannabis has analgesic, muscle relaxant, and appetite stimulant effects and reduces intra-ocular pressure. Anecdotal reports exist of benefit from cannabis in a variety of disorders including glaucoma, multiple sclerosis, and wasting in patients with AIDS and malignant neoplasms.

◊ References to the potential medical uses of cannabis.

1. Doyle E, Spence AA. Cannabis as a medicine? *Br J Anaesth* 1995; **74:** 359–61.
2. Gray C. Cannabis—the therapeutic potential. *Pharm J* 1995; **254:** 771–3.
3. Grinspoon L, Bakalar JB. Marihuana as a medicine: a plea for reconsideration. *JAMA* 1995; **273:** 1875–6.
4. Voth EA, Schwartz RH. Medicinal applications of delta-9-tetrahydrocannabinol and marijuana. *Ann Intern Med* 1997; **126:** 791–8.
5. British Medical Association. *Therapeutic uses of cannabis.* Amsterdam: Harwood Academic, 1997.
6. Robson P. Cannabis as medicine: time for the phoenix to rise? *BMJ* 1998; **316:** 1034–5.
7. Robson P. Therapeutic aspects of cannabis and cannabinoids. *Br J Psychiatry* 2001; **178:** 107–15.
8. Mechoulam R, *et al.* Cannabidiol: an overview of some pharmacological aspects. *J Clin Pharmacol* 2002; **42** (11 suppl): 11S–19S.
9. Zajicek J, *et al.* Cannabinoids for treatment of spasticity and other symptoms related to multiple sclerosis (CAMS study): multicentre randomised placebo-controlled trial. *Lancet* 2003; **362:** 1517–26.
10. Killestein J, *et al.* Cannabinoids in multiple sclerosis: do they have a therapeutic role? *Drugs* 2004; **64:** 1–11.

## Canola Oil

Cánola, aceite de.

*CAS — 120962-03-0.*

### Profile

Canola oil is a form of rape oil (p.1737) from strains selected for low erucic acid content. It is used as an edible oil and in pharmaceutical manufacturing and cosmetics.

### Preparations

**Proprietary Preparations** (details are given in Part 3)

**Multi-ingredient:** ***NZ:*** Mr Nits.

## Cantharides

Blistering Beetle; Cantáridas; Cantharis; Insectes Coléoptères Hétéromères; Lytta; Méloides; Russian Flies; Spanish Fly.

### Adverse Effects

Following ingestion of cantharides there is burning pain in the throat and stomach, difficulty in swallowing, nausea, vomiting, haematemesis, abdominal pain, bloody diarrhoea, tenesmus, renal pain, frequent micturition, haematuria, uraemia, severe hypotension, and circulatory failure. Oral doses of cantharidin (the active ingredient of cantharides) of less than 65 mg have been lethal. A dose of 1 mg or contact with one insect can produce distressing symptoms. Skin contact results in blisters.

◊ References.

1. Hundt HKL, *et al.* Post-mortem serum concentration of cantharidin in a fatal case of cantharides poisoning. *Hum Exp Toxicol* 1990; **9:** 35–40.

## Uses and Administration

Cantharides is the dried beetle *Cantharis vesicatoria* (*Lytta vesicatoria*) (Meloidae) or other spp., containing not less than 0.6% of cantharidin. Preparations of cantharides have been employed externally as rubefacients, counter-irritants, and vesicants. They should not be taken internally or applied over large surfaces owing to the risk of absorption. The use of cantharides in cosmetic products is prohibited in the UK by law.

Cantharides is used in homoeopathic medicine.

Mylabris (Chinese blistering beetle; Chinese cantharides; Indian blistering beetle), the dried beetles of the species *Mylabrus sidae* (= *M. phalerata*), *M. cichorii*, and *M. pustulator*, has been used as a substitute for cantharides and as a source of cantharidin (see below) in the East.

---

# Cantharidin

Cantaridina. Hexahydro-3aα,7aα-dimethyl-4β,7β-epoxyisobenzofuran-1,3-dione.

$C_{10}H_{12}O_4$ = 196.2.

*CAS — 56-25-7.*

## Profile

Cantharidin is obtained from cantharides or mylabris (see under Cantharides, above). Cantharidin in flexible collodion has been applied for the removal of warts and molluscum contagiosum. It has also been used in veterinary medicine. Owing to the high toxicity of cantharidin it has been recommended that preparations containing it should not be used medicinally. Adverse effects are those described for cantharides (see above).

## Preparations

**Proprietary Preparations** (details are given in Part 3)
***Canad.:*** Canthacur; Cantharone; ***Singapore:*** Canthacur†.

**Multi-ingredient: *Canad.:*** Canthacur-PS; Cantharone Plus.

---

# Capsicum

Capsic.; Capsici Fructus; Capsicum frutescens; Chillies; Piment Rouge; Pimentão; Spanischer Pfeffer.

NOTE. Ground cayenne pepper of commerce is normally a blend of varieties of capsicum. Paprika is from *Capsicum annuum* var. *longum*; it is milder than capsicum.

**Pharmacopoeias.** In *Eur.* (see p.vi), *Jpn*, and *US*.
*US* also includes capsicum oleoresin (capsicin).

**Ph. Eur. 5.0** (Capsicum). The dried ripe fruits of *Capsicum annuum* var. *minimum* and small-fruited varieties of *C. frutescens*. It contains a minimum of 0.4% of total capsaicinoids expressed as capsaicin, calculated with reference to the dried drug. Protect from light.

**USP 27** (Capsicum). The dried ripe fruits of *Capsicum frutescens*, known in commerce as African Chillies, or of *C. annuum* var. *connoides*, known in commerce as Tabasco Pepper, or *C. annuum* var. *longum*, known in commerce as Louisiana Long Pepper, or of a hybrid between the Honka variety of Japanese Capsicum and the Old Louisiana Sport Capsicum, known in commerce as Louisiana Sport Pepper.

**USP 27** (Capsicum Oleoresin). An alcoholic extract of the dried ripe fruits of *Capsicum annum* var. *minimum* and small fruited varieties of *C. fruiscons* (Solanaceae). It contains not less than 8% of total capsaicins. It is a dark red oily liquid. Soluble in alcohol, in acetone, in chloroform, in ether, and in volatile oils; soluble with opalescence in fixed oils. Store in airtight containers.

## Profile

Capsicum has a carminative action but it is mainly used externally, often in the form of capsicum oleoresin, as a counter-irritant (see Rubefacients and Topical Analgesia, p.4). It is also included in preparations for the management of cough and cold symptoms. However, preparations of capsicum and capsicum oleoresin can be very irritant. Capsaicin (p.24), the active ingredient of capsicum, is also used in topical preparations in the treatment of painful skin conditions.

Capsicum oleoresin is used in 'pepper sprays' for law enforcement and self defence.

Capsicum is also used in homoeopathic medicine and in cookery.

**Effects on the gastrointestinal tract.** The initial response to the ingestion of a hot pepper is a hot or burning sensation in the mouth which is attributed to the binding of capsaicin to receptors in the oral cavity.[1] Casein-containing substances such as milk can reverse this burning sensation, apparently by displacing capsaicin, this being due to their lipophilicity.

Spicy meals have long been associated with gastrointestinal discomfort and ingestion of meals containing 1.5 g of red or black pepper has been shown to cause signs of gastric mucosal damage comparable with those caused by a 625-mg dose of aspirin.[2] However, other studies in *animals*[3] and humans[4,5] suggest that capsaicin may have a protective effect on gastric mucosa. Ingestion of about 30 g of jalapeño peppers (a capsicum fruit) caused no visible damage to the duodenal or gastric mucosa of 12 healthy subjects[6] and daily ingestion of meals containing a total of 3 g of chilli powder did not affect the clinical progress of patients with duodenal ulcers given antacids.[7]

1. Henkin R. Cooling the burn from hot peppers. *JAMA* 1991; **266:** 2766.
2. Myers BM, *et al.* Effect of red pepper and black pepper on the stomach. *Am J Gastroenterol* 1987; **82:** 211–14.
3. Holzer P. Peppers, capsaicin, and the gastric mucosa. *JAMA* 1989; **261:** 3244–5.
4. Kang JY, *et al.* Chili—protective factor against peptic ulcer? *Dig Dis Sci* 1995; **40:** 576–9.
5. Yeoh KG, *et al.* Chili protects against aspirin-induced gastroduodenal mucosal injury in humans. *Dig Dis Sci* 1995; **40:** 580–3.
6. Graham DY, *et al.* Spicy food and the stomach: evaluation by videoendoscopy. *JAMA* 1988; **260:** 3473–5.
7. Kumar N, *et al.* Do chillies influence healing of duodenal ulcer? *BMJ* 1984; **288:** 1803–4.

**Pepper sprays.** References to the toxic effects of 'pepper sprays' containing capsicum oleoresin.

1. Zollman TM, *et al.* Clinical effects of oleoresin capsicum (pepper spray) on the human cornea and conjunctiva. *Ophthalmology* 2000; **107:** 2186–9.
2. Chan TC, *et al.* The effect of oleoresin capsicum "pepper" spray inhalation on respiratory function. *J Forensic Sci* 2002; **47:** 299–304.

## Preparations

**Proprietary Preparations** (details are given in Part 3)
***Arg.:*** Redol; ***Austral.:*** Shingles Pain Relief†; ***Austria:*** ABC; Capsiplast†; ***Chile:*** Dolorub; Parche Leon Fortificante; ***Ger.:*** ABC Warme-Pflaster; Capsamol; Dolenon; Kneipp Rheuma Salbe†; Rheumaplast N†; Thermo Burger; ***Ital.:*** Cerotto Bertelli Arnikos; Dolpyc; Thermogene; ***UK:*** Fiery Jack.

**Multi-ingredient: *Arg.:*** Infrarub; Veracolate; ***Austral.:*** APR Cream; Bioglan Joint Mobility†; Bioglan The Blue One†; Capsolin†; For Peripheral Circulation Herbal Plus Formula 5†; Gingo A†; Goanna Heat Cream†; Lifesystem Herbal Formula 6 For Peripheral Circulation†; Radian-B; Thermalife C†; Valerian†; ***Austria:*** Biokosma Red Point-Massagecreme; Mentopin; Salhumin; Trauma-Salbe warmend; Traumasalbe; ***Belg.:*** Dolpyc†; Rado-Salil; Stilene; Thermocream; ***Braz.:*** Pilulas Ross; ***Canad.:*** Absorbine Arthritis; Cayenne Plus; Herbalax Forte†; Phytolax†; Rheumalan; Rhumatisme; ***Fr.:*** Baume Saint-Bernard†; Capsic†; Disalgyl; Dolpyc†; Kamol; Le Thermogene; ***Ger.:*** Caye Balsam; Finalgon N Schmerzpflaster†; Gothaplast Rheumamed AC; ***Hong Kong:*** LEAN Formula w/ Advantra; ***India:*** Algipan; Relaxyl; ***Israel:*** Mento-O-Cap; Radian-B; Rublex Massage Cream; ***Ital.:*** Capso; Capsolin; Remy; Sloan; ***Neth.:*** Sloan's balsem; ***Port.:*** Balsamo Analgesico; Balsamo Analgesico Sanitas; Caroid; Dologel†; Medalginan; ***S.Afr.:*** Radian†; Sportsman Rub†; ***Spain:*** Balsamo Midalgan†; Dolokey; Killpan†; Linimento Naion; Linimento Sloan†; Pomada Revulsiva†; ***Switz.:*** Capsolin†; Embropax†; Emplatre Croix D†; Incutin†; Massorax; Midalgan; Sloan Baume†; Sloan Liniment†; ***Thai.:*** Flatulence Gastulence; Meloids; Veracolate; ***UK:*** Algipan†; Allcock's Porous Capsicum Plaster†; Allens Dry Tickly Cough; Balmosa; Buttercup Syrup; Catarrh Mixture; Cremalgin; Fiery Jack; Hactos; Hansaplast Herbal Heat Plaster; Herbal Indigestion Naturtabs; Honey & Molasses; Indian Brandee; Indigestion and Flatulence; Indigestion and Flatulence Tablets†; Indigestion Relief; Jamaican Sarsaparilla; Kilkof; Life Drops; Potters Strong Bronchial Catarrh Pastilles; Potters Sugar Free Cough Pastilles; Radian-B; Ralgex; Rheumatic Pain Relief; Sanderson's Throat Specific; Vegetable Cough Remover; ***USA:*** Throat Discs; Veracolate†.

---

# Caraway

Alcaravea; Alcaravia; Caraway Fruit; Caraway Seed; Carum; Cumin des Prés; Fructus Carvi; Kümmel.

**Pharmacopoeias.** In *Eur.* (see p.vi) and *Pol.* Also in *USNF*.

**Ph. Eur. 5.0** (Caraway Fruit; Caraway BP 2003). The whole, dried fruits of *Carum carvi*. It contains not less than 3.0% v/w of essential oil, calculated with reference to the dried drug. It has an odour reminiscent of carvone. Protect from light.

The BP 2003 directs that when Powdered Caraway is prescribed or demanded, material containing not less than 2.5% v/w of essential oil shall be dispensed or supplied.

**USNF 22** (Caraway). The dried, ripe fruit of *Carum carvi* (Apiaceae). Preserve against attack by insects.

## Profile

Caraway is an aromatic carminative, and is used in gastrointestinal disorders and as a flavour. The seeds are used in cookery. It is the source of caraway oil (below).

## Preparations

***USNF 22:*** Compound Cardamom Tincture.

**Proprietary Preparations** (details are given in Part 3)

**Multi-ingredient: *Austria:*** Abbiofort; Absimed; Aktiv milder Magen- und Darmtee; Aponatura Wind; Apotheker Bauer's Magentee; Bio-Garten Tee fur den Magen; Bio-Garten Tee gegen Blahungen; Bio-Garten Tropfen gegen Blahungen; Bioreform-Magentee; Bioreform-Windtreibender Tee; Carminative; Karvisin; Krauterdoktor Magen-Darmtropfen; Krauterhaus Mag Kottas Babytee; Krauterhaus Mag Kottas Tee fur die Verdauung; Krauterhaus Mag Kottas Tee gegen Blahungen; Mag Kottas Baby-Tee; Mag Kottas Blahungs-Verdauungstee; Mag Kottas Krauterexpress-Blahungs-Verdauungstee; Mag Kottas Krauterexpress-Tee fur stillende Mutter; Mag Kottas Tee fur stillende Mutter; Magentee†; Midro Tee; Montana; Myrtilen; Naturland Verdauungs; Nesthakchen; Neuners Krautertee Nr 107 - Blahungstee; Neuners Krautertee Nr 126 - Starkungstee fur stillende Mutter; Neuners Krautertee Nr 14 - Verdauungstee; Neuners Krautertee Nr 17 - Lebertee; Neuners Krautertee Nr 217 - Krauterhexlein Kinder-Blahungstee; Sidroga Leber-Galle-Tee; Species Carvi comp; St Radegunder Blahungstreibender Tee; St Radegunder Verdauungstee; ***Braz.:*** Balsamo Branco†; ***Fr.:*** Santane $C_6$†; Santane $D_5$†; Santane $F_{10}$†; Santane $O_1$†; Tisane des Familles†; Tisane Digestive Weleda†; ***Ger.:*** Agamadon N†; Carminativum-Hetterich N; Carminativum-Pascoe; Cholosom-Tee; Echtroferment-N†; Floradix Multipretten N; Gastrol S; Gastrosecur; Hevert-Carmin symbio†; Iberogast; Kneipp Flatuol†; Kneipp Magen-Tee†; Lomatol; Majocarmin-Tee; Meteophyt S†; Montana N; Presselin Blahungs K 4 N; Presselin Dyspeptikum; Stomachicon N†; Stovalid N; ***Israel:*** Jungborn; Lido Tea; Midro-Tea; ***Ital.:*** Anice (Specie Composta); Cadifen; Cadimint; Camomilla (Specie Composta); Florelax; Midro; Tarassaco (Specie Composta); ***Spain:*** Natusor Aerofane; ***Switz.:*** Adistop Lax†; Ajaka†; Kernosan Heidelberger Poudre; Phytomed Gastro†; Tisane favorisant l'allaitement; Tisane laxative Natterman no 13†; ***UK:*** Carminative Tea†.

---

# Caraway Oil

Alcaravea, aceite esencial de; Kümmelöl; Oleum Cari; Oleum Carui; Oleum Carvi.

**Pharmacopoeias.** In *Br.* and *Ger.* Also in *USNF*.

**BP 2003** (Caraway Oil). A clear, colourless or pale yellow liquid, visibly free from water, with an odour of caraway. It is obtained by distillation from caraway. It contains 53 to 63% w/w of ketones calculated as carvone ($C_{10}H_{14}O$). At 20° it is soluble 1 in 7 of alcohol (80%). Store at a temperature not exceeding 25° in well-filled containers. Protect from light.

**USNF 22** (Caraway Oil). The volatile oil distilled from caraway. It contains not more than 50% v/v of carvone ($C_{10}H_{14}O$). Soluble 1 in 8 of alcohol (80%). Store in airtight containers. Protect from light.

## Profile

Caraway oil is an aromatic carminative and is used in gastrointestinal disorders and as a flavour. It is also employed as caraway water for infant colic (see Gastrointestinal Spasm, p.1242).

## Preparations

***BP 2003:*** Aromatic Cardamom Tincture; Compound Cardamom Tincture.

**Proprietary Preparations** (details are given in Part 3)

**Multi-ingredient: *Austria:*** Benium; Nesthakchen; Parodontax; Pascopankreat†; Sabatif; Sanvita Magen; Sigman-Haustropfen; Spasmo Claim; ***Ger.:*** Aspasmon N; Benium†; Enteroplant; Euflat I; Floradix Multipretten N; Galloselect M; Gastricard; Grunlicht Magenbalsam Tropfen†; Hevert-Carmin symbio†; Hevert-Gall S†; Kneipp Rheuma Stoffwechsel-Bad Heublumen-Aquasan†; Lomatol; Majocarmin forte; Neo-Ballistol; Pascopankreat novo; Pascopankreat S†; ratioGast; Roflatol Phyto (Rowo-146)†; Sirmia Abfuhrkapseln†; ***India:*** Bestozyme; Catazyme-P; Neopeptine; Vitazyme; ***Switz.:*** Ajaka†; Capsules laxatives Nattermann Nr. 13†; Flatulex; Huile Po-Ho A. Vogel; ***Thai.:*** Gas-Nep; Gripe Mixture; ***UK:*** Atkinson & Barker's Gripe Mixture; Nurse Harvey's Gripe Mixture.

---

# Carbon-13

Carbono 13.

*CAS — 14762-74-4.*

## Profile

Carbon-13 is a naturally occurring, non-radioactive, stable isotope of carbon. It has been used to label organic compounds, such as urea (p.1162), for use in diagnostic tests, including breath and blood tests for the diagnosis of *Helicobacter pylori* infection.

## Preparations

***USP 27:*** Urea C 13 for Oral Solution.

**Proprietary Preparations** (details are given in Part 3)
***Fr.:*** Heli-Kit; ***Gr.:*** Pylobactel; ***Ital.:*** Breathquality-UBT; Citredici UBT Kit; Helicokit; Pylobactell; ***Mex.:*** Alitest; ***Spain:*** Pylori Chek; Tau Kit; Ubtest; ***Swed.:*** Diabact UBT; ***Switz.:*** Pylori 13; ***UK:*** Diabact UBT; Pylobactell; ***USA:*** Meretek UBT.

**Multi-ingredient: *USA:*** Ez-HBT.

---

# Cardamom

Cardamomi; Cardamomo, fruto del.

**Pharmacopoeias.** In *Br.* and *Jpn.* Also in *USNF*.

**BP 2003** (Cardamom Fruit). The dried, nearly ripe fruit of *Elettaria cardamomum* var. *minuscula*. Only the seeds are used in making preparations of cardamom and they are used immediately after removal from the fruit. The seeds should not be stored after removal from the fruit. They have a strongly aromatic odour and taste and contain not less than 4% v/w of volatile oil.

**USNF 22** (Cardamom Seed). The dried ripe seed of *Elettaria cardamomum* (Zingiberaceae), recently removed from the capsule. Preserve against attack by insects.

## Profile

Preparations of cardamom are used as carminatives and as flavours. The seeds are used in cookery. Cardamom seeds are the source of cardamom oil (below).

## Preparations

***USNF 22:*** Compound Cardamom Tincture.

**Proprietary Preparations** (details are given in Part 3)

**Multi-ingredient: *Austral.:*** Peritone†; Travelaide†; ***Austria:*** Mariazeller; ***Ger.:*** Gallexier; Montana N; Presselin Dyspeptikum; Schwedentrunk Elixier; ***India:*** Carmicide; ***Ital.:*** Sedobex†; ***S.Afr.:*** Alma; Enterodyne; ***Spain:*** Digestovital; ***Switz.:*** Stomacine; ***Thai.:*** Carmicide; ***UK:*** Aluminium Free Indigestion†; Indian Brandee; Pegina.

## Cardamom Oil

Cardamomo, aceite esencial de; Ol. Cardamom.

**Pharmacopoeias.** In *Br.* Also in *USNF.*

**BP 2003** (Cardamom Oil). A clear, colourless or pale yellow liquid, visibly free from water, with an odour of cardamom fruit. It is distilled from crushed cardamom fruit. At 20° it is soluble 1 in 6 of alcohol (70%). Store at a temperature not exceeding 25° in well-filled containers. Protect from light.

**USNF 22** (Cardamom Oil). The volatile oil obtained from cardamom seed. Soluble 1 in 5 of alcohol (70%). Store in airtight containers. Protect from light.

### Profile

Preparations of cardamom oil are used as carminatives and as flavours.

### Preparations

***BP 2003:*** Aromatic Cardamom Tincture; Compound Cardamom Tincture; Compound Rhubarb Tincture.

**Proprietary Preparations** (details are given in Part 3)

**Multi-ingredient:** ***India:*** Catazyme-P; Digeplex; Vitazyme; ***Thai.:*** Gas-Nep.

## Carglumic Acid *(rINN)*

Carglutamic Acid. *N*-Carbamoyl-L-glutamic acid.

$C_6H_{10}N_2O_5$ = 190.2.

*CAS — 1188-38-1.*

*ATC — A16AA05.*

### Profile

Carglumic acid is used for the treatment of hyperammonaemia in patients with *N*-acetylglutamate synthase deficiency. The initial daily dose ranges from 100 to 250 mg/kg, adjusted thereafter to maintain normal plasma levels of ammonia. Individual responsiveness to carglumic acid should be tested before starting long-term therapy; daily maintenance doses range from 10 to 100 mg/kg. The total daily dose should preferably be taken as 2 to 4 divided doses before food.

### Preparations

**Proprietary Preparations** (details are given in Part 3)

***Austria:*** Carbaglu; ***Denm.:*** Carbaglu; ***Fr.:*** Carbaglu; ***UK:*** Carbaglu.

## Carnauba Wax

Brazil Wax; Caranda Wax; Cera Carnauba; Cera Coperniciae; Cera de carnauba; E903.

*CAS — 8015-86-9.*

**Pharmacopoeias.** In *Eur.* (see p.vi), *Int.*, and *Jpn.* Also in *USNF.*

**Ph. Eur. 5.0** (Carnauba Wax). It is obtained from the leaves of *Copernicia cerifera.* Pale yellow or yellow powder, flakes, or hard masses. It has a relative density of about 0.97. M.p. 80° to 88°. Practically insoluble in water and in alcohol; soluble on heating in ethyl acetate and in xylene. Protect from light.

**USNF 22** (Carnauba Wax). It is obtained from the leaves of *Copernicia cerifera* (Palmae). A light brown to pale yellow, moderately coarse powder or flakes, possessing a characteristic bland odour, and free from rancidity. Sp. gr. about 0.99. M.p. 80° to 86°. Insoluble in water; slightly soluble in boiling alcohol; soluble in warm chloroform and in warm toluene; freely soluble in warm benzene.

### Profile

Carnauba wax is used in pharmacy as a coating agent. Its use is also permitted in certain foods. Various types and grades are used industrially in the manufacture of polishes.

## Caroverine *(pINN)*

Caroverina. 1-[2-(Diethylamino)ethyl]-3-(*p*-methoxybenzyl)-2(1*H*)-quinoxalinone.

$C_{22}H_{27}N_3O_2$ = 365.5.

*CAS — 23465-76-1.*

*ATC — A03AX11.*

### Profile

Caroverine is a smooth muscle relaxant with calcium-channel blocking and glutamate-antagonist properties. It is used as the base or the hydrochloride in conditions associated with painful smooth muscle spasm. Typical doses (expressed as the base) are 20 to 40 mg by mouth three or four times daily, or 40 to 80 mg by slow intravenous or intramuscular injection, up to a maximum of 200 mg daily; it has also been given rectally. It is also used in cerebral circulatory disorders and in tinnitus.

◊ References.


1. Denk DM, *et al.* Caroverine in tinnitus treatment: a placebo-controlled blind study. *Acta Otolaryngol* 1997; **117:** 825–30.
2. Ehrenberger K. Clinical experience with caroverine in inner ear diseases. *Adv Otorhinolaryngol* 2002; **59:** 156–62.
3. Quint C, *et al.* The quinoxaline derivative caroverine in the treatment of sensorineural smell disorders: a proof-of-concept study. *Acta Otolaryngol* 2002; **122:** 877–81.


### Preparations

**Proprietary Preparations** (details are given in Part 3)

***Austria:*** Delirex; Spasmium; Tinnitin; ***Switz.:*** Calmaverine.

**Multi-ingredient:** ***Austria:*** Spagall; Spasmium comp.

## Carzenide *(rINN)*

Carzenida. *p*-Sulphamoylbenzoic acid.

$C_7H_7NO_4S$ = 201.2.

*CAS — 138-41-0.*

### Profile

Carzenide is an antispasmodic that has been used in the treatment of dysmenorrhoea.

## Cassia Oil

Canela de la China, aceite de; Chinese Cinnamon Oil; Cinnamomi Cassiae Aetheroleum; Oleum Cassiae; Oleum Cinnamomi; Oleum Cinnamomi Cassiae.

**Pharmacopoeias.** In *Chin., Eur.* (see p.vi), and *Jpn.*

*Chin.* and *Jpn* also include cassia bark which may be known as cinnamon bark. In some countries cassia oil is known as cinnamon oil.

**Ph. Eur. 5.0** (Cassia Oil). The oil obtained by steam distillation of the leaves and young branches of *Cinnamomum cassia* (*C. aromaticum*). It contains 70 to 90% of cinnamaldehyde. A clear, mobile, yellow to reddish-brown liquid, with a characteristic odour of cinnamaldehyde. Store in well-filled airtight containers. Protect from light and heat.

### Profile

Cassia oil has properties resembling those of cinnamon oil (p.1672) and is used similarly as a carminative and flavour. Hypersensitivity to cinnamaldehyde, the main constituent of cassia oil, has been reported.

### Preparations

**Proprietary Preparations** (details are given in Part 3)

**Multi-ingredient:** ***Ger.:*** Grunlicht Hingfong Essenz†; ***UK:*** Dragon Balm.

## Castor Oil

Aceite de Ricino; Huile de Ricin; Ol. Ricin.; Oleum Ricini; Ricini Oleum Virginale; Ricino, aceite de; Rizinusöl.

*ATC — A06AB05.*

NOTE. CASOIL is a code approved by the BP 2003 for use on single unit doses of eye drops containing castor oil where the individual container may be too small to bear all the appropriate labelling information.

**Pharmacopoeias.** In *Chin., Eur.* (see p.vi), *Jpn,* and *US.*

*Eur.* and *USNF* also include hydrogenated castor oil.

**Ph. Eur. 5.0** (Castor Oil, Virgin). The fatty oil obtained by cold expression from the seeds of *Ricinus communis.* Relative density about 0.958. It is a clear, almost colourless or slightly yellow, viscous, hygroscopic liquid. Miscible with alcohol and with glacial acetic acid; slightly soluble in petroleum spirit. Store in well-filled airtight containers. Protect from light.

**Ph. Eur. 5.0** (Castor Oil, Hydrogenated; Ricini Oleum Hydrogenatum). The oil obtained by hydrogenation of castor oil. It consists mainly of the triglyceride of 12-hydroxystearic acid. Almost white to pale yellow fine powder, masses, or flakes. M.p. 83° to 88°. Practically insoluble in water; very slightly soluble in dehydrated alcohol; freely soluble in dichloromethane; slightly soluble in petroleum spirit. Store in well-filled containers.

**USP 27** (Castor Oil). The fixed oil obtained from the seed of *Ricinus communis* (Euphorbiaceae). It is a pale yellowish or almost colourless, transparent, viscid liquid. Has a faint, mild odour; is free from foreign and rancid odour; and has a bland, characteristic taste. Soluble in alcohol; miscible with dehydrated alcohol, with chloroform, with ether, and with glacial acetic acid. Store in airtight containers at a temperature not exceeding 40°.

**USNF 22** (Hydrogenated Castor Oil). Refined, bleached, hydrogenated, and deodorised castor oil, consisting mainly of the triglyceride of hydroxystearic acid. A white, crystalline wax. M.p. 85° to 88°. Insoluble in water and in most common organic solvents. Store in airtight containers at a temperature not exceeding 40°.

### Adverse Effects and Precautions

Oral administration of castor oil, particularly in large doses, may produce nausea, vomiting, colic, and severe purgation. Castor oil should not be given when intestinal obstruction is present.

The seeds of *Ricinus communis* contain a toxic protein, ricin (p.1738). Allergic reactions have been reported in subjects handling the seeds.

### Uses and Administration

Castor oil is used externally for its emollient effect. It has also been used topically to allay irritation due to foreign bodies in the eye. Castor oil may be employed as the solvent in some injections.

Hydrogenated castor oil is used as a stiffening agent. Polyoxyl castor oils (p.1414) are used as emulsifying and solubilising agents.

Castor oil has been used as a laxative, but such use is obsolete.

### Preparations

***BP 2003:*** Chloroxylenol Solution; Flexible Collodion; Zinc and Castor Oil Ointment;

***USP 27:*** Aromatic Castor Oil; Castor Oil Capsules; Castor Oil Emulsion; Flexible Collodion.

**Proprietary Preparations** (details are given in Part 3)

***Arg.:*** Capsulas Handel; ***Braz.:*** Laxol; ***Canad.:*** Neoloid; Unisoil†; ***Ger.:*** Laxopol; ***Gr.:*** Kikelaio EF 3; ***Israel:*** Laxopol; ***Spain:*** Palmil†; Ricino Koki†; ***Switz.:*** Herbapharm Rical; ***USA:*** Emulsoil; Neoloid; Purge.

**Multi-ingredient:** ***Arg.:*** Calculina; ***Austral.:*** Seda-Rash†; ***Braz.:*** Steitonit†; ***Ital.:*** Bal Tar†; Herbatar†; ***Mex.:*** Nutegen G; ***Spain:*** Otocerum; ***UK:*** Exzem Oil†; Panda Baby Cream†; ***USA:*** Dermuspray; Dr Dermi-Heal; Granulderm; Granulex; GranuMed; Mammol; Medicone Rectal; Proderm.

## Catalase

Caperase; Catalasa; Equilase; Optidase.

### Profile

Catalase is an enzyme obtained from a wide variety of biological sources including animal liver (hepatocatalase) and certain bacteria and fungi. It is a protein composed of 4 polypeptide subunits, the precise composition of which varies according to the source, and has a molecular weight of about 240 000. Catalase has the ability to promote the decomposition of hydrogen peroxide to water and oxygen.

It has been applied to wounds and skin ulcers and has also been used in the treatment of eczema. It has sometimes been used with glucose oxidase (p.1694) in food preservation to break down hydrogen peroxide produced during oxidation of glucose, and is also included in preparations for contact lens care to neutralise hydrogen peroxide.

Catalase is a free-radical scavenger and has been investigated for its ability to limit reperfusion injury thought to be related to free-radical production. Combinations of catalase with superoxide dismutase have also been investigated.

◊ References.


1. Greenwald RA. Superoxide dismutase and catalase as therapeutic agents for human diseases: a critical review. *Free Radic Biol Med* 1990; **8:** 201–9.


### Preparations

**Proprietary Preparations** (details are given in Part 3)

***Austria:*** Lensan B†; Les Yeux 2†; Titmus Losung 2†; ***Ital.:*** Citrizan; ***Spain:*** Biocatalase.

**Multi-ingredient:** ***Arg.:*** One Step; ***Belg.:*** Pulvo 47†; Pulvo Neomycine†; ***Canad.:*** UltraCare; ***Fr.:*** Pulvo 47; Pulvo 47 Neomycine; ***Ger.:*** Oxysept Comfort†; Pulvo; Pulvo Neomycin; ***Israel:*** Omnicare†; Oxysept†; ***Ital.:*** Citrizan Antibiotico; ***Neth.:*** Rheumajecta†; ***NZ:*** Omnicare 1 Step; ***Thai.:*** Pulvo 47; ***USA:*** UltraCare.

## Catechu

Gambier; Gambir; Pale Catechu.

*CAS — 8001-48-7.*

NOTE. Distinguish from Black Catechu (p.1661).

**Pharmacopoeias.** In *Jpn.* Also in *BP(Vet).*

*Chin.* and *Jpn* include Ramulus Uncariae cum Uncis, the thorn, from various species of *Uncaria.*

**BP(Vet) 2003** (Catechu). A dried aqueous extract of the leaves and young shoots of *Uncaria gambier* occurring as dull pale greyish-brown to dark reddish-brown cubes. Odourless or almost odourless.

### Profile

Catechu is an astringent and has been given in preparations for the treatment of diarrhoea and other gastrointestinal disorders.

### Preparations

**Proprietary Preparations** (details are given in Part 3)

**Multi-ingredient:** ***Austral.:*** Chemists Own Diarrhoea Mixture; Diarcalm†; ***Fr.:*** Elixir Bonjean; ***Ital.:*** Flavion; ***S.Afr.:*** Enterodyne; ***UK:*** Chesty Cough Relief; Spanish Tummy Mixture.

## CD4 Antibodies

Anti-CD4 Monoclonal Antibodies; Anticuerpos CD4; CD4mAb; Monoclonal CD4 Antibodies.

### Profile

Monoclonal antibodies raised against CD4 receptors are under investigation in the treatment of immunologically mediated disorders, such as rheumatoid arthritis, multiple sclerosis, inflammatory bowel disease, asthma, cutaneous T-cell lymphoma and various other skin disorders, with the aim of decreasing and eliminating circulating helper T lymphocytes. They have also been tried in transplantation. CD4 antibodies investigated include clenoliximab, keliximab, and priliximab.

◊ References.


1. Robinet E, *et al.* CD4 monoclonal antibody administration in atopic dermatitis. *J Am Acad Dermatol* 1997; **36:** 582–8.

2. van Oosten BW, *et al.* Treatment of multiple sclerosis with the monoclonal anti-CD4 antibody cM-T412: results of a randomized, double-blind, placebo-controlled, MR-monitored phase II trial. *Neurology* 1997; **49:** 351–7.
3. Stronkhorst A, *et al.* CD4 antibody treatment in patients with active Crohn's disease: a phase I dose finding study. *Gut* 1997; **40:** 320–7.
4. Cooperative Clinical Trials in Transplantation Research Group. Murine OKT4A immunosuppression in cadaver donor renal allograft recipients: a cooperative clinical trials in transplantation pilot study. *Transplantation* 1997; **15:** 1243–51.
5. Kon OM, *et al.* Randomised, dose-ranging, placebo-controlled study of chimeric antibody to CD4 (keliximab) in chronic severe asthma. *Lancet* 1998; **352:** 1109–13.
6. Yocum DE, *et al.* Clinical and immunologic effects of a PRIMATIZED anti-CD4 monoclonal antibody in active rheumatoid arthritis: results of a phase I, single dose, dose escalating trial. *J Rheumatol* 1998; **25:** 1257–62.
7. Wendling D, *et al.* A randomized, double blind, placebo controlled multicenter trial of murine anti-CD4 monoclonal antibody therapy in rheumatoid arthritis. *J Rheumatol* 1998; **25:** 1457–61.
8. Gottlieb AB, *et al.* Anti-CD4 monoclonal antibody treatment of moderate to severe psoriasis vulgaris: results of a pilot, multicenter, multiple-dose, placebo-controlled study. *J Am Acad Dermatol* 2000; **43:** 595–604.

## Celery

Apio; Apium; Celery Fruit; Celery Seed.

*CAS — 8015-90-5 (celery oil).*

### Profile

Celery consists of the dried ripe fruits of *Apium graveolens* (Umbelliferae). Other parts of the plant are also used. Celery is reported to have diuretic properties and has been included in herbal preparations for rheumatic disorders. Celery oil has also been used similarly. Allergic and photoallergic reactions have been reported.

Celery is also used in homoeopathic medicine and in cookery.

◊ References.

1. Houghton P. Bearberry, dandelion and celery. *Pharm J* 1995; **255:** 272–3.

**Interactions.** For a report of severe phototoxicity occurring in a patient who had consumed celery soup before undergoing PUVA therapy, see Interactions under Methoxsalen, p.1153.

### Preparations

**Proprietary Preparations** (details are given in Part 3)

**Multi-ingredient:** ***Arg.:*** Calmtabs; ***Austral.:*** Arthriforte†; Arthritic Pain Herbal Formula 1†; Bioglan Arthri Plus†; Devils Claw Plus†; Fluid Loss†; Lifesystem Herbal Formula 1 Arthritic Aid†; ***UK:*** Mixed Vegetable Tablets; Modern Herbals Rheumatic Pain; Rheumatic Pain; Rheumatic Pain Relief; Rheumatic Pain Tablets†; Vegetex.

## Cellobiose

Glucobiosa. 4-*O*-β-D-Glucopyranosyl-D-glucose.

$C_{12}H_{22}O_{11}$ = 342.3.

*CAS — 528-50-7.*

### Profile

Cellobiose is an indigestible disaccharide that has been used to assess intestinal permeability. It has been used as an alternative to lactulose in the differential sugar absorption test (p.1269).

◊ References.

1. Hodges S, *et al.* Cellobiose: mannitol differential permeability in small bowel disease. *Arch Dis Child* 1989; **64:** 853–5.
2. Juby LD, *et al.* Cellobiose/mannitol sugar test—a sensitive tubeless test for coeliac disease: results on 1010 unselected patients. *Gut* 1989; **30:** 476–80.

## Cellulase *(USAN)*

Celulasa.

*CAS — 9012-54-8.*

### Profile

Cellulase is a concentrate of cellulose-splitting (cellulolytic) enzymes derived from *Aspergillus niger* or other sources. It is used in food processing and has been given orally with other digestive enzymes for its supposed benefit in minor digestive disorders such as dyspepsia and flatulence. Hemicellulase has been given for similar purposes.

### Preparations

**Proprietary Preparations** (details are given in Part 3)

**Multi-ingredient:** ***Arg.:*** Biletan Enzimatico; Biluen Enzimatico; Dom-Polienzim; Gastridin-E; Gastron Fuerte; Pakinase; Pankreon Total; Polienzim; ***Austria:*** Arca-Enzym; Gallo Merz†; Ora-Gallin; ***Belg.:*** Digestomen; ***Braz.:*** Dasc; Digeplus; Espasmo Novozyme†; Essen; Normopride Enzimatico†; Sintozima; ***Chile:*** Onoton; ***Fr.:*** Pancrelase†; ***Hong Kong:*** Topase; ***India:*** Dipep; Farizym; Panolase; ***Ital.:*** Digestopan; Essen Enzimatico; Luizym†; ***Mex.:*** Dixiflen; Espaven Enzimatico; Ochozim; Onoton; ***Port.:*** Colerin-F; Espasmo Canulase; ***S.Afr.:*** Spasmo-Canulase; ***Spain:*** Espasmo Digestomen†; Lidobama Complex†; Paidozim; Polidasa†; ***Switz.:*** Spasmo-Canulase; Zymoplex; ***Thai.:*** Sanzyme-S; ***USA:*** Arco-Lase Plus†; Arco-Lase†; Enzyme; Gustase Plus†; Gustase†.

## Centaury

Centáurea menor; Centaurii Minoris Herba; Petite Centaurée; Tausendgüldenkraut.

**Pharmacopoeias.** In *Eur.* (see p.vi).

**Ph. Eur. 5.0** (Centaury). The whole or cut dried flowering tops of *Centaurium erythraea* (*C. minus*; *C. umbellatum*; *Erythraea centaurium*). It has a very bitter taste. Protect from light.

### Profile

Centaury is used as a bitter, including for appetite loss and dyspepsia.

**Hepatotoxicity.** A report[1] of hepatotoxicity possibly associated with the use of Copaltra, a herbal preparation marketed as an adjunct in the treatment of diabetes mellitus and containing centaury and *Coutarea latiflora* (copalchi) (Rubiaceae). A further 5 cases had been reported to the French pharmacovigilance network.

1. Wurtz A-S, *et al.* Possible hepatotoxicity from Copaltra, an herbal medicine. *Ann Pharmacother* 2002; **36:** 941–2.

### Preparations

**Proprietary Preparations** (details are given in Part 3)

**Multi-ingredient:** ***Austria:*** Amylatin; Aponatura Starkungs; Apotheker Bauer's Magentee; China-Eisenwein; Eryval; Gewusst wie Leber-Gallentee; Grippogran; Kneipp Verdauungs-Tee; Krauterdoktor Erkaltungstropfen; Krauterdoktor Harnstein- und Nieren-griesstropfen; Krauterdoktor Verdauungsfordernde Tropfen; Krauterpfarrer Weidinger Tee bei Sodbrennen; Mag Kottas Blahungs-Verdauungstee; Mag Kottas Krauterexpress-Blahungs-Verdauungstee; Mag Kottas Krauterexpress-Magen-Darm-Tee; Magentee EF-EM-ES; Mariazeller; Neuners Krautertee Nr 14 - Verdauungstee; Neuners Krautertee Nr 17 - Lebertee; Neuners Krautertee Nr 20 - Kreislauftee; Neuners Krautertee Nr 9 - Magentee; Sidroga Magen-Darm-Tee; Solisan; St Radegunder Verdauungstee; ***Braz.:*** Camomila†; ***Fr.:*** Copaltra†; Diacure; Tisane Hepatique de Hoerdt; Tisanes de l'Abbe Hamon no 16†; ***Ger.:*** Alsicur†; Amara-Tropfen; Aranidorm-S†; Canephron; Cefagastrin†; Hevert-Magen-Galle-Leber-Tee†; JuGrippan†; Kneipp Verdauungs-Tee N†; Leber-Galle-Tropfen 83; Montana N; Phonix Gastriphon†; Stullmaton; ***Hong Kong:*** Canephron N†; ***Ital.:*** Assenzio (Specie Composta); Centaurea (Specie Composta); Fluxoten†; Genziana (Specie Composta); ***Spain:*** Digestol Sanatorium†; Natusor Hepavesical; Odisor; ***Switz.:*** Gastrosan; Phytomed Gastro†; Tisane pour l'estomac; ***UK:*** Digest†.

## Cereus

Cactus; Night-blooming Cereus.

### Profile

Cereus, the flowers and stems of night-blooming cereus (*Selenicereus grandiflorus*; *Cactus grandiflorus*) (Cactaceae), is thought to have cardiac stimulant actions and has been used in various cardiovascular disorders. It has also been used as an anthelmintic and in the treatment of rheumatism.

It is also used in homoeopathic medicine.

### Preparations

**Proprietary Preparations** (details are given in Part 3)

**Multi-ingredient:** ***Ger.:*** Cardibisana; Oxacant N; Oxacant-forte N; Oxacant-Khella N.

## Ceruletide *(BAN, USAN, rINN)*

Caerulein; Cerulein; Ceruletida; FI-6934; 883-S.

$C_{58}H_{73}N_{13}O_{21}S_2$ = 1352.4.

*CAS — 17650-98-5 (ceruletide); 71247-25-1 (ceruletide diethylamine).*

*ATC — V04CC04.*

NOTE. The name Ceruleinum has been applied to Indigo Carmine (p.1700).

**Description.** Ceruletide is a decapeptide amide originally isolated from the skin of the Australian frog, *Hyla caerulea*, and other amphibians. Ceruletide may exist as a salt with 1 to 3 moles of diethylamine (ceruletide diethylamine).

### Adverse Effects

Ceruletide stimulates gallbladder contraction and gastrointestinal muscle and may give rise to abdominal discomfort. Hypotensive reactions may also occur.

### Uses and Administration

Ceruletide is structurally related to pancreozymin (p.1727) and has similar actions. When given parenterally it stimulates gallbladder contraction and relaxes the sphincter of Oddi; it also causes an increase in the secretion of pancreatic enzymes and stimulates intestinal muscle.

As ceruletide diethylamine it is used as an aid to diagnostic radiology and in the management of paralytic ileus. It is also used in tests of pancreatic exocrine function, sometimes with secretin (p.1742); these studies generally require duodenal intubation of the patient and examination of duodenal aspirate and are rarely performed.

For most radiographic procedures of the biliary and digestive tracts ceruletide diethylamine is given by intramuscular injection in a dose equivalent to 300 nanograms/kg of ceruletide. Doses equivalent to 1 to 2 nanograms/kg per minute are given by intravenous infusion in pancreatic function tests and in the treatment of paralytic ileus.

◊ References.

1. Vincent ME, *et al.* Pharmacology, clinical uses, and adverse effects of ceruletide, a cholecystokinetic agent. *Pharmacotherapy* 1982; **2:** 223–34.
2. Gullo L, *et al.* Caerulein induced plasma amino acid decrease: a simple, sensitive, and specific test of pancreatic function. *Gut* 1990; **31:** 926–9.

### Preparations

**Proprietary Preparations** (details are given in Part 3)
***Ger.:*** Takus.

## Chamomile

Manzanilla.

**Description.** The name Chamomile is used for the dried flowerheads from 2 species of *Compositae* having similar medicinal properties:

- Chamomile from *Anthemis nobilis* (*Chamaemelum nobile*) is known as Chamomile Flowers, Chamomillae Romanae Flos, Manzanilla Romana, or Roman Chamomile Flower.
- Chamomile from *Matricaria recutita* (*Chamomilla recutita*) is known as Camomile Allemande, Camomilla, Chamomilla, Chamomillae Anthodium, Flos Chamomillae, Flos Chamomillae Vulgaris, German Chamomile, Hungarian Chamomile, Kamillenblüten, Manzanilla Ordinaria, Matricaria Flower, or Matricariae Flos

**Pharmacopoeias.** *Eur.* (see p.vi) includes chamomile from *Anthemis nobilis* and *Matricaria recutita*. *Pol.* and *USNF* include chamomile from *Matricaria recutita*.

*Eur.* also includes Matricaria Oil.

**Ph. Eur. 5.0** (Chamomile Flower, Roman; Chamomile Flowers BP 2003). The dried flowerheads obtained from the cultivated double variety of *Anthemis nobilis* (*Chamaemelum nobile*), containing not less than 0.7% v/w of essential oil. It has a strong characteristic odour. Protect from light.

**Ph. Eur. 5.0** (Matricaria Flower; Matricaria Flowers BP 2003). The dried flowerheads obtained from *Matricaria recutita* (*Chamomilla recutita*), containing not less than 0.4% v/w of blue essential oil and 0.25% of apigenin-7-glucoside, calculated with reference to the dried drug. It has a characteristic, pleasant and aromatic odour. Protect from light.

**Ph. Eur. 5.0** (Matricaria Oil). The blue essential oil obtained by steam distillation from the fresh or dried flower-heads or flowering tops of *Matricaria recutita* (*Chamomilla recutita*). There are 2 types of matricaria oil which are characterised as rich in bisabolol oxides, or rich in levomenol. Store in a well-filled, airtight container, protected from light at a temperature not exceeding 25°.

**USNF 22** (Chamomile). The dried flowerheads of *Matricaria recutita* (*Matricaria chamomilla*, *Matricaria chamomilla* var. *courrantiana*, *Chamomilla recutita*) (Asteraceae alt. Compositae). It contains not less than 0.4% of blue volatile oil, not less than 0.3% of apigenin-7-glucoside, and not less than 0.15% of bisabolan derivatives, calculated as levomenol. Protect from light.

### Profile

Chamomile has been applied externally as a poultice in the early stages of inflammation, and preparations containing chamomile or extracts of chamomile (including the oil or a constituent, chamazulene), have been used for skin disorders, including the prevention and treatment of cracked nipples and nappy rash. It is also used in homoeopathic medicine. 'Chamomile tea' is a domestic remedy for indigestion and has also been reported to have hypnotic properties.

There have been reports of contact sensitivity and anaphylaxis.

◊ Reviews.

1. Berry M. The chamomiles. *Pharm J* 1995; **254:** 191–3.

**Hypersensitivity.** References.

1. Van Ketel WG. Allergy to Matricaria chamomilla. *Contact Dermatitis* 1987; **16:** 50–1.
2. McGeorge BC, Steele MC. Allergic contact dermatitis of the nipple from Roman chamomile ointment. *Contact Dermatitis* 1991; **24:** 139–40.
3. Rodriguez-Serna M, *et al.* Allergic and systemic contact dermatitis from Matricaria chamomilla tea. *Contact Dermatitis* 1998; **39:** 192–3.
4. Jensen-Jarolim E, *et al.* Fatal outcome of anaphylaxis to camomile-containing enema during labor: a case study. *J Allergy Clin Immunol* 1998; **102:** 1041–2.
5. Giordano-Labadie F, *et al.* Allergic contact dermatitis from camomile used in phytotherapy. *Contact Dermatitis* 2000; **42:** 247.
6. Foti C, *et al.* Contact urticaria from Matricaria chamomilla. *Contact Dermatitis* 2000; **42:** 360–1.

### Preparations

***Ph. Eur.:*** Matricaria Liquid Extract.

**Proprietary Preparations** (details are given in Part 3)
***Austral.:*** Camoderm†; ***Austria:*** Chamillamont; Kamillat; Kamillen; Kamillomed; Kamillosan; Markalakt; ***Belg.:*** Kamillosan; ***Braz.:*** Kamillosan; ***Chile:*** Kamillosan; ***Fr.:*** Cefamig; ***Ger.:*** APS Balneum†; Azulon; Chamo S; Eukamillat; Galenat Kamill N; Kamillan supra; Kamille N; Kamillen; Kamillen-Bad N Ritsert; Kamillenbad Intradermi; Kamillencreme N; Kamillenextract; Kamillin; Kamilloderm; Kamillosan; Markalakt; Matmille; PC 30 N; Perkamillon†; Sagitta Kamillbad†; Soledum med; ***India:*** Kamillosan; ***Irl.:*** Kamillosan; ***Ital.:*** Ceru Spray; Milla; ***Mex.:*** Kamillosan; ***NZ:*** Kamillosan; ***Spain:*** Kamillosan†; ***Switz.:*** Edmilla†; Kamillen-Bad; Kamillin Medipharm;

Kamillofluid; Kamillosan; Perkamillon†; **UK:** Ashton & Parsons Infants Powders; Kamillosan.

**Multi-ingredient:** numerous preparations are listed in Part 3.

## Chaparral

### Profile

Chaparral is derived from the creosote bush, *Larrea tridentata* (Zygophyllaceae). It has been included in various herbal preparations but such use has been associated with severe hepatotoxicity. Recommendations that products containing chaparral should not be consumed have been made in several countries.

Masoprocol (p.566) is an antineoplastic isolated from creosote bush.

**Hepatotoxicity.** References.

1. Gordon DW, *et al.* Chaparral ingestion: the broadening spectrum of liver injury caused by herbal medications. *JAMA* 1995; **273:** 489–90.
2. Batchelor WB, *et al.* Chaparral-induced hepatic injury. *Am J Gastroenterol* 1995; **90:** 831–3.
3. Sheikh NM, *et al.* Chaparral-associated hepatotoxicity. *Arch Intern Med* 1997; **157:** 913–19.

### Preparations

**Proprietary Preparations** (details are given in Part 3)

**Multi-ingredient: Austral.:** Proyeast†.

## Chenodeoxycholic Acid *(BAN, rINN)*

Ácido quenodeoxicólico; Acidum Chenodeoxycholicum; CDCA; Chenic Acid; Chenodiol *(USAN)*. 3α,7α-Dihydroxy-5β-cholan-24-oic acid.

$C_{24}H_{40}O_4$ = 392.6.

*CAS — 474-25-9.*

*ATC — A05AA01.*

**Pharmacopoeias.** In *Eur.* (see p.vi).

**Ph. Eur. 5.0** (Chenodeoxycholic Acid). A white or almost white powder. Very slightly soluble in water; freely soluble in alcohol; soluble in acetone; slightly soluble in dichloromethane.

### Adverse Effects and Precautions

As for Ursodeoxycholic Acid, p.1761. Diarrhoea may occur more frequently than with ursodeoxycholic acid. A transient rise in liver-function test values and hypercholesterolaemia (low-density lipoprotein) have been reported with chenodeoxycholic acid.

Chenodeoxycholic acid is embryotoxic in some *animals*.

### Interactions

As for Ursodeoxycholic Acid, p.1761.

### Pharmacokinetics

Chenodeoxycholic acid is absorbed from the gastrointestinal tract and undergoes first-pass metabolism and enterohepatic recycling. It is partly conjugated in the liver before being excreted into the bile and, under the influence of intestinal bacteria, the free and conjugated forms undergo 7α-dehydroxylation to lithocholic acid. Some lithocholic acid is excreted directly in the faeces and the rest absorbed, mainly to be conjugated and sulfated by the liver before excretion in the faeces. Chenodeoxycholic acid also undergoes epimerisation to ursodeoxycholic acid.

◊ References.

1. Crosignani A, *et al.* Clinical pharmacokinetics of therapeutic bile acids. *Clin Pharmacokinet* 1996; **30:** 333–58.

### Uses and Administration

Chenodeoxycholic acid is a naturally occurring bile acid (p.1660). When given orally it reduces hepatic synthesis of cholesterol and provides additional bile salts to the pool available for solubilisation of cholesterol and lipids. It has been used for the dissolution of cholesterol-rich gallstones (p.1761) in patients with a functioning gallbladder, in usual doses of about 15 mg/kg daily. The daily dose may be divided unequally and the larger dose given before bedtime to counteract the increase in biliary cholesterol concentrations seen overnight. Treatment may need to be given for up to 2 years, depending on the size of the stone. It should be continued for about 3 months after radiological disappearance of the stones. Chenodeoxycholic acid is also used in reduced doses with ursodeoxycholic acid.

### Preparations

**Proprietary Preparations** (details are given in Part 3)

***Austria:*** Chenofalk; ***Belg.:*** Chenofalk; ***Braz.:*** Fluibil†; ***Ger.:*** Chenofalk; ***Hong Kong:*** Chenofalk; ***Irl.:*** Chendol†; Chenofalk†; ***Israel:*** Soluston; ***Mex.:*** Chenofalk; Sulobil; ***Neth.:*** Chenofalk; ***Port.:*** Chebil; ***Spain:*** Quenobilan; Quenocol; ***Switz.:*** Chenofalk†.

**Multi-ingredient: *Austria:*** Lithofalk; ***Ger.:*** Lithofalk; Urso Mix; Ursofalk + Chenofalk†; ***Ital.:*** Bilenor; Litobile†; ***Switz.:*** Lithofalk†.

## Chloroacetophenone

Cloroacetofenona; CN; Phenacyl Chloride. 2-Chloroacetophenone.

$C_8H_7ClO$ = 154.6.

*CAS — 532-27-4.*

NOTE. The name mace is applied to solutions of chloroacetophenone.

### Profile

Chloroacetophenone is a lachrymatory which is irritant to the skin and eyes. It has been used in a riot-control gas.

◊ References.

1. Hu H, *et al.* Tear gas—harassing agent or toxic chemical weapon? *JAMA* 1989; **262:** 660–3.
2. Treudler R, *et al.* Occupational contact dermatitis due to 2-chloroacetophenone tear gas. *Br J Dermatol* 1999; **140:** 531–4.

## Chloroplatinic Acid

Cloroplatínico, ácido; Kloroplatinasyra. Hexachloroplatinic acid hexahydrate.

$H_2PtCl_6,6H_2O$ = 517.9.

*CAS — 16941-12-1 (anhydrous chloroplatinic acid); 18497-13-7 (chloroplatinic acid hexahydrate).*

### Profile

Aqueous solutions of platinic chloride ($PtCl_4$ = 336.9) are used in corneal tattooing solutions.

## Chondroitin Sulfate Sodium

Chondroitin 4-Sulfate (chondroitin sulfate A); Chondroitin Sulphate Sodium; CSA (chondroitin sulfate A); Sodium Chondroitin Sulfate.

$(C_{14}H_{19}NO_{14}SNa_2)_n$.

*CAS — 9007-28-7 (chondroitin sulfate); 9082-07-9 (chondroitin sulfate sodium); 24967-93-9 (chondroitin sulfate A); 39455-18-0 (chondroitin sulfate A sodium); 25322-46-7 (chondroitin sulfate C); 12678-07-8 (chondroitin sulfate C sodium).*

*ATC — M01AX25.*

**Pharmacopoeias.** In *USNF.*

**USNF 22** (Chondroitin Sulfate Sodium). The sodium salt of the sulfated linear glycosaminoglycan obtained from bovine, porcine, or avian cartilages of healthy and domestic animals used for food by humans. It consists mostly of the sodium salt of the sulfate ester of *N*-acetylchondrosamine (2-acetamido-2-deoxy-β-D-galactopyranose) and D-glucuronic acid copolymer. These hexoses are alternately linked β-1,4 and β-1,3 in the polymer. Chondrosamine moieties in the prevalent glycosaminoglycan are monosulfated primarily on position 4 and less so on position 6. Chondroitin sulfate sodium is extremely hygroscopic once dried. Store in airtight containers.

### Profile

Chondroitin sulfate is an acid mucopolysaccharide that is a constituent of most cartilaginous tissues. It is used as the sodium salt, chondroitin sodium sulfate. It is given orally in reactive arthritides (see under Spondyloarthropathies, p.11), such as gonococcal arthritis, and is sometimes given with glucosamine for its supposed chondroprotective action in bone, joint, and connective tissue disorders. It is also used for its visco-elastic properties as an adjunct to ocular surgical procedures, including cataract extraction and intra-ocular lens implantation, and has been used for the relief of dry eye. A medium containing chondroitin sulfate A has been used to preserve corneas for transplantation. Chondroitin sulfate sodium has also been used as a means of replacing the glycosaminoglycan layer in the bladder in the treatment of interstitial cystitis (p.1473). Chondroitin sulfate A and C are components of the heparinoid danaparoid (p.891).

**Osteoarthritis.** For references to the use of chondroitin in the treatment of osteoarthritis, see under Glucosamine, p.1694.

### Preparations

***USNF 22:*** Chondroitin Sulfate Sodium Tablets; Glucosamine and Chondroitin Sulfate Sodium Tablets.

**Proprietary Preparations** (details are given in Part 3)

***Arg.:*** Bioflogil; Condroitina; Condrosulf; Structum; ***Austria:*** Condrosulf; ***Braz.:*** Dunason; ***Canad.:*** Uracyst-S; ***Chile:*** Condrosulf; ***Fr.:*** Chondrosulf; Lacrypos; Structum; ***Port.:*** Ossin; ***Switz.:*** Condrosulf; Structum.

**Multi-ingredient: *Arg.:*** Asotrex; Optilac; Viscoat; ***Austral.:*** Duovisc; Viscoat; ***Belg.:*** Viscoat†; ***Canad.:*** Uracyst-S Test Kit; ***Fr.:*** Viscoat; ***Ger.:*** Duovisc; Viscoat; ***Hong Kong:*** Duovisc; Viscoat; ***Ital.:*** Joint Support; Viscoat; ***Malaysia:*** Viscoat; ***NZ:*** Viscoat; ***S.Afr.:*** Duovisc; Viscoat; ***Singapore:*** Duovisc; Flexeze; Viscoat; ***Switz.:*** Viscoat†; ***Thai.:*** Duovisc; Viscoat; ***UK:*** Jointace; Viscoat†; ***USA:*** Viscoat.

## Chrome Alum

Chromium Potassium Sulfate; Chromium Potassium Sulphate; Cromo, alumbre de.

$KCr(SO_4)_2,12H_2O$ = 499.4.

*CAS — 10141-00-1 (anhydrous chrome alum); 7788-99-0 (chromium potassium sulfate dodecahydrate).*

### Profile

Chrome alum is used in tanning, as a mordant in dyeing, and for hardening gelatin in photographic materials. It has been used as a sclerosant in medicine.

### Preparations

**Proprietary Preparations** (details are given in Part 3)

**Multi-ingredient: *Arg.:*** Skleremo; ***Braz.:*** Varikromo; ***Fr.:*** Scleremo.

## Chromium Trioxide

Anhídrido Crómico; Chromic Acid; Chromic Anhydride; Cromo, trióxido de.

$CrO_3$ = 99.99.

*CAS — 1333-82-0.*

### Profile

Chromium trioxide and other chromium compounds are used in industry. Solutions of chromium trioxide are corrosive, acting by oxidation. Repeated contact with chromium and its salts may cause eczematous dermatitis, particularly in hypersensitive persons and can also cause deep perforating ulcers known as 'chrome holes'. If inhaled, chromic dusts cause rhinitis and painless ulcers which may perforate the nasal septum; inhalation may cause severe lung damage and inflammation of the eyes. There may also be involvement of the CNS and there is an increased risk of lung cancer. Hexavalent chromium compounds are more dangerous than di- or trivalent compounds.

Acute symptoms of poisoning from the ingestion of chromium salts include intense thirst, dizziness, abdominal pain with vomiting and diarrhoea, hepatic injury, anuria or oliguria, and peripheral vascular collapse. Kidney damage may lead to fatal uraemia. Treatment is symptomatic and supportive. Protective measures should be taken when handling or working with chromium and its salts.

Chromium trioxide was formerly used as a caustic and astringent.

Chromium is an essential trace element as described on p.1425.

**Adverse effects.** General references[1-4] to chromium toxicity including reports of poisoning with ammonium dichromate,[5] chromium tripicolinate,[6] chromium trioxide,[7] potassium dichromate,[8-10] and sodium dichromate.[11]

1. Chromium. *Environmental Health Criteria 61.* Geneva: WHO, 1988.
2. Health and Safety Executive. The toxicity of chromium and inorganic chromium compounds. *Toxicity Review 21.* London: HMSO, 1989.
3. Barceloux DG. Chromium. *J Toxicol Clin Toxicol* 1999; **37:** 173–94.
4. Dayan AD, Paine AJ. Mechanisms of chromium toxicity, carcinogenicity and allergenicity: review of the literature from 1985 to 2000. *Hum Exp Toxicol* 2001; **20:** 439–51.
5. Meert KL, *et al.* Acute ammonium dichromate poisoning. *Ann Emerg Med* 1994; **24:** 748–50.
6. Cerulli J, *et al.* Chromium picolinate toxicity. *Ann Pharmacother* 1998; **32:** 428–31.
7. Matey P, *et al.* Chromic acid burns: early aggressive excision is the best method to prevent systemic toxicity. *J Burn Care Rehabil* 2000; **21:** 241–5.
8. Michie CA, *et al.* Poisoning with a traditional remedy containing potassium dichromate. *Hum Exp Toxicol* 1991; **10:** 129–31.
9. Stift A, *et al.* Liver transplantation for potassium dichromate poisoning. *N Engl J Med* 1998; **338:** 766–7.
10. Kolacinski Z, *et al.* Acute potassium dichromate poisoning: a toxicokinetic case study. *J Toxicol Clin Toxicol* 1999; **37:** 785–91.
11. Ellis EN, *et al.* Effects of hemodialysis and dimercaprol in acute dichromate poisoning. *J Toxicol Clin Toxicol* 1982; **19:** 249–58.

**Handling.** Chromium trioxide is a powerful oxidising agent and is liable to explode in contact with small quantities of alcohol, ether, glycerol, and other organic substances.

## Chromocarb Diethylamine *(rINNM)*

Cromocarbo, dietilamina de. The diethylamine salt of 4-oxo-4*H*-1-benzopyran-2-carboxylic acid .

$C_{14}H_{17}O_4N$ = 263.3.

*CAS — 4940-39-0 (chromocarb).*

### Profile

Chromocarb diethylamine is used to reduce capillary haemorrhage (including conjunctival haemorrhage) associated with various disorders, and for venous insufficiency. It is given by mouth in doses of 0.6 to 1.2 g daily in divided doses. It is also used as eye drops; 1 or 2 drops of a 10% solution have been instilled up to 6 times daily.

### Preparations

**Proprietary Preparations** (details are given in Part 3)

***Arg.:*** Angioftal; ***Belg.:*** Angiophtal†; ***Fr.:*** Angiophtal; Campel; ***Ital.:*** Fludarene; ***Port.:*** Fradilen; ***Spain:*** Activadone.

## Chrysoidine Hydrochloride Citrate

Crisoidina, hidrocloruro del citrato de. 4-Phenylazobenzene-1,3-diamine hydrochloride citrate; Azobenzene-2,4-diamine hydrochloride citrate.

$C_{12}H_{12}N_4,HCl,C_6H_8O_7$ = 440.8.

*CAS — 532-82-1 (chrysoidine hydrochloride); 5909-04-6 (chrysoidine hydrochloride citrate).*

### Profile

Chrysoidine hydrochloride citrate has been used as a dye but has been associated with tumours of the bladder.

**Carcinogenicity.** The development of tumours of the urinary bladder in anglers was possibly associated with the use of chrysoidine hydrochloride (chrysoidine Y; CI Basic Orange 2; Colour Index No. 11270) for colouring the maggots used as bait.[1-3]

1. Searle CE, Teale J. Chrysoidine-dyed bait: a possible carcinogenic hazard to anglers? *Lancet* 1982; **i:** 564.

2. Sole GM. Maggots dyed with chrysoidine: a possible risk to anglers. *BMJ* 1984; **289:** 1043–4.
3. Massey JA, *et al.* Maggots dyed with chrysoidine. *BMJ* 1984; **289:** 1451–2.


## Chymopapain *(BAN, USAN, rINN)*

BAX-1526; NSC-107079; Quimopapaína; Quimopapaina.

*CAS — 9001-09-6.*

*ATC — M09AB01.*

**Description.** Chymopapain is a proteolytic enzyme isolated from the latex of papaya (*Carica papaya*), differing from papain in electrophoretic mobility, solubility, and substrate specificity. Molecular weight approximately 27 000.

### Units

One nanokatal (nKat) is defined as the amount of chymopapain which produces 1 nanomole of *p*-nitroaniline per second from DL-benzoylarginine-*p*-nitroanilide substrate at pH 6.4 and 37°.

In some countries CTE units have been used, defined as the amount of chymopapain which produces a hydrolysate from acid-denatured haemoglobin at pH 4.0 in one minute with an optical density at 275 nm equivalent to that of a tyrosine solution 0.0001%.

### Adverse Effects

The most important adverse effect of chymopapain is anaphylaxis, which can occur in up to about 1% of patients. It has resulted in fatalities and restricts use to a single treatment session per patient. Typical symptoms include angioedema, hypotension, laryngeal oedema and bronchospasm, shock, and cardiac arrest. Allergic skin reactions may also occur. Other reported reactions include headache, nausea and vomiting, paralytic ileus, urinary retention, thrombophlebitis, paraesthesias, foot-drop, and discitis. Severe muscle spasm and an increase in back pain are common. Paraplegia, acute transverse myelitis, and intracerebral and subarachnoid haemorrhage have occurred.

**Incidence of adverse effects.** A 1984 postmarketing surveillance study on a US chymopapain preparation for intradiscal injection (Chymodiactin) involved data from 29 075 patients (representing about 50% of the total number of vials sold).[1] Anaphylactic reactions were confirmed in 194 patients (0.67%), 2 of whom died. The incidence was higher in women than in men. In 52 cases the reaction occurred after the test dose. Serious neurological reactions reported were: cerebral haemorrhage (6 cases, 3 fatal; autopsy revealed that they had underlying cerebrovascular abnormalities); paraplegia (11 cases, 5 of which may have been due to incorrect needle placement); transverse myelitis with paraplegia (2 cases, after 2 and 3 weeks, with subsequent recovery); and seizures (2 cases on injection and 1 several days after the procedure). Twenty-two patients had discitis with severe back pain and spasm. In 9 cases bacteria could be cultured, and 1 patient subsequently developed fatal *Staphylococcus aureus* meningitis.

Another review[2] of serious reactions associated with chymopapain between 1982 and 1991 (including data from the earlier postmarketing study) involved 121 reports among about 135 000 patients. They included fatal anaphylaxis (7), infections (24), haemorrhage (32), and neurological reactions (32).

Both reviews concluded that careful attention to proper patient selection and correct techniques of intradiscal needle placement are the most important factors in avoiding adverse effects with chymopapain.


1. Agre K, *et al.* Chymodiactin postmarketing surveillance: demographic and adverse experience data in 29075 patients. *Spine* 1984; **9:** 479–85.
2. Nordby EJ, *et al.* Safety of chemonucleolysis: adverse effects reported in the United States, 1982–1991. *Clin Orthop* 1993; **293:** 122–34.


### Precautions

Chymopapain should not be used in those patients with a known sensitivity to papaya proteins or in patients with progressive paralysis, or tumours of the spinal cord, or lesions of the cauda equina. Severe spondylolisthesis is also a contra-indication. It should not be given to patients with heart failure, coronary artery disease, or respiratory failure who may be at increased risk if anaphylaxis occurs, nor to patients receiving beta blockers.

Care is required in administering chymopapain to ensure that the injection is into the disc and not intrathecal. However, discography is not recommended since the use of contrast media may exacerbate neurotoxicity and may inactivate the enzyme.

The risk of allergic reactions associated with chymopapain is so high that no patient should ever receive it more than once. Tests to identify those most at risk and pretreatment with antihistamines ($H_1$ and $H_2$) and corticosteroids may be used, but facilities for the emergency management of anaphylactic reactions should always be to hand when giving patients chymopapain. The risk of anaphylaxis is higher in women.

Injection of more than one disc is associated with an increased frequency of neurological reactions; therefore, such injection should only be carried out following confirmation of definite further disc involvement.

### Uses and Administration

Chymopapain is used as an injection into the intervertebral disc in the treatment of sciatic pain and other symptoms secondary to herniation of intervertebral discs of the lumbar spine (chemonucleolysis).

Chymopapain injection should preferably be given under local, rather than general, anaesthesia. The dose for a single intervertebral disc is 2 to 4 nanokatals, with a maximum dose per patient of 8 nanokatals.

**Chemonucleolysis.** The use of chymopapain for the treatment of lumbar disc herniation remains controversial. While some clinicians consider it when conservative management of low back pain (p.7) has failed and before proceeding to surgery[1] others are reported to have largely abandoned the technique in view of its serious adverse effects.[2] The safety and efficacy of chemonucleolysis with chymopapain continues to be debated; it is still considered by some[3-6] to be a useful alternative to surgery in correctly selected patients and with strict adherence to preparation and technique.


1. Williams F. Chemonucleolysis for treating sciatica. *Br J Hosp Med* 1994; **52:** 52.
2. Bush K. Chemonucleolysis for treating sciatica. *Br J Hosp Med* 1994; **52:** 52–3.
3. Nordby EJ, *et al.* Chemonucleolysis. *Spine* 1996; **21:** 1102–5.
4. Brown MD. Update on chemonucleolysis. *Spine* 1996; **21** (24 suppl): 62S–68S.
5. Poynton AR, *et al.* Chymopapain chemonucleolysis: a review of 105 cases. *J R Coll Surg Edinb* 1998; **43:** 407–9.
6. Wittenberg RH, *et al.* Five-year results from chemonucleolysis with chymopapain or collagenase: a prospective randomized study. *Spine* 2001; **26:** 1835–41.


### Preparations

**Proprietary Preparations** (details are given in Part 3)
***Austral.:*** Chymodiactin; ***Belg.:*** Discase†; ***Canad.:*** Chymodiactin†; ***Fr.:*** Chymodiactine†; ***Irl.:*** Chymodiactin†; ***Spain:*** Chymodiactin; ***UK:*** Chymodiactin†; ***USA:*** Chymodiactin†.

## Chymotrypsin *(BAN, rINN)*

α-Chymotrypsin; Chymotrypsinum; Quimotripsina.

*CAS — 9004-07-3.*

*ATC — B06AA04; S01KX01.*

**Pharmacopoeias.** In *Chin., Eur.* (see p.vi), and *US.*

**Ph. Eur. 5.0** (Chymotrypsin). A proteolytic enzyme obtained by the activation of chymotrypsinogen extracted from the pancreas of beef. It contains not less than 5 microkatals in each mg. A white crystalline or amorphous powder; the amorphous form is hygroscopic. Sparingly soluble in water. A 1% solution in water has a pH of 3.0 to 5.0. Solutions have a maximum stability at pH 3 and a maximum activity at about pH 8. Store at 2° to 8° in airtight containers. Protect from light.

**USP 27** (Chymotrypsin). A proteolytic enzyme crystallised from an extract of the pancreas gland of the ox, *Bos taurus* (Bovidae). It contains not less than 1000 USP units in each mg, calculated on the dried basis. A white to yellowish-white, crystalline or amorphous, odourless powder. An amount equivalent to 100 000 USP units is soluble in 10 mL of water and in 10 mL of sodium chloride 0.9%. Store in airtight containers at a temperature not exceeding 40°.

### Units

Various methods have been used to assay the potency of chymotrypsin. Ph. Eur. 5.0 expresses activity in terms of microkatals while USP 27 expresses in terms of USP units. Other units that may be encountered are FIP units, Armour units, and Denver (or Wallace or Wampole) units.

### Uses and Administration

Chymotrypsin is a proteolytic enzyme that has been used in ophthalmology for the dissection of the zonule of the lens, thus facilitating intracapsular cataract extraction and reducing trauma to the eye. For this purpose a solution of chymotrypsin in a sterile diluent such as sodium chloride 0.9% has been injected to irrigate the posterior chamber.

Chymotrypsin has also been given, usually by mouth or topically, for its supposed action in reducing soft-tissue inflammation and oedema associated with surgery or traumatic injuries, and in patients suffering from upper respiratory-tract disorders.

Hypersensitivity reactions have been reported.

### Preparations

***USP 27:*** Chymotrypsin for Ophthalmic Solution.

**Proprietary Preparations** (details are given in Part 3)
***Fr.:*** Alphacutanee; ***Ger.:*** Alpha-Chymocutan†; Alpha-Chymotrase†; ***Spain:*** Quimotrase†.

**Multi-ingredient:** ***Austria:*** Wobenzym; ***Braz.:*** Parenzyme; Parenzyme Ampicilina; Parenzyme Analgesico; Parenzyme Tetraciclina; Probenzima Ampicilina†; Probenzima Analgesico†; Thiomucase; ***Fr.:*** Alphintern†; ***Ger.:*** Enzym-Wied; Wobe-Mugos E; ***India:*** Alfapsin; Soluzyme; ***Ital.:*** Essen Enzimatico; ***Mex.:*** Ochozim; Ribotripsin; Wobe-Mugos; Wobenzym; ***Port.:*** Chimar; ***Spain:*** Bristaciclina Dental; Dertrase; Dosil Enzimatico; Doxiten Enzimatico; Epixian†; Quimodril; Solupen Enzimatico†; Terranilo†.

## Cicloxilic Acid *(rINN)*

Ácido cicloxílico. *cis*-2-Hydroxy-2-phenylcyclohexanecarboxylic acid.

$C_{13}H_{16}O_3$ = 220.3.

*CAS — 57808-63-6.*

### Profile

Cicloxilic acid has been used in the treatment of hepatic disorders.

## Ciliary Neurotrophic Factor

CNTF; Factor neurotrófico ciliar.

### Profile

Ciliary neurotrophic factor is a nerve growth factor produced in neural tissues and released in response to injury. Recombinant ciliary neurotrophic factor has been investigated in motor neurone disease (p.1739) and peripheral neuropathy. It has also been tried in obesity.

◊ References.


1. Miller RG, *et al.* A placebo-controlled trial of recombinant human ciliary neurotrophic (rhCNTF) factor in amyotrophic lateral sclerosis. *Ann Neurol* 1996; **39:** 256–60.
2. Ettinger MP, *et al.* Recombinant variant of ciliary neurotrophic factor for weight loss in obese adults: a randomized, dose-ranging study. *JAMA* 2003; **289:** 1826–32.


## Cimicifuga

Black Cohosh; Black Snakeroot; Bugbane; Cimicífuga.

NOTE. Distinguish from Blue Cohosh, p.1661.

**Pharmacopoeias.** *Chin.* includes the rhizome of *Cimicifuga heracleifolia, C. dahurica,* and *C. foetida. Jpn* includes the rhizome of *C. simplex, C. heracleifolia, C. dahurica,* and *C. foetida.*

### Profile

Cimicifuga, the roots of *Cimicifuga racemosa* (*Actaea racemosa*) (Ranunculaceae), is used for menopausal and gynaecological disorders and is included in preparations for coughs. It has been reported that it may cause vertigo, headache, prostration, and gastrointestinal irritation when taken in large doses.

It is used in homoeopathic medicine as Actaea racemosa or Actaea rac.

◊ Reviews.


1. Pepping J. Black cohosh: Cimicifuga racemosa. *Am J Health-Syst Pharm* 1999; **56:** 1400–2.
2. Jacobson JS, *et al.* Randomized trial of black cohosh for the treatment of hot flashes among women with a history of breast cancer. *J Clin Oncol* 2001; **19:** 2739–45.
3. Borrelli F, Ernst E. Cimicifuga racemosa: a systematic review of its clinical efficacy. *Eur J Clin Pharmacol* 2002; **58:** 235–41.
4. Huntley A, Ernst E. A systematic review of the safety of black cohosh. *Menopause* 2003; **10:** 58–64.


### Preparations

**Proprietary Preparations** (details are given in Part 3)
***Arg.:*** Herbaccion Menopausia; Menofem; ***Austria:*** Agnukliman; ***Braz.:*** Clifemin; Mencirax; Menofem†; ***Chile:*** Ginemaxim; Mensifem; ***Fr.:*** Cimipax; ***Ger.:*** Cefakliman mono; Cimisan; Cirkufemal†; Evalin; Femikliman uno; Femilla N; Feminon C; Herbagyn†; Indianische Frauenwurzel; Jinda; Klimadynon; Kytta-Kliman†; Natu-fem; Remifemin; Valverde Traubensilberkerze; ***Hong Kong:*** Klimadynon; ***Malaysia:*** Remifemin; ***Mex.:*** Mensifem; ***Singapore:*** Klimadynon; Remifemin; ***Spain:*** Avala; Remifemin; ***Switz.:*** Cimifemine; Femicin; Maxifem; Menofem†; Remifemin†; ***Thai.:*** Remifemin.

**Multi-ingredient:** ***Austral.:*** Dong Quai Complex†; Extralife Meno-Care†; Extralife PMS-Care†; Harpagophytum Complex†; Herbal PMS Formula†; Lifesystem Herbal Formula 4 Women's Formula†; Medinat Esten†; PMT Complex†; Proesten†; Salagesic†; Soy Forte with Block Cohosh†; Viburnum Complex†; Women's Formula Herbal Formula 3†; ***Ger.:*** Femisana; Presselin Dysmen Olin 3 N†; Remifemin plus; ***Hong Kong:*** Phytoestrin; ***Ital.:*** Climil Complex; Climil-80; Hiperogyn; ***S.Afr.:*** Bronchicough; Bronchicum; ***UK:*** Biophylin†; Gerard House Helonias Compound†; Gerard House Ligvites†; Gerard House Reumalex; Modern Herbals Rheumatic Pain; St Johnswort Compound; Super Mega B+C; Vegetable Cough Remover; Vegetex; ***USA:*** Estrocare.

## Cinametic Acid *(rINN)*

Ácido cinamético; Acidum Cinameticum. 4-(2-Hydroxyethoxy)-3-methoxycinnamic acid.

$C_{12}H_{14}O_5$ = 238.2.

*CAS — 35703-32-3.*

### Profile

Cinametic acid is used as a choleretic in doses of 750 mg daily by mouth in divided doses.

### Preparations

**Proprietary Preparations** (details are given in Part 3)
***Fr.:*** Transoddi†.

## Cinchona Bark

Chinae Cortex; Chinarinde; Cinchona; Cinchonae Cortex; Cinchonae Succirubrae Cortex; Jesuit's Bark; Peruvian Bark; Quina; Quina Vermelha; Quino, corteza del; Quinquina; Quinquina Rouge; Red Cinchona Bark.

**Pharmacopoeias.** In *Eur.* (see p.vi).

**Ph. Eur. 5.0** (Cinchona Bark). The whole or cut, dried bark of *Cinchona pubescens* (*Cinchona succirubra*), of *C. calisaya,* of *C. ledgeriana,* or of its varieties or hybrids. It contains a minimum of 6.5% of total alkaloids, of which 30 to 60% are quinine-type alkaloids. It has an intensely bitter, somewhat astringent taste. Protect from light.

### Profile

Cinchona contains a number of alkaloids, including two pairs of optical isomers: quinine (p.460) and quinidine, (p.991) and cinchonine and cinchonidine. Cinchona alkaloids have long been used for their antimalarial activity either singly, as quinine or quinidine, or in mixtures, such as totaquine. Quinidine is also used for its antiarrhythmic properties.

Cinchona bark is used as a bitter and is also employed in herbal remedies and in homoeopathic medicine.

### Preparations

**Proprietary Preparations** (details are given in Part 3)
***Ital.:*** Venustas Antiforfora.

**Multi-ingredient:** ***Austria:*** Amara; Brady's-Magentropfen; China Eisenwein†; China-Eisenwein; Ferrovin-Chinaeisenwein; Mariazeller; ***Belg.:*** Aperop†; ***Braz.:*** Gastrogenol†; Vinho Reconstituinte†; ***Fr.:*** Quinimax; Quintonine; ***Ger.:*** Amara-Tropfen-Pascoe; Cardibisana; Gastrol S; Hepaticum-Medice H; Hicoton; Majocarmin forte; Majocarmin mite; ***Ital.:*** Bitteridina†; Chinoidina; Rabarbaroni†; ***Port.:*** Solucao Stago†; ***Spain:*** Pildoras Ferrug Sanatori†; ***Switz.:*** Phytomed Rhino†; Vin Tonique de Vial.

---

## Cineole

Cajuputol; Cineol; Cineolum; Eucaliptol; Eucalyptol *(USAN)*. 1,8-Epoxy-*p*-menthane; 1,3,3-Trimethyl-2-oxabicyclo[2.2.2]octane.

$C_{10}H_{18}O$ = 154.2.

*CAS — 470-82-6.*

**Description.** Cineole is a colourless liquid, with an aromatic camphoraceous odour, obtained from eucalyptus oil, cajuput oil, and other oils.

**Pharmacopoeias.** In *Eur.* (see p.vi), *US*, and *Viet.*

**Ph. Eur. 5.0** (Cineole). A clear colourless liquid. It solidifies at about 0.5°. Practically insoluble in water; miscible with alcohol and with dichloromethane. Store in airtight containers. Protect from light.

**USP 27** (Eucalyptol). It is obtained from eucalyptus oil and from other sources. Store in airtight containers.

### Profile

Cineole has the actions and uses of eucalyptus oil (p.1686). It has been used in counter-irritant ointments and in dental products. It has also been used in nasal preparations, but oily solutions inhibit ciliary movement and may cause lipoid pneumonia. Preparations containing cineole with other volatile substances have been used in the treatment of renal and biliary calculi.

### Preparations

**Proprietary Preparations** (details are given in Part 3)
***Ger.:*** Soledum; Soledum Balsam.

**Multi-ingredient:** ***Arg.:*** Aseptobron; Aseptobron Ampicilina; Atomo Desinflamante G; Atomo Desinflamante Familiar; Bano Liquido con Eucalipto; Bronco Etersan; Di-Neumobron; Hebert Caramelos; Listerine Clasico; Listerine Cool Mint; Listerine Fresh Burst; No-Tos Adultos; Otorinazol; Refenax Caramelos Expectorantes; ***Austral.:*** BFI†; Euky Bear Nasex†; Euky Bearub†; Extra-life Nasex; Methyl Salicylate Ointment Compound†; Nasex†; Tixylix Chest Rub; Vasylox; Vicks Sinex; ***Austria:*** Endrine Mild†; Endrine†; Rhinospray Plus; Rowachol; Rowatinex; Wick Sinex; ***Belg.:*** Balsoclase Expectorans; Balsoclase†; Endrine; Endrine Doux; Eucalyptine Le Brun; Eucalyptine Pholcodine Le Brun; Inhalene; ***Braz.:*** Algice; Angi-a-Mid†; Angino-Rub; Axol†; Baldin-CE†; Benzotal Balsamico†; Binotine Balsamico†; Bromil; Broncopinol; Canfomenol†; Cortagrip†; Durapen Balsamico†; Eucaliptan; Eucaliptol Composto†; Eucaliptol†; Eucalyptine†; Expectocilin Balsamico†; Fluomint; Gargotan†; Gargotrat†; Gripanil; Gripefago C†; Gripol C Capuride†; Gripomatine; Griponia; Gripsay; Inalobel†; Inatrex Balsamico†; Inhadrina†; Inhalante Yatropan; Inhalosam†; Killgrip; Listerine†; Mentalol†; Mentolatum†; Morrugripe†; Napiro†; Novalgrip†; Optacilin Balsamico†; Ozonyl; Ozonyl Aquoso; Ozonyl Expectorante; Pastilhas Valda†; Pectal; Penetro; Piritosse†; Plenogripe†; Pulmodex-C†; Pulmogripe†; Quelodin; Rinofen†; Soma Balsamico†; Tabletes Valda†; Tetrapulmo; Tetratoss†; Transpulmin; Transpulmin Balsamo; Transpulmin Xarope; Tripulmin; Tripulmin Balsamico; Tripulmin†; Valda†; Vick Pastilhas†; Yatropan†; ***Canad.:*** Alsirub; Antiseptic Mouthwash; Balminil Camphorub; Balminil Nasal Ointment; Bentasil†; Cal Mo Dol; Calmomusc†; Camphre Compose†; Carboseptol; Creo Grippe†; Demo-Cineol; Inarub†; Infraline†; Jack & Jill Rub†; Listerine; Listerine Antisptic Tartar Control; Marco Rub Camphorated†; Mielocol; Pastilles Valda†; Physio-Rub; Pommade au The des Bois†; Thermo Rub; Valda; Vaporisateur Medicamente; ***Chile:*** Listerine; Rowatinex; ***Denm.:*** Otrivin Menthol; ***Fin.:*** Otrivin Menthol; ***Fr.:*** Bi-Qui-Nol†; Biolau; Bismurectol†; Broncho-Tulisan Eucalyptol†; Bronchospray†; Campho-Pneumine†; Dinacode; Dinacode avec codeine; Essence Algerienne; Eucalyptine; Eucalyptine Le Brun; Eucalyptine Pholcodine†; Hexapneumine; Neo-Codion; Pectoderme; Pholcones Bismuth; Pholcones†; Pinorhinol†; Pulmocod†; Pulmofluide Simple; Rectophedrol†; Valda; Valda Septol†; Vapo-Myrtol†; Vegebom; ***Ger.:*** Denosol†; Eufimenth-Balsam N; Parodontal F5 med†; Pinimenthol Oral N†; Rhinospray Plus; Rowachol; Rowachol comp; Rowachol-Digestiv; Rowatinex; Sedotussin Expectorans†; Transpulmin Balsam; Wick Vaporub†; ***Hong Kong:*** Biocalyptol; Neo-Rowachol; Neo-Rowatinex; Rowachol; Rowatinex; Valda; ***India:*** Dristan Nasal Drops; Endrine; Endrine Mild; Karvol Plus; Sinarest Vapocaps; ***Irl.:*** Listerine†; Rowachol; Rowatinex; Valda; ***Israel:*** Gargol; Rowachol; Rowatinex; ***Ital.:*** Abiostil; Balsamico (Unguento); Balta Intimo; Broncopulmin†; Calyptol; Codetilina-Eucaliptolo He†; Fluirespir; Lacrime†; Lipobalsamo; Neo Soluzione Sulfo Balsamica†; Paidorinovit; Pastiglie Valda; Pulmarin; Pumilene Vapo; Rinogutt Eucalipto-Fher; Rinos†; Rinovit; Transpulmina Gola; Transpulmina Tosse; Vicks Sinex; ***Malaysia:*** Purporent; Rowachol; Rowatinex; ***Mex.:*** Andociclina Balsamica; Cholex; Eucalin; Guayalin-Plus; Numonyl; ***Mon.:*** Bronchodermine; Calyptol; Glyco-Thymoline; ***Neth.:*** Balsoclase Compositum†; Balsoclase-E; Otrivin Menthol; Rhinocaps†; ***NZ:*** Listerine; Listerine Tartar Control; Tixylix Chest Rub; Vicks Sinex; ***Port.:*** Fluidin Nocturno†; Halitol; Listerine; Rectopulmo Adultos; Rectopulmo Infantil; Transpulmina; Valda; ***S.Afr.:*** Respisniffers†; Woodwards Inhalant; ***Spain:*** Balsamo Kneipp; Broncovital; Bronquimar Vit A†; Bronquimar†; Brota Rectal Bals; Caltoson Balsamico; Caramelos Agua del Carmen; Caramelos Balsam†; Dimayon†; Diminex Antitusigeno; Diminex Balsamico†; Doctomitil; Dolmitin; Edusan Fte Rectal†; Etro Balsamico†; Eucalyptospirine; Eucalyptospirine Lact†; Eupnol; Kneipp Balsamo†; Maboterpen†; Mentobox; Orto Nasal†; Pastillas Juanola; Pastillas Pectoral Kely; Piorlis; Pomada Balsamica†; Pulmo Grey Balsam†; Pulmofasa; Pulmofasa Antihist†; Pulmonilo Synergium†; Queratil†; Respir Balsamico†; Retarpen Balsamico; Rinobanedif; Rowachol; Rowanefrin; Sinus Inhalaciones; Tifell; Trophires; Vitavox Pastillas; ***Swed.:*** Otrivin Menthol; ***Switz.:*** Bisolvex†; Bronchol N†; Neo-Bronchol; Olbas†; Rectoquintyl-Promethazine†; Rectoquintyl†; Rectoseptal-Neo bismuthe; Rectoseptal-Neo Pholcodine†; Rectoseptal-Neo simple; Resorbane; Sedasept; Sedotussin; Vicks Sinex; ***Thai.:*** Dexalin; Olympic Balm; Rowachol; Rowatinex; Sore Mouth Gel; ***UK:*** Dubam; Listerine Antiseptic Mouthwash; Lockets; Nostroline; Nowax; Rowachol; Rowatinex†; ***USA:*** Babee; BFI; Cool-Mint Listerine; FreshBurst Listerine; Listerine; Pfeiffer's Cold Sore; Rid-a-Pain; Saratoga; Sting-Eze.

---

## Cinnamedrine *(USAN, rINN)*

*N*-Cinnamylephedrine. α-{1-[Methyl(3-phenyl-2-propenyl)amino]ethyl}benzenemethanol hydrochloride.

$C_{19}H_{23}NO$ = 281.4.

*CAS — 90-86-8.*

## Cinnamedrine Hydrochloride *(rINNM)*

*N*-Cinnamylephedrine Hydrochloride.

$C_{19}H_{23}NO,HCl$ = 317.9.

### Profile

Cinnamedrine hydrochloride is reported to have sympathomimetic actions resembling those of ephedrine. It was formerly used in combination with analgesics in the symptomatic relief of dysmenorrhoea.

### Preparations

**Proprietary Preparations** (details are given in Part 3)

**Multi-ingredient:** ***Braz.:*** Sanacol†; ***Canad.:*** Midol Original†; ***Chile:*** Tapal-2; ***Hong Kong:*** Midol†.

---

## Cinnamon

Canela; Canela do Ceilão; Cannelle Dite de Ceylan; Ceylon Cinnamon; Ceylonzimt; Cinnam.; Cinnamomi Cortex; Cinnamon Bark; Zimt.

**Pharmacopoeias.** In *Eur.* (see p.vi).

**Ph. Eur. 5.0** (Cinnamon). The dried bark of the shoots of coppiced trees of *Cinnamomum zeylanicum* containing not less than 1.2% v/w of essential oil. It has a characteristic, aromatic odour. Protect from light.

The BP 2003 directs that when Powdered Cinnamon is prescribed or demanded, material containing not less than 1.0% v/w of essential oil shall be dispensed or supplied.

### Profile

Cinnamon is carminative and slightly astringent and is included in some preparations for gastrointestinal disorders. It is also used as a flavour. It is a source of cinnamon oil (below).

### Preparations

***Ph. Eur.:*** Cinnamon Tincture;
***USNF 22:*** Compound Cardamom Tincture.

**Proprietary Preparations** (details are given in Part 3)

**Multi-ingredient:** ***Austria:*** Brady's-Magentropfen; China-Eisenwein; Mariazeller; Montana; Naturland Heilkrautermundwasser; Synpharma Aromatische Tinktur; Teekanne Magen- und Darmtee; ***Braz.:*** Balsamo Branco†; Formitonicum†; Licor de Cacau†; ***Fr.:*** Elixir Grez; Quintonine; Santane $D_5$†; Santane $F_{10}$†; Santane $R_8$†; ***Ger.:*** Amara-Tropfen-Pascoe; Doppelherz Melissengeist; Gastrosecur; Majocarmin forte; Melissengeist; Montana N; Schwedentrunk Elixier; Sedovent; ***Hong Kong:*** Gl†; ***India:*** Carmicide; ***Israel:*** Davilla; ***Ital.:*** Assenzio (Specie Composta); Dam; ***Spain:*** Agua del Carmen; Vigortonic; ***Switz.:*** Baume; ***Thai.:*** Carmicide; Meloids; ***UK:*** Aluminium Free Indigestion†; Melissa Comp..

---

## Cinnamon Oil

Aetheroleum Cinnamomi Zeylanici; Canela, aceite esencial de; Ceylon Cinnamon Bark Oil; Cinnam. Oil; Cinnamoni Zeylanicii Corticus Aetheroleum; Esencia de Canela; Essence de Cannelle de Ceylan; Oleum Cinnamomi; Zimtöl.

**Pharmacopoeias.** *Eur.* (see p.vi) includes oil from both the bark and the leaf. *Jpn* specifies oil from either *Cinnamomum cassia* or *Cinnamomum zeylanicum*.

Cinnamon oil has been used as the name for cassia oil in some countries.

**Ph. Eur. 5.0** (Cinnamon Bark Oil, Ceylon). The oil obtained by steam distillation of the bark of the shoots of *Cinnamomum zeylanicum* (*C. verum*). It contains 55 to 75% of cinnamaldehyde and less than 7.5% of eugenol. A clear, mobile, light yellow liquid becoming reddish over time, with a characteristic odour of cinnamaldehyde. Store in well-filled airtight containers. Protect from light and heat.

**Ph. Eur. 5.0** (Cinnamon Leaf Oil, Ceylon). The oil obtained by steam distillation of the leaves of *C. zeylanicum* (*C. verum*). It contains less than 3% of cinnamaldehyde, and 70 to 85% of eugenol. A clear, mobile, reddish brown to dark brown liquid, with a characteristic odour of eugenol. Store in well-filled airtight containers. Protect from light and heat.

### Profile

Cinnamon bark oil has properties and uses similar to those of cinnamon (above). It is also included in preparations for musculoskeletal and joint disorders and for respiratory-tract disorders. There have been a number of reports of hypersensitivity to cinnamaldehyde and other constituents of cinnamon oil. Cinnamon leaf oil has also been used, although the amounts of eugenol and cinnamaldehyde are different from the bark oil.

### Preparations

***BP 2003:*** Aromatic Cardamom Tincture; Compound Cardamom Tincture; Concentrated Cinnamon Water; Tolu-flavour Solution.

**Proprietary Preparations** (details are given in Part 3)

**Multi-ingredient:** ***Austria:*** Melissengeist; Tiger Balsam Rot; ***Belg.:*** Calmant Martou†; ***Braz.:*** Axol†; Ovariusedan†; ***Canad.:*** Tiger Balm Red; ***Chile:*** Agua Del Carmen; Agua Melisa Carminativa; ***Fr.:*** Aromasol; Gouttes aux Essences; Tigridol; ***Ger.:*** Amol Heilkrautergeist N; Melissengeist; Salviathymol N; ***Hong Kong:*** Magesto; ***India:*** Bestozyme; Catazyme-P; Digeplex; Vitazyme; ***Israel:*** Karvol; ***NZ:*** Karvol; ***S.Afr.:*** Enterodyne; Karvol; ***Singapore:*** Karvol; ***Spain:*** Depurativo Richelet; ***Switz.:*** Baume de Chine Temple of Heaven blanc; Pirom; Spagyrom; ***Thai.:*** Magesto; Mesto-Of; ***UK:*** Slippery Elm Stomach Tablets; Tiger Balm Liquid†.

---

## Citicoline *(pINN)*

CDP-Choline; Citicolina; Citidoline; Cytidine Diphosphate Choline; Cytidine diphosphocholine; IP-302. Choline cytidine-5′-pyrophosphate.

$C_{14}H_{26}N_4O_{11}P_2$ = 488.3.

*CAS — 987-78-0.*

*ATC — N06BX06.*

## Citicoline Sodium *(USAN, pINNM)*

Cytidine 5′-{sodium *P*′-[2-(trimethylammonio)-ethyl] hydrogen diphosphate}, inner salt.

$C_{14}H_{25}N_4NaO_{11}P_2$ = 510.3.

*CAS — 33818-15-4.*

### Profile

Citicoline is a derivative of choline and cytidine that is involved in the biosynthesis of lecithin. It is claimed to increase blood flow and oxygen consumption in the brain and has been given in the treatment of cerebrovascular disorders (including ischaemic stroke, p.836), parkinsonism, and head injury. It is given by intravenous or intramuscular injection in doses of up to 1 g daily or by mouth in divided doses of 200 to 600 mg daily.

Citicoline sodium has also been used.

**Cerebrovascular disorders.** Citicoline has shown some short- to medium-term benefit for disturbances of memory and behaviour associated with cerebrovascular disorders.[1]

1. Fioravanti M, Yanagi M. Cytidinediphosphocholine (CDP choline) for cognitive and behavioural disturbances associated with chronic cerebral disorders in the elderly. Available in The Cochrane Library; Issue 2. Chichester: John Wiley; 2004.

**Strabismus.** Experimental studies have shown that centrally-acting drugs such as citicoline may improve vision in patients with amblyopia (see Strabismus, p.1487). However, their role in clinical practice remains to be established.[1]

1. Chatzistefanou KI, Mills MD. The role of drug treatment in children with strabismus and amblyopia. *Paediatr Drugs* 2000; **2:** 91–100.

### Preparations

**Proprietary Preparations** (details are given in Part 3)
***Arg.:*** Complegel Novo; Neuriclor; Reagin; Somazina; ***Austria:*** Startonyl; ***Braz.:*** Axion†; Somazina; ***Chile:*** Somazina; ***Fr.:*** Rexort; ***Ital.:*** Acticolin†; Actomin†; Brassel; Cebroton; Cidilin; Citidel†; Citifar; Cition; Citsav†; Difosfocin; Encelin†; Flussorex; Gerolin; Kemodyn; Link; Logan; Neurex; Neuroton; Nicholin; Nicolsint; Polineural†; Sinkron; Sintoclar; ***Jpn:*** Nicholin; ***Mex.:*** Somazina†; ***Port.:*** Hipercol; Somazina; Startonyl; Trausan; ***Spain:*** Numatol; Sauran†; Somazina.

**Multi-ingredient:** ***Arg.:*** Neuriclor Vascular; Nimodilat Plus; Nimoreagin; Nivas Plus; Reagin Vascular.

---

## Citiolone *(rINN)*

BO-714; Citiolona. *N*-(Perhydro-2-oxo-3-thienyl)acetamide.

$C_6H_9NO_2S$ = 159.2.

*CAS — 1195-16-0.*

*ATC — A05BA04.*

### Profile

Citiolone has been used in the treatment of hepatic disorders and as a mucolytic. Hypersensitivity reactions have been reported.

◊ References.

1. de Barrio M, *et al.* Recurrent fixed drug eruption caused by citiolone. *J Investig Allergol Clin Immunol* 1997; **7:** 193–4.

### Preparations

**Proprietary Preparations** (details are given in Part 3)
***Ital.:*** Citiolase†; ***Spain:*** Mucorex.

**Multi-ingredient:** ***Spain:*** Hubergrip; Mucorex Ampicilina†; Mucorex Ciclin†; Sulquibron†; Tosdetan†.

## Anhydrous Citric Acid

Acidum Citricum Anhydricum; Cítrico anhidro, ácido; Citronensäure; E330. 2-Hydroxypropane-1,2,3-tricarboxylic acid.

$C_6H_8O_7$ = 192.1.

*CAS — 77-92-9.*

*ATC — A09AB04.*

**Pharmacopoeias.** In *Eur.* (see p.vi) and *Jpn. US* allows either the anhydrous or monohydrate form.

**Ph. Eur. 5.0** (Citric Acid, Anhydrous). Colourless crystals or granules or a white crystalline powder. Very soluble in water; freely soluble in alcohol.

**USP 27** (Citric Acid). It is anhydrous or contains one molecule of water of hydration. Colourless, translucent crystals, or a white, granular to fine, crystalline powder. Soluble 1 in 0.5 of water, 1 in 2 of alcohol, and 1 in 30 of ether. Store in airtight containers.

## Citric Acid Monohydrate

Acido del Limón; Acidum Citricum Monohydricum; Cítrico monohidrato, ácido; Hydrous Citric Acid.

$C_6H_8O_7,H_2O$ = 210.1.

*CAS — 5949-29-1.*

*ATC — A09AB04.*

**Pharmacopoeias.** In *Chin., Eur.* (see p.vi), *Jpn, Pol.,* and *Viet. US* allows either the anhydrous or monohydrate form.

**Ph. Eur. 5.0** (Citric Acid Monohydrate). Efflorescent, colourless crystals or granules, or a white crystalline powder. Very soluble in water; freely soluble in alcohol. Store in airtight containers.

**USP 27** (Citric Acid). It is anhydrous or contains one molecule of water of hydration. Colourless, translucent crystals, or a white, granular to fine, crystalline powder. The hydrous form is efflorescent in dry air. Soluble 1 in 0.5 of water, 1 in 2 of alcohol, and 1 in 30 of ether. Store in airtight containers.

### Adverse Effects and Precautions

Citric acid ingested frequently or in large quantities may cause erosion of the teeth and have a local irritant action.

### Interactions

**Aluminium hydroxide.** Intestinal absorption of aluminium ions may be enhanced by oral administration of citrates. Caution is needed in patients with chronic renal disease receiving aluminium hydroxide as a phosphate binder who are given a calcium supplement in the form of effervescent tablets that contain citric acid.[1]

1. Mees EJD, Basçi A. Citric acid in calcium effervescent tablets may favour aluminium intoxication. *Nephron* 1991; **59:** 322.

### Uses and Administration

Citric acid is used in effervescing mixtures; the monohydrate is used in the preparation of effervescent granules.

Citric acid monohydrate is used as a synergist to enhance the effectiveness of antoxidants.

Preparations containing citric acid are used in the management of dry mouth (p.1576) and to dissolve renal calculi, alkalinise the urine, and prevent encrustation of urinary catheters. Citric acid is an ingredient of citrated anticoagulant solutions. Citric acid has also been used in preparations for the treatment of coughs, gastrointestinal disturbances, and metabolic acidosis.

### Preparations

***BP 2003:*** Lemon Syrup; Paediatric Compound Tolu Linctus; Paediatric Simple Linctus; Potassium Citrate Mixture; Simple Linctus;
***Ph. Eur.:*** Anticoagulant Acid-Citrate-Glucose Solutions (ACD); Anticoagulant Citrate-Phosphate-Glucose Solution (CPD);
***USP 27:*** Anticoagulant Citrate Dextrose Solution; Anticoagulant Citrate Phosphate Dextrose Adenine Solution; Anticoagulant Citrate Phosphate Dextrose Solution; Citric Acid, Magnesium Oxide, and Sodium Carbonate Irrigation; Magnesium Carbonate and Citric Acid for Oral Solution; Magnesium Citrate Oral Solution; Potassium and Sodium Bicarbonates and Citric Acid Effervescent Tablets for Oral Solution; Potassium Citrate And Citric Acid Oral Solution; Sodium Citrate and Citric Acid Oral Solution; Tricitrates Oral Solution.

**Proprietary Preparations** (details are given in Part 3)
***Ger.:*** Citrosteril†; ***S.Afr.:*** Crystacit.

**Multi-ingredient:** ***Arg.:*** Alikal; Uvasal; ***Austral.:*** Alka-Seltzer; Citralite; Citravescent; Durolax X-Pack; Eno; Picolax; Picoprep; Ural; Uricalm; Uricosal; ***Austria:*** Alka-Seltzer; Duplotrast Z; Helo-acid; Kalioral; ***Belg.:*** Alka-Seltzer; Andrews†; ***Braz.:*** Alka-Seltzer†; Citrosodine; Digestbem; Estomazil†; Frubiase†; Licor de Cacau†; Regulador Xavier n-2†; Solucao Anticoagulante†; Sonrisal; ***Canad.:*** Alka-Seltzer; Bromo Madelon; Citrocarbonate†; PMS-Dicitrate; ***Chile:*** Disfruta; Fenokomp 39; Justegas; Kanacitrin; Sal De Fruta Eno; Summer's Eve Hierbas; Uroalquine; Yasta; ***Denm.:*** Fenwal ACD†; ***Fin.:*** Alka-Seltzer; ***Fr.:*** Alka-Seltzer; Citrocholine; Elixir Grez; Foncitril; Hepargitol; Ornitaine; Sphingogel; ***Ger.:*** Alka-Seltzer; Barilux Brausetabletten; Blemaren N; Citropepsin; Lithurex S; Pepzitrat; Retterspitz Ausserlich†; Retterspitz Gelee†; Retterspitz Innerlich†; Unibaryt†; Uronor; ***Gr.:*** Gastrovison; ***Hong Kong:*** Alka-Seltzer; Eno; ***India:*** Carmicide; Coscopin; Coscopin Plus; Dristan Expectorant; ***Irl.:*** Andrews; Carbex; Cymalon; Mictral; ***Israel:*** Eno; Pico-Salax†; Urikal; ***Ital.:*** Alka-Seltzer; Citroepatina; Duogas; Eno†; Gastrovison†; Geffer; Lavanda Sofar; Limonal†; Roget†; ***Malaysia:*** Alka-Seltzer; Citravescent; Picroprep; Potcit; Ural; ***Mex.:*** Kaposalt; Korifen; ***Neth.:*** Alka-Seltzer; Hexoll†; ***Norw.:*** Pico-Salax†; ***NZ:*** Alka-Seltzer; Lemsip Dry Cough; Picoprep; Ural; ***Port.:*** Alka-Seltzer; Creme Laser Hidrante; Eno; Sais Andrews†; ***S.Afr.:*** Adco-Sodasol; Alkafizz; Betasoda; Citro-Soda; Citrocit; Effersol; Pneucid; Quatro-Soda; Uri-Alk; ***Singapore:*** Alka-Seltzer; Dicitrate; ***Spain:*** Alka-Seltzer; Justegas; Pastillas Antisep Garg L; Sal de Fruta Eno; Salcedogen†; Sales de Frutas P G; Uralyt Urato; ***Swed.:*** Alka-Seltzer; Pico-Salax†; Renapur; ***Switz.:*** Alka-Seltzer; E-Z-Gas II; Pico-Salax†; Siesta-1; Uro-Tainer Solutio R†; Uro-Tainer Suby G†; ***Thai.:*** Alka-Seltzer; Carmicide; ***UK:*** Alka-Seltzer; Alka-Seltzer XS; Allens Junior Cough; Andrews; Carbex; Collins Elixir Pastilles†; Cymalon; Effercitrate; Eno; Hill's Balsam Chesty Cough for Children; Lemsip Cough & Cold Dry Cough; Melissin†; Mictral†; Potters Children's Cough Pastilles; Resolve; Uriflex G; Uriflex R; Uro-Tainer Solution R; Uro-Tainer Suby G; Zubes Blackcurrant; Zubes Honey & Lemon; ***USA:*** Alka-Seltzer Antacid; Alka-Seltzer Effervescent Tablets; Alka-Seltzer with Aspirin; Bicitra; Bromo Seltzer Effervescent Granules; Cytra-2; Cytra-3; Cytra-K; Cytra-LC; Extra Strength Alka-Seltzer Effervescent Tablets; Gold Alka-Seltzer; Oracit; Original Alka-Seltzer Effervescent Tablets; Polycitra; Polycitra-K; Polycitra-LC; Renacidin; Sparkles; Summers Eve Disposable; Zee-Seltzer.

## Citronella Oil

Citronela, aceite esencial de; Citronellae Aetheroleum; Oleum Citronellae.

**Pharmacopoeias.** In *Eur.* (see p.vi).

**Ph. Eur. 5.0** (Citronella Oil). The oil obtained by steam distillation from the fresh or partially dried aerial parts of *Cymbopogon winterianus*. It contains 30.0 to 45.0% citronellal, 9.0 to 15.0% citronellol, 2.0 to 4.0% citronellyl acetate, less than 2.0% geranial, 20.0 to 25.0% geraniol, 3.0 to 8.0% geranyl acetate, 1.0 to 5.0% limonene, and less than 2.0% neral. A pale yellow to brownish-yellow liquid with a very strong odour of citronellal. Store in well-filled containers. Protect from light.

### Profile

Citronella oil is used as a perfume and insect repellent. Hypersensitivity has been reported.

### Preparations

**Proprietary Preparations** (details are given in Part 3)
***Arg.:*** Aulo Gelio Repelente; Repelente Rep; ***Ger.:*** Kneipp Beruhigungs-Bad spezial†; Schupps Melissen Olbad; Valmarin Bad N†; ***UK:*** Mozzie Patch; Natrapel.

**Multi-ingredient:** ***Arg.:*** Repelente Rep; ***Austral.:*** Goanna Bite-Eze†; ***Austria:*** Biokosma Embrocation; Biokosma Medizinalbad; Biokosma Red Point-Massagecreme; Melissengeist; Valin Baldrian; ***Fr.:*** Ysol 206; ***Ger.:*** Kneipp Krauter Taschenkur Nerven und Schlaf N†; Melissengeist; Schupps Baldrian Sedativbad†; ***Ital.:*** Air Citronella; Citrosystem; Mistick Verde; Natural Zanzy†; Punginо†; ***S.Afr.:*** No-Bite; ***Switz.:*** Novital; Saltrates; ***UK:*** Snowfire; ***USA:*** Treo.

## Clivers

Amor de hortelano; Cleavers; Galii Aparinis Herba; Galium; Goosegrass.

### Profile

Clivers is the dried aerial parts of *Galium aparine* (Rubiaceae). It has been used in herbal medicine, principally as a diuretic.

### Preparations

**Proprietary Preparations** (details are given in Part 3)

**Multi-ingredient:** ***Austral.:*** Galium Complex†; Herbal Cleanse†; Uva-Ursi Complex†; ***UK:*** Antitis; Athera; Backache; Boldo†; Cascade; Gerard House Buchu Compound†; Gerard House Water Relief Tablets; HealthAid Boldo-Plus; Heath & Heather Water Relief Tablets†; Kas-Bah; Modern Herbals Menopause; Modern Herbals Water Retention; Psorasolv; Sciargo; Skin Cleansing; Tabritis; Water Naturtabs; Watershed.

## Clove

Caryoph.; Caryophylli Flos; Caryophyllum; Clavo; Clou de Girofle; Cloves; Cravinho; Cravo-da-India; Gewürznelke; Giroflier; Tropical Myrtle.

**Pharmacopoeias.** In *Chin., Eur.* (see p.vi), and *Jpn.*

**Ph. Eur. 5.0** (Clove). The whole flower buds of *Syzygium aromaticum* (*Eugenia caryophyllus*), containing not less than 15% v/w of volatile oil, dried until they become reddish-brown, and with a characteristic aromatic odour. Protect from light.

The BP 2003 directs that when Powdered Clove is prescribed or demanded, material containing not less than 12.0% v/w of essential oil shall be dispensed or supplied.

### Profile

Clove is a carminative and is used as a flavour. It is the source of clove oil (below).

Clove and clove oil have been abused in the form of cigarettes.

**Abuse.** Smoking of cigarettes composed of a mixture of tobacco and cloves is a habit that originated in Indonesia and has spread to the USA. There have been reports of severe and sometimes fatal respiratory illness related to smoking clove cigarettes and there is also evidence from *animal* studies that clove cigarette smoke and eugenol (the principal constituent of clove oil) have harmful pulmonary effects. The Council on Scientific Affairs of the American Medical Association considers that in addition to the hazards associated with smoking tobacco, clove cigarettes may also produce severe lung injury in certain susceptible individuals and could also induce pulmonary aspiration in healthy individuals due to diminution of the gag reflex produced by the local anaesthetic action of eugenol.[1] The American Academy of Pediatrics has also alerted paediatricians in the USA to clove-cigarette smoking by young people and warned of the risks.[2]

1. American Medical Association Council on Scientific Affairs. Evaluation of the health hazard of clove cigarettes. *JAMA* 1988; **260:** 3641–4.
2. Committee on Substance Abuse. Hazards of clove cigarettes. *Pediatrics* 1991; **88:** 395–6.



### Preparations

**Proprietary Preparations** (details are given in Part 3)

**Multi-ingredient:** ***Austria:*** Apotheker Bauer's Kindertee; Drovitol; Mariazeller; Naturland Heilkrautermundwasser; Synpharma Aromatische Tinktur; ***Belg.:*** Eugiron†; ***Braz.:*** Balsamo Branco†; Fargestium†; ***Fr.:*** Tisane Clairo†; ***Ger.:*** Discmigon†; Doppelherz Melissengeist; Inconturina; Melissengeist; ***Hong Kong:*** Gl†; ***Ital.:*** Promix; Saugella Uomo; ***Port.:*** Midro; ***UK:*** Aluminium Free Indigestion†; Clairo Tea†; Melissa Comp.; Revitonil.

## Clove Oil

Caryophylli Floris Aetheroleum; Clavo, aceite esencial de; Esencia de Clavo; Essence de Girofle; Nelkenöl; Ol. Caryoph.; Oleum Caryophylli.

**Pharmacopoeias.** In *Eur.* (see p.vi) and *Jpn.* Also in *USNF.*

**Ph. Eur. 5.0** (Clove Oil). A clear yellow liquid obtained by steam distillation from clove containing 75.0 to 88.0% of eugenol. It becomes brown on exposure to air. Miscible with dichloromethane, with toluene, and with fatty oils. Store in well-filled airtight containers. Protect from light and heat.

**USNF 22** (Clove Oil). The volatile oil distilled with steam from clove. It contains not less than 85.0% of phenolic substances, chiefly eugenol. Soluble 1 in 2 of alcohol (70%). Store in well-filled airtight containers.

**Incompatibility.** PVC bottles softened and distorted fairly rapidly in the presence of clove oil, which should not be stored or dispensed in such bottles.[1]

1. Department of Pharmaceutical Sciences of the Pharmaceutical Society of Great Britain. Plastics medicine bottles of rigid PVC. *Pharm J* 1973; **210:** 100.

### Profile

Clove oil is a carminative that is sometimes used in the treatment of flatulent colic. It is also used as a flavour.

Applied externally clove oil is irritant but can produce local anaesthesia. It is used as a domestic remedy for toothache, a plug of cotton wool soaked in the oil being inserted in the cavity of the carious tooth; repeated application may damage the gingival tissues. Mixed with zinc oxide, it is used as a temporary anodyne dental filling, although eugenol (p.1686), one of its constituents, is often preferred. Clove oil is included as a counter-irritant in preparations for musculoskeletal and joint disorders.

Eugenol may cause hypersensitivity.

**Adverse effects.** A report of severe toxicity following ingestion of clove oil by a child.[1] Adverse effects included coma, acidosis, a generalised seizure, disordered blood clotting, and acute liver damage.

For reference to the harmful effects of smoking clove cigarettes, see under Clove, above.

1. Hartnoll G, *et al.* Near fatal ingestion of oil of cloves. *Arch Dis Child* 1993; **69:** 392–3.

### Preparations

***BP 2003:*** Aromatic Cardamom Tincture.

**Proprietary Preparations** (details are given in Part 3)
***UK:*** Dentogen; Soothake Toothache Gel.

**Multi-ingredient:** ***Austral.:*** Silver Clove Medicated Balm†; ***Austria:*** China-Balsam; Fittydent; Melissengeist; Neo-Angin; Parodontax; Tiger Balsam Rot; ***Braz.:*** Algidente; Anestesiol; ***Canad.:*** Dentalgar†; Gouttes Dentaires†; Tiger Balm Red; Tiger Balm White; ***Chile:*** Agua Del Carmen; Agua Melisa Carminativa; Hustagil; ***Fr.:*** Aromasol; Baume Aroma; Gouttes aux Essences; Tigridol; ***Ger.:*** Amol Heilkrautergeist N; China-Balsam; Erkaltungsbalsam forte Salbe†; GA-301-Redskin 301†; Hustagil Erkaltungsbalsam; Hustagil Inhalationsol†; Melissengeist; Nur 1 Tropfen medizinisches Mundwasser; Parodontal F5 med†; Repha-Os; Rheuma-Salbe†; Salviathymol N; ***Hong Kong:*** Magesto; ***Ital.:*** Dentosan Azione Intensiva; Dentosan Mese; Fialetta Odontalgica Dr Knapp; Ondroly-A; ***NZ:*** Electric Blue Headlice; Toothache Drops; ***S.Afr.:*** Enterodyne; ***Spain:*** Dentol Topico; Otogen Calmante; ***Switz.:*** Baume de Chine Temple of Heaven blanc; Olbas†; Osa Gel de dentition aux plantes†; Spagyrom; ***Thai.:*** Magesto; Masaga; Mesto-Of; ***UK:*** Eftab†; Hactos; Nine Rubbing Oils; Olbas; Olbas for Children; Potters Sugar Free Cough Pastilles; Red Oil; Snowfire; Soothake Toothache Tincture; Teenstick; Tiger Balm; Tiger Balm Liquid†; ***USA:*** Dentapaine; Numzit; Toothache Gel.

## Cnicus Benedictus

Blessed Thistle; Cardo Santo; Carduus Benedictus; Chardon Bénit; Holy Thistle; Kardobenediktenkraut.

### Profile

Cnicus benedictus, the flowering tops of *Cnicus benedictus* (*Carbenia benedicta; Carduus benedictus*) (Compositae), has been used as a bitter. It has also been used in homoeopathic medicine.

### Preparations

**Proprietary Preparations** (details are given in Part 3)

**Multi-ingredient:** ***Austria:*** Aponatura Galle; Mag Kottas Leber-Gallentee; Mariazeller; ***Belg.:*** Tisane Antibiliaire et Stomachique†; ***Braz.:*** Digestron; ***Ger.:*** Bomagall forte S†; Carvomin; Cheiranthol; Gallexier; Gastritol; Hevert-Gall S†; ***Switz.:*** Gastrosan; ***UK:*** Bio-Strath Artichoke Formula; Gerard House Gladlax†; Sure-Lax (Herbal).

## Cobalt Chloride

Cobalto, cloruro de; Cobaltous Chloride.
$CoCl_2,6H_2O = 237.9$.
*CAS — 7646-79-9 (anhydrous cobalt chloride); 7791-13-1 (cobalt chloride hexahydrate).*

### Adverse Effects

Reactions to cobalt have included anorexia, nausea and vomiting, diarrhoea, precordial pain, cardiomyopathy, flushing of the face and extremities, skin rashes, tinnitus, temporary nerve deafness, renal injury, diffuse thyroid enlargement, and hypothyroidism. In large doses it may reduce the production of erythrocytes.

◊ References.


1. Kennedy A, *et al.* Fatal myocardial disease associated with industrial exposure to cobalt. *Lancet* 1981; **i:** 412–4.
2. Cugell DW, *et al.* The respiratory effects of cobalt. *Arch Intern Med* 1990; **150:** 177–83.
3. Evans P, *et al.* Cobalt and cobalt compounds. *Toxicity Review 29.* London: HMSO, 1993.


### Uses and Administration

Cobalt chloride, when given to both normal and anaemic subjects, produces reticulocytosis and a rise in the erythrocyte count. This property suggested its use in the treatment of certain types of anaemia, but its general therapeutic use is, however, unjustified and not without danger.

In veterinary medicine, cobalt chloride has been given as a dietary supplement to ruminants.

## Cobalt Oxide

Cobalto, óxido de; Tricobalt Tetroxide.
$Co_3O_4 = 240.8$.
*CAS — 1308-06-1.*

**Pharmacopoeias.** In *BP(Vet).*

**BP(Vet) 2003** (Cobalt Oxide). It consists of cobalt (II, III) oxide (tricobalt tetroxide) with a small proportion of cobalt (III) oxide (dicobalt trioxide). A black, odourless or almost odourless, powder. Practically insoluble in water; dissolves in mineral acids and in solutions of alkali hydroxides.

### Profile

Cobalt oxide is used in veterinary practice for the prevention of cobalt deficiency in ruminants. The chloride and sulfate have been used similarly. For the adverse effects of cobalt, see Cobalt Chloride, above.

## Coccidioidin

Coccidioidina.

**Pharmacopoeias.** In *US.*

**USP 27** (Coccidioidin). A sterile solution containing the antigens obtained from the byproducts of mycelial growth or from the spherules of the fungus *Coccidioides immitis*; it contains a suitable antimicrobial. A clear, practically colourless or amber-coloured liquid. Store at 2° to 8°. Any dilutions should be stored at 2° to 8° and used within 24 hours. The expiry date is not later than 3 years (mycelial product) or 18 months (spherule-derived product) after release from the manufacturer's cold storage.

### Profile

Coccidioidin is used as an aid to the diagnosis of coccidioidomycosis and, in conjunction with other antigens, to assess the status of cell-mediated immunity. The usual dose is 0.1 mL of a 1 in 100 dilution by intradermal (intracutaneous) injection.

### Preparations

***USP 27:*** Coccidioidin.

**Proprietary Preparations** (details are given in Part 3)
***USA:*** BioCox†; Spherulin.

## Co-dergocrine Mesilate

Codergocrina, mesilato de; Co-dergocrine Mesylate *(BAN)*; Co-dergocrine Methanesulphonate; Codergocrini Mesilas; Dihydroergotoxine Mesylate; Dihydroergotoxine Methanesulphonate; Dihydrogenated Ergot Alkaloids; Ergoloid Mesylates *(USAN)*; Hydrogenated Ergot Alkaloids.
*CAS — 11032-41-0 (co-dergocrine); 8067-24-1 (co-dergocrine mesilate).*
*ATC — C04AE01.*

**Pharmacopoeias.** In *Eur.* (see p.vi), *Jpn*, and *US.*

**Ph. Eur. 5.0** (Codergocrine Mesilate). A mixture of dihydroergocornine mesilate ($C_{31}H_{41}N_5O_5,CH_4O_3S = 659.8$), dihydroergocristine mesilate, α-dihydroergocryptine mesilate, and β-dihydroergocryptine mesilate (epicriptine mesilate). It contains 30 to 35% of dihydroergocornine, 30 to 35% of dihydroergocristine, 20 to 25% of α-dihydroergocryptine, and 10 to 13% of β-dihydroergocryptine. A white or yellowish powder. Sparingly soluble in water; sparingly soluble to soluble in alcohol; slightly soluble in dichloromethane. A 0.5% solution in water has a pH of 4.2 to 5.2. Protect from light.

**USP 27** (Ergoloid Mesylates). A mixture of the methanesulfonate salts of the three hydrogenated alkaloids, dihydroergocristine, dihydroergocornine, and dihydroergocryptine, in an approximate weight ratio of 1:1:1. Dihydroergocryptine mesilate exists as a mixture of alpha- and beta-isomers. The ratio of alpha- to beta-isomers is not less than 1.5:1.0 and not more than 2.5:1.0. A white to off-white, microcrystalline or amorphous, practically odourless powder. Slightly soluble in water; soluble in alcohol and in methyl alcohol; sparingly soluble in acetone. A 0.5% solution in water has a pH of 4.2 to 5.2. Store in airtight containers. Protect from light.

### Adverse Effects

Side-effects occasionally reported with co-dergocrine mesilate include abdominal cramps, nausea, vomiting, headache, blurred vision, skin rashes, nasal congestion, flushing of the skin, dizziness, bradycardia, and orthostatic hypotension.

Local irritation has been reported following sublingual use.

**Effects on the cardiovascular system.** Of 8 patients given co-dergocrine mesilate 1.5 mg three times daily for the treatment of dementia, 3 developed severe sinus bradycardia associated with general deterioration in their condition, necessitating withdrawal of the treatment.[1] However, no sinus bradycardia had been observed in 40 elderly patients in whom the dose was built up to 1.5 mg three times daily over 3 weeks.[2]


1. Cayley ACD, *et al.* Sinus bradycardia following treatment with Hydergine for cerebrovascular insufficiency. *BMJ* 1975; **4:** 384–5.
2. Cohen C. Sinus bradycardia following treatment with Hydergine. *BMJ* 1975; **4:** 581.


### Precautions

Co-dergocrine mesilate should be used with caution in patients with severe bradycardia.

### Pharmacokinetics

Bioavailability of co-dergocrine after oral administration is low; this has been attributed to incomplete absorption from the gastrointestinal tract and extensive first-pass metabolism. Elimination is biphasic with a short half-life of 1.5 to 2.5 hours (α phase) and a longer half-life of 13 to 15 hours (β phase). Co-dergocrine is mainly excreted with bile in the faeces, although small amounts are eliminated in the urine.

### Uses and Administration

Unlike the natural ergot alkaloids, co-dergocrine mesilate has only limited vasoconstrictor effects.

It is used as an adjunct in treating symptoms of mild to moderate dementia in the elderly, in doses of 3 or 4.5 mg daily by mouth, preferably before meals. Higher doses have also been used. It is also given sublingually in similar doses. Doses of 300 to 600 micrograms once or twice daily have been given intramuscularly; it has also been given subcutaneously or by intravenous infusion.

In some countries, co-dergocrine mesilate has been used in the treatment of hypertension (p.825), migraine (p.464), and in peripheral vascular disease (p.831).

Co-dergocrine esilate has been used similarly to the mesilate.

**Dementia.** Co-dergocrine has been used for many years in dementia (p.1484) but its value is not established.[1-3] Originally its effects were thought to be mediated through peripheral and cerebral vasodilatation but it is now classified as a metabolic enhancer.


1. Wadworth AN, Chrisp P. Co-dergocrine mesylate: a review of its pharmacodynamic and pharmacokinetic properties and therapeutic use in age-related cognitive decline. *Drugs Aging* 1992; **2:** 153–73.
2. Schneider LS, Olin JT. Overview of clinical trials of Hydergine in dementia. *Arch Neurol* 1994; **51:** 787–98.
3. Olin J, *et al.* Hydergine for dementia. Available in The Cochrane Library; Issue 2. Chichester: John Wiley; 2004.


**Erectile dysfunction.** For reference to the use of creams containing co-dergocrine mesilate, isosorbide dinitrate, and either aminophylline or testosterone in the treatment of erectile dysfunction, see under Glyceryl Trinitrate, p.925.

### Preparations

***BP 2003:*** Co-dergocrine Tablets;
***USP 27:*** Ergoloid Mesylates Capsules; Ergoloid Mesylates Oral Solution; Ergoloid Mesylates Tablets.

**Proprietary Preparations** (details are given in Part 3)
***Arg.:*** CCK; Coplexina; Ergoxina; Hydergina; Somoblon; Vimotadine; ***Austria:*** Aramexe; Dorehydrin; Ergomed; Hydergin; ***Belg.:*** Hydergine; Ibexone; Stofilan; ***Braz.:*** Hydergine; ***Canad.:*** Hydergine; ***Chile:*** Geroplus; Hydergina; ***Fin.:*** Artergin; Hydergin; ***Fr.:*** Capergyl; Ergodose; Hydergine; Optamine†; Perenan†; Zenium†; ***Ger.:*** Circanol; Dacoren†; DCCK; Defluina N; Enirant†; Ergodesit; ergoplus†; ergotox; Hydergin; Hydro-Cebral; Nehydrin N†; Orphol; Sponsin; ***Hong Kong:*** Hydergine; Perenan; Stofilan†; Trigogine; ***India:*** Cereloid; ***Irl.:*** Hydergine†; ***Israel:*** Hydergine; ***Ital.:*** Hydergina; Ischelium; ***Malaysia:*** Beagocrine; Headgen; Hydergine; Vasculin; ***Mex.:*** Hydergina; Progeril†; ***Neth.:*** Hydergine; ***Port.:*** Hydergine; Redergot; Secamin; ***Singapore:*** Headgen; Hydergine; Perenan†; Trigogine; ***Spain:*** Ergodilat; Hydergina; ***Swed.:*** Hydergin; ***Switz.:*** Ergohydrine; Hydergine; Progeril†; ***Thai.:*** Codergine; Coergot†; Helcon; Hycereal; Hydergine; Hydrine; Hymed; Naline; Perenan; Redergin; Togine; Trigogine; Vaculin†; Vasculin; Vasian; ***UK:*** Hydergine; ***USA:*** Gerimal; Hydergine.

**Multi-ingredient:** ***Arg.:*** CCK Flunarizina; Difusil; Neuriclor Vascular; Neuronal Vascular; Reagin Vascular; ***Austria:*** Pontuc; ***Braz.:*** Vincetron; ***Ger.:*** Pontuc†; Sinedyston†; ***Ital.:*** Ischelium Papaverina†; Visergil†; ***Port.:*** Euvifor; Projuvex†; ***Spain:*** Clinadil Compositum; Piracetam Complex; Visergil†.

## Coenzyme A

CoA; CoASH; Coenzima A. 5′-O-{3-Hydroxy-3-[2-(2-mercaptoethylcarbamoyl)ethylcarbamoyl]-2,2-dimethylpropyl}adenosine-3′-dihydrogenphosphate-5′-trihydrogendiphosphate.
$C_{21}H_{36}N_7O_{16}P_3S = 767.5$.
*CAS — 85-61-0.*

### Profile

Formed from adenosine triphosphate, cysteine, and pantothenic acid, coenzyme A is involved in the body in many physiological roles, including the formation of citrate, the oxidation of pyruvate, the oxidation and synthesis of fatty acids, the synthesis of triglycerides, cholesterol, and phospholipids, and the acetylation of amines, choline, and glucosamine. It has been given by injection in a variety of metabolic disorders. Coenzyme A is contra-indicated in acute myocardial infarction.

### Preparations

**Proprietary Preparations** (details are given in Part 3)
***Ital.:*** Coalip†; ***Spain:*** Aluzime†.
**Multi-ingredient:** ***Ital.:*** Bio-Biol†.

## Cogalactoisomerase Sodium

Cogalactoisomerasa sódica; UDPG; Uridine-5′-diphosphoglucose Sodium.
$C_{15}H_{22}N_2Na_2O_{17}P_2,3H_2O = 664.3$.
*CAS — 133-89-1 (cogalactoisomerase).*

### Profile

Cogalactoisomerase sodium is used in various hepatic disorders.

### Preparations

**Proprietary Preparations** (details are given in Part 3)
***Ital.:*** Bivitox; Epatoxil; Liverasi; Toxepasi.

## Colforsin *(USAN, rINN)*

Boforsin; Colforsina; Forscolin; Forskolin; HL-362; L-75-1362B. (3R,4aR,5S,6S,6aS,10S,10aR,10bS)-Dodecahydro-5,6,10,10b-tetrahydroxy-3,4a,7,7,10a-pentamethyl-3-vinyl-1*H*-naphtho[2,1-*b*]pyran-1-one, 5-acetate.
$C_{22}H_{34}O_7 = 410.5$.
*CAS — 66575-29-9.*

### Profile

Colforsin is an adenylate cyclase stimulator derived from the plant *Plectranthus barbatus* (*Coleus forskohlii*) (Labiatae). It has been investigated for a number of conditions, including glaucoma and impotence. It is reported to have positive inotropic and bronchodilator effects. It has been used in the form of colforsin daropate hydrochloride.

### Preparations

**Proprietary Preparations** (details are given in Part 3)
***Jpn:*** Adehl.

## Collagen

Colágeno.
*ATC — B02BC07; G04BX11.*

### Profile

Collagen is a fibrous protein component of mammalian connective tissue making up almost one third of the total body protein.

Collagen, processed in a variety of ways, has been used in surgery as a haemostatic and as a repair and suture material. For cosmetic purposes it has been injected into the dermis to correct scars and other contour deformities of the skin. Collagen implants have been used to block tear outflow in the management of dry eye (p.1576).

Intraurethral administration of collagen has been used in the treatment of stress incontinence (p.476). There has also been interest in the use of collagen by mouth to suppress the inflammatory process in rheumatoid arthritis (p.9) and scleroderma (p.1348).

◊ References.


1. Herschorn S, *et al.* Early experience with intraurethral collagen injections for urinary incontinence. *J Urol (Baltimore)* 1992; **148:** 1797–1800.
2. Sieper J, *et al.* Oral type II collagen treatment in early rheumatoid arthritis: a double-blind, placebo-controlled, randomized trial. *Arthritis Rheum* 1996; **39:** 41–51.
3. Stanton SL, Monga AK. Incontinence in elderly women: is periurethral collagen an advance? *Br J Obstet Gynaecol* 1997; **104:** 154–7.
4. Anonymous. GAX collagen for genuine stress incontinence. *Drug Ther Bull* 1997; **35:** 86–7.
5. Hamraoui K, *et al.* Efficacy and safety of percutaneous treatment of iatrogenic femoral artery pseudoaneurysm by biodegradable collagen injection. *J Am Coll Cardiol* 2002; **39:** 1297–1304.


### Preparations

**Proprietary Preparations** (details are given in Part 3)
***Arg.:*** Hidroplus CL; Membracel; Proteita; Zyplast; ***Austral.:*** Ionil Rinse; Zyderm; Zyplast; ***Austria:*** Avitene†; Instat†; Zyderm†; Zyplast†; ***Belg.:*** Colgen†; ***Fr.:*** Collafilm†; Collatamp G; Lenidermyl†; Pangen; Zyderm†; Zyplast†; ***Ger.:*** Hemocol; Medifome; Opragen†; Pangen; Porcoll; Promogran; Surgicoll; Tachotop N; TissuCone; TissuFleece; TissuFoil; TissuVlies†; Tutoplast Dura; Tutoplast Fascia lata; Zyderm; Zyplast;

**Hong Kong:** Avitene; Zyderm; Zyplast; **Israel:** Zyderm†; Zyplast†; **Ital.:** Alfagen; Condress; Idroskin; Instat†; Neopelle; Skinat; Stimtes; **Mex.:** Fibroquel; **Neth.:** Willospon Forte; **NZ:** Ionil Rinse; **Port.:** Catrix; **Singapore:** Articolase; Zyderm; Zyplast; **Switz.:** Instat†; Lyostypt†; **UK:** Contigen; Fibracol†; Instat†; Lyostypt†; **USA:** Avitene; Hemotene.

**Multi-ingredient: Arg.:** Amenite E; Aspergun; Celuvital; Hidroplus Nieve; Hidrosam T; Medicreme; Rep-Cartil; Totalos Plus; **Austral.:** John Plunketts Protective Day Cream†; John Plunketts Super Wrinkle Cream†; **Austria:** TachoComb; **Belg.:** Duracoll; **Chile:** Acnoxyl Gel Humectante; **Fr.:** Promogran; Taido; **Ger.:** Septocoll; TachoComb; **Hong Kong:** TachoComb; **Ital.:** Artrodue; Unidermo; **Port.:** Estriagel†; **Singapore:** Articolase (w/glucosamine); **Switz.:** Gorgonium; **Thai.:** TachoComb; **USA:** PDP Liquid Protein.

## Collagenase

Clostridiopeptidase A; Colagenasa.

*CAS — 9001-12-1.*

### Profile

Collagenase is a proteolytic enzyme derived from the fermentation of *Clostridium histolyticum* and has the ability to break down collagen. Preparations containing collagenase are used topically for the debridement of dermal ulcers and burns, and possibly other necrotic lesions, to facilitate granulation and epithelialisation. It has also been given by injection into the intervertebral disc for chemonucleolysis in the treatment of low back pain (p.7). Collagenase is under investigation for use in Dupuytren's disease and Peyronie's disease.

Hypersensitivity reactions may occur. Local burning, erythema, and pain have been reported at the site of application. It has been suggested that debridement of infected wounds may increase the risk of bacteraemia and that patients should be watched for signs of systemic bacterial infection. The activity of collagenase may be reduced by antiseptics containing detergents, hexachlorophene, and heavy metal ions.

Collagenase potency is expressed in units based on the amount of enzyme required to degrade a standard preparation of undenatured collagen.

**Chemonucleolysis.** Collagenase has been studied as an alternative to chymopapain (p.1671) for chemonucleolysis because of the risk of anaphylaxis with the latter. Although early trials with collagenase reported benefit, there were also reports of back pain and muscle spasm.[1] Collagenase was not as effective as chymopapain in a comparative trial,[2] and further study may be warranted before a firm recommendation can be made.

1. Brown MD. Update on chemonucleolysis. *Spine* 1996; **21** (24 suppl): 62S–68S.
2. Wittenberg RH, *et al.* Five-year results from chemonucleolysis with chymopapain or collagenase: a prospective randomized study. *Spine* 2001; **26:** 1835–41.

**Peyronie's disease.** Beneficial effects have been reported with intralesional collagenase in men with Peyronie's disease.[1,2]

1. Gelbard MK, *et al.* The use of collagenase in the treatment of Peyronie's disease. *J Urol (Baltimore)* 1985; **134:** 280–3.
2. Gelbard MK, *et al.* Collagenase versus placebo in the treatment of Peyronie's disease: a double-blind study. *J Urol (Baltimore)* 1993; **149:** 56–8.

### Preparations

**Proprietary Preparations** (details are given in Part 3)
**Belg.:** Varilisin†; **Braz.:** Kollagenase; **Canad.:** Santyl; **Hong Kong:** Iruxol Mono; **Ital.:** Noruxol; **Neth.:** Novuxol; **Port.:** Ulcerase†; **USA:** Santyl.

**Multi-ingredient: Arg.:** Iruxol; **Braz.:** Gyno Iruxol; Iruxol; Kollagenase com cloranfenicol; **Fin.:** Iruxol; Iruxol Mono; **Ger.:** Iruxol N; **Irl.:** Iruxol Mono; **Ital.:** Iruxol; **Mex.:** Ulcoderma; **S.Afr.:** Iruxol Mono; **Spain:** Iruxol Mono; Iruxol Neo; **Switz.:** Iruxol Mono.

## Colophony

Colofonia; Coloph.; Colophane; Colophonium; Resin; Resina Pini; Resina Terebinthinae; Rosin.

**Pharmacopoeias.** In *Eur.* (see p.vi) and *Jpn.*

**Ph. Eur. 5.0** (Colophony). The residue remaining after distillation of the volatile oil from the oleoresin obtained from various species of *Pinus*. Translucent, pale yellow to brownish-yellow, angular, irregularly shaped, brittle, glassy pieces of different sizes the surfaces of which bear conchoidal markings. Do not reduce to a fine powder.

### Profile

Colophony is an ingredient of some collodions and plaster-masses. It has been used as an ingredient of ointments and dressings for wounds and minor skin disorders. Skin sensitisation and allergic respiratory symptoms have been reported.

**Hypersensitivity.** Reviews.

1. Downs AM, Sansom JE. Colophony allergy: a review. *Contact Dermatitis* 1999; **41:** 305–10.

### Preparations

**BP 2003:** Flexible Collodion.

**Proprietary Preparations** (details are given in Part 3)
**Multi-ingredient: Austral.:** Zam-Buk†; **Austria:** Ehrenhofer-Salbe; Vulpuran; **Braz.:** Basilicao; **Hong Kong:** Zam-Buk†; **Ital.:** Fialetta Odontalgica Dr Knapp; **Singapore:** Zam-Buk†; **Spain:** Empapol†; **UK:** Dispello; Herbheal Ointment; Pickles Corn Caps.

## Comfrey

Boneset; Comfrey Root; Consolidae Radix; Consuelda; Symphytum.

NOTE. Boneset is also a common name used for *Eupatorium perfoliatum* (see p.1661).

### Profile

Comfrey consists of the dried root and rhizome of *Symphytum officinale* (Boraginaceae); the leaf has also been used. It contains about 0.7% of allantoin, large quantities of mucilage, and some tannin. It may also contain pyrrolizidine alkaloids.

Comfrey was formerly used as an application to wounds and ulcers to stimulate healing and was also given systemically for gastric ulceration. It has been applied topically in the treatment of inflammatory disorders. The healing action of comfrey has been attributed to the presence of allantoin (p.1141). Comfrey is used in homoeopathic medicine.

There are reports of hepatotoxicity attributed to pyrrolizidine alkaloids present in comfrey preparations and such preparations have been withdrawn or banned in a number of countries.

◊ Review.

1. Stickel F, Seitz HK. The efficacy and safety of comfrey. *Public Health Nutr* 2000; **3:** 501–8.

**Adverse effects.** Toxic pyrrolizidine alkaloids have been isolated from several species of comfrey plants including common comfrey (*Symphytum officinale*), prickly comfrey (*S. asperum*), and Russian comfrey (*S. uplandicum*). Ingestion of plants containing pyrrolizidine alkaloids is a common cause of hepatic veno-occlusive disease in developing countries[1] and pyrrolizidine alkaloid hepatotoxicity presumably due to comfrey has been reported in North America and Europe.[1,2] Pulmonary endothelial hyperplasia and carcinogenic activity have also been reported in *animals*.[1,2]

1. Ridker PM, McDermott WV. Comfrey herb tea and hepatic veno-occlusive disease. *Lancet* 1989; **i:** 657–8.
2. Bach N, *et al.* Comfrey herb tea-induced hepatic veno-occlusive disease. *Am J Med* 1989; **87:** 97–9.

### Preparations

**Proprietary Preparations** (details are given in Part 3)
**Austria:** Traumaplant; **Canad.:** Procomfrin†; **Ger.:** Kytta-Plasma f; Kytta-Salbe f; Traumaplant.

**Multi-ingredient: Fr.:** Tisanes de l'Abbe Hamon no 15†; **Ger.:** Kytta-Balsam f; Rhus-Rheuma-Gel N; Syviman N; **Israel:** Comfrey Plus; **Port.:** Solucao Stago†; **Switz.:** Alpina Gel a la consoude†; Gel a la consoude; Keppur; Kytta Baume; Kytta Pommade; **UK:** Arnileve.

## Complement Blockers

Inhibidores del complemento.

### Profile

A number of compounds are under investigation for their ability to inhibit activation of the complement system. Such compounds include soluble forms of the complement receptors such as TP-10 (sCR1) or its derivatives such as mirococept (APT-070, SCR1-3), naturally-occurring complement blockers such as CD59, synthetic complement blockers, and the monoclonal antibodies pexelizumab and eculizumab. The potential clinical applications of such compounds are being investigated in various conditions, including the prevention of acute respiratory distress syndrome, reperfusion injury following myocardial infarction, or post-transplantation graft dysfunction. They are also being investigated as adjunctive therapy following acute myocardial infarction, and for the treatment of paroxysmal nocturnal haemoglobinuria.

◊ References.

1. Makrides SC. Therapeutic inhibition of the complement system. *Pharmacol Rev* 1998; **50:** 59–87.
2. McGeer EG, McGeer PL. The future use of complement inhibitors for the treatment of neurological diseases. *Drugs* 1998; **55:** 739–46.

## Complement C1 Esterase Inhibitor

$C_1$ Esterase Inhibitor; Inhibidor de la C1 esterasa.

### Profile

Complement C1 esterase inhibitor is a protein that plays a role in regulation of the complement system. It is prepared from human plasma and is given by intravenous infusion as replacement therapy in hereditary angioedema (p.761), both for short-term prophylaxis, and treatment of acute life-threatening attacks. Typical doses are about 25 units/kg, given by slow intravenous injection, adjusted according to symptoms and plasma concentration of the inhibitor, and repeated if necessary.

A recombinant complement C1 esterase inhibitor is under investigation.

◊ Complement C1 esterase inhibitor may be effective in both the prevention and treatment of acute hereditary angioedema.[1] It has also been tried in the management of other conditions including sepsis (p.144) and capillary leak syndrome.[2] It is under investigation for the treatment of pancreatitis and for use in allogeneic lung transplantation, thermal injury, and shock.[2] It is also being studied as a means of limiting reperfusion injury in patients with acute myocardial infarction.[3]

1. Waytes AT, *et al.* Treatment of hereditary angioedema with a vapor-heated C1 inhibitor concentrate. *N Engl J Med* 1996; **334:** 1630–4.
2. Caliezi C, *et al.* C1-esterase inhibitor: an anti-inflammatory agent and its potential use in the treatment of diseases other than hereditary angioedema. *Pharmacol Rev* 2000; **52:** 91–112.
3. de Zwaan C, *et al.* Continuous 48-h C1-inhibitor treatment, following reperfusion therapy, in patients with acute myocardial infarction. *Eur Heart J* 2002; **23:** 1670–7.

### Preparations

**Proprietary Preparations** (details are given in Part 3)
**Arg.:** Angioneurina; **Austria:** Berinert; **Fr.:** Esterasine; **Ger.:** Berinert; **Ital.:** C1 Inattivatore Umano; **Switz.:** Berinert HS; **UK:** Berinert P†.

## Condurango

Condurango Bark; Eagle-vine Bark.

**Pharmacopoeias.** In *Jpn* and *Swiss.*

### Profile

Condurango, the dried stem bark of *Marsdenia condurango* (*Gonolobus condurango*) (Asclepiadaceae), has been used as a bitter. It has also been used in homoeopathic medicine.

### Preparations

**Proprietary Preparations** (details are given in Part 3)
**Multi-ingredient: Austria:** Pascopankreat†; Sigman-Haustropfen; **Braz.:** Camomila†; Estomafitino†; **Ger.:** Majocarmin forte; Nervogastrol N; Pankreaplex Neu; Pascopankreat; Pascopankreat novo; **Switz.:** Padma-Lax; Stomacine.

## Congo Red

CI Direct Red 28; Colour Index No. 22120; Rojo Congo; Rubrum Congoensis. Disodium 3,3′-[biphenyl-4,4′-diylbis(azo)]bis[4-aminonaphthalene-1-sulphonate].

$C_{32}H_{22}N_6Na_2O_6S_2 = 696.7.$

*CAS — 573-58-0.*

### Profile

Congo red is used as a stain in the diagnosis of amyloidosis. It causes amyloid in tissue samples to fluoresce under polarised light.

## Convallaria

Convalaria; Lily of the Valley; Maiblume; Maiglöckchenkraut; May Lily; Muguet.

*CAS — 3253-62-1 (convallatoxol); 13473-51-3 (convalloside); 13289-19-5 (convallatoxoloside); 508-75-8 (convallatoxin).*

**Pharmacopoeias.** In *Ger.* and *Pol.* (from *C. majalis* or closely related species).

### Profile

Convallaria consists of the dried flowers, herb, or the rhizomes and roots of lily of the valley, *Convallaria majalis* (Liliaceae). Several crystalline glycosides have been obtained from the plant including convallarin, convalloside, convallatoxoloside, and convallatoxin.

Convallaria contains cardiac glycosides and has actions on the heart similar to those of digoxin (p.895). Convallaria is used in herbal and homoeopathic medicine.

◊ *Convallaria majalis* has been designated unsafe for inclusion in foods, beverages, or drugs by the FDA in the USA.[1]

1. Larkin T. *FDA Consumer* 1983; **17** (Oct.): 5.

### Preparations

**Proprietary Preparations** (details are given in Part 3)
**Ger.:** Convacard; Valdig-N Burger.

**Multi-ingredient: Arg.:** Passacanthine; **Austria:** Cardiofrik†; Omega; **Fr.:** Tisanes de l'Abbe Hamon no 16†; Tisanes de l'Abbe Hamon no 3†; **Ger.:** Aesrutal S†; Cardibisana; Cefascillan†; Convallocor-SL†; Convastabil; Cor-loges; Cor-Vel N†; Corguttin N plus†; Goldtropfen-Hetterich†; Guttacor†; Hypercard†; Lacoerdin-N†; Miroton; Miroton N; Oxacant N; Oxacant-forte N; Oxacant-Khella N; Raufuncton N†; Viscorapas duo; **Spain:** Uralyt†.

## Corbadrine *(rINN)*

Corbadrina; l-3,4-Dihydroxynorephedrine; Levonordefrin; l-Nordefrin. (−)-2-Amino-1-(3,4-dihydroxyphenyl)propan-1-ol.

$C_9H_{13}NO_3 = 183.2.$

*CAS — 829-74-3 (corbadrine); 6539-57-7 (nordefrin); 61-96-1 (nordefrin hydrochloride).*

**Pharmacopoeias.** In *US.*

**USP 27** (Levonordefrin). A white to buff-coloured, odourless, crystalline solid. Practically insoluble in water; slightly soluble in alcohol, in acetone, in chloroform, and in ether; freely soluble in aqueous solutions of mineral acids.

### Profile

Corbadrine is a sympathomimetic (see Adrenaline, p.852) that has been added to local anaesthetic preparations in dentistry to diminish absorption and to localise the effect; a concentration of 1 in 20 000 has been used.

### Preparations

*USP 27:* Mepivacaine Hydrochloride and Levonordefrin Injection; Procaine and Tetracaine Hydrochlorides and Levonordefrin Injection; Propoxycaine and Procaine Hydrochlorides and Levonordefrin Injection.

**Proprietary Preparations** (details are given in Part 3)

*Used as an adjunct in: **Canad.:*** Polocaine; ***S.Afr.:*** Carbocaine; ***USA:*** Carbocaine with Neo-Cobefrin; Isocaine; Polocaine.

## Coriander

Coentro; Coriand.; Coriander Fruit; Coriander Seed; Coriandri Fructus; Fruto del cilantro.

**Pharmacopoeias.** In *Eur.* (see p.vi) and *Pol.*

**Ph. Eur. 5.0** (Coriander). The dried cremocarp of *Coriandrum sativum*, containing not less than 0.3% v/w of essential oil, calculated with reference to the dried substance. Protect from light. The BP 2003 directs that when Powdered Coriander is prescribed or demanded material containing not less than 0.2% v/w of essential oil shall be dispensed or supplied.

### Profile

Coriander is the source of coriander oil (below). It is a carminative and is used as a flavour.

### Preparations

**Proprietary Preparations** (details are given in Part 3)

**Multi-ingredient: *Arg.:*** Salutaris; ***Austria:*** Apotheker Bauer's Blahungstee; Bio-Garten Tropfen gegen Blahungen; Brady's-Magentropfen; Carminative; Carminativum Babynos; Dr. Ernst Richter's Abfuhrtee-Filterbeutel†; Krauterpfarrer Weidinger Tee bei Sodbrennen; Mariazeller; Planta Lax; ***Belg.:*** Tamarine†; ***Braz.:*** Fitolax; Florlax; Fontolax; Frutalax; Laxarine; Laxtam; Novolax†; Sene Composta†; Tamaril; Tamarine; Tamarix; ***Fr.:*** Mediflor Tisane Digestive No 3; Tisane Grande Chartreuse†; ***Ger.:*** Carminativum Babynos; Floradix Multipretten N; Gastrol S; Presselin Dyspeptikum; Ramend Krauter; ***Ital.:*** Cadifen; Cadimint; Dicalmir; Tamarine; Tisana Cisbey†; ***Mex.:*** Naturetti; ***Spain:*** Agua del Carmen; Jarabe Manceau; Jarabe Manzanas Siken†; Pruina; Vegetalin†; ***Switz.:*** Boldoflorine†; Tamarine†; Tisane laxative Natterman no 13†; ***UK:*** Melissa Comp..

## Coriander Oil

Cilantro, aceite esencial de; Coriandri Aetheroleum; Ol. Coriand; Oleum Coriandri.

**Pharmacopoeias.** In *Eur.* (see p.vi). Also in *USNF.*

**Ph. Eur. 5.0** (Coriander Oil). An essential oil obtained by steam distillation from the fruits of *Coriandrum sativum*. A clear colourless or pale yellow liquid, with the characteristic spicy odour. It contains not less than 65% and not more than 78% of linalol. Relative density 0.860 to 0.880. Store in well-filled airtight containers at a temperature not exceeding 25°. Protect from light.

**USNF 22** (Coriander Oil). The volatile oil obtained by steam distillation from coriander. Specific gravity 0.863 to 0.875. Soluble 1 in 3 of alcohol (70%). Store in airtight containers at a temperature not exceeding 40°. Protect from light.

### Profile

Coriander oil is aromatic and carminative and is used as a flavour.

### Preparations

*BP 2003:* Compound Orange Spirit; Compound Rhubarb Tincture;
*USNF 22:* Compound Orange Spirit.

**Proprietary Preparations** (details are given in Part 3)

**Multi-ingredient: *Ger.:*** Floradix Multipretten N; Gastricard.

## Corn Silk

Maíz, barba del; Stigma Maydis; Zea.

**Pharmacopoeias.** In *Fr.*

### Profile

Corn silk, the stigma and style of maize (*Zea mays*) (Gramineae), has diuretic properties and is used for urinary-tract disorders including renal calculi.

Maize is widely used as a food and has also been used in herbal medicine.

### Preparations

**Proprietary Preparations** (details are given in Part 3)

***Braz.:*** Insadol†; ***Fr.:*** Insadol; ***Switz.:*** Insadol; ***UK:*** Protat.

**Multi-ingredient: *Austral.:*** Althaea Complex†; Urinase†; ***Fr.:*** Antigoutteux Rezall†; Tisane Orientale Soker†; Tisanes de l'Abbe Hamon no 3†; ***Spain:*** Diurinat; Renusor; ***UK:*** Elixir Damiana and Saw Palmetto.

## Cottonseed Oil

Aceite de Algodon; Algodón, aceite de; Cotton Oil; Ol. Gossyp. Sem.; Oléo de Algodoeiro; Oleum Gossypii Seminis.

*CAS — 8001-29-4.*

**Pharmacopoeias.** In *USNF,* which also includes hydrogenated cottonseed oil.

*Eur.* (see p.vi) includes only the hydrogenated oil.

**Ph. Eur. 5.0** (Cottonseed Oil, Hydrogenated; Gossypii Oleum Hydrogenatum). Obtained by refining and hydrogenation of oil obtained from seeds of cultivated plants of various varieties of *Gossypium hirsutum* or of other species of *Gossypium*. It consists mainly of triglycerides of palmitic and stearic acids. It is a white mass or powder which melts to a clear pale yellow liquid when heated. M.p. 57° to 70°. Practically insoluble in water; very slightly soluble in alcohol; freely soluble in dichloromethane and in toluene. Protect from light.

**USNF 22** (Cottonseed Oil). The refined fixed oil obtained from the seed of plants of various varieties of *Gossypium hirsutum* or of other species of *Gossypium* (Malvaceae). It is a pale yellow, oily liquid, odourless or nearly so. Slightly soluble in alcohol; miscible with carbon disulfide, with chloroform, with ether, and with petroleum spirit. Store in airtight containers at a temperature not exceeding 40°. Protect from light. At temperatures below 10° particles of solid fat may separate from the oil and at about 0° to −5° the oil becomes a solid or nearly so.

**USNF 22** (Hydrogenated Cottonseed Oil). It is obtained by hydrogenating Cottonseed Oil and consists mainly of triglycerides of palmitic and stearic acids. A white mass or powder that melts to a clear, pale yellow liquid when heated. M.p. 57° to 70°. Practically insoluble in water; very slightly soluble in alcohol; freely soluble in dichloromethane and in toluene. Store in airtight containers at a temperature not exceeding 40°. Protect from light and moisture. Do not allow to freeze.

### Profile

Cottonseed oil is used as an oily vehicle.

An extract of cottonseed oil, gossypol (p.1695), has been tried as a contraceptive in males.

## Couch-grass

Agropyron; Chiendent; Dogs Grass; Grama; Graminis Rhizoma; Quackgrass; Triticum; Twitch.

NOTE. The plant has also been known as *Triticum repens*.

**Pharmacopoeias.** In *Eur.* (see p.vi) and *Pol.*

**Ph. Eur. 5.0** (Couch Grass Rhizome). The whole or cut, washed and dried rhizome of *Agropyron repens* (*Elymus repens*); the adventitious roots are removed. Protect from light.

### Profile

Couch-grass is a mild diuretic that has been used in herbal medicine in the treatment of urinary-tract disorders. It contains glucose, mannitol, inositol, and triticin (a carbohydrate resembling inulin).

### Preparations

**Proprietary Preparations** (details are given in Part 3)

***Ger.:*** Acorus.

**Multi-ingredient: *Austria:*** Abfuhrtee; Brostalin; Krauterhaus Mag Kottas Blasentee; Krauterhaus Mag Kottas Entwasserungstee; Naturland Entschlackungstee; Neuners Krautertee Nr 2 - Fruhjahrskurtee; Sidroga Nieren- und Blasentee; ***Fr.:*** Herbesan; Mediflor Tisane Antirhumatismale No 2; Mediflor Tisane No 4 Diuretique; Mediflor Tisane Pectorale d'Alsace†; Obeflorine; Tisane Hepatique de Hoerdt; Tisane Orientale Soker†; Tisanes de l'Abbe Hamon no 11†; ***Ger.:*** Blasen-Nieren-Tee Stada†; Harntee 400; Hevert-Blasen-Nieren-Tee N; Presselin Stoffwechsel-Tee Hapeka 225 N; Renob Blasen- und Nierentee; ***Ital.:*** Betulla (Specie Composta); Depurativo†; Emmenoiasi; Gramigna (Specie Composta); Tisana Arnaldi†; Tisana Cisbey†; Tisana Kelemata; ***Spain:*** Diurinat; Renusor; ***Switz.:*** The Franklin†; ***UK:*** Antitis; Kas-Bah.

## Coumarin

1,2-Benzopyrone; 5,6-Benzo-α-pyrone; Cumarin; Cumarina; Tonka Bean Camphor. 2*H*-1-Benzopyran-2-one.

$C_9H_6O_2$ = 146.1.

*CAS — 91-64-5.*

**Pharmacopoeias.** In *Ger.*

### Profile

Coumarin is the odorous principle of Tonka seed (Tonka or Tonquin bean); it may be prepared synthetically. Coumarin has been given to reduce excess tissue protein and associated fluid in the treatment of lymphoedema (see below). It has also been used as a fixative in perfumery and as a flavour. It is reported to be an immunostimulant and has been tried in the treatment of malignant neoplasms.

Coumarin derivatives are used as anticoagulants; coumarin itself is not an active anticoagulant.

**Effects on the liver.** Coumarin has been classified as hepatotoxic based on studies in *animals*. Liver toxicity ranging from elevated liver enzymes to serious organ damage has been reported in humans. Seventeen of 2173 patients enrolled in a clinical/toxicological study of coumarin developed elevated liver enzyme values;[1] the majority of patients were given 100 mg coumarin daily for 1 month followed by 50 mg daily for 2 years. However, none of the patients developed permanent liver damage and liver enzyme values returned to normal in 5 patients who continued taking coumarin. Results from 5 studies supported by the Lymphoedema Association of Australia, in which patients received 400 mg daily for a mean duration of 14.6 months, showed 2 cases of hepatotoxicity among 1106 patients.[2] In the period of 14 months up to May 1995, the Australian Drug Evaluation Committee received 10 reports of suspected adverse reactions to coumarin,[3] including 6 cases of jaundice in women who had taken 400 mg daily for 1 to 4 months. Periportal and lobular necrosis were found on biopsy in 1 case and another had a fatal outcome due to massive hepatic necrosis.

Reports of hepatotoxicity have led to the withdrawal of coumarin in a number of countries.


1. Cox D, *et al.* The rarity of liver toxicity in patients treated with coumarin (1,2-benzopyrone). *Hum Toxicol* 1989; **8:** 501–6.
2. Casley-Smith JR, Casley-Smith JR. Frequency of coumarin hepatotoxicity. *Med J Aust* 1995; **162:** 391.
3. Anonymous. Lodema and the liver. *Aust Adverse Drug React Bull* 1995; **14:** 11. Also available at http://www.health.gov.au/tga/docs/html/aadrbltn/v14n3.htm (accessed 04/12/03)


**Lymphoedema.** Benzopyrones such as coumarin are reported to reduce excess protein in tissues with high-protein oedema, hence the use of coumarin in lymphoedema of various causes, including postmastectomy, and filarial lymphoedema and elephantiasis.[1-5] Evidence for its efficacy is, however, conflicting;[4-6] at best the action is slow and treatment may need to be given for 6 months to 2 years before any benefit is seen.


1. Jamal S, *et al.* The effects of 5,6 benzo-[a]-pyrone (coumarin) and DEC on filaritic lymphoedema and elephantiasis in India: preliminary results. *Ann Trop Med Parasitol* 1989; **83:** 287–90.
2. Turner CS. Congenital lymphedema. *JAMA* 1990; **264:** 518.
3. Casley-Smith JR, *et al.* Treatment of lymphedema of the arms and legs with 5,6-benzo-[α]-pyrone. *N Engl J Med* 1993; **329:** 1158–63.
4. Casley-Smith JR, *et al.* Treatment of filarial lymphoedema and elephantiasis with 5,6-benzo-α-pyrone (coumarin). *BMJ* 1993; **307:** 1037–41.
5. Casley-Smith JR. Benzo-pyrones in the treatment of lymphoedema. *Int Angiol* 1999; **18:** 31–41.
6. Loprinzi CL, *et al.* Lack of effect of coumarin in women with lymphedema after treatment for breast cancer. *N Engl J Med* 1999; **340:** 346–50.


### Preparations

**Proprietary Preparations** (details are given in Part 3)

***Arg.:*** Esberiven; ***Fr.:*** Lysedem†; ***Ger.:*** Venalot mono; ***Switz.:*** Lymphex†; Venalot†; Venium†.

**Multi-ingredient: *Arg.:*** Esberiven; ***Braz.:*** Flebotrat†; Micotox†; Venalot; Venalot H; ***Ger.:*** Caye Balsam; Kneipp Rheuma Stoffwechsel-Bad Heublumen-Aquasan†; Venalot; Venalot N; ***Mex.:*** Venalot.

## Coutarea Latiflora

Copalchi.

NOTE. The name copalchi has also been applied to *Croton niveus* (Euphorbiaceae).

### Profile

*Coutarea latiflora* is an ingredient of herbal remedies used in the management of diabetes mellitus. For a report of hepatotoxicity associated with a preparation containing *Coutarea latiflora* see Centaury, p.1669.

**Adverse Effects.** Rhabdomyolysis and haemolysis occurred in a 58-year-old man 2 days after starting treatment with *Coutarea latiflora*.[1] The patient had a similar reaction 4 years earlier after taking the same product.


1. Roca B. Rhabdomyolysis and hemolysis after use of Coutarea latiflora. *Am J Med* 2003; **115:** 677.


### Preparations

**Proprietary Preparations** (details are given in Part 3)

***Ger.:*** Sucontral.

**Multi-ingredient: *Fr.:*** Copaltra†.

## Cowberry

Arándano rojo; Red Whortleberry.

**Pharmacopoeias.** In *Pol.*

### Profile

The leaves of the cowberry, *Vaccinium vitis-idaea* (Ericaceae), have astringent properties and have been used as a domestic remedy for diarrhoea.

## CR Gas

EA-3547; Gas CR. Dibenz[*b,f*][1,4]oxazepine.

$C_{13}H_9NO$ = 195.2.

*CAS — 257-07-8.*

### Profile

A riot-control gas with irritant and lachrymatory properties similar to those of CS gas (p.1677); it is described as a tear gas. CR gas is reported not to be hydrolysed by water and therefore to be suitable for use in water cannons.

## Cranberry

Arándano.

**Pharmacopoeias.** *USNF* includes a liquid preparation.

**USNF 22** (Cranberry Liquid Preparation). The bright red juice derived from the fruits of *Vaccinium macrocarpon* or *V. oxycoccos* (Ericaceae). It contains no added substances and is for manufacturing purposes only. pH between 2.4 and 2.6. Store at 2° to 8°.

### Profile

Cranberry consists of the fruit of *Vaccinium macrocarpon*, the

American cranberry or *V. oxycoccus*, the European cranberry. Cranberry juice has been reported to reduce the incidence of urinary-tract infections.

**Interactions.** For a report of interactions between cranberry juice and *warfarin*, see p.1026.

**Urinary-tract infections.** Cranberries and cranberry juice have been used widely for many years for both the prevention and treatment of urinary-tract infections. A systematic review[1] of available data concluded that there was some evidence that cranberry juice for prevention may decrease the number of symptomatic urinary-tract infections in women over a 12 month period but further trials were needed. However, another such review[2] assessing the effectiveness of cranberry for treatment concluded that there was no good quality evidence to suggest that it is effective.


1. Jepson RG, *et al.* Cranberries for preventing urinary tract infections. Available in The Cochrane Library; Issue 2. Chichester: John Wiley; 2004.
2. Jepson RG, *et al.* Cranberries for treating urinary tract infections. Available in The Cochrane Library; Issue 2. Chichester: John Wiley; 2004.


### Preparations

**Proprietary Preparations** (details are given in Part 3)

**Multi-ingredient:** ***Austral.:*** Bioglan Cranbiotic Super†; Cranberry Complex†; Extralife Uri-Care†; ***Canad.:*** Prostease.

## Crataegus

Aubépine; Biancospino; English Hawthorn; Haw; Pilriteiro; Weissdorn; Whitethorn.

*ATC — C01EB04.*

**Pharmacopoeias.** In *Chin., Eur.* (see p.vi), and *Pol.* Also in *USNF.*

**Ph. Eur. 5.0** (Hawthorn Berries; Crataegi Fructus). The dried false fruits of *Crataegus oxyacantha* (*C. laevigata*), or *C. monogyna*, or their hybrids or a mixture of these false fruits. They contain not less than 1% of procyanidins, calculated as cyanidin chloride ($C_{15}H_{11}ClO_6$ = 322.7) with reference to the dried drug. Protect from light.

**Ph. Eur. 5.0** (Hawthorn Leaf and Flower; Crataegi Folium cum Flore). The whole or cut, dried flower bearing branches of *Crataegus oxyacantha* (*C. laevigata*), or *C. monogyna*, or their hybrids or, more rarely, other European *Crataegus* species including *C. pentagyna*, *C. nigra*, and *C. azarolus*. It contains not less than 1.5% of flavonoids, calculated as hyperoside ($C_{21}H_{20}O_{12}$ = 464.4) calculated with reference to the dried drug. Protect from light.

**USNF 22** (Hawthorn Leaf with Flower). The dried tips of the flower-bearing branches up to 7 cm in length of *Crataegus monogyna* or *C. laevigata*, also known as *C. oxyacantha* (Rosaceae). It contains not less than 0.6% of *C*-glycosylated flavones, expressed as vitexin ($C_{21}H_{20}O_{10}$ = 432.4), and not less than 0.45% of *C*-glycosylated flavones, expressed as hyperoside, calculated with reference to the dried drug. Protect from light.

### Profile

Crataegus contains flavonoid glycosides with cardiotonic properties similar to those of digoxin (p.895). Crataegus is used in herbal and homoeopathic medicine.

◊ References.


1. Rigelsky JM, Sweet BV. Hawthorn: pharmacology and therapeutic uses. *Am J Health-Syst Pharm* 2002; **59:** 417–22.
2. Chang Q, *et al.* Hawthorn. *J Clin Pharmacol* 2002; **42:** 605–12.
3. Pittler MH, *et al.* Hawthorn extract for treating chronic heart failure: meta-analysis of randomized trials. *Am J Med* 2003; **114:** 665–74.


### Preparations

***Ph. Eur.:*** Hawthorn Leaf and Flower Dry Extract.

**Proprietary Preparations** (details are given in Part 3)

***Austria:*** Aponatura Herz; Bericard; Biogelat Herzstarkungs; Cardiofort; Cardiphyt; Crataegan; Crataegutt; Esbericard; Neo-Cratylen; Sanadorn; Vitalin; ***Braz.:*** Dekatin; ***Chile:*** Cratenox; ***Fr.:*** Aubeline; Cardiocalm; Crataegol†; Spasmosedine; ***Ger.:*** Adenylocrat; Arte-Rutin C†; Basticrat; Bomacorin; Born†; Chronocard N; Cordapur Novo; Corocrat; Coronator†; Craegium; Cratae-Loges; Crataegutt; Crataegysat F; Crataepas; Crataezyma†; Cratecor; Craviscum mono†; Esbericard novo; Faros; Herz-Tropfen Eu Rho†; Kneipp Pflanzen-Dragees Weissdorn†; Kneipp Weissdorn-Pflanzensaft Sebastianeum†; Kneipp Weissdorn-Tee†; Koro-Nyhadin; Kyaugutt†; Kytta-Cor; Liquicard†; Naranocor†; Natucor; Neo-Cratylen†; Normotin V1†; Optocor†; Orthangin N†; Orthangin novo; Orthocardon-N†; Oxacant-mono; Poikilocard Mono; Regulacor-POS; Rephacratin†; Senicor; Steicorton; Tensitruw†; Tonoplantin Mono†; Vitalin†; ***Neth.:*** Crataegutt†; ***Spain:*** Crataegutt†; Elusanes Espino Albar†; ***Switz.:*** Cardiplant; Crataegisan; Crataegitan; Esbericard†; Eurhyton†; Faros; Sedosan N.

**Multi-ingredient:** ***Arg.:*** Hepatodirectol; Passacanthine; Sequals G; ***Austral.:*** Asa Tones†; Bioglan Bioage Peripheral†; Crataegus Complex†; For Peripheral Circulation Herbal Plus Formula 5†; Gingo A†; Ginkgo Biloba Plus†; Ginkgo Complex†; Lifechange Circulation Aid†; Lifesystem Herbal Formula 6 For Peripheral Circulation†; Multi-Vitamin Day & Night†; ***Austria:*** Apotheker Bauer's Grippetee; Belisir; Biovital Weissdorn; Cardalept; Cardiofrik†; Corodyn; Doppelherz Tonikum†; Heli-Sal; Herz- und Kreislauftonikum Bioflora; Kneipp Herz- und Kreislauf-Unterstutzungs-Tee; Krauterpfarrer Weidinger Tee fur das Altersherz; Mag Kottas Herz- und Kreislauftee; Naturland Herz-Kreislauf; Neuners Krautertee Nr 20 - Kreislauftee; Neuners Krautertee Nr 32 - Kreislaufregulierungstee; Neuners Krautertee Nr 44 - Kreislaufanregender Tee; Omega; Rutiviscal; Sidroga Herz-Kreislauf-Tee; St Radegunder Herz-Kreislauf-Tonikum; St Radegunder Herz-Kreislauf-unterstutzender Tee; Teekanne Herz- und Kreislauftee; Virgilocard; Wechseltee EF-EM-ES; ***Belg.:*** Natudor; Sedinal; Seneuval†; Spasmosedine†; Tisane Contre la Tension†; Tisane pour Dormir†; ***Braz.:*** Akhauma†; Anevrase; Calman; Calmazin†; Calmiplan; Maracugina†; Neurosedol†; Pasalix; Passi Catha†; Passicarbone†; Passiflora Composta†; Passiflorine; Sedalin†; Serenus; Sominex; Sonotabs†; ***Chile:*** Armonyl; ***Fr.:*** Actisane Nervosite†; Actisane Troubles du Sommeil†; Anxoral; Astressane†; Biocarde; Euphytose; Germose; Lenicalm; Mediflor Tisane Calmante Troubles du Sommeil No 12; Mediflor Tisane Circulation du Sang No 12; Natudor; Neuroflorine; Neurotensyl†; Nicoprive; Noctisan†; Nocvalene; Nuidor†; Passiflorine; Passinevryl; Phytocalm; Quinisedine; Santane $H_7$†; Santane $N_9$†; Santane $V_3$†; Sedalozia†; Sedatif Tiber; Sedatonyl†; Sedibaine†; Sedopal; Spasmidenal†; Spasmine; Sympaneurol; Sympathyl; Sympavagol; Tranquital; Vagostabyl; Vericardine†; ***Ger.:*** Aesrutal S†; Antihypertonicum S; Antisklerosin S†; Ardeycordal N; Asgoviscum N; Biovital Aktiv; Biovital Classic; Biovital N†; Biovital Weissdorn Tonikum†; Cardibisana; Cardio-Longoral; Chlorophyl liquid "Schuh"; Convallocor-SL†; Convastabil; Cor-Select; Cor-Vel N†; Corguttin N plus†; Coroverlan†; Crataelanat†; Diawern†; Dr. Hotz Vollbad†; Euvalon†; Fovysat; Ginseng-Complex "Schuh"; Goldtropfen-Hetterich†; Guttacor†; Herz-Starkung N; Heusin; Ilja Rogoff; JuViton; Kneipp Drei-Pflanzen-Dragees N†; Kneipp Herz- und Kreislauf-Tee†; Korodin; Kreislauftropen†; Lacoerdin Mg Plus; Lacoerdin-N†; Nephrisan P; Nitro-Crataegutt; Nitro-cum†; Oxacant N; Oxacant-forte N; Oxacant-Khella N; Oxacant-sedativ; Passin; Passiorin N†; Presselin Arterien K 5 P; Protecor; Rauwoplant†; Salus Herz-Schutz-Kapseln; Salusan†; Septacord; Stenocrat; Szillosan forte†; Tornix; Vasesana-Vasoregulans†; Viscorapas duo; ***Hong Kong:*** Ginkgo Plus Vivo-Livo; ***Israel:*** Nerven-Dragees; Passiflora; ***Ital.:*** Anevrasi; Bianco Val; Blandonal†; Lenicalm; Mirtiros†; Nicoprive†; Noctis; Parvisedil; Passiflorine; Prexene†; Quietan†; Relaten†; Sedatol; Sedofit; Sedopuer F; Tauma†; ***Mex.:*** Ifupasil; ***Mon.:*** Neuropax; ***Port.:*** Calmo†; Gabisedil; Neurocardol; ***Singapore:*** Noricaven; ***Spain:*** Natusor High Blood Pressure; Natusor Somnisedan; Passiflorine†; Sedasor; Sedonat; Sonofit†; Tensiben; ***Switz.:*** Arterosan Plus; Cardiaforce; Dragees pour le coeur et les nerfs; Gouttes pour le coeur et les nerfs Concentrees; Korodin†; Phytomed Cardio; Sirop Passi-Par; Tai Ginseng N†; Tisane pour le coeur et la circulation; Valverde Dragees pour le coeur; Valverde Gouttes pour le coeur; ***UK:*** Tranquil.

## Creatine

*N*-(Aminoiminomethyl)-*N*-methylglycine.

$C_4H_9N_3O_2$ = 131.1.

*CAS — 57-00-1 (creatine); 6020-87-7 (creatine monohydrate).*

## Creatine Phosphate

Creatina, fosfato de; Creatine Phosphoric Acid; Fosfocreatine; Phosphocreatine. *N*-[Imino(phosphonoamino)-methyl]-*N*-methylglycine.

$C_4H_{10}N_3O_5P$ = 211.1.

*CAS — 67-07-2 (creatine phosphate); 922-32-7 (creatine phosphate disodium).*

*ATC — C01EB06.*

### Profile

Creatine is an endogenous substance found mainly in skeletal muscle of vertebrates. Creatine phosphate has been tried in the treatment of cardiac disorders and has been added to cardioplegic solutions. Creatine monohydrate has been tried in metabolic disorders and used as a dietary supplement. It is also under investigation for the treatment of motor neurone disease.

◊ References.


1. Pedone V, *et al.* An assessment of the activity of creatine phosphate (Neoton) on premature ventricular beats by continuous ECG monitoring in patients with coronary cardiac disease. *Clin Trials J* 1984; **21:** 91.
2. Ferraro S, *et al.* Acute and short-term efficacy of high doses of creatine phosphate in the treatment of cardiac failure. *Curr Ther Res* 1990; **47:** 917–23.
3. Mastroberto P, *et al.* Creatine phosphate protection of the ischemic myocardium during cardiac surgery. *Curr Ther Res* 1992; **51:** 37–45.
4. Stöckler S, *et al.* Creatine replacement therapy in guanidinoacetate methyltransferase deficiency, a novel inborn error of metabolism. *Lancet* 1996; **348:** 789–90.
5. Mujika I, Padilla S. Creatine supplementation as an ergogenic aid for sports performance in highly trained athletes: a critical review. *Int J Sports Med* 1997; **18:** 491–6.
6. Juhn MS, Tarnopolsky M. Oral creatine supplementation and athletic performance: a critical review. *Clin J Sport Med* 1998; **8:** 286–97. Correction. *ibid.* 1999; **9:** 62.
7. Benzi G. Is there a rationale for the use of creatine either as nutritional supplementation or drug administration in humans participating in a sport? *Pharmacol Res* 2000; **41:** 255–64.
8. Mazzini L, *et al.* Effects of creatine supplementation on exercise performance and muscular strength in amyotrophic lateral sclerosis: preliminary results. *J Neurol Sci* 2001; **191:** 139–44.
9. Groeneveld JG, *et al.* A randomized sequential trial of creatine in amyotrophic lateral sclerosis. *Ann Neurol* 2003; **53:** 437–45.
10. Persky AM, *et al.* Pharmacokinetics of the dietary supplement creatine. *Clin Pharmacokinet* 2003; **42:** 557–74.


### Preparations

**Proprietary Preparations** (details are given in Part 3)

***Arg.:*** Musashi Creatina; ***Ital.:*** Creatile.

## Creatinine

Creatinina. 2-Amino-1-methyl-4-imidazolidinone.

$C_4H_7N_3O$ = 113.1.

*CAS — 60-27-5.*

**Pharmacopoeias.** In *Ger.* Also in *USNF.*

**USNF 22** (Creatinine). White, odourless, crystals or crystalline powder. Soluble in water; slightly soluble in alcohol; practically insoluble in acetone, in chloroform, and in ether.

### Profile

Creatinine is used as a bulking agent for freeze-drying.

Plasma concentrations or clearance of endogenous creatinine are used as an index of renal function.

## Creatinolfosfate Sodium *(rINNM)*

Creatinolfosfato sódico. The sodium salt of 1-(2-hydroxyethyl)-1-methylguanidine *O*-phosphate .

$C_4H_{11}N_3NaO_4P$ = 219.1.

*CAS — 6903-79-3 (creatinolfosfate).*

*ATC — C01EB05.*

### Profile

Creatinolfosfate has been used as an adjuvant in the treatment of cardiac disorders.

### Preparations

**Proprietary Preparations** (details are given in Part 3)

***Ital.:*** Aplodan†; ***Spain:*** Dragosil†.

## Crotalaria

### Profile

Crotalaria spp. have been used in herbal teas but liver damage has been reported following their ingestion, possibly due to their content of pyrrolizidine alkaloids.

## CS Gas

CS Spray; Gas CS.

$C_{10}H_5ClN_2$ = 188.6.

*CAS — 2698-41-1.*

### Profile

CS gas (more properly CS spray) is the name commonly given to a particulate dispersion of α-(*o*-chlorobenzylidene) malonitrile, used as a riot-control agent or 'tear gas'. Its toxic effects include irritation of the eyes and nose, with copious lachrymation and rhinorrhoea; blepharospasm; a burning sensation of the mouth and throat; tightness in the chest, with difficulty in breathing; coughing; an increase in salivation; and retching and vomiting. These effects usually disappear a few minutes after exposure ends. The effects of pre-existing disease of the respiratory tract may be exacerbated. Erythema and blistering of the skin may occur.

Exposed persons should be removed to a well ventilated area. Treatment is symptomatic. Contaminated skin may be washed with soap and water, but only if symptoms persist since exposure to water may initially exacerbate symptoms. If contamination of the eyes has been severe they should be irrigated with physiological saline or water and a local anaesthetic instilled to relieve pain.

◊ References.


1. Hu H, *et al.* Tear gas—harassing agent or toxic chemical weapon? *JAMA* 1989; **262:** 660–3.
2. Yih J-P. CS gas injury to the eye. *BMJ* 1995; **311:** 276.
3. Gray PJ. Treating CS gas injuries to the eye: exposure at close range is particularly dangerous. *BMJ* 1995; **311:** 871.
4. Jones GRN. CS sprays: antidote and decontaminant. *Lancet* 1996; **347:** 968–9.
5. Anderson PJ, *et al.* Acute effects of the potent lacrimator o-chlorobenzylidene malonitrile (CS) tear gas. *Hum Exp Toxicol* 1996; **15:** 461–5.
6. Anonymous. "Safety" of chemical batons. *Lancet* 1998; **352:** 159.
7. Varma S, Holt PJ. Severe cutaneous reaction to CS gas. *Clin Exp Dermatol* 2001; **26:** 248–50.
8. Nathan R, *et al.* Long-term psychiatric morbidity in the aftermath of CS spray trauma. *Med Sci Law* 2003; **43:** 98–104.


## Cucurbita

Abóbora; Calabaza, semillas de; Kürbissamen; Melon Pumpkin Seeds; Pepo; Semence de Courge.

**Pharmacopoeias.** In *Ger.*

### Profile

Cucurbita consists of the seeds of *Cucurbita pepo* (Cucurbitaceae) or related species. It was formerly used for the expulsion of tapeworms (*Taenia*).

It is an ingredient of several herbal preparations used in urinary-tract disorders.

### Preparations

**Proprietary Preparations** (details are given in Part 3)

***Chile:*** Lefkur; ***Fr.:*** ViTiX; ***Ger.:*** Cysto-Urgenin; Granu Fink Kurbiskern; Nomon mono; Prosta Fink forte; Prostalog†; Turiplex†; Urgenin Cucurbitae oleum; Uvirgan mono; Vesiherb.

**Multi-ingredient:** ***Arg.:*** Clean-AC; Cleanance; ***Austral.:*** Lifechange Mens Complex with Saw Palmetto†; ***Canad.:*** Prostease; ProstGard; ***Chile:*** Clean-AC; Cleanance; ***Fr.:*** Salucur†; ***Ger.:*** Alsicur†; Cysto Fink†; Granu Fink Kurbiskern N; Granu Fink Prosta; Prosta Fink N†; Prostamed; Prostata-Kurbis S†; Uvirgan N; ***Hong Kong:*** Sawmetto Vivo-Livo; ***Port.:*** Bioclin Sebo Care; Prostamed; ***Switz.:*** Cysto-Caps Chassot†; Granu Fink Prosta; Prosta-Caps Chassot N; Prosta-Caps Fink†.

## Cusparia

Angostura; Angostura Bark; Carony Bark; Cusparia Bark.

NOTE. 'Angostura Bitters' (*Dr. J.G.B. Siegert & Sons Ltd*) contains gentian and various aromatic ingredients but no cusparia; it is named after the town in which it was first made.

### Profile

Cusparia, the bark of *Galipea officinalis* (Rutaceae), has been used as a bitter.

## Cyanoacrylate Adhesives

Cianoacrilato, adhesivos de.

*CAS — 1069-55-2 (bucrilate); 6606-65-1 (enbucrilate); 137-05-3 (mecrilate); 6701-17-3 (ocrilate);.*

### Profile

A number of cyanoacrylate compounds have been used as surgical tissue adhesives. They include:

- bucrilate (bucrylate; isobutyl 2-cyanoacrylate, $C_8H_{11}NO_2 = 153.2$)
- enbucrilate (butyl 2-cyanoacrylate, $C_8H_{11}NO_2 = 153.2$),
- mecrilate (mecrylate; methyl 2-cyanoacrylate, $C_5H_5NO_2 = 111.1$)
- ocrilate (ocrylate; octil 2-cyanoacrylate, $C_{12}H_{19}NO_2 = 209.3$).

Some cyanoacrylates are used for household purposes and as nail fixatives and others have been investigated as tubal occlusive agents for female sterilisation, for sclerotherapy in bleeding gastric varices (p.1716), and for embolisation of intracranial vascular lesions.

**Adverse effects.** Reports of inadvertent application of cyanoacrylate adhesives to the eyes,[1,2] mouth,[3] and ears.[4,5]


1. Lyons C, *et al.* Superglue inadvertently used as eyedrops. *BMJ* 1990; **300:** 328.
2. DeRespinis PA. Cyanoacrylate nail glue mistaken for eye drops. *JAMA* 1990; **263:** 2301.
3. Cousin GCS. Accidental application of cyanoacrylate to the mouth. *Br Dent J* 1990; **169:** 293–4.
4. O'Donnell JJ, *et al.* Cyanoacrylate adhesive mistaken for ear drops. *J Accid Emerg Med* 1997; **14:** 199.
5. Persaud R. A novel approach to the removal of superglue from the ear. *J Laryngol Otol* 2001; **115:** 901–2.


**Treatment of adverse effects.** In the event of accidental adhesion of the skin the bonded surfaces may be separated following application of acetone, prolonged soaking in warm (not hot) soapy water, and/or mixtures of alcohol and water. If necessary, the surfaces may be peeled or rolled apart with the aid of a spatula; attempts should not be made to pull the surfaces directly apart. Acetone and alcohol should not be used near or in the eyes. Solvents such as nitromethane, toluene, or xylene may be used to aid skin detachment from solid objects. Solvents should be used with care and should not be introduced into the oropharynx. Eyelids stuck together or bonded to the eyeball should be washed thoroughly with saline or water at room temperature and a gauze patch applied; the eye will open without further action in 1 to 4 days. Manipulative attempts to open the eyes should not be made. Although cyanoacrylate introduced into the eyes may cause double vision and lachrymation there is usually no residual damage. If lips are accidentally stuck together plenty of warm water should be applied and maximum wetting and pressure from saliva inside the mouth encouraged. Lips should be peeled or rolled apart and not pulled. Adhesive introduced into the mouth solidifies and adheres, but saliva will lift the adhesive in ½ to 2 days. Care should be taken to avoid choking.

Heat is evolved on solidification of cyanoacrylate and in rare cases may cause burns.

**Uses.** References to the use of bucrilate,[1,2] enbucrilate,[3,4] and ocrilate.[5-9]


1. Kind R, *et al.* Bucrylate treatment of bleeding gastric varices: 12 years' experience. *Endoscopy* 2000; **32:** 512–9.
2. Shepler TR, Seiff SR. Use of isobutyl cyanoacrylate tissue adhesive to stabilize external eyelid weights in temporary treatment of facial palsies. *Ophthal Plast Reconstr Surg* 2001; **17:** 169–73.
3. Schonauer F, *et al.* Use of Indermil tissue adhesive for closure of superficial skin lacerations in children. *Minerva Chir* 2001; **56:** 427–9.
4. Sinha S, *et al.* A single blind, prospective, randomized trial comparing n-butyl 2-cyanoacrylate tissue adhesive (Indermil) and sutures for skin closure in hand surgery. *J Hand Surg* 2001; **26:** 264–5.
5. Kutcher MJ, *et al.* Evaluation of a bioadhesive device for the management of aphthous ulcers. *J Am Dent Assoc* 2001; **132:** 368–76.
6. Puri P. Tissue glue aided lid repositioning in temporary management of involutional entropion. *Eur J Ophthalmol* 2001; **11:** 211–4.
7. Bernard L, *et al.* A prospective comparison of octyl cyanoacrylate tissue adhesive (dermabond) and suture for the closure of excisional wounds in children and adolescents. *Arch Dermatol* 2001; **137:** 1177–80.
8. Mattick A, *et al.* A randomised, controlled trial comparing a tissue adhesive (2-octylcyanoacrylate) with adhesive strips (Steristrips) for paediatric laceration repair. *Emerg Med J* 2002; **19:** 405–7.
9. Magee WP, *et al.* Use of octyl-2-cyanoacrylate in cleft lip repair. *Ann Plast Surg* 2003; **50:** 1–5.


### Preparations

**Proprietary Preparations** (details are given in Part 3)
***UK:*** Dermabond; Histoacryl; Indermil; LiquiBand; SuperSkin.
**Multi-ingredient:** ***Ger.:*** Epiglu; ***UK:*** Epiglu.

## Cyclobutyrol Sodium *(rINNM)*

Ciclobutirol sódico. Sodium 2-(1-hydroxycyclohexyl)butyrate.

$C_{10}H_{17}NaO_3 = 208.2.$

*CAS — 512-16-3 (cyclobutyrol); 1130-23-0 (cyclobutyrol sodium).*

*ATC — A05AX03.*

### Profile

Cyclobutyrol sodium is a choleretic that has been given by mouth. Cyclobutyrol betaine, cyclobutyrol calcium, and cyclobutyrol nicotinamide have been used similarly.

### Preparations

**Proprietary Preparations** (details are given in Part 3)
***Fr.:*** Hebucol†; ***Ital.:*** Epa-Bon†.
**Multi-ingredient:** ***Austria:*** Trommgallol; ***Spain:*** Levaliver†; Liberbil†; Lidobama Complex†; Menabil Complex; Prodessal†; Salcemetic; Sugarbil.

## Cyclodextrins

Ciclodextrinas.

## Alfadex *(BAN, rINN)*

Alfadexum; Alphacyclodextrin; α-Cyclodextrin. Cyclomaltohexaose.

$C_{36}H_{60}O_{30} = 972.8.$

*CAS — 10016-20-3.*

**Pharmacopoeias.** In *Eur.* (see p.vi).

**Ph. Eur. 5.0** (Alfadex). A white or almost white, amorphous or crystalline powder. Freely soluble in water and in propylene glycol; practically insoluble in dehydrated alcohol and in dichloromethane. Store in airtight containers.

## Betadex *(BAN, USAN, rINN)*

Betadexum; β-Cyclodextrin; E459. Cyclo-α-(1→4)-D-heptaglucopyranoside.

$C_{42}H_{70}O_{35} = 1135.$

*CAS — 7585-39-9.*

**Pharmacopoeias.** In *Chin.* and *Eur.* (see p.vi). Also in *USNF.*

**Ph. Eur. 5.0** (Betadex). A white or almost white, amorphous or crystalline powder. Sparingly soluble in water; practically insoluble in alcohol and in dichloromethane; freely soluble in propylene glycol. Store in airtight containers.

**USNF 22** (Betadex). A nonreducing cyclic compound composed of seven alpha-(1-4) linked D-glucopyranosyl units. It is a white, practically odourless, fine crystalline powder. Soluble 1 in 54 of water. Store in airtight containers.

## Hydroxypropylbetadex

Hydroxypropylbetadexum; 2-Hydroxypropyl-β-cyclodextrin.

**Pharmacopoeias.** In *Eur.* (see p.vi).

**Ph. Eur. 5.0** (Hydroxypropylbetadex). A white or almost white, amorphous or crystalline powder. Freely soluble in water and in propylene glycol.

### Profile

Cyclodextrins, such as alfadex and betadex, are produced by the enzymatic degradation of starch and are used as carrier molecules for drug delivery systems. Hydroxypropylbetadex, a derivative of betadex, is also used.

◊ References.


1. Ridgway K. Drug release rates: cyclodextrin complexes. *Pharm J* 1990; **245:** 344–5.
2. Szejtli J. Cyclodextrins: properties and applications. *Drug Invest* 1990; **2** (suppl 4): 11–21.
3. El Shaboury MH. Physical properties and dissolution profiles of tablets directly compressed with β-cyclodextrin. *Int J Pharmaceutics* 1990; **63:** 95–100.
4. Stella VJ, Rajewski RA. Cyclodextrins: their future in drug formulation and delivery. *Pharm Res* 1997; **14:** 556–67.
5. Loftsson T, Olafsson JH. Cyclodextrins: new drug delivery systems in dermatology. *Int J Dermatol* 1998; **37:** 241–6.
6. Redenti E, *et al.* Drug/cyclodextrin/hydroxy acid multicomponent systems: properties and pharmaceutical applications. *J Pharm Sci* 2000; **89:** 1–8.
7. Loftsson T, Masson M. Cyclodextrins in topical drug formulations: theory and practice. *Int J Pharm* 2001; **225:** 15–30.
8. Loftsson T, Stefansson E. Cyclodextrins in eye drop formulations: enhanced topical delivery of corticosteroids to the eye. *Acta Ophthalmol Scand* 2002; **80:** 144–50.


## Cyclovalone *(rINN)*

Ciclovalona. 2,6-Divanillylidenecyclohexanone.

$C_{22}H_{22}O_5 = 366.4.$

*CAS — 579-23-7.*

### Profile

Cyclovalone is a choleretic that has been given by mouth.

### Preparations

**Proprietary Preparations** (details are given in Part 3)
***Belg.:*** Vanidene†; ***Fr.:*** Vanilone†.

## Cynara

Alcachofa; Alcachôfra; Artichaut; Artichoke Leaf.

**Pharmacopoeias.** In *Fr.*

### Profile

Cynara, the leaves of the globe artichoke, *Cynara scolymus* (Compositae), is reputed to have diuretic and choleretic properties. It may also have some hypolipidaemic activity.

### Preparations

**Proprietary Preparations** (details are given in Part 3)
***Arg.:*** Chofitol; Cynarex; ***Austria:*** Cynarix; Hepa-S†; Hepactiv; Heparstad; Regulin; ***Belg.:*** Cynarol†; ***Braz.:*** Chophytol; ***Fr.:*** Chophytol; Gallexier; Hepanephrol; ***Ger.:*** aar gamma N; Carminagal N; Cefacynar; Cyna Bilisan; Cynacur; Cynafol†; Cynarix N; Hekbilin Kapseln†; Hepagallin N; Hepar SL; Hepar-POS; Heparstad; Hewechol Artischockendragees; Lipei; Losapan; Maquil†; ratioHepar; ***Port.:*** Hepanephrol; ***Switz.:*** Chophytol†; Hepa-S.

**Multi-ingredient:** ***Arg.:*** Arceligasol; Bagohepat; Bilidren; Biliosan Compuesto; Dioxicolagol; Hepacur; Hepatalgina; Hepatodirectol; Herbaccion Dig Fresh; Herbaccion Digestivo; Palatrobil; ***Austral.:*** Extralife Liva-Care†; Lifesystem Herbal Formula 7 Liver Tonic†; Liver Tonic Herbal Formula 6†; ***Austria:*** Agnuchol; Aponatura Leber; Bio-Strath Leber-Galle; Cynarix comp; Gallesyn neu; Mag Doskar's Leber-Galletonikum; Magentropen N Legastol†; Sanvita Leber-Galle; Tiroler Adler Leber- und Gallentee; Tiroler Adler Schwedenbitter; ***Belg.:*** Tisane pour le Foie†; ***Braz.:*** Alcafelol; Boldigan†; Chofranina; Colachofra; Composto Emagrecedor; Cynarobil†; Digestron; Emagrevit; Epagogo†; Epatovis†; Figadosan†; Figatil†; Gotas Hepaticas†; Gotas Preciosas†; Hecrosine B12†; Hepachofril Solution†; Hepachofril†; Hepacholan†; Hepasedan†; Hepatilon†; Hepatophil†; Hepatoregius; Hepavirmo†; Jurubileno†; Kop Hepar†; Lisotox†; Litrison†; Metionina Composta†; Necrohepat†; Olocynan†; Prinachol; Solvobil; ***Canad.:*** Milk Thistle; ***Fr.:*** Actibil; Actisane Digestion†; Aromabyl†; Canol; Elixir Spark; Gastralsan†; Hepaclem; Hepax; Romarinex-Choline†; Tisane des Familles†; Vegelax; ***Ger.:*** Artischocke plus Legastol†; Bilicura Forte†; Carmol Magen-Galle-Darm; Cynarzym N; Gallexier; Galloselect M; Hepatofalk Neu†; Pascobilin novo; Salus Leber-Galle-Tee Nr.18†; Sirmia Artischockenelixier N†; Ullus Galle-Tee N†; ***Hong Kong:*** Hepatofalk; ***Ital.:*** Colax; Digelax; Epagest; Florerbe Lassativa†; Fluend†; Lievistar†; Vadolax; Vegebyl†; ***Mex.:*** Chofabol; Ifuchol; ***Spain:*** Cinaro Bilina†; Cynaro Bilina; Lipograsil; Menabil Complex; Nico Hepatocyn; ***Switz.:*** Bilifuge; Boldocynara; Demonatur Gouttes pour le foie et la bile; Phytomed Hepato; Stago†; Tisane hepatique et biliaire; ***UK:*** Bio-Strath Artichoke Formula.

## Cynarine

Cinarina; Cynarin; 1,5-Dicaffeoylquinic Acid. 1-Carboxy-4,5-dihydroxy-1,3-cyclohexylene bis(3,4-dihydroxycinnamate).

$C_{25}H_{24}O_{12} = 516.5.$

*CAS — 1182-34-9; 1884-24-8.*

### Profile

Cynarine is an active ingredient of cynara (above). It has been used as a choleretic.

### Preparations

**Proprietary Preparations** (details are given in Part 3)
***Braz.:*** Cynaron†.
**Multi-ingredient:** ***Austria:*** Trommgallol; ***Braz.:*** Colagolen†.

## Cytochrome C

Citocromo C.

**Pharmacopoeias.** *Chin.* includes Cytochrome C Solution and preparations for injection.

### Profile

Cytochrome C is a haemoprotein occurring in the body and involved in electron and hydrogen transport in biological oxidation processes. It has been given intravenously in various hypoxic conditions.

Cytochrome C is an ingredient of some eye drops used for the treatment of cataract but its actions, if any, are unclear.

### Preparations

**Proprietary Preparations** (details are given in Part 3)
**Multi-ingredient:** ***Fr.:*** Vitaphakol†; ***Ger.:*** Vitreolent plus†; ***Port.:*** Vitaphakol†; ***Spain:*** Vitaphakol; ***Switz.:*** Vitaphakol†.

## Cytokines

Citocinas.

### Profile

Cytokines are a group of endogenous peptide regulatory molecules with the ability to affect cellular differentiation and/or proliferation. In contrast to peptide hormones, cytokines tend to act locally. Most cytokines are multifunctional molecules with a range of biological effects; they act primarily as mediators of inflammation or as growth factors. Cytokines that are used clinically include thrombopoietin (p.760), granulocyte and granulocyte-macrophage colony-stimulating factors such as filgrastim (p.753) and molgramostim (p.756), interferons (p.640), interleukin-2 (p.562), oprelvekin (p.757), tumour necrosis factor (p.590), somatomedins (p.1338), and urogastrone (p.1294); those under investigation include interleukin-1 (p.1701), interleukin-3 (p.755), interleukin-12 (p.1701), and other interleukins, fibroblast growth factor, keratinocyte growth factor, nerve growth factor, platelet-derived growth factor, and transforming growth factor. Some cytokines are involved in the pathophysiology of diseases and a number of cytokine antagonists are also being studied.

◊ References.


1. Lambiase A, *et al.* Topical treatment with nerve growth factor for corneal neurotrophic ulcers. *N Engl J Med* 1998; **338:** 1174–80.
2. Fu X, *et al.* Randomised placebo-controlled trial of use of topical recombinant bovine basic fibroblast growth factor for second-degree burns. *Lancet* 1998; **352:** 1661–4.
3. Wieman TJ, *et al.* Efficacy and safety of a topical gel formulation of recombinant human platelet-derived growth factor-BB (becaplermin) in patients with chronic neuropathic diabetic ulcers: a phase III randomized placebo-controlled double-blind study. *Diabetes Care* 1998; **21:** 822–7.
4. Anonymous. Platelet-derived growth factor for diabetic ulcers. *Med Lett Drugs Ther* 1998; **40:** 73–4.
5. Bernabei R, *et al.* Effect of topical application of nerve-growth factor on pressure ulcers. *Lancet* 1999; **354:** 307.
6. Kuter DJ. Future directions with platelet growth factors. *Semin Hematol* 2000; **37:** 41–9.
7. Apfel SC, *et al.* Efficacy and safety of recombinant human nerve growth factor in patients with diabetic polyneuropathy: a randomized controlled trial. *JAMA* 2000; **284:** 2215–21.
8. Xing Z, Wang J. Consideration of cytokines as therapeutics agents or targets. *Curr Pharm Des* 2000; **6:** 599–611.
9. Schooltink H, Rose-John S. Cytokines as therapeutic drugs. *J Interferon Cytokine Res* 2002; **22:** 505–16.
10. Andreakos ET, *et al.* Cytokines and anti-cytokine biologicals in autoimmunity: present and future. *Cytokine Growth Factor Rev* 2002; **13:** 299–313.
11. Stevceva L. Cytokines and their antagonists as therapeutic agents. *Curr Med Chem* 2002; **9:** 2201–7.


## Damiana

Turnera.

### Profile

Damiana is the dried leaves and stem of *Turnera diffusa* var. *aphrodisiaca* (Turneraceae) and possibly other species of *Turnera*. Damiana is drunk as a tea, and is used in herbal medicine for a variety of indications. It has a reputation as an aphrodisiac, but there is no evidence for this. It is also used in homoeopathic medicine.

### Preparations

**Proprietary Preparations** (details are given in Part 3)
***UK:*** Gerard House Curzon†.

**Multi-ingredient: *Austral.:*** Bioglan Mens Super Soy/Clover†; Bioglan The Blue One†; Medinat Esten†; ***Canad.:*** Damiana-Sarsaparilla Formula; ***Ital.:*** Dam; Four-Ton; ***Spain:*** Energysor; ***UK:*** Daily Fatigue Relief; Damiana and Kola Tablets; Elixir Damiana and Saw Palmetto; Regina Royal Concorde; Strength; Zotrim.

## Dapiprazole Hydrochloride *(USAN, rINNM)*

AF-2139; Hidrocloruro de dapiprazol. 5,6,7,8-Tetrahydro-3-[2-(4-*o*-tolyl-1-piperazinyl)ethyl]-s-triazolo[4,3-*a*]pyridine monohydrochloride.

$C_{19}H_{27}N_5,HCl = 361.9.$

*CAS — 72822-12-9 (dapiprazole); 72822-13-0 (dapiprazole hydrochloride).*

*ATC — S01EX02.*

### Profile

Dapiprazole hydrochloride is an alpha blocker administered as eye drops to reverse mydriasis; it is also used in some countries in the management of glaucoma. Dapiprazole may also have antipsychotic activity.

**Reversal of mydriasis.** Dapiprazole is used to reverse the effects of mydriatics (sympathomimetics, and to some extent tropicamide) following surgery or ophthalmoscopic examination (p.1487). It also appears to enhance recovery of accommodation after the use of cycloplegics and may be effective for reversing mydriasis after cataract extraction.

References.


1. Allinson RW, *et al.* Reversal of mydriasis by dapiprazole. *Ann Ophthalmol* 1990; **22:** 131–8.
2. Ponte F, *et al.* Intraocular dapiprazole for the reversal of mydriasis after extracapsular cataract extraction with intraocular lens implantation: Part II: comparison with acetylcholine. *J Cataract Refract Surg* 1991; **17:** 785–9.
3. Johnson ME, *et al.* Efficacy of dapiprazole with hydroxyamphetamine hydrobromide and tropicamide. *J Am Optom Assoc* 1993; **64:** 629–33.
4. Molinari JF, *et al.* Dapiprazole clinical efficacy for counteracting tropicamide 1%. *Optom Vis Sci* 1994; **71:** 319–22.
5. Wilcox CS, *et al.* Comparison of the effects on pupil size and accommodation of three regimens of topical dapiprazole. *Br J Ophthalmol* 1995; **79:** 544–8.


### Preparations

**Proprietary Preparations** (details are given in Part 3)
***Austria:*** Benglau; ***Ger.:*** Remydrial†; ***Israel:*** Glamidolo; ***Ital.:*** Glamidolo; ***USA:*** Rev-Eyes.

## Dehydrocholic Acid *(BAN, rINN)*

Ácido dehidrocólico; Chologon; Triketocholanic Acid. 3,7,12-Trioxo-5β-cholan-24-oic acid.

$C_{24}H_{34}O_5 = 402.5.$

*CAS — 81-23-2 (dehydrocholic acid); 145-41-5 (sodium dehydrocholate).*

**Pharmacopoeias.** In *Chin., It., Jpn,* and *US.*

**USP 27** (Dehydrocholic Acid). A white, fluffy, odourless powder. Practically insoluble in water; soluble 1 in 100 of alcohol, 1 in 135 of acetic acid at 15°, 1 in 130 of acetone at 15°, 1 in 35 of chloroform, 1 in 2200 of ether at 15°, 1 in 135 of ethyl acetate at 15°, and 1 in 960 of benzene at 15°; solutions in alcohol and in chloroform are usually slightly turbid; soluble in glacial acetic acid and in solutions of alkali hydroxides and carbonates.

### Profile

Dehydrocholic acid is a semisynthetic bile acid (p.1660) that is used for its hydrocholeretic properties, increasing the volume and water content of the bile without appreciably altering the content of bile acids. It has been used to improve biliary drainage and has also been given for the temporary relief of constipation. Usual doses of 250 to 500 mg three times daily by mouth after meals have been employed.

Dehydrocholic acid is contra-indicated in significant cholelithiasis, complete mechanical biliary obstruction, and in severe hepatic impairment.

### Preparations

***USP 27:*** Dehydrocholic Acid Tablets.

**Proprietary Preparations** (details are given in Part 3)
***Braz.:*** Decholin†; ***Canad.:*** Dycholium†; ***USA:*** Cholan-HMB; Decholin.

**Multi-ingredient: *Arg.:*** Bagohepat; Bibol Leloup; Bil 13; Bil 13 Enzimatico; Bilagol; Carbogasol Digestivo; Digenorflat; Hepadigenor; Hepatalgina; Novodig; Pakinase; Palatrobil; Pankreon Compuesto; Pankreon Total; ***Austria:*** Gallo Merz†; ***Braz.:*** B-Vesil; Colagolen†; Colagotil†; Digeplus; Digestron; Dioctosal†; Espasmo Novozyme†; Essen; Filogaster; Hepatobyl†; Plasil Enzimatico; Sintozima; Vonil Enzimatico†; ***Canad.:*** Regubil†; ***Fin.:*** Fellesan†; ***Hong Kong:*** Bilsan; ***Ital.:*** Certobil†; ***Mex.:*** Plasil Enzimatico; ***Port.:*** Drenomade†; Espasmo Canulase; ***S.Afr.:*** Spasmo-Canulase; ***Spain:*** Nulacin Fermentos; ***Swed.:*** Fellesan†; ***Switz.:*** Gillazyme plus†; Gillazyme†; Spasmo-Canulase.

## Denatonium Benzoate *(BAN, USAN, rINN)*

Benzoato de denatonio; NSC-157658. Benzyldiethyl(2,6-xylylcarbamoylmethyl)ammonium benzoate monohydrate.

$C_{28}H_{34}N_2O_3,H_2O = 464.6.$

*CAS — 3734-33-6 (anhydrous denatonium benzoate); 86398-53-0 (denatonium benzoate monohydrate).*

**Pharmacopoeias.** In *USNF.*

**USNF 22** (Denatonium Benzoate). When dried at 105° for 2 hours, it contains one molecule of water of hydration or is anhydrous. Soluble 1 in 20 of water, 1 in 2.4 of alcohol, 1 in 2.9 of chloroform, and 1 in 5000 of ether; very soluble in methyl alcohol. pH of a 3% solution in water is between 6.5 and 7.5. Store in airtight containers.

### Profile

Denatonium benzoate is used where an intensely bitter taste is required for medicinal or industrial purposes and as a partial denaturant for alcohol in toiletries. It is known commercially as Bitrex.

## Deoxyribonucleic Acid

ADN; Animal Nucleic Acid; Desoxirribonucleico, ácido; Desoxypentose Nucleic Acid; Desoxyribonucleic Acid; Desoxyribose Nucleic Acid; DNA; Thymus Nucleic Acid.

### Profile

Deoxyribonucleic acid is a nucleotide polymer, and 1 of the 2 distinct varieties of nucleic acid (p.1722). It is found in the cell nuclei of living tissues. Proprietary preparations of deoxyribonucleic acid are marketed in some countries and are advocated for a variety of debilitated and convalescent conditions. The sodium and magnesium salts are also used.

### Preparations

**Proprietary Preparations** (details are given in Part 3)
***Ital.:*** Placentex; Polides†.

**Multi-ingredient: *Fr.:*** Adena C; Nutrigene†; Osteogen†; ***India:*** Placentrex.

## Dextran Sulfate

Dextran Sulfate Sodium; Dextran Sulphate; Dextran Sulphate Sodium; Dextrano, sulfato de.

*CAS — 9011-18-1.*

*ATC — B05AA05.*

**Pharmacopoeias.** In *Jpn.*

### Profile

Dextran sulfate is the sodium salt of sulfuric acid esters of dextran. It has been used as an anticoagulant and as a lipid regulating drug, and has been investigated for its antiviral activity. Dextran sulfate potassium has also been used.

**Interactions.** As mentioned on p.844, anaphylactoid reactions have occurred in patients receiving ACE inhibitors during low-density lipoprotein apheresis using a dextran sulfate-cellulose column.[1,2] Withdrawal of the ACE inhibitor for 1 to 3 days before apheresis may prevent the reaction.[2]


1. Olbricht CJ, *et al.* Anaphylactoid reactions, LDL apheresis with dextran sulphate, and ACE inhibitors. *Lancet* 1992; **340:** 908–9.
2. Agishi T. Anion-blood contact reaction (ABC reaction) in patients treated by LDL apheresis with dextran sulfate-cellulose column while receiving ACE inhibitors. *JAMA* 1994; **271:** 195–6.


### Preparations

**Proprietary Preparations** (details are given in Part 3)

**Multi-ingredient: *Arg.:*** Dirosea; ***Austral.:*** VR; ***Fr.:*** Avene Antirougeurs; Creme au Melilot Composee; Dextrarine Phenylbutazone; Diroseal; ***Ger.:*** Phlebodril N; ***Ital.:*** Stranoval; ***Port.:*** Cicapost; Doxivenil; ***Switz.:*** Doxivenil.

## Dextrorphan *(BAN, pINN)*

Dextrorfano. 17-Methyl-9α,13α,14α-morphinan-3-ol.

$C_{17}H_{23}NO = 257.4.$

*CAS — 125-73-5.*

## Dextrorphan Hydrochloride *(BANM, USAN, pINNM)*

Ro-01-6794/706.

$C_{17}H_{23}NO,HCl = 293.8.$

*CAS — 69376-27-8.*

### Profile

Dextrorphan, a metabolite of dextromethorphan (p.1117), is an antagonist of the excitatory neurotransmitter *N*-methyl-D-aspartate (NMDA). It possesses some cough suppressant activity and has been investigated as a neuroprotective agent in the management of stroke.

◊ References.


1. Albers GW, *et al.* Safety, tolerability, and pharmacokinetics of the N-methyl-D-aspartate antagonist dextrorphan in patients with acute stroke. *Stroke* 1995; **26:** 254–8.


## Dibutyl Sebacate

Sebacato de dibutilo.

$C_{18}H_{34}O_4 = 314.5.$

*CAS — 109-43-3.*

**Pharmacopoeias.** In *USNF.*

**USNF 22** (Dibutyl Sebacate). It consists of esters of *n*-butyl alcohol and saturated dibasic acids, principally sebacic acid. A colourless, oily liquid of very mild odour. Practically insoluble in water and in glycerol; soluble in alcohol, in isopropyl alcohol, and in liquid paraffin; very slightly soluble in propylene glycol. Store in airtight containers.

### Profile

Dibutyl sebacate is a plasticiser used in pharmaceutical formulation of tablets (including modified release), beads, and granules, and microcapsule preparations. It is also used as a food flavouring.

## Dichlorodiethylsulfide

Dichlorodiethylsulphide; Gas mostaza; Mustard Gas; Sulfur Mustard; Yellow Cross Liquid; Yperite. Bis(2-chloroethyl)sulphide.

$C_4H_8Cl_2S = 159.1.$

*CAS — 505-60-2.*

### Profile

Dichlorodiethylsulfide was developed for use in chemical warfare and has even more severe vesicant and irritant properties than its nitrogen analogue, chlormethine (p.537). It was formerly used topically in the treatment of psoriasis.

◊ Reviews of the toxicology of dichlorodiethylsulfide,[1,2] and debate on the management of casualties injured by dichlorodiethylsulfide and other chemical warfare agents.[3-9] Most patients exposed to dichlorodiethylsulfide recover completely and only a small proportion will have long-term eye or lung damage,[10] although death from respiratory, renal, and bone-marrow failure may occur.[9]

Eleven fishermen who accidentally retrieved corroded and leaking gas shells containing dichlorodiethylsulfide from underwater dumps, presented with very inflamed skin, especially in the axillary and genitofemoral regions, yellow blisters on the hands and legs, painful irritation of the eyes, and transient blindness. Two developed pulmonary oedema.[11] There was evidence of a mutagenic effect and in view of the increased risk of lung cancer in soldiers and workers exposed to the gas it is reasonable to assume that fishermen heavily exposed to dichlorodiethylsulfide also have an increased cancer risk.


1. Smith KJ, *et al.* Sulfur mustard: its continuing threat as a chemical warfare agent, the cutaneous lesions induced, progress in understanding its mechanism of action, its long-term health effects, and new developments for protection and therapy. *J Am Acad Dermatol* 1995; **32:** 765–76.
2. Dacre JC, Goldman M. Toxicology and pharmacology of the chemical warfare agent sulfur mustard. *Pharmacol Rev* 1996; **48:** 289–326.

3. Heyndrickx A, Heyndrickx B. Management of war gas injuries. *Lancet* 1990; **ii:** 1248–9.
4. Fouyn T, *et al.* Management of chemical warfare injuries. *Lancet* 1991; **337:** 121.
5. Willems JL, *et al.* Management of chemical warfare injuries. *Lancet* 1991; **337:** 121–2.
6. Maynard RL, *et al.* Management of chemical warfare injuries. *Lancet* 1991; **337:** 122.
7. Newman-Taylor AJ, Morris AJR. Experience with mustard gas casualties. *Lancet* 1991; **337:** 242.
8. Heyndrickx A. Chemical warfare injuries. *Lancet* 1991; **337:** 430.
9. Rees J, *et al.* Mustard gas casualties. *Lancet* 1991; **337:** 430.
10. Murray VSG, Volans GN. Management of injuries due to chemical weapons. *BMJ* 1991; **302:** 129–30.
11. Wulf HC, *et al.* Sister chromatid exchanges in fishermen exposed to leaking mustard gas shells. *Lancet* 1985; **i:** 690–1.


## Digitalin

Amorphous Digitalin; Digitalina; Digitalinum Purum Germanicum.

NOTE. Distinguish from Digitaline Cristallisée (digitoxin, p.894) which is very much more potent.

### Profile

Digitalin is a standardised mixture of glycosides from *Digitalis purpurea*. It has actions similar to those of digoxin (p.895). Because of its ready solubility in water it was formerly used for the preparation of solutions for injection. It is also present in some ophthalmic preparations.

### Preparations

**Proprietary Preparations** (details are given in Part 3)
***Ger.:*** Augentonikum N.

**Multi-ingredient:** ***Ital.:*** Digifar.

## Dihydroergocristine Mesilate *(BANM)*

Dihidroergocristina, mesilato de; Dihydroergocristine Mesylate; Dihydroergocristine Methanesulphonate; Dihydroergocristini Mesilas. (6a*R*,9*R*,10a*R*)-*N*-[(2*R*,5*S*,10a*S*,10b*S*)-5-Benzyl-10b-hydroxy-2-isopropyl-3,6-dioxooctahydro-8*H*-[1,3]oxazolo[3,2-*a*]pyrrolo[2,1-*c*]pyrazin-2-yl]-7-methyl-4,6,6a,7,8,9,10,10a-octahydroindolo[4,3-*fg*]quinoline-9-carboxamide methanesulphonate.

$C_{35}H_{41}N_5O_5,CH_4O_3S$ = 707.8.

*CAS — 17479-19-5 (dihydroergocristine); 24730-10-7 (dihydroergocristine mesilate).*

*ATC — C04AE04.*

**Pharmacopoeias.** In *Eur.* (see p.vi).

**Ph. Eur. 5.0** (Dihydroergocristine Mesilate). A white or almost white, fine crystalline powder. Slightly soluble in water; soluble in methyl alcohol. A 0.5% solution in water has a pH of 4.0 to 5.0. Protect from light.

### Profile

Dihydroergocristine mesilate is a component of co-dergocrine mesilate (p.1674) and has similar actions. In some countries it has been given by mouth in the symptomatic treatment of mental deterioration associated with cerebrovascular insufficiency and in peripheral vascular disease. It has also been given by intramuscular injection.

◊ References.


1. Franciosi A, Zavattini G. Dihydroergocristine in the treatment of elderly patients with cognitive deterioration: a double-blind, placebo-controlled, dose-response study. *Curr Ther Res* 1994; **55:** 1391–1401.


### Preparations

**Proprietary Preparations** (details are given in Part 3)
***Austria:*** Diertina†; Nehydrin; ***Braz.:*** Iskemil; Iskevert; ***Ital.:*** Defluina; Diertina; Difluid; Ergocris†; Gral†; Unergol†; Vasoton†; ***Mex.:*** Decme†; ***Port.:*** Diertina; ***Spain:*** Diertine; Ergodavur; ***Switz.:*** Diertina†.

**Multi-ingredient:** ***Arg.:*** Cervilane; Cinacris; Micerfin; ***Austria:*** Brinerdin; Defluina; Pressimedin†; Sandoven†; Supergan†; ***Braz.:*** Isketam; Norogil; Vasofluina†; Vertizine D; ***Chile:*** Cervilane; ***Fr.:*** Cervilane†; Iskedyl; ***Ital.:*** Brinerdina; ***Mex.:*** Cervilan; ***Port.:*** Brinerdine; Cervilane; ***S.Afr.:*** Brinerdin; ***Spain:*** Brinerdina; Clinadil; Diemil; Dipervina†; Iskedyl†; Isquebral†; ***Switz.:*** Brinerdine; Pressimed†; ***Thai.:*** Bedin; Brinerdin; Hyperdine.

## Dihydroergocryptine Mesilate

Dihidroergocriptina, mesilato de; Dihydroergocryptine Mesylate; Dihydroergocryptine Methanesulphonate; Dihydroergokryptine Mesylate.

$C_{32}H_{43}N_5O_5,CH_4O_3S$ = 673.8.

*CAS — 25447-66-9 (dihydroergocryptine, α-isomer); 19467-62-0 (dihydroergocryptine, β-isomer); 14271-05-7 (dihydroergocryptine mesilate, α-isomer); 65914-79-6 (dihydroergocryptine mesilate, β-isomer).*

*ATC — N04BC03.*

### Profile

Dihydroergocryptine mesilate is a component of co-dergocrine mesilate (p.1674) and has similar actions. It has been given by mouth in doses of up to 20 mg daily for migraine and age-related dementia, and in maintenance doses up to 60 to 120 mg daily for parkinsonism. It has also been used to inhibit lactation. In some countries it has also been given with caffeine for cerebrovascular and peripheral vascular disorders.

◊ References.


1. Faglia G, *et al.* Dihydroergocriptine in management of microprolactinomas. *J Clin Endocrinol Metab* 1987; **65:** 779–84.
2. Martignoni E, *et al.* Dihydroergocryptine in the treatment of Parkinson's disease: a six months' double-blind clinical trial. *Clin Neuropharmacol* 1991; **14:** 78–83.
3. Scarzella L, *et al.* Dihydroergocryptine in the management of senile psycho-organic syndrome. *Int J Clin Pharmacol Res* 1992; **12:** 37–46.
4. Battistin L, *et al.* Alpha-dihydroergocryptine in Parkinson's disease: a multicentre randomized double blind parallel group study. *Acta Neurol Scand* 1999; **99:** 36–42.
5. Bergamasco B, *et al.* Alpha-dihydroergocryptine in the treatment of de novo parkinsonian patients: results of a multicentre, randomized, double-blind, placebo-controlled study. *Acta Neurol Scand* 2000; **101:** 372–80.
6. Micieli G, *et al.* Alpha-dihydroergocryptine and predictive factors in migraine prophylaxis. *Int J Clin Pharmacol Ther* 2001; **39:** 144–51.
7. Tergau F, *et al.* Treatment of restless legs syndrome with the dopamine agonist alpha-dihydroergocryptine. *Mov Disord* 2001; **16:** 731–5.


### Preparations

**Proprietary Preparations** (details are given in Part 3)
***Ger.:*** Almirid; Cripar; ***Ital.:*** Daverium; Myrol†; ***Switz.:*** Cripar.

**Multi-ingredient:** ***Fr.:*** Vasobral; ***Hong Kong:*** Vasobral; ***Ital.:*** Vasobral.

## Dihydroxydibutylether

Dihidroxidibutiléter; Hydroxybutyloxide. 4,4′-Oxybis(butan-2-ol).

$C_8H_{18}O_3$ = 162.2.

*CAS — 821-33-0.*

### Profile

Dihydroxydibutylether is a choleretic.

### Preparations

**Proprietary Preparations** (details are given in Part 3)
***Fr.:*** Dyskinebyl†; ***Hong Kong:*** Diskinebyl†; ***Ital.:*** Dis-Cinil Ilfi†; Diskin.

**Multi-ingredient:** ***Arg.:*** Binvex; ***Ital.:*** Dis-Cinil Complex.

## Diisopropanolamine

Diisopropanolamina. 1,1′-Iminobis(propan-2-ol).

$C_6H_{15}NO_2$ = 133.2.

*CAS — 110-97-4.*

### Profile

Diisopropanolamine is an organic base that is used as a neutralising agent in cosmetics and toiletries.

## Dill

Aneth; Anethum; Eneldo.

NOTE. Indian Dill is the dried ripe fruits of *Anethum sowa*.

**Pharmacopoeias.** *Fr.* includes dill fruit.

### Profile

Dill (*Anethum graveolens*, Apiaceae) is a culinary herb and has also been used in herbal medicine. It is the source of dill oil (see below).

### Preparations

**Proprietary Preparations** (details are given in Part 3)

**Multi-ingredient:** ***Austral.:*** Herb-a-Lax†; ***Fr.:*** Calmosine.

## Dill Oil

Eneldo, aceite esencial de; European Dill Seed Oil; Oleum Anethi.

*CAS — 8016-06-6.*

**Pharmacopoeias.** In *Br.*

**BP 2003** (Dill Oil). A clear colourless or pale yellow liquid, visibly free from water, obtained by distillation from the dried ripe fruits of *Anethum graveolens*. It darkens with age and has a characteristic odour of the crushed fruit. It contains 43 to 63% of carvone. At 20°, soluble 1 in 1 or more of alcohol (90%) and 1 in 10 or more of alcohol (80%). Store at a temperature not exceeding 25° in well-filled containers. Protect from light.

### Profile

Dill oil, usually in the form of dill water, is used as an aromatic carminative, although the efficacy of such traditional remedies in infant colic is considered dubious (see Gastrointestinal Spasm, p.1242).

### Preparations

**Proprietary Preparations** (details are given in Part 3)

**Multi-ingredient:** ***Canad.:*** Babys Own Gripe Water†; Chase Kolik Gripe Water; Woodwards Gripe Water; ***India:*** Bestozyme; Neopeptine; ***Israel:*** Dentinox; Nurse Harvey's Gripe Mixture; Woodwards Gripe Water; ***Singapore:*** Dentinox; ***Thai.:*** Baby Gripe; Bebidol; Gripe Mixture; ***UK:*** Atkinson & Barker's Gripe Mixture; Neo Gripe Mixture; Nurse Harvey's Gripe Mixture; Woodwards Gripe Water.

## Dimecrotic Acid *(rINN)*

2,4-Dimethoxy-β-methylcinnamic acid.

$C_{12}H_{14}O_4$ = 222.2.

*CAS — 7706-67-4.*

### Profile

Dimecrotic acid has been used as the magnesium salt as a choleretic.

### Preparations

**Proprietary Preparations** (details are given in Part 3)
***Fr.:*** Hepadial; ***Port.:*** Hepadoddi; ***Spain:*** Fisiobil.

## Dimethoxymethane

Dimetoximetano; Formal; Formaldehyde Dimethyl Acetal; Methylal.

$CH_2(OCH_3)_2$ = 76.09.

*CAS — 109-87-5.*

### Profile

Dimethoxymethane has been used in perfumery. It has been included in preparations for topical analgesia.

### Preparations

**Proprietary Preparations** (details are given in Part 3)

**Multi-ingredient:** ***UK:*** PR Freeze Spray.

## *p*,α-Dimethylbenzyl Alcohol

Tolinol; *p*-Tolylmethylcarbinol; Tolynolum. 1-(*p*-Tolyl)ethanol.

$C_9H_{12}O$ = 136.2.

*CAS — 536-50-5.*

NOTE. The name tolynol has been applied to both *p*,α-dimethylbenzyl alcohol and mephenesin (p.1394).

### Profile

*p*,α-Dimethylbenzyl alcohol has been used as a choleretic in the treatment of hepatic disorders and is an ingredient of preparations for gastrointestinal disorders. *p*,α-Dimethylbenzyl alcohol nicotinate has also been used.

### Preparations

**Proprietary Preparations** (details are given in Part 3)

**Multi-ingredient:** ***Austria:*** Claim; Galle-Donau; Spagall; Spasmo Claim.

## Dimethyltryptamine

Businessman's Trip; *N*,*N*-Dimethyltryptamine; Dimetiltriptamina; DMT. 3-(2-Dimethylaminoethyl)indole.

$C_{12}H_{16}N_2$ = 188.3.

*CAS — 61-50-7.*

### Profile

Dimethyltryptamine is an active principle obtained from the seeds and leaves of *Piptadenia peregrina* (Mimosaceae) from which the hallucinogenic snuff cohoba is prepared. It may also be obtained from other South American plants. It has been reported to be present in the tropical legume *Mucuna pruriens*.

Dimethyltryptamine produces hallucinogenic and sympathomimetic effects that are similar to those of lysergide (p.1708), but of shorter duration. It has no therapeutic use. Diethyltryptamine (DET) and dipropyltryptamine (DPT) are related synthetic hallucinogens with longer actions but are less potent than dimethyltryptamine.

## 2,4-Dinitrochlorobenzene

2,4-Dinitroclorobenceno; DNCB. 1-Chloro-2,4-dinitrobenzene.

$C_6H_3ClN_2O_4$ = 202.6.

*CAS — 97-00-7.*

### Profile

2,4-Dinitrochlorobenzene is a potent sensitiser and has been applied topically in the evaluation of delayed hypersensitivity. It has also been used as an immunostimulant in various conditions including leprosy, HIV infection, and some forms of cancer, and in the treatment of alopecia and warts.

2,4-Dinitrochlorobenzene has been reported to be mutagenic *in vitro*.

◊ References.


1. Happle R. The potential hazards of dinitrochlorobenzene. *Arch Dermatol* 1985; **121:** 330–2.
2. Stricker RB, Goldberg B. Host-directed therapy for AIDS. *Ann Intern Med* 1995; **123:** 471–2.
3. Todd DJ. Topical treatment with dinitrochlorobenzene. *Lancet* 1995; **346:** 975.
4. Stricker RB, Goldberg B. Safety of topical dinitrochlorobenzene. *Lancet* 1995; **346:** 1293.
5. Strobbe LJ, *et al.* Topical dinitrochlorobenzene combined with systemic dacarbazine in the treatment of recurrent melanoma. *Melanoma Res* 1997; **7:** 507–12.
6. Traub A, *et al.* Topical immune modulation with dinitrochlorobenzene in HIV disease: a controlled trial from Brazil. *Dermatology* 1997; **195:** 369–73.

7. Yoshizawa Y, *et al.* Successful immunotherapy of chronic nodular prurigo with topical dinitrochlorobenzene. *Br J Dermatol* 1999; **141:** 387–9.
8. Yoshizawa Y, *et al.* Topical dinitrochlorobenzene therapy in the treatment of refractory atopic dermatitis: systemic immunotherapy. *J Am Acad Dermatol* 2000; **42:** 258–62.

## Diolamine *(pINN)*

Diaethanolamin; Diethanolamine; Diolamina. Bis(2-hydroxyethyl)amine; 2,2′-Iminobisethanol.

$C_4H_{11}NO_2$ = 105.1.

*CAS — 111-42-2.*

**Pharmacopoeias.** In *USNF.*

**USNF 22** (Diethanolamine). It is a mixture of olamines, consisting largely of diolamine. White or clear, colourless crystals, deliquescing in moist air, or a colourless liquid. Miscible with water, with alcohol, with acetone, with chloroform, and with glycerol; slightly soluble to insoluble in ether, in petroleum spirit, and in benzene. Store in airtight containers. Protect from light.

### Profile

Diolamine is an organic base which is used as an emulsifier and dispersant.

It is used to solubilise fusidic acid and sulfafurazole by the formation of the diolamine salt. It has been used for the preparation of salts of iodinated organic acids used as contrast media. It may be irritating to the skin and mucous membranes.

## Dioxins

Dioxinas.

NOTE. The name Dioxin has also been applied to dimethoxane.

### Profile

The term 'dioxins' encompasses a large group of closely related chemicals known as polychlorinated dibenzo-*p*-dioxins (PCDDs) and polychlorinated dibenzofurans (PCDFs). The most toxic is 2,3,7,8-tetrachlorodibenzo-*p*-dioxin (TCDD).

Dioxins are byproducts in the manufacture of commercial chemical products such as chlorinated phenols and polychlorinated biphenyls (PCBs), and can also be produced in smaller quantities by combustion processes and industrial waste. They first came to public attention during the Vietnam war, when they were found to be present in the herbicide Agent Orange used as a defoliant. They are incriminated as causing chloracne (a severe and persistent acne caused by chlorinated compounds). They are potent teratogens and carcinogens in *animals*. An increased incidence of cancer at different organs due to dioxins has been claimed but this has not been substantiated by clinical and follow-up studies. An effect on cell-mediated immunity has been observed.

Exposure should be limited to the lowest feasible concentration.

**Adverse effects.** The impact of dioxins in food and the environment has been reviewed.[1-3]

An excess of soft tissue sarcomas was found in workers exposed to chlorophenoxy herbicides including those contaminated with TCDD,[4] but cautious interpretation of these results was advised.[5] In Vietnam veterans the risk of non-Hodgkin's lymphoma was about 50% higher than control subjects, but was not related to exposure to Agent Orange, nor was there evidence for an increase in other cancers.[6] Exposure to TCDD was implicated in an increase in cancer mortality in chemical workers,[7,8] but confounding factors such as smoking may have been present.[8,9] Other studies[10,11] have not shown an association between dioxin exposure and an increase in the incidence of human cancer, and epidemiological studies following occupational or accidental exposures have found no clear persistent systemic effects, except for chloracne, and no clear association with carcinogenesis or reproductive disorders.[1,2] Decreased plasma immunoglobulin G concentrations were measured in people following exposure to TCDD 20 years earlier as a result of accidental environmental contamination in Seveso, Italy.[12]

In the USA, the National Academy of Sciences' Institute of Medicine is reported to have carried out an evaluation of publications on herbicide exposure, largely in industrial and agricultural workers.[13] They concluded that exposure to herbicides or dioxin was associated with soft-tissue sarcomas, Hodgkin's disease, non-Hodgkin lymphoma, chloracne, and porphyria cutanea tarda, and that there was limited evidence of an association with respiratory and prostate cancers and multiple myeloma. An update to the report has also suggested a link between Agent Orange exposure and spina bifida in veterans' offspring.[14] There is some evidence that exposure of men to TCDD is associated with a decreased male to female sex ratio in their offspring.[15] Results from studies[16-18] suggest that prenatal exposure to PCBs has an effect on mental and motor development in early childhood, although this may be counteracted by an advantageous home environment. However, virtually no adverse effects in relation to postnatal exposure to PCBs present in breast milk were demonstrated.[18]

1. Polychlorinated dibenzo-para-dioxins and dibenzofurans. *Environmental Health Criteria 88.* Geneva: WHO, 1989.
2. Department of the Environment. Dioxins in the environment. *Pollution Paper 27.* London: HMSO, 1989.
3. MAFF. Dioxins in food. *Food Surveillance Paper 31.* London: HMSO, 1992.
4. Saracci R, *et al.* Cancer mortality in workers exposed to chlorophenoxy herbicides and chlorophenols. *Lancet* 1991; **338:** 1027–32.
5. Peto R. Occupational exposure to chlorophenoxy herbicides and chlorophenols. *Lancet* 1991; **338:** 1392.
6. Suskind R. The association of selected cancers with service in the US military in Vietnam. *Arch Intern Med* 1990; **150:** 2449–50.
7. Manz A, *et al.* Cancer mortality among workers in chemical plant contaminated with dioxin. *Lancet* 1991; **338:** 959–64.
8. Fingerhut MA, *et al.* Cancer mortality in workers exposed to 2,3,7,8-tetrachlorodibenzo-p-dioxin. *N Engl J Med* 1991; **324:** 212–18.
9. Triebig G. Is dioxin carcinogenic? *Lancet* 1991; **338:** 1592.
10. Coggon O, *et al.* Mortality and incidence of cancer at four factories making phenoxy herbicides. *Br J Ind Med* 1991; **48:** 173–8.
11. Green LM. A cohort mortality study of forestry workers exposed to phenoxy acid herbicides. *Br J Ind Med* 1991; **48:** 234–8.
12. Baccarelli A, *et al.* Immunologic effects of dioxin: new results from Seveso and comparison with other studies. *Environ Health Perspect* 2002; **110:** 1169–73.
13. McCarthy M. Agent Orange. *Lancet* 1993; **342:** 362.
14. Stephenson J. New IOM report links Agent Orange Exposure to risk of birth defect in Vietnam vets' children. *JAMA* 1996; **275:** 1066–7.
15. Mocarelli P, *et al.* Paternal concentrations of dioxin and sex ratio of offspring. *Lancet* 2000; **355:** 1858–63.
16. Walkowiak J, *et al.* Environmental exposure to polychlorinated biphenyls and quality of the home environment: effects on psychodevelopment in early childhood. *Lancet* 2001; **358:** 1602–7.
17. Vreugdenhil HJ, *et al.* Effects of prenatal PCB and dioxin background exposure on cognitive and motor abilities in Dutch children at school age. *J Pediatr* 2002; **140:** 48–56.
18. Jacobson JL, Jacobson SW. Association of prenatal exposure to an environmental contaminant with intellectual function in childhood. *J Toxicol Clin Toxicol* 2002; **40:** 467–75.

## Diphenyl

Difenilo; E230; Phenylbenzene. Biphenyl.

$C_{12}H_{10}$ = 154.2.

*CAS — 92-52-4.*

### Profile

Diphenyl is fungistatic against a limited number of moulds and has been employed for impregnating the material used for wrapping citrus fruits.

**Adverse effects.** Workers exposed to high concentrations of diphenyl (up to 128 mg/m$^3$) developed toxic symptoms that included irritation of the throat and eyes, headache, nausea, diffuse abdominal pain, numbness, aching of limbs, and general fatigue.[1] One of the workers, who also had somnolence, icterus, ascites, and oedema of the legs, died; at autopsy, the liver showed necrosis. Chronic hepatitis was reported in a woman exposed over a 25-year period to diphenyl in the paper used to pack citrus fruit.[2]

1. Häkkinen I, *et al.* Diphenyl poisoning in fruit paper production. *Arch Environ Health* 1973; **26:** 70–4.
2. Carella G, Bettolo PM. Reversible hepatotoxic effects of diphenyl: report of a case and a review of the literature. *J Occup Med* 1994; **36:** 575–6.

## Dipivefrine *(BAN, rINN)*

Dipivalyl Epinephrine; Dipivefrin *(USAN)*; DPE.

$C_{19}H_{29}NO_5$ = 351.4.

*CAS — 52365-63-6.*

*ATC — S01EA02.*

## Dipivefrine Hydrochloride *(BANM, rINNM)*

Dipivalyl Adrenaline Hydrochloride; Dipivalyl Epinephrine Hydrochloride; Dipivefrin Hydrochloride; Dipivefrini Hydrochloridum; Hidrocloruro de dipivefrina. (*RS*)-4-[1-Hydroxy-2-(methylamino)ethyl]-*o*-phenylene dipivalate hydrochloride.

$C_{19}H_{29}NO_5,HCl$ = 387.9.

*CAS — 64019-93-8.*

*ATC — S01EA02.*

**Pharmacopoeias.** In *Eur.* (see p.vi) and *US.*

**Ph. Eur. 5.0** (Dipivefrine Hydrochloride). A white or almost white crystalline powder. Freely soluble in water, in alcohol, and in dichloromethane; very soluble in methyl alcohol.

**USP 27** (Dipivefrin Hydrochloride). White, crystalline powder or small crystals, having a faint odour. Very soluble in water. Store in airtight containers.

### Profile

Dipivefrine is an ester and prodrug of adrenaline (p.852). A 0.1% solution of the hydrochloride is used topically as eye drops to reduce intra-ocular pressure in patients with open-angle glaucoma or ocular hypertension (p.1485).

◊ References.

1. Parrow KA, *et al.* Is it worthwhile to add dipivefrin HCl 0.1% to topical $\beta_1$-, $\beta_2$-blocker therapy? *Ophthalmology* 1989; **96:** 1338–41.
2. Drake MV, *et al.* Levobunolol compared to dipivefrin in African American patients with open angle glaucoma. *J Ocul Pharmacol* 1993; **9:** 91–5. Correction. *ibid.*; 385.
3. Albracht DC, *et al.* A double-masked comparison of betaxolol and dipivefrin for the treatment of increased intraocular pressure. *Am J Ophthalmol* 1993; **116:** 307–13.
4. Widengard I, *et al.* Effects of latanoprost and dipivefrin, alone or combined, on intraocular pressure and on blood-aqueous barrier permeability. *Br J Ophthalmol* 1998; **82:** 404–6.

### Preparations

***BP 2003:*** Dipivefrine Eye Drops;
***USP 27:*** Dipivefrin Hydrochloride Ophthalmic Solution.

**Proprietary Preparations** (details are given in Part 3)
***Arg.:*** Propine; ***Austral.:*** Dipoquin; Propine; ***Austria:*** Glaucothil; ***Belg.:*** Propine; ***Braz.:*** Propine; ***Canad.:*** DPE†; Propine; ***Denm.:*** Diprin†; Oftapinex; Propine; ***Fin.:*** Oftapinex; Propine; ***Fr.:*** Propine; ***Ger.:*** d Epifrin; Glaucothil; ***Gr.:*** Diopine; Thilodrin; ***Hong Kong:*** Propine; ***Irl.:*** Propine; ***Israel:*** Difrin; Prodren; Propine; ***Ital.:*** Propine; ***Malaysia:*** Propine; ***Mex.:*** Diopine; Dipine†; ***Norw.:*** Oftapinex; Propine; ***NZ:*** Dipoquin†; Propine†; ***Port.:*** Propine; ***S.Afr.:*** Propine; ***Singapore:*** Propine; ***Spain:*** Diopine; Glaudrops; ***Swed.:*** Diprin†; Oftapinex; Propine; ***Switz.:*** Diopine; Diphemin†; ***Thai.:*** Propine; ***UK:*** Propine; ***USA:*** AkPro; Propine.

**Multi-ingredient:** ***Austria:*** Thiloadren; Thilodigon; ***Canad.:*** Probeta; ***Ger.:*** Thiloadren N; Thilodigon; ***Gr.:*** Thilocombin.

## Disodium Guanylate

Disodium Guanosine-5′-monophosphate; E627; Guanilato disódico; Sodium 5′-Guanylate. Guanosine 5′-(disodium phosphate).

$C_{10}H_{12}N_5Na_2O_8P,xH_2O$.

*CAS — 5550-12-9 (anhydrous disodium guanylate).*

### Profile

Disodium guanylate has been used as a flavour enhancer in foods. It has also been used in eye drops containing other nucleosides in the treatment of corneal damage. The term sodium 5′-ribonucleotide has been used to refer to a mixture of disodium guanylate with disodium inosinate (below).

### Preparations

**Proprietary Preparations** (details are given in Part 3)
**Multi-ingredient:** ***Austria:*** Vitasic†; ***Fr.:*** Vitacic.

## Disodium Inosinate

Disodium Inosine-5′-monophosphate; E631; Inosinato disódico; Sodium 5′-Inosinate. Inosine 5′-(disodium phosphate).

$C_{10}H_{11}N_4Na_2O_8P,xH_2O$.

*CAS — 4691-65-0 (anhydrous disodium inosinate).*

### Profile

Disodium inosinate has been used as a flavour enhancer in foods. It has also been given by mouth and been applied topically in the treatment of visual disturbance.

### Preparations

**Proprietary Preparations** (details are given in Part 3)
***Arg.:*** Lumiclar; ***Fr.:*** Correctol; ***Ger.:*** Antikataraktikum N; ***Switz.:*** Catacol†.

**Multi-ingredient:** ***Arg.:*** Antikatarata.

## Disulfiram *(BAN, rINN)*

Dissulfiramo; Disulfiramum; Éthyldithiourame; TTD. Tetraethylthiuram disulphide; Bis(diethylthiocarbamoyl) disulfide.

$C_{10}H_{20}N_2S_4$ = 296.5.

*CAS — 97-77-8.*

*ATC — P03AA04; N07BB01.*

**Pharmacopoeias.** In *Eur.* (see p.vi), *Jpn, Pol.,* and *US.*

**Ph. Eur. 5.0** (Disulfiram). A white or almost white, crystalline powder. M.p. 70° to 73°. Practically insoluble in water; sparingly soluble in alcohol; freely soluble in dichloromethane. Protect from light.

**USP 27** (Disulfiram). A white to off-white, odourless crystalline powder. M.p. 69° to 72°. Very slightly soluble in water; soluble 1 in 30 of alcohol and 1 in 15 of ether; soluble in acetone, in carbon disulfide, and in chloroform. Store in airtight containers. Protect from light.

**Stability.** Studies on the stability of disulfiram preparations.

1. Gupta VD. Stability of aqueous suspensions of disulfiram. *Am J Hosp Pharm* 1981; **38:** 363–4.
2. Philips M, *et al.* Stability of an injectable disulfiram formulation sterilized by gamma irradiation. *Am J Hosp Pharm* 1985; **42:** 343–5.

### Adverse Effects and Treatment

Drowsiness and fatigue are common during initial treatment with disulfiram. Other side-effects reported include a garlic-like or metallic aftertaste, gastrointestinal upsets, body odour, bad breath, headache, impotence, and allergic dermatitis. Peripheral and optic neuropathies, psychotic reactions, and hepatotoxicity may occur.

***Disulfiram-alcohol reaction*.** The use of disulfiram in the management of alcoholism is based on the extremely unpleasant, but generally self-limiting, systemic effects which occur when a patient receiving the drug ingests alcohol. These effects begin with flushing of the face and, as vasodilatation spreads, throbbing in the head and neck and a pulsating headache may develop. Respiratory difficulties, nausea, copious vomiting, sweating, thirst, chest pain, tachycardia, palpitations, marked hypotension, giddiness, weakness, blurred vision, and confusion may follow. The intensity and duration of symptoms is very variable and even small quantities of alcohol may result in alarming reactions. In addition to the above effects, severe reactions have included respiratory depression, cardiovascular collapse, cardiac arrhythmias, myocardial infarction, acute heart failure, unconsciousness, convulsions, and sudden death.

Severe reactions require intensive supportive therapy; oxygen and intravenous fluids may be necessary. Potassium concentrations should be monitored. The intravenous administration of ascorbic acid, ephedrine sulfate, or antihistamines has been suggested.

◊ Reviews.

1. Chick J. Safety issues concerning the use of disulfiram in treating alcohol dependence. *Drug Safety* 1999; **20:** 427–35.

**Effects on the blood.** There were isolated reports of blood dyscrasias associated with disulfiram in the 1960s. The US manufacturer recommends that blood counts should be performed during treatment.

**Effects on the liver.** A review of 18 cases of hepatitis in patients receiving disulfiram.[1] Symptoms have appeared between 10 days and 6 months after initiating disulfiram, and clinical improvement has been seen within 2 weeks of discontinuing disulfiram although liver enzyme values may not return to normal for several months. Fatal hepatic coma had been reported in 7 patients. The clinical picture of disulfiram-induced hepatitis is consistent with a hypersensitivity reaction.

1. Mason NA. Disulfiram-induced hepatitis: case report and review of the literature. *DICP Ann Pharmacother* 1989; **23:** 872–4.

**Effects on the nervous system.** ENCEPHALOPATHY. A 2% incidence of reversible toxic encephalopathy has been reported in patients receiving disulfiram.[1] Onset varies from days to months following the start of therapy and early signs include impaired concentration, memory deficits, anxiety, depression, and somnolence. Confusion and disorientation follow, often accompanied by paranoid delusions and sometimes hallucinations. Other symptoms may include ataxia, loss of fine motor coordination, slurred speech, and intention tremor. The encephalopathy usually resolves within 3 days to 2 weeks of stopping disulfiram, although symptoms may persist for 6 weeks. There are conflicting opinions on whether this psychosis is a toxic reaction to disulfiram or a response to abstinence from alcohol, but the authors suspected that most cases represent a toxic encephalopathy. However, psychosis without any suggestion of encephalopathy has been reported.[2]

1. Hotson JR, Langston JW. Disulfiram-induced encephalopathy. *Arch Neurol* 1976; **33:** 141–2.
2. Rossiter SK. Psychosis with disulfiram prescribed under probation order. *BMJ* 1992; **305:** 763.

PERIPHERAL NEUROPATHY. Reports of peripheral neuropathy associated with disulfiram and reference to previously reported cases.[1,2] Onset of neuropathy varied from days to months after starting disulfiram treatment and could develop with doses of 250 or 500 mg daily. The most common symptom reported was pins and needles, but numbness, pain/burning, and weakness were frequently described; usually both muscle weakness and sensory loss were noted. Optic atrophy has also been described. Although there might be some improvement immediately after disulfiram withdrawal, the neurological deficit only improved slowly and symptoms might persist for as long as 2 years.[1]

1. Watson CP, *et al.* Disulfiram neuropathy. *Can Med Assoc J* 1980; **123:** 123–6.
2. Frisoni GB, Di Monda V. Disulfiram neuropathy: a review (1971-1988) and report of a case. *Alcohol Alcohol* 1989; **24:** 429–37.

**Effects on the respiratory tract.** Bronchospasm and hypertension were observed in an asthmatic patient taking disulfiram following an alcohol challenge test.[1]

1. Zapata E, Orwin A. Severe hypertension and bronchospasm during disulfiram-ethanol test reaction. *BMJ* 1992; **305:** 870.

**Effects on the skin.** Orange-coloured palms and soles, provoking an initial diagnosis of jaundice, developed in a 55-year-old man who had been taking disulfiram for about 2 months.[1] It was postulated that the discoloration was due to accumulation of carotenes in the skin as a result of inhibition of vitamin A metabolism by disulfiram. The discoloration disappeared soon after disulfiram was stopped.

1. Santonastaso M, *et al.* Yellow palms with disulfiram. *Lancet* 1997; **350:** 266.

**Overdosage.** There has been a report of a 6-year-old boy who experienced disulfiram intoxication after receiving disulfiram 250 mg four times daily to a total of 13 doses but who later recovered.[1] Of 6 previous reports one child died and 3 had moderate or severe brain damage. The syndrome of disulfiram intoxication in children is distinct from the disulfiram-alcohol interaction or acute disulfiram intoxication in adults. It is characterised by lethargy or somnolence, weakness, hypotonia, and vomiting, beginning approximately 12 hours after ingestion and progressing to stupor or coma. Dehydration, moderate tachycardia, and marked tachypnoea occur frequently, muscle tone is greatly decreased, and deep-tendon reflexes may be weak or absent.

Severe neurological damage has also been reported[2] in a 5-year-old girl following acute disulfiram intoxication which was initially diagnosed as diabetic ketoacidosis.

1. Benitz WE, Tatro DS. Disulfiram intoxication in a child. *J Pediatr* 1984; **105:** 487–9.
2. Mahajan P, *et al.* Basal ganglion infarction in a child with disulfiram poisoning. *Pediatrics* 1997; **99:** 605–8.

## Precautions

Disulfiram is contra-indicated in the presence of cardiovascular disease or psychosis or severe personality disorders, and should not be given to patients known to be hypersensitive to it or to other thiuram compounds, such as those used in rubber vulcanisation or pesticides. It should be used with caution in the presence of diabetes mellitus, epilepsy, impaired hepatic or renal function, respiratory disorders, cerebral damage, or hypothyroidism. Caution is also advised when giving disulfiram to those who are addicted to other drugs in addition to alcohol. It is probably best avoided in pregnancy.

Disulfiram should not be given until at least 24 hours after the last ingestion of alcohol. Patients beginning therapy should be fully aware of the disulfiram-alcohol reaction and should be warned to avoid alcohol in any form, including alcohol-containing medicines and alcohol-based topical preparations. Reactions to alcohol may occur as long as 2 weeks after the cessation of disulfiram.

The US manufacturers have recommended that regular blood counts and liver function tests should be performed during long-term therapy.

**Pregnancy.** A report of 2 infants with severe limb-reduction anomalies whose mothers had taken disulfiram during pregnancy.[1] Only 2 similar cases had previously been reported.

1. Nora AH, *et al.* Limb-reduction anomalies in infants born to disulfiram-treated alcoholic mothers. *Lancet* 1977; **ii:** 664.

## Interactions

Disulfiram inhibits hepatic enzymes and may interfere with the metabolism of other drugs taken at the same time. It enhances the effects of phenytoin and coumarin anticoagulants and their dosage may need to be reduced. It also inhibits the metabolism and excretion of rifampicin. Toxic reactions have occurred following the concomitant administration of disulfiram and isoniazid or metronidazole. Disulfiram may inhibit the metabolism of paraldehyde leading to an accumulation of acetaldehyde and these drugs should not be given concomitantly.

◊ In a study[1] to evaluate the effects of disulfiram on cytochrome P450 isoenzymes, the results suggested that disulfiram-mediated inhibition is predominantly selective for CYP2E1 after both acute and chronic administration.

1. Frye RF, Branch RA. Effect of chronic disulfiram administration on the activities of CYP1A2, CYP2C19, CYP2D6, CYP2E1, and N-acetyltransferase in healthy human subjects. *Br J Clin Pharmacol* 2002; **53:** 155–62.

**Analgesics.** The potential of disulfiram to impair drug metabolism was demonstrated[1] when it was found to prolong the plasma half-life of *phenazone*, probably by inhibiting the hepatic microsomal mixed function oxidases. It was also suggested[1] that disulfiram alters catecholamine metabolism since urinary excretion of vanilmandelic acid was significantly reduced and that of homovanillic acid was increased.

1. Vesell ES, *et al.* Impairment of drug metabolism by disulfiram in man. *Clin Pharmacol Ther* 1971; **12:** 785–92.

**Antidepressants.** It has been reported[1] that *amitriptyline* appeared to enhance the disulfiram-alcohol reaction. There is the potential for serious interactions during the disulfiram-alcohol reaction with drugs having CNS actions mediated by noradrenaline or dopamine, such as *tricyclic antidepressants* or those inhibiting the same enzymes as disulfiram, such as *MAOIs*.[2]

1. MacCallum WAG. Drug interactions in alcoholism treatment. *Lancet* 1969; **i:** 313.
2. Sellers EM, *et al.* Drugs to decrease alcohol consumption. *N Engl J Med* 1981; **305:** 1255–62.

**Antiprotozoals.** For reference to toxicity associated with *metronidazole* given to alcoholic patients who were also receiving disulfiram, see Alcohol, under Interactions of Metronidazole, p.608.

**Antipsychotics.** Although *chlorpromazine* was formerly given to reduce the nausea and vomiting associated with the disulfiram-alcohol reaction,[1] it has been suggested[2] that phenothiazine antiemetics such as chlorpromazine might increase hypotension because of their α-adrenoceptor blocking activity and should therefore be contra-indicated. There is the potential for serious interactions during the disulfiram-alcohol reaction with drugs having CNS actions mediated by noradrenaline or dopamine, such as *phenothiazines*.[3]

1. Cummins JF, Friend DG. Use of chlorpromazine in chronic alcoholics. *Am J Med Sci* 1954; **227:** 561–4.
2. Kwentus J, Major LF. Disulfiram in the treatment of alcoholism: a review. *J Stud Alcohol* 1979; **40:** 428–46.
3. Sellers EM, *et al.* Drugs to decrease alcohol consumption. *N Engl J Med* 1981; **305:** 1255–62.

**Benzodiazepines.** *Diazepam* was reported[1] to reduce the intensity of the disulfiram-alcohol reaction.

1. MacCallum WAG. Drug interactions in alcoholism treatment. *Lancet* 1969; **i:** 313.

**Cannabis.** For a suggestion that a combination of disulfiram and *cannabis* may produce a hypomanic state, see p.1666.

**Cardiovascular drugs.** Clinically serious pharmacodynamic interactions might be anticipated during the disulfiram-alcohol reaction in patients taking other drugs that impair blood pressure regulation, such as *alpha blockers*, *beta blockers*, or *vasodilators*.[1]

1. Sellers EM, *et al.* Drugs to decrease alcohol consumption. *N Engl J Med* 1981; **305:** 1255–62.

**Macrolides.** Fatal toxic epidermal necrolysis and fulminant hepatitis have been reported[1] after starting *clarithromycin* treatment in a patient who was receiving disulfiram.

1. Masiá M, *et al.* Fulminant hepatitis and fatal toxic epidermal necrolysis (Lyell disease) coincident with clarithromycin administration in an alcoholic patient receiving disulfiram therapy. *Arch Intern Med* 2002; **162:** 474–6.

## Pharmacokinetics

Disulfiram is absorbed variably from the gastrointestinal tract and is rapidly reduced to diethyldithiocarbamate (ditiocarb, p.1038), principally by the glutathione reductase system in the erythrocytes; reduction may also occur in the liver. Diethyldithiocarbamate is metabolised in the liver to its glucuronide and methyl ester and to diethylamine, carbon disulfide, and sulfate ions. Metabolites are excreted primarily in the urine; carbon disulfide is exhaled in the breath.

◊ There was marked intersubject variability in plasma concentrations of disulfiram and its metabolites in a study of 15 male alcoholics given single 250-mg doses of disulfiram by mouth and repeated dosing with 250 mg daily for 12 days.[1] Variability might result from the marked lipid solubility of disulfiram, differences in plasma protein binding, or enterohepatic cycling. Average times to reach peak plasma concentrations after single or repeated doses were 8 to 10 hours for disulfiram, diethyldithiocarbamate, diethyldithiocarbamate-methyl ester, and diethylamine, and for carbon disulfide in breath; peak plasma concentrations of carbon disulfide occurred after 5 to 6 hours. Plasma concentrations of disulfiram were negligible within 48 hours of a dose, although concentrations of some metabolites were still raised. In urine, 1.7 and 8.3% of a disulfiram dose was eliminated as diethyldithiocarbamate-glucuronide in the 24 hours after a single and repeated dose respectively, while diethylamine accounted for 1.6 and 5.7%, respectively. In the 24 hours after a single and repeated dose 22.4 and 31.3%, respectively, was eliminated as carbon disulfide in the breath.

1. Faiman MD, *et al.* Elimination kinetics of disulfiram in alcoholics after single and repeated doses. *Clin Pharmacol Ther* 1984; **36:** 520–6.

## Uses and Administration

Disulfiram is used as an adjunct in the treatment of chronic alcoholism (see Alcohol Withdrawal and Abstinence, p.1166). Disulfiram is not a cure and the treatment is likely to be of little value unless it is undertaken with the willing cooperation of the patient and is used with supportive psychotherapy.

Disulfiram inhibits aldehyde dehydrogenase, the enzyme responsible for the oxidation of acetaldehyde, a metabolite of alcohol. The resulting accumulation of acetaldehyde in the blood is widely believed to be responsible for many of the unpleasant symptoms of the disulfiram-alcohol reaction which occur when alcohol is taken, even in small quantities, after the administration of disulfiram (see Adverse Effects and Treatment, above). Symptoms can arise within 10 minutes of the ingestion of alcohol and last from half an hour in mild cases to several hours in severe cases. It is advisable to carry out the initial treatment in hospital or in a specialised unit where the patient can be kept under close supervision.

Disulfiram is given by mouth. The dose is 800 mg, taken as a single dose, on the first day of treatment, reduced by 200 mg daily to a maintenance dose which is usually 100 to 200 mg daily. In the USA, where doses above 500 mg daily are not recommended, an initial dose of 500 mg daily for 1 to 2 weeks is given, followed by a maintenance dose of 250 mg daily or within the range of 125 to 500 mg daily. Treatment should be reviewed after no longer than 6 months. Maintenance therapy with disulfiram may need to be continued for months or years, until the patient is fully recovered socially and a basis for permanent self-control has been established.

A test dose of alcohol has been given under close supervision when the patient is receiving maintenance doses of disulfiram, in order to demonstrate the nature of the disulfiram-alcohol reaction. However, these challenge tests are not routinely recommended, and should not in any case be used in patients over 50 years of age. Many authorities consider that an explicit description of the reaction is sufficient.

Disulfiram implants have been used in an attempt to overcome problems of patient compliance but have been largely abandoned due to lack of clinical efficacy.

**Alcoholism.** References.

1. Wright C, Moore RD. Disulfiram treatment of alcoholism. *Am J Med* 1990; **88:** 647–55.
2. Hughes JC, Cook CCH. The efficacy of disulfiram: a review of outcome studies. *Addiction* 1997; **92:** 381–95.
3. O'Shea B. Disulfiram revisited. *Hosp Med* 2000; **61:** 849–51.
4. Brewer C, *et al.* Does disulfiram help to prevent relapse in alcohol abuse? *CNS Drugs* 2000; **14:** 329–341.

## Preparations

***BP 2003:*** Disulfiram Tablets;
***USP 27:*** Disulfiram Tablets.

**Proprietary Preparations** (details are given in Part 3)

***Arg.:*** Abstensyl; Vandisul; ***Austral.:*** Antabuse; ***Austria:*** Antabus; ***Belg.:*** Antabuse; ***Braz.:*** Antietanol†; Sarcoton; ***Canad.:*** Antabuse†; ***Chile:*** Tolerane; ***Denm.:*** Antabus; ***Fin.:*** Antabus; ***Fr.:*** Esperal; ***Ger.:*** Antabus; ***India:*** Esperal; ***Irl.:*** Antabuse; ***Israel:*** Antabuse; ***Ital.:*** Antabuse; Etiltox; ***Mex.:*** Etabus†; ***Neth.:*** Refusal; ***Norw.:*** Antabus†; ***NZ:*** Antabuse; ***Port.:*** Tetradin; **S.Afr.:** Antabuse; **Spain:** Antabus; **Swed.:** Antabus; **Switz.:** Antabus; **Thai.:** Antabuse; Difiram; **UK:** Antabuse; **USA:** Antabuse†.

**Multi-ingredient: Fr.:** TTD-$B_3$-$B_4$; **Swed.:** Tenutex.

## Dizocilpine Maleate *(USAN, rINNM)*

Maleato de dizocilpina; MK-801. (+)-10,11-Dihydro-5-methyl-5*H*-dibenzo[*a*,*d*]-cyclohepten-5,10-imine maleate.

$C_{16}H_{15}N,C_4H_4O_4$ = 337.4.

*CAS — 77086-21-6 (dizocilpine); 77086-22-7 (dizocilpine maleate).*

### Profile

Dizocilpine is an antagonist of the excitatory neurotransmitter *N*-methyl-D-aspartate (NMDA). It has been investigated for its antiepileptic properties as well as for a potential role in various other neurological disorders including the prevention of damage due to cerebral ischaemia.

◊ Dizocilpine has good anticonvulsant activity but as it causes alarming psychotropic effects it was abandoned as a possible therapy for epilepsy.[1] Interest in its use as a possible therapy for stroke continued.

1. Richens A. New antiepileptic drugs. *Br J Hosp Med* 1990; **44:** 241.

## Drosera

Droserae Herba; Herba Rorellae; Rorela; Ros Solis; Sundew.

### Profile

Drosera consists of the air-dried entire plant *Drosera rotundifolia* (Droseraceae) and other *Drosera* spp. Preparations of drosera have been used for its reputed value in respiratory disorders.

It has been used in homoeopathic medicine.

### Preparations

**Proprietary Preparations** (details are given in Part 3)
**Ger.:** Makatussin Saft Drosera; Makatussin Tropfen Drosera.

**Multi-ingredient: Austral.:** Asa Tones†; **Austria:** Erkaltungstee; Grippetee Dr Zeidler; Krauterdoktor Krampf- und Reizhustensirup; Neuners Krautertee Nr 211 - Krauterhexlein Kinder-Hustentee; Pilka; Pilka Forte; **Belg.:** Sirop Toux du Larynx†; **Braz.:** Broncotussan†; **Chile:** Fitotos; Gotas Nican; Notosil; Pectoral Pasteur; Pulmagol; Ramistos; Sedotus; **Fr.:** Pastilles Monleon; Pulmonase†; Sirop Pectoral adulte†; Sirop Pectoral enfant†; Tussidoron; **Ger.:** Bronchicum Pflanzlicher; Drosithym-N; Lomal; Makatussin Tropfen forte; Mintetten Truw†; Tussiflorin Hustenstiller; **Israel:** Pilka; **Neth.:** Abdijsiroop (Akker-Siroop)†; **Port.:** Fluidin Infantil†; Lactucol†; Pilka F; **Spain:** Broncovital; Mentobox†; Pazbronquial; Pilka; **Switz.:** Bromocod N; Bronchalin†; Bronchofluid N; Bronchofluid†; Demo elixir pectoral N; Demo gouttes contre la toux†; Demo pates pectorales†; Demo sirop contre la toux†; Demotussil; Drosinula; Escotussin; Famel; Gouttes contre la toux "S"; Makatussin forte†; Makatussin†; Nican; Pastilles pectorales Demo N; Pastilles pectorales formule 541†; Pilka; Sirop S contre la toux et la bronchite; Thymodrosin N; Thymodrosin†; Tussanil Compositum.

## Drotaverine *(rINN)*

Drotaverina. 1-(3,4-Diethoxybenzylidene)-6,7-diethoxy-1,2,3,4-tetrahydroisoquinoline.

$C_{24}H_{31}NO_4$ = 397.5.

*CAS — 14009-24-6 (drotaverine); 985-12-6 (drotaverine hydrochloride).*

*ATC — A03AD02.*

**Pharmacopoeias.** *Pol.* includes Drotaverine Hydrochloride.

### Profile

Drotaverine is used as an antispasmodic in the management of biliary-tract, urinary-tract, and gastrointestinal spasm, in usual doses of 120 to 240 mg daily by mouth in divided doses. It has also been given by intramuscular or intravenous injection.

◊ References.

1. Bolaji OO, *et al.* Pharmacokinetics and bioavailability of drotaverine in humans. *Eur J Drug Metab Pharmacokinet* 1996; **21:** 217–21.
2. Romics I, *et al.* The effect of drotaverine hydrochloride in acute colicky pain caused by renal and ureteric stones. *BJU Int* 2003; **92:** 92–6.

**Porphyria.** Drotaverine has been associated with acute attacks of porphyria and is considered unsafe in porphyric patients.

### Preparations

**Proprietary Preparations** (details are given in Part 3)
**Arg.:** Proconfial; **Hung.:** No-Spa; **India:** Drotin; **Thai.:** Deolin; No-Spa; Spablock; Toverine.

**Multi-ingredient: Hung.:** Bispan; Neotroparin; Quarelin; Triospan.

## Dulcamara

Bittersüss; Bittersweet; Douce-Amère; Dulcamarae Caulis; Woody Nightshade.

### Profile

Dulcamara consists of the dried stems and branches of *Solanum dulcamara* (Solanaceae). It was formerly a popular remedy for chronic rheumatism and skin eruptions and was given as an infusion. It has been used in homoeopathic medicine.

All parts of the plant are poisonous due to the presence of solanaceous alkaloids. The berries have caused poisoning in children. Adverse effects are treated as described under Atropine, p.477.

### Preparations

**Proprietary Preparations** (details are given in Part 3)
**Ger.:** Cefabene; Dolexaderm H†; Solapsor.

**Multi-ingredient: Austria:** Dermatodoron; **Fr.:** Elixir Contre La Toux Weleda†; **Ger.:** Dermatodoron; Kneipp Rheuma Tee N†; **Ital.:** Depurativo†; Tisana Arnaldi†.

## Ebselen *(rINN)*

DR-3305; Ebseleno; PZ-51. 2-Phenyl-1,2-benzisoselenazolin-3-one.

$C_{13}H_9NOSe$ = 274.2.

*CAS — 60940-34-3.*

### Profile

Ebselen has antoxidant activity and inhibits lipid peroxidation. It has been investigated as a neuroprotectant in stroke.

◊ References.

1. Yamaguchi T, *et al.* Ebselen is acute ischemic stroke: a placebo-controlled, double-blind clinical trial. *Stroke* 1998; **29:** 12–17.
2. Saito I, *et al.* Neuroprotective effect of an antioxidant, ebselen, in patients with delayed neurological deficits after aneurysmal subarachnoid hemorrhage. *Neurosurgery* 1998; **42:** 269–78.

## Echinacea

Black Sampson; Brauneria; Coneflower; Equinácea; Rudbeckia; Sonnenhutkraut.

**Pharmacopoeias.** In *USNF* which has separate monographs for different species. Also included are monographs for the powdered form and for the powdered extract of each species.

**USNF 22** (Echinacea Angustifolia). It consists of the dried rhizome and roots of *Echinacea angustifolia* (Asteraceae), harvested in the autumn after 3 or more years of growth. It contains not less than 0.5% of total phenols. Protect from light.

**USNF 22** (Echinacea Pallida). It consists of the dried rhizome and roots of *Echinacea pallida* (Asteraceae), harvested in the autumn after 3 or more years of growth. It contains not less than 0.5% of total phenols. Protect from light.

**USNF 22** (Echinacea Purpurea Root). It consists of the dried rhizome and roots of *Echinacea purpurea* (Asteraceae), harvested in the autumn after 3 or more years of growth. It contains not less than 0.5% of total phenols. Protect from light.

### Profile

Echinacea is reported to have immunostimulant properties and is used in herbal preparations for the prophylaxis of bacterial and viral infections. It is also used in homoeopathic medicine.

**Respiratory disorders.** Echinacea is widely used in herbal preparations to treat upper respiratory-tract infections such as the common cold. Studies have produced conflicting results, but meta-analyses suggest that most have methodological flaws rendering evidence of efficacy unconvincing. Evaluation of specific preparations is also difficult because of varying composition. Hypersensitivity reactions including anaphylaxis have been reported.

References.

1. Houghton P. Echinacea. *Pharm J* 1994; **253:** 342–3.
2. Pepping J. Echinacea. *Am J Health-Syst Pharm* 1999; **56:** 121–2.
3. Melchart D, *et al.* Echinacea for preventing and treating the common cold. Available in The Cochrane Library; Issue 2. Chichester: John Wiley; 2004.
4. Turner RB, *et al.* Ineffectiveness of echinacea for prevention of experimental rhinovirus colds. *Antimicrob Agents Chemother* 2000; **44:** 1708–9.
5. Giles JT, *et al.* Evaluation of echinacea for treatment of the common cold. *Pharmacotherapy* 2000; **20:** 690–7.
6. Schulten B, *et al.* Efficacy of Echinacea purpurea in patients with a common cold: a placebo-controlled, randomised, double-blind clinical trial. *Arzneimittelforschung* 2001; **51:** 563–8.
7. Mullins RJ, Heddle R. Adverse reactions associated with echinacea: the Australian experience. *Ann Allergy Asthma Immunol* 2002; **88:** 42–51.
8. Schwarz E, *et al.* Oral administration of freshly expressed juice of Echinacea purpurea herbs fail to stimulate the nonspecific immune response in healthy young men: results of a double-blind, placebo-controlled crossover study. *J Immunother* 2002; **25:** 413–20.
9. Anonymous. Echinacea for prevention and treatment of upper respiratory infections. *Med Lett Drugs Ther* 2002; **44:** 29–30.
10. Barrett BP, *et al.* Treatment of the common cold with unrefined echinacea: a randomized, double-blind, placebo-controlled trial. *Ann Intern Med* 2002; **137:** 939–46.
11. Taylor JA, *et al.* Efficacy and safety of echinacea in treating upper respiratory tract infections in children: a randomized controlled trial. *JAMA* 2003; **290:** 2824–30.

### Preparations

**Proprietary Preparations** (details are given in Part 3)
**Austral.:** Echinacin†; **Austria:** Echinacin; Echinaforce†; Myo-Echinacin; **Belg.:** Echinacin; **Braz.:** Equinacea; **Canad.:** Citranacea; Echina Pro†; **Ger.:** aar vir; Berubi†; Bilgast echinac†; Cefasept; Cefasept mono†; Cefatox; Dore Immun†; Echan; Echifit; Echiherb; Echinacin; Echinaforce; Echinapur; Echinatur; Episcorit; Esberitox mono; Fudimun†; Immunopret†; Lymphozil; Mentopin Echinacea†; Pascotox forte-Injektopas; Pascotox mono; Resplant; Wiedimmun; **Ital.:** EuMunil; **Spain:** Echinacin; **Switz.:** Drosana Resiston; Echinacin; Echinaforce; EchinaMed; **UK:** Benylin Active Response; Echinacea; Echinaforce; Phytocold; Skin Clear.

**Multi-ingredient: Austral.:** Cold and Flu Relief†; Cough Relief†; Echinacea & Antioxidants†; Echinacea 4000†; Echinacea ACE + Zinc†; Echinacea ACE Plus Zinc†; Echinacea Complex†; Echinacea Herbal Plus Formula†; Echinacea Lozenge†; Echinacea Plus†; Flavons†; Galium Complex†; Gartech†; Herbal Cleanse†; Herbal Cold & Flu Relief†; Lifesystem Herbal Plus Formula 8 Echinacea†; Logicin Natural Lozenges; Odourless Garlic†; Proyeast†; Relief Rub†; Respatona Plus Bronchial Cough Relief†; Sambucus Complex†; Urgenin†; Urinase†; Vita-Minis Cold & Flu†; **Austria:** Parodontax; Spasmo-Urgenin; Urgenin; **Belg.:** Urgenin; **Braz.:** Infantoss; Parodontax†; **Canad.:** Bentasil Licorice with Echinacea; Benylin First Defense; **Chile:** Paltomiel Plus; **Ger.:** Alsicur†; Bagnisan med Heilbad†; Bomagall forte S†; Cefaktivon†; Ermsech; Esberitox N; Hewenephron duo; JuGrippan†; Pascotox†; **Hong Kong:** Urgenin; **Israel:** Parodontax; Urgenin; **Ital.:** Aclon Lievit†; Allergenid†; Bodyguard; Dermilia Flebozin; Enertonic†; Golatux; Immumil; Influ-Zinc; Probigol; Promix; Promix 3; Ribovir; Sanaderm†; **NZ:** Lice Blaster; Strepsils Echinacea Defence; **Port.:** Neo Urgenin†; Spasmo-Urgenin; Vitace; **S.Afr.:** Spasmo-Urgenin; **Singapore:** Noricaven; **Spain:** Neo Urgenin; Spasmo-Urgenin; Uralyt†; Urgenin; **Switz.:** Alpina Gel a la consoude†; Demonatur Capsules contre les refroidissements; Demonatur Dragees pour les reins et la vessie; Esberitop; Esberitox N†; Gel a la consoude; Phytomed Prosta; Phytomed Rhino†; Prosta-Caps Chassot N; Spagymun; Spagyrom; Urgenine†; **Thai.:** Spasmo-Urgenin; **UK:** Antifect; Beechams for Natural Relief†; Buttercup Pol'N'Count†; Cold-eeze†; Echinacea; Goodypops; Hay Fever & Sinus Relief; Hayfever & Sinus Relief; Kleer†; Modern Herbals Cold & Catarrh; Revitonil; Savlon Natural First Aid for Burns; Savlon Natural First Aid for Insect Bites & Stings; Sinotar.

## Eledoisin *(rINN)*

ELD-950; Eledoisina. 5-Oxo-Pro-Pro-Ser-Lys-Asp-Ala-Phe-Ile-Gly-Leu-Met-$NH_2$.

$C_{54}H_{85}N_{13}O_{15}S$ = 1188.4.

*CAS — 69-25-0 (eledoisin); 10129-92-7 (eledoisin trifluoroacetate).*

### Profile

Eledoisin is a peptide extracted from the posterior salivary glands of certain small octopuses (*Eledone* spp., Mollusca), or obtained by synthesis. Its actions resemble those of substance P; it is a potent vasodilator and increases capillary permeability. It has been given as the trifluoroacetate in eye drops to stimulate lachrymal secretion in Sjögren's syndrome and other dry eye conditions.

### Preparations

**Proprietary Preparations** (details are given in Part 3)
**Spain:** Eloisin.

## Entsufon Sodium *(USAN, rINNM)*

Entsufón sódico. Sodium 2-{2-[2-(*p*-1,3,3-tetramethylbutylphenoxy)ethoxy]ethoxy}ethanesulfonate.

$C_{20}H_{33}NaO_6S$ = 424.5.

*CAS — 55837-16-6 (entsufon); 2917-94-4 (entsufon sodium).*

### Profile

Entsufon sodium is a detergent used as a soap substitute for cleansing the skin.

### Preparations

**Proprietary Preparations** (details are given in Part 3)
**Hong Kong:** pHisoDerm†.

**Multi-ingredient: Canad.:** pHisoHex; **USA:** pHisoHex.

## Epomediol

1,8-Epoxy-4-isopropyl-1-methylcylohexane-2,6-diol.

$C_{10}H_{18}O_3$ = 186.2.

*ATC — A05BA05.*

### Profile

Epomediol has been given by mouth in the treatment of hepatic disorders.

◊ References.

1. Capurso L, *et al.* Activity of epomediol in the treatment of hepatopathies: a double-blind multi-centre study. *J Int Med Res* 1987; **15:** 134–47.

### Preparations

**Proprietary Preparations** (details are given in Part 3)
**Ital.:** Clesidren†.

## Epostane *(BAN, USAN, rINN)*

Epostano; Win-32729. 4α,5α-Epoxy-3,17β-dihydroxy-4β,17α-dimethyl-5α-androst-2-ene-2-carbonitrile.

$C_{22}H_{31}NO_3$ = 357.5.

*CAS — 80471-63-2.*

### Profile

Epostane has antiprogestogenic activity and has been investigated for use with prostaglandins in the termination of pregnancy, and as a uterine stimulant for the induction of labour.

## Equisetum

Cola de Caballo; Equiseti Herba; Equiseto; Herba Equiseti; Horsetail; Prêle; Schachtelhalmkraut.

**Pharmacopoeias.** In *Eur.* (see p.vi) and *Pol.*

**Ph. Eur. 5.0** (Equisetum Stem; Horsetail BP 2003). The whole or cut, dried sterile aerial parts of *Equisetum arvense*. It contains a minimum of 0.3% of total flavonoids expressed as isoquercitroside ($C_{21}H_{20}O_{12}$ = 464.4), calculated with reference to the dried drug.

### Profile

Equisetum is an ingredient of herbal preparations that have been used in the treatment of genito-urinary and respiratory disorders. Similar preparations have been used in the treatment of cardiovascular disorders, rheumatic disorders, liver disorders, constipation, and as a tonic.

Equisetum is used in homoeopathic medicine.

The related species *Equisetum hiemale* is used in China for the treatment of eye disorders.

### Preparations

**Proprietary Preparations** (details are given in Part 3)

***Austral.:*** Bioglan Silica-Vite†; ***Austria:*** Bio Equisan; ***Fr.:*** Siliprele; ***Ger.:*** Biolavan†; Kneipp Zinnkraut-Pflanzensaft†; Prodiuret; Pulvhydrops Mono; Redaxa fit; Salus Zinnkraut†; Zinnkraut-Tropfen; ***Ital.:*** Bioequiseto; Osteosil.

**Multi-ingredient: *Arg.:*** Arceligasol; Centella Queen Complex; ***Austral.:*** Cal Alkyline†; Extralife Fluid-Care†; Medinat Esten†; Serenoa Complex†; Silicic Complex†; ***Austria:*** Aurita-Nieren-Blasentee; Bio-Garten Tee fur Niere und Blase; Bio-Garten Tropfen fur Niere und Blase; Bioreform-Blasen- und Nierentee; Blasen- und Nierentee; Blasentee EF-EM-ES; Bogumil-tassenfertiger milder Abfurtee; Drogimed; Droxitop; Ehrmann's Entschlackungstee; Entschlackender Abfuhrtee EF-EM-ES; Kneipp Nieren- und Blasen-Tee; Krauterdoktor Entwasserungs-Elixier; Krauterhaus Mag Kottas Entwasserungstee; Krauterhaus Mag Kottas Fruhjahrs- und Herbstkurtee; Krauterhaus Mag Kottas Nierentee; Krauterpfarrer Weidinger Tee bei Nieren- und Blasenbeschwerden; Mag Doskar's Nieren- und Blasentonikum; Mag Kottas Entwasserungstee; Mag Kottas Krauterexpress-Entwasserungstee; Mag Kottas Krauterexpress-Nieren-Blasentee; Mag Kottas Nieren-Blasentee; Naturland Rheuma Tee; Neuners Krautertee Nr 3 - Blasentee; Neuners Krautertee Nr 32 - Kreislafregulierungstee; Neuners Krautertee Nr 4 - Nierentee; Nierentee EF-EM-ES; Pneumopan; St Bonifatius-Tee; St Radegunder Entwasserungs-Elixier; St Radegunder Entwasserungstee; St Radegunder Nierentee; Synpharma Instant-Blasen- und Nierentee; Teekanne Blasen- und Nierentee; Uropurat; ***Fr.:*** Arterase; Circulatonic; Obeflorine; Tisane des Familles†; Tisanes de l'Abbe Hamon no 3†; ***Ger.:*** Agamadon†; Cystinol; Equisil N; Eviprostat N; Harntee 400; Harntee STADA; Hernia-Tee†; Hevert-Blasen-Nieren-Tee N; Kneipp Blasen- und Nieren-Tee†; nephro-loges; Nephroselect M; Nieron-Tee N; Presselin Nieren-Blasen K 3; Presselin Stoffwechsel-Tee Hapeka 225 N; Salus Rheuma-Tee Krautertee Nr. 12†; Salusan†; Solidagoren N; Tonsilgon; Tussiflorin N†; ***Hong Kong:*** Eviprostat†; ***Ital.:*** Nosenil†; ***Jpn:*** Eviprostat; ***Singapore:*** Eviprostat; ***Spain:*** Diurinat; Natusor Artilane; Natusor Harpagosinol; Natusor Infenol; Natusor Renal; Resolutivo Regium; Uralyt†; ***Switz.:*** Enveloppements ECR†; Eviprostat†; Nephrosolid; Tisane Diuretique; Urinex; ***UK:*** Antiglan; Antitis; Aqualette; Gerard House Waterlex†; Kas-Bah.

---

## Ergometrine Maleate *(BANM, rINNM)*

Ergobasine Maleate; Ergometrinhydrogenmaleat; Ergometrini Maleas; Ergonovine Bimaleate; Ergonovine Maleate; Ergostetrine Maleate; Ergotocine Maleate; Maleato de ergometrina; Maleato de Ergonovina. *N*-[(*S*)-2-Hydroxy-1-methylethyl]-D-lysergamide hydrogen maleate; 9,10-Didehydro-*N*-[(*S*)-2-hydroxy-1-methylethyl]-6-methylergoline-8β-carboxamide hydrogen maleate.

$C_{19}H_{23}N_3O_2,C_4H_4O_4$ = 441.5.

*CAS — 60-79-7 (ergometrine); 129-51-1 (ergometrine maleate).*

*ATC — G02AB03.*

**Pharmacopoeias.** In *Chin., Eur.* (see p.vi), *Int., Jpn,* and *US.*

**Ph. Eur. 5.0** (Ergometrine Maleate). A white or slightly coloured crystalline powder. Sparingly soluble in water; slightly soluble in alcohol. A 1% solution in water has a pH of 3.6 to 4.4. Store in airtight glass containers at a temperature of 2° to 8°. Protect from light.

**USP 27** (Ergonovine Maleate). A white to greyish-white or faintly yellow, odourless, microcrystalline powder. It darkens with age and on exposure to light. Sparingly soluble in water; slightly soluble in alcohol; insoluble in chloroform and in ether. Store in airtight containers at a temperature not exceeding 8°. Protect from light.

**Stability.** Reports of deterioration and degradation of ergometrine-containing injections when exposed to high temperatures in the tropics.[1-4] The mean loss in one study[3] of ergometrine injection under shipment to the tropics was 5.8%, but in some individual samples the loss was more marked: 18 of 80 test samples contained less than 80% of the stated content, and in 3 cases the content was less than 60% of the stated amount. A similar but much less significant pattern was seen with methylergometrine: the content varied from 98.6 to 99.5% of the labelled amount. Tablets of ergometrine and methylergometrine were also shown to be unstable under simulated tropical conditions, with humidity as the main adverse factor.[5]

1. Walker GJA, *et al.* Potency of ergometrine in tropical countries. *Lancet* 1988; **ii:** 393.
2. Abu-Reid IO, *et al.* Stability of drugs in the tropics. *Int Pharm J* 1990; **4:** 6–10.
3. Hogerzeil HV, *et al.* Stability of essential drugs during shipment to the tropics. *BMJ* 1992; **304:** 210–12.
4. Hogerzeil HV, Walker GJ. Instability of (methyl)ergometrine in tropical climates: an overview. *Eur J Obstet Gynecol Reprod Biol* 1996; **69:** 25–9.
5. de Groot ANJA, *et al.* Ergometrine and methylergometrine tablets are not stable under simulated tropical conditions. *J Clin Pharm Ther* 1995; **20:** 109–13.

### Adverse Effects and Treatment

Nausea and vomiting, abdominal pain, diarrhoea, headache, dizziness, tinnitus, chest pain, palpitations, bradycardia and other cardiac arrhythmias, myocardial infarction, dyspnoea, and pulmonary oedema have been reported after use of ergometrine. Hypertension may occur, particularly after rapid intravenous administration; hypotension has also been reported. Hypersensitivity reactions, including shock, have occurred. Ergometrine shows less tendency to produce gangrene than ergotamine, but ergotism has been reported and symptoms of acute poisoning are similar (see p.467).

Adverse effects should be treated as for ergotamine, p.467.

**Effects on the respiratory system.** Bronchospasm has been reported after use of ergometrine.[1] Although studies *in vitro* on *canine* bronchi have suggested a direct action on smooth muscle, this could not be confirmed in studies using human bronchi.

1. Hill H, *et al.* Ergometrine and bronchospasm. *Anaesthesia* 1987; **42:** 1115–16.

**Overdosage.** There have been reports[1-5] of accidental administration of adult doses of ergometrine maleate to neonates, sometimes instead of vitamin K. Symptoms have included peripheral vasoconstriction, encephalopathy, convulsions, respiratory failure, acute renal failure, and temporary lactose intolerance. After administration of ergometrine with oxytocin, water intoxication has also been reported.[1] In all of these cases, recovery occurred after intensive symptomatic treatment including assisted ventilation and anticonvulsants. However, deaths have also been recorded.[5] The long-term outcome of ergometrine overdosage has been reported for 6 infants.[5] Their ages at follow-up ranged from 18 months to 5 years; all had normal physical and behavioural development and neurological outcomes.

1. Whitfield MF, Salfield SAW. Accidental administration of Syntometrine in adult dosage to the newborn. *Arch Dis Child* 1980; **55:** 68–70.
2. Pandey SK, Haines CI. Accidental administration of ergometrine to newborn infant. *BMJ* 1982; **285:** 693.
3. Mitchell AA, *et al.* Accidental administration of ergonovine to a newborn. *JAMA* 1983; **250:** 730–1.
4. Donatini B, *et al.* Inadvertent administration of uterotonics to neonates. *Lancet* 1993; **341:** 839–40.
5. Dargaville PA, Campbell NT. Overdose of ergometrine in the newborn infant: acute symptomatology and long-term outcome. *J Paediatr Child Health* 1998; **34:** 83–9.

### Precautions

As for Ergotamine Tartrate, p.467. Ergometrine maleate is contra-indicated for the induction of labour or for use during the first stage of labour. If used at the end of the second stage of labour, before delivery of the placenta, there must be expert obstetric supervision. Its use should be avoided in patients with pre-eclampsia, eclampsia, or threatened spontaneous abortion.

**Porphyria.** Ergometrine maleate has been associated with acute attacks of porphyria and is considered unsafe in porphyric patients.

### Interactions

As for Ergotamine Tartrate, p.468. The vasoconstrictor effects of ergometrine are enhanced by sympathomimetics. Halothane has been considered to diminish the effects of ergometrine on the uterus.

**Sympathomimetics.** Use of *dopamine* in a patient treated with ergometrine was associated with subsequent development of gangrene in both hands and feet.[1]

1. Buchanan N, *et al.* Symmetrical gangrene of the extremities associated with the use of dopamine subsequent to ergometrine administration. *Intensive Care Med* 1977; **3:** 55–6.

### Pharmacokinetics

Ergometrine is reported to be rapidly absorbed after administration by mouth and by intramuscular injection, with onset of uterine contractions in about 5 to 15 minutes and 2 to 7 minutes respectively. Elimination appears to be principally by hepatic metabolism.

### Uses and Administration

Ergometrine has a much more powerful action on the uterus than most other ergot alkaloids, especially on the puerperal uterus. Its main action is the production of intense contractions, which at higher doses are sustained, in contrast to the more physiological rhythmic uterine contractions induced by oxytocin; its action is more prolonged than that of oxytocin.

Ergometrine maleate is used in the active management of the third stage of labour, and to prevent or treat postpartum or postabortal haemorrhage caused by uterine atony; by maintaining uterine contraction and tone, blood vessels in the uterine wall are compressed, and blood flow reduced.

In the active management of the third stage of labour, ergometrine maleate and oxytocin are given together under full obstetric supervision. A dose of ergometrine maleate 500 micrograms and oxytocin 5 units is injected intramuscularly after delivery of the anterior shoulder of the infant; contractions are reported to occur within 2 to 3 minutes. Delivery of the placenta is actively assisted while the uterus is firmly contracted.

In the prevention or treatment of postpartum haemorrhage, a similar dose of ergometrine maleate with oxytocin is given intramuscularly following delivery of the placenta or when bleeding occurs. Intravenous administration of a combined preparation of ergometrine maleate with oxytocin has been used but is no longer recommended. Ergometrine maleate alone is used for prevention or treatment of postpartum or postabortal haemorrhage in a usual intramuscular dose of 200 micrograms. In emergencies such as excessive uterine bleeding, ergometrine maleate has been given intravenously in a dose of 200 micrograms. This dose may be repeated every 2 to 4 hours as needed, or for up to 5 doses. Single doses of 250 to 500 micrograms have also been used. Intravenous doses should be administered slowly to reduce the risk of adverse effects, particularly hypertension. Parenteral treatment of haemorrhage may be followed by ergometrine maleate 200 to 400 micrograms by mouth two to four times daily for up to 7 days, until the danger of atony and haemorrhage has passed.

In the treatment of mild secondary postpartum haemorrhage, ergometrine maleate has been given by mouth in a dose of 500 micrograms three times daily for 2 to 7 days.

Ergometrine maleate has been administered by the sublingual and rectal routes.

Ergometrine tartrate was formerly used.

**Diagnosis and testing.** Ergometrine maleate[1-6] or methylergometrine maleate[2,7] have been used in a provocation test for the diagnosis of Prinzmetal's angina (variant angina) (p.813). Ergometrine maleate has also been used in the diagnosis of oesophageal spasm.[8]

1. Waters DD, *et al.* Ergonovine testing in a coronary care unit. *Am J Cardiol* 1980; **46:** 922–30.
2. Anonymous. Provocation of coronary spasm: research or diagnostic test? *Lancet* 1982; **ii:** 805.
3. Health and Public Policy Committee, American College of Physicians. Performance of ergonovine provocative testing for coronary artery spasm. *Ann Intern Med* 1984; **100:** 151–2.
4. Song J-K, *et al.* Safety and clinical impact of ergonovine stress echocardiography for diagnosis of coronary vasospasm. *J Am Coll Cardiol* 2000; **35:** 1850–6.
5. Kashima K, *et al.* Long-term outcome of patients with ergonovine induced coronary constriction not associated with ischemic electrocardiographic changes. *J Cardiol* 2001; **37:** 301–8.
6. Palinkas A, *et al.* Safety of ergot stress echocardiography for non-invasive detection of coronary vasospasm. *Coron Artery Dis* 2001; **12:** 649–54.
7. Bertrand ME, *et al.* Frequency of provoked coronary arterial spasm in 1089 consecutive patients undergoing coronary arteriography. *Circulation* 1982; **65:** 1299–1306.
8. Richter JE, *et al.* Esophageal chest pain: current controversies in pathogenesis, diagnosis, and therapy. *Ann Intern Med* 1989; **110:** 66–78.

**Postpartum haemorrhage.** If the uterus fails to contract adequately after delivery (uterine atony), or if retained placental remnants prevent retraction of the placental bed, postpartum haemorrhage may occur. These two causes account for about 80% of cases of postpartum haemorrhage; in the remainder it is usually due to trauma of the genital tract.

Postpartum haemorrhage may be fatal to the mother unless promptly dealt with, and **management** generally involves:

- removal of the placenta if it has not been expelled
- the use of oxytocics to contract the uterus
- transfusion if blood loss is severe

Intravenous oxytocin injection, followed by intravenous ergometrine injection and oxytocin infusion has been recommended for the treatment of bleeding due to uterine atony. Prostaglandins such as carboprost, dinoprostone, or sulprostone may be used for primary postpartum haemorrhage that has not been controlled by oxytocin and ergot preparations. Rectal misoprostol has also been shown to be effective,[1] and a subsequent review[2] suggested that it might be a possible first-line treatment, although it was acknowledged that the original study was not large enough to evaluate the effects on maternal mortality, serious morbidity, or hysterectomy rates.

Secondary postpartum haemorrhage occurs between 24 hours and 12 weeks after delivery and although associated with maternal morbidity rather than death in developed countries, it is a major contributor to maternal death in developing countries. Antibacterials, oxytocics, hormone therapy and a variety of surgical treatments are used, but a systematic review[3] concluded that evidence for the best treatment is lacking.

**Prophylactic** management of postpartum haemorrhage is favoured in some countries but in others may be reserved for women at greater risk, including those who have undergone prolonged labour, those who have an overdistended uterus (for example in multiple pregnancy), or after antepartum haemorrhage, or deep general anaesthesia. Active management of the third stage of labour involves prophylactic use of an oxytocic, cord clamping before placental delivery, and cord traction.

Studies[4,5] and a subsequent meta-analysis[6] including additional trials of actively managed labour found that routine oxytocics (usually with crowning of the head, delivery of the anterior shoulder, or after delivery of the placenta) reduced blood loss, the risk of postpartum haemorrhage, and the risk of prolonged third stage of labour. Oxytocin and ergot alkaloids seem to be of similar efficacy in decreasing postpartum haemorrhage, but oxytocin is less likely to predispose to delayed placental delivery and also less likely to cause hypertension.[7] The timing of prophylactic oxytocin (before or after placental delivery) does not seem to make a difference.[8] Syntometrine (ergometrine and oxytocin) and ergot alkaloids also appear to be of similar efficacy, but Syntometrine may be less likely to be associated with a prolonged third stage of labour.[7] Syntometrine may be associated with a small reduction in the risk of postpartum haemorrhage compared with oxytocin,[9] but a higher incidence of nausea, vomiting, and hypertension. A systematic review[10] concluded that there seemed little evidence in favour of ergot alkaloids alone compared with either oxytocin alone or with Syntometrine, although the data were sparse and more studies were required in domiciliary deliveries in developing countries where the incidence of third stage complications is greatest. Misoprostol has also been investigated as an alternative for routine management of the third stage of labour because it may be given orally or rectally and is inexpensive, therefore offering advantages in developing countries, especially in tropical regions where parenteral ergometrine formulations suffer from problems of instability. However, systematic reviews[11,12] of studies including a large multicentre WHO study[13] involving 9 countries concluded that neither oral misoprostol[11,12] nor intramuscular prostaglandins[11] were preferable to conventional injectable uterotonics for the management of the third stage of labour, especially for women at low risk; it was suggested[11] that there was insufficient evidence to justify use of prophylactic misoprostol even when other uterotonics were unavailable.


1. Lokugamage AU, *et al.* A randomized study comparing rectally administered misoprostol versus Syntometrine combined with an oxytocin infusion for the cessation of primary post partum hemorrhage. *Acta Obstet Gynecol Scand* 2001; **80:** 835–9.
2. Mousa HA, Alfirevic Z. Treatment for primary postpartum haemorrhage. Available in The Cochrane Library: Issue 2. Chichester: John Wiley; 2004.
3. Alexander J, *et al.* Treatments for secondary postpartum haemorrhage. Available in The Cochrane Library: Issue 2. Chichester: John Wiley; 2004.
4. Prendiville WJ, *et al.* The Bristol third stage trial: active versus physiological management of third stage of labour. *BMJ* 1988; **297:** 1295–1300.
5. Rogers J, *et al.* Active versus expectant management of third stage of labour: the Hinchingbrooke randomised controlled trial. *Lancet* 1998; **351:** 693–9.
6. Prendiville WJ, *et al.* Active versus expectant management in the third stage of labour. Available in The Cochrane Library; Issue 2. Chichester: John Wiley; 2004.
7. Elbourne D, *et al.* Choice of oxytocic preparation for routine use in the management of the third stage of labour: an overview of the evidence from controlled trials. *Br J Obstet Gynaecol* 1988; **95:** 17–30.
8. Jackson KW, *et al.* A randomized controlled trial comparing oxytocin administration before and after placental delivery in the prevention of postpartum hemorrhage. *Am J Obstet Gynecol* 2001; **185:** 873–7.
9. McDonald S, *et al.* Prophylactic ergometrine-oxytocin versus oxytocin for the third stage of labour. Available in The Cochrane Library; Issue 2. Chichester: John Wiley; 2004.
10. Elbourne DR, *et al.* Prophylactic use of oxytocin in the third stage of labour. Available in The Cochrane Library: Issue 2. Chichester: John Wiley; 2004.
11. Gülmezoglu AM, *et al.* Prostaglandins for prevention of postpartum haemorrhage. Available in The Cochrane Library; Issue 2. Chichester: John Wiley; 2004.
12. Villar J, *et al.* Systematic review of randomized controlled trials of misoprostol to prevent postpartum hemorrhage. *Obstet Gynecol* 2002; **100:** 1301–12.
13. Gülmezoglu AM, *et al.* WHO multicentre randomised trial of misoprostol in the management of the third stage of labour. *Lancet* 2001; **358:** 689–95.


### Preparations

***BP 2003:*** Ergometrine and Oxytocin Injection; Ergometrine Injection; Ergometrine Tablets;
***USP 27:*** Ergonovine Maleate Injection; Ergonovine Maleate Tablets.

**Proprietary Preparations** (details are given in Part 3)
***Arg.:*** Evina; Metrergina; ***Braz.:*** Ergotrate; ***Canad.:*** Ergotrate†; ***Ger.:*** Secalysat EM†; ***Gr.:*** Mitrotan; ***Mex.:*** Cryovin†; Ergofar†; Ergotrate; ***Thai.:*** Gynaemine; ***USA:*** Ergotrate.

**Multi-ingredient:** ***Austral.:*** Syntometrine; ***Hong Kong:*** Syntometrine; ***Irl.:*** Syntometrine; ***Israel:*** Syntometrine†; ***Malaysia:*** Syntometrine; ***NZ:*** Syntometrine; ***S.Afr.:*** Syntometrine; ***UK:*** Syntometrine.

## Ergot

Cornezuelo del centeno; Secale Cornutum.

**Description.** Ergot consists of the sclerotium of the fungus *Claviceps purpurea* (Hypocreaceae) developed in the ovary of the rye, *Secale cereale* (Gramineae), containing not less than 0.15% of total alkaloids, calculated as ergotoxine, and not less than 0.01% of water-soluble alkaloids, calculated as ergometrine. Some authorities have expressed alkaloidal content in terms of ergotamine and ergometrine.

### Adverse Effects and Treatment

As for Ergotamine Tartrate, p.467.

Epidemic ergot poisoning, arising from the ingestion of ergotised rye bread, is now seldom seen. Two forms of epidemic toxicity, which rarely occur together, have been described: a gangrenous form characterised by agonising pain of the extremities of the body followed by dry gangrene of the peripheral parts, and a rarer nervous type giving rise to paroxysmal epileptiform convulsions.

**Poisoning.** A report of an outbreak of ergotism, attributed to the ingestion of infected wild oats (*Avena abyssinica*), in Ethiopia.[1]


1. King B. Outbreak of ergotism in Wollo, Ethiopia. *Lancet* 1979; **ii:** 1411.


### Uses and Administration

Ergot has the vasoconstricting and oxytocic actions of its constituent alkaloids, especially ergotamine (p.467) and ergometrine (above). A liquid extract or tablets of prepared ergot were formerly used as an oxytocic. Preparations containing ergot extracts have been promoted for use in dyspepsia and nervous disorders.

### Preparations

**Proprietary Preparations** (details are given in Part 3)
***India:*** Ergotab.

## Ergotoxine

Ergotoxina.

*CAS — 8006-25-5 (ergotoxine); 8047-28-7 (ergotoxine esilate); 8047-29-8 (ergotoxine phosphate); 564-36-3 (ergocornine); 511-08-0 (ergocristine); 511-09-1 (ergocryptine).*

### Profile

Ergotoxine is a mixture of naturally occurring ergot alkaloids. It contains equal proportions of ergocornine ($C_{31}H_{39}N_5O_5$ = 561.7), ergocristine ($C_{35}H_{39}N_5O_5$ = 609.7), and ergocryptine($C_{32}H_{41}N_5O_5$ = 575.7), as the α- and β-isomers. The esilate was formerly used as an oxytocic and in the treatment of migraine. Ergotoxine phosphate has also been used.

### Preparations

**Proprietary Preparations** (details are given in Part 3)
**Multi-ingredient:** ***Thai.:*** Belloid†.

## Etaden

Ethaden. 2-[(6-Amino-1*H*-purin-8-yl)amino]ethanol.

$C_7H_{10}N_6O$ = 194.2.

*CAS — 66813-29-4.*

### Profile

Etaden is used in the form of eye drops to stimulate epithelial regrowth.

## Ethaverine Hydrochloride *(rINNM)*

Hidrocloruro de etaverina. 6,7-Diethoxy-1-(3,4-diethoxybenzyl)isoquinoline hydrochloride.

$C_{24}H_{29}NO_4,HCl$ = 432.0.

*CAS — 486-47-5 (ethaverine); 985-13-7 (ethaverine hydrochloride).*

### Profile

Ethaverine is the tetraethoxy analogue of papaverine (p.1728) and has been used as the hydrochloride as an antispasmodic in respiratory-tract, biliary, gastrointestinal, and genito-urinary disorders. It has also been used in migraine, vascular disorders and as an antiarrhythmic.

Ethaverine sulfamate has also been used.

### Preparations

**Proprietary Preparations** (details are given in Part 3)
**Multi-ingredient:** ***Austria:*** Asthma Efeum; Gastripan; Hylakombun†; Oddispasmol; ***Braz.:*** Eufermen; ***Ger.:*** Migrane-Kranit Kombi†; ***Switz.:*** Elzym†; ***Thai.:*** Elzym.

## Ethoxyphenyldiethylphenylbutylamine Hydrochloride

Etoxifenildietilfenilbutilamina, hidrocloruro de. 1-(4-Ethoxyphenyl)-*N*,*N*-diethyl-3-phenylbutylamine hydrochloride.

$C_{22}H_{31}NO,HCl$ = 361.9.

*CAS — 13988-32-4 (ethoxyphenyldiethylphenylbutylamine); 10535-87-2 (ethoxyphenyldiethylphenylbutylamine hydrochloride).*

### Profile

Ethoxyphenyldiethylphenylbutylamine hydrochloride has been used as an antispasmodic.

## Ethyl Cinnamate

Cinamato de etilo. Ethyl (*E*)-3-phenylprop-2-enoate.

$C_{11}H_{12}O_2$ = 176.2.

*CAS — 103-36-6.*

**Pharmacopoeias.** In *Br.*

**BP 2003** (Ethyl Cinnamate). A clear, colourless or almost colourless liquid with a fruity, balsamic odour. Practically insoluble in water; miscible with most organic solvents.

### Profile

Ethyl cinnamate is used as a flavour and perfume; it is an ingredient of Tolu-flavour Solution (BP 2003).

### Preparations

***BP 2003:*** Tolu-flavour Solution.

## Ethyl Oleate

Aethylis Oleas; Ethylis Oleas; Oleato de etilo.

$C_{20}H_{38}O_2$ = 310.5.

*CAS — 111-62-6.*

**Pharmacopoeias.** In *Eur.* (see p.vi). Also in *USNF.*

**Ph. Eur. 5.0** (Ethyl Oleate). A clear, pale yellow or colourless liquid. It consists of the ethyl esters of fatty acids, mainly oleic acid. It may contain a suitable antoxidant. Practically insoluble in water; miscible with alcohol, with dichloromethane, and with petroleum spirit (40° to 60°). Protect from light.

**USNF 22** (Ethyl Oleate). It consists of esters of ethyl alcohol and high-molecular-weight fatty acids, principally oleic acid. A mobile, practically colourless liquid. Insoluble in water; miscible with alcohol, with vegetable oils, with liquid paraffin, and with most organic solvents. Store in airtight containers. Protect from light.

**Incompatibility.** Ethyl oleate dissolves some types of rubber and causes others to swell.

### Profile

Ethyl oleate is used as an oily vehicle.

## Ethyl Vanillin

Etilvanilina. 3-Ethoxy-4-hydroxybenzaldehyde.

$C_9H_{10}O_3$ = 166.2.

*CAS — 121-32-4.*

**Pharmacopoeias.** In *USNF.*

**USNF 22** (Ethyl Vanillin). Fine, white or slightly yellowish crystals with a vanilla-like odour. M.p. is between 76° and 78°. Soluble 1 in 100 of water at 50° and 1 in 2 of alcohol; freely soluble in chloroform, in ether, and in solutions of alkali hydroxides. Its solutions are acid to litmus. Store in airtight containers. Protect from light.

### Profile

Ethyl vanillin is used as a flavour and in perfumery to impart the odour and taste of vanilla.

## Ethylene Glycol

Ethylene Alcohol; Etilenglicol; Glycol. Ethane-1,2-diol.

$C_2H_6O_2$ = 62.07.

*CAS — 107-21-1.*

### Adverse Effects

Toxic effects arising from ingestion of ethylene glycol result from its major metabolites: aldehydes, glycolate, lactate, and oxalate. Clinical features may be divided into three stages depending on the time elapsed since ingestion. In the first 12 hours, the patient may show signs of drunkenness and experience nausea and vomiting. Convulsions and neurological defects may occur. From 12 to 24 hours, there may be tachycardia, mild hypertension, pulmonary oedema, and heart failure. Between 24 and 72 hours, patients with severe ethylene glycol poisoning may experience flank pain and renal involvement with associated decreased plasma concentrations of calcium and bicarbonate, metabolic acidosis, deposition of oxalate in tissues and kidney tubules, proteinuria, oxaluria, haematuria, and renal failure. There may be respiratory failure, cardiovascular collapse, and sometimes coma and death. The fatal dose is reported to be about 100 mL.

Skin irritation and penetration have been reported following topical application.

Diethylene glycol produces similar toxicity, except that there is no conversion to oxalate and there is greater nephrotoxicity. Poisoning has followed adulteration of medicinal products with diethylene glycol.

◊ References.


1. Anonymous. Some wine to break the ice. *Lancet* 1985; **ii:** 254.
2. Vale JA, Buckley BM. Metabolic acidosis in diethylene glycol poisoning. *Lancet* 1985; **ii:** 394.
3. Buckley BM, Vale JA. Poisoning by alcohols and ethylene glycol. *Prescribers' J* 1986; **26:** 110–15.
4. Hanif M, *et al.* Fatal renal failure caused by diethylene glycol in paracetamol elixir: the Bangladesh epidemic. *BMJ* 1995; **311:** 88–91.
5. Lewis LD, *et al.* Delayed sequelae after acute overdoses or poisonings: cranial neuropathy related to ethylene glycol ingestion. *Clin Pharmacol Ther* 1997; **61:** 692–9.
6. O'Brien KL, *et al.* Epidemic of pediatric deaths from acute renal failure caused by diethylene glycol poisoning. *JAMA* 1998; **279:** 1175–80.
7. Singh J, *et al.* Diethylene glycol poisoning in Gurgaon, India, 1998. *Bull WHO* 2001; **79:** 88–95.


### Treatment of Adverse Effects

The stomach should be emptied by lavage if ingestion of ethylene glycol was within the preceding hour. Severe metabolic acidosis should be corrected with sodium bicarbonate intravenously and hypocalcaemia corrected with calcium gluconate. Haemodialysis or peritoneal dialysis may be of value. Alcohol may be given by mouth or intravenously as it is a competitor of the metabolism of ethylene glycol. Alternatively fomepizole (p.1039), an alcohol-dehydrogenase inhibitor, may be used for the treatment of ethylene glycol poisoning.

◊ References.


1. Harry P, *et al.* Ethylene glycol poisoning in a child treated with 4-methylpyrazole. *Pediatrics* 1998; **102:** E31.
2. Barceloux DG, *et al.* American Academy of Clinical Toxicology practice guidelines on the treatment of ethylene glycol poisoning. *Clin Toxicol* 1999; **37:** 537–60.
3. Brent J, *et al.* Fomepizole for the treatment of ethylene glycol poisoning. *N Engl J Med* 1999; **340:** 832–8.

4. Borron SW, *et al.* Fomepizole in treatment of uncomplicated ethylene glycol poisoning. *Lancet* 1999; **354:** 831.
5. Baum CR, *et al.* Fomepizole treatment of ethylene glycol poisoning in an infant. *Pediatrics* 2000; **106:** 1489–91.
6. Brent J. Current management of ethylene glycol poisoning. *Drugs* 2001; **61:** 979–88.
7. Battistella M. Fomepizole as an antidote for ethylene glycol poisoning. *Ann Pharmacother* 2002; **36:** 1085–9.

### Pharmacokinetics

Ethylene glycol is absorbed from the gastrointestinal tract and is metabolised, chiefly in the liver, by alcohol dehydrogenase. Its breakdown products account for its toxicity and include aldehydes, glycolate, lactate, and oxalate.

◊ References.

1. Sivilotti ML, *et al.* Toxicokinetics of ethylene glycol during fomepizole therapy: implications for management. *Ann Emerg Med* 2000; **36:** 114–25.

### Uses

Ethylene glycol is commonly encountered in antifreeze solutions and has been used illicitly to sweeten some wines. Diethylene glycol has been used similarly.

## Ethylenediamine

Edamine *(USAN, pINN)*; Edamina; Ethylendiaminum.

$C_2H_8N_2 = 60.10.$

*CAS — 107-15-3 (anhydrous ethylenediamine); 6780-13-8 (ethylenediamine monohydrate).*

**Pharmacopoeias.** In *Eur.* (see p.vi), *Jpn*, and *US*.

**Ph. Eur. 5.0** (Ethylenediamine). A clear, colourless or slightly yellow, hygroscopic liquid. On exposure to air, white fumes are evolved. On heating it evaporates completely. Miscible with water and with alcohol. Store in airtight containers. Protect from light.

**USP 27** (Ethylenediamine). A clear, colourless or only slightly yellow liquid having an ammonia-like odour. It is strongly alkaline and may readily absorb carbon dioxide from the air to form a non-volatile carbonate. Miscible with water and with alcohol. Store in well-filled, airtight, glass containers.

### Adverse Effects

Ethylenediamine is irritant to the skin and to mucous membranes. Severe exfoliative dermatitis has been reported following systemic use of preparations containing ethylenediamine. Hypersensitivity reactions are common. Concentrated solutions cause skin burns. Headache, dizziness, shortness of breath, nausea, and vomiting have also been reported following exposure to fumes. Ethylenediamine splashed onto the skin or eyes should be removed by flooding with water for a prolonged period.

**Hypersensitivity.** A review of allergy to ethylenediamine and aminophylline.[1]

1. Anonymous. Allergy to aminophylline. *Lancet* 1984; **ii :** 1192–3.

### Precautions

Skin reactions may occur in patients given aminophylline after they have become sensitised to ethylenediamine. Cross-sensitivity with edetic acid and with some antihistamines has been reported.

**Cross-sensitivity.** It was reported that some topical corticosteroid creams, including Tri-Adcortyl in the UK,[1] and Kenacomb, Halcicomb, and Viaderm in Canada,[2] contained ethylenediamine and could cause unexpected cross-sensitivity reactions with piperazine[1] or aminophylline.[2]

1. Wright S, Harman RRM. Ethylenediamine and piperazine sensitivity. *BMJ* 1983; **287**: 463–4.
2. Hogan DJ. Excipients in topical corticosteroid preparations in Canada. *Can Med Assoc J* 1989; **141**: 1032.

### Uses and Administration

Ethylenediamine or ethylenediamine hydrate forms a stable mixture with theophylline to produce aminophylline or aminophylline hydrate. Ethylenediamine is widely used in the chemical and pharmaceutical industries and as an ingredient of some topical creams.

### Preparations

**Proprietary Preparations** (details are given in Part 3)

**Multi-ingredient:** ***Braz.:*** Narizima Adulto†.

## Eucalyptus Leaf

Eucalypti Folium; Eucalyptusblätter.

**Pharmacopoeias.** In *Eur.* (see p.vi).

**Ph. Eur.** (Eucalyptus Leaf). It consists of the whole or cut dried leaves of older branches of *Eucalyptus globulus*. The whole drug contains not less than 2% v/w of essential oil and the cut drug not less than 1.5% v/w of essential oil, both calculated with reference to the anhydrous drug. It has an aromatic odour of cineole. Protect from light.

### Profile

Eucalyptus leaf has been used in oral preparations for coughs and associated respiratory-tract disorders. It is also used as a flavour. It is a source of eucalyptus oil (see below).

### Preparations

**Proprietary Preparations** (details are given in Part 3)

**Multi-ingredient:** ***Austral.:*** Arthrirub; Goanna Bite-Eze†; ***Austria:*** Euka; Gewusst wie Husten-Bronchialtee; Krauterpfarrer Weidinger Tee bei Husten und Heiserkeit; St Radegunder Bronchialtee; ***Belg.:*** Eugiron†; ***Braz.:*** Axol†; Broncol; Calmante Creosotado†; Pulmoiodo†; Tosseina†; Tussifen; Xarope de Eucalipto†; ***Canad.:*** Beech Nut Cough Drops; ***Chile:*** Codetol PM; Paltomiel; Paltomiel Plus; Pulmosina; ***Fr.:*** Balsofumine; Balsofumine Mentholee; Santane $O_1$†; Tisanes de l'Abbe Hamon no 15†; ***Ger.:*** Cefabronchin†; Em-eukal; Hevertopect N; ***Israel:*** Gingisan; ***Ital.:*** Fosfoguaiacol; Ingro†; ***NZ:*** Otrivine Menthol; ***Spain:*** Bronpul; Calyptol Inhalante†; Diabesor; Llantusil; Natusor Broncopul; Natusor Gripotul; Pastillas Antisep Garg M; Vapores Pyt; ***UK:*** Calrub; Collins Elixir Decongesant Pasilles; Nasal Inhaler†; No-Sor Nose Balm; Revitonil.

## Eucalyptus Oil

Esencia de Eucalipto; Essence d'Eucalyptus Rectifiée; Eucalipto, aceite esencial de; Eucalypti Aetheroleum; Oleum Eucalypti.

**Pharmacopoeias.** In *Chin.*, *Eur.* (see p.vi), *Jpn*, and *Pol.*

**Ph. Eur. 5.0** (Eucalyptus Oil). A colourless or pale yellow liquid with a characteristic aromatic camphoraceous odour and a pungent camphoraceous taste. It is obtained by steam distillation and rectification from the fresh leaves or terminal branches of various species of *Eucalyptus* rich in cineole. The species mainly used are *E. globulus*, *E. polybractea*, and *E. smithii*. It contains not less than 70% w/w of cineole. Relative density 0.906 to 0.927. Soluble 1 in 5 of alcohol (70%). Store in well-filled airtight containers at a temperature not exceeding 25°. Protect from light.

### Adverse Effects and Precautions

The symptoms of poisoning with eucalyptus oil include gastrointestinal symptoms such as epigastric burning, nausea and vomiting, and CNS depression, including coma. Cyanosis, ataxia, miosis, pulmonary damage, delirium, and convulsions may occur. Deaths have been reported.

Oily solutions of eucalyptus oil were formerly used in nasal preparations, but this use is now considered unsuitable as the vehicle inhibits ciliary movements and may cause lipoid pneumonia.

◊ References.

1. Patel S, Wiggins J. Eucalyptus oil poisoning. *Arch Dis Child* 1980; **55:** 405.
2. Spoerke DG, *et al.* Eucalyptus oil: 14 cases of exposure. *Vet Hum Toxicol* 1989; **31:** 166–8.
3. Webb NJA, Pitt WR. Eucalyptus oil poisoning in childhood: 41 cases in south-east Queensland. *J Paediatr Child Health* 1993; **29:** 368–71.
4. Tibballs J. Clinical effects and management of eucalyptus oil ingestion in infants and young children. *Med J Aust* 1995; **163:** 177–80.
5. Anpalahan M, Le Couteur DG. Deliberate self-poisoning with eucalyptus oil in an elderly woman. *Aust N Z J Med* 1998; **28:** 58.
6. Darben T, *et al.* Topical eucalyptus oil poisoning. *Australas J Dermatol* 1998; **39:** 265–7.

### Uses and Administration

Eucalyptus oil has been taken by mouth for catarrh and coughs and is an ingredient of many preparations. It has been used as an inhalation often in combination with other volatile substances. Eucalyptus oil has also been applied as a rubefacient and is used as a flavour.

### Preparations

**Proprietary Preparations** (details are given in Part 3)

***Austral.:*** Bosisto's Eucalyptus Spray†; ***Austria:*** Luuf Bronchial; ***Ger.:*** Aspecton Eukaps; Bronchodurat Eucalyptusol†; Bronchomed†; Eucalyptrol L†; Exeu; Gelodurat; Nasivin gegen Erkaltung Kinderbad†; Pinimenthol Erkaltungsbad fur Kinder; Pinimenthol Erkaltungskapseln; Tussidermil N.

**Multi-ingredient:** numerous preparations are listed in Part 3.

## Eugenol

4-Allylguaiacol; Eugen.; Eugenic Acid; Eugenolum. 4-Allyl-2-methoxyphenol.

$C_{10}H_{12}O_2 = 164.2.$

*CAS — 97-53-0.*

**Pharmacopoeias.** In *Eur.* (see p.vi), *Pol.*, *US*, and *Viet.*

**Ph. Eur. 5.0** (Eugenol). A colourless or pale yellow liquid with a strong odour of clove. Practically insoluble in water and in glycerol; freely soluble in alcohol (70%); miscible with alcohol, with glacial acetic acid, with dichloromethane, and with fatty oils. Eugenol darkens in colour on exposure to air. Store in well-filled containers. Protect from light.

**USP 27** (Eugenol). It is obtained from clove oil or from other sources. A colourless or pale yellow liquid having a strongly aromatic odour of clove. Upon exposure to air, it darkens and thickens. Slightly soluble in water; miscible with alcohol, with chloroform, with ether, and with fixed oils. Store in airtight containers. Protect from light.

### Profile

Eugenol is a constituent of clove oil (p.1673) and some other essential oils. It is employed in dentistry, often mixed with zinc oxide, as a temporary anodyne dental filling, and is an ingredient in oral hygiene preparations. Eugenol has been used as a flavour.

Eugenol is an irritant and sensitiser and can produce local anaesthesia. It is reported to inhibit prostaglandin synthesis.

For the pulmonary effects of eugenol inhalation from clove cigarettes, see Abuse, under Clove, p.1673.

◊ References.

1. Sarrami N, *et al.* Adverse reactions associated with the use of eugenol in dentistry. *Br Dent J* 2002; **193:** 257–9.

### Preparations

**Proprietary Preparations** (details are given in Part 3)

***Ital.:*** Bastoncino†; ***USA:*** Red Cross Toothache.

**Multi-ingredient:** ***Arg.:*** Sicadentol Plus; ***Austria:*** Ledermix; ***Belg.:*** Calmant Martou†; Dentophar; ***Braz.:*** Passaja†; Relampago†; UM Instante†; Um Segundo†; ***Canad.:*** Jiffy Toothache Drops†; ***Chile:*** Listermint Con Fluor; ***Denm.:*** Ledermix; ***Fr.:*** Alodont; Pectoderme; ***Hong Kong:*** Counterpain; ***Irl.:*** Ledermix†; ***Israel:*** Dentin; ***Ital.:*** Creosoto Composto; Eugenol-Guaiacolo Composto; Odongi; Odontalgiche (Dentali); ***Malaysia:*** Flanil; ***S.Afr.:*** Counterpain; Ledermix†; ***Singapore:*** Begesic; Flanil; ***Spain:*** Alvogil; Neodesfila†; Piorlis; Pomada Revulsiva†; Tangenol; Tifell; ***Switz.:*** Alodont; Alvogyl; Benzocaine PD; Dental-Phenjoca†; Endomethasone†; Ledermix; Rocanal Permanent Gangrene†; Rocanal Permanent Vital†; Spirogel†; ***Thai.:*** Begesic; Counterpain; Flanil; Heat Cream; Masa Balm†; Muscalax; Neotica; Nox-Pain; Olympic Balm; Painza; Reduxpain; Sancago; Stopain; ***UK:*** Aezodent†; Ledermix.

## Euphorbia

Euforbia; Pill-bearing Spurge; Snake Weed.

**Pharmacopoeias.** *Chin.* includes monographs for *Euphorbia humifusa* or *E. maculata* herb and *E. pekinensis* root.

### Profile

Euphorbia, the aerial parts of *Euphorbia hirta* (*E. pilulifera*, *Chamaesyce hirta*) (Euphorbiaceae), has sedative and expectorant properties and is used in the treatment of asthma and other respiratory-tract disorders. It has also been used for intestinal amoebiasis.

Other *Euphorbia* spp. are used for a variety of disorders. The seeds and latex of *E. lathyrus* (caper spurge) have been used as a purgative but are too toxic for general use. Many species have been used as arrow poisons.

### Preparations

**Proprietary Preparations** (details are given in Part 3)

**Multi-ingredient:** ***Austral.:*** Asa Tones†; Euphorbia Complex†; Procold†; Sambucus Complex†; ***Canad.:*** Sirop Cocillana Codeine; ***Fr.:*** Tisanes de l'Abbe Hamon no 14†; ***Hong Kong:*** Cocillana Compound; Mefedra-N; ***UK:*** Antibron.

## Euphrasia

Eufrasia; Eyebright.

### Profile

Euphrasia, the aerial parts of various *Euphrasia* spp. including *E. rostkoviana* and *E. officinalis* (Scrophulariaceae), has been used topically for blepharitis, conjunctivitis, and other eye disorders. However, such use is not generally recommended. Euphrasia has also been used for nasal catarrh and sinusitis, and to prevent snoring.

It is also used in homoeopathic medicine.

### Preparations

**Proprietary Preparations** (details are given in Part 3)

***UK:*** Snore Calm.

**Multi-ingredient:** ***Austral.:*** Bilberry Plus†; Eye Health Herbal Plus Formula 4†; Lifesystem Herbal Plus Formula 5 Eye Relief†; Sambucus Complex†; ***Ital.:*** Eulux; ***Switz.:*** Collypan; Oculosan; ***UK:*** Se-Power; Vital Eyes.

## Evening Primrose

King's Cureall.

### Profile

Evening primrose, the aerial parts of *Oenothera biennis* (Onagraceae) and related species of *Oenothera*, is reported to have sedative and astringent properties. It has been used in herbal preparations for respiratory and gastrointestinal disorders.

Evening primrose seed is the source of evening primrose oil (below), which is a source of essential fatty acids.

## Evening Primrose Oil

Onagra, aceite de.

**Description.** Evening primrose oil is a fixed oil obtained from the seeds of *Oenothera biennis* or other spp. (Onagraceae) and contains linoleic acid with some gamolenic acid.

**Pharmacopoeias.** In *Pol.*

### Adverse Effects and Precautions

See Gamolenic Acid, p.1690.

**Effects on the nervous system.** Temporal lobe epilepsy was diagnosed following treatment with evening primrose oil in 3 patients who had previously been diagnosed as schizophrenic.[1] Tonic-clonic (grand mal) seizures occurred in 2 additional schizophrenic patients during treatment with evening primrose oil.[2]

All of these patients had received or were taking phenothiazine antipsychotics.


1. Vaddadi KS. The use of gamma-linolenic acid and linoleic acid to differentiate between temporal lobe epilepsy and schizophrenia. *Prostaglandins Med* 1981; **6:** 375–9.
2. Holman CP, Bell AFJ. A trial of evening primrose oil in the treatment of chronic schizophrenia. *J Orthomol Psychiatry* 1983; **12:** 302–4.


## Uses and Administration

Evening primrose oil is a source of linoleic and gamolenic acid which are essential fatty acids of the omega-6 series that act as prostaglandin precursors (see p.1690). Evening primrose oil has been given by mouth for the symptomatic relief of atopic eczema in usual doses of up to 3 grams twice daily; it is also used topically as a cream for the relief of dry or inflamed skin. Evening primrose oil has also been given by mouth for mastalgia. Evening primrose oil has been investigated in a variety of other disorders including multiple sclerosis, rheumatoid arthritis, and the premenstrual syndrome. Mixtures of essential fatty acids (including EF-4, EF-12, and EF-27) derived from evening primrose oil and other oils have also been investigated in various conditions, including diabetic neuropathy, restenosis following angioplasty, and skin damage following radiotherapy.

◊ General references.


1. Kleijnen J. Evening primrose oil. *BMJ* 1994; **309:** 824–5.


**Eczema.** For the use of evening primrose oil as a source of essential fatty acids for the management of eczema, see under Gamolenic Acid, p.1690.

**Mastalgia.** For the use of evening primrose oil as a source of gamolenic acid for the management of mastalgia, see p.1690.

**Menopausal disorders.** Although there are anecdotal reports of benefit, a controlled study[1] found that evening primrose oil was no more effective than placebo for managing menopausal vasomotor symptoms (p.1540).


1. Chenoy R, *et al.* Effect of oral gamolenic acid from evening primrose oil on menopausal flushing. *BMJ* 1994; **308:** 501–3.


**Multiple sclerosis.** For the use of evening primrose oil in the management of multiple sclerosis, see under Gamolenic Acid, p.1690.

**Premenstrual syndrome.** For conflicting results from the use of evening primrose oil in premenstrual syndrome see under Gamolenic Acid, p.1690.

**Rheumatoid arthritis.** For the use of evening primrose oil as a source of gamolenic acid for the management of rheumatoid arthritis, see p.1690.

## Preparations

**Proprietary Preparations** (details are given in Part 3)
***Arg.:*** Efamol; ***Austral.:*** Bioglan Primrose Micelle†; Epogam†; Naudicelle†; ***Canad.:*** Efalex Focus†; Efamol; Gamma Oil†; Naudicelle†; Onagre†; Primanol; ***Fr.:*** Bioleine; Bionagrol; ***Ger.:*** Epogam; Gammacur; Linola gamma; Neobonsen; Unigamol; ***India:*** Simrose; ***Irl.:*** Epogam; Naudicelle; ***Ital.:*** Epogam†; ***Malaysia:*** Quest Gamma Oil; ***NZ:*** Efamol; ***Switz.:*** Cremol-P†; Efamol; Epogam; ***UK:*** E.P.O. & E†; Efamast†; Efamol; Epogam†; Evening Gold; Evoprim; Galanol GLX†; Gamma Oil†; Gammaderm; GammaOil Premium†; Naudicelle†.

**Multi-ingredient:** ***Austral.:*** Bioglan Arthri Plus†; Bioglan Ginger-Vite Forte†; Bioglan Primrose-E†; Bioglan Zellulean with Escin†; Efacal†; Efalex; Efamarine; Epo + Maxepa + Vitamin E Herbal Plus Formula 8†; For Women Multi Plus EPO†; Lifesystem Herbal Plus Formula 9 Fatty Acids And Vitamin E†; Maxepa & EPO†; Medinat PMT-Eze†; Naudicelle Marine†; PMS Support†; ***Canad.:*** Efamol Fortify†; Primanol-Borage; Super Gamma Oil with Vitamin E†; ***Fr.:*** Bionagrol Plus; Dioptec; ***NZ:*** Efacal; Efamarine; Efamax; Mr Nits; ***Port.:*** Atopic; ***Singapore:*** VitaEPA Plus; ***UK:*** Efacal†; Efalex; Efamarine; Efamol Plus Coenzyme Q10†; Efamol PMP; Efamol Safflower & Linseed†; Epopa†; Exzem Oil†; Galanol Gold†; Galmarin†; Gamma Marine†; Naudicelle Plus†; PMT Formula; Royal Galanol†; Super GammaOil Marine†; ***USA:*** Eucerin Itch-Relief.

---

# Febuprol *(rINN)*

Febuproll. 1-Butoxy-3-phenoxy-2-propanol.

$C_{13}H_{20}O_3$ = 224.3.

*CAS — 3102-00-9.*

## Profile

Febuprol is a choleretic used in the treatment of biliary-tract disorders in a dose of 100 mg three times daily by mouth.

## Preparations

**Proprietary Preparations** (details are given in Part 3)
***Ger.:*** Valbil; ***Port.:*** Valbil.

---

# Fencibutirol *(USAN, rINN)*

Mg-4833. 2-(1-Hydroxy-4-phenylcyclohexyl)butyric acid.

$C_{16}H_{22}O_3$ = 262.3.

*CAS — 5977-10-6.*

## Profile

Fencibutirol is a choleretic that has been used in the treatment of constipation and biliary-tract disorders.

## Preparations

**Proprietary Preparations** (details are given in Part 3)

**Multi-ingredient:** ***Ital.:*** Hepasil Composto†; Magisbile; Neo-Heparbil†; Sintobil†.

---

# Fenclonine *(USAN, rINN)*

CP-10188; Fenclonina; NSC-77370; Parachlorophenylalanine. 2-Amino-3-(4-chlorophenyl)propionic acid; DL-3-(*p*-Chlorophenyl)alanine.

$C_9H_{10}ClNO_2$ = 199.6.

*CAS — 7424-00-2.*

## Profile

Fenclonine is an inhibitor of the biosynthesis of serotonin. It has been used for the relief of symptoms of carcinoid syndrome, especially flushing and diarrhoea. Hypothermia, bone marrow depression, and psychiatric side-effects such as confusion and depression have occurred during treatment.

---

# Fenipentol *(rINN)*

1-Phenylpentan-1-ol; α-Butylbenzyl alcohol.

$C_{11}H_{16}O$ = 164.2.

*CAS — 583-03-9.*

## Profile

Fenipentol is a choleretic that has been given by mouth for the treatment of hepatic and biliary-tract disorders in doses of 100 to 200 mg three times daily. The hemisuccinate and sodium hemisuccinate have also been used.

## Preparations

**Proprietary Preparations** (details are given in Part 3)
***Ger.:*** Febichol; ***Ital.:*** Pentabil.

**Multi-ingredient:** ***Chile:*** Digezin; ***Ital.:*** Critichol; ***Port.:*** Cholipin†; ***Spain:*** Menabil Complex.

---

# Fennel

Fenchel; Fennel Fruit; Fennel Seed; Fenouil; Fenouil Amer; Foeniculum; Fruto de Hinojo; Funcho; Hinojo.

**Pharmacopoeias.** In *Chin., Eur.* (see p.vi), *Jpn,* and *Pol.*

**Ph. Eur. 5.0** (Fennel, Bitter; Foeniculi Amari Fructus). It consists of the dry, cremocarps and mericarps of *Foeniculum vulgare*, subsp. *vulgare*, var. *vulgare*. It contains not less than 4.0% v/w of essential oil, calculated with reference to the anhydrous drug. The oil contains not less than 60.0% of anethole and not less than 15.0% of fenchone. Bitter fennel is greenish-brown, brown, or green. Protect from light and moisture.

**Ph. Eur. 5.0** (Fennel, Sweet; Foeniculi Dulcis Fructus). It consists of the dry, cremocarps and mericarps of *Foeniculum vulgare*, subsp. *vulgare*, var. *dulce*. It contains not less than 2.0% v/w of essential oil, calculated with reference to the anhydrous drug. The oil contains not less than 80.0% of anethole. Sweet fennel is pale green or pale yellowish-brown. Protect from light and moisture.

## Profile

Fennel is the source of fennel oil (below). It is used as a flavour and carminative, although the efficacy of such traditional remedies in infant colic is considered dubious (see Gastrointestinal Spasm, p.1242). It is also used in herbal remedies for respiratory-tract disorders.

## Preparations

**Proprietary Preparations** (details are given in Part 3)
***Ger.:*** roha-Fenchel-Tee†.

**Multi-ingredient:** ***Arg.:*** Arceligasol; ***Austral.:*** Digestive Aid†; ***Austria:*** Aktiv Leber- und Gallentee; Aktiv milder Magen- und Darmtee; Anifer Fenchelhonig; Aponatura Wind; Apotheker Bauer's Blahungstee; Apotheker Bauer's Brust- und Hustentee; Apotheker Bauer's Kindertee; Aurita-Verdauungstee; Bio-Garten Tee gegen Blahungen; Bio-Garten Tee gegen Verstopfung; Bioreform-Windtreibender Tee; Brady's-Magentropfen; Carminativum Babynos; Euka; Gewusst wie Darmtee; Gewusst wie Gruner Fastentee; Gewusst wie Leber-Gallentee; Granobil; Illings Bozner May-cur-Tee; Karvisin; Kneipp Husten- und Bronchial-Tee; Kneipp Verdauungs-Tee; Krauterdoktor Hustentropfen; Krauterhaus Mag Kottas Babytee; Krauterhaus Mag Kottas milder Abfuhrtee; Krauterhaus Mag Kottas Tee gegen Blahungen; Krauterpfarrer Weidinger Tee bei Vollegefuhl und Blahungen; Krauterpfarrer Weidinger Tee fur Leber und Galle; Laxalpin; Mag Kottas Baby-Tee; Mag Kottas Blahungs-Verdauungstee; Mag Kottas Krauterexpress-Blahungs-Verdauungstee; Mag Kottas Krauterexpress-Magen-Darm-Tee; Mag Kottas Krauterexpress-Tee fur stillende Mutter; Mag Kottas May-Cur-Tee; Mag Kottas Tee fur stillende Mutter; Nesthakchen; Neuners Krautertee Nr 10 - Grippetee; Neuners Krautertee Nr 11 - zur Unterstutzung der Tatigkeit der Bronchien und Atemwege; Neuners Krautertee Nr 126 - Starkungstee fur stillende Mutter; Neuners Krautertee Nr 14 - Verdauungstee; Neuners Krautertee Nr 217 - Krauterhexlein Kinder-Blahungstee; Neuners Krautertee Nr 8 - Magentee gegen Ubersauerung; Neuners Krautertee Nr 9 - Magentee; Pascopankreat†; Planta Lax; Sidroga Kindertee; Sinolax-Milder; Species Carvi comp; St Radegunder Abfuhrtee mild; St Radegunder Blahungstreibender Tee; St Radegunder Bronchialtee; St Radegunder Magenberuhigungstee; St Radegunder Reizmildernder Magentee; St Radegunder Tee gegen Durchfall; Teekanne Herz- und Kreislauftee; Teekanne Husten- und Brusttee; Teekanne Leber- und Galletee; Tiroler Adler Schwedenbitter; ***Belg.:*** Eugiron†; Tisane Antibiliaire et Stomachique†; Tisane Depurative "les 12 Plantes"†; Tisane Diuretique†; Tisane Purgative†; ***Braz.:*** Puersan†; ***Canad.:*** Thunas Laxative; ***Fr.:*** Bolcitol; Colominthe†; Mediflor Tisane Contre la Constipation Passagere No 7; Mediflor Tisane Digestive No 3; Mediflor Tisane No 4 Diuretique; Santane $D_5$†; Santane $H_7$†; Tisane des Familles†; Tisane Digestive Weleda†; ***Ger.:*** Brust- und Husten-Tee Stada N†; Carminativum Babynos; Carminativum-Hetterich N; Cefabronchin†; Cefagastrin†; Echtroferment-N†; Em-eukal; Em-eukal Husten- und Brusttee; Floradix Maskam†; Floradix Multipretten N; Gallexier; Gastricholan-L; Gastrol S; Grunlicht Hingfong Essenz†; Harntee 400; Hevert-Magen-Galle-Leber-Tee†; Kneipp Flatuol†; Kneipp Husten- und Bronchial-Tee†; Kneipp Magen-Tee†; Kneipp Verdauungs-Tee N†; Leber-Galle-Tropfen 83; Lomatol; Magentee†; Majocarmin-Tee; Pascopankreat novo; Presselin Blahungs K 4 N; Presselin Dyspeptikum; Presselin Stoffwechsel-Tee Hapeka 225 N; Ramend Krauter; Salus Abfuhr-Tee Nr. 2†; Salus Bronchial-Tee Nr.8†; Salus Leber-Galle-Tee Nr.18†; Salus Nerven-Schlaf-Tee Nr.22†; Salus Rheuma-Tee Krautertee Nr. 12†; Stovalid N; Ullus Magen-Tee N†; Urodil Blasen-Nieren Arzneitee†; ***Hong Kong:*** Gl†; ***Israel:*** Jungborn; ***Ital.:*** Altea (Specie Composta); Anice (Specie Composta); Cadifen; Cadimint; Colimil; Dicalmir; Epagest; Evamilk; Normalax†; Senna-Specie Composta; Timo (Specie Composta); Tisana Cisbey†; Tonactiv†; ***Spain:*** Crislaxo; Himelan; Jarabe Manzanas Siken†; Natusor Aerofane; Natusor Malvasen; Senalsor; ***Switz.:*** Adistop Lax†; Ajaka†; Caved-S†; Kernosan Elixir; Kernosan Heidelberger Poudre; The Brioni†; The Franklin†; Tisane antiflatulente pour nourissons et enfants; Tisane favorisant l'allaitement; Tisane laxative; Tisane laxative Natterman no 13†; Tisane pectorale et antitussive; Tisane pour les enfants†; ***UK:*** Carminative Tea†; Cleansing Herbs; Gerard House Gladlax†; Herbal Indigestion Naturtabs; Indigestion and Flatulence; Lion Cleansing Herbs; Lustys Herbalene; Out-of-Sorts; Revitonil; Sure-Lax (Herbal).

---

# Fennel Oil

Aetheroleum Foeniculi; Esencia de Hinojo; Essência de Funcho; Hinojo, aceite esencial; Oleum Foeniculi.

**Pharmacopoeias.** In *Eur.* (see p.vi), *Jpn,* and *Pol.* Also in *USNF.*

**Ph. Eur. 5.0** (Bitter-Fennel Fruit Oil; Foeniculi Amari Fructus Aetheroleum). The essential oil obtained by steam distillation from the ripe fruits of *Foeniculum vulgare*, subsp. *vulgare*, var. *vulgare*. It contains 12.0 to 25.0% fenchone and 55.0 to 75.0% anethole. A clear, colourless or pale yellow liquid with a characteristic odour. Store in well-filled, airtight containers at a temperature not exceeding 25°. Protect from light.

**USNF 22** (Fennel Oil). The volatile oil distilled with steam from the dried, ripe fruit of *Foeniculum vulgare* (Apiaceae). Congealing temperature not lower than 3°. Soluble 1 in 1 of alcohol (90%). If solid matter has separated, carefully warm the oil until it is completely liquefied, and mix before using. Store in airtight containers.

## Profile

Fennel oil is used as an aromatic flavour and carminative (but see the comment under Fennel, above); the German expert committee for herbal drugs and preparations (Commission E) considers that the use of fennel oil in infants and toddlers is contra-indicated. It is also used in herbal remedies for respiratory-tract disorders.

## Preparations

**Proprietary Preparations** (details are given in Part 3)
***Austria:*** Stern Biene Fenchelhonig†; ***Ger.:*** Fenchelsaft N†; Stern Biene Fenchelhonig†; Stern Biene Fenchelsirup.

**Multi-ingredient:** ***Austria:*** Benium; Eucarbon; Luuf-Hustentee; Nesthakchen; Sabatif; Solubitrat; Spasmo Claim; Thierry†; Zeller-Augenwasser; ***Belg.:*** Eucarbon†; ***Canad.:*** Babys Own Gripe Water†; Chase Kolik Gripe Water Alcohol-Free; ***Ger.:*** Benium†; Bronchicum Hustentee†; Cystium-wern; Em-eukal Husten- und Brusttee; Ephepect-Pastillen N; Ephepect†; Euflat I; Floradix Multipretten N; Gastricard; Grunlicht Hingfong Essenz†; Grunlicht Magenbalsam Tropfen†; Hevert-Carmin symbio†; Hevertopect N; Hingfong-Essenz Hofmanns; Infantussin N†; Majocarmin forte; Neo-Lapitrypsin†; Nierentee 2000; Pulmocordio mite SL; ratioGast; Roflatol Phyto (Rowo-146)†; Salviathymol N; ***Hong Kong:*** Magesto; ***Israel:*** Novicarbon; ***Switz.:*** Ajaka†; Eucarbon†; Flatulex; Huile Po-Ho A. Vogel; Laxasan; Pastilles pectorales formule 541†; ***Thai.:*** Gas-Nep; Magesto; ***UK:*** Indigestion and Flatulence Tablets†.

---

# Fenoverine *(rINN)*

Fenoverina. 10-[(4-Piperonyl-1-piperazinyl)acetyl]phenothiazine.

$C_{26}H_{25}N_3O_3S$ = 459.6.

*CAS — 37561-27-6.*

*ATC — A03AX05.*

## Profile

Fenoverine has been used as an antispasmodic but has been withdrawn in some countries following reports of rhabdomyolysis.

**Adverse effects.** Reports of rhabdomyolysis associated with fenoverine,[1,2] including a fatality.[1] A genetic predisposition has been suggested.[2]


1. Chariot P, *et al.* Fenoverine-induced rhabdomyolysis. *Hum Exp Toxicol* 1995; **14:** 654–6.
2. Jouglard J, *et al.* Research into individual predisposition to develop acute rhabdomyolysis attributed to fenoverine. *Hum Exp Toxicol* 1996; **15:** 815–20.


## Preparations

**Proprietary Preparations** (details are given in Part 3)
***Mex.:*** Spasmopriv; ***Singapore:*** Spasmopriv; ***Thai.:*** Spasmopriv.

---

# Fenpipramide Hydrochloride *(BANM, rINNM)*

Hidrocloruro de fenpipramida. 2,2-Diphenyl-4-piperidinobutyramide hydrochloride.

$C_{21}H_{26}N_2O,HCl$ = 358.9.

*CAS — 77-01-0 (fenpipramide); 14007-53-5 (fenpipramide hydrochloride).*

## Profile

Fenpipramide hydrochloride has been used as an antispasmodic. It is also used for its antimuscarinic actions in veterinary medicine.

## Fenpiverinium Bromide (rINN)

Bromuro de fenpiverinio; Fenpipramide Methobromide; Fenpipramide Methylbromide. 1-(3-Carbamoyl-3,3-diphenylpropyl)-1-methylpiperidinium bromide; 2,2-Diphenyl-4-piperidinobutyramide methyl bromide.

$C_{22}H_{29}BrN_2O$ = 417.4.

*CAS — 125-60-0.*

*ATC — A03AB21.*

### Profile

Fenpiverinium bromide has been used as an antispasmodic.

---

## Fenugreek

Bockshornsame; Faenum-Graecum; Fenogreco; Greek hay; Semen Foenugraeci; Semen Trigonellae.

**Pharmacopoeias.** In *Chin.* and *Eur.* (see p.vi).

**Ph. Eur. 5.0** (Fenugreek). The dried ripe seeds of *Trigonella foenum-graecum*. It has a strong characteristic odour. Protect from light.

### Profile

Fenugreek has been used as an appetite stimulant and as an ingredient in preparations for respiratory disorders. It also has emollient properties.

**Adverse effects.** Loss of consciousness occurred in a 5-week-old infant following ingestion of a herbal tea containing fenugreek.[1] On recovery the infant and his urine had an aroma characteristic of that found in 'maple syrup urine disease', an inborn condition involving defective metabolism of branched-chain amino acids. Further investigation revealed that the infant did not have the disease; the aroma was due to the presence of sotolone in the fenugreek seeds used to prepare the tea.

1. Sewell AC, *et al.* False diagnosis of maple syrup urine disease owing to ingestion of herbal tea. *N Engl J Med* 1999; **341:** 769.

### Preparations

**Proprietary Preparations** (details are given in Part 3)
***Fr.:*** Fenugrene.

**Multi-ingredient:** ***Austral.:*** Bilberry Plus†; Garlic and Horseradish + C Complex†; Panax Complex†; Sinus and Hayfever†; ***Fr.:*** Sthenorex; ***UK:*** Fenulin†.

---

## Ferric Chloride

Ferr. Perchlor.; Ferri Chloridum Hexahydricum; Férrico, cloruro; Ferrum Sesquichloratum; Iron Perchloride; Iron Sesquichloride; Iron Trichloride.

$FeCl_3,6H_2O$ = 270.3.

*CAS — 7705-08-0 (anhydrous ferric chloride); 10025-77-1 (ferric chloride hexahydrate).*

**Pharmacopoeias.** In *Eur.* (see p.vi).

**Ph. Eur. 5.0** (Ferric Chloride Hexahydrate). A very hygroscopic, crystalline mass or orange-yellow to brownish-yellow crystals. Very soluble in water and in alcohol; freely soluble in glycerol. Store in airtight containers. Protect from light.

### Profile

Ferric chloride has the general properties of iron salts (p.1434) but is exceptionally astringent. It has been used mainly by local application for its styptic and astringent properties. Local application of ferric chloride or other iron salts may cause permanent discoloration of the skin.

### Preparations

**Proprietary Preparations** (details are given in Part 3)
***Ital.:*** Cotone Emostatico.

**Multi-ingredient:** ***Belg.:*** Ouate Hemostatique; ***UK:*** Glykola.

---

## Fibronectin

Cold-insoluble Globulin; Fibronectina.

### Profile

Fibronectin is an endogenous polypeptide with a molecular weight of 440 000 to 550 000 whose roles include attachment of cells to the extracellular matrix and stimulation of phagocytosis. It is used in combination with other blood products in wound-sealant preparations. Infusion of fibronectin or fibronectin-rich plasma has been tried in patients with sepsis, infection, burns or other trauma, or severe malnutrition. Eye drops of fibronectin have been used in the treatment of corneal erosions.

◊ References.

1. Anonymous. Fibronectins and vitronectin. *Lancet* 1989; **i:** 474–6.
2. Gipson IK, *et al.* Corneal wound healing and fibronectin. *Int Ophthalmol Clin* 1993; **33:** 149–63.

### Preparations

**Proprietary Preparations** (details are given in Part 3)

**Multi-ingredient:** ***Arg.:*** Tissucol Duo Quick; ***Austral.:*** Tisseel Duo; ***Austria:*** Tissucol; Tissucol Duo Quick; ***Canad.:*** Tisseel; ***Denm.:*** Tisseel Duo Quick; ***Fin.:*** Tisseel Duo Quick; ***Fr.:*** Biocol†; Tissucol; ***Ger.:*** Tissucol Duo S; Tissucol Fibrinkleber tiefgefroren†; Tissucol-Kit; ***Hong Kong:*** Tisseel; ***Israel:*** Tisseel; ***Spain:*** Tissucol Duo; ***Swed.:*** Tisseel Duo Quick; ***Switz.:*** Tissucol; Tissucol Duo S; ***UK:*** Tisseel.

---

## Flavonoid Compounds

Bioflavonoids; Flavonoides; Vitamin P Substances.

## Benzquercin (rINN)

Benzquercina. 3,3′,4′,5,7-Pentakis(benzyloxy)flavone.

$C_{50}H_{40}O_7$ = 752.8.

*CAS — 13157-90-9.*

## Diosmin (BAN, rINN)

Barosmin; Buchu Resin; Diosmetin 7-Rutinoside; Diosmina; Diosminum. 3′,5,7-Trihydroxy-4′-methoxyflavone 7-[6-*O*-(6-deoxy-α-L-mannopyranosyl)-β-D-glucopyranoside].

$C_{28}H_{32}O_{15}$ = 608.5.

*CAS — 520-27-4.*

*ATC — C05CA03.*

**Pharmacopoeias.** In *Eur.* (see p.vi).

**Ph. Eur. 5.0** (Diosmin). A greyish-yellow or light yellow hygroscopic powder. Practically insoluble in water and in alcohol; soluble in dimethyl sulfoxide. It dissolves in dilute solutions of alkali hydroxides. Store in airtight containers.

## Ethoxazorutoside (rINN)

Aethoxazorutin; Aethoxazorutoside; Ethoxazorutin; Etoxazorutósido.

$C_{33}H_{41}NO_{17}$ = 723.7.

*CAS — 30851-76-4.*

## Flavodate Sodium (rINNM)

Flavodate Disodium; Flavodato sódico. Disodium (4-oxo-2-phenyl-4*H*-chromene-5,7-diyldioxy)diacetate.

$C_{19}H_{12}Na_2O_8$ = 414.3.

*CAS — 37470-13-6 (flavodic acid); 13358-62-8 (flavodate disodium).*

## Hesperidin

Hesperidina. 5-Hydroxy-2-(3-hydroxy-4-methoxyphenyl)-4-oxo-4*H*-chromen-7-yl rutinoside.

$C_{28}H_{34}O_{15}$ = 610.6.

*CAS — 520-26-3 (hesperidin); 24292-52-2 (hesperidin methyl chalcone).*

**Description.** Hesperidin is a flavonoid isolated from the rind of certain citrus fruits.

## Leucocianidol (rINN)

Leucocyanidin; Leucocyanidol. 2-(3,4-Dihydroxyphenyl)chroman-3,4,5,7-tetrol.

$C_{15}H_{14}O_7$ = 306.3.

*CAS — 480-17-1.*

## Monoxerutin (rINN)

Monohydroxyethylrutosides; Monoxerutina. 7-(β-Hydroxyethyl)rutoside.

$C_{29}H_{34}O_{17}$ = 654.6.

*CAS — 23869-24-1.*

*ATC — C05CA02.*

## Oxerutins (BAN)

Hydroxyethylrutosides; Oxerutinas.

**Description.** Oxerutins consist of a mixture of 5 different *O*-(β-hydroxyethyl)rutosides, not less than 45% of which is troxerutin (trihydroxyethylrutoside, below), but which also includes monohydroxyethylrutoside, dihydroxyethylrutoside, and tetrahydroxyethylrutoside.

## Quercetin

3,3′,4′,5,7-Pentahydroxyflavone; Quercetina. 2-(3,4-Dihydroxyphenyl)-3,5,7-trihydroxy-4*H*-1-benzopyran-4-one.

$C_{15}H_{10}O_7$ = 302.2.

*CAS — 117-39-5.*

## Rutoside (BAN, rINN)

Rutin; Rutósido; Rutosidum. 2-(3,4-Dihydroxyphenyl)-3,5,7-trihydroxy-4-oxo-4*H*-chromen-3-yl rutinoside trihydrate; 2-(3,4-Dihydroxyphenyl)-5,7-dihydroxy-4-oxo-4*H*-chromen-3-yl 6-*O*-(α-L-rhamnosyl)-β-D-glucoside.

$C_{27}H_{30}O_{16},3H_2O$ = 664.6.

*CAS — 153-18-4 (anhydrous rutoside).*

*ATC — C05CA01.*

**Description.** Rutoside is a flavonoid obtained from buckwheat, *Fagopyrum esculentum* (Polygonaceae), or from other sources which include the flower buds of the Japanese pagoda-tree, *Sophora japonica*, and the leaves of several species of *Eucalyptus*.

**Pharmacopoeias.** In *Eur.* (see p.vi), *Pol.*, and *Viet.*

**Ph. Eur. 5.0** (Rutoside Trihydrate). A yellow or greenish-yellow crystalline powder. Practically insoluble in water; sparingly soluble in dehydrated alcohol; practically insoluble in dichloromethane; soluble in methyl alcohol. It dissolves in solutions of alkali hydroxides. Protect from light.

## Troxerutin (BAN, rINN)

THR; Trihydroxyethylrutoside; Trioxyethylrutin; Troxerutina. 3′,4′,7-Tris[*O*-(2-hydroxyethyl)]rutin; 5-Hydroxy-7-(2-hydroxyethoxy)-2-[3,4-bis(2-hydroxyethoxy)phenyl]-4-oxo-4*H*-chromen-3-yl rutinoside.

$C_{33}H_{42}O_{19}$ = 742.7.

*CAS — 7085-55-4.*

*ATC — C05CA04.*

**Description.** Troxerutin is the principal component of oxerutins, above.

**Pharmacopoeias.** In *Ger.*

### Profile

Flavonoids are naturally occurring antoxidants that are widely distributed in plants. Preparations containing natural or semisynthetic flavonoids are thought to improve capillary function by reducing abnormal leakage. They have been given to relieve capillary impairment and venous insufficiency of the lower limbs, and for haemorrhoids.

It has been suggested that flavonoids present in some foods, such as fruit, vegetables, tea, and red wine may protect against the development of atherosclerosis (p.815).

◊ References.

1. Knekt P, *et al.* Flavonoid intake and coronary mortality in Finland: a cohort study. *BMJ* 1996; **312:** 478–81.
2. Hertog MGL, *et al.* Antioxidant flavonols and coronary heart disease risk. *Lancet* 1997; **349:** 699.
3. Youdim KA, *et al.* Dietary flavonoids as potential neuroprotectants. *Biol Chem* 2002; **383:** 503–19.
4. Lopez-Lazaro M. Flavonoids as anticancer agents: structure-activity relationship study. *Curr Med Chem Anti-Canc Agents* 2002; **2:** 691–714.
5. Lyseng-Williamson KA, Perry CM. Micronised purified flavonoid fraction: a review of its use in chronic venous insufficiency, venous ulcers and haemorrhoids. *Drugs* 2003; **63:** 71–100.

### Preparations

**Proprietary Preparations** (details are given in Part 3)
***Arg.:*** Flebon; Flebotropin; Flerox; Jatamansin; Venoruton; Venosmil; ***Austral.:*** Paroven; ***Austria:*** Venoruton; ***Belg.:*** Veinamitol; Ven-Detrex; Venoruton; ***Braz.:*** Daflon; Venoruton; ***Chile:*** Flebopex; Insuven; Venoruton; ***Denm.:*** Venoruton; ***Fr.:*** Daflon; Diamoril; Dio; Diosmil; Diovenor; Endium; Flavan; Flebosmil; Intercyton; Litosmil†; Mediveine; Preparation H Veinotonic; Relvene; Rheoflux; Squad†; Veinamitol; Veineva; Venirene; ***Ger.:*** Drisi-Ven; Pherarutin†; Posorutin; Rutinion; Tovene; Trirutin N†; Troxeven; Vastribil; Veno SL; Venoruton; ***Hong Kong:*** Venoruton; ***India:*** Venusmin; ***Irl.:*** Paroven†; ***Israel:*** Novorutin†; Veinamitol; Venoruton; Vridol; ***Ital.:*** Alven; Arvenum; Diosven; Doven; Flebil†; Pericel; Venolen; Venoruton; Venosmine; ***Mex.:*** Sies; Teboven; ***Neth.:*** Venoruton; ***NZ:*** Paroven†; ***Port.:*** Fleboton†; Hepacalmina; Venex; Veno-V; Venoruton; Venosmil; Veroven; ***S.Afr.:*** Paroven; Varemoid†; ***Spain:*** Daflon†; Diosminil†; Insuven†; Intercyton†; Pentovena; Venolep; Venoruton; Venosmil; Viodenum†; ***Switz.:*** Hemerven; Neorutin; Pur-Rutin; Varemoid†; Veniten†; Venoruton; Venutabs; ***Thai.:*** Flavon; Heteroid; Varemoid†; Venoruton; ***UK:*** Paroven; ***USA:*** Citro-Flav.

**Multi-ingredient:** ***Arg.:*** Ajomast Circulatorio; CVP B1 B6 B12; CVP Duo; CVP Flebo; CVP Forte; Cyclo 3; Daflon; Epiteliol-C; Esberiven; Escina Forte; Escina Omega; Flebitol; Flebotropin; Kacerutin; Mimixin; Phlogenzym; Troxeven; Ulcevarin; Vefluxan; Veraldid; Vitamina C-Complex; ***Austral.:*** B-Complex Threshold†; Beta A-C†; Bio C†; Bio-C Complex†; Bioglan Cirflo†; Bioglan Fingers & Toes†; Bioglan Mega C†; Bioglan Super Cal C†; Bioglan The Blue One†; Bioglan Zellulean with Escin†; Bioglan Zn-A-C†; Biosor-C†; C Supa + Bioflavonoids†; Child Chew C†; Cold & Flu Tablets Non Drowsy†; Crataegus Complex†; Devils Claw Plus†; Ethical Nutrients Bioflavonoids Plus†; Extralife Leg-Care†; Eye Health Herbal Plus Formula 4†; Flavonoid Complex†; Flavons†; For Peripheral Circulation Herbal Plus Formula 5†; Gentle C with Bioflavonoids†; Hamamelis Complex†; Harpagophytum Complex†; Lifesystem Herbal Formula 6 For Peripheral Circulation†; Lifesystem Herbal Plus Formula 5 Eye Relief†; Macro C; Natures Way Total C†; Proflo†; Rubus Complex†; Super Cal-C Bio†; Sustained Release Buffered C†; Vita-Minis Vitamin C Plus†; Z-Acne†; ***Austria:*** Aesrutan†; Calcipot C; Daflon; Helopyrin; Influvidon; Phlebodril; Phlogenzym; Ruticalzon; Rutiscorbin; Rutiviscal; Sandoven†; Sklerovitol; Sterofundin R†; Tetesept; Trimedil; Veno†; Venotop; Vit-C-Lutsch; Wallerox; Wobenzym; ***Belg.:*** Daflon; Ex'ail†; ***Braz.:*** Castanha de India Composta†; Dactil OB; Flebotrat†; Frenovex†; Gingilone; Gripen; Hemoaenus†; Hemodotti; Hemorroidex; Hemorrol†; Hermodotti†; Manolio†; Mirorroidin; Novaboin†; Novarrutina; Panvitrop†; Phlogenzym†; Trimedal; Varizol; Venalot; Venocur Triplex; ***Canad.:*** Duo-CVP; ***Chile:*** Daflon 500; Duo-CVP; Hemoplex; Phyto Corrective Gel; Primacy Phyto +; Venartel; ***Denm.:*** Capiven; ***Fr.:*** Cemaflavone; Cepevit†; Circularine†; Cirkan; Cyclo 3 Fort; Ercevit†; Esberiven Fort; Ex'ail†; Gel a l'Acetotartrate d'Alumine Defresne; Ginkor; Ginkor Fort; Ophtadil; Rheobral; Solurutine Papaverine F. Retard†; Trisolvit†; Vascocitrol; Veliten; Venyl; Video†; Vita 3†; Vitarutine; Vivene; ***Ger.:*** Aescorin N†; Antihypertonicum S; Antimyopikum†; Antisklerosin S†; Calcium-Rutinion; Cycloven Forte N; Echtrovit-K†; Emocrat forte; Enzym-Wied; Essaven N; Essaven ultra; Eukalisan forte†; Eukalisan N; Euvitan†; Fagorutin Buchweizen; Fagorutin Rosskastanien-Balsam N; Intradermi; Lindigoa S; Movicard; Perivar; Phlebodril; Phlogenzym; Posti N; Ruticalzon VC; Tornix; Vaso-E-Bion; Venalot; Venalot N; Venelbin†; Veno-Hexanicit†; Veno-Tebonin N; Vitosal; Wobenzym N; ***Hong Kong:*** Daflon; Essaven†; Ginkor Fort; Haemosol†; Poly C; ***India:*** Cadisper C; CVP; Gynae-CVP; Kalpastic; Styptocid; ***Ital.:*** Angioton; Blunorm†; Bo-Gum†; CVP†; Daflon 500; Dermoangiopan; Digifar; Emortrofine; Flavone 500†; Fleboside; Ginkoftal; Neomyrt Plus; Pulsalux; RepaVen; Rutisan CE; Traumal; Varicofit; Venactive; ***Malaysia:*** Daflon 500; Ginkor Fort; Hemorid; ***Mex.:*** Cal-Rutina; Daflon; Fabroven; Flavit; Phlogenzym; Variton; Venalot; Wobenzym; ***Mon.:*** Vincarutine; ***NZ:*** Botanica Hayfever; ***Port.:*** Actilam; Cegripe; Cyclo 3; Daflon; Projuvex†; Rutinice Fortissimo; ***S.Afr.:*** Essaven; ***Singapore:*** Cyclo 3 Fort; Daflon 500; ***Spain:*** Caprofides Hemostatico; Circovenil Fuerte†; Citroflavona Mag†; Citroflavona†; Daflon 500; Epistaxol; Esberiven; Fabroven; Flebeside; Gingilone; Nasopomada; Quercetol Hemostatico†; Quercetol K†; Rutice Fuerte†; Venosan†; Vitaendil C K P†; ***Switz.:*** Daflon 500; Demoven N; Flavovenyl; No Grip†; Optazine†; Phlebodril N; Phlebodril†; Venosan†; Video-Net; Vita 3†; ***Thai.:*** Biocalron; Cyclo 3 Fort; Daflon; Essaven; Ginkor Fort; Heroid; Siduol; ***UK:*** Flavorola C†; ***USA:*** Amino-Opti-C; C Factors "1000" Plus; Cholinoid; Citrus-flav C; Ester-C Plus; Ester-C Plus

Multi-Mineral; Flavons; Lipoflavonoid; Pan C; Peridin-C; Proflavanol; Pycnogenol Plus; Span C.

## Flopropione (rINN)

Flopropiona; Fluropropiofenone; Phloropropiophenone; RP-13907. 2′,4′,6′-Trihydroxypropiophenone.

$C_9H_{10}O_4$ = 182.2.

*CAS — 2295-58-1.*

**Pharmacopoeias.** In *Jpn.*

### Profile

Flopropione is an antispasmodic that has been given by mouth in doses of 40 to 80 mg three times daily.

### Preparations

**Proprietary Preparations** (details are given in Part 3)
***Hong Kong:*** Cospanon†; ***Jpn:*** Cospanon.

**Multi-ingredient:** ***Spain:*** Espasmo Digestomen†.

## Fluorescein (BAN)

Fluoresceína. 3′,6′-Dihydroxyspiro[isobenzofuran-1(3*H*),9′(9*H*)-xanthen]-3-one.

$C_{20}H_{12}O_5$ = 332.3.

*CAS — 2321-07-5.*

*ATC — S01JA01.*

**Pharmacopoeias.** In *US.*

**USP 27** (Fluorescein). A yellowish-red to red, odourless powder. Insoluble in water; soluble in dilute alkali hydroxides. Store in airtight containers.

## Fluorescein Dilaurate (BANM)

Fluoresceína, dilaurato de.

$C_{44}H_{56}O_7$ = 696.9.

*CAS — 7308-90-9.*

*ATC — S01JA01.*

## Fluorescein Sodium (BANM)

CI Acid Yellow 73; Colour Index No. 45350; D & C Yellow No. 8; Fluorescein Natrium; Fluoresceína sódica; Fluoresceinum Natricum; Obiturin; Resorcinolphthalein Sodium; Sodium Fluorescein; Soluble Fluorescein; Uranin. Disodium fluorescein.

$C_{20}H_{10}Na_2O_5$ = 376.3.

*CAS — 518-47-8.*

*ATC — S01JA01.*

NOTE. FLN is a code approved by the BP 2003 for use on single unit doses of eye drops containing fluorescein sodium where the individual container may be too small to bear all the appropriate labelling information. LIDFLN is a similar code approved for eye drops containing lidocaine hydrochloride and fluorescein sodium and PROXFLN a code for eye drops containing proxymetacaine hydrochloride and fluorescein sodium.

**Pharmacopoeias.** In *Chin., Eur.* (see p.vi), *Int., Jpn,* and *US.*

**Ph. Eur. 5.0** (Fluorescein Sodium). An orange-red, fine hygroscopic powder. Freely soluble in water; soluble in alcohol; practically insoluble in dichloromethane and in hexane. A 2% solution in water has a pH of 7.0 to 9.0. Store in airtight containers. Protect from light.

**USP 27** (Fluorescein Sodium). An orange-red, hygroscopic, odourless powder. Freely soluble in water; sparingly soluble in alcohol. Store in airtight containers.

### Adverse Effects and Precautions

The intravenous injection of fluorescein sodium may produce nausea and vomiting. Extravasation is painful. Hypersensitivity reactions range from urticaria to occasional instances of severe anaphylaxis. Cardiac arrests and fatalities have occurred rarely. Concern that impurities or a defect in manufacturing processes might be responsible for the serious reactions led to a review of the BP specification in the early 1980s and a reduction in the permitted level of impurities. Facilities for resuscitation should be available whenever fluorescein sodium is used intravenously.

The skin and urine may be coloured yellow but this is transient. Fluorescein sodium can stain skin, clothing, and soft contact lenses on contact. Intraocular fluorescein can produce transient blurring of vision.

Oral fluorescein dilaurate should not be given to patients with acute necrotising pancreatitis. Sulfasalazine may interfere with estimations of fluorescein in the fluorescein dilaurate test.

◊ Two large studies have examined the incidence of adverse reactions following intravenous fluorescein angiography. An international survey[1] collected information concerning 594 687 angiographic procedures; the incidence of serious reactions was 1 in 18 020, and that of fatal reactions, 1 in 49 557. Reactions included anaphylactic shock, cardiac arrest, myocardial infarction, and shock with hypotension or respiratory distress. A USA survey of 221 781 fluorescein angiograms[2] reported frequency rates of 1 in 63 for a moderate reaction (urticaria, syncope, thrombophlebitis, pyrexia, tissue necrosis, or nerve palsy) and 1 in 1900 for severe reactions (respiratory or cardiac events or tonic-clonic seizures); there was one death.

Individual reports of adverse reactions to intravenous fluorescein sodium include pancreatitis,[3] painful crises in patients with sickle-cell disease,[4] psoriasiform drug eruption,[5] and photoallergy[6] and phototoxicity.[7]


1. Zografos L. Enquête internationale sur l'incidence des accidents graves ou fatals pouvant survenir lors d'une angiographie fluoresceinique. *J Fr Ophtalmol* 1983; **6:** 495–506.
2. Yannuzzi LA, *et al.* Fluorescein angiography complication survey. *Ophthalmology* 1986; **93:** 611–17.
3. Morgan LH, Martin JM. Acute pancreatitis after fluorescein. *BMJ* 1983; **287:** 1596.
4. Acheson R, Serjeant G. Painful crises in sickle cell disease after fluorescein angiography. *Lancet* 1985; **i:** 1222.
5. Mayama M, *et al.* Psoriasiform drug eruption induced by fluorescein sodium used for fluorescein angiography. *Br J Dermatol* 1999; **140:** 982–4.
6. Hochsattel R, *et al.* Photoallergic reaction to fluorescein. *Contact Dermatitis* 1990; **22:** 42–4.
7. Kearns GL, *et al.* Fluorescein phototoxicity in a premature infant. *J Pediatr* 1985; **107:** 796–8.


**Breast feeding.** The American Academy of Pediatrics[1] states that there have been no reports of any clinical effect on the infant associated with the use of fluorescein by breast-feeding mothers, and that therefore it may be considered to be usually compatible with breast feeding.


1. American Academy of Pediatrics. The transfer of drugs and other chemicals into human milk. *Pediatrics* 2001; **108:** 776–89. Correction. *ibid.*; 1029. Also available at: http://aappolicy.aappublications.org/cgi/content/full/pediatrics%3b108/3/776 (accessed 02/06/04)


### Uses and Administration

Fluorescein sodium stains damaged cornea and ocular fluids and is applied to the eye for the detection of corneal lesions and foreign bodies, as an aid to the fitting of hard contact lenses, and in various other diagnostic ophthalmic procedures. It is applied as a 1 or 2% solution as eye drops or as sterile papers impregnated with fluorescein sodium. It may also be given in combination with a local anaesthetic, typically as a 0.25% solution with lidocaine hydrochloride, oxybuprocaine hydrochloride, or proxymetacaine hydrochloride.

Fluorescein sodium may be given by rapid intravenous injection, usually as a solution equivalent to fluorescein 10 or 25% for the examination of the ophthalmic vasculature by retinal angiography. The usual dose is the equivalent of 500 mg of fluorescein. A dose of 7.5 mg/kg has been suggested for children. The oral route has also been tried for angiography. Other uses of intravenous fluorescein sodium have included the differentiation of healthy from diseased or damaged tissue and visualisation of the biliary tract.

Fluorescein dilaurate is given by mouth for the assessment of exocrine pancreatic function (see below). Pancreatic enzymes hydrolyse the ester and the amount of free fluorescein excreted in the urine can therefore be taken as a measure of pancreatic activity. A dose of 348.5 mg of fluorescein dilaurate, equivalent to 0.5 mmol of fluorescein, is given with a standard meal, and urine collected for the following 10 hours. The manufacturers give instructions concerning the type and amount of liquid and food which may be taken during this period. A control dose of 188.14 mg of fluorescein sodium, also equivalent to 0.5 mmol of fluorescein, is given on the following day under the same conditions.

**Pancreatic function test.** Studies of the fluorescein dilaurate test have considered it to be a useful noninvasive screening test for the exclusion of pancreatic exocrine failure in outpatients, particularly those presenting with steatorrhoea.[1-3] The need for tests such as the pancreozymin-secretin test, which requires duodenal intubation, may thus be avoided. However, low specificity (a relatively high rate of false-positive responses) has been reported with the fluorescein dilaurate test in some patient populations,[2,4] and the need for careful patient instruction in performance of the test has been emphasised.[3] In order to avoid the prolonged collection of urine necessary in the standard test, serum concentrations of fluorescein may be measured several hours after taking the test substance.[5]

The test has been used successfully in children,[6] particularly when the doses of fluorescein dilaurate and fluorescein sodium are reduced and fluid intake modified,[7] although the manufacturers recommend that the commercially available test is not used for this age group. In children, a simplified, single-day test using dual markers, fluorescein dilaurate and mannitol, has been investigated with encouraging results.[8] The fluorescein dilaurate test was found to be more sensitive than the faecal elastase 1 test for the diagnosis of mild-to-moderate exocrine pancreatic insufficiency in a study involving 40 patients.[9]


1. Barry RE, *et al.* Fluorescein dilaurate—tubeless test for pancreatic exocrine failure. *Lancet* 1982; **ii:** 742–4.
2. Boyd EJS, *et al.* Prospective comparison of the fluorescein-dilaurate test with the secretin-cholecystokinin test for pancreatic exocrine function. *J Clin Pathol* 1982; **35:** 1240–3.
3. Gould SR, *et al.* Evaluation of a tubeless pancreatic function test in patients with steatorrhoea in a district general hospital. *J R Soc Med* 1988; **81:** 270–3.
4. Braganza JM. Fluorescein dilaurate test. *Lancet* 1982; **ii:** 927–8.
5. Dimagno EP. A perspective on the use of tubeless pancreatic function tests in diagnosis. *Gut* 1998; **43:** 2–3.
6. Cumming JGR, *et al.* Diagnosis of exocrine pancreatic insufficiency in cystic fibrosis by use of fluorescein dilaurate test. *Arch Dis Child* 1986; **61:** 573–5.
7. Dalzell AM, Heaf DP. Fluorescein dilaurate test of exocrine pancreatic function in cystic fibrosis. *Arch Dis Child* 1990; **65:** 788–9.
8. Green MR, *et al.* Dual marker one day pancreolauryl test. *Arch Dis Child* 1993; **68:** 649–52.
9. Leodolter A, *et al.* Comparison of two tubeless function tests in the assessment of mild-to-moderate exocrine pancreatic insufficiency. *Eur J Gastroenterol Hepatol* 2000; **12:** 1335–8.


**Pediculosis.** Infestation of the eye lashes or brows with pubic lice (p.1499) has been successfully treated with a single application of a 20% solution of fluorescein.[1]


1. Mathew M, *et al.* A new treatment of pthiriasis palpebrarum. *Ann Ophthalmol* 1982; **14:** 439–41.


**Retinal angiography.** Fluorescein is usually given intravenously for retinal angiography, but a study in 20 healthy subjects concluded that an oral dose of fluorescein sodium 25 mg/kg could produce good quality retinal angiograms in the majority of subjects.[1] This study used specially prepared 500-mg capsules of fluorescein sodium; the authors commented that previous oral studies had used the liquid preparation intended for intravenous use. Only mild reactions, possibly due to hypersensitivity, appear to have been reported with oral fluorescein.


1. Watson AP, Rosen ES. Oral fluorescein angiography: reassessment of its relative safety and evaluation of optimum conditions with use of capsules. *Br J Ophthalmol* 1990; **74:** 458–61.


### Preparations

***BP 2003:*** Fluorescein Eye Drops; Fluorescein Injection;
***USP 27:*** Fluorescein Injection; Fluorescein Sodium and Benoxinate Hydrochloride Ophthalmic Solution; Fluorescein Sodium and Proparacaine Hydrochloride Ophthalmic Solution; Fluorescein Sodium Ophthalmic Strips.

**Proprietary Preparations** (details are given in Part 3)
***Arg.:*** Angiofluor; Fluorescite; RFG-Kit; ***Austral.:*** Disclo-Plaque†; Fluorescite; Fluorets; Ful-Glo†; ***Austria:*** Fluoftal; ***Canad.:*** Diofluor; Fluor-I-Strip AT†; Fluorescite; Fluorets; Funduscein†; ***Hong Kong:*** Fluorescite; Fluorets; ***India:*** Fluore Stain Strips; ***Irl.:*** Fluorets; ***Ital.:*** Fluoralfa; Pancreolauryl-Test†; ***Malaysia:*** Fluorescite; ***Mex.:*** Optifluor; ***NZ:*** Fluorescite; Fluorets; Ful-Glo†; ***S.Afr.:*** Fluorescite; Fluorets; ***Singapore:*** Fluorescite; Fluorets; ***Thai.:*** Fluorescite; ***UK:*** Fluorets; ***USA:*** Ak-Fluor; Fluor-I-Strip; Fluorescite; Fluorets; Ful-Glo; Funduscein; Ophthifluor.

**Multi-ingredient:** ***Austral.:*** Fluress; ***Austria:*** Flurekain; Pancreolauryl-Test; ***Canad.:*** Fluoracaine; Fluress†; ***Fin.:*** Oftan Flurekain; ***Ger.:*** Pancreolauryl-Test N; Thilorbin; ***Ital.:*** Healon Yellow†; ***NZ:*** Fluress; ***Port.:*** Fluotest; ***Spain:*** Fluotest; Pancreolauryl; ***Swed.:*** Fluress; ***UK:*** Pancreolauryl-Test†; ***USA:*** Flu-Oxinate; Fluoracaine; Fluorocaine; Fluorox; Flurate; Fluress; Flurox; Healon Yellow.

## Formic Acid

Ameisensäure; Aminic Acid; E236; E238 (calcium formate); E237 (sodium formate); Fórmico, ácido.

$CH_2O_2$ = 46.03.

*CAS — 64-18-6.*

**Pharmacopoeias.** In *Pol.*

### Profile

Formic acid resembles acetic acid in its properties (see p.1645) but is more irritating and pungent. The acid and its sodium and calcium salts are used as preservatives in food. Solutions containing about 60% formic acid have been marketed for the removal of lime scale from kettles. Formic acid has also been used for the removal of tattoos. It is an ingredient of some external preparations promoted for the relief of musculoskeletal and joint disorders, and has been used with benzyl alcohol to aid the removal of nits.

◊ In a report of 3 patients who swallowed descaling agents containing 40 or 55% formic acid, the major complications included local corrosive effects, metabolic acidosis, derangement of blood-clotting mechanisms, and acute onset of respiratory and renal failure.[1] All 3 patients died between 5 and 14 days after admission to hospital. A further report of 53 cases of formic acid ingestion included 15 fatalities.[2]


1. Naik RB, *et al.* Ingestion of formic acid-containing agents — report of three fatal cases. *Postgrad Med J* 1980; **56:** 451–6.
2. Rajan N, *et al.* Formic acid poisoning with suicidal intent: a report of 53 cases. *Postgrad Med J* 1985; **61:** 35–6.


### Preparations

**Proprietary Preparations** (details are given in Part 3)

**Multi-ingredient:** ***Austria:*** Aciforin; Berggeist; ***Belg.:*** Euphon; ***Fr.:*** Euphon†; ***Ger.:*** Discmigon†; ***Ital.:*** Rubistenol†; Rubjovit; ***Switz.:*** Fortalis.

## Fosfocreatinine (rINN)

Fosfocreatinina; Phosphocreatinine. (1-Methyl-4-oxo-2-imidazolidinylidene)phosphoramidic acid.

$C_4H_8N_3O_4P$ = 193.1.

*CAS — 5786-71-0 (fosfocreatinine); 19604-05-8 (fosfocreatinine sodium).*

### Profile

Fosfocreatinine or fosfocreatinine sodium has been used in muscle disorders.

### Preparations

**Proprietary Preparations** (details are given in Part 3)
***Ital.:*** Sustenium.

## Fosforylcholine

Fosforilcolina; Phosphorylcholine. (2-Hydroxyethyl)trimethylammonium chloride dihydrogen phosphate.

$C_5H_{15}ClNO_4P$ = 219.6.

*CAS — 107-73-3.*

### Profile

Fosforylcholine is a choleretic that has been used in the treatment of hepatic disorders. The calcium and magnesium salts have also been used.

### Preparations

**Proprietary Preparations** (details are given in Part 3)

***Fr.:*** Heparexine†.

## Frankincense

Olibanum.

NOTE. Distinguish from Indian Frankincense, below.

### Profile

Frankincense is the aromatic gum resin of *Boswellia sacra* (*B. carteri*) (Burseraceae) or other species of *Boswellia*. It is used in incense and as a fumigant.

Frankincense (Ru Xiang) is also used in Chinese medicine.

## Indian Frankincense

Indian Olibanum.

NOTE. Distinguish from Frankincense (above).

### Profile

Indian frankincense is the gum resin of *Boswellia serrata* (*B. glabra*) (Burseraceae). It has anti-inflammatory activity and is included in herbal preparations for musculoskeletal and joint disorders. It is also under investigation for use in inflammatory bowel disease and asthma.

Frankincense (see above), obtained from other species of *Boswellia*, is used for its aromatic properties.

◊ References.


1. Gupta I, *et al.* Effects of Boswellia serrata gum resin in patients with ulcerative colitis. *Eur J Med Res* 1997; **2:** 37–43.
2. Gupta I, *et al.* Effects of Boswellia serrata gum resin in patients with bronchial asthma: results of a double-blind, placebo-controlled, 6-week clinical study. *Eur J Med Res* 1998; **3:** 511–14.
3. Gupta I, *et al.* Effects of gum resin of Boswellia serrata in patients with chronic colitis. *Planta Med* 2001; **67:** 391–5.
4. Kimmatkar N, *et al.* Efficacy and tolerability of Boswellia serrata extract in treatment of osteoarthritis of knee—a randomized double blind placebo controlled trial. *Phytomedicine* 2003; **10:** 3–7.


### Preparations

**Proprietary Preparations** (details are given in Part 3)

**Multi-ingredient:** ***Austral.:*** Bioglan Joint Mobility†; ***Singapore:*** Artrex; ***UK:*** NatraFlex.

## Fumitory

Erdrauchkraut; Fumaria; Herba Fumariae.

**Pharmacopoeias.** In *Ger.*

### Profile

Fumitory comprises the dried or fresh flowering plant *Fumaria officinalis* (Papaveraceae) and is used in herbal medicine. It is an ingredient of preparations used mainly for gastrointestinal and biliary-tract disorders. Fumitory is also used in homoeopathic medicine.

### Preparations

**Proprietary Preparations** (details are given in Part 3)

***Austria:*** Bilobene; Oddibil; ***Braz.:*** Oddibil; ***Fr.:*** Oddibil; ***Ger.:*** Bilobene; Bomagall mono; Oddibil; ***Mex.:*** Oddibil†; ***Spain:*** Colambil†.

**Multi-ingredient:** ***Austria:*** Hepabene; Oddispasmol; ***Belg.:*** Tisane Depurative "les 12 Plantes"†; ***Fr.:*** Actibil; Actisane Digestion†; Bolcitol; Depuratif Parnel; Depuratum; Gastralsan†; Schoum; ***Ital.:*** Depurativo†; Soluzione Schoum; ***Spain:*** Natusor Hepavesical; Odisor; Solucion Schoum; ***UK:*** Echinacea; Skin Cleansing.

## Gabexate Mesilate *(rINNM)*

Gabexate Mesylate; Mesilato de gabexato. Ethyl 4-(6-guanidinohexanoyloxy)benzoate methanesulphonate.

$C_{16}H_{23}N_3O_4,CH_4SO_3$ = 417.5.

*CAS — 39492-01-8 (gabexate); 56974-61-9 (gabexate mesilate).*

**Pharmacopoeias.** In *Jpn.*

### Profile

Gabexate mesilate is a proteolytic enzyme inhibitor that has been tried in the treatment of pancreatitis (p.1726), and in the prevention of pancreatitis following endoscopic retrograde cholangiopancreatography. It has also been tried as an anticoagulant for haemodialysis. Hypersensitivity reactions including anaphylaxis have occurred.

◊ References.


1. Scuro LA, *et al.* Gabexate mesilate (Foy) treatment of acute pancreatitis: an Italian multicentre pilot study. *Clin Trials J* 1990; **27:** 39–49.
2. Messori A, *et al.* Effectiveness of gabexate mesilate in acute pancreatitis: a metaanalysis. *Dig Dis Sci* 1995; **40:** 734–8.
3. Cavallini G, *et al.* Gabexate for the prevention of pancreatic damage related to endoscopic retrograde cholangiopancreatography. *N Engl J Med* 1996; **335:** 919–23.
4. Matsukawa Y, *et al.* Anaphylaxis induced by gabexate mesylate. *BMJ* 1998; **317:** 1563.
5. Ranucci M, *et al.* Gabexate mesilate and antithrombin III for intraoperative anticoagulation in heparin pretreated patients. *Perfusion* 1999; **14:** 357–62.
6. Andriulli A, *et al.* Gabexate or somatostatin administration before ERCP in patients at high risk for post-ERCP pancreatitis: a multicenter, placebo-controlled, randomized clinical trial. *Gastrointest Endosc* 2002; **56:** 488–95.
7. Matsukawa Y, *et al.* Fatal cases of gabexate mesilate-induced anaphylaxis. *Int J Clin Pharmacol Res* 2002; **22:** 81–3.


### Preparations

**Proprietary Preparations** (details are given in Part 3)

***Ital.:*** Foy; ***Jpn:*** Foy.

## Gall

Agallas de roble; Aleppo Galls; Blue Galls; Galla; Galläpfel; Galls; Noix de Galle; Nutgall.

**Pharmacopoeias.** In *Chin.*

### Profile

Gall is the excrescences on the twigs of *Quercus infectoria* (Fagaceae), resulting from the stimulus given to the tissues of the young twigs by the development of the larvae of the gall-wasp, *Adleria gallae-tinctoriae* (*Cynips gallae-tinctoriae*) (Cynipidae). It contains about 50 to 70% of gallotannic acid.

Gall is an astringent and has been used in ointments and suppositories for the treatment of haemorrhoids. It is a source of tannic acid (p.1751).

### Preparations

**Proprietary Preparations** (details are given in Part 3)

***Spain:*** Litiax.

## Gamma-aminobutyric Acid

γ-Aminobutírico, ácido; Aminobutyric Acid; GABA; Piperidic Acid. 4-Aminobutyric acid.

$C_4H_9NO_2$ = 103.1.

*CAS — 56-12-2.*

*ATC — N03AG03.*

### Profile

Gamma-aminobutyric acid is a principal inhibitory neurotransmitter in the CNS. It has been claimed to be of value in cerebral disorders and to have an antihypertensive effect.

### Preparations

**Proprietary Preparations** (details are given in Part 3)

***Braz.:*** Gammar; ***Hong Kong:*** Gammalon; ***Port.:*** Mielomade; ***Thai.:*** Bainto; Gammalon.

**Multi-ingredient:** ***Arg.:*** Cadencial Plus; ***Braz.:*** Complevit†; Gaba; Gabax; Gabormon†; Id Sedin; ***Chile:*** Actebral; Gamalate B6; ***Spain:*** Cefabol; Gamalate B6.

## Gamolenic Acid *(BAN, rINN)*

Ácido gamolénico; GLA; γ-Linolenic Acid. (Z,Z,Z)-Octadeca-6,9,12-trienoic acid.

$C_{18}H_{30}O_2$ = 278.4.

*CAS — 506-26-3.*

*ATC — D11AX02.*

## Linoleic Acid

Linoleico, ácido; Linolic Acid. (Z,Z)-Octadeca-9,12-dienoic acid.

$C_{18}H_{32}O_2$ = 280.4.

### Adverse Effects and Precautions

Gamolenic and linoleic acids from evening primrose oil, and presumably other sources, can produce minor gastrointestinal disturbances and headache. They can precipitate symptoms of undiagnosed temporal lobe epilepsy, and should be used with caution in patients with a history of epilepsy or those taking epileptogenic drugs, in particular phenothiazines. Hypersensitivity reactions may also occur.

### Uses and Administration

Gamolenic and linoleic acid are essential fatty acids of the omega-6 series that act as prostaglandin precursors. Endogenous gamolenic acid is derived from linoleic acid, which is present in many vegetable oils and is an essential constituent of the diet. The most widely-used source of these acids is evening primrose oil (see p.1686). Gamolenic and linoleic acids have been used in skin disorders and mastalgia, and have been investigated in a variety of other disorders including multiple sclerosis, rheumatoid arthritis, and the premenstrual syndrome.

Products containing gamolenic-acid rich plant oils are promoted in many countries as dietary supplements, often in combination with fish oils or other sources of omega-3 triglycerides (see p.976).

A derivative of gamolenic acid, lithium gamolenate, has been investigated in pancreatic cancer.

**Eczema.** Atopic eczema (p.1135) may be due to a defect in essential fatty acid metabolism[1,2] and some beneficial symptomatic effects have been reported with evening primrose oil.[1,3] Meta-analysis of 9 studies involving 311 patients[4] has reported improvement in disease symptoms, especially itching, but a subsequent study in 123 patients found no therapeutic effect of evening primrose oil, alone or with fish oil.[5] Although the design and interpretation of this study has been criticised by the manufacturers of evening primrose oil,[6] the authors consider such criticism invalid,[7] and point out that an earlier large study yielded similar results.[8] No difference was found between placebo and evening primrose oil in a further study[9] in children with eczema, and there was also no effect on asthma symptoms in those patients suffering from both disorders. Studies[10,11] of borage oil (another source of gamolenic acid) also found no overall efficacy in adults or children with atopic eczema, although one study noted a suggestion of benefit in a subgroup of patients.[10] In a study[12] of a group of formula-fed infants with a high maternal familial risk of developing atopic eczema, borage oil supplementation did not prevent the expression of atopy, although it showed a tendency to alleviate the severity of the condition later in infancy.

Benefit has been reported in infants with seborrhoeic dermatitis from local application of borage oil.[13]


1. Wright S. Essential fatty acids and the skin. *Br J Dermatol* 1991; **125:** 503–15.
2. Horrobin DF. Essential fatty acid metabolism and its modification in atopic eczema. *Am J Clin Nutr* 2000; **71** (suppl): 367S–372S.
3. Rustin MHA. Dermatology. *Postgrad Med J* 1990; **66:** 894–905.
4. Morse PF, *et al.* Meta-analysis of placebo-controlled studies of the efficacy of Epogam in the treatment of atopic eczema: relationship between plasma essential fatty acid changes and clinical response. *Br J Dermatol* 1989; **121:** 75–90.
5. Berth-Jones J, Graham-Brown RAC. Placebo-controlled trial of essential fatty acid supplementation in atopic dermatitis. *Lancet* 1993; **341:** 1557–60. Correction. *ibid.*; **342:** 564.
6. Shield MJ, *et al.* Essential fatty acid supplementation in atopic dermatitis. *Lancet* 1993; **342:** 377.
7. Berth-Jones J, *et al.* Essential fatty acid supplementation in atopic dermatitis. *Lancet* 1993; **342:** 377–8. Correction. *ibid.*; 752.
8. Bamford JTM, *et al.* Atopic eczema unresponsive to evening primrose oil (linoleic and gamma-linolenic acids). *J Am Acad Dermatol* 1985; **13:** 959–65.
9. Hederos C-A, Berg A. Epogam evening primrose oil treatment in atopic dermatitis and asthma. *Arch Dis Child* 1996; **75:** 494–7.
10. Henz BM, *et al.* Double-blind, multicentre analysis of the efficacy of borage oil in patients with atopic eczema. *Br J Dermatol* 1999; **140:** 685–8.
11. Takwale A, *et al.* Efficacy and tolerability of borage oil in adults and children with atopic eczema: randomised, double blind, placebo controlled, parallel group trial. *BMJ* 2003; **327:**1385–7.
12. van Gool CJ, *et al.* γ-Linolenic acid supplementation for prophylaxis of atopic dermatitis—a randomized controlled trial in infants at high familial risk. *Am J Clin Nutr* 2003; **77:** 943–51.
13. Tollesson A, Frithz A. Borage oil, an effective new treatment for infantile seborrhoeic dermatitis. *Br J Dermatol* 1993; **129:** 95.


**Mastalgia.** Gamolenic acid (usually given in the form of evening primrose oil) has fewer adverse effects than drugs such as danazol or bromocriptine and has been preferred for mastalgia (p.1546), especially in patients with less severe symptoms or those who require prolonged or repeated treatment. However, there is no clear evidence of efficacy.

**Multiple sclerosis.** There is some evidence that modifying the intake of dietary fats and supplementing the diet with omega-6 polyunsaturated fatty acids, such as linoleic acid, could influence the clinical course of multiple sclerosis (p.646) and many patients practise dietary modification, including taking evening primrose oil. One study[1] has shown a reduction in severity and duration of relapse in patients taking linoleic acid supplements (as sunflower oil), and another[2] has reported benefit in patients who limited their intake of dietary saturated fatty acids and supplemented their diet with polyunsaturated fatty acids. However, the relationship between dietary fat and multiple sclerosis cannot be considered proven.


1. Millar JHD, *et al.* Double-blind trial of linoleate supplementation of the diet in multiple sclerosis. *BMJ* 1973; **1:** 765–8.
2. Swank RL, Dugan BB. Effect of low saturated fat diet in early and late cases of multiple sclerosis. *Lancet* 1990; **336:** 37–9.


**Premenstrual syndrome.** Progressive improvement in premenstrual syndrome (p.1551) was reported over 5 cycles in an open pilot study in 19 patients receiving evening primrose oil.[1] However, subsequent results have not demonstrated any benefit.[2-4] Evening primrose oil has been considered for cyclical mastalgia (see above).


1. Larsson B, *et al.* Evening primrose oil in the treatment of premenstrual syndrome: a pilot study. *Curr Ther Res* 1989; **46:** 58–63.
2. Khoo SK, *et al.* Evening primrose oil and treatment of premenstrual syndrome. *Med J Aust* 1990; **153:** 189–92.
3. Collins A, *et al.* Essential fatty acids in the treatment of premenstrual syndrome. *Obstet Gynecol* 1993; **81:** 93–8.
4. Budeiri DJ, *et al.* Is evening primrose oil of value in the treatment of premenstrual syndrome? *Control Clin Trials* 1996; **17:** 60–8.


**Rheumatoid arthritis.** Patients with rheumatoid arthritis (p.9) taking NSAIDs have shown subjective improvement following 12 months' treatment with evening primrose oil, with or without fish oil, when compared with placebo.[1] A clinically important reduction in signs and symptoms of disease activity has also been seen in patients treated with gamolenic acid in the form of borage oil.[2] It has been demonstrated[3] that during treatment with evening primrose oil patients with rheumatoid arthritis have increased plasma concentrations of gamolenic, dihomo-gamma-linolenic, and arachidonic acids, and decreased plasma concentrations of oleic and eicosapentaenoic acids and apolipoprotein B. The increase in plasma-arachidonic acid and decrease in eicosapentaenoic acid may be unfavourable in patients with rheumatoid arthritis, since arachidonic acid is the precursor of inflammatory prostaglandins and eicosapentaenoic acid may have an anti-inflammatory role. A systematic review[4] of these and other studies concluded that there does appear to be some potential benefit for the use of gamolenic acid in rheumatoid arthritis, although optimum dosage and duration of treatment remains to be established.


1. Belch JJF, *et al.* Effects of altering dietary essential fatty acids on requirements for non-steroidal anti-inflammatory drugs in patients with rheumatoid arthritis: a double blind placebo controlled study. *Ann Rheum Dis* 1988; **47:** 96–104.
2. Leventhal LJ, *et al.* Treatment of rheumatoid arthritis with gammalinolenic acid. *Ann Intern Med* 1993; **119:** 867–73.
3. Jäntti J, *et al.* Evening primrose oil in rheumatoid arthritis: changes in serum lipids and fatty acids. *Ann Rheum Dis* 1989; **48:** 124–7.
4. Little C, Parsons T. Herbal therapy for treating rheumatoid arthritis. Available in The Cochrane Library; Issue 2. Chichester: John Wiley; 2004.


### Preparations

**Proprietary Preparations** (details are given in Part 3)
***Denm.:*** Epogam†; ***Ger.:*** Linola-Fett 2000; ***Hong Kong:*** Efamast†; ***Ital.:*** Ictage 6; Normogam; ***NZ:*** Epogam†; ***S.Afr.:*** Epogam†; ***Spain:*** Epogam†; ***UK:*** PowerLean†; Super GLA.

**Multi-ingredient:** ***Arg.:*** Exomega; Quelodin F; ***Braz.:*** Gamaline-V; Glavit; Oleo de Primula; Primoris; ***Canad.:*** Bionagre plus E; Efalex; Gamma Oil Marine†; ***Chile:*** Ureadin Pediatrics; ***Fr.:*** Exomega; ***Ger.:*** Linola; Linola-Fett; Unguentacid; ***Hong Kong:*** Aderma Exomega; ***Ital.:*** Derman-Oil; Dermana Pasta; Efagel; Errevit Forte Gamma†; Granoleina; Topialyse; Trofinerv Antiox; ***NZ:*** Efalex; Efamast; ***Port.:*** Geriso; ***S.Afr.:*** Efamol G; ***Switz.:*** Acne-Med Wolff Simplex; Linola; Linola gras; Linola mi-gras; Linoladiol; Vitafissan N.

## Gangliosides

Gangliósidos.

### Profile

Gangliosides are endogenous substances present in mammalian cell membranes, especially in the cortex of the brain. They are glycosphingolipids composed of a hydrophilic oligosaccharide chain, characterised by sialic acid residues, attached to a lipophilic moiety. The four major gangliosides found in the mammalian brain are referred to as $G_{M1}$, $G_{D1a}$, $G_{D1b}$, and $G_{T1b}$.

Experimental studies have reported that gangliosides may have a neuroprotective effect on the central and peripheral nervous systems. Preparations of gangliosides from bovine brain were given for peripheral neuropathies and cerebrovascular disorders and their role in spinal cord injury has also been investigated. The modified ganglioside siagoside is being studied in patients with Parkinson's disease.

Concern has been expressed by several authorities about the development of Guillain-Barré syndrome and other motor neurone disorders in some patients and it was suggested that gangliosides were contra-indicated in Guillain-Barré syndrome and all autoimmune disorders. Subsequently these concerns over safety as well as of efficacy led to the withdrawal of ganglioside preparations in many countries.

◊ References.


1. Geisler FH, *et al.* Recovery of motor function after spinal-cord injury—a randomized, placebo-controlled trial with GM-1 ganglioside. *N Engl J Med* 1991; **324:** 1829–38.
2. Raschetti R, *et al.* Guillain-Barré syndrome and ganglioside therapy in Italy. *Lancet* 1992; **340:** 60.
3. Figueras A, *et al.* Bovine gangliosides and acute motor polyneuropathy. *BMJ* 1992; **305:** 1330–1.
4. Roberts JW, *et al.* Iatrogenic hyperlipidaemia with GM-1 ganglioside. *Lancet* 1993; **342:** 115.
5. Landi G, *et al.* Guillain-Barré syndrome after exogenous gangliosides in Italy. *BMJ* 1993; **307:** 1463–4.
6. Nobile-Orazio E, *et al.* Gangliosides: their role in clinical neurology. *Drugs* 1994; **47:** 576–85.
7. Candelise L, Ciccone A. Gangliosides for acute ischaemic stroke. Available in The Cochrane Library; Issue 2. Chichester: John Wiley; 2004.


### Preparations

**Proprietary Preparations** (details are given in Part 3)
***Braz.:*** Sinaxial; Sygen; ***Thai.:*** Cronassial†.

## Garlic

Aglio; Ail; Ajo; Allium; Knoblauch.
*CAS — 8008-99-9 (garlic extract).*

**Pharmacopoeias.** In *USNF,* which also includes Garlic Fluidextract, Powdered Garlic, and Powdered Garlic Extract. *Eur.* (see p.vi) includes Garlic Powder.
*Eur.* also includes Garlic for Homoeopathic Preparations.

**Ph. Eur. 5.0** (Garlic Powder). It is produced from garlic that has been cut, freeze-dried or dried at a temperature not exceeding 65°, and powdered. It contains not less than 0.45% of allicin, calculated with reference to the dried drug. It is a light yellowish powder. Protect from light.

**Ph. Eur. 5.0** (Garlic for Homoeopathic Preparations). The fresh bulb of *Allium sativum*. Store in airtight containers. Protect from light.

**USNF 22** (Garlic). The fresh or dried compound bulbs of *Allium sativum* (Liliaceae). It contains not less than 0.5% of alliin and not less than 0.2% of γ-glutamyl-(*S*)-allyl-L-cysteine, calculated on the dried basis. Store in a dry place at a temperature of 8° to 15°. Protect from light.

**USNF 22** (Powdered Garlic). It is produced from garlic that has been cut, freeze-dried or dried at a temperature not exceeding 65°, and powdered. It contains not less than 0.3% of alliin and not less than 0.1% of γ-glutamyl-(*S*)-allyl-L-cysteine, calculated on the dried basis. Store in a dry place at a temperature of 8° to 15°. Protect from light.

### Adverse Effects

◊ Reports of burns or skin lesions following topical application of garlic to children,[1,2] and to adults,[3,4] including self-inflicted injury.[5]


1. Garty B-Z. Garlic burns. *Pediatrics* 1993; **91:** 658–9.
2. Canduela V, *et al.* Garlic: always good for the health? *Br J Dermatol* 1995; **132:** 161–2.
3. Farrell AM, Staughton RCD. Garlic burns mimicking herpes zoster. *Lancet* 1996; **347:** 1195.
4. Eming SA, *et al.* Severe toxic contact dermatitis caused by garlic. *Br J Dermatol* 1999; **141:** 391–2.
5. Lachter J, *et al.* Garlic: a way out of work. *Mil Med* 2003; **168:** 499–500.


### Uses and Administration

The constituents of garlic include alliin, allicin, diallyl disulfide, and ajoene. It has traditionally been reported to have expectorant, diaphoretic, disinfectant, and diuretic properties. More recently, it has been investigated for antimicrobial, antihypertensive, lipid-lowering, fibrinolytic, antiplatelet, and cancer protective effects. It is used in homoeopathic medicine. Garlic oil has also been used.

◊ References.


1. Kleijnen J, *et al.* Garlic, onions and cardiovascular risk factors: a review of the evidence from human experiments with emphasis on commercially available preparations. *Br J Clin Pharmacol* 1989; **28:** 535–44.
2. Mansell P, Reckless JPD. Garlic. *BMJ* 1991; **303:** 379–80.
3. McElnay JC, Po ALW. Garlic. *Pharm J* 1991; **246:** 324–6.
4. Kiesewetter H, *et al.* Effect of garlic on platelet aggregation in patients with increased risk of juvenile ischaemic attack. *Eur J Clin Pharmacol* 1993; **45:** 333–6.
5. Deshpande RG, *et al.* Inhibition of Mycobacterium avium complex isolates from AIDS patients by garlic (Allium sativum). *J Antimicrob Chemother* 1993; **32:** 623–6.
6. Dorant E, *et al.* Garlic and its significance for the prevention of cancer in humans: a critical review. *Br J Cancer* 1993; **67:** 424–9.
7. Ackermann RT, *et al.* Garlic shows promise for improving some cardiovascular risk factors. *Arch Intern Med* 2001; **161:** 813–24.


**Hyperlipidaemia.** Garlic has been widely promoted for use in the treatment of hyperlipidaemia (p.823). Several early placebo-controlled trials[1,2] and meta-analyses[3,4] showed that garlic significantly decreased total serum-cholesterol concentrations. However, more recent data suggest that the effect is at best modest[5] or that there is no significant difference[6-8] when compared with placebo.


1. Jain AK, *et al.* Can garlic reduce levels of serum lipids? A controlled clinical study. *Am J Med* 1993; **94:** 632–5.
2. Kenzelmann R, Kade F. Limitation of the deterioration of lipid parameters by a standardized garlic-ginkgo combination product: a multicenter placebo-controlled double-blind study. *Arzneimittelforschung* 1993; **43:** 978–81.
3. Warshafsky S, *et al.* Effect of garlic on total serum cholesterol: a meta-analysis. *Ann Intern Med* 1993; **119:** 599–605.
4. Silagy C, Neil A. Garlic as a lipid lowering agent—a meta-analysis. *J R Coll Physicians Lond* 1994; **28:** 39–45.
5. Stevinson C, *et al.* Garlic for treating hypercholesterolemia: a meta-analysis of randomized clinical trials. *Ann Intern Med* 2000; **133:** 420–9.
6. Neil HAW, *et al.* Garlic powder in the treatment of moderate hyperlipidaemia: a controlled trial and a meta-analysis. *J R Coll Physicians Lond* 1996; **30:** 329–34.
7. Berthold HK, *et al.* Effect of a garlic oil preparation on serum lipoproteins and cholesterol metabolism: a randomized controlled trial. *JAMA* 1998; **279:** 1900–2.
8. Isaacsohn JL, *et al.* Garlic powder and plasma lipids and lipoproteins: a multicenter, randomized, placebo-controlled trial. *Arch Intern Med* 1998; **158:** 1189–94.


### Preparations

***USNF 22:*** Garlic Delayed-Release Tablets.

**Proprietary Preparations** (details are given in Part 3)
***Arg.:*** Ajomast; Alliocaps Oligoplex; Kyolic Super Formula; ***Austral.:*** Garlix†; Macro Garlic†; ***Austria:*** Allio Vital; Kwai; ***Canad.:*** Kwai; Kyolic; ***Fr.:*** Past Ail†; Thirial†; ***Ger.:*** Alliosan; Beni-cur†; Carisano; Ilja Rogoff Forte; Kneipp Knoblauch Dragees N†; Kneipp Knoblauch-Pflanzensaft†; Kwai; Quam†; Ravalgen; Sapec; Sirmia Knoblauchsaft N†; Strongus; Tegra†; Vitagutt Knoblauch; ***Ital.:*** Aglio; Kwai; ***Port.:*** Alho Rogoff; ***Switz.:*** A Vogel Capsules a l'ail; Kwai; Sanhelios 333†; ***UK:*** Garlimega; Kwai; Kyolic.

**Multi-ingredient:** ***Arg.:*** Ajolip; Ajomast Circulatorio; ***Austral.:*** Crataegus Complex†; Echinacea & Antioxidants†; Echinacea ACE Plus Zinc†; Ethical Nutrients Antioxidant Fish Oil Garlic Plus†; Garlic Allium Complex†; Garlic and Horseradish + C Complex†; Garlic, Horseradish, A & C Capsules†; Gartech†; Herbal Cold & Flu Relief†; Horse Radish and Garlic Tablets†; Lifesystem Herbal Formula 7 Liver Tonic†; Liver Tonic Herbal Formula 6†; Odourless Garlic†; Procold†; Proesten†; Protol†; Proyeast†; Silybum Complex†; ***Austria:*** Heli-Sal; Rutiviscal; ***Belg.:*** Ex'ail†; ***Braz.:*** Neo Sativan†; ***Canad.:*** Kyolic 101; Kyolic 102; Kyolic 103; Kyolic 104; Kyolic 106; ***Fr.:*** Arterase; Ex'ail†; ***Ger.:*** Asgoviscum N; Discmigon†; Ilja Rogoff; Kneipp Drei-Pflanzen-Dragees N†; Lipidavit; Presselin Arterien K 5 P; ***Hong Kong:*** Ginkgo Plus Vivo-Livo; ***Ital.:*** Prexene†; ***Switz.:*** Allium Plus; Arterosan Plus; Keli-med; ***UK:*** Antifect; Beechams for Natural Relief†; Brewers Yeast with Garlic†; Buttercup Pol'N'Count†; Clogar; Coldeeze†; Fishogar; Garlodex†; Hay Fever & Sinus Relief; Hayfever & Sinus Relief; Kincare†; Liqufruta Garlic Cough Medicine.

## Gavestinel *(BAN, USAN, rINN)*

GV-150526X. 4,6-Dichloro-3-[(*E*)-2-(phenylcarbamoyl)vinyl]indole-2-carboxylic acid.
$C_{18}H_{12}Cl_2N_2O_3$ = 375.2.
*CAS — 153436-22-7.*

### Profile

Gavestinel is a glycine antagonist that has been investigated as a neuroprotectant in stroke.

**Stroke.** Gavestinel has been tried for its supposed neuroprotective properties in acute stroke, but two major multicentre, randomised controlled studies have failed to demonstrate any benefit over placebo.[1,2]


1. Lees KR, *et al.* Glycine antagonist (gavestinel) in neuroprotection (GAIN International) in patients with acute stroke: a randomised controlled trial. *Lancet* 2000; **355:** 1949–54.
2. Sacco RL, *et al.* Glycine antagonist in neuroprotection for patients with acute stroke: GAIN Americas: a randomized controlled trial. *JAMA* 2001; **285:** 1719–28.


## Gelsemium

Gelsemium Root; Jessamine; Yellow Jasmine Root.
*CAS — 509-15-9 (gelsemine).*

### Profile

Gelsemium consists of the dried rhizome and roots of *Gelsemium sempervirens* (Loganiaceae). It contains toxic indole alkaloids including gelsemine ($C_{20}H_{22}N_2O_2$ = 322.4). It depresses the CNS and has been used mainly in neuralgic conditions, particularly trigeminal neuralgia and migraine.

Gelsemium is used in homoeopathic medicine.

### Preparations

**Proprietary Preparations** (details are given in Part 3)
**Multi-ingredient:** ***Fr.:*** Coquelusedal; Coquelusedal Paracetamol.

## Gene Therapy

Terapéutica génica.

### Profile

Gene therapy is a product of the increasing knowledge of genetic function and the availability of methods to examine and manipulate the genome. Exogenous genetic material is introduced into body cells (transfection) in such a way that the cells are able to express the products of the new genes. It should be distinguished from the administration of products themselves derived from organisms (usually micro-organisms) whose genome has been manipulated by similar recombinant DNA technology, for example the use of recombinant cytokines, monoclonal antibodies, or antisense products.

Gene therapy is under investigation in three main areas:

- the replacement of abnormal or defective genes in patients with inherited disease
- the alteration of the characteristics of cells to change their relative susceptibility to other therapies (for example by making haematopoietic stem cells more resistant to the adverse effects of antineoplastics, or by making tumour cells selectively express an enzyme which converts an otherwise non-toxic prodrug into a cytotoxic agent)
- for localised production of a biologically active substance that cannot be administered directly or would have unacceptable effects following systemic administration.

To date, all gene therapy in humans has been of differentiated somatic cells; alteration of the human genome in a manner transmissible to offspring, either by treating the germ cells or the early embryo, is considered at present to pose insuperable ethical problems.

Various methods for delivery of genetic material have been investigated, none of which is yet completely satisfactory. Although removal of donor cells from the patient followed by *ex vivo* transfer of the new gene (by physical or viral methods) and return of the modified cells may be feasible for modifying haematopoietic stem cells, for most tissues, methods of *in vivo* transfer are required. Modified viruses rendered incapable of replicating have been widely studied as vectors for gene therapy. Retroviruses have the advantage that the DNA they carry is integrated into the host genome, resulting in permanent expression of the gene, but there has been some concern that they may disrupt existing genetic material with possibly oncogenic effect; in addition, their small size limits the size of gene that they can carry, and they are largely ineffective in infecting non-dividing cells. Adenoviruses are more stable and can infect non-dividing as well as dividing cells, but their genetic freight is not integrated into the chromosome and transmitted to the cell's progeny, and the gene products are therefore only expressed transiently; they are also highly immunogenic which limits repeated administration. Some other viral types, including herpes simplex viruses, adeno-associated viruses, and lentiviruses, are also under investigation. Viruses with tropisms for a particular tissue may be useful in producing localised effects.

Chemical or physical methods for DNA delivery have been extensively investigated *in vitro* and in *animals*, and have been studied in small numbers of patients. Such methods include direct injection of DNA, the use of DNA complexes bound to a ligand which can be taken up by cells, formulation of DNA in liposomes which can fuse with cell membranes and allow the DNA to enter the cell, and more exotic methods such as 'gene guns', in which DNA-coated gold particles are fired into the cells. Although gene expression can be achieved following such methods, it is again transient because the new genetic material is not integrated with that of the host, and physical methods are currently less efficient and more limited in scope than viral ones.

Numerous clinical studies are being carried out although, at present, relatively few patients have actually received gene therapy. The first successful therapy was for severe combined immunodeficiency, a single-gene disorder due to deficiency of the enzyme adenosine deaminase. Transfection of the gene for this enzyme into the patient's T-cells *ex vivo* and re-infusion of the modified T-cells has been shown to produce substantial clinical improvement, although therapy must be repeated periodically because of the limited lifespan of the lymphocytes.

Studies in patients with cystic fibrosis have also shown some success, and a number of other single-gene disorders, including $alpha_1$ antitrypsin deficiency, familial hypercholesterolaemia, Gaucher disease, the haemoglobinopathies and haemophilias, and Duchenne muscular dystrophy are being studied or have been proposed as possible candidates.

Gene therapy is also under investigation in various acquired diseases, particularly in the management of various types of cancer. Strategies being studied include modification of tumour cells either to increase their immunogenicity or to render them selectively sensitive to antineoplastics, and transfection of tumour cells with tumour suppressor genes. Other disorders being studied clinically include HIV infection, rheumatoid arthritis, and atherosclerosis.

◊ Some reviews and references concerning gene therapy are listed below. See also under the discussions of individual diseases for comments on gene therapy in the context of their conventional treatment.

1. Coutelle C. Gene therapy approaches for cystic fibrosis. *Biologicals* 1995; **23:** 21–5.
2. Hoeben RC. Gene therapy for the haemophilias: current status. *Biologicals* 1995; **23:** 27–9.
3. Lever AML, Goodfellow P, eds. Gene therapy. *Br Med Bull* 1995; **51:** 1–242.
4. Hanania EG, *et al.* Recent advances in the application of gene therapy to human disease. *Am J Med* 1995; **99:** 537–52.
5. Blau HM, Springer ML. Gene therapy—a novel form of drug delivery. *N Engl J Med* 1995; **333:** 1204–7.
6. Whartenby KA, *et al.* Gene therapy: clinical potential and relationships to drug treatment. *Drugs* 1995; **50:** 951–8.
7. Dorin J. Somatic gene therapy. *BMJ* 1996; **312:** 323–4.
8. Southern KW. Gene therapy for cystic fibrosis: current issues. *Br J Hosp Med* 1996; **55:** 495–9.
9. Weichselbaum RR, Kufe D. Gene therapy of cancer. *Lancet* 1997; **349** (suppl II): 10–12.
10. Alton EWFW, Geddes DM. Prospects for respiratory gene therapy. *Br J Hosp Med* 1997; **58:** 47–9.
11. Knoell DL, Yiu IM. Human gene therapy for hereditary diseases: a review of trials. *Am J Health-Syst Pharm* 1998; **55:** 899–904.
12. Smith AE. Gene therapy—where are we? *Lancet* 1999; **354** (suppl): 1–4.
13. Hu WS, Pathak VK. Design of retroviral vectors and helper cells for gene therapy. *Pharmacol Rev* 2000; **52:** 493–511.
14. Mah C, *et al.* Virus-based gene delivery systems. *Clin Pharmacokinet* 2002; **41:** 901–11.
15. WHO. Gene transfer medicinal products. *WHO Drug Inf* 2002; **16:** 275–82.
16. Medicines and Healthcare Regulatory Agency. Recommendations of the GTAC/CSM working party on retroviruses. Internet Document: Apr 2003. Available at: http://www.mhra.gov.uk/news/2003/retroviruses.pdf (accessed 03/06/04)

## Genistein

CI-75610; Genisteol; Prunetol. 4′,5,7-Trihydroxyisoflavone; 5,7-Dihydroxy-3-(4-hydroxyphenyl)-4*H*-1-benzopyran-4-one.

$C_{15}H_{10}O_5 = 270.2.$

*CAS — 446-72-0.*

### Profile

Genistein is a soya isoflavone that inhibits tyrosine kinase. It is a phytoestrogen that has been tried for the relief of menopausal symptoms. It is also being investigated for its beneficial effect on blood lipids and for its proposed tumour-suppressing activity.

◊ References.

1. Squadrito F, *et al.* The effect of the phytoestrogen genistein on plasma nitric oxide concentrations, endothelin-1 levels and endothelium dependent vasodilation in postmenopausal women. *Atherosclerosis* 2002; **163:** 339–47.
2. Morabito N, *et al.* Effects of genistein and hormone-replacement therapy on bone loss in early postmenopausal women: a randomized double-blind placebo-controlled study. *J Bone Miner Res* 2002; **17:** 1904–12.
3. Squadrito F, *et al.* Effect of genistein on endothelial function in postmenopausal women: a randomized, double-blind, controlled study. *Am J Med* 2003; **114:** 470–6.

### Preparations

**Proprietary Preparations** (details are given in Part 3)
**Multi-ingredient:** ***Ital.:*** Evestrel; ***Port.:*** Afron; Femnet.

## Gentian

Bitter Root; Enzianwurzel; Genciana; Gentian Root; Gentiana; Gentianae Radix; Genziana; Raiz de Genciana.

**Pharmacopoeias.** In *Eur.* (see p.vi), *Jpn*, and *Pol.*
*Jpn* includes Japanese Gentian, from *G. scabra* and other species. *Chin.* also specifies *G. scabra* and other species.

**Ph. Eur. 5.0** (Gentian Root; Gentian BP 2003). The dried, fragmented underground organs of *Gentiana lutea* yielding not less than 33% of water-soluble extractive. It has a characteristic odour. Protect from light.

### Profile

Gentian is used as a bitter. An alcoholic infusion of gentian, bitter-orange peel, and lemon peel has been used as an ingredient in a number of bitter mixtures.

Gentian has been used in homoeopathic medicine.

### Preparations

***BP 2003:*** Acid Gentian Mixture; Alkaline Gentian Mixture; Compound Gentian Infusion; Concentrated Compound Gentian Infusion.

**Proprietary Preparations** (details are given in Part 3)
***Ger.:*** Digestivum-Hetterich S; Enziagil Magenplus.

**Multi-ingredient:** ***Austral.:*** Calmo†; Digestaid†; Digestive Aid†; Extralife Sleep-Care†; Pacifenity†; Relaxaplex†; Sinulin; ***Austria:*** Abdomilon N; Amara; Bio-Garten Tee zur Starkung und Kraftigung; Brady's-Magentropfen; China-Eisenwein; Digestol; Krauterelixier; Magentee†; Mariazeller; Montana; Naturland Magentonikum; Naturland Verdauungs; Neuners Krautertee Nr 20 - Kreislauftee; Sanvita Magen; Sigman-Haustropfen; Sinupret; Sinusol; St Radegunder Verdauungstee; ***Braz.:*** Camomila†; Digestar†; Estomafitino†; Fargestium†; Fideine†; Formitonicum†; Gotas Digestivas; Gotas Preciosas†; Lactifero†; Xarope Iodo-Suma; ***Canad.:*** Herbal Laxative; Herbal Nerve; ***Fr.:*** Elixir Grez; Quintonine; Triogene†; ***Ger.:*** Abdomilon N; Amara-Tropfen; Amara-Tropfen-Pascoe; Anore X N; Discmigon†; Dr. Hotz Vollbad†; Gallexier; Gastralon N; Gastrol S; Gastrosecur; Hepaticum-Medice H; Infi-tract; Kneipp Flatuol†; Leber-Galle-Tropfen 83; Majocarmin forte; Majocarmin mite; Montana N; Phonix Gastriphon†; Schwedentrunk Elixier; Schwedentrunk mit Ginseng†; Schwedentrunk†; Sedovent; Sinupret; Stovalid N; Unex Amarum; ventri-loges N; Ventrimarin novo†; ***Hong Kong:*** Sinupret; ***Ital.:*** Amaro Medicinale; Amaro Padil†; Assenzio (Specie Composta); Caramelle alle Erbe Digestive; Centaurea (Specie Composta); Chinoidina; Depurativo†; Elisir Depurativo Ambrosiano†; Frerichs Maldifassi; Genziana (Specie Composta); ***Singapore:*** Sinupret; ***Spain:*** Depurativo Richelet; Digestol Sanatorium†; ***Switz.:*** Demonatur Gouttes pour le foie et la bile; Gastrosan; Padma-Lax; Sinupret; ***Thai.:*** Pepsitase; Sinupret; ***UK:*** Acidosis; Appetiser Mixture; Indigestion Mixture; Kalms; Quiet Tyme; Scullcap & Gentian Tablets; Stomach Mixture.

## Gentisic Acid Ethanolamide

Etanolamida del ácido gentísico. 2,5-Dihydroxybenzoic acid ethanolamide.

$C_9H_{11}NO_4 = 197.2.$

### Profile

Gentisic acid ethanolamide has been used as a complexing agent in the manufacture of pharmaceutical preparations.

## Geranium Oil

Aetheroleum Pelargonii; Geranio, aceite esencial de; Oleum Geranii; Pelargonium Oil; Rose Geranium Oil.

### Profile

Geranium oil is a volatile oil obtained by distillation from the aerial parts of various species and hybrid forms of *Pelargonium* (Geraniaceae). It contains geraniol. It is used to perfume various preparations and has been included in insect repellent preparations. Hypersensitivity reactions have been associated with geraniol.

**Postherpetic neuralgia.** A study[1] involving 30 patients has indicated that topically applied geranium oil is of benefit in the management of the pain of postherpetic neuralgia. Pain relief was obtained within a few minutes but further study is required to determine the duration of effect beyond 1 hour. Adverse effects were considered to be minor and included burning in the eye, skin rash, and lightheadedness.

1. Greenway FL, *et al.* Temporary relief of postherpetic neuralgia pain with topical geranium oil. *Am J Med* 2003; **115:** 586–7.

### Preparations

**Proprietary Preparations** (details are given in Part 3)
***Ital.:*** Entom Nature.

**Multi-ingredient:** ***Fr.:*** Acarcid; Euvanol†; ***Ital.:*** Air Citronella; Dentosan Azione Intensiva; Dentosan Mese; Mistick Verde; Natural Zanzy†; Otosan Natural Ear Drops; Sanaderm†; Vapor Flay†; ***NZ:*** Mr Nits; ***UK:*** Medicated Extract of Rosemary; Nostroline; Teenstick.

## Germanium

Germanio.

Ge = 72.64.

*CAS — 7440-56-4.*

### Profile

Germanium compounds have been used in dietary supplements promoted as beneficial in a wide range of conditions including cancer, chronic fatigue syndrome, and immunodeficiency disorders. However, germanium compounds can produce severe renal damage and their use should be discouraged.

Germanium has also been used in dental alloys and has various industrial uses.

**Effects on the kidneys.** In the UK the Department of Health has recommended that germanium should not be taken as a dietary supplement due to a significant incidence of renal toxicity. There have been a number of reports of severe renal damage, including fatalities, resulting from germanium ingestion.

References.

1. Okada K, *et al.* Renal failure caused by long-term use of a germanium preparation as an elixir. *Clin Nephrol* 1989; **31:** 219–24.
2. van der Spoel JI, *et al.* Dangers of dietary germanium supplements. *Lancet* 1990; **336:** 117. Correction. *ibid.* 1991; **337:** 864.
3. Schauss AG. Nephrotoxicity in humans by the ultratrace element germanium. *Ren Fail* 1991; **13:** 1–4.
4. Hess B, *et al.* Tubulointerstitial nephropathy persisting 20 months after discontinuation of chronic intake of germanium lactate citrate. *Am J Kidney Dis* 1993; **21:** 548–52.
5. Tao SH, Bolger PM. Hazard assessment of germanium supplements. *Regul Toxicol Pharmacol* 1997; **25:** 211–19.
6. Swennen B, *et al.* Epidemiological survey of workers exposed to inorganic germanium compounds. *Occup Environ Med* 2000; **57:** 242–8.

## Ginkgo Biloba

EGB-761; Fossil Tree; GBE-761; Ginkgo biloba; Kew Tree; Maidenhair Tree; *Salisburia adiantifolia.*

*ATC — N06DX02.*

**Pharmacopoeias.** In *Chin.* and *Eur.* (see p.vi). Also in *USNF.*

**Ph. Eur. 5.0** (Ginkgo Leaf). The whole or fragmented dried leaf of *Ginkgo biloba* containing not less than 0.5% of flavonoids, calculated as flavone glycosides with reference to the dried drug. The leaf is greyish or yellowish-green or yellowish-brown.

**USNF 22** (Ginkgo). The dried leaf of *Ginkgo biloba* (Ginkgoaceae) containing not less than 0.5% of flavonoids, calculated as flavonol glycosides, with a mean molecular mass of 756.7, and not less than 0.1% of terpene lactones, both on the dried basis. The leaf is khaki green to greenish-brown. Protect from light and moisture.

### Adverse Effects

Adverse effects include headaches, dizziness, palpitations, gastrointestinal disturbances, bleeding disorders, and skin hypersensitivity reactions.

**Poisoning.** Reports[1,2] of convulsions induced by ingestion of large amounts of ginkgo seeds. Convulsions were thought to be due to the presence of 4-metoxypyridoxine, a competitive antagonist of pyridoxine; administration of suitable quantities of a vitamin-$B_6$ source may be of benefit in preventing such convulsions.[2]

1. Miwa H, *et al.* Generalized convulsions after consuming a large amount of gingko nuts. *Epilepsia* 2001; **42:** 280–1.
2. Kajiyama Y, *et al.* Ginkgo seed poisoning. *Pediatrics* 2002; **109:** 325–7.

### Interactions

It has been suggested that *Ginkgo biloba* should be used with caution in patients receiving anticoagulants or drugs that affect platelet aggregation.

### Uses and Administration

An extract from the leaves of *Ginkgo biloba* has been used in cerebrovascular and peripheral vascular disorders. It is also being investigated in Alzheimer's disease, multi-infarct dementia, and in tinnitus. *Ginkgo biloba* is used in homoeopathic medicine.

*Ginkgo biloba* is a source of ginkgolides (below).

**Dementia.** *Ginkgo biloba* extracts have been tried in the treatment of dementia including Alzheimer's disease (p.1484). Meta-analyses[1-3] have found the extracts to be more effective than placebo but the authors of all analyses commented that further investigation is needed to establish any clinical value.

1. Oken BS, *et al.* The efficacy of ginkgo biloba on cognitive function in Alzheimer disease. *Arch Neurol* 1998; **55:** 1409–15.
2. Ernst E, Pittler MH. Ginkgo biloba for dementia: a systematic review of double-blind, placebo-controlled trials. *Clin Drug Invest* 1999; **17:** 301–8.
3. Birks J, Grimley Evans J. Ginkgo biloba for cognitive impairment and dementia. Available in The Cochrane Library; Issue 2. Chichester: John Wiley; 2004.

**Peripheral vascular disorders.** *Ginkgo biloba* extracts have been tried in the treatment of peripheral vascular disorders (p.831). A meta-analysis[1] found the extracts to be more effective than placebo in the symptomatic treatment of intermittent claudication, although the authors considered the size of the effect to be modest and of uncertain clinical relevance.

1. Pittler MH, Ernst E. Ginkgo biloba extract for the treatment of intermittent claudication: a meta-analysis of randomized trials. *Am J Med* 2000; **108:** 276–81.

**Tinnitus.** *Ginkgo biloba* extracts have been tried in the treatment of tinnitus (p.1381). A systematic review[1] of 5 randomised controlled trials cautiously concluded that these results were favourable, although a later double-blind placebo-controlled study[2] failed to show benefit.

1. Ernst E, Stevinson C. Ginkgo biloba for tinnitus: a review. *Clin Otolaryngol* 1999; **24:** 164–7.
2. Drew S, Davies E. Effectiveness of Ginkgo biloba in treating tinnitus: double blind, placebo controlled trial. *BMJ* 2001; **322:** 73.

## Preparations

**Proprietary Preparations** (details are given in Part 3)

***Arg.:*** Clarvix; Herbaccion Cerebral; Kalter; Tanakan; ***Austral.:*** Progink-go†; Tavonin; ***Austria:*** Cerebokan; Ceremin; Gingohexal; Gingol; Tebofortan; Tebonin; ***Belg.:*** Memfit; ***Braz.:*** Clibium; Dinaton; Equitam; Gibilon; Ginbiloba; Gincolin; Ginkoba; Ginkobil†; Ginkoplus; Kiadon; Kirsan; Mensana; Tanakan; Tebonin; ***Chile:*** Kiadon; Ment Vital; Nokatar; Rokan; Tebokan; ***Fr.:*** Ginkogink; Tanakan; Tramisal; ***Ger.:*** Duogink; Gingiloba; Gingium; Gingobeta; Gingopret; Ginkobil; Ginkodilat; Ginkopur; Isoginkgo; Kaveri; Rokan; Tebonin; ***Hong Kong:*** Ebamin; Exormin†; Tanakan; ***Ital.:*** Ginkoba; Novel Ginkgo; ***Malaysia:*** Gincare; Ginkocer; Memocap; Tanakan; ***Mex.:*** Tanakan; Tebonin; Vasodil; ***Neth.:*** Tavonin; ***Port.:*** Abolibe; Biloban; Gincoben; Vasactife; ***Singapore:*** Gincare; Ginexin-F; Ginkapran; Ginkosen; Oxivel†; Tanakan; Tebokan†; ***Spain:*** Fitokey Ginkgo; Normocir; Tanakene; ***Switz.:*** Demonatur Ginkgo; Geriaforce; Gingosol; Ginkoba†; Oxivel; Symfona N; Tanakene; Tebofortin; Tebokan; Valverde Vitalite; ***Thai.:*** Tanakan; ***UK:*** Ginkovital; Mentor†; ***USA:*** BioGinkgo.

**Multi-ingredient: *Arg.:*** Flebitol; Garcinol Max; Top Life Memory; Venoful; ***Austral.:*** Bilberry Plus Eye Health†; Bioglan Fingers & Toes†; Bioglan Vision-Eze†; Bioglan Zellulean with Escin†; Extralife Extra-Brite†; Extralife Eye-Care†; Extralife Leg-Care†; Eye Health Herbal Plus Formula 4†; For Peripheral Circulation Herbal Plus Formula 5†; Gingo A†; Ginkgo Biloba Plus†; Ginkgo Complex†; Ginkgo Plus Herbal Plus Formula 10†; Ginzing G†; Herbal Arthritis Formula†; Herbal Capillary Care†; Lifechange Circulation Aid†; Lifechange Multi Plus Antioxidant†; Lifesystem Herbal Formula 6 For Peripheral Circulation†; Lifesystem Herbal Plus Formula 11 Ginkgo†; Lifesystem Herbal Plus Formula 5 Eye Relief†; Prophthal†; Vig†; ***Braz.:*** Composto Anticelulitico†; Derm'attive Solaire; Traumed; ***Canad.:*** Ginkoba M/E; ***Chile:*** Gincosan; Gingo-Ther; Mentania; ***Fr.:*** Ginkor; Ginkor Fort; Parogencyl anti-age gencives; ***Ger.:*** Perivar; Veno-Tebonin N; ***Hong Kong:*** Ginkgo Plus Vivo-Livo; Ginkgo-PS; Ginkor Fort; ***Ital.:*** Alvear Sport†; Angioton; Enertonic†; Forticrin; Ginkgo Plus†; Ginkoftal; Ginkoret; Memoactive; Memorandum; Nosenil†; Nutrex†; Pik-Gel†; Pollingel con Ginkgo Biloba; Pulsalux; Varicoft; Vasobrain; Vasopt; Vertigingo; ***Malaysia:*** Cerestar; Ginkor Fort; ***Singapore:*** Memoloba; ***Switz.:*** Allium Plus; Arterosan Plus; Capsules-vital; Gincosan; ***Thai.:*** Ginkor Fort; ***USA:*** Dorofen; Gentaplex.

# Ginkgolides

Ginkgólidos.

*CAS — 15291-75-5 (ginkgolide A); 15291-77-7 (ginkgolide B); 15291-76-6 (ginkgolide C).*

**Description.** Ginkgolides A, B, and C (BN-52020, BN-52021, and BN-52022 respectively) are isolated from *Ginkgo biloba* (Ginkgoaceae) (see above).

## Profile

Ginkgolides are terpenoid molecules isolated from *Ginkgo biloba* (above), with platelet-activating factor (PAF) antagonist properties. They have been investigated as BN-52063, a mixture of ginkgolides A (BN-52020), B (BN-52021), and C (BN-52022), for asthma and other inflammatory and allergic disorders, and also in immune disorders such as endotoxic shock and graft rejection; ginkgolide B, which has the most potent PAF antagonist properties, has been investigated in similar conditions administered alone.

Other ginkgolides, including ginkgolide M (BN-52023) and ginkgolide J (BN-52024), have also been identified.

◊ References.


1. Braquet P. The ginkgolides: potent platelet- activating factor antagonists isolated from Ginkgo biloba L: chemistry, pharmacology and clinical applications. *Drugs Of The Future* 1987; **12:** 643–99.
2. Chung KF, *et al.* Effect of a ginkgolide mixture (BN 52063) in antagonising skin and platelet responses to platelet activating factor in man. *Lancet* 1987; **i:** 248–51.
3. Roberts NM, *et al.* Effect of a PAF antagonist, BN52063, on PAF-induced bronchoconstriction in normal subjects. *Br J Clin Pharmacol* 1988; **26:** 65–72.
4. Kleijnen J, Knipschild P. Ginkgo biloba. *Lancet* 1992; **340:** 1136–9.
5. Houghton P. Ginkgo. *Pharm J* 1994; **253:** 122–3.


# Ginseng

Ginseng Radix; Jintsam; Ninjin; Panax; Pannag; Renshen; Schinsent.

**Description.** Ginseng is the dried root of *Panax ginseng* (*P. schinseng*) (Araliaceae). Other varieties of ginseng include *Panax quinquefolius* (American Ginseng) and *P. pseudoginseng*. The root commonly known as Siberian or Russian ginseng belongs to the same family, Araliaceae, but is an entirely different plant, *Eleutherococcus senticosus* (see Siberian Ginseng, p.1744). Brazilian ginseng is reported to be derived from another unrelated plant, *Pfaffia paniculata*.

Ginseng contains complex mixtures of saponins termed ginsenosides or panaxosides. At least 13 saponins have been isolated from extracts of *P. ginseng* roots.

**Pharmacopoeias.** In *Chin., Eur.* (see p.vi), and *Jpn*. Also in *USNF* (as Asian Ginseng and American Ginseng). *USNF* includes additionally powdered forms of these two varieties of ginseng.

*Jpn* also includes Red Ginseng, the dried root of *P. ginseng* which has been steamed.

*Chin.* and *Jpn* also include Rhizoma Panacis Japonica from *Panax japonicus*. *Chin.* also includes Radix Notoginseng from *P. notoginseng*, and Rhizoma Panacis Majoris from *P. japonicus* var. *major* and *P. japonicus* var. *bipinnatifidus*.

**Ph. Eur. 5.0** (Ginseng). The whole or cut dried root of *Panax ginseng*. It contains not less than 0.4% of combined ginsenosides,
Rg1 ($C_{42}H_{72}O_{14}$,$2H_2O$ = 837.0) and
Rb1 ($C_{54}H_{92}O_{23}$,$3H_2O$ = 1163.3),
calculated with reference to the dried drug. Protect from light.

**USNF 22** (Asian Ginseng). The dried roots of *Panax ginseng* (Araliaceae). It contains not less than 0.2% of ginsenoside $Rg_1$ and not less than 0.1% of ginsenoside $Rb_1$, both calculated on the dried basis. Store in a dry place at a temperature of 8° to 15°.

**USNF 22** (American Ginseng). The dried roots of *Panax quinquefolius* (Araliaceae). It contains not less than 4.0% of total ginsenosides, calculated on the dried basis. Store in airtight containers. Protect from light and heat.

## Adverse Effects

◊ A 2-year study[1] of ginseng in 133 subjects who had used a wide variety of commercial preparations including roots, capsules, tablets, teas, extracts, cigarettes, chewing gum, and candies reported that the majority of preparations were taken by mouth, but a few subjects had experimented with intranasal and parenteral routes, and topical preparations had also been used. The stimulant effects of ginseng were confirmed but there was also a high incidence of side-effects including 47 cases of morning diarrhoea, 33 of skin eruptions, 26 of sleeplessness, 25 of nervousness, 22 of hypertension, 18 of euphoria, and 14 of oedema. The 'ginseng abuse syndrome' defined as hypertension together with nervousness, sleeplessness, skin eruptions, and morning diarrhoea was experienced by 14 subjects who took ginseng by mouth in an average daily dose of 3 g. Abrupt withdrawal precipitated hypotension, weakness, and tremor in 1 user. About 50% of the subjects had discontinued the use of ginseng within the 2 years. Oestrogenic effects have also been reported from the use of ginseng,[2-4] and a case of Stevens-Johnson syndrome has also occurred.[5]

A systematic review[6] of some of these and other studies and case reports concluded that single-ingredient preparations of ginseng were well tolerated when data from clinical trials were examined. Adverse effects were generally mild and reversible, the most common being headache, sleep disturbances, and gastrointestinal disorders. It was more difficult to determine causality from the evidence given in isolated case reports; likewise, interpretation of data involving combination products was difficult.


1. Siegel RK. Ginseng abuse syndrome: problems with the panacea. *JAMA* 1979; **241:** 1614–15.
2. Palmer BV, *et al.* Gin Seng and mastalgia. *BMJ* 1978; **1:** 1284.
3. Punnonen R, Lukola A. Oestrogen-like effect of ginseng. *BMJ* 1980; **281:** 1110.
4. Greenspan EM. Ginseng and vaginal bleeding. *JAMA* 1983; **249:** 2018.
5. Dega H, *et al.* Ginseng as a cause for Stevens-Johnson syndrome? *Lancet* 1996; **347:** 1344.
6. Coon JT, Ernst E. Panax ginseng: a systematic review of adverse effects and drug interactions. *Drug Safety* 2002; **25:** 323–44.


## Interactions

◊ For reports of interactions between *phenelzine* and ginseng, see p.315. For details of an interaction between *warfarin* and ginseng, see p.1027. For a suggestion that ginseng may interfere with *digoxin* assays, see p.896.

## Uses and Administration

Ginseng is reported to enhance the natural resistance and recuperative power of the body and to reduce fatigue. It is available commercially as roots, powdered roots, tablets, capsules, teas, oils, or extracts.

## Preparations

***USNF 22:*** Asian Ginseng Tablets.

**Proprietary Preparations** (details are given in Part 3)

***Arg.:*** Ginsana; Herbaccion Bioenergizante; Juvitan; Transformal; Vitagenol; ***Austral.:*** Ginzing†; Herbal Stress Relief†; ***Austria:*** Ginsana; ***Belg.:*** Ginsana; ***Braz.:*** Ginsana; Ginsex; ***Canad.:*** Ginsana; ***Fr.:*** Gerimax Tonique; Ginsana; Ginsatonic†; ***Ger.:*** Ardey-aktiv; Coriosta Vitaltonikum N; Gerivit†; Ginroy†; Ginsana; Herz-Punkt Starkungstonikum mit Ginseng N†; Hevert-Aktivon Mono; Kneipp Ginsenetten†; Orgaplasma; ***Ital.:*** Gi-Sen; Ginsana; Novel 1000†; ***Malaysia:*** Ginsana; ***Mex.:*** Gincaps; Sanjin Royal Jelly; ***Port.:*** Ginsana; Neo Vitalisan†; ***S.Afr.:*** Ginsana†; ***Singapore:*** Ginsana; ***Spain:*** Bio Star; Ginsana; ***Switz.:*** Ginsana; ***Thai.:*** Ginsana; Ginsroy; ***UK:*** Korseng; Red Kooga.

**Multi-ingredient: *Arg.:*** Inteligen Ginseng; Optimina Plus; Top Life Memory; ***Austral.:*** Bioglan Ginsynergy†; Extralife Extra-Brite†; Ginkgo Biloba Plus†; Ginkgo Complex†; Ginzing E†; Ginzing G†; Glycyrrhiza Complex†; Infant Tonic†; Irontona†; Nervatona Plus†; Panax Complex†; Trillium Complex†; Vig†; Vitatona†; ***Braz.:*** Gerin; Poliseng; ***Canad.:*** Damiana-Sarsaparilla Formula; Energy Plus; Ginkoba M/E; ***Chile:*** Gincosan; Mentania; ***Fr.:*** Actisane Fatigue Passagere†; Gintonal; Nostress; Toncatil; Tonisan†; ***Ger.:*** Alsiroyal†; Cardibisana; Ginseng-Complex "Schuh"; Hypercard†; Peking Ginseng Royal Jelly N; Schwedentrunk mit Ginseng†; ***Hong Kong:*** GinsengSure; ***Ital.:*** Alvear con Ginseng; Apergan; Bio-Real Complex†; Bio-Real Plus†; Bioton; Cocktail Reale†; Fitostress†; Fon Wan Ginsenergy; Fon Wan Pocket Energy†; Fon Wan Pollen†; Forticrin; Fosfarsile Forte; Four-Ton; Gincola†; Ginsana Ton; Neoplus; Ottovis; Pollingel Ginseng; ***Malaysia:*** 30 Plus; Adult Citrex Multivitamin + Ginseng + Omega 3; Cerestar; ***S.Afr.:*** Activex 40 Plus; ***Spain:*** Energysor; Esforza; Farmacola†; Minadex Mix Ginseng†; Ton Was; Vigortonic; ***Switz.:*** Biorganic Geri†; Biovital Ginseng; Burgerstein TopVital; Geri; Gincosan; Imuvit; Supradyn Vital 50+; Tai Ginseng N†; Vigoran; ***Thai.:*** Imugins; Imuvit†; Multilim RG; Revitan; ***UK:*** Red Kooga Co-Q-10 and Ginseng; Regina Royal Concorde.

# Glatiramer Acetate *(BAN, USAN)*

COP-1; Copolymer 1; Glatiramer, acetato de. L-Glutamic acid polymer with L-alanine, L-lysine and L-tyrosine, acetate.

*CAS — 28704-27-0; 147245-92-9.*
*ATC — L03AX13.*

## Adverse Effects and Precautions

The most commonly seen side-effects following injection of glatiramer acetate are chest pain, palpitations or tachycardia, dyspnoea, asthenia, flushing (vasodilatation), nausea, arthralgia, hypertonia, and anxiety. Many of these occur as an immediate post-injection reaction. Convulsions and anaphylactoid reactions have been reported rarely. Antibodies to the drug develop with chronic therapy but are of unknown clinical significance. Pain, erythema, pruritus, and induration may occur at the injection site.

Glatiramer acetate should be given with caution to patients with pre-existing cardiac disorders; such patients should be followed up regularly during treatment.

◊ References.


1. Ziemssen T, *et al.* Risk-benefit assessment of glatiramer acetate in multiple sclerosis. *Drug Safety* 2001; **24:** 979–90.


**Effects on the skin.** Localised lipoatrophy at the injection site developed in 6 patients receiving glatiramer acetate.[1]


1. Drago F, *et al.* Localized lipoatrophy after glatiramer acetate injection in patients with remitting-relapsing multiple sclerosis. *Arch Dermatol* 1999; **135:** 1277–8.


## Interactions

The UK manufacturer reports that an increased incidence of injection-site reactions to glatiramer acetate has been seen in patients receiving corticosteroids concurrently.

## Uses and Administration

Glatiramer acetate, a random polymer of L-alanine, L-glutamic acid, L-lysine, and L-tyrosine, is a peptide that has some structural resemblance to myelin basic protein, and is used to reduce the frequency of relapses in the management of relapsing-remitting multiple sclerosis (p.646). It is administered by subcutaneous injection in a dose of 20 mg daily. It should not be given by the intravenous or intramuscular route. An oral formulation is under investigation.

**Multiple sclerosis.** References.[1-8] A systematic review failed to find evidence to support the routine use of glatiramer acetate in multiple sclerosis.[8]


1. La Mantia L, *et al.* Meta-analysis of clinical trials with copolymer 1 in multiple sclerosis. *Eur Neurol* 2000; **43:** 189–93.
2. Anonymous. Glatiramer acetate for multiple sclerosis. *Drug Ther Bull* 2001; **39:** 41–3.
3. Francis DA. Glatiramer acetate (Copaxone). *Int J Clin Pract* 2001; **55:** 394–8.
4. Sela M, Teitelbaum D. Glatiramer acetate in the treatment of multiple sclerosis. *Expert Opin Pharmacother* 2001; **2:** 1149–65.
5. Simpson D, *et al.* Glatiramer acetate: a review of its use in relapsing-remitting multiple sclerosis. *CNS Drugs* 2002; **16:** 825–50.
6. Dhib-Jalbut S. Glatiramer acetate (Copaxone) therapy for multiple sclerosis. *Pharmacol Ther* 2003; **98:** 245–55.
7. Boneschi FM, *et al.* Effects of glatiramer acetate on relapse rate and accumulated disability in multiple sclerosis: meta-analysis of three double-blind, randomized, placebo-controlled clinical trials. *Multiple Sclerosis* 2003; **9:** 349–55.
8. Munari L, *et al.* Therapy with glatiramer acetate for multiple sclerosis. Available in The Cochrane Library; Issue 2. Chichester: John Wiley; 2004.


## Preparations

**Proprietary Preparations** (details are given in Part 3)

***Arg.:*** Copaxone; ***Austral.:*** Copaxone; ***Braz.:*** Copaxone; ***Canad.:*** Copaxone; ***Denm.:*** Copaxone; ***Fin.:*** Copaxone; ***Irl.:*** Copaxone; ***Israel:*** Copaxone; ***Ital.:*** Copaxone; ***Neth.:*** Copaxone; ***Norw.:*** Copaxone; ***Port.:*** Copaxone; ***Spain:*** Copaxone; ***Swed.:*** Copaxone; ***Switz.:*** Copaxone; ***UK:*** Copaxone; ***USA:*** Copaxone.

# Glicofosfopeptical

Fosfoglicopeptical.

## Profile

Glicofosfopeptical is reported to possess immunostimulant properties and has been given in doses of 1 g by mouth every eight hours.

## Preparations

**Proprietary Preparations** (details are given in Part 3)

***Mex.:*** Inmunoferon†; Inmunol; ***Port.:*** Imunoferon; ***Spain:*** Inmunoferon.

# Glucomannan

E425; Glucomanano; Konjac Flour; Konjac Mannan.

## Profile

Glucomannan, a powdered extract from the tubers of *Amorphophallus konjac*, has been promoted as an anorectic. It has been claimed to reduce the appetite by absorbing liquid in the gastrointestinal tract. It is also used in the treatment of constipation and hyperlipidaemia. Glucomannan has been investigated as a dietary adjunct in the management of diabetes mellitus.

There is a risk of intestinal or oesophageal obstruction and faecal impaction, especially if it is swallowed dry. Therefore, it should always be taken with sufficient fluid and should not be taken immediately before going to bed. It should be avoided in patients who have difficulty swallowing.

◊ References.

1. Henry DA, *et al.* Glucomannan and risk of oesophageal obstruction. *BMJ* 1986; **292:** 591–2.
2. Renard E, *et al.* Noninsulin-dependent diabetes and glucose intolerance: effect of glucomannan fibre on blood glucose and serum insulin. *Sem Hop Paris* 1991; **67:** 153–7.
3. Vuksan V, *et al.* Beneficial effects of viscous dietary fiber from konjac-mannan in subjects with the insulin resistance syndrome: results of a controlled metabolic trial. *Diabetes Care* 2000; **23:** 9–14.
4. Staiano A, *et al.* Effect of the dietary fiber glucomannan on chronic constipation in neurologically impaired children. *J Pediatr* 2000; **136:** 41–5.

## Preparations

**Proprietary Preparations** (details are given in Part 3)

***Arg.:*** Modekal; ***Chile:*** Redicres Rapido; ***Fr.:*** Konjax†; Muraligne; ***India:*** Dietmann; ***Ital.:*** Dicoplus; Dietoman; NormaLine; ***Mex.:*** Dietoman; Esbeltex; ***Port.:*** Bioregime; Florilax.

**Multi-ingredient:** ***Arg.:*** KLB6 Fruit Diet; ***Fr.:*** AMK†; Filigel; ***Ital.:*** Dimalosio†; Ecamannan; Fibrovit†; Glucoman; Lactomannan; ***Port.:*** Bioregime Fort; Bioregime SlimKit.

---

# Glucosamine *(USAN, rINN)*

Chitosamine; Glucosamina; NSC-758. 2-Amino-2-deoxy-β-D-glucopyranose.

$C_6H_{13}NO_5$ = 179.2.

*CAS — 3416-24-8.*

*ATC — M01AX05.*

**Pharmacopoeias.** *USNF* includes Glucosamine Hydrochloride, Glucosamine Sulfate Potassium Chloride, and Glucosamine Sulfate Sodium Chloride.

## Profile

Glucosamine is a natural substance found in chitin, mucoproteins, and mucopolysaccharides. It is involved in the manufacture of glycosaminoglycan, which forms cartilage tissue in the body; glucosamine is also present in tendons and ligaments. Glucosamine must be synthesised by the body but the ability to do this declines with age. Glucosamine and its salts have therefore been advocated in the treatment of rheumatic disorders including osteoarthritis. Glucosamine may be isolated from chitin or prepared synthetically; glucosamine sulfate and hydriodide, have also been used.

**Effects on glucose metabolism.** Glucosamine has a role in glucose metabolism, increasing insulin resistance in skeletal muscle,[1,2] which has raised concerns about its safety profile in diabetic patients.[3] However, alteration of glycaemic homoeostasis was not demonstrated in a 3-year randomised controlled trial in patients without diabetes.[4]

1. Adams ME. Hype about glucosamine. *Lancet* 1999; **354:** 353–4.
2. Chan NN, *et al.* Drug-related hyperglycemia. *JAMA* 2002; **287:** 714–15.
3. Chan NN, *et al.* Glucosamine sulphate and osteoarthritis. *Lancet* 2001; **357:** 1618–9.
4. Reginster JY, *et al.* Long-term effects of glucosamine sulphate on osteoarthritis progression: a randomised, placebo-controlled clinical trial. *Lancet* 2001; **357:** 251–6.

**Osteoarthritis.** Glucosamine and its salts are widely available as licensed products or so-called 'health supplements' used for the management of osteoarthritis; it may be combined with other substances supposed to be of benefit, including chondroitin, vitamins, and various herbs. A systematic review[1] of the use of glucosamine for osteoarthritis (p.9) has concluded that it is generally both safe and superior to placebo, but that further research is still necessary to confirm its long-term value, and particularly its long-term toxicity. Similarly, meta-analyses[2,3] of randomised placebo-controlled studies concluded that while there was some evidence for efficacy of glucosamine and chondroitin in the treatment of osteoarthritis, methodological flaws and publication bias had led to exaggeration of its potential benefit,[2] and that further studies are needed to fully characterise their disease-modifying properties.[3]

1. Towheed TE, *et al.* Glucosamine therapy for treating osteoarthritis. Available in The Cochrane Library; Issue 2. Chichester: John Wiley; 2004.
2. McAlindon TE, *et al.* Glucosamine and chondroitin for treatment of osteoarthritis: a systematic quality assessment and meta-analysis. *JAMA* 2000; **283:** 1469–75.
3. Richy F, *et al.* Structural and symptomatic efficacy of glucosamine and chondroitin in knee osteoarthritis: a comprehensive meta-analysis. *Arch Intern Med* 2003; **163:** 1514–22.

## Preparations

**Proprietary Preparations** (details are given in Part 3)

***Arg.:*** Adaxil; Artrilase; Baliartrin; Belmalen Plus; Mecanyl; Ostatac; Vartalon Complemento; ***Braz.:*** Dinaflex; ***Chile:*** Artridol; Bioflex; Dinaflex; Viartril; ***Ger.:*** Dona 200-S; Progona†; ***Hong Kong:*** MarinEx; Viartril S; Viartril†; ***Irl.:*** Dona; ***Ital.:*** Dona; Viartril S; ***Malaysia:*** Viartril S; ***Mex.:*** Vartalon; Viartril; ***Port.:*** Viartril S; ***Singapore:*** Artril; Glutilage; Kudona; Viartril S; Vital; ***Spain:*** Cartisorb; Hespercorbin; Xicil; ***Thai.:*** Viartril.

**Multi-ingredient:** ***Arg.:*** Asotrex; ***Austral.:*** Bioglan Joint Mobility†; ***Chile:*** Dinaflex Duo; Hiperflex; ***Hong Kong:*** Procosamine; ***Ital.:*** Artrosan†; Joint Support; ***Singapore:*** Articolase (w/glucosamine); Flexeze; ***Spain:*** Anartril†; ***UK:*** BackOsamine; Healtheries Musseltone & Glucosamine; Joint Action; Jointace; ***USA:*** Dorofen.

---

# Glucose Oxidase

Corylophyline; β-D-Glucopyranose aerodehydrogenase; Glucosa oxidasa; Microcide; Notatin; P-FAD.

*CAS — 9001-37-0.*

## Profile

Glucose oxidase is an enzyme obtained from certain fungi which catalyses the oxidation of glucose to gluconic acid, with the concomitant production of hydrogen peroxide. It is used for its preservative properties as an additive in certain foods, sometimes in combination with catalase (p.1668). It is also used in fertility tests and tests of diabetic control. It has been used as an ingredient of toothpastes for its supposed benefits in the prophylaxis of dental caries.

## Preparations

**Proprietary Preparations** (details are given in Part 3)

**Multi-ingredient:** ***Braz.:*** Bromelin; Expectoral; ***Singapore:*** Biotene; ***UK:*** Biotene Dry Mouth; Biotene Oralbalance.

---

# Glucose Tests

Glucosa, pruebas de.

## Profile

Several tests are available so that patients with diabetes mellitus (p.324) can monitor their disease. Tests can be employed to detect the presence of glucose in the urine and some of the preparations are used to detect several substances in the urine. These tests are easy to carry out but are not considered reliable enough for insulin-dependent patients who should ideally check their blood-glucose concentrations using one of the available blood tests. Diabetic clinics often measure the degree of haemoglobin glycosylation as an indicator of mean blood-glucose control over a period of weeks or months.

Urine tests generally use either the copper-reduction method or the glucose-oxidase method and both produce a colour change in the presence of glucose. Blood tests generally use the glucose-oxidase method; they may be read visually or by means of a meter. A meter gives the more precise reading. Patients should be properly trained in the use of these tests and in the interpretation of the results; they should be aware that concomitant drug therapy might affect the result.

## Preparations

***USP 27:*** Glucose Enzymatic Test Strip.

**Proprietary Preparations** (details are given in Part 3)

***Arg.:*** Accutrend Glucosa; Dextrostix; Diastix; Glucometer Elite; Glucostix; Glucotide; Glucotrend; Glukotest; Haemo-Glukotest 20-800; One Touch; Precision Plus; ***Austral.:*** Accu-Chek; Accutrend Glucose; Advantage; Ascensia; Betachek; BM-Test BG; BM-Test Glycemie 20-800; Clinistix; Clinitest; Diabur-Test 5000; Diascreen Glucose; Diastix; Esprit; ExacTech; Excel ET†; Glucofilm†; Glucoflex-R; Glucometer; Glucostix; Glucostrip†; Glucotrend†; Medi-Test Glucose; MediSense Sof-Tact; Omnitest; Optium; Precision Plus; Tes-Tape; ***Braz.:*** Glico-Fita; ***Canad.:*** Accu-Check III/Chemstrip bG†; Accutrend GC; Advantage; Chemstrip bG†; Chemstrip uG; Clinistix†; Clinitest; Companion 2†; Diastix; Glucofilm†; Glucostix†; Tes-Tape; ***Chile:*** Accu-Chek; Accutrend Glucosa; Glukotest; ***Fr.:*** Accu-Chek†; BM-Test Glycemie; Clinistix; Clinitest; Dextrostix†; Glucofilm†; Glucostix†; Glucotide; One Touch; Tracer Glucose†; ***India:*** Diastix; ***Irl.:*** BM-Accutest; BM-Test 1-44; Clinistix; Clinitest; Combina Glucose; Compact; Dextrostix†; Diabur-Test 5000; Diastix; Glucomen; Glucometer Elite; Glucostix; Glucotide; Glucotrend†; Hypoguard; Medisense; One Touch; PocketScan; Tes-Tape†; ***Israel:*** Clinistix; Clinitest; ***Ital.:*** Accu-Chek; Accutrend Glucose; BM-Test BG†; Clinistix; Clinitest; Dextrostix†; Diabur-Test 5000; Diastix; Glico Test†; Glico Urine B†; Glucofilm; Glucometer; Glucosan; Glucostix; Glucotrend; Glukurtest; Haemoglukotest 20-800; Reflocheck†; Tes-Tape†; Uni-Check; ***Mex.:*** Accutrend Glucose; Clinitest; Dextrostix; Diabur-Test 5000; Diastix; Gluco-Cinta; Glucostix; Glucotide; Haemo-Glukotest 20-800; ***NZ:*** Accutrend Glucose; Advantage; BM-Test 1-44; Clinistix; Clinitest; Diabur-5000; Diastix; Exatech†; Glucocard; Glucofilm†; Glucometer Elite; Glucometer Esprit; Glucostix; Precision Plus; Tes-Tape†; ***Port.:*** Clinistix; Elite; Euroflash; Glucocard; Glucostix†; Glucotouch; One Touch; ***S.Afr.:*** Tes-Tape†; ***Switz.:*** Tes-Tape†; ***UK:*** Ascensia Glucodisc; BM-Accutest; BM-Test 1-44; BM-Test BG†; Clinistix; Clinitest; Diabur-Test 5000; Diastix; Easistix BG†; Easistix UG†; Exactech; Glucostix; Glucotide; Hypoguard Supreme Plus; Medi-Test Glucose; Medi-Test Glycaemie C; Medisense G2; ***USA:*** Accu-Check Advantage; Chemstrip bG; Chemstrip uG; Clinistix; Clinitest; Dextrostix†; Diascan; Diastix; First Choice; Glucofilm; Glucostix; One Touch.

---

# Gluten

## Profile

Gluten is a mixture of 2 proteins, gliadin and glutenin, and is present in wheat flour and to a lesser extent in barley and rye. Gliadin is a prolamine, one of the 2 chief groups of plant proteins, and glutenin belongs to the other main group termed glutelins.

Gluten is of medicinal and pharmaceutical interest in that patients with coeliac disease (p.1417) are sensitive to the gliadin fraction of gluten contained in the normal diet. Treatment consists of the use of gluten-free diets; gluten-free foods are available.

A gluten-free diet may also be beneficial in patients with dermatitis herpetiformis (p.1134).

---

# Glycerol *(rINN)*

E422; Glicerol; Glycerin; Glycerine; Glycerolum. Propane-1,2,3-triol.

$C_3H_8O_3$ = 92.09.

*CAS — 56-81-5.*

*ATC — A06AG04; A06AX01.*

**Pharmacopoeias.** In *Chin., Eur.* (see p.vi), *Int., Jpn, US,* and *Viet.*

*Eur.* and *Int.* also include Glycerol (85 per cent).

*Pol.* includes Glycerol (86 per cent).

**Ph. Eur. 5.0** (Glycerol). A clear, colourless or almost colourless, very hygroscopic, syrupy liquid, unctuous to the touch. Miscible with water and with alcohol; slightly soluble in acetone; practically insoluble in fixed oils and in essential oils. Store in airtight containers.

**USP 27** (Glycerin). A clear, colourless, hygroscopic, syrupy liquid. Has not more than a slight characteristic odour, which is neither harsh nor disagreeable. Miscible with water and with alcohol; insoluble in chloroform, in ether, and in fixed and volatile oils. Its solutions are neutral to litmus. Store in airtight containers.

**Incompatibility.** Strong oxidising agents form explosive mixtures with glycerol. Black discoloration has been reported with glycerol and bismuth subnitrate or zinc oxide when exposed to light.

## Adverse Effects and Precautions

The adverse effects of glycerol are primarily due to its dehydrating action.

When taken by mouth glycerol may cause headache, nausea, and vomiting; diarrhoea, thirst, dizziness, and mental confusion may occur less frequently. Cardiac arrhythmias have been reported.

Glycerol increases plasma osmolality resulting in the withdrawal of water from the extravascular spaces. The consequent expansion of extracellular fluid, especially if sudden, can lead to circulatory overload, pulmonary oedema, and heart failure; glycerol must therefore be used with caution in patients at risk, such as those with hypervolaemia, cardiac failure, or renal disease. Severe dehydration can occur and glycerol should be used cautiously in dehydrated patients. Patients with diabetes mellitus may additionally develop hyperglycaemia and glycosuria following metabolism of glycerol. Nonketotic hyperosmolar hyperglycaemic coma is rare, but fatalities have been reported.

Haemolysis, haemoglobinuria, and acute renal failure have also been associated with glycerol when given intravenously (see Raised Intracranial Pressure, below).

Glycerol can cause irritation when given topically or rectally. A local anaesthetic may be used before application of glycerol to the cornea to reduce the likelihood of a painful response.

For incompatibilities with glycerol, including the risk of explosive mixtures, see above.

**Effects on the cardiovascular system.** A 73-year-old man, free of cardiac complaints but who had previously experienced an acute myocardial infarction, developed severe pulmonary oedema following the administration of glycerol by mouth for elevated intra-ocular pressure.[1] The necessity for detailed cardiac evaluation before the use of oral glycerol was emphasised.

1. Almog Y, *et al.* Pulmonary edema as a complication of oral glycerol administration. *Ann Ophthalmol* 1986; **18:** 38–9.

**Effects on the ears.** A 56-year-old man given 100 mL of glycerol and 100 mL of sodium chloride 0.9% as part of a test for Ménière's disease developed temporary hearing loss in the non-involved ear. Two previous reports of deterioration in hearing associated with the glycerol test were reviewed by the author.[1]

1. Mattox DE, Goode RL. Temporary loss of hearing after a glycerin test. *Arch Otolaryngol* 1978; **104:** 359–61.

**Effects on the eyes.** Caution in applying glycerol to the cornea has been recommended. Studies in *animals*[1] and in man[2] have indicated that the topical application of glycerol to the eye can damage the endothelial cells of the cornea.

1. Sherrard ES. The corneal endothelium in vivo: its response to mild trauma. *Exp Eye Res* 1976; **22:** 347–57.
2. Goldberg MH, *et al.* The effects of topically applied glycerin on the human corneal endothelium. *Cornea* 1982; **1:** 39–44.

**Hyperosmolar nonketotic coma.** Hyperosmolar nonketotic coma has been associated with the oral use of glycerol[1] and deaths have occurred.[2] The most susceptible patients are maturity-onset elderly diabetics with acute or chronic disease predisposing to fluid deprivation, and in these patients oral glycerol may be best avoided.[1] If glycerol is used in patients with predisposing conditions, adequate measures should be taken to recognise the development of hyperosmolar nonketotic hyperglycaemia and prevent dehydration.[1,2]

1. Oakley DE, Ellis PP. Glycerol and hyperosmolar nonketotic coma. *Am J Ophthalmol* 1976; **81:** 469–72.
2. Sears ES. Nonketotic hyperosmolar hyperglycemia during glycerol therapy for cerebral edema. *Neurology* 1976; **26:** 89–94.

## Pharmacokinetics

Glycerol is readily absorbed from the gastrointestinal tract and undergoes extensive metabolism, principally in the liver; it may be used in the synthesis of lipids, metabolised to glucose or glycogen, or oxidised to carbon dioxide and water. It may also be excreted in the urine unchanged.

◊ References.


1. Nahata MC, *et al.* Variations in glycerol kinetics in Reye's syndrome. *Clin Pharmacol Ther* 1981; **29:** 782–7.
2. Heinemeyer G. Clinical pharmacokinetic considerations in the treatment of increased intracranial pressure. *Clin Pharmacokinet* 1987; **13:** 1–25.


## Uses and Administration

Glycerol is an osmotic dehydrating agent with hygroscopic and lubricating properties. When given orally or parenterally, glycerol increases the plasma osmolality, resulting in the movement of water by osmosis from the extravascular spaces into the plasma.

Glycerol is given by mouth for the short-term reduction of vitreous volume and intra-ocular pressure before and after ophthalmic surgery, and as an adjunct in the management of acute glaucoma (p.1485). Its onset of action is rapid, with a maximal reduction in intra-ocular pressure occurring about 1 to 1½ hours after a dose; the duration of action is about 5 hours. The usual initial dose of glycerol is 1 to 1.8 g/kg given as a 50% solution. There can be problems of palatability when glycerol solutions are given orally; chilling or flavouring the solutions may help.

Glycerol may be applied topically to reduce corneal oedema, but as the effect is only transient its use is primarily limited to facilitating ocular examination and diagnosis. Glycerol eye drops can be painful on instillation and the prior application of a local anaesthetic has been recommended.

Glycerol has also been given by mouth or intravenously to reduce intracranial pressure (see below).

Glycerol may be used rectally as suppositories or a solution in single doses to promote faecal evacuation in the management of constipation (p.1240). It usually acts within 15 to 30 minutes. Glycerol is commonly classified as an osmotic laxative but may act additionally or alternatively through its local irritant effects; it may also have lubricating and faecal softening actions.

Glycerol is used as a demulcent in cough preparations (p.1112).

Glycerol has a wide range of applications in pharmaceutical formulation; these include its use as a vehicle and solvent, as a sweetening agent, as a preservative in some liquid medications, as a plasticiser in tablet film-coating, and as a tonicity adjuster. It is often included in topical preparations such as eye drops, creams, and lotions as a lubricant and also for its moisturising properties since, when absorbed, its hygroscopic action may enhance moisture retention. Ear drops for the removal of ear wax often contain glycerol as a lubricating and softening agent.

Glycerol is also used as a cryoprotectant in cryopreservation.

**Diagnosis of Ménière's disease.** Glycerol has been used[1] in the diagnosis of Ménière's disease (p.422) to distinguish potentially reversible cochlear dysfunction from the relatively irreversible pathology of advanced disease, or to predict the results of endolymphatic sac surgery. Glycerol is given by mouth to reduce the endolymphatic fluid volume and pressure and any transient improvement in hearing is measured. However, the side-effects of glycerol such as headache, nausea, and vomiting can be a problem and the test has been reported to have low sensitivity and to give false-positive results. See also under Effects on the Ears, above.


1. Skalabrin TA, Mangham CA. Analysis of the glycerin test for Meniere's disease. *Otolaryngol Head Neck Surg* 1987; **96:** 282–8.


**Raised intracranial pressure.** Glycerol has been given intravenously or by mouth for its osmotic diuretic effect to reduce cerebral oedema and hence decrease the intracranial pressure (p.833). It is also reported to be able to increase blood flow to areas of brain ischaemia. It has been used in a variety of clinical conditions[1] including cerebral infarction or stroke,[2] Reye's syndrome,[3] and meningitis;[4] it has been reported to be ineffective in hepatic coma.[5] Some patients have experienced serious adverse effects including haemolysis, haemoglobinuria, and renal failure.[6,7]


1. Frank MSB, *et al.* Glycerol: a review of its pharmacology, pharmacokinetics, adverse reactions, and clinical use. *Pharmacotherapy* 1981; **1:** 147–60.
2. Righetti E, *et al.* Glycerol for acute stroke. Available in The Cochrane Library; Issue 2. Chichester: John Wiley; 2004.
3. Nahata MC, *et al.* Variations in glycerol kinetics in Reye's syndrome. *Clin Pharmacol Ther* 1981; **29:** 782–7.
4. Kilpi T, *et al.* Oral glycerol and intravenous dexamethasone in preventing neurologic and audiologic sequelae of childhood bacterial meningitis. *Pediatr Infect Dis J* 1995; **14:** 270–8.
5. Record CO, *et al.* Glycerol therapy for cerebral oedema complicating fulminant hepatic failure. *BMJ* 1975; **ii:** 540.
6. Hägnevik K, *et al.* Glycerol-induced haemolysis with haemoglobinuria and acute renal failure: report of three cases. *Lancet* 1974; **i:** 75–7.
7. Welch KMA, *et al.* Glycerol-induced haemolysis. *Lancet* 1974; **i:** 416–17.


**Trigeminal neuralgia.** Selective destruction of pain-bearing nerves is reserved for patients who do not respond to conventional drug therapy for trigeminal neuralgia (p.8). This may be achieved by the instillation of glycerol among the trigeminal rootlets (percutaneous retrogasserian glycerol rhizolysis).[1-5] The efficacy and safety of this procedure have been debated,[1,4] but some centres report good long-term results in the majority of patients.[5] It has been suggested that variations in viscosity and osmolality may influence results.[2]


1. Sweet WH. The treatment of trigeminal neuralgia (tic douloureux). *N Engl J Med* 1986; **315:** 174–7.
2. Waltz TA, Copeland BR. Treatment of trigeminal neuralgia. *N Engl J Med* 1987; **316:** 693.
3. Young RF. Glycerol rhizolysis for treatment of trigeminal neuralgia. *J Neurosurg* 1988; **69:** 39–45.
4. Burchiel KJ. Percutaneous retrogasserian glycerol rhizolysis in the management of trigeminal neuralgia. *J Neurosurg* 1988; **69:** 361–6.
5. Jho H-D, Lunsford LD. Percutaneous retrogasserian glycerol rhizotomy: current technique and results. *Neurosurg Clin N Am* 1997; **8:** 63–74.


### Preparations

***BP 2003:*** Glycerol Eye Drops; Glycerol Suppositories; Phenol and Glycerol Injection;
***USP 27:*** Calamine Lotion; Glycerin Ophthalmic Solution; Glycerin Oral Solution; Glycerin Suppositories.

**Proprietary Preparations** (details are given in Part 3)
***Arg.:*** Micronema; Vixorfit; ***Austral.:*** Bausch & Lomb Computer Eye Drops†; ***Braz.:*** Glicel†; ***Canad.:*** Alpha Keri†; Gly-Rectal†; ***Chile:*** Fleet Babylax; ***Fr.:*** Bebegel; Glycerotone†; ***Ger.:*** Babylax†; Glycerosteril; Glycilax; Milax; Nene-Lax; ***Gr.:*** Glicerolo microclismi; ***Hong Kong:*** Glyceol; ***Irl.:*** Babylax; ***Israel:*** Minilax; ***Ital.:*** Verolax; Zetalax; ***Jpn:*** Glyceol; ***Malaysia:*** Fleet Babylax; ***Mex.:*** BB Fleet†; Neutro Bar; Supositorios Senosiain; ***Port.:*** Bebegel; Rectiole†; Verolax; ***S.Afr.:*** Regard; ***Singapore:*** Fleet Babylax; ***Spain:*** Adulax; Gely; Glicerotens; Paidolax; Supo Gliz; Supo Kristal†; Verolax; Vitrosups; ***Swed.:*** Miniderm; ***Switz.:*** Bulboid; Cristal†; Practomil; ***Thai.:*** Glyceol; Glycerosteril; ***UAE:*** Laxolyne; ***UK:*** Benylin Tickly Coughs; Boots Cough Syrup 3 Months Plus; Neutrogena Norwegian Formula Dermatological Cream; Nirolex Dry Cough; Senokot Direct Relief; Tixylix Baby Syrup; ***USA:*** Colace Infant/Child; Computer Eye Drops; Eye-Lube-A; Fleet Babylax; Listermint Arctic Mint Mouthwash; Ophthalgan†; Osmoglyn; Sani-Supp.

**Multi-ingredient:** ***Arg.:*** Irix Lagrimas; Skleremo; ***Austral.:*** Aci-Jel; Anusol; Auralgan; Egopsoryl TA; Hamilton Body Lotion; Hamilton Cleansing Lotion; Hamilton Dry Skin; Magnoplasm; Murine Contact†; Nutrasorb†; SM-33; Soothe'n Heal†; Visine True Tears; ***Belg.:*** Aloplastine; Laxavit; ***Braz.:*** Bluderm; Dermamina; Estomafitino†; Mentoval†; Narizima Adulto†; Narizima Pediatrico†; Pasta d'Agua; Varikromo; ***Canad.:*** Agarol Plain; Agarol†; Auralgan; Bronchex; Bronchisaft†; Collyrium†; Epi-Lyt; Moisture Drops; Rhinedrine Moisturizing; Swim-Ear; Tucks; ***Chile:*** Acnoxyl Jabon Liquido; ***Denm.:*** Analka; Glyoktyl; Pectyl; ***Fr.:*** Aloplastine; Charlieu Topicrem; Dexeryl; Ictyane; Pharmatex; Rectopanbiline; Scleremo; Taido; ***Ger.:*** Lacrisic; Lubrikano; Norgalax Miniklistier; Zinksalbe; ***Hong Kong:*** Aderma Dermalibour; Aderma Exomega; Baby Cough with Antihistamine; Ego Skin Cream; Visine for Contacts; ***India:*** Neotomic; Otogesic; ***Irl.:*** Micolette; ***Israel:*** Kamil Blue; Microlet; Taro Gel; ***Ital.:*** Dropyal; Evasen Dischetti; Evasen Liquido; Glicerolax; Microclisma Evacuante AD-BB†; Microclismi Marco Viti; Microclismi Sella; Naturalass; Novilax; Salviette H; Solecin; ***Malaysia:*** Egozite Baby Cream; ***Mex.:*** Nutegen G; Nutrasorb; ***Mon.:*** Glyco-Thymoline; ***NZ:*** Aci-Jel; Auralgan; Ego Skin Cream; Karicare Breast and Body Cream; Karicare Ointment; Lemsip Dry Cough; Rosken Skin Repair; Silic; ***Port.:*** Antiacneicos Niacex; Cicapost; Dagragel; Hidratante VG; Lubrificante Anestesico; Multi-Mam Compressas; Nutraisdin; Ureadin Facial; Ureadin Maos; ***S.Afr.:*** Moisture Drops; ***Singapore:*** Egozite Baby Cream; Topicrem; Tropex; ***Switz.:*** Lacrycon; Neo-Decongestine; Realderm; ***Thai.:*** Baby Cough Syrup; Baby Cough with Antihistamine; Tussis†; ***UK:*** Allens Junior Cough; Beehive Balsam; Codella†; Collins Elixir Pastilles†; Earex Plus; Honey & Molasses; Imuderm; Jackson's Lemon Linctus; Jackson's Troublesome Coughs; Lemsip Cough & Cold Dry Cough; Lockets; Lockets Medicated Linctus; Melissin†; Meltus Honey & Lemon; Micolette; Relaxit; Swim-Ear; ***USA:*** Aci-Jel†; Allergen; Astroglide; Auralgan; Clearasil Antibacterial; Collyrium Fresh; Entertainer's Secret; Epi-Lyt; Formulation R; Hemorid For Women; Maxilube; Moisture Drops; N'ice; Numzit; Surgel; Swim-Ear; Therevac Plus; Therevac SB; Trimo-San; Tucks.

## Glycerophosphoric Acid

Glicerofosfórico, ácido; Glycerylphosphoric Acid; Monoglycerylphosphoric Acid.

$C_3H_9O_6P$ = 172.1.

*CAS — 27082-31-1; 57-03-4 (α-glycerophosphoric acid); 17181-54-3 (β-glycerophosphoric acid); 5746-57-6 (L-α-glycerophosphoric acid); 1509-81-5 (DL-α-glycerophosphoric acid).*

## Sodium Glycerophosphate

Natrii Glycerophosphas; Natrium Glycerophosphoricum; Sodium Glycerylphosphate.

$C_3H_7Na_2O_6P,xH_2O$.

*CAS — 1555-56-2 (anhydrous α-sodium glycerophosphate); 819-83-0 (β-sodium glycerophosphate, anhydrous).*

*ATC — B05XA14.*

**Pharmacopoeias.** In *Chin.* and *Eur.* (see p.vi).

### Profile

Glycerophosphoric acid and various glycerophosphates have been used in tonics. They were once considered as a suitable means of providing phosphorus. Calcium and magnesium glycerophosphates (see p.1225 and p.1228, respectively) may be considered as a source of calcium or magnesium.

◊ Reference to the use of sodium glycerophosphate as a source of phosphorus in infant parenteral nutrition.[1]


1. Costello I, *et al.* Sodium glycerophosphate in the treatment of neonatal hypophosphataemia. *Arch Dis Child* 1995; **73:** F44–5.


### Preparations

**Proprietary Preparations** (details are given in Part 3)
***Austria:*** Glycophos; ***Fin.:*** Glycophos†; ***Gr.:*** Glycophos; ***Port.:*** Glycophos; ***Swed.:*** Glycophos; ***Switz.:*** Glycophos; ***UK:*** Glycophos.

**Multi-ingredient:** ***Arg.:*** Antikatarata; ***Belg.:*** Verrulyse-Methionine†; ***Fr.:*** Biotone; Ionyl; Phosphore-Medifa; Verrulyse-Methionine; ***Israel:*** Babyzim; ***Ital.:*** Calciofix; Glicero-Valerovit; Neuroftal; Neurol; ***S.Afr.:*** Nervade†.

## Glyceryl Palmitostearate

Glicerol, palmitoestearato de. A mixture of mono-, di-, and triglycerides of $C_{16}$ and $C_{18}$ fatty acids.

*CAS — 8067-32-1.*

### Profile

Glyceryl palmitostearate is used in pharmaceutical manufacturing as a diluent and lubricant for tablets and capsules.

## Gold

E175; Oro.

Au = 196.96655.

*CAS — 7440-57-5.*

### Profile

Gold is a bright-yellow, malleable, and ductile metal; the finely divided powder may be black, ruby, or purple. The main use of metallic gold in health care is now in dentistry. Gold may also be employed as a colouring agent for some foodstuffs. In the treatment of rheumatoid arthritis, gold is used in the form of compounds such as auranofin (p.19), aurothioglucose (p.19), and sodium aurothiomalate (p.88). The radionuclide gold-198 is described in the chapter on radiopharmaceuticals (p.1523). There have been rare reports of hypersensitivity reactions to metallic gold.

Gold is used (as Aurum or Aurum Met.) in homoeopathic medicine. Gold salts are also used in homoeopathy.

◊ References.


1. Merchant B. Gold, the noble metal and the paradoxes of its toxicology. *Biologicals* 1998; **26:** 49–59.
2. Ehrlich A, Belsito DV. Allergic contact dermatitis to gold. *Cutis* 2000; **65:** 323–6.


### Preparations

**Proprietary Preparations** (details are given in Part 3)
**Multi-ingredient:** ***Ger.:*** Cefassin.

## Gossypol

Gosipol. 2,2′-Bis(1,6,7-trihydroxy-3-methyl-5-isopropylnaphthalene-8-carboxaldehyde).

$C_{30}H_{30}O_8$ = 518.6.

*CAS — 303-45-7.*

### Profile

Gossypol is a pigment extracted from cottonseed oil (p.1676). It possesses antispermatogenic activity and has been studied, especially in China, as a male contraceptive. It has also been investigated for its antineoplastic, antiprotozoal, antiviral, and spermicidal activity and has been studied in women in the treatment of certain gynaecological disorders.

Side-effects have included fatigue, changes in appetite, gastrointestinal effects, burning sensation of the face and hands, some loss of libido, and persistent oligospermia. Hypokalaemia has occurred.

◊ The pharmacology and therapeutic potential of gossypol have been reviewed.[1] Although controlled studies[2,3] have shown gossypol to be an effective male contraceptive, WHO concluded[4] that gossypol would not be acceptable as a male antifertility drug because of the occurrence of adverse effects such as hypokalaemia and irreversible testicular damage resulting in azoospermia or severe oligozoospermia.


1. Wu D. An overview of the clinical pharmacology and therapeutic potential of gossypol as a male contraceptive agent and in gynaecological disease. *Drugs* 1989; **38:** 333–41.
2. Coutinho EM, *et al.* Antispermatogenic action of gossypol in men. *Fertil Steril* 1984; **42:** 424–30.
3. Liu G, *et al.* Clinical trial of gossypol as a male contraceptive drug part I: efficacy study. *Fertil Steril* 1987; **48:** 459–61.
4. Waites GMH, *et al.* Gossypol: reasons for its failure to be accepted as a safe, reversible male antifertility drug. *Int J Androl* 1998; **21:** 8–12.


## Gravel Root

Joe Pye Weed; Queen of the Meadow; Raíz de eupatorio.

### Profile

Gravel root is the root of *Eupatorium purpureum* (Compositae) and has diuretic, antilithic, and antirheumatic properties. It is used for renal and urinary calculus and other urinary-tract disorders, and has also been used for gout and rheumatism.

### Preparations

**Proprietary Preparations** (details are given in Part 3)
**Multi-ingredient:** ***UK:*** Backache.

## Greater Celandine

Celidonia; Chelidonii Herba; Chelidonium; Schöllkraut; Tetterwort.

**Pharmacopoeias.** In *Eur.* (see p.vi) and *Pol.*

**Ph. Eur. 5.0** (Greater Celandine). The dried, whole, or cut aerial parts of *Chelidonium majus* collected during flowering. It contains a minimum of 0.6% of total alkaloids expressed as chelidonine ($C_{20}H_{19}NO_5$ = 353.4), calculated with reference to the dried drug.

### Profile

Greater celandine has sedative and spasmolytic properties and the aerial parts are used for liver, biliary, and gastrointestinal disorders, and have also been used for respiratory-tract disorders. The latex has been used externally for warts and other skin conditions.

Greater celandine is also used in homoeopathic medicine.

It has been reported to cause hepatotoxicity.

**Effects on the liver.** References.

1. Benninger J, *et al.* Acute hepatitis induced by greater celandine (Chelidonium majus). *Gastroenterology* 1999; **117:** 1234–7.
2. Stickel F, *et al.* Acute hepatitis induced by Greater Celandine (Chelidonium majus). *Scand J Gastroenterol* 2003; **38:** 565–8.

### Preparations

**Proprietary Preparations** (details are given in Part 3)
***Ger.:*** Ardeycholan N†; Chelidophyt†; Chol 4000†; Cholarist; Cholspasmin Phyto; Gallopas; Panchelidon N†; Paverysat forte N; Siosol†; ***Switz.:*** Virulex.

**Multi-ingredient:** ***Arg.:*** Quelodin F; ***Austral.:*** Berberis Complex†; Extralife Liva-Care†; Lexat†; ***Austria:*** Aristochol†; Choleodoron; ***Belg.:*** Aporil; ***Braz.:*** Quelodin; ***Fr.:*** Nitrol; ***Ger.:*** Aristochol; Aristochol CC; Aristochol N; Bilisan C3†; Cefachol†; Chol-Kugeletten Neu; Chol-Truw S†; Cholagogum F; Cholagogum N; Cholagutt-N; Cholapret†; Cholhepan N; Cholosom Phyto N; Cholosom SL; Cynarzym N; Femisana; Gallemolan forte; Gallemolan G; Galloselect M; Hepar-Pasc N†; Hepaticum-Medice H; Hepatofalk Neu†; Hevert-Gall S†; Hevert-Magen-Galle-Leber-Tee†; Horvilan N; Iberogast; Infi-tract; JuCholan S†; Legapas comp†; Marianon; Nervogastrol N; Neurochol C; Novo Mandrogallan N†; Opobylphyto; Pascohepan novo†; Presselin Hepaticum P; Schwohepan S; spasmo gallo sanol; Steigal†; ***Hong Kong:*** Hepatofalk; Hepatofalk Planta; ***Ital.:*** Tisana Arnaldi†; ***Port.:*** Cholagutt; ***Singapore:*** Hepatofalk Planta; ***Spain:*** Menstrunat; Natusor Hepavesical; Nitroina; ***Switz.:*** Demonatur Gouttes pour le foie et la bile; Iberogast; Stago†.

## Green-lipped Mussel

Extracto de mejillón de labios verdes.

### Profile

An extract from the green-lipped mussel *Perna canaliculus* (Mytilidae), stated to contain amino acids, fats, carbohydrates, and minerals, has been promoted for the treatment of rheumatic disorders including rheumatoid arthritis (p.9). It has also been tried in asthma.

**Rheumatic disorders.** A review of the investigation of green-lipped mussel in the treatment of arthritis has not revealed conclusive evidence of its usefulness.[1]

1. Li Wan Po A, Maguire T. Green-lipped mussel. *Pharm J* 1990; **244:** 640–1.

### Preparations

**Proprietary Preparations** (details are given in Part 3)
***UK:*** Healtheries Musseltone; Lyprinol; Mobilyzer; Oceantone; Seatone; Supplex.

**Multi-ingredient:** ***Austral.:*** Prost-1†; ***UK:*** Healtheries Musseltone & Glucosamine.

## Griffonia Simplicifolia

### Profile

The leaf, stem, and twigs of *Griffonia simplicifolia* (Fabaceae) have been used for a variety of disorders in its native West Africa. It is included in herbal and nutritional supplements. It is a source of lectins and has insecticidal properties.

### Preparations

**Proprietary Preparations** (details are given in Part 3)

**Multi-ingredient:** ***Fr.:*** Prosatietil; ***Ital.:*** Climil Complex.

## Grindelia

Gum Plant; Gumweed; Tar Weed.

**Pharmacopoeias.** In *Fr.* which allows *Grindelia camporum, G. humilis, G. robusta*, and *G. squarrosa*.

### Profile

Various *Grindelia* spp. (Asteraceae) have been included in herbal preparations used for respiratory-tract disorders. It is also used in homoeopathic medicine.

### Preparations

**Proprietary Preparations** (details are given in Part 3)

**Multi-ingredient:** ***Arg.:*** Expectosan Hierbas y Miel; ***Austral.:*** Asa Tones†; Breathe Eazy Chest Rub†; Euphorbia Complex†; ***Austria:*** Paracodin; ***Belg.:*** Paracodine; ***Braz.:*** Broncmel†; Broncotussan†; Calmatoss; Gotas Nican; Infantoss; Limao Bravo†; Lobelia Composta†; Pectal; Pectoss†; Pulmoformil†; Xarope de Caraguata; Xarope de Limao Bravo†; Xarope Grindelia de Oliveira Junior†; Xarope Peitoral de Ameixa Composto; Xpe SPC; ***Canad.:*** Herbal Cold Relief; ***Chile:*** Gotas Nican; Ramistos; ***Fr.:*** Coquelusedal; Coquelusedal Paracetamol; Dinacode; Ephydion; Germose; Glottyl†; Neo-Codion; Niver†; Vegetoserum; ***Ger.:*** Asthma 6-N; Bronchicum Elixir N; Melrosum Hustensirup N†; ***Ital.:*** Broncosedina; Sedobex†; Tussanyl; ***Neth.:*** Bronchicum; ***Port.:*** Lactucol†; ***S.Afr.:*** Bronchicough; Bronchicum; ***Spain:*** Pazbronquial; ***Switz.:*** Famel; Neo-Codion N; Nican.

## Ground Ivy

Hiedra terrestre; Lierre Terrestre.

**Pharmacopoeias.** In *Chin.* and *Fr.*

### Profile

Ground ivy, the aerial parts of *Glechoma hederacea* (*Nepeta hederacea*) (Labiatae) has been used for respiratory-tract and gastrointestinal disorders.

It is also used in homoeopathic medicine.

### Preparations

**Proprietary Preparations** (details are given in Part 3)

**Multi-ingredient:** ***Belg.:*** Tisane Pectorale†; ***Fr.:*** Mediflor Tisane Pectorale d'Alsace†; ***Switz.:*** Demo gouttes bronchiques†; ***UK:*** Gerard House Water Relief Tablets; Heath & Heather Water Relief Tablets†; Water Naturtabs.

## Guaiacum Resin

Guaiac; Guaiacum; Guajakharz; Resina de guayaco.

*CAS — 9000-29-7.*

### Profile

Guaiacum resin is obtained from guaiacum wood (lignum vitae; *Guaiacum officinale* or *G. sanctum*) (Zygophyllaceae) and has been used in the treatment of rheumatism. It is used in herbal and homoeopathic medicine.

Guaiacum resin is used in the detection of occult blood in the faeces. The accuracy of the guaiacum test has been questioned and some drugs may interfere with the result.

◊ References.

1. Ko CW, *et al.* Fecal occult blood testing in a general medical clinic: comparison between guaiac-based and immunochemical-based tests. *Am J Med* 2003; **115:** 111–14.

### Preparations

**Proprietary Preparations** (details are given in Part 3)

**Multi-ingredient:** ***UK:*** Gerard House Ligvites†; Gerard House Reumalex; Rheumasol†; Rheumatic Pain; Rheumatic Pain Relief; Rheumatic Pain Remedy; Rheumatic Pain Tablets†.

## Guaiazulene

Guayazuleno. 1,4-Dimethyl-7-isopropylazulene.

$C_{15}H_{18}$ = 198.3.

*CAS — 489-84-9.*

*ATC — S01XA01.*

### Profile

Guaiazulene has been reported to have anti-allergic, anti-inflammatory, antipyretic, and antiseptic properties.

### Preparations

**Proprietary Preparations** (details are given in Part 3)
***Arg.:*** Azulon; ***Austria:*** Azulen; Azulenal; Garmastan; ***Fr.:*** Azulene; ***Ger.:*** Garmastan†.

**Multi-ingredient:** ***Arg.:*** Sodorant; ***Austria:*** Piniment; Spasmo Claim; Tampositorien mit Belladonna; Thrombocid; ***Fr.:*** Cicatryl; Pepsane; ***Ger.:*** Azupanthenol; Thrombocid; ***Hong Kong:*** Thrombocid; ***Israel:*** Aronal Forte; ***Ital.:*** Collyria; ***Port.:*** Thrombocid; ***Spain:*** Balneogel†; Predni Azuleno; ***Switz.:*** Bain extra-doux dermatologique Nouvelle Formule; Phlogidermil†; Phytoberidin†; Thrombocid.

## Gutta Percha

Gummi Plasticum; Gutapercha; Gutt. Perch.

**Pharmacopoeias.** In *US.*

**USP 27** (Gutta Percha). The coagulated, dried, purified latex of the trees of the genera *Palaquium* and *Payena* and most commonly *Palaquium gutta* (Sapotaceae). It occurs in lumps or blocks of variable size; externally brown or greyish-brown to greyish-white in colour; internally reddish-yellow or reddish-grey and having a laminated or fibrous appearance. It is flexible but only slightly elastic. Has a slight, characteristic odour. Insoluble in water; partly soluble in carbon disulfide, in turpentine oil, and in benzene; about 90% soluble in chloroform. Store under water. Protect from light.

### Profile

Gutta percha has been used in various dressings. In dentistry, gutta percha has been used as a filling material and as the basis of compounds for taking dental impressions.

## Haematoporphyrin

Hematoporfirina.

$C_{34}H_{38}N_4O_6$ = 598.7.

*CAS — 14459-29-1.*

### Profile

Haematoporphyrin is a red pigment, free from iron, obtained from haematin. It is an ingredient of preparations promoted as tonics, particularly for the elderly, and has been used in the treatment of depression. Derivatives of haematoporphyrin are used as photosensitisers in the photodynamic therapy of malignant neoplasms (see Porfimer Sodium, p.580).

### Preparations

**Proprietary Preparations** (details are given in Part 3)
***Fr.:*** Hemedonine†.

**Multi-ingredient:** ***Austria:*** KH3; ***Chile:*** Actebral; KH3; KH3-Vit; ***Fr.:*** Novitan†; ***Ger.:*** KH3; Revicain comp plus; ***Hong Kong:*** KH3; ***Ital.:*** Porfirin 12; Tonogen; Vit-Porphyrin; ***NZ:*** KH3; ***Port.:*** KH3†; ***S.Afr.:*** Revaton†; ***Spain:*** Actilevol Orex†; KH3 Powel†; ***Thai.:*** KH3; ***UK:*** KH3†.

## Hamamelis

Amamelide; Hamamelidis; Witch Hazel.

**Pharmacopoeias.** In *Eur.* (see p.vi) and *US.*

**Ph. Eur. 5.0** (Hamamelis Leaf). The whole or cut dried leaves of *Hamamelis virginiana* containing not less than 7% tannins, expressed as pyrogallol ($C_6H_6O_3$ = 126.1), calculated with reference to the dried drug. Protect from light.

**USP 27** (Witch Hazel). A clear, colourless distillate prepared from recently cut and partially dried dormant twigs of *Hamamelis virginiana.* pH between 3.0 and 5.0. Store in airtight containers at a temperature not exceeding 40°.

### Profile

Hamamelis has astringent properties and contains gallic acid, a bitter principle, and a trace of volatile oil. It is used in preparations for the symptomatic relief of haemorrhoids (p.1243). Hamamelis water is used as a cooling application and has been applied as a haemostatic.

Hamamelis is used in herbal or homoeopathic preparations for a variety of disorders.

### Preparations

***USP 27:*** Witch Hazel.

**Proprietary Preparations** (details are given in Part 3)
***Austral.:*** Optrex; Witch Doctor†; ***Austria:*** Hametum; Sperti Praparation H; ***Canad.:*** Optrex; Preparation H Cleansing Pads†; Snap Skin Cleanser Sensitive†; ***Chile:*** Similia; Sperti (Preparacion H) Clear Gel; ***Fr.:*** Optrex; ***Ger.:*** F 99 Sulgan N†; Fiamelis; Haemo Duoform; Hamasana; Hametum; Pellit Sonnenbrand†; Posterine; Tampositorien H; Venoplant top; Virgamelis†; ***Irl.:*** Optrex†; ***Ital.:*** Acqua Virginiana; Optrex; ***Malaysia:*** Optrex; ***Neth.:*** Venoplant†; ***NZ:*** Optrex; ***Port.:*** Optrex; ***Singapore:*** Optrex; ***Spain:*** Derminiol; Hemo Derminiol; Optrex; ***Switz.:*** Hametum-N†; Hametum†; Optrex; ***Thai.:*** Hametum†; Optrex; ***UK:*** I-Doc†; Optrex; Preparation H Clear Gel; Witch Doctor; Witch Sunsore; ***USA:*** A-E-R; Fleet Medicated Pads; Neutrogena Drying.

**Multi-ingredient:** numerous preparations are listed in Part 3.

## Harmaline

Harmalina. 3,4-Dihydroharmine.

$C_{13}H_{14}N_2O$ = 214.3.

*CAS — 304-21-2.*

**Description.** Harmaline is an alkaloid obtained from peganum, the dried seeds of *Peganum harmala* (Zygophyllaceae).

## Harmine

Harmina; 7-Methoxy-1-methyl-9*H*-pyrido[3,4-*b*]indole.

$C_{13}H_{12}N_2O$ = 212.2.

*CAS — 442-51-3.*

**Description.** Harmine is an alkaloid obtained from peganum, the dried seeds of *Peganum harmala* (Zygophyllaceae).

Harmine is identical with an alkaloid known as banisterine or telepathine obtained from *Banisteria caapi* (Malpighiaceae).

### Profile

Harmine and harmaline are the main active principles of a hallucinogenic drink, known in South American regions as 'ayahuasca', 'caapi', or 'yagé', that is made from closely related plants of the family Malpighiaceae. They have no therapeutic use.

## Helonias

Blazing Star; Chamaelirium; False Unicorn; Starwort.

### Profile

Helonias is the root of *Chamaelirium luteum* (*Helonias dioica*) (Liliaceae). It is used in herbal medicine particularly for gynaecological disorders. It is also used in homoeopathic preparations.

### Preparations

**Proprietary Preparations** (details are given in Part 3)

**Multi-ingredient:** ***Austral.:*** Nervatona Plus†; Nervatona†; ***UK:*** Gerard House Helonias Compound†; Period Pain Relief.

## Henna

Henna Leaf; Lawsonia.

### Profile

Henna is the dried leaves of *Lawsonia inermis* (*L. alba*) (Lythraceae), containing lawsone (p.1705). Powdered henna is used for dyeing the hair, skin, and nails.

**Adverse effects.** Allergic skin reactions to henna used to dye the skin have been reported.[1] Such reactions were usually due to additives used to shorten the application time of the dye and allergic reactions to 'plain' henna were rare. Similar reactions have been reported[2-6] following henna tattoos on the skin. The adulterant, which is added to natural henna to darken it ('black henna'), was identified[2,5] as paraphenylenediamine (p.1728).

The suggestion that henna may cause neonatal hyperbilirubinaemia is discussed under Lawsone, p.1705.

1. Lestringant GG, *et al.* Cutaneous reactions to henna and associated additives. *Br J Dermatol* 1999; **141:** 598–600.

2. Brancaccio RR, *et al.* Identification and quantification of para-phenylenediamine in a temporary black henna tattoo. *Am J Contact Dermat* 2002; **13:** 15–8.
3. Marcoux D, *et al.* Sensitization to para-phenylenediamine from a streetside temporary tattoo. *Pediatr Dermatol* 2002; **19:** 498–502.
4. Neri I, *et al.* Childhood allergic contact dermatitis from henna tattoo. *Pediatr Dermatol* 2002; **19:** 503–5.
5. Bowling JC, Groves R. An unexpected tattoo. *Lancet* 2002; **359:** 649.
6. Leggiadro RJ, *et al.* Temporary tattoo dermatitis. *J Pediatr* 2003; **142:** 586.


## Heptaminol Hydrochloride *(BANM, rINNM)*

Heptaminoli Hydrochloridum; Hidrocloruro de heptaminol; RP-2831. 6-Amino-2-methylheptan-2-ol hydrochloride.

$C_8H_{19}NO,HCl = 181.7.$

*CAS — 372-66-7 (heptaminol); 543-15-7 (heptaminol hydrochloride).*

*ATC — C01DX08.*

**Pharmacopoeias.** In *Eur.* (see p.vi).

**Ph. Eur. 5.0** (Heptaminol Hydrochloride). A white or almost white crystalline powder. Freely soluble in water; soluble in alcohol; practically insoluble in dichloromethane.

### Profile

Heptaminol hydrochloride is a cardiac stimulant and vasodilator and has been given in the treatment of cardiovascular disorders. Heptaminol and heptaminol adenosine phosphate have also been used.

### Preparations

**Proprietary Preparations** (details are given in Part 3)
***Belg.:*** Hept-A-Myl†; ***Fr.:*** Ampecyclal; Hept-A-Myl; ***Ital.:*** Coreptil; ***Port.:*** Heptylon†.

**Multi-ingredient:** ***Arg.:*** Flebitol; ***Austria:*** Thilocombin†; ***Fr.:*** Debrumyl; Ginkor Fort; ***Ger.:*** Normotin-R; Perivar; Veno-Hexanicit†; Veno-Tebonin N; ***Hong Kong:*** Ginkor Fort; ***Malaysia:*** Ginkor Fort; ***Port.:*** Debrumyl; Forticol; ***Spain:*** Denubil; Largatrex; ***Thai.:*** Ginkor Fort.

## Herniaria

Bruchkraut; Herba Herniariae; Herniary; Rupture-wort.

### Profile

Herniaria consists of the dried leaves and flowering tops of various species of rupture-wort, chiefly *Herniaria glabra* and *H. hirsuta* (Caryophyllaceae). It has astringent and diuretic properties and has been given in urinary-tract disorders. It is also used in homoeopathic medicine.

### Preparations

**Proprietary Preparations** (details are given in Part 3)

**Multi-ingredient:** ***Austria:*** Blasen-Tee†; Blasentee EF-EM-ES; Krauterhaus Mag Kottas Blasentee; Krauterhaus Mag Kottas Nierentee; Mag Kottas Entwasserungstee; Mag Kottas Krauterexpress-Entwasserungstee; Mag Kottas Krauterexpress-Nieren-Blasentee; Mag Kottas Nieren-Blasentee; St Radegunder Nierentee; Uropurat; ***Ger.:*** Hernia-Tee†; Herniol†.

## Hexylene Glycol

Hexilenglicol. 2-Methyl-2,4-pentanediol.

$C_6H_{14}O_2 = 118.2.$

*CAS — 107-41-5.*

**Pharmacopoeias.** In *USNF.*

**USNF 22** (Hexylene Glycol). A clear, colourless, viscous liquid. Absorbs moisture when exposed to moist air. Miscible with water and with many organic solvents including alcohol, acetone, chloroform, ether, and hexanes. Store in airtight containers.

### Profile

Hexylene glycol has properties similar to those of propylene glycol (p.1735). It is used as a pharmaceutical aid.

## Histamine

Histamina. 2-(Imidazol-4-yl)ethylamine.

$C_5H_9N_3 = 111.1.$

*CAS — 51-45-6.*

*ATC — V04CG03.*

## Histamine Hydrochloride

Histamina, hidrocloruro de; Histamine Dihydrochloride *(USAN)*; Histamini Dihydrochloridum.

$C_5H_9N_3,2HCl = 184.1.$

*CAS — 56-92-8.*

*ATC — V04CG03.*

**Pharmacopoeias.** In *Eur.* (see p.vi).

**Ph. Eur. 5.0** (Histamine Dihydrochloride). Hygroscopic, colourless crystals or white crystalline powder. Very soluble in water; soluble in alcohol. A 5% solution in water has a pH of 2.85 to 3.60. Protect from light.

## Histamine Phosphate

Histamina, fosfato de; Histamine Acid Phosphate; Histamine Diphosphate; Histamini Phosphas.

$C_5H_9N_3,2H_3PO_4,H_2O = 325.2.$

*CAS — 51-74-1 (anhydrous histamine phosphate).*

*ATC — V04CG03.*

**Pharmacopoeias.** In *Eur.* (see p.vi). *Chin.* and *US* specify the anhydrous substance.

**Ph. Eur. 5.0** (Histamine Phosphate). Colourless, long prismatic crystals. Freely soluble in water; slightly soluble in alcohol. A 5% solution in water has a pH of 3.75 to 3.95. Protect from light.

**USP 27** (Histamine Phosphate). Anhydrous histamine phosphate occurs as colourless, odourless, long prismatic crystals. Is stable in air but is affected by light. Soluble 1 in 4 of water. Its solutions are acid to litmus. Store in airtight containers. Protect from light.

**Stability.** A study concluded that solutions of histamine phosphate could be sterilised by heating in an autoclave with little degradation.[1] Autoclaved solutions could be stored for a minimum of 4 months.

1. McDonald C, *et al.* Stability of solutions of histamine acid phos.phate after sterilization by heating in an autoclave. *J Clin Pharm Ther* 1990; **15:** 41–4.

### Adverse Effects and Treatment

Injection of histamine salts can produce a range of adverse effects that includes headache, flushing of the skin, general vasodilatation with a fall in blood pressure, tachycardia, bronchial constriction and dyspnoea, visual disturbances, vomiting, diarrhoea, and other gastrointestinal effects. These reactions may be serious and excessive dosage can produce collapse and shock, and may be fatal. Reactions may occur at the injection site.

Some of these effects may be relieved by an antihistamine, but adrenaline may be required and should always be available.

### Precautions

Histamine salts should be used with care in patients with asthma or other hypersensitivity disorders, in elderly patients, and in patients with cardiovascular disorders.

### Pharmacokinetics

Histamine salts exert a rapid, though transient, effect when given parenterally. Histamine is rapidly metabolised by methylation and oxidation; the metabolites are excreted in the urine.

◊ References.

1. Middleton M, *et al.* Pharmacokinetics of histamine dihydrochloride in healthy volunteers and cancer patients: implications for combined immunotherapy with interleukin-2. *J Clin Pharmacol* 2002; **42:** 774–81.

### Uses and Administration

Histamine causes stimulation of smooth muscle, especially of the bronchioles, and lowers blood pressure by dilating the arterioles and capillaries. It also stimulates exocrine gland secretion, especially the gastric glands.

Intradermal injection of histamine produces the characteristic 'triple response' of erythema, flare, and wheal. This is utilised as a control response in skin testing for hypersensitivity. Also, since it is mediated in part by axon reflexes, it has been used to test the integrity of sensory nerves, for example in leprosy.

Inhalation of histamine causes bronchoconstriction and is used as a test of bronchial reactivity.

Histamine has also been given subcutaneously to identify the causes of achlorhydria and intravenously in the diagnosis of phaeochromocytoma, but safer tests are generally preferred.

Histamine is included in some combination topical preparations for musculoskeletal disorders.

Histamine hydrochloride is under investigation as an adjunct in the management of acute myeloid leukaemia and malignant melanoma. It has also been tried as an adjunct to interferons and other drugs in the management of hepatitis C.

### Preparations

***USP 27:*** Histamine Phosphate Injection.

**Proprietary Preparations** (details are given in Part 3)
***Mex.:*** Destamin.

**Multi-ingredient:** ***Arg.:*** Histaglobin; Infrarub; ***Austria:*** Histaglobin; ***Braz.:*** Infrarub†; ***Canad.:*** Midalgan; ***Fr.:*** Algipan; Pneumoplasme a l'Histamine†; ***Ger.:*** GA-301-Redskin 301†; Histadestal; Midysalb†; ***India:*** Algipan; Histaglobulin; ***Port.:*** Midalgan; ***S.Afr.:*** Histaglobin; ***Switz.:*** Midalgan; Radalgin; ***Thai.:*** Histaglobin†.

## Histoplasmin

Histoplasmina.

**Pharmacopoeias.** In *US.*

**USP 27** (Histoplasmin). A clear, colourless, sterile solution containing standardised culture filtrates of *Histoplasma capsulatum* grown on liquid synthetic medium. It may contain a suitable antimicrobial. Store at 2° to 8°. The expiry date is not later than 2 years after release from the manufacturer's cold storage.

### Profile

Histoplasmin, in an intradermal (intracutaneous) dose of 0.1 mL of a 1 in 100 dilution, may be used as an aid to the diagnosis of histoplasmosis. However, the diagnostic value of the test has been questioned and it may interfere with serological tests for histoplasmosis.

Histoplasmin has also been used, in conjunction with other antigens, to assess cell-mediated immunity.

### Preparations

***USP 27:*** Histoplasmin.

**Proprietary Preparations** (details are given in Part 3)
***USA:*** Histolyn-CYL.

## Horseradish

Armoracia; Rábano rusticano.

### Profile

Horseradish, the root of *Cochlearia armoracia* (*Armoracia rusticana*; *Nasturtium armoracia*; *Radicula armoracia*) (Cruciferae), has diuretic and antiseptic properties and stimulates the digestion. It is used in gastrointestinal, respiratory-tract, and urinary-tract disorders, and has also been used externally.

It is also used in homoeopathic medicine.

Horseradish is widely used as a food flavouring and condiment.

### Preparations

**Proprietary Preparations** (details are given in Part 3)

**Multi-ingredient:** ***Austral.:*** Garlic and Horseradish + C Complex†; Garlic, Horseradish, A & C Capsules†; Horse Radish and Garlic Tablets†; Procold†; Sinus and Hayfever†; ***Braz.:*** Infantoss; ***Ger.:*** Angocin Anti-Infekt N; ***Switz.:*** Kernosan Elixir; ***UK:*** Mixed Vegetable Tablets.

## Hyaluronic Acid *(BAN)*

Hialurónico, ácido. (1→3)-*O*-(2-Acetamido-2-deoxy-β-D-glucopyranosyl)-(1→4)-*O*-β-D-glucopyranosiduronan.

*CAS — 9004-61-9.*

*ATC — D03AX05; M09AX01; S01KA01.*

NOTE. The term Hyaluronan is used to cover both hyaluronic acid and sodium hyaluronate.

## Sodium Hyaluronate *(BANM)*

Hialuronato sódico; Hyaluronate Sodium *(USAN)*; Natrii Hyaluronas.

*CAS — 9067-32-7.*

*ATC — D03AX05; M09AX01; S01KA01.*

**Pharmacopoeias.** In *Eur.* (see p.vi).

**Ph. Eur. 5.0** (Sodium Hyaluronate). The sodium salt of hyaluronic acid, a glycosaminoglycan consisting of D-glucuronic acid and *N*-acetyl-D-glucosamine disaccharide units. It is extracted from cocks' combs or obtained by fermentation from streptococci (Lancefield Groups A and C). A white or almost white, very hygroscopic powder or a fibrous aggregate. Sparingly soluble to soluble in water; practically insoluble in dehydrated alcohol and in acetone. A 0.5% solution in water has a pH of 5.0 to 8.5. Store in airtight containers. Protect from light and humidity.

### Adverse Effects

There have been reports of a transient rise in intra-ocular pressure following the administration of sodium hyaluronate into the eye. When injected into the knee, pain and inflammation may occur at the injection site. There have also been occasional reports of hypersensitivity, including, rarely, anaphylaxis.

**Effects on the eyes.** Crystalline deposits on intra-ocular lenses have been reported in patients following the use of a high viscosity sodium hyaluronate preparation during cataract surgery.[1]

1. Jensen MK, *et al.* Crystallization on intraocular lens surfaces associated with the use of Healon GV. *Arch Ophthalmol* 1994; **112:** 1037–42.

**Inflammatory reaction.** Severe peritoneal inflammation has been reported[1] following use of a sodium hyaluronate-based bioresorbable membrane to prevent postoperative adhesion formation.

1. Klingler PJ, *et al.*. Seprafilm®-induced peritoneal inflammation: a previously unknown complication: report of a case. *Dis Colon Rectum* 1999; **42:** 1639–43.

### Uses and Administration

Hyaluronic acid is widely distributed in body tissues and intracellular fluids, including the aqueous and vitreous humour, and synovial fluid; it is a component of the ground substance or tissue cement surrounding cells.

A viscous solution of sodium hyaluronate is used during surgical procedures on the eye, for example for cataract extraction. Introduction of the solution into the anterior or posterior chamber via a fine cannula or needle allows tissues to be separated during surgery and protects them from trauma.

Sodium hyaluronate is given by intra-articular injection in the treatment of osteoarthritis of the knee. Doses vary according to the preparation used, but are of the order of 20 to 25 mg once weekly for 5 weeks or up to 30 mg once weekly for 3 or 4 weeks; it is generally recommended that the treatment course for any individual joint should not be repeated within 6 months.

Hyaluronic acid is applied topically to promote wound healing. Zinc hyaluronate has also been used. A film containing sodium hyaluronate and carmellose is used to prevent surgical adhesion. Sodium hyaluronate has also been used in the management of lesions of the oral mucosa.

Hylans, which are polymers derived from hyaluronic acid, are used similarly.

Sodium hyaluronate instilled intravesically has been used as a temporary replacement of the glycosaminoglycan layer in the bladder for the symptomatic treatment of interstitial cystitis.

Topical formulations of diclofenac in hyaluronic acid (CT-1101, AT-2101) are under investigation in the treatment of actinic keratoses.

◊ Reviews.


1. Goa KL, Benfield P. Hyaluronic acid: a review of its pharmacology and use as a surgical aid in ophthalmology, and its therapeutic potential in joint disease and wound healing. *Drugs* 1994; **47:** 536–66.
2. Adams ME, *et al.* A risk-benefit assessment of injections of hyaluronan and its derivatives in the treatment of osteoarthritis of the knee. *Drug Safety* 2000; **23:** 115–30.


**Actinic keratoses.** For references to the use of diclofenac in a hyaluronic acid gel in the treatment of actinic keratoses, see p.33.

**Dry eye.** The usual management of dry eye (p.1576) is with artificial tears. Sodium hyaluronate has also been reported to be of some benefit. Alleviation of symptoms[1-3] and an increase in tear film stability[1,2] has been demonstrated following the topical application of sodium hyaluronate solution (0.1 or 0.2%) compared with saline-based placebo solutions. However, another study[4] failed to demonstrate any advantage over placebo, although it has been suggested[4,5] that sodium hyaluronate might play a role in maintaining a healthy corneal epithelium.


1. Mengher LS, *et al.* Effect of sodium hyaluronate (0.1%) on break-up time (NIBUT) in patients with dry eyes. *Br J Ophthalmol* 1986; **70:** 442–7.
2. Sand BB, *et al.* Sodium hyaluronate in the treatment of keratoconjunctivitis sicca: a double masked clinical trial. *Acta Ophthalmol (Copenh)* 1989; **67:** 181–3.
3. Condon PI, *et al.* Double blind, randomised, placebo controlled, crossover, multicentre study to determine the efficacy of a 0.1% (w/v) sodium hyaluronate solution (Fermavisc) in the treatment of dry eye syndrome. *Br J Ophthalmol* 1999; **83:** 1121–4.
4. Shimmura S, *et al.* Sodium hyaluronate eyedrops in the treatment of dry eyes. *Br J Ophthalmol* 1995; **79:** 1007–11.
5. Aragona P, *et al.* Long term treatment with sodium hyaluronate-containing artificial tears reduces ocular surface damage in patients with dry eye. *Br J Ophthalmol* 2002; **86:** 181–4.


**Osteoarthritis.** In osteoarthritis, the size and concentration of hyaluronic acid molecules naturally present in synovial fluid is reduced. Thus, one approach in the management of osteoarthritis (p.9) of the knee is viscosupplementation of the synovial fluid by the intra-articular injection of hyaluronic acid or its derivatives. Such injections may reduce pain over 1 to 6 months but may be associated with a short-term increase in knee inflammation. Some studies suggest that this may be an effective option for patients who are unable to take oral NSAIDs or have regular intra-articular corticosteroids, and who are unsuitable candidates for joint replacement surgery, although the evidence of benefit has been questioned.

References.


1. Altman RD, Moskowitz R. Intraarticular sodium hyaluronate (Hyalgan) in the treatment of patients with osteoarthritis of the knee: a randomized clinical trial. *J Rheumatol* 1998; **25:** 2203–12. Correction. *ibid.* 1999; **26:** 1216.
2. Anonymous. Hyaluronan or hylans for knee osteoarthritis? *Drug Ther Bull* 1999; **37:** 71–2.
3. Huskisson EC, Donnelly S. Hyaluronic acid in the treatment of osteoarthritis of the knee. *Rheumatology (Oxford)* 1999; **38:** 602–7.
4. Wobig M, *et al.* The role of elastoviscosity in the efficacy of viscosupplementation for osteoarthritis of the knee: a comparison of hylan G-F 20 and a lower-molecular-weight hyaluronan. *Clin Ther* 1999; **21:** 1549–62.
5. Felson DT, Anderson JJ. Hyaluronate sodium injections for osteoarthritis: hope, hype, and hard truths. *Arch Intern Med* 2002; **162:** 245–7.


**Wound healing.** Hyaluronic acid has been used to aid wound healing,[1,2] the overall management of which is discussed on p.1139.


1. Soldati D, *et al.* Mucosal wound healing after nasal surgery: a controlled clinical trial on the efficacy of hyaluronic acid containing cream. *Drugs Exp Clin Res* 1999; **25:** 253–61.
2. Harris PA, *et al.* Use of hyaluronic acid and cultured autologous keratinocytes and fibroblasts in extensive burns. *Lancet* 1999; **353:** 35–6.


### Preparations

**Proprietary Preparations** (details are given in Part 3)

***Arg.:*** Artflex; Dropstar; Gengigel; Hyalart; Hyasol; Lacripharma; Provisc; Synvisc; ***Austral.:*** AMO Vitrax; Fermathron; Healon; Ophthalin; Provisc; Synvisc; Vismed; ***Austria:*** Amvisc†; Artzal; Connettivina; Etamucin; Healonid; Hyalgan; ***Belg.:*** Healon; Provisc†; ***Braz.:*** Biolon†; Healon; Hyaludermin; Polireumin; Synvisc; ***Canad.:*** Biolon; Cystistat; Eyestil; Healon; Hylashield†; NeoVisc; Suplasyn†; Synvisc; ***Chile:*** Healon; Hyalgan; Lagricel Ofteno; Synvisc; ***Denm.:*** Artz; Hyalgan; ***Fin.:*** Artzal; Healon; Hyalgan; ***Fr.:*** Arthrum H; Healon†; Hyal-Drop; Hyalgan†; Hyalofill; Hyalugel; Hylo-Comod; Hylocomod; Ialuset; Ostenil; Provisc; Synvisc; Vismed; Vitrax†; ***Ger.:*** Arthrease; Biolon; Dispasan; Go-On; Healon; Hy-GAG; Hya-ject; Hya-Ophtal; Hyal-System; Hyalart; Hyalform; Hylo-COMOD; Hysan; Jossalind†; Laservis; Orthovisc†; Ostenil; Provisc; Suplasyn; Synvisc; Viscoseal; Vislube; Vismed; ***Gr.:*** Hyalart; ***Hong Kong:*** Connettivina; Healon; Hialid; Hyalgan; Hyruan; Ial†; Ophthalin†; Provisc; Synvisc†; Vismed; ***India:*** Halonix; ***Irl.:*** Healonid†; Hyalgan; Ophthalin; Provisc; ***Israel:*** Adant; Amvisc†; Arthrease; Biolon; Eyecon; Healon; Hylo-Comod; Ophthalin; Orthovisc; Synvisc; ***Ital.:*** Artz; Biolon†; Connettivina; Dropstar; Go-On; Healon†; Hy-Drop; Hyalart; Hyalgan; Hyalistil; Ial; Ialect; Ialum; Ialurex; Irilens; Ocustil; Ophtalin; Otoial†; Provisc; Vismed; ***Jpn:*** Hyalein; ***Malaysia:*** Healon; Hyalgan; Provisc; Synvisc; ***Mex.:*** Biolon; Lagricel; Synvisc; ***Norw.:*** Healon†; ***NZ:*** AMO Vitrax; Healon; Ophthalin; Provisc; Synvisc; ***Port.:*** Gengigel; Hyalart; Hyalofill; ***S.Afr.:*** AMO Vitrax; Amvisc†; Biolone; Healon; Provisc; Synvisc†; ***Singapore:*** AMO Vitrax; Healon; Hialid; Hyalgan; Hylaform; Ophthalin†; Provisc; Restylane; Synvisc; ***Spain:*** Hyalgan; Iiyalgon†; ***Swed.:*** AMO Vitrax†; Amvisc†; Artzal; Healon†; Hyalgan; Synvisc; ***Switz.:*** AMO Vitrax†; Biolon†; Fermavisc; Healon; Hyal-Drop; Ial; Ialugen; Laservis; Ostenil; Rhinogen; Synvisc; Viscoseal; Vislube; Vismed; ***Thai.:*** AMO Vitrax†; Connettivina; Healon; Ial; Ophthalin; Provisc; Synvisc; ***UK:*** Arthrease; Cystistat; Fermathron; Gengigel; Healonid; Hyalgan; Hyalofill; Ophthalin; Orthovisc; Ostenil; Provisc†; Supartz; Suplasyn; Synvisc; ***USA:*** AMO Vitrax; Amvisc; Coease; Healon; Hyalgan; Orthovisc; Shellgel; Supartz; Synvisc.

**Multi-ingredient:** ***Arg.:*** Cremisona; Hyalcrom; Hyanac; Maxus; Panoxi; Viscoat; ***Austral.:*** Duovisc; Viscoat; ***Belg.:*** Viscoat†; ***Chile:*** Hydrating B5 Gel; ***Fr.:*** Hyalogran; Mucogyne; Viscoat; ***Ger.:*** Duovisc; Viscoat; ***Hong Kong:*** Duovisc; Viscoat; ***Ital.:*** Altergen; Connettivina Plus; Dropyal; Healon Yellow†; Idroskin C; Osmogel; Trofo 5; Viscoat; ***Malaysia:*** Viscoat; ***NZ:*** Viscoat; ***Port.:*** Synchrorose; Synchrovit; ***S.Afr.:*** Duovisc; Viscoat; ***Singapore:*** Duovisc; Viscoat; ***Swed.:*** Provisc†; ***Switz.:*** Alphastria; Ialugen Plus; Lacrycon; Viscoat†; ***Thai.:*** Duovisc; Viscoat; ***UK:*** Gelclair; Seprafilm; Viscoat†; ***USA:*** Healon Yellow; Seprafilm; Viscoat.

## Hyaluronidase *(BAN, rINN)*

Hialuronidasa; Hyaluronidasum.

*CAS — 9001-54-1.*

*ATC — B06AA03.*

**Pharmacopoeias.** In *Chin.* and *Eur.* (see p.vi). *US* includes as an injectable form.

**Ph. Eur. 5.0** (Hyaluronidase). An enzyme capable of hydrolysing mucopolysaccharides of the hyaluronic acid type. It is prepared from the testes of mammals by a method that has been shown to reduce contamination by known infectious agents to acceptable limits; a suitable stabilising agent may be added to the purified preparation. A white or yellowish-white, amorphous powder; it contains not less than 300 international units of hyaluronidase activity per mg, calculated with reference to the dried substance. Soluble in water; practically insoluble in alcohol and in acetone. A 0.3% solution in water has a pH of 4.5 to 7.5. Store at 2° to 8° in airtight containers.

### Units

The international and USP units are equivalent. One international or USP unit is equivalent to one turbidity-reducing unit or about 3.3 viscosity-reducing units.

### Adverse Effects and Precautions

Sensitivity to hyaluronidase occasionally occurs. Hyaluronidase should be used with caution in patients with infections; because of the danger of spreading infection, the enzyme generally should not be injected into or around an infected area. It has been suggested that the presence of malignancy may similarly be a contra-indication to the use of hyaluronidase. It should not be given by intravenous injection nor should it be used for anaesthetic procedures in cases of unexplained premature labour. Hyaluronidase should not be applied directly to the cornea. It should not be used to reduce the swelling of bites or stings.

### Uses and Administration

Hyaluronidase is an enzyme that reversibly depolymerises hyaluronic acid (above), a component of the ground substance or tissue cement surrounding cells, thereby temporarily reducing its viscosity and rendering the tissues more readily permeable to injected fluids.

Hyaluronidase is used to increase the speed of absorption and to diminish discomfort due to subcutaneous or intramuscular injection of fluids, to promote resorption of excess fluids and extravasated blood in the tissues, and to increase the effectiveness of local anaesthesia.

In the UK, the usual dose of hyaluronidase to facilitate subcutaneous or intramuscular injection is 1500 units, added directly to the injection. To aid the dispersal of extravasated fluids or blood, the same dose is given in 1 mL of Water for Injections or 0.9% sodium chloride into the affected area. Lower doses of hyaluronidase are used in some countries; in the USA, the usual dose is 150 units.

In hypodermoclysis, hyaluronidase is used to aid the subcutaneous administration of relatively large volumes of fluids, especially in infants and young children, where intravenous injection is difficult. Care should be taken in the treatment of children and the elderly to control the speed and total volume administered and to avoid overhydration. Hyaluronidase may be added to the injection fluid or may be injected into the site before the fluid is given. In the UK, 1500 units of hyaluronidase is generally used for each 500 to 1000 mL of fluid for subcutaneous administration, but in the USA, 150 units of hyaluronidase is considered adequate for each litre of hypodermoclysis solution.

The diffusion of local anaesthetics is accelerated by the addition of 1500 units (in the USA, 150 units) of hyaluronidase to the anaesthetic solution. This is of value in the reduction of fractures and in pudendal block in midwifery. It has also been used in ophthalmology as an aid to local anaesthesia at recommended doses of 15 units/mL of local anaesthetic solution. Intravitreal hyaluronidase injection is under investigation in the management of vitreous haemorrhage.

Hyalosidase (GL enzyme) is a highly purified form of hyaluronidase that has been studied.

◊ General references.


1. Watson D. Hyaluronidase. *Br J Anaesth* 1993; **71:** 422–5.


**Ophthalmic surgery.** In a study[1] involving 150 consecutive patients undergoing surgery for senile cataract, retrobulbar anaesthesia with lidocaine 2% solution plus adrenaline 1:100 000 and hyaluronidase 15 units/mL produced successful anaesthesia in 69 of 75 cases (92%), which was significantly better than 42 of 75 treated with lidocaine plus adrenaline alone. Although poor results have been reported from hyaluronidase and a local anaesthetic without adrenaline to restrict local anaesthetic absorption, the use of the enzyme and adrenaline was recommended as an aid to achieving complete ocular akinesia and anaesthesia in cataract surgery. Hyaluronidase has also been used with a mixture of bupivacaine and lidocaine for peribulbar anaesthesia, but results have been conflicting. In a study[2] in 50 patients, addition of hyaluronidase 25 units/mL of local anaesthetic mixture had no significant effect on time to satisfactory anaesthesia. However, in a second study[3] involving 200 patients, addition of hyaluronidase 50 or 300 units/mL improved the quality of the peribulbar block and, in the case of the higher concentration, also increased the speed of onset.


1. Thomson I. Addition of hyaluronidase to lignocaine with adrenaline for retrobulbar anaesthesia in the surgery of senile cataract. *Br J Ophthalmol* 1988; **72:** 700–2.
2. Prosser DP, *et al.* Re-evaluation of hyaluronidase in peribulbar anaesthesia. *Br J Ophthalmol* 1996; **80:** 827–30.
3. Dempsey GA, *et al.* Hyaluronidase and peribulbar block. *Br J Anaesth* 1997; **78:** 671–4.


### Preparations

***BP 2003:*** Hyaluronidase Injection;
***USP 27:*** Hyaluronidase for Injection; Hyaluronidase Injection.

**Proprietary Preparations** (details are given in Part 3)

***Arg.:*** Unidasa; ***Austral.:*** Hyalase; ***Austria:*** Neopermease†; Permease†; ***Braz.:*** Hyalozima; ***Canad.:*** Wydase†; ***Chile:*** Wydase; ***Ger.:*** Hylase; ***India:*** Hynidase; ***Israel:*** Hyalase; ***Ital.:*** Jaluran; ***Neth.:*** Hyason; ***NZ:*** Hyalase; ***S.Afr.:*** Hyalase; ***UK:*** Hyalase; ***USA:*** Wydase†.

**Multi-ingredient:** ***Arg.:*** Nilflux; ***Austria:*** Lemuval; ***Braz.:*** Oto Xilodase; Xilodase; ***Fr.:*** Lasonil†; ***Israel:*** Lasonil†; ***Ital.:*** Jalovis†; Lasonil H†; Lasoproct†; Lido-Hyal; ***NZ:*** Lasonil; ***Spain:*** Lasonil; Oto Difusor†; ***Switz.:*** Lido-Hyal.

## Hydrangea

Hidrangea; Seven Barks; Smooth Hydrangea; Wild Hydrangea.

### Profile

Hydrangea, the root of *Hydrangea arborescens* (Hydrangeaceae), has diuretic and litholytic properties and is used for genitourinary disorders including renal and urinary calculi. It has also been used in homoeopathic preparations.

### Preparations

**Proprietary Preparations** (details are given in Part 3)

**Multi-ingredient:** ***UK:*** Antiglan; Backache.

## Hydrastine Hydrochloride

Hidrastina, hidrocloruro de. 6,7-Dimethoxy-3-(5,6,7,8-tetrahydro-6-methyl-1,3-dioxolo[4,5-g]isoquinolin-5-yl)isobenzofuran-1(3*H*)-one hydrochloride.

$C_{21}H_{21}NO_6,HCl = 419.9.$

*CAS — 118-08-1 (hydrastine); 5936-28-7 (hydrastine hydrochloride).*

### Profile

Hydrastine hydrochloride, the hydrochloride of an alkaloid obtained from *Hydrastis canadensis* (Ranunculaceae) (see Hydrastis, below), has been reputed to cause uterine contractions and arrest uterine haemorrhage but it is of doubtful value. It was also formerly used in gastrointestinal disorders. Toxic doses are reported to cause strychnine-like convulsions and relaxation of the gut.

## Hydrastis

Golden Seal; Goldenseal; Hidraste; Hidrastis; Hydrast.; Hydrastis Rhizoma; Idraste; Yellow Root.

**Pharmacopoeias.** In *Eur.* (see p.vi). Also in *USNF.*

**Ph. Eur. 5.0** (Goldenseal Rhizome). The whole or cut, dried rhizome and root of *Hydrastis canadensis* containing not less than 2.5% of hydrastine and not less than 3.0% of berberine, calculated on the dried basis. Protect from light.

**USNF 22** (Goldenseal). The dried roots and rhizomes of *Hydrastis canadensis* (Ranunculaceae), containing not less than 2.0% of hydrastine and not less than 2.5% of berberine, calculated on the dried basis. Store in airtight containers. Protect from light, moisture, and heat.

### Profile

Hydrastis was formerly used to arrest excessive uterine haemorrhage. It is included in some herbal preparations for gastrointestinal disorders and peripheral vascular disorders. It is used in homoeopathic medicine. The pharmacological activity of hydrastis is attributed primarily to 2 of its constituent alkaloids, berberine (p.1659) and hydrastine (above).

### Preparations

**Proprietary Preparations** (details are given in Part 3)

***Ger.:*** Gingivitol N.

**Multi-ingredient:** ***Austral.:*** Bilberry Plus†; Herbal Cleanse†; Hydrastis Complex†; Sambucus Complex†; Trillium Complex†; Urapro†; Urinase†; ***Braz.:*** Bromidrastina†; Uterovarol†; ***Fr.:*** Climaxol; Curoveinyl†; ***Spain:*** Proctosor; Solucion Schoum; ***UK:*** Digestive; Fenulin†; Gerard House

Golden Seal Compound†; HRI Golden Seal Digestive; Papaya Plus†; Wind & Dyspepsia Relief.

## Hydrazine Sulfate

Hidrazina, sulfato de; Hydrazine Sulphate.

$H_6N_2O_4S$ = 130.1.

*CAS — 302-01-2 (hydrazine); 10034-93-2 (hydrazine sulfate).*

### Profile

Hydrazine sulfate is employed in various industrial processes. It is used in the preparation of hydrazine hydrate which is applied after a solution of platinic chloride for corneal tattooing. It has been tried, but with little if any benefit, in the management of cancer-related anorexia and cachexia.

**Adverse effects and treatment.** References to adverse effects resulting from exposure to hydrazine.[1-5] Pyridoxine has been used in the management of hydrazine intoxication.[6-8]


1. Albert DM, Puliafito CA. Choroidal melanoma: possible exposure to industrial toxins. *N Engl J Med* 1977; **296:** 634–5.
2. Durant PJ, Harris RA. Hydrazine and lupus. *N Engl J Med* 1980; **303:** 584–5.
3. Hydrazine. *Environmental Health Criteria 68.* Geneva: WHO, 1987. Available at: http://www.inchem.org/documents/ehc/ehc/ehc68.htm (accessed 16/06/04)
4. Hydrazine health and safety guide. *IPCS Health and Safety Guide 56.* Geneva: WHO, 1991. Available at: http://www.inchem.org/documents/hsg/hsg/hsg056.htm (accessed 16/06/04)
5. Hainer MI, *et al.* Fatal hepatorenal failure associated with hydrazine sulfate. *Ann Intern Med* 2000; **133:** 877–80.
6. Kirklin JK, *et al.* Treatment of hydrazine-induced coma with pyridoxine. *N Engl J Med* 1976; **294:** 938–9.
7. Harati Y, Niakan E. Hydrazine toxicity, pyridoxine therapy, and peripheral neuropathy. *Ann Intern Med* 1986; **104:** 728–9.
8. Nagappan R, Riddell T. Pyridoxine therapy in a patient with severe hydrazine sulfate toxicity. *Crit Care Med* 2000; **28:** 2116–18.


**Anorexia and cachexia.** References[1-3] to the use of hydrazine sulfate in patients with anorexia or cachexia associated with cancer.


1. Tayek JA, *et al.* Effect of hydrazine sulphate on whole-body protein breakdown measured by $^{14}$C-lysine metabolism in lung cancer patients. *Lancet* 1987; **ii:** 241–4.
2. Loprinzi CL, *et al.* Cancer-associated anorexia and cachexia: implications for drug therapy. *Drugs* 1992; **43:** 499–506.
3. Kaegi E. Unconventional therapies for cancer: hydrazine sulfate. *Can Med Assoc J* 1998; **158:** 1327–30.


## Hydrochloric Acid

Acidum Hydrochloridum; Clorhídrico, ácido; E507; Salzsäure.

HCl = 36.46.

*CAS — 7647-01-0.*

*ATC — A09AB03; B05XA13.*

NOTE. The impure acid of commerce is known as Spirits of Salt and as Muriatic Acid.

**Pharmacopoeias.** *Chin., Eur.* (see p.vi), *Int., Jpn, Pol., Swiss,* and *Viet.* include various concentrations. Also in *USNF.*

**Ph. Eur. 5.0** (Hydrochloric Acid, Concentrated; Acidum Hydrochloridum Concentratum; Hydrochloric Acid BP 2003). It contains 35.0 to 39.0% w/w of HCl. A clear, colourless, fuming liquid. Miscible with water. Store below 30° in stoppered containers of glass or other inert material.

**Ph. Eur. 5.0** (Hydrochloric Acid, Dilute; Acidum Hydrochloridum Dilutum). It contains 9.5 to 10.5% w/w of HCl prepared by mixing hydrochloric acid 274 g with water 726 g.

**USNF 22** (Hydrochloric Acid). It contains 36.5 to 38.0% w/w of HCl. A colourless, fuming liquid having a pungent odour. It ceases to fume when it is diluted with 2 volumes of water. Store in airtight containers.

**USNF 22** (Diluted Hydrochloric Acid). It contains 9.5 to 10.5% w/v of HCl and may be prepared by mixing hydrochloric acid 226 mL with sufficient water to make 1000 mL. A colourless, odourless liquid. Store in airtight containers.

### Adverse Effects

Hydrochloric acid is highly irritant and corrosive and ingestion has proved fatal. The corrosive effect causes chemical burns and severe pain. There may be violent vomiting, haematemesis, and circulatory collapse; acids can also produce intravascular coagulation and haemolysis. Ulceration may lead to perforation and patients can suffer strictures and pyloric stenosis. Asphyxiation may result from laryngeal oedema. Inhalation of acid fumes or aspiration of ingested acids may cause pneumonitis.

◊ References.


1. Chlorine and hydrogen chloride. *Environmental Health Criteria 21.* Geneva: WHO, 1982. Available at: http://www.inchem.org/documents/ehc/ehc/ehc21.htm (accessed 16/06/04)
2. Munoz Munoz E, *et al.* Massive necrosis of the gastrointestinal tract after ingestion of hydrochloric acid. *Eur J Surg* 2001; **167:** 195–8.


### Treatment of Adverse Effects

Treatment following ingestion is mainly symptomatic. Gastric lavage and activated charcoal are not generally appropriate and emetics must *not* be used. Small amounts of water or milk may be given to dilute the acid but larger volumes may increase the risk of emesis and hence of further damage. Neutralising agents are not recommended because of the possibility of heat being produced during exothermic reactions, which may increase the injury further. Opioid analgesia may be required for pain. Endoscopy should be performed and surgical intervention may be necessary. There is little evidence to support the value of corticosteroids in preventing stricture formation.

Acid burns of the skin should be flooded immediately with water and the washing should be copious and prolonged. Any affected clothing should be removed while flooding is being carried out. For burns in the eye, the lids should be kept open and the eye flushed with a steady stream of water at room temperature or sodium chloride 0.9%. A few drops of a local anaesthetic solution will relieve lid spasm and facilitate irrigation.

### Uses and Administration

Hydrochloric acid has been used as an escharotic. It has been used in the diluted form for the treatment of achlorhydria and other gastrointestinal disorders. It has also been given intravenously in the management of metabolic alkalosis (p.1217). An acid perfusion test using hydrochloric acid has been used in the diagnosis of oesophageal disorders. When taken orally, it should be sipped through a straw to protect the teeth.

Hydrochloride acid (muriaticum acidum) is used in homoeopathic medicine.

**Diagnosis and testing.** References and comments on the use of an acid perfusion test in the diagnosis of oesophageal disorders,[1-5] such as gastro-oesophageal reflux disease (p.1242) and oesophageal motility disorders (p.1246). The test involves intra-oesophageal perfusion of 0.1M hydrochloric acid; subsequent development of pain indicates an acid-sensitive oesophagus. This test has also been used in the differential diagnosis of angina.[2]


1. Sladen GE, *et al.* Oesophagoscopy, biopsy, and acid perfusion test in diagnosis of "reflux oesophagitis". *BMJ* 1975; **1:** 71–6.
2. Anonymous. Angina and oesophageal disease. *Lancet* 1986; **i:** 191–2.
3. Hewson EG, *et al.* Acid perfusion test: does it have a role in the assessment of non cardiac chest pain? *Gut* 1989; **30:** 305–10.
4. de Caestecker JS, Heading RC. Acid perfusion in the assessment of non-cardiac chest pain. *Gut* 1989; **30:** 1795–7.
5. Howard PJ, *et al.* Acid perfusion is a good screening test for symptomatic oesophageal reflux. *Gut* 1989; **30:** A1445.


**Pregnancy.** Heartburn during pregnancy may be due to reflux of alkaline duodenal contents. A dilute solution of hydrochloric acid (pH 2) taken after meals and at bedtime produced improvements in heartburn in pregnant women.[1]


1. Anonymous. Heartburn in pregnancy. *Drug Ther Bull* 1990; **28:** 11–12.


### Preparations

**Proprietary Preparations** (details are given in Part 3)
**Multi-ingredient:** ***Ital.:*** Gastro-Pepsin.

## Hydrofluoric Acid

Fluohydric Acid; Fluorhídrico, ácido; Fluoric Acid.

HF = 20.01.

*CAS — 7664-39-3.*

**Description.** Hydrofluoric acid is a solution of hydrogen fluoride in water. Various strengths are used. It attacks glass strongly.

### Adverse Effects

As for Hydrochloric Acid, above. Although the corrosive effects of hydrofluoric acid tend to predominate, absorption may produce systemic fluoride poisoning as described under Sodium Fluoride, p.1444.

The pain from contact with weak solutions may be delayed, so that the patient is not aware of being burnt until some hours later, when the area begins to smart; intense pain then sets in and this may persist for several days. Destruction of tissue proceeds under the toughened coagulated skin, so that the ulcers extend deeply, heal slowly, and leave a scar.

The fumes of hydrofluoric acid are highly irritant.

### Treatment of Adverse Effects

The initial treatment of poisoning following oral exposure to hydrofluoric acid is similar to that described for hydrochloric acid, see above. Calcium gluconate should also be given intravenously to correct known or suspected hypocalcaemia. Burns in the eye are also managed as for hydrochloric acid, although irrigation of the eye may be continued with calcium gluconate solution 2% after initial flood with water or sodium chloride 0.9%.

In the event of skin burns with hydrofluoric acid, contaminated clothing or articles should be removed and the skin washed with copious cold water or sodium chloride 0.9%. Irrigation with a solution of a calcium salt, e.g. 1% calcium gluconate, is carried out to convert the fluoride to an insoluble form and so prevent absorption. Milk may be tried if such solutions are not available. A calcium gluconate gel is sometimes used and it may be necessary to infiltrate the affected areas with calcium gluconate intradermally or subcutaneously. Hydrofluoric acid passes through finger- and toe-nails without causing any apparent damage; nails will therefore have to be removed or perforated to be able to treat the underlying tissues. Other first-aid measures reported to be effective include prolonged soaks in iced solutions of benzalkonium chloride or benzethonium chloride; iced water has sometimes been used as has iced magnesium sulfate solution. Local, or even general, anaesthesia may be needed. Burn eschars should be excised and necrotic tissue debrided. Absorption may lead to systemic fluoride toxicity and the need for intravenous calcium gluconate to manage hypocalcaemic symptoms.

◊ References to the treatment of hydrofluoric acid burns.


1. Browne TD. The treatment of hydrofluoric acid burns. *J Soc Occup Med* 1974; **24:** 80–9.
2. MacKinnon MA. Hydrofluoric acid burns. *Dermatol Clin* 1988; **6:** 67–74.
3. McIvor ME. Acute fluoride toxicity: pathophysiology and management. *Drug Safety* 1990; **5;** 79–85.
4. Kirkpatrick JJR, *et al.* Hydrofluoric acid burns: a review. *Burns* 1995; **21:** 483–93.
5. Sanz-Gallen P, *et al.* Hypocalcaemia and hypomagnesaemia due to hydrofluoric acid. *Occup Med (Lond)* 2001; **51:** 294–5.
6. Martin HCO, Muller MJ. Hydrofluoric acid burns from a household rust remover. *Med J Aust* 2002; **176:** 296.
7. Foster KN, *et al.* Hydrofluoric acid burn resulting from ignition of gas from a compressed air duster. *J Burn Care Rehabil* 2003; **24:** 234–8.


### Uses

Hydrofluoric acid is used in industry. Its main use has been for the production of fluorocarbons for use as refrigerants and propellants. It has also been used as an ingredient of preparations for glass etching and rust removal.

Hydrofluoric acid (fluoricum acidum) is used in homoeopathic medicine.

## Hydroquinine Hydrobromide

Dihydrochinin Hydrobromide; Dihydroquinine Hydrobromide; Hidroquinina, hidrobromuro de; Hydrochinin Hydrobromide; Methylhydrocupreine Hydrobromide. 8α,9R-10,11-Dihydro-6′-methoxycinchonan-9-ol hydrobromide.

$C_{20}H_{26}N_2O_2$,HBr = 407.3.

*CAS — 522-66-7 (hydroquinine).*

*ATC — M09AA01.*

NOTE. Do not confuse with Hydroquinone (p.1148).

### Profile

Hydroquinine is a derivative of quinine (p.460) used similarly in the treatment of nocturnal muscle cramps. It is given as the hydrobromide in a dose of 200 mg with the evening meal and a further 100 mg at bedtime for 14 days.

**Muscle spasm.** Quinine and its derivatives such as hydroquinine have traditionally been used for the prevention of nocturnal cramps (p.1386) but there has been concern over their efficacy and potential for adverse effects, especially in the elderly.

References.


1. Jansen PHP, *et al.* Randomised controlled trial of hydroquinine in muscle cramps. *Lancet* 1997; **349:** 528–32.
2. van Kan HJM, *et al.* Hydroquinine pharmacokinetics after oral administration in adult patients with muscle cramps. *Eur J Clin Pharmacol* 2000; **56:** 263–7.


### Preparations

**Proprietary Preparations** (details are given in Part 3)
***Neth.:*** Inhibin.

## Hydroxyamfetamine Hydrobromide

*(BANM, rINNM)*

Bromhidrato de Hidroxianfetamina; Hidrobromuro de hidroxianfetamina; Hydroxyamphetamine Hydrobromide; Oxamphetamine Hydrobromide. (±)-4-(2-Aminopropyl)phenol hydrobromide.

$C_9H_{13}NO$,HBr = 232.1.

*CAS — 103-86-6 (hydroxyamfetamine); 1518-86-1 ((±)-hydroxyamfetamine); 306-21-8 (hydroxyamfetamine hydrobromide); 140-36-3 ((±)-hydroxyamfetamine hydrobromide).*

**Pharmacopoeias.** In *US.*

**USP 27** (Hydroxyamphetamine Hydrobromide). A white, crystalline powder. Freely soluble in water and in alcohol; slightly soluble in chloroform; practically insoluble in ether. Its solutions in water are slightly acid to litmus, having a pH of about 5. Protect from light.

### Profile

Hydroxyamfetamine hydrobromide is a sympathomimetic with an action similar to that of ephedrine (p.1120), but it has little or no stimulant effect on the CNS. It was formerly used as a vasopressor and in the management of some cardiac disorders.

In ophthalmology, hydroxyamfetamine hydrobromide has been used in a 1% solution as a mydriatic and in the diagnosis of Horner's syndrome.

### Preparations

***USP 27:*** Hydroxyamphetamine Hydrobromide Ophthalmic Solution.

**Proprietary Preparations** (details are given in Part 3)
***USA:*** Paredrine.

**Multi-ingredient:** ***USA:*** Paremyd.

## Hydroxyapatite *(BAN)*

542 (edible bone phosphate); Durapatite *(USAN)*; Hidroxiapatito; Hydroxylapatite; Win-40350. Decacalcium dihydroxide hexakis(orthophosphate).

$3Ca_3(PO_4)_2,Ca(OH)_2$ = 1004.6.

*CAS — 1306-06-5.*

### Profile

Hydroxyapatite is a natural mineral with composition similar to that of the mineral in bone. Hydroxyapatite for therapeutic purposes is prepared from bovine bone and contains, in addition to calcium and phosphate, trace elements, fluoride and other ions, proteins, and glycosaminoglycans. It is given by mouth to patients requiring both calcium and phosphorus supplementation. Hydroxyapatite with tricalcium phosphate has been used in bone grafts.

Hydroxyapatite derived from marine coral has been used in the construction of orbital implants for use following surgical removal of the eye.

**Adverse effects.** Reference to problems associated with the use of coral-derived orbital implants.[1]

1. Shields CL, *et al.* Problems with the hydroxyapatite orbital implant: experience with 250 consecutive cases. *Br J Ophthalmol* 1994; **78:** 702–6.

**Uses.** A mixture of calcium phosphates with calcium carbonate could be combined to form a paste which could be injected into acute fractures;[1] under physiological conditions the paste hardened within minutes, due to the formation of dahllite, a carbonated apatite, and held the bones in place as it was progressively replaced by living bone.

1. Constantz BR, *et al.* Skeletal repair by in situ formation of the mineral phase of bone. *Science* 1995; **267:** 1796–9.

### Preparations

**Proprietary Preparations** (details are given in Part 3)
***Austria:*** Ossopan; Osteogenon; ***Braz.:*** Ossopan; ***Fr.:*** Ossopan; ***Ger.:*** Ossopan; ***India:*** Ossopan; ***Irl.:*** Ossopan; ***Ital.:*** Apagen; ***Mex.:*** Ossopan; ***Port.:*** Ossopan; ***Singapore:*** Ossopan; ***Spain:*** Ossopan; Osteopor; ***Switz.:*** Ossopan; ***Thai.:*** Ossopan; ***UK:*** Ossopan†; Osteo Support.
**Multi-ingredient:** ***Arg.:*** Totalos Plus.

## Hydroxymethylnicotinamide

Hidroximetilnicotinamida; *N*-Hydroxymethylnicotinamide; Nicotinylmethylamide. *N*-Hydroxymethylpyridine-3-carboxamide.
$C_7H_8N_2O_2$ = 152.2.
*CAS — 3569-99-1.*

**Pharmacopoeias.** In *Pol.*

### Profile

Hydroxymethylnicotinamide is a cholagogue and has been used in the treatment of various disorders of the gallbladder.

### Preparations

**Proprietary Preparations** (details are given in Part 3)
***India:*** Bilamide.
**Multi-ingredient:** ***Spain:*** Sambil†.

## Hydroxyquinoline Sulfate

Chinosolum; Hidroxiquinolina, sulfato de; Hydroxyquinoline Sulphate; Oxichinolini Sulfas; Oxine Sulphate; Oxyquinol; Oxyquinoline Sulfate *(USAN)*; Sulfate d'Orthoxyquinoléine. Quinolin-8-ol sulphate; 8-Quinolinol sulphate.
$(C_9H_7NO)_2,H_2SO_4$ = 388.4.
*CAS — 148-24-3 (hydroxyquinoline); 134-31-6 (hydroxyquinoline sulfate).*

**Pharmacopoeias.** In *Fr.* and *Swiss.* Also in *USNF.*

**USNF 22** (Oxyquinoline Sulfate). A yellow powder. Very soluble in water; slightly soluble in alcohol; practically insoluble in acetone and in ether; freely soluble in methyl alcohol.

### Profile

Hydroxyquinoline sulfate has properties similar to those of potassium hydroxyquinoline sulfate (p.1734) and has been used similarly in the topical treatment of skin, oropharyngeal, and vaginal disorders.

Derivatives of hydroxyquinoline including the salicylate, benzoate, borate, hydrofluoride, iodochloride, silicofluoride, and sodium hydroxyquinoline sulfate have been used similarly.

### Preparations

**Proprietary Preparations** (details are given in Part 3)
***Braz.:*** Oto-Cer†; ***Ger.:*** Leioderm; ***Ital.:*** Aftir Shampoo; ***Neth.:*** Superol.
**Multi-ingredient:** ***Arg.:*** Curisept; ***Austral.:*** Aci-Jel; ***Austria:*** Racestyptin†; ***Braz.:*** Andolba; Cerumin; Colpolase; Gynaseptol†; Higienex†; Lacto Vagin; Lacto-Gin†; Leucocida; Lisofenicol†; Lisoquinol†; Nestosyl†; Pan-Emecort; Senol; Varigerm†; ***Canad.:*** Dermoplast†; ***Chile:*** Diproquin; ***Fr.:*** Chromargon; Dermacide; Nestosyl; ***Ger.:*** Chinosol; Chinosol S Vaseline†; Leioderm P; ***Ital.:*** Leucorsan†; Ustiosan; Viderm; ***NZ:*** Aci-Jel; ***Port.:*** Apyrol; ***S.Afr.:*** Cuticura; ***Spain:*** Neodesfila†; ***Switz.:*** Benzocaine PD; Racestyptine†; ***USA:*** Aci-Jel†; Auroguard Otic; Fem pH; Medicone Derma; Medicone Rectal; Oxyzal; Stypto-Caine; Trimo-San; Triv.

## Hymecromone *(BAN, USAN, rINN)*

Himecromona; Hymecromonum; Imecromone; LM-94. 7-Hydroxy-4-methylcoumarin.
$C_{10}H_8O_3$ = 176.2.
*CAS — 90-33-5.*
*ATC — A05AX02.*

**Pharmacopoeias.** In *Chin., Eur.* (see p.vi), and *Jpn.*

**Ph. Eur. 5.0** (Hymecromone). An almost white crystalline powder. Very slightly soluble in water; slightly soluble in dichloromethane; sparingly soluble in methyl alcohol. It dissolves in dilute solutions of ammonia. Protect from light.

### Profile

Hymecromone is a choleretic and biliary antispasmodic. It has been given with fluid in doses of 400 mg three times daily at mealtimes. It has also been given as the sodium salt by slow intravenous injection as an adjunct to diagnostic procedures. Diarrhoea may occasionally occur.

### Preparations

**Proprietary Preparations** (details are given in Part 3)
***Austria:*** Cholonerton; Unichol; ***Belg.:*** Cantabiline; ***Fr.:*** Bilicante†; Cantabiline; ***Ger.:*** Chol-Spasmoletten; Cholspasmin; Gallo Merz Spasmo; ***Ital.:*** Cantabilin; ***Spain:*** Bilicanta.

## Hypoglycin A

Hipoglicina A. L-2-Amino-3-(2-methylenecyclopropyl)propionic acid.
$C_7H_{11}NO_2$ = 141.2.
*CAS — 156-56-9.*

### Profile

Hypoglycin A is a toxic substance present in the arillus of unripe ackee (akee), the fruit of *Blighia sapida* (Sapindaceae). It is responsible for Jamaican vomiting sickness, with symptoms of acute and severe vomiting, hypoglycaemia, muscular weakness, CNS depression, convulsions, and coma, frequently fatal. Glycine (p.1433) has been suggested for the management of hypoglycin A toxicity.

## Hypophosphorous Acid

Acidum Hypophosphorosum; Hipofosforoso, ácido; Phosphinic Acid.
$H_3PO_2$ = 66.0.
*CAS — 6303-21-5; 14332-09-3.*

**Pharmacopoeias.** In *USNF.*

**USNF 22** (Hypophosphorous Acid). It contains 30 to 32% of $H_3PO_2$. A colourless or slightly yellow, odourless liquid. Store in airtight containers.

### Profile

Hypophosphorous acid is used as an antoxidant. Hypophosphates were used in tonics; like the glycerophosphates they are not a suitable source of phosphorus.

### Preparations

**Proprietary Preparations** (details are given in Part 3)
**Multi-ingredient:** ***UK:*** Dispello.

## Ibogaine

Ibogaina; NIH-10567. 12-Methoxyibogamine.
$C_{20}H_{26}N_2O$ = 310.4.
*CAS — 83-74-9.*

### Profile

Ibogaine is a hallucinogenic indole alkaloid extracted from the West African shrub *Tabernanthe iboga* (Apocynaceae). It has been investigated as an aid to withdrawal from drug addiction.

◊ References.

1. Popik P, *et al.* 100 years of ibogaine: neurochemical and pharmacological actions of a putative anti-addictive drug. *Pharmacol Rev* 1995; **47:** 235–53.
2. Alper KR, *et al.* Treatment of acute opioid withdrawal with ibogaine. *Am J Addict* 1999; **8:** 234–42.

## Idazoxan Hydrochloride *(BANM, pINNM)*

Hidrocloruro de idazoxano; RX-781094. 2-(2,3-Dihydro-1,4-benzodioxin-2-yl)-2-imidazoline hydrochloride.
$C_{11}H_{12}N_2O_2,HCl$ = 240.7.
*CAS — 79944-58-4 (idazoxan); 79944-56-2 (idazoxan hydrochloride).*

### Profile

Idazoxan hydrochloride is an alpha$_2$-adrenoceptor antagonist that has been investigated in neurological disorders including depression, dementia, and parkinsonism.

◊ References.

1. Ghika J, *et al.* Idazoxan treatment in progressive supranuclear palsy. *Neurology* 1991; **41:** 986–91.
2. Litman RE, *et al.* Idazoxan, an alpha2 antagonist, augments fluphenazine in schizophrenic patients: a pilot study. *J Clin Psychopharmacol* 1993; **13:** 264–7.
3. Grossman F, *et al.* A double-blind study comparing idazoxan and bupropion in bipolar depressed patients. *J Affect Disord* 1999; **56:** 237–43.
4. Manson AJ, *et al.* Idazoxan is ineffective for levodopa-induced dyskinesias in Parkinson's disease. *Mov Disord* 2000; **15:** 336–7.
5. Rascol O, *et al.* Idazoxan, an alpha-2 antagonist, and L-DOPA-induced dyskinesias in patients with Parkinson's disease. *Mov Disord* 2001; **16:** 708–13.

## Idebenone *(rINN)*

CV-2619; Idebenona. 2-(10-Hydroxydecyl)-5,6-dimethoxy-3-methyl-*p*-benzoquinone.
$C_{19}H_{30}O_5$ = 338.4.
*CAS — 58186-27-9.*
*ATC — N06BX13.*

### Profile

Idebenone has been used in the treatment of mental impairment associated with cerebrovascular disorders. A dose of 90 mg daily, in divided doses after food, has been given by mouth. Idebenone has also been tried in Alzheimer's disease and in Friedreich's ataxia.

**Dementia.** Idebenone was found to be safe and effective in patients with mild to moderate Alzheimer's disease (p.1484) when followed for up to 2 years.[1,2] In a further study, its safety and efficacy were comparable to tacrine[3].

1. Weyer G, *et al.* Efficacy and safety of idebenone in the long-term treatment of Alzheimer's disease: a double-blind, placebo controlled multicentre study. *Hum Psychopharmacol Clin Exp* 1996; **11:** 53–65.
2. Gutzmann H, Hadler D. Sustained efficacy and safety of idebenone in the treatment of Alzheimer's disease: update on a 2-year double-blind multicentre study. *J Neural Transm* 1998; **54** (suppl): 301–10.
3. Gutzmann H, *et al.* Safety and efficacy of idebenone versus tacrine in patients with Alzheimer's disease: results of a randomized, double-blind, parallel-group multicenter study. *Pharmacopsychiatry* 2002; **35:** 12–18.

**Friedreich's ataxia.** Preliminary studies of idebenone in the treatment of Friedreich's ataxia.[1-5]

1. Hausse AO, *et al.* Idebenone and reduced cardiac hypertrophy in Friedreich's ataxia. *Heart* 2002; **87:** 346–9.
2. Artuch R, *et al.* Friedreich's ataxia: idebenone treatment in early stage patients. *Neuropediatrics* 2002; **33:** 190–3.
3. Mariotti C, *et al.* Idebenone treatment in Friedreich patients: one-year-long randomized placebo-controlled trial. *Neurology* 2003; **60:** 1676–9.
4. Buyse G, *et al.* Idebenone treatment in Friedreich's ataxia: neurological, cardiac, and biochemical monitoring. *Neurology* 2003; **60:** 1679–81.
5. Rustin P, *et al.* Idebenone treatment in Friedreich patients: one-year-long randomized placebo-controlled trial. *Neurology* 2004; **62:** 524–5.

### Preparations

**Proprietary Preparations** (details are given in Part 3)
***Arg.:*** Esanic; Geniceral; Idesole; Nemocebral; Pavertrin; Sicoplus; Ulcourona; ***Ital.:*** Daruma; Mnesis; ***Mex.:*** Lucebanol; ***Port.:*** Amizal; Cerestabon; Idecortex.
**Multi-ingredient:** ***Arg.:*** Idesole Plus.

## Ilodecakin *(USAN, rINN)*

Ilodecakina; Sch-52000.
*CAS — 149824-15-7.*

### Profile

Ilodecakin is a recombinant human interleukin-10. It is under investigation for its anti-inflammatory properties in several diseases including psoriasis, inflammatory bowel disease, and hepatitis C.

◊ References.

1. Asadullah K, *et al.* Interleukin-10 therapy—review of a new approach. *Pharmacol Rev* 2003; **55:** 241–69.

## Indeloxazine Hydrochloride *(USAN, rINNM)*

CI-874; Hidrocloruro de indeloxazina. (±)-2-[(Inden-7-yloxy)methyl]morpholine hydrochloride.
$C_{14}H_{17}NO_2,HCl$ = 267.8.
*CAS — 60929-23-9 (indeloxazine); 65043-22-3 (indeloxazine hydrochloride).*

### Profile

Indeloxazine hydrochloride has been reported to improve cerebral function. It has been promoted for the treatment of hypobulia (a lack of volition or drive) and for emotional disturbances associated with cerebrovascular disorders.

## Indigo Carmine

Blue X; Ceruleinum; CI Food Blue 1; Colour Index No. 73015; Disodium Indigotin-5,5′-disulphonate; E132; FD & C Blue No. 2; Indicarminum; Indigotina; Indigotindisulfonate Sodium; Indigotine; Sodium Indigotindisulphonate. Disodium 3,3′-dioxo-2,2′-bi-indolinylidene-5,5′-disulphonate.
$C_{16}H_8N_2Na_2O_8S_2$ = 466.4.
*CAS — 483-20-5 (indigotin-5,5′-disulphonic acid); 860-22-0 (indigo carmine).*
*ATC — V04CH02.*

NOTE. The name Caerulein has been applied to Ceruletide (p.1669).

**Pharmacopoeias.** In *It., Jpn,* and *US.*

**USP 27** (Indigotindisulfonate Sodium). A dusky, purplish-blue powder, or blue granules having a coppery lustre. Soluble 1 in 100 of water; slightly soluble in alcohol; practically insoluble in most other organic solvents. Its solutions have a blue or bluish-purple colour. Store in airtight containers at a temperature of 25°, excursions permitted between 15° and 30°. Protect from light.

### Adverse Effects and Precautions

Indigo carmine may cause nausea, vomiting, hypertension, and bradycardia, and occasionally, hypersensitivity reactions such as skin rash, pruritus, and bronchoconstriction. Skin discoloration may occur after administration of large parenteral doses.

**Hypersensitivity.** Cardiac arrest following the administration of indigo carmine 80 mg intravenously resulted in the deaths of 2 elderly patients.[1] Both had a history of asthmatic bronchitis. A life-threatening anaphylactoid reaction associated with indigo carmine use has also been reported, although the authors commented that such events are rare.[2]

1. Voiry AM, *et al.* Deux accidents mortels lors d'une injection peropératoire de carmin d'indigo. *Ann Med Nancy* 1976; **15:** 413–19.
2. Gousse AE, *et al.* Life-threatening anaphylactoid reaction associated with indigo carmine intravenous injection. *Urology* 2000; **56:** 508.

### Uses and Administration

Following intravenous injection indigo carmine is rapidly excreted, principally by the kidneys. It has been used in a test of renal function, but has largely been replaced by agents that give more precise results. It is used as a marker dye, particularly in urological procedures, when it is administered in a usual dose of 40 mg, preferably by intravenous injection but sometimes intramuscularly. It has also been used as a marker dye in amniocentesis.

Indigo carmine has been used as a blue dye in medicinal preparations but it is relatively unstable. It has also been investigated as a dye-spray in the detection of colorectal adenomas. It is used as a food colour.

### Preparations

***USP 27:*** Indigotindisulfonate Sodium Injection.

## Indocyanine Green

Verde de indocianina. Sodium 2-{7-[1,1-dimethyl-3-(4-sulphobutyl)benz[e]indolin-2-ylidene]hepta-1,3,5-trienyl}-1,1-dimethyl-1*H*-benz[e]indolio-3-(butyl-4-sulphonate).

$C_{43}H_{47}N_2NaO_6S_2$ = 775.0.
*CAS — 3599-32-4.*

**Pharmacopoeias.** In *US.*

**USP 27** (Indocyanine Green). An olive-brown, dark green, blue-green, dark blue, or black powder. Is odourless or has a slight odour. It contains not more than 5.0% of sodium iodide, calculated on the dried basis. Soluble in water and in methyl alcohol; practically insoluble in most other organic solvents. Its solutions are deep emerald-green in colour. pH of a 0.5% solution in water is about 6. Its aqueous solutions are stable for about 8 hours. Store at a temperature of 25°, excursions permitted between 15° and 30°.

### Adverse Effects and Precautions

Indocyanine green is reported to be well tolerated. Solutions contain a small amount of sodium iodide and should be used with caution in patients hypersensitive to iodine. Clearance of indocyanine green may be altered by drugs that interfere with liver function.

**Hypersensitivity.** A report of anaphylactoid reactions to indocyanine green in 3 patients.[1] The authors commented that of 20 reactions that had been reported 9 involved anaphylactoid shock (with 2 subsequent deaths) and 11 involved hypotension or bronchospasm; they suggested that such reactions were dose-dependent and had a non-immune mechanism.

1. Speich R, *et al.* Anaphylactoid reactions after indocyanine-green administration. *Ann Intern Med* 1988; **109:** 345–6.

### Pharmacokinetics

After intravenous injection indocyanine green is rapidly bound to plasma protein. It is taken up by the liver and is rapidly excreted unchanged into the bile.

### Uses and Administration

Indocyanine green is an indicator dye used for assessing cardiac output and liver function, and for examining the choroidal vasculature in ophthalmic angiography. It is also used to assess blood flow and haemodynamics in various organs including the liver.

The usual dose for cardiac assessment is 5 mg injected rapidly via a cardiac catheter. A suggested dose for children is 2.5 mg, and for infants 1.25 mg. Several doses need to be given to obtain a number of dilution curves. However, the total dose should not exceed 2 mg/kg.

The usual dose of indocyanine green for testing liver function is 500 micrograms/kg intravenously.

**Diagnostic use.** Indocyanine green has been employed to assess blood flow to various organs and in other haemodynamic studies. However, some methods of determination of indocyanine green clearance as a measure of liver blood flow have been questioned on the grounds that extraction of the dye by the liver is not complete as is often assumed.[1] Interindividual variability in indocyanine clearance may introduce further error.[2]

There have been reports of the use of indocyanine green to assess cerebral blood flow in children during cardiopulmonary bypass[3] and to measure plasma volume in neonates.[4] In ophthalmology, indocyanine green angiography is used to visualise the choroidal circulation.[5]

1. Skak C, Keiding S. Methodological problems in the use of indocyanine green to estimate hepatic blood flow and ICG clearance in man. *Liver* 1987; **7:** 155–62.
2. Bauer LA, *et al.* Variability of indocyanine green pharmacokinetics in healthy adults. *Clin Pharm* 1989; **8:** 54–5.
3. Roberts I, *et al.* Estimation of cerebral blood flow with near infrared spectroscopy and indocyanine green. *Lancet* 1993; **342:** 1425.
4. Anthony MY, *et al.* Measurement of plasma volume in neonates. *Arch Dis Child* 1992; **67:** 36–40.
5. Owens SL. Indocyanine green angiography. *Br J Ophthalmol* 1996; **80:** 263–6.

### Preparations

***USP 27:*** Indocyanine Green for Injection.

**Proprietary Preparations** (details are given in Part 3)
***Ger.:*** Cardio-Green†; ICG-Pulsion; ***Israel:*** IC Green; ICG-Pulsion; ***USA:*** Cardio-Green; IC Green.

## Inhibin

Inhibina.

### Profile

Inhibin is a glycoprotein secreted by the testes and ovaries and because of its ability to suppress secretion of follicle-stimulating hormone by the pituitary it has been investigated as a potential contraceptive in both men and women.

## Inosine *(rINN)*

Hypoxanthine Riboside; Inosina. 6,9-Dihydro-9-β-D-ribofuranosyl-1*H*-purin-6-one.

$C_{10}H_{12}N_4O_5$ = 268.2.
*CAS — 58-63-9.*
*ATC — D06BB05; G01AX02; S01XA10.*

### Profile

Inosine has been used in the treatment of anaemias and cardiovascular, liver, and skin disorders and has been used as a tonic.

### Preparations

**Proprietary Preparations** (details are given in Part 3)
***Braz.:*** Troficardil†; ***Spain:*** Tebertin†.

**Multi-ingredient:** ***Austria:*** Laevadosin†; ***Ital.:*** For Liver†; Fruttocal†; Neo-Eparbiol; ***Spain:*** Boldosal†; Nutracel; Rubrocortin.

## Inositol

*i*-Inositol; *meso*-Inositol. *myo*-Inositol.

$C_6H_{12}O_6$ = 180.2.
*CAS — 87-89-8.*
*ATC — A11HA07.*

**Pharmacopoeias.** In *Fr.*

### Profile

Inositol, an isomer of glucose, has traditionally been considered to be a vitamin B substance although it has an uncertain status as a vitamin and a deficiency syndrome has not been identified in man. Sources of inositol include whole-grain cereals, fruits, and plants, in which it occurs as the hexaphosphate, fytic acid. It also occurs in both vegetables and meats in other forms. The usual daily intake of inositol from the diet is about 1 g. It is an ingredient of numerous vitamin preparations and dietary supplements, and of preparations promoted for a wide variety of disorders.

Inositol appears to be involved physiologically in lipid metabolism and has been tried, with little evidence of efficacy, in disorders associated with fat transport and metabolism. It has been investigated in the treatment of depression and anxiety, in diabetic neuropathy, and in neonatal respiratory distress syndrome and retinopathy of prematurity.

**Neonatal respiratory distress syndrome.** Inositol supplementation has been tried in premature infants with respiratory distress syndrome (p.1084). A meta-analysis[1] found that infants given inositol had improved survival and lower rates of bronchopulmonary dysplasia and retinopathy of prematurity than those given placebo.

1. Howlett A, Ohlsson A. Inositol for respiratory distress syndrome in preterm infants. Available in The Cochrane Library; Issue 2. Chichester: John Wiley; 2004.

### Preparations

**Proprietary Preparations** (details are given in Part 3)
***Hong Kong:*** Inositat†.

**Multi-ingredient:** ***Austral.:*** Hair and Skin Formula†; Liv-Detox†; ***Austria:*** Aslavital; Lemazol; ***Braz.:*** Hecrosine B12†; Hepatogenol†; Hormo Hepatico; Infiltran B12†; Metiocolin B12; Metionina Composta†; Necrohepat†; Xantinon Complex; ***Canad.:*** Amino-Cerv; ***Chile:*** Hepabil; ***Fr.:*** Hepagrume; ***Ger.:*** Hepalipon N†; Lipovitan; ***Hong Kong:*** Bilsan; Lipochol; ***India:*** Delphicol; ***Ital.:*** Digelax; Hepatos B12; Porfirin 12; Stimolfit; ***Port.:*** Metionina†; ***S.Afr.:*** Hepavite; Prohep; ***Spain:*** Complidermol; Dertrase; Policolinosil; Tri Hachemina; ***Thai.:*** Lipochol; Liporon; Proheparum†; ***UK:*** Fat-Solv†; Lipotropic Factors; ***USA:*** Amino-Cerv.

## Interleukin-1

Catabolin; Endogenous Pyrogen; Haematopoietin-1; IL-1; Interleucina 1; Leucocyte Endogenous Mediator; Lymphocyte Activating Factor.

### Profile

Interleukin-1 is one of a number of polypeptides produced by lymphocytes, monocytes, and other cells which are involved in the complex hormonal regulation of immune response, and which are known collectively as cytokines (p.1678). It may also be produced by recombinant DNA technology. Two distinct forms, interleukin-1α and interleukin-1β, are known to exist, which interact with the same receptor and appear to have similar biological activities. The term lymphokines has also been used to describe these compounds but is more properly restricted to products of the various lymphocyte subsets, such as interleukin-2.

It has been suggested that interleukin-1 may be of value in a wide variety of conditions including burn and wound healing, as an adjuvant to enhance the response to vaccines, and as an adjunct to cancer chemotherapy, antiviral therapy, or radiotherapy for its haematopoietic and possible antitumour activity. Adverse effects include fever, chills, headache, gastrointestinal disturbances, local erythema at the injection site, hypotension, and CNS effects.

Interleukin-2 is described in the chapter on Antineoplastics (p.562). Other interleukins under investigation include interleukin-3 (p.755) as a haematopoietic; interleukin-4 (IL-4) and interleukin-6 (IL-6) for malignant neoplasms and thrombocytopenia; ilodecakin (p.1700) is a recombinant interleukin-10 for inflammatory disorders; and interleukin-12 (p.1701) for malignant neoplasms and infections. Oprelvekin (p.757) is a recombinant interleukin-11 used in thrombocytopenia.

◊ Pharmacokinetics of some interleukins.

1. Bocci V. Interleukins: clinical pharmacokinetics and practical implications. *Clin Pharmacokinet* 1991; **21:** 274–84.

## Interleukin-1 Receptor Antagonists

Antagonista del Receptor de la Interleucina 1; IL-1ra; IL-1i; Interleukin-1 Inhibitors.

### Profile

Interleukin-1 (see above) is a cytokine that is involved in the hormonal regulation of immune response. Interleukin-1 receptor antagonists are being investigated or used in a range of inflammatory and immune-modulated disorders. The recombinant interleukin-1 receptor antagonist anakinra (p.14) is used in the treatment of rheumatoid arthritis.

## Interleukin-2 Fusion Toxins

Toxinas de fusión de interleucina 2.

### Profile

Recombinant technology has permitted the production of a number of products in which protein sequences from natural growth factors or cytokines are combined with a toxin. Such products include fusion toxins in which the receptor binding domain of diphtheria toxin is replaced with sequences from interleukin-2, thus producing specific cytotoxicity in cells expressing the interleukin-2 receptor. The interleukin-2 fusion toxin denileukin diftitox (p.546) is used in the treatment of cutaneous T-cell lymphoma, and both this and the related compound $DAB_{486}$ interleukin-2 have been investigated in a variety of disorders including diabetes mellitus, psoriasis, rheumatoid arthritis, cutaneous T-cell lymphoma and other malignancies, and HIV infection.

## Interleukin-6 Antibodies

IL-6 Antibody.

## Elsilimomab *(rINN)*

Immunoglobulin G1, anti-(human interleukin 6) (mouse monoclonal B-E8 heavy chain), disulfide with mouse monoclonal B-E8 κ-chain, dimer.

*CAS — 468715-71-1.*

### Profile

Monoclonal antibodies to interleukin-6 are under investigation for the treatment of various disorders including post-transplant lymphoproliferative disorders and renal cell carcinoma.

## Interleukin-12

IL-12.

## Edodekin Alfa *(USAN, rINN)*

Ro-24-7472/000.
*CAS — 187348-17-0.*

**Description.** A recombinant human interleukin-12.

### Profile

Recombinant human interleukin-12 (edodekin alfa) is under

investigation in a number of disorders including various cancers such as renal cell carcinoma.

## Inulin (BAN)

Alant Starch; Inulina.
*CAS — 9005-80-5.*

**Pharmacopoeias.** In *Br.* and *US.*

**BP 2003** (Inulin). A polysaccharide obtained from the tubers of *Dahlia variabilis, Helianthus tuberosus*, and other genera of the family Compositae. It is a white, odourless or almost odourless, hygroscopic, amorphous, granular powder. Slightly soluble in cold water, but freely soluble in hot water; slightly soluble in organic solvents.

**USP 27** (Inulin). A polysaccharide which, on hydrolysis, yields mainly fructose. A white, friable, chalk-like, amorphous, odourless powder. Soluble in hot water; slightly soluble in cold water and in organic solvents. A 10% solution in water has a pH of 4.5 to 7.0. Store at a temperature of 25°, excursions permitted between 15° and 30°.

### Pharmacokinetics

Inulin is rapidly removed from the circulation following intravenous administration but is not metabolised. A trace may be found in the bile and may cross the placenta, but it is predominantly eliminated in the urine by glomerular filtration without secretion or reabsorption in the renal tubule.

### Uses and Administration

Inulin is used intravenously as a diagnostic agent to measure the glomerular filtration rate. Although an accurate test, it is complex to perform and is generally reserved for research purposes. Crystals of inulin may be deposited on storage of the injection; they should be dissolved by heating for not more than 15 minutes before use and the injection cooled to a suitable temperature before administration.

Polyfructosan, an inulin analogue of lower average molecular weight, has been used similarly.

### Preparations

***BP 2003:*** Inulin Injection;
***USP 27:*** Inulin in Sodium Chloride Injection.

**Proprietary Preparations** (details are given in Part 3)
***Austria:*** Inutest; ***Swed.:*** Inutest†.

**Multi-ingredient: *Ital.:*** Lactolas; Naturalass; Snell'it.

## Iris Versicolor

Blue Flag; Iris versicolor; Iris Virginica.

### Profile

The rhizomes of *Iris versicolor* (Iridaceae) are used in herbal preparations for skin and gastrointestinal disorders, and also in homoeopathic medicine.

### Preparations

**Proprietary Preparations** (details are given in Part 3)

**Multi-ingredient: *UK:*** Blue Flag Root Compound†; Catarrh Mixture; HRI Clear Complexion; Skin Eruptions Mixture.

## Isometheptene Hydrochloride (BANM, rINNM)

Hidrocloruro de isometepteno. 1,5,N-Trimethylhex-4-enylamine hydrochloride; 1,5-Dimethylhex-4-enyl(methyl)amine hydrochloride.
$C_9H_{19}N,HCl = 177.7.$
*CAS — 503-01-5 (isometheptene); 6168-86-1 (isometheptene hydrochloride).*
*ATC — A03AX10.*

## Isometheptene Mucate (BANM, rINNM)

Mucato de isometepteno. Isometheptene galactarate.
$(C_9H_{19}N)_2,C_6H_{10}O_8 = 492.6.$
*CAS — 7492-31-1.*
*ATC — A03AX10.*

**Pharmacopoeias.** In *Br.* and *US.*

**BP 2003** (Isometheptene Mucate). A white crystalline powder. Very soluble in water; slightly soluble in dehydrated alcohol; very slightly soluble in chloroform; practically insoluble in ether. A 5% solution in water has a pH of 5.4 to 6.6. Store in airtight containers. Protect from light.

**USP 27** (Isometheptene Mucate). A white crystalline powder. Freely soluble in water; soluble in alcohol; practically insoluble in chloroform and in ether. pH of a 5% solution in water is between 6.0 and 7.5.

### Adverse Effects and Precautions

For the adverse effects of sympathomimetics such as isometheptene, and precautions to be observed, see under Adrenaline, p.852.

**Porphyria.** Isometheptene mucate has been associated with acute attacks of porphyria and is considered unsafe in porphyric patients.

### Interactions

For the interactions of sympathomimetics in general, see under Adrenaline, p.853. Isometheptene has been reported to produce severe hypertensive reactions in patients receiving MAOIs.

**Bromocriptine.** For a report of hypertension and life-threatening complications following concomitant use of isometheptene and *bromocriptine*, see under Sympathomimetics, p.1202.

### Uses and Administration

Isometheptene is an indirect-acting sympathomimetic (see under Adrenaline, p.854). It is included for its vasoconstrictor effect, usually as the mucate, in some analgesic combination products used to treat acute migraine attacks (p.464). Typical doses of isometheptene mucate in migraine are 130 mg at the beginning of an attack, with 65 mg hourly thereafter as necessary, up to a total maximum dose of 325 mg in a 12-hour period.

Isometheptene hydrochloride has also been used in the management of migraine and smooth muscle spasm; it has been given by mouth, as well as intramuscular, or occasionally subcutaneous, or slow intravenous, injection. The mucate has also been used in the management of muscle spasms.

### Preparations

***USP 27:*** Isometheptene Mucate, Dichloralphenazone, and Acetaminophen Capsules.

**Proprietary Preparations** (details are given in Part 3)
***Switz.:*** Octinum†.

**Multi-ingredient: *Braz.:*** Cefaldina; Doralgina; Doridina; Dorsedin; Neomigran; Neosaldina; Sedalgina; Sedol; Sulindor†; Tensaldin; ***Hong Kong:*** Midrid; ***UK:*** Midrid; ***USA:*** Duradrin; Isocom†; Isopap†; Midchlor†; Midrin; Migratine.

## Isospaglumic Acid (rINN)

Ácido isospaglúmico. N-(N-Acetyl-L-α-aspartyl)-L-glutamic acid.
$C_{11}H_{16}N_2O_8 = 304.3.$
*CAS — 3106-85-2.*

### Profile

Isospaglumic acid has been used as the sodium or the magnesium salt. It is given as eye drops for allergic eye conditions and in nasal solutions for allergic rhinitis.

### Preparations

**Proprietary Preparations** (details are given in Part 3)
***Austria:*** Rhinaaxia; ***Braz.:*** Naabak; Naaxia; ***Fr.:*** Naabak; Naaxia; Rhinaaxia; ***Hong Kong:*** Naaxia; ***Singapore:*** Naabak; ***Spain:*** Naaxia; ***Switz.:*** Rhinaaxia.

**Multi-ingredient: *Gr.:*** Naaxia; ***S.Afr.:*** Naaxia; ***Switz.:*** Naaxia.

## Isoxsuprine Hydrochloride (BANM, rINNM)

Caa-40; Hidrocloruro de isoxsuprina; Isoxsuprini Hydrochloridum; Phenoxyisopropylnorsuprifen. 1-(4-Hydroxyphenyl)-2-(1-methyl-2-phenoxyethylamino)propan-1-ol hydrochloride.
$C_{18}H_{23}NO_3,HCl = 337.8.$
*CAS — 395-28-8 (isoxsuprine); 579-56-6 (isoxsuprine hydrochloride).*
*ATC — C04AA01.*

**Pharmacopoeias.** In *Eur.* (see p.vi) and *US.*

**Ph. Eur. 5.0** (Isoxsuprine Hydrochloride). A white or almost white crystalline powder. Sparingly soluble in water and in alcohol; practically insoluble in dichloromethane. A 1% solution in water has a pH of 4.5 to 6.0. Protect from light.

**USP 27** (Isoxsuprine Hydrochloride). A white, odourless, crystalline powder. Soluble 1 in 500 of water, 1 in 100 of alcohol and of 0.1N sodium hydroxide solution, and 1 in 2500 of 0.1N hydrochloric acid; practically insoluble in chloroform and in ether. pH of a 1% solution in water is between 4.5 and 6.0. Store in airtight containers.

### Adverse Effects

Isoxsuprine may cause transient flushing, hypotension, tachycardia, rashes, and gastrointestinal disturbances. Maternal pulmonary oedema and fetal tachycardia have been reported following intravenous administration in premature labour.

**Pulmonary oedema.** Pulmonary oedema has been reported in mothers given isoxsuprine for premature labour.[1,2]

1. Nagey DA, Crenshaw MC. Pulmonary complications of isoxsuprine therapy in the gravida. *Obstet Gynecol* 1982; **59** (suppl): 38S–42S.
2. Nimrod C, *et al.* Pulmonary edema associated with isoxsuprine therapy. *Am J Obstet Gynecol* 1984; **148:** 625–9.

### Precautions

Isoxsuprine is contra-indicated after recent arterial haemorrhage. It should not be given immediately post partum, nor should it be used for premature labour if there is infection.

In women being treated for premature labour, the risk of pulmonary oedema means that extreme caution is required and the precautions and risk factors discussed under Salbutamol Sulfate, p.792, apply.

**Pregnancy.** Ileus was found to be more common in the offspring of mothers who received isoxsuprine than in matched controls.[1] The incidence of respiratory distress syndrome also rose as the isoxsuprine concentration in cord blood exceeded 10 nanograms/mL; likewise the incidence of hypocalcaemia and hypotension rose progressively with increasing concentrations. The cord concentrations correlated inversely with the drug-free interval before delivery and it was suggested that with frequent assessment of uterine response it should be possible to avoid delivering infants at a time when they have high plasma-isoxsuprine concentrations.[1]

In another study[2] of the association between ruptured membranes, beta-adrenergic therapy, and respiratory distress syndrome, it was found that both therapy with isoxsuprine and premature rupture of membranes were individually associated with a lowered incidence of respiratory distress syndrome, but when present together they resulted in an increased risk of respiratory distress syndrome. It was suggested that therapy with beta-adrenergic drugs including isoxsuprine should be restricted to patients with intact membranes.[1]

1. Brazy JE, *et al.* Isoxsuprine in the perinatal period II: relationships between neonatal symptoms, drug exposure, and drug concentration at the time of birth. *J Pediatr* 1981; **98:** 146–51.
2. Curet LB, *et al.* Association between ruptured membranes, tocolytic therapy, and respiratory distress syndrome. *Am J Obstet Gynecol* 1984; **148:** 263–8.

### Pharmacokinetics

Isoxsuprine hydrochloride is well absorbed from the gastrointestinal tract. The peak plasma concentration occurs about 1 hour after administration by mouth. A plasma half-life of about 1.5 hours has been reported. Isoxsuprine is excreted in the urine mainly as conjugates.

### Uses and Administration

Isoxsuprine is a vasodilator that also stimulates beta-adrenergic receptors. It causes direct relaxation of vascular and uterine smooth muscle and its vasodilating action is greater on the arteries supplying skeletal muscles than on those supplying skin. Isoxsuprine also produces positive inotropic and chronotropic effects.

Isoxsuprine hydrochloride has been used to arrest premature labour (p.794), but drugs with a more selective action are now preferred. It has also been given in the treatment of cerebral and peripheral vascular disease.

For use as a vasodilator, isoxsuprine hydrochloride is given by mouth in doses of 10 to 20 mg 3 or 4 times daily.

To arrest premature labour, isoxsuprine hydrochloride is given initially by intravenous infusion in doses of 200 to 500 micrograms/minute, adjusted according to the patient's response, until control is achieved. It is now common practice to administer beta agonists by syringe pump when using them to delay premature labour. Maternal blood pressure and hydration, and maternal and fetal heart rates should be monitored during the infusion. Subsequent treatment when labour has been arrested consists of intramuscular injections of 10 mg every 3 to 8 hours for several days. Prophylaxis may be continued by mouth with 30 to 90 mg daily in divided doses.

The resinate has also been used similarly.

### Preparations

***USP 27:*** Isoxsuprine Hydrochloride Injection; Isoxsuprine Hydrochloride Tablets.

**Proprietary Preparations** (details are given in Part 3)
***Arg.:*** Duvadilan; Fadaespasmol; Isodilan; Isotenk; Uterine; ***Austria:*** Xuprin; ***Belg.:*** Duvadilan†; ***Braz.:*** Inibina; ***Gr.:*** Duvadilan; ***Hong Kong:*** Duvadilan†; ***India:*** Duvadilan; ***Irl.:*** Duvadilan†; ***Israel:*** Vasolan; ***Ital.:*** Duvadilan†; Fenam†; Vasosuprina Ilfi; ***Mex.:*** Vadosilan; ***Neth.:*** Duvadilan†; ***Port.:*** Dilum; ***Spain:*** Duvadilan†; ***Thai.:*** Duvadilan; ***USA:*** Vasodilan; Voxsuprine.

## Jamaica Dogwood

Fish Poison Bark; Piscidia.

### Profile

Jamaica dogwood, the root bark of *Piscidia erythrina* (*P. piscipula*; *Ichthyomethia piscipula*) (Leguminosae), has analgesic, antispasmodic, and sedative properties. It is mainly used for insomnia due to neuralgia or nervous tension. The bark and twigs of Jamaica dogwood have been used as a fish poison.

### Preparations

**Proprietary Preparations** (details are given in Part 3)

**Multi-ingredient: *Braz.:*** Regran†; ***Fr.:*** Bronpax†; Jouvence de l'Abbe Soury; Schoum; ***Ital.:*** Sedatol; Soluzione Schoum; ***Spain:*** Solucion Schoum; ***UK:*** Anased; Biophylin†; Gerard House Valerian Compound†; HRI Calm Life; Nodoff; Nytol Herbal; Slumber.

## Java Tea

Orthosiphonblätter; Orthosiphonis Folium; Ortosifón.

**Pharmacopoeias.** In *Eur.* (see p.vi).

**Ph. Eur. 5.0** (Java Tea). The fragmented, dried leaves and tops of stems of *Orthosiphon stamineus* (*O. aristatus*; *O. spicatus*). Protect from light.

### Profile

Java tea is used in herbal medicine mainly for the treatment of urinary-tract disorders.

### Preparations

**Proprietary Preparations** (details are given in Part 3)
***Austria:*** Carito mono; ***Fr.:*** Urosiphon†; ***Ger.:*** Aquacaps†; Carito mono; Diurevit Mono; Nephronorm med; Orthosiphonblatter Indischer Nierentee; Repha Orphon.

**Multi-ingredient: *Austria:*** Apotheker Bauer's Harntreibender Tee; Apotheker Bauer's Nieren- und Blasentee; Blasen- und Nierentee; Droxitop; Gewusst wie Entschlackungstee; Krauterhaus Mag Kottas Blasentee;

Krauterhaus Mag Kottas Nierentee; Mag Kottas Entwasserungstee; Mag Kottas Krauterexpress-Entwasserungstee; Mag Kottas Krauterexpress-Nieren-Blasentee; Mag Kottas Nieren-Blasentee; Neuners Krautertee Nr 31 - Harnwegstee; Sidroga Nieren- und Blasentee; Solubitrat; **Belg.:** Tisane Contre la Tension†; **Fr.:** Actisane Minceur†; Aminsane†; Dellova; Promincil; Tealine; **Ger.:** Aqualibra; BioCyst; Canephron novo; Cysto Fink†; Etmoren†; Harntee 400; Harntee 450†; Harntee STADA; Harntee-Steiner; Heumann Blasen- und Nierentee Solubitrat S; Hevert-Blasen-Nieren-Tee N; Heweberberol-Tee; Nephro-Pasc; Nephronorm med; Nephropur tri; Nephrubin-N; Nierentee 2000; Nieron Blasen- und Nieren-Tee VI; Presselin Arterien K 5 P; Presselin Nieren-Blasen K 3; Uro Fink†; Urodil Blasen-Nieren Arzneitee†; Urodil phyto; Urostei†; **Spain:** Lepisor; Urisor; **Switz.:** Bilifuge; Demonatur Dragees pour les reins et la vessie; Dragees pour reins et vessie S†; Phytomed Nephro; Prosta-Caps Chassot N; Tisane pour les reins et la vessie.

## Jin Bu Huan

### Profile

Jin bu huan is a traditional Chinese remedy used as a sedative and analgesic and variously stated to contain *Lycopodium serratum* or *Polygala chinensis*. Adverse effects including CNS depression and acute hepatotoxicity have been attributed to its alkaloidal content of L-tetrahydropalmatine.

**Adverse effects.** Acute hepatitis has been reported in 7 previously healthy patients following ingestion of jin bu huan; symptoms occurred again in 2 following re-use.[1] It was noted that the content of plant material did not seem to correspond to the labelled species. Hepatitis and extreme fatigue have also been reported in 3 adults after taking jin bu huan for periods ranging from 6 days to 6 months.[2]

Accidental ingestion of jin bu huan by 3 children[2] produced profound lethargy and muscle weakness. Two of the children also developed respiratory depression and bradycardia.


1. Woolf GM, *et al.* Acute hepatitis associated with the Chinese herbal product jin bu huan. *Ann Intern Med* 1994; **121:** 729–35.
2. Horowitz RS, *et al.* The clinical spectrum of jin bu huan toxicity. *Arch Intern Med* 1996; **156:** 899–903.


## Juniper

Baccae Juniperi; Enebro; Genièvre; Iuniperi Pseudo-fructus; Juniper Berry; Juniper Fruit; Juniperi Fructus; Juniperi Galbulus; Wacholderbeeren; Zimbro.

**Pharmacopoeias.** In *Eur.* (see p.vi) and *Pol.*

**Ph. Eur. 5.0** (Juniper). The dried ripe cone berry of *Juniperus communis*. It contains not less than 1% v/w of essential oil, calculated with reference to the anhydrous drug. It has a strongly aromatic odour, especially if crushed. Protect from light.

### Profile

Juniper is the source of juniper oil (below). It has carminative, diuretic, antiseptic, and anti-inflammatory properties. It is used in herbal and homoeopathic medicine and as a flavour in gin.

### Preparations

**Proprietary Preparations** (details are given in Part 3)
**Ger.:** Kneipp Wacholderbeer-Pflanzensaft†.

**Multi-ingredient: Arg.:** Water Pill c Potasio; **Austral.:** Arthritic Pain Herbal Formula 1†; Fluid Loss†; Lifesystem Herbal Formula 1 Arthritic Aid†; Profluid†; Protemp†; **Austria:** Aktiv Blasen- und Nierentee; Aponatura Entwasserungs; Apotheker Bauer's Harntreibender Tee; Aurita-Nieren-Blasentee; Blasen-Tee†; Kneipp Entwasserungstee; Mariazeller; Neuners Krautertee Nr 18 - Stoffwechseltee; Neuners Krautertee Nr 19 - Harntreibender Stoffwechseltee; Neuners Krautertee Nr 29 - Stoffwechseltee mild; Neuners Krautertee Nr 30 - Stoffwechseltee stark; Neuners Krautertee Nr 4 - Nierentee; St Bonifatius-Tee; **Belg.:** Tisane Diuretique†; **Braz.:** Pilulas De Witt's; **Canad.:** Arthrisan†; Herbal Laxative; **Fr.:** Depuratum; Mediflor Tisane Antirhumatismale No 2; Santane $A_4$†; Santane $R_8$†; **Ger.:** Amara-Tropfen; Befelka-Tinktur†; Discmigon†; Gastrol S; Harntee 400; Hevert-Entwasserungs-Tee†; Hevert-Gicht-Rheuma-Tee comp†; Imbak†; Junisana; Kneipp Entschlackungs-Tee†; Kneipp Rheuma Tee N†; Presselin Stoffwechsel-Tee Hapeka 225 N; Salus Rheuma-Tee Krautertee Nr. 12†; **Ital.:** Broncosedina; Depurfat†; **Switz.:** Ajaka†; Kernosan Heidelberger Poudre; Phytomed Nephro; Tisane laxative Natterman no 13†; Tisane pour les reins et la vessie; **UK:** Backache; Watershed.

## Juniper Oil

Enebro, aceite esencial de; Essence de Genièvre; Juniper Berry Oil; Juniperi Aetheroleum; Oleum Juniperi; Wacholderöl.

**Pharmacopoeias.** In *Eur.* (see p.vi).

**Ph. Eur. 5.0** (Juniper Oil). The essential oil obtained by steam distillation from the ripe, non-fermented berry cones of *Juniperus communis*. A suitable antioxidant may be added. A mobile, colourless to yellowish liquid with a characteristic odour. Store in well-filled airtight containers at a temperature not exceeding 25°. Protect from light.

### Profile

Juniper oil has been used as a carminative and as an ingredient of herbal remedies for urinary-tract disorders and muscle and joint pain. Prolonged use may cause gastrointestinal irritation and there may be a risk of renal damage from high doses.

### Preparations

**Proprietary Preparations** (details are given in Part 3)
**Ger.:** Leukona-Stoffwechsel-Bad; Roleca Wacholder; **Switz.:** Roleca-S†.

**Multi-ingredient: Austral.:** Medinat PMT-Eze†; **Austria:** Apotheker Bauer's Inhalationsmischung; Berggeist; **Braz.:** Solvobil; **Ger.:** Dolo-cyl; GA-301-Redskin 301†; Kneipp Rheuma-Bad†; Neo-Lapitrypsin†; Nierentee 2000; Nieroxin N; Olbas; Schupps Heilkrauter Rheumabad†; Schupps Latschenkiefer Olbad†; **Ital.:** Otosan Natural Ear Drops; **Spain:** Emolytar; Polytar; **Switz.:** Ajaka†; Baby Liberol†; Bain antirhumatismal; Caprisana†; Demo pommade contre les refroidissements pour bebes†; Huile Po-Ho A. Vogel; Liberol Baby N; Olbas†; Spagyrom; **UK:** Diuretabs; HealthAid Boldo-Plus; Juno Junipah†; Olbas; Olbas for Children; Sciargo; St Johnswort Compound; Watershed.

## Kallidinogenase *(BAN, rINN)*

Callicrein; Kalidinogenasa; Kalléone; Kallikrein.
*CAS — 9001-01-8.*
*ATC — C04AF01.*

**Pharmacopoeias.** In *Jpn.*

### Profile

Kallidinogenase is an enzyme isolated from the pancreas and urine of mammals. It converts kininogen into the kinin, kallidin. Kallidinogenase has been used in male infertility (p.1316) since the kallikrein-kinin system has a physiological role in the male genital tract. It also has vasodilating properties and has been used in the treatment of peripheral vascular disease (p.831).

### Preparations

**Proprietary Preparations** (details are given in Part 3)
**Austria:** Padutin; **Ger.:** Padutin†.

## Kava

Kava-Kava.
*CAS — 500-64-1 (kawain); 495-85-2 (methysticin); 500-62-9 (yangonin).*

### Profile

Kava is the rhizome of *Piper methysticum* (Piperaceae), a shrub indigenous to islands of the South Pacific. It contains pyrones including kawain, methysticin, and yangonin. Kava has been used in the South Pacific to produce an intoxicating beverage used for recreational purposes and during convalescence. It is reported to have sedative, skeletal muscle relaxant, and anaesthetic properties. It is given in some anxiety- and stress-related disorders. It was formerly used as an antiseptic and diuretic in inflammatory conditions of the genito-urinary tract in the form of a liquid extract. Kawain has also been used for nervous disorders and as a tonic. Kava has been used in homoeopathic medicine.

A characteristic rash resembling that of pellagra occurs in some heavy consumers of kava. Extrapyramidal effects and cases of hepatitis have been reported. Preparations of kava for internal use have been withdrawn in the UK and some other Western countries on account of its potential for serious hepatotoxic effects.

◊ References.


1. Anonymous. Kava. *Lancet* 1988; **ii:** 258–9.
2. Anonymous. Tonga trouble. *Pharm J* 1990; **245:** 288.
3. Ruze P. Kava-induced dermopathy: a niacin deficiency? *Lancet* 1990; **335:** 1442–5.
4. Schelosky L, *et al.* Kava and dopamine antagonism. *J Neurol Neurosurg Psychiatry* 1995; **58:** 639–40.
5. Spillane PK, *et al.* Neurological manifestations of kava intoxication. *Med J Aust* 1997; **167:** 172–3.
6. Pepping J. Kava: piper methysticum. *Am J Health-Syst Pharm* 1999; **56:** 957–60.
7. Anonymous. Kava extract linked to hepatitis. *WHO Drug Inf* 2000; **14:** 98.
8. Escher M, *et al.* Hepatitis associated with kava, a herbal remedy for anxiety. *BMJ* 2001; **322:** 139.
9. Stevinson C, *et al.* A systematic review of the safety of kava extract in the treatment of anxiety. *Drug Safety* 2002; **25:** 251–61.
10. Anonymous. Hepatic toxicity possibly associated with kava-containing products—United States, Germany, and Switzerland, 1999-2002. *MMWR* 2002; **51:** 1065–7. Also available at: http://www.cdc.gov/mmwr/preview/mmwrhtml/mm5147a1.htm (accessed 15/07/04)
11. Stickel F, *et al.* Hepatitis induced by Kava (Piper methysticum rhizoma). *J Hepatol* 2003; **39:** 62–7.
12. Pittler MH, Ernst E. Kava extract for treating anxiety. Available in The Cochrane Library; Issue 2. Chichester: John Wiley; 2004.


### Preparations

**Proprietary Preparations** (details are given in Part 3)
**Austria:** Laitan†; Largon; **Braz.:** Ansiopax; Calmiton; Calmonex; Kavakan; Kavalac; Kavasedon; Laitan; Natuzilium; **Chile:** Laikan 100; **Ger.:** Aigin†; Antares†; Ardeydystin†; Cefakava†; Eukavan†; Jakava†; Ka-Sabona†; Kava-Phyton†; Kavacur†; Kavaform N†; Kavain Harras N†; Kavasedon†; Kavatino†; Kavosporal forte†; Kytta-Kava†; Laitan†; Limbao†; Maoni†; Nervonocton N†; Neuronika; Sedalint Kava†; **Mex.:** Laiken; **Switz.:** Kavasedon†; Kavasol†; Kavetten†; Laitan†; Songha Day†.

**Multi-ingredient: Austria:** Kavaform; Kavavit; **Ger.:** Bilicura Forte†; Cysto Fink†; Hewepsychon duo†; Hyposedon N†; Kavain Harras Plus†; Kavosporal comp†; Somnuvis S†; **Ital.:** Ansiderm†; **Switz.:** Cysto-Caps Chassot†; Kawaform; Yakona N†.

## Keracyanin *(rINN)*

Cyaninoside; Keracianina. 3-[6-O-(6-Deoxy-α-L-mannopyranosyl)-β-D-glucopyranosyloxy]-3′,4′,5,7-tetrahydroxyflavylium chloride.
$C_{27}H_{31}ClO_{15}$ = 631.0.
*CAS — 18719-76-1.*

### Profile

Keracyanin is claimed to improve visual function in poor light conditions. It has been given by mouth in usual doses of 400 to 600 mg daily.

### Preparations

**Proprietary Preparations** (details are given in Part 3)
**Fr.:** Meralops†; **Ital.:** Meralop; **Spain:** Meralop.

## Keratinase

Queratinasa.
*CAS — 9025-41-6.*

### Profile

Keratinase is a proteolytic enzyme that has been obtained from cultures of *Streptomyces fradiae*. It can digest keratin, which is resistant to most proteolytic enzymes, in the presence of trace amounts of metal ions. It is used in the commercial separation of hair from animal hides, and has been tried as a depilatory; it has also been included in some topical antibacterial ointments, presumably to aid penetration of the active substances.

## Kinkeliba

Combreti Folium; Combretum.

**Pharmacopoeias.** In *Fr.*

### Profile

Kinkeliba is the dried leaves of *Combretum micranthum* (*C. altum*; *C. raimbaultii*) (Combretaceae), a shrub indigenous to West Africa. It has been used as an ingredient of herbal remedies given for the treatment of biliary, liver, and gastrointestinal disorders. Other species of *Combretum* are also used.

Kinkeliba is used in homoeopathic medicine.

### Preparations

**Proprietary Preparations** (details are given in Part 3)

**Multi-ingredient: Belg.:** Tisane pour le Foie†; **Fr.:** Hepaclem; Hepax; Jecopeptol; Mediflor Tisane Hepatique No 5; Romarene; Romarinex; Romarinex-Choline†; Solution Stago Diluee; Uremiase†; **Switz.:** Bilifuge.

## Klebsiella pneumoniae Glycoprotein

Glucoproteína de Klebsiella pneumoniae; RU-41740.

### Profile

*Klebsiella pneumoniae* glycoprotein has been used for its immunomodulating activity in the management of respiratory-tract infections, wounds, burns, and soft-tissue disorders. It has also been used in immunotherapy.

### Preparations

**Proprietary Preparations** (details are given in Part 3)
**Braz.:** Biostim†; **Fr.:** Biostim; **Ital.:** Acintor; Biostim; **Mex.:** Biostim; **Port.:** Biostim.

## Krebiozen

Crebiocén.
*CAS — 9008-19-9.*

### Profile

Krebiozen is the name of a preparation that was formerly promoted as a 'cancer cure' in the USA, but totally discredited by the FDA. It was stated to be obtained from the blood of horses previously injected with an extract of *Actinomyces bovis*.

## Kveim Antigen

Antígeno de Kveim.

### Profile

Kveim antigen is a fine suspension in physiological saline of sarcoid tissue prepared from spleens taken from patients with active sarcoidosis. It is used as an intradermal injection in the Kveim (Kveim-Siltzbach) test for the diagnosis of sarcoidosis (p.1087).

◊ References.


1. James DG, Williams WJ. Kveim-Siltzbach test revisited. *Sarcoidosis* 1991; **8:** 6–9.


◊ The safety of the Kveim test has been questioned, particularly with reference to the risk of transmission of sarcoidosis, and of hepatitis B, HIV, and Creutzfeldt-Jakob disease.[1] However, the procedure to identify acceptable sarcoid spleens and the method of preparation were considered sufficient to reduce the risk of transmission of infections[2] and of Creutzfeldt-Jakob disease.[3]


1. Wigly RD. Moratorium on Kveim tests. *Lancet* 1993; **341:** 1284.
2. du Bois RM, *et al.* Moratorium on Kveim tests. *Lancet* 1993; **342:** 173.
3. de Silva RN, Will RG. Moratorium on Kveim tests. *Lancet* 1993; **342:** 173.


## Laburnum

Golden Chain; Golden Rain; Lluvia de oro.

### Profile

All parts of laburnum, *Laburnum anagyroides* (*L. vulgare*;

*Cytisus laburnum*) (Leguminosae), are toxic. The toxic principle is cytisine which has actions similar to nicotine.

## Lactic Acid

Acidum Lacticum; E270; E326 (potassium lactate); Láctico, ácido; Milchsäure. 2-Hydroxypropionic acid.

$C_3H_6O_3$ = 90.08.

*CAS — 50-21-5; 79-33-4 ((+)-lactic acid); 10326-41-7 ((−)-lactic acid); 598-82-3 ((±)-lactic acid).*

*ATC — G01AD01.*

**Pharmacopoeias.** In *Chin.*, *Int.*, *Jpn*, *Pol.*, and *US*.

*Eur.* (see p.vi) includes monographs for the racemate and the (*S*)-enantiomer.

**Ph. Eur. 5.0** (Lactic Acid). A mixture of lactic acid, its condensation products, such as lactoyl-lactic acid and other polylactic acids, and water. The equilibrium between lactic acid and polylactic acids depends on the concentration and temperature. It is usually the racemate (*RS*-lactic acid), and contains the equivalent of 88 to 92% w/w of $C_3H_6O_3$. A colourless or slightly yellow, syrupy liquid. Miscible with water and with alcohol.

**Ph. Eur. 5.0** ((*S*)-Lactic Acid). A mixture of (*S*)-lactic acid, its condensation products, such as lactoyl-lactic acid and other polylactic acids, and water. The equilibrium between lactic acid and polylactic acids depends on the concentration and temperature. It contains the equivalent of 88 to 92% w/w of $C_3H_6O_3$, of which not less than 95% is the (*S*)-enantiomer. A colourless or slightly yellow, syrupy liquid. Miscible with water and with alcohol.

**USP 27** (Lactic Acid). A mixture of lactic acid and lactic acid lactate equivalent to a total of 88 to 92% w/w of $C_3H_6O_3$. It is obtained by the lactic fermentation of sugars or is prepared synthetically. Lactic acid obtained by fermentation of sugars is laevorotatory, while that prepared synthetically is racemic.

A colourless or yellowish, hygroscopic, practically odourless, syrupy liquid. When it is concentrated by boiling, lactic acid lactate is formed. Miscible with water, with alcohol, and with ether; insoluble in chloroform. Store in airtight containers.

### Adverse Effects and Treatment

As for Hydrochloric Acid, p.1699, although in the concentrations used it is less corrosive.

**Neonates.** There was evidence that neonates had difficulty in metabolising *R*-(−)-lactic acid and this isomer and the racemate should not be used in foods for infants less than 3 months old.[1]

1. FAO/WHO. Toxicological evaluation of certain food additives with a review of general principles and of specifications: seventeenth report of the joint FAO/WHO expert committee on food additives. *WHO Tech Rep Ser 539* 1974.

### Uses and Administration

Lactic acid has actions similar to those of acetic acid (p.1645) and has been used similarly in the treatment of infective skin and vaginal disorders. It has been used in the preparation of lactate injections and infusions to provide a source of bicarbonate for the treatment of metabolic acidosis (for the problems of using lactate in metabolic acidosis, see p.1217). It is also employed topically in the treatment of warts (p.1139), often with salicylic acid, and in emollient creams. Other uses include the treatment of severe aphthous stomatitis in terminally ill, immunocompromised patients.

Lactic acid has also been used as a food preservative and as an ingredient of cosmetics.

◊ References to the use of lactic acid in the treatment of bacterial vaginosis,[1,2] warts,[3] and dry[4,5] or photodamaged[6] skin.

1. Andersch B, *et al.* Treatment of bacterial vaginosis with an acid cream: a comparison between the effect of lactate-gel and metronidazole. *Gynecol Obstet Invest* 1986; **21:** 19–25.
2. Holst E, Brandberg Å. Treatment of bacterial vaginosis in pregnancy with a lactate gel. *Scand J Infect Dis* 1990; **22:** 625–6.
3. Bunney MH, *et al.* An assessment of methods of treating viral warts by comparative treatment trials based on a standard design. *Br J Dermatol* 1976; **94:** 667–79.
4. Dahl MV, Dahl AC. 12% Lactate lotion for the treatment of xerosis: a double-blind clinical evaluation. *Arch Dermatol* 1983; **119:** 27–30.
5. Rogers RS, *et al.* Comparative efficacy of 12% ammonium lactate lotion and 5% lactic acid lotion in the treatment of moderate to severe xerosis. *J Am Acad Dermatol* 1989; **21:** 714–16.
6. Stiller MJ, *et al.* Topical 8% glycolic acid and 8% L-lactic acid creams for the treatment of photodamaged skin: a double-blind vehicle-controlled clinical trial. *Arch Dermatol* 1996; **132:** 631–6.

### Preparations

***BP 2003:*** Lactic Acid Pessaries;
***USP 27:*** Compound Clioquinol Topical Powder.

**Proprietary Preparations** (details are given in Part 3)
***Arg.:*** Celucrem; ***Austral.:*** Avecyde†; ***Austria:*** Espritin; Warzin; ***Belg.:*** Lacta-Gynecogel; ***Canad.:*** Lubriderm AHA; Penederm; ***Chile:*** Eucerin; ***Fr.:*** Ictyoderm; Lactacyd Femina; ***Ger.:*** Lactisan; Lactisol; RMS; Tampovagan c Acid lact†; Unguentum Lactisol†; ***Irl.:*** Relact; ***Ital.:*** Saugella Intilac; Unigyn; ***Malaysia:*** Avecyde; ***Mex.:*** Acid-Lac; Avecyde; Eucerin Piel con Tendencia Acneica; ***NZ:*** BK; ***Port.:*** Atopic; ***Singapore:*** Avecyde; Lachydrin; ***Spain:*** Keratisdin; ***Switz.:*** Vagoclyss; ***USA:*** Lactinol; Lactrex.

**Multi-ingredient:** ***Arg.:*** Akerat; Callicida; Caminol; Coltix; Dermocridin; Duofilm; Hidrolac; Lacticare; Nutrafilm; Opoenterol; Pasem; Verruclean; Verrutopic; ***Austral.:*** Aussie Tan Skin Moisturiser†; Calmurid; Cornkil; Dermadrate; Dermatech Wart Treatment; Duofilm; ***Austria:*** Apotheker Bauer's Huhneraugentinktur; Calmurid; Calmurid HC; Duofilm; Helo-acid; Hylak; Hylak forte; Lavagin; ***Belg.:*** Aporil; Calmurid; ***Braz.:*** Calope; Calotrat†; Colpacid†; Colpolase; Dermacyd†; Duofilm; Higienex†; Kalostop; Lacticare; Lacto Vagin; Lacto-Gin†; Salic; Tirakallos†; Varigerm†; Vulgix†; ***Canad.:*** Calmurid HC†; Calmurid†; Cuplex†; Duofilm; Duoplant; Epi-Lyt; Lacticare; Penederm; Tiacid; Viron Wart Lotion; ***Chile:*** Akerat; Duofilm; Lactacyd; Lacticare; Primacy C+AHA; ***Denm.:*** Verucid; ***Fin.:*** Calmuril; Wicnelact; ***Fr.:*** Akerat; Duofilm; Geliofil; Kerafilm; Lactacyd Derma; Lactacyd Femina; Lacticare; Propy-Lacticare; Saugella; Verrufilm; Verrupan; ***Ger.:*** Akaderm N; Aknederm N†; Anthozym N†; Calmurid; Calmurid HC†; Clabin; Collomack; Dr. Hotz Vollbad†; Duofilm; Efasit N†; Gehwol Huhneraugen Pflaster; Kneipp Milch-Molke-Bad†; Sagrosept; Sol-co-Derman; Vagisan; W-Tropfen; Warzen-Alldahin; ***Hong Kong:*** Collomack; Duofilm; Lactacyd; Lacticare; Roidhemo†; Solcoderm; Verrufilm†; ***India:*** Cotaryl; Lacgel; ***Irl.:*** Calmurid; Calmurid HC; Cuplex; Duofilm; Lacticare; Salactol; Salatac; ***Israel:*** Babyzim; Calmurid; Calmurid HC; Salatac; U-Lactin Foot Cream; U-Lactin Forte; ***Ital.:*** Aflogine†; Bruciaporri; Duofilm; Eudermico; Gastro-Pepsin; Geliofil; Geroderm Zolfo; Ginil; Lactacyd Derma; Lactacyd Intimo; Lactocol; Pluriderm†; Saugella Salviettine; Sensigel; Sensiquell; Unidermo; Verel; Verucid†; Verunec; Violgen†; ***Malaysia:*** Collomack; Duofilm; Lactacyd; Lacticare; Solcoderm; ***Mex.:*** Duofilm; Lacticare; ***Neth.:*** Calmurid; Tintorine†; ***Norw.:*** Verucid; ***NZ:*** Calmurid; Dermadrate; Duofilm; ***Port.:*** Atopic; Bioclin Sebo Care; Calicida Indiano; Calmurid; Creme Laser Hidrante; Despigmentante; Duofilm; Hidro-Lact†; Lactacyd; Lecia; Pansebase; Pansebase Composto; Secpel; Secpel Composto; Ureadin Maos; Verrucare; ***S.Afr.:*** Duofilm; ***Singapore:*** Collomack; Dermadrate; Dermatech Wart Treatment; Duofilm; High Potency Lightening Serum†; Lactacyd; Lacticare; ***Spain:*** Antiverrugas; Callicida Brujo†; Callicida Cor Pik; Callicida Durcall†; Callix; Cusiter†; Euzymina Lisina I; Ginejuvent; Roidhemo; Unguento Callicida Naion; Verufil; ***Swed.:*** Calmuril; Lactal†; ***Switz.:*** Acne Lotion; Calmurid; Calmurid HC; Clabin; Coruzol; Duofilm; Elle-care†; Solcoderm; Vin Tonique de Vial; Waruzol; Warz-ab Extor; ***Thai.:*** Collomack; Duofilm; Lactacyd; Lacticare; ***UK:*** Bazuka; Calmurid; Calmurid HC; Cuplex; Duofilm; Lacticare; Salactol; Salatac Gel; Tampovagan†; ***USA:*** AmLactin AP; Epi-Lyt; Feminique; Lacticare; Lactinol-E; Massengill; Massengill Disposable; SLT.

## Lactic-acid-producing Organisms

Láctico, organismos productores de ácido.

### Profile

Lactic-acid-producing organisms were introduced as therapeutic agents with the idea of acidifying the intestinal contents and thus preventing the growth of putrefactive organisms. Live cultures designed to restore or maintain a healthy microbial flora have been referred to as probiotics. *Lactobacillus bulgaricus*, which occurs in naturally soured milk, was the organism originally used but it can be difficult to obtain growth of this organism in the intestines and *L. acidophilus*, which is an inhabitant of the human intestine, is preferred by many.

Preparations containing various *Lactobacillus* spp. and other lactic-acid-producing organisms have been used in the treatment of vaginal and gastrointestinal disorders but evidence to support this use is limited. Other organisms that have been tried include *Bifidobacterium bifidum*, *Enterococcus* and *Streptococcus* spp., and the yeast *Saccharomyces boulardii*. Natural yogurt is a common source of lactic-acid-producing organisms.

A vaccine produced from strains of lactobacillus found in women with trichomoniasis has been used in the prophylaxis of recurrent trichomoniasis (see p.1642).

◊ Reviews[1-5] concerning the use of lactic-acid-producing organisms including *Lactobacillus* spp., *Bifidobacterium bifidum*, and *Streptococcus thermophilus* have been published. However, some preparations have been found to contain smaller quantities or different species of organisms to those specified on the label.[6]

Metabolic acidosis has occurred following use of tablets containing *Lactobacillus acidophilus*.[7] Cases of infection associated with the use of lactic-acid-producing organisms seem to be very rare,[8] although fungaemia associated with the use of *Saccharomyces boulardii* has been reported.[9]

1. Scott E, Li Wan Po A. Lactobacillus. *Pharm J* 1990; **245:** 698–9.
2. Fuller R. Probiotics in human medicine. *Gut* 1991; **32:** 439–42.
3. Drutz DJ. Lactobacillus prophylaxis for Candida vaginitis. *Ann Intern Med* 1992; **116:** 419–20.
4. Roffe C. Biotherapy for antibiotic-associated and other diarrhoeas. *J Infect* 1996; **32:** 1–10.
5. Van Niel CW, *et al.* Lactobacillus therapy for acute infectious diarrhea in children: a meta-analysis. *Pediatrics* 2002; **109:** 678–84.
6. Hamilton-Miller JMT, *et al.* "Probiotic" remedies are not what they seem. *BMJ* 1996; **312:** 55–6.
7. Oh MS, *et al.* D-lactic acidosis in a man with short-bowel syndrome. *N Engl J Med* 1979; **301:** 249–52.
8. Borriello SP, *et al.* Safety of probiotics that contain lactobacilli or bifidobacteria. *Clin Infect Dis* 2003; **36:** 775–80.
9. Piarroux R, *et al.* Are live saccharomyces yeasts harmful to patients? *Lancet* 1999; **353:** 1851–2.

### Preparations

**Proprietary Preparations** (details are given in Part 3)
***Arg.:*** Acidofilofago; Flevic; Floratil; Tropivag; ***Austral.:*** Acidophilus Tablets†; Bioglan Acidophilus†; Bioglan Superdophilus†; Ethical Nutrients Inner Health Powder†; Ethical Nutrients Maxi Bifidus†; Ethical Nutrients Maxi Dophilus†; Mega Acidophilus†; ***Austria:*** Antibiophilus; Bioflorin; Doederlein; Lactofit; Reflor; Symbioflor I; ***Belg.:*** Lacteol; Perenterol†; ***Braz.:*** Bac Resistente†; Camboacy†; Floratil; Leiba; ***Canad.:*** Bacid; ***Chile:*** Bio-Flora; Biolactus; Gastrofloral; Lacteol Forte; Perenteryl; Perocur; ***Denm.:*** Paraghurt; Precosa; ***Fin.:*** Lactophilus; Precosa; ***Fr.:*** Bacilor; Bioprotus; Diarlac; Lacteol; Lyo-Bifidus; Rhino-Lacteol†; Ultra-Levure; Ultra-derme; ***Ger.:*** Acidophilus; Diarrhoesan SC†; Hamadin; Hylak N; Hylak Plus; Infectodiarrstop GG; Lacteol; Omniflora Akut; Omnisept; Paidoflor; Perenterol; Perocur; Santax S; Symbioflor I; Vagiflor; ***Gr.:*** Ultra-Levure; ***Hong Kong:*** Bioflor; Lacteol; Solco-Trichovac†; ***India:*** Myconip; Sporlac; ***Ital.:*** Bioflorin; Codex; Dicoflor; Ecoflorina; Hygine In†; Inulac; Lab/A; Lacteol; Lactonorm; Ramno Fix; Ramno-Flor; Regolact Plus; ***Mex.:*** Floratil; Lacteol Fort; Sinuberase; ***Norw.:*** Precosa†; ***NZ:*** Blis K12 Throat Guard; ***Port.:*** Antibiophilus; Enterol; Lacteol; UL 250; ***S.Afr.:*** Inteflora; ***Singapore:*** Lacteol; ***Spain:*** Casenfilus; Lacteol; Lactofilus; Lactoliofil†; Ultra-Levura; ***Swed.:*** Precosa; ***Switz.:*** Bioflorin; Fiormil; Lacteol; Lactoferment†; Perenterol; Solco-Trichovac; Ultra-Levure; Ventrux; ***Thai.:*** Lacbon; Lacteol; ***UK:*** Bio Acidophilus; Biodophilus; Culturelle LCG†; ***USA:*** Bacid; Kala; Lactinex; MoreDophilus; Pro-Bionate; Superdophilus.

**Multi-ingredient:** ***Arg.:*** Biol Preo; Faelac; Nilflux; Totalflora; Tropivag Plus; ***Austral.:*** Acidophilus Bifidus†; Acidophilus Complex†; Acidophilus Plus†; Cyto-Bifidus†; Enterocare†; Lactobac†; Natures Own Acidophilus Plus†; Natures Way Acidophilus Plus†; Ultra Strength Megadophilus†; ***Austria:*** Gynoflor; Hylak; Hylak forte; Hylakombun†; Infloran; Omniflora; Prosymbioflor; Trevis; ***Belg.:*** Gynoflor; ***Braz.:*** Lactipan†; ***Canad.:*** Fermalac Vaginal; Fermalac†; ***Fr.:*** Ampho-Vaccin intestinal†; Biolactyl; Florgynal; Imudon; IRS 19; Ophidus; Triphidus; Trophigil; ***Ger.:*** Antiprurit; Eksalb Simplex†; Eksalb†; Gynoflor; Hylak forte N†; Imbak†; IRS 19; Pro-Symbioflor; ***Hong Kong:*** Gyno-Flor E†; Infloran; Shin-Biofermin S; ***India:*** Amplus; Ampoxin-LB; Bicidal Plus; Lactisyn; Nutrolin-B; Vitazyme; Vizylac; ***Ital.:*** Al-Flor; Alvear Complex†; Bifilact; Bio Flora; Biolactine; Colifagina S; Ecoendocilli Testimonia†; Ecofermenti; Endolac; Enteroseven; Fermentur-to-Lio; Flar†; Florbiox; Florelax; Floridral; Gastroenterol; Giflorex; Ginil; Infloran; Kiri; Lactipan; Lactisporin; Lactivis; Lactogermine; Lactolife; Lactovit†; Liozim; Neo Lactoflorene; Pentaglucano†; Probiox†; Prontomix-in†; Vaxitiol; Yovis; Yovita; ***Mex.:*** Neo-Panlacticos; Neo-Panlacticos Plus; ***Port.:*** Benflorene†; Coli-Fagina S; Infloran; ***Spain:*** Antibiofilus†; Infloran; ***Switz.:*** Gynoflor; Infloran; Ribolac†; ***Thai.:*** Infloran; ***UK:*** Acidophilus Plus; Beneflora; Culture Care; Fibre Dophilus; Natudophilus.

## Laetrile

*CAS — 1332-94-1 (laetrile); 29883-15-6 (amygdalin).*

### Profile

Laetrile is the term used for a product consisting chiefly of amygdalin, which is the major cyanogenic glycoside of apricot kernels. Amygdalin is *R*-α-cyanobenzyl-6-*O*-β-D-glucopyranosyl-β-D-glucopyranoside ($C_{20}H_{27}NO_{11}$ = 457.4). Laetrile is also used as a term for *R*-α-cyanobenzyl-6-*O*-β-D-glucopyranosiduronic acid ($C_{14}H_{15}NO_7$ = 309.3).

Laetrile was claimed to be preferentially hydrolysed in cancer cells by β-glucosidases to benzaldehyde and hydrogen cyanide, which killed the cell, but amygdalin does not appear to be absorbed from the gastrointestinal tract, and both normal and malignant cells contain only traces of β-glucosidases. Laetrile has also been claimed to be 'vitamin $B_{17}$', the deficiency of which is said to result in cancer; there is no evidence for accepting this view and laetrile is of no known value in human nutrition.

There have been several reports of cyanide poisoning and other adverse reactions associated with the use of laetrile, especially when taken by mouth.

◊ A review of the sources, chemistry, metabolism, claims for efficacy, and toxicity of laetrile.[1]

1. Chandler RF, *et al.* Controversial laetrile. *Pharm J* 1984; **232:** 330–2.

## Laminaria

Stipites Laminariae; Styli Laminariae; Thallus Eckloniae; Thallus Laminariae.

**Pharmacopoeias.** In *Chin.*

### Profile

Laminaria is the dried stalks of the seaweeds *Laminaria japonica*, *L. digitata*, and possibly other species of *Laminaria*. The stalks swell in water to about 6 times their volume and have been used surgically to dilate cavities and to dilate the cervix in labour or abortion induction.

An extract of various species of *Laminaria* has been used as a dietary supplement (see Seaweeds, Kelps, and Wracks, p.1742).

**Adverse effects.** Anaphylaxis[1-3] and toxic shock syndrome[4] have been reported following the insertion of laminaria for cervical dilatation.

1. Nguyen MT, Hoffman DR. Anaphylaxis to laminaria. *J Allergy Clin Immunol* 1995; **95:** 138–9.
2. Cole DS, Bruck LR. Anaphylaxis after laminaria insertion. *Obstet Gynecol* 2000; **95:** 1025.
3. Chanda M, *et al.* Hypersensitivity reactions following laminaria placement. *Contraception* 2000; **62:** 105–6.
4. Sutkin G, *et al.* Toxic shock syndrome after laminaria insertion. *Obstet Gynecol* 2001; **98:** 959–61.

### Preparations

**Proprietary Preparations** (details are given in Part 3)
**Multi-ingredient:** ***Ger.:*** Cetraria Salbe†; ***Spain:*** Fucusor.

## Lappa

Bardana; Bardanae Radix; Bardane (Grande); Burdock; Burdock Root; Lappa Root.

**Pharmacopoeias.** In *Fr.*
*Chin.* and *Jpn* include the fruits.

### Profile

Lappa is the dried root of the great burdock, *Arctium lappa* (*A. majus*), and other species of *Arctium* (Compositae). It was formerly used in the form of a decoction as a diuretic and diaphoretic but there is little evidence of its efficacy. Herbal preparations containing lappa have been used in the treatment of skin, musculoskeletal, and gastrointestinal disorders. The leaves and fruits of *Arctium* spp. have also been used.

Lappa is used in homoeopathic medicine.

### Preparations

**Proprietary Preparations** (details are given in Part 3)
***Fr.:*** Anthraxivore†; ***Port.:*** Saforelle.

**Multi-ingredient:** ***Austral.:*** Acne Oral Spray†; Herbal Cleanse†; Trifolium Complex†; ***Belg.:*** Stanno-Bardane†; Tisane Depurative "les 12 Plantes"†; ***Fr.:*** Arbum; Aromabyl†; Depuratif Parnel; Fitacnol; Tisanes de l'Abbe Hamon no 16†; Zeniac; Zeniac LP; ***Ital.:*** Depurativo†; ***Port.:*** Erpecalm; ***Spain:*** Diabesor; ***UK:*** Backache; Blue Flag Root Compound†; Cascade; Catarrh Mixture; GB Tablets; Gerard House Skin; Gerard House Water Relief Tablets; Heath & Heather Skin Tablets†; Heath & Heather Water Relief Tablets†; Hofels White Willow and Burdock†; HRI Clear Complexion; Kleer†; Modern Herbals Water Retention; Rheumatic Pain Remedy; Skin Cleansing; Skin Eruptions Mixture; Tabritis; Water Naturtabs.

## Laronidase *(USAN, rINN)*

Alpha-L-iduronidase. 8-L-Histidine-α-L-iduronidase (human).
*CAS — 210589-09-6.*
*ATC — A16AB05.*

### Adverse Effects, Treatment, and Precautions

Infusion reactions have been reported in patients given laronidase. Common symptoms include flushing, fever, headache, and rash; symptoms reported less commonly include cough, bronchospasm, dyspnoea, urticaria, angioedema, and pruritus. Antihistamines and/or antipyretics (e.g. paracetamol or ibuprofen) may relieve symptoms; a reduction in the rate of infusion should also be considered for mild reactions, but if severe, the infusion should be stopped and restarted once symptoms have subsided. Adrenaline should be used with caution because there is a greater incidence of coronary artery disease in patients with mucopolysaccharidosis I. Pre-treatment with antihistamines and/or antipyretics about 60 minutes before infusion is recommended to prevent reactions. IgG antibodies to laronidase are expected to develop within 3 months of initiation of treatment in the majority of patients, although the effect of this on safety and efficacy is not clear. However, such patients may be at increased risk of hypersensitivity reactions and should be treated with caution. Injection site reactions have also been reported.

### Interactions

The manufacturers of laronidase recommend that it should not be given with chloroquine or procaine because of the potential risk of interference with the intracellular uptake of the enzyme.

### Uses and Administration

Laronidase is recombinant human α-L-iduronidase used as enzyme replacement therapy for the treatment of the non-neurological manifestations of mucopolysaccharidosis I (see below). It is given by intravenous infusion in a dose of 100 units/kg each week. The initial infusion rate should be 2 units/kg per hour, increased every 15 minutes during the first hour, as tolerated, to a maximum of 43 units/kg per hour such that the infusion is completed in about 3 to 4 hours (but see also under Adverse Effects, Treatment, and Precautions, above). In some countries, the dose is expressed as mg/kg: 100 units is equivalent to approximately 0.58 mg of laronidase.

**Mucopolysaccharidosis I.** Mucopolysaccharidosis I is a progressive disorder characterised by deficiency of the enzyme α-L-iduronidase, which is necessary to catalyse the hydrolysis of terminal α-L-iduronic residues of the glycosaminoglycans, dermatan sulfate and heparan sulfate, resulting in their accumulation in tissues. Enzyme replacement therapy with laronidase has been reported to confer benefit on the systemic manifestations of the disease such as hepatomegaly, joint stiffness, pulmonary disease, and eye disease; beneficial effect on neurological manifestations has not yet been reported.

References.


1. Kakkis ED, *et al.* Enzyme-replacement therapy in mucopolysaccharidosis I. *N Engl J Med* 2001; **344:** 182–8.
2. Wraith JE. Enzyme replacement therapy in mucopolysaccharidosis type I: progress and emerging difficulties. *J Inherit Metab Dis* 2001; **24:** 245–50.
3. Kakkis ED. Enzyme replacement therapy for the mucopolysaccharide storage disorders. *Expert Opin Invest Drugs* 2002; **11:** 675–85.
4. Kakavanos R, *et al.* Immune tolerance after long-term enzyme-replacement therapy among patients who have mucopolysaccharidosis I. *Lancet* 2003; **361:** 1608–13.
5. Anonymous. Alpha-L-iduronidase (laronidase; aldurazyme). *Med Lett Drugs Ther* 2003; **45:** 88.


### Preparations

**Proprietary Preparations** (details are given in Part 3)
***USA:*** Aldurazyme.

## Lavender

English Lavender; Lavendelblüten.

**Pharmacopoeias.** *Eur.* (see p.vi) and *Pol.* include lavender flower.

**Ph. Eur. 5.0** (Lavender Flower; Lavandulae flos). It consists of the dried flower of *Lavandula angustifolia* (*L. officinalis*). It contains not less than 1.3% v/w of essential oil, calculated with reference to the anhydrous drug. Protect from light.

### Profile

Lavender flower is used as a sedative. It has also been used as a cholagogue. It is an ingredient of herbal remedies used for a variety of disorders.

Lavender flowers are the source of lavender oil (below).

### Preparations

**Proprietary Preparations** (details are given in Part 3)

**Multi-ingredient:** ***Austria:*** Baldrian-Krautertonikum; Bio-Garten Tee zur Beruhigung; Bioreform-Beruhigungstee; Euka; Herz- und Kreislauftonikum Bioflora; Mentopin; Neuners Krautertee Nr 1 - Nerventee; Neuners Krautertee Nr 141 - Schlaftee; Neuners Krautertee Nr 201 - Krauterhexlein Kinder-Beruhigungstee; St Radegunder Herz-Kreislauf-unterstutzender Tee; Teekanne Schlaf- und Nerventee; ***Braz.:*** Balsamo Branco†; Rinofen†; Traumac; ***Fr.:*** Mediflor Tisane Digestive No 3; Santane $N_9$†; Santane $R_8$†; Tisane Sedative Weleda†; ***Ger.:*** Aranidorm-S†; Presselin Dyspeptikum; Salus Nerven-Schlaf-Tee Nr.22†; ***NZ:*** Botanica Hayfever; ***Port.:*** Cholagutt; Erpecalm; ***Spain:*** Linimento Naion; ***Switz.:*** Tisane relaxante N; ***UK:*** Vital Eyes.

## Lavender Oil

English Lavender Oil (from *L. intermedia*); Esencia de Alhucema; Esencia de Espliego; Essência de Alfazema; Foreign Lavender Oil (from *L. officinalis*); Huile Essentielle de Lavande; Lavanda, aceite esencial de; Lavandulae Aetheroleum; Lavendelöl; Lavender Flower Oil; Oleum Lavandulae.

**Pharmacopoeias.** In *Eur.* (see p.vi).

**Ph. Eur. 5.0** (Lavender Oil). An essential oil obtained by steam distillation from the flowering tops of *Lavandula angustifolia* (*L. officinalis*). A colourless or pale yellow clear liquid with a characteristic odour. Relative density 0.878 to 0.892. Store in well-filled airtight containers at a temperature not exceeding 25°. Protect from light.

### Profile

Lavender oil has been used as a carminative and as a flavour. It is sometimes applied externally as an insect repellent. Its chief use is in perfumery and it is occasionally used in ointments and other pharmaceutical preparations to cover disagreeable odours. It has been suggested that lavender oil may have sedative properties following inhalation.

Lavender oil has been reported to produce nausea, vomiting, headache, and chills when inhaled or absorbed through the skin. It may cause contact allergy and phototoxicity.

**Adverse effects.** There have been reports of contact dermatitis associated with lavender oil in a shampoo,[1] and facial dermatitis following application of the oil to pillows for its sedative properties.[2]


1. Brandão FM. Occupational allergy to lavender oil. *Contact Dermatitis* 1986; **15:** 249–50.
2. Coulson IH, Khan ASA. Facial 'pillow' dermatitis due to lavender oil allergy. *Contact Dermatitis* 1999; **41:** 111.


**Insomnia.** Ambient exposure to lavender oil produced similar sleep patterns to conventional sedatives in 4 elderly patients.[1]


1. Hardy M, *et al.* Replacement of drug treatment for insomnia by ambient odour. *Lancet* 1995; **346:** 701.


### Preparations

**Proprietary Preparations** (details are given in Part 3)

**Multi-ingredient:** ***Arg.:*** Deca-Scab; ***Austral.:*** Neutralice†; ***Austria:*** Berggeist; Inno Rheuma; Naturland Sportmassageol; Rowalind; ***Braz.:*** Analgen; Benegel†; Gelflex; Gelol†; Gelonevral; Inhalante Yatropan; Mentalol†; Mialgex; Nevrol; Salimetin; Vulgix†; Yatropan†; ***Fr.:*** Aromasol; Balsofumine; Balsofumine Mentholee; Bronchospray†; Citrosil†; Ephydrol; Gouttes aux Essences; Paps; Pectoderme; Perubore; ***Ger.:*** Amol Heilkrautergeist N; Dolo-cyl; Leber-Galle-Tropfen 83; ***Irl.:*** Rowalind†; ***Ital.:*** Citrosystem; Mistick Verde; Natural Zanzy†; Sanaderm†; ***NZ:*** Electric Blue Headlice; ***Port.:*** Solubeol; Vaporil; ***Singapore:*** Vapex†; ***Spain:*** Dolokey; Termosan; ***Switz.:*** Baume du Chalet; Demo baume†; Dolo-Arthrosenex sine Heparino; Dolorex†; Embropax†; Hygiodermil; Kernosan Huile de Massage†; Kytta Pommade; Liberol Bain; Massorax; Muco-Sana; Nasobol; Oculosan; Perubare; Phlogidermil†; Pulmex; Saltrates; Seracalm†; Spagyrom; ***UK:*** Arnica Massage Balm; Eucanol; Larch Resin comp.; Massage Balm with Calendula; Migrastick; ***USA:*** Nasal Jelly.

## Lawsone

Lawsonia. 2-Hydroxy-1,4-naphthoquinone.
$C_{10}H_6O_3 = 174.2.$
*CAS — 83-72-7.*

### Profile

Lawsone is a dye present in henna (p.1696), the leaves of *Lawsonia* spp., and may also be prepared synthetically. It has been used with dihydroxyacetone in sunscreen preparations. There appears to be no evidence that it has any sunscreening properties when used alone.

**Adverse effects.** Observation that lawsone causes oxidative damage to red blood cells *in vitro* supported a suggestion that percutaneous absorption of henna could contribute to unexplained neonatal hyperbilirubinaemia in countries where the ceremonial use of henna is widespread.[1]


1. Zinkham WH, Oski FA. Henna: a potential cause of oxidative hemolysis and neonatal hyperbilirubinemia. *Pediatrics* 1996; **97:** 707–9.


## Lead

Plomo.
Pb = 207.2.
*CAS — 7439-92-1.*

**Description.** Lead is a grey, malleable and ductile metal.

### Adverse Effects

Lead poisoning (plumbism) may be due to inorganic or organic lead and may be acute or, more often, chronic. It has followed exposure to a wide range of compounds and objects from which lead may be absorbed following ingestion or inhalation. Some of those that have been incriminated include paint, pottery glazes, crystal glassware, domestic water supplies, petrol, poteen, cosmetics, herbal or folk remedies, newsprint, and retained bullets. Children are often the victims of accidental poisoning and may be vulnerable to chronic exposure to lead from environmental pollution.

Acute effects of lead poisoning include metallic taste, abdominal pain, diarrhoea, vomiting, hypotension, muscle weakness and cramps, fatigue, abnormal liver function tests, and acute interstitial nephritis. Encephalopathy may occur and is more common in children. Symptoms of chronic poisoning with inorganic lead include anorexia, abdominal pain, constipation, anaemia, headache, fatigue, irritability, peripheral neuropathy, and encephalopathy with convulsions and coma. There may be kidney damage and impairment of mental function. Children with elevated lead concentrations may be asymptomatic apart from intellectual deficits and behavioural disorders.

Organic lead poisoning produces mainly CNS symptoms; there can be gastrointestinal and cardiovascular effects, and renal and hepatic damage.

◊ General references.


1. WHO. Recommended health-based limits in occupational exposure to heavy metals: report of a WHO study group. *WHO Tech Rep Ser 647* 1980.
2. Ibels LS, Pollock CA. Lead intoxication. *Med Toxicol* 1986; **1:** 387–410.
3. Lead—environmental aspects. *Environmental Health Criteria 85.* Geneva: WHO, 1989. Available at: http://www.inchem.org/documents/ehc/ehc/ehc85.htm (accessed 17/06/04)
4. Inorganic lead. *Environmental Health Criteria 165.* Geneva: WHO, 1995. Available at: http://www.inchem.org/documents/ehc/ehc/ehc165.htm (accessed 17/06/04)


### Treatment of Adverse Effects

Gastric lavage may be considered within one hour of acute ingestion of inorganic lead salts. The main aim in the management of both acute and chronic lead poisoning is to control the symptoms and reduce the concentration of lead in the body. Patients should be removed from the source of exposure and iron and calcium deficiencies corrected. Chelation therapy may be required, depending on the levels of lead in the blood. Sodium calcium edetate (p.1051) is given for the initial management of symptomatic lead poisoning; because of fears that symptoms might initially be exacerbated by mobilisation of stored lead, it may be given with dimercaprol (p.1037). Sodium calcium edetate, succimer (p.1054), or penicillamine (p.1046) are used for chelation therapy in asymptomatic patients. Renal and hepatic function should also be monitored and convulsions controlled with a benzodiazepine.

◊ Treatment of lead poisoning is aimed primarily at alleviating acute symptoms, and then at reducing the body-lead stores.[1,2] Initial therapy of acute symptomatic poisoning entails supportive therapy including intravenous fluids and anticonvulsants if necessary. Encephalopathy is rare in adults but more common in children and requires urgent treatment; combined therapy with sodium calcium edetate in combination with dimercaprol has substantially reduced mortality rates.[3] In this case, only the minimum fluid should be administered to avoid overload. Chelation therapy with both sodium calcium edetate and dimercaprol should be continued for 5 days and may be repeated if necessary.[1,3-5] For symptomatic patients without encephalopathy it may be possible to discontinue the dimercaprol after 3 days. The value of adding dimercaprol to chelation therapy with sodium calcium edetate has been questioned;[6] combination with succimer has also been used in moderate symptomatic toxicity.[2] Patients who are asymptomatic may be treated with sodium calcium edetate alone[1,4,5] or succimer.[5] Penicillamine may be used as an alternative.[5] Long-term management involves eliminating environmental exposure.[7] Continued chelation with oral penicillamine may be necessary until the desired tissue levels are achieved.[3,4] Results from one study[8] indicated that succimer did not improve scores on tests of cognition, behaviour, or neuropsychological function despite lowering blood levels of lead in children who had initial levels of less than 450 nanograms/mL. The authors suggested that, since succimer is as effective a chelator as any other currently available, chelation therapy in general may not be beneficial in children with these blood-lead levels.

A provocation test that measures urinary excretion of lead following administration of a standard dose of sodium calcium edetate has been widely used as a means of assessing the need for therapy. However, sodium calcium edetate is associated with nephrotoxicity and the test is cumbersome to perform, thus guidelines recommend blood-lead concentrations as a guide to treatment.[5] Children with blood-lead concentrations above 250 nanograms/mL may require chelation therapy, although there is no consensus; chelation therapy is recommended at blood-lead concentrations above 450 nanograms/mL.

Finally, it should be noted that chelation therapy is not a substitute for environmental controls in those suffering occupational exposure.[9] Chelation therapy is generally not appropriate for long-term lead exposure in asymptomatic individuals in whom a significant proportion of the total body lead is tightly bound to compact bone and brain. A provocation test may be useful in identifying patients with mild symptoms who may respond to chelation therapy.[9]


1. Ibels LS, Pollock CA. Lead intoxication. *Med Toxicol* 1986; **1:** 387–410.
2. Gordon JN, *et al.* Lead poisoning: case studies. *Br J Clin Pharmacol* 2002; **53:** 451–8.
3. Chisholm JJ. The use of chelating agents in the treatment of acute and chronic lead intoxication in childhood. *J Pediatr* 1968; **73:** 1–38.
4. Chisholm JJ, Barltrop D. Recognition and management of children with increased lead absorption. *Arch Dis Child* 1979; **54:** 249–62.
5. Committee on Environmental Health of the American Academy of Pediatrics. Screening for elevated blood lead levels. *Pediatrics* 1998; **101:** 1072–8. Also available at: http://aappolicy.aappublications.org/cgi/content/full/pediatrics;101/6/1072 (accessed 17/06/04)
6. O'Connor ME. CaEDTA vs CaEDTA plus BAL to treat children with elevated blood lead levels. *Clin Pediatr (Phila)* 1992; **31:** 386–90.
7. Committee on Environmental Health of the American Academy of Pediatrics. Lead poisoning: from screening to primary prevention. *Pediatrics* 1993; **92:** 176–83.
8. Rogan WJ, *et al.* The effect of chelation therapy with succimer on neuropsychological development in children exposed to lead. *N Engl J Med* 2001; **344:** 1421–6.
9. Rempel D. The lead-exposed worker. *JAMA* 1989; **262:** 532–4.


### Lead in the Environment

Many countries have taken action to reduce lead exposure from environmental sources, including food, paint, and petrol, by limiting or banning altogether the use of lead compounds in such sources. Such measures have been of value in reducing childhood exposure to lead. Screening of all children to detect those at risk of chronic lead poisoning and developmental deficit has been advocated, but selective screening in areas perceived as high risk may be appropriate in countries where the overall level of lead contamination is low.

### Pharmacokinetics

Lead is absorbed from the gastrointestinal tract. It is also absorbed by the lungs from dust particles or fumes.

Inorganic lead is not absorbed through intact skin, but organic lead compounds may be absorbed rapidly.

Lead is distributed in the soft tissues, with higher concentrations in the liver and kidneys. In the blood it is associated with the erythrocytes. Over a period of time lead accumulates in the body and is deposited in calcified bone, hair, and teeth. Lead crosses the placental barrier. It is excreted in the faeces, urine, and sweat, and also appears in breast milk.

### Uses and Administration

Lead compounds were formerly employed as astringents, but the medicinal use of preparations containing lead is no longer recommended. The lead salts or compounds that have been used have included lead acetate and lead subacetate (for lead lotion, still known sometimes as lotio plumbi), lead carbonate, lead monoxide, and lead oleate (for lead plaster-mass).

### Preparations

**Proprietary Preparations** (details are given in Part 3)

**Multi-ingredient:** ***Austria:*** Vulpuran; ***Mex.:*** Emplasto Monopolis.

## Lecithin

E322; E442 (ammonium phosphatides); Lecitina.

**Pharmacopoeias.** In *Ger.* Also in *USNF.*

**USNF 22** (Lecithin). A complex mixture of acetone-insoluble phosphatides, which consists chiefly of phosphatidyl choline, phosphatidyl olamine, phosphatidyl serine, and phosphatidyl inositol, combined with various amounts of other substances such as triglycerides, fatty acids, and carbohydrates, as separated from the crude vegetable oil source. It contains not less than 50% of acetone-insoluble matter.

The consistency of both natural grades and refined grades of lecithin may vary from plastic to fluid, depending upon the content of free fatty acid and oil, and upon the presence or absence of other diluents. Its colour varies from light yellow to brown, depending on the source, on crop variations, and on whether it is bleached or unbleached.

It is odourless or has a characteristic, slight nutlike odour. It is partially soluble in water, but readily hydrates to form emulsions. The oil-free phosphatides are soluble in fatty acids, but are practically insoluble in fixed oils. When all phosphatide fractions are present, lecithin is partially soluble in alcohol and practically insoluble in acetone.

### Profile

Lecithin is an emulsifying and stabilising agent used in both the pharmaceutical and the food industries.

Lecithin has also been used as a source of choline and tried in the treatment of dementia (p.1484) but with little evidence of clinical benefit. It has also been tried in various extrapyramidal disorders. Phosphatidyl serine (p.1731) has been used similarly. Other constituents of lecithin such as phosphatidyl olamine and phosphatidyl inositol may be found in natural pulmonary surfactants (p.1736).

◊ References.


1. Higgins JPT, Flicker L. Lecithin for dementia and cognitive impairment. Available in The Cochrane Library; Issue 2. Chichester: John Wiley; 2004.


### Preparations

**Proprietary Preparations** (details are given in Part 3)

***Arg.:*** Reducin; ***Austral.:*** Buerlecithin†; ***Austria:*** Buerlecithin Compact; Dermo WAS; ***Ger.:*** Buerlecithin; ***India:*** Essentiale-L; ***Ital.:*** Misura†; ***Mex.:*** Leciderm; ***Port.:*** Pansebase Solido; ***Switz.:*** Buerlecithin Compact.

**Multi-ingredient:** ***Arg.:*** Ayton; Cholesterol Reducing Plan; KLB6 Fruit Diet; ***Austral.:*** Berberis Complex†; Bioglan Zellulean with Escin†; Extralife Arthri-Care†; Extralife Extra-Brite†; Extralife Liva-Care†; ML 20†; Plantiodine Plus†; ***Austria:*** Aponatura Leber; Bilatin; Buerlecithin; Colagain†; Lecikur; Lecivital; ***Canad.:*** Complex 15; Kyolic 104; ***Fr.:*** Arkotonic†; Cholegerol; ***Ger.:*** Haut-Vital N†; Hicoton; Kola-Dallmann mit Lecithin†; Lipidavit; Vita Buerlecithin; ***Hong Kong:*** Ginkgo-PS; Wari-Procomil; ***Ital.:*** Lemivit†; Nutrigel; Ottovis; Solecin; Tricortin; ***Mex.:*** Lecifar-K; ***Port.:*** Pansebase; Pansebase Composto; Secpel; Secpel Composto; ***Switz.:*** Biovital Ginseng; Vita Buerlecithin; ***Thai.:*** Wari-Procomil; ***UK:*** All In One Plus Grapefruit†; Kelp Plus 3; Naudicelle SL†; S.P.H.P.; ***USA:*** KLB6.

## Leishmanin

Leishmanina.

### Profile

Leishmanin is a suspension of *Leishmania* promastigotes used in an intradermal test to indicate previous exposure to leishmanial antigens. Its chief use is in epidemiological studies of leishmaniasis (p.597). The leishmanin skin test has also been known as the Montenegro test.

## Lemon

**Pharmacopoeias.** *Br.* includes dried lemon peel and *Swiss* includes fresh lemon peel.

**BP 2003** (Dried Lemon Peel). The dried outer part of the pericarp of the ripe, or nearly ripe, fruit of *Citrus limon*. It contains not less than 2.5% v/w of volatile oil.

### Profile

Lemon, *Citrus limon* (*Citrus limonum*) (Rutaceae), is an ingredient of herbal remedies used for gastrointestinal disorders and as tonics. The juice is traditionally included in preparations for colds and coughs. Lemon is a source of bioflavonoids used to improve capillary function (see Flavonoid Compounds, p.1688). The peel is the source of lemon oil (p.1706). Citrus fruits are a source of vitamin C (p.1460).

Photosensitivity is associated with citrus oils.

### Preparations

***BP 2003:*** Concentrated Compound Gentian Infusion;
***USNF 22:*** Lemon Tincture.

**Proprietary Preparations** (details are given in Part 3)

**Multi-ingredient:** ***Austria:*** Everon†; Gencydo; ***Braz.:*** Balsamo Brancot†; ***Ger.:*** Doppelherz Melissengeist; Gencydo; Salusan†; ***Port.:*** Erpecalm.

## Lemon Oil

Aetheroleum Citri; Citronenöl; Esencia de Cidra; Essence de Citron; Essência de Limão; Limón, aceite esencial de; Limonis Aetheroleum; Ol. Limon.; Oleum Citri; Oleum Limonis.

**Pharmacopoeias.** In *Eur.* (see p.vi) and *Pol.* Also in *USNF.*

**Ph. Eur. 5.0** (Lemon Oil). The essential oil obtained by suitable mechanical means without the aid of heat from the fresh peel of *Citrus limon*. It contains a maximum of 0.5% β-caryophyllene, 0.5 to 2.3% geranial, 0.1 to 0.8% geranyl acetate, 56.0 to 78.0% limonene, 0.3 to 1.5% neral, 0.2 to 0.9% neryl acetate, 7.0 to 17.0% β-pinene, 1.0 to 3.0% sabinene, 6.0 to 12.0% γ-terpinene, and a maximum of 0.6% α-terpineol.

A clear mobile pale yellow to greenish-yellow liquid with a characteristic odour. It may become cloudy at low temperatures. Store in well-filled airtight containers at a temperature not exceeding 25°. Protect from light. Where applicable the label should state that the contents are Italian-type lemon oil.

**USNF 22** (Lemon Oil). The volatile oil obtained by expression, without the aid of heat, from the fresh peel of the fruit of *Citrus* × *limon* (Rutaceae), with or without the previous separation of the pulp and the peel. The total aldehyde content, calculated as citral, is not less than 2.2% and not more than 3.8% for California-type lemon oil, and not less than 3.0% and not more than 5.5% for Italian-type lemon oil. Store in well-filled airtight containers.

### Profile

Lemon oil is chiefly used in perfumery and as a flavour. It is used in the preparation of terpeneless lemon oil (below). It has also been used with other volatile agents in rubefacient preparations and preparations for respiratory-tract disorders.

Photosensitivity reactions and contact dermatitis have been reported.

### Preparations

***BP 2003:*** Aromatic Ammonia Spirit;
***USNF 22:*** Compound Orange Spirit.

**Proprietary Preparations** (details are given in Part 3)

**Multi-ingredient:** ***Austral.:*** Austral-Balm†; Genuine Australian Eucalyptus Drops†; ***Austria:*** Spasmo Claim; ***Chile:*** Agua Del Carmen; Agua Melisa Carminativa; ***Fr.:*** Citrosil†; Ephydrol; ***Ger.:*** Amol Heilkrautergeist N; Babix-Wundsalbe N; Ceprovit†; Melissengeist; Tachynerg N†; ***Israel:*** Garonsept; ***NZ:*** Electric Blue Headlice; Lemsip Dry Cough; ***Switz.:*** Neo-Angin au miel et citron; Pommade Po-Ho N A Vogel†; ***UK:*** Collins Elixir Pastilles†; Melissa Comp.; ***USA:*** Mexsana.

## Terpeneless Lemon Oil

Limón exento de terpeno, aceite esencial de; Oleum Limonis Deterpenatum.

**Pharmacopoeias.** In *Br.*

**BP 2003** (Terpeneless Lemon Oil). A clear colourless or pale yellow liquid, visibly free from water, with the characteristic odour and taste of lemon, prepared by concentrating lemon oil under reduced pressure until most of the terpenes have been removed, or by solvent partition. It contains not less than 40% w/w of aldehydes calculated as citral. Soluble 1 in 1 of alcohol (80%). Store in well-filled containers at a temperature not exceeding 25°. Protect from light.

### Profile

Terpeneless lemon oil is used as a flavour. It has the advantages of being stronger in taste and odour and more readily soluble than the natural oil and is used in the preparation of lemon spirit and lemon syrup.

Photosensitivity is associated with citrus oils.

### Preparations

***BP 2003:*** Compound Orange Spirit; Lemon Spirit; Lemon Syrup.

**Proprietary Preparations** (details are given in Part 3)

**Multi-ingredient:** ***UK:*** Lemsip Cough & Cold Dry Cough; Meltus Honey & Lemon.

## Lemon Grass Oil

Essência de Capim-Limão; Indian Melissa Oil; Indian Verbena Oil; Lemongrass, aceite de; Lemongrass Oil; Oleum Graminis Citrati.

### Profile

Lemon grass oil is the volatile oil obtained by distillation from *Cymbopogon flexuosus* or *C. citratus* (Gramineae). It contains citral and citronellal.

Lemon grass oil was formerly given as a carminative. It has been used in perfumery and as a flavour.

### Preparations

**Proprietary Preparations** (details are given in Part 3)

**Multi-ingredient:** ***Ger.:*** Kneipp Krauter Taschenkur Nerven und Schlaf N†.

## Lemon Verbena

Herba Lippiae Citriodorae; Herba Verbenae Odoratae; Hierba luisa; Verveine Odorante.

**Pharmacopoeias.** In *Fr.*

### Profile

Lemon verbena, the flowering tops or leaves of *Lippia citriodora* (*Aloysia triphylla*; *Verbena triphylla*) (Verbenaceae), has antispasmodic and sedative actions and has been used for gastrointestinal disorders and as a tonic. It is most commonly used as an ingredient of herbal teas.

### Preparations

**Proprietary Preparations** (details are given in Part 3)

**Multi-ingredient:** ***Fr.:*** Tisanes de l'Abbe Hamon no 14†; ***Spain:*** Agua del Carmen.

## Lentinan

LC-33; Lentinano.

*CAS — 37339-90-5.*
*ATC — L03AX01.*

### Profile

Lentinan is a glucan extracted from the mushroom *Lentinus edodes*. It appears to act as an immunostimulant. It has been tried in the treatment of malignant neoplasms and in HIV infection.

## Lepromin

Lepromina.

### Profile

Lepromin is a suspension of killed *Mycobacterium leprae* prepared from the skin of heavily infected patients suffering from lepromatous leprosy (lepromin H) or from armadillo tissue infected with *M. leprae* (lepromin A). It is used in an intradermal skin test for the classification of leprosy (p.133) and the assessment of immune responsiveness to *M. leprae*. The test is not diagnostic for leprosy.

◊ The original lepromin (of Mitsuda and Hayashi), a suspension of the whole autoclaved homogenised leproma including some tissue elements, is sometimes called integral lepromin, whereas purified bacillary suspensions are sometimes called bacillary lepromins.[1] Leprolins are the soluble proteins of the bacilli with or without proteins of the lepra, not coagulated by heating, and do not elicit the early reaction. The Dharmendra antigen is neither a lepromin nor a leprolin and is used especially for testing the early reactions; it gives only a weak late reaction. Purified protein derivatives of *Mycobacterium leprae*, such as leprosin A,[2] have also been developed.

1. Abe M, *et al*. Immunological problems in leprosy research. *Lepr Rev* 1974; **45:** 244–72.
2. Stanford JL. Skin testing with mycobacterial reagents in leprosy. *Tubercle* 1984; **65:** 63–74.

## Leptin

Leptina.

### Profile

Leptin is an endogenous protein that is involved in the control of body-weight. A recombinant form is under investigation in the management of obesity (p.1583); it has also been tried in diabetic lipodystrophy. Leptin has also been reported to have effects on other biological processes.

◊ General references.

1. Veniant MM, LeBel CP. Leptin: from animals to humans. *Curr Pharm Des* 2003; **9:** 811–8.

**Obesity.** Leptin is a 167-amino acid peptide hormone, secreted by adipose tissue, that acts either directly or via specific receptors in the CNS to decrease food intake, increase energy expenditure, and influence glucose and fat metabolism and neuroendocrine function. Although there is some evidence that subcutaneous administration results in loss of body fat it is not clear whether leptin will prove a suitable treatment for most obese patients.

References.

1. Auwerx J, Staels B. Leptin. *Lancet* 1998; **351:** 737–42.
2. Mantzoros CS. The role of leptin in human obesity and disease: a review of current evidence. *Ann Intern Med* 1999; **130:** 671–80.
3. Heymsfield SB, *et al*. Recombinant leptin for weight loss in obese and lean adults: a randomized, controlled, dose-escalation trial. *JAMA* 1999; **282:** 1568–75.
4. Hukshorn CJ, *et al*. Weekly subcutaneous pegylated recombinant native human leptin (PEG-OB) administration in obese men. *J Clin Endocrinol Metab* 2000; **85:** 4003–4009.
5. Wilding JP. Leptin and the control of obesity. *Curr Opin Pharmacol* 2001; **1:** 656–61.
6. Salvador J, *et al*. Perspectives in the therapeutic use of leptin. *Expert Opin Pharmacother* 2001; **2:** 1615–22.
7. Lee DW, *et al*. Leptin and the treatment of obesity: its current status. *Eur J Pharmacol* 2002; **440:** 129–39.
8. El-Haschimi K, Lehnert H. Leptin resistance—or why leptin fails to work in obesity. *Exp Clin Endocrinol Diabetes* 2003; **111:** 2–7.
9. Proietto J, Thorburn AW. The therapeutic potential of leptin. *Expert Opin Invest Drugs* 2003; **12:** 373–8.

## Lerdelimumab *(rINN)*

*CAS — 285985-06-0.*

### Profile

Lerdelimumab is a human monoclonal antibody specific for transforming growth factor β2 that is under investigation for the prevention of excessive postoperative scarring following glaucoma surgery.

## Levomenol *(rINN)*

(−)-α-Bisabolol. (−)-6-Methyl-2-(4-methyl-3-cyclohexen-1-yl)-5-hepten-2-ol.

$C_{15}H_{26}O$ = 222.4.

*CAS — 23089-26-1.*

### Profile

Levomenol is a sesquiterpene isolated from the volatile oil of chamomile. (p.1669) It has been tried as a transepidermal penetration enhancer and is present in many emollient preparations.

◊ References.

1. Kadir R, Barry BW. α-Bisabolol, a possible safe penetration enhancer for dermal and transdermal therapeutics. *Int J Pharmaceutics* 1991; **70:** 87–94.

### Preparations

**Proprietary Preparations** (details are given in Part 3)

**Multi-ingredient:** ***Arg.:*** Confortel; ***Chile:*** Eucerin; Suavigel; ***Fr.:*** Alpha 5 DS; Apaisance; Dermophil Indien; Epiphane; ***Ger.:*** Mirfulan Spray N; Sensicutan; ***Hong Kong:*** Camoderm†; Kamillosan; Oat Milk Treatment Cream†; ***Ital.:*** Biothymus DS; Broxo al Fluoro; Intim; ***Mex.:*** Aveendix; ***Port.:*** Hidratante VV; Lactonico; ***Switz.:*** Antidry; Dermophil Indien Nouvelle formule; ***Thai.:*** Kamillosan.

## Lexipafant *(BAN, USAN, rINN)*

BB-882; DO-6. Ethyl *N*-methyl-*N*-[α-(2-methylimidazo[4,5-*c*]pyridin-1-yl)tosyl]-L-leucinate.

$C_{23}H_{30}N_4O_4S$ = 458.6.

*CAS — 139133-26-9.*

### Profile

Lexipafant is a platelet-activating factor antagonist that is being investigated in the prevention of neurological and renal complications following cardiac surgery. It has also been studied for possible applications in asthma, sepsis, and pancreatitis.

## Linseed

Flaxseed; Leinsamen; Lin; Linaza; Linho; Lini Semen; Lini Semina; Linum; Semilla de Lino.

*ATC — A06AC05.*

**Pharmacopoeias.** In *Chin., Eur.* (see p.vi), and *Pol.*

**Ph. Eur. 5.0** (Linseed). The dried ripe seeds of *Linum usitatissimum*. Protect from light.

### Profile

Preparations of linseed have been administered for their demulcent and laxative actions. Crushed linseed has been used as a poultice. Linseed is the source of linseed oil, below.

### Preparations

**Proprietary Preparations** (details are given in Part 3)

***Austria:*** Linusit Gold†; ***Ger.:*** Linusit Creola†; Linusit Darmaktiv Leinsament†.

**Multi-ingredient:** ***Chile:*** Aloelax; ***Ger.:*** Dralinsa†; Duoventrin; Pascomag; ***Switz.:*** Enveloppements ECR†; Linoforce; Optilax†.

## Linseed Oil

Aceite de Linaza; Flaxseed Oil; Huile de Lin; Leinöl; Linaza, aceite de; Oleum Lini.

*ATC — A06AC05.*

**Pharmacopoeias.** In *Eur.* (see p.vi).

**Ph. Eur. 5.0** (Linseed Oil, Virgin). The oil obtained by cold expression from ripe seeds of *Linum usitatissimum*. A suitable antoxidant may be added. A clear, yellow or brownish-yellow liquid. It turns dark and gradually thickens on exposure to air. When cooled, it becomes a soft mass at about −20°. Relative density about 0.931. Very slightly soluble in alcohol; miscible with petroleum spirit. Store in airtight containers. Protect from light.

### Profile

Linseed oil is used in veterinary medicine as a purgative for horses and cattle. In man, linseed oil is included in topical preparations for a variety of skin disorders. It has been tried as a vegetable source of omega-3 fatty acids (p.976).

Boiled linseed oil ('boiled oil') is linseed oil heated with litharge, manganese resinate, or other driers, to a temperature of about 150° so that metallic salts of the fatty acids are formed and cause the oil to dry more rapidly. It must not be used for medicinal purposes.

### Preparations

**Proprietary Preparations** (details are given in Part 3)

***Chile:*** Linna-Oil.

**Multi-ingredient:** ***Austria:*** Dermowund; ***Fr.:*** Huile de Haarlem†; ***India:*** Buta-Proxyvon; Duoflam Gel; Nimulid Nugel; ***Switz.:*** Malvedrin; ***UK:*** Efamol Safflower & Linseed†; Nine Rubbing Oils.

## Lithium Benzoate

Litio, benzoato de.

$C_7H_5LiO_2$ = 128.1.

*CAS — 553-54-8.*

### Profile

Lithium benzoate has been used as a diuretic and urinary disinfectant. Its use cannot be recommended because of the pharmacological effect of the lithium ion (p.301). Each g contains 7.8 mmol of lithium.

### Preparations

**Proprietary Preparations** (details are given in Part 3)

**Multi-ingredient:** ***Fr.:*** Antigoutteux Rezall†; ***Port.:*** Urocrasina†.

## Lobenzarit Sodium *(USAN, rINNM)*

CCA; Lobenzarit sódico. 4-Chloro-2,2′-iminodibenzoate disodium.

$C_{14}H_8ClNNa_2O_4$ = 335.7.

*CAS — 63329-53-3 (lobenzarit); 64808-48-6 (lobenzarit sodium).*

### Profile

Lobenzarit sodium has been used as an immunomodulator in rheumatoid arthritis.

## Lodoxamide Trometamol *(BANM, rINNM)*

Lodoxamida trometamol; Lodoxamide Tromethamine *(USAN)*; U-42585 (lodoxamide); U-42718 (lodoxamide ethyl); U-42585E (lodoxamide trometamol). *N,N′*-(2-Chloro-5-cyano-*m*-phenylene)dioxamic acid compound with trometamol.

$C_{11}H_6ClN_3O_6,2C_4H_{11}NO_3$ = 553.9.

*CAS — 53882-12-5 (lodoxamide); 53882-13-6 (lodoxamide ethyl); 63610-09-3 (lodoxamide trometamol).*

*ATC — S01GX05.*

NOTE. Lodoxamide Ethyl is also *USAN*.

### Adverse Effects

Lodoxamide eye drops may cause local irritation. Reported effects include burning or stinging, and itching. Flushing and dizziness have also been reported.

### Uses and Administration

Lodoxamide has a stabilising action on mast cells resembling that of sodium cromoglicate (p.795). Lodoxamide trometamol is used in eye drops for allergic conjunctivitis (p.421), particularly vernal keratoconjunctivitis; a concentration equivalent to 0.1% of lodoxamide is used, one or two drops usually being instilled into the eye four times daily.

Lodoxamide has also been studied for its prophylactic effect in the treatment of asthma, but has not proved to be of benefit; it has usually been given by mouth as the ethyl ester or by inhalation as the trometamol salt.

**Conjunctivitis.** Lodoxamide is an effective treatment for vernal keratoconjunctivitis.[1,2] There is some evidence that it may be more effective than sodium cromoglicate for this purpose (see p.797).

1. Anonymous. Lodoxamide for vernal keratoconjunctivitis. *Med Lett Drugs Ther* 1994; **36:** 26.
2. Lee S, Allard TRFK. Lodoxamide in vernal keratoconjunctivitis. *Ann Pharmacother* 1996; **30:** 535–7.

### Preparations

**Proprietary Preparations** (details are given in Part 3)

***Arg.:*** Alomide; ***Austral.:*** Lomide; ***Austria:*** Alomide; Lomide; ***Belg.:*** Alomide; ***Braz.:*** Alomide; ***Canad.:*** Alomide; ***Chile:*** Alomide; ***Denm.:*** Alomide; ***Fin.:*** Alomide; ***Fr.:*** Almide; ***Ger.:*** Alomide; InfectoTop†; ***Gr.:*** Alomide; Thilomide; ***Hong Kong:*** Alomide; ***Irl.:*** Alomide; ***Israel:*** Alomide; ***Ital.:*** Alomide; ***Malaysia:*** Alomide; ***Mex.:*** Alomide†; ***Norw.:*** Alomide; ***NZ:*** Lomide; ***Port.:*** Alomide; ***S.Afr.:*** Alomide; ***Singapore:*** Alomide; ***Spain:*** Alomide; ***Switz.:*** Alomide; ***Thai.:*** Alomide; ***UK:*** Alomide; ***USA:*** Alomide.

## Lorenzo's Oil

Lorenzo, aceite de.

### Profile

Lorenzo's oil is a liquid containing glyceryl trierucate (a source of erucic acid) and glyceryl trioleate (a source of oleic acid), in the ratio 1 part to 4 parts respectively. It has been used with dietary modification for the treatment of adrenoleucodystrophy, a genetic disorder characterised by demyelination, adrenal cortical insufficiency, and accumulation of saturated 'very-long-chain fatty acids'.

**Adrenoleucodystrophy.** Adrenoleucodystrophy is a rare X-linked metabolic disorder in which accumulation of saturated very-long-chain fatty acids results in diffuse and multifocal demyelination of the nervous system and adrenocortical insufficiency. The most common form usually affects children and is characterised primarily by cerebral demyelination; it is usually fatal within a few years. In the adult variant, called adrenomyeloneuropathy, demyelination of the spinal cord and peripheral neuropathy progress slowly over many years.[1]

There appears to be no effective treatment for adrenoleucodystrophy or its variants. A high dietary intake of long-chain monounsaturated fatty acids, as provided by the mixture Lorenzo's oil (glyceryl trierucate with glyceryl trioleate), has been tried, the idea being to monopolise the specific enzyme involved in the conversion of long-chain fatty acids to very-long-chain fatty acids. Although dietary therapy with Lorenzo's oil has reduced plasma concentrations of saturated very-long-chain fatty acids, there is no evidence that this improves or delays progression of adrenoleucodystrophy or adrenomyeloneuropathy.[2-5] However, it has been suggested that these disorders may not respond to correction of the biochemical abnormality once neurological damage has occurred.[4] The effectiveness of treatment before the appearance of neurological symptoms is currently being studied.[1,6] There is some evidence to suggest that the childhood form may have an immunological component, but results using immunosuppressants or immunoglobulins have been reported to be disappointing.[4] Bone marrow transplants may improve symptoms but should only be tried in those with mild cerebral involvement.[1] Lovastatin can also reduce plasma concentrations of very-long-chain fatty acids.[7]

1. van Geel BM, *et al*. X linked adrenoleukodystrophy: clinical presentation, diagnosis, and therapy. *J Neurol Neurosurg Psychiatry* 1997; **63:** 4–14.
2. Aubourg P, *et al*. A two-year trial of oleic and erucic acids ("Lorenzo's oil") as treatment for adrenomyeloneuropathy. *N Engl J Med* 1993; **329:** 745–52.
3. Kaplan PW, *et al*. Visual evoked potentials in adrenoleukodystrophy: a trial with glycerol trioleate and Lorenzo oil. *Ann Neurol* 1993; **34:** 169–74.
4. Rizzo WB. Lorenzo's oil—hope and disappointment. *N Engl J Med* 1993; **329:** 801–2.

5. van geel BM, *et al.* Progression of abnormalities in adrenomyeloneuropathy and neurologically asymptomatic X-linked adrenoleukodystrophy despite treatment with "Lorenzo's oil". *J Neurol Neurosurg Psychiatry* 1999; **67:** 290–9.
6. Moser HW. Treatment of X-linked adrenoleukodystrophy with Lorenzo's oil. *J Neurol Neurosurg Psychiatry* 1999; **67:** 279–80.
7. Pai GS, *et al.* Lovastatin therapy for X-linked adrenoleukodystrophy: clinical and biochemical observations on 12 patients. *Mol Genet Metab* 2000; **69:** 312–22.

**Adverse effects.** Thrombocytopenia has been reported in patients receiving Lorenzo's oil, although patients are often asymptomatic.[1] It is possible that giant platelets which retain most of their function are produced and that these are not counted by automatic counting procedures giving a false impression of thrombocytopenia.[2]

Lymphocytopenia with an increased incidence of infection has also been reported in few patients.[3]

1. Zinkham WH, *et al.* Lorenzo's oil and thrombocytopenia in patients with adrenoleukodystrophy. *N Engl J Med* 1993; **328:** 1126–7.
2. Stöckler S, *et al.* Giant platelets in erucic acid therapy for adrenoleukodystrophy. *Lancet* 1993; **341:** 1414–15.
3. Unkrig CJ, *et al.* Lorenzo's oil and lymphocytopenia. *N Engl J Med* 1994; **330:** 577.

### Preparations

**Proprietary Preparations** (details are given in Part 3)

**Multi-ingredient:** ***UK:*** Lorenzo's Oil.

## Lovage Root

Levistici Radix; Levístico.

**Pharmacopoeias.** In *Eur.* (see p.vi) and *Pol.*

**Ph. Eur. 5.0** (Lovage Root). The whole or cut, dried rhizome and root of *Levisticum officinale*. The whole drug contains not less than 0.4% v/w of essential oil and the cut drug not less than 0.3% v/w of essential oil, calculated with reference to the dried drug. Protect from light.

### Profile

Lovage root is used in herbal medicine for gastrointestinal and urinary-tract disorders.

### Preparations

**Proprietary Preparations** (details are given in Part 3)

**Multi-ingredient:** ***Austria:*** Aponatura Entwasserungs; Aponatura Verdauungs; Ehrenhofer-Salbe; Kneipp Stoffwechsel-Unterstutzungs-Tee; Neuners Krautertee Nr 19 - Harntreibender Stoffwechseltee; Neuners Krautertee Nr 2 - Fruhjahrskurtee; Neuners Krautertee Nr 31 - Harnwegstee; ***Ger.:*** Canephron; Hevert-Entwasserungs-Tee†; Nephroselect M; Presselin Nieren-Blasen K 3; ***Hong Kong:*** Canephron N†; ***Switz.:*** Tisane pour les reins et la vessie.

## Lupulus

Hop Strobile; Hopfenzapfen; Hops; Houblon; Humulus; Lupuli Flos; Lupuli Strobulus; Lúpulo; Strobili Lupuli.

**Pharmacopoeias.** In *Eur.* (see p.vi) and *Pol.*

**Ph. Eur. 5.0** (Hop Strobile). The dried, generally whole, female inflorescences (strobiles) of the hop plant *Humulus lupulus*. It has a characteristic aromatic odour. Protect from light.

### Profile

Lupulus has been used as a bitter, and supplies the characteristic flavour of beers. It is used in herbal and folk medicine as a sedative. It is also used in homoeopathic medicine.

### Preparations

**Proprietary Preparations** (details are given in Part 3)

***Austria:*** Zirkulin Beruhigungs-Tee; ***Ger.:*** Bonased-L†; Lactidorm.

**Multi-ingredient:** ***Arg.:*** Calmtabs; ***Austral.:*** Extralife Sleep-Care†; Pacifenity†; Passiflora Complex†; Passionflower Plus†; Prosed-X†; ReDormin; Relaxaplex†; ***Austria:*** Aktiv Nerven- und Schlaftee; Aponatura Beruhigungs; Aponatura Einschlaf; Bakanasan Einschlaf; Baldracin; Baldrian AMA; Baldrian Dispert Compositum; Baldrian-Elixier; Baldrian-Krautertonikum; Baldriparan Beruhigungs; Belisir; Bio-Garten Tee zur Beruhigung; Bio-Garten Tropfen zur Beruhigung; Biogelat Schlaf; Bioreform-Beruhigungstee; Doppelherz Tonikum†; Einschlafkapseln; Hova; Klosterfrau-Beruhigungskapseln; Krauterdoktor Beruhigungstropfen; Krauterdoktor Entspannungs- und Einschlaftropfen; Krauterdoktor Nerven-Tonikum; Krauterhaus Mag Kottas Nerven- und Schlaftee; Krauterpfarrer Weidinger Tee bei Schlafstorungen; Luvased; Mag Doskar's Nerventonikum; Mag Kottas Krauterexpress-Nerven-Schlaf-Tee; Mag Kottas Schlaftee; Montana; Nervendragees; Nervenruh; Nerventee EF-EM-ES; Nervifloran; Neuners Krautertee Nr 1 - Nerventee; Neuners Krautertee Nr 141 - Schlaftee; Neuners Krautertee Nr 16 - Beruhigungstee bei Wechselbeschwerden; Neuners Krautertee Nr 201 - Krauterhexlein Kinder-Beruhigungstee; Phytogran; Sanhelios Einschlaf; Seda-Grandelat; Sedadom; Sidroga Nerven- und Schlaftee; St Radegunder Beruhigungs- und Einschlaftee; St Radegunder Nerven-Tonikum; St Radegunder Nerventee; Vivinox; Wechseltee EF-EM-ES; ***Canad.:*** Herbal Sleep Aid; Relax and Sleep; ***Chile:*** Valupass; ***Fr.:*** Nostress; Santane $D_5$†; Santane $N_9$†; ***Ger.:*** Aranidorm-S†; Ardeysedon N; Avedorm duo; Avedorm N†; Baldrian-Dispert Nacht; Baldrianox S†; Baldriparan N Stark; Baldriparan N†; Biosedon S†; Boxocalm; Cefasedativ; Cysto Fink†; Discmigon†; Dormeasan; Dormoverlan; Einschlaf-Kapseln biologisch†; Gutnacht; Hicoton; Hovaletten N†; Ilja Rogoff; Ivel Schlaf†; JuDorm; JuNeuron S†; Kneipp Baldrian + Hopfen†; Kytta-Sedativum f; Leukona-Beruhigungsbad; Leukona-Sedativ-Bad sine Chloralhydrat†; Leukona-Sedativ-Bad†; Lomasleep; Luvased; Luvased-Tropfen N†; Moradorm S; Nervendragees; Nervinetten†; Nervinfant N; Nervoregin forte; Pascosedon; Phytogran; Presselin Nerven K 1 N; Salus Nerven-Schlaf-Tee Nr.22†; Salusan†; Schlaf- und Nerventee; Schupps Baldrian Sedativbad†; Seda Kneipp N†; Seda-Plantina; Sedacur; Sedaselect D; Sedasyx; Sedatruw S†; Selon; Sensinerv forte; Somnuvis S†; Stomasal Med; Valdispert comp; Valeriana mild; Visinal†; Vivinox N; Vivinox-Schlafdragees†; ***Israel:*** Nerven-Dragees; ***Ital.:*** Emmenoiasi; Melissa (Specie Composta); Valeriana (Specie Composta); ***Mex.:*** Ivel; ***Switz.:*** Baldriparan; Cysto-Caps Chassot†; Dicalm; Dormeasan; Dragees pour le coeur et les nerfs; Dragees pour le sommeil nouvelle formule; Hova; Hyperiforce comp; Nervinetten; Phytoberidin†; Phytomed Nervo; Phytomed Somni; ReDormin; Soporin; Tisane calmante pour les enfants; Tisane pour le sommeil et les nerfs; Valverde Dragees pour le coeur; Valverde Dragees pour le sommeil; ***UK:*** Anased; Avena Sativa Comp; Gerard 99†; Gerard House Serenity; Gerard House Somnus; Gerard House Valerian Compound†; Heath & Heather Becalm†; Heath & Heather Quiet Night†; HRI Calm Life; HRI Night; Kalms; Natrasleep; Newrelax; Night Time†; Nodoff; Nytol Herbal; Quiet Days; Quiet Life; Quiet Nite; Quiet Tyme; Relax B⁺; Slumber; Stressless; Super Mega B+C; Unwind Herbal Nytol; Valerina Night-Time.

## Lysergide *(BAN, rINN)*

Lisergida; LSD; LSD-25; Lysergic Acid Diethylamide. (+)-*NN*-Diethyl-D-lysergamide; (6a*R*,9*R*)-*NN*-Diethyl-4,6,6a,7,8,9-hexahydro-7-methylindolo[4,3-*fg*]quinoline-9-carboxamide.

$C_{20}H_{25}N_3O = 323.4.$

*CAS — 50-37-3.*

### Profile

Lysergide was formerly used therapeutically but is now encountered as a drug of abuse for its hallucinogenic and psychedelic properties.

There is considerable variation in individual reaction to lysergide. Disorders of visual perception are among the first and most constant reactions to lysergide. Subjects may be hypersensitive to sound. Extreme alterations of mood, depression, distortion of body image, depersonalisation, disorders of thought and time sense, and synaesthesias may be experienced. Anxiety, often amounting to panic, may occur (a 'bad trip'). The effects of lysergide may recur months after ingestion of lysergide; the recurrence or 'flashback' may be spontaneous or induced by alcohol, other drugs, stress, or fatigue.

The subjective effects of lysergide may be preceded or accompanied by somatic effects that are mainly sympathomimetic in nature and include mydriasis, tremor, hyperreflexia, hyperthermia, piloerection, muscle weakness, and ataxia. There may be nausea and vomiting and increased heart rate and blood pressure. Derangement of blood clotting mechanisms has been described. In addition, respiratory arrest, convulsions, and coma may result from overdoses. There is no evidence of fatal reactions to lysergide in man, although accidental deaths, suicides, and homicides have occurred during lysergide intoxication.

Tolerance develops to the behavioural effects of lysergide after several days and may be lost over a similar period. There is cross-tolerance between lysergide, mescaline, and psilocybine and psilocin, but not to amfetamine or to cannabis.

Physical dependence on lysergide does not seem to occur.

## Mace Oil

Macis, aceite de.

NOTE. Mace has also been used as a name for solutions of chloroacetaphenone (p.1670), a tear gas.

### Profile

Mace oil is a volatile oil obtained by distillation from mace, the arillus of the seed of *Myristica fragrans* (Myristicaceae).

Nutmeg (p.1722) is the dried kernel of the seed of *M. fragrans*.

Mace is used as a flavour and carminative similarly to nutmeg (p.1722). It has also been used with herbal substances and other volatile agents in preparations for musculoskeletal and respiratory-tract disorders. As with nutmeg, large doses of mace may cause epileptiform convulsions and hallucinations.

### Preparations

**Proprietary Preparations** (details are given in Part 3)

**Multi-ingredient:** ***Austria:*** China-Eisenwein.

## Macrogols *(BAN, rINN)*

Macrogola; Macrogoles; PEGs; Polyethylene Glycols; Polyoxyethylene Glycols.

$CH_2(OH)(CH_2OCH_2)_mCH_2OH$. Alternatively some authorities use the general formula $H(OCH_2CH_2)_nOH$ when the number assigned to *n* for a specified macrogol is 1 more than that of *m* in the first formula.

*CAS — 25322-68-3 (macrogols); 37361-15-2 (macrogol 300).*

*ATC — A06AD15.*

**Pharmacopoeias.** Macrogols of various molecular weights are included in many pharmacopoeias.

*Eur.* (see p.vi) has a general monograph describing macrogol 300, 400, 600, 1000, 1500, 3000, 3350, 4000, 6000, 8000, 20 000, and 35 000. *USNF* has a general monograph describing Polyethylene Glycol which requires that it be labelled with the average nominal molecular weight as part of the official title.

**Ph. Eur. 5.0** (Macrogols). Mixtures of polymers with the general formula $H(OCH_2CH_2)_nOH$, where *n* represents the average number of oxyethylene groups. The type of macrogol is defined by a number that indicates the average relative molecular mass. A suitable stabiliser may be added.

Macrogol 300, 400, and 600 are clear, viscous, colourless or almost colourless, hygroscopic liquids. Miscible with water; very soluble in alcohol, in acetone, and in dichloromethane.

Macrogol 1000 is a white or almost white, hygroscopic solid with a waxy or paraffin-like appearance. Very soluble in water; freely soluble in alcohol and in dichloromethane.

Macrogol 1500 is a white or almost white solid with a waxy or paraffin-like appearance. Very soluble in water and in dichloromethane; freely soluble in alcohol.

Macrogol 3000 and 3350 are white or almost white solids with a waxy or paraffin-like appearance. Very soluble in water and in dichloromethane; very slightly soluble in alcohol.

Macrogol 4000, 6000, and 8000 are white or almost white solids with a waxy or paraffin-like appearance. Very soluble in water and in dichloromethane; practically insoluble in alcohol.

Macrogol 20 000 and 35 000 are white or almost white solids with a waxy or paraffin-like appearance. Very soluble in water; practically insoluble in alcohol; soluble in dichloromethane.

All macrogols are practically insoluble in fatty oils and in mineral oils. All macrogols should be stored in airtight containers.

**USNF 22** (Polyethylene Glycol). Addition polymers of ethylene oxide and water, represented by the formula $H(OCH_2CH_2)_nOH$, in which *n* represents the average number of oxyethylene groups. They may contain a suitable antioxidant. Each macrogol is usually designated by a number that corresponds approximately to its average molecular weight. As the average molecular weight increases, the water solubility, hygroscopicity, and solubility in organic solvents decrease, while the viscosity increases.

Liquid grades occur as clear to slightly hazy, colourless or practically colourless, slightly hygroscopic, viscous liquids, having a slight, characteristic odour. Solid grades occur as practically odourless, white, waxy, plastic material having a consistency similar to beeswax, or as creamy-white flakes, beads, or powders. Liquid grades are miscible with water; solid grades are freely soluble in water; all grades are soluble in alcohol, in acetone, in chloroform, in ethoxyethanol, in ethyl acetate, and in toluene; all grades are insoluble in ether and in hexane. The pH of a 5% solution of a macrogol in water is between 4.5 and 7.5. Store in airtight containers.

**Incompatibility.** Macrogols can demonstrate oxidising activity leading to incompatibilities. The activity of bacitracin or benzylpenicillin may be reduced in a macrogol base. Some plastics are softened by macrogols.

### Adverse Effects and Precautions

Macrogols appear to have relatively low toxicity, although any toxicity appears to be greatest with the macrogols of low molecular weight. They may cause stinging when administered topically, especially to mucous membranes, and have been associated with hypersensitivity reactions such as urticaria. Hyperosmolality, metabolic acidosis, and renal failure have been reported following the topical application of macrogols to burn patients. Topical preparations with a macrogol base should therefore be used with caution in patients with renal impairment and/or large areas of raw surfaces, burns, or open wounds.

Patients undergoing bowel cleansing with mixtures of macrogols (3350 or 4000) and electrolytes commonly experience local gastrointestinal discomfort, bloating, and nausea. Abdominal cramps, vomiting, and anal irritation may also occur and there have been rare reports of possible hypersensitivity reactions. These colonic lavage solutions are contra-indicated in gastrointestinal obstruction or perforation, ileus, gastric retention, peptic ulcer disease, and toxic megacolon; caution is advisable in patients with ulcerative colitis. Since aspiration may be a problem, they should be used with caution in patients with an impaired gag reflex, reflux oesophagitis, or diminished levels of consciousness. They should be given with caution to diabetic patients. Drugs taken within one hour of starting colonic lavage with an orally administered macrogol and electrolyte mixture may be flushed from the gastrointestinal tract unabsorbed.

**Effects on fluid and electrolyte homoeostasis.** A syndrome of elevated total serum calcium (with a concomitant decrease in ionised calcium), hyperosmolality, metabolic acidosis, and renal failure has been observed in *animals*[1] and in burn patients[2] following the topical application of preparations with a macrogol base. The FDA has recommended that topical preparations containing macrogols should be used with caution in burn patients with known or suspected renal impairment, as macrogols absorbed through denuded skin and not excreted normally by a compromised kidney could lead to symptoms of progressive renal impairment.[3]

The use of macrogol and electrolyte solutions for bowel preparation has also been associated with sodium and water retention, resulting in exacerbation of heart failure in a patient with diabetic gastroparesis,[4] and with the development of pulmonary oedema possibly due to aspiration in a child without cardiac or renal disease.[5]

1. Herold DA, *et al.* Toxicity of topical polyethylene glycol. *Toxicol Appl Pharmacol* 1982; **65:** 329–35.
2. Bruns DE, *et al.* Polyethylene glycol intoxication in burn patients. *Burns* 1982; **9:** 49–52.
3. Anonymous. Topical PEG in burn ointments. *FDA Drug Bull* 1982; **12:** 25–6.
4. Granberry MC, *et al.* Exacerbation of congestive heart failure after administration of polyethylene glycol-electrolyte lavage solution. *Ann Pharmacother* 1995; **29:** 1232–5.
5. Paap CM, Ehrlich R. Acute pulmonary edema after polyethylene glycol intestinal lavage in a child. *Ann Pharmacother* 1993; **27:** 1044–7.

**Effects on the kidneys.** Macrogol 400 which was present in a lorazepam injection could have contributed to renal damage suggestive of acute tubular necrosis in a patient who received large doses (averaging lorazepam 95 mg daily) for 43 days.[1] The cumulative dose of macrogol 400 during this period was about 220 mL.

1. Laine GA, *et al.* Polyethylene glycol nephrotoxicity secondary to prolonged high-dose intravenous lorazepam. *Ann Pharmacother* 1995; **29:** 1110–14.

**Hypersensitivity.** Hypersensitivity to macrogols is uncommon but both immediate urticarial reactions and delayed allergic contact dermatitis have been reported following the topical application of preparations with a macrogol vehicle or base.[1] An anaphylactic reaction has been associated with the ingestion of macrogols in a multivitamin tablet.[2] The manufacturers of preparations containing macrogols and electrolytes for bowel cleansing have reported isolated instances of skin reactions and rhinorrhoea.

1. Fisher AA. Immediate and delayed allergic contact reactions to polyethylene glycol. *Contact Dermatitis* 1978; **4:** 135–8.
2. Kwee YN, Dolovich J. Anaphylaxis to polyethylene glycol (PEG) in a multivitamin tablet. *J Allergy Clin Immunol* 1982; **69:** 138.

**Overdosage.** Ingestion of 2 litres of a colonic lavage solution containing macrogol 400 instead of macrogol 4000 resulted in a patient developing severe metabolic acidosis and rapidly becoming comatose due to systemic absorption of the macrogol.[1] The patient was successfully treated with intravenous bicarbonate and dialysis.

1. Bélaïche J, *et al.* Coma acidosique après préparation colique par du polyèthylène glycol. *Gastroenterol Clin Biol* 1983; **7:** 426–7.

## Pharmacokinetics

Liquid macrogols may be absorbed when taken by mouth but macrogols of high molecular weight, such as macrogol 3350, are not significantly absorbed from the gastrointestinal tract. There is evidence of absorption of macrogols when applied to damaged skin. Macrogols entering the systemic circulation are predominantly excreted unchanged in the urine; low-molecular-weight macrogols may be partly metabolised.

◊ References.

1. DiPiro JT, *et al.* Absorption of polyethylene glycol after administration of a PEG-electrolyte lavage solution. *Clin Pharm* 1986; **5:** 153–5.

## Uses and Administration

Macrogols are relatively stable, non-toxic compounds which have a range of properties depending on their molecular weight. They are widely used in pharmaceutical manufacturing as water-soluble bases for topical preparations and suppositories, as solvents and vehicles, and as solubilising agents, tablet binders, plasticisers in film coating, and tablet lubricants. They have also been reported to have antibacterial properties.

A mixture of macrogol 3350 or 4000 with electrolytes is used to empty the bowel before colonoscopy, radiological procedures, or surgery. These preparations have been formulated so that the osmotic activity of the macrogol and concentrations of the electrolytes result in a minimum net effect on the fluid and electrolyte balance. Adults are given 200 to 300 mL of the reconstituted aqueous solution (containing about 59 g or 60 g or 105 g of the macrogol per litre), which they have to swallow rapidly, and this is repeated every 10 to 15 minutes until the rectal effluent is clear, or until a total of 4 litres of the solution has been consumed. A dose for children is 25 to 40 mL/kg per hour. Bowel evacuation usually begins about 1 hour after starting administration and is complete in about 4 hours. Patients should fast for at least 2 or 3 hours before drinking the solution. Additional flavouring ingredients, sugar, or other sweeteners should not be added to the solution. If distension or pain occur, administration should be temporarily stopped or the interval between drinks extended. For administration by nasogastric tube, a rate of 20 to 30 mL per minute has been used.

Similar preparations are used in patients 12 years of age and over for the treatment of chronic constipation in a usual dose of 125 mL of a solution containing 105 g of the macrogol per litre two or three times daily. The maximum course is 2 weeks, which may be repeated if necessary. In the management of faecal impaction, 8 doses of 125 mL of solution should be consumed within 6 hours for a maximum of 3 days. Patients with impaired cardiovascular function should take no more than 2 doses in any one hour. Children may be treated for faecal impaction in an escalating dose over 7 days until disimpaction occurs; the total daily dose should be divided and consumed within a 12 hour period. Those aged 2 to 4 years should start with two doses of 62.5 mL of solution daily increasing steadily to a maximum of 8 doses on days 6 and 7; children aged 5 to 11 years should start with four doses of 62.5 mL of solution daily increasing steadily to a maximum of 12 doses on days 5 to 7.

Macrogols of high molecular weight such as macrogol 4000 have been used as inert markers in studies on intestinal absorption and excretion.

Conjugation of drugs and therapeutic proteins with macrogols (pegylation) has been tried in an attempt to improve their pharmacokinetic profiles and to reduce their adverse effects. Pegylation may also reduce the immunogenicity of therapeutic proteins. Examples of pegylated proteins include pegademase (p.1729), pegaspargase (p.528), and peginterferon alfa (p.643).

**Drug delivery systems.** References to the use of macrogols in delivery systems for drugs and proteins.

1. Reddy KR. Controlled-release, pegylation, liposomal formulations: new mechanisms in the delivery of injectable drugs. *Ann Pharmacother* 2000; **34:** 915–23.
2. Harris JM, *et al.* Pegylation: a novel process for modifying pharmacokinetics. *Clin Pharmacokinet* 2001; **40:** 539–51.

**Phenol poisoning.** Washing with liquid macrogols has been recommended in the emergency treatment of skin contamination with phenol, see p.1188.

## Preparations

***USP 27:*** PEG 3350 and Electrolytes for Oral Solution.

**Proprietary Preparations** (details are given in Part 3)
***Belg.:*** Forlax; ***Canad.:*** Visine True Tears; ***Fr.:*** Forlax; ***Ger.:*** Forlax; Laxofalk; ***Hong Kong:*** Forlax; ***Ital.:*** Pergidal; ***Malaysia:*** Forlax; ***Thai.:*** Forlax; ***UK:*** Idrolax; ***USA:*** MiraLax.

**Multi-ingredient:** ***Arg.:*** Adital; Barex; Irix Lagrimas; Transipeg; ***Austral.:*** Colonic Lavage Powder; Colonlytely; Colonprep; Glycoprep; Glycoprep-C; GoLytely†; Movicol; Prep Kit-C; Visine Advanced Relief; Visine Revive†; Visine True Tears; ***Austria:*** Klean-Prep; Movicol; Transipeg; ***Belg.:*** Colopeg; Klean-Prep; Movicol; Precosol; Transipeg; ***Braz.:*** Blinkene†; Nu-Lytely†; ***Canad.:*** Aquasite†; CoLyte; GoLytely; Klean-Prep; Peglyte; Pro-Lax†; Rhinaris; Salinol; Secaris; Visine Moisturizing; ***Denm.:*** Klean-Prep; Ledermix; Movicol; ***Fin.:*** Colonsteril; Klean-Prep; Movicol; ***Fr.:*** Colopeg; Fortrans; Klean-Prep; Movicol; SST; Transipeg; ***Ger.:*** Colonorm N; Delcoprep; Endofalk; Isomol; Klean-Prep; Lens Fresh†; Movicol; Oralav; ***Gr.:*** Klean-Prep; ***Hong Kong:*** Fortrans†; Hypotears; Klean-Prep; Movicol; Visine Moisturizing; ***Irl.:*** Klean-Prep; Movicol; ***Israel:*** Hypotears PF†; Meroken New; ***Ital.:*** Gofreely†; Hypotears; Isocolan; Klean-Prep; Macro-P; Movicol; Selg; Selg-Esse; ***Malaysia:*** Fortrans; Hypotears; ***Mex.:*** NuLytely; Transipeg†; Visine Extra; ***Neth.:*** Klean-Prep; Movicolon; ***Norw.:*** Klean-Prep; Laxabon; Movicol; ***NZ:*** Glycoprep; GoLytely†; Klean-Prep; Movicol; Revive†; Visine Advanced Relief; ***Port.:*** Klean-Prep; ***S.Afr.:*** GoLytely; Klean-Prep; Movicol; ***Singapore:*** Fortrans; Klean-Prep; Movicol; ***Spain:*** Evacuante; Klean-Prep; Movicol; ***Swed.:*** Klean-Prep; Laxabon; Movicol; ***Switz.:*** Colo-Sol; Cololyt; Fordtran; Gleitmittel; Hypotears; Isocolan; Klean-Prep; Movicol; Tracheo Fresh; Transipeg; ***Thai.:*** Unison Enema; ***UK:*** Hypotears; Klean-Prep; Movicol; SST; ***USA:*** Advanced Relief Visine; Aquasite; Co-Lav†; CoLyte; Go-Evac†; GoLytely; Hypotears; Nu-Tears II; NuLytely; OCL; Tetrasine Extra; Visine Moisturizing.

# Magnesium Glutamate Hydrobromide

Glutamato magnésico, hidrobromuro de; Magnesium α-Aminoglutarate Hydrobromide; Magnesium Bromoglutamate.

$(C_5H_8NO_4)_2Mg,HBr = 397.5.$

## Profile

Magnesium glutamate hydrobromide has been used as a sedative and hypnotic in the treatment of insomnia, neuroses, and behavioural disorders. The use of bromides is generally deprecated.

## Preparations

**Proprietary Preparations** (details are given in Part 3)

**Multi-ingredient:** ***Chile:*** Gamalate B6; ***Spain:*** Cefabol; Gamalate B6; Psicosoma Solucion.

# Maleic Acid

Acidum Maleicum; Maleico, ácido; Toxilic Acid. *cis*-Butenedioic acid.

$C_2H_2(CO_2H)_2 = 116.1.$

*CAS — 110-16-7.*

**Pharmacopoeias.** In *Eur.* (see p.vi).

**Ph. Eur. 5.0** (Maleic Acid). A white crystalline powder. Freely soluble in water and in alcohol. A 5% solution in water has a pH of less than 2. Store in glass containers. Protect from light.

## Profile

Maleic acid is used in the preparation of Ergometrine Injection (BP 2003) and Ergometrine and Oxytocin Injection (BP 2003).

# Malic Acid

Apple Acid; E296; Hydroxysuccinic Acid; Málico, ácido. Hydroxybutanedioic acid.

$C_4H_6O_5 = 134.1.$

*CAS — 6915-15-7 (malic acid); 636-61-3 ((+)-malic acid); 97-67-6 ((−)-malic acid); 617-48-1 ((±)-malic acid).*

**Pharmacopoeias.** In *Eur.* (see p.vi). Also in *USNF.*

**Ph. Eur. 5.0** (Malic Acid). A white crystalline powder. Freely soluble in water and in alcohol, sparingly soluble in acetone.

**USNF 22** (Malic Acid). A white or practically white, crystalline powder or granules. Very soluble in water; freely soluble in alcohol.

## Profile

Malic acid is used in pharmaceutical formulations as an acidifier, flavour, and as an alternative to citric acid in effervescent powders. It is used with butylated hydroxytoluene as an antioxidant in vegetable oils. It is used topically with benzoic acid and salicylic acid for desloughing of ulcers, burns, and wounds, and systemically with arginine (p.1421) in preparations for the treatment of liver disorders. Pastilles containing malic acid are also used in the management of dry mouth (p.1576).

## Preparations

**Proprietary Preparations** (details are given in Part 3)

**Multi-ingredient:** ***Austria:*** Acerbine; Leberinfusion; Rocmaline; ***Chile:*** Secand; ***Fin.:*** Xerodent; ***Fr.:*** Rocmaline; Sphingogel; Squaphane; SST; ***Ger.:*** Infumal†; ***Ital.:*** Keraflex; ***Port.:*** Hyfac AHA†; Squaphane†; ***S.Afr.:*** Aserbine; ***Spain:*** Acerbiol; ***Swed.:*** Xerodent; ***Switz.:*** Acerbine; ***UK:*** Aserbine; Salivix; SST.

# Mallow

Malvenblätter (mallow leaf); Malvenblüten (mallow flower); Mauve des Bois (*Malva silvestris*).

**Pharmacopoeias.** *Eur.* (see p.vi) includes the dried flowers. *Pol.* and *Swiss* include Mallow Leaf (Malvae Folium) which may be *Malva sylvestris* or *M. neglecta*.

**Ph. Eur. 5.0** (Mallow Flower; Malvae sylvestris flos). The whole or fragmented dried flower of *Malva sylvestris* or its cultivated varieties. Protect from light.

## Profile

Mallow flower and leaf act as demulcents and are ingredients of herbal remedies for coughs and cold symptoms. Mallow flower is also used to enhance the colour of herbal teas and other foodstuffs. Mallow is also included in herbal remedies for gastrointestinal disorders.

## Preparations

**Proprietary Preparations** (details are given in Part 3)
***Braz.:*** Mictasol; ***Switz.:*** Malvedrin.

**Multi-ingredient:** ***Arg.:*** Acnetrol; KW; Mictasol Azul; Prurigel; ***Austral.:*** Neo-Cleanse†; ***Austria:*** Anifer Hustentee; Aponatura Hustenlosende; Apotheker Bauer's Magentee; Gewusst wie Darmtee; Gewusst wie Magentee mild; Gewusst wie Nerven-Schlaftee; Krauterhaus Mag Kottas Babytee; Krauterhaus Mag Kottas Fruhjahrs- und Herbstkurtee; Krauterhaus Mag Kottas Gallen- und Lebertee; Krauterhaus Mag Kottas Husten- und Bronchialtee; Krauterhaus Mag Kottas Magen- und Darmtee; Krauterhaus Mag Kottas milder Abfuhrtee; Krauterhaus Mag Kottas Tee fur die Verdauung; Krauterhaus Mag Kottas Tee gegen Blahungen; Krauterhaus Mag Kottas Tee gegen Durchfall; Mag Kottas Baby-Tee; Mag Kottas Beruhigungstee; Mag Kottas Blahungs-Verdauungstee; Mag Kottas Krauterexpress-Beruhigungstee; Mag Kottas Krauterexpress-Blahungs-Verdauungstee; Mag Kottas Krauterexpress-Magen-Darm-Tee; Mag Kottas Krauterexpress-Tee fur stillende Mutter; Mag Kottas Leber-Gallentee; Mag Kottas Magen- und Darmtee; Mag Kottas Tee fur stillende Mutter; Midro Tee; St Radegunder Abfuhrtee mild; St Radegunder Hustentee; St Radegunder Magenberuhigungstee; St Radegunder Reizmildernder Magentee; ***Belg.:*** Mictasol; Tisane Antibiliaire et Stomachique†; Tisane Depurative "les 12 Plantes"†; Tisane Pectorale†; Tisane Purgative†; ***Braz.:*** Forsalil†; Malva Composta†; Malvodon; Malvol†; Malvosulfam†; Mictasol com Sulfa; Peitoral Angico Pelotense; Varigerm†; ***Canad.:*** Swiss Herb Cough Drops; ***Fr.:*** Mediflor Tisane Hepatique No 5; Mediflor Tisane Pectorale d'Alsace†; Mictasol; Mictasol Bleu†; Mucogyne; Niver†; Santane $C_6$†; Santane $O_1$†; Tisane Sedative Weleda†; ***Israel:*** Midro-Tea; ***Ital.:*** Alkagin; Glicerolax; Microclisma Evacuante AD-BB†; Microclismi Marco Viti; Microclismi Sella; Mictasol Bleu; Mictasone; Nevril; Piodermina; Proctonet; Tisana Cisbey†; ***Port.:*** Alkagin; Midro; ***Switz.:*** Malvedrin; Malveol.

# Malotilate *(USAN, rINN)*

Malotilato; NKK-105. Diisopropyl 1,3-dithiole-$\Delta^{2,\alpha}$-malonate.

$C_{12}H_{16}O_4S_2 = 288.4.$

*CAS — 59937-28-9.*

## Profile

Malotilate has been investigated for its reported protective effects on liver function in patients with chronic hepatic disease.

◊ References.

1. A European Multicentre Study Group. The results of a randomized double blind controlled trial evaluating malotilate in primary biliary cirrhosis. *J Hepatol* 1993; **17:** 227–35.

# Mammalian Tissue Extracts

Mamíferos, extractos tisulares.

## Profile

Many medicinal preparations with definite pharmacological activity and valid clinical uses are of mammalian origin and are described under their appropriate monographs—for example, calcitonin, corticotropin, hydrocortisone (cortisol), some enzymes, heparin, insulin, parathyroid hormone, pituitary hormones, some sex hormones, and thyroid.

Many other preparations of animal origin have been promoted for a wide variety of disorders. Evidence of pharmacological activity is often lacking, and such preparations are often of doubtful benefit.

## Preparations

**Proprietary Preparations** (details are given in Part 3)
***Arg.:*** Bros; ***Austria:*** Ambotonin; Cerebrolysin; Cerebrotonin; Epiphysan†; ***Ger.:*** Cerebrolysin; ***Hong Kong:*** Cerebrolysin; ***Ital.:*** Liposom; ***Thai.:*** Cerebrolysin.

**Multi-ingredient:** ***Arg.:*** Pat-Chobet; ***Canad.:*** Revitonus C; ***Fr.:*** Pro-Nat†; ***Ger.:*** AntiFocal; NeyChondrin N (Revitorgan-Dilutionen N Nr 68); NeyTumorin (Revitorgan-Lingual Nr 66); NeyTumorin N (Revitorgan-Dilutionen N Nr 66); Ribo-Wied; ***UK:*** S.P.H.P..

# Manuka

New Zealand Tea Tree.

## Profile

The oil of manuka (*Leptospermum scoparium*) is used for its antimicrobial properties as an alternative to melaleuca oil (p.1710). Manuka honey has also been used as a wound dressing (p.1434).

◊ References.


1. Cooper RA, *et al.* The sensitivity to honey of Gram-positive cocci of clinical significance isolated from wounds. *J Appl Microbiol* 2002; **93:** 857–63.
2. Cooper RA, *et al.* The efficacy of honey in inhibiting strains of Pseudomonas aeruginosa from infected burns. *J Burn Care Rehabil* 2002; **23:** 366–70.
3. English HK, *et al.* The effects of manuka honey on plaque and gingivitis: a pilot study. *J Int Acad Periodontol* 2004; **6:** 63–7.


## Mastic

Almáciga; Mastiche; Mastix.

**Pharmacopoeias.** In *Eur.* (see p.vi).

**Ph. Eur. 5.0** (Mastic). The dried resinous exudate obtained from stems and branches of *Pistacia lentiscus* var. *latifolius*. It contains a minimum of 1% v/w of essential oil, calculated with reference to the anhydrous drug. It should not be powdered.

### Profile

Solutions of mastic in alcohol, chloroform, or ether have been used, applied on cotton wool, as temporary fillings for carious teeth. Compound Mastic Paint (BP 1980) was formerly used as a protective covering for wounds and to hold gauze in position.

Mastic gum has been used in the management of peptic ulcer disease.

**Peptic ulcer disease.** Mastic may be effective in the treatment of peptic ulcer disease possibly due to an antibacterial action on *Helicobacter pylori*.[1] However, one small clinical study found no benefit.[2]


1. Huwez FU, *et al.* Mastic gum kills Helicobacter pylori. *N Engl J Med* 1998; **339:** 1946. Correction. *ibid.*: **340:** 576 [dose].
2. Bebb JR, *et al.* Mastic gum has no effect on Helicobacter pylori load in vivo. *J Antimicrob Chemother* 2003; **52:** 522–3.


### Preparations

**Proprietary Preparations** (details are given in Part 3)
***UK:*** Mastika.

## Meadowsweet

Filipendulae Ulmariae; Queen of the Meadows; Reina de los prados; Reine des Prés; Spiraeae Herba; Ulmaria.

**Pharmacopoeias.** In *Eur.* (see p.vi).

**Ph. Eur. 5.0** (Meadowsweet). The whole or cut, dried flowering tops of *Filipendula ulmaria* (*Spiraea ulmaria*). It contains a minimum of 0.1% v/w of steam-volatile substances (dried drug). It has an aromatic odour of methyl salicylate after crushing.

### Profile

Meadowsweet is used in herbal medicine as a diuretic and in gastrointestinal and rheumatic disorders. It is also used in homoeopathic medicine.

### Preparations

**Proprietary Preparations** (details are given in Part 3)

**Multi-ingredient: *Belg.:*** Tisane Diuretique†; ***Fr.:*** Actisane Douleurs Articulaires†; Actisane Minceur†; Aminsane†; Artrosan†; Mediflor Tisane Antirhumatismale No 2; Mediflor Tisane No 4 Diuretique; Mediflor Tisane Pectorale d'Alsace†; Polypirine; Santane $A_4$†; Santane $O_1$†; Santane $R_8$†; Tisane des Familles†; Tisane Touraine†; Tisanes de l'Abbe Hamon no 3†; ***Ital.:*** Artoxan†; Sambuco (Specie Composta); Tiglio (Specie Composta); ***Spain:*** Dolosul; Natusor Harpagosinol; Natusor Renal; ***Switz.:*** Urinex; ***UK:*** Acidosis; Indigestion Mixture; Natraleze†; ***USA:*** Amerigel.

## Meclofenoxate Hydrochloride *(BANM, rINNM)*

Centrophenoxine Hydrochloride; Clofenoxine Hydrochloride; Clophenoxate Hydrochloride; Deanol 4-Chlorophenoxyacetate Hydrochloride; Hidrocloruro de meclofenoxato; Meclofenoxane Hydrochloride. 2-Dimethylaminoethyl 4-chlorophenoxyacetate hydrochloride.

$C_{12}H_{16}ClNO_3,HCl = 294.2.$

*CAS — 51-68-3 (meclofenoxate); 3685-84-5 (meclofenoxate hydrochloride).*

*ATC — N06BX01.*

**Pharmacopoeias.** In *Chin.* and *Jpn.*

### Profile

Meclofenoxate hydrochloride has been claimed to aid cellular metabolism in the presence of diminished oxygen concentrations. It has been given mainly for mental changes in the elderly, or following strokes or head injury.

### Preparations

**Proprietary Preparations** (details are given in Part 3)
***Austria:*** Lucidril; ***Fr.:*** Lucidril†; ***Ger.:*** Cerutil; Helfergin.

## Meglumine *(BAN, rINN)*

Meglumina; Megluminum. *N*-Methylglucamine; 1-Methylamino-1-deoxy-D-glucitol.

$C_7H_{17}NO_5 = 195.2.$

*CAS — 6284-40-8.*

**Pharmacopoeias.** In *Chin., Eur.* (see p.vi), *Int., Jpn,* and *US.*

**Ph. Eur. 5.0** (Meglumine). A white or almost white, crystalline powder. Freely soluble in water; sparingly soluble in alcohol; practically insoluble in dichloromethane.

**USP 27** (Meglumine). White to faintly yellowish-white, odourless crystals or powder. Freely soluble in water; sparingly soluble in alcohol.

### Profile

Meglumine is an organic base used for the preparation of salts of organic acids including many used as contrast media.

## Melaleuca Oil

Australian Tea Tree Oil; Melaleuca, aceite de; Melaleucae Aetheroleum; Oleum Melaleucae; Tea Tree Oil.

*CAS — 68647-73-4; 8022-72-8.*

NOTE. Though the synonym Ti-tree Oil has been used for melaleuca oil (e.g. in BPC 1949), the name Ti-tree is also applied to species of *Cordyline* (Liliaceae) indigenous to New Zealand.

**Pharmacopoeias.** In *Eur.* (see p.vi).

**Ph. Eur. 5.0** (Tea Tree Oil). The essential oil obtained by steam distillation from the foliage and terminal branchlets of *Melaleuca alternifolia, M. linariifolia, M. dissitiflora,* and/or other species of *Melaleuca*. It contains less than 7.0% aromadendrene, less than 15% cineole, 0.5 to 12.0% *p*-cymene, 0.5 to 4.0% limonene, 1.0 to 6.0% α-pinene, less than 3.5% sabinene, 5.0 to 13.0% α-terpinene, 10.0 to 28.0% γ-terpinene, minimum of 30% terpinen-4-ol, 1.5 to 8.0% α-terpineol, and 1.5 to 5.0% terpinolene.

A clear, mobile, colourless to pale yellow liquid with a characteristic odour. Store in well-filled airtight containers at a temperature not exceeding 25°. Protect from light.

### Profile

Melaleuca oil has been reported to have bactericidal and fungicidal properties and is used topically for various skin disorders.

◊ References.


1. Bassett IB, *et al.* A comparative study of tea-tree oil versus benzoylperoxide in the treatment of acne. *Med J Aust* 1990; **153:** 455–8.
2. Blackwell AL. Tea tree oil and anaerobic (bacterial) vaginosis. *Lancet* 1991; **337:** 300.
3. Carson CF, *et al.* Susceptibility of methicillin-resistant Staphylococcus aureus to the essential oil of melaleuca alternifolia. *J Antimicrob Chemother* 1995; **35:** 421–4.
4. Carson CF, *et al.* Efficacy and safety of tea tree oil as a topical antimicrobial agent. *J Hosp Infect* 1998; **40:** 175–8.
5. Allen P. Tea tree oil: the science behind the antimicrobial hype. *Lancet* 2001; **358:** 1245.
6. Satchell AC, *et al.* Treatment of interdigital tinea pedis with 25% and 50% tea tree oil solution: a randomized, placebo-controlled, blinded study. *Australas J Dermatol* 2002; **43:** 175–8.
7. Hammer KA, *et al.* In vitro activity of Melaleuca alternifolia (tea tree) oil against dermatophytes and other filamentous fungi. *J Antimicrob Chemother* 2002; **50:** 195–9.
8. Satchell AC, *et al.* Treatment of dandruff with 5% tea tree oil shampoo. *J Am Acad Dermatol* 2002; **47:** 852–5.
9. Koh KJ, *et al.* Tea tree oil reduces histamine-induced skin inflammation. *Br J Dermatol* 2002; **147:** 1212–7.
10. Mozelsio NB, *et al.* Immediate systemic hypersensitivity reaction associated with topical application of Australian tea tree oil. *Allergy Asthma Proc* 2003; **24:** 73–5.
11. Perrett CM, *et al.* Tea tree oil dermatitis associated with linear IgA disease. *Clin Exp Dermatol* 2003; **28:** 167–70.


### Preparations

**Proprietary Preparations** (details are given in Part 3)
***Austral.:*** Clean Skin Anti Acne†; Rapaid Antiseptic; Rapaid First Aid†; ***Chile:*** Acnoxyl Gel Cuidado Intensivo; Acnoxyl Gel De Limpieza; Acnoxyl Stick Corrector; Sebolic; ***Fr.:*** Myleuca; ***UK:*** Amber Gold†; Burnshield Gel; Melavir; Savlon Natural Antiseptic.

**Multi-ingredient: *Arg.:*** Aveno; ***Austral.:*** APR Cream; Austral-Balm†; Burnaid First Aid Burn Gel†; Clean Skin Face Wash†; Curaderm; Neutralice†; Rapaid Medicated†; Rapaid Rash-Relief; Relief Rub†; SP Cream; VR; ***Chile:*** Acnoxyl Abrasivo; Acnoxyl Gel Humectante; Acnoxyl Jabon; Acnoxyl Jabon Liquido; Acnoxyl Locion Tonica; Acnoxyl Shampoo Cabello Graso; ***Fr.:*** Dermocica; Mycogel; ***Ital.:*** Proctopure; ***NZ:*** Electric Blue Headlice; Lice Blaster; ***Port.:*** Emopads†; Mycogel†; Peliphane†; ***Singapore:*** Burnaid; Tinasolve; ***UK:*** Kleer Cream†; Skin Clear; Tea Tree & Witch Hazel Cream; Teenstick.

## Melatonin

*N*-Acetyl-5-methoxytryptamine; Melatonina. *N*-[2-(5-Methoxyindol-3-yl)ethyl]acetamide.

$C_{13}H_{16}N_2O_2 = 232.3.$

*CAS — 73-31-4.*

### Profile

Melatonin is a hormone produced in the pineal gland from the amino acid tryptophan. Results mainly from *animal* studies indicate that melatonin increases the concentration of aminobutyric acid and serotonin in the midbrain and hypothalamus and enhances the activity of pyridoxal-kinase, an enzyme involved in the synthesis of aminobutyric acid, dopamine, and serotonin. Melatonin is involved in the inhibition of gonadal development and in the control of oestrus. It is also involved in protective changes in skin coloration. There appears to be a diurnal rhythm of melatonin secretion; it is secreted during hours of darkness and may affect sleep pattern. Because of its possible role in influencing circadian rhythm, melatonin has been tried in the alleviation of jet lag and other disorders resulting from delay of sleep. It has also been studied in various depressive disorders including seasonal affective disorder, and in large doses for its contraceptive activity.

A number of melatonin analogues are being developed.

**Adverse effects.** An increase in seizure activity was noted in 4 of 6 children with severe neurological deficits during treatment with melatonin for sleep disorders.[1] Seizure activity returned to baseline values when melatonin was stopped and recurred on rechallenge.


1. Sheldon SH. Pro-convulsant effects of oral melatonin in neurologically disabled children. *Lancet* 1998; **351:** 1254.


**Uses.** Melatonin has been tried in a number of disorders[1] including, in large doses, as an adjunct to conventional chemotherapy for malignant neoplasms[2,3] and, with norethisterone, as a contraceptive.[4] It is possible that contraceptive use of melatonin may be associated with a reduced risk of breast cancer.[5] For mention of response to melatonin in 2 patients with sarcoidosis, see p.1087. Preliminary studies have also suggested that melatonin may be beneficial in hyperlipidaemias,[6] cluster headaches,[7] and tinnitus.[8] Repeated bedtime doses may also play a part in reducing nocturnal blood pressure in patients with essential hypertension.[9] Claims for its value as an anti-ageing treatment and for use in conditions such as Alzheimer's disease and AIDS are unfounded.[2,10] The effects of long-term use of melatonin have yet to be assessed.


1. Wetterberg L. Melatonin and clinical application. *Reprod Nutr Dev* 1999; **39:** 367–82.
2. Pepping J. Melatonin. *Am J Health-Syst Pharm* 1999; **56:** 2520–7.
3. Lissoni P, *et al.* Decreased toxicity and increased efficacy of cancer chemotherapy using the pineal hormone melatonin in metastatic solid tumour patients with poor clinical status. *Eur J Cancer* 1999; **35:** 1688–92.
4. Short RV. Melatonin. *BMJ* 1993; **307:** 952–3.
5. Cohen M, *et al.* Hypotheses: melatonin/steroid combination contraceptives will prevent breast cancer. *Breast Cancer Res Treat* 1995; **33:** 257–64.
6. Pittalis S, *et al.* Effect of a chronic therapy with the pineal hormone melatonin on cholesterol levels in idiopathic hypercholesterolemic patients. *Recenti Prog Med* 1997; **88:** 401–2.
7. Leone M, *et al.* Melatonin versus placebo in the prophylaxis of cluster headache; a double-blind pilot study with parallel groups. *Cephalalgia* 1996; **16:** 494–6.
8. Rosenberg SI, *et al.* Effect of melatonin on tinnitus. *Laryngoscope* 1998; **108:** 305–10.
9. Scheer FAJL, *et al.* Daily nighttime melatonin reduces blood pressure in male patients with essential hypertension. *Hypertension* 2004; **43:** 192–7.
10. Brzezinski A. Melatonin in humans. *N Engl J Med* 1997; **336:** 186–95.


INSOMNIA. Although melatonin is considered[1-6] to be potentially useful in the management of various forms of insomnia (p.667), especially those associated with circadian rhythm disturbances, there is little evidence of efficacy from large studies and its long-term safety remains to be established. In healthy subjects melatonin has been reported[7,8] to reduce the time to onset of sleep and to increase the time spent asleep. Whether this is due to adjustment of the 'body clock' or any hypnotic action of melatonin is unclear. Improved quality of sleep has been reported in elderly patients treated with melatonin for insomnia,[9] and it might be of use in delayed sleep phase syndrome[10] and insomnia in shift workers and totally blind people, although some[11,12] have found no beneficial effects of melatonin in night shift workers or emergency medicine employees. There has also been a report[13] of a patient with somnolence associated with melatonin deficiency after pinealectomy who responded to treatment with melatonin. A preliminary report[14] has suggested that use of melatonin may enable benzodiazepine therapy for insomnia to be discontinued without impairing the quality of sleep. However, melatonin might have a deleterious effect on sleep patterns in some circumstances.[15]


1. Haimov I, Lavie P. Potential of melatonin replacement therapy in older patients with sleep disorders. *Drugs Aging* 1995; **7:** 75–8.
2. Brown GM. Melatonin in psychiatric and sleep disorders: therapeutic implications. *CNS Drugs* 1995; **3:** 209–26.
3. Anonymous. Melatonin. *Med Lett Drugs Ther* 1995; **37:** 111–12.
4. Arendt J. Melatonin. *BMJ* 1996; **312:** 1242–3.
5. Lamberg L. Melatonin potentially useful but safety, efficacy remain uncertain. *JAMA* 1996; **276:** 1011–14.
6. Skene DJ, *et al.* Use of melatonin in the treatment of phase shift and sleep disorders. *Adv Exp Med Biol* 1999; **467:** 79–84.
7. Zhdanova IV, *et al.* Sleep-inducing effects of low doses of melatonin ingested in the evening. *Clin Pharmacol Ther* 1995; **57:** 552–8.
8. Attenburrow MEJ, *et al.* Low dose melatonin improves sleep in middle-aged subjects. *Psychopharmacology (Berl)* 1996; **126:** 179–81.
9. Garfinkel D, *et al.* Improvement of sleep quality in elderly people by controlled-release melatonin. *Lancet* 1995; **346:** 541–4.
10. Nagtegaal JE, *et al.* Effects of melatonin on the quality of life in patients with delayed sleep phase syndrome. *J Psychosom Res* 2000; **48:** 45–50.
11. Wright SW, *et al.* Randomized clinical trial of melatonin after night-shift work: efficacy and neuropsychologic effects. *Ann Emerg Med* 1998; **32:** 334–40.
12. Jockovich M, *et al.* Effect of exogenous melatonin on mood and sleep efficiency in emergency medicine residents working night shifts. *Acad Emerg Med* 2000; **7:** 955–8.
13. Lehmann ED, *et al.* Somnolence associated with melatonin deficiency after pinealectomy. *Lancet* 1996; **347:** 323.
14. Garfinkel D, *et al.* Facilitation of benzodiazepine discontinuation by melatonin: a new clinical approach. *Arch Intern Med* 1999; **159:** 2456–60.
15. Middleton BA, *et al.* Melatonin and fragmented sleep patterns. *Lancet* 1996; **348:** 551–2.


JET LAG. Melatonin has been reported to alleviate jet lag following long flights.[1-3] The most appropriate dosing schedule has yet to be determined but will depend on both the direction of travel and the distance travelled. A systematic review[4] has concluded that melatonin is effective in preventing or reducing jet lag in those travelling across 5 or more time zones, particularly in an easterly direction, and especially if jet lag has been experienced previously; travellers crossing 2 to 4 time zones may also derive benefit.


1. Waterhouse J, *et al.* Jet-lag. *Lancet* 1997; **350:** 1611–16.
2. Arendt J. Jet-lag. *Lancet* 1998; **351:** 293–4.
3. Arendt J. Jet-lag and shift work: (2) therapeutic use of melatonin. *J R Soc Med* 1999; **92:** 402–5.
4. Herxheimer A, Petrie KJ. Melatonin for the prevention and treatment of jet lag. Available in The Cochrane Library; Issue 2. Chichester: John Wiley; 2004.


### Preparations

**Proprietary Preparations** (details are given in Part 3)
***Arg.:*** Buenas Noches; Melatol; Repentil; ***Chile:*** Novel; ***Hong Kong:*** HT903†; Melapure; ***Mex.:*** Benedorm; Cronocaps; Revenox; ***USA:*** Transzone.

**Multi-ingredient:** ***India:*** Eternex; ***UK:*** Rapi-snooze†; ***USA:*** Bevitamel; Melagesic PM.

## Melissa

Balm; Lemon Balm; Melisa; Melissae Folium; Melissenblatt.

**Pharmacopoeias.** In *Eur.* (see p.vi) and *Pol.*

**Ph. Eur. 5.0** (Melissa Leaf). The dried leaf of *Melissa officinalis*. It contains not less than 4% of total hydroxycinnamic derivatives expressed as rosmarinic acid ($C_{18}H_{16}O_8$ = 360.3), calculated with reference to the dried drug. It has an odour reminiscent of lemon. Protect from light.

### Profile

Melissa has been used as a carminative and sedative. It is an ingredient of herbal remedies used for a variety of disorders. It is also reported to have virustatic activity. The chief constituent of melissa is citral. Hypersensitivity reactions to melissa have been reported. It is used in homoeopathic medicine.

Melissa is the source of melissa oil (see below).

◊ References.


1. Ballard CG, *et al.* Aromatherapy as a safe and effective treatment for the management of agitation in severe dementia: the results of a double-blind, placebo-controlled trial with melissa. *J Clin Psychiatry* 2002; **63:** 553–8.


### Preparations

**Proprietary Preparations** (details are given in Part 3)
***Austria:*** Aponatura Herz; Lomaherpan; ***Chile:*** Citromel; ***Ger.:*** Gastrovegetalin; Kneipp Melisse Pflanzensaft†; Lomaherpan; ***Switz.:*** Valverde boutons de fievre creme.

**Multi-ingredient:** ***Arg.:*** Dr Calm; Erbonda Noche; Nervocalm; Sedante Arceli; Valeriana Oligoplex; ***Austria:*** Abdomilon N; Absimed; Aktiv Nerven- und Schlaftee; Aponatura Beruhigungs; Aponatura Einschlaf; Aurita-Nerventee; Baldracin; Baldrian-Elixier; Baldrian-Krautertonikum; Baldriparan Beruhigungs; Belisir; Bio-Garten Tee zur Beruhigung; Bio-Garten Tropfen zur Beruhigung; Bioreform-Beruhigungstee; Cardalept; Doppelherz Tonikum†; Erbesil; Gastregan; Gewusst wie Nerven-Schlaftee; Herz- und Kreislauftonikum Bioflora; Kneipp Nerven- und Schlaf-Tee; Krauterdoktor Beruhigungstropfen; Krauterdoktor Entspannungs- und Einschlaftropfen; Krauterdoktor Magen-Darmtropfen; Krauterdoktor Nerven-Tonikum; Krauterdoktor Rosmarin-Wein; Krauterhaus Mag Kottas Babytee; Krauterhaus Mag Kottas Magen- und Darmtee; Krauterhaus Mag Kottas Nerven- und Schlaftee; Krauterhaus Mag Kottas Wechseltee; Krauterpfarrer Weidinger Tee bei Schlafstorungen; Krauterpfarrer Weidinger Tee bei Verstimmungen und Erregungszustanden; Krauterpfarrer Weidinger Tee bei Vollegefuhl und Blahungen; Krauterpfarrer Weidinger Tee bei Wetterfuhligkeit und Kreislaufstorungen; Krauterpfarrer Weidinger Tee fur das Altersherz; Mag Doskar's Magentonikum; Mag Doskar's Nerventonikum; Mag Kottas Beruhigungstee; Mag Kottas Krauterexpress-Beruhigungstee; Mag Kottas Krauterexpress-Nerven-Schlaf-Tee; Mag Kottas Krauterexpress-Tee fur stillende Mutter; Mag Kottas Krauterexpress-Wechseltee; Mag Kottas Magen- und Darmtee; Mag Kottas Nerven-Beruhigungstee; Mag Kottas Schlaftee; Mag Kottas Tee fur stillende Mutter; Mag Kottas Wechseltee; Mariazeller; Nervendragees; Nervifloran; Neuners Krautertee Nr 1 - Nerventee; Neuners Krautertee Nr 141 - Schlaftee; Neuners Krautertee Nr 16 - Beruhigungstee bei Wechselbeschwerden; Neuners Krautertee Nr 201 - Krauterhexlein Kinder-Beruhigungstee; Neuners Krautertee Nr 209 - Krauterhexlein Kinder-Magentee; Neuners Krautertee Nr 9 - Magentee; Passedan; Passelyt; Phytogran; Seda-Grandelat; Sedogelat; Sedogelat forte; Sidroga Herz-Kreislauf-Tee; Sidroga Kindertee; Sidroga Magen-Darm-Tee; Sidroga Nerven- und Schlaftee; Songha; Species nervinae; St Radegunder Beruhigungs- und Einschlaftee; St Radegunder Fiebertee; St Radegunder Herz-Kreislauf-Tonikum; St Radegunder Herz-Kreislauf-unterstutzender Tee; St Radegunder Magenberuhigungstee; St Radegunder Nerven-Tonikum; St Radegunder Nerventee; St Radegunder Reizmildernder Magentee; St Radegunder Rosmarin-Wein; Synpharma Instant-Nerventee; Teekanne Magen- und Darmtee; Teekanne Schlaf- und Nerventee; The Chambard-Tee; Wechseltee EF-EM-ES; ***Belg.:*** Songha; Tisane pour le Foie†; Tisane Purgative†; ***Braz.:*** Anevrase; Balsamo Branco†; Calmapax; Camomila†; Elixir de Passiflora†; Especies Calmantes†; Fargestium†; Passaneuro; Passiflora Composta†; Passilex; Sedantol†; Sonhare†; ***Canad.:*** Nyrene†; ***Chile:*** Melipass; ***Fr.:*** Biocarde; Colominthe†; Dystolise; Elixir Bonjean; Mediflor Tisane Calmante Troubles du Sommeil No 14; Mediflor Tisane Circulation du Sang No 12; Mediflor Tisane Pectorale d'Alsace†; Santane $D_5$†; Santane $N_9$†; Tisane des Familles†; Tisane Grande Chartreuse†; Tisane Touraine†; Vagostabyl; ***Ger.:*** Abdomilon N; Aranidorm-S†; Avedorm†; Baldriparan N Stark; Befelka-Tinktur†; Doppelherz Melissengeist; Dormarist; Euvegal Entspannungs- und Einschlafdragees; Euvegal Entspannungs- und Einschlaftropfen; Euvegal forte†; Euvegal N†; Gastrol S; Gutnacht; Heumann Beruhigungstee Tenerval N; Iberogast; JuDorm; JuNeuron S†; Kneipp Krauter Taschenkur Nerven und Schlaf N†; Kneipp Nerven- und Schlaf-Tee N†; Lindofluid N; Luvased-Tropfen N†; Melissengeist; Nerven-Tee Stada N†; Nervosana; Oxacant N; Oxacant-sedativ; Pascosedon; Phytonoctu; Plantival novo; Presselin Blahungs K 4 N; Pronervon Phyto; RubieSed; Salus Nerven-Schlaf-Tee Nr.22†; Salusan†; Schlaf- und Nerventee; Seda-Plantina; Sedacur; Sedariston; Sedasyx; Sedatruw S†; Sedinfant N; Sirmiosta Nervenelixier N†; Stullmaton; SX Valeriana comp†; ***Israel:*** Songha Night; ***Ital.:*** Colimil; Cura†; Emmenoiasi; Fluxoten†; Melissa (Specie Composta); Sedatol; Tisana Arnaldi†; Tisana Cisbey†; Tisana Kelemata; Valeriana (Specie Composta); ***Mex.:*** Plantival; ***NZ:*** Botanica Hayfever; Mr Nits; ***Port.:*** Songha; ***Spain:*** Agua del Carmen; Caramelos Agua del Carmen; Digestol Sanatorium†; Himelan; Jaquesor; Mesatil; Natusor Aerofane; Natusor Jaquesan; Nervikan; Resolutivo Regium; Solucion Schoum; ***Switz.:*** Arterosan Plus; Baldriparan; Cardiaforce; Dormiplant; Dragees pour la detente nerveuse; Gastrosan; Hyperiforce comp; Iberogast; Melissa Tonic†; Phytoberidin†; Phytomed Nervo; Relax; Seracalm†; Songha Night†; Soporin; The Brioni†; The Franklin†; Tisane antiflatulente pour nourissons et enfants; Tisane calmante pour les enfants; Tisane favorisant l'allaitement; Tisane pour l'estomac; Tisane pour le coeur et la circulation; Tisane pour le sommeil et les nerfs; Tisane pour les enfants†; Tisane relaxante N; Valverde Dragees pour la detente; ***UK:*** Melissa Comp.; Melissin†; Valerina Day Time; Valerina Night-Time.

## Melissa Oil

Balm Oil; Esencia de Melisa; Lemon Balm Oil.

*CAS — 8014-71-9.*

### Profile

Melissa oil is the essential oil obtained from melissa (*Melissa officinalis*), above. It is used in preparations with other essential oils in a variety of disorders.

### Preparations

**Proprietary Preparations** (details are given in Part 3)

**Multi-ingredient:** ***Austria:*** Opino; ***Belg.:*** Calmant Martou†; ***Chile:*** Agua Del Carmen; Agua Melisa Carminativa; ***Ger.:*** Amol Heilkrautergeist N; Cor-Select; Neo-Lapitrypsin†; Thrombocid; ***Ital.:*** Dentosan Azione Intensiva; Dentosan Mese; ***Port.:*** Thrombocid; ***Switz.:*** Anal-Gen; Baume du Chalet; Thrombocid.

## Memantine Hydrochloride *(BANM, USAN, rINNM)*

1-Amino-3,5-dimethyladamantane Hydrochloride; D-145 (memantine); 3,5-Dimethyl-1-adamantanamine hydrochloride; DMAA (memantine); Hidrocloruro de memantina. 3,5-Dimethyltricyclo[3.3.1.1$^{3,7}$]decan-l-amine hydrochloride.

$C_{12}H_{21}N,HCl$ = 215.8.

*CAS — 19982-08-2 (memantine); 41100-52-1 (memantine hydrochloride).*

*ATC — N06DX01.*

### Adverse Effects and Precautions

Common adverse effects with memantine include hallucinations, confusion, dizziness, headache, and tiredness. Less common reactions such as anxiety, hypertonia, vomiting, cystitis, and increased libido have also occurred.

Treatment with memantine is not recommended in patients with severe renal impairment as no data are available for such patients. A reduced dose is required in those with moderate renal impairment (see below).

Only limited clinical data are available for patients with recent myocardial infarction, uncompensated congestive heart failure, and uncontrolled hypertension and use of memantine in these patients should be closely monitored. Caution is also recommended in patients with epilepsy.

### Interactions

Use of other *N*-methyl-D-aspartate antagonists such as amantadine, ketamine, or dextromethorphan with memantine may increase both the incidence and severity of adverse effects and should be avoided. The effects of dopaminergics and antimuscarinics may also be enhanced whereas memantine may reduce the actions of barbiturates and antipsychotics.

Memantine may alter the effects of the antispasmodics baclofen and dantrolene.

### Pharmacokinetics

Memantine is well absorbed after oral administration. Plasma protein binding is about 45%. Memantine undergoes only limited metabolism; the main metabolites are *N*-3,5-dimethyl-gludantan and 1-nitroso-3,5-dimethyl-adamantane. The majority of a dose is excreted unchanged via the kidney; some active renal tubular secretion and reabsorption occurs. The terminal half-life ranges from 60 to 100 hours although under alkaline conditions the rate of elimination is reduced.

### Uses and Administration

Memantine is a derivative of amantadine (p.1197) and is likewise an antagonist of *N*-methyl-D-aspartate receptors. It is given in the treatment of moderately severe to severe Alzheimer's disease (see Dementia, below). Memantine has also been given in the treatment of parkinsonism (p.1196) and central spasticity (p.1386), and has been used in other disorders such as brain injury or comatose states. It is given by mouth as the hydrochloride.

In the treatment of **Alzheimer's disease**, the initial dose of memantine hydrochloride is 5 mg daily in the morning for the first week; this should be increased in weekly increments of 5 mg to a maximum dose of 20 mg daily. Doses of 10 mg and over should be taken in 2 divided doses. Reduced doses are recommended in patients with renal impairment (see below). Clinical benefit should be reassessed on a regular basis.

Memantine hydrochloride has also been given by slow intravenous injection.

Memantine is also under investigation in the treatment of glaucoma and peripheral neuropathy.

**Administration in renal impairment.** The manufacturers have advised that no dose adjustment is needed when memantine hydrochloride is given for Alzheimer's disease in patients with mild renal impairment; however, in those with moderate impairment (creatinine clearance 40 to 60 mL/minute per 1.73m$^2$) the maximum dose should be reduced to 10 mg daily. No data is available for patients with severe impairment.

**Dementia.** A systematic review[1] of the use of memantine in dementia concluded that although it did have a beneficial effect on cognitive decline in patients with moderate to severe Alzheimer's disease, and in those with mild to moderate vascular dementia, the effects were not clinically discernible and more studies were needed to assess the role of memantine in such conditions.


1. Areosa Sastre A, Sherriff F. Memantine for dementia. Available in The Cochrane Library; Issue 2. Chichester: John Wiley; 2004.


### Preparations

**Proprietary Preparations** (details are given in Part 3)
***Arg.:*** Akatinol; Conexine; Neuroplus; ***Austral.:*** Ebixa; ***Braz.:*** Akatinol; ***Fr.:*** Ebixa; ***Ger.:*** Axura; ***Irl.:*** Ebixa; ***Norw.:*** Ebixa; ***UK:*** Ebixa; ***USA:*** Namenda.

## Menbutone *(BAN, rINN)*

Menbutona; SC-1749 (menbutone sodium). 4-(4-Methoxy-1-naphthyl)-4-oxobutyric acid.

$C_{15}H_{14}O_4$ = 258.3.

*CAS — 3562-99-0.*

### Profile

Menbutone is used as a choleretic to stimulate gastrointestinal function in veterinary medicine.

## Menthol

Hexahydrothymol; Mentholum; Mentol. *p*-Menthan-3-ol; 2-Isopropyl-5-methylcyclohexanol.

$C_{10}H_{20}O$ = 156.3.

*CAS — 1490-04-6 (menthol); 15356-60-2 ((+)-menthol); 2216-51-5 ((−)-menthol); 89-78-1((±)-menthol).*

**Description.** Menthol is either the laevo-isomer, levomenthol (*BAN, rINN*), or a racemic mixture, racementhol (*BAN, rINN*). The laevo-isomer may be obtained from the volatile oils of various species of *Mentha* (Labiatae) or it may be prepared synthetically.

**Pharmacopoeias.** In *Chin., Eur.* (see p.vi), *Jpn, Pol., US,* and *Viet.*

*Eur.* and *Jpn* have separate monographs for laevo-menthol (levomenthol) and racemic menthol (racementhol).

**Ph. Eur. 5.0** (Levomenthol). It occurs as colourless, acicular or prismatic shiny crystals. M.p. about 43°. Practically insoluble in water; very soluble in alcohol and in petroleum spirit; freely soluble in fatty oils and in liquid paraffin; very slightly soluble in glycerol.

**Ph. Eur. 5.0** (Menthol, Racemic; Racementhol BP 2003). It occurs as colourless, acicular or prismatic shiny crystals or as a free-flowing or agglomerated crystalline powder. M.p. about 34°. Practically insoluble in water; very soluble in alcohol and in petroleum spirit; freely soluble in fatty oils and in liquid paraffin; very slightly soluble in glycerol.

**USP 27** (Menthol). An alcohol obtained from diverse mint oils or prepared synthetically. It may be laevorotatory (*l*-menthol), from natural or synthetic sources, or racemic (*dl*-menthol). It occurs as colourless, hexagonal crystals, usually needle-like, or in fused masses, or crystalline powder. Has a pleasant, peppermint-like odour. M.p. of *l*-menthol 41° to 44°. Slightly soluble in water; very soluble in alcohol, in chloroform, in ether, and in petroleum spirit; freely soluble in glacial acetic acid, in fixed and volatile oils, and in liquid paraffin. Store in airtight containers preferably at a temperature of 15° to 30°.

**Compounding.** A liquid or soft mass is formed when menthol is triturated with camphor, cloral hydrate, phenol, and many other substances.

### Adverse Effects, Treatment, and Precautions

Menthol may give rise to hypersensitivity reactions including contact dermatitis. Ingestion of significant quantities of menthol is reported to cause symptoms similar to those seen after ingestion of camphor (p.1665), including severe abdominal pain, nausea, vomiting, vertigo, ataxia, drowsiness, and coma; they may be managed similarly. There have been reports (below) of apnoea and instant collapse in infants following the local application of menthol to their nostrils.

**Administration to infants.** Instillation of decongestant preparations containing menthol directly into the nostrils of infants and young children has resulted in acute respiratory distress with cyanosis[1] and respiratory arrest,[2] and must be avoided. In one case,[1] nasal application was associated with concurrent chemical conjunctivitis.


1. Wyllie JP, Alexander FW. Nasal instillation of 'Olbas Oil' in an infant. *Arch Dis Child* 1994; **70:** 357–8.
2. Blake KD. Dangers of common cold treatments in children. *Lancet* 1993; **341:** 640.


**Effects on the nervous system.** Ataxia, confusion, euphoria, nystagmus, and diplopia developed in a 13-year-old boy following the inhalation of 5 mL of Olbas oil instead of the recommended few drops.[1] It was considered probable that the menthol in the preparation was responsible for the symptoms; the amount of menthol inhaled was approximately 200 mg.

1. O'Mullane NM, *et al.* Adverse CNS effects of menthol-containing Olbas oil. *Lancet* 1982; **i:** 1121.

### Pharmacokinetics

After absorption, menthol is excreted in the urine and bile as a glucuronide.

### Uses and Administration

Menthol is chiefly used to relieve symptoms of bronchitis, sinusitis, and similar conditions. For this purpose it may be used as an inhalation, usually with benzoin or eucalyptus oil, as pastilles, or as an ointment with camphor and eucalyptus oil for application to the chest or nostrils (but see Adverse Effects above). However, as mentioned under the section on the management of cough (p.1112), the use of menthol in inhalations is unlikely to provide any additional benefit.

When applied to the skin menthol dilates the blood vessels, causing a sensation of coldness followed by an analgesic effect. It relieves itching and is used in creams, lotions, or ointments in pruritus and urticaria.

In small doses by mouth menthol has a carminative action.

**Action.** It has been suggested that the apparent benefits of menthol in nasal congestion may be due to an effect on calcium channels of sensory nerves.[1] This mechanism has also been implicated in its muscle relaxant action on the gastrointestinal tract when used as peppermint oil (p.1283).

1. Anonymous. How does menthol work? *Pharm J* 1993; **251:** 480.

### Preparations

***BP 2003:*** Menthol and Benzoin Inhalation;
***USP 27:*** Benzocaine and Menthol Topical Aerosol; Menthol Lozenges; Tetracaine and Menthol Ointment.

**Proprietary Preparations** (details are given in Part 3)
***Arg.:*** Flex-All; Rati Salil Ice; Robitussin Caramelos; ***Austral.:*** Dencorub Arthritis Ice; Ice Gel†; Vicks Throat Drops†; Vicks Vapodrops with Butter and Menthol†; ***Austria:*** Nifint; Wick Vapo Syrup; ***Braz.:*** Analgen; ***Canad.:*** Absorbine Jr; Absorbine Power Gel; Antiphlogistine Rub A-535 Ice; Ben-Gay Ice; Bentasil Black Currant; Big V Cough Lozenge†; Celestial Seasonings†; Certified Ice; Cough Drops; Cough Lozenges; Deep Cold; Fisherman's Friend; Flex-All; Honey Lemon Cough Lozenges; Ice Gel; Ice Gel Therapy; Life Brand Cough Lozenges†; Meggezones; Myoflex Ice†; No Name Cough Lozenge†; Obus Form Therapeutic Ice†; Physiomenthol; Polar Ice; Safeway Cough Lozenges†; Soothing Ice Rub; Vicks Throat Drops; Vicks Vaposyrup†; ***Fr.:*** Matiga†; ***Ger.:*** Nifint; Novopin MIG; Wick Vaposyrup†; ***Hong Kong:*** Perskindol†; ***Spain:*** Icespray†; Prulit; ***Switz.:*** Perskindol†; ***Thai.:*** Counterpain Cool; Stopain; ***UK:*** 4Head; Avoca Menthol Cone†; Deep Freeze Cold Gel; Happinose; Ice Cool Stress & Tension Relief; Meggezones; Quool; Vicks Vaposyrup for Tickly Coughs; ***USA:*** Absorbine Jr; Ben-Gay Patch; Ben-Gay Vanishing; Extra Strength Vicks Cough Drops; Halls-Plus Maximum Strength; Kof-Eze; N'ice; N'ice 'n Clear; Sportscreme Ice; Therapeutic Mineral Ice; Vicks Cough Drops; Wonder Ice.

**Multi-ingredient:** numerous preparations are listed in Part 3.

---

## Menyanthes

Bitterklee; Bogbean; Buckbean; Folia Trifoli Fibrini; Marsh Trefoil; Menyanthidis Trifoliatae Folium; Trébol de agua; Trèfle d'Eau.

NOTE. Bog myrtle (see p.1661) has also been used as a common name for *Menyanthes trifoliata*.

**Pharmacopoeias.** In *Eur.* (see p.vi) and *Pol.*

**Ph. Eur. 5.0** (Bogbean Leaf). The dried, entire or fragmented leaf of *Menyanthes trifoliata*. It has a very bitter and persistent taste.

### Profile

Menyanthes has been used as a bitter. It is used in herbal medicine for rheumatic, gastrointestinal, and biliary-tract disorders. It is also used in homoeopathic and folk medicine.

### Preparations

**Proprietary Preparations** (details are given in Part 3)

**Multi-ingredient:** ***Austria:*** Krauterhaus Mag Kottas Gallen- und Lebertee; Mag Kottas Krauterexpress-Leber-Gallentee; Mag Kottas Leber-Gallentee; Mageentee†; Mariazeller; Neuners Krautertee Nr 9 - Mageentee; ***Fr.:*** Tisane Hepatique de Hoerdt; ***Ger.:*** Cefaktivon†; Gallexier; ***UK:*** Modern Herbals Rheumatic Pain; Rheumatic Pain; Rheumatic Pain Relief; Rheumatic Pain Remedy; Rheumatic Pain Tablets†; Vegetex.

---

## Mercaptamine *(BAN, rINN)*

Cysteamine *(USAN)*; L-1573; MEA; Mercamine; Mercaptamina. 2-Aminoethanethiol.

$C_2H_7NS$ = 77.15.

*CAS — 60-23-1.*

*ATC — A16AA04.*

## Mercaptamine Bitartrate *(BANM, rINNM)*

Bitartrato de mercaptamina; Cysteamine Bitartrate.

$C_2H_7NS, C_4H_6O_6$ = 227.2.

*CAS — 27761-19-9.*

*ATC — A16AA04.*

## Mercaptamine Hydrochloride *(BANM, rINNM)*

Cl-9148; Cysteamine Hydrochloride *(USAN)*; Hidrocloruro de mercaptamina.

$C_2H_7NS,HCl$ = 113.6.

*CAS — 156-57-0.*

*ATC — A16AA04.*

### Adverse Effects and Precautions

Mercaptamine can be unpalatable and may cause breath and body odour. It may cause gastrointestinal disturbances including anorexia, nausea, vomiting, diarrhoea, and abdominal pain; rarely, there may be gastrointestinal ulceration or bleeding. Other adverse effects may include drowsiness, malaise, rashes, fever, flushing, and ventricular tachycardia. Mercaptamine may cause increases in liver enzyme values and precipitate hepatic coma in patients with overt hepatic damage. Interstitial nephritis has also occurred rarely. Nervousness, depression, and, rarely, hallucinations, have been reported.

◊ Three patients with nephropathic cystinosis developed fever, maculopapular eruption, leucopenia, or headache within 2 weeks of starting mercaptamine at doses of 53, 67, and 75 mg/kg daily by mouth, respectively.[1] These side-effects resolved within 48 hours of drug withdrawal and all 3 patients were able to tolerate mercaptamine when restarted at a dose of 10 mg/kg daily, slowly increased to therapeutic levels over 2 to 3 months. Higher doses of mercaptamine had been associated with lethargy and seizures.

1. Schneider JA, *et al.* Cysteamine therapy in nephropathic cystinosis. *N Engl J Med* 1981; **304:** 1172.

### Pharmacokinetics

◊ Results of a pharmacokinetic-pharmacodynamic study[1] in paediatric patients with nephropathic cystinosis showed that although mercaptamine is rapidly cleared from plasma, dosing every 6 hours was sufficient to maintain the content of cystine in the white blood cells below the target value (see below).

1. Belldina EB, *et al.* Steady-state pharmacokinetics and pharmacodynamics of cysteamine bitartrate in paediatric nephropathic cystinosis patients. *Br J Clin Pharmacol* 2003; **56:** 520–5.

### Uses and Administration

Mercaptamine reduces intracellular cystine levels and is given by mouth as the bitartrate in the treatment of cystinosis (see below); it has also been given as the hydrochloride. Doses are expressed in terms of the base; 2.94 g of the bitartrate or 1.47 g of the hydrochloride are each equivalent to 1 g of mercaptamine. Mercaptamine bitartrate is given in an initial dose that is one-sixth to one-quarter of the expected maintenance dose, and is then increased gradually over 4 to 6 weeks. The usual maintenance dose in adults is 2 g daily in 4 divided doses with or after food. Children up to 12 years of age are given 1.3 g/$m^2$ daily in 4 divided doses. Doses are given in conjunction with monitoring of leucocyte-cystine levels which should be kept below 1 nanomol of hemicystine per mg of protein.

Phosphocysteamine, a phosphorothioester of mercaptamine, is more palatable being odourless and tasteless, and is used similarly.

Mercaptamine facilitates glutathione synthesis and was formerly used intravenously in the treatment of severe paracetamol poisoning to prevent hepatic damage, but other forms of treatment are now preferred (see p.76).

**Cystinosis.** Mercaptamine and phosphocysteamine (which appears to be rapidly hydrolysed to mercaptamine after administration) have been reported to be of benefit in children with cystinosis, a rare autosomal recessive metabolic disorder characterised by the intracellular accumulation of cystine. Cystinosis is marked by growth retardation, rickets, Fanconi syndrome, and renal failure; acute episodes of acidosis and dehydration may develop, and there may be photophobia associated with deposition of cystine in the eye.[1] Use of mercaptamine, which results in a reduction in the concentrations of cystine in leucocytes, has been shown to be effective in controlling many of the symptoms,[2-4] especially if begun early, although it is not clear from the present contradictory results[4,5] how much benefit is seen on renal function. Compliance may be a problem, due to the unpalatable taste and odour of mercaptamine, and the more palatable prodrug phosphocysteamine has been developed as an alternative;[6,7] more palatable formulations of mercaptamine are also being investigated. Mercaptamine eye drops are reportedly of benefit in reversing or preventing deposition of corneal cystine crystals.[8] Renal transplantation may be necessary if renal failure develops.

1. Gahl WA, *et al.* Cystinosis. *N Engl J Med* 2002; **347:** 111–21.
2. Yudkoff M, *et al.* Effects of cysteamine therapy in nephropathic cystinosis. *N Engl J Med* 1981; **304:** 141–5.
3. Gahl WA, *et al.* Cysteamine therapy for children with nephropathic cystinosis. *N Engl J Med* 1987; **316:** 971–7.
4. Reznik VM, *et al.* Treatment of cystinosis with cysteamine from early infancy. *J Pediatr* 1991; **119:** 491–3.
5. Markello TC, *et al.* Improved renal function in children with cystinosis treated with cysteamine. *N Engl J Med* 1993; **328:** 1157–62.
6. Gahl WA, *et al.* Cystinosis: progress in a prototypic disease. *Ann Intern Med* 1988; **109:** 557–69.
7. van't Hoff WG, *et al.* Effects of oral phosphocysteamine and rectal cysteamine in cystinosis. *Arch Dis Child* 1991; **66:** 1434–7.
8. Kaiser-Kupfer MI, *et al.* A randomized placebo-controlled trial of cysteamine eye drops in nephropathic cystinosis. *Arch Ophthalmol* 1990; **108;** 689–93.

### Preparations

**Proprietary Preparations** (details are given in Part 3)
***Austral.:*** Cystagon; ***Denm.:*** Cystagon; ***Fin.:*** Cystagon; ***Fr.:*** Cystagon; ***Ger.:*** Cystagon; ***Ital.:*** Cystagon; ***Spain:*** Cystagon; ***Swed.:*** Cystagon; ***UK:*** Cystagon.

---

## Mercuric Chloride

Bicloruro de Mercurio; Cloreto Mercúrico; Corrosive Sublimate; Hydrarg. Perchlor.; Hydrargyri Dichloridum; Hydrargyri Perchloridum; Hydrargyrum Bichloratum; Mercuric Chlor.; Mercúrico, cloruro; Mercurique (Chlorure); Mercury Bichloride; Mercury Perchloride; Quecksilberchlorid.

$HgCl_2$ = 271.5.

*CAS — 7487-94-7.*

*ATC — D08AK03.*

**Pharmacopoeias.** In *Eur.* (see p.vi).

**Ph. Eur. 5.0** (Mercuric Chloride). A white crystalline powder, or colourless or white crystals or heavy crystalline masses. Soluble in water and in glycerol; freely soluble in alcohol. Protect from light.

### Profile

The use of mercuric chloride as an antibacterial substance is limited by its toxicity, its precipitating action on proteins, its irritant action on raw surfaces, its corrosive action on metals, and by the fact that its activity is greatly reduced in the presence of excreta or body fluids.

Details of the adverse effects of inorganic mercury compounds are provided under Mercury, below.

### Preparations

**Proprietary Preparations** (details are given in Part 3)
**Multi-ingredient:** ***Spain:*** Oxido Amarit†; Pantenil.

---

## Yellow Mercuric Oxide

Gelbes Quecksilberoxyd; Hydrargyri Oxidum Flavum; Hydrargyri Oxydum Flavum; Mercúrico amarillo, óxido; Mercurique (Oxyde) Jaune; Oxido Amarillo de Mercurio; Yellow Precipitate.

$HgO$ = 216.6.

*CAS — 21908-53-2.*

**Pharmacopoeias.** In *Fr.* and *It.*

### Profile

Yellow mercuric oxide has been used in eye ointments for the local treatment of minor infections including the eradication of pubic lice from the eyelashes. Absorption can occur and produce the adverse effects of inorganic mercury (see Mercury, below).

**Pediculosis.** Yellow mercuric oxide 1% eye ointment was considered to be a safe and effective treatment in pediculosis (p.1499) of the eyelashes caused by pubic lice (pthiriasis palpebrarum).[1]

1. Ashkenazi I, *et al.* Yellow mercuric oxide: a treatment of choice for phthiriasis palpebrarum. *Br J Ophthalmol* 1991; **75:** 356–8.

**Porphyria.** Mercuric oxide has been associated with acute attacks of porphyria and is considered unsafe in porphyric patients.

### Preparations

**Proprietary Preparations** (details are given in Part 3)
***Austral.:*** Golden Eye Ointment; ***Fr.:*** Pommade Maurice; ***USA:*** Stye.

**Multi-ingredient:** ***India:*** Bell Diono Resolvent; Bell Resolvent; ***Spain:*** Oxido Amarit†.

---

## Mercurous Chloride

Calomel; Calomelanos; Cloreto Mercuroso; Hydrarg. Subchlor.; Hydrargyri Subchloridum; Hydrargyrosi Chloridum; Hydrargyrum Chloratum (Mite); Mercureux (Chlorure); Mercurioso, cloruro; Mercurius Dulcis; Mercury Monochloride; Mercury Subchloride; Mild Mercurous Chloride; Protocloruro de Mercurio; Quecksilberchlorür.

$HgCl$ = 236.0; $Hg_2Cl_2$ = 472.1.

*CAS — 7546-30-7 (HgCl); 10112-91-1 ($Hg_2Cl_2$).*

NOTE. Precipitated Mercurous Chloride (Hydrargyri Subchloridum Praecipitatum), is a white amorphous powder, for which the synonym 'White Precipitate' (Praecipitatum Album) has been used. White Precipitate has also been used as a name for Ammoniated Mercury.

**Pharmacopoeias.** In *Chin.* as $Hg_2Cl_2$.

### Profile

Mercurous chloride was formerly given as a laxative and was applied topically as an antibacterial. It was one of the mercury compounds employed in the management of syphilis in the pre-antibiotic era.

The mercurous form of mercury does not possess the corrosive properties of the mercuric form and is not absorbed to any great extent. However, the mercurous form can be converted to the mercuric with consequent toxicity as described under Mercury (see below).

## Mercury

Hydrarg.; Hydrargyrum; Hydrargyrum Depuratum; Mercure; Mercurio; Quecksilber; Quicksilver.

Hg = 200.59.

*CAS — 7439-97-6.*

*ATC — D08AK05.*

**Description.** Mercury is a shining, silvery white, very mobile liquid, easily divisible into globules, which readily volatilises on heating.

### Adverse Effects

Poisoning with liquid mercury or inorganic mercury salts has arisen from a variety of sources such as batteries, cosmetics, dental materials, medical equipment, and jewellery manufacture. Barometers, sphygmomanometers, and thermometers are still sources of liquid mercury. Trace amounts of organic and inorganic mercury may also be ingested in the diet.

The effects of **acute** exposure depend on the nature of the compound.

- *Liquid mercury* if ingested is poorly absorbed and, unless there is aspiration or pre-existing gastrointestinal disorders, is not considered to be a severe toxicological hazard. The greatest dangers from liquid mercury arise from the inhalation of mercury vapour, which can cause various gastrointestinal effects including nausea, vomiting, and diarrhoea; more importantly it is toxic to the respiratory system and this effect can be fatal. Some CNS involvement has also been reported. Adverse effects have also been reported after accidental or intentional parenteral administration.
- *Inorganic salts* such as mercuric chloride are corrosive when ingested causing severe nausea, vomiting, pain, bloody diarrhoea, and necrosis. The kidney is also involved and tubular necrosis may develop. Mercurous salts are considered to be less hazardous, but the mercurous form can be converted to the mercuric.
- *Organic mercurial compounds* produce similar toxic effects to inorganic compounds, but they have a more selective action on the CNS that has proved difficult to treat. The degree of toxicity varies with the different groups of organic mercurials; those used as preservatives or disinfectants being less toxic than the ethyl or methyl compounds that are not used pharmaceutically or clinically. Methylmercury is notorious for its toxicity; there have been cases of fetal neurotoxicity during outbreaks of methylmercury poisoning.

**Chronic mercury poisoning** may result from inhalation of mercury vapour, skin contact with mercury or mercury compounds, or ingestion of mercury salts over prolonged periods. It is characterised by many symptoms including tremor, motor and sensory disturbances, mental deterioration, gastrointestinal symptoms, dermatitis, kidney damage, salivation, and gingivitis. A blue line may be present on the gums. There is little difference between acute and chronic poisoning with organic mercurials.

The syndrome of *acrodynia* (pink disease), with symptoms of sweat, rash, erythema of the extremities, photophobia, wasting, weakness, hypertension, tachycardia, and diminished reflexes, occurred in children given mercury in teething powders or in ointments or dusting powders. Such preparations have long since been withdrawn from use. However, the syndrome is still a feature of mercury poisoning from other sources.

Hypersensitivity to mercury and mercurial compounds has been reported.

Mercurialentis has been reported in patients treated with eye drops containing an organomercurial preservative.

**Chronic exposure.** Acute *occupational exposure* to mercury vapour in 53 men resulted in an initial phase described as metal fume fever, an intermediate phase of severe symptoms with CNS, gastrointestinal, respiratory, and urological involvement, and a late phase with persistent CNS symptoms, dysuria, and pain on ejaculation.[1,2] Although persistent hyperchloraemia was noted in the 11 patients with the highest mercury levels, renal impairment tended to be temporary.[2] Long-term follow-up of a patient who had an intravenous injection of mercury 12 years previously also revealed no persistent renal impairment,[3] despite the presence of mercury microemboli in lungs, kidneys, liver, and subcutaneous tissues and high concentrations in the urine. At this time, the patient had residual reductions in respiratory function, polyneuropathy, and marked asthenozoospermia. Spermatozoal abnormalities may also have contributed to his wife's miscarriage.

Fetal neurotoxicity following *maternal exposure* to methylmercury is well recognised, and there has been widespread concern about the effect of maternal diets on the developing fetus because of mercury concentrations in freshwater and marine organisms. Results from a study in the Faroe Islands demonstrated an association between delays in neurological development in children and maternal consumption of pilot whale meat.[4] However, data from a study conducted in a fish-consuming population in the Seychelles failed to find a similar connection.[5]

There has been considerable concern over the systemic absorption of mercury from *dental amalgam*, which typically contains between 40 and 70% of mercury. However, the quantities absorbed from amalgam fillings is reported to be relatively small[6,7] and current evidence suggests that the use of dental amalgam for tooth restoration is both safe and effective.[8,9] The main risks appear to be occupational exposure of dental staff and environmental concerns. Some patients with hypersensitivity to mercury (manifest most commonly as local lichenoid reactions) may benefit from removal of amalgam fillings.[10,11]

Ethylmercury is contained in thiomersal, which is used as a preservative in routine vaccines for infants and children, thus representing a potential source of mercury exposure.[12,13] Measurement of mercury blood concentrations in infants at intervals up to 28 days following vaccination did not, however, demonstrate levels above the recognised limits of safety; moreover, data suggest that the half-life of ethylmercury might be shorter than that of methylmercury.[12] Critics[14,15] of this study suggested that blood samples should have been drawn within hours of vaccination when mercury levels could potentially have exceeded safety limits.

The symptoms of *acrodynia* have been mistaken for those of phaeochromocytoma.[16-19]


1. Bluhm RE, *et al.* Elemental mercury vapour toxicity, treatment, and prognosis after acute, intensive exposure in chloralkali plant workers part I: history, neuropsychological findings and chelator effects. *Hum Exp Toxicol* 1992; **11:** 201–10.
2. Bluhm RE, *et al.* Elemental mercury vapour toxicity, treatment, and prognosis after acute, intensive exposure in chloralkali plant workers part II: hyperchloraemia and genitourinary symptoms. *Hum Exp Toxicol* 1992; **11:** 211–15.
3. dell'Omo M, *et al.* Long-term toxicity of intravenous mercury injection. *Lancet* 1996; **348:** 64.
4. Grandjean P, *et al.* Cognitive deficit in 7-year-old children with prenatal exposure to methylmercury. *Neurotoxicol Teratol* 1997; **19:** 417–28.
5. Myers GJ, *et al.* Prenatal methylmercury exposure from ocean fish consumption in the Seychelles child development study. *Lancet* 2003; **361:** 1686–92.
6. Eley BM. The future of dental amalgam: a review of the literature. Part 3: mercury exposure from amalgam restorations in dental patients. *Br Dent J* 1997; **182:** 333–8.
7. Eley BM. The future of dental amalgam: a review of the literature. Part 4: mercury exposure hazards and risk assessment. *Br Dent J* 1997; **182:** 373–81.
8. FDI/WHO. Consensus statement on dental amalgam. *FDI World* 1995; **4** (July/Aug): 9–10.
9. Eley BM. The future of dental amalgam: a review of the literature. Part 6: possible harmful effects of mercury from dental amalgam. *Br Dent J* 1997; **182:** 455–9.
10. Ibbotson SH, *et al.* The relevance and effect of amalgam replacement in subjects with oral lichenoid reactions. *Br J Dermatol* 1996; **134:** 420–3.
11. McGivern B, *et al.* Delayed and immediate hypersensitivity reactions associated with the use of amalgam. *Br Dent J* 2000; **188:** 73–6.
12. Pichichero ME, *et al.* Mercury concentrations and metabolism in infants receiving vaccines containing thiomersal: a descriptive study. *Lancet* 2002; **360:** 1737–41.
13. Clarkson TW, *et al.* The toxicology of mercury—current exposures and clinical manifestations. *N Engl J Med* 2003; **349:** 1731–7.
14. Colman E. Mercury in infants given vaccines containing thiomersal. *Lancet* 2003; **361:** 698.
15. Halsey NA, Goldman LR. Mercury in infants given vaccines containing thiomersal. *Lancet* 2003; **361:** 698–9.
16. Henningsson C, *et al.* Acute mercury poisoning (acrodynia) mimicking pheochromocytoma in an adolescent. *J Pediatr* 1993; **122:** 252–3.
17. Velzeboer SCJM, *et al.* A hypertensive toddler. *Lancet* 1997; **349:** 1810.
18. Wößmann W, *et al.* Mercury intoxication presenting with hypertension and tachycardia. *Arch Dis Child* 1999; **80:** 556–7.
19. Torres AD, *et al.* Mercury intoxication and arterial hypertension: report of two patients and review of the literature. Abstract: *Pediatrics* 2000; **105:** 627. Full version: http://pediatrics.aappublications.org/cgi/content/full/105/3/e34 (accessed 17/06/04)


**Effects on the kidneys.** The kidneys are one of the primary sites for the accumulation of mercury in the body. All forms of mercury (liquid mercury, inorganic mercury, and organic mercury) may be toxic to the kidney although the inorganic forms are the most nephrotoxic.[1]


1. Zalups RK. Molecular interactions with mercury in the kidney. *Pharmacol Rev* 2000; **52:** 113–43.


### Treatment of Adverse Effects

The treatment of **acute** mercury toxicity depends on the form of mercury, the route of exposure, and the dose. Supportive measures may be needed with all types of toxicity. Ingestion of liquid mercury seldom requires active treatment since it is poorly absorbed by this route. Acute oral poisoning due to inorganic mercury salts should be treated if appropriate by activated charcoal or gastric lavage to reduce absorption. Acute exposure via inhalation or injection mainly requires supportive therapy although excision of the affected area has been recommended following subcutaneous administration. In severe cases chelation therapy may be required to facilitate the removal of mercury from the body. Chelating agents that may be used include dimercaprol (p.1037), penicillamine (p.1049), succimer (p.1054), or unithiol (p.1055). Some centres institute haemodialysis early in the course of treatment; others wait until renal failure develops.

Poisoning due to organic mercury is difficult to treat. The same measures as above should be adopted, except that it is recommended by some that dimercaprol should not be used since *animal* evidence indicates that it may increase the brain concentrations of mercury. An additional measure that has been tried is the administration of a thiol resin complex to prevent the reabsorption of mercury from the bile.

Mercurials on the skin should be removed by copious washing with soap and water.

The management of **chronic** toxicity is generally symptomatic although chelation therapy has been used in some patients.

◊ References.


1. Kostyniak PJ, *et al.* Extracorporeal regional complexing haemodialysis treatment of acute inorganic mercury intoxication. *Hum Exp Toxicol* 1990; **9:** 137–41.
2. Ferguson L, Cantilena LR. Enhanced mercury clearance during hemodialysis with chelating agents. *Clin Pharmacol Ther* 1991; **49:** 131.
3. Florentine MJ, Sanfilippo DJ. Elemental mercury poisoning. *Clin Pharm* 1991; **10:** 213–21.
4. Bluhm RE, *et al.* Elemental mercury vapour toxicity, treatment, and prognosis after acute, intensive exposure in chloralkali plant workers part I: history, neuropsychological findings and chelator effects. *Hum Exp Toxicol* 1992; **11:** 201–10.
5. Toet AE, *et al.* Mercury kinetics in a case of severe mercuric chloride poisoning treated with dimercapto-1-propane sulphonate (DMPS). *Hum Exp Toxicol* 1994; **13:** 11–16.
6. Houeto P, *et al.* Elemental mercury vapour toxicity: treatment and levels in plasma and urine. *Hum Exp Toxicol* 1994; **13:** 848–52.
7. Aaseth J, *et al.* Treatment of mercury and lead poisonings with dimercaptosuccinic acid and sodium dimercaptopropanesulfonate: a review. *Analyst* 1995; **120:** 853–4.
8. Isik S, *et al.* Subcutaneous metallic mercury injection: early, massive excision. *Ann Plast Surg* 1997; **38:** 645–8.
9. Baum CR. Treatment of mercury intoxication. *Curr Opin Pediatr* 1999; **11:** 265–8.


### Pharmacokinetics

There is little absorption of liquid mercury from globules in the gastrointestinal tract. The main hazard of liquid mercury is from absorption following inhalation of mercury vapour; this mercury is widely distributed before being oxidised to the mercuric form. Concentrations can be detected in the brain.

Soluble inorganic mercuric salts are absorbed from the gastrointestinal tract and can also be absorbed through the skin. The mercury is distributed throughout the soft tissues with high concentrations in the kidneys; it is mainly excreted in the urine and faeces with an elimination half-life of about 60 days, although it may take years to eliminate mercury from the brain; elimination from other tissues may take several months.

Organic alkyl mercury compounds are more readily absorbed from both the gastrointestinal and the respiratory tracts. They are widely distributed and can produce high concentrations in the brain. Alkyl mercury compounds are excreted in urine and in the faeces with extensive enterohepatic recycling. The biological half-life varies but is longer than that of inorganic mercury.

Organic mercury, and to some extent inorganic mercury, diffuse across the placenta and are distributed into breast milk.

### Uses and Administration

The hazards associated with mercury generally outweigh any therapeutic benefit and its clinical use has largely been abandoned. The use of mercurial diuretics such as mersalyl (p.952) has generally been superseded by other diuretics. Ointments containing mercurials, such as ammoniated mercury (p.1152) have also generally been replaced by less toxic preparations. Mercurials were formerly used as spermicides.

Some ionisable inorganic mercury salts and certain organic compounds of mercury have been used as disinfectants, and some mercury salts are effective parasiticides and fungicides. Organic mercurials such as phenylmercuric acetate, borate, and nitrate are also used as preservatives (p.1189). Mercury is a component of dental amalgams.

Other mercury salts that have been used for their antibacterial activity include mercuric chloride, yellow mercuric oxide, and mercurous chloride (above).

Some mercury compounds have been used in homoeopathic medicine.

### Preparations

**Proprietary Preparations** (details are given in Part 3)
***Arg.:*** Lagrimas de Santa Lucia; ***Ger.:*** Farco-Oxicyanid-Tupfer†.

**Multi-ingredient:** ***Austria:*** Coldophthal; ***Spain:*** Oftalmol Dexa†; Oftalmol Ocular.

## Mescaline

Mescalina. 3,4,5-Trimethoxyphenethylamine.

$C_{11}H_{17}NO_3$ = 211.3.

*CAS — 54-04-6.*

### Profile

Mescaline is an alkaloid obtained from the cactus *Lophophora williamsii* (*Anhalonium williamsii, A. lewinii*) (Cactaceae), which grows in the northern regions of Mexico. The cactus is known in those areas by the Aztec name 'peyote' or 'peyotl' and dried slices of the cactus are called 'mescal buttons'.

Mescaline produces hallucinogenic and sympathomimetic effects similar to those produced by lysergide (see p.1708), but it is less potent. Its effects last for up to 12 hours. It has no therapeutic use. Both Mexican and North American Indians have used peyote in religious ceremonies on account of its hallucinogenic activity.

**Botulism.** Peyote consumed during a ceremonial ritual was believed to have caused botulism in three men.[1] The sample was found to contain type B botulinum toxin when assayed.


1. Hashimoto H, *et al.* Botulism from peyote. *N Engl J Med* 1998; **339:** 203–4.

## Mesoglycan Sodium

Mesoglicano sódico.

### Profile

Mesoglycan sodium is a mucopolysaccharide complex (glycosaminoglycan) extracted from calf aorta, containing mainly suleparoid (heparan sulfate) (p.1009) and dermatan sulfate (p.892). It has been claimed to have antithrombotic, antiplatelet, and antihyperlipidaemic properties.

◊ References.

1. Forconi S, *et al.* A randomized, ASA-controlled trial of mesoglycan in secondary prevention after cerebral ischemic events. *Cerebrovasc Dis* 1995; **5:** 334–41.

### Preparations

**Proprietary Preparations** (details are given in Part 3)
***Ital.:*** Perclar; Prisma; ***Port.:*** Prisma.

## Metamfepramone Hydrochloride *(rINNM)*

Dimepropion Hydrochloride *(BANM)*; Hidrocloruro de metanfepramona; Metamfepyramone Hydrochloride. 2-Dimethylaminopropiophenone hydrochloride.

$C_{11}H_{15}NO,HCl = 213.7.$

*CAS — 15351-09-4 (metamfepramone); 10105-90-5 (metamfepramone hydrochloride).*

### Profile

Metamfepramone, the dimethyl analogue of diethylpropion (p.1587), is a sympathomimetic that has been used as the hydrochloride in the treatment of hypotension and in preparations for the symptomatic relief of the common cold. It was formerly used as an anorectic agent.

### Preparations

**Proprietary Preparations** (details are given in Part 3)
**Multi-ingredient: *Ger.:*** Tempil N.

## Metesculetol Sodium *(rINNM)*

Metesculetol sódico. [(7-Hydroxy-4-methyl-2-oxo-2*H*-1-benzopyran-6-yl)oxy]acetate sodium.

$C_{12}H_9NaO_6 = 272.2.$

*CAS — 52814-39-8 (metesculetol); 53285-61-3 (metesculetol sodium).*

### Profile

Metesculetol is included in preparations for peripheral vascular disorders and haemorrhoids. Metescufylline is a compound of metesculetol and etamiphylline (p.785) that has been given by mouth for its reputed vasoprotectant effect.

### Preparations

**Proprietary Preparations** (details are given in Part 3)
**Multi-ingredient: *Chile:*** Parogencyl Bi-Actif; ***Fr.:*** Fluon; Intrait de Marron D'Inde P; Parogencyl gencives fragilisees; Parogencyl sensibilite gencives; Veinotonyl; ***Hong Kong:*** Pyodontyl; ***Ital.:*** Parogencyl.

## Methiosulfonium Chloride

Methylmethionine Sulfonium Chloride; Metiosulfonio, cloruro de; Vitamin U. (3-Amino-3-carboxypropyl)dimethylsulphonium chloride.

$C_6H_{14}ClNO_2S = 199.7.$

*CAS — 1115-84-0.*

*ATC — A02BX04.*

### Profile

Methiosulfonium chloride has been used for its reputed protective effect on the liver and gastrointestinal mucosa.

### Preparations

**Proprietary Preparations** (details are given in Part 3)
**Multi-ingredient: *Hong Kong:*** Crema-U†; Rudd-U; ***Singapore:*** Weisen-U.

## Methyl Fluorosulfate

Fluorosulfato, metilo de; Magic Methyl; Methyl Fluorosulphate; Methyl Fluorosulphonate.

$CH_3FO_3S = 114.1.$

*CAS — 421-20-5.*

### Profile

Methyl fluorosulfate has been used as a laboratory methylating agent. Pulmonary oedema has occurred after inhalation, and concern has been expressed concerning possible carcinogenicity.

## Methylergometrine Maleate *(BANM, rINNM)*

Maleato de metilergometrina; Methylergobasine Maleate; Methylergonovine Maleate. *N*-[(*S*)-1-(Hydroxymethyl)propyl]-D-lysergamide hydrogen maleate; 9,10-Didehydro-*N*-[(*S*)-1-(hydroxymethyl)propyl]-6-methylergoline-8β-carboxamide hydrogen maleate.

$C_{20}H_{25}N_3O_2,C_4H_4O_4 = 455.5.$

*CAS — 113-42-8 (methylergometrine); 57432-61-8 (methylergometrine maleate).*

*ATC — G02AB01.*

**Pharmacopoeias.** In *Jpn* and *US.*

**USP 27** (Methylergonovine Maleate). A white to pinkish-tan, odourless, microcrystalline powder. Soluble 1 in 100 of water, 1 in 175 of alcohol, 1 in 1900 of chloroform, and 1 in 8400 of ether. pH of a 0.02% solution in water is between 4.4 and 5.2. Store in airtight containers at a temperature not exceeding 8°. Protect from light.

**Stability.** For mention of slight variations in the methylergometrine content of the injection following transport to a tropical climate, see under Ergometrine Maleate, p.1684.

### Adverse Effects, Treatment, and Precautions

As for Ergometrine Maleate, p.1684.

**Poisoning.** References.

1. Aeby A, *et al.* Methylergometrine poisoning in children: review of 34 cases. *J Toxicol Clin Toxicol* 2003; **41:** 249–53.

### Pharmacokinetics

Methylergometrine maleate is reported to be rapidly absorbed after administration by mouth and by intramuscular injection. Oral bioavailability may show considerable interindividual variation. It undergoes extensive first-pass hepatic metabolism and only small amounts of unchanged drug are excreted in the urine. The elimination half-life is reported to be about 2 to 3 hours.

◊ The pharmacokinetics of methylergometrine maleate has been studied following oral administration in healthy subjects[1,2] and in postpartum women.[3] Small amounts of methylergometrine have been detected in breast milk.[4]

1. Mäntylä R, *et al.* Methylergometrine (methylergonovine) concentrations in the human plasma and urine. *Int J Clin Pharmacol Biopharm* 1978; **16:** 254–7.
2. de Groot ANJA, *et al.* Comparison of the bioavailability and pharmacokinetics of oral methylergometrine in men and women. *Int J Clin Pharmacol Ther* 1995; **33:** 328–32.
3. Allonen H, *et al.* Methylergometrine: comparison of plasma concentrations and clinical response of two brands. *Int J Clin Pharmacol Biopharm* 1978; **16:** 340–2.
4. Erkkola R, *et al.* Excretion of methylergometrine (methylergonovine) into the human breast milk. *Int J Clin Pharmacol Biopharm* 1978; **16:** 579–80.

### Uses and Administration

Methylergometrine maleate has an action on the uterus similar to that of ergometrine maleate (p.1684) and is used similarly in the prevention and treatment of postpartum or postabortal haemorrhage. It is given after delivery of the anterior shoulder or on completion of the third stage of labour in a dose of 200 micrograms intramuscularly, repeated for up to 5 doses if necessary at intervals of 2 to 4 hours. In emergencies 200 micrograms may be given by slow intravenous injection over at least 60 seconds. In the USA its use before delivery of the placenta is not generally recommended. During the puerperium 200 to 400 micrograms has been given by mouth 2 to 4 times daily for up to 7 days.

Methylergometrine is a metabolite of methysergide (p.469).

**Diagnosis and testing.** For reference to the use of methylergometrine maleate in the diagnosis of variant angina, see Ergometrine Maleate, p.1684.

### Preparations

***USP 27:*** Methylergonovine Maleate Injection; Methylergonovine Maleate Tablets.

**Proprietary Preparations** (details are given in Part 3)
***Arg.:*** Basofortina; ***Austria:*** Methergin; ***Belg.:*** Methergin; ***Braz.:*** Methergin; ***Chile:*** Methergin; ***Denm.:*** Methergin; ***Fin.:*** Methergin; ***Fr.:*** Methergin; ***Ger.:*** Methergin; Methylergobrevin; ***Gr.:*** Demergin; Methergin; ***Hong Kong:*** Methergin; ***India:*** Ingagen-M; Methergin; Utergin; ***Israel:*** Methergin; ***Ital.:*** Methergin; ***Malaysia:*** Methergin; ***Mex.:*** Methergin; ***Neth.:*** Methergin; ***Port.:*** Methergin; ***Spain:*** Methergin; ***Swed.:*** Methergin; ***Switz.:*** Methergin; ***Thai.:*** Ergotyl; Metrine; Nathergen; ***USA:*** Methergine.

**Multi-ingredient: *Ger.:*** Syntometrin.

## Methylhydroxyquinoline Metilsulfate

Methylhydroxyquinoline Methylsulphate; Metilhidroxiquinolina, metilsulfato de. 1-Methyl-8-hydroxyquinolinium methyl sulphate.

$C_{10}H_{10}NO,CH_3O_4S = 271.3.$

### Profile

Methylhydroxyquinoline metilsulfate has been used topically to treat eye irritation.

### Preparations

**Proprietary Preparations** (details are given in Part 3)
***Belg.:*** Uvestat†; ***Fr.:*** Uveline†; ***Spain:*** Chibro Uvelina†.

## Methylmethacrylate

Metacrilato de metilo. Methyl 2-methylacrylate; Methyl 2-methylpropenoate.

$C_5H_8O_2 = 100.1.$

*CAS — 80-62-6.*

### Adverse Effects

Occupational exposure to methylmethacrylate monomer vapour during preparation of the bone cement may irritate the respiratory tract, eyes, and skin. Cases of occupational asthma have been reported. Contact dermatitis, dizziness, nausea and vomiting may also occur. Methylmethacrylate monomer may be harmful to the liver.

Methylmethacrylate monomer acts as a peripheral vasodilator and has caused hypotension and, rarely, cardiac arrest and death when absorbed during the use of polymethylmethacrylate (PMMA) as a bone cement during orthopaedic surgery. Other adverse effects associated with the use of polymethylmethacrylate as a bone cement include thrombophlebitis, pulmonary embolism, haemorrhage, haematoma, short-term irregularities in cardiac conduction, and cerebrovascular accident.

**Effects on the nervous system.** Sensory polyneuropathy has been reported in a dental technician following occupational exposure to methylmethacrylate monomer.[1]

1. Sadoh DR, *et al.* Occupational exposure to methyl methacrylate monomer induces generalised neuropathy in a dental technician. *Br Dent J* 1999; **186:** 380–1.

### Uses and Administration

Methylmethacrylate forms the basis of acrylic bone cements used in orthopaedic surgery. A liquid consisting chiefly of methylmethacrylate monomer with a polymerisation initiator is mixed with a powder consisting of polymethylmethacrylate (PMMA) or a methylmethacrylate ester copolymer. The reaction is exothermic. Barium sulfate or zirconium dioxide may be added as a contrast medium. Polymethylmethacrylate beads containing gentamicin have been implanted for the prophylaxis and treatment of bone infections and some soft-tissue infections. Bone cements containing antibacterials such as gentamicin or erythromycin are also available.

Polymethylmethacrylate has also been used as a material for intra-ocular lenses, for denture bases, as a cement for dental prostheses, and in composite resins for dental restoration.

A number of polymers based on methacrylic acid are used in pharmaceutical technology mainly as film coating agents and binders. The Ph. Eur. 5.0 includes Ammonio Methacrylate Copolymer (Type A) and Ammonio Methacrylate Copolymer (Type B) (copolymers of acrylic and methacrylic acid esters), Basic Butylated Methacrylate Copolymer, Methacrylic Acid-Methyl Methacrylate Copolymer (1:1), Methacrylic Acid-Ethyl Acrylate Copolymer (1:1), Methacrylic Acid-Ethyl Acrylate Copolymer (1:1) Dispersion 30 per cent, Methacrylic Acid-Methyl Methacrylate Copolymer (1:2), and Polyacrylate Dispersion 30 per cent (a dispersion of an ethylacrylate-methyl methacrylate copolymer in water). USNF 22 includes Methacrylic Acid Copolymer (a copolymer of methacrylic acid and an acrylic or methacrylic ester), Ammonio Methacrylate Copolymer, and Ammonio Methacrylate Copolymer Dispersion.

**Bone disorders.** Percutaneous vertebral injection of methylmethacrylate bone cement has been used successfully to relieve the pain of metastatic vertebral bone lesions (p.513) and vertebral compression fractures due to osteoporosis[1,2]

1. Kaemmerlen P, *et al.* Percutaneous injection of orthopedic cement in metastatic vertebral lesions. *N Engl J Med* 1989; **321:** 121.
2. Barr JD, *et al.* Percutaneous vertebroplasty for pain relief and spinal stabilization. *Spine* 2000; **25:** 923–8.

### Preparations

**Proprietary Preparations** (details are given in Part 3)
***Austria:*** Knochenzement†; Sulfix†; ***Chile:*** Palacos R; ***Ger.:*** CMW; flint; Hansaplast Spruhpflaster†; Palacos R; Palamed; ***Neth.:*** Palacos; ***Port.:*** Palacos R†; ***Singapore:*** Palacos R; ***Switz.:*** Palacos†; ***Thai.:*** Palacos R; ***UK:*** Palacos R.

**Multi-ingredient: *Arg.:*** Septopal; ***Austral.:*** Palacos E with Garamycin; Palacos R with Garamycin; Septopal; ***Austria:*** AKZ†; Refobacin-Palacos R†; Septopal; ***Belg.:*** Palacos LV avec Gentamicine; Palacos R avec Gentamicine; Septopal†; ***Braz.:*** Septopal; ***Chile:*** Palacos R con Gentamicina; Perlas de PMMA con Gentamicina; ***Denm.:*** Antibiotic Simplex†; Palacos cum Gentamicin†; Septopal; ***Fin.:*** Palacos R cum Gentamicin; Septopal; ***Fr.:*** Palacos LV avec Gentamicine; Palacos R avec Gentamicine; ***Ger.:*** CMW mit Gentamicin; Copal; Epiglu; Palamed G; Refobacin-Palacos R; Septopal; ***Gr.:*** Palacos-R with Gentamycin; Septopal; ***Hong Kong:*** Septopal; ***India:*** Septopal; ***Irl.:*** Palacos R with Gentamicin†; Septopal†; ***Malaysia:*** Septopal; ***Neth.:*** Palacos met gentamicine; Septopal; ***Norw.:*** Palacos cum Gentamicin†; Septopal; ***NZ:*** Palacos with Garamycin; ***Port.:*** Palacos R com Gentamicina†; ***S.Afr.:*** Palacos R with Garamycin; Septopal; ***Singapore:*** Refobacin-Palacos R; Septopal; ***Swed.:*** Palacos cum Gentamicin†; Septopal; ***Switz.:*** AKZ†; Palacos avec Garamycin†; Septopal; ***Thai.:*** Refobacin-Palacos R; Septopal; ***UK:*** Epiglu; Palacos LV with Gentamicin; Palacos R with Gentamicin; Septopal.

## Metochalcone *(rINN)*

CB-1314; Methochalcone; Metocalcona; Trimethoxychalcone. 2′,4,4′-Trimethoxychalcone.

$C_{18}H_{18}O_4 = 298.3.$

*CAS — 18493-30-6.*

### Profile

Metochalcone has been used as a choleretic.

### Preparations

**Proprietary Preparations** (details are given in Part 3)
**Multi-ingredient:** ***Spain:*** Neocolan.

## Metyrapone *(BAN, USAN, rINN)*

Metirapona; Su-4885 (metyrapone tartrate). 2-Methyl-1,2-di(3-pyridyl)propan-1-one.
$C_{14}H_{14}N_2O$ = 226.3.
*CAS — 54-36-4.*
*ATC — V04CD01.*

**Pharmacopoeias.** In *Br., Jpn,* and *US.*

**BP 2003** (Metyrapone). A white to light amber crystalline powder with a characteristic odour. M.p. 50° to 53°. Sparingly soluble in water; freely soluble in alcohol and in chloroform; it dissolves in dilute mineral acids. Protect from light.

**USP 27** (Metyrapone). A white to light amber, fine, crystalline powder, having a characteristic odour. It darkens on exposure to light. Sparingly soluble in water; soluble in chloroform and in methyl alcohol; forms water-soluble salts with acids. Store in airtight containers. Protect from heat and light.

### Adverse Effects

Metyrapone may give rise to nausea and vomiting, abdominal pain, headache, sedation, dizziness, hypotension, and hypersensitivity rashes. Hypoadrenalism, hirsutism, and bone marrow depression may occur rarely. Long-term use of metyrapone can cause hypertension.

**Alopecia.** Reports of alopecia[1,2] associated with administration of metyrapone for Cushing's syndrome.

1. Harris PL. Alopecia associated with long-term metyrapone use. *Clin Pharm* 1986; **5:** 66–8.
2. Harries-Jones R, Overstall P. Metyrapone-induced alopecia. *Postgrad Med J* 1990; **66:** 584.

### Precautions

Metyrapone should be used with extreme caution, if at all, in patients with gross hypopituitarism or with reduced adrenal secretory activity because of the risk of precipitating acute adrenal failure. Thyroid dysfunction or liver cirrhosis may alter the response to metyrapone.

Dizziness and sedation may affect the performance of skilled tasks such as driving.

**Porphyria.** Metyrapone is considered to be unsafe in patients with porphyria because it has been shown to be porphyrinogenic in *in-vitro* systems.

### Interactions

Phenytoin is reported to increase the metabolism of metyrapone; doubling the dose of metyrapone may counteract the interaction. However, as many other drugs may interfere with steroid assessment, medication is best avoided where possible during the metyrapone test. Drugs reported to interfere with the metyrapone test include antidepressants such as amitriptyline, antithyroid drugs, antipsychotics such as chlorpromazine, barbiturates, corticosteroids, cyproheptadine, and hormones that affect the hypothalamic-pituitary axis such as oestrogens and progestogens.

### Pharmacokinetics

Metyrapone is rapidly absorbed from the gastrointestinal tract. It is metabolised by rapid reduction to metyrapol and excreted in the urine as glucuronide conjugates of metyrapone and metyrapol.

### Uses and Administration

Metyrapone inhibits the enzyme 11β-hydroxylase responsible for the synthesis of the glucocorticoids cortisone and hydrocortisone (cortisol) as well as aldosterone from their precursors. The consequent fall in the plasma concentrations of circulating glucocorticoids stimulates the anterior pituitary gland to produce more corticotropin. This, in turn, stimulates the production of more 11-deoxycortisol and other precursors which are metabolised in the liver and excreted in the urine where they can be measured. Metyrapone is therefore used as a test of the feedback hypothalamic-pituitary mechanism in the diagnosis of Cushing's syndrome, although the dexamethasone suppression test (p.1098) may be preferred.

After demonstration of the responsiveness of the adrenal cortex, metyrapone is given by mouth, usually in a dose of 750 mg every 4 hours for 6 doses. Administration with milk or after a meal may minimise the gastrointestinal side-effects of metyrapone. A suggested dose by mouth for children is 15 mg/kg, with a minimum dose of 250 mg, every 4 hours for 6 doses. In patients with a normally functioning pituitary gland excretion of 17-hydroxycorticosteroids is increased two- to fourfold and that of 17-ketosteroids about twofold.

Metyrapone is also used in the management of Cushing's syndrome (p.1313) when doses may range from 250 mg to 6 g daily.

Since metyrapone inhibits the synthesis of aldosterone it has been used to treat some cases of resistant oedema; it is given with a glucocorticoid to suppress the normal corticotropin response to low plasma concentrations of glucocorticoids. The suggested usual dosage of metyrapone in resistant oedema is 3 g daily in divided doses.

Metyrapone tartrate has also been used.

◊ References.

1. Atkinson AB. The treatment of Cushing's syndrome. *Clin Endocrinol (Oxf)* 1991; **34:** 507–13.
2. Avgerinos PC, *et al.* The metyrapone and dexamethasone suppression tests for the differential diagnosis of the adrenocorticotropin-dependent Cushing syndrome: a comparison. *Ann Intern Med* 1994; **121:** 318–27.
3. Avgerinos PC, *et al.* A comparison of the overnight and the standard metyrapone test for the differential diagnosis of adrenocorticotrophin-dependent Cushing's syndrome. *Clin Endocrinol (Oxf)* 1996; **45:** 483–91.

### Preparations

***BP 2003:*** Metyrapone Capsules;
***USP 27:*** Metyrapone Tablets.

**Proprietary Preparations** (details are given in Part 3)
***Austral.:*** Metopirone; ***Fr.:*** Metopirone; ***Irl.:*** Metopirone; ***Neth.:*** Metopiron; ***NZ:*** Metopirone†; ***Swed.:*** Metopiron; ***Switz.:*** Metopirone; ***UK:*** Metopirone; ***USA:*** Metopirone.

## Miglustat *(BAN, USAN, rINN)*

Butyldeoxynojirimycin; *n*-Butyl-deoxynojirimycin; OGT-918; OXAIDS; SC-48334. 1,5-(Butylimino)-1,5-dideoxy-D-glucitol; (2*R*,3*R*,4*R*,5*S*)-1-Butyl-2-(hydroxymethyl)piperidine-3,4,5-triol.
$C_{10}H_{21}NO_4$ = 219.3.
*CAS — 72599-27-0.*
*ATC — A16AX06.*

### Adverse Effects and Precautions

Diarrhoea and other gastrointestinal disturbances, weight loss, tremor, dizziness, headache, cramps, and visual disturbances are frequent in patients receiving miglustat, and some patients may experience paraesthesias, peripheral neuropathy, or cognitive dysfunction. Neurological and cognitive function should be assessed before and periodically during treatment. Studies in *animals* have indicated an effect on spermatogenesis; male patients should not attempt conception during, or for 3 months after stopping, treatment. Care is required in renal impairment.

### Uses and Administration

Miglustat is an inhibitor of the enzyme glucosylceramide synthase, responsible for the first step in the synthesis of glucosylceramide and most other glycolipids. It is used to help prevent the accumulation of glucosylceramide in patients with mild to moderate type 1 Gaucher disease (p.1649) who cannot be treated with enzyme replacement therapy. The initial dose is 100 mg by mouth 3 times daily; reduction to 100 mg once or twice daily may be necessary in some patients because of diarrhoea.

◊ Reviews.

1. McCormack PL, Goa KL. Miglustat. *Drugs* 2003; **63:** 2427–34.

**Administration in renal impairment.** The initial dose of miglustat should be reduced in renal impairment according to the patient's creatinine clearance (CC):

- CC 50 to 70 mL/minute per 1.73 m$^2$: 100 mg twice daily
- CC 30 to 50 mL/minute per 1.73 m$^2$: 100 mg daily
- CC less than 30 mL/minute per 1.73 m$^2$: not recommended

### Preparations

**Proprietary Preparations** (details are given in Part 3)
***UK:*** Zavesca; ***USA:*** Zavesca.

## Dementholised Mint Oil

Menta, aceite esencial desmentolado de; Menthae Arvensis Aetheroleum Partim Mentholi Privum.

**Pharmacopoeias.** In *Eur.* (see p.vi).
Mint oil or Mentha oil is in *Ger.* and *Jpn.*

**Ph. Eur. 5.0** (Mint Oil, Partly Dementholised; Dementholised Mint Oil BP 2003). The essential oil obtained by steam distillation from the fresh, flowering aerial parts, recently gathered from *Mentha canadensis* (*M. arvensis* var. *glabrata*; *M. arvensis* var. *piperascens*) followed by partial separation of menthol by crystallisation. A colourless or pale yellow to greenish-yellow liquid with a characteristic odour. Store in well-filled airtight containers at a temperature not exceeding 25°. Protect from light.

### Profile

Dementholised mint oil is used as a flavour. *Mentha arvensis* is used in herbal medicine as a febrifuge and for rheumatic disorders. Peppermint oil (p.1283) and spearmint oil (p.1749) are used as carminatives and flavours.

### Preparations

**Proprietary Preparations** (details are given in Part 3)
***Austria:*** Carmol; Physiomint; ***Ger.:*** Japanol; JHP Rodler; Kneipp Minzol Trost Tropfen†.

**Multi-ingredient:** ***Austria:*** Parodontax; ***Belg.:*** Calmant Martou†; ***Ger.:*** Dreierlei; Parodontal F5 med†; Trachiform; ***Ital.:*** Broncosedina; ***Switz.:*** Acidodermil†; Huile analgesique "Temple of Heaven" contre les maux de tete; Kernosan Huile de Massage†; Malveol; Neo-Angin au miel et citron; Neo-Angin exempt de sucre; Novital; Onguent nasal Ruedi; Osa Gel de dentition aux plantes†; Pastilles pectorales Demo N; Pommade nasale Ruedi†; Roliwol†; Tonex†; Tyrothricin; ***UK:*** Olbas; Olbas for Children.

## Miracle Fruit

Fruta milagrosa.

### Profile

Miracle fruit is the fruit of *Synsepalum dulcificum* (*Richardella dulcifica*) (Sapotaceae). It contains a glycoprotein 'miraculin' with no apparent taste of its own but which is able to make sour substances taste sweet and to improve the flavour of foods. Its activity is reduced by heating.

## Mistletoe

European Mistletoe; Gui; Mistelkraut; Muérdago; Tallo de Muérdago; Visci Caulis; Viscum; Viscum Album.

**Pharmacopoeias.** In *Ger.*

### Profile

Mistletoe is the dried, evergreen, dioecious semi-parasite, *Viscum album* (Loranthaceae), which grows on the branches of deciduous trees, chiefly apple, poplar, and plum. It occurs as a mixture of broken stems and leaves and occasional fruits. Mistletoe has a vasodilator action and has been used in herbal preparations for hypertension and cardiovascular disorders although its activity when taken orally is questionable. It has also been used in nervous disorders and in homoeopathic medicine.

Mistletoe contains lectins with cytotoxic and immunomodulatory actions *in vitro* and preparations have been given by injection in a number of neoplastic diseases.

Ingestion of the berries and other parts has been reported to cause nausea, vomiting, diarrhoea, and bradycardia.

◊ A review of mistletoe.[1] There are about 1300 species of mistletoe representing 36 genera of the Loranthaceae, and what is called the "common mistletoe" varies from country to country: in Europe the term describes *Viscum album* while in the USA it describes *Phoradendron flavescens*. The toxicity of aqueous extracts of mistletoe has been found to depend upon the nature of the host plant. Three classes of cytotoxic compounds are present in the leaves and stems of *V. album* although the berries are generally considered to be the most toxic part of the plant. These are alkaloids, viscotoxins, and lectins. The viscotoxins have been shown to cause hypotension, bradycardia, arterial vasoconstriction, and a negative inotropic effect, and may act as acetylcholine agonists. The lectins show toxic effects in *animals* similar to those seen with ricin.

1. Anderson LA, Phillipson JD. Mistletoe—the magic herb. *Pharm J* 1982; **229:** 437–9.

**Adverse effects.** Reports of hepatitis following the ingestion of herbal remedies containing mistletoe.[1,2]

1. Harvey J, Colin-Jones DG. Mistletoe hepatitis. *BMJ* 1981; **282:** 186–7.
2. Weeks GR, Proper JS. Herbal medicines—gaps in our knowledge. *Aust J Hosp Pharm* 1989; **19:** 155–7.

**Malignant neoplasms.** Reviews[1-3] of the use of mistletoe for the treatment of malignant neoplasms. Studies have been of variable quality, and have produced conflicting results; it has been suggested that the more rigorous trials do not demonstrate benefit.[3]

1. Mansky PJ. Mistletoe and cancer: controversies and perspectives. *Semin Oncol* 2002; **29:** 589–94.
2. Kienle GS, *et al.* Mistletoe in cancer—a systematic review on controlled clinical trials. *Eur J Med Res* 2003; **8:** 109–19.
3. Ernst E, *et al.* Mistletoe for cancer? A systematic review of randomised clinical trials. *Int J Cancer* 2003; **107:** 262–7.

### Preparations

**Proprietary Preparations** (details are given in Part 3)
***Austria:*** Apotheker Bauer's Misteltinktur; Eurixor; Helixor; Iscador; Isorel; Isugran; ***Ger.:*** Abnobaviscum; Cefalektin; Eurixor; Helixor; Iscador; Kneipp Mistel-Pflanzensaft†; Kneipp Pflanzen-Dragees Mistel†; Lektinol; Mistel Curarina; Mistel-Krautertabletten; Mistelol-Kapseln; Misteltropfen; Misteltropfen Hofmanns; Plenosol N†; Salus Mistel-Tropfen; Viscysat; Vysorel†; ***Switz.:*** Iscador.

**Multi-ingredient:** ***Austral.:*** Calmo†; Pacifenity†; ***Austria:*** Heli-Sal; Herz- und Kreislauftonikum Bioflora; Mag Kottas Nerven-Beruhigungstee; Neuners Krautertee Nr 20 - Kreislauftee; Neuners Krautertee Nr 32 - Kreislafregulierungstee; Rutiviscal; Vivinox; Wechseltee EF-EM-ES; ***Belg.:*** Tisane Contre la Tension†; ***Fr.:*** Mediflor Tisane Circulation du Sang No 12; Santane H$_7$†; Tisanes de l'Abbe Hamon no 6†; ***Ger.:*** Antihypertonicum S; Antisklerosin S†; Asgoviscum N; Heusin; Hypercard†; Ilja Rogoff; Kneipp Drei-Pflanzen-Dragees N†; Presselin Arterien K 5 P; Salusan†; Syviman N; Vasesana-Vasoregulans†; Viscophyll.

## Monoctanoin *(BAN, USAN)*

Monoctanoína; Monooctanoin; Mono-octanoin.
*CAS — 26402-26-6 (glyceryl mono-octanoate).*

**Description.** Monoctanoin is a semisynthetic mixture of glycerol esters, containing:
80 to 85% of glyceryl mono-octanoate ($C_{11}H_{22}O_4$ = 218.3),
10 to 15% of glyceryl mono-decanoate ($C_{13}H_{26}O_4$ = 246.3) and glyceryl di-octanoate ($C_{19}H_{36}O_5$ = 344.5),
and a maximum of 2.5% of free glycerol ($C_3H_8O_3$ = 92.09).

### Adverse Effects and Precautions

Abdominal pain, nausea, vomiting, and diarrhoea may occur particularly if monoctanoin is infused rapidly or in large doses; it has been recommended that perfusion pressure should not exceed 20 cm of water. Minor irritation of the gastric and duodenal mucosa has been reported. Acidosis may occur, particularly in patients with hepatic impairment, and leucopenia has been reported. Monoctanoin should not be given to patients with hepatic impairment, biliary tract infection, cholestatic jaundice, jejunitis, duodenal ulcer, or pancreatitis. It should not be given by the intravenous or intramuscular routes.

**Incidence of adverse effects.** Adverse effects[1] occurred in 67% of 343 patients treated with monoctanoin perfusion, with multiple side-effects in 41%. Abdominal pain was most common, occurring in 40% of patients. Nausea, vomiting, and diarrhoea were usually dose related, occurring in 25%, 15%, and 16% of patients respectively. Fever, attributed to cholangitis, was noted in 5%. Severe side-effects occurred in 12 patients; a patient with cirrhosis developed acidosis and encephalopathic signs.

1. Palmer KR, Hofmann AF. Intraductal mono-octanoin for the direct dissolution of bile duct stones: experience in 343 patients. *Gut* 1986; **27:** 196–202.

## Uses and Administration

Monoctanoin is used to dissolve cholesterol gallstones (p.1761) retained following cholecystectomy. It is administered by continuous perfusion through a catheter inserted directly into the common bile duct at a rate of 3 to 5 mL per hour. Perfusion may be suspended during meals. The solution should be warmed prior to perfusion, and the temperature should be maintained at 37° during administration. Treatment is continued for 2 to 10 days. If no reduction in the size of the stones is detectable after 7 to 10 days of treatment, further treatment is unlikely to be effective.

◊ References.

1. Palmer KR, Hofmann AF. Intraductal mono-octanoin for the direct dissolution of bile duct stones: experience in 343 patients. *Gut* 1986; **27:** 196–202.
2. Stock SE, *et al.* Treatment of common bile duct stones using mono-octanoin. *Br J Surg* 1992; **79:** 653–4.

## Preparations

**Proprietary Preparations** (details are given in Part 3)
***USA:*** Moctanin.

# Monoethanolamine

2-Hydroxyethylamine; 2-Aminoethanol.

$C_2H_7NO = 61.08$.

*CAS — 141-43-5.*

**Pharmacopoeias.** In *Br.* Also in *USNF.*

**BP 2003** (Ethanolamine). A clear, colourless, or pale yellow liquid with a slight odour. It is alkaline to litmus. Miscible with water and with alcohol; slightly soluble in ether.

**USNF 22** (Monoethanolamine). A clear, colourless, moderately viscous liquid having a distinctly ammoniacal odour. Miscible with water, with alcohol, with acetone, with chloroform, and with glycerol; immiscible with ether, with petroleum spirit, and with fixed oils, although it dissolves many essential oils. Store in airtight containers. Protect from light.

# Monoethanolamine Oleate *(rINN)*

Ethanolamine Oleate *(USAN)*; Oleato de monoetanolamina. 2-Hydroxyethylamine compound with oleic acid; 2-Aminoethanol compound with oleic acid.

$C_2H_7NO,C_{18}H_{34}O_2 = 343.5$.

*CAS — 2272-11-9.*
*ATC — C05BB01.*

## Adverse Effects and Precautions

Monoethanolamine oleate is irritant to skin and mucous membranes. Local injection may cause sloughing, ulceration, and, in severe cases, necrosis. Pain may occur at the site of injection. Patients receiving treatment for oesophageal varices may develop pleural effusion or infiltration. Hypersensitivity reactions have been reported.

Sclerotherapy should not be used to treat varicose veins of the legs in patients with thrombosis or a tendency to thrombosis, or with acute phlebitis, marked arterial, cardiac, or renal disease, local or systemic infections, or uncontrolled metabolic disorders such as diabetes mellitus.

**Effects on the kidneys.** Acute renal failure, which cleared spontaneously within 3 weeks, occurred in 2 obese women given sclerosing injections of 15 to 20 mL of a solution containing monoethanolamine oleate 5% and benzyl alcohol 2%.[1]

1. Maling TJB, Cretney MJ. Ethanolamine oleate and acute renal failure. *N Z Med J* 1975; **82:** 269–70.

## Uses and Administration

Monoethanolamine oleate is used as a sclerosant in the treatment of varicose veins and oesophageal varices. For sclerotherapy of varicose veins, 2 to 5 mL of a 5% solution of monoethanolamine oleate is injected slowly into empty isolated sections of vein, divided between 3 or 4 sites. Injection into full veins is also possible. For sclerotherapy of oesophageal varices, the dose is 1.5 to 5 mL of a 5% solution per varix to a maximum total dose of 20 mL per treatment session. Treatment may be given in the initial management of bleeding varices, then repeated at intervals until the varices are occluded.

**Variceal haemorrhage.** Portal hypertension may occur in many conditions that affect the liver, and leads to the development of collateral channels linking the portal and systemic circulations. Enlargement of such blood vessels beneath the oesophageal and gastric mucosa produces varices which have about a 30% risk of rupture and bleeding. Oesophageal varices are more often a cause of haemorrhage than gastric varices. Capillaries and veins in the gastric mucosa may also become swollen, a condition known as portal hypertensive gastropathy, and clinically important bleeding may occur in severe cases.

Variceal haemorrhage is usually severe, with mortality as high as 50% for the initial episode; the recurrence rate may be as high as 100% in patients who survive without treatment. Bleeding may stop spontaneously, but in those who continue to bleed, control of haemorrhage is difficult and patients should be referred to a centre with appropriate specialist facilities. Treatment to stabilise the patient may be necessary before they can be safely transferred.

**Acute management**. Initial treatment is supportive and requires measures to prevent aspiration and maintain a clear airway, and volume replacement with colloid and blood. Emergency endoscopy should be performed to establish the site of haemorrhage and exclude non-variceal sources of bleeding. The choice of treatment depends on the site of haemorrhage.[1-9] ***Endoscopic methods*** have been favoured for initial management. Injection sclerotherapy or banding ligation are used for bleeding oesophageal varices but the optimum management of bleeding gastric varices remains to be defined; the value of injection sclerotherapy varies with their location. Intravariceal injection of bovine or human thrombin, or cyanoacrylate tissue adhesives, has been used in gastric varices. Where the source of haemorrhage is non-variceal and due to gastropathy, portal decompressive surgery is effective, although it is associated with a high incidence of encephalopathy in cirrhotic patients. Small studies have shown propranolol to be effective in arresting haemorrhage.[10]

***Injection sclerotherapy*** for variceal haemorrhage may be performed during the emergency endoscopy procedure. Intravariceal injection, paravariceal injection, or a combination of the two have been used. The most widely used sclerosants are monoethanolamine oleate and sodium tetradecyl sulfate for intravariceal injection and lauromacrogol 400 for paravariceal injection. Sclerotherapy controls bleeding in up to 95% of cases. Ulceration and stricture formation occur frequently following injection sclerotherapy.

An alternative technique is ***endoscopic banding ligation***, where elastic bands are placed around the varices. The tissue subsequently necroses to leave a superficial ulcer. This technique has a similar efficacy to injection sclerotherapy, but may be more difficult to perform if active bleeding is occurring. Procedures may be repeated if bleeding continues or restarts.

Where endoscopy is unavailable, drug therapy or balloon tamponade may be used until the patient can be transferred to a specialist centre. These techniques may also have a role when sclerotherapy fails and some have suggested that initial drug therapy may be preferable to sclerotherapy.[11]

***Drug therapy*** is aimed at controlling portal venous pressure, although it is ineffective in massive haemorrhage and its effects cease once the drug is stopped. Two meta-analyses[11,12] have examined data from studies comparing drug therapy with endoscopic methods for the treatment of acute variceal bleeding. Sclerotherapy did not appear to be superior to vasoactive drugs as the first single treatment, and was associated with more frequent adverse effects.[11] Adjunctive drug therapy improved the efficacy of endoscopic therapy (injection sclerotherapy or band ligation) compared with endoscopic methods alone, although overall mortality was not affected; severe adverse effects were similar in both groups.[12]

Drugs used include vasopressin and its analogue terlipressin and, more recently, somatostatin and its analogue octreotide. Vasopressin controls haemorrhage in about 50% of patients. It is given by continuous intravenous infusion, together with glyceryl trinitrate, which counteracts the adverse cardiac effects of vasopressin, while potentiating its reduction of portal pressure. Terlipressin has the advantage of a longer therapeutic action, enabling bolus doses to be given. A comparison[13] of terlipressin and sclerotherapy found them to be equally effective for the control of acute variceal bleeding. A meta-analysis[14] of studies comparing terlipressin with placebo, or other drugs or interventions, also gave favourable results. However, somatostatin,[2] and particularly octreotide,[2,15,16] which may be given by bolus injection, are now generally preferred as they are thought to have similar efficacy to vasopressin but fewer adverse effects. A meta-analysis[17] of studies comparing somatostatin or its analogues octreotide and vapreotide with either placebo or no drug treatment suggested a small benefit in controlling bleeding; however, no mortality benefit has yet been shown.

***Balloon tamponade*** controls bleeding by direct pressure on the varices. Although it is a very effective means of controlling haemorrhage, there is a high incidence of rebleeding once pressure is removed and the incidence of complications is high. It is useful in cases of massive haemorrhage when drug therapy is ineffective and sclerotherapy is difficult.

***Surgery***, such as the formation of a shunt or oesophageal transection, may be necessary if the above measures fail to control the bleeding. However, such techniques have been associated with high mortality in some series. Formation of a transjugular intrahepatic portal-systemic shunt is now generally preferred.[4] It may be particularly useful in candidates for liver transplantation.

Short-term ***antibacterial prophylaxis*** has been proposed[18] for cirrhotic patients with gastrointestinal bleeding, including variceal bleeding, because reduced rates of infection and improved short-term survival have been reported in a few studies.

**Long-term management**. Once the acute bleeding has been controlled measures are needed to prevent rebleeding. Endoscopic therapy is widely used, with injection sclerotherapy or banding ligation being repeated until the varices are obliterated. Banding ligation is now the treatment of choice; it eradicates varices in fewer treatment sessions than injection sclerotherapy and reduces the risk of ulceration and stricture formation.[19] Sucralfate has been given following sclerotherapy as it may reduce the frequency of stricture formation and reduce bleeding from treatment-related ulcers. It seems to have no influence on ulcer healing following banding ligation.[20] Some practitioners carry out regular endoscopic checks and repeat sclerotherapy or banding ligation when varices reappear, although this approach is no more effective in terms of improving survival than giving treatment once bleeding occurs. Drug therapy is an alternative to endoscopic methods. Beta blockers (mainly propranolol) reduce the incidence of recurrent variceal bleeding and may improve survival.[21] A combination of nadolol with isosorbide mononitrate has been reported to reduce the risk of rebleeding more than repeated sclerotherapy, although there was no significant effect on mortality.[22] Drug therapy has also been used as an adjunct to endoscopic methods to control rebleeding in the period before variceal obliteration has occurred, or for long-term management following endoscopic therapy. However, studies comparing endoscopic band ligation with combination drug therapy have produced variable results.[23] Long-term octreotide therapy following sclerotherapy has also been investigated and may reduce recurrent variceal bleeding.[24] Several studies[25-27] have compared transjugular intrahepatic portosystemic shunting with endoscopic treatment, but no clear benefit has been demonstrated and there may be an increased risk of encephalopathy with the use of shunts. Surgery, including liver transplantation, should be considered in patients with recurrent life-threatening haemorrhage. Propranolol may also have a role in patients with portal hypertensive gastropathy. In a controlled study, propranolol reduced the incidence of recurrent bleeding from portal hypertensive gastropathy in patients with cirrhosis.[28]

**Prophylaxis** of a first bleed in patients with portal hypertension is controversial since about 70% of patients who have varices will never bleed, but should probably be given to patients with cirrhosis and varices thought to be at high risk of bleeding. A reliable system that will identify those at high risk of haemorrhage has yet to be devised. The NIEC (North Italian Endoscopic Club) system is probably the best so far.[29] Sclerotherapy had been considered as a method of prophylaxis, but its value has not been clearly established. Studies show that beta blockers decrease the incidence of a first bleed[30] and are probably the treatment of choice if prophylaxis is to be given. Banding ligation may be a suitable alternative for patients who are unable to take beta blockers.[31] Others consider banding ligation to be the standard therapy for prophylaxis.[9]

It is postulated that a reduction in portal pressure to below 12 mmHg is necessary to reduce the incidence of variceal bleeding and that treatment with beta blockers alone does not achieve this. More effective drugs are being sought, and isosorbide mononitrate[9,32,33] (as adjunctive therapy with a beta blocker) and clonidine[34] have been investigated for the prophylaxis of a first bleed and prevention of recurrent haemorrhage in patients with portal hypertension.

1. Williams SGJ, Westaby D. Management of variceal haemorrhage. *BMJ* 1994; **308:** 1213–17.
2. Roberts LR, Kamath PS. Pathophysiology and treatment of variceal hemorrhage. *Mayo Clin Proc* 1996; **71:** 973–83.
3. Sung JJY. Non-surgical treatment of variceal haemorrhage. *Br J Hosp Med* 1997; **57:** 162–6.
4. Stanely AJ, Haynes PC. Portal hypertension and variceal haemorrhage. *Lancet* 1997; **350:** 1235–9.
5. McCormack G, McCormick PA. A practical guide to the management of oesophageal varices. *Drugs* 1999; **57:** 327–35.
6. Dagher L, *et al.* Management of oesophageal varices. *Hosp Med* 2000; **61:** 711–17.
7. Anonymous. Early management of bleeding oesophageal varices. *Drug Ther Bull* 2000; **38:** 37–40.
8. Krige JEJ, Beckingham IJ. ABC of diseases of liver, pancreas, and biliary system. Portal hypertension—1: varices. *BMJ* 2001; **322:** 348–51.
9. Sharara AI, Rockey DC. Gastroesophageal variceal hemorrhage. *N Engl J Med* 2001; **345:** 669–81.
10. Anonymous. Portal hypertensive gastropathy. *Lancet* 1991; **338:** 1045–6.
11. D'Amico G, *et al.* Emergency sclerotherapy versus medical interventions for bleeding oesophageal varices in cirrhotic patients. Available in The Cochrane Library; Issue 2. Chichester: John Wiley; 2004.
12. Bañares R, *et al.* Endoscopic treatment versus endoscopic plus pharmacologic treatment for acute variceal bleeding: a meta-analysis. *Hepatology* 2002; **35:** 609–15.
13. Escorsell À, *et al.* Multicenter randomized controlled trial of terlipressin versus sclerotherapy in the treatment of acute variceal bleeding: the TEST study. *Hepatology* 2000; **32:** 471–6.
14. Ioannou G, *et al.* Terlipressin for acute esophageal variceal hemorrhage. Available in The Cochrane Library; Issue 2. Chichester: John Wiley; 2004.
15. Erstad BL. Octreotide for acute variceal bleeding. *Ann Pharmacother* 2001; **35:** 618–26.
16. Corley DA, *et al.* Octreotide for acute esophageal variceal bleeding: a meta-analysis. *Gastroenterology* 2001; **120:** 946–54.
17. Gøtzsche PC. Somatostatin analogues for acute bleeding oesophageal varices. Available in The Cochrane Library; Issue 2. Chichester: John Wiley; 2004.
18. Bernard B, *et al.* Antibiotic prophylaxis for the prevention of bacterial infections in cirrhotic patients with gastrointestinal bleeding: a meta-analysis. *Hepatology* 1999; **29:** 1655–61.
19. Laine L, Cook D. Endoscopic ligation compared with sclerotherapy for treatment of esophageal variceal bleeding: a meta-analysis. *Ann Intern Med* 1995; **123:** 280–7.
20. Nijhawan S, Rai RR. Does post-ligation oesophageal ulcer healing require treatment? *Lancet* 1994; **343:** 116–17.
21. Bernard B, *et al.* Beta-adrenergic antagonists in the prevention of gastrointestinal rebleeding in patients with cirrhosis: a meta-analysis. *Hepatology* 1997; **25:** 63–70.

22. Villanueva C, *et al.* Nadolol plus isosorbide mononitrate compared with sclerotherapy for the prevention of variceal rebleeding. *N Engl J Med* 1996; **334:** 1624–9.
23. Groszmann RJ, Garcia-Tsao G. Endoscopic variceal banding vs. pharmacological therapy for the prevention of recurrent variceal hemorrhage: what makes the difference? *Gastroenterology* 2002; **123:** 1388–91.
24. Jenkins SA, *et al.* Randomised trial of octreotide for long term management of cirrhosis after variceal haemorrhage. *BMJ* 1997; **315:** 1338–41.
25. Sanyal AJ, *et al.* Transjugular intrahepatic portosystemic shunts compared with endoscopic sclerotherapy for the prevention of recurrent variceal hemorrhage: a randomized, controlled trial. *Ann Intern Med* 1997; **126:** 849–57.
26. Cello JP, *et al.* Endoscopic sclerotherapy compared with percutaneous transjugular intrahepatic portosystemic shunt after initial sclerotherapy in patients with acute variceal hemorrhage: a randomized, controlled trial. *Ann Intern Med* 1997; **126:** 858–65.
27. Rössle M, *et al.* Randomised trial of transjugular-intrahepatic-portosystemic shunt versus endoscopy plus propranolol for prevention of variceal rebleeding. *Lancet* 1997; **349:** 1043–9.
28. Pérez-Ayuso RM, *et al.* Propranolol in prevention of recurrent bleeding from severe portal hypertensive gastropathy in cirrhosis. *Lancet* 1991; **337:** 1431–4.
29. The North Italian Endoscopic Club for the Study and Treatment of Esophageal Varices. Prediction of the first variceal hemorrhage in patients with cirrhosis of the liver and esophageal varices: a prospective multicenter study. *N Engl J Med* 1988; **319:** 983–9.
30. Pagliaro L, *et al.* Prevention of first bleeding in cirrhosis: a meta-analysis of randomised trials of nonsurgical treatment. *Ann Intern Med* 1992; **117:** 59–70.
31. Burroughs AK, Patch D. Primary prevention of bleeding from esophageal varices. *N Engl J Med* 1999; **340:** 1033–5.
32. Angelico M, *et al.* Isosorbide-5-mononitrate versus propranolol in the prevention of first bleeding in cirrhosis. *Gastroenterology* 1993; **104:** 1460–5.
33. Merkel C, *et al.* Randomised trial of nadolol alone or with isosorbide mononitrate for primary prophylaxis of variceal bleeding in cirrhosis. *Lancet* 1996; **348:** 1677–81.
34. Blendis LM. Clonidine for portal hypertension: a sympathetic solution? *Ann Intern Med* 1992; **116:** 515–17.

**Varicose veins.** Varicose veins are tortuous, protruding veins in the legs, that occur when weak vein walls and valve incompetence result in venous reflux and dilatation. Symptoms associated with varicose veins include heaviness, tension, aching, and itching of the legs. Complications include oedema, thrombophlebitis, deep venous thrombosis, lipodermatosclerosis, and venous ulceration. Risk factors for varicose veins include increasing age, pregnancy, and occupations that involve prolonged standing.

Conservative management using compression hosiery may be effective for relief of symptoms in some patients. Surgery or sclerotherapy are other treatment options, depending on the veins affected. In sclerotherapy, a sclerosant is injected into the affected vein where it irritates and damages the lining of the vein causing local thrombosis, fibrosis, and stenosis. Graduated compression dressings are usually applied after sclerotherapy to minimise the time taken for the surrounding tissue to absorb the damaged segment of vein. Compression may also help to reduce complications of sclerotherapy including hyperpigmentation, oedema, aching, thrombophlebitis, and deep venous thrombosis. Various agents have been used as sclerosants: detergent sclerosants include monoethanolamine oleate, sodium tetradecyl sulfate, lauromacrogol 400, and sodium morrhuate; osmotic sclerosants include hypertonic sodium chloride solutions, and hypertonic mixtures of sodium chloride and glucose; caustic sclerosants include chromated glycerol, and a mixture of iodine and sodium iodide.

References.

1. Drake LA, *et al.* American Academy of Dermatology. Guidelines of care for sclerotherapy treatment of varicose veins and telangiectatic leg veins. *J Am Acad Dermatol* 1996; **34:** 523–8.
2. Green D. Sclerotherapy for the permanent eradication of varicose veins: theoretical and practical considerations. *J Am Acad Dermatol* 1998; **38:** 461–75.
3. London NJ, Nash R. ABC of arterial and venous disease: varicose veins. *BMJ* 2000; **320:** 1391–4.
4. Tisi PV, Beverley CA. Injection sclerotherapy for varicose veins. Available in The Cochrane Library; Issue 2. Chichester: John Wiley; 2004.

### Preparations

***BP 2003:*** Ethanolamine Oleate Injection.

**Proprietary Preparations** (details are given in Part 3)
***Braz.:*** Ethamolin; ***Canad.:*** Ethamolin†; ***Jpn:*** Oldamin; ***USA:*** Ethamolin.

## Motherwort

Agripalma; Leonuri Cardiacae Herba; Leonurus; Motherwort Herb.

**Pharmacopoeias.** In *Eur.* (see p.vi). *Chin.* includes the fruit.

**Ph. Eur. 5.0** (Motherwort). The whole or cut, dried, flowering aerial parts of *Leonurus cardiaca*. It contains not less than 0.2% of flavonoids, expressed as hyperoside ($C_{21}H_{20}O_{12}$ = 464.4) calculated with reference to the dried drug. Protect from light.

### Profile

Motherwort is given in herbal medicine for nervous and cardiac disorders; it is also used in products promoted for mild hyperthyroidism.

### Preparations

**Proprietary Preparations** (details are given in Part 3)
***Ger.:*** Thyreogutt mono.

***Multi-ingredient: Austral.:*** Pacifenity†; Valerian†; ***Austria:*** Thyreogutt; ***Canad.:*** Thunas Tab for Menstrual Pain; ***Fr.:*** Biocarde; ***Ger.:*** Biovital Aktiv; Biovital Classic; Biovital N†; Biovital Weissdorn Tonikum†; Kneipp Herz- und Kreislauf-Tee†; Mutellon; Oxacant N; Oxacant-sedativ; ***Switz.:*** Tisane pour le coeur et la circulation; ***UK:*** Daily Menopause Relief; Gerard House Motherwort Compound†; Modern Herbals Stress; Period Pain Relief; Prementaid; Quiet Life; SuNerven; Wellwoman.

## Moxaverine Hydrochloride *(BANM, rINNM)*

Hidrocloruro de moxaverina; Meteverine Hydrochloride. 1-Benzyl-3-ethyl-6,7-dimethoxyisoquinoline hydrochloride.

$C_{20}H_{21}NO_2,HCl$ = 343.8.

*CAS — 10539-19-2 (moxaverine); 1163-37-7 (moxaverine hydrochloride).*

*ATC — A03AD30.*

### Profile

Moxaverine hydrochloride has a similar structure to papaverine (p.1728) and has been given by mouth and injection as an antispasmodic and in vascular disorders. The base is also used as an antispasmodic.

Doses of moxaverine hydrochloride of up to 300 mg three times daily by mouth have been suggested for the treatment of vasospastic disorders, although much lower doses have been recommended for the treatment of gastrointestinal and biliary-tract spasm.

### Preparations

**Proprietary Preparations** (details are given in Part 3)
***Ger.:*** Certonal; Kollateral.

***Multi-ingredient: Austria:*** Hedonin; ***Ger.:*** Kollateral A + E†.

## Mulungu

Erythrina mulungu.

### Profile

The bark of the mulungu tree (*Erythrina verna*, Fabaceae) has traditionally been used in South America as a sedative and as a hypotensive.

### Preparations

**Proprietary Preparations** (details are given in Part 3)

***Multi-ingredient: Braz.:*** Anevrase; Calmapax; Elixir de Maracuja Composto†; Elixir de Passiflora†; Especies Calmantes†; Maracugina†; Neurosedol†; Passaneuro; Passicalm; Passiflora Composta†; Passilex; Ritmoneuran†; Sedalin†; Serenase†; Tolusil†; Vidcalm†; Xarope Sao Joao.

## Mumps Skin Test Antigen

Parotiditis, prueba cutánea contra el antígeno de la.

**Pharmacopoeias.** In *US.*

**USP 27** (Mumps Skin Test Antigen). A sterile suspension of formaldehyde-inactivated mumps virus prepared from the extra-embryonic fluid of virus-infected chick embryos, concentrated and purified by differential centrifugation, and diluted with isotonic sodium chloride solution. It contains a preservative and glycine as a stabilising agent. Each mL contains not less than 20 complement-fixing units. It should be stored at 2° to 8°. The expiry date is not later than 18 months after date of manufacture or of release from manufacturer's cold storage.

### Profile

Recovery from mumps produces skin hypersensitivity to mumps virus. Mumps skin test antigen, has been used with other antigens to assess the status of cell-mediated immunity. A positive reaction may indicate previous infection with mumps virus but it is not considered to be very reliable. It should not be given to patients hypersensitive to egg protein.

**Anergy testing.** For reference to the use of mumps skin test antigen for anergy testing in HIV-positive patients, see Tuberculins, p.1759.

### Preparations

***USP 27:*** Mumps Skin Test Antigen.

**Proprietary Preparations** (details are given in Part 3)
***Canad.:*** MSTA†; ***USA:*** MSTA†.

## Muramidase Hydrochloride

N-Acetylmuramide Glycanohydrolase Hydrochloride; E1105 (muramidase); Globulin $G_1$ Hydrochloride; Lysozyme Hydrochloride; Muramidasa, hidrocloruro de.

*CAS — 9001-63-2 (muramidase); 9066-59-5 (muramidase hydrochloride).*

**Pharmacopoeias.** In *Jpn.*

### Profile

Muramidase is a mucopolysaccharidase normally present in saliva and other tissues and secretions. It is active against Gram-positive bacteria, possibly by transforming the insoluble polysaccharides of the cell wall to soluble mucopeptides. It is also thought to be active against some viruses and some Gram-negative bacteria.

Muramidase has been given, usually as the hydrochloride, to patients with herpes zoster and other painful viral infections, and for mouth and respiratory-tract disorders. It has been used with antibacterials in an attempt to enhance their activity. Sensitivity reactions have been reported.

**Adverse effects.** A report[1] of a toxic epidermal necrolysis-type drug eruption in a patient who took an oral cold preparation containing muramidase chloride, which was considered to be the probable cause. The patient's condition improved following intravenous corticosteroid therapy.

1. Kobayashi M, *et al.* A case of toxic epidermal necrolysis-type drug eruption induced by oral lysozyme chloride. *J Dermatol* 2000; **27:** 401–4.

### Preparations

**Proprietary Preparations** (details are given in Part 3)
***Belg.:*** Murazyme; ***Braz.:*** Murazyme; ***Hong Kong:*** Eurozyme; Flemizyme; Jemizym; Neuzym; ***Ital.:*** Immunozima; ***Jpn:*** Leftose; Neuzym; ***Malaysia:*** Leftose; Neuzym; Noflux; ***Singapore:*** Leftose; Lyzyme; Neuflo; Neuzyme; ***Thai.:*** Leftose.

***Multi-ingredient: Arg.:*** Bim; Factus; Gammanova; ***Austria:*** Sanoral; Tongill; ***Braz.:*** Cifrantil†; Colpistar; Eritrosima†; Floregin Composto†; Floregin†; Lisofenicol†; Lisoquinol†; Munolan†; Narizima Adulto†; Narizima Pediatrico†; Trinotrex; Trisdazol†; Velutrix†; ***Fr.:*** Cantalene; Glossithiase; Hexalyse; Lyso-6; Lysocalm†; Lysopaine; Oroseptol Lysozyme†; ***Ger.:*** Frubienzym; ***Hong Kong:*** Haemosol†; Hexalyse; Quadezyme; ***Ital.:*** Narlisim; ***Port.:*** Narizima; ***Singapore:*** Biotene; ***Spain:*** Egarone; Espectral; Espectral Balsamico†; Inexfal†; Lizipaina; Normo Nar; Pulmotropic; Rino Dexa; Trofalgon; ***Switz.:*** Arbid-top; Lyso-6; Lysopaine; Mebucasol f; Sangerol; ***Thai.:*** Siduol; ***UK:*** Biotene Dry Mouth; BioXtra.

## Poisonous Mushrooms or Toadstools

Setas venenosas.

*CAS — 23109-05-9 (α-amanitin); 21150-22-1 (β-amanitin); 21150-23-2 (γ-amanitin); 58919-61-2 (coprine); 16568-02-8 (gyromitrin); 2552-55-8 (ibotenic acid); 60-34-4 (methylhydrazine); 300-54-9 (muscarine); 2763-96-4 (muscimol); 37338-80-0 (orellanine); 17466-45-4 (phalloidin); 28227-92-1 (phalloin); 39412-56-1 (phallolysin).*

### Classification

This monograph describes poisonous mushrooms often known as toadstools, their toxins, toxic effects, and the treatment of those effects. Their only use is in homoeopathic medicine, which employs *Amanita muscaria* as Agaricus muscarius. *A. muscaria* and *Psilocybe* spp. are abused for their psychoactive properties (see also Psilocin, p.1736).

Mushrooms can be classified into 8 groups according to their principal toxins and toxic effects:

- *Group I.* Most deaths due to mushroom poisoning follow the ingestion of mushrooms containing cyclopeptides and among these mushrooms *Amanita phalloides* ('death cap') has been reported to be responsible for 90% of all mushroom fatalities. The cyclopeptides are a group of heat-stable cyclic polypeptides with molecular weights ranging from 800 to 1100 and include the amatoxins (α-, β-, γ-amanitin) and phallotoxins (phalloidin, phaloin, phallolysin). Other mushrooms containing cyclopeptides include *A. verna* ('deadly agaric', 'fool's mushroom'), *A. virosa*, ('destroying angel') and *A. bisporigera* ('white destroying angel'), and *Galerina autumnalis*, *G. marginata*, and *G. venenata*.
- *Group II.* Although *A. muscaria* ('fly agaric') and *A. pantherina* ('panther cap', 'false blusher') may contain small amounts of muscarine, the antimuscarinic effects of the hallucinogenic agent muscimol and the insecticidal agent ibotenic acid usually predominate.
- *Group III.* Many species of *Gyromitra* contain toxins known as gyromitrins that decompose to release methylhydrazine (monomethylhydrazine; MMH) an inhibitor of the coenzyme pyridoxal phosphate.
- *Group IV.* Mushrooms whose principal toxin is muscarine include many of the *Clitocybe* and *Inocybe* spp. *A. muscaria* and *A. pantherina* (see above) may also contain small amounts.
- *Group V. Coprinus atramentarius* ('ink cap') contains the compound coprine, one of whose metabolites is an inhibitor of acetaldehyde dehydrogenase and it may therefore produce 'disulfiram-like' symptoms after drinking alcohol.
- *Group VI.* Mushrooms that may contain the hallucinogenic indoles psilocin and psilocybine include species of *Psilocybe*, *Panaeolus*, *Gymnopilus*, *Stropharia*, and *Conocybe*.
- *Group VII.* Many mushrooms that only act as gastrointestinal irritants and do not produce systemic effects are included in this group.
- *Group VIII.* A further group has sometimes been used to classify some species of *Cortinarius* that contain a renal toxin thought by some to be orellanine, but whose exact nature remains to be determined.

### Adverse Effects

The clinical course of poisoning due to mushrooms is related to their principal toxins:

- *Group I.* The manifestations of poisoning with mushrooms containing cyclopeptides may be divided into three phases. Initial symptoms may occur 6 to 24 hours after ingestion and usually consist of gastrointestinal effects such as abdominal pain, nausea, severe vomiting, and profuse diarrhoea similar to that in cholera. The patient may then appear to recover and be symptom-free for 2 to 3 days, but liver-enzyme values may be increasing. Following this phase, the more serious toxic effects of the amatoxins become apparent and there are signs of hepatic, renal, cardiac, and CNS toxicity. Symptoms include jaundice, oliguria, anuria, hypoglycaemia, coagulopathies, circulatory collapse, convulsions, and coma. The mortality rate is high in this phase with death usually being due to hepatic failure following hepatic necrosis. Up to 90% of untreated patients may die, though the rate may be as low as 15 to 30% following treatment.

- *Group II.* The adverse effects of mushrooms containing ibotenic acid and muscimol usually occur within 2 hours of ingestion. Symptoms may include ataxia, euphoria, delirium, and hallucinations associated with other antimuscarinic effects. Fatalities are rare.
- *Group III.* Patients who have ingested mushrooms containing gyromitrins usually develop symptoms of poisoning within 6 to 24 hours. These consist initially of nausea, vomiting, abdominal pain, and muscle cramps, headache, dizziness and fatigue. Delirium, convulsions, coma, methaemoglobinaemia and haemolysis may also occur. Occasionally jaundice and hepatic necrosis may lead to hepatic failure and death. Up to 40% of patients may die.
- *Group IV.* Symptoms typical of 'cholinergic crisis' (see Adverse Effects of Neostigmine, p.1492) may appear about 30 minutes to 2 hours after ingestion of mushrooms containing muscarine. These may include bradycardia, bronchospasm, salivation, perspiration, lachrymation, rhinorrhoea, involuntary urination and defaecation, and diarrhoea. Miosis, hypotension, and cardiac arrhythmias may also occur. Rarely death may follow due to cardiac arrest or respiratory-tract obstruction.
- *Group V.* Since one of the metabolites of coprine is an acetaldehyde dehydrogenase inhibitor, drinking alcohol, even up to several days after ingestion of mushrooms containing this compound, will produce symptoms similar to those of the 'disulfiram-alcohol' interaction (see Disulfiram, Adverse Effects, p.1681). Fatalities are rare.
- *Group VI.* The adverse effects of ingestion of mushrooms containing psilocin and psilocybine are similar to those described under lysergide (p.1708). Symptoms usually occur within about 30 minutes to 2 hours. Fatalities are rare.
- *Group VII.* Generally no treatment is required for adverse gastrointestinal effects seen with this group of mushrooms.
- *Group VIII.* There may be a delay of as long as 14 to 20 days before symptoms of poisoning due to *Cortinarius* appear. Patients will develop an intense thirst. Other symptoms usually include nausea, vomiting, diarrhoea, and anorexia. Muscle aching and spasms and a feeling of coldness may also occur. In severe cases renal failure may lead to death. It has been reported that up to 15% of patients may die.

**Pregnancy.** α-Amanitine does not appear to cross the placental barrier, even during the acute phase of intoxication.[1]

1. Belliardo F, *et al.* Amatoxins do not cross the placental barrier. *Lancet* 1983; **i:** 1381.

### Treatment of Adverse Effects

As there are no specific antidotes for the majority of cases of mushroom poisoning and which species is involved is often unknown, treatment consists primarily of symptomatic and supportive measures. The stomach may be emptied by gastric lavage if the patient has not already vomited spontaneously. However, if presentation is delayed because of the slow onset of symptoms seen with some types of mushrooms measures to empty the stomach are unlikely to be productive. Activated charcoal may be of use in binding toxins in the gastrointestinal tract and preventing absorption. Determining the interval between ingestion and the onset of symptoms often helps to identify the type of mushrooms ingested. If possible specimens of the mushrooms or a sample of the stomach contents should be sent to an expert mycologist for identification. Particular attention should be paid to intravenous replacement of fluids and electrolytes especially if vomiting and diarrhoea are severe. If the ingestion of hepatotoxic or nephrotoxic mushrooms is suspected liver and renal function should be monitored.

Since some mushrooms contain a wide range of toxins and patients may have ingested more than one species, specific therapy should only be instituted following positive identification.

- *Group I.* There is little clinical evidence to support the efficacy of specific agents or treatments for the management of cyclopeptide poisoning. A variety of agents including benzylpenicillin and silymarin or silybin (silibinin) have been given to try to protect the liver against the hepatotoxic effects of the amatoxins. Exchange transfusions, haemodialysis, or charcoal haemoperfusion have been tried to facilitate amatoxin removal. The removal of bile via a duodenal tube left *in situ* has been suggested to reduce enterohepatic circulation of amatoxins. Forced diuresis has also been advocated. Liver transplantation may be required for progressive hepatic failure. A radio-immunoassay for the detection of amatoxins is available in some countries to confirm a diagnosis of cyclopeptide poisoning.
- *Group II.* Specific treatment is usually only required if symptoms are severe. Physostigmine has been used to treat antimuscarinic symptoms. As mushrooms containing ibotenic acid and muscimol may also contain small amounts of muscarine, atropine may be required to control muscarinic symptoms.
- *Group III.* Pyridoxine hydrochloride has been given as an intravenous infusion as specific therapy to overcome the inhibition of pyridoxal phosphate by methylhydrazine, but the use of large doses of pyridoxine might itself produce adverse neurological effects. Methylthioninium chloride may be required if methaemoglobinaemia is severe.
- *Group IV.* Atropine sulfate may be required to control the symptoms of muscarine poisoning but it should only be used if definite muscarinic symptoms are present.
- *Group V.* There is no specific treatment for the 'disulfiram-alcohol' reaction except for the maintenance of blood pressure.
- *Group VI.* If symptoms are severe some patients may require sedation with diazepam.

◊ General reviews.

1. Köppel C. Clinical symptomatology and management of mushroom poisoning. *Toxicon* 1993; **31:** 1513–40.

**Amanita phalloides.** The use of specific antidotes in the treatment of poisoning due to *Amanita phalloides* remains controversial. Benzylpenicillin, sulfamethoxazole, thioctic acid, cytochrome C, ascorbic acid, insulin, growth hormone, silymarin or silybin, and corticosteroids have all been used or suggested. However, at present there is limited clinical evidence to support the use of only benzylpenicillin and silymarin or silybin.[1,2] Liver transplantation should be considered in patients with progressive hepatic failure.[2]

1. Floersheim GL. Treatment of human amatoxin mushroom poisoning: myths and advances in therapy. *Med Toxicol* 1987; **2:** 1–9.
2. Klein AS, *et al.* Amanita poisoning: treatment and the role of liver transplantation. *Am J Med* 1989; **86:** 187–93.

## Musk

Almíscar; Almizcle; Deer Musk; Mosc.; Moschus.
*CAS — 541-91-3 (muskone).*

**Pharmacopoeias.** In *Chin.*

### Profile

Musk is the dried secretions from the preputial follicles of the musk deer, *Moschus moschiferus* or some other spp. of *Moschus* (Cervidae). It is used as a fragrance and fixative in perfumery.

A series of nitrated tertiary butyl toluenes or xylenes, or related compounds, are used as artificial musks. Musk ambrette, a synthetic nitromusk compound used in perfumery and as a food flavour, has been reported to cause contact dermatitis and photosensitivity.

Musk is used in homoeopathic medicine.

◊ References.

1. Schmeiser HH, *et al.* Evaluation of health risks caused by musk ketone. *Int J Hyg Environ Health* 2001; **203:** 293–9.

## Black Mustard

Graine de Moutarde Noire; Mostarda Preta; Mostaza negra; Moutarde Jonciforme; Schwarzer Senfsame; Semen Sinapis; Semilla de Mostaza; Sinapis Nigra.

**Description.** Black mustard is the dried ripe seeds of *Brassica nigra* (*B. sinapioides*) (Cruciferae).

**Pharmacopoeias.** In *Swiss* which allows *B. nigra, B. juncea,* and other species.

## White Mustard

Mostaza blanca; Sinapis Alba.

**Description.** White mustard is the dried ripe seeds of *Brassica alba* (Cruciferae).

**Pharmacopoeias.** *Chin.* allows *B. alba* or *B. juncea.*

## Volatile Mustard Oil

Allylsenföl; Essence of Mustard; Mostaza, aceite esencial de; Oleum Sinapis Volatile.

## Allyl Isothiocyanate *(USAN)*

Isothiocyanato-l-propene.
$C_4H_5NS = 99.15$.
*CAS — 57-06-7.*

**Pharmacopoeias.** *Fr.* and *US*

**USP 27** (Allyl Isothiocyanate). A colourless to pale yellow, very refractive, liquid with a pungent, irritating odour and an acrid taste. Slightly soluble in water; miscible with alcohol, with carbon disulfide, and with ether. Store in airtight containers.

### Profile

Black and white mustard seeds have been used as emetics, in counter-irritant and rubefacient preparations, and as condiments. Volatile mustard oil, prepared from black mustard seeds, is largely composed of allyl isothiocyanate. It is an extremely powerful irritant that has been used as a counter-irritant and rubefacient. Expressed mustard oil contains a smaller proportion of volatile oil and has been used as a less powerful counter-irritant.

**Adverse effects.** A report of 2 cases of IgE-mediated anaphylaxis to mustard condiment.[1]

1. Vidal C, *et al.* Anaphylaxis to mustard. *Postgrad Med J* 1991; **67:** 404.

**Handling.** Allyl isothiocyanate is a potent lachrymator, with a pungent irritating odour. Care should be taken to protect the eyes, to prevent inhalation of fumes, and to avoid tasting.

### Preparations

**Proprietary Preparations** (details are given in Part 3)
***Fr.:*** Autoplasme Vaillant; Pneumoplasme†; Sinapisme Rigollot.

**Multi-ingredient:** ***Austria:*** Biokosma Red Point-Massagecreme; ***Braz.:*** Analgen; Benegel†; Gelflex; Gelol†; Gelonevral; Mialgex; Mostardina†; Nevrol; ***Canad.:*** Kinot†; Penetrating Rub†; Rheumalan; ***Fr.:*** Pneumoplasme a l'Histamine†; ***Ger.:*** Cor-Select; ***Spain:*** Dolokey; ***Switz.:*** Liberol†; ***UK:*** Nine Rubbing Oils; Radian-B Red Oils; Red Oil; ***USA:*** Dermolin; Methalgen; Musterole Extra.

## Myristyl Alcohol

Alcohol miristilo; NSC-8549; 1-Tetradecanol.
$C_{14}H_{30}O = 214.4$.
*CAS — 112-72-1.*

**Pharmacopoeias.** In *USNF.*

**USNF 22** (Myristyl Alcohol). M.p. 36° to 42°.

### Profile

Myristyl alcohol is used as an oleaginous vehicle. Contact dermatitis has been associated with its use.

## Myrrh

Gum Myrrh; Mirra; Myrrha.

**Pharmacopoeias.** In *Eur.* (see p.vi) and *US.*

**Ph. Eur. 5.0** (Myrrh). A gum-resin, hardened in air, obtained from the stem and branches of *Commiphora molmol* and/or other species of *Commiphora.* Protect from light.

**USP 27** (Myrrh). The oleo-gum resin obtained from the stems and branches of *Commiphora molmol* and other related species of *Commiphora* (Burseraceae) other than *C. mukul.* Store in airtight containers in a dry place.

### Profile

Myrrh is astringent to mucous membranes; the tincture is used in mouthwashes and gargles for inflammatory disorders of the mouth and pharynx. It has also been used as a carminative. Myrrh has been tried in the treatment of schistosomiasis and fascioliasis.

Contact dermatitis has been reported.

◊ References.

1. Massoud A, *et al.* Preliminary study of therapeutic efficacy of a new fasciolicidal drug derived from Commiphora molmol (myrrh). *Am J Trop Med Hyg* 2001; **65:** 96–9.
2. Sheir Z, *et al.* A safe, effective, herbal antischistosomal therapy derived from myrrh. *Am J Trop Med Hyg* 2001; **65:** 700–4.

### Preparations

***USP 27:*** Myrrh Topical Solution.

**Proprietary Preparations** (details are given in Part 3)
***Ger.:*** Inspirol P; Lomasatin M†.

**Multi-ingredient:** ***Austria:*** Brady's-Magentropfen; Dentinox; Drovitol; Paradenton; Parodontax; ***Braz.:*** Malvosulfam†; Parodontax†; ***Canad.:*** Chase Coldsorex; Cold Sore Lotion; Lotion pour Feux Sauvages; ***Denm.:*** Dolodent; ***Ger.:*** Ad-Muc; Infi-tract; Mint-Lysoform; Myrrhinil-Intest; Repha-Os; Schwedentrunk mit Ginseng†; Schwedentrunk†; ***Israel:*** Parodontax; ***Ital.:*** Gengivario; ***Spain:*** Buco Regis; ***Switz.:*** Baume; Eubucal; ***UK:*** Allcock's Porous Capsicum Plaster†; Herbal Indigestion Naturtabs; HRI Golden Seal Digestive; Indigestion and Flatulence; Vocalzone; Wind & Dyspepsia Relief.

## Myrtillus

Baccae Myrtilli; Bilberry; Blaeberry; Heidelbeere; Huckleberry; Hurtleberry; Mirtilo; Myrtilli Fructus; Whortleberry.

**Pharmacopoeias.** In *Eur.* (see p.vi).

**Ph. Eur. 5.0** (Bilberry Fruit, Dried; Dried Bilberry BP 2003; Bilberry Fruit, Fresh; Fresh Bilberry BP 2003). The ripe fruit of *Vaccinium myrtillus.* The dried fruit contains a minimum of 1.0% of tannins, expressed as pyrogallol, calculated with reference to the dried drug. The fresh or frozen fruit contains a minimum of 0.30% of anthocyanins, expressed as cyanidin-3-glucoside chloride (chrysanthemin, $C_{21}H_{21}ClO_{11} = 484.8$), calculated with reference to the dried drug. The frozen fruit should be stored at or below −18°.

### Profile

Myrtillus has diuretic and astringent properties. It has been used for ophthalmic and circulatory disorders and for diarrhoea.

Myrtillus is used in homoeopathic medicine.

### Preparations

**Proprietary Preparations** (details are given in Part 3)
***Arg.:*** Mirtilene Forte; ***Austral.:*** Herbal Eye Care Formula†; ***Braz.:*** Miralis; ***Ger.:*** Difrarel; ***Ital.:*** Alcodin; Angiorex; Antocin†; Mirtilene Forte; Retinol; Tegens; ***Port.:*** Difrarel; Varison; ***Spain:*** Difrarel†; Largitor†; ***Switz.:*** Myrtaven.

**Multi-ingredient:** ***Austral.:*** Bilberry Plus Eye Health†; Bilberry Plus†; Bioglan Pygno-Vite†; Bioglan Vision-Eze†; Extralife Eye-Care†; Extralife Leg-Care†; Herbal PMS Formula†; Pine OPC†; Prophthal†; Pykno†; St Mary's

Thistle Plus†; **Austria:** Amersan; Aponatura Durchfall; Krauterhaus Mag Kottas Tee gegen Durchfall; Luuf-Halspastillen fur Kinder; Myrtilen; **Braz.:** Antomiopic; **Chile:** Gingo-Ther; **Fr.:** Diacure; Difrarel; Difrarel E; Flebior; Santane $H_7$†; **Ger.:** Salus Augenschutz-Kapseln NA; **Ital.:** Alvear con Ginseng; Alvear Sport†; Angioton; Api Baby; Bebimix; Biolactine; Biophil†; Capill; Dermilia Flebozin; Evamilk; Fluiven†; Lactovit†; Memovisus; Mirtilene; Mirtiros†; Neomyrt Plus; Nerex; Promix 3; Retinovit; Tussol; Ultravisin; Varicofit; **Spain:** Antomiopic; Difrarel E†; Mirtilus; **UK:** Se-Power.

## Nadide *(BAN, USAN, rINN)*

Codehydrogenase I; Coenzyme I; Co-I; Diphosphopyridine Nucleotide; DPN; NAD; Nadida; Nicotinamide Adenine Dinucleotide; NSC-20272. 1-(3-Carbamoylpyridinio)-β-D-ribofuranoside 5-(adenosine-5′-pyrophosphate).

$C_{21}H_{27}N_7O_{14}P_2$ = 663.4.

*CAS — 53-84-9.*

### Profile

Nadide is a naturally occurring coenzyme claimed to be of value in the treatment of alcohol and opioid addiction. The reduced form of nadide, NADH, has been used in the management of chronic fatigue syndrome.

**Parkinsonism.** The reduced form of nadide, NADH (β-NADH; reduced DPN) and its phosphate derivative (NADPH) have been given in the management of Parkinson's disease in an attempt to enhance endogenous dopamine synthesis by stimulating the enzyme tyrosine hydroxylase. Although some beneficial effects have been reported in several case series, a placebo-controlled study failed to find any evidence of efficacy and the routine use of NADH has not been recommended.[1]

1. Swerdlow RH. Is NADH effective in the treatment of Parkinson's disease? *Drugs Aging* 1998; **13:** 263–8.

### Preparations

**Proprietary Preparations** (details are given in Part 3)
**S.Afr.:** DPN; **Spain:** Nad; **UK:** Enada†.

## Nafamostat Mesilate *(rINNM)*

FUT-175; Nafamostat Mesylate *(USAN)*. 6-Amidino-2-naphthyl *p*-guanidinobenzoate dimethanesulfonate.

$C_{21}H_{25}N_5O_8S_2$ = 539.6.

*CAS — 81525-10-2 (nafamostat); 82956-11-4 (nafamostat mesilate).*

### Profile

Like aprotinin (p.742) nafamostat is a proteolytic enzyme inhibitor. The mesilate is used in the treatment of acute pancreatitis and disseminated intravascular coagulation, and as an anticoagulant in haemodialysis.

Hyperkalaemia has been reported.

◊ References.

1. Yanamoto H, *et al.* Therapeutic trial of cerebral vasospasm with the serine protease inhibitor, FUT-175, administered in the acute stage after subarachnoid hemorrhage. *Neurosurgery* 1992; **30:** 358–63.
2. Akizawa T, *et al.* Nafamostat mesilate: a regional anticoagulant for haemodialysis in patients at high risk for bleeding. *Nephron* 1993; **64:** 376–81.
3. Miyata T, *et al.* Effectiveness of nafamostat mesilate on glomerulonephritis in immune-complex diseases. *Lancet* 1993; **341:** 1353.
4. Murase M, *et al.* Nafamostat mesilate reduces blood loss during open heart surgery. *Circulation* 1993; **88:** 432–6.
5. Kitagawa H, *et al.* Hyperkalaemia due to nafamostat mesylate. *N Engl J Med* 1995; **332:** 687.

## Naphthylacetic Acid

Naftilacético, ácido; 1-Naphthaleneacetic Acid; 1-Naphthylacetic Acid.

$C_{12}H_{10}O_2$ = 186.2.

*CAS — 86-87-3.*

### Profile

Naphthylacetic acid has been used as a choleretic.

### Preparations

**Proprietary Preparations** (details are given in Part 3)
**Multi-ingredient: Austria:** Galle-Donau; Spagall; **Switz.:** Bilipax.

## Natalizumab *(rINN)*

*CAS — 189261-10-7.*

### Profile

Natalizumab is an alpha-4 integrin-specific humanised monoclonal antibody under investigation for the treatment of multiple sclerosis, Crohn's disease, and ulcerative colitis.

◊ References.

1. Gordon FH, *et al.* A pilot study of treatment of active ulcerative colitis with natalizumab, a humanized monoclonal antibody to alpha-4 integrin. *Aliment Pharmacol Ther* 2002; **16:** 699–705.
2. Miller DH, *et al.* A controlled trial of natalizumab for relapsing multiple sclerosis. *N Engl J Med* 2003; **348:** 15–23.
3. Ghosh S, *et al.* Natalizumab for active Crohn's disease. *N Engl J Med* 2003; **348:** 24–32.

## Nebracetam *(rINN)*

WEB-1881. (±)-4-(Aminomethyl)-1-benzyl-2-pyrrolidinone.

$C_{12}H_{16}N_2O$ = 204.3.

*CAS — 116041-13-5; 97205-34-0.*

### Profile

Nebracetam acts on the CNS and has been investigated as a cognition adjuvant in the treatment of Alzheimer's disease.

## Nefiracetam *(rINN)*

DM-9384; DZL-221. 2-Oxo-1-pyrrolidineaceto-2′,6′-xylidide.

$C_{14}H_{18}N_2O_2$ = 246.3.

*CAS — 77191-36-7.*

### Profile

Nefiracetam acts on the CNS and has been described as a 'nootropic'. It has been investigated in some cerebrovascular disorders and for the treatment of Alzheimer's disease.

## Neroli Oil

Aurantii Amari Floris Aetheroleum; Azahar, aceite esencial de; Bitter-Orange Flower Oil; Esencia de Azahar; Essência de Flor de Laranjeira; Oleum Neroli; Orange Flower Oil; Orange-flower Oil.

**Pharmacopoeias.** In *Eur.* (see p.vi).

**Ph. Eur. 5.0** (Bitter-orange-flower Oil). A clear, pale yellow or dark yellow liquid with a characteristic odour reminiscent of bitter-orange flowers, obtained by steam distillation from the fresh flowers of *Citrus aurantium* subsp. *aurantium* (*C. aurantium* subsp. *amara*). Miscible with alcohol, with liquid paraffin, with petroleum spirit, and with fatty oils. Store in well-filled airtight containers. Protect from light and heat.

### Profile

Neroli oil is used as a flavour and in perfumery. Photosensitivity reactions have been reported.

### Preparations

**Proprietary Preparations** (details are given in Part 3)
**Multi-ingredient: Braz.:** Thiodeol†; **Chile:** Agua Melisa Carminativa; **Switz.:** Hygiodermil; Kemeol; Kemerhine†; Oculosan; Seracalm†.

## Nerve Agents

Gases nerviosos.

### Sarin

GB; Sarín. Isopropyl methylphosphonofluoridate.

$C_4H_{10}FO_2P$ = 140.1.

*CAS — 107-44-8.*

### Soman

GD; Somán. Pinacolyl methylphosphonofluoridate.

$C_7H_{16}FO_2P$ = 182.2.

*CAS — 96-64-0.*

### Tabun

GA; Tabún. Ethyl *N*-dimethylphosphoramidocyanidate.

$C_5H_{11}N_2O_2P$ = 162.1.

*CAS — 77-81-6.*

### VX

Methylphosphonothioic acid S-{2-[bis(1-methylethyl)amino]-ethyl} *O*-ethyl ester.

$C_{11}H_{26}NO_2PS$ = 267.4.

*CAS — 50782-69-9.*

### Profile

The nerve agents, sarin, soman, tabun, and VX (also referred to as 'nerve gases') used in chemical warfare are extremely potent inhibitors of cholinesterase. The effects of poisoning due to these agents, and their treatment, are similar to those for organophosphorus insecticides (p.1507) but as the nerve agents have a much greater intrinsic toxicity the symptoms of poisoning are more severe. Pyridostigmine has been administered prophylactically to personnel at risk from exposure to nerve agents (see p.1496).

◊ References.

1. Ministry of Defence. *Medical manual of defence against chemical agents.* London: HMSO, 1987. (JSP312)
2. World MJ. Toxic gas trauma. *Lancet* 1995; **346:** 260–1.
3. Nozaki H, *et al.* A case of VX poisoning and the difference from sarin. *Lancet* 1995; **346:** 698–9.
4. Okumura T, *et al.* Report on 640 victims of the Tokyo subway sarin attack. *Ann Emerg Med* 1996; **28:** 129–35.
5. Suzuki J, *et al.* Eighteen cases exposed to sarin in Matsumoto, Japan. *Intern Med* 1997; **36:** 466–70.
6. Holstege CP, *et al.* Chemical warfare: nerve agent poisoning. *Crit Care Clin* 1997; **13:** 923–42.
7. United States Army. *Medical Management of Chemical Casualties Handbook*, 3rd ed. Aberdeen, Maryland: Medical Research Institute of Chemical Defense; 1999. Also available at: http://www.vnh.org/CHEMCASU/titlepg.html (accessed 17/06/04)
8. Weinbroum AA, *et al.* Anaesthesia and critical care considerations in nerve agent warfare trauma casualties. *Resuscitation* 2000; **47:** 113–23.
9. Anonymous. Prevention and treatment of injury from chemical warfare agents. *Med Lett Drugs Ther* 2002; **44:** 1–3.
10. Janowsky DS. Central anticholinergics to treat nerve-agent poisoning. *Lancet* 2002; **359:** 265–6.
11. Lee EC. Clinical manifestations of sarin nerve gas exposure. *JAMA* 2003; **290:** 659–62.
12. Rotenberg JS, Newmark J. Nerve agent attacks on children: diagnosis and management. *Pediatrics* 2003; **112:** 648–58.

## Neutral Red

CI Basic Red 5; Colour Index No. 50040; Neutral Red Chloride; Nuclear Fast Red; Rojo neutro; Toluylene Red. 3-Amino-7-dimethylamino-2-methylphenazine hydrochloride.

$C_{15}H_{16}N_4$,HCl = 288.8.

*CAS — 553-24-2.*

### Profile

Neutral red is used as an indicator for alkalinity and for preparing neutral-red paper. It is also used as a stain in microscopy.

It is a photoactive dye that has been tried in photodynamic therapy of recurrent herpes simplex infections, but with limited success.

## Niaouli Oil

Essence de Niaouli; Gomenol.

**Pharmacopoeias.** In *It.*

### Profile

Niaouli oil is a volatile oil, obtained by distillation from the fresh leaves of *Melaleuca viridiflora* or *Melaleuca quinquenervia* (Myrtaceae). It contains cineole and has similar actions to eucalyptus oil (p.1686). It is an ingredient of many preparations. Typical indications include respiratory tract congestion. Cajuput oil (p.1664) and melaleuca oil (p.1710) are also prepared from *Melaleuca* spp.

### Preparations

**Proprietary Preparations** (details are given in Part 3)
**Fr.:** Gomenol; Gomenoleo; Huile Gomenolee.
**Multi-ingredient: Arg.:** Aseptobron; Aseptobron Ampicilina; Di-Neumobron; Medex Rub; No-Tos Adultos; Otorinazol; Refenax Caramelos Expectorantes; **Austria:** Biokosma Medizinalbad; Biokosma Red Point-Massagecreme; Expigen; **Braz.:** Algice; Baldin-CE†; Benzotal Balsamico†; Binotine Balsamico†; Canfomenol†; Cortagrip†; Durapen Balsamico†; Gripanil; Gripefago C†; Griponia; Gripsay; Inalobel†; Inatrex Balsamico†; Killgrip; Mentalol†; Optacilin Balsamico†; Ozonyl; Ozonyl Aquoso; Ozonyl Expectorante; Plenogripe†; Pulmogripe†; Soma Balsamico†; Tetrapulmo; **Canad.:** Balminil Suppositories; **Fr.:** Balsolene; Biogaze; Coquelusedal; Coquelusedal Paracetamol; Dinacode; Euvanol†; Gomenol-Syner-Penicilline†; Hexaquine; Terpone; Thiopon Balsamique†; Vapo-Myrtol†; Vaseline Gomenolee; **Ger.:** Palatol; Palatol N†; **Ital.:** Broncopulmin†; Paidorinovit; Rinantipiol; Rinobalsamiche; Rinofomentil; Rinopaidolo; Rinovit; Rinovit Nube†; **Port.:** Creodermol†; Recto Bronco Tosse†; Rectopulmo Adultos; Rectopulmo Infantil; **Spain:** Brisfirina Balsamica†; Broncovital; Bronquimar Vit A†; Bronquimar†; Brota Rectal Bals; Dimayon†; Diminex Balsamico†; Edusan Fte Rectal†; Electopen Balsam Retard†; Etro Balsamico†; Maboterpen†; Pastillas Pectoral Kely; Pulmo Grey Balsam†; Pulmonilo Synergium†; Rinobanedif; Sanaden Reforzado†; Ultrabion Balsamico†; Vapores Pyt; Vitavox Pastillas; Xibornol Prodes†; **Switz.:** Bisolvex†; Demo baume†; Liberol Bain; Pulmex; Resorbane.

## Nicaraven *(rINN)*

Nicaravén. (±)-*N*,*N*′-Propylenebis[nicotinamide].

$C_{15}H_{16}N_4O_2$ = 284.3.

*CAS — 79455-30-4.*

### Profile

Nicaraven is under investigation as a cerebral vasodilator.

## Nicergoline *(BAN, USAN, rINN)*

FI-6714; Nicergolina; Nicergolinum. 10α-Methoxy-1,6-dimethylergolin-8β-ylmethyl 5-bromonicotinate.

$C_{24}H_{26}BrN_3O_3$ = 484.4.

*CAS — 27848-84-6.*
*ATC — C04AE02.*

**Pharmacopoeias.** In *Eur.* (see p.vi).

**Ph. Eur. 5.0** (Nicergoline). A fine to granular white or yellowish powder. It exhibits polymorphism. Practically insoluble in water; soluble in alcohol; freely soluble in dichloromethane.

### Adverse Effects and Precautions

Adverse effects which may occur after nicergoline include gastrointestinal disturbances and, particularly after parenteral administration, hypotension.

**Incidence of adverse effects.** Adverse effects occurred in 25 of 359 patients with cerebrovascular insufficiency treated with nicergoline for 1 month;[1] the drug had to be withdrawn in 11. The reactions included 6 cases of hot flushes, 8 of general malaise, 2 of agitation, 3 of hyperacidity, 1 of nausea, 3 of diarrhoea, and 2 of dizziness and somnolence.

1. Dauverchain J. Bedeutung von Nicergolin bei der symptomatischen Behandlung des arteriellen Hochdrucks und der chronischen, zerebro-vaskulären Insuffizienz. *Arzneimittelforschung* 1979; **29:** 1308–10.

**Porphyria.** Nicergoline is considered to be unsafe in patients with porphyria because it has been shown to be porphyrinogenic in *in-vitro* systems, although there is conflicting evidence of porphyrinogenicity.

### Interactions

◊ For a study indicating that nicergoline enhances the cardiac depressant action of propranolol, see Ergot Derivatives, in Interactions of Beta Blockers, p.871.

### Uses and Administration

Nicergoline is an ergot derivative. It has been used similarly to co-dergocrine mesilate (p.1674) to treat symptoms of mental deterioration associated with cerebrovascular insufficiency (see Dementia, p.1484) and has also been used in peripheral vascular disease (p.831). Nicergoline has been given in doses of up to 60 mg daily by mouth in divided doses, and by intramuscular injection in doses of 2 to 4 mg twice daily; 4 to 8 mg daily has been given by slow intravenous infusion. Nicergoline tartrate has been used in preparations for parenteral administration.

◊ References.


1. Ronchi F, *et al.* Symptomatic treatment of benign prostatic obstruction with nicergoline: a placebo controlled clinical study and urodynamic evaluation. *Urol Res* 1982; **10:** 131–4.
2. Bousquet J, *et al.* Double-blind, placebo-controlled study of nicergoline in the treatment of pruritus in patients receiving maintenance hemodialysis. *J Allergy Clin Immunol* 1989; **83:** 825–8.
3. Saletu B, *et al.* Nicergoline in senile dementia of Alzheimer type and multi-infarct dementia: a double-blind, placebo-controlled, clinical and EEG/ERP mapping study. *Psychopharmacology (Berl)* 1995; **117:** 385–95.
4. Herrmann WM, *et al.* A multicenter randomized double-blind study on the efficacy and safety of nicergoline in patients with multi-infarct dementia. *Dementia Geriatr Cogn Disord* 1997; **8:** 9–17.
5. Fioravanti M, Flicker L. Nicergoline for dementia and other age associated forms of cognitive impairment. Available in The Cochrane Library; Issue 3. Chichester: John Wiley; 2004.


### Preparations

**Proprietary Preparations** (details are given in Part 3)
***Arg.:*** Cergodun; Nicergolent; Sermion; ***Austria:*** Ergotop; Sermion; ***Braz.:*** Sermion; ***Chile:*** Sermion; ***Fr.:*** Sermion; ***Ger.:*** Circo-Maren; duracebrol†; ergobel; Memoq†; Nicergobeta; Nicerium; Sermion; ***Hong Kong:*** Sermion; ***Ital.:*** Cebran; Ergolin†; Neugen†; Nicer; Sermion; ***Mex.:*** Sermion; ***Port.:*** Erg XXI; Sermion; ***Spain:*** Fisifax; Sermion; Varson; ***Switz.:*** Sermion; ***Thai.:*** Sermion.

**Multi-ingredient:** ***Arg.:*** Angiolit; Sibelium Plus.

## Nicotine

Nicotina; Nicotinum. (S)-3-(1-Methylpyrrolidin-2-yl)pyridine.
$C_{10}H_{14}N_2$ = 162.2.
*CAS — 54-11-5.*
*ATC — N07BA01.*

**Description.** Nicotine is a liquid alkaloid obtained from the dried leaves of the tobacco plant, *Nicotiana tabacum* and related species (Solanaceae). Tobacco leaves contain 0.5 to 8% of nicotine combined as malate or citrate.

**Pharmacopoeias.** In *Eur.* (see p.vi) and *US.*

**Ph. Eur. 5.0** (Nicotine). A colourless or brownish, volatile, hygroscopic, viscous liquid. Soluble in water; miscible with dehydrated alcohol. Store under nitrogen in airtight containers. Protect from light.

**USP 27** (Nicotine). It should be stored under nitrogen at a temperature below 25°. Protect from light and moisture.

## Nicotine Polacrilex *(USAN)*

*CAS — 96055-45-7.*
*ATC — N07BA01.*

**Pharmacopoeias.** In *US.*

**USP 27** (Nicotine Polacrilex). A weak carboxylic cation-exchange resin prepared from methacrylic acid and divinylbenzene, in complex with nicotine. Store in airtight containers.

## Nicotine Resinate

*ATC — N07BA01.*

**Pharmacopoeias.** In *Eur.* (see p.vi).

**Ph. Eur. 5.0** (Nicotine Resinate). A complex of nicotine with a weak cationic exchange resin. It may contain glycerol. A white or slightly yellowish powder. Practically insoluble in water. Store in airtight containers. Protect from light.

## Nicotine Tartrate

Nicotine Bitartrate *(USAN).*
$C_{10}H_{14}N_2,2C_4H_6O_6,2H_2O$ = 498.4.
*CAS — 65-31-6 (anhydrous nicotine tartrate).*
*ATC — N07BA01.*

### Dependence and Withdrawal

Nicotine dependence is most commonly associated with cigarette smoking. It is characterised by a strong desire to continue taking the agent, a physical and psychological need for it, and a characteristic abstinence syndrome on withdrawal. Common symptoms seen on nicotine withdrawal include irritability, anxiety, depression, restlessness, poor concentration, increased appetite, weight gain, and insomnia. The management of smoking cessation is discussed under Uses and Administration, below.

Mild withdrawal symptoms have been reported from nicotine replacement preparations used to aid smoking cessation.

◊ References.


1. Hatsukami D, *et al.* Physical dependence on nicotine gum: effect of duration of use. *Psychopharmacology (Berl)* 1993; **111:** 449–56.
2. Benowitz NL, Henningfield JE. Establishing a nicotine threshold for addiction: the implications for tobacco regulation. *N Engl J Med* 1994; **331:** 123–5.
3. Keenan RM, *et al.* Pharmacodynamic effects of cotinine in abstinent cigarette smokers. *Clin Pharmacol Ther* 1994; **55:** 581–90.
4. Slade J, *et al.* Nicotine and addiction: the Brown and Williamson documents. *JAMA* 1995; **274:** 225–33.
5. Kessler DA. Nicotine addiction in young people. *N Engl J Med* 1995; **333:** 186–9.
6. Doll R, Crofton J, eds. Tobacco and health. *Br Med Bull* 1996; **52:** 1–223.
7. Benowitz NL. Nicotine addiction. *Prim Care* 1999; **26:** 611–31.
8. Colby SM, *et al.* Are adolescent smokers dependent on nicotine? A review of the evidence. *Drug Alcohol Depend* 2000; **59** (suppl 1): S83–S95.
9. Royal College of Physicians. *Nicotine addiction in Britain: a report of the Tobacco Advisory Group of the Royal College of Physicians.* London: Royal College of Physicians, 2000. Also available at: http://www.rcplondon.ac.uk/pubs/books/nicotine/index.htm (accessed 02/07/04)
10. West R, *et al.* A comparison of the abuse liability and dependence potential of nicotine patch, gum, spray and inhaler. *Psychopharmacology (Berl)* 2000; **149:** 198–202.


### Adverse Effects and Treatment

Nicotine is a highly toxic substance and in acute poisoning death may occur within minutes due to respiratory failure arising from paralysis of the muscles of respiration. The fatal oral dose of nicotine for an adult is from 40 to 60 mg.

Less severe poisoning causes initial stimulation followed by depression of the autonomic nervous system. Typical symptoms include burning of the mouth and throat, nausea and salivation, abdominal pain, vomiting, diarrhoea, dizziness, weakness, hypertension followed by hypotension, mental confusion, headache, hearing and visual disturbances, dyspnoea, faintness, convulsions, sweating, and prostration. Transient cardiac standstill or paroxysmal atrial fibrillation may occur.

Nicotine is rapidly absorbed through the skin or by inhalation as well as by ingestion and nicotine poisoning may occur due to careless handling when it is used as a horticultural insecticide.

Prompt treatment of nicotine poisoning is essential. If contact was with the skin, contaminated clothing should be removed and the skin washed thoroughly with cold water without rubbing. If the patient has swallowed nicotine, gastric lavage and activated charcoal may be beneficial. Treatment is supportive and includes support of respiration and control of convulsions. Atropine may be used to suppress features of parasympathomimetic stimulation.

Apart from effects such as dizziness, headache, and gastrointestinal disturbances mentioned above, adverse effects associated with *nicotine replacement preparations* have also included cold and flu-like symptoms, palpitations, insomnia, vivid dreams, myalgia, chest pain, blood pressure changes, anxiety, irritability, somnolence, and dysmenorrhoea. Allergic reactions have been reported. Adverse effects associated with specific preparations include skin reactions with transdermal patches; nasal irritation, epistaxis, lachrymation, and sensations in the ear with the nasal spray; throat irritation with the spray, inhalator, sublingual tablets, lozenges, or chewing gum; aphthous ulceration with the inhalator, sublingual tablets, lozenges, or chewing gum; increased salivation and sometimes swelling of the tongue with chewing gum; cough, rhinitis, stomatitis, sinusitis, and dry mouth with the inhalator; and unpleasant taste with the sublingual tablets or lozenges. Excessive swallowing of nicotine released from oral replacement preparations may cause hiccups in the first few days of treatment.

◊ References.


1. Greenland S, *et al.* A meta-analysis to assess the incidence of adverse effects associated with the transdermal nicotine patch. *Drug Safety* 1998; **18:** 297–308.
2. Gourlay SG, *et al.* Predictors and timing of adverse experiences during transdermal nicotine therapy. *Drug Safety* 1999; **20:** 545–55.


**Adverse effects of tobacco products.** Chronic use of tobacco is linked to a variety of diseases. By the mid-1960s, epidemiological data established tobacco smoking as a cause of lung cancer (p.519). Smoking is also associated with cancers of the larynx, mouth, cervix, bladder, pancreas, oesophagus, stomach, and kidneys, and with leukaemia.[1] Smoking is a risk factor in cardiovascular, respiratory, and peripheral and cerebral vascular diseases.[1,2] Smoking also increases the risk of developing peptic ulcer disease and may affect other gastrointestinal disorders.

Maternal smoking in pregnancy is associated with low birth-weight infants and increased risk of abortion, still-birth, and neonatal death (see also Pregnancy under Precautions, below).

Passive smoking refers to inhalation of secondhand tobacco smoke or environmental tobacco smoke. Risks to health from passive exposure are lower than those from active smoking. However, studies have established passive smoking as a cause of lung cancer;[3] passive smoking is also associated with increased risk of heart disease[4] and chronic respiratory disease.[5,6] Smokeless tobacco products also carry risks to health, for example the association of cancers of the head and neck (see p.517) with the use of snuff or chewing tobacco.


1. Wald NJ, Hackshaw AK. Cigarette smoking: an epidemiological overview. *Br Med Bull* 1996; **52:** 3–11.
2. Ashton H. Adverse effects of nicotine. *Adverse Drug React Bull* 1991; **149:** 560–3.
3. Lam TH. Passive smoking in perspective. *Med Toxicol Adverse Drug Exp* 1989; **4:** 153–62.
4. Steenland K. Passive smoking and the risk of heart disease. *JAMA* 1992; **267:** 94–9.
5. Law MR, Hackshaw AK. Environmental tobacco smoke. *Br Med Bull* 1996; **52:** 22–34.
6. DiFranza JR, Lew RA. Mortality and morbidity in children associated with the use of tobacco products by other people. *Pediatrics* 1996; **97:** 560–8.


**Effects on carbohydrate metabolism.** Hyperinsulinaemia and insulin resistance have been associated with long-term use of nicotine gum.[1]


1. Eliasson B, *et al.* Long-term use of nicotine gum is associated with hyperinsulinemia and insulin resistance. *Circulation* 1996; **94:** 878–81.


**Effects on the cardiovascular system.** As mentioned above, nicotine from tobacco products is associated with increased risk of cardiovascular disease. It would not be surprising, therefore, if nicotine replacement preparations were also associated with cardiovascular adverse effects, and there are anecdotal reports of cardiovascular events, including myocardial infarction,[1,2] stroke,[3] and cerebral haematoma,[4] associated with use of such products. However, in studies in patients with cardiovascular disease, 5- or 10-week courses of transdermal nicotine were not associated with an increase in cardiovascular events compared with placebo.[5,6]


1. Warner JG, Little WC. Myocardial infarction in a patient who smoked while wearing a nicotine patch. *Ann Intern Med* 1994; **120:** 695.
2. Arnaot MR. Nicotine patches may not be safe. *BMJ* 1995; **310:** 663–4.
3. Pierce JR. Stroke following application of a nicotine patch. *Ann Pharmacother* 1994; **28:** 402.
4. Riche G, *et al.* Intracerebral haematoma after application of nicotine patch. *Lancet* 1995; **346:** 777–8.
5. Working Group for the Study of Transdermal Nicotine in Patients with Coronary Artery Disease. Nicotine replacement therapy for patients with coronary artery disease. *Arch Intern Med* 1994; **154:** 989–95.
6. Joseph AM, *et al.* The safety of transdermal nicotine as an aid to smoking cessation in patients with cardiac disease. *N Engl J Med* 1996; **335:** 1792–8.


**Vasculitis.** Vasculitis occurring in 2 patients was associated with transdermal nicotine patches.[1]


1. van der Klauw MM, *et al.* Vasculitis attributed to the nicotine patch (Nicotinell). *Br J Dermatol* 1996; **134:** 361–4.


### Precautions

Nicotine preparations should not be used in patients who have experienced recent cerebrovascular accident. They should be used with caution in patients with cardiovascular disease and should be avoided in severe cardiovascular disease, including during the immediate postmyocardial infarction period, and in patients with severe arrhythmias or unstable angina pectoris. They should be used with caution in those with peripheral vascular disease, in endocrine disorders including phaeochromocytoma, hyperthyroidism, and diabetes mellitus, in peptic ulcer disease, or renal or hepatic impairment. Their use is contra-indicated during pregnancy or breast feeding (but see below).

Nicotine preparations should not be used in patients who continue to smoke. Combined use of different preparations is not recommended (but see under Smoking Cessation, below).

Skin patches should not be used on broken skin.

**Breast feeding.** The American Academy of Pediatrics[1] notes that there have been reports of decreased milk production in breast-feeding mothers who smoke, and of decreased weight gain in the infant. There is, however, controversy regarding the effects of nicotine on infant size at 1 year of age. Although nicotine and its metabolite cotinine have been shown to be distributed into breast milk there are hundreds of compounds in tobacco smoke; nicotine is not necessarily the only component that might be detrimental to the breast-fed infant. Nicotine is present in breast milk in concentrations between 1.5 to 3 times the maternal plasma concentration, but there is no evidence documenting whether this amount of nicotine presents a health risk to the infant. Indeed, one study reported that the incidence of acute respiratory illness in infants whose mothers smoked was decreased in those who were breast fed when compared with those infants who were bottle fed.


1. American Academy of Pediatrics. The transfer of drugs and other chemicals into human milk. *Pediatrics* 2001; **108:** 776–89. Correction. *ibid.*; 1029. Also available at: http://aappolicy.aappublications.org/cgi/content/full/pediatrics%3b108/3/776 (accessed 02/07/04)


**Exercise.** Physical exercise increased mean peak plasma concentrations of nicotine in 8 healthy subjects treated with a transdermal nicotine patch.[1] The effect was thought to be most likely due to increased skin perfusion resulting in increased uptake.


1. Klemsdal TO, *et al.* Physical exercise increases plasma concentrations of nicotine during treatment with a nicotine patch. *Br J Clin Pharmacol* 1995; **39:** 677–9.


**Myasthenia gravis.** A patient with myasthenia gravis noted worsening of his symptoms following application of transdermal nicotine patches, the effects being most severe about 1 hour after application, and resolving within 3 hours once the patch was removed.[1] Previous heavy smoking had not produced similar adverse effects, despite the fact that blood-nicotine concentrations are typically higher just after finishing a cigarette than when using the patch.[2]


1. Moreau T, *et al.* Nicotine-sensitive myasthenia gravis. *Lancet* 1994; **344:** 548–9.
2. Pethica D. Nicotine-sensitive myasthenia gravis. *Lancet* 1994; **344:** 961.


**Pregnancy.** Cigarette smoking during pregnancy is associated with an increased risk of low birthweight, spontaneous abortion, and perinatal mortality.[1] There is also some evidence of a possible association between smoking during pregnancy and the sudden infant death syndrome (SIDS).[2] In addition to nicotine, cigarette smoke contains many other chemicals, which are also fetal toxins, including carbon monoxide and lead.[3] Although smoking poses a far greater risk than pure nicotine, nicotine replacement therapy (NRT) is not without potential risks and should be reserved for mothers unable to quit with behavioural therapy alone.[3] It has been suggested that where NRT is required, the intermittent delivery formulations such as nicotine gum or inhalator, which expose the fetus to a lower total dose of nicotine, are preferable to continuous use formulations such as patches.[3]


1. British Medical Association. *Smoking and reproductive life: the impact of smoking on sexual, reproductive and child health.* London: British Medical Association, 2004. Available at: http://www.bma.org/ap.nsf/Content/SmokingReproductiveLife/$file/Smoking.pdf (accessed 02/07/04)
2. Wisborg K, *et al.* A prospective study of smoking during pregnancy and SIDS. *Arch Dis Child* 2000; **83:** 203–6. Corrections. *ibid.* 2001; **84:** 93 and 187.
3. Dempsey DA, Benowitz NL. Risks and benefits of nicotine to aid smoking cessation in pregnancy. *Drug Safety* 2001; **24:** 277–322.


## Interactions

Tobacco smoking induces hepatic metabolic enzymes and the pharmacokinetics of many drugs are altered. Drugs such as methoxsalen which inhibit the cytochrome P450 isoenzyme CYP2A6 may decrease the metabolism of nicotine, resulting in increased plasma concentrations.

◊ References.


1. Miller LG. Cigarettes and drug therapy: pharmacokinetic and pharmacodynamic considerations. *Clin Pharm* 1990; **9:** 125–35.
2. Zevin S, Benowitz NL. Drug interactions with tobacco smoking: an update. *Clin Pharmacokinet* 1999; **36:** 425–38.
3. Sellers EM, *et al.* Inhibition of cytochrome P450 2A6 increases nicotine's oral bioavailability and decreases smoking. *Clin Pharmacol Ther* 2000; **68:** 35–43.


**Nicotinic acid.** As described on p.1441, a possible interaction between nicotinic acid and nicotine from a transdermal patch has been reported.

## Pharmacokinetics

Nicotine is readily absorbed through mucous membranes and the skin; bioavailability of oral nicotine is low due to extensive first-pass metabolism. Nicotine is widely distributed; it crosses the blood-brain barrier and the placenta and is found in breast milk. The elimination half-life is about 1 to 2 hours. Nicotine is metabolised mainly in the liver via the cytochrome P450 isoenzyme CYP2A6 to cotinine and nicotine-*N*-oxide. Nicotine and its metabolites are excreted in the urine.

◊ References.


1. Gorsline J, *et al.* Steady-state pharmacokinetics and dose relationship of nicotine delivered from Nicoderm (nicotine transdermal system). *J Clin Pharmacol* 1993; **33:** 161–8.
2. Gupta SK, *et al.* Bioavailability and absorption kinetics of nicotine following application of a transdermal system. *Br J Clin Pharmacol* 1993; **36:** 221–7.
3. Schneider NG, *et al.* Clinical pharmacokinetics of nasal nicotine delivery: a review and comparison to other nicotine systems. *Clin Pharmacokinet* 1996; **31:** 65–80.
4. Benowitz NL, *et al.* Sources of variability in nicotine and cotinine levels with the use of nicotine nasal spray, transdermal nicotine and cigarette smoking. *Br J Clin Pharmacol* 1997; **43:** 259–67.
5. Zins BJ, *et al.* Pharmacokinetics of nicotine tartrate after single-dose liquid enema, oral, and intravenous administration. *J Clin Pharmacol* 1997; **37:** 426–36.
6. Schneider NG, *et al.* The nicotine inhaler: clinical pharmacokinetics and comparison with other nicotine treatments. *Clin Pharmacokinet* 2001; **40:** 661–84.


## Uses and Administration

The main physiological action of nicotine is paralysis of all autonomic ganglia, preceded by stimulation. Centrally, small doses cause respiratory stimulation, while larger doses produce convulsions and arrest of respiration. The effects on skeletal muscle are similar to those on ganglia.

Nicotine chewing gum, transdermal patches, lozenges, sublingual tablets, nasal spray, or inhalator are used as aids for smoking cessation (below).

- *Chewing gum* is available in strengths of 2 mg and 4 mg; the nicotine may be present in the gum in the form of a complex with methacrylic acid polymer (nicotine polacrilex). Individuals who smoke 20 cigarettes or less per day should start with the 2-mg strength gum chewed slowly over about 30 minutes when the urge to smoke occurs. Those who smoke over 20 cigarettes a day or require more than 15 pieces daily of the 2-mg gum should receive the 4-mg strength. Not more than 15 pieces should be used per day.
- *Sublingual tablets* containing the equivalent of 2 mg of nicotine as a β-cyclodextrin complex may also be used: the recommended dose is 1 or 2 tablets sublingually every hour, increased to a maximum of 40 tablets daily if necessary, for at least 3 months. The dose should then be gradually reduced until it can be withdrawn.
- *Lozenges* containing 1 or 2 mg of nicotine (as the polacrilex or as the tartrate) are also available. The initial dose is 1 lozenge every 1 to 2 hours increased to a maximum daily dose of 30 of the 1-mg lozenges or 15 of the 2-mg lozenges. Treatment should continue for at least 3 months, after which the dose should be gradually reduced and then withdrawn.
- Adhesive *transdermal patches* are designed to be worn for 16 or 24 hours and are available in different strengths that deliver from 5 to 21 mg during the recommended wearing time. One patch should be applied daily, on waking, to a dry, non-hairy area of skin on the hip, trunk, or upper arm, usually beginning with the highest strength or with a dose determined by the previous daily consumption of cigarettes. A different site of application should be used each day with several days elapsing before the patch is applied to the same area of skin. Treatment is usually withdrawn gradually by reducing the dose every 2 to 8 weeks.
- A suggested initial dosage for a *nasal spray* containing 500 micrograms per spray is one spray administered into each nostril up to twice hourly as required up to a maximum of 80 sprays daily for the first 8 weeks and reduced gradually thereafter. Treatment for more than 3 months is not recommended.
- Nicotine *inhalator cartridges* contain nicotine 10 mg for use in an appropriate inhaler mouthpiece. The initial dose is 6 to 16 cartridges daily for up to 12 weeks and is reduced gradually over a further 6 to 12 weeks.

It has been recommended that the use of nicotine therapy for smoking cessation should be reviewed if abstinence has not been achieved in 3 months and that the total treatment period should not exceed 6 months.

Nicotine has been used as a horticultural insecticide.

**Alzheimer's disease.** The use of nicotine as a cholinergic agonist is one of a number of methods being studied[1] to overcome brain cholinergic deficits in patients with Alzheimer's disease (see Dementia, p.1484). Preliminary studies[2,3] using nicotine patches have been of limited duration and were inconclusive. Transdermal nicotine has been used for the control of behavioural symptoms such as agitation in a small number of patients with Alzheimer's disease.[4] A systematic review[5] was unable to present any conclusions on the efficacy and safety of nicotine in Alzheimer's disease because of a lack of adequate randomised controlled trials.


1. Baldinger SL, Schroeder DJ. Nicotine therapy in patients with Alzheimer's disease. *Ann Pharmacother* 1995; **29:** 314–15.
2. Wilson AL, *et al.* Nicotine patches in Alzheimer's disease: pilot study on learning, memory, and safety. *Pharmacol Biochem Behav* 1995; **51:** 509–14.
3. Snaedal J, *et al.* The effects of nicotine in dermal plaster on cognitive functions in patients with Alzheimer's disease. *Dementia* 1996; **7:** 47–52.
4. Rosin RA, *et al.* Transdermal nicotine for agitation in dementia. *Am J Geriatr Psychiatry* 2001; **9:** 443–4.
5. López-Arrieta JLA, Sanz FJ. Nicotine for Alzheimer's disease. Available in The Cochrane Library; Issue 2. Chichester: John Wiley; 2004.


**Blepharospasm.** Nicotine nasal spray was reported to be of benefit in a patient with blepharospasm (p.1390) refractory to botulinum A toxin.[1] However, a subsequent study in 4 patients with blepharospasm reported no improvement with the use of nicotine nasal spray.[2]


1. Dursun SM, *et al.* Treatment of blepharospasm with nicotine nasal spray. *Lancet* 1996; **348:** 60.
2. Dressler D, *et al.* Nicotine nasal spray is not reliable treatment for blepharospasm: results of a pilot study. *Mov Disord* 1998; **13:** 190.


**Extrapyramidal disorders.** Nicotine transdermal patches have been reported to produce beneficial effects[1] in schizophrenic patients with antipsychotic-induced akathisia (p.677).


1. Anfang MK, Pope HG. Treatment of neuroleptic-induced akathisia with nicotine patches. *Psychopharmacology (Berl)* 1997; **134:** 153–6.


**Skin disorders.** There have been anecdotal reports of nicotine producing beneficial effects in various skin disorders, including pyoderma gangrenosum,[1] and dermatitis due to fluorouracil therapy.[2]


1. Kanekura T, *et al.* Nicotine for pyoderma gangrenosum. *Lancet* 1995; **345:** 1058.
2. Kingsley EC. 5-Fluorouracil dermatitis prophylaxis with a nicotine patch. *Ann Intern Med* 1994; **120:** 813.


**Smoking cessation.** Smoking is the single most important cause of preventable illness and premature death in the UK and USA; it is estimated that around 1 in 5 deaths are due to smoking-related illnesses. The financial burden of smoking-related diseases on health care providers is also substantial. Many governments have undertaken initiatives to promote smoking cessation.

Nicotine dependence and the development of a characteristic withdrawal syndrome (see Dependence and Withdrawal, above) make stopping smoking very difficult. Many individuals relapse when trying to give up or need several attempts before successfully stopping. Both nonpharmacological and pharmacological treatments can improve the abstinence rate and are most effective when the two approaches are combined.[1-8]

Nonpharmacological methods include counselling, training in coping skills, and support groups; although the abstinence rate increases with the intensity of the support, even brief advice is effective in encouraging cessation.

The first-line pharmacological intervention is *nicotine replacement therapy* (NRT) which is an effective treatment for reducing the cravings associated with stopping smoking. NRT is available in numerous formulations: chewing gum, transdermal patches, inhalators, and nasal spray and, more recently, sublingual tablets and lozenges. A systematic review[8] of NRT found abstinence was approximately doubled when compared with controls, regardless of the intensity of any additional nonpharmacological support.

Choice of formulation is based on patient preference, tolerance, and previous treatments, if any. The transdermal patch is easiest to use and compliance is greatest with this route but local effects may be troublesome. The gum has an unpleasant taste initially and some find the chewing action difficult. The sublingual tablet may be useful for those who have difficulty chewing the gum. The nasal spray has a fast onset of action but may cause local irritation. The inhalator has the advantage of simulating cigarette smoking but may cause local irritation of the mouth and throat. The lozenge has the advantage that it can be sucked discreetly. Patients who are unable to tolerate one type of NRT may benefit from a course of an alternative NRT preparation.

Combination therapy with different types of NRT (patches with either the nasal spray, inhalator, or chewing gum) has also been tried as a means of increasing efficacy although combination therapy is not recommended by the manufacturers of NRT preparations.

NRT is usually continued for about 3 months before being withdrawn. Although the manufacturers advise gradual withdrawal, others[4,6] have found that this offers no advantage and recommend abrupt withdrawal. NRT has also been used long-term and may be of particular benefit in those patients who feel they would relapse if NRT was stopped or in those who have persistent withdrawal symptoms.

There has been concern over the use of NRT in patients with cardiovascular disease (see Effects on the Cardiovascular System, p.1720) but clinical experience and studies have shown that NRT can be used with caution in these patients. The use of NRT in those who have suffered a recent myocardial infarction or those with severe arrhythmias or unstable angina is, however, contra-indicated as such patients have not been adequately studied.

A number of other drugs have also been used to achieve abstinence from smoking. *Bupropion* is effective and recommended by some as a first-line alternative to NRT; its action is said to be independent of its antidepressant activity. Bupropion in combination with NRT has been used successfully. *Clonidine* is also effective but adverse effects limit its usefulness and it is reserved as a second-line treatment. The antidepressant *nortriptyline* is another second-line drug. Preliminary investigations suggest that *selegiline* may also be effective. There is little or no evidence to support the efficacy of other treatments such as *silver acetate, mecamylamine, lobeline*, or *anxiolytics* such as *buspirone*, and their use is not recommended. A *vaccine* for the prevention of smoking relapse is under investigation.


1. American Society of Health-System Pharmacists. ASHP therapeutic position statement on smoking cessation. *Am J Health-Syst Pharm* 1999; **56:** 460–4. Also available at: http://www.ashp.org/bestpractices/tps/Therapeutic%20Position%20Statement%20Smoking%20Cessation.pdf (accessed 02/07/04)
2. Anonymous. Nicotine replacement to aid smoking cessation. *Drug Ther Bull* 1999; **37:** 52–4.
3. West R, *et al.* Smoking cessation guidelines for health professionals: an update. *Thorax* 2000; **55:** 987–99.
4. Royal College of Physicians. *Nicotine addiction in Britain: a report of the Tobacco Advisory Group of the Royal College of Physicians.* London: Royal College of Physicians, 2000. Also available at: http://www.rcplondon.ac.uk/pubs/books/nicotine/index.htm (accessed 02/07/04)
5. Fiore MC, *et al.* A clinical practice guideline for treating tobacco use and dependence: a US public health service report. *JAMA* 2000; **283:** 3244–54.
6. Simpson D. Smoking cessation. In: *Doctors and tobacco: medicine's big challenge.* London: Tobacco Control Resource Centre, British Medical Association, 2000. Available at: http://www.bma.org.uk/tcrc.nsf/ (accessed 02/07/04)
7. Covey LS, *et al.* Advances in non-nicotine pharmacotherapy for smoking cessation. *Drugs* 2000; **59:** 17–31.
8. Silagy C, *et al.* Nicotine replacement therapy for smoking cessation. Available in The Cochrane Library; Issue 2. Chichester: John Wiley; 2004.


**Spasticity.** There have been anecdotal reports[1] of beneficial responses to nicotine in spastic dystonia.


1. Vaughan CJ, *et al.* Treatment of spastic dystonia with transdermal nicotine. *Lancet* 1997; **350:** 565.


**Tics.** Tourette's syndrome (see Tics, p.664) is characterised by motor and vocal tics and behavioural disturbances. Nicotine[1-5] has been reported to be of benefit when used alone or with the more usual treatment of haloperidol in patients with Tourette's syndrome whose symptoms were not satisfactorily controlled with haloperidol alone. It is hoped that the use of transdermal nicotine patches will avoid the reported problems of compliance associated with the taste and gastrointestinal effects of nicotine gum.


1. McConville BJ, *et al.* The effects of nicotine plus haloperidol compared to nicotine only and placebo nicotine only in reducing tic severity and frequency to Tourette's disorder. *Biol Psychiatry* 1992; **31:** 832–40.

2. Silver AA, Sanberg PR. Transdermal nicotine patch and potentiation of haloperidol in Tourette's syndrome. *Lancet* 1993; **342:** 182.
3. Dursun SM, *et al.* Longlasting improvement of Tourette's syndrome with transdermal nicotine. *Lancet* 1994; **344:** 1577.
4. Sanberg PR, *et al.* Nicotine for the treatment of Tourette's syndrome. *Pharmacol Ther* 1997; **74:** 21–5.
5. Silver AA, *et al.* Transdermal nicotine and haloperidol in Tourette's disorder: a double-blind placebo-controlled study. *J Clin Psychiatry* 2001; **62:** 707–14.

**Ulcerative colitis.** Investigation of the use of nicotine in ulcerative colitis (see Inflammatory Bowel Disease, p.1243) has been prompted by the observation that this condition is rare in smokers.[1] Results from 2 studies[2,3] suggested that transdermal nicotine added to conventional therapy could improve symptoms in active disease. However another study[4] found that transdermal nicotine was no more effective than placebo in maintaining disease remission. Some consider[5] that the adverse effects of nicotine are likely to limit its use in some patients, particularly those who have never smoked. Local delivery to the colon, in the form of enemas[6] and oral modified-release capsules,[7] is under investigation as a means of reducing the adverse effects of nicotine.

1. Guslandi M. Nicotine treatment for ulcerative colitis. *Br J Clin Pharmacol* 1999; **48:** 481–4.
2. Pullan RD, *et al.* Transdermal nicotine for active ulcerative colitis. *N Engl J Med* 1994; **330:** 811–15.
3. Sandborn WJ, *et al.* Transdermal nicotine for mildly to moderately active ulcerative colitis: a randomized, double-blind, placebo-controlled trial. *Ann Intern Med* 1997; **126:** 364–71.
4. Thomas GAO, *et al.* Transdermal nicotine as maintenance therapy for ulcerative colitis. *N Engl J Med* 1995; **332:** 988–92.
5. Rhodes J, Thomas G. Nicotine treatment in ulcerative colitis. *Drugs* 1995; **49:** 157–60.
6. Sandborn WJ, *et al.* Nicotine tartrate liquid enemas for mildly to moderately active left-sided ulcerative colitis unresponsive to first-line therapy: a pilot study. *Aliment Pharmacol Ther* 1997; **11:** 663–71.
7. Green JT, *et al.* An oral formulation of nicotine for release and absorption in the colon: its development and pharmacokinetics. *Br J Clin Pharmacol* 1999; **48:** 485–93.

### Preparations

***USP 27:*** Nicotine Polacrilex Gum; Nicotine Transdermal System.

**Proprietary Preparations** (details are given in Part 3)
***Arg.:*** Nicorette; Nicotinell TTS; ***Austral.:*** Nicabate; Nicorette; Nicotinell; QuitX; ***Austria:*** Nicolan†; Nicorette; Nicotinell; Nicotrol; ***Belg.:*** Nicorette; Nicotinell; NiQuitin; ***Braz.:*** Nicolan†; Nicorette†; Nicotinell TTS; NiQuitin†; ***Canad.:*** Habitrol; Nicoderm; Nicorette; Nicotrol; Prostep; ***Chile:*** Nicorette; Nicotinell; ***Denm.:*** Nicorette; Nicotinell; NiQuitin; ***Fin.:*** Nicorette; Nicotinell; ***Fr.:*** Nicogum; Nicopatch; Nicorette; Nicotinell; NiQuitin; ***Ger.:*** Nicorette; Nicotinell; nikofrenon; NiQuitin; ***Hong Kong:*** Nicorette; Nicotinell; ***India:*** Nicotinell TTS; ***Irl.:*** Niconil†; Nicorette; Nicotinell; NiQuitin; ***Israel:*** Nicorette; Nicotinell; NiQuitin; ***Ital.:*** Nicorette; Nicotinell TTS; Nicotrans†; ***Malaysia:*** Nicorette; Nicotinell; ***Mex.:*** Nicorette†; Nicotinell TTS; NiQuitin; ***Neth.:*** Nicorette; Nicotinell; ***Norw.:*** Nicorette; Nicotinell; ***NZ:*** Nicabate; Nicorette; Nicotinell; Nicotrol; ***Port.:*** Nicorette; Nicotinell TTS; ***S.Afr.:*** Nicorette; Nicotinell TTS†; Quit; ***Singapore:*** Nicorette; Nicotinell; ***Spain:*** Nicodisc†; Nicomax; Nicorette; Nicotinell; Nicotrans†; Nicotrol; ***Swed.:*** Nicolan†; Nicorette; Nicotinell; Nikotugg; NiQuitin; ***Switz.:*** Nicorette; Nicostop TTS†; Nicotinell; ***Thai.:*** Nicorette; Nicotinell; ***UK:*** Nicorette; Nicotinell; NiQuitin; Stoppers†; ***USA:*** Commit; Habitrol; Nicoderm; Nicorette; Nicotrol; Prostep.

**Multi-ingredient: *UK:*** Resolution†.

## Nitisinone *(USAN, rINN)*

NTBC; SC-0735. 2-(α,α,α-Trifluoro-2-nitro-*p*-toluoyl)-1,3-cyclohexanedione.

$C_{14}H_{10}F_3NO_5$ = 329.2.

*CAS — 104206-65-7.*

*ATC — A16AX04.*

### Profile

Nitisinone is a 4-hydroxyphenylpyruvate dioxygenase inhibitor that is used in the management of hereditary tyrosinaemia. It has also been tried in alkaptonuria, another hereditary metabolic disorder.

◊ References.

1. Holme E, Lindstedt S. Tyrosinaemia type I and NTBC (2-(2-nitro-4-trifluoromethylbenzoyl)-1,3-cyclohexanedione). *J Inherit Metab Dis* 1998; **21:** 507–17.
2. Ros J, *et al.* NTBC as palliative treatment in chronic tyrosinaemia type I. *J Inherit Metab Dis* 1999; **22:** 665–6.
3. Phornphutkul C, *et al.* Natural history of alkaptonuria. *N Engl J Med* 2002; **347:** 2111–21.
4. Gissen P, *et al.* Ophthalmic follow-up of patients with tyrosinaemia type I on NTBC. *J Inherit Metab Dis* 2003; **26:** 13–16.

## Nitric Acid

Acidum Nitricum; Aqua Fortis; Azotic Acid; Nit. Acid; Nítrico, ácido; Salpetersäure.

$HNO_3$ = 63.01.

*CAS — 7697-37-2.*

**Pharmacopoeias.** In *Eur.* (see p.vi) (68 to 70%) and *Pol.* (10%). Also in *USNF* (69 to 71%).

**Ph. Eur. 5.0** (Nitric Acid). A clear, colourless to almost colourless liquid. Miscible with water. It contains 68.0 to 70.0% w/w of $HNO_3$. Protect from light.

**USNF 22** (Nitric Acid). A highly corrosive fuming liquid, having a characteristic, highly irritating odour. It contains 69.0 to 71.0% w/w of $HNO_3$. Store in airtight containers.

### Adverse Effects and Treatment

As for Hydrochloric Acid, p.1699.

There may be methaemoglobinaemia. Nitric acid stains the skin yellow.

**Effects on the respiratory system.** Respiratory failure due to pulmonary oedema occurred in a 56-year-old man after inhaling nitric acid which he had used as a metal cleaner.[1] The man died despite extensive ventilatory support.

1. Bur A, *et al.* Fatal pulmonary edema after nitric acid inhalation. *Resuscitation* 1997; **35:** 33–6.

### Uses and Administration

Nitric acid has a powerful corrosive action and has been used to remove warts (p.1139), but it should be applied with caution, and less corrosive substances are available. It has also been used for the removal of tattoos.

### Preparations

**Proprietary Preparations** (details are given in Part 3)

**Multi-ingredient: *Ger.:*** Solco-Derman; ***Hong Kong:*** Solcoderm; ***Malaysia:*** Solcoderm; ***Switz.:*** Solcoderm; Solcogyn.

## Nitrobenzene

Nitrobenceno; Nitrobenzol; Oil of Mirbane.

$C_6H_5NO_2$ = 123.1.

*CAS — 98-95-3.*

### Adverse Effects

Nitrobenzene is highly toxic and the ingestion of 1 g may be fatal. Poisoning may occur from absorption through the skin, by inhalation, or by ingestion. Toxic effects are usually delayed for several hours and may include nausea, prostration, burning headache, methaemoglobinaemia with cyanosis, haemolytic anaemia, vomiting (with characteristic odour), convulsions, and coma, ending in death after a few hours.

### Treatment of Adverse Effects

After ingestion of nitrobenzene the stomach should be emptied. Methaemoglobinaemia may be treated with methylthioninium chloride. Blood transfusions or haemodialysis may be necessary. Oxygen should be given if cyanosis is severe.

If the skin or eyes are splashed with nitrobenzene, contaminated clothing should be removed immediately and the affected areas washed thoroughly with water at room temperature for at least 15 minutes.

### Uses

Nitrobenzene is used in the manufacture of aniline, as a preservative in polishes, and in perfumery and soaps.

## Nizofenone *(rINN)*

Nizofenona; Y-9179. 2′-Chloro-2-[2-[(diethylamino)methyl]imidazol-1-yl]-5-nitrobenzophenone.

$C_{21}H_{21}ClN_4O_3$ = 412.9.

*CAS — 54533-85-6.*

*ATC — N06BX10.*

### Profile

Nizofenone has been investigated for its nootropic actions.

## Nucleic Acid

Acide Zymonucléique; Acidum Nucleicum; Nucleico, ácido; Nucleinic Acid.

### Profile

Nucleic acids are a complex mixture of phosphorus-containing organic acids present in living cells. Nucleic acids are of 2 types, ribonucleic acids (RNA, see p.1738) and deoxyribonucleic acids (DNA, see p.1679). They are composed of chains of nucleotides (phosphate esters of purine or pyrimidine bases and pentose sugars).

Since the administration of nucleic acid gives rise to a marked temporary leucocytosis (usually preceded by a short period of leucopenia) it was formerly given in the treatment of a variety of bacterial infections in the hope of enhancing the natural defence mechanisms. Its therapeutic value, however, was never established.

### Preparations

**Proprietary Preparations** (details are given in Part 3)
***India:*** Nulip.

## Nutmeg

Muscade; Myristica; Noz Moscada; Nuez Moscada; Nuez moscada; Nux Moschata.

**Description.** Nutmeg consists of the dried kernels of the seeds of *Myristica fragrans* (Myristicaceae), containing not less than 5% v/w of volatile oil; the powdered drug contains not less than 4% v/w. Mace (see Mace Oil, p.1708) is the dried arillus of the seed of *M. fragrans*.

**Pharmacopoeias.** In *Chin.*

### Adverse Effects

Nutmeg, taken in large doses, may cause nausea and vomiting, flushing, dry mouth, tachycardia, stimulation of the CNS possibly with epileptiform convulsions, miosis or occasionally mydriasis, euphoria, and hallucinations. Myristicin and elimicin are thought to be the constituents responsible for the psychotic effects of nutmeg, possibly following metabolism to amfetamine-like compounds.

◊ Some references to the adverse effects of nutmeg.

1. Panayotopoulos DJ, Chisholm DD. Hallucinogenic effect of nutmeg. *BMJ* 1970; **1:** 754.
2. Venables GS, *et al.* Nutmeg poisoning. *BMJ* 1976; **1:** 96.
3. Dietz WH, Stuart MJ. Nutmeg and prostaglandins. *N Engl J Med* 1976; **294:** 503.
4. Faguet RA, Rowland KF. "Spice cabinet" intoxication. *Am J Psychiatry* 1978; **135:** 860–1.
5. Abernethy MK, Becker LB. Acute nutmeg intoxication. *Am J Emerg Med* 1992; **10:** 429–30.
6. Brenner N, *et al.* Chronic nutmeg psychosis. *J R Soc Med* 1993; **86:** 179–80.
7. Quin GI, *et al.* Nutmeg intoxication. *J Accid Emerg Med* 1998; **15:** 287–8.
8. Sangalli BC, Chiang W. Toxicology of nutmeg abuse. *J Toxicol Clin Toxicol* 2000; **38:** 671–8.
9. Stein U, *et al.* Nutmeg (myristicin) poisoning—report on a fatal case and a series of cases recorded by a poison information centre. *Forensic Sci Int* 2001; **118:** 87–90.

### Uses and Administration

Nutmeg is the source of nutmeg oil (below). It is aromatic and carminative and is used as a flavour. Nutmeg has been reported to inhibit prostaglandin synthesis.

It is used in homoeopathic medicine.

### Preparations

**Proprietary Preparations** (details are given in Part 3)

**Multi-ingredient: *Austria:*** Mariazeller; ***Ger.:*** Doppelherz Melissengeist; Melissengeist; ***Spain:*** Agua del Carmen; ***UK:*** Aluminium Free Indigestion†; Melissa Comp..

## Nutmeg Oil

Ätherisches Muskatöl; Esencia de Nuez Moscada; Essence de Muscade; Essência de Moscada; Myristica Oil; Myristicae Fragrantis Aetheroleum; Nuez moscada, aceite esencial de; Oleum Myristicae.

**Pharmacopoeias.** In *Eur.* (see p.vi).

**Ph. Eur. 5.0** (Nutmeg Oil). The oil obtained by steam distillation of the dried and crushed kernels of *Myristica fragrans*. A colourless to pale yellow liquid with a spicy odour. Store in well-filled, airtight containers. Protect from light and heat.

### Profile

Nutmeg oil is aromatic and carminative and is used as a flavour. Nutmeg oil and expressed nutmeg oil, a solid fat, are rubefacient.

### Preparations

***BP 2003:*** Aromatic Ammonia Spirit.

**Proprietary Preparations** (details are given in Part 3)

**Multi-ingredient: *Austral.:*** Vicks Vaporub†; ***Austria:*** Emser Nasensalbe; Expectal-Balsam; Melissengeist; Pe-Ce; Wick Vaporub; ***Belg.:*** Vicks Vaporub; ***Braz.:*** Vick Vaporub; ***Canad.:*** Vaporizing Ointment; ***Chile:*** Agua Melisa Carminativa; ***Fr.:*** Vegebom; Vicks Vaporub; ***Ger.:*** Emser Nasensalbe N; ***NZ:*** Vicks Vaporub; ***S.Afr.:*** Enterodyne; ***Swed.:*** Vicks Vaporub; ***Switz.:*** Roliwol†; Vicks Vaporub N; ***Thai.:*** Tiffyrub; ***UK:*** Dragon Balm; No-Sor Vapour Rub; Nowax.

## Nux Vomica

Brechnuss; Noce Vomica; Noix Vomique; Nuez vómica; Strychni Semen.

*CAS — 357-57-3 (anhydrous brucine).*

**Pharmacopoeias.** In *Chin.* and *Jpn.*

### Profile

Nux vomica consists of the dried ripe seeds of *Strychnos nux-vomica* (Loganiaceae). It has the actions of strychnine (see p.1750). As well as containing strychnine, nux vomica contains brucine which has similar properties.

Nux vomica (Nux vom.) is used in herbal and homoeopathic medicine for a wide variety of disorders including those of digestion or debility. Ignatia, the dried seed of *Strychnos ignatii*, is also used in homoeopathic medicine where it is known as Ignatia amara or Iamara.

### Preparations

**Proprietary Preparations** (details are given in Part 3)
***Braz.:*** Cessagripe†.

**Multi-ingredient: *Belg.:*** Aperop†; Sanicolax†; ***Braz.:*** Estomafitino†; Fargestium†; Gotas Digestivas; Kola Fosfatada Soel†; ***Chile:*** Fenokomp 39; Fenolftaleina Compuesta; Homeofortin III; ***Fr.:*** Curoveinyl†; ***Ital.:*** Lassatina; ***Mex.:*** Bigenol; ***Spain:*** Alofedina; ***Switz.:*** Padma-Lax; ***Thai.:*** Flatulence Gastulence.

## Oak Bark

Common Oak; Corteza de roble; Durmast Oak; Écorce de Chêne; Eichenrinde; Quercus; Quercus Cortex.

**Pharmacopoeias.** In *Eur.* (see p.vi) and *Pol.*

**Ph. Eur. 5.0** (Oak Bark). The cut and dried bark from the fresh young branches of *Quercus robur*, *Q. petraea*, and *Q. pubescens*. It contains a minimum of 3.0% of tannins, expressed as pyrogallol, calculated with reference to the dried drug.

### Profile

Oak bark contains quercitannic acid. It has astringent properties and is used in some herbal and homoeopathic preparations for a variety of disorders. It was formerly used for haemorrhoids and as a gargle.

### Preparations

**Proprietary Preparations** (details are given in Part 3)
***Ger.:*** Traxaton; ***Hong Kong:*** Urocalun; ***Singapore:*** Urocalun; ***USA:*** Amerigel.

**Multi-ingredient:** ***Austria:*** Menodoron; ***Fr.:*** Tisanes de l'Abbe Hamon no 14†; ***Ger.:*** Tonsilgon; ***Spain:*** Natusor Astringel; ***Switz.:*** Kernosan Elixir; ***UK:*** Peerless Composition Essence; ***USA:*** Amerigel.

## Octanoic Acid *(USAN, rINN)*

Ácido octanoico; Acidum Caprylicum; Caprylic Acid.

$CH_3.(CH_2)_6.CO_2H = 144.2.$

*CAS — 124-07-2.*

**Pharmacopoeias.** In *Eur.* (see p.vi).
**Ph. Eur. 5.0** (Caprylic Acid; Octanoic Acid BP 2003). A clear, colourless or slightly yellowish, oily liquid. Very slightly soluble in water; very soluble in alcohol and in acetone. It dissolves in dilute solutions of alkali hydroxides.

## Sodium Octanoate

Natrii Caprylas; Octanoato sódico; Sodium Caprylate.

$C_8H_{15}NaO_2 = 166.2.$

*CAS — 1984-06-1.*

**Pharmacopoeias.** In *Eur.* (see p.vi).
**Ph. Eur. 5.0** (Sodium Caprylate). A white crystalline powder. Very soluble or freely soluble in water; sparingly soluble in alcohol; freely soluble in acetic acid; practically insoluble in acetone. A 10% solution in water has a pH of 8.0 to 10.5.

### Profile

Octanoic acid and its salts have antifungal activity.

Sodium octanoate is used to stabilise albumin solution against the effects of heat. Octanoic acid labelled with carbon-13 has been used in a breath test to measure gastric emptying.

### Preparations

**Proprietary Preparations** (details are given in Part 3)
***Canad.:*** Capricin†.

**Multi-ingredient:** ***Austral.:*** Caprilate†.

## Olaquindox *(BAN, rINN)*

Bay-Va-9391. 2-(2-Hydroxyethylcarbamoyl)-3-methylquinoxaline 1,4-dioxide.

$C_{12}H_{13}N_3O_4 = 263.2.$

*CAS — 23696-28-8.*

### Profile

Olaquindox is an antibacterial added to animal feedstuffs as a growth promotor. Photoallergic reactions in animal handlers have been reported following exposure to olaquindox.

## Oleander

Adelfa; Common Oleander; Oleanderblätter; Oleandri Folium; Rose Bay.

### Profile

Oleander is the dried leaves of the shrub *Nerium oleander* (Apocynaceae), which contain cardioactive glycosides, including oleandrin. It has been used in the treatment of heart disorders. The flowers and bark have been used similarly. Toxicity, similar to that seen with digoxin, may occur following ingestion of any part of the plant; fatalities have been reported. Yellow oleander (*Thevetia peruviana*) also contains cardiac glycosides and exhibits similar toxicity to oleander.

Oleander has also been used in homoeopathic medicine.

**Treatment of adverse effects.** References to the treatment of oleander poisoning or yellow oleander poisoning.


1. Shumaik GM, *et al.* Oleander poisoning: treatment with digoxin-specific Fab antibody fragments. *Ann Emerg Med* 1988; **17:** 732–5.
2. Safadi R, *et al.* Beneficial effect of digoxin-specific Fab antibody fragments in oleander intoxication. *Arch Intern Med* 1995; **155:** 2121–5.
3. Eddleston M, *et al.* Anti-digoxin Fab fragments in cardiotoxicity induced by ingestion of yellow oleander: a randomised controlled trial. *Lancet* 2000; **355:** 967–72.
4. Fonseka MM, *et al.* Yellow oleander poisoning in Sri Lanka: outcome in a secondary care hospital. *Hum Exp Toxicol* 2002; **21:** 293–5.
5. de Silva HA, *et al.* Multiple-dose activated charcoal for treatment of yellow oleander poisoning: a single-blind, randomised, placebo-controlled trial. *Lancet* 2003; **361:** 1935–8.


### Preparations

**Proprietary Preparations** (details are given in Part 3)
**Multi-ingredient:** ***Ger.:*** Miroton.

## Olive Oil

Aceite de oliva; Azeite; Olivae Oleum.

**Pharmacopoeias.** In *Jpn.* Also in *USNF.*
*Eur.* (see p.vi) includes monographs for virgin olive oil and refined olive oil. *Eur.* also includes olive leaf.
**Ph. Eur. 5.0** (Olive Oil, Virgin; Olivae Oleum Virginale). The fatty oil obtained by cold expression or other suitable mechanical means from the ripe drupes of *Olea europaea*. It is a clear, yellow or greenish-yellow, transparent liquid with a characteristic odour. When cooled it begins to become cloudy at 10° and becomes a butter-like mass at 0°. Practically insoluble in alcohol; miscible with petroleum spirit (50° to 70°). Store in well-filled containers at a temperature not exceeding 25°. Protect from light.
**Ph. Eur. 5.0** (Olive Oil, Refined; Olivae Oleum Raffinatum). The fatty oil obtained by refining of crude olive oil. A suitable antioxidant may be added. It is a clear, colourless, or greenish-yellow, transparent liquid. When cooled it begins to become cloudy at 10° and becomes a butter-like mass at about 0°. Practically insoluble in alcohol; miscible with petroleum spirit (50° to 70°). Store in well-filled containers at a temperature not exceeding 25°. Protect from light. Store under an inert gas if intended for use in the manufacture of parenteral dosage forms.
**USNF 22** (Olive Oil). The fixed oil obtained from the ripe fruits of *Olea europaea* (Oleaceae). It is a pale yellow, or light greenish-yellow, oily liquid, having a slight characteristic odour. Slightly soluble in alcohol; miscible with carbon disulfide, with chloroform, and with ether. Store in airtight containers at a temperature not exceeding 40°.

### Profile

When taken internally, olive oil is nutrient, demulcent, and mildly laxative. It may also be given rectally (100 to 500 mL warmed to about 32°) to soften impacted faeces (p.1240).

Externally, olive oil is emollient and soothing to inflamed surfaces, and is employed to soften the skin and crusts in eczema (p.1135) and psoriasis (p.1137), and as a lubricant for massage. It is used to soften ear wax (p.1262).

Olive oil is used in the preparation of liniments, ointments, plasters, and soaps; it is also used as a vehicle for oily suspensions for injection.

Epidemiological evidence points to the cardiovascular benefits of olive oil in the diet. An extract of olive leaves has been promoted as a dietary supplement and herbal medicine.

### Preparations

***BP 2003:*** Olive Oil Ear Drops.

**Proprietary Preparations** (details are given in Part 3)
**Multi-ingredient:** ***Arg.:*** Calculina; Clinoleic; ***Austral.:*** Gold Cross BOZ Ointment; ***Austria:*** Clinoleic; ***Belg.:*** Clinoleic†; ***Braz.:*** Quelodin; Steitonit†; ***Denm.:*** Clinoleic; ***Fin.:*** Clinoleic; ***Fr.:*** Clinoleic; Oliclinomel; ***Ger.:*** Baran-mild N†; Befelka-Oel; Clinoleic; Dr. Hotz Vollbad†; ***Gr.:*** Clinoleic; ***Israel:*** Clinoleic; ***Ital.:*** Clinoleic; Prexene†; ***Mex.:*** Clinoleic; ***NZ:*** Snorenz; ***Spain:*** Aceite Acalorico; Clinoleic; Natusor High Blood Pressure; Oliclinomel; Tensiben; ***Swed.:*** Clinoleic; ***Switz.:*** Clinoleic; ***UK:*** Clinoleic; Exzem Oil†; OlioClinomel; Snor-Away; Snorenz†.

## Ololiuqui

*CAS — 2889-26-1 (isoergine); 478-94-4 (ergine); 2390-99-0 (chanoclavine); 548-43-6 (elymoclavine); 602-85-7 (lysergol).*

### Profile

Ololiuqui consists of the seeds of *Rivea corymbosa* or *Ipomoea tricolor* (*I. violacea*) both convolvulaceous plants similar to the garden plant 'morning glory', *Ipomoea purpurea*. The brown seeds of *R. corymbosa* are known as 'badoh' and the black seeds of *I. tricolor* as 'badoh negro'.

Ololiuqui has hallucinogenic properties and is considered to be sacred by some Mexican Indians. Alkaloidal fractions contain at least 5 closely related individual components, namely D-isolysergic acid amide (isoergine), D-lysergic acid amide (ergine), chanoclavine, elymoclavine, and lysergol.

The name 'ololiuqui' has been erroneously applied to seeds of *Datura meteloides* (Solanaceae).

## Onion

Cebolla.

### Profile

Onion is the bulb of *Allium cepa* (Liliaceae). It has been reported to reduce platelet aggregation, lower serum cholesterol, and to enhance fibrinolysis. It has been used in preparations for the treatment of urinary-tract disorders and in topical preparations for scars and contractures.

Onion is used in homoeopathic medicine.

**Cardiovascular disease.** A review of controlled studies purporting to show beneficial effects of garlic and/or onion on cardiovascular risk factors found those studies to have severe methodological failings.[1]


1. Kleijnen J, *et al.* Garlic, onions and cardiovascular risk factors: a review of the evidence from human experiments with emphasis on commercially available preparations. *Br J Clin Pharmacol* 1989; **28:** 535–44.


**Stings.** An onion bulb was used to treat the wound caused by a blue-spotted stingray (*Dasyatis kuhlii*).[1] Pain relief occurred within 30 minutes.


1. Whiting SD, Guinea ML. Treating stingray wounds with onions. *Med J Aust* 1998; **168:** 584.


### Preparations

**Proprietary Preparations** (details are given in Part 3)
***Austral.:*** Mederma; ***Malaysia:*** Mederma; ***Singapore:*** Mederma; ***USA:*** Mederma.

**Multi-ingredient:** ***Arg.:*** Contractubex; ***Austral.:*** Garlic Allium Complex†; ***Austria:*** Contractubex; ***Belg.:*** Pelvo Magnesium†; ***Ger.:*** Contractubex; ***Hong Kong:*** Contractubex; ***Switz.:*** Contractubex.

## Ononis

Arrête-Boeuf; Gatuña; Hauhechelwurzel; Ononidis Radix; Racine de Bugrane; Radix Ononidis; Restharrow Root; Spiny Restharrow.

**Pharmacopoeias.** In *Eur.* (see p.vi).
**Ph. Eur. 5.0** (Restharrow Root). The whole or cut, dried root of *Ononis spinosa.*

### Profile

Ononis has diuretic activity. It has been used in herbal preparations for the treatment of oedema, urinary-tract disorders, rheumatic disorders, and constipation.

### Preparations

**Proprietary Preparations** (details are given in Part 3)
**Multi-ingredient:** ***Austria:*** Aktiv Blasen- und Nierentee; Aponatura Entwasserungs; Aurita-Nieren-Blasentee; Bio-Garten Tee zur Erhohung der Harnmenge; Bioreform-Harntreibender Tee; Blasen-Tee†; Gewusst wie Entschlackungstee; Kneipp Nieren- und Blasen-Tee; Krauter Hustensaft; Krauterdoktor Harnstein- und Nieren-griesstropfen; Krauterhaus Mag Kottas Blasentee; Krauterhaus Mag Kottas Entschlackungstee; Krauterhaus Mag Kottas Nierentee; Krauterpfarrer Weidinger Rheumatee; Krauterpfarrer Weidinger Tee zur Entwasserung; Mag Kottas Krauterexpress-Nieren-Blasentee; Naturland Entschlackungstonikum; Neuners Krautertee Nr 18 - Stoffwechseltee; Neuners Krautertee Nr 204 - Krauterhexlein Kinder Nieren- und Blasentee; Neuners Krautertee Nr 25 - Entschlackungstee; Neuners Krautertee Nr 30 - Stoffwechseltee stark; Nierentee EF-EM-ES; Solisan; St Radegunder Entwasserungstee; St Radegunder Nierentee; Teekanne Blasen- und Nierentee; Uropurat; ***Fr.:*** Depuratum; Schoum; ***Ger.:*** Alasenn; Aqualibra; Befelka-Tinktur†; Blasen-Nieren-Tee Stada†; Harntee 400; Hevert-Blasen-Nieren-Tee N; Hevert-Entwasserungs-Tee†; Hevert-Gicht-Rheuma-Tee comp†; Heweberberol-Tee; Kneipp Blasen- und Nieren-Tee†; nephro-loges; Nephronorm med; Nephroselect M; Nephrubin-N; Nieron Blasen- und Nieren-Tee VI; Nieron-Tee N; Presselin Nieren-Blasen K 3; Reducelle†; Renob Blasen- und Nierentee; Ullus Blasen-Nieren-Tee N†; Urodil Blasen-Nieren Arzneitee†; Uvirgan N; ***Ital.:*** Gramigna (Specie Composta); Soluzione Schoum; ***Switz.:*** Demonatur Dragees pour les reins et la vessie; Dragees pour reins et vessie S†; Nephrosolid; Phytomed Nephro; Prosta-Caps Chassot N.

## Bitter Orange

Bigaradier; Naranja Amarga; Naranja amarga, corteza de; Pomeranze; Seville Orange.

**Pharmacopoeias.** *Eur.* includes the dried peel and flowers. *Jpn* and *Pol.* include the peel.
**Ph. Eur. 5.0** (Bitter-orange Epicarp and Mesocarp; Aurantii amari epicarpium et mesocarpium; Dried Bitter-Orange Peel BP 2003). The dried epicarp and mesocarp of the ripe fruit of *Citrus aurantium*, partly freed from the white spongy tissue of the mesocarp and endocarp, containing a minimum of 2.0% v/w of essential oil, calculated with reference to the anhydrous drug. It has an aromatic odour and a spicy bitter taste.
**Ph. Eur. 5.0** (Bitter-orange Flower; Aurantii amari flos). The whole, dried, unopened flower of *C. aurantium* ssp. *aurantium* containing a minimum of 8.0% of total flavonoids, expressed as naringin ($C_{27}H_{32}O_{14} = 580.5$), calculated with reference to the dried drug.

### Profile

The dried peel of the bitter orange, *Citrus aurantium* ssp. *aurantium* (*Citrus aurantium* ssp. *amara*) (Rutaceae) is used as a flavour and for its bitter and carminative properties. An essential oil is prepared from fresh bitter-orange peel (bitter orange oil) and is similar to sweet orange oil (p.1724).

The flowers are an ingredient of herbal remedies used for nervous and sleep disorders. Bitter-orange flower is the source of Neroli Oil (p.1719).

The whole dried immature fruit is used similarly to the dried peel. In Chinese medicine, the dried immature fruits are known as Zhi Shi and Zhi Qiao.

Photosensitivity is associated with citrus oils.

◊ *Citrus aurantium* was one of the most frequently used herbal remedies in Puerto Rico.[1] Indications included sleep disorders, gastrointestinal disorders, respiratory ailments, and raised blood pressure.

The volatile oil of dried bitter-orange peel has shown antifungal activity.[2]


1. Hernández L, *et al.* Use of medicinal plants by ambulatory patients in Puerto Rico. *Am J Hosp Pharm* 1984; **41:** 2060–4.
2. Ramadan W, *et al.* Oil of bitter orange: new topical antifungal agent. *Int J Dermatol* 1996; **35:** 448–9.


### Preparations

***BP 2003:*** Concentrated Compound Gentian Infusion; Concentrated Orange Peel Infusion; Orange Peel Infusion; Orange Syrup;
***Ph. Eur.:*** Bitter-Orange-Epicarp and Mesocarp Tincture.

**Proprietary Preparations** (details are given in Part 3)
***Ger.:*** Carvomin Magentropfen mit Pomeranze.

**Multi-ingredient:** ***Arg.:*** Calmtabs; Hepatodirectol; ***Austria:*** Aktiv Nerven- und Schlaftee; Aponatura Starkungs; Apotheker Bauer's Kindertee; Aurita-Nerventee; Baldrian-Krautertonikum; Bio-Garten Tee fur Leber und Galle; Bio-Garten Tee zur Beruhigung; Bio-Garten Tee zur Starkung und Kraftigung; Bioreform-Beruhigungstee; Bioreform-Leber- und Galletee; Bronchiplant; Bronchiplant light; China-Eisenwein; Digestol; Expectal-Tropfen; Ferrovin-Chinaeisenwein; Ferrovin-Eisenelixier; Gewusst wie Nerven-Schlaftee; Krauterdoktor Beruhigungstropfen; Krauterdoktor Entschlackungs-Elixier; Krauterhaus Mag Kottas Nerven- und Schlaftee; Krauterhaus Mag Kottas Tee fur die Verdauung; Krauterhaus Mag Kottas Tee gegen Durchfall; Luuf Krauter-Hustensaft; Mag Kottas Beruhigungstee; Mag Kottas Herz- und Kreislauftee; Mag Kottas Krauterexpress-Beruhigungstee; Mag Kottas Krauterexpress-Nerven-Schlaf-Tee; Mag Kottas Nerven-Beruhigungstee; Mag Kottas Schlaftee; Mariazeller; Montana; Nervifloran; Neuners Krautertee Nr 16 - Beruhigungstee bei Wechselbeschwerden; Neuners Krautertee Nr 201 - Krauterhexlein Kinder-Beruhigungstee; Neuners Krautertee Nr 209 - Krauterhexlein Kinder-Magentee; Neuners Krautertee Nr 210 - Krauterhexlein Kinder-Schweisstreibender Tee; Neuners Krautertee Nr 217 - Krauterhexlein Kinder-Blahungstee; Psychobald; Seda-Grandelat; Sidroga Brust-Husten-Tee; Sidroga Herz-Kreislauf-Tee; Sidroga Nerven- und Schlaftee; Sigman-Haustropfen; St Bonifatius-Tee; St Radegunder Beruhigungs- und Einschlaftee; St Radegunder Entschlackungs-Elixier; St Radegunder Herz-Kreislauf-Tonikum; St Radegunder Verdauungstee; Synpharma Instant-Nerventee; ***Belg.:*** Aperop†; Calmant Martou†; Tisane pour Dormir†; ***Braz.:*** Catuaba†; ***Fr.:*** Antigoutteux Rezall†; Calmophytum; Elixir Bonjean; Elixir Grez; Mediflor Tisane Calmante Troubles du Sommeil No 14; Quintonine; Santane $A_4$†; Santane $N_9$†; Santane $O_1$†; Santane $V_3$†; Tisanes de l'Abbe Hamon no 6†; Vegetoserum; ***Ger.:*** Carminativum-Hetterich N; Doppelherz Melissengeist; Gallexier; Gastrosecur; Meteophyt S†; Montana N; Salusan†; Sedovent; Stomachicon N†; ***Hong Kong:*** LEAN Formula w/ Advantra; ***India:*** Toniazol; ***Israel:*** Passiflora; ***Ital.:*** Assenzio (Specie Composta); Depurativo†; Fluend†; Gastro-Pepsin; Genziana (Specie Composta); Rabarbaro-ni†; Valeriana (Specie Composta); ***Spain:*** Agua del Carmen; Euzymina Lisina I; Euzymina Lisina II; Jaquesor; Natusor Jaquesan; Sedonat; ***Switz.:*** Demo pates pectorales†; Pastilles pectorales Demo N; Phytomed Nervo; Tisane calmante pour les enfants; Tisane pour le sommeil et les nerfs; ***UK:*** Vital Eyes.

## Sweet Orange

Naranja.

**Pharmacopoeias.** *Chin.* includes the fruit.

### Profile

Sweet orange, *Citrus sinensis* (*Citrus aurantium* var. *dulcis*) (Rutaceae), is an ingredient of herbal remedies used for nervous and sleep disorders. The peel is the source of sweet orange oil (below). Citrus fruits are a source of vitamin C (p.1460). Photosensitivity is associated with citrus oils.

### Preparations

***USNF 22:*** Orange Syrup; Sweet Orange Peel Tincture.

**Proprietary Preparations** (details are given in Part 3)

**Multi-ingredient:** ***Austria:*** Kneipp Nerven- und Schlaf-Tee; Krauterpfarrer Weidinger Tee bei Schlafstorungen; Krauterpfarrer Weidinger Tee bei Verstimmungen und Erregungszustanden; Magentee EF-EM-ES; Tussimont; ***Fr.:*** Santane $H_7$†; Santane $V_3$†; ***Ger.:*** Majocarmin forte; Salus Nerven-Schlaf-Tee Nr.22†.

## Sweet Orange Oil

Arancia Dolce Essenza; Aurantii Dulcis Aetheroleum; Essence of Orange; Essence of Portugal; Essência de Laranja; Naranja, aceite esencial de; Orange Oil.

NOTE. The oil from the flowers of *Citrus aurantium* var. *amara* is known as neroli oil or orange flower oil (p.1719).

**Pharmacopoeias.** In *Eur.* (see p.vi) and *Jpn.* Also in *USNF.*

**Ph. Eur. 5.0** (Sweet Orange Oil). An essential oil obtained without heating, by suitable mechanical treatment from the fresh peel of the fruit of *Citrus sinensis* (*Citrus aurantium* var. *dulcis*). A suitable antoxidant may be added. It contains 0.4 to 0.6% α-pinene, 0.02 to 0.3% β-pinene, 0.2 to 1.1% sabinene, 1.7 to 2.5% β-myrcene, 92.0 to 97.0% limonene, 0.1 to 0.4% octanal, 0.1 to 0.4% decanal, 0.2 to 0.7% linalol, 0.02 to 0.10% neral, 0.02 to 0.5% valencene, and 0.03 to 0.02% geranial.

A clear, pale yellow to orange, mobile liquid, which may become cloudy when chilled. It has a characteristic odour of fresh orange peel. Relative density 0.842 to 0.850. Store in well-filled airtight containers at a temperature not exceeding 25°. Protect from light.

**USNF 22** (Orange Oil). The volatile oil obtained by expression from the fresh peel of the ripe fruit of *Citrus sinensis* (Rutaceae), containing not less than 1.2% w/v and not more than 2.5% w/v of aldehydes, calculated as decanal ($C_{10}H_{20}O$ = 156.3). It may be California-type or Florida-type orange oil. Store in well-filled airtight containers.

### Profile

Sweet orange oil is used as a flavour and in perfumery. It is used in the preparation of terpeneless orange oil. Photosensitivity reactions have been reported with citrus oils.

### Preparations

***USNF 22:*** Compound Orange Spirit.

**Proprietary Preparations** (details are given in Part 3)

**Multi-ingredient:** ***Hong Kong:*** Magesto; ***Switz.:*** Pinimenthol; ***Thai.:*** Magesto.

## Terpeneless Orange Oil

Naranja sin terpeno, aceite esencial de; Oleum Aurantii Deterpenatum.

**Pharmacopoeias.** In *Br.*

**BP 2003** (Terpeneless Orange Oil). A clear yellow or orange-yellow liquid, visibly free from water, with the odour and taste of orange, prepared by concentrating orange oil under reduced pressure until most of the terpenes have been removed, or by solvent partition. It contains not less than 18% w/w of aldehydes calculated as decanal ($C_{10}H_{20}O$ = 156.3). Soluble 1 in 1 of alcohol (90%). Store in well-filled containers at a temperature not exceeding 25°. Protect from light.

### Profile

Terpeneless orange oil consists chiefly of the free alcohols (+)-linalol and (+)-terpineol. It is used as a flavour. It is stronger in flavour and more readily soluble than the natural oil. Photosensitivity is associated with citrus oils.

### Preparations

***BP 2003:*** Compound Orange Spirit.

## Orazamide *(rINN)*

AICA Orotate; Orazamida; Oroxamide. 5-Aminoimidazole-4-carboxamide orotate dihydrate.

$C_9H_{10}N_6O_5,2H_2O$ = 318.2.

*CAS — 2574-78-9 (anhydrous orazamide); 60104-30-5 (orazamide dihydrate).*

### Profile

Orazamide has been given by mouth in the treatment of liver disorders.

### Preparations

**Proprietary Preparations** (details are given in Part 3)
***Belg.:*** Aicamin†; ***Port.:*** Aicamin.

**Multi-ingredient:** ***Port.:*** Oraica.

## Orlistat *(BAN, USAN, rINN)*

Orlipastat; Ro-18-0647; Ro-18-0647/002; Tetrahydrolipstatin. *N*-Formyl-L-leucine, ester with (3*S*,4*S*)-3-hexyl-4-[(2*S*)-2-hydroxytridecyl]-2-oxetanone; (*S*)-1-[(2*S*,3*S*)-3-Hexyl-4-oxo-oxetan-2-ylmethyl]dodecyl *N*-formyl-L-leucinate.

$C_{29}H_{53}NO_5$ = 495.7.

*CAS — 96829-58-2.*

*ATC — A08AB01.*

### Adverse Effects

Gastrointestinal disturbances, including faecal urgency and incontinence, flatulence, and fatty stools or discharge, are the most frequently reported adverse effects during treatment with orlistat. They may be minimised by limiting the amount of fat in the diet. Other reported effects have included headache, anxiety, fatigue, and menstrual irregularities. There have been concerns about an increased risk of breast cancer in patients taking orlistat but the manufacturers consider that there is no evidence of a causal link.

**Effects on the cardiovascular system.** A report of hypertension associated with orlistat therapy.[1] Blood pressure decreased on discontinuing orlistat and increased again on rechallenge. The authors noted that 13 cases of hypertension associated with orlistat had been reported to the manufacturers.


1. Persson M, *et al.* Orlistat associated with hypertension. *BMJ* 2000; **321:** 87.


### Precautions

Orlistat should not be given to patients with chronic malabsorption syndrome or cholestasis and should be given with caution to patients with a history of hyperoxaluria or calcium oxalate nephrolithiasis. Adjustments to dosage of hypoglycaemics may be necessary in patients with type II diabetes because of improved metabolic control following weight loss in these patients. Supplements of fat-soluble vitamins may be necessary during long-term therapy, but they should be taken at least 2 hours before or after an orlistat dose or at bedtime.

### Interactions

Orlistat may reduce the absorption of fat-soluble vitamins. The manufacturer recommends that it not be taken with acarbose. In patients receiving warfarin, international normalised ratio should be monitored during treatment with orlistat. A reduction in ciclosporin concentrations to subtherapeutic levels has been reported in transplant recipients given orlistat (see p.1356).

### Pharmacokinetics

Orlistat is minimally absorbed following oral administration.

### Uses and Administration

Orlistat is a gastric and pancreatic lipase inhibitor that limits the absorption of dietary fat. It is used together with dietary modification in the management of obesity (p.1583), i.e. in patients with a body mass index of 30 kg/m$^2$ or greater. It may also be used in overweight patients with a body mass index of 28 kg/m$^2$ or more if there are associated risk factors. Treatment with orlistat should only be started once the patient has achieved a weight loss of at least 2.5 kg over 4 consecutive weeks as a result of diet alone. Orlistat is given in a usual dose of 120 mg by mouth three times daily, immediately before, during, or up to 1 hour after meals. If a meal is missed or contains no fat, the dose should be omitted. Orlistat therapy should be stopped if the patient does not lose at least 5% of their body-weight during the first 12 weeks of therapy.

◊ References.


1. Davidson MH, *et al.* Weight control and risk factor reduction in obese subjects treated for 2 years with orlistat: a randomized controlled trial. *JAMA* 1999; **281:** 235–42. Correction. *ibid.*; 1174.
2. Hvizdos KM, Markham A. Orlistat: a review of its use in the management of obesity. *Drugs* 1999; **58:** 743–60.
3. Heymsfield SB, *et al.* Effects of weight loss with orlistat on glucose tolerance and progression to type 2 diabetes in obese adults. *Arch Intern Med* 2000; **160:** 1321–6.
4. Finer N, *et al.* One-year treatment of obesity: a randomized, double-blind, placebo-controlled, multicentre study of orlistat, a gastrointestinal lipase inhibitor. *Int J Obes Relat Metab Disord* 2000; **24:** 306–13.
5. Rossner S, *et al.* Weight loss, weight maintenance, and improved cardiovascular risk factors after 2 years treatment with orlistat for obesity. *Obes Res* 2000; **8:** 49–61.
6. Heck AM, *et al.* Orlistat, a new lipase inhibitor for the management of obesity. *Pharmacotherapy* 2000; **20:** 270–9.
7. National Institute for Clinical Excellence. Guidance on the use of orlistat for the treatment of obesity in adults. Available at: http://www.nice.org.uk/pdf/orlistatguidance.pdf (accessed 02/07/04)
8. Lucas KH, Kaplan-Machlis B. Orlistat—a novel weight loss therapy. *Ann Pharmacother* 2001; **35:** 314–28.
9. Keating GM, Jarvis B. Orlistat: in the prevention and treatment of type 2 diabetes mellitus. *Drugs* 2001; **61:** 2107–21.
10. Snider LJ, Malone M. Orlistat use in type 2 diabetes. *Ann Pharmacother* 2002; **36:** 1210–18.
11. Torgerson JS, *et al.* XENical in the prevention of diabetes in obese subjects (XENDOS) study: a randomized study of orlistat as an adjunct to lifestyle changes for the prevention of type 2 diabetes in obese patients. *Diabetes Care* 2004; **27:** 155–61.


### Preparations

**Proprietary Preparations** (details are given in Part 3)
***Arg.:*** Xenical; ***Austral.:*** Xenical; ***Austria:*** Xenical; ***Belg.:*** Xenical; ***Braz.:*** Xenical; ***Canad.:*** Xenical; ***Chile:*** Xenical; ***Denm.:*** Xenical; ***Fin.:*** Xenical; ***Fr.:*** Xenical; ***Ger.:*** Xenical; ***Gr.:*** Xenical; ***Hong Kong:*** Xenical; ***Irl.:*** Xenical; ***Israel:*** Xenical; ***Ital.:*** Xenical; ***Mex.:*** Xenical; ***Neth.:*** Xenical; ***Norw.:*** Xenical; ***NZ:*** Xenical; ***Port.:*** Xenical; ***S.Afr.:*** Xenical; ***Singapore:*** Xenical; ***Spain:*** Xenical; ***Swed.:*** Xenical; ***Switz.:*** Xenical; ***Thai.:*** Xenical; ***UK:*** Xenical; ***USA:*** Xenical.

## Orotic Acid *(BAN, pINN)*

Ácido orótico; Animal Galactose Factor; Uracil-6-carboxylic Acid; Whey Factor. 1,2,3,6-Tetrahydro-2,6-dioxopyrimidine-4-carboxylic acid.

$C_5H_4N_2O_4$ = 156.1.

*CAS — 65-86-1 (anhydrous orotic acid); 50887-69-9 (orotic acid monohydrate).*

### Profile

Orotic acid occurs naturally in the body; it is found in milk. It is an intermediate in the biosynthesis of pyrimidine nucleotides. Orotic acid and its calcium, carnitine, choline, lithium, lysine, magnesium, and potassium salts have been used in liver disorders. Some of these salts, as well as chromium orotate, cyproheptadine orotate, and deanol orotate, have been given as tonics or dietary supplements. Magnesium, ferrous, and zinc orotates have been used as mineral sources.

### Preparations

**Proprietary Preparations** (details are given in Part 3)
***Ger.:*** magnerot Classic; Magnesorot; Power Orot; Zinkorot.

**Multi-ingredient:** ***Arg.:*** Bil 13; ***Austral.:*** Bioglan Bioage Peripheral†; Mag-Oro†; Magnesium Plus†; ***Austria:*** Kavaform; Lemazol; ***Ger.:*** Antisklerosin S†; Hepatofalk Neu†; Hepatofalk†; Neuro-Wied; ***Hong Kong:*** Hepatofalk; Lipochol; Tres Orix Forte; ***Ital.:*** Epa-Treis†; Oro B12†; ***Mex.:*** Lipovitasi-Or; ***Port.:*** Oraica; ***S.Afr.:*** Hepabionta†; ***Spain:*** Antibiofilus†; Hepadif; Hepato Fardi; Tres Orix Forte; ***Switz.:*** Kawaform; Magnesium Complexe; Vigoran; ***Thai.:*** Lipochol; ***UK:*** Cardeymin†; Sugar Bloc.

## Orthodichlorobenzene

Ortodiclorobenceno. 1,2-Dichlorobenzene.

$C_6H_4Cl_2$ = 147.0.

*CAS — 95-50-1.*

### Profile

Orthodichlorobenzene has been used as a wood and furniture preservative. It has also been used as an ingredient of solutions for dissolving ear wax. It is an irritant volatile liquid; lens opacities have occurred.

### Preparations

**Proprietary Preparations** (details are given in Part 3)

**Multi-ingredient:** ***Austral.:*** Cerumol; ***Switz.:*** Cerumenol.

## Oryzanol

Gamma Oryzanol; Orizanol; γ-Oryzanol; γ-OZ. Triacontanyl 3-(4-hydroxy-3-methoxyphenyl)prop-2-enoate.

$C_{40}H_{58}O_4$ = 602.9.

*CAS — 11042-64-1.*

### Profile

Oryzanol is a substance extracted from rice bran oil and rice embryo bud oil. It has been given by mouth in the treatment of hyperlipidaemias. It has also been used for its supposed effects on autonomic and endocrine function.

◊ References.


1. Cicero AF, Gaddi A. Rice bran oil and gamma-oryzanol in the treatment of hyperlipoproteinaemias and other conditions. *Phytother Res* 2001; **15:** 277–89.


### Preparations

**Proprietary Preparations** (details are given in Part 3)
***Hong Kong:*** Gammariza†.
**Multi-ingredient:** ***Ital.:*** Lenirose; Mavipiu.

## Osalmid *(rINN)*

L-1718; Osalmida; Oxaphenamide. 4′-Hydroxysalicylanilide.

$C_{13}H_{11}NO_3$ = 229.2.

*CAS — 526-18-1.*

### Profile

Osalmid has been used as a choleretic.

## Otilonium Bromide *(BAN, rINN)*

Bromuro de otilonio; Octylonium Bromide; SP-63. Diethylmethyl{2-[4-(2-octyloxybenzamido)benzoyloxy]ethyl}ammonium bromide.

$C_{29}H_{43}BrN_2O_4$ = 563.6.

*CAS — 26095-59-0.*
*ATC — A03AB06.*

### Profile

Otilonium bromide is used in the symptomatic treatment of gastrointestinal disorders associated with smooth muscle spasms in doses up to 120 mg daily by mouth. It has also been administered rectally and by nebuliser.

◊ References.


1. Battaglia G, *et al.* Otilonium bromide in irritable bowel syndrome: a double-blind, placebo-controlled, 15-week study. *Aliment Pharmacol Ther* 1998; **12:** 1003–10.


### Preparations

**Proprietary Preparations** (details are given in Part 3)
***Arg.:*** Pasminox; Spasmoctyl; ***Belg.:*** Spasmomen; ***Gr.:*** Doralin; ***Hong Kong:*** Spasmomen; ***Ital.:*** Spasen; Spasmomen; ***Spain:*** Spasmoctyl.
**Multi-ingredient:** ***Arg.:*** Pasminox Somatico; ***Ital.:*** Spasen Somatico; Spasen†; Spasmomen Somatico.

## Oxaceprol *(rINN)*

Acetylhydroxyproline; C061. (−)-1-Acetyl-4-hydroxy-L-proline.

$C_7H_{11}NO_4$ = 173.2.

*CAS — 33996-33-7.*
*ATC — D11AX09; M01AX24.*

### Profile

Oxaceprol is reported to affect connective tissue metabolism and has been used in dermatology, to promote wound healing, and in rheumatic disorders. Adverse effects have included gastric pain, nausea, diarrhoea, dizziness, headache, and skin rashes.

◊ References.


1. Bauer HW, *et al.* Oxaceprol is as effective as diclofenac in the therapy of osteoarthritis of the knee and hip. *Clin Rheumatol* 1999; **18:** 4–9.
2. Herrmann G, *et al.* Oxaceprol is a well-tolerated therapy for osteoarthritis with efficacy equivalent to diclofenac. *Clin Rheumatol* 2000; **19:** 99–104.


### Preparations

**Proprietary Preparations** (details are given in Part 3)
***Arg.:*** Joint; ***Fr.:*** Jonctum; ***Ger.:*** AHP 200; ***Spain:*** Tejuntivo.
**Multi-ingredient:** ***Spain:*** Robervital.

## Oxalic Acid

Oxálico, ácido.

$HO_2C.CO_2H,2H_2O$ = 126.1.

*CAS — 144-62-7 (anhydrous oxalic acid); 6153-56-6 (oxalic acid dihydrate).*

### Adverse Effects

Following ingestion, severe gastroenteritis is produced by the corrosive action of oxalic acid and its soluble salts on the gastrointestinal tract. Burning of the mouth, throat, and oesophagus with ulceration may also occur. Hypoxia may occur in the presence of laryngeal oedema, and shock and hypotension may arise in severe cases. Oxalates can chelate body calcium following systemic absorption, and may produce symptoms of hypocalcaemia such as tetany, convulsions, and, in some cases, ventricular fibrillation. Oxalate crystals may be deposited in the blood vessels, heart, liver, and lungs; deposition in the renal tubules leads to acute renal failure. The mean fatal dose of oxalates has been reported to be about 15 to 30 g, although death has occurred with much lower doses. Death may occur within a few hours of ingestion.

◊ Fatalities have resulted from intravenous administration of sodium oxalate[1] or ingestion of oxalic acid.[2]

Crystals of calcium oxalate present in the sap of daffodils[3] or *Agave tequilana* plants[4] have been reported to contribute to the rash experienced by workers coming into contact with these plants.


1. Dvořáčková I. Tödliche Vergiftung nach intravenöser Verabreichung von Natriumoxalat. *Arch Toxikol* 1966; **22:** 63–7.
2. Farré M, *et al.* Fatal oxalic acid poisoning from sorrel soup. *Lancet* 1989; **ii:** 1524.
3. Julian CG, Bowers PW. The nature and distribution of daffodil pickers' rash. *Contact Dermatitis* 1997; **37:** 259–62.
4. Salinas ML, *et al.* Irritant contact dermatitis caused by needle-like calcium oxalate crystals, raphides, in Agave tequilana among workers in tequila distilleries and agave plantations. *Contact Dermatitis* 2001; **44:** 94–6.


### Treatment of Adverse Effects

Following ingestion of oxalic acid, a dilute solution of any soluble calcium salt should be given to precipitate the oxalate; alternatively milk may be given. Oral activated charcoal has also been suggested if ingestion has occurred within 1 hour. Gastric lavage is contra-indicated by some centres given the corrosive nature of oxalic acid. However, others have recommended that if mucosal corrosion has not occurred the stomach may be carefully emptied by lavage using large quantities of diluted lime water or dilute solutions of other calcium salts. Calcium gluconate 10% should be given intravenously in doses of 10 mL to prevent tetany. Acute renal failure should be anticipated in surviving patients and calls for careful fluid management. Haemodialysis or peritoneal dialysis have also been suggested for the removal of oxalate in primary oxalosis in an attempt to prevent acute renal failure and correct hypocalcaemia.

### Uses

Oxalic acid has varied industrial uses and has been used in escharotic preparations. Oxalic acid salts have been administered by mouth and the urinary excretion of oxalate used as a screening test for lipid malabsorption.

**Diagnostic use.** References.


1. Rampton DS, *et al.* Screening for steatorrhoea with an oxalate loading test. *BMJ* 1984; **288:** 1419. Correction. *ibid.*; 1728.
2. Sangaletti O, *et al.* Urinary oxalate recovery after oral oxalic acid load: an alternative method to the quantitative determination of stool fat for the diagnosis of lipid malabsorption. *J Int Med Res* 1989; **17:** 526–31.


### Preparations

**Proprietary Preparations** (details are given in Part 3)
**Multi-ingredient:** ***Ger.:*** Solco-Derman; ***Hong Kong:*** Solcoderm; ***Malaysia:*** Solcoderm; ***Switz.:*** Solcoderm; Solcogyn.

## Oxiracetam *(BAN, rINN)*

CGP-21690E; CT-848; ISF-2522. 4-Hydroxy-2-oxo-1-pyrrolidineacetamide.

$C_6H_{10}N_2O_3$ = 158.2.

*CAS — 62613-82-5.*
*ATC — N06BX07.*

### Profile

Oxiracetam has been used as a nootropic in organic brain syndromes and senile dementia.

**Dementia.** Clinical benefit has been reported in patients with dementia (p.1484) given oxiracetam,[1] but in the USA it was withdrawn from phase II clinical studies in patients with Alzheimer's disease due to lack of efficacy.[2]


1. Maina G, *et al.* Oxiracetam in the treatment of primary degenerative and multi-infarct dementia: a double-blind, placebo-controlled study. *Neuropsychobiology* 1990; **21:** 141–5.
2. Parnetti L. Clinical pharmacokinetics of drugs for Alzheimer's disease. *Clin Pharmacokinet* 1995; **29:** 110–29.


### Preparations

**Proprietary Preparations** (details are given in Part 3)
***Ital.:*** Neuractiv†; Neuromet†.

## Ozagrel *(rINN)*

OKY-046 (ozagrel hydrochloride). (*E*)-*p*-(imidazol-1-ylmethyl)cinnamic acid.

$C_{13}H_{12}N_2O_2$ = 228.2.

*CAS — 82571-53-7.*

### Profile

Ozagrel is a thromboxane synthetase inhibitor that has been used as the hydrochloride and as the sodium salt in the treatment of asthma and of cerebrovascular disorders.

◊ References.


1. Nagatsuka K, *et al.* A new approach to antithrombotic therapy—evaluation of combined therapy of thromboxane synthetase inhibitor and very low dose of aspirin. *Stroke* 1985; **16:** 806–9.
2. Fujimura M, *et al.* Effects of aerosol administration of a thromboxane synthetase inhibitor (OKY-046) on bronchial responsiveness to acetylcholine in asthmatic subjects. *Chest* 1990; **98:** 276–9.
3. Fujimura M, *et al.* Attenuating effect of a thromboxane synthetase inhibitor (OKY-046) on bronchial responsiveness to methacholine is specific to bronchial asthma. *Chest* 1990; **98:** 656–60.
4. Oishi M, *et al.* Effects of sodium ozagrel on hemostatic markers and cerebral blood flow in lacunar infarction. *Clin Neuropharmacol* 1996; **19:** 526–31.
5. Kato H, *et al.* Treatment of branch retinal arterial occlusion with sodium ozagrel, a thromboxane A2 synthetase inhibitor. *J Int Med Res* 1997; **25:** 108–11.
6. Kunitoh H, *et al.* A double-blind, placebo-controlled trial of the thromboxane synthetase blocker OKY-046 on bronchial hypersensitivity in bronchial asthma patients. *J Asthma* 1998; **35:** 355–60.
7. Seki H, *et al.* Trial of prophylactic administration of TXA2 synthetase inhibitor, ozagrel hydrochloride, for preeclampsia. *Hypertens Pregnancy* 1999; **18:** 157–64.


### Preparations

**Proprietary Preparations** (details are given in Part 3)
***Jpn:*** Cataclot; Domenan; Xanbon.

## Palmidrol *(rINN)*

*N*-(2-Hydroxyethyl)palmitamide.

$C_{18}H_{37}NO_2$ = 299.5.

*CAS — 544-31-0.*

### Profile

Palmidrol is a naturally occurring lipid compound that has been used as an immunostimulant. It is given by mouth in doses of 1 g two or three times daily for the treatment of respiratory-tract infections.

### Preparations

**Proprietary Preparations** (details are given in Part 3)
***Chile:*** Palmitan.

# Pancreatic Enzymes

## Pancreatin *(BAN)*

Pancreatina; Pancreatinum.

*CAS — 8049-47-6.*

**Pharmacopoeias.** In *Chin., Eur.* (see p.vi), *Jpn,* and *US* as pancreatin or another pancreatic exocrine extract or both.

**Ph. Eur. 5.0** (Pancreas Powder; Pancreatis Pulvis; Pancreatic Extract BP 2003). It is prepared from the fresh or frozen pancreases of mammals. It contains various enzymes having proteolytic, lipolytic, and amylolytic activities. Each mg of pancreas powder contains not less than 1 Ph. Eur. unit of total proteolytic activity, not less than 15 Ph. Eur. units of lipolytic activity, and not less than 12 Ph. Eur. units of amylolytic activity. A slightly brown, amorphous powder. Partly soluble in water; practically insoluble in alcohol. Store in airtight containers at a temperature not exceeding 15°.

**BP 2003** (Pancreatin). A preparation of mammalian pancreas containing enzymes having protease, lipase, and amylase activity. Each mg of pancreatin contains not less than 1.4 FIP units of free protease activity, not less than 20 FIP units of lipase activity, and not less than 24 FIP units of amylase activity. It may contain sodium chloride. A white or buff amorphous powder, free from unpleasant odour. Soluble or partly soluble in water forming a slightly turbid solution; practically insoluble in alcohol and in ether. Store at a temperature not exceeding 15°.

**USP 27** (Pancreatin). A substance containing enzymes, principally amylase, lipase, and protease, obtained from the pancreas of the hog or of the ox. It is a cream-coloured, amorphous powder, having a faint, characteristic, but not offensive odour. Its greatest activities are in neutral or faintly alkaline media; more than traces of mineral acids or large amounts of alkali hydroxides make it inert. An excess of alkali carbonate also inhibits its action.

Pancreatin contains, in each mg, not less than 25 USP units of amylase activity, not less than 2 USP units of lipase activity, and not less than 25 USP units of protease activity. Pancreatin of a higher digestive power may be labelled as a whole-number multiple of the 3 minimum activities, or may be diluted with lactose, or with sucrose containing not more than 3.25% of starch, or with pancreatin of lower digestive power. Store in airtight containers at a temperature not exceeding 30°.

## Pancrelipase *(USAN)*

Pancrelipasa.

*CAS — 53608-75-6.*

**Pharmacopoeias.** In *US.*

**USP 27** (Pancrelipase). A substance containing enzymes, principally lipase, with amylase and protease, obtained from the pancreas of the hog. It is a cream-coloured, amorphous powder having a faint characteristic, but not offensive odour. Its greatest activities are in neutral or faintly alkaline media; more than traces of mineral acids or large amounts of alkali hydroxides make it inert. An excess of alkali carbonate also inhibits its action. Pancrelipase contains, in each mg, not less than 24 USP units of lipase activity, not less than 100 USP units of amylase activity, and not less than 100 USP units of protease activity. Store in airtight containers preferably at a temperature not exceeding 25°.

### Units

The Ph. Eur. and USP units of protease activity depend upon the rate of hydrolysis of casein, those of lipase activity depend upon the rate of hydrolysis of olive oil, and those of amylase activity depend upon the rate of hydrolysis of starch. Because of differences in the assay conditions, the Ph. Eur. and USP units are not readily comparable.

FIP units of protease, lipase, and amylase activity are approximately equivalent to Ph. Eur. units.

### Adverse Effects and Precautions

Pancreatic enzyme supplements commonly cause gastrointestinal side-effects such as abdominal discomfort and nausea and vomiting. They may also cause buccal and perianal irritation, particularly in infants. Colonic strictures (fibrosing colonopathy) have occurred, mainly in children with cystic fibrosis receiving high doses of pancreatin preparations; the use of high doses in patients with cystic fibrosis should preferably be avoided (see Effects on the Gastrointestinal Tract, below). Adequate hydration should be maintained at all times in patients receiving higher strength preparations.

Hypersensitivity reactions have been reported; these may be sneezing, lachrymation, or skin rashes. Hyperuricaemia or hyperuricosuria have occurred with high doses. There have been occasional reports of the contamination of pancreatin preparations with *Salmonella* spp.

**Effects on folic acid.** Pancreatic extract significantly inhibited folate absorption in healthy subjects and in pancreatic insufficient patients.[1] Testing *in vitro* showed that pancreatic extract formed insoluble complexes with folate. It was suggested[1] that patients being treated for pancreatic insufficiency should be monitored for folate status or given folic acid supplementation, particularly if pancreatic enzymes and bicarbonate (or cimetidine) were being used together in the treatment regimen.

1. Russell RM, *et al.* Impairment of folic acid absorption by oral pancreatic extracts. *Dig Dis Sci* 1980; **25:** 369–73.

**Effects on the gastrointestinal tract.** FIBROSING COLONOPATHY. Following the introduction of high-strength pancreatic enzyme preparations, there were a number of reports[1-6] of colonic strictures in children with cystic fibrosis who received these formulations, and the problem, now dubbed fibrosing colonopathy, was reviewed.[7,8] Fibrosing colonopathy has also been reported[9] in an adult who was not thought to have cystic fibrosis, but who had been taking high doses of pancreatic enzyme supplements, including two with methylacrylic acid copolymer (MAC) coatings, for 5 years following surgical removal of the pancreas.

The pathogenesis and aetiology of this condition still remain unclear. Dose-related thickening of the colon wall has been described,[10] and an inflammatory or immune-mediated mechanism has been suggested.[11,12] It has also been suggested that the type of preparation used may have a role. An analysis[13] of cases of fibrosing colonopathy occurring in the UK between 1984 and 1994 demonstrated that there was a dose-related association between the high-strength preparations and this adverse effect although there was some criticism and debate surrounding the methodology of this particular analysis.[14-16] A subsequent case-control study[17] of patients in the US presenting between 1990 and 1994 concluded that there was a strong association between high daily doses of pancreatic enzymes, in any form, and the development of fibrosing colonopathy; no significant differences were observed between the various high- and low-strength preparations used. Re-analysis[18] of the UK data found a highly statistically significant association with the intake of preparations using MAC for enteric coating, but no evidence that a high intake of lipase in the absence of MAC was a risk factor for the disease. However, at least one case has been reported with a preparation that did not contain this material.[19]

As a result of these problems, high-strength preparations were withdrawn in the USA, while in the UK, the Committee on Safety of Medicines recommended[20] that unless special reasons exist, patients with cystic fibrosis should not use high-strength pancreatin preparations, and that all patients treated with these products should be monitored carefully for gastrointestinal obstruction. The Committee subsequently elaborated on these recommendations:[21] they advised that Nutrizym 22, Pancrease HL, and Panzytrat 25 000 should not be used in children with cystic fibrosis who were aged 15 years or less; that the total daily dose of pancreatic enzyme supplements for patients with cystic fibrosis should not exceed a lipase activity of 10 000 units/kg; and that patients on any pancreatin preparation should be reviewed to exclude colonic damage if new abdominal symptoms or a change in symptoms occurred. Other risk factors identified were male sex, more severe cystic fibrosis, and the concomitant use of laxatives.[21] The US Cystic Fibrosis Foundation has made recommendations for the management of patients who do not respond adequately to moderate doses of pancreatic enzymes,[22] and similar recommendations have been made in the UK.[23]

1. Smyth RL, *et al.* Strictures of ascending colon in cystic fibrosis and high-strength pancreatic enzymes. *Lancet* 1994; **343:** 85–6.
2. Oades PJ, *et al.* High-strength pancreatic enzyme supplements and large-bowel stricture in cystic fibrosis. *Lancet* 1994; **343:** 109.
3. Campbell CA, *et al.* High-strength pancreatic enzyme supplements and large-bowel stricture in cystic fibrosis. *Lancet* 1994; **343:** 109–110.
4. Mahony MJ, Corcoran M. High-strength pancreatic enzymes. *Lancet* 1994; **343:** 599–600.
5. Knabe N, *et al.* Extensive pathological changes of the colon in cystic fibrosis and high-strength pancreatic enzymes. *Lancet* 1994; **343:** 1230.
6. Pettei MJ, *et al.* Pancolonic disease in cystic fibrosis and high-dose pancreatic enzyme therapy. *J Pediatr* 1994; **125:** 587–9.
7. Taylor CJ. Colonic strictures in cystic fibrosis. *Lancet* 1994; **343:** 615–16. Correction. *ibid.*; 1108.
8. Taylor CJ. The problems with high dose pancreatic enzyme preparations. *Drug Safety* 1994; **11:** 75–9.
9. Bansi DS, *et al.* Fibrosing colonopathy in an adult owing to over use of pancreatic enzyme supplements. *Gut* 2000; **46:** 283–5.
10. MacSweeney EJ, *et al.* Relationship of thickening of colon wall to pancreatic-enzyme treatment in cystic fibrosis. *Lancet* 1995; **345:** 752–6.
11. Croft NM, *et al.* Gut inflammation in children with cystic fibrosis on high-dose enzyme supplements. *Lancet* 1995; **346:** 1265–7.
12. Lee J, *et al.* Is fibrosing colonopathy an immune mediated disease? *Arch Dis Child* 1997; **77:** 66–70.
13. Smyth RL, *et al.* Fibrosing colonopathy in cystic fibrosis: results of a case-control study. *Lancet* 1995; **346:** 1247–51.
14. Dodge JA. Concern about records of fibrosing colonopathy study. *Lancet* 2001; **357:** 1526–7.
15. Dodge JA. Further comments on fibrosing colonopathy study. *Lancet* 2001; **358:** 1546.
16. O'Hara D, Talbot IC. Further comments on fibrosing colonopathy study. *Lancet* 2001; **358:** 1546.
17. FitzSimmons SC, *et al.* High-dose pancreatic-enzyme supplements and fibrosing colonopathy in children with cystic fibrosis. *N Engl J Med* 1997; **336:** 1283–9.
18. Prescott P, Bakowski MT. Pathogenesis of fibrosing colonopathy: the role of methacrylic acid copolymer. *Pharmacoepidemiol Drug Safety* 1999; **8:** 377–84.
19. Taylor CJ, Steiner GM. Fibrosing colonopathy in a child on low-dose pancreatin. *Lancet* 1995; **345:** 1106–7.
20. Committee on Safety of Medicines/Medicines Control Agency. Update: bowel strictures and high-potency pancreatins. *Current Problems* 1994; **20:** 13.
21. Committee on Safety of Medicines/Medicines Control Agency. Fibrosing colonopathy associated with pancreatic enzymes. *Current Problems* 1995; **21:** 11.
22. Borowitz DS, *et al.* Use of pancreatic enzyme supplements for patients with cystic fibrosis in the context of fibrosing colonopathy. *J Pediatr* 1995; **127:** 681–4.
23. Littlewood JM. Fibrosing colonopathy in cystic fibrosis: commentary, implications of the Committee on Safety of Medicines 10 000 IU lipase/kg/day recommendation for use of pancreatic enzymes in cystic fibrosis. *Arch Dis Child* 1996; **74:** 466–8.

MOUTH ULCERATION. In 3 children taking preparations of pancreatic extracts (Pancrex V powder, Pancrex V Forte), severe mouth ulceration and angular stomatitis, causing dysphagia, loss of weight, and pyrexia, were attributed to digestion of the mucous membrane due to retention of the preparations in the mouth before swallowing.[1]

1. Darby CW. Pancreatic extracts. *BMJ* 1970; **2:** 299–300.

**Hypersensitivity.** A successful desensitisation regimen has been described[1] for a child with cystic fibrosis who vomited within 1 to 2 hours after ingestion of pancreatic enzymes, suggestive of a type I hypersensitivity reaction.

1. Chamarthy LM, *et al.* Desensitization to pancreatic enzyme intolerance in a child with cystic fibrosis. Abstract: *Pediatrics* 1998; **102:** 134–5. Full version: http://pediatrics.aappublications.org/cgi/content/full/102/1/e13 (accessed 02/07/04)

### Uses and Administration

Pancreatic enzymes (as pancreatin or pancrelipase) hydrolyse fats to glycerol and fatty acids, break down protein into peptides, proteoses and derived substances, and convert starch into dextrins and sugars. They are given by mouth in conditions of pancreatic exocrine deficiency such as pancreatitis and cystic fibrosis. They are available in the form of powder, capsules containing powder or enteric-coated granules (which may be opened before use and the contents sprinkled on soft food), enteric-coated tablets, or granules. If pancreatic enzymes are mixed with liquids or food the resulting mixture should not be allowed to stand for more than 1 hour prior to use. Histamine $H_2$-receptor antagonists, such as cimetidine or ranitidine, have been given an hour before a dose in an attempt to lessen destruction of the pancreatic enzymes by gastric acid; alternatively, antacids may be given with the dose.

The dose of pancreatic enzymes is adjusted according to the needs of the individual patient and will also depend on the dosage form. In the UK, proprietary preparations generally provide about 5 000 to 10 000 units of lipase activity per dose-unit and usual doses, given with each meal, range from about 10 000 to 56 000 units of lipase activity (with varying proportions of protease and amylase activity, depending on the preparation). In the USA, doses providing up to 40 000 USP units of lipase activity may be given with each meal. So-called high-strength or high-potency preparations are available for those receiving high doses, and typically contain about 20 000 to 40 000 units of lipase activity per dose unit, but their use has been associated with the development of fibrosing colonopathy in children with cystic fibrosis (see above). Such preparations are consequently not recommended for children in the UK and authorities there consider the total daily dose of pancreatic supplements for patients with cystic fibrosis should not exceed a lipase activity of 10 000 units/kg.

Pancreatin is also used to remove protein deposits from the surface of soft contact lenses (p.1164).

**Cystic fibrosis.** Patients with cystic fibrosis (p.123) suffer from pancreatic insufficiency and consequent malabsorption. Pancreatin or pancrelipase may therefore play a role in the management of the disorder, being taken before or with each meal or snack.

**Generic substitution.** Three patients with cystic fibrosis whose gastrointestinal symptoms had been well controlled with pancrelipase developed symptoms following substitution of generic pancrelipase for their previous brand.[1] The generic product had a different lipase content and was almost inactive at stomach pH *in vitro*, apparently because of a defective enteric coating. Different brands of pancrelipase may not be therapeutically equivalent and should not be routinely substituted.

1. Hendeles L, *et al.* Treatment failure after substitution of generic pancrelipase capsules: correlation with in vitro lipase activity. *JAMA* 1990; **263:** 2459–61.

**Pancreatitis.** Pancreatitis is an inflammatory process affecting the pancreas. Acute pancreatitis comprises necrosis of pancreatic tissue occurring in an otherwise healthy gland, whereas chronic pancreatitis is the manifestation of pathological processes resulting in inflammation and progressive fibrosis of pancreatic tissue. Acute disease may be superimposed on a background of chronic pancreatitis.

**Acute pancreatitis** is frequently associated with either biliary tract disorders (such as gallstones or cholecystitis) or the intake of large amounts of alcohol, or less frequently with abdominal surgery, pancreatic trauma, hyperparathyroidism, hyperlipidaemia, infection, or the adverse effects of drugs. Symptoms include pain, which ranges from mild to extremely severe and which typically persists for several days, nausea and vomiting, ileus, and hypovolaemic shock. In severe disease, pulmonary, renal, and hepatic failure, encephalopathy, and death may ensue. A mortality rate of about 10% has been reported.

The management of acute disease is essentially supportive.[1] Adequate analgesia for pain is important (see Pancreatic Pain, p.7); in mild cases, analgesia, adequate hydration, and temporary interruption of oral intake of food to 'rest' the pancreas may be adequate. Since most patients suffer from hypoxaemia it has been recommended that they should receive additional humidified oxygen by mask, with mechanical ventilation if blood gases indicate the development of severe pulmonary failure. Shock should be managed with blood or plasma, and electrolyte solutions, while insulin may be required for disturbances of glucose homoeostasis.

The value of other interventions is mostly doubtful. As an extension of the concept of 'pancreatic rest', inhibitors of pancreatic secretion such as somatostatin or octreotide have been tried but without significant effect, while protease inhibitors such as aprotinin or gabexate mesilate have also proven disappointing,[2] perhaps because activation of pancreatic proteases (thought to play a significant role in pathogenesis) has already taken place by the time therapy is begun.[2] Gabexate and somatostatin may, however, have roles in the prevention of acute pancreatitis following endoscopic retrograde cholangiopancreatography (ERCP).[3] Preliminary studies of the platelet-activating factor antagonist lexipafant were initially promising but were not supported by subsequent larger studies.[1]

Although prophylactic antibacterials are often given, there has been some uncertainty about their value.[4,5] However, a study in patients with acute necrotising pancreatitis indicated markedly reduced mortality in those given prophylactic antibacterials (initially cefuroxime),[6] and a retrospective study[7] reported a reduction in the incidence, but not in the time of onset, of infection in those receiving such drugs. In a review[8] of the treatment of acute necrotising pancreatitis, it was pointed out that early studies that failed to demonstrate any benefit of prophylactic antibacterials had also included patients with interstitial oedematous acute pancreatitis. The authors emphasised that the prevention of infection is critical in acute necrotising pancreatitis, since the development of infected necrosis substantially increases mortality, and concluded that use of antibacterials is the mainstay of management in such patients.

Peritoneal dialysis reduces early complications of acute pancreatitis but increases the risk of subsequent infection and has no overall effect on survival.[4] The role of surgery continues to be somewhat controversial; it is accepted for complications or when a potential surgical emergency exists. Surgery to remove gallstones may be carried out once pancreatitis has resolved, but surgical intervention during acute episodes may increase morbidity and mortality. Early endoscopic decompression of the obstructed bile duct may be beneficial in patients with cholangitis or progressive jaundice but not in those without biliary obstruction.[9]

**Chronic pancreatitis** is frequently associated with high alcohol-intake although a tropical form, associated with malnutrition, also exists, and some cases are idiopathic. Symptoms include recurrent episodes of pain (often less excruciating and of shorter duration than in acute pancreatitis) which normally become less severe and frequent over the years with the inexorable progression of fibrosis. Loss of exocrine tissue eventually leads in many patients to pancreatic exocrine insufficiency, with maldigestion and steatorrhoea, and in some to diabetes mellitus due to islet cell loss. Other symptoms may include cholestatic jaundice, fatty degeneration of the liver, stenosis of the bile duct, and hepatic cirrhosis (although this may also be due to alcohol intake). It has been estimated that more than 50% of patients die within 20 years of diagnosis, with those who continue to drink alcohol being at greatest risk.

Adequate analgesia with opioids is essential (see Pancreatic Pain, p.7). Nerve blocks of the coeliac plexus with phenol or alcohol have generally proved disappointing, although coeliac plexus blocks using corticosteroids and local anaesthetic may be effective.[5] Patients should be advised to abstain from alcohol, which can exacerbate the frequency and severity of painful episodes. Steatorrhoea requires replacement of pancreatic enzymes with preparations of pancreatin or pancrelipase. Because the enzymes are inactivated by gastric acid they may be taken after histamine $H_2$ antagonists or with a sodium-containing antacid such as sodium bicarbonate (magnesium-, calcium-, and possibly aluminium-containing antacids may further interfere with fat absorption). Alternatively, enteric-coated enzyme preparations may be used. In some patients with mild disease pancreatic enzyme replacement may also improve pain. Supplements of fat-soluble vitamins are not normally necessary, but may be given intravenously if required. Diabetes should be managed appropriately once steatorrhoea is under control.

Surgery, up to and including total pancreatectomy, has an important role in the relief of intractable pain, and may also be necessary for the management of complications. Endoscopic decompression using contrast media containing prednisolone and ulinastatin has been reported to produce beneficial responses.[10] Anecdotal results suggest that some patients with pancreatic pseudocysts, which usually require surgical drainage, may respond to octreotide.[11]


1. Nam JH, Murthy S. Acute pancreatitis—the current status in management. *Expert Opin Pharmacother* 2003; **4**: 235–41.
2. Steinberg W, Tenner S. Acute pancreatitis. *N Engl J Med* 1994; **330**: 1198–1210.
3. Pande H, Thuluvath PJ. Pharmacological prevention of post-endoscopic retrograde cholangiopancreatography pancreatitis. *Drugs* 2003; **63**: 1799–812.
4. Fernández-del Castillo C, *et al.* Acute pancreatitis. *Lancet* 1993; **342**: 475–9.
5. Mitchell RMS, *et al.* Pancreatitis. *Lancet* 2003; **361**: 1447–55.
6. Sainio V, *et al.* Early antibiotic treatment in acute necrotising pancreatitis. *Lancet* 1995; **346**: 663–7.
7. Ho HS, Frey CF. The role of antibiotic prophylaxis in severe acute pancreatitis. *Arch Surg* 1997; **132**: 487–93.
8. Baron TH, Morgan DE. Acute necrotizing pancreatitis. *N Engl J Med* 1999; **340**: 1412–17. Correction. *ibid.*; **341**: 460.
9. Baillie J. Treatment of acute biliary pancreatitis. *N Engl J Med* 1997; **336**: 286–7.
10. Ohwada M, *et al.* New endoscopic treatment for chronic pancreatitis, using contrast media containing ulinastatin and prednisolone. *J Gastroenterol* 1997; **32**: 216–21.
11. Gullo L, Barbara L. Treatment of pancreatic pseudocysts with octreotide. *Lancet* 1991; **338**: 540–1.


### Preparations

***BP 2003:*** Pancreatin Granules; Pancreatin Tablets;
***USP 27:*** Pancreatin Tablets; Pancrelipase Capsules; Pancrelipase Delayed-release Capsules; Pancrelipase Tablets.

**Proprietary Preparations** (details are given in Part 3)
***Arg.:*** Creon; Pancrecura; Pankreozym; Prolipase; ***Austral.:*** Bioglan Panazyme†; Cotazym S Forte; Creon; Opti-Free Enzymatic†; Opti-Plus†; Pancenz†; Pancrease; Panzytrat; Polyzym†; Viokase†; ***Austria:*** Kreon; Opti-Free†; Pancrin; Pankreon forte; Panzynorm; Polyzym†; Prolipase†; ***Belg.:*** Creon; Pancrease; Viokase†; ***Braz.:*** Cotazym; Opti-Free Enzimatica; Opti-free Supraclens; Pancrease; Pankreon†; Panzytrat; Polyzym; Ultrase†; ***Canad.:*** Cotazym; Creon; Digess†; Opti-Zyme; Pancrease; Ultrase; Viokase; ***Chile:*** Creon; ***Denm.:*** Pancrease; Pankreon; ***Fin.:*** Pancrease; Pankreon; ***Fr.:*** Alipase†; Creon; Licrease; Opti-Plus†; Pancreal Kirchner†; Polyzym; ***Ger.:*** Bilipeptal Mono; Carzodelan; Cholspasminase N; Cotazym; Euflat-E; Fermento duodenal; Hevertozym; Kreon; Lipazym; Meteophyt forte; Mezym F; Nutrizym N; Ozym; Pancholtruw N†; Pangrol; Pankreatan; Pankreon; Panpeptal N; Panpur; Panzynorm forte-N; Panzytrat; Tryptoferm; Unexym mono; ***Gr.:*** Creon; Pancrease; Panzytrat; ***Hong Kong:*** Creon; ***India:*** Festal N; Panzynorm-N; ***Irl.:*** Creon; Nutrizym; Pancrease; Pancrex; Panzytrat†; ***Israel:*** Creon; Pancrease; ***Ital.:*** Creon; Enzipan; Festal N†; Krebsilasi; Luitase; Pancrease; Pancreon†; Pancrex; Pancrin†; Pancrotanon†; Pankreaden†; ***Malaysia:*** Creon; ***Mex.:*** Creon; Pancrease; Polyzym†; Selecto; ***Neth.:*** Creon; Pancrease; Pancrease HL; Panzytrat; ***Norw.:*** Pancrease; Pankreon; ***NZ:*** Cotazym; Creon; Pancrease; Pancrex; Panzytrat; Viokase†; ***Port.:*** Kreon; ***S.Afr.:*** Creon; Pankrease; Viokase; ***Singapore:*** Creon; ***Spain:*** Kreon; Pancrease; Pankreon†; ***Swed.:*** Pancrease; Pankreon; ***Switz.:*** Creon; Panzytrat; Prolipase; ***Thai.:*** Creon; ***UK:*** Clen-Zym; Creon; Nutrizym; Pancrease; Pancrease HL; Pancrex; ***USA:*** Cotazym†; Creon; Donnazyme†; Enzymatic Cleaner; Ilozyme†; Ku-Zyme HP; Lipram; Opti-Zyme; Pancrease; Protilase†; Ultrase; Viokase; Vision Care Enzymatic Cleaner; Zymase†.

**Multi-ingredient:** ***Arg.:*** Bibol Leloup; Bil 13 Enzimatico; Biletan Enzimatico; Biluen Enzimatico; Carbogasol Digestivo; Digenorflat; Digesplen; Facilgest; Faradil Enzimatico; Gastridin-E; Gastrimet Enzimatico; Gastron Fuerte; Hepadigenor; Homocisteon Compuesto; Moperidona Enzimatica; Novodig; Pakinase; Pankreoflat; Pankreoflat Sedante; Pankreon Compuesto; Pankreon Total; Praxis; Pulsar Enzimatico; Tridigestivo Soubeiran; ***Austral.:*** Digestaid†; Enzyme†; Lexat†; Natures Own Digestive Enzymes†; Prozyme†; ***Austria:*** Arca-Enzym; Aristochol†; Combizym; Combizym Compositum; Digestif Rennie; Enzyflat; Gallo Merz†; Gingivan; Helopanflat; Helopanzym; Intestinol; Nutrizym†; Ora-Gallin; Pankreoflat; Pankreon compositum†; Paspertase; Wobenzym; ***Belg.:*** Combizym†; Digestomen; ***Braz.:*** Azime; Combizym Composto; Combizym†; Dasc; Digecap-Zimatico; Digeplus; Digestal†; Elozima; Espasmo Novozyme†; Essen; Filogaster; Hepatoregius; Nutrizim; Pankreoflat; Peptopancreasi; Plasil Enzimatico; Sintozima; Vonil Enzimatico†; ***Canad.:*** Alsilax†; Vesilax†; ***Chile:*** Combizym Compositum; Digenil; Flapex E; Hepabil; Neopankreoflat; Nutrizima; Onoton; ***Fin.:*** Combizym; Combizym Compositum; ***Fr.:*** Hepatoum†; Pancrelase†; ***Ger.:*** Arbuz; Chol-Arbuz N; Combizym; Combizym Compositum; Enzym-Lefax; Enzym-Wied; Helopanflat N†; Hevert Enzym Novo†; Meteozym; Pankreoflat; Pascopankreat; Paspertase; Stacho-Zym N†; Unexym MD S; Ventracid N; Wobenzym N; ***Hong Kong:*** Combizym; Pankreoflat; Topase; ***India:*** Digeplex-T; Dispeptal; Hepa-Merz; Merckenzyme; Pankreoflat; Panolase; Papytazyme; ***Israel:*** Encypalmed; Pankreoflat; ***Ital.:*** Combizym; Digestopan; Ede 6; Eudigestio; Pancreoflat; Pancreon Compositum†; Pancresil; Pepto-Pancreasi; ***Mex.:*** Difarben; Dirfaben; Dixiflen; Espaven Enzimatico; Onoton; Pankreoflat; Plasil Enzimatico; Selecto-D; Wobenzym; ***Neth.:*** Combizym; Combizym Compositum†; ***Norw.:*** Combizym; ***NZ:*** Combizym; Combizym Compositum†; ***Port.:*** Colerin-F; Combizym; Combizym Compositum; Espasmo Canulase; Fermetone Composto; Helopanflat†; Nutrizym†; Pankreoflat; ***S.Afr.:*** Pankreoflat; Spasmo-Canulase; ***Spain:*** Digestomen Complex; Edym Sedante†; Espasmo Digestomen†; Lidobama Complex†; Nulacin Fermentos; Paigastrol†; Pankreoflat; Wobenzimal; ***Swed.:*** Combizym; Combizym Compositum; ***Switz.:*** Combizym; Combizym Compositum†; Fermento duodenal; Gillazyme plus†; Gillazyme†; Helopanflat; Spasmo-Canulase; ***Thai.:*** Combizym; Combizym Compositum; Enzymet; Gaszym; Papytazyme; Pepsitase; Polyenzyme-I; Polyenzyme-N; Proctase-P; Sanzyme-S; ***UK:*** Digezyme†; ***USA:*** Digepepsin; Hi-Vegi-Lip; Pancrezyme 4X†.

## Pancreozymin *(BAN)*

CCK-PZ; Pancreocimina.
*ATC — V04CK02.*

NOTE. The endogenous hormone is known as cholecystokinin (CCK).

### Units

The potency of pancreozymin may be expressed as Crick-Harper-Raper units based on the pancreatic secretion in *cats* or as Ivy *dog* units based on the increase in gallbladder pressure. One Ivy dog unit is considered to be approximately equivalent to 1 Crick-Harper-Raper unit.

### Profile

Pancreozymin is a polypeptide hormone prepared from the duodenal mucosa of *pigs*. When administered by intravenous injection it causes an increase in the secretion of pancreatic enzymes and stimulates gallbladder contraction.

Pancreozymin has been used, usually with secretin, as a test for exocrine pancreatic function and in the diagnosis of biliary-tract disorders; these tests generally involved duodenal intubation of the patient and examination of duodenal aspirate. Pancreozymin has also been used as an adjunct to cholecystography. Vasomotor reactions, abdominal discomfort, and hypersensitivity have been reported.

◊ It was concluded that cholecystokinin provocation testing was ineffective in predicting which patients with acalculous biliary pain would receive symptomatic relief from cholecystectomy in a study involving 58 patients.[1]


1. Smythe A, *et al.* A requiem for the cholecystokinin provocation test? *Gut* 1998; **43**: 571–4.


## Pangamic Acid

Pangámico, ácido.

### Profile

The name pangamic acid has been applied variously to gluconic acid 6-[bis(diisopropylamino)acetate] ($C_{20}H_{40}N_2O_8$ = 436.5), gluconic acid, 6-ester with N,N-dimethylglycine ($C_{10}H_{19}NO_8$ = 281.3), gluconic acid, 6-ester with N,N-diisopropylglycine ($C_{14}H_{27}NO_8$ = 337.4), and a substance or mixture of substances isolated from apricot kernels and rice bran. It has also been known as vitamin $B_{15}$ although there is no evidence that pangamic acid is a vitamin. Preparations containing the vasoactive substance di-isopropylammonium dichloroacetate (p.900) have sometimes been described as pangamic acid or vitamin $B_{15}$. There is much uncertainty about the identity of products sold in health food stores as 'vitamin $B_{15}$', pangamic acid, or sodium or calcium pangamate and different brands have been reported to have completely different compositions.

Claims for the activity of pangamic acid as a promotor of tissue oxygenation and its alleged value in numerous disorders have not been substantiated.

### Preparations

**Proprietary Preparations** (details are given in Part 3)
***Arg.:*** B15; ***Ger.:*** Oyo; ***Port.:*** Pulsor.
**Multi-ingredient:** ***Mex.:*** B1-12-15; ***Spain:*** Policolinosil.

## Panthenol *(BAN, USAN)*

*dl*-Panthenol; ±-Pantothenyl Alcohol.
$C_9H_{19}NO_4$ = 205.3.
*CAS — 16485-10-2.*

**Pharmacopoeias.** In *US.*

**USP 27** (Panthenol). A racemic mixture of the dextrorotatory and laevorotatory isomers of panthenol. A white to creamy white, crystalline powder with a slight, characteristic odour. Freely soluble in water, in alcohol, and in propylene glycol; soluble in chloroform and in ether; slightly soluble in glycerol. Store in airtight containers.

## Dexpanthenol *(BAN, USAN, rINN)*

Dexpantenol; Dexpanthenolum; Dextro-Pantothenyl Alcohol; Pantothenol. (*R*)-2,4-Dihydroxy-*N*-(3-hydroxypropyl)-3,3-dimethylbutyramide.
$C_9H_{19}NO_4$ = 205.3.
*CAS — 81-13-0.*
*ATC — A11HA30; D03AX03; S01XA12.*

**Pharmacopoeias.** In *Eur.* (see p.vi), *US,* and *Viet.*

**Ph. Eur. 5.0** (Dexpanthenol). A colourless or slightly yellowish, hygroscopic, viscous liquid, or a white or almost white, crystalline powder. Very soluble in water; freely soluble in alcohol. A 5% solution in water has a pH not greater than 10.5. Store in airtight containers.

**USP 27** (Dexpanthenol). A clear, viscous, somewhat hygroscopic liquid, having a slight characteristic odour. Some crystallisation may occur on standing. Freely soluble in water, in alcohol, in methyl alcohol, and in propylene glycol; soluble in chloroform and in ether; slightly soluble in glycerol. Store in airtight containers.

### Adverse Effects and Precautions

There have been a few reports of allergic reactions possibly associated with the administration of dexpanthenol. Dexpanthenol is contra-indicated in haemophiliacs and in patients with ileus due to mechanical obstruction.

### Uses and Administration

Dexpanthenol is the alcoholic analogue of D-pantothenic acid (p.1442). It has been given intramuscularly in doses of 250 to 500 mg to prevent or control gastrointestinal atony but its value has not been established. It has also been given by slow intravenous infusion.

Dexpanthenol and the racemate panthenol have been used topically in strengths of 2 or 5% for the treatment of various minor skin disorders. They are also included in some vitamin preparations.

◊ References.


1. Kehrl W, Sonnemann U. Verbesserung der Wundheilung nach Nasenoperationen durch kombinierte Anwendung von Xylometazolin und Dexpanthenol. *Laryngorhinootologie* 2000; **79**: 151–4.
2. Gehring W, Gloor M. Effect of topically applied dexpanthenol on epidermal barrier function and stratum corneum hydration: results of a human in vivo study. *Arzneimittelforschung* 2000; **50**: 659–63.
3. Ebner F, *et al.* Topical use of dexpanthenol in skin disorders. *Am J Clin Dermatol* 2002; **3**: 427–33.


### Preparations

***USP 27:*** Dexpanthenol Preparation.

**Proprietary Preparations** (details are given in Part 3)
***Arg.:*** Nutraisdin; Recugel; ***Austria:*** Bepanthen; Dex-Panol; Pantothen; ***Belg.:*** Bepanthene†; ***Braz.:*** Bepantol; ***Chile:*** Bepantol; ***Fin.:*** Bepanthen; ***Fr.:*** Bepanthen; Pan-Sun; ***Ger.:*** Bepanthen; Corneregel; Cutemul†; Dexpanol†; Marolderm†; Nasicur; Otriven mit Dexpanthenol; Pan-Ophtal; Panthenol; Panthogenat; Pelina; Rhinoclir; Ucee D; Urupan; Wund- und Heilsalbe N; ***Israel:*** Bepanthen; ***Ital.:*** Bepanten; ***NZ:*** Bepanthen; ***Port.:*** Bepanthene; ***S.Afr.:*** Bepantol; ***Spain:*** Bepanthene; ***Switz.:*** Bepanthene; Unathen; ***UAE:*** Dexipan; ***UK:*** Bepanthen†; ***USA:*** Ilopan; Panthoderm.

**Multi-ingredient:** ***Arg.:*** Dermocridin; Heduline; Mucobase; Nutraisdin; Sebulex; Talowin; ***Austral.:*** Macro Natural Vitamin E Cream; Sebirinse†; Superfade†; ***Austria:*** Beneuran Vit B-Komplex; Bepanthen; Bepanthen Plus; Colda; Coldistan; Dolobene; Felix; Halset plus Dexpanthenol; Keratosis; Keratosis forte; Mar Plus; Oleovit; Panto Liquid; Pelsana Med; Siccaprotect; Sigman-Haustropfen; Sunsan-Heillotion; Venobene; ***Braz.:*** Babyglos†; Capel; Dolobene; Naridrin; Nasopan†; Nazobio; Nitronasal†; Perlax†; Rinatrol†; Rinozin†; Solucao Nasal de Nafazolina†; Varizol; ***Canad.:*** Aquasol A†; Selsun with Provitamin $B_5$; ***Chile:*** Acnoxyl Shampoo Cabello Graso; Eucerin; Panthoderm-A; Pomada Vitaminica; ***Fin.:*** Oftan A-Pant; Pantyson; Wicaran; Wicarba; Wicnevit; ***Ger.:*** Brand- und Wund-Gel Eu Rho; Dispatenol; Dolobene; Essaven Tri-Complex; Hermalind; Hewekzem novo N; Hydro Cordes; Lipo Cordes; Lipovitan; Mar Plus; Nasic; Pantederm; PC 30 V; Remederm; Siccaprotect; Wund- und Brand-Gel Eu Rho†; ***Hong Kong:*** Dolobene; Egozite Baby Cream; ***India:*** Optineuron; Sioneuron; Vitneurin; ***Israel:*** Bepanthen Plus; Kamil Blue; Panthisone; Pedisol; ***Ital.:*** Alfa Acid; Emazian B12; Emoantitossina; Herbavit†; Lenirose; Rinopanteina; ***Malaysia:*** Egozite Baby Cream; ***NZ:*** Sebirinse; ***Port.:*** Bepanthene; Bepanthene Plus; Bexident; Carmitol; Cicapost; Efluvium Anti-seborreico; Eucerin Pele com tendencia para o acne creme antiborbulhas†; Lactigriet; Nutraisdin; Ureadin 10 Plus; ***S.Afr.:*** Broncol; ***Singapore:*** Egozite Baby Cream; ***Spain:*** Anasilpiel; Neo Visage†; ***Switz.:*** Alphastria; Bepanthene Plus; Carbamide + VAS; Carbamide Creme; Cortimycine; Demostan N; Dermacalm-d; Dolobene; Galamila; Gorgonium; Hepathrombine; Leniderm; Lyman; Nastop†; Pelsano; Pigmanorm; Remexal; Roll-bene†; Siccalix; Sportium; Sportusal; Sportusal Spray sine heparino; Stilex; Turexan Capilla; Turexan Lotion; Unatol; Venucreme; Venugel; ***Thai.:*** Detuss†; Romilar; ***UK:*** Vipsogal†; ***USA:*** Ilopan-Choline†.

## Papain

Papaína; Papayotin.
*CAS — 9001-73-4.*

**Pharmacopoeias.** In *US.*

**USP 27** (Papain). A purified proteolytic substance derived from *Carica papaya* (Caricaceae). It contains not less than 6000 USP units per mg. A white to light tan, amorphous powder. Soluble in water, the solution being colourless to light yellow and more or less opalescent; practically insoluble in alcohol, in chloroform, and in ether. pH of a 2% solution in water is between 4.8 and 6.2. Store in airtight containers at a temperature of 8° to 15°. Protect from light.

### Units

USP 27 defines the USP unit of papain activity as the activity that releases the equivalent of 1 microgram of tyrosine from a specified casein substrate under the conditions of the assay, using the enzyme concentration that liberates 40 micrograms of tyrosine per mL of test solution.

One FIP unit of papain is defined as the enzyme activity which under specified conditions hydrolyses 1 micromol of *N*-benzoyl-L-arginine ethyl ester per minute.

The Warner-Chilcott unit, based on the quantity of enzyme required to clot 2.64 microlitre of milk substrate in 2 minutes at 40°, under specified conditions, has also been used for papain.

### Adverse Effects

Hypersensitivity reactions have occurred.

**Effects on the eyes.** Ocular and periorbital angioedema occurring within 4 hours of use of a contact lens cleansing solution containing papain has been reported.[1]

1. Bernstein DI, *et al.* Local ocular anaphylaxis to papain enzyme contained in a contact lens cleansing solution. *J Allergy Clin Immunol* 1984; **74:** 258–60.

**Oesophageal perforation.** Extensive destruction of the oesophageal wall, with perforation, resulted from the use of a papain suspension given to treat an obstruction caused by impacted meat.[1] The patient had been given 1.2 g of papain over a 12-hour period. Ten days after a thoracotomy, the descending thoracic aorta ruptured, and she died from haemorrhage.

1. Holsinger JW, *et al.* Esophageal perforation following meat impaction and papain ingestion. *JAMA* 1968; **204:** 734–5.

### Uses and Administration

Papain consists chiefly of a mixture of papain and chymopapain, proteolytic enzymes that hydrolyse polypeptides, amides, and esters, especially at bonds involving basic amino acids, or leucine or glycine, yielding peptides of lower molecular weight. It is used as a topical debriding agent in conjunction with urea. It is also used for the removal of protein deposits from the surface of soft contact lenses (p.1164).

Preparations of papain, alone or combined with antibacterial agents and/or other substances, have been taken by mouth for their supposed anti-inflammatory properties, and it has also been used as an ingredient of various mixtures claimed to aid digestion.

Papain is widely used as a meat tenderiser and in the clarification of beverages.

**Malignant neoplasms.** Papain has been included in proteolytic enzyme preparations used in oncology to reduce the adverse effects of chemotherapy and radiotherapy. Although the number of clinical studies on which to judge efficacy is limited, a review[1] of such studies suggested that systemic enzyme therapy might be beneficial. Clinical studies have used a preparation containing papain, trypsin, and chymotrypsin in a weight ratio of 5:2:2, and the beneficial effect seems to be based on its anti-inflammatory potential.

1. Leipner J, Saller R. Systemic enzyme therapy in oncology: effect and mode of action. *Drugs* 2000; **59:** 769–80.

### Preparations

***USP 27:*** Papain Tablets for Topical Solution.

**Proprietary Preparations** (details are given in Part 3)
***Arg.:*** Tromasin; ***Austral.:*** Hydrocare Enzymatic Protein Remover†; Stop Itch†; ***Canad.:*** Hydrocare Protein Remover†; Solarcaine Stop Itch†; Stop Itch; ***Chile:*** Papenzima; ***Ger.:*** Vermizym; ***Hong Kong:*** Eurolase; ***Malaysia:*** Beazyme; ***NZ:*** Hydrocare Fizzy Protein Remover†; Stop Itch; ***Spain:*** Cacital†; ***USA:*** Allergan Enzymatic; ProFree.

**Multi-ingredient:** ***Arg.:*** Butimerin; Homocisteon Compuesto; Opoenterol; Pakinase; Pankreon Total; Solustres; Tromasin con Aspirina; Vulnofilin Compuesto; ***Austral.:*** Betaine Digestive Aid†; Bio-Disc†; Bioglan Discone†; Digestaid†; Digestive Aid†; Enzyme†; Natures Own Digestive Enzymes†; Prost-1†; Prozyme†; ***Austria:*** Digestif Rennie; Wobe-Mugos; Wobenzym; ***Belg.:*** Digestomen; ***Braz.:*** Fideine†; Filogaster; ***Canad.:*** Herbalax Forte†; Phytolax†; Vesilax†; ***Ger.:*** Arbuz; Chol-Arbuz N; Enzym-Wied; Mulsal N; Wobe-Mugos E; Wobe-Mugos Th†; Wobenzym N; ***India:*** Bestozyme; Catazyme-P; Dipep; Molzyme; Neopeptine; Papytazyme; Unienzyme c MPS; ***Ital.:*** Digestopan; ***Mex.:*** Dermobion; Digenor Plus; Wobe-Mugos; Wobenzym; ***Port.:*** Caroid; ***Spain:*** Digestomen Complex; Espasmo Digestomen†; Lizipaina; Nasotic Oto†; ***Switz.:*** Lysopaine; ***Thai.:*** Papytazyme; Pepsitase; Polyenzyme-I; ***UK:*** Enzyme Digest; Herbal Indigestion Naturtabs; Indigestion and Flatulence; Papaya Plus†; ***USA:*** Accuzyme; Ethezyme; Gladase; Panafil; Panafil-White; Papaya Enzyme.

---

## Papaverine *(BAN)*

Papaverina. 6,7-Dimethoxy-1-(3,4-dimethoxybenzyl)isoquinoline.

$C_{20}H_{21}NO_4$ = 339.4.
*CAS — 58-74-2.*
*ATC — A03AD01; G04BE02.*

NOTE. Papaverine should not be confused with papaveretum (p.74).

## Papaverine Hydrochloride *(BAN)*

Papaverina, hidrocloruro de; Papaverini Hydrochloridum; Papaverinii Chloridum; Papaverinium Chloride. 6,7-Dimethoxy-1-(3,4-dimethoxybenzyl)isoquinoline hydrochloride.

$C_{20}H_{21}NO_4,HCl$ = 375.8.
*CAS — 63817-84-5 (papaverine cromesilate); 61-25-6 (papaverine hydrochloride); 39024-96-9 (papaverine monophosadenine); 2053-26-1 (anhydrous papaverine sulfate).*
*ATC — A03AD01; G04BE02.*

**Pharmacopoeias.** In *Chin., Eur.* (see p.vi), *Int., Jpn, Pol., US,* and *Viet.*

**Ph. Eur. 5.0** (Papaverine Hydrochloride). White or almost white crystals or crystalline powder. Sparingly soluble in water; slightly soluble in alcohol. A 2% solution in water has a pH of 3.0 to 4.0.

**USP 27** (Papaverine Hydrochloride). Odourless white crystals or white, crystalline powder. Soluble 1 in 30 of water and 1 in 120 of alcohol; soluble in chloroform; practically insoluble in ether. pH of a 2% solution in water is between 3.0 and 4.5. Store in airtight containers at a temperature of 25°, excursions permitted between 15° and 30°. Protect from light.

### Adverse Effects and Precautions

Adverse effects of papaverine given by mouth include gastrointestinal disturbance, flushing of the face, headache, malaise, drowsiness, skin rash, sweating, orthostatic hypotension, and dizziness. Jaundice, eosinophilia, and signs of altered liver function may occur, sometimes due to hypersensitivity. In addition parenteral administration of high doses can result in cardiac arrhythmias; a slow rate of intravenous or intramuscular administration is recommended. Thrombosis has been reported at the injection site.

Intracavernosal injection can cause dose-related priapism and local fibrosis has been reported following long-term therapy.

Papaverine should be given with caution to patients with reduced gastrointestinal motility. Caution is also advised in the presence of cardiac conduction disorders or unstable cardiovascular disease, especially when papaverine is administered parenterally. Intravenous administration is contra-indicated in patients with complete atrioventricular block.

**Glaucoma.** There appeared to be no basis for the manufacturers' recommendation that papaverine should be used with caution in patients with glaucoma.[1] There was no obvious mechanism to support such a warning and only 1 report of an adverse reaction had been received by the FDA. The author had given papaverine intracavernosally to patients with glaucoma and had observed no deterioration.

1. Swartz DA, Todd MW. Intracavernous papaverine and glaucoma. *JAMA* 1990; **264:** 570.

**Intracavernosal administration.** Systemic adverse effects occurring after intracavernosal injection of papaverine are infrequent but include dizziness and syncope,[1,2] probably related to the hypotensive effects of papaverine; abnormal liver function test results have also occurred.[1-3]

The most serious acute adverse effect is priapism[1,2,4] and patients should be instructed to seek medical help if an erection lasts for more than 4 hours. Detumescence can be effected by aspiration of blood from the corpus or by local injection of an alpha-adrenergic agonist such as adrenaline, metaraminol, or phenylephrine (see Priapism under Alprostadil, p.1513). Other local effects include haematoma, infection, and, on long-term therapy, fibrosis and penile distortion.[1,2]

Dispensing errors have resulted in inadvertent injection of *papaveretum* with potentially fatal consequences.[2,5,6]

1. Krane RJ, *et al.* Impotence. *N Engl J Med* 1989; **321:** 1648–59.
2. Bénard F, Lue TF. Self-administration in the pharmacological treatment of impotence. *Drugs* 1990; **39:** 394–8.
3. Levine SB, *et al.* Side effects of self-administration of intracavernous papaverine and phentolamine for the treatment of impotence. *J Urol (Baltimore)* 1989; **141:** 54–7.
4. Virag R. About pharmacologically induced prolonged erection. *Lancet* 1985; **i:** 519–20.
5. Robinson LQ, Stephenson TP. Self injection treatment for impotence. *BMJ* 1989; **299:** 1568.
6. Gregoire A. Self injection treatment for impotence. *BMJ* 1990; **300:** 537.

### Interactions

**Levodopa.** For a report of papaverine decreasing the effectiveness of levodopa, see p.1208.

### Pharmacokinetics

The biological half-life of papaverine given by mouth is reported to be between one and two hours, but there is wide interindividual variation. It is extensively bound (about 90%) to plasma proteins.

Papaverine is mainly metabolised in the liver and excreted in the urine, almost entirely as glucuronide-conjugated phenolic metabolites.

The reports of infrequent systemic effects after intracavernosal injection of papaverine indicate that there is some distribution to the systemic circulation from the corpus cavernosum.

### Uses and Administration

Papaverine is an alkaloid present in opium, although it is not related chemically or pharmacologically to the other opium alkaloids. Papaverine has a direct relaxant effect on smooth muscle which is attributed in part to its ability to inhibit phosphodiesterase. It has been given in the management of cerebral, peripheral, and coronary vascular disorders; it is also given as an antispasmodic for gastrointestinal disorders and coughs. However, there is little evidence to justify its clinical use in these conditions.

Papaverine has been given by mouth as the hydrochloride in doses of up to 600 mg daily. Sustained-release preparations have been used. The codecarboxylase derivative, cromesilate, hydrobromide, monophosadenine, nicotinate, sulfate, and teprosilate have also been used. Papaverine hydrochloride has also been given in doses of 30 to 120 mg by slow intramuscular or intravenous injection (but see Adverse Effects and Precautions, above).

Papaverine hydrochloride has been given by injection into the corpus cavernosum of the penis for the diagnosis and treatment of erectile dysfunction (p.1745). Phentolamine may be added if the response is inadequate.

### Preparations

***USP 27:*** Papaverine Hydrochloride Injection; Papaverine Hydrochloride Tablets.

**Proprietary Preparations** (details are given in Part 3)
***Arg.:*** Mesotina; Ova; ***Braz.:*** Dipaverina; ***Fr.:*** Oxadilene†; ***USA:*** Pavabid.

**Multi-ingredient:** ***Arg.:*** Antipasmol; Antispasmina; Gastranil; Hepatodirectol; Saltos; Trixol; ***Austria:*** Androskat; Asthma 23 D; Asthma†; Myocardon; Normensan†; Ora-Gallin compositum; Perphyllon†; ***Braz.:*** Analgosedan†; Antispasmin†; Atroveran†; Atrovex†; Calmazin†; Calmovarin†; Codeverin; Colinex†; Diarona†; Dipirol; Ductoveran; Espasmalgon; Espasmobel†; Espasmocron; Espasmolex†; Espasmosan Composto†; Espasmosan†; Gaba; Melpaz†; Metilsedor†; Monotrean; Monotrean B6†; Nicopaverina; Nicopaverina B6; Pasmalgin†; Plenocedan†; Regran†; Revulsan; Sedalene; Somasedin†; Spasmotropin; Tebasedan†; Uroseptin†; Vagostesyl; ***Chile:*** Belupan; Buton; Dipatropin; Dolospam; Papatropin; ***Fr.:*** Acticarbine; Solurutine Papaverine F. Retard†; ***Hong Kong:*** Bromhexine Compound; Codomex Orange; Codomex Purple; Codoplex; Metoplex; ***India:*** Brovon; ***Israel:*** Patropin; Spasmalgin; ***Ital.:*** Antispasmina Colica; Farmospasmina†; Ischelium Papaverina†; Monotrean; ***Mex.:*** Acilin; Ayoral; ***Neth.:*** Androskat; ***Port.:*** Antispasmina Colica; Cosmaxil; ***Spain:*** Analgilasa†; Angiosedante†; Rubia Paver†; Sulmetin Papaver; Sulmetin Papaverina; ***Swed.:*** Spasmofen; ***Switz.:*** Dolopyrine; Spasmosol; ***UK:*** Brovon.

---

## Paradichlorobenzene

Dichlorbenzol; Paradiclorobenceno. 1,4-Dichlorobenzene.

$C_6H_4Cl_2$ = 147.0.
*CAS — 106-46-7.*

### Profile

Paradichlorobenzene has general properties similar to those of orthodichlorobenzene (see p.1724) but is considered to be less toxic. It is present in several preparations intended for the removal of ear wax (see p.1262). It has been used as a furniture preservative and in mothballs and lavatory deodorant blocks. Abuse of preparations containing paradichlorobenzene has been reported.

### Preparations

**Proprietary Preparations** (details are given in Part 3)

**Multi-ingredient:** ***Austral.:*** Cerumol; ***Canad.:*** Cerumol; ***Hong Kong:*** Cerumol†; ***India:*** Waxolve; ***Irl.:*** Cerumol†; ***Israel:*** Cerumol; ***Malaysia:*** Cerumol; ***Port.:*** Otoceril; ***S.Afr.:*** Cerumol; ***Singapore:*** Cerumol; ***Switz.:*** Cerumenol; ***UK:*** Cerumol.

---

## Paraphenylenediamine

Parafenilendiamina.

$C_6H_4(NH_2)_2$ = 108.1.
*CAS — 106-50-3.*

NOTE. Commonly known in the hairdressing trade as *'para'*.

### Profile

Paraphenylenediamine is used in hair colour preparations.

It is estimated that about 4% of apparently normal subjects are sensitive to paraphenylenediamine, and 1% acutely sensitive; oedema and severe dermatitis may follow application in such persons. Effects on the eye may include chemosis, lachrymation, exophthalmos, and sometimes permanent blindness. For references to hypersensitivity following skin tattoos with henna adulterated with paraphenyldiamine, see p.1696.

Following ingestion, severe angioedema-like symptoms with respiratory difficulty and dyspnoea may occur and may require emergency tracheostomy; vomiting, massive oedema, gastritis, rise in blood pressure, vertigo, tremors, convulsions, and coma have been reported.

Some studies have linked hair dyes with mutagenicity and carcinogenicity, although such findings have often been refuted.

---

## Paratoluenediamine

Paratoluendiamina. 2-Methyl-1,4-phenylenediamine.

$C_7H_{10}N_2$ = 122.2.
*CAS — 95-70-5.*

### Profile

Paratoluenediamine is used in hair colour preparations.

Like paraphenylenediamine, above, paratoluenediamine may be associated with sensitivity reactions.

---

## Parsley

Perejil; Persil; Petroselinum.

### Profile

Parsley (*Petroselinum crispum*, Umbelliferae) is used in herbal medicine, where it is mainly given as a diuretic. It is also used as a culinary herb and flavour.

### Preparations

**Proprietary Preparations** (details are given in Part 3)
***Ger.:*** Kneipp Petersilie N†.

**Multi-ingredient:** ***Arg.:*** Water Pill c Potasio; ***Austral.:*** Extralife Fluid-Care†; Fluid Loss†; Medinat PMT-Eze†; Odourless Garlic†; Uva-Ursi Plus†; ***Austria:*** Apotheker Bauer's Harntreibender Tee; Blasen-Tee†; Krauterhaus Mag Kottas Entwasserungstee; Krauterpfarrer Weidinger Tee zur Entwasserung; Magentee†; Naturland Entschlackungstonikum; Neuners Krautertee Nr 126 - Starkungstee fur stillende Mutter; Neuners Krautertee Nr 18 - Stoffwechseltee; Neuners Krautertee Nr 25 - Entschlackungstee; Neuners Krautertee Nr 3 - Blasentee; Neuners Krautertee Nr 4 - Nierentee; ***Braz.:*** Tintura de Salsa Caroba e Manaca†; ***Canad.:*** Herbal Throat; ***Ger.:*** Asparagus-P; nephro-loges; ***UK:*** Athera; Digest†; Fre-bre; Garlodex†; Gerard House Helonias Compound†; Kincare†; Mixed Vegetable Tablets; Modern Herbals Menopause.

---

## Parsley Piert

Alquimila arvense; Aphanes.

### Profile

Parsley piert, the aerial parts of *Aphanes arvensis* (*Alchemilla arvensis*) (Rosaceae) has astringent, diuretic, and demulcent properties. It is used for urinary-tract disorders, including renal and urinary calculi.

### Preparations

**Proprietary Preparations** (details are given in Part 3)

**Multi-ingredient:** ***Austral.:*** Profluid†; Protemp†; ***Canad.:*** Swiss Herb Cough Drops; ***Fr.:*** Gonaxine; ***UK:*** Backache Relief; Diuretabs; HRI Water Balance; Watershed.

## Passion Flower

Grenadille; May-pop; Pasiflora; Pasionari; Passiflora; Passiflorae Herba.

**Pharmacopoeias.** In *Eur.* (see p.vi).

**Ph. Eur. 5.0** (Passion Flower). The fragmented or cut, dried aerial parts of *Passiflora incarnata*; it may also contain flowers and/or fruits. It contains not less than 1.5% of total flavonoids expressed as vitexin ($C_{21}H_{20}O_{10}$ = 432.4), calculated with reference to the dried drug. Protect from light.

### Profile

Passion flower is reputed to have antispasmodic and sedative properties and has been used as an ingredient of herbal remedies, chiefly in the form of a liquid extract tincture.

Passion flower is also used in homoeopathic medicine.

### Preparations

**Proprietary Preparations** (details are given in Part 3)
***Arg.:*** Sedante Noche; ***Austria:*** Passiflorin; ***Ger.:*** Passiflora Curarina; ***UK:*** Modern Herbals Sleep Aid; Natracalm; Naturest; Nodoff; Phytocalm.

**Multi-ingredient:** ***Arg.:*** Armonil; Calmtabs; Herbaccion Sedante; Insomnal; Nervocalm; No-Nerviol; Passacanthine; Sedante Arceli; Sedante Dia; Serenil; Top Life Relax; ***Austral.:*** Calmo†; Euphorbia Complex†; Executive B†; Extralife Sleep-Care†; Goodnight Formula†; Herbal Anxiety Formula†; Infant Calm†; Lifesystem Herbal Plus Formula 2 Valerian†; Multi-Vitamin Day & Night†; Naturest†; Nervatona Plus†; Nervatona†; Pacifenity†; Passiflora Complex†; Passionflower Plus†; Proesten†; Prosed-X†; Relaxaplex†; Valerian Plus Herbal Plus Formula 12†; ***Austria:*** Nervenruh; Passedan; Passelyt; Sedogelat; Wechseltee EF-EM-ES; ***Belg.:*** Sedinal; Seneuval†; Tisane Contre la Tension†; ***Braz.:*** A Saude da Mulher; Akhuma†; Anevrase; Benzomel; Bronquiogem; Calman; Calmapax; Calmazin†; Calmiplan; Composto Emagrecedor; Elixir de Maracuja Composto†; Elixir de Passiflora†; Emagrevit; Especies Calmantes†; Gotas Nican; Maracugina†; Neurosedol†; Pasalix; Passaneuro; Passi Catha†; Passicalm; Passicarbone†; Passiflora Composta†; Passiflorine; Passilex; Ritmoneuran†; Sedalin†; Sedantol†; Serenase†; Serenus; Sominex; Sonotabs†; Vagostesyl; Vidcalm†; ***Canad.:*** Herbal Sleep Aid; Relax and Sleep; ***Chile:*** Armonyl; ***Fr.:*** Actisane Nervosite†; Anxoral; Astressane†; Biocarde; Euphytose; Mediflor Tisane Calmante Troubles du Sommeil No 14; Natisedine†; Natudor; Neuroflorine; Neurotensyl†; Nocvalene; Nuidor†; Panxeol; Passiflorine; Passinevryl; Phytocalm; Phytotherapie Boribel no 8†; Sedatif Tiber; Sympaneurol; Sympavagol; Tisanes de l'Abbe Hamon no 6†; Vericardine†; ***Ger.:*** Aranidorm-S†; Avedorm†; Biosedon S†; Biral†; Dormo-Sern; Dormoverlan; Euvegal N†; Gutnacht; Habstal-Nerv N; Hyposedon N†; JuNeuron S†; Kytta-Sedativum f; Luvased-Tropfen N†; Moradorm; Moradorm S; Nerven-Tee Stada N†; Nervendragees; Nervinfant N; Nervoregin forte; Neurapas; Passin; Passiorin N†; Phytonoctu; Presselin Nerven K 1 N; Pronervon Phyto; RubieSed; Salusan†; Seda-Plantina; Sedinfant N; Sirmiosta Nervenelixier N†; Somnuvis S†; Tornix; Valena N†; Valeriana mild; Visinal†; Vivinox N; ***Hong Kong:*** Epizon; ***Israel:*** Calmanervin; Nerven-Dragees; Passiflora; Passiflora Compound; ***Ital.:*** Anevrasi; Bio-Strath†; Biocalm; Blandonal†; Fitosonno; Noctis; Parvisedil; Passiflorine; Quietan†; Reve; Sedatol; Sedofit; Sedopuer F; Tauma†; Val-Plus; ***Mex.:*** Ifupasil; ***Mon.:*** Neuropax; ***Port.:*** Bio-Strath No 8†; Calmo†; Gabisedil; Neurocardol; Valesono; ***S.Afr.:*** Biral; ***Spain:*** Baldrian†; Brevilon†; Passiflorine†; Sedasor; Sedonat; Sonofit†; Valdispert Complex; ***Switz.:*** Dicalm; Dragees antirhumatismales; Dragees pour la detente nerveuse; Dragees pour le coeur et les nerfs; Drosana Hyperflorin†; Gouttes pour le coeur et les nerfs Concentrees; Melissa Tonic†; Phytoberidin†; Phytomed Cardio; Phytomed Nervo; Phytomed Somni; Plantival†; Relax; Sirop Passi-Par; Soporin; Tisane antirhumatismale; Tisane calmante pour les enfants; Tisane relaxante N; Valverde Dragees pour la detente; Valverde Dragees pour le coeur; Valverde Gouttes pour le coeur; ***UK:*** Anased; Avena Sativa Comp; Bio-Strath Valerian Formula; Daily Tension & Strain Relief; Gerard 99†; Gerard House Motherwort Compound†; Gerard House Serenity; Gerard House Valerian Compound†; Heath & Heather Becalm†; Heath & Heather Quiet Night†; Herbal Pain Relief; HRI Night; Modern Herbals Stress; Night Time†; Nodoff; Nytol Herbal; PMT Formula; Quiet Life; Quiet Nite; Quiet Tyme; Relax B⁺; Slumber; SuNerven; Super Mega B+C.

## Patent Blue V

Acid Blue 3; Azul Patente V; CI Food Blue 5; Colour Index No. 42051; E131. Calcium α-(4-diethylaminophenyl)-α-(4-diethyliminiocyclohexa-2,5-dienylidene)-5-hydroxytoluene-2,4-disulphonate.

$(C_{27}H_{31}N_2O_7S_2)_2Ca$ = 1159.4.
*CAS — 3536-49-0.*

NOTE. The name Patent Blue V is also used as a synonym for Sulphan Blue (CI No. 42045) (see p.1750).

**Pharmacopoeias.** In *Fr.*

### Adverse Effects and Precautions

Hypersensitivity reactions may occur immediately or a few minutes after injection of patent blue V; on rare occasions they may be severe and include shock, dyspnoea, laryngeal spasm, and oedema. Nausea, hypotension, and tremor have been reported. Administration of a small dose to test for hypersensitivity has been suggested.

**Hypersensitivity.** An urticarial rash occurred in a 5-year-old girl after use of tablets containing patent blue V to disclose the presence of dental plaque.[1] Anaphylactic shock has been reported.[2,3]

1. Chadwick BL, *et al.* Allergic reaction to the food dye patent blue. *Br Dent J* 1990; **168:** 386–7.
2. Woltsche-Kahr I, *et al.* Anaphylactic shock following peritumoral injection of patent blue in sentinel lymph node biopsy procedure. *Eur J Surg Oncol* 2000; **26:** 313–14.
3. Adverse Drug Reactions Advisory Committee (ADRAC). Patent blue V and anaphylaxis. *Aust Adverse Drug React Bull* 2002; **21:** 10. Also available at: http://www.tga.health.gov.au/adr/aadrb/aadr0208.htm (accessed 02/07/04)

### Uses and Administration

Patent blue V is injected subcutaneously to colour the lymph vessels so that they can be injected with a contrast medium. A dose of 0.25 mL of the 2.5% solution diluted with an equal volume of sodium chloride 0.9% or lidocaine hydrochloride 1% injected subcutaneously in each interdigital web space has been used. Additional injections at different sites may be required when the lower limbs are to be examined. The bluish skin colour which may develop after injection usually disappears after 24 to 48 hours.

Patent blue V is used as a food colour.

**Malignant neoplasms of the breast.** Intradermal injection of patent blue V at the site of a primary breast tumour has been used to identify the associated lymph nodes,[1] but concern has been expressed regarding possible long-term staining of the skin.[2]

1. Borgstein PJ, *et al.* Intradermal blue dye to identify sentinel lymphnode in breast cancer. *Lancet* 1997; **349:** 1668–9.
2. Giuliano AE. Intradermal blue dye to identify sentinel lymph node in breast cancer. *Lancet* 1997; **350:** 958.

## Pegademase (rINN)

PEG-ADA; Pegademasa; PEG-Adenosine Deaminase.
*ATC — L03AX04.*

NOTE. Pegademase Bovine is *USAN*.

### Profile

Pegademase is a conjugate of adenosine deaminase, an endogenous enzyme that converts adenosine to inosine, with a macrogol (polyethylene glycol). Pegademase bovine is used in the treatment of severe combined immunodeficiency disease (SCID) associated with a deficiency of adenosine deaminase in patients who are not suitable for bone marrow transplantation or in whom the transplantation has failed. It is given by intramuscular injection once every 7 days, in an initial dose of 10 units/kg; increments of 5 units/kg are then given weekly up to a usual weekly maintenance dose of 20 units/kg. A single dose of 30 units/kg should not be exceeded. Pegademase should be administered with caution to patients with thrombocytopenia and avoided if the latter is severe.

◊ References.

1. Hershfield MS, *et al.* Treatment of adenosine deaminase deficiency with polyethylene glycol-modified adenosine deaminase. *N Engl J Med* 1987; **316:** 589–96.
2. Anonymous. Pegademase. *Med Lett Drugs Ther* 1990; **32:** 87–8.
3. Lee CR, *et al.* Pegademase bovine: replacement therapy for severe combined immunodeficiency disease. *DICP Ann Pharmacother* 1991; **25:** 1092–5.
4. Shovlin CL, *et al.* Adult presentation of adenosine deaminase deficiency. *Lancet* 1993; **341:** 1471.
5. Hershfield MS. Adenosine deaminase deficiency: clinical expression, molecular basis, and therapy. *Semin Hematol* 1998; **35:** 291–8.

### Preparations

**Proprietary Preparations** (details are given in Part 3)
***USA:*** Adagen.

## Penicilloyl-polylysine

Benzylpenicilloyl-polylysine; Peniciloil polilisina; PO-PLL; PPL.
*CAS — 53608-77-8.*

**Description.** Penicilloyl-polylysine is a polypeptide compound formed by the interaction of a penicillanic acid and polylysine of an average degree of polymerisation of 20 lysine residues per molecule.

**Pharmacopoeias.** *US* includes a concentrated form.

**USP 27** (Benzylpenicilloyl Polylysine Concentrate). It has a molar concentration of benzylpenicilloyl moiety of not less than 0.0125 M and not more than 0.020 M. It contains one or more suitable buffers. It is not intended for direct administration. pH of the concentrate is between 6.5 and 8.5. Store in airtight containers.

### Adverse Effects and Precautions

Severe hypersensitivity reactions have occasionally been reported following administration of penicilloyl-polylysine; a scratch test is recommended before intradermal administration.

### Uses and Administration

Penicilloyl-polylysine is used to detect penicillin hypersensitivity. It is generally indicated only for adults with a history of penicillin hypersensitivity. After a preliminary scratch test it may then be given by intradermal injection. The development, usually within 5 to 15 minutes, of a wheal, erythema, and pruritus is generally judged a positive reaction. The incidence of penicillin hypersensitivity is stated to be less than 5% in patients showing a negative reaction. Penicilloyl-polylysine does not detect those liable to suffer late reactions or reactions due to minor antigen determinants; these reactions require other tests. False-positive reactions to penicilloyl-polylysine also occur.

### Preparations

***USP 27:*** Benzylpenicilloyl Polylysine Injection.

**Proprietary Preparations** (details are given in Part 3)
***Canad.:*** Pre-Pen†; ***Swed.:*** Pre-Pen†; ***USA:*** Pre-Pen.

## Pentagastrin (BAN, USAN, rINN)

AY-6608; ICI-50123; Pentagastrina. *tert*-Butyloxycarbonyl-[β-Ala[13]]gastrin-(13-17)-pentapeptide amide; Boc-βAla-Trp-Met-Asp-Phe—$NH_2$.

$C_{37}H_{49}N_7O_9S$ = 767.9.
*CAS — 5534-95-2.*
*ATC — V04CG04.*

**Pharmacopoeias.** In *Br.* and *Chin.*

**BP 2003** (Pentagastrin). A white or almost white powder. Practically insoluble in water; slightly soluble in alcohol; soluble in dimethylformamide and in 5M ammonia. Protect from light.

### Adverse Effects

Pentagastrin may cause a number of gastrointestinal effects including nausea and abdominal cramps. Cardiovascular effects including flushing of the skin, tachycardia, bradycardia, and hypotension have occasionally been reported. There may be headache, drowsiness, dizziness, and altered sensations in the extremities. Hypersensitivity reactions are rare.

### Precautions

Pentagastrin should be given with care to patients with acute peptic ulceration or with active pancreatic, hepatic, or biliary-tract disease.

### Uses and Administration

Pentagastrin is a synthetic pentapeptide that is not active when given by mouth but when given parenterally has effects similar to those of natural gastrin. Since it stimulates the secretion of gastric acid, pepsin, and intrinsic factor, it is used as a diagnostic agent to test the secretory action of the stomach. It has been used to diagnose disorders associated with increased or decreased gastric acid secretion and in the evaluation of gastric acid secretion following vagotomy or gastric resection. The usual dose is 6 micrograms/kg by subcutaneous injection; by intravenous infusion the dose is 600 nanograms/kg per hour, in sodium chloride 0.9%. It has also been given intramuscularly and by nasal inhalation.

Pentagastrin stimulates the secretion of pancreatic enzymes and thus has been used as a test for pancreatic function. It has also been tried in the diagnosis of medullary carcinoma of the thyroid.

### Preparations

***BP 2003:*** Pentagastrin Injection.

**Proprietary Preparations** (details are given in Part 3)
***Canad.:*** Peptavlon†; ***Fr.:*** Peptavlon†; ***Switz.:*** Peptavlon†; ***USA:*** Peptavlon†.

## Pepsin

Pepsina; Pepsini Pulvis.
*CAS — 9001-75-6.*
*ATC — A09AA03.*

**Pharmacopoeias.** In *Chin., Eur.* (see p.vi), and *Viet.* In *Jpn* as Saccharated Pepsin.

**Ph. Eur. 5.0** (Pepsin Powder; Pepsin BP 2003). It is prepared from the gastric mucosa of pigs, cattle, or sheep. It contains gastric proteinases active in acid medium (pH 1 to 5). It has an activity of not less than 0.5 Ph. Eur. units/mg, calculated with reference to the dried substance. A hygroscopic, white or slightly yellow, crystalline or amorphous powder. Soluble in water; practically insoluble in alcohol. A solution in water may be slightly opalescent with a weak acidic reaction. Store at 2° to 8° in airtight containers. Protect from light.

### Uses and Administration

Pepsin contains proteolytic enzymes secreted by the stomach, which control the degradation of proteins into proteoses and peptones. It hydrolyses polypeptides including those with bonds adjacent to aromatic or dicarboxylic L-amino-acid residues.

Pepsin has been given with dilute hydrochloric acid, or with substances such as glutamic acid hydrochloride, or betaine hydrochloride, as an adjunct in the treatment of gastric hypochlorhydria, or to treat deficiencies of digestive enzyme secretion. It has also been given for its supposed benefit as an ingredient of mixtures for dyspepsia and other gastrointestinal disorders.

### Preparations

**Proprietary Preparations** (details are given in Part 3)
***Canad.:*** Fermentol.

**Multi-ingredient:** ***Arg.:*** Gastridin-E; Opoenterol; Tridigestivo Soubeiran; ***Austral.:*** Bepep†; Betaine Digestive Aid†; Bioglan Digestive Zyme†; Digestaid†; Enzyme†; Natures Own Digestive Enzymes†; Prozyme†; ***Austria:*** Everon†; Helo-acid; Helopanzym; Oroacid; Pansan†; Pepsiton; Vinopepsin; ***Belg.:*** Digestomen; ***Braz.:*** Digeplus; Espasmo Novozyme†;

Essen; Filogaster; Hepatoregius; Pantopept; Peptopancreasi; Primeral; ***Chile:*** Flapex E; ***Fr.:*** Hepatoum†; ***Ger.:*** Citropepsin; Pepzitrat; ***India:*** Digeplex; Digeplex-T; Dipep; Lupizyme; Papytazyme; ***Israel:*** Babyzim; Betazim; ***Ital.:*** Digestopan; Essen Enzimatico; Eudigestio; Gastro-Pepsin; Pepto-Pancreasi; ***Mex.:*** Ochozim; ***Port.:*** Espasmo Canulase; Modulanzime; ***S.Afr.:*** Spasmo-Canulase; ***Spain:*** Digestomen Complex; Espasmo Digestomen†; Euzymina Lisina I; Euzymina Lisina II; Paigastrol†; Troforex Pepsico; ***Switz.:*** Spasmo-Canulase; Stomacine; ***Thai.:*** Papytazyme; Pepsitase; ***UK:*** Digezyme†; Enzyme Plus; ***USA:*** Digepepsin.

## Perflubron *(USAN, rINN)*

Perflubrón; Perfluorooctylbromide; PFOB. 1-Bromoheptadecafluorooctane.

$C_8BrF_{17}$ = 499.0.

*CAS — 423-55-2.*

*ATC — V08CX01.*

**Pharmacopoeias.** In *US.*

**USP 27** (Perflubron). A clear, colourless, practically odourless liquid. Store in airtight containers. Protect from light.

### Profile

Perfluorocarbons can absorb, transport, and release oxygen and carbon dioxide. Perflubron is a perfluorocarbon tried as an alternative to red blood cell preparations to improve gaseous transport, in particular oxygen supply, to the tissues. It may also be instilled directly to the lungs for use in partial liquid ventilation as an adjunct to mechanical ventilation in patients with respiratory failure.

Perflubron is in clinical trials for use as an intravenous contrast medium in computed tomography and ultrasound. It has also been given by mouth to enhance delineation of the bowel during magnetic resonance imaging.

Other perfluorocarbons have also been used. A mixture of perfluamine (perfluorotripropylamine) and perflunafene (p.1730) has been used to prevent myocardial ischaemia during percutaneous transluminal coronary angioplasty.

Perfluorocarbons such as perflunafene and perfluorooctane (p.1730) have been used in eye surgery.

**Blood substitutes.** References to the use of perflubron and other perfluorocarbons as oxygen carriers.


1. Garrelts JC. Fluosol: an oxygen-delivery fluid for use in percutaneous transluminal coronary angioplasty. *DICP Ann Pharmacother* 1990; **24:** 1105–12.
2. Ravis WR, *et al.* Perfluorochemical erythrocyte substitutes: disposition and effects on drug distribution and elimination. *Drug Metab Rev* 1991; **23:** 375–411.
3. Urbaniak SJ. Artificial blood. *BMJ* 1991; **303:** 1348–50.
4. Jones JA. Red blood cell substitutes: current status. *Br J Anaesth* 1995; **74:** 697–703.
5. Remy B, *et al.* Red blood cell substitutes: fluorocarbon emulsions and haemoglobin solutions. *Br Med Bull* 1999; **55:** 277–98.
6. Lowe KC. Perfluorinated blood substitutes and artificial oxygen carriers. *Blood Rev* 1999; **13:** 171–84.
7. Prowse CV. Alternatives to standard blood transfusion: availability and promise. *Transfus Med* 1999; **9:** 287–99.
8. Matsumoto S, Kuroda Y. Perfluorocarbon for organ preservation before transplantation. *Transplantation* 2002; **74:** 1804–9.
9. Jahr JS, *et al.* Blood substitutes and oxygen therapeutics: an overview and current status. *Am J Ther* 2002; **9:** 437–43.


**Respiratory distress syndrome.** References to the use of perfluorocarbons, including perflubron, for partial liquid ventilation in neonatal respiratory distress syndrome (p.1084) and acute respiratory distress syndrome (p.1075).


1. Hirschl RB, *et al.* Liquid ventilation in adults, children, and full-term neonates. *Lancet* 1995; **346:** 1201–2.
2. Leach CL, *et al.* Partial liquid ventilation with perflubron in premature infants with severe respiratory distress syndrome. *N Engl J Med* 1996; **335:** 761–7.
3. Hirschl RB, *et al.* Initial experience with partial liquid ventilation in adult patients with acute respiratory distress syndrome. *JAMA* 1996; **275:** 383–9.
4. Wolfson MR, Shaffer TH. Liquid assisted ventilation update. *Eur J Pediatr* 1999; **158:** S27–S31.
5. Davies M. Liquid ventilation. *J Paediatr Child Health* 1999; **35:** 434–7.
6. Weis CM, Fox WW. Current status of liquid ventilation. *Curr Opin Pediatr* 1999; **11:** 126–32.
7. Kacmarek RM. Liquid ventilation. *Respir Care Clin N Am* 2002; **8:** 187–209.


### Preparations

**Proprietary Preparations** (details are given in Part 3)
***USA:*** Imagent GI; LiquiVent.

## Perflunafene *(BAN, rINN)*

Perfluorodecahydronaphthalene; Perfluorodecalin.

$C_{10}F_{18}$ = 462.1.

*CAS — 306-94-5.*

### Profile

Perflunafene is a perfluorocarbon with similar properties to perflubron (above). Intraocular injection of perlunafene is used to provide temporary tamponade in ophthalmic procedures such as retinal re-attachment. Perflunafene and perfluamine have been used together for their oxygen-carrying properties in blood substitute preparations and to prevent myocardial ischaemia during percutaneous transluminal coronary angioplasty.

### Preparations

**Proprietary Preparations** (details are given in Part 3)
***Israel:*** Adato-Deca; ***Neth.:*** Eftiar Decalin.

## Perfluorooctane

Octadecafluorooctane; Perfluoro-n-octane; Perfluoro-octa.

$C_8F_{18}$ = 438.1.

*CAS — 307-34-6.*

### Profile

Perfluorooctane is a perfluorocarbon with similar properties to perflubron (above). Intraocular injection of perfluorooctane is used to provide temporary tamponade in ophthalmic procedures such as retinal re-attachment.

◊ References.


1. Scott IU, *et al.* Outcomes of surgery for retinal detachment associated with proliferative vitreoretinopathy using perfluoro-n-octane: a multicenter study. *Am J Ophthalmol.* 2003; **136:** 454–63.


### Preparations

**Proprietary Preparations** (details are given in Part 3)
***Israel:*** Adato-Octa; ***Neth.:*** Eftiar Octane; ***USA:*** Perfluoron.

## Persic Oil

Melocotón, aceite de; Oleum Persicorum; Peach or.

**Pharmacopoeias.** *Chin.* and *Jpn* include Peach Kernel (Persicae Semen) and also Apricot Kernel (Armeniacae Semen).

### Profile

Persic oil is the fixed oil expressed from the kernels of varieties of *Prunus persica* (peach) or *P. armeniaca* (apricot) (Rosaceae). It closely resembles almond oil (p.1651) in its general characteristics and is used as an oily vehicle.

## Peru Balsam

Bals. Peruv.; Bálsamo del Perú; Balsamum Peruvianum; Baume du Pérou; Baume du San Salvador; Peruvian Balsam.

**Pharmacopoeias.** In *Eur.* (see p.vi).

**Ph. Eur. 5.0** (Peru Balsam). The balsam obtained from the scorched and wounded trunk of *Myroxylon balsamum* var. *pereirae*. It contains not less than 45.0% w/w and not more than 70.0% w/w of esters, mainly benzyl benzoate and benzyl cinnamate.

A dark brown, viscous liquid which is not sticky, is non-drying, and does not form threads. It is transparent and yellowish-brown when viewed in a thin layer. Practically insoluble in water, freely soluble in dehydrated alcohol; not miscible with fatty oils except for castor oil. Protect from light.

### Profile

Peru balsam has a very mild antiseptic action by virtue of its content of cinnamic and benzoic acids. Diluted with an equal part of castor oil, it has been used as an application to bedsores and chronic ulcers; it has also been used in topical preparations for the treatment of superficial skin lesions and pruritus. It is an ingredient of some rectal preparations used for the symptomatic relief of haemorrhoids (see p.1243).

Peru balsam is an ingredient of some preparations used in the treatment of respiratory congestion.

Skin sensitisation has been reported.

### Preparations

**Proprietary Preparations** (details are given in Part 3)
***Austria:*** Perudent†; ***Belg.:*** Tulle Gras Lumiere†; ***Fr.:*** Tulle Gras Lumiere; ***Ger.:*** Branolind N†; Tulle Gras Lumiere†.

**Multi-ingredient:** ***Arg.:*** Anusol; Anusol Duo S; Anusol-A; ***Austral.:*** Anusol; Ayrton's Chilblain†; ***Austria:*** Mamellin; Pudan-Lebertran-Zinksalbe; Pulmex; Rombay; Vulpuran; ***Belg.:*** Oxyplastine†; Perubore; Pulmex; Pulmex Baby; Rectovasol; ***Braz.:*** Anusol-HC; Balmex; Calminex H; Claudemor; Pomada Martel†; ***Chile:*** Pulmex; ***Fr.:*** Agathol; Anaxeryl; Balsofumine; Balsofumine Mentholee; Brulex; Dermophil Indien; Oxyperol; Perubore; Pommade Lelong; Pulmax†; ***Ger.:*** Anusol; derma-loges N†; Peru-Lenicet; ***Hong Kong:*** Anusol; Anusol-HC†; Cortison Kemicetine†; ***Irl.:*** Anugesic-HC; Anusol; Anusol-HC; ***Israel:*** Anusol; Contra Combustiones†; Hemo; Pulmex; ***Ital.:*** Anusol; Fomentil; ***Malaysia:*** Anusol; ***NZ:*** Anusol; ***Port.:*** Anucet; Claudemor; ***S.Afr.:*** Anugesic; Anusol-HC†; Ung Vernleigh; ***Singapore:*** Anusol; ***Spain:*** Antigrietun; Balsamo Kneipp; Cicatral; Grietalgen; Kneipp Balsamo†; Linitul; Vapores Pyt; Vitamina F99 Topica; ***Switz.:*** Anginol†; Demo pommade contre les refroidissements; Demo pommade contre les refroidissements pour bebes†; Dermophil Indien Nouvelle formule; Euproctol N; Furodermil†; Haemocortin; Haemolan; HEC; Nasobol; Perubare; Pulmex; Pulmex Baby; Rapura; ***Thai.:*** Anusol; ***UK:*** Anugesic-HC; Anusol; Anusol-HC, Plus HC; Dragon Balm; ***USA:*** Anumed; Anumed HC; Balmex Baby; Dermuspray; Dr Dermi-Heal; Flanders Buttocks; Granulderm; Granulex; GranuMed; Hemril; Mammol; Medicone Rectal; Proderm; Saratoga.

## Phencyclidine Hydrochloride *(BANM, USAN, rINNM)*

CI-395; CN-25253-2; GP-121; Hidrocloruro de fenciclidina; NSC-40902; PCP. 1-(1-Phenylcyclohexyl)piperidine hydrochloride.

$C_{17}H_{25}N,HCl$ = 279.8.

*CAS — 77-10-1 (phencyclidine); 956-90-1 (phencyclidine hydrochloride).*

NOTE. The name PCP has also been used as a synonym for pentachlorophenol.

Phencyclidine used illicitly has been known as: angel dust, angel hair, angel mist, crystal, cyclone, dust, elephant tranquilliser, embalming fluid, goon, hog, horse tranquilliser, killer weed, KW, mint weed, mist, monkey dust, monkey gland, peace pills, peace weed, rocket fuel, scuffle, sheets, super weed, surfer, and T.

### Adverse Effects, Treatment, and Precautions

Phencyclidine can induce a psychosis clinically indistinguishable from schizophrenia. Adverse effects reported include bizarre and violent behaviour, hallucinations, euphoria, agitation, catatonic rigidity, disorientation, incoordination, nystagmus, hypersalivation, vomiting, convulsions, numbness, hypertension, tachycardia, rhabdomyolysis leading to renal failure, acidosis, and, occasionally, malignant hyperthermia. Severe intoxication may result in respiratory depression, coma, and death.

Treatment of the adverse effects of phencyclidine is symptomatic; if agitated the patient should be kept quiet in a darkened room, and diazepam given if necessary. Hyperthermia should be treated. Activated charcoal should preferably be given within 1 hour of ingestion; multiple doses may be of benefit since phencyclidine is actively secreted into the gastrointestinal tract. Renal excretion should be promoted by hydration and use of diuretics if necessary. Acidification of the urine is no longer recommended since acidosis may be exacerbated and renal failure precipitated. Severe behavioural problems or psychoses may require administration of antipsychotics such as haloperidol, but phenothiazines, which may provoke an anticholinergic reaction or lower the seizure threshold, should be avoided.

**Breast feeding.** The American Academy of Pediatrics[1] has stated that, when used as a drug of abuse by a breast-feeding mother, phencyclidine has caused hallucinogenic effects in the infant.


1. American Academy of Pediatrics. The transfer of drugs and other chemicals into human milk. *Pediatrics* 2001; **108:** 776–89. Correction. *ibid.*; 1029. Also available at: http://aappolicy.aappublications.org/cgi/content/full/pediatrics%3b108/3/776 (accessed 02/07/04)


### Uses and Administration

Phencyclidine is related chemically to ketamine (see p.1302) and is a potent analgesic and anaesthetic. It was formerly given intravenously to produce an amnesic trance-like state, with analgesia, but severe adverse effects, especially postoperative psychoses, precluded its use. It was formerly used in veterinary medicine as an immobilising agent. Phencyclidine is widely abused in some countries for its hallucinogenic effects and has been taken by mouth, sniffed, injected or smoked.

Numerous analogues of phencyclidine have been similarly abused and include PHP (rolicyclidine; 1-(1-phenylcyclohexyl)pyrrolidine), PCC (1-piperidinocyclohexanecarbonitrile), PCE (*N*-ethyl-1-phenylcyclohexylamine), and TCP (1-[1-(2-thienyl)cyclohexyl]piperidine).

## Phenolsulfonphthalein

Fenolsolfonftaleina; Fenolsulfonftaleína; Phenol Red; Phenolsulfonphthaleinum; Phenolsulphonphthalein *(BAN)*; PSP. 4,4′-(3*H*-2,1-Benzoxathiol-3-ylidene)diphenol *S,S*-dioxide.

$C_{19}H_{14}O_5S$ = 354.4.

*CAS — 143-74-8.*

*ATC — V04CH03.*

**Pharmacopoeias.** In *Chin., Eur.* (see p.vi), and *Jpn.*

**Ph. Eur. 5.0** (Phenolsulfonphthalein; Phenolsulphonphthalein BP 2003). A bright to dark red, crystalline powder. Very slightly soluble in water; slightly soluble in alcohol.

### Adverse Effects and Precautions

Hypersensitivity reactions to phenolsulfonphthalein may occasionally occur. Excretion may be altered in patients with gout.

### Interactions

Excretion of phenolsulfonphthalein may be affected in patients taking aminohippuric acid, atropine, contrast media, diuretics, penicillin, probenecid, salicylates, sulfinpyrazone, or some sulfonamides.

### Pharmacokinetics

After intravenous injection, phenolsulfonphthalein is in part bound to plasma proteins, and in a patient with normal kidney function is rapidly excreted, mainly in the urine; some is excreted by the liver. Renal clearance is predominantly by tubular secretion, only a small amount being eliminated by glomerular filtration.

### Uses and Administration

Phenolsulfonphthalein has been used as a test of renal function by estimating the rate of urinary excretion after intravenous administration. It has also been given intramuscularly.

Alkaline urine is coloured red to violet.

Phenolsulfonphthalein has also been used as a drug ingestion indicator, a marker in drug absorption studies, and in a test of residual urine.

## 4-Phenylpiracetam

BRN-5030440; Carphedon; Karfedon. 2-Oxo-4-phenyl-1-pyrrolidineacetamide.

$C_{12}H_{14}N_2O_2 = 218.3$.

*CAS — 77472-70-9.*

### Profile

4-Phenylpiracetam is a nootropic that has been abused in sport.

## Phenylpropanol

Ethyl Phenyl Carbinol; Fenilpropanol; α-Hydroxypropylbenzene; SH-261. 1-Phenylpropan-1-ol; α-Ethylbenzyl alcohol.

$C_9H_{12}O = 136.2$.

*CAS — 93-54-9.*

**Pharmacopoeias.** In *Chin.*

### Profile

Phenylpropanol is a choleretic used for the treatment of biliary-tract and gastrointestinal disorders.

### Preparations

**Proprietary Preparations** (details are given in Part 3)
***Austria:*** Gallenperlen.

**Multi-ingredient:** ***Austria:*** Hedonin; ***Braz.:*** Quelodin.

## Phloroglucinol

Floroglucinol; Phloroglucin. Benzene-1,3,5-triol.

$C_6H_6O_3 = 126.1$.

*CAS — 108-73-6.*

*ATC — A03AX12.*

**Pharmacopoeias.** In *Fr.* which also includes the dihydrate.

### Profile

Phloroglucinol is used as an antispasmodic sometimes in combination with trimethylphloroglucinol. It has been given by mouth, intravenous or intramuscular injection, and rectally.

### Preparations

**Proprietary Preparations** (details are given in Part 3)
***Fr.:*** Spasfon-Lyoc; Spassirex; ***Ital.:*** Spasmex.

**Multi-ingredient:** ***Arg.:*** Nero; ***Belg.:*** Spasfon; ***Fr.:*** Meteoxane; Spasfon; ***Gr.:*** Spasfon; ***Ital.:*** Spasmex; ***Mex.:*** Panclasa.

## Phosgene

Carbonic Dichloride; Carbonyl Chloride; Chloroformyl Chloride; Fosgeno.

$COCl_2 = 98.92$.

*CAS — 75-44-5.*

### Adverse Effects

Poisoning may occur from industrial use or from the generation of phosgene from chlorinated compounds such as dichloromethane, chloroform, or carbon tetrachloride in the presence of heat. Symptoms of poisoning, which may be delayed for up to 24 (rarely 72) hours, include burning of the eyes and throat, cough, dyspnoea, cyanosis, and pulmonary congestion and oedema. Death may result from anoxia. Exposure to 50 ppm may be rapidly fatal. Massive exposure may cause intravascular haemolysis, thrombus formation, and immediate death. Exertional dyspnoea may persist for months following exposure to high concentrations.

### Treatment of Adverse Effects

After inhalation of phosgene or absorption from the skin, treatment consists of complete rest and inhalation of oxygen. The mouth, eyes, nose, and skin should be irrigated with copious amounts of water. Oral or parenteral corticosteroids have been used for bronchospasm but the role of inhaled corticosteroids is considered to be controversial. Antibacterials may reduce respiratory infections. Further treatment is symptomatic.

### Uses and Administration

Phosgene is used in the chemical industry. It has been used as a war gas.

◊ References.

1. Borak J, Diller WF. Phosgene exposure: mechanisms of injury and treatment strategies. *J Occup Environ Med* 2001; **43:** 110–9.

## Phosphatidyl Choline

Fosfatidilcolina; Phosphatidylcholine.

### Profile

Phosphatidyl choline is a phospholipid and a constituent of lecithin (p.1706). Phosphatidyl choline is an ingredient of preparations that have been promoted for liver disorders, peripheral vascular disorders, and hyperlipidaemias.

### Preparations

**Proprietary Preparations** (details are given in Part 3)
***Ital.:*** Essentiale; Lipostabil; ***USA:*** PhosChol.

**Multi-ingredient:** ***Austral.:*** Tyroseng†; ***Ital.:*** Essaven; Zeroac; ***Singapore:*** Memoloba.

## Phosphatidyl Serine

Fosfatidilserina; Phosphatidylserine.

### Profile

Phosphatidyl serine is a phospholipid that has been tried in the treatment of organic psychiatric syndromes and investigated as a cognition adjuvant. Phosphatidyl serine is a constituent of lecithin (p.1706).

◊ References.

1. Pepping J. Phosphatidylserine. *Am J Health-Syst Pharm* 1999; **56:** 2038, 2043–4.

### Preparations

**Proprietary Preparations** (details are given in Part 3)
***Braz.:*** Bros; ***Ital.:*** Senefor†; ***UK:*** Cognito.

**Multi-ingredient:** ***Ital.:*** NeoBros; NeoBros 10; NeoBros C.

## Phosphoric Acid

Acido Fosfórico; Concentrated Phosphoric Acid; E338; Fosfórico, ácido; Orthophosphoric Acid; Phosph. Acid; Phosphorsäure.

$H_3PO_4 = 98.00$.

*CAS — 7664-38-2.*

**Pharmacopoeias.** *Eur.* (see p.vi) and *Pol.* include various concentrations. Also in *USNF.*

**Ph. Eur. 5.0** (Phosphoric Acid, Concentrated; Phosphoric Acid BP 2003). It contains 84 to 90% w/w of $H_3PO_4$. A clear, colourless, corrosive, syrupy liquid. When stored at a low temperature it may solidify, forming a mass of colourless crystals which do not melt until the temperature reaches 28°. Miscible with water and with alcohol. Store in glass containers.

**Ph. Eur. 5.0** (Phosphoric Acid, Dilute). It contains 9.5 to 10.5% w/w $H_3PO_4$ and is prepared by mixing phosphoric acid 115 g with water 885 g.

**USNF 22** (Phosphoric Acid). It contains 85 to 88% w/w of $H_3PO_4$. A colourless, odourless liquid of syrupy consistency. Miscible with water and with alcohol. Store in airtight containers.

**USNF 22** (Diluted Phosphoric Acid). It contains 9.5 to 10.5% w/v $H_3PO_4$ and may be prepared by mixing phosphoric acid 69 mL with purified water to 1000 mL. A clear, colourless, odourless liquid. Store in airtight containers.

### Adverse Effects and Treatment

As for Hydrochloric Acid, p.1699.

### Uses and Administration

Phosphoric acid has industrial uses. Dilute phosphoric acid has been used well diluted in preparations intended for the management of nausea and vomiting (p.1245); it has also been included in preparations for vaginal infections. Phosphoric acid is used in dentistry to etch tooth enamel.

Phosphoric acid is used in homoeopathic medicine.

### Preparations

***USP 27:*** Sodium Fluoride and Phosphoric Acid Gel; Sodium Fluoride and Phosphoric Acid Topical Solution.

**Proprietary Preparations** (details are given in Part 3)
***Fr.:*** Phosoforme.

**Multi-ingredient:** ***Arg.:*** Plus & White; ***Austral.:*** Emetrol; Floraquin†; ***Braz.:*** Biotonico Fontoura†; Teutonico†; Tonico No 1†; ***Chile:*** Homeofortin III; ***Fr.:*** Acti 5†; Actiphos; Biotone; Ionyl; Marinol; Phosphoneuros; ***Israel:*** Peptical; ***S.Afr.:*** Emetrol; Emex; ***Spain:*** Oximen; ***Switz.:*** Frubiose Calcium†; ***Thai.:*** Floraquin†; Quinradon-N; Quinradon†; ***USA:*** Emetrol; Formula EM.

## Phosphorus

Fósforo; White Phosphorus; Yellow Phosphorus.

P = 30.973761.

*CAS — 7723-14-0.*

**Handling.** Phosphorus has been used for the illicit preparation of explosives or fireworks; care is required with its supply.

**Stability and storage.** Phosphorus is unstable in air and should be stored under water.

### Adverse Effects

Acute poisoning by phosphorus, a general protoplasmic poison, occurs in three distinct stages. The first stage represents local gastrointestinal irritation with intense thirst, pain, nausea, vomiting, and diarrhoea. The breath may smell of garlic and vomitus and excreta are luminescent. Shock, delirium, convulsions, coma, and death may occur. In patients who survive, a second, asymptomatic stage may be present lasting for up to several days or even weeks. The third stage represents systemic toxicity and is characterised by hepatic and renal damage, haemorrhage due to hypoprothrombinaemia and low fibrinogen concentrations, cardiovascular collapse, and CNS involvement including confusion, convulsions, and coma. Death may occur during either the first or third stages.

The fatal dose is about 1 mg/kg.

Symptoms of chronic poisoning are very slow in onset and are associated with lowered resistance to infection and defective tissue repair. They include periostitis and necrosis of the mandible ('phossy jaw').

Externally, phosphorus causes severe burns to the skin. Phosphorus is absorbed following skin contamination and systemic symptoms may occur.

### Treatment of Adverse Effects

After ingestion of phosphorus the stomach should be washed out with copious amounts of water; alternatives that have been suggested include potassium permanganate solution 1 in 5000 or hydrogen peroxide 2%.

Liquid paraffin or a solution of sodium sulfate may be introduced into the stomach following lavage and left there. Activated charcoal may be given by mouth. The use of digestible fats and oils should be avoided.

Further treatment is symptomatic and supportive and may include: fluid and electrolyte replacement; blood transfusion or vitamin K to correct coagulation disorders; and management of convulsions and renal and hepatic dysfunctions. Contaminated areas on skin should be immersed in water or irrigated with copious amounts of warm water; warm solutions of sodium bicarbonate 1% or copper sulfate 1% have also been suggested. It is essential that all particles of unoxidised phosphorus are removed from the skin.

### Uses and Administration

Elemental phosphorus is no longer used in medicine. Inorganic phosphates are given in deficiency states and bone diseases (see under Uses and Administration of Sodium Phosphate, p.1231). Phosphorus has been used in the manufacture of rat and cockroach poisons.

It is used in homoeopathic medicine.

## Physalis

Alkekengi; Alquequenje; Bladder Cherry; Chinese Lantern; Ground Cherry; Strawberry Tomato; Winter Cherry.

**Pharmacopoeias.** In *Chin.*

### Profile

The berries of *Physalis alkekengi* (Solanaceae) are reputed to have diuretic properties.

Cape gooseberry is the edible fruit of *P. peruviana.*

## Picibanil

OK-432.

### Profile

Picibanil, which is derived from *Streptococcus pyogenes*, is an immunomodulator that has been tried in the treatment of malignant neoplasms and viral infections.

◊ References.

1. Shirai M, *et al.* Intratumoural injection of OK-432 and lymphokine-activated killer activity in peripheral blood of patients with hepatocellular carcinoma. *Eur J Cancer* 1990; **26:** 965–9.
2. Imarura T, *et al.* Intrapericardial OK-432 instillation for the management of malignant pericardial effusion. *Cancer* 1991; **68:** 259–63.
3. Tanaka N, *et al.* Intratumoral injection of a streptococcal preparation, OK-432, before surgery for gastric cancer: a randomized trial. *Cancer* 1994; **74:** 3097–3103.
4. Katano M, Morisaki T. The past, the present and future of the OK-432 therapy for patients with malignant effusions. *Anticancer Res* 1998; **18:** 3917–25.
5. Luzzatto C, *et al.* Sclerosing treatment of lymphangiomas with OK-432. *Arch Dis Child* 2000; **82:** 316–18.
6. Giguere CM, *et al.* Treatment of lymphangiomas with OK-432 (Picibanil) sclerotherapy: a prospective multi-institutional trial. *Arch Otolaryngol Head Neck Surg* 2002; **128:** 1137–44.

## Pidotimod *(rINN)*

(*R*)-3-[(*S*)-5-Oxoprolyl]-4-thiazolidinecarboxylic acid.

$C_9H_{12}N_2O_4S = 244.3$.

*CAS — 121808-62-6.*

*ATC — L03AX05.*

### Profile

Pidotimod is an immunostimulant used in patients with cell-mediated immunodepression during respiratory- and urinary-tract infections. It is given by mouth in usual doses of 800 mg twice daily.

◊ References.

1. Various. Pidotimod: a new biological response modifier. *Arzneimittelforschung* 1994; **44** (12a): 1399–1530.
2. Guerra B, *et al.* Pidotimod in the management of vulvar papillomatosis: double-blind clinical trial versus placebo. *Am J Ther* 1998; **5:** 147–52.

### Preparations

**Proprietary Preparations** (details are given in Part 3)
***Ital.:*** Onaka; Pigitil; Polimod; ***Mex.:*** Adimod.

## Pilewort

Celidonia menor; Ficaire; Ficaria Ranunculoides; Ficaria Verna; Lesser Celandine.

**Pharmacopoeias.** In *Fr.*

### Profile

Pilewort, the aerial parts of *Ranunculus ficaria* (Ranunculaceae), has astringent and demulcent properties and is used topically for the treatment of haemorrhoids.

### Preparations

**Proprietary Preparations** (details are given in Part 3)

**Multi-ingredient:** ***Arg.:*** Confortel; ***Fr.:*** Apaisance; Avenoc†; Hemorrogel; ***UK:*** Piletabs; Pilewort Compound†.

## Pinaverium Bromide *(rINN)*

Bromuro de pinaverio. 4-(6-Bromoveratryl)-4-{2-[2-(6,6-dimethyl-2-norpinyl)ethoxy]ethyl}morpholinium bromide.

$C_{26}H_{41}Br_2NO_4$ = 591.4.

*CAS — 59995-65-2 (pinaverium); 53251-94-8 (pinaverium bromide).*

*ATC — A03AX04.*

### Profile

Pinaverium bromide is a calcium-channel blocker with some antimuscarinic-like effects. It is used for the relief of gastrointestinal spasm in usual doses of 50 mg by mouth three times daily at mealtimes.

**Effects on the gastrointestinal tract.** Two patients experienced heartburn and dysphagia after taking pinaverium bromide by mouth between meals; endoscopy revealed acute oesophageal ulceration which healed on discontinuation of treatment.[1] The manufacturer's recommendation to take pinaverium bromide during meals was emphasised.

1. André J-M, *et al.* Ulcères oesophagiens après prise de bromure de pinaverium. *Acta Endosc* 1980; **10:** 289–91.

### Preparations

**Proprietary Preparations** (details are given in Part 3)

***Arg.:*** Dicetel; ***Austria:*** Dicetel; ***Belg.:*** Dicetel; ***Braz.:*** Dicetel; ***Canad.:*** Dicetel; ***Chile:*** Eldicet; Laudil; ***Fr.:*** Dicetel; ***Gr.:*** Dicetel; ***Hong Kong:*** Dicetel†; ***India:*** Eldicet; ***Ital.:*** Dicetel; ***Mex.:*** Dicetel; ***Neth.:*** Dicetel†; ***Port.:*** Dicetel; ***Spain:*** Eldicet; ***Switz.:*** Dicetel; ***Thai.:*** Dicetel.

## Pipoxolan *(BAN, pINN)*

Pipoxolán. 5,5-Diphenyl-2-(2-piperidinoethyl)-1,3-dioxolan-4-one.

$C_{22}H_{25}NO_3$ = 351.4.

*CAS — 23744-24-3.*

## Pipoxolan Hydrochloride *(BANM, USAN, pINNM)*

*CAS — 18174-58-8.*

### Profile

Pipoxolan is used as a smooth muscle relaxant in usual doses of 10 to 30 mg by mouth three times daily. Pipoxolan hydrochloride has also been used.

### Preparations

**Proprietary Preparations** (details are given in Part 3)

***Ger.:*** Rowapraxin; ***Hong Kong:*** Rowapraxin; ***Irl.:*** Rowapraxin†; ***Malaysia:*** Rowapraxin.

**Multi-ingredient:** ***Irl.:*** Migranat.

## Piracetam *(BAN, USAN, rINN)*

CI-871; Piracetamum; Pyrrolidone Acetamide; UCB-6215. 2-(2-Oxopyrrolidin-1-yl)acetamide.

$C_6H_{10}N_2O_2$ = 142.2.

*CAS — 7491-74-9.*

*ATC — N06BX03.*

**Pharmacopoeias.** In *Eur.* (see p.vi).

**Ph. Eur. 5.0** (Piracetam). A white or almost white powder. It exhibits polymorphism. Freely soluble in water; soluble in alcohol. Protect from light.

### Adverse Effects and Precautions

Piracetam is reported to produce insomnia or somnolence, weight gain, hyperkinesia, nervousness, and depression. Diarrhoea and rashes may occur at a lower frequency. Piracetam should not be given to patients with hepatic impairment or severe renal impairment; dosage reductions are recommended for patients with lesser degrees of renal impairment. Therapy with piracetam should not be withdrawn abruptly.

### Interactions

**Anticoagulants.** For reference to the effect of piracetam on warfarin, see p.1027.

### Uses and Administration

Piracetam acts on the CNS and has been described as a 'nootropic'; it is said to protect the cerebral cortex against hypoxia. It is also reported to inhibit platelet aggregation and reduce blood viscosity at high doses. Piracetam is used as an adjunct in the treatment of myoclonus of cortical origin. It has also been used in dementia. Other disorders or states in which it has been tried (on the basis of a supposed 'cerebrocortical insufficiency' responsive to piracetam) include alcoholism, vertigo, cerebrovascular accidents, dyslexia, behavioural disorders in children, and after trauma or surgery.

In cortical myoclonus, piracetam is given in doses of 7.2 g daily increasing by 4.8 g daily every 3 or 4 days up to a maximum of 20 g daily. It is given by mouth in 2 or 3 divided doses. Once the optimal dose of piracetam has been established, attempts should be made to reduce the dose of other drugs. For dosage in renal impairment see below.

Piracetam has been given for various other disorders in doses of 0.8 to 1 g three times daily by mouth. In severe disorders it has been given by intramuscular or intravenous injection.

**Administration in renal impairment.** Dosage should be reduced in patients with mild to moderate renal impairment according to creatinine clearance (CC):

- CC between 60 and 40 mL/minute: half the usual dose
- CC between 40 and 20 mL/minute: one-quarter of the usual dose

**Dementia.** Although piracetam is used in some countries in the management of cognitive impairment and dementia (p.1484), a recent systematic review[1] concluded that the evidence from the published literature did not support this use.

1. Flicker L, Grimley Evans J. Piracetam for dementia or cognitive impairment. Available in The Cochrane Library; Issue 2. Chichester: John Wiley; 2004.

**Myoclonus.** A review[1] of 62 case reports, 3 open studies, and 2 double-blind studies concluded that piracetam is beneficial in the treatment of disabling myoclonus (p.353), either as adjunctive treatment or as monotherapy. Similar conclusions were made in another review[2] in which experience of 12 patients with progressive myoclonus epilepsy, 8 of whom benefited from piracetam in doses of up to 45 g daily without significant adverse effects, was described.

1. Van Vleymen B, Van Zandijcke M. Piracetam in the treatment of myoclonus: an overview. *Acta Neurol Belg* 1996; **96:** 270–80.
2. Genton P, *et al.* Piracetam in the treatment of cortical myoclonus. *Pharmacopsychiatry* 1999; **32** (suppl): 49–53.

**Stroke.** Piracetam did not influence the outcome if given within 12 hours of the onset of acute ischaemic stroke in a multicentre, randomised, double-blind trial,[1] although post hoc analyses suggested that it might confer benefit when given within 7 hours of onset, particularly in patients with stroke of moderate to severe degree. Further analyses of the same data concluded that piracetam did not produce significant adverse effects when given in high doses to patients with acute stroke,[2] and significantly more patients had recovered from aphasia on piracetam than placebo.[3] The results of two further randomised, double-blind, placebo-controlled trials supporting the role of piracetam as an adjunct to intensive speech therapy in improving aphasia following stroke were also reported.[3] In contrast, a review of the first study considered that the trend towards an increased risk of early death in patients allocated to piracetam was of concern, and concluded that the data did not support routine use of piracetam in acute ischaemic stroke.[4]

1. De Deyn PP, *et al.* Treatment of acute and ischemic stroke with piracetam. *Stroke* 1997; **28:** 2347–52.
2. De Reuck J, Van Vleyman B. The clinical safety of high-dose piracetam—its use in the treatment of acute stroke. *Pharmacopsychiatry* 1999; **32** (suppl 1): 33–7.
3. Huber W. The role of piracetam in the treatment of acute and chronic aphasia. *Pharmacopsychiatry* 1999; **32** (suppl 1): 38–43.
4. Ricci S, *et al.* Piracetam for acute ischaemic stroke. Available in The Cochrane Library; Issue 2. Chichester: John Wiley; 2004.

**Vertigo.** Piracetam has been reported to be of benefit in patients with vertigo (p.423) of both central or peripheral origin.[1]

1. Oosterveld WJ. The effectiveness of piracetam in vertigo. *Pharmacopsychiatry.* 1999; **32** (suppl 1): 54–60.

### Preparations

**Proprietary Preparations** (details are given in Part 3)

***Arg.:*** Noostan; ***Austria:*** Cerebryl; Nootropil; Novocephal; Pirabene; ***Belg.:*** Braintop; Geratam; Noodis; Nootropil; ***Braz.:*** Cintilan; Nootrofic; Nootron; Nootropil†; ***Chile:*** Nootropyl; ***Fin.:*** Nootropil; ***Fr.:*** Axonyl; Gabacet; Geram; Nootropyl; ***Ger.:*** Avigilen; Cerebroforte; Cerepar N; Cuxabrain; durapitrop†; Encetrop†; Memo-Puren; Nootrop; Normabrain; Novocetam†; Piracebral; Piracetrop; Sinapsan; ***Hong Kong:*** Nootropil; ***India:*** Piratam; ***Ital.:*** Cerebropan; Cleveral†; Flavis†; Nootropil; Norzetam; Psycoton; ***Malaysia:*** Cebrotonin; Knowful; Nootropil; ***Mex.:*** Dinagen; Nootropil; ***Neth.:*** Nootropil; ***Norw.:*** Nootropil; ***Port.:*** Acetar; Noostan; Nootropil; Oxibran; Stimubral; ***S.Afr.:*** Nootropil; ***Singapore:*** Cebrotonin; Cetam; Nootropil; Piratam; Racetam; ***Spain:*** Ciclofalina; Genogris†; Nootropil; ***Swed.:*** Nootropil; ***Switz.:*** Nootropil; Pirax; ***Thai.:*** Embol; Mempil; Noocetam; Nootropil; ***UK:*** Nootropil.

**Multi-ingredient:** ***Braz.:*** Energiclin; Energivit; Exit; Isketam; Psicoglut†; Vincetron; ***Port.:*** Anacervix; Centracetam; Euvifor; Stimilfar; ***Spain:*** Anacervix; Devincal; Diemil; Memorino†; Piracetam Complex.

## Pirenoxine Sodium *(rINNM)*

Catalin Sodium; Pirenoxina sódica; Pirfenoxone Sodium. Sodium 1-hydroxy-5-oxo-5*H*-pyrido[3,2-*a*]phenoxazine-3-carboxylate.

$C_{16}H_7N_2NaO_5$ = 330.2.

*CAS — 1043-21-6 (pirenoxine); 51410-30-1 (pirenoxine sodium).*

**Pharmacopoeias.** *Jpn* includes Pirenoxine.

### Profile

Pirenoxine sodium is used in the treatment of cataracts, usually as 0.005% eye drops.

### Preparations

**Proprietary Preparations** (details are given in Part 3)

***Arg.:*** Catalin; ***Braz.:*** Clarvisol; ***Ger.:*** Clarvisor; ***Hong Kong:*** Catalin; Kary Uni; ***India:*** Catalin; ***Ital.:*** Clarvisan; Pirfalin; ***Jpn:*** Catalin; ***Malaysia:*** Catalin; ***Mex.:*** Clarvisan; ***Port.:*** Clarvisan; ***Singapore:*** Catalin; Kary Uni; ***Spain:*** Clarvisan; ***Thai.:*** Catalin.

## Pirfenidone *(USAN, rINN)*

AMR-69; Pirfenidona. 5-Methyl-1-phenyl-2(1*H*)-pyridone.

$C_{12}H_{11}NO$ = 185.2.

*CAS — 53179-13-8.*

### Profile

Pirfenidone is an antifibrotic drug under investigation in disorders such as idiopathic pulmonary fibrosis, multiple sclerosis, and familial adenomatous polyposis.

◊ References.

1. Nicod LP. Pirfenidone in idiopathic pulmonary fibrosis. *Lancet* 1999; **354:** 268–9.
2. Walker JE, Margolin SB. Pirfenidone for chronic progressive multiple sclerosis. *Multiple Sclerosis* 2001; **7:** 305–12.
3. Nagai S, *et al.* Open-label compassionate use one year-treatment with pirfenidone to patients with chronic pulmonary fibrosis. *Intern Med* 2002; **41:** 1118–23.
4. Bowen JD, *et al.* Open-label study of pirfenidone in patients with progressive forms of multiple sclerosis. *Multiple Sclerosis* 2003; **9:** 280–3.
5. Lindor NM, *et al.* Desmoid tumors in familial adenomatous polyposis: a pilot project evaluating efficacy of treatment with pirfenidone. *Am J Gastroenterol* 2003;**98:** 1868–74.

## Pirglutargine

Arginina, piroglutamato de; Arginine Pidolate; Arginine Pyroglutamate. L-Arginine DL-pyroglutamate.

$C_{11}H_{21}N_5O_5$ = 303.3.

*CAS — 64855-91-0.*

### Profile

Pirglutargine has been used for its reputed cerebral stimulant effect.

### Preparations

**Proprietary Preparations** (details are given in Part 3)

***Ital.:*** Adiuvant.

**Multi-ingredient:** ***Port.:*** Detoxergon.

## Piridoxilate *(BAN, rINN)*

Piridoxilato; Pyridoxine $\alpha_5$-Hemiacetal Glyoxylate; Pyridoxylate. The reciprocal salt of 2-(5-hydroxy-4-hydroxymethyl-6-methyl-3-pyridylmethoxy)glycolic acid with 2-[4,5-bis(hydroxymethyl)-2-methyl-3-pyridyloxy]glycolic acid (1:1).

$C_{10}H_{13}NO_6,C_{10}H_{13}NO_6$ = 486.4.

*CAS — 24340-35-0.*

### Profile

Piridoxilate was formerly used in the treatment of various circulatory disorders. It has been associated with the development of the kidney stones and renal impairment.

## Pirisudanol Maleate *(rINNM)*

Dimaleato de pirisudanol; Pyrisuccideanol Maleate. 2-Dimethylaminoethyl 5-hydroxy-4-hydroxymethyl-6-methyl-3-pyridylmethyl succinate maleate.

$C_{16}H_{24}N_2O_6,(C_4H_4O_4)_2$ = 572.5.

*CAS — 33605-94-6 (pirisudanol); 53659-00-0 (pirisudanol maleate).*

*ATC — N06BX08.*

### Profile

Pirisudanol is the succinic acid ester of pyridoxine and of deanol. It has been given as the maleate in the treatment of cerebrovascular and similar disorders in doses of up to 1.2 g daily.

### Preparations

**Proprietary Preparations** (details are given in Part 3)

***Belg.:*** Nadex†; ***Fr.:*** Stivane†; ***Ital.:*** Mentium; ***Port.:*** Pridana; ***Spain:*** Mentis; ***Switz.:*** Nadex†.

## Pitofenone Hydrochloride *(rINNM)*

Hidrocloruro de pitofenona. Methyl 2-[4-(2-piperidinoethoxy)benzoyl]benzoate hydrochloride.

$C_{22}H_{25}NO_4,HCl$ = 403.9.

*CAS — 54063-52-4 (pitofenone); 1248-42-6 (pitofenone hydrochloride).*

### Profile

Pitofenone hydrochloride has been used as an antispasmodic.

### Preparations

**Proprietary Preparations** (details are given in Part 3)

**Multi-ingredient:** ***Fin.:*** Litalgin.

## Plantain

Llantén.

NOTE. Plantain herb has also been used as a synonym for Ribwort Plantain (Plantago lanceolata).

**Pharmacopoeias.** In *Chin.* and *Jpn.*, which also have separate monographs for the seed. *Chin* also permits *P. depressa*.
*Fr.* includes the leaves.

### Profile

Plantain consists of the seeds or leaves of *Plantago major* var. *asiatica*. It is reported to possess diuretic and antihaemorrhagic properties. It is used in homoeopathic medicine and herbal preparations.

### Preparations

**Proprietary Preparations** (details are given in Part 3)
***Fr.:*** Sensivision au plantain.
**Multi-ingredient:** ***Austral.:*** Hamamelis Complex†; ***Fr.:*** Ephydrol; ***Port.:*** Erpecalm; ***Switz.:*** Kernosan Elixir; Pastilles pectorales Demo N; Pectoral N; Sirop pectoral DP1†; Sirop pectoral DP2, DP3†; Tisane pectorale pour les enfants.

## Plastics

Plásticos.

**Pharmacopoeias.** Many pharmacopoeias include standards for plastic containers and closures.

### Adverse Effects

Plastic materials used in medicine and pharmacy may give rise to adverse effects, either by direct contact of the plastic with tissues or by indirect contact (for example, when a solution stored in a plastic container, such as a disposable syringe, is injected). Adverse effects may also arise among workers through handling the materials or by inhaling fumes during manufacture.

Pure polymeric plastics appear to be of low toxicity, though carcinogenic effects have been produced by some on prolonged implantation. However, some monomers are toxic, as may be substances added during manufacture to impart specific physical properties. These additives include plasticisers added to reduce brittleness, ultraviolet-ray absorbers to prevent degradation by light, and antioxidants and lubricants which are sometimes needed for satisfactory processing. Monomer residues or additives can leach out from the finished plastic materials and have been the main causes of adverse effects. These may include haemolysis of blood cells, thrombosis, hypersensitivity reactions, precancerous changes, and local tissue necrosis. Silicone particles have been shed from dialysis tubing resulting in hypersplenism, pancytopenia, and occasionally in the production of a granulomatous hepatitis.

See also under Vinyl Chloride, p.1764, Methylmethacrylate, p.1714, and Polytef, below.

## Pleurisy Root

Asclepia tuberosa; Butterfly Weed.

### Profile

The root of *Asclepias tuberosa* (Asclepiadaceae) has traditionally been used for pleurisy and other respiratory-tract disorders.

### Preparations

**Proprietary Preparations** (details are given in Part 3)
**Multi-ingredient:** ***Austral.:*** Verbascum Complex†; ***UK:*** Antibron; Chest Mixture; Horehound and Aniseed Cough Mixture; Vegetable Cough Remover.

## Pokeroot

Fitolaca; Poke Root.

**Pharmacopoeias.** In *Chin.*

### Profile

Pokeroot, the root of *Phytolacca decandra* (*P. americana*) (Phytolaccaceae) has emetic, purgative, anti-inflammatory, and anti-infective actions. It has been used for rheumatic and arthritic disorders, and for respiratory-tract infections, but is highly toxic in large doses and is not generally recommended. It has also been used externally for skin disorders.

It is used in homoeopathic medicine.

The related species, *P. dodecandra*, is the source of the molluscicide endod (p.1504).

### Preparations

**Proprietary Preparations** (details are given in Part 3)
***Braz.:*** Tyll†.
**Multi-ingredient:** ***Braz.:*** Fucus Composto†; ***Chile:*** Homeoplasmina; ***Fr.:*** Homeoplasmine; ***UK:*** Psorasolv.

## Polacrilin Potassium *(USAN, rINNM)*

Polacrilina potásica; Polacrilinum Kalii.

*CAS — 54182-62-6 (polacrilin); 50602-21-6 (polacrilin).*

**Pharmacopoeias.** In *USNF.*

**USNF 22** (Polacrilin Potassium). The potassium salt of a unifunctional low-cross-linked carboxylic cation-exchange resin prepared from methacrylic acid and divinylbenzene. A white to off-white, free-flowing powder. Has a faint odour or is odourless. Insoluble in water and in most liquids.

### Profile

Polacrilin potassium is used as a tablet and capsule disintegrant.

## Poly A.poly U

Poli (A). poli (U); Polyadenylic-polyuridylic Acid.

*CAS — 24936-38-7.*

### Profile

Poly A.poly U is a double-stranded polyribonucleotide comprising polyadenylic and polyuridylic acids, and is believed to be a stimulant of the immune system. It has been studied as an adjuvant in the management of operable solid tumours.

## Poly I.poly C

Poli (I). poli (C); Polyinosinic-polycytidylic Acid.

*CAS — 24939-03-5.*
*ATC — L03AX07.*

### Profile

Poly I.poly C is a synthetic double-stranded polyribonucleotide complex of equimolar concentrations of polyinosinic and polycytidylic acids, described as a mismatched double-strand RNA.

Poly I.poly C and the complex of poly I.poly C stabilised with poly-L-lysine in carmellose (carboxymethylcellulose) [poly(ICLC)] have been found to induce the production of interferon and have been investigated in the treatment of malignant neoplasms and viral infections. Poly I.poly C has been investigated for the treatment of AIDS, SARS, chronic fatigue syndrome, renal cell carcinoma, and invasive metastatic melanoma, and poly(ICLC) for the treatment of primary brain tumours.

### Preparations

**Proprietary Preparations** (details are given in Part 3)
***USA:*** Ampligen.

## Polysaccharide-K

Polisacárido-K; PSK; PS-K.

### Profile

Polysaccharide-K is a protein-bound polysaccharide isolated from a fungus, *Coriolus versicolor*. It is claimed to have immunostimulant and antineoplastic properties.

◊ References.


1. Tsukagoshi S, *et al.* Krestin (PSK). *Cancer Treat Rev* 1984; **11:** 131–55.
2. Go P, Chung C-H. Adjuvant PSK immunotherapy in patients with carcinoma of the nasopharynx. *J Int Med Res* 1989; **17:** 141–9.
3. Torisu M, *et al.* Significant prolongation of disease-free period gained by oral polysaccharide K (PSK) administration after curative surgical operation of colorectal cancer. *Cancer Immunol Immunother* 1990; **31:** 261–8.
4. Nakazato H, *et al.* Efficacy of immunochemotherapy as adjuvant treatment after curative resection of gastric cancer. *Lancet* 1994; **343:** 1122–6.
5. Hayakawa K, *et al.* Effect of Krestin as adjuvant treatment following radical radiotherapy in non-small cell lung cancer patients. *Cancer Detect Prev* 1997; **21:** 71–7.
6. Fisher M, Yang LX. Anticancer effects and mechanisms of polysaccharide-K (PSK): implications of cancer immunotherapy. *Anticancer Res* 2002; **22:** 1737–54.
7. Ohwada S, *et al.* Adjuvant therapy with protein-bound polysaccharide K and tegafur uracil in patients with stage II or III colorectal cancer: randomized, controlled trial. *Dis Colon Rectum* 2003; **46:** 1060–8.


## Polytef *(USAN)*

Politef *(pINN)*; Politefo; PTFE. Poly(tetrafluoroethylene).

$(C_2F_4)_n$.

*CAS — 9002-84-0.*

### Profile

Polytef has numerous industrial applications. As 'Teflon' it is used on 'non-stick' cooking utensils.

A paste of polytef has been used for a variety of purposes including the treatment of aphonia, for replacement grafts in vascular surgery, and in the correction of some forms of urinary incontinence (p.476). The main concern with these procedures is migration of polytef particles. It has also been applied to the skin as a barrier paste with perfluoroalkylpolyether to reduce exposure to chemical warfare agents.

**Adverse effects.** Brain injury in a child was possibly associated with migration of polytef particles from a periureteral injection performed 1 year earlier.[1] Three cases of polytef adenopathy and one case of giant granuloma have been reported[2] in children who had previously undergone subureteral polytef injection for the treatment of vesicoureteral reflux.


1. Borgatti R, *et al.* Brain injury in a healthy child one year after periureteral injection of Teflon. *Pediatrics* 1996; **98:** 290–1.
2. Aragona F, *et al.* Polytetrafluoroethylene giant granuloma and adenopathy: long-term complications following subureteral polytetrafluoroethylene injection for the treatment of vesicoureteral reflux in children. *J Urol (Baltimore)* 1997; **158:** 1539–42.


**Uses.** References.


1. Polley JW, *et al.* The use of Teflon in orbital floor reconstruction following blunt facial trauma: a 20-year experience. *Plast Reconstr Surg* 1987; **79:** 39–43.
2. Puri P. Endoscopic correction of primary vesicoureteric reflux by subureteric injection of polytetrafluoroethylene. *Lancet* 1990; **335:** 1320–2.
3. Maskell R, *et al.* Correction of vesicoureteric reflux by endoscopic injection. *Lancet* 1991; **338:** 1460–1.
4. Anonymous. Use of Teflon preparations for urinary incontinence and vesicoureteral reflux. *JAMA* 1993; **269:** 2975–80.
5. Duckett JRA. The use of periurethral injectables in the treatment of genuine stress incontinence. *Br J Obstet Gynaecol* 1998; **105:** 390–6.
6. Su TH, *et al.* Injection therapy for stress incontinence in women. *Int Urogynecol J* 1999; **10:** 200–6.
7. Chaffange P, *et al.* Traitement endoscopique du réflux vésicorénal chez l'enfant: résultats à court et à long terme des injections de polytétrafluoroéthylene (Téflon). *Prog Urol* 2001; **11:** 546–51.
8. Meschia M, *et al.* Injection therapy for the treatment of stress urinary incontinence in women. *Gynecol Obstet Invest* 2002; **54:** 67–72.
9. Huber TS, *et al.* Patency of autogenous and polytetrafluoroethylene upper extremity arteriovenous hemodialysis accesses: a systematic review. *J Vasc Surg* 2003; **38:** 1005–11.
10. Klinkert P, *et al.* Saphenous vein versus PTFE for above-knee femoropopliteal bypass: a review of the literature. *Eur J Vasc Endovasc Surg* 2004; **27:** 357–62.


## Poplar Buds

Álamo, brotes de; Balm of Gilead Buds.

**Pharmacopoeias.** *Pol.* includes the leaves from *Populus nigra.*

### Profile

The buds of various species of *Populus*, including *P. nigra*, *P. candicans*, *P. gileadensis*, and *P. tacamahacca* (*P. balsamifera*), have been used for the analgesic effect of their salicin content, as well as in preparations for a variety of other disorders. They also contain volatile oil, resin, and other substances. The resin from poplar buds is one of the major sources of propolis (p.1735).

### Preparations

**Proprietary Preparations** (details are given in Part 3)
**Multi-ingredient:** ***Austral.:*** Valerian†; ***Austria:*** Phytodolor; Prostagutt; ***Braz.:*** Eviprostat†; ***Canad.:*** Mielocol; Wampole Bronchial Cough Syrup; ***Ger.:*** Eviprostat N; Phytodolor; Prostamed; ***Hong Kong:*** Eviprostat†; ***Jpn:*** Eviprostat; ***Port.:*** Prostamed; ***Singapore:*** Eviprostat; ***Switz.:*** Eviprostat†; Phytomed Prosta; ***UK:*** Balm of Gilead; Gerard House Ligvites†; Gerard House Reumalex; Hofels White Willow and Burdock†; Peerless Composition Essence; Tabritis.

## Poppy-seed Oil

Adormidera, aceite de semilla de; Huile d'Oeillette; Maw Oil; Oleum Papaveris; Oleum Papaveris Seminis.

### Profile

Poppy-seed oil is the fixed oil expressed from the ripe seeds of the opium poppy, *Papaver somniferum* (Papaveraceae). It is used as a substitute for olive oil for culinary and pharmaceutical purposes. It is also used in the preparation of Iodised Oil Fluid Injection (BP 2003). Commercial grades are used in making soaps, paints, and varnishes.

## Potassium Aminobenzoate

Aminobenzoate Potassium; Aminobenzoato potásico. Potassium 4-aminobenzoate.

$C_7H_6KNO_2$ = 175.2.

*CAS — 138-84-1.*

**Pharmacopoeias.** In *US.*

**USP 27** (Aminobenzoate Potassium). A white crystalline powder. Very soluble in water; soluble in alcohol; practically insoluble in ether. A 1% solution in water has a pH of about 7, while a 5% solution has a pH of 8.0 to 9.0.

### Adverse Effects and Precautions

Anorexia, nausea, fever, and skin rash have been reported.

Potassium aminobenzoate should be given with caution to patients with renal impairment. The manufacturers recommend that treatment should be interrupted during periods of fasting, anorexia, or low food intake, to avoid the possible development of hypoglycaemia.

### Interactions

Potassium aminobenzoate can inactivate sulfonamides.

### Uses and Administration

Potassium aminobenzoate has been used in the treatment of various disorders associated with excessive fibrosis, such as scleroderma (p.1348) and Peyronie's disease, in usual doses of 12 g daily by mouth in 4 to 6 divided doses.

**Peyronie's disease.** Variable results have been reported with potassium aminobenzoate in the treatment of Peyronie's disease,[1-3] but evidence from well controlled trials is lacking. It has been suggested that a successful response is more likely if treatment is started in the acute stage.[2]


1. Gingell JC, Desai KM. Peyronie's disease. *BMJ* 1988; **298:** 1489–90.
2. Mohanty KC, Strachan RG. Peyronie's disease. *BMJ* 1989; **298:** 254.
3. Carson CC. Potassium aminobenzoate for the treatment of Peyronie's disease: is it effective? *Tech Urol* 1997; **3:** 135–9.


### Preparations

***USP 27:*** Aminobenzoate Potassium Capsules; Aminobenzoate Potassium for Oral Solution; Aminobenzoate Potassium Tablets.

**Proprietary Preparations** (details are given in Part 3)
***Austria:*** Potaba; ***Canad.:*** Potaba; ***Ger.:*** Potaba; ***Hong Kong:*** Potaba†; ***Mex.:*** Potabex†; ***Switz.:*** Potaba†; ***UK:*** Potaba; ***USA:*** Potaba.

## Potassium Borotartrate

Borotartrato potásico; Potassium Sodium Borotartrate; Soluble Cream of Tartar.
*CAS — 12001-68-2.*

### Profile

Potassium borotartrate is reported to have similar properties to those of bromides. It has been used in nervous disorders and has been used in photography as a retarder for alkaline developers. Chronic boron poisoning (see under Boric Acid, p.1662) has been reported following the use of potassium borotartrate internally.

### Preparations

**Proprietary Preparations** (details are given in Part 3)
**Multi-ingredient:** ***Fr.:*** Dinacode.

## Potassium Bromate

924; Bromato potásico.
$KBrO_3$ = 167.0.
*CAS — 7758-01-2.*

### Adverse Effects

Nausea, vomiting, severe abdominal pains, diarrhoea, and lethargy are common after ingestion of potassium bromate. Acute renal failure arising from tubular necrosis usually presents with oliguria or anuria within 1 to 3 days of significant ingestion, and is the most frequent cause of death. Ototoxicity may present as tinnitus or hearing loss within hours of ingestion, and can progress to sensorineural deafness in some patients. Ototoxicity and nephrotoxicity may be irreversible.

Potassium bromate poisoning an also produce hypotension, myocarditis, hepatitis, and encephalopathy characterised by agitation, delirium, convulsions, and coma. Microangiopathic anaemia has also been reported.

Potassium bromate is carcinogenic in *animals*.

**Acute toxicity.** Reports of bromate poisoning.


1. Lue JN, *et al.* Bromate poisoning from ingestion of professional hair-care neutralizer. *Clin Pharm* 1988; **7:** 66–70.
2. Lichtenberg R, *et al.* Bromate poisoning. *J Pediatr* 1989; **114:** 891–4.
3. De Vriese A, *et al.* Severe acute renal failure due to bromate intoxication: report of a case and discussion of management guidelines based on a review of the literature. *Nephrol Dial Transplant* 1997; **12:** 204–9.


### Treatment of Adverse Effects

After the ingestion of potassium bromate the stomach should be emptied by lavage; use of a 2 to 5% solution of sodium bicarbonate has been suggested to reduce bromate absorption and prevent hydrobromic acid production. Activated charcoal has also been recommended as an adsorbent. Attention to the patient's fluid, acid-base, and electrolyte status is important, particularly in the presence of acute renal failure. Pain is relieved by the injection of pethidine. An intravenous infusion of 100 to 500 mL of a 1% sodium thiosulfate solution has sometimes been given. Oxygen may be indicated. The prompt use of haemodialysis or peritoneal dialysis has been suggested.

**Thiosulfate.** Although the use of intravenous sodium thiosulfate is an accepted practice in the treatment of bromate poisoning, convincing evidence that it reduces bromate to bromide is lacking.[1,2] Oral sodium thiosulfate solutions have also been used but are no longer recommended because hydrogen sulfide, itself a powerful irritant and toxic agent, may be evolved in the presence of hydrochloric acid.[2]


1. McElwee NE, Kearney TE. Sodium thiosulfate unproven as bromate antidote. *Clin Pharm* 1988; **7:** 570–2.
2. De Vriese A, *et al.* Severe acute renal failure due to bromate intoxication: report of a case and discussion of management guidelines based on a review of the literature. *Nephrol Dial Transplant* 1997; **12:** 204–9.


### Uses

Potassium bromate is an oxidising agent. It has no therapeutic uses but it has been widely used as the 'neutraliser' of thioglycollate hair-waving lotions. It has been used in the preparation of barley malt for beer. It has also been used as a flour-maturing agent but such use is no longer considered appropriate and is prohibited in some countries.

**Food additive.** Potassium bromate is a genotoxic carcinogen and should not be present in foods as consumed. Its use for the treatment of flour for bread-making is not appropriate.


1. FAO/WHO. Evaluation of certain food additives and contaminants: forty-fourth report of the joint FAO/WHO expert committee on food additives. *WHO Tech Rep Ser 859* 1995.


## Potassium Chlorate

Clorato potásico; Kalium Chloricum; Potassii Chloras.
$KClO_3$ = 122.5.
*CAS — 3811-04-9.*

**Pharmacopoeias.** In *Swiss.*

**Handling and storage.** Potassium chlorate is unstable and, in contact with organic or readily oxidisable substances such as charcoal, phosphorus, or sulfur it is liable to explode especially if heated or subjected to friction or percussion. It should not be allowed to come into contact with matches or surfaces containing phosphorus compounds. Reasonable steps should be taken before supplying potassium chlorate to ensure that it will not be used for the illicit preparation of explosives or fireworks.

### Profile

Potassium chlorate has been used as an astringent, usually as a mouthwash or gargle. Concentrated solutions are irritant.

Acute poisoning from ingestion requires prompt symptomatic treatment. Symptoms include nausea, vomiting, diarrhoea, abdominal pain, haemolytic anaemia, haemorrhage, methaemoglobinaemia, hyperkalaemia, and renal failure. There may be liver damage and central effects with convulsions and coma.

If methaemoglobinaemia is severe, patients may require exchange transfusion with whole blood. Several authorities consider that methylthioninium chloride should be given intravenously if methaemoglobinaemia is greater than 30%, although some advise against such use for fear of converting chlorate to the more toxic hypochlorite.

### Preparations

**Proprietary Preparations** (details are given in Part 3)
**Multi-ingredient:** ***Canad.:*** Fletchers Sore Mouth Medicine; ***Spain:*** Cloroboral†; Edifaringen; Solurrinol; Tyroneomicin†.

## Potassium Hydroxide

Ätzkali; Caustic Potash; E525; Hidróxido potásico; Kalii Hydroxidum; Kalii Hydroxydum; Kalium Hydroxydatum; Potash Lye.
KOH = 56.11.
*CAS — 1310-58-3.*

**Pharmacopoeias.** In *Eur.* (see p.vi) and *Jpn.* Also in *USNF.*

**Ph. Eur. 5.0** (Potassium Hydroxide). White, crystalline, hard masses, supplied as sticks, pellets, or irregularly shaped pieces; it is deliquescent in air, hygroscopic, and absorbs carbon dioxide. Very soluble in water; freely soluble in alcohol. Store in airtight, nonmetallic containers.

**USNF 22** (Potassium Hydroxide). It contains not less than 85% of total alkali, calculated as KOH, including not more than 3.5% of $K_2CO_3$. White or practically white, fused masses, or small pellets, or flakes, or sticks, or other forms. It is hard and brittle and shows a crystalline fracture. Exposed to air, it rapidly absorbs carbon dioxide and moisture, and deliquesces. Soluble 1 in 1 of water, 1 in 3 of alcohol, and 1 in 2.5 of glycerol; very soluble in boiling alcohol. Store in airtight containers.

### Adverse Effects and Treatment

As for Sodium Hydroxide, p.1748.

### Uses and Administration

Potassium hydroxide is a powerful caustic that has been used to remove warts. A 2.5% solution in glycerol has been used as a cuticle solvent. An escharotic preparation of potassium hydroxide and calcium hydroxide was known as Vienna paste. Potassium hydroxide is used to adjust the pH of solutions in pharmaceutical formulations.

### Preparations

***BP 2003:*** Chloroxylenol Solution; Potassium Hydroxide Solution.

**Proprietary Preparations** (details are given in Part 3)
***Spain:*** Cerumenol; Kuson†.

**Multi-ingredient:** ***Austria:*** Leberinfusion; ***Ger.:*** Acarex; Glutarsin E; Kalium-Magnesium-Asparaginat; KMA†; Sekudrill; ***Ital.:*** Sekudrill.

## Potassium Hydroxyquinoline Sulfate

Oxiquinol potásico; Oxyquinol Potassium; Potassii Hydroxyquinolini Sulphas; Potassium Hydroxyquinoline Sulphate; Potassium Oxyquinoline Sulphate.

**Pharmacopoeias.** In *Br., Fr.,* and *Ger.*

**BP 2003** (Potassium Hydroxyquinoline Sulphate). An equimolecular mixture of potassium sulfate and quinolin-8-ol sulfate monohydrate. It contains 50.6 to 52.6% of quinolin-8-ol and 29.5 to 32.5% of potassium sulfate, calculated with reference to the anhydrous substance. A pale yellow, odourless or almost odourless, microcrystalline powder. Freely soluble in water; insoluble in ether. On extraction with hot dehydrated alcohol a residue of potassium sulfate and a solution of quinolin-8-ol sulfate are obtained.

### Profile

Potassium hydroxyquinoline sulfate has antibacterial, antifungal, and deodorant properties and is used, often with benzoyl peroxide, in the topical treatment of fungal infections, minor bacterial infections, and acne.

### Preparations

***BP 2003:*** Potassium Hydroxyquinoline Sulphate and Benzoyl Peroxide Cream.

**Proprietary Preparations** (details are given in Part 3)
**Multi-ingredient:** ***Belg.:*** Aseptosyl; ***Irl.:*** Quinocort; Quinoderm; Valderma; ***S.Afr.:*** Auralgicin†; Oto-Phen Forte; Quinoderm; Quinoderm-H†; Universal Earache Drops†; ***Spain:*** Stoma Anestesia Dental†; ***Switz.:*** Quinoderm†; Rectoseptal-Neo bismuthe; Rectoseptal-Neo simple; ***UK:*** Quinocort†; Quinoderm; Quinoped†; Valderma.

## Potassium Metaphosphate

E452 (potassium polyphosphates); Polifosfato potásico; Potassium Kurrol's Salt; Potassium Polymetaphosphate.
$(KPO_3)_x$.
*CAS — 7790-53-6.*

**Pharmacopoeias.** In *USNF.*

**USNF 22** (Potassium Metaphosphate). A straight-chain polyphosphate, having a high degree of polymerisation. It contains the equivalent of 59 to 61% of $P_2O_5$. A white, odourless powder. Insoluble in water; soluble in dilute solutions of sodium salts.

### Profile

Potassium metaphosphate is used as a buffer.

## Pramiracetam Sulfate *(USAN, rINNM)*

Amacetam Sulphate; CI-879; Pramiracetam Sulphate; Sulfato de pramiracetam. *N*-[2-(Diisopropylamino)ethyl]-2-oxo-1-pyrrolidineacetamide sulphate.
$C_{14}H_{27}N_3O_2,H_2SO_4$ = 367.5.
*CAS — 68497-62-1 (pramiracetam); 72869-16-0 (pramiracetam sulfate).*
*ATC — N06BX16.*

### Profile

Pramiracetam sulfate is used in age-related memory impairment and senile dementia (p.1484), in doses equivalent to 600 mg of pramiracetam twice daily by mouth. It has also been tried, without much success, as an adjunct to ECT in severe depression.

◊ References.


1. McLean A, *et al.* Placebo-controlled study of pramiracetam in young males with memory and cognitive problems resulting from head injury and anoxia. *Brain Inj* 1991; **5:** 375–80.
2. Auteri A, *et al.* Pharmacokinetics of pramiracetam in healthy volunteers after oral administration. *Int J Clin Pharmacol Res* 1992; **12:** 129–32.
3. Scarpazza P, *et al.* Multicenter evaluation of pramiracetam for the treatment of memory impairment of probable vascular origin. *Adv Therapy* 1993; **10:** 217–25.


### Preparations

**Proprietary Preparations** (details are given in Part 3)
***Ital.:*** Neupramir; Pramistar†; Rement†.

## Pramiverine Hydrochloride *(BANM, rINNM)*

EMD-9806 (pramiverine); Hidrocloruro de pramiverina; HSP-2986 (pramiverine). *N*-Isopropyl-4,4-diphenylcyclohexylamine hydrochloride.
$C_{21}H_{27}N,HCl$ = 329.9.
*CAS — 14334-40-8 (pramiverine); 14334-41-9 (pramiverine hydrochloride).*

### Profile

Pramiverine hydrochloride has been used as an antispasmodic.

### Preparations

**Proprietary Preparations** (details are given in Part 3)
**Multi-ingredient:** ***Chile:*** Sistalgina.

## Pregnancy and Fertility Tests

Pruebas de embarazo y de fertilidad.

### Profile

There are a number of kits available for simple pregnancy and fertility testing. A common method of detecting pregnancy is to use specific antibodies to measure the increase in chorionic gonadotrophin in the urine. The period of ovulation can be detected by measuring luteinising hormone excretion in similar ways.

These tests can give false results. Those carrying out the tests should be aware of this and of problems such as contaminated specimens, concomitant drug therapy, or other factors that could affect the result.

### Preparations

**Proprietary Preparations** (details are given in Part 3)
***Arg.:*** Evaplan; Evatest; Gestatest; Gravitest; Mater Test; Nueve Lunas; Ovutest; PG/53; Si o No; Tea Test; Very-Test; ***Austral.:*** Answer; Clearblue One Step; Clearplan One Step; Clearview HCG; Clinitek HCG; Crystal Clear; Discover Onestep Ovulation Prediction; Discover Onestep†;

Dotest; Evaplan†; Evatest One Step†; First Response†; Fortel; Nimbus; Ovuplan; Predictor†; Pregnosis; **Braz.:** Clearblue Easy; Detect Baby; Fertility Day; Predictor; **Canad.:** Answer Now; Clearblue; Clearplan; Conceive†; Confidelle; Confirm; Fact Plus; First Response; Simplicity; **Chile:** Clearplan; **Fr.:** Babycheck-Plus; BB Test; Bluetest; Clearblue; Clearplan; Elle-Test; Emotion; G.Test; Indicatest; Predictor; Primacard†; Primastick; Primatime; Revelatest; **Irl.:** Fertility Score†; Testpack hCG-Urine; Today Ovulation Test; Uni-Gold hCG; **Israel:** Clearblue; Gravindex; Predictor; Pregnosticon; Prepurex; **Ital.:** Advisor†; Clearblue; Clearplan; Conferma 3 Plus; Confidelle Progress; Diagnosis; Gravitest Crual; PG 53†; Predictor; Rivela†; **Mex.:** Intimide; **NZ:** Cards HCG-Urine; Clearblue; Clearplan; Crystal Clear; Discover One Step; LH Predict; MDS Quick; **Port.:** Bluetest†; Clearview HCG†; **Switz.:** Clearplan; **UK:** Auratek hCG; Calista; Check-Mate; Clearblue; Clearplan†; Clearview HCG; Concept; Discover; Early Bird; First Response; Neo-Planotest; Ovukit†; Ovuquick; Predictor; Pregna-Cert†; Pregna-Sure HCG†; Pregnospia Duoclon; Prepurex†; Quick N Easy; Ramp†; Reveal; Tandem Icon†; Test Pack Plus; **USA:** Advance; Answer; Clearblue Easy; Clearplan Easy; Clearview HCG; Conceive Ovulation Predictor; Conceive Pregnancy; ept Stick Test; Fact Plus; First Response; Fortel; Nimbus; OvuGen; Ovukit; Ovuquick; Pregnosis; QTest; QTest Ovulation; QuickVue; RapidVue; TestPack Plus hCG-Urine; UCG-Slide; Unistep hCG.

## Prenylamine *(BAN, USAN, rINN)*

B-436; Hoechst-12512. 2-Benzhydrylethyl(α-methylphenethyl)amine.

$C_{24}H_{27}N = 329.5$.

*CAS — 390-64-7.*

*ATC — C01DX02.*

## Prenylamine Lactate *(BANM, rINNM)*

Lactato de prenilamina; Prenylaminii Lactas.

$C_{24}H_{27}N,C_3H_6O_3 = 419.6$.

*CAS — 69-43-2.*

*ATC — C01DX02.*

### Profile

Prenylamine depletes myocardial catecholamine stores and has some calcium-channel blocking activity. It was formerly used in the treatment of angina pectoris but has been superseded by less toxic drugs. Administration of prenylamine has been associated with the development of ventricular arrhythmias and ECG abnormalities. Tremor and extrapyramidal symptoms have also occurred.

**Porphyria.** Prenylamine is considered to be unsafe in patients with porphyria because it has been shown to be porphyrinogenic in *in-vitro* systems.

## Primula Root

Primelwurzel; Prímula; Racine de Primevére; Schlüsselblumenwurzel.

**Pharmacopoeias.** *Eur.* (see p.vi) includes Primula root.

**Ph. Eur. 5.0** (Primula Root; Primulae Radix). Consists of the whole or cut, dried rhizome and root of *Primula veris* [cowslip] or *P. elatior* [oxlip]. It has a bitter taste. Protect from light.

### Profile

Primula root has expectorant properties and is used for cough and other respiratory-tract disorders.

Cowslip, the flowers, leaves, and roots of *Primula veris* (*P. officinalis*) (Primulaceae), is widely used in herbal medicine. The flowers have sedative properties and are used for insomnia, hyperactivity, and anxiety disorders. The flowers and leaves have also been used similarly to primula root. Cowslip is also used in homoeopathic medicine.

Oxlip flowers and root (*P. elatior*) and primrose root (*P. vulgaris*) have also been used.

### Preparations

**Proprietary Preparations** (details are given in Part 3)
**Ger.:** Ipalat†.

**Multi-ingredient:** **Arg.:** Expectosan Hierbas y Miel; **Austria:** Anifer Hustentropfen; Apotheker Bauer's Brust- und Hustentee; Apotheker Bauer's Grippetee; Bio-Strath Husten; Bronchithym; Cardiodoron; Egmovit; Granobil; Heumann's Bronchialtee; Hustensaft-Dr Schmidgall†; Kneipp Husten- und Bronchial-Tee; Krauter Hustensaft; Krauterdoktor Hustentropfen; Krauterpfarrer Weidinger Tee bei Fruhjahrsmudigkeit; Krauterpfarrer Weidinger Tee bei Husten und Heiserkeit; Krauterpfarrer Weidinger Tee bei Wetterfuhligkeit und Kreislaufstorungen; Sinupret; Sinusol; Sinusol-Schleimlosender Tee; St Radegunder Thorasan-Krauterhustensaft; Synpharma Instant-Brust- und Hustentee; Thymoval; **Canad.:** Pectothymin†; **Ger.:** Bronchicum Elixir N; Bronchicum Elixir Plus; Bronchicum Sekret-Loser; Bronchicum Thymian; Bronchipret; Bronchitten forte K†; Brust- und Hustentee; Cardiodoron; Drosithym-N; Ephepect†; Equisil N; Expectysat N; Guttae 20 Hustentropfen N†; Harzer Hustenloser; Heumann Bronchialtee Solubifix; JuViton; Kinder Em-eukal Hustensaft; Kneipp Husten- und Bronchial-Tee†; Kneipp Krauter Hustensaft N Kneipp Tannolsaft†; Melrosum Hustensirup N†; Mintetten Truw†; Perdiphen phyto†; Phytobronchin; Primotussan†; Salus Bronchial-Tee Nr.8†; Sinuforton; Sinupret; Tussiflorin forte; Tussiflorin Hustensaft; Tussiflorin Hustentropfen; Tussiflorin N†; TUSSinfant N; **Hong Kong:** Pectoral; Sinupret; **Neth.:** Abdijsiroop (Akker-Siroop)†; Bronchicum; **Port.:** Bio-Strath No 1†; Bio-Strath No 5†; Codeisan†; Fluidin Infantil†; **S.Afr.:** Bronchicough; Bronchicum; **Singapore:** Sinupret; **Switz.:** Demo sirop bronchique N†; Demo-Pectol; Kernosan Elixir; Pectoral N; Perpector; Sinupret; Sirop S contre la toux et la bronchite; Tisane pectorale pour les enfants; **Thai.:** Sinupret; Solvopret TP; **UK:** Bio-Strath Willow Formula; Onopordon Comp B.

## Proadifen Hydrochloride *(USAN, rINNM)*

Hidrocloruro de proadifeno; NSC-39690; Propyladiphenine Hydrochloride; RP-5171; SKF-525A; SKF-525-A. 2-Diethylaminoethyl 2,2-diphenylvalerate hydrochloride.

$C_{23}H_{31}NO_2,HCl = 390.0$.

*CAS — 302-33-0 (proadifen); 62-68-0 (proadifen hydrochloride).*

### Profile

Proadifen has been found to enhance the effects of a large number of drugs, possibly by inhibiting metabolism.

## Procodazole *(rINN)*

Procodazol; Propazol; Propazole. 3-(Benzimidazol-2-yl)propionic acid.

$C_{10}H_{10}N_2O_2 = 190.2$.

*CAS — 23249-97-0 (procodazole); 6315-23-7 (procodazole ethyl ester); 59345-72-1 (procodazole sodium).*

### Profile

Procodazole is reported to have immunostimulant properties. The ethyl ester and the sodium salt have been used.

### Preparations

**Proprietary Preparations** (details are given in Part 3)
**Spain:** Estimulocel†.

## Promelase *(pINN)*

Promelasa; Seaprose S.

*CAS — 9074-07-1.*

### Profile

Promelase is an alkaline protease derived from *Aspergillus melleus*. It has been taken by mouth in doses of 30 to 90 mg daily for its supposed benefit in oedema and inflammation associated with trauma, infection, and surgical procedures.

### Preparations

**Proprietary Preparations** (details are given in Part 3)
**Ital.:** Altan; Flaminase; Mezen; **Port.:** Onoprose; **Thai.:** Korynase.

## Propolis

Bee Glue; Propóleo.

### Profile

Propolis is a resinous substance collected by bees, primarily, at least in Europe, from poplar buds (see also p.1733), and used by them to seal their hives. It has been traditionally used for a wide variety of disorders, and in cosmetics and varnishes. Propolis has been reported to have anti-inflammatory and antimicrobial properties. It has been used as an ointment for the relief of symptoms of herpes labialis. Hypersensitivity reactions have been reported.

◊ References.

1. Grange JM, Davey RW. Antibacterial properties of propolis (bee glue). *J R Soc Med* 1990; **83:** 159–60.
2. Krol W, *et al.* Synergistic effect of ethanolic extract of propolis and antibiotics on the growth of Staphylococcus aureus. *Arzneimittelforschung* 1993; **43:** 607–9.
3. Volpert R, Elstner EF. Interactions of different extracts of propolis with leukocytes and leukocytic enzymes. *Arzneimittelforschung* 1996; **46:** 47–51.
4. Murray MC, *et al.* A study to investigate the effect of a propolis-containing mouthrinse on the inhibition of de novo plaque formation. *J Clin Periodontol* 1997; **24:** 796–8.
5. Burdock GA. Review of the biological properties and toxicity of bee propolis (propolis). *Food Chem Toxicol* 1998; **36:** 347–63.

### Preparations

**Proprietary Preparations** (details are given in Part 3)
**Arg.:** Propoleos; **Austral.:** Helastop†; **Ger.:** Propolisept-Salbe; **Ital.:** Golapiol; Oral Spray; Pro-30C; Pro-Gola; Propolcream; **UK:** Buttercup Lozenges†; **USA:** Probax.

**Multi-ingredient:** **Braz.:** Calmatoss; Infantoss; Proplax†; **Fr.:** Pollen Royal; Propargile; **Ital.:** Ap stress; Biogreen; Bodyguard; Cocktail Reale†; Fosfarsile Forte; Golapiol C; Immumil; Keratolip; Neo-Stomygen; Orostick†; Otosan Natural Ear Drops; Probigol; Promix; Promix 3; Propast; Propomill; **Switz.:** Osa Gel de dentition aux plantes†; **UK:** Beeline†.

## Propylene Glycol

E1520; Glicol Propilênico; Propilenglicol; Propilenoglicol; Propylenglycolum. (±)-Propane-1,2-diol.

$C_3H_8O_2 = 76.09$.

*CAS — 57-55-6 ((±)-propylene glycol); 4254-16-4 ((±)-propylene glycol); 4254-14-2 ((−)-propylene glycol); 4254-15-3 ((+)-propylene glycol);.*

**Pharmacopoeias.** In *Chin., Eur.* (see p.vi), *Jpn, Pol.,* and *US.*

**Ph. Eur. 5.0** (Propylene Glycol). A clear, colourless, viscous, hygroscopic liquid. Miscible with water and with alcohol. Store in airtight containers.

**USP 27** (Propylene Glycol). A clear, colourless, practically odourless, viscous liquid. It absorbs moisture when exposed to moist air. Miscible with water, with acetone, and with chloroform; soluble in ether; will dissolve in many essential oils but is immiscible with fixed oils. Store in airtight containers.

### Adverse Effects and Precautions

Systemic toxicity of propylene glycol is considered to be low after oral doses unless large quantities have been ingested, or when preparations containing propylene glycol are given to neonates or to patients in renal failure. Systemic toxicity is manifested most commonly by CNS depression, especially in neonates and children. Other reported adverse effects include hepatic or renal impairment, intravascular haemolysis, seizures, coma, arrhythmias, and cardiorespiratory arrest. Hyperosmolality has occurred, particularly in small infants and in patients with renal impairment; lactic acidosis may also be a greater problem in the latter group.

After topical use, propylene glycol may produce some local irritation, particularly if applied under occlusive dressings or to mucous membranes; toxicity may occur following application to burns. Hypersensitivity reactions have also been reported. Local sensitivity has been reported following use of ear drops containing propylene glycol as the vehicle. Injections of preparations containing high concentrations of propylene glycol may produce pain or irritation.

### Interactions

**Anticoagulants.** Propylene glycol has been reported to decrease the effect of *heparin*.[1]

1. Col J, *et al.* Propylene glycol-induced heparin resistance during nitroglycerin infusion. *Am Heart J* 1985; **110:** 171–3.

### Pharmacokinetics

Propylene glycol is rapidly absorbed from the gastrointestinal tract. There is evidence of topical absorption when applied to damaged skin.

It is extensively metabolised in the liver primarily by oxidation to lactic and pyruvic acid and is also excreted in the urine unchanged.

◊ References.

1. Yu DK, *et al.* Pharmacokinetics of propylene glycol in humans during multiple dosing regimens. *J Pharm Sci* 1985; **74:** 876–9.
2. Speth PAJ, *et al.* Propylene glycol pharmacokinetics and effects after intravenous infusion in humans. *Ther Drug Monit* 1987; **9:** 255–8.

### Uses and Administration

Propylene glycol is widely used in pharmaceutical manufacturing as a solvent and vehicle especially for drugs unstable or insoluble in water. It may also be used as a stabiliser in vitamin preparations, as a plasticiser, and as a preservative. Propylene glycol is used extensively in foods and cosmetics.

Propylene glycol has humectant properties and is used similarly to glycerol in topical moisturising preparations.

Propylene glycol is used in veterinary medicine as a glucose precursor.

### Preparations

**Proprietary Preparations** (details are given in Part 3)

**Multi-ingredient:** **Austral.:** Dermatech Liquid; **Austria:** Acerbine; **Canad.:** Episec; Gyne-Moistrin; Rhinaris; Rhinedrine Lubricant†; Rhinedrine Moisturizing; Salinol; Secaris; **Fr.:** Intrasite; Propy-Lacticare; **Ger.:** Sekudrill; **Israel:** Taro Gel; **Ital.:** Dopo Pik; Sekudrill; **Port.:** Emopads†; **S.Afr.:** Aserbine; **Spain:** Acerbiol; **Switz.:** Acerbine; **UK:** Aserbine; **USA:** Astroglide; Massengill Disposable; Surgel; Zonite.

## Protoporphyrin IX Disodium

Protoporfirina IX disódica; Protoporphyrin Disodium. Disodium 7,12-diethenyl-3,8,13,17-tetramethyl-21*H*,23*H*-porphine-2,18-dipropanoate.

$C_{34}H_{32}N_4Na_2O_4 = 606.6$.

*CAS — 50865-01-5 (protoporphyrin IX disodium); 553-12-8 (protoporphyrin IX).*

### Profile

Protoporphyrin IX disodium has been given by mouth for the treatment of impaired hepatic function associated with gallstones and cholecystitis.

### Preparations

**Proprietary Preparations** (details are given in Part 3)
**Hong Kong:** Prolmon†.

## Proxazole Citrate *(USAN, rINNM)*

AF-634; Citrato de proxazol; Propaxoline Citrate; PZ-17105. *NN*-Diethyl-3-(1-phenylpropyl)-1,2,4-oxadiazole-5-ethanamine citrate.

$C_{17}H_{25}N_3O,C_6H_8O_7 = 479.5$.

*CAS — 5696-09-3 (proxazole); 132-35-4 (proxazole citrate).*

*ATC — A03AX07.*

### Profile

Proxazole citrate is used as an antispasmodic and in vascular disorders and has been used in veterinary medicine.

### Preparations

**Proprietary Preparations** (details are given in Part 3)
**Ital.:** Toness.

## Prozapine Hydrochloride *(rINNM)*

Hexadiphane Hydrochloride; Hidrocloruro de prozapina. 1-(3,3-Diphenylpropyl)cyclohexamethyleneimine hydrochloride.

$C_{21}H_{27}N,HCl = 329.9$.

*CAS — 3426-08-2 (prozapine); 13657-24-4 (prozapine hydrochloride).*

### Profile

Prozapine hydrochloride is an antispasmodic that has been given orally with sorbitol in biliary and gastrointestinal disorders.

### Preparations

**Proprietary Preparations** (details are given in Part 3)

**Multi-ingredient:** ***Fr.:*** Norbiline†; ***Ital.:*** Norbiline†.

---

## Psilocin

4-Hydroxy-*NN*-dimethyltryptamine; Psilocina; Psilocyn. 3-(2-Dimethylaminoethyl)indol-4-ol.

$C_{12}H_{16}N_2O = 204.3$.

*CAS — 520-53-6.*

## Psilocybine *(BAN, rINN)*

CY-39; 4-Phosphoryloxy-*NN*-dimethyltryptamine; Psilocibina; Psilocybin. 3-(2-Dimethylaminoethyl)indol-4-yl dihydrogen phosphate.

$C_{12}H_{17}N_2O_4P = 284.2$.

*CAS — 520-52-5.*

### Profile

Psilocin is an indole alkaloid obtained from the sacred Mexican mushroom (teonanácatl), *Psilocybe mexicana* (Agaricaceae). The main indole alkaloid present in this mushroom, however, is psilocybine.

In the UK, psilocybine is present in the indigenous mushroom *Psilocybe semilanceata* (magic mushroom; liberty cap). Psilocybine is also present in other species of mushrooms including *Stropharia cubensis* and *Conocybe* spp.

Psilocybine has hallucinogenic and sympathomimetic properties similar to those of lysergide (p.1708). It is less potent than lysergide and its hallucinogenic effects last for up to 6 hours. There is evidence to suggest that psilocybine is converted to the active form psilocin in the body. It has no therapeutic use.

---

## Pulegium Oil

Pennyroyal Oil; Poleo, aceite esencial de.

### Profile

Pulegium oil is a volatile oil distilled from pennyroyal herb, *Mentha pulegium* (Labiatae), containing pulegone ($C_{10}H_{16}O = 152.2$). It was formerly used as an emmenagogue. Severe toxic effects have followed its use as an abortifacient with convulsions, hepatotoxicity, and death. It is reported to have insect repellent activity.

**Adverse effects.** Severe hepatotoxicity accompanied by seizures occurred in 2 infants each of whom had received herbal teas containing pulegium oil.[1] In one of the infants multiple organ failure developed, and fulminant hepatic failure with hepatocellular necrosis and cerebral oedema proved fatal. A further 4 cases of toxicity associated with ingestion of pulegium oil have been reported;[2] three of the cases were adult patients who had ingested either herbal teas to induce menses (2 cases) or a herbal extract as an abortifacient (1 fatality), and the fourth was a 22-month old child who had ingested the oil.


1. Bakerink JA, *et al.* Multiple organ failure after ingestion of pennyroyal oil from herbal tea in two infants. *Pediatrics* 1996; **98:** 944–7.
2. Anderson IB, *et al.* Pennyroyal toxicity: measurement of toxic metabolite levels in two cases and review of the literature. *Ann Intern Med* 1996; **124:** 726–34.


### Preparations

**Proprietary Preparations** (details are given in Part 3)

**Multi-ingredient:** ***Fr.:*** Santane O₁†.

---

## Pulmonary Surfactants

Tensioactivos pulmonares.

**Description.** Pulmonary surfactants are mixtures consisting mainly of phospholipids and surfactant proteins that are used to replace deficient endogenous lung surfactants. A number of preparations have been studied including:

- natural human surfactant obtained from amniotic fluid or biosynthetic material
- natural animal-derived surfactants, which are bovine or porcine lung extracts that may be modified by the addition of synthetic surfactants, as in the case of beractant, or unmodified, as in the case of bovactant and calfactant
- synthetic or semisynthetic preparations, which may contain the phospholipid colfosceril palmitate, a major constituent of natural lung surfactants, in combination with other substances that aid spreading and absorption such as the synthetic peptide sinapultide.

## Beractant *(BAN, USAN)*

A-60386X.

*CAS — 108778-82-1.*

**Description.** Beractant is a modified bovine lung extract containing mostly phospholipids, modified by the addition of colfosceril palmitate, palmitic acid, and tripalmitin.

The term Surfactant TA has been applied to a modified bovine lung surfactant.

## Bovactant *(BAN)*

SF-R11.

**Description.** Bovactant is an extract of bovine lung containing about 92% of phospholipids, 3.2% of cholesterol, 0.6% of surfactant-associated hydrophobic proteins, and 0.4% of free fatty acid.

## Calfactant *(BAN, USAN)*

*CAS — 183325-78-2.*

**Description.** Calfactant is an unmodified calf lung extract that includes mostly phospholipids and hydrophobic surfactant-specific proteins (SP-B and SP-C).

## Colfosceril Palmitate *(BAN, USAN, rINN)*

Dipalmitoylphosphatidylcholine; DPPC; Palmitato de colfoscerilo; 129Y83. 1,2-Dipalmitoyl-*sn*-glycero(3)phosphocholine.

$C_{40}H_{80}NO_8P = 734.0$.

*CAS — 63-89-8.*

*ATC — R07AA01.*

**Description.** Colfosceril palmitate is a phospholipid which forms an important constituent of natural and many synthetic pulmonary surfactant compounds.

## Lucinactant *(USAN)*

ATI-02; $KL_4$-surfactant.

**Description.** Lucinactant is a mixture of sinapultide, colfosceril palmitate, sodium palmitoyloleaylphosphatidyl glycerol, and palmitic acid.

## Poractant Alfa *(BAN)*

*CAS — 129069-19-8.*

**Description.** Poractant alfa is an extract of porcine lung containing not less than 90% of phospholipids, about 1% of hydrophobic proteins (SP-B and SP-C), and about 9% of other lipids.

## Pumactant *(BAN)*

Artificial Lung Expanding Compound.

**Description.** Pumactant is a mixture of colfosceril palmitate and phosphatidyl glycerol (2-oleoyl-1-palmitoyl-*sn*-glycero(3)phospho(1)-*sn*-glycerol) in the proportion 7:3.

## Sinapultide *(USAN, rINN)*

ATI-01.

*CAS — 138531-07-4.*

**Description.** Sinapultide is a synthetic peptide that mimics the actions of human surfactant protein B, an important constituent of natural pulmonary surfactant compounds.

### Adverse Effects and Precautions

Surfactant therapy may be associated with an increased risk of pulmonary haemorrhage, especially in more premature infants. Therapy should only be given where there are adequate facilities for ventilation and monitoring. Rapid chest expansion and improvement of oxygenation may follow successful treatment, and peak ventilatory pressure and inspired oxygen concentration may need to be reduced promptly to avoid the risk of pneumothorax and hyperoxaemia. A transient decrease in brain electrical activity has been reported in neonates given surfactant but its significance is unknown. Transient bradycardia has also been reported. Giving surfactant has occasionally been associated with obstruction of the endotracheal tube by mucus.

◊ While surfactant therapy is clearly associated with an increased risk of pulmonary haemorrhage,[1-4] meta-analysis suggests that the risk is small compared with the benefits.[1] However, neonates who do develop moderate or severe pulmonary haemorrhage after surfactant therapy are at increased risk of death or short-term morbidity.[5] Haemodynamic changes associated with surfactant therapy or consequent pulmonary haemorrhage may also predispose premature infants to intracranial (periventricular) haemorrhage.[5,6] Early preventive use of surfactant in very low birth-weight infants may be associated with a poorer neurodevelopmental outcome,[7] although a long-term follow-up study[8] of premature infants born in the surfactant era concluded that these children had similar neurodevelopmental outcomes to such children born before the introduction of surfactant therapy. Decreased brain electrical activity has been reported after surfactant treatment.[9]

The rate of instillation of surfactant may be significant: one study,[10] in which the apparatus was adapted so that mechanical ventilation could continue while giving surfactant, found that rapid instillation over a 5-minute period provoked a transient increase in cerebral blood flow velocity associated with an increase in carbon dioxide tension, compared with slow instillation over 15 minutes. Although the authors acknowledged that such changes are likely to be related to several factors, particularly the type of surfactant, they recommended that, until further data are available, instillation should take place slowly, over at least 15 to 20 minutes.


1. Raju TNK, Langenberg P. Pulmonary hemorrhage and exogenous surfactant therapy: a metaanalysis. *J Pediatr* 1993; **123:** 603–10.
2. Majeed-Saidan MA, *et al.* Pulmonary haemorrhage in low-birth-weight babies. *Lancet* 1993; **341:** 120.
3. Rogers D. Pulmonary haemorrhage, surfactant, and low-birth-weight babies. *Lancet* 1993; **341:** 698.
4. Pappin A, *et al.* Extensive intraalveolar pulmonary hemorrhage in infants dying after surfactant therapy. *J Pediatr* 1994; **124:** 621–6.
5. Pandit PB, *et al.* Outcome following pulmonary haemorrhage in very low birthweight neonates treated with surfactant. *Arch Dis Child Fetal Neonatal Ed* 1999; **81:** F40–F44.
6. Gunkel JH, Banks PLC. Surfactant therapy and intracranial hemorrhage: review of the literature and results of new analyses. *Pediatrics* 1993; **92:** 775–86.
7. Vaucher YE, *et al.* Outcome at twelve months of adjusted age in very low birthweight infants with lung immaturity: a randomized placebo-controlled trial of human surfactant. *J Pediatr* 1993; **122:** 126–32.
8. D'Angio CT, *et al.* Longitudinal, 15-year follow-up of children born at less than 29 weeks' gestation after introduction of surfactant therapy into a region: neurologic, cognitive, and educational outcomes. *Pediatrics* 2002; **110:** 1094–1102.
9. Hellström-Westas L, *et al.* Cerebroelectrical depression following surfactant treatment in preterm neonates. *Pediatrics* 1992; **89:** 643–7.
10. Saliba E, *et al.* Instillation rate effects of Exosurf on cerebral and cardiovascular haemodynamics in preterm neonates. *Arch Dis Child* 1994; **71:** F174–8.


### Uses and Administration

Pulmonary surfactants are compounds with surface active properties similar to those natural substances in the lung that help to maintain the patency of the airways by reducing the surface tension of pulmonary fluids. Exogenous pulmonary surfactants are used in the treatment of neonatal respiratory distress syndrome (p.1084) in premature infants, and may also be given for prevention in infants considered to be at risk of developing the syndrome. Doses vary, but most pulmonary surfactants are given in recommended doses of 100 to 200 mg phospholipids per kg birth-weight; a suggested dose for colfosceril palmitate is 67.5 mg/kg. For the treatment of overt neonatal respiratory distress syndrome, the initial dose is given as soon as possible after diagnosis, while for prevention it is given as soon as possible after birth. It is given as a suspension via an endotracheal tube to intubated neonates receiving mechanical ventilation. Manufacturers may recommend regimens with or without disconnection from the ventilator. Repeat doses may be given if necessary, although the number of doses and the dosage interval varies.

Pulmonary surfactants have also been tried in acute respiratory distress syndrome and for meconium aspiration syndrome.

**Acute respiratory distress syndrome.** Pulmonary surfactants have been investigated for acute respiratory distress syndrome (p.1075). In adults, they have been given by intrabronchial instillation[1] or nebulisation[2-4] but results have been largely disappointing. Sequential bronchopulmonary segmental lavage with a synthetic surfactant has also been tried[5] and appeared to be well tolerated. Endotracheal poractant alfa moderately improved oxygenation in some children with severe acute respiratory distress syndrome secondary to pulmonary or systemic disease.[6]


1. Haslam PL, *et al.* Surfactant replacement therapy in late-stage adult respiratory distress syndrome. *Lancet* 1994; **343:** 1009–11.
2. do Campo JL, *et al.* Natural surfactant aerosolisation in adult respiratory distress syndrome. *Lancet* 1994; **344:** 413–14.
3. Weg JG, *et al.* Safety and potential efficacy of an aerosolized surfactant in human sepsis-induced adult respiratory distress syndrome. *JAMA* 1994; **272:** 1433–8.
4. Anzueto A, *et al.* Aerosolized surfactant in adults with sepsis-induced respiratory distress syndrome. *N Engl J Med* 1996; **334:** 1417–21.
5. Wiswell TE, *et al.* Bronchopulmonary segmental lavage with Surfaxin ($KL_4$-Surfactant) for acute respiratory distress syndrome. *Am J Respir Crit Care Med* 1999; **160:** 1188–95.
6. López-Herce J, *et al.* Surfactant treatment for acute respiratory distress syndrome. *Arch Dis Child* 1999; **80:** 248–52.


**Drowning.** Reference to the use of colfosceril palmitate in the management of a 9-year-old rescued after near drowning.[1]


1. McBrien M, *et al.* Artificial surfactant in the treatment of near drowning. *Lancet* 1993; **342:** 1485–6.


**Meconium aspiration syndrome.** Results from a pilot study[1] of beractant as a tracheobronchial lavage fluid for the treatment of infants with severe meconium aspiration syndrome were promising, and a small comparative trial[2] found that bronchoalveolar lavage with diluted beractant, with or without intravenous dexamethasone, significantly improved oxygenation in neonates when compared with standard therapy. Systematic review[3] of two randomised controlled trials evaluating the effect of intratracheal administration of beractant also found encouraging results, although comparison with other established treatments for meconium aspiration syndrome remains to be done.


1. Lam BCC, Yeung CY. Surfactant lavage for meconium aspiration syndrome: a pilot study. *Pediatrics* 1999; **103:** 1014–18.
2. Salvia-Roigés MD, *et al.* Efficacy of three treatment schedules in severe meconium aspiration syndrome. *Acta Paediatr* 2004; **93:** 60–5.
3. Soll RF, Dargaville P. Surfactant for meconium aspiration syndrome in full term infants. Available in The Cochrane Library; Issue 2. Chichester: John Wiley, 2004.

### Preparations

**Proprietary Preparations** (details are given in Part 3)
***Arg.:*** Baby Fact B; Exosurf; Natsurf; Surfactante B; Survanta; ***Austral.:*** Exosurf; Survanta; ***Austria:*** Alveofact; Curosurf; Exosurf; Survanta; ***Belg.:*** Alvofact; Exosurf†; Survanta; ***Braz.:*** Alveofact†; Curosurf; Exosurf; Survanta; ***Canad.:*** Exosurf; Survanta; ***Chile:*** Exosurf; ***Denm.:*** Curosurf; Exosurf†; ***Fin.:*** Curosurf; Exosurf†; ***Fr.:*** Curosurf; Surfexo Neonatal†; Survanta; ***Ger.:*** Alveofact; Curosurf; Exosurf†; Survanta; ***Hong Kong:*** Exosurf; Survanta; ***Irl.:*** Curosurf; Exosurf; ***Israel:*** Curosurf; Exosurf; Infasurf; ***Ital.:*** Alveofact†; Curosurf; Exosurf; ***Jpn:*** Surfacten; ***Mex.:*** Exosurf; Survanta; ***Neth.:*** Alvofact; Curosurf; Exosurf; Survanta; ***Norw.:*** Curosurf; Survanta-Vent; ***NZ:*** Survanta; ***Port.:*** Curosurf†; ***S.Afr.:*** Curosurf; Exosurf†; Survanta; ***Singapore:*** Exosurf†; Survanta; ***Spain:*** Curosurf; Exosurf†; Survanta; ***Swed.:*** Curosurf; Exosurf†; Survanta-Vent; ***Switz.:*** Curosurf; Exosurf†; Survanta; ***Thai.:*** Alvofact†; Exosurf†; Survanta; ***UK:*** Alec†; Curosurf; Exosurf†; Survanta; ***USA:*** Curosurf; Exosurf; Infasurf; Survanta.

## Pulsatilla

Meadow Anemone; Pasque Flower.
*CAS — 62887-80-3.*

### Profile

Pulsatilla is the whole flowering plant of *Pulsatilla vulgaris* (*Anemone pulsatilla*) or *Pulsatilla pratensis* (Ranunculaceae). It has been used in herbal preparations for the treatment of conditions including nervous disorders, circulatory disorders, and gynaecological disorders and benign prostatic hyperplasia. It is also used in homoeopathic medicine.

### Preparations

**Proprietary Preparations** (details are given in Part 3)
***USA:*** Yeast-X.

**Multi-ingredient:** ***Austral.:*** Bioglan Cirflo†; Calmo†; Lifesystem Herbal Formula 4 Women's Formula†; Proflo†; Viburnum Complex†; Women's Formula Herbal Formula 3†; ***Braz.:*** Eviprostat†; ***Fr.:*** Cicaderma†; Hepatoum; Histo-Fluine P; ***Ger.:*** Eviprostat N; ***Hong Kong:*** Eviprostat†; ***Jpn:*** Eviprostat; ***Singapore:*** Eviprostat; ***Switz.:*** Eviprostat†; ***UK:*** Anased; Daily Menopause Relief; Nytol Herbal; Period Pain Relief; Prementaid.

## Pumilio Pine Oil

Dwarf Pine Needle Oil; Essence de Pin de Montagne; Latschenöl; Oleum Pini Pumilionis; Olio di Mugo; Pino mugo, aceite esencial de.
*CAS — 8016-46-4.*

**Pharmacopoeias.** In *Swiss.*

### Profile

Pumilio pine oil is a volatile oil obtained by distillation from the fresh leaves of *Pinus mugo* var. *pumilio* (Pinaceae). It has been inhaled with steam, sometimes with other essential oils, to relieve cough and nasal congestion and has been applied externally as a rubefacient. It has also been used as a perfume.

### Preparations

**Proprietary Preparations** (details are given in Part 3)

**Multi-ingredient:** ***Austral.:*** Biosal; Goanna Heat Cream†; Goanna Liniment†; Goanna Salve†; Karvol†; Menalation†; Vicks Inhaler†; ***Austria:*** Allgauer; Anifer Hustenbalsam; Anifer Krauterol; Apotheker Bauer's Inhalationsmischung; Babix; Berggeist; Bronchostop; Colda; Emser Nasensalbe; Erkaltungsbad; Erkaltungsbalsam; Expectal-Balsam; Jopinol; Leukona-Rheuma-Bad; Luuf Balsam; Luuf-Erkaltungsol; Mentopin; Nasanal; Opino; Piniment; Resol†; Tetesept†; ***Belg.:*** Eucalytux; ***Canad.:*** Vap Air; ***Ger.:*** Aerosol Spitzner N; Cefarheumin N†; Dolo-cyl; Em-eukal; Emser Erkaltungsgel†; Emser Nasensalbe N; Euflux-N; Franzbranntwein; Hevertopect N; Hustagil Inhalationsol†; Inspirol Mundwasser konzentrat†; Ipalat†; Klosterfrau Franzbranntwein Latschenkiefer; Kneipp Erkaltungs-Balsam N†; Kneipp Krauter Hustensaft N Kneipp Tannolsaft†; Nasentropfen-ratiopharm; Neo-Lapitrypsin†; Nervfluid S†; Night-Care†; Pinimenthol Oral N†; Pumilen-N†; Retterspitz Aerosol†; Retterspitz Heilsalbe†; Rosarthron; Schupps Latschenkiefer Olbad†; Thrombocid; ***Irl.:*** Karvol; ***Israel:*** Karvol; Mentholatum Balm; ***Ital.:*** Antipulmina; Broncosedina; Pinedrin; Pumilene Vapo; ***Malaysia:*** Purporent; ***NZ:*** Vicks Inhaler; ***Port.:*** Thrombocid; ***Switz.:*** Baby Liberol†; Eau-de-vie de France avec huile de pin nain du Tirol; Liberol Baby N; Liberol Bain; Liberol N; Liberol†; Makatussin†; Pinimenthol; Thrombocid; ***UK:*** Allens Pine & Honey; Boots Vapour Rub†; Catarrh Pastilles†; Karvol; Mentholatum Rub; Nasal Inhaler†; Original Cabdrivers Expectorant; Potter's Catarrh Pastilles.

## Punarnava

Punarnaba.

### Profile

Punarnava is the fresh or dried plant *Boerhaavia diffusa* (*B. repens*) (Nyctaginaceae), containing an alkaloid, punarnavine. It has been used in India as a diuretic and for liver disorders, usually in the form of a liquid extract.

## Pyricarbate *(rINN)*

Piricarbato; Pyridinolcarbamate. 2,6-Pyridinediyldimethylene bis(methylcarbamate).
$C_{11}H_{15}N_3O_4$ = 253.3.
*CAS — 1882-26-4.*

### Profile

Pyricarbate has been given by mouth in the treatment of atherosclerosis and other vascular disorders, hyperlipidaemias, and thromboembolic disorders. Adverse effects have included gastrointestinal disturbances and liver damage.

### Preparations

**Proprietary Preparations** (details are given in Part 3)
***Hong Kong:*** Anginin†; ***Ital.:*** Cicloven; ***Port.:*** Anginin; ***Spain:*** Colesterinex†; Esteribol†; ***Thai.:*** Anginin†.

**Multi-ingredient:** ***Braz.:*** Davistar†.

## Pyritinol Hydrochloride *(BANM, rINNM)*

Hidrocloruro de piritinol; Pyrithioxine Hydrochloride. 5,5-Dihydroxy-6,6-dimethyl-3,3-dithiodimethylenebis(4-pyridylmethanol) dihydochloride monohydrate.
$C_{16}H_{20}N_2O_4S_2,2HCl,H_2O$ = 459.4.
*CAS — 1098-97-1 (pyritinol); 10049-83-9 (anhydrous pyritinol hydrochloride).*
*ATC — N06BX02.*

**Pharmacopoeias.** In *Chin.* and *Pol.*

### Profile

Pyritinol hydrochloride has been described as a nootropic that promotes the uptake of glucose by the brain. It has been used in the treatment of various cerebrovascular and mental function disorders. It has been given by mouth in a usual dose of 600 mg daily. Pyritinol hydrochloride has also been given as an alternative to penicillamine in rheumatoid arthritis.

◊ References.


1. Knezevic S, *et al.* Pyritinol treatment of SDAT patients: evaluation by psychiatric and neurological examination, psychometric testing and rCBF measurements. *Int Clin Psychopharmacol* 1989; **4:** 25–38.
2. Lemmel EM. Comparison of pyritinol and auranofin in the treatment of rheumatoid arthritis. *Br J Rheumatol* 1993; **32:** 375–82.
3. Straumann A, *et al.* Acute pancreatitis due to pyritinol: an immune-mediated phenomenon. *Gastroenterology* 1998; **115:** 452–4.
4. Maria V, *et al.* Severe cholestatic hepatitis induced by pyritinol. *BMJ* 2004; **328:** 572–4.


### Preparations

**Proprietary Preparations** (details are given in Part 3)
***Arg.:*** Epocan; ***Austria:*** Encephabol; ***Braz.:*** Encefabol†; ***Chile:*** Encefabol; ***Fr.:*** Encephabol†; ***Ger.:*** Ardeyceryl P; Encephabol; ***Hong Kong:*** Encephabol; ***India:*** Encephabol; ***Ital.:*** Encefabol†; ***Malaysia:*** Encephabol; Pyritil; ***Mex.:*** Bonifen; Encephabol; ***Port.:*** Bonifen; Cerbon; ***S.Afr.:*** Encephabol; ***Singapore:*** Encephabol; ***Thai.:*** Encephabol; Memonol; Pyritil.

**Multi-ingredient:** ***Arg.:*** Gabimex Plus; ***Spain:*** Memorino†; Refulgin†; Viadetres.

## Quassia

Bitter Wood; Cuasia; Leño de Cuasia; Quassia Wood; Quassiae Lignum; Quassiaholz.
*CAS — 76-78-8 (quassin); 76-77-7 (neoquassin).*
*ATC — P03AX04.*

**Pharmacopoeias.** In *Jpn.*

### Profile

Quassia is the dried stem wood of Jamaica quassia, *Picrasma excelsa* (*Aeschrion excelsa; Picraena excelsa*) (Simaroubaceae), or of Surinam quassia, *Quassia amara* (Simaroubaceae). It has been used as a bitter. It was formerly given as an enema for the expulsion of threadworms and was applied for pediculosis. It may also be used as a flavour in food, drinks, and confectionery. Extracts of quassia or preparations containing its triterpenoid bitter principle quassin are used to denature alcohol.

### Preparations

**Proprietary Preparations** (details are given in Part 3)

**Multi-ingredient:** ***Braz.:*** Camomila†; Fargestium†; ***Fr.:*** Quintonine; Spevin†; ***Ital.:*** Cura†; Dekar 2; ***Switz.:*** Stomacine; ***UK:*** Sanderson's Throat Specific.

## Quinine and Urea Hydrochloride

Carbamidated Quinine Dihydrochloride; Chininum Dihydrochloricum Carbamidatum; Quinina y urea, hidrocloruro de; Urea-Quinine.
$C_{20}H_{24}N_2O_2,CH_4N_2O,2HCl,5H_2O$ = 547.5.
*CAS — 549-52-0 (anhydrous quinine and urea hydrochloride).*

### Profile

Quinine and urea hydrochloride has been used for the treatment of haemorrhoidal bleeding and anal fissure. It was formerly used as a local anaesthetic and for the therapeutic actions of quinine.

### Preparations

**Proprietary Preparations** (details are given in Part 3)
***Fr.:*** Kinurea H.

## Quinine Ascorbate *(USAN)*

Ascorbato de quinina; Quinine Biascorbate.
$C_{20}H_{24}N_2O_2,2C_6H_8O_6$ = 676.7.
*CAS — 146-40-7.*

### Profile

Quinine ascorbate is a compound (2 : 1) of ascorbic acid with quinine. It has been used as an ingredient of preparations promoted as smoking deterrents.

### Preparations

**Proprietary Preparations** (details are given in Part 3)
**Multi-ingredient:** ***Ital.:*** Nicoprive†.

## Rape Oil

Colza, aceite de; Colza Oil; Oleum Rapae; Rapeseed Oil.

**Pharmacopoeias.** In *Eur.* (see p.vi) and *Jpn.*

**Ph. Eur. 5.0** (Rapeseed Oil, Refined). The fatty oil obtained from the seeds of *Brassica napus* and *Brassica campestris* by mechanical expression or extraction and then refined. A suitable antoxidant may be added. It contains not more than 2% of erucic acid. A clear light yellow liquid. Practically insoluble in water and in alcohol; miscible with petroleum spirit. Store in well-filled airtight containers. Protect from light.

### Profile

Rape oil has been used in liniments in place of olive oil. It is used in some countries as an edible oil but the erucic acid ($C_{22}H_{42}O_2$ = 338.6) content of the oil has been implicated in muscle damage. The erucic acid content of oils and fats intended for human consumption and of foodstuffs containing oil or fat is subject to legal control. Contaminated rape oil was the cause of the toxic oil syndrome that affected thousands of Spanish citizens in early 1981. Rape oil is also used in industrial manufacturing.

There has been some debate whether the frequency of allergic respiratory symptoms in sensitive individuals is increased in areas in which oilseed rape is cultivated.

## Raspberry Leaf

Frambuesa, hoja de; Rubi Idaei Folium.

### Profile

Raspberry leaf consists of the dried leaflets of *Rubus idaeus* (Rosaceae). It contains a principle, readily extracted with hot water, which relaxes the smooth muscle of the uterus and intestine of some *animals.*

Raspberry 'tea' has been a traditional remedy for painful and profuse menstruation and for use before and during labour. The infusion has also been used as an astringent gargle.

◊ References.


1. Simpson M, *et al.* Raspberry leaf in pregnancy: its safety and efficacy in labor. *J Midwifery Womens Health* 2001; **46:** 51–9.


### Preparations

**Proprietary Preparations** (details are given in Part 3)

**Multi-ingredient:** ***Austral.:*** Rubus Complex†; ***Austria:*** Bio-Garten Tee gegen Durchfall; Bioreform-Tee gegen Durchfall; ***Belg.:*** Eugiron†; ***Ger.:*** Salus Bronchial-Tee Nr.8†; ***UK:*** Gerard House Helonias Compound†.

## Red Clover

Cow Clover; Meadow Clover; Purple Clover; Trébol rojo; Trefoil.

**Pharmacopoeias.** In *USNF*, which also includes the powdered form and powdered extract.

**USNF 22** (Red Clover). The dried inflorescence of *Trifolium pratense* (Fabaceae). It contains not less than 0.5% of isoflavones, calculated on the dried basis as the sum of daidzein, genistein (p.1692), formononetin, and biochanin A. Protect from light and moisture.

### Profile

The flowerheads of red clover have been used in herbal medicine. The isoflavones present in red clover have been investigated, similarly to other phytoestrogens, for their potential endocrine effects.

### Preparations

***USNF 22:*** Red Clover Tablets.

**Proprietary Preparations** (details are given in Part 3)
***Austral.:*** Promensil; ***Braz.:*** Climadil; ***UK:*** Menoflavon.

**Multi-ingredient:** ***Austral.:*** Bioglan Mens Super Soy/Clover†; Bioglan Soy Power Plus†; Lifechange Menopause Formula†; Trifolium Complex†.

## Relaxin

Relaxina.
*CAS — 9002-69-1.*

### Profile

Relaxin is a polypeptide hormone that has been extracted from the corpus luteum of the ovaries of pregnant sows, although a human recombinant form is also now available. It is reported to be related structurally to insulin and has a molecular weight of about 6000.

Relaxin is secreted by the human corpus luteum during pregnancy and is thought to interact with other reproductive hormones. It acts on connective tissue, including collagen, and causes relaxation of the pubic symphysis and softening of the uterine cervix. In many *animal* species relaxin appears to play a major part in cervical ripening before parturition; significant species difference is shown. It has been studied for cervical ripening in humans. Recombinant human relaxin has also been investigated in infertility, cardiovascular disorders, and scleroderma (p.1348).

◊ References.

1. Seibold JR, *et al.* Safety and pharmacokinetics of recombinant human relaxin in systemic sclerosis. *J Rheumatol* 1998; **25:** 302–7.
2. Seibold JR, *et al.* Recombinant human relaxin in the treatment of scleroderma: a randomized, double-blind, placebo-controlled trial. *Ann Intern Med* 2000; **132:** 871–9.
3. Kelly AJ, *et al.* Relaxin for cervical ripening and induction of labour. Available in The Cochrane Library; Issue 2. John Wiley: Chichester; 2004.

## Rhamnose

Ramnosa; L-Rhamnose. 6-Deoxy-L-mannose.

$C_6H_{12}O_5$ = 164.2.

*CAS — 3615-41-6.*

### Profile

Rhamnose is a monosaccharide used to assess intestinal permeability.

For reference to the use of rhamnose in the differential sugar absorption test, see Lactulose, p.1269.

◊ References.

1. van Nieuwenhoven MA, *et al.* The sensitivity of the lactulose/rhamnose gut permeability test. *Eur J Clin Invest* 1999; **29:** 160–5.
2. Haase AM, *et al.* Dual sugar permeability testing in diarrheal disease. *J Pediatr* 2000; **136:** 232–7.
3. van Nieuwenhoven MA, *et al.* Effects of pre- and post-absorptive factors on the lactulose/rhamnose gut permeability test. *Clin Sci* 2000; **98:** 349–53.

## Rhatany Root

Krameria; Krameria Root; Ratanhiae Radix; Ratania, raíz de.

**Pharmacopoeias.** In *Eur.* (see p.vi).

**Ph. Eur. 5.0** (Rhatany Root). The dried, usually fragmented, underground organs of *Krameria triandra*. It contains not less than 5% of tannins, expressed as pyrogallol, calculated with reference to the dried drug. It is known as Peruvian rhatany. Protect from light.

### Profile

Rhatany root has astringent properties and is used in herbal and homoeopathic preparations for a variety of disorders, including oropharyngeal inflammation.

### Preparations

***Ph. Eur.:*** Rhatany Tincture.

**Proprietary Preparations** (details are given in Part 3)
***Austria:*** ratioSept; ***Ger.:*** ratioSept; Salvibest†.

**Multi-ingredient:** ***Arg.:*** Esculeol P; ***Austria:*** Curol; Parodontax; ***Braz.:*** Parodontax†; ***Chile:*** Hemorrol; ***Ger.:*** Repha-Os; ***Israel:*** Parodontax; ***Ital.:*** Gengivario; ***Spain:*** Encialina; ***Switz.:*** Eubucal.

## Rhus

Sumach Berries; Zumaque.

### Profile

Rhus consists of the dried fruits of the smooth or Pennsylvanian sumach, *Rhus glabra* (Anacardiaceae). It has astringent and reputed diuretic properties. *R. aromatica* has been used similarly to *R. glabra*.

Poison ivy (*R. radicans*) and poison oak (*R. toxicodendron*), species growing in the USA, contain irritant poisons, such as urushiol, that produce severe contact dermatitis. Extracts of poison ivy and poison oak have been used for the prophylaxis of poison ivy dermatitis but their effectiveness has not been proved.

Some *Rhus* spp. are used in homoeopathic medicine. The spice sumac is prepared from the berries of *R. coriaria*.

### Preparations

**Proprietary Preparations** (details are given in Part 3)
**Multi-ingredient:** ***Chile:*** Rhus Opodeldoc; ***Ger.:*** Cysto Fink†; Hicoton; Rhus-Rheuma-Gel N; ***Switz.:*** Cysto-Caps Chassot†.

## Ribonuclease

Ribonucleasa; RNase.

*CAS — 9001-99-4.*

### Profile

Ribonuclease is an enzyme present in most mammalian tissue, and it is involved in the catalytic cleavage of ribonucleic acid. It has been applied, alone or with other drugs, for its supposed anti-inflammatory properties.

### Preparations

**Proprietary Preparations** (details are given in Part 3)
***Mex.:*** Cro 50†.

**Multi-ingredient:** ***Braz.:*** Bromelin; Expectoral; ***Fr.:*** Ribatran; ***Mex.:*** Ridasa.

## Ribonucleic Acid

ARN; Plant Nucleic Acid; Ribonucleico, ácido; Ribose Nucleic Acid; RNA; Yeast Nucleic Acid.

### Profile

Ribonucleic acid is a nucleotide polymer, and 1 of the 2 distinct varieties of nucleic acid (see p.1722). It is found in the cytoplasm and in small amounts in the cell nuclei of living tissues and is directly involved in protein synthesis. Therapeutically, it has been tried in the treatment of mental retardation and to improve memory in senile dementia, and proprietary preparations containing various salts of ribonucleic acid have been advocated for a variety of asthenic and convalescent conditions. Ribonucleic acid may have a role in enteral feeds under some circumstances. Gene suppression by RNA interference, using specific double-stranded ribonucleic acid sequences, is under investigation.

Immune RNA (extracted from the spleens and lymph nodes of immunised animals) has been tried in the immunotherapy of hepatitis and cancer.

### Preparations

**Proprietary Preparations** (details are given in Part 3)
***Ger.:*** AU 4 Regeneresen; Osteochondrin S; Regeneresen; RN13 Regeneresen.

**Multi-ingredient:** ***Fr.:*** Nutrigene†; ***India:*** Placentrex; ***Spain:*** Dertrase; Nucleserina; Policolinosil.

## Ribwort Plantain

Plantaginis Lanceolatae; Plantain Herb; Spitzwegerich; Spitzwegerichkraut.

**Pharmacopoeias.** *Eur.* (see p.vi) and *Pol.* include the leaf.

**Ph. Eur. 5.0** (Ribwort Plantain; Plantaginis Lanceolatae Folium). The whole or fragmented, dried leaf and scape of *Plantago lanceolata*. It contains not less than 1.5% of total *ortho*-dihydroxycinnamic acid derivatives expressed as acteoside ($C_{29}H_{36}O_{15}$ = 624.6) with reference to the dried drug. Protect from light.

### Profile

Ribwort plantain is an ingredient in herbal remedies used for catarrh and inflammation of the upper respiratory tract.

### Preparations

**Proprietary Preparations** (details are given in Part 3)
***Austria:*** Tetesept; ***Ger.:*** Broncho-Sern; Harzer Hustenelixier†; Kneipp Hustensaft Spitzwegerich†; Kneipp Spitzwegerich-Pflanzensaft Hustentrost†; Proguval.

**Multi-ingredient:** ***Austria:*** Aktiv Husten- und Bronchialtee; Anifer Hustentee; Anitos; Aponatura Hustenstillende; Aurita-Bronchialtee; Bio-Garten Tee gegen Erkaltung; Bio-Garten Tropfen gegen Husten; Bioreform-Erkaltungstee; Breston; Brust- und Hustentee EF-EM-ES; Egmovit; Erkaltungstee; Gewusst wie Husten-Bronchialtee; Grippetee EF-EM-ES; Hustensaft-Dr Schmidgall†; Jutussin neo; Kneipp Grippe-Tee; Kneipp Husten- und Bronchial-Tee; Krauterhaus Mag Kottas Grippetee; Krauterhaus Mag Kottas Husten- und Bronchialtee; Luuf-Halspastillen; Mag Kottas Grippe-Tee; Mag Kottas Husten-Bronchialtee; Mag Kottas Krauterexpress-Grippe-Tee; Mag Kottas Krauterexpress-Husten-Bronchialtee; Neuners Krautertee Nr 11 - zur Unterstutzung der Tatigkeit der Bronchien und Atemwege; Neuners Krautertee Nr 124 - zur Entspannung vor der Geburt; Neuners Krautertee Nr 7 - Bronchial- und Lungentee; Pneumopan; Scottopect; Sidroga Brust-Husten-Tee; St Radegunder Hustentee; St Radegunder Thorasan-Krauterhustensaft; Tussimont; ***Ger.:*** Bronchicum Elixir Plus; Brust- und Husten-Tee Stada N†; Equisil N; Eucabal; Kneipp Husten- und Bronchial-Tee†; Pulmonium N†; ***Hong Kong:*** Pectoral; ***Ital.:*** Altea (Specie Composta); Timo (Specie Composta); ***Spain:*** Llantusil; Natusor Farinol; Natusor Gastrolen; Natusor Infenol; ***Switz.:*** Bronchofluid N; Bronchofluid†; Demo pates pectorales†; Gouttes contre la toux "S"; Neo-DP; Nican; Thymodrosin N; Thymodrosin†; Tisane pectorale et antitussive.

## Ricin

Ricino.

*CAS — 9009-86-3.*

NOTE. The title ricin is used for the castor seed in *Chin.* and *Fr.*

### Profile

Ricin is a lectin present in castor seeds, the seeds of *Ricinus communis* (Euphorbiaceae). It is extremely toxic when given parenterally and the fatal dose by injection has been reported to be around 1 microgram/kg. The toxicity of orally ingested beans depends on how thoroughly they are chewed since the hard seed coat prevents absorption. Ingestion of as few as 3 castor seeds by a child and 4 by an adult may be fatal. Ricin may also be absorbed through abraded skin. It has potential use in aerosol form as an agent of chemical warfare. Toxic effects may be delayed for several days following exposure by any route. Early symptoms include severe gastrointestinal irritation, haemorrhage, vomiting, and diarrhoea, which may result in circulatory collapse. Abnormal liver function tests and pulmonary oedema have been reported. Ophthalmological disturbances ranging from irritation and conjunctivitis to optic nerve damage may occur; miosis and mydriasis have also been reported. Proteinuria, haematuria, and renal impairment may develop and serum creatinine levels may be raised. In severe cases haemolysis of the red blood cells with subsequent acute renal failure may occur. Fatalities due to multi-organ failure have occurred. If the patient presents within 1 hour of ingestion any seeds may be removed by gastric lavage and activated charcoal given. Treatment thereafter is symptomatic.

After expression of the oil from castor seeds (see p.1668), the ricin remaining in the seed cake or 'pomace' is destroyed by steam treatment. The detoxified pomace is used as a fertiliser.

Ricin conjugated with monoclonal or polyclonal antibodies is being studied in the treatment of cancers; zolimomab aritox is an example of such a conjugate. Some of these conjugates have been investigated for various malignancies, particularly leukaemias and lymphomas.

**Toxicity.** A report of ricin toxicity following partial chewing and ingestion of 10 to 15 castor oil seeds.[1] Reviews[2,3] of ricin toxicity, including its potential as an agent of chemical warfare.

1. Aplin PJ, Eliseo T. Ingestion of castor oil plant seeds. *Med J Aust* 1997; **167:** 260–1.
2. Bradberry SM, *et al.* Ricin poisoning. *Toxicol Rev* 2003; **22:** 65–70.
3. Lord MJ, *et al.* Ricin: mechanisms of cytotoxicity. *Toxicol Rev* 2003; **22:** 53–64.

**Uses.** References to the use of ricin conjugates with monoclonal antibodies in the treatment of cancer.

1. Byers VS, *et al.* Phase I study of monoclonal antibody-ricin A chain immunotoxin XomaZyme-791 in patients with metastatic colon cancer. *Cancer Res* 1989; **49:** 6153–60.
2. Oratz R, *et al.* Antimelanoma monoclonal antibody-ricin A chain immunoconjugate (XMMME-001-RTA) plus cyclophosphamide in the treatment of metastatic malignant melanoma: results of a phase II trial. *J Biol Response Mod* 1990; **9:** 345–54.
3. Anonymous. Application considered for immunotoxin in treatment of graft-vs-host disease. *JAMA* 1991; **265:** 2041–2.
4. Amlot PL, *et al.* A phase I study of an anti-CD22-deglycosylated ricin A chain immunotoxin in the treatment of B-cell lymphomas resistant to conventional therapy. *Blood* 1993; **82:** 2624–33.
5. Senderowicz AM, *et al.* Complete sustained response of a refractory, post-transplantation, large B-cell lymphoma to an anti-CD22 immunotoxin. *Ann Intern Med* 1997; **126:** 882–5.
6. Multani PS, *et al.* Phase II clinical trial of bolus infusion anti-B4 blocked ricin immunoconjugate in patients with relapsed B-cell non-Hodgkin's lymphoma. *Clin Cancer Res* 1998; **4:** 2599–2604.

## Ricinoleic Acid

Ricinoleico, ácido.

*CAS — 141-22-0.*

### Profile

Ricinoleic acid is a mixture of fatty acids obtained by the hydrolysis of castor oil. It is an ingredient of some proprietary vaginal jellies used to maintain or restore normal vaginal acidity.

### Preparations

**Proprietary Preparations** (details are given in Part 3)
**Multi-ingredient:** ***Austral.:*** Aci-Jel; ***Israel:*** Glovan; ***NZ:*** Aci-Jel; ***USA:*** Aci-Jel†.

## Riluzole *(BAN, USAN, rINN)*

PK-26124; Riluzol; RP-54274. 2-Amino-6-(trifluoromethoxy)benzothiazole; 6-Trifluoromethoxy-1,3-benzothiazol-2-ylamine.

$C_8H_5F_3N_2OS$ = 234.2.

*CAS — 1744-22-5.*

*ATC — N07XX02.*

### Adverse Effects and Treatment

Adverse effects associated most commonly with riluzole are asthenia, nausea, elevations in liver enzyme values, headache, and abdominal pain. Other gastrointestinal effects may include diarrhoea or constipation, anorexia, and vomiting. There may be tachycardia, dizziness, vertigo, or somnolence. Circumoral paraesthesia has been reported and decreased lung function and rhinitis may occur. Anaphylactoid reactions, angioedema, pancreatitis, and neutropenia have all been reported rarely.

**Effects on the blood.** See under Overdosage, below.

**Effects on the kidneys.** A 44-year-old patient developed renal tubular impairment 3 months after starting riluzole treatment for amyotrophic lateral sclerosis.[1] Tubular function recovered 1 month after discontinuation of riluzole.

1. Poloni TE, *et al.* Renal tubular impairment during riluzole therapy. *Neurology* 1999; **52:** 670.

**Effects on the liver.** Icteric toxic hepatitis, with jaundice and elevated liver enzyme values, has been reported[1] in an elderly woman receiving riluzole for amyotrophic lateral sclerosis (ALS). Acute hepatitis developed in 2 patients several weeks after starting therapy with riluzole for ALS.[2] Liver histology showed hepatocellular damage with inflammatory infiltration and microvesicular steatosis without fibrosis. Hepatotoxicity was reversed in all these cases when riluzole was stopped.

1. Castells LI, *et al.* Icteric toxic hepatitis associated with riluzole. *Lancet* 1998; **351:** 648.
2. Remy A-J, *et al.* Acute hepatitis after riluzole administration. *J Hepatol* 1999; **30:** 527–30.

**Effects on the pancreas.** Riluzole was cited[1] as the most likely cause of severe pancreatitis that developed in a 77-year-old woman 6 months after starting therapy for sporadic amyotrophic lateral sclerosis; pancreatic symptoms improved when riluzole was stopped.

1. Drory VE, *et al.* Riluzole-induced pancreatitis. *Neurology* 1999; **52:** 892–3.

**Overdosage.** Severe neutropenia developed in a 63-year-old woman receiving riluzole for amyotrophic lateral sclerosis

10 days after inadvertent dose increase to 200 mg daily (twice the standard recommended dose).[1]

Methaemoglobinaemia has been reported[2] in a 43-year-old patient with amyotrophic lateral sclerosis following intentional overdose with 2.8 g of riluzole. The patient was treated with gastric lavage followed by activated charcoal; intravenous methylthioninium chloride successfully reversed the methaemoglobinaemia. However, the patient died of respiratory failure related to her underlying disease 7 days after the overdose.

1. North WA, *et al.* Reversible granulocytopenia in association with riluzole therapy. *Ann Pharmacother* 2000; **34:** 322–4.
2. Viallon A, *et al.* Methemoglobinemia due to riluzole. *N Engl J Med* 2000; **343:** 665–6.

## Precautions

Riluzole is contra-indicated in patients with hepatic disease or markedly raised liver enzyme values. Liver function tests should be performed before and throughout treatment with riluzole. In the UK, riluzole is not recommended in patients with renal impairment although the US manufacturer states that the pharmacokinetics are not significantly different in renal impairment. Extreme caution should be exercised in those with a history of liver disorders. Patients or their carers should be told how to recognise signs of neutropenia and should be advised to seek immediate medical attention if symptoms such as fever develop; white blood cell counts should be determined in febrile illness and riluzole stopped if neutropenia occurs. Riluzole may cause dizziness or vertigo and patients should be warned not to drive or operate machinery if these symptoms occur.

Riluzole has been reported to impair fertility in *animals*.

## Pharmacokinetics

Riluzole is rapidly absorbed from the gastrointestinal tract following oral administration with peak plasma concentrations occurring after 1 to 1½ hours. The rate and extent of absorption are decreased when riluzole is given with a high-fat meal. Riluzole is widely distributed throughout the body and is about 97% bound to plasma proteins. It crosses the blood-brain barrier. Riluzole is extensively metabolised to several metabolites in the liver, mainly by the cytochrome P450 isoenzyme CYP1A2, and subsequent glucuronidation. Riluzole is excreted mainly in the urine predominantly as glucuronides with an elimination half-life of about 12 hours. About 2% is excreted unchanged in the urine. Small amounts are excreted in faeces. There is some evidence that clearance of riluzole is reduced in Japanese patients.

◊ References.

1. Le Liboux A, *et al.* Single- and multiple-dose pharmacokinetics of riluzole in white subjects. *J Clin Pharmacol* 1997; **37:** 820–7.
2. Le Liboux A, *et al.* A comparison of the pharmacokinetics and tolerability of riluzole after repeat dose administration in healthy elderly and young volunteers. *J Clin Pharmacol* 1999; **39:** 480–6.

## Uses and Administration

Riluzole is a glutamate antagonist used in the management of amyotrophic lateral sclerosis, a form of motor neurone disease. Riluzole is indicated to slow progression of early disease but efficacy has not been demonstrated in its late stages. The precise mechanism of action is unknown but it may inhibit presynaptic glutamate release and interfere with its postsynaptic effects. The usual adult dose of riluzole is 50 mg twice daily by mouth on an empty stomach.

**Motor neurone disease.** Motor neurone disease (motoneuron disease) represents a group of fatal progressive degenerative disorders that affect upper and/or lower motor neurones in the brain and spinal cord. The most common form of motor neurone disease is amyotrophic lateral sclerosis (known in the USA as Lou Gehrig's disease), which involves both upper and lower motor neurones. It produces muscular atrophy and weakness and symptoms of progressive bulbar palsy such as slowness of movement and speech disturbances. Most patients die within 2 to 5 years of disease onset, usually from respiratory failure. There is no completely effective treatment and management remains largely supportive with appropriate symptomatic management of spasticity (p.1386), neuropathic pain (p.7), and sialorrhoea. Tricyclic antidepressants are widely used for their multiple beneficial effects. Occupational and speech therapy also play a crucial role in maximising function. Pathological crying or laughing (pseudobulbar affect) may occur in as many as 50% of patients and has been treated with amitriptyline or fluvoxamine. Dysphagia may eventually compromise food and fluid intake necessitating enteral nutrition as an alternative or supplemental route for oral nutrition. Respiratory support will ultimately be necessary, initially with non-invasive ventilation but progressing eventually to tracheostomy.

Although the pathogenesis of motor neurone disease is still uncertain, it is thought that accumulation of the excitatory neurotransmitter glutamate in the CNS may be involved. Clinical studies have shown riluzole, a glutamate antagonist, to be modestly effective in prolonging survival and delaying the time to use of tracheostomy. However, there is still insufficient data to be able to assess which patients would derive greatest benefit. Additionally, questions have been raised about the clinical usefulness of riluzole in terms of cost-benefit, and there are concerns about adverse effects, notably hepatotoxicity.

Also under study for the treatment of motor neurone disease are somatomedins, in particular mecasermin (insulin-like growth factor I). Neurotrophic factors have been investigated including brain-derived neurotrophic factor (BDNF) and recombinant ciliary neurotrophic factor (CNTF), but results have been generally inconclusive. Glial-cell-derived neurotrophic factor (GDNF) is also under investigation. There has also been some interest in the antiepileptic drug gabapentin, which may inhibit glutamate formation in the CNS from branched-chain amino acids. Lamotrigine and topiramate have also been tried but with disappointing results. Dextromethorphan has also been studied in amyotrophic lateral sclerosis. Immunoglobulins have been tried in some forms of motor neurone disease such as multifocal motor neuropathy.

A small percentage of patients with familial amyotrophic lateral sclerosis have been shown to have a mutation in the gene encoding for the enzyme copper-zinc superoxide dismutase but there has been no consensus as to whether patients with this mutation should be given superoxide dismutase supplements.

References.

1. Bryson HM, *et al.* Riluzole: a review of its pharmacodynamic and pharmacokinetic properties and therapeutic potential in amyotrophic lateral sclerosis. *Drugs* 1996; **52:** 549–63.
2. Wagner ML, Landis BE. Riluzole: a new agent for amyotrophic lateral sclerosis. *Ann Pharmacother* 1997; **31:** 738–44.
3. Anonymous. Riluzole for amyotrophic lateral sclerosis. *Drug Ther Bull* 1997; **35:** 11–12.
4. Quality Standards Subcommittee of the American Academy of Neurology. Practice advisory on the treatment of amyotrophic lateral sclerosis with riluzole: report of the Quality Standards Subcommittee of the American Academy of Neurology. *Neurology* 1997; **49:** 657–9.
5. Walling AD. Amyotrophic lateral sclerosis: Lou Gehrig's disease. *Am Fam Physician* 1999; **59:** 1489–96.
6. Mackin GA. Optimizing care of patients with ALS: steps to early detection and improved quality of life. *Postgrad Med* 1999; **105:** 143–56.
7. Parton MJ, *et al.* Motor neuron disease and its management. *J R Coll Physicians Lond* 1999; **33:** 212–8.
8. Miller RG, *et al.* Practice parameter: the care of the patient with amyotrophic lateral sclerosis (an evidence-based review): report of the Quality Standards Subcommittee of the American Academy of Neurology. *Neurology* 1999; **52:** 1311–23.
9. Shaw PJ. Motor neurone disease. *BMJ* 1999; **318:** 1118–21.
10. Ludolph AC, Riepe MW. Do the benefits of currently available treatments justify early diagnosis and treatment of amyotrophic lateral sclerosis? — Arguments against. *Neurology* 1999; **53** (suppl 5): S46–S49.
11. Cashman NR. Do the benefits of currently available treatments justify early diagnosis and announcement? — Arguments for. *Neurology* 1999; **53** (suppl 5): S50–S52.
12. Miller RG, *et al.* Riluzole for amyotrophic lateral sclerosis (ALS)/motor neuron disease (MND). Available in The Cochrane Library; Issue 2. Chichester: John Wiley; 2004.
13. Rowland LP, Shneider NA. Amyotrophic lateral sclerosis. *N Engl J Med* 2001; **344:** 1688–1700.
14. Dib M. Amyotrophic lateral sclerosis: progress and prospects for treatment. *Drugs* 2003; **63:** 289–310.
15. Mitchell JD, *et al.* Recombinant human insulin-like growth factor I (rhIGF-I) for amyotrophic lateral sclerosis/motor neuron disease. Available in The Cochrane Library; Issue 2. Chichester: John Wiley; 2004.

**Movement disorders.** Beneficial results have been obtained with riluzole in small studies of patients with Huntington's chorea[1,2] and levodopa-induced dyskinesias in advanced Parkinson's disease.[3] Riluzole has also been tried in a small number of patients with early Parkinson's disease but no evidence of benefit was observed.[4]

1. Rosas HD, *et al.* Riluzole therapy in Huntington's disease (HD). *Mov Disord* 1999; **14:** 326–30.
2. Huntington Study Group. Dosage effects of riluzole in Huntington's disease: a multicenter placebo-controlled study. *Neurology* 2003; **61:** 1551–6.
3. Merims D, *et al.* Riluzole for levodopa-induced dyskinesias in advanced Parkinson's disease. *Lancet* 1999; **353:** 1764–5.
4. Jankovic J, Hunter C. A double-blind, placebo-controlled and longitudinal study of riluzole in early Parkinson's disease. *Parkinsonism Relat Disord* 2002; **8:** 271–6.

## Preparations

**Proprietary Preparations** (details are given in Part 3)

***Arg.:*** Rilutek; ***Austral.:*** Rilutek; ***Austria:*** Rilutek; ***Belg.:*** Rilutek; ***Braz.:*** Rilutek; ***Canad.:*** Rilutek; ***Denm.:*** Rilutek; ***Fin.:*** Rilutek; ***Fr.:*** Rilutek; ***Ger.:*** Rilutek; ***Gr.:*** Rilutek; ***Hong Kong:*** Rilutek; ***Irl.:*** Rilutek; ***Israel:*** Rilutek; ***Ital.:*** Rilutek; ***Jpn:*** Rilutek; ***Mex.:*** Rilutek; ***Neth.:*** Rilutek; ***Norw.:*** Rilutek; ***Port.:*** Rilutek; ***S.Afr.:*** Rilutek; ***Singapore:*** Rilutek; ***Spain:*** Rilutek; ***Swed.:*** Rilutek; ***Switz.:*** Rilutek; ***Thai.:*** Rilutek; ***UK:*** Rilutek; ***USA:*** Rilutek.

---

# Ritodrine Hydrochloride *(BANM, USAN, rINNM)*

DU-21220 (ritodrine); Hidrocloruro de ritodrina. *erythro*-2-(4-Hydroxyphenethylamino)-1-(4-hydroxyphenyl)propan-1-ol hydrochloride.

$C_{17}H_{21}NO_3,HCl = 323.8.$

*CAS — 26652-09-5 (ritodrine); 23239-51-2 (ritodrine hydrochloride).*

*ATC — G02CA01.*

**Pharmacopoeias.** In *Br.* and *US.*

**BP 2003** (Ritodrine Hydrochloride). A white or almost white, crystalline powder. Freely soluble in water; soluble in dehydrated alcohol; practically insoluble in acetone and in ether. A 2% solution in water has a pH of 4.5 to 6.0. Store in airtight containers.

**USP 27** (Ritodrine Hydrochloride). A white to nearly white, odourless or practically odourless, crystalline powder. Freely soluble in water and in alcohol; practically insoluble in ether; soluble in propyl alcohol. pH of a 2% solution in water is between 4.5 and 6.0. Store in airtight containers at a temperature of 25°, excursions permitted between 15° and 30°.

## Adverse Effects and Precautions

As for Salbutamol Sulfate, p.791. Leucopenia or agranulocytosis has been reported occasionally with prolonged intravenous use.

In women given ritodrine for premature labour, the risk of pulmonary oedema means that extreme caution is required and the precautions and risk factors discussed under Salbutamol Sulfate, p.792, apply.

**Effects on the eyes.** Ritodrine and to a lesser extent salbutamol have been implicated in retinopathy in the premature infant when used for premature labour.[1]

1. Michie CA, *et al.* Do maternal β-sympathomimetics influence the development of retinopathy in the premature infant? *Arch Dis Child* 1994; **71:** F149.

**Effects on the heart.** Myocardial ischaemia or signs of myocardial ischaemia have been reported in patients given ritodrine.[1,2]

1. Brosset P, *et al.* Cardiac complications of ritodrine in mother and baby. *Lancet* 1982; **i:** 1468.
2. Ben-Shlomo I, *et al.* Myocardial ischaemia during intravenous ritodrine treatment: is it so rare? *Lancet* 1986; **ii:** 917–18.

**Pulmonary oedema.** Several cases of pulmonary oedema have been reported in patients given a $beta_2$ agonist, including ritodrine, for premature labour.[1-4] In 1995 the UK Committee on Safety of Medicines[4] (CSM) commented that it had received 10 reports of pulmonary oedema, fatal in 2 patients. The CSM considered that fluid overload was the most important predisposing factor. Other risk factors included multiple pregnancies, a history of cardiac disease, and maternal infection. For further discussion of the precautions necessary in the use of $beta_2$ agonists to treat premature labour, and the risk factors involved, see p.792.

1. Hawker F. Pulmonary oedema associated with $\beta_2$-sympathomimetic treatment of premature labour. *Anaesth Intensive Care* 1984; **12:** 143–51.
2. Pisani RJ, Rosenow EC. Pulmonary edema associated with tocolytic therapy. *Ann Intern Med* 1989; **110:** 714–18.
3. Clesham GJ, *et al.* β Adrenergic agonists and pulmonary oedema in preterm labour. *BMJ* 1994; **308:** 260–2.
4. Committee on Safety of Medicines/Medicines Control Agency. Reminder: ritodrine and pulmonary oedema. *Current Problems* 1995; **21:** 7.

## Interactions

As for Salbutamol Sulfate, p.792.

## Pharmacokinetics

Ritodrine is rapidly absorbed from the gastrointestinal tract but is subject to fairly extensive first-pass metabolism; about 30% of an oral dose is bioavailable. It is metabolised in the liver primarily by conjugation with glucuronic acid or sulfate and excreted in urine as unchanged drug and metabolites. About 70 to 90% of a dose is reported to be excreted in the urine within 10 to 12 hours. It crosses the placenta.

◊ References.

1. Gandar R, *et al.* Serum level of ritodrine in man. *Eur J Clin Pharmacol* 1980; **17:** 117–22.
2. Gross AS, Brown KF. Plasma protein binding of ritodrine at parturition and in nonpregnant women. *Eur J Clin Pharmacol* 1985; **28:** 479–81.
3. Pacifici GM, *et al.* Sulphation and glucuronidation of ritodrine in human foetal and adult tissues. *Eur J Clin Pharmacol* 1993; **44:** 259–64.
4. Pacifici GM, *et al.* Ritodrine sulphation in the human liver and duodenal mucosa: interindividual variability. *Eur J Drug Metab Pharmacokinet* 1998; **23:** 67–74.

## Uses and Administration

Ritodrine hydrochloride is a direct-acting sympathomimetic with predominantly beta-adrenergic activity and a selective action on $beta_2$ receptors (a $beta_2$ agonist). It has general properties similar to those of salbutamol (see p.793). It decreases uterine contractility and is used to arrest premature labour (p.794).

Ritodrine hydrochloride is usually given by intravenous infusion. Where possible this should be with the aid of a **syringe pump**, when the concentration should be 3 mg/mL, using glucose 5% as the diluent. A recommended initial rate of infusion is 50 micrograms/minute increased at intervals of 10 minutes by 50-microgram increments until there is evidence of patient response, which is usually at a rate of 150 to 350 micrograms/minute, the latter figure being the maximum recommended rate. If no syringe pump is available then the infusion may be made using a **controlled infusion device** to deliver a more dilute solution of 300 micrograms/mL, with glucose 5% being used once again as the diluent. The same dose is employed as with the syringe pump.

The maternal pulse should be monitored throughout the infusion and the rate adjusted to avoid a maternal heart rate of more than 140 beats per minute. A close watch should also be kept on the patient's state of hydration since fluid overload is considered to be a key risk factor for pulmonary oedema. The infusion should be continued for 12 to 48 hours after the contractions have stopped. Ritodrine hydrochloride may subsequently be given **by mouth** in an initial dose of 10 mg every 2 hours for 24 hours, starting 30 minutes before the end of the intravenous infusion. Thereafter, 10 to 20 mg may be given every 4 to 6 hours according to the patient's response. The total daily dose by mouth should not exceed 120 mg.

If intravenous infusion is inappropriate, 10 mg may be given **intramuscularly** every 3 to 8 hours and continued for 12 to 48 hours after the contractions have stopped.

### Preparations

**BP 2003:** Ritodrine Injection; Ritodrine Tablets;
**USP 27:** Ritodrine Hydrochloride Injection; Ritodrine Hydrochloride Tablets.

**Proprietary Preparations** (details are given in Part 3)
***Arg.:*** Ritopar; ***Austral.:*** Yutopar†; ***Belg.:*** Pre-Par†; ***Braz.:*** Miodrina; ***Canad.:*** Yutopar†; ***Chile:*** Materlac; ***Fr.:*** Pre-Par†; ***Ger.:*** Pre-Par†; ***Gr.:*** Yutopar; ***Hong Kong:*** Yutopar; ***India:*** Yutopar; ***Irl.:*** Yutopar†; ***Israel:*** Ritopar; ***Ital.:*** Miolene; Pre-Par†; ***Neth.:*** Pre-Par†; ***Port.:*** Pre-Par; ***Singapore:*** Yutopar†; ***Spain:*** Pre-Par; ***Thai.:*** Yutopar†; ***UK:*** Yutopar; ***USA:*** Yutopar†.

## Rociverine *(rINN)*

LG-30158; Rociverina. 2-Diethylamino-1-methylethyl *cis*-1-hydroxy(bicyclohexyl)-2-carboxylate.

$C_{20}H_{37}NO_3$ = 339.5.
*CAS — 53716-44-2.*
*ATC — A03AA06.*

### Profile

Rociverine is an antispasmodic that has been given by mouth in doses of 30 to 40 mg or rectally in doses of 50 to 75 mg daily. It has also been given by injection.

### Preparations

**Proprietary Preparations** (details are given in Part 3)
***Ital.:*** Rilaten.

## Rose Bengal Sodium

CI Acid Red 94; Colour Index No. 45440; Rosa de bengala sódico; Rose Bengal; Sodium Rose Bengal. The disodium salt of 4,5,6,7-tetrachloro-2′,4′,5′,7′-tetraiodofluorescein .

$C_{20}H_2Cl_4I_4Na_2O_5$ = 1017.6.
*CAS — 11121-48-5 (rose bengal); 632-69-9 (rose bengal disodium).*
*ATC — S01JA02.*

NOTE. The name Rose Bengale has been applied to the substance described in this monograph as well as to dichlorotetraiodofluorescein (CI Acid Red 93; Ext. D & C Reds Nos. 5 and 6; Colour Index No. 45435), a compound used as its disodium or dipotassium salt as a colouring agent.

ROS is a code approved by the BP 2003 for use on single unit doses of eye drops containing rose bengal sodium where the individual container may be too small to bear all the appropriate labelling information.

### Profile

Rose bengal sodium stains devitalised conjunctival and corneal epithelial cells as well as mucus and is used as an aid in the diagnosis of dry eye. It is used to detect or assess ocular damage resulting from Sjögren's syndrome or from ill-fitting contact lenses, and for keratitis, squamous cell carcinomas, and detection of foreign bodies. Rose bengal sodium is applied as 1% eye drops or as sterile papers impregnated with the dye.

Instillation of this dye may be painful, especially in dry eyes. Rose bengal sodium can stain exposed skin, clothing, and soft contact lenses.

Rose bengal sodium is taken up by the liver and excreted in the bile; the iodine-131-labelled compound (p.1524) has been used as a diagnostic aid in the determination of hepato-biliary function.

### Preparations

**Proprietary Preparations** (details are given in Part 3)
***Canad.:*** Ak-Rose; ***USA:*** Rosets.

## Rose Fruit

Brier Fruit; Cynosbati Fructus; Cynosbati Pseudofructus; Dog Rose Fruits; Églantier; Escaramujo; Hips; Hypanthium Rosae; Rosae Fructus; Rosae Pseudo-fructus; Rose Hips.

**Pharmacopoeias.** In *Eur.* (see p.vi) and *Jpn.*

**Ph. Eur. 5.0** (Dog Rose). The rose hips made up by the receptacle and the remains of the dried sepals of *Rosa canina*, *R. pendulina*, and other *Rosa* spp., with the achenes removed. It contains not less than 0.3% of ascorbic acid, calculated with reference to the dried drug. Protect from light.

### Profile

The fruits of various *Rosa* species, in particular the dog rose, *R. canina*, are used as a source of Vitamin C (p.1460). Rose fruit is included in herbal preparations for constipation and urinary-tract disorders.

### Preparations

**Proprietary Preparations** (details are given in Part 3)

**Multi-ingredient:** ***Arg.:*** Vitamina C-Complex; ***Austral.:*** Bio C†; Bioglan Mega C†; Bioglan Super Cal C†; C Supa + Bioflavonoids†; Flavons†; Glycyrrhiza Complex†; Plantiodine Plus†; Sustained Release Buffered C†; ***Austria:*** Amersan; Apotheker Ehrmanns Grippekapseln; Bio-Garten Entschlackungstee; Bio-Garten Tee zur Starkung und Kraftigung; Bioreform-Entschlackungstee; Gewusst wie Gruner Fastentee; Grippetee Dr Zeidler; Krauterdoktor Entschlackungs-Elixier; Krauterhaus Mag Kottas Grippetee; Krauterhaus Mag Kottas milder Abfuhrtee; Krauterhaus Mag Kottas Nierentee; Krauterpfarrer Weidinger Tee bei Nieren- und Blasenbeschwerden; Krauterpfarrer Weidinger Tee fur Leber und Galle; Krauterpfarrer Weidinger Tee zur Starkung der Abwehrkrafte; Mag Kottas Beruhigungstee; Mag Kottas Grippe-Tee; Mag Kottas Krauterexpress-Beruhigungstee; Mag Kottas Krauterexpress-Grippe-Tee; Neuners Krautertee Nr 207 - Krauterhexlein Kinder-Brusttee; Neuners Krautertee Nr 25 - Entschlackungstee; Neuners Krautertee Nr 4 - Nierentee; Sidroga Erkaltungstee; St Radegunder Entschlackungs-Elixier; ***Chile:*** Calcio 520; ***Ger.:*** Hevert-Entwasserungs-Tee†; Nephronorm med; Salus Abfuhr-Tee Nr. 2†; Urodil Blasen-Nieren Arzneitee†; ***Ital.:*** Fluend†; Golapiol C; Longevital; Sambuco (Specie Composta); ***Switz.:*** A Vogel Capsules polyvitaminees; Tisane contre les refroidissements; ***UK:*** Top C; ***USA:*** Amino-Opti-C; C Factors "1000" Plus; Ester-C Plus; Ester-C Plus Multi-Mineral.

## Rose Oil

Attar of Rose; Esencia de Rosa; Oleum Rosae; Otto of Rose; Rosa, aceite esencial de.

**Pharmacopoeias.** In *USNF.*

**USNF 22** (Rose Oil). A volatile oil distilled with steam from the fresh flowers of *Rosa gallica*, *R. damascena*, *R. alba*, *R. centifolia*, and varieties of these species (Rosaceae). It is a colourless or yellow liquid, having the characteristic odour of rose. At 25° it is a viscous liquid. On gradual cooling, it changes to a translucent, crystalline mass, easily liquefied by warming. Miscible with an equal volume of chloroform. Store in well-filled airtight containers.

### Profile

Rose oil is largely employed in perfumery and toilet preparations and has been used as a flavour. It contains citronellol. Hypersensitivity reactions have been reported.

### Preparations

**USNF 22:** Stronger Rose Water;
**USP 27:** Rose Water Ointment.

**Proprietary Preparations** (details are given in Part 3)
**Multi-ingredient:** ***Port.:*** Cicapost.

## Rosemary

Roris Marini.

**Pharmacopoeias.** *Eur.* (see p.vi) includes the dried leaf.

**Ph. Eur. 5.0** (Rosemary Leaf; Rosmarini Folium). The whole, dried leaf of *Rosmarinus officinalis*. It contains not less than 1.2% v/w of essential oil and not less than 3% of total hydroxycinnamic derivatives, expressed as rosmarinic acid ($C_{18}H_{16}O_8$ = 360.3) both with reference to the anhydrous drug.

### Profile

Rosemary (*Rosmarinus officinalis*, Lamiaceae) has rubefacient and mild analgesic activity when applied topically, and is included in external preparations for rheumatic and circulatory disorders. It is also reported to have carminative, spasmolytic, and diuretic effects and is included in herbal preparations for gastrointestinal, cardiovascular, and urinary-tract disorders.

Rosemary is a source of rosemary oil (below).

### Preparations

**Proprietary Preparations** (details are given in Part 3)
***Ger.:*** Kneipp Rosmarin-Pflanzensaft†.

**Multi-ingredient:** ***Arg.:*** Acnetrol; Sequals G; ***Austral.:*** Avena Complex†; Garlic Allium Complex†; ***Austria:*** Aponatura Kreislauf; Apotheker Bauer's Magentee; Bio-Garten Tee zur Starkung und Kraftigung; Cardalept; Euka; Herz- und Kreislauftonikum Bioflora; Kneipp Herz- und Kreislauf-Unterstutzungs-Tee; Krauterdoktor Rosmarin-Wein; Krauterpfarrer Weidinger Tee bei Fruhjahrsmudigkeit; Krauterpfarrer Weidinger Tee fur das Altersherz; Krauterpfarrer Weidinger Tee zur Entwasserung; Mag Kottas Herz- und Kreislauftee; Naturland Herz-Kreislauf; Naturland Rheuma Tee; Nervifloran; Neuners Krautertee Nr 20 - Kreislauftee; Neuners Krautertee Nr 29 - Stoffwechseltee mild; Neuners Krautertee Nr 3 - Blasentee; Neuners Krautertee Nr 30 - Stoffwechseltee stark; Sidroga Herz-Kreislauf-Tee; St Radegunder Herz-Kreislauf-Tonikum; St Radegunder Herz-Kreislauf-unterstutzender Tee; St Radegunder Rosmarin-Wein; Teekanne Herz- und Kreislauftee; ***Belg.:*** Tisane Antibiliaire et Stomachique†; ***Chile:*** Rhus Opodeldoc; ***Fr.:*** Boldoflorine†; Depuratum; Hepax; Mediflor Tisane Contre la Constipation Passagere No 7; Mediflor Tisane Digestive No 3; Mediflor Tisane Hepatique No 5; Romarene; Romarinex-Choline†; Santane $D_5$†; Santane $F_{10}$†; Santane $O_1$†; Santane $R_8$†; Tisane Mexicaine†; ***Ger.:*** Canephron; Hevert-Entwasserungs-Tee†; JuViton; Kneipp Herz- und Kreislauf-Tee†; Melissengeist; Salusan†; Seda-Plantina; ***Hong Kong:*** Canephron N†; ***Ital.:*** Depurfat†; ***Spain:*** Killpan†; Linimento Naion; Mesatil; Natusor Hepavesical; Natusor Low Blood Pressure; Natusor Sinulan; Resolutivo Regium; ***Switz.:*** Boldoflorine†; Melissa Tonic†; Phytomed Cardio.

## Rosemary Oil

Esencia de Romero; Essence de Romarin; Essência de Alecrim; Oleum Roris Marini; Oleum Rosmarini; Romero, aceite esencial de; Rosmarini Aetheroleum; Rosmarinöl.

**Pharmacopoeias.** In *Eur.* (see p.vi).

**Ph. Eur. 5.0** (Rosemary Oil). The essential oil obtained by steam distillation from the flowering aerial parts of *Rosmarinus officinalis*. It is available as Spanish type rosemary oil and Moroccan and Tunisian type rosemary oil. Spanish type rosemary oil contains 2.0 to 4.5% borneol, 0.5 to 2.5% bornyl acetate, 8.0 to 12.0% camphene, 13.0 to 21.0% camphor, 16.0 to 25.0% cineole, 1.0 to 2.2% *p*-cymene, 2.5 to 5.0% limonene, 1.5 to 5.0% β-myrcene, 18 to 26% α-pinene, 2.0 to 6.0% β-pinene, 1.0 to 3.5% α-terpineol, and 0.7 to 2.5% verbenone. Moroccan and Tunisian type rosemary oil contains 1.5 to 5.0% borneol, 0.1 to 1.5% bornyl acetate, 2.5 to 6.0% camphene, 5.0 to 15.0% camphor, 38.0 to 55.0% cineole, 0.8 to 2.5% *p*-cymene, 1.5 to 4.0% limonene, 1.0 to 2.0% β-myrcene, 9.0 to 14.0% α-pinene, 4.0 to 9.0% β-pinene, 1.0 to 2.6% α-terpineol, and a maximum of 0.4% verbenone.

A clear, mobile, colourless to pale yellow liquid with a characteristic odour. Store in well-filled airtight containers at a temperature not exceeding 25°. Protect from light.

### Profile

Rosemary oil is carminative and mildly irritant. It is used in perfumery and as a flavour and has been employed in hair lotions, inhalations, and liniments.

### Preparations

**Proprietary Preparations** (details are given in Part 3)
***Ger.:*** Perozon Rosmarin-Olbad mono†.

**Multi-ingredient:** ***Arg.:*** Bano Liquido con Eucalipto; ***Austral.:*** Bioglan Fingers & Toes†; Euky Bearub†; Tixylix Chest Rub; ***Austria:*** Berggeist; Biokosma Embrocation; Biokosma Medizinalbad; Biokosma Red Point-Massagecreme; Bronchiplant; Carl Baders Divinal; Criniton; Dracodermalin; Inno Rheuma; Naturland Sportcreme; Naturland Sportmassageol; Opino; Pulmex; Rheuma; Rowalind; Salhumin; Tetesept†; ***Belg.:*** Perubore; Pulmex; Pulmex Baby; ***Braz.:*** Analgen; Benegel†; Gelflex; Gelol†; Gelonevral; Mialgex; Nevrol; ***Chile:*** Agua Del Carmen; Agua Melisa Carminativa; Lefkaflam; Pulmex; ***Fr.:*** Aromasol; Dinacode; Perubore; Pulmax†; ***Ger.:*** Arthrodeformat P; Arthrodynat P; Balnostim Bad N†; Cefarheumin N†; Cor-Vel; Criniton; Dolexamed N†; Dolo-cyl; Dr. Hotz Vollbad†; Eucafluid N†; Grunlicht Hingfong Essenz†; Guttacor-Balsam N†; Hingfong-Essenz Hofmanns; Histajodol N†; Kneipp Erkaltungs-Balsam N†; Kneipp Herzsalbe Unguentum Cardiacum Kneipp†; Kneipp Kreislauf-Bad Rosmarin-Aquasan†; Leukona-Kreislauf-Bad; Leukona-Rheumasalbe; Retterspitz Ausserlich†; Retterspitz Gelee†; Retterspitz Quick†; Rheuma-Pasc N†; Rosarthron; Rosarthron forte†; Schupps Heilkrauter Rheumabad†; thermo-loges†; Thrombocid; Togal Mobil Rheuma-Bad†; Top-Sabona; Vaxicum NA; Weleda-Rheumasalbe M; ***Irl.:*** Rowalind†; ***Ital.:*** Calyptol; ***Malaysia:*** Purporent; ***Mon.:*** Calyptol; ***NZ:*** Electric Blue Headlice; Tixylix Chest Rub; ***Port.:*** Thrombocid; ***Spain:*** Beta Romero; Calyptol Inhalante†; Dolokey; Linimento Klari; Masagil; Tonimax; ***Switz.:*** Acidodermil†; Caprisana†; Frigoplasma; Incutin†; Kernosan Huile de Massage†; Liberol Bain; Novital; Perubare; Pulmex; Pulmex Baby; Spagyrom; Thrombocid; ***UK:*** Adiantine; Arnica Massage Balm; Medicated Extract of Rosemary; Soothol.

## Roxarsone *(BAN, USAN, rINN)*

NSC-2101; Roxarsona. 4-Hydroxy-3-nitrophenylarsonic acid.

$C_6H_6AsNO_6$ = 263.0.
*CAS — 121-19-7.*

**Pharmacopoeias.** In *US* for veterinary use only.

**USP 27** (Roxarsone). A pale yellow, crystalline powder. Slightly soluble in cold water; soluble in boiling water; freely soluble in dehydrated alcohol, in acetic acid, in acetone, in methyl alcohol, and in alkalis; insoluble in ether and in ethyl acetate; sparingly soluble in dilute mineral acids. It puffs up and deflagrates on heating.

### Profile

Roxarsone has been used as a growth promotor in animal feeds.

## Royal Jelly

Jalea real; Queen Bee Jelly.

### Profile

Royal jelly is a milky-white viscid secretion from the salivary glands of the worker honey bee, *Apis mellifera* (Apidae); it is essential for the development of queen bees. Royal jelly has been used as a general 'tonic', to ward off the effects of old age, and to ease sufferers from chronic degenerative diseases, but of the many and diverse claims made for its therapeutic value, none has been substantiated.

Royal jelly is also incorporated in some cosmetic preparations for its supposed beneficial effect on skin tissue.

**Hypersensitivity.** There have been a number of cases of anaphylactoid reactions and acute severe exacerbations of asthma[1-4] (one fatal[2]) in atopic individuals who took royal jelly.


1. Thien FCK, *et al.* Royal jelly-induced asthma. *Med J Aust* 1993; **159:** 639.
2. Bullock RJ, *et al.* Fatal royal jelly-induced asthma. *Med J Aust* 1994; **160:** 44.
3. Peacock S, *et al.* Respiratory distress and royal jelly. *BMJ* 1995; **311:** 1472.
4. Thien FCK, *et al.* Asthma and anaphylaxis induced by royal jelly. *Clin Exp Allergy* 1996; **26:** 216–22.


### Preparations

**Proprietary Preparations** (details are given in Part 3)
***Fr.:*** Apiserum; ***Ital.:*** Alvear; Biogel; Biovital; Clinvit; Gelamel; Natura Vivа†; Novel Jelly; Opalia†; Pa-Real; Ritmogel; Roburvit; Telergon II; Theogel†; Trefovital†; Trofomed†; ***UK:*** Biobees; Regina Royal One Hundred; Rojema.

**Multi-ingredient:** ***Fr.:*** Arkotonic†; Gintonal; Pollen Royal; ***Ger.:*** Alsiroyal†; Peking Royal Jelly N; ***Ital.:*** Alvear Complex†; Alvear con Ginseng; Alvear Sport†; Apergan; Api Baby; Apiserum con Telergon 1; Apistress; Bebimix; Bio-200; Bio-Real Complex†; Bio-Real Plus†; Bio-Real†; Bioton; Biotrefon Plus; Biovigor†; Cocktail Reale†; Eurogel; Fon Wan Ginsenergy; Fon Wan Pollen†; Fosfarsile Forte; Fosfarsile Junior; Four-Ton; Granvit; Longevital; Miegel†; Neoplus; Nerex; Novogel†; Nutrex†; Nutrigel; Ottovis; Pollingel; Provitamin A-E; Ribovir; Royal E; Vigogel†; ***Thai.:*** Multilim RG; ***UK:*** Arthrotone†; Beeline†; Regina Royal Concorde; Regina Royal Five; Royal Galanol†.

## Rubber

Caoutchouc; Caucho; India-Rubber.

### Profile

Rubber consists of the prepared latex of *Hevea brasiliensis* and other species of *Hevea* (Euphorbiaceae). It is used as a component of many medical devices such as catheters, syringes, enema tips, ostomy bags, balloons, and surgical gloves. Hypersensitivity reactions have occurred after direct contact of skin and mucous membranes with rubber components of such products and also after indirect contact with preparations stored in or given by them; deaths have been reported. Reactions have been attributed either to protein components of the rubber or to additives such as preservatives or vulcanisation accelerators. For references to glove starch powder as a possible risk factor in the development of rubber latex allergy, see Adverse Effects of Starch, p.1449. Cross-sensitivity between rubber proteins and those of certain fruits, including bananas and chestnuts, has been reported.

◊ References.


1. Landwehr LP, Boguniewicz M. Current perspectives on latex allergy. *J Pediatr* 1996; **128:** 305–12.
2. Senst BL, Johnson RA. Latex allergy. *Am J Health-Syst Pharm* 1997; **54:** 1071–5.
3. Woods JA, *et al.* Natural rubber latex allergy: spectrum, diagnostic approach, and therapy. *J Emerg Med* 1997; **15:** 71–85.
4. Zaidi Z, *et al.* Latex allergy: a life-threatening complication. *Hosp Med* 1998; **59:** 505–7.
5. Smith CC. Risk of latex allergy from medication vial closures. *Ann Pharmacother* 1999; **33:** 373–4.
6. Wakelin SH, White IR. Natural rubber latex allergy. *Clin Exp Dermatol* 1999; **24:** 245–8.
7. Bowyer RVStL. Latex allergy: how to identify it and the people at risk. *J Clin Nurs* 1999; **8:** 144–9.
8. Levy DA, Leynadier F. Latex allergy: review of recent advances. *Curr Allergy Rep* 2001; **1:** 32–8.
9. Hamann CP, *et al.* Management of dental patients with allergies to natural rubber latex. *Gen Dent* 2002; **50:** 526–36.
10. Bernstein DI. Management of natural rubber latex allergy. *J Allergy Clin Immunol* 2002; **110** (suppl 2): S111–S116.
11. Nieto A, *et al.* Efficacy of latex avoidance for primary prevention of latex sensitization in children with spina bifida. *J Pediatr* 2002; **140:** 370–2.
12. Hourihane JO'B, *et al.* Impact of repeated surgical procedures on the incidence and prevalence of latex allergy: a prospective study of 1263 children. *J Pediatr* 2002; **140:** 479–82.
13. Cullinan P, *et al.*. British Society of Allergy and Clinical Immunology. Latex allergy: a position paper of the British Society of Allergy and Clinical Immunology. *Clin Exp Allergy* 2003; **33:** 1484–99.


## Rubidium Iodide

Rubidio, ioduro de.

RbI = 212.4.

*CAS — 7790-29-6.*

### Profile

Rubidium iodide has the actions of iodine and the iodides (see p.1598). It is an ingredient of several proprietary ophthalmic preparations promoted for the treatment of eye disorders.

### Preparations

**Proprietary Preparations** (details are given in Part 3)

**Multi-ingredient:** ***Ital.:*** Facovit; Jodo Calcio Vitaminico; Polijodurato; Rubidiosin Compostо†; Rubistenol†; Rubjovit.

## Rue Oil

Oleum Rutae; Ruda, aceite esencial de.

### Profile

Rue oil is a volatile oil obtained from rue, *Ruta graveolens* (Rutaceae). Rue oil and infusions of rue were formerly used as antispasmodics and emmenagogues and are reported to have abortifacient properties. Rue is a photosensitiser and the oil is a powerful local irritant.

Rue (Ruta grav.) is used in homoeopathic medicine.

### Preparations

**Proprietary Preparations** (details are given in Part 3)

**Multi-ingredient:** ***Austral.:*** Joint & Muscle Relief Cream†; ***Braz.:*** Piolin†; ***Singapore:*** Noricaven; ***UK:*** Arnileve.

## Ruscogenin

Ruscogenina. (25*R*)-Spirost-5-ene-1β,3β-diol.

$C_{27}H_{42}O_4$ = 430.6.

*CAS — 472-11-7.*

### Profile

Ruscogenin is a sapogenin obtained from butcher's broom, *Ruscus aculeatus* (Liliaceae). It has been applied in the local treatment of haemorrhoids as rectal ointment or suppositories. It has also been tried in peripheral vascular disorders.

### Preparations

**Proprietary Preparations** (details are given in Part 3)

***Arg.:*** Flebopom; ***Ger.:*** Ruscorectal†; ***Spain:*** Hemodren Simple†; Ruscorectal.

**Multi-ingredient:** ***Arg.:*** Miopropan Proctologico; ***Fr.:*** Calmoroide†; Proctolog; ***Ital.:*** Ruscoroid; ***Port.:*** Proctolog; ***Singapore:*** Proctolog; ***Spain:*** Abrasone Rectal; Hemodren Compuesto; Neo Analsona; Proctolog; Ruscus; Venacol.

## Sabeluzole *(BAN, USAN, rINN)*

R-58735; Sabeluzol. (±)-4-(2-Benzothiazolylmethylamino)-α-[(4-fluorophenoxy)methyl]-1-piperidineethanol.

$C_{22}H_{26}FN_3O_2S$ = 415.5.

*CAS — 104153-38-0; 104383-17-7;.*

### Profile

Sabeluzole is a benzothiazole derivative with anticonvulsant and antihypoxic properties. It has been investigated in the treatment of Alzheimer's disease and of sleep apnoea.

## Sacrosidase *(USAN)*

Sacrosidasa.

*CAS — 85897-35-4.*

### Profile

Sacrosidase is a therapeutic enzyme used for sucrase replacement therapy in congenital sucrase-isomaltase deficiency. It is given with each meal or snack in usual doses of 8 500 international units for patients up to 15 kg, or 17 000 international units for patients over 15 kg.

◊ References.


1. Treem WR, *et al.* Sacrosidase therapy for congenital sucrase-isomaltase deficiency. *J Pediatr Gastroenterol Nutr* 1999; **28:** 137–42.


### Preparations

**Proprietary Preparations** (details are given in Part 3)

***USA:*** Sucraid.

## Sage

Feuilles de Sauge; Salbeiblätter; Salvia.

**Pharmacopoeias.** In *Eur.* (see p.vi) and *Pol. Eur.* also includes three-lobed sage.

**Ph. Eur. 5.0** (Sage Leaf (Salvia officinalis); Salviae Officinalis Folium). The whole or cut dried leaves of *Salvia officinalis*. The whole drug contains not less than 1.5% v/w and the cut drug not less than 1.0% v/w of essential oil, both calculated with reference to the anhydrous drug. Sage leaf oil is rich in thujone. Protect from light.

**Ph. Eur. 5.0** (Sage Leaf, Three-lobed; Salviae Trilobae Folium). The whole or cut, dried leaves of *Salvia fructicosa* (*S. triloba*). The whole drug contains not less than 1.8% v/w of essential oil, and the cut drug not less than 1.2% v/w of essential oil, both calculated with reference to the anhydrous drug. It has a spicy odour when ground, similar to eucalyptus oil. Protect from light.

### Profile

Sage has carminative, antispasmodic, antiseptic, and astringent properties and is used as a flavour. It is used in preparations for a wide variety of purposes, including respiratory-tract disorders, gastrointestinal disorders, and in mouthwashes and gargles for disorders of the mouth and throat. It is also used in homoeopathic medicine. Three-lobed sage leaf (Greek sage) is also used; it is sometimes found as an adulterant of sage.

Sage is the source of sage leaf oil (see below).

### Preparations

**Proprietary Preparations** (details are given in Part 3)

***Austria:*** Aperisan; Nosweat; Salvysat; ***Ger.:*** Aperisan; Fichtensirup N; Salbei Curarina; Salvysat; Sweatosan N; Viru-Salvysat.

**Multi-ingredient:** ***Arg.:*** Acnetrol; Sedante Arceli; ***Austral.:*** Feminine Herbal Complex†; ***Austria:*** Apotheker Bauer's Blahungstee; Bio-Strath Schleimhaut; Bronchostop; Cional; Dynexan; Erbesil; Krauterhaus Mag Kottas Wechseltee; Luuf-Halspastillen; Mentopin; Neuners Krautertee Nr 10 - Grippetee; Neuners Krautertee Nr 107 - Blahungstee; Neuners Krautertee Nr 16 - Beruhigungstee bei Wechselbeschwerden; Neuners Krautertee Nr 311 - Bronchialtee zur Inhalation; Neuners Krautertee Nr 8 - Magentee gegen Ubersauerung; Paradenton; Teekanne Husten- und Brusttee; ***Belg.:*** Tisane pour Dormir†; ***Chile:*** Eciclean; ***Fr.:*** Bolcitol; Gonaxine; Santane $V_3$†; Saugella; Tisane Hepatique de Hoerdt; Tisanes de l'Abbe Hamon no 6†; ***Ger.:*** Agamadon†; Amara-Tropfen; Helago-Pflege-Oel; Leber-Galle-Tropfen 83; Melissengeist; Mycatox; Odala wern†; Parodontal; Presselin Blahungs K 4 N; Presselin Dyspeptikum; Vitosal; ***Israel:*** Baby Paste + Chamomile; Kamilotract; Kamiltract Baby†; ***Ital.:*** Donalg; Saugella Salviettine; ***Port.:*** Emopads†; ***S.Afr.:*** Dynexan; ***Spain:*** Diabesor; Menstrunat; Natusor Farinol; Natusor Low Blood Pressure; Vegetalin†; ***Switz.:*** Anginesin; Dynexan†; Tisane pectorale et antitussive; Tonex†; ***UK:*** Catarrh†.

## Sage Oil

NOTE. The oil of three-lobed sage (see above), which is sometimes found as an adulterant, has a lower thujone content than oil from *Salvia officinalis*

**Pharmacopoeias.** In *Swiss. Eur.* (see p.vi) includes Clary Sage Oil from *Salvia sclarea.*

### Profile

Sage oil is used similarly to sage (see above).

### Preparations

**Proprietary Preparations** (details are given in Part 3)

***Fr.:*** Node G; ***Ger.:*** Buchol†; Fichtensirup N.

**Multi-ingredient:** ***Austria:*** Anifer Hustenbalsam; Colda; Coldistan; Fittydent; Parodontax; Piniment; Salbei-Halspastillen; Tetesept†; ***Ger.:*** Dr. Hotz Vollbad†; Hoemarin Derma†; Kneipp Rheuma Stoffwechsel-Bad Heublumen-Aquasan†; Parodontal F5 med†; Pernionin N; Salviathymol N; Schupps Heilkrauter Rheumabad†; Trauma-cyl; Varicylum-S; ***Israel:*** Parodontax; ***Ital.:*** Pluriderm†; ***Switz.:*** Bismorectal; Demo pommade contre les refroidissements pour bebes†; Kernosan Huile de Massage†; Osa Gel de dentition aux plantes†; Pastilles pectorales formule 541†.

## Salverine Hydrochloride *(rINNM)*

Hidrocloruro de salverina; M-811 (salverine). 2-[2-(Diethylamino)ethoxy]-benzanilide hydrochloride.

$C_{19}H_{24}N_2O_2,HCl$ = 348.9.

*CAS — 6376-26-7 (salverine).*

### Profile

Salverine hydrochloride has been used as an antispasmodic in combination preparations for the treatment of biliary-tract disorders, respiratory-tract disorders, and pain.

### Preparations

**Proprietary Preparations** (details are given in Part 3)

**Multi-ingredient:** ***Austria:*** Cynarix comp; Montamed; Novipec.

## Sambucus

Elder Flowers; Fleurs de Sureau; Holunderblüten; Sabugueiro; Sambuc.; Sambuci Flos; Saúco.

**Pharmacopoeias.** In *Eur.* (see p.vi) and *Pol.*

**Ph. Eur. 5.0** (Elder Flower). The dried flowers of *Sambucus nigra*. It contains not less than 0.8% of flavonoids, calculated as isoquercitroside with reference to the dried drug. Protect from light.

### Profile

Sambucus has astringent, diaphoretic, and anticatarrhal properties and is used in herbal and homoeopathic preparations for a variety of disorders, particularly respiratory-tract disorders. Elder-flower water has been used as a vehicle for eye and skin lotions. Elder-flower ointment has been used as a basis for pomades and cosmetic ointments.

### Preparations

**Proprietary Preparations** (details are given in Part 3)

***Port.:*** Sambucol†.

**Multi-ingredient:** ***Austral.:*** Sambucus Complex†; ***Austria:*** Apotheker Bauer's Grippetee; Aurita-Erkaltungstee; Bio-Garten Entschlackungstee; Bogumil-tassenfertiger milder Abfuhrtee; Entschlackender Abfuhrtee EF-EM-ES; Grippetee Dr Zeidler; Grippetee EF-EM-ES; Grippogran; Krauter Hustensaft; Krauterdoktor Erkaltungstropfen; Krauterhaus Mag Kottas Grippetee; Krauterpfarrer Weidinger Tee zur Entschlackung; Laxalpin; Mag Kottas Grippe-Tee; Mag Kottas Krauterexpress-Grippe-Tee; Neuners Krautertee Nr 10 - Grippetee; Neuners Krautertee Nr 2 - Fruhjahrskurtee; Neuners Krautertee Nr 210 - Krauterhexlein Kinder-Schweisstreibender Tee; Sidroga Erkaltungstee; Sinupret; Sinusol-Schleimlosender Tee; St Radegunder Fiebertee; Teekanne Erkaltungstee; Tuscalman; ***Fr.:*** Tisane des Familles†; ***Ger.:*** Hevert-Erkaltungs-Tee†; Hevert-Gicht-Rheuma-Tee comp†; Kneipp Erkaltungs-Tee†; Kneipp Rheuma Tee N†; Sinupret; ***Hong Kong:*** Sinupret; ***Ital.:*** Sambuco (Specie Composta); Tiglio (Specie Composta); ***Singapore:*** Sinupret; ***Spain:*** Natusor Gripotul; Natusor Sinulan; ***Switz.:*** Sinupret; The Brioni†; Tisane contre les refroidissements; ***Thai.:*** Sinupret; ***UK:*** Cleansing Herbs; EP&C Essence; Hay Fever & Sinus Relief; Hayfever & Sinus Relief; Herb and Honey Cough Elixir; Life Drops; Lifedrops†; Lion Cleansing Herbs; Lustys Herbalene; Modern Herbals Cold & Catarrh; Sinotar; Tabritis.

## Sanguinaria

Bloodroot; Red Puccoon; Sanguinaria canadensis; Sanguinarine canadensis; Sanguinaris canadensis.

### Profile

Sanguinaria consists of the dried rhizome of *Sanguinaria canadensis* (Papaveraceae). Sanguinarine, an alkaloid extracted from sanguinaria, has been used as an antiplaque agent in toothpaste and mouthwash preparations. Sanguinaria was formerly used as an expectorant but fell into disuse because of its toxicity. Sanguinaria has also been classified by the FDA as a herb that is unsafe for use in foods, beverages, or drugs.

Sanguinaria is used in homoeopathic medicine.

◊ Reviews.


1. Karlowsky JA. Bloodroot: Sanguinaria canadensis L. *Can Pharm J* 1991; **124:** 260, 262–3, 267.
2. Grenby TH. The use of sanguinarine in mouthwashes and toothpaste compared with some other antimicrobial agents. *Br Dent J* 1995; **178:** 254–8.
3. Tenenbaum H, *et al.* Effectiveness of a sanguinarine regimen after scaling and root planing. *J Periodontol* 1999; **70:** 307–11.


### Preparations

**Proprietary Preparations** (details are given in Part 3)

***Canad.:*** Viadent†; ***Ital.:*** Periogard†; ***Port.:*** Periogard†.

**Multi-ingredient:** ***Arg.:*** Clematis Ill Oligoplex; ***Austral.:*** Lexat†; ***Canad.:*** Mielocol; Viadent; Wampole Bronchial Cough Syrup; ***Ital.:*** Dentosan Carie & Alito; Eudent con Glysan; Periogard†; ***Port.:*** Periogard†.

## Sapropterin Hydrochloride *(rINNM)*

Dapropterin Hydrochloride; Hidrocloruro de sapropterina; SUN-0588 (sapropterin or sapropterin hydrochloride); (6*R*)-5,6,7,8-Tetrahydrobiopterin Hydrochloride. (−)-(6*R*)-2-Amino-6-[(1*R*,2*S*)-1,2-dihydroxypropyl]- 5,6,7,8-tetrahydro-4(3*H*)-pteridinone dihydrochloride.

$C_9H_{15}N_5O_3,2HCl = 314.2.$

*CAS — 62989-33-7 (sapropterin); 69056-38-8 (sapropterin hydrochloride).*

### Profile

Sapropterin, the active form of tetrahydrobiopterin, has been tried as the hydrochloride for the correction of hyperphenylalaninaemia that may be responsible for neurological symptoms seen in patients receiving treatment for leukaemia, and in other conditions associated with tetrahydrobiopterin ($BH_4$) deficiency.

◊ References.

1. Blau N, *et al.* Hyperphenylalaninemia caused by dihydropteridine reductase deficiency in children receiving chemotherapy for acute lymphoblastic leukemia. *J Pediatr* 1989; **115:** 661–2.
2. Hyland K, *et al.* Reply. *J Pediatr* 1989; **115:** 662.
3. Ueda S, *et al.* Tetrahydrobiopterin restores endothelial function in long-term smokers. *J Am Coll Cardiol* 2000; **35:** 71–5.
4. Thony B, *et al.* Tetrahydrobiopterin biosynthesis, regeneration and functions. *Biochem J* 2000; **347:** 1–16.
5. Muntau AC, *et al.* Tetrahydrobiopterin as an alternative treatment for mild phenylketonuria. *N Engl J Med* 2002; **347:** 2122–32.

## Sarsaparilla

Salsaparilha; Salsepareille; Sarsa; Sarsaparilla Root; Smilacis Rhizoma; Zarzaparrilla.

**Pharmacopoeias.** In *Chin.* and *Jpn.* which specify *Smilax glabra.*

### Profile

Sarsaparilla is the dried root of various species of *Smilax* (Liliaceae). It has been used, usually in the form of a decoction or extract, as a vehicle and flavour for medicaments. It is also an ingredient of herbal and homoeopathic preparations.

### Preparations

**Proprietary Preparations** (details are given in Part 3)

**Multi-ingredient:** ***Arg.:*** Urinefrol; ***Austral.:*** Herbal Cleanse†; Proesten†; ***Belg.:*** Tisane Depurative "les 12 Plantes"†; ***Braz.:*** Elixir de Inhame†; Elixir de Marinheiro†; Licor de Tayuya†; Tintura de Salsa Caroba e Manaca†; ***Canad.:*** Damiana-Sarsaparilla Formula; ***Ger.:*** Pankreaplex Neu; ***Ital.:*** Depurativo†; Tisana Kelemata; ***Port.:*** Solucao Stago†; ***UK:*** Blue Flag Root Compound†; Gerard House Ligvites†; Gerard House Reumalex; HRI Clear Complexion; Jamaican Sarsaparilla; Skin Eruptions Mixture.

## Sassafras Oil

Oleum Sassafras; Sasafrás, aceite esencial de.

### Profile

Sassafras oil is a volatile oil distilled from the root or root bark of *Sassafras albidum* (Lauraceae), or from the wood of certain species of *Ocotea* (Lauraceae). It contains safrole.

Sassafras oil has rubefacient properties and was formerly used as a pediculicide. Neither sassafras nor the oil should be taken internally; the use of herb teas of sassafras may lead to a large dose of safrole. The use of safrole in foods has been banned because of carcinogenic and hepatotoxic risks. The use of safrole in toilet preparations is also controlled.

**Poisoning.** A 47-year-old woman experienced 'shakiness', vomiting, anxiety, tachycardia, and raised blood pressure after ingestion of a potentially fatal dose of sassafras oil (5 mL). She was given activated charcoal and symptomatic management.[1]

1. Grande GA, Dannewitz SR. Symptomatic sassafras oil ingestion. *Vet Hum Toxicol* 1987; **29:** 447.

### Preparations

**Proprietary Preparations** (details are given in Part 3)

**Multi-ingredient:** ***Arg.:*** Inhalador Medex; ***Austral.:*** Urinase†; Zam-Buk†; ***Braz.:*** Tintura de Salsa Caroba e Manaca†; ***Fr.:*** Vegebom; ***S.Afr.:*** Zam-Buk; ***Spain:*** Inhalador†; Linimento Klari; Linimento Sloan†; ***Switz.:*** Dental-Phenjoca†; Spirogel†.

## Saxitoxin

Saxitoxina.

*CAS — 35523-89-8.*

### Profile

Saxitoxin is a neurotoxin associated with paralytic shellfish poisoning. It is an endotoxin produced by species of dinoflagellate plankton present in infected molluscs.

◊ References.

1. Halstead BW, Schantz EJ. *Paralytic shellfish poisoning.* Geneva: WHO, 1984.
2. Aquatic (marine and freshwater) biotoxins. *Environmental Health Criteria 37.* Geneva: WHO, 1984. Available at: http://www.inchem.org/documents/ehc/ehc/ehc37.htm (accessed 08/07/04)
3. Hartigan-Go K, Bateman DN. Redtide in the Philippines. *Hum Exp Toxicol* 1994; **13:** 824–30.
4. Gessner BD, *et al.* Hypertension and identification of toxin in human urine and serum following a cluster of mussel-associated paralytic shellfish poisoning outbreaks. *Toxicon* 1997; **35:** 711–22.
5. de Carvalho M, *et al.* Paralytic shellfish poisoning: clinical and electrophysiological observations. *J Neurol* 1998; **245:** 551–4.
6. Lehane L. Paralytic shellfish poisoning: a potential public health problem. *Med J Aust* 2001; **175:** 29–31.
7. Garcia C, *et al.* Paralytic shellfish poisoning: post-mortem analysis of tissue and body fluid samples from human victims in the Patagonia fjords. *Toxicon* 2004; **43:** 149–58.

## Schick Test

Prueba de Schick.

**Pharmacopoeias.** *Br.* and *US* include standards for Schick test toxin and control.

**BP 2003** (Schick Test Toxin). It is prepared from a toxigenic strain of *Corynebacterium diphtheriae*. It contains a suitable antimicrobial preservative. Store at 2° to 8°.

**BP 2003** (Schick Control). It is Schick Test Toxin that has been heated at a temperature not lower than 70° and not higher than 85° for not less than 5 minutes. It is prepared from the same batch of Schick Test Toxin as that with which it is to be used. Store at 2° to 8°.

**USP 27** (Diphtheria Toxin for Schick Test ). It is a sterile solution of the diluted, standardised toxic products of the growth of the diphtheria bacillus (*Corynebacterium diphtheriae*). Store at 2° to 8°.

**USP 27** (Schick Test Control). It is Diphtheria Toxin for Schick Test that has been inactivated by heat. Store at 2° to 8°.

### Profile

The Schick test has been used for the diagnosis of susceptibility to diphtheria and, more importantly, to detect patients who might experience an adverse reaction to diphtheria vaccines. Children up to the age of about 8 to 10 years rarely suffer from such reactions and therefore the Schick test is not usually performed in this age group. In older children and adults a Schick test was formerly used before the use of standard diphtheria vaccines. However, diphtheria vaccines for use in adults and adolescents (p.1612) are now formulated with lesser amounts of toxoid so Schick testing is unnecessary.

A dose of 0.2 mL of the Schick toxin was administered intradermally (intracutaneously) into the flexor surface of the forearm. A similar dose of Schick control was injected into the other forearm. The reaction to the injections was read after 24 to 48 hours, and again after 5 to 7 days to detect late reactors and to confirm a reading taken earlier.

- a *negative reaction*, indicating that the patient is immune to diphtheria, occurs when there is no redness at either injection site
- a *positive reaction*, indicating susceptibility to diphtheria, occurs as a red flush about 10 mm or more in diameter at the site of injection of the test dose with no reaction to the control injection
- a *negative-and-pseudo reaction*, also indicating immunity, is shown by a flush which develops rapidly at each injection site but the reaction fades more rapidly than a positive reaction; the reaction is due to non-specific constituents of the injection
- a *combined* or *positive-and-pseudo reaction*, also indicating susceptibility, is shown by a flush which develops rapidly at each injection site, but as it fades a positive reaction develops at the site of the test dose.

### Preparations

***BP 2003:*** Schick Control; Schick Test Toxin;
***USP 27:*** Diphtheria Toxin for Schick Test; Schick Test Control.

## Scoparium

Broom Tops; Genêt; Genêt à Balai; Planta Genista; Retama negra; Scoparii Cacumina.

**Pharmacopoeias.** In *Fr.*

### Profile

Scoparium is the dried tops of broom, *Sarothamnus scoparius* (*Cytisus scoparius*) (Leguminosae). It is a mild diuretic, haemostatic, and vasoconstrictor and has been given as a decoction or alcoholic extract. It has oxytocic properties and should be avoided in pregnancy. It contains sparteine (p.1749).

### Preparations

**Proprietary Preparations** (details are given in Part 3)
***Ger.:*** Cefacor†; Repowine mono; Spartiol.

**Multi-ingredient:** ***Fr.:*** Creme Rap; Curoveinyl†; Santane $H_7$†; Santane $R_8$†; Santane $V_3$†; Tisanes de l'Abbe Hamon no 16†; ***Ger.:*** Goldtropfen-Hetterich†; JuPhlebon S†; Oxacant N; Venacton.

## Sea Buckthorn

Argousier; Sallowthorn; Sea-buckthorn.

NOTE. Distinguish from Buckthorn (p.1254).

### Profile

Sea buckthorn (*Hippophae rhamnoides*, Eleagnaceae) is the source of sea buckthorn oil, below.

### Preparations

**Proprietary Preparations** (details are given in Part 3)
***Fr.:*** Hippophan†.

## Sea Buckthorn Oil

### Profile

Sea buckthorn oil is extracted from the seeds and berries of sea buckthorn (above) and has been taken orally for skin and mucous membrane disorders and as a tonic. It has also been investigated in liver fibrosis.

### Preparations

**Proprietary Preparations** (details are given in Part 3)
***UK:*** Omega 7.

## Seaweeds, Kelps, and Wracks

**Pharmacopoeias.** In *Eur.* (see p.vi).

**Ph. Eur. 5.0** (Kelp; Fucus vel Ascophyllum; Fucus BP 2003). The fragmented dried thallus of *Fucus vesiculosus* or *F. serratus* or *Ascophyllum nodosum*. It contains not less than 0.03% and not more than 0.2% of total iodine, calculated with reference to the dried drug. It has a salty and mucilaginous taste, and an unpleasant marine odour. Protect from light.

The Ph. Eur. title was formerly Bladderwrack and the BP 2003 gives Bladderwrack as an approved synonym.

### Profile

Dried seaweeds of various species are ingredients of a number of herbal preparations.

The terms kelps and wracks have been used indiscriminately for each other and other brown seaweeds. For example, Kelp (Ph. Eur. 5.0) refers to a preparation of various species of wrack and was formerly titled Bladderwrack.

Bladder wrack (*Fucus vesiculosus*), toothed wrack (*F. serratus*), or knotted wrack (*Ascophyllum nodosum*) are included in preparations given for various disorders including obesity, constipation, and iodine deficiency. *F. vesiculosus* is also used in homoeopathic medicine.

Kelps refer properly to species of *Laminaria* and *Macrocystis*. They are present as an ingredient of several dietary supplements and herbal preparations, including for use in obesity; they have also been used as a source of iodine. Laminaria stalks (p.1704) are used for dilation of cavities or the cervix.

**Adverse effects and precautions.** Kelp can concentrate various heavy metals; auto-immune thrombocytopenic purpura with dyserythropoiesis occurring in a patient who had been taking kelp tablets for 6 weeks was attributed to the arsenic content of the preparation.[1]

Clinical hyperthyroidism has also been reported in patients taking kelp-containing preparations as part of a slimming regimen[2] or a dietary supplement.[3]

The FDA has advised that preparations containing compounds such as kelp, which may be taken by mouth in bulk laxatives or weight-control preparations, should be taken with a full glass of water or, if the patient has difficulty in swallowing, they should be avoided. Such compounds swell into masses that may obstruct the oesophagus if not taken with sufficient water.

1. Pye KG, *et al.* Severe dyserythropoiesis and autoimmune thrombocytopenia associated with ingestion of kelp supplements. *Lancet* 1992; **339:** 1540.
2. de Smet PA, *et al.* Hyperthyreoidie tijdens het gebruik van kelp tabletten. *Ned Tijdschr Geneeskd* 1990; **134:** 1058–9.
3. Eliason BC. Transient hyperthyroidism in a patient taking dietary supplements containing kelp. *J Am Board Fam Pract* 1998; **11:** 478–80.

### Preparations

**Multi-ingredient:** numerous preparations are listed in Part 3.

## Secretin *(BAN, rINN)*

Secretina.

*CAS — 17034-35-4.*
*ATC — V04CK01.*

**Pharmacopoeias.** In *Jpn.*

### Units

The potency of secretin may be expressed as Crick-Harper-Raper (CHR) units based on the pancreatic secretion in *cats* or as clinical units, the value of which was amended in the 1960s. One clinical unit is considered to be approximately equivalent to 4 CHR units. One clinical unit is equivalent to 200 nanograms of a purified synthetic preparation of secretin.

### Adverse Effects

Hypersensitivity reactions may occasionally occur. Diarrhoea has occurred in patients given high doses by intravenous infusion.

### Precautions

The secretin test should be avoided in patients with acute pancreatitis. A test dose has been suggested for patients at particular risk of hypersensitivity reactions.

### Uses and Administration

Secretin is a polypeptide hormone involved in the regulation of gastric function. It is prepared from the duodenal mucosa of *pigs*; a synthetic version is also available. On intravenous injection it causes an increase in the secretion by the pancreas of water and bicarbonate into the duodenum.

Secretin is used alone, or in conjunction with pancreozymin (p.1727) or other cholecystokinetic agents such as ceruletide (p.1669) or sincalide (p.1746), as a test for exocrine pancreatic function. The test usually involves duodenal intubation of the patient and examination of duodenal aspirate. The dose of secretin used has varied but common doses have been 1 clinical unit/kg given by slow intravenous injection.

Patients with the Zollinger-Ellison syndrome (p.1247) show an increase in gastrin when given secretin; this is in contrast to a small change or no effect in subjects without the disorder. The usual dose of secretin for the diagnosis of Zollinger-Ellison syndrome is 2 clinical units/kg by slow intravenous injection. Serum-gastrin concentrations are measured for up to 30 minutes following the test dose.

Secretin is also used in a dose of 1 clinical unit/kg by slow intravenous injection as an aid in the identification of the pancreatic ducts in patients undergoing endoscopic retrograde cholangiopancreatography.

**Autism.** There have been anecdotal reports of improvement in behaviour in autistic children given porcine secretin. However, a double-blind placebo-controlled study[1] involving 60 children with autism or pervasive developmental disorder noted no benefit over 4 weeks following a single infusion of 400 micrograms/kg of synthetic human secretin. A randomised, placebo-controlled study[2] in 64 children with autism has similarly found no evidence of efficacy from 2 repeated doses of porcine secretin.

1. Sandler AD, *et al.* Lack of benefit of a single dose of synthetic human secretin in the treatment of autism and pervasive developmental disorder. *N Engl J Med* 1999; **341:** 1801–6.
2. Roberts W, *et al.* Repeated doses of porcine secretin in the treatment of autism: a randomized, placebo-controlled trial. Abstract: *Pediatrics* 2001; **107:** e71. Full version: http://pediatrics.aappublications.org/cgi/content/full/107/5/e71 (accessed 08/07/04)

### Preparations

**Proprietary Preparations** (details are given in Part 3)
***Ger.:*** Secrelux; Sekretolin†; ***USA:*** SecreFlo.

## Selfotel *(USAN, rINN)*

CGS-19755. *cis*-4-(Phosphonomethyl)pipecolic acid.
$C_7H_{14}NO_5P = 223.2$.
*CAS — 110347-85-8.*

### Profile

Selfotel is an *N*-methyl-D-aspartate (NMDA) antagonist that has been investigated for use in ischaemic stroke and head trauma.

◊ References.

1. Davis SM, *et al.* Termination of acute stroke studies involving selfotel treatment. *Lancet* 1997; **349:** 32.
2. Yenari MA, *et al.* Dose escalation safety and tolerance study of the competitive NMDA antagonist selfotel (CGS 19755) in neurosurgery patients. *Clin Neuropharmacol* 1998; **21:** 28–34.
3. Stewart L, *et al.* First observations of the safety and tolerability of a competitive antagonist to the glutamate NMDA receptor (CGS 19755) in patients with severe head injury. *J Neurotrauma* 1999; **16:** 843–50.
4. Morris GF, *et al.* Failure of the competitive N-methyl-D-aspartate antagonist Selfotel (CGS 19755) in the treatment of severe head injury: results of two phase III clinical trials. *J Neurosurg* 1999; **91:** 737–43.
5. Davis SM, *et al.* Selfotel in acute ischemic stroke: possible neurotoxic effects of an NMDA antagonist. *Stroke* 2000; **31:** 347–54.

## Senecio

### Profile

The ragwort, *Senecio jacobaea*, and, in the USA, the golden ragwort (golden senecio; liferoot; squaw weed) *S. aureus* (Compositae), have been used in the form of extracts as emmenagogues but are of doubtful value. Ragwort, in the form of a decoction or ointment, has also been applied externally to aid wound healing and in the treatment of peripheral vascular disorders. *S. aureus* is also used in homoeopathic preparations.

Many species of the genus *Senecio*, which includes the ragworts and groundsels, are poisonous and have been found to contain pyrrolizidine alkaloids which produce hepatic necrosis. The ragwort, *S. jacobaea*, which is abundant throughout the British Isles, is poisonous to livestock when eaten in quantity. Poisoning has also been reported in humans following ingestion of herbal teas containing pyrrolizidine alkaloids.

### Preparations

**Proprietary Preparations** (details are given in Part 3)
**Multi-ingredient:** ***Canad.:*** Thunas Tab for Menstrual Pain; ***Ger.:*** Senecion†; ***USA:*** Succus Cineraria Maritima.

## Senlizumab *(BAN)*

Bay-10-3356; Bay-w-3356; CDP-571.
*CAS — 336128-48-4.*

### Profile

Senlizumab is a humanised monoclonal antibody to tumour necrosis factor. It has been investigated in the treatment of Crohn's disease, ulcerative colitis, and rheumatoid arthritis.

◊ References.

1. Rankin EC, *et al.* The therapeutic effects of an engineered human anti-tumour necrosis factor alpha antibody (CDP571) in rheumatoid arthritis. *Br J Rheumatol* 1995; **34:** 334–42.
2. Evans RC, *et al.* Treatment of ulcerative colitis with an engineered human anti-TNF alpha antibody CDP571. *Aliment Pharmacol Ther* 1997; **11:** 1031–5.
3. Stack WA, *et al.* Randomised controlled trial of CDP571 antibody to tumour necrosis factor-α in Crohn's disease. *Lancet* 1997; **349:** 521–4.
4. Anonymous. CDP 571: anti-TNF monoclonal antibody, BAY 103356, BAY W 3356, Humicade. *Drugs R D* 2003; **4:** 174–8.

## Sepia

### Profile

Sepia is the dried inky secretion of the cuttle fish. It is used in homoeopathic medicine.

## Serotonin

Enteramine; 5-HT; 5-Hydroxytryptamine; Serotonina. 3-(2-Aminoethyl)-1*H*-indol-5-ol.
$C_{10}H_{12}N_2O = 176.2$.
*CAS — 50-67-9.*

### Profile

Serotonin is found in the brain, blood platelets, and throughout the gastrointestinal tract. Its roles include involvement in CNS neurotransmission, haemostasis, vascular spasm, and gastrointestinal motility. Many drugs have some action on serotonin receptors. Several types and subtypes of serotonin receptors have been identified and drugs with serotonin-agonist activity and those displaying serotonin-antagonist activity may both be used to treat the same condition, as in migraine or depression.

Serotonin itself may be of value in the treatment of posthypoxic myoclonus (p.353). Serotonin *precursors* have been given for the treatment of depression (see Oxitriptan, p.311 and Tryptophan, p.320). *Selective serotonin reuptake inhibitors* are used in depression (see Fluoxetine Hydrochloride, p.292); also *MAOIs* and *tricyclic antidepressants* have some serotonin-agonist activity. *Sumatriptan* (p.471) is an agonist used in migraine.

Among the drugs exhibiting serotonin-antagonist activity are the antimigraine *ergot alkaloids*; *antihistamines* such as cyproheptadine (p.430), and pizotifen (p.470); *antihypertensives* such as ketanserin (p.943); and *antiemetics* such as ondansetron (p.1281). *Other drugs* with recognised serotonin-antagonist activity include fenclonine (p.1687), dexfenfluramine (p.1586), fenfluramine (p.1588), chlorpromazine (p.675), and the tetracyclic antidepressant mianserin (p.306).

Serotonin also occurs in stinging nettles (*Urtica dioica*) (p.1762), bananas, and other fruit, and in the stings of wasps and scorpions.

◊ References.

1. Hindle AT. Recent developments in the physiology and pharmacology of 5-hydroxytryptamine. *Br J Anaesth* 1994; **73:** 395–407.
2. Hoyer D, *et al.* International Union of Pharmacology classification of receptors for 5-hydroxytryptamine (serotonin). *Pharmacol Rev* 1994; **46:** 157–203.

## Serrapeptase *(rINN)*

Serrapeptasa; Serratia Extracellular Proteinase; Serratiopeptidase.
*CAS — 37312-62-2.*

### Profile

Serrapeptase is a proteolytic enzyme derived from *Serratia* spp. It has been taken by mouth for its supposed action in relieving inflammation and oedema associated with trauma, infection, respiratory-tract congestion, or chronic venous insufficiency, in usual doses of 5 to 10 mg (10 000 to 20 000 units) up to three times daily.

◊ References.

1. Tachibana M, *et al.* A multi-centre, double-blind study of serrapeptase versus placebo in post-antrotomy buccal swelling. *Pharmatherapeutica* 1984; **3:** 526–30.
2. Paparella P, *et al.* Serratia peptidase and acute phase protein behavior following vaginal hysterectomy: results of a randomized double-blind, placebo-controlled trial. *Curr Ther Res* 1989; **45:** 664–76.
3. Shimizu H, *et al.* A case of serratiopeptidase-induced subepidermal bullous dermatosis. *Br J Dermatol* 1999; **141:** 1139–40.

### Preparations

**Proprietary Preparations** (details are given in Part 3)
***Arg.:*** Danzen; ***Braz.:*** Danzen†; ***Fr.:*** Dazen; ***Ger.:*** Aniflazym; ***Hong Kong:*** Danzen; Unizen; ***India:*** Bidanzen; Flanzen; Infladase; Kineto; Seraim; ***Ital.:*** Danzen; ***Jpn:*** Dasen; ***Malaysia:*** Danzen; Unizen; ***Mex.:*** Danzen; ***Port.:*** Aniflazime; ***Singapore:*** Danzen; Korzen; Septirose†; Serrazyme; Sinsia; Unizen; ***Thai.:*** Dailat; Danzen; Danzyme; Denzo; Medizyme; Podase; Rodase; Seramed; Serradase; Serrano; Serrao; Serrapep; Serrason; Serrin; Sumidin; Unizen.

## Sesame Oil

Aceite de Ajonjolí; Benne Oil; Gingelly Oil; Oleum Sesami; Refined Sesame Oil; Sésamo, aceite de; Teel Oil.
*CAS — 8008-74-0.*

**Pharmacopoeias.** In *Chin., Eur.* (see p.vi), and *Jpn.* Also in *USNF.*

**Ph. Eur. 5.0** (Sesame Oil, Refined; Sesami Oleum Raffinatum). The fatty oil obtained from the ripe seeds of *Sesamum indicum* by expression or extraction and subsequent refining. It may contain a suitable antioxidant. It is a clear, light yellow, almost colourless liquid. It solidifies to a soft mass at about –4°. Practically insoluble in alcohol; miscible with petroleum spirit. Store in well-filled, airtight containers. Protect from light. Refined sesame oil for use in the manufacture of parenteral dosage forms should be stored under an inert gas in airtight containers.

**USNF 22** (Sesame Oil). The refined fixed oil obtained from the seed of one or more cultivated varieties of *Sesamum indicum* (Pedaliaceae). A pale yellow, practically odourless, oily liquid. Slightly soluble in alcohol; miscible with carbon disulfide, with chloroform, with ether, and with petroleum spirit. Store in airtight containers at a temperature not exceeding 40°. Protect from light.

### Profile

Sesame oil has been used in the preparation of liniments, plasters, ointments, and soaps. Because it is relatively stable, it is a useful solvent and vehicle for parenteral products. Hypersensitivity reactions have been observed.

◊ Reports of hypersensitivity reactions[1-4] and subcutaneous nodules[5] associated with sesame administration.

1. Kanny G, *et al.* Sesame seed and sesame seed oil contain masked allergens of growing importance. *Allergy* 1996; **51:** 952–7.
2. Stern A, Wuthrich B. Non-IgE-mediated anaphylaxis to sesame. *Allergy* 1998; **53:** 325–6.
3. Pecquet C, *et al.* Immediate hypersensitivity to sesame in foods and cosmetics. *Contact Dermatitis* 1998; **39:** 313.
4. Asero R, *et al.* A case of sesame seed-induced anaphylaxis. *Allergy* 1999; **54:** 526–7.
5. Darsow U, *et al.* Subcutaneous oleomas induced by self-injection of sesame seed oil for muscle augmentation. *J Am Acad Dermatol* 2000; **42:** 292–4.

### Preparations

**Proprietary Preparations** (details are given in Part 3)
**Multi-ingredient:** ***NZ:*** Snorenz; ***UK:*** Goodnight StopSnore; Snor-Away; Snorenz†.

## Shellac

E904; Goma laca; Gomme Laque; Lacca; Lacca in Tabulis; Schellack.
*CAS — 9000-59-3.*

**Pharmacopoeias.** In *Eur.* (see p.vi). Also in *USNF.*
*Jpn* includes Purified Shellac and White Shellac (Bleached).

**Ph. Eur. 5.0** (Shellac). It is obtained by purification of the resinous secretion of the female insect *Kerria lacca* (Kerr) Lindinger (*Laccifer lacca* Kerr). There are 4 types of shellac depending on the nature of the treatment of crude secretion (seedlac): Wax-containing Shellac; Bleached Shellac; Dewaxed Shellac; and Bleached, Dewaxed Shellac.

Brownish-orange or yellow, shining, translucent, hard or brittle more or less thin flakes (Wax-containing Shellac; Dewaxed Shellac), or a creamy-white or brownish-yellow powder (Bleached Shellac; Bleached, Dewaxed Shellac).

Practically insoluble in water. With dehydrated alcohol it gives a more or less opalescent solution (Wax-containing Shellac; Bleached Shellac) or a clear solution (Dewaxed Shellac; Bleached, Dewaxed Shellac). When warmed, it is sparingly soluble or soluble in alkaline solutions. Protect from light. Store Bleached Shellac and Bleached, Dewaxed Shellac at a temperature not exceeding 15°.

**USNF 22** (Shellac). It is obtained by purification of lac, the resinous secretion of the insect *Laccifer lacca kerr* (Coccidae). There are 4 varieties: Orange Shellac, Dewaxed Orange Shellac, Regular Bleached (White) Shellac, and Refined Bleached Shellac. Orange Shellac occurs as thin, hard, brittle, transparent, pale lemon-yellow to brownish-orange flakes, having little or no odour. Bleached Shellac occurs as opaque, amorphous, cream to yellow granules or coarse powder, having little or no odour.

Insoluble in water; very slowly soluble in alcohol, 85 to 95% (w/w); soluble in ether, 13 to 15%, in petroleum spirit, 2 to 6%, in benzene, 10 to 20%, and in aqueous solutions of ethanolamines, alkalis, and borax; sparingly soluble in turpentine oil. Store preferably at a temperature not exceeding 8°.

### Profile

Shellac is used as an enteric coating for pills and tablets, but disintegration time has been reported to increase markedly on storage.

### Preparations

**USNF 22:** Pharmaceutical Glaze.

## Shepherd's Purse

Bolsa de pastor; Capsella; Herba Bursae Pastoris; Shepherds Burse Herb.

**Pharmacopoeias.** In *Fr.*

### Profile

Shepherd's purse, the aerial parts of *Capsella bursa-pastoris* (*Thlaspi bursa-pastoris*) (Cruciferae) has antihaemorrhagic and astringent properties. It is used to prevent or arrest bleeding, and has been specifically used for menorrhagia. It is also used for urinary-tract disorders and diarrhoea.

It is also used in homoeopathic medicine.

### Preparations

**Proprietary Preparations** (details are given in Part 3)
***Ger.:*** Styptysat.

**Multi-ingredient:** ***Austria:*** Menodoron; ***Fr.:*** Hemoluol†; Histo-Fluine P; Tisanes de l'Abbe Hamon no 14†; ***Ger.:*** Bomagall forte S†; Presselin Dysmen Olin 3 N†; Rhoival; ***Spain:*** Proctosor; ***UK:*** Antitis; Sciargo.

## Siam Benzoin

Benjoin du Laos; Benjuí de Siam; Benzoe Tonkinensis.
*CAS — 9000-72-0.*

**Pharmacopoeias.** In *Chin., Fr., It.,* and *Swiss.* Also in many pharmacopoeias under the title benzoin and should not be confused with Sumatra benzoin. *Jpn* and *US* allow both Siam benzoin and Sumatra benzoin under the title Benzoin.

**USP 27** (Benzoin). A balsamic resin from *Styrax tonkinensis*, or other species of the *Anthostyrax* section of the genus *Styrax* (Styracaceae). It yields not less than 90% of alcohol-soluble extractive. It occurs as pebble-like tears of variable size and shape, compressed, yellowish-brown to rusty brown externally, milky white on fracture, separate or very slightly agglutinated, hard and brittle at ordinary temperatures but softened by heat. It has an agreeable, balsamic, vanilla-like odour.

### Profile

Siam benzoin has been used similarly to Sumatra benzoin (p.1751). It has also been used as a preservative and was formerly used in the preparation of benzoinated lard.

### Preparations

***USP 27:*** Compound Benzoin Tincture; Podophyllum Resin Topical Solution.

**Proprietary Preparations** (details are given in Part 3)

**Multi-ingredient:** ***Braz.:*** Dermol; ***Canad.:*** Cold Sore Lotion†; ***Fr.:*** Balsolene; Borostyrol; Homeoplasmine; Inotyol; ***Israel:*** Inotyol; Kank-A; ***Ital.:*** Ondroly-A; ***Switz.:*** Borostyrol N.

## Siberian Ginseng

*Acanthopanax senticosus*; *Eleutherococcus senticosus* (Araliaceae); Ciwujia; Eleuthero.

NOTE. The name Russian Ginseng has been applied to *Eleutherococcus senticosus*.
The name Ginseng usually refers to *Panax ginseng* and related species (see p.1693).
Some material supplied as Siberian ginseng may be *Periploca sepium* (Asclepiadaceae), a plant unrelated to *Eleutherococcus senticosus*, due to the similarity of the Chinese names for these plants.

**Pharmacopoeias.** In *Chin.* and *Eur.* (see p.vi). Also in *USNF.*
**Ph. Eur. 5.0** (Eleutherococcus; Eleutherococci Radix). The dried, whole or cut underground organs of *Eleutherococcus senticosus*. It contains not less than 0.08% for the sum of eleutheroside B and eleutheroside E.

**USNF 22** (Eleuthero). The dried rhizome with roots of *Eleutherococus senticosus* (Araliaceae) (*Acanthopanax senticosus*) (Araliaceae). It contains not less than 0.08% of the sum of eleutheroside B and eleutheroside E, calculated on the dried basis. Protect from light.

### Profile

Siberian ginseng is reported to enhance natural resistance and to improve performance under stress. It is used similarly to ginseng (*Panax ginseng*) (see p.1693) although the constituents of the two herbs are different. It is also used in traditional Chinese medicine.

◊ Reviews.

1. Davydov M, Krikorian AD. Eleutherococcus sentiosus (Rupr. & Maxim.) Maxim. (Araliaceae) as an adaptogen: a closer look. *J Ethnopharmacol* 2000; **72:** 345–93.

**Interactions.** For a report of raised serum-digoxin concentrations in a patient taking *digoxin* and Siberian ginseng, see Interference with Digoxin Assays, p.896.

### Preparations

**Proprietary Preparations** (details are given in Part 3)
***Ger.:*** Eleu; Eleu-Kokk; Eleu-Twardypharm; Eleutheroforce; Eleutherokokk; Eleutherokokk-Aktiv-Kapseln SenticoMega†; Konstitutin; Lebensenergie-Kapseln; Vital-Kapseln; ***Switz.:*** Eleu-Kokk†; ***UK:*** Elagen.

**Multi-ingredient:** ***Austral.:*** Bioglan Ginsynergy†; Gingo A†; Ginkgo Biloba Plus†; Medinat Esten†; Tyroseng†; ***Chile:*** Gingo-Ther; ***Ital.:*** Enertonic†; Fon Wan Eleuthero; Nosenil†; Nutrex†; ***Spain:*** Energysor; Esforza; Natusor Low Blood Pressure; Tonimax.

## Sildenafil Citrate *(BANM, USAN, rINNM)*

Citrato de sildenafilo; UK-92480-10. 5-[2-Ethoxy-5-(4-methylpiperazin-1-ylsulfonyl)phenyl]-1,6-dihydro-1-methyl-3-propylpyrazolo[4,3-*d*]pyrimidin-7-one citrate; 1-{[3-(6,7-Dihydro-1-methyl-7-oxo-3-propyl-1*H*-pyrazolo[4,3-*d*]pyrimidin-5-yl)-4-ethoxyphenyl]sulfonyl}-4-methylpiperazone citrate.
$C_{22}H_{30}N_6O_4S,C_6H_8O_7 = 666.7.$
*CAS — 139755-83-2 (sildenafil); 171599-83-0 (sildenafil citrate).*
*ATC — G04BE03.*

### Adverse Effects

Adverse effects most commonly reported from sildenafil are headache, flushing, and dyspepsia. There may be visual disturbances, dizziness, and nasal congestion. Other adverse effects reported include diarrhoea, vomiting, swelling of the eyelids, pain and redness of the eyes, muscle pain, skin rashes, and urinary-tract infection. Priapism has also occurred. There have also been reports of palpitations and serious cardiovascular events, including sudden cardiac death, associated with the use of sildenafil.

◊ Reviews.

1. Vitezic D. A risk-benefit assessment of sildenafil in the treatment of erectile dysfunction. *Drug Safety* 2001; **24:** 255–65.
2. Padma-nathan H, *et al.* A 4-year update on the safety of sildenafil citrate (Viagra). *Urology* 2002; **60** (suppl 2): 67–90.

**Convulsions.** A report[1] of 2 patients who experienced a first tonic-clonic seizure shortly after taking sildenafil.

1. Gilad R, *et al.* Tonic-clonic seizures in patients taking sildenafil. *BMJ* 2002; **325:** 869.

**Effects on the cardiovascular system.** There has been considerable uncertainty about the potential cardiovascular risk associated with sildenafil treatment. Minor effects associated with vasodilatation, such as headache and flushing are relatively common, but in patients without pre-existing cardiovascular risk factors the risk of serious cardiovascular events associated with the drug appears to be low. However, there has been a report of myocardial infarction in a patient who had no apparent risk factors,[1] and a consensus document issued by the American College of Cardiology and the American Heart Association (ACC/AHA) has pointed out that patients with erectile dysfunction are mostly over 45 years of age and are more likely to have risk factors predisposing them to cardiovascular disease.[2] As of November 1998, 130 deaths in US patients taking sildenafil had been reported to the FDA; 3 of these were due to stroke and 77 to some other cardiovascular event.[3] The nature of the relationship between drug and event was considered unclear, but some of these patients were also receiving nitrates, a combination now contra-indicated because of the greatly increased risk of potentially life-threatening hypotension.[2] The Australian Adverse Drug Reactions Advisory Committee[4] stated in June 2002 that it had received 773 reports of adverse reactions associated with the use of sildenafil. There were 20 reports of myocardial infarction, including 4 fatalities; 9 of these 20 patients had pre-existing cardiovascular disease or diabetes or were considered to be at high risk of cardiovascular disease, and 1 patient was taking nitrates. Other cardiovascular effects reported included 26 reports of chest pain and 10 other fatalities (6 sudden unexplained deaths, 2 strokes, and 2 subarachnoid haemorrhages). However, it was pointed out that the timing of these adverse effects in relation to sildenafil ingestion was often not reported and that, since sildenafil is taken in the context of sexual activity and, in some cases, underlying coronary disease, the contribution of sildenafil to cardiac events was difficult to assess.

It is still uncertain whether patients with **pre-existing** cardiovascular disease are at increased risk when taking sildenafil without concomitant nitrates. The ACC/AHA consensus statement noted that the evidence was scanty and suggested that sildenafil could be used, but with caution, in patients with stable coronary artery disease provided that nitrates were not taken.[2] Evidence to assess the risk in other cardiovascular disorders is even less extensive, although a case report of a patient with hypertrophic cardiomyopathy who experienced cardiovascular adverse effects following a dose of sildenafil suggested that the drug may precipitate an unstable haemodynamic state in this condition.[5] A later review,[6] however, concluded that sildenafil appeared to be well tolerated in most patients with chronic stable cardiovascular disease.

1. Feenstra J, *et al.* Acute myocardial infarction associated with sildenafil. *Lancet* 1998; **352:** 957–8.
2. Cheitlin MD, *et al.* Use of sildenafil (Viagra) in patients with cardiovascular disease. ACC/AHA Expert Consensus Document. *J Am Coll Cardiol* 1999; **33:** 273–82. Correction. *ibid.*; **34:** 1850.
3. US Food and Drug Administration. Postmarketing safety of sildenafil citrate (Viagra): summary of reports of death in Viagra users received from marketing (late March) through mid-November 1998. Available at: http://www.fda.gov/cder/consumerinfo/viagra/safety3.htm (accessed 08/07/04)
4. Adverse Drug Reactions Advisory Committee (ADRAC). Sildenafil—three years experience. *Aust Adverse Drug React Bull* 2002; **21:** 6. Also available at: http://www.tga.health.gov.au/docs/html/aadrbltn/aadr0206.htm (accessed 08/07/04)
5. Stauffer J-C, *et al.* Subaortic obstruction after sildenafil in a patient with hypertrophic cardiomyopathy. *N Engl J Med* 1999; **341:** 700–701.
6. Tran D, Howes LG. Cardiovascular safety of sildenafil. *Drug Safety* 2003; **26:** 453–60.

**Effects on the eyes.** The Australian Adverse Drug Reactions Advisory Committee[1] stated in June 2002 that it had received 65 reports of abnormal vision from a total of 773 adverse reactions associated with use of sildenafil reported over 3 years. A bluish tinge or haze to vision and some increased light sensitivity has been reported by patients taking sildenafil, with the percentage of reports increasing with increasing dose.[2] The visual symptoms usually peak after 1 to 2 hours following ingestion and resolve about 3 to 4 hours later. The effects of a single dose of sildenafil 100 mg were studied in 5 healthy volunteers.[3] Electroretinogram measurements showed significant changes that correlated well with plasma-sildenafil concentrations, peaking at 1 hour after administration and showing complete recovery at the 6-hour measurements. Inhibition of phosphodiesterase type-6 in rod photoreceptors is the most likely mechanism of sildenafil-associated retinal dysfunction. However, there is as yet no clear evidence of retinal toxic effects or whether repeated dosing with sildenafil causes prolonged or further retinal dysfunction.[2,3] Likewise, it remains to be determined whether recovery of function as plasma-sildenafil concentrations subside also occurs in older patients or those with retinal degenerative disorders such as retinitis pigmentosa.

Other visual disturbances reported in patients taking sildenafil have included temporary loss of vision and increased intra-ocular pressure.[4] A 69-year-old man who experienced permanent loss of vision in one eye a few hours after taking sildenafil 100 mg was found to have an occlusion in a retinal artery.[5] Several cases of nonarteritic anterior ischaemic optic neuropathy associated with sildenafil use have also been reported.[6,7]

1. Adverse Drug Reactions Advisory Committee (ADRAC). Sildenafil—three years experience. *Aust Adverse Drug React Bull* 2002; **21:** 6. Also available at: http://www.tga.health.gov.au/docs/html/aadrbltn/aadr0206.htm (accessed 08/07/04)
2. Marmor MF. Sildenafil (Viagra) and ophthalmology. *Arch Ophthalmol* 1999; **117:** 518–19.
3. Vobig MA, *et al.* Retinal side-effects of sildenafil. *Lancet* 1999; **353:** 375.
4. Committee on Safety of Medicines/Medicines Control Agency. Sildenafil (Viagra). *Current Problems* 1999; **25:** 16. Also available at: http://www.mca.gov.uk/ourwork/monitorsafequalmed/currentproblems/volume25nov.htm (accessed 08/07/04)
5. Tripathi A, O'Donnell N. Branch retinal artery occlusion; another complication of sildenafil. *Br J Ophthalmol* 2000; **84:** 934–5.
6. Boshier A, *et al.* A case of nonarteritic ischemic optic neuropathy (NAION) in a male patient taking sildenafil. *Int J Clin Pharmacol Ther* 2002; **40:** 422–3.
7. Pomeranz HD, *et al.* Sildenafil-associated nonarteritic anterior ischemic optic neuropathy. *Ophthalmology* 2002; **109:** 584–7.

### Precautions

Caution is required in patients with hepatic or severe renal impairment, and dosage reduction of sildenafil may be necessary. Care is also needed in patients with anatomical or haematological disorders which may predispose them to priapism. Patients who experience dizziness or visual disturbances should not drive or operate hazardous machinery.

The safety of sildenafil is uncertain in patients with severe hepatic impairment, bleeding disorders, active peptic ulceration, hypotension, a recent history of stroke, myocardial infarction, or life-threatening arrhythmia, unstable angina, heart failure, or retinal disorders such as retinitis pigmentosa (a minority of whom have genetic disorders of retinal phosphodiesterases). The manufacturers advise that it should not be used in these groups.

**Cardiovascular disease.** For mention of a consensus statement on the use of sildenafil in patients with cardiovascular disease, see above.

### Interactions

Sildenafil or other phosphodiesterase type-5 inhibitors may potentiate the hypotensive effects of organic nitrates, and are therefore contra-indicated in patients receiving such drugs. Standard doses of sildenafil should not be given within 4 hours of an alpha blocker as such use may lead to symptomatic hypotension; similarly an interval of 6 hours is recommended with vardenafil; use of tadalafil with an alpha blocker is not recommended. Sildenafil may also enhance the hypotensive effect of nicorandil and use of the two drugs together should be avoided. Use of sildenafil with drugs that inhibit the cytochrome P450 isoenzyme CYP3A4, such as cimetidine, erythromycin, itraconazole, ketoconazole, and HIV-protease inhibitors, may reduce sildenafil clearance necessitating a reduction in dosage. Furthermore, plasma concentrations of sildenafil are significantly increased by ritonavir, requiring even greater dosage reduction, and these two drugs should not be given together unless absolutely essential. Grapefruit juice should be avoided with sildenafil or other phosphodiesterase type-5 inhibitors as it may increase their plasma concentrations.

**Antivirals.** Rises in sildenafil concentrations after administration of *saquinavir* or *ritonavir* were consistent[1] with inhibition of metabolism mediated by the cytochrome P450 isoenzyme CYP3A4. The larger increases seen with ritonavir may be due to its additional inhibition of the isoenzyme CYP2C9. Fatal myocardial infarction has been reported[2] in a 47-year-old patient who took sildenafil 25 mg with ritonavir and saquinavir.

1. Muirhead GJ, *et al.* Pharmacokinetic interactions between sildenafil and saquinavir/ritonavir. *Br J Pharmacol* 2000; **50:** 99–107.
2. Hall MCS, Ahmad S. Interaction between sildenafil and HIV-1 combination therapy. *Lancet* 1999; **353:** 2071–2.

**Dihydrocodeine.** The use of dihydrocodeine with sildenafil was associated with priapism in 2 men who had previously been treated successfully with sildenafil.[1] The first patient had two prolonged erections, lasting 4 and 5 hours, and the effect did not recur when the dihydrocodeine was stopped. The second patient experienced priapism on 3 occasions in the first week of dihydrocodeine treatment, but not in the subsequent 2 weeks despite continuing both drugs.

1. Goldmeier D, Lamba H. Prolonged erections produced by dihydrocodeine and sildenafil. *BMJ* 2002; **324:** 1555.

**Food.** Grapefruit juice has been shown to increase bioavailability but delay absorption of sildenafil in healthy subjects.[1]

1. Jetter A, *et al.* Effects of grapefruit juice on the pharmacokinetics of sildenafil. *Clin Pharmacol Ther* 2002; **71:** 21–9.

**Nitrates.** Administration of sildenafil 50 mg to patients receiving isosorbide mononitrate or glyceryl trinitrate 1 hour after sildenafil, resulted in substantially greater decreases in blood pressure than when the nitrate was administered alone in 2 crossover studies in patients with angina.[1] Treatment-related adverse effects were reported in 8 of 16 patients who took sildenafil with isosorbide mononitrate and 3 of 15 who received sildenafil with glyceryl trinitrate. The authors confirmed that sildenafil should not be taken with nitrates.

1. Webb DJ, *et al.* Sildenafil citrate potentiates the hypotensive effects of nitric oxide donor drugs in male patients with stable angina. *J Am Coll Cardiol* 2000; **36:** 25–31.

## Pharmacokinetics

Sildenafil is rapidly absorbed after a dose by mouth, with a bioavailability of approximately 40%. Peak plasma concentrations are attained within 30 to 120 minutes; the rate of absorption is reduced when sildenafil is given with food.

Sildenafil is widely distributed into tissues and is approximately 96% bound to plasma proteins. It is metabolised in the liver primarily by cytochrome P450 isoenzymes CYP3A4 (the major route) and CYP2C9. The major metabolite, *N*-desmethylsildenafil, also has some activity. The terminal half-lives of sildenafil and the *N*-desmethyl metabolite are about 4 hours.

Sildenafil is excreted as metabolites, predominantly in the faeces, and to a lesser extent the urine. Clearance may be reduced in the elderly and in patients with hepatic or severe renal impairment.

◊ References.

1. Muirhead GJ, *et al.* Pharmacokinetics of sildenafil (VIAGRA™), a selective cGMP PDE5 inhibitor, after single oral doses in fasted and fed healthy volunteers. *Br J Clin Pharmacol* 1996; **42:** 268P.
2. Muirhead GJ, *et al.* The effects of age and renal and hepatic impairment on the pharmacokinetics of sildenafil. *Br J Clin Pharmacol* 2002; **53** (suppl 1): 21S–30S.

## Uses and Administration

Sildenafil is a phosphodiesterase type-5 inhibitor used in the management of erectile dysfunction (see below). It is given by mouth as the citrate although doses are expressed in terms of the base. The usual dose is 50 mg about one hour before sexual intercourse. The dose may be increased or decreased depending on response. The maximum recommended dose is 100 mg, and sildenafil should not be taken more than once in 24 hours. An initial dose of 25 mg is recommended in elderly patients; for doses in hepatic and renal impairment, see below. An initial dose of no more than 25 mg daily is also advised in patients taking sildenafil with inhibitors of cytochrome P450 isoenzyme CYP3A4; the manufacturers advise that the dose should not exceed 25 mg every 48 hours if given with ritonavir, although such a combination is best avoided entirely (see under Interactions, above). Standard doses should not be taken within 4 hours of an alpha blocker because of the risk of symptomatic hypotension.

◊ References.

1. Goldstein I, *et al.* Oral sildenafil in the treatment of erectile dysfunction. *N Engl J Med* 1998; **338:** 1397–1404. Correction. *ibid.*; **339:** 59.
2. Anonymous. Sildenafil: an oral drug for impotence. *Med Lett Drugs Ther* 1998; **40:** 51–2.
3. Anonymous. Sildenafil for erectile dysfunction. *Drug Ther Bull* 1998; **36:** 81–4.
4. Derry FA, *et al.* Efficacy and safety of oral sildenafil (Viagra) in men with erectile dysfunction caused by spinal cord injury. *Neurology* 1998; **51:** 1629–33.
5. Langtry HD, Markham A. Sildenafil: a review of its use in erectile dysfunction. *Drugs* 1999; **57:** 967–89.
6. Montorsi F, *et al.* Efficacy and safety of fixed-dose oral sildenafil in the treatment of erectile dysfunction of various etiologies. *Urology* 1999; **53:** 1011–18.
7. Rendell MS, *et al.* Sildenafil for treatment of erectile dysfunction in men with diabetes: a randomized controlled trial. *JAMA* 1999; **281:** 421–6.
8. Kedia S, *et al.* Treatment of erectile dysfunction with sildenafil citrate (Viagra) after radiation therapy for prostate cancer. *Urology* 1999; **54:** 308–12.
9. Zippe CD, *et al.* Role of Viagra after radical prostatectomy. *Urology* 2000; **55:** 241–5.
10. Fink HA, *et al.* Sildenafil for male erectile dysfunction: a systematic review and meta-analysis. *Arch Intern Med* 2002; **162:** 1349–60.

**Administration in hepatic impairment.** An initial dose of 25 mg of sildenafil is recommended in patients with hepatic impairment.

**Administration in renal impairment.** An initial dose of 25 mg of sildenafil is recommended in patients with renal impairment (creatinine clearance less than 30 mL/minute).

**Erectile dysfunction.** Erectile dysfunction (impotence) signifies inability of a male to achieve satisfactory erection of the penis during sexual intercourse. Estimates of prevalence depend to some extent upon the definitions that are used, but the problem is thought to be not uncommon, particularly in older men. The causes of erectile dysfunction may be psychological, organic, or a combination of both. Psychological factors include stress, mental depression, and anxieties about sexual performance. Organic causes include androgen deficiency as a result of hypogonadism, neurological dysfunction (including central or peripheral lesions due to malignancy or trauma), peripheral vascular disorders, and penile abnormalities such as Peyronie's disease or microphallus. Sometimes organic dysfunction may be secondary to another disease, such as diabetes mellitus in which neurological and vascular damage lead to erectile dysfunction in over one-third of all patients. In addition, erectile dysfunction may be drug-induced.

Approaches to the management of erectile dysfunction depend to some extent upon the causative factors.

In those few patients in whom erectile dysfunction is secondary to androgen deficiency in hypogonadism, androgen replacement, preferably by the intramuscular injection or transdermal application of a suitable testosterone ester, may be of value. Androgen replacement therapy is inappropriate in patients with normal testosterone concentrations and may carry significant health risks. In patients with hypogonadism secondary to hyperprolactinaemia addition of bromocriptine is often effective in improving sexual function.

Psychotherapy or behavioural therapy alone may be adequate in patients in whom no organic cause is detected, but even when organic factors play a role psychosocial factors are also important and should be addressed by appropriate counselling.

When causes of erectile dysfunction are partly or primarily organic, the main options are:

- use of a vacuum pump to induce erection by negative pressure, followed by constriction of the base of the penis with a band to maintain tumescence
- oral or sublingual therapy
- injection of vasoactive substances into the corpora cavernosa
- transurethral administration of vasoactive substances
- implantation of a penile prosthesis is generally reserved for patients in whom other therapy has failed or is refused, but it may also be a suitable first-line choice for some patients

Vascular surgery may have a limited application, in vasogenic dysfunction, but its role is not clearly defined and there are some doubts about its long-term effectiveness.

**Oral therapy** for erectile dysfunction has had a chequered history, and most of the drugs tried have proved little more effective than placebo. However, with the advent of sildenafil and other inhibitors of phosphodiesterase type-5, oral therapy is now established in erectile dysfunction. Data from randomised controlled trials have shown efficacy of sildenafil in erectile dysfunction compared with placebo, including in men with diabetes mellitus and spinal-cord injury; it has no effect on the penis in the absence of sexual stimulation. It is generally more effective in erectile dysfunction of psychogenic origin and in mild to moderate cases of organic origin. There has, however, been concern about cardiac-related deaths associated with the use of sildenafil, although causality has not been firmly established. Visual disturbances have also been reported. Other phosphodiesterase type-5 inhibitors also used are tadalafil and vardenafil.

Yohimbine, an $\alpha_2$-adrenoceptor antagonist, may have some benefit, although more in erectile dysfunction of psychological than organic origin. Oral phentolamine is available for the treatment of erectile dysfunction in some countries and has been reported to be of benefit. Trazodone, a serotonin antagonist and reuptake inhibitor used in the treatment of depression, may rarely cause priapism and has therefore been investigated for the treatment of erectile dysfunction. Beneficial effects have been reported either alone or with yohimbine. Oral L-arginine, the precursor of nitric oxide, has also shown some promise in studies.

**Sublingual** apomorphine, a dopaminergic ($D_1$ or $D_2$) agonist, has also demonstrated efficacy, but nausea may be a problem.

**Intracavernosal injection** therapy is the most effective pharmacological method of treating erectile dysfunction and, until the advent of effective oral therapy, was the most widely used. Unfortunately, one major disadvantage of this method is the need for repeated self-injection of the penis, and studies suggest that the long-term drop-out rate is high. However, it is still a valuable option in men unresponsive to, or unable to take, oral therapy. The drugs most commonly used for intracavernosal injection therapy are alprostadil, papaverine, and phentolamine. Alprostadil is the preferred drug because it is superior in efficacy to papaverine (with or without phentolamine), and is associated with a lower incidence of priapism and fibrosis. However, the erection is frequently painful. Papaverine, a non-specific phosphodiesterase inhibitor, has been used alone or in combination with phentolamine, an α-adrenoceptor antagonist. Erectile dysfunction of neurogenic or psychogenic origin generally responds better to papaverine than dysfunction of vascular origin. However, long-term use of intracavernosal papaverine may result in fibrosis, and it has been suggested that it should not be used more than three times a week or on two successive days. Priapism may also be a problem. Triple therapy, involving the combination of alprostadil, papaverine, and phentolamine, has been reported to be effective and to have a relatively low incidence of adverse effects. Other drugs that have been used for intracavernosal therapy include aviptadil, a smooth muscle relaxant used with phentolamine, ketanserin used with alprostadil, and moxisylyte.

The **transurethral route** is a less invasive but also less effective option than intracavernosal therapy. A transurethral pellet of alprostadil is reported to be effective, although efficacy is inconsistent; common side-effects include penile pain and urethral pain or burning. Transurethral alprostadil as a cream or gel has also shown promise.

A number of studies have also investigated **transcutaneous** therapy. Results from pilot studies investigating transcutaneous delivery of glyceryl trinitrate, papaverine, minoxidil, or alprostadil from creams, gels, or pastes have been variable. Topical treatment with a cream containing co-dergocrine mesilate, isosorbide dinitrate, and either aminophylline or testosterone has also been tried, with mixed results.

References.

1. Dinsmore W, Evans C. ABC of sexual health: Erectile dysfunction. *BMJ* 1999; **318:** 387–90.
2. Burnett AL. Oral pharmacotherapy for erectile dysfunction: current perspectives. *Urology* 1999; **54:** 392–400.
3. Meinhardt W, *et al.* Comparative tolerability and efficacy of treatments for impotence. *Drug Safety* 1999; **20:** 133–46.
4. Langford N. Adverse reactions to drugs used for erectile dysfunction. *Adverse Drug React Bull* 1999; (Apr): 743–6.
5. Nehra A, *et al.* Pharmacotherapeutic advances in the treatment of erectile dysfunction. *Mayo Clin Proc* 1999; **74:** 709–21.
6. Cummings MH, Alexander WD. Erectile dysfunction in patients with diabetes. *Hosp Med* 1999; **60:** 638–44.
7. Morgentaler A. Male impotence. *Lancet* 1999; **354:** 1713–18.
8. Williams G. Male erectile dysfunction. *Prescribers' J* 2000; **40:** 49–58.
9. Lue TF. Erectile dysfunction. *N Engl J Med* 2000; **342:** 1802–13.
10. Wespes E, *et al.* European Association of Urology. Guidelines on erectile dysfunction. *Eur Urol* 2002; **41:** 1–5. Also available at: http://www.uroweb.nl/files/uploaded_files/guidelines/updateEdysfunction.pdf (accessed 08/07/04)
11. Guay AT, *et al.* American Association of Clinical Endocrinologists medical guidelines for clinical practice for the evaluation and treatment of male sexual dysfunction: a couple's problem—2003 update. *Endocr Pract* 2003; **9:** 77–95. Also available at: http://www.aace.com/clin/guidelines/sexdysguid.pdf (accessed 08/07/04)

**Oesophageal motility disorders.** Preliminary studies[1-3] have investigated the use of sildenafil in patients with oesophageal motility disorders (p.1246) such as achalasia or nutcracker oesophagus. Although some benefit has been reported, further studies are needed.

1. Bortolotti M, *et al.* Effects of sildenafil on esophageal motility of patients with idiopathic achalasia. *Gastroenterology* 2000; **118:** 253–7.
2. Eherer AJ, *et al.* Effect of sildenafil on oesophageal motor function in healthy subjects and patients with oesophageal motor disorders. *Gut* 2002; **50:** 758–64.
3. Lee JI, *et al.* The effect of sildenafil on oesophageal motor function in healthy subjects and patients with nutcracker oesophagus. *Neurogastroenterol Motil* 2003; **15:** 617–23.

**Premature ejaculation.** Early reports have suggested that sildenafil may be effective in the management of premature ejaculation and the rationale for such use has been reviewed.[1]

1. Abdel-Hamid IA. Phosphodiesterase 5 inhibitors in rapid ejaculation: potential use and possible mechanisms of action. *Drugs* 2004; **64:** 13–26.

**Priapism.** Sildenafil has been reported to be effective in the treatment of priapism in 3 patients with sickle-cell disease.[1] In 2 of these patients, sildenafil was also successful in preventing further episodes of priapism when it was taken at the onset of symptoms.

1. Bialecki ES. Sildenafil relieves priapism in patients with sickle cell disease. *Am J Med* 2002; **113:** 252.

**Pulmonary hypertension.** Oral sildenafil, either alone[1-5] or with inhaled iloprost[1] or inhaled nitric oxide,[6] has produced beneficial responses in patients with primary or secondary pulmonary hypertension (p.832).

1. Ghofrani HA, *et al.* Combination therapy with oral sildenafil and inhaled iloprost for severe pulmonary hypertension. *Ann Intern Med* 2002; **136:** 515–22.
2. Ghofrani HA, *et al.* Sildenafil for treatment of lung fibrosis and pulmonary hypertension: a randomised controlled trial. *Lancet* 2002; **360:** 895–900.
3. Watanabe H, *et al.* Sildenafil for primary and secondary pulmonary hypertension. *Clin Pharmacol Ther* 2002; **71:** 398–402.
4. Carroll WD, Dhillon R. Sildenafil as a treatment for pulmonary hypertension. *Arch Dis Child* 2003; **88:** 827–8.
5. Sastry BKS, *et al.* Clinical efficacy of sildenafil in primary pulmonary hypertension: a randomized, placebo-controlled, double-blind, crossover study. *J Am Coll Cardiol* 2004; **43:** 1149–53.
6. Michelakis E, *et al.* Oral sildenafil is an effective and specific pulmonary vasodilator in patients with pulmonary arterial hypertension: comparison with inhaled nitric oxide. *Circulation* 2002; **105:** 2398–2403.

## Preparations

**Proprietary Preparations** (details are given in Part 3)

***Arg.:*** Anaus; Bifort; File; Firmel; Lumix; Magnus; Segurex; Sildefil; Vimax; Vorst; ***Austral.:*** Viagra; ***Austria:*** Viagra; ***Belg.:*** Viagra; ***Braz.:*** Viagra; ***Canad.:*** Viagra; ***Chile:*** Alfin; Dirtop; Erosfil; Helpin; Ripol; Seler; ***Denm.:*** Viagra; ***Fin.:*** Viagra; ***Fr.:*** Viagra; ***Ger.:*** Viagra; ***Gr.:*** Viagra; ***Hong Kong:*** Viagra; ***India:*** Caverta; Penegra; ***Irl.:*** Viagra; ***Israel:*** Viagra; ***Ital.:*** Viagra; ***Jpn:*** Viagra; ***Malaysia:*** Viagra; ***Mex.:*** Viagra; ***Norw.:*** Viagra; ***NZ:*** Viagra;

**Port.:** Viagra; **S.Afr.:** Viagra; **Singapore:** Viagra; **Spain:** Viagra; **Swed.:** Viagra; **Switz.:** Viagra; **Thai.:** Viagra; **UK:** Viagra; **USA:** Viagra.

## Silver

E174; Plata.

Ag = 107.8682.

*CAS — 7440-22-4.*

*ATC — D08AL30.*

**Pharmacopoeias.** In *Swiss*.

### Profile

Silver is a pure white, malleable and ductile metal. It possesses antibacterial properties and is used topically either as the metal or as silver salts. It is not absorbed to any great extent and the main problem associated with the metal is argyria, a grey discoloration of the tissues. Silver is also present as the core in some copper-wound plastic intra-uterine contraceptive devices. Silver is used as a colouring agent for some types of confectionery. It is also used as Argentum Metallicum in homoeopathy.

Numerous salts or compounds of silver have been used therapeutically, including silver acetate (p.1746), silver allantoinate and silver zinc allantoinate, silver borate, silver carbonate, silver chloride, silver chromate, silver glycerolate, colloidal silver iodide, silver lactate, silver manganite, silver nitrate (p.1746), silver-nylon polymers, silver protein (p.1746), and sulfadiazine silver (p.259).

**Catheter care.** The benefits of silver coated or impregnated catheters in preventing or reducing urinary-tract infection are uncertain, and studies have provided conflicting evidence. Some[1] consider that the benefits are statistically insignificant. However, a meta-analysis[2] involving 8 trials with a total of 2355 patients concluded, despite some concerns about the quality and heterogeneity of the studies, that there was a benefit, but that silver alloy coated catheters were significantly more effective in preventing urinary-tract infections than were those coated with silver oxide.

1. Reiche T, *et al.* A prospective, controlled, randomized study of the effect of a slow-release silver device on the frequency of urinary tract infection in newly catheterized patients. *BJU Int* 2000; **85:** 54–9.
2. Saint S, *et al.* The efficacy of silver alloy-coated urinary catheters in preventing urinary tract infection: a meta-analysis. *Am J Med* 1998; **105:** 236–41.

### Preparations

**Proprietary Preparations** (details are given in Part 3)
**Austral.:** Micropur†; **Braz.:** Ultradina†; **Denm.:** CuNova T†; **Fr.:** Micropur; **Ital.:** Katomed; **UK:** Avance; Contreet.

**Multi-ingredient: Arg.:** Efodil; **Canad.:** Nova-T; **Chile:** Nova-T; **Fr.:** Actisorb Plus; Nova-T; Oligorhine; **Ger.:** Actisorb Silver; Grune Salbe "Schmidt" N†; Nova-T; **Hong Kong:** Nova-T; **Irl.:** Actisorb Silver; **Israel:** Nova-T; **Ital.:** Actisorb Plus; Agipiu; Katoxyn; Nova-T; Vulnopur; **Malaysia:** Nova-T; **Mex.:** Nova-T; **Neth.:** Nova-T; **NZ:** Nova-T; **S.Afr.:** Nova-T; **Singapore:** Nova-T; **Spain:** Argentocromo; **Switz.:** Argent; Gyrosan; Nova-T; **Thai.:** Nova-T; **UK:** Actisorb Silver; Nova-T†.

## Silver Acetate

Argenti Acetas; Plata, acetato de.

$C_2H_3AgO_2$ = 166.9.

*CAS — 563-63-3.*

### Profile

Silver acetate has been used similarly to silver nitrate as an antiseptic. It has also been used in antismoking preparations.

**Smoking cessation.** References.

1. Lancaster T, Stead LF. Silver acetate for smoking cessation. Available in The Cochrane Library; Issue 2. Chichester: John Wiley; 2004.

### Preparations

**Proprietary Preparations** (details are given in Part 3)
**Canad.:** Smokerette†.

## Silver Nitrate

Argenti Nitras; Nitrato de Plata; Nitrato de Prata; Plata, nitrato de.

$AgNO_3$ = 169.9.

*CAS — 7761-88-8.*

*ATC — D08AL01.*

**Pharmacopoeias.** In *Eur.* (see p.vi), *Int., Jpn, Pol., US,* and *Viet.*

**Ph. Eur. 5.0** (Silver Nitrate). A white crystalline powder or transparent colourless crystals. Very soluble in water; soluble in alcohol. Store in nonmetallic containers. Protect from light.

**USP 27** (Silver Nitrate). Colourless or white crystals. On exposure to light in the presence of organic matter, it becomes grey or greyish-black. Soluble 1 in 0.4 of water, 1 in 0.1 of boiling water, 1 in 30 of alcohol, and 1 in 6.5 of boiling alcohol; slightly soluble in ether. Its solutions in water have a pH of about 5.5. Store in airtight containers. Protect from light.

**Incompatibility.** Silver nitrate is incompatible with a range of substances. Although it is unlikely that there will be a need to add any of the interacting substances to silver nitrate solutions considering its current uses, pharmacists should be aware of the potential for incompatibility.

The reported yellow-brown discoloration of samples of silver nitrate bladder irrigation (1 in 10 000) probably arose from the reaction of the silver nitrate with alkali released from the glass bottle which appeared to be soda-glass.[1]

1. *PSGB Lab Report P/80/6* 1980.

### Adverse Effects

Symptoms of poisoning stem from the corrosive action of silver nitrate and include pain in the mouth, sialorrhoea, abdominal pain, diarrhoea, vomiting, coma, and convulsions.

Short-term mild conjunctivitis is common in infants given silver nitrate eye drops; repeated use or the use of high concentrations produces severe damage and even blindness. Chronic application to the conjunctiva, mucous surfaces, or open wounds leads to argyria (see Silver, above), which though difficult to treat is mainly a cosmetic hazard.

Although silver nitrate is not readily absorbed, absorption of nitrite following reduction of nitrate may cause methaemoglobinaemia. There is also a risk of electrolyte disturbances.

**Effects on the eyes.** Silver nitrate from a stick containing 75% was applied to the eyes of a newborn infant instead of a 1% solution.[1] After 1 hour there was a thick purulent secretion, the eyelids were red and oedematous, and the conjunctiva markedly injected. The corneas had a blue-grey bedewed appearance with areas of corneal opacification. After treatment by lavage and topical application of antibacterials and homatropine 2% there was a marked improvement and after 1 week topical application of corticosteroids was started. Residual damage was limited to slight corneal opacity.

1. Hornblass A. Silver nitrate ocular damage in newborns. *JAMA* 1975; **231:** 245.

### Uses and Administration

Silver nitrate possesses antiseptic properties and is used in many countries as a 1% solution for the prophylaxis of gonococcal ophthalmia neonatorum (see Neonatal Conjunctivitis, p.136). However, as it can cause irritation, other drugs are often used.

In stick form it has been used as a caustic to destroy warts (p.1139) and other small skin growths. Compresses soaked in a 0.5% solution of silver nitrate have been applied to severe burns to reduce infection. Solutions have also been used as topical antiseptics and astringents in other conditions.

Silver nitrate (Argentum Nitricum; Argent. Nit.) is used in homoeopathic medicine. It has also been used in cosmetics to dye eyebrows and eye lashes.

### Preparations

**BP 2003:** Sterile Silver Nitrate Solution;
**USP 27:** Silver Nitrate Ophthalmic Solution; Toughened Silver Nitrate.

**Proprietary Preparations** (details are given in Part 3)
**Denm.:** Helvedstensstifter; **Ger.:** Mova Nitrat; **Port.:** Argenpal; **Spain:** Argenpal.

**Multi-ingredient: Austral.:** Super Banish; **Hong Kong:** Biscasil†; **Spain:** Argentofenol; **Switz.:** Grafco batonnets de bois†; **UK:** Avoca.

## Silver Protein

Albumosesilber; Argentoproteinum; Argentum Proteinicum; Plata, proteína de; Protargolum; Proteinato de Plata; Proteinato de Prata; Strong Protargin; Strong Protein Silver; Strong Silver Protein.

*CAS — 7440-22-4 (colloidal silver); 9015-51-4 (silver protein).*

NOTE. Synonyms for mild silver protein include: Argentoproteinum Mite; Argentum Vitellinicum; Mild Protargin; Mild Silver Proteinate; Silver Nucleinate; Silver Vitellin; Vitelinato de Plata and Vitelinato de Prata.

**Pharmacopoeias.** In *It., Jpn, Pol.,* and *Viet.*

### Profile

Silver protein solutions have antibacterial properties, due to the presence of low concentrations of ionised silver, and have been used as eye drops and for application to mucous membranes. The mild form of silver protein is considered to be less irritating, but less active.

Colloidal silver, which is also a preparation of silver in combination with protein, has also been used topically for its antibacterial activity.

### Preparations

**Proprietary Preparations** (details are given in Part 3)
**Braz.:** Argirol; Colirio de Argyrol†; **Fr.:** Stillargol; Vitargenol†; **Ger.:** Rhinoguttae Argenti diacetylotannici proteinici; Rhinoguttae pro Infantibus N.

**Multi-ingredient: Austria:** Coldargan; **Belg.:** Argyrophedrine; **Braz.:** Argyrophedrine†; **Ger.:** Gastrarctin N; **Ital.:** Argirofedrina; Argisone; Argotone; Arscolloid; Bio-Arscolloid; Corti-Arscolloid; Rinantipiol; Rinofomentil; Rinovit Nube†; **Port.:** Naso-Calma.

## Sincalide *(BAN, USAN, rINN)*

CCK-OP; Sincalida; SQ-19844. De-1-(5-oxo-L-proline)-de-2-L-glutamine-5-methionine-caerulein.

$C_{49}H_{62}N_{10}O_{16}S_3$ = 1143.3.

*CAS — 25126-32-3.*

*ATC — V04CC03.*

**Pharmacopoeias.** *US* includes Sincalide for Injection.

### Adverse Effects

Sincalide stimulates gallbladder contraction and gastrointestinal muscle and may give rise to abdominal discomfort. Dizziness, nausea, and flushing may also occur.

### Uses and Administration

Sincalide is the synthetic C-terminal octapeptide of cholecystokinin (see pancreozymin, p.1727) and when given by intravenous injection it stimulates gallbladder contraction; it also stimulates intestinal muscle.

Sincalide is used for testing gallbladder function and as an adjunct to cholecystography. It is usually given in doses of 20 nanograms/kg by intravenous injection over 30 to 60 seconds. It is also used as a diagnostic agent, often with secretin (p.1742), for testing the functional capacity of the pancreas; this test generally requires duodenal intubation of the patient and examination of duodenal aspirate. A suggested procedure is to give a 1-hour intravenous infusion of secretin, and 30 minutes after starting this infusion, to start a separate infusion of sincalide 20 nanograms/kg over a 30-minute period. A dose of 40 nanograms/kg may be given to accelerate the transit time of a barium meal through the small bowel; it should be given after the barium meal has passed the proximal jejunum.

### Preparations

**USP 27:** Sincalide for Injection.

**Proprietary Preparations** (details are given in Part 3)
**Canad.:** Kinevac; **USA:** Kinevac.

## Sivelestat *(USAN, rINN)*

EI-546; LY-544349; ONO-5046. *o*-(*p*-Hydroxybenzenesulfonamido)hippuric acid pivalate.

$C_{20}H_{22}N_2O_7S$ = 434.5.

*CAS — 127373-66-4.*

## Sivelestat Sodium *(USAN, rINNM)*

$C_{20}H_{21}N_2NaO_7S,4H_2O$ = 528.5.

*CAS — 201677-61-4.*

### Profile

Sivelestat is an elastase inhibitor that primarily inhibits neutrophil elastase. It is given by intravenous infusion as the sodium salt in the treatment of acute lung injury associated with systemic inflammatory response syndrome.

◊ References.

1. Zeiher BG, *et al.* Neutrophil elastase and acute lung injury: prospects for sivelestat and other neutrophil elastase inhibitors as therapeutics. *Crit Care Med* 2002; **30** (suppl): S281–S287.

### Preparations

**Proprietary Preparations** (details are given in Part 3)
**Jpn:** Elaspol.

## Skullcap

Escutelaria; Scullcap; Scutellaria.

**Pharmacopoeias.** *Chin.* includes Herba Scutellariae Barbatae (Barbated Skullcap Herb; *Scutellaria barbata*) and Radix Scutellariae (Baical Skullcap Root; *S. baicalensis*). *Jpn* includes Scutellaria Root (*S. baicalensis*).

### Profile

Skullcap, the aerial parts of *Scutellaria lateriflora* (Labiatae) and other *Scutellaria* spp., has sedative and antispasmodic properties. It is used as a nerve tonic, and for insomnia and menstrual disorders.

Baical skullcap (*S. baicalensis*) is used in Chinese herbal medicine.

### Preparations

**Proprietary Preparations** (details are given in Part 3)
**Multi-ingredient: Austral.:** Calmo†; Feminine Herbal Complex†; Goodnight Formula†; Lifesystem Herbal Formula 12 Willowbark†; Naturest†; Pacifenity†; Passiflora Complex†; Passionflower Plus†; Relaxaplex†; Valerian†; Willowbark Plus Herbal Formula 11†; **Canad.:** Herbal Nerve; **UK:** Biophylin†; Gerard House Valerian Compound†; Herbal Indigestion Naturtabs; HRI Calm Life; Newrelax; Nodoff; Quiet Days; Quiet Tyme; Scullcap & Gentian Tablets; St Johnswort Compound; Stressless; Super Mega B+C; Vegetable Cough Remover; Wellwoman.

## Skunk Cabbage

Col apestosa; Skunkweed.

### Profile

Skunk cabbage, the root and rhizome of *Symplocarpus foetidus* (*Dracontium foetidum*) (Araceae), has expectorant properties and is used in respiratory-tract disorders.

### Preparations

**Proprietary Preparations** (details are given in Part 3)
**Multi-ingredient: UK:** Horehound and Aniseed Cough Mixture; Vegetable Cough Remover.

## Slippery Elm

Elm Bark; Olmo resbaladizo; Slippery Elm Bark; Ulmus; Ulmus Fulva.

**Pharmacopoeias.** In *US.*

**USP 27** (Elm). The dried inner bark of *Ulmus rubra* (*U. fulva*) (Ulmaceae). Store in a dry place at a temperature of 8° to 15°.

### Profile

Slippery elm contains a considerable amount of mucilage and has been used as a demulcent.

### Preparations

**Proprietary Preparations** (details are given in Part 3)

**Multi-ingredient:** ***Austral.:*** Bioglan Psylli-Mucil Plus†; Cal Alkyline†; Digestive Aid†; Enterocare†; Herbal Cleanse†; PC Regulax†; Travelaide†; ***Canad.:*** Herbal Cough Expectorant†; Herbal Throat; ***UK:*** Biobalm†; Fenulin†; Modern Herbals Pile; Natraleze†; Papaya Plus†; Pileabs; Slippery Elm Stomach Tablets.

## Soda Lime

Cal Sodada; Cal sodada; Calcaria absorbens; Calcaria Compositio; Calx Sodica; Chaux Sodée.

*CAS — 8006-28-8.*

**Pharmacopoeias.** In *Br.* Also in *USNF.*

**BP 2003** (Soda Lime). A mixture of sodium hydroxide, or sodium hydroxide and potassium hydroxide, with calcium hydroxide. White or greyish-white granules, or it may be coloured with an indicator to show when its absorptive capacity is exhausted. It absorbs about 20% of its weight of carbon dioxide. Partially soluble in water; almost completely soluble in 1M acetic acid. A suspension in water is strongly alkaline to litmus.

**USNF 22** (Soda Lime). A mixture of calcium hydroxide and sodium or potassium hydroxide or both. It may contain an indicator that is inert and that changes colour when the soda lime can no longer absorb carbon dioxide. White or greyish-white granules. May have a colour if an indicator is added.

**Incompatibility.** Soda lime is incompatible with trichloroethylene.

### Profile

Soda lime is used to absorb carbon dioxide, for instance in closed-circuit anaesthetic apparatus, and in the determination of the basal metabolic rate. Limits are specified for particle size, and particles should be free from dust.

Soda lime must not be used with trichloroethylene, since this is decomposed by warm alkali to produce a toxic end product that gives rise to lesions of the nervous system.

Soda lime is irritating and corrosive to skin, mucous membranes, and eyes.

## Sodium Aminobenzoate

Aminobenzoate Sodium. Sodium 4-aminobenzoate.

$C_7H_6NNaO_2$ = 159.1.

**Pharmacopoeias.** In *US.*

**USP 27** (Aminobenzoate Sodium). pH of a 5% solution in water is between 8.0 and 9.0.

### Profile

Sodium aminobenzoate has been used in analgesic preparations.

### Preparations

**Proprietary Preparations** (details are given in Part 3)

**Multi-ingredient:** ***Ital.:*** Fotofil; Neo-Ustiol; ***Spain:*** Tri Hachemina; ***USA:*** Pabalate†.

## Sodium Arsenate

Arseniato de sodio; Natrium Arsenicicum; Sodium Arseniate.

$Na_2HAsO_4,7H_2O$ = 312.0.

*CAS — 7778-43-0 (anhydrous sodium arsenate); 10048-95-0 (sodium arsenate heptahydrate).*

### Profile

Sodium arsenate was formerly used in the treatment of chronic skin diseases, in parasitic diseases of the blood, and in some forms of anaemia. It has the adverse effects of Arsenic Trioxide, p.1657.

### Preparations

**Proprietary Preparations** (details are given in Part 3)

**Multi-ingredient:** ***Fr.:*** Aromabyl†; ***Mex.:*** Iodarsolo B12.

## Sodium Carbonate Anhydrous

Carbonato de sodio anhidro; Cenizas de Soda; E500; Exsiccated Sodium Carbonate; Natrii Carbonas Anhydricus; Natrium Carbonicum Calcinatum; Natrium Carbonicum Siccatum.

$Na_2CO_3$ = 106.0.

*CAS — 497-19-8.*

NOTE. Soda ash is a synonym for the technical grade of sodium carbonate anhydrous.

**Pharmacopoeias.** In *Eur.* (see p.vi) and *Jpn. USNF* allows the anhydrous substance or the monohydrate.

**Ph. Eur. 5.0** (Sodium Carbonate, Anhydrous). A white or almost white, slightly granular, hygroscopic powder. Freely soluble in water; practically insoluble in alcohol. A 10% solution in water is strongly alkaline. Store in airtight containers.

**USNF 22** (Sodium Carbonate). Colourless crystals, or white, crystalline powder or granules. Soluble 1 in 3 of water and 1 in 1.8 of boiling water.

## Sodium Carbonate Decahydrate

Carbonato de sodio decahidratado; Cristales de Sosa; E500; Natrii Carbonas; Natrii Carbonas Decahydricus; Natrium Carbonicum Crystallisatum.

$Na_2CO_3,10H_2O$ = 286.1.

*CAS — 6132-02-1.*

NOTE. Washing soda is a synonym for the technical grade of sodium carbonate decahydrate.

**Pharmacopoeias.** In *Eur.* (see p.vi) and *Jpn.*

**Ph. Eur. 5.0** (Sodium Carbonate Decahydrate). Colourless, efflorescent, transparent crystals or white crystalline powder. Freely soluble in water; practically insoluble in alcohol. A 10% solution in water is strongly alkaline. Store in airtight containers.

## Sodium Carbonate Monohydrate

Carbonato de sodio monohidratado; E500; Natrii Carbonas Monohydricus.

$Na_2CO_3,H_2O$ = 124.0.

*CAS — 5968-11-6.*

**Pharmacopoeias.** In *Eur.* (see p.vi). *USNF* allows the anhydrous substance or the monohydrate.

**Ph. Eur. 5.0** (Sodium Carbonate Monohydrate). A white, crystalline powder or colourless crystals. Freely soluble in water; practically insoluble in alcohol. A 10% solution in water is strongly alkaline. Store in airtight containers.

**USNF 22** (Sodium Carbonate). Colourless crystals, or white, crystalline powder or granules. When exposed to dry air above 50°, it effloresces and at 100° it becomes anhydrous. Soluble 1 in 3 of water and 1 in 1.8 of boiling water.

### Profile

Sodium carbonate is used in antacid preparations. Anhydrous sodium carbonate and the monohydrate are also used as reagents. The decahydrate has been used in alkaline baths. Sodium carbonate in its anhydrous or hydrated form is also used as a water softener.

Sodium carbonate may be irritating or mildly corrosive to skin, mucous membranes, and eyes.

### Preparations

***BPC 1973:*** Surgical Chlorinated Soda Solution;
***USP 27:*** Citric Acid, Magnesium Oxide, and Sodium Carbonate Irrigation.

**Proprietary Preparations** (details are given in Part 3)

**Multi-ingredient:** ***Arg.:*** Mylanta Reflux; Otoclean Gotas Oticas; Sal de Fruta Eno; Sincerum; Yasta; ***Austral.:*** Eno; ***Braz.:*** Albicon; Digestbem; Estomazil†; Sal de Fruta Eno; Sonrisal; ***Fr.:*** Bactident; Hydralin; ***Hong Kong:*** Eno; Hydralin; ***Irl.:*** Cymalon; ***Israel:*** Urikal; ***Ital.:*** Eno†; ***Port.:*** Eno; Sais de Frutos†; Sais Zitos†; ***Spain:*** Cloritines†; Sal de Fruta Eno; Tanasid; ***Switz.:*** Saltrates Rodell; ***UK:*** Cymalon; Eno; Resolve.

## Sodium Chlorate

Clorato de potasio; Natrium Chloricum; Sodii Chloras.

$NaClO_3$ = 106.4.

*CAS — 7775-09-9.*

### Profile

Sodium chlorate closely resembles potassium chlorate (p.1734) in its properties and has been used as an astringent. Its main use is as a weedkiller and it is therefore a common household chemical. Poor storage conditions can lead to explosions.

### Preparations

**Proprietary Preparations** (details are given in Part 3)

**Multi-ingredient:** ***Spain:*** Co Bucal.

## Sodium Dichloroacetate *(USAN)*

CPC-211; DCA; Dicloroacetato de sodio.

$C_2HCl_2NaO_2$ = 150.9.

*CAS — 2156-56-1 (sodium dichloroacetate); 79-43-6 (dichloroacetic acid).*

### Profile

Dichloroacetic acid activates pyruvate dehydrogenase, a mitochondrial enzyme which catalyses metabolism of pyruvate and lactate, and it inhibits glycolysis. It also stimulates myocardial contractility. Sodium dichloroacetate has been used for the treatment of congenital lactic acidosis, lactic acidosis in patients with severe malaria, homozygous familial hypercholesterolaemia, and for severe brain injury. It is also under investigation for stroke.

**Adverse effects.** Adverse effects reported to date with sodium dichloroacetate have mainly involved the central and peripheral nervous systems.[1] Anxiolytic or sedative effects are common. Reversible polyneuropathy has been reported after chronic use, as has asymptomatic elevation of serum transaminases. Reduced urate clearance and elevated serum urate levels have been reported in patients with type 2 diabetes mellitus.

1. Stacpoole PW, *et al.* Pharmacokinetics, metabolism, and toxicology of dichloroacetate. *Drug Metab Rev* 1998; **30:** 499–539.

**Pharmacokinetics.** References.

1. Henderson GN, *et al.* Pharmacokinetics of dichloroacetate in adult patients with lactic acidosis. *J Clin Pharmacol* 1997; **37:** 416–25.
2. Shangraw RE, Fisher DM. Pharmacokinetics and pharmacodynamics of dichloroacetate in patients with cirrhosis. *Clin Pharmacol Ther* 1999 **66:** 380–90.

**Use in metabolic acidosis.** In a study[1] in 29 patients with lactic acidosis (p.1217), sodium dichloroacetate 50 mg/kg given by intravenous infusion over 30 minutes, followed by a second dose 2 hours after beginning the first infusion, produced a metabolic response in 23 patients with a short-term increase in survival. However, a subsequent study[2] found that, while dichloroacetate infusion did reduce blood-lactate concentrations, it did not alter haemodynamics or survival in patients with severe lactic acidosis. A review[3] of these and other controlled studies in the treatment of acquired and congenital lactic acidosis concluded that the maximum lactate-lowering effect is dose-dependent but independent of time following administration. Whether lowering lactate levels contributes to reducing morbidity and mortality in hyperlactataemia remains controversial, although data from recent studies suggest that treatment in mild cases may reduce the risk of death. A review[4] of the treatment of children with dichloroacetate for congenital lactic acidosis hypothesised that it might improve quality of life by reducing the frequency of acid-base decompensations, improving neurological function, and stimulating linear growth.

In a randomised, double-blind, placebo-controlled study[5] in 124 West African children with severe *Plasmodium falciparum* malaria, a single intravenous infusion of sodium dichloroacetate in a dose of 50 mg/kg given at the same time as quinine increased the rate and magnitude of fall in blood-lactate levels without compromising the plasma kinetics of quinine.

Sodium dichloroacetate has also been studied[6] in patients with traumatic brain injury for its lactate-lowering effect in cerebrospinal fluid.

1. Stacpoole PW, *et al.* Dichloroacetate in the treatment of lactic acidosis. *Ann Intern Med* 1988; **108:** 58–63.
2. Stacpoole PW, *et al.* A controlled clinical trial of dichloroacetate for treatment of lactic acidosis in adults. *N Engl J Med* 1992; **327:** 1564–9.
3. Stacpoole PW, *et al.* Efficacy of dichloroacetate as a lactate-lowering drug. *J Clin Pharmacol* 2003; **43:** 683–91.
4. Stacpoole PW, *et al.* Treatment of congenital lactic acidosis with dichloroacetate. *Arch Dis Child* 1997; **77:** 535–41.
5. Agbenyega T, *et al.* Population kinetics, efficacy, and safety of dichloroacetate for lactic acidosis due to severe malaria in children. *J Clin Pharmacol* 2003; **43:** 386–96.
6. Williams PJ, Dichloroacetate: population pharmacokinetics with a pharmacodynamic sequential link model. *J Clin Pharmacol* 2001; **41:** 259–67.

## Sodium Dithionite

Ditionito de sodio; Sodium Hydrosulfite; Sodium Hydrosulphite; Sodium Sulphoxylate.

$Na_2S_2O_4$ = 174.1.

*CAS — 7775-14-6.*

NOTE. The name sodium hydrosulfite is also applied to $NaHSO_2$ = 88.06.

**Pharmacopoeias.** In *Pol.*

### Profile

Sodium dithionite is used as a reducing agent. It may be used in the form of a simple urine test in the detection of paraquat poisoning. A 0.25% solution has been used to remove phenazopyridine stains from fabric. It is irritant to the skin.

## Sodium Gluconate

E576; Gluconato de sodio. Monosodium D-gluconate.

$C_6H_{11}NaO_7$ = 218.1.

*CAS — 527-07-1.*

**Pharmacopoeias.** In *US.*

### Profile

Sodium gluconate is a food additive.

Gluconates act as acceptors of hydrogen ions produced by metabolic processes and are an indirect source of bicarbonate ions.

## Sodium Hydroxide

Ätznatron; Caustic Soda; E524; Hidróxido de sodio; Natrii Hydroxidum; Natrium Hydricum; Natrium Hydroxydatum; Soda Lye.

NaOH = 40.00.

*CAS — 1310-73-2.*

**Pharmacopoeias.** In *Chin., Eur.* (see p.vi), *Int.,* and *Jpn.* Also in *USNF.*

**Ph. Eur. 5.0** (Sodium Hydroxide). White, crystalline masses supplied as pellets, sticks, or slabs. It is deliquescent and readily absorbs carbon dioxide. Very soluble in water; freely soluble in alcohol. A 0.01% solution in water has a pH of not less than 11.0. Store in airtight, nonmetallic containers.

**USNF 22** (Sodium Hydroxide). White or practically white fused masses, small pellets, flakes, sticks, or other forms. It is hard and brittle and shows a crystalline fracture. When exposed to air it rapidly absorbs moisture and carbon dioxide. Soluble 1 in 1 of water; freely soluble in alcohol. Store in airtight containers.

### Adverse Effects

Sodium hydroxide is strongly alkaline and corrosive, and rapidly destroys organic tissues.

The ingestion of caustic alkalis causes immediate burning pain in the mouth, throat, substernal region, and epigastrium, and the lining membranes become swollen and detached. There is dysphagia, hypersalivation, vomiting with the vomitus becoming blood-stained, diarrhoea, and shock. In severe cases, abdominal pain, asphyxia due to oedema of the glottis, circulatory failure, oesophageal or gastric perforation, peritonitis, or pneumonia may occur. Stricture of the oesophagus can develop weeks or months later.

Caustic alkalis on contact with the skin can produce full thickness burns leading to extensive damage. Alkali burns to the eyes cause conjunctival oedema and corneal destruction; damage may be irreversible.

### Treatment of Adverse Effects

Ingestion should not be treated by lavage or emesis. Dilution with water or milk is generally considered controversial for management of corrosive ingestion. However, early dilution therapy of alkalis may reduce oesophageal injury; large volumes of fluid should be avoided. Neutralisation of alkalis is contra-indicated. The airway should be maintained and shock and pain alleviated.

In cases of skin contamination, clothing should be removed immediately and the skin flooded with copious amounts of water for at least 15 minutes. Excision or skin grafting of burnt areas may be necessary in severe cases. Contaminated eyes should be irrigated thoroughly with water or 0.9% sodium chloride until the conjunctival sac pH is normal, which may require irrigation for up to an hour.

### Uses and Administration

Sodium hydroxide is a powerful caustic. A 2.5% solution in glycerol has been used as a cuticle solvent. An escharotic preparation of sodium hydroxide and calcium oxide was known as London paste. Sodium hydroxide is also used for adjusting the pH of solutions.

**Disinfection.** For reference to the possible use of sodium hydroxide for the disinfection of material contaminated by the agent causing Creutzfeldt-Jakob disease, see p.1164.

### Preparations

**Proprietary Preparations** (details are given in Part 3)
**Multi-ingredient:** ***Austria:*** Leberinfusion; Sulfo-Schwefelbad; ***Ger.:*** Glutarsin E; Infumal†; ***Spain:*** Alucol†; ***Switz.:*** Saltrates.

## Sodium Iodoheparinate

Iodoheparinate Sodium; Iodoheparinato de sodio.

### Profile

Sodium iodoheparinate is a derivative of heparin (p.927) used topically for the treatment of corneal burns and ulceration.

### Preparations

**Proprietary Preparations** (details are given in Part 3)
***Fr.:*** Dioparine†; ***Switz.:*** Dioparine†.

## Sodium Methylarsinate

Metilarsinato de sodio; Natrium Methylarsonicum; Sodium Metharsinite. Disodium monomethylarsonate hexahydrate.

$CH_3AsNa_2O_3,6H_2O = 292.0.$

*CAS — 5967-62-4.*

### Profile

Sodium methylarsinate is an organic arsenic compound with adverse effects similar to those of arsenic trioxide (p.1657). It was formerly included in some vitamin and mineral preparations. It has also been used as a herbicide.

### Preparations

**Proprietary Preparations** (details are given in Part 3)
**Multi-ingredient:** ***Braz.:*** Carneferrol†.

## Sodium Morrhuate *(rINN)*

Morrhuate Sodium; Morruato de sodio.

*CAS — 8031-09-2.*

**Pharmacopoeias.** *Chin.* and *US* include the injection.

### Profile

Sodium morrhuate consists of the sodium salts of the fatty acids of cod-liver oil. It is a sclerosant that has been used in the treatment of varicose veins (p.1717). Usual doses are 50 to 100 mg for small or medium veins or 150 to 250 mg for large veins given as a 5% solution by intravenous injection.

### Preparations

***USP 27:*** Morrhuate Sodium Injection.

**Proprietary Preparations** (details are given in Part 3)
***USA:*** Scleromate.

## Sodium Phenylacetate *(USAN)*

Fenilacetato de sodio.

$C_8H_7NaO_2 = 158.1.$

*CAS — 114-70-5.*

### Profile

Sodium phenylacetate is used for hyperammonaemia in patients with enzymatic deficiencies in the urea cycle (p.1421). Sodium phenylbutyrate (see below) is a prodrug for sodium phenylacetate.

◊ References.

1. The Urea Cycle Disorders Conference Group. Consensus statement from a conference for the management of patients with urea cycle disorders. *J Pediatr* 2001; **138** (suppl 1): S1–S5.
2. Summar M. Current strategies for the management of neonatal urea cycle disorders. *J Pediatr* 2001; **138** (suppl 1): S30–S39.
3. Batshaw ML, *et al.* Alternative pathway therapy for urea cycle disorders: twenty years later. *J Pediatr* 2001; **138** (suppl 1): S46–S55. Correction. *ibid.* 2002; **140:** 490.

### Preparations

**Proprietary Preparations** (details are given in Part 3)
**Multi-ingredient:** ***USA:*** Ucephan.

## Sodium Phenylbutyrate *(BAN, USAN)*

Fenilbutirato de sodio. Sodium 4-Phenylbutyrate.

$C_{10}H_{11}NaO_2 = 186.2.$

*CAS — 1716-12-7.*

*ATC — A16AX03.*

### Profile

Sodium phenylbutyrate is a prodrug for sodium phenylacetate (see above) and is used in the treatment of hyperammonaemia in patients with urea cycle disorders (p.1421). It is given by mouth in equally divided doses with meals. The total daily dose for patients weighing under 20 kg is 450 to 600 mg/kg, and for those weighing over 20 kg, 9.9 to 13.0 g/m$^2$.

Sodium phenylbutyrate is also under investigation for the treatment of some sickle-cell disorders (p.734) and for use as a potential differentiation-inducing agent in malignant glioma and acute myeloid leukaemia.

◊ References.

1. Batshaw ML, *et al.* Alternative pathway therapy for urea cycle disorders: twenty years later. *J Pediatr* 2001; **138** (suppl 1): S46–S55. Correction. *ibid.* 2002; **140:** 490.

### Preparations

**Proprietary Preparations** (details are given in Part 3)
***Fr.:*** Ammonaps; ***Ger.:*** Ammonaps; ***Ital.:*** Ammonaps; ***Spain:*** Ammonaps; ***UK:*** Ammonaps; ***USA:*** Buphenyl.

## Sodium Polymetaphosphate

E452 (sodium polyphosphates); Polimetafosfato de sodio.

*CAS — 50813-16-6.*

NOTE. Although Sodium hexametaphosphate has been used as a synonym for the polymetaphosphate, the latter also exists in much higher degrees of polymerisation.

### Profile

Sodium polymetaphosphate has been used as a 5% dusting powder in hyperhidrosis and bromhidrosis, and as a prophylactic against athlete's foot.

Sodium polymetaphosphate combines with calcium and magnesium ions to form complex soluble compounds and is used as a water softener.

## Sodium Pyruvate

Piruvato de sodio. Sodium α-ketopropionate; sodium 2-oxopropanoate.

$C_3H_3NaO_3 = 111.1.$

*CAS — 127-17-3 (pyruvic acid); 113-24-6 (sodium pyruvate).*

### Profile

Sodium pyruvate has been given intravenously in the diagnosis of disorders of pyruvate metabolism.

◊ Relative serum concentrations of lactate and pyruvate following a 10-minute intravenous infusion of sodium pyruvate 500 mg/kg have been used as an aid to the diagnosis of disorders of pyruvate metabolism.[1] Death shortly after pyruvate loading in a 9-year-old child with restrictive cardiomyopathy suggests that the test should not be performed when cardiac function is decreased.[2]

1. Dijkstra U, *et al.* Friedreich's ataxia: intravenous pyruvate load to demonstrate a defect in pyruvate metabolism. *Neurology* 1984; **34:** 1493–7.
2. Matthys D, *et al.* Fatal outcome of pyruvate loading test in child with restrictive cardiomyopathy. *Lancet* 1991; **338:** 1020–1.

## Sodium Silicate

Silicato de sodio; Soluble Glass; Water Glass.

*CAS — 1344-09-8.*

### Profile

Concentrated aqueous solutions of sodium silicate are commercially available and have many industrial uses. The solutions vary in composition, viscosity, and density; the greater the ratio of $Na_2O$ to $SiO_2$ the more tacky and alkaline the solution.

## Sodium Succinate

E363 (succinic acid); Succinato de sodio.

$C_4H_4Na_2O_4,6H_2O = 270.1.$

*CAS — 150-90-3 (anhydrous sodium succinate); 6106-21-4 (sodium succinate hexahydrate).*

### Profile

Sodium succinate is an ingredient of topical preparations tried for the treatment of cataract. It is also used as a food additive.

### Preparations

**Proprietary Preparations** (details are given in Part 3)
**Multi-ingredient:** ***Fr.:*** Cristopal; Vitaphakol†; ***Port.:*** Vitaphakol†; ***Spain:*** Vitaphakol; ***Switz.:*** Vitaphakol†.

## Solidago

Echtes Goldrutenkraut (*S. virgaurea*); European Goldenrod (*S. virgaurea*); Golden Rod; Goldrutenkraut (*S. gigantea* or *S. canadensis*); Herba Virgaureae (*S. virgaurea*); Solidage; Solidaginis Herba (*S. gigantea* or *S. canadensis*); Solidaginis Virgaureae Herba (*S. virgaurea*); Solidago Virga Aurea (*S. virgaurea*).

NOTE. The name Aaron's Rod has been applied to a number of plants including *Solidago* spp., *Verbascum* spp., and *Sempervivum tectorum.*

**Pharmacopoeias.** In *Eur.* (see p.vi) and *Pol.*

**Ph. Eur. 5.0** (Goldenrod, European; Solidaginis virgaureae herba). The whole or cut dried, flowering aerial parts of *Solidago virgaurea*. It contains not less than 1.0% of flavonoids, expressed as hyperoside ($C_{21}H_{20}O_{12} = 464.4$) with reference to the dried drug.

**Ph. Eur. 5.0** (Goldenrod; Solidaginis herba). The whole or cut dried, flowering aerial parts of *Solidago gigantea* or *S. canadensis*. It contains not less than 2.5% of flavonoids, expressed as hyperoside ($C_{21}H_{20}O_{12} = 464.4$) with reference to the dried drug.

### Profile

*Solidago virgaurea* (Asteraceae) has diuretic and anti-inflammatory activity. It is mainly used in inflammatory disorders of the bladder and kidneys and for the treatment of renal stones. It is also included in herbal preparations used for a variety of disorders.

*S. gigantea* (Early golden-rod) and *S. canadensis* were once considered to be adulterants of *S. virgaurea* but are now recognised as having similar activity.

Solidago is used in homoeopathic medicine.

### Preparations

**Proprietary Preparations** (details are given in Part 3)
***Ger.:*** Calcufel Aqua; Canephron S; Cystinol Long; Cystium Solidago; Cysto Fink Mono; Kalkurenal Goldrute; Nephrisol mono; Nephrolith mono; Nieral; Solidago M†; Stromic; Urodyn†; Urol mono; Uroplant.

**Multi-ingredient:** ***Austral.:*** Bioglan Cranbiotic Super†; Extralife Fluid-Care†; ***Austria:*** Apotheker Bauer's Harntreibender Tee; Apotheker Bauer's Nieren- und Blasentee; Droxitop; Kneipp Nieren- und Blasen-Tee; Krauterhaus Mag Kottas Entwasserungstee; Krauterpfarrer Weidinger Tee bei Nieren- und Blasenbeschwerden; Krauterpfarrer Weidinger Tee zur Entschlackung; Naturland Entschlackungstee; Neuners Krautertee Nr 2 - Fruhjahrskurtee; Neuners Krautertee Nr 204 - Krauterhexlein Kinder Nieren- und Blasentee; Neuners Krautertee Nr 3 - Blasentee; Neuners Krautertee Nr 4 - Nierentee; Phytodolor; Sidroga Nieren- und Blasentee; Solubitrat; Teekanne Blasen- und Nierentee; Urelium Neu; ***Canad.:*** Arthrisan†; ***Fr.:*** Solution Stago Diluee; ***Ger.:*** Aqualibra; BioCyst; Blasen-Nieren-Tee Stada†; Canephron novo; Cefanephrin†; Cefasabal; Cystinol; Cysto Fink†; Etmoren†; Harntee 400; Harntee 450†; Harntee STADA; Harntee-Steiner; Heumann Blasen- und Nierentee Solubitrat S; Heweberol-Tee; Hewenephron duo; Inconturina; Kneipp Blasen- und Nieren-Tee†; nephro-loges; Nephro-Pasc; Nephronorm med; Nephropur tri; Nephroselect M; Nephrubin-N; Nieron Blasen- und Nieren-Tee VI; Nieron S; Nieroxin N; Phytodolor; Presselin Nieren-Blasen K 3; Prostamed; Renob Blasen- und Nierentee; Rhoival; Solidagoren N; Ullus Blasen-Nieren-Tee N†; Uro Fink†; Uro-Pasc†; Urodil Blasen-Nieren Arzneitee†; Urodil phyto; Urosteí†; ***Ital.:*** Flavion; Gramigna (Specie Composta); ***Port.:*** Prostamed; ***Spain:*** Natusor Artilane; Natusor Renal; Renusor; Uralyt†; ***Switz.:*** Demonatur Dragees pour les reins et la vessie; Dragees pour reins et vessie S†; Nephrosolid; Phytomed Nephro; Phytomed Prosta; Phytomed Rhino†; Urinex.

## Sorrel

Acedera Común; Azeda-Brava; Garden Sorrel; Herba Rumicis Acetosae; Oseille; Sorrel Dock; Sour Dock; Vinagrera; Wiesensauerampfer.

NOTE. The name sour dock has also been used for yellow dock (p.1766).

### Profile

Sorrel (*Rumex acetosa*, Polygonaceae) has been used for respiratory-tract disorders. It is also used as a culinary herb.

### Preparations

**Proprietary Preparations** (details are given in Part 3)

**Multi-ingredient:** ***Austria:*** Sinupret; ***Ger.:*** Sinupret; ***Hong Kong:*** Sinupret; ***Singapore:*** Sinupret; ***Switz.:*** Sinupret; ***Thai.:*** Sinupret.

## Sparteine Sulfate *(USAN, rINNM)*

Spart. Sulph.; Sparteine Sulphate; (−)-Sparteine Sulphate; *l*-Sparteine Sulphate; Sparteinum Sulfuricum; Sulfato de esparteína. Dodecahydro-7,14-methano-2*H*,6*H*-dipyrido[1,2-*a*:1′,2′-e][1,5]diazocine sulphate pentahydrate.

$C_{15}H_{26}N_2,H_2SO_4,5H_2O = 422.5.$

*CAS — 90-39-1 (sparteine); 299-39-8 (anhydrous sparteine sulfate); 6160-12-9 (sparteine sulfate pentahydrate).*

*ATC — C01BA04.*

**Pharmacopoeias.** In *Fr.* and *Viet.*

### Profile

Sparteine sulfate is a salt of the dibasic alkaloid, sparteine, which is obtained from scoparium (p.1742). Sparteine sulfate has been reported to lessen the irritability and conductivity of cardiac muscle and has been used in the treatment of cardiac arrhythmias. Small doses stimulate and large doses paralyse the autonomic ganglia. Peripherally, it has a fairly strong curare-like action, arresting respiration by paralysing the phrenic endings.

The metabolic oxidation of sparteine exhibits genetic polymorphism and this property has been exploited in *in-vitro* screening tests to identify other drugs that may be subject to similar genetic variations in their metabolism.

**Precautions.** Sparteine present in a herbal slimming preparation might cause adverse effects in slow metabolisers if excessive doses were ingested; pregnant women might be particularly at risk.[1]

1. Galloway JH, *et al.* Potentially hazardous compound in a herbal slimming remedy. *Lancet* 1992; **340:** 179.

### Preparations

**Proprietary Preparations** (details are given in Part 3)

**Multi-ingredient:** ***Braz.:*** Belacodid; Bromosedan†.

## Spearmint

Menta; Mentha Viridis; Menthae Crispae Folium; Mint.

### Profile

Spearmint consists of the dried leaves and flowering tops of common spearmint, *Mentha spicata* (*M. viridis*) or of scotch spearmint (*M. cardiaca*) (Labiatae). Spearmint is the source of spearmint oil (below). It has carminative properties and is used as a flavour.

### Preparations

**Proprietary Preparations** (details are given in Part 3)

***Braz.:*** Giamebil.

**Multi-ingredient:** ***Austria:*** Carminative; Mag Kottas Baby-Tee; Mag Kottas Beruhigungstee; Mag Kottas Krauterexpress-Beruhigungstee; Sidroga Herz-Kreislauf-Tee; Sidroga Magen-Darm-Tee; Sidroga Nerven- und Schlaftee; Sidroga Stoffwechseltee; Teekanne Herz- und Kreislauftee; ***Fr.:*** Mediflor Tisane Digestive No 3; Tisanes de l'Abbe Hamon no 17†; ***Switz.:*** Alpina Gel a la consoude†; Gel a la consoude; Tisane antirhumatismale; Tisane pour l'estomac; Tisane pour le coeur et la circulation; Tisane pour le sommeil et les nerfs.

## Spearmint Oil

Huile Essentielle de Menthe Crépue; Menta, aceite esencial de; Oleum Menthae Crispae; Oleum Menthae Viridis.

**Pharmacopoeias.** In *Br.* and *Fr.*

**BP 2003** (Spearmint Oil). It is obtained by distillation from fresh flowering plants of *Mentha spicata* or *Mentha × cardiaca*. A clear colourless, pale yellow or greenish-yellow liquid when freshly distilled, visibly free from water and with the odour of spearmint. It becomes darker and viscous on keeping. It contains not less than 55% w/w of carvone. Soluble 1 in 1 of alcohol (80%) at 20°; the solution may become cloudy when diluted. Store at a temperature not exceeding 25° in well-filled containers. Protect from light.

### Profile

Spearmint oil has similar properties to peppermint oil (p.1283) and is used as a carminative and as a flavour.

**Allergy.** Allergic contact cheilitis in a patient has been attributed to the spearmint oil present in tooth paste.[1]

1. Skrebova N, *et al.* Allergic contact cheilitis from spearmint oil. *Contact Dermatitis* 1998; **39:** 35.

### Preparations

**Proprietary Preparations** (details are given in Part 3)

**Multi-ingredient:** ***Austria:*** Euka; ***Ital.:*** Dentosan Azione Intensiva; Dentosan Mese; ***Switz.:*** Alvogyl; ***UK:*** Eftab†; Fre-bre.

## Spike Lavender

### Profile

Spike lavender, *Lavandula latifolia* (Lamiaceae), is used similarly to lavender (p.1705) as a sedative and for biliary disorders. It is the source of spike lavender oil (below).

### Preparations

**Proprietary Preparations** (details are given in Part 3)

**Multi-ingredient:** ***Ger.:*** Cholagutt-N; ***Spain:*** Natusor Somnisedan; Sedasor.

## Spike Lavender Oil

Alhucema, aceite esencial de; Huile Essentielle d'Aspic; Ol. Lavand. Spic.; Oleum Lavandulae Spicatae; Spicae Aetheroleum; Spike Oil.

**Pharmacopoeias.** In *Fr.*

### Profile

Spike lavender oil is the volatile oil from *Lavandula latifolia* (*L. spica*) (Labiatae). It resembles lavender oil (above) in its properties and is mainly used in perfumery. Hypersensitivity reactions may occur.

### Preparations

**Proprietary Preparations** (details are given in Part 3)

***Austria:*** Tavipec; ***Ger.:*** Bronchobest; ***Thai.:*** Tavipec.

**Multi-ingredient:** ***Austria:*** Novipec; Tussamag; ***Ger.:*** Neo-Lapitrypsin†; ***Switz.:*** Baume du Chalet; Fortalis.

## Spirulina

Espirulina.

### Profile

Spirulina is a species of blue-green algae that has been promoted as an anorectic, but there is no convincing evidence that it is safe or effective for this indication.

### Preparations

**Proprietary Preparations** (details are given in Part 3)

***Fr.:*** Phycocyane; ***UK:*** Biolina.

**Multi-ingredient:** ***Austral.:*** Cal Alkyline†; Rubus Complex†; ***India:*** Vitexid.

## Stearic Acid

Acido Esteárico; Acidum Stearicum; Esteárico, ácido; Octadecanoic Acid; Stearinsäure.

*CAS — 57-11-4 (stearic acid); 57-10-3 (palmitic acid).*

NOTE. Stearic acid is sometimes incorrectly called 'stearine' in commerce.

**Pharmacopoeias.** In *Chin.*, *Eur.* (see p.vi), *Jpn*, and *Pol.* Also in *USNF.*

*USNF* also includes a purified form.

**Ph. Eur. 5.0** (Stearic Acid). It is obtained from fat or oils from a vegetable or animal source and is a mixture consisting mainly of stearic acid ($C_{18}H_{36}O_2 = 284.5$) and palmitic acid ($C_{16}H_{32}O_2 = 256.4$). Stearic Acid 50 contains 40 to 60% stearic acid, the sum of the contents of stearic and palmitic acids being a minimum 90%. Stearic Acid 70 contains 60 to 80% stearic acid, the sum of the contents of stearic and palmitic acids being a minimum 90%. Stearic Acid 95 contains a minimum of 90% stearic acid, the sum of the contents of stearic and palmitic acids being a minimum 96%. White, waxy, flaky crystals, white hard masses, or a white or yellowish-white powder. Practically insoluble in water; soluble in alcohol and in petroleum spirit (50° to 70°).

**USNF 22** (Stearic Acid). A mixture of stearic acid and palmitic acid, the content of stearic acid being not less than 40%, and the sum of the two not less than 90%. Congealing point not lower than 54°. Hard, white or faintly yellowish, somewhat glossy and crystalline solid, or white or yellowish-white powder, with a slight odour, suggesting tallow. Practically insoluble in water; soluble 1 in 20 of alcohol, 1 in 2 of chloroform, and 1 in 3 of ether.

**USNF 22** (Purified Stearic Acid). It contains not less than 90% stearic acid and not less than 96% of stearic and palmitic acids. Congealing point 66° to 69°.

### Profile

Stearic acid is used as a lubricant in making tablets and capsules. It is also used as an emulsifying and solubilising agent. Various stearates are also used as pharmaceutical aids (see Nonionic Surfactants, p.1411, and Soaps and other Anionic Surfactants, p.1574).

## Stone Root

Collinsonia; Collinsonia del Canadá; Hardhack; Heal-all; Knob Root.

### Profile

Stone root, the root and rhizome of *Collinsonia canadensis* (Labiatae), has diuretic and litholytic properties and is used in the treatment of renal and urinary calculi. It is also used as an astringent for gastrointestinal disorders. It has also been included in herbal preparations for haemorrhoids,

It is used in homoeopathic medicine.

### Preparations

**Proprietary Preparations** (details are given in Part 3)

**Multi-ingredient:** ***Austral.:*** Hamamelis Complex†; ***UK:*** Piletabs.

## Storax

Balsamum Styrax Liquidus; Estoraque; Estoraque Líquido; Liquid Storax; Styrax.

**Pharmacopoeias.** In *Chin.* and *US.*

**USP 27** (Storax). The balsam obtained from the trunk of *Liquidambar orientalis* (Levant storax) or *L. styraciflua* (American storax) (Hamamelidaceae). It is a semiliquid greyish to greyish-brown, sticky, opaque mass depositing on standing a heavy dark brown layer (Levant storax), or semisolid, sometimes a solid mass, softened by gently heating (American storax). It is transparent in thin layers, has a characteristic odour, and is more dense than water.

Insoluble in water; soluble, usually incompletely, in an equal weight of warm alcohol; soluble in acetone, in carbon disulfide, and in ether, some insoluble residue usually remaining.

### Profile

Storax has actions similar to those of Peru balsam (p.1730). Purified storax or prepared storax was formerly applied as an ointment in the treatment of parasitic skin diseases. Storax has a mild antiseptic action and is an ingredient of some preparations for upper respiratory-tract disorders and for application to skin and mucous membranes. Skin sensitisation has been reported.

### Preparations

***BP 2003:*** Benzoin Inhalation; Compound Benzoin Tincture;
***BPC 1954:*** Compound Iodoform Paint;
***USP 27:*** Compound Benzoin Tincture.

**Proprietary Preparations** (details are given in Part 3)

**Multi-ingredient:** ***Fr.:*** Phytolithe; ***Ital.:*** Lacrime†; ***NZ:*** Frador; ***UK:*** Frador.

## Streptodornase *(BAN, rINN)*

Estreptodornasa; Streptococcal Deoxyribonuclease.

*CAS — 37340-82-2.*

### Profile

Streptodornase is an enzyme obtained from cultures of various strains of *Streptococcus haemolyticus*. It catalyses the depolymerisation of polymerised deoxyribonucleoproteins. It liquefies the viscous nucleoprotein of dead cells; it has no effect on living cells. It is used with streptokinase in the topical treatment of lesions, wounds, and other conditions that require the removal of clots or purulent matter; the combination may also be used to dissolve clots in the bladder or in urinary catheters.

It has also been given by mouth with streptokinase and sometimes with antibacterials, for its supposed benefit in reducing oedema and inflammation associated with trauma and infection.

### Preparations

**Proprietary Preparations** (details are given in Part 3)

**Multi-ingredient:** ***Arg.:*** Varidasa; ***Austral.:*** Varidase; ***Austria:*** Varidase; ***Belg.:*** Varidase†; ***Denm.:*** Varidase; ***Fin.:*** Varidase; ***Ger.:*** Varidase; ***Irl.:*** Varidase; ***Israel:*** Varidase†; ***Ital.:*** Varidase; ***Mex.:*** Varidasa; ***Neth.:*** Varidase†; ***Norw.:*** Varidase†; ***NZ:*** Varidase†; ***Port.:*** Varidasa; ***S.Afr.:*** Varidase†; ***Spain:*** Ernodasa; Varibiotic†; Varidasa; ***Swed.:*** Varidase; ***UK:*** Varidase.

## Strontium Chloride

Estroncio, cloruro de.

$SrCl_2,6H_2O = 266.6.$

*CAS — 10476-85-4 (anhydrous strontium chloride).*

### Profile

Strontium chloride is used as a 10% toothpaste for the relief of dental hypersensitivity. Strontium acetate has been used similarly.

### Preparations

**Proprietary Preparations** (details are given in Part 3)

***Austria:*** Sensodyne med; ***Braz.:*** Sensodyne Formula Original; ***Canad.:*** Sensodyne; ***Chile:*** Dentoxil; ***Switz.:*** Sensodent; ***UK:*** Sensodyne Mint; Sensodyne Original; ***USA:*** Sensodyne-SC.

**Multi-ingredient:** ***Arg.:*** Esme Topico; ***Canad.:*** Reversa UV.

## Strychnine

Estricnina; Strychnina. Strychnidin-10-one.
$C_{21}H_{22}N_2O_2$ = 334.4.
*CAS — 57-24-9.*

**Description.** Strychnine is an alkaloid obtained from the seeds of nux vomica (p.1722) and other species of *Strychnos.*

## Strychnine Hydrochloride

Estricnina, hidrocloruro de; Strych. Hydrochlor.; Strychninae Hydrochloridum.
$C_{21}H_{22}N_2O_2,HCl,2H_2O$ = 406.9.
*CAS — 1421-86-9 (anhydrous strychnine hydrochloride); 6101-04-8 (strychnine hydrochloride dihydrate).*

## Strychnine Nitrate

Azotato de Estricnina; Estricnina, nitrato de; Nitrato de Estricnina; Strychninae Nitras; Strychninum Nitricum.
$C_{21}H_{22}N_2O_2,HNO_3$ = 397.4.
*CAS — 66-32-0.*

**Pharmacopoeias.** In *Chin.*

## Strychnine Sulfate

Estricnina, sulfato de; Strychninae Sulphas; Strychnine Sulphate; Strychninum Sulfuricum; Sulfato de Estricnina.
$(C_{21}H_{22}N_2O_2)_2,H_2SO_4,5H_2O$ = 857.0.
*CAS — 60-41-3 (anhydrous strychnine sulfate); 60491-10-3 (strychnine sulfate pentahydrate).*

**Pharmacopoeias.** In *Fr.* and *Viet.*

### Adverse Effects

The symptoms of strychnine poisoning are mainly those arising from stimulation of the CNS. Early signs occurring within 15 to 30 minutes of ingestion include tremors, slight twitching, and stiffness of the face and limbs. Painful convulsions develop and may be triggered by minor sensory stimuli; since consciousness is not impaired patients may be extremely distressed. All forms of sensation are heightened. The body becomes arched backwards in hyperextension with the head retracted, arms and legs extended, fists clenched, and the feet turned inward. The jaw is rigidly clamped and contraction of the facial muscles produces a characteristic grinning expression known as 'risus sardonicus'. The convulsions may recur repeatedly and are interspersed with periods of relaxation. If not treated adequately, few patients survive more than 5 episodes of convulsions, death usually occurring due to respiratory arrest. Fatalities have occurred with doses as little as 16 mg.

Secondary effects arising from the severe spasms include lactic acidosis, rhabdomyolysis, renal failure, hyperthermia, hyperkalaemia, and dehydration.

**Poisoning.** References.


1. O'Callaghan WG, *et al.* Unusual strychnine poisoning and its treatment: report of eight cases. *BMJ* 1982; **285:** 478.
2. Blain PG, *et al.* Strychnine poisoning: abnormal eye movements. *J Toxicol Clin Toxicol* 1982; **19:** 215–17.
3. Boyd RE, *et al.* Strychnine poisoning: recovery from profound lactic acidosis, hyperthermia, and rhabdomyolysis. *Am J Med* 1983; **74:** 507–12.
4. Burn DJ, *et al.* Strychnine poisoning as an unusual cause of convulsions. *Postgrad Med J* 1989; **65:** 563–4.
5. Yamarick W, *et al.* Strychnine poisoning in an adolescent. *J Toxicol Clin Toxicol* 1992; **30:** 141–8.
6. Heiser JM, *et al.* Massive strychnine intoxication: serial blood levels in a fatal case. *J Toxicol Clin Toxicol* 1992; **30:** 269–83.
7. Nishiyama T, Nagase M. Strychnine poisoning: natural course of a nonfatal case. *Am J Emerg Med* 1995; **13:** 172–3.
8. Katz J, *et al.* Strychnine poisoning from a Cambodian traditional remedy. *Am J Emerg Med* 1996; **14:** 475–7.
9. Hernandez AF, *et al.* Acute chemical pancreatitis associated with nonfatal strychnine poisoning. *J Toxicol Clin Toxicol* 1998; **36:** 67–71.
10. Greene R, Meatherall R. Dermal exposure to strychnine. *J Anal Toxicol* 2001; **25:** 344–7.
11. Wood D, *et al.* Case report: survival after deliberate strychnine self-poisoning, with toxicokinetic data. *Crit Care* 2002; **6:** 456–9.


### Treatment of Adverse Effects

The main aim of therapy in strychnine poisoning is the prompt prevention or control of convulsions and asphyxia. Activated charcoal should be given if the patient presents within 1 hour of ingestion. Convulsions should be controlled or prevented by diazepam. Intubation and assisted respiration may be required. Should diazepam fail then phenobarbital may be tried. All unnecessary external stimuli should be avoided and if possible the patient should be kept at rest in a quiet darkened room. Patients should be monitored for any secondary effects such as metabolic acidosis so that appropriate symptomatic treatment can be given.

### Uses and Administration

Strychnine competes with glycine, which is an inhibitory neurotransmitter; it thus exerts a central stimulant effect by blocking an inhibitory activity.

Strychnine was formerly used as a bitter and analeptic but is now mainly used under strict control as a rodenticide, or as a mole poison. It has been used in multi-ingredient preparations for the treatment of ophthalmic and urinary-tract disorders. It has also been tried in the treatment of nonketotic hyperglycinaemia.

**Nonketotic hyperglycinaemia.** Nonketotic hyperglycinaemia (also known as glycine encephalopathy) is an inborn defect in the enzyme system responsible for the metabolism of glycine. It is characterised by raised concentrations of glycine in plasma, CSF, and urine. Symptoms of glycine accumulation include respiratory distress, muscular hypotonia, seizures, vomiting, and extreme lethargy. Mental retardation and early infant death are common.

Sodium benzoate can reduce plasma-glycine concentrations to near normal but is relatively ineffective in reducing CSF levels or in preventing mental retardation.[1] Strychnine, a glycine antagonist, has been of some benefit in counteracting the effects of high concentrations of glycine in the CNS.[2-4] However, even treatment with both may be ineffective in severe cases[5] and may ultimately have little effect on the course of the disease.[6] Glycine is reported to stimulate *N*-methyl-D-aspartate (NMDA) receptors in the CNS and the combination of strychnine and ketamine (an NMDA receptor antagonist) was of some benefit in a newborn infant with severe nonketotic hyperglycinaemia.[7] Addition of low-dose dextromethorphan (an NMDA receptor antagonist) to treatment with sodium benzoate, arginine, carnitine, diazepam, and phenobarbital in an infant with nonketotic hyperglycinaemia[8] was associated with resolution of nystagmus and improvement in eye contact and interactive behaviour, without altering serum- or CSF-glycine concentrations. Dextromethorphan with sodium benzoate alone may also be helpful, although the combination is not uniformly effective.[9] Treatment with sodium benzoate and dextromethorphan was beneficial in a 6-month-old child with mild atypical nonketotic hyperglycinaemia,[10] although it was later shown that it was sodium benzoate that had the greatest effect on EEG and behavioural changes. A partial response to low-protein diet and sodium benzoate was demonstrated in a patient with late-onset nonketotic hyperglycinaemia; there was a more dramatic response when imipramine was added to therapy.[11]


1. Krieger I, *et al.* Cerebrospinal fluid glycine in nonketotic hyperglycinemia: effect of treatment with sodium benzoate and a ventricular shunt. *Metabolism* 1977; **26:** 517–24.
2. Ch'ien LT, *et al.* Glycine encephalopathy. *N Engl J Med* 1978; **298:** 687.
3. Gitzelmann R, *et al.* Strychnine for the treatment of nonketotic hyperglycinaemia. *N Engl J Med* 1978; **298:** 1424.
4. Arneson D, *et al.* Strychnine therapy in nonketotic hyperglycinemia. *Pediatrics* 1979; **63:** 369–73.
5. Sankaran K, *et al.* Glycine encephalopathy in a neonate. *Clin Pediatr (Phila)* 1982; **21:** 636–7.
6. MacDermot KD, *et al.* Attempts at use of strychnine sulfate in the treatment of nonketotic hyperglycinemia. *Pediatrics* 1980; **65:** 61–4.
7. Tegtmeyer-Metzdorf H, *et al.* Ketamine and strychnine treatment of an infant with nonketotic hyperglycinaemia. *Eur J Pediatr* 1995; **154:** 649–53.
8. Alemzadeh R, *et al.* Efficacy of low-dose dextromethorphan in the treatment of nonketotic hyperglycinemia. *Pediatrics* 1996; **97:** 924–6.
9. Hamosh A, *et al.* Long-term use of high-dose benzoate and dextromethorphan for the treatment of nonketotic hyperglycinemia. *J Pediatr* 1998; **132:** 709–13.
10. Neuberger JM, *et al.* Effect of sodium benzoate in the treatment of atypical nonketotic hyperglycinaemia. *J Inherit Metab Dis* 2000; **23:** 22–6.
11. Wiltshire EJ, *et al.* Treatment of late-onset nonketotic hyperglycinaemia: effectiveness of imipramine and benzoate. *J Inherit Metab Dis* 2000; **23:** 15–21.


### Preparations

**Proprietary Preparations** (details are given in Part 3)
**Multi-ingredient:** ***Austria:*** Dysurgal†; ***Chile:*** Vigofortal; ***Israel:*** Tesopalmed Forte cum Yohimbine; ***Ital.:*** Neuroftal; ***Thai.:*** Hemo-Cyto-Serum.

## Suanzaorentang

Ziziphus Soup.

### Profile

Suanzaorentang is an ancient Chinese remedy for anxiety and insomnia. It contains five herbs: suanzaoren (*Zizyphus spinosus*, Rhamnaceae), fuling (*Poria cocos*, Polyporaceae), gancao (*Glycyrrhiza uralensis*, Leguminosae), zhimu (*Anemarrhena asphodeloides*, Liliaceae), and chuanxiong (*Ligusticum chuanxiong*, Umbelliferae).

## Succinimide

Butanimide; Succinimida. Pyrrolidine-2,5-dione.
$C_4H_5NO_2$ = 99.09.
*CAS — 123-56-8.*
*ATC — G04BX10.*

### Profile

Succinimide has been claimed to inhibit the formation of oxalic acid calculi in the kidney and to reduce hyperoxaluria.

## Sucrose Octa-acetate

Sacarosa, octaacetato de; Sucrose Octaacetate.
$C_{28}H_{38}O_{19}$ = 678.6.
*CAS — 126-14-7.*

**Pharmacopoeias.** In *USNF.*

**USNF 22** (Sucrose Octaacetate). A white, practically odourless, hygroscopic powder. M.p. not lower than 78°. Soluble 1 in 1100 of water, 1 in 11 of alcohol, 1 in 0.3 of acetone, 1 in 0.5 of toluene, and 1 in 0.6 of benzene; very soluble in chloroform and in methyl alcohol; soluble in ether. Store in airtight containers.

### Profile

Sucrose octa-acetate has been used as an alcohol denaturant. It is also incorporated into preparations intended to deter nail biting.

### Preparations

**Proprietary Preparations** (details are given in Part 3)
**Multi-ingredient:** ***Spain:*** Morde X.

## Sulfobromophthalein Sodium

Bromsulfophthalein Sodium; Bromsulphthalein Sodium; BSP; SBP; Sodium Sulfobromophthalein; Sulfobromoftaleína sódica; Sulphobromophthalein Sodium *(BANM)*. Disodium 4,5,6,7-tetrabromophenolphthalein-3′,3″-disulphonate; Disodium 5,5′-(4,5,6,7-tetrabromophthalidylidene)bis(2-hydroxybenzenesulphonate).
$C_{20}H_8Br_4Na_2O_{10}S_2$ = 838.0.
*CAS — 297-83-6 (sulfobromophthalein); 71-67-0 (sulfobromophthalein sodium).*
*ATC — V04CE02.*

**Pharmacopoeias.** In *Chin., It.,* and *Jpn.*

### Profile

In patients with normal hepatic function sulfobromophthalein sodium is rapidly extracted, conjugated, and excreted in bile. It was formerly used intravenously as a diagnostic agent for testing the functional capacity of the liver but may cause severe hypersensitivity reactions.

## Sulfuric Acid

Acid. Sulph.; Acid. Sulph. Dil.; E513; Oil of Vitriol; Sulfúrico, ácido; Sulphuric Acid; Verdünnte Schwefelsäure (dilute sulfuric acid).
$H_2SO_4$ = 98.08.
*CAS — 7664-93-9.*

NOTE. Concentrated oil of vitriol of commerce, 'COV', contains about 95 to 98% w/w, and brown oil of vitriol, 'BOV', contains 75 to 85% w/w of $H_2SO_4$.

Nordhausen or fuming sulfuric acid, 'Oleum', is sulfuric acid containing $SO_3$.

Battery or accumulator acid is sulfuric acid diluted with distilled water to a specific gravity of 1.2 to 1.26.

**Pharmacopoeias.** *Br., Eur.* (see p.vi), and *Pol.,* include various concentrations. Also in *USNF.*

**BP 2003** (Dilute Sulphuric Acid). It contains 9.5 to 10.5% w/w of $H_2SO_4$ and is prepared by adding 104 g of sulfuric acid to 896 g of water, with constant stirring and cooling.

**Ph. Eur. 5.0** (Sulphuric Acid). It contains 95.0 to 100.5% w/w of $H_2SO_4$. A colourless, very hygroscopic, oily liquid. Miscible with water and with alcohol producing intense heat. Store in airtight containers.

**USNF 22** (Sulfuric Acid). It contains 95.0 to 98.0% w/w of $H_2SO_4$. A clear, colourless, oily liquid. Is very caustic and corrosive. Miscible with water and with alcohol with the generation of much heat. Store in airtight containers.

**Dilution.** When sulfuric acid is mixed with other liquids, it should always be added slowly, with constant stirring, to the diluent.

### Adverse Effects and Treatment

As for Hydrochloric Acid, p.1699.

### Uses and Administration

Sulfuric acid has various industrial uses. Dilute sulfuric acid has been used as an astringent in diarrhoea and it has occasionally been prescribed in mixtures with vegetable bitters to stimulate appetite.

### Preparations

**Proprietary Preparations** (details are given in Part 3)
**Multi-ingredient:** ***USA:*** Debacterol.

## Sulphan Blue *(BAN)*

Azul sulfán; Blue VRS; Isosulfan Blue *(USAN)*; P-1888; P-4125; Sulfan Blue. Sodium α-(4-diethylaminophenyl)-α-(4-diethyliminiocyclo-hexa-2,5-dienylidene)toluene-2,5-disulfonate.
$C_{27}H_{31}N_2NaO_6S_2$ = 566.7.
*CAS — 68238-36-8 (2,5-disulfonate isomer); 129-17-9 (2,4-disulfonate isomer).*

NOTE. Sulphan blue was formerly described in *BPC 1954* as the 2,4-disulfonate isomer and the following synonyms have been applied to this 2,4-isomer: Acid Blue 1; Alphazurine 2G; Colour Index No. 42045; Patent Blue V; Sulphanum Caeruleum. The name Patent Blue V, however, is mainly used for CI No. 42051 (p.1729).

### Profile

Intravenous doses of sulphan blue produce staining of the skin and have been used as a direct visual test of the state of the circulation in healthy and damaged tissues, particularly in assessing tissue viability in burns and soft-tissue trauma. It has also been used subcutaneously in lymphangiography to outline the lymph vessels.

Hypersensitivity reactions including anaphylaxis and attacks of asthma have been reported with sulphan blue. It has also been reported to interfere with blood tests for protein and iron.

### Preparations

**Proprietary Preparations** (details are given in Part 3)
***USA:*** Lymphazurin.

## Sumatra Benzoin

Benjoim; Benjuí, bálsamo de; Benzoë; Benzoin; Gum Benjamin; Gum Benzoin.

*CAS — 9000-05-9 (.*

**Pharmacopoeias.** In *Br.* and *Jpn.*

*US* allows both Siam benzoin and Sumatra benzoin under the title Benzoin.

**BP 2003** (Sumatra Benzoin). A balsamic resin obtained from the incised stem of *Styrax benzoin* and of *S. paralleloneurus*. It contains not less than 25% of total balsamic acids, calculated as cinnamic acid and with reference to the dried material, and not more than 20% of alcohol (90%)-insoluble matter.

Hard brittle masses of whitish tears embedded in a greyish-brown to reddish-brown translucent matrix, known in commerce as block benzoin. It also occurs in the form of tears with cream-coloured surfaces and, when broken, exhibiting surfaces having a milky-white colour. It has an agreeable balsamic odour. Store at a temperature not exceeding 25°. Protect from light.

**USP 27** (Benzoin). A balsamic resin from *Styrax paralleloneurus* or *S. benzoin* (Styracaceae). It yields not less than 75% of alcohol-soluble extractive. It occurs as blocks or lumps of variable size made up of tears, compacted together, with a reddish-brown, reddish-grey, or greyish-brown resinous mass. The tears are externally yellowish or rusty brown, milky white on fresh fracture, hard and brittle at ordinary temperatures but softened by heat. It has an aromatic and balsamic odour. When heated it does not emit a pinaceous odour. When digested with boiling water, the odour suggests cinnamates or storax.

### Profile

Sumatra benzoin is an ingredient of inhalations which are used in the treatment of catarrh of the upper respiratory tract. Sumatra benzoin is also used in topical preparations for its antiseptic and protective properties. Skin sensitisation has been reported.

### Preparations

***BP 2003:*** Benzoin Inhalation; Compound Benzoin Tincture;
***BPC 1954:*** Compound Iodoform Paint;
***USP 27:*** Compound Benzoin Tincture; Podophyllum Resin Topical Solution.

**Proprietary Preparations** (details are given in Part 3)

**Multi-ingredient:** ***Austral.:*** Nappy-Mate†; Nyal Cold Sore†; ***Belg.:*** Borostyrol†; ***Braz.:*** Axol†; Inalobel†; Inhadrina†; Inhalante Yatropan; Micotissim†; Micoz; Rinofen†; Yatropan†; ***Canad.:*** Chase Coldsorex; Cold Sore Lotion; Lotion pour Feux Sauvages; ***Fr.:*** Balsofumine; Balsofumine Mentholee; ***Ger.:*** Nur 1 Tropfen medizinisches Mundwasser; ***Ital.:*** Citrosil Nubesan; Fomentil; ***NZ:*** Cold Sore; ***Port.:*** Kemphor; Vaporil; ***Switz.:*** Baume; ***UK:*** Allens Dry Tickly Cough; Frador; Kilkof; Potters Strong Bronchial Catarrh Pastilles; Potters Sugar Free Cough Pastilles; Snowfire; Sunspot†; Throaties Pastilles; ***USA:*** Pfeiffer's Cold Sore.

## Surgibone *(USAN)*

### Profile

Surgibone is sterile, specially processed mature bovine bone, that has been used for grafting procedures in orthopaedic and reconstructive surgery.

## Sutilains *(BAN, USAN, rINN)*

BAX-1515; Sutilaína.

*CAS — 12211-28-8.*

### Profile

Sutilains contains enzymes derived from *Bacillus subtilis*. It has proteolytic actions in most conditions, and has been used for the debridement of wounds, burns, and decubitus ulcers.

## Tadalafil *(USAN, rINN)*

GF-196960; IC-351; Tadalafilo. (6*R*,12a*R*)-2,3,6,7,12,12a-Hexahydro-2-methyl-6-[3,4-(methylenedioxy)phenyl]pyrazino-[1′,2′:1,6]pyrido[3,4-*b*]indole-1,4-dione.

$C_{22}H_{19}N_3O_4$ = 389.4.

*CAS — 171596-29-5.*

*ATC — G04BE08.*

### Adverse Effects

As for Sildenafil, p.1744. Visual disturbances may occur less frequently with tadalafil than with sildenafil.

**Effects on the cardiovascular system.** References.

1. Kloner RA, *et al.* Cardiovascular effects of tadalafil. *Am J Cardiol* 2003; **92:** 37M–46M.

### Precautions

As for Sildenafil, p.1744. Dosage reductions may be required in patients with hepatic or renal impairment (see under Uses and Administration, below); a careful individual benefit/risk evaluation should be carried out in patients with severe hepatic impairment.

### Interactions

As for Sildenafil, p.1744. Rifampicin, an inducer of the cytochrome P450 isoenzyme CYP3A4, has been shown to decrease the plasma concentrations of tadalafil.

### Pharmacokinetics

Tadalafil is well absorbed after a dose by mouth. Peak plasma concentrations are attained within 2 hours; the rate of absorption is not affected by food.

Tadalafil is widely distributed into tissues and is approximately 94% bound to plasma proteins. It is metabolised in the liver primarily by the cytochrome P450 isoenzyme CYP3A4. The major metabolite, the methylcatechol glucuronide, is inactive. The mean half-life of tadalafil is about 17.5 hours.

Tadalafil is excreted, predominantly as metabolites, in the faeces (61% of the dose), and to a lesser extent the urine (36% of the dose). Clearance may be reduced in the elderly and in patients with renal impairment.

### Uses and Administration

Tadalafil is a phosphodiesterase type-5 inhibitor with actions and uses similar to those of sildenafil (p.1745). It is used in the management of erectile dysfunction (see p.1745). Tadalafil is given by mouth in a usual dose of 10 mg at least 30 minutes before sexual intercourse and may be taken with or without food; the daily dose may be increased to 20 mg, or decreased to 5 mg, if necessary. Efficacy may persist for up to 36 hours after dosing. Tadalafil should not be taken more than once in 24 hours; the manufacturers in fact discourage continuous daily use because of inadequate safety data for long-term use. Dosage adjustments are not necessary in elderly patients; for recommendations in hepatic or renal impairment, see below.

◊ References.

1. Brock GB, *et al.* Efficacy and safety of tadalafil for the treatment of erectile dysfunction: results of integrated analyses. *J Urol (Baltimore)* 2002; **168:** 1332–6.
2. Brock GB. Tadalafil: a new agent for erectile dysfunction. *Can J Urol* 2003; **10** (suppl 1): 17–22.
3. Bella AJ, Brock GB. Tadalafil in the treatment of erectile dysfunction. *Curr Urol Rep* 2003; **4:** 472–8.
4. Curran MP, Keating GM. Tadalafil. *Drugs* 2003; **63:** 2203–12. Correction. *ibid.*; 2703.
5. Meuleman EJ. Review of tadalafil in the treatment of erectile dysfunction. *Expert Opin Pharmacother* 2003; **4:** 2049–56.
6. Padma-Nathan H. Efficacy and tolerability of tadalafil, a novel phosphodiesterase 5 inhibitor, in treatment of erectile dysfunction. *Am J Cardiol* 2003; **92** (suppl 1): 19M–25M.

**Administration in hepatic impairment.** The manufacturers recommend a maximum dose of 10 mg of tadalafil in patients with mild to moderate hepatic impairment; there are no available data for higher doses in this patient population. See also Precautions, above.

**Administration in renal impairment.** The dose of tadalafil may need to be reduced in patients with renal impairment. In the UK, the manufacturers recommend a maximum dose of 10 mg in patients with severe renal impairment. In the USA, for patients with moderate renal impairment (creatinine clearance 31 to 50 mL/minute), the manufacturers recommend an initial dose of 5 mg, and a maximum dose of 10 mg in 48 hours; patients with severe renal impairment (creatinine clearance less than 30 mL/minute) may be given a maximum dose of 5 mg.

### Preparations

**Proprietary Preparations** (details are given in Part 3)
***Austral.:*** Cialis; ***Denm.:*** Cialis; ***Fr.:*** Cialis; ***Ger.:*** Cialis; ***Irl.:*** Cialis; ***Port.:*** Cialis; ***Swed.:*** Cialis; ***UK:*** Cialis; ***USA:*** Cialis.

## Tannic Acid

Acidum Tannicum; Gallotannic Acid; Gerbstoff; Tánico, ácido; Tanin; Tann. Acid; Tannin; Tanninum.

*CAS — 1401-55-4.*

NOTE. In pharmaceutical literature, the name digallic acid is frequently confused with tannic acid.

Commercial grades of tannic acid may contain gallic acid and being less soluble are not suitable for medicinal use.

**Pharmacopoeias.** In *Eur.* (see p.vi), *Jpn, Pol.,* and *US.*

**Ph. Eur. 5.0** (Tannic Acid). A mixture of esters of glucose with gallic acid and 3-galloylgallic acid. A yellowish-white or slightly brown amorphous light powder or shiny plates. Very soluble in water; freely soluble in alcohol, in acetone, and in glycerol (85%); practically insoluble in dichloromethane. Protect from light.

**USP 27** (Tannic Acid). A tannin usually obtained from nutgalls (see Gall, p.1690), the excrescences produced on the young twigs of *Quercus infectoria* and allied species of *Quercus*, from the seed pods of tara (*Caesalpinia spinosa*), or from the nutgalls or leaves of sumac (any of a genus *Rhus*).

Amorphous powder, glistening scales, or spongy masses, varying in colour from yellowish-white to light brown. Is odourless or has a faint, characteristic odour. Very soluble in water, in alcohol, and in acetone; freely soluble in diluted alcohol; slightly soluble in dehydrated alcohol; practically insoluble in chloroform, in ether, in petroleum spirit, and in benzene; soluble 1 in about 1 of warm glycerol. Store in airtight containers. Protect from light.

### Profile

Tannic acid has been used as an astringent for the mucous membranes of the mouth and throat, and in suppositories for tannic acid have been used in the treatment of haemorrhoids. It is an ingredient in a number of dermatological preparations.

Former uses of tannic acid include application to burns, addition to barium sulfate enemas to improve the quality of radiological pictures of the colon, and as an ingredient of 'Universal Antidote'. However, tannic acid has been associated with liver toxicity, sometimes fatal.

**Tattoo removal.** Although tannic acid may be used by plastic surgeons and dermatologists to produce a controlled partial-thickness burn in tattoo removal[1] it has been pointed out that in unskilled or amateur hands this procedure has resulted in full thickness burns requiring skin grafting to obtain satisfactory healing.[2]

1. Mercer NSG, Davies DM. Tattoos. *BMJ* 1991; **303:** 380.
2. Scott M, Ridings P. Tattoos. *BMJ* 1991; **303:** 720.

### Preparations

**Proprietary Preparations** (details are given in Part 3)
***Ger.:*** Tannosynt; ***Spain:*** Tanagel Papeles.

**Multi-ingredient:** ***Austral.:*** SM-33; ***Austria:*** Haemanal; Onycho Phytex†; Paradenton; Phytex†; Tebege-Tannin†; ***Belg.:*** Aperop†; ***Braz.:*** Anapyon†; Boralina†; Lacto Vagin; Lacto-Gin†; ***Canad.:*** Bunion Salve†; Outgro†; Tanac; ***Fr.:*** Allerbiocid S; Eau Precieuse; HEC; Marinol; ***Ger.:*** Bioget; Tannolil; ***Hong Kong:*** Cortison Kemicetine†; ***Irl.:*** Phytex; ***Israel:*** Rectozorin; ***Ital.:*** Blefarolin; Neo Emocicatrol; ***S.Afr.:*** Burn-A-Sept†; ***Singapore:*** HEC†; ***Spain:*** Antihemorroidal; Depurativo Richelet; Dextricea; Queratil†; Sabanotropico; Talkosona†; Talquissar†; Tanagel; Tangenol; ***Switz.:*** HEC; ***UK:*** Colsor; Phytex; TCP; ***USA:*** Dermasept Antifungal; Orasept; Outgro; Tanac; Tanac Dual Core.

## Tansy

Tanaceto.

### Profile

Tansy, the flowering tops of *Tanacetum vulgare* (*Chrysanthemum vulgare*) (Compositae), has been used as an anthelmintic and to stimulate menstruation. The oil is highly toxic and use of tansy is generally not recommended.

### Preparations

**Proprietary Preparations** (details are given in Part 3)
**Multi-ingredient:** ***Austral.:*** Calmo†.

## Taraxacum

Dandelion Root; Diente de León; Löwenzahnwurzel; Pissenlit; Taraxacum Root.

**Pharmacopoeias.** In *Pol.*

*Chin.* specifies Taraxacum Herb from other species of *Taraxacum.*

### Profile

Taraxacum is the fresh or dried root of the common dandelion, *Taraxacum officinale* (Compositae). It has been used as a bitter, as a diuretic, and as a mild laxative. It has also been used in homoeopathic medicine.

◊ References.

1. Houghton P. Bearberry, dandelion and celery. *Pharm J* 1995; **255:** 272–3.

### Preparations

**Proprietary Preparations** (details are given in Part 3)
***Ger.:*** Carvicum; Galleb S†; Justogen mono†; Kneipp Lowenzahn-Pflanzensaft†; Taraleon.

**Multi-ingredient:** ***Arg.:*** Quelodin F; ***Austral.:*** Berberis Complex†; Biglan Cranbiotic Super†; Extralife Fluid-Care†; Extralife Liva-Care†; Feminine Herbal Complex†; Fluid Loss†; Glycoplex†; Herbal Cleanse†; Herbal Diuretic Formula†; Lifesystem Herbal Formula 7 Liver Tonic†; Liver Tonic Herbal Formula 6†; Profluid†; Silybum Complex†; St Mary's Thistle Plus†; Trifolium Complex†; Uva-Ursi Complex†; Uva-Ursi Plus†; ***Austria:*** Agnuchol; Apotheker Hoyers Brennesseltonikum; Aurita-Leber-Galletee; Bio-Garten Entschlackungstee; Bio-Garten Tee zur Erhohung der Harnmenge; Bio-Garten Tropfen fur Galle und Leber; Bio-Strath Nieren-Blasen; Bioreform-Entschlackungstee; Bioreform-Harntreibender Tee; Brennesseltonikum; Citochol; Digestol; Ehrmann's Entschlackungstee; Felidon neu; Fruhjahrs-Elixier ohne Alkohol; Gallen- und Lebertee EF-EM-ES; Gallesyn neu; Gallogran; Gewusst wie Darmtee; Gewusst wie Entschlackungstee; Gewusst wie Gruner Fastentee; Gewusst wie Leber-Gallentee; Kneipp Galle- und Leber-Tee; Kneipp Stoffwechsel-Unterstutzungs-Tee; Krauterdoktor Entschlackungs-Elixier; Krauterdoktor Gallentreibende Tropfen; Krauterdoktor Harnstein- und Nieren-griesstropfen; Krauterhaus Mag Kottas Entschlackungstee; Krauterhaus Mag Kottas Gallen- und Lebertee; Krauterpfarrer Weidinger Tee zur Entschlackung; Mag Doskar's Leber-Galletonikum; Mag Kottas Entschlackungstee; Mag Kottas Entwasserungstee; Mag Kottas Krauterexpress-Entschlackungstee; Mag Kottas Krauterexpress-Entwasserungstee; Mag Kottas Krauterexpress-Leber-Gallentee; Mag Kottas Leber-Gallentee; Magentee EF-EM-ES; Magentropen N Legastol†; Montana; Naturland Entschlackungstee; Naturland Rheuma Tee; Neuners Krautertee Nr 17 - Lebertee; Neuners Krautertee Nr 20 - Kreislauftee; Neuners Krautertee Nr 25 - Entschlackungstee; Neuners Krautertee Nr 29 - Stoffwechseltee mild; Sanvita Leber-Galle; Sidroga Leber-Galle-Tee; Sidroga Stoffwechseltee; Solisan; St Radegunder Entschlackungs-Elixier; St Radegunder Leber-Galle-Tee; Teekanne Leber- und Galletee; Tiroler Adler Leber- und Gallentee; Urelium Neu; ***Canad.:*** Milk Thistle Formula; ***Fr.:*** Diacure; Maxidraine; Romarene; Romarenex-Choline†; ***Ger.:*** Agrimonas N†; Alasenn; Amara-Tropfen; Aristochol N;

Artischocke plus Legastol†; Carmol Magen-Galle-Darm; Cefachol†; Cholosom SL; Cholosom-Tee; Gallemolan forte; Gallemolan G; Gallexier; Galloselect M; Hepatofalk Neu†; Hevert-Entwasserungs-Tee†; Hevert-Gall S†; JuCholan S†; Kneipp Galle- und Leber-Tee N†; Legapas comp†; Neurochol C; Nieron S; Nieron-Tee N; Novo Mandrogallan N†; Pascobilin novo; Pascohepan novo†; Presselin Hepaticum P; Salus Leber-Galle-Tee Nr. 18†; Salus Rheuma-Tee Krautertee Nr. 12†; Sirmia Artischockenelixier N†; Tonsilgon; Ullus Galle-Tee N†; Uro-Pasc†; ***Hong Kong:*** Hepatofalk; ***Ital.:*** Centaurea (Specie Composta); Depurfat†; Tarassaco (Specie Composta); Varicofit; ***Switz.:*** Boldocynara; Demonatur Gouttes pour le foie et la bile; Gastrosan; Phytomed Hepato; Phytomed Nephro; Tisane hepatique et biliaire; ***UK:*** Adios; Aqualette; Backache; Boldex; Boldo†; Califig†; Gerard House Buchu Compound†; Gerard House Golden Seal Compound†; Gerard House Waterlex†; HealthAid Boldo-Plus; Herbulax; HRI Water Balance; Natural Herb Tablets; Out-of-Sorts; Rheumatic Pain; Stomach Mixture; Uvacin; Weight Loss Aid; Wind & Dyspepsia Relief.

## Targinine *(BAN)*

Tilarginine *(pINN)*; BW-546C88; 546C88; L-NMMA; Targinina. $N^{\omega}$-Methyl-L-arginine.

$C_7H_{16}N_4O_2$ = 188.2.

*CAS — 17035-90-4.*

### Profile

Targinine is a nitric oxide synthase inhibitor under investigation in the treatment of septic shock and migraine.

◊ References.

1. Lassen LH, *et al.* Nitric oxide synthase inhibition in migraine. *Lancet* 1997; **349:** 401–2.
2. Hussein Z, *et al.* Pharmacokinetics of the nitric oxide synthase inhibitor L-$N^{G}$-methylarginine hydrochloride in patients with septic shock. *Clin Pharmacol Ther* 1999; **65:** 1–9.

## Tartaric Acid

Acidum Tartaricum; E334; E353 (metatartaric acid); Tart. Acid; Tartárico, ácido; Tartrique (Acide); Weinsäure. (+)-L-Tartaric acid; (2R,3R)-2,3-Dihydroxybutane-1,4-dioic acid.

$C_4H_6O_6$ = 150.1.

*CAS — 87-69-4; 526-83-0.*

**Pharmacopoeias.** In *Eur.* (see p.vi), *Jpn,* and *Pol.* Also in *USNF.*

**Ph. Eur. 5.0** (Tartaric Acid). A white or almost white, crystalline powder or colourless crystals. Very soluble in water; freely soluble in alcohol.

**USNF 22** (Tartaric Acid). Colourless or translucent crystals or a white, fine to granular, crystalline powder. Is odourless. Soluble 1 in 0.8 of water, 1 in 0.5 of boiling water, 1 in 3 of alcohol, 1 in 250 of ether, and 1 in 1.7 of methyl alcohol.

### Adverse Effects

Strong solutions of tartaric acid are mildly irritant and if ingested undiluted may cause violent vomiting and diarrhoea, abdominal pain, and thirst. Cardiovascular collapse or acute renal failure may follow.

### Pharmacokinetics

Tartaric acid is absorbed from the gastrointestinal tract but up to 80% of an ingested dose is probably destroyed by micro-organisms in the lumen of the intestine before absorption occurs. Absorbed tartaric acid is excreted unchanged in the urine.

### Uses and Administration

Tartaric acid is used in the preparation of effervescent powders, granules, and tablets, as an ingredient of cooling drinks, and as a saline purgative. If not neutralised, it must be taken well diluted. Tartaric acid or metatartaric acid are used in wine-making as de-acidifying agents to assist in the removal of excess malic acid by forming an insoluble double salt with calcium carbonate.

### Preparations

**Proprietary Preparations** (details are given in Part 3)

**Multi-ingredient:** ***Arg.:*** Alikal; Sal de Fruta Eno; Uvasal; ***Austral.:*** Citralite; Citravescent; Dexsal; Salvital†; Ural; Uricalm; ***Austria:*** Helo-acid; Lactolavol; ***Belg.:*** Zoru; ***Canad.:*** E-Z-Gas II; Unik-Zoru†; ***Chile:*** Frunalia; Frutasal Knop; Uroknop; ***Fr.:*** Dermacide; Zeniac LP Fort; ***Ger.:*** Bourget†; Retterspitz Ausserlich†; Retterspitz Geleet†; Retterspitz Innerlich†; ***Hong Kong:*** Floxil†; ***Israel:*** Eno; ***Ital.:*** Antimicotica Solforata; Geffer; Magnesia Effervescente Sella; Non Acid†; ***Malaysia:*** Citravescent; Ural; ***NZ:*** Solucol†; Ural; ***Port.:*** Sais de Frutos†; Sais Zitos†; Thiospot; ***S.Afr.:*** Adco-Sodasol; Alkafizz; Citro-Soda; Quatro-Soda; Uri-Alk; ***Spain:*** Citinoides; Hectonona; Mucorex Ciclin†; Salcedol; Sales de Frutas P G; Sales Fruta Mag Viviar; Salmagne; Starlep†; ***Swed.:*** Gastroluft†; ***Switz.:*** Gastroluft†; Gynasol†; Siesta-1; ***UK:*** Jaaps Health Salt; ***USA:*** Baros†.

## Taurine *(rINN)*

Taurina. 2-Aminoethanesulphonic acid.

$C_2H_7NO_3S$ = 125.1.

*CAS — 107-35-7.*

**Pharmacopoeias.** In *Chin.* and *US.*

**USP 27** (Taurine). White crystals or crystalline powder. Soluble in water.

### Profile

Taurine is an amino acid known to be involved in bile acid conjugation as well as other physiological functions. It has been included in preparations for parenteral nutrition of low-birth-weight infants and in infant formulas but its role as an essential nutrient has not been established.

Taurine is included in some preparations for cardiovascular and metabolic disorders.

### Preparations

**Proprietary Preparations** (details are given in Part 3)
***Ital.:*** O-Due.

**Multi-ingredient:** ***Port.:*** Detoxergon; ***Spain:*** Taurobetina.

## Terpineol

$C_{10}H_{18}O$ = 154.2.

*CAS — 8000-41-7 (terpineol); 98-55-5 (α-terpineol).*

**Pharmacopoeias.** In *Br.*

**BP 2003** (Terpineol). A mixture of structural isomers in which α-terpineol predominates. It is a colourless, slightly viscous liquid which may deposit crystals; it has a pleasant characteristic odour. Very slightly soluble in water; freely soluble in alcohol (70%); soluble in ether.

### Profile

Terpineol has disinfectant and solvent properties. It is used with other volatile agents in preparations for respiratory-tract disorders.

### Preparations

***BP 2003:*** Chloroxylenol Solution.

**Proprietary Preparations** (details are given in Part 3)

**Multi-ingredient:** ***Arg.:*** Aseptobron; Aseptobron Ampicilina; Atomo Desinflamante G; Atomo Desinflamante Familiar; Bronco Etersan; Di-Neumobron; ***Austral.:*** Karvol†; Tixylix Chest Rub; ***Austria:*** Resol†; ***Braz.:*** Bromil; Eucaliptan; Eucaliptol Composto†; Mentalol†; Mentolatun†; Napiro†; Penetro; Tabletes Valda†; Valda†; ***Canad.:*** Iba-Cide†; ***Fr.:*** Pectoderme; Valda; ***Hong Kong:*** Valda; ***India:*** Dettol Obstetric; Fairgenol; Karvol Plus; Sinarest Vapocaps; ***Irl.:*** Karvol; Valda; ***Israel:*** Gargol; Karvol; Rexitol; ***Ital.:*** Calyptol; Rikospray; ***Mon.:*** Calyptol; ***Neth.:*** Rhinocaps†; ***NZ:*** Tixylix Chest Rub; ***Port.:*** Valda; ***S.Afr.:*** AF; Karvol; ***Singapore:*** Karvol; ***Spain:*** Caltoson Balsamico; Calyptol Inhalante†; Empapol†; Eupnol; Pastillas Juanola; ***Switz.:*** Sedotussin; ***UK:*** Biocream†; Chymol; Jacksons Mentholated Balm; Karvol; Nowax; Waxwane.

## Tetrabenazine *(BAN, rINN)*

Ro-1-9569; Tetrabenazina. 1,3,4,6,7,11b-Hexahydro-3-isobutyl-9,10-dimethoxybenzo-[*a*]quinolizin-2-one.

$C_{19}H_{27}NO_3$ = 317.4.

*CAS — 58-46-8.*
*ATC — N05AK01.*

### Adverse Effects

Drowsiness is the most frequent side-effect of tetrabenazine. Orthostatic hypotension, symptoms of extrapyramidal dysfunction, gastrointestinal disturbances, and depression may also occur. Neuroleptic malignant syndrome and parkinsonism have been reported rarely. Overdosage has produced sedation, sweating, hypotension, and hypothermia.

**Effects on mental function.** Depression is well documented as an adverse effect of tetrabenazine, and occurs in about 15% of patients; it has been reported to respond to reboxetine.[1] Florid psychiatric symptoms such as panic attacks and obsessive-compulsive symptoms may be precipitated or exacerbated by tetrabenazine.[2]

1. Schreiber W, *et al.* Reversal of tetrabenazine induced depression by selective noradrenaline (norepinephrine) reuptake inhibition. *J Neurol Neurosurg Psychiatry* 1999; **67:** 550.
2. Bruneau MA, *et al.* Catastrophic reactions induced by tetrabenazine. *Can J Psychiatry* 2002; **47:** 683.

**Extrapyramidal disorders.** Dysphagia and choking were associated with tetrabenazine in the treatment of Huntington's chorea.[1] Fatal pneumonia, probably as a consequence of aspiration, had also been reported.

1. Snaith RP, Warren H de B. Treatment of Huntington's chorea with tetrabenazine. *Lancet* 1974; **i:** 413–14.

**Overdosage.** A patient who swallowed approximately 1 g (40 tablets) of tetrabenazine became drowsy 2 hours later and marked sweating occurred.[1] Her state of consciousness improved after 24 hours and she talked rationally and gained full control of micturition after 72 hours.

1. Kidd DW, McLellan DL. Self-poisoning with tetrabenazine. *Br J Clin Pract* 1972; **26:** 179–80.

### Precautions

Tetrabenazine may exacerbate the symptoms of parkinsonism. It may cause drowsiness; affected patients should not drive or operate machinery.

### Interactions

Tetrabenazine has been reported to block the action of reserpine. It may also diminish the effects of levodopa and exacerbate the symptoms of parkinsonism. Use of tetrabenazine immediately after a course of an MAOI may lead to confusion, restlessness, and disorientation; tetrabenazine should not be given with, or within 14 days of stopping, such therapy.

### Pharmacokinetics

Absorption of tetrabenazine is poor and erratic following oral doses. It appears to be extensively metabolised by first-pass metabolism. Its major metabolite, hydroxytetrabenazine, which is formed by reduction, is reported to be as active as the parent compound. It is excreted in the urine mainly in the form of metabolites.

### Uses and Administration

Tetrabenazine is used in the management of movement disorders including chorea (p.664), ballism (p.664), dystonias (p.1209), tardive dyskinesia (see under Extrapyramidal Disorders, p.677), and similar symptoms of CNS dysfunction.

For the treatment of chorea, ballism, and other organic CNS movement disorders, a starting dose of 25 mg three times daily by mouth has been recommended, although a dose of 12.5 mg twice daily may be more appropriate initially as it is less likely to cause excessive sedation. The dose may be gradually increased according to response up to a maximum of 200 mg daily. If the patient does not respond within 7 days of receiving the maximum dose further treatment with tetrabenazine is unlikely to be of benefit. An initial starting dose of 12.5 mg daily has been suggested for elderly patients.

For moderate to severe tardive dyskinesia, a dose of 12.5 mg daily is recommended initially, subsequently titrated according to response.

**Extrapyramidal disorders.** In a long-term study[1] of the use of tetrabenazine in 400 patients with movement disorders, the best responses seemed to be in tardive dyskinesia, tardive dystonia, and Huntington's disease but benefit was also obtained in some patients with idiopathic dystonia, segmental myoclonus, and Tourette's syndrome. Others have commented that in severe dystonia unresponsive to other drugs a combination of tetrabenazine with trihexyphenidyl and pimozide is sometimes effective.[2]

1. Jankovic J, Beach J. Long-term effects of tetrabenazine in hyperkinetic movement disorders. *Neurology* 1997; **48:** 358–62.
2. Marsden CD, Quinn NP. The dystonias. *BMJ* 1990; **300:** 139–44.

### Preparations

**Proprietary Preparations** (details are given in Part 3)
***Austral.:*** Nitoman†; ***Canad.:*** Nitoman; ***Denm.:*** Nitoman; ***India:*** Revocon; ***NZ:*** Xenazine; ***UK:*** Xenazine.

## Tetrachlorodecaoxide

TCDO; Tetrachlorodecaoxygen Anion Complex; Tetraclorodecaóxido; WF-10.

$Cl_4O_{10}$ = 301.8.

*CAS — 92047-76-2.*

### Profile

Tetrachlorodecaoxide is a water-soluble anion complex containing oxygen in a chlorite matrix. Active oxygen is only released in the presence of biological material. It has been applied as a solution for the stimulation of wound healing.

**Wounds.** Tetrachlorodecaoxide was reported to promote wound healing compared with saline in a double-blind study of 271 patients,[1] but a smaller study failed to show any benefit over glycerol.[2]

1. Hinz J, *et al.* Rationale for and results from a randomised, double-blind trial of tetrachlorodecaoxygen anion complex in wound healing. *Lancet* 1986; **i:** 825–8.
2. Hughes LE, *et al.* Failure of tetrachlorodecaoxygen anion complex to assist wound healing. *Lancet* 1989; **ii:** 1271.

### Preparations

**Proprietary Preparations** (details are given in Part 3)
***Austria:*** Oxilium; ***Switz.:*** Oxilium; ***Thai.:*** Immunokine; Oxoferin.

## Tetramethylammonium Iodide

Tetrametilamonio, ioduro de.

$C_4H_{12}IN$ = 201.0.

*CAS — 75-58-1.*

### Profile

Tetramethylammonium iodide is a quaternary ammonium compound that has been used for the emergency disinfection of drinking water. It has also been employed for its ganglion-blocking properties.

## Thalidomide *(BAN, USAN, rINN)*

K-17; NSC-66847; Talidomida. 2-Phthalimidoglutarimide.

$C_{13}H_{10}N_2O_4$ = 258.2.

*CAS — 50-35-1.*
*ATC — L04AX02.*

**Pharmacopoeias.** In *US.*

**USP 27** (Thalidomide). A white to off-white powder. Sparingly soluble in water, in dehydrated alcohol, in acetone, in butyl acetate, in ethyl acetate, in glacial acetic acid, and in methyl alcohol; practically insoluble in chloroform, in ether, and in benzene; very soluble in dimethylformamide, in dioxan, and in pyridine. Store in airtight containers. Protect from light.

### Adverse Effects and Precautions

Thalidomide was withdrawn from use as a hypnotic in the early 1960s after it was discovered that it produced teratogenic effects when given in early pregnancy. These effects involved mainly malformations of the limbs and defects of the ears, eyes, and internal organs, and could develop following a single dose. Further abnormalities and problems, including effects on the CNS, developed in later life.

In consequence, thalidomide should not be used in women of child-bearing potential, or if such use is absolutely essential then stringent contraceptive measures must be used, including the simultaneous use of 2 reliable forms of contraception for at least 4 weeks before, during, and for 4 weeks after, thalidomide therapy. Regular pregnancy testing is mandatory. If pregnancy occurs during thalidomide therapy the drug must be stopped immediately and the patient given appropriate evaluation and counselling. As thalidomide is present in semen, male patients receiving thalidomide should use barrier methods of contraception if their partner is of child-bearing potential. Patients should not donate blood or sperm during thalidomide therapy.

The other major adverse effect of thalidomide is peripheral neuropathy, which can be severe and irreversible.

Other common adverse effects include constipation, dizziness, and orthostatic hypotension. Drowsiness or somnolence occur frequently and, if affected, patients should not drive or operate machinery. Hypersensitivity reactions have occurred. An erythematous macular rash may develop, usually 2 to 10 days after initiation of therapy. Stevens-Johnson syndrome and toxic epidermal necrolysis have also been reported, and therefore thalidomide should be stopped if skin rash develops and only restarted after appropriate clinical evaluation. Thalidomide therapy should not be resumed if the rash is exfoliative, purpuric, or bullous, or if Stevens-Johnson syndrome or toxic epidermal necrolysis is suspected. Bradycardia, neutropenia, and an increase in the viral load in HIV-infected patients have also been reported.

◊ Reviews.


1. Günzler V. Thalidomide in human immunodeficiency virus (HIV) patients: a review of safety considerations. *Drug Safety* 1992; **7:** 116–34.
2. Clark TE, *et al.* Thalomid® (thalidomide) capsules: a review of the first 18 months of spontaneous postmarketing adverse event surveillance, including off-label prescribing. *Drug Safety* 2001; **24:** 87–117.


**Effects on the cardiovascular system.** Use of thalidomide in patients with malignant neoplastic disease has been associated with an increased risk of deep-vein thrombosis. There were 27 spontaneous reports of thromboembolic events in the first 18 months of thalidomide returning to the US market in July 1998; 26 of these were in patients with malignancies.[1] A review[2] of thromboembolic events associated with thalidomide identified 67 such reports from a total of 2075 adverse events reported to the FDA between October 1998 and June 2001; a further 29 cases were identified from clinical trial data. Deep-vein thrombosis occurred in 48 of these patients, pulmonary embolism in 25, and 23 developed both. The most common primary diagnoses among these patients were multiple myeloma and renal cell carcinoma. However, it should be noted that patients with cancer are known to be at increased risk of venous thromboembolism and some chemotherapeutic regimens may further increase this risk. The contribution of thalidomide to the development of venous thromboembolism remains to be fully evaluated in controlled trials.

It has been suggested that in those patients who develop thromboembolism, thalidomide may be continued once appropriate anticoagulant therapy has begun.[1]


1. Clark TE, *et al.* Thalomid® (thalidomide) capsules: a review of the first 18 months of spontaneous postmarketing adverse event surveillance, including off-label prescribing. *Drug Safety* 2001; **24:** 87–117.
2. Bennett CL, *et al.* Thalidomide-associated deep vein thrombosis and pulmonary embolism. *Am J Med* 2002; **113:** 603–6.


**Effects on the endocrine system.** Amenorrhoea has been reported[1,2] in women taking thalidomide for severe dermatological conditions; menses resumed 2 to 3 months after stopping thalidomide.[2]

Hypothyroidism has been associated with thalidomide use in patients with multiple myeloma,[3] and it was suggested that some adverse effects of thalidomide, such as bradycardia and constipation, may be manifestations of hypothyroidism.


1. Passeron T, *et al.* Thalidomide-induced amenorrhoea: two cases. *Br J Dermatol* 2001; **144:** 1292–3.
2. Francès C, *et al.* Transient secondary amenorrhea in women treated by thalidomide. *Eur J Dermatol* 2002; **12:** 63–5.
3. Badros AZ, *et al.* Hypothyroidism in patients with multiple myeloma following treatment with thalidomide. *Am J Med* 2002; **112:** 412–13.


**Effects on mental function.** Symptoms of dementia appeared in a patient who had been taking thalidomide for about 2 months for the treatment of multiple myeloma.[1] Dementia later resolved completely within 48 hours of stopping thalidomide.


1. Morgan AE, *et al.* Reversible dementia due to thalidomide therapy for multiple myeloma. *N Engl J Med* 2003; **348:** 1821–2.


**Effects on sexual function.** Dose-related sexual dysfunction, including loss of libido, loss of penile rigidity, and premature ejaculation, was associated with thalidomide use in 2 male patients.[1]


1. Pouaha J, *et al.* Thalidomide and sexual dysfunction in men. *Br J Dermatol* 2002; **146:** 1112–13.


**Effects on the skin.** Toxic epidermal necrolysis has been reported[1] in a 62-year-old woman approximately 5 weeks after starting thalidomide therapy for the treatment of a glioblastoma. Although the patient was taking several other drugs, including dexamethasone, thalidomide was considered responsible since its administration had the closest temporal relationship to the adverse effect. Toxic epidermal necrolysis has also been reported[2] in a 64-year-old patient 24 days after initiation of thalidomide and dexamethasone therapy for myeloma. The authors in this case postulated that there may be an adverse interaction between thalidomide and dexamethasone.

Thalidomide had previously been investigated in a randomised placebo-controlled trial[3] for the treatment of toxic epidermal necrolysis, but the trial was prematurely terminated because of significantly higher mortality in the thalidomide group; the causes of death were those usually attributed to the disease itself. Thalidomide had been chosen as an investigative drug because it is a potent inhibitor of tumour necrosis factor (TNF)-α, which has been implicated in the pathogenesis of this condition. However, the authors noted that there was a tendency for plasma concentrations of TNF-α to increase after treatment with thalidomide compared with the placebo group, and postulated that thalidomide might paradoxically enhance TNF-α production in these patients.


1. Horowitz SB, Stirling AL. Thalidomide-induced toxic epidermal necrolysis. *Pharmacotherapy* 1999; **19:** 1177–80.
2. Rajkumar SV, *et al.* Life-threatening toxic epidermal necrolysis with thalidomide therapy for myeloma. *N Engl J Med* 2000; **343:** 972–3.
3. Wolkenstein P, *et al.* Randomised comparison of thalidomide versus placebo in toxic epidermal necrolysis. *Lancet* 1998; **352:** 1586–9.


**Migraine.** Migraine attacks were associated with thalidomide administration in a 36-year-old man.[1]


1. García-Albea E, *et al.* Jaqueca típica y talidomida. *Med Clin (Barc)* 1993; **100:** 557.


**Mutagenicity.** Reports of the birth of 3 malformed infants to parents who had themselves been exposed to thalidomide *in utero*[1,2] have provoked fears that thalidomide may be a mutagen. However, the limb malformations seen in the infants are not typical of mutagenesis[3] and the teratogenic effect of thalidomide is likely to be associated with interference with angiogenesis in the fetus rather than mutation.[4]


1. McBride WG. Thalidomide may be a mutagen. *BMJ* 1994; **308:** 1635–6.
2. Tenconi R, *et al.* Amniotic band sequence in child of thalidomide victim. *BMJ* 1994; **309:** 1442.
3. Read AP. Thalidomide may be a mutagen. *BMJ* 1994; **308:** 1636.
4. D'Amato RJ, *et al.* Thalidomide is an inhibitor of angiogenesis. *Proc Natl Acad Sci U S A* 1994; **91:** 4082–5.


## Interactions

The sedative activity of barbiturates, alcohol, chlorpromazine, and reserpine has been reported to be enhanced by thalidomide. Use with other drugs that have the potential to cause peripheral neuropathy should be undertaken cautiously.

**Antineoplastics.** There may be an increased risk of deep-vein thrombosis from the use of thalidomide with *doxorubicin* (see p.549). See also Effects on the Cardiovascular System, above.

**Corticosteroids.** For reference to a possible interaction between thalidomide and *dexamethasone*, see under Effects on the Skin, above.

**Hormonal contraceptives.** Thalidomide does *not* alter the metabolism of ethinylestradiol and norethisterone,[1,2] and so the efficacy of oral contraceptives should not be affected by thalidomide therapy. Nevertheless, 2 reliable forms of contraception should always be used simultaneously when taking thalidomide (see under Adverse Effects and Precautions, above), bearing in mind that the reliability of hormonal contraceptives may be compromised by drugs other than thalidomide (see p.1534).


1. Trapnell CB, *et al.* Thalidomide does not alter the pharmacokinetics of ethinyl estradiol and norethindrone. *Clin Pharmacol Ther* 1998; **64:** 597–602.
2. Scheffler MR, *et al.* Thalidomide does not alter estrogen-progesterone hormone single-dose pharmacokinetics. *Clin Pharmacol Ther* 1999; **65:** 483–90.


## Pharmacokinetics

Thalidomide is slowly absorbed from the gastrointestinal tract; peak plasma concentrations are reached within about 3 to 6 hours of an oral dose. It crosses the placenta and is distributed into the semen. The exact metabolic fate of thalidomide is unknown, however, it appears to undergo non-enzymatic hydrolysis in plasma. The elimination half-life is about 5 to 7 hours.

◊ References.


1. Aweeka F, *et al.* Pharmacokinetics and pharmacodynamics of thalidomide in HIV patients treated for oral aphthous ulcers: ACTG protocol 251. *J Clin Pharmacol* 2001; **41:** 1091–7.
2. Wohl DA, *et al.* Safety, tolerability, and pharmacokinetic effects of thalidomide in patients infected with human immunodeficiency virus: AIDS Clinical Trials Group 267. *J Infect Dis* 2002; **185:** 1359–63.
3. Teo SK, *et al.* Clinical pharmacokinetics of thalidomide. *Clin Pharmacokinet* 2004; **43:** 311–27.


## Uses and Administration

Thalidomide has immunomodulating activity. It should always be given under appropriately supervised and controlled conditions because of the teratogenic risks and other potential adverse effects (see under Adverse Effects and Precautions, above).

Thalidomide is used for the treatment of acute cutaneous manifestations of moderate to severe type 2 (erythema nodosum leprosum) lepra reactions (see Leprosy, p.133), but should not be given as monotherapy if moderate to severe neuritis is present; in such cases, corticosteroid therapy should also be given and continued until neuritis improves. Thalidomide may also be used for maintenance therapy for prevention and suppression of the cutaneous manifestations of recurrent type 2 lepra reactions. It is of no value in type 1 lepra reactions. It is given by mouth in usual doses of 100 to 300 mg once daily, preferably at bedtime. In severe cases up to 400 mg daily may be given. The dose should be reduced gradually by 50 mg every 2 to 4 weeks once a satisfactory response has been achieved.

Thalidomide is also used in the treatment of multiple myeloma (p.511) refractory to standard therapies. It is given in an initial dose of 200 mg once daily and, according to patient tolerance, the dose may be increased by 100 mg at weekly intervals up to a maximum dose of 800 mg daily.

Thalidomide has been used in several other conditions whose aetiology may involve the immune system, such as treatment and prevention of graft-versus-host disease, treatment and prevention of recurrent aphthous stomatitis in severely and terminally immunocompromised patients, treatment of the clinical manifestations of both tuberculous and non-tuberculous mycobacterial infection, and treatment of HIV-associated wasting syndrome, Kaposi's sarcoma, and Crohn's disease. It has also been used in the treatment of primary brain malignancies. Thalidomide is being investigated in some other malignancies.

◊ Guidelines on the clinical use of thalidomide.


1. Powell RJ, Gardner-Medwin JMM. Guideline for the clinical use and dispensing of thalidomide. *Postgrad Med J* 1994; **70:** 901–4.
2. Lary JM, *et al.* The return of thalidomide: can birth defects be prevented? *Drug Safety* 1999; **21:** 161–9.


**Action.** The mechanism of action of thalidomide is not completely understood, although investigations have shown that it has various anti-inflammatory and immunomodulating effects, including inhibition of the synthesis of tumour necrosis factor (TNF)-α. However, this inhibition is incomplete and selective, and increased plasma-TNF-α concentrations have been observed in some patient groups. Other immunomodulatory and anti-inflammatory properties include inhibition of leucocyte chemotaxis into the site of inflammation and reduction of phagocytosis by polymorphonuclear leucocytes. Thalidomide also appears to modulate interleukins, although results of investigations into its effect on specific interleukins and interferon gamma have so far been equivocal. Effects on CD4+ cells and variable effects on other mediators of intercellular reactions have also been implicated. Thalidomide also inhibits angiogenesis, which may have implications in solid tumours and other diseases.

References.


1. Schuler U, Ehninger G. Thalidomide: rationale for renewed use in immunological disorders. *Drug Safety* 1995; **12:** 364–9.
2. Calabrese L, Fleischer AB. Thalidomide: current and potential clinical applications. *Am J Med* 2000; **108:** 487–95.
3. Peuckmann V, *et al.* Potential novel uses of thalidomide: focus on palliative care. *Drugs* 2000; **60:** 273–92.


**Behçet's syndrome.** Thalidomide was effective for the treatment of oral and genital ulceration and follicular lesions in a randomised, double-blind, placebo-controlled trial[1] in 96 male patients with Behçet's syndrome (p.1076). It was also noted that the development of new oral and genital ulcers was prevented, although relapses may occur on cessation of therapy. Thalidomide has also been reported[2,3] to be of benefit for severe oral and genital ulceration in children with Behçet's syndrome unresponsive to other treatments. Thalidomide also improved symptoms in a woman with Behçet's syndrome who had recurrent perforating intestinal ulcers.[4]


1. Hamuryudan V, *et al.* Thalidomide in the treatment of the mucocutaneous lesions of the Behçet syndrome: a randomized, double-blind, placebo-controlled trial. *Ann Intern Med* 1998; **128:** 443–50.
2. Shek LP-C, *et al.* Thalidomide responsiveness in an infant with Behçet's syndrome. *Pediatrics* 1999; **103:** 1295–7.
3. Kari JA, *et al.* Thalidomide use in childhood Behçet's syndrome. *Arch Dis Child* 2000; **82** (suppl 1): A46.
4. Sayarlioglu M, *et al.* Treatment of recurrent perforating intestinal ulcers with thalidomide in Behçet's disease. *Ann Pharmacother* 2004; **38:** 808–11.


**Graft-versus-host disease.** Beneficial responses to thalidomide have been reported[1-6] in graft-versus-host disease (p.1344) in bone marrow transplant recipients, including children.


1. Lim SH, *et al.* Successful treatment with thalidomide of acute graft-versus-host disease after bone-marrow transplantation. *Lancet* 1988; **i:** 117.
2. McCarthy DM, *et al.* Thalidomide for graft-versus-host disease. *Lancet* 1988; **ii:** 1135.
3. Heney D, *et al.* Thalidomide for chronic graft-versus-host disease in children. *Lancet* 1988; **ii:** 1317.
4. Vogelsang GB, *et al.* Thalidomide for the treatment of chronic graft-versus-host disease. *N Engl J Med* 1992; **326:** 1055–8.
5. Cole CH, *et al.* Thalidomide in the management of chronic graft-versus-host disease in children following bone marrow transplantation. *Bone Marrow Transplant* 1994; **14:** 937–42.
6. Mehta P, *et al.* Thalidomide in children undergoing bone marrow transplantation: series at a single institution and review of the literature. Abstract: *Pediatrics* 1999; **103:** 806. Full version: http://pediatrics.aappublications.org/cgi/content/full/103/4/e44 (accessed 08/07/04)


**HIV-associated complications.** It has been proposed that thalidomide's inhibitory activity against tumour necrosis factor (TNF)-α may explain its anti-HIV effect. However, there are conflicting reports as both decreased and increased TNF-α levels, as well as unchanged levels, have been observed in HIV-patients.[1] Nevertheless, thalidomide has shown some promise as a therapeutic agent for some AIDS-related diseases. It is an effective treatment for severe ulceration of the mouth (p.1245), oropharynx, and oesophagus in patients with HIV-infection.[2-4] It has also proved to be of benefit in HIV-associated wasting[5] (p.623), and has shown promise in high doses for the treatment of Kaposi's sarcoma[6] (p.524). However, of concern is the finding that modest increases in plasma HIV RNA levels have been observed in some patients, which correlated with increases in TNF-α levels.[2,4]


1. Ravot E, *et al.* New uses for old drugs in HIV infection: the role of hydroxyurea, cyclosporin and thalidomide. *Drugs* 1999; **58:** 953–63.
2. Jacobson JM, *et al.* Thalidomide for the treatment of oral aphthous ulcers in patients with human immunodeficiency virus infection. *N Engl J Med* 1997; **336:** 1487–93.
3. Ramirez-Amador VA, *et al.* Thalidomide as therapy for human immunodeficiency virus-related oral ulcers: a double-blind placebo-controlled clinical trial. *Clin Infect Dis* 1999; **28:** 892–4.
4. Jacobson JM, *et al.* Thalidomide for the treatment of esophageal aphthous ulcers in patients with human immunodeficiency virus infection. *J Infect Dis* 1999; **180:** 61–7.
5. Reyes-Terán G, *et al.* Effects of thalidomide on HIV-associated wasting syndrome: a randomized, double-blind, placebo-controlled trial. *AIDS* 1996; **10:** 1501–7.
6. Little RF, *et al.* Activity of thalidomide in AIDS-related Kaposi's sarcoma. *J Clin Oncol* 2000; **18:** 2593–2602.


**Inflammatory bowel disease.** Small open-label studies[1-3] have shown efficacy of thalidomide in patients with refractory Crohn's disease (see under Inflammatory Bowel Disease, p.1243). In many of those patients already receiving corticosteroids the dosage could be reduced and in some corticosteroids could be withdrawn completely.


1. Ehrenpreis ED, *et al.* Thalidomide therapy for patients with refractory Crohn's disease: an open-label trial. *Gastroenterology* 1999; **117:** 1271–7.
2. Vasiliauskas EA, *et al.* An open-label pilot study of low-dose thalidomide in chronically active, steroid-dependent Crohn's disease. *Gastroenterology* 1999; **117:** 1278–87.
3. Bariol C, *et al.* Early studies on the safety and efficacy of thalidomide for symptomatic inflammatory bowel disease. *J Gastroenterol Hepatol* 2002; **17:** 135–9.


**Kaposi's sarcoma.** See under HIV-associated complications, above.

**Lupus erythematosus.** Thalidomide has been found to be of benefit in lupus erythematosus, including chronic discoid lupus erythematosus,[1] lupus erythematosus profundus,[2] systemic lupus erythematosus[3] (p.1088), and cutaneous lupus erythematosus.[4-7]


1. Knop J, *et al.* Thalidomide in the treatment of sixty cases of chronic discoid lupus erythematosus. *Br J Dermatol* 1983; **108:** 461–6.
2. Burrows NP, *et al.* Lupus erythematosus profundus with partial C4 deficiency responding to thalidomide. *Br J Dermatol* 1991; **125:** 62–7.
3. Bessis D, *et al.* Thalidomide for systemic lupus erythematosus. *Lancet* 1992; **339:** 549–50.
4. Atra E, Sato EI. Treatment of the cutaneous lesions of systemic lupus erythematosus with thalidomide. *Clin Exp Rheumatol* 1993; **11:** 487–93.
5. Stevens RJ, *et al.* Thalidomide in the treatment of the cutaneous manifestations of lupus erythematosus: experience in sixteen consecutive patients. *Br J Rheumatol* 1997; **36:** 353–9.
6. Duong DJ, *et al.* American experience with low-dose thalidomide therapy for severe cutaneous lupus erythematosus. *Arch Dermatol* 1999; **135:** 1079–87.
7. Pelle MT, Werth VP. Thalidomide in cutaneous lupus erythematosus. *Am J Clin Dermatol* 2003; **4:** 379–87.


**Malignant neoplasms.** Thalidomide has shown benefit in the treatment of patients with relapsed advanced multiple myeloma[1-4] (p.511) and has also produced encouraging results in patients with newly diagnosed disease, either alone or in combination with dexamethasone.[4-6] Thalidomide has also shown promise in patients with recurrent high-grade gliomas[7] (p.513) and is under investigation for metastatic melanoma[8] (p.522).


1. Singhal S, *et al.* Antitumor activity of thalidomide in refractory multiple myeloma. *N Engl J Med* 1999; **341:** 1565–71.
2. Rajkumar SV, *et al.* Thalidomide in the treatment of relapsed multiple myeloma. *Mayo Clin Proc* 2000; **75:** 897–901.
3. Kumar S, *et al.* Response rate, durability of response, and survival after thalidomide therapy for relapsed multiple myeloma. *Mayo Clin Proc* 2003; **78:** 34–9.
4. Cavenagh JD, *et al.* Thalidomide in multiple myeloma: current status and future prospects. *Br J Haematol* 2003; **120:** 18–26.
5. Rajkumar SV, *et al.* Combination therapy with thalidomide plus dexamethasone for newly diagnosed myeloma. *J Clin Oncol* 2002; **20:** 4319–23.
6. Weber D, *et al.* Thalidomide alone or with dexamethasone for previously untreated multiple myeloma. *J Clin Oncol* 2003; **21:** 16–19.
7. Fine HA, *et al.* Phase II trial of the antiangiogenic agent thalidomide in patients with recurrent high-grade gliomas. *J Clin Oncol* 2000; **18:** 708–15.
8. Danson S, *et al.* Randomized phase II study of temozolomide given every 8 hours or daily with either interferon alfa-2b or thalidomide in metastatic malignant melanoma. *J Clin Oncol* 2003; **21:** 2551–7.


**Mouth ulceration.** See under Behçet's syndrome and under HIV-associated complications, above.

**Oesophageal ulceration.** Thalidomide has been shown to be of benefit in the treatment of idiopathic oesophageal ulcers in patients with AIDS (see under HIV-associated complications, above). Thalidomide has also been reported[1] to have healed an oesophageal ulcer refractory to other treatments in an immunocompetent patient.


1. Ollivier S, *et al.* Idiopathic giant oesophageal ulcer in an immunocompetent patient: the efficacy of thalidomide treatment. *Gut* 1999; **45:** 463–4.


**Rheumatic disorders.** Beneficial responses to thalidomide have been reported in the treatment of refractory rheumatoid arthritis[1] and adult-onset Still's disease.[2] Thalidomide also improved symptoms in 2 children with systemic onset juvenile rheumatoid arthritis, in whom other therapy, including the tumour necrosis factor inhibitor etanercept, had been ineffective.[3]


1. Gutiérrez-Rodríguez O, *et al.* Treatment of refractory rheumatoid arthritis—the thalidomide experience. *J Rheumatol* 1989; **16:** 158–63.
2. Stambe C, Wicks IP. TNFα and response of treatment-resistant adult-onset Still's disease to thalidomide. *Lancet* 1998; **352:** 544–5.
3. Lehman TJA, *et al.* Thalidomide therapy for recalcitrant systemic onset juvenile rheumatoid arthritis. *J Pediatr* 2002; **140:** 125–7.


**Sarcoidosis.** Beneficial responses to thalidomide have been reported[1,2] in the treatment of sarcoidosis.


1. Carlesimo M, *et al.* Treatment of cutaneous and pulmonary sarcoidosis with thalidomide. *J Am Acad Dermatol* 1995; **32:** 866–9.
2. Baughman RP, *et al.* Thalidomide for chronic sarcoidosis. *Chest* 2002; **122:** 227–32.


**Skin disorders.** Beneficial responses to thalidomide have been reported in dermatological disorders including erythema multiforme[1,2] (p.1135), pruritus associated with uraemia,[3] Langerhans-cell histiocytosis[4] (p.505), epidermolysis bullosa,[5] prurigo nodularis,[6] pyoderma gangrenosum[7] (p.1138), and Schnitzler's syndrome.[8]


1. Bahmer FA, *et al.* Thalidomide treatment of recurrent erythema multiforme. *Acta Derm Venereol (Stockh)* 1982; **62:** 449–50.
2. Moisson YF, *et al.* Thalidomide for recurrent erythema multiforme. *Br J Dermatol* 1992; **126:** 92–3.
3. Silva SRB, *et al.* Thalidomide for the treatment of uremic pruritus: a crossover randomized double-blind trial. *Nephron* 1994; **67:** 270–3.
4. Meunier L, *et al.* Adult cutaneous Langerhans cell histiocytosis: remission with thalidomide treatment. *Br J Dermatol* 1995; **132:** 168.
5. Goulden V, *et al.* Linear prurigo simulating dermatitis artefacta in dominant dystrophic epidermolysis bullosa. *Br J Dermatol* 1993; **129:** 443–6.
6. Ferrándiz C, *et al.* Sequential combined therapy with thalidomide and narrow-band (TL01) UVB in the treatment of prurigo nodularis. *Dermatology* 1997; **195:** 359–61.
7. Federman GL, Federman DG. Recalcitrant pyoderma gangrenosum treated with thalidomide. *Mayo Clin Proc* 2000; **75:** 842–4.
8. Worm M, Kolde G. Schnitzler's syndrome: successful treatment of two patients using thalidomide. *Br J Dermatol* 2003; **148:** 601–2.


### Preparations

***USP 27:*** Thalidomide Capsules.

**Proprietary Preparations** (details are given in Part 3)
***USA:*** Thalomid.

## Thallium Acetate

Talio, acetato de; Thallous Acetate.

$C_2H_3O_2Tl$ = 263.4.

*CAS — 563-68-8.*

### Adverse Effects

Thallium salts are toxic when inhaled, ingested, or absorbed through the skin. Symptoms of poisoning may appear within 12 to 24 hours of a single toxic dose and include severe abdominal pain, nausea and vomiting, diarrhoea, gastrointestinal haemorrhage, salivation, metallic taste, paralytic ileus, pancreatic damage, and in severe cases cardiovascular collapse, tremors, delirium, convulsions, paralysis, and coma, leading to death in 1 to 2 days. However, the acute reaction may subside, to be followed within about 10 days by the development of neurological effects including paraesthesia, myalgia, myopathy, motor neuropathy, and visual disturbances due to optic neuropathy, psychosis, delirium, convulsions, and other signs of encephalopathy, tachycardia, hypertension, skin eruptions, and hepatorenal injury. Recovery from neurological damage is slow and may be incomplete. Alopecia occurs within 15 to 20 days; stomatitis and a bluish line in the gums may also develop. Death may result from respiratory failure; patients are also predisposed for several weeks to cardiac arrhythmias and sudden death. Fatalities have occurred after ingestion of 1 g or less in adults, although the UK Poisons Information Service consider the usual lethal dose by ingestion to be in the range 3 to 10 g in adults.

Smaller repeated doses are also toxic, with symptoms appearing over several weeks. Constipation is a common feature of less severe poisoning.

**Poisoning.** References.


1. Moeschlin S. Thallium poisoning. *Clin Toxicol* 1980; **17:** 133–46.
2. Heyl T, Barlow RJ. Thallium poisoning: a dermatological perspective. *Br J Dermatol* 1989; **121:** 787–92.
3. Luckit J, *et al.* Thrombocytopenia associated with thallium poisoning. *Hum Exp Toxicol* 1990; **9:** 47–8.
4. Moore D, *et al.* Thallium poisoning. *BMJ* 1993; **306:** 1527–9.
5. Tabandeh H, Thompson GM. Visual function in thallium toxicity. *BMJ* 1993; **307:** 324.
6. Questel F, *et al.* Thallium-contaminated heroin. *Ann Intern Med* 1996; **124:** 616.
7. Tromme I, *et al.* Skin signs in the diagnosis of thallium poisoning. *Br J Dermatol* 1998; **138:** 321–5.
8. Hoffman RS. Thallium poisoning during pregnancy: a case report and comprehensive literature review. *J Toxicol Clin Toxicol* 2000; **38:** 767–75.
9. Misra UK, *et al.* Thallium poisoning: emphasis on early diagnosis and response to haemodialysis. *Postgrad Med J* 2003; **79:** 103–5.
10. Hoffman RS. Thallium toxicity and the role of Prussian blue in therapy. *Toxicol Rev* 2003; **22:** 29–40.


### Treatment of Adverse Effects

After the acute ingestion of thallium, gastric lavage should be considered within 1 hour of ingestion; a saline purgative such as magnesium sulfate may be given. Intensive supportive therapy is necessary.

Various methods have been employed in an attempt to increase the faecal and urinary excretion of thallium. A suspension of activated charcoal has been given to reduce intestinal absorption and enteric recycling, but is less successful than Prussian blue (p.1051) by mouth or duodenal tube. The administration of potassium chloride by mouth may mobilise thallium from the tissues but is hazardous, especially if given during the early stage; signs of poisoning may be transiently aggravated.

Haemoperfusion, haemodialysis, or peritoneal dialysis have been reported to be effective in eliminating absorbed thallium, although clinical benefit doubtful.

### Uses and Administration

Thallium acetate was formerly used by mouth for depilation in ringworm and as an ingredient of depilatory creams but both systemic and local treatments have caused deaths, and it is no longer used for such purposes. It has also been used as a rodenticide and insecticide, although its use is strictly regulated in many countries. However, it is used in industry and is therefore still a hazard. Cases of malicious poisoning are still encountered occasionally.

## Theobroma

Cacao or Cocoa Powder; Chocolate; Teobroma; Theobrom.

**Pharmacopoeias.** In *USNF.*

**USNF 22** (Chocolate). A powder prepared from the roasted, cured kernels of the ripe seed of *Theobroma cacao* (Sterculiaceae).

### Profile

Theobroma is used as a flavoured basis for tablets and lozenges. Theobroma oil (p.1482) is used as a basis for suppositories.

**Breast feeding.** The American Academy of Pediatrics[1] states that irritability or increased bowel activity have been reported in infants whose mothers consumed excessive amounts of chocolate (16 ounces (approximately 450 g) or more daily).


1. American Academy of Pediatrics. The transfer of drugs and other chemicals into human milk. *Pediatrics* 2001; **108:** 776–89. Correction. *ibid.* 1029. Also available at http://aappolicy.aappublications.org/cgi/content/full/pediatrics%3b108/3/776 (accessed 08/07/04)


### Preparations

***USNF 22:*** Chocolate Syrup.

**Proprietary Preparations** (details are given in Part 3)

***Multi-ingredient: Austria:*** Asthmatee EF-EM-ES; ***Braz.:*** Licor de Cacau†.

## Theodrenaline Hydrochloride *(BANM, rINNM)*

H-8352; Hidrocloruro de teodrenalina; Noradrenaline Theophylline Hydrochloride. 7-[2-(3,4,β-Trihydroxyphenethylamino)ethyl]theophylline hydrochloride.

$C_{17}H_{21}N_5O_5,HCl$ = 411.8.

*CAS — 13460-98-5 (theodrenaline); 2572-61-4 (theodrenaline hydrochloride).*

*ATC — C01CA23.*

### Profile

Theodrenaline is mainly used as the hydrochloride in preparations with cafedrine promoted for the treatment of hypotension.

### Preparations

**Proprietary Preparations** (details are given in Part 3)

***Multi-ingredient: Austria:*** Akrinor; ***Fr.:*** Praxinor; ***Ger.:*** Akrinor; ***S.Afr.:*** Akrinor; ***Spain:*** Bifort; ***Switz.:*** Akrinor†.

## Thioctic Acid

Alpha Lipoic Acid; Lipoic Acid; α-Liponic Acid; Tióctico, ácido. 5-(1,2-Dithiolan-3-yl)valeric acid.

$C_8H_{14}O_2S_2$ = 206.3.

*CAS — 62-46-4.*

**Pharmacopoeias.** In *USNF.*

**USNF 22** (Alpha Lipoic Acid). M.p. 60.0° to 62.0°.

### Profile

Thioctic acid is used for its antioxidant effects in the treatment of diabetic neuropathy. It has been tried in the treatment of liver dysfunction and in subacute necrotising encephalopathy. Beneficial results have been claimed in amanitin poisoning following ingestion of the mushroom *Amanita phalloides,* but such use is controversial (see under Poisonous Mushrooms or Toadstools, p.1718). Ethylenediamine thioctate, sodium thioctate, thioctic acid amide (thioctamide), and trometamol thioctate have been used similarly.

**Diabetic neuropathy.** Some evidence[1-4] suggests that thioctic acid may be of benefit in diabetic neuropathy.


1. Ziegler D, *et al.* Effects of treatment with the antioxidant α-lipoic acid on cardiac autonomic neuropathy in NIDDM patients: a 4-month randomized controlled multicenter trial (DEKAN study). *Diabetes Care* 1997; **20:** 369–73.
2. Ziegler D, *et al.* Treatment of symptomatic diabetic polyneuropathy with the antioxidant α-lipoic acid: a 7-month multicenter randomized controlled trial (ALADIN III study). *Diabetes Care* 1999; **22:** 1296–1301.
3. Ametov AS, *et al.* The sensory symptoms of diabetic polyneuropathy are improved with alpha-lipoic acid: the SYDNEY trial. *Diabetes Care* 2003; **26:** 770–6. Correction. *ibid.*; 2227.
4. Ziegler D, *et al.* Treatment of symptomatic diabetic polyneuropathy with the antioxidant α-lipoic acid: a meta-analysis. *Diabet Med* 2004; **21:** 114–21.


### Preparations

***USNF 22:*** Alpha Lipoic Acid Capsules; Alpha Lipoic Acid Tablets.

**Proprietary Preparations** (details are given in Part 3)
***Arg.:*** Biletan; Ciagen; Neurotioct; Neutracol; Tioctan; ***Austria:*** Thioctacid; Tioctan; ***Ger.:*** Alpha-Lipogamma; Alpha-Lipon; alpha-Vibolex; Alphaflam; Azulipont; Berlithion†; Biomo-lipon; duralipon; espa-lipon; Fenint; Neurium; Neurothioct†; Pleomix-Alpha; Thioctacid; Thiogamma; Tromlipon; Verla-Lipon; ***Hong Kong:*** Lipoicin†; ***Jpn:*** Tioctan; ***Thai.:*** Lipoicin.

**Multi-ingredient:** ***Arg.:*** Biletan Enzimatico; Carbogasol Digestivo; Co-Tioctan; Nervomax TB12; ***Hong Kong:*** Lipochol; ***Ital.:*** Byodinoral; Tiobec; ***Spain:*** Policolinosil; Sugarceton†; ***Thai.:*** Lipochol.

## Thiomucase

C-84-04; Chondroitinsulphatase; Tiomucasa.

### Profile

Thiomucase is a mucopolysaccharidase with general properties similar to those of hyaluronidase, p.1698, but which also depolymerises chondroitin sulfate. It has been given to assist the diffusion of local anaesthetic injections.

### Preparations

**Proprietary Preparations** (details are given in Part 3)

**Multi-ingredient:** ***Braz.:*** Thiomucase.

## Thiram *(USAN, rINN)*

NSC-1771; SQ-1489; Tiram; TMT; TMTD. Tetramethylthiuram disulphide.

$C_6H_{12}N_2S_4$ = 240.4.
*CAS — 137-26-8.*
*ATC — P03AA05.*

### Profile

Thiram, the methyl analogue of disulfiram (p.1681), has antibacterial and antifungal activity. It is applied topically as an aerosol in the treatment of wounds and other skin disorders. It has been used as a fungicide in agriculture, and in industry as a rubber accelerator. Occupational exposure to thiram may cause irritation of mucous membranes and skin.

### Preparations

**Proprietary Preparations** (details are given in Part 3)
***Belg.:*** Nobecutane†; ***Ger.:*** Nobecutan†.

**Multi-ingredient:** ***Spain:*** Sulfiselen†.

## Thorium Dioxide

Thorium Oxide; Torio, dióxido de.

$ThO_2$ = 264.0.
*CAS — 1314-20-1.*

### Profile

Colloidal solutions of thorium dioxide were formerly used as X-ray contrast media for examination of the liver and spleen, for arteriography, and occasionally for outlining the cerebral ventricles. Its elimination is very slow and incomplete. It accumulates in the reticuloendothelial system, especially in the liver and spleen. As it is radioactive (half-life: $1.41 \times 10^{10}$ years), this accumulation is dangerous and there is strong evidence that the ensuing prolonged exposure to its radiation is a contributing factor in the development of malignant diseases and blood disorders often 20 to 30 years after its use.

## Thuja

Tuya.

### Profile

Thuja consists of the fresh leaves and twigs of *Thuja occidentalis* (Cupressaceae). It is included in some topical preparations for warts and in herbal antiseptic preparations. It is also used in herbal preparations for respiratory-tract disorders, and in homoeopathic medicine.

### Preparations

**Proprietary Preparations** (details are given in Part 3)
***Chile:*** Thujaderm.

**Multi-ingredient:** ***Austria:*** Colda; ***Belg.:*** Aporil; ***Braz.:*** Calope; ***Fr.:*** Nitrol; Verrupan; ***Ger.:*** Esberitox N; ***Port.:*** Erpecalm; ***Spain:*** Nitroina; ***Switz.:*** Esberitop; Esberitox N†.

## Thymalfasin *(USAN, rINN)*

Thymosin α1; Timalfasina.
*CAS — 62304-98-7; 69521-94-4.*

### Profile

Thymalfasin is a thymus hormone (p.1756) found in thymosin fraction 5 (a crude thymus gland extract) now produced by synthesis. Thymalfasin is used alone or in combination with interferon as an immunomodulator for the treatment of chronic hepatitis B and C (p.618). It is given by subcutaneous injection in a dose of 1.6 mg twice weekly for up to 12 months. It is also used to enhance the effectiveness of influenza vaccines in immunocompromised or elderly patients and of influenza and hepatitis B vaccines in chronic haemodialysis patients.

Thymalfasin is under investigation for a number of other diseases, including hepatitis D, hepatocellular carcinoma, non-small cell lung cancer, melanoma, and HIV infection and AIDS.

◊ References.


1. Garaci E, *et al.* Sequential chemoimmunotherapy for advanced non-small cell lung cancer using cisplatin, etoposide, thymosin-α1 and interferon-α2a. *Eur J Cancer* 1995; **31A:** 2403–5.
2. Rasi G, *et al.* Combination thymosin $\alpha_1$ and lymphoblastoid interferon treatment in chronic hepatitis C. *Gut* 1996; **39:** 679–83.
3. Zavaglia C, *et al.* A pilot study of thymosin-α1 therapy for chronic hepatitis D. *J Clin Gastroenterol* 1996; **23:** 162–3.
4. Andreone P, *et al.* A randomized controlled trial of thymosin-$\alpha_1$ versus interferon alfa treatment in patients with hepatitis B e antigen antibody- and hepatitis B virus DNA-positive chronic hepatitis B. *Hepatology* 1996; **24:** 774–7.
5. Sherman KE, *et al.* Combination therapy with thymosin α1 and interferon for the treatment of chronic hepatitis C infection: a randomized, placebo-controlled double-blind trial. *Hepatology* 1998; **27:** 1128–35.
6. Chien R-N, *et al.* Efficacy of thymosin α1 in patients with chronic hepatitis B: a randomized, controlled trial. *Hepatology* 1998; **27:** 1383–7.
7. Rasi G, *et al.* Combined treatment with thymosin-α1 and low dose interferon-α after dacarbazine in advanced melanoma. *Melanoma Res* 2000; **10:** 189–92.
8. Ancell CD, *et al.* Thymosin alpha-1. *Am J Health-Syst Pharm* 2001; **58:** 879–85.


### Preparations

**Proprietary Preparations** (details are given in Part 3)
***Arg.:*** Zadaxin; ***Ital.:*** Timosin†; Zadaxin; ***Malaysia:*** Zadaxin; ***Mex.:*** Zadaxin; ***Singapore:*** Zadaxin; ***Thai.:*** Zadaxin.

## Thyme

Common Thyme; French Thyme; Garden Thyme; Rubbed Thyme; Thymi Herba; Timo; Tomillo.

**Pharmacopoeias.** In *Eur.* (see p.vi) and *Pol.*

**Ph. Eur. 5.0** (Thyme). The whole leaves and flowers separated from the previously dried stems of *Thymus vulgaris*, or *T. zygis*, or a mixture of both species. It contains not less than 12 mL/kg of essential oil, of which a minimum of 40% is thymol and carvacrol, both calculated with reference to the anhydrous drug. It has a strong aromatic odour reminiscent of thymol.

### Profile

Thyme is the source of thyme oil (below). It has carminative, antiseptic, antitussive, and expectorant properties and is used chiefly in preparations for respiratory-tract disorders and as a flavour.

### Preparations

**Proprietary Preparations** (details are given in Part 3)
***Austria:*** Scottopect; ***Chile:*** Hustagil; ***Ger.:*** Anastil; Antussan†; Aspecton; Biotuss; Bronchicum Pastillen; Bronchipret; Bronchitten†; Expectal N; Fichtensirup N; Gelobronchial; Hustagil Thymian-Hustensaft; Hustagil Thymiantropfen; Husties; Isephca S; Kolton bronchiale Erkaltungssaft†; Makatussin Saft; Melrosum Hustensirup; Menthymin mono; Mirfusot; Nimopect; Pertussin; Sanopinwern; Soledum Hustensaft; Soledum Hustentropfen N; Thymi-Fips†; Thymipin N; Thymiverlan; Tussamag Hustensaft N; Tussamag Hustentropfen N; ***Israel:*** Thymi Syrup; ***Neth.:*** Daro Thijm†.

**Multi-ingredient:** ***Arg.:*** Expectosan Hierbas y Miel; ***Austral.:*** Bronchilin; Cough Relief†; Euphorbia Complex†; Respatona Decongestant Formula†; Respatona Plus Bronchial Cough Relief†; ***Austria:*** Aktiv Husten- und Bronchialtee; Anifer Hustentee; Anifer Hustentropfen; Anitos; Aponatura Hustenstillende; Apotheker Bauer's Brust- und Hustentee; Aurita-Bronchialtee; Bio-Garten Tee gegen Erkaltung; Bio-Garten Tropfen gegen Husten; Bio-Strath Husten; Bioreform-Erkaltungstee; Breston; Bronchiplant; Bronchiplant light; Bronchipret; Bronchithym; Bronchosan; Bronchostop; Bronchostop sine; Brust- und Hustentee EF-EM-ES; Codelum; Egmovit; Erbesil; Erkaltungstee; Expectal-Tropfen; Gewusst wie Husten-Bronchialtee; Granobil; Grippetee Dr Zeidler; Hustensaft-Dr Schmidgall†; Jutussin neo; Kneipp Grippe-Tee; Kneipp Husten- und Bronchial-Tee; Krauter Hustensaft; Krauterdoktor Hustentropfen; Krauterdoktor Krampf- und Reizhustensirup; Krauterhaus Mag Kottas Husten- und Bronchialtee; Luuf Krauter-Hustensaft; Luuf-Hustentee; Mag Kottas Husten-Bronchialtee; Mag Kottas Krauterexpress-Husten-Bronchialtee; Mediplant Krauter; Naturland Heilkrautermundwasser; Neuners Krautertee Nr 10 - Grippetee; Neuners Krautertee Nr 126 - Starkungstee fur stillende Mutter; Neuners Krautertee Nr 211 - Krauterhexlein Kinder-Hustentee; Neuners Krautertee Nr 311 - Bronchialtee zur Inhalation; Neuners Krautertee Nr 7 - Bronchial- und Lungentee; Paracodin; Pilka; Pilka Forte; Pneumopan; Pneumopect†; Scottopect; Sidroga Brust-Husten-Tee; Spasmo-Granobil-Krampf- und Reizhusten; St Radegunder Bronchialtee; St Radegunder Thorasan-Krauterhustensaft; Synpharma Instant-Brust- und Hustentee; Teekanne Erkaltungstee; Teekanne Husten- und Brusttee; Thymoval; Tussamag; Tussimont; ***Belg.:*** Balsoclase†; Colimax; Thymoseptine; ***Braz.:*** Broncmel†; Pectoss†; ***Canad.:*** Herbal Throat; Pectothymin†; Swiss Herb Cough Drops; ***Chile:*** Phyto Corrective Gel; Primacy Phyto +; Rhus Opodeldoc; ***Fin.:*** Katapekt; ***Fr.:*** Depuratum; Elixir Contre La Toux Weleda†; Germose; Niver†; Santane $D_5$†; Santane $R_8$†; Saugella; Tussidoron; ***Ger.:*** Anastil N†; Aspecton N†; Bronchialtee N†; Bronchicum Elixir N; Bronchicum Elixir Plus; Bronchicum Hustentee†; Bronchicum Pflanzlicher; Bronchicum Sekret-Loser; Bronchicum Thymian; Bronchicum Tropfen N; Bronchipret; Bronchitten forte K†; Bronchosyx N; Brust- und Husten-Tee Stada N†; Brust- und Hustentee; Cefabronchin†; Cefadrin; Cito-Guakalin; Drosithym-N; Em-eukal; Ephepect-Pastillen N; Ephepect†; Equisil N; Eucabal; Eupatal; Expectysat N; Guttae 20 Hustentropfen N†; Harzer Hustenloser; Hevert-Erkaltungs-Tee†; Hevert-Magen-Galle-Leber-Tee†; Hevertopect N; Infantussin N†; Junisana; Kinder Em-eukal Hustensaft; Kneipp Erkaltungs-Tee†; Kneipp Husten- und Bronchial-Tee†; Kneipp Krauter Hustensaft N Kneipp Tannolsaft†; Lomal; Makatussin Tropfen; Melissengeist; Melrosum Hustensirup N†; Mintetten Truw†; Muc-Sabona; Original Schneckensirup; Perdiphen phyto†; Phytobronchin; Primotussan†; Pulmocordio forte†; Pulmocordio mite SL; Pulmotin; Salus Bronchial-Tee Nr.8†; Schneckensaft N†; Schneckensirup†; Sedotussin Expectorans†; Sinuforton; Thymipin N; Tussiflorin forte; Tussiflorin Hustenstiller; TUSSinfant N; ***Hong Kong:*** Pectoral; ***Israel:*** Pilka; ***Ital.:*** Altea (Specie Composta); Broncosedina; Fluend†; Immumil; Pinedrin; Piodermina; Pluriderm†; Sciroppo Merck all'Efetonina†; Sebacnol; Timo (Specie Composta); Tussol; ***Neth.:*** Balsoclase Compositum†; Bronchicum; ***Port.:*** Calmarum; Fluidin Antiasmatico†; ***S.Afr.:*** Bronchicough; Bronchicum; ***Spain:*** Mentobox†; Natusor Asmaten; Natusor Farinol; Natusor Gripotul; Natusor Infenol; Natusor Renal; Natusor Sinulan; Pazbronquial; Pilka; Wobenzimal; ***Switz.:*** Bronchalin†; Bronchofluid N; Bronchofluid†; Bronchosan Nouvelle formule; Codipront cum Expectorans; Demo gouttes bronchiques†; Demo sirop bronchique N†; Demo sirop contre la toux†; DemoPectol; Dinacode N; Dragees contre la toux no 536†; Expectoran Codein; Liberol Dragees contre la toux; Liberol Pastilles contre la toux; Liberol Sirop contre la toux; Makatussin forte†; Makatussin†; Neo-DP; Nican; Pastilles pectorales formule 541†; Pectoral N; Pilka; Sedotussin†; Sirop pectoral DP1†; Sirop pectoral DP2, DP3†; Thymodrosin N; Thymodrosin†; Tisane pectorale et antitussive; Tisane pectorale pour les enfants; ***Thai.:*** Solvopret; Solvopret TP; ***UK:*** Herb and Honey Cough Elixir; Snowfire.

## Thyme Oil

Esencia de Tomillo; Essência de Tomilho; Ol. Thym.; Oleum Thymi; Thymi Aetheroleum; Tomillo, aceite esencial de.

**Pharmacopoeias.** In *Eur.* (see p.vi) and *Pol.*

**Ph. Eur. 5.0** (Thyme Oil). The essential oil obtained by steam distillation from the fresh flowering aerial parts of *Thymus vulgaris*, *T. zygis*, or a mixture of both species. A clear, yellow or very dark reddish-brown, mobile liquid with a characteristic aromatic, spicy odour, reminiscent of thymol. Miscible with dehydrated alcohol and with petroleum spirit. It contains between 36 and 55% of thymol. Store in well-filled, airtight containers at a temperature not exceeding 25°. Protect from light.

### Profile

Thyme oil is used similarly to thyme (above).

### Preparations

**Proprietary Preparations** (details are given in Part 3)
***Ger.:*** Bronchicum Medizinal-Bad; Fichtensirup N; Kneipp Erkaltungs-Bad†; Penaten; Thymian Erkaltungs-Bad.

**Multi-ingredient:** ***Austral.:*** Breathe Eazy Chest Rub†; Efalex; Relief Rub†; Tixylix Chest Rub; Zam-Buk†; ***Austria:*** Biokosma Medizinalbad; Biokosma Red Point-Massagecreme; Bronchostop; Expectal-Balsam; Expigen; Heumann's Bronchialtee; Luuf-Hustentee; Perozon Heublumen; Sanvita Bronchial; Scottopect; Synpharma Bronchial; ***Belg.:*** Perubore; ***Canad.:*** Efalex; ***Chile:*** Hustagil; ***Fr.:*** Acarcid; Balsofumine; Balsofumine Mentholee; Biogaze; Citrosil†; Gouttes aux Essences; Otylol†; Perubore; Vapo-Myrtol†; ***Ger.:*** Antitussivum Burger N; Aspecton-Balsam; Em-eukal; Grunlicht Hingfong Essenz†; Heumann Bronchialtee Solubifix; Hoepixin N†; Hustagil Erkaltungsbalsam; Hustagil Inhalationsol†; Kneipp Erkaltungs-Balsam N†; Kneipp Rheuma Stoffwechsel-Bad Heublumen-Aquasan†; Makatussin Balsam mit Menthol†; Melrosum Medizinalbad; Nasivin gegen Erkaltung N†; Nasivin Intensiv-Bad N†; Nasulind; Night-Care†; Pulmotin; Retterspitz Aerosol†; Retterspitz Innerlich†; Schupps Heilkrauter Erkaltungsbad†; ***Hong Kong:*** Zam-Buk†; ***Ital.:*** Calyptol; Fomentil; Neo Zeta-Foot†; Sanaderm†; Vegetallumina; ***Mon.:*** Calyptol; ***NZ:*** Efalex; Tixylix Chest Rub; ***Port.:*** Creodermol†; Erpecalm; Vaporil; ***S.Afr.:*** Zam-Buk; ***Singapore:*** Zam-Buk†; ***Spain:*** Calyptol Inhalante†; H Tussan; Termosan; ***Switz.:*** Brosol†; Caprisana†; Demo gouttes contre la toux†; Demo pommade contre les refroidissements; Demo pommade contre les refroidissements pour bebes†; Demonatur Capsules contre les refroidissements; Dolo-Arthrosenex sine Heparino; Dolorex†; Frigoplasma; Kernosan Huile de Massage†; Liberol Bain; Liberol N; Liberol†; Makatussin†; Perubare; Pulmex; Sedasept; Spagyrom; ***Thai.:*** St Luke's Oil; ***UK:*** Efalex; Nine Rubbing Oils; Snowfire; Snufflebabe; ***USA:*** Maximum Strength Flexall 454; Unguentine.

## Thymidine

NSC-21548; Thymine 2-Desoxyriboside; Timidina. 1-(2-Deoxy-β-D-ribofuranosyl)-5-methyluracil; 1-(2-Deoxy-β-D-ribofuranosyl)-1,2,3,4-tetrahydro-5-methylpyrimidine-2,4-dione.

$C_{10}H_{14}N_2O_5$ = 242.2.
*CAS — 50-89-5.*

### Profile

Thymidine is a nucleoside constituent of cells. It was formerly given by intravenous infusion to modulate the toxicity of methotrexate but is not considered to be a substitute for calcium folinate; it may also have an antineoplastic action of its own.

Thymidine is given topically with other nucleosides in preparations for the treatment of corneal damage.

### Preparations

**Proprietary Preparations** (details are given in Part 3)

**Multi-ingredient:** ***Austria:*** Vitasic†; ***Fr.:*** Vitacic.

## Thymus Hormones

Timo, hormonas del.

*CAS — 69558-55-0 (thymopentin); 60529-76-2 (thymopoietin); 63340-72-7 (thymic humoral factor).*

### Profile

The thymus gland controls the development of T-lymphocytes and thereby plays a central role in cell-mediated immunity and the regulation of immune responses. Several polypeptides characterised in the thymus or serum are able to induce lymphocyte differentiation *in vitro* and *in vivo*. They include: thymosin fraction 5, a crude thymus gland extract; thymalfasin (p.1755); thymic humoral factor (THF), isolated from crude thymic extract dialysate; nonathymulin (thymulin, serum thymic factor, Facteur Thymique Serique, FTS), a synthetic nonapeptide; thymomodulin, a partially purified extract from calf thymus; thymogene A, extracted from calf thymus; thymopoietin, a polypeptide of known amino acid sequence; thymopentin (thymopoietin pentapeptide, TP-5), a fragment of thymopoietin with 5 amino acids; and thymostimulin (TP-1), extracted from calf thymus.

Various preparations, including crude extracts from calf thymus gland, thymomodulin, thymopentin, and thymostimulin have been tried as immunomodulators in auto-immune and immunodeficiency disorders and as adjuncts in the treatment of malignant disease.

**Uses.** Thymus hormones have been tried in the treatment of numerous conditions including rheumatoid arthritis,[1-4] diabetes mellitus,[5,6] immunodeficiency disorders,[7-12] skin disorders[13-16], malignant neoplasms,[17-20] and some infections.[21,22]


1. Amor B, *et al.* Nonathymulin in rheumatoid arthritis: two double blind, placebo controlled trials. *Ann Rheum Dis* 1987; **46:** 549–54.
2. Lemmel EM, *et al.* Immunmodulierende Therapie der chronischen Polyarthritis mit Thymopentin: eine multizentrische placebokontrollierte Studie an 119 Patienten. *Dtsch Med Wochenschr* 1988; **113:** 172–6.
3. Kantharia BK, *et al.* Thymopentin (TP-5) in the treatment of rheumatoid arthritis. *Br J Rheumatol* 1989; **28:** 118–23.
4. Sundal E, Bertelletti D. Thymopentin treatment of rheumatoid arthritis. *Arzneimittelforschung* 1994; **44:** 1145–9.
5. Giordano C, *et al.* Early administration of an immunomodulator and induction of remission in insulin-dependent diabetes mellitus. *J Autoimmun* 1990; **3:** 611–17.
6. Moncada E, *et al.* Insulin requirements and residual beta-cell function 12 months after concluding immunotherapy in type I diabetic patients treated with combined azathioprine and thymostimulin administration for one year. *J Autoimmun* 1990; **3:** 625–38.
7. Terrizzi A, *et al.* Thymomodulin prevents post-operative immunodepression measured by means of skin tests. *Int J Immunother* 1988; **4:** 193–8.
8. Skotnicki AB. Thymic hormones and lymphokines. *Drugs Today* 1989; **25:** 337–62.
9. Beyer WEP, *et al.* Effect of immunomodulator thymopentin on impaired seroresponse to influenza vaccine in patients on haemodialysis. *Nephron* 1990; **54:** 296–301.
10. Beall G, *et al.* A double-blind, placebo-controlled trial of thymostimulin in symptomatic HIV-infected patients. *AIDS* 1990; **4:** 679–81.
11. Brivio F, *et al.* Effect of thymopentin administered perioperatively on the surgery-induced increase in soluble interleukin-2 receptor blood levels in colon cancer patients. *Curr Ther Res* 1991; **50:** 293–7.
12. Hassner A, Adelman DC. Biologic response modifiers in primary immunodeficiency disorders. *Ann Intern Med* 1991; **115:** 294–307.
13. David TJ. Recent developments in the treatment of childhood atopic eczema. *J R Coll Physicians Lond* 1991; **25:** 95–101.
14. Harper JI, *et al.* A double-blind placebo-controlled study of thymostimulin (TP-1) for the treatment of atopic eczema. *Br J Dermatol* 1991; **125:** 368–72.
15. Giordano N, *et al.* Efficacy and safety of thymopentin in patients suffering from progressive systemic sclerosis. *Curr Ther Res* 1991; **49:** 731–9.
16. Hsieh K-H, *et al.* Thymopentin treatment in severe atopic dermatitis—clinical and immunological evaluations. *Arch Dis Child* 1992; **67:** 1095–1102.
17. Cascinelli N, *et al.* Perinodular injection of thymopentine (TP5) in cutaneous and subcutaneous metastases of melanoma. *Melanoma Res* 1993; **3:** 471–6.
18. Pavesi L, Italian Cooperative Trials Group. Fluorouracil (F), with and without high dose folinic acid (HDFA) plus epirubicin (E) and cyclophosphamide (C): FEC versus HDFA-FEC plus or minus thymostimulin (TS) in metastatic breast cancer: results of a multicenter study. *Eur J Cancer* 1993; **29A:** S77.
19. Mustacchi G, Italian Cooperative Trials Group. High dose folinic acid (HDFA) and fluorouracil (Fu) plus or minus thymostimulin (TS) for treatment of metastatic colorectal cancer (MCRC): a randomized multicentric study. *Eur J Cancer* 1993; **29A:** S89.
20. Bodey B, *et al.* Review of thymic hormones in cancer diagnosis and treatment. *Int J Immunopharmacol* 2000; **22:** 261–73.
21. Periti P, *et al.* Antimicrobial chemoimmunoprophylaxis in colorectal surgery with cefotetan and thymostimulin: prospective, controlled multicenter study. *J Chemother* 1993; **5:** 37–42.
22. Sundal E, Bertelletti D. Management of viral infections with thymopentin. *Arzneimittelforschung* 1994; **44:** 866–71.


### Preparations

**Proprietary Preparations** (details are given in Part 3)
***Arg.:*** Leucotrofina; ***Austral.:*** Thymunes†; ***Braz.:*** Leucogen; Timosan†; TP-1†; ***Ger.:*** Neythymun; Thym-Uvocal; Thymo-Glanduretten; Thymoject; Thymophysin; Thymowied; ***Ital.:*** Biothymus†; Sintomodulina; Timunox†; ***Mex.:*** Himus†; Leucotrofina†; ***Spain:*** TP-1†.

**Multi-ingredient:** ***Austria:*** Wobe-Mugos; ***Ger.:*** AntiFocal; Wobe-Mugos Th†; ***Ital.:*** Biothymus F Urto; Biothymus M Urto.

## Tibezonium Iodide *(rINN)*

Ioduro de tibezonio; Rec-15/0691. Diethylmethyl{2-[4-(4-phenylthiophenyl)-3*H*-1,5-benzodiazepin-2-ylthio]ethyl}ammonium iodide.

$C_{28}H_{32}IN_3S_2 = 601.6.$
*CAS — 54663-47-7.*
*ATC — A01AB15.*

### Profile

Tibezonium iodide has been used in the treatment of infections of the mouth and throat.

### Preparations

**Proprietary Preparations** (details are given in Part 3)
***Gr.:*** Riposon; ***Ital.:*** Antoral; ***Mex.:*** Maxoral; ***Port.:*** Maxius.

## Tilactase *(rINN)*

β-Galactosidase; β-D-Galactosidase; β-D-Galactoside Galactohydrolase; Lactase; Tilactasa.
*CAS — 9031-11-2.*
*ATC — A09AA04.*

**Pharmacopoeias.** In *Jpn* (from *Aspergillus oryzae* or *Penicillium multicolor*) and *US* (from *Aspergillus oryzae*).

**USP 27** (Lactase). A hydrolytic enzyme derived from *Aspergillus oryzae*. Each g contains not less than 30 000 USP units. Store in airtight containers at room temperature.

### Profile

Tilactase hydrolyses lactose into glucose and galactose. It has been added to milk and milk products, or taken by mouth with a meal containing dairy products, in order to prevent the symptoms of lactose intolerance (p.1439) in persons deficient in the endogenous enzyme.

### Preparations

**Proprietary Preparations** (details are given in Part 3)
***Arg.:*** Lac-Tas; ***Austral.:*** Lact-Easy†; Lactaid†; ***Canad.:*** Dairyaid; Lactaid; Lactrase; ***Irl.:*** Colief; Lactaid†; ***Ital.:*** Lactaid†; Silact; ***Jpn:*** Galantase; ***Port.:*** Lisolac; ***S.Afr.:*** Galantase†; ***Switz.:*** Lacdigest; ***UK:*** Colief; Lactaid†; ***USA:*** Dairy Ease; Lactaid; Lactrase; SureLac.

**Multi-ingredient:** ***Spain:*** Lactored†; Polidasa†.

## Tilia

Lime Flower; Linden; Tiliae Flos; Tilleul; Tilo.

**Pharmacopoeias.** *Eur.* (see p.vi) and *Pol.* include the flowers.
*Fr.* also includes the bark.

**Ph. Eur. 5.0** (Lime Flower). The whole dried inflorescences of *Tilia cordata*, *Tilia platyphyllos*, *Tilia* × *vulgaris* (=[*Tilia* × *europaea*]), or a mixture of these species. It has a faint aromatic odour. Protect from light.

### Profile

Tilia is mildly astringent and is reputed to have antispasmodic and diaphoretic properties. Lime-flower 'tea' is a traditional domestic remedy.

Various species of tilia are used in herbal and homoeopathic preparations for a variety of disorders.

### Preparations

**Proprietary Preparations** (details are given in Part 3)
***Belg.:*** Vibtil; ***Canad.:*** Hepamig†; ***Fr.:*** Vibtil.

**Multi-ingredient:** ***Arg.:*** Armonil; Dr Calm; Herbaccion Sedante; Insomnal; Nervocalm; No-Nerviol; Sedante Arceli; Sedante Dia; Serenil; Top Life Relax; ***Austral.:*** Crataegus Complex†; ***Austria:*** Aponatura Erkaltungs; Apotheker Bauer's Grippetee; Aurita-Erkaltungstee; Bogumil-tassenfertiger milder Abfurtee; Gewusst wie Husten-Bronchialtee; Grippefloran; Grippetee Dr Zeidler; Grippetee EF-EM-ES; Grippogran; Kneipp Grippe-Tee; Krauterdoktor Erkaltungstropfen; Krauterhaus Mag Kottas Grippetee; Mag Kottas Grippe-Tee; Mag Kottas Krauterexpress-Grippe-Tee; Neuners Krautertee Nr 10 - Grippetee; Neuners Krautertee Nr 210 - Krauterhexlein Kinder-Schweisstreibender Tee; Sidroga Erkaltungstee; Sidroga Kindertee; St Bonifatius-Tee; St Radegunder Fiebertee; Teekanne Erkaltungstee; ***Belg.:*** Eugiron†; Natudor; Tisane Antibiliaire et Stomachique†; Tisane Pectorale†; Tisane pour le Foie†; ***Fr.:*** Actisane Troubles du Sommeil†; Apaisance; Calmophytum; Lenicalm; Mediflor Tisane Antirhumatismale No 2; Mediflor Tisane Calmante Troubles du Sommeil No 14; Noctisan†; Phytotherapie Boribel no 8†; Santane $N_9$†; Santane $O_1$†; Tisane des Familles†; Tisanes de l'Abbe Hamon no 6†; Vigilia; ***Ger.:*** Grunlicht Hingfong Essenz†; Kneipp Erkaltungs-Tee†; Nervosana; Salus Bronchial-Tee Nr.8†; ***Israel:*** Jungborn; ***Ital.:*** Alkagin; Fluend†; Lenicalm; Sambuco (Specie Composta); Sebacnol; Sedofit; Tiglio (Specie Composta); Tussol; Videorelax; ***Port.:*** Alkagin; ***Spain:*** Agua del Carmen; Jaquesor; Mesatil; Natusor Gripotul; Natusor Jaquesan; Natusor Sinulan; Natusor Somnisedan; ***Switz.:*** Tisane antiflatulente pour nourissons et enfants; Tisane contre les refroidissements; Tisane pour les enfants†; ***UK:*** Daily Menopause Relief; Gerard House Motherwort Compound†; Tranquil; Wellwoman.

## Timonacic *(rINN)*

ATC; NSC-25855; Thioproline; Timonácico. Thiazolidine-4-carboxylic acid.

$C_4H_7NO_2S = 133.2.$
*CAS — 444-27-9.*

NOTE. The name ATC has also been used for a combination of paracetamol and trichloroethanol (4-acetamidophenyl 2,2,2-trichloroethyl carbonate).

### Profile

Timonacic is used as an adjuvant in the treatment of acute and chronic hepatic disorders.

Timonacic methyl hydrochloride (carbolidine hydrochloride) has been used as a mucolytic.

### Preparations

**Proprietary Preparations** (details are given in Part 3)
***Ital.:*** Ciliar†; Muvial; Tiazolidin†; ***Switz.:*** Heparegen.

## Tin

Estaño.
Sn = 118.71.
*CAS — 7440-31-5.*

### Profile

Tin is a silver-white, lustrous, malleable, ductile metal. Owing to their low solubility, tin and tin oxide are very poorly absorbed from the gastrointestinal tract have low toxicity. Chronic inhalation causes a benign form of pneumoconiosis.

Organic compounds of tin are highly toxic and may cause liver and kidney damage as well as severe neurological damage associated with oedema of the white matter of the brain. Treatment has been symptomatic. Contamination of the skin with organic tin compounds can cause severe burning; suitable precautions should be taken to prevent absorption of organic tin compounds through the skin.

Tin and tin oxide have been given in the treatment of boils, but there is little evidence of effectiveness; they were also formerly used in some countries for the treatment of tapeworm. Organic tin compounds, especially tributyltin oxide (TBTO), are used as molluscicides; they are highly toxic.

**Tin in food.** Excess amounts of tin in food tend to arise from tin-coated cans, especially unlacquered ones, and may produce gastric irritation. Concentrations as low as 150 micrograms/g in canned beverages and 250 micrograms/g in other canned foods have produced adverse effects in certain individuals, but some foods containing up to 700 micrograms/g have not produced any detectable effects. Further studies were required to identify the chemical forms of tin that cause acute gastric irritation and any possible potentiating or moderating factors. It appeared likely that infants and small children consumed proportionally greater amounts of tin than adults. Consumers should be advised not to store foods in opened cans.[1]

The previously recommended acceptable daily intake for chronic exposure to tin was re-affirmed as a provisional tolerable weekly intake of 14 mg/kg.[1] The UK Tin in Food Regulations 1992 limit the maximum amount of tin in foods sold in the UK to 200 mg/kg of such food.[2]


1. FAO/WHO. Evaluation of certain food additives and contaminants: thirty-third report of the joint FAO/WHO expert committee on food additives. *WHO Tech Rep Ser 776* 1989.
2. MAFF. The Tin in Food Regulations 1992. *Statutory Instrument 1992 No. 496*. London: HMSO, 1992. Also available at: http://www.hmso.gov.uk/si/si1992/UKsi_19920496_en_1.htm (accessed 09/07/04)


### Preparations

**Proprietary Preparations** (details are given in Part 3)
**Multi-ingredient:** ***Belg.:*** Stanno-Bardane†.

## Tin-protoporphyrin

Protoporfirina-Estaño; (Sn)-protoporphyrin.

### Profile

Tin-protoporphyrin and the related compound tin-mesoporphyrin are metalloporphyrins which inhibit haem oxygenase, an enzyme involved in the breakdown of haem to bile pigments. They have been investigated as inhibitors of bilirubin production in hyperbilirubinaemia of various causes, and have been tried in porphyria (p.1040).

◊ References.


1. Rubaltelli FF, *et al.* Tin-protoporphyrin in the management of children with Crigler-Najjar disease. *Pediatrics* 1989; **84:** 728–31.
2. McDonagh AF. Tin-protoporphyrin in the management of children with Crigler-Najjar disease. *Pediatrics* 1990; **86:** 151–2.
3. Berglund L, *et al.* Studies with the haeme oxygenase inhibitor Sn-protoporphyrin in patients with primary biliary cirrhosis and idiopathic haemochromatosis. *Gut* 1990; **31:** 899–904.
4. Dover SB, *et al.* Tin-protoporphyrin combined with haem arginate—an improved treatment for acute hepatic porphyria. *Gut* 1991; **32:** A597.
5. Dover SB, *et al.* Haem-arginate plus tin-protoporphyrin for acute hepatic porphyria. *Lancet* 1991; **338:** 263.
6. Kappas A, *et al.* Direct comparison of Sn-mesoporphyrin, an inhibitor of bilirubin production, and phototherapy in controlling hyperbilirubinemia in term and near-term newborns. *Pediatrics* 1995; **95:** 468–74.
7. Rubaltelli FF, *et al.* Congenital nonobstructive, nonhemolytic jaundice: effect of tin-mesoporphyrin. *Pediatrics* 1995; **95:** 942–4.
8. Valaes T, *et al.* Control of hyperbilirubinemia in glucose-6-phosphate dehydrogenase-deficient newborns using an inhibitor of bilirubin production, Sn-mesoporphyrin. Abstract: *Pediatrics* 1998; **101:** 915. Full version: http://pediatrics.aappublications.org/cgi/content/full/101/5/e1 (accessed 09/07/04)

9. Martinez JC, *et al.* Control of severe hyperbilirubinemia in full-term newborns with the inhibitor of bilirubin production Sn-mesoporphyrin. *Pediatrics* 1999; **103:** 1–5.
10. Kappas A, *et al.* A single dose of Sn-mesoporphyrin prevents development of severe hyperbilirubinemia in glucose-6-phosphate dehydrogenase-deficient newborns. *Pediatrics* 2001; **108:** 25–30.
11. Kappas A, *et al.* Sn-mesoporphyrin interdiction of severe hyperbilirubinemia in Jehovah's Witness newborns as an alternative to exchange transfusion. *Pediatrics* 2001; **108:** 1374–7.

## Tiquizium Bromide *(pINN)*

Bromuro de tiquizio; HSR-902. *trans*-3-(Di-2-thienylmethylene)octahydro-5-methyl-2*H*-quinolizinium bromide.
$C_{19}H_{24}BrNS_2$ = 410.4.
*CAS — 71731-58-3.*

### Profile

Tiquizium bromide has been used as an antispasmodic.

## Tiropramide Hydrochloride *(rINNM)*

Hidrocloruro de tiropramida. DL-α-Benzamido-*p*-[2-(diethylamino)ethoxy]-*N*,*N*-dipropylhydrocinnamamide hydrochloride.
$C_{28}H_{41}N_3O_3,HCl$ = 504.1.
*CAS — 55837-29-1 (tiropramide); 57227-16-4 (tiropramide hydrochloride).*
*ATC — A03AC05.*

### Profile

Tiropramide hydrochloride is used as an antispasmodic. Doses of 100 mg have been given two or three times daily by mouth. It has also been given rectally and parenterally.

### Preparations

**Proprietary Preparations** (details are given in Part 3)
***Ger.:*** Alfospas†; ***Ital.:*** Alfospas; Maiorad; ***Port.:*** Maiorad; ***Thai.:*** Maiorad.

## Titanium

Titanio.
Ti = 47.867.
*CAS — 7440-32-6.*

### Profile

Titanium has been used in the repair of skull damage and for implantation in dental surgery.

◊ References.

1. Brown D. All you wanted to know about titanium, but were afraid to ask. *Br Dent J* 1997; **182:** 393–4.
2. Williams D. The golden anniversary of titanium biomaterials. *Med Device Technol* 2001; **12:** 8–11.

## Tocilizumab *(USAN, pINN)*

Atlizumab; MRA; R-1569. Immunglobulin G1, anti-(human interleukin 6 receptor) (human-mouse monoclonal MRA heavy chain), disulfide with human-mouse monoclonal MRA κ-chain, dimer.
*CAS — 375823-41-9.*

### Profile

Tocilizumab, an interleukin-6 receptor monoclonal antibody, is under investigation for the treatment of various disorders including lymphoproliferative disease and rheumatoid arthritis.

◊ References.

1. Ito H, *et al.* A pilot randomized trial of a human anti-interleukin-6 receptor monoclonal antibody in active Crohn's disease. *Gastroenterology* 2004; **126:** 989–96.

## Tolonium Chloride *(rINN)*

CI Basic Blue 17; Cloruro de tolonio; Colour Index No. 52040; Toluidine Blue O. 3-Amino-7-dimethylamino-2-methylphenazathionium chloride.
$C_{15}H_{16}ClN_3S$ = 305.8.
*CAS — 92-31-9.*

NOTE. Distinguish from Toluidine Blue, Colour Index No. 63340.

### Profile

Tolonium chloride is a thiazine dye chemically related to methylthioninium chloride (p.1042). It has been used to stain oral and gastric neoplasms and was given intravenously to stain the parathyroid glands. Other uses have included the treatment of menstrual disorders and methaemoglobinaemia.

Tolonium chloride should be avoided in patients with G6PD deficiency as haemolysis may occur.

### Preparations

**Proprietary Preparations** (details are given in Part 3)
***Canad.:*** Orascan†; ***Ger.:*** Toluidinblau.

## Tonzonium Bromide *(rINN)*

Bromuro de tonzonio; NC-1264; NSC-5648; Thonzonium Bromide *(USAN)*. Hexadecyl[2-(*N*-*p*-methoxybenzyl-*N*-pyrimidin-2-ylamino)ethyl]dimethylammonium bromide.
$C_{32}H_{55}BrN_4O$ = 591.7.
*CAS — 553-08-2.*

### Profile

Tonzonium bromide is a cationic surfactant. As an additive in ear drops and aerosol sprays it has been claimed to promote tissue contact by dispersion and penetration of cellular debris and exudate.

### Preparations

**Proprietary Preparations** (details are given in Part 3)
**Multi-ingredient:** ***Ital.:*** Rinedrone†; ***NZ:*** Coly-Mycin S Otic†; ***USA:*** Coly-Mycin S Otic; Cortisporin-TC.

## Tormentil

Consolda Vermelha; Erect Cinquefoil; Tormentilla; Tormentillae Rhizoma.

**Pharmacopoeias.** In *Eur.* (see p.vi) and *Pol.*

**Ph. Eur. 5.0** (Tormentil). The whole or cut, dried rhizome, freed from the roots, of *Potentilla erecta* (*P. tormentilla*). It contains not less than 7% of tannins expressed as pyrogallol, calculated with reference to the dried drug. Protect from light.

### Profile

Tormentil has astringent properties and is used in herbal preparations for diarrhoea and other indications. Gastrointestinal irritation and vomiting have occasionally occurred.

◊ References.

1. Subbotina MD, *et al.* Effect of oral administration of tormentil root extract (Potentilla tormentilla) on rotavirus diarrhea in children: a randomized, double blind, controlled trial. *Pediatr Infect Dis J* 2003; **22:** 706–11.

### Preparations

**Proprietary Preparations** (details are given in Part 3)
***Austria:*** Diaro; ***Ger.:*** Herbatorment†; ratioGast.
**Multi-ingredient:** ***Austria:*** Aponatura Durchfall; Bio-Garten Tee gegen Durchfall; Bioreform-Tee gegen Durchfall; Drovitol; Eogran; Krauterhaus Mag Kottas Tee gegen Durchfall; Krauterpfarrer Weidinger Tee zur Entwasserung; ***Ger.:*** Mundra†; Repha-Os; ***Switz.:*** Baume.

## Transfer Factor

Transferencia, factor de.

### Profile

Transfer factor is a peptide constituent of dialysable leucocyte extracts prepared from the leucocytes of a sensitised donor, that can passively transfer cell-mediated immunity to a non-sensitised recipient.

Transfer factor has been suggested for use in infections due to bacteria, fungi, and viruses, inflammatory disorders, skin disorders such as eczema, nervous system disorders, immunodeficiency diseases, and malignancies, although the response when it has been tried in some of these conditions has not always been satisfactory.

◊ References.

1. Fudenberg HH, Fudenberg HH. Transfer factor: past, present and future. *Annu Rev Pharmacol Toxicol* 1989; **29:** 475–516.
2. AUSTIMS Research Group. Interferon-α and transfer factor in the treatment of multiple sclerosis: a double-blind, placebo-controlled trial. *J Neurol Neurosurg Psychiatry* 1989; **52:** 566–74.
3. McBride SJ, McCluskey DR. Treatment of chronic fatigue syndrome. *Br Med Bull* 1991; **47:** 895–907.
4. Hassner A, Adelman DC. Biologic response modifiers in primary immunodeficiency disorders. *Ann Intern Med* 1991; **115:** 294–307.

## Transforming Growth Factor Antibodies

### Profile

A human monoclonal antibody specific for transforming growth factor β1 is under investigation for the treatment of systemic sclerosis.

Lerdelimumab (p.1707) is a human monoclonal antibody specific for transforming growth factor β2.

## Trepibutone *(rINN)*

AA-149; Trepibutona; Trepionate. 3-(2,4,5-Triethoxybenzoyl)propionic acid.
$C_{16}H_{22}O_6$ = 310.3.
*CAS — 41826-92-0.*
*ATC — A03AX09.*

**Pharmacopoeias.** In *Jpn.*

### Profile

Trepibutone has been reported to have spasmolytic and choleretic activity and is used in biliary-tract disorders and pancreatitis.

### Preparations

**Proprietary Preparations** (details are given in Part 3)
***Port.:*** Choliatron.

## Tribenoside *(BAN, USAN, rINN)*

21401-Ba; Ba-21401; Tribenósido; Tribenosidum. Ethyl 3,5,6-tri-*O*-benzyl-D-glucofuranoside.
$C_{29}H_{34}O_6$ = 478.6.
*CAS — 10310-32-4.*
*ATC — C05AX05; C05CX01.*

**Pharmacopoeias.** In *Eur.* (see p.vi).

**Ph. Eur. 5.0** (Tribenoside). A yellowish to pale yellow, clear, viscous liquid. Practically insoluble in water; very soluble in acetone, in dichloromethane, and in methyl alcohol. Store under nitrogen in airtight containers.

### Profile

Tribenoside has been used in inflammatory and varicose disorders of the veins, including haemorrhoids (p.1243). It has been given by mouth in usual doses of 800 mg daily. It has also been given rectally and topically.

### Preparations

**Proprietary Preparations** (details are given in Part 3)
***Austria:*** Glyvenol†; ***Belg.:*** Glyvenol; ***Braz.:*** Glyvenol; ***Hong Kong:*** Glyvenol†; ***Ital.:*** Venalisin†; Venodin†; ***Mex.:*** Glyvenol; ***Switz.:*** Glyvenol†; ***Thai.:*** Glyvenol†.
**Multi-ingredient:** ***Austria:*** Procto-Glyvenol†; ***Braz.:*** Procto-Glyvenol; Rectanus†; ***Chile:*** Euproct; Procto-Glyvenol; Proctogel; ***Israel:*** Procto-Glyvenol; ***Mex.:*** Procto-Glyvenol; ***Port.:*** Procto-Glyvenol; ***Switz.:*** Procto-Glyvenol; ***UAE:*** Haemoproct.

## Tributyl Acetylcitrate

Tributylis Acetylcitras. Tributyl 2-(acetyloxy)propane-1,2,3-tricarboxylate.
$C_{20}H_{34}O_8$ = 402.5.
*CAS — 77-90-7.*

**Pharmacopoeias.** In *Eur.* (see p.vi). Also in *USNF.*

**Ph. Eur. 5.0** (Tributyl Acetylcitrate). A clear oily liquid. Immiscible with water; miscible with alcohol and with dichloromethane.

**USNF 22** (Acetyltributyl Citrate). A clear, practically colourless, oily liquid. Insoluble in water; freely soluble in alcohol, in isopropyl alcohol, in acetone, and in toluene. Store in airtight containers.

### Profile

Tributyl acetylcitrate is a plasticiser and flavour used in pharmaceutical manufacturing and in the food industry.

## Tricarbaurinium

Aluminon; Triammonium Aurintricarboxylate; Tricarbaurinio. 3-(3,3′-Dicarboxy-4,4′-dihydroxybenzhydrylidene)-6-oxocyclohexa-1,4-diene-1-carboxylic acid, triammonium salt.
$C_{22}H_{23}N_3O_9$ = 473.4.
*CAS — 569-58-4.*

### Profile

Tricarbaurinium has been used topically in the treatment of oropharyngeal disorders.

## Triethyl Citrate

E1505; Triethylis Citras; Trietilo, citrato de. 2-Hydroxy-1,2,3-propanetricarboxylic acid triethyl ester.
$C_{12}H_{20}O_7$ = 276.3.
*CAS — 77-93-0.*

**Pharmacopoeias.** In *Eur.* (see p.vi). Also in *USNF.*

**Ph. Eur. 5.0** (Triethyl Citrate). A clear, viscous, colourless or almost colourless, hygroscopic liquid. Soluble in water; miscible with alcohol; slightly soluble in fatty oils. Store in airtight containers.

**USNF 22** (Triethyl Citrate). A practically colourless oily liquid. Soluble in water; miscible with alcohol and with ether. Store in airtight containers.

### Profile

Triethyl citrate is a plasticiser used in pharmaceutical manufacturing and in the food and cosmetics industries.

## Trilostane *(BAN, USAN, pINN)*

Trilostano; Win-24540. 4α,5α-Epoxy-17β-hydroxy-3-oxoandrostane-2α-carbonitrile.
$C_{20}H_{27}NO_3$ = 329.4.
*CAS — 13647-35-3.*
*ATC — H02CA01.*

### Adverse Effects

Side-effects associated with trilostane have included flushing, nausea, vomiting, diarrhoea, rhinorrhoea, and oedema of the palate. Skin rashes may occur and, rarely, granulocytopenia in immunocompromised patients.

### Precautions

Trilostane is contra-indicated in pregnancy and should be used with caution in patients with renal or hepatic impairment. Circulating corticosteroids and blood electrolytes should be monitored. During severe stress, the drug may have to be discontinued and corticosteroid supplements may be required.

### Interactions

Trilostane may interfere with the activity of oral contraceptives. Hyperkalaemia may occur if trilostane is given with potassium-sparing diuretics.

### Uses and Administration

Trilostane is an adrenocortical suppressant that inhibits the enzyme system essential for the production of glucocorticoids and mineralocorticoids. It has been used in the treatment of Cushing's syndrome (p.1313) and primary aldosteronism.

The usual daily dose is 240 mg by mouth in divided doses for at least 3 days and then adjusted, according to the patient's response, within the range of 120 to 480 mg daily. Doses of 960 mg daily have been given.

Trilostane with glucocorticoid replacement therapy has also been used in postmenopausal women with breast cancer who relapse following initial oestrogen receptor antagonist therapy. In these patients, the maintenance dose is 960 mg daily, or 720 mg daily if side-effects occur.

### Preparations

**Proprietary Preparations** (details are given in Part 3)
***UK:*** Modrenal.

## Trimebutine Maleate *(BANM, rINNM)*

Maleato de trimebutina. 2-Dimethylamino-2-phenylbutyl 3,4,5-trimethoxybenzoate hydrogen maleate.

$C_{22}H_{29}NO_5,C_4H_4O_4$ = 503.5.

*CAS — 39133-31-8 (trimebutine); 34140-59-5 (trimebutine maleate).*

*ATC — A03AA05.*

**Pharmacopoeias.** In *Jpn.*

### Profile

Trimebutine maleate has been used as an antispasmodic in gastrointestinal disorders in doses of up to 600 mg daily by mouth. It has also been given by injection and rectally. Trimebutine base has also been used.

**Irritable bowel syndrome.** Trimebutine has been reported[1-3] to be effective in the treatment of irritable bowel syndrome (p.1244) although a considerable placebo response has been observed.[1] Its action is thought to be mediated both via gastrointestinal opioid receptors and modulation of the release of gastrointestinal peptides.[4]

1. Ghidini O, *et al.* Single drug treatment for irritable colon: rociverine versus trimebutine maleate. *Curr Ther Res* 1986; **39:** 541–8.
2. Schaffstein W, *et al.* Comparative safety and efficacy of trimebutine versus mebeverine in the treatment of irritable bowel syndrome. *Curr Ther Res* 1990; **47:** 136–45.
3. Kountouras J, *et al.* Efficacy of trimebutine therapy in patients with gastroesophageal reflux disease and irritable bowel syndrome. *Hepatogastroenterology* 2002; **49:** 193–7.
4. Delvaux M, Wingate D. Trimebutine: mechanism of action, effects on gastrointestinal function and clinical results. *J Int Med Res* 1997; **25:** 225–46.

### Preparations

**Proprietary Preparations** (details are given in Part 3)
***Arg.:*** Debridat; Fenatrop; Miopropan; ***Austria:*** Debridat; ***Braz.:*** Debridat; ***Canad.:*** Modulon; ***Chile:*** Debridat; Dolpic Forte; Trim; ***Fr.:*** Debridat; Modulon; Transacalm; ***Gr.:*** Garapepsin; Ibutin; ***Hong Kong:*** Cerekinon; ***Ital.:*** Debridat; Digerent; Kaliust†; Trimedat; ***Jpn:*** Cerekinon; ***Malaysia:*** Cerekinon; ***Mex.:*** Debridat; Espabion; Libertrim; Prescol; ***Port.:*** Debridat; ***Singapore:*** Cerekinon; Debridat; ***Spain:*** Polibutin; ***Switz.:*** Debridat; ***Thai.:*** Cerekinon.

**Multi-ingredient:** ***Arg.:*** Debridat B; Fenatrop-A; Miopropan Proctologico; Miopropan-T; ***Fr.:*** Proctolog; ***Ital.:*** Debrum; ***Port.:*** Proctolog; ***Singapore:*** Proctolog; ***Spain:*** Proctolog.

## Trinitrophenol

Carbazotic Acid; Picric Acid; Picrinic Acid; Trinitrofenol. 2,4,6-Trinitrophenol.

$C_6H_3N_3O_7$ = 229.1.

*CAS — 88-89-1.*

**Pharmacopoeias.** In *Fr.*

**Storage and hazards.** Trinitrophenol burns readily and explodes when heated rapidly or when subjected to percussion.

For safety in handling trinitrophenol is usually supplied mixed with not less than half its weight of water. It should be stored in a cool place. It must not be stored in glass-stoppered bottles.

Trinitrophenol combines with metals to form salts, some of which are very explosive.

### Profile

Trinitrophenol has disinfectant properties and was formerly used in the treatment of burns. It is now chiefly used in manufacturing and as a laboratory reagent.

Dermatitis, skin eruptions, severe itching, and yellow staining of the skin may occur following contact with trinitrophenol. Systemic toxicity may follow ingestion or absorption through the skin or lungs; symptoms may include vomiting, pain, and diarrhoea, progressing to haemolysis, hepatitis, anuria, convulsions, unconsciousness, and death. The metabolic rate is increased, causing pyrexia.

It has been used in homoeopathy.

### Preparations

**Proprietary Preparations** (details are given in Part 3)

**Multi-ingredient:** ***Chile:*** Agua Sulfatada Picrica; ***Spain:*** Oftalmol Dexa†; Oftalmol Ocular; Queratil†.

## Trolamine *(pINN)*

Triethanolamine; Trolamina; Trolaminum.

*CAS — 102-71-6.*

**Description.** Trolamine is a variable mixture of bases containing mainly 2,2′,2″-nitrilotriethanol (trolamine $(CH_2OH.CH_2)_3N$), together with 2,2′-iminobisethanol (diolamine) and smaller amounts of 2-aminoethanol (monoethanolamine).

**Pharmacopoeias.** In *Eur.* (see p.vi). Also in *USNF.*

**Ph. Eur. 5.0** (Trolamine; Triethanolamine BP 2003). A clear, viscous, colourless or slightly yellow, very hygroscopic liquid. Miscible with water and with alcohol; soluble in dichloromethane. Store in airtight containers. Protect from light.

**USNF 22** (Trolamine). A mixture of alkanolamines consisting largely of trolamine containing some diolamine and monoethanolamine. A colourless to pale yellow, viscous, hygroscopic liquid having a slight ammoniacal odour. Miscible with water and with alcohol; soluble in chloroform. Store in airtight containers. Protect from light.

### Adverse Effects

Trolamine salts may be irritating to the skin and mucous membranes. Contact dermatitis has been reported following the use of ear drops containing trolamine polypeptide oleate-condensate.

**Carcinogenicity.** Following concern of the possible production of carcinogenic nitrosamines in the stomach, the Swiss authorities restricted the use of trolamine to preparations for external use.[1]

1. Anonymous. Trolamine: concerns regarding potential carcinogenicity. *WHO Drug Inf* 1991; **5:** 9.

### Uses and Administration

Trolamine is used combined with fatty acids such as stearic and oleic acids as an emulsifier and as an alkalinising agent. It has also been used to reduce dithranol-induced staining of the skin.

Ear drops containing trolamine polypeptide oleate-condensate 10% are used for the removal of impacted ear wax.

Trolamine salicylate (p.95) has also been used.

### Preparations

**Proprietary Preparations** (details are given in Part 3)
***Arg.:*** Biafine; Orla-Wax; Solucer; ***Austral.:*** Neutrogena†; ***Belg.:*** Xerumenex; ***Braz.:*** Rapid Gel†; ***Canad.:*** Cerumenex; ***Chile:*** Biafine; ***Fr.:*** Biafine; Lamiderm; ***Ger.:*** Cerumenex N; ***Israel:*** Biafine; ***Ital.:*** Cerumenex†; ***Neth.:*** Xerumenex; ***Port.:*** Biafine; ***S.Afr.:*** Cerumenex†; ***Switz.:*** Biafine; Cerumenex; ***USA:*** Cerumenex.

**Multi-ingredient:** ***Arg.:*** Onixol; ***Braz.:*** Benzilol†; Cerumin; Paraqueimol; ***Canad.:*** Soropon; ***Ital.:*** Dopo Pik; ***Port.:*** Transbronquina†; ***USA:*** Maxilube.

## Trometamol *(BAN, rINN)*

NSC-6365; THAM; Trihydroxymethylaminomethane; TRIS; Tris(hydroxymethyl)aminomethane; Trometamolum; Tromethamine *(USAN)*. 2-Amino-2-(hydroxymethyl)propane-1,3-diol.

$C_4H_{11}NO_3$ = 121.1.

*CAS — 77-86-1.*

*ATC — B05BB03; B05XX02.*

**Pharmacopoeias.** In *Eur.* (see p.vi) and *US.*

**Ph. Eur. 5.0** (Trometamol). A white crystalline powder or colourless crystals. Freely soluble in water; sparingly soluble in alcohol; very slightly soluble in ethyl acetate. A 5% solution in water has a pH of 10.0 to 11.5.

**USP 27** (Tromethamine). A white, crystalline powder having a slight characteristic odour. Soluble 1 in 1.8 of water and 1 in 45.5 of alcohol; freely soluble in low-molecular-weight aliphatic alcohols; practically insoluble in carbon tetrachloride, in chloroform, and in benzene. pH of a 5% solution in water is between 10.0 and 11.5. Store in airtight containers.

### Adverse Effects and Precautions

Great care must be taken to avoid extravasation at the injection site as solutions may cause tissue damage. Local irritation, venospasm and phlebitis have occurred.

Respiratory depression can occur and mechanical ventilation may be required. Hypoglycaemia may also occur. Trometamol is contra-indicated in anuria and uraemia, and should be used cautiously in patients with renal impairment as hyperkalaemia has been reported in such patients. Trometamol is not recommended for use in patients with respiratory acidosis alone. If it is used in patients with respiratory acidosis accompanying metabolic acidosis, ventilation should be maintained mechanically. Trometamol is contra-indicated in chronic respiratory acidosis.

Blood concentrations of bicarbonate, glucose, and electrolytes, partial pressure of carbon dioxide, and blood pH should be monitored during infusion of trometamol.

### Uses and Administration

Trometamol is an organic amine proton acceptor used as an alkalinising agent in the treatment of metabolic acidosis (p.1217). It also acts as a weak osmotic diuretic. Trometamol is mainly used during cardiac bypass surgery and during cardiac arrest. It may also be used to reduce the acidity of citrated blood for use in bypass surgery.

The dose used should be the minimum required to increase the pH of the blood to within normal limits and is based on the body-weight and the base deficit. Trometamol is given by slow intravenous infusion as a 0.3M solution; it should not be given for longer than a day except in life-threatening emergencies.

Trometamol citrate is given by mouth for the management of urinary calculi and acidosis. Trometamol acefyllinate has also been used for acidosis.

◊ References.

1. Nahas GG, *et al.* Guidelines for the treatment of acidaemia with THAM. *Drugs* 1998; **55:** 191–224.

### Preparations

***USP 27:*** Tromethamine for Injection.

**Proprietary Preparations** (details are given in Part 3)
***Austral.:*** Tham; ***Austria:*** Tris; ***Fr.:*** Thamacetat†; ***Ger.:*** Tham; Tris; ***Ital.:*** Thamesol; ***Swed.:*** Addex-THAM.

**Multi-ingredient:** ***Fr.:*** Alcaphor; ***Ger.:*** Complete†; ***Israel:*** Complete All-In-One†; ***Norw.:*** Tribonat; ***Spain:*** Sugarceton†; ***Swed.:*** Tribonat; ***Switz.:*** Saltrates.

## Trypan Blue

CI Direct Blue 14; Colour Index No. 23850; Trypanum Caeruleum. Tetrasodium 3,3′-[(3,3′-dimethylbiphenyl-4,4′-diyl)bisazo]bis[5-amino-4-hydroxynaphthalene-2,7-disulphonate].

$C_{34}H_{24}N_6Na_4O_{14}S_4$ = 960.8.

*CAS — 72-57-1.*

### Profile

Trypan blue solutions are used as stains in microscopy and for visualisation of various tissues as an aid to ophthalmic surgery.

### Preparations

**Proprietary Preparations** (details are given in Part 3)
***Fr.:*** Parkipan†; ***Neth.:*** MembraneBlue; VisionBlue.

**Multi-ingredient:** ***Fr.:*** Parkipan.

## Trypsin *(BAN)*

Tripsina; Trypsinum.

*CAS — 9002-07-7.*

*ATC — B06AA07; D03BA01.*

**Pharmacopoeias.** In *Chin., Eur.* (see p.vi), and *US.*

**Ph. Eur. 5.0** (Trypsin). A proteolytic enzyme obtained by the activation of trypsinogen extracted from mammalian pancreas. It has an activity of not less than 0.5 microkatals/mg, calculated with reference to the dried substance. A white or almost white, crystalline or amorphous powder; the amorphous form is hygroscopic. Sparingly soluble in water. A 1% solution in water has a pH of 3.0 to 6.0. Solutions have a maximum stability at pH 3 and a maximum activity at pH 8. Store at 2° to 8° in airtight containers. Protect from light.

**USP 27** (Crystallized Trypsin). A proteolytic enzyme crystallised from an extract of the pancreas gland of the ox. It contains not less than 2500 USP units in each mg, calculated on the dried basis. A white to yellowish-white, odourless, crystalline or amorphous powder. Store in airtight containers at temperature not exceeding 40°.

### Profile

Trypsin is a proteolytic enzyme that has been applied for the debridement of wounds. It has also been taken by mouth, usually with chymotrypsin (p.1671), and sometimes with antibacterial or other drugs, for its supposed benefit in relieving oedema and inflammation associated with infection or trauma. Trypsin solutions have been inhaled for the liquefaction of viscous sputum, and trypsin is also an ingredient of mixtures intended to relieve various gastrointestinal disorders. Trypsin has been used in oncology in a combination preparation with chymotrypsin and papain (see under Uses and Administration of Papain, p.1728).

Hypersensitivity reactions may occasionally occur.

### Preparations

**Proprietary Preparations** (details are given in Part 3)

**Multi-ingredient:** ***Arg.:*** Phlogenzym; ***Austria:*** Leukase; Leukase-Kegel; Phlogenzym; Wobenzym; ***Braz.:*** Parenzyme; Parenzyme Ampicilina; Parenzyme Analgesico; Parenzyme Tetraciclina; Phlogenzym†; Probenzima Ampicilina†; Probenzima Analgesico†; ***Fr.:*** Alphintern†; Ribatran; ***Ger.:*** Enzym-Wied; Hevert Enzym Novo†; Mulsal N; Phlogenzym; Wobe-Mugos E; Wobe-Mugos Th†; Wobenzym N; ***India:*** Alfapsin; Soluzyme; ***Ital.:*** Essen Enzimatico; ***Mex.:*** Ochozim; Phlogenzym; Ribotripsin; Wobe-

Mugos; Wobenzym; **Port.:** Chimar; **Spain:** Bristaciclina Dental; Dertrase; Dosil Enzimatico; Doxiten Enzimatico; Epixian†; Kanapomada†; Naso Pekamin; Oxidermiol Enzima; Quimodril; Solupen Enzimatico†; **USA:** Dermuspray; Granulderm; Granulex; GranuMed.

## Tuberculins

Tuberculinas.

*ATC — V04CF01.*

**Pharmacopoeias.** In *Eur.* (see p.vi) and *US.*

**Ph. Eur. 5.0** (Tuberculin for Human Use, Old). It consists of a filtrate, concentrated by heating, containing the soluble products of the culture and lysis of one or more strains of *Mycobacterium tuberculosis* and/or *M. bovis*. It contains a suitable preservative that does not give rise to false-positive reactions. In concentrated form, it is a transparent, viscous, yellow or brown liquid. Protect from light.

**Ph. Eur. 5.0** (Tuberculin Purified Protein Derivative for Human Use). A preparation obtained by precipitation from the heated products of the culture and lysis of *Mycobacterium tuberculosis* and/or *M. bovis*. It contains a suitable preservative that does not give rise to false-positive reactions. It is a colourless or pale yellow liquid; the diluted preparation may be a freeze-dried powder which upon dissolution gives a colourless or pale yellow liquid. Protect from light.

**USP 27** (Tuberculin). A sterile solution derived from the concentrated, soluble products of growth of the tubercle bacillus (*Mycobacterium tuberculosis* or *M. bovis*) prepared in a special medium. It is provided either as Old Tuberculin, a culture filtrate adjusted to the standard potency by the addition of glycerol and isotonic sodium chloride solution, or as Purified Protein Derivative (PPD), a further purified protein fraction. Store at 2° to 8°.

### Adverse Effects

Pain and pruritus may occur at the injection site, occasionally with vesiculation, ulceration, or necrosis in highly sensitive persons. Granuloma has been reported.

Nausea, headache, dizziness, malaise, rash, urticaria, oedema, and pyrexia have been reported occasionally; immediate systemic hypersensitivity, including anaphylaxis, has been reported rarely. There have also been rare reports of lymphangitis.

**Hypersensitivity.** There are rare reports[1-3] of severe anaphylactic or anaphylactoid reactions, occasionally fatal,[1] to tuberculin.


1. DiMaio VJM, Froede RC. Allergic reactions to the tine test. *JAMA* 1975; **233:** 769.
2. Spiteri MA, *et al.* Life threatening reaction to tuberculin testing. *BMJ* 1986; **293:** 243–4.
3. Wright DN, *et al.* Systemic and local allergic reactions to the tine test purified protein derivative. *JAMA* 1989; **262:** 2999–3000.


**Lymphangitis.** Lymphangitis has been reported on 5 occasions after the Mantoux test and on 7 occasions after the Heaf test.[1] However, it was noted that a tuberculin test may have been inappropriate in some of these patients, particularly older subjects and those with evidence of healed tuberculous lesions.[2]


1. Morrison JB. Lymphangitis after tuberculin tests. *BMJ* 1984; **289:** 413.
2. Festenstein F. Lymphangitis after tuberculin tests. *BMJ* 1984; **289:** 625–6.


### Precautions

Tuberculin should be given with caution to patients who have, or are suspected of having, active tuberculosis; although severe local reactions may occur in patients with active tuberculosis, sensitivity may be diminished if it is particularly severe. Sensitivity to tuberculin may also be diminished in the following conditions: viral or severe bacterial infection including HIV infection and infectious mononucleosis; neoplastic disease particularly lymphoma; sarcoidosis; corticosteroid or immunosuppressive therapy; recent administration of live virus vaccines; ultraviolet light treatment; chronic renal failure; dehydration; and malnutrition.

Tuberculins may be adsorbed onto the surface of syringes and should therefore be administered immediately.

### Uses and Administration

Tuberculin skin tests are used to detect tuberculoprotein hypersensitivity when BCG vaccination is being considered or as an aid to diagnosis of tuberculosis. A person showing a specific sensitivity to tuberculin is considered to have been infected with the tubercle bacillus, though the infection may be inactive. Administration of tuberculin for sensitivity testing is by intradermal injection (as in the Mantoux test) or by multiple-puncture devices (such as the Heaf test or tine tests). The term tine test is generally used for disposable multiple-puncture devices coated with dried old tuberculin or purified protein derivative. However, some consider tine tests to be unreliable and they are not recommended for use in the UK.

In the UK, it is recommended that tuberculin testing should always be performed, except in neonates, when BCG vaccination is being considered; either the Mantoux test or the Heaf test is recommended.

For a routine **Mantoux** test, 0.1 mL (10 units) of a diluted solution of tuberculin purified protein derivative (PPD), containing 100 units/mL, is injected intradermally. Results should be read after 48 to 72 hours but may, if necessary, be read for up to 96 hours after the test, and are graded by the degree of induration:

- negative: induration of 0 to 4 mm diameter
- positive: palpable in duration of at least 5 mm diameter
- strongly positive result: palpable induration of at least 15 mm diameter

If a patient is suspected of having tuberculosis or is known to be hypersensitive to tuberculin, 0.1 mL (1 unit) of a solution of tuberculin PPD containing 10 units/mL should be used. A solution containing 1000 units/mL is also available; it may be used if there is doubt about interpretation when the 100 units/mL solution is used.

For the **Heaf** test, a solution of tuberculin purified protein derivative, containing 100 000 units/mL, is used. The solution is applied to the forearm and a multiple-puncture gun (Heaf gun) is used; a puncture of 1 mm depth is recommended for children under 2 years of age and a puncture of 2 mm for older children and adults. Results may be read 3 to 10 days after the test and the reaction graded:

- grade 0 (negative): no induration at the puncture sites
- grade 1 (negative): discrete induration at 4 or more needle sites
- grade 2 (positive): an indurated ring formed by confluent papules with a clear centre
- grade 3 (positive): one uniform circle of induration 5 to 10 mm wide
- grade 4 (positive): solid induration over 10 mm wide, possibly with accompanying vesiculation or ulceration.

Grade 3 and 4 reactions are regarded as strongly positive equivalent to an induration of 15 mm or more in the Mantoux test. Individuals with grade 0 or 1 reactions who have not previously received BCG vaccines may be offered BCG vaccination; a grade 1 reaction is not usually related to infection with *Mycobacterium tuberculosis*. Patients with a grade 2 reaction or more (or an induration of 5 to 14 mm in the Mantoux test) are considered to be hypersensitive to tuberculoprotein and should not be vaccinated.

Investigation for the presence of active tuberculosis is generally only indicated for patients showing a strongly positive reaction to a Mantoux or Heaf test. However, there are many factors that should be considered when interpreting the results of a tuberculin skin test; in addition to those listed under Precautions (see above), there are the effects of previous BCG vaccination, repeated tuberculin testing, and age. In some areas, a positive reaction may be a result of cross-sensitivity of the test to non-tuberculous mycobacteria (see below).

In some other countries the population tested, the procedures used, and grading of reactions may differ slightly from that outlined above.

Tuberculins are also used, in conjunction with other antigens, to assess the status of cell-mediated immunity (see Anergy Testing, below).

**Anergy testing.** Patients with HIV infection are at an increased risk of developing tuberculosis but often show a diminished reactivity to antigens (anergy), making the interpretation of negative tuberculin skin tests difficult. Anergy testing has therefore been recommended in patients with HIV infection when tuberculin testing is used in the diagnosis of tuberculosis. However, the Centers for Disease Control (CDC) in the USA[1] no longer recommend routine anergy testing in HIV patients because of problems with standardisation and reproducibility of the test, amongst other factors limiting the test's usefulness. They do suggest, however, that anergy testing may be of benefit in guiding individual therapeutic decisions in selected situations. In general, the CDC recommend two additional skin test antigens, *Candida* and mumps, in conjunction with tuberculin purified protein derivative. The test antigens are given concurrently with tuberculin, usually by the Mantoux method (see above). Other antigens may be administered, and tetanus antigens are frequently used for anergy testing. In some cases more than two control antigens may be required to avoid misclassifying immunocompetent patients as anergic. Variations on the usual definitions of positive and negative response to the Mantoux test have also been employed.


1. Centers for Disease Control. Anergy skin testing and preventive therapy for HIV-infected persons: revised recommendations. *MMWR* 1997; **46** (RR-15): 1–10. Corrected title online at: http://www.cdc.gov/mmwr/preview/mmwrhtml/00049386.htm (accessed 09/07/04)


**Latent tuberculosis.** Full eradication of tuberculosis from developed countries requires identification of latent as well as active cases.[1] Tuberculin testing has been in use for over 100 years and, while still considered a useful diagnostic agent for tuberculosis, the problems of false-positive reactions or reduced sensitivity to the test are well recognised.[1] Use of the test to identify latent disease has evolved with experience.[2] Previous BCG vaccination is one factor that significantly increases the likelihood of a false-positive reaction to tuberculin testing, which makes the diagnosis of latent tuberculosis particularly difficult.[3] Interpretation of the skin test should therefore be made by considering the induration size in the context of the individual clinical profile, including other risk factors for infection.[2,3] It has been suggested[2] that it is not necessary for low-risk persons in the general population of the USA to receive routine tuberculin testing for tuberculosis; high-risk groups of adults and children for whom screening might be warranted have been defined, and consensus recommendations made. An opinion has also been ventured[4] that tuberculin testing before BCG vaccination is not necessary in children in the UK.


1. Lee E, Holzman RS. Evolution and current use of the tuberculin test. *Clin Infect Dis* 2002; **34:** 365–70.
2. American Thoracic Society. Targeted tuberculin testing and treatment of latent tuberculosis infection. 1999. Available at: http://www.thoracic.org/adobe/statements/latenttbl-27.pdf (accessed 09/07/04)
3. Wang L, *et al.* A meta-analysis of the effect of Bacille Calmette Guérin vaccination on tuberculin skin test measurements. *Thorax* 2002; **57:** 804–9. Correction: *ibid.* 2003; **58:** 188.
4. Bothamley GH, *et al.* Tuberculin testing before BCG vaccination. *BMJ* 2003; **327:** 243–4.


**Malignant disease.** Benefit has been reported[1] in 2 patients with adult T-cell leukaemia/lymphoma predominantly involving the skin following local treatment with tuberculin purified protein derivative.


1. Kanekura T, *et al.* Purified protein derivative treatment for skin lesions of adult T-cell leukaemia/lymphoma. *Br J Dermatol* 1999; **140:** 767–8.


**Non-tuberculous mycobacterial infection.** The tuberculin skin test is not specific for *Mycobacterium tuberculosis*, but can also represent a cross-reaction caused by antigens on other non-tuberculous mycobacteria. Re-examination[1] of results from children with non-tuberculous mycobacterial infection concluded that the avian Mantoux test (avian tuberculin purified protein derivative (PPD) prepared from *M. avium*) was more sensitive than the human Mantoux test (tuberculin PPD prepared from *M. tuberculosis*) in the detection of non-tuberculous mycobacteria in regions with a low incidence of tuberculosis, and may be a useful aid to differential diagnosis in areas where tuberculosis is prevalent.


1. Daley AJ, Isaacs D. Differential avian and human tuberculin skin testing in non-tuberculous mycobacterial infection. *Arch Dis Child* 1999; **80:** 377–9.


### Preparations

**Ph. Eur.:** Old Tuberculin for Human Use; Tuberculin Purified Protein Derivative for Human Use;
**USP 27:** Tuberculin.

**Proprietary Preparations** (details are given in Part 3)
**Austria:** Monotest; **Belg.:** Monovacc-Test; **Braz.:** Multitest†; **Canad.:** Tubersol; **Fr.:** Monotest; Neotest†; Tubertest; **Ger.:** Tubergen-Test; **Ital.:** Biocine Test PPD; Monotest; **NZ:** Monotest; Tubersol; **S.Afr.:** Biocine Test; Japan Freeze-Dried Tuberculin†; Monotest; PPD Tine Test†; **Spain:** Tubersol PPD; **Swed.:** Monotest; **USA:** Aplisol; Aplitest†; Mono-Vacc Test (O.T.)†; Tine Test PPD†; Tubersol.

**Multi-ingredient: Austral.:** Multitest CMI; **Austria:** Multitest; **Belg.:** Multitest†; **Canad.:** Multitest CMI†; **Fr.:** Multitest IMC†; **Ger.:** Immignost†; Multitest; **Israel:** Multitest CMI; **Ital.:** Multitest IMC†; **Neth.:** Multitest CMI†; **NZ:** Multitest CMI; **S.Afr.:** Multitest CMI; **Spain:** Multitest IMC†; **USA:** Multitest CMI†.

## Tucaresol *(BAN, rINN)*

BW-589C; 589C; 589C80. α-(2-Formyl-3-hydroxyphenoxy)-*p*-toluic acid.

$C_{15}H_{12}O_5 = 272.3$.

*CAS — 84290-27-7.*

### Profile

Tucaresol is reported to interact with haemoglobin to increase oxygen affinity. It has been investigated as an oral drug for the treatment of sickle-cell disease (p.734). Tucaresol is also reported to have immunostimulant properties and is under investigation in HIV infection and hepatitis B. Hypersensitivity reactions have occurred.

◊ References.


1. Rolan PE, *et al.* The pharmacokinetics, tolerability and pharmacodynamics of tucaresol (589C80; 4[2-formyl-3-hydroxyphenoxymethyl]benzoic acid), a potential anti-sickling agent, following oral administration to healthy subjects. *Br J Clin Pharmacol* 1993; **35:** 419–25.
2. Arya R, *et al.* Tucaresol increases oxygen affinity and reduces haemolysis in subjects with sickle cell anaemia. *Br J Haematol* 1996; **93:** 817–21.
3. Peck RW, *et al.* Effect of food and gender on the pharmacokinetics of tucaresol in healthy volunteers. *Br J Clin Pharmacol* 1998; **46:** 83–6.


## Tuftsin

$N^2$-[1-($N^2$-L-threonyl-L-lysyl)-L-prolyl]-L-arginine.

$C_{21}H_{40}N_8O_6 = 500.6$.

*CAS — 9063-57-4.*

### Profile

Tuftsin is a naturally occurring tetrapeptide and has been investigated as the acetate for its immunostimulant activity.

## Javanese Turmeric

Curcuma Zanthorrhiza; Curcumae Javanicae; Curcumae Xanthorrhizae Rhizoma.

**Pharmacopoeias.** In *Eur.* (see p.vi).

**Ph. Eur. 5.0** (Turmeric, Javanese). It consists of the dried rhizome, cut in slices, of *Curcuma xanthorrhiza*. It contains not less than 5% v/w of essential oil and not less than 1% of dicinnamoyl methane derivatives expressed as curcumin, both calculated with reference to the anhydrous drug. It has an aromatic odour. Protect from light.

### Profile

Javanese turmeric is an ingredient of preparations indicated for biliary and gastrointestinal disorders.

### Preparations

**Proprietary Preparations** (details are given in Part 3)
***Ger.:*** Bilagit Mono; Curcu-Truw; Curcumen; Infi-tract.

**Multi-ingredient:** ***Austria:*** Aristochol†; Choleodoron; Teekanne Leber- und Galletee; ***Belg.:*** Tisane Contre la Tension†; Tisane pour le Foie†; ***Fr.:*** Hepaclem; ***Ger.:*** Bilisan C3†; Bilisan Duo; Chol-Truw S†; Cholapret†; Cholosom SL; Cholosom-Tee; Divalol W; Enzym-Harongan; Gallexier; Hepaticum novo; Hepatofalk Neu†; Hepatofalk Planta N†; Infi-tract; ***Hong Kong:*** Hepatofalk; ***Singapore:*** Hepatofalk Planta.

## Turpentine Oil

Aetheroleum Terebinthinae; Esencia de Trementina; Essence de Térébenthine; Oleum Terebinthinae; Oleum Terebinthinae Depuratum; Rectified Turpentine Oil; Spirits of Turpentine; Trementina, aceite esencial de.

**Pharmacopoeias.** In *Chin., Eur.* (see p.vi), and *Jpn.*

**Ph. Eur. 5.0** (Turpentine Oil, Pinus Pinaster Type; Terebinthini Aetheroleum ab Pinum Pinastrum). An essential oil obtained by steam distillation, followed by rectification at a temperature below 180°, from the oleoresin obtained by tapping *Pinus pinaster*. A suitable antoxidant may be added. It contains 70.0 to 85.0% α-pinene, 0.5 to 1.5% camphene, 11.0 to 20.0% β-pinene, maximum 1% car-3-ene, 0.4 to 1.5% β-myrcene, 1.0 to 7.0% limonene, 0.2 to 2.5% longifolene, 0.1 to 3.0% β-caryophyllene, and maximum 1.0% caryophyllene oxide.

A clear, colourless or pale yellow liquid with a characteristic odour. Relative density 0.856 to 0.872. Store in well-filled airtight containers at a temperature not exceeding 25°. Protect from light.

### Adverse Effects

In poisoning with turpentine oil there may be local burning and gastrointestinal upset, coughing and choking, pulmonary oedema, excitement, coma, fever, tachycardia, liver damage, haematuria, and albuminuria. Fatalities have occurred.

The application to the skin of liniments containing turpentine oil may cause irritation and absorption of large amounts may cause some of the effects listed above. Hypersensitivity reactions and local irritation have been reported.

### Uses and Administration

Turpentine oil is widely used as a solvent. It is applied topically as a rubefacient. It is an ingredient of many preparations used in respiratory-tract disorders, but is now judged to be neither safe nor effective.

### Preparations

***BP 2003:*** White Liniment.

**Proprietary Preparations** (details are given in Part 3)
***Fr.:*** Ozothine; ***Ger.:*** Terpestrol H†.

**Multi-ingredient:** ***Arg.:*** Atomo Desinflamante C; Bronco Etersan; Notoxin; Otocalmia; Rati Salil Crema; ***Austral.:*** Capsolin†; Goanna Heat Cream†; Goanna Liniment†; Goanna Salve†; Relief Rub†; Turpentine White Liniment†; Vicks Vaporub†; ***Austria:*** Aciforin; Baby Luuf; Bronchostop; Carl Baders Divinal; Dolex†; Dracodermalin; Emser Nasensalbe; Ilon Abszess; Kinder Erkaltungsbalsam; Kinder Luuf; Leukona-Rheuma-Bad; Luuf Balsam; Pe-Ce; Piniment; Rubriment; Salhumin; Scottopect; Tetesept†; Trauma-Salbe warmend; Traumasalbe; Tussamag; Vulpuran; Wick Vaporub; ***Belg.:*** Reflexspray; Vicks Vaporub; ***Braz.:*** A Curitybina; Analgen; Angino-Rub; Benegel†; Frixopel; Gelflex; Gelofrix; Gelogel†; Gelol†; Gelonevral; Massageol; Massubal†; Mentalol†; Mialgex; Nevrol; Oleo Eletrico; Prontoalivio†; Salimetin; Sanador†; Traumac; Traumagel; Vick Vaporub; ***Canad.:*** Cal Mo Dol; Cerumol; ***Chile:*** Balsamo Leon; Hansaplast Descongestionante; ***Fin.:*** Vicks Vaporub; ***Fr.:*** Dinacode; Huile de Haarlem†; Lao-Dal†; Lumbalgine; Ozothine; Ozothine a la Diprophylline; Vicks Vaporub; ***Ger.:*** Angocin percutan†; Bartelin N†; Em-eukal; Emser Nasensalbe N; Erkaltungsbalsam-ratiopharm E Salbe; Hevertopect N; Hoemarin Rheuma†; Ilon Abszess; Kneipp Erkaltungs-Balsam N†; Kneipp Tonikum-Bad Fichtennadel-Aquasan†; Leukona-Rheuma-Bad N; Leukona-Rheumasalbe; Ozothin; Plantmobil†; Rheumaliment N†; Schupps Latschenkiefer Olbad†; Trauma-Salbe Rodler 302 N; Wick Vaporub; ***India:*** Waxolve; ***Irl.:*** Cerumol†; Vicks Vaporub†; ***Israel:*** Deep Heat Rub; Mento-O-Cap; ***Ital.:*** Capsolin; Vicks Vaporub; ***Malaysia:*** Thermorub; ***Neth.:*** Vicks Vaporub; ***NZ:*** Vicks Vaporub; ***Port.:*** Balsamo Nostrum; Freimax; Lauromentol; Linimento de Sloan†; ***S.Afr.:*** Respisniffers†; Warm-Up†; Woodwards Inhalant; ***Spain:*** Dologex; Embrocacion Gras; Killpan†; Linimento Klari; Linimento Sloan†; Masagil; Otocerum; Pomada Revulsiva†; Reflex; Termosan; ***Swed.:*** Vicks Vaporub; ***Switz.:*** Alginex; Artragel†; Baume du Chalet; Caprisana†; Capsolin†; Cerumenol; Embropax†; Kernosan Huile de Massage†; Liberol†; Makatussin†; Massorax; Olbas†; Pinimenthol; Roliwol†; Schwefelbad Dr Klopfer†; Sloan Baume†; Sloan Liniment†; Tumarol†; Vicks Vaporub N; ***Thai.:*** Stopain; Tiffyrub; ***UK:*** BN†; Boots Vapour Rub†; Deep Heat Rub; Dragon Balm; Ellimans; Goddards Embrocation; Gonne Balm; Modern Herbals Muscular Pain; Nasciodine; Nine Rubbing Oils; Tixycolds Cold and Hayfever†; Vicks Vaporub; Waxwane; Woodwards Baby Chest Rub†.

## Tyramine Hydrochloride

Tiramina, hidrocloruro de; *p*-Tyramine Hydrochloride; Tyrosamine Hydrochloride. 4-Hydroxyphenethylamine hydrochloride; 4-(2-Aminoethyl)phenol hydrochloride.

$C_8H_{11}NO,HCl = 173.6.$

*CAS — 51-67-2 (tyramine); 60-19-5 (tyramine hydrochloride).*

### Profile

Tyramine hydrochloride is a sympathomimetic with indirect effects on adrenergic receptors. It has been given by mouth or injection in the tyramine pressor test, for the investigation of monoamine oxidase inhibitory activity or amine uptake blocking activity, as well as of various physiological and disease states.

It has also been tried in the diagnosis of migraine and phaeochromocytoma.

The hazards of taking foods rich in tyramine while under treatment with MAOIs are described in the chapter on Antidepressants (see Phenelzine, p.314).

### Preparations

**Proprietary Preparations** (details are given in Part 3)
**Multi-ingredient:** ***Ger.:*** Mydrial-Atropin.

## Ubidecarenone *(BAN, rINN)*

Coenzyme Q10; Ubidecarenona; Ubidecarenonum; Ubiquinone-10. 2-Deca(3-methylbut-2-enylene)-5,6-dimethoxy-3-methyl-*p*-benzoquinone.

$C_{59}H_{90}O_4 = 863.3.$

*CAS — 303-98-0.*

*ATC — C01EB09.*

**Pharmacopoeias.** In *Chin., Eur.* (see p.vi), and *Jpn.* Also in *USNF.*

**Ph. Eur. 5.0** (Ubidecarenone). A yellow or orange crystalline powder. It gradually decomposes and darkens on exposure to light. M.p. about 48°. Practically insoluble in water; very slightly soluble in dehydrated alcohol; soluble in acetone. Store in airtight containers. Protect from light.

**USNF 22** (Ubidecarenone). A yellow to orange, crystalline powder. M.p. about 48°. Practically insoluble in water; very slightly soluble in dehydrated alcohol; soluble in ether. Protect from light.

### Profile

Ubidecarenone is a naturally occurring coenzyme involved in electron transport in the mitochondria. It is claimed to be a free radical scavenger and to have antoxidant and membrane stabilising properties. It has been given by mouth as an adjunct in cardiovascular disorders, including mild or moderate heart failure. It has also been tried in other conditions associated with coenzyme deficiency, and is promoted as a dietary supplement. Ubidecarenone is under investigation for the management of Huntington's chorea and parkinsonism.

◊ For a report of the use of ubidecarenone in muscle weakness, see Effects on Skeletal Muscle, under Simvastatin, p.997.

◊ References.


1. Greenberg S, Frishman WH. Co-enzyme $Q_{10}$: a new drug for cardiovascular disease. *J Clin Pharmacol* 1990; **30:** 596–608.
2. Spigset O. Reduced effect of warfarin caused by ubidecarenone. *Lancet* 1994; **344:** 1372–3.
3. Garcia Silva MT, *et al.* Improvement of refractory sideroblastic anaemia with ubidecarenone. *Lancet* 1994; **343:** 1039.
4. Gattermann N, *et al.* No improvement of refractory sideroblastic anaemia with ubidecarenone. *Lancet* 1995; **345:** 1121–2.
5. Nagao T, *et al.* Treatment of warfarin-induced hair loss with ubidecarenone. *Lancet* 1995; **346:** 1104–5.
6. Pepping J. Coenzyme $Q_{10}$. *Am J Health-Syst Pharm* 1999; **56:** 519–21.
7. Khatta M, *et al.* The effect of coenzyme $Q_{10}$ in patients with congestive heart failure. *Ann Intern Med* 2000; **132:** 636–40.
8. Tran MT, *et al.* Role of coenzyme Q10 in chronic heart failure, angina, and hypertension. *Pharmacotherapy* 2001; **21:** 797–806.
9. Huntington Study Group. A randomized, placebo-controlled trial of coenzyme Q10 and remacemide in Huntington's disease. *Neurology* 2001; **57:** 397–404.
10. Rahman S, *et al.* Neonatal presentation of coenzyme Q10 deficiency. *J Pediatr* 2001; **139:** 456–8.
11. Shults CW, *et al.* Effects of coenzyme Q10 in early Parkinson disease: evidence of slowing of the functional decline. *Arch Neurol* 2002; **59:** 1541–50.


### Preparations

***USNF 22:*** Ubidecarenone Capsules; Ubidecarenone Tablets.

**Proprietary Preparations** (details are given in Part 3)
***Braz.:*** Coex; Vinocard Q10; ***Canad.:*** Co-Q-10; ***Fr.:*** Bio-Quinon Q10 Super; ***Hong Kong:*** CoQuinone; Eiquinon; Salcotan†; ***Ital.:*** Caomet†; Cardioton†; Coedieci; Decafar; Decorenone; Dymion†; Iuvacor; Miodene; Miotyn; Mitocor; Roburis†; Ubicarden†; Ubicardio; Ubicor; Ubidenone; Ubidex; Ubifactor†; Ubimaior; Ubisint†; Ubiten; Ubivis; ***Jpn:*** Neuquinon; ***Malaysia:*** Bio-Quinone; Neuquinon; ***Port.:*** Q 10; Ubenzima; Ubicondrial; ***Thai.:*** Bio-Quinone; Decaquinon; ***UK:*** Co-Q-10; ***USA:*** Co-Q-10; Co-Quinone.

**Multi-ingredient:** ***Canad.:*** Mega AO; ***Ital.:*** Agedin Plus; Ener-E; Visu Q10; ***UK:*** Efamol Plus Coenzyme Q10†; Red Kooga Co-Q-10 and Ginseng.

## Ulinastatin *(rINN)*

Ulinastatina; Urinastatin.

*CAS — 80449-31-6; 80449-32-7.*

**Pharmacopoeias.** In *Jpn.*

### Profile

Ulinastatin is a glycoprotein proteolytic enzyme inhibitor isolated from human urine. It has been given by injection in acute pancreatitis (p.1726) and in acute circulatory insufficiency.

◊ References.


1. Ohwada M, *et al.* New endoscopic treatment for chronic pancreatitis, using contrast media containing ulinastatin and prednisolone. *J Gastroenterol* 1997; **32:** 216–21.


### Preparations

**Proprietary Preparations** (details are given in Part 3)
***Jpn:*** Miraclid.

## Urazamide

5-Aminoimidazole-4-carboxamide ureidosuccinate.

$C_9H_{14}N_6O_6 = 302.2.$

### Profile

Urazamide has been used in the treatment of hepatic disorders in doses of 400 to 800 mg daily by mouth. It has also been given by intramuscular and intravenous injection.

### Preparations

**Proprietary Preparations** (details are given in Part 3)
***Ital.:*** Carbaica.

## Uridine

Uracil Riboside; Uridina. 1-β-D-Ribofuranosyluracil; 1-β-D-Ribofuranosylpyrimidine-2,4(1*H*,3*H*)-dione.

$C_9H_{12}N_2O_6 = 244.2.$

*CAS — 58-96-8.*

### Profile

Uridine is one of the four nucleosides present in ribonucleic acid. Uridine has been used in patients with hereditary orotic aciduria.

### Preparations

**Proprietary Preparations** (details are given in Part 3)
**Multi-ingredient:** ***Austria:*** Laevadosin†; Vitasic†; ***Fr.:*** Vitacic; ***Ital.:*** Centrum; Cituridina†; For Liver†; ***Spain:*** Inexfal†; Prodessal†.

## Uridine Triphosphate

Ins-316; Uridina trifosfato; Uridine Triphosphoric Acid; UTP. Uridine 5′-(tetrahydrogen triphosphate).

$C_9H_{15}N_2O_{15}P_3 = 484.1.$

*CAS — 63-39-8.*

### Profile

Uridine triphosphate has been investigated for the treatment of cystic fibrosis (p.123) and as an aid to the diagnosis of lung cancer. It has also been claimed to be of value in muscular atrophy and muscular weakness, and has been included in preparations for neuralgia, neuritis, and muscular disorders; trisodium uridine triphosphate has also been used.

**Uses.** Uridine triphosphate has been reported to be effective in stimulating chloride secretion in the nasal epithelium of patients with cystic fibrosis.[1] It has been suggested that correction of the ion-transport abnormalities in cystic fibrosis patients may reduce the viscosity of the secretions in the early stages of the disease,[2] and selected nucleotides such as uridine triphosphate should be investigated as therapeutic agents.[1]

The suggestion that uridine might produce improvement in patients with galactosaemia has not been confirmed.[3]

Uridine triphosphate has been investigated to improve sputum expectoration.[4,5]


1. Knowles MR, *et al.* Activation by extracellular nucleotides of chloride secretion in the airway epithelia of patients with cystic fibrosis. *N Engl J Med* 1991; **325:** 533–8.
2. Davis PB. Cystic fibrosis from bench to bedside. *N Engl J Med* 1991; **325:** 575–77.
3. Holton JB, Leonard JV. Clouds still gathering over galactosaemia. *Lancet* 1994; **344:** 1242–3.
4. Bennett WD, *et al.* Effect of aerosolized uridine 5′-triphosphate on mucociliary clearance in mild chronic bronchitis. *Am J Respir Crit Care Med* 2001; **164:** 302–6.
5. Johnson FL, *et al.* Improved sputum expectoration following a single dose of INS316 in patients with chronic bronchitis. *Chest* 2002; **122:** 2021–9.


### Preparations

**Proprietary Preparations** (details are given in Part 3)
***Fr.:*** Uteplex; ***Ital.:*** Miocuril.

**Multi-ingredient:** ***Arg.:*** Nucleo CMP; ***Braz.:*** Nucleo CMP; ***Chile:*** Citoneuron; ***Ger.:*** Keltican N; ***Ital.:*** Fosfoutipi Vitaminico; ***Spain:*** Cefabol; Nucleo CMP; Taurobetina.

## Ursodeoxycholic Acid *(BAN, rINN)*

Ácido ursodeoxicólico; Acidum Ursodeoxycholicum; UDCA; Ursodesoxycholic Acid; Ursodiol *(USAN)*. 3α,7β-Dihydroxy-5β-cholan-24-oic acid.

$C_{24}H_{40}O_4 = 392.6.$

*CAS — 128-13-2.*

*ATC — A05AA02.*

**Pharmacopoeias.** In *Chin., Eur.* (see p.vi), *Jpn,* and *US.*

**Ph. Eur. 5.0** (Ursodeoxycholic Acid). A white or almost white powder. Very slightly soluble in water; freely soluble in alcohol; slightly soluble in acetone and in dichloromethane.

**USP 27** (Ursodiol). A white or almost white, crystalline powder.

Practically insoluble in water; freely soluble in alcohol and in glacial acetic acid; sparingly soluble in chloroform; slightly soluble in ether. Store in airtight containers.

**Stability.** References.


1. Mallett MS, *et al.* Stability of ursodiol 25 mg/mL in an extemporaneously prepared oral liquid. *Am J Health-Syst Pharm* 1997; **54:** 1401–4.
2. Johnson CE, Streetman DD. Stability of oral suspensions of ursodiol made from tablets. *Am J Health-Syst Pharm* 2002; **59:** 361–3.


## Adverse Effects and Precautions

Ursodeoxycholic acid may cause nausea, vomiting, and other gastrointestinal disturbances; diarrhoea is reported to occur less frequently than with chenodeoxycholic acid. Increased liver enzyme values are also less likely. Pruritus may occur. Treatment with ursodeoxycholic acid may cause more calcification of cholesterol stones than chenodeoxycholic acid.

Ursodeoxycholic acid should not be given to patients with peptic ulcer disease, inflammatory bowel disease, or chronic liver disease (but see below). It is ineffective for the dissolution of calcified and pigment gallstones and is of no value in patients without a patent and functioning gallbladder. Its use should be avoided in pregnancy.

## Interactions

Ursodeoxycholic acid should not be used with drugs, such as oestrogenic hormones, that increase bile cholesterol. Use with bile-acid binding drugs including antacids, charcoal, and colestyramine should be avoided since this may reduce the effectiveness of therapy with ursodeoxycholic acid.

## Pharmacokinetics

Ursodeoxycholic acid is absorbed from the gastrointestinal tract and undergoes enterohepatic recycling. It is partly conjugated in the liver before being excreted into the bile. Under the influence of intestinal bacteria the free and conjugated forms undergo 7α-dehydroxylation to lithocholic acid, some of which is excreted directly in the faeces and the rest absorbed and mainly conjugated and sulfated by the liver before excretion in the faeces. However, in comparison with chenodeoxycholic acid, less ursodeoxycholic acid undergoes such bacterial degradation.

◊ References.


1. Crosignani A, *et al.* Clinical pharmacokinetics of therapeutic bile acids. *Clin Pharmacokinet* 1996; **30:** 333–58.


## Uses and Administration

Ursodeoxycholic acid is a naturally occurring bile acid (see p.1660) present in small quantities in human bile. Ursodeoxycholic acid suppresses the synthesis and secretion of cholesterol by the liver and inhibits intestinal absorption of cholesterol. It is used for the dissolution of cholesterol-rich **gallstones** in patients with functioning gallbladders (see below). The usual dose is 6 to 12 mg/kg daily as a single bedtime dose or in 2 or 3 divided doses; obese patients may require up to 15 mg/kg daily. The daily dose may be divided unequally and the larger dose given before bedtime to counteract the increase in biliary cholesterol concentration seen overnight. The time required for dissolution of gallstones is likely to be between 6 and 24 months depending on stone size and composition. Treatment should be continued for 3 to 4 months after radiological disappearance of the stones. A dose of 300 mg twice daily has been suggested for the *prevention* of gallstones in patients undergoing rapid weight loss. Ursodeoxycholic acid has also been given in reduced doses in combination with chenodeoxycholic acid (p.1670).

Ursodeoxycholic acid is also used in **primary biliary cirrhosis**. The usual dose is 10 to 15 mg/kg daily in 2 to 4 divided doses.

Ursodeoxycholic acid has been tried in the treatment of primary sclerosing cholangitis.

The more hydrophilic derivative, tauroursodeoxycholic acid, has also been used.

**Chronic liver disease.** The use of ursodeoxycholic acid in chronic liver diseases has been summarised.[1-4] There have been differing opinions of its value in primary biliary cirrhosis (below). Response has been reported in liver disease in cystic fibrosis,[5-7] cholestasis associated with pregnancy,[8] sclerosing cholangitis,[9] chronic active hepatitis,[10] and viral hepatitis.[11,12] Ursodeoxycholic acid had initially shown some promise in the treatment of nonalcoholic steatohepatitis,[13] but a randomised, controlled study[14] failed to confirm this. There has also been some interest in the use of ursodeoxycholic acid to treat refractory graft-versus-host disease of the liver in transplant patients,[15] and possibly as an adjuvant to immunosuppressant therapy[16-18] after orthotopic liver transplantation (p.1346). It may also be of benefit in the prevention of hepatic complications following allogeneic bone marrow transplantation.[19,20]


1. de Caestecker JS, *et al.* Ursodeoxycholic acid in chronic liver disease. *Gut* 1991; **32:** 1061–5.
2. Rubin RA, *et al.* Ursodiol for hepatobiliary disorders. *Ann Intern Med* 1994; **121:** 207–18.
3. Kowdley KV. Ursodeoxycholic acid therapy in hepatobiliary disease. *Am J Med* 2000; **108:** 481–6.
4. Trauner M, Graziadei IW. Review article: mechanisms of action and therapeutic applications of ursodeoxycholic acid in chronic liver diseases. *Aliment Pharmacol Ther* 1999; **13:** 979–95.
5. Colombo C, *et al.* Effects of ursodeoxycholic acid therapy for liver disease associated with cystic fibrosis. *J Pediatr* 1990; **117:** 482–9.
6. Cotting J, *et al.* Effects of ursodeoxycholic acid treatment on nutrition and liver function in patients with cystic fibrosis and longstanding cholestasis. *Gut* 1990; **31:** 918–21.
7. Scher H, *et al.* Ursodeoxycholic acid improves cholestasis in infants with cystic fibrosis. *Ann Pharmacother* 1997; **31:** 1003–5.
8. Palma J, *et al.* Ursodeoxycholic acid in the treatment of cholestasis of pregnancy: a randomized, double-blind study controlled with placebo. *J Hepatol* 1997; **27:** 1022–8.
9. Lindor KD, *et al.* Ursodiol for primary sclerosing cholangitis. *N Engl J Med* 1997; **336:** 691–5.
10. Rolandi E, *et al.* Effects of ursodeoxycholic acid (UDCA) on serum liver damage indices in patients with chronic active hepatitis: a double-blind controlled study. *Eur J Clin Pharmacol* 1991; **40:** 473–6.
11. Puoti C, *et al.* Ursodeoxycholic acid and chronic hepatitis C infection. *Lancet* 1993; **341:** 1413–14.
12. Angelico M, *et al.* Recombinant interferon-α and ursodeoxycholic acid versus interferon-α alone in the treatment of chronic hepatitis C: a randomized clinical trial with long-term follow-up. *Am J Gastroenterol* 1995; **90:** 263–9.
13. Laurin J, *et al.* Ursodeoxycholic acid or clofibrate in the treatment of non-alcohol-induced steatohepatitis: a pilot study. *Hepatology* 1996; **23:** 1464–7.
14. Lindor KD, *et al.* Ursodeoxycholic acid for treatment of nonalcoholic steatohepatitis: results of a randomized trial. *Hepatology* 2004; **39:** 770–8.
15. Fried RH, *et al.* Ursodeoxycholic acid treatment of refractory chronic graft-versus-host disease of the liver. *Ann Intern Med* 1992; **116:** 624–9.
16. Persson H, *et al.* Ursodeoxycholic acid for prevention of acute rejection in liver transplant recipients. *Lancet* 1990; **ii:** 52–3.
17. Friman S, *et al.* Adjuvant treatment with ursodeoxycholic acid reduces acute rejection after liver transplantation. *Transplant Proc* 1992; **24:** 389–90.
18. Clavien P-A, *et al.* Evidence that ursodeoxycholic acid prevents steroid-resistant rejection in adult liver transplantation. *Clin Transplant* 1996; **10:** 658–62.
19. Essell JH, *et al.* Ursodiol prophylaxis against hepatic complications of allogeneic bone marrow transplantation: a randomized, double-blind, placebo-controlled trial. *Ann Intern Med* 1998; **128:** 975–81.
20. Ruutu T, *et al.* Ursodeoxycholic acid for the prevention of hepatic complications in allogeneic stem cell transplantation. *Blood* 2002; **100:** 1977–83.


PRIMARY BILIARY CIRRHOSIS. Primary biliary cirrhosis (PBC) is a chronic liver disease of unknown aetiology that develops due to progressive destruction of small and intermediate bile ducts within the liver, subsequently evolving to fibrosis and cirrhosis. Over 90% of patients are female, usually aged between 40 and 60 years. The disease is thought to be auto-immune in nature. Most patients develop antimitochondrial antibodies that may be evident even before disease is clinically apparent.[1,2] Genetic factors and hormonal stimulation may play a role in precipitating PBC.[1,2] Infectious agents such as *Chlamydophila pneumoniae* (*Chlamydia pneumoniae*)[2] or retroviruses[3] may be involved in the pathogenesis.

Clinical manifestations include pruritus, fatigue, jaundice, hepatomegaly, hypercholesterolaemia leading to xanthoma formation, and in late disease portal hypertension, bleeding oesophageal varices and liver failure may develop. Impaired calcium and vitamin D absorption may result in osteomalacia or osteoporosis, and fat-soluble vitamin deficiencies may occur. There may be accumulation of copper in the liver.[4] Various other disorders including rheumatoid arthritis, scleroderma, thyroiditis, and Sjögren's syndrome may be associated with PBC.[1,5]

The disease is slowly progressive, with a mean survival of 8 years for symptomatic patients, and 16 years for asymptomatic individuals.[1,6] Despite its presumed auto-immune aetiology, few immunosuppressive drugs have shown any benefit,[5,7] although newer drugs such as mycophenolate mofetil, sirolimus, and tacrolimus have yet to be fully evaluated.[7] The best-studied treatment for PBC is ursodeoxycholic acid, which is thought to replace toxic endogenous bile acids, stimulate bile acid secretion, and exert local immunosuppressive and cytoprotective effects.[1,4,5,7,8] The value of ursodeoxycholic acid is controversial: although it improves serum bilirubin and liver enzyme concentrations,[9] its reported therapeutic benefits in terms of delaying disease progression and the need for liver transplantation[5,10] have not been confirmed by meta-analysis or systematic review.[9,11] In consequence, some do not recommend its use,[11,12] although others still believe it to be the treatment of choice.[1,7] Both penicillamine and azathioprine have been used in PBC, but trials have failed to show any benefit from treatment[5-7] and their use has declined. Corticosteroids, colchicine, ciclosporin, chlorambucil, and methotrexate have also been tried with more success, but toxicity has restricted their use.[5,7] They may be of benefit[2,4,6,7] when used with ursodeoxycholic acid, although some guidelines[5] do not recommend their use. Budesonide[7] and bezafibrate[1,7] have also been tried.

Symptomatic treatment includes the use of bile acid sequestrants, such as colestyramine, to treat both pruritus and hypercholesterolaemia. Ursodeoxycholic acid may also improve pruritus in up to 40% of patients, and rifampicin, phenobarbital, and opioid antagonists are used as second-line therapies.[1,4,5,8] Vitamin D and calcium supplementation will prevent osteomalacia; supplementation with vitamins A, E, and K may also be necessary.[1,4,5,8] Liver transplantation is recommended for liver failure,[1,2,5] although PBC can recur in the allograft.[5]


1. Nishio A, *et al.* Primary biliary cirrhosis: lessons learned from an organ-specific disease. *Clin Exp Med* 2001; **1:** 165–78.
2. Kaplan MM. Primary biliary cirrhosis: past, present, and future. *Gastroenterology* 2002; **123:** 1392–4.
3. Mason A, Nair S. Primary biliary cirrhosis: new thoughts on pathophysiology and treatment. *Curr Gastroenterol Rep* 2002; **4:** 45–51.
4. Poupon R, Poupon RE. Treatment of primary biliary cirrhosis. *Baillieres Best Pract Res Clin Gastroenterol* 2000; **14:** 615–28.
5. Heathcote EJ. Management of primary biliary cirrhosis. *Hepatology* 2000; **31:** 1005–13.
6. Heathcote EJ. Evidence-based therapy of primary biliary cirrhosis. *Eur J Gastroenterol Hepatol* 1999; **11:** 607–15.
7. Holtmeier J, Leuschner U. Medical treatment of primary biliary cirrhosis and primary sclerosing cholangitis. *Digestion* 2001; **64:** 137–50.
8. Prince MI, Jones DE. Primary biliary cirrhosis: new perspectives in diagnosis and treatment. *Postgrad Med J* 2000; **76:** 199–206.
9. Gluud C, Christensen E. Ursodeoxycholic acid for primary biliary cirrhosis. Available in The Cochrane Library; Issue 2. Chichester: John Wiley; 2004.
10. Lindor KD, *et al.* Ursodeoxycholic acid for primary biliary cirrhosis. *Lancet* 2000; **355:** 657–8.
11. Goulis J, *et al.* Randomised controlled trials of ursodeoxycholic-acid therapy for primary biliary cirrhosis: a meta-analysis. *Lancet* 1999; **354:** 1053–60.
12. Anonymous. Ursodeoxycholic acid for primary biliary cirrhosis. *Drug Ther Bull* 1999; **37:** 30–2.


**Gallstones.** Gallstones (cholelithiasis) occur when mechanisms for the solubilisation of cholesterol or bilirubin fail or are overcome. They may be divided into those formed of pure cholesterol, which are usually solitary; pigment stones, largely made up of bilirubin or its derivatives; and mixed stones of cholesterol, bile pigment, and calcium salts, which form the great majority of cases seen in the West.

Gallstones are generally more common in women than in men. The prevalence also increases with age and obesity, although rapid weight loss as a result of dieting or surgery is associated with an increased risk.

As many as two-thirds of patients with gallstones are asymptomatic. Symptoms usually relate to the site of the stone although biliary colic is often present regardless of whether the stone is in the gallbladder or biliary tract. If the stone blocks the exit from the gallbladder, inflammation and bacterial infection may follow (acute cholecystitis), sometimes leading to perforation and subsequent peritonitis. Less commonly, obstruction of the common bile duct by gallstones (choledocholithiasis) may lead to cholestasis and jaundice; infection of the bile ducts and septicaemia may follow. Pancreatitis may also be associated with gallstone disease, and there may be an increased risk of developing malignant neoplasms of the gallbladder.

**Treatment.** Asymptomatic gallstones discovered during other investigations should not be treated, and even mildly symptomatic patients may be managed with analgesics and subsequent observation. Potent analgesics such as morphine or pethidine may be needed in more severe cases (see Biliary and Renal Colic, p.4). In symptomatic patients the preferred treatment for gallstones is surgical removal of the gallbladder; 'keyhole surgery' (laparoscopic cholecystectomy) causes less postoperative morbidity than open surgery, and has largely replaced other methods of treatment.

In patients unsuited to, or unwilling to undergo, surgery for gallbladder stones, drug therapy, alone or with lithotripsy, may be considered.

Exogenous bile acids have been tried in an attempt to dissolve the cholesterol component of gallstones. Ursodeoxycholic acid is more effective and is associated with fewer adverse effects than chenodeoxycholic acid. Combination therapy has also been tried but this is no more effective than ursodeoxycholic acid alone. Dissolution of gallstones is slow but can be achieved in about one-third of cases with the best results seen with small stones. However, about half of all successfully treated patients will develop further gallstones within 10 years. Studies of prophylactic bile acid therapy have mostly yielded disappointing results, although such therapy may be of benefit in patients on very-low-calorie diets, after surgery for weight loss, and in those receiving treatment with octreotide.

Somewhat larger stones may respond to extracorporeal shock-wave lithotripsy, or fluoroscopically guided laser lithotripsy, which may be more effective. Oral bile acids should then be given to dissolve the stone fragments.

Another method is the direct instillation of a solvent (usually methyl *tert*-butyl ether) into the gallbladder. This dissolves stones within a matter of hours, and is effective against almost all cholesterol-based stones regardless of size and number. Care is required to avoid overflow of the solvent into the common bile duct or the duodenum, where it can cause inflammation. Other solvents, such as ethyl propionate have been investigated as potentially less toxic alternatives, and edetic acid has been suggested as a possible solvent for non-cholesterol gallstones. As with all non-surgical methods, recurrence is likely.

Patients with **stones in the common bile duct** or **acute cholecystitis** require prompt therapy because of the risk of serious complications; endoscopic sphincterotomy and physical retrieval of the stones with a basket or balloon appears to be the preferred treatment, with open surgery as an alternative. A biliary stent to allow bile flow around the stone has been used as a temporary measure in patients with stones too large to remove by endoscopic sphincterotomy. Lithotripsy or infusion of a solvent such as monoctanoin or methyl *tert*-butyl ether are possible alternatives in patients unfit for surgery.

In patients who develop cholecystitis or cholangitis antibacterial therapy may be required (see Biliary-tract Infections, p.121).

References.


1. Johnston DE, Kaplan MM. Pathogenesis and treatment of gallstones. *N Engl J Med* 1993; **328:** 412–21.
2. Ransohoff DF, Gracie WA. Treatment of gallstones. *Ann Intern Med* 1993; **119:** 606–19.
3. May GR, *et al.* Efficacy of bile acid therapy for gallstone dissolution: a meta-analysis of randomized trials. *Aliment Pharmacol Ther* 1993; **7:** 139–48.

4. Hofmann AF, *et al.* Pathogenesis and treatment of gallstones. *N Engl J Med* 1993; **328:** 1854–5.
5. Anonymous. Managing patients with gallstones. *Drug Ther Bull* 1994; **32:** 33–5.
6. Lanzini A, Northfield TC. Pharmacological treatment of gallstones: practical guidelines. *Drugs* 1994; **47:** 458–70.
7. Tait N, Little JM. The treatment of gall stones. *BMJ* 1995; **311:** 99–105.
8. Jakobs R, *et al.* Fluoroscopically guided laser lithotripsy versus extracorporeal shock wave lithotripsy for retained bile duct stones: a prospective randomised study. *Gut* 1997; **40:** 678–82.
9. Toouli J, Wright TA. Gallstones. *Med J Aust* 1998; **169:** 166–71.
10. Bateson MC. Gallbladder disease. *BMJ* 1999; **318:** 1745–8.
11. Ahmed A, *et al.* Management of gallstones and their complications. *Am Fam Physician* 2000; **61:** 1673–80.


### Preparations

***BP 2003:*** Ursodeoxycholic Acid Capsules; Ursodeoxycholic Acid Tablets; ***USP 27:*** Ursodiol Capsules.

**Proprietary Preparations** (details are given in Part 3)
***Arg.:*** Dexo; Solutrat; UDCA; Urzac; ***Austral.:*** Ursofalk; ***Austria:*** Ursofalk; ***Belg.:*** Ursochol; Ursofalk; ***Braz.:*** Ursacol; ***Canad.:*** Urso; Ursofalk†; ***Chile:*** Solvobil; Ursofalk; ***Fin.:*** Adursal; ***Fr.:*** Arsacol†; Delursan; Destolit†; Ursolvan; ***Ger.:*** Cholacid†; Cholit-Ursan; Cholofalk; UDC; Urso; Ursochol; Ursofalk; ***Gr.:*** Ursofalk; ***Hong Kong:*** Ursofalk; Ursolvan†; Urososan; ***India:*** Udiliv; ***Irl.:*** Ursofalk; ***Israel:*** Ursofalk; Ursolit; ***Ital.:*** Benursil; Biliepar; Coledos; Desocol; Desoxil; Deursil; Dissolursil; Epasol; Fraurs; Galmax; Lentorsil; Litoff; Litursol; Tauro; Tudcabil; Urdes; Ursacol; Ursilon; Ursobil; Ursodamor; Ursodexil; Ursodiol; Ursofalk; Ursoflor; Ursolac; Ursolisin; Urson†; Ursoproge; ***Jpn:*** Urso; Ursosan; ***Malaysia:*** Ursofalk; ***Mex.:*** Ursofalk; ***Neth.:*** Ursochol; Ursofalk; ***Norw.:*** Ursofalk; ***NZ:*** Actigall; ***Port.:*** Destolit; Ursofalk; ***S.Afr.:*** Ursotan; ***Singapore:*** Ursofalk; Ursolvan†; ***Spain:*** Ursobilane; Ursochol; Ursolite†; ***Swed.:*** Ursofalk; ***Switz.:*** Deursil; Ursochol; Ursofalk; ***Thai.:*** Ursofalk; Ursolin; ***UK:*** Destolit; Urdox; Ursofalk; Ursogal; ***USA:*** Actigall; Urso.

**Multi-ingredient:** ***Austria:*** Lithofalk; ***Ger.:*** Lithofalk; Urso Mix; Ursofalk + Chenofalk†; ***Ital.:*** Bilenor; Litobile†; ***Switz.:*** Lithofalk†.

## Urtica

Ortiga; Stinging Nettle.

**Pharmacopoeias.** In *Ger., Pol.,* and *Swiss.* Also in *USNF.*

*Eur.* (see p.vi) includes a form for homoeopathic preparations.

**Ph. Eur. 5.0** (Common Stinging Nettle for Homoeopathic Preparations). The whole, fresh, flowering plant of *Urtica dioica.* Protect from light.

**USNF 22** (Stinging Nettle). The dried roots and rhizomes of *Urtica dioica* (Urticaceae), and may contain *Urtica urens*, known in commerce as dwarf nettle, as a minor component. It contains not less than 0.8% of total amino acids, not less than 0.05% of sitosterol, and not less than 0.003% scopoletin ($C_{10}H_8O_4$ = 192.2), calculated on the dried basis. Store in airtight containers. Protect from light.

### Profile

Urtica (*Urtica dioica*) has been used in herbal medicine, mainly for urinary-tract and rheumatic disorders. *Urtica urens* has been used similarly.

*Urtica dioica* and *U.urens* have also been used in homoeopathy.

### Preparations

**Proprietary Preparations** (details are given in Part 3)
***Austria:*** Urtica Plus; ***Braz.:*** Bazoton†; ***Ger.:*** Arthrodynat N; Azuprostat Urtica; Bazoton; Cirkuprostan†; Dr Grandel Brennessel Vital Tonikum†; Flexal Brennessel; Hostid†; Hox Alpha; Kneipp Brennesselkraut Pflanzensaft Kneippianum†; Kneipp Pflanzen-Dragees Brennessel†; Pro-Sabona Uno; Prostaforton; Prostagalen; Prostaherb N; Prostamed Urtica; Prostaneurin; Prostata; Prostawern; Reumaless†; Rheuma-Hek; Serless; Uriginex Urtica†; Uro-POS; Urtica Plus N†; Urticaprostat uno; Urticur†; Urtipret; Urtivit; utk; ***Ital.:*** Venustas Shampoo per Capelli con Forfora e/o Grassi†; ***Switz.:*** Simic†; Valverde prostate capsules; ***Thai.:*** Urtipret†.

**Multi-ingredient:** ***Austral.:*** Cough Relief†; Extralife Flow-Care†; Infant Tonic†; Irontona†; Respatona Decongestant Formula†; Respatona Plus Bronchial Cough Relief†; Urapro†; Vitatona†; ***Austria:*** Anaemodoron; Apotheker Bauer's Harntreibender Tee; Apotheker Bauer's Nieren- und Blasentee; Apotheker Hoyers Brennesseltonikum; Berggeist; Bio-Garten Tee zur Erhohung der Harnmenge; Bioreform-Harntreibender Tee; Bogumil-tassenfertiger milder Abfurtee; Brennesseltonikum; Brostalin; Ehrmann's Entschlackungstee; Florissamol; Fruhjahrs-Elixier ohne Alkohol; Gewusst wie Gruner Fastentee; Krauterdoktor Entwasserungs-Elixier; Krauterhaus Mag Kottas Entschlackungstee; Krauterhaus Mag Kottas Entwasserungstee; Krauterhaus Mag Kottas Fruhjahrs- und Herbstkurtee; Krauterpfarrer Weidinger Rheumatee; Krauterpfarrer Weidinger Tee zur Entschlackung; Mag Doskar's Nieren- und Blasentonikum; Mag Kottas Entschlackungstee; Mag Kottas Krauterexpress-Entschlackungstee; Menodoron; Mentopin; Naturland Entschlackungstee; Naturland Rheuma Tee; Neuners Krautertee Nr 19 - Harntreibender Stoffwechseltee; Neuners Krautertee Nr 8 - Magentee gegen Ubersauerung; Prostagutt; Prostatonin; Sidroga Stoffwechseltee; Species Carvi comp; St Radegunder Entwasserungs-Elixier; St Radegunder Entwasserungstee; Synpharma Instant-Blasen- und Nierentee; ***Braz.:*** Lactifero†; Prostem Plus; ***Fr.:*** Fitacnol; Salucur†; ***Ger.:*** Befelka-Tinktur†; Combudoron; Presselin Nieren-Blasen K 3; Prostagutt forte; Prostatin F; Salus Rheuma-Tee Krautertee Nr. 12†; Uvirgan N; Vollmers praparierter gruner N; Winar; ***Ital.:*** Biothymus DS; Herbavit†; Nosenil†; Omadine†; Sebacnol; Shamday Antiforfora; ***Malaysia:*** Prostakan; ***Mex.:*** Prosgutt; ***Spain:*** Natusor Artilane; ***Switz.:*** Prostagutt-F; Prostatonin; Tisane Diuretique; ***UK:*** Kleer†; Savlon Natural First Aid for Burns.

## Usnea Barbata

Barba de capuchino.

*CAS — 125-46-2 (usnic acid).*

### Profile

*Usnea barbata* is a lichen. It contains usnic acid, which is reported to have antimicrobial activity. *Usnea barbata* extract, usnic acid, and copper usnate have been used in topical preparations.

### Preparations

**Proprietary Preparations** (details are given in Part 3)
***Ger.:*** Dr Grandel Granobil; ***Ital.:*** Vidermina; Zeta N.

**Multi-ingredient:** ***Ital.:*** Aseptil†; Foot Zeta; Micofoot; Neo Zeta-Foot†; Steril Zeta.

## Valepotriates

Valepotriatos.

## Acevaltrate *(rINN)*

4-Acetoxymethyl-(1 or 6)-3-(acetoxy-3-methylbutyryloxy)-1,6,-7,7a-tetrahydro-(6 or 1)-isovaleryloxycyclopenta[*c*]pyran-7-spiro-2′-oxiran.

$C_{24}H_{32}O_{10}$ = 480.5.

*CAS — 25161-41-5.*

## Didrovaltrate *(rINN)*

6-Acetoxy-1,4a,5,6,7,7a-hexahydro-1-isovaleryloxy-4-isovaleryloxymethylcyclopenta[*c*]pyran-7-spiro-2′-oxiran.

$C_{22}H_{32}O_8$ = 424.5.

*CAS — 18296-45-2.*

## Valtrate *(pINN)*

4-Acetoxymethyl-1,6-di-isovaleryloxy-1,6,7,7a-tetrahydrocyclopenta[*c*]pyran-7-spiro-2′-oxiran.

$C_{22}H_{30}O_8$ = 422.5.

*CAS — 18296-44-1.*

### Profile

Valepotriates are epoxy-iridoid esters, isolated from valerian (see below). They include acevaltrate, didrovaltrate, and valtrate. On prolonged storage and drying they are hydrolysed to yield isovaleric acid.

A mixture stated to contain acevaltrate, didrovaltrate, and valtrate has been used as a sedative and as an anxiolytic. Concern has been expressed over the potential toxicity of valepotriates which have been reported to have cytotoxic properties *in vitro*.

### Preparations

**Proprietary Preparations** (details are given in Part 3)
***Austria:*** Valmane.

## Valerian

Baldrianwurzel; Valer; Valerian Rhizome; Valerian Root; Valeriana; Valerianae Radix.

*CAS — 8057-49-6 (valerian extract).*

*ATC — N05CM09.*

**Pharmacopoeias.** In *Eur.* (see p.vi) and *Pol.* Also in *USNF. Jpn* has Japanese Valerian from *V. fauriei.*

**Ph. Eur. 5.0** (Valerian Root; Valerian BP 2003). The yellowish-grey to pale brownish-grey whole underground parts of *Valeriana officinalis*, including the rhizome surrounded by the roots and stolons, or by fragments of these parts. It contains not less than 0.5% v/w of essential oil for the whole drug and not less then 0.3% v/w for the cut drug, both calculated with reference to the dried drug. Protect from light.

**USNF 22** (Valerian). The subterranean parts of *Valeriana officinalis* (Valerianaceae), including the rhizome, roots, and stolons. It contains not less than 0.5% of volatile oil and not less than 0.05% of valerenic acid, calculated on the dried basis. Store in airtight containers. Protect from light.

### Profile

Valerian has sedative properties and is used as an extract, infusion, or tincture, or occasionally as the dried root, in preparations for anxiety states. It has also been used as a carminative. The odour of valerian may be removed from the skin and from hard surfaces with sodium bicarbonate.

◊ Reviews.


1. Houghton P. Valerian. *Pharm J* 1994; **253:** 95–6.
2. Houghton PJ. The scientific basis for the reputed activity of valerian. *J Pharm Pharmacol* 1999; **51:** 505–12.
3. Plushner SL. Valerian: valeriana officinalis. *Am J Health-Syst Pharm* 2000; **57:** 328–35.
4. Stevinson C, Ernst E. Valerian for insomnia: a systematic review of randomized clinical trials. *Sleep Med* 2000; **1:** 91–9.


**Adverse effects.** Liver damage[1] was reported in 4 patients who took herbal stress remedies that contained valerian. Cardiac complications and delirium in a 58-year-old man may have been caused by the withdrawal of prolonged therapy with a valerian root extract preparation.[2]


1. MacGregor FB, *et al.* Hepatotoxicity of herbal remedies. *BMJ* 1989; **299:** 1156–7.
2. Garges HP, *et al.* Cardiac complications and delirium associated with valerian root withdrawal. *JAMA* 1998; **280:** 1566–7.


### Preparations

***USNF 22:*** Valerian Tablets.

**Proprietary Preparations** (details are given in Part 3)
***Arg.:*** Sedante Nativa; ***Austral.:*** Herbal Sleep Formula†; ***Austria:*** Baldrinetten; Cirkulin Baldrian†; Hovasin; ***Belg.:*** Relaxine; Valdispert; Valerial; ***Braz.:*** Sonoripan; Valerin; Valerix; Valezen; Valmane; ***Canad.:*** Nytol Natural Source; Sleep-Eze V Natural; Unisom Natural Source; ***Chile:*** Sominex; ***Fin.:*** Valrian; ***Fr.:*** Relaxine†; ***Ger.:*** Baldriparan Stark; Baldrisedon Mono†; Baldurat; Benedorm†; Euvegal Balance; Hewedormir†; Kneipp Baldrian Pflanzensaft Nerventrost†; Kneipp Baldrian†; Melival†; Nervipan†; Phytodorma; Recvalysat; Sedalint Baldrian†; Sedonium; Valdispert; Valmane†; ***Hong Kong:*** Cirku Sed; ***Israel:*** Valeton; ***Ital.:*** Ticalma; Val-Uno; ***Neth.:*** Valdispert; ***Port.:*** Valdispert; ***S.Afr.:*** Calmettes; ***Spain:*** Ansiokey; Cirkused; Coenrelax; Tauval†; Valdispert; Valeriana Orto; ***Swed.:*** Baldrian-Dispert; Neurol; Valerecen; ***Switz.:*** Baldriparan pour la nuit; Baldrisedon; ReDormin; Sedasol eco natura; Sedonium; Sirop pour le sommeil; Valdispert†; Valverde Sirop pour le sommeil; ***UK:*** Phytorelax; Sedonium.

**Multi-ingredient:** ***Arg.:*** Armonil; Calmtabs; Dioxicolagol; Erbonda Noche; Herbaccion Sedante; Insomnal; Nervocalm; Sedante Arceli; Sedante Dia; Serenil; Top Life Relax; Trixol; Valeriana Oligoplex; ***Austral.:*** Calmo†; Executive B†; Extralife Sleep-Care†; Goodnight Formula†; Lifesystem Herbal Plus Formula 2 Valerian†; Macro Anti-Stress†; Multi-Vitamin Day & Night†; Naturest†; Pacifenity†; Passiflora Complex†; Passionflower Plus†; Prosed-X†; ReDormin; Relaxaplex†; Valerian Plus Herbal Plus Formula 12†; Valerian†; ***Austria:*** Absimed; Aktiv Nerven- und Schlaftee; Aponatura Einschlaf; Aurita-Nerventee; Bakanasan Einschlaf; Baldracin; Baldrian AMA; Baldrian Dispert Compositum; Baldrian-Elixier; Baldrian-Krautertonikum; Baldriparan Beruhigungs; Bio-Garten Tee fur den Magen; Bio-Garten Tee zur Beruhigung; Bio-Garten Tropfen fur Magen und Darm; Biogelat Schlaf; Bioreform-Beruhigungstee; Bioreform-Magentee; Cardiofrik†; Einschlafkapseln; Eryval; Gewusst wie Nerven-Schlaftee; Hova; Klosterfrau-Beruhigungskapseln; Kneipp Nerven- und Schlaf-Tee; Krauterdoktor Entspannungs- und Einschlaftropfen; Krauterdoktor Magen-Darmtropfen; Krauterdoktor Nerven-Tonikum; Krauterhaus Mag Kottas Nerven- und Schlaftee; Krauterhaus Mag Kottas Wechseltee; Krauterpfarrer Weidinger Rheumatee; Luvased; Mag Doskar's Nerventonikum; Mag Kottas Beruhigungstee; Mag Kottas Krauterexpress-Beruhigungstee; Mag Kottas Krauterexpress-Nerven-Schlaf-Tee; Mag Kottas Krauterexpress-Wechseltee; Mag Kottas Nerven-Beruhigungstee; Mag Kottas Schlaftee; Mag Kottas Wechseltee; Nervendragees; Nervenruh; Nerventee EF-EM-ES; Nervifloran; Neuners Krautertee Nr 1 - Nerventee; Neuners Krautertee Nr 124 - zur Entspannung vor der Geburt; Neuners Krautertee Nr 141 - Schlaftee; Neuners Krautertee Nr 9 - Magentee; Phytogran; Psychobald; Sanhelios Einschlaf; Sedadom; Sedogelat; Sedogelat forte; Sidroga Nerven- und Schlaftee; Songha; Species nervinae; St Bonifatius-Tee; St Radegunder Beruhigungs- und Einschlaftee; St Radegunder Nerven-Tonikum; St Radegunder Nerventee; Synpharma Instant-Nerventee; Teekanne Schlaf- und Nerventee; Thymoval; Valin Baldrian; Vivinox; Wechseltee EF-EM-ES; ***Belg.:*** Natudor; Seneuval†; Songha; ***Braz.:*** Anevrase; Antispasmin†; Colinex†; Passicalm; Regran†; Sedantol†; Sominex; Sonhare†; Uterovarol†; Vidcalm†; ***Canad.:*** Herbal Nerve; Herbal Sleep Aid; Nyrene†; Relax and Sleep; ***Chile:*** Armonyl; Valupass; ***Fr.:*** Actisane Troubles du Sommeil†; Anxoral; Biocarde; Euphytose; Mediflor Tisane Calmante Troubles du Sommeil No 14; Mediflor Tisane Circulation du Sang No 12; Neuroflorine; Neurotensyl†; Noctisan†; Palpipax; Passinevryl; Phytocalm; Phytotherapie Boribel no 8†; Sedalozia†; Sedibaine†; Spasmidenal†; Spasmine; Sympaneurol; Tisane Sedative Weleda†; Tranquital; Valerbe†; Vericardine†; ***Ger.:*** Aranidorm-S†; Ardeysedon N; Avedorm duo; Avedorm†; Baldrian-Dispert Nacht; Baldrianox S†; Baldriparan N Stark; Baldriparan N†; Biosedon S†; Biral†; Boxocalm; Cefasedativ; Cor-Select; Diawern†; Dormarist; Dormeasan; Dormo-Sern; Dormoverlan; Dreierlei; Einschlaf-Kapseln biologisch†; Euvalon†; Euvegal Entspannungs- und Einschlafdragees; Euvegal Entspannungs- und Einschlaftropfen; Euvegal forte†; Euvegal N†; Euvitan†; Goldtropfen-Hetterich†; Grunlicht Dreierlei Tropfen†; Grunlicht Hingfong Essenz†; Gutnacht; Guttacor†; Habstal-Nerv N; Heumann Beruhigungstee Tenerval N; Hingfong-Essenz Hofmanns; Hovaletten N†; Hyperesa; Ivel Schlaf†; JuDorm; JuNeuron S†; Kavosporal comp†; Kneipp Baldrian + Hopfen†; Kneipp Krauter Taschenkur Nerven und Schlaf N†; Kneipp Nerven- und Schlaf-Tee N†; Kytta-Sedativum f; Leukona-Beruhigungsbad; Leukona-Sedativ-Bad sine Chloralhydrat†; Leukona-Sedativ-Bad†; Lomasleep; Luvased; Luvased-Tropfen N†; Majocarmin mite; Moradorm; Moradorm S; Mutellon; Nerven-Tee Stada N†; Nervendragees; Nervinetten†; Nervoregin forte; Nervosana; Neurapas; Nitrangin compositum; Nitro-cum†; Oxacant N; Oxacant-sedativ; Pascosedon; Phytonoctu; Plantival novo; Presselin Nerven K 1 N; Pronervon Phyto; Psychotonin-sed†; Rhoival; RubieSed; Salusan†; Schlaf- und Nerventee; Schupps Baldrian Sedativbad†; Schwedentrunk Elixier; Seda Kneipp N†; Seda-Plantina; Sedacur; Sedariston; Sedariston Konzentrat; Sedaselect D; Sedasyx; Sedatruw S†; Sedinfant N; Selon; Sensinerv forte; Sirmiosta Nervenelixier N†; Somnuvis S†; SX Valeriana comp†; Tornix; Valdispert comp; Valena N†; Valeriana comp novum; Valeriana forte N; Valeriana mild; Visinal†; Vivinox N; Vivinox-Schlafdragees†; ***Hong Kong:*** Epizon; ***Israel:*** Calmanervin; Nerven-Dragees; Passiflora; Passiflora Compound; Songha Night; ***Ital.:*** Anevrasi; Bianco Val; Bio-Strath†; Biocalm; Bitteridina†; Camomilla (Specie Composta); Fitosonno; Florelax; Glicero-Valerovit; Melissa (Specie Composta); Noctis; Parvisedil; Quietan†; Reve; Sedatol; Sedopuer F; Val-Plus; Valeriana (Specie Composta); ***Mex.:*** Ivel; Plantival; ***Port.:*** Antispasmina Colica; Bio-Strath No 8†; Gabisedil; Neurocardol; Songha; Valesono; ***S.Afr.:*** Biral; Restin; ***Spain:*** Baldrian†; Brevilon†; Natusor Somnisedan; Nervikan; Sedasor; Sedonat; Valdispert Complex; ***Switz.:*** Baldriparan; Dicalm; Dormeasan; Dormiplant; Dragees pour la detente nerveuse; Dragees pour le coeur et les nerfs; Dragees pour le sommeil nouvelle formule; Hova; Melissa Tonic†; Nervinetten; Perpector; Phytoberidin†; Phytomed Somni; Plantival†; ReDormin; Relax; Seracalm†; Songha Night†; Soporin; Tisane calmante pour les enfants; Tisane pour le sommeil et les nerfs; Tisane relaxante N; Valverde Dragees pour la detente; Valverde Dragees pour le coeur; Valverde Dragees pour le sommeil; ***UK:*** Avena Sativa Comp; Bio-Strath Valerian Formula; Biophylin†; Daily Menopause Relief; Daily Tension & Strain Relief; Digestive; Gerard 99†; Gerard House Gladlax†; Gerard House Serenity; Gerard House Somnus; Gerard House Valerian Compound†; Heath & Heather Becalm†; Heath & Heather Quiet Night†; Herbal Indigestion Naturtabs; Herbal Pain Relief; HRI Calm Life; HRI Golden Seal Digestive; HRI Night; Indigestion and Flatulence; Kalms; Laxative Tablets; Modern Herbals Stress; Natrasleep; Natural Herb Tablets; Newrelax; Night Time†; Nodoff; Period Pain Relief; PMT Formula; Prementaid; Quiet Days; Quiet Life; Quiet Nite; Quiet Tyme; Rapi-snooze†; Relax B+; Scullcap & Gentian Tablets; Stressless; SuNerven; Super Mega B+C; Sure-Lax (Herbal); Unwind Herbal Nytol; Valerina Day Time; Valerina Night-Time; Vegetable Cough Remover; Wellwoman; Wind & Dyspepsia Relief.

## Vanilla

Baunilha; Vainilla; Vanilla Beans; Vanilla Pods.

**Pharmacopoeias.** In *USNF.*

**USNF 22** (Vanilla). The cured, full-grown, unripe fruit of *Vanilla planifolia*, often known in commerce as Mexican, Bourbon, or Madagascar vanilla, or of *V. tahitensis*, known in commerce as Tahitian vanilla (Orchidaceae). Vanilla that has become brittle should not be used. Store in airtight containers at a temperature not exceeding 8°.

**Profile**
Vanilla is used as a flavour and in perfumery. However, the odour and flavour of vanilla are not entirely due to vanillin (see below) but depend on the presence of other aromatic substances.

**Preparations**

***USNF 22:*** Vanilla Tincture.

## Vanillin

Vainillina; Vanillic Aldehyde; Vanillinum. 4-Hydroxy-3-methoxybenzaldehyde.
$C_8H_8O_3$ = 152.1.
*CAS — 121-33-5.*

**Pharmacopoeias.** In *Eur.* (see p.vi), *Pol.*, and *Viet.* Also in *USNF.*
**Ph. Eur. 5.0** (Vanillin). White or slightly yellowish crystalline needles or powder. M.p. 81° to 84°. Slightly soluble in water; freely soluble in alcohol and in methyl alcohol; it dissolves in dilute solutions of alkali hydroxides. Protect from light.
**USNF 22** (Vanillin). Fine, white to slightly yellow crystals, usually needle-like, having an odour and taste suggestive of vanilla. M.p. 81° to 83°. Soluble 1 in 100 of water at 25°, 1 in 20 of water at 80°, 1 in 20 of glycerol; freely soluble in alcohol, in chloroform, in ether, and in solutions of fixed alkali hydroxides. Its solutions are acid to litmus. Store in airtight containers. Protect from light.

**Profile**
Vanillin is used as a flavour and in perfumery.

**Preparations**

***BP 2003:*** Tolu-flavour Solution.

## Vardenafil *(rINN)*

1-{[3-(3,4-Dihydro-5-methyl-4-oxo-7-propylimidazo[5,1-*f*]-*as*-triazin-2-yl)-4-ethoxyphenyl]sulfonyl}-4-ethylpiperazine.
$C_{23}H_{32}N_6O_4S$ = 488.6.
*CAS — 224785-90-4.*
*ATC — G04BE09.*

## Vardenafil Dihydrochloride *(USAN, rINNM)*

$C_{23}H_{32}N_6O_4S,2HCl$ = 561.5.
*CAS — 224789-15-5.*
*ATC — G04BE09.*

## Vardenafil Hydrochloride *(USAN, rINNM)*

Bay-38-9456; Vardenafil Monohydrochloride.
$C_{23}H_{32}N_6O_4S,HCl$ = 525.1.
*CAS — 224785-91-5.*
*ATC — G04BE09.*

**Adverse Effects**
As for Sildenafil, p.1744. Photosensitivity has been reported with vardenafil.

**Effects on the cardiovascular system.** References.

1. Thadani U, *et al.* The effect of vardenafil, a potent and highly selective phosphodiesterase-5 inhibitor for the treatment of erectile dysfunction, on the cardiovascular response to exercise in patients with coronary artery disease. *J Am Coll Cardiol* 2002; **40:** 2006–12.

**Precautions**
As for Sildenafil, p.1744.

The UK manufacturer has reported that vardenafil may prolong the QT interval and is best avoided in patients with relevant risk factors such as hypokalaemia and congenital QT prolongation.

**Interactions**
As for Sildenafil, p.1744. Drugs such as erythromycin that inhibit the cytochrome P450 isoenzyme CYP3A4 may reduce vardenafil clearance necessitating a reduction in dosage. Use of vardenafil with potent CYP3A4 inhibitors such as ritonavir, indinavir, ketoconazole, and itraconazole is contra-indicated. An enhanced hypotensive effect may be seen if vardenafil is taken with nifedipine. The UK manufacturer has reported that vardenafil may prolong the QT interval and recommends that its use with antiarrhythmics should be avoided.

**Pharmacokinetics**
Vardenafil is rapidly absorbed after a dose by mouth, with a bioavailability of approximately 15%. Peak plasma concentrations are attained within 30 to 120 minutes; the rate of absorption is reduced when vardenafil is given with a high-fat meal.

Vardenafil is widely distributed into tissues and is approximately 95% bound to plasma proteins. It is metabolised in the liver primarily by cytochrome P450 isoenzymes CYP3A4 (the major route) as well as CYP3A5 and CYP2C isoforms. The major metabolite produced by desethylation of vardenafil also has some activity. The terminal half-life is about 4 to 5 hours.

Vardenafil is excreted as metabolites predominantly in the faeces (91 to 95%), and to a lesser extent in the urine (2 to 6%). Clearance may be reduced in the elderly and in patients with hepatic or severe renal impairment.

◊ References.

1. Rajagopalan P, *et al.* Effect of high-fat breakfast and moderate-fat evening meal on the pharmacokinetics of vardenafil, an oral phosphodiesterase-5 inhibitor for the treatment of erectile dysfunction. *J Clin Pharmacol* 2003; **43:** 260–7.

**Uses and Administration**
Vardenafil is a phosphodiesterase type-5 inhibitor with actions and uses similar to those of sildenafil (p.1745). It is used in the management of erectile dysfunction (see p.1745). Vardenafil is given by mouth as the hydrochloride trihydrate although doses are expressed in terms of the base; vardenafil hydrochloride trihydrate 11.85 mg is approximately equivalent to 10 mg of vardenafil. The usual dose is 10 mg taken about 25 minutes to one hour before sexual intercourse. The dose may be increased or decreased depending on response. The maximum recommended dose is 20 mg, and vardenafil should not be taken more than once in 24 hours. The dose may be taken with or without food, but onset of activity may be delayed if taken with a high-fat meal. An initial dose of 5 mg is recommended in elderly patients, which may be increased to 10 mg and then to 20 mg if necessary; for doses in hepatic or renal impairment, see below. A maximum daily dose of 5 mg is advised in patients taking vardenafil with erythromycin (see under Interactions, above).

◊ Reviews.

1. Keating GM, Scott LJ. Vardenafil: a review of its use in erectile dysfunction. *Drugs* 2003; **63:** 2673–2703.
2. Crowe SM, Streetman DS. Vardenafil treatment for erectile dysfunction. *Ann Pharmacother* 2004; **38:** 77–85.
3. Kendirci M, *et al.* Vardenafil: a novel type 5 phosphodiesterase inhibitor for the treatment of erectile dysfunction. *Expert Opin Pharmacother* 2004; **5:** 923–32.

**Administration in hepatic impairment.** An initial dose of 5 mg of vardenafil is recommended in patients with mild to moderate hepatic impairment, which may be increased if necessary, according to response and tolerability. The maximum dose recommended in patients with moderate hepatic impairment is 10 mg.

**Administration in renal impairment.** In the UK, an initial dose of 5 mg of vardenafil is recommended in patients with a creatinine clearance of less than 30 mL/minute, which may be increased to 10 mg and then to 20 mg if necessary, according to response and tolerability. US licensing information does not consider adjustment to be necessary.

**Preparations**

**Proprietary Preparations** (details are given in Part 3)
***UK:*** Levitra; ***USA:*** Levitra.

## Varenicline *(rINN)*

7,8,9,10-Tetrahydro-6*H*-6,10-methanoazepino[4,5-*g*]quinoxaline.
$C_{13}H_{13}N_3$ = 211.3.
*CAS — 249296-44-4.*

## Varenicline Tartrate *(USAN, rINNM)*

CP-526555-18.
$C_{13}H_{13}N_3,C_4H_6O_6$ = 361.3.
*CAS — 375815-87-5.*

**Profile**
Varenicline is a selective nicotinic receptor agonist that is under investigation as an aid for smoking cessation.

## Vascular Endothelial Growth Factor

**Profile**
Vascular endothelial growth factor is a protein that stimulates angiogenesis. A gene therapy product supplying the gene for vascular endothelial growth factor via an adenoviral vector is under investigation for intimal hyperplasia.

## Vasoactive Intestinal Peptide

Péptido vasoactivo intestinal; VIP.
*CAS — 37221-79-7.*

## Aviptadil *(BAN, rINN)*

Vasoactive Intestinal Octacosapeptide (Swine).
$C_{147}H_{238}N_{44}O_{42}S$ = 3325.8.
*CAS — 40077-57-4.*

**Profile**
Vasoactive intestinal peptide acts as a hormone and neurotransmitter in various parts of the body; it is a potent relaxant of smooth muscle and has vasodilator and bronchodilator properties as well as stimulating the gastrointestinal tract to increased secretion. It has been tried in the management of acute oesophageal food impaction, and for the treatment of acute respiratory distress syndrome, pulmonary arterial hypertension, and chronic thromboembolic pulmonary hypertension. Its analogue aviptadil has been used as a combination product with phentolamine for erectile dysfunction (p.1745).

## Vegetable Fatty Oils

Olea Herbaria.

**Pharmacopoeias.** In *Eur.* (see p.vi).
**Ph. Eur. 5.0** (Vegetable Fatty Oils). Vegetable fatty oils are mainly solid or liquid triglycerides of fatty acids that may contain small amounts of other lipids such as waxes, free fatty acids, partial glycerides, or unsaponifiable matters. They are obtained from the seeds or fruits of plants by expression and/or solvent extraction, and may then be refined or hydrogenated with the addition of a suitable antoxidant if necessary. The following are defined:

- *virgin oil*: the oil obtained from raw materials of special quality by mechanical procedures such as cold expression or centrifugation.
- *refined oil*: the oil obtained by expression and/or solvent extraction, and subsequently, either alkali refining (followed by bleaching and deodorisation) or physical refining.
- *hydrogenated oil*: an oil obtained by expression and/or solvent extraction, and subsequently, either alkali refining or physical refining, then possible bleaching, followed by drying, hydrogenation, and subsequently bleaching and deodorisation.

Only phosphoric acid and alkali refined oils may be used in the preparation of parenteral dosage forms.

## Hydrogenated Vegetable Oil

Aceite vegetal hidrogenado.

**Pharmacopoeias.** In *Br.* and *Jpn.* Also in *USNF.*
**BP 2003** (Hydrogenated Vegetable Oil). A mixture of triglycerides of fatty acids of vegetable origin. An almost white, fine powder at room temperature and a pale yellow, oily liquid above its m.p. of 57° to 70°. Practically insoluble in water; soluble in chloroform, in hot isopropyl alcohol, and in petroleum spirit. Store at a temperature of 8° to 25°.
**USNF 22** (Hydrogenated Vegetable Oil). Type 1 Hydrogenated Vegetable Oil occurs as a fine, white powder, beads, or small flakes; m.p. 57° to 85°. Type 2 Hydrogenated Vegetable Oil occurs as a plastic (semi-solid) or flakes, having a softer consistency than Type 1; m.p. 20° to 50°.
Insoluble in water; soluble in chloroform, in hot isopropyl alcohol, and in petroleum spirit. Store in airtight containers at a temperature of 8° to 15°.

**Profile**
Vegetable fatty oils are generally solid or liquid triglycerides of fatty acids that may contain small amounts of other lipids. They are obtained from the seeds or fruits of plants by expression and/or solvent extraction, and may then be refined or hydrogenated with the addition of a suitable antoxidant if necessary. They are fixed oils (expressed oils) and do not evaporate on warming as opposed to essential oils (ethereal oils, volatile oils), which evaporate readily and are usually obtained from their aromatic plant source by distillation. Some fixed vegetable oils are used to modify the consistency of ointments and for their emollient properties. They have also been used as vehicles for fat-soluble substances such as vitamins.

Hydrogenated vegetable oil is refined, bleached, hydrogenated, and deodorised vegetable oil stearins consisting mainly of the triglycerides of stearic and palmitic acids. It is used as a tablet lubricant and as an ointment or suppository basis.

**Preparations**

**Proprietary Preparations** (details are given in Part 3)
***Spain:*** Blodex.

## Veratrine

Veratrina.
*CAS — 8051-02-3 (veratrine mixture); 71-62-5 (veratrine amorphous); 62-59-9 (veratrine crystallised, cevadine).*

**Description.** Veratrine is a mixture of alkaloids from the dried ripe seeds of *Schoenocaulon officinale* (Liliaceae) (sabadilla). Veratrine should be distinguished from protoveratrines obtained from veratrum.

**Adverse Effects, Treatment, and Precautions**
Veratrine resembles aconite (p.1646) in its action on the peripheral nerve endings and poisoning should be treated similarly. It is an intense local irritant and has a powerful direct stimulating action on all muscle tissues. It has a violent irritant action on mucous membranes, even in minute doses, and must be handled with great care. When ingested it causes violent vomiting, purging, an intense burning sensation in the mouth and throat, and general muscular weakness.

**Uses and Administration**
Veratrine should not be used internally. It was formerly applied externally for its analgesic properties and as a parasiticide, especially for head lice, but even when used in this way there is danger of systemic poisoning from absorption.

## Green Veratrum

American Hellebore; American Veratrum; Eléboro verde; Green Hellebore; Green Hellebore Rhizome; Veratro Verde; Veratrum Viride.

*CAS — 8002-39-9.*

*ATC — C02KA01.*

**Description.** Green veratrum consists of the dried rhizome and roots of *Veratrum viride* (Liliaceae) from which are derived the alkaloidal mixtures alkavervir and cryptenamine.

## White Veratrum

Eléboro blanco; European Hellebore; Veratrum Album; White Hellebore; White Hellebore Rhizome.

*ATC — C02KA01.*

**Description.** White veratrum consists of the dried rhizome and roots of *Veratrum album* (Liliaceae) from which are derived the alkaloids protoveratrine A and B.

### Adverse Effects

Veratrum alkaloids may cause nausea and vomiting at conventional therapeutic doses. Other adverse effects include epigastric and substernal burning, sweating, mental confusion, bradycardia or cardiac arrhythmias, dizziness, and hiccup. Profound hypotension and respiratory depression can occur at high doses.

**Sneezing powder.** Various symptoms of intoxication occurred in 7 patients due to the use of a sneezing powder containing white veratrum alkaloids.[1]

1. Fogh A, *et al.* Veratrum alkaloids in sneezing-powder: a potential danger. *J Toxicol Clin Toxicol* 1983; **20:** 175–9.

### Treatment of Adverse Effects

Following oral ingestion of veratrum alkaloids the stomach should be emptied by aspiration and lavage; activated charcoal may be considered within 1 hour of ingestion. Excessive hypotension with bradycardia or cardiac arrhythmias can be treated with atropine. The patient should be placed in a supine position with the feet raised.

### Uses and Administration

White and green veratrum contain a number of pharmacologically active alkaloids that produce centrally mediated peripheral vasodilatation and bradycardia. They have been used in the treatment of hypertension but are generally considered to produce an unacceptably high incidence of adverse effects and have largely been replaced by less toxic antihypertensives.

Both green and white veratrum have also been used as insecticides.

White veratrum has been used, as Veratrum Album, in homoeopathy.

## Verbascum

Aaron's Rod (*Verbascum thapsus*); Bouillon Blanc; Great Mullein (*Verbascum thapsus*); Mullein; Orange Mullein (*Verbascum phlomoides*); Wollblumen.

NOTE. The name Aaron's Rod has been applied to a number of plants including *V. densiflorum*, *Solidago* spp., and *Sempervivum tectorum*.

**Pharmacopoeias.** *Eur.* (see p.vi) includes the dried flowers.

**Ph. Eur. 5.0** (Mullein Flower; Verbasci flos). The dried flowers, reduced to the corolla and the androecium, of *Verbascum thapsus*, *V. densiflorum*, and *V. phlomoides*. Store in airtight containers.

### Profile

Verbascum flower is an ingredient of herbal remedies for coughs and cold symptoms. The dried leaves and stems have also been used.

### Preparations

**Proprietary Preparations** (details are given in Part 3)
***Ger.:*** Eres N.

**Multi-ingredient:** ***Austral.:*** Procold†; Verbascum Complex†; ***Austria:*** Apotheker Bauer's Brust- und Hustentee; Bio-Garten Tee gegen Erkaltung; Bioreform-Erkaltungstee; Brust- und Hustentee EF-EM-ES; Erkaltungstee; Jutussin neo; Krauterhaus Mag Kottas Husten- und Bronchialtee; Krauterpfarrer Weidinger Tee bei Husten und Heiserkeit; Mag Kottas Husten-Bronchialtee; Neuners Krautertee Nr 211 - Krauterhexlein Kinder-Hustentee; St Radegunder Bronchialtee; ***Fr.:*** Mediflor Tisane Pectorale d'Alsace†; ***Ger.:*** Equisil N; Hevertopect N; Salus Bronchial-Tee Nr.8†; ***Spain:*** Bronpul; Natusor Broncopul.

## Vervain

Herba Columbariae; Herba Verbenae; Shop Vervain Wort; Verbena.

**Pharmacopoeias.** In *Chin.*

### Profile

Vervain, the aerial parts of *Verbena officinalis* (Verbenaceae), has been used for a wide range of disorders. It is a bitter and has been used for digestive disorders. It also has sedative properties and has been used for anxiety disorders and as a tonic during convalescence from chronic illness.

### Preparations

**Proprietary Preparations** (details are given in Part 3)

**Multi-ingredient:** ***Austral.:*** Avena Complex†; Calmo†; Naturest†; ***Austria:*** Krauterpfarrer Weidinger Tee bei Fruhjahrsmudigkeit; Krauterpfarrer Weidinger Tee bei Wetterfuhligkeit und Kreislaufstorungen; Sinupret; Sinusol; Sinusol-Schleimlosender Tee; ***Belg.:*** Tisane pour le Foie†; ***Fr.:*** Calmophytum; Santane $A_4$†; Santane $C_5$†; Santane $H_7$†; Tisane des Familles†; Tisane Touraine†; Vigilia; ***Ger.:*** Sinupret; ***Hong Kong:*** Sinupret; ***Singapore:*** Sinupret; ***Switz.:*** Sinupret; Tisane antiflatulente pour nourissons et enfants; Tisane pour les enfants†; ***Thai.:*** Sinupret; ***UK:*** Athera; Catarrh†; HRI Night; Modern Herbals Menopause; Modern Herbals Stress; Newrelax; Period Pain Relief; Prementaid; Scullcap & Gentian Tablets; Stressless; SuNerven.

## Vetrabutine Hydrochloride *(BANM, rINNM)*

Dimophebumine Hydrochloride; Hidrocloruro de vetrabutina; Sp-281. *N,N*-Dimethyl-α-(3-phenylpropyl)veratrylamine hydrochloride.

$C_{20}H_{27}NO_2,HCl = 349.9.$

*CAS — 3735-45-3 (vetrabutine); 5974-09-4 (vetrabutine hydrochloride).*

### Profile

Vetrabutine hydrochloride is used as a uterine relaxant in veterinary medicine.

## Vinburnine *(rINN)*

CH-846; (−)-Eburnamonine; 3α,16α-Eburnamonine; Vinburnina; Vincamone. (3α,16α)-Eburnamenin-14(15*H*)-one.

$C_{19}H_{22}N_2O = 294.4.$

*CAS — 4880-88-0.*

*ATC — C04AX17.*

### Profile

Vinburnine is an alkaloid related to vincamine (below) and has been used in conditions associated with cerebral circulatory insufficiency.

Vinburnine phosphate has been used similarly.

### Preparations

**Proprietary Preparations** (details are given in Part 3)
***Fr.:*** Cervoxan; ***Ital.:*** Eburnal; Scleramin†; Tensiplex; ***Port.:*** Cervoxan; ***Spain:*** Cervoxan; Eburnoxin†.

## Vincamine *(BAN, rINN)*

Vincamina. Methyl (3α,16α)-14,15-dihydro-14β-hydroxyeburnamenine-14-carboxylate.

$C_{21}H_{26}N_2O_3 = 354.4.$

*CAS — 1617-90-9.*

*ATC — C04AX07.*

**Pharmacopoeias.** In *Fr.*

### Profile

Vincamine is an alkaloid obtained from *Vinca minor* (Apocynaceae). It is claimed to increase cerebral circulation and utilisation of oxygen and has been used in a variety of cerebral disorders. Vincamine may have adverse effects on the cardiovascular system and care should be taken in patients with hypertension or cardiac dysfunction.

Vincamine salts including vincamine hydrochloride, oxoglurate, teprosilate, and hydrogen tartrate have also been used.

### Preparations

**Proprietary Preparations** (details are given in Part 3)
***Arg.:*** Cincuental; Vinkhum; ***Austria:*** Aethroma; Cetal; Oxygeron†; ***Belg.:*** Cerebroxine; ***Braz.:*** Vincagil†; ***Fr.:*** Vinca; Vincafor†; Vincimax†; ***Ger.:*** Cetal†; Equipur†; Ophdilvas N; Vinca-Tablinen†; Vincapront†; ***Hong Kong:*** Aethroma; ***Ital.:*** Anasclerol†; Ausomina†; Vasonett; Vinca-Ri; Vinca-Tre-is; Vincadar; Vincafolina†; Vinsal†; Vraap; ***Mex.:*** Cetovinca†; Vincapan; ***Port.:*** Arteriovinca; Cervinca; Vincagil; ***Spain:*** Arteriovinca; Cetovinca†; Dilarterial†; Domeni; Tefavinca; Vadicate; Vincacen; Vincaminol; ***Switz.:*** Aethroma†; Cetal; Oxygeron; ***Thai.:*** Oxygeron†.

**Multi-ingredient:** ***Arg.:*** Ribex; ***Fr.:*** Rheobral; ***Mon.:*** Vincarutine; ***Port.:*** Anacervix; Centracetam; Stimilfar; ***Spain:*** Anacervix; Arteriobrate†; Devincal; Dipervina†.

## Vinpocetine *(USAN, rINN)*

AY-27255; Ethyl Apovincaminate; Ethyl Apovincaminoate; RGH-4405; Vinpocetina. Ethyl (3α,16α)-eburnamenine-14-carboxylate.

$C_{22}H_{26}N_2O_2 = 350.5.$

*CAS — 42971-09-5.*

*ATC — N06BX18.*

### Profile

Vinpocetine is a derivative of vincamine (above). It has been used in cerebrovascular disorders in doses of 15 to 30 mg daily by mouth in divided doses. It has also been tried in cognitive impairment although good evidence to support this is lacking.

◊ References.

1. Grandt R, *et al.* Vinpocetine pharmacokinetics in elderly subjects. *Arzneimittelforschung* 1989; **39:** 1599–1602.
2. Blaha L, *et al.* Clinical evidence of the effectiveness of vinpocetine in the treatment of organic psychosyndrome. *Hum Psychopharmacol Clin Exp* 1989; **4:** 103–11.
3. Bereczki D, Fekete I. A systematic review of vinpocetine therapy in acute ischaemic stroke. *Eur J Clin Pharmacol* 1999; **55:** 349–52.
4. Szatmari SZ, Whitehouse PJ. Vinpocetine for cognitive impairment and dementia. Available in The Cochrane Library; Issue 2. Chichester: John Wiley; 2004.

### Preparations

**Proprietary Preparations** (details are given in Part 3)
***Arg.:*** Cavinton; ***Ger.:*** Cavinton; ***Jpn:*** Calan†; ***Mex.:*** Cavinton†; ***Port.:*** Cavinton; DC Vin†; Ultra-Vinca; Vipocem; ***Singapore:*** Cavinton; ***Thai.:*** Cavinton.

## Vinyl Chloride

VCM; Vinilo, cloruro de; Vinyl Chloride Monomer. Chloroethylene.

$C_2H_3Cl = 62.50.$

*CAS — 75-01-4.*

### Profile

Vinyl chloride is used in the manufacture of polyvinyl chloride (PVC) and other vinyl polymers. Occupational exposure to vinyl chloride in polymerisation plants has been associated with acro-osteolysis, especially in the terminal phalanges of the fingers, a condition resembling Raynaud's phenomenon, and sclerodermatous skin changes. Liver damage and hepatic angiosarcoma, splenomegaly, thrombocytopenia, impaired respiratory function, and chromosomal abnormalities have also occurred.

◊ References.

1. Infante PF, *et al.* Genetic risks of vinyl chloride. *Lancet* 1976; **i:** 734–5.
2. Black CM, *et al.* Genetic susceptibility to scleroderma-like syndrome induced by vinyl chloride. *Lancet* 1983; **i:** 53–5.
3. Piratsu R, *et al.* La mortalità dei produttori di cloruro di vinile in Italia. *Med Lav* 1991; **82:** 388–423.
4. Riordan SM, *et al.* Vinyl chloride related hepatic angiosarcoma in a polyvinyl chloride autoclave cleaner in Australia. *Med J Aust* 1991; **155:** 125–8.
5. Mur JM, *et al.* Spontaneous abortion and exposure to vinyl chloride. *Lancet* 1992; **339:** 127–8.
6. McLaughlin JK, Lipworth L. A critical review of the epidemiologic literature on health effects of occupational exposure to vinyl chloride. *J Epidemiol Biostat* 1999; **4:** 253–75.

## Viquidil Hydrochloride *(rINNM)*

Hidrocloruro de viquidil; LM-192; Mequiverine Hydrochloride; Quinicine Hydrochloride. 1-(6-Methoxy-4-quinolyl)-3-(3-vinyl-4-piperidyl)propan-1-one hydrochloride.

$C_{20}H_{24}N_2O_2,HCl = 360.9.$

*CAS — 84-55-9 (viquidil); 52211-63-9 (viquidil hydrochloride).*

### Profile

Viquidil hydrochloride has been used in various cerebrovascular disorders.

### Preparations

**Proprietary Preparations** (details are given in Part 3)
***Ger.:*** Desclidium†.

## Water

Agua; Aqua; Aqua Communis; Aqua Fontana; Aqua Potabilis; Eau Potable; Wasser.

$H_2O = 18.02.$

*CAS — 7732-18-5.*

## Purified Water

Agua purificada; Purified water.

**Pharmacopoeias.** In *Chin.*, *Eur.* (see p.vi), *Int.*, *Jpn*, *Pol.*, *US*, and *Viet.*

*Eur.* also includes Highly Purified Water. *US* also includes Sterile Purified Water.

Some pharmacopoeias only include distilled water or have additional monographs for demineralised water or distilled water.

**Ph. Eur. 5.0** (Water, Purified; Aqua Purificata). It is water for the preparation of medicines other than those that are required to be both sterile and apyrogenic, unless otherwise justified and authorised. It is prepared from suitable potable water either by distillation, by ion exchange, by reverse osmosis, or by any other suitable method. Store in conditions designed to prevent growth of micro-organisms and to avoid any other contamination. Submonographs cover Purified Water in Bulk and Purified Water in Containers.

**Ph. Eur. 5.0** (Water, Highly Purified; Aqua Valde Purificata). It is water intended for the preparation of medicinal products where water of high biological quality is needed, except where Water for Injections is required.

**USP 27** (Purified Water). It is prepared from potable water by a suitable process.

**Preparation.** DEIONISATION. By passing potable water through columns of anionic and cationic ion-exchange resins, ionisable substances can be removed, producing a water of high specific resistance. Colloidal and non-ionisable impurities such as pyrogens may not be removed by this process.

DISTILLATION. In this process water is separated as vapour from non-volatile impurities and is subsequently condensed. In practice, non-volatile impurities may be carried into the distillate by entrainment unless a suitable baffle is fitted to the still.

## Water for Injections

Agua para inyecciones; Aq. pro Inj.; Aqua ad Iniectabilia; Aqua ad Injectionem; Aqua Injectabilis; Aqua pro Injectione; Aqua pro Injectionibus; Eau pour Préparations Injectables; Wasser für Injektionszwecke; Water for Injection.

**Pharmacopoeias.** In *Chin., Eur.* (see p.vi), *Int., Jpn, Pol., US,* and *Viet.*
*US* also includes Sterile Water for Injection, Sterile Water for Inhalation, Sterile Water for Irrigation, and Bacteriostatic Water for Injection.
**Ph. Eur. 5.0** (Water for Injections). It is water for the preparation of medicines for parenteral administration when water is used as the vehicle, and for dissolving or diluting substances or preparations for parenteral administration. It is prepared by distillation of potable water or purified water from a neutral glass, quartz, or suitable metal still fitted with an effective device for preventing the entrainment of droplets; the first portion of the distillate is discarded and the remainder collected. Store in conditions designed to prevent growth of micro-organisms and to avoid any other contamination. Sub-monographs cover Water for Injections in Bulk and Sterilised Water for Injections.
**USP 27** (Water for Injection). It is purified by distillation or a purification process that is equivalent or superior to distillation in the removal of chemicals and micro-organisms. When used for the preparation of parenteral solutions it should be sterilised first or the final preparation should be sterilised after preparation. Sterile Water for Injection, Inhalation, or Irrigation and Bacteriostatic Water for Injection are the subjects of separate monographs.

### Profile

There are international standards for the quality of water intended for human consumption. Toxic substances such as arsenic, barium, cadmium, chromium, copper, cyanide, lead, and selenium may constitute a danger to health if present in drinking water in excess of the recommended concentrations. Water-borne infections are also a hazard.

Fluoride is regarded as an essential constituent of drinking water but may endanger health if present in excess—see Sodium Fluoride, p.1444. Ingestion of water containing large quantities of nitrates may cause methaemoglobinaemia in infants; many countries have standards for nitrates in water.

The use of tap water containing metal ions (such as aluminium, copper, and lead), fluoride, or tosylchloramide sodium, for dialysis may be hazardous.

Hard water contains soluble calcium and magnesium salts, which form scale and sludge in boilers, water pipes, and autoclaves; they also cause the precipitation of soap and prevent its lathering. Temporary hardness in water is due to the presence of bicarbonates which are converted to insoluble carbonates on heating. Permanent hardness is due to dissolved chlorides, nitrates, and sulfates, which do not form a precipitate on heating. The presence or absence of such salts can play a part in cardiovascular health.

Without further purification, potable water may be unsuitable for certain pharmaceutical purposes. In such instances, purified water should always be used. Most pharmacopoeias include monographs on various preparations of water, such as water suitable for injections. Potable water should not be used when such preparations of water are specified.

Excessive ingestion of water can lead to water intoxication with disturbances of the electrolyte balance.

◊ References.


1. Manz F, *et al.* The most essential nutrient: defining the adequate intake of water. *J Pediatr* 2002; **141:** 587–92.


### Preparations

**Proprietary Preparations** (details are given in Part 3)
***Fin.:*** Aquasteril; ***UK:*** Aquasol; Sterac†; Uriflex W.

## Wild Carrot

Dauci Herba; Daucus; Queen Anne's Lace; Zanahoria silvestre.

NOTE. The name Queen Anne's lace has also been used for cow parsley (*Anthriscus sylvestris*), another umbellifer.

**Pharmacopoeias.** In *Chin.*

### Profile

The fruits of the wild carrot, *Daucus carota* (Umbelliferae) have been used as a diuretic and anthelmintic, and are included in herbal preparations for various indications. Other parts of the plant have been used in folk medicine. The root of the cultivated form, *D. carota* ssp. *sativus*, is a culinary item and a source of carotenoids in the diet.

### Preparations

**Proprietary Preparations** (details are given in Part 3)
**Multi-ingredient:** ***Arg.:*** Hepatalgina; Palatrobil; ***Ital.:*** Evamilk; Pluriderm†; ***UK:*** Sciargo; Watershed.

## Wild Cherry Bark

Corteza de cerezo silvestre; Prunus Serotina; Virginian Prune; Virginian Prune Bark; Wild Black Cherry Bark; Wild Cherry.

### Profile

Wild cherry bark is the dried bark of the wild or black cherry, *Prunus serotina* (Rosaceae), known in commerce as Thin Natural Wild Cherry Bark, containing not less than 10% of water-soluble extractive. It has a slight odour and an astringent, aromatic, bitter taste, recalling that of bitter almonds. It contains (+)-mandelonitrile glucoside (prunasin) and an enzyme system, which interact in the presence of water yielding benzaldehyde, hydrocyanic acid, and glucose.

Wild cherry bark, in the form of the syrup, has been used in the treatment of cough but it has little therapeutic value. It has also been used as a flavour.

### Preparations

**Proprietary Preparations** (details are given in Part 3)
**Multi-ingredient:** ***Canad.:*** Mielocol; Rophelin; Wampole Bronchial Cough Syrup; ***UK:*** Potters Day & Night Cough Pastilles†.

## Wild Lettuce

Herba Lactucae Virosae; Lechuga silvestre.

### Profile

The wild lettuce, *Lactuca virosa* (Compositae), has been given in herbal medicine as a sedative and antitussive. The dried latex extract (lactucarium; lettuce opium) is also used.

### Preparations

**Proprietary Preparations** (details are given in Part 3)
**Multi-ingredient:** ***Canad.:*** Sirop Cocillana Codeine; ***UK:*** Anased; Antibron; Gerard House Somnus; Gerard House Valerian Compound†; HRI Night; Nytol Herbal; Quiet Life; Quiet Nite; Slumber; Unwind Herbal Nytol.

## Xanthine-containing Beverages

Xantina, bebidas con.

### Adverse Effects

The adverse effects of xanthine-containing beverages are largely due to their caffeine (p.782), theophylline (p.798), and theobromine (p.798) content. Common side-effects are sleeplessness, anxiety, tremor, palpitations, and withdrawal headache.

**Breast feeding.** For references to the effects of caffeinated beverages in breast feeding, see under Caffeine, p.782.

**Effects on the heart.** A meta-analysis of published studies found no evidence of an association between coffee consumption and the development of coronary heart disease,[1] and a large cohort study in women also found no evidence of a link.[2] Expert opinion in the UK[3] has been that the evidence that caffeine or coffee consumption contributes to coronary heart disease development is inconsistent. Coffee prepared by boiling, as is the practice in Scandinavia for example, does raise serum cholesterol concentrations due to the presence of the diterpenes cafestol and kahweol, and coffee made in a cafetière has a similar effect, but filtered coffee does not, as the hypercholesterolaemic fraction does not pass a paper filter.[4] A case-control study has suggested a relationship between consumption of boiled, but not filtered, coffee and incidence of a first non-fatal myocardial infarction.[5] Others have raised concern that the potential pressor effect of caffeine itself may be a cardiovascular risk factor,[6] but as mentioned above there is little evidence for this.

Tea drinking has not been associated with increased cardiovascular risk[3]—indeed, its polyphenol content has been suggested to have beneficial antoxidant effects.[7,8]


1. Myers MG, Basinski A. Coffee and coronary heart disease. *Arch Intern Med* 1992; **152:** 1767–72.
2. Willett WC, *et al.* Coffee consumption and coronary heart disease in women: a ten-year follow-up. *JAMA* 1996; **275:** 458–62.
3. Department of Health. Nutritional aspects of cardiovascular disease. Report of the cardiovascular review group committee on medical aspects of food policy. Report on health and social subjects no. 46. London: HMSO, 1994.
4. Urgert R, *et al.* Comparison of effect of cafetière and filtered coffee on serum concentrations of liver aminotransferases and lipids: six month randomised controlled trial. *BMJ* 1996; **313:** 1362–6.
5. Hammar N, *et al.* Association of boiled and filtered coffee with incidence of first nonfatal myocardial infarction: the SHEEP and the VHEEP study. *J Intern Med* 2003; **253:** 653–9.
6. James JE. Is habitual caffeine use a preventable cardiovascular risk factor? *Lancet* 1997; **349:** 279–81.
7. Luo M, *et al.* Inhibition of LDL oxidation by green tea extract. *Lancet* 1997; **349:** 360–1.
8. Geleijnse JM, *et al.* Tea flavonoids may protect against atherosclerosis: the Rotterdam study. *Arch Intern Med* 1999; **159:** 2170–4.


**Effects on the muscles.** Severe myositis in an elderly man who drank around 14 litres of tea daily was attributed to hypokalaemia produced by the xanthine content of the beverage.[1] The patient improved following intravenous potassium replacement and subsequently remained well following a reduction in tea intake.


1. Trewby PN, *et al.* Teapot myositis. *Lancet* 1998; **351:** 1248.


**Malignant neoplasms.** A review of available data did not suggest a clinically significant association between the regular use of coffee and the development of cancer of the lower urinary tract in men or women.[1]


1. Viscoli CM, *et al.* Bladder cancer and coffee drinking: a summary of case-control research. *Lancet* 1993; **341:** 1432–7.


### Interactions

The possibility of synergistic effects in patients receiving xanthines who consume large amounts of xanthine-containing beverages should be borne in mind.

**Antipsychotics.** Xanthine-containing beverages have been reported to precipitate some antipsychotic drugs from solution *in vitro*, but do not appear to alter antipsychotic concentrations *in vivo*. For references, see p.680.

### Uses and Administration

Xanthine-containing beverages including chocolate, coffee, cocoa, cola, maté, and tea are widely consumed and have a mild stimulant effect on the CNS. The primary xanthine constituent is caffeine (p.782) but other xanthine derivatives such as theobromine (p.798) and theophylline (p.798) may also be present; cocoa and chocolate contain significant amounts of theobromine.

Coffee is the kernel of the dried ripe seeds of *Coffea arabica, C. liberica, C. canephora* (robusta coffee), and other species of *Coffea* (Rubiaceae), roasted until it acquires a deep brown colour and a pleasant characteristic aroma. It contains about 1 to 2% of caffeine. Coffee has been used in the form of an infusion or decoction as a stimulant and as a flavour in some pharmaceutical preparations. A decoction is used as a beverage containing up to about 100 mg of caffeine per 100 mL. Preparations of instant coffee may contain up to 40% less caffeine while decaffeinated preparations may contain only up to about 3 mg per 100 mL.

Kola (cola, cola seeds, kola nuts) is the dried cotyledons of *Cola nitida* and *C. acuminata* (Sterculiaceae), containing up to about 2.5% of caffeine and traces of theobromine. Kola is used in the preparation of cola drinks which may contain up to 20 mg of caffeine per 100 mL. Kola has been used to treat migraine in homoeopathic medicine.

Maté (Paraguay Tea) is the dried leaves of *Ilex paraguensis* (Aquifoliaceae), containing 0.2 to 2% of caffeine and traces of theobromine. Maté is less astringent than tea and is extensively used as a beverage in South America.

Tea (thea, chá, thé, tee) is the prepared young leaves and leaf-buds of *Camellia sinensis* (=*C. thea*) (Theaceae). It contains 1 to 5% of caffeine, up to 24% of tannin, and small amounts of theobromine and theophylline. Tea is used in an infusion as a beverage containing up to about 60 mg of caffeine per 100 mL.

Guarana consists of the crushed seeds of *Paullinia cupana* var *sorbilis* (Sapindaceae). Caffeine appears to be its major active ingredient which was once termed guaranine. Herbal preparations include a beverage or liquid extract and may contain 5% caffeine.

### Preparations

**Proprietary Preparations** (details are given in Part 3)
***Fr.:*** Camiline; Exolise†; ***Ger.:*** Bioday†; Carbo Konigsfeld; ***Spain:*** Exolise†; ***UK:*** Yariba; ***USA:*** Tegreen.

**Multi-ingredient:** ***Austral.:*** Avena Complex†; Bioglan 3B Beer Belly Buster†; Infant Tonic†; Irontona†; T & T Antioxidant†; Vig Recovery†; Vig†; Vitatona†; ***Austria:*** Aponatura Kreislauf; Blasen- und Nierentee; Colagain†; Gewusst wie Gruner Fastentee; Kneipp Herz- und Kreislauf-Unterstutzungs-Tee; Mag Kottas Herz- und Kreislauftee; ***Belg.:*** Aperop†; ***Braz.:*** Astenol†; Catuaba†; Catuama†; Derm'attive; Gastrogenol†; Geripan†; Iofoscal†; Kola Fosfatada Soel†; Salutina†; ***Canad.:*** Energy Plus; ***Fr.:*** Actisane Fatigue Passagere†; Biotone; Filigel; Kola Astier†; Maxidraine; Mincifit; Promincil; Quintonine; Santane $V_3$†; Tealine; Tonactil; Tonisan†; Triogene†; Uromil; YSE; ***Ger.:*** Cardibisana; Kola-Dallmann mit Lecithin†; Kola-Dallmann†; Myrrhinil-Intest; Nieroxin N; Ramend Krauter; Repursan ST†; ***Hong Kong:*** LEAN Formula w/ Advantra; Wari-Procomil; ***Ital.:*** Chinoidina; Dam; Enertonic†; Fitostress†; Four-Ton; Gincola†; Memorandum; Nosenil†; ***Port.:*** Lipoforte; ***Spain:*** Elingrip†; Fitosvelt; Rimagrip; Vigortonic; ***Switz.:*** Dragees contre les maux de tete†; Ganavit†; ***Thai.:*** Wari-Procomil; ***UK:*** Biofreeze; Chlorophyll; Cleansing Herbs; Daily Fatigue Relief; Damiana and Kola Tablets; Glykola; Koladex†; Labiton; Lion Cleansing Herbs; S.P.H.P.; Strength; Zotrim.

## Xantofyl Palmitate *(rINN)*

Heleniene; Palmitato de xantofila; Xanthophyl Dipalmitate.
β,ε-Carotene-3,3′-diyl dipalmitate.
$C_{72}H_{116}O_4$ = 1045.7.
*CAS — 547-17-1.*

### Profile

Xantofyl palmitate has been used by mouth in the treatment of some visual disturbances.

## Xylazine *(BAN, rINN)*

Xilazina. *N*-(5,6-Dihydro-4*H*-1,3-thiazin-2-yl)-2,6-xylidine.
$C_{12}H_{16}N_2S$ = 220.3.
*CAS — 7361-61-7.*

**Pharmacopoeias.** In *US.*
**USP 27** (Xylazine). Colourless to white crystals. Sparingly soluble in acetone, in chloroform, and in dilute acid; insoluble in dilute alkali. Store in airtight containers at a temperature of 25°, excursions permitted between 15° and 30°.

## Xylazine Hydrochloride *(BANM, USAN, rINNM)*

Bay-Va-1470; Hidrocloruro de xilazina.

$C_{12}H_{16}N_2S,HCl = 256.8.$

*CAS — 23076-35-9.*

**Pharmacopoeias.** In *US.*

*Eur.* (see p.vi) includes for veterinary use only.

**Ph. Eur. 5.0** (Xylazine Hydrochloride for Veterinary Use). A white or almost white, crystalline, hygroscopic powder. Freely soluble in water and in dichloromethane; very soluble in methyl alcohol. A 10% solution in water has a pH of 4.0 to 5.5. Store in airtight containers. Protect from light.

**USP 27** (Xylazine Hydrochloride). Colourless to white crystals. Sparingly soluble in acetone, in methyl alcohol, and in dilute acid; insoluble in dilute alkali. A 1% solution in water has a pH of 4.0 to 6.0. Store in airtight containers at a temperature of 25°, excursions permitted between 15° and 30°.

### Profile

Xylazine is a sedative, analgesic, and muscle relaxant used in veterinary medicine. The hydrochloride is used similarly. Abuse has been reported.

**Adverse effects.** Reports[1-5] of toxicity and abuse associated with xylazine. Bradycardia, hypotension, and coma was associated with the self-administration of 200 mg of xylazine. Treatment was supportive.[1]

1. Samanta A, *et al.* Accidental self administration of xylazine in a veterinary nurse. *Postgrad Med J* 1990; **66:** 244–5.
2. Mittleman RE, *et al.* Xylazine toxicity—literature review and report of two cases. *J Forensic Sci* 1998; **43:** 400–2.
3. Hoffmann U, *et al.* Severe intoxication with the veterinary tranquilizer xylazine in humans. *J Anal Toxicol* 2001; **25:** 245–9.
4. Capraro AJ, *et al.* Severe intoxication from xylazine inhalation. *Pediatr Emerg Care* 2001; **17:** 447–8.
5. Elejalde JI, *et al.* Drug abuse with inhaled xylazine. *Eur J Emerg Med* 2003; **10:** 252–3.

## Xylose

Wood Sugar; Xilosa; D-Xylose; Xylosum. α-D-Xylopyranose.

$C_5H_{10}O_5 = 150.1.$

*CAS — 58-86-6; 6763-34-4.*

**Pharmacopoeias.** In *Eur.* (see p.vi) and *US.*

**Ph. Eur. 5.0** (Xylose). A white or almost white crystalline powder or colourless needles. Freely soluble in water; soluble in hot alcohol.

**USP 27** (Xylose). Odourless, colourless needles or white crystalline powder. Very soluble in water; slightly soluble in alcohol. Store in airtight containers at a temperature of 15° to 30°.

### Profile

Xylose has been used for the investigation of absorption from the gastrointestinal tract. In the absence of malabsorption, about 35% of a 5-g oral dose and about 25% of a 25-g oral dose are reported to be excreted in the urine within 5 hours. It has been given by mouth, usually in a dose of either 5 or 25 g, with up to 700 mL of water. The amount recovered in the urine is estimated and used to assess any malabsorption. Adjustment may have to be made for renal impairment. Xylose may cause some gastrointestinal discomfort with large doses. Other drugs may affect the absorption of xylose and interfere with the xylose test.

The test has been adapted to use blood-xylose concentrations.

◊ References.

1. Craig RM, Ehrenpreis ED. D-xylose testing. *J Clin Gastroenterol* 1999; **29:** 143–50.

### Preparations

**Proprietary Preparations** (details are given in Part 3)
***Canad.:*** Xylo-Pfan†; ***UK:*** Xylose-BMS†; ***USA:*** Xylo-Pfan†.

## Yellow Dock

Curly Dock; Lengua de vaca; Sour Dock.

NOTE. The name sour dock has also been used for sorrel (p.1749).

### Profile

Yellow dock, the root of *Rumex crispus* (Polygonaceae) has laxative and choleretic properties. It is used for constipation, jaundice, and chronic skin disorders.

It is also used in homoeopathic medicine.

### Preparations

**Proprietary Preparations** (details are given in Part 3)

**Multi-ingredient:** ***Austral.:*** Herbal Cleanse†; Trifolium Complex†; ***Canad.:*** Herborex; ***Fr.:*** Tisanes de l'Abbe Hamon no 11†; ***UK:*** Savlon Natural First Aid for Insect Bites & Stings; Skin Eruptions Mixture.

## Yohimbine Hydrochloride *(rINNM)*

Aphrodine Hydrochloride; Chlorhydrate de Québrachine; Corynine Hydrochloride; Hidrocloruro de yohimbina. Methyl 17α-hydroxy-yohimban-16α-carboxylate hydrochloride.

$C_{21}H_{26}N_2O_3,HCl = 390.9.$

*CAS — 146-48-5 (yohimbine); 65-19-0 (yohimbine hydrochloride).*

**Pharmacopoeias.** In *US.*

**USP 27** (Yohimbine Hydrochloride). A white to yellow powder. Slightly soluble in water and in alcohol; soluble in boiling water. Store in airtight containers.

### Profile

Yohimbine is the principal alkaloid of the bark of the yohimbe tree, *Pausinystalia yohimbe* (*Corynanthe yohimbi*) (Rubiaceae); it is also found in *Rauwolfia serpentina.* It is an $\alpha_2$-adrenoceptor blocker with a short duration of action. It has an antidiuretic effect and produces increases in heart rate and blood pressure, and orthostatic hypotension. It has been reported to cause anxiety and manic reactions. It has been given by mouth in the treatment of erectile dysfunction (p.1745) and for its alleged aphrodisiac properties but convincing evidence of such an effect is lacking. It is contra-indicated in renal or hepatic disease.

**Adverse effects.** A warning about the potential adverse effects, including anxiety, manic reactions, bronchospasm and a lupus-like syndrome, associated with yohimbine taken in health food products.[1] Interactions with tricyclic antidepressants and with phenothiazines might also occur.

1. De Smet PAGM, Smeets OSNM. Potential risks of health food products containing yohimbe extracts. *BMJ* 1994; **309:** 958.

**Uses.** References to the use of yohimbine in erectile dysfunction.

1. Ernst E, Pittler MH. Yohimbine for erectile dysfunction: a systematic review and meta-analysis of randomised clinical trials. *J Urol (Baltimore)* 1998; **159:** 433–6.
2. Tam SW, *et al.* Yohimbine: a clinical review. *Pharmacol Ther* 2001; **91:** 215–43.
3. Lebret T, *et al.* Efficacy and safety of a novel combination of L-arginine glutamate and yohimbine hydrochloride: a new oral therapy for erectile dysfunction. *Eur Urol* 2002; **41:** 608–13.
4. Guay AT, *et al.* Yohimbine treatment of organic erectile dysfunction in a dose-escalation trial. *Int J Impot Res* 2002; **14:** 25–31.

### Preparations

***USP 27:*** Yohimbine Injection.

**Proprietary Preparations** (details are given in Part 3)
***Arg.:*** Yohimex; ***Austria:*** Yocon; ***Braz.:*** Yohydrol†; Yomax; ***Canad.:*** Yocon; ***Chile:*** Yocon; ***Denm.:*** Virigen; ***Fr.:*** Yocoral; ***Ger.:*** Pluriviron mono; Yocon; ***Hong Kong:*** Yocon†; ***Port.:*** Zumba; ***Singapore:*** Urobine; ***UK:*** Prowess Plain; ***USA:*** Aphrodyne; Dayto Himbin†; Yocon; Yohimex†.

**Multi-ingredient:** ***Arg.:*** Ferona; Optimina Plus; ***Austria:*** Pasuma-Dragees; ***Braz.:*** Geravitine†; Gerosenil†; Ioimbina Composta†; Libiplus; Lupercaina†; Renovator†; Sexormom†; Testofran†; Tonaton; ***Fin.:*** Potentol; ***Hong Kong:*** Wari-Procomil; ***Israel:*** Tesopalmed Forte cum Yohimbine; ***Thai.:*** Wari-Procomil; ***UK:*** Prowess†.

## Yucca

Yuca.

### Profile

Various species of *Yucca* (Liliaceae), including Mohave yucca (*Y. schidigera*; *Y. mohavensis*), the Joshua tree (*Y. brevifolia*; *Y. arborescens*), and bear grass (*Y. filamentosa*) have been used in herbal medicine and as foods.

### Preparations

**Proprietary Preparations** (details are given in Part 3)

**Multi-ingredient:** ***Austral.:*** Prost-1†; ***Braz.:*** Bronquiogem.

## Zanthoxylum Fruit

Prickly Ash Berries; Zanthoxylum, fruto de.

**Pharmacopoeias.** In *Chin.* and *Jpn.*

### Profile

Zanthoxylum fruit is the pericarp of the ripe fruit of *Zanthoxylum piperitum* (*Xanthoxylum piperitum*) (Rutaceae) or other species of *Zanthoxylum.* It contains about 3.3% v/w of essential oil.

Zanthoxylum (BPC 1934) (Toothache Bark; Xanthoxylum) is the dried bark of the northern prickly ash, *Z. americanum*, or the southern prickly ash, *Z. clavaherculis.* Both varieties contain a complex mixture of components, including benzophenanthridine alkaloids; northern prickly ash also contains coumarins.

Zanthoxylum fruit has carminative properties and has been used for rheumatic disorders. Zanthoxylum bark has been used similarly, but there is some concern about the potential toxicity of the benzophenanthridine alkaloids which it contains, and some authorities consider that it should not be recommended.

### Preparations

**Proprietary Preparations** (details are given in Part 3)

**Multi-ingredient:** ***Austral.:*** For Peripheral Circulation Herbal Plus Formula 5†; Lifesystem Herbal Formula 6 For Peripheral Circulation†; Uva-Ursi Plus†; ***UK:*** Daily Overwork & Mental Fatigue Relief; Hofels White Willow and Burdock†; Peerless Composition Essence; Rheumasol†; Tabritis.

## Zein

Zeína.

*CAS — 9010-66-6 (zeins).*

**Pharmacopoeias.** In *USNF.*

**USNF 22** (Zein). A prolamine derived from corn, *Zea mays* (Gramineae). A white to yellow powder. Insoluble in water and in acetone; readily soluble in acetone-water mixtures between the limits of 60% and 80% of acetone by volume; soluble in aqueous alcohols, in ethoxyethanol; in glycols, in furfuryl alcohol, in tetrahydrofurfuryl alcohol, and in aqueous alkaline solutions of pH 11.5 and above; insoluble in all anhydrous alcohols except methyl alcohol. Store in airtight containers.

### Profile

Zein is used as a tablet binder and coating agent for pharmaceutical preparations and foodstuffs. It has been used as a substitute for shellac.

## Zirconium

Zirconio.

Zr = 91.224.

*CAS — 7440-67-7 (zirconium); 1314-23-4 (zirconium dioxide); 60676-90-6 (zirconium lactate); 7699-43-6 (zirconium oxychloride);.*

### Profile

Zirconium and its compounds e.g. zirconium dioxide, zirconium lactate, and zirconium oxychloride, have been used in deodorant preparations; the dioxide is also used in dentistry. There have been reports of hypersensitivity reactions with granulomas. Zirconium dioxide has also been used as a contrast medium.

**Adverse effects.** A report[1] of pulmonary fibrosis associated with inhalation of a polishing agent containing mainly zirconium dioxide with quartz.

1. Bartter T, *et al.* Zirconium compound-induced pulmonary fibrosis. *Arch Intern Med* 1991; **151:** 1197–1201.

# Part 3

# Preparations

This part of Martindale contains brief details of proprietary preparations available in a number of countries and includes those supplied on prescription as well as those sold directly to the public. They are provided to help the reader identify preparations and to suggest their uses. Inclusion is not an endorsement of the activity of any ingredient nor of the preparation's indications.

For this edition we have covered Argentina, Australia, Austria, Belgium, Brazil, Canada, Chile, Denmark, Finland, France, Germany, Greece, Hong Kong, India, Ireland, Israel, Italy, Malaysia, Mexico, the Netherlands, New Zealand, Norway, Portugal, Singapore, South Africa, Spain, Sweden, Switzerland, Thailand, the United Arab Emirates, UK, and USA. We have also included some proprietary preparations from Japan.

Generally each entry consists of: the proprietary name; manufacturer or source of supply and country; ingredients usually listed by the manufacturer as being active; and a guide to the manufacturer's indications. Where possible, entries from different countries but with the same name and active ingredients have been amalgamated for clarity. We have tried to highlight instances where preparations are available with the same name, but significantly different ingredients.

An entry may cover a range of dosage forms and strengths. Dosage forms are only specified when different forms have the same proprietary name but different active ingredients. Specifying all dosage forms and the quantity of each active ingredient would have vastly increased the number of entries. Furthermore, Part 3 is not intended as a guide to prescribing; where a preparation is to be supplied the dose should be appropriate for that preparation and that particular patient, and authoritative local sources should be consulted.

The ingredients have usually been translated into English. Almost all the ingredients listed are described in the monographs in Parts 1 and 2, and readers are directed to an appropriate monograph by the page number provided after the ingredient.

We have tried to include preparations that were available in the last few years since they may still be in circulation and their names may still be referred to in the literature and in practice. Such preparations that have been withdrawn from the market or are no longer being actively marketed may be identified by the symbol †. Readers should be aware that since Part 3 was prepared other preparations are likely to have been withdrawn or introduced; also ingredients may change, as may indications.

The manufacturer's full name and address can be found in the Directory of Manufacturers.

Each preparation title is also listed in the General Index. Where thought helpful, preparation titles have also been listed at the end of the relevant monograph. However, it should be noted that the absence of such a list at the end of a monograph is no indication as to the availability of a substance as many drugs are marketed as generic or unbranded preparations.

**2-4-2** *Medipharma, Hong Kong.*
Coal tar (p.1159·2); salicylic acid (p.1157·1); sulfur (p.1158·2).
*Keratinisation disorders; psoriasis.*

**44** *Procter & Gamble, Mex.*
Dextromethorphan hydrobromide (p.1117·3); guaifenesin (p.1122·1).
*Coughs.*

**50:50** *BCM, UK.*
White soft paraffin (p.1479·3); liquid paraffin (p.1479·1).
*Dry skin.*

**217** *Frosst, Canad.†.*
Aspirin (p.15·1); caffeine citrate (p.782·1).
*Fever; inflammation; pain.*

**222** *Johnson & Johnson, Canad.*
Aspirin (p.15·1); caffeine citrate (p.782·1); codeine phosphate (p.27·1).
*Fever; inflammation; pain.*

**282** *Lioh, Canad.*
Aspirin (p.15·1); caffeine citrate (p.782·1); codeine phosphate (p.27·1).
*Fever; inflammation; pain.*

**292** *Lioh, Canad.*
Aspirin (p.15·1); caffeine citrate (p.782·1); codeine phosphate (p.27·1).
*Fever; inflammation; pain.*

**642** *Lioh, Canad.*
Dextropropoxyphene hydrochloride (p.28·3).
*Pain.*

**692** *Frosst, Canad.†.*
Dextropropoxyphene hydrochloride (p.28·3); aspirin (p.15·1); caffeine (p.782·1).
*Pain.*

**3-A** *Sophia, Mex.*
Diclofenac sodium (p.32·1).
*Pain and inflammation associated with eye surgery; prevention of cystoid macular oedema; prevention of miosis during cataract surgery.*

**A-200** *Shalpharm, Israel.*
Pyrethrins (p.1509·3); piperonyl butoxide (p.1509·2).
*Pediculosis.*

**A 313** *Pharmadevelopppement, Fr.*
*Capsules:* Vitamin A palmitate (p.1453·1).
*Vitamin A deficiency.*
*Ointment:* Vitamin A (p.1451·2).
Formerly contained vitamin A and tyrothricin.
*Dermatitis.*

**A Acido** *Dominguez, Arg.*
Tretinoin (p.1161·1).

**A + B Balsam N** *Mickan, Ger.†.*
Menthol (p.1711·3); camphor (p.1665·3); eucalyptus oil (p.1686·2).
*Respiratory-tract disorders.*

**A Curitybina** *Uniao Quimica, Braz.*
*Paste; plaster:* Salicylic acid (p.1157·1).
*Topical liquid:* Salicylic acid (p.1157·1); glacial acetic acid (p.1645·2); turpentine oil (p.1760·1).
*Keratinisation disorders.*

**A & D** *Swiss Herbal, Canad.*
Vitamin A (p.1451·2); vitamin D (p.1461·2).

**A + D + E-Vicotrat** *Heyl, Ger.†.*
Vitamin A palmitate (p.1453·1); colecalciferol (p.1461·3); alpha tocoferil acetate (p.1465·1).
*Deficiency of fat-soluble vitamins.*

**A and D Medicated** *Schering-Plough, USA.*
Zinc oxide (p.1163·2); cod-liver oil (p.1425·2); vitamin A (p.1451·2); vitamin D (p.1461·2).
*Nappy rash.*

**A & D Ointment** *Schering-Plough, Canad.; National Care, Canad.*
Vitamin A (p.1451·2); vitamin D (p.1461·2).
*Minor skin disorders.*

**A + $D_3$-Vicotrat** *Heyl, Ger.†.*
Vitamin A palmitate (p.1453·1); colecalciferol (p.1461·3).
*Vitamin A and $D_3$ deficiency.*

**A + E Thilo** *Alcon, Ger.*
Vitamin A acetate (p.1453·1); alpha tocoferil acetate (p.1465·1).
*Vitamin A and E deficiency.*

**A Grin** *Grin, Mex.*
Vitamin A palmitate (p.1453·1).
*Vitamin A deficiency.*

**3A Ofteno** *SMB, Chile.*
Diclofenac sodium (p.32·1).
*Cystoid macular oedema; eye inflammation; inhibition of miosis during surgery.*

**A Saude da Mulher** *Novamed, Braz.*
Sodium salicylate (p.90·1); plumeria lancifolia; passion flower (p.1729·1).
*Pain; sedative.*

**A Vogel Capsules a l'ail** *Bioforce, Switz.*
Garlic (p.1691·1).
*Cerebrovascular disorders.*

**A Vogel Capsules polyvitaminees** *Bioforce, Switz.*
Halibut-liver oil (p.1434·1); rose fruit (p.1740·1); acerola; dried yeast (p.1469·1); safflower oil (p.1443·3).
*Tonic.*

**A to Z** *Hall, Canad.*
Multivitamin and mineral preparation (p.1417·1).

**AA Cold** *General Drugs, Thai.†.*
Brompheniramine maleate (p.426·1); phenylephrine hydrochloride (p.1126·3); phenylpropanolamine hydrochloride (p.1127·3).
*Nasal congestion.*

**AAA**
*Note. This name is used for preparations of different composition.*
*Roche Consumer, S.Afr.*
Benzocaine (p.1370·3); cetalkonium chloride (p.1172·1).
*Mouth and throat disorders.*

*Manx, UK.*
Benzocaine (p.1370·3).
*Sore throat.*

**Aacidexam** *Organon, Belg.*
Dexamethasone sodium phosphate (p.1097·2).
*Corticosteroid.*

**Aacifemine** *Organon, Belg.*
Estriol (p.1552·3).
*Oestrogen deficiency.*

**AA-HC Otic** *Schein, USA†.*
Hydrocortisone (p.1103·3); glacial acetic acid (p.1645·2); propylene glycol diacetate (p.1415·3); benzethonium chloride (p.1169·2).
*Ear infection.*

**aar brain N** *aar, Ger.*
Hypericum (p.299·1).
*Depression.*

**aar gamma N** *aar, Ger.*
Cynara (p.1678·3).
*Dyspepsia.*

**aar os** *aar, Ger.*
Putamen ovi.
*Bone and teeth disorders; calcium deficiency.*

**aar vir** *aar, Ger.*
Echinacea pallida (p.1683·2).
*Influenza.*

**Aarane**
*Sanova, Austria†; Aventis, Switz.*
Sodium cromoglicate (p.795·3); reproterol hydrochloride (p.791·2).
*Obstructive airways disease.*

**Aarane N** *Aventis, Ger.*
Sodium cromoglicate (p.795·3); reproterol hydrochloride (p.791·2).
*Obstructive airways disease.*

**AAS**
*Sanofi Synthelabo, Braz.; Sinterapico, Braz.; Brasterapica, Braz.; GlaxoSmithKline, Port.; Sanofi Synthelabo, Spain.*
Aspirin (p.15·1).
*Fever; inflammation; pain; thromboembolism prophylaxis.*

**AB** *Saval, Chile.*
Chlorhexidine hydrochloride (p.1173·3).
*Mouth and throat disorders.*

**AB Antitusivo** *Saval, Chile.*
Chlorhexidine hydrochloride (p.1173·3); noscapine (p.1125·3).
*Coughs.*

**AB FE** *Camps, Spain.*
Aspirin (p.15·1); caffeine (p.782·1); phenazone (p.82·3).
*Fever; pain.*

**Abacateirol** *Regius, Braz.†.*
Persea persea; sodium salicylate (p.90·1); methenamine (p.230·1); theophylline (p.798·3).
*Kidney disorders.*

**Abacin** *Benedetti, Ital.*
Co-trimoxazole (p.199·3).
*Bacterial infections; Pneumocystis carinii pneumonia.*

**Abacten** *Andromaco, Chile.*
Azithromycin (p.159·1).
*Bacterial infections.*

**Abactrim** *Andreu, Spain†.*
Co-trimoxazole (p.199·3).
*Bacterial infections; Pneumocystis carinii pneumonia.*

**Abacus** *Pharmaland, Thai.*
Hydroxyzine hydrochloride (p.434·3).
*Anxiety; hypersensitivity reactions; pruritus; tension.*

**Abaktal**
*Lek, Hong Kong†; Lek, Thai.*
Pefloxacin mesilate (p.241·3).
*Bacterial infections.*

**Abalgin**
*Note. This name is used for preparations of different composition.*
*Laboratorios Chile, Chile.*
*Oral drops:* Adiphenine (p.1648·1); phenobarbital (p.367·3).
*Suppositories:* Propyphenazone (p.85·3); adiphenine (p.1648·1).
*Muscle spasm; pain.*

*Nycomed, Denm.; Nycomed, Fin.*
Dextropropoxyphene hydrochloride (p.28·3).
*Musculoskeletal and joint disorders; pain.*

**Abaprim** Gentili, Ital.†.
Trimethoprim (p.272·2).
*Bacterial infections.*

**Abba** Medichrom, Gr.
Ketoconazole (p.403·3).
*Fungal scalp infections.*

**Abbiofort** Synpharma, Austria.
Caraway (p.1667·2); psyllium seed (p.1268·1).
*Constipation; stool softener.*

**Abbocalcijex** Abbott, Gr.
Calcitriol (p.1461·2).
*Renal osteodystrophy; vitamin D deficiency.*

**Abbocillin-V** Sigma, Austral.
Benzathine phenoxymethylpenicillin (p.163·2).
*Bacterial infections.*

**Abbocillin-VK** Sigma, Austral.
Phenoxymethylpenicillin potassium (p.242·1).
*Bacterial infections.*

**Abboderm** Abbott, Chile.
Erythromycin (p.208·1); alcohol (p.1166·1).
*Acne.*

**Abbodop**
Abbott, Denm.; Abbott, Fin.; Abbott, Norw.; Abbott, Swed.
Dopamine hydrochloride (p.907·1).
*Heart failure; oliguria; shock.*

**Abbokinase**
Abbott, Austria; Abbott, Canad.†; Abbott, Israel; Abbott, Spain†; Abbott, Swed.; Abbott, USA.
Urokinase (p.1018·2).
*Thromboembolic disorders.*

**Abbolipid** Abbott, Ger.
Safflower oil (p.1443·3); soya oil (p.1447·2).
*Lipid infusion for parenteral nutrition.*

**Abboplegisol** Abbott, Spain.
Electrolyte infusion (p.1217·1).
*Adjunct to open-heart surgery.*

**Abbosynagis** Abbott, Israel.
Palivizumab (p.1637·2).
*Respiratory syncytial virus infections.*

**Abboticin**
Abbott, Denm.; Abbott, Fin.; Abbott, Norw.; Abbott, Swed.
Erythromycin (p.208·1), erythromycin ethyl succinate (p.208·1), erythromycin lactobionate (p.208·2), or erythromycin stearate (p.208·2).
*Bacterial infections.*

**Abboticine** Abbott, Fr.
Erythromycin ethyl succinate (p.208·1).
*Bacterial infections.*

**Abbottracurium** Abbott, Braz.
Atracurium besilate (p.1399·1).
*Competitive neuromuscular blocker.*

**Abbottselsun** Abbott, Spain.
Selenium sulfide (p.1157·3).
*Scalp disorders.*

**ABC** Beiersdorf, Austria.
Capsicum (p.1667·1).
*Muscle and joint pain.*

**ABC Warme-Pflaster** Beiersdorf, Ger.
Cayenne pepper (p.1667·1).
ABC Warme-Pflaster N formerly contained arnica flowers and cayenne pepper.
*Musculoskeletal and joint disorders.*

**ABC Warme-Pflaster Sensitive** Beiersdorf, Ger.
Nonivamide (p.67·2).
*Musculoskeletal, joint, peri-articular, and soft-tissue disorders.*

**ABC Warme-Salbe** Beiersdorf, Ger.
Diethylamine salicylate (p.34·1); benzyl nicotinate (p.21·2); nonivamide (p.67·2).
*Musculoskeletal, joint, and soft-tissue disorders; neuralgia.*

**ABC to Z** Nature's Bounty, USA.
Ferrous fumarate (p.1427·3); folic acid (p.1429·1); multivitamins and minerals (p.1417·1).
*Iron-deficiency anaemias.*

**ABCDin** Ferrosan, Denm.
Multivitamin preparation (p.1417·1).

**Abdijsiroop (Akker-Siroop)** Alfaco, Neth.†.
Belladonna tincture (p.479·1); drosera (p.1683·1); ipecacuanha tincture (p.1122·3); cowslip tincture (p.1735·1); ephedrine hydrochloride (p.1120·1).
*Coughs.*

**Abdine Cold Relief** Bell, UK.
Paracetamol (p.76·2).
*Cold and influenza symptoms.*

**Abdomilon N**
Caesaro, Austria.
Absinthium (p.1645·1); angelica (p.1655·1); calamus (p.1664·1); gentian (p.1692·2); melissa (p.1711·1).
Abdomilon formerly contained absinthium, angelica, calamus, frangula bark, gentian, melissa, and rhubarb.
*Dyspepsia.*

Cesra, Ger.
Absinthium (p.1645·1); angelica root (p.1655·1); calamus root (p.1664·1); gentian root (p.1692·2); melissa leaves (p.1711·1).
*Gastrointestinal disorders.*

**Abdominol** Medea, Spain.
Atropine methobromide (p.476·3); caffeine (p.782·1); propyphenazone (p.85·3).
*Pain due to smooth muscle spasm.*

**Abdoscan**
Nycomed, Austria†; Nycomed Imaging, Denm.†; Nycomed, Fin.†; Nycomed, Ger.†; Nycomed Imaging, Norw.†; Amersham, Spain†; Nycomed Amersham, Swed.†; Nycomed, Switz.†; Nycomed Amersham, UK†.
Ferristene (p.1061·3).
*Contrast medium for magnetic resonance imaging.*

**Abduce** Pharmanik (Φαρμανικ), Gr.
Aciclovir (p.626·1).
*Labial and genital herpes simplex infections.*

**Abecidin A C D** Pasteur, Chile.
Vitamin A palmitate; ergocalciferol; vitamin C (p.1417·1).
*Vitamin supplement.*

**Abelcet**
Gautier, Arg.; Amgen, Austral.; Liposome Company, Austria; Wyeth Lederle, Belg.; Merck Bago, Braz.; Liposome Company, Canad.; Elan, Denm.; Wyeth Lederle, Fin.; Elan, Fr.; Liposome, Gr.; Liposome Company, Hong Kong†; Liposome Company, Irl.; Segix, Ital.; Liposome Company, Norw.; Esteve, Port.; Liposome Company, Singapore; Pacific Biosciences, Singapore; Elan, Spain; Wyeth Lederle, Swed.; Liposome Company, Switz.; Elan, UK; Enzon, USA.
Amphotericin B phospholipid complex (p.391·2) (p.391·2).
*Fungal infections.*

**Abenol** GlaxoSmithKline, Canad.
Paracetamol (p.76·2).
*Fever; pain.*

**Abentel** Atlantic, Thai.
Albendazole (p.101·2).
*Worm infections.*

**Aberel** Janssen-Cilag, Fr.†.
Tretinoin (p.1161·1).
*Keratinisation disorders.*

**Aberela**
Janssen-Cilag, Norw.; Janssen-Cilag, Swed.
Tretinoin (p.1161·1).
*Acne; photoageing of the skin.*

**Aberten** Menarini, Gr.
Theophylline (p.798·3).
*Asthma; chronic obstructive pulmonary disease; neonatal apnoea and bradycardia.*

**Abesira** Clariana, Spain.
Vitamin B substances and amino acids (p.1417·1).
*Anaemias; metabolic disorders; tonic.*

**Abetol** CT, Ital.†.
Labetalol hydrochloride (p.943·3).
*Hypertension.*

**Abflex** Xeragen, S.Afr.
Paracetamol (p.76·2); doxylamine succinate (p.432·3); caffeine (p.782·1); codeine phosphate (p.27·1).
*Pain with tension.*

**Abfuhrdragees** Sanochemia, Austria.
Aloes (p.1248·2); phenolphthalein (p.1284·1); hard soap (p.1575·2).
*Bowel evacuation; constipation.*

**Abfuhrdragees mild** Sanochemia, Austria.
Aloes (p.1248·2); frangula bark (p.1266·3); hard soap (p.1575·2).
*Constipation.*

**Abfuhrtee** Sanochemia, Austria.
Couch-grass (p.1676·2); chamomile (p.1669·3); centaurea cyanus; frangula bark (p.1266·3); rhubarb (p.1287·3); senna (p.1288·2).
*Constipation.*

**Abfuhrtee EF-EM-ES** Smetana, Austria.
Achillea (p.1646·2); peppermint leaf (p.1283·2); senna (p.1288·2).
Formerly contained frangula bark, hypericum, peppermint leaf, and senna.
*Constipation.*

**Abfuhrtee N** Bad Heilbrunner, Ger.
Senna (p.1288·2).
*Constipation.*

**Abfuhrtropfen** Ratiopharm, Ger.†.
Sodium picosulfate (p.1289·3).
*Constipation.*

**Abidec**
Warner-Lambert, Irl.; Teofarma, Ital.; Pfizer Consumer, UK.
Multivitamin preparation (p.1417·1).

**Abilify**
Bristol-Myers Squibb, Austral.; Bristol-Myers Squibb, UK; Otsuka, UK; Bristol-Myers Squibb, USA; Otsuka, USA.
Aripiprazole (p.671·1).
*Schizophrenia.*

**Abine** Dosa, Arg.
Gemcitabine (p.558·2).
*Malignant neoplasms.*

**Abinol** Recalcine, Chile.
Lorazepam (p.704·1).
*Anxiety; childhood behaviour disorders; insomnia; premedication.*

**Abiocef** Ibi, Ital.
Cefonicid sodium (p.174·2).
Lidocaine hydrochloride (p.1377·3) is included in this preparation to alleviate the pain of injection.
*Bacterial infections.*

**Abiolex** Andromaco, Chile.
Amoxicillin (p.155·3).
*Bacterial infections.*

**Abiostil** Deca, Ital.
Neomycin sulfate (p.235·1); cineole (p.1672·1); oleum pini sylvestris; camphor (p.1665·3); menthol (p.1711·3).
*Nasopharyngeal infections.*

**Abiotyl** Biocrom, Arg.
Amoxicillin (p.155·3).
*Bacterial infections.*

**Abiplatin**
Sanova, Austria; Teva, Israel; Teva, S.Afr.; Abic-Teva, Thai.
Cisplatin (p.538·1).
*Malignant neoplasms.*

**Abiposid** Sanova, Austria†.
Etoposide (p.551·3).
*Malignant neoplasms.*

**Abitren**
Teva, Hong Kong†; Abic, Israel; Abic, Thai.†.
Diclofenac sodium (p.32·1).
*Gout; inflammation; musculoskeletal, joint, peri-articular, and soft-tissue disorders; pain.*

**Abitrexate**
Sanova, Austria; Teva, Israel; Teva, S.Afr.; Abic-Teva, Thai.
Methotrexate sodium (p.568·3).
*Malignant neoplasms; psoriasis; rheumatoid arthritis.*

**Ablock** Biolab Sanus, Braz.
Atenolol (p.865·2).
*Hypertension.*

**Ablock Plus** Biolab Sanus, Braz.
Atenolol (p.865·2); hydrochlorothiazide (p.933·2).
*Hypertension.*

**Abnobaviscum** Abnoba, Ger.
Mistletoe (p.1715·3).
*Malignant neoplasms.*

**Abolibe** Sidefarma, Port.
Ginkgo biloba (p.1692·3).
*Mental function disorders; vascular disorders.*

**Abopur** Norton Healthcare, Denm.
Allopurinol (p.412·2).
*Gout; renal calculi.*

**Abrasone** Seid, Spain.
Fluocinolone acetonide (p.1101·2); framycetin sulfate (p.215·1).
*Infected skin disorders.*

**Abrasone Rectal** Seid, Spain.
Fluocinolone acetonide (p.1101·2); hexetidine (p.1182·1); ruscogenin (p.1741·1).
*Anorectal disorders.*

**Abreva** SmithKline Beecham Consumer, USA.
Docosanol (p.632·1).
*Herpes labialis.*

**Abrilar**
Note. This name is used for preparations of different composition.
Roemmers, Arg.
Salmeterol xinafoate (p.795·1).
*Asthma.*

Pharma Investi, Chile.
Alfa-hederina.
*Coughs; respiratory-tract congestion.*

**Abrol** Rekah, Israel.
Paracetamol (p.76·2).
*Fever; pain.*

**Abrolen** Specifar (Σπεσιφαρ), Gr.
Ambroxol hydrochloride (p.1114·3).
*Respiratory disorders associated with viscous mucus.*

**Abrolet** Rekah, Israel.
Paracetamol (p.76·2).
*Fever; pain.*

**Absenor**
Orion, Fin.; Orion, Swed.
Sodium valproate (p.380·1).
*Epilepsy; mania.*

**Absimed** Synpharma, Austria.
Caraway (p.1667·2); melissa (p.1711·1); valerian (p.1762·2).
*Gastrointestinal disorders.*

**Absint** Medochemie, Hong Kong.
Flunitrazepam (p.698·2).
*Insomnia.*

**Absorbase** Carolina, USA.
Vehicle for topical preparations.

**Absorber HFV** Arteva, Ger.
Dimeticone (p.1289·2).
*Reduction of gastrointestinal gas.*

**Absorbine Analgesic** Young, Canad.
Methyl salicylate (p.59·3); camphor (p.1665·3); menthol (p.1711·3); eucalyptus oil (p.1686·2).

**Absorbine Antifungal** Young, Canad.†.
Tolnaftate (p.410·1).
*Tinea pedis.*

**Absorbine Antifungal Foot Powder** Young, USA.
Miconazole nitrate (p.405·3).
*Fungal skin infections.*

**Absorbine Arthritis** Young, Canad.
Menthol (p.1711·3); capsicum (p.1667·1).

**Absorbine Athletes Foot Care** Young, USA.
Tolnaftate (p.410·1); menthol (p.1711·3).
*Fungal infections.*

**Absorbine Jr**
Young, Canad.; Young, USA.
Menthol (p.1711·3).
*Muscle, joint, and soft-tissue pain; neuralgia.*

**Absorbine Jr Antifungal** Young, Canad.
Tolnaftate (p.410·1).
Formerly contained tolnaftate and menthol.
*Tinea pedis.*

**Absorbine Power Gel** Young, Canad.
Menthol (p.1711·3).

**Absorlent** Esteve, Spain.
Estradiol (p.1550·1).
*Menopausal disorders; osteoporosis.*

**Absorlent Plus** Esteve, Spain.
Patch A, estradiol (p.1550·1); patch B, estradiol; norethisterone acetate (p.1562·2).
*Menopausal disorders; osteoporosis.*

**Abstem** Wyeth, Irl.†.
Calcium carbimide (p.1664·2).
*Alcoholism.*

**Absten S** Medley, Braz.
Mazindol (p.1589·1).
*Obesity.*

**Abstensyl** Sintesina, Arg.
Disulfiram (p.1681·3).
*Alcoholism.*

**Abtrim** Ashbourne, UK.
Clotrimazole (p.396·2).
*Fungal skin infections; vaginal candidiasis.*

**Abufene** Bouchara-Recordati, Fr.
Beta-alanine.
*Menopausal disorders.*

**Abuglib** Pharmacos Abug, Mex.
Glibenclamide (p.331·2).
*Diabetes mellitus.*

**Abutiroi** Pharmacos Abug, Mex.
Levothyroxine sodium (p.1600·1).
*Thyroid hormone.*

**Abutol** Nettopharma, Denm.†.
Acebutolol hydrochloride (p.848·1).
*Angina pectoris; arrhythmias; hypertension.*

**AC & C** WestCan, Canad.
Aspirin (p.15·1); caffeine (p.782·1); codeine phosphate (p.27·1).
*Fever; inflammation; pain.*

**AC Vascular** Biotenk, Arg.
Nimodipine (p.972·3).
*Cerebrovascular disorders.*

**Aca**
Atlantic, Malaysia; Atlantic, Thai.
Trihexyphenidyl hydrochloride (p.490·2).
*Parkinsonism.*

**Acabel**
Grunenthal, Arg.; Grunenthal, Chile; Euro-Labor, Port.; Grunenthal, Port.; Andromaco, Spain.
Lornoxicam (p.54·2).
*Inflammation; musculoskeletal and joint disorders; pain.*

**Acacin** Fustery, Mex.
Cefalexin (p.168·1).
*Bacterial infections.*

**Acadione** Aventis, Fr.
Tiopronin (p.1054·3).
*Cystinuric lithiasis; polyarthritis.*

**Acalix** Roemmers, Arg.
Diltiazem hydrochloride (p.900·1).
*Arrhythmias; hypertension; ischaemic heart disease.*

**Acalka**
Gross, Braz.; Silesia, Chile; Helsinn, Port.; Robert, Spain.
Potassium citrate (p.1223·1).
*Alkalinisation of urine; renal calculi.*

**Acamed** Medifive, Thai.
Trihexyphenidyl hydrochloride (p.490·2).
*Parkinsonism.*

**Acamol**
Volta, Chile; Teva, Israel.
Paracetamol (p.76·2).
*Fever; pain.*

**Acamol Compuesto** Volta, Chile.
Paracetamol (p.76·2); pseudoephedrine hydrochloride (p.1129·2); chlorphenamine maleate (p.427·3).

**Acamol Tsinun Day** Teva, Israel.
Paracetamol (p.76·2); pseudoephedrine hydrochloride (p.1129·2).
*Cold symptoms.*

**Acamol Tsinun Night** Teva, Israel.
Paracetamol (p.76·2); pseudoephedrine hydrochloride (p.1129·2); chlorphenamine maleate (p.427·3).
*Cold symptoms.*

**Acamoli** Teva, Israel.
Paracetamol (p.76·2).
*Fever; pain.*

**Acamoli Cold** Teva, Israel.
Paracetamol (p.76·2); pseudoephedrine hydrochloride (p.1129·2); chlorphenamine maleate (p.427·3).
*Cold symptoms.*

**Acanol** Sanofi Synthelabo, Mex.
Loperamide (p.1271·2).
*Diarrhoea.*

**Acantex**
Roche, Arg.
Ceftriaxone (p.183·3).
*Bacterial infections.*

Roche, Chile.
Ceftriaxone sodium (p.182·3).
*Bacterial infections.*

**Acarcid** Pierre Fabre Sante, Fr.
Acetamide; crotamiton (p.1145·1); benzalkonium chloride (p.1168·3); thyme oil (p.1755·3); geranium oil (p.1692·2); myrtle oil.
*Elimination of house dust mites.*

**Acarcid perles** Pierre Fabre Sante, Fr.†.
Piperonyl butoxide (p.1509·2); permethrin (p.1508·3); carbaryl (p.1501·2); methoprene (p.1507·2).
*Acaricide.*

**Acardi** Boehringer Ingelheim, Jpn.
Pimobendan (p.983·1).
*Heart failure.*

**Acardust**
*Raymos, Arg.; Pharmygiene, Fr.; Scat, Israel; Geymonat, Ital.†; SCAT, Switz.†.*
Esdepallethrine (p.1505·1); piperonyl butoxide (p.1509·2).
*Acaricide.*

**Acarex** *Allergopharma, Ger.*
Potassium hydroxide (p.1734·2); methyl alcohol (p.1475·2).
*Test for detection of house dust mite excretae.*

**Acaril** *Allergopharma, Ger.*
Benzyl benzoate (p.1500·2).
*Elimination of house dust mites.*

**Acarilbial** *Bial, Port.*
Benzyl benzoate (p.1500·2).

**Acarosan** *Allergopharma, Ger.*
Benzyl benzoate (p.1500·2).
*Elimination of house-dust mites.*

**Acarsan** *Biosintetica, Braz.*
Benzyl benzoate (p.1500·2).
*Pediculosis; scabies.*

**Acasmul** *Pharma Investi, Chile.*
Diltiazem hydrochloride (p.900·1).
*Angina pectoris; ischaemic heart disease.*

**Acatar** *SMB, Belg.*
Dextromethorphan hydrobromide (p.1117·3); guaifenesin (p.1122·1).
*Coughs.*

**ACB**
*Pacific, NZ.*
Acebutolol hydrochloride (p.848·1).
*Angina pectoris; arrhythmias; hypertension.*
*Merck, Singapore; Pacific, Singapore.*
Acebutolol (p.848·1).
*Angina pectoris; arrhythmias; hypertension.*

**ACC**
*Hexal, Arg.; Hexal, Austria; Hexal, Ger.; Hexal, S.Afr.; Ecosol, Switz.*
Acetylcysteine (p.1112·3) or acetylcysteine sodium (p.1113·1).
*Paracetamol overdosage; respiratory-tract congestion.*

**Accolate**
*AstraZeneca, Arg.; AstraZeneca, Austral.; AstraZeneca, Belg.; AstraZeneca, Braz.; AstraZeneca, Canad.; AstraZeneca, Chile; AstraZeneca, Fin.; AstraZeneca, Hong Kong; AstraZeneca, Irl.; AstraZeneca, Israel; AstraZeneca, Mex.; AstraZeneca, Port.; AstraZeneca, S.Afr.; AstraZeneca, Singapore; AstraZeneca, Spain; AstraZeneca, Switz.; AstraZeneca, Thai.; AstraZeneca, UK; AstraZeneca, USA.*
Zafirlukast (p.807·1).
*Asthma.*

**Accoleit** *AstraZeneca, Ital.*
Zafirlukast (p.807·1).
*Asthma.*

**Accomin** *Whitehall, Austral.†.*
Vitamin B substances with lysine and iron (p.1417·1).

**Accomin Centrum** *Whitehall, Austral.†.*
Vitamin B substances with lysine and iron (p.1417·1).

**Accomin Vitamin** *Whitehall, Austral.†.*
Amino-acid, vitamin, and iron preparation (p.1417·1).

**Accu-Check Advantage** *Boehringer Mannheim, USA.*
Test for glucose in blood (p.1694·2).

**Accu-Check III/Chemstrip bG** *Boehringer Mannheim, Canad.†.*
Test for glucose in blood (p.1694·2).

**Accu-Chek**
*Roche Diagnostics, Austral.; Roche, Chile; Boehringer Mannheim, Fr.†; Roche Diagnostics, Ital.*
Test for glucose in blood (p.1694·2).

**Accuhist** *Pediamed, USA.*
Pseudoephedrine hydrochloride (p.1129·2); brompheniramine maleate (p.426·1).

**Accuhist DM Pediatric** *Pediamed, USA.*
*Oral drops:* Pseudoephedrine hydrochloride (p.1129·2); brompheniramine maleate (p.426·1); dextromethorphan hydrobromide (p.1117·3).
*Syrup:* Pseudoephedrine hydrochloride (p.1129·2); brompheniramine maleate (p.426·1); dextromethorphan hydrobromide (p.1117·3); guaifenesin (p.1122·1).
*Upper respiratory-tract disorders.*

**Accuhist LA** *Pediamed, USA.*
Phenylephrine hydrochloride (p.1126·3); chlorphenamine maleate (p.427·3); hyoscyamine sulfate (p.485·1); atropine sulfate (p.477·1); hyoscine hydrobromide (p.483·3).

**Accuhist PDX** *Pediamed, USA.*
*Oral drops:* Pseudoephedrine hydrochloride (p.1129·2); brompheniramine maleate (p.426·1); dextromethorphan hydrobromide (p.1117·3).
*Syrup:* Phenylephrine hydrochloride (p.1126·3); brompheniramine maleate (p.426·1); dextromethorphan hydrobromide (p.1117·3); guaifenesin (p.1122·1).
*Upper respiratory-tract disorders.*

**Accuneb** *Dey, USA.*
Salbutamol sulfate (p.791·3).
*Asthma.*

**Accupaque**
*Nycomed, Austria; Amersham, Ger.; Nycomed Amersham, Switz.*
Iohexol (p.1064·2).
*Contrast medium for radiography and computerised tomography.*

**AccuPeel**
*ICN, Hong Kong; ICN, Singapore.*
Trichloroacetic acid (p.1162·1).
*Dyschromia; facial wrinkles.*

**Accupep** *Sherwood, USA.*
Preparation for enteral nutrition (p.1417·1).
*Gastrointestinal disorders.*

**Accupril**
*Parke, Davis, Arg.; Pfizer, Austral.; Pfizer, Belg.; Pfizer, Braz.; Pfizer, Canad.; Parke, Davis, Chile; Pfizer, Hong Kong; Pfizer, Malaysia; Pfizer, NZ; Pfizer, S.Afr.; Pfizer, Singapore; Pfizer, Thai.; Parke, Davis, USA.*
Quinapril hydrochloride (p.991·1).
*Heart failure; hypertension.*

**Accuprin** *Parke, Davis, Ital.*
Quinapril hydrochloride (p.991·1) or quinaprilat (p.991·2).
*Heart failure; hypertension.*

**Accupro**
*Pfizer, Austria; Pfizer, Denm.; Pfizer, Fin.; Godecke, Ger.; Parke, Davis, Ger.; Parke, Davis, Irl.; Pfizer, Swed.; Pfizer, Switz.; Pfizer, UK.*
Quinapril hydrochloride (p.991·1) or quinaprilat (p.991·2).
*Heart failure; hypertension.*

**Accupro Comp**
*Pfizer, Fin.; Pfizer, Swed.*
Quinapril hydrochloride (p.991·1); hydrochlorothiazide (p.933·2).
*Hypertension.*

**Accupron** *Pfizer, Gr.*
Quinapril (p.991·2).
*Heart failure; hypertension; myocardial infarction.*

**Accurbron** *Marion Merrell Dow, USA.*
Theophylline (p.798·3).
*Asthma; bronchospasm.*

**Accure** *Alphapharm, Austral.*
Isotretinoin (p.1148·3).
*Acne.*

**Accuretic**
*Parke, Davis, Arg.; Pfizer, Austral.; Pfizer, Belg.; Warner-Lambert, Braz.†; Pfizer, Canad.; Parke, Davis, Chile; Parke, Davis, Irl.; Parke, Davis, Ital.; Pfizer, NZ; Pfizer, S.Afr.; Pfizer, Switz.; Pfizer, UK; Parke, Davis, USA.*
Quinapril hydrochloride (p.991·1); hydrochlorothiazide (p.933·2).
*Hypertension.*

**Accutane**
*Roche, Canad.; Roche, USA.*
Isotretinoin (p.1148·3).
*Acne.*

**Accutest Fecal** *Marco, Austral.*
Test for haemoglobin in faeces.

**Accutest Multi-Drug** *Marco, Austral.*
Test for amfetamine, benzoylecgonine, methamfetamine, morphine, or THC in urine.

**Accutin** *Durascan, Denm.*
Isotretinoin (p.1148·3).
*Acne.*

**Accutrend Cholesterol**
*Roche Diagnostics, Ital.; Roche, Mex.; Roche Diagnostics, UK.*
Test for cholesterol in blood.

**Accutrend Colesterol**
*Roche, Arg.; Roche, Chile.*
Test for cholesterol in blood.

**Accutrend GC** *Roche Diagnostics, Canad.*
Test for glucose and cholesterol in blood (p.1694·2).

**Accutrend Glucosa**
*Roche, Arg.; Roche, Chile.*
Test for glucose in blood (p.1694·2).

**Accutrend Glucose**
*Roche Diagnostics, Austral.; Roche Diagnostics, Ital.; Roche, Mex.; Roche Diagnostics, NZ.*
Test for glucose in blood (p.1694·2).

**Accutrend Trigliceridos** *Roche, Chile.*
Test for triglycerides in blood.

**Accuvit** *Ache, Braz.*
Multivitamin preparation (p.1417·1).

**Accuzide**
*Pfizer, Austria; Godecke, Ger.; Parke, Davis, Ger.*
Quinapril hydrochloride (p.991·1); hydrochlorothiazide (p.933·2).
*Hypertension.*

**Accuzyme** *Healthpoint, USA.*
Papain (p.1727·3); urea (p.1162·2).
*Debridement of necrotic tissue.*

**ACD** *Gobbi, Arg.*
Vitamin A; vitamin C; vitamin D (p.1417·1).

**Ac-De** *Lemery, Mex.*
Dactinomycin (p.545·1).
*Malignant neoplasms.*

**Acea** *Adams, UK.*
Metronidazole (p.607·2).
*Rosacea.*

**Aceclofar** *Julphar, UAE.*
Aceclofenac (p.11·2).
*Musculoskeletal and joint disorders; pain.*

**Acecol** *Boehringer Ingelheim, Jpn.*
Temocapril hydrochloride (p.1010·2).
*Hypertension.*

**Acecomb** *AstraZeneca, Austria.*
Hydrochlorothiazide (p.933·2); lisinopril (p.946·3).
*Hypertension.*

**Acecor**
*Note. This name is used for preparations of different composition.*
*Sankyo, Austria.*
Temocapril hydrochloride (p.1010·2).
*Hypertension.*
*SPA, Ital.†.*
Acebutolol hydrochloride (p.848·1).
*Arrhythmias; heart failure; hypertension.*

**Acecromol** *Wolff, Ger.*
Sodium cromoglicate (p.795·3).
*Asthma.*

**Acedicone** *Boehringer Ingelheim, Belg.*
Thebacon hydrochloride (p.1131·2).
*Coughs.*

**Acediur**
*Note. This name is used for preparations of different composition.*
*Menarini, Ital.*
Captopril (p.879·2); hydrochlorothiazide (p.933·2).
*Hypertension.*
*Sigma-Tau, Spain.*
Enalapril maleate (p.909·2); hydrochlorothiazide (p.933·2).
*Hypertension.*

**Acef** *KG, Ital.*
Cefazolin sodium (p.170·3).
Lidocaine hydrochloride (p.1377·3) is included in this preparation to alleviate the pain of injection.
*Bacterial infections.*

**Aceflan** *Uniao Quimica, Braz.*
Aceclofenac (p.11·2).
*Inflammation; pain.*

**ACE-Hemmer** *Ratiopharm, Ger.*
Captopril (p.879·2).
*Heart failure; hypertension.*

**ACE-Hemmer comp** *Ratiopharm, Ger.*
Captopril (p.879·2); hydrochlorothiazide (p.933·2).
*Hypertension.*

**Aceite Acalorico** *Ordesa, Spain.*
Olive oil (p.1723·2); betacarotene (p.1422·3); liquid paraffin (p.1479·1).
*Constipation; obesity.*

**Aceite Esmeralda Moone** *Gordon, Arg.*
Camphor (p.1665·3); methyl salicylate (p.59·3); phenol (p.1188·1).
*Musculoskeletal and joint disorders.*

**Aceite Geve Concentrado** *Teofarma, Spain.*
Cod-liver oil (p.1425·2).
*Deficiency of vitamins A and D.*

**Acekapton** *Strallhofer, Austria.*
Aspirin (p.15·1).
*Fever; pain.*

**Acel-Imune**
*Lederle, Switz.†; Wyeth-Ayerst, USA†.*
A diphtheria, tetanus, and acellular pertussis vaccine (p.1613·3).
*Active immunisation of infants and young children.*

**Acelluvax**
*Chiron, Ital.†; Chiron, Thai.†.*
An acellular pertussis vaccine (p.1631·2).
*Active immunisation.*

**Acelluvax DTP**
*Chiron, Israel; Chiron, Thai.†.*
A diphtheria, tetanus, and acellular pertussis vaccine (p.1613·3).
*Active immunisation of infants and young children.*

**Acel-P**
*Wyeth-Ayerst, Canad.†; Lederle, Ger.†; Lederle, Switz.†.*
An adsorbed acellular pertussis vaccine (p.1631·2).
*Active immunisation.*

**Acemedrox** *Bunker, Braz.*
Medroxyprogesterone acetate (p.1557·2).
*Progestogenic.*

**Acemetadoc** *Docpharm, Ger.*
Acemetacin (p.11·3).
*Gout; inflammation; musculoskeletal, joint, and periarticular disorders.*

**Acemin** *AstraZeneca, Austria.*
Lisinopril (p.946·3).
*Diabetic nephropathy; heart failure; hypertension; myocardial infarction.*

**Acemix** *Bioprogress, Ital.*
Acemetacin (p.11·3).
*Musculoskeletal and joint disorders.*

**Acemuc** *Betapharm, Ger.*
Acetylcysteine (p.1112·3).
*Respiratory-tract disorders with viscous mucus.*

**Acemucol** *Streuli, Switz.*
Acetylcysteine (p.1112·3).
*Respiratory-tract disorders associated with excess or viscous mucus.*

**Acemuk** *Hexal, Arg.*
Acetylcysteine (p.1112·3).
*Respiratory-tract disorders with increased or viscous mucus.*

**Acemycin** *Elpen (Ελπεν), Gr.*
Cefamandole nafate (p.169·3).
*Bacterial infections.*

**Acenorm**
*Alphapharm, Austral.; Azupharma, Ger.*
Captopril (p.879·2).
*Diabetic nephropathy; heart failure; hypertension; myocardial infarction.*

**Acenorm HCT** *Azupharma, Ger.*
Captopril (p.879·2); hydrochlorothiazide (p.933·2).
*Hypertension.*

**Acenox** *Pasteur, Chile.*
Acenocoumarol (p.848·3).
*Thromboembolic disorders.*

**Acenterine** *Christiaens, Belg.*
Aspirin (p.15·1).
*Musculoskeletal and joint disorders.*

**Aceomel** *Clonmel, Irl.*
Captopril (p.879·2).
*Heart failure; hypertension.*

**Aceon** *Solvay, USA.*
Perindopril erbumine (p.980·2).
*Hypertension.*

**Aceoto** *Zambon, Spain; Salvat, Spain.*
Ciprofloxacin (p.188·2) or ciprofloxacin hydrochloride (p.188·2).
*Bacterial infections.*

**Aceoto Plus** *Zambon, Spain.*
Ciprofloxacin (p.188·2); fluocinolone acetonide (p.1101·2).
*Otitis externa.*

**Acephen** *G & W, USA.*
Paracetamol (p.76·2).
*Pain.*

**Acephlogont** *Azupharma, Ger.*
Acemetacin (p.11·3).
*Gout; inflammation, musculoskeletal, joint, and soft-tissue disorders.*

**Aceplus**
*Note. This name is used for preparations of different composition.*
*Bristol-Myers Squibb, Austria.*
Fosinopril sodium (p.919·1); hydrochlorothiazide (p.933·2).
*Hypertension.*
*Bristol-Myers Squibb, Ital.; Bristol-Myers Squibb, Neth.†.*
Captopril (p.879·2); hydrochlorothiazide (p.933·2).
*Hypertension.*

**Acepran** *Andromaco, Chile.*
Clonazepam (p.359·1).
*Epilepsy; panic attacks.*

**Acepress** *Bristol-Myers Squibb, Ital.*
Captopril (p.879·2).
*Diabetic nephropathy; heart failure; hypertension; myocardial infarction.*

**Acepril**
*Note. This name is used for preparations of different composition.*
*United Nordic, Denm.; Duopharma, Hong Kong.*
Lisinopril (p.946·3).
*Heart failure; hypertension.*
*Spirig, Switz.*
Enalapril maleate (p.909·2).
*Heart failure; hypertension.*
*Bristol-Myers Squibb, UK.*
Captopril (p.879·2).
*Diabetic nephropathy; heart failure; hypertension; myocardial infarction.*

**Aceprilex** *Uno, Ital.*
Captopril (p.879·2).

**Acequide** *Recordati, Ital.*
Quinapril hydrochloride (p.991·1); hydrochlorothiazide (p.933·2).
*Hypertension.*

**Acequin** *Recordati, Ital.*
Quinapril hydrochloride (p.991·1) or quinaprilat (p.991·2).
*Heart failure; hypertension.*

**Aceratun** *Delta, Braz.*
Urea hydrogen peroxide (p.1195·3).
*Cleansing of external ear.*

**Acerbine**
*Note. This name is used for preparations of different composition.*
*Montavit, Austria.*
Benzoic acid (p.1169·3); malic acid (p.1709·2); propylene glycol (p.1735·2); propylene glycol malate (p.1735·3); salicylic acid (p.1157·1).
*Bruises; burns; sunburn; ulcers; wounds.*
*Interdelta, Switz.*
*Ointment:* Benzoic acid (p.1169·3); malic acid (p.1709·2); salicylic acid (p.1157·1); propylene glycol (p.1735·2); propylene glycol malate (p.1735·3); hexachlorophene (p.1181·2).
*Topical solution; topical gel:* Benzoic acid (p.1169·3); malic acid (p.1709·2); salicylic acid (p.1157·1); propylene glycol (p.1735·2); propylene glycol malate (p.1735·3).
*Burns; wounds.*

**Acerbiol** *Vitafarma, Spain.*
Benzyl alcohol (p.1170·2); benzoic acid (p.1169·3); malic acid (p.1709·2); propylene glycol malate (p.1735·3); propylene glycol (p.1735·2); salicylic acid (p.1157·1).
*Burns; skin ulcers; wounds.*

**Acerbon** *AstraZeneca, Ger.; Promed, Ger.*
Lisinopril (p.946·3).
*Heart failure; hypertension.*

**Acercomp**
*AstraZeneca, Fin.; AstraZeneca, Ger.; Promed, Ger.*
Lisinopril (p.946·3); hydrochlorothiazide (p.933·2).
*Hypertension.*

**Acerdil** *Drugtech, Chile.*
Lisinopril (p.946·3).
*Hypertension.*

**Acerdil-D** *Drugtech, Chile.*
Lisinopril (p.946·3); hydrochlorothiazide (p.933·2).
*Hypertension.*

**Aceren** *Nycomed, Denm.*
Enalapril maleate (p.909·2).
*Heart failure; hypertension.*

**Aceril** *Dexcel, Israel.*
Captopril (p.879·2).
*Diabetic nephropathy; heart failure; hypertension; myocardial infarction.*

**Acerpes**
*Hexal, Arg.; Bioglan, Ger.; Ecosol, Switz.*
Aciclovir (p.626·1).
*Herpesvirus infections.*

**Acertil** *Servier, Hong Kong.*
Perindopril (p.980·2).
*Heart failure; hypertension.*

**Acertol** *Lacer, Spain.*
Paracetamol (p.76·2).
*Fever; pain.*

**Aces** *Carlson, USA.*
Betacarotene; calcium ascorbate; *d*-alpha tocoferol; selenomethionine (p.1417·1).
*Nutritional supplement.*

**Acesal**
*OPW, Ger.; Roland, Ger.; Geymonat, Ital.*
Aspirin (p.15·1).
*Fever; musculoskeletal, joint, and soft-tissue disorders; pain; thrombosis prophylaxis.*

**Acesal Calcium** *OPW, Ger.†; Roland, Ger.†.*
Aspirin (p.15·1).
Calcium carbonate (p.1254·2) is included in this preparation in an attempt to limit adverse effects on the gastrointestinal mucosa.
*Fever; pain; rheumatism; thromboembolic disorders.*

**Acesistem** *Sigma-Tau, Ital.*
Enalapril maleate (p.909·2); hydrochlorothiazide (p.933·2).
*Hypertension.*

**Acestrol** *Probios, Port.*
Megestrol acetate (p.1558·2).
*Malignant neoplasms.*

**Acet**
*Pharmascience, Canad.; Pharmascience, Malaysia; Pharmascience, Singapore.*
Paracetamol (p.76·2).
*Fever; pain.*

**Acet-2, Acet-3** *Pharmascience, Canad.†.*
Paracetamol (p.76·2); codeine phosphate (p.27·1); caffeine (p.782·1).
*Fever; pain.*

**Acet Codeine** *Pharmascience, Canad.†.*
Paracetamol (p.76·2); codeine phosphate (p.27·1).
*Fever; pain.*

**Aceta** *Century, USA.*
Paracetamol (p.76·2).
*Fever; pain.*

**Aceta with Codeine** *Century, USA.*
Paracetamol (p.76·2); codeine phosphate (p.27·1).
*Pain.*

**Acetab** *Romilo, Canad.†.*
Paracetamol (p.76·2).

**Acetabs** *Krewel, Ger.*
Acetylcysteine (p.1112·3).
*Respiratory-tract disorders with viscous mucus.*

**Acetacol** *PP Lab, Thai.*
Paracetamol (p.76·2); chlorphenamine maleate (p.427·3).
Formerly contained paracetamol, phenylpropanolamine hydrochloride, and chlorphenamine maleate.
*Cold symptoms; hay fever; nasal congestion.*

**Acetadiazol** *Grin, Mex.*
Acetazolamide (p.849·1).
*Epilepsy; glaucoma; oedema.*

**Acetadote** *Cumberland, USA.*
Acetylcysteine (p.1112·3).
*Paracetamol poisoning.*

**Acetafen** *Rayere, Mex.*
Paracetamol (p.76·2).
*Fever; pain.*

**Aceta-Gesic** *Rugby, USA.*
Phenyltoloxamine citrate (p.439·1); paracetamol (p.76·2).
*Upper respiratory-tract symptoms.*

**Acetalgine** *Streuli, Switz.*
Paracetamol (p.76·2).
*Fever; pain.*

**Acetaminophen with Codeine** *Pharmascience, Canad.*
Paracetamol (p.76·2); caffeine (p.782·1); codeine phosphate (p.27·1).
*Coughs; fever; pain.*

**Acetamol**
*Bergamo, Braz.†; Abiogen, Ital.*
Paracetamol (p.76·2).
*Fever; pain.*

**Acetan** *Kwizda, Austria.*
Lisinopril (p.946·3).
*Diabetic nephropathy; heart failure; hypertension; myocardial infarction.*

**Aceta-P** *PP Lab, Thai.*
Paracetamol (p.76·2).
*Fever; pain.*

**Acetapyrin-C** *PP Lab, Thai.*
Paracetamol (p.76·2); chlorphenamine maleate (p.427·3).
*Cold symptoms; hay fever.*

**Acetar**
*Note. This name is used for preparations of different composition.*
*Clintex, Port.*
Piracetam (p.1732·1).
*Cerebrovascular disorders; chronic alcoholism; mental function impairment; Raynaud's syndrome.*

*Thai Otsuka, Thai.*
Electrolyte infusion with or without glucose (p.1217·1).
*Carbohydrate source; fluid and electrolyte disorders.*

**Acetard** *Nycomed, Denm.†.*
Aspirin (p.15·1).
*Fever; inflammation; pain.*

**Acetasil** *Silom, Thai.*
Paracetamol (p.76·2).
*Fever; pain.*

**Acetasol** *Barre-National, USA.*
Acetic acid (p.1645·2); propylene glycol acetate (p.1415·3); benzethonium chloride (p.1169·2).
*Ear infection.*

**Acetasol HC** *Barre-National, USA.*
Hydrocortisone (p.1103·3); acetic acid (p.1645·2); propylene glycol diacetate (p.1415·3); benzethonium chloride (p.1169·2).
*Ear infection.*

**Acetat-Haemodialyse** *Alte Kreis, Austria†.*
Sodium chloride; potassium chloride; magnesium chloride; calcium chloride; sodium acetate; with or without glucose (p.1221·1).
*Haemodialysis solutions.*

**Acetazone Forte** *Technilab, Canad.*
Chlorzoxazone (p.1392·3); paracetamol (p.76·2).
*Pain; skeletal muscle spasm.*

**Acetazone Forte C8** *Technilab, Canad.*
Chlorzoxazone (p.1392·3); paracetamol (p.76·2); codeine phosphate (p.27·1).
*Pain; skeletal muscle spasm.*

**Acetec** *Biolab, Malaysia.*
Enalapril maleate (p.909·2).
*Heart failure; hypertension.*

**Aceten**
*Wockhardt, India; Biotech, S.Afr.*
Captopril (p.879·2).
*Diabetic nephropathy; heart failure; hypertension; myocardial infarction.*

**Acetensil** *Andromaco, Spain.*
Enalapril maleate (p.909·2).
*Heart failure; hypertension.*

**Acetensil Plus** *Andromaco, Spain.*
Enalapril maleate (p.909·2); hydrochlorothiazide (p.933·2).
*Hypertension.*

**Acetest**
*Bayer, Canad.; Bayer Diagnostics, Fr.; Bayer Diagnostics, Irl.; Bayer Diagnostics, Mex.; Bayer Diagnostics, UK; Bayer, USA.*
Test for ketones in urine, plasma, or serum.
In the UK these are described in the Drug Tariff as Nitroprusside Reagent Tablets (Rothera's Tablets).

**Aceticil** *Cazi, Braz.*
Aspirin (p.15·1).
*Fever; inflammation; pain; thromboembolism prophylaxis.*

**Acetif** *Novag, Mex.*
Paracetamol (p.76·2).
*Fever; pain.*

**Acetin**
*Note. This name is used for preparations of different composition.*
*Millet Roux, Braz.†; IQFA, Mex.*
Aspirin (p.15·1).
*Fever; inflammation; pain; thromboembolism prophylaxis.*

*LBS, Thai.*
Acetylcysteine (p.1112·3).
*Respiratory-tract disorders.*

**Acetocaustin** *Temmler, Ger.*
Monochloroacetic acid (p.1154·2).
*Verrucas.*

**Acetocaustine** *Asta Medica, Switz.*
Monochloroacetic acid (p.1154·2).
*Warts.*

**Acetofen** *Medley, Braz.*
Paracetamol (p.76·2).
*Fever; pain.*

**Acetoflux** *EMS, Braz.*
Medroxyprogesterone acetate (p.1557·2).
*Progestogenic.*

**Acetolit** *Mertens, Arg.*
Paracetamol (p.76·2).
*Fever; pain.*

**Acetolyt**
*Madaus, Austria; Combustin, Ger.*
Calcium-sodium-hydrogencitrate.
*Acidosis.*

**Acetonal** *Brady, Austria.*
Aluminium acetotartrate (p.1652·3); trichlorisobutyl salicylate.
*Anorectal disorders.*

**Acetopt**
*Sigma, Austral.; Sigma, NZ.*
Sulfacetamide sodium (p.257·3).
*Bacterial eye infections.*

**Acetosal** *Rekah, Israel.*
Aspirin (p.15·1).
*Fever; inflammation; pain.*

**Acetoxyl** *Stiefel, Canad.*
Benzoyl peroxide (p.1143·2).
*Acne.*

**Acetuber** *Teofarma, Spain.*
Cocarboxylase (p.1455·2); dimenhydrinate (p.431·1); glucose (p.1432·2); pyridoxine (p.1457·2); potassium chloride (p.1232·2).
Formerly contained cocarboxylase, dimenhydrinate, glucose, pyridoxine, potassium chloride, and dibasic sodium phosphate.
*Acetonaemia; vomiting in pregnancy.*

**Acetylcodone** *UCB, Belg.*
Acetyldihydrocodeine hydrochloride (p.1114·2).
*Coughs.*

**Acetylin** *Bristol-Myers Squibb, Ger.*
Aspirin (p.15·1).
*Fever; pain.*

**Acetyst** *Ritsert, Ger.*
Acetylcysteine (p.1112·3).
*Respiratory-tract disorders associated with increased or viscous mucus.*

**Acevit** *Recalcine, Chile.*
Vitamin A palmitate; ergocalciferol; ascorbic acid (p.1417·1).
*Vitamin supplement.*

**Acevor** *Help, Gr.*
Roxithromycin (p.254·2).
*Bacterial infections.*

**Acezide** *Bristol-Myers Squibb, UK.*
Captopril (p.879·2); hydrochlorothiazide (p.933·2).
These ingredients can be described by the British Approved Name Co-zidocapt.
*Hypertension.*

**AC-FA** *Pharmasant, Thai.†.*
Ketoconazole (p.403·3).
*Fungal skin infections.*

**Acfol**
*Cazi, Braz.; ITF, Port.; Italfarmaco, Spain.*
Folic acid (p.1429·1).
*Folic acid deficiency; prevention of neural tube defects in pregnancy.*

**Aches/Pains** *Homeocan, Canad.*
Homoeopathic preparation.

**Achromide** *Propan, S.Afr.*
Merbromin (p.1185·3); acriflavinium chloride (p.1165·3); sulfanilamide (p.263·2); zinc oxide (p.1163·2); cod-liver oil (p.1425·2).
*Burns; ulcers; wounds.*

**Achromycin**
*Sigma, Austral.; Wyeth Lederle, Austria; Wyeth-Ayerst, Canad.†; Wyeth Lederle, Denm.†; Lederle, Ger.; Wyeth Lederle, India; Lederle, Irl.†; Lederle, S.Afr.†; Wyeth Lederle, Swed.†; Wyeth-Ayerst, Thai.; Wyeth, UK†.*
Tetracycline hydrochloride (p.266·2).
*Amoebiasis; bacterial infections.*

**Achromycin V**
*Sigma, Austral.; Wyeth-Ayerst, Canad.†; Lederle, Hong Kong†; Lederle, USA.*
Tetracycline hydrochloride (p.266·2).
*Bacterial infections.*

**Achromycine** *Lederle, Switz.†.*
Tetracycline hydrochloride (p.266·2).
*Bacterial infections.*

**Aci Tip** *Roemmers, Arg.*
Magaldrate (p.1271·3); simeticone (p.1289·2).
*Gastric hyperacidity.*

**Aciben** *Mavi, Mex.†.*
Aspirin (p.15·1).

**Acic**
*Hexal, Austria; Hexal, Ger.*
Aciclovir (p.626·1) or aciclovir sodium (p.626·1).
*Herpesvirus infections.*

**Aciclin** *Fidia, Ital.*
Aciclovir (p.626·1).
*Herpesvirus infections.*

**Aciclo** *Ahimsa, Arg.*
Aciclovir (p.626·1).

**Aciclobene** *Ratiopharm, Austria.*
Aciclovir (p.626·1) or aciclovir sodium (p.626·1).
*Herpesvirus infections.*

**Aciclobeta** *Betapharm, Ger.*
Aciclovir (p.626·1).
*Herpesvirus infections.*

**Aciclodan** *Pharmacodane, Denm.*
Aciclovir (p.626·1).
*Herpesvirus infections.*

**Aciclomed** *Cimed, Braz.*
Aciclovir (p.626·1).

**Aciclor** *Hertz, Braz.†.*
Aciclovir (p.626·1).
*Herpesvirus infections.*

**Aciclosina** *Cipan, Port.*
Aciclovir (p.626·1).
*Herpesvirus infections.*

**Aciclostad**
*Stada, Austria; Stada, Ger.; Ciclum, Spain.*
Aciclovir (p.626·1).
*Herpesvirus infections.*

**Aciclotyrol** *Tyrol, Austria.*
Aciclovir (p.626·1) or aciclovir sodium (p.626·1).
*Herpes simplex infections; varicella zoster infections.*

**Acic-Ophtal** *Winzer, Ger.*
Aciclovir (p.626·1).
*Herpes simplex eye infections.*

**Acicvir** *Pacific, NZ.*
Aciclovir (p.626·1).
*Herpesvirus infections.*

**Acid A Vit** *Pierre Fabre, Neth.†.*
Tretinoin (p.1161·1).
*Acne.*

**Acid Control** *Novopharm, Canad.; Stanley, Canad.*
Famotidine (p.1265·2).

**Acid Halt** *Wampole, Canad.*
Famotidine (p.1265·2).

**Acid Mantle**
*Darier, Mex.*
Emollient.
*Skin irritation.*

*Sandoz Consumer, USA.*
An ointment base.

**Acid Reducer** *Genpharm, Canad.; Stanley, Canad.*
Ranitidine hydrochloride (p.1285·2).

**Acide acetylsalicylique comp. "Radix"** *Streuli, Switz.*
Aspirin (p.15·1); paracetamol (p.76·2); codeine hydrochloride (p.27·1); lidocaine hydrochloride (p.1377·3).
*Fever; pain.*

**Aciderm** *Sanval, Braz.*
Ketoconazole (p.403·3).
*Fungal infections.*

**Acidern** *Sanval, Braz.†.*
Undecenoic acid (p.410·3); triacetin (p.410·2); lidocaine hydrochloride (p.1377·3).
*Fungal skin infections.*

**Acidex**
*Note. This name is used for preparations of different composition.*
*Armstrong, Arg.*
Ranitidine hydrochloride (p.1285·2).
*Gastritis; gastro-oesophageal reflux; gastrointestinal haemorrhage; peptic ulcer; Zollinger-Ellison syndrome.*

*Heralds, Braz.†.*
Aluminium hydroxide (p.1249·2); magnesium hydroxide (p.1272·2); aluminium hydroxide-magnesium carbonate co-dried gel (p.1250·1); dimethicone (p.1289·2).
*Flatulence; gastrointestinal hyperacidity.*

*Pinewood, Irl.; Pinewood, UK.*
Sodium alginate (p.1577·1); sodium bicarbonate (p.1223·2); calcium carbonate (p.1254·2).
*Flatulence; gastro-oesophageal reflux; heartburn.*

*Salters, S.Afr.†.*
Aluminium hydroxide gel (p.1249·2).
*Dyspepsia; heartburn.*

**Acid-Eze** *Norton, UK†.*
Cimetidine (p.1255·3).
*Dyspepsia; heartburn.*

**Acidin** *East India Pharma, India.*
Aluminium hydroxide (p.1249·2); magnesium hydroxide (p.1272·2); simeticone (p.1289·2).
*Flatulence; gastritis; gastrointestinal hyperacidity; peptic ulcer.*

**Acidine** *Upha, Malaysia.*
Famotidine (p.1265·2).
*Peptic ulcer; Zollinger-Ellison syndrome.*

**Acidion** *Inibsa, Spain.*
Aluminium hydroxide (p.1249·2); dimethicone (p.1289·2); magnesium carbonate (p.1272·1); magnesium hydroxide (p.1272·2).
*Dyspepsia; flatulence; gastrointestinal hyperacidity.*

**Acidix** *Solfran, Mex.*
Nalidixic acid (p.234·1).
*Urinary-tract infections.*

**Acid-Lac** *Remexa, Mex.*
Lactic acid (p.1704·1).
*Maintenance of normal skin pH.*

**Acidodermil** *Vifor, Switz.†.*
Bornyl salicylate (p.21·2); mint oil (p.1715·2); rosemary oil (p.1740·2).
*Skin disorders.*

**Acidofilofago** *Roux-Ocefa, Arg.*
*Lactobacillus acidophilus* (p.1704·2).
*Diarrhoea; enterocolitis.*

**Acidophilus** *Novartis Consumer, Ger.*
*Lactobacillus acidophilus* (p.1704·2).
*Gastrointestinal disorders.*

**Acidophilus Bifidus** *Blackmores, Austral.†.*
*Lactobacillus acidophilus* (p.1704·2); *Bifidobacterium bifidum* (p.1704·2).
*Maintenance of normal gastrointestinal flora.*

**Acidophilus Complex** *Neo-Life, Austral.†.*
*Lactobacillus acidophilus* (p.1704·2); *Lactobacillus bulgaricus* (p.1704·2); *Bifidobacterium bifidum* (*Bacillus bifidus*) (p.1704·2).
*Digestive disorders.*

**Acidophilus Plus**
*Note. This name is used for preparations of different composition.*
*GNLD, Austral.†.*
*Lactobacillus acidophilus* (p.1704·2); *Bifidobacterium bifidum* (p.1704·2); *Lactobacillus bulgaricus* (p.1704·2); *Lactobacillus casei*; *Streptococcus thermophilus* (p.1704·2).
*Digestive disorders.*

*Quest, UK.*
*Lactobacillus acidophilus* (p.1704·2); *Lactobacillus rhamnosus* (p.1704·2); *Bifidobacterium bifidum* (p.1704·2); *Enterococcus faecium* (p.1704·2).

**Acidophilus Tablets** *Vitaglow, Austral.†.*
*Lactobacillus acidophilus* (p.1704·2).
*Digestive disorders.*

**Acidosis** *Potter's, UK.*
*Oral liquid:* Meadowsweet (p.1710·1); compound gentian infusion (p.1692·2); euonymus (p.1265·2).
*Dyspepsia; flatulence; heartburn.*
*Tablets:* Meadowsweet (p.1710·1); vegetable charcoal (p.1030·3); rhubarb (p.1287·3).
*Dyspepsia; gastric hyperacidity; heartburn.*

**Acidovert** *Klein, Ger.*
Calcium citrate (p.1225·1); magnesium citrate (p.1272·1).
*Acid-base regulation; metabolic acidosis.*

**Acidown** *Brunel, S.Afr.†.*
Cimetidine (p.1255·3).
*Gastrointestinal disorders.*

**Acidrina** *Solvay, Spain†.*
Aluminium hydroxide (p.1249·2); dimethicone (p.1289·2); magnesium hydroxide (p.1272·2).
*Dyspepsia; flatulence; gastrointestinal hyperacidity.*

**Acidrine**
*Teofarma, Austria†; Solvay, Belg.†; Teofarma, Fr.; Cheplapharm, Ger.; Teofarma, Ital.*
Myrtecaine laurilsulfate (p.1381·3); aluminium glycinate (p.1249·1); galactane sulfate.
*Gastrointestinal disorders.*

**Acidum phosphoricum Med Complex** *Dynamit, Austria.*
Homoeopathic preparation.

**Acidum picrinicum Med Complex** *Dynamit, Austria.*
Homoeopathic preparation.

**Acidumphos-Gastreu** *Reckeweg, Ger.*
Homoeopathic preparation.
Formerly known as Diabetes-Gastreu S R40.

**Acid-X** *BDI, USA.*
Paracetamol (p.76·2); calcium carbonate (p.1254·2).
*Gastrointestinal disorders.*

**Acidylina** *Fermenti, Ital.†.*
Ascorbic acid (p.1460·2).

**Aciflux**
*Note. This name is used for preparations of different composition.*
*Andromaco, Chile.*
Ranitidine hydrochloride (p.1285·2).
*Dyspepsia; gastric hyperacidity.*

*SmithKline Beecham, Neth.*
Cimetidine (p.1255·3); alginic acid (p.1576·3).
*Gastro-oesophageal reflux.*

**Acifol**
*Note. This name is used for preparations of different composition.*
*Dominguez, Arg.*
Folic acid (p.1429·1).

*Fustery, Mex.*
Propranolol (p.990·1).

**Acifolico** *Elofar, Braz.†.*
Folic acid (p.1429·1).
*Anaemias.*

**Aciforin** *Pharmonta, Austria.*
Formic acid (p.1689·3); methyl salicylate (p.59·3); turpentine oil (p.1760·1).
*Musculoskeletal pain.*

**Acifugan**
*Henning, Ger.†; Jaba, Port.; Lacer, Spain; Synthelabo, Switz.†.*
Allopurinol (p.412·2); benzbromarone (p.414·3).
*Gout; hyperuricaemia.*

**Acifur** *Fustery, Mex.*
Aciclovir (p.626·1).
*Herpesvirus infections.*

**Acigon** *Nicholas Piramal, India.*
Alginic acid (p.1576·3) or sodium alginate (p.1577·1); aluminium hydroxide (p.1249·2); magnesium trisilicate (p.1272·3); sodium bicarbonate (p.1223·2).
*Gastro-oesophageal reflux.*

**Acihexal** *Hexal, Austral.*
Aciclovir (p.626·1).
*Herpesvirus infections.*

**Aci-Jel**
*Note. This name is used for preparations of different composition.*
*Janssen-Cilag, Austral.; Janssen-Cilag, NZ; Ortho McNeil, USA†.*
Glacial acetic acid (p.1645·2); hydroxyquinoline sulfate (p.1700·1); ricinoleic acid (p.1738·3); glycerol (p.1694·3).
*Maintenance of vaginal acidity.*

*Janssen-Cilag, Irl.; Janssen-Cilag, UK.*
Acetic acid (p.1645·2).
*Vaginal infections.*

**Acilac**
*Note. This name is used for preparations of different composition.*
*Euroderm, Arg.*
Alpha hydroxyacid; vitamin E (p.1464·3); urea (p.1162·2).
*Dry skin.*

*Technilab, Canad.*
Lactulose (p.1269·1).
*Constipation; hepatic encephalopathy.*

**Acilax** *Jean-Marie, Hong Kong.*
Aciclovir (p.626·1).
*Herpesvirus infections.*

**Acilen** *IFI, Ital.†.*
Acetylcarnitine or acetylcarnitine hydrochloride (p.1646·1).
*Cerebrovascular disorders; peripheral neuropathy.*

**Acilin** *Berman, Mex.*
Charcoal (p.1030·2); iodochloride; papaverine (p.1728·1).
*Gastrointestinal astringent.*

**Aciloc**
*Note. This name is used for preparations of different composition.*
*Orion, Denm.; Orion, Swed.†.*
Cimetidine (p.1255·3).
*Acid aspiration; gastro-oesophageal reflux; gastrointestinal haemorrhage; peptic ulcer; Zollinger-Ellison syndrome.*

*Cadila Pharma, India; Cadila, Thai.*
Ranitidine hydrochloride (p.1285·2).
*Dyspepsia; gastro-oesophageal reflux; gastrointestinal hyperacidity; peptic ulcer; Zollinger-Ellison syndrome.*

**Acimax** *Alphapharm, Austral.*
Omeprazole magnesium (p.1278·2).
*Gastro-oesophageal reflux; peptic ulcer; Zollinger-Ellison syndrome.*

**Acimed** *Sanitas, Arg.*
*Note. A similar name is used for preparations of different composition (see below).*
Omeprazole (p.1278·2).
*Acid aspiration; gastro-oesophageal reflux; peptic ulcer; Zollinger-Ellison syndrome.*

**Aci-Med** *Triomed, S.Afr.*
*Note. A similar name is used for preparations of different composition (see above).*
Cimetidine (p.1255·3).
*Gastro-oesophageal reflux; peptic ulcer; upper gastrointestinal haemorrhage; Zollinger-Ellison syndrome.*

**Acimethin**
*Madaus, Austria; Gry, Ger.; Vifor, Switz.*
Methionine (p.1042·1).
*Adjunct in antibiotic therapy; paracetamol overdosage; renal calculi; urinary-tract disorders.*

**Acimol** *Pfleger, Ger.*
Methionine (p.1042·1).
*Renal calculi; urine acidification.*

**Acimox** *Diba, Mex.*
Amoxicillin trihydrate (p.155·3).
*Bacterial infections.*

**Acimox-Ex** *Diba, Mex.*
Amoxicillin trihydrate (p.155·3); ambroxol hydrochloride (p.1114·3).
*Respiratory-tract infections.*

**Acimpil** *Farcoral, Mex.†.*
Ampicillin (p.157·1).
*Bacterial infections.*

**Acinal** *Tegur, Mex.†.*
Nalidixic acid (p.234·1).

**Acinil**
*Gea, Denm.; Gea, Norw.†; Gea, Swed.*
Cimetidine (p.1255·3).
*Acid aspiration; gastro-oesophageal reflux; gastrointestinal haemorrhage; peptic ulcer; Zollinger-Ellison syndrome.*

**Acintor** *Lepetit, Ital.*
*Klebsiella pneumoniae* glycoprotein (p.1703·3).
*Respiratory-tract infections.*

**Acipem** *Caber, Ital.*
Pipemidic acid (p.243·1).
*Urinary-tract infections.*

**Acipen** *Yamanouchi, Neth.*
Phenoxymethylpenicillin potassium (p.242·1).
*Bacterial infections.*

**Acipen-V** *Yamanouchi, Neth.*
Phenoxymethylpenicillin (p.242·1).
*Bacterial infections.*

**Aciphex** *Eisai, USA.*
Rabeprazole sodium (p.1285·1).
*Gastro-oesophageal reflux; peptic ulcer; Zollinger-Ellison syndrome.*

**Aciril** *Molteni, Ital.†.*
Ibuprofen lysine (p.46·3).
*Musculoskeletal and joint disorders.*

**Acirufan** *Laetitia, Ger.*
Homoeopathic preparation.

**Aci-Sanorania** *Sanorania, Ger.†.*
Aciclovir (p.626·1).
*Herpesvirus infections.*

**Acistin** *Piam, Ital.†.*
Infant feed (p.1417·1).
*Cystinosis.*

**Acitab** *Mavi, Mex.*
Aspirin (p.15·1).
*Pain.*

**Acitak** *Trinity, UK.*
Cimetidine (p.1255·3).
*Acid aspiration; gastro-oesophageal reflux; peptic ulcer; Zollinger-Ellison syndrome.*

**Aci-Tip** *Pharma Investi, Chile.*
Magaldrate (p.1271·3); simeticone (p.1289·2).
*Flatulence; gastric hyperacidity; gastritis; gastro-oesophageal reflux.*

**Acitop** *Cipla-Medpro, S.Afr.*
Aciclovir (p.626·1).
*Herpes labialis.*

**Acitra** *Procter & Gamble, Braz.†.*
Benzethonium chloride (p.1169·2); vitamin C (p.1460·2).
*Mouth disinfection.*

**Acitrom** *Sarabhai Piramal, India.*
Acenocoumarol (p.848·3).
*Thromboembolic disorders.*

**Acival** *Geminis, Arg.*
Nimodipine (p.972·3).
*Cerebrovascular disorders.*

**Aciveral** *Bunker, Braz.*
Aciclovir (p.626·1).

**Acivir**
*Curasan, Ger.; Cipla, India; Cipla, Israel.*
Aciclovir (p.626·1) or aciclovir sodium (p.626·1).
*Herpes simplex infections.*

**Acks** *BPL, India.*
Ibuprofen (p.45·3); mephenesin (p.1394·3); methyl salicylate (p.59·3); menthol (p.1711·3).
*Musculoskeletal, joint, and soft-tissue disorders.*

**Aclacin** *Medac, UK†.*
Aclarubicin hydrochloride (p.525·2).
*Acute myeloid leukaemia.*

**Aclaplastin** *Medac, Ger.†.*
Aclarubicin hydrochloride (p.525·2).
*Myeloid leukaemia.*

**Aclav** *Disprovent, Arg.*
Amoxicillin (p.155·3); clavulanic acid (p.193·3).
*Bacterial infections.*

**Aclimafel** *AF, Mex.*
Veralipride (p.727·2).
*Menopausal disorders.*

**Aclin**
*Alphapharm, Austral; Alphapharm, Hong Kong; Alphapharm, Malaysia; Merck, Malaysia.*
Sulindac (p.91·2).
*Musculoskeletal and joint disorders; pain with inflammation.*

**Aclinda** *Azupharma, Ger.*
Clindamycin hydrochloride (p.194·2).
*Bacterial infections.*

**Aclon Lievit** *Geymonat, Ital.†.*
Dried yeast (p.1469·1); vitamins (p.1417·1); echinacea (p.1683·2); betacarotene (p.1422·3).
*Acne; seborrhoea.*

**Aclonium** *SmithKline Beecham, Ital.†.*
Gabapentin (p.362·2).
*Epilepsy.*

**Aclophen** *Nutripharm, USA.*
Phenylephrine hydrochloride (p.1126·3); paracetamol (p.76·2); chlorphenamine maleate (p.427·3).
*Upper respiratory-tract symptoms.*

**Acloral** *Liomont, Mex.*
Ranitidine hydrochloride (p.1285·2).
*Acid aspiration; gastro-oesophageal reflux; gastrointestinal haemorrhage; peptic ulcer; Zollinger-Ellison syndrome.*

**Aclorisan** *Dovalle, Braz.*
Aluminium hydroxide (p.1249·2); magnesium hydroxide (p.1272·2); dimethicone (p.1289·2).
*Flatulence; gastrointestinal hyperacidity.*

**Aclosan** *Gobbi, Arg.*
Tamsulosin hydrochloride (p.1009·2).
*Benign prostatic hyperplasia.*

**Aclosone**
*Schering-Plough, Fr.†; Schering-Plough, Neth.; Schering-Plough, S.Afr.†.*
Alclometasone dipropionate (p.1090·3).
*Skin disorders.*

**Aclotan** *Piam, Ital.*
Dermatan sulfate sodium (p.892·2).
*Thrombosis prophylaxis.*

**Aclotine** *Lab Francais du Fractionnement, Fr.*
Antithrombin (human) (p.742·2).
*Thromboembolic disorders.*

**Aclovate** *Glaxo Wellcome, USA.*
Alclometasone dipropionate (p.1090·3).
*Skin disorders.*

**Aclovir** *Ratiopharm, Fin.*
Aciclovir (p.626·1).
*Herpes simplex infections; varicella-zoster infections.*

**ACM 20** *ACM, Fr.*
Multivitamin, mineral, and amino-acid preparation (p.1417·1).

**Acnacyl**
*Rosken, Hong Kong; Pfizer Consumer, Singapore.*
Benzoyl peroxide (p.1143·2).
*Acne.*

**Acnaid** *Stiefel, Chile.*
*Cream:* Sulfur (p.1158·2); resorcinol (p.1156·3); chloroxylenol (p.1177·2).
*Soap:* Sulphonated rice bran oil; sulfonated mustard oil; liquid paraffin (p.1479·1).
*Acne.*

**Acnase** *Zurita, Braz.*
Benzoyl peroxide (p.1143·2); sulfur (p.1158·2).
*Acne.*

**Acnaveen**
*Note. This name is used for preparations of different composition.*
*Rydelle, Fr.†; Dermoteca, Port.†.*
Avena (p.1658·2); salicylic acid (p.1157·1); carbocisteine (p.1116·2).
*Acne; seborrhoea.*

*Johnson & Johnson, Ital.*
Avena (p.1658·2); salicylic acid (p.1157·1).
*Acne; seborrhoea.*

*Bioglan, UK†.*
Sulfur (p.1158·2); salicylic acid (p.1157·1).
*Acne.*

**Acne** *Homeocan, Canad.*
Homoeopathic preparation.

**Acne Blemish Cream** *Bonne Bell, Canad.†.*
Sulfur (p.1158·2).
*Acne.*

**Acne Creme** *Widmer, Switz.*
Salicylic acid (p.1157·1); colloidal sulfur (p.1158·2); colloidal silicon dioxide (p.1581·3); triclosan (p.1195·2).
*Acne.*

**Acne Creme Plus** *Widmer, Switz.*
Benzoyl peroxide (p.1143·2); miconazole nitrate (p.405·3).
*Acne.*

**Acne Derm** *Fischer, Israel.*
Benzoyl peroxide (p.1143·2).
*Acne.*

**Acne Gel** *Widmer, Switz.*
Colloidal sulfur (p.1158·2); pyridoxine hydrochloride (p.1456·3); triclosan (p.1195·2); urea (p.1162·2).
*Acne.*

**Acne Hermal** *Olvos, Gr.*
Erythromycin (p.208·1).
*Acne.*

**Acne Lotion** *Widmer, Switz.*
Salicylic acid (p.1157·1); lactic acid (p.1704·1); triclosan (p.1195·2); zinc sulfate (p.1469·3); magnesium sulfate dihydrate (p.1228·2).
*Acne.*

**Acne Lotion 10** *C & M, USA.*
Sulfur (p.1158·2).
*Acne.*

**Acne Mask** *Neutrogena, Israel.*
Benzoyl peroxide (p.1143·2).
*Acne.*

**Acne Oral Spray** *Brauer, Austral.†.*
Lappa (p.1704·3); artemisia abrotanum; bellis perennis; fumaria; hepar sulf; juglans reg.; kali brom.; nat. mur.; rhus ven.; saponaria; selenium; sulfur; sulfur iod.; viola tric.
*Acne.*

**Acne & Pimple Gel** *Curacel, Austral.*
Sulfur (p.1158·2); allantoin (p.1141·3); zinc oxide (p.1163·2); resorcinol (p.1156·3); *dl*-alpha tocoferil acetate; vitamin A palmitate; eicosapentaenoic acid.
*Acne.*

**Acne Plus**
*Widmer, Austria; Widmer, Ger.*
Miconazole nitrate (p.405·3); benzoyl peroxide (p.1143·2).
*Acne.*

**Acne-Aid**
*Note. This name is used for preparations of different composition.*
*Stiefel, Arg.; Stiefel, Austral.; Stiefel, Braz.†; Stiefel, Canad.; Stiefel, Hong Kong; Stiefel, Israel; Stiefel, Malaysia; Stiefel, Mex.; Stiefel, Singapore; Stiefel, Thai.*
Soap.
*Acne.*

*Stiefel, Canad.†.*
*Topical gel:* Sulfur (p.1158·2); resorcinol (p.1156·3); chloroxylenol (p.1177·2).
*Acne.*

*Stiefel, Hong Kong; Stiefel, Malaysia; Stiefel, Singapore.*
*Cream:* Sulfur (p.1158·2); resorcinol (p.1156·3); chloroxylenol (p.1177·2).
*Acne.*

**Acnecide**
*Galderma, Irl.; Galderma, UK†.*
Benzoyl peroxide (p.1143·2).
*Acne.*

**Acneclear** *Janpharm, S.Afr.*
*Cleansing bar:* Triclosan (p.1195·2).
*Cream:* Miconazole nitrate (p.405·3); benzoyl peroxide (p.1143·2).
*Acne.*

**Acneclin** *ICN, Arg.*
Minocycline hydrochloride (p.231·3).
*Bacterial infections.*

**Acnecolor** *Spirig, Switz.*
Clotrimazole (p.396·2).
*Acne.*

**Acnecure** *Taxandria, Neth.*
Miconazole nitrate (p.405·3); benzoyl peroxide (p.1143·2).
*Acne.*

**Acnederm**
*Note. This name is used for preparations of different composition.*
*Ego, Austral.†; Ego, Hong Kong; Ego, Malaysia; Ego, Singapore.*
Sulfur (p.1158·2); ichthammol (p.1148·2); undecenoic acid monoethanolamide (p.411·1); zinc oxide (p.1163·2).
*Acne.*

*Ego, NZ.*
*Lotion:* Azelaic acid (p.1142·3); phenoxyethanol (p.1189·1).
*Ointment:* Sulfur (p.1158·2); ammoniumsulfobitol (p.1148·2); undecylenic alkanolamide (p.411·1); zinc oxide (p.1163·2); alcloxa (p.1141·2).
*Acne.*

**Acnederm Foaming Wash** *Ego, NZ.*
Cetrimide (p.1172·1); chlorhexidine gluconate (p.1173·2); phenoxyethanol (p.1189·1).
*Acne.*

**Acnederm Wash**
*Note. This name is used for preparations of different composition.*
*Ego, Austral.†; Ego, Malaysia; Ego, Singapore.*
Cetrimide (p.1172·1).
*Acne.*

*Ego, NZ.*
Cetrimide (p.1172·1); chlorhexidine gluconate (p.1173·2); propylene phenoxyethanol.
*Acne.*

**Acnefuge** *Spirig, Switz.*
Benzoyl peroxide (p.1143·2).
*Acne.*

**Acne-Med Wolff Simplex** *Medika, Switz.*
Hexachlorophene (p.1181·2); linoleic acid (p.1690·2); alpha tocoferil acetate (p.1465·1).
*Acne.*

**Acneryne** *Galderma, Belg.*
Erythromycin (p.208·1).
*Acne.*

**Acnesan**
*Note. This name is used for preparations of different composition.*
*Fortbenton, Arg.; QIF, Braz.†.*
Benzoyl peroxide (p.1143·2).
*Acne.*
*Novogaleno, Ital.*
Sulfur (p.1158·2); zinc sulfate (p.1469·3); glycolic acid (p.1147·3); enoxolone (p.36·2).
*Seborrhoea.*

**Acnesoap** *Stiefel, Braz.*
Soap substitute.
*Acne.*

**Acnesol** *Systopic, India.*
Erythromycin (p.208·1).
*Acne.*

**Acnestop** *Euroderm, Arg.*
Clindamycin (p.194·2).
*Acne.*

**Acnetrim**
*Trima, Israel; Trima, Singapore†; Unipharm, Singapore†.*
Erythromycin (p.208·1).
*Acne.*

**Acnetrol** *Lagos, Arg.*
*Lotion:* Mallow (p.1709·3); calendula (p.1665·2); rosemary (p.1740·2); enebro (p.1159·2).
*Topical gel:* Chamomile (p.1669·3); trepadora; sage (p.1741·2); rosemary (p.1740·2).
*Skin disorders.*

**Acnex**
*Note. This name is used for preparations of different composition.*
*Dermtek, Canad.*
Salicylic acid (p.1157·1).
*Acne.*
*Rafa, Israel.*
Hexachlorophene (p.1181·2); tyrothricin (p.275·1); resorcinol (p.1156·3); sulfur (p.1158·2); zinc oxide (p.1163·2).
*Acne; dermatitis; eczema.*

**Acnexyl** *Pharmasant, Thai.*
Benzoyl peroxide (p.1143·2).
*Acne.*

**Acnezaic** *Pfizer Consumer, Ital.*
Azelaic acid (p.1142·3).
*Acne.*

**Acnidazil**
*Janssen-Cilag, Austria†; Janssen-Cilag, Belg.†; Janssen-Cilag, Denm.†; Janssen-Cilag, Ger.†; Italchimici, Ital.; Janssen-Cilag, Neth.; Janssen-Cilag, S.Afr.; Johnson & Johnson MSD Consumer, UK†.*
Miconazole nitrate (p.405·3); benzoyl peroxide (p.1143·2).
*Acne.*

**Acnisal**
*Dermapharm, Irl.; Dermapharm, UK.*
Salicylic acid (p.1157·1).
*Acne.*

**Acnisdin** *Isdin, Spain.*
Sulfur (p.1158·2); calcium dobesilate (p.1664·2); resorcinol (p.1156·3).
*Acne.*

**Acnisdin Retinoico** *Isdin, Spain.*
Calcium dobesilate (p.1664·2); tretinoin (p.1161·1).
*Acne; psoriasis.*

**Acno** *Baker Cummins, USA.*
Sulfur (p.1158·2); salicylic acid (p.1157·1).
*Acne.*

**Acno Cleanser** *Baker Cummins, USA.*
Skin cleanser.

**Acnoil Free** *Dermoteca, Port.*
Magnesium silicate (p.1580·2); aluminium silicate (p.1250·2).
*Acne.*

**Acnomel**
*Note. This name is used for preparations of different composition.*
*Key, Arg.*
Resorcinol (p.1156·3); sulfur (p.1158·2).
*Acne.*
*Chattem, Canad.†.*
*Cream:* Resorcinol (p.1156·3); sulfur (p.1158·2); isopropyl alcohol (p.1184·3).
*Vanishing cream:* Resorcinol (p.1156·3); sulfur (p.1158·2).
*Acne.*
*Numark, USA.*
Resorcinol (p.1156·3); sulfur (p.1158·2); titanium dioxide (p.1160·3).
*Acne.*

**Acnomel Acne Mask** *Chattem, Canad.†.*
Resorcinol (p.1156·3); sulfur (p.1158·2).
Formerly contained salicylic acid.
*Acne.*

**Acnosan** *Bescansa, Spain†.*
Camphor (p.1665·3); boric acid (p.1662·1); resorcinol (p.1156·3); salicylic acid (p.1157·1); undecenoic acid (p.410·3); zinc sulfate (p.1469·3); copper sulfate (p.1426·1).
*Acne.*

**Acnosil** *Heralds, Braz.†.*
Benzoyl peroxide (p.1143·2); sulfur (p.1158·2).
*Acne.*

**Acnotex** *C & M, USA.*
Sulfur (p.1158·2); salicylic acid (p.1157·1); methylbenzethonium chloride (p.1186·1).
*Acne.*

**A1cNOW** *Metrika, USA.*
Test for glycosylated haemoglobin in blood.

**Acnoxin** *Andromaco, Arg.*
Salicylic acid (p.1157·1); resorcinol monoacetate (p.1156·3); chloramphenicol (p.185·1).
*Acne.*

**Acnoxyl Abrasivo** *Koni-Cofarm, Chile.*
Essential fatty acids; melaleuca oil (p.1710·2).
*Acne.*

**Acnoxyl Gel Cuidado Intensivo** *Koni-Cofarm, Chile.*
Melaleuca oil (p.1710·2).
*Acne.*

**Acnoxyl Gel De Limpieza** *Koni-Cofarm, Chile.*
Melaleuca oil (p.1710·2).
*Acne.*

**Acnoxyl Gel Humectante** *Koni-Cofarm, Chile.*
Melaleuca oil (p.1710·2); collagen (p.1674·3).
*Acne.*

**Acnoxyl Jabon** *Koni-Cofarm, Chile.*
Palmitic acid; oleic acid (p.1481·3); docosahexaenoic acid (p.976·1); liquid paraffin (p.1479·1); melaleuca oil (p.1710·2).
*Acne.*

**Acnoxyl Jabon Liquido** *Koni-Cofarm, Chile.*
Melaleuca oil (p.1710·2); alfa hydroxy acids; glycerol (p.1694·3).
*Acne.*

**Acnoxyl Locion Tonica** *Koni-Cofarm, Chile.*
Melaleuca oil (p.1710·2); alfa hydroxy acids; alcohol (p.1166·1); menthol (p.1711·3).
*Acne.*

**Acnoxyl Shampoo Cabello Graso** *Koni-Cofarm, Chile.*
Melaleuca oil (p.1710·2); dexpanthenol (p.1727·2); menthol (p.1711·3).
*Seborrhoeic dermatitis.*

**Acnoxyl Stick Corrector** *Koni-Cofarm, Chile.*
Melaleuca oil (p.1710·2).
*Acne.*

**ACNU**
*Baxter Oncology, Ger.; Viatris, Neth.; Asta Medica, Switz.*
Nimustine hydrochloride (p.576·3).
*Malignant neoplasms.*

**Acobiotic** *Heralds, Braz.†.*
Tetracycline hydrochloride (p.266·2); thiamphenicol (p.269·2).
*Bacterial infections.*

**Acocontin** *Modi-Mundipharma, India.*
Ambroxol hydrochloride (p.1114·3).
*Respiratory-tract disorders associated with viscous mucus.*

**Acodon** *Nakorn, Thai.*
Dipyrone (p.35·3).
*Fever; pain.*

**Acoflam** *Goldshield, UK.*
Diclofenac sodium (p.32·1).
*Gout; inflammation; musculoskeletal, joint, and periarticular disorders; pain.*

**Acoin** *Combustin, Ger.*
Tetracaine hydrochloride (p.1385·1); lauromacrogol 400 (p.1412·3).
*Local anaesthesia.*

**Acolitium** *Igefarma, Braz.†.*
Lithium carbonate (p.301·1).
*Nutritional supplement.*

**Acolyt** *Modi-Mundipharma, India.*
Ambroxol hydrochloride (p.1114·3).
*Respiratory-tract disorders associated with viscous mucus.*

**Acon** *Aventis, Mex.*
Vitamin A palmitate (p.1453·1).
*Vitamin A deficiency.*

**Acondicionador Labial** *Rider, Chile.*
*SPF 15:* Padimate o (p.1155·1); oxybenzone (p.1154·3).
*Sunscreen.*

**Aconeurin** *Heralds, Braz.†.*
Vitamin B substances (p.1417·1).
*Vitamin B deficiency.*

**Aconex** *Agepha, Austria.*
Naphazoline hydrochloride (p.1124·3).
*Conjunctivitis.*

**Aconit Schmerzol** *Wala, Ger.*
Homoeopathic preparation.

**Aconitum**
*Truw, Ger.†; Weleda, Ger.*
Homoeopathic preparation.

**Aconitum Med Complex** *Dynamit, Austria.*
Homoeopathic preparation.

**Aconitum-Homaccord** *Peithner, Austria.*
Homoeopathic preparation.

**Acordin** *Mepha, Switz.*
Isosorbide dinitrate (p.941·1).
*Angina pectoris; heart failure; myocardial infarction.*

**Acorus** *Zeppenfeldt, Ger.*
Couch-grass (p.1676·2).
*Urinary-tract disorders.*

**Acotoss** *Neckerman, Braz.†.*
Diphenhydramine hydrochloride (p.431·3); sodium citrate (p.1223·2); ammonium chloride (p.1115·2).
*Coughs and cold symptoms.*

**Acovil** *Aventis, Spain.*
Ramipril (p.994·1).
*Diabetic nephropathy; heart failure following myocardial infarction; hypertension; myocardial infarction prevention.*

**Acpan** *Gray, Arg.*
Glycopyrronium bromide (p.482·3).

**Acqta** *Rayere, Mex.*
Loperamide (p.1271·2).
*Diarrhoea.*

**Acqua di Sirmione** *Terme Sirmione, Ital.*
Sulfurous thermal water (p.1158·2).
*Catarrh; cold symptoms; rhinitis; sinusitis.*

**Acqua Virginiana** *Kelemata, Ital.*
Hamamelis (p.1696·3).
*Skin irritation.*

**Acridin** *Legrand, Braz.*
Acriflavinium chloride (p.1165·3); methenamine (p.230·1); methylthioninium chloride (p.1042·2); belladonna (p.479·1).
*Urinary-tract infections.*

**Acriflex** *SSL, UK.*
Chlorhexidine gluconate (p.1173·2).
*Burns; scalds; wounds.*

**Acrisuxin**
*Chemomedica, Austria†; Geistlich, Switz.†.*
Ethosuximide (p.360·1); mepacrine hydrochloride (p.606·3).
*Absence seizures.*

**Acromax**
*Note. This name is used for preparations of different composition.*
*Agepha, Austria.*
Sodium cromoglicate (p.795·3).
*Allergic conjunctivitis; allergic rhinitis.*
*Climax, Braz.*
Adenosine; methionine; betaine; choline; pyridoxine; cyanocobalamin; sorbitol (p.1417·1).
*Digestive disorders; liver disorders.*

**Acromicina**
*Cyanamid, Ital.†; Wyeth, Mex.*
Tetracycline hydrochloride (p.266·2).
*Bacterial infections.*

**Acrosin** *Climax, Braz.*
Liver extract.
*Liver disorders.*

**Acroxil** *Sons, Mex.*
Amoxicillin trihydrate (p.155·3).
*Bacterial infections.*

**Acrylarm** *Poen, Arg.*
Carbomer 940 (p.1577·2).
*Dry eyes.*

**Acsacea** *Chemomedica, Austria.*
Metronidazole (p.607·2).
*Rosacea.*

**Ac-Sal** *Andromaco, Chile.*
Salicylic acid (p.1157·1); triclosan (p.1195·2); aloe vera (p.1141·3).
*Acne.*

**Acset** *Bio-Transfusion, Fr.†.*
Activated factor VII (p.750·3).
*Haemophilias A and B.*

**ACT** *Johnson & Johnson Medical, USA.*
*Note. A similar name is used for preparations of different composition (see below).*
Sodium fluoride (p.1444·3).
*Dental caries prophylaxis.*

**ACT-3**
*Note. A similar name is used for preparations of different composition (see above).*
*Whitehall Consumer, Austral.; Whitehall, NZ.*
Ibuprofen (p.45·3).
*Fever; inflammation; musculoskeletal and joint disorders; pain.*

**Acta**
*Jean-Marie, Hong Kong; Jean-Marie, Singapore†.*
Tretinoin (p.1161·1).
*Acne.*

**Actacel**
*Aventis Pasteur, Arg.; Aventis Pasteur, Chile; Aventis Pasteur, Singapore; Aventis Pasteur, Thai.*
A diphtheria, tetanus, pertussis, and haemophilus influenzae vaccine (p.1614·2).
*Active immunisation.*

**Actacode** *Sigma, Austral.*
Codeine phosphate (p.27·1).
*Coughs.*

**Actagen** *Goldline, USA.*
Pseudoephedrine hydrochloride (p.1129·2); triprolidine hydrochloride (p.442·3).
*Upper respiratory-tract symptoms.*

**Actagen-C Cough** *Goldline, USA.*
Pseudoephedrine hydrochloride (p.1129·2); codeine phosphate (p.27·1); triprolidine hydrochloride (p.442·3).
*Coughs and cold symptoms.*

**Actal**
*Note. This name is used for preparations of different composition.*
*ICN, Hong Kong; ICN, Malaysia; ICN, Singapore; ICN, Thai.; Merck Consumer, UK.*
Alexitol sodium (p.1248·1).
*Dyspepsia; gastric hyperacidity; heartburn; peptic ulcer.*
*Merck Consumer, UK†.*
*Pastilles:* Hydrotalcite (p.1267·3).
*Dyspepsia; heartburn.*

**Actal Plus**
*Note. This name is used for preparations of different composition.*
*ICN, Hong Kong; ICN, Singapore.*
Aluminium hydroxide (p.1249·2); magnesium hydroxide (p.1272·2); simeticone (p.1289·2).
*Gastric hyperacidity; heartburn; peptic ulcer.*
*ICN, Malaysia.*
Alexitol sodium (p.1248·1); magnesium hydroxide (p.1272·2); simeticone (p.1289·2).
*Gastric hyperacidity; heartburn; peptic ulcer.*

**Actan**
*Note. This name is used for preparations of different composition.*
*Saval, Chile.*
Fluoxetine (p.296·3).
*Bulimia; depression; obsessive-compulsive disorder.*
*Restan, S.Afr.†.*
Alexitol sodium (p.1248·1).
*Hyperchlorhydria; peptic ulcer, gastro-oesophageal reflux.*

**Actapront** *Purissimus, Arg.*
Isothipendyl hydrochloride (p.435·2).
*Pruritus.*

**Actapulgite**
*Ipsen, Belg.; Beaufour, Fr.; Beaufour, Switz.*
Attapulgite (p.1251·1).
*Gastrointestinal disorders.*

**Actebral**
*Note. This name is used for preparations of different composition.*
*Menarini, Belg.*
Cyprodenate (p.1585·3).
*Cerebral disorders.*
*Recalcine, Chile.*
Dedietilaminoetil-p-aminobenzoato hydrochloride; gamma-aminobutyric acid (p.1690·2); haematoporphyrin hydrochloride (p.1696·2).
*Mental function impairment.*

**Acthar**
*Aventis, Irl.; Roche, S.Afr.†; Rorer, UK†; Rhone-Poulenc Rorer, USA.*
Corticotropin (p.1322·1).
Available on a named-patient basis only in the UK.
*Corticosteroid release stimulant; diagnostic testing of adrenocortical function.*

**Acthelea** *Elea, Arg.*
Corticotropin (p.1322·1).
*Corticosteroid release stimulant; diagnostic testing of adrenocortical function.*

**Act-HIB**
*Pasteur Merieux, Austria; Aventis Pasteur, Belg.; Aventis Pasteur, Braz.; Aventis Pasteur, Canad.; Aventis Pasteur, Chile; Aventis Pasteur, Denm.; Aventis Pasteur, Fr.; Aventis Pasteur, Ger.; Vianex (Βιανέξ), Gr.; Aventis Pasteur, Hong Kong; Aventis Pasteur, Irl.; Pasteur Merieux, Israel; Aventis Pasteur, Ital.; Aventis Pasteur, Malaysia; Aventis Pasteur, Neth.; Aventis Pasteur, Norw.; Aventis, S.Afr.; Aventis Pasteur, Singapore; Aventis Pasteur, Spain; Aventis Pasteur, Swed.; Pro Vaccine, Switz.†; Aventis Pasteur, Thai.; Aventis Pasteur, UK†; Pasteur Merieux, USA.*
A haemophilus influenzae conjugate vaccine (tetanus toxoid conjugate) (p.1616·1).
*Active immunisation.*

**Act-HIB DTP** *Aventis Pasteur, UK.*
A diphtheria, tetanus, pertussis, and haemophilus influenzae vaccine (p.1614·2).
*Active immunisation.*

**Act-HIB plus DPT** *Pasteur Merieux, Austria.*
Haemophilus influenzae conjugate vaccine (tetanus toxoid conjugate); diphtheria, tetanus, and pertussis vaccine (p.1614·2).
*Active immunisation.*

**Act-HIB Polio**
*Aventis Pasteur, Norw.; Pasteur Merieux, Swed.†.*
A haemophilus influenzae conjugate vaccine (tetanus toxoid conjugate) and an injectable inactivated poliomyelitis vaccine (types I, II and III) (p.1616·3).
*Active immunisation.*

**Acthrel** *Ferring, USA.*
Corticorelin triflutate (p.1321·3).
*Determination of ACTH production in Cushing's syndrome.*

**Acti 5** *Pierre Fabre, Fr.†.*
*Syrup:* Deanol glutamate; lysine hydrochloride (p.1439·2); calcium gluconogluceptate; phosphoric acid (p.1731·2).
*Pierre Fabre Sante, Fr.*
*Oral liquid:* Deanol glutamate or deanol pidolate (p.1585·3); sodium ascorbate (p.1460·2); magnesium aminobenzoate.
Formerly contained deanol glutamate, sodium ascorbate, magnesium aminobenzoate, and hesperidin methyl chalcone.
*Tonic.*

**Acti Valda Diet** *Canonne, Braz.†.*
Enoxolone (p.36·2); cyclomenol; lidocaine hydrochloride (p.1377·3).

**Acti-B$_{12}$** *Sabex, Canad.*
Hydroxocobalamin (p.1458·2); amino acids (p.1417·1).
*Anaemia.*

**ActiBath** *Jergens, USA.*
Avena (p.1658·2).
*Dry skin; pruritus.*

**Actibil** *Arkopharma, Fr.*
Cynara (p.1678·3); fumitory (p.1690·1).
*Gastrointestinal and urinary-tract disorders.*

**Actibrush** *Colgate-Palmolive, UK†.*
Triclosan (p.1195·2); gantrez.
*Dental hygiene.*

**ActiCal Plus** *Usana, Canad.*
A vitamin D and mineral preparation (p.1417·1).

**Acticalcin** *TRB, Braz.*
Calcitonin (salmon) (p.768·2).
*Bone pain due of malignancy; hypercalcaemia; osteoporosis; Paget's disease of bone; sympathetic pain syndromes.*

**Acticarbine** *Elerte, Fr.*
Papaverine hydrochloride (p.1728·1); activated charcoal (p.1030·2).
*Gastrointestinal disorders.*

**Actichlor** *Adams, Hong Kong.*
Sodium dichloroisocyanurate (p.1191·3).
*Disinfection of surfaces and equipment.*

**Acticillin** *British Dispensary, Thai.*
Amoxicillin trihydrate (p.155·3).
*Bacterial infections.*

**Acticin**
*Note. This name is used for preparations of different composition.*
*Strakan, UK†.*
Tretinoin (p.1161·1).
*Acne.*

*Penederm, USA; Alpharma, USA.*
Permethrin (p.1508·3).
*Scabies.*

**Acticinco** *Robapharm, Spain†.*
Calcium gluceptate (p.1225·2); lysine hydrochloride (p.1439·2); deanol pyroglutamate (p.1585·3).
*Tonic.*

**Acticolin** *Upsamedica, Ital.†.*
Citicoline sodium (p.1672·3).
*Cerebrovascular disorders; parkinsonism.*

**Acticort** *Baker Cummins, USA.*
Hydrocortisone (p.1103·3).
*Skin disorders.*

**Acticrom** *Francia, Ital.*
Sodium cromoglicate (p.795·3).
*Allergic conjunctivitis; keratoconjunctivitis.*

**Actidil**
*Glaxo Wellcome, Austria†; Warner-Lambert, Ital.*
Triprolidine hydrochloride (p.442·3).
*Hypersensitivity reactions.*

**Actidine** *Daewon, Hong Kong†.*
Famotidine (p.1265·2).
*Gastro-oesophageal reflux; gastrointestinal haemorrhage; peptic ulcer; Zollinger-Ellison syndrome.*

**Actidose with Sorbitol** *Paddock, USA.*
Activated charcoal (p.1030·2); sorbitol (p.1446·3).
*Emergency treatment of poisoning.*

**Actidose-Aqua**
*Cambridge, UK; Paddock, USA.*
Activated charcoal (p.1030·2).
*Emergency treatment of poisoning.*

**Actidox** *Saninter, Port.*
Doxycycline (p.206·2).
*Bacterial infections.*

**Actidue** *Warner-Lambert, Ital.*
Yellow tablets (daytime), paracetamol (p.76·2); phenylpropanolamine hydrochloride (p.1127·3); blue tablets (night-time) paracetamol; diphenhydramine hydrochloride (p.431·3).
*Cold and influenza symptoms.*

**Actifed**
*Note. This name is used for preparations of different composition.*
*Pfizer Consumer, Austral.; GlaxoSmithKline, Belg.; Pfizer Consumer, Canad.; Warner-Lambert, Ger.†; GlaxoSmithKline, Hong Kong; Pfizer Consumer, Irl.; GlaxoSmithKline, Israel; Warner-Lambert, Ital.; GlaxoSmithKline, Malaysia; Pfizer, NZ; Pfizer Consumer, Port.; GlaxoSmithKline, S.Afr.; GlaxoSmithKline, Singapore; GlaxoSmithKline, Thai.; Wellcome, USA.*
Triprolidine hydrochloride (p.442·3); pseudoephedrine hydrochloride (p.1129·2).
*Allergic rhinitis; cold symptoms; upper respiratory-tract congestion.*

*GlaxoSmithKline, Belg.*
*Syrup:* Dextromethorphan hydrobromide (p.1117·3).
Formerly contained triprolidine hydrochloride, codeine phosphate, pseudoephedrine hydrochloride, and guaifenesin.
*Coughs.*

*Pfizer Sante, Fr.*
Triprolidine hydrochloride (p.442·3); pseudoephedrine hydrochloride (p.1129·2); paracetamol (p.76·2).
*Cold symptoms; upper respiratory-tract congestion.*

*GlaxoSmithKline, India.*
Triprolidine hydrochloride (p.442·3); phenylpropanolamine (p.1127·3).
*Respiratory-tract congestion.*

**Actifed Allergy** *Wellcome, USA.*
White daytime caplets, pseudoephedrine (p.1129·2); blue night time caplets, pseudoephedrine; diphenhydramine hydrochloride (p.431·3).

**Actifed CC Chesty** *Pfizer, NZ.*
Guaifenesin (p.1122·1).
Formerly contained guaifenesin, pseudoephedrine hydrochloride, and triprolidine hydrochloride.
*Coughs and cold symptoms.*

**Actifed CC Dry**
*Pfizer Consumer, Austral.*
Pholcodine (p.1128·3).
*Coughs.*

*Pfizer, NZ.*
Pholcodine (p.1128·3).
Formerly contained dextromethorphan hydrobromide, pseudoephedrine hydrochloride, and triprolidine hydrochloride.
*Coughs.*

**Actifed CC Junior**
*Warner-Lambert, Austral.†; Warner-Lambert, NZ†.*
Dextromethorphan hydrobromide (p.1117·3); triprolidine hydrochloride (p.442·3).
*Coughs.*

**Actifed Chesty**
*Note. This name is used for preparations of different composition.*
*Pfizer Consumer, Irl.*
Triprolidine hydrochloride (p.442·3); pseudoephedrine hydrochloride (p.1129·2); guaifenesin (p.1122·1).
*Coughs; upper respiratory-tract congestion.*

*Pfizer, NZ.*
Guaifenesin (p.1122·1); pseudoephedrine hydrochloride (p.1129·2).
Formerly known as Actifed CC Chesty.
*Coughs and cold symptoms.*

**Actifed Chesty Cough & Nasal Congestion**
*Pfizer Consumer, Austral.*
Guaifenesin (p.1122·1); pseudoephedrine hydrochloride (p.1129·2).
*Coughs; respiratory-tract congestion.*

**Actifed Cold & Allergy** *Warner-Lambert, USA.*
Triprolidine hydrochloride (p.442·3); pseudoephedrine hydrochloride (p.1129·2).
*Upper respiratory-tract congestion.*

**Actifed Cold & Fever** *GlaxoSmithKline, S.Afr.*
Triprolidine hydrochloride (p.442·3); pseudoephedrine hydrochloride (p.1129·2); paracetamol (p.76·2).
Formerly known as Actigesic.
*Cold and influenza symptoms.*

**Actifed Cold & Sinus** *Warner-Lambert, USA.*
Triprolidine hydrochloride (p.442·3); pseudoephedrine hydrochloride (p.1129·2); paracetamol (p.76·2).
*Cold symptoms.*

**Actifed Composto** *Warner-Lambert, Ital.*
Triprolidine hydrochloride (p.442·3); pseudoephedrine hydrochloride (p.1129·2); dextromethorphan hydrobromide (p.1117·3).
*Coughs; respiratory-tract congestion.*

**Actifed Compound**
*Note. This name is used for preparations of different composition.*
*GlaxoSmithKline, Hong Kong; GlaxoSmithKline, Israel; GlaxoSmithKline, Singapore; GlaxoSmithKline, Thai.*
Triprolidine hydrochloride (p.442·3); pseudoephedrine hydrochloride (p.1129·2); codeine phosphate (p.27·1).
*Coughs and cold symptoms.*

*Pfizer Consumer, Irl.*
Triprolidine hydrochloride (p.442·3); pseudoephedrine hydrochloride (p.1129·2); dextromethorphan hydrobromide (p.1117·3).
*Coughs; upper respiratory-tract congestion.*

**Actifed DM**
*Note. This name is used for preparations of different composition.*
*Warner-Lambert, Canad.†; GlaxoSmithKline, Hong Kong; GlaxoSmithKline, Israel; GlaxoSmithKline, Malaysia; GlaxoSmithKline, Singapore; GlaxoSmithKline, Thai.*
Triprolidine hydrochloride (p.442·3); pseudoephedrine hydrochloride (p.1129·2); dextromethorphan hydrobromide (p.1117·3).
*Coughs and cold symptoms.*

*GlaxoSmithKline, India.*
Triprolidine hydrochloride (p.442·3); phenylpropanolamine (p.1127·3); dextromethorphan hydrobromide (p.1117·3).
*Respiratory-tract congestion.*

**Actifed Dry** *Pfizer, NZ.*
Dextromethorphan hydrobromide (p.1117·3); pseudoephedrine hydrochloride (p.1129·2).
Formerly known as Actifed CC Dry.
*Coughs.*

**Actifed Dry Cough & Nasal Congestion** *Pfizer Consumer, Austral.*
Pseudoephedrine hydrochloride (p.1129·2); dextromethorphan hydrobromide (p.1117·3).
*Upper respiratory-tract disorders.*

**Actifed Dry Cough Regular** *GlaxoSmithKline, S.Afr.*
Triprolidine hydrochloride (p.442·3); pseudoephedrine hydrochloride (p.1129·2); codeine phosphate (p.27·1).
Formerly known as Actifed Co.
*Coughs.*

**Actifed Dry Cough Sugar Free** *GlaxoSmithKline, S.Afr.*
Triprolidine hydrochloride (p.442·3); pseudoephedrine hydrochloride (p.1129·2); dextromethorphan hydrobromide (p.1117·3).
Formerly known as Actifed DM.
*Coughs.*

**Actifed Expectorant**
*Note. This name is used for preparations of different composition.*
*Pfizer Sante, Fr.*
Carbocisteine (p.1116·2).
*Respiratory-tract congestion.*

*GlaxoSmithKline, Israel; GlaxoSmithKline, Malaysia; GlaxoSmithKline, Singapore.*
Triprolidine hydrochloride (p.442·3); pseudoephedrine hydrochloride (p.1129·2); guaifenesin (p.1122·1).
*Coughs.*

**Actifed jour et nuit** *Pfizer Sante, Fr.*
White tablets, paracetamol (p.76·2); pseudoephedrine hydrochloride (p.1129·2); blue tablets, paracetamol; diphenhydramine hydrochloride (p.431·3).
The white tablets replaced yellow tablets which contained paracetamol and phenylpropanolamine hydrochloride.
*Cold symptoms.*

**Actifed Nasale** *Warner-Lambert, Ital.*
Oxymetazoline hydrochloride (p.1126·1).
*Nasal congestion.*

**Actifed Plus**
*Note. This name is used for preparations of different composition.*
*Pfizer Consumer, Canad.; Wellcome, USA.*
Triprolidine hydrochloride (p.442·3); pseudoephedrine hydrochloride (p.1129·2); paracetamol (p.76·2).
*Cold symptoms.*

*GlaxoSmithKline, India.*
Triprolidine hydrochloride (p.442·3); phenylpropanolamine (p.1127·3); paracetamol (p.76·2).
*Respiratory-tract congestion associated with pain or fever.*

**Actifed Sinus Daytime** *Wellcome, USA.*
Pseudoephedrine hydrochloride (p.1129·2); paracetamol (p.76·2).
*Upper respiratory-tract symptoms.*

**Actifed Sinus Nighttime** *Wellcome, USA.*
Pseudoephedrine hydrochloride (p.1129·2); diphenhydramine hydrochloride (p.431·3); paracetamol (p.76·2).
*Upper respiratory-tract symptoms.*

**Actifed Toux Seche** *Pfizer Sante, Fr.*
Triprolidine hydrochloride (p.442·3); dextromethorphan hydrobromide (p.1117·3).
*Coughs.*

**Actifedrin**
*GlaxoSmithKline, Arg.; Zest, Braz.; GlaxoSmithKline, Chile.*
Triprolidine hydrochloride (p.442·3); pseudoephedrine hydrochloride (p.1129·2).
*Cold symptoms; rhinitis.*

**Actifedrin Antitusivo** *GlaxoSmithKline, Chile.*
Triprolidine hydrochloride (p.442·3); pseudoephedrine hydrochloride (p.1129·2); codeine phosphate (p.27·1).
*Upper respiratory-tract disorders.*

**Actifen** *Gebro, Austria.*
Dexibuprofen (p.46·1).
*Fever; inflammation; pain.*

**Actiferrine** *Mepha, Switz.*
Ferrous sulfate (p.1428·2); DL-serine.
*Iron deficiency; iron-deficiency anaemia.*

**Actiferrine-F Nouvelle formule** *Mepha, Switz.*
Ferrous sulfate (p.1428·2); DL-serine; folic acid (p.1429·1).
*Pregnancy- or lactation-induced anaemia.*

**Actiferro** *Lampugnani, Ital.*
Sodium ferric gluconate complex (p.1444·3).
*Iron-deficiency disorders.*

**Actifluor** *Byk Gulden, Ital.*
Sodium fluoride (p.1444·3); stannous fluoride (p.1448·3).
*Dental caries prophylaxis.*

**Actigall**
*Novartis, NZ; Watson, USA.*
Ursodeoxycholic acid (p.1760·3).
*Gallstones; primary biliary cirrhosis; primary sclerosing cholangitis.*

**Actigeron** *Bago, Chile.*
Acetylcarnitine hydrochloride (p.1646·1).
*Dementia.*

**Actigrip** *Warner-Lambert, Ital.*
Triprolidine hydrochloride (p.442·3); pseudoephedrine hydrochloride (p.1129·2); paracetamol (p.76·2).
*Influenza symptoms; respiratory-tract congestion.*

**Actihaemyl** *Solco, Ger.; Stulln, Ger.*
Protein-free bovine blood extract.
*Burns; eye disorders; peripheral and cerebral vascular disorders; wounds.*

**Actihist** *Hovid, Malaysia.*
Pseudoephedrine hydrochloride (p.1129·2); triprolidine hydrochloride (p.442·3).
*Cold symptoms; rhinitis.*

**Actihist Expectorant** *Hovid, Malaysia.*
Guaifenesin (p.1122·1); pseudoephedrine hydrochloride (p.1129·2); triprolidine hydrochloride (p.442·3).
*Coughs and cold symptoms.*

**Actihist-Co**
*Hovid, Hong Kong; Hovid, Malaysia.*
Dextromethorphan hydrobromide (p.1117·3); pseudoephedrine hydrochloride (p.1129·2); triprolidine hydrochloride (p.442·3).
*Coughs; nasal congestion.*

**Actil** *Masa, Thai.*
Triprolidine hydrochloride (p.442·3); pseudoephedrine hydrochloride (p.1129·2).
*Allergic rhinitis; cold symptoms; hay fever; nasal congestion.*

**Actilam** *Sofex, Port.*
Hesperidin (p.1688·2); deanol acetamidobenzoate (p.1585·3); magnesium glycerophosphate (p.1228·1).
*Mental function disorders; vascular disorders.*

**Actilax** *Alphapharm, Austral.*
Lactulose (p.1269·1).
*Constipation; hepatic encephalopathy.*

**Actilevol Orex** *Wasserman, Spain†.*
Vitamins (p.1417·1); carnosine; cyproheptadine hydrochloride (p.430·1); haematoporphyrin hydrochloride (p.1696·2).
*Tonic.*

**Actilife** *Lifeplan, UK†.*
Vitamins, minerals, fish oils, ginseng, and betacarotene (p.1417·1).
*Nutritional supplement.*

**Actilis** *Pautrat, Fr.*
Barrier cream.

**Actilyse**
*Boehringer Ingelheim, Arg.; Boehringer Ingelheim, Austral.; Boehringer Ingelheim, Austria; Boehringer Ingelheim, Belg.; Boehringer de Angeli, Braz.; Boehringer Ingelheim, Chile; Boehringer Ingelheim, Denm.; Boehringer Ingelheim, Fin.; Boehringer Ingelheim, Fr.; Boehringer Ingelheim, Ger.; Boehringer Ingelheim, Gr.; Boehringer Ingelheim, Hong Kong; German Remedies, India; Boehringer Ingelheim, Irl.; Boehringer Ingelheim, Israel; Boehringer Ingelheim, Ital.; Boehringer Ingelheim, Malaysia; Boehringer Ingelheim, Mex.; Boehringer Ingelheim, Neth.; Boehringer Ingelheim, Norw.; Boehringer Ingelheim, NZ; Boehringer Ingelheim, Port.; Boehringer Ingelheim, S.Afr.; Boehringer Ingelheim, Singapore; Boehringer Ingelheim, Spain; Boehringer Ingelheim, Swed.; Boehringer Ingelheim, Switz.; Boehringer Ingelheim, Thai.; Boehringer Ingelheim, UK.*
Alteplase (p.857·1).
*Myocardial infarction; pulmonary embolism; stroke.*

**Actimag**
*Vita, Ital.; Iquinosa, Spain.*
Magnesium pidolate (p.1228·2).
*Magnesium depletion.*

**Actiment** *Tecnonat, Arg.*
Nutritional supplement (p.1417·1).

**Actimidol** *Sterling Health, Spain†.*
Ibuprofen (p.45·3).
*Fever; musculoskeletal and joint disorders; pain.*

**Actimmune** *Genentech, USA.*
Interferon gamma-1b (p.647·2).
*Infections in chronic granulomatous disease; osteopetrosis.*

**Actimol** *Pharmed, India.*
Diclofenac sodium (p.32·1); paracetamol (p.76·2).
*Rheumatoid arthritis.*

**Actimoxi** *Clariana, Spain.*
Amoxicillin trihydrate (p.155·3).
*Bacterial infections.*

**Actin** *The Forty-Two, Thai.*
Co-trimoxazole (p.199·3).
*Bacterial infections.*

**Actinac**
*Hoechst Marion Roussel, Canad.†; Hoechst Marion Roussel, Irl.†; Peckforton, UK.*
Chloramphenicol (p.185·1); hydrocortisone acetate (p.1103·3); nicoboxil (p.66·3); allantoin (p.1141·3); precipitated sulfur (p.1158·2).
*Acne.*

**Actinerval** *Bago, Arg.*
Carbamazepine (p.353·3).
*Epilepsy; neuralgia.*

**Actino-Hermal** *Hermal, Ger.†.*
Fluorouracil (p.554·2).
*Skin cancer.*

**Action** *Sante Naturelle, Canad.*
Ascorbic acid (p.1460·2).

**Action Chewable** *Bayer, Austral.†.*
Chlorphenamine maleate (p.427·3); phenylephrine tartrate (p.1126·3).
*Cold symptoms; hay fever.*

**Action Cold & Flu** *Bayer, Austral.*
Chlorphenamine maleate (p.427·3); phenylephrine acid tartrate (p.1126·3); aspirin (p.15·1); ascorbic acid (p.1460·2).
*Cold and influenza symptoms.*

**Actiphos** *Teofarma, Fr.*
Phosphoric acid salts (p.1731·2).
*Tonic.*

**Actiplas** *Dompe Biotec, Ital.†.*
Alteplase (p.857·1).
*Myocardial infarction.*

**Actipram** *Laboratorios Chile, Chile.*
Citalopram hydrobromide (p.289·1).
*Depression.*

**Actiprofen**
*GlaxoSmithKline Consumer, Austral.; Sanofi Synthelabo, Braz.; Bayer, Canad.†.*
Ibuprofen (p.45·3).
*Fever; inflammation; musculoskeletal and joint disorders; pain.*

**Actiq**
*Orphan, Austral.; Lafon, Fr.; Elan, Ger.; Ferrer, Spain; Swedish Orphan, Swed.; Cephalon, UK; Cephalon, USA.*
Fentanyl citrate (p.40·1).
*Pain.*

**Actiquim** *Quimica y Farmacia, Mex.*
Naproxen (p.65·1).
*Inflammation; musculoskeletal and joint disorders.*

**Actira**
*Bayer, Austria; Bayer, Spain.*
Moxifloxacin hydrochloride (p.233·1).
*Bacterial infections.*

**Actireuma** *Farmila, Ital.†.*
Multivitamin preparation with omega-3 and omega-6 triglycerides and herbal extracts (p.1417·1).
*Nutritional supplement in joint disorders.*

**Actisac** *Polipharm, Thai.*
Fluoxetine (p.296·3).
*Depression.*

**Actisane Constipation Occasionnelle** *Dolisos, Fr.†.*
Senna (p.1288·2); tamarind (p.1293·2).
*Constipation.*

**Actisane Digestion** *Dolisos, Fr.†.*
Cynara (p.1678·3); boldo (p.1661·2); fumitory (p.1690·1).
*Biliary-tract disorders.*

**Actisane Douleurs Articulaires** *Dolisos, Fr.†.*
Devil's claw root (p.28·2); meadowsweet (p.1710·1).
*Joint disorders.*

**Actisane Fatigue Passagere** *Dolisos, Fr.†.*
Ginseng (p.1693·1); tea (p.1765·3).
*Tonic.*

**Actisane Hemorroides, Jambes Lourdes** Dolisos, Fr.†.
Aesculus (p.1648·2); melilotus officinalis; red vine.
*Haemorrhoids; venous insufficiency.*

**Actisane Minceur** Dolisos, Fr.†.
Bladderwrack (p.1742·3); java tea (p.1702·3); meadowsweet (p.1710·1).
*Obesity.*

**Actisane Nervosite** Dolisos, Fr.†.
Crataegus (p.1677·1); red-poppy petal (p.1058·1); passion flower (p.1729·1).
*Cardiac disorders.*

**Actisane Troubles du Sommeil** Dolisos, Fr.†.
Crataegus (p.1677·1); tilia (p.1756·2); valerian (p.1762·2).
Formerly known as Achisane Troubles du Sommeil.
*Insomnia.*

**Actisens** Byk Gulden, Ital.
Sodium fluoride (p.1444·3); potassium nitrate (p.1190·1).
*Gum hypersensitivity.*

**Actisite**
Willvonseder, Austria; Meda, Denm.†; Wybert, Ger.†; Solco, Ital.; Dentaid, Spain; Solco, Swed.†; Solco, Switz.; Alza, USA.
Tetracycline hydrochloride (p.266·2).
*Bacterial mouth infections.*

**Actiskenan** UPSA, Fr.
Morphine sulfate (p.60·2).
*Pain.*

**Actisorb** Johnson & Johnson Medical, Fr.†.
Activated charcoal (p.1030·2).
*Infected wounds.*

**Actisorb Plus**
Johnson & Johnson Medical, Fr.; Ethicon, Ital.
Activated charcoal (p.1030·2); silver (p.1746·1).
*Infected or malodorous wounds.*

**Actisorb Silver**
Johnson & Johnson, Ger.; Johnson & Johnson, Irl.; Johnson & Johnson Medical, UK.
Activated charcoal (p.1030·2); silver (p.1746·1).
Formerly known as Actisorb Plus in *Irl.* and *UK.*
*Infected or malodorous wounds.*

**Actisoufre** Grimberg, Fr.
Sodium sulfate (p.1290·1); dried yeast (p.1469·1).
*Rhinitis; upper respiratory-tract inflammation.*

**Actisson** Urgo, Fr.†.
Dietary fibre preparation (p.1417·1).
*Constipation.*

**Actithiol** Almirall, Spain.
Carbocisteine (p.1116·2).
*Respiratory-tract disorders.*

**Actithiol Antihist** Almirall, Spain.
Carbocisteine (p.1116·2); promethazine hydrochloride (p.439·1).
*Respiratory-tract disorders.*

**Actitonic** Amido, Fr.
*Solution for adults:* Amino-acid and mineral preparation (p.1417·1).
*Solution for children*†: Amino-acid preparation (p.1417·1).
*Tonic.*

**Activadone**
Alcon Cusi, Spain.
*Eye drops:* Chromocarb diethylamine (p.1670·3).
*Adjunct in eye surgery; conjunctival capillary fragility.*
Thea, Spain†.
*Capsules:* Chromocarb diethylamine (p.1670·3).
*Capillary haemorrhage; venous insufficiency.*

**Activarol**
Monot, Fr.†.
Glycine; arginine (p.1417·1).
*Tonic.*
Carlo Erba OTC, Ital.
Haematoporphyrin hydrochloride; glycine; cyanocobalamin; calcium gluconate (p.1417·1).
*Tonic.*
Azevedos, Port.
Haematoporphyrin hydrochloride; glycine; cyanocobalamin (p.1417·1).
*Tonic.*

**Activase**
Roche, Canad.; Genentech, USA.
Alteplase (p.857·1).
*Maintenance of central venous catheter patency; myocardial infarction; pulmonary embolism; stroke.*

**Activator** Andromaco, Chile.
Magnesium oxide (p.1272·3); pyridoxine hydrochloride (p.1456·3).
*Magnesium deficiency disorders.*

**Active C** Roche-Posay, Braz.
Ascorbic acid (p.1460·2).
*Vitamin C supplement.*

**Active Dry Lotion** Norwood, Canad.
*SPF 15*†: Octinoxate (p.1154·3); oxybenzone (p.1154·3).
*SPF 30:* Octinoxate (p.1154·3); oxybenzone (p.1154·3); octisalate (p.1154·3).
*Sunscreen.*

**Active Multi** Quest, Canad.†.
Multivitamin and mineral preparation (p.1417·1).

**Activella** Novo Nordisk, USA.
Estradiol (p.1550·1); norethisterone acetate (p.1562·2).
*Menopausal disorders; osteoporosis.*

**Activelle**
Elea, Arg.; Novo Nordisk, Austria; Novo Nordisk, Belg.; Medley, Braz.; Silesia, Chile; Novo Nordisk, Denm.; Novo Nordisk, Fin.; Novo Nordisk, Fr.; Novo Nordisk, Ger.; Novo Nordisk, Gr.; Novo Nordisk, Hong Kong; Novo Nordisk, Irl.; Novo Nordisk, Israel; Novo Nordisk, Ital.; Novo Nordisk, Malaysia; Novo Nordisk, Neth.; Novo Nordisk, Norw.; Isdin, Port.; Novo Nordisk, S.Afr.; Novo Nordisk, Singapore; Isdin, Spain; Novo Nordisk, Swed.; Novo Nordisk, Switz.; Novo Nordisk, Thai.
Estradiol (p.1550·1); norethisterone acetate (p.1562·2).
*Menopausal disorders; osteoporosis.*

**Activex 40 Plus** Propan, S.Afr.
Ginseng (p.1693·1); muira puama; vitamins (p.1417·1); minerals; kelp (p.1742·3); lysine hydrochloride.

**Activir**
GlaxoSmithKline, Austria; Allen, Austria; GlaxoSmithKline, Fr.; GlaxoSmithKline, S.Afr.
Aciclovir (p.626·1).
*Herpes labialis.*

**Activital** ECR, Switz.
Arginine aspartate (p.1421·1); calcium gluconate (p.1225·2); magnesium gluconate (p.1228·1).
*Tonic.*

**Activon** Drossapharm, Switz.
Etofenamate (p.38·1).
*Soft-tissue disorders.*

**Activox** Arkopharma, Fr.
Erysimum; chamomile (p.1669·3).
*Mouth and throat disorders.*

**Actizyme** Willvonseder, Austria†.
Subtilisin-A; poloxamer 338 (p.1414·2) (p.1164·2).
*Cleaning of contact lenses.*

**Actocortina** Altana, Spain.
Hydrocortisone sodium phosphate (p.1104·1).
*Corticosteroid.*

**Actol** Mayrhofer, Austria†.
Niflumic acid (p.67·1).
*Inflammation; pain.*

**Actomin** GNR, Ital.†.
Citicoline sodium (p.1672·3).
*Cerebrovascular disorders; parkinsonism.*

**Actomite** Ceuta, UK.
Bioallethrin (p.1500·3).
*Elimination of house dust mite.*

**Actonel**
Aventis, Arg.; Aventis, Austral.; Aventis, Austria; Procter & Gamble, Belg.; Aventis, Braz.; Procter & Gamble, Canad.; Aventis, Chile; Procter & Gamble, Fr.; Procter & Gamble, Ger.; Aventis, Ger.; Aventis, Hong Kong; Aventis, Irl.; Aventis, Israel; Procter & Gamble, Ital.; Procter & Gamble, Neth.; Aventis, Port.; Aventis, S.Afr.; Aventis, Singapore; Aventis, Spain; Aventis, Switz.; Aventis, Thai.; Aventis, UK; Procter & Gamble, UK; Procter & Gamble, USA.
Risedronate sodium (p.774·3).
*Osteoporosis; Paget's disease of bone.*

**Actonorm** Wallace Mfg Chem., UK.
*Oral gel:* Aluminium hydroxide (p.1249·2); magnesium hydroxide (p.1272·2); simeticone (p.1289·2).
*Oral powder:* Magnesium carbonate (p.1272·1); aluminium hydroxide (p.1249·2); atropine sulfate (p.477·1); calcium carbonate (p.1254·2); magnesium trisilicate (p.1272·3); sodium bicarbonate (p.1223·2); peppermint oil (p.1283·2).
*Dyspepsia; flatulence; gastric hyperacidity.*

**Actophlem** Covan, S.Afr.
Theophylline (p.798·3); etofylline (p.785·1); diphenylpyraline hydrochloride (p.432·3); ammonium chloride (p.1115·2); sodium citrate (p.1223·2).
*Coughs.*

**Actopril** Ergha, Irl.
Captopril (p.879·2).
*Heart failure; hypertension.*

**Actos**
Abbott, Arg.; Lilly, Austral.; Abbott, Braz.; Lilly, Canad.; Abbott, Chile; Takeda, Denm.; Lilly, Fin.; Takeda, Fr.; Takeda, Ger.; Takeda, Gr.; Takeda, Hong Kong; Takeda, Ital.; Takeda, Jpn; Takeda, Norw.; Lilly, NZ; Lilly, Port.; Lilly, S.Afr.; Lilly, Spain; Lilly, Swed.; Takeda, Switz.; Takeda, Thai.; Takeda, UK; Takeda, USA; Lilly, USA.
Pioglitazone hydrochloride (p.344·1).
*Diabetes mellitus.*

**Actosolv**
Aventis, Austria; Aventis, Belg.; Aventis, Fr.†; Hoechst Marion Roussel, Ger.†; Hoechst Marion Roussel, Israel†; Aventis, Ital.
Urokinase (p.1018·2).
*Thromboembolic disorders.*

**Actospect** Covan, S.Afr.
Guaifenesin (p.1122·1).
*Coughs.*

**Actovegin**
Nycomed, Austria; Nycomed, Ger.; Nycomed, Hong Kong; Nycomed, Thai.
Protein-free bovine blood extract.
*Burns; cerebral circulatory and metabolic disorders; eye disorders; peripheral vascular disorders; ulcers; wounds.*

**Actraphane HM**
Novo Nordisk, Gr.
Mixtures of insulin injection (human, recombinant) and isophane insulin (human, recombinant) in varying proportions (p.333·3).
*Diabetes mellitus.*
Novo Nordisk, S.Afr.
Mixture of soluble insulin injection (human, biosynthetic) 30% and isophane insulin injection (human, biosynthetic) 70% (p.333·3).
*Diabetes mellitus.*

**Actraphane HM 10/90, 20/80, 30/70, 40/60, 50/50**
Novo Nordisk, Ger.; Novo Nordisk, Ital.
Mixtures of neutral insulin injection (human, monocomponent) and isophane insulin injection (human, monocomponent) respectively in the proportions indicated (p.333·3).
*Diabetes mellitus.*

**Actrapid**
Novo Nordisk, Austral; Novo Nordisk, Denm.; Novo Nordisk, Fin.; Novo Nordisk, Ger.; Novo Nordisk, Irl.; Novo Nordisk, Malaysia; Novo Nordisk, Neth.; Novo Nordisk, Norw.; Novo Nordisk, NZ; Novo Nordisk, Port.; Novo Nordisk, Spain; Novo Nordisk, Swed.; Novo Nordisk, UK.
Neutral insulin injection (human, monocomponent) (p.333·3).
Formerly known as Human Actrapid in the *UK.*
*Diabetes mellitus.*
Pentafarma, Chile; Knoll, India.
Insulin injection (porcine, highly purified) (p.333·3).
*Diabetes mellitus.*

**Actrapid HM**
Novo Nordisk, Arg.; Novo Nordisk, Austria; Novo Nordisk, Belg.; Pentafarma, Chile; Novo Nordisk, Fr.; Novo Nordisk, Gr.; Novo Nordisk, Hong Kong; Novo Nordisk, Ital.; Novo Nordisk, S.Afr.; Novo Nordisk, Singapore; Novo Nordisk, Switz.; Novo Nordisk, Thai.
Neutral insulin injection (human, monocomponent) (p.333·3).
*Diabetes mellitus.*

**Actrapid MC**
Novo Nordisk, Arg.; Novo Nordisk, Braz.; Novo Nordisk, Hong Kong; Novo Nordisk, Switz.
Neutral insulin injection (porcine, monocomponent) (p.333·3).
*Diabetes mellitus.*

**Actron**
Note. This name is used for preparations of different composition.
Bayer, Austria; Bayer, USA†.
Ketoprofen (p.51·2).
*Fever; musculoskeletal and joint disorders; pain.*
Bayer, Fr.
Aspirin (p.15·1); paracetamol (p.76·2); caffeine (p.782·1).
*Fever; pain.*
Bayer, Spain.
Paracetamol (p.76·2).
*Fever; pain.*

**Actron Compuesto** Bayer, Spain.
Aspirin (p.15·1); caffeine (p.782·1); paracetamol (p.76·2).
*Fever; pain.*

**Actroneffix** Bayer, Fr.†.
Ketoprofen (p.51·2).
*Fever; pain.*

**Actualene** Carlo Erba OTC, Ital.
Cabergoline (p.1203·3).
*Hyperprolactinaemia; lactation suppression; prolactinoma.*

**Actuss** Sigma, Austral.
Pholcodine (p.1128·3).
*Coughs.*

**Actymine** Codifra, Fr.
Vitamins; minerals; vegetable oils; bioflavonoids; anthocyanosides (p.1417·1).
*Dry skin; sun-induced skin damage.*

**Actypral** Codifra, Fr.
Bioflavonoids; vitamins; minerals; lycopene (p.1417·1).
*Skin ageing.*

**Acuaderm** Bajer, Arg.
Calamine (p.1144·1); diphenhydramine hydrochloride (p.431·3); camphor (p.1665·3); aloe vera (p.1141·3).
*Pruritus.*

**Acuafil** Sophia, Mex.
Wool fat (p.1483·1); liquid paraffin (p.1479·1).
*Dry eyes.*

**Acuafil Ofteno** Sophia, Mex.
Polyvinyl alcohol (p.1581·1).
*Dry eyes.*

**Acuatim** Otsuka, Jpn.
Nadifloxacin (p.233·3).
*Acne.*

**Acubiron** Bohm, Spain.
Pygeum africanum (p.1568·2).
*Benign prostatic hyperplasia.*

**Acucil** Apotex, S.Afr.†.
Amoxicillin trihydrate (p.155·3).
*Bacterial infections.*

**Acuco** Apotex, S.Afr.†.
Co-trimoxazole (p.199·3).
*Bacterial infections.*

**Acudor** Ferring, Port.
Etodolac (p.37·3).
*Gout; musculoskeletal, joint, and peri-articular disorders; pain.*

**ACU-dyne** Acme, USA.
Povidone-iodine (p.1190·3).
*Skin disinfection; vaginal disorders.*

**Acu-Erylate S** Apotex, S.Afr.†.
Erythromycin estolate (p.208·1).
*Bacterial infections.*

**Acuflex** Apotex, S.Afr.†.
Indometacin (p.47·3).
*Gout; musculoskeletal and joint disorders.*

**Acuflu-P** Apotex, S.Afr.†.
Triprolidine hydrochloride (p.442·3); pseudoephedrine hydrochloride (p.1129·2); paracetamol (p.76·2).
*Cold and influenza symptoms.*

**Acugesic** Duopharma, Hong Kong.
Tramadol hydrochloride (p.94·3).
*Pain.*

**Acugesil** Apotex, S.Afr.†.
Paracetamol (p.76·2); codeine phosphate (p.27·1); caffeine (p.782·1); meprobamate (p.706·2).
*Pain with tension.*

**Acugest** Apotex, S.Afr.†.
Triprolidine hydrochloride (p.442·3); pseudoephedrine hydrochloride (p.1129·2).
*Cold and influenza symptoms.*

**Acugest Co** Apotex, S.Afr.†.
Triprolidine hydrochloride (p.442·3); pseudoephedrine hydrochloride (p.1129·2); codeine phosphate (p.27·1).
*Coughs.*

**Acugest Expect** Apotex, S.Afr.†.
Triprolidine hydrochloride (p.442·3); pseudoephedrine hydrochloride (p.1129·2); guaifenesin (p.1122·1).
*Coughs.*

**Acuilix** Pfizer, Fr.
Hydrochlorothiazide (p.933·2); quinapril hydrochloride (p.991·1).
*Hypertension.*

**Acuitel** Pfizer, Fr.
Quinapril hydrochloride (p.991·1).
*Heart failure; hypertension.*

**Acular**
Allergan, Arg.; Allergan, Austral.; Allergan, Austria; Allergan, Braz.; Allergan, Canad.; Allergan, Chile; Allergan, Denm.; Allergan, Fin.; Allergan, Fr.; Allergan, Ger.; Allergan, Hong Kong; Allergan, Irl.; Allergan, Ital.; Allergan, Malaysia; Allergan, NZ; Allergan, Port.; Allergan, S.Afr.; Allergan, Singapore; Allergan, Spain; Allergan, Switz.; Allergan, Thai.; Allergan, UK; Allergan, USA.
Ketorolac trometamol (p.52·1).
*Allergic conjunctivitis; inflammation, pain, and photophobia following ocular surgery.*

**Aculare** Allergan, Belg.
Ketorolac trometamol (p.52·1).
*Allergic conjunctivitis; ocular inflammation following cataract surgery.*

**Acularen** Allergan, Mex.
Ketorolac trometamol (p.52·1).
*Allergic conjunctivitis; postoperative ocular inflammation.*

**Aculfin** Apsen, Braz.†.
Sulfasalazine (p.1291·1).
*Ankylosing spondylitis; rheumatoid arthritis; ulcerative colitis.*

**Aculoid** Apotex, S.Afr.†.
Cyclizine hydrochloride (p.429·3).
*Nausea; vestibular disorders; vomiting.*

**Acumet** Apotex, S.Afr.†.
Metoclopramide hydrochloride (p.1274·3).
*Gastrointestinal disorders.*

**Acumod** Apotex, S.Afr.†.
Amiloride hydrochloride (p.858·2); hydrochlorothiazide (p.933·2).
*Hypertension; oedema.*

**Acunaso** Apotex, S.Afr.†.
Pseudoephedrine hydrochloride (p.1129·2).
*Upper respiratory-tract congestion.*

**Acuode** Recalcine, Chile.
Colecalciferol (p.1461·3).
*Hypoparathyroidism; osteomalacia; rickets; tetanus; vitamin D deficiency.*

**Acuolens** Alcon Cusi, Spain.
Hypromellose (p.1579·3).
*Dry eyes.*

**Acu-Oxytet** Apotex, S.Afr.†.
Oxytetracycline hydrochloride (p.241·1).
*Bacterial infections.*

**Acupan**
3M, Belg.; Biocodex, Fr.; 3M, Irl.; 3M, Israel; 3M, NZ; CEPA, Spain†; 3M, Switz.; 3M, UK.
Nefopam hydrochloride (p.66·2).
*Pain.*

**Acuphlem** Apotex, S.Afr.†.
Carbocisteine (p.1116·2).
*Respiratory-tract disorders with excess mucus.*

**Acupillin** Apotex, S.Afr.†.
Ampicillin trihydrate (p.157·2).
*Bacterial infections.*

**Acuprel** Pfizer, Spain.
Quinapril hydrochloride (p.991·1).
*Heart failure; hypertension.*

**Acupril**
Parke, Davis, Mex.; Parke, Davis, Neth.; Pfizer, Port.
Quinapril hydrochloride (p.991·1) or quinaprilat (p.991·2).
*Heart failure; hypertension.*

**Acurate** Apotex, S.Afr.
Paracetamol (p.76·2); doxylamine succinate (p.432·3); caffeine (p.782·1); codeine phosphate (p.27·1).
*Pain with tension.*

**Acuretic**
Pfizer, Port.; Binesa, Spain.
Quinapril hydrochloride (p.991·1); hydrochlorothiazide (p.933·2).
*Hypertension.*

**Acusprain** Apotex, S.Afr.†.
Naproxen (p.65·1).
*Dysmenorrhoea; gout; musculoskeletal and joint disorders.*

**Acustat** Transpen, UK.
Skin patch.
*Musculoskeletal, joint, and soft-tissue injury.*

**Acustop** Apotex, S.Afr.†.
Paracetamol (p.76·2); codeine phosphate (p.27·1); promethazine hydrochloride (p.439·1).
*Fever; pain.*

**Acustop Cataplasma** *Emerging Pharma, Singapore.*
Flurbiprofen (p.43·3).
*Musculoskeletal, joint, peri-articular, and soft-tissue disorders.*

**AcuTect** *Diatide, USA.*
Technetium-99m apcitide (p.1525·2).
*Scintigraphic imaging of acute venous thrombosis.*

**Acutil Fosforo** *Angelini, Ital.*
Aceglutamide (p.1645·2) or glutamine (p.1433·2); L-asparagine (p.1422·1); DL-phosphoserine; pyridoxine (p.1457·2) or pyridoxine hydrochloride (p.1456·3).
*Tonic.*

**Acutrim** *Ciba, USA†; Heritage Consumer, USA†.*
Phenylpropanolamine hydrochloride (p.1127·3).
*Obesity.*

**Acutussive** *Apotex, S.Afr.†.*
Triprolidine hydrochloride (p.442·3); pseudoephedrine hydrochloride (p.1129·2); guaifenesin (p.1122·1); codeine phosphate (p.27·1).
*Coughs.*

**Acuzide** *Parke, Davis, Neth.*
Quinapril hydrochloride (p.991·1); hydrochlorothiazide (p.933·2).
*Hypertension.*

**Acuzole** *Apotex, S.Afr.†.*
Metronidazole (p.607·2).
*Anaerobic bacterial infections; protozoal infections.*

**ACV** *Greater Pharma, Thai.*
Aciclovir (p.626·1).
*Herpes simplex infections.*

**ACWY Vax** *GlaxoSmithKline, UK.*
A meningococcal vaccine (groups A, C, $W_{135}$, and Y) (p.1626·1).
*Active immunisation.*

**Acxen** *Loren, Mex.*
Paracetamol (p.76·2); naproxen (p.65·1).
*Inflammation; pain.*

**ACY** *Ecobi, Ital.*
Aciclovir (p.626·1).
*Herpesvirus infections.*

**Acyclostad** *Berner, Fin.*
Aciclovir (p.626·1).
*Herpesvirus infections.*

**Acyclo-V** *Alphapharm, Austral.*
Aciclovir (p.626·1).
*Herpesvirus infections; HIV infection.*

**Acydona** *Pliva, Spain.*
Povidone-iodine (p.1190·3).
*Disinfection of burns, skin, and wounds.*

**Acyflox** *Pliva, Spain.*
Aspirin (p.15·1); ascorbic acid (p.1460·2).
*Fever; pain.*

**Acylene** *UCB, Spain.*
Aluminium hydroxide (p.1249·2); magnesium hydroxide (p.1272·2); aluminium hydroxide-magnesium carbonate co-dried gel (p.1250·1).
*Gastrointestinal hyperacidity.*

**Acyprin** *Collins, Mex.*
Allopurinol (p.412·2).
*Hyperuricaemia.*

**Acypront** *Mack, Malaysia.*
Acetylcysteine (p.1112·3).
*Respiratory-tract congestion.*

**Acyrax** *Orion, Fin.*
Aciclovir (p.626·1) or aciclovir sodium (p.626·1).
*Herpesvirus infections.*

**Acyvir**
*Merck, Hong Kong; Glaxo Allen, Ital.; Pharmasant, Thai.*
Aciclovir (p.626·1).
*Herpesvirus infections.*

**AD Pabyrn** *LPB, Ital.*
Vitamin A palmitate (p.1453·1); colecalciferol (p.1461·3).
*Vitamin A and D deficiency.*

**AD Shock** *Mertens, Arg.*
Vitamin A (p.1451·2); ergocalciferol (p.1462·1).
*Hypocalcaemia; hypoparathyroidism; osteoarthritis; osteomalacia; renal osteodystrophy; rickets; tetanus.*

**ADA** *Estedi, Spain.*
Phenylephrine hydrochloride (p.1126·3).
*Nasal congestion; sinus congestion.*

**Adacel** *Aventis Pasteur, Canad.*
An adsorbed diphtheria, tetanus, and pertussis vaccine (p.1613·3).
*Active immunisation.*

**Adaferin**
*Lavipharm, Gr.; Galderma, India; Galderma, Israel; Galderma, Mex.*
Adapalene (p.1141·1).
*Acne.*

**Adagen** *Enzon, USA.*
Pegademase bovine (p.1729·2).
*Adenosine deaminase deficiency.*

**Adalat**
*Bayer, Arg.; Bayer, Austral.; Bayer, Austria; Bayer, Belg.; Bayer, Braz.; Bayer, Canad.; Bayer, Chile; Bayer, Denm.; Bayer, Fin.; Bayer, Ger.; Bayer, Gr.; Bayer, Hong Kong; Bayer, Irl.; Bayer, Ital.; Bayer, Jpn; Bayer, Malaysia; Bayer, Mex.; Bayer, Neth.; Bayer, Norw.; Bayer, NZ; Bayer, Port.; Bayer, S.Afr.; Bayer, Singapore; Bayer, Spain; Bayer, Swed.; Bayer, Switz.; Bayer, Thai.; Bayer, UK; Bayer, USA.*
Nifedipine (p.966·2).
*Angina pectoris; hypertension; Raynaud's syndrome.*

**Adalate** *Bayer, Fr.*
Nifedipine (p.966·2).
*Angina pectoris; hypertension; Raynaud's syndrome.*

**Adalgen** *Andromaco, Chile.*
Paracetamol (p.76·2); chlormezanone (p.675·1).
*Musculoskeletal, joint, peri-articular, and soft-tissue disorders; pain.*

**Adalgur** *Aventis, Spain.*
Paracetamol (p.76·2); thiocolchicoside (p.1395·2).
*Pain; skeletal muscle spasm.*

**Adalgur N** *Aventis, Port.*
Paracetamol (p.76·2); thiocolchicoside (p.1395·2).
*Musculoskeletal and joint pain.*

**Adalken** *Kendrick, Mex.*
Penicillamine (p.1046·3).
*Heavy metal poisoning; Wilson's disease.*

**Adamon**
*Note. This name is used for preparations of different composition.*
*Kampel Martian, Arg.; Asta Medica, Austria.*
Tramadol hydrochloride (p.94·3).
*Pain.*

*Asta Medica, Thai.*
Ciclonium bromide (p.480·2).
*Dysmenorrhoea; gastro-intestinal, biliary, and urinary-tract spasm.*

**Adancor** *Lipha Sante, Fr.*
Nicorandil (p.965·3).
*Angina pectoris.*

**Adant** *Tedec Meiji, Israel.*
Sodium hyaluronate (p.1697·3).
*Osteoarthritis of the knee; shoulder pain.*

**Adapettes**
*Alcon, Braz.†.*
Cleaning solution for contact lenses (p.1164·2).

*Alcon, Mex.*
Disodium edetate (p.1037·3); sorbic acid (p.1192·3) (p.1164·2).
*Wetting solution for contact lenses.*

*Alcon, USA.*
Range of solutions for contact lenses (p.1164·2).

**Adapine** *Amrad, Austral.†.*
Nifedipine (p.966·2).
*Hypertension.*

**Adaptic** *Ethicon, Ital.*
White soft paraffin (p.1479·3).
*Burns; wounds.*

**Adasept** *Odan, Canad.*
*Cleanser:* Triclosan (p.1195·2).
*Skin cleanser.*

*Topical gel:* Triclosan (p.1195·2); salicylic acid (p.1157·1); sodium thiosulfate (p.1053·3).
*Acne.*

**Adaspor** *IMS, Ital.*
Adazone; peracetic acid (p.1187·3).
*Instrument disinfection.*

**Adato-Cel** *Chiron, Israel.*
Hypromellose (p.1579·3) in sodium chloride.
*Aid in eye surgery and gonioscopy.*

**Adato-Deca** *Chiron, Israel.*
Perflunafene (p.1730·1).
*Aid in eye surgery.*

**Adato-Octa** *Chiron, Israel.*
Perfluorooctane (p.1730·2).
*Ophthalmic tamponade.*

**Adato-Sil Ol** *Chiron, Israel.*
Dimethicone (p.1482·1).
*Aid in eye surgery.*

**Adavite** *Hudson, USA.*
A range of vitamin preparations (p.1417·1).

**Adax** *Saval, Chile.*
Alprazolam (p.668·3).
*Anxiety; mixed anxiety depressive states; panic attacks.*

**Adaxil** *Byk, Arg.*
Glucosamine sulfate (p.1694·1).
Lidocaine hydrochloride (p.1377·3) is included in the intramuscular injection to alleviate the pain of injection.
*Musculoskeletal and joint disorders.*

**A-D-C** *Mertens, Arg.*
Vitamin A palmitate (p.1453·1); ergocalciferol (p.1462·1); ascorbic acid (p.1460·2).
*Vitamin A, D, and C supplement.*

**ADC Fluor** *Mertens, Arg.*
Vitamin A; vitamin D; vitamin C (p.1417·1) sodium fluoride (p.1444·3).
*Nutritional supplement.*

**Adcal** *Strakan, UK.*
Calcium carbonate (p.1254·2).
*Calcium supplement; hyperphosphataemia; osteoporosis.*

**Adcal-$D_3$** *Strakan, UK.*
Calcium carbonate (p.1254·2); colecalciferol (p.1461·3).
*Calcium and vitamin D deficiency; osteoporosis.*

**Adco-Amoclav** *Ranbaxy, S.Afr.*
Amoxicillin (p.155·3); clavulanic acid (p.193·3).
*Bacterial infections.*

**Adco-Ciprin** *Ranbaxy, S.Afr.*
Ciprofloxacin (p.188·2).
*Bacterial infections.*

**Adco-Dermed** *Adcock Ingram, S.Afr.*
Ketoconazole (p.403·3).
*Pityriasis versicolor; seborrhoeic dermatitis.*

**Adco-Dol** *Adcock Ingram, S.Afr.*
Paracetamol (p.76·2); codeine phosphate (p.27·1); caffeine (p.782·1); doxylamine succinate (p.432·3).
*Fever; pain.*

**Adco-Flupain** *Adcock Ingram, S.Afr.*
Triprolidine hydrochloride (p.442·3); pseudoephedrine hydrochloride (p.1129·2); paracetamol (p.76·2).
*Cold and influenza symptoms.*

**Adco-Indogel** *Adcock Ingram, S.Afr.*
Indometacin (p.47·3).
*Musculoskeletal and joint disorders.*

**Adco-Kiddipayne** *Adcock Ingram, S.Afr.*
Paracetamol (p.76·2); codeine phosphate (p.27·1); promethazine hydrochloride (p.439·1).
*Fever; pain.*

**Adco-Linctopent** *Adcock Ingram, S.Afr.*
Bromhexine hydrochloride (p.1115·3); orciprenaline sulfate (p.790·2).
*Coughs.*

**Adco-Liquilax** *Adcock Ingram, S.Afr.*
Lactulose (p.1269·1).
*Constipation; hepatic encephalopathy.*

**Adco-Loten** *Adcock Ingram, S.Afr.*
Atenolol (p.865·2); chlortalidone (p.882·3).
*Hypertension.*

**Adco-Muco Expect** *Adcock Ingram Generics, S.Afr.†.*
Triprolidine hydrochloride (p.442·3); pseudoephedrine hydrochloride (p.1129·2); guaifenesin (p.1122·1).
*Coughs.*

**Adco-Payne** *Adcock Ingram, S.Afr.*
Paracetamol (p.76·2); codeine phosphate (p.27·1); caffeine (p.782·1); meprobamate (p.706·2).
*Pain and tension.*

**Adco-Phenobarbitone Vitalet** *Adcock Ingram, S.Afr.*
Phenobarbital (p.367·3); vitamin B substances (p.1417·1).
*Epilepsy; insomnia; sedative.*

**Adcor** *Pharmus, Braz.†.*
Nifedipine (p.966·2).
*Angina pectoris; hypertension.*

**Adco-Retic** *Adcock Ingram, S.Afr.*
Amiloride hydrochloride (p.858·2); hydrochlorothiazide (p.933·2).
*Hypertension; oedema.*

**Adcortyl**
*Bristol-Myers Squibb, Irl.; Bristol-Myers Squibb, Israel; Bristol-Myers Squibb, UK.*
Triamcinolone acetonide (p.1110·2).
*Inflammatory disorders; musculoskeletal and joint disorders; skin disorders.*

**Adcortyl with Graneodin** *Bristol-Myers Squibb, UK†.*
Triamcinolone acetonide (p.1110·2); neomycin sulfate (p.235·1); gramicidin (p.220·2).
*Infected skin disorders.*

**Adcortyl in Orabase**
*Bristol-Myers Squibb, Irl.; Bristol-Myers Squibb, UK.*
Triamcinolone acetonide (p.1110·2).
*Inflammatory disorders of the mouth; lesions of the oral mucosa.*

**Adco-Sinal Co** *Adcock Ingram, S.Afr.*
Paracetamol (p.76·2); phenylpropanolamine hydrochloride (p.1127·3); phenyltoloxamine citrate (p.439·1); codeine phosphate (p.27·1).
*Cold and influenza symptoms.*

**Adco-Sodasol** *Adcock Ingram, S.Afr.*
Sodium citrate (p.1223·2); sodium bicarbonate (p.1223·2); anhydrous citric acid (p.1673·1); tartaric acid (p.1752·1).
*Gastric hyperacidity; urinary alkalinisation.*

**Adco-Sufedrin** *Adcock Ingram, S.Afr.*
Pseudoephedrine hydrochloride (p.1129·2).
*Upper respiratory-tract congestion.*

**Adco-Tussend** *Adcock Ingram, S.Afr.*
Triprolidine hydrochloride (p.442·3); pseudoephedrine hydrochloride (p.1129·2); codeine phosphate (p.27·1).
*Coughs.*

**Addamel** *Fresenius Kabi, Spain.*
Electrolyte (p.1217·1) and trace-element preparation (p.1417·1).
*Parenteral nutrition.*

**Addamel N**
*Fresenius Kabi, Gr.; Fresenius Kabi, Hong Kong; Pharmacia Upjohn, Israel; Fresenius Kabi, Ital.; Fresenius Kabi, Malaysia; Fresenius Kabi, Neth.; Fresenius Kabi, NZ; Baxter, NZ; Fresenius Kabi, Port.; Fresenius Kabi, Singapore; Fresenius Kabi, Switz.; Fresenius Kabi, Thai.*
Electrolyte (p.1217·1) and trace element preparation (p.1417·1).
*Parenteral nutrition.*

**Addamel Novum** *Pharmacia Upjohn, Belg.†.*
Electrolyte (p.1217·1) and trace element (p.1417·1) preparation.
*Parenteral nutrition.*

**Addel N** *Baxter, Ger.*
Electrolyte (p.1217·1) and trace element (p.1417·1) preparation.
*Parenteral nutrition.*

**Addera** *Semper, Fin.*
Nutritional supplement (p.1417·1).

**Adderall** *Shire Richwood, USA.*
Dexamfetamine sulfate (p.1585·3); dexamfetamine saccharate (p.1586·3); amfetamine sulfate (p.1584·3); amfetamine aspartate (p.1584·3).
Formerly known as Obetrol.
*Attention deficit hyperactivity disorder; narcoleptic syndrome.*

**Addex**
*Fresenius Kabi, Fin.; Fresenius Kabi, Norw.; Fresenius Kabi, Swed.*
A range of electrolyte preparations (p.1217·1).

**Addex-THAM** *Fresenius Kabi, Swed.*
Trometamol (p.1758·2).
*Acute metabolic acidosis; acute respiratory acidosis.*

**Addigrip**
*Aventis Pasteur, Austria; Aventis Pasteur, Belg.; Aventis Pasteur, Ger.*
An inactivated influenza vaccine (surface antigen) (p.1620·2).
*Active immunisation.*

**Addi-K**
*Leo, Hong Kong; Leo, Singapore; Leo, Thai.*
Potassium chloride (p.1232·2).
*Hypokalaemia.*

**Addiphos**
*Fresenius Kabi, Denm.; Pharmacia, Irl.; Fresenius Kabi, Neth.; Fresenius Kabi, Swed.†; Fresenius Kabi, UK.*
Electrolyte preparation (p.1217·1).
*Parenteral nutrition.*

**Additene** *Novartis, Fin.†.*
Nutritional supplement (p.1417·1).

**Additrace**
*Pharmacia, Irl.; Fresenius Kabi, S.Afr.†; Fresenius Kabi, UK.*
Trace element preparation (p.1417·1).
*Parenteral nutrition.*

**Addivita** *Scheffler, Ital.*
Ascorbic acid (p.1460·2).
*Vitamin C deficiency.*

**ADE 2 (Adedois)** *Prodotti, Braz.*
Vitamin A acetate (p.1453·1); ergocalciferol (p.1462·1).
*Vitamin A and D deficiency.*

**Adecaps** *Medicopharm, Austria.*
Cod-liver oil (p.1425·2).
*Vitamin A and D deficiency.*

**Adecur**
*Tecnofarma, Chile.*
Terazosin (p.1011·1).
*Benign prostatic hyperplasia; hypertension.*

*Asofarma, Mex.*
Terazosin hydrochloride (p.1010·3).
*Benign prostatic hyperplasia; hypertension.*

**Adecut** *Takeda, Jpn.*
Delapril hydrochloride (p.892·2).
*Hypertension.*

**Adeflor M** *Upjohn, USA.*
Multivitamin and mineral preparation with fluoride (p.1444·3) and iron (p.1417·1).
*Dental caries prophylaxis; dietary supplement.*

**Adeforte** *Gross, Braz.*
Vitamin A palmitate (p.1453·1); colecalciferol (p.1461·3); tocoferil acetate (p.1465·1).
*Vitamin supplement.*

**Adeglos** *Ortoquimica, Braz.†.*
Zinc oxide (p.1163·2); boric acid (p.1662·1); dogfish-liver oil.
*Skin disorders.*

**Adegrip** *Heralds, Braz.†.*
Dipyrone (p.35·3); caffeine (p.782·1); guaifenesin (p.1122·1) ascorbic acid (p.1460·2).
*Cold and influenza symptoms.*

**Adegripan** *Heralds, Braz.†.*
Dipyrone (p.35·3); sodium camsilate; guaifenesin (p.1122·1); vitamin C (p.1460·2); mepyramine maleate (p.437·1).
*Cold and influenza symptoms.*

**Adehl** *Kayaku, Jpn.*
Colforsin daropate hydrochloride (p.1674·3).

**Adek** *Falk, Ger.†.*
Vitamins A, D, E, and K (p.1417·1).

**Adekin** *Desitin, Ger.*
Amantadine hydrochloride (p.1197·2).
*Influenza A; parkinsonism.*

**Adekon** *Aventis, Mex.*
Vitamin A palmitate (p.1453·1); ergocalciferol (p.1462·1).
*Vitamin A and D deficiency.*

**Adekon C** *Aventis, Mex.*
Vitamin A palmitate (p.1453·1); ergocalciferol (p.1462·1); ascorbic acid (p.1460·2).
*Vitamin A, D, and C deficiency.*

**Adeks**
*Axcan, Canad.*
Multivitamin preparation with zinc (p.1417·1).

*Scandipharm, USA.*
Multivitamin and mineral preparation (p.1417·1).

**Adel** *Senosiain, Mex.*
Clarithromycin (p.192·2).
*Bacterial infections.*

**Adelcort** *Adelco, Gr.*
Prednisolone (p.1108·1).
*Corticosteroid.*

**Ad-Element** *Darrow, Braz.*
Trace-element preparation (p.1417·1).
*Parenteral nutrition.*

**Adelfan-Esidrex**
*Novartis, Braz.; Novartis, Spain.*
Reserpine (p.995·1); dihydralazine sulfate (p.899·3); hydrochlorothiazide (p.933·2).
*Hypertension.*

**Adelheid-Jodquelle, Tolzer** *Jodquellen, Ger.*
Sodium iodide (p.1598·1); potassium; sodium; ammonium; calcium; magnesium; iron; chloride; sodium bromide; bicarbonate.
*Iodine-deficiency disorders.*

**Adelone** *Cooper (Κοπερ), Gr.*
Prednisolone acetate (p.1108·1).
*Inflammatory eye disorders.*

**Adeloren** *Loren, Mex.*
Vitamin A (p.1451·2); colecalciferol (p.1461·3).

**Adelphane** *Novartis, India.*
Reserpine (p.995·1); dihydralazine sulfate (p.899·3).
*Hypertension.*

**Adelphane-Esidrex**
*Novartis, Hong Kong; Novartis, India.*
Reserpine (p.995·1); dihydralazine sulfate (p.899·3); hydrochlorothiazide (p.933·2).
*Hypertension.*

**Adelphan-Esidrex**
*Novartis, Austria; Novartis, Switz.*
Reserpine (p.995·1); dihydralazine sulfate (p.899·3); hydrochlorothiazide (p.933·2).
*Hypertension.*

**Adelphan-Esidrix** *Novartis, Ger.*
Reserpine (p.995·1); dihydralazine sulfate (p.899·3); hydrochlorothiazide (p.933·2).
*Hypertension.*

**Adena C** *Innotech, Fr.*
Pink tablets, deoxyribonucleic acid (p.1679·2); white tablets, ascorbic acid (p.1460·2).
*Tonic.*

**Adenas** *Eagle, Austral.†.*
Vitamins; minerals; ginseng; eleutherococcus senticosis root (p.1417·1).
*Tonic.*

**Adenil** *Adesil, Arg.*
Betamethasone valerate (p.1093·2); gentamicin sulfate (p.217·1); miconazole nitrate (p.405·3).
*Infected skin disorders.*

**Adenobeta** *Salus, Ital.*
Cocarboxylase chloride (p.1455·2); cyanocobalamin (p.1458·2).
*Neuritis.*

**Adenocard**
*Libbs, Braz.; Fujisawa, Canad.; Fujisawa, USA.*
Adenosine (p.851·2).
*Diagnosis of arrhythmias; paroxysmal supraventricular tachycardia.*

**Adenocor**
*Sanofi Synthelabo, Austral.; Sanofi Synthelabo, Belg.; Sanofi Winthrop, Denm.; Sanofi Synthelabo, Fin.; Sanofi Synthelabo, Gr.; Sanofi Synthelabo, Irl.; Sanofi Winthrop, Israel; Sanofi Synthelabo, Malaysia; Sanofi Synthelabo, Neth.; Sanofi Synthelabo, Norw.; Sanofi Synthelabo, NZ; Sanofi Synthelabo, Port.†; Sanofi Synthelabo, S.Afr.; Sanofi Synthelabo, Singapore; Sanofi Synthelabo, Spain; Sanofi Synthelabo, Thai.; Sanofi Synthelabo, UK.*
Adenosine (p.851·2).
*Diagnosis of arrhythmias; paroxysmal supraventricular tachycardia.*

**Adenoject** *Sun, India.*
Adenosine (p.851·2).
*Coronary vasodilator in diagnostic procedures; paroxysmal supraventricular tachycardia.*

**Adenoplex Forte** *EG, Ital.*
Cocarboxylase (p.1455·2); pyridoxine hydrochloride (p.1456·3); cyanocobalamin (p.1458·2).
*Neuritis.*

**Adenoprostal** *IBSA, Switz.*
Pollen extract.
*Micturition disorders associated with benign prostatic hyperplasia.*

**Adenosan** *Pharmanik (Φαρμανικ), Gr.*
Ketoconazole (p.403·3).
*Fungal skin infections.*

**Adenoscan**
*Sanofi Synthelabo, Austral.; Sanofi Synthelabo, Austria.; Sanofi Synthelabo, Fin.; Sanofi Synthelabo, Fr.; Sanofi Synthelabo, Ger.; Sanofi Synthelabo, Hong Kong; Sanofi Synthelabo, Ital.; Sanofi Synthelabo, Neth.; Sanofi Synthelabo, Spain; Sanofi Synthelabo, UK; Fujisawa, USA.*
Adenosine (p.851·2).
*Coronary vasodilator during radionuclide myocardial perfusion imaging.*

**Adenovit** *NCSN, Ital.*
Cyanocobalamin (p.1458·2); cocarboxylase hydrochloride (p.1455·2); pyridoxine hydrochloride (p.1456·3).
*Neuropathies.*

**Adenyl** *Medipha, Fr.*
Adenosine phosphate (p.1647·3).
*Haemorrhoids; venous insufficiency.*

**Adenylocrat** *Godecke, Ger.*
Crataegus (p.1677·1).
*Cardiac disorders.*

**Adepal** *Wyeth Lederle, Fr.*
Levonorgestrel (p.1563·2); ethinylestradiol (p.1553·2).
*Biphasic oral contraceptive.*

**Adepril**
*Note. This name is used for preparations of different composition.*
*Teofarma, Ital.*
Amitriptyline hydrochloride (p.280·3).
*Depression.*

*Wayne, Mex.†.*
Carbamazepine (p.353·3).

**Adepsique** *Psicofarma, Mex.*
Amitriptyline hydrochloride (p.280·3); diazepam (p.690·1); perphenazine (p.714·2).
*Insomnia; mixed anxiety depressive states.*

**Adept** *Shire, UK.*
Icodextrin (p.1427·1).
*Prevention of surgical adhesions.*

**Adeptolon** *Godecke, Ger.†.*
Prednisolone (p.1108·1); *N*-(4-bromobenzyl)-*N'*-ethyl-*N'*-methyl-*N*-(2-pyridyl)ethylenediamine maleate.
*Hypersensitivity disorders; pruritus.*

**Aderan** *Roemmers, Arg.*
Sibutramine hydrochloride (p.1593·1).
*Obesity.*

**Aderm** *Sigma, Austral.*
Aqueous Cream BP.

**Aderma Dermalibour** *Bio-Merieux, Hong Kong; Pierre Fabre, Hong Kong.*
Avena (p.1658·2); zinc oxide (p.1163·2); zinc sulfate (p.1469·3); copper sulfate (p.1426·1); glycerol (p.1694·3).
*Dry skin; eczema; nappy rash.*

**Aderma Epitheliale** *Bio-Merieux, Hong Kong; Pierre Fabre, Hong Kong.*
Avena (p.1658·2); vitamin A (p.1451·2); vitamin E (p.1464·3).
*Skin abrasions; sunburn; wounds.*

**Aderma Exomega** *Bio-Merieux, Hong Kong; Pierre Fabre, Hong Kong.*
Avena (p.1658·2); omega 6 fatty acids (p.1690·2); glycerol (p.1694·3).
*Eczema.*

**A-Derma Lait Ecran** *Ducray, Fr.*
*SPF 25:* Avena (p.1658·2); zinc oxide (p.1163·2); titanium dioxide (p.1160·3).
*Sunscreen.*

**A-Derma Pain Salicylique** *Ducray, Fr.*
Salicylic acid (p.1157·1).
*Skin disorders.*

**Aderma Ultra High Protection** *Bio-Merieux, Hong Kong; Pierre Fabre, Hong Kong.*
Titanium dioxide (p.1160·3); zinc oxide (p.1163·2); avena (p.1658·2).
*Sunscreen.*

**Adermicina** *Gramon, Arg.*
Neomycin sulfate (p.235·1); vitamin A (p.1451·2); ergocalciferol (p.1462·1); zinc oxide (p.1163·2); benzocaine (p.1370·3).

**Adermicina A** *Gramon, Arg.*
Vitamin A (p.1451·2); zinc oxide (p.1163·2); benzocaine (p.1370·3).

**Adermina** *Koni-Cofarm, Chile.*
Fluocinolone (p.1101·2).
*Skin disorders.*

**Adermykon** *Terramin, Austria†.*
Chlorphenesin (p.396·1).
*Fungal and bacterial infections.*

**Adermykon-C** *Allergan-Frumtost, Braz.†.*
Chlorphenesin (p.396·1); chloramphenicol (p.185·1); lidocaine (p.1377·3).
*Ear infections.*

**Aderofix D3** *Precifarma, Braz.†.*
Vitamin A (p.1451·2); colecalciferol (p.1461·3).
*Vitamin deficiencies.*

**Aderogil D3** *Aventis, Braz.*
Colecalciferol (p.1461·3); vitamin A acetate (p.1453·1).
*Vitamin deficiencies.*

**Aderogyl**
*GlaxoSmithKline, Arg.*
Vitamin A palmitate; ergocalciferol; acetomenaphthone (p.1417·1).
*Vitamin A, D, and K supplement.*

*Aventis, Mex.*
Vitamin preparation (p.1417·1).

**Aderplus spezial Dr Hagedorn** *Naturarzneimittel, Ger.*
Homoeopathic preparation.

**Adesinon-P** *Wakamoto, Hong Kong†.*
Adenosine triphosphate, disodium salt (p.1648·1).
*Cardiac disorders; cerebral disorders; deafness; eczema; eye strain; muscle weakness.*

**Adesipress-TTS** *Pharmacia Upjohn, Ital.*
Clonidine (p.885·2).
*Hypertension.*

**Adesitrin** *Pharmacia Upjohn, Ital.*
Glyceryl trinitrate (p.923·2).
*Angina pectoris.*

**Adex** *Dexxon, Israel.*
Ibuprofen (p.45·3).
*Fever; musculoskeletal and joint disorders; pain.*

**Adexolin** *Seven Seas, UK†.*
Multivitamin preparation (p.1417·1).

**Adexone** *Rekah, Israel.*
Dexamethasone (p.1097·1); salicylic acid (p.1157·1).
*Skin disorders.*

**Adezan** *Adelco, Gr.*
Dipyridamole (p.903·1).
*Thromboembolic disorders.*

**Adezio** *Xepa-Soul Pattinson, Malaysia.*
Cetirizine hydrochloride (p.427·1).
*Allergic rhinitis; urticaria.*

**Adfen** *Adcock Ingram Self Medication, S.Afr.†.*
Ibuprofen (p.45·3).
*Fever; inflammation; musculoskeletal and joint disorders; pain.*

**AD-Furp** *Furp, Braz.†.*
Vitamin A palmitate (p.1453·1); colecalciferol (p.1461·3); zinc oxide (p.1163·2); cod-liver oil (p.1425·2).
*Skin disorders.*

**Adgyn Combi** *Strakan, UK†.*
16 Tablets, estradiol (p.1550·1); 12 tablets, estradiol; norethisterone (p.1562·2).
*Menopausal disorders.*

**Adgyn Estro** *Strakan, UK†.*
Estradiol (p.1550·1).
*Menopausal disorders.*

**Adgyn Medro** *Strakan, UK†.*
Medroxyprogesterone acetate (p.1557·2).
*Adjunct in hormone replacement therapy; amenorrhoea; dysfunctional uterine bleeding; endometriosis.*

**Adhaegon** *Ratiopharm, Austria.*
Dihydroergotamine mesilate (p.465·3).
*Chronic venous insufficiency; hypotension; migraine; varicose veins.*

**Adiantine** *Potter's, UK.*
Hamamelis (p.1696·3); rosemary oil (p.1740·2); bay oil (p.1659·1).
*Scalp disorders.*

**Adiaril** *Gallia, Fr.*
Glucose; sucrose; potassium gluconate; sodium citrate; sodium chloride (p.1222·2).
*Diarrhoea; oral rehydration therapy.*

**Adiazine**
*Bouchara-Recordati, Fr.; IFET (ΙΦΕΤ), Gr.*
Sulfadiazine (p.258·2).
*Bacterial infections; nocardiosis; toxoplasmosis.*

**Adibal** *Diba, Mex.*
Vitamin A palmitate (p.1453·1); ergocalciferol (p.1462·1).
*Vitamin A and D deficiency.*

**Adiboran AD** *Eurospital, Ital.†.*
Vitamin A palmitate (p.1453·1); colecalciferol (p.1461·3).
*Vitamin A and D deficiency.*

**Adicanil** *Pharmaten (Φαρματεν), Gr.*
Lisinopril (p.946·3).
*Heart failure; hypertension; myocardial infarction.*

**Adiclair** *Ardeypharm, Ger.*
Nystatin (p.406·3).
*Fungal infections.*

**Adiecal** *Francia, Ital.*
Calcium carbonate (p.1254·2).
*Calcium deficiency.*

**Adiefim Calcium** *Francia, Ital.†.*
Calcium carbonate; fluorine; colecalciferol; malt (p.1417·1).
*Nutritional supplement.*

**Adifen**
*Note. This name is used for preparations of different composition.*
*Adipharm (Αδηφαρμ), Gr.*
Tamoxifen citrate (p.584·1).
*Breast cancer.*

*Raza, Malaysia.*
Nifedipine (p.966·2).
*Angina pectoris; hypertension.*

**Adifteper** *ISM, Ital.†.*
A diphtheria, tetanus, and pertussis vaccine (p.1613·3).
*Active immunisation.*

**Adilox** *David, India.*
Ampicillin (p.157·1); cloxacillin (p.198·2).
*Bacterial infections.*

**Adimod** *Armstrong, Mex.*
Pidotimod (p.1731·3).
*Immunostimulant.*

**Adinol** *Teva, Israel.*
Zinc oxide (p.1163·2); Burrow's solution; wool alcohols (p.1482·3); silicon dioxide (p.1581·3).
*Barrier preparation; eczema; nappy rash; skin irritation.*

**Adiod** *Teofarma, Spain.*
Colecalciferol (p.1461·3); vitamin A (p.1451·2); iodine (p.1598·1).
*Deficiency of vitamins A and D.*

**Adios** *Dendron, UK.*
Bladderwrack (p.1742·3); boldo (p.1661·2); butternut; taraxacum (p.1751·3).
*Obesity.*

**Adipex**
*Gerot, Austria†; Gerot, Malaysia; Gerot, Switz.*
Phentermine polystyrene sulfonate (p.1592·2).
*Obesity.*

**Adipex-P** *Gate, USA.*
Phentermine hydrochloride (p.1592·2).
*Obesity.*

**Adipine** *Trinity, UK.*
Nifedipine (p.966·2).
*Angina pectoris; hypertension.*

**Adipodiet** *Frandiet, Fr.*
Nutritional supplement (p.1417·1).

**Adiporell** *Sanorell, Ger.*
Homoeopathic preparation.

**Adiporetic** *Frandiet, Fr.*
Nutritional supplement (p.1417·1).

**Adipost** *Ascher, USA†.*
Phendimetrazine tartrate (p.1592·1).
*Obesity.*

**Adiro**
*Bayer, Arg.; Bayer, Mex.; Bayer, Spain.*
Aspirin (p.15·1).
*Fever; inflammation; pain; thromboembolism prophylaxis.*

**Adisar** *Pharma Investi, Chile.*
Sibutramine hydrochloride (p.1593·1).
*Obesity.*

**Adisterolo** *Abiogen, Ital.*
Vitamin A (p.1451·2); colecalciferol (p.1461·3).
*Vitamin A and D deficiency.*

**Adistop** *Phyteia, Switz.†.*
Cathine hydrochloride (p.1585·2).
*Obesity.*

**Adistop Lax** *Phyteia, Switz.†.*
Frangula (p.1266·3); aloes (p.1248·2); senna (p.1288·2); peppermint leaf (p.1283·2); caraway (p.1667·2); fennel (p.1687·2).
*Constipation.*

**Adital** *Gobbi, Arg.*
Macrogol (p.1708·2); electrolytes (p.1217·1).
*Bowel evacuation; constipation.*

**Adiugrip** *Aventis Pasteur, Ital.*
An influenza vaccine (p.1620·2).
*Active immunisation.*

**Adiuvant** *Manetti Roberts, Ital.*
Pirglutargine (p.1732·3).
*Mental function disorders.*

**Adivon** *Ederka, Mex.†.*
Ibuprofen (p.45·3).

**Adizem**
*Napp, Irl.; Rafa, Israel; Napp, UK.*
Diltiazem hydrochloride (p.900·1).
*Angina pectoris; hypertension.*

**ADL** *Bencard, Ger.†.*
Allergen extracts (p.1650·1).
*Allergen immunotherapy.*

**Admag** *TP, Thai.†.*
Aluminium hydroxide (p.1249·2); magnesium hydroxide (p.1272·2); simeticone (p.1289·2).
*Flatulence; gastric hyperacidity.*

**Admag-M** *TP, Thai.†.*
Dried aluminium hydroxide gel (p.1249·2); magnesium trisilicate (p.1272·3).
*Gastric hyperacidity; gastritis; peptic ulcer.*

**Admiral** *Chrispa (Χρισπα), Gr.*
Tenoxicam (p.93·1).
*Dysmenorrhoea; gout; inflammation; osteoarthritis; pain; rheumatoid arthritis; spondyloarthropathies.*

**Admon** *Esteve, Spain.*
Nimodipine (p.972·3).
*Mental function impairment; neurological deficit following subarachnoid haemorrhage.*

**Ad-Muc** *Merz, Ger.*
Chamomile (p.1669·3); myrrh (p.1718·3).
*Inflammatory disorders of the mouth and gums.*

**ADN**
*Braun, Arg.; Braun, Chile.*
A range of preparations for enteral nutrition (p.1417·1).

**Adnax** *DM, Braz.†.*
Naphazoline hydrochloride (p.1124·3); diphenhydramine hydrochloride (p.431·3).
*Nasal congestion.*

**Adnemic** *Nakorn, Thai.*
Multivitamin and mineral preparation with ferrous fumarate (p.1427·3) (p.1417·1).
*Iron-deficiency anaemia; vitamin deficiency.*

**Adnemic F** *Nakorn, Thai.*
Multivitamin and mineral preparation with ferrous fumarate (p.1427·3) and folic acid (p.1429·1) (p.1417·1).
*Iron-deficiency anaemia; vitamin deficiency.*

**Ado C** *Kwizda, Austria.*
Paracetamol (p.76·2); ascorbic acid (p.1460·2).
*Fever; pain.*

**Adocante Docura** *Bravir, Braz.†.*
Sodium cyclamate (p.1426·2); saccharin (p.1443·2).
*Sugar substitute.*

**Adocomp** *TAD, Ger.*
Captopril (p.879·2); hydrochlorothiazide (p.933·2).
*Hypertension.*

**Adocor** *TAD, Ger.*
Captopril (p.879·2).
*Heart failure; hypertension.*

**Adocyl C** *Virtus, Braz.†.*
Sodium cyclamate (p.1426·2); saccharin (p.1443·2).
*Sugar substitute.*

**Adofen** *Ferrer, Spain.*
Fluoxetine hydrochloride (p.292·1).
*Bulimia nervosa; depression; obsessive-compulsive disorder.*

**Adol** *Julphar, UAE.*
Paracetamol (p.76·2).
*Fever; pain.*

**Adol Allergy Sinus** *Julphar, UAE.*
Paracetamol (p.76·2); pseudoephedrine hydrochloride (p.1129·2); chlorphenamine maleate (p.427·3).
*Hay fever; sinusitis; upper respiratory-tract disorders.*

**Adol Cold** *Julphar, UAE.*
Paracetamol (p.76·2); pseudoephedrine hydrochloride (p.1129·2); dextromethorphan hydrobromide (p.1117·3).
*Cold and influenza symptoms.*

**Adol Compound** *Julphar, UAE.*
Salicylamide (p.87·3); paracetamol (p.76·2); caffeine (p.782·1); codeine phosphate (p.27·1).
*Fever; pain.*

**Adol Extra** *Julphar, UAE.*
Paracetamol (p.76·2); caffeine (p.782·1).
*Fever; pain.*

**Adol PM** *Julphar, UAE.*
Paracetamol (p.76·2); diphenhydramine hydrochloride (p.431·3).
*Cold symptoms; insomnia.*

**Adol Sinus** *Julphar, UAE.*
Paracetamol (p.76·2); pseudoephedrine hydrochloride (p.1129·2).
*Nasal congestion; sinus headache.*

**Adolan** *Abic, Israel.*
Methadone hydrochloride (p.57·2).
*Opioid withdrawal syndrome; pain.*

**Adolcas** *Casasco, Arg.*
Monofluoride phosphate; calcium carbonate (p.1254·2).
*Osteoporosis.*

**Adolkin** *Prodes, Spain†.*
Metamizole magnesium (p.36·1).
*Fever; pain.*

**Adolonta** *Grunenthal, Spain.*
Tramadol hydrochloride (p.94·3).
*Pain.*

**Adolorin** *Kwizda, Austria.*
Propyphenazone (p.85·3); paracetamol (p.76·2); caffeine (p.782·1).
*Fever; pain.*

**Adolorin ASS/Vit C** *Kwizda, Austria.*
Aspirin (p.15·1); ascorbic acid (p.1460·2).
*Cold and influenza symptoms.*

**Adolphs Salt Substitute** *Adolphs, USA.*
Sodium-free dietary salt substitute (p.1417·1).

**Adolquir** *Kin, Spain.*
Dexketoprofen trometamol (p.51·2).
*Pain.*

**Adoluron CC** *Kwizda, Austria.*
Propyphenazone (p.85·3); paracetamol (p.76·2); codeine hydrochloride (p.27·1).
*Fever; pain.*

**Adona**
*Note. This name is used for preparations of different composition.*
*Silesia, Chile.*
Paracetamol (p.76·2); ibuprofen (p.45·3).
*Fever; inflammation; pain.*

*Tanabe, Hong Kong; SIT, Ital.; Tanabe, Jpn.*
Carbazochrome sodium sulfonate (p.745·1).
*Haemorrhagic disorders.*

**Adop-Tar** *ICN, Arg.*
Fluocinolone acetonide (p.1101·2); salicylic acid (p.1157·1); coal tar (p.1159·2).
*Psoriasis.*

**Adoquick Vit C**
*Kwizda, Austria.*
Aspirin (p.15·1); ascorbic acid (p.1460·2).
*Cold and influenza symptoms.*

**Adormix** *Sanofi Synthelabo, Chile.*
Zolpidem tartrate (p.728·3).
*Insomnia.*

**Adovit C** *Kwizda, Austria†.*
Aspirin (p.15·1); ascorbic acid (p.1460·2).
*Fever; pain.*

**Adoxa** *Bioglan, USA.*
Doxycycline (p.206·2).
*Bacterial infections.*

**Adprex** *Hebron, Braz.*
Hypericum (p.299·1).
*Depression.*

**Adprin-B** *Pfeiffer, USA.*
Aspirin (p.15·1).
Calcium carbonate (p.1254·2), magnesium carbonate (p.1272·1), and magnesium oxide (p.1272·3) are included in this preparation in an attempt to limit adverse effects on the gastrointestinal mucosa.
*Pain.*

**Adrebloc** *Beta, Arg.*
Amlodipine (p.862·2); benazepril hydrochloride (p.867·2).
*Hypertension.*

**Adrecort** *Allen, Mex.*
Dexamethasone (p.1097·1).
*Corticosteroid.*

**Adrectal** *Vifor, Switz.†.*
*Ointment:* Ephedrine hydrochloride (p.1120·1); lidocaine hydrochloride (p.1377·3); peppermint oil (p.1283·2); thymol (p.1194·2); zinc stearate (p.1575·3).
*Suppositories:* Ephedrine hydrochloride (p.1120·1); lidocaine hydrochloride (p.1377·3); tetracaine hydrochloride (p.1385·1); peppermint oil (p.1283·2); thymol (p.1194·2); zinc stearate (p.1575·3).
*Anorectal disorders.*

**Adreject** *ALK, Spain.*
Adrenaline (p.852·2).
*Anaphylaxis.*

**Adrekar**
*Sanofi Synthelabo, Austria; Sanofi Synthelabo, Ger.*
Adenosine (p.851·2).
*Arrhythmias.*

**Adrenam** *NAM, Ger.*
Etilefrine hydrochloride (p.914·1).
*Hypotension.*

**Adrenol** *Fabra, Arg.*
Co-trimoxazole (p.199·3).
*Bacterial infections.*

**Adrenoplasma** *Climax, Braz.*
Carbazochrome (p.745·1).
*Haemorrhage.*

**Adrenor**
*Samarth, India; Llorens, Spain†.*
Noradrenaline acid tartrate (p.974·3).
*Adjunct in cardiac arrest; glaucoma; hypotension.*

**Adrenoxil**
*Climax, Braz.; CPH, Port.*
Carbazochrome (p.745·1).
*Haemorrhagic disorders.*

**Adrenoxyl** *Sanofi Synthelabo, Ger.*
Carbazochrome (p.745·1).
*Haemorrhage.*

**Adreson** *Organon, Belg.*
Cortisone acetate (p.1096·1).
*Corticosteroid.*

**Adrevil** *Novartis Consumer, Ger.†.*
Butalamine hydrochloride (p.878·2).
*Peripheral and cerebral vascular disorders.*

**Adrexan** *Mayoly-Spindler, Fr.*
Propranolol hydrochloride (p.989·3).
*Cardiovascular disorders.*

**Adrezon** *Ono, Hong Kong†.*
Carbazochrome (p.745·1).
*Haemorrhage.*

**Adriblastin**
*Pharmacia, Austria; Pharmacia, Ger.; Pharmacia, Switz.*
Doxorubicin hydrochloride (p.547·3).
*Malignant neoplasms.*

**Adriblastina**
*Pharmacia, Arg.; Pharmacia, Belg.; Pharmacia, Braz.; Pharmacia, Chile; Pharmacia-Upjohn, Gr.; Pharmacia Upjohn, Israel; Pharmacia Upjohn, Ital.; Pharmacia Upjohn, Mex.; Pharmacia, Neth.; Pharmacia, Port.; Pharmacia Upjohn, S.Afr.†; Pharmacia, Thai.*
Doxorubicin hydrochloride (p.547·3).
*Malignant neoplasms.*

**Adriblastine** *Pharmacia, Fr.*
Doxorubicin hydrochloride (p.547·3).
*Malignant neoplasms.*

**Adrigyl** *Bouchara-Recordati, Fr.*
Colecalciferol (p.1461·3).
*Vitamin D deficiency.*

**Adrim**
*Dabur, India; Dabur, Thai.*
Doxorubicin hydrochloride (p.547·3).
*Malignant neoplasms.*

**Adrimedac** *Medac, Ger.*
Doxorubicin hydrochloride (p.547·3).
*Malignant neoplasms.*

**Adrinex** *Medical, Port.*
Adrenaline (p.852·2); benzyl nicotinate (p.21·2).
*Musculoskeletal, joint, peri-articular, and soft-tissue disorders.*

**Adrocil** *Oftalder, Port.*
Trifluridine (p.655·3).
*Viral eye infections.*

**Adro-derm** *Adroka, Switz.†.*
Propyl alcohol (p.1191·2); alcohol (p.1166·1); chlorhexidine gluconate (p.1173·2).
*Skin disinfection.*

**Adronat**
*Neopharmed, Ital.; Tecnifar, Port.*
Alendronate sodium (p.765·3).
*Osteoporosis.*

**Adroxef** *Laboratorios Chile, Chile.*
Cefadroxil (p.167·2).
*Bacterial infections.*

**Adroyd** *Parke, Davis, India.*
Oxymetholone (p.1565·2).
*Aplastic anaemia.*

**Adrucil**
*Pharmacia, Canad.; Gensia, USA.*
Fluorouracil (p.554·2).
*Malignant neoplasms.*

**Adrusen**
*SIFI, Ital.*
Lycopene; vitamins; minerals (p.1417·1).

*SIFI, Singapore.*
Food supplement with vitamins and minerals (p.1417·1).

**Ad-Sorb** *Key, Austral.*
Activated charcoal (p.1030·2).
*Flatulence.*

**Adsorbed DT Coq** *Aventis Pasteur, Hong Kong.*
An adsorbed diphtheria, tetanus, and pertussis vaccine (p.1613·3).
*Active immunisation.*

**Adsorbed DT Vax** *Pasteur Merieux, Hong Kong†.*
An adsorbed diphtheria and tetanus vaccine (p.1613·1).
*Active immunisation.*

**Adsorbocarpine** *Alcon, USA.*
Pilocarpine hydrochloride (p.1495·1).
*Glaucoma; raised intra-ocular pressure; reversal of mydriasis.*

**Adsorbonac**
*Alcon, Ger.; Alcon, Hong Kong†; Alcon, Ital.; Alcon, Singapore†; Alcon, USA.*
Sodium chloride (p.1233·3).
*Corneal oedema.*

**ADT**
*Note. This name is used for preparations of different composition.*
*CSL, Austral; CSL, NZ†.*
An adsorbed diphtheria and tetanus vaccine (p.1613·1).
*Active immunisation.*

*Zimaia, Port.*
Amitriptyline hydrochloride (p.280·3).
*Depression; nocturnal enuresis.*

**AD-Til** *Altana, Braz.*
Colecalciferol (p.1461·3); vitamin A acetate (p.1453·1).
*Vitamin deficiencies.*

**Aduar** *Vannier, Arg.*
Mebendazole (p.108·2); tinidazole (p.617·1).

**Aducin** *Nettopharma, Denm.*
Ranitidine hydrochloride (p.1285·2).
*Acid aspiration; gastro-oesophageal reflux; peptic ulcer; Zollinger-Ellison syndrome.*

**Adulax** *Casen Fleet, Spain.*
Glycerol (p.1694·3).
*Constipation.*

**Adult Chesty Cough** *Numark, UK.*
Diphenhydramine (p.431·3).
*Coughs.*

**Adult Chesty Cough Non Drowsy** *Numark, UK.*
Guaifenesin (p.1122·1).
*Coughs.*

**Adult Citrex** *Raza, Malaysia.*
Multivitamin preparations with zinc (p.1469·2) (p.1417·1).

**Adult Citrex Cal-Mag-D3** *Raza, Malaysia; Pharmaniaga, Malaysia.*
Calcium (p.1225·1); colecalciferol (p.1461·3); magnesium (p.1227·3).
*Vitamin D and mineral supplement.*

**Adult Citrex Multivitamin + Ginseng + Omega 3** *Raza, Malaysia.*
Multivitamin preparation with ginseng (p.1693·1) and omega-3 marine triglycerides (p.976·2).

**Adult Dry Cough** *Numark, UK.*
Dextromethorphan (p.1117·3).
*Coughs.*

**Adult Ideal Quota** *Larkhall Laboratories, UK†.*
Multivitamin and mineral preparation (p.1417·1).

**Adult Meltus for Chesty Coughs & Catarrh**
*SSL, UK†.*
Guaifenesin (p.1122·1); cetylpyridinium chloride (p.1173·1); honey (p.1434·2).
*Catarrh; coughs.*

**Adumbran**
*Boehringer Ingelheim, Austria; Boehringer Ingelheim, Ger.; Boehringer Ingelheim, Spain.*
Oxazepam (p.712·2).
*Anxiety; insomnia.*

**Adurix** *Nycomed, Denm.*
Clopamide (p.888·2).
*Diabetes insipidus; hypertension; oedema.*

**Adursal** *Leiras, Fin.*
Ursodeoxycholic acid (p.1760·3).
*Biliary-tract disorders; chronic active hepatitis; gallstones.*

**Advair**
*GlaxoSmithKline, Canad.; Glaxo Wellcome, USA.*
Fluticasone propionate (p.1102·3); salmeterol xinafoate (p.795·1).
*Obstructive airways disease.*

**Advance**
*Note. This name is used for preparations of different composition.*
*Avon, Canad.*
Pyrithione zinc (p.1156·2).
*Scalp disorders.*

*Advanced Care, USA.*
Pregnancy test (p.1734·3).

**Advanced Antioxidants Formula** *Solgar, UK†.*
Multivitamin and mineral preparation with superoxide dismutase inducers and proanthocyanidin complex (p.1417·1).
*Dietary supplement.*

**Advanced Formula Di-Gel** *Schering-Plough, USA.*
Magnesium hydroxide (p.1272·2); calcium carbonate (p.1254·2); simeticone (p.1289·2).
*Hyperacidity.*

**Advanced Formula Multibionta** *Seven Seas, UK†.*
Vitamins; minerals; *Lactobacillus acidophilus*; *Bifidobacterium bifidum*; *Bifidobacterium longum* (p.1417·1).
*Tonic.*

**Advanced Formula Plax** *Pfizer, USA.*
Sodium pyrophosphate.

**Advanced Formula Tegrin** *Block, USA†.*
Coal tar (p.1159·2).
*Scalp disorders.*

**Advanced Formula Zenate** *Solvay, USA.*
Multivitamin and mineral preparation with iron and folic acid (p.1417·1).
Formerly called Zenate.
*Nutritional supplement in pregnancy and lactation.*

**Advanced Relief Visine** *Pfizer Consumer, USA.*
Tetryzoline hydrochloride (p.1131·2); macrogol 400 (p.1709·1); povidone (p.1581·2); dextran 70 (p.746·2).
*Dry eyes; eye irritation.*

**Advanced-RF Natal Care** *Ethex, USA.*
Vitamin and mineral preparation (p.1417·1).

**Advantage**
*Note. This name is used for preparations of different composition.*
*Roche Diagnostics, Austral.; Roche Diagnostics, Canad.; Roche Diagnostics, NZ.*
Test for glucose in blood (p.1694·2).

*Allergan, Canad.†.*
Subtilisin (p.1164·2).
*Protein and lipid remover for contact lenses.*

**Advantage 24**
*Note. A similar name is used for preparations of different composition (see above).*
*Wellspring, Canad.; Lake, USA.*
Nonoxinol 9 (p.1413·3).
*Contraceptive.*

**Advantan**
*Schering, Arg.; CSL, Austral.; Schering, Austria; Schering, Belg.; Schering, Braz.; Schering, Fin.; Asche, Ger.; Schering, Ger.; Shepa, Gr.; Schering, Hong Kong; Schering, Ital.; Schering, Mex.; CSL, NZ; Schering, Port.; Schering, S.Afr.; Schering, Switz.*
Methylprednisolone aceponate (p.1106·3).
*Skin disorders.*

**Advate**
*Baxter BioScience, UK; Baxter, USA.*
A factor VIII preparation (p.751·1).
*Haemorrhagic disorders.*

**Adventan** *Schering, Spain.*
Methylprednisolone aceponate (p.1106·3).
*Skin disorders.*

**Advera**
*Abbott, Arg.; Abbott, Austral.; Abbott, Braz.; Abbott, Canad.†; Abbott, Fin.†; Abbott, Fr.†; Ross, Israel; Abbott, Ital.†; Abbott, Mex.; Ross, USA.*
Preparation for enteral nutrition in immunocompromised patients (p.1417·1).

**Adversuten** *AWD, Ger.*
Prazosin hydrochloride (p.985·1).
*Heart failure; hypertension; Raynaud's syndrome.*

**Advicor** *KOS, USA.*
Nicotinic acid (p.1441·1); lovastatin (p.949·1).
*Hypercholesterolaemia.*

**Advil**
*Wyeth Lederle, Austria; Whitehall, Braz.; Whitehall-Robins, Canad.; Wyeth Consumer, Chile; Whitehall, Fr.; Whitehall, Hong Kong; Whitehall, Irl.; Whitehall, Israel; Wyeth, Mex.; Wyeth Consumer, Neth.; Wyeth, Spain; Wyeth Consumer, UK; Wyeth-Ayerst, USA; Whitehall, USA.*
Ibuprofen (p.45·3).
Fever; inflammation; pain.

**Advil Allergy Sinus** *Wyeth Consumer, USA.*
Pseudoephedrine hydrochloride (p.1129·2); chlorphenamine maleate (p.427·3); ibuprofen (p.45·3).
*Upper respiratory-tract disorders.*

**Advil Cold** *Wyeth Lederle, Austria.*
Ibuprofen (p.45·3); pseudoephedrine hydrochloride (p.1129·2).
*Cold and influenza symptoms.*

**Advil Cold & Flu** *Whitehall, Irl.*
Ibuprofen (p.45·3); pseudoephedrine (p.1129·2).
*Cold and influenza symptoms.*

**Advil Cold & Sinus**
*Whitehall-Robins, Canad.; Whitehall, UK†; Whitehall, USA.*
Ibuprofen (p.45·3); pseudoephedrine hydrochloride (p.1129·2).
Formerly known as Coadvil in the *USA*.
*Cold and influenza symptoms; sinus congestion.*

**Advil CS** *Whitehall, S.Afr.*
Ibuprofen (p.45·3); pseudoephedrine hydrochloride (p.1129·2).
*Cold and influenza symptoms.*

**Advil Mono** *Whitehall, Belg.†.*
Ibuprofen (p.45·3).
*Fever; pain.*

**Advisor** *Abbott, Ital.†.*
Pregnancy test (p.1734·3).

**AD-vitamin** *ACO, Swed.*
Vitamin A palmitate (p.1453·1); colecalciferol (p.1461·3).
*Vitamin supplement.*

**AD-Vitan** *Janssen-Cilag, Belg.†.*
Vitamin A acetate (p.1453·1); colecalciferol (p.1461·3).
*Osteomalacia; rickets; vitamin A and D deficiency.*

**Adyston** *Krewel, Ger.*
Pholedrine sulfate (p.982·3); norfenefrine hydrochloride (p.975·3).
*Hypotension.*

**Aedolac**
*Guieu, Fr.†; Rottapharm, Ital.*
Emollient.
*Dry skin; eczema.*

**Aegrosan** *Opfermann, Ger.*
Dimeticone (p.1289·2).
*Reduction of gastrointestinal gas.*

**A-E-Mulsin**
*Mucos, Austria; Mucos, Ger.*
Vitamin A palmitate (p.1453·1); alpha tocoferil acetate (p.1465·1).
*Vitamin A and E deficiency.*

**Aequalyre** *Boehringer Ingelheim, Fr.†.*
Sodium chloride (p.1233·3).
*Conjunctival irrigation; eyelid cleansing.*

**Aequamen** *Byk Gulden, Ger.*
Betahistine mesilate (p.1660·1).
*Ménière's syndrome; vestibular disorders.*

**Aequifusine** *Braun, Switz.*
Electrolyte infusion with glucose (p.1217·1).
*Fluid and electrolyte disorders.*

**Aequiseral** *Streuli, Switz.†.*
Electrolyte and glucose solution (p.1217·1).
*Dehydration.*

**Aequiton-P** *Sudmedica, Ger.*
Phenazone (p.82·3).
*Fever; pain.*

**A-E-R** *Birchwood, USA.*
Hamamelis (p.1696·3).
*Anorectal disorders; vaginal irritation.*

**Aerflu** *Pulitzer, Ital.*
Flunisolide (p.1101·1).
*Respiratory-tract hypersensitivity; rhinitis.*

**Aerius**
*White, Arg.; Schering-Plough, Belg.; Schering, Canad.; Schering-Plough, Chile; SP, Denm.; Schering-Plough, Fin.; Schering-Plough, Fr.; Essex, Ger.; Schering-Plough, Gr.; Schering-Plough, Hong Kong; Scher-*

ing-Plough, Neth.; Schering-Plough, Norw.; Schering-Plough, Port.; Schering-Plough, Singapore; Schering-Plough, Spain; Schering-Plough, Swed.; Essex, Switz.; Schering-Plough, Thai.
Desloratadine (p.431·1).
*Allergic rhinitis; urticaria.*

**Aero Helpp Forte** ISA, Arg.
Permethrin (p.1508·3); piperonyl butoxide (p.1509·2); malathion (p.1507·1).
*Pediculosis.*

**Aero Itan** Saval, Chile.
Dimeticone (p.1482·1); metoclopramide (p.1274·3); chlordiazepoxide (p.674·2).
*Dyspepsia; flatulence; gastrointestinal motility disorders; meteorism.*

**Aero Plus** Upsamedica, Spain.
Dimethicone (p.1289·2); metoclopramide hydrochloride (p.1274·3).
*Aerophagia; delayed gastric emptying.*

**Aero Red** Uriach, Spain.
Dimethicone (p.1289·2).
*Flatulence.*

**Aero Red Antiacido** Uriach, Spain.
Calcium carbonate (p.1254·2); simeticone (p.1289·2); magnesium hydroxide (p.1272·2).
*Flatulence; gastric hyperacidity.*

**Aero Red Complex** Uriach, Spain.
Dimethicone (p.1289·2); lipolytic enzymes; amylolytic enzymes; proteolytic enzymes; cellulolytic enzymes.
Formerly known as Aero Red Eupeptico.
*Digestive system disorders.*

**Aeroaid** Health & Medical, USA; Graham-Field, USA.
Thiomersal (p.1194·1).
*Skin disinfection; wounds.*

**AeroBec**
3M, Denm.; 3M, Fin.; 3M, Ger.; Asta Medica, Ger.; 3M, Irl.; Riker, Mex.†; 3M, Neth.; 3M, Norw.; 3M, S.Afr.; 3M, Switz.; 3M, UK.
Beclometasone dipropionate (p.1091·1).
*Obstructive airways disease.*

**AeroBid** Forest Pharmaceuticals, USA.
Flunisolide (p.1101·1).
*Asthma.*

**Aerobin**
Farmasan, Ger.; Farmasan, Thai.; TTN, Thai.
Theophylline (p.798·3) or theophylline sodium glycinate (p.804·3).
*Obstructive airways disease.*

**Aero-Bud** Andromaco, Chile.
Budesonide (p.1094·2).
*Asthma.*

**Aerocaine** Aeroceuticals, USA.
Benzocaine (p.1370·3); benzethonium chloride (p.1169·2).
*Skin disorders.*

**Aerocef** Klinge, Austria.
Cefixime (p.172·3).
*Bacterial infections.*

**Aerocid** Aerocid, Fr.†.
Pancreas powder (porcine); simeticone (p.1289·2).
Formerly contained adrenaline, pancreatin, liver extract, and ergot.
*Dyspepsia.*

**Aero-Clenil** Farmalab, Braz.†.
Salbutamol (p.791·3).
*Obstructive airways disease.*

**Aerocort** Cipla, India.
Salbutamol (p.791·3) or salbutamol sulfate (p.791·3); beclometasone dipropionate (p.1091·1).
*Asthma.*

**Aerocrom**
Rhone-Poulenc Rorer, Mex.†; Castlemead, UK†.
Sodium cromoglicate (p.795·3); salbutamol sulfate (p.791·3).
*Asthma.*

**Aeroderm** Seid, Spain.
Lidocaine hydrochloride (p.1377·3).
*Burns; insect stings; skin irritation.*

**Aerodesin** Lysoform, Ger.
Propyl alcohol (p.1191·2); alcohol (p.1166·1); glutaral (p.1180·3).
*Surface disinfection.*

**Aerodine**
Note. This name is used for preparations of different composition.
Teuto, Braz.
Salbutamol (p.791·3) or salbutamol sulfate (p.791·3).
*Obstructive airways disease.*

Graham-Field, USA†.
Povidone-iodine (p.1190·3).
*Skin disinfection.*

**Aerodiol**
Servier, Arg.; Servier, Austral.; Servier, Belg.; Servier, Braz.; Servier, Denm.; Servier, Fr.; Servier, Ger.; Servier, Hong Kong; Servier, Ital.; Servier, Neth.; Servier, UK.
Estradiol (p.1550·1).
*Menopausal disorders.*

**Aerodur** Stern, Ger.; AstraZeneca, Ger.
Terbutaline sulfate (p.797·2).
*Obstructive airways disease.*

**Aerodyne** Klinge, Austria.
Theophylline (p.798·3) or theophylline sodium glycinate (p.804·3).
*Obstructive airways disease.*

**Aerofagil** Geymonat, Ital.
Sodium citrate (p.1223·2); dimeticone (p.1289·2).
*Aerophagia; meteorism.*

**Aeroflat**
Roche, Chile; Biosarto, Spain.
Simeticone (p.1289·2); metoclopramide (p.1274·3).
*Aid in gastrointestinal radiology; gastrointestinal disorders; nausea and vomiting.*

**Aeroflux** Glaxo Wellcome, Mex.
Salbutamol sulfate (p.791·3); ambroxol hydrochloride (p.1114·3).
*Asthma; bronchitis; respiratory-tract disorders with increased mucus.*

**Aeroflux Edulito** GlaxoSmithKline, Braz.
Salbutamol (p.791·3); guaifenesin (p.1122·1); sodium citrate (p.1223·2).
*Obstructive airways disease.*

**Aerofreeze** Graham-Field, USA.
Dichlorodifluoromethane (p.1236·1); trichlorofluoromethane (p.1236·1).
*Topical anaesthesia.*

**Aerogal** Galien, Arg.
Silicone oil (p.1482·1).
*Barrier preparation.*

**Aerogastrol** Medipharm, Chile.
Metoclopramide (p.1274·3); simeticone (p.1289·2); chlordiazepoxide (p.674·2).
*Dyspepsia; flatulence; gastrointestinal motility disorders; meteorism.*

**Aerogel** Upsamedica, Spain.
Aluminium hydroxide (p.1249·2); dimethicone (p.1289·2).
*Dyspepsia; flatulence; gastrointestinal hyperacidity.*

**AeroHist Plus** Aero, USA.
Phenylephrine hydrochloride (p.1126·3); chlorphenamine maleate (p.427·3); hyoscine methonitrate (p.483·3).
*Upper respiratory-tract disorders.*

**Aero-Jet** Farmalab, Braz.
Salbutamol (p.791·3).
*Obstructive airways disease.*

**AeroKid** Aero, USA.
Phenylephrine hydrochloride (p.1126·3); chlorphenamine maleate (p.427·3); hyoscine methonitrate (p.483·3).
*Upper respiratory-tract disorders.*

**Aerolate** Fleming, USA.
Theophylline (p.798·3).
*Obstructive airways disease.*

**Aerolid** Piam, Ital.
Flunisolide (p.1101·1).
*Respiratory-tract hypersensitivity; rhinitis.*

**Aerolin**
GlaxoSmithKline, Braz.; GlaxoSmithKline, Chile; Glaxo Wellcome, Gr.; 3M, Irl.; 3M, Israel; 3M, Neth.; 3M, UK†.
Salbutamol (p.791·3) or salbutamol sulfate (p.791·3).
*Obstructive airways disease; premature labour.*

**Aerolind** TAD, Ger.†.
Salbutamol (p.791·3).
*Obstructive airways disease.*

**Aeromax** GlaxoSmithKline, Ger.
Salmeterol xinafoate (p.795·1).
*Obstructive airways disease.*

**Aeromicrosona C** ICN, Arg.
Ketoconazole (p.403·3); hydrocortisone acetate (p.1103·3); gentamicin sulfate (p.217·1).
*Infected skin disorders.*

**Aeromuc** Klinge, Austria.
Acetylcysteine (p.1112·3).
*Respiratory-tract disorders.*

**Aeronix** Menarini, Spain.
Zafirlukast (p.807·1).
*Asthma.*

**Aero-Om** OM, Port.
Simeticone (p.1289·2).
*Adjunct in gastrointestinal radiology; aerophagia; gastrointestinal distension; infant colic; meteorism.*

**Aeropax**
Orion, Denm.; Ercopharm, Switz.†.
Dimethicone (p.1289·2).
*Aid in radiography and gastroscopy; infant colic; meteorism.*

**Aeropaxyn** Lannacher, Austria.
Sodium cromoglicate (p.795·3).
*Asthma; bronchitis.*

**Aero-Ped** Stiefel, Braz.
Salbutamol sulfate (p.791·3).
*Obstructive airways disease.*

**Aero-Plus** Andromaco, Chile.
Salbutamol (p.791·3); beclometasone dipropionate (p.1091·1).
*Obstructive airways disease.*

**Aero-Sal** Andromaco, Chile.
Salbutamol (p.791·3).
*Obstructive airways disease.*

**Aeroseb** Panalab, Arg.
*Shampoo:* Pyrithione zinc (p.1156·2); cade oil (p.1159·2).
*Scalp disorders.*

*Soap:* Pyrithione zinc (p.1156·2).
*Seborrhoea.*

**Aeroseb-Dex** Allergan Herbert, USA.
Dexamethasone (p.1097·1).
*Skin disorders.*

**Aerosil** Degussa, UK.
Colloidal silicon dioxide (p.1581·3).
*Pharmaceutical formulation aid.*

**Aerosol Spitzner N** Spitzner, Ger.
Oleum pini sylvestris; pumilio pine oil (p.1737·1); eucalyptus oil (p.1686·2); siberian fir oil; noble pine oil.
*Respiratory-tract disorders.*

**Aerosolv** Klinge, Austria.
Acetylcysteine (p.1112·3).
*Respiratory-tract disorders with viscous mucus.*

**Aerosoma** Etex, Chile.
Salbutamol (p.791·3); beclometasone dipropionate (p.1091·1).
*Obstructive airways disease.*

**Aerosporin** Glaxo Wellcome, Canad.†.
Polymyxin B sulfate (p.245·1).
*Gram-negative infections.*

**Aerotamol** Royton, Braz.
Salbutamol (p.791·3).
*Obstructive airways disease.*

**Aerotec** Sanofi Synthelabo, Ital.
Salbutamol sulfate (p.791·3).
*Obstructive airways disease.*

**Aerotherm** Aeroceuticals, USA†.
Benzocaine (p.1370·3); benzethonium chloride (p.1169·2).
*Skin disorders.*

**Aerotide** GlaxoSmithKline, Braz.
Beclometasone dipropionate (p.1091·1); salbutamol (p.791·3).
*Asthma.*

**Aerotina** Raffo, Arg.
Loratadine (p.436·1).
*Hypersensitivity reactions.*

**Aerotrat** Cazi, Braz.
Salbutamol sulfate (p.791·3).
*Obstructive airways disease.*

**Aerovac** Sankyo, Austria.
Lysates of *Staphylococcus aureus*; *Streptococcus mitis*; *Streptococcus pyogenes*; *Streptococcus pneumoniae*; *Klebsiella pneumoniae*; *Moraxella catarrhalis*; *Haemophilus influenzae*.
*Respiratory-tract infections.*

**Aerovac G** Casasco, Arg.
*Haemophilus influenzae*; *Streptococcus pneumoniae*; *Klebsiella pneumoniae*; *Moraxella catarrhalis*; streptococcus.
*Respiratory-tract infections.*

**Aerovacuna** Nezel, Spain†.
Lysates of *diplococcus*; *streptococcus*; *Micrococcus pyogenes*; *Gaffkya anaerobia*; *Neisseria*; *Haemophilus influenzae*; *Klebsiella pneumoniae*; *Moraxella*.
*Respiratory-tract infections.*

**Aerovent** Teva, Israel.
Ipratropium bromide (p.787·1).
*Obstructive airways disease.*

**Aerovial** Recalcine, Chile.
Budesonide (p.1094·2).
*Asthma.*

**Aeroxina** Elea, Arg.
Clarithromycin (p.192·2).
*Bacterial infections.*

**Aerozoin** Graham-Field, USA.
Compound benzoin tincture.
*Barrier preparation.*

**AErrane**
Baxter, Austral.; Pharmacia Upjohn, Belg.†; Pharmacia Upjohn, Irl.†; Zeneca, Israel; Baxter, Ital.; Baxter, Neth.; Baxter, NZ; Zeneca, S.Afr.; Baxter, Spain; AstraZeneca, Thai.†; Baxter Anaesthesia, UK.
Isoflurane (p.1301·1).
*General anaesthesia.*

**Aescorin Forte** Steigerwald, Ger.
Aesculus (p.1648·2).
*Soft-tissue injury; venous insufficiency.*

**Aescorin N** Steigerwald, Ger.
*Injection*†: Rutoside sodium sulfate (p.1688·3); esculoside (p.1648·2).
*Ointment:* Aesculus (p.1648·2); hamamelis (p.1696·3).
*Haemorrhoids; vascular disorders.*

**Aescosulf N** Truw, Ger.
Homoeopathic preparation.

**Aesculaforce**
Bio-Garten, Austria; Bioforce, Switz.
Aesculus (p.1648·2).
*Venous insufficiency.*

**Aesculaforce N** Bioforce, Switz.†.
Homoeopathic preparation.

**AesculaMed** Bioforce, Switz.
Aesculus (p.1648·2).
*Venous insufficiency.*

**Aesculo Gel L** Engelhard, Ger.
Coconut oil (p.1481·1).
*Pediculosis.*

**Aesculus Med Complex** Dynamit, Austria.
Homoeopathic preparation.

**Aescusan**
Jenapharm, Ger.
*Delayed-release tablets; tablets:* Aesculus (p.1648·2).
*Venous insufficiency.*

Riemser, Ger.
*Cream:* Aesculus (p.1648·2); hamamelis (p.1696·3).
*Soft-tissue inflammation; venous insufficiency.*

**Aescuven** Cesra, Ger.
Aesculus (p.1648·2).
*Soft-tissue inflammation; venous insufficiency.*

**Aesim** Frasca, Arg.
Simeticone (p.1289·2).
*Flatulence.*

**Aesol** Leiras, Fin.
Vitamin A palmitate (p.1453·1); alpha tocoferil acetate (p.1465·1).
*Vitamins A and E deficiency; vitamins A and E supplement.*

**Aesrutal S** Steigerwald, Ger.†.
Convallaria (p.1675·3); crataegus (p.1677·1); ammi visnaga fruit (p.1653·3).
*Circulatory insufficiency; heart failure.*

**Aesrutan** Engelshof, Austria†.
Rutoside (p.1688·2); aesculus (p.1648·2).
*Chronic venous insufficiency; haemorrhoids.*

**Aet** Craveri, Arg.
Lauromacrogol 400 (p.1412·3).
*Varices.*

**Aethoxysclerol**
BSN, Austral; Teuto, Braz.
Lauromacrogol 400 (p.1412·3).
*Varices.*

**Aethoxysklerol**
Nycomed, Austria; Codali, Belg.; Kreussler, Denm.; Kreussler, Fin.; Kreussler, Ger.; Sigma-Tau, Neth.; Inverdia, Swed.; Kreussler, Switz.; Kreussler, Thai.
Lauromacrogol 400 (p.1412·3).
*Dilated cutaneous veins; haemorrhoids; varices.*

**Aethroma**
Ratiopharm, Austria; Mepha, Hong Kong; Mepha, Switz.†.
Vincamine (p.1764·2).
*Cerebrovascular disorders; hearing disorders; tinnitus.*

**Aetoxisclerol** Kreussler, Fr.
Lauromacrogol 400 (p.1412·3).
Formerly known as Veinosclerol.
*Varices.*

**Aetoxy Sklerol** Dominguez, Arg.
Lauromacrogol 400 (p.1412·3).
*Varices.*

**Aezodent** Associated Dental, UK†.
Chlorobutanol (p.1176·3); methyl salicylate (p.59·3); benzocaine (p.1370·3); menthol (p.1711·3); eugenol (p.1686·2).
*Denture irritation.*

**AF**
Note. This name is used for preparations of different composition.
Valdecasas, Mex.
Folic acid (p.1429·1).
*Folic acid deficiency.*

Aspen, S.Afr.
Zinc undecenoate (p.411·1); undecenoic acid (p.410·3); terpineol (p.1752·2).
*Fungal skin infections.*

**222 AF** Johnson & Johnson, Canad.†.
Paracetamol (p.76·2).
*Fever; pain.*

**AF Anacin** Whitehall-Robins, Canad.†.
Paracetamol (p.76·2).
*Fever; pain.*

**Afalpi Tiptipot** CTI, Israel.
Pseudoephedrine hydrochloride (p.1129·2).
*Upper respiratory-tract congestion.*

**Afazol** Grin, Mex.
Naphazoline hydrochloride (p.1124·3).
*Eye irritation.*

**Afazol Z** Grin, Mex.
Naphazoline hydrochloride (p.1124·3); zinc sulfate (p.1469·3).
*Eye disorders.*

**Afebrin**
Note. This name is used for preparations of different composition.
Legrand, Braz.
Phenylpropanolamine hydrochloride (p.1127·3); phenylephrine hydrochloride (p.1126·3); phenyltoloxamine citrate (p.439·1); carbinoxamine maleate (p.426·3).
*Cold and influenza symptoms.*

Westmont, Hong Kong.
Paracetamol (p.76·2).
*Fever; pain.*

Inkeysa, Spain†.
Dipyrone (p.35·3).
*Fever; pain.*

**Afebryl**
SMB, Belg.; Galephar, Fr.; Azevedos, Port.†.
Aspirin (p.15·1); paracetamol (p.76·2); ascorbic acid (p.1460·2).
*Fever; inflammation; pain.*

**Afecton** Help, Gr.
Cefaclor (p.167·1).
*Bacterial infections.*

**Afeditab** Watson, USA.
Nifedipine (p.966·2).
*Angina pectoris; hypertension.*

**Afeksin** United Nordic, Denm.
Fluoxetine hydrochloride (p.292·1).
*Bulimia; depression.*

**Afeme** Cetus, Arg.
Dexchlorpheniramine (p.428·1).
*Hypersensitivity reactions.*

**Afenil**
Note. This name is used for preparations of different composition.
Vianex (Βιανέξ), Gr.
Trandolapril (p.1016·1).
*Hypertension.*

Piam, Ital.
Food for special diets (p.1417·1).
*Phenylketonuria.*

**Afenoxin** Faran, Gr.
Ciprofloxacin hydrochloride (p.188·2).
*Bacterial infections.*

**Aferadol** Oberlin, Fr.†.
Paracetamol (p.76·2).
*Fever; pain.*

**Affectine** Galpharma, Israel.
Fluoxetine hydrochloride (p.292·1).
*Depression; obsessive-compulsive disorder.*

**Affex** Klinge, Irl.
Fluoxetine (p.296·3).
*Bulimia; depression; obsessive-compulsive disorder.*

**AFI-B$_6$** Nycomed, Norw.†.
Pyridoxine hydrochloride (p.1456·3).
*Peripheral neuritis; pyridoxine deficiency; sideroblastic anaemia.*

**AFI-B-Total** Nycomed, Norw.
Vitamin B substances (p.1417·1).

**AFI-C** Nycomed, Norw.†.
Ascorbic acid (p.1460·2).
*Vitamin C deficiency.*

**AFI-D$_2$** Nycomed, Norw.
Ergocalciferol (p.1462·1).
*Hypoparathyroid tetany.*

**Afid Plus** Fresenius Kabi, Ger.
Bis(3-aminopropyl)-dodecylamine; cocospropylenediamineguanidinium diacetate.
*Instrument disinfection.*

**AFI-E** Nycomed, Norw.†.
Alpha tocoferil acetate (p.1465·1).
*Vitamin E deficiency.*

**A-Fil** GenDerm, USA.
Methyl anthranilate (p.1154·1); titanium dioxide (p.1160·3).
*Sunscreen.*

**Afilan** Merck, Arg.
Mazindol (p.1589·1).
*Obesity.*

**Afilite** Argiletz, Fr.
Nutritional supplement (p.1417·1).

**Afipran** Nycomed, Norw.
Metoclopramide (p.1274·3) or metoclopramide hydrochloride (p.1274·3).
*Gastrointestinal disorders.*

**Aflamid** Boehringer Ingelheim, Mex.
Meloxicam (p.56·1).
*Ear, nose, and throat inflammation.*

**Aflamin** Hexal, S.Afr.
Indometacin (p.47·3).
*Gout; musculoskeletal and joint disorders.*

**Aflamina** Boehringer Ingelheim, Mex.†.
Phenylbutazone piperazine (p.84·1).

**Aflarex** Alcon, Chile.
Fluorometholone acetate (p.1102·2).
*Inflammatory eye disorders.*

**Aflat** Omega, Arg.
Simeticone (p.1289·2).
*Flatulence; infant colic.*

**Aflen** Galenica, Gr.
Triflusal (p.1017·3).
*Thrombosis prophylaxis.*

**Afloben** Esseti, Ital.
Benzydamine hydrochloride (p.21·1).
*Puerperal vaginal hygiene; vaginitis.*

**Aflodac** Biotekfarma, Ital.†.
Sulindac (p.91·2).
*Gout; musculoskeletal and joint disorders.*

**Aflogen** Faran, Gr.
Nimesulide (p.67·1).
*Inflammation; musculoskeletal disorders; pain.*

**Aflogine** Deverge, Ital.†.
Cetrimonium tosilate (p.1173·1); allantoin (p.1141·3); lactic acid (p.1704·1); sodium adipate.
*Personal hygiene; vaginal douche.*

**Aflogol** Instituto Sanitas, Chile.
Calcium aminosalicylate (p.155·1).
*Skin and hair disorders.*

**Aflogos** Biomedica, Ital.†.
Diflunisal arginine (p.34·3).
*Pain.*

**Afloxan**
Rottapharm, Chile; Rotta, Hong Kong; Rotta, Ital.; Rotta, Thai.
Proglumetacin maleate (p.85·2).
*Gout; inflammation; musculoskeletal, joint, peri-articular, and soft-tissue disorders; pain.*

**Afloyan** Farmabion, Spain†.
Etofibrate (p.914·2).
*Hyperlipidaemias.*

**Aflubin** Bittner, Austria.
Homoeopathic preparation.

**Aflukin C** IPS, Neth.†.
Quinine sulfate (p.460·2); ascorbic acid (p.1460·2).
*Cold and influenza symptoms.*

**Aflumycin** Agis, Israel.
Prednisolone (p.1108·1); gentamicin sulfate (p.217·1).
*Infected skin disorders.*

**Afluon** Viatris, Spain.
Azelastine hydrochloride (p.425·2).
*Allergic conjunctivitis; allergic rhinitis.*

**Afluta** Kwizda, Austria.
Flutamide (p.556·2).
*Prostatic cancer.*

**Afluvit** IPS, Neth.†.
Paracetamol (p.76·2); ascorbic acid (p.1460·2).
*Cold and influenza symptoms.*

**Afongan**
AB-Consult, Austria; Galderma, Ital.†; Alcon, Mex.†; Galderma, Port.
Omoconazole nitrate (p.407·2).
*Fungal and Gram-positive bacterial infections; fungal infections of the skin and mucous membranes.*

**Afonilum**
Ebewe, Austria; Abbott, Ger.
Theophylline (p.798·3).
*Obstructive airways disease.*

**Afonilum novo** Abbott, Ger.
Theophylline sodium glycinate (p.804·3).
*Obstructive airways disease.*

**Afonina** Farmatrading, Port.†.
Benzocaine (p.1370·3); tyrothricin (p.275·1).
*Mouth and throat disorders.*

**Afonisan** Purissimus, Arg.
Sulfadiazine (p.258·2); allantoin (p.1141·3).
*Mouth and throat disorders.*

**Afopic** Teuto, Braz.
Folic acid (p.1429·1).

**Aforinol** Rekah, Israel.
Mepyramine maleate (p.437·1); xylometazoline hydrochloride (p.1132·2); hamamelis (p.1696·3).
*Nasal congestion.*

**Afos** Salus, Ital.
Fosfomycin calcium (p.214·2).
*Bacterial infections.*

**afpred-DEXA** Hefa, Ger.
Dexamethasone sodium metasulfobenzoate (p.1097·2).
Formerly known as afpred-1.
*Obstructive airways disease.*

**afpred-THEO** Hefa, Ger.
Theophylline (p.798·3).
Formerly known as afpred-2.
*Cor pulmonale; neonatal apnoea; obstructive airways disease.*

**Afrazine** Schering-Plough, UK.
Oxymetazoline hydrochloride (p.1126·1).
*Nasal congestion.*

**African Gold** Strickland, Canad.
Hydroquinone (p.1148·1).

**Afrin**
Note. This name is used for preparations of different composition.
Schering-Plough, Braz.; Schering-Plough, Hong Kong; Schering-Plough, Malaysia; Schering-Plough, Mex.; Schering-Plough, Singapore.
Oxymetazoline hydrochloride (p.1126·1).
*Ear disorders; nasal congestion; ocular congestion.*

Schering-Plough, USA.
*Nasal drops; nasal spray:* Oxymetazoline hydrochloride (p.1126·1).
*Tablets:* Pseudoephedrine sulfate (p.1129·2).
*Nasal congestion.*

**Afrin Moisturizing Saline Mist** Schering-Plough, USA.
Sodium chloride (p.1233·3).
Formerly called Afrin Saline Mist.
*Inflammation and dryness of nasal membranes.*

**Afrin Natural** Schering-Plough, Braz.
Sodium chloride (p.1233·3).
*Nasal congestion.*

**Afrinex** Schering-Plough, Mex.
Dexbrompheniramine maleate (p.426·1); pseudoephedrine sulfate (p.1129·2).
*Nasal congestion.*

**Afrinex Infantil** Schering-Plough, Mex.
Aspirin (p.15·1); phenylephrine hydrochloride (p.1126·3); chlorphenamine maleate (p.427·3).
*Allergic rhinitis; fever; nasal congestion; pain.*

**Afrodor**
Note. This name is used for preparations of different composition.
Farco, Ger.
Quebracho; acecarbromal; vitamin E (p.1417·1).
*Tonic.*

Medinova (Μεντνοβα), Gr.
Ambroxol hydrochloride (p.1114·3).
*Respiratory disorders associated with viscous mucus.*

**Afrolate** Bayer, Spain†.
Etofenamate (p.38·1).
*Peri-articular disorders; soft-tissue disorders.*

**Afron** Neves, Port.
Genistein (p.1692·1); daidzein; glicitein.
*Menopausal disorders; menstrual disorders.*

**Aftab**
Rottapharm, Fin.; Opfermann, Ger.†; Rottapharm, Ital.
Triamcinolone acetonide (p.1110·2).
*Aphthous ulcer; gingivitis; stomatitis.*

**Aftach**
Teijin, Jpn; Helsinn, Port.
Triamcinolone acetonide (p.1110·2).
*Aphthous ulcer.*

**Af-Taf** Sam-On, Israel.
Phenylephrine hydrochloride (p.1126·3).
*Nasal congestion.*

**Aftagel** Cooperation Pharmaceutique, Fr.
Lidocaine hydrochloride (p.1377·3); zinc sulfate (p.1469·3).
*Inflammatory mouth disorders.*

**Aftajuventus** Ern, Spain.
Benzalkonium chloride (p.1168·3); hydrocortisone hydrogen succinate (p.1104·1).
Formerly known as Afta.
*Stomatitis.*

**Aftasone** Vinas, Spain.
Hydrocortisone hydrogen succinate (p.1104·1).
*Mouth ulcers.*

**Aftasone B C** Vinas, Spain.
Ascorbic acid (p.1460·2); hydrocortisone hydrogen succinate (p.1104·1); pyridoxine (p.1457·2); riboflavin (p.1456·1).
Formerly known as Oralsone B C.
*Mouth ulcers.*

**Aftate**
Schering-Plough, Hong Kong; Schering-Plough, USA.
Tolnaftate (p.410·1).
*Fungal skin infections.*

**After Bite**
Tender, Canad.; Tender, Israel†; Pensa, Spain; Ardern, UK.
Ammonia (p.1653·3).
*Insect bites; stings.*

**After Burn** Tender, Israel.
Lidocaine (p.1377·3).
*Pain and minor skin irritation.*

**After Sun** Dermoteca, Port.
Moisturiser.

**Afterburn** Tender, Canad.
Lidocaine hydrochloride (p.1377·3).

**After-Work** Hamilton, Austral.†.
Emollient.
*Dry skin.*

**Aftir Gel** Biochimici, Ital.
Malathion (p.1507·1).
*Pediculosis.*

**Aftir Shampoo** Biochimici, Ital.
Hydroxyquinoline sulfate (p.1700·1).
*For use after Aftir Gel; pediculosis.*

**Aftosium** Ferrier, Fr.
Homoeopathic preparation.

**Aftsinun** Sam-On, Israel†.
Diphenhydramine hydrochloride (p.431·3); pseudoephedrine hydrochloride (p.1129·2).
*Cold symptoms; coughs; nasal congestion; sinusitis.*

**Aftsinun Veshiul** Sam-On, Israel†.
Diphenhydramine hydrochloride (p.431·3); pseudoephedrine hydrochloride (p.1129·2); codeine phosphate (p.27·1).
*Cold symptoms; coughs; nasal congestion; sinusitis.*

**Afungil** Senosiain, Mex.
Fluconazole (p.398·1).
*Fungal infections.*

**Agaffin** Merck, Austria.
Sodium picosulfate (p.1289·3).
*Bowel evacuation; constipation.*

**Agamadon** Agamadon, Ger.†.
Aquilegia; sedi telephii; teucrii scor; equisetum (p.1684·1); sanicula; chamomile (p.1669·3); sage (p.1741·2); birch leaves (p.1660·3).
*Gastrointestinal disorders.*

**Agamadon N** Agamadon, Ger.†.
Chamomile (p.1669·3); peppermint leaf (p.1283·2); caraway (p.1667·2).
*Dyspepsia.*

**Agapurin**
Medphano, Ger.; Slovakofarma, Singapore; Slovakofarma, Thai.
Pentoxifylline (p.979·3).
*Cerebral and peripheral vascular disorders.*

**Agarol**
Note. This name is used for preparations of different composition.
Parke, Davis, Arg.
*Capsules; oral liquid:* Liquid paraffin (p.1479·1); sodium picosulfate (p.1289·3); agar (p.1576·3).
*Chewing gum:* Sodium picosulfate (p.1289·3).
*Constipation.*

Parke, Davis, Austral.; Pfizer, Hong Kong.
Liquid paraffin (p.1479·1).
*Constipation.*

Ache, Braz.; Parke, Davis, India; Warner-Lambert, Irl.†; Aspen Consumer, S.Afr.†; Warner-Lambert Consumer, Switz.†; Warner-Lambert, UK†.
Liquid paraffin (p.1479·1); phenolphthalein (p.1284·1); agar (p.1576·3).
*Constipation.*

Warner-Lambert, Canad.†.
Liquid paraffin (p.1479·1); glycerol (p.1694·3); phenolphthalein (p.1284·1); agar (p.1576·3).
*Constipation.*

Warner-Lambert, Spain†; Pfizer, Thai.
Liquid paraffin (p.1479·1); phenolphthalein (p.1284·1).
*Constipation.*

**Agarol CM** Warner-Lambert, Ital.
Liquid paraffin (p.1479·1).
*Constipation.*

**Agarol Extra** Numark, Canad.
Senna (p.1288·2).
*Constipation.*

**Agarol Fibras Naturales** Parke, Davis, Arg.
Ispaghula (p.1268·1).
*Constipation.*

**Agarol N** Pfizer Consumer, Ger.
Liquid paraffin (p.1479·1).
Agarol formerly contained liquid paraffin and phenolphthalein.
*Constipation.*

**Agarol Plain**
Note. This name is used for preparations of different composition.
Numark, Canad.
Liquid paraffin (p.1479·1); glycerol (p.1694·3).
*Constipation.*

Pfizer, Gr.
Liquid paraffin (p.1479·1).
*Constipation.*

**Agarol with Sennosides** Numark, Canad.
Senna (p.1288·2).
*Constipation.*

**Agarol Soft** Pfizer, Switz.
Fig (p.1266·3); sorbitol (p.1446·3).
*Constipation.*

**Agaroletten** Pfizer Consumer, Ger.
Bisacodyl (p.1251·3).
*Bowel evacuation; constipation.*

**Agasten** Novartis, Braz.
Clemastine fumarate (p.429·1).
*Hypersensitivity.*

**Agastrin** Rottapharm, Ital.†.
Trihydroxyaluminium magnesium carbonate.
*Gastrointestinal disorders associated with hyperacidity.*

**Agathol** Iderne, Fr.
Zinc oxide (p.1163·2); titanium dioxide (p.1160·3); peru balsam (p.1730·2).
*Burns.*

**AGB** Cassara, Arg.
A hepatitis B vaccine (recombinant) (p.1618·1).
*Active immunisation.*

**Age Block** Avon, Canad.
Avobenzone (p.1142·3); octinoxate (p.1154·3); oxybenzone (p.1154·3).
*Sunscreen.*

**Agedin Plus** GD, Ital.
Eicosapentaenoic acid (p.976·2); ubidecarenone (p.1760·2); methionine (p.1042·1); betacarotene (p.1422·3).
*Nutritional supplement.*

**A-Gel**
Pharmatel, Austral.†; Pharmatel, NZ.
Lubricating gel.
*Personal and surgical lubricant.*

**Agelan**
Antigen, Hong Kong; Antigen, Irl.
Indapamide (p.938·2).
*Hypertension.*

**Agelmin** Kleva, Gr.
Cetirizine hydrochloride (p.427·1).
*Allergic conjunctivitis; allergic rhinitis; pruritus.*

**A-gen 53**
Note. This name is used for preparations of different composition.
Solco, Austria.
Polysaccharide polysulfuric acid ester.
*Contraceptive.*

Herbrand, Ger.; Chefaro, Ger.
Cellulose poly(sulfuric acid ester), trisodium salt; nonoxinol 9 (p.1413·3).
*Contraceptive.*

**Agenerase**
GlaxoSmithKline, Arg.; GlaxoSmithKline, Austral.; GlaxoSmithKline, Belg.; GlaxoSmithKline, Braz.; GlaxoSmithKline, Canad.; GlaxoSmithKline, Chile; GlaxoSmithKline, Denm.; GlaxoSmithKline, Fin.; GlaxoSmithKline, Fr.; GlaxoSmithKline, Ger.; Glaxo Wellcome, Gr.; GlaxoSmithKline, Israel; GlaxoSmithKline, Ital.; Glaxo Wellcome, Mex.; GlaxoSmithKline, Norw.; GlaxoSmithKline, NZ; Glaxo Wellcome, Port.; Glaxo Wellcome, Spain; GlaxoSmithKline, Swed.; GlaxoSmithKline, Switz.; GlaxoSmithKline, UK; Glaxo Wellcome, USA.
Amprenavir (p.628·2).
*HIV infection.*

**Agermin** Andromaco, Chile.
Chlorhexidine (p.1173·2).
*Disinfection of skin and wounds.*

**Ageroplas** Farma Lepori, Spain.
Ditazole (p.905·3).
*Thromboembolism prophylaxis.*

**Agerpen** Reig Jofre, Spain.
Amoxicillin trihydrate (p.155·3).
*Bacterial infections.*

**Agerpen Mucolitico** I Farmacologia, Spain†.
Amoxicillin trihydrate (p.155·3); bromhexine hydrochloride (p.1115·3).
*Respiratory-tract infections.*

**Agevit** Stafford-Miller, Fr.†.
A range of vitamin and mineral supplements (p.1417·1).

**Agglad Ofteno** SMB, Chile.
Brimonidine tartrate (p.876·3).
*Glaucoma; ocular hypertension.*

**Aggrastat**
Merck Sharp & Dohme, Austral.; Merck Sharp & Dohme, Austria; Merck Sharp & Dohme, Belg.; Merck Frosst, Canad.; Merck Sharp & Dohme, Denm.; Merck Sharp & Dohme, Fin.; Merck Sharp & Dohme, Ger.; Vianex (Βιανεξ), Gr.; Merck Sharp & Dohme, Hong Kong; Merck Sharp & Dohme, Irl.; Merck Sharp & Dohme, Israel; Merck Sharp & Dohme, Ital.; Merck Sharp & Dohme, Malaysia; Merck Sharp & Dohme, Neth.; Merck Sharp & Dohme, Norw.; Merck Sharp & Dohme, NZ; Merck Sharp & Dohme, Singapore; Merck Sharp & Dohme, Swed.; Merck Sharp & Dohme, Switz.; Merck Sharp & Dohme, UK; Merck, USA.
Tirofiban hydrochloride (p.1013·3).
*Myocardial infarction; prevention of ischaemic cardiac complications during angioplasty or atherectomy; unstable angina.*

**Aggrastet** Merck Sharp & Dohme, S.Afr.
Tirofiban hydrochloride (p.1013·3).
*Prevention of cardiac ischaemia in angioplasty or atherectomy.*

**Aggrenox**
Boehringer Ingelheim, Belg.; Boehringer Ingelheim, Canad.; Boehringer Ingelheim, Gr.; Boehringer Ingelheim, Port.; Boehringer Ingelheim, USA.
Dipyridamole (p.903·1); aspirin (p.15·1).
*Thromboembolic disorders.*

**Aggripal S1** Chiron, Singapore; Pacific Biosciences, Singapore.
An influenza vaccine (surface antigen) (p.1620·2).
*Active immunisation.*

**Agilan** Klinge, Austria.
Dihydroergotamine mesilate (p.465·3); etilefrine hydrochloride (p.914·1).
*Hypotension.*

**Agilex** Mertens, Arg.
Indometacin (p.47·3).
*Fever; inflammation; pain.*

**Agilisin** Sankyo, Braz.
Indometacin (p.47·3).
*Fever; gout; musculoskeletal, joint, and peri-articular disorders; pain.*

**Agilo** Klinge, Austria.
Etilefrine hydrochloride (p.914·1).
*Hypotension.*

**Agilona** Vinas, Spain.
Benzydamine flufenamate.
*Inflammation; pain; peri-articular and soft-tissue disorders.*

**Aginax** Biogyne, Fr.
Soap substitute.
*Skin irritation.*

**Agiobulk** Byk Madaus, S.Afr.
Ispaghula (p.1268·1).
*Constipation; diarrhoea.*

**Agiocur**
Madaus, Austria; Madaus, Fin.; Madaus, Ger.; Madaus, Hong Kong; Madaus, Israel; Neo-Farmaceutica, Port.; Madaus, Thai.
Ispaghula (p.1268·1).
*Colostomy management; constipation; diarrhoea; diverticular disease; inflammatory bowel disease; irritable bowel syndrome; stool softener.*

**Agiofibe** Knoll, Austral.
Ispaghula (p.1268·1).
*Dietary fibre supplement.*

**Agiofibra**
Altana, Braz.; Byk Gulden, Mex.
Ispaghula (p.1268·1).
*Constipation; diarrhoea; dietary fibre supplement.*

**Agiolax**
Phoenix, Arg.; Knoll, Austral.; Madaus, Austria; Madaus, Belg.; Altana, Braz.; Madaus, Fin.; Madaus, Fr.; Madaus, Ger.; Madaus, Hong Kong; Madaus, Israel; Madaus, Ital.; Byk Gulden, Mex.; Byk, Neth.; Neo-Farmaceutica, Port.; Byk Madaus, S.Afr.; Madaus, Spain; Biomed, Switz.; Madaus, Thai.
Ispaghula (p.1268·1); senna (p.1288·2).
Formerly contained ispaghula, senna, and guaiazulene in *Belg.*
*Constipation; stool softener.*

**Agiolax Ballast** Madaus, Ger.†.
Ispaghula (p.1268·1).
*Constipation; stool softener.*

**Agiolax mite** Biomed, Switz.
Ispaghula (p.1268·1).
*Constipation; irritable bowel syndrome; stool softener.*

**Agiolax Pico** Madaus, Ger.
Sodium picosulfate (p.1289·3).
*Constipation.*

**Agiolind** Madaus, Austria.
Ispaghula (p.1268·1).
*Constipation; stool softener.*

**Agiopic** Madaus, Austria.
Sodium picosulfate (p.1289·3).
*Bowel evacuation; constipation.*

**AgioPico Plus** Madaus, Ger.†.
Sodium picosulfate (p.1289·3).
*Constipation.*

**Agioten** Gerolimatos (Γερολυματος), Gr.
Enalapril maleate (p.909·2).
*Heart failure; hypertension.*

**Agipiu** Candioli, Ital.
Silver carbonate (p.1746·1); alkylbenzyldimethylammonium saccharinate (p.1169·1).
*Burn and wound disinfection.*

**Agiserc** Agis, Israel.
Betahistine (p.1660·1).
*Vestibular disorders.*

**Agisolvan** Agis, Israel†.
Acetylcysteine (p.1112·3).
*Respiratory-tract disorders associated with viscous mucus.*

**Agispor** Agis, Israel.
Bifonazole (p.395·1).
*Fungal skin infections; seborrhoeic dermatitis.*

**Agispor Onychoset** Agis, Israel.
Bifonazole (p.395·1); urea (p.1162·2).
*Fungal nail infections.*

**Agisten** Agis, Israel.
Clotrimazole (p.396·2).
*Fungal skin infections; vaginitis.*

**Agit** Sanol, Ger.
Dihydroergotamine mesilate (p.465·3).
*Hypotension; migraine and other vascular headaches; varices.*

**Agit plus** Sanol, Ger.
Dihydroergotamine mesilate (p.465·3); etilefrine hydrochloride (p.914·1).
*Hypotension.*

**Aglio** Wassen, Ital.
Garlic (p.1691·1).
*Nutritional supplement.*

**Aglucide** Beta, Arg.
Gliclazide (p.332·1).
*Diabetes mellitus.*

**Aglucil** Elofar, Braz.
Glibenclamide (p.331·2).
*Diabetes mellitus.*

**Aglutella**
Plasmon, Ital.
Range of gluten-free food for special diets (p.1417·1).
Ultrapharm, UK†.
Low-protein food for special diets (p.1417·1).

**Agnesin** Hevert, Ger.
Homoeopathic preparation.

**Agnofem** Madaus, Austria.
Agnus castus (p.1649·1).
*Mastalgia; menstrual disorders.*

**Agnolyt**
Madaus, Ger.; Biomed, Switz.; Natural Touch, UK†.
Vitex agnus castus (p.1649·1).
*Mastalgia; menstrual disorders.*

**Agno-Sabona** Sabona, Ger.
Agnus castus (p.1649·1).
*Mastalgia; menstrual disorders.*

**Agnucaston**
Bionorica, Ger.; Bionorica, Hong Kong†; Bionorica, Thai.
Vitex agnus castus (p.1649·1).
*Mastalgia; menstrual disorders.*

**Agnuchol** Gebro, Austria.
Cynara (p.1678·3); taraxacum (p.1751·3); peppermint leaf (p.1283·2).
*Digestive disorders; gallbladder disorders.*

**Agnufemil** Steigerwald, Ger.
Agnus castus (p.1649·1).
*Mastalgia; premenstrual syndrome.*

**Agnukliman** Smetana, Austria.
Cimicifuga (p.1671·3).
*Menopausal disorders.*

**Agnumens** Smetana, Austria.
Agnus castus (p.1649·1).
*Menstrual disorders; premenstrual syndrome.*

**Agnurell** Sanorell, Ger.
Homoeopathic preparation.

**Agnus castus** Hevert, Ger.
Homoeopathic preparation.

**Agofell** Janssen-Cilag, S.Afr.
Diisopromine hydrochloride (p.1261·2); sorbitol (p.1446·3).
*Biliary-tract disorders.*

**Agofenac** Ogera, Switz.
Diclofenac sodium (p.32·1).
*Gout; inflammation; musculoskeletal and joint disorders; pain.*

**Agon**
Therapharm, Austral.; Aventis, NZ†.
Felodipine (p.914·3).
*Angina pectoris; hypertension.*

**Agoprim** Ogera, Switz.
Co-trimoxazole (p.199·3).
*Bacterial infections; Pneumocystis carinii pneumonia.*

**Agopton**
Takeda, Austria; Takeda, Ger.; Takeda, Switz.
Lansoprazole (p.1269·3).
*Gastro-oesophageal reflux; gastrointestinal hyperacidity; peptic ulcer; Zollinger-Ellison syndrome.*

**Agoral** Warner-Lambert, USA.
Liquid paraffin (p.1479·1); phenolphthalein (p.1284·1); agar (p.1576·3).
*Constipation.*

**Agorex** Ogera, Switz.
Amiloride hydrochloride (p.858·2); hydrochlorothiazide (p.933·2).
*Hypertension; oedema.*

**Agorhino** Ogera, Switz.
Phenylephrine hydrochloride (p.1126·3); dimenhydrinate (p.431·1); caffeine (p.782·1).
*Cold symptoms; nasal and sinus congestion; rhinitis.*

**Agpisen** Alpharma, Mex.
Ranitidine (p.1285·2).
*Peptic ulcer.*

**A/G-Pro** Miller, USA.
Multivitamin, mineral, and amino-acid preparation (p.1417·1).

**Agradil** Sanofi Synthelabo, Ital.
Veralipride (p.727·2).
*Menopausal disorders.*

**A-Gram** Inava, Fr.
Amoxicillin trihydrate (p.155·3) or amoxicillin sodium (p.155·3).
*Bacterial infections.*

**Agrastat**
Merck Sharp & Dohme, Arg.; Merck Sharp & Dohme, Braz.; Merck Sharp & Dohme, Chile; Merck Sharp & Dohme-Chibret, Fr.; Merck Sharp & Dohme, Mex.; Merck Sharp & Dohme, Spain.
Tirofiban hydrochloride (p.1013·3).
*Myocardial infarction; prevention of ischaemic cardiac complications during angioplasty or atherectomy; unstable angina.*

**Agreal**
Sanofi Synthelabo, Belg.; Sanofi Synthelabo, Braz.; Sanofi Synthelabo, Chile; Grunenthal, Fr.; Synthelabo, Hong Kong†; Sanofi Synthelabo, Port.; Sanofi Synthelabo, Spain.
Veralipride (p.727·2).
*Menopausal disorders.*

**Agre-Gola** Vemedia, Neth.
Cetylpyridinium chloride (p.1173·1); phenol (p.1188·1); menthol (p.1711·3).
*Sore throat.*

**Agremol** Eurodrug, Thai.
Dipyridamole (p.903·1).
*Angina pectoris; thromboembolic disorders.*

**Agrenox** Boehringer Ingelheim, Arg.
Dipyridamole (p.903·1); aspirin (p.15·1).
*Cerebrovascular ischaemia.*

**Agrimel** Ortoquimica, Braz.†.
Aconite (p.1646·3); rorippa nasturtium aquaticum; tolu (p.1131·3); ipecacuanha (p.1122·3).
*Coughs.*

**Agrimonas N** Niedermaier, Ger.†.
Taraxacum (p.1751·3); celandine; absinthium (p.1645·1).
*Dyspepsia.*

**Agrippal**
Socopharm, Fr.; Gerolimatos (Γερολυματος), Gr.; Chiron Vaccines, Ital.; Fustery, Mex.; Biovac, S.Afr.; Meda, Swed.; Chiron, Thai.; Wyeth, UK.
An influenza vaccine (surface antigen) (p.1620·2).
*Active immunisation.*

**Agrumina** Also, Ital.
Ascorbic acid (p.1460·2).
*Vitamin C deficiency; vitamin C supplement.*

**Agruvit** Aventis, Ital.
Ascorbic acid (p.1460·2); calcium ascorbate (p.1460·2).
*Vitamin C deficiency; vitamin C supplement.*

**Agrylin**
Orphan, Austral.; Shire, Canad.; Roberts, Israel; Tema, S.Afr.; Roberts, USA.
Anagrelide hydrochloride (p.1654·3).
*Essential thrombocythaemia.*

**Agua del Carmen**
Note. This name is used for preparations of different composition.
Pasteur, Chile.
Melissa oil (p.1711·2); lemon oil (p.1706·2); rosemary oil (p.1740·2); peppermint oil (p.1283·2); clove oil (p.1673·3); cinnamon oil (p.1672·2).
*Insomnia; nervous disorders.*
Fardi, Spain.
Coriander seeds (p.1676·1); matricaria (p.1669·3); melissa (p.1711·1); dried bitter-orange peel (p.1723·3); tilia (p.1756·2); lemon verbena (p.1706·3); cinnamon (p.1672·2); angelica (p.1655·1); nutmeg (p.1722·2); hyssopus officinalis.
*Menstrual disorders; nervous disorders.*

**Agua Inglesa** Granado, Braz.
Broom; cinchona; pear.
Formerly contained cassau, chamomile, broom, cinnamon, centaury, bitter orange, absinthium, and cinchona.
*Reduced appetite.*

**Agua Melisa Carminativa** Instituto Sanitas, Chile.
Melissa oil (p.1711·2); lemon oil (p.1706·2); clove oil (p.1673·3); nutmeg oil (p.1722·3); peppermint oil (p.1283·2); rosemary oil (p.1740·2); neroli oil (p.1719·2); cinnamon oil (p.1672·2).
*Anxiety; dyspepsia; excess gastrointestinal gas.*

**Agua Sulfatada Picrica** Volta, Chile.
Copper sulfate (p.1426·1); zinc sulfate (p.1469·3); camphorated alcohol; trinitrophenol (p.1758·1).

**Aguala** Alpes Chemie, Chile.
Sodium picosulfate (p.1289·3).
*Bowel evacuation; constipation.*

**Agudil** Sigma-Tau, Spain.
Glutamine (p.1433·2); asparagine (p.1422·1); pyridoxine hydrochloride (p.1456·3); phosphoserine.
*Tonic.*

**Agufam** ST, Thai.
Famotidine (p.1265·2).
*Gastro-oesophageal reflux; peptic ulcer; Zollinger-Ellison syndrome.*

**Agurin** Recalcine, Chile.
Algestone acetophenide (p.1541·3); estradiol enantate (p.1550·1).
*Combined oral contraceptive; dysmenorrhoea.*

**Agyr** Tyrol, Austria.
Ciprofloxacin hydrochloride (p.188·2).
*Bacterial infections.*

**Agyrax**
UCB, Belg.
Meclozine hydrochloride (p.436·3).
Formerly contained buclizine hydrochloride, hydroxyzine hydrochloride, and buphenine hydrochloride.
*Nausea; vertigo; vomiting.*
Vedim, Fr.
Meclozine hydrochloride (p.436·3).
Formerly contained buphenine hydrochloride, meclozine hydrochloride, and hydroxyzine hydrochloride.
*Motion sickness; vertigo.*

**AH 3 N** Rodleben, Ger.
Hydroxyzine hydrochloride (p.434·3).
*Pruritus.*

**AHA Skin Lightening Gel** Therapeutic-Ocean, Singapore†.
Kojic acid (p.1151·2); hydroquinone (p.1148·1); glycolic acid (p.1147·3).
*Skin hyperpigmentation.*

**AH-chew** WE, USA.
Phenylephrine hydrochloride (p.1126·3); chlorphenamine maleate (p.427·3); hyoscine methonitrate (p.483·3).
*Upper respiratory-tract symptoms.*

**AH-chew D** WE, USA.
Phenylephrine hydrochloride (p.1126·3).
*Nasal congestion.*

**AHD 2000** Lysoform, Ger.
Alcohol (p.1166·1).
*Hand disinfection; skin disinfection.*

**Ahecan** Marrero, Spain†.
Hydrogen peroxide (p.1182·2).
*Epistaxis; mouth, skin, and wound disinfection.*

**AHF**
CSL, Austral.; CSL, NZ.
A factor VIII preparation (p.751·1).
*Factor VIII deficiency; von Willebrand's disease.*

**Ahiston** Teva, Israel.
Chlorphenamine maleate (p.427·3).
*Hypersensitivity reactions.*

**Ahiston Compound** Teva, Israel.
Chlorphenamine maleate (p.427·3); phenylephrine hydrochloride (p.1126·3).
*Hypersensitivity reactions.*

**AHP 200** Chephasaar, Ger.
Oxaceprol (p.1725·1).
*Musculoskeletal, joint, peri-articular, and soft-tissue disorders.*

**A-Hydrocort**
Abbott, Canad.; Abbott, USA.
Hydrocortisone sodium succinate (p.1104·1).
*Corticosteroid.*

**Aicamin**
Sanofi Winthrop, Belg.†; Esfar, Port.
Orazamide (p.1724·2).
*Liver disorders.*

**Aid III MSUD** SHS, Fr.†.
Food for special diets (p.1417·1).
*Leucinosis.*

**Aida**
Paraphar, Fr.†; Paraphar, Singapore†.
Hydroquinone (p.1148·1).
*Skin hyperpigmentation.*

**Aidar** Pharmaland, Thai.
Cimetidine (p.1255·3).
*Peptic ulcer; Zollinger-Ellison syndrome.*

**Aid-Lax** Nobel, Canad.†.
Aloin (p.1248·3); cascara (p.1255·1); phenolphthalein (p.1284·1); bile salts (p.1660·3).

**Aidol** Pharmanik (Φαρμανικ), Gr.
Mefenamic acid (p.55·2).
*Dysmenorrhoea; inflammation; musculoskeletal and joint disorders; pain.*

**Aigin** Hevert, Ger.†.
Kava (p.1703·2).
*Anxiety.*

**Aiglonyl** Fumouze, Fr.
Sulpiride (p.722·2).
*Behaviour disorders in children; neuroses.*

**Ailax**
Galen, Irl.; Galen, UK†.
Dantron (p.1261·1); poloxamer 188 (p.1414·2).
These ingredients can be described by the British Approved Name Co-danthramer.
*Constipation.*

**Aima-Calcin** ISI, Ital.†.
Elcatonin (p.768·3).
*Hypercalcaemia; osteoporosis; Paget's disease of bone; reflex sympathetic dystrophy.*

**Aimafix**
Scott-Cassara, Arg.; Kedrion, Ital.
Factor IX (p.752·2).
*Haemorrhagic disorders.*

**Ainedif** Richmond, Arg.
Diclofenac (p.32·1).
*Inflammation.*

**Ainex**
Note. This name is used for preparations of different composition.
Schering-Plough, Chile.
Nimesulide (p.67·1).
*Fever; inflammation; pain.*
Promeco, Mex.†.
Ibuprofen (p.45·3).

**Ainscrid** Ethypharm, Fr.†.
Indometacin (p.47·3).
*Fever; inflammation.*

**Air Citronella** Antipiol, Ital.
Citronella oil (p.1673·2); geranium oil (p.1692·2).
*Insect repellent.*

**Air Salonpas** Hisamitsu, NZ; Pharmaco, NZ.
Camphor (p.1665·3); menthol (p.1711·3); methyl salicylate (p.59·3).

**Airbeclosona** Northia, Arg.
Beclometasone (p.1092·1).
*Asthma.*

**Airbronal** Baliarda, Arg.
Theophylline (p.798·3); ketotifen fumarate (p.788·1).
*Obstructive airways disease.*

**Aircort** Italchimici, Ital.
Budesonide (p.1094·2).
*Asthma; nasal polyps; rhinitis.*

**Airest** Caber, Ital.
Bamifylline hydrochloride (p.781·3).
*Asthma; bronchospasm.*

**Airol**
Pierre Fabre, Ger.; Pierre Fabre, Gr.; Pierre Fabre, Israel; Pierre Fabre, Ital.; Roche, Mex.†; Orient, Singapore†; Pierre Fabre, Singapore†; Pierre Fabre, Switz.
Tretinoin (p.1161·1).
*Acne.*

**Airomet** Masa, Thai.
Omeprazole (p.1278·2).
*Peptic ulcer; Zollinger-Ellison syndrome.*

**Airomir**
3M, Arg.; 3M, Austral.; UCB, Belg.; 3M, Canad.; 3M, Chile; 3M, Denm.; 3M, Fin.; 3M, Fr.; 3M, Hong Kong; 3M, Irl.; 3M, Malaysia; 3M, Neth.; 3M, Norw.; 3M, NZ; 3M, S.Afr.; 3M, Singapore; 3M, Swed.; 3M, Switz.; 3M, Thai.; Ivax, UK.
Salbutamol (p.791·3) or salbutamol sulfate (p.791·3).
*Obstructive airways disease.*

**Airsalbu** Northia, Arg.
Salbutamol (p.791·3).
*Obstructive airways disease.*

**Air-Tal** Almirall, Belg.
Aceclofenac (p.11·2).
*Inflammation; musculoskeletal, joint, and peri-articular disorders.*

**Airtal**
Grunenthal, Chile; Rowex, Irl.†; Probios, Port.; Almirall, Spain.
Aceclofenac (p.11·2).
*Gout; musculoskeletal, joint, peri-articular, and soft-tissue disorders; pain.*

**Airtal Difucrem** Almirall, Spain.
Aceclofenac (p.11·2).
*Peri-articular and soft-tissue disorders.*

**Airum** Pharmafina, Chile.
Clenbuterol (p.784·2).
*Bronchospasm.*

**Airvitess** Farmasan, Ger.†.
Ketotifen fumarate (p.788·1).
*Asthma; hypersensitivity disorders.*

**Air-X** RX, Thai.
Simeticone (p.1289·2).
*Aid to gastroscopy and X-ray examination; flatulence.*

**Ajaka** Streuli, Switz.†.
Aloes (p.1248·2); aloin (p.1248·3); belladonna (p.479·1); caraway (p.1667·2); fennel (p.1687·2); juniper (p.1703·1); caraway oil (p.1667·3); fennel oil (p.1687·3); juniper oil (p.1703·1).
*Constipation.*

**Ajan** 3M, Ger.
Nefopam hydrochloride (p.66·2).
*Pain.*

**Ajolip** Natufarma, Arg.
Garlic (p.1691·1); bearberry (p.1659·2).
*Dietary supplement.*

**Ajomast** Monserrat, Arg.
Garlic (p.1691·1).
*Hyperlipidaemia.*

**Ajomast Circulatorio** Monserrat, Arg.
Garlic (p.1691·1); rutoside (p.1688·2).
*Circulatory disorders; haemorrhoids; venous insufficiency.*

**Ajuta** Hermes, Ger.
Devil's claw root (p.28·2).
*Musculoskeletal and joint disorders.*

**Akabar** AF, Mex.
Nifuroxazide (p.237·2).
*Bacterial infections of the gastrointestinal tract.*

**Akacin**
Diba, Mex.; Atlantic, Thai.
Amikacin sulfate (p.154·1).
*Gram-negative bacterial infections.*

**Akaderm N** Gepepharm, Ger.
Salicylic acid (p.1157·1); lactic acid (p.1704·1).
*Skin disorders.*

**Akamin** Alphapharm, Austral.
Minocycline hydrochloride (p.231·3).
*Bacterial infections.*

**Akamon**
Medochemie, Hong Kong; Medochemie, Malaysia.
Bromazepam (p.671·3).
*Anxiety.*

**Akarin** Nycomed, Denm.
Citalopram hydrobromide (p.289·1) or citalopram hydrochloride (p.289·1).
*Depression; panic attacks.*

**Akarpine** Akorn, USA.
Pilocarpine hydrochloride (p.1495·1).
*Glaucoma; raised intra-ocular pressure; reversal of mydriasis.*

**Akatinol**
Phoenix, Arg.
Memantine hydrochloride (p.1711·2).
*Mental function impairment; movement disorders.*

Searle, Braz.†.
Memantine (p.1711·2).
*Parkinsonism.*

**Ak-Beta** Akorn, USA.
Levobunolol hydrochloride (p.946·2).
*Glaucoma; ocular hypertension.*

**Ak-Chlor** Akorn, USA.
Chloramphenicol (p.185·1).
*Eye infections.*

**Ak-Cide** Akorn, USA†.
Prednisolone acetate (p.1108·1); sulfacetamide sodium (p.257·3).
*Infected eye disorders.*

**Ak-Con**
Akorn, Canad.; Akorn, USA.
Naphazoline hydrochloride (p.1124·3).
*Minor eye irritation.*

**Ak-Dex** Akorn, USA†.
Dexamethasone sodium phosphate (p.1097·2).
*Eye inflammation.*

**Ak-Dilate**
Akorn, Canad.; Akorn, USA.
Phenylephrine hydrochloride (p.1126·3).
*Funduscopy; open-angle glaucoma; ophthalmic examination; pupil dilatation during surgery; refraction without cycloplegia; uveitis.*

**AKE**
Fresenius Kabi, Ger.; Fresenius Kabi, Switz.; Fresenius, Thai.†.
Amino-acid, carbohydrate, and electrolyte infusion (p.1417·1).
*Parenteral nutrition.*

**Akeral** IPFI, Ital.†.
Vitamin A acetate (p.1453·1).
*Vitamin A deficiency disorders.*

**Akerat**
Note. This name is used for preparations of different composition.
Pierre Fabre Dermo-Cosmetique, Arg.; Avene, Fr.
Urea (p.1162·2); salicylic acid (p.1157·1); lactic acid (p.1704·1).
*Dry skin; keratinisation disorders.*

Silesia, Chile.
Urea (p.1162·2); salicylic acid (p.1157·1); lactic acid (p.1704·1); almond oil (p.1651·1).
*Skin disorders.*

**Akevir** Kener, Mex.†.
Aciclovir (p.626·1).

**Akezol** Kener, Mex.†.
Acetazolamide (p.849·1).

**Akfen** Wyeth, Irl.†.
Guanfacine hydrochloride (p.927·2).
*Hypertension.*

**Ak-Fluor** Akorn, USA.
Fluorescein sodium (p.1689·1).
*Ophthalmic diagnostic agent.*

**Akhauma** Gilton, Braz.†.
Crataegus (p.1677·1); hamamelis (p.1696·3); passion flower (p.1729·1); salix (p.87·3).
*Sedative.*

**Akicin** General Drugs, Thai.
Amikacin sulfate (p.154·1).
*Bacterial infections.*

**Akila mains et peau** Adam, Mon.†.
Chlorhexidine gluconate (p.1173·2); hydrogen peroxide (p.1182·2); propyl alcohol (p.1191·2).
*Skin disinfection.*

**Akila spray** Adam, Mon.†.
Glutaral (p.1180·3); benzalkonium chloride (p.1168·3); bromonitrodioxan; alcohol (p.1166·1); propyl alcohol (p.1191·2).
*Surface disinfection.*

**Akildia** Asepta, Mon.
Centella (p.1144·3); karite.
*Foot care in diabetes.*

**Akileine** Asepta, Mon.
A range of preparations for foot disorders.

**Akilen**
Medochemie, Hong Kong; Medochemie, Malaysia.
Verapamil hydrochloride (p.1019·1).
*Angina pectoris; arrhythmias; heart failure; hypertension.*

**Akindex**
Fournier, Belg.†; Urgo, Fr.; Freda, Port.†.
Dextromethorphan hydrobromide (p.1117·3).
*Coughs.*

**Akindol** Fournier, Spain†.
Paracetamol (p.76·2).
*Fever; pain.*

**Akineton**
Abbott, Arg.; Abbott, Austral.; Ebewe, Austria; Knoll, Belg.; Abbott, Braz.; Abbott, Canad.; Abbott, Chile; Abbott, Denm.; Abbott, Fin.; Knoll, Fr.; Abbott, Ger.; Vianex (Βιανέξ), Gr.; Abbott, Irl.; Abbott, Ital.; Knoll, Mex.; Knoll, Neth.; Abbott, Norw.; Abbott, Port.; Knoll, S.Afr.; Knoll, Singapore†; Abbott, Spain; Abbott, Swed.; Knoll, Switz.; Knoll, Thai.†; Abbott, UK†; Knoll, USA.
Biperiden (p.479·3), biperiden hydrochloride (p.479·3), or biperiden lactate (p.479·3).
*Bronchospasm; drug-induced extrapyramidal disorders; head injury; nicotine poisoning; nocturnal cramps; parkinsonism; phosphorus poisoning; spasticity; trigeminal neuralgia.*

**Akinspray** Urgo, Belg.
Benzalkonium chloride (p.1168·3); lidocaine hydrochloride (p.1377·3).
*Mouth and throat disorders.*

**Akipic** Asepta, Mon.
Calendula (p.1665·2); aloes (p.1248·2).
*Bites and stings; insect repellent.*

**Akirol** Sedabel, Braz.
Sulfur (p.1158·2); benzoyl peroxide (p.1143·2).
*Acne.*

**Akistin** Nycomed, Austria.
Diethylamine salamidacetate (p.87·3).
*Musculoskeletal and joint disorders; neuralgias.*

**Aklonin** Wernigerode, Ger.†.
Phenamazide hydrochloride (p.487·3).
*Smooth muscle cramp; vomiting.*

**Ak-NaCl** Akorn, USA.
Sodium chloride (p.1233·3).
*Corneal oedema.*

**Akne** Ichthyol, Austria.
Erythromycin (p.208·1).
*Acne.*

**Akne Cordes** Ichthyol, Ger.
Erythromycin (p.208·1).
*Acne.*

**Aknecin** Dermopen, Braz.†.
Salicylic acid (p.1157·1); sulfur (p.1158·2).
*Acne.*

**Aknederm Ery** Gepepharm, Ger.
Erythromycin (p.208·1).
*Acne.*

**Aknederm N** Gepepharm, Ger.†.
Salicylic acid (p.1157·1); lactic acid (p.1704·1).
*Skin disorders.*

**Aknederm Neu** Gepepharm, Ger.
Ictasol (p.1148·3); zinc oxide (p.1163·2).
*Skin disorders.*

**Aknederm Oxid** Gepepharm, Ger.
Benzoyl peroxide (p.1143·2).
*Acne.*

**Ak-Nefrin** Akorn, USA†.
Phenylephrine hydrochloride (p.1126·3).
*Minor eye irritation.*

**Aknefug simplex** Wolff, Ger.
Hexachlorophene (p.1181·2).
*Acne; rosacea.*

**Aknefug-EL** Wolff, Ger.
Erythromycin (p.208·1).
*Acne.*

**Aknefug-Emulsion** Wolff, Ger.
Estradiol (p.1550·1); hexachlorophene (p.1181·2).
*Acne.*

**Aknefug-liquid** Wolff, Ger.
Salicylic acid (p.1157·1).
*Acne; seborrhoeic eczema.*

**Aknefug-oxid** Wolff, Ger.
Benzoyl peroxide (p.1143·2).
*Acne.*

**aknemago** Strathmann, Ger.†.
Erythromycin (p.208·1).
*Acne.*

**Aknemin**
Merck, Neth.†; Crookes Healthcare, UK.
Minocycline hydrochloride (p.231·3).
*Bacterial infections.*

**Aknemycin**
Note. This name is used for preparations of different composition.
Hermal, Austria†; Boots Healthcare, Belg.; Hermal, Ger.; Hermal, Hong Kong; Hermal, Malaysia; Boots Healthcare, Neth.; Hermal, Singapore; Boots Healthcare, Switz.
Erythromycin (p.208·1).
*Acne.*

Hermal, Ger.; Hermal, Israel; Boots Healthcare, Switz.
*Topical emulsion:* Erythromycin (p.208·1); ichthammol (p.1148·2).
*Acne.*

**Akne-Mycin**
Boots Healthcare, Port.; Healthpoint, USA.
Erythromycin (p.208·1).
*Acne.*

**Aknemycin compositum** Hermal, Austria.
Erythromycin (p.208·1); light ammonium bituminosulphonate (p.1148·2).
*Acne.*

**Aknemycin Plus**
Hermal, Ger.; Hermal, Israel; Hermal, Malaysia; Hermal, Singapore; Crookes Healthcare, UK.
Erythromycin (p.208·1); tretinoin (p.1161·1).
*Acne.*

**Ak-Neo-Dex** Akorn, USA.
Neomycin sulfate (p.235·1); dexamethasone sodium phosphate (p.1097·2).
*Eye inflammation with bacterial infection.*

**Akne-Puren** Alpharma-Isis, Ger.
Minocycline hydrochloride (p.231·3).
*Acne.*

**Aknereduct** Azupharma, Ger.†.
Minocycline hydrochloride (p.231·3).
*Acne.*

**Akneroxid**
Hermal, Austria; Boots Healthcare, Belg.; Hermal, Ger.; Hermal, Malaysia; Boots Healthcare, Neth.; Hermal, Singapore; Boots Healthcare, Switz.
Benzoyl peroxide (p.1143·2).
*Acne.*

**Aknex** Gebro, Switz.
Benzoyl peroxide (p.1143·2).
*Acne.*

**Aknicare**
General Topics, Ital.; Dermoteca, Port.
Pyruvic acid; triclosan (p.1195·2).
*Soap substitute for acne-prone skin.*

**Aknichthol** Ichthyol, Austria.
Ictasol (p.1148·3); salicylic acid (p.1157·1); colloidal sulfur (p.1158·2).
*Acne.*

**Aknichthol Creme** Ichthyol, Ger.
Ictasol (p.1148·3).
*Acne.*

**Aknichthol N**
Ichthyol, Ger.
Ictasol (p.1148·3); salicylic acid (p.1157·1).
*Acne; rosacea.*

Ichthyol, Switz.
Sodium bituminosulphonate (p.1148·3); salicylic acid (p.1157·1).
*Acne.*

**Aknilox** Drossapharm, Switz.
Erythromycin (p.208·1).
*Acne.*

**Aknin** Sanofi Synthelabo, Ger.†.
*Lotion:* Erythromycin (p.208·1).
*Ointment:* Sulfur (p.1158·2); salicylic acid (p.1157·1).
*Acne.*

**Aknin-Mino** Sanofi Synthelabo, Ger.
Minocycline hydrochloride (p.231·3).
*Acne.*

**Aknin-N** Sanofi, Switz.
Minocycline hydrochloride (p.231·3).
*Acne.*

**Aknoral** IBSA, Switz.
Minocycline hydrochloride (p.231·3).
*Acne.*

**Aknosan** Hermal, Ger.
Minocycline hydrochloride (p.231·3).
*Acne.*

**Akorazol** Collins, Mex.
Ketoconazole (p.403·3).
*Fungal infections.*

**Ak-Pentolate** Akorn, USA.
Cyclopentolate hydrochloride (p.480·3).
*Production of mydriasis and cycloplegia.*

**Ak-Poly-Bac** Akorn, USA.
Polymyxin B sulfate (p.245·1); bacitracin zinc (p.161·3).
*Eye infections.*

**Ak-Pred** Akorn, USA.
Prednisolone sodium phosphate (p.1108·1).
*Eye inflammation.*

**AkPro** Akorn, USA.
Dipivefrine hydrochloride (p.1681·2).
*Glaucoma.*

**Akratol** Rafarm, Gr.
Nabumetone (p.63·3).
*Inflammation; musculoskeletal and joint disorders; pain.*

**Akrinor**
Asta Medica, Austria; AWD, Ger.; Adcock Ingram, S.Afr.; Asta Medica, Switz.†.
Cafedrine hydrochloride (p.878·2); theodrenaline hydrochloride (p.1754·3).
*Circulatory disorders; hypotension.*

**Ak-Rinse** Akorn, USA.
Electrolytes (p.1217·1).
*Eye irrigation.*

**Ak-Rose** Akorn, Canad.
Rose bengal sodium (p.1740·1).
*Ophthalmic diagnostic agent.*

**Akrotherm** Gepepharm, Ger.†.
Benzyl nicotinate (p.21·2); nonivamide (p.67·2).
*Peripheral vascular disorders; soft-tissue injury.*

**Ak-Spore** Akorn, USA.
*Eye drops†:* Polymyxin B sulfate (p.245·1); neomycin sulfate (p.235·1); gramicidin (p.220·2).
*Eye ointment:* Polymyxin B sulfate (p.245·1); neomycin sulfate (p.235·1); bacitracin zinc (p.161·3).
*Eye infections.*

**Ak-Spore HC** Akorn, USA†.
*Ear drops:* Hydrocortisone (p.1103·3); neomycin sulfate (p.235·1); polymyxin B (p.245·2).
*Bacterial ear infections.*
*Eye drops; eye ointment:* Polymyxin B sulfate (p.245·1); neomycin sulfate (p.235·1); hydrocortisone (p.1103·3).
*Eye inflammation with bacterial infection.*

**Ak-Sulf** Akorn, USA.
Sulfacetamide sodium (p.257·3).
*Eye infections.*

**Akt-3** Lupin, India.
1 Capsule, rifampicin (p.250·2); 1 tablet, ethambutol (p.212·2); isoniazid (p.222·2).
*Tuberculosis.*

**Akt-4** Lupin, India.
1 Capsule, rifampicin (p.250·2); 2 tablets, pyrazinamide (p.246·3); 1 tablet, ethambutol (p.212·2); isoniazid (p.222·2).
*Tuberculosis.*

**Ak-Taine**
Akorn, Canad.; Akorn, USA.
Proxymetacaine hydrochloride (p.1384·1).
*Local anaesthesia.*

**Aktiferrin** Ratiopharm, Austria.
Ferrous sulfate (p.1428·2); DL-serine.
*Iron deficiency; iron deficiency anaemia.*

**Aktiferrin compositum** Ratiopharm, Austria.
Ferrous sulfate (p.1428·2); DL-serine; folic acid (p.1429·1).
*Iron and folic acid deficiency.*

**Aktiferrin N** Merckle, Ger.
Ferrous sulfate (p.1428·2).
*Iron deficiency.*

**Aktiferrin-F** Mepha, Israel.
Ferrous sulfate (p.1428·2); folic acid (p.1429·1); DL-serine.
*Iron and folic acid deficiency.*

**Aktiosan** Hexal, Arg.
Diclofenac sodium (p.32·1).
*Gout; musculoskeletal, joint, and soft-tissue disorders.*

The symbol † denotes a preparation no longer actively marketed

**Aktipar** Orion, Fin.†.
Levodopa (p.1205·2); benserazide hydrochloride (p.1200·2).
*Parkinsonism.*

**Aktiv Blasen- und Nierentee** Apotheke Heiligen Josef, Austria.
Birch leaf (p.1660·3); juniper (p.1703·1); ononis (p.1723·3); bearberry (p.1659·2); peppermint leaf (p.1283·2).
*Renal and urinary-tract disorders.*

**Aktiv Husten- und Bronchialtee** Apotheke Heiligen Josef, Austria.
Plantago lanceolata (p.1738·2); aniseed (p.1655·2); thyme (p.1755·2); althaea (p.1651·3).
*Catarrh; coughs.*

**Aktiv Leber- und Gallentee** Apotheke Heiligen Josef, Austria.
Peppermint leaf (p.1283·2); achillea (p.1646·2); fennel (p.1687·2); turmeric (p.1058·3).
*Liver and gallbladder disorders.*

**Aktiv milder Magen- und Darmtee** Apotheke Heiligen Josef, Austria.
Aniseed (p.1655·2); fennel (p.1687·2); caraway (p.1667·2); chamomile (p.1669·3); achillea (p.1646·2).
*Gastrointestinal disorders.*

**Aktiv Nerven- und Schlaftee** Apotheke Heiligen Josef, Austria.
Lupulus (p.1708·1); valerian (p.1762·2); melissa (p.1711·1); peppermint leaf (p.1283·2); orange flowers (p.1723·3).
*Nervous disorders; sleep disorders.*

**Aktivakid** Hoechst Marion Roussel, S.Afr.†.
Liver extracts; vitamin $B_{12}$; yeast extract; ferric glycerophosphate; lysine (p.1417·1).
*Tonic.*

**Aktivanad**
Nycomed, Austria.
*Oral liquid:* Liver extract; yeast; rose fruit; caffeine (p.1417·1).
*Syrup:* Liver extract; yeast; rose fruit; ferric glycerophosphate; lysine (p.1417·1).
*Tonic.*
Aventis, S.Afr.
*Syrup:* Haematoporphyrin; liver extracts; caffeine; yeast extract (p.1417·1).
*Tablets:* Haematoporphyrin; liver extracts; amino acids; vitamins; caffeine; yeast extract; ferric glycerophosphate (p.1417·1).
*Tonic.*

**Aktivanad-N** Rentschler, Ger.
*Oral liquid:* Liver extract; yeast extract; caffeine (p.1417·1).
*Tablets:* Vitamin B substances; vitamin C; caffeine (p.1417·1).
*Tonic.*

**Aktivin** Michallik, Ger.
Isopropyl alcohol (p.1184·3).
*Skin disinfection.*

**Aktiv-Puder** Klosterfrau, Ger.†.
Colloidal silicon dioxide (p.1581·3).
*Burns; skin disorders.*

**AkTob** Akorn, USA.
Tobramycin (p.271·2).

**Akton** Exel, Belg.
Cloxazolam (p.685·3).
*Anxiety; premedication; sleep disorders.*

**Ak-Tracin** Akorn, USA.
Bacitracin (p.161·3).
*Eye infections.*

**Aktren** Bayer, Ger.
Ibuprofen (p.45·3).
*Fever; pain.*

**Ak-Trol** Akorn, USA.
Dexamethasone (p.1097·1); neomycin sulfate (p.235·1); polymyxin B sulfate (p.245·1).
*Eye inflammation with bacterial infection.*

**Akudol** Wassermann, Ital.†.
Naproxen sodium (p.65·1).
*Fever; musculoskeletal and joint disorders; pain.*

**Ak-Vernacon** Akorn, Canad.
Pheniramine maleate (p.438·3); phenylephrine hydrochloride (p.1126·3).
*Antihistamine; decongestant.*

**Akwa Tears**
Note. This name is used for preparations of different composition.
Akorn, Canad.
Wool fat (p.1483·1); liquid paraffin (p.1479·1); white soft paraffin (p.1479·3).
Akorn, USA.
*Eye drops:* Polyvinyl alcohol (p.1581·1).
*Eye ointment:* White soft paraffin (p.1479·3); liquid paraffin (p.1479·1); wool fat (p.1483·1).
*Dry eyes.*

**AKZ**
Pfizer, Austria†; Howmedica, Switz.†.
Erythromycin gluceptate (p.208·2); colistimethate sodium (p.199·1); polymethylmethacrylate/methylmethacrylate copolymer (p.1714·3).
*Bone cement for orthopaedic surgery.*

**al 110**
Nestle, Braz.; Nestle, Fr.; Nestle, Ital.; Nestle, Port.; Nestle, Switz.†; Nestle, UK†.
Food for special diets (p.1417·1).
*Lactose intolerance.*

**Alacetan** Asconex, Ger.
Aspirin (p.15·1); paracetamol (p.76·2); caffeine (p.782·1).
*Fever; inflammation; pain.*

**Alacol DM** Ballay, USA.
Dextromethorphan hydrobromide (p.1117·3); brompheniramine maleate (p.426·1); phenylephrine hydrochloride (p.1126·3).
*Upper respiratory-tract disorders.*

**Alacor** Durascan, Denm.
Enalapril maleate (p.909·2).
*Heart failure; hypertension.*

**Ala-Cort** Del-Ray, USA.
Hydrocortisone (p.1103·3).
*Skin disorders.*

**Alacramyn** Bioclon, Mex.
Scorpion venom antisera (p.1638·3).
*Scorpion stings.*

**Alacta-NF** Mead Johnson Nutritionals, Thai.
Food supplement with vitamins and minerals (p.1417·1).

**Alaidol** Byk, Arg.
Proglumetacin maleate (p.85·2).
*Musculoskeletal, joint, peri-articular, and soft-tissue disorders; pain.*

**Alamag** Goldline, USA.
Aluminium hydroxide (p.1249·2); magnesium hydroxide (p.1272·2).
*Hyperacidity.*

**Alamag Plus** Goldline, USA.
Aluminium hydroxide (p.1249·2); magnesium hydroxide (p.1272·2); simeticone (p.1289·2).
*Hyperacidity.*

**Alamast** Santen, USA.
Pemirolast potassium (p.790·3).
*Allergic conjunctivitis.*

**Alamil** Biochimico, Braz.†.
Terbinafine hydrochloride (p.408·2).
*Fungal infections.*

**Alamin** David, India.
Amino-acid infusion (p.1417·1).
*Parenteral nutrition.*

**Alanase** Pacific, NZ.
Beclometasone dipropionate (p.1091·1).
*Nasal polyps; rhinitis.*

**Alandiem** Zimaia, Port.
Diltiazem hydrochloride (p.900·1).
*Angina pectoris; hypertension.*

**Alantomicina Complex** Cantabria, Spain†.
Allantoin (p.1141·3); bacitracin (p.161·3); hydrocortisone acetate (p.1103·3); neomycin (p.235·1); zinc oxide (p.1163·2).
*Infected skin disorders.*

**Alapren**
Chibret, Denm.†; Ranbaxy, S.Afr.
Enalapril (p.909·2) or enalapril maleate (p.909·2).
*Heart failure; hypertension.*

**Alapril** Mediolanum, Ital.
Lisinopril (p.946·3).
*Heart failure; hypertension; myocardial infarction.*

**Alapryl** Menarini, Spain.
Halazepam (p.701·2).
*Anxiety.*

**Alasenn** Schworer, Ger.
Senna (p.1288·2); ononis (p.1723·3); achillea (p.1646·2); taraxacum (p.1751·3).
*Constipation.*

**Alastik** Grunenthal, Chile.
*Cream; lotion:* Glycolic acid (p.1147·3).
*Acne; dry skin; eye contour disorders; photoageing of the skin; seborrhoea; skin pigmentation disorders.*
*Topical gel:* Glycolic acid (p.1147·3); hydroquinone (p.1148·1); kojic acid (p.1151·2).
*Skin pigmentation disorders.*

**Alasulf** Major, USA.
Sulfanilamide (p.263·2); aminoacridine hydrochloride (p.1165·3); allantoin (p.1141·3).
*Vaginal infections.*

**Alavac-S**
Artu, Neth.†.
Allergen extracts (p.1650·1).
*Allergen immunotherapy.*
Teomed, Switz.
House-dust mite allergen extracts (p.1650·1) (p.1650·2).
*Allergen immunotherapy.*

**Alavert** Wyeth-Ayerst, USA.
Loratadine (p.436·1).
*Hypersensitivity reactions.*

**Alavert Allergy & Sinus D** Wyeth Consumer, USA.
Loratadine (p.436·1); pseudoephedrine hydrochloride (p.1129·2).
*Upper respiratory-tract disorders.*

**Alaxa** Angelini, Ital.
Bisacodyl (p.1251·3).
*Constipation.*

**Alaxan** Great Eastern, Thai.; Therapharma, Thai.
Carisoprodol (p.1392·1); phenylbutazone calcium (p.84·1).
*Musculoskeletal and joint disorders.*

**Alaxan Pl** Therapharma, Thai.; Great Eastern, Thai.
Ibuprofen (p.45·3); paracetamol (p.76·2).
*Musculoskeletal pain.*

**Alba**
Note. A similar name is used for preparations of different composition (see below).
SNBTS, UK.
Albumin (p.740·3).
*Plasma volume expansion.*

**Alba-3**
Note. A similar name is used for preparations of different composition (see above).
IQB, Braz.
Albendazole (p.101·2).
*Worm infections.*

**Albalon**
Allergan, Austral.; Allergan, Belg.; Allergan, Canad.; Allergan, Hong Kong; Allergan, Malaysia; Allergan, NZ; Allergan, S.Afr.†; Allergan, Switz.; Allergan, Thai.; Allergan, USA.
Naphazoline hydrochloride (p.1124·3).
*Eye irritation.*

**Albalon Relief**
Allergan, Austral.; Allergan, NZ.
Phenylephrine hydrochloride (p.1126·3).
*Eye irritation.*

**Albalon-A**
Allergan, Austral.; Allergan, Canad.; Allergan, NZ; Allergan, S.Afr.
Naphazoline hydrochloride (p.1124·3); antazoline phosphate (p.424·2).
*Allergic inflammatory eye conditions; eye irritation.*

**Albamycin** Upjohn, USA†.
Novobiocin sodium (p.239·2).
*Bacterial infections.*

**Albasol** Allergan, Chile.
Naphazoline hydrochloride (p.1124·3).
*Eye congestion.*

**Albasol A** Allergan, Chile.
Naphazoline hydrochloride (p.1124·3); antazoline phosphate (p.424·2).
*Eye disorders.*

**Albassol** Allergan-Frumtost, Braz.†.
Antazoline phosphate (p.424·2); naphazoline hydrochloride (p.1124·3).
*Ocular congestion.*

**Albatel** TO-Chemicals, Thai.
Albendazole (p.101·2).
*Worm infections.*

**Albay**
Thomson, Austral.; Ebos, NZ; Bayer, S.Afr.†; Miles, USA.
Venoms of bee (p.1650·2), wasp (p.1650·2), hornet, yellow jacket, and mixed vespids (p.1650·1).
*Allergen immunotherapy of insect stings; diagnosis of hypersensitivity to insect stings.*

**Albego** Daker Farmasimes, Spain†.
Camazepam (p.674·1).
*Anxiety; insomnia.*

**Alben**
Infabra, Braz.†; Biolab, Thai.
Albendazole (p.101·2).
*Worm infections.*

**Albenda**
Milano, Thai.; Julphar, UAE.
Albendazole (p.101·2).
*Worm infections.*

**Albendrox** Royton, Braz.
Albendazole (p.101·2).
*Worm infections.*

**Albendy** Galenogal, Braz.†.
Albendazole (p.101·2).
*Worm infections.*

**Albensil** Arlex, Mex.†.
Albendazole (p.101·2).

**Albentel** Teuto, Braz.
Albendazole (p.101·2).
*Worm infections.*

**Albenza** SmithKline Beecham, USA.
Albendazole (p.101·2).
*Cysticercosis; echinococcosis.*

**Albenzonil** Ducto, Braz.
Albendazole (p.101·2).
*Worm infections.*

**Albeoler** Andromaco, Chile.
Fluticasone propionate (p.1102·3).
*Asthma.*

**Alber T**
Unison, Hong Kong; Unison, Thai.
Tolnaftate (p.410·1); triacetin (p.410·2).
*Fungal skin infections.*

**Albert Tiafen** Aventis, Canad.
Tiaprofenic acid (p.93·3).
*Osteoarthritis; rheumatoid arthritis.*

**Albesine Biotic** Indeco, Arg.
Amoxicillin (p.155·3); diclofenac (p.32·1).

**Albetol** Leiras, Fin.
Labetalol hydrochloride (p.943·3).
*Angina pectoris; hypertension.*

**Albey**
Dome-Hollister-Stier, Fr.; Medi Challenge, S.Afr.
Bee venom (p.1650·2) or wasp venom (p.1650·2) (p.1650·1).
Formerly known as Albay in *Fr.*
*Allergen immunotherapy of bee or wasp stings; diagnosis of hypersensitivity to bee or wasp stings.*

**Albezole** Khandelwal, India.
Albendazole (p.101·2).
*Worm infections.*

**Albicansan** Sanum-Kehlbeck, Ger.
Homoeopathic preparation.

**Albicar** Casasco, Arg.
Levocarnitine (p.1423·3).
*Carnitine deficiency.*

**Albicon** Formalab, Braz.
Borax (p.1661·3); potassium chloride (p.1232·2); benzocaine (p.1370·3); sodium carbonate (p.1747·1).
*Local disinfection and anaesthesia.*

**Albicort**
Sanofi Synthelabo, Belg.; Sanofi Synthelabo, Neth.
Triamcinolone acetonide (p.1110·2).
*Corticosteroid.*

**Albicort Compositum**
Sanofi Synthelabo, Belg.†; Sanofi Synthelabo, Neth.
Triamcinolone acetonide (p.1110·2); salicylic acid (p.1157·1).
*Keratinisation disorders; psoriasis.*

**Albicort Oticum** Sanofi Synthelabo, Belg.†.
Triamcinolone acetonide (p.1110·2); salicylic acid (p.1157·1).
*Otitis externa.*

**Albintil** Solvay, Spain.
Multivitamin preparation (p.1417·1).

**Albios** Giuliani, Ital.
Dietary fibre supplement with minerals (p.1417·1).

**Albiotic** Pharmacia, Ger.
Lincomycin hydrochloride (p.226·2).
*Bacterial infections.*

**Albistat** Janssen-Cilag, Belg.†.
Miconazole nitrate (p.405·3).
*Vulvovaginal yeast infections.*

**Albistin** Cazi, Braz.
Nystatin (p.406·3).
*Fungal infections.*

**Albital**
Note. This name is used for preparations of different composition.
Cristalia, Braz.
Acetyltryptophan sodium; potassium caprylate; protein (p.1417·1).
*Parenteral nutrition.*
Nuovo ISM, Ital.; Serono, Mex.
Albumin (p.740·3).
*Hypoalbuminaemia.*

**Albocresil**
Byk, Arg.; Altana, Braz.; Grunenthal, Chile.
Policresulen (p.1190·1).
*Haemorrhage; mucous membrane inflammation in the mouth; skin ulcers and burns; vaginal infections.*

**Alboral** Silanes, Mex.
Diazepam (p.690·1).
*Alcohol withdrawal syndrome; anxiety disorders; epilepsy; insomnia; premedication; skeletal muscle spasm; tetany.*

**Albothyl**
Byk Gulden, Ger.; Altana, Hong Kong; Altana, Malaysia; Byk Gulden, Mex.; Byk Gulden, Singapore; Pacific Biosciences, Singapore; Byk Gulden, Thai.†.
Metacresolsulfonic acid-formaldehyde (p.756·1).
*Burns; gynaecological disorders; skin and mucous membrane disorders; ulcers; wounds.*

**Alboz** Collins, Mex.
Omeprazole (p.1278·2).
*Peptic ulcer.*

**Albraton** Steigerwald, Ger.
Homoeopathic preparation.

**Albucid**
Chauvin ankerpharm, Ger.; Allergan, India.
Sulfacetamide sodium (p.257·3).
*Chlamydial eye infections.*

**Albulin** Cibran, Braz.†.
Salbutamol (p.791·3).
*Obstructive airways disease.*

**Albumaid Preparations** Scientific Hospital Supplies, UK†.
A range of amino-acid preparations for special diets (p.1417·1).
*Homocystinuria; phenylketonuria; protein malabsorption syndromes.*

**Albuman**
Berna, Belg.†; Berna, Ital.; Berna, Switz.; Berna, Thai.†.
Albumin (p.740·3).
*Burns; hypoalbuminaemia; hypovolaemic shock.*

**Albumar** Grossman, Mex.
Albumin (p.740·3).
*Plasma volume expansion; shock.*

**Albumarc** American Red Cross, USA.
Albumin (p.740·3).

**Albumax** Blausiegel, Braz.
Albumin (p.740·3).
*Plasma volume expansion.*

**Albumex**
CSL, Austral.; CSL, NZ.
Albumin (p.740·3).
*Adult respiratory distress syndrome; burns; haemodialysis; hypoproteinaemia; plasma exchange; plasma volume expansion; shock.*

**Albuminar**
Aventis Behring, Braz.; Aventis Behring, Hong Kong; Centeon, Irl.†; Centeon, Israel; Centeon, USA.
Albumin (p.740·3).
*Hypoproteinaemia; hypovolaemia.*

**Albumyn** Bioclon, Mex.
Albumin (p.740·3).
*Hypoproteinaemia; plasma volume expansion.*

**Albunex** Mallinckrodt, Braz.†.
Albumin (p.740·3).

**Alburone** *Nestle, Fr.†.*
Food for special diets (p.1417·1).

**Albusol** *NBI, S.Afr.*
Albumin (p.740·3).
*Hypoproteinaemia; hypovolaemia.*

**Albustix**
*Bayer, Austral.†; Bayer Diagnostics, Fr.; Bayer Diagnostics, Irl.; Bayer Diagnostici, Ital.; Bayer, NZ; Bayer Diagnostics, UK; Bayer, USA.*
Test for protein in urine.

**Albutamol** *Centaur, India.*
Etofylline (p.785·1); salbutamol (p.791·3); bromhexine (p.1115·3).
*Obstructive airways disease.*

**Albutein**
*Alpha, Hong Kong; Alpha Therapeutic, Ital.; Alpha Therapeutic, Malaysia; Alpha Therapeutic, Singapore; Alpha Therapeutic, Thai.; Grifols, UK; Alpha Therapeutic, USA.*
Albumin (p.740·3).
*Burns; cardiopulmonary bypass procedures; hyperbilirubinaemia; hypoproteinaemia; hypovolaemia; shock.*

**Albyl** *Leo, Denm.†.*
Aspirin (p.15·1).
*Fever; inflammation; pain.*

**Albyl minor** *Recip, Swed.*
Aspirin (p.15·1).
*Fever; pain.*

**Albyl-E** *Nycomed, Norw.*
Aspirin (p.15·1).
Magnesium oxide (p.1272·3) is included in the 500 mg tablets in an attempt to limit adverse effects on the gastrointestinal mucosa.
*Fever; pain; rheumatism; thrombosis prophylaxis.*

**Albym-Test**
*Boehringer Mannheim Diagnostics, Irl.†; Roche Diagnostics, NZ†; Roche Diagnostics, UK†.*
Test for protein in urine.

**Alca-C** *Novartis Consumer, Switz.*
Carbasalate calcium (p.25·1); ascorbic acid (p.1460·2).
*Cold symptoms.*

**Alcacat** *Baxter, Mex.*
Sodium chloride (p.1233·3).

**Alcacyl** *Novartis Consumer, Switz.*
Carbasalate calcium (p.25·1).
Aluminium hydroxide (p.1249·2) is included in this preparation in an attempt to limit adverse effects on the gastrointestinal mucosa.
*Fever; inflammation; pain.*

**Alcacyl instant** *Novartis Consumer, Switz.*
Lysine aspirin (p.54·3).
*Fever; inflammation; pain.*

**Alcafelol** *Luper, Braz.*
Choline citrate (p.1424·3); cynara (p.1678·3); boldo (p.1661·2); magnesium sulfate (p.1228·2).
*Liver disorders.*

**Alcaine**
*Alcon, Austral.; Alcon, Canad.; Alkon (Αλκον), Gr.; Alcon, Hong Kong; Alcon, Malaysia; Alcon, Mex.; Alcon, Norw.; Alcon, Singapore; Alcon, Switz.; Alcon, USA.*
Proxymetacaine hydrochloride (p.1384·1).
*Local anaesthesia.*

**Alcalinos Gelos** *Gelos, Spain.*
Calcium carbonate (p.1254·2); magnesium hydroxide (p.1272·2); sodium bicarbonate (p.1223·2); dibasic sodium phosphate (p.1231·1).
*Gastrointestinal hyperacidity.*

**Alcalinos Vita** *Vita, Spain†.*
Aluminium hydroxide (p.1249·2); calcium carbonate (p.1254·2); magnesium hydroxide (p.1272·2).
*Gastrointestinal hyperacidity.*

**Alcalone Plus** *Bunker, Braz.*
Magnesium hydroxide (p.1272·2); aluminium hydroxide (p.1249·2); simeticone (p.1289·2).
*Flatulence; gastrointestinal hyperacidity.*

**Alcalosio** *SIT, Ital.*
Anhydrous glucose (p.1432·2); potassium citrate (p.1223·1); pyridoxine hydrochloride (p.1456·3); sodium bicarbonate (p.1223·2); sodium citrate (p.1223·2).
*Acetonaemia; gastrointestinal hyperacidity; vomiting.*

**Alca-Luftal** *Bristol-Myers Squibb, Braz.*
Simeticone (p.1289·2); magnesium hydroxide (p.1272·2); aluminium hydroxide (p.1249·2).
*Flatulence; gastrointestinal hyperacidity.*

**Alcamag** *Laborsil, Braz.†.*
Aluminium hydroxide (p.1249·2); magnesium hydroxide (p.1272·2); calcium carbonate (p.1254·2).
*Gastrointestinal hyperacidity.*

**Alcamex** *Cooper (Κοπερ), Gr.*
Calcium carbonate (p.1254·2).
*Prevention and treatment of calcium deficiency.*

**Alcan** *Sons, Mex.*
Chloramphenicol (p.185·1).
*Bacterial infections.*

**Alcaphor** *Pharmadeveloppement, Fr.*
Trometamol citrate (p.1758·3); sodium acid citrate (p.1223·2); dipotassium citrate (p.1224·1).
*Metabolic acidosis; renal calculi.*

**Alcare** *Calgon Vestal, USA.*
Alcohol (p.1166·1).
*Antiseptic.*

**Alcasedine** *Will-Pharma, Neth.*
Algeldrate (p.1249·2); magnesium trisilicate (p.1272·3).
*Dyspepsia; heartburn.*

**Alcasol** *Viatris, Belg.*
Sodium bicarbonate (p.1223·2); borax (p.1661·3); sodium chloride (p.1233·3).
*Eye disorders.*

**Alcaten** *Ariston, Braz.†.*
Fentetramin.
*Sympathomimetic.*

**Alcatex** *Medix, Mex.*
Cimetidine (p.1255·3).

**Alcelam** *Pharmasant, Thai.*
Alprazolam (p.668·3).
*Anxiety; insomnia.*

**Alchera** *Aspen, S.Afr.*
Zopiclone (p.729·3).
*Insomnia.*

**Alcinal** *Rekah, Israel.*
Dextromethorphan hydrobromide (p.1117·3); guaifenesin (p.1122·1); chlorphenamine maleate (p.427·3); phenylpropanolamine hydrochloride (p.1127·3).
*Coughs and cold symptoms.*

**Alcinal New** *Rekah, Israel.*
Dextromethorphan hydrobromide (p.1117·3); guaifenesin (p.1122·1); chlorphenamine maleate (p.427·3).
*Coughs and cold symptoms.*

**Alcinal Plus** *Rekah, Israel.*
Dextromethorphan hydrobromide (p.1117·3); guaifenesin (p.1122·1); chlorphenamine maleate (p.427·3); phenylpropanolamine hydrochloride (p.1127·3); paracetamol (p.76·2).
*Coughs and cold symptoms.*

**Alcis** *Chiesi, Spain.*
Estradiol (p.1550·1).
*Menopausal disorders; osteoporosis.*

**Alciton** *Kleva, Gr.*
Calcitonin (p.768·2).
*Osteoporosis.*

**Alcobon**
*Roche, Irl.†; ICN, NZ; Pacific, NZ.*
Flucytosine (p.399·3).
*Fungal infections.*

**Alcoderm**
*Note. This name is used for preparations of different composition.*
*Bajer, Arg.*
Coal tar (p.1159·2).
*Skin disorders.*

*Galderma, Irl.*
Liquid paraffin (p.1479·1).
*Dry skin.*

*Galderma, UK†.*
Moisturiser.
*Dry skin.*

**Alcodin** *Alcon, Ital.*
Myrtillus (p.1718·3).
*Capillary fragility; eye disorders.*

**Alcohcan** *Marrero, Spain†.*
Alcohol (p.1166·1); benzalkonium chloride (p.1168·3).
*Skin and wound disinfection.*

**Alcohocel** *Calmante Vitaminado, Spain.*
Alcohol (p.1166·1); cetylpyridinium chloride (p.1173·1).
*Skin disinfection.*

**Alcohol Benzalconio** *Viviar, Spain.*
Alcohol (p.1166·1); benzalkonium chloride (p.1168·3).
*Skin, wound, and surface disinfection.*

**Alcohol Cetil** *Noriega, Spain.*
Alcohol (p.1166·1); cetylpyridinium chloride (p.1173·1).
*Skin disinfection.*

**Alcohol Cetilpi Cuve** *Perez Gimenez, Spain.*
Alcohol (p.1166·1); cetylpyridinium chloride (p.1173·1).
*Skin disinfection.*

**Alcohol CL Benz** *Betamadrileno, Spain.*
Alcohol (p.1166·1); benzalkonium chloride (p.1168·3).
*Skin, wound, and surface disinfection.*

**Alcohol Poten** *Maxfarma, Spain.*
Alcohol (p.1166·1); benzethonium chloride (p.1169·2).
*Skin, wound, and surface disinfection.*

**Alcohol Potenciado** *Viviar, Spain.*
Alcohol (p.1166·1); benzalkonium chloride (p.1168·3).
*Skin, wound, and surface disinfection.*

**Alcohol Reforzado** *PQS, Spain†.*
Alcohol (p.1166·1); benzalkonium chloride (p.1168·3).
*Skin, wound, and surface disinfection.*

**Alcohol Sanit Cuve** *Calmante Vitaminado, Spain†.*
Alcohol (p.1166·1); cetylpyridinium chloride (p.1173·1).
*Skin disinfection.*

**Alcohten** *Marrero, Spain†.*
Alcohol (p.1166·1).
*Skin disinfection.*

**Alcojel** *Wellspring, Canad.*
Isopropyl alcohol (p.1184·3).
*Skin disorders.*

**Alcolex** *Labomed, Chile.*
Benzoxonium chloride (p.1170·2); alcohol (p.1166·1).
*Disinfection of instruments, skin, and wounds.*

**Alcomicin** *Alcon, Canad.*
Gentamicin sulfate (p.217·1).
*Eye infections.*

**Alcon Adequad** *Alcon, Belg.*
Dextran 70 (p.746·2); hypromellose (p.1579·3).
*Dry eyes.*

**Alcon AE** *Alcon, Arg.*
Vitamin A; vitamin E (p.1417·1).
*Dietary supplement.*

**Alcon Eye Gel** *Alcon, Belg.*
Carbomer (p.1577·2).
*Dry eyes.*

**Alcon Lagrimas** *Alcon, Arg.*
Dextran 70 (p.746·2); hypromellose (p.1579·3).
*Dry eyes.*

**Alcontar** *Galderma, Arg.*
Coal tar (p.1159·2).
*Eczema; psoriasis.*

**Alcopac Reforzado** *Agua del Carmen, Spain†.*
Alcohol (p.1166·1); benzalkonium chloride (p.1168·3).
*Skin, wound, and surface disinfection.*

**Alcophyllex** *Propan, S.Afr.*
Theophylline (p.798·3); etofylline (p.785·1); diphenhydramine hydrochloride (p.431·3); ammonium chloride (p.1115·2); sodium citrate (p.1223·2).
*Bronchospasm.*

**Alcophyllin** *Propan, S.Afr.*
Theophylline (p.798·3).
*Obstructive airways disease.*

**Alcos-Anal**
*Note. This name is used for preparations of different composition.*
*Bristol-Myers Squibb, Ger.; Meda, Norw.*
Sodium oleate (p.1574·3); lauromacrogol 400 (p.1412·3); chlorocarvacrol.
*Anorectal disorders.*

*Meda, Swed.*
Sodium oleate (p.1574·3); 2-hydroxy-5-chlorothymol.
*Anorectal disorders.*

**Alco-Screen**
*Marco, Austral.; Aptus, NZ.*
Test for alcohol in saliva.

**Alcover**
*Gerot, Austria; CT, Ital.*
Sodium oxybate (p.1308·3).
*Alcohol withdrawal syndrome.*

**Alcowipe** *SSL, UK.*
Isopropyl alcohol (p.1184·3).
*Hard surface disinfection.*

**Alcoxidine** *Vitamed, Israel.*
Chlorhexidine gluconate (p.1173·2).
*Skin disinfection.*

**Alcur** *Gea, Denm.*
Acetylcysteine (p.1112·3).
*Respiratory-tract congestion.*

**Alcusal** *Mentholatum, Austral.*
Copper salicylate.
*Musculoskeletal and joint disorders; sports injuries.*

**Alda** *Nakorn, Thai.*
Albendazole (p.101·2).
*Worm infections.*

**Aldactacine** *Pharmacia, Spain.*
Altizide (p.858·1); spironolactone (p.1003·1).
*Ascites; hypertension; oedema.*

**Aldactazide**
*Pharmacia, Canad.; SPA, Ital.; Searle, USA.*
Spironolactone (p.1003·1); hydrochlorothiazide (p.933·2).
*Heart failure; hypertension; liver cirrhosis with oedema and/or ascites; nephrotic syndrome.*

**Aldactazine**
*Pharmacia, Belg.; Pharmacia, Fr.; Pharmacia, Port.*
Altizide (p.858·1); spironolactone (p.1003·1).
*Hypertension; nephrotic syndrome; oedema.*

**Aldactide**
*Pharmacia, Irl.; Pharmacia, UK.*
Spironolactone (p.1003·1); hydroflumethiazide (p.937·2).
These ingredients can be described by the British Approved Name Co-flumactone.
*Heart failure; hypertension.*

**Aldactone**
*Pharmacia, Arg.; Pharmacia, Austral.; Roche, Austria; Pharmacia, Belg.; Pharmacia, Braz.; Pharmacia, Canad.; Pharmacia, Fin.; Pharmacia, Fr.; Roche, Ger.; Pharmacia-Upjohn, Gr.; Pharmacia, Hong Kong; RPG, India; Pharmacia, Irl.; Searle, Israel; Lepetit, Ital.; Searle, Mex.; Pharmacia, Neth.; Pharmacia, Norw.; Pharmacia, NZ; Pharmacia, Port.; Pharmacia, S.Afr.; Pharmacia, Singapore; Pharmacia, Spain; Pharmacia, Swed.; Pharmacia, Switz.; Pharmacia, Thai.; Pharmacia, UK; Searle, USA.*
Spironolactone (p.1003·1) or potassium canrenoate (p.984·2).
*Heart failure; hirsutism in females; hyperaldosteronism; hypertension; hypokalaemia; hypomagnesaemia; liver cirrhosis with ascites or oedema; malignant ascites; myasthenia gravis; nephrotic syndrome; oedema.*

**Aldactone Saltucin**
*Roche, Austria; Roche, Ger.*
Spironolactone (p.1003·1); butizide (p.878·2).
*Heart failure; hyperaldosteronism; hypertension; liver cirrhosis and ascites; nephrotic syndrome; oedema.*

**Aldalix** *Pharmacia, Fr.*
Spironolactone (p.1003·1); furosemide (p.919·3).
*Heart failure.*

**Aldar** *Mavi, Mex.†.*
Nifedipine (p.966·2).

**Aldara**
*3M, Arg.; 3M, Austral.; 3M, Belg.; 3M, Canad.; 3M, Chile; 3M, Denm.; 3M, Fin.; 3M, Fr.; 3M, Ger.; 3M, Gr.; 3M, Hong Kong; 3M, Irl.; 3M, Israel; 3M, Ital.; 3M, Malaysia; 3M, Mex.; 3M, Neth.; 3M, Norw.; 3M, NZ; 3M, S.Afr.; 3M, Singapore; 3M, Spain; 3M, Swed.; 3M, Switz.; 3M, Thai.; 3M, UK; 3M, USA.*
Imiquimod (p.638·1).
*Actinic keratosis; anogenital warts.*

**Aldarone** *Cadila Pharma, India.*
Amiodarone hydrochloride (p.859·2).
*Arrhythmias.*

**Aldazida**
*Note. This name is used for preparations of different composition.*
*Pharmacia, Arg.; Pharmacia, Braz.*
Spironolactone (p.1003·1); hydrochlorothiazide (p.933·2).
*Heart failure; hyperaldosteronism; hypertension; hypokalaemia; liver cirrhosis with ascites and oedema; nephrotic syndrome; oedema.*

*Searle, Mex.*
Spironolactone (p.1003·1); butizide (p.878·2).
*Hypertension; oedema.*

**Aldazide** *Pharmacia, S.Afr.*
Spironolactone (p.1003·1); butizide (p.878·2).
*Hypertension; nephrotic syndrome; oedema.*

**Aldazine**
*Alphapharm, Austral.; Alphapharm, Malaysia; Merck, Malaysia; Pacific, NZ.*
Thioridazine hydrochloride (p.724·2).
*Agitation; anxiety; behaviour disorders in children; psychoses.*

**Aldecin**
*Schering-Plough, Austral.; Byk, Belg.†; Schering-Plough, Denm.†; Schering-Plough, Hong Kong; Schering-Plough, NZ†; Byk, Switz.†.*
Beclometasone dipropionate (p.1091·1).
*Nasal polyps; obstructive airways disease; rhinitis.*

**Aldecina**
*Schering-Plough, Braz.†; Byk, Port.*
Beclometasone dipropionate (p.1091·1).
*Obstructive airways disease; rhinitis.*

**Aldic** *Shiwa, Thai.*
Furosemide (p.919·3).
*Barbiturate poisoning; hypertension; oedema; renal impairment.*

**Al-Dim** *Francia, Ital.†.*
Citric acid; chromium tripicolinate (p.1417·1).
*Nutritional supplement.*

**Aldipin** *Helvepharm, Switz.*
Nifedipine (p.966·2).
*Angina pectoris; hypertension; Raynaud's syndrome.*

**Aldira** *Novartis Consumer, Spain†.*
Terfenadine (p.441·1).
*Hypersensitivity reactions.*

**Aldo Asma** *Aldo, Spain.*
Ascorbic acid; phenylephrine hydrochloride (p.1126·3); isoprenaline hydrochloride (p.940·2).
*Obstructive airways disease.*

**Aldo Otico** *Aldo, Spain.*
Framycetin sulfate (p.215·1); lidocaine hydrochloride (p.1377·3); triamcinolone acetonide (p.1110·2); choline salicylate (p.26·2).
*External ear disorders; otitis media.*

**Aldoacne** *Aldo, Spain†.*
Benzoyl peroxide (p.1143·2).
*Acne.*

**Aldobronquial** *Aldo, Spain.*
Salbutamol sulfate (p.791·3).
*Obstructive airways disease.*

**Aldoclor** *Merck, USA.*
Methyldopa (p.953·2); chlorothiazide (p.882·1).
*Hypertension.*

**Aldocumar** *Aldo, Spain.*
Warfarin sodium (p.1022·2).
*Thromboembolic disorders; thrombosis prophylaxis.*

**Aldoderma** *Aldo, Spain.*
Framycetin sulfate (p.215·1); triamcinolone acetonide (p.1110·2).
*Infected skin disorders.*

**Aldoleo** *Altana, Spain.*
Chlortalidone (p.882·3); spironolactone (p.1003·1).
*Hypertension; oedema.*

**Aldolor** *CTI, Israel.*
Paracetamol (p.76·2).
*Fever; pain.*

**Aldomet**
*Sidus, Arg.; Merck Sharp & Dohme, Austral.; Merck Sharp & Dohme, Belg.; Prodome, Braz.; Merck Frosst, Canad.; Merck Sharp & Dohme, Denm.; Merck Sharp & Dohme-Chibret, Fr.; Vianex (Βιανεξ), Gr.; Merck Sharp & Dohme, Hong Kong; Merck Sharp & Dohme, Irl.; Merck Sharp & Dohme, Ital.; Merck Sharp & Dohme, Malaysia; Merck Sharp & Dohme, Mex.; Merck Sharp & Dohme, Neth.; Merck Sharp & Dohme, Norw.; Merck Sharp & Dohme, NZ†; Merck Sharp & Dohme, Port.; Merck Sharp & Dohme, S.Afr.; Biopat, Spain; Merck Sharp & Dohme, Swed.; Merck Sharp & Dohme, Switz.; Merck Sharp & Dohme, Thai.; Merck Sharp & Dohme, UK; Merck, USA†.*
Methyldopa (p.953·2) or methyldopate hydrochloride (p.953·2).
*Hypertension.*

**Aldometil** *Merck Sharp & Dohme, Austria.*
Methyldopa (p.953·2).
*Hypertension.*

**Aldomin** *Merck Sharp & Dohme, Israel.*
Methyldopa (p.953·2).
*Hypertension.*

**Aldonar** *Upsifarma, Port.*
Spironolactone (p.1003·1).
*Hypertension.*

**Aldopren** *Amrad, Austral.†.*
Methyldopa (p.953·2).
*Hypertension.*

**Aldopur**
Kwizda, Austria; Hormosan, Ger.†.
Spironolactone (p.1003·1).
*Cor pulmonale; heart failure; hyperaldosteronism; hypertension; liver cirrhosis with ascites and oedema; nephrotic syndrome.*

**Aldoretic**
Merck Sharp & Dohme, Austria; Chibret, Port.; Merck Sharp & Dohme, S.Afr.†; Merck Sharp & Dohme, Switz.†.
Amiloride hydrochloride (p.858·2); hydrochlorothiazide (p.933·2); methyldopa (p.953·2).
*Hypertension.*

**Aldoril**
Merck Sharp & Dohme, Canad.†; Merck, USA.
Methyldopa (p.953·2); hydrochlorothiazide (p.933·2).
*Hypertension.*

**Aldoron** Armstrong, Arg.
Nimesulide (p.67·1).
*Gout; musculoskeletal, joint, and peri-articular disorders.*

**Aldo-Silverderma** Aldo-Union, Hong Kong.
Sulfadiazine silver (p.259·1).
*Burns; pressure sores and skin ulcers.*

**Aldosomnil** Aldo, Spain.
Lormetazepam (p.705·2).
*Insomnia; premedication.*

**Aldospirone** Teva, Israel.
Spironolactone (p.1003·1).
*Heart failure; hyperaldosteronism; hypertension; hypokalaemia; liver cirrhosis; oedema.*

**Aldospray Analgesico** Aldo, Spain.
Mabuprofen (p.46·3).
*Peri-articular and soft-tissue disorders.*

**Aldotensin** Teuto, Braz.
Methyldopa (p.953·2).
*Hypertension.*

**Aldozone** Pharmacia, Switz.
Spironolactone (p.1003·1); butizide (p.878·2).
*Heart failure; hypertension; liver cirrhosis with ascites; nephrotic syndrome; oedema.*

**Aldrox**
Note. This name is used for preparations of different composition.
Whitehall, Braz.†.
Aluminium hydroxide (p.1249·2).
*Gastrointestinal hyperacidity.*

Pasteur, Chile.
Alendronate sodium (p.765·3).
*Osteoporosis.*

**Aldurazyme**
Genzyme, UK; Genzyme, USA.
Laronidase (p.1705·1).
*Mucopolysaccharidosis I.*

**Alec** Britannia Pharmaceuticals, UK†.
Pumactant (p.1736·2).
*Respiratory distress syndrome.*

**Aledin** Nestle, Switz.†.
Preparation for enteral nutrition (p.1417·1).
*Coeliac disease; diarrhoea.*

**Aledron** IQFA, Mex.
Oxolamine citrate (p.1126·1).
*Coughs.*

**Aleevex** Food Supplement, UK†.
Eucalyptus oil (p.1686·2); camphor (p.1665·3); menthol (p.1711·3).
*Cold symptoms.*

**Alegysal** Nikken, Jpn.
Pemirolast potassium (p.790·3).
*Allergic rhinitis; asthma.*

**Alembicol D** Alembic Products, UK.
Fractionated coconut oil (p.1440·3).
*Food for special diets; malabsorption syndromes.*

**Alemelano** Elvetium, Arg.
Bifemelane hydrochloride (p.1660·2).

**Al-En** Francia, Ital.†.
Creatine; carnitine bitartrate; magnesium oxide; vitamins (p.1417·1).
*Nutritional supplement.*

**Alenato** ICN, Arg.
Alendronate sodium (p.765·3).
*Osteoporosis.*

**Alenbit** Chrispa (Χρισπα), Gr.
Norfloxacin (p.238·3).
*Urinary tract infections.*

**Alencast** Chrispa (Χρισπα), Gr.
Nimesulide (p.67·1).
*Inflammation; musculoskeletal disorders; pain.*

**Alendil** Farmoquimica, Braz.
Alendronate sodium (p.765·3).
*Osteoporosis.*

**Alendros** Abiogen, Ital.
Alendronate sodium (p.765·3).
*Osteoporosis.*

**Alenic Alka** Rugby, USA.
*Oral liquid:* Aluminium hydroxide (p.1249·2); magnesium carbonate (p.1272·1).
*Tablets:* Aluminium hydroxide (p.1249·2); magnesium trisilicate (p.1272·3); sodium bicarbonate (p.1223·2).
*Hyperacidity.*

**Alenstran** Chrispa (Χρισπα), Gr.
Cetirizine hydrochloride (p.427·1).
*Allergic conjunctivitis; allergic rhinitis; pruritus.*

**Alental** Chobet, Arg.
Fluoxetine hydrochloride (p.292·1).
*Depression.*

**Alenzantyl** Chrispa (Χρισπα), Gr.
Azelaic acid (p.1142·3).
*Acne.*

**Aleot** Apomedica, Austria.
Chlorphenesin (p.396·1); diphenhydramine hydrochloride (p.431·3); chlorobutanol (p.1176·3); benzalkonium chloride (p.1168·3); urea (p.1162·2).
*Ear disorders.*

**Alepa** Duopharm, Ger.
Silybum marianum (p.1043·3).
*Liver disorders.*

**Alepam** Alphapharm, Austral.
Oxazepam (p.712·2).
*Alcohol withdrawal syndrome; anxiety.*

**Aleprozil** Diba, Mex.
Omeprazole (p.1278·2).
*Aspiration syndrome; gastro-oesophageal reflux; peptic ulcer; Zollinger-Ellison syndrome.*

**Alepsal**
Note. This name is used for preparations of different composition.
Spedrog, Arg.; Rudefsa, Mex.
Phenobarbital (p.367·3).
*Epilepsy.*

Genevrier, Fr.
Phenobarbital (p.367·3); caffeine (p.782·1).
*Epilepsy; febrile convulsions.*

**Alepsal Compuesto** Rudefsa, Mex.
Phenobarbital (p.367·3); phenytoin sodium (p.370·2).
*Epilepsy.*

**Alercortil** Allergan, Arg.
Hydrocortisone (p.1103·3); naphazoline hydrochloride (p.1124·3).
*Conjunctivitis.*

**Alercrom** Grin, Mex.
Sodium cromoglicate (p.795·3).
*Allergic conjunctivitis.*

**Alerdil** Diba, Mex.
Chlorphenamine (p.428·1).
*Hypersensitivity.*

**Aler-Dryl** Reese, USA.
Diphenhydramine hydrochloride (p.431·3).

**Alerfedine** Lazar, Arg.
Fexofenadine hydrochloride (p.433·3).
*Allergic rhinitis.*

**Alerfedine D** Lazar, Arg.
Fexofenadine hydrochloride (p.433·3); pseudoephedrine hydrochloride (p.1129·2).
*Allergic rhinitis.*

**Alerfrin** Allergan, Spain.
Oxymetazoline hydrochloride (p.1126·1).
*Ocular congestion and irritation.*

**Alerfur** Fustery, Mex.
Astemizole (p.424·2).
*Hypersensitivity.*

**Alerg** 1A, Ger.
Sodium cromoglicate (p.795·3).
*Allergic conjunctivitis; allergic rhinitis.*

**Alergaliv** Sigma, Braz.
Loratadine (p.436·1).
*Hypersensitivity reactions.*

**Alergan** Chemopharma, Chile.
Loratadine (p.436·1).
*Allergic eye disorders; allergic rhinitis; allergic skin disorders; urticaria.*

**Alergi** Raymos, Arg.
Dexamethasone (p.1097·1); chlorphenamine (p.428·1).
*Hypersensitivity reactions.*

**Alergibon**
Galderma, Braz.; Galderma, Mex.
Emollient; soap substitute.
*Barrier preparation; dry skin.*

**Alergical**
Iquinosa, Spain.
*Cream:* Betamethasone valerate (p.1093·2); fluocinolone acetonide (p.1101·2).
*Skin disorders.*

Juventus, Spain.
*Syrup:* Chlorphenamine maleate (p.427·3); prednisolone metasulfobenzoate sodium (p.1108·1).
*Tablets:* Ascorbic acid (p.1460·2); chlorphenamine maleate (p.427·3); prednisolone (p.1108·1).
*Hypersensitivity reactions; skin disorders.*

**Alergical Expect** Juventus, Spain.
Chlorphenamine maleate (p.427·3); diprophylline (p.784·3); guaifenesin (p.1122·1); paracetamol (p.76·2).
*Bronchospasm; fever; pain.*

**Alergiderm** Prodotti, Braz.
Promethazine hydrochloride (p.439·1).
*Hypersensitivity reactions.*

**Alergidryl** Klonal, Arg.
Chlorphenamine (p.428·1).
*Hypersensitivity reactions.*

**Alergiftalmina** Davi, Port.
Antazoline phosphate (p.424·2); naphazoline hydrochloride (p.1124·3).
*Blepharospasm; conjunctivitis.*

**Alergin** Cipla, India.
Ephedrine hydrochloride (p.1120·1); theophylline (p.798·3); phenobarbital (p.367·3).
*Asthma; bronchospasm.*

**Alergist** Almirall, Spain†.
Terfenadine (p.441·1).
*Hypersensitivity reactions.*

**Alergitanil** Prodotti, Braz.
Mepyramine maleate (p.437·1).
*Hypersensitivity reactions.*

**Alergitrat**
Note. This name is used for preparations of different composition.
Fecofar, Arg.
Chlorphenamine (p.428·1).
*Hypersensitivity reactions.*

Medley, Braz.†.
Mepyramine maleate (p.437·1); tripelennamine hydrochloride (p.442·3); strontium bromide (p.1663·1); calcium pantothenate; magnesium thiosulfate.
*Hypersensitivity reactions.*

**Alergo Filinal** Eurofarma, Braz.
Diphenhydramine hydrochloride (p.431·3); aminophylline (p.780·2); guaifenesin (p.1122·1); pyridoxine hydrochloride (p.1456·3).
*Respiratory-tract disorders.*

**Alergo Glucalbet** Dansk-Flama, Braz.
Mepyramine maleate (p.437·1); pentoxyverine citrate (p.1126·2); calcium gluconate (p.1225·2); ammonium chloride (p.1115·2).
*Coughs.*

**Alergocrom** Aldo, Spain.
Sodium cromoglicate (p.795·3).
*Asthma; bronchospasm.*

**Alergoftal**
Alcon Cusi, Malaysia; Cusi, Singapore†; Alcon Cusi, Spain.
Antazoline phosphate (p.424·2); naphazoline hydrochloride (p.1124·3).
*Eye irritation.*

**Alergogel** Laborsil, Braz.†.
Diphenhydramine hydrochloride (p.431·3); ammonium chloride (p.1115·2).
*Respiratory-tract congestion.*

**Alergoliber** Recordati, Spain.
Rupatadine fumarate (p.440·3).
*Allergic rhinitis.*

**Alergolon** Biolab Sanus, Braz.
Methylprednisolone (p.1106·1).
*Corticosteroid.*

**Alergomed** Alergomed, Braz.†.
Allergen preparation (p.1650·1).
*Allergen immunotherapy.*

**Alergoral** Darrow, Braz.
Allergen preparation (p.1650·1).
*Allergen immunotherapy.*

**Alergosan** Klinger, Braz.
Promethazine (p.439·1).
*Hypersensitivity reactions.*

**Alergotox** Makros, Braz.†.
Diphenhydramine hydrochloride (p.431·3); theophylline (p.798·3); aminophylline (p.780·2).
*Hypersensitivity.*

**Alergotox Efedrina** Makros, Braz.†.
Diphenhydramine hydrochloride (p.431·3); ephedrine hydrochloride (p.1120·1); liver antitoxin.
*Hypersensitivity.*

**Alergotox Expectorante** Makros, Braz.†.
Diphenhydramine hydrochloride (p.431·3); guaifenesin (p.1122·1); aminophylline (p.780·2); liver antitoxin.
*Respiratory-tract congesion.*

**Alergotox Nasal** Makros, Braz.†.
Diphenhydramine hydrochloride (p.431·3); naphazoline hydrochloride (p.1124·3).
*Nasal congestion.*

**Alergotox Pastilhas** Makros, Braz.†.
Diphenhydramine hydrochloride (p.431·3); cetylpyridinium chloride (p.1173·1); benzocaine (p.1370·3).
*Mouth and throat disorders.*

**Alergovalle** Dovalle, Braz.
Dexchlorpheniramine (p.428·1).
*Hypersensitivity reactions.*

**Alergyo** Sanval, Braz.
Dexchlorpheniramine maleate (p.427·3).
*Hypersensitivity reactions.*

**Alerid**
UCB, Austria; Asche, Ger.; Cipla, India.
Cetirizine hydrochloride (p.427·1).
*Hypersensitivity reactions.*

**Alerjon** Edol, Port.
Oxymetazoline hydrochloride (p.1126·1).
*Eye irritation.*

**Alerken** Kener, Mex.†.
Astemizole (p.424·2).

**Alerlisin** Menarini, Spain.
Cetirizine hydrochloride (p.427·1).
*Hypersensitivity reactions.*

**Alermine** Royton, Braz.
Dexchlorpheniramine maleate (p.427·3).
*Hypersensitivity reactions.*

**Alermizol**
Pharmacia, Arg.; Reig Jofre, Spain.
Astemizole (p.424·2).
*Hypersensitivity reactions.*

**Alernex** Dabur, India.
Fexofenadine hydrochloride (p.433·3).
*Allergic rhinitis; urticaria.*

**Alerpriv** Montpellier, Arg.
Loratadine (p.436·1).
*Hypersensitivity reactions.*

**Alerpriv D** Montpellier, Arg.
Loratadine (p.436·1); pseudoephedrine sulfate (p.1129·2).
*Cold and influenza symptoms; otitis; rhinitis; sinusitis.*

**Aler-Releaf** Reese, USA†.
Chlorphenamine maleate (p.427·3); phenylpropanolamine hydrochloride (p.1127·3).

**Alersan** Hexal, Braz.
Betamethasone dipropionate (p.1093·1).
Formerly contained mepyramine maleate and magnesium thiosulfate.
*Hypersensitivity.*

**Alertal** Sintofarma, Braz.†.
Loratadine (p.436·1).
*Hypersensitivity.*

**Alertec** Draxis, Canad.
Modafinil (p.1591·1).
*Narcoleptic syndrome.*

**Alertonic**
Sigma, Austral.
Pipradrol hydrochloride (p.1592·3); vitamin B substances; minerals; trace elements (p.1417·1).
*Tonic.*

Aventis, Canad.
Pipradrol hydrochloride (p.1592·3); vitamin B substances (p.1417·1).
*Tonic.*

Mer-National, S.Afr.
Pipradrol hydrochloride (p.1592·3); vitamin B substances (p.1417·1); minerals.
*Tonic.*

**Alertop** Laboratorios Chile, Chile.
Cetirizine hydrochloride (p.427·1).
*Hypersensitivity reactions.*

**Alertrin** Helsinn, Port.†.
Loratadine (p.436·1).
*Allergic rhinitis; eye irritation; urticaria.*

**Alerzona** Silesia, Chile.
Mepyramine maleate (p.437·1); prednisone acetate (p.1109·3).
*Skin disorders.*

**Alesion** Boehringer Ingelheim, Jpn.
Epinastine hydrochloride (p.433·3).
*Allergic rhinitis; asthma; pruritus.*

**Alesse**
Wyeth-Ayerst, Canad.; Wyeth-Ayerst, USA.
Levonorgestrel (p.1563·2); ethinylestradiol (p.1553·2).
28-Day packs also contain 7 inert tablets.
*Combined oral contraceptive.*

**Aletir** Bunker, Braz.
Cetirizine hydrochloride (p.427·1).
*Hypersensitivity reactions.*

**Aletris Oligoplex** Madaus, Ger.
Homoeopathic preparation.

**Aleucin** Piam, Ital.
Food for special diets (p.1417·1).
*Maple syrup urine disease.*

**Aleudrina** Boehringer Ingelheim, Spain.
Isoprenaline sulfate (p.940·2).
*Cardiac disorders; shock.*

**Aleve**
Roche, Arg.; Roche Consumer, Austral.; Roche, Austria; Roche, Belg.; Nicholas, Fr.; Roche Nicholas, Ger.; Roche, Ital.; Roche Consumer, Neth.; Roche Consumer, S.Afr.; Roche, Spain; Roche, Switz.; Procter & Gamble, USA.
Naproxen sodium (p.65·1).
*Fever; gout; musculoskeletal and joint disorders; pain.*

**Alex** Glenmark, India.
Dextromethorphan hydrobromide (p.1117·3); phenylpropanolamine hydrochloride (p.1127·3); chlorphenamine maleate (p.427·3); paracetamol (p.76·2); caffeine (p.782·1).
*Cold symptoms; coughs.*

**Alex Cough** Glenmark, India.
*Lozenges:* Dextromethorphan hydrobromide (p.1117·3).
*Coughs; sore throat.*
*Syrup:* Dextromethorphan hydrobromide (p.1117·3); phenylpropanolamine hydrochloride (p.1127·3); chlorphenamine maleate (p.427·3); guaifenesin (p.1122·1).
*Coughs.*

**Alex Paediatric** Glenmark, India.
Phenylpropanolamine hydrochloride (p.1127·3); chlorphenamine maleate (p.427·3).
*Nasal congestion; nasal hypersensitivity reactions.*

**Alexan**
Pfizer, Austria; Pharmacia Upjohn, Braz.†; Pharmacia, Chile; Mack, Illert., Ger.; Mack, Hong Kong; Mack, Israel; Pharmacia Upjohn, Mex.; Ferraz, Lynce, Port.; Bodene, S.Afr.; Mack, Singapore; Nycomed, Swed.†; Mack, Switz.†; Mack, Thai.
Cytarabine (p.543·1).
Formerly known as Cytovis in *Israel*.
*Leukaemias; non-Hodgkins lymphomas.*

**Alexia** Saval, Chile.
Fexofenadine hydrochloride (p.433·3).
*Allergic rhinitis; allergic skin disorders.*

**Alexia D** Saval, Chile.
Fexofenadine hydrochloride (p.433·3); pseudoephedrine sulfate (p.1129·2).
*Allergic rhinitis.*

**Alexin**
Note. This name is used for preparations of different composition.
Dabur, India.
Cefalexin (p.168·1).
*Bacterial infections.*

Jaba, Port.
Lansoprazole (p.1269·3).
*Gastro-oesophageal reflux; peptic ulcer; Zollinger-Ellison syndrome.*

**Alex-P** *Glenmark, India.*
Dextromethorphan hydrobromide (p.1117·3); phenylpropanolamine hydrochloride (p.1127·3); chlorphenamine maleate (p.427·3); paracetamol (p.76·2).
*Cold symptoms; coughs.*

**Aleztem** *Rayere, Mex.*
Astemizole (p.424·2).
*Hypersensitivity.*

**Alfa**
*Note. This name is used for preparations of different composition.*
*Bergamon, Ital.*
Didecyldimethylammonium chloride (p.1178·3).
*Disinfection of burns, mucous membranes, and wounds.*
*Pfizer Lambert, Spain.*
Naphazoline nitrate (p.1124·3).
*Eye irritation.*

**Alfa Acid** *Euroderm, Ital.*
Ammonium lactate (p.1142·3); salicylic acid (p.1157·1); dexpanthenol (p.1727·2).
*Scalp disorders.*

**Alfa C** *Bracco, Ital.*
Benzalkonium chloride (p.1168·3).
*Eye irritation.*

**Alfa Calcimax** *Gador, Arg.*
Alfacalcidol (p.1461·2).
*Osteomalacia; osteoporosis; renal osteodystrophy; rickets; vitamin D deficiency.*

**Alfa D** *Osteolab, Chile.*
Alfacalcidol (p.1461·2).
*Vitamin D supplement.*

**Alfa Kappa** *Kedrion, Ital.*
Amino-acid preparation (p.1417·1).
*Nutritional supplement in renal failure.*

**Alfabase** *Cassara, Arg.*
Emollient.

**Alfabase 8** *Cassara, Arg.*
Glycolic acid (p.1147·3).
*Photoageing of skin.*

**Alfabetal** *Mitim, Ital.†.*
Labetalol hydrochloride (p.943·3).
*Hypertension.*

**Alfabios** *Biotekfarma, Ital.†.*
Fluocinolone acetonide (p.1101·2).
*Corticosteroid.*

**Alfacaina** *Dentsply, Ital.*
Articaine hydrochloride (p.1370·3).
Adrenaline (p.852·2) is included in this preparation as a vasoconstrictor to diminish absorption and localise the effect of the local anaesthetic.
*Local anaesthesia.*

**Alfacid** *Grunenthal, Ger.*
Rifabutin (p.249·1).
*Mycobacterium-avium complex infections in AIDS patients; tuberculosis.*

**Alfacort**
*Cassara, Arg.; Julphar, UAE.*
Hydrocortisone (p.1103·3) or hydrocortisone acetate (p.1103·3).
*Inflammatory eye disorders; skin disorders.*

**Alfacortone** *Spirig, Switz.*
Hydrocortisone acetate (p.1103·3).
*Skin disorders.*

**Alfad**
*Biosintetica, Braz.; Byk Gulden, Mex.*
Alfacalcidol (p.1461·2).
*Hyperparathyroidism; hypoparathyroidism; osteomalacia; osteoporosis; renal osteodystrophy; rickets; vitamin D deficiency.*

**AlfaD** *Berk, UK†.*
Alfacalcidol (p.1461·2).
*Vitamin D deficiency.*

**Alfadelta** *Farmacusi, Spain†.*
Alfacalcidol (p.1461·2).
*Hypoparathyroidism; osteomalacia; renal osteodystrophy; vitamin D deficiency.*

**Alfadil** *Pfizer, Swed.*
Doxazosin mesilate (p.908·3).
*Benign prostatic hyperplasia; hypertension.*

**Alfadoxin** *Laboratorios Chile, Chile.*
Doxazosin mesilate (p.908·3).
*Benign prostatic hyperplasia; hypertension.*

**Alfaferone** *Wassermann, Ital.*
Interferon alfa (p.640·3).
*Anogenital warts; hepatitis B; hepatitis C; malignant neoplasms.*

**Alfaflor** *INTES, Ital.*
Bottle A, betamethasone sodium phosphate (p.1093·1); naphazoline nitrate (p.1124·3); bottle B, tetracycline hydrochloride (p.266·2).
*Inflammatory eye disorders.*

**Alfa-Fluorone** *New Farma, Ital.†.*
*Lotion:* Fluocinolone acetonide (p.1101·2).
*Skin disorders.*
*Vaginal solution:* Fluocinolone acetonide (p.1101·2); benzalkonium chloride (p.1168·3).
*Vulvovaginal infections.*

**Alfagamma** *Humana, Ital.*
Essential fatty acids; vitamin E; vitamin $B_6$ (p.1417·1).
*Nutritional supplement.*

**Alfagen** *Wassermann, Ital.*
Collagen (p.1674·3).
*Ulcers; wounds.*

**Alfaken** *Kendrick, Mex.*
Lisinopril (p.946·3).
*Hypertension.*

**Alfakinasi** *Wassermann, Ital.*
Urokinase (p.1018·2).
*Thromboembolic disorders.*

**Alfalfa Sativa Compuesta** *Hochstetter, Chile.*
Alfalfa; avena sativa; papaya (p.1417·1).
*Tonic.*

**Alfalfa Tonic**
*Boiron, Canad.; Homeocan, Canad.*
Homoeopathic preparation.

**Alfamox** *Teofarma, Ital.*
Amoxicillin trihydrate (p.155·3).
*Bacterial infections.*

**Alfan** *Alpharma, Mex.*
Dextromethorphan hydrobromide (p.1117·3); chlorphenamine maleate (p.427·3); ephedrine hydrochloride (p.1120·1).
*Coughs; nasal congestion.*

**Alfapsin** *Lyka, India.*
Trypsin (p.1758·3); chymotrypsin (p.1671·2).
*Inflammation; oedema.*

**Alfare**
*Nestle, Austral.; Nestle, Braz.; Nestle, Fr.; Nestle, Ital.; Nestle, Mex.; Nestle, Port.; Nestle, Switz.; Nestle, UK†.*
Preparation for enteral nutrition (p.1417·1).
*Cow's milk and soya intolerance; diarrhoea; malabsorption disorders.*

**Alfarol**
*Chugai, Hong Kong†; Chugai, Jpn.*
Alfacalcidol (p.1461·2).
*Hypoparathyroidism; osteomalacia; osteoporosis; renal failure; rickets.*

**Alfasin** *Sintofarma, Braz.*
Finasteride (p.1554·2).
*Alopecia; benign prostatic hyperplasia.*

**Alfason** *Yamanouchi, Ger.*
Hydrocortisone butyrate (p.1104·1).
*Skin disorders.*

**Alfast** *Cristalia, Braz.*
Alfentanil hydrochloride (p.12·2).

**Alfater** *Nuovo ISM, Ital.*
Interferon alfa (p.640·3).
*Anogenital warts; hepatitis B; hepatitis non-A non-B; malignant neoplasms.*

**Alfatil** *Lilly, Fr.*
Cefaclor (p.167·1).
*Bacterial infections.*

**Alfavit** *Medgenix, Belg.*
Ephedrine tartrate (p.1120·3); vitamins (p.1417·1).
*Tonic.*

**Alfavitil** *DNR, Arg.*
Pronalen.
*Cellulitis.*

**Alfazina** *Salus, Ital.†.*
Propyphenazone (p.85·3); caffeine (p.782·1).
*Fever; pain.*

**Alfazol** *IQFA, Mex.*
Albendazole (p.101·2).
*Worm infections.*

**Alfener** *Vilco, Gr.*
Diltiazem (p.901·3).
*Angina; hypertension.*

**Alfenta**
*Janssen-Ortho, Canad.; Taylor, USA.*
Alfentanil hydrochloride (p.12·2).
*Analgesia during anaesthesia.*

**Alferm** *Schoning-Berlin, Ger.*
*Ointment:* Prednisolone (p.1108·1); thymol (p.1194·2).
*Suppositories:* Prednisolone (p.1108·1); thymol (p.1194·2); menthol (p.1711·3).
*Anorectal disorders.*

**Alferon** *Cryopharma, Mex.*
Interferon alfa-2a (recombinant) (p.640·3).
*Hepatitis B; malignant neoplasms.*

**Alferon N** *Interferon Sciences, USA.*
Interferon alfa-n3 (p.640·3).
*Genital warts.*

**Alferos** *Berenguer Infale, Spain†.*
Azelastine hydrochloride (p.425·2).
*Allergic rhinitis.*

**Alfetim** *Beecham, Spain.*
Alfuzosin hydrochloride (p.856·2).
*Benign prostatic hyperplasia.*

**Alficetin** *Bristol-Myers Squibb, Arg.*
Colistimethate sodium (p.199·1).
*Bacterial infections.*

**Alfin** *Instituto Sanitas, Chile.*
Sildenafil citrate (p.1744·2).
*Erectile dysfunction.*

**Alfitar** *Fardi, Spain.*
Coal tar (p.1159·2).
*Psoriasis; seborrhoeic dermatitis.*

**Al-Flor** *Francia, Ital.*
Lactic-acid producing bacteria (p.1704·2); yeast; anise; lime; vitamin C; vitamin B substances (p.1417·1).
*Restoration of gastrointestinal flora.*

**Alfospas**
*Opfermann, Ger.†; Rottapharm, Ital.*
Tiropramide hydrochloride (p.1757·1).
*Smooth muscle spasm.*

**Alfuca** *Kenyaku, Thai.*
Albendazole (p.101·2).
*Worm infections.*

**Algafan** *Darrow, Braz.†.*
Dextropropoxyphene (p.28·3); paracetamol (p.76·2).
*Pain.*

**Alganex** *Roche, Swed.*
Tenoxicam (p.93·1).
*Dysmenorrhoea; inflammation; musculoskeletal, joint, and peri-articular disorders; postoperative pain.*

**Algedol** *Pharmacia, Arg.*
Morphine sulfate (p.60·2).
*Pain.*

**Algedrox** *De Mayo, Braz.*
Aluminium hydroxide (p.1249·2); magnesium hydroxide (p.1272·2); dimeticone (p.1289·2).
*Flatulence; gastrointestinal hyperacidity.*

**Algefit** *Nycomed, Austria.*
Diclofenac sodium (p.32·1).
*Soft-tissue and peri-articular disorders.*

**Algenac** *Ofimex, Mex.†.*
Diclofenac (p.32·1).

**Algesal**
*Note. This name is used for preparations of different composition.*
*Raffo, Arg.; Solvay, Austria; Pharmaselect, Ger.; Byk Gulden, Mex.; Solvay, Port.; Solvay, Spain; Solvay, Switz.*
Diethylamine salicylate (p.34·1); myrtecaine (p.1381·3) or myrtecaine laurilsulfate (p.1381·3).
*Musculoskeletal, joint, peri-articular, and soft-tissue disorders; neuralgia.*
*Solvay, Belg.; Solvay, Canad.†; Solvay, Fin.; Solvay, Ital.; LTM, Neth.; Nycomed, Norw.; Solvay, Swed.; Zeroderma, UK.*
Diethylamine salicylate (p.34·1).
*Musculoskeletal, joint, peri-articular, and soft-tissue disorders; neuralgias.*

**Algesal Forte** *LTM, Neth.*
Diethylamine salicylate (p.34·1); myrtecaine (p.1381·3).
*Muscle and joint pain.*

**Algesal Suractive** *Solvay, Fr.†.*
Diethylamine salicylate (p.34·1); myrtecaine (p.1381·3).
*Soft-tissue disorders.*

**Algesalona**
*Solvay, Ger.; Solvay, Switz.*
Diethylamine salicylate (p.34·1); myrtecaine (p.1381·3); flufenamic acid (p.43·2).
*Musculoskeletal, joint, peri-articular, and soft-tissue disorders.*

**Algesalona E** *Solvay, Ger.*
Etofenamate (p.38·1).
*Musculoskeletal, joint, peri-articular, and soft-tissue disorders.*

**Algexin** *Cimed, Braz.*
Hyoscine butylbromide (p.483·3).
*Smooth muscle spasm.*

**Algho** *Rhone-Poulenc Rorer, Spain†.*
Aspirin (p.15·1).
*Fever; inflammation; pain; thromboembolism prophylaxis.*

**Algi** *Mabo, Spain.*
Metamizole magnesium (p.36·1).
*Fever; pain.*

**Algiasdin** *Isdin, Spain.*
Ibuprofen (p.45·3).
*Fever; inflammation; musculoskeletal, joint, and peri-articular disorders; pain.*

**Algi-Butazolon** *Dovalle, Braz.*
*Oral solution:* Diclofenac (p.32·1); paracetamol (p.76·2).
*Tablets:* Diclofenac (p.32·1); paracetamol (p.76·2); carisoprodol (p.1392·1); caffeine (p.782·1).

**Algice** *Cazi, Braz.*
Green tablets, dipyrone (p.35·3); sodium camsilate; cineole (p.1672·1); guaifenesin (p.1122·1); niaouli oil (p.1719·3); yellow tablets, vitamin C (p.1460·2).
*Cold and influenza symptoms.*

**Algicon**
*Note. This name is used for preparations of different composition.*
*Rhone-Poulenc Rorer, Austral.†; Aventis, Irl.; Aventis, Neth.*
*Oral suspension:* Magnesium alginate (p.1577·1); aluminium hydroxide-magnesium carbonate co-dried gel (p.1250·1); magnesium carbonate (p.1272·1); potassium bicarbonate (p.1223·1); calcium carbonate (p.1254·2).
*Gastro-oesophageal reflux.*
*Rhone-Poulenc Rorer, Austral.†; Rhone-Poulenc Rorer, Irl.†; Aventis, Neth.*
*Tablets:* Magnesium alginate (p.1577·1); aluminium hydroxide-magnesium carbonate co-dried gel (p.1250·1); magnesium carbonate (p.1272·1); potassium bicarbonate (p.1223·1).
*Gastro-oesophageal reflux.*
*Aventis, Mex.*
*Oral suspension:* Magnesium alginate (p.1577·1); aluminium hydroxide-magnesium carbonate co-dried gel (p.1250·1); magnesium carbonate (p.1272·1); calcium carbonate (p.1254·2).
*Tablets:* Magnesium alginate (p.1577·1); aluminium hydroxide-magnesium carbonate co-dried gel (p.1250·1); magnesium carbonate (p.1272·1).
*Gastrointestinal hyperacidity.*
*Rhone-Poulenc Rorer, Norw.†; Aventis, UK.*
Aluminium hydroxide-magnesium carbonate co-dried gel (p.1250·1); magnesium alginate (p.1577·1); magnesium carbonate (p.1272·1); potassium bicarbonate (p.1223·1).
*Gastric hyperacidity; gastro-oesophageal reflux.*

**Algicote**
*Note. This name is used for preparations of different composition.*
*Rhodia, Braz.†.*
Aluminium hydroxide-magnesium carbonate co-dried gel (p.1250·1); magnesium alginate (p.1577·1); magnesium carbonate (p.1272·1).
*Gastrointestinal hyperacidity.*
*Aventis, Chile.*
*Chewable tablets:* Magnesium alginate (p.1577·1); aluminium hydroxide-magnesium carbonate co-dried gel (p.1250·1); magnesium carbonate (p.1272·1); potassium bicarbonate (p.1223·1).
*Oral suspension:* Magnesium alginate (p.1577·1); aluminium hydroxide-magnesium carbonate co-dried gel (p.1250·1); magnesium carbonate (p.1272·1); calcium carbonate (p.1254·2); potassium bicarbonate (p.1223·1).
*Gastro-oesophageal reflux.*

**Algi-Danilon** *Allergan-Frumtost, Braz.†.*
Ibuprofen (p.45·3); paracetamol (p.76·2).
*Fever; inflammation; pain.*

**Algidente** *Sedabel, Braz.*
Phenol (p.1188·1); procaine hydrochloride (p.1383·2); clove oil (p.1673·3).
Formerly contained chloroform, phenol, procaine hydrochloride, and clove oil.
*Mouth disorders.*

**Algiderm** *Finadiet, Arg.*
Erythromycin ethyl succinate (p.208·1).
*Bacterial infections.*

**Algiderma** *Davi, Port.*
Diethylamine salicylate (p.34·1).
*Musculoskeletal, joint, and soft-tissue disorders.*

**Algidol**
*Note. This name is used for preparations of different composition.*
*Sintesa, Belg.†; Almirall, Spain.*
Paracetamol (p.76·2); codeine phosphate (p.27·1); ascorbic acid (p.1460·2).
*Pain.*
*Vitae, Mex.†.*
Ibuprofen (p.45·3).
*Pain.*

**Algidrin** *Fardi, Spain.*
Ibuprofen lysine (p.46·3).
*Inflammation; pain.*

**Algifemin** *Instituto Sanitas, Chile.*
Mefenamic acid (p.55·2).
*Pain.*

**Algifen** *Sintofarma, Braz.*
Ibuprofen (p.45·3); paracetamol (p.76·2).
*Fever; inflammation; pain.*

**Algifene**
*Note. This name is used for preparations of different composition.*
*Roche Nicholas, Fr.†.*
Ibuprofen (p.45·3).
*Fever; pain.*
*Ferraz, Lynce, Port.*
*Injection:* Dextropropoxyphene hydrochloride (p.28·3).
*Tablets†:* Dextropropoxyphene (p.28·3); paracetamol (p.76·2).
*Pain.*

**Algiflamanil** *Neo Quimica, Braz.†.*
Oxyphenbutazone (p.76·1); paracetamol (p.76·2).
*Fever; inflammation; pain.*

**Algiflex**
*Note. This name is used for preparations of different composition.*
*EMS, Braz.*
Ibuprofen (p.45·3).
*Gilton, Braz.†.*
Orphenadrine (p.486·2); dipyrone (p.35·3); caffeine (p.782·1).
*Skeletal muscle spasm.*

**Algifor** *Vifor, Switz.*
Ibuprofen (p.45·3) or ibuprofen lysine (p.46·3).
*Fever; pain.*

**Algi-Itamanil** *Neo Quimica, Braz.*
Ibuprofen (p.45·3); paracetamol (p.76·2).
*Fever; inflammation; pain.*

**Algik** *Azevedos, Port.*
Paracetamol (p.76·2); caffeine (p.782·1).
*Fever; pain.*

**Algikey** *Inkeysa, Spain.*
Ketorolac trometamol (p.52·1).
*Pain.*

**Algimate** *Bonafarma, Port.*
Clonixin lysine (p.26·3).
*Pain.*

**Algimesil** *Francia, Ital.*
Nimesulide (p.67·1).
*Musculoskeletal and joint disorders.*

**Alginex** *Sanopharm, Switz.*
Ethyl salicylate (p.37·3); camphor (p.1665·3); menthol (p.1711·3); turpentine oil (p.1760·1).
*Musculoskeletal, joint, and peri-articular disorders; sports injuries.*

**Alginflan** *Teuto, Braz.†.*
Phenylbutazone (p.83·2); paracetamol (p.76·2).
*Fever; inflammation; pain.*

**Alginor** *Boehringer Ingelheim, Ital.*
Cimetropium bromide (p.480·2).
*Adjunct in gastrointestinal examinations and surgical procedures; gastrointestinal disorders.*

**Algin-Vek** Faran, Gr.
Tenoxicam (p.93·1).
*Dysmenorrhoea; gout; inflammation; osteoarthritis; pain; rheumatoid arthritis; spondyloarthropathies.*

**Algio Nervomax** TRB, Arg.
Ampoule 1, thiamine hydrochloride (p.1455·1); pyridoxine hydrochloride (p.1456·3); cyanocobalamin (p.1458·2); ampoule 2, diclofenac sodium (p.32·1).
*Pain; peri-articular and soft-tissue disorders.*

**Algio Nervomax Fuerte** TRB, Arg.
Ampoule 1, thiamine hydrochloride (p.1455·1); pyridoxine hydrochloride (p.1456·3); cyanocobalamin (p.1458·2); ampoule 2, diclofenac sodium (p.32·1); betamethasone sodium phosphate (p.1093·1).
*Musculoskeletal and joint disorders.*

**Algio-Bladuril** Casasco, Arg.
Flavoxate hydrochloride (p.482·2); propyphenazone (p.85·3).
*Bladder disorders; female genital-tract spasm.*

**Algion** Saval, Chile.
Hyoscine butylbromide (p.483·3); paracetamol (p.76·2).
*Smooth muscle spasm.*

**Algiopiret** Fada, Arg.
Dipyrone (p.35·3).
*Fever; pain.*

**Algioprofen** Lazar, Arg.
Ibuprofen (p.45·3).
*Fever; musculoskeletal and joint disorders; pain.*

**Algioprux** Sidus, Arg.
Naproxen (p.65·1).
*Inflammation; pain.*

**Algiospray** Novag, Mex.†.
Peridilmethylamine.

**Algio-Truxa** Raffo, Arg.
Paracetamol (p.76·2); piroxicam (p.84·2).
*Inflammation; pain.*

**Algioxib** Dupomar, Arg.
Rofecoxib (p.86·3).
*Osteoarthritis; pain.*

**Algipan**
Note. This name is used for preparations of different composition.
Qualiphar, Belg.
Methyl nicotinate (p.59·2); glycol salicylate (p.44·3); mephenesin (p.1394·3).
*Musculoskeletal pain; skeletal muscle spasm.*

UCB, Fr.
Methyl nicotinate (p.59·2); glycol salicylate (p.44·3); histamine hydrochloride (p.1697·1); mephenesin (p.1394·3).
*Muscle pain.*

Wyeth, India.
Methyl nicotinate (p.59·2); glycol salicylate (p.44·3); capsicum oleoresin (p.1667·1); histamine hydrochloride (p.1697·1).
*Muscle and joint pain; neuralgia.*

Whitehall, Irl.
Methyl nicotinate (p.59·2); glycol salicylate (p.44·3); capsaicin (p.24·2).
*Musculoskeletal and joint pain.*

Whitehall, UK†.
Methyl nicotinate (p.59·2); glycol salicylate (p.44·3); capsicum oleoresin (p.1667·1).
*Muscle and joint pain.*

**Algi-Ped** Stiefel, Braz.†.
Diphenhydramine hydrochloride (p.431·3); dipyrone (p.35·3).
*Hypersensitivity reactions.*

**Algi-Peralgin** Infabra, Braz.†.
Oxyphenbutazone (p.76·1); paracetamol (p.76·2).
*Fever; inflammation; pain.*

**Algiprofen** Euroforma, Braz.†.
Ketoprofen (p.51·2).
*Gout; musculoskeletal, joint, and peri-articular disorders; pain.*

**Algi-Reumac** Windson, Braz.†.
Oxyphenbutazone (p.76·1); paracetamol (p.76·2).
*Fever; inflammation; pain.*

**Algi-Reumatril** Galenogal, Braz.†.
Paracetamol (p.76·2); ibuprofen (p.45·3).
*Inflammation; pain.*

**Algirona** Bunker, Braz.
Dipyrone (p.35·3).
*Fever; pain.*

**Algisan** Prodes, Spain†.
Ibuprofen (p.45·3).
*Fever; inflammation; musculoskeletal and joint disorders; pain.*

**Algiseda** Sanitas, Arg.
Carisoprodol (p.1392·1); paracetamol (p.76·2).
*Musculoskeletal, joint, and peri-articular disorders.*

**Algisedal** Viatris, Fr.
Paracetamol (p.76·2); codeine phosphate (p.27·1).
*Pain.*

**Algiseptico** Fada, Arg.
Piperacillin (p.243·1).
*Bacterial infections.*

**Algispray** Casasco, Arg.
Dichlorodifluoromethane (p.1236·1); trichlorofluoromethane (p.1236·1).
*Local anaesthesia; pain.*

**Algist** Hoechst Marion Roussel, S.Afr.†.
Paracetamol (p.76·2); caffeine (p.782·1); chlorphenamine maleate (p.427·3); phenylephrine hydrochloride (p.1126·3).
*Cold symptoms.*

**Algi-Tanderil** Klinger, Braz.
Diclofenac sodium (p.32·1); paracetamol (p.76·2); carisoprodol (p.1392·1); caffeine (p.782·1).
*Inflammation; pain.*

**Algitec** SmithKline Beecham, Irl.†.
Sodium alginate (p.1577·1); cimetidine (p.1255·3).
*Gastro-oesophageal reflux.*

**Algitrin** Schering-Plough, Mex.
Ibuprofen (p.45·3); paracetamol (p.76·2).
*Fever; pain.*

**Algizolin** Luper, Braz.†.
Oxyphenbutazone (p.76·1); paracetamol (p.76·2).
*Fever; inflammation; pain.*

**Algobene** Ratiopharm, Austria†.
Aspirin (p.15·1).
*Fever; pain.*

**Algoceanic** Proceane, Fr.
Sea water; bladderwrack (p.1742·3); chondrus crispus; ascophyllum nodosum.
*Mineral supplement.*

**Algoced** Pharmascience, Fr.†.
Dextropropoxyphene hydrochloride (p.28·3); paracetamol (p.76·2).
*Pain.*

**Algocetil** Francia, Ital.
Sulindac (p.91·2).
*Gout; musculoskeletal, joint, and peri-articular disorders; neuritis.*

**Algocor** Teofarma, Ital.
Gallopamil hydrochloride (p.922·3).
*Angina pectoris; myocardial infarction.*

**Algofen** Pfizer Consumer, Ital.
Ibuprofen (p.45·3).
*Pain.*

**Algofina** Strallhofer, Austria.
Aspirin (p.15·1); paracetamol (p.76·2).
*Fever; pain.*

**Algoflex Same** Savoma, Ital.†.
Diethylamine salicylate (p.34·1).
*Musculoskeletal and joint disorders.*

**Algofren** Unipharma, Gr.
Ibuprofen (p.45·3).
*Dysmenorrhoea; inflammation; musculoskeletal and joint disorders; pain.*

**Algogen** Nakornpatana, Thai.
Paracetamol (p.76·2).
*Pain.*

**Algolider** Garant, Ital.
Nimesulide (p.67·1).
*Fever; inflammation; pain.*

**Algolisina** Polifarma, Ital.
Pridinol mesilate (p.1395·2); benzydamine hydrochloride (p.21·1); lidocaine hydrochloride (p.1377·3).
*Musculoskeletal, joint, peri-articular, and soft-tissue disorders.*

**Algolysin** Teva, Israel.
Dextropropoxyphene hydrochloride (p.28·3); paracetamol (p.76·2).
*Pain.*

**Algonapril** Francia, Ital.
Naproxen (p.65·1).
*Gout; inflammation; musculoskeletal, joint, and soft-tissue disorders; pain.*

**Algo-Nevriton** Sciencex, Fr.†.
Acetiamine hydrochloride (p.1454·3); aspirin (p.15·1).
*Musculoskeletal and joint disorders; neuralgia; pain.*

**Algophene** SMB, Belg.
Paracetamol (p.76·2); dextropropoxyphene hydrochloride (p.28·3).
*Pain.*

**Algopirina** Medisint, Ital.
Aspirin (p.15·1); paracetamol (p.76·2).
*Cold and influenza symptoms; pain.*

**Algoplaque**
Urgo, Fr.
A hydrocolloid dressing.
*Burns; ulcers; wounds.*

Urgo, Ger.
Carmellose sodium (p.1577·3).
*Ulcers; wounds.*

**Algopriv** Interdelta, Switz.†.
Diproqualone camsilate (p.35·3); ethenzamide (p.37·2).
*Inflammation; pain.*

**Algo-Prolixan** Jacoby, Austria.
Azapropazone (p.20·1); dextropropoxyphene hydrochloride (p.28·3).
*Musculoskeletal and joint disorders.*

**Algosenac** Senese, Ital.
Diclofenac sodium (p.32·1).
*Musculoskeletal and joint disorders; painful smooth muscle spasm.*

**Algosfar** Medifarma, Mex.
Hyoscine butylbromide (p.483·3); dipyrone (p.35·3).
*Smooth muscle spasm.*

**Algostase** SMB, Belg.
Paracetamol (p.76·2); caffeine (p.782·1).
*Fever; pain.*

**Algosteril**
Brothier, Fr.; Johnson & Johnson, Ger.; Johnson & Johnson, Ital.†; Smith & Nephew, UK.
Calcium alginate (p.745·1).
*Haemostatic dressing; wounds.*

**Algotropyl** Alpharma, Fr.
Paracetamol (p.76·2); promethazine hydrochloride (p.439·1).
*Cold symptoms.*

**Algoxam** Boniscontro & Gazzone, Ital.
Piroxicam (p.84·2).
*Musculoskeletal and joint disorders.*

**Alho Rogoff** Crefar, Port.
Garlic (p.1691·1).
*Cardiovascular disorders; rheumatic disorders; senility; stress.*

**Alho-Arthrosan N** Wiedemann, Ger.
Homoeopathic preparation.

**Alho-Sedosan** Wiedemann, Ger.
Homoeopathic preparation.

**Alhydrate**
Nestle, Fr.; Nestle, Ital.
Oral rehydration solution (p.1222·2).
*Diarrhoea.*

**Alhydrox** Stallergenes, Ital.†.
An allergen extract (p.1650·1).
*Allergen immunotherapy.*

**Ali Veg** SmithKline Beecham, Spain.
Cimetidine (p.1255·3).
*Acid aspiration; gastro-oesophageal reflux; gastrointestinal haemorrhage; gastrointestinal hyperacidity; peptic ulcer; short-bowel syndrome; Zollinger-Ellison syndrome.*

**Alib** Ibfarma, Braz.†.
Albendazole (p.101·2).
*Worm infections.*

**A-Lices** Hoe, Singapore.
Malathion (p.1507·1).
*Pediculosis.*

**Alicura** Catarinense, Braz.
Aspirin (p.15·1); caffeine (p.782·1).
*Fever; pain.*

**Alidase** Microsules Bernabo, Arg.
Naproxen (p.65·1) or naproxen sodium (p.65·1).
*Fever; gout; musculoskeletal, joint, and peri-articular disorders; pain.*

**Alidol** Syntex, Mex.
Ketorolac trometamol (p.52·1).
*Pain.*

**Alidor** Aventis, Braz.†.
Aspirin (p.15·1).
*Fever; inflammation; pain; thromboembolism prophylaxis.*

**Aliflus** Glaxo Allen, Ital.
Salmeterol xinafoate (p.795·1); fluticasone propionate (p.1102·3).
*Asthma.*

**Aligest** Schering-Plough, Spain†.
Aluminium hydroxide (p.1249·2); dimethicone (p.1289·2); magnesium hydroxide (p.1272·2).
*Gastrointestinal hyperacidity and flatulence.*

**Aligest Plus** Schering-Plough, Spain†.
Aluminium hydroxide (p.1249·2); calcium carbonate (p.1254·2); magnesium hydroxide (p.1272·2); simeticone (p.1289·2).
*Flatulence; gastrointestinal hyperacidity.*

**Alikal** GlaxoSmithKline, Arg.
Aspirin (p.15·1); caffeine (p.782·1); sodium bicarbonate (p.1223·2); tartaric acid (p.1752·1); citric acid (p.1673·1); magnesium sulfate (p.1228·2).
*Dyspepsia; headache.*

**Alimentum**
Abbott, Canad.; Abbott, Fin.†; Ross, USA.
Protein hydrolysate infant feed (p.1417·1).
*Fat malabsorption; food hypersensitivity; protein maldigestion; protein sensitivity.*

**Alimix**
Janssen-Cilag, Ger.†; JC Healthcare, Ital.†.
Cisapride (p.1259·2).
*Dyspepsia; gastro-oesophageal reflux; gastroparesis.*

**Alimta** Lilly, USA.
Pemetrexed (p.579·1).
*Malignant pleural mesothelioma.*

**Alin**
Note. This name is used for preparations of different composition.
Millet Roux, Braz.
Albendazole (p.101·2).
*Worm infections.*

Chinoin, Mex.
Dexamethasone (p.1097·1), dexamethasone isonicotinate (p.1097·2), or dexamethasone sodium phosphate (p.1097·2).
*Corticosteroid.*

**Alin Nasal** Chinoin, Mex.
Dexamethasone sodium phosphate (p.1097·2); neomycin sulfate (p.235·1); phenylephrine hydrochloride (p.1126·3).
*Rhinitis; sinusitis.*

**Alin Oftalmico** Chinoin, Mex.
Dexamethasone sodium phosphate (p.1097·2); neomycin sulfate (p.235·1).
*Eye disorders.*

**Alinamin B12**
Takeda, Malaysia; Takeda, Singapore.
Fursultiamine (p.1454·3); vitamin $B_{12}$ (p.1458·2).
Procaine hydrochloride (p.1383·2) is included in this preparation to alleviate the pain of injection.
*Anaemias; neuritis.*

Takeda, Thai.
Fursultiamine hydrochloride (p.1455·2); vitamin $B_{12}$ (p.1458·2).
*Macrocytic anaemia; megaloblastic anaemia; neuritis.*

**Alinamin-F**
Note. This name is used for preparations of different composition.
Takeda, Hong Kong; Takeda, Singapore.
Fursultiamine (p.1454·3) or fursultiamine hydrochloride (p.1455·2); riboflavin (p.1456·1).
*Arthralgia; beri-beri; CNS disorders; gastrointestinal motility disorders; myalgia; myocardial metabolic disorders; neuralgia; peripheral nerve paralysis; peripheral neuritis; vitamin $B_1$ deficiency; Wernicke's encephalopathy.*

Takeda, Jpn.
Fursultiamine hydrochloride (p.1455·2).
*Vitamin $B_1$ deficiency; vitamin $B_1$ supplement.*

Takeda, Thai.
*Injection:* Fursultiamine hydrochloride (p.1455·2).
*Tablets:* Fursultiamine hydrochloride (p.1455·2); riboflavin (p.1456·1).
*Vitamin $B_1$ deficiency.*

**Alindrin** Astra, Swed.
Ibuprofen (p.45·3).
*Fever; pain.*

**Alinia** Romark, USA.
Nitazoxanide (p.612·1).
*Cryptosporidiosis; giardiasis.*

**Alinol** Pharmasant, Thai.
Allopurinol (p.412·2).
*Gout; hyperuricaemia; renal calculi.*

**Alinor** Alpharma, Norw.
Atenolol (p.865·2).
*Angina pectoris; arrhythmias; hypertension; hyperthyroidism; migraine; myocardial infarction.*

**Alinvit** Collins, Mex.
Multivitamin preparation (p.1417·1).

**Alipase** Janssen-Cilag, Fr.†.
Pancrelipase (p.1725·3).
*Pancreatic insufficiency.*

**Alipride** Centaur, India.
Cisapride (p.1259·2).
*Delayed gastric emptying; gastro-oesophageal reflux.*

**Aliseum** Formenti, Ital.
Diazepam (p.690·1).
*Anxiety disorders; epilepsy; insomnia.*

**Alitest** Columbia, Mex.
Carbon-13 (p.1667·3).
*Diagnostic agent.*

**Alitraq**
Abbott, Arg.; Abbott, Austral.; Abbott, Braz.; Abbott, Fin.†; Abbott, Hong Kong; Abbott, Irl.; Ross, Israel; Abbott, Mex.; Abbott, NZ; Abbott, Singapore; Abbott Nutrition, UK.
Preparation for enteral nutrition (p.1417·1).

**Aliucillin** Aliud, Austria.
Phenoxymethylpenicillin potassium (p.242·1).
*Bacterial infections.*

**Aliudox** Aliud, Austria.
Doxycycline hyclate (p.206·2).
*Bacterial infections.*

**Aliviador** Biologia, Braz.†.
Methyl salicylate (p.59·3); camphor (p.1665·3); menthol (p.1711·3).
*Musculoskeletal and joint disorders.*

**Alivian** Cazi, Braz.
Meloxicam (p.56·1).

**Alivioderm** Hexal, Braz.
Nitrofurazone (p.238·2).
*Infected burns; skin infections.*

**Aliviomas** Alacan, Spain.
Naproxen (p.65·1).
*Fever; gout; musculoskeletal and joint disorders; pain.*

**Aliviosin** Alacan, Spain.
Indometacin (p.47·3).
*Gout; inflammation; musculoskeletal, joint, and peri-articular disorders; pain.*

**ALK**
Scherax, Ger.
A range of allergen extracts (p.1650·1).
*Allergen immunotherapy.*

Trimedal, Switz.
A range of grass and tree pollen allergen extracts (p.1650·1).
*Allergen immunotherapy.*

**Alka** Bayer Consumer, UK.
Aspirin (p.15·1).
*Pain.*

**Alka XS Go** Bayer Consumer, UK.
Aspirin (p.15·1); paracetamol (p.76·2); caffeine (p.782·1).
*Pain.*

**Alkafizz** Xeragen, S.Afr.
Sodium citrate (p.1223·2); sodium bicarbonate (p.1223·2); anhydrous citric acid (p.1673·1); tartaric acid (p.1752·1).
*Gastric hyperacidity; urinary alkalinisation.*

**Alkagin**
Note. This name is used for preparations of different composition.
Ganassini, Ital.
Calendula (p.1665·2); mallow (p.1709·3); tilia (p.1756·2).
*Personal hygiene.*

Dermoteca, Port.
*Topical gel:* Calendula (p.1665·2); mallow (p.1709·3); tilia (p.1756·2); aloe (p.1141·3); chlorhexidine gluconate (p.1173·2).
*Topical solution:* Calendula (p.1665·2); mallow (p.1709·3); tilia (p.1756·2); triclosan (p.1195·2).
*Personal hygiene.*

**Alkala N** *Sanum-Kehlbeck, Ger.*
Sodium citrate (p.1223·2); potassium bicarbonate (p.1223·1); sodium bicarbonate (p.1223·2).
*Gastrointestinal hyperacidity.*

**Alkala T** *Sanum-Kehlbeck, Ger.*
Sodium bicarbonate (p.1223·2).
*Metabolic acidosis.*

**Alkalite D** *Garec, S.Afr.*
Dicycloverine hydrochloride (p.481·2); dried aluminium hydroxide gel (p.1249·2); light magnesium oxide (p.1272·3).
*Gastric hyperacidity.*

**Alkamine** *ANB, Thai.*
Aluminium hydroxide gel (p.1249·2); magnesium trisilicate (p.1272·3); kaolin (p.1268·3); atropine sulfate (p.477·1).
*Gastric hyperacidity; peptic ulcer.*

**Alka-Mints** *Bayer, USA.*
Calcium carbonate (p.1254·2).
*Hyperacidity.*

**Alkanil** *Inga, India.*
Sodium acid citrate (p.1223·2); dipotassium hydrogen citrate.
*Adjunct to sulfonamide therapy; dysuria; metabolic acidosis; systemic alkaliniser.*

**Alka-Seltzer**
*Note. This name is used for preparations of different composition.*
*Bayer, Austral.; Bayer, Austria; Bayer, Belg.; Bayer, Braz.†; Bayer Consumer, Canad.; Bayer, Fin.; Bayer, Fr.; Bayer, Ger.; Bayer, Hong Kong; Bayer, Irl.; Bayer Consumer, Malaysia; Bayer, Neth.; Bayer, NZ; Bayer Consumer, Singapore; Bayer, Swed.; Bayer, Switz.; Bayer, Thai.; Bayer Consumer, UK.*
Aspirin (p.15·1); citric acid (p.1673·1); sodium bicarbonate (p.1223·2).
*Gastric discomfort; pain.*

*Agis, Israel.*
Aspirin (p.15·1).
*Fever; musculoskeletal and joint disorders; pain; thrombosis prophylaxis.*

*Bayer, Port.; Bayer, Spain.*
Aspirin (p.15·1); calcium phosphate (p.1225·3); citric acid (p.1673·1); sodium bicarbonate (p.1223·2).
*Dyspepsia; fever; pain.*

**Alka-Seltzer Antacid** *Miles Consumer Healthcare, USA.*
Sodium bicarbonate (p.1223·2); citric acid (p.1673·1); potassium bicarbonate (p.1223·1).
*Gastrointestinal disorders.*

**Alka-Seltzer with Aspirin** *Miles Consumer Healthcare, USA.*
Aspirin (p.15·1); citric acid (p.1673·1); sodium bicarbonate (p.1223·2).
*Arthritis; fever; gastrointestinal disorders; myocardial infarction; pain.*

**Alka-Seltzer Effervescent Tablets** *Miles, USA.*
Sodium bicarbonate (p.1223·2); citric acid (p.1673·1); aspirin (p.15·1).
*Hyperacidity.*

**Alka-Seltzer Plus Cold**
*Note. This name is used for preparations of different composition.*
*Bayer, Canad.†.*
Aspirin (p.15·1); phenylpropanolamine bitartrate (p.1128·2); chlorphenamine maleate (p.427·3).
*Cold symptoms.*

*Miles Consumer Healthcare, USA.*
*Capsules:* Chlorphenamine maleate (p.427·3); pseudoephedrine hydrochloride (p.1129·2); paracetamol (p.76·2).
*Tablets†:* Phenylpropanolamine bitartrate (p.1128·2); chlorphenamine maleate (p.427·3); aspirin (p.15·1).
*Cold symptoms; nasal congestion.*

**Alka-Seltzer Plus Cold & Cough**
*Miles, USA†.*
*Tablets:* Phenylpropanolamine bitartrate (p.1128·2); chlorphenamine maleate (p.427·3); dextromethorphan hydrobromide (p.1117·3); aspirin (p.15·1).
*Coughs and cold symptoms.*

*Miles Consumer Healthcare, USA.*
*Capsules:* Dextromethorphan (p.1117·3); pseudoephedrine hydrochloride (p.1129·2); chlorphenamine maleate (p.427·3); paracetamol (p.76·2).

**Alka-Seltzer Plus Cold & Sinus** *Bayer, USA.*
*Capsules:* Pseudoephedrine hydrochloride (p.1129·2); paracetamol (p.76·2).
*Effervescent tablets†:* Aspirin (p.15·1); phenylpropanolamine bitartrate (p.1128·2).
*Cold symptoms; nasal congestion.*

**Alka-Seltzer Plus Night-Time Cold** *Miles Consumer Healthcare, USA.*
*Capsules:* Doxylamine succinate (p.432·3); dextromethorphan (p.1117·3); pseudoephedrine hydrochloride (p.1129·2); paracetamol (p.76·2).
*Tablets†:* Phenylpropanolamine bitartrate (p.1128·2); brompheniramine maleate (p.426·1); dextromethorphan hydrobromide (p.1117·3); aspirin (p.15·1).
*Coughs and cold symptoms.*

**Alka-Seltzer Plus Nose & Throat** *Bayer, USA.*
Paracetamol (p.76·2); chlorphenamine maleate (p.427·3); dextromethorphan hydrobromide (p.1117·3); phenylephrine hydrochloride (p.1126·3).
*Upper respiratory-tract disorders.*

**Alka-Seltzer Plus Sinus** *Bayer, USA†.*
Phenylpropanolamine tartrate (p.1128·2); aspirin (p.15·1).
*Upper respiratory-tract congestion.*

**Alka-Seltzer Plus Sinus Allergy** *Miles, USA†.*
Phenylpropanolamine bitartrate (p.1128·2); brompheniramine maleate (p.426·1); aspirin (p.15·1).
*Upper respiratory-tract symptoms.*

**Alka-Seltzer XS** *Bayer Consumer, UK.*
Aspirin (p.15·1); paracetamol (p.76·2); caffeine (p.782·1); citric acid (p.1673·1); sodium bicarbonate (p.1223·2).
*Gastric discomfort; pain.*

**Alkasid**
*Leo, Denm.; Julphar, UAE.*
Aluminium magnesium silicate (p.1577·1); simeticone (p.1289·2).
*Dyspepsia; flatulence; gastritis; gastro-oesophageal reflux; heartburn; peptic ulcer.*

**Alkasol** *Stadmed, India.*
Sodium acid citrate (p.1223·2).
*Dysuria; fever; metabolic acidosis; systemic alkaliniser.*

**Alkasol-P** *Stadmed, India.*
Sodium acid citrate (p.1223·2); paracetamol (p.76·2); sorbitol (p.1446·3).
*Alkali depletion; cold symptoms; fever; pain.*

**Alkasolve** *Sam-On, Israel.*
Potassium citrate (p.1223·1); sodium citrate (p.1223·2).
*Diabetic acidosis; urinary alkalisation.*

**Alkavite** *Vitality, USA.*
A multivitamin and mineral preparation (p.1417·1).

**Alkenide** *Zambon, Fr.*
Poloxamer 188 (p.1414·2).
*Skin cleanser.*

**Alkeran**
*GlaxoSmithKline, Austral.; GlaxoSmithKline, Austria; GlaxoSmithKline, Belg.; GlaxoSmithKline, Braz.; GlaxoSmithKline, Canad.; GlaxoSmithKline, Chile; GlaxoSmithKline, Denm.; GlaxoSmithKline, Fin.; GlaxoSmithKline, Fr.; GlaxoSmithKline, Ger.; Glaxo Wellcome, Gr.; IFET (ΙΦΕΤ), Gr.; GlaxoSmithKline, Hong Kong; GlaxoSmithKline, India; Wellcome, Irl.; GlaxoSmithKline, Israel; GlaxoSmithKline, Ital.; GlaxoSmithKline, Malaysia; Glaxo Wellcome, Mex.; GlaxoSmithKline, Neth.; GlaxoSmithKline, Norw.; GlaxoSmithKline, NZ; Wellcome, Port.; GlaxoSmithKline, S.Afr.; GlaxoSmithKline, Singapore; GlaxoSmithKline, Swed.; GlaxoSmithKline, Switz.; GlaxoSmithKline, Thai.; GlaxoSmithKline, UK; Celgene, USA.*
Melphalan (p.566·1) or melphalan hydrochloride (p.566·3).
*Malignant neoplasms; polycythaemia vera.*

**Alkerana** *GlaxoSmithKline, Arg.*
Melphalan (p.566·1).
*Malignant neoplasms; polycythaemia vera.*

**Alket** *Ripari-Gero, Ital.*
Ketoprofen (p.51·2).
*Gout; musculoskeletal, joint, peri-articular, and soft-tissue disorders; pain; phlebitis.*

**Alkets** *Roberts, USA; Hauck, USA.*
Calcium carbonate (p.1254·2).
*Hyperacidity.*

**Alko Isol** *Marc-O, Canad.†.*
Isopropyl alcohol (p.1184·3).

**Alkocean** *Proceane, Fr.*
Shark-liver oil.
*Tonic.*

**Alkyloxan** *Choongwae, Singapore†.*
Cyclophosphamide (p.540·2).
*Malignant neoplasms.*

**All Clear** *Bausch & Lomb, USA.*
Naphazoline hydrochloride (p.1124·3).
*Eye irritation.*

**All In One Plus Grapefruit** *Solgar, UK†.*
Soya lecithin (p.1706·1); grapefruit powder concentrate; cider vinegar.
*Dietary supplement.*

**All Pecium** *Dermoteca, Port.*
Pyrithione zinc (p.1156·2); sulfur (p.1158·2).
*Seborrhoeic dermatitis.*

**Allamin** *Kyorin, Thai.*
Amino-acid preparation (p.1417·1).
*Nutritional supplement.*

**Allbee** *Robins, USA.*
A range of vitamin preparations (p.1417·1).

**Allbee with C**
*Whitehall-Robins, Canad.†; Whitehall, Irl.†.*
Vitamin B substances with ascorbic acid (p.1417·1).

**Allbee C-550** *Whitehall-Robins, Canad.†.*
Vitamin B substances with ascorbic acid (p.1417·1).

**Allbee C-800** *Whitehall-Robins, Canad.†.*
Vitamin B substances, ascorbic acid, and vitamin E (p.1417·1).

**Allbee C-800 plus Iron** *Whitehall-Robins, Canad.†.*
Vitamin B substances, ascorbic acid, vitamin E, folic acid, and iron (p.1417·1).

**Allcock's Porous Capsicum Plaster** *Richards & Appleby, UK†.*
Burgundy pitch; frankincense; orris; capsicum (p.1667·1); camphor (p.1665·3); elemi; myrrh (p.1718·3).

**Alleal** *Pierre Fabre, Ital.*
Ketotifen fumarate (p.788·1).
*Asthma; bronchitis.*

**Alledryl** *Prater, Chile.*
Loratadine (p.436·1).
*Hypersensitivity reactions.*

**Allegra**
*Aventis, Arg.; Aventis, Braz.; Aventis, Canad.; Aventis, Chile; Aventis, India; Aventis, Mex.; Hoechst Marion Roussel, USA.*
Fexofenadine hydrochloride (p.433·3).
*Allergic rhinitis; allergic skin disorders; eye irritation.*

**Allegra-D**
*Aventis, Arg.; Aventis, Braz.; Aventis, Canad.; Aventis, Chile; Aventis, Mex.; Aventis, USA.*
Fexofenadine hydrochloride (p.433·3); pseudoephedrine hydrochloride (p.1129·2).
*Allergic rhinitis.*

**Allegro** *Trima, Israel.*
Fluticasone propionate (p.1102·3).
*Allergic rhinitis.*

**Allegron**
*Aspen, Austral.; Lilly, NZ†; King, UK.*
Nortriptyline hydrochloride (p.310·2).
*Depression; nocturnal enuresis.*

**Allens Chesty Cough** *Allens, UK.*
Ammonium chloride (p.1115·2); tolu tincture (p.1131·3); squill tincture (p.1130·3); menthol (p.1711·3); marrubium (p.1124·1).
*Coughs.*

**Allens Dry Tickly Cough** *Allens, UK.*
Benzoin tincture (p.1751·1); ipecacuanha tincture (p.1122·3); capsicum tincture (p.1667·1); cetylpyridinium chloride (p.1173·1).
*Coughs.*

**Allens Junior Cough** *Allens, UK.*
Glycerol (p.1694·3); anhydrous citric acid (p.1673·1).
*Coughs; sore throat.*

**Allens Pine & Honey** *Allens, UK.*
Ipecacuanha (p.1122·3); liquorice (p.1270·2); pumilio pine oil (p.1737·1); squill oxymel.
*Bronchitis; cold symptoms; coughs.*

**Allent** *Ascher, USA.*
Brompheniramine maleate (p.426·1); pseudoephedrine hydrochloride (p.1129·2).
*Allergic rhinitis; nasal congestion.*

**Aller-Aide** *Technilab, Canad.*
Diphenhydramine hydrochloride (p.431·3).

**Allerbiocid S** *Allerbio, Fr.*
Benzyl benzoate (p.1500·2); tannic acid (p.1751·2).
*Insecticide for bedding and upholstery.*

**Allercalm** *Amnol, Ital.*
Zinc orotate; vitamin A (p.1417·1).
*Nutritional supplement.*

**Aller-Chlor** *Rugby, USA.*
Chlorphenamine maleate (p.427·3).
*Hypersensitivity reactions.*

**Allercon** *Parmed, USA.*
Pseudoephedrine hydrochloride (p.1129·2); triprolidine hydrochloride (p.442·3).
*Upper respiratory-tract symptoms.*

**Allercreme** *Carme, USA.*
Emollient and moisturiser.

**Allercrom** *Rhone-Poulenc Rorer, Austria†.*
Sodium cromoglicate (p.795·3).
*Allergic conjunctivitis; allergic rhinitis.*

**Allerdine** *LBS, Thai.*
Loratadine (p.436·1).
*Allergic rhinitis; allergic skin disorders.*

**Allerdryl** *ICN, Canad.*
Diphenhydramine hydrochloride (p.431·3).
*Hypersensitivity.*

**Allerest** *Fisons, USA.*
Naphazoline hydrochloride (p.1124·3).
*Minor eye irritation.*

**Allerest Allergy & Sinus Relief** *Heritage Consumer, USA.*
Pseudoephedrine hydrochloride (p.1129·2); paracetamol (p.76·2).

**Allerest Headache Strength** *Ciba, USA.*
Pseudoephedrine hydrochloride (p.1129·2); chlorphenamine maleate (p.427·3); paracetamol (p.76·2).
*Upper respiratory-tract symptoms.*

**Allerest 12 Hour** *Ciba, USA†.*
Phenylpropanolamine hydrochloride (p.1127·3); chlorphenamine maleate (p.427·3).
*Upper respiratory-tract symptoms.*

**Allerest 12 Hour Nasal** *Ciba Consumer, USA.*
Oxymetazoline hydrochloride (p.1126·1).
*Nasal congestion.*

**Allerest Maximum Strength** *Ciba, USA.*
Pseudoephedrine hydrochloride (p.1129·2); chlorphenamine maleate (p.427·3).
*Upper respiratory-tract symptoms.*

**Allerest Sinus Pain Formula** *Ciba, USA.*
Pseudoephedrine hydrochloride (p.1129·2); chlorphenamine maleate (p.427·3); paracetamol (p.76·2).
*Upper respiratory-tract symptoms.*

**Aller-Eze** *Novartis Consumer, UK.*
*Cream†:* Diphenhydramine hydrochloride (p.431·3).
*Hypersensitivity reactions of the skin; insect bites and stings.*
*Eye drops; nasal spray:* Azelastine hydrochloride (p.425·2).
*Allergic conjunctivitis; allergic rhinitis.*
*Tablets†:* Clemastine hydrogen fumarate (p.429·1).
*Hypersensitivity reactions; insect bites and stings.*

**Aller-Eze Plus** *Novartis Consumer, UK†.*
Clemastine hydrogen fumarate (p.429·1); phenylpropanolamine hydrochloride (p.1127·3).
*Hay fever.*

**Allerfen** *Sella, Ital.*
Promethazine hydrochloride (p.439·1).
*Hypersensitivity reactions; insomnia.*

**Allerfre** *Boots Healthcare, Neth.*
Loratadine (p.436·1).
*Allergic rhinitis; urticaria.*

**Allerfrim** *Rugby, USA.*
Pseudoephedrine hydrochloride (p.1129·2); triprolidine hydrochloride (p.442·3).
*Upper respiratory-tract symptoms.*

**Allerfrim with Codeine** *Rugby, USA.*
Pseudoephedrine hydrochloride (p.1129·2); codeine phosphate (p.27·1); triprolidine hydrochloride (p.442·3).
*Coughs and cold symptoms.*

**Allergan** *Bouty, Ital.*
Diphenhydramine hydrochloride (p.431·3).
*Insect bites; pruritus; sunburn.*

**Allergan Enzymatic** *Allergan, USA.*
Papain (p.1727·3) (p.1164·2).
*Cleansing solution for soft contact lenses.*

**Allergefon** *Lafon, Fr.*
Carbinoxamine maleate (p.426·3).
*Hypersensitivity reactions.*

**Allergen** *Goldline, USA.*
Benzocaine (p.1370·3); phenazone (p.82·3); glycerol (p.1694·3).
*Ear pain.*

**Allergenid** *Herbaline, Ital.†.*
Agrimony (p.1649·1); black currant (p.1661·1); echinacea (p.1683·2).
*Hypersensitivity reactions.*

**Allergex** *Propan, S.Afr.*
Chlorphenamine maleate (p.427·3).
*Hypersensitivity reactions.*

**Allergie-Injektopas** *Pascoe, Ger.*
Homoeopathic preparation.

**Allergies** *Homeocan, Canad.*
Homoeopathic preparation.

**Allergika** *Illa, Ger.*
*Bath additive:* Soya oil (p.1447·2).
*Cream; ointment:* White soft paraffin (p.1479·3); liquid paraffin (p.1479·1).
*Skin disorders.*

**Allergin**
*Note. This name is used for preparations of different composition.*
*Propan, S.Afr.*
Diphenhydramine hydrochloride (p.431·3); ammonium chloride (p.1115·2); sodium citrate (p.1223·2); menthol (p.1711·3).
*Coughs.*

*PP Lab, Thai.*
Chlorphenamine maleate (p.427·3).
*Hypersensitivity.*

**Allergipuran N** *Scheurich, Ger.†.*
Bufexamac (p.21·3).
*Inflammatory skin disorders.*

**Allergocomod** *Ioltech, Fr.*
Sodium cromoglicate (p.795·3).
*Eye disorders.*

**Allergo-COMOD** *Ursapharm, Ger.*
Sodium cromoglicate (p.795·3).
*Allergic conjunctivitis; allergic rhinitis.*

**Allergocrom**
*Ursapharm, Ger.; Ursapharm, Malaysia; Ursapharm, Neth.†.*
Sodium cromoglicate (p.795·3).
*Allergic conjunctivitis; allergic rhinitis.*

**Allergodil**
*Sidus, Arg.; Asta Medica, Austria; Viatris, Belg.; Grunenthal, Chile; AstraZeneca, Denm.; Viatris, Fr.; Viatris, Ger.; Asta Medica, Ital.; Viatris, Neth.; Viatris, Port.; Asta Medica, Switz.*
Azelastine hydrochloride (p.425·2).
*Allergic conjunctivitis; allergic rhinitis.*

**Allergofact** *Doctum, Gr.*
Loratadine (p.436·1).
*Allergic rhinitis; pruritus.*

**Allergoid-HAL** *Hal, Neth.†.*
Aluminium hydroxide adsorbed modified allergens (p.1650·1).
*Allergen immunotherapy.*

**Allergojovis** *Biomedica-Chemica, Gr.*
Sodium cromoglicate (p.795·3).
*Allergic conjunctivitis; allergic rhinitis.*

**Allergokatt** *Kattwiga, Ger.*
Homoeopathic preparation.

**Allergo-Loges** *Loges, Ger.*
Homoeopathic preparation.

**Allergopos N** *Ursapharm, Ger.*
Antazoline phosphate (p.424·2); tetryzoline hydrochloride (p.1131·2).
*Eye disorders.*

**Allergospasmin**
*Asta Medica, Austria†; Viatris, Ger.*
Sodium cromoglicate (p.795·3); reproterol hydrochloride (p.791·2).
*Obstructive airways disease.*

**Allergospasmine** *Asta Medica, Switz.*
Sodium cromoglicate (p.795·3); reproterol hydrochloride (p.791·2).
*Obstructive airways disease.*

**Allergosyx** *Syxyl, Ger.*
Homoeopathic preparation.

**Allergotin** *Cooper (Κοπερ), Gr.*
Sodium cromoglicate (p.795·3).
*Allergic conjunctivitis; allergic rhinitis.*

**Allergoval** *Kohler-Pharma, Ger.*
Sodium cromoglicate (p.795·3).
*Hypersensitivity reactions.*

**Allergovit**
*Allergopharma, Ger.; Allergopharma, Switz.*
Allergen extracts (p.1650·1).
*Allergen immunotherapy.*

**Allergy** *Parmed, USA.*
Chlorphenamine maleate (p.427·3).

**Allergy Drops**
*Bausch & Lomb, Canad.; Bausch & Lomb, USA.*
Naphazoline hydrochloride (p.1124·3).
*Eye irritation.*

**Allergy Elixir** *Tanta, Canad.*
Diphenhydramine hydrochloride (p.431·3).

**Allergy Eyes** *Abbott, Austral.†.*
Antazoline sulfate (p.424·2); xylometazoline hydrochloride (p.1132·2).
*Allergic and inflammatory eye disorders.*

**Allergy Formula** *Stanley, Canad.*
Diphenhydramine hydrochloride (p.431·3).

**Allergy Relief**
*Note. This name is used for preparations of different composition.*
*Brauer, Austral.†.*
Homoeopathic preparation.
Formerly known as Allergy Symptoms Relief.

*Apotex, Canad.*
Cetirizine hydrochloride (p.427·1).

*JCP, Canad.†.*
Terfenadine (p.441·1).

*Unichem, UK; Zee, USA.*
Chlorphenamine maleate (p.427·3).
*Hypersensitivity reactions.*

**Allergy Sinus** *WestCan, Canad.*
Pseudoephedrine hydrochloride (p.1129·2); chlorphenamine maleate (p.427·3); paracetamol (p.76·2).

**Allergy Tablets** *Tanta, Canad.*
Diphenhydramine hydrochloride (p.431·3).

**Allerief** *Orbis Consumer, UK.*
Chlorphenamine maleate (p.427·3).
*Hypersensitivity reactions.*

**Allerin**
*Note. This name is used for preparations of different composition.*
*United American, Singapore.*
Diphenhydramine hydrochloride (p.431·3); guaifenesin (p.1122·1); phenylephrine hydrochloride (p.1126·3).
Formerly contained diphenhydramine hydrochloride, guaifenesin, phenylpropanolamine hydrochloride, and sodium citrate.
*Allergic rhinitis; cold symptoms; sinusitis; sore throat.*

*Great Eastern, Thai.; United American, Thai.*
Diphenhydramine hydrochloride (p.431·3); guaifenesin (p.1122·1); sodium citrate (p.1223·2).
Formerly contained diphenhydramine hydrochloride, guaifenesin, sodium citrate, and phenylpropanolamine hydrochloride.
*Coughs and cold symptoms.*

**AllerMax**
*Note. This name is used for preparations of different composition.*
*Schering-Plough, Austral.*
Mometasone furoate (p.1107·2).
*Allergic rhinitis.*

*Pfeiffer, USA.*
Diphenhydramine hydrochloride (p.431·3).
*Insomnia; motion sickness; parkinsonism.*

**Allermed** *Murdock, USA.*
Pseudoephedrine hydrochloride (p.1129·2).
*Nasal congestion.*

**Allernix** *Technilab, Canad.*
Diphenhydramine hydrochloride (p.431·3).
*Antihistamine.*

**Allerphed** *Great Southern, USA.*
Pseudoephedrine hydrochloride (p.1129·2); triprolidine hydrochloride (p.442·3).
*Upper respiratory-tract symptoms.*

**Allerphen** *Malayan, Singapore.*
Chlorphenamine maleate (p.427·3).
*Hay fever; hypersensitivity reactions; insect bites; pruritus.*

**Allersan** *Europharm, Hong Kong.*
Betamethasone (p.1093·1); dexchlorpheniramine maleate (p.427·3).
*Hypersensitivity reactions.*

**Allerset**
*Hal, Ger.†.*
Allergen extracts of pollen, fungi, house dust mites (p.1650·2), and skin (p.1650·2) (p.1650·1).
*Allergen immunotherapy.*

*Hal, Neth.†.*
Aqueous allergen extracts (p.1650·1).
*Allergen immunotherapy.*

**Allersil** *Silom, Thai.*
Loratadine (p.436·1).
*Allergic rhinitis; allergic skin disorders; hay fever.*

**Allersol** *Ocusoft, USA†.*
Naphazoline hydrochloride (p.1124·3).

**Aller-Tab** *Silom, Thai.*
Loratadine (p.436·1).
*Allergic rhinitis; allergic skin disorders; hay fever.*

**Allertac** *Propan, S.Afr.†.*
Atropine sulfate (p.477·1); hyoscine hydrobromide (p.483·3); hyoscyamine sulfate (p.485·1); phenylpropanolamine hydrochloride (p.1127·3); pheniramine maleate (p.438·3); chlorphenamine maleate (p.427·3).
*Congestion and hypersecretion of the nasal and paranasal sinuses.*

**AllerTek** *Ratiopharm, UK.*
Cetirizine (p.427·2).
*Allergic rhinitis; urticaria.*

**AlleRx** *Adams, USA.*
*Suspension:* Phenylephrine tannate (p.1127·2); chlorphenamine tannate (p.428·1); mepyramine tannate (p.437·1).
*Upper respiratory-tract disorders.*
*Tablets:* AM Tablets, pseudoephedrine hydrochloride (p.1129·2); hyoscine methonitrate (p.483·3); PM tablets, chlorphenamine maleate (p.427·3); hyoscine methonitrate.
*Cold symptoms; rhinitis; sinusitis.*

**Allerzil** *Bruno, Ital.*
Terfenadine (p.441·1).
*Allergic conjunctivitis; allergic rhinitis; allergic skin disorders.*

**Allevyn**
*Smith & Nephew, Ger.; Smith & Nephew, Irl.; Smith & Nephew, UK.*
Hydrophilic polyurethane dressing.
*Ulcers; wounds.*

**Allfen** *MCR, USA.*
Guaifenesin (p.1122·1).
*Coughs.*

**Allfen-DM** *MCR, USA.*
Dextromethorphan hydrobromide (p.1117·3); guaifenesin (p.1122·1).
*Coughs.*

**Allgauer** *Allga, Austria.*
Pumilio pine oil (p.1737·1); eucalyptus oil (p.1686·2); peppermint oil (p.1283·2).
*Cold and influenza symptoms.*

**Allio Vital** *Agepha, Austria.*
Garlic (p.1691·1).
*Tonic.*

**Alliocaps Oligoplex** *Madaus, Arg.*
Garlic (p.1691·1).

**Alliosan** *Allmedica, Ger.*
Garlic (p.1691·1).
*Atherosclerosis; hyperlipidaemias.*

**Allium Cepa Compose** *Boiron, Fr.*
Homoeopathic preparation.

**Allium Plus** *Zeller, Switz.*
Ginkgo biloba (p.1692·3); garlic (p.1691·1).
*Cerebrovascular disorders; tonic.*

**All-Nite Cold Formula** *Major, USA.*
Pseudoephedrine hydrochloride (p.1129·2); dextromethorphan hydrobromide (p.1117·3); doxylamine succinate (p.432·3); paracetamol (p.76·2).
*Coughs and cold symptoms.*

**Allnol** *Merck, Hong Kong.*
Allopurinol (p.412·2).
*Gout; hyperuricaemia; renal calculi.*

**Allo** *CT, Ger.; ABZ, Ger.; 1A, Ger.*
Allopurinol (p.412·2).
*Gout; hyperuricaemia; renal calculi.*

**allo-basan** *Schonenberger, Switz.*
Allopurinol (p.412·2).
*Gout; hyperuricaemia; renal calculi.*

**Allobenz** *Merck, Austria; Arcana, Austria.*
Allopurinol (p.412·2); benzbromarone (p.414·3).
*Gout; hyperuricaemia; renal calculi.*

**Allobeta** *Betapharm, Ger.*
Allopurinol (p.412·2).
*Gout; hyperuricaemia; renal calculi.*

**Alloboxal** *Hexal, Arg.*
Allopurinol (p.412·2).
*Gout; hyperuricaemia; renal calculi.*

**Allochrysine**
*Solvay, Belg.; Solvay, Fr.*
Aurotioprol (p.20·1).
*Rheumatoid arthritis.*

**Allo.comp.** *Ratiopharm, Ger.*
Allopurinol (p.412·2); benzbromarone (p.414·3).
*Gout; hyperuricaemia.*

**Allo-Efeka** *Riemser, Ger.*
Allopurinol (p.412·2).
*Gout; hyperuricaemia; renal calculi.*

**Alloferin**
*ICN, Austria; ICN, Ger.; ICN, Hong Kong; Roche, Israel†; ICN, Malaysia; Pharmaco, S.Afr.; ICN, Singapore; ICN, Thai.†.*
Alcuronium chloride (p.1398·3).
*Competitive neuromuscular blocker.*

**Alloferine** *ICN, Braz.*
Alcuronium chloride (p.1398·3).
*Competitive neuromuscular blocker.*

**Allohexal**
*Hexal, Austral.; Hexal, Ger.†.*
Allopurinol (p.412·2).
*Gout; hyperuricaemia; renal calculi.*

**Allomaron**
*Aventis, Ger.; Aventis, S.Afr.; Aventis, Thai.*
Allopurinol (p.412·2); benzbromarone (p.414·3).
*Gout; hyperuricaemia; renal calculi.*

**Allonol** *Ratiopharm, Fin.*
Allopurinol (p.412·2).
*Gout; hyperuricaemia; uric acid nephropathy.*

**Allopin** *General Drugs, Thai.*
Allopurinol (p.412·2).
*Gout; hyperuricaemia.*

**Allopur**
*Nycomed, Norw.; Gea, Switz.*
Allopurinol (p.412·2).
*Gout; hyperuricaemia; renal calculi; uric acid nephropathy.*

**Allo-Puren** *Alpharma-Isis, Ger.*
Allopurinol (p.412·2).
*Gout; hyperuricaemia; renal calculi.*

**Alloril** *Dexxon, Israel.*
Allopurinol (p.412·2).
*Gout; hyperuricaemia; renal calculi; uric acid nephropathy.*

**Allorin**
*Douglas, Austral.; Douglas, Hong Kong†; Douglas, NZ; Douglas, Singapore†; Douglas, Thai.†; TTN, Thai.†.*
Allopurinol (p.412·2).
*Gout; hyperuricaemia; renal calculi.*

**Allostad** *Stada, Austria.*
Allopurinol (p.412·2).
*Gout; hyperuricaemia; renal calculi; uric acid nephropathy.*

**Allo-300-Tablinen** *Sanorania, Ger.†.*
Allopurinol (p.412·2).
*Gout; hyperuricaemia; renal calculi.*

**Allotyrol** *Tyrol, Austria.*
Allopurinol (p.412·2).
*Gout; hyperuricaemia; renal calculi; uric acid nephropathy.*

**Allpargin** *Merz, Ger.†.*
Allopurinol (p.412·2).
*Gout; hyperuricaemia.*

**All-Pro** *Solgar, UK†.*
Amino-acid preparation (p.1417·1).

**Allpyral**
*Thomson, Austral.; Dome-Hollister-Stier, Fr.†; Ebos, NZ; Miles, USA.*
Range of allergen extracts (p.1650·1).
*Allergen immunotherapy.*

**Allpyral Pure Mite** *Medi Challenge, S.Afr.*
*D. pteronyssinus* extracts (p.1650·2)(p.1650·1).
*Hyposensitisation.*

**Allpyral Special Grass** *Medi Challenge, S.Afr.*
Grass pollen extracts(p.1650·1).
*Hyposensitisation.*

**Allsan** *Biomed, Switz.*
A range of vitamin preparations with or without minerals (p.1417·1).

**Allstam** *Biostam (Βιοσταμ), Gr.*
Carbocisteine (p.1116·2).
*Respiratory disorders associated with viscous mucus.*

**Alltotal**
*Allergan, Austria†.*
Cleaning, wetting, and storage solution for hard and gas permeable contact lenses (p.1164·2).

*Allergan, Ger.†.*
Polyvinyl alcohol (p.1581·1) (p.1164·2).
*Storage and wetting solution for contact lenses.*

**Alltracel P** *Synapse, Irl.*
Calcium cellulose (p.757·2).
*Haemorrhage.*

**Alltracel S** *Synapse, Irl.*
Calcium cellulose (p.757·2); chlorhexidine (p.1173·2).
*Haemorrhage.*

**Allural** *Britisfarma, Spain†.*
Allopurinol (p.412·2).
*Gout; hyperuricaemia; renal calculi; uric acid nephropathy.*

**Allurit** *Aventis, Ital.*
Allopurinol (p.412·2).
*Gout; hyperuricaemia; renal calculi.*

**Allvoran** *TAD, Ger.*
Diclofenac sodium (p.32·1).
*Inflammation; musculoskeletal, joint, and soft-tissue disorders; pain.*

**Allya** *Pascoe, Ger.*
*Injection:* Homoeopathic preparation.
*Ointment:* Hypericum oil (p.299·2); camphor (p.1665·3).
*Musculoskeletal, joint, peri-articular, and soft-tissue disorders.*
*Tablets:* Devil's claw root (p.28·2).
*Musculoskeletal and joint disorders.*

**Alma** *Restan, S.Afr.*
Peppermint oil (p.1283·2); cardamom (p.1667·3).
*Carminative.*

**Almac** *Hovid, Singapore†.*
Aluminium hydroxide (p.1249·2); magnesium hydroxide (p.1272·2); simeticone (p.1289·2).
*Dyspepsia; flatulence; gastric hyperacidity; heartburn.*

**Almacone** *Rugby, USA.*
Aluminium hydroxide (p.1249·2); magnesium hydroxide (p.1272·2); simeticone (p.1289·2).
*Hyperacidity.*

**Almag**
*CT, Ger.; Hua, Thai.*
Aluminium hydroxide (p.1249·2); magnesium hydroxide (p.1272·2) or magnesium trisilicate (p.1272·3).
*Gastric hyperacidity; gastritis; peptic ulcer.*

**Almagel** *Atlas, Canad.*
Aluminium hydroxide (p.1249·2); magnesium hydroxide (p.1272·2).

**Almagel Plus** *Atlas, Canad.*
Aluminium hydroxide (p.1249·2); magnesium hydroxide (p.1272·2); simeticone (p.1289·2).

**Almarion** *Chew, Thai.*
Theophylline (p.798·3).
*Obstructive airways disease.*

**Almarl** *Sumitomo, Jpn.*
Arotinolol hydrochloride (p.865·1).
*Angina pectoris; hypertension; tachycardia; tremor.*

**Almarytm** *3M, Ital.*
Flecainide acetate (p.916·2).
*Arrhythmias.*

**Almasal** *Chew, Thai.*
Theophylline (p.798·3); salbutamol sulfate (p.791·3).
*Obstructive airways disease.*

**Almax** *Almirall, Spain.*
Almagate (p.1248·2).
*Dyspepsia; gastritis; gastro-oesophageal reflux; peptic ulcer.*

**Almaxane** *Siam Bheasach, Thai.†.*
*Suspension:* Dried aluminium hydroxide gel (p.1249·2); magnesium hydroxide (p.1272·2); simeticone (p.1289·2).
*Tablets:* Dried aluminium hydroxide gel (p.1249·2); aluminium magnesium silicate (p.1577·1); magnesium hydroxide (p.1272·2); simeticone (p.1289·2).
*Flatulence; gastric hyperacidity; peptic ulcer.*

**Almebex Plus B$_{12}$** *Dayton, USA.*
Vitamin B substances (p.1417·1).

**Almevax**
*Wellcome, Irl.†; Chiron Vaccines, UK.*
A rubella vaccine (Wistar RA 27/3 strain) (p.1637·3).
*Active immunisation.*

**Almide** *Alcon, Fr.*
Lodoxamide trometamol (p.1707·3).
*Allergic eye disorders.*

**Almigastrico** *Labesfal, Port.†.*
Aluminium hydroxide (p.1249·2).
*Antacid.*

**Almigripe** *Labesfal, Port.*
Paracetamol (p.76·2); caffeine (p.782·1).
*Fever; pain.*

**Alminox** *Nycomed, Denm.*
Aluminium glycinate (p.1249·1); magnesium oxide (p.1272·3).
*Gastritis; gastro-oesophageal reflux; peptic ulcer.*

**Almiral**
*Medochemie, Hong Kong; Medochemie, Malaysia; Medochemie, Singapore; Medochemie, Thai.*
Diclofenac diethylamine (p.32·1) or diclofenac sodium (p.32·1).
*Gout; inflammation; musculoskeletal, joint, and periarticular disorders; pain.*

**Almirid** *Desitin, Ger.*
Dihydroergocryptine mesilate (p.1680·1).
*Parkinsonism.*

**Almiron** *Nutricia, Thai.*
Infant feed (p.1417·1).
*Lactase deficiency; lactose intolerance.*

**Almiron Pepti** *Nutricia, Fin.*
Infant feed (p.1417·1).
*Cow's milk and soya protein allergy.*

**Almitil** *Almirall, Spain†.*
Enoxacin (p.207·2).
*Urinary-tract infections.*

**Almodan** *Berk, UK†.*
Amoxicillin (p.155·3) or amoxicillin sodium (p.155·3).
*Bacterial infections.*

**Almogran**
*Almirall, Belg.; Almirall, Denm.; Lundbeck, Fin.; Pharmafarm, Fr.; Bayer, Ger.; Lundbeck, Irl.; Almirall, Norw.; Almirall, Spain; Lundbeck, Swed.; Lundbeck, UK.*
Almotriptan malate (p.465·2).
*Migraine.*

**Almora**
*Note. This name is used for preparations of different composition.*
*Elpen (Ελπεν), Gr.*
Potassium chloride; sodium bicarbonate; sodium chloride (p.1222·2).
*Oral rehydration solution.*

*Forest Pharmaceuticals, USA.*
Magnesium gluconate (p.1228·1).
*Dietary supplement.*

**Almorsan** *TRB, Arg.*
Amoxicillin trihydrate (p.155·3).
*Bacterial infections.*

**Almotrex** *Solvay, Ital.*
Almotriptan malate (p.465·2).
*Migraine.*

**Almyrol** *Lysoform, Ger.*
Guanidine derivative; alkylamine; didecyldimethylammonium chloride (p.1178·3).
*Instrument disinfection.*

**Alna**
*Boehringer Ingelheim, Austria; Boehringer Ingelheim, Ger.*
Tamsulosin hydrochloride (p.1009·2).
*Benign prostatic hyperplasia.*

**Alnase** *Taro, Israel.*
Phenylephrine hydrochloride (p.1126·3); naphazoline hydrochloride (p.1124·3); mepyramine maleate (p.437·1).
*Cold symptoms; rhinitis; sinusitis.*

**Alnax** *Masa, Thai.*
Alprazolam (p.668·3).
*Anxiety; mixed anxiety depressive states.*

**Alnex** *Pisa, Mex.*
Dipyrone (p.35·3).
*Fever; pain.*

**Alnok** *Durascan, Denm.*
Cetirizine hydrochloride (p.427·1).
*Allergic rhinitis; hay fever; urticaria.*

**Aloclair** *Forest Laboratories, UK.*
Povidone (p.1581·2).
*Mouth pain.*

**Alocril** *Allergan, Canad.; Allergan, USA.*
Nedocromil sodium (p.789·3).
*Allergic conjunctivitis.*

**Alodan** *Gerot, Austria.*
Pethidine hydrochloride (p.80·2).
*Pain.*

**Alodont** *Pfizer Sante, Fr.; Uhlmann-Eyraud, Switz.*
Cetylpyridinium chloride (p.1173·1); chlorobutanol (p.1176·3); eugenol (p.1686·2).
*Mouth and throat disorders.*

**Alodorm** *Alphapharm, Austral.*
Nitrazepam (p.710·1).
*Insomnia.*

**Aloe Complex** *Dolisos, Canad.*
Homoeopathic preparation.

**Aloe Grande** *Gordon, USA.*
Vitamin A (p.1451·2); vitamin E (p.1464·3); aloe vera (p.1141·3).
*Skin disorders.*

**Aloe Vera Plus** *GNLD, Austral.†.*
Aloe vera (p.1141·3); ascorbic acid; chamomile; eleutherococcus senticosis; passion flower (p.1417·1).
*Digestive disorders; tonic.*

**Aloe Vesta** *Calgon Vestal, USA.*
Skin cleanser.

**Aloebel** *Fortbenton, Arg.*
Aloe vera (p.1141·3); urea (p.1162·2).

**Aloelax** *Knop, Chile.*
Cape aloes (p.1248·2); linseed (p.1707·2).
*Constipation.*

**Alofedina** *Coll, Spain.*
Aloes (p.1248·2); belladonna (p.479·1); ipecacuanha (p.1122·3); nux vomica (p.1722·3); podophyllum (p.1155·2).
Formerly contained aloin, belladonna, phenolphthalein, ipecacuanha, nux vomica, and podophyllum.
*Constipation.*

**Alofresh** *Garden House, Arg.*
Sunflower oil (p.1451·1); parsley oil.
*Dietary supplement; halitosis.*

**Alogesia** *Seid, Spain.*
Ibuprofen lysine (p.46·3).
*Fever; pain.*

**Aloid** *Cilag, Mex.*
Miconazole nitrate (p.405·3).
*Fungal skin and nail infections.*

**Aloinophen** *Streuli, Switz.†.*
Aloes (p.1248·2); belladonna (p.479·1); bisacodyl (p.1251·3); ipecacuanha (p.1122·3).
*Constipation.*

**Alomen** *Benedetti, Ital.*
Ceftezole sodium (p.182·1).
Lidocaine hydrochloride (p.1377·3) is included in this preparation to alleviate the pain of injection.
*Bacterial infections.*

**Alomide**
*Alcon, Arg.; Alcon, Austria; Alcon, Belg.; Alcon, Braz.; Alcon, Canad.; Alcon, Chile; Alcon, Denm.; Alcon, Fin.; Alcon, Ger.; Alkon (Αλκον), Gr.; Alcon, Hong Kong; Alcon, Irl.; Alcon, Israel; Alcon, Ital.; Alcon, Malaysia; Alcon, Mex.†; Alcon, Norw.; Alcon, Port.; Alcon, S.Afr.; Alcon, Singapore; Alcon Cusi, Spain; Alcon, Switz.; Alcon, Thai.; Alcon, UK; Alcon, USA.*
Lodoxamide trometamol (p.1707·3).
*Allergic conjunctivitis.*

**Alonet** *Pharmachemie, Singapore.*
Atenolol (p.865·2).
*Angina pectoris; arrhythmias; hypertension; myocardial infarction.*

**Alongamicina Balsa** *Synthelabo, Spain†.*
Ampicillin sodium (p.157·1); ampicillin benzathine (p.158·1); bromhexine hydrochloride (p.1115·3); guaifenesin (p.1122·1).
*Respiratory-tract infections.*

**Alopam**
*Alpharma, Denm.; Alpharma, Fin.; Alpharma, Norw.*
Oxazepam (p.712·2).
*Anxiety; insomnia.*

**Alopate** *Wolfs, Belg.*
Zinc oxide (p.1163·2); titanium oxide (p.1160·3); kaolin (p.1268·3).
*Skin disorders.*

**Aloperidin** *Janssen-Cilag, Gr.*
Haloperidol (p.701·2) or haloperidol decanoate (p.701·3).
*Huntington's chorea; psychoses; tics.*

**Alopexy**
*Pierre Fabre, Fr.; Pierre Fabre, Switz.*
Minoxidil (p.960·1).
*Alopecia androgenetica.*

**Alophen**
*Note. This name is used for preparations of different composition.*
*Numark, Canad.; Numark, USA.*
Bisacodyl (p.1251·3).
*Constipation.*

*Warner-Lambert, Irl.†; Warner-Lambert, UK†.*
Phenolphthalein (p.1284·1); aloin (p.1248·3).
Formerly contained phenolphthalein, aloin, belladonna, and ipecacuanha.
*Constipation.*

**Aloplastine**
*Wolfs, Belg.; Biologiques de l'Ile-de-France, Fr.*
Zinc oxide (p.1163·2); glycerol (p.1694·3); purified talc (p.1159·1).
*Skin disorders.*

**Alopon** *Resinag, Switz.*
Aluminium chlorohydrate (p.1142·1).
*Anorectal disorders.*

**Alopresin** *Sanofi Synthelabo, Spain.*
Captopril (p.879·2).
*Diabetic nephropathy; heart failure; hypertension; myocardial infarction.*

**Alopresin Diu** *Sanofi Synthelabo, Spain.*
Hydrochlorothiazide (p.933·2); captopril (p.879·2).
*Hypertension.*

**Aloprim** *Nabi, USA.*
Allopurinol sodium (p.413·3).
*Hyperuricaemia during cancer chemotherapy.*

**Alor** *Atley, USA.*
Hydrocodone tartrate (p.45·1); aspirin (p.15·1).
*Pain.*

**Alora** *Procter & Gamble, USA.*
Estradiol (p.1550·1).
*Menopausal disorders; oestrogen deficiency.*

**Aloral** *Lagap, UK†.*
Allopurinol (p.412·2).
*Gout; hyperuricaemia.*

**Alorin** *Essex, Ital.*
Loratadine (p.436·1).
*Allergic rhinitis; allergic skin disorders.*

**Aloset** *Recalcine, Chile.*
Methyldopa (p.953·2).
*Carcinoid syndrome; hypertension.*

**Alosfar** *Esfar, Port.*
Allopurinol (p.412·2).
*Gout; hyperuricaemia; renal calculi.*

**Alosol** *Aventis, Mex.*
Polymyxin B sulfate (p.245·1); neomycin sulfate (p.235·1); lidocaine hydrochloride (p.1377·3).
*Mouth and throat infections.*

**Alostil** *Pharmacia, Fr.*
Minoxidil (p.960·1).
*Alopecia androgenetica.*

**Alovir** *Caber, Ital.*
Aciclovir (p.626·1).
*Herpesvirus infections.*

**Alox** *Andromaco, Chile.*
Oxcarbazepine (p.366·3).
*Epilepsy.*

**Aloxan Derma** *Resinag, Israel.*
Aluminium chlorohydrate (p.1142·1).
*Burns; skin disorders; skin ulceration; wounds.*

**Aloxi** *MGI, USA.*
Palonosetron hydrochloride (p.1282·3).
*Nausea and vomiting associated with chemotherapy.*

**Aloxidil** *IDI, Ital.*
Minoxidil (p.960·1).
*Alopecia androgenetica.*

**Al-Oxin** *Francia, Ital.†.*
Carnitine; betacarotene; sodium glutathione; ginkgo; yeast; vitamin C; vitamin E (p.1417·1).
*Nutritional supplement.*

**Alpagelle** *Pharmadeveloppement, Fr.*
Miristalkonium chloride (p.1186·3).
*Contraceptive.*

**Alpare** *Stallergenes, Ital.†.*
An allergen extract (p.1650·1).
*Allergen immunotherapy.*

**Alpaz** *Royal, Chile.*
Zopiclone (p.729·3).
*Insomnia.*

**l-Alpha** *Leo, Belg.*
Alfacalcidol (p.1461·2).
*Hypoparathyroidism; osteoporosis; renal osteodystrophy; rickets.*

**Alpha Cade** *Dermoteca, Port.*
Salicylic acid (p.1157·1); cade oil (p.1159·2); cedar oil.
*Psoriasis; seborrhoeic dermatitis.*

**Alpha D3**
*Sidus, Arg.; Gerolimatos (Γερολυματος), Gr.; Teva, Hong Kong; GlaxoSmithKline, India; Teva, Israel; Segix, Ital.; Novopharm, Singapore; Pharmachemie, Singapore; Teva, Singapore; Teva, Thai.*
Alfacalcidol (p.1461·2).
*Hyperparathyroidism; hypoparathyroidism; neonatal hypocalcaemia; osteomalacia; osteoporosis; renal osteodystrophy; rickets.*

**Alpha 5 DS** *Liphaderm, Fr.*
Glycolic acid (p.1147·3); piroctone olamine (p.1155·2); alpha hydroxy acid esters; levomenol (p.1707·1); allantoin (p.1141·3); vitamin A palmitate (p.1453·1); vitamin E acetate (p.1465·1).
*Skin disorders.*

**Alpha Fraction** *Dome-Hollister-Stier, Fr.†.*
Modified coca extract (p.1650·1).
*Allergen immunotherapy.*

**Alpha Keri**
*Note. This name is used for preparations of different composition.*
*Bristol-Myers Squibb, Austral.; Bristol-Myers Squibb, Canad.; Bristol-Myers Squibb, Hong Kong; Bristol-Myers Squibb, NZ; Westwood, Singapore†; Bristol-Myers Squibb, UK; Westwood, USA.*
Liquid paraffin (p.1479·1); lanolin oil (p.1483·1).
*Bath additive; dry skin disorders; pruritus.*

*Bristol-Myers Squibb, Canad.†.*
*Soap:* Glycerol (p.1694·3).

*Bristol-Myers Squibb, USA.*
*Cleansing bar:* Skin cleanser.

**Alpha Keri Silky Smooth** *Bristol-Myers, Austral.†.*
Vitamin E (p.1464·3).
*Emollient.*

**Alpha Keri Tar** *Bristol-Myers, Austral.†.*
*Bath oil:* Coal tar (p.1159·2); oil-soluble, dewaxed lanolin fraction (p.1483·1); liquid paraffin (p.1479·1).
*Bath additive; skin disorders.*

*Shampoo:* Coal tar (p.1159·2); salicylic acid (p.1157·1); sulfur (p.1158·2).
*Scalp disorders.*

*Topical gel:* Coal tar (p.1159·2).
*Skin disorders.*

**Alpha Septol** *Dermoteca, Port.†.*
Pyrithione zinc (p.1156·2); piroctone olamine (p.1155·2); salicylic acid (p.1157·1).
*Seborrhoeic dermatitis.*

**Alpha UV** *LED, Fr.*
*SPF 15; SPF 30:* Avobenzone (p.1142·3); octinoxate (p.1154·3); titanium dioxide (p.1160·3).
*Sunscreen.*

**Alpha-Amoxyclav** *Alpha, NZ†.*
Amoxicillin trihydrate (p.155·3); potassium clavulanate (p.193·3).
*Bacterial infections.*

**Alphacaine**
*Dentsply, Fr.; Heck, Switz.*
Articaine hydrochloride (p.1370·3).
Adrenaline hydrochloride (p.852·3) is included in this preparation as a vasoconstrictor to diminish absorption and localise the effect of the local anaesthetic.
*Local anaesthesia.*

**Alphacedre** *Dermoteca, Port.*
Vitamin B substances (p.1417·1); chlorhexidine gluconate (p.1173·2); cedar oil.
*Scalp disorders.*

**Alpha-Chymocutan** *Strathmann, Ger.†.*
Chymotrypsin (p.1671·2).
*Soft-tissue inflammation and oedema.*

**Alpha-Chymotrase** *Strathmann, Ger.†.*
Chymotrypsin (p.1671·2).
*Respiratory-tract disorders; soft-tissue inflammation and oedema.*

**Alphacin** *Alphapharm, Austral.*
Ampicillin trihydrate (p.157·2).
*Bacterial infections.*

**Alphacortison** *Procter & Gamble, Neth.†.*
Hydrocortisone (p.1103·3); urea (p.1162·2).
*Skin disorders.*

**Alphacutanee** *Leurquin, Fr.*
Chymotrypsin (p.1671·2).
*Oedema.*

**Alpha-Depressan** *OPW, Ger.†.*
Urapidil (p.1018·1).
*Hypertension.*

**Alphaderm**
*Procter & Gamble, Belg.†; Procter & Gamble, Irl.; Alliance, UK.*
Hydrocortisone (p.1103·3); urea (p.1162·2).
*Dry skin disorders.*

**Alphadinal** *Alpharma, Mex.*
Naphazoline hydrochloride (p.1124·3).
*Nasal congestion.*

**Alphadine**
*Note. This name is used for preparations of different composition.*
*Minerva (Μινερβα), Gr.*
Ranitidine hydrochloride (p.1285·2).
*Conditions where gastric acid reduction is beneficial; gastric hypersecretion including Zollinger-Ellison syndrome; peptic ulcer.*

*Nicholas Piramal, India.*
Povidone-iodine (p.1190·3).
*Bacterial and fungal infections of the skin and mucous membranes; skin disinfection.*

**Alphadopa** *Wockhardt, India.*
Methyldopa (p.953·2).
*Hypertension.*

**Alphadrate** *Procter & Gamble, Neth.†.*
Urea (p.1162·2).
*Dry skin disorders.*

**Alphaflam** *Lichtenstein, Ger.*
Thioctic acid (p.1754·3).
*Diabetic polyneuropathy.*

**Alphagan**
*Allergan, Arg.; Allergan, Austral.; Allergan, Austria; Allergan, Belg.; Allergan, Braz.; Allergan, Canad.; Allergan, Chile; Allergan, Denm.; Allergan, Fin.; Allergan, Fr.; Allergan, Ger.; Alvia (Αλβια), Gr.; Allergan, Hong Kong; Allergan, Irl.; Allergan, Israel; Allergan, Ital.; Allergan, Malaysia; Allergan, Mex.; Allergan, NZ; Allergan, Port.; Allergan, S.Afr.; Allergan, Singapore; Allergan, Spain; Allergan, Swed.; Allergan, Switz.; Allergan, Thai.; Allergan, UK; Allergan, USA.*
Brimonidine tartrate (p.876·3).
*Glaucoma; ocular hypertension.*

**Alphaglobin**
*Alpha Therapeutic, Ger.†; Grifols, Ital.†.*
A normal immunoglobulin (p.1627·2).
*Chronic lymphocytic leukaemia; idiopathic thrombocytopenic purpura; immunodeficiencies; passive immunisation.*

**Alphakeptol** *Dermoteca, Port.*
Pyrithione zinc (p.1156·2); salicylic acid (p.1157·1); piroctone olamine (p.1155·2).
*Scalp disorders.*

**Alphakinase** *Alpha Therapeutic, Ger.†.*
Urokinase (p.1018·2).
*Thromboembolic disorders.*

**Alpha-Lipogamma** *Worwag, Ger.*
Thioctic acid (p.1754·3) or meglumine thioctate.
*Diabetic polyneuropathy.*

**Alpha-Lipon** *Aliud, Ger.; Stada, Ger.*
Thioctic acid (p.1754·3).
*Diabetic polyneuropathy.*

**Alphalox-D** *Alpharma, Mex.*
Aluminium hydroxide (p.1249·2); magnesium hydroxide (p.1272·2); dicycloverine hydrochloride (p.481·2).
*Gastrointestinal hyperacidity.*

**Alphamox** *Alphapharm, Austral.*
Amoxicillin trihydrate (p.155·3).
*Bacterial infections.*

**Alphanate**
*Alpha, Hong Kong; Alpha Therapeutic, Ital.; Alpha Therapeutic, Malaysia; Alpha Therapeutic, Singapore; Alpha Therapeutic, Thai.; Grifols, UK; Alpha Therapeutic, USA.*
A factor VIII preparation (p.751·1).
*Haemorrhagic disorders.*

**Alphane** *Bailleul, Fr.†.*
Zinc sulfate (p.1469·3); pyridoxine hydrochloride (p.1456·3).
*Seborrhoea.*

**Alphanine**
*Alpha Therapeutic, Ger.†; Alpha, Hong Kong; Alpha Therapeutic, Ital.; Alpha Therapeutic, Malaysia; Alpha Therapeutic, Singapore; Alpha Therapeutic, Thai.; Grifols, UK; Alpha Therapeutic, USA.*
Factor IX (p.752·2).
*Factor IX deficiency.*

**Alphaparin** *Grifols, UK.*
Certoparin sodium (p.882·1).
*Venous thromboembolism prophylaxis.*

**Alphapress**
*Alphapharm, Austral.; Unipharm, Israel.*
Hydralazine hydrochloride (p.931·2).
*Hypertension.*

**Alphapril** *Alphapharm, Austral.*
Enalapril maleate (p.909·2).
*Heart failure; hypertension.*

**Alphastria** *Inpharzam, Switz.*
Sodium hyaluronate (p.1697·3); vitamin A palmitate (p.1453·1); alpha tocoferil acetate (p.1465·1); dexpanthenol (p.1727·2); allantoin (p.1141·3); camphor (p.1665·3); menthol (p.1711·3).
*Prevention of skin striae.*

**Alphatrex** *Savage, USA.*
Betamethasone dipropionate (p.1093·1).
*Skin disorders.*

**Alphavase** *Ashbourne, UK†.*
Prazosin hydrochloride (p.985·1).
*Heart failure; hypertension.*

**alpha-Vibolex** *Chephasaar, Ger.*
Thioctic acid (p.1754·3).
*Diabetic polyneuropathy.*

**Alpha-Zedex** *Wockhardt, India.*
Terfenadine (p.441·1); bromhexine hydrochloride (p.1115·3); guaifenesin (p.1122·1).
*Cold symptoms; coughs.*

**Alphazole** *Dermoteca, Port.*
Climbazole (p.396·2); salicylic acid (p.1157·1); cedar oil.
*Scalp disorders.*

**Alphexine** *Lilly, Fr.*
Cefaclor (p.167·1).
*Bacterial infections.*

**Alphintern** *Leurquin, Fr.†.*
Chymotrypsin (p.1671·2); trypsin (p.1758·3).
*Oedema.*

**Alphosyl**
*Note. This name is used for preparations of different composition.*
*Stafford-Miller, Austral.; Block, Austria; GlaxoSmithKline Consumer, Belg.†; Reed & Carnrick, Canad.†; Stafford-Miller, Fin.†; GlaxoSmithKline Sante, Fr.; Stafford-Miller, Irl.; Stafford-Miller, Israel; GlaxoSmithKline, Port.†; Genop, S.Afr.; Stafford-Miller, Spain; Meda, Swed.; Stafford-Miller, Switz.; GlaxoSmithKline Consumer, UK†.*
Allantoin (p.1141·3); coal tar (p.1159·2).
*Psoriasis.*

*Stafford-Miller, Austral.; Stafford-Miller, Spain.*
*Shampoo:* Coal tar (p.1159·2).
*Scalp disorders.*

**Alphosyl 2 in 1**
*Stafford-Miller, Israel; GlaxoSmithKline Consumer, UK.*
Coal tar (p.1159·2).
*Scalp disorders.*

**Alphosyl HC**
*Stafford-Miller, Irl.; Stafford-Miller, Israel; GlaxoSmithKline, Port.†; GlaxoSmithKline Consumer, UK.*
Allantoin (p.1141·3); coal tar (p.1159·2); hydrocortisone (p.1103·3).
*Psoriasis.*

**Alphosyle** *Monsanto, Ital.*
Allantoin (p.1141·3); coal tar (p.1159·2).
*Psoriasis.*

**Alpicort**
*Note. This name is used for preparations of different composition.*
*Montavit, Austria.*
Prednisolone (p.1108·1); salicylic acid (p.1157·1); coal tar (p.1159·2); colloidal sulfur (p.1158·2); thymol (p.1194·2).
*Scalp disorders.*

*Wolff, Ger.; Cimex, Switz.†.*
Prednisolone (p.1108·1); salicylic acid (p.1157·1).
*Scalp disorders.*

**Alpicort F**
*Wolff, Ger.; Medika, Switz.*
Prednisolone (p.1108·1); salicylic acid (p.1157·1); estradiol benzoate (p.1550·1).
*Scalp disorders.*

**Alpin** *Arlex, Mex.†.*
Hyoscine butylbromide (p.483·3).

**Alpina Gel a la consoude** *Alpinamed, Switz.†.*
Comfrey (p.1675·2); hypericum (p.299·1); calendula (p.1665·2); spearmint (p.1749·1); echinacea purpurea (p.1683·2).
*Soft-tissue injury.*

**Alpina Gel a l'arnica avec spilanthes** *Alpinamed, Switz.†.*
Arnica (p.1656·3); spilantes oleracea.
*Musculoskeletal and joint pain; soft-tissue disorders.*

**Alpina Pommade au souci** *Alpinamed, Switz.†.*
Calendula (p.1665·2); calendula oil (p.1665·2).
*Burns; wounds.*

**Alpirex** *Berman, Mex.*
Paracetamol (p.76·2).
*Fever; pain.*

**Alplax** *Gador, Arg.*
Alprazolam (p.668·3).
*Anxiety; panic attacks.*

**Alplax Digest** *Gador, Arg.*
Alprazolam (p.668·3); sulpiride (p.722·2).
*Somatic disorders.*

**Alplax Net** *Gador, Arg.*
Alprazolam (p.668·3); domperidone (p.1263·2); simeticone (p.1289·2).
*Anxiety with gastrointestinal disorders.*

**Alpovex** *Rivero, Arg.*
Ampicillin (p.157·1).
*Bacterial infections.*

**Alpoxen**
*Alpharma, Denm.†; Alpharma, Fin.; Alpharma, Norw.; Alpharma, Swed.*
Naproxen (p.65·1).
*Fever; gout; inflammation; musculoskeletal and joint disorders; pain.*

**Alpralid** *CTI, Israel.*
Alprazolam (p.668·3).
*Anxiety; panic disorders.*

**Alpratyrol** *Tyrol, Austria.*
Alprazolam (p.668·3).
*Anxiety disorders.*

**Alprax**
*Arrow, Austral.; Torrent, India.*
Alprazolam (p.668·3).
*Anxiety; mixed anxiety depressive states.*

**Alpraz** *SMB, Belg.*
Alprazolam (p.668·3).
*Anxiety disorders; depression; nervous tension.*

**Alprazig** *Baldacci, Ital.*
Alprazolam (p.668·3).
*Anxiety disorders.*

**Alpress** *Pfizer, Fr.*
Prazosin hydrochloride (p.985·1).
*Hypertension.*

**Alprim**
*Alphapharm, Austral.; Alphapharm, Malaysia; Merck, Malaysia; Alphapharm, Singapore; Merck, Singapore.*
Trimethoprim (p.272·2).
*Bacterial infections of the urinary tract.*

**Alprocontin** *Modi-Mundipharma, India.*
Alprazolam (p.668·3).
*Anxiety; mixed anxiety depressive states.*

**Alpronax** *Merck, Port.*
Alprazolam (p.668·3).
*Anxiety disorders.*

**Alprostapint**
*Pint, Austria; Pint, Israel.*
Alprostadil (p.1512·3).
*Maintenance of patent ductus arteriosus.*

**Alprostar** *Recordati, Ital.*
Alprostadil alfadex (p.1512·3).
*Thromboangiitis obliterans.*

**Alprox**
*Orion, Denm.; Orion, Fin.; Orion, Irl.; Rafa, Israel.*
Alprazolam (p.668·3).
*Alcohol withdrawal syndrome; anxiety; panic attacks.*

**Alquen** *GlaxoSmithKline, Spain.*
Ranitidine hydrochloride (p.1285·2).
*Acid aspiration; gastro-oesophageal reflux; gastrointestinal hyperacidity; peptic ulcer; Zollinger-Ellison syndrome.*

**Alra** *Medi-Test, Fr.*
A range of skin-care preparations containing aloe vera (p.1141·3) for use in oncology patients.

**Alrac** *Eurofarma, Braz.†.*
Aluminium hydroxide (p.1249·2); magnesium hydroxide (p.1272·2).
*Gastrointestinal hyperacidity.*

**Alramucil** *Alra, USA†.*
Psyllium hydrophilic mucilloid (p.1268·1).
*Constipation.*

**Alramucil Instant Mix** *Alra, USA†.*
Ispaghula (p.1268·1).

**Alrex**
*BL, Braz.†; Bausch & Lomb, USA.*
Loteprednol etabonate (p.1105·3).
*Allergic conjunctivitis.*

**Alrheumun** *Teofarma, Ger.*
Ketoprofen (p.51·2).
*Gout; inflammation; musculoskeletal and joint disorders; pain.*

**Alrin** *Teva, Israel.*
Oxymetazoline hydrochloride (p.1126·1).
*Nasal congestion.*

**Alrof** *David, India.*
Rofecoxib (p.86·3).
*Osteoarthritis; pain; rheumatoid arthritis.*

**Alserine** *Samakeephaesaj, Thai.*
Cimetidine (p.1255·3).
*Gastric hyperacidity; gastro-oesophageal reflux; peptic ulcer; Zollinger-Ellison syndrome.*

**Alsicur** *Alsitan, Ger.†.*
Cucurbita (p.1677·3); cucurbita oil (p.1677·3); pollen; centaury (p.1669·2); echinacea (p.1683·2); vitamin E (p.1464·3).
*Urinary-tract disorders.*

**Alsidexten** *Lemery, Mex.*
Diclofenac sodium (p.32·1).
*Inflammation; pain.*

**Alsidrine** *Alsi, Canad.*
Ammonium chloride (p.1115·2); cocillana (p.1117·2).

**Alsilax** *Alsi, Canad.†.*
Magnesium sulfate (p.1228·2); cascara (p.1255·1); boldo (p.1661·2); pancreatin (p.1725·3); peptone.

**Alsiline** *Alsi, Canad.†.*
Aloin (p.1248·3); cascara (p.1255·1); phenolphthalein (p.1284·1); bile salts (p.1660·3).

**Alsimine with Vitamins A & D** *Alsi, Canad.*
Multivitamins with calcium and iron (p.1417·1).

**Alsiphene** *Alsi, Canad.*
Paracetamol (p.76·2).

**Alsiroyal** *Alsitan, Ger.†.*
Royal jelly (p.1740·3); vitamin E (p.1464·3); ginseng (p.1693·1).
*Tonic.*

**Alsirub** *Alsi, Canad.*
Methyl salicylate (p.59·3); menthol (p.1711·3); cineole (p.1672·1).

**Alsogil** *Also, Ital..*
*Suppositories†:* Aspirin (p.15·1); paracetamol (p.76·2).
*Cold symptoms; pain.*
*Tablets:* Aspirin (p.15·1); paracetamol (p.76·2); caffeine (p.782·1).
*Cold and influenza symptoms; pain.*

**Alsol**
*Note. This name is used for preparations of different composition.*
*Athenstaedt, Ger.*
Basic aluminium acetotartrate (p.1652·3).
*Hyperhidrosis; soft-tissue injury.*

*Also, Ital.†.*
Cetylpyridinium chloride (p.1173·1).
Formerly contained bisdequalinium diacetate.
*Mouth and throat infections.*

**Alsol N** *Athenstaedt, Ger.*
Basic aluminium acetotartrate (p.1652·3).
*Napkin rash; skin disorders; wounds.*

**Alsoy**
*Nestle, Braz.; Nestle, Canad.; Nestle, Ital.; Nestle, Thai.*
Soya infant feed (p.1417·1).
*Cow's milk intolerance; lactose intolerance.*

**Alstat** *David, India.*
Etamsylate (p.749·3).
*Haemorrhage; menorrhagia.*

**Alsucral**
*Orion, Fin.; Orion, Malaysia; Orion, Singapore.*
Sucralfate (p.1290·2).
*Gastro-oesophageal reflux; peptic ulcer.*

**Alsylax** *Boehringer Ingelheim, Chile.*
Bisacodyl (p.1251·3).
*Bowel evacuation; constipation.*

**Altace**
*Aventis, Canad.; Monarch, USA.*
Ramipril (p.994·1).
*Heart failure following myocardial infarction; hypertension; primary prophylaxis of atherosclerotic complications.*

**Altacite**
*Hoechst Marion Roussel, S.Afr.†; Peckforton, UK†.*
Hydrotalcite (p.1267·3).
*Gastrointestinal hyperacidity.*

**Altacite Plus**
*Hoechst Marion Roussel, Irl.†; Peckforton, UK.*
Hydrotalcite (p.1267·3); simeticone (p.1289·2).
These ingredients can be described by the British Approved Name Co-simalcite.
*Gastrointestinal disorders.*

**Altan** *Rottapharm, Ital.*
Promelase (p.1735·2).
*Respiratory-system disorders.*

**Altat** *Teikoku, Jpn.*
Roxatidine acetate hydrochloride (p.1288·1).
*Gastritis; gastro-oesophageal reflux; gastrointestinal haemorrhage; peptic ulcer; premedication; Zollinger-Ellison syndrome.*

**Altea (Specie Composta)** *Dynacren, Ital.*
Althaea (p.1651·3); thyme (p.1755·2); fennel (p.1687·2); plantago lanceolata (p.1738·2); liquorice (p.1270·2); iceland moss.
*Herbal tea; respiratory-tract congestion.*

**Altemol** *Andromaco, Mex.*
Interferon alfa-n3 (p.640·3).
*Anogenital warts.*

**Alten**
*Medochemie, Hong Kong; Medochemie, Malaysia; Medochemie, Singapore†.*
Tretinoin (p.1161·1).
*Acne.*

**Alteporina** *Alter, Spain†.*
Cefminox sodium (p.174·1).
*Bacterial infections.*

**Altergen** *IBSA, Ital.*
Sodium hyaluronate (p.1697·3); sulfadiazine silver (p.259·1).
*Burns; ulcers; wounds.*

**Alter-H$_2$** *Carter-Wallace, Mex.†.*
Ranitidine hydrochloride (p.1285·2).
*Gastro-oesophageal reflux; peptic ulcer; Zollinger-Ellison syndrome.*

**Altermon** *Faran, Gr.*
Menotrophin (p.1330·1).
*Male and female infertility.*

**Alterna** *Abbott, Arg.*
Preparation for enteral nutrition (p.1417·1).

**ALternaGEL** *J&J-Merck, USA.*
Dried aluminium hydroxide gel (p.1249·2).
*Hyperacidity symptoms.*

**Alternus** *Lafi, Chile.*
Haloperidol (p.701·2).

**Altersol** *IBSA, Ital.*
Acetylcysteine (p.1112·3).
*Respiratory-tract congestion.*

**Altesona** *Alter, Spain†.*
Cortisone acetate (p.1096·1).
*Corticosteroid.*

**Althaea Complex** *Blackmores, Austral.†.*
Maize (p.1676·1); althaea (p.1651·3); buchu (p.1663·1); bearberry (p.1659·2); *d*-alpha tocoferil acid succinate (p.1465·1); vitamin A acetate (p.1453·1).
*Urinary-tract disorders.*

**Althrocin** *Alembic, India.*
Erythromycin estolate (p.208·1).
*Bacterial infections.*

**Altiazem**
*Menarini, Hong Kong; Lusofarmaco, Ital.; Menarini, Singapore†; Menarini, Thai.*
Diltiazem hydrochloride (p.900·1).
*Angina pectoris; hypertension; myocardial infarction.*

**Alticort** *Silesia, Chile.*
Clobetasol propionate (p.1095·2).
*Skin disorders.*

**Alti-CPA** *Altimed, Canad.*
Cyproterone acetate (p.1544·1).

**Altim** *Aventis, Fr.*
Cortivazol (p.1096·2).
*Corticosteroid.*

**Alti-MPA** *Altimed, Canad.*
Medroxyprogesterone acetate (p.1557·2).

**Altinac** *Upsher-Smith, USA†.*
Tretinoin (p.1161·1).
*Acne.*

**Altior** *Pensa, Spain.*
Ibuprofen (p.45·3).
*Fever; pain.*

**Altocel** *Irex, Fr.*
Loperamide hydrochloride (p.1271·1).
*Diarrhoea.*

**Altocor** *Aura, USA.*
Lovastatin (p.949·1).
*Hyperlipidaemias.*

**Altodor** *OM, Ger.†.*
Etamsylate (p.749·3).
*Haemorrhagic disorders.*

**Altone** *Pharmasant, Thai.*
Spironolactone (p.1003·1).
*Heart failure; liver cirrhosis with ascites; oedema.*

**Altosone** *Essex, Ital.*
Mometasone furoate (p.1107·2).
*Skin disorders.*

**Altracart II** *Althin, Swed.†.*
Sodium bicarbonate (p.1221·1).
*Haemodialysis.*

**Altramet**
*Asta Medica, Ger.†; Lek, Hong Kong†.*
Cimetidine (p.1255·3) or cimetidine hydrochloride (p.1255·3).
*Aspiration syndromes; gastro-oesophageal reflux; gastrointestinal haemorrhage; gastrointestinal hyperacidity; hypersensitivity reactions; peptic ulcer; Zollinger-Ellison syndrome.*

**Altruline**
*Roerig, Chile.*
Sertraline (p.317·3).
*Depression.*

*Pfizer, Mex.*
Sertraline hydrochloride (p.317·2).
*Depression; mixed anxiety depressive states; obsessive-compulsive disorder; panic disorder.*

**Alu-3** *Germania, Austria.*
Aluminium tyrosinate.
*Gastrointestinal disorders; hyperphosphataemia.*

**Alubifar** *Rottapharm, Spain.*
Almasilate (p.1248·2).
*Dyspepsia; gastritis; gastro-oesophageal reflux; peptic ulcer.*

**Alubron-Saar** *CPF, Ger.†.*
Aluminium chloride (p.1142·1).
*Mouth and throat inflammation.*

**Alu-Cap**
*IFET (ΙΦΕΤ), Gr.; 3M, Israel; 3M, UK†; 3M, USA.*
Aluminium hydroxide (p.1249·2).
*Gastric hyperacidity; hyperphosphataemia; peptic ulcer.*

**Alucid**
*Note. This name is used for preparations of different composition.*
*Labima, Belg.*
Aluminium glycinate (p.1249·1); calcium carbonate (p.1254·2); magnesium trisilicate (p.1272·3); sodium bicarbonate (p.1223·2).
*Gastrointestinal disorders.*

*Upha, Malaysia.*
Aluminium hydroxide (p.1249·2); magnesium hydroxide (p.1272·2); simeticone (p.1289·2).
*Flatulence; gastric hyperacidity.*

**Alucinol** *Franco-Indian, India.*
Aluminium hydroxide (p.1249·2); magnesium hydroxide (p.1272·2); simeticone (p.1289·2).
*Dyspepsia; gastrointestinal hyperacidity; heartburn; peptic ulcer.*

**Alucol**
*Note. This name is used for preparations of different composition.*
*Sanova, Austria; Melisana, Switz.*
Dried aluminium hydroxide gel (p.1249·2); magnesium hydroxide (p.1272·2).
*Gastric hyperacidity; gastric irritation; gastro-oesophageal reflux.*

*Farmasierra, Spain†.*
Dimeticone (p.1289·2); magnesium hydroxide (p.1272·2); sodium hydroxide (p.1747·3); polyethylene glycol.
*Dyspepsia; flatulence; hyperacidity.*

**Alucol Silicona** *Farmasierra, Spain.*
Aluminium hydroxide (p.1249·2); dimethicone (p.1289·2); magnesium hydroxide (p.1272·2).
*Gastrointestinal hyperacidity and flatulence.*

**Aluctyl**
*Monal, Fr.†; Yamanouchi, Ital.*
Aluminium lactate (p.1653·1).
*Mouth and throat disorders.*

**Aludal** *Teva Tuteur, Arg.*
Granisetron (p.1267·2).
*Nausea and vomiting.*

**Aludrox**
*Note. This name is used for preparations of different composition.*
*Riemser, Ger.; Wyeth, India; Pfizer Consumer, Irl.*
Aluminium hydroxide (p.1249·2).
*Gastrointestinal hyperacidity; heartburn; hyperphosphataemia; peptic ulcer.*

*Wyeth, Gr.*
*Oral suspension:* Aluminium hydroxide (p.1249·2); magnesium oxide (p.1272·3).
*Tablets:* Aluminium hydroxide (p.1249·2); magnesium hydroxide (p.1272·2).
*Antacid.*

*Pfizer Consumer, UK.*
*Oral liquid:* Aluminium hydroxide (p.1249·2).
*Tablets†:* Aluminium hydroxide-magnesium carbonate co-dried gel (p.1250·1); magnesium hydroxide (p.1272·2).
*Dyspepsia; hyperphosphataemia.*

*Wyeth-Ayerst, USA.*
Aluminium hydroxide (p.1249·2); magnesium hydroxide (p.1272·2); simeticone (p.1289·2).
*Hyperacidity.*

**Aludrox II** *Bago, Arg.*
Aluminium hydroxide (p.1249·2); magnesium hydroxide (p.1272·2); simeticone (p.1289·2).
*Flatulence; gastric hyperacidity.*

**Aludrox AC** *Bago, Arg.*
Ranitidine hydrochloride (p.1285·2).
*Gastric hyperacidity.*

**Aludrox Forte** *Bago, Arg.*
Aluminium hydroxide (p.1249·2); magnesium hydroxide (p.1272·2).
*Gastric hyperacidity.*

**Aludrox MH** *Wyeth, India.*
Aluminium hydroxide (p.1249·2); magnesium hydroxide (p.1272·2).
*Gastrointestinal hyperacidity; peptic ulcer.*

**Aludroxil** *Sanval, Braz.*
Aluminium hydroxide (p.1249·2).
*Antacid.*

**Alugel**
*Atlas, Canad.; Pharmacia, Spain.*
Aluminium hydroxide (p.1249·2).
Formerly known as Alugelibys in *Spain.*
*Dyspepsia; gastritis; gastro-oesophageal reflux; gastrointestinal hyperacidity; hyperphosphataemia.*

**Alugel Magnesiado** *Pharmacia, Spain.*
*Chewable tablets:* Aluminium hydroxide (p.1249·2); magnesium oxide (p.1272·3).
Formerly known as Alugelibys Magnesiado.
*Oral suspension:* Aluminium hydroxide (p.1249·2); magnesium hydroxide (p.1272·2).
*Dyspepsia; gastrointestinal hyperacidity.*

**Alukon** *Apotex, S.Afr.†.*
Aluminium hydroxide (p.1249·2).
*Gastric hyperacidity.*

**Alum Milk** *Aventis, Thai.*
Aluminium hydroxide (p.1249·2); magnesium hydroxide (p.1272·2).
*Dyspepsia; gastritis; peptic ulcer.*

**Alumadrine** *Fleming, USA†.*
Phenylpropanolamine hydrochloride (p.1127·3); chlorphenamine maleate (p.427·3); paracetamol (p.76·2).
*Upper respiratory-tract symptoms.*

**Alu-Mag** *Kanda, Braz.†.*
Aluminium hydroxide (p.1249·2); magnesium hydroxide (p.1272·2).
*Gastrointestinal hyperacidity.*

**Alumag**
Trianon, Canad.; Teva, Israel.
Aluminium hydroxide (p.1249·2); magnesium hydroxide (p.1272·2).
*Flatulence; gastrointestinal hyperacidity; peptic ulcer.*

**Alumagall** Interdelta, Switz.
Dried aluminium hydroxide gel (p.1249·2); magnesium hydroxide (p.1272·2); allantoin (p.1141·3).
*Gastric hyperacidity.*

**Aluminium Free Indigestion** Larkhall Laboratories, UK†.
Calcium carbonate (p.1254·2); cinnamon (p.1672·2); nutmeg (p.1722·2); clove (p.1673·2); cardamom seed (p.1667·3).

**Alumite** Xixia, S.Afr.
Dicycloverine hydrochloride (p.481·2); aluminium hydroxide (p.1249·2); magnesium oxide (p.1272·3).
*Gastrointestinal disorders.*

**Alumpak** ICN, Arg.
Aluminium chloride (p.1142·1).
*Hyperhidrosis.*

**Alupent**
Boehringer Ingelheim, Austral.; Boehringer Ingelheim, Austria; Boehringer Ingelheim, Belg.†; Boehringer Ingelheim, Canad.; Boehringer Ingelheim, Fr.†; Boehringer Ingelheim, Ger.; Boehringer Ingelheim, Gr.; German Remedies, India; Boehringer Ingelheim, Irl.; Boehringer Ingelheim, Ital.; Promeco, Mex.†; Boehringer Ingelheim, NZ†; Boehringer Ingelheim, S.Afr.†; Boehringer Ingelheim, Spain†; Boehringer Ingelheim, Switz.†; Boehringer Ingelheim, Thai.; Boehringer Ingelheim, UK; Boehringer Ingelheim, USA.
Orciprenaline sulfate (p.790·2).
*Beta blocker overdosage; digitalis intoxication; obstructive airways disease; Stokes-Adams attacks.*

**Alupent Expectorant** Boehringer Ingelheim, Irl.
Orciprenaline sulfate (p.790·2); bromhexine hydrochloride (p.1115·3).
*Obstructive airways disease.*

**Alupep** Sriprasit, Thai.
Aluminium hydroxide (p.1249·2); magnesium trisilicate (p.1272·3); kaolin (p.1268·3); atropine sulfate (p.477·1).
*Gastrointestinal disorders.*

**Alupir** Pharma Line, Ital.†.
Aluminium aspirin (p.14·1).
*Cold symptoms; musculoskeletal disorders; neuritis.*

**Aluprim** Zimaia, Port.†.
Aluminium aspirin (p.14·1).
*Fever; pain.*

**Alurate** Roche, USA†.
Aprobarbital (p.670·3).
*Insomnia; sedative.*

**Alusil** Salters, S.Afr.†.
Magnesium trisilicate (p.1272·3); aluminium hydroxide (p.1249·2).
*Gastrointestinal hyperacidity.*

**Alusorb** DHA, Singapore†.
Dried aluminium hydroxide gel (p.1249·2); simeticone (p.1289·2).
*Flatulence; gastric hyperacidity; heartburn; peptic ulcer.*

**Alu-Tab**
3M, Austral.; 3M, Canad.; 3M, Hong Kong; 3M, Malaysia; 3M, NZ; 3M, Singapore; 3M, USA.
Aluminium hydroxide (p.1249·2).
*Gastric hyperacidity; hyperphosphataemia; peptic ulcer.*

**Alutard** ALK, Norw.
Allergen extracts from timothy (*Phleum pratense*) or birch (*Betula verrucosa*) (p.1650·1).
*Allergen immunotherapy.*

**Alutard SQ**
ALK, Denm.; ALK, Fin.; ALK, Swed.; Trimedal, Switz.
Allergen extracts (p.1650·1).
*Allergen immunotherapy.*

**Alutop** General Drugs, Thai.
*Oral gel:* Dried aluminium hydroxide gel (p.1249·2); magnesium hydroxide (p.1272·2); simeticone (p.1289·2).
*Flatulence; gastric hyperacidity; peptic ulcer.*
*Tablets:* Dried aluminium hydroxide gel (p.1249·2); magnesium hydroxide (p.1272·2).
*Gastric hyperacidity; peptic ulcer.*

**Aluzime** Alter, Spain†.
Coenzyme A (p.1674·3).
*Glomerular kidney disease; metabolic disorders.*

**Alvadermo Fuerte** Inexfa, Spain†.
Fluocinolone acetonide (p.1101·2).
*Skin disorders.*

**Alvear** SIT, Ital.
Royal jelly (p.1740·3).
*Nutritional supplement.*

**Alvear Complex** Whitehall, Ital.†.
Royal jelly (p.1740·3); pollen; dried yeast (p.1469·1); lactic-acid-producing organisms (p.1704·2).
*Nutritional supplement.*

**Alvear con Ginseng** SIT, Ital.
Ginseng (p.1693·1); honey (p.1434·2); royal jelly (p.1740·3); myrtillus (p.1718·3).
*Nutritional supplement.*

**Alvear Sport** Whitehall, Ital.†.
Yellow capsules: royal jelly (p.1740·3); pollen; red capsules: ginkgo biloba (p.1692·3); myrtillus (p.1718·3); tablets: glucose (p.1432·2); royal jelly.
*Nutritional supplement.*

**Alvedon**
Astra, Norw.†; Astra, Swed.; AstraZeneca, UK.
Paracetamol (p.76·2).
*Fever; pain.*

**Alvedrin** Offenbach, Mex.
Ampicillin trihydrate (p.157·2).
*Bacterial infections.*

**Alven** Wassermann, Ital.
Diosmin (p.1688·2).
*Peripheral vascular disorders.*

**Alvent** Farmalab, Braz.
Ipratropium bromide (p.787·1).
*Obstructive airways disease.*

**Alveofact**
Boehringer Ingelheim, Austria; Boehringer de Angeli, Braz.†; Boehringer Ingelheim, Ger.; Boehringer Ingelheim, Ital.†.
Bovactant (p.1736·2).
*Neonatal respiratory distress syndrome.*

**Alveofen** Prieto, Arg.
Fenoterol (p.785·2).
*Obstructive airways disease.*

**Alveolex** Klinge, Irl.†.
Acetylcysteine (p.1112·3).
*Cystic fibrosis; respiratory-tract disorders with excess or viscous mucus.*

**Alveoten** Ibi, Ital.
Neltenexine (p.1125·2).
*Respiratory-tract disorders.*

**Alvercol**
Norgine, Austral.; Norgine, Hong Kong†; Norgine, Irl.†; Norgine, S.Afr.
Sterculia (p.1290·2); alverine citrate (p.1250·2).
*Hypertonic constipation; irritable bowel syndrome.*

**Alvesco** Altana, Austral.
Ciclesonide (p.1095·2).
*Asthma.*

**Alvesin** Berlin-Chemie, Ger.
Amino-acid and electrolyte infusion (p.1417·1).
*Parenteral nutrition.*

**Alvidina** Farcoral, Mex.
Ranitidine hydrochloride (p.1285·2).
*Peptic ulcer; Zollinger-Ellison syndrome.*

**Alvis** Novartis Ophthalmics, Arg.
Pilocarpine hydrochloride (p.1495·1).
*Ocular hypertension; production of miosis.*

**Alvityl** Solvay, Fr.
Multivitamin preparation (p.1417·1).

**Alvium** Columbia, Mex.
Loratadine (p.436·1); pseudoephedrine (p.1129·2).
*Cold symptoms.*

**Alvo Nasal** Lafedar, Arg.
Diphenhydramine hydrochloride (p.431·3); naphazoline hydrochloride (p.1124·3); phenylephrine hydrochloride (p.1126·3).
*Nasal congestion.*

**Alvofact**
Boehringer Ingelheim, Belg.; Boehringer Ingelheim, Neth.; Boehringer Ingelheim, Thai.†.
Bovactant (p.1736·2).
*Neonatal respiratory distress syndrome.*

**Alvogil** Prats, Spain.
Butyl aminobenzoate (p.1373·1); eugenol (p.1686·2); iodoform (p.1184·2).

**Alvogyl** Septodont, Switz.
Butyl aminobenzoate (p.1373·1); iodoform (p.1184·2); eugenol (p.1686·2); spearmint oil (p.1749·1); penghawar djambi fibra.
*Pain following tooth extraction.*

**Alxen** Ofimex, Mex.†.
Naproxen (p.65·1).

**Alymphon** Iso, Ger.
Homoeopathic preparation.

**Alyostal**
Stallergenes, Fr.; Stallergenes, Switz.
A range of allergan extracts (p.1650·1).
*Allergen immunotherapy; diagnosis of hypersensitivity.*

**Alyrane**
Zeneca, Austral.†; Pharmacia Upjohn, Belg.†; Pharmacia Upjohn, Denm.†; Zeneca, Israel; Pharmacia Upjohn, Neth.†; Zeneca, S.Afr.†; Pharmacia Upjohn, Swed.†; Baxter Anaesthesia, UK†.
Enflurane (p.1298·1).
*General anaesthesia.*

**Alzaimax** Rontag, Arg.
Donepezil hydrochloride (p.1489·2).
*Alzheimer's disease.*

**Alzam** Parke-Med, S.Afr.
Alprazolam (p.668·3).
*Anxiety disorders; panic disorder.*

**Alzaten** Ariston, Arg.
Phenylephrine hydrochloride (p.1126·3); caffeine (p.782·1).
*Hypotension.*

**Alzen** Tecnifar, Port.
Quetiapine fumarate (p.718·2).
*Schizophrenia.*

**Alzental** Shin Poong, Singapore.
Albendazole (p.101·2).
*Worm infections.*

**Alzol** Pharmasant, Thai.
Albendazole (p.101·2).
*Worm infections.*

**Alzolam** Sun, Singapore†.
Alprazolam (p.668·3).
*Anxiety; mixed anxiety depressive states; panic disorders; phobias.*

**Alzomed-F** Farcoral, Mex.
Benzonatate (p.1115·3).
*Coughs.*

**AM** New Vision, Canad.
Multivitamin preparation (p.1417·1).

**AM Treatment** Avon, Canad.
*SPF 15:* Octinoxate (p.1154·3); oxybenzone (p.1154·3).
*Sunscreen.*

**Ama** Atlantic, Thai.
Chlorpromazine hydrochloride (p.675·2); amobarbital (p.670·1).
*Anxiety; psychoses; tension.*

**Amabagyl** Hoechst Marion Roussel, Mex.†.
Diiodohydroxyquinoline (p.603·3).

**Amace-BP** Systopic, India.
Amlodipine besilate (p.862·1); benazepril (p.867·2).
*Hypertension.*

**Amacin** Asian Pharm, Thai.
Amoxicillin trihydrate (p.155·3).
*Bacterial infections.*

**Amacone** Hua, Thai.
Aluminium hydroxide (p.1249·2); magnesium hydroxide (p.1272·2) or magnesium trisilicate (p.1272·3); simeticone (p.1289·2).
*Flatulence; gastric hyperacidity; peptic ulcer.*

**Amadol** TAD, Ger.; Viatris, Ger.
Tramadol hydrochloride (p.94·3).
*Pain.*

**Amagesan** Ritsert, Ger.
Amoxicillin trihydrate (p.155·3).
*Bacterial infections.*

**Amalium** Janssen-Cilag, Austria.
Flunarizine hydrochloride (p.434·1).
*Migraine.*

**Aman**
Note. A similar name is used for preparations of different composition (see below).
Hexal, Ger.
Amantadine sulfate (p.1197·2).
*Drug-induced extrapyramidal disorders; influenza A; parkinsonism.*

**Am-An**
Note. A similar name is used for preparations of different composition (see above).
Berman, Mex.
Ampicillin sodium (p.157·1) or ampicillin trihydrate (p.157·2).
*Bacterial infections.*

**Amanta**
ABZ, Ger.; Azupharma, Ger.
Amantadine hydrochloride (p.1197·2) or amantadine sulfate (p.1197·2).
*Influenza A; parkinsonism.*

**Amantagamma** Worwag, Ger.
Amantadine hydrochloride (p.1197·2).
*Drug-induced extrapyramidal disorders; parkinsonism.*

**Amantan** Byk, Belg.
Amantadine hydrochloride (p.1197·2).
*Influenza A; parkinsonism.*

**Amantrel** Cipla, India.
Amantadine (p.1198·2).
*Herpes zoster infections; influenza A; parkinsonism.*

**Amaphen** Trimen, USA†.
Paracetamol (p.76·2); caffeine (p.782·1); butalbital (p.673·3).
*Pain.*

**Amaphen with Codeine** Trimen, USA.
Codeine phosphate (p.27·1); paracetamol (p.76·2); caffeine (p.782·1); butalbital (p.673·3).
*Pain.*

**Amara** Koch, Austria.
Gentian tincture (p.1692·2); cinchona bark tincture (p.1671·3); absinthium tincture (p.1645·1).
*Gastrointestinal disorders.*

**Amara-Tropfen** Weleda, Ger.
Absinthium (p.1645·1); cichorium intybus; centaury (p.1669·2); gentian (p.1692·2); imperatoria; juniper (p.1703·1); achillea (p.1646·2); sage (p.1741·2); taraxacum (p.1751·3).
*Gastrointestinal disorders.*

**Amara-Tropfen-Pascoe** Pascoe, Ger.
Gentian (p.1692·2); cinchona bark (p.1671·3); absinthium (p.1645·1); cinnamon bark (p.1672·2).
*Gastrointestinal disorders.*

**Amarel** Aventis, Fr.
Glimepiride (p.332·2).
*Diabetes mellitus.*

**Amaro Medicinale** Giuliani, Ital.
Rhubarb (p.1287·3); cascara (p.1255·1); gentian (p.1692·2); boldo (p.1661·2).
*Appetite loss; constipation; digestive disorders.*

**Amaro Padil** Pfizer, Ital.†.
Cascara (p.1255·1); gentian (p.1692·2).
*Constipation.*

**Amaryl**
Aventis, Arg.; Aventis, Austral.; Hoechst Marion Roussel, Austria; Aventis, Braz.; Aventis, Chile; Aventis, Denm.; Aventis, Fin.; Aventis, Ger.; Aventis, Hong Kong; Aventis, India; Aventis, Irl.; Hoechst, Ital.; Aventis, Malaysia; Aventis, Mex.; Aventis, Neth.; Aventis, Norw.; Aventis, Port.; Aventis, S.Afr.; Aventis, Singapore; Aventis, Spain; Aventis, Swed.; Aventis, Switz.; Aventis, Thai.; Aventis, UK; Hoechst Marion Roussel, USA.
Glimepiride (p.332·2).
*Diabetes mellitus.*

**Amarylle** Aventis, Belg.
Glimepiride (p.332·2).
*Diabetes mellitus.*

**Amasulin** Takeda, Jpn.
Carumonam sodium (p.166·3).
Mepivacaine hydrochloride (p.1381·2) is included in the intramuscular injection to alleviate the pain of injection.
*Bacterial infections.*

**Amatine** Shire, Canad.
Midodrine hydrochloride (p.959·2).
*Idiopathic orthostatic hypotension.*

**Amazyl** Christiaens, Belg.†.
Bismuth subnitrate (p.1252·2); magnesium trisilicate (p.1272·3); borax (p.1661·3).
*Cracked nipples.*

**Ambacamp** Pharmacia, Ger.
Bacampicillin hydrochloride (p.161·2).
*Bacterial infections.*

**Ambamida** Sintesina, Arg.
Erythromycin (p.208·1).
*Bacterial infections.*

**Ambatrol** SmithKline Beecham, Fr.†.
Nifuroxazide (p.237·2).
*Diarrhoea.*

**Ambaxino** Pharmacia, Spain.
Bacampicillin hydrochloride (p.161·2).
*Bacterial infections.*

**Ambe 12** Merckle, Ger.
Cyanocobalamin (p.1458·2).
*Vitamin $B_{12}$ deficiency.*

**Amben** Medochemie, Hong Kong.
Cefadroxil (p.167·2).
*Bacterial infections.*

**Ambenat** Ratiopharm, Austria.
Glycol salicylate (p.44·3); benzyl nicotinate (p.21·2); heparin sodium (p.928·1).
*Muscle, nerve, and joint pain.*

**Ambene**
Note. This name is used for preparations of different composition.
Ratiopharm, Austria.
Ampoule A, phenylbutazone sodium (p.84·1); sodium salamidacetate (p.87·3); dexamethasone (p.1097·1); ampoule B, cyanocobalamin (p.1458·2).
Lidocaine hydrochloride (p.1377·3) is included in both ampoules to alleviate the pain of injection.
*Arthritis; degenerative spinal disorders; neuralgias; neuritis.*

Merckle, Ger.
Phenylbutazone (p.83·2) or phenylbutazone sodium (p.84·1).
Lidocaine hydrochloride (p.1377·3) is included in the injection to alleviate the pain of injection.
*Gout; musculoskeletal and joint disorders.*

**Ambene Comp** Merckle, Ger.
Ampoule 1, phenylbutazone sodium (p.84·1); ampoule 2, cyanocobalamin (p.1458·2).
Lidocaine hydrochloride (p.1377·3) is included in each ampoule to alleviate the pain of injection.
*Gout; musculoskeletal and joint-disorders.*

**Ambene N**
Note. This name is used for preparations of different composition.
Ratiopharm, Austria.
*Suppositories:* Phenylbutazone (p.83·2); cyanocobalamin (p.1458·2).
*Tablets:* Phenylbutazone (p.83·2); thiamine hydrochloride (p.1455·1); cyanocobalamin (p.1458·2).
Aluminium glycinate (p.1249·1) is included in this preparation in an attempt to limit adverse effects on the gastrointestinal mucosa.
*Gout; musculoskeletal, joint, soft-tissue, and peri-articular disorders; neuritis; superficial thrombophlebitis.*

Merckle, Ger.
Glycol salicylate (p.44·3); benzyl nicotinate (p.21·2).
*Musculoskeletal, joint, and soft-tissue disorders.*

**Ambenyl** Parke, Davis, Canad.†.
Codeine phosphate (p.27·1); bromazine hydrochloride (p.425·3); diphenhydramine hydrochloride (p.431·3); ammonium chloride (p.1115·2); sulfogaiacol (p.1131·1).
*Coughs.*

**Ambenyl Cough Syrup** Forest Pharmaceuticals, USA.
Codeine phosphate (p.27·1); bromazine hydrochloride (p.425·3).
*Allergic upper respiratory symptoms; coughs and cold symptoms.*

**Ambenyl-D** Forest Pharmaceuticals, USA.
Guaifenesin (p.1122·1); pseudoephedrine hydrochloride (p.1129·2); dextromethorphan hydrobromide (p.1117·3).
*Coughs; nasal congestion.*

**Amber Gold** Larkhall Laboratories, UK†.
Melaleuca oil (p.1710·2).

**Ambezetal** Cimed, Braz.
Ampicillin benzathine (p.158·1); ampicillin sodium (p.157·1).
*Bacterial infections.*

**Ambi 10** Kiwi, USA.
*Cream:* Benzoyl peroxide (p.1143·2).
*Acne.*
*Soap:* Triclosan (p.1195·2).

**AMBI 60/580** AMBI, USA.
Pseudoephedrine hydrochloride (p.1129·2); guaifenesin (p.1122·1).
*Respiratory-tract congestion.*

**AMBI 60/580/30** AMBI, USA.
Pseudoephedrine hydrochloride (p.1129·2); guaifenesin (p.1122·1); dextromethorphan hydrobromide (p.1117·3).
*Coughs; respiratory-tract congestion.*

**AMBI 1000/55** AMBI, USA.
Guaifenesin (p.1122·1); dextromethorphan hydrobromide (p.1117·3).
*Coughs.*

**Ambi Skin Tone** Kiwi, USA†.
Hydroquinone (p.1148·1); padimate O (p.1155·1).
*Hyperpigmentation.*

**Ambidrin** Collins, Mex.
Ampicillin (p.157·1).
*Bacterial infections.*

**Ambien** Sanofi, USA.
Zolpidem tartrate (p.728·3).
*Insomnia.*

**Ambilan**
Note. This name is used for preparations of different composition.
Laboratorios Chile, Chile.
Amoxicillin trihydrate (p.155·3); potassium clavulanate (p.193·3).
*Bacterial infections.*
Orion, Fin.
Emollient.

**Ambilan Bid** Laboratorios Chile, Chile.
Amoxicillin trihydrate (p.155·3); potassium clavulanate (p.193·3).
*Bacterial infections.*

**Ambiosol** Solfran, Mex.
Ampicillin (p.157·1).
*Bacterial infections.*

**Ambirix** GlaxoSmithKline, Swed.
An inactivated hepatitis A and recombinant hepatitis B vaccine (p.1620·1).
*Active immunisation.*

**AmBisome**
Gador, Arg.; Gilead, Austral.; Calea, Austria; Nexstar, Belg.†; United Medical, Braz.†; Fujisawa, Canad.; Gilead, Denm.; Orphan, Fin.; Gilead, Fr.; Gilead, Ger.; Gilead, Gr.; Gilead, Hong Kong; Gilead, Irl.; Nexstar, Israel; Gilead, Ital.; Gilead, Neth.; Gilead, Norw.; Baxter, NZ; Gilead, NZ; Gilead, Spain; Swedish Orphan, Swed.; Fresenius Kabi, Switz.; Gilead, Thai.; Gilead, UK; Fujisawa, USA.
Liposomal amphotericin B (p.391·2) (p.391·2).
*Fungal infections; leishmaniasis.*

**Ambistryn-S** Sarabhai Piramal, India.
Streptomycin sulfate (p.256·2).
*Tuberculosis.*

**Ambi-Wolff** Wolff, Ger.†.
Barrier cream.

**Ambiz** Unichem, India.
Zolpidem (p.729·2).
*Insomnia.*

**Ambodil** Arlex, Mex.†.
Ambroxol (p.1114·3).

**Amboneural** Arcana, Austria.
Selegiline hydrochloride (p.1214·1).
*Parkinsonism.*

**Amboral** Remek, Gr.
Ambroxol hydrochloride (p.1114·3).
*Respiratory disorders associated with viscous mucus.*

**Ambotetra** Cilag, Mex.
Tetracycline hydrochloride (p.266·2).
*Bacterial infections.*

**Ambotonin** Ebewe, Austria.
Proteolytic peptide from porcine brain (Cerebrolysin) (p.1709·3).
*Alzheimer's disease; cerebral disorders.*

**Ambra Med Complex** Dynamit, Austria.
Homoeopathic preparation.

**Ambra Oligoplex** Madaus, Arg.
Mineral preparation (p.1417·1).

**Ambral** Beige, S.Afr.†.
Metronidazole (p.607·2).
*Amoebiasis; anaerobic bacterial infections; giardiasis; trichomoniasis.*

**Ambramicina** Scharper, Ital.
Tetracycline hydrochloride (p.266·2).
*Bacterial infections.*

**Ambra-Sinto T** Medley, Braz.
Tetracycline hydrochloride (p.266·2).
*Bacterial infections.*

**Ambre Solaire** Garnier, UK.
Avobenzone (p.1142·3); enzacamene (p.1147·1); ecamsule (p.1146·3); titanium dioxide (p.1160·3).
*Sunscreen.*

**Ambredin** Solco, Austria.
Theophylline (p.798·3); aceverine hydrochloride; octodrine phosphate (p.975·3).
*Obstructive airways disease.*

**Ambrexin** Fustery, Mex.
Amoxicillin trihydrate (p.155·3); bromhexine hydrochloride (p.1115·3).
*Respiratory-tract infections.*

**Ambril**
Merck, Arg.; Cascan, Ger.; GlaxoSmithKline, Ger.
Ambroxol hydrochloride (p.1114·3).
*Respiratory-tract disorders associated with increased or viscous mucus.*

**Ambritan** Daker Farmasimes, Spain†.
Cobamamide (p.1459·1).
*Tonic.*

**Ambro** ABZ, Ger.; Hemopharm, Ger.
Ambroxol hydrochloride (p.1114·3).
*Respiratory-tract disorders with viscous mucus.*

**Ambrobene** Ratiopharm, Austria.
Ambroxol hydrochloride (p.1114·3).
*Respiratory-tract disorders with viscous mucus.*

**Ambrobeta** Betapharm, Ger.
Ambroxol hydrochloride (p.1114·3).
*Respiratory-tract disorders with viscous mucus.*

**Ambrobion** Medicus, Gr.
Ambroxol hydrochloride (p.1114·3).
*Respiratory disorders associated with viscous mucus.*

**Ambrodoc** Docpharm, Ger.
Ambroxol hydrochloride (p.1114·3).
*Respiratory-tract disorders with viscous mucus.*

**Ambrodoxy** Hexal, Ger.
Doxycycline hyclate (p.206·2); ambroxol hydrochloride (p.1114·3).
*Respiratory-tract infections with increased or viscous mucus.*

**Ambrofur** Fustery, Mex.
Ambroxol hydrochloride (p.1114·3).
*Respiratory-tract disorders with viscous mucus.*

**Ambrohexal**
Hexal, Austria; Hexal, Ger.
Ambroxol hydrochloride (p.1114·3).
*Respiratory-tract disorders associated with increased or viscous mucus.*

**Ambroinfant** Rubiepharm, Ger.
Ambroxol hydrochloride (p.1114·3).
*Respiratory-tract disorders with viscous mucus.*

**Ambrol** Shiwa, Thai.
Ambroxol hydrochloride (p.1114·3).
*Respiratory-tract disorders associated with increased or viscous mucus.*

**Ambrolan** Lannacher, Austria.
Ambroxol hydrochloride (p.1114·3).
*Respiratory-tract disorders.*

**Ambrolitic** Chiesi, Spain.
Ambroxol hydrochloride (p.1114·3).
*Respiratory-tract disorders.*

**Ambrolos**
Hexal, Austria; Hexal, Ger.
Ambroxol hydrochloride (p.1114·3).
*Respiratory-tract disorders with viscous mucus.*

**Ambrolytic** Samakeephaesaj, Thai.
Ambroxol hydrochloride (p.1114·3).
*Respiratory-tract disorders associated with increased or viscous mucus.*

**Ambromucil** Malesci, Ital.
Ambroxol acefyllinate (p.1114·3).
*Obstructive airways disease.*

**Ambromyc** Pharmedia (Φαρμεντια), Gr.
Ambroxol hydrochloride (p.1114·3).
*Respiratory disorders associated with viscous mucus.*

**Ambropp** Dermapharm, Ger.
Ambroxol hydrochloride (p.1114·3).
*Respiratory-tract disorders with increased or viscous mucus.*

**Ambro-Puren** Alpharma-Isis, Ger.
Ambroxol hydrochloride (p.1114·3).
*Respiratory-tract disorders with viscous mucus.*

**Ambroten** Marjan, Braz.
Ambroxol (p.1114·3).
*Respiratory-tract congestion.*

**Ambrotos** Recalcine, Chile.
Ambroxol hydrochloride (p.1114·3); ammonium citrate (p.1654·1).
*Respiratory-tract disorders.*

**Ambrowel** Welfer, Mex.†.
Ambroxol (p.1114·3).

**Ambrox** Nakorn, Thai.
Ambroxol hydrochloride (p.1114·3).
*Respiratory-tract disorders associated with increased or viscous mucus.*

**Ambroxan** M & H, Thai.
Ambroxol hydrochloride (p.1114·3).
*Respiratory-tract disorders associated with increased or viscous mucus.*

**Ambroxol AL comp** Aliud, Ger.
Ambroxol hydrochloride (p.1114·3); doxycycline hyclate (p.206·2).
*Respiratory-tract infections.*

**Ambroxol comp** Ratiopharm, Ger.
Ambroxol hydrochloride (p.1114·3); doxycycline hyclate (p.206·2).
*Respiratory-tract infections.*

**Ambroxolvan** Bergamo, Braz.†.
Ambroxol hydrochloride (p.1114·3).
*Respiratory-tract congestion.*

**Ambufen** Macrophar, Thai.
Ibuprofen (p.45·3).
*Musculoskeletal and joint disorders.*

**Amchafibrin** Fides Ecopharma, Spain.
Tranexamic acid (p.760·3).
*Haemorrhage; hereditary angioedema.*

**Amciderm**
Hermal, Ger.; Pharmasant, Thai.
Amcinonide (p.1091·1).
*Skin disorders.*

**Amcidil** Macrophar, Thai.
Dicloxacillin (p.205·2).
*Gram-positive bacterial infections.*

**Amcillin** Dumex-Alpharma, Thai.
Ampicillin sodium (p.157·1) or ampicillin trihydrate (p.157·2).
*Bacterial infections.*

**Amcinafal** Relyo, Gr.
Tenoxicam (p.93·1).
*Dysmenorrhoea; gout; inflammation; osteoarthritis; pain; rheumatoid arthritis; spondyloarthropathies.*

**Amcinil** Crosara, Ital.†.
Amcinonide (p.1091·1).
*Skin disorders.*

**Amclo** Nicholas Piramal, India.
Amoxicillin trihydrate (p.155·3); cloxacillin sodium (p.198·2).
*Bacterial infections.*

**Amco** Polipharm, Thai.
Magnesium trisilicate (p.1272·3); aluminium hydroxide (p.1249·2); magnesium hydroxide (p.1272·2); simeticone (p.1289·2).
*Dyspepsia; flatulence; gastric hyperacidity; peptic ulcer.*

**Amcopan** Macrophar, Thai.
Hyoscine butylbromide (p.483·3).
*Smooth muscle spasm.*

**Amcopan Plus** Macrophar, Thai.
Hyoscine butylbromide (p.483·3); paracetamol (p.76·2).
*Smooth muscle spasm and pain.*

**Amcort** Keene, USA.
Triamcinolone diacetate (p.1110·2).
*Corticosteroid.*

**Amc-Puren** Alpharma-Isis, Ger.
Amoxicillin trihydrate (p.155·3).
*Bacterial infections.*

**AMD**
Seroyal, Canad.†.
Trace element preparation with vitamin C (p.1417·1).
NBF-Lanes, Ital.†.
Lutein; betacarotene; vitamin C; vitamin E; nicotinic acid; licophene; carrot extract (p.1417·1).
*Macular degeneration in the elderly.*

**Amdipin** Labomed, Chile.
Amlodipine besilate (p.862·1).
*Hypertension; ischaemic heart disease.*

**Amdox-Puren** Alpharma-Isis, Ger.
Doxycycline hyclate (p.206·2); ambroxol hydrochloride (p.1114·3).
*Respiratory-tract infections with viscous mucus.*

**Amebamagma** John Wyeth, India.
Tinidazole (p.617·1).
*Amoebiasis; giardiasis; trichomoniasis.*

**Ameblin** Berman, Mex.
Metronidazole benzoate (p.607·2).
*Amoebiasis; anaerobic bacterial infections; giardiasis; trichomoniasis.*

**Amebyl** Offenbach, Mex.
Metronidazole (p.607·2); diiodohydroxyquinoline (p.603·3).
*Amoebiasis; bacterial infections; giardiasis.*

**Amebysol** Rayere, Mex.
Tinidazole (p.617·1).
*Amoebiasis; giardiasis; trichomoniasis.*

**Ameclina** Offenbach, Mex.
Amoxicillin trihydrate (p.155·3).
*Bacterial infections.*

**Amedran** Pharmedia (Φαρμεντια), Gr.
Gemfibrozil (p.923·1).
*Hyperlipidaemias.*

**Amefin** Searle, Mex.
Quinfamide (p.615·2).
*Amoebiasis.*

**Amefur** Fustery, Mex.
Quinfamide (p.615·2).
*Amoebiasis.*

**Amekrin**
Pfizer, Denm.; Pfizer, Fin.; Warner-Lambert, Norw.†; Pfizer, Swed.
Amsacrine (p.527·3).
*Acute leukaemias.*

**Amen** Carnrick, USA.
Medroxyprogesterone acetate (p.1557·2).
*Abnormal uterine bleeding; secondary amenorrhoea.*

**Amender** Serral, Mex.
Methyldopa (p.953·2).
*Hypertension.*

**Amenicil** Phoenix, Arg.
Hypericum (p.299·1).
*Depression.*

**Amenite A** Amenite, Arg.
Vitamin A (p.1451·2).
*Skin disorders.*

**Amenite Cap** Amenite, Arg.
Pyrithione zinc (p.1156·2).
*Scalp disorders.*

**Amenite E** Amenite, Arg.
Collagen (p.1674·3); elastin.
*Skin disorders.*

**Amenox** Sanofi Synthelabo, Mex.
Quinfamide (p.615·2).
*Amoebiasis.*

**Amerge**
GlaxoSmithKline, Canad.; Glaxo Wellcome, USA.
Naratriptan hydrochloride (p.470·1).
*Migraine.*

**Americaine** Novartis Consumer, USA.
Benzocaine (p.1370·3).
*Anorectal disorders.*

**Americaine Anesthetic** Celltech, USA.
Benzocaine (p.1370·3).
*Local anaesthesia; lubrication.*

**Americaine First Aid** Fisons, USA.
Benzocaine (p.1370·3); benzethonium chloride (p.1169·2).
*Skin disorders.*

**Americaine Otic** Celltech, USA.
Benzocaine (p.1370·3).
*Pain and pruritus in otitis.*

**Americet** MCR, USA.
Paracetamol (p.76·2); caffeine (p.782·1); butalbital (p.673·3).
*Pain.*

**Ameride** Bristol-Myers Squibb, Spain.
Amiloride hydrochloride (p.858·2); hydrochlorothiazide (p.933·2).
*Hepatic cirrhosis with ascites; hypertension; oedema.*

**Amerifed** AMBI, USA.
Pseudoephedrine hydrochloride (p.1129·2); chlorphenamine maleate (p.427·3).

**Amerigel** Amerx, USA.
*Lotion:* Oak (p.1722·3).
*Nappy rash.*
*Ointment:* Oak bark (p.1722·3); meadowsweet (p.1710·1); zinc acetate (p.1469·2).
*Skin disorders.*

**Amerituss AD** AMBI, USA.
Dextromethorphan hydrobromide (p.1117·3); chlorphenamine maleate (p.427·3); phenylephrine hydrochloride (p.1126·3).

**Amermycin** Unison, Thai.
Doxycycline (p.206·2).
*Bacterial infections.*

**Amersan** Austroplant, Austria.
Agrimony herb (p.1649·1); achillea (p.1646·2); peppermint oil (p.1283·2); rose fruit (p.1740·1); berberis; black currant (p.1661·1); myrtillus (p.1718·3).
*Liver and biliary tract disorders.*

**Amerscan DMSA** Nycomed Amersham, UK.
Technetium-99m succimer (p.1525·2).
*Radionuclide imaging of the kidney.*

**Amerscan Hepatate**
Activa, Braz.†.
Technetium-99m stannous fluoride (p.1525·2).
*Diagnostic agent.*
Nycomed Amersham, UK.
Technetium-99m colloidal tin (p.1525·2).
*Radionuclide imaging of the liver and spleen.*

**Amerscan Medronate** Nycomed Amersham, UK.
Technetium-99m medronate (p.1525·2).
*Bone scintigraphy.*

**Amerscan Pentetate** Nycomed Amersham, UK.
Technetium-99m pentetate (p.1525·2).
*Assessment of renal function; radionuclide imaging of the brain and lungs; studies of gastro-oesophageal reflux and gastric emptying.*

**Amerscan Pulmonate** Nycomed Amersham, UK.
Technetium-99m (p.1525·2) labelled albumin aggregates.
*Scintigraphic imaging of the lung.*

**Amerscan Stannous** Nycomed Amersham, UK.
Technetium-99m stannous medronate (p.1525·2).
*Red blood cell labelling for blood pool scintigraphy.*

**Amertec** Nycomed Amersham, UK.
Technetium-99m (p.1525·2) as sodium pertechnetate.
*Radionuclide imaging.*

**A-Methapred**
Abbott, Israel.
Methylprednisolone (p.1106·1).
*Corticosteroid.*
Abbott, USA.
Methylprednisolone sodium succinate (p.1106·2).
*Corticosteroid.*

**Ametic** Aspen, S.Afr.†.
Metoclopramide hydrochloride (p.1274·3).
*Gastrointestinal disorders.*

**Ametionin** Piam, Ital.†.
Food for special diets (p.1417·1).
*Homocystinuria.*

**Ametop**
Smith & Nephew, Canad.
Tetracaine hydrochloride (p.1385·1).
*Local anaesthesia.*
Smith & Nephew, Hong Kong; Smith & Nephew, Irl.; Smith & Nephew, NZ; Smith & Nephew, S.Afr.†; Smith & Nephew Healthcare, UK.
Tetracaine (p.1385·1).
*Local anaesthesia.*

**Ametricid** Medix, Mex.
Tinidazole (p.617·1).
*Amoebiasis; giardiasis; trichomoniasis.*

**Ametycine**
Sanofi Synthelabo, Fr.; Biosyn, Ger.
Mitomycin (p.573·3).
*Malignant neoplasms.*

**Ameu** Democal, Switz.
Omega-3 triglycerides (p.976·1).
*Hyperlipidaemias.*

**Amevive** Biogen, USA.
Alefacept (p.1141·2).
*Psoriasis.*

**Amfamox** Amrad, Austral.
Famotidine (p.1265·2).
*Gastro-oesophageal reflux; peptic ulcer; Zollinger-Ellison syndrome.*

**Amfipen**
Yamanouchi, Irl.†; Yamanouchi, UK†.
Ampicillin (p.157·1).
*Bacterial infections.*

**Amfostat**
Bristol-Myers Squibb, Arg.; Bristol-Myers Squibb, Mex.
Amphotericin B (p.391·2).
*Fungal infections; leishmaniasis.*

**Amgenal Cough** *Goldline, USA.*
Bromazine hydrochloride (p.425·3); codeine phosphate (p.27·1).
*Coughs and cold symptoms.*

**Amgrip** *Collins, Mex.*
Caffeine (p.782·1); dextromethorphan (p.1117·3); phenylephrine (p.1126·3); chlorphenamine (p.428·1); moroxydine hydrochloride (p.649·3).
*Cold and influenza symptoms.*

**Amias** *AstraZeneca, UK; Takeda, UK.*
Candesartan cilexetil (p.878·3).
*Hypertension.*

**Amicacil** *Teuto, Braz.*
Amikacin sulfate (p.154·1).
*Bacterial infections.*

**Amicalin** *Royton, Braz.*
Amikacin (p.154·1).
*Bacterial infections.*

**Amicaliq** *Tanabe, Jpn.*
Amino-acid, carbohydrate, and electrolyte infusion (p.1417·1).
*Parenteral nutrition.*

**Amicar**
*Wyeth, Austral.; Wyeth-Ayerst, Canad.; Wyeth, Mex.; Wyeth, NZ; Wyeth, S.Afr.†; Immunex, USA.*
Aminocaproic acid (p.741·3).
*Fibrinolysis.*

**Amicasil**
*Phoinix Pharm (Φοινιξ Φαρμ), Gr.; Pharmatex, Ital.*
Amikacin sulfate (p.154·1).
*Bacterial infections.*

**Amicel** *Salus, Ital.†.*
Econazole nitrate (p.397·2).
*Fungal infections.*

**Amicic**
*Novartis Ophthalmics, Fr.; Ciba Vision, Switz.†.*
Amino-acid preparation (p.1417·1).
*Corneal ulcers.*

**Amicilon** *Ariston, Braz.*
Amikacin sulfate (p.154·1).
*Bacterial infections.*

**Amicin** *Biochem, India.*
Amikacin sulfate (p.154·1).
*Bacterial infections.*

**Amicla** *Wyeth Lederle, Belg.*
Amcinonide (p.1091·1).
*Skin disorders.*

**Amiclair** *Abatron, UK.*
Enzymatic contact lens cleanser (p.1164·2).

**Amiclav** *Ashbourne, UK.*
Amoxicillin trihydrate (p.155·3); potassium clavulanate (p.193·3).
These ingredients can be described by the British Approved Name Co-amoxiclav.
*Bacterial infections.*

**Amico** *SIT, Ital.*
Amino-acid preparation with cobamamide (p.1417·1).
*Tonic.*

**Amico-L** *TO-Chemicals, Thai.*
Aluminium hydroxide (p.1249·2); magnesium hydroxide (p.1272·2); simeticone (p.1289·2).
*Dyspepsia; flatulence; gastric hyperacidity; peptic ulcer.*

**Amicose** *Igefarma, Braz.†.*
Miconazole nitrate (p.405·3).
*Fungal infections.*

**Amicrobin** *Quimifar, Spain.*
Norfloxacin (p.238·3).
*Genito-urinary tract infections.*

**Amidal** *Douglas, Austral.†.*
Amiloride hydrochloride (p.858·2).
*Hepatic cirrhosis with ascites; hypertension; oedema.*

**Amidalin** *Hexal, Braz.*
Tyrothricin (p.275·1); benzocaine (p.1370·3).
*Mouth and throat disorders.*

**Amidate** *Abbott, USA.*
Etomidate (p.1299·1).
*General anaesthesia.*

**Amidiaz** *Richmond, Arg.*
Morphine (p.60·1).
*Pain.*

**Amidona** *Grunenthal, Chile.*
Methadone hydrochloride (p.57·2).
*Opioid withdrawal; pain.*

**Amidonal** *PCR, Ger.†.*
Aprindine hydrochloride (p.864·2).
*Arrhythmias.*

**Amidox** *Berk, UK†.*
Amiodarone hydrochloride (p.859·2).
*Arrhythmias.*

**Amidrin** *Fardi, Spain.*
Xylometazoline hydrochloride (p.1132·2).
Formerly contained ephedrine hydrochloride and sulfanilamide.
*Nasal congestion; sinus congestion.*

**Amigdagen** *Prodotti, Braz.*
Neomycin sulfate (p.235·1); tyrothricin (p.275·1); benzocaine (p.1370·3); menthol (p.1711·3).
*Mouth and throat disorders.*

**Amigdalol** *Delta, Braz.*
Tyrothricin (p.275·1); cetrimonium bromide (p.1173·1); vitamin C (p.1460·2); lidocaine (p.1377·3).
*Mouth and throat disorders.*

**Amigdamicin** *Sedabel, Braz.*
Neomycin sulfate (p.235·1); tyrothricin (p.275·1); benzocaine (p.1370·3); menthol (p.1711·3).
*Mouth and throat disorders.*

**Amigdobis** *Chinoin, Mex.*
Acetic acid (p.1645·2).

**Amigesic** *Amide, USA.*
Salsalate (p.88·1).
*Fever; inflammation; pain.*

**Ami-Hydrotride** *Upha, Malaysia.*
Amiloride hydrochloride (p.858·2); hydrochlorothiazide (p.933·2).
*Hypertension; oedema.*

**Amikafur** *Fustery, Mex.*
Amikacin sulfate (p.154·1).
*Bacterial infections.*

**Amikal** *Gea, Denm.*
Amiloride hydrochloride (p.858·2).
*Hypertension; oedema.*

**Amikalem** *Lemery, Mex.*
Amikacin sulfate (p.154·1).
*Bacterial infections.*

**Amikan**
*Anpharm (Ανφαρμ), Gr.; SoSe, Ital.*
Amikacin sulfate (p.154·1).
*Bacterial infections.*

**Amikasol** *Samakeephaesaj, Thai.*
Amikacin sulfate (p.154·1).
*Bacterial infections.*

**Amikasons** *Sons, Mex.*
Amikacin sulfate (p.154·1).
*Bacterial infections.*

**Amikavi** *Mavi, Mex.*
Amikacin (p.154·1).
*Bacterial infections.*

**Amikayect** *Grossman, Mex.*
Amikacin sulfate (p.154·1).
*Bacterial infections.*

**Amikin**
*Bristol-Myers Squibb, Austral.; Cibran, Braz.†; Bristol, Canad.; Bristol-Myers Squibb, Hong Kong; Bristol-Myers Squibb, Irl.; Bristol-Myers Squibb, Israel; Bristol-Myers Squibb, Malaysia; Bristol-Myers Squibb, Mex.; Bristol-Myers Squibb, NZ; Bristol-Myers Squibb, S.Afr.; Bristol-Myers Squibb, Singapore; Bristol-Myers Squibb, Thai.; Bristol-Myers Squibb, UK; Apothecon, USA.*
Amikacin sulfate (p.154·1).
*Bacterial infections.*

**Amikine** *Bristol-Myers Squibb, Switz.*
Amikacin sulfate (p.154·1).
*Bacterial infections.*

**Amiklin** *Bristol-Myers Squibb, Fr.*
Amikacin sulfate (p.154·1).
*Bacterial infections.*

**Amilamont** *Rosemont, UK.*
Amiloride hydrochloride (p.858·2).
*Heart failure; hepatic cirrhosis with ascites; hypertension.*

**Amilande** *Sanofi Synthelabo, Spain.*
Amisulpride (p.669·3).
*Schizophrenia.*

**Amilco**
*OBA, Denm.; Ivax, Hong Kong; Ivax, Irl.*
Amiloride hydrochloride (p.858·2); hydrochlorothiazide (p.933·2).
*Hepatic cirrhosis with ascites; hypertension; oedema.*

**Amil-Co** *Ivax, UK.*
Amiloride hydrochloride (p.858·2); hydrochlorothiazide (p.933·2).
These ingredients can be described by the British Approved Name Co-amilozide.
*Ascites; heart failure; hepatic cirrhosis; hypertension.*

**Amilene** *Tecnofarma, Chile.*
Ondansetron (p.1281·1).
*Nausea and vomiting.*

**Amilhydrozide** *Douglas, Thai.†; TTN, Thai.†.*
Amiloride hydrochloride (p.858·2); hydrochlorothiazide (p.933·2).
*Hepatic cirrhosis with ascites and oedema; hypertension; oedema.*

**Amilide** *Ranbaxy, Thai.†.*
Amiloride hydrochloride (p.858·2); hydrochlorothiazide (p.933·2).
*Heart failure; hypertension.*

**Amilin** *Hua, Thai.*
Ampicillin trihydrate (p.157·2).
*Bacterial infections.*

**Amilit-IFI** *IFI, Ital.†.*
Amitriptyline hydrochloride (p.280·3).
*Depression.*

**Amilmaxco** *Ashbourne, UK†.*
Amiloride hydrochloride (p.858·2); hydrochlorothiazide (p.933·2).
These ingredients can be described by the British Approved Name Co-amilozide.
*Ascites; heart failure; hypertension.*

**Amilo-basan** *Schonenberger, Switz.*
Amiloride hydrochloride (p.858·2); hydrochlorothiazide (p.933·2).
*Hypertension; liver cirrhosis with ascites; oedema.*

**Amilocomp beta** *Betapharm, Ger.*
Amiloride hydrochloride (p.858·2); hydrochlorothiazide (p.933·2).
*Hypertension; oedema.*

**Amiloferm** *Nordic, Swed.*
Amiloride hydrochloride (p.858·2); hydrochlorothiazide (p.933·2).
*Hypertension; liver cirrhosis with ascites; oedema.*

**Amilohyd** *Gerard, Denm.†.*
Amiloride (p.858·3); hydrochlorothiazide (p.933·2).
*Hypertension; oedema.*

**Amiloral/HCT** *Aliud, Austria.*
Amiloride hydrochloride (p.858·2); hydrochlorothiazide (p.933·2).
*Heart failure; hypertension; liver cirrhosis with ascites; oedema.*

**Amiloretic** *Aspen, S.Afr.*
Amiloride hydrochloride (p.858·2); hydrochlorothiazide (p.933·2).
*Hypertension; oedema.*

**Amiloretik**
*Hexal, Austria; Hexal, Ger.*
Amiloride hydrochloride (p.858·2); hydrochlorothiazide (p.933·2).
*Hypertension; liver cirrhosis with ascites; oedema.*

**Amilorid comp**
*Genericon, Austria; Heumann, Ger.; Ratiopharm, Ger.; Upsamedica, Switz.†.*
Amiloride hydrochloride (p.858·2); hydrochlorothiazide (p.933·2).
*Hypertension; liver cirrhosis with ascites; oedema.*

**Amiloride Composto** *Ratiopharm, Port.*
Amiloride hydrochloride (p.858·2); hydrochlorothiazide (p.933·2).

**Amilorid/HCT**
*Tyrol, Austria; Aliud, Ger.; Atid, Ger.*
Amiloride hydrochloride (p.858·2); hydrochlorothiazide (p.933·2).
*Heart failure; hypertension; liver cirrhosis with ascites; oedema.*

**Amilostad HCT** *Stada, Austria.*
Amiloride hydrochloride (p.858·2); hydrochlorothiazide (p.933·2).
*Hypertension; liver cirrhosis with ascites; oedema.*

**Amilozid** *CT, Ger.*
Amiloride hydrochloride (p.858·2); hydrochlorothiazide (p.933·2).
*Hypertension; oedema.*

**Amimox**
*Tika, Norw.†.*
Amoxicillin (p.155·3).
*Bacterial infections.*

*Tika, Swed.*
Amoxicillin trihydrate (p.155·3).
*Bacterial infections; peptic ulcer associated with Helicobacter pylori.*

**Amin 21 K** *Italfarmacia, Ital.*
Amino-acid preparation with potassium (p.1417·1).
*Nutritional supplement.*

**Amin-Aid**
*McGaw, NZ†; R&D, USA.*
Preparation for enteral nutrition in renal failure (p.1417·1).

**Amindan** *Desitin, Ger.*
Selegiline hydrochloride (p.1214·1).
*Parkinsonism.*

**Aminess**
*Recip, Denm.†; Pharmacia Upjohn, Neth.†; Clintec, USA.*
Amino-acid infusion (p.1417·1).
*Parenteral nutrition in renal impairment.*

*Pharmacia, Hong Kong; Recip, Norw.; Recip, Swed.*
Amino-acid preparation (p.1417·1).
*Nutritional supplement in renal failure.*

**Aminess-N** *Recip, Fin.*
Amino-acid preparation (p.1417·1).
*Dietary supplement.*

**Amineurin** *Hexal, Ger.*
Amitriptyline hydrochloride (p.280·3).
*Depression; pain.*

**Amino** *Natural Life, Arg.*
Amino-acid preparation (p.1417·1).
*Dietary supplement.*

**Amino 3** *Fiori, Ital.*
Amino-acid preparation (p.1417·1).

**Amino MS** *Larkhall Laboratories, UK†.*
Alanine (p.1421·1); lysine hydrochloride (p.1439·2); glutamic acid hydrochloride (p.1433·2); tyrosine (p.1451·1).

**Amino PG** *Cantassium Co., UK†.*
Amino-acid and zinc preparation (p.1417·1).

**Amino-Cerv**
*Milex, Canad.; Milex, USA.*
Cystine (p.1426·3); inositol (p.1701·2); methionine (p.1042·1); sodium propionate (p.408·1); urea (p.1162·2).
*Cervicitis; post cauterisation; post conisation; post cryosurgery; postpartum cervical tears.*

**Aminocid** *Faria, Braz.*
Dipyrone (p.35·3); thiamine (p.1455·2); pyridoxine (p.1457·2); cyanocobalamin (p.1458·2).
*Neuritis.*

**Aminocina** *Biochimico, Braz.*
Amikacin sulfate (p.154·1).
*Bacterial infections.*

**Aminocont** *Mundipharma, Fin.*
Aminophylline hydrate (p.780·2).
*Obstructive airways disease.*

**Aminodrip** *Wockhardt, India.*
Amino-acid infusion (p.1417·1).
*Parenteral nutrition.*

**Aminoefedrison NF** *Rhein, Mex.*
Theophylline (p.798·3); ambroxol hydrochloride (p.1114·3).
*Respiratory-tract disorders with viscous mucus.*

**Aminofilin** *Phoenix, Arg.*
Theophylline (p.798·3).
*Obstructive airways disease.*

**Aminoflex** *Braun, Switz.†.*
Amino-acid and electrolyte infusion (p.1417·1).
*Parenteral nutrition.*

**Aminofluid** *Otsuka, Jpn.*
Amino-acid, carbohydrate, and electrolyte infusion (p.1417·1).
*Parenteral nutrition.*

**Aminofusin Hepar** *Baxter, Ger.*
Amino-acid and electrolyte infusion (p.1417·1).
*Parenteral nutrition in liver disorders.*

**Aminofusin L kohlenhydratfrei** *Fresenius Kabi, Austria†.*
Amino-acid, electrolyte, and pyridoxine hydrochloride infusion (p.1417·1).
*Parenteral nutrition.*

**Aminofusin N** *Baxter, Ger.*
Amino-acid, xylitol, and electrolyte infusion (p.1417·1).
*Parenteral nutrition.*

**Aminofusin 10% Plus** *Baxter, Ger.*
Amino-acid and electrolyte infusion (p.1417·1).
*Parenteral nutrition.*

**Aminogran**
*UCB, Austral.; UCB, Irl.; Euromed, Ital.; Pharmabroker, NZ; UCB, Swed.; UCB, UK.*
Food for special diets (p.1417·1).
*Phenylketonuria.*

**Aminogran Mineral Mixture**
*UCB, Austral.; UCB, Irl.*
Mineral preparation (p.1417·1).
*Mineral supplement; phenylketonuria (in conjunction with Aminogran).*

**Aminoima** *IMA, Braz.*
Aminophylline (p.780·2).
*Obstructive airways disease.*

**Aminoleban**
*Otsuka, Hong Kong; Otsuka, Jpn; Thai Otsuka, Thai.*
Amino-acid infusion (p.1417·1).
*Parenteral nutrition in hepatic encephalopathy and liver disorders.*

**Aminoleban EN**
*Otsuka, Hong Kong; Otsuka, Jpn; Thai Otsuka, Thai.*
Preparation for enteral nutrition (p.1417·1).
*Hepatic encephalopathy; liver failure.*

**Aminoliv** *Teuto, Braz.*
Aminophylline (p.780·2).
*Obstructive airways disease.*

**Aminomal**
*Malesci, Ital.*
*Delayed-release tablets; injection; suppositories; tablets:* Aminophylline (p.780·2).
Lidocaine hydrochloride (p.1377·3) is included in the intramuscular injection to alleviate the pain of injection; lidocaine (p.1377·3) is also included in the suppositories.
*Elixir:* Theophylline (p.798·3).
*Obstructive airways disease.*

*Menarini, Switz.†.*
Aminophylline (p.780·2).
*Obstructive airways disease.*

**Aminomega** *Larkhall Laboratories, UK†.*
Amino-acid preparation (p.1417·1).

**Aminomel** *Baxter, Ger.†.*
Amino-acid infusion (p.1417·1).
*Parenteral nutrition.*

**Aminomel E** *Baxter, Ger.†.*
Amino-acid and electrolyte infusion (p.1417·1).
*Parenteral nutrition.*

**Aminomel X-E** *Baxter, Ger.*
Amino-acid, carbohydrate, and electrolyte infusion (p.1417·1).
*Parenteral nutrition.*

**Amino-Mel G** *Fresenius Kabi, Austria.*
Amino-acid, electrolyte, and glucose infusion (p.1417·1).
*Parenteral nutrition.*

**Amino-Mel hepa** *Fresenius Kabi, Austria.*
Amino-acid and electrolyte infusion (p.1417·1).
*Parenteral nutrition in liver disease.*

**Amino-Mel nephro** *Fresenius Kabi, Austria.*
Amino-acid infusion (p.1417·1).
*Parenteral nutrition in renal disease.*

**Aminomel nephro** *Baxter, Ger.*
Amino-acid infusion (p.1417·1).
*Parenteral nutrition in renal impairment.*

**Amino-Min-D** *Tyson, USA.*
Calcium with vitamin D and minerals (p.1417·1).
*Calcium deficiency; dietary supplement.*

**Aminomix**
*Fresenius Kabi, Austria; Fresenius Kabi, Fr.; Fresenius-Klinik, Ger.; Fresenius Kabi, Norw.; Fresenius Kabi, Spain; Meda, Swed.†; Fresenius Kabi, Switz.*
A range of amino-acid and carbohydrate infusions with or without electrolytes (p.1417·1).
*Parenteral nutrition.*

*Fresenius Kabi, Gr.*
Amino-acid infusion (p.1417·1).
*Parenteral nutrition.*

Fresenius Kabi, Port.
Amino-acid and electrolyte infusion (p.1417·1).
*Parenteral nutrition.*

**Aminomux** Gador, Arg.
Disodium pamidronate (p.773·3).
*Hypercalcaemia of malignancy; osteolysis of malignancy; osteoporosis; Paget's disease of bone.*

**Amino-Opti-C** Tyson, USA.
Lemon bioflavonoids (p.1688·2); rutoside (p.1688·2); hesperidin (p.1688·2); vitamin C (p.1460·2); rose hips (p.1740·1).
*Capillary bleeding.*

**Amino-Opti-E** Tyson, USA†.
Vitamin E (p.1464·3).
*Vitamin E deficiency.*

**Aminopad**
Fresenius Kabi, Austria; Baxter, Ger.
Amino-acid infusion (p.1417·1).
*Parenteral nutrition.*

**Aminopan** UCB, Ger.
Somatostatin acetate (p.1339·3).
*Gastrointestinal haemorrhage; postoperative pancreatic disorders.*

**Aminoped** Fresenius, Braz.†.
Amino-acid infusion (p.1417·1).
*Parenteral nutrition.*

**Aminoplasmal**
Braun, Arg.; Braun, Austria; Braun, Chile; Braun, Denm.; Braun, Fin.; Braun, Hong Kong; Braun, Irl.†; Braun, Israel; Braun Melsungen, Ital.; Braun, Norw.†; Braun, Port.; Braun, Singapore; Braun, Spain; Braun, Swed.; Braun, Thai.; Braun, UK.
A range of amino-acid infusions with or without electrolytes (p.1417·1).
*Parenteral nutrition.*

**Aminoplasmal E kohlenhydratfrei** Braun, Ger.
Amino-acid and electrolyte infusion (p.1417·1).
*Parenteral nutrition.*

**Aminoplasmal elektrolyt- und kohlenhydratfrei** Braun, Ger.
Amino-acid infusion (p.1417·1).
*Parenteral nutrition.*

**Aminoplasmal Hepa**
Braun, Ger.; Bioser (Βιοσερ), Gr.
Amino-acid infusion (p.1417·1).
*Parenteral nutrition.*

**Aminoplasmal L-5, L-10** Bioser (Βιοσερ), Gr.
Amino-acid infusion (p.1417·1).
*Parenteral nutrition.*

**Aminoplasmal PO** Braun, Ger.
Amino-acid and electrolyte infusion (p.1417·1).
*Parenteral nutrition.*

**Aminoplex** Sidus, Arg.
Amino acids; vitamin B substances (p.1417·1).
*Dietary supplement.*

**Aminoplex 12** Geistlich, UK†.
Amino acid and electrolyte infusion (p.1417·1).
*Parenteral nutrition.*

**Aminoplex 24** Geistlich, UK†.
Amino-acid infusion with or without electrolytes (p.1417·1).
*Parenteral nutrition.*

**Aminopt** Sigma, Austral.
Aminoacridine hydrochloride (p.1165·3).
*Eye infections.*

**Aminoram** Fresenius Kabi, Ital.
Food for special diets (p.1417·1).
*Liver disorders.*

**Aminorell** Sanorell, Ger.†.
Amino-acid and trace element preparation (p.1417·1).

**Aminosol**
Abbott, Mex.; Thai Otsuka, Thai.
Amino-acid infusion with or without electrolytes (p.1417·1).
*Parenteral nutrition.*

**Aminosolut** DeltaSelect, Ger.
Amino-acid, carbohydrate, and electrolyte infusion (p.1417·1).
*Parenteral nutrition.*

**Aminostab** Fresenius Kabi, Fr.
Amino-acid infusion (p.1417·1).
*Parenteral nutrition.*

**Aminosteril**
Roux-Ocefa, Arg.; Fresenius Kabi, Austria; Fresenius, Braz.†; Fresenius Kabi, Denm.†; Baxter, Fin.; Fresenius Kabi, Mex.; Fresenius Kabi, Spain; Fresenius Kabi, Switz.; Fresenius Kabi, Thai.; Fresenius Kabi, UK†.
A range of amino-acid infusions with or without electrolytes (p.1417·1).
*Parenteral nutrition.*

**Aminosteril 15%** Fresenius Kabi, Ger.†.
Amino-acid infusion (p.1417·1).
*Parenteral nutrition.*

**Aminosteril KE elektrolyt- u. kohlenhydratfreiM** Fresenius Kabi, Ger.†.
Amino-acid infusion (p.1417·1).
*Parenteral nutrition.*

**Aminosteril KE kohlenhydratfrei** Fresenius Kabi, Ger.†.
Amino-acid and electrolyte infusion (p.1417·1).
*Parenteral nutrition.*

**Aminosteril N-Hepa**
Fresenius Kabi, Ger.
Amino-acid infusion (p.1417·1).
*Parenteral nutrition in liver disease.*

Fresenius Kabi, Hong Kong.
Amino-acid infusion (p.1417·1).
*Parenteral nutrition in liver failure.*

**Aminosteril plus** Fresenius Kabi, Ger.
Amino-acid and electrolyte infusion (p.1417·1).
*Parenteral nutrition.*

**Aminostress** Lafare, Ital.
Nutritional supplement (p.1417·1).

**Aminosyn**
Abbott, Canad.†; Abbott, USA.
A range of amino-acid infusions with or without glucose and electrolytes (p.1417·1).
*Parenteral nutrition.*

**Aminoterapia** Defuen, Arg.
*Cream:* Vitamin A; vitamin E acetate; ceramide; amino acids (p.1417·1).
*Nail disorders.*

*Tablets:* Cystine; gelatin; cellulose (p.1417·1).
*Skin, hair, and nail disorders.*

**Aminoterapia M** Defuen, Arg.
Cystine; gelatin (p.1417·1).
*Skin, hair, and nail disorders.*

**Aminotool** Volchem, Ital.
Amino-acid preparation (p.1417·1).

**Aminotox** Teuto, Braz.
Adenosine (p.851·2); methionine (p.1042·1); betaine hydrochloride (p.1660·2); choline citrate (p.1424·3); pyridoxine hydrochloride (p.1456·3).
*Liver disorders.*

**Aminotrans** GHP, Thai.
Amino-acid infusion (p.1417·1).
*Parenteral nutrition.*

**Aminotril** Progest, Ital.†.
*Lotion:* Triaminodil; vitamin A palmitate (p.1453·1).
*Shampoo:* Pyrithione zinc (p.1156·2); Triaminodil.
*Hair loss; seborrhoeic dermatitis.*

**Aminotripa** Otsuka, Jpn.
Amino-acid, carbohydrate, and electrolyte infusion (p.1417·1).
*Parenteral nutrition.*

**Aminovac** Nikkho, Braz.
Allergen preparation (p.1650·1).
*Allergen immunotherapy.*

**Aminoveinte** Madariaga, Spain.
Multivitamin and amino-acid preparation (p.1417·1).
*Tonic.*

**Aminoven**
Fresenius Kabi, Austria; Fresenius Kabi, Fin.; Fresenius Kabi, Ital.; Fresenius Kabi, Port.; Fresenius Kabi, Switz.; Fresenius Kabi, UK.
Amino-acid infusion (p.1417·1).
*Parenteral nutrition.*

**Aminoven Infant**
Fresenius Kabi, Ger.; Fresenius Kabi, Switz.
Amino-acid infusion (p.1417·1).
Formerly known as Aminovenos Pad and Aminovenos Infant in *Switz.*
*Parenteral nutrition.*

**Aminovenoes N-Paed** Fresenius Kabi, Thai.
Amino-acid infusion (p.1417·1).
Formerly known as Aminovenos N-Pad.
*Parenteral nutrition.*

**Aminovenos Pad**
Fresenius, Belg.†; Fresenius-Klinik, Ger.†.
Amino-acid infusion (p.1417·1).
*Parenteral nutrition.*

**Aminovit con Carnosina** FAMA, Ital.†.
Carbohydrate, amino acids, minerals, and vitamins (p.1417·1).
*Nutritional supplement.*

**Aminoxidin**
Fada, Arg.
Ampicillin (p.157·1).
*Bacterial infections.*

**Aminoxidin Sulbactam** Fada, Arg.
Ampicillin (p.157·1); sulbactam (p.257·2).
*Bacterial infections.*

**Aminozim** Monsanto, Ital.
Amino-acid preparation (p.1417·1).
*Tonic.*

**Aminozyme** Stadmed, India.
Protein hydrolysate; vitamin B substances; zinc sulfate (p.1417·1).
*Burns; enzyme deficiency; hypoproteinaemia; nutritional supplement.*

**Aminsane** Dolisos, Fr.†.
Bladderwrack (p.1742·3); java tea (p.1702·3); meadowsweet (p.1710·1).
*Obesity.*

**Amiobal** Baldacci, Braz.
Amiodarone hydrochloride (p.859·2).
*Arrhythmias.*

**Amiobeta** Betapharm, Ger.
Amiodarone hydrochloride (p.859·2).
*Arrhythmias.*

**Amiocar** Klonal, Arg.
Amiodarone (p.859·2).
*Arrhythmias.*

**Amiod** 1A, Ger.
Amiodarone hydrochloride (p.859·2).
*Arrhythmias.*

**Amiodacore** CTI, Israel.
Amiodarone hydrochloride (p.859·2).
*Arrhythmias; heart failure.*

**Amiodar** Sigma-Tau, Ital.
Amiodarone hydrochloride (p.859·2).
*Angina pectoris; arrhythmias.*

**Amiodarex** Sanofi Synthelabo, Ger.
Amiodarone hydrochloride (p.859·2).
*Arrhythmias.*

**Amiodura** Merck dura, Ger.
Amiodarone hydrochloride (p.859·2).
*Arrhythmias.*

**Amiogamma** Worwag, Ger.
Amiodarone hydrochloride (p.859·2).
*Arrhythmias.*

**Amiohexal** Hexal, Ger.
Amiodarone hydrochloride (p.859·2).
*Arrhythmias.*

**Amiopia** Medical, Spain.
Vitamins, minerals, amino acids (p.1417·1); isoniazid (p.222·2).
*Eye disorders.*

**Amiorel** Boehringer Ingelheim, Arg.
Bromhexine hydrochloride (p.1115·3).
*Respiratory-tract disorders with increased or viscous mucus.*

**Amiorel Compuesto DM** Boehringer Ingelheim, Arg.
Bromhexine hydrochloride (p.1115·3); diphenhydramine hydrochloride (p.431·3); dextromethorphan hydrobromide (p.1117·3); ephedrine hydrochloride (p.1120·1).
*Respiratory-tract disorders.*

**Amioxid** Neuraxpharm, Ger.
Amitriptylinoxide (p.285·2).
*Depression.*

**Amiparen**
Otsuka, Jpn; Thai Otsuka, Thai.
Amino-acid infusion (p.1417·1).
*Parenteral nutrition.*

**Amiphos** Dabur, India.
Amifostine (p.1031·3).
*Radiation-associated xerostomia; reduction of nephrotoxicity due to cisplatin; reduction of neutropenia due to cyclophosphamide and cisplatin therapy for ovarian cancer.*

**Amipress** Salus, Ital.†.
Labetalol hydrochloride (p.943·3).
*Hypertension.*

**Amiretic** Biolab Sanus, Braz.
Amiloride hydrochloride (p.858·2); hydrochlorothiazide (p.933·2).
*Hypertension.*

**Amirone** Julphar, UAE.
Amiodarone hydrochloride (p.859·2).
*Arrhythmias.*

**Amisol** Medica Korea, Singapore.
Clobetasone butyrate (p.1095·3).
*Skin disorders.*

**Amitacon** Egis, Thai.
Glyceryl trinitrate (p.923·2).
*Angina pectoris.*

**Ami-Tex LA** Amide, USA†.
Phenylpropanolamine hydrochloride (p.1127·3); guaifenesin (p.1122·1).
*Coughs.*

**Amithiazide** Jean-Marie, Hong Kong.
Amiloride hydrochloride (p.858·2); hydrochlorothiazide (p.933·2).
*Hypertension; oedema.*

**Amitone**
Note. This name is used for preparations of different composition.
Unison, Hong Kong.
Ketotifen fumarate (p.788·1).
*Allergic rhinitis; asthma.*

Menley & James, USA.
Calcium carbonate (p.1254·2).
*Hyperacidity.*

**Amitrex** Sanofi Synthelabo, Port.
Amisulpride (p.669·3).
*Schizophrenia.*

**Amitrid** Leiras, Fin.
Amiloride hydrochloride (p.858·2); hydrochlorothiazide (p.933·2).
*Heart failure; hypertension; oedema.*

**Amitrip** Pacific, NZ.
Amitriptyline hydrochloride (p.280·3).
*Depression; nocturnal enuresis.*

**Amitrol** Douglas, Austral.†.
Amitriptyline hydrochloride (p.280·3).
*Depression; nocturnal enuresis.*

**Amitron** Torlan, Spain.
Amoxicillin sodium (p.155·3) or amoxicillin trihydrate (p.155·3).
*Bacterial infections.*

**Amivia** Coloplast, Fr.
Calcium alginate (p.745·1); carmellose sodium (p.1577·3).
*Ulcers; wounds.*

**Amix**
Note. A similar name is used for preparations of different composition (see below).
Ashbourne, UK.
Amoxicillin trihydrate (p.155·3).
*Bacterial infections.*

**Amixen** Microsules Bernabo, Arg.
Amoxicillin (p.155·3).
*Bacterial infections.*

**Amixen Plus** Microsules Bernabo, Arg.
Amoxicillin trihydrate (p.155·3); diclofenac potassium (p.32·1).
*Bacterial infections.*

**Amixx**
Note. A similar name is used for preparations of different composition (see above).
Krewel, Ger.
Amantadine hydrochloride (p.1197·2).
*Drug-induced extrapyramidal disorders; parkinsonism.*

**Amiyec** IQFA, Mex.
Amikacin sulfate (p.154·1).
*Bacterial infections.*

**Amiyodazol** Rimsa, Mex.†.
Metronidazole (p.607·2).

**Amiyu** Ajinomoto, Thai.
Amino-acid preparation (p.1417·1).
*Renal failure.*

**Amizal** Vida, Port.
Idebenone (p.1700·3).
*Mental impairment associated with cerebrovascular disorders.*

**Amizet 10** Tanabe, Jpn.
Amino-acid infusion (p.1417·1).
*Parenteral nutrition.*

**Amizet 10X** Tanabe, Jpn.
Amino-acid and carbohydrate infusion (p.1417·1).
*Parenteral nutrition.*

**Amizide**
Alphapharm, Austral.; Alphapharm, Malaysia; Merck, Malaysia; Pacific, NZ.
Amiloride hydrochloride (p.858·2); hydrochlorothiazide (p.933·2).
*Hypertension; liver cirrhosis with ascites; oedema.*

**AMK**
Note. This name is used for preparations of different composition.
Plantes Tropicales, Fr.†.
Glucomannan (p.1693·3); bladderwrack (p.1742·3).
*Slimming aid.*

Pisa, Mex.
Amikacin sulfate (p.154·1).
*Bacterial infections.*

**Amlactin**
Note. A similar name is used for preparations of different composition (see below).
Upsher-Smith, USA.
Ammonium lactate (p.1142·3).
*Dry skin.*

**AmLactin AP**
Note. A similar name is used for preparations of different composition (see above).
Upsher-Smith, USA.
Pramocaine hydrochloride (p.1382·2); lactic acid (p.1704·1).

**Amloc**
Pfizer, Arg.
Amlodipine besilate (p.862·1).
*Angina pectoris; hypertension.*

Bago, Chile.
Amlodipine (p.862·2).
*Angina pectoris; hypertension.*

**Amlodac** Zydus, India.
Amlodipine besilate (p.862·1).
*Angina pectoris; hypertension.*

**Amlodin** Sumitomo, Jpn.
Amlodipine besilate (p.862·1).
*Angina pectoris; hypertension.*

**Amlodine** Quesada, Arg.
Amlodipine (p.862·2).
*Angina pectoris; hypertension.*

**Amlopine** Berlin Pharm, Thai.
Amlodipine besilate (p.862·1).
*Angina pectoris; congestive heart failure; hypertension.*

**Amloprax** Teuto, Braz.
Amlodipine besilate (p.862·1).
*Hypertension.*

**Amlopres** Cipla, India.
Amlodipine besilate (p.862·1).
*Angina pectoris; hypertension.*

**Amlor**
Pfizer, Belg.; Pfizer, Fr.
Amlodipine besilate (p.862·1).
*Angina pectoris; hypertension.*

**Amlotens** Klonal, Arg.
Amlodipine (p.862·2).
*Angina pectoris; hypertension.*

**Amlovasc** Hexal, Braz.
Amlodipine besilate (p.862·1).
*Angina; hypertension.*

**Ammeltz** Kobayashi, Thai.
Methyl salicylate (p.59·3); menthol (p.1711·3); camphor (p.1665·3).
*Musculoskeletal pain; soft-tissue disorders.*

**Ammidene** Macrophar, Thai.
Piroxicam (p.84·2).
*Gout; musculoskeletal and joint disorders.*

**Ammiformin** Macrophar, Thai.
Metformin hydrochloride (p.342·3).
*Diabetes mellitus.*

**Ammi-Indocin** Macrophar, Thai.
Indometacin (p.47·3).
*Gout; musculoskeletal and joint disorders.*

**Ammilazo** *Macrophar, Thai.*
Phenazopyridine hydrochloride (p.83·1).
*Urinary-tract pain.*

**Amminac** *Macrophar, Thai.*
Diclofenac sodium (p.32·1).
*Inflammation; musculoskeletal and joint disorders; pain.*

**Ammirox** *Macrophar, Thai.*
Roxithromycin (p.254·2).
*Bacterial infections.*

**Ammitram** *Macrophar, Thai.*
Tramadol hydrochloride (p.94·3).
*Pain.*

**Ammi-Votara** *Macrophar, Thai.*
Diclofenac sodium (p.32·1).
*Musculoskeletal, joint, peri-articular, and soft-tissue disorders.*

**Ammonaps**
*Orphan, Fr.; Orphan, Ger.; Orphan, Ital.; Orphan, Spain; Orphan, UK.*
Sodium phenylbutyrate (p.1748·2).
*Urea cycle disorders.*

**Amnesteem** *Bertek, USA.*
Isotretinoin (p.1148·3).
*Acne.*

**Amniex** *Mastelli, Ital.†.*
Amniotic membrane (human) (p.1654·2).
*Skin substitute.*

**Amniolina** *Reig Jofre, Spain.*
Talc (p.1159·1); zinc oxide (p.1163·2).
*Nappy rash.*

**Amnivent** *Ashbourne, UK.*
Aminophylline (p.780·2).
*Bronchospasm.*

**AMO Endosol**
*Advanced Medical Optics, Austral.; Allergan, Braz.; Allergan, USA.*
Electrolytes (p.1217·1).
*Irrigation solution during surgery.*

**Amo Resan** *Alacan, Spain.*
Amoxicillin trihydrate (p.155·3); bromhexine hydrochloride (p.1115·3).
*Respiratory-tract infections.*

**AMO Vitrax**
*Advanced Medical Optics, Austral.; Advanced Medical Optics, NZ; Allergan, S.Afr.; AMO, Singapore; Allergan, Swed.†; Allergan, Switz.†; Allergan, Thai.†; Allergan, USA.*
Sodium hyaluronate (p.1697·3).
*Aid in ophthalmic surgery.*

**Amobay** *Bayer, Mex.*
Amoxicillin trihydrate (p.155·3).
*Bacterial infections.*

**Amobiotic** *Laboratorios Chile, Chile.*
Amoxicillin (p.155·3).
*Bacterial infections.*

**Amobronc** *Ist. Chim. Inter., Ital.*
Ambroxol hydrochloride (p.1114·3).
*Respiratory-system disorders.*

**Amocasin** *Northia, Arg.*
Salbutamol (p.791·3).
*Asthma.*

**Amocetin** *Remedina, Gr.*
Nimesulide (p.67·1).
*Inflammation; musculoskeletal disorders; pain.*

**Amocid** *Lysoform, Ger.*
Orthophenylphenol (p.1187·2).
*Surface disinfection.*

**Amocillin** *Caps, S.Afr.*
Amoxicillin sodium (p.155·3).
*Bacterial infections.*

**Amocla** *Kuhnil, Singapore.*
Amoxicillin trihydrate (p.155·3); potassium clavulanate (p.193·3).
*Bacterial infections.*

**Amoclan** *Hexal, Austria.*
Amoxicillin trihydrate (p.155·3); potassium clavulanate (p.193·3).
*Bacterial infections.*

**Amoclav**
*Hexal, Ger.*
Amoxicillin trihydrate (p.155·3); potassium clavulanate (p.193·3).
*Bacterial infections.*

*Rolab, S.Afr.*
Amoxicillin (p.155·3); clavulanic acid (p.193·3).
*Bacterial infections.*

**Amoclavam** *Merck, Port.*
Amoxicillin trihydrate (p.155·3); potassium clavulanate (p.193·3).
*Bacterial infections.*

**Amoclave** *Bial, Spain.*
Amoxicillin trihydrate (p.155·3); potassium clavulanate (p.193·3).
*Bacterial infections.*

**Amoclax** *Hexal, Austria.*
Amoxicillin trihydrate (p.155·3); potassium clavulanate (p.193·3).
*Bacterial infections.*

**Amocol** *Offenbach, Mex.*
Ambroxol (p.1114·3).
*Respiratory-tract congestion.*

**Amodex** *Bouchara-Recordati, Fr.*
Amoxicillin trihydrate (p.155·3) or amoxicillin sodium (p.155·3).
*Bacterial infections.*

**Amodivyr** *Copernico, Ital.*
Aciclovir (p.626·1).
*Herpesvirus infections.*

**Amofat** *Protein, Mex.†.*
Famotidine (p.1265·2).

**Amofil** *Veripalvelu, Fin.*
A factor VIII preparation (p.751·1).
*Factor VIII deficiency; haemophilia A.*

**Amoflamisan** *Beecham, Spain†.*
Amoxicillin trihydrate (p.155·3).
*Bacterial infections.*

**Amoflux** *Lampugnani, Ital.*
Amoxicillin trihydrate (p.155·3).
*Bacterial infections.*

**Amohexal** *Hexal, Austral.*
Amoxicillin trihydrate (p.155·3).
*Bacterial infections.*

**Amoksiklav**
*Lek, Hong Kong; Lek, Thai.*
Amoxicillin trihydrate (p.155·3); potassium clavulanate (p.193·3).
*Bacterial infections.*

**Amol Heilkrautergeist N** *Altana, Ger.*
Melissa oil (p.1711·2); clove oil (p.1673·3); cinnamon oil (p.1672·2); lemon oil (p.1706·2); peppermint oil (p.1283·2); lavender oil (p.1705·2); menthol (p.1711·3).
*Capillary disorders; gastrointestinal disorders.*

**Amolex** *Andromaco, Chile.*
Amoxicillin (p.155·3); clavulanic acid (p.193·3).
*Bacterial infections.*

**Amolgen** *Solfran, Mex.*
Paracetamol (p.76·2).
*Fever; pain.*

**Amolin**
*Note. A similar name is used for preparations of different composition (see below).*
*Ergha, Irl.*
Atenolol (p.865·2).
*Angina pectoris; arrhythmias; hypertension; myocardial infarction.*

**Am-O-Lin**
*Note. A similar name is used for preparations of different composition (see above).*
*Bayer, NZ.*
Almond oil (p.1651·1); calamine (p.1144·1); salicylic acid (p.1157·1).
*Nappy rash; skin irritation.*

**Amopen** *Yorkshire Pharmaceuticals, UK†.*
Amoxicillin (p.155·3).
*Bacterial infections.*

**Amophar** *Irex, Fr.†.*
Amoxicillin trihydrate (p.155·3).
*Bacterial infections.*

**Amoram** *Eastern Pharmaceuticals, UK.*
Amoxicillin trihydrate (p.155·3).
*Bacterial infections.*

**Amorion** *Orion, Fin.*
Amoxicillin trihydrate (p.155·3).
*Bacterial infections.*

**Amosan**
*Note. This name is used for preparations of different composition.*
*Oral-B, Austral.*
Sodium perborate (p.1192·2); sodium bitartrate.
*Inflammatory mouth disorders.*

*Oral-B, Canad.; Oral-B, USA.*
Sodium perborate (p.1192·2).
*Oral lesions.*

*Oral-B, Mex.†.*
Urea hydrogen peroxide (p.1195·3).

**Amosol** *SoSe, Ital.*
Amoxicillin trihydrate (p.155·3).
*Bacterial infections.*

**Amosyt** *Abigo, Swed.*
Dimenhydrinate (p.431·1).
*Ménière's syndrome; nausea; vertigo.*

**Amotein** *Chiesi, Spain.*
Metronidazole (p.607·2).
*Anaerobic bacterial infections.*

**Amoval** *Saval, Chile.*
Amoxicillin (p.155·3).
*Bacterial infections.*

**Amoval Duo** *Saval, Chile.*
Amoxicillin (p.155·3).
*Bacterial infections.*

**Amox**
*EMS, Braz.; KG, Ital.; Berenguer Infale, Spain†; SM, Thai.*
Amoxicillin (p.155·3) or amoxicillin trihydrate (p.155·3).
*Bacterial infections.*

**Amoxa**
*Atlantic, Hong Kong; Atlantic, Singapore; Atlantic, Thai.*
Amoxicillin trihydrate (p.155·3).
*Bacterial infections.*

**Amoxal** *Hexal, Austria.*
Amoxicillin trihydrate (p.155·3).
*Bacterial infections.*

**Amoxapen**
*Remedica, Hong Kong; Remedica, Singapore.*
Amoxicillin (p.155·3).
*Bacterial infections.*

**Amoxaren** *Areu, Spain.*
Amoxicillin trihydrate (p.155·3).
*Bacterial infections.*

**Amoxcillin** *Greater Pharma, Thai.*
Amoxicillin (p.155·3).
*Bacterial infections.*

**Amox-G** *Klonal, Arg.*
Amoxicillin (p.155·3).
*Bacterial infections.*

**Amox-G Bronquial** *Klonal, Arg.*
Amoxicillin (p.155·3); bromhexine (p.1115·3).
*Bacterial infections.*

**Amoxi**
*Arion, Arg.; Mar, Arg.; SMB, Belg.; CT, Ger.; ABZ, Ger.; 1A, Ger.; Rubiepharm, Ger.; Sanol, Ger.; Generics, Israel.*
Amoxicillin (p.155·3) or amoxicillin trihydrate (p.155·3).
*Bacterial infections.*

**Amoxi Gobens** *Normon, Spain.*
Amoxicillin sodium (p.155·3) or amoxicillin trihydrate (p.155·3).
*Bacterial infections.*

**Amoxi Gobens Mucol** *Normon, Spain.*
Amoxicillin trihydrate (p.155·3); bromhexine hydrochloride (p.1115·3).
*Respiratory-tract infections.*

**Amoxi Respiratorio** *Mar, Arg.*
Amoxicillin (p.155·3); ambroxol (p.1114·3).
*Respiratory-tract infections.*

**Amoxibacter** *Rubio, Spain.*
Amoxicillin trihydrate (p.155·3).
*Bacterial infections.*

**amoxi-basan** *Schonenberger, Switz.*
Amoxicillin (p.155·3).
*Bacterial infections.*

**Amoxibeta** *Betapharm, Ger.*
Amoxicillin trihydrate (p.155·3).
*Bacterial infections.*

**Amoxibiocin** *Orion, Ger.†.*
Amoxicillin (p.155·3).
*Bacterial infections.*

**Amoxibiot** *Hexal, Arg.*
Amoxicillin (p.155·3) or amoxicillin trihydrate (p.155·3).
*Bacterial infections.*

**Amoxibron** *Sanfer, Mex.*
Amoxicillin trihydrate (p.155·3); bromhexine hydrochloride (p.1115·3).
*Respiratory-tract infections.*

**Amoxicap** *Hovid, Singapore.*
Amoxicillin trihydrate (p.155·3).
*Bacterial infections.*

**Amoxicina** *Oriental, Arg.*
Amoxicillin (p.155·3).
*Bacterial infections.*

**Amoxiclav**
*CT, Ger.; Teva, Israel; Hovid, Malaysia; Columbia, Mex.*
Amoxicillin trihydrate (p.155·3); potassium clavulanate (p.193·3).
*Bacterial infections.*

**Amoxi-Clavulan** *Stada, Ger.*
Amoxicillin trihydrate (p.155·3); potassium clavulanate (p.193·3).
*Bacterial infections.*

**Amoxicler** *Monserrat, Arg.*
Amoxicillin trihydrate (p.155·3).
*Bacterial infections.*

**Amoxi-Cophar** *Cophar, Switz.*
Amoxicillin trihydrate (p.155·3).
*Bacterial infections.*

**Amoxid** *Kwizda, Austria†.*
Amoxicillin trihydrate (p.155·3).
*Bacterial infections.*

**Amoxidal** *Roemmers, Arg.*
Amoxicillin (p.155·3).
*Bacterial infections.*

**Amoxidal Duo** *Roemmers, Arg.*
Amoxicillin trihydrate (p.155·3).
*Bacterial infections.*

**Amoxidal Respiratorio** *Roemmers, Arg.*
Amoxicillin sodium (p.155·3) or amoxicillin trihydrate (p.155·3); ambroxol hydrochloride (p.1114·3).
*Respiratory-tract infections.*

**Amoxidal Respiratorio Duo** *Roemmers, Arg.*
Amoxicillin trihydrate (p.155·3); ambroxol hydrochloride (p.1114·3).
*Respiratory-tract infections.*

**Amoxidel** *Sanofi Synthelabo, Spain†.*
Amoxicillin trihydrate (p.155·3).
*Bacterial infections.*

**Amoxidel Bronquial** *Synthelabo, Spain†.*
Amoxicillin trihydrate (p.155·3); brovanexine hydrochloride (p.1116·1).
*Respiratory-tract infections.*

**Amoxident** *Eastern Pharmaceuticals, UK.*
Amoxicillin (p.155·3).
*Bacterial infections.*

**Amoxidil** *Cifarma, Braz.†.*
Amoxicillin (p.155·3).
*Bacterial infections.*

**Amoxi-Diolan** *Brahms, Ger.*
Amoxicillin trihydrate (p.155·3).
*Bacterial infections.*

**Amoxidoc** *Docpharm, Ger.*
Amoxicillin trihydrate (p.155·3).
*Bacterial infections.*

**Amoxidura Plus** *Merck dura, Ger.*
Amoxicillin trihydrate (p.155·3); potassium clavulanate (p.193·3).
*Bacterial infections.*

**Amoxifar** *Zambon, Braz.*
Amoxicillin trihydrate (p.155·3).
*Bacterial infections.*

**Amoxifar Balsamico** *Farmoquimica, Braz.†.*
Amoxicillin (p.155·3); bromhexine (p.1115·3).
*Bacterial infections.*

**Amoxifur** *Fustery, Mex.*
Amoxicillin trihydrate (p.155·3).
*Bacterial infections.*

**Amoxigran** *Hovid, Singapore†.*
Amoxicillin trihydrate (p.155·3).
*Bacterial infections.*

**Amoxigrand** *Ahimsa, Arg.*
Amoxicillin (p.155·3).
*Bacterial infections.*

**Amoxigrand Bronquial** *Ahimsa, Arg.*
Amoxicillin (p.155·3); ambroxol (p.1114·3).
*Respiratory-tract infections.*

**Amoxigrand Compuesto** *Ahimsa, Arg.*
Amoxicillin (p.155·3); clavulanic acid (p.193·3).
*Bacterial infections.*

**Amoxi-Hefa** *Hefa, Ger.*
Amoxicillin trihydrate (p.155·3).
*Bacterial infections.*

**Amoxihexal**
*Hexal, Austria; Hexal, Ger.*
Amoxicillin trihydrate (p.155·3).
*Bacterial infections.*

**Amoxil**
*GlaxoSmithKline, Austral.; GlaxoSmithKline, Braz.; Wyeth-Ayerst, Canad.†; SmithKline Beecham, Gr.; SmithKline Beecham, Hong Kong†; German Remedies, India; GlaxoSmithKline, Irl.; Sanfer, Mex.; GlaxoSmithKline, NZ; GlaxoSmithKline, S.Afr.; GlaxoSmithKline, Singapore; GlaxoSmithKline, Thai.; GlaxoSmithKline, UK; GlaxoSmithKline, USA.*
Amoxicillin (p.155·3), amoxicillin sodium (p.155·3), or amoxicillin trihydrate (p.155·3).
*Bacterial infections.*

**Amoxilan** *Lannacher, Austria.*
Amoxicillin trihydrate (p.155·3).
*Bacterial infections.*

**Amoxillat** *Azupharma, Ger.*
Amoxicillin trihydrate (p.155·3).
*Bacterial infections.*

**Amoxillat-Clav** *Azupharma, Ger.*
Amoxicillin trihydrate (p.155·3); potassium clavulanate (p.193·3).
*Bacterial infections.*

**Amoxillin**
*Esseti, Ital.; Alpharma, Norw.*
Amoxicillin trihydrate (p.155·3).
*Bacterial infections.*

**Amoximedical** *Medical, Spain.*
Amoxicillin trihydrate (p.155·3).
*Bacterial infections.*

**Amoxi-Mepha** *Mepha, Switz.*
Amoxicillin trihydrate (p.155·3).
*Bacterial infections.*

**Amoximerck** *Merck dura, Ger.*
Amoxicillin trihydrate (p.155·3).
*Bacterial infections.*

**Amoximex** *Medika, Switz.*
Amoxicillin trihydrate (p.155·3).
*Bacterial infections.*

**Amoxin** *Ratiopharm, Fin.*
Amoxicillin trihydrate (p.155·3).
*Bacterial infections.*

**Amoxin Comp** *Ratiopharm, Fin.*
Amoxicillin trihydrate (p.155·3); potassium clavulanate (p.193·3).
*Bacterial infections.*

**Amoxina**
*Hexal, Braz.;*
Amoxicillin (p.155·3).
*Bacterial infections.*

*Aesculapius, Ital.*
Amoxicillin trihydrate (p.155·3).
*Bacterial infections.*

**Amoxinovag** *Novag, Mex.*
Amoxicillin trihydrate (p.155·3).
*Bacterial infections.*

**Amoxi-Ped** *Stiefel, Braz.*
Amoxicillin (p.155·3).
*Bacterial infections.*

**Amoxipen**
*Biochimico, Braz.; Metopharma, Ital.†.*
Amoxicillin trihydrate (p.155·3).
*Bacterial infections.*

**Amoxipenil**
*Montpellier, Arg.; Bago, Chile.*
Amoxicillin trihydrate (p.155·3).
*Bacterial infections.*

**Amoxipenil Bronquial** *Montpellier, Arg.*
Amoxicillin trihydrate (p.155·3); ambroxol hydrochloride (p.1114·3).
*Respiratory-tract infections.*

**Amoxiplus** *Ratiopharm, Austria.*
Amoxicillin trihydrate (p.155·3); potassium clavulanate (p.193·3).
*Bacterial infections.*

**Amoxipoten** *Del Bel, Arg.*
Amoxicillin (p.155·3).
*Bacterial infections.*

**Amoxi-Puren** *Alpharma-Isis, Ger.*
Amoxicillin trihydrate (p.155·3).
*Bacterial infections.*

**Amoxisol** *Rimsa, Mex.*
Amoxicillin trihydrate (p.155·3).
*Bacterial infections.*

**Amoxistad** *Stada, Austria.*
Amoxicillin trihydrate (p.155·3).
*Bacterial infections.*

**Amoxitab** *Hovid, Singapore†.*
Amoxicillin trihydrate (p.155·3).
*Bacterial infections.*

**Amoxi-Tablinen** *Lichtenstein, Ger.*
Amoxicillin trihydrate (p.155·3).
*Bacterial infections.*

**Amoxitan** *Bunker, Braz.*
Amoxicillin (p.155·3).
*Bacterial infections.*

**Amoxitenk** *Biotenk, Arg.*
Amoxicillin (p.155·3) or amoxicillin trihydrate (p.155·3).
*Bacterial infections.*

**Amoxitenk Plus** *Biotenk, Arg.*
Amoxicillin (p.155·3); clavulanic acid (p.193·3).
*Bacterial infections.*

**Amoxitenk Respiratorio** *Biotenk, Arg.*
Amoxicillin (p.155·3); ambroxol hydrochloride (p.1114·3).
Lidocaine hydrochloride (p.1377·3) is included in the injection to alleviate the pain of injection.
*Respiratory-tract infections.*

**Amoxivan** *Khandelwal, India.*
Amoxicillin (p.155·3) or amoxicillin trihydrate (p.155·3).
*Bacterial infections.*

**Amoxivet** *ICN, Mex.*
Amoxicillin trihydrate (p.155·3).
*Bacterial infections.*

**Amoxi-Wolff** *Wolff, Ger.*
Amoxicillin trihydrate (p.155·3).
*Bacterial infections.*

**Amoxtiol** *Daker Farmasimes, Spain†.*
Amoxicillin trihydrate (p.155·3); carbocisteine (p.1116·2).
*Respiratory-tract infections.*

**Amoxy** *Shiwa, Thai.; Hua, Thai.; M & H, Thai.; PP Lab, Thai.*
Amoxicillin (p.155·3) or amoxicillin trihydrate (p.155·3).
*Bacterial infections.*

**Amoxyfizz** *Schwulst, S.Afr.†.*
Amoxicillin (p.155·3).
*Bacterial infections.*

**Amoxylin** *Biomedis, Thai.; Great Eastern, Thai.*
Amoxicillin trihydrate (p.155·3).
*Bacterial infections.*

**Amoxypen** *Grunenthal, Ger.*
Amoxicillin trihydrate (p.155·3).
*Bacterial infections.*

**Amoxyplus** *Novag, Spain.*
Amoxicillin trihydrate (p.155·3); potassium clavulanate (p.193·3).
*Bacterial infections.*

**Ampamet** *Menarini, Ital.*
Aniracetam (p.1655·1).
*Mental function impairment.*

**Amparax** *Wyeth, Chile.*
Lorazepam (p.704·1).
*Anxiety; insomnia.*

**Ampat** *Asian Pharm, Thai.†.*
Ampicillin trihydrate (p.157·2).
*Bacterial infections.*

**Ampavit** *ANB, Thai.*
Vitamin $B_{12}$ (p.1458·2).
*Megaloblastic anaemia.*

**Ampecyclal** *Sarget, Fr.; Asta Medica, Fr.*
Heptaminol adenosine phosphate (p.1697·1).
*Haemorrhoids; metrorrhagia; peripheral vascular disorders.*

**Ampex** *Pharmacos, Mex.*
Ampicillin trihydrate (p.157·2).
*Bacterial infections.*

**Ampexin** *Biolab, Thai.†.*
Ampicillin trihydrate (p.157·2).
*Bacterial infections.*

**Amphisept** *Goldschmidt, Switz.*
Alcohol (p.1166·1).
*Hand disinfection.*

**Amphisept E** *Bode, Ger.*
Alcohol (p.1166·1).
*Hand disinfection.*

**Amphocil**
*Mayne, Austral.; Torrex, Austria; Zodiac, Braz.; Alza, Denm.†; Genesis, Gr.; Mayne, Hong Kong; Alza, Irl.; Sequus, Israel; Zeneca, Ital.†; Faulding, Malaysia; Lemery, Mex.; AstraZeneca, Neth.†; Zeneca, Port.†; Alza, Singapore; Almirall, Spain; Zeneca, Swed.†; Cambridge, UK.*
Amphotericin B-sodium cholesteryl sulfate complex (p.391·2) (p.391·2).
*Fungal infections; leishmaniasis.*

**Amphocycline** *Bristol-Myers Squibb, Fr.*
Amphotericin B (p.391·2); tetracycline (p.266·2).
*Bacterial and fungal infections.*

**Amphodyn**
*Klinge, Austria.*
Etilefrine hydrochloride (p.914·1); aescin (p.1648·2).
*Circulatory disorders; hypotension.*

*Fujisawa, Ger.*
Etilefrine hydrochloride (p.914·1); aesculus (p.1648·2).
*Circulatory disorders; hypotension.*

**Amphojel**
*Whitehall, Austral.†; Axcan, Canad.; Whitehall, NZ; Aspen Consumer, S.Afr.†; Wyeth-Ayerst, USA.*
Aluminium hydroxide (p.1249·2).
*Gastrointestinal hyperacidity; hyperphosphataemia.*

**Amphojel 500** *Axcan, Canad.†.*
Aluminium hydroxide (p.1249·2); magnesium hydroxide (p.1272·2).
*Antacid.*

**Amphojel Plus** *Axcan, Canad.†.*
*Oral liquid:* Aluminium hydroxide (p.1249·2); magnesium hydroxide (p.1272·2); simeticone (p.1289·2).
*Tablets:* Aluminium hydroxide-magnesium carbonate co-dried gel (p.1250·1); magnesium hydroxide (p.1272·2); simeticone (p.1289·2).
*Antacid; flatulence.*

**Ampholysine Plus** *Peters, Fr.†.*
Polihexanide (p.1190·1); mixed amphoteric and quaternary ammonium salts.
*Instrument disinfection.*

**Ampho-Moronal**
*Bristol-Myers Squibb, Austria; Bristol-Myers Squibb, Ger.; Bristol-Myers Squibb, Switz.*
Amphotericin B (p.391·2).
*Fungal infections.*

**Ampho-Moronal V** *Bristol-Myers Squibb, Ger.†.*
Amphotericin B (p.391·2); triamcinolone acetonide (p.1110·2).
*Fungal skin infections.*

**Ampho-Moronal V L** *Bristol-Myers Squibb, Ger.†.*
Amphotericin B (p.391·2); triamcinolone acetonide (p.1110·2).
Formerly known as Ampho-Moronal V N.
*Skin disorders with fungal infection.*

**Amphosca a l'orchitine** *Lehning, Fr.*
Homoeopathic preparation.

**Amphosca a l'ovarine** *Lehning, Fr.*
Homoeopathic preparation.

**Amphosca Orchitine** *Homeocan, Canad.*
Homoeopathic preparation.

**Amphosca Ovarine** *Homeocan, Canad.*
Homoeopathic preparation.

**Amphosept BV** *Anios, Fr.†.*
Didecyldimethylammonium chloride (p.1178·3); alkylbenzylammonium chloride; alkylethylbenzylammonium chloride; alkylaminoalkyl glycine.
*Instrument disinfection.*

**Amphotec**
*Raffo, Arg.; Sequus, USA.*
Amphotericin B (p.391·2).
*Fungal infections.*

**Ampho-Vaccin intestinal** *Sanofi Winthrop, Fr.†.*
*Bifidobacterium bifidum* (p.1704·2); *Escherichia coli*; *Enterococcus faecalis* (p.1704·2); *Proteus vulgaris*; *Pseudomonas aeruginosa.*
*Diarrhoea.*

**Ampi**
*Arion, Arg.*
Ampicillin (p.157·1).
*Bacterial infections.*

*ABZ, Ger.†.*
Ampicillin trihydrate (p.157·2).
*Bacterial infections.*

**Ampibac** *CT, Ital.*
Bacampicillin hydrochloride (p.161·2).
*Bacterial infections.*

**Ampibal** *Collins, Mex.*
Ampicillin (p.157·1).
*Bacterial infections.*

**Ampi-Bis** *Northia, Arg.*
Ampicillin (p.157·1).
*Bacterial infections.*

**Ampi-Bis Plus** *Northia, Arg.*
Ampicillin (p.157·1); sulbactam (p.257·2).
*Bacterial infections.*

**Ampicap** *Hovid, Singapore†.*
Ampicillin trihydrate (p.157·2).
*Bacterial infections.*

**Ampicidar** *Columbia, Mex.*
Ampicillin (p.157·1).
*Bacterial infections.*

**Ampiciflan** *Bunker, Braz.*
Ampicillin (p.157·1).
*Bacterial infections.*

**Ampicil** *Medley, Braz.*
Ampicillin (p.157·1) or ampicillin sodium (p.157·1).
*Bacterial infections.*

**Ampicilase** *Teuto, Braz.*
Ampicillin (p.157·1) or ampicillin sodium (p.157·1).
*Bacterial infections.*

**Ampicilib** *Ibfarma, Braz.†.*
Ampicillin (p.157·1).
*Bacterial infections.*

**Ampicilon** *Delta, Braz.*
Ampicillin (p.157·1).
*Bacterial infections.*

**Ampicimax** *Royton, Braz.*
Ampicillin (p.157·1).
*Bacterial infections.*

**Ampicin** *Bristol, Canad.†.*
Ampicillin sodium (p.157·1).
*Bacterial infections.*

**Ampicler**
*Monserrat, Arg.; Heralds, Braz.†.*
Ampicillin trihydrate (p.157·2).
*Bacterial infections.*

**Ampicler com Probenecide** *Heralds, Braz.†.*
Ampicillin (p.157·1).
Probenecid (p.416·3) is included in this preparation to reduce renal tubular excretion of the antibiotic.
*Bacterial infections.*

**Ampiclox**
*GlaxoSmithKline, Hong Kong; GlaxoSmithKline, S.Afr.; GlaxoSmithKline, Thai.*
Ampicillin (p.157·1); cloxacillin (p.198·2).
*Bacterial infections.*

*GlaxoSmithKline, Irl.*
Ampicillin sodium (p.157·1) or ampicillin trihydrate (p.157·2); cloxacillin sodium (p.198·2).
*Bacterial infections.*

**Ampiclox-D** *Sanfer, Mex.*
Ampicillin (p.157·1); dicloxacillin (p.205·2).
*Bacterial infections.*

**Ampicrom** *Brasifa, Braz.†.*
Ampicillin (p.157·1).
*Bacterial infections.*

**Ampicyn**
*Aspen, Austral.*
Ampicillin sodium (p.157·1).
*Bacterial infections.*

*Siam Bheasach, Thai.*
Ampicillin (p.157·1).
*Bacterial infections.*

**Ampidrat** *Collins, Mex.*
Ampicillin (p.157·1).
*Bacterial infections.*

**Ampifar** *Farmoquimica, Braz.*
Ampicillin (p.157·1).
*Bacterial infections.*

**Ampifar Balsamico** *Farmoquimica, Braz.†.*
Ampicillin sodium (p.157·1); ampicillin benzathine (p.158·1).
Lidocaine hydrochloride (p.1377·3) is included in this preparation to alleviate the pain of injection.
*Bacterial infections.*

**Ampifen** *Malayan, Singapore.*
Ibuprofen (p.45·3).
*Musculoskeletal, joint, and soft-tissue disorders; pain.*

**Ampigen** *Fabra, Arg.*
Ampicillin sodium (p.157·1) or ampicillin trihydrate (p.157·2).
*Bacterial infections.*

**Ampigen SB** *Fabra, Arg.*
*Injection:* Ampicillin sodium (p.157·1); sulbactam sodium (p.257·2).
*Tablets:* Sultamicillin tosilate (p.264·2).
*Bacterial infections.*

**Ampigran** *Legrand, Braz.*
Ampicillin (p.157·1).
*Bacterial infections.*

**Ampigrand** *Ahimsa, Arg.*
Ampicillin (p.157·1).
*Bacterial infections.*

**Ampigrin** *Collins, Mex.*
Ampicillin (p.157·1).
*Bacterial infections.*

**Ampilevel** *Ern, Spain.*
Ampicillin benzathine (p.158·1); ampicillin sodium (p.157·1).
*Bacterial infections.*

**Ampilin**
*Atlantic, Hong Kong†; Lyka, India; Atlantic, Malaysia; Atlantic, Singapore; Atlantic, Thai.*
Ampicillin sodium (p.157·1) or ampicillin trihydrate (p.157·2).
*Bacterial infections.*

**Ampilisa** *Lisapharma, Ital.*
Ampicillin sodium (p.157·1) or ampicillin trihydrate (p.157·2).
*Bacterial infections.*

**Ampillin** *PP Lab, Thai.*
Ampicillin trihydrate (p.157·2).
*Bacterial infections.*

**Ampilon** *Loren, Mex.*
Ampicillin trihydrate (p.157·2).
*Bacterial infections.*

**Ampilong** *Uniao Quimica, Braz.†.*
Ampicillin (p.157·1).
*Bacterial infections.*

**Ampilox** *Biochem, India.*
Ampicillin (p.157·1), ampicillin sodium (p.157·1), or ampicillin trihydrate (p.157·2); cloxacillin (p.198·2) or cloxacillin sodium (p.198·2).
*Bacterial infections.*

**Ampilux** *Tubilux, Ital.*
Ampicillin sodium (p.157·1).
*Eye infections.*

**Ampimax** *Hexal, S.Afr.†.*
Ampicillin trihydrate (p.157·2).
*Bacterial infections.*

**Ampimex** *Arlex, Mex.†.*
Ampicillin (p.157·1).
*Bacterial infections.*

**Ampina** *Richmond, Arg.*
Nimodipine (p.972·3).
*Cerebrovascular disorders.*

**Ampipen**
*Wyeth, India; Caps, S.Afr.*
Ampicillin (p.157·1).
*Bacterial infections.*

**Ampiplus**
*Note. This name is used for preparations of different composition.*
*Menarini, Ital.*
Ampicillin sodium (p.157·1); dicloxacillin sodium (p.205·2).
*Bacterial infections.*

*Tecefarma, Spain.*
Ampicillin trihydrate (p.157·2).
*Bacterial infections.*

**Ampiplus Simplex** *Menarini, Ital.*
Ampicillin sodium (p.157·1).
*Bacterial infections.*

**Ampi-Quim** *Quimica y Farmacia, Mex.*
Ampicillin (p.157·1).
*Bacterial infections.*

**Ampiretard** *Cibran, Braz.†.*
Benzathine benzylpenicillin (p.162·3).
*Bacterial infections.*

**Ampiset** *Collins, Mex.*
Ampicillin (p.157·1).
*Bacterial infections.*

**Ampispectrin** *QIF, Braz.†.*
Ampicillin (p.157·1).
*Bacterial infections.*

**Ampisuspen** *Medifarma, Mex.†.*
Ampicillin (p.157·1).
*Bacterial infections.*

**Ampitab** *Hovid, Singapore†.*
Ampicillin trihydrate (p.157·2).
*Bacterial infections.*

**Ampi-Tecno** *Tecnofarma, Mex.*
Ampicillin (p.157·1).
*Bacterial infections.*

**Ampitenk** *Biotenk, Arg.*
Ampicillin (p.157·1) or ampicillin trihydrate (p.157·2).
*Bacterial infections.*

**Ampitotal** *Eurofarma, Braz.†.*
Ampicillin (p.157·1).
*Bacterial infections.*

**Ampival** *Sanval, Braz.*
Ampicillin (p.157·1).
*Bacterial infections.*

**Ampixen** *Oriental, Arg.*
Ampicillin (p.157·1).
*Bacterial infections.*

**Ampizan** *Allergan-Frumtost, Braz.†.*
Ampicillin benzathine (p.158·1); ampicillin sodium (p.157·1).
*Bacterial infections.*

**Amplacilina** *Eurofarma, Braz.*
Ampicillin sodium (p.157·1).
*Bacterial infections.*

**Amplal** *Gallia, Braz.†.*
Amoxicillin (p.155·3).
*Bacterial infections.*

**Amplamox**
*Biolab Sanus, Braz.; Tecnifar, Port.*
Amoxicillin trihydrate (p.155·3).
*Bacterial infections.*

**Amplavit** *Cimed, Braz.*
Multivitamin preparation (p.1417·1).

**Amplexol** *Sanofi Synthelabo, Port.*
Isosorbide mononitrate (p.942·1).
*Angina pectoris; heart failure; myocardial infarction.*

**Ampliactil** *Aventis, Arg.*
Chlorpromazine hydrochloride (p.675·2).
*Behaviour disorders; hiccups; nausea and vomiting; psychoses.*

**Ampliar** *Casasco, Arg.*
Atorvastatin calcium (p.866·1).
*Hypercholesterolaemia.*

**Amplibenzatin Bronquial** *Armstrong, Arg.*
1 Ampoule, ampicillin sodium (p.157·1); ampicillin benzathine (p.158·1); 1 ampoule, clonixin lysine (p.26·3); chlorphenamine maleate (p.427·3); bromhexine hydrochloride (p.1115·3).
Lidocaine hydrochloride (p.1377·3) is included in this preparation to alleviate the pain of injection.
*Respiratory-tract infections.*

**Amplictil** *Aventis, Braz.*
Chlorpromazine hydrochloride (p.675·2).
*Nausea and vomiting; premedication; psychoses; tetanus.*

**Amplidermis** *Medea, Spain.*
Acedoben (p.1645·2); allantoin (p.1141·3); chlorquinaldol (p.187·3); dexamethasone (p.1097·1); mepyramine maleate (p.437·1); vitamin F.
*Infected burns, skin ulcers, and wounds; infected skin disorders.*

**Amplifar** *Tecnifar, Port.*
Ampicillin trihydrate (p.157·2).
*Bacterial infections.*

**Ampligen**
*Note. This name is used for preparations of different composition.*
*Natus, Braz.†.*
Gentamicin (p.219·1).
*Bacterial infections.*

*HemispheRx, USA.*
Poly I.poly C (p.1733·2).
*AIDS and HIV infection; chronic fatigue syndrome; invasive metastatic melanoma; renal cell carcinoma.*

**Amplimed** *Medquimica, Braz.†.*
Ampicillin (p.157·1).
*Bacterial infections.*

**Ampliron** *Rhein, Mex.*
Amoxicillin trihydrate (p.155·3).
*Bacterial infections.*

**Amplital** *Pharmacia Upjohn, Ital.*
Ampicillin (p.157·1), ampicillin sodium (p.157·1), or ampicillin trihydrate (p.157·2).
*Bacterial infections.*

**Amplitor** *Cibran, Braz.†.*
Ampicillin (p.157·1).
*Bacterial infections.*

**Amplium**
*Note. This name is used for preparations of different composition.*
*Farmasa, Braz.*
Tinidazole (p.617·1).
*Anaerobic bacterial infections; protozoal infections.*

*Sigma-Tau, Ital.*
Ampicillin sodium (p.157·1) or ampicillin trihydrate (p.157·2); cloxacillin sodium (p.198·2).
*Bacterial infections.*

**Amplium-G** *Farmasa, Braz.*
Tinidazole (p.617·1); miconazole nitrate (p.405·3).
*Vulvovaginal infections.*

**Amplizer** *OFF, Ital.*
Ampicillin trihydrate (p.157·2).
*Bacterial infections.*

**Amplofen** *Merck, Braz.*
Ampicillin (p.157·1).
*Bacterial infections.*

**Amplomicina** *Cibran, Braz.†.*
Gentamicin sulfate (p.217·1).
*Bacterial infections.*

**Amplospec** *Biochimico, Braz.*
Ceftriaxone (p.183·3).
*Bacterial infections.*

**Amplotal** *Medley, Braz.*
Ampicillin benzathine (p.158·1); ampicillin sodium (p.157·1).
*Bacterial infections.*

**Amplozol** *Sigma, Braz.†.*
Albendazole (p.101·2).
*Worm infections.*

**Amplus**
*Note. This name is used for preparations of different composition.*
*Szama, Arg.*
Salicylic acid (p.1157·1); pilocarpine hydrochloride (p.1495·1); dexpanthenol; vitamin $B_6$.
*Scalp disorders.*

*Jagson, India.*
*Capsules; tablets:* Ampicillin trihydrate (p.157·2); cloxacillin sodium (p.198·2); lactic-acid-producing organisms (p.1704·2).
*Injection:* Ampicillin (p.157·1); cloxacillin (p.198·2).
*Bacterial infections.*

**Ampoxin** *Unichem, India.*
Ampicillin (p.157·1); cloxacillin (p.198·2).
*Bacterial infections.*

**Ampoxin-LB** *Unichem, India.*
Ampicillin trihydrate (p.157·2); cloxacillin sodium (p.198·2); lactic-acid-producing organisms (p.1704·2).
*Bacterial infections.*

**Ampra** *M & H, Thai.*
Ampicillin sodium (p.157·1) or ampicillin trihydrate (p.157·2).
*Bacterial infections.*

**Amprace** *Amrad, Austral.*
Enalapril maleate (p.909·2).
*Heart failure; hypertension.*

**Amprexyl**
*Unison, Hong Kong.*
Ampicillin trihydrate (p.157·2).
*Bacterial infections.*

*Unison, Thai.*
Ampicillin (p.157·1).
*Bacterial infections.*

**Ampro** *Nakorn, Thai.*
Ampicillin trihydrate (p.157·2).
*Bacterial infections.*

**AMS** *Salters, S.Afr.†.*
Sulfanilamide (p.263·2); acriflavinium chloride (p.1165·3); merbromin (p.1185·3).
*Wounds.*

**Amsa P-D** *Pfizer, Canad.*
Amsacrine (p.527·3).
*Acute leukaemias.*

**Amsapen** *Antibioticos, Mex.*
Ampicillin sodium (p.157·1).
*Bacterial infections.*

**Amsidine**
*Pfizer, Belg.; Parke, Davis, Fr.†; Goldshield, Irl.; Parke, Davis, Neth.; Goldshield, UK.*
Amsacrine (p.527·3).
*Acute leukaemias.*

**Amsidyl**
*Pfizer, Austral.; Godecke, Ger.; Parke, Davis, NZ†; Pfizer, Switz.*
Amsacrine (p.527·3).
*Acute leukaemias.*

**Amsupros** *Pharmacia, Arg.*
Estramustine sodium phosphate (p.551·1).
*Prostatic cancer.*

**AMT** *Acis, Ger.*
Amantadine sulfate (p.1197·2).
*Influenza; parkinsonism.*

**Amuchina** *Pisa, Mex.*
Sodium hypochlorite (p.1192·1); sodium chloride (p.1233·3).
*Mucous membrane, skin, surface, and wound disinfection.*

**Amuchina Med** *Galephar, Switz.*
Sodium chloride (p.1233·3).
*Hand, skin, and wound disinfection.*

**Amuclan** *Wolff, Ger.*
Amoxicillin trihydrate (p.155·3); potassium clavulanate (p.193·3).
*Bacterial infections.*

**Amuclean** *Amuchina, Ital.*
Benzalkonium chloride (p.1168·3).
*Burn and wound disinfection.*

**Amuctol** *Grunenthal, Arg.*
Erdosteine (p.1121·1).
*Respiratory-tract disorders with viscous mucus.*

**Amukin**
*Bristol-Myers Squibb, Belg.; Bristol-Myers Squibb, Neth.*
Amikacin sulfate (p.154·1).
*Bacterial infections.*

**Amukine** *Gifrer Barbezat, Fr.*
Sodium hypochlorite (p.1192·1); sodium chloride (p.1233·3).
*Skin, mucous membrane and wound cleansing.*

**Amukine Med** *Amuchina, Ital.*
Sodium hypochlorite (p.1192·1).
*Disinfection of burns, skin, wounds, and mucous membranes.*

**A-Mulsin** *Mucos, Ger.*
Vitamin A palmitate (p.1453·1).
*Adjunct in cytotoxic therapy or radiotherapy; keratinisation disorders; vitamin A deficiency.*

**A-Mulsion** *Seroyal, Canad.†.*
Vitamin A palmitate (p.1453·1).

**Amuno** *Merck Sharp & Dohme, Ger.†.*
Indometacin (p.47·3).
*Gout; inflammation; musculoskeletal, joint, peri-articular, and soft-tissue disorders; pain.*

**Amunovax** *Aventis Pasteur, Spain.*
A measles vaccine (Schwarz strain) (p.1623·1).
*Active immunisation.*

**Amvey** *Merck, Hong Kong.*
Zopiclone (p.729·3).
*Insomnia.*

**Amvisc**
*Johnson & Johnson, Austria†; Iolab, Israel†; MCM, S.Afr.†; Johnson & Johnson, Swed.†; Bausch & Lomb, USA.*
Sodium hyaluronate (p.1697·3).
*Aid in ophthalmic surgery.*

**AMX** *Pisa, Mex.*
Amoxicillin (p.155·3).
*Bacterial infections.*

**Amxol**
*Biolab, Hong Kong; Biolab, Malaysia; Biolab, Singapore; Biolab, Thai.*
Ambroxol hydrochloride (p.1114·3).
*Respiratory-tract disorders associated with increased or viscous mucus.*

**Amyben** *Lexon, UK.*
Amiodarone hydrochloride (p.859·2).
*Tachyarrhythmias.*

**Amycil** *Rimsa, Mex.†.*
Mebendazole (p.108·2).

**Amycor** *Lipha Sante, Fr.*
Bifonazole (p.395·1).
*Fungal skin infections.*

**Amycor Onychoset** *Lipha Sante, Fr.*
Bifonazole (p.395·1); urea (p.1162·2).
*Fungal nail infections.*

**Amydramine** *Julphar, UAE.*
Diphenhydramine hydrochloride (p.431·3); ammonium chloride (p.1115·2); sodium citrate (p.1223·2); menthol (p.1711·3).
*Coughs.*

**Amydramine II** *Julphar, UAE.*
Diphenhydramine hydrochloride (p.431·3).
*Cold symptoms; coughs; hypersensitivity reactions.*

**Amydramine Paediatric** *Julphar, UAE.*
Diphenhydramine hydrochloride (p.431·3); sodium citrate (p.1223·2); menthol (p.1711·3).
*Coughs.*

**Amygdol** *Knoll, Fr.†.*
Chlorhexidine gluconate (p.1173·2); amylocaine hydrochloride (p.1370·2).
*Mouth and throat disorders.*

**Amygdorectol**
*Merck Medication Familiale, Fr.; Merck-Lipha, Switz.*
Bismuth camphocarbonate (p.1253·1).
*Mouth and throat disorders.*

**Amygdospray** *Monot, Fr.†.*
Hexamidine isetionate (p.1181·3); tetracaine hydrochloride (p.1385·1).
*Mouth and throat disorders.*

**Amykon** *Engelhard, Ger.*
Miconazole nitrate (p.405·3).
*Fungal skin infections.*

**Amylatin** *Synpharma, Austria.*
Angelica (p.1655·1); centaury (p.1669·2); absinthium (p.1645·1).
*Gastrointestinal disorders.*

**Amylodiastase** *SERP, Mon.*
Amylase (cereal extract) (p.1654·2).
*Dyspepsia.*

**Amytal**
*Lilly, Austral.; Lilly, Canad.; Flynn, Irl.†; Flynn, UK; Lilly, USA.*
Amobarbital (p.670·1) or amobarbital sodium (p.670·1).
*Insomnia; status epilepticus.*

**Amytril** *Cristalia, Braz.*
Amitriptyline hydrochloride (p.280·3).
*Depression.*

**Amze** *Richmond, Arg.*
Amlodipine (p.862·2).
*Angina pectoris; hypertension.*

**Amzepril** *Richmond, Arg.*
Amlodipine (p.862·2); benazepril (p.867·2).
*Hypertension.*

**AN 1** *Krugmann, Ger.*
Amfetaminil (p.1584·3).
*Narcoleptic syndrome.*

**Anabact**
*Bioglan, Irl.; Bioglan, Singapore†; Bioglan, Thai.†; Cambridge Healthcare, UK.*
Metronidazole (p.607·2).
*Malodorous fungating tumours; malodorous skin ulcers; rosacea.*

**Anabar** *Lunsco, USA.*
Paracetamol (p.76·2); salicylamide (p.87·3); phenyltoloxamine citrate (p.439·1).

**Anabet** *Bristol-Myers Squibb, Port.*
Nadolol (p.963·1).
*Hypertension.*

**Anabol** *British Dispensary, Thai.*
Methandienone (p.1559·3).
*Anabolic.*

**Anabol-Hevert** *Hevert, Ger.†.*
Homoeopathic preparation.

**Anaboline Depot** *Adelco, Gr.*
Nandrolone decanoate (p.1561·2).
*Anabolic.*

**anabol-loges** *Loges, Ger.*
Alpha tocoferil acetate (p.1465·1); magnesium hydrogen phosphate; terra silicea; hypericum (p.299·1).
*Bone and connective tissue disorders.*

**Anabron** *Millet Roux, Braz.*
Ambroxol hydrochloride (p.1114·3).
*Respiratory-tract congestion.*

**Anacal**
*Note. This name is used for preparations of different composition.*
*Sankyo, Port.*
A heparinoid (p.931·1); lauromacrogol 400 (p.1412·3); prednisolone (p.1108·1); hexachlorophene (p.1181·2).
*Anorectal disorders.*

*Sankyo, UK.*
A heparinoid (p.931·1); lauromacrogol 400 (p.1412·3).
*Anorectal disorders.*

**Anacalcit** *Belmac, Spain.*
Sodium cellulose phosphate (p.1052·1).
*Hypercalcaemia; hypercalciuria; osteopetrosis; vitamin D intoxication.*

**Anacaps** *Ducray, Fr.*
Soya isoflavones; bamboo extract; watercress extract; vitamins; zinc (p.1417·1).
*Hair and scalp disorders.*

**Anacervix**
*Lepori, Port.; Farma Lepori, Spain.*
Piracetam (p.1732·1); vincamine (p.1764·2).
*Cerebral trauma; cerebrovascular disorders.*

**Anacidol**
*Note. This name is used for preparations of different composition.*
*Menarini, Ital.*
Aluminium hydroxide (p.1249·2); magnesium hydroxide (p.1272·2); dimeticone (p.1289·2); milk powder.
*Gastrointestinal disorders.*

*Spirig, Switz.*
Calcium carbonate (p.1254·2); aluminium hydroxide-magnesium carbonate co-dried gel (p.1250·1).
*Gastric disorders.*

**Anacidron** *Bergamo, Braz.†.*
Dicycloverine hydrochloride (p.481·2); magnesium hydroxide (p.1272·2); aluminium hydroxide (p.1249·2); simeticone (p.1289·2).
*Flatulence; gastrointestinal disorders.*

**Anacidron-H** *Bergamo, Braz.†.*
Aluminium hydroxide (p.1249·2).
*Gastrointestinal hyperacidity.*

**Anacin**
*Whitehall-Robins, Canad.; Wyeth Consumer, Chile; Whitehall, Hong Kong; Whitehall, Israel; ICC, Israel; Wyeth Consumer, Singapore; Robins, USA.*
Aspirin (p.15·1); caffeine (p.782·1).
*Fever; pain.*

**Anacin with Codeine** *Whitehall-Robins, Canad.†.*
Aspirin (p.15·1); caffeine (p.782·1); codeine phosphate (p.27·1).
*Fever; pain.*

**Anaclosil**
*IFET (ΙΦΕΤ), Gr.; Antibioticos, Spain.*
Cloxacillin sodium (p.198·2).
*Bacterial infections.*

**Anacrodyne** *Rekah, Israel.*
Vitamin $B_6$ (p.1456·3).
*Vitamin $B_6$ deficiency.*

**Anacyclin**
*Novartis, Braz.; Geigy, Ger.†.*
Lynestrenol (p.1557·1); ethinylestradiol (p.1553·2).
28-Day packs also contain 6 inert tablets.
*Combined oral contraceptive.*

**Anadekin** *Collins, Mex.*
Vitamins A, D, and K (p.1417·1).

**Anadent** *Taro, Israel.*
*Topical gel:* Benzocaine (p.1370·3).
*Topical solution:* Benzocaine (p.1370·3); phenylephrine hydrochloride (p.1126·3).
*Mouth disorders.*

**Anadermin** *Ecobi, Ital.†.*
Chlorhexidine gluconate (p.1173·2); precipitated sulfur (p.1158·2).
*Skin disinfection.*

**Anadin**
*Note. This name is used for preparations of different composition.*
*Whitehall, Irl.*
Aspirin (p.15·1); caffeine (p.782·1); quinine sulfate (p.460·2).
*Cold symptoms; pain.*

*Wyeth Consumer, UK.*
Aspirin (p.15·1); caffeine (p.782·1).
*Pain.*

**Anadin Cold Control** *Whitehall, UK†.*
Paracetamol (p.76·2); caffeine (p.782·1); phenylephrine hydrochloride (p.1126·3).
*Cold and influenza symptoms.*

**Anadin Cold Control Flu Strength** *Whitehall, UK†.*
Paracetamol (p.76·2); phenylephrine hydrochloride (p.1126·3).
*Cold and influenza symptoms.*

**Anadin Extra**
*Whitehall, Irl.; Wyeth Consumer, Port.; Wyeth Consumer, UK.*
Aspirin (p.15·1); paracetamol (p.76·2); caffeine (p.782·1).
*Fever; pain.*

**Anadin Ibuprofen** *Wyeth Consumer, UK.*
Ibuprofen (p.45·3).
*Fever; pain.*

**Anadin Paracetamol** *Wyeth Consumer, UK.*
Paracetamol (p.76·2).
*Fever; pain.*

**Anadin Ultra** *Wyeth Consumer, UK.*
Ibuprofen (p.45·3).
*Fever; pain.*

**Anadol** *TO-Chemicals, Thai.*
Tramadol hydrochloride (p.94·3).
*Pain.*

**Anador** *Boehringer de Angeli, Braz.*
Dipyrone (p.35·3).
*Fever; pain.*

**Anadrol** *Unimed, USA.*
Oxymetholone (p.1565·2).
*Anaemias.*

**Anadvil** *Whitehall, Fr.*
Ibuprofen (p.45·3).
*Fever; pain.*

**Anadvil Rhume** *Whitehall, Fr.*
Ibuprofen (p.45·3); pseudoephedrine hydrochloride (p.1129·2).
*Cold symptoms.*

**Anaebell** *Bell, India.*
Acriflavinium chloride (p.1165·3); lidocaine (p.1377·3); thymol (p.1194·2).
*Skin disorders.*

**Anaemodoron** *Weleda, Austria.*
Fragaria vesca; urtica dioica (p.1762·1).
*Iron-deficiency anaemia.*

**Anaerobex** *Gerot, Austria.*
Metronidazole (p.607·2).
*Anaerobic bacterial infections; Helicobacter pylori infections.*

**Anaeromet** *GlaxoSmithKline, Belg.*
Metronidazole (p.607·2).
*Anaerobic bacterial infections; protozoal infections.*

**Anaestalgin** *Streuli, Switz.*
Procaine hydrochloride (p.1383·2); caffeine (p.782·1).
*Pain.*

**Anaesthecomp N** *Ritsert, Ger.*
Lidocaine hydrochloride (p.1377·3); diphenhydramine hydrochloride (p.431·3).
*Allergic rashes; insect stings; sunburn.*

**Anaestherit** *Sanova, Austria.*
Benzocaine (p.1370·3).
*Anorectal disorders; skin disorders.*

**Anaesthesin** *Ritsert, Ger.*
Benzocaine (p.1370·3).
*Local anaesthesia.*

**Anaesthesin N** *Ritsert, Ger.*
Benzocaine (p.1370·3).
*Local anaesthesia.*

**Anaesthesin-Rivanol** *Ritsert, Ger.*
Benzocaine (p.1370·3); ethacridine lactate (p.1165·3).
*Painful throat infections.*

**Anaesthesulf** *Ritsert, Ger.*
Lauromacrogol 400 (p.1412·3).
Formerly known as Anaesthesulf P and contained lauromacrogol 400 and zinc oxide.
*Pruritic skin disorders.*

**Anaesthetic Ear Drops** *Vitamed, Israel.*
Tetracaine (p.1385·1); phenazone (p.82·3).
*Otitis.*

**Anaesthol** *Merz, Ger.†.*
Lidocaine hydrochloride (p.1377·3).
Adrenaline (p.852·2) and noradrenaline (p.974·3) are included in this preparation as vasoconstrictors to diminish absorption and localise the effect of the local anaesthetic.
*Local anaesthesia.*

**Anafen**
*Note. This name is used for preparations of different composition.*
*Pacific, NZ†.*
Ibuprofen (p.45·3).
*Musculoskeletal, joint, peri-articular, and soft-tissue disorders; pain.*
*TO-Chemicals, Thai.†.*
Tiaprofenic acid (p.93·3).
*Pain.*

**Anafertin** *Armstrong, Mex.*
Algestone acetophenide (p.1541·3); estradiol enantate (p.1550·1).
*Injectable contraceptive; menstrual disorders.*

**Anaflam** *David, India.*
Ibuprofen (p.45·3); paracetamol (p.76·2).
*Fever; inflammation; musculoskeletal and joint disorders; pain.*

**Ana-Flex**
*Note. A similar name is used for preparations of different composition (see below).*
*Gunther, Braz.*
Diclofenac sodium (p.32·1).
*Gout; inflammation; musculoskeletal, joint, and peri-articular disorders; pain.*

**Anaflex**
*Note. A similar name is used for preparations of different composition (see above).*
*Geistlich, Singapore; Geistlich, UK.*
Polynoxylin (p.1190·1).
*Skin infections.*

**Anaflin** *Ehlinger, Mex.†.*
Naproxen (p.65·1).

**Anafortan** *Khandelwal, India.*
*Injection:* Camylofin (p.1666·1).
*Tablets:* Camylofin (p.1666·1); paracetamol (p.76·2).
*Smooth muscle spasm.*

**Anafranil**
*Novartis, Arg.; Novartis, Austral.; Novartis, Austria; Novartis, Belg.; Novartis, Braz.; Novartis, Canad.; Novartis, Chile; Novartis, Denm.; Novartis, Fin.; Novartis, Fr.; Novartis, Ger.; Novartis, Gr.; Novartis, Hong Kong; Novartis, India; Novartis, Irl.; Novartis, Israel; Novartis, Ital.; Novartis, Malaysia; Novartis, Mex.; Novartis, Neth.; Novartis, Norw.; Novartis, NZ; Novartis, Port.; Novartis, S.Afr.; Novartis, Singapore; Novartis, Spain; Novartis, Swed.; Novartis, Switz.; Novartis, Thai.; Novartis, UK; Novartis, USA.*
Clomipramine hydrochloride (p.289·3).
*Depression; narcoleptic syndrome; nocturnal enuresis; obsessive-compulsive disorder; pain; panic attacks; phobic states.*

**Anagastra** *Madaus, Spain.*
Pantoprazole sodium (p.1283·1).
*Gastro-oesophageal reflux; peptic ulcer.*

**Anagen** *Rydelle, Fr.†.*
Amino-acid, vitamin, and mineral preparation (p.1417·1).
*Hair and nail disorders.*

**Anagregal** *Gentili, Ital.*
Ticlopidine hydrochloride (p.1011·2).
*Thrombosis prophylaxis.*

**Ana-Guard** *Bayer, S.Afr.†.*
Adrenaline hydrochloride (p.852·3).
*Anaphylaxis.*

**Anahelp** *Stallergenes, Fr.*
Adrenaline (p.852·2).
*Anaphylaxis.*

**Ana-Kit**
*Bayer, Canad.†; Ebos, NZ†; Bayer, USA.*
*Combination pack:* Injection, adrenaline hydrochloride (p.852·3); 4 chewable tablets, chlorphenamine maleate (p.427·3).
*Anaphylaxis.*

**Anakit** *Dome-Hollister-Stier, Fr.†.*
Adrenaline (p.852·2).
*Anaphylaxis.*

**Analab** *Biolab, Thai.*
Tramadol hydrochloride (p.94·3).
*Pain.*

**Analept** *Faran, Gr.*
Enalapril maleate (p.909·2).
*Heart failure; hypertension.*

**Analeric** *Vianex (Βιανέξ), Gr.*
Diflunisal (p.34·1).
*Inflammation; pain.*

**Analfin** *Tecnofarma, Mex.*
Morphine sulfate (p.60·2).
*Pain.*

**Analgen**
*Note. This name is used for preparations of different composition.*
*Johnson & Johnson, Braz.*
*Ointment:* Turpentine oil (p.1760·1); methyl salicylate (p.59·3); camphor (p.1665·3); mustard oil (p.1718·2); rosemary oil (p.1740·2); lavender oil (p.1705·2); menthol (p.1711·3).
*Topical gel:* Menthol (p.1711·3).
*Musculoskeletal and joint disorders.*
*Aventis, S.Afr.*
*Tablets:* Aspirin (p.15·1); paracetamol (p.76·2); codeine phosphate (p.27·1); caffeine (p.782·1).
*Fever; pain.*

**Anal-Gen**
*Note. A similar name is used for preparations of different composition (see above).*
*BCL, Switz.*
Hamamelis water (p.1696·3); melissa oil (p.1711·2).
*Anogenital skin disorders.*

**Analgen-SA** *Aventis, S.Afr.*
Aluminium aspirin (p.14·1); paracetamol (p.76·2); codeine phosphate (p.27·1); caffeine (p.782·1); chlorphenoxamine hydrochloride (p.428·3); phenobarbital (p.367·3).
*Fever; pain.*

**Analgesia Creme** *Rugby, USA.*
Trolamine salicylate (p.95·3).
*Muscle, joint, and soft-tissue pain; neuralgia.*

**Analgesic Balm**
*Note. This name is used for preparations of different composition.*
*DC Labs, Canad.*
Menthol (p.1711·3); methyl salicylate (p.59·3); cloral hydrate (p.684·1).
*Pfizer Consumer, Canad.; Goldline, USA; Major, USA; URL, USA.*
Menthol (p.1711·3); methyl salicylate (p.59·3).
*Muscle, joint, and soft-tissue pain; neuralgia.*
*Stanley, Canad.†.*
Menthol (p.1711·3); methyl salicylate (p.59·3); eucalyptus oil (p.1686·2); guaiacol (p.1122·1).

**Analgesic/Calmative** *Biochemie, Austral.*
Paracetamol (p.76·2); codeine phosphate (p.27·1); doxylamine succinate (p.432·3).
*Pain.*

**Analgesico Ut Asens Fn** *Asens, Spain†.*
Camphor (p.1665·3); alcohol (p.1166·1); ammonia (p.1653·3); menthol (p.1711·3).
*Soft-tissue disorders.*

**Analgesil** *Kinder, Braz.*
Dipyrone (p.35·3).
*Pain.*

**Analgesin** *Teuto, Braz.*
Aspirin (p.15·1).
*Fever; inflammation; pain.*

**Analgex** *Uniao Quimica, Braz.*
Dipyrone (p.35·3).
*Fever; pain.*

**Analgex C** *Uniao Quimica, Braz.†.*
*Injection:* Ampoule 1, dipyrone (p.35·3); guaifenesin (p.1122·1); caffeine (p.782·1); mepyramine maleate (p.437·1); ampoule 2, vitamin C (p.1460·2).
Lidocaine hydrochloride (p.1377·3) is included in this preparation to alleviate the pain of injection.
*Tablets:* Green tablets, dipyrone (p.35·3); caffeine (p.782·1); mepyramine maleate (p.437·1); orange tablets, vitamin C (p.1460·2).
*Cold and influenza symptoms.*

**Analgil** *Azevedos, Port.*
Methyl salicylate (p.59·3); menthol (p.1711·3); camphor (p.1665·3); guaiacol (p.1122·1).
*Musculoskeletal and joint disorders.*

**Analgilasa** *Ipsen, Spain.*
*Tablets:* Caffeine (p.782·1); codeine phosphate (p.27·1); paracetamol (p.76·2).
*Suppositories†:* Caffeine (p.782·1); codeine phosphate (p.27·1); papaverine hydrochloride (p.1728·1); paracetamol (p.76·2).
*Pain.*

**Analgin**
*Note. This name is used for preparations of different composition.*
*Medphano, Ger.*
Dipyrone (p.35·3).
*Fever; pain.*
*Sam-On, Israel†.*
Aspirin (p.15·1); codeine phosphate (p.27·1).
*Influenza symptoms; pain.*

**Analgin C-R** *EMS, Braz.*
Green tablets, dipyrone (p.35·3); chlorphenamine maleate (p.427·3); orange tablets, vitamin C (p.1460·2).
*Cold and influenza symptoms.*

**Analgina** *Apsen, Braz.†.*
Dipyrone (p.35·3).
*Fever; pain.*

**Analgine** *Sterop, Belg.*
Dipyrone (p.35·3).
*Fever; pain.*

**Analgiol** *Abello, Spain†.*
Codeine phosphate (p.27·1).
*Pain.*

**Analgiplus** *Ipsen, Spain.*
Paracetamol (p.76·2); codeine phosphate (p.27·1).
*Pain.*

**Analgit** *Krewel, Ger.†.*
Dipyrone (p.35·3).
*Fever; pain.*

**Analgosedan** *Brasmedica, Braz.†.*
Dipyrone (p.35·3); homatropine methylbromide (p.483·2); adiphenine (p.1648·1); papaverine hydrochloride (p.1728·1).
*Smooth muscle spasm.*

**Analip** *Iketon, Ital.†.*
Pantethine (p.978·3).
*Hyperlipidaemias.*

**Analka** *Medic, Denm.*
Docusate (p.1262·1); glycerol (p.1694·3).
*Bowel evacuation; constipation.*

**Analmex** *Ofimex, Mex.†.*
Paracetamol (p.76·2).
*Fever; pain.*

**Analmorph** *Gray, Arg.*
Morphine hydrochloride (p.60·1).
*Pain.*

**Analog LCP** *Scientific Hospital Supplies, Irl.*
Food for special diets (p.1417·1).
*Phenylketonuria.*

**Analog MSUD**
*SHS, Fr.; Scientific Hospital Supplies, UK.*
Food for special diets (p.1417·1).
*Maple syrup urine disease.*

**Analog RVHB** *Scientific Hospital Supplies, UK.*
Food for special diets (p.1417·1).
*Homocystinuria; hypermethioninaemia.*

**Analog XLEU** *SHS, Fr.*
Food for special diets (p.1417·1).
*Isovaleric acidaemia.*

**Analog XLYS** *SHS, Fr.*
Food for special diets (p.1417·1).
*Hyperlysinaemia.*

**Analog XLYS Low Try** *SHS, Fr.*
Food for special diets (p.1417·1).
*Glutaric aciduria.*

**Analog XMET** *SHS, Fr.*
Food for special diets (p.1417·1).
*Homocystinuria.*

**Analog XMET, Cys** *SHS, Fr.*
Food for special diets (p.1417·1).
*Sulfite oxidase deficiency.*

**Analog XMTVI**
*SHS, Fr.; Scientific Hospital Supplies, UK.*
Food for special diets (p.1417·1).
Formerly known as Analog Xmet, Thre, Val, Isoleu in the *UK.*
*Methylmalonic or propionic acidaemia.*

**Analog XP** *Scientific Hospital Supplies, UK.*
Food for special diets (p.1417·1).
*Phenylketonuria.*

**Analog Xphen, Tyr**
*SHS, Fr.; Scientific Hospital Supplies, UK.*
Food for special diets (p.1417·1).
*Tyrosinaemia.*

**Analog XPTM** *SHS, Fr.*
Food for special diets (p.1417·1).
*Tyrosinaemia.*

**Analpan** *Duopharma, Hong Kong.*
Diclofenac sodium (p.32·1).
*Inflammation; musculoskeletal and joint disorders; pain.*

**Analpram-HC** *Ferndale, USA.*
Hydrocortisone acetate (p.1103·3); pramocaine hydrochloride (p.1382·2).
*Anorectal disorders.*

**Analter** *Alter, Spain†.*
Paracetamol (p.76·2).
*Fever; pain.*

**Analtrix** *Faria, Braz.*
Oxyphenbutazone (p.76·1); paracetamol (p.76·2).
Aluminium hydroxide (p.1249·2) is included in this preparation in an attempt to limit adverse effects on the gastrointestinal mucosa.
*Fever; inflammation; pain.*

**Analux**
*Cusi, Hong Kong†; Alcon Cusi, Malaysia; Cusi, Singapore†; Alcon Cusi, Spain.*
Phenylephrine hydrochloride (p.1126·3).
*Eye irritation.*

**Analverin** *Dovalle, Braz.*
Hyoscyamine hydrobromide (p.485·1); dipyrone (p.35·3).
*Pain; smooth muscle spasm.*

**Analverin Composto** *Dovalle, Braz.*
Dipyrone (p.35·3); hyoscine (p.483·3).
*Muscle spasm; pain.*

**Analverin Plus** *Dovalle, Braz.*
Paracetamol (p.76·2); hyoscine (p.483·3).
*Muscle spasm; pain.*

**Anamai** *Nakorn, Thai.*
21 Tablets, norethisterone (p.1562·2); mestranol (p.1559·2); 7 tablets, inert.
*Combined oral contraceptive.*

**AnaMantle HC** *Bradley, USA.*
Hydrocortisone acetate (p.1103·3); lidocaine hydrochloride (p.1377·3).

**Anamine** *Mayrand, USA†.*
Pseudoephedrine hydrochloride (p.1129·2); chlorphenamine maleate (p.427·3).
*Cold symptoms.*

**Anamorph** *Fawns & McAllan, Austral.*
Morphine sulfate (p.60·2).
*Pain.*

**Ananase**
*Rhone-Poulenc Rorer, Hong Kong†; Rottapharm, Ital.; Delta, Port.; Aventis, S.Afr.†.*
Bromelains (p.1662·2).
*Inflammation; oedema.*

**Ananase Forte** *Aventis, Chile.*
Bromelains (p.1662·2).
*Episiotomy; inflammation.*

**Anandron**
*Aventis, Arg.; Aventis, Austral.; Aventis, Braz.; Aventis, Canad.; Aventis, Denm.†; Hoechst Marion Roussel, Fin.†; Aventis, Fr.; Hoechst Marion Roussel, Gr.; Aventis, Mex.; Aventis, Neth.; Hoechst Marion Roussel, Norw.†; Aventis, Port.; Aventis, Swed.*
Nilutamide (p.576·2).
*Prostatic cancer.*

**Anapen**
*Note. This name is used for preparations of different composition.*
*Allerbio, Fr.; Decomed, Port.†; Celltech, UK.*
Adrenaline (p.852·2).
*Anaphylaxis.*
*CEPA, Spain†.*
Benzylpenicillin sodium (p.163·2); clemizole penicillin (p.194·1).
*Bacterial infections.*

**Anapenil** *Grossman, Mex.*
*Injection:* Clemizole penicillin (p.194·1); benzylpenicillin sodium (p.163·2).
*Tablets; oral solution:* Phenoxymethylpenicillin potassium (p.242·1).
*Bacterial infections.*

**Anaphase**
*Pierre Fabre Dermo-Cosmetique, Arg.; Ducray, Fr.*
Tocoferil nicotinate (p.1015·1); vitamin B substances (p.1417·1).
*Hair disorders.*

**Anaphyl** *Sam-On, Israel.*
Chlorphenamine maleate (p.427·3).
*Hypersensitivity reactions.*

**Anaphylaxie-Besteck** *Bencard, Ger.†.*
Adrenaline hydrochloride (p.852·3).
*Anaphylactic shock.*

**Anapirol** *Dinafarma, Braz.†.*
Dipyrone (p.35·3); caffeine (p.782·1); orphenadrine citrate (p.486·1).
*Smooth muscle spasm.*

**Anaplex** *ECR, USA.*
Pseudoephedrine hydrochloride (p.1129·2); chlorphenamine maleate (p.427·3).
*Cold symptoms.*

**Anaplex DM** *ECR, USA.*
Dextromethorphan hydrobromide (p.1117·3); brompheniramine maleate (p.426·1); pseudoephedrine hydrochloride (p.1129·2).
*Coughs.*

**Anaplex HD** *ECR, USA.*
Hydrocodone tartrate (p.45·1); pseudoephedrine hydrochloride (p.1129·2); brompheniramine maleate (p.426·1).
Formerly contained hydrocodone tartrate, phenylephrine hydrochloride, and chlorphenamine maleate.
*Coughs and cold symptoms.*

**Anapolon** *Syntex, UK†.*
Oxymetholone (p.1565·2).
*Anaemias.*

**Anapres** *Lemery, Mex.*
Prazosin (p.986·1).
*Hypertension.*

**Anapril**
*Merck, Hong Kong; Berlin Pharm, Singapore; Berlin Pharm, Thai.*
Enalapril maleate (p.909·2).
*Heart failure; hypertension.*

**Anaprol** *Provit, Mex.*
Dipyrone (p.35·3).
*Fever; inflammation; pain.*

**Anaprolina** *Silesia, Chile.*
Nandrolone decanoate (p.1561·2).
*Anabolic; breast cancer; osteoporosis.*

**Anaprox**
*Roche, Austral.; Roche, Canad.; Minerva (Μινερβα), Gr.; Roche, Spain†; Roche, USA.*
Naproxen sodium (p.65·1).
*Fever; inflammation; musculoskeletal, joint, and peri-articular disorders; pain.*

**Anapsique** *Psicofarma, Mex.*
Amitriptyline hydrochloride (p.280·3).
*Depression; hyperactivity in children; nocturnal enuresis.*

**Anapsyl** *Novag, Mex.*
Naproxen sodium (p.65·1).
*Inflammation; musculoskeletal and joint disorders; pain.*

**Anaptivan** *Help, Gr.*
Cefuroxime sodium (p.184·1).
*Bacterial infections.*

**Anapyon** *DM, Braz.†.*
Tyrothricin (p.275·1); chlorophyll (p.1057·1); tannic acid (p.1751·2).
*Mouth and throat infections.*

**Anara** *Chinoin, Mex.*
Sodium picosulfate (p.1289·3).
*Bowel evacuation; constipation.*

**Anarex**
*Upha, Malaysia; Beacons, Singapore.*
Orphenadrine citrate (p.486·1); paracetamol (p.76·2).
*Skeletal muscle spasm; pain.*

**Angril**
*Medochemie, Hong Kong; Medochemie, Malaysia; Medochemie, Thai.*
Danazol (p.1545·2).
*Benign breast disorders; endometriosis; female infertility; gynaecomastia; hereditary angioedema; menorrhagia; precocious puberty.*

**Anaribes** *Farmachimici, Ital.*
Black currant; betacarotene; vitamin E (p.1417·1).
*Nutritional supplement.*

**Anartril** *Farma Lepori, Spain†.*
Glucosamine sulfate (p.1694·1); glucosamine hydriodide (p.1694·1).
*Inflammation; osteomyelitis.*

**Anartrit**
*Note. This name is used for preparations of different composition.*
*Garden House, Arg.*
Calcium (p.1225·1); magnesium (p.1227·3); colecalciferol (p.1461·3).
*Calcium supplement; osteoporosis.*

*Hexal, Braz.*
Piroxicam (p.84·2).
*Dysmenorrhoea; gout; musculoskeletal, joint, and peri-articular disorders.*

**Anasclerol** *Expharma, Ital.†.*
Vincamine hydrochloride (p.1764·2).
*Cerebrovascular disorders.*

**Anased** *Potter's, UK.*
Lupulus (p.1708·1); Jamaica dogwood (p.1702·3); wild lettuce (p.1765·2); passion flower (p.1729·1); pulsatilla (p.1737·1).
*Pain; tension.*

**Anaseptil** *Farmasa, Braz.*
Polymyxin B sulfate (p.245·1); bacitracin zinc (p.161·3); neomycin sulfate (p.235·1); zinc peroxide (p.1195·3).
Formerly contained polymyxin B sulfate, neomycin sulfate, zinc peroxide, and zinc oxide.
*Bacterial skin infections.*

**Anasilpiel** *Euroexim, Spain.*
*Ointment:* Dexpanthenol (p.1727·2); neomycin undecenoate (p.235·2); triamcinolone acetonide (p.1110·2).
*Topical aerosol:* Neomycin undecylenate (p.235·2); triamcinolone acetonide (p.1110·2).
*Infected skin disorders.*

**Anasma** *Alter, Spain.*
Salmeterol xinafoate (p.795·1); fluticasone propionate (p.1102·3).
*Asthma.*

**Anaspaz** *Ascher, USA.*
Hyoscyamine sulfate (p.485·1).
*Smooth muscle spasm.*

**Anastase** *Motima, Fr.*
Vegetable extracts from phaseolus vulgaris; cyprus; hamamelis; watercress; lemon; pineapple (p.1417·1).

**Anasten** *Errekappa, Ital.*
Magnesium; potassium; levocarnitine; ubidecarenone; vitamin C (p.1417·1).
*Nutritional supplement.*

**Anastil** *Eberth, Ger..*
*Injection†:* Guaiacol (p.1122·1).
*Bronchitis; pneumonia.*
*Oral drops:* Thyme (p.1755·2).
*Bronchitis; catarrh; coughs.*

**Anastil N** *Eberth, Ger.†.*
Thyme (p.1755·2); camphor (p.1665·3); guaifenesin (p.1122·1).
*Bronchitis; catarrh; coughs.*

**Anastim con RTH** *Pierre Fabre Dermo-Cosmetique, Arg.*
RTH extract; α-pinene; saw palmetto (p.1569·1); crotamiton (p.1145·1); enoxolone (p.36·2).
*Scalp disorders.*

**Anatac** *UCB, Spain.*
Carbocisteine (p.1116·2).
*Respiratory-tract disorders.*

**Anatensol**
*Bristol-Myers Squibb, Austral.; Bristol-Myers Squibb, Braz.†; Sarabhai Piramal, India; Bristol-Myers Squibb, Ital.; Bristol-Myers Squibb, Neth.; Bristol-Myers Squibb, Port.*
Fluphenazine decanoate (p.699·3), fluphenazine enantate (p.699·3), or fluphenazine hydrochloride (p.699·3).
*Psychoses.*

**Anatetall**
*Chiron Vaccines, Ital.; Chiron, Thai.*
An adsorbed tetanus vaccine (p.1640·3).
*Active immunisation.*

**Anatine** *Pharmacia, Arg.*
Finasteride (p.1554·2).
*Benign prostatic hyperplasia.*

**Anatopic** *Martin, Spain†.*
Fluocinolone acetonide (p.1101·2).
*Skin disorders.*

**Anatoxal Di** *Berna, Switz.†.*
An adsorbed diphtheria vaccine (p.1612·3).
*Active immunisation.*

**Anatoxal Di Te**
*Kwizda, Austria; Berna, Belg.†; Berna, Ital.; Berna, Port.†; Berna, Spain; Berna, Switz.*
An adsorbed diphtheria and tetanus vaccine (p.1613·1). Separate preparations are available for infants and young children and for older children and adults.
*Active immunisation.*

**Anatoxal Di Te Berna** *Faran, Gr.*
An adsorbed diphtheria and tetanus vaccine (p.1613·1).
*Active immunisation.*

**Anatoxal Di Te Per**
*Kwizda, Austria; Berna, Ital.†; Berna, Port.†; Berna, Spain; Berna, Switz.†.*
An adsorbed diphtheria, tetanus, and pertussis vaccine (p.1613·3).
*Active immunisation of infants.*

**Anatoxal Te**
*Berna, Belg.†; Berna, Port.†; Berna, Spain; Berna, Switz.*
An adsorbed tetanus vaccine (p.1640·3).
*Active immunisation.*

**Anatoxal Te Di** *Berna, Spain.*
An adsorbed diphtheria and tetanus vaccine (p.1613·1).
*Active immunisation of children and adults.*

**Anatoxal-TE-Berna** *Faran, Gr.*
An adsorbed tetanus vaccine (p.1640·3).
*Active immunisation.*

**Anatoxina Estafilococica** *Butantan, Braz.†.*
A staphylococcal vaccine (p.1640·2).
*Active immunisation.*

**Anatrast** *Lafayette, USA.*
Barium sulfate (p.1061·1).
*Contrast medium for gastrointestinal radiography.*

**Anatuss** *Mayrand, USA†.*
*Syrup:* Phenylpropanolamine hydrochloride (p.1127·3); dextromethorphan hydrobromide (p.1117·3); guaifenesin (p.1122·1).
*Tablets:* Phenylpropanolamine hydrochloride (p.1127·3); dextromethorphan hydrobromide (p.1117·3); guaifenesin (p.1122·1); paracetamol (p.76·2).
*Coughs.*

**Anatuss DM** *Merz, USA†.*
Guaifenesin (p.1122·1); pseudoephedrine hydrochloride (p.1129·2); dextromethorphan hydrobromide (p.1117·3).

**Anatuss LA** *Merz, USA†.*
Guaifenesin (p.1122·1); pseudoephedrine hydrochloride (p.1129·2).
*Coughs.*

**Anatyl** *Sanval, Braz.*
Paracetamol (p.76·2).
*Fever; pain.*

**Anauran** *Zambon, Ital.*
Polymyxin B sulfate (p.245·1); neomycin sulfate (p.235·1); lidocaine hydrochloride (p.1377·3).
*External ear disorders.*

**Anaus** *Beta, Arg.*
Sildenafil citrate (p.1744·2).
*Erectile dysfunction.*

**Anausin** *Viatris, Fr.*
Metoclopramide hydrochloride (p.1274·3).
*Nausea and vomiting.*

**Anavix** *Demo, Gr.*
Ambroxol hydrochloride (p.1114·3).
*Respiratory disorders associated with viscous mucus.*

**Anax** *Whan In, Singapore†.*
Naproxen sodium (p.65·1).
*Gout; musculoskeletal, joint, and peri-articular disorders; pain.*

**Anaxeryl** *Bailly, Fr.*
Dithranol (p.1146·1); ichthammol (p.1148·2); salicylic acid (p.1157·1); resorcinol (p.1156·3); peru balsam (p.1730·2).
Formerly contained dithranol, ichthammol, salicylic acid, resorcinol, peru balsam, and birch tar oil.
*Alopecia; psoriasis.*

**Anazo** *Progress, Thai.*
Phenazopyridine hydrochloride (p.83·1).
*Urinary-tract pain.*

**Anbesol**
*Note. This name is used for preparations of different composition.*
*Whitehall-Robins, Canad.*
*Topical gel:* Benzocaine (p.1370·3); phenol (p.1188·1).
*Topical liquid:* Benzocaine (p.1370·3); phenol (p.1188·1); camphor (p.1665·3); menthol (p.1711·3).
*Minor skin abrasions; mouth pain.*

*Wyeth Consumer, Chile.*
Benzocaine (p.1370·3).
*Mouth pain.*

*SSL, Irl.; SSL, UK.*
Lidocaine hydrochloride (p.1377·3); chlorocresol (p.1177·1); cetylpyridinium chloride (p.1173·1).
*Denture irritation; mouth ulcers; teething.*

*Whitehall, USA.*
*Topical gel:* Benzocaine (p.1370·3); phenol (p.1188·1).
*Oral lesions.*
*Topical liquid:* Benzocaine (p.1370·3); phenol (p.1188·1); menthol (p.1711·3); camphor (p.1665·3); povidone-iodine (p.1190·3).
*Mouth and throat disorders.*

**Anbesol Baby** *Whitehall-Robins, Canad.*
Benzocaine (p.1370·3).
*Teething.*

**Anbifen** *ANB, Thai.*
Ibuprofen (p.45·3).
*Fever; pain.*

**Anbikan** *ANB, Thai.*
Kanamycin (p.225·2).
*Gram-negative bacterial infections.*

**Anbikin** *ANB, Thai.*
Amikacin sulfate (p.154·1).
*Bacterial infections.*

**Anbin**
*Grifols, Ital.; Grifols, Spain.*
Antithrombin III (p.742·2).
*Antithrombin III deficiency.*

**Anbycin** *ANB, Thai.†.*
Lincomycin (p.226·2).
*Gram-positive bacterial infections.*

**Ancamin** *PP Lab, Thai.*
Calamine (p.1144·1); zinc oxide (p.1163·2); chlorphenamine maleate (p.427·3).
*Insect bites; pruritus; skin irritation.*

**Ancef**
*SmithKline Beecham, Canad.†.*
Cefazolin sodium (p.170·3).
*Bacterial infections.*

*SmithKline Beecham, USA.*
Cefazolin sodium (p.170·3).
*Bacterial infections.*

**Anceron** *Schering-Plough, S.Afr.*
Beclometasone dipropionate (p.1091·1).
*Rhinitis.*

**Ancet** *C & M, USA.*
Skin cleanser.

**Anchocalm** *Genepharm, Gr.*
Buspirone hydrochloride (p.672·2).
*Generalised anxiety.*

**Ancid** *Hexal, Ger.*
Hydrotalcite (p.1267·3).
*Gastrointestinal hyperacidity; heartburn; peptic ulcer.*

**Ancivin** *Padro, Spain.*
Famciclovir (p.633·2).
*Herpesvirus infections.*

**Anclomax** *Blausiegel, Braz.*
Aciclovir (p.626·1).

**Anco** *BASF, Ger.†.*
Ibuprofen (p.45·3).
*Inflammation; musculoskeletal, joint, and soft-tissue disorders; pain.*

**Ancobon** *ICN, USA.*
Flucytosine (p.399·3).
*Candidiasis; cryptococcosis.*

**Anconevron** *Pharmanik (Φαρμανικ), Gr.*
Bromazepam (p.671·3).
*Anxiety disorders.*

**Ancopir**
*Grossmann, Hong Kong; Grossmann, Switz.*
Vitamin B substances (p.1417·1).
Lidocaine hydrochloride (p.1377·3) is included in the intramuscular injection to alleviate the pain of injection.
*Adjuvant in radiation therapy; alcoholism; lumbago; neuralgia; neuritis; sciatica; vitamin B deficiency.*

**Ancoren** *Sanitas, Port.*
Atenolol (p.865·2).
*Angina pectoris; arrhythmias; hypertension; myocardial infarction.*

**Ancoron** *Libbs, Braz.*
Amiodarone hydrochloride (p.859·2).
*Arrhythmias.*

**Ancotil**
*ICN, Austral; ICN, Austria; Roche, Braz.†; ICN, Denm.; CSP, Fr.; ICN, Ger.; ICN, Hong Kong; ICN, Irl.; ICN, Ital.; ICN, Malaysia; ICN, Neth.; Medilink, Norw.†; ICN, Singapore†; Medilink, Swed.; ICN, Switz.; ICN, UK.*
Flucytosine (p.399·3).
Formerly known as Alcobon in the *UK*.
*Fungal infections.*

**Andante** *Boehringer Ingelheim, Ger.*
Bunazosin hydrochloride (p.878·1).
*Hypertension.*

**Andantol**
*Viatris, Belg.†; Asta Medica, Braz.; Sanfer, Mex.*
Isothipendyl hydrochloride (p.435·2).
*Allergic skin disorders.*

**Andapsin** *Orion, Swed.*
Sucralfate (p.1290·2).
*Gastrointestinal haemorrhage; peptic ulcer.*

**Andehist** *Cypress, USA.*
*Oral drops:* Carbinoxamine maleate (p.426·3); pseudoephedrine hydrochloride (p.1129·2).
*Rhinitis.*
*Syrup:* Pseudoephedrine hydrochloride (p.1129·2); brompheniramine maleate (p.426·1).
*Upper respiratory-tract disorders.*

**Andehist DM**
*Cypress, USA.*
*Syrup:* Pseudoephedrine hydrochloride (p.1129·2); brompheniramine maleate (p.426·1); dextromethorphan hydrobromide (p.1117·3).
*Coughs.*

*Silarx, USA.*
*Oral drops:* Carbinoxamine maleate (p.426·3); pseudoephedrine hydrochloride (p.1129·2); dextromethorphan hydrobromide (p.1117·3).
*Coughs and cold symptoms.*

**Andergin** *Searle, Ital.†.*
Miconazole nitrate (p.405·3).
*Fungal infections.*

**Andil** *Recalcine, Chile.*
Paracetamol (p.76·2); adiphenine hydrochloride (p.1648·1).
*Colic; fever; pain.*

**Andilex** *CT, Ital.*
Nicorandil (p.965·3).
*Angina pectoris.*

**Andion** *Gea, Denm.†.*
Beclometasone dipropionate (p.1091·1).
*Asthma.*

**Andociclina Balsamica** *Andromaco, Mex.*
Oxytetracycline (p.241·1); guaifenesin (p.1122·1); cineole (p.1672·1).
Lidocaine (p.1377·3) is included in this preparation to alleviate the pain of injection.
*Respiratory-tract disorders.*

**Andolba** *Eurofarma, Braz.*
Benzocaine (p.1370·3); benzethonium chloride (p.1169·2); menthol (p.1711·3); hydroxyquinoline benzoate (p.1700·1).
*Gynaecological disorders.*

**Andolex**
*3M, Denm.; 3M, S.Afr.; 3M, Swed.*
Benzydamine hydrochloride (p.21·1).
*Mouth and throat disorders.*

**Andolex-C** *3M, S.Afr.*
Benzydamine hydrochloride (p.21·1); chlorhexidine gluconate (p.1173·2).
*Inflammation and infection of the mouth and throat.*

**Andolor** *Krewel, Ger.*
Tilidine hydrochloride (p.94·1).
Naloxone hydrochloride (p.1044·3) is included in this preparation to discourage abuse.
*Pain.*

**Andopan** *Atlantis, Mex.*
Paracetamol (p.76·2).
*Fever; pain.*

**Andoprim** *Andromaco, Mex.*
Co-trimoxazole (p.199·3).
*Bacterial infections.*

**Andox** *Atlantis, Mex.*
Paracetamol (p.76·2).
*Fever; pain.*

**Andractim**
*Besins, Belg.; Besins, Fr.; Piette, Thai.*
Androstanolone (p.1541·3).
*Gynaecomastia; lichen sclerosus; male hypogonadism.*

**Andre** *Andre, India.*
Boric acid (p.1662·1); chlorphenamine maleate (p.427·3); sodium chloride (p.1233·3); zinc sulfate (p.1469·3); chlorobutanol (p.1176·3); naphazoline hydrochloride (p.1124·3).
*Conjunctivitis.*

**Andreafol** *Andreabal, Switz.*
Folic acid (p.1429·1).
*Neural tube defect prophylaxis.*

**Andregen** *Andre, India.*
Gentamicin sulfate (p.217·1).
*Bacterial eye infections.*

**Andre-I-Kul** *Andre, India.*
Phenylephrine hydrochloride (p.1126·3); naphazoline hydrochloride (p.1124·3); menthol (p.1711·3); camphor (p.1665·3).
*Eye irritation.*

**Andrews**
*SmithKline Beecham, Belg.†; GlaxoSmithKline, Irl.; GlaxoSmithKline Consumer, UK.*
Citric acid (p.1673·1); magnesium sulfate (p.1228·2); sodium bicarbonate (p.1223·2).
*Constipation; dyspepsia.*

**Andrews Answer** *SmithKline Beecham Consumer, UK†.*
Paracetamol (p.76·2); caffeine (p.782·1).
*Dyspepsia; headache.*

**Andrews Antacid**
*GlaxoSmithKline, Irl.; GlaxoSmithKline Consumer, UK.*
Calcium carbonate (p.1254·2); magnesium carbonate (p.1272·1).
*Gastric hyperacidity; heartburn.*

**Andrews Tums Antacid** *GlaxoSmithKline Consumer, Austral.*
Calcium carbonate (p.1254·2).
*Calcium supplement; dyspepsia; heartburn.*

**Andrioderma** *Andromaco, Arg.*
Vitamin A (p.1451·2).
*Skin disorders.*

**Andriodermol** *Uniao Quimica, Braz.*
*Topical liquid:* Undecenoic acid (p.410·3); sodium undecenoate (p.411·1); propionic acid (p.407·3); sodium propionate (p.408·1); hexylresorcinol (p.1182·1).
*Topical paint:* Undecenoic acid (p.410·3); zinc undecenoate (p.411·1); calcium propionate (p.408·1); hexylresorcinol (p.1182·1).
*Skin infections.*

**Andriol**
*Organon, Austral.; Organon, Austria; Organon, Canad.; Organon, Ger.; Organon, Hong Kong; Organon, Ital.; Organon, Malaysia; Organon, Mex.; Organon, Neth.; Organon, Port.; Organon, Singapore; Organon, Switz.; Organon, Thai.*
Testosterone undecylate (p.1570·1).
*Male hypogonadism; osteoporosis.*

**Androbloc** *Torrex, Austria.*
Flutamide (p.556·2).
*Prostatic cancer.*

**Androcur**
*Gobbi, Arg.; Schering, Austral.; Schering, Austria; Schering, Belg.; Schering, Braz.; Berlex, Canad.; Schering, Denm.; Schering, Fin.; Schering, Fr.; Schering, Ger.; Shepa, Gr.; Schering, Hong Kong; Schering, Irl.; Schering, Israel; Schering, Ital.; Schering, Malaysia; Schering, Mex.; Schering, Neth.; Schering, Norw.; Schering, NZ; Schering, Port.; Schering, S.Afr.; Schering, Singapore; Schering, Spain; Schering, Swed.; Schering, Switz.; Schering, Thai.; Schering, UK.*
Cyproterone acetate (p.1544·1).
*Androgen-dependent acne, alopecia, hirsutism, and seborrhoea in females; prostatic cancer; sexual deviation and hypersexuality in males.*

**Androderm**
*Mayne, Austral.; Paladin, Canad.; AstraZeneca, Ger.; Promed, Ger.; Schwarz, Ital.; CEPA, Spain; AstraZeneca, Switz.; SmithKline Beecham, USA.*
Testosterone (p.1569·3).
*Testosterone deficiency.*

**Andro-Diane** *Schering, Austria.*
Cyproterone acetate (p.1544·1).
*Androgen-dependent hirsutism, alopecia, acne, and seborrhoea in females.*

**Androdor** *Andromaco, Chile.*
Flutamide (p.556·2).
*Prostatic cancer.*

**Androfemon** *Jenapharm, Ger.*
Estradiol valerate (p.1550·2); testosterone enantate (p.1570·1).
*Menopausal disorders.*

**AndroGel** *Unimed, USA.*
Testosterone (p.1569·3).
*Hypogonadism.*

**Android** *ICN, USA.*
Methyltestosterone (p.1559·3).
*Breast cancer; cryptorchidism; male hypogonadism.*

**Androlic** *British Dispensary, Thai.*
Oxymetholone (p.1565·2).
*Anaemias; cachexia.*

**Androlip** *Teuto, Braz.*
Simvastatin (p.997·1).
*Hyperlipdaemias.*

**Androlistica** *Holistica, Fr.*
Cucurbita oil; palm-nut oil; onion; omega-3 marine triglycerides; borage oil; yam extract; sea lettuce (p.1417·1).
*Male menopause.*

**Androlone-D** *Keene, USA.*
Nandrolone decanoate (p.1561·2).
*Anaemia in renal disease.*

**Andropatch**
*GlaxoSmithKline, Irl.; GlaxoSmithKline, UK.*
Testosterone (p.1569·3).
*Hypogonadism.*

**Andropel** *Fortbenton, Arg.*
Finasteride (p.1554·2).
*Alopecia.*

**Andropository** *Rugby, USA†.*
Testosterone enantate (p.1570·1).
*Breast cancer; delayed puberty (males); male hypogonadism.*

**Androskat**
*Byk, Austria; Byk, Neth.*
Papaverine hydrochloride (p.1728·1); phentolamine mesilate (p.982·1).
*Erectile dysfunction.*

**Androstat** *Gautier, Arg.*
Cyproterone acetate (p.1544·1).
*Prostatic cancer.*

**Androsteron** *Bergamo, Braz.†.*
Cyproterone acetate (p.1544·1).

**Androtardyl** *Schering, Fr.*
Testosterone enantate (p.1570·1).
*Male hypogonadism.*

**Androvite** *Optimox, USA.*
Multivitamin and mineral preparation with iron and folic acid (p.1417·1).

**Androxicam** *Andromaco, Mex.*
Piroxicam (p.84·2).
*Gout; musculoskeletal, joint and peri-articular disorders; pain.*

**Androxinon** *Schering, Arg.*
Bicalutamide (p.530·1).
*Prostatic cancer.*

**Androxon**
*Organon, Braz.; Organon, Israel; Organon, Norw.; Donmed, S.Afr.*
Testosterone undecylate (p.1570·1).
*Male hypogonadism.*

**Androxyl** *Duopharma, Hong Kong.*
Cefadroxil (p.167·2).
*Bacterial infections.*

**Andrumin** *Janssen-Cilag, Austral.†.*
Dimenhydrinate (p.431·1).
*Motion sickness; vestibular disorders.*

**Andursil**
*Novartis, Braz.; Sanopharm, Switz.*
Aluminium hydroxide-magnesium carbonate co-dried gel (p.1250·1); simeticone (p.1289·2).
*Flatulence; gastro-oesophageal reflux; gastrointestinal hyperacidity.*

**Andursil N** *Zyma, Ger.†.*
Heavy magnesium carbonate (p.1272·1); dried aluminium hydroxide gel (p.1249·2).
*Gastrointestinal disorders.*

**Anebron** *Protein, Mex.†.*
Salbutamol (p.791·3).

**Anectine**
*Glaxo Wellcome, Canad.†; Wellcome, Irl.; Glaxo Wellcome, Mex.; GlaxoSmithKline, Spain; GlaxoSmithKline, UK; Glaxo Wellcome, USA.*
Suxamethonium chloride (p.1406·2).
*Depolarising neuromuscular blocker.*

**Anekron** *EMS, Braz.*
Choline citrate (p.1424·3); betaine hydrochloride (p.1660·2); methionine (p.1042·1); adenosine (p.851·2); vitamin $B_6$ (p.1456·3); sorbitol (p.1446·3).
*Liver disorders.*

**Anemagen** *Ethex, USA.*
Ferrous fumarate (p.1427·3); cyanocobalamin (p.1458·2); stomach extract.
Ascorbic acid (p.1460·2) is included in this preparation to increase the absorption and availability of iron.
*Anaemias.*

**Anemagen OB** *Ethex, USA.*
Ferrous fumarate (p.1427·3); calcium; vitamins (p.1417·1).
Docusate sodium (p.1262·2) is included in this preparation to reduce the constipating effects of iron.

**Anemet** *Aventis, Ger.*
Dolasetron mesilate (p.1262·3).
*Nausea and vomiting.*

**Anemidox**
*Note. This name is used for preparations of different composition.*
*Merck, Arg.*
Folic acid; thiamine; riboflavine; pyridoxine; cyanocobalamin (p.1417·1).
*Anaemias; vitamin B deficiency.*

*Merck, India.*
Ferrous fumarate (p.1427·3); folic acid (p.1429·1); vitamin $B_{12}$ (p.1458·2); calcium carbonate (p.1254·2); vitamin D (p.1461·2).
Vitamin C (p.1460·2) is included to increase the absorption and availability of iron.
*Iron-deficiency anaemias.*

**Anemidox-Ferrum** *Merck, Arg.*
Ferrous fumarate (p.1427·3); cyanocobalamin (p.1458·2); folic acid (p.1429·1).
Ascorbic acid (p.1460·2) is included in this preparation to increase the absorption and availability of iron.
*Anaemias.*

**Anemital** *Basi, Port.*
Ferrous gluconate (p.1428·1).
*Anaemias.*

**Anemix** *Hebron, Braz.*
Ferrous sulfate (p.1428·2); vitamin B substances (p.1417·1).
*Anaemias.*

**Anemofer** *Marjan, Braz.*
Cyanocobalamin (p.1458·2); ferrous sulfate (p.1428·2); folic acid (p.1429·1).
Ascorbic acid (p.1460·2) is included in the tablet preparation to increase the absorption and availability of iron.
*Anaemias.*

**Anemokol** *Biologia, Braz.†.*
Liver extract; malt extract (p.1439·2); ferric ammonium citrate (p.1427·2).
*Anaemias.*

**Anemul mono** *Medopharm, Ger.†.*
Dexamethasone (p.1097·1).
*Skin disorders.*

**Anerex** *AF, Mex.*
Vitamin B substances with iron (p.1417·1).
*Anaemias; tonic.*

**Anergan** *Forest Pharmaceuticals, USA†.*
Promethazine hydrochloride (p.439·1).
*Hypersensitivity reactions; motion sickness; nausea; postoperative pain (adjunct); sedative; vomiting.*

**Anervan**
*Recip, Fin.; Recip, Norw.; Recip, Swed.*
Ergotamine tartrate (p.467·2); chlorcyclizine hydrochloride (p.427·2); caffeine (p.782·1); meprobamate (p.706·2).
*Cluster headache; migraine.*

**Anesdente do Bebe** *Loprofar, Braz.*
Tetracaine hydrochloride (p.1385·1); menthol (p.1711·3).
*Teething pain.*

**Anespas** *Rudefsa, Mex.*
Prifinium bromide (p.488·2).
*Muscle spasm; pain.*

**Anest Compuesto** *Llorens, Spain†.*
Tetracaine (p.1385·1).
Naphazoline nitrate (p.1124·3) is included in this preparation as a vasoconstrictor to diminish absorption and localise the effect of the local anaesthetic.
*Local anaesthesia.*

**Anestacon** *PolyMedica, USA.*
Lidocaine hydrochloride (p.1377·3).
*Urethral pain.*

**Anestalcon**
*Alcon, Arg.; Alcon, Braz.; Alcon, Chile.*
Proxymetacaine hydrochloride (p.1384·1).
*Local anaesthesia.*

**Anestesi Doble** *Alcon Cusi, Spain.*
Oxybuprocaine hydrochloride (p.1382·1); tetracaine hydrochloride (p.1385·1).
*Local anaesthesia.*

**Anestesia Loc Braun C/A** *Braun, Spain†.*
Procaine hydrochloride (p.1383·2).
Adrenaline (p.852·2) is included in this preparation as a vasoconstrictor to diminish absorption and localise the effect of the local anaesthetic.
*Local anaesthesia.*

**Anestesia Loc Braun S/A** *Braun, Spain.*
Cinchocaine hydrochloride (p.1373·2); procaine hydrochloride (p.1383·2).
*Local anaesthesia.*

**Anestesia Topi Braun C/A** *Braun, Spain.*
Tetracaine hydrochloride (p.1385·1).
Adrenaline (p.852·2) is included in this preparation as a vasoconstrictor to diminish absorption and localise the effect of the local anaesthetic.
*Local anaesthesia.*

**Anestesia Topi Braun S/A** *Braun, Spain.*
Tetracaine (p.1385·1).
*Local anaesthesia.*

**Anestesico**
*Allergan, Braz.*
Tetracaine hydrochloride (p.1385·1).
Phenylephrine hydrochloride (p.1126·3) is included in this preparation as a vasoconstrictor to diminish absorption and localise the effect of the local anaesthetic.
*Local anaesthesia.*

*Alcon Cusi, Spain.*
Tetracaine hydrochloride (p.1385·1).
Naphazoline hydrochloride (p.1124·3) is included in this preparation as a vasoconstrictor to diminish absorption and localise the effect of the local anaesthetic.
*Local anaesthesia.*

**Anestesiol** *Loprofar, Braz.*
Thymol (p.1194·2); menthol (p.1711·3); camphor (p.1665·3); tetracaine hydrochloride (p.1385·1); phenazone (p.82·3); clove oil (p.1673·3).
*Mouth disorders.*

**Anesthal** *Jagson, India.*
Thiopental sodium (p.1309·1).
*General anaesthesia; status epilepticus.*

**Anesthesique Double** *Asta Medica, Belg.†.*
Oxybuprocaine hydrochloride (p.1382·1); tetracaine hydrochloride (p.1385·1).
*Local anaesthesia.*

**Anestina Braun** *Palex, Spain†.*
Lidocaine hydrochloride (p.1377·3); procaine hydrochloride (p.1383·2); tetracaine hydrochloride (p.1385·1).
*Local anaesthesia.*

**Anestocil**
*DM, Braz.†; Edol, Port.*
Oxybuprocaine hydrochloride (p.1382·1).
*Local anaesthesia.*

**Anethaine**
*Rhone-Poulenc Rorer, S.Afr.†; Torbet Laboratories, UK.*
Tetracaine hydrochloride (p.1385·1).
*Local anaesthesia.*

**Anetin** *Ibirn, Ital.†.*
Carnitine (p.1423·3).
*Carnitine deficiency; myocardial ischaemia.*

**Aneural** *Merck dura, Ger.†.*
Maprotiline hydrochloride (p.306·1).
*Depression.*

**Aneurin** *Teva, Ger.*
Thiamine hydrochloride (p.1455·1).
*Vitamin $B_1$ deficiency.*

**Aneurol**
*Note. This name is used for preparations of different composition.*
*Sanico, Belg.†.*
Thiamine hydrochloride (p.1455·1).
*Neurogenic pain; rheumatic pain; vitamin $B_1$ deficiency.*

*Lacer, Spain.*
Diazepam (p.690·1).
Contains pyridoxine hydrochloride.
*Alcohol withdrawal syndrome; anxiety; febrile convulsions; insomnia; skeletal muscle spasm.*

**Anevrase** *Cazi, Braz.*
*Oral solution:* Passion flower (p.1729·1); mulungu (p.1717·2); valerian (p.1762·2); melmendro; crataegus (p.1677·1); melissa (p.1711·1).
*Tablets:* Passion flower (p.1729·1); mulungu (p.1717·2); valerian (p.1762·2); melmendro; crataegus (p.1677·1).
*Sedative.*

**Anevrasi** *Donini, Ital.*
Passion flower (p.1729·1); crataegus (p.1677·1); valerian (p.1762·2).
*Insomnia.*

**Anew** *Avon, Canad.*
*SPF 15 cream; SPF 15 lotion:* Octinoxate (p.1154·3); oxybenzone (p.1154·3).
*SPF 15 eye cream:* Octinoxate (p.1154·3); titanium dioxide (p.1160·3).
*Sunscreen.*

**Anew Day Force** *Avon, Canad.*
*SPF 15:* Avobenzone (p.1142·3); octinoxate (p.1154·3); oxybenzone (p.1154·3).
*Sunscreen.*

**Anew Luminosity** *Avon, Canad.*
*SPF 15:* Avobenzone (p.1142·3); octinoxate (p.1154·3); oxybenzone (p.1154·3).
*Sunscreen.*

**Anew Positivity** *Avon, Canad.*
*SPF 15:* Avobenzone (p.1142·3); octinoxate (p.1154·3); oxybenzone (p.1154·3).
*Sunscreen.*

**Anexa** *Microsules, Arg.*
Amlodipine besilate (p.862·1).
*Angina pectoris; hypertension.*

**Anexate**
*Roche, Austral.; Roche, Austria; Roche, Belg.; Roche, Canad.; Roche, Fr.; Roche, Ger.; Roche, Gr.; Roche, Hong Kong; Roche, Irl.; Roche, Israel; Roche, Ital.; Roche, Neth.; Roche, Norw.; Roche, NZ; Roche, Port.; Roche, S.Afr.; Roche, Singapore; Roche, Spain; Roche, Switz.; Roche, Thai.; Roche, UK.*
Flumazenil (p.1038·3).
*Benzodiazepine overdosage; reversal of benzodiazepine-induced sedation.*

**Anexsia** *Andrx, USA.*
Hydrocodone tartrate (p.45·1); paracetamol (p.76·2).
*Pain.*

**Anfagladin** *Anpharm (Ανφαρμ), Gr.*
Propylene glycol cefatrizine (p.170·3).
*Bacterial infections.*

**Anfenax** *Douglas, NZ†.*
Diclofenac sodium (p.32·1).
*Osteoarthritis; rheumatoid arthritis.*

**Anfertil** *Wyeth, Braz.*
Norgestrel (p.1563·2); ethinylestradiol (p.1553·2).
*Combined oral contraceptive.*

**Anflat** *Cazi, Braz.*
Simeticone (p.1289·2).
*Flatulence.*

**Anflene** *Teuto, Braz.*
Piroxicam (p.84·2).

**Anfocort** *Bristol-Myers Squibb, Ital.*
Halcinonide (p.1103·2); amphotericin B (p.391·2).
*Infected skin disorders.*

**Anfokali** *Bano, Austria.*
Homoeopathic preparation.

**Anfomicin** *Windson, Braz.†.*
Neomycin sulfate (p.235·1); sulfadiazine (p.258·2); tyrothricin (p.275·1); benzocaine (p.1370·3).
*Mouth and throat disorders.*

**Anforicin B** *Cristalia, Braz.*
Amphotericin B (p.391·2).

**Anfoterin** *Teuto, Braz.*
Tetracycline hydrochloride (p.266·2); amphotericin B (p.391·2).
*Vaginal infections.*

**Anfozan** *Proel, Gr.*
Disodium etidronate (p.771·2).
*Osteoporosis; Paget's disease of bone.*

**Angass** *Medice, Ger.*
Bismuth subnitrate (p.1252·2); bismuth aluminate (p.1252·1).
*Peptic ulcer.*

**Angass S** *Medice, Ger.*
Bismuth subnitrate (p.1252·2).
*Peptic ulcer.*

**Ange** *Teikoku, Jpn.*
Levonorgestrel (p.1563·2); ethinylestradiol (p.1553·2).
28-Day packs contain 7 inert tablets.
*Triphasic oral contraceptive.*

**Angenol** *Merck, Hong Kong.*
Paracetamol (p.76·2).
*Fever; pain.*

**Angettes** *Bristol-Myers Squibb, UK.*
Aspirin (p.15·1).
*Thrombosis prophylaxis.*

**Angeze** *Opus, UK.*
Isosorbide mononitrate (p.942·1).
*Angina pectoris.*

**Anghostan-100** *Biostam (Βιοσταμ), Gr.*
Ticlopidine (p.1012·1).
*Thromboembolic disorders.*

**Angiact** *Nycomed, Denm.†.*
Diltiazem hydrochloride (p.900·1).
*Angina pectoris; hypertension.*

**Angi-a-Mid** *Sibras, Braz.†.*
Tyrothricin (p.275·1); neomycin sulfate (p.235·1); sodium salicylate (p.90·1); cineole (p.1672·1); menthol (p.1711·3); thymol (p.1194·2); camphor (p.1665·3).

**Angicon** *Royal, Chile.*
Doxazosin mesilate (p.908·3).
*Benign prostatic hyperplasia; hypertension.*

**Angicontin** *Norpharma, Denm.†.*
Diltiazem hydrochloride (p.900·1).
*Angina pectoris; hypertension.*

**Angicor** *Aventis, Denm.*
Nicorandil (p.965·3).
*Angina pectoris.*

**Angidil** *Errekappa, Ital.*
Diltiazem hydrochloride (p.900·1).
*Angina pectoris; hypertension.*

**Angidine** *Vifor, Switz.*
Gramicidin (p.220·2); benzethonium chloride (p.1169·2); tetracaine hydrochloride (p.1385·1).
*Mouth and throat disorders.*

**Angifebrine** *Pharmacal, Switz.†.*
Propyphenazone (p.85·3); paracetamol (p.76·2).
*Fever; pain.*

**Angifonil** *Diviser Aquilea, Spain.*
Cetylpyridinium chloride (p.1173·1).
*Bacterial mouth infections.*

**Angil** *Sanval, Braz.*
Isosorbide (p.941·1).
*Angina pectoris.*

**Angileptol** *Sigma-Tau, Spain.*
Enoxolone (p.36·2); benzocaine (p.1370·3); chlorhexidine hydrochloride (p.1173·3).
Formerly contained enoxolone, benzocaine, and sulfaguanidine.
*Mouth and throat disorders.*

**Angilol**
*Douglas, Hong Kong†; Douglas, NZ†; DDSA Pharmaceuticals, UK.*
Propranolol hydrochloride (p.989·3).
*Angina pectoris; arrhythmias; essential tremor; hypertension; hyperthyroidism; migraine; myocardial infarction; obstructive cardiomyopathy.*

**Angimon** *Dexcel, UK†.*
Verapamil hydrochloride (p.1019·1).
*Angina pectoris; hypertension.*

**Angina MCC** *Streuli, Switz.*
Cetylpyridinium chloride (p.1173·1); lidocaine hydrochloride (p.1377·3); menthol (p.1711·3).
*Mouth and throat disorders.*

**Angina-Gastreu S R1** *Reckeweg, Ger.*
Homoeopathic preparation.

**Anginamide** *Medgenix, Belg.*
Sulfacetamide sodium (p.257·3).
*Infections of the mouth and throat.*

**Anginasin N** Opfermann, Ger.†.
Hexetidine (p.1182·1); camphor (p.1665·3); menthol (p.1711·3).
*Mouth and throat disorders.*

**Anginazol** DP-Medica, Switz.
Dichlorobenzyl alcohol (p.1178·3); cetylpyridinium chloride (p.1173·1); chlorquinaldol (p.187·3); lidocaine hydrochloride (p.1377·3).
*Mouth and throat infections.*

**Anginesin** Grossmann, Switz.
Aluminium acetotartrate (p.1652·3); sage (p.1741·2).
*Mouth and throat pain.*

**Anginin**
Banyu, Hong Kong†; Delta, Port.; Banyu, Thai.†.
Pyricarbate (p.1737·1).
*Thromboembolic disorders; vascular disorders.*

**Anginine**
Sigma, Austral.; GlaxoSmithKline, NZ.
Glyceryl trinitrate (p.923·2).
*Angina pectoris.*

**Angino Tricin** Sanval, Braz.
Neomycin sulfate (p.235·1); tyrothricin (p.275·1); benzocaine (p.1370·3); sodium perborate (p.1192·2).
*Mouth and throat disorders.*

**Anginol**
Note. This name is used for preparations of different composition.
Labima, Belg.
Dequalinium chloride (p.1178·1).
*Mouth and throat disorders.*

Streuli, Switz.†.
Ethacridine lactate (p.1165·3); levomenthol (p.1711·3); camphor (p.1665·3); peru balsam (p.1730·2).
*Mouth and throat disorders.*

**Anginol-Lidocaine** Labima, Belg.
Dequalinium chloride (p.1178·1); lidocaine hydrochloride (p.1377·3).
*Mouth and throat disorders.*

**Anginomycin** MIP, Ger.
Tyrothricin (p.275·1); bacitracin (p.161·3).
*Mouth and throat infections.*

**Anginor** Vesta, S.Afr.†.
Nifedipine (p.966·2).
*Angina pectoris; hypertension.*

**Angino-Rub** Eurofarma, Braz.
Benzydamine hydrochloride (p.21·1); cineole (p.1672·1); turpentine oil (p.1760·1); camphor (p.1665·3); thymol (p.1194·2); menthol (p.1711·3).
Formerly contained camphor, cineole, sassafras, sodium salicylate, turpentine, thymol, tyrothricin, menthol, and neomycin.
*Mouth and throat disorders.*

**Anginotrat** Purissimus, Arg.
Gentamicin embonate (p.219·1); sulfadiazine (p.258·2); benzocaine (p.1370·3).
*Mouth and throat disorders.*

**Anginova**
Note. This name is used for preparations of different composition.
Medinova, Port.
Dequalinium chloride (p.1178·1); benzocaine (p.1370·3).
*Mouth and throat disorders.*

Medinova, Switz.
Dequalinium chloride (p.1178·1); lidocaine hydrochloride (p.1377·3).
*Mouth and throat disorders.*

**Anginovag** Novag, Spain.
Dequalinium chloride (p.1178·1); enoxolone (p.36·2); hydrocortisone acetate (p.1103·3); lidocaine hydrochloride (p.1377·3); tyrothricin (p.275·1).
*Mouth and throat disorders.*

**Anginovin H** Pfluger, Ger.
Homoeopathic preparation.

**Anginozetes** Gilton, Braz.†.
Tyrothricin (p.275·1); benzocaine (p.1370·3).
*Mouth and throat disorders.*

**Angiocardyl N** Rhenomed, Ger.†.
Atropine sulfate (p.477·1); glyceryl trinitrate (p.923·2); theobromine and sodium salicylate (p.798·2).
Formerly contained atropine sulfate, glyceryl trinitrate, phenobarbital, and theobromine and sodium salicylate.
*Cardiac disorders.*

**Angiocine** Wolfs, Belg.
Lidocaine hydrochloride (p.1377·3); chlorhexidine hydrochloride (p.1173·3).
*Mouth and throat disorders.*

**Angiocis** Schering, UK.
Technetium-99m stannous pyrophosphate (p.1525·2).
*Red blood cell labelling for blood pool scintigraphy.*

**Angio-Conray** Bracco, Ital.†.
Sodium iotalamate (p.1065·3).
*Radiographic contrast medium.*

**Angiodarona** Cazi, Braz.
Amiodarone (p.859·2).
*Arrhythmias.*

**Angiodrox** Solvay, Spain.
Diltiazem hydrochloride (p.900·1).
*Angina pectoris; hypertension.*

**Angiofilina** Fabra, Arg.
Amlodipine besilate (p.862·1).
*Angina pectoris; hypertension.*

**Angiofluor** Poen, Arg.
Fluorescein sodium (p.1689·1).
*Adjunct in eye examination.*

**Angioflux** Mitim, Ital.
A heparinoid (p.931·1).
*Thrombosis prophylaxis.*

**Angioftal** Allergan, Arg.
Chromocarb diethylamine (p.1670·3).
*Conjunctivitis.*

**Angiografin**
Schering, Austral.; Schering, Ger.†; Schering, Neth.; Schering, S.Afr.†.
Meglumine amidotrizoate (p.1060·2).
*Radiographic contrast medium.*

**Angiografina** Schering, Arg.
Meglumine amidotrizoate (p.1060·2).
*Radiographic contrast medium.*

**Angiolingual** Royal, Chile.
Glyceryl trinitrate (p.923·2).
*Angina pectoris.*

**Angiolit** Pharmacia, Arg.
Nicergoline (p.1719·3); flunarizine (p.434·2).
*Cerebral and peripheral vascular disorders; circulatory disorders of the ear and eye.*

**Angiolong** Farmalab, Braz.
Diltiazem hydrochloride (p.900·1).
*Angina pectoris; arrhythmias; hypertension.*

**Angiomax**
CSL, NZ; Medicines Company, USA.
Bivalirudin (p.875·2).
*Thromboembolism prophylaxis in patients with unstable angina undergoing coronary angioplasty.*

**Angioneurina** Baxter, Arg.
$C_1$ esterase inhibitor (p.1675·2).

**Angionorm** Farmasan, Ger.
Dihydroergotamine mesilate (p.465·3).
*Chronic venous insufficiency; hypotension; migraine and other vascular headache.*

**Angiopas** Pascoe, Ger.
Homoeopathic preparation.

**Angiophtal**
Bournonville, Belg.†; Merck Sharp & Dohme-Chibret, Fr.
Chromocarb diethylamine (p.1670·3).
*Capillary fragility in the eye.*

**Angiopine** Ashbourne, UK.
Nifedipine (p.966·2).
*Angina pectoris; hypertension; Raynaud's syndrome.*

**Angiopril** Diffucap, Braz.
Enalapril maleate (p.909·2).
*Hypertension.*

**Angiorex** Lampugnani, Ital.
Myrtillus (p.1718·3).
*Capillary disorders.*

**Angiosedante** Unifarma, Spain†.
Aminophylline (p.780·2); papaverine hydrochloride (p.1728·1).
*Biliary colic; cardiac stimulation; obstructive airways disease.*

**Angioton** GD, Ital.
*Cream:* Ginkgo biloba (p.1692·3); centella (p.1144·3); menthol (p.1711·3); bioflavonoids (p.1688·2).
*Peripheral vascular disorders.*
*Tablets:* Centella (p.1144·3); myrtillus (p.1718·3); rutoside (p.1688·2); ginkgo biloba (p.1692·3); vitamins (p.1417·1).
*Venous disorders.*

**Angioton S** DHU, Ger.
Homoeopathic preparation.

**Angiotrofin** Armstrong, Mex.
Diltiazem hydrochloride (p.900·1).
*Angina pectoris; hypertension.*

**Angiovist** Schering, Chile.
Sodium amidotrizoate (p.1060·2); meglumine amidotrizoate (p.1060·2).
*Radiographic contrast medium.*

**Angiozem** Ashbourne, UK.
Diltiazem hydrochloride (p.900·1).
*Angina pectoris; hypertension.*

**Angipress**
Note. This name is used for preparations of different composition.
Biosintetica, Braz.
Atenolol (p.865·2).
*Angina pectoris; arrhythmias; hypertension; myocardial infarction.*

Crinos, Ital.
Diltiazem hydrochloride (p.900·1).
*Angina pectoris; hypertension.*

**Angipress CD** Biosintetica, Braz.
Atenolol (p.865·2); chlortalidone (p.882·3).
*Hypertension.*

**Angised**
GlaxoSmithKline, Hong Kong; GlaxoSmithKline, India; Wellcome, Irl.†; GlaxoSmithKline, Israel; GlaxoSmithKline, S.Afr.; Glaxo Wellcome, Singapore†; GlaxoSmithKline, Thai.
Glyceryl trinitrate (p.923·2).
*Angina pectoris.*

**Angispray**
Note. A similar name is used for preparations of different composition (see below).
Monot, Fr.†.
Hexetidine (p.1182·1); propionic acid (p.407·3); chlorobutanol (p.1176·3).
*Mouth and throat disorders.*

**Angi-Spray**
Note. A similar name is used for preparations of different composition (see above).
Aspen, S.Afr.
Isosorbide dinitrate (p.941·1).
*Angina pectoris; heart failure; myocardial infarction.*

**Angitak** Eastern Pharmaceuticals, UK.
Isosorbide dinitrate (p.941·1).
*Angina pectoris.*

**Angitil** Trinity, UK.
Diltiazem hydrochloride (p.900·1).
*Angina pectoris; hypertension.*

**Angitrate** Aspen, S.Afr.
Isosorbide mononitrate (p.942·1).
*Angina pectoris.*

**Angitrit** Ranbaxy, Thai.
Isosorbide dinitrate (p.941·1).
*Angina pectoris.*

**Angizem**
Inverni della Beffa, Ital.; Sun, Singapore†; Sun, Thai.
Diltiazem hydrochloride (p.900·1).
*Angina pectoris; hypertension.*

**Anglix** Novartis, Mex.
Glyceryl trinitrate (p.923·2).
*Angina pectoris.*

**Anglopen** Liomont, Mex.
Ampicillin (p.157·1), ampicillin sodium (p.157·1), or ampicillin trihydrate (p.157·2).
*Bacterial infections.*

**Anglucid** Collins, Mex.
Metformin (p.342·3).
*Diabetes mellitus.*

**Angocin Anti-Infekt N** Repha, Ger.
Tropaeolum majus (p.1659·3); horseradish (p.1697·3).
*Respiratory-tract infections; urinary-tract infections.*

**Angocin Bronchialtropfen** Repha, Ger.
Marrubium vulgare (p.1124·1).
*Catarrh.*

**Angocin percutan** Repha, Ger.†.
Camphor (p.1665·3); eucalyptus oil (p.1686·2); turpentine oil (p.1760·1).
*Muscle and joint pain; respiratory-tract disorders.*

**Angoron** Sanofi Synthelabo, Gr.
Amiodarone hydrochloride (p.859·2).
*Arrythmias; wolff-Parkinson-White syndrome.*

**Angoten** Microsules, Arg.
Amiodarone hydrochloride (p.859·2).
*Arrhythmias.*

**Angstrom Corpo** Pfizer Consumer, Ital.
Octinoxate (p.1154·3); avobenzone (p.1142·3).
*Sunscreen.*

**Angstrom Viso** Pfizer Consumer, Ital.
*Cream:* Octinoxate (p.1154·3); avobenzone (p.1142·3); vitamin E acetate (p.1465·1); dimethicone (p.1482·1); betacarotene (p.1422·3); allantoin (p.1141·3); sodium pidolate (p.1158·1); triclosan (p.1195·2).
*Stick:* Octinoxate (p.1154·3); avobenzone (p.1142·3); vitamin E acetate (p.1465·1); betacarotene (p.1422·3).
*Barrier preparation; sunscreen.*

**Anguilce** TRB, Arg.
Elcatonin (p.768·3).
*Hypercalcaemia; osteoporosis; Paget's disease of bone; reflex sympathetic dystrophy.*

**Angular** Fada, Arg.
Bromazepam (p.671·3).
*Anxiety.*

**Angurate Magentee** Alsitan, Ger.
Mentzelia cordifolia.
*Gastrointestinal disorders.*

**Angyton** Royton, Braz.
Amiodarone hydrochloride (p.859·2).
*Arhythmias.*

**Anhidrot** Stiefel, Arg.
Aluminium chloride (p.1142·1).
*Hyperhidrosis.*

**Anhisnon** Polipharm, Thai.†.
Astemizole (p.424·2).
*Hypersensitivity reactions.*

**Anhista** Sriprasit, Thai.
Chlorphenamine maleate (p.427·3); paracetamol (p.76·2).
*Cold symptoms.*

**Anhydrol Forte**
Dermal Laboratories, Irl.; Dermal, Israel; Dermal Laboratories, UK.
Aluminium chloride (p.1142·1).
*Hyperhidrosis.*

**Anhypen** Yamanouchi, Denm.†.
Ampicillin sodium (p.157·1).
*Bacterial infections.*

**Anice (Specie Composta)** Dynacren, Ital.
Aniseed (p.1655·2); chamomile (p.1669·3); caraway (p.1667·2); peppermint leaf (p.1283·2); fennel (p.1687·2).
*Gastrointestinal disorders; herbal tea.*

**Anidrosan** Cesam, Port.†.
Aluminium chloride (p.1142·1).
*Hyperhidrosis.*

**Aniduv** Kampel Martian, Arg.
Nimodipine (p.972·3).
*Cerebrovascular disorders.*

**Anifed** Formenti, Ital.†.
Nifedipine (p.966·2).
*Hypertension; ischaemic heart disease.*

**Anifer Fenchelhonig** Hofmann, Austria.
Fennel (p.1687·2); honey (p.1434·2).
*Coughs and cold symptoms.*

**Anifer Hustenbalsam** Hofmann, Austria.
Eucalyptus oil (p.1686·2); pumilio pine oil (p.1737·1); sage oil (p.1741·2).
*Respiratory-tract disorders.*

**Anifer Hustentee** Anifer, Austria.
Althaea (p.1651·3); aniseed (p.1655·2); thyme (p.1755·2); plantago lanceolata leaf (p.1738·2); mallow flowers (p.1709·3).
*Respiratory-tract disorders.*

**Anifer Hustentropfen** Hofmann, Austria.
Thyme (p.1755·2); cowslip rhizome (p.1735·1).
*Coughs.*

**Anifer Krauterol** Hofmann, Austria.
Eucalyptus oil (p.1686·2); oleum pini sylvestris; pumilio pine oil (p.1737·1).
*Respiratory-tract disorders.*

**Aniflazime** Seber, Port.
Serrapeptase (p.1743·2).
*Inflammation; respiratory-tract congestion.*

**Aniflazym** Takeda, Ger.
Serrapeptase (p.1743·2).
*Inflammation.*

**Anikef** Duopharma, Hong Kong.
Cefuroxime (p.184·1).
*Bacterial infections.*

**Anilar** Kampel Martian, Arg.
Sertraline (p.317·3).
*Depression.*

**Anilid** Kener, Mex.†.
Chlortalidone (p.882·3).

**Anilusin** Cryopharma, Mex.†.
Insulin (p.333·3).
*Diabetes mellitus.*

**Animal Shapes** Major, USA.
Multivitamin preparation (p.1417·1).

**Animal Shapes + Iron** Major, USA.
Multivitamin preparation with iron (p.1417·1).

**Animativ** Biosaude, Port.
Multivitamin preparation with iron (p.1417·1).

**Animex-On** Microsules Bernabo, Arg.
Fluoxetine hydrochloride (p.292·1).
*Bulimia; depression.*

**Animic** Vinas, Spain.
Hypericum (p.299·1).
*Sleep disorders; tonic.*

**Animine**
Note. This name is used for preparations of different composition.
McGloin, Austral.†.
*Cream:* Benzocaine (p.1370·3); benzalkonium chloride (p.1168·3).
*Lotion:* Lidocaine hydrochloride (p.1377·3); benzalkonium chloride (p.1168·3); calamine (p.1144·1).
*Bites; pruritus; stings.*

Sanofi Synthelabo, Belg.†.
Trimethylxanthine sodium alphanaphthylacetate.
*Mental function impairment; tonic.*

**Anionen-Spurenelement** Fresenius Kabi, Austria.
Electrolytes for infusion (p.1217·1).
*Parenteral nutrition.*

**Aniospray** Anios, Fr.
Formaldehyde (p.1179·3); glyoxal (p.1181·1); glutaral (p.1180·3); didecyldimethylammonium chloride (p.1178·3).
*Disinfection of instruments and surfaces.*

**Anisan** Pascoe, Ger.
Menthol (p.1711·3); bismuth subgallate (p.1252·2); aluminium acetate tartrate (p.1652·3); hypericum oil (p.299·2); hamamelis (p.1696·3); liver oil.
*Anorectal disorders.*

**Anisimol** Medipharm, Chile.
Fluoxetine (p.296·3).
*Bulimia; depression.*

**Anistal** Silanes, Mex.
Ranitidine hydrochloride (p.1285·2).
*Acid aspiration; gastro-oesophageal reflux; gastrointestinal haemorrhage; peptic ulcer; Zollinger-Ellison syndrome.*

**Anitos** Bittner, Austria.
Senega (p.1130·2); plantago lanceolata (p.1738·2); thyme (p.1755·2); anise oil (p.1655·2).
*Coughs and cold symptoms.*

**Anitrim** Italmex, Mex.
Co-trimoxazole (p.199·3).
*Bacterial infections.*

**Anivy** Roberts, Canad.†.
Chlorphenesin (p.396·1); benzocaine (p.1370·3).
*Insect bites; poison ivy; skin irritation.*

**Anlodibal** Baldacci, Braz.
Amlodipine besilate (p.862·1).
*Angina pectoris; hypertension.*

**Anna** Nakorn, Thai.
21 Tablets, levonorgestrel (p.1563·2); ethinylestradiol (p.1553·2); 7 tablets, inert.
*Combined oral contraceptive.*

**Annadine** Unison, Thai.
Povidone-iodine (p.1190·3).
*Skin disinfection.*

**Anningzochin** Laves, Ger.†.
*Mycobacterium chelonae* subsp. *chelonae*.
*Immunotherapy.*

**Annoxen** Siam Bheasach, Thai.
Naproxen sodium (p.65·1).
*Acute gout; musculoskeletal, joint, and peri-articular disorders.*

**Anodan-HC** Odan, Canad.
Hydrocortisone acetate (p.1103·3); zinc sulfate (p.1469·3).
*Anorectal disorders.*

**Anodesyn** Thornton & Ross, UK.
Lidocaine hydrochloride (p.1377·3); allantoin (p.1141·3).
*Anorectal disorders.*

**Anolor** Blansett, USA.
Butalbital (p.673·3); paracetamol (p.76·2); caffeine (p.782·1).

**Anoquan** Roberts, USA†.
Paracetamol (p.76·2); caffeine (p.782·1); butalbital (p.673·3).
*Pain.*

**Anoran** Labima, Belg.†.
Phendimetrazine hydrochloride (p.1592·1).
*Obesity.*

**Anore Dolor** Schwarzwalder, Ger.
Homoeopathic preparation.

**Anore rheumatic N** Schwarzwalder, Ger.
Homoeopathic preparation.

**Anore X N** Schwarzwalder, Ger.
Absinthium (p.1645·1); gentian (p.1692·2); angelica (p.1655·1).
*Appetite loss; dyspepsia; meteorism.*

**Anoreine**
Note. This name is used for preparations of different composition.
Janssen-Cilag, Austria.
Carrageenan (p.1578·2); titanium dioxide (p.1160·3); zinc oxide (p.1163·2).
*Anorectal disorders.*
Martin, Fr.
Carrageenan (p.1578·2); bismuth subgallate (p.1252·2); zinc oxide (p.1163·2).
*Anorectal disorders.*

**Anoreine mit Lidocain** Janssen-Cilag, Austria.
Carrageenan (p.1578·2); titanium dioxide (p.1160·3); zinc oxide (p.1163·2); lidocaine (p.1377·3).
*Anorectal disorders.*

**Anorfin** Geo, Denm.
Buprenorphine hydrochloride (p.21·3).
*Pain.*

**Anorsia** Asian Pharm, Thai.
Pizotifen malate (p.470·3).
*Anorexia; vascular headache.*

**102 Anos** ISA, Arg.
Dietary supplement (p.1417·1).

**Anosedil** Heralds, Braz.†.
Lorazepam (p.704·1).
*Alcohol withdrawal syndrome; anxiety; epilepsy; insomnia; nausea and vomiting; premedication.*

**Anovate** USV, India.
Beclometasone dipropionate (p.1091·1); phenylephrine hydrochloride (p.1126·3); lidocaine hydrochloride (p.1377·3).
*Anorectal disorders.*

**Anovulatorio Micro-Dosis** Laboratorios Chile, Chile; Mintlab, Chile.
Levonorgestrel (p.1563·2); ethinylestradiol (p.1553·2).
*Combined oral contraceptive.*

**Anovulatorios** Laboratorios Chile, Chile.
Lynestrenol (p.1557·1); mestranol (p.1559·2).
*Combined oral contraceptive; menstrual disorders.*

**Anoxant** Eagle, Austral.†.
A vitamin, mineral, amino-acid, and herbal antoxidant preparation (p.1417·1).

**Anoxid** Volchem, Ital.
Vitamins A, C, and E (p.1417·1).
Formerly contained vitamins A, C, and E with selenium.
*Nutritional supplement.*

**Anpec**
Alphapharm, Austral.; Alphapharm, Malaysia; Merck, Malaysia.
Verapamil hydrochloride (p.1019·1).
*Angina pectoris; arrhythmias; hypertension.*

**Anplag** Mitsubishi, Jpn.
Sarpogrelate hydrochloride (p.996·3).
*Thromboembolic disorders.*

**Anposel** Medipharm, Chile.
Meloxicam (p.56·1).
*Osteoarthritis; pain; rheumatoid arthritis.*

**Anpress** Condrugs, Thai.
Alprazolam (p.668·3).
*Anxiety; mixed anxiety depressive states.*

**Anquil**
Janssen-Cilag, Irl.; Concord, UK†.
Benperidol (p.671·2).
*Deviant sexual behaviour.*

**Ansaid**
Pharmacia, Canad.; Pharmacia, Chile; Pharmacia Upjohn, Mex.; Upjohn, USA.
Flurbiprofen (p.43·3).
*Gout; inflammation; musculoskeletal, joint, peri-articular, and soft-tissue disorders; pain.*

**Ansar** Bioclon, Mex.
Benzyl benzoate (p.1500·2).
*Pediculosis; scabies.*

**Ansatipin**
Pharmacia, Fin.; Kenfarma, Spain; Pharmacia, Swed.
Rifabutin (p.249·1).
*Opportunistic mycobacterial infections; tuberculosis.*

**Ansatipine** Pharmacia, Fr.
Rifabutin (p.249·1).
*Mycobacterial infections; tuberculosis.*

**Anselol**
Douglas, Austral.; Douglas, NZ.
Atenolol (p.865·2).
*Angina pectoris; arrhythmias; hypertension; myocardial infarction.*

**Ansentron** Biosintetica, Braz.
Ondansetron hydrochloride (p.1281·1).
*Vomiting.*

**Anseren** Novartis, Ital.
Ketazolam (p.703·1).
*Anxiety disorders.*

**Ansial** Pharmacia, Arg.
Buspirone hydrochloride (p.672·2).
*Anxiety.*

**Ansiderm** IDI, Ital.†.
Magnesium (p.1227·3); kava (p.1703·2).
*Nutritional supplement.*

**Ansienon** Cazi, Braz.
Buspirone hydrochloride (p.672·2).
*Anxiety.*

**Ansieten** Elvetium, Arg.
Ketazolam (p.703·1).
*Anxiety.*

**Ansietil** Tecnofarma, Chile.
Ketazolam (p.703·1).
*Anxiety.*

**Ansilan** Cosmopharm, Gr.
Famotidine (p.1265·2).
*Conditions where gastric acid reduction is beneficial; gastric hypersecretion including Zollinger-Ellison syndrome; peptic ulcer.*

**Ansilive** Libbs, Braz.
Diazepam (p.690·1).
*Alcohol withdrawal syndrome; anxiety; epilepsy; insomnia; premedication; sedative; skeletal muscle spasm.*

**Ansilor** Cavalheiro, Port.
Lorazepam (p.704·1).
*Anxiety; insomnia.*

**Ansimar** ABC, Ital.
Doxofylline (p.785·1).
*Obstructive airways disease.*

**Ansiokey** Inkeysa, Spain.
Valerian (p.1762·2).
*Insomnia; nervous disorders.*

**Ansiolin** Rhone-Poulenc Aventis, Ital.
Diazepam (p.690·1).
*Anxiety; epilepsy; insomnia; premedication.*

**Ansiopax** Hebron, Braz.
Kava (p.1703·2).
*Sedative.*

**Ansiotex** Cimed, Braz.
Pimethixene (p.439·1).
*Hypersensitivity reactions.*

**Ansitec** Libbs, Braz.
Buspirone hydrochloride (p.672·2).
*Anxiety.*

**Ansiten** Azevedos, Port.
Buspirone hydrochloride (p.672·2).
*Anxiety disorders.*

**Ansium** Lesvi, Spain.
Diazepam (p.690·1); sulpiride (p.722·2).
*Anxiety.*

**Ansiven** Abbott, Switz.
Propofol (p.1305·3).
*General anaesthesia; sedative.*

**Anso**
Lacer, Hong Kong.
Hexetidine (p.1182·1); lidocaine hydrochloride (p.1377·3); triamcinolone acetonide (p.1110·2); pentosan polysulfate (p.979·2).
*Anorectal disorders.*
Lacer, Spain.
Hexetidine (p.1182·1); lidocaine hydrochloride (p.1377·3); triamcinolone acetonide (p.1110·2); pentosan polysulfate sodium (p.979·2).
*Anorectal disorders.*

**Ansudor** Galderma, Ger.
Aluminium chlorohydrate (p.1142·1); triclocarban (p.1195·1).
*Hyperhidrosis; intertrigo; wound exudate.*

**Answer**
Carter-Wallace, Austral.
Pregnancy test (p.1734·3).
Carter-Wallace, USA.
Fertility test or pregnancy test (p.1734·3).

**Answer Now** Carter Horner, Canad.
Pregnancy test (p.1734·3).

**Anta** Pharmasant, Thai.
Lorazepam (p.704·1).
*Anxiety; epilepsy; insomnia; muscle relaxation.*

**Antabus**
Chemomedica, Austria; Alpharma, Denm.; Alpharma, Fin.; Byk Gulden, Ger.; Byk Tosse, Ger.; Dumex, Norw.†; Bohm, Spain; Alpharma, Swed.; Alpharma, Switz.
Disulfiram (p.1681·3).
*Chronic alcoholism.*

**Antabuse**
Orphan, Austral.; Sanofi Synthelabo, Belg.; Wyeth-Ayerst, Canad.†; Dumex, Irl.; Wyeth-Ayerst, Israel; Crinos, Ital.; CSL, NZ; Dumex, NZ; Aspen, S.Afr.; Dumex-Alpharma, Thai.; Alpharma, UK; Odyssey, USA†.
Disulfiram (p.1681·3).
*Chronic alcoholism.*

**Antacal** Errekappa, Ital.
Amlodipine besilate (p.862·1).
*Angina pectoris; hypertension.*

**Antacia** The Forty-Two, Thai.
Aluminium hydroxide (p.1249·2); magnesium hydroxide (p.1272·2); simeticone (p.1289·2).
*Flatulence; gastric hyperacidity; gastritis; peptic ulcer.*

**Antacid**
Note. This name is used for preparations of different composition.
DC Labs, Canad.
Aluminium hydroxide (p.1249·2); magnesium hydroxide (p.1272·2).
Geneva, USA.
*Oral suspension:* Aluminium hydroxide (p.1249·2); magnesium hydroxide (p.1272·2).
*Tablets:* Calcium carbonate (p.1254·2).
*Hyperacidity.*

**Antacid Chewable Tablets** Vitelle, Austral.†.
Calcium carbonate (p.1254·2); magnesium carbonate (p.1272·1).
*Dyspepsia; gastro-oesophageal reflux; heartburn.*

**Antacid Liquid** Shoppers Drug Mart, Canad.†.
Aluminium hydroxide (p.1249·2); magnesium hydroxide (p.1272·2); simeticone (p.1289·2).

**Antacid Plus Antiflatulant** Stanley, Canad.; DC Labs, Canad.
Aluminium hydroxide (p.1249·2); magnesium hydroxide (p.1272·2); simeticone (p.1289·2).

**Antacid Suspension** Pharmel, Canad.
Aluminium hydroxide (p.1249·2); magnesium hydroxide (p.1272·2).

**Antacid Tablet**
Note. This name is used for preparations of different composition.
Stanley, Canad.
Aluminium hydroxide (p.1249·2); magnesium hydroxide (p.1272·2); simeticone (p.1289·2).
Swiss Herbal, Canad.
Magnesium hydroxide (p.1272·2); calcium carbonate (p.1254·2).

**Antacide Suspension** Therapex, Canad.
Aluminium hydroxide (p.1249·2); magnesium hydroxide (p.1272·2).

**Antacide Suspension avec Antiflatulent** Therapex, Canad.
Aluminium hydroxide (p.1249·2); magnesium hydroxide (p.1272·2); simeticone (p.1289·2).

**Antacidum** Pfizer, Austria.
Dihydroxyaluminum sodium carbonate (p.1261·2).
*Dyspepsia; hyperacidity; peptic ulcer.*

**Antacidum OPT** Optimed, Ger.†.
Aluminium hydroxide (p.1249·2).
*Gastric hyperacidity; hyperphosphaturia.*

**Antacidum Rennie** Roche, Austria.
Calcium carbonate (p.1254·2); magnesium carbonate (p.1272·1).
*Hyperacidity.*

**Antacil** Nakorn, Thai.
*Oral suspension:* Aluminium hydroxide gel (p.1249·2); magnesium hydroxide (p.1272·2); simeticone (p.1289·2).
*Flatulence; gastric hyperacidity; peptic ulcer.*
*Tablets:* Magnesium trisilicate (p.1272·3); dried aluminium hydroxide gel (p.1249·2); kaolin (p.1268·3).
*Gastric hyperacidity; peptic ulcer.*

**Antacsal** Alpharma, Mex.
Aspirin (p.15·1).
*Fever; pain; thromboembolism prophylaxis.*

**Antaderm** Darier, Mex.
Allantoin (p.1141·3); coal tar (p.1159·2).
*Psoriasis; seborrhoeic dermatitis.*

**Antadine** Sanofi Omnimed, S.Afr.
Amantadine hydrochloride (p.1197·2).
*Drug-induced extrapyramidal disorders; influenza A; parkinsonism.*

**Antadys** Theramex, Mon.
Flurbiprofen (p.43·3).
*Dysmenorrhoea; musculoskeletal and joint disorders.*

**Antafit** Polipharm, Thai.
Carbamazepine (p.353·3).
*Epilepsy; trigeminal neuralgia.*

**Antagon**
Note. This name is used for preparations of different composition.
Ativus, Braz.
Ranitidine hydrochloride (p.1285·2).
*Gastro-oesophageal reflux; gastrointestinal haemorrhage; peptic ulcer; Zollinger-Ellison syndrome.*
Organon, USA.
Ganirelix acetate (p.1325·1).
*Inhibition of premature luteinising hormone surges in controlled ovarian hyperstimulation.*

**Antagon I**
Note. A similar name is used for preparations of different composition (see above).
Liomont, Mex.
Astemizole (p.424·2).
*Hypersensitivity.*

**Antagonil** Novartis, Ger.; Yamanouchi, Ger.
Nicardipine hydrochloride (p.965·1).
*Angina pectoris; hypertension.*

**Antagosan**
Aventis, Fr.†; Hoechst Marion Roussel, Ger.†; Hoechst Marion Roussel, Ital.†.
Aprotinin (p.742·3).
*Haemorrhagic disorders; shock.*

**Antak** GlaxoSmithKline, Braz.
Ranitidine hydrochloride (p.1285·2).
*Acid aspiration; gastro-oesophageal reflux; gastrointestinal haemorrhage; peptic ulcer; Zollinger-Ellison syndrome.*

**Antalgic** Caps, S.Afr.
Paracetamol (p.76·2).
*Fever; pain.*

**Antalgil** Centra, Ital.
Ibuprofen (p.45·3).
*Pain.*

**Antalgin**
Note. This name is used for preparations of different composition.
Medix, Mex.
Indometacin (p.47·3).
*Gout; inflammation; musculoskeletal, joint and periarticular disorders; pain.*
Roche, Spain.
Naproxen sodium (p.65·1).
*Fever; gout; musculoskeletal and joint disorders; pain.*

**Antalgo** Selvi, Ital.
Nimesulide (p.67·1).
*Fever; inflammation; pain.*

**Antalin** Saval, Chile.
Amitriptyline hydrochloride (p.280·3); chlordiazepoxide (p.674·2).
*Mixed anxiety-depressive disorders.*

**Antalisin** Centra, Ital.
Ibuprofen lysine (p.46·3).
*Fever; pain.*

**Antalon** Dresden, Ger.†.
Pimozide (p.715·1).
*Schizophrenia.*

**Antalvic** Aventis, Fr.†.
Dextropropoxyphene hydrochloride (p.28·3).
*Pain.*

**Antalyre** Boehringer Ingelheim, Fr.
Chlorhexidine gluconate (p.1173·2); oxedrine tartrate (p.977·3).
*Conjunctival irritation.*

**Antanazol** Shin Poong, Singapore.
Ketoconazole (p.403·3).
*Fungal infections; seborrhoeic dermatitis.*

**Antanidina** Bergamo, Braz.†.
Ranitidine (p.1285·2).
*Gastro-oesophageal reflux; gastrointestinal haemorrhage; peptic ulcer; Zollinger-Ellison syndrome.*

**Antarene** Elerte, Fr.
Ibuprofen (p.45·3).
*Fever; pain.*

**Antares** Krewel, Ger.†.
Kava (p.1703·2).
*Anxiety; nervous disorders.*

**Antarol** Antigen, Hong Kong†.
Propranolol hydrochloride (p.989·3).
*Angina pectoris; anxiety; arrhythmias; hypertension; hyperthyroidism; migraine; myocardial infarction.*

**Antassa** Medical Industries, Austral.†.
Calcium carbonate (p.1254·2); chamomile (p.1669·3).
*Gastrointestinal hyperacidity.*

**Antasten** Cetus, Arg.
Captopril (p.879·2).
*Hypertension.*

**Antasten-Privin** Novartis Ophthalmics, Swed.
Antazoline sulfate (p.424·2); naphazoline nitrate (p.1124·3); boric acid (p.1662·1); borax (p.1661·3).
*Allergic conjunctivitis.*

**Antaxone**
Zambon, Braz.†; Zambon, Ital.; Zambon, Port.; Pharmazam, Spain.
Naltrexone hydrochloride (p.1046·1).
*Alcohol withdrawal syndrome; opioid withdrawal syndrome.*

**Antazallerge** Siam Bheasach, Thai.
Antazoline hydrochloride (p.424·2); tetryzoline hydrochloride (p.1131·2).
*Conjunctivitis.*

**Antazoline-V** Rugby, USA.
Naphazoline hydrochloride (p.1124·3); antazoline phosphate (p.424·2).
*Eye irritation.*

**Antebor**
Wolfs, Belg.; Biologiques de l'Ile-de-France, Fr.
Sulfacetamide sodium (p.257·3).
*Skin infections.*

**Antebor $B_6$** Biologiques de l'Ile-de-France, Fr.†.
Sulfacetamide sodium (p.257·3); pyridoxine hydrochloride (p.1456·3).
*Bacterial skin infections.*

**Antebor N** Sanofi, Switz.
Chlorhexidine (p.1173·2); triclosan (p.1195·2).
*Acne.*

**Antelepsin** Desitin, Ger.
Clonazepam (p.359·1).
*Epilepsy.*

**Antelmina** Gerda, Fr.†.
Piperazine hydrate (p.111·2).
*Intestinal nematode infections.*

**Antemesyl** Molteni, Ital.†.
*Injection:* Mepyramine hydrochloride (p.437·1); pyridoxine hydrochloride (p.1456·3).
*Suppositories:* Mepyramine hydrochloride (p.437·1).
*Nausea and vomiting.*

**Antemin** Streuli, Switz.
Dimenhydrinate (p.431·1).
*Nausea and vomiting.*

**Antemin compositum** Streuli, Switz.
Dimenhydrinate (p.431·1); caffeine (p.782·1); pyridoxine hydrochloride (p.1456·3).
*Nausea and vomiting.*

**Anten** Pacific, NZ.
Doxepin hydrochloride (p.291·2).
*Depression.*

**Antenex** Alphapharm, Austral.
Diazepam (p.690·1).
*Alcohol withdrawal syndrome; anxiety disorders; skeletal muscle spasm; spasticity.*

**Antepan**
Sanofi Synthelabo, Austria; Henning, Ger.
Protirelin (p.1337·3).
*Assessment of pituitary and thyroid function.*

**Antepar** Glaxo Wellcome, Thai.†.
Piperazine hydrate (p.111·2).
*Ascariasis; enterobiasis.*

**Antepsin**
Boehringer Ingelheim, Arg.; Whitehall, Braz.†; Orion, Denm.; Orion, Fin.; Wyeth, Irl.; Baldacci, Ital.; Orion, Norw.; Chugai, UK; Merck, UK.
Sucralfate (p.1290·2).
*Gastritis; gastrointestinal haemorrhage; gastro-oesophageal reflux; peptic ulcer.*

**Antergan** Nakorn, Thai.
Hydrocortisone acetate (p.1103·3); mepyramine maleate (p.437·1).
*Pruritus; skin irritation.*

**Anthel**
Note. This name is used for preparations of different composition.
Alphapharm, Austral.
Pyrantel embonate (p.113·2).
*Worm infections.*

Shiwa, Thai.
Albendazole (p.101·2).
*Worm infections.*

**Anthelios**
Note. This name is used for preparations of different composition.
Roche-Posay, Arg.
*SPF 10; SPF 20; SPF 40; SPF 50; SPF 60:* Drometrizole trisiloxane; ecamsule (p.1146·3); avobenzone (p.1142·3); octocrilene (p.1154·3); titanium dioxide (p.1160·3).
*Sunscreen.*

Cosmair, Canad.
*SPF 30; SPF 60:* Avobenzone (p.1142·3); enzacamene (p.1147·1); ecamsule (p.1146·3); titanium dioxide (p.1160·3).
*Sunscreen.*

Roche-Posay, Fr.
*SPF 10†:* Octocrilene (p.1154·3); avobenzone (p.1142·3); drometrizole trisiloxane; ecamsule (p.1146·3).
*SPF 20; SPF 30; SPF 40; SPF 50; SPF 60;:* Octocrilene (p.1154·3); titanium dioxide (p.1160·3); avobenzone (p.1142·3); drometrizole trisiloxane; ecamsule (p.1146·3).
*Sunscreen.*

Roche-Posay, Irl.
Octocrilene (p.1154·3); avobenzone (p.1142·3); ecamsule (p.1146·3); titanium dioxide (p.1160·3).
*Sunscreen.*

**Anthelios Stick** Cosmair, Canad.†.
Avobenzone (p.1142·3); enzacamene (p.1147·1).
*Sunscreen.*

**Anthelios T** Roche-Posay, Fr.†.
*SPF 30:* Titanium dioxide (p.1160·3).
*Sunscreen.*

**Antherpos**
Note. This name is used for preparations of different composition.
Roche-Posay, Arg.
*SPF 50:* Ecamsule (p.1146·3); avobenzone (p.1142·3); titanium dioxide (p.1160·3).
*Sunscreen.*

Roche-Posay, Braz.
Drometrizole trisiloxane; ecamsule (p.1146·3); avobenzone (p.1142·3); octocrilene (p.1154·3); titanium dioxide (p.1160·3).
*Sunscreen.*

Cosmair, Canad.
*SPF 50:* Avobenzone (p.1142·3); enzacamene (p.1147·1); ecamsule (p.1146·3); titanium dioxide (p.1160·3).
*Sunscreen.*

Roche-Posay, Fr.
*SPF 50:* Octocrilene (p.1154·3); titanium dioxide (p.1160·3); avobenzone (p.1142·3); ecamsule (p.1146·3).
*Sunscreen.*

Roche-Posay, Irl.
Enzacamene (p.1147·1); avobenzone (p.1142·3); titanium dioxide (p.1160·3).
*Lip protectant; sunscreen.*

**Anthex** Rolab, S.Afr.
Mebendazole (p.108·2).
*Worm infections.*

**Anthisan**
Rhone-Poulenc Rorer, Austral.†; Aventis, Hong Kong; Aventis, Irl.; Aventis, NZ; Aventis, S.Afr.; Aventis, UK.
Mepyramine maleate (p.437·1).
*Allergic skin disorders; pruritus.*

**Anthisan Plus** Aventis, UK.
Mepyramine maleate (p.437·1); benzocaine (p.1370·3).
*Bites and stings.*

**Anthozym** Petrasch, Austria.
Beta vulgaris; lactic acid; ferrous lactate; ascorbic acid; calcium lactate; potassium aspartate; magnesium aspartate; black currant juice (p.1417·1).
*Tonic.*

**Anthozym N** Reith & Petrasch, Ger.†.
Beetroot; lactic acid (p.1704·1).
*Tonic.*

**Anthraderm**
Note. A similar name is used for preparations of different composition (see below).
Gerot, Austria.
Dithranol (p.1146·1); salicylic acid (p.1157·1).
*Psoriasis.*

**Anthra-Derm**
Note. A similar name is used for preparations of different composition (see above).
Dermik, USA.
Dithranol (p.1146·1).
*Psoriasis.*

**Anthraforte** Medican, Canad.
Dithranol (p.1146·1).
*Psoriasis.*

**Anthranol**
Medican, Canad.; Stiefel, Mex.†; Stiefel, Spain†.
Dithranol (p.1146·1).
*Psoriasis.*

**Anthrascalp** Medican, Canad.
Dithranol (p.1146·1).
*Psoriasis.*

**Anthraxiton** Chrispa (Χρισπα), Gr.
Diclofenac sodium (p.32·1).
*Dysmenorrhoea; inflammation; musculoskeletal and joint disorders; pain.*

**Anthraxivore** Picot, Fr.†.
Arctium lappa (p.1704·3).
*Skin infections.*

**Anti Anorex Triple** Lesvi, Spain.
Cyproheptadine hydrochloride (p.430·1); deanol aceglumate (p.1585·3); metoclopramide hydrochloride (p.1274·3).
*Tonic.*

**Anti B** Biogam, Arg.
A hepatitis B immunoglobulin (p.1617·2).
*Passive immunisation.*

**Anti CD3** Butantan, Braz.†.
Muromonab-CD3 (p.1360·3).
*Transplant rejection.*

**Anti Itch** Medibrands, Israel.
Pramocaine hydrochloride (p.1382·2).
*Pain; pruritus; skin irritation.*

**Anti-Ac** Clement-Thekan, Fr.
Pirimiphos-methyl (p.1509·2); permethrin (p.1508·3); piperonyl butoxide (p.1509·2).
*House dust mite acaricide.*

**Antiacid**
Note. This name is used for preparations of different composition.
Garden House, Arg.
Magnesium carbonate (p.1272·1); menthol (p.1711·3); calcium carbonate (p.1254·2).
*Antacid; dietary supplement.*

Shabba, Arg.
Aluminium hydroxide (p.1249·2); magnesium hydroxide (p.1272·2).
*Antacid.*

**Antiacide** Marc-O, Canad.†.
Aluminium hydroxide (p.1249·2); magnesium hydroxide (p.1272·2).

**Anti-Acido** Giuliani, Ital.
Aluminium hydroxide dried gel (p.1249·2); magnesium hydroxide (p.1272·2); dimeticone (p.1289·2).
*Aerophagia; gastric hyperacidity; meteorism.*

**Antiacido Eno** SmithKline Beecham, Spain†.
Calcium carbonate (p.1254·2); magnesium carbonate (p.1272·1).
*Gastrointestinal hyperacidity.*

**Antiacido Salud** Boots Healthcare, Spain†.
Aluminium hydroxide (p.1249·2); calcium carbonate (p.1254·2); magnesium hydroxide (p.1272·2).
*Gastrointestinal hyperacidity.*

**Antiacil** Sedabel, Braz.
Aluminium hydroxide (p.1249·2); magnesium hydroxide (p.1272·2); magnesium trisilicate (p.1272·3).
*Antacid.*

**Antiacne** Drag, Chile.
Sulfur (p.1158·2); resorcinol (p.1156·3).
*Acne.*

**Anti-Acne**
Note. This name is used for preparations of different composition.
MDM, Ital.
Sublimed sulfur (p.1158·2); meclocycline sulfosalicylate (p.229·1); nicoboxil (p.66·3).
*Acne.*

Byk Leo, Spain†.
Alcohol; sulfur (p.1158·2); resorcinol (p.1156·3); triclosan (p.1195·2).
*Acne.*

**Anti-Acne Control Formula** Clinique, Canad.
Salicylic acid (p.1157·1).
*Acne.*

**Anti-Acne Formula for Men** Clinique, Canad.†.
Salicylic acid (p.1157·1); sulfur (p.1158·2).
*Acne.*

**Anti-Acne Spot Treatment** Clinique, Canad.
Salicylic acid (p.1157·1).
*Acne.*

**Antiacneicos Ac-Sal** Isdin, Port.
Salicylic acid (p.1157·1); triclosan (p.1195·2); aloe vera (p.1141·3); polyglyceryl methacrylate.
*Acne.*

**Antiacneicos Niacex** Isdin, Port.
Niseiramida; glycerol (p.1694·3); sodium carbomer.
*Acne.*

**Antiadipositum X-112** Hanseler, Switz.
Cathine hydrochloride (p.1585·2).
*Obesity.*

**Antiadipositum X-112 N** Riemser, Ger.
Phenylpropanolamine hydrochloride (p.1127·3); thiamine hydrochloride; pyridoxine hydrochloride; ascorbic acid (p.1417·1).
*Obesity.*

**Antiadipositum X-112 S** Hanseler, Ger.†.
Cathine hydrochloride (p.1585·2).
*Obesity.*

**Antiadiposo** Teofarma, Ital.
Iodocasein (p.1598·3); thiamine nitrate (p.1455·1).
*Metabolic activator.*

**Anti-Ageing Kalmia** Homeocan, Canad.
Homoeopathic preparation.

**Anti-Algos** Truw, Ger.†.
Paracetamol (p.76·2).
*Fever; pain.*

**Anti-Asmatico** CPH, Port.
Aminophylline (p.780·2); phenobarbital (p.367·3); ephedrine hydrochloride (p.1120·1).
*Asthma.*

**Antiax** Saval, Chile.
Magaldrate (p.1271·3); simeticone (p.1289·2).
*Dyspepsia; gastric hyperacidity; gastritis; gastro-oesophageal reflux; peptic ulcer.*

**Antibacin** Elpen (Ελπεν), Gr.
Ceftriaxone sodium (p.182·3).
*Bacterial infections.*

**Antibacter** Biol, Arg.
Sodium hypochlorite (p.1192·1); magnesium hypochlorite.
*Disinfection.*

**Antibex** Raza, Malaysia; Pharmaniaga, Malaysia.
Chlorhexidine gluconate (p.1173·2).
*Skin and wound disinfection.*

**Antibio-Aberel** Janssen-Cilag, Fr.†.
Tretinoin (p.1161·1); erythromycin (p.208·1).
*Acne.*

**Antibiocilina** Fada, Arg.
Amoxicillin (p.155·3).
*Bacterial infections.*

**Antibiocin** Orion, Ger.†.
Phenoxymethylpenicillin potassium (p.242·1).
*Bacterial infections.*

**Antibiocort** Eczane, Arg.
Hydrocortisone (p.1103·3); naphazoline (p.1124·3); neomycin (p.235·1); gramicidin (p.220·2).
*Infected eye disorders.*

**Antibiofilus** Llorente, Spain†.
*Lactobacillus acidophilus* (p.1704·2); choline orotate (p.1724·3); vitamins (p.1417·1).
*Gastrointestinal disorders; restoration of the gastrointestinal flora.*

**Antibiopen** Antibioticos, Spain.
Ampicillin sodium (p.157·1) or ampicillin trihydrate (p.157·2).
*Bacterial infections.*

**Antibiophilus**
Germania, Austria; Azevedos, Port.
*Lactobacillus rhamnosus* (p.1704·2).
*Diarrhoea.*

**Antibioptal**
Note. This name is used for preparations of different composition.
Poen, Arg.
Tobramycin (p.271·2); phenylephrine hydrochloride (p.1126·3).
*Bacterial eye infections.*

Farmila, Ital.
Chloramphenicol (p.185·1); neomycin sulfate (p.235·1).
*Bacterial eye infections.*

**Antibio-Synalar** Aventis, Fr.
Fluocinolone acetonide (p.1101·2); polymyxin B sulfate (p.245·1); neomycin sulfate (p.235·1).
*Otitis.*

**Antibi-Otic**
Note. A similar name is used for preparations of different composition (see below).
Seng, Thai.
Chloramphenicol (p.185·1).
*Bacterial ear infections.*

**AntibiOtic**
Note. A similar name is used for preparations of different composition (see above).
Parnell, USA†.
Hydrocortisone (p.1103·3); neomycin sulfate (p.235·1); polymyxin B (p.245·2).
*Bacterial ear infections.*

**Antibiotic Cold Sore Ointment** Novartis Consumer, Canad.
Polymyxin B sulfate (p.245·1); tyrothricin (p.275·1); camphor (p.1665·3); menthol (p.1711·3); benzocaine (p.1370·3).
*Herpes labialis.*

**Antibiotic Cream** Technilab, Canad.
Gramicidin (p.220·2); polymyxin B sulfate (p.245·1).

**Antibiotic Ointment** Stanley, Canad.; Technilab, Canad.
Bacitracin (p.161·3); polymyxin B sulfate (p.245·1).

**Antibiotic Simplex** Pfizer, Denm.†.
Erythromycin gluceptate (p.208·2); colistimethate sodium (p.199·1); polymethylmethacrylate/methylmethacrylate copolymer (p.1714·3).
*Bone cement for orthopaedic surgery.*

**Antibiotique Onguent** Prodemdis, Canad.
Bacitracin (p.161·3); polymyxin B sulfate (p.245·1).

**Antibiotrex** Stiefel, Fr.
Isotretinoin (p.1148·3); erythromycin (p.208·1).
*Acne.*

**Antibiotulle Lumiere**
Solvay, Fr.; Hefa, Ger.
Neomycin sulfate (p.235·1); polymyxin B sulfate (p.245·1).
*Infected leg ulcers; infected wounds and burns.*

**Antiblef Eczem** Ciba Vision, Spain†.
Clioquinol (p.196·3); hydrocortisone acetate (p.1103·3).
*Infected eye disorders.*

**Antiblefarica** Novartis, Spain†.
Bismuth loretinate; chlortetracycline hydrochloride (p.187·3); cortisone acetate (p.1096·1).
*Eye disorders.*

**Antiblut** Genepharm, Gr.
Nifedipine (p.966·2).
*Angina; hypertension.*

**Antibron** Potter's, UK.
Lobelia (p.1589·1); wild lettuce (p.1765·2); coltsfoot (p.1117·2); euphorbia (p.1686·3); pleurisy root (p.1733·1); senega (p.1130·2).
*Coughs.*

**Anticatarral** Edigen, Spain.
Chlorphenamine maleate (p.427·3); phenylephrine hydrochloride (p.1126·3); paracetamol (p.76·2).
Formerly contained chlorphenamine maleate, phenylephrine hydrochloride, guaiazulene, muramidase hydrochloride, and paracetamol.
*Cold and influenza symptoms.*

**Anticerumen** Liade, Spain.
Sodium laurilsulfate (p.1574·2).
*Removal of ear wax.*

**Antichloric** Therabel, Belg.
Calcium carbonate (p.1254·2); heavy magnesium carbonate (p.1272·1).
Formerly contained light calcium carbonate, heavy magnesium carbonate, belladonna, and liquorice.
*Peptic ulcer.*

**Anticholium**
Kohler, Austria; Kohler, Ger.
Physostigmine salicylate (p.1494·1).
*Alcohol withdrawal syndrome; antimuscarinic poisoning; central anticholinergic syndrome.*

**Anticold** Andromaco, Chile.
Paracetamol (p.76·2); chlorphenamine maleate (p.427·3); pseudoephedrine sulfate (p.1129·2).
*Cold and influenza symptoms.*

**Anticon** Uniderm, Israel.
Copper-wound plastic (p.1425·3).
*Intra-uterine contraceptive device.*

**Anticongestiva** Sanofi Synthelabo, Spain.
Zinc oxide (p.1163·2).
*Skin irritation.*

**Anticorizza** Ogna, Ital.
Paracetamol (p.76·2); salicylamide (p.87·3); caffeine (p.782·1); tripelennamine hydrochloride (p.442·3).
*Cold and influenza symptoms.*

**Anticude** UCB, Spain.
Edrophonium bromide (p.1490·3).
*Diagnosis of myasthenia gravis; reversal of competitive neuromuscular blockade.*

**Anti-D**
Upha, Malaysia; Beacons, Singapore.
Chlorpropamide (p.330·3).
*Diabetes mellitus.*

**Anti-Dandruff Shampoo** Avant Garde, Canad.†.
Pyrithione zinc (p.1156·2).

**Antidep**
Torrent, India; Torrent, Thai.†.
Imipramine hydrochloride (p.300·1).
*Depression; narcoleptic syndrome; nocturnal enuresis.*

**Anti-Dessechement** Lierac, Fr.
Urea (p.1162·2).
*Dry skin.*

**Antidia** Daewon, Hong Kong†.
Nifuroxazide (p.237·2).
*Diarrhoea.*

**Antidiar**
Note. This name is used for preparations of different composition.
Ahimsa, Arg.
Phthalylsulfathiazole (p.242·3); menadione (p.1466·3).
*Diarrhoea.*

Aerocid, Fr.†.
Loperamide hydrochloride (p.1271·1).
*Diarrhoea.*

**Anti-Diarrheal** Stanley, Canad.
Loperamide hydrochloride (p.1271·1).

**Antidifar** Alpharma, Mex.
Diiodohydroxyquinoline (p.603·3).
*Amoebiasis.*

**Antidin** Teuto, Braz.
Ranitidine hydrochloride (p.1285·2).
*Peptic ulcer.*

**Antidol**
*Note. This name is used for preparations of different composition.*
*Elvetium, Arg.*
Rofecoxib (p.86·3).
*Osteoarthritis; pain.*
*Gerbex, Canad.*
Aspirin (p.15·1); caffeine (p.782·1).
*Quimica y Farmacia, Mex.; Cinfa, Spain.*
Paracetamol (p.76·2).
*Fever; pain.*

**Antidoloroso Rudol** *Bayer, Spain†.*
Aspirin (p.15·1); caffeine (p.782·1).
*Fever; pain.*

**Antidote Anti-Digitale BM** *Roche, Switz.†.*
Digoxin-specific antibody fragments (p.1036·3).
*Digitalis poisoning.*

**Antidoto Arvin** *Knoll, Spain†.*
Ancrod antisera.
*Overdosage with ancrod.*

**Antidotum Thallii-Heyl** *Heyl, Ger.*
Prussian blue (p.1051·2).
*Thallium poisoning.*

**Antidrasi** *Visufarma, Ital.*
Diclofenamide (p.894·1) or diclofenamide sodium (p.894·1).
*Control of intra-ocular pressure during eye surgery; glaucoma.*

**Antidry** *Adroka, Switz.*
*Bath oil:* Liquid paraffin (p.1479·1); almond oil (p.1651·1).
*Ointment:* Pansy; zinc oxide (p.1163·2); almond oil (p.1651·1).
*Shower oil:* Liquid paraffin (p.1479·1); soya oil (p.1447·2); levomenol (p.1707·1).
*Topical lotion:* Sodium lactate (p.1223·2); almond oil (p.1651·1).
*Skin disorders.*

**Antiedema** *Alcon Cusi, Spain.*
Sodium chloride (p.1233·3).
*Corneal oedema.*

**Antiemorroidali** *Ogna, Ital.; AFOM, Ital.*
Ichthammol (p.1148·2); zinc oxide (p.1163·2); bismuth subgallate (p.1252·2); belladonna (p.479·1).
*Haemorrhoids.*

**Antiespasmodico** *Veinfar, Arg.*
Homatropine (p.483·2).
*Smooth muscle spasm.*

**Antiestrias** *Isdin, Port.*
Centella (p.1144·3); borage oil (p.1661·3); *dl*-alpha tocoferil acetate (p.1465·1); jojoba oil.
*Firming cream.*

**Antietanol** *Aventis, Braz.†.*
Disulfiram (p.1681·3).
*Chronic alcoholism.*

**Antifebrin** *Royton, Braz.*
Aspirin (p.15·1).
*Fever; inflammation; pain.*

**Antifect**
*Note. This name is used for preparations of different composition.*
*Schulke & Mayr, Ger.†.*
Alcohol (p.1166·1); propyl alcohol (p.1191·2); glyoxal (p.1181·1).
*Surface disinfection.*
*Potter's, UK.*
Garlic (p.1691·1); garlic oil (p.1691·2); echinacea (p.1683·2).
*Catarrh; nasal congestion; rhinitis.*

**Antiflam** *Rolab, S.Afr.*
Ibuprofen (p.45·3).
*Fever; pain.*

**Anti-Flamme** *Natures Kiss, Austral.†.*
Arnica (p.1656·3); calendula (p.1665·2); hypericum (p.299·1); peppermint oil (p.1283·2).
*Local pain and injury.*

**Antiflog** *FIRMA, Ital.*
Piroxicam (p.84·2).
*Musculoskeletal, joint, and peri-articular disorders.*

**Antiflogil** *Farmasa, Braz.*
Nimesulide (p.67·1).
*Fever; inflammation; pain.*

**Antiflogol** *Poen, Arg.*
Betamethasone (p.1093·1); tetryzoline hydrochloride (p.1131·2); chloramphenicol (p.185·1).
*Infected eye disorders.*

**Antifloxil** *Alter, Spain†.*
Nimesulide (p.67·1).
*Fever; inflammation; pain.*

**Antiflu**
*Note. This name is used for preparations of different composition.*
*Byk Gulden, Ital.*
Paracetamol (p.76·2); chlorphenamine maleate (p.427·3); caffeine (p.782·1).
*Cold and influenza symptoms.*
*Pharmco, S.Afr.*
Paracetamol (p.76·2); mepyramine maleate (p.437·1); diphenhydramine hydrochloride (p.431·3); caffeine (p.782·1); codeine phosphate (p.27·1); phenylephrine hydrochloride (p.1126·3).
*Cold and influenza symptoms.*

**Antiflu Forte** *Synco, Hong Kong.*
Paracetamol (p.76·2); salicylamide (p.87·3); phenylpropanolamine hydrochloride (p.1127·3); phenylephrine hydrochloride (p.1126·3); chlorphenamine maleate (p.427·3); caffeine (p.782·1).
*Cold and influenza symptoms; rhinitis.*

**Antiflu-Des** *Chinoin, Mex.*
Amantadine hydrochloride (p.1197·2); chlorphenamine maleate (p.427·3); paracetamol (p.76·2).
Formerly contained amantadine hydrochloride, chlorphenamine maleate, phenylpropanolamine hydrochloride, and paracetamol.
*Influenza symptoms.*

**Antiflu-N-Forte** *Synco, Hong Kong.*
Paracetamol (p.76·2); salicylamide (p.87·3); ephedrine hydrochloride (p.1120·1); phenylephrine hydrochloride (p.1126·3); dexchlorpheniramine maleate (p.427·3); caffeine (p.782·1).
*Cold and influenza symptoms; rhinitis.*

**AntiFocal** *Vitorgan, Ger.*
Animal tissue extract: diencephalon; cerebellum (p.1709·3); cort. cerebri; cerebrum fet.; medulla spinal; hepar.; pancreas; lien; thyreoidea (p.1604·2); thymus juv. (p.1756·1); placenta; mucosa misc.
*Nervous system disorders.*

**AntiFocal N** *Vitorgan, Ger.*
Metenolone acetate (p.1559·2); liothyronine hydrochloride (p.1602·2); chorionic gonadotrophin (p.1320·3); pyridoxine hydrochloride (p.1456·3); cyanocobalamin (p.1458·2).
*Nervous system disorders.*

**Antifohnon-N** *Sudmedica, Ger.†.*
Ephedrine hydrochloride (p.1120·1); ethenzamide (p.37·2).
*Circulatory disorders.*

**Antifungal**
*YSP, Malaysia; Yung Shin, Singapore.*
Miconazole nitrate (p.405·3).
*Fungal skin and vulvovaginal infections.*

**Antifungal Foot Deodorant** *Or-Dov, Austral.†.*
Tolnaftate (p.410·1).
*Tinea pedis.*

**Antifungol** *Hexal, Ger.*
Clotrimazole (p.396·2).
*Fungal infections of the skin and genito-urinary tract.*

**Antigeron** *Farmasa, Braz.*
Cinnarizine (p.428·3).
*Peripheral vascular disorders; vestibular disorders.*

**Anti-Geruchs** *Twardy, Ger.†.*
Chlorophyllin (p.1057·1).
*Body odour; metabolic disorders.*

**Antiglan** *Potter's, UK.*
Saw palmetto (p.1569·1); equisetum (p.1684·1); hydrangea (p.1698·3).
Formerly contained kava, saw palmetto, equisetum, and hydrangea.
*Bladder discomfort.*

**Antigoutteux Rezall** *Medecine Vegetale, Fr.†.*
Lithium benzoate (p.1707·2); lithium salicylate (p.54·2); colchicum (p.416·3); maize (p.1676·1); bitter-orange (p.1723·3).
*Gout; rheumatism.*

**Antigreg**
*Piam, Ital.; Piam, Singapore.*
Ticlopidine hydrochloride (p.1011·2).
*Thrombosis prophylaxis.*

**Antigrietun** *Casen Fleet, Spain.*
Allantoin (p.1141·3); aminoacridine (p.1165·3); peru balsam (p.1730·2); prednisolone (p.1108·1).
*Allergic skin disorders; cracked nipples; mastitis; superficial burns.*

**Antigripal Compuesto** *Vent-3, Arg.*
Paracetamol (p.76·2); chlorphenamine maleate (p.427·3); pseudoephedrine hydrochloride (p.1129·2); dextromethorphan hydrobromide (p.1117·3).
*Cold and influenza symptoms.*

**Anti-Gripe** *Plough, Port.*
Aconite (p.1646·3); belladonna (p.479·1); codeine (p.27·1); caffeine (p.782·1); paracetamol (p.76·2).
*Cold symptoms; fever; pain.*

**Antigriphine** *GlaxoSmithKline Consumer, Belg.*
Paracetamol (p.76·2); caffeine (p.782·1).
*Fever; pain.*

**Antigripine** *Sanofi Winthrop, Braz.†.*
Paracetamol (p.76·2); caffeine (p.782·1); cresotamide.
*Cold and influenza symptoms.*

**Antigrippine**
*Note. This name is used for preparations of different composition.*
*SmithKline Beecham Consumer, Neth.*
Paracetamol (p.76·2); caffeine (p.782·1); ascorbic acid (p.1460·2).
*Fever; pain.*
*GlaxoSmithKline Consumer, Port.*
Dextromethorphan hydrobromide (p.1117·3); phenylpropanolamine hydrochloride (p.1127·3); paracetamol (p.76·2).
Formerly contained aspirin, codeine phosphate, and vitamin C.
*Fever; pain.*
*SmithKline Beecham Consumer, Switz.†.*
Paracetamol (p.76·2); ascorbic acid (p.1460·2).
*Cold symptoms.*

**Antigrippine a l'Aspirine** *SmithKline Beecham Sante, Fr.†.*
Aspirin (p.15·1); ascorbic acid (p.1460·2); caffeine hydrate (p.782·1).
*Fever; pain.*

**Antigrippine Midy** *SmithKline Beecham, Belg.†.*
Paracetamol (p.76·2); 3-methylsalicylamide; codeine phosphate (p.27·1); caffeine (p.782·1); ascorbic acid (p.1460·2).
*Cold symptoms.*

**Anti-H** *Biodim, Fr.*
Aluminium sodium silicate (p.1250·2); kaolin (p.1268·3); sodium bicarbonate (p.1223·2); calcium carbonate (p.1254·2).
*Flatulence; gastrointestinal pain.*

**Anti-Hemorroidaires** *Aventis, Fr.†.*
*Rectal ointment:* Hydrocortisone (p.1103·3); cinchocaine hydrochloride (p.1373·2).
*Suppositories:* Hydrocortisone acetate (p.1103·3); esculoside (p.1648·2); benzocaine (p.1370·3).
Formerly contained hydrocortisone acetate, benzocaine, esculoside, framycetin sulfate, heparin, and butyl amino benzoate.
*Anorectal disorders.*

**Antihemorroidal**
*Note. This name is used for preparations of different composition.*
*Denver, Arg.*
Lidocaine (p.1377·3); betamethasone (p.1093·1); phenylephrine (p.1126·3).
*Haemorrhoids.*
*Cinfa, Spain.*
Benzocaine (p.1370·3); hydrocortisone acetate (p.1103·3); neomycin sulfate (p.235·1); tannic acid (p.1751·2).
*Anorectal disorders.*
*ICN, Spain.*
*Ointment:* Hydrocortisone acetate (p.1103·3); neomycin sulfate (p.235·1); promethazine hydrochloride (p.439·1); vitamin A (p.1451·2).
*Suppositories†:* Hydrocortisone acetate (p.1103·3); promethazine hydrochloride (p.439·1); vitamin A (p.1451·2).
*Anorectal disorders.*

**Anti-Hist**
*Note. A similar name is used for preparations of different composition (see below).*
*Clonmel, Irl.†.*
Chlorphenamine maleate (p.427·3).
*Hypersensitivity reactions.*

**Antihist-1**
*Note. A similar name is used for preparations of different composition (see above).*
*Goldline, USA†; Major, USA†; Rugby, USA†.*
Clemastine fumarate (p.429·1).

**Antihistamine Forte** *Unichem, UK†.*
Terfenadine (p.441·1).
*Hay fever; hypersensitivity reactions.*

**Antihistaminico** *Llorens, Spain.*
Chlorphenamine maleate (p.427·3).
*Hypersensitivity reactions of the eye.*

**Antihist-D** *Goldline, USA†.*
Clemastine fumarate (p.429·1); phenylpropanolamine hydrochloride (p.1127·3).
*Upper respiratory-tract disorders.*

**Anti-Homocysteine Factor** *Eagle, Austral.†.*
Amino acids, vitamin B substances; minerals (p.1417·1).
*Elevated homocysteine levels.*

**Antihydral**
*Schmidgall, Austria†; Robugen, Ger.; Iromedica, Switz.*
Methenamine (p.230·1).
*Hyperhidrosis; skin infections.*

**Antihydral M**
*Schmidgall, Austria†; Robugen, Ger.; Robugen, Hong Kong; Medipharm, Switz.†.*
Methenamine (p.230·1); sulfur (p.1158·2).
*Fungal skin infections; hyperhidrosis.*

**Antihypertonicum Forte** *Hevert, Ger.*
Homoeopathic preparation.

**Antihypertonicum S** *Schuck, Ger.*
Betula (p.1660·3); crataegus (p.1677·1); mistletoe (p.1715·3); olive; rhododendron leaf; rutoside (p.1688·2); proxyphylline (p.791·2).
*Arteriosclerosis; hypertension.*

**Antihypertonicum-Weliplex** *Weber & Weber, Ger.*
Homoeopathic preparation.

**Antihypertonikum-Tropfen N** *Schuck, Ger.*
Homoeopathic preparation.

**Anti-inhibitor Coagulant Complex** *Baxter, UK†.*
A factor VIII inhibitor bypassing fraction (p.752·2).
*Haemorrhage in patients with inhibitors to factor VIII.*

**Anti-Inhibitor Coagulant Complex (Autoplex T)** *Baxter, Israel†.*
A factor VIII inhibitor bypassing fraction (p.752·2).
*Haemorrhage in patients with inhibitors to factor VIII.*

**Anti-Kalium** *Medice, Ger.*
Calcium polystyrene sulfonate (p.1032·3).
*Hyperkalaemia.*

**Antikataraktikum N** *Ursapharm, Ger.*
Disodium inosinate (p.1681·3).
*Visual disturbances.*

**Antikataraktikum N oral** *Ursapharm, Ger.†.*
Disodium uridine 5′-monophosphate.
*Cataracts.*

**Antikatarata** *Novartis Ophthalmics, Arg.*
Disodium inosinate (p.1681·3); nicotinamide (p.1441·2); magnesium aspartate (p.1227·3); sodium glycerophosphate (p.1695·2).
*Cataracts.*

**Antikeloides Creme** *Widmer, Switz.*
Dexamethasone (p.1097·1); urea (p.1162·2); vitamin A palmitate (p.1453·1).
*Scars.*

**Antil** *Carnot, Mex.†.*
Cimetidine (p.1255·3).

**Antilerg** *ICN, Arg.*
Ketotifen fumarate (p.788·1).
*Allergic conjunctivitis.*

**Antilergal** *Medix, Mex.*
Loratadine (p.436·1).
*Hypersensitivity reactions; rhinitis.*

**Antilipid** *Kleva, Gr.*
Gemfibrozil (p.923·1).
*Hyperlipidaemias.*

**Antilirium** *Forest Pharmaceuticals, USA.*
Physostigmine salicylate (p.1494·1).
*Reversal of drug-induced CNS antimuscarinic effects.*

**Antimast N** *Selz, Ger.*
Homoeopathic preparation.

**Antimast T** *Selz, Ger.*
Homoeopathic preparation.

**Antimet** *Antigen, Irl.*
Metoclopramide hydrochloride (p.1274·3).
*Gastrointestinal disorders.*

**Antimic** *Klinger, Braz.†.*
Salicylic acid (p.1157·1); potassium iodide (p.1598·1); iodine (p.1598·1) boric acid (p.1662·1); magenta (p.1185·1).
*Skin infections.*

**Anti-Micot** *Neckerman, Braz.†.*
Undecenoic acid (p.410·3).
*Fungal infections.*

**Antimicotica Solforata** *AFOM, Ital.*
Sodium thiosulfate (p.1053·3); tartaric acid (p.1752·1).
*Fungal skin infections.*

**Antimicotico**
*IFI, Ital.†.*
*Ointment:* Benzoxiquine (p.1170·2); dexamethasone (p.1097·1); pyridoxine (p.1457·2); polyenacid.
*Fungal skin infections.*
*Savoma, Ital.*
*Cream:* Clotrimazole (p.396·2).
*Fungal infections.*

**Antimigrin** *Gebro, Austria.*
Naratriptan hydrochloride (p.470·1).
*Migraine.*

**Antiminth**
*Note. This name is used for preparations of different composition.*
*Costec, Arg.*
*Shampoo:* Pyrithione zinc (p.1156·2).
*Scalp disorders.*
*Soap:* Chlorhexidine gluconate (p.1173·2).
*Skin cleanser.*
*Pfizer, USA.*
Pyrantel embonate (p.113·2).
*Worm infections.*

**Antimyk** *Pfleger, Ger.†.*
Clotrimazole (p.396·2).
*Fungal infections.*

**Antimyopikum** *Ursapharm, Ger.†.*
Troxerutin (p.1688·3); alpha tocoferil acetate (p.1465·1).
*Progressive shortsightedness.*

**Antinaus** *Pacific, NZ.*
Prochlorperazine maleate (p.716·3).
*Anxiety; Ménière's disease; nausea and vomiting; psychoses; vertigo.*

**Anti-Nauseant** *Stanley, Canad.*
Dimenhydrinate (p.431·1).
*Nausea.*

**Antinephrin M** *Hanosan, Ger.*
Homoeopathic preparation.

**Antinerveux Lesourd** *Lesourd, Fr.*
Lotus petal; melilot.
*Insomnia; irritability.*

**Antineuralgica** *Alpharma, Norw.*
Caffeine (p.782·1); phenazone (p.82·3).
*Pain.*

**Antineuralgicum (Rowo-633)** *Pharmakon, Ger.†.*
Homoeopathic preparation.
Lidocaine hydrochloride (p.1377·3) is included in this preparation to alleviate the pain of injection.

**Antineurina** *Mabo, Spain.*
Cyanocobalamin (p.1458·2); pyridoxine hydrochloride (p.1456·3); thiamine hydrochloride (p.1455·1).
*Neuritis; vitamin B deficiency.*

**Antinevralgico Dr Knapp** *Montefarmaco, Ital.*
Paracetamol (p.76·2); aspirin (p.15·1); caffeine (p.782·1).
*Fever; pain.*

**Antinevralgico Penegal** *FAMA, Ital.†.*
Paracetamol (p.76·2); aspirin (p.15·1).
*Fever; pain.*

**Antinicoticum sine (Rowo-100)** *Pharmakon, Ger.*
Homoeopathic preparation.

**Antio** *Pentamedical, Ital.*
Zinc ricinoleate.
*Body odour.*

**Antiobes** *Novartis Consumer, Spain†.*
Fenproporex hydrochloride (p.1588·3).
*Obesity.*

**Antiobiocilina** *Fada, Arg.*
Amoxicillin (p.155·3).
*Bacterial infections.*

**Antiopiaz** *Richmond, Arg.*
Naloxone (p.1045·1).
*Opioid withdrawal.*

**Antiotic** Grossmann, Switz.
Amoxicillin trihydrate (p.155·3).
*Bacterial infections.*

**Antiox** Mayrand, USA†.
Betacarotene (p.1422·3); ascorbic acid (p.1460·2).

**Antioxidans E** Hevert, Ger.
*dl*-Alpha tocoferil acetate (p.1465·1).
*Vitamin E deficiency.*

**Antioxidant Forte Tablets** Vitelle, Austral.†.
Betacarotene (p.1422·3); riboflavin (p.1456·1); ascorbic acid (p.1460·2); sodium ascorbate (p.1460·2); *d*-alpha tocoferil acid succinate (p.1465·1); zinc amino acid chelate (p.1469·3); folic acid (p.1429·1); silybum marianum (p.1043·3); vitis vinifera.
*Anti-oxidant; vitamin A, C, E, and $B_2$, folic acid, and zinc deficiencies.*

**Antioxidant Nutrients** Solgar, UK†.
Multivitamin preparation with amino acids and zinc (p.1417·1).
*Dietary supplement.*

**Antioxidant Tablets** Cenovis, Austral.†; Vitelle, Austral.†.
Ascorbic acid (p.1460·2); sodium ascorbate (p.1460·2); betacarotene (p.1422·3); *d*-alpha tocoferil acid succinate (p.1465·1); zinc amino acid chelate (p.1469·3); riboflavin (p.1456·1).
*Anti-oxidant; vitamin A, C, E, $B_2$, and zinc deficiencies.*

**Antioxidante Vital** AM, Arg.
Vitamin and mineral preparation (p.1417·1).

**Antioxirell** Sanorell, Ger.†.
Vitamin C; vitamin E; betacarotene; vitamin A; selenium (p.1417·1).
*Dietary supplement.*

**Antipanin N** Michallik, Ger.†.
Paracetamol (p.76·2).
Formerly contained ethenzamide and paracetamol.
*Pain.*

**Antipanin P** Michallik, Ger.†.
Paracetamol (p.76·2).
*Pain.*

**Antiparkin** Viatris, Ger.
Selegiline hydrochloride (p.1214·1).
Formerly known as Movergan.
*Parkinsonism.*

**Antipasmol** Monserrat, Arg.
Belladonna (p.479·1); papaverine hydrochloride (p.1728·1).
*Smooth muscle spasm.*

**Antipeol**
Note. This name is used for preparations of different composition.
Restan, S.Afr.
Zinc oxide (p.1163·2); ichthammol (p.1148·2); salicylic acid (p.1157·1).
*Skin disorders.*

Medico-Biological Laboratories, UK.
Zinc oxide (p.1163·2); ichthammol (p.1148·2); salicylic acid (p.1157·1); urea (p.1162·2).
*Skin disorders.*

**Antiphlogistine**
Note. This name is used for preparations of different composition.
CIF, Braz.
Boric acid (p.1662·1); salicylic acid (p.1157·1); iodine (p.1598·1); peppermint oil (p.1283·2); sweet birch oil (p.60·1); eucalyptus oil (p.1686·2).
*Inflammation.*

Fumouze, Fr.
Kaolin (p.1268·3); salicylic acid (p.1157·1).
*Muscle and connective tissue pain.*

Carter-Wallace, Switz.
Salicylic acid (p.1157·1); methyl salicylate (p.59·3); eucalyptus oil (p.1686·2); peppermint oil (p.1283·2).
*Inflammation; pain.*

**Antiphlogistine Rub A-535** Carter Horner, Canad.
Methyl salicylate (p.59·3); camphor (p.1665·3); menthol (p.1711·3); eucalyptus oil (p.1686·2).
*Musculoskeletal pain.*

**Antiphlogistine Rub A-535 Capsaicin** Carter Horner, Canad.
Capsaicin (p.24·2).
*Musculoskeletal and joint disorders.*

**Antiphlogistine Rub A-535 Ice** Carter Horner, Canad.
Menthol (p.1711·3).
*Musculoskeletal pain.*

**Antiphlogistine Rub A-535 No Odour** Carter Horner, Canad.
Trolamine salicylate (p.95·3).
*Musculoskeletal pain.*

**Anti-Phosphat**
Brady, Austria; Gry, Ger.
Aluminium hydroxide (p.1249·2).
*Hyperphosphataemia.*

**Anti-Phosphate** Bichsel, Switz.
Dried aluminium hydroxide (p.1249·2).
*Hyperphosphataemia.*

**Anti-Plaque Chewing Gum** Or-Dov, Austral.†.
Chlorhexidine acetate (p.1173·2).
*Dental plaque.*

**Antipressan**
Teva, Hong Kong; Berk, UK.
Atenolol (p.865·2).
*Angina pectoris; arrhythmias; hypertension; myocardial infarction.*

**Antiprex** Elpen (Ελπεν), Gr.
Enalapril maleate (p.909·2).
*Heart failure; hypertension.*

**Antiprotin** Julphar, UAE.
Bromocriptine mesilate (p.1200·3).
*Acromegaly; benign breast disorders; female infertility; hyperprolactinaemia; menstrual disorders; parkinsonism.*

**Antiprurit** Kade, Ger.
Cell components and metabolic products of *Staphylococcus aureus*; *Enterococcus faecalis* (p.1704·2); *Pseudomonas aeruginosa*; and *Escherichia coli*; hydrocortisone (p.1103·3).
*Skin disorders.*

**Antipsichos** Proel, Gr.
Buspirone hydrochloride (p.672·2).
*Generalised anxiety.*

**Antipulmina** Lisapharma, Ital.
Peppermint oil (p.1283·2); pumilio pine oil (p.1737·1); eucalyptus oil (p.1686·2).
*Respiratory-tract disorders.*

**Antipyn** Garec, S.Afr.
Paracetamol (p.76·2); codeine phosphate (p.27·1); caffeine (p.782·1).
*Fever; pain.*

**Antipyn Forte** Garec, S.Afr.
Paracetamol (p.76·2); codeine phosphate (p.27·1); caffeine (p.782·1); meprobamate (p.706·2).
*Pain associated with tension.*

**Antireumina** Kedrion, Ital.
Aspirin (p.15·1); paracetamol (p.76·2); caffeine (p.782·1).
*Fever; pain.*

**Antirrinum** Reig Jofre, Spain.
Oxymetazoline hydrochloride (p.1126·1).
*Nasal congestion; sinus congestion.*

**Anti-rugas C** Dermoteca, Port.
Ascorbic acid (p.1460·2).
*Sun-induced skin damage.*

**Antis** Gerolimatos (Γερολυματος), Gr.
Butamirate citrate (p.1116·2).
*Cough.*

**Antiscabbia Candioli al DDT Terapeutico**
Candioli, Ital.
Benzyl benzoate (p.1500·2); benzocaine (p.1370·3); clofenotane (p.1502·1).
*Scabies.*

**Antiscabiosum** Strathmann, Ger.
Benzyl benzoate (p.1500·2).
*Scabies.*

**Antisept** Salud, Spain†.
Chlorhexidine gluconate (p.1173·2).
*Skin and wound disinfection.*

**Antisepthic Hexil** Florida, Arg.
Benzalkonium chloride (p.1168·3); chlorhexidine (p.1173·2).
*Disinfection.*

**Antiseptic Foot Balm**
Scholl, Israel†; Scholl, UK†.
Menthol (p.1711·3); halquinol (p.220·3); methyl salicylate (p.59·3).
*Sore feet.*

**Antiseptic Lozenges** Mentholatum, UK†.
Menthol (p.1711·3); eucalyptus oil (p.1686·2); amylmetacresol (p.1168·2).
*Cold symptoms; coughs; nasal congestion; sore throat.*

**Antiseptic Mouthwash**
Note. This name is used for preparations of different composition.
Scott, Canad.; Sutton, Canad.
Cineole (p.1672·1); menthol (p.1711·3); thymol (p.1194·2).

Thornton & Ross, UK.
Sodium salicylate (p.90·1); thymol (p.1194·2); menthol (p.1711·3).
*Mouth disorders.*

**Antiseptic Ointment** National Care, Canad.
Chloroxylenol (p.1177·2).
*Skin protection.*

**Antiseptic Skin Cream**
Note. This name is used for preparations of different composition.
National Care, Canad.
Benzalkonium chloride (p.1168·3).

National Care, Canad.
Benzethonium chloride (p.1169·2); vitamin A (p.1451·2); vitamin D (p.1461·2).
*Ostomy care; skin irritation.*

**Antiseptic Throat Lozenges**
Note. This name is used for preparations of different composition.
Sutton, Canad.
Hexylresorcinol (p.1182·1).
Formerly known as Antiseptic Sore Throat Lozenges.

Unichem, UK.
Amylmetacresol (p.1168·2).
*Sore throat.*

**Antiseptico Hertz** Hertz, Braz.†.
Lidocaine (p.1377·3); benzethonium.

**Antiseptin**
Note. This name is used for preparations of different composition.
Hertz, Braz.†.
Bacitracin (p.161·3); neomycin (p.235·1); zinc (p.1469·2).
*Skin infections.*

Instituto Sanitas, Chile.
Triclosan (p.1195·2).
*Disinfection of hands; skin infection.*

**Antiseptique Pastilles** Prodemdis, Canad.
Domiphen bromide (p.1179·1).

**Antiseptique-Calmante** Chauvin, Fr.†.
Methylthioninium chloride (p.1042·2); methylrosanilinium chloride (p.1186·1); boric acid (p.1662·1); procaine hydrochloride (p.1383·2).
*Corneal and conjunctival trauma.*

**Antisettico Astringente Sedativo** Bruschettini, Ital.
Zinc phenolsulfonate (p.1163·3); sulfacetamide sodium (p.257·3); naphazoline hydrochloride (p.1124·3); lidocaine hydrochloride (p.1377·3).
*Conjunctivitis.*

**Antisklerosin S** Medopharm, Ger.†.
Crataegus (p.1677·1); mistletoe (p.1715·3); nicotinic acid (p.1441·1); magnesium orotate (p.1724·3); rutoside (p.1688·2).
*Arteriosclerosis; circulatory disorders; hyperlipidaemias.*

**Anti-Smoking Tablets** Potter's, UK†.
Lobelia (p.1589·1).
*Aid to smoking withdrawal.*

**Antisol** Raza, Malaysia; Pharmaniaga, Malaysia.
Chlorhexidine gluconate (p.1173·2).
*Skin disinfection.*

**Antispa** TP, Thai.
Hyoscine butylbromide (p.483·3).
*Smooth muscle spasm.*

**Antispas** Keene, USA.
Dicycloverine hydrochloride (p.481·2).
*Functional bowel syndrome; irritable bowel syndrome.*

**Antispasmin** QIF, Braz.†.
Belladonna (p.479·1); papaverine hydrochloride (p.1728·1); valerian (p.1762·2).
*Smooth muscle spasm.*

**Antispasmina** Hexa-Medinova, Arg.
Dipyrone (p.35·3); papaverine hydrochloride (p.1728·1); homatropine methylbromide (p.483·2).
*Pain; smooth muscle spasm.*

**Antispasmina Colica**
Note. This name is used for preparations of different composition.
Recordati, Ital.
Papaverine hydrochloride (p.1728·1); belladonna (p.479·1); hyoscyamine (p.485·1).
*Gastrointestinal spasm.*

Lepori, Port.
Papaverine (p.1728·1); belladonna (p.479·1); valerian (p.1762·2).
*Smooth muscle spasm.*

**Antispasmodic Elixir** Morton Grove, USA.
Phenobarbital (p.367·3); hyoscyamine sulfate (p.485·1); atropine sulfate (p.477·1); hyoscine hydrobromide (p.483·3).

**Antisseptico** Furp, Braz.†.
Povidone-iodine (p.1190·3).
*Disinfection.*

**Antistax**
Boehringer Ingelheim, Austria; Pharmaton, Ger.; Fher, Spain; Pharmaton, Switz.; Boehringer Ingelheim, UK.
Red vine leaf.
*Venous insufficiency.*

**Antistina-Privin** Novartis, Denm.
Antazoline sulfate (p.424·2); naphazoline nitrate (p.1124·3).
*Conjunctivitis.*

**Antistine-Privine** Novartis, Austral.
Antazoline sulfate (p.424·2); naphazoline nitrate (p.1124·3).
*Allergic conjunctivitis; eye irritation.*

**Antistin-Privin**
Novartis, Fin.; Novartis Ophthalmics, Ger.; Ciba Vision, Israel; Adcock Ingram, S.Afr.; Novartis Ophthalmics, Singapore; Novartis Ophthalmics, Switz.
Antazoline sulfate (p.424·2); naphazoline nitrate (p.1124·3).
*Allergic conjunctivitis.*

**Antistin-Privina** Ciba Vision, Ital.
Antazoline sulfate (p.424·2); naphazoline nitrate (p.1124·3).
*Allergic conjunctivitis.*

**Antitensin** Teuto, Braz.
Propranolol hydrochloride (p.989·3).
*Hypertension.*

**Antitis** Potter's, UK.
Buchu leaf (p.1663·1); clivers (p.1673·2); couch-grass (p.1676·2); equisetum (p.1684·1); shepherd's purse (p.1744·1); bearberry (p.1659·2).
*Cystitis; urinary or bladder discomfort.*

**Antitoxikon** Sanofi Synthelabo, Braz.†.
Liver extract.
*Liver disorders.*

**Antituss**
Note. A similar name is used for preparations of different composition (see below).
Pharmco, S.Afr.†.
Promethazine hydrochloride (p.439·1); codeine phosphate (p.27·1); ephedrine hydrochloride (p.1120·1).
*Cold symptoms; coughs.*

**Anti-Tuss**
Note. A similar name is used for preparations of different composition (see above).
Century, USA.
Guaifenesin (p.1122·1).
*Coughs.*

**Antitussive Decongestant Antihistamine Syrup** Prodemdis, Canad.†.
Phenylpropanolamine hydrochloride (p.1127·3); pheniramine maleate (p.438·3); mepyramine maleate (p.437·1); dextromethorphan hydrobromide (p.1117·3).

**Antitussivum Burger** Ysatfabrik, Ger.
Codeine phosphate (p.27·1).
*Coughs.*

**Antitussivum Burger N** Ysatfabrik, Ger.
Dihydrocodeine tartrate (p.34·3); thyme oil (p.1755·3).
*Coughs.*

**Antivenin** Wyeth-Ayerst, Canad.†.
Crotalidae antiserum (p.1639·1).
*Snake envenomation.*

**Antivenin (Latrodectus Mactans)** Merck Frosst, Canad.
Black widow spider antiserum (p.1640·1).
*Black widow spider bite.*

**Antiverrugas** Isdin, Spain.
Lactic acid (p.1704·1); salicylic acid (p.1157·1).
*Warts.*

**Antivert**
Pfizer, Canad.†; Pfizer, USA.
Meclozine hydrochloride (p.436·3).
*Motion sickness; vertigo.*

**Anti-Ves** Novartis, Ital.
Soya oil; vitamins (p.1417·1).
*Nutritional supplement.*

**Antivipmyn** Bioclon, Mex.
Polyvalent crotalidae antiserum (p.1639·1).
*Snake envenomation.*

**Antivirax** EMS, Braz.
Aciclovir (p.626·1).
*Herpesvirus infections.*

**Antivom** Unipharma, Gr.
Betahistine hydrochloride (p.1660·1).
*Menière's disease; vertigo.*

**Antizid** Lilly, S.Afr.
Nizatidine (p.1277·2).
*Heartburn; hyperacidity.*

**Antizine** Pharmasant, Thai.
Hydroxyzine hydrochloride (p.434·3).
*Hypersensitivity reactions; sedative.*

**Antizol**
Paladin, Canad.; Orphan Medical, Israel; IDIS, UK; Orphan Medical, USA.
Fomepizole (p.1039·2).
Available on a named patient basis only in the *UK*.
*Ethylene glycol poisoning; methanol poisoning.*

**Antizona** Alonga, Spain†.
Idoxuridine (p.637·3) in dimethyl sulfoxide.
*Herpesvirus skin infections.*

**Antocin** Tubilux, Ital.†.
Myrtillus (p.1718·3).
*Capillary disorders.*

**Antomiopic**
Allergan, Braz.; Novartis, Spain.
Vitamins and amino acids (p.1417·1); myrtillus (p.1718·3).
*Eye disorders.*

**Antopal** Bama, Spain.
Binifibrate (p.875·1).
*Hyperlipidaemias.*

**Antopar** Lek, Hong Kong†.
Benzoyl peroxide (p.1143·2).
*Acne.*

**Antoral** Recordati, Ital.
Tibezonium iodide (p.1756·2).
*Mouth and throat disinfection.*

**Antoril** Teva Tuteur, Arg.
Gemcitabine (p.558·2).
*Malignant neoplasms.*

**Antoxymega** Larkhall Laboratories, UK†.
Multivitamin and mineral preparation (p.1417·1).

**Antra**
AstraZeneca, Austria; AstraZeneca, Ger.; AstraZeneca, Ital.; AstraZeneca, Switz.
Omeprazole (p.1278·2), omeprazole magnesium (p.1278·2), or omeprazole sodium (p.1278·2).
*Acid aspiration; gastro-oesophageal reflux; peptic ulcer; Zollinger-Ellison syndrome.*

**Antral** Carnot, Mex.†.
Metronidazole (p.607·2).
*Amoebiasis; giardiasis; trichomoniasis.*

**Antramups** AstraZeneca, Switz.
Omeprazole magnesium (p.1278·2).
*Gastro-oesophageal reflux; peptic ulcer; Zollinger-Ellison syndrome.*

**Antran** Solfran, Mex.
Multivitamin and mineral preparation (p.1417·1).

**Antranol** Stiefel, Braz.†.
Dithranol (p.1146·1).
*Psoriasis.*

**Antrenyl** Novartis, India.
Oxyphenonium bromide (p.487·2).
*Adjunct in diarrhoea; gastritis; gastrointestinal hyperacidity; gastrointestinal hypermotility; peptic ulcer.*

**Antrex** Orion, Fin.
Calcium folinate (p.1431·1).
*Adjunct to fluorouracil in colorectal cancer; megaloblastic leukaemia; reduction of methotrexate toxicity.*

**Antrizine** Major, USA.
Meclozine hydrochloride (p.436·3).
*Motion sickness; vertigo.*

**Antrocol** Poythress, USA†.
Atropine sulfate (p.477·1); phenobarbital (p.367·3).
*Gastrointestinal disorders.*

**Antroquoril** Essex, Austral.
Betamethasone valerate (p.1093·2).
*Skin disorders.*

**Antup R** Teijin, Jpn.
Isosorbide dinitrate (p.941·1).
*Angina pectoris; ischaemic heart disease; myocardial infarction.*

**Anturan**
Novartis, Austral.†; Novartis, Austria†; Novartis, Israel†; Novartis, NZ†; Geigy, Switz.†; Novartis, UK.
Sulfinpyrazone (p.417·3).
*Gout; hyperuricaemia; myocardial infarction; thromboembolic disorders.*

**Anturane** Novartis, USA.
Sulfinpyrazone (p.417·3).
*Gouty arthritis.*

**Antussan** Dolorgiet, Ger.†.
*Oral drops; oral liquid:* Thyme (p.1755·2).
Formerly contained menthol, camphor, benzoic acid, ephedrine hydrochloride, sodium dibunate, thyme, and primula rhizome.
*Catarrh; coughs.*

*Tablets:* Ambroxol hydrochloride (p.1114·3).
*Respiratory-tract disorders with increased or viscous mucus.*

**Antussia** Asian Pharm, Thai.
*Capsules:* Dextromethorphan hydrobromide (p.1117·3); guaifenesin (p.1122·1); pseudoephedrine hydrochloride (p.1129·2); diphenhydramine hydrochloride (p.431·3).

*Syrup:* Dextromethorphan hydrobromide (p.1117·3); guaifenesin (p.1122·1); phenylephrine hydrochloride (p.1126·3).
Formerly contained dextromethorphan hydrobromide, guaifenesin, phenylpropanolamine hydrochloride, and phenylephrine hydrochloride.

*Hypersensitivity reactions.*

**Antust** Progress, Thai.
Dextromethorphan hydrobromide (p.1117·3); chlorphenamine maleate (p.427·3); terpin hydrate (p.1131·1).
*Coughs.*

**Antux** Ache, Braz.
Levodropropizine (p.1119·3).
*Coughs.*

**Anu-Aide** Technilab, Canad.
Zinc sulfate (p.1469·3).
*Haemorrhoids.*

**Anuar**
Note. This name is used for preparations of different composition.
Pharmacia, Arg.
*Injection:* Chloramphenicol sodium succinate (p.185·1); colistimethate sodium (p.199·1); cinchocaine hydrochloride (p.1373·2); dipyrone (p.35·3); guaifenesin (p.1122·1); chlorphenamine (p.427·3).

*Tablets:* Roxithromycin (p.254·2).

*Bacterial infections.*

Tecnoforma, Chile.
Cyproterone acetate (p.1544·1); ethinylestradiol (p.1553·2).
*Androgen-induced acne, alopecia, and hirsutism in women.*

**Anucet** Sanobia, Port.
*Ointment:* Hydrocortisone acetate (p.1103·3); phenylephrine hydrochloride (p.1126·3); lidocaine hydrochloride (p.1377·3); tetracaine hydrochloride (p.1385·1); belladonna (p.479·1); peru balsam (p.1730·2).

*Suppositories:* Hydrocortisone acetate (p.1103·3); phenylephrine hydrochloride (p.1126·3); lidocaine hydrochloride (p.1377·3); tetracaine hydrochloride (p.1385·1); belladonna (p.479·1).

*Anorectal disorders.*

**Anucort-HC** G & W, USA.
Hydrocortisone acetate (p.1103·3).

**Anugesic** Pfizer Consumer, S.Afr.
*Ointment:* Pramocaine hydrochloride (p.1382·2).

*Suppositories:* Bismuth subgallate (p.1252·2); bismuth oxide (p.1252·1); resorcinol (p.1156·3); bismuth oxyiodide (p.1253·1); peru balsam (p.1730·2); benzyl benzoate (p.1500·2); zinc oxide (p.1163·2); boric acid (p.1662·1); pramocaine hydrochloride (p.1382·2).

*Anorectal disorders.*

**Anugesic-HC**
Note. This name is used for preparations of different composition.
Pfizer, Canad.
Pramocaine hydrochloride (p.1382·2); hydrocortisone acetate (p.1103·3); zinc sulfate (p.1469·3).
*Anorectal disorders.*

Pfizer, Irl.
*Cream:* Pramocaine hydrochloride (p.1382·2); hydrocortisone acetate (p.1103·3); zinc oxide (p.1163·2); peru balsam (p.1730·2); benzyl benzoate (p.1500·2); bismuth oxide (p.1252·1); resorcinol (p.1156·3).

*Suppositories:* Pramocaine hydrochloride (p.1382·2); hydrocortisone acetate (p.1103·3); zinc oxide (p.1163·2); bismuth subgallate (p.1252·2); peru balsam (p.1730·2); benzyl benzoate (p.1500·2); bismuth oxide (p.1252·1).

*Anorectal disorders.*

Pfizer, UK.
*Cream:* Pramocaine hydrochloride (p.1382·2); hydrocortisone acetate (p.1103·3); bismuth oxide (p.1252·1); peru balsam (p.1730·2); zinc oxide (p.1163·2); benzyl benzoate (p.1500·2).

*Suppositories:* Pramocaine hydrochloride (p.1382·2); hydrocortisone acetate (p.1103·3); zinc oxide (p.1163·2); bismuth subgallate (p.1252·2); bismuth oxide (p.1252·1); Peru balsam (p.1730·2); benzyl benzoate (p.1500·2).

*Anorectal disorders.*

**Anulbet** Alpes Chemie, Chile.
Famotidine (p.1265·2).
*Gastro-oesophageal reflux; peptic ulcer; Zollinger-Ellison syndrome.*

**Anulette** Silesia, Chile.
Levonorgestrel (p.1563·2); ethinylestradiol (p.1553·2).
*Combined oral contraceptive; menstrual disorders.*

**Anumed** Major, USA.
Bismuth subgallate (p.1252·2); bismuth resorcinol compound (p.1253·1); benzyl benzoate (p.1500·2); zinc oxide (p.1163·2); peru balsam (p.1730·2).
*Anorectal disorders.*

**Anumed HC** Major, USA.
Hydrocortisone acetate (p.1103·3); bismuth subgallate (p.1252·2); bismuth resorcinol compound (p.1253·1); benzyl benzoate (p.1500·2); peru balsam (p.1730·2); zinc oxide (p.1163·2).
*Anorectal disorders.*

**Anumedin** Kade, Ger.
Prednisolone acetate (p.1108·1); cinchocaine hydrochloride (p.1373·2).
*Anorectal disorders.*

**Anurin** Abbott, Mex.†.
Pipemidic acid (p.243·1).

**Anusept** Lichtenstein, Ger.†.
Bismuth subnitrate (p.1252·2); zinc oxide (p.1163·2); benzocaine (p.1370·3).
*Anorectal disorders.*

**Anusol**
Note. This name is used for preparations of different composition.
Parke, Davis, Arg.
Bismuth resorcinol compound (p.1253·1); zinc oxide (p.1163·2); bismuth subgallate (p.1252·2); peru balsam (p.1730·2); bismuth oxyiodide (p.1253·1).
*Haemorrhoids.*

Parke, Davis, Austral.
*Suppositories; ointment:* Zinc oxide (p.1163·2); peru balsam (p.1730·2); benzyl benzoate (p.1500·2).

*Wipes:* Hamamelis water (p.1696·3); glycerol (p.1694·3).

*Anorectal disorders.*

Pfizer Consumer, Canad.
Zinc sulfate (p.1469·3).
*Anorectal disorders.*

Pfizer Sante, Fr.
Bismuth oxide (p.1252·1); bismuth subgallate (p.1252·2); zinc oxide (p.1163·2).
*Anorectal disorders.*

Pfizer Consumer, Ger.
Bismuth oxide-bismuthoxyiodide-1,3-bis-(ammoniumoxy)-benzol-4,5-(bismuthylsulfonate); zinc oxide (p.1163·2); peru balsam (p.1730·2).
*Anorectal disorders.*

Pfizer, Hong Kong.
Peru balsam (p.1730·2); bismuth oxide (p.1252·1); bismuth subgallate (p.1252·2); zinc oxide (p.1163·2).
*Anorectal disorders.*

Pfizer Consumer, Irl.
*Cream:* Zinc oxide (p.1163·2); bismuth oxide (p.1252·1); peru balsam (p.1730·2).

*Suppositories; ointment:* Bismuth subgallate (p.1252·2); bismuth oxide (p.1252·1); peru balsam (p.1730·2); zinc oxide (p.1163·2).

*Anorectal disorders.*

Parke, Davis, Israel.
Bismuth subgallate (p.1252·2); bismuth oxide (p.1252·1); peru balsam (p.1730·2); zinc oxide (p.1163·2).
*Anorectal disorders.*

Warner-Lambert, Ital.
Resorcinol (p.1156·3); yellow bismuth oxide (p.1252·1); bismuth subgallate (p.1252·2); bismuth oxyiodide (p.1253·1); peru balsam (p.1730·2); zinc oxide (p.1163·2).
*Anorectal disorders.*

Pfizer, Malaysia; Parke, Davis, Malaysia.
Zinc oxide (p.1163·2); peru balsam (p.1730·2); benzyl benzoate (p.1500·2).
*Anorectal disorders.*

Warner-Lambert, Neth.
Bismuth subgallate (p.1252·2); zinc oxide (p.1163·2).
*Anorectal disorders.*

Pfizer, NZ.
Zinc oxide (p.1163·2); peru balsam (p.1730·2); benzyl benzoate (p.1500·2).
*Anorectal disorders.*

Pfizer Consumer, S.Afr.
Bismuth subgallate (p.1252·2); bismuth oxide (p.1252·1); zinc oxide (p.1163·2).
*Anorectal disorders.*

Pfizer Consumer, Singapore.
*Ointment:* Peru balsam (p.1730·2); benzyl benzoate (p.1500·2); bismuth oxide (p.1252·1); bismuth subgallate (p.1252·2); bismuth oxyiodide (p.1253·1); resorcinol (p.1156·3).

*Suppositories:* Peru balsam (p.1730·2); benzyl benzoate (p.1500·2); bismuth oxide (p.1252·1); bismuth subgallate (p.1252·2); resorcinol (p.1156·3); zinc oxide (p.1163·2).

*Haemorrhoids.*

Pfizer, Thai.
Peru balsam (p.1730·2); benzyl benzoate (p.1500·2); bismuth oxide (p.1252·1); bismuth subgallate (p.1252·2); resorcinol (p.1156·3); zinc oxide (p.1163·2).
*Haemorrhoids; pruritus ani.*

Pfizer Consumer, UK.
*Cream:* Bismuth oxide (p.1252·1); peru balsam (p.1730·2); zinc oxide (p.1163·2).

*Ointment; suppositories:* Bismuth subgallate (p.1252·2); bismuth oxide (p.1252·1); peru balsam (p.1730·2); zinc oxide (p.1163·2).

*Anorectal disorders.*

Warner-Lambert, USA.
*Ointment:* Zinc oxide (p.1163·2); pramocaine hydrochloride (p.1382·2).

*Suppositories:* Benzyl alcohol (p.1170·2); soybean oil (p.1447·2); tocoferil acetate (p.1465·1).
Formerly contained bismuth subgallate, bismuth resorcinol compound, benzyl benzoate, zinc oxide, and peru balsam.

*Anorectal disorders.*

**Anusol Duo** Parke, Davis, Arg.
Hydrocortisone acetate (p.1103·3); pramocaine hydrochloride (p.1382·2).
*Anorectal disorders.*

**Anusol Duo S** Parke, Davis, Arg.
Pramocaine hydrochloride (p.1382·2); hydrocortisone acetate (p.1103·3); benzyl benzoate (p.1500·2); bismuth oxide (p.1252·1); bismuth subgallate (p.1252·2); peru balsam (p.1730·2); zinc oxide (p.1163·2).
*Anorectal disorders.*

**Anusol Plus** Pfizer Consumer, Canad.
Pramocaine hydrochloride (p.1382·2); zinc sulfate (p.1469·3).
*Anorectal disorders.*

**Anusol-A** Parke, Davis, Arg.
Pramocaine hydrochloride (p.1382·2); zinc oxide (p.1163·2); peru balsam (p.1730·2); benzyl benzoate (p.1500·2); kaolin (p.1268·3); calcium phosphate (p.1225·3).
*Haemorrhoids.*

**Anusol-HC**
Note. This name is used for preparations of different composition.
Parke, Davis, Arg.; Monarch, USA.
Hydrocortisone acetate (p.1103·3).
*Anorectal disorders; skin disorders.*

Pfizer, Braz.
Hydrocortisone acetate (p.1103·3); bismuth resorcinol compound (p.1253·1); zinc oxide (p.1163·2); bismuth subgallate (p.1252·2); peru balsam (p.1730·2); benzyl benzoate (p.1500·2).
*Anorectal disorders.*

Pfizer, Canad.
Zinc sulfate (p.1469·3); hydrocortisone acetate (p.1103·3).
*Anorectal disorders.*

Warner-Lambert, Hong Kong†.
*Ointment:* Peru balsam (p.1730·2); benzyl benzoate (p.1500·2); bismuth oxide (p.1252·1); bismuth subgallate (p.1252·2); zinc oxide (p.1163·2); hydrocortisone acetate (p.1103·3).

*Suppositories:* Peru balsam (p.1730·2); benzyl benzoate (p.1500·2); bismuth subgallate (p.1252·2); zinc oxide (p.1163·2); hydrocortisone acetate (p.1103·3).

*Anorectal disorders.*

Pfizer Consumer, Irl.
Hydrocortisone acetate (p.1103·3); benzyl benzoate (p.1500·2); bismuth subgallate (p.1252·2); bismuth oxide (p.1252·1); peru balsam (p.1730·2); zinc oxide (p.1163·2); resorcinol (p.1156·3).
*Anorectal disorders.*

Parke, Davis, S.Afr.†.
Bismuth subgallate (p.1252·2); bismuth oxide (p.1252·1); bismuth oxyiodide (p.1253·1); resorcinol (p.1156·3); peru balsam (p.1730·2); benzyl benzoate (p.1500·2); zinc oxide (p.1163·2); boric acid (p.1662·1); hydrocortisone acetate (p.1103·3).
*Anorectal disorders.*

**Anusol-HC, Plus HC** Pfizer Consumer, UK.
Bismuth subgallate (p.1252·2); bismuth oxide (p.1252·1); peru balsam (p.1730·2); zinc oxide (p.1163·2); hydrocortisone acetate (p.1103·3); benzyl benzoate (p.1500·2).
Anusol HC formerly contained bismuth subgallate, bismuth oxide, peru balsam, zinc oxide, hydrocortisone acetate, benzyl benzoate, and resorcinol.
*Anorectal disorders.*

**Anuzinc**
Note. This name is used for preparations of different composition.
Sabex, Canad.
Zinc sulfate (p.1469·3).
*Anorectal disorders.*

Technilab, Hong Kong†.
*Ointment:* Zinc sulfate (p.1469·3).

*Suppositories:* Bismuth oxide (p.1252·1); bismuth subgallate (p.1252·2); zinc oxide (p.1163·2).

*Anorectal disorders.*

**Anuzinc HC** Sabex, Canad.
Zinc sulfate (p.1469·3); hydrocortisone acetate (p.1103·3).
*Anorectal disorders.*

**Anuzinc HC Plus** Sabex, Canad.
Zinc sulfate (p.1469·3); hydrocortisone acetate (p.1103·3); pramocaine hydrochloride (p.1382·2).
*Anorectal disorders.*

**Anvitoff**
Abbott, Ger.; Knoll, Switz.
Tranexamic acid (p.760·3).
*Haemorrhagic disorders.*

**Anvitol** Azevedos, Port.
Haematoporphyrin hydrochloride; glycine; cyanocobalamin (p.1417·1).
*Tonic.*

**Anxer**
Unison, Hong Kong; Unison, Thai.
Cefalexin (p.168·1).
*Bacterial infections.*

**Anxicalm** Clonmel, Irl.
Diazepam (p.690·1).
*Anxiety; epilepsy; insomnia; premedication; skeletal muscle spasm.*

**Anxielax** Macrophar, Thai.
Dipotassium clorazepate (p.685·1).
*Anxiety; insomnia.*

**Anxietum** Ferrier, Fr.
Homoeopathic preparation.

**Anxiety/Stress L72** Homeocan, Canad.
Homoeopathic preparation.

**Anxiolan** Medochemie, Thai.
Buspirone hydrochloride (p.672·2).
*Anxiety.*

**Anxiolit**
Gerot, Austria; Medichemie, Switz.
Oxazepam (p.712·2).
*Anxiety disorders; insomnia.*

**Anxiolit plus** Gerot, Austria.
Oxazepam (p.712·2); methylbenactyzium bromide (p.485·3).
*Anxiety disorders.*

**Anxipress-D** Pharmaland, Thai.
Perphenazine (p.714·2); amitriptyline hydrochloride (p.280·3).
*Depression.*

**Anxira** Condrugs, Thai.
Lorazepam (p.704·1).
*Anxiety.*

**Anxirid** Aspen, S.Afr.
Alprazolam (p.668·3).
*Anxiety disorders; mixed anxiety depressive states.*

**Anxium** Knop, Chile.
Hypericum (p.299·1).
*Depression.*

**Anxoral** IPRAD, Fr.
Crataegus (p.1677·1); passion flower (p.1729·1); valerian (p.1762·2).
Formerly contained crataegus, passion flower, valerian, and phenobarbital.
*Anxiety; insomnia.*

**Anxut** Eisai, Ger.
Buspirone hydrochloride (p.672·2).
*Anxiety.*

**Anxyrex** Irex, Fr.
Bromazepam (p.671·3).
*Alcohol withdrawal syndrome; anxiety.*

**Any** Homme de Fer, Fr.
Mequinol (p.1151·3).
*Hyperpigmentation.*

**Anzac** Bangkok Lab & Cosmetic, Thai.
Fluoxetine hydrochloride (p.292·1).
*Mixed anxiety depressive states; obsessive-compulsive disorder.*

**Anzatax**
Mayne, Austral.; Mayne, Hong Kong; Faulding, Malaysia; Faulding, Singapore; DBL, Thai.; Faulding, Thai.
Paclitaxel (p.577·3).
*Breast cancer; non-small cell lung cancer; ovarian cancer.*

**Anzemet**
Aventis, Arg.; Aventis, Austral.; Hoechst Marion Roussel, Austria; Aventis, Braz.; Aventis, Canad.; Aventis, Fin.; Aventis, Fr.; Hoechst Marion Roussel, Gr.; Aventis, Ital.; Aventis, Mex.; Aventis, Switz.; Amdipharm, UK; Hoechst Marion Roussel, USA.
Dolasetron mesilate (p.1262·3).
*Nausea and vomiting.*

**Anzion** Farmaline, Thai.
Alprazolam (p.668·3).
*Anxiety.*

**Anzopac** UCI, Braz.
Capsules, lansoprazole (p.1269·3); tablets, clarithromycin (p.192·2); capcules, amoxicillin trihydrate (p.155·3).
*Peptic ulcer.*

**Aodrops** Ciba Vision, Canad.
Lubricant for contact lenses (p.1164·2).

**Aofen** Progress, Thai.
Griseofulvin (p.400·3).
*Fungal infections of skin, hair, and nails.*

**Aoflow** Ciba Vision, Canad.
Cleansing solution for contact lenses (p.1164·2).

**A-O-Q10 MaxiPower Formula** Solgar, UK†.
Multivitamin and mineral preparation with amino acids, coenzyme Q-10, and fibre (p.1417·1).
*Dietary supplement.*

**Aorinyl** Progress, Thai.†.
Phenylephrine hydrochloride (p.1126·3); brompheniramine maleate (p.426·1); phenylpropanolamine hydrochloride (p.1127·3).
*Allergic respiratory-tract disorders; nasal congestion.*

**Aorten** Brasterapica, Braz.†.
Captopril (p.879·2).
*Hypertension.*

**Aosept**
Ciba Vision, Austral.†; Novartis, Austria†; Ciba Vision, Braz.; Ciba Vision, Canad.; Ciba Vision, NZ; Ciba Vision, USA.
Hydrogen peroxide (p.1182·2) (p.1164·2).
*Disinfecting solution for soft contact lenses.*

**Aotal** Lipha Sante, Fr.
Acamprosate calcium (p.668·1).
*Alcoholism.*

**Aova** *Velka, Gr.*
Ranitidine hydrochloride (p.1285·2).
*Conditions where gastric acid reduction is beneficial; gastric hypersecretion including Zollinger-Ellison syndrome; peptic ulcer.*

**AP** *Steigerwald, Ger.*
A range of homoeopathic preparations.

**AP Inyec Cloruro Potasic** *Fresenius Kabi, Spain.*
Potassium chloride (p.1232·2).
*Hypokalaemia.*

**APA**
*Note. This name is used for preparations of different composition.*
*Lannacher, Austria.*
*Suppositories:* Paracetamol (p.76·2); propyphenazone (p.85·3).
*Fever; pain.*
*Tablets:* Paracetamol (p.76·2); dextropropoxyphene hydrochloride (p.28·3).
*Pain.*
*Merck, Hong Kong†.*
Paracetamol (p.76·2); propyphenazone (p.85·3).
*Fever; pain.*

**Apacef**
*AstraZeneca, Belg.; AstraZeneca, Fr.*
Cefotetan disodium (p.177·1).
*Bacterial infections.*

**Apacet**
*Merck, Austria†; Parmed, USA.*
Paracetamol (p.76·2).
*Fever; pain.*

**Apagen** *Stomygen, Ital.*
Hydroxyapatite (p.1699·3).
*Dental disorders.*

**Apain** *AstraZeneca, Denm.*
Ibuprofen (p.45·3).
*Pain.*

**Apaisac** *Saninter, Port.†.*
Emollient.

**Apaisance** *Lierac, Fr.*
*Cream:* Tilia (p.1756·2); enoxolone (p.36·2); helichrysum; pilewort (p.1732·1).
*Topical spray:* Tilia (p.1756·2); levomenol (p.1707·1); chamomile (p.1669·3).
*Skin disorders.*

**Apaisyl** *Monot, Fr.†.*
Isothipendyl hydrochloride (p.435·2).
*Hypersensitivity.*

**Apalin** *Duopharma, Hong Kong.*
Amikacin sulfate (p.154·1).
*Bacterial infections.*

**Apamid**
*Pfizer, Fin.; Weifa, Norw.; Parke, Davis, Swed.; Weifa, Thai.*
Glipizide (p.332·2).
*Diabetes mellitus.*

**Apamox** *F5 Profas, Spain.*
Amoxicillin trihydrate (p.155·3).
*Bacterial infections.*

**Apap**
*CPC, Hong Kong†; Cypress, USA.*
Paracetamol (p.76·2).
*Fever; pain.*

**A-Par** *Pharmygiene, Fr.*
Esdepallethrine (p.1505·1); piperonyl butoxide (p.1509·2).
*Destruction of scabies mite, fleas and lice in textiles and adjunct to treatment.*

**A-Parkin** *Dexxon, Israel.*
Amantadine sulfate (p.1197·2).
*Influenza A; parkinsonism.*

**Aparoxal** *Veyron-Froment, Fr.*
Phenobarbital (p.367·3).
*Epilepsy.*

**Aparsonin N** *Merckle, Ger.*
Bromhexine hydrochloride (p.1115·3).
*Respiratory-tract disorders associated with increased mucus.*

**Apasmil** *Cordoba, Arg.*
An antilymphocyte immunoglobulin (p.1348·3).

**Apasmo** *Sidus, Arg.*
Camylofin hydrochloride (p.1666·1); dipyrone (p.35·3).
*Muscle spasm; pain.*

**Apasmo Compuesto** *Sidus, Arg.*
Pargeverine (p.487·3); dipyrone (p.35·3).
*Smooth muscle spasm.*

**Apatate** *Kenwood, USA.*
Vitamin B complex (p.1417·1).

**Apatate with Fluoride** *Kenwood, USA.*
Vitamin B substances (p.1417·1) with sodium fluoride (p.1444·3).

**Apatef**
*Wyeth, Austral.; AstraZeneca, Ital.; Lederle, NZ; AstraZeneca, Port.*
Cefotetan disodium (p.177·1).
*Bacterial infections.*

**Apatite** *Weleda, UK.*
Homoeopathic preparation.

**Apecitab** *Dosa, Arg.*
Capecitabine (p.533·2).
*Malignant neoplasms.*

**Apefer** *Teuto, Braz.†.*
Ferrous gluconate (p.1428·1); vitamins (p.1417·1).
Ascorbic acid (p.1460·2) is included in this preparation to increase the absorption and availability of iron.
*Anaemias.*

**Apegmone** *Lipha Sante, Fr.†.*
Tioclomarol (p.1013·2).
*Thromboembolic disorders.*

**Apekumarol** *Pharmacia Upjohn, Swed.†.*
Dicoumarol (p.894·2).
*Thromboembolic disorders.*

**A-Pen**
*Note. A similar name is used for preparations of different composition (see below).*
*Orion, Fin.*
Ampicillin sodium (p.157·1).
*Bacterial infections.*

**Apen**
*Note. A similar name is used for preparations of different composition (see above).*
*Xixia, S.Afr.*
Ampicillin (p.157·1); cloxacillin (p.198·2).
*Bacterial infections.*

**Apeplus** *Mediderm.*
Finasteride (p.1554·2).
*Alopecia.*

**Aperamid** *Ardeypharm, Ger.†.*
Loperamide hydrochloride (p.1271·1).
*Diarrhoea.*

**Aperdan** *ABC, Ital.*
Naproxen cetrimonium (p.65·3).
*Vulvovaginal disorders.*

**Apergan** *Panzera, Ital.*
Royal jelly (p.1740·3); glucose (p.1432·2); ginseng (p.1693·1).
*Nutritional supplement.*

**Aperisan**
*Byk, Austria; Dentinox, Ger.*
Sage (p.1741·2).
*Catarrh; mouth and throat inflammation.*

**Aperop** *Pharmacobel, Belg.†.*
Nux vomica (p.1722·3); kola (p.1765·3); orange peel (p.1723·3); cinchona bark (p.1671·3); haemoglobin (p.755·2); iodine (p.1598·1); tannic acid (p.1751·2); calcium phosphate hydrochloride.
*Tonic.*

**Apertia** *Lundbeck, Austria.*
Citalopram hydrobromide (p.289·1) or citalopram hydrochloride (p.289·1).
*Anxiety; depression; obsessive-compulsive disorder; panic attacks.*

**Apetibe** *Luper, Braz.*
Buclizine (p.426·3); amino acids; vitamins (p.1417·1).
*Reduced appetite; tonic.*

**Apetil**
*Note. This name is used for preparations of different composition.*
*Bunker, Braz.*
Buclizine hydrochloride (p.426·3); amino acids; vitamin B substances (p.1417·1).
*Reduced appetite; tonic.*
*Ram, USA.*
Multivitamin and mineral preparation (p.1417·1).

**Apetin** *Gilton, Braz.†.*
Carnitine; vitamin B substances (p.1417·1).
*Reduced appetite; tonic.*

**Apetinil-Depo** *Syntex, Switz.†.*
Etilamfetamine hydrochloride (p.1588·1).
*Obesity.*

**Apetitol Forte** *Mertens, Arg.*
Cyproheptadine hydrochloride (p.430·1); vitamins (p.1417·1).
*Reduced appetite.*

**Apetrol** *Medipharm, Chile.*
Cyproheptadine hydrochloride (p.430·1); vitamins (p.1417·1).
*Reduced appetite.*

**Apevitin BC** *EMS, Braz.*
Cyproheptadine hydrochloride (p.430·1); vitamin B substances; ascorbic acid (p.1417·1).
*Reduced appetite; tonic.*

**ApexiCon** *PharmaDerm, USA.*
Diflorasone diacetate (p.1099·3).
*Skin disorders.*

**APF** *Cypress, USA.*
Sodium fluoride (p.1444·3).
*Dental caries prophylaxis.*

**Aphenylbarbit** *Streuli, Switz.*
Phenobarbital (p.367·3).
*Epilepsy; febrile convulsions; sedative.*

**Aphilan** *UCB, Fr.*
*Cream:* Hydrocortisone (p.1103·3).
*Skin disorders.*
*Tablets:* Buclizine hydrochloride (p.426·3).
*Allergic conjunctivitis; allergic rhinitis; motion sickness; urticaria.*

**Aphloine P** *DB, Fr.*
Aphloia; hamamelis (p.1696·3); viburnum; esculoside (p.1648·2).
*Haemorrhoids; peripheral vascular insufficiency.*

**Aphrodyne** *Star, USA.*
Yohimbine hydrochloride (p.1766·2).

**Aphthasol** *Block, USA.*
Amlexanox (p.781·1).
*Aphthous ulcers.*

**Aphtiria** *Debat, Fr.†.*
Lindane (p.1506·3).
*Disinfection of clothes and bedding; pediculosis.*

**Aphtoral** *Pierre Fabre Sante, Fr.*
Chlorhexidine gluconate (p.1173·2); tetracaine hydrochloride (p.1385·1); ascorbic acid (p.1460·2).
Formerly known as Eludril.
*Mouth and throat disorders.*

**Api Baby** *Sanitalia, Ital.*
Pollen; royal jelly (p.1740·3); fructose; myrtillus (p.1718·3).
*Nutritional supplement.*

**Apifortyl** *Mack, Thai.†.*
Multivitamin and mineral preparation (p.1417·1).

**Apihepar** *Asta Medica, Austria; Madaus, Austria.*
Silybum marianum (p.1043·3).
*Liver disorders.*

**Apilaxe** *Cooperation Pharmaceutique, Fr.*
Sorbitol (p.1446·3); althaea leaf (p.1651·3).
*Constipation.*

**Apilcav** *Libbs, Braz.*
Alprostadil (p.1512·3).
*Erectile dysfunction.*

**Apimid** *Apogepha, Ger.*
Flutamide (p.556·2).
*Prostatic cancer.*

**Apiocolina** *Bruschettini, Ital.*
*Escherichia coli* lysate.
*Anorectal inflammation.*

**Apir Bicarbonato Sod** *Fresenius Kabi, Spain†.*
Sodium bicarbonate (p.1223·2).
*Metabolic acidosis.*

**Apir Clorurado** *Fresenius Kabi, Spain.*
Sodium chloride (p.1233·3).
*Fluid and electrolyte disorders.*

**Apir Cloruro Amonico** *Fresenius Kabi, Spain†.*
Ammonium chloride (p.1115·2).
*Hypochloraemia; metabolic alkalosis.*

**Apir Glucoibys** *Pharmacia Upjohn, Spain†.*
Glucose (p.1432·2).
*Carbohydrate source; fluid and electrolyte disorders.*

**Apir Glucopotasico** *Fresenius Kabi, Spain†.*
Glucose (p.1432·2); potassium chloride (p.1232·2).
*Hypokalaemia.*

**Apir Glucosado** *Fresenius Kabi, Spain.*
Glucose (p.1432·2).
*Fluid and electrolyte disorders; parenteral nutrition.*

**Apir Glucosalino** *Fresenius Kabi, Spain.*
Glucose (p.1432·2); sodium chloride (p.1233·3).
*Fluid and electrolyte disorders.*

**Apir Ringer** *Fresenius Kabi, Spain.*
Electrolyte infusion (p.1217·1).
*Fluid and electrolyte depletion.*

**Apir Ringer Lactato** *Fresenius Kabi, Spain.*
Electrolyte infusion with sodium lactate (p.1217·1).
*Fluid and electrolyte depletion.*

**Apiretal** *Ern, Spain.*
Paracetamol (p.76·2).
*Fever; pain.*

**Apiretal Codeina** *Ern, Spain.*
Paracetamol (p.76·2); codeine (p.27·1).
*Pain.*

**Apiroflex Clorurado** *Fresenius Kabi, Spain†.*
Sodium chloride (p.1233·3).
*Fluid and electrolyte disorders.*

**Apiroflex Glucosada** *Fresenius Kabi, Spain†.*
Glucose (p.1432·2).
*Fluid and electrolyte disorders; parenteral nutrition.*

**Apiroflex Glucosalina** *Fresenius Kabi, Spain†.*
Glucose (p.1432·2); sodium chloride (p.1233·3).
*Fluid and electrolyte disorders.*

**Apirol** *Merck Sharp & Dohme, Israel.*
Norfloxacin (p.238·3).
*Bacterial infections.*

**Apiron** *Delta, Braz.*
Dipyrone (p.35·3).
*Fever; pain.*

**Apis** *Brauer, Austral.†.*
Homoeopathic preparation.

**Apiserum** *DB, Fr.*
Royal jelly (p.1740·3).
*Tonic.*

**Apiserum con Telergon I** *Medicafarm, Ital.*
Wine; acacia honey (p.1434·2); royal jelly (p.1740·3).
*Nutritional supplement.*

**Apisgel** *Dolisos, Canad.*
Homoeopathic preparation.

**Apis-Homaccord** *Peithner, Austria.*
Homoeopathic preparation.

**Apistress** *Sanitalia, Ital.*
Royal jelly (p.1740·3); pollen; propolis (p.1735·2).
*Nutritional supplement.*

**Apixol** *Columbia, Mex.*
Dipyrone (p.35·3).
*Fever; pain.*

**APL**
*Wyeth-Ayerst, Austral.†; Wyeth-Ayerst, Canad.†; Wyeth, Chile; Aspen, S.Afr.†; Wyeth-Ayerst, USA†.*
Chorionic gonadotrophin (p.1320·3).
*Male and female infertility; male hypogonadism; prepubertal cryptorchidism.*

**Aplacasse** *Kirby, Arg.*
Lorazepam (p.704·1).
*Anxiety.*

**Aplace** *Kyorin, Jpn.*
Troxipide (p.1294·2).
*Gastritis; peptic ulcer.*

**Aplacid** *ITF, Chile.*
Sulpiride (p.722·2).
*Depression.*

**Aplactin** *Upsa, Ital.*
Pravastatin sodium (p.984·3).
*Atherosclerosis; hyperlipidaemias.*

**Aplaket**
*Rotta, Hong Kong; Rottapharm, Ital.; Rotta, Malaysia; Delta, Port.; Rotta, Singapore; Rotta, Thai.*
Ticlopidine hydrochloride (p.1011·2).
*Thrombosis prophylaxis.*

**A-Plex** *Lemery, Mex.†.*
Tretinoin (p.1161·1).

**Aplexil** *Rhone-Poulenc Rorer, Austria†.*
Oxomemazine (p.438·2); guaifenesin (p.1122·1); paracetamol (p.76·2); sodium benzoate (p.1169·3).
*Respiratory-tract disorders.*

**Aplical** *Grunenthal, Chile.*
Calcium carbonate (p.1254·2).
*Calcium deficiency; osteoporosis.*

**Aplical-D** *Grunenthal, Chile.*
Calcium carbonate (p.1254·2); colecalciferol (p.1461·3).
*Calcium deficiency; osteomalacia; osteoporosis.*

**Apligraf** *Novartis, USA.*
Bioengineered human skin equivalent (p.1158·1).
*Diabetic foot ulcers; venous leg ulcers.*

**Aplisol** *Parkedale, USA.*
Tuberculin purified protein derivative (p.1759·1).
*Diagnosis of tuberculosis.*

**Aplitest** *Parke, Davis, USA†.*
Tuberculin purified protein derivative (p.1759·1).
*Diagnosis of tuberculosis.*

**Aplodan** *AstraZeneca, Ital.†.*
Creatinolfosfate (p.1677·3).
*Muscle disorders.*

**Aplona** *Athenstaedt, Ger.*
Apple powder; colloidal silicon dioxide (p.1581·3).
*Diarrhoea.*

**Aplosyn-Otic** *Pascual, Hong Kong.*
Neomycin sulfate (p.235·1); polymyxin B sulfate (p.245·1); fluocinolone acetonide (p.1101·2).
*Otitis externa; otitis media.*

**Apnol** *Pharmaland, Thai.*
Allopurinol (p.412·2).
*Gout; hyperuricaemia.*

**Apoacor** *Curex, Israel.*
Verapamil hydrochloride (p.1019·1).
*Angina pectoris; arrhythmias; hypertension.*

**Apo-Alpraz**
*Apotex, Canad.; Apotex, Malaysia; Apotex, Singapore.*
Alprazolam (p.668·3).
*Anxiety; sedative.*

**Apo-Amilzide**
*Apotex, Canad.; Apotex, Hong Kong; Apotex, Malaysia; Apotex, Singapore.*
Amiloride hydrochloride (p.858·2); hydrochlorothiazide (p.933·2).
*Hepatic cirrhosis with ascites; hypertension; oedema.*

**Apo-Amoxi**
*Apotex, Canad.; Apotex, NZ†; Apotex, Singapore.*
Amoxicillin trihydrate (p.155·3).
*Bacterial infections.*
*Apotex, Hong Kong.*
Amoxicillin (p.155·3).
*Bacterial infections.*

**Apo-Ampi** *Apotex, Canad.*
Ampicillin trihydrate (p.157·2).
*Bacterial infections.*

**Apo-Atenol**
*Apotex, Canad.; Apotex, Hong Kong; Apotex, Malaysia; Apotex, Singapore.*
Atenolol (p.865·2).
*Angina pectoris; arrhythmias; hypertension.*

**Apobase** *Alpharma, Fin.*
Emollient.

**Apo-C** *Apotex, Canad.†.*
Ascorbic acid (p.1460·2).
*Vitamin supplement.*

**Apo-Cal**
*Apotex, Canad.; Apotex, Hong Kong; Apotex, Malaysia.*
Calcium carbonate (p.1254·2).
*Calcium deficiency; calcium supplement.*

**Apocanda** *Apogepha, Ger.†.*
Clotrimazole (p.396·2).
*Fungal infections.*

**Apocapen** *Curex, Israel†.*
Captopril (p.879·2).
*Diabetic nephropathy; heart failure; hypertension; myocardial infarction.*

**Apo-Capto**
*Apotex, Canad.; Apotex, Hong Kong; Apotex, Malaysia; Apotex, Singapore.*
Captopril (p.879·2).
*Heart failure; hypertension.*

**Apocard**
*3M, Port.†; 3M, Spain.*
Flecainide acetate (p.916·2).
*Arrhythmias.*

**Apo-Cepalex** *Apotex, Hong Kong†.*
Cefalexin (p.168·1).
*Bacterial infections.*

**Apo-Cephalex** *Apotex, Canad.*
Cefalexin (p.168·1).
*Bacterial infections.*

**Apo-Chlorax**
Apotex, Canad.; Apotex, Malaysia; Apotex, Singapore.
Chlordiazepoxide hydrochloride (p.674·2); clidinium bromide (p.480·2).
*Gastrointestinal disorders with associated anxiety.*

**Apociclina** Protein, Mex.†.
Doxycycline (p.206·2).

**Apocillin** Alpharma, Norw.
Phenoxymethylpenicillin potassium (p.242·1).
*Bacterial infections.*

**Apo-Cloxi**
Apotex, Canad.; Apotex, Hong Kong.
Cloxacillin sodium (p.198·2).
*Bacterial infections.*

**Apocort** Alpharma, Fin.
Hydrocortisone acetate (p.1103·3).
*Skin disorders.*

**Apocortal** Alpharma, Norw.†.
Hydrocortisone acetate (p.1103·3).
*Skin disorders.*

**Apo-Cromolyn** Apotex, Canad.
Sodium cromoglicate (p.795·3).
*Allergic rhinitis; asthma.*

**Apocyclin** Alpharma, Fin.
Tetracycline hydrochloride (p.266·2).
*Bacterial infections.*

**Apoderm** Nycomed, Austria.
Deproteinised derivative of calf blood.
*Burns; ulcers; wounds.*

**Apo-Diclo**
Apotex, Canad.; Apotex, Hong Kong; Apotex, Malaysia; Apotex, NZ.
Diclofenac (p.32·1), diclofenac potassium (p.32·1), or diclofenac sodium (p.32·1).
*Inflammation; musculoskeletal and joint disorders; pain.*

**Apo-Diltiaz**
Apotex, Canad.; Apotex, Hong Kong.
Diltiazem hydrochloride (p.900·1).
*Angina pectoris; arrhythmias; hypertension.*

**Apodorm**
Alpharma, Denm.; Alpharma, Norw.; Alpharma, Swed.
Nitrazepam (p.710·1).
*Epilepsy; infantile spasm; insomnia.*

**Apodoxin** Alpharma, Fin.
Doxycycline (p.206·2).
*Bacterial infections.*

**Apo-Doxy**
Apotex, Canad.; Apotex, Singapore.
Doxycycline (p.206·2) or doxycycline hyclate (p.206·2).
*Bacterial infections.*

**Apodoxy** Curex, Israel†.
Doxycycline (p.206·2).
*Bacterial infections; malaria.*

**Apo-Erythro**
Apotex, Canad.; Apotex, Hong Kong.
Erythromycin (p.208·1), erythromycin ethyl succinate (p.208·1), or erythromycin stearate (p.208·2).
*Bacterial infections.*

**Apo-Feno** Apotex, Canad.
Fenofibrate (p.915·2).
*Hyperlipidaemias.*

**Apo-Feno-Micro** Apotex, Hong Kong.
Fenofibrate (p.915·2).
*Hyperlipidaemias.*

**Apofin** Chiesi, Ital.
Apomorphine hydrochloride (p.1199·1).
*Parkinsonism.*

**Apo-Gain**
Apotex, Canad.; Apotex, Hong Kong; Apotex, Malaysia; Apotex, NZ†.
Minoxidil (p.960·1).
*Alopecia androgenetica.*

**Apogastine** Curex, Israel.
Famotidine (p.1265·2).
*Gastro-oesophageal reflux; peptic ulcer; Zollinger-Ellison syndrome.*

**APO-go** Britannia Pharmaceuticals, UK.
Apomorphine hydrochloride (p.1199·1).
*Parkinsonism.*

**APO-go Pen** Italfarmaco, Spain.
Apomorphine hydrochloride (p.1199·1).
*Parkinsonism.*

**Apohair** Curex, Israel†.
Minoxidil (p.960·1).
*Alopecia.*

**Apo-Hepat** Pekana, Ger.
Homoeopathic preparation.

**Apo-Hexa** Apotex, Canad.†.
Multivitamin preparation (p.1417·1).

**Apo-Hydro**
Apotex, Canad.; Apotex, Malaysia; Apotex, Singapore.
Hydrochlorothiazide (p.933·2).
*Hypertension; oedema.*

**Apo-Infekt** Pekana, Ger.
Homoeopathic preparation.

**Apo-Ipravent** Apotex, Canad.
Ipratropium bromide (p.787·1).
*Bronchodilator.*

**Apo-ISDN**
Apotex, Canad.; Apotex, Hong Kong; Apotex, Malaysia; Apotex, Singapore.
Isosorbide dinitrate (p.941·1).
*Angina pectoris; heart failure.*

**Apo-K**
Apotex, Canad.; Apotex, Hong Kong; Apotex, Malaysia.
Potassium chloride (p.1232·2).
*Hypokalaemia.*

**Apo-Keto**
Apotex, Canad.; Apotex, Hong Kong†; Apotex, Malaysia; Apotex, Singapore.
Ketoprofen (p.51·2).
*Inflammation; musculoskeletal, joint, and peri-articular disorders; pain.*

**Apokinon**
Rontag, Arg.; Aguettant, Fr.
Apomorphine hydrochloride (p.1199·1).
*Parkinsonism.*

**Apokyn** Bertek, USA.
Apomorphine hydrochloride (p.1199·1).
*Parkinsonism.*

**Apolar**
Alpharma, Fin.; Alpharma, Norw.; Alpharma, Swed.
Desonide (p.1096·3).
*Skin disorders.*

**Apolar med dekvalon** Alpharma, Norw.
Desonide (p.1096·3); dequalinium chloride (p.1178·1).
*Infected skin disorders.*

**Apo-Levocarb**
Apotex, Canad.; Apotex, Hong Kong; Apotex, Malaysia; Apotex, NZ†.
Levodopa (p.1205·2); carbidopa (p.1204·3).
*Parkinsonism.*

**Apolide** Protein, Mex.†.
Nimesulide (p.67·1).

**Apollonset** Pharmanik (Φαρμανικ), Gr.
Diazepam (p.690·1).
*Alcohol withdrawal syndrome; anxiety disorders; premedication; skeletal muscle spasm; sleep disorders; status epilepticus; tetanus.*

**Apo-Methazide** Apotex, Canad.
Methyldopa (p.953·2); hydrochlorothiazide (p.933·2).
*Hypertension.*

**Apo-Methoprazine** Apotex, Canad.
Levomepromazine maleate (p.703·2).

**Apo-Metoclop**
Apotex, Canad.; Apotex, Hong Kong†.
Metoclopramide hydrochloride (p.1274·3).
*Gastrointestinal disorders; nausea and vomiting.*

**Apomex** Curex, Israel†.
Selegiline hydrochloride (p.1214·1).
*Parkinsonism.*

**Apomin** Merck, Hong Kong.
Chlorphenamine maleate (p.427·3).
*Hypersensitivity reactions.*

**Apomine**
Mayne, Austral.; Baxter, NZ; Faulding, NZ.
Apomorphine hydrochloride (p.1199·1).
*Parkinsonism.*

**Apominolin** Curex, Israel†.
Minocycline hydrochloride (p.231·3).
*Bacterial infections.*

**Apomoxyn** Curex, Israel†.
Amoxicillin (p.155·3).
*Bacterial infections.*

**Aponacin** Curex, Israel†.
Naproxen (p.65·1).
*Musculoskeletal and joint disorders; pain.*

**Apo-Nadol**
Apotex, Canad.; Apotex, Hong Kong.
Nadolol (p.963·1).
*Angina pectoris; arrhythmias; hypertension; hyperthyroidism; migraine.*

**Aponal** Roche, Ger.
Doxepin hydrochloride (p.291·2).
*Anxiety; depression; insomnia; withdrawal syndromes.*

**Apo-Napro-Na**
Apotex, Canad.; Apotex, Hong Kong; Apotex, Malaysia; Apotex, Singapore.
Naproxen sodium (p.65·1).
*Inflammation; musculoskeletal and joint disorders; pain.*

**Aponatura Beruhigungs** Terralife, Austria.
Lupulus (p.1708·1); melissa (p.1711·1) with or without vitamin C (p.1460·2).
*Sedative.*

**Aponatura Durchfall** Terralife, Austria.
*Capsule:* Tormentil (p.1757·2); myrtillus (p.1718·3).
*Oral drops:* Tormentil (p.1757·2); myrtillus (p.1718·3); strawberry leaf.
*Diarrhoea.*

**Aponatura Einschlaf** Terralife, Austria.
Valerian (p.1762·2); lupulus (p.1708·1); melissa (p.1711·1).
*Sleep disorders.*

**Aponatura Entwasserungs** Terralife, Austria.
*Capsules:* Juniper (p.1703·1); ononis (p.1723·3).
*Oral drops:* Juniper (p.1703·1); ononis (p.1723·3); lovage (p.1708·1).
*Urinary-tract disorders.*

**Aponatura Erkaltungs** Terralife, Austria.
Tilia (p.1756·2); absinthium (p.1645·1); vitamin C (p.1460·2).
*Cold and influenza symptoms.*

**Aponatura Galle** Terralife, Austria.
Absinthium (p.1645·1); peppermint leaf (p.1283·2); cnicus benedictus (p.1673·3).
*Gallbladder disorders.*

**Aponatura Herz** Terralife, Austria.
Crataegus (p.1677·1); melissa (p.1711·1); peppermint leaf (p.1283·2).
*Cardiac disorders.*

**Aponatura Hustenlosende** Terralife, Austria.
Althaea (p.1651·3); mallow leaf (p.1709·3); ammonium chloride (p.1115·2).
*Coughs.*

**Aponatura Hustenstillende** Terralife, Austria.
Plantago lanceolata (p.1738·2); thyme (p.1755·2); wild thyme.
*Coughs.*

**Aponatura Kreislauf** Terralife, Austria.
Rosemary (p.1740·2); maté (p.1765·3).
*Circulatory disorders.*

**Aponatura Leber** Terralife, Austria.
Lecithin (p.1706·1); cynara (p.1678·3); absinthium (p.1645·1).
*Liver disorders.*

**Aponatura Nieren- und Blasen** Terralife, Austria.
Java tea; peppermint leaf (p.1283·2).
*Kidney and bladder disorders.*

**Aponatura Starkungs** Terralife, Austria.
Centaury (p.1669·2); bitter orange peel (p.1723·3); calamus root (p.1664·1).
*Tonic.*

**Aponatura Verdauungs** Terralife, Austria.
*Capsules:* Angelica (p.1655·1); absinthium (p.1645·1).
*Oral drops:* Angelica (p.1655·1); absinthium (p.1645·1); lovage (p.1708·1).
*Gastrointestinal disorders.*

**Aponatura Wind** Terralife, Austria.
Aniseed (p.1655·2); fennel (p.1687·2); caraway (p.1667·2).
*Gastrointestinal disorders.*

**Apo-Nifed**
Apotex, Canad.; Apotex, Singapore.
Nifedipine (p.966·2).
*Angina pectoris; hypertension.*

**Aponil** Glaxo Allen, Ital.
Lacidipine (p.944·2).
*Hypertension.*

**Apo-Norflox** Apotex, Canad.
Norfloxacin (p.238·3).
*Urinary-tract infections.*

**Aponorm** Curex, Israel†.
Atenolol (p.865·2).
*Angina pectoris; hypertension.*

**Apo-Oflox**
Apotex, Canad.; Apotex, Malaysia.
Ofloxacin (p.239·3).
*Bacterial infections.*

**Apo-Paradex** Apotex, NZ†.
Paracetamol (p.76·2); dextropropoxyphene napsilate (p.28·3).
*Pain.*

**Apo-Pen-VK** Apotex, Canad.
Phenoxymethylpenicillin potassium (p.242·1).
*Bacterial infections.*

**Apophage** Curex, Israel.
Metformin hydrochloride (p.342·3).
*Diabetes mellitus.*

**Apo-Pindol** Apotex, Canad.
Pindolol (p.983·2).
*Angina pectoris; hypertension.*

**Apopiran** Protein, Mex.†.
Piroxicam (p.84·2).

**Apoplectal** Klinge, Austria†.
Etofylline (p.785·1); aesculus (p.1648·2); buphenine hydrochloride (p.1663·2).
*Cerebrovascular disorders.*

**Apoplectal N** Fujisawa, Ger.
Aesculus (p.1648·2); buphenine hydrochloride (p.1663·2).
Formerly contained aesculus, buphenine hydrochloride, and etofylline.
*Cerebrovascular disorders.*

**Apo-Prazo**
Apotex, Canad.; Apotex, Hong Kong.
Prazosin hydrochloride (p.985·1).
*Hypertension.*

**Apoprin** Protein, Mex.†.
Ranitidine (p.1285·2).

**Apo-Pulm** Pekana, Ger.
Homoeopathic preparation.

**A-Por** Aspen, S.Afr.
Clotrimazole (p.396·2).
*Fungal skin infections; vulvovaginal fungal infections.*

**Aporex** Alpharma, Norw.
Dextropropoxyphene hydrochloride (p.28·3); paracetamol (p.76·2).
*Pain.*

**Aporil** Qualiphar, Belg.
Salicylic acid (p.1157·1); acetic acid (p.1645·2); lactic acid (p.1704·1); thuja (p.1755·1); greater celandine (p.1695·3).
*Warts.*

**Apo-Salvent**
Apotex, Canad.; Apotex, Hong Kong.
Salbutamol (p.791·3) or salbutamol sulfate (p.791·3).
*Obstructive airways disease.*

**Apo-Sulfatrim**
Apotex, Canad.; Apotex, Hong Kong†; Apotex, NZ; Apotex, Singapore.
Co-trimoxazole (p.199·3).
*Bacterial infections; Pneumocystis carinii pneumonia.*

**Apo-Sulin**
Apotex, Canad.; Apotex, Malaysia.
Sulindac (p.91·2).
*Inflammation; musculoskeletal, joint, and peri-articular disorders; pain.*

**Apo-Tamox**
Apotex, Canad.; Apotex, Hong Kong; Apotex, Singapore.
Tamoxifen citrate (p.584·1).
*Anovulatory infertility; breast cancer; endometrial cancer.*

**Apotel** Unipharma, Gr.
Paracetamol (p.76·2).
*Fever; pain.*

**Apoterfin** Curex, Israel†.
Terfenadine (p.441·1).
*Allergic rhinitis; allergic skin disorders.*

**Apo-Tetra**
Apotex, Canad.; Apotex, Hong Kong†.
Tetracycline hydrochloride (p.266·2).
*Bacterial infections.*

**Apotheker Bauer's Blahungstee** Jauntal, Austria.
Angelica (p.1655·1); fennel (p.1687·2); chamomile (p.1669·3); coriander (p.1676·1); sage (p.1741·2).
*Flatulence.*

**Apotheker Bauer's Brust- und Hustentee**
Jauntal, Austria.
Fennel (p.1687·2); Iceland moss; cowslip flowers (p.1735·1); thyme leaf (p.1755·2); verbascum flowers (p.1764·1).
*Catarrh.*

**Apotheker Bauer's Franzbranntwein-Gel**
Jauntal, Austria.
Brandy (p.1166·1); concentrated ammonia (p.1653·3).
*Insect bites; minor injuries.*

**Apotheker Bauer's Grippetee** Jauntal, Austria.
Cowslip rhizome (p.1735·1); pimpinella; sambucus (p.1741·3); tilia (p.1756·2); crataegus (p.1677·1).
*Cold and influenza symptoms.*

**Apotheker Bauer's Harntreibender Tee**
Jauntal, Austria.
Urtica (p.1762·1); java tea (p.1702·3); parsley root (p.1728·3); solidago virgaurea (p.1748·3); juniper (p.1703·1).
*Renal calculi.*

**Apotheker Bauer's Huhneraugentinktur**
Jauntal, Austria.
Salicylic acid (p.1157·1); lactic acid (p.1704·1); resorcinol (p.1156·3); flexible collodion.
*Corns and callouses.*

**Apotheker Bauer's Inhalationsmischung**
Jauntal, Austria.
Eucalyptus oil (p.1686·2); juniper oil (p.1703·1); pumilio pine oil (p.1737·1).
*Respiratory-tract disorders.*

**Apotheker Bauer's Kindertee** Jauntal, Austria.
Orange flowers (p.1723·3); fennel (p.1687·2); clove (p.1673·2); hibiscus flowers; pansy.
*Gastrointestinal disorders.*

**Apotheker Bauer's Magentee** Jauntal, Austria.
Angelica (p.1655·1); caraway (p.1667·2); mallow leaf (p.1709·3); rosemary leaf (p.1740·2); centaury (p.1669·2); calendula (p.1665·2).
*Gastrointestinal disorders.*

**Apotheker Bauer's Misteltinktur** Jauntal, Austria.
Mistletoe (p.1715·3).
*Circulatory disorders.*

**Apotheker Bauer's Nieren- und Blasentee**
Jauntal, Austria.
Birch leaf (p.1660·3); urtica (p.1762·1); java tea (p.1702·3); solidago virgaurea (p.1748·3); bearberry (p.1659·2).
*Kidney and bladder disorders.*

**Apotheker Ehrmanns Grippekapseln** Adler, Austria.
Salix bark (p.87·3); rose fruit (p.1740·1).
*Cold and influenza symptoms.*

**Apotheker Hoyers Brennesseltonikum** St Valentinus Apotheke, Austria.
Urtica (p.1762·1); taraxacum (p.1751·3); birch leaf (p.1660·3).
*Tonic.*

**Apo-Theo**
Apotex, Canad.; Apotex, Hong Kong†; Apotex, Malaysia; Apotex, Singapore.
Theophylline (p.798·3).
*Obstructive airways disease.*

**Apotil** Curex, Israel†.
Timolol maleate (p.1012·2).
*Glaucoma; ocular hypertension.*

**Apo-Timol**
Apotex, Canad.; Apotex, NZ†.
Timolol maleate (p.1012·2).
*Angina pectoris; arrhythmias; hypertension; migraine; myocardial infarction.*

**Apo-Timop**
Apotex, Canad.; Apotex, Hong Kong; Apotex, NZ.
Timolol maleate (p.1012·2).
*Glaucoma; ocular hypertension.*

**Apo-Triazide**
Apotex, Canad.; Apotex, Hong Kong; Apotex, Malaysia; Apotex, Singapore.
Hydrochlorothiazide (p.933·2); triamterene (p.1016·2).
*Hypertension; oedema.*

**Apo-Triazo** *Apotex, Canad.*
Triazolam (p.725·3).
*Insomnia.*

**Apo-Trihex**
*Apotex, Canad.; Apotex, Hong Kong; Apotex, Malaysia; Apotex, Singapore.*
Trihexyphenidyl hydrochloride (p.490·2).
*Drug-induced extrapyramidal disorders; parkinsonism.*

**Apo-Trimip**
*Apotex, Canad.; Apotex, Hong Kong†.*
Trimipramine maleate (p.320·2).
*Depression.*

**Apotrin** *Ridupharm, Switz.†.*
Betacarotene (p.1422·3); canthaxanthin (p.1056·3).
*Photodermatoses; protoporphyria.*

**Apo-Tuss** *Pekana, Ger.*
Homoeopathic preparation.

**Apoven** *Douglas, Austral.*
Ipratropium bromide (p.787·1).
*Obstructive airways disease.*

**Apovent** *Curex, Israel.*
Ipratropium bromide (p.787·1).
*Obstructive airways disease.*

**Apo-Verap** *Apotex, Canad.*
Verapamil hydrochloride (p.1019·1).
*Angina; arrhythmias; hypertension.*

**Apox** *Curex, Israel†.*
Alprazolam (p.668·3).
*Anxiety; panic disorders.*

**Apozan** *Curex, Israel†.*
Ranitidine hydrochloride (p.1285·2).
*Gastro-oesophageal reflux; gastrointestinal hyperacidity; peptic ulcer; zollinger Ellison syndrome.*

**Apozepam**
*Alpharma, Denm.; Alpharma, Swed.*
Diazepam (p.690·1).
*Alcohol withdrawal syndrome; anxiety; insomnia; premedication; restlessness; skeletal muscle spasm.*

**Appearex** *Merz, USA.*
Biotin (p.1423·2).
*Nail disorders.*

**Appedrine**
*Note. This name is used for preparations of different composition.*
*Chattem, Canad.*
Benzocaine (p.1370·3); ferrous fumarate (p.1427·3); carmellose sodium (p.1577·3); vitamins (p.1417·1).
*Obesity.*

*Thompson, USA†.*
Phenylpropanolamine hydrochloride (p.1127·3); multivitamins and minerals.

**Appelin-B12** *Pharos, Singapore.*
Benzoic acid; inositol; lysine; sorbitol; vitamin $B_{12}$; vitamin C (p.1417·1).
*Tonic.*

**Appetiser Mixture** *Potter's, UK.*
Chamomile (p.1669·3); calumba (p.1665·2); compound gentian infusion (p.1692·2).
*Flatulence; tonic.*

**Appeton** *Kotra, Malaysia.*
A range of vitamin preparations with or without minerals, ginseng, lysine, or taurine (p.1417·1).

**Appeton Weight Gain** *Kotra, Malaysia.*
A preparation for enteral nutrition (p.1417·1).

**Appetrol** *Covan, S.Afr.†.*
Cathine hydrochloride (p.1585·2).
*Obesity.*

**Applicaine**
*Carter-Wallace, Austral.; ICN, NZ†.*
*Oral gel:* Choline salicylate (p.26·2).
*Oral pain; teething.*

*Carter-Wallace, Austral.; ICN, NZ†.*
*Topical liquid:* Benzocaine (p.1370·3).
*Mouth ulcers; oral pain; teething.*

**APR Cream** *Curacel, Austral.*
Methyl salicylate (p.59·3); camphor (p.1665·3); menthol (p.1711·3); capsicum oleoresin (p.1667·1); copper sulfate (p.1426·1); eicosapentaenoic acid (p.976·2); melaleuca oil (p.1710·2); zinc sulfate (p.1469·3).
*Musculoskeletal and joint disorders.*

**Apra** *Altaire, USA.*
Paracetamol (p.76·2).
*Fever; pain.*

**Apracur**
*Note. This name is used for preparations of different composition.*
*Serch, Arg.*
Paracetamol (p.76·2); phenylephrine (p.1126·3); clemizole (p.429·2).
*Influenza symptoms.*

*Schering, Austria†.*
Paracetamol (p.76·2); phenylephrine hydrochloride (p.1126·3); clemizole hydrochloride (p.429·2).
*Cold and influenza symptoms.*

*Virtus, Braz.†.*
Chlorphenamine maleate (p.427·3); ascorbic acid (p.1460·2); dipyrone (p.35·3).
*Cold and influenza symptoms.*

*Trahan, Thai.*
Paracetamol (p.76·2); phenylephrine hydrochloride (p.1126·3); clemizole hydrochloride (p.429·2); salicylamide (p.87·3).
*Cold symptoms.*

**Apracur Antifebril** *Serch, Arg.*
Paracetamol (p.76·2).
*Fever; pain.*

**Apracur Biotic** *Serch, Arg.*
Amoxicillin (p.155·3).
*Bacterial infections.*

**Apracur Bucofaringeo** *Serch, Arg.*
Hexylresorcinol (p.1182·1); benzocaine (p.1370·3).

**Apracur Expectorante** *Serch, Arg.*
Ambroxol (p.1114·3).
*Respiratory-tract congestion.*

**Apracur Nasal** *Serch, Arg.*
Oxymetazoline (p.1126·2).
*Nasal congestion.*

**Apra-Gel** *Roche, Belg.†.*
Naproxen (p.65·1).
*Musculoskeletal, joint, and peri-articular disorders.*

**Apranax**
*Roche, Belg.; Roche, Fr.; Syntex, Ger.†; Roche, Ger.†; Roche, Switz.*
Naproxen (p.65·1) or naproxen sodium (p.65·1).
*Gout; inflammation; musculoskeletal, joint, and peri-articular disorders; pain.*

**Apraz** *Schering-Plough, Braz.*
Alprazolam (p.668·3).
*Anxiety.*

**Aprednislon** *Merck, Austria.*
Prednisolone (p.1108·1).
*Corticosteroid.*

**Apresazide** *Novartis, USA.*
Hydralazine hydrochloride (p.931·2); hydrochlorothiazide (p.933·2).
*Hypertension.*

**Apresolin**
*Novartis, Denm.†; Novartis, Norw.; Novartis, Swed.*
Hydralazine hydrochloride (p.931·2).
*Heart failure; hypertension.*

**Apresolina**
*Novartis, Braz.; Novartis, Mex.*
Hydralazine hydrochloride (p.931·2).
*Heart failure; hypertension.*

**Apresoline**
*Novartis, Austral.; Novartis, Canad.; Novartis, Hong Kong; Novartis, Irl.; Novartis, Neth.; Novartis, NZ; Novartis, S.Afr.; Novartis, Thai.; Sovereign, UK; Novartis, USA.*
Hydralazine hydrochloride (p.931·2).
*Heart failure; hypertension.*

**Apri** *Duramed, USA.*
Desogestrel (p.1547·2); ethinylestradiol (p.1553·2).
28-Day packs also contain 7 inert tablets.
*Combined oral contraceptive.*

**Aprical**
*Shire, Ger.; Rentschler, Israel†.*
Nifedipine (p.966·2).
*Angina pectoris; hypertension; Raynaud's syndrome.*

**April** *Gador, Arg.*
Levonorgestrel (p.1563·2); ethinylestradiol (p.1553·2).
*Combined oral contraceptive.*

**Aprinol** *Anpharm (Ανφαρμ), Gr.*
Ambroxol hydrochloride (p.1114·3).
*Respiratory disorders associated with viscous mucus.*

**Aprinox**
*Abbott, Austral.; Sovereign, UK.*
Bendroflumethiazide (p.867·3).
*Hypertension; oedema; suppression of lactation.*

**Aprix-DN** *Recalcine, Chile.*
Yellow tablets, paracetamol (p.76·2); pseudoephedrine hydrochloride (p.1129·2); blue tablets, paracetamol; pseudoephedrine hydrochloride; chlorphenamine maleate (p.427·3).
*Influenza symptoms.*

**Aprodine** *Major, USA.*
Pseudoephedrine hydrochloride (p.1129·2); triprolidine hydrochloride (p.442·3).
*Upper respiratory-tract symptoms.*

**Aprodine with Codeine** *Major, USA.*
Pseudoephedrine hydrochloride (p.1129·2); codeine phosphate (p.27·1); triprolidine hydrochloride (p.442·3).
*Coughs and cold symptoms.*

**Aprofen** *Progress, Thai.*
Ibuprofen (p.45·3).
*Fever; musculoskeletal, joint, and soft-tissue disorders; pain.*

**Aproten**
*Diet Erba, NZ; Ultrapharm, UK.*
Low-protein, gluten-free foods for special diets (p.1417·1).

**Aprovel**
*Sanofi Synthelabo, Arg.; Sanofi Synthelabo, Belg.; Sanofi Synthelabo, Braz.; Sanofi Synthelabo, Chile; Sanofi Synthelabo, Denm.; Sanofi Synthelabo, Fin.; Bristol-Myers Squibb, Fin.; Bristol-Myers Squibb, Fr.; Sanofi Synthelabo, Ger.; Sanofi Synthelabo, Gr.; Sanofi Synthelabo, Hong Kong; Sanofi Synthelabo, Irl.; Bristol-Myers Squibb, Irl.; Sanofi Synthelabo, Ital.; Sanofi Synthelabo, Malaysia; Sanofi Synthelabo, Mex.; Sanofi Winthrop, Neth.; Bristol-Myers Squibb, Neth.; Sanofi Synthelabo, Norw.; Bristol-Myers Squibb, Norw.; Bristol-Myers Squibb, Port.; Sanofi Synthelabo, Port.; Sanofi Synthelabo, S.Afr.; Sanofi Synthelabo, Singapore; Sanofi Synthelabo, Spain; Sanofi Synthelabo, Swed.; Bristol-Myers Squibb, Swed.; Sanofi, Switz.; Bristol-Myers Squibb, Switz.; Sanofi Synthelabo, Thai.; Sanofi Synthelabo, UK; Bristol-Myers Squibb, UK.*
Irbesartan (p.940·1).
*Diabetic nephropathy; hypertension.*

**Aprovel HCT**
*Sanofi Synthelabo, Hong Kong; Sanofi Synthelabo, Thai.*
Irbesartan (p.940·1); hydrochlorothiazide (p.933·2).
*Hypertension.*

**Aproxal** *Elpen (Ελπεν), Gr.*
Amoxicillin trihydrate (p.155·3).
*Bacterial infections.*

**Aprozide** *Sanofi Synthelabo, Braz.*
Irbesartan (p.940·1); hydrochlorothiazide (p.933·2).
*Hypertension.*

**APS Balneum** *APS, Ger.†.*
Chamomile oil (p.1669·3).
*Bath additive; skin disorders.*

**Apsomol** *Farmasan, Ger.*
Salbutamol sulfate (p.791·3).
*Obstructive airways disease.*

**Apsor**
*Note. This name is used for preparations of different composition.*
*Lipha Sante, Fr.*
Tacalcitol (p.1158·3).
*Psoriasis.*

*IDI, Ital.†.*
Betamethasone valero-acetate (p.1093·2); tretinoin (p.1161·1); salicylic acid (p.1157·1).
Formerly contained betamethasone valero-acetate, tretinoin, precipitated sulfur, salicylic acid, camphor, and allantoin.
*Psoriasis.*

**Aptamil AR** *Milupa, Port.*
Infant feed (p.1417·1).
*Gastro-oesophageal reflux.*

**Aptamil HA** *Milupa, Port.*
Infant feed (p.1417·1).
*Milk intolerance.*

**Aptamil HA 2** *Milupa, Ital.†.*
Infant feed (p.1417·1).
*Cow's milk intolerance.*

**Aptamil HA con LCP Milupan** *Milupa, Ital.†.*
Infant feed (p.1417·1).
*Milk intolerance.*

**APT-Ampicloxa** *Merck, Hong Kong.*
Ampicillin trihydrate (p.157·2); cloxacillin sodium (p.198·2).
*Bacterial infections.*

**Aptin**
*Astra, Denm.†; Astra, Norw.†.*
Alprenolol benzoate (p.856·3).
*Angina pectoris; arrhythmias; hypertension; hyperthyroidism; myocardial infarction; tremor.*

*Astra, Ger.†.*
Alprenolol hydrochloride (p.856·3).
*Angina pectoris; arrhythmias; heart failure; hypertension; myocardial infarction.*

**Aptin N** *Hassle, Swed.†.*
Alprenolol benzoate (p.856·3).
*Angina pectoris; arrhythmias; hypertension; myocardial infarction.*

**Aptine** *Astra, Belg.†.*
Alprenolol benzoate (p.856·3).
*Angina pectoris; arrhythmias; hypertension; myocardial infarction.*

**Aptodin Plus** *GD, Ital.*
Vitamin, mineral, and amino-acid preparation (p.1417·1).

**Apton** *Delta, Port.*
Pantoprazole (p.1283·1).
*Gastro-oesophageal reflux; peptic ulcer.*

**Aptus Amphetamine** *Aptus, NZ.*
Test for amfetamine in urine.

**Aptus Benzodiazepine** *Aptus, NZ.*
Test for benzodiazepines in urine.

**Aptus Cannabis** *Aptus, NZ.*
Test for THC in urine.

**Aptus Cocaine** *Aptus, NZ.*
Test for cocaine in urine.

**Aptus Methadone** *Aptus, NZ.*
Test for methadone in urine.

**Aptus Methamphetamine** *Aptus, NZ.*
Test for methamfetamine in urine.

**Aptus Opiate** *Aptus, NZ.*
Test for opiates in urine.

**Apurin**
*Fresenius Kabi, Austria; Gea, Denm.; Gea, Fin.*
Allopurinol (p.412·2) or allopurinol sodium (p.413·3).
*Gout; hyperuricaemia; renal calculi.*

**Apurol** *Siegfried, Thai.*
Allopurinol (p.412·2).
*Gout; hyperuricaemia.*

**Apurone**
*3M, Belg.†; Substipharm, Fr.*
Flumequine (p.214·2).
*Bacterial infections of the urinary tract.*

**Apuzin** *YSP, Malaysia.*
Captopril (p.879·2).
*Diabetic nephropathy; heart failure; hypertension; myocardial infarction.*

**Apydan**
*Desitin, Denm.; Algol, Fin.*
Oxcarbazepine (p.366·3).
*Epilepsy.*

**Apyrol** *Salusif, Port.*
Sodium hydroxyquinoline sulfate (p.1700·1); camphor (p.1665·3).
*Muscular pain; soft-tissue disorders; wounds.*

**Aqium Active Defence** *Ego, Austral.†.*
Barrier cream and emollient.

**Aqsia** *Chauvin, UK†.*
Electrolyte solution (p.1217·1).
*Eye irrigation.*

**Aqua Ban**
*Lane, UK; Thompson, USA.*
Ammonium chloride (p.1115·2); caffeine (p.782·1).
*Premenstrual water retention.*

**Aqua Ban Plus** *Thompson, USA.*
Ammonium chloride (p.1115·2); caffeine (p.782·1); ferrous sulfate (p.1428·2).
*Premenstrual water retention.*

**Aqua Dermis** *American Remedies, Malaysia; Bio-Pharmaceuticals, Malaysia.*
Soap substitute.

**Aqua Ear** *Whitehall, NZ.*
Glacial acetic acid (p.1645·2); isopropyl alcohol (p.1184·3).
*Otitis externa.*

**Aqua Emoform** *Byk Gulden, Ital.*
Sodium monofluorophosphate (p.1446·2); sodium fluoride (p.1444·3).
*Gingival inflammation; oral hygiene.*

**Aqua Lub** *Probifasa, Mex.*
Lubricant for vaginal and rectal use.

**Aqua Soap** *Remexa, Mex.*
Soap substitute.

**AquaBalm** *Quintessa, USA.*
Emollient.
*Dry skin.*

**Aquabase**
*Westbrook, UK†.*
A non ionic emulsifying wax.

*Paddock, USA.*
Vehicle for topical preparations.

**Aquacaps** *Muller Goppingen, Ger.†.*
Java tea (p.1702·3).
*Urinary-tract disorders.*

**Aquacare**
*Allergan, Austral.; Allergan, NZ; Menley & James, USA.*
Urea (p.1162·2).
*Dry skin; eczema; keratinisation disorders.*

**Aquacel**
*Bristol-Myers Squibb, Arg.; Convatec, Austral.; Convatec, Fr.; Convatec, Port.*
Carmellose sodium (p.1577·3).
*Burns; ulcers; wounds.*

**Aquachloral** *PolyMedica, USA.*
Cloral hydrate (p.684·1).
*Sedative.*

**Aquacort** *Spectropharm, Canad.†.*
Hydrocortisone (p.1103·3).
*Skin disorders.*

**Aquaderm**
*Note. This name is used for preparations of different composition.*
*Baker Cummins, Canad.†.*
*SPF 15:* Octisalate (p.1154·3); avobenzone (p.1142·3); octinoxate (p.1154·3); titanium dioxide (p.1160·3).
*SPF 30:* Avobenzone (p.1142·3); octocrilene (p.1154·3); octinoxate (p.1154·3); titanium dioxide (p.1160·3).
*Sunscreen.*

*Paladin, Canad.*
Emollient.

*Baker Cummins, USA.*
*SPF 15:* Octinoxate (p.1154·3); oxybenzone (p.1154·3).
*Sunscreen.*

**Aquadon** *Rekah, Israel.*
Chlortalidone (p.882·3).
*Hypertension; oedema.*

**Aquadrate**
*Alliance, Irl.; Alliance, UK.*
Urea (p.1162·2).
*Dry skin disorders.*

**Aquae**
*Hamilton, Austral.; Hamilton, Hong Kong.*
Carmellose sodium (p.1577·3); sorbitol (p.1446·3); electrolytes (p.1217·1).
*Artificial saliva.*

**Aquaear** *Whitehall, Austral.†.*
Glacial acetic acid (p.1645·2); isopropyl alcohol (p.1184·3).
*Prevention of otitis externa.*

**Aquafilme** *Sofex, Port.*
Emollient.

**Aquafor** *Asta Medica, Ital.*
Xipamide (p.1029·2).
*Hypertension.*

**Aquaform** *Maersk, UK.*
Hydrogel dressing.
*Ulcers; wounds.*

**Aquagel** *Adams, Hong Kong.*
Lubricating jelly.

**Aquagen SQ**
*ALK, Denm.; ALK, Fin.; ALK, Swed.*
Allergen extracts (p.1650·1).
*Allergen immunotherapy; diagnosis of hypersensitivity.*

**Aqualan** *Orion, Fin.*
Emollient.

**Aqualane** *Roux-Ocefa, Arg.*
Beeswax (p.1480·1); liquid paraffin (p.1479·1); white soft paraffin (p.1479·3).
*Barrier cream.*

**Aqualarm** *Chauvin, Fr.*
Carbomer 980 (p.1577·2).
*Dry eyes.*

**Aqualcium** Aqualab, Fr.†
Mineral preparation (p.1417·1).
*Calcium deficiency.*

**Aqualette** Lichtwer, UK.
Taraxacum (p.1751·3); equisetum (p.1684·1).

**Aqualibra** Medice, Ger.
Ononis (p.1723·3); java tea (p.1702·3); solidago (p.1748·3).
*Urinary-tract disorders.*

**Aquamag** Aqualab, Fr.†
Mineral preparation (p.1417·1).
*Magnesium deficiency.*

**Aquamephyton** Merck, USA.
Phytomenadione (p.1467·1).
*Coagulation disorders associated with vitamin K deficiency, due to faulty formation of factors II, VII, IX, and X.*

**Aquamycetin-N** Winzer, Ger.
Chloramphenicol (p.185·1).
*Bacterial eye infections.*

**Aquanil**
Note. This name is used for preparations of different composition.
Dispolab, Chile.
Soap-free skin cleanser.
Novartis, Denm.; Novartis, Fin.; Novartis, Norw.; Novartis Ophthalmics, Swed.
Timolol maleate (p.1012·2).
*Glaucoma; ocular hypertension.*
Darier, Mex.
Sodium lauril sulfate (p.1574·2).
*Skin disorders.*
Person & Covey, USA.
Emollient and moisturiser.

**Aquanil HC**
Dispolab, Chile; Darier, Mex.; Person & Covey, USA.
Hydrocortisone (p.1103·3).
*Skin disorders.*

**Aquaphilic** Medco, USA.
Vehicle for topical preparations.

**Aquaphor**
Note. This name is used for preparations of different composition.
Smith & Nephew, Canad.†
White soft paraffin (p.1479·3).
*Dry skin; ointment base.*
Lilly, Ger.
Xipamide (p.1029·2).
*Hypertension; oedema.*
Beiersdorf, USA.
Yellow soft paraffin; liquid paraffin; mineral wax; wool wax alcohol.
*Barrier ointment; ointment base.*

**Aquaphor Healing Ointment** Beiersdorf, USA.
Soft paraffin; liquid paraffin; ceresin; wool alcohols; panthenol; bisabolol.
*Dry skin disorders.*

**Aquaphoril** Asta Medica, Austria.
Xipamide (p.1029·2).
*Hypertension; oedema.*

**Aquaphyllin** Ferndale, USA.
Theophylline (p.798·3).
*Asthma; bronchospasm.*

**Aquapred** Winzer, Ger.
Chloramphenicol (p.185·1); prednisolone sodium phosphate (p.1108·1).
*Inflammatory disorders and infections of the eye.*

**Aquareduct** Azupharma, Ger.
Spironolactone (p.1003·1).
*Ascites; hyperaldosteronism; oedema.*

**Aquaretic** Azupharma, Ger.
Amiloride hydrochloride (p.858·2); hydrochlorothiazide (p.933·2).
*Hypertension; oedema.*

**Aquarhine** Monot, Fr.†
Sodium chloride (p.1233·3).

**Aquarid** Alliance, S.Afr.
Furosemide (p.919·3).
*Oedema.*

**Aquarius** Demo, Gr.
Ketoconazole (p.403·3).
*Fungal scalp infections.*

**Aquasalina** Bruschettini, Ital.
Sodium chloride (p.1233·3); borax (p.1661·3); boric acid (p.1662·1).
*Eye and nasal irrigation.*

**Aquasept** SSL, UK.
Triclosan (p.1195·2).
*Skin disinfection.*

**Aquasite**
Note. This name is used for preparations of different composition.
Ciba Vision, Canad.†
Macrogol 400 (p.1709·1); dextran 70 (p.746·2).
Novartis Ophthalmics, USA.
Macrogol 400 (p.1709·1); dextran 70 (p.746·2); polycarbophil (p.1284·2).
*Dry eyes.*

**Aquasol** SSL, UK.
Purified water (p.1764·3).

**Aquasol A**
Note. This name is used for preparations of different composition.
Dermik, Canad.†
Vitamin A palmitate (p.1453·1); dexpanthenol (p.1727·2).
*Skin disorders.*
Rhone-Poulenc Rorer, Hong Kong†; Astra, USA.
Vitamin A (p.1451·2).
*Vitamin A deficiency.*

**Aquasol A+D** Minerva (Μινερβα), Gr.
Retinol (p.1451·2); ergocalciferol (p.1417·1).
*Vitamin A and D deficiency.*

**Aquasol E**
Novartis Consumer, Canad.; Astra, USA†.
Vitamin E (p.1464·3).
*Vitamin E deficiency.*

**Aquasport** Also, Ital.
Mineral preparation (p.1417·1).

**Aquasteril** Baxter, Fin.
Water for injections (p.1765·1).

**Aquasun** Pfizer, NZ.
*Aquababy SPF 30+; Aquabloc SPF 30+:* Octinoxate (p.1154·3); zinc oxide (p.1163·2).
*Lotion SPF 18; sports gel SPF 22:* Octinoxate (p.1154·3); avobenzone (p.1142·3); oxybenzone (p.1154·3); octocrilene (p.1154·3).
*SPF 30+ lotion; SPF 30+ cream:* Octinoxate (p.1154·3); avobenzone (p.1142·3); octil triazone (p.1154·3).
*SPF 4; SPF 8:* Octinoxate (p.1154·3); avobenzone (p.1142·3).
*Stick SPF 30:* Octinoxate (p.1154·3); avobenzone (p.1142·3); enzacamene (p.1147·1).
*Sunscreen.*

**Aquasun Sports** Pfizer, NZ†.
*SPF 15:* Octinoxate (p.1154·3); avobenzone (p.1142·3); oxybenzone (p.1154·3); octil triazone (p.1154·3).
*Sunscreen.*

**Aquasun Stick** Pfizer, NZ†.
*SPF 15:* Octinoxate (p.1154·3); avobenzone (p.1142·3); oxybenzone (p.1154·3); octil triazone (p.1154·3).
*Sunscreen.*

**Aquatab C** Adams, USA.
Guaifenesin (p.1122·1); pseudoephedrine hydrochloride (p.1129·2); dextromethorphan hydrobromide (p.1117·3).
Formerly contained guaifenesin, phenylpropanolamine hydrochloride, and dextromethorphan hydrobromide.
*Coughs.*

**Aquatab D** Adams, USA.
Guaifenesin (p.1122·1); pseudoephedrine hydrochloride (p.1129·2).
Formerly contained guaifenesin and phenylpropanolamine hydrochloride.
*Nasal congestion.*

**Aquatab DM** Adams, USA.
Guaifenesin (p.1122·1); dextromethorphan hydrobromide (p.1117·3).
*Coughs.*

**Aquatabs**
Sovedis, Fr.; Medentech, Irl.†; Rudefsa, Mex.†
Sodium dichloroisocyanurate (p.1191·3).
*Water purification.*

**Aquatain** Whitehall-Robins, Canad.
Emollient.

**AquaTar** Allergan Herbert, USA†.
Coal tar (p.1159·2).
*Skin disorders.*

**AquaTears** Novartis, Austria.
Carbomer 974P (p.1577·2).
*Dry eyes.*

**Aquatensen** Wallace, USA.
Methyclothiazide (p.953·2).
*Hypertension; oedema.*

**Aquaviron** Nicholas Piramal, India.
Testosterone (p.1569·3).
*Cryptorchidism; delayed puberty; hypogonadotrophic hypogonadism; osteoporosis.*

**Aquavit-E** Cypress, USA.
*dl*-Alpha tocoferil acetate (p.1465·1).
*Vitamin E deficiency.*

**Aqua-Vite Super Kelp** Bio-Health, UK†.
Multivitamins; ascophyllum nodosum (p.1417·1).

**Aqucilina** Antibioticos, Spain.
Procaine benzylpenicillin (p.246·1).
*Bacterial infections.*

**Aqucilina D A** Antibioticos, Spain.
Benzylpenicillin potassium (p.163·2); procaine benzylpenicillin (p.246·1).
*Bacterial infections.*

**Aquedux** Sanofi Synthelabo, Port.
Furosemide (p.919·3).
*Hypertension; oedema.*

**Aquella** Lifeplan, UK.
Boldo; kelp; cider vinegar; lappa; taraxacum (p.1417·1).
*Herbal supplement.*

**Aqueous Charcodote** Pharmascience, Singapore.
Activated charcoal (p.1030·2).
*Emergency treatment of poisoning.*

**Aquim** Ego, NZ.
Dimethicone (p.1482·1).
*Barrier preparation.*

**Aquitol** Teva, Israel.
Vitamin A palmitate (p.1453·1); ergocalciferol (p.1462·1).
*Vitamin A and D supplement.*

**Aquo-Cytobion** Merck, Ger.
Hydroxocobalamin acetate (p.1458·2).
*Vitamin $B_{12}$ deficiency.*

**Aquomin** Belmac, Spain†.
Ciclopirox olamine (p.396·1).
*Fungal skin and nail infections.*

**Aquo-Trinitrosan** Merck, Ger.
Glyceryl trinitrate (p.923·2).
*Angina pectoris; controlled hypotension; heart failure; hypertension; myocardial infarction.*

**Aqupla** Shionogi, Jpn.
Nedaplatin (p.576·2).
*Malignant neoplasms.*

**Arabine**
Faulding, Denm.; Baxter, Fin.; Baxter, Swed.
Cytarabine (p.543·1).
*Acute leukaemias.*

**Aracaf** Nakorn, Thai.
Diphenhydramine hydrochloride (p.431·3); ammonium chloride (p.1115·2); sodium citrate (p.1223·2).
*Cold symptoms; cough; nasal congestion.*

**ARA-cell** Cell Pharm, Ger.
Cytarabine (p.543·1).
*Acute leukaemias; non-Hodgkins lymphoma.*

**Arachitol** Solvay, India.
Colecalciferol (p.1461·3).
*Hypoparathyroidism; rickets, osteomalacia.*

**Aracmyn Plus** Bioclon, Mex.
Spider venom antiserum (p.1640·1).
*Spider bites (Latrodectus mactans, Loxosceles).*

**Aracytin**
Janssen-Cilag, Arg.; Pharmacia, Braz.; Pharmacia, Chile; Pharmacia-Upjohn, Gr.; Pharmacia Upjohn, Ital.
Cytarabine (p.543·1).
*Malignant neoplasms.*

**Aracytine** Pharmacia, Fr.
Cytarabine (p.543·1).
*Leukaemias; myelodysplasia.*

**Aradix** Recalcine, Chile.
Methylphenidate (p.1590·3).

**Aradois** Biolab Sanus, Braz.
Losartan potassium (p.947·2).
*Hypertension.*

**Aradois H** Biolab Sanus, Braz.
Losartan potassium (p.947·2); hydrochlorothiazide (p.933·2).
*Hypertension.*

**Aragest** Dexxon, Israel.
Medroxyprogesterone acetate (p.1557·2).
*Endometriosis; menstrual disorders.*

**Aralast** Alpha Therapeutic, USA.
Alpha$_1$-proteinase inhibitor (p.1651·2).
*Alpha$_1$-proteinase deficiency.*

**Aralen**
Sanofi Synthelabo, Canad.; Sanofi Winthrop, Israel†; Sanofi Synthelabo, Mex.; Sanofi Winthrop, USA.
Chloroquine (p.448·2), chloroquine hydrochloride (p.448·2), or chloroquine phosphate (p.448·2).
*Amoebiasis; malaria.*

**Aralia Med Complex** Dynamit, Austria.
Homoeopathic preparation.

**Aramexe** Ratiopharm, Austria.
Co-dergocrine mesilate (p.1674·1).
*Cerebrovascular disorders; cervical syndrome; hypertension; migraine; peripheral vascular disease.*

**Aramin** Cristalia, Braz.
Metaraminol tartrate (p.952·2).
*Hypotension.*

**Aramine**
Merck Sharp & Dohme, Austral.; Merck Sharp & Dohme, Belg.†; IFET (ΙΦΕΤ), Gr.; Merck Sharp & Dohme, Hong Kong†; Merck Sharp & Dohme, Norw.; Merck Sharp & Dohme, NZ; Merck Sharp & Dohme, Thai.; Merck Sharp & Dohme, UK†; Merck, USA.
Metaraminol tartrate (p.952·2).
*Hypotension.*

**Aranesp**
Amgen, Austral.; Amgen, Austria; Amgen, Denm.; Amgen, Fin.; Amgen, Fr.; Amgen, Ger.; Amgen, Gr.; Amgen, Irl.; Amgen, Israel; Amgen, Neth.; Amgen, Norw.; Amgen, Port.; Amgen, Spain; Amgen, Swed.; Amgen, UK; Amgen, USA.
Darbepoetin alfa (p.745·2).
*Anaemia associated with cancer chemotherapy; anaemia in renal failure.*

**Aranidorm-S** Weber & Weber, Ger.†
Centaury (p.1669·2); chamomile (p.1669·3); passion flower (p.1729·1); valerian (p.1762·2); lavender (p.1705·1); lupulus (p.1708·1); melissa (p.1711·1); atropa bellad.; avena sat.; coffeinum; datura stram.; eschscholtzia calif.; hyoscyamus nig.; lactuca vir.; papaver dub.; zincum isovalerianicum.
*Hyperactivity; insomnia.*

**Araniforce-forte** Weber & Weber, Ger.
Homoeopathic preparation.

**Aranisan-N** Weber & Weber, Ger.
Homoeopathic preparation.

**Aratac**
Alphapharm, Austral.; Alphapharm, Malaysia; Merck, Malaysia; Pacific, NZ; Alphapharm, Singapore; Merck, Singapore; Merck, Thai.
Amiodarone hydrochloride (p.859·2).
*Arrhythmias.*

**Aratan** Andromaco, Chile.
Losartan potassium (p.947·2).
*Hypertension.*

**Aratan D** Andromaco, Chile.
Losartan potassium (p.947·2); hydrochlorothiazide (p.933·2).
*Hypertension.*

**Arava**
Aventis, Arg.; Aventis, Austral.; Aventis, Belg.; Aventis, Braz.; Aventis, Canad.; Aventis, Chile; Aventis, Denm.; Aventis, Fin.; Aventis, Fr.; Aventis, Ger.; Hoechst Marion Roussel, Gr.; Aventis, Hong Kong; Aventis, India; Aventis, Irl.; Aventis, Israel; Lepetit, Ital.; Aventis, Malaysia; Aventis, Mex.; Aventis, Neth.; Aventis, Norw.; Aventis, NZ; Aventis, Port.; Aventis, S.Afr.; Aventis, Singapore; Aventis, Spain; Aventis, Swed.; Aventis, Switz.; Aventis, Thai.; Aventis, UK; Hoechst Marion Roussel, USA.
Leflunomide (p.53·2).
*Rheumatoid arthritis; psoriatic arthritis.*

**Arbe-Plus** Helfarma, Port.†
Arginine hydrochloride; vitamin B substances (p.1417·1).
*Tonic.*

**Arbid**
Kolassa, Austria; Medichemie, Switz.
Buphenine hydrochloride (p.1663·2); diphenylpyraline hydrochloride (p.432·3).
*Rhinitis; sinusitis.*

**Arbid N** Gepepharm, Ger.
Diphenylpyraline hydrochloride (p.432·3).
*Cold symptoms.*

**Arbid-top** Medichemie, Switz.
Phenylephrine hydrochloride (p.1126·3); dequalinium chloride (p.1178·1); muramidase hydrochloride (p.1717·2).
*Nasal congestion.*

**Arbil** Ranbaxy, UK.
Carbamazepine (p.353·3).
*Bipolar disorder; epilepsy; trigeminal neuralgia.*

**Arbralene** Berk, UK†.
Metoprolol tartrate (p.957·1).
*Angina pectoris; arrhythmias; hypertension; hyperthyroidism; migraine; myocardial infarction.*

**Arbum** Joldes, Fr.
Lappa (p.1704·3); zinc gluconate (p.1469·2); pyridoxine hydrochloride (p.1456·3); biotin (p.1423·2).
*Seborrhoea.*

**Arbuz** Bittermedizin, Ger.
Papain (p.1727·3); pancreatin (p.1725·3).
*Digestive disorders.*

**Arca-Be** Arcana, Austria.
Thiamine disulfide (p.1455·2); pyridoxine hydrochloride (p.1456·3); cyanocobalamin (p.1458·2).
*Neuralgias; neuritis.*

**Arcablock** Arcana, Austria.
Atenolol (p.865·2).
*Angina pectoris; arrhythmias; hypertension; myocardial infarction.*

**Arcablock comp** Arcana, Austria.
Atenolol (p.865·2); chlortalidone (p.882·3).
*Hypertension.*

**Arca-Enzym** Arcana, Austria.
Pancreatin (p.1725·3); cellulase (p.1669·1); ox bile (p.1660·3); bromelains (p.1662·2).
*Digestive disorders.*

**Arcafen** Merck, Hong Kong†.
Clomifene citrate (p.1542·2).
*Anovulatory infertility.*

**Arcalion**
Servier, Braz.; Therval, Fr.; Servier, Hong Kong; Serdia, India; Servier, Malaysia; Servier, Port.; Servier, Singapore; Servier, Spain; Servier, Switz.; Servier, Thai.
Sulbutiamine (p.1455·1).
*Asthenia.*

**Arcana Expectorant** Arcana, S.Afr.†
Triprolidine hydrochloride (p.442·3); pseudoephedrine hydrochloride (p.1129·2); codeine phosphate (p.27·1); guaifenesin (p.1122·1).
*Coughs.*

**Arcanacycline** Arcana, S.Afr.†
Tetracycline hydrochloride (p.266·2).
*Bacterial infections.*

**Arcanacysteine** Arcana, S.Afr.†
Carbocisteine (p.1116·2).
*Respiratory-tract disorders with increased or viscous mucus.*

**Arcanafed** Arcana, S.Afr.†
Triprolidine hydrochloride (p.442·3); pseudoephedrine hydrochloride (p.1129·2).
*Cold and influenza symptoms.*

**Arcanafenac** Arcana, S.Afr.†
Diclofenac sodium (p.32·1).
*Gout; inflammation; musculoskeletal and joint disorders; pain.*

**Arcanaflex** Arcana, S.Afr.†
Paracetamol (p.76·2); chlormezanone (p.675·1).
*Pain with tension.*

**Arcanaflu** Arcana, S.Afr.†
*Capsules:* Paracetamol (p.76·2); vitamin C (p.1460·2); phenylephrine hydrochloride (p.1126·3); chlorphenamine maleate (p.427·3); caffeine (p.782·1).
*Syrup:* Paracetamol (p.76·2); phenylpropanolamine hydrochloride (p.1127·3); dextromethorphan hydrobromide (p.1117·3).
*Cold and influenza symptoms.*

**Arcanagesic** Arcana, S.Afr.†
*Syrup:* Paracetamol (p.76·2).
*Tablets:* Paracetamol (p.76·2); codeine phosphate (p.27·1).
*Fever; pain.*

**Arcanamycin** Arcana, S.Afr.†
Erythromycin estolate (p.208·1) or erythromycin stearate (p.208·2).
*Bacterial infections.*

**Arcanaprim** Arcana, S.Afr.†
Co-trimoxazole (p.199·3).
*Bacterial infections.*

**Arcasin**
Note. This name is used for preparations of different composition.
Brahms, Ger.; Cimex, Switz.†.
Phenoxymethylpenicillin potassium (p.242·1).
*Bacterial infections.*

Esteve, Spain.
Cisapride (p.1259·2).
*Gastro-oesophageal reflux; gastroparesis.*

**Arcavit A** Merck, Austria.
Vitamin A acetate (p.1453·1).
*Vitamin A deficiency.*

**Arcavit A/E** Arcana, Austria.
Vitamin A palmitate (p.1453·1); dl-alpha tocoferil acetate (p.1465·1).
*Vitamin A and E deficiency.*

**Arceligasol** Gezzi, Arg.
Hyssopus officinalis; bladderwrack (p.1742·3); fennel (p.1687·2); coltsfoot (p.1117·2); cynara (p.1678·3); equisetum (p.1684·1); peppermint (p.1283·2).

**Arcental** FS Profas, Spain.
Ketoprofen (p.51·2).
*Gout; inflammation; musculoskeletal, joint, peri-articular, and soft-tissue disorders; pain.*

**Archidex** TP, Thai.
Dexamethasone phosphate (p.1097·2); neomycin (p.235·1).
*Infected eye or ear disorders.*

**Archifen** Archifar, Thai.
*Ear drops:* Chloramphenicol (p.185·1); lidocaine hydrochloride (p.1377·3).
*Bacterial ear infections.*
*Eye drops:* Chloramphenicol (p.185·1).
*Bacterial eye infections.*

**Architex** Cooperation Pharmaceutique, Fr.†.
Sodium monofluorophosphate (p.1446·2); calcium carbonate (p.1254·2).
*Osteoporosis.*

**Arcid** Diafarm, Spain.
Ranitidine hydrochloride (p.1285·2).
*Acid aspiration; gastro-oesophageal reflux; gastrointestinal hyperacidity; peptic ulcer; short-bowel syndrome; Zollinger-Ellison syndrome.*

**Arclonac** Condrugs, Thai.
Diclofenac sodium (p.32·1).
*Musculoskeletal and joint disorders.*

**Arco Pain** Romilo, Canad.†.
Aspirin (p.15·1); caffeine citrate (p.782·1).

**Arcobee with C** Nature's Bounty, USA.
Vitamin B substances with vitamin C (p.1417·1).

**Arcoiran** Alter, Spain.
Sumatriptan succinate (p.471·2).
*Cluster headache; migraine.*

**Arcolan** Galderma, Braz.
Ketoconazole (p.403·3).
*Seborrhoeic dermatitis.*

**Arcolane** Galderma, Chile.
Ketoconazole (p.403·3).
*Pityriasis versicolor; seborrhoeic dermatitis.*

**Arco-Lase** Arco, USA†.
Amylolytic enzymes (p.1654·2); proteolytic enzymes; cellulolytic enzymes (p.1669·1); lipase.
*Digestion disorders.*

**Arco-Lase Plus** Arco, USA†.
Amylolytic enzymes (p.1654·2); proteolytic enzymes; cellulolytic enzymes (p.1669·1); lipase; hyoscyamine sulfate (p.485·1); atropine sulfate (p.477·1); phenobarbital (p.367·3).
*Gastrointestinal disorders.*

**Arcosal** Rosco, Denm.
Tolbutamide (p.348·1).
*Diabetes mellitus.*

**Arcostrong** Arcolab, Switz.†.
Vitamins; minerals; ginseng; lecithin; choline; inositol; methionine (p.1417·1).
*Tonic.*

**Arcoxia**
Merck Sharp & Dohme, Irl.; Merck Sharp & Dohme, NZ; Merck Sharp & Dohme, UK.
Etoricoxib (p.38·2).
*Gouty arthritis; osteoarthritis; rheumatoid arthritis.*

**Arctuvan** Fujisawa, Ger.
Bearberry leaves (p.1659·2).
Formerly contained methenamine, salol, and bearberry leaves.
*Urinary-tract infections.*

**Ardey-aktiv** Ardeypharm, Ger.
Ginseng (p.1693·1).
*Tonic.*

**Ardeyceryl P** Ardeypharm, Ger.
Pyritinol hydrochloride (p.1737·2).
*Mental function disorders.*

**Ardeycholan N** Ardeypharm, Ger.†.
Greater celandine (p.1695·3).
*Smooth muscle spasm.*

**Ardeycordal N** Ardeypharm, Ger.
Crataegus (p.1677·1); potassium aspartate (p.1233·1); magnesium aspartate (p.1227·3).
Formerly contained ethaverine, crataegus, valerian, potassium aspartate, magnesium aspartate, and sparteine sulfate.
*Arrhythmias.*

**Ardeydorm** Ardeypharm, Ger.
Tryptophan (p.320·3).
*Sleep disorders.*

**Ardeydystin** Ardeypharm, Ger.†.
Kava (p.1703·2).
Formerly contained valerian root, kavain, and crataegus.
*Nervous disorders.*

**Ardeyhepan N** Ardeypharm, Ger.
Silybum marianum (p.1043·3).
*Liver disorders.*

**Ardeysedon N** Ardeypharm, Ger.
Valerian root (p.1762·2); lupulus (p.1708·1).
*Nervous disorders; sleep disorders.*

**Ardeytropin** Ardeypharm, Ger.
Tryptophan (p.320·3).
*Depression; sleep disorders.*

**Ardin** Korea Pharma, Singapore.
Loratadine (p.436·1).
*Allergic rhinitis; urticaria.*

**Ardine**
Disprovent, Arg.; Columbia, Mex.; Antibioticos, Spain.
Amoxicillin trihydrate (p.155·3).
*Bacterial infections.*

**Ardine Bronquial** Antibioticos, Spain.
Amoxicillin trihydrate (p.155·3); bromhexine hydrochloride (p.1115·3).
*Respiratory-tract infections.*

**Ardineclav** Antibioticos, Spain.
Amoxicillin trihydrate (p.155·3); potassium clavulanate (p.193·3).
*Bacterial infections.*

**Ardinex**
Ebewe, Austria; Abbott, Fin.; Mundipharma, Swed.
Ibuprofen (p.45·3); codeine phosphate (p.27·1).
*Pain.*

**Ardoral** Cinfa, Spain.
Ranitidine hydrochloride (p.1285·2).
*Acid aspiration; gastro-oesophageal reflux; gastrointestinal hyperacidity; peptic ulcer; short-bowel syndrome; Zollinger-Ellison syndrome.*

**Arduan**
Organon Teknika, Ital.†; Organon, USA†.
Pipecuronium bromide (p.1405·2).
*Competitive neuromuscular blocker.*

**Arecamin** Northia, Arg.
Cefalotin (p.168·3).
*Bacterial infections.*

**Aredia**
Novartis, Austral.; Novartis, Austria; Novartis, Belg.; Novartis, Braz.; Novartis, Canad.; Novartis, Chile; Novartis, Denm.; Novartis, Fin.; Novartis, Fr.; Novartis, Ger.; Novartis, Gr.; Novartis, Hong Kong; Novartis, Irl.; Novartis, Israel; Novartis, Ital.; Novartis, Malaysia; Novartis, Mex.; Novartis, Neth.; Novartis, Norw.; Novartis, NZ; Novartis, Port.; Novartis, S.Afr.; Novartis, Singapore†; Novartis, Spain; Novartis, Swed.; Novartis, Switz.; Novartis, Thai.; Novartis, UK; Novartis, USA.
Disodium pamidronate (p.773·3).
*Hypercalcaemia of malignancy; osteolytic lesions and bone pain in multiple myeloma and in bone metastases associated with breast cancer; Paget's disease of bone.*

**Aredronet** Sun, India.
Disodium pamidronate (p.773·3).
*Hypercalcaemia of malignancy; osteolytic lesions and bone pain in multiple myeloma and in bone metastases associated with breast cancer; Paget's disease of bone.*

**Arelcant** Boehringer Ingelheim, Austria.
Fenoterol hydrobromide (p.785·2); ipratropium bromide (p.787·1).
*Obstructive airways disease.*

**Arelix**
Aventis, Austria; Aventis, Braz.; Aventis, Ger.; Aventis, Irl.; Sanofi Synthelabo, S.Afr.; Aventis, Switz.
Piretanide (p.983·3) or piretanide sodium (p.983·3).
*Forced diuresis; heart failure; hypertension; oedema; renal failure.*

**Arelix ACE** Aventis, Ger.
Piretanide (p.983·3); ramipril (p.994·1).
*Hypertension.*

**Arem** Aspen, S.Afr.
Nitrazepam (p.710·1).
*Insomnia.*

**Aremin** Boniscontro & Gazzone, Ital.
Suleparoid (p.1009·1).
*Soft-tissue injury; thromboembolic disorders.*

**Aremis** Esteve, Spain.
Sertraline hydrochloride (p.317·2).
*Depression; obsessive-compulsive disorder; panic attacks.*

**Arendal**
Armstrong, Arg.; Pharma Investi, Chile.
Alendronate sodium (p.765·3).
*Osteoporosis.*

**Arestal**
Janssen-Cilag, Austria†; Janssen-Cilag, Fr.; Norgine, Neth.
Loperamide oxide (p.1271·1).
*Diarrhoea.*

**Arestin** OraPharma, USA.
Minocycline hydrochloride (p.231·3).
*Periodontitis.*

**Aretensin** Takeda, Ger.
Ramipril (p.994·1); piretanide (p.983·3).
*Hypertension.*

**Areuma** Ecobi, Ital.
Nimesulide (p.67·1).
*Fever; inflammation; pain.*

**Areuzolin** Areu, Spain.
Cefazolin sodium (p.170·3).
*Bacterial infections.*

**Arfarel** Pharmanik (Φαρμανικ), Gr.
Clindamycin phosphate (p.194·2).
*Acne.*

**Arfen**
Note. This name is used for preparations of different composition.
Medochemie, Hong Kong; Medochemie, Malaysia.
Paracetamol (p.76·2).
*Fever; pain.*

Lisapharma, Ital.
Ibuprofen lysine (p.46·3).
*Gynaecological inflammatory disorders; musculoskeletal and joint disorders; radiculitis.*

Medinfar, Port.
Ibuprofen (p.45·3).
*Fever; inflammation; musculoskeletal, joint, peri-articular, and soft-tissue disorders; pain.*

**Arfen Plus** Medochemie, Hong Kong.
Paracetamol (p.76·2); caffeine (p.782·1).
*Fever; pain.*

**Arfloxina** Arlex, Mex.†.
Ciprofloxacin (p.188·2).
*Bacterial infections.*

**Arflur** FDC, India.
Flurbiprofen (p.43·3).
*Musculoskeletal and joint disorders; pain.*

**Argatroban** SmithKline Beecham, USA.
Argatroban (p.864·3).
*Heparin-induced thrombocytopenia.*

**Argeal** Ducray, Fr.
Kaolin (p.1268·3); saw palmetto (p.1569·1).
*Seborrhoeic dermatitis.*

**Argeflox** Bristol-Myers Squibb, Arg.
Ciprofloxacin hydrochloride (p.188·2).
*Bacterial infections.*

**Argenpal**
Braun, Port.; Braun, Spain.
Silver nitrate (p.1746·1).
*Aphthous ulcers; skin disorders; verrucas; wounds.*

**Argent** Katadyn, Switz.
Heavy kaolin (p.1268·3); silver (p.1746·1).
*Burns; wounds.*

**Argental** Liferpal, Mex.
Sulfadiazine silver (p.259·1).
*Infected skin disorders.*

**Argent-Eze** Lennon, S.Afr.†.
Sulfadiazine silver (p.259·1).
*Burns.*

**Argentocromo** Bucca, Spain.
Merbromin (p.1185·3); silver (p.1746·1).
*Gingivitis; mouth infection.*

**Argentofenol** Bucca, Spain.
Phenol (p.1188·1); methylthioninium chloride (p.1042·2); silver nitrate (p.1746·1).
*Aphthous stomatitis; oral bleeding; tonsillitis.*

**Argentum Med Complex** Dynamit, Austria.
Homoeopathic preparation.

**Argesic** Econo Med, USA.
Methyl salicylate (p.59·3).
*Muscle, joint, and soft-tissue pain; neuralgia.*

**Argesic-SA** Econo Med, USA.
Salsalate (p.88·1).
*Fever; inflammation; pain.*

**Argicilline** Monot, Fr.†.
Gramicidin (p.220·2).
*Nose and throat infections.*

**Argidam** Terapeutico, Ital.
L-arginine; damiana; muira puama; zinc gluconate; vitamin E (p.1417·1).
*Nutritional supplement.*

**Argiletz** Argiletz, Fr.
Nutritional supplement (p.1417·1).

**Argin** Volchem, Ital.
Protein supplement (p.1417·1).
*Arginine deficiency.*

**Arginaid Extra** Novartis Nutrition, USA.
Preparation for enteral nutrition (p.1417·1).

**Arginotri-B**
Bouchara-Recordati, Fr.
Arginine hydrochloride (p.1421·1); thiamine hydrochloride; pyridoxine hydrochloride (p.1417·1).
*Tonic.*

Bouchara, Switz.
Arginine hydrochloride (p.1421·1); vitamin B substances (p.1417·1).
*Pain; vitamin B deficiency.*

**Argirofedrina** Vaillant, Ital.
Ephedrine sulfate (p.1120·1); anhydrous sodium sulfate (p.1290·1); mild silver protein (p.1746·2).
*Nasal congestion.*

**Argirol** Allergan, Braz.
Mild silver protein (p.1746·2).
*Eye infections.*

**Argisone** Teofarma, Ital.
Hydrocortisone acetate (p.1103·3); mild silver protein (p.1746·2).
*Bacterial eye infections.*

**Argital** ISA, Arg.
Multivitamin and mineral preparation (p.1417·1).

**Argivit** Aesculapius, Ital.
Amino-acid, vitamin, and mineral preparation (p.1417·1).
*Nutritional supplement.*

**Argocian** Biol, Arg.
Hexoprenaline sulfate (p.786·3).
*Premature labour.*

**Argotone** Merck, Ital.
Ephedrine hydrochloride (p.1120·1); mild silver protein (p.1746·2).
*Nasal congestion.*

**Argun** Merckle, Ger.
Lonazolac calcium (p.54·2).
*Inflammation; musculoskeletal, joint, and soft-tissue disorders; pain.*

**Argyrophedrine**
Merck, Belg.
Ephedrine levulinate (p.1120·3); mild silver protein (p.1746·2).
*Respiratory-tract congestion.*

Sanofi Synthelabo, Braz.†.
Ephedrine sulfate (p.1120·1); mild silver protein (p.1746·2).
*Nasal congestion.*

**Arhemapectine Antihemorragique** Aerocid, Fr.
Pectin (p.1580·3).
*Haemorrhage.*

**Aria** Lichtwer, UK.
Soya isoflavones; calcium; folic acid; B vitamins; selenium (p.1417·1).
*Nutritional supplement.*

**Arial** Dompe, Ital.
Salmeterol xinafoate (p.795·1).
*Obstructive airways disease.*

**Arianna** Schering, Ital.
Gestodene (p.1556·1); ethinylestradiol (p.1553·2).
*Combined oral contraceptive.*

**Aricept**
Pfizer, Austral.; Pfizer, Austria; Pfizer, Belg.; Pfizer, Canad.; Pfizer, Denm.; Pfizer, Fin.; Eisai, Fr.; Eisai, Ger.; Pfizer, Ger.; Pfizer, Gr.; Eisai, Hong Kong; Pfizer, Irl.; Pfizer, Israel; Pfizer, Ital.; Eisai, Jpn; Eisai, Malaysia; Pfizer, Norw.; Pfizer, NZ; Pfizer, Port.; Pfizer, S.Afr.; Eisai, Singapore; Pfizer, Spain; Pfizer, Swed.; Pfizer, Switz.; Eisai, Thai.; Pfizer, UK; Eisai, USA; Pfizer, USA.
Donepezil hydrochloride (p.1489·2).
*Alzheimer's disease.*

**Aricodiltosse** Menarini, Ital.
Dextromethorphan hydrobromide (p.1117·3).
*Coughs.*

**Aridil** CP Pharmaceuticals, UK.
Furosemide (p.919·3); amiloride hydrochloride (p.858·2).
These ingredients can be described by the British Approved Name Co-amilofruse.
*Ascites; oedema.*

**Arifenicol** Ariston, Braz.
Chloramphenicol (p.185·1).
*Bacterial infections.*

**Arilin**
Wolff, Ger.; Medika, Switz.
Metronidazole (p.607·2).
*Anaerobic bacterial infections; protozoal infections.*

**Ariline** Montavit, Austria.
Metronidazole (p.607·2).
*Anaerobic bacterial infections; protozoal infections.*

**Arilvax**
Evans, Fin.; Evans, Irl.; Evans Medical, Israel; Evans, Neth.; Medpro, S.Afr.; Celltech, Singapore; SBL, Swed.; Medeva, Switz.; Chiron Vaccines, UK.
A yellow fever vaccine (17D strain) (p.1644·2).
*Active immunisation.*

**Arima** Alphapharm, Austral.
Moclobemide (p.308·2).
*Depression.*

**Arimidex**
AstraZeneca, Arg.; AstraZeneca, Austral.; AstraZeneca, Austria; AstraZeneca, Belg.; AstraZeneca, Braz.; AstraZeneca, Canad.; AstraZeneca, Chile; AstraZeneca, Denm.; AstraZeneca, Fin.; AstraZeneca, Fr.; AstraZeneca, Ger.; Astra-Zeneca, Gr.; AstraZeneca, Hong Kong; AstraZeneca, Irl.; Zeneca, Israel; AstraZeneca, Ital.; AstraZeneca, Malaysia; Zeneca, Mex.; AstraZeneca, Neth.; AstraZeneca, Norw.; AstraZeneca, NZ; AstraZeneca, Port.; AstraZeneca, S.Afr.; AstraZeneca, Singapore; AstraZeneca, Spain; AstraZeneca, Swed.; AstraZeneca, Switz.; AstraZeneca, Thai.; AstraZeneca, UK; AstraZeneca, USA.
Anastrozole (p.528·1).
*Breast cancer.*

**Aripax** Erfar, Gr.
Lorazepam (p.704·1).
*Anxiety disorders; insomnia; status epilepticus.*

**Aristaloe** Neo Dermos, Arg.
Aloe vera (p.1141·3); elastin.

**Aristamed** Nordmark, Thai.
Sulfisomidine (p.264·1).
*Bacterial skin infections.*

**Aristin-C** Anpharm (Ανφαρμ), Gr.
Ciprofloxacin (p.188·2) or ciprofloxacin hydrochloride (p.188·2).
*Bacterial infections.*

**Aristo** Steiner, Ger.
Hypericum (p.299·1).
*Depression.*

**Aristo L** Steiner, Ger.†.
Aloes (p.1248·2).
*Constipation.*

**Aristochol**
Note. This name is used for preparations of different composition.
Linobion, Austria†.
Greater celandine (p.1695·3); Javanese turmeric (p.1759·3); silybum marianum (p.1043·3); aloes (p.1248·2); pancreatin (p.1725·3).

Steiner, Ger.
Greater celandine (p.1695·3); cape aloe (p.1248·2).
*Constipation.*

**Aristochol CC** *Steiner, Ger.*
Greater celandine (p.1695·3); turmeric (p.1058·3).
*Gastrointestinal spasm.*

**Aristochol N** *Steiner, Ger.*
Greater celandine (p.1695·3); achillea (p.1646·2); taraxacum (p.1751·3); gnaphalii flowers; absinthium (p.1645·1).
*Biliary disorders.*

**Aristocor** *Kwizda, Austria.*
Flecainide acetate (p.916·2).
*Arrhythmias.*

**Aristocort**
*Sigma, Austral.; Stiefel, Canad.; Lederle, Hong Kong; Sigma, NZ; Wyeth-Ayerst, Thai.; Fujisawa, USA.*
Triamcinolone (p.1110·2), triamcinolone acetonide (p.1110·2), or triamcinolone diacetate (p.1110·2).
*Corticosteroid.*

**Aristoforat** *Steiner, Ger.*
Hypericum (p.299·1).
*Depression.*

**Aristogyl** *Aristo, India.*
Metronidazole (p.607·2) or metronidazole benzoate (p.607·2).
*Amoebiasis; giardiasis.*

**Aristomycin** *Pharmanik (Φαρμανικ), Gr.*
Roxithromycin (p.254·2).
*Bacterial infections.*

**Aristopramida** *Ariston, Braz.*
Metoclopramide (p.1274·3).
*Nausea and vomiting.*

**Aristospan**
*Stiefel, Canad.; Fujisawa, USA.*
Triamcinolone hexacetonide (p.1110·2).
*Corticosteroid.*

**Aritmina** *Solvay, Ital.†.*
Ajmaline (p.856·1).
*Arrhythmias.*

**Arixtra**
*Sanofi Synthelabo, Austral.; Sanofi Synthelabo, Fr.; Sanofi Synthelabo, Hong Kong; Sanofi Synthelabo, NZ; Sanofi Synthelabo, Port.; Sanofi Synthelabo, Spain; Sanofi Synthelabo, Switz.; Sanofi Synthelabo, UK; Organon, USA; Sanofi Synthelabo, USA.*
Fondaparinux sodium (p.918·3).
*Thromboembolism prophylaxis following orthopaedic surgery.*

**Arkamin** *Unichem, India.*
Clonidine hydrochloride (p.885·2).
*Hypertension.*

**Arkamin-H** *Unichem, India.*
Clonidine hydrochloride (p.885·2); hydrochlorothiazide (p.933·2).
*Hypertension.*

**Arkocaps** *Arkopharma, Switz.*
Frangula bark (p.1266·3).
*Constipation.*

**Arkocapsulas Carbon Veg** *Arkochim, Spain.*
Activated charcoal (p.1030·2).
*Diarrhoea.*

**Arkocapsulas Hiperico** *Arkochim, Spain.*
Hypericum (p.299·1).
*Tonic.*

**Arkogelules** *Arkopharma, Fr.*
A range of herbal preparations.

**Arkonsol** *Romilo, Canad.†.*
Benzalkonium chloride (p.1168·3).

**Arkonutril MM** *Arkopharma, Fr.†.*
Preparation for enteral nutrition (p.1417·1).

**Arkophytum** *Arkopharma, Fr.*
Devil's claw root (p.28·2); black currant (p.1661·1); salix (p.87·3).
*Painful joint disorders.*

**Arkotonic** *Arkopharma, Fr.†.*
Pollen; carnitine (p.1423·3); vitamin E (p.1464·3); ascorbic acid (p.1460·2); royal jelly (p.1740·3); soya lecithin (p.1706·1).
*Tonic.*

**Arkovital** *Arkopharma, Fr.†.*
A range of vitamin, mineral, and trace element supplements (p.1417·1).

**Arkovital C** *Arkopharma, Fr.†.*
Ascorbic acid (p.1460·2).
*Cold symptoms; tonic; vitamin C deficiency.*

**Arlette 28** *Osteolab, Chile.*
Desogestrel (p.1547·2).
*Progestogen-only oral contraceptive.*

**Arlevert** *Hennig, Ger.*
Cinnarizine (p.428·3); dimenhydrinate (p.431·1).
*Vertigo.*

**Arlexicam** *Arlex, Mex.†.*
Piroxicam (p.84·2).

**Arlidin**
*Aventis, Canad.; USV, India; Grossman, Mex.*
Buphenine hydrochloride (p.1663·2).
*Cerebral and peripheral vascular disorders.*

**Arlitene** *Asta Medica, Ital.†.*
Moxisylyte hydrochloride (p.962·2).
*Cardiovascular disorders.*

**ARM** *Ascher, USA†.*
Phenylpropanolamine hydrochloride (p.1127·3); chlorphenamine maleate(p.427·3).
*Upper respiratory-tract symptoms.*

**Armaya** *Centrum, Spain.*
Polypodium leucotomos.
*Eczema; psoriasis.*

**Armil** *Squibb, Spain.*
Benzalkonium chloride (p.1168·3).
*Skin and mucous membrane disinfection.*

**Arminol** *Krewel, Ger.*
Sulpiride (p.722·2).
*Depression; schizophrenia; vestibular disorders.*

**Armocur** *Agis, Israel.*
Cyproterone acetate (p.1544·1).
*Prostatic cancer; sexual disorders.*

**Armoglobulina** *Aventis Behring, Braz.*
A normal immunoglobulin (p.1627·2).
*Hypogammaglobulinaemia; idiopathic thrombocytopenic purpura; passive immunisation.*

**Armonil**
*Note. This name is used for preparations of different composition.*
*Elvetium, Arg.*
Tilia (p.1756·2); passion flower (p.1729·1); valerian (p.1762·2).
*Insomnia.*

*Recordati, Ital.*
Estradiol (p.1550·1).
*Menopausal disorders; osteoporosis.*

**Armonyl** *Maver, Chile.*
Valerian (p.1762·2); passiion flower (p.1729·1); crataegus (p.1677·1).
*Insomnia.*

**Arnecrem** *Casasco, Arg.*
Permethrin (p.1508·3); benzyl benzoate (p.1500·2); benzocaine (p.1370·3).
*Pediculosis.*

**Arnela** *Andromaco, Chile.*
Clotrimazole (p.396·2).
*Fungal skin and nail infections.*

**Arnica Comp**
*DHU, Ger.*
Homoeopathic preparation.

*Bio-Pharmaceuticals, Malaysia.*
Arnica (p.1656·3); calendula (p.1665·2).
*Minor wounds; soft-tissue disorders.*

**Arnica comp/Apis Salbe** *Weleda, Ger.*
Homoeopathic preparation.

**Arnica Hamamelis Compuesta** *Knop, Chile.*
Homoeopathic preparation.

**Arnica Kneipp Salbe** *Kneipp, Ger.†.*
Arnica oil (p.1656·3); heparin (p.927·3).
*Peripheral vascular disorders; skin trauma.*

**Arnica Komplex** *Richter, Austria.*
Homoeopathic preparation.

**Arnica Massage Balm** *Weleda, UK.*
Arnica flower oil; birch leaf oil (p.60·1); lavender oil (p.1705·2); rosemary oil (p.1740·2).
*Rheumatic and muscular pain.*

**Arnica Med Complex** *Dynamit, Austria.*
Homoeopathic preparation.

**Arnica Oligoplex** *Madaus, Ger.*
Homoeopathic preparation.

**Arnica Plus** *Homeocan, Canad.*
Homoeopathic preparation.

**Arnicadol** *Phytomedica, Fr.*
Arnica (p.1656·3); menthol (p.1711·3).
*Soft-tissue injury.*

**Arnicaid** *Hylands, Canad.*
Homoeopathic preparation.

**Arnicalm** *Boiron, Canad.*
Homoeopathic preparation.

**Arnica-loges** *Loges, Ger.†.*
Arnica (p.1656·3).
*Boils; insect bites; musculoskeletal, joint, and soft-tissue disorders; superficial phlebitis.*

**Arnican** *Cooperation Pharmaceutique, Fr.*
Arnica (p.1656·3).
*Soft-tissue disorders.*

**Arnicet** *Metochem, Austria.*
Arnica (p.1656·3); hamamelis (p.1696·3).
*Muscle pain; skin irritation; soft-tissue disorders.*

**Arnicon** *Pan Quimica, Spain.*
Arnica (p.1656·3); methyl salicylate (p.59·3); menthol (p.1711·3).
*Musculoskeletal and joint pain.*

**Arniflor** *VSM, Neth.†.*
Arnica (p.1656·3).
*Bruising; haematoma; muscle pain; sprain.*

**Arniflor-N** *Spitzner, Ger.†; Schwabe, Ger.†.*
Arnica (p.1656·3).
*Boils; insect bites; musculoskeletal and joint disorders; superficial phlebitis; wounds.*

**Arnigel**
*Note. This name is used for preparations of different composition.*
*Boiron, Fr.*
Homoeopathic preparation.

*Boiron, Port.*
Arnica (p.1656·3).
*Muscle pain; soft-tissue injuries.*

**Arnika plus** *Ratiopharm, Ger.†.*
Arnica (p.1656·3); heparin sodium (p.928·1); aesculus (p.1648·2).
*Soft-tissue injury; venous disorders.*

**Arnikaderm** *Knop, Chile.*
Arnica (p.1656·3).
*Inflammation; oedema.*

**Arnikamill** *Biomo, Ger.*
Chamomile (p.1669·3); arnica flowers (p.1656·3).
*Haemorrhoids; skin disorders; soft-tissue inflammation; wounds.*

**Arnikatinktur** *Hetterich, Ger.*
Arnica (p.1656·3).
*Inflammation; musculoskeletal, joint, and soft-tissue disorders.*

**Arnileve** *Nelson, UK.*
Arnica (p.1656·3); hypericum (p.299·1); rue (p.1741·1); comfrey (p.1675·2).
*Musculoskeletal and soft-tissue disorders.*

**Arnilose** *AJC, Fr.†.*
Arginine hydrochloride (p.1421·1); ornithine hydrochloride (p.1442·3); sorbitol (p.1446·3); fructose (p.1431·3).
*Dyspepsia.*

**Arobon**
*Sanova, Austria; Nestle, Ital.; Nestle, Norw.†.*
Ceratonia (p.1579·1).
*Diarrhoea.*

**Arocin** *Modern Health Products, UK†.*
Betacarotene (p.1422·3).

**Arofexx** *Neopharmed, Ital.*
Rofecoxib (p.86·3).
*Osteoarthritis; rheumatoid arthritis.*

**Arola Rosebalm** *Pharmaceutical Enterprises, S.Afr.*
Bismuth subnitrate (p.1252·2); dimethicone (p.1482·1); allantoin (p.1141·3); zinc oxide (p.1163·2).
*Skin disorders.*

**Arolac** *IPRAD, Fr.*
Lisuride maleate (p.1210·3).
*Hyperprolactinaemia; lactation inhibition.*

**Aroltex** *Kampel Martian, Arg.*
Pergolide (p.1211·3).
*Parkinsonism.*

**Aromabyl** *Plantes et Medecines, Fr.†.*
Cynara (p.1678·3); lappa (p.1704·3); cascara (p.1255·1); juglans regia; sodium salicylate (p.90·1); sodium arsenate (p.1747·1); boldo (p.1661·2).
*Constipation; dyspepsia.*

**Aromacin** *Pharmacia-Upjohn, Gr.*
Exemestane (p.552·3).
*Breast cancer.*

**Aromasil** *Pharmacia, Spain.*
Exemestane (p.552·3).
*Breast cancer.*

**Aromasin**
*Pharmacia, Arg.; Pharmacia, Austral.; Pharmacia, Austria; Pharmacia, Belg.; Pharmacia, Braz.; Pharmacia, Canad.; Pharmacia, Chile; Pharmacia, Denm.; Pharmacia, Fin.; Pharmacia, Ger.; Pharmacia, Hong Kong; Pharmacia, Irl.; Pharmacia Upjohn, Israel; Pharmacia Upjohn, Ital.; Pharmacia, Neth.; Pharmacia, Norw.; Pharmacia, Port.; Pharmacia, Singapore; Pharmacia, Swed.; Pharmacia, Switz.; Pharmacia, Thai.; Pharmacia, UK; Pharmacia Upjohn, USA.*
Exemestane (p.552·3).
*Breast cancer.*

**Aromasine** *Pharmacia, Fr.*
Exemestane (p.552·3).
*Breast cancer.*

**Aromasol** *Dolisos, Fr.*
Clove oil (p.1673·3); peppermint oil (p.1283·2); pine oil; lavender oil (p.1705·2); cinnamon oil (p.1672·2); rosemary oil (p.1740·2); wild thyme oil.
*Respiratory-tract congestion.*

**Aronal Forte** *Teva, Israel.*
Vitamin A (p.1451·2); guaiazulene (p.1696·2); aluminium lactate (p.1653·1); aldioxa (p.1141·2).
*Sensitive gums; toothpaste.*

**Aropax**
*GlaxoSmithKline, Arg.; GlaxoSmithKline, Austral.; GlaxoSmithKline, Belg.; GlaxoSmithKline, Braz.; Novartis, Mex.; GlaxoSmithKline, NZ; GlaxoSmithKline, S.Afr.*
Paroxetine hydrochloride (p.311·2).
*Depression; generalised anxiety disorder; obsessive-compulsive disorder; panic disorders; post-traumatic stress disorder; social phobia.*

**Aroselin** *Leovan, Gr.*
Nitrendipine (p.973·3).
*Hypertension.*

**Arovit**
*Roche, Arg.; Roche, Braz.; Bio-Sante, Canad.; Roche Nicholas, Fr.; Roche, Ital.; Roche Consumer, S.Afr.; Roche, Swed.; Roche, Switz.*
Vitamin A acetate (p.1453·1) or vitamin A palmitate (p.1453·1).
*Keratinisation disorders; vitamin A deficiency.*

**Aroxat** *GlaxoSmithKline, Chile.*
Paroxetine hydrochloride (p.311·2).
*Depression; obsessive-compulsive disorder; panic attacks; social phobia.*

**Aroxin**
*DHA, Hong Kong; DHA, Singapore.*
Amoxicillin trihydrate (p.155·3).
*Bacterial infections.*

**Arpamyl LP** *GNR, Fr.†.*
Verapamil hydrochloride (p.1019·1).
*Hypertension.*

**Arpha** *Urgo, Fr.†.*
Paracetamol (p.76·2); chlorphenamine maleate (p.427·3).
*Cold symptoms.*

**Arpha Hustensirup** *Urgo, Ger.*
Dextromethorphan hydrobromide (p.1117·3).
*Coughs.*

**Arphos** *Fournier, Fr.*
Calcium glycerophosphate; magnesium gluconate (p.1417·1).
Formerly contained cyanocobalamin, phosphoric acid, and calcium gluceptate.
*Tonic.*

**Arpicolin** *Rosemont, UK.*
Procyclidine hydrochloride (p.488·2).
*Drug-induced extrapyramidal disorders; parkinsonism.*

**Arpilon** *Enzypharm, Austria.*
Pipecuronium bromide (p.1405·2).
*Competitive neuromuscular blocker.*

**Arpimycin** *Rosemont, UK†.*
Erythromycin ethyl succinate (p.208·1).
*Bacterial infections.*

**Arrestin** *Vortech, USA†.*
Trimethobenzamide hydrochloride (p.442·2).
*Nausea and vomiting.*

**Arret**
*Janssen-Cilag, Irl.; Johnson & Johnson MSD Consumer, UK.*
Loperamide hydrochloride (p.1271·1).
*Diarrhoea.*

**Arretin** *ICN, Mex.*
Tretinoin (p.1161·1).
*Acne.*

**Arritlan** *QIF, Braz.†.*
Endralazine mesilate (p.910·3).
*Hypertension.*

**Arrumalon** *Sidus, Arg.*
Glycosaminoglycans; peptides; cartilage; bone marrow.
*Osteoarthritis.*

**Arsacol** *Zambon, Fr.†.*
Ursodeoxycholic acid (p.1760·3).
*Gallstones.*

**Arscolloid** *SIT, Ital.*
Dichlorobenzyl alcohol (p.1178·3); silver protein (p.1746·2).
*Oral disinfection.*

**Arsiquinoforme** *Synthelabo, Fr.†.*
Quinine acetarsolate (p.462·1); quinine formate (p.462·1).
*Malaria.*

**Art**
*Negma, Fr.; Negma, Israel.*
Diacerein (p.30·1).
*Osteoarthritis.*

**Artagen**
*Ranbaxy, India; Ranbaxy, Thai.†.*
Naproxen (p.65·1).
*Gout; musculoskeletal, joint, and soft-tissue disorders; pain.*

**Artal** *Pharmia, Fin.*
Pentoxifylline (p.979·3).
*Peripheral and cerebral vascular disorders; vascular eye disorders.*

**Artamin**
*Biochemie, Austria; Biochemie, Malaysia; Biochemie, Singapore†.*
Penicillamine (p.1046·3).
*Benign hyperglobulinaemic purpura; chronic active hepatitis; cystinosis; cystinuria; heavy metal poisoning; primary biliary cirrhosis; rheumatoid arthritis; scleroderma; Wilson's disease.*

**Artandyl** *Synco, Hong Kong.*
Trihexyphenidyl hydrochloride (p.490·2).
*Drug-induced extrapyramidal disorders; parkinsonism.*

**Artane**
*Wyeth, Arg.; Wyeth, Austral.; Wyeth Lederle, Austria; Wyeth Lederle, Belg.; Wyeth, Braz.; Wyeth-Ayerst, Canad.†; Wyeth, Chile; Wyeth Lederle, Fin.†; Aventis, Fr.; Wyeth, Ger.; Wyeth, Gr.; Wyeth, Hong Kong; Wyeth, Irl.; Lederle, Israel; Wyeth Lederle, Ital.; Wyeth, Mex.; Teofarma, Neth.; Teofarma, Port.; Wyeth, S.Afr.†; Teofarma, Spain; Lederle, Switz.†; Wyeth-Ayerst, Thai.; Lederle, USA†.*
Trihexyphenidyl hydrochloride (p.490·2).
*Drug-induced extrapyramidal disorders; parkinsonism.*

**Artaxan** *Malesci, Ital.*
Nabumetone (p.63·3).
*Musculoskeletal, joint, peri-articular, and soft-tissue disorders.*

**Arte Rautin forte S** *Maurer, Ger.†.*
Rauwolfia serpentina (p.994·3).
Formerly contained rauwolfia serpentina, olive leaf, crataegus, mistletoe, juniper, valerian, rutoside, and etofylline.
*Anxiety disorders; hypertension.*

**Artedin** *GD, Ital.*
Garlic; ginkgo biloba; vitamin C; vitamin E (p.1417·1).
*Nutritional supplement.*

**Artelac**
*Bausch & Lomb, Arg.; Riel, Austria; Tramedico, Belg.; Bausch & Lomb, Braz.; Santen, Fin.; Chauvin, Fr.; Mann, Ger.; Mann, Irl.; Santen, Norw.; Lepori, Port.; Santen, Swed.; Pharma-Global, UK.*
Hypromellose (p.1579·3).
*Dry eyes.*

**Arteolol** *Lacer, Spain.*
Carteolol hydrochloride (p.880·3).
*Angina pectoris; arrhythmias; hypertension.*

**Arteopilo** *Bausch & Lomb, Switz.*
Carteolol hydrochloride (p.880·3); pilocarpine hydrochloride (p.1495·1).
*Glaucoma; ocular hypertension.*

**Arteoptic**
*Novartis, Denm.; Novartis, Fin.; Novartis Ophthalmics, Ger.; Otsuka, Hong Kong; OM, Port.; Novartis Ophthalmics, Swed.; Bausch & Lomb, Switz.; Otsuka, Thai.*
Carteolol hydrochloride (p.880·3).
*Glaucoma; ocular hypertension.*

**Arterase** *Clement Thionville, Fr.*
Equisetum (p.1684·1); garlic (p.1691·1); cupressus sempervirens; aesculus (p.1648·2).
*Capillary fragility; venous insufficiency.*

**Arterenol** *Aventis, Ger.*
Noradrenaline hydrochloride (p.975·1).
*Shock.*

**Artergin** *Orion, Fin.*
Co-dergocrine mesilate (p.1674·1).
*Mental function disorders in the elderly.*

**Arteria-cyl Ho-Len-Complex** *Liebermann, Ger.*
Homoeopathic preparation.

**Arteriobrate** *Farma Lepori, Spain†.*
Aluminium clofibrate (p.884·3); vincamine (p.1764·2).
*Exudative diabetic retinopathy; hyperlipidaemias.*

**Arterioflexin** *Lannacher, Austria.*
Clofibrate (p.884·3).
*Hyperlipidaemias.*

**Arteriol** *Gador, Arg.*
Buflomedil (p.877·2).
*Cerebral and peripheral vascular disorders; Raynaud's syndrome.*

**Arteriovinca**
*Lepori, Port.; Farma Lepori, Spain.*
Vincamine (p.1764·2).
*Cerebral trauma; cerebrovascular disorders; circulatory disorders of the eye, ear, nose, and throat; vestibular disorders.*

**Arterium** *Llorens, Spain†.*
Nicofibrate hydrochloride (p.965·3).
*Hyperlipidaemias.*

**Arterodiet** *Yves Ponroy, Fr.*
Fish oil (p.1417·1).
*Nutritional supplement.*

**Arterosan** *Royal, Chile.*
Simvastatin (p.997·1).
*Hypercholesterolaemia.*

**Arterosan Plus** *Mavena, Switz.*
Crataegus (p.1677·1); melissa (p.1711·1); garlic oil (p.1691·2); ginkgo biloba (p.1692·3).
*Cerebrovascular disorders.*

**Arte-Rutin C** *Maurer, Ger.†.*
Crataegus (p.1677·1).
Formerly contained rutoside, crataegus, olive leaf, valerian, lupulus, and mistletoe.
*Heart failure.*

**Artesol** *Drugtech, Chile.*
Cilostazol (p.884·1).

**Arteven** *Boehringer Ingelheim, Ital.*
Suleparoid (p.1009·1).
*Thrombosis prophylaxis.*

**Artevil** *Drugtech, Chile.*
Clopidogrel (p.888·3).

**Artex**
*Servier, Belg.†; Therval, Fr.; Servier, Neth.; Servier, Port.*
Tertatolol hydrochloride (p.1011·1).
*Hypertension.*

**Artexal**
*Servier, Braz.†; Servier, Denm.; Servier, Irl.*
Tertatolol hydrochloride (p.1011·1).
*Hypertension.*

**Artflex** *Elvetium, Arg.*
Sodium hyaluronate (p.1697·3).
*Osteoarthritis of the knee; shoulder pain.*

**Arth-A Oligocan** *Homeocan, Canad.*
Homoeopathic preparation.

**Artha-G** *Williams, USA.*
Salsalate (p.88·1).
*Fever; inflammation; pain.*

**Arthaxan** *SmithKline Beecham, Ger.†.*
Nabumetone (p.63·3).
*Musculoskeletal and joint disorders.*

**Arth-B Oligocan** *Homeocan, Canad.*
Homoeopathic preparation.

**Arthotec** *Heumann, Ger.; Aventis, Ger.; Pharmacia, Ger.*
Diclofenac sodium (p.32·1).
Misoprostol (p.1519·2) is included in this preparation in an attempt to limit adverse effects on the gastrointestinal mucosa.
*Musculoskeletal and joint disorders.*

**Arthrabas** *Tosse, Ger.†.*
Chloroquine phosphate (p.448·2).
*Arthritis; lupus erythematosus.*

**Arthrease**
*DePuy, Ger.; Biotechnology, Israel; DePuy, UK.*
Sodium hyaluronate (p.1697·3).
*Osteoarthritis of the knee.*

**Arthrex** *BASF, Ger.†.*
Diclofenac sodium (p.32·1).
*Gout; inflammation; musculoskeletal, joint, and soft-tissue disorders; pain.*

**Arthrex Duo** *BASF, Ger.†.*
Diclofenac sodium (p.32·1).
*Gout; inflammation; musculoskeletal, joint, and soft-tissue disorders; pain.*

**Arthrexin**
*Alphapharm, Austral.; Alphapharm, Malaysia; Merck, Malaysia; Pacific, NZ; Aspen, S.Afr.*
Indometacin (p.47·3).
*Gout; inflammation; musculoskeletal, joint, peri-articular, and soft-tissue disorders; pain.*

**Arthribosan B 31** *Bock, Ger.†.*
Homoeopathic preparation.

**Arthricare Double Ice** *Del, USA; Commerce, USA.*
Menthol (p.1711·3); camphor (p.1665·3).
*Muscle and joint pain.*

**Arthricare Hand & Body** *Del, Canad.*
Capsaicin (p.24·2).

**Arthricare Odor Free**
*Del, Canad.; Del, USA; Commerce, USA.*
Menthol (p.1711·3); methyl nicotinate (p.59·2); capsaicin (p.24·2).
*Muscle and joint pain.*

**Arthricare Triple Medicated**
*Del, Canad.; Del, USA; Commerce, USA.*
Methyl salicylate (p.59·3); menthol (p.1711·3); methyl nicotinate (p.59·2).
*Muscle and joint pain.*

**Arthricare Ultra** *Del, Canad.*
Menthol (p.1711·3); capsaicin (p.24·2).

**Arthrifid S** *Fides, Ger.†.*
Homoeopathic preparation.

**Arthriforte** *Blackmores, Austral.†.*
Fish oil (p.976·2); eicosapentaenoic acid (p.976·2); vitamin A (p.1451·2); turmeric (p.1058·3); devil's claw root (p.28·2); celery seed oil (p.1669·1); vitamin E (p.1464·3).
*Arthritis; inflammation; rheumatism.*

**Arthrirub** *Slimax, Austral.*
Camphor (p.1665·3); eucalyptus (p.1686·1); methyl salicylate (p.59·3); menthol (p.1711·3); alisma plantago aquatica oil.
*Cold symptoms; hay fever; headache; musculoskeletal and joint disorders.*

**Arthrisan** *Planta, Canad.†.*
*Capsules:* Salix (p.87·3); juniper (p.1703·1).
*Oral drops:* Salix (p.87·3); juniper (p.1703·1); solidago canadensis (p.1748·3).
*Arthritis.*

**Arthriselect** *Dreluso, Ger.*
Homoeopathic preparation.

**Arthritic Pain** *Homeocan, Canad.*
Homoeopathic preparation.

**Arthritic Pain Herbal Formula I** *Vitelle, Austral.†.*
Celery (p.1669·1); juniper (p.1703·1); devil's claw root (p.28·2); salix alba (p.87·3).
*Arthritis; rheumatism.*

**Arthritic Pain L10** *Homeocan, Canad.*
Homoeopathic preparation.

**Arthritic Pain Relief** *Mentholatum, Canad.†.*
Capsaicin (p.24·2).

**Arthritis Foundation Pain Reliever** *McNeil Consumer, USA†.*
Aspirin (p.15·1).
*Fever; musculoskeletal and joint disorders; myocardial infarction; pain; transient ischaemic attacks.*

**Arthritis Hot Creme** *Thompson, USA.*
Methyl salicylate (p.59·3); menthol (p.1711·3).
*Muscle, joint, and soft-tissue pain; neuralgia.*

**Arthritis Pain Formula**
*Note. This name is used for preparations of different composition.*
*Hylands, Canad.*
Homoeopathic preparation.

*Whitehall, USA.*
Aspirin (p.15·1).
Aluminium hydroxide (p.1249·2) and magnesium hydroxide (p.1272·2) are included in this preparation in an attempt to limit adverse effects on the gastrointestinal mucosa.
*Arthritis; fever; pain.*

**Arthritis Pain Formula Aspirin Free** *Whitehall, USA.*
Paracetamol (p.76·2).
*Fever; pain.*

**Arthritis Relief** *Brauer, Austral.†.*
Homoeopathic preparation.

**Arthrixyl N** *Syxyl, Ger.*
Homoeopathic preparation.

**arthro akut** *Byk Tosse, Ger.; Byk Gulden, Ger.*
Lonazolac calcium (p.54·2).
*Inflammation; musculoskeletal and joint disorders; pain.*

**Arthrocine** *Merck Sharp & Dohme-Chibret, Fr.*
Sulindac (p.91·2).
*Musculoskeletal, joint, and peri-articular disorders.*

**Arthrodeformat P** *Ziethen, Ger.*
Pituitary extract (p.1110·1); rosemary oil (p.1740·2).
*Rheumatic disorders.*

**Arthrodestal N** *Krugmann, Ger.*
Glycol salicylate (p.44·3); camphor (p.1665·3); benzyl nicotinate (p.21·2).
*Musculoskeletal, joint, and soft-tissue disorders; neuralgia.*

**Arthrodont** *Veyron-Froment, Fr.*
Enoxolone (p.36·2).
*Gum disorders.*

**Arthrodynat N** *Ziethen, Ger.*
Urtica (p.1762·1).
*Rheumatic disorders.*

**Arthrodynat P** *Ziethen, Ger.*
Rosemary oil (p.1740·2); camphor (p.1665·3); hypericum oil (p.299·2).
*Rheumatic disorders.*

**Arthrofen** *Ashbourne, UK.*
Ibuprofen (p.45·3).
*Inflammation; musculoskeletal and joint disorders; pain.*

**Arthrokehlan A** *Sanum-Kehlbeck, Ger.*
Formoltoxoid from *Propionibacterium acnes* (p.540·2).
*Musculoskeletal and joint disorders.*

**Arthrokehlan U** *Sanum-Kehlbeck, Ger.*
Formol toxoid from Corynebacterium spp.
*Tonic.*

**Arthropan** *Purdue Frederick, USA.*
Choline salicylate (p.26·2).
*Fever; inflammation; pain.*

**Arthropas K** *Pascoe, Ger.†.*
Homoeopathic preparation.

**Arthrorell** *Sanorell, Ger.*
Homoeopathic preparation.

**Arthrose-Echtroplex** *Weber & Weber, Ger.*
Homoeopathic preparation.

**Arthrose-Gastreu R73** *Reckeweg, Ger.*
Homoeopathic preparation.

**Arthrosenex AR** *Riemser, Ger.*
Arnica (p.1656·3).
*Musculoskeletal and joint disorders.*

**Arthrosetten H** *Riemser, Ger.*
Devil's claw root (p.28·2).
*Musculoskeletal and joint disorders.*

**Arthrosin** *Ashbourne, UK†.*
Naproxen (p.65·1).
*Dysmenorrhoea; gout; musculoskeletal and joint disorders.*

**Arthrotabs** *Duopharm, Ger.*
Devil's claw root (p.28·2).
*Musculoskeletal and joint disorders.*

**Arthrotec**
*Pharmacia, Austral.; Sanova, Austria; Pharmacia, Belg.; Pharmacia, Canad.; Pharmacia, Denm.; Pharmacia, Fin.; Pharmacia, Hong Kong; Pharmacia, Irl.; Searle, Israel; Searle, Neth.; Pharmacia, Norw.; Pharmacia, Port.; Pharmacia, S.Afr.; Searle, Singapore†; Pharmacia, Swed.; Pharmacia, Switz.; Pharmacia, Thai.; Pharmacia, UK; Searle, USA.*
Diclofenac sodium (p.32·1).
Misoprostol (p.1519·2) is included in this preparation in an attempt to limit adverse effects on the gastrointestinal mucosa.
*Musculoskeletal and joint disorders.*

**Arthrotone** *Pharmadass, UK†.*
Devil's claw root (p.28·2); royal jelly (p.1740·3).

**Arthroxen** *CP Pharmaceuticals, UK.*
Naproxen (p.65·1).
*Musculoskeletal and joint disorders.*

**Arthrum H** *LCA, Fr.*
Sodium hyaluronate (p.1697·3).
*Joint disorders.*

**Arthryl** *Rottapharm, Fin.*
Glucosamine sulfate.
*Musculoskeletal and joint disorders.*

**Articaina C/E** *Inibsa, Spain.*
Articaine hydrochloride (p.1370·3).
Adrenaline acid tartrate (p.852·2) is included in this preparation as a vasoconstrictor to diminish absorption and localise the effect of the local anaesthetic.
*Local anaesthesia.*

**Articlox** *Unipharma, Gr.*
Hydroxocobalamin (p.1458·2).
*Megaloblastic anaemia; vitamin B12 deficiency.*

**Articolase** *SIRC, Singapore.*
Collagen (p.1674·3).
*Peri-articular disorders.*

**Articolase (w/glucosamine)** *SIRC, Singapore.*
Collagen (p.1674·3); glucosamine sulfate (p.1694·1).
*Joint disorders.*

**Articulan** *Tecnimede, Port.*
Etodolac (p.37·3).
*Musculoskeletal and joint disorders.*

**Articurell** *Sanorell, Ger.*
Homoeopathic preparation.

**Artifene** *Northia, Arg.*
Dextropropoxyphene (p.28·3); dipyrone (p.35·3).
*Pain.*

**Artificial Tears**
*Note. This name is used for preparations of different composition.*
*Rivex, Canad.*
Polyvinyl alcohol (p.1581·1).
*Dry eyes.*

*Bausch & Lomb, USA.*
Hypromellose (p.1579·3).
*Dry eyes.*

**Artiflam** *Tramedico, Belg.†.*
Tiaprofenic acid (p.93·3) or tiaprofenic acid, trometamol salt (p.94·1).
*Inflammation.*

**Artilog** *Pharmacia Upjohn, Ital.*
Celecoxib (p.25·2).
*Osteoarthritis; rheumatoid arthritis.*

**Artin** *Sanova, Austria.*
Aloes (p.1248·2); frangula bark (p.1266·3).
*Constipation; stool softener.*

**Artinizona** *Teuto, Braz.*
Prednisone (p.1109·3).
*Corticosteroid.*

**Artinor** *ICN, Mex.*
Piroxicam (p.84·2).
*Inflammation; pain.*

**Artischocke plus Legastol** *Twardy, Ger.†.*
Peppermint leaf (p.1283·2); cynara (p.1678·3); taraxacum (p.1751·3).
*Biliary disorders.*

**Artisial**
*Note. This name is used for preparations of different composition.*
*Jouveinal, Canad.†.*
Electrolyte preparation (p.1217·1).
*Saliva substitute.*

*Pfizer, Fr.; Cell Pharm, Ger.†.*
Electrolytes (p.1217·1); carmellose sodium (p.1577·3); sorbitol (p.1446·3).
*Saliva substitute.*

**Artistry** *Amway, Canad.*
*SPF 8:* Octinoxate (p.1154·3); oxybenzone (p.1154·3).
*Sunscreen.*

**Artocoron** *Abbott, Ger.*
Naftidrofuryl oxalate (p.964·1).
*Peripheral vascular disorders.*

**Artofen**
*Biogal, Israel; Democal, Switz.*
Ibuprofen (p.45·3).
*Musculoskeletal, joint, peri-articular, and soft-tissue disorders.*

**Artoid** *Artu, Neth.†.*
Pollen extracts(p.1650·1).
*Allergen immunotherapy.*

**Artok** *Nycomed, Austria.*
Lornoxicam (p.54·2).
*Musculoskeletal and joint disorders; pain.*

**Artonil** *Gea, Swed.*
Ranitidine hydrochloride (p.1285·2).
*Gastro-oesophageal reflux; peptic ulcer; Zollinger-Ellison syndrome.*

**Artosin**
*Boehringer Mannheim, Ger.†; Boehringer Mannheim, Neth.†.*
Tolbutamide (p.348·1).
*Diabetes mellitus.*

**Artotec** *Pharmacia, Fr.*
Diclofenac sodium (p.32·1).
Misoprostol (p.1519·2) is included in this preparation in an attempt to limit adverse effects on the gastrointestinal mucosa.
*Musculoskeletal and joint disorders.*

**Artoxan** *Herbaline, Ital.†.*
Devil's claw root (p.28·2); silver birch (p.1660·3); fraxinus excelsior; meadowsweet (p.1710·1).
*Musculoskeletal, joint, and peri-articular disorders; myalgia.*

**Artragel** *Interdelta, Switz.†.*
Glycol salicylate (p.44·3); benzyl nicotinate (p.21·2); camphor (p.1665·3); levomenthol (p.1711·3); turpentine oil (p.1760·1).
*Musculoskeletal and joint pain.*

**Artragil** *Faes, Spain.*
Piroxicam (p.84·2).
*Gout; musculoskeletal, joint, and peri-articular disorders; pain.*

**Artrait** *TRB, Arg.*
Methotrexate (p.568·2) or methotrexate sodium (p.568·3).
*Malignant neoplasms; psoriasis; rheumatoid arthritis.*

**Artren**
*Merck, Braz.; Merck, Chile.*
Diclofenac (p.32·1), diclofenac resinate (p.33·1), or diclofenac sodium (p.32·1).
*Fever; gout; inflammation; musculoskeletal, joint, peri-articular, and soft-tissue disorders; pain.*

**Artrenac** *Merck, Mex.*
Diclofenac sodium (p.32·1).
*Inflammation; musculoskeletal, joint and peri-articular disorders; pain.*

**Artrenac Pro** *Merck, Mex.*
Diclofenac sodium (p.32·1).
Misoprostol (p.1519·2) is included in this preparation in an attempt to limit adverse effects on the gastrointestinal mucosa.
*Osteoarthritis; rheumatoid arthritis.*

**Artrex**
*Note. This name is used for preparations of different composition.*
*Spedrog, Arg.*
Allopurinol (p.412·2); colchicine (p.415·1).
*Gout; hyperuricaemia.*

*AyurCore, Singapore.*
Withania somnifera; boswellia serrata (p.1690·1); turmeric (p.1058·3); ginger (p.1267·1).
*Musculoskeletal, joint, and soft-tissue disorders.*

**Artri** *Medical, Spain.*
Adenosine phosphate (p.1647·3); indometacin (p.47·3).
*Fever; inflammation; pain.*

**Artribid** *Merck Sharp & Dohme, Port.*
Sulindac (p.91·2).
*Gout; musculoskeletal, joint, and peri-articular disorders.*

**Artricam** *Pfizer, Braz.†.*
Ampiroxicam (p.14·2).

**Artriden** *Berman, Mex.*
Mefenamic acid (p.55·2).
*Inflammation; pain.*

**Artridol**
*Note. This name is used for preparations of different composition.*
*Laboratorios Chile, Chile.*
Glucosamine sulfate (p.1694·1).
*Degenerative joint disorders.*

*Rimsa, Mex.*
Indometacin (p.47·3); betamethasone (p.1093·1); methocarbamol (p.1395·1).
*Gout; musculoskeletal, joint, and peri-articular disorders.*

*Merck, Port.*
Hydroxymethoxy ethyl benzoate; phenylpropyl salicylate.
*Musculoskeletal, joint, peri-articular, and soft-tissue disorders.*

**Artril**
*Note. This name is used for preparations of different composition.*
*Farmasa, Braz.*
Ibuprofen (p.45·3).
*Fever; inflammation; pain.*

*Advance, Singapore.*
Glucosamine sulfate (p.1694·1).
*Osteoarthritis.*

**Artrilan** *Offenbach, Mex.*
Prednisolone (p.1108·1); salicylamide (p.87·3); meprobamate (p.706·2).
*Musculoskeletal and joint disorders.*

**Artrilase** *Bago, Arg.*
Glucosamine sulfate (p.1694·1).
*Musculoskeletal and joint disorders.*

**Artrinid** *Biolab Sanus, Braz.*
Ketoprofen (p.51·2).
*Gout; musculoskeletal, joint, and peri-articular disorders; pain.*

**Artrinovo** *Llorens, Spain.*
Indometacin (p.47·3).
*Gout; inflammation; musculoskeletal, joint, and peri-articular disorders; pain.*

**Artritol** *Bio-Sante, Canad.*
*Capsules:* Paracetamol (p.76·2).
*Cream:* Methyl salicylate (p.59·3); menthol (p.1711·3).

**Artriunic** *Novag, Spain.*
Tenoxicam (p.93·1).
*Gout; musculoskeletal, joint and peri-articular disorders.*

**Artrizona** *Silesia, Chile.*
Diacerein (p.30·1).
*Degenerative joint disorders.*

**Artrocaptin** *Estedi, Spain.*
Tolmetin sodium (p.94·2).
*Musculoskeletal, joint, and peri-articular disorders; pain.*

**Artrocur** *Wyeth Lederle, Ital.†.*
A heparinoid (p.931·1); aminopropylone (p.14·2).
*Muscle and joint pain.*

**Artrodar**
*TRB, Arg.; TRB, Braz.; Ecupharma, Ital.†.*
Diacerein (p.30·1).
*Osteoarthritis.*

**Artrodesmol Extra** *Reig Jofre, Spain.*
Dimethyl sulfoxide (p.1473·2); phenylbutazone (p.83·2); fluocinolone acetonide (p.1101·2); methyl salicylate (p.59·3).
*Peri-articular and soft-tissue disorders.*

**Artrodol** *AGIPS, Ital.*
Diflunisal (p.34·1).
*Musculoskeletal, joint, and soft-tissue disorders; pain.*

**Artrodue** *MDM, Ital.*
Collagen (p.1674·3); mucopolysaccharides; vitamins; copper (p.1417·1).
*Joint disorders.*

**Artrofenac** *SoSe, Ital.*
Diclofenac sodium (p.32·1).
*Musculoskeletal and joint disorders; painful smooth muscle spasm.*

**Artrofene** *Sankyo, Port.*
Ketoprofen lysine (p.51·3).
*Musculoskeletal, joint, peri-articular, and soft-tissue disorders; neuralgia.*

**Artroglobina** *Elvetium, Arg.*
Diacerein (p.30·1).
*Musculoskeletal and joint disorders.*

**Artrogota** *Teofarma, Spain†.*
Diethylamine salicylate (p.34·1).
*Peri-articular and soft-tissue disorders.*

**Artrolyt** *Neo-Farmaceutica, Port.†.*
Diacerein (p.30·1).
*Osteoarthrosis.*

**Artromed** *Medosan, Ital.*
Amtolmetin guacil (p.14·3).
*Musculoskeletal and joint disorders; pain.*

**Artron** *Liomont, Mex.*
Naproxen (p.65·1).
*Musculoskeletal, joint, and peri-articular disorders; pain.*

**Artroplex** *Knop, Chile.*
Homoeopathic preparation.

**Artroreuma** *Teofarma, Ital.†.*
Tiaprofenic acid (p.93·3).
*Inflammation; pain.*

**Artrosal** *OTC, Spain†.*
Ethyl vanillin; phenylpropanol salicylate.
*Rheumatic and muscle pain.*

**Artrosan**
*Note. This name is used for preparations of different composition.*
*Dolisos, Fr.†.*
Devil's claw root (p.28·2); meadowsweet (p.1710·1).
*Joint disorders.*

*Provita, Ital.†.*
Multivitamin and mineral preparation with glucosamine sulfate (p.1694·1) (p.1417·1).
*Joint disorders.*

**Artrosil** *Ache, Braz.*
Ketoprofen lysine (p.51·3).

**Artrosilene** *Dompe, Ital.*
Ketoprofen lysine (p.51·3).
*Inflammation; musculoskeletal, joint, and peri-articular disorders.*

**Artrotec**
*Monsanto, Ital.; Searle, Mex.; Pharmacia, Spain.*
Diclofenac sodium (p.32·1).
Misoprostol (p.1519·2) is included in this preparation in an attempt to limit adverse effects on the gastrointestinal mucosa.
*Inflammation; musculoskeletal and joint disorders; pain.*

**Artroxen** *Errekappa, Ital.†.*
Naproxen (p.65·1).
*Musculoskeletal and joint disorders.*

**Artroxicam**
*Note. This name is used for preparations of different composition.*
*Medichrom, Gr.*
Tenoxicam (p.93·1).
*Dysmenorrhoea; gout; inflammation; osteoarthritis; pain; rheumatoid arthritis; spondyloarthropathies.*

*Fonten, Ital.*
Piroxicam (p.84·2).
*Musculoskeletal, joint, peri-articular, and soft-tissue disorders.*

**Artruic** *IFET (ΙΦΕΤ), Gr.*
Tenoxicam (p.93·1).
*Dysmenorrhoea; gout; inflammation; osteoarthritis; pain; rheumatoid arthritis; spondyloarthropathies.*

**Arturic**
*Alpharma, Fin.; Alpharma, Norw.*
Allopurinol (p.412·2).
*Gout; hyperuricaemia; renal calculi; uric acid nephropathy.*

**Artyflam** *Rayere, Mex.*
Piroxicam (p.84·2).
*Inflammation; musculoskeletal and joint disorders.*

**Artz**
*AstraZeneca, Denm.; Sankyo, Ital.*
Sodium hyaluronate (p.1697·3).
*Osteoarthritis of the knee.*

**Artzal**
*Sankyo, Austria; AstraZeneca, Fin.; Astra, Swed.*
Sodium hyaluronate (p.1697·3).
*Arthrosis of the knee.*

**Aru C** *Chauvin ankerpharm, Ger.*
Clotrimazole (p.396·2).
*Corynebacterium skin infections; fungal skin infections.*

**Arubendol**
*Note. This name is used for preparations of different composition.*
*Alpharma-Isis, Ger.*
Terbutaline sulfate (p.797·2).
*Obstructive airways disease.*

*Klinge, Ger.†.*
Salbutamol (p.791·3).
*Obstructive airways disease.*

**Aruclonin** *Chauvin ankerpharm, Ger.*
Clonidine hydrochloride (p.885·2).
*Glaucoma; ocular hypertension.*

**Arudel** *Alter, Spain.*
Simvastatin (p.997·1).
*Hyperlipidaemias; secondary prophylaxis of ischaemic heart disease.*

**Arufil** *Chauvin ankerpharm, Ger.*
Povidone (p.1581·2).
*Dry eyes.*

**Arutimol** *Chauvin ankerpharm, Ger.*
Timolol maleate (p.1012·2).
*Glaucoma; ocular hypertension.*

**Arutrin** *Chauvin ankerpharm, Ger.*
Triamcinolone acetonide (p.1110·2).
*Skin disorders.*

**Arvekap** *Ipsen, Gr.*
Triptorelin (p.1341·2) or triptorelin embonate (p.1341·2).
*Endometriosis; female infertility; prostatic cancer; uterine fibroids.*

**Arvenum** *Stroder, Ital.*
Diosmin (p.1688·2).
*Peripheral vascular disorders.*

**Arvin**
*Knoll, Canad.†; Knoll, Spain†.*
Ancrod (p.863·2).
*Peripheral vascular disorders; thromboembolic disorders.*

**Arwin** *Ebewe, Austria.*
Ancrod (p.863·2).
*Peripheral vascular disorders.*

**Arythmol**
*Abbott, Irl.; Abbott, UK.*
Propafenone hydrochloride (p.988·3).
*Arrhythmias.*

**Arzepam** *Solfran, Mex.*
Diazepam (p.690·1).

**Arzide** *David, India.*
Rifampicin (p.250·2); isoniazid (p.222·2).
*Tuberculosis.*

**Arzimol** *Belmac, Spain.*
Cefprozil (p.179·2).
*Bacterial infections.*

**Arzomicin** *Grunenthal, Arg.*
Azithromycin (p.159·1).
*Bacterial infections.*

**Arzomicina** *APS, Port.*
Azithromycin (p.159·1).
*Bacterial infections.*

**AS/85** *Aesculapius, Ital.†.*
Naproxen aminobutanol (p.65·3).
*Gynaecological disorders.*

**AS Cor** *SmithKline Beecham, Mex.*
Norfenefrine hydrochloride (p.975·3).
*Hypotension.*

**AS 101 VA N** *Staufen, Ger.*
Homoeopathic preparation.

**ASA**
*German Remedies, India; Liomont, Mex.†.*
Aspirin (p.15·1).
*Fever; pain; thromboembolism prophylaxis.*

**Asa Right Powder** *Eagle, Austral.†.*
Vitamin and mineral preparation with equisetum and ginger (p.1417·1).
*Respiratory congestion.*

**Asa Tones** *Eagle, Austral.†.*
Grindelia camporum (p.1696·1); hedera helix; potassium iodide (p.1598·1); crataegus (p.1677·1); euphorbia hirta (p.1686·3); liquorice (p.1270·2); polygala tenuifolia (p.1130·2); drosera longifolia (p.1683·1).
*Upper respiratory-tract symptoms.*

**Asacol**
*Byk, Belg.; Procter & Gamble, Canad.; Leiras, Denm.; Leiras, Fin.; Faran, Gr.; Tillotts, Hong Kong; Tillotts, Israel; Giuliani, Ital.; Schering-Plough, Mex.; Byk, Neth.; Schering, Norw.; Baxter, NZ; Tillotts, NZ; Helsinn, Port.; Aventis, S.Afr.; Tillotts, Singapore; Schering, Swed.; Sanofi Synthelabo, Switz.; Tillotts, Thai.; Procter & Gamble, UK; Procter & Gamble, USA.*
Mesalazine (p.1273·2).
*Inflammatory bowel disease.*

**Asacolitin** *Henning, Ger.*
Mesalazine (p.1273·2).
*Ulcerative colitis.*

**Asacolon** *Medeva, Irl.*
Mesalazine (p.1273·2).
*Proctitis; proctosigmoiditis; ulcerative colitis.*

**ASAD**
*Stallergenes, Fr.; Stallergenes, Switz.*
Allergen extracts (p.1650·1).
*Allergen immunotherapy.*

**Asafen**
*Note. This name is used for preparations of different composition.*
*Sanofi Synthelabo, Braz.†.*
Paracetamol (p.76·2); ephedrine hydrochloride (p.1120·1); thenyldiamine (p.442·1); caffeine (p.782·1).
*Cold and influenza symptoms.*

*Sanofi Synthelabo, Mex.*
Paracetamol (p.76·2); caffeine (p.782·1); phenylephrine (p.1126·3); chlorphenamine (p.428·1).
*Pain.*

**Asafen Nueva Formula** *Sanofi Synthelabo, Chile.*
Paracetamol (p.76·2); chlorphenamine maleate (p.427·3); pseudoephedrine hydrochloride (p.1129·2); caffeine (p.782·1).
*Nasal congestion; upper respiratory-tract disorders.*

**Asaflow** *Sandipro, Belg.*
Aspirin (p.15·1).
*Cardiovascular and cerebrovascular disorders.*

**Asalazin** *Medichrom, Gr.*
Mesalazine (p.1273·2).
*Inflammatory bowel disease.*

**Asalen** *Covan, S.Afr.*
Phenylephrine hydrochloride (p.1126·3); chlorphenamine maleate (p.427·3); paracetamol (p.76·2); caffeine (p.782·1).
*Cold symptoms.*

**Asalex** *Chiesi, Ital.*
Mesalazine (p.1273·2).
*Inflammatory bowel disease.*

**Asalit** *Merck, Braz.*
Mesalazine (p.1273·2).
*Inflammatory bowel disease.*

**Asamax** *Yamanouchi, Ital.*
Mesalazine (p.1273·2).
*Crohn's disease; ulcerative colitis.*

**Asaphen** *Pharmascience, Canad.*
Aspirin (p.15·1).
*Fever; inflammation; pain.*

**ASA-ratio** *Ratiopharm, Ital.*
Aspirin (p.15·1).
*Fever; pain.*

**Asarid** *Boehringer Ingelheim, Belg.*
Aspirin (p.15·1).
*Cardiovascular disorders; fever; pain.*

**Asarum Med Complex** *Dynamit, Austria.*
Homoeopathic preparation.

**Asasantin**
*Boehringer Ingelheim, Austral.; Boehringer Ingelheim, Austria; Boehringer Ingelheim, Fin.; Boehringer Ingelheim, Ger.; Boehringer Ingelheim, Irl.; Boehringer Ingelheim, Mex.; Boehringer Ingelheim, Neth.; Boehringer Ingelheim, Norw.; Boehringer Ingelheim, S.Afr.; Boehringer Ingelheim, Spain†; Boehringer Ingelheim, Swed.; Boehringer Ingelheim, UK.*
Aspirin (p.15·1); dipyridamole (p.903·1).
*Thromboembolism prophylaxis.*

**Asasantine**
*Boehringer Ingelheim, Canad.†; Boehringer Ingelheim, Fr.; Boehringer Ingelheim, Switz.*
Dipyridamole (p.903·1); aspirin (p.15·1).
*Thromboembolic disorders.*

**ASAtard** *Boehringer Ingelheim, S.Afr.†.*
Aspirin (p.15·1).
*Thrombosis prophylaxis.*

**Asaurex** *Cryopharma, Mex.†.*
Cimetidine (p.1255·3).

**Asawin** *Sanofi Winthrop, Mex.†.*
Aspirin (p.15·1).

**Asax** *Pasteur, Chile.*
Furosemide (p.919·3).
*Hypertension; oedema.*

**Asazine** *Tillotts, Switz.*
Mesalazine (p.1273·2).
*Ulcerative colitis.*

**Asba** *Medirel, Switz.†.*
Calcium carbonate (p.1254·2); camphor (p.1665·3); peppermint oil (p.1283·2).
*Mouth and throat disorders.*

**Ascabiol**
*Note. This name is used for preparations of different composition.*
*Aventis, Austral.; Aventis, Irl.; Aspen, S.Afr.; Aventis, UK.*
Benzyl benzoate (p.1500·2).
*Pediculosis; scabies.*

*Zambon, Fr.*
Benzyl benzoate (p.1500·2); sulfiram (p.1510·1).
*Scabies.*

*Nicholas Piramal, India.*
Lindane (p.1506·3).
*Pediculosis; scabies.*

**Ascal**
*Viatris, Neth.; Farmasierra, Spain.*
Carbasalate calcium (p.25·1).
*Fever; pain; thromboembolism prophylaxis.*

**Ascarical** *Farmoquimica, Braz.*
Pyrantel embonate (p.113·2).
*Worm infections.*

**Ascaridil** *Janssen-Cilag, Braz.*
Levamisole hydrochloride (p.107·2).
*Ascariasis.*

**Ascarin** *Iodo Suma, Braz.†.*
Piperazine hydrate (p.111·2).
*Ascariasis; enterobiasis.*

**Ascarinase** *Ibefar, Braz.†.*
Piperazine hydrate (p.111·2).
*Worm infections.*

**Ascariobel** *Sedabel, Braz.*
Mebendazole (p.108·2).
*Worm infections.*

**Ascaritor** *Kanda, Braz.†.*
Mebendazole (p.108·2).
*Worm infections.*

**Ascarobex** *Opofarm, Braz.†.*
Mebendazole (p.108·2).
*Worm infections.*

**Ascarotrat** *Medley, Braz.†.*
Tetramisole hydrochloride (p.114·1).
*Nematode infections.*

**Ascaverm** *Gemballa, Braz.†.*
Tetramisole (p.114·1).
*Nematode infections.*

**Ascencyl** *Theraplix, Fr.†.*
Adenosine phosphate; cyanocobalamin; magnesium aspartate; manganese gluconate (p.1417·1).
*Tonic.*

**Ascensia** *Roche Diagnostics, Austral.*
Test for glucose in blood (p.1694·2).

**Ascensia Glucodisc** *Bayer Diagnostics, UK.*
Test for glucose in blood (p.1694·2).

**Ascocid** *Volchem, Ital.*
Peptide, lipid, and carbohydrate preparation with vitamin C (p.1417·1).
*Nutritional supplement.*

**Ascodyne** *Chemedica, Switz.*
Multivitamin preparation with amino acids (p.1417·1).
*Tonic.*

**Ascofer**
*Desbergers, Canad.†; Gerda, Fr.*
Ferrous ascorbate (p.1427·3).
*Iron-deficiency anaemias.*

**Ascomed** *Ripari-Gero, Ital.†.*
Ascorbic acid (p.1460·2).
*Vitamin C deficiency.*

**Ascomp with Codeine** *Breckenridge, USA.*
Codeine phosphate (p.27·1); aspirin (p.15·1); caffeine (p.782·1); butalbital (p.673·3).
*Pain.*

**Ascor** *McGuff, USA.*
Ascorbic acid (p.1460·2).
*Vitamin C supplement.*

**Ascorbex** *Sante Naturelle, Canad.*
Ascorbic acid (p.1460·2).

**Ascorbin**
*Montavit, Austria; Orion, Fin.; Leiras, Fin.; Orion, Malaysia; Orion, Singapore.*
Ascorbic acid (p.1460·2).
*Vitamin C deficiency.*

**Ascorbisal** *Lannacher, Austria.*
Aspirin (p.15·1); ascorbic acid (p.1460·2).
*Fever; musculoskeletal and joint disorders; pain.*

**Ascorell** *Sanorell, Ger.*
Ascorbic acid (p.1460·2).
*Vitamin C deficiency.*

**Ascortil** *UCI, Braz.†.*
Vitamin C (p.1460·2).
*Vitamin C supplement.*

**Ascortonyl** *Gerda, Fr.*
Ascorbic acid (p.1460·2); magnesium potassium aspartate.
Formerly contained ascorbic acid, magnesium potassium aspartate, and cyanocobalamin.
*Tonic.*

**Ascorvit** *Jenapharm, Ger.*
Ascorbic acid (p.1460·2).
*Vitamin C deficiency.*

**Ascosal** *Grossmann, Switz.*
Aspirin (p.15·1); ascorbic acid (p.1460·2).
*Cold symptoms.*

**Ascot** *Polipharm, Thai.*
Aspirin (p.15·1).
*Inflammation; pain; thromboembolic disorders.*

**Ascotodin** *Bruschettini, Ital.*
Mebechinium metilsulfate; thonzylamine hydrochloride (p.442·2).
*Eye disorders.*

**AscoTop** *AstraZeneca, Ger.; Promed, Ger.*
Zolmitriptan (p.473·3).
*Migraine.*

**Ascoxal**
Note. This name is used for preparations of different composition.
*AstraZeneca, Arg.*
Ascorbic acid (p.1460·2); sodium percarbonate (p.1192·3).
*Gingivitis.*
*AstraZeneca, Austral.†; AstraZeneca, Fin.; Astra, Mex.; AstraZeneca, Norw.; Astra, Swed.*
Ascorbic acid (p.1460·2); sodium percarbonate (p.1192·3); copper sulfate (p.1426·1).
*Mouth and throat disorders.*

**Ascredar** *Roche, Austria.*
Disodium clodronate (p.770·2).
*Hypercalcaemia of malignancy; osteolytic bone metastases; Paget's disease of bone.*

**Ascriptin**
*Rhone-Poulenc Rorer, Hong Kong†; Rhone-Poulenc Rorer, Irl.†; Aventis, Israel; Aventis, Ital.; Aventis, Mex.*
Aspirin (p.15·1).
Aluminium hydroxide (p.1249·2) and magnesium hydroxide (p.1272·2) are included in this preparation in an attempt to limit adverse effects on the gastrointestinal mucosa.
*Fever; inflammation; pain; thromboembolic disorders.*
*Rhone-Poulenc Rorer, USA.*
Aspirin (p.15·1).
Aluminium hydroxide (p.1249·2), calcium carbonate (p.1254·2), and magnesium hydroxide (p.1272·2) are included in this preparation in an attempt to limit adverse effects on the gastrointestinal mucosa.
*Fever; inflammation; myocardial infarction; pain; transient ischaemic attacks.*

**Asdron** *Marjan, Braz.*
Ketotifen fumarate (p.788·1).
*Allergic conjunctivitis; allergic rhinitis; asthma; urticaria.*

**Aselli** *Weifa, Norw.*
*Cream:* Cetylpyridinium chloride (p.1173·1); zinc tannate.
*Minor skin disorders; skin disinfection; sunburn.*
*Ointment:* Zinc tannate; zinc oxide (p.1163·2); titanium dioxide (p.1160·3); cod-liver oil (p.1425·2).
*Minor skin disorders.*

**Asendin**
*Wyeth-Ayerst, Canad.†; Wyeth, NZ†; Lederle, USA.*
Amoxapine (p.286·3).
*Depression.*

**Asendis**
*Wyeth, Irl.†; Goldshield, UK.*
Amoxapine (p.286·3).
*Depression.*

**Asenlix** *Aventis, Mex.*
Clobenzorex hydrochloride (p.1585·3).
*Obesity.*

**Asenta** *Agis, Israel.*
Donepezil hydrochloride (p.1489·2).
*Alzheimer's disease.*

**ASEP** *Galen, UK.*
Glutaral (p.1180·3).
*Instrument disinfection.*

**Asepsal** *Magis, Ital.†.*
Ibuprofen isobutanolammonium (p.46·3).
*Gynaecological disorders.*

**Aseptalum** *ICN, Arg.*
Aluminium subacetate (p.1652·3).
*Astringent.*

**Aseptiderm** *Pharmethic, Belg.†.*
Cetrimonium bromide (p.1173·1).
*Disinfection of skin and instruments.*

**Aseptil** *SmithKline Beecham, Ital.†.*
Copper usnate (p.1762·1); diazolidinyl urea; zinc oxide (p.1163·2); alcloxa (p.1141·2).
*Skin and wound disinfection.*

**Aseptisol** *Bode, Ger.*
Glutaral (p.1180·3); formaldehyde (p.1179·3); didecylmethyloxethylammonium propionate.
*Instrument disinfection.*

**Aseptobron** *Temis, Arg.*
*Inhalation:* Menthol (p.1711·3); cineole (p.1672·1); niaouli (p.1719·3); camphor (p.1665·3); terpinol (p.1752·2); pinus pinaster oil.
*Injection:* Camphor (p.1665·3); cineole (p.1672·1); niaouli (p.1719·3); guaiacol (p.1122·1); iodoform (p.1184·2).
*Syrup:* Dextromethorphan (p.1117·3); chlorphenamine (p.428·1).
*Respiratory-tract disorders.*

**Aseptobron Ampicilina** *Temis, Arg.*
Ampicillin sodium (p.157·1); clonixin lysine (p.26·3); cineole (p.1672·1); niaouli oil (p.1719·3); terpineol (p.1752·2).
Lidocaine hydrochloride (p.1377·3) is included in this preparation to alleviate the pain of injection.
*Respiratory-tract infections.*

**Aseptobron Antigripal** *Temis, Arg.*
Levophenylephrine hydrochloride (p.1127·2); paracetamol (p.76·2); vitamin C (p.1460·2).
*Cold and influenza symptoms.*

**Aseptobron Bromexina** *Temis, Arg.*
Oxeladin citrate (p.1126·1); bromhexine hydrochloride (p.1115·3).
*Coughs.*

**Aseptobron C** *Temis, Arg.*
Oxeladin citrate (p.1126·1); carbinoxamine maleate (p.426·3).

**Aseptobron Caramelos** *Temis, Arg.*
Tyrothricin (p.275·1); benzocaine (p.1370·3).
*Mouth and throat disorders.*

**Aseptobron Expectorante** *Temis, Arg.*
Bromhexine hydrochloride (p.1115·3).
*Respiratory-tract disorders with increased or viscous mucus.*

**Aseptobron N** *Temis, Arg.*
Benzocaine (p.1370·3); gramicidin (p.220·2); neomycin (p.235·1) or neomycin sulfate (p.235·1).
*Mouth and throat disorders.*

**Aseptobron Respiratorio** *Temis, Arg.*
Amoxicillin trihydrate (p.155·3); ambroxol hydrochloride (p.1114·3).
*Respiratory-tract infections.*

**Aseptobron Unicap** *Temis, Arg.*
Hydrocodone resinate; chlorphenamine resinate.

**Asepto-Glutaral** *Preston, Arg.*
Glutaral (p.1180·3).
*Disinfection.*

**Aseptoman** *Geistlich, Switz.†.*
Isopropyl alcohol (p.1184·3); 1,3-butanediol.
*Hand disinfection.*

**Aseptone 1** *Rougier, Canad.†.*
Clorophene sodium (p.1177·3); sodium *o*-phenylphenol (p.1187·2).
*Surface disinfection for clean surfaces.*

**Aseptone 2** *Rougier, Canad.†.*
Clorophene sodium (p.1177·3); sodium *o*-phenylphenol (p.1187·2); sodium lauril ether sulfate (p.1574·3).
*Surface disinfection.*

**Aseptone 5** *Rougier, Canad.†.*
Clorophene sodium (p.1177·3); sodium *o*-phenylphenol (p.1187·2); sodium alkyl-polyether sulfate.
*Surface disinfection.*

**Aseptone Quat** *Rougier, Canad.†.*
*n*-Alkyldimethylbenzylammonium chlorides (p.1168·3); *n*-alkyldimethylethylbenzylammonium chlorides; octoxinols (p.1414·1).
*Surface disinfection.*

**Aseptosyl** *Sanofi Synthelabo, Belg.*
Potassium hydroxyquinoline sulfate (p.1734·2); lidocaine hydrochloride (p.1377·3).
*Mouth and throat disorders.*

**Aserbine**
*Pharmaco, S.Afr.; Goldshield, UK.*
Benzoic acid (p.1169·3); malic acid (p.1709·2); salicylic acid (p.1157·1); propylene glycol (p.1735·2).
*Burns; skin ulcers; wounds.*

**Asercit** *Serono, Mex.†.*
Dacarbazine (p.544·2).

**Aseroprim** *Serono, Mex.†.*
Azathioprine (p.1349·1).

**Asestor** *Spedrog, Arg.*
Simeticone (p.1289·2); homatropine methylbromide (p.483·2).
*Flatulence; gastrointestinal spasm.*

**Asfeina** *Bial, Port.*
Aspirin (p.15·1); caffeine (p.782·1).
*Fever; pain.*

**Asgoviscum N** *AstraZeneca, Ger.*
Mistletoe (p.1715·3); crataegus (p.1677·1); garlic (p.1691·1).
*Cardiac disorders.*

**Ashbourne Emollient Medicinal Bath Oil** *Ashbourne, UK.*
Liquid paraffin (p.1479·1); acetylated wool alcohols (p.1483·1).
*Skin disorders.*

**Ashton & Parsons Infants Powders** *SSL, UK.*
Chamomile (p.1669·3).
*Colic; teething.*

**Asialax** *Asian Pharm, Thai.*
Carisoprodol (p.1392·1); phenylbutazone (p.83·2).
*Musculoskeletal and joint disorders.*

**Asialum** *Asian Pharm, Thai.*
Aluminium hydroxide (p.1249·2); magnesium hydroxide (p.1272·2).
*Dyspepsia; gastric hyperacidity; peptic ulcer.*

**Asiamox** *Asian Pharm, Thai.*
Amoxicillin trihydrate (p.155·3).
*Bacterial infections.*

**Asianbron** *Asian Pharm, Thai.*
Theophylline (p.798·3); guaifenesin (p.1122·1).
*Obstructive airways disease.*

**Asiatapp** *Asian Pharm, Thai.*
Brompheniramine maleate (p.426·1); phenylephrine hydrochloride (p.1126·3).
Formerly contained brompheniramine maleate, phenylephrine hydrochloride, and phenylpropanolamine hydrochloride.
*Asthma; cold symptoms.*

**Asiazole** *Asian Pharm, Thai.*
Metronidazole (p.607·2).
*Amoebiasis; trichomoniasis.*

**Asiazole-TN** *Asian Pharm, Thai.*
Tinidazole (p.617·1).
*Amoebiasis; giardiasis; trichomoniasis.*

**Asic**
Note. This name is used for preparations of different composition.
*Cesam, Port.†.*
Bearberry (p.1659·2); carboxyethylgermanium; titanium dioxide (p.1160·3); methoxycinnamate.
*Hyperpigmentation.*
*Pharmaceutical Enterprises, S.Afr.*
Dicycloverine hydrochloride (p.481·2); doxylamine succinate (p.432·3); pyridoxine hydrochloride (p.1456·3).
*Nausea and vomiting in pregnancy.*

**Asig** *Sigma, Austral.*
Quinapril hydrochloride (p.991·1).
*Heart failure; hypertension.*

**Asilone**
Note. This name is used for preparations of different composition.
*Daudt, Braz.*
*Oral suspension:* Aluminium hydroxide (p.1249·2); magnesium hydroxide (p.1272·2); simeticone (p.1289·2).
*Dyspepsia; flatulence.*
*Daudt, Braz.; Knoll, Irl.†; Thornton & Ross, UK.*
*Tablets:* Aluminium hydroxide (p.1249·2); simeticone (p.1289·2).
*Dyspepsia; flatulence; gastritis; gastro-oesophageal reflux; hiatus hernia; peptic ulcer.*
*Knoll, Irl.†; Thornton & Ross, UK.*
*Oral suspension; oral gel:* Aluminium hydroxide (p.1249·2); light magnesium oxide (p.1272·3); simeticone (p.1289·2).
*Dyspepsia; flatulence; gastritis; gastro-oesophageal reflux; hiatus hernia; peptic ulcer.*
*Roche, S.Afr.*
Aluminium hydroxide (p.1249·2); simeticone (p.1289·2).
*Gastric hyperacidity.*

**Asilone Heartburn** *Thornton & Ross, UK.*
Alginic acid (p.1576·3) or sodium alginate (p.1577·1); aluminium hydroxide (p.1249·2); magnesium trisilicate (p.1272·3); sodium bicarbonate (p.1223·2).
*Dyspepsia; heartburn.*

**Asilone Windcheaters** *Thornton & Ross, UK.*
Simeticone (p.1289·2).
*Flatulence.*

**Asimil B12** *Torlan, Spain†.*
Mecobalamin (p.1459·1).
*Vitamin B12 deficiency.*

**Asinis** *Bittner, Austria.*
Homoeopathic preparation.

**Asiolex** *Pharmacia, Arg.*
Anastrozole (p.528·1).
*Breast cancer.*

**Asipral** *Labomed, Chile.*
Azithromycin (p.159·1).
*Bacterial infections.*

**Asisdun** *Duncan, Arg.*
Cyproterone (p.1544·3).

**Askina**
Note. This name is used for preparations of different composition.
*Braun, Fr.*
Hydrogel dressing.
*Ulcers; wounds.*
*Braun, UK.*
Sodium chloride (p.1233·3).
*Wound cleansing and irrigation.*

**Askina Biofilm** *Braun, Fr.*
Carmellose (p.1577·3).
*Wounds.*

**Askina Sorb** *Braun, Fr.*
Calcium alginate (p.745·1); carmellose sodium (p.1577·3).
*Wounds.*

**Askit** *Askit, UK.*
Aspirin (p.15·1); aloxiprin (p.14·1); caffeine citrate (p.782·1).
*Fever; pain.*

**ASL** *Normon, Spain.*
Lysine aspirin (p.54·3).
*Fever; inflammation; pain; thromboembolism prophylaxis.*

**Aslanvital** *Vitamed, Braz.†.*
Multivitamin and mineral preparation (p.1417·1).

**Aslavital** *Sanova, Austria.*
*Injection:* Procaine hydrochloride (p.1383·2); glutamic acid (p.1433·2).
*Tablets:* Procaine hydrochloride (p.1383·2); pyridoxine hydrochloride (p.1456·3); inositol (p.1701·2).
*Tonic.*

**Asmabec**
*Celltech, Fr.; Celltech, Irl.; Celltech, Spain; Celltech, UK.*
Beclometasone dipropionate (p.1091·1).
*Asthma.*

**Asmabiol** *Biol, Arg.*
Theophylline (p.798·3).
*Obstructive airways disease.*

**Asmacortone** *NCSN, Ital.*
Methylprednisolone sodium succinate (p.1106·2).
*Corticosteroid.*

**Asmafen**
*Xepa-Soul Pattinson, Hong Kong; Xepa-Soul Pattinson, Malaysia; Pacific, NZ; Xepa-Soul Pattinson, Singapore.*
Ketotifen fumarate (p.788·1).
*Allergic bronchitis; allergic conjunctivitis; allergic rhinitis; allergic skin disorders; asthma; hay fever.*

**Asmafin** *Cazi, Braz.*
Aminophylline hydrate (p.780·2).
*Obstructive airways disease.*

**Asmaflu** *Max Farma, Ital.*
Flunisolide (p.1101·1).
*Allergic disorders of the respiratory tract.*

**Asmafort** *Julphar, UAE.*
Ketotifen fumarate (p.788·1).
*Allergic conjunctivitis; allergic rhinitis; asthma; urticaria.*

**Asmalene** *FIRMA, Ital.†.*
Bitolterol mesilate (p.781·3).
*Obstructive airways disease.*

**Asmalergin** *Merck, Braz.*
Ketotifen fumarate (p.788·1).
*Allergic conjunctivitis; allergic rhinitis; asthma; urticaria.*

**Asmaline** *Polipharm, Thai.*
Terbutaline sulfate (p.797·2).
*Obstructive airways disease.*

**Asmaliv** *Legrand, Braz.*
Salbutamol sulfate (p.791·3).
*Obstructive airways disease.*

**Asmalix** *Century, USA.*
Theophylline (p.798·3).
*Obstructive airways disease.*

**Asmanex** *Schering-Plough, UK.*
Mometasone furoate (p.1107·2).
*Asthma.*

**Asmanoc** *Shiwa, Thai.*
Ketotifen fumarate (p.788·1).
*Asthma; bronchitis; hay fever.*

**Asmanon** *Cazi, Braz.*
Ketotifen fumarate (p.788·1).
*Hypersensitivity reactions.*

**Asmapax** *Nicholas Piramal, India.*
Ephedrine (p.1120·1); theophylline (p.798·3); phenobarbital (p.367·3).
*Obstructive airways disease.*

**Asmapen** *Neo Quimica, Braz.*
Aminophylline (p.780·2).
*Obstructive airways disease.*

**Asmaral-K** *Serral, Mex.*
Ketotifen (p.788·2).
*Asthma.*

**Asmasal**
*Celltech, Fr.; Celltech, Irl.; Celltech, Spain; Silom, Thai.; Celltech, UK.*
Salbutamol (p.791·3) or salbutamol sulfate (p.791·3).
*Obstructive airways disease.*

**Asmasal Expectorant** *Silom, Thai.*
Salbutamol (p.791·3); guaifenesin (p.1122·1).
*Bronchospasm associated with respiratory-tract congestion.*

**Asmasolon** *Great Eastern, Thai.; Westmont, Thai.*
Theophylline (p.798·3).
*Obstructive airways disease.*

**Asmatec** *UCB, Port.*
Formoterol fumarate (p.786·1).
*Obstructive airways disease.*

**Asmaten** *Duopharma, Hong Kong.*
Ketotifen fumarate (p.788·1).
*Allergic bronchitis; allergic rhinitis; allergic skin disorders; asthma.*

**Asmatil** *Alodial, Port.*
Fluticasone propionate (p.1102·3).
*Asthma.*

**Asmatiron** *Ibefar, Braz.†.*
Theophylline (p.798·3); ephedrine hydrochloride (p.1120·1); homatropine methylbromide (p.483·2); diphenhydramine hydrochloride (p.431·3); lobelia (p.1589·1); stramonium (p.489·2).
*Obstructive airways disease.*

**Asmatol** *Roux-Ocefa, Arg.*
Salbutamol sulfate (p.791·3).
*Obstructive airways disease.*

**Asmaven** *Berk, UK†.*
Salbutamol sulfate (p.791·3).
*Obstructive airways disease; premature labour.*

**Asmavent**
*Technilab, Canad.†.*
Salbutamol sulfate (p.791·3).
*Obstructive airways disease.*

*Mintlab, Chile.*
Salbutamol (p.791·3).
*Obstructive airways disease.*

**Asmavent-B** *Mintlab, Chile.*
Salbutamol (p.791·3); beclometasone dipropionate (p.1091·1).
*Obstructive airways disease.*

**Asmax** *Ativus, Braz.*
Ketotifen fumarate (p.788·1).
*Allergic conjunctivitis; allergic rhinitis; asthma; urticaria.*

**Asmen** *Farmalab, Braz.*
Ketotifen fumarate (p.788·1).
*Allergic conjunctivitis; allergic rhinitis; asthma; urticaria.*

**Asmeren** *Labomed, Chile.*
Clenbuterol (p.784·2).
*Obstructive airways disease.*

**Asmeton**
*Sankyo, Hong Kong; Sankyo, Thai.*
Methoxyphenamine hydrochloride (p.1124·2); aminophylline (p.780·2); chlorphenamine maleate (p.427·3); noscapine (p.1125·3).
*Asthma; bronchitis; coughs.*

**Asmifen** *Bunker, Braz.*
Ketotifen fumarate (p.788·1).
*Hypersensitivity reactions.*

**Asmodrin** *Sanval, Braz.*
Aminophylline (p.780·2).
*Obstructive airways disease.*

**Asmofen** *Teuto, Braz.*
Ketotifen fumarate (p.788·1).
*Hypersensitivity reactions.*

**Asmol**
*Alphapharm, Austral.*
Salbutamol sulfate (p.791·3).
*Obstructive airways disease.*
*Pacific, NZ.*
Salbutamol (p.791·3).
*Obstructive airways disease.*

**Asmo-Lavi** *Vitoria, Port.*
Fluticasone propionate (p.1102·3).
*Asthma.*

**Asmopul** *Asmopul, Arg.*
Atropine (p.476·3); adrenaline (p.852·2).
*Asthma.*

**Asmoquinol** *Ducto, Braz.*
Aminophylline (p.780·2).
*Obstructive airways disease.*

**Asmosterona** *Zambon, Braz.†.*
Prednisolone (p.1108·1); tripelennamine hydrochloride (p.442·3); ephedrine hydrochloride (p.1120·1).
*Asthma.*

**Asmotone Plus** *East India Pharma, India.*
Bromhexine hydrochloride (p.1115·3); terbutaline sulfate (p.797·2); guaifenesin (p.1122·1).
*Obstructive airways disease.*

**Asmovent** *Raza, Malaysia; Pharmaniaga, Malaysia.*
Salbutamol sulfate (p.791·3).
*Obstructive airways disease.*

**Asmovent Expectorant** *Raza, Malaysia; Pharmaniaga, Malaysia.*
Guaifenesin (p.1122·1); salbutamol sulfate (p.791·3).
*Respiratory-tract disorders.*

**Aso DDI** *Raffo, Arg.*
Didanosine (p.630·3).
*HIV infection.*

**Asodal** *Sandipro, Belg.*
Paracetamol (p.76·2); codeine phosphate (p.27·1); caffeine (p.782·1); tiemonium iodide (p.489·3).
*Colic; muscle spasm and pain.*

**Asodocel** *Raffo, Arg.*
Docetaxel (p.547·1).
*Malignant neoplasms.*

**Asoflut** *Raffo, Arg.*
Flutamide (p.556·2).

**Asofurtal** *Raffo, Arg.*
Tegafur (p.586·2); uracil.
*Malignant neoplasms.*

**Asoifos** *Asofarma, Arg.*
Ifosfamide (p.561·1).
*Malignant neoplasms.*

**Asolmicina** *Defuen, Arg.*
Minocycline (p.231·3).
*Bacterial infections.*

**A-Solmicina-C** *Richet, Arg.*
Chloramphenicol palmitate (p.185·1).
*Bacterial infections.*

**Asomutan** *Raffo, Arg.*
Mitomycin (p.573·3).
*Malignant neoplasms.*

**Asonacor** *Ebewe, Austria.*
Propafenone hydrochloride (p.988·3).
*Arrhythmias.*

**Asotax**
*Raffo, Arg.; Asofarma, Mex.*
Paclitaxel (p.577·3).
*Malignant neoplasms.*

**Asotecan** *Raffo, Arg.*
Topotecan (p.589·1).
*Malignant neoplasms.*

**Asoteron** *Raffo, Arg.*
Cyproterone (p.1544·3).
*Prostatic cancer.*

**Asotrex** *Raffo, Arg.*
Glucosamine sulfate (p.1694·1); chondroitin sulfate sodium (p.1670·2).
*Musculoskeletal and joint disorders.*

**Asovon** *Progress, Thai.*
Bromhexine hydrochloride (p.1115·3).
*Respiratory-tract disorders associated with increased or viscous mucus.*

**Asovorin** *Raffo, Arg.*
Calcium levofolinate (p.1431·1).
*Malignant neoplasms.*

**ASP** *Merck, Port.†.*
Aspirin (p.15·1).
*Fever; pain.*

**Aspac** *Inexfa, Spain†.*
Paracetamol (p.76·2).
*Fever; pain.*

**Aspagin** *Proel, Gr.*
Tenoxicam (p.93·1).
*Dysmenorrhoea; gout; inflammation; osteoarthritis; pain; rheumatoid arthritis; spondyloarthropathies.*

**Aspalgin** *Fawns & McAllan, Austral.*
Aspirin (p.15·1); codeine phosphate (p.27·1).
*Fever; inflammation; pain.*

**Asparagus-P** *Plantina, Ger.*
Asparagus; parsley (p.1728·3).
*Oedema; renal calculi.*

**Aspartamins** *Solgar, UK†.*
Mineral aspartate preparation (p.1417·1).

**Aspartatol** *Eagle, Austral.†.*
Potassium aspartate (p.1233·1); magnesium aspartate (p.1227·3); glutamine (p.1433·2).
*Tonic.*

**Asparten** *Euro-Labor, Port.*
Arginine aspartate (p.1421·1).
*Fatigue.*

**Aspartina** *Bouty, Ital.*
Aspartame (p.1422·1).
*Sugar substitute.*

**Aspartono** *Medix, Spain†.*
Adenosine triphosphate; glucose; magnesium aspartate; potassium aspartate (p.1417·1).
*Cardiopathies; liver disorders; muscular dystrophies; tonic.*

**A-Spas** *Hyrex, USA.*
Hyoscyamine sulfate (p.485·1).
*Gastrointestinal disorders.*

**Aspaserine B6 Tranq** *UCB, Spain.*
Diazepam (p.690·1).
Contains pyridoxine.
*Alcohol withdrawal syndrome; anxiety; febrile convulsions; insomnia; skeletal muscle spasm.*

**Aspasmine** *Sterop, Belg.*
Hyoscine butylbromide (p.483·3).
*Smooth muscle spasm.*

**Aspasmon N** *Norgine, Ger.*
Peppermint oil (p.1283·2); anise oil (p.1655·2); caraway oil (p.1667·3).
*Catarrh; gastrointestinal disorders.*

**Aspav** *Alpharma, UK.*
Aspirin (p.15·1); papaveretum (p.74·3).
*Pain.*

**Aspec** *PSM, NZ.*
Aspirin (p.15·1).
*Fever; inflammation; pain.*

**Aspecton** *Krewel, Ger.*
Thyme (p.1755·2).
*Catarrh; coughs.*

**Aspecton Eukaps** *Krewel, Ger.*
Eucalyptus oil (p.1686·2).
*Respiratory-tract catarrh.*

**Aspecton N** *Krewel, Ger.†.*
Thyme (p.1755·2); gypsophila saponins.
*Respiratory-tract disorders.*

**Aspecton-Balsam** *Krewel, Ger.*
Camphor (p.1665·3); thyme oil (p.1755·3); eucalyptus oil (p.1686·2).
*Cold symptoms; coughs.*

**Aspectonetten N** *Krewel, Ger.*
Gypsophila saponins.
Formerly contained butetamate citrate.
*Respiratory-tract catarrh.*

**Aspegic**
*Sanofi Synthelabo, Belg.; Sanofi Synthelabo, Fr.; Sanofi Synthelabo, Ital.; Sanofi Synthelabo, Malaysia; Sanofi Synthelabo, Neth.; Sanofi Synthelabo, Port.; Sanofi Synthelabo, Switz.*
Lysine aspirin (p.54·3).
*Fever; gout; inflammation; musculoskeletal and joint disorders; pain; thrombosis prophylaxis.*

**Aspellin** *Fisons, UK†.*
Methyl salicylate (p.59·3); ethyl salicylate (p.37·3); ammonium salicylate (p.14·2); menthol (p.1711·3); camphor (p.1665·3).
*Pain.*

**Aspent** *Ranbaxy, Thai.*
Aspirin (p.15·1).
*Myocardial infarction; osteoarthritis; rheumatoid arthritis; transient ischaemic attacks.*

**Aspercreme**
*Note. This name is used for preparations of different composition.*
*Stella, Canad.; Thompson, USA.*
Trolamine salicylate (p.95·3).
*Muscle, joint, and soft-tissue pain; neuralgia.*

*Roche, Ital.†.*
Diethylamine salicylate (p.34·1); methyl nicotinate (p.59·2).
*Musculoskeletal disorders.*

**Aspergum**
*Heritage Consumer, Canad.; Schering-Plough, USA.*
Aspirin (p.15·1).
*Fever; inflammation; myocardial infarction; pain; transient ischaemic attacks.*

**Aspergun** *ICN, Arg.*
Piroctone olamine (p.1155·2); collagen (p.1674·3).
*Dandruff.*

**Asperivo** *Rivopharm, Switz.*
Aspirin (p.15·1).
*Fever; pain.*

**Aspex** *Rekah, Israel.*
Aspirin (p.15·1); caffeine (p.782·1).
*Fever; pain.*

**Asphaline** *Vifor, Switz.*
Camphor (p.1665·3); thymol (p.1194·2); paraformaldehyde (p.1187·3); zinc oxide (p.1163·2).
*Root canal infections.*

**Aspi-C** *Eurofarma, Braz.†.*
Aspirin (p.15·1); ascorbic acid (p.1460·2).
*Fever; pain.*

**Aspicot** *Concept, India.*
Aspirin (p.15·1).
*Thromboembolism prophylaxis.*

**Aspidol** *Piam, Ital.*
Lysine aspirin (p.54·3).
*Pain.*

**Aspiglicina** *Antonetto, Ital.*
Aspirin (p.15·1).
Glycine (p.1433·3) is included in this preparation in an attempt to limit adverse effects on the gastrointestinal mucosa.
*Neuralgia.*

**Aspilets**
*United American, Hong Kong; United American, Thai.; Great Eastern, Thai.*
Aspirin (p.15·1).
*Fever; pain; thromboembolic disorders.*

**Aspinfantil** *Diviser Aquilea, Spain.*
Aspirin (p.15·1).
*Fever; musculoskeletal, joint, and peri-articular disorders; pain; thromboembolism prophylaxis.*

**Aspiricor** *Bayer, Austria.*
Aspirin (p.15·1).
*Migraine; thromboembolism prophylaxis.*

**Aspirin Backache** *Bayer Consumer, Canad.*
Aspirin (p.15·1); methocarbamol (p.1395·1).
*Back pain.*

**Aspirin C**
*Bayer, Fin.; Bayer, Israel.*
Aspirin (p.15·1); ascorbic acid (p.1460·2).
*Fever; musculoskeletal and joint disorders; pain; thrombosis prophylaxis.*

**Aspirin + C** *Bayer, Austria.*
Aspirin (p.15·1); ascorbic acid (p.1460·2).
*Fever; pain.*

**Aspirin Cardio** *Bayer, Fin.*
Aspirin (p.15·1).
*Thromboembolism prophylaxis.*

**Aspirin forte** *Bayer, Ger.*
Aspirin (p.15·1); caffeine (p.782·1).
*Inflammation; pain.*

**Aspirin Free Anacin** *Robins, USA.*
Paracetamol (p.76·2).
Formerly known as Anacin-3.

**Aspirin Free Anacin PM** *Whitehall, USA.*
Paracetamol (p.76·2); diphenhydramine hydrochloride (p.431·3).
*Insomnia; pain.*

**Aspirin Free Excedrin** *Bristol-Myers Squibb, USA.*
Paracetamol (p.76·2); caffeine (p.782·1).
*Pain.*

**Aspirin Free Excedrin Dual** *Bristol-Myers Squibb, USA†.*
Paracetamol (p.76·2); calcium carbonate (p.1254·2); magnesium carbonate (p.1272·1); magnesium oxide (p.1272·3).

**Aspirin Free Pain Relief** *Hudson, USA.*
Paracetamol (p.76·2).
*Fever; pain.*

**Aspirin plus C** *Bayer, Ger.*
Aspirin (p.15·1); ascorbic acid (p.1460·2).
*Cold symptoms; fever; pain.*

**Aspirin with Stomach Guard** *Bayer Consumer, Canad.*
Aspirin (p.15·1).
Calcium carbonate (p.1254·2), magnesium carbonate (p.1272·1), and magnesium oxide (p.1272·3) are included in this preparation in an attempt to limit adverse effects on the gastrointestinal mucosa.
*Fever; inflammation; pain.*

**Aspirina**
*Bayer, Braz.; Bayer, Chile; Bayer, Ital.; Bayer, Mex.; Bayer, Port.; Bayer, Spain.*
Aspirin (p.15·1).
Calcium carbonate (p.1254·2) may be included in the chewable tablets in an attempt to limit adverse effects on the gastrointestinal mucosa.
*Fever; inflammation; musculoskeletal, joint, and peri-articular disorders; pain; thromboembolism prophylaxis.*

**Aspirina 03 and 05** *Bayer, Ital.*
Aspirin (p.15·1).
Magnesium hydroxide (p.1272·2) and aluminium glycinate (p.1249·1) are included in this preparation in an attempt to limit adverse effects on the gastrointestinal mucosa.
*Fever; pain.*

**Aspirina 05** *Bayer, Ital.†.*
Aspirin (p.15·1).
Calcium carbonate (p.1254·2) is included in this preparation in an attempt to limit adverse effects on the gastrointestinal mucosa.
*Fever; pain.*

**Aspirina C**
*Bayer, Braz.; Bayer, Chile; Bayer, Ital.; Bayer, Port.; Bayer, Spain.*
Aspirin (p.15·1); ascorbic acid (p.1460·2).
*Fever; musculoskeletal disorders; pain.*

**Aspirina Complex** *Bayer, Spain.*
Aspirin (p.15·1); phenylephrine acid tartrate (p.1126·3); chlorphenamine maleate (p.427·3).
Formerly contained aspirin, phenylpropanolamine tartrate, and chlorphenamine maleate.
*Cold and influenza symptoms.*

**Aspirina Forte** *Bayer, Braz.*
Aspirin (p.15·1); caffeine (p.782·1).
*Fever; pain.*

**Aspirina Plus** *Bayer, Spain.*
Aspirin (p.15·1); caffeine (p.782·1).
*Fever; pain.*

**Aspirine**
*Bayer, Belg.; Bayer, Fr.; Bristol-Myers Squibb, Fr.*
Aspirin (p.15·1).
*Fever; pain; thromboembolism prophylaxis.*

**Aspirine C**
*Bayer, Belg.; Bayer, Neth.; Bayer, Switz.*
Aspirin (p.15·1); ascorbic acid (p.1460·2).
*Fever; pain.*

**Aspirine Duo** *Bayer, Belg.*
Aspirin (p.15·1); caffeine (p.782·1).
*Fever; pain.*

**Aspirine pH8** *3M, Fr.*
Aspirin (p.15·1).
*Fever; pain.*

**Aspirine Protect** *Bayer, Neth.*
Aspirin (p.15·1).
*Thrombosis prophylaxis.*

**Aspirine vitamine C** *Bayer, Fr.; Oberlin, Fr.; UPSA, Fr.*
Aspirin (p.15·1); ascorbic acid (p.1460·2).
*Fever; pain.*

**Aspirinetas** *Bayer, Arg.*
Aspirin (p.15·1).
*Fever; pain.*

**Aspirinetta** *Bayer, Ital.*
Aspirin (p.15·1).
*Fever; pain.*

**Aspirinetta C** *Bayer, Ital.†.*
Aspirin (p.15·1); ascorbic acid (p.1460·2).
*Fever; inflammation; pain.*

**Aspirin-Free Bayer Select Allergy Sinus** *Sterling Health, USA.*
Pseudoephedrine hydrochloride (p.1129·2); chlorphenamine maleate (p.427·3); paracetamol (p.76·2).

**Aspirin-Free Bayer Select Head & Chest Cold** *Sterling Health, USA.*
Pseudoephedrine hydrochloride (p.1129·2); dextromethorphan hydrobromide (p.1117·3); guaifenesin (p.1122·1); paracetamol (p.76·2).

**Aspirisan** *Sanval, Braz.†.*
Aspirin (p.15·1); caffeine (p.782·1).
*Fever; pain.*

**Aspirisucre** *Arkomedika, Fr.*
Aspirin (p.15·1).
*Fever; pain.*

**Aspi-Rub** *Sidus, Arg.*
Methyl salicylate (p.59·3).

**Aspisin** *Farmasa, Braz.†.*
Aspirin (p.15·1).
*Fever; inflammation; pain; thromboembolism prophylaxis.*

**Aspisol** *Bayer, Ger.*
Lysine aspirin (p.54·3).
*Fever; pain; rheumatism; thromboembolic disorders.*

**Aspitopic** *Bayer, Spain.*
Etofenamate (p.38·1).
*Inflammation; pain.*

**Asplin** *Diafarm, Spain†.*
Paracetamol (p.76·2).
*Fever; pain.*

**Asporin 0.5** *MC, Ital.†.*
Sodium phenolate; glutaral (p.1180·3).
*Instrument sterilisation.*

**Asporin 2** *MC, Ital.†.*
Glutaral (p.1180·3).
*Instrument sterilisation.*

**Asprimox** *Invamed, USA.*
Aspirin (p.15·1).
Aluminium hydroxide (p.1249·2), calcium carbonate (p.1254·2), and magnesium hydroxide (p.1272·2) are included in this preparation in an attempt to limit adverse effects on the gastrointestinal mucosa.

**Aspro**
*Roche Consumer, Austral.; Roche, Austria; Roche, Belg.; Roche Nicholas, Fr.; Roche Nicholas, Ger.; Roche, Hong Kong†; Roche Consumer, Irl.; Roche, Ital.; Roche Consumer, Neth.; Roche, NZ; Roche, Port.;*

Roche, S.Afr.†; Roche Consumer, Singapore; Roche Nicholas, Spain†; Roche, Switz.; Roche Consumer, UK.
Aspirin (p.15·1).
*Fever; inflammation; musculoskeletal and joint disorders; pain; thromboembolism prophylaxis.*

**Aspro C**
Roche, Ital.; Roche, Switz.†.
Aspirin (p.15·1); ascorbic acid (p.1460·2).
*Fever; pain.*

**Aspro + C** Roche, Belg.†.
Aspirin (p.15·1); ascorbic acid (p.1460·2).
*Fever; pain.*

**Aspro mit Vitamin C** Roche, Austria.
Aspirin (p.15·1); ascorbic acid (p.1460·2).
*Fever; pain.*

**Aspro vitamine C** Roche Nicholas, Fr.
Aspirin (p.15·1); ascorbic acid (p.1460·2).
*Fever; pain.*

**Asproaccel** Roche Nicholas, Fr.
Aspirin (p.15·1); caffeine (p.782·1).
*Fever; pain.*

**Aspylin** QIF, Braz.†.
Aspirin (p.15·1).
*Fever; inflammation; pain; thromboembolism prophylaxis.*

**ASS**
Genericon, Austria; Ratiopharm, Austria; Hexal, Ger.; CT, Ger.; Ratiopharm, Ger.; Stada, Ger.; Worwag, Ger.; Azupharma, Ger.; Heumann, Ger.; Aliud, Ger.; Merck dura, Ger.; Atid, Ger.; Alpharma-Isis, Ger.; RAN, Ger.; 1A, Ger.; Mepha, Switz.
Aspirin (p.15·1).
*Fever; inflammation; pain; rheumatism; thromboembolic disorders.*

**ASS + C** Ratiopharm, Ger.; Hexal, Ger.
Aspirin (p.15·1); ascorbic acid (p.1460·2).
*Cold symptoms; fever; pain.*

**ASS OPT** Optimed, Ger.†.
Aspirin (p.1460·2).
*Fever; musculoskeletal and joint disorders; pain; thromboembolic disorders.*

**Assal** Salus, Mex.
Salbutamol (p.791·3) or salbutamol sulfate (p.791·3).

**Assalix** Bionorica, Ger.
Salix (p.87·3).
*Fever; pain; rheumatism.*

**Assan** Permamed, Switz.
Flufenamic acid (p.43·2); glycol salicylate (p.44·3); heparin sodium (p.928·1).
*Musculoskeletal and joint pain; peripheral vascular disorders; soft-tissue injury.*

**Assan-Thermo** Permamed, Switz.
Flufenamic acid (p.43·2); glycol salicylate (p.44·3); benzyl nicotinate (p.21·2); heparin sodium (p.928·1).
*Musculoskeletal and joint disorders.*

**ASSbene** Ratiopharm, Austria.
Aspirin (p.15·1).
*Fever; pain.*

**Assenzio (Specie Composta)** Dynacren, Ital.
Absinthium (p.1645·1); gentian (p.1692·2); dried bitter-orange peel (p.1723·3); centaury (p.1669·2); cinnamon (p.1672·2).
*Appetite loss; herbal tea.*

**Assepium** Gross, Braz.
Co-trimoxazole (p.199·3).
*Bacterial infections; Pneumocystis carinii pneumonia; protozoal infections.*

**Assepium Balsamico** Gross, Braz.
Co-trimoxazole (p.199·3); guaifenesin (p.1122·1); ammonium chloride (p.1115·2).
*Respiratory-tract infections.*

**Asseptobron** Eurofarma, Braz.†.
Oxytetracycline (p.241·1); sodium camsilate; guaifenesin (p.1122·1).
*Bacterial infections.*

**Assieme**
Simesa, Ital.; Tecnifar, Port.
Budesonide (p.1094·2); formoterol fumarate (p.786·1).
*Asthma.*

**Assist** GD, Ital.
Soya oil; lutein; zinc (p.1417·1).
*Nutritional supplement.*

**Assist Energetico** Ledi, Ital.†.
Vitamin preparation (p.1417·1).

**Assist Reintegratore** Ledi, Ital.†.
Nutritional supplement (p.1417·1).
*Fluid and electrolyte imbalance.*

**Assival** Teva, Israel.
Diazepam (p.690·1).
*Anxiety; epilepsy; insomnia; skeletal muscle spasm.*

**ASS-Kombi** Ratiopharm, Ger.†.
Paracetamol (p.76·2); aspirin (p.15·1); ascorbic acid (p.1460·2).
*Pain.*

**Assocort** Bristol-Myers Squibb, Ital.
Triamcinolone acetonide (p.1110·2); nystatin (p.406·3).
*Infected skin disorders.*

**Assogen** Metapharma, Ital.†.
Cloricromen hydrochloride (p.889·1).
*Thrombosis prophylaxis.*

**Assoral** Savio, Ital.
Roxithromycin (p.254·2).
*Bacterial infections.*

**Assplant** Robugen, Ger.
Salix (p.87·3).
*Rheumatism.*

**Assy Espuma** Andromaco, Chile.
Permethrin (p.1508·3).
*Pediculosis.*

**Astahis** Siam Bheasach, Thai.†.
Astemizole (p.424·2).
*Hypersensitivity reactions.*

**Astaplatin** Asta Oncologia, Braz.
Cisplatin (p.538·1).
*Malignant neoplasms.*

**Astat** Tsumura, Jpn.
Lanoconazole (p.405·2).
*Fungal skin infections.*

**Astelin**
Sanfer, Mex.; Wallace, USA.
Azelastine hydrochloride (p.425·2).
*Allergic rhinitis.*

**Astem** Asian Pharm, Thai.†.
Astemizole (p.424·2).
*Hypersensitivity reactions.*

**Astemina** Diba, Mex.
Astemizole (p.424·2).
*Hypersensitivity.*

**Astenol** Farmabraz, Braz.†.
Erythroxylon catuaba; guarana (p.1765·3); thiamine; pepsin (p.1417·1).
*Tonic.*

**Astenolit** Altana, Spain.
Vitamin, mineral and amino-acid preparation (p.1417·1).
*Tonic.*

**Astergyl** Aster, Braz.
Metronidazole (p.607·2).

**Asteriodine** Aster, Braz.
Povidone-iodine (p.1190·3).
*Skin disinfection.*

**Astesen** Senosiain, Mex.
Astemizole (p.424·2).
*Allergic conjunctivitis; allergic rhinitis; urticaria.*

**Astezol** ICN, Arg.
Astemizole (p.424·2).
*Hypersensitivity reactions.*

**Asthalin** Cipla, India.
Salbutamol (p.791·3) or salbutamol sulfate (p.791·3).
*Obstructive airways disease.*

**Asthalin Expectorant** Cipla, India.
Salbutamol sulfate (p.791·3); guaifenesin (p.1122·1).
*Obstructive airways disease.*

**Asthamsian** Asian Pharm, Thai.
Terbutaline sulfate (p.797·2).
*Obstructive airways disease.*

**Asthavent** Cipla-Medpro, S.Afr.
Salbutamol (p.791·3).
*Obstructive airways disease.*

**Asthenal** Grossmann, Switz.
Sodium dimethyl aminophenylphosphinate; glutamic acid; thiamine hydrochloride; ascorbic acid (p.1417·1).
*Tonic.*

**Asthenopin** Mann, Ger.†.
Pilocarpine hydrochloride (p.1495·1).
*Eye disorders.*

**Asthma**
Note. This name is used for preparations of different composition.
Disperga, Austria†.
Papaverine hydrochloride (p.1728·1); ephedrine hydrochloride (p.1120·1); propyphenazone (p.85·3); hyoscine hydrobromide (p.483·3).
*Obstructive airways disease.*

Upha, Malaysia.
Ephedrine hydrochloride (p.1120·1); theophylline (p.798·3).
*Bronchial asthma; chronic bronchitis.*

**Asthma & Catarrh Relief** Herbal Concepts, UK.
Ipecacuanha (p.1122·3); lobelia (p.1589·1); marrubium (p.1124·1); liquorice (p.1270·2).
*Asthma; catarrh.*

**Asthma 23 D** Sanova, Austria.
Ephedrine hydrochloride (p.1120·1); belladonna (p.479·1); papaverine hydrochloride (p.1728·1); caffeine-naphthylacetic sodium; theophylline (p.798·3).
*Obstructive airways disease.*

**Asthma Efeum** Apomedica, Austria.
Proxyphylline (p.791·2); phenazone (p.82·3); ethaverine sulfamate (p.1685·2); ephedrine hydrochloride (p.1120·1); diphenhydramine hydrochloride (p.431·3).
*Obstructive airways disease.*

**Asthma H** Pfluger, Ger.
Homoeopathic preparation.

**Asthma 6-N** Hobein, Ger.
Ephedrine hydrochloride (p.1120·1); grindelia (p.1696·1); senega root (p.1130·2).
*Obstructive airways disease.*

**Asthma T** Sam-On, Israel†.
Theophylline (p.798·3).
*Asthma.*

**Asthma-Bomin H** Pfluger, Ger.
Homoeopathic preparation.

**AsthmaHaler Mist** Numark, USA.
Adrenaline acid tartrate (p.852·2).
*Bronchospasm.*

**Asthma-Hilfe** Agepha, Austria.
Aminophylline (p.780·2); theobromine (p.798·2); ephedrine hydrochloride (p.1120·1); sulfogaiacol (p.1131·1).
*Obstructive airways disease.*

**Asthmakhell N** Steigerwald, Ger.
Homoeopathic preparation.

**Asthmalgine** Cochon, Fr.†.
Sodium benzoate (p.1169·3); ephedrine hydrochloride (p.1120·1); caffeine (p.782·1); hyoscyamus (p.485·2). The oral solution also contains Desessartz syrup.
*Asthma.*

**Asthmalitan** MIT, Ger.
Salbutamol sulfate (p.791·3).
*Obstructive airways disease.*

**Asthmalyticum-Ampullen N (Rowo-210)**
Pharmakon, Ger.†.
Homoeopathic preparation.
Lidocaine hydrochloride (p.1377·3) is included in this preparation to alleviate the pain of injection.

**AsthmaNefrin** Menley & James, USA.
Racepinefrine hydrochloride (p.854·1).
*Obstructive airways disease.*

**Asthma-Spray** CT, Ger.†.
Salbutamol (p.791·3).
*Obstructive airways disease.*

**Asthmatee EF-EM-ES** Smetana, Austria.
Enulae root; marrubium vulgare (p.1124·1); origanum; aniseed (p.1655·2); arnica (p.1656·3); cacao husk (p.1754·3).
*Obstructive airways disease.*

**Asthmavowen-N** Weber & Weber, Ger.
Homoeopathic preparation.

**Asthmaxine** Synco, Hong Kong.
Bromhexine hydrochloride (p.1115·3).
*Respiratory-tract congestion.*

**Asthmino** Jagson, India.
Theophylline (p.798·3); ephedrine hydrochloride (p.1120·1); phenobarbital (p.367·3).
*Obstructive airways disease.*

**Asthmo-Kranit Mono** Krewel, Ger.†.
Terbutaline sulfate (p.797·2).
Formerly contained ethaverine hydrochloride, ephedrine hydrochloride, phenobarbital, and theophylline.
*Obstructive airways disease.*

**Asthmolin** Pharmasant, Thai.
Salbutamol sulfate (p.791·3).
*Obstructive airways disease.*

**Asthmolysin** Kade, Ger.†.
Diprophylline (p.784·3).
*Asthma; bronchial disorders.*

**Asthmoprotect** Azupharma, Ger.
Terbutaline sulfate (p.797·2).
*Obstructive airways disease.*

**Asthmotrat** Unipharma, Gr.
Salbutamol sulfate (p.791·3).
*Asthma; chronic respiratory failure.*

**Astho-Med** Schonenberger, Switz.
Dextromethorphan hydrobromide (p.1117·3).
Formerly contained diphenhydramine hydrochloride, diprophylline, guaifenesin, and phenylpropanolamine hydrochloride.
*Coughs.*

**Asticol** Clinced, Austria†.
Paracetamol nicotinate (p.78·3); propyphenazone (p.85·3); caffeine (p.782·1).

**Astidin** Piam, Ital.†.
Infant feed (p.1417·1).
*Histidinaemia.*

**Astifat** Fatol, Ger.
Ketotifen fumarate (p.788·1).
*Asthma; bronchitis; hypersensitivity reactions.*

**Astin** Galen, Mex.
Pravastatin sodium (p.984·3).
*Atherosclerosis; hypercholesterolaemia.*

**Astmazol** Pharmasant, Thai.†.
Astemizole (p.424·2).
*Hypersensitivity reactions.*

**Astomera** Bittner, Austria.
Homoeopathic preparation.

**Astone** Ramelco, Canad.†.
Aspirin (p.15·1); caffeine (p.782·1).

**Astonin** Merck, Spain.
Fludrocortisone (p.1100·2).
*Adrenocortical insufficiency; hypotension.*

**Astonin H**
Merck, Austria; Merck, Ger.
Fludrocortisone (p.1100·2).
*Adrenocortical insufficiency; congenital adrenal hyperplasia; hypotension.*

**Astracaine** AstraZeneca, Canad.
Articaine hydrochloride (p.1370·3).
Adrenaline (p.852·2) is included in this preparation as a vasoconstrictor to diminish absorption and localise the effect of the local anaesthetic.
*Local anaesthesia.*

**Astramorph** AstraZeneca, Braz.†.
Morphine sulfate (p.60·2).
*Pain.*

**Astramorph PF** Astra, USA.
Morphine sulfate (p.60·2).
*Pain.*

**Astratonil** Astra, Swed.†.
Multivitamin preparation (p.1417·1).

**Astreptine** Darci, Belg.†.
Sulfanilamide (p.263·2).
*Infected wounds.*

**Astressane** Dolisos, Fr.†.
Crataegus (p.1677·1); red-poppy petal (p.1058·1); passion flower (p.1729·1).
*Cardiac irritability.*

**Astrexine** UCB, Belg.
Chlorhexidine hydrochloride (p.1173·3).
*Wounds and skin disinfection.*

**Astriderm** Remexa, Mex.†.
Resorcinol (p.1156·3).
*Seborrhoeic dermatitis.*

**Astrin** Elan, Spain.
Fluoxetine hydrochloride (p.292·1).
*Bulimia nervosa; depression; obsessive-compulsive disorder.*

**Astrix**
Faulding, Austral.; Mayne, Hong Kong; Faulding, Singapore.
Aspirin (p.15·1).
*Thromboembolic disorders.*

**Astrocast** Chrispa (Χρισπα), Gr.
Budesonide (p.1094·2).
*Topical corticosteroid.*

**Astroglide** Biofilm, USA.
Glycerol (p.1694·3); propylene glycol (p.1735·2); polyquaternium-5.
*Vaginal lubricant.*

**Astronautal** Strallhofer, Austria.
Diphenylpyraline hydrochloride (p.432·3); pyridoxine hydrochloride (p.1456·3).
*Motion sickness; nausea; vertigo.*

**Astudal** Almirall, Spain.
Amlodipine besilate (p.862·1).
*Angina pectoris; hypertension.*

**Astyl** Lophal, Fr.
Deanol bisorcate (p.1585·3).
*Tonic.*

**Astymin-3** Tablets, India.
Amino-acid infusion (p.1417·1).
*Parenteral nutrition.*

**Astymin Forte** Tablets, India.
Amino-acids and multivitamin preparation (p.1417·1).
*Hypoproteinaemia; tonic.*

**Asucrose** Wockhardt, India.
Acarbose (p.328·3).
*Diabetes mellitus.*

**Asulblan** Fada, Arg.
Amiodarone (p.859·2).
*Arrhythmias.*

**Asumalife** YSP, Malaysia.
Ketotifen fumarate (p.788·1).
*Allergic rhinitis; allergic skin disorders; asthma.*

**Asverin** Tanabe, Jpn.
Tipepidine hibenzate (p.1131·3).
*Coughs.*

**AT III** Baxter, Ger.
Antithrombin III (p.742·2).
*Antithrombin III deficiency.*

**AT 10**
Sanofi Synthelabo, Austral.†; Merck, Austria; Merck, Belg.; Bayer, Ger.; Bayer, Switz.; Intrapharm, UK.
Dihydrotachysterol (p.1461·3).
*Hypoparathyroidism; osteomalacia; pseudohypoparathyroidism; renal osteodystrophy; tetany; vitamin D-resistant rickets.*

**Atacand**
AstraZeneca, Arg.; AstraZeneca, Austral.; AstraZeneca, Austria; AstraZeneca, Belg.; AstraZeneca, Braz.; AstraZeneca, Canad.; AstraZeneca, Chile; AstraZeneca, Denm.; AstraZeneca, Fin.; AstraZeneca, Fr.; AstraZeneca, Ger.; Promed, Ger.; Astra-Zeneca, Gr.; AstraZeneca, Irl.; Teva, Israel; AstraZeneca, Malaysia; AstraZeneca, Mex.; AstraZeneca, Neth.; AstraZeneca, Norw.; AstraZeneca, NZ; AstraZeneca, Port.; AstraZeneca, S.Afr.; AstraZeneca, Singapore; AstraZeneca, Spain; Hassle, Swed.; AstraZeneca, Switz.; Astra, USA.
Candesartan cilexetil (p.878·3).
*Hypertension.*

**Atacand HCT**
AstraZeneca, Braz.; AstraZeneca, USA.
Candesartan cilexetil (p.878·3); hydrochlorothiazide (p.933·2).
*Hypertension.*

**Atacand Plus**
AstraZeneca, Austral.; AstraZeneca, Austria; AstraZeneca, Belg.; AstraZeneca, Fin.; AstraZeneca, Ger.; Promed, Ger.; AstraZeneca, Irl.; Teva, Israel; AstraZeneca, Neth.; AstraZeneca, Norw.; AstraZeneca, S.Afr.; AstraZeneca, Singapore; AstraZeneca, Spain; Hassle, Swed.; AstraZeneca, Switz.
Candesartan cilexetil (p.878·3); hydrochlorothiazide (p.933·2).
*Hypertension.*

**Atacand-D** AstraZeneca, Arg.
Candesartan cilexetil (p.878·3); hydrochlorothiazide (p.933·2).
*Hypertension.*

**AtacandZid** AstraZeneca, Denm.
Candesartan cilexetil (p.878·3); hydrochlorothiazide (p.933·2).
*Hypertension.*

**Ataclor** Errekappa, Ital.†.
Atenolol (p.865·2); chlortalidone (p.882·3).
*Hypertension.*

**Atacoly** Profarb, Braz.†.
Neomycin sulfate (p.235·1); clioquinol (p.196·3); attapulgite (p.1251·1); pectin (p.1580·3).
*Diarrhoea.*

**Atagripe** Windson, Braz.†.
Aspirin (p.15·1); mepyramine maleate (p.437·1); caffeine (p.782·1); vitamin C (p.1460·2).
*Cold and influenza symptoms.*

**Atalin** Gemballa, Braz.
Kaolin (p.1268·3); pectin (p.1580·3).
*Diarrhoea.*

**Ataline**
Medochemie, Hong Kong; Medochemie, Malaysia; Medochemie, Singapore†; Medochemie, Thai.†.
Terbutaline sulfate (p.797·2).
*Obstructive airways disease.*

**Atamet** Athena Neurosciences, USA.
Carbidopa (p.1204·3); levodopa (p.1205·2).
*Parkinsonism.*

**Atamir** Biochemie, Denm.
Penicillamine (p.1046·3).
*Cystinuria; heavy metal poisoning; rheumatoid arthritis; Wilson's disease.*

**Atano** Milano, Thai.
Hydroxyzine hydrochloride (p.434·3).
*Anxiety disorders; hypersensitivity reactions; pruritus.*

**Atapec** Gemballa, Braz.
Homatropine methylbromide (p.483·2); furazolidone (p.605·2); pectin (p.1580·3).
*Diarrhoea.*

**Atapryl** Athena Neurosciences, USA.
Selegiline hydrochloride (p.1214·1).

**Atarax**
Pfizer, Austral.†; UCB, Austria; UCB, Belg.; Pfizer, Canad.; UCB, Denm.; UCB, Fin.; UCB, Fr.; UCB, Ger.; UCB, Gr.; UCB, Hong Kong; UCB, India; Pfizer, Irl.†; UCB, Ital.; UCB, Malaysia; Riker, Mex.†; UCB, Neth.; UCB, Norw.; UCB, Port.; UCB, Singapore; UCB, Spain; UCB, Swed.; UCB, Switz.; UCB, Thai.; Pfizer, UK; Pfizer, USA.
Hydroxyzine (p.435·1), hydroxyzine embonate (p.434·3), or hydroxyzine hydrochloride (p.434·3).
*Alcohol withdrawal syndrome; anxiety; insomnia; motion sickness; nausea and vomiting; premedication; pruritus; senile agitation; urticaria.*

**Ataraxone** Lazar, Arg.
Hydroxyzine hydrochloride (p.434·3).
*Allergic conjunctivitis; allergic rhinitis; allergic skin disorders; anxiety; premedication.*

**Atarin** Leiras, Fin.
Amantadine hydrochloride (p.1197·2).
*Influenza A; parkinsonism.*

**Atarone** Vinas, Spain†.
Pantethine (p.978·3).
*Hyperlipidaemias.*

**Atarviton** Erfar, Gr.
Diazepam (p.690·1).
*Alcohol withdrawal syndrome; anxiety disorders; premedication; skeletal muscle spasm; sleep disorders; status epilepticus; tetanus.*

**Atasol** Carter Horner, Canad.
Paracetamol (p.76·2).
*Fever; pain.*

**Atasol-8, -15, -30** Carter Horner, Canad.
Paracetamol (p.76·2); codeine phosphate (p.27·1); caffeine citrate (p.782·1).
*Fever; pain.*

**Atassol** Solfran, Mex.
Dextromethorphan (p.1117·3).
*Coughs.*

**Atatosse Balsamico** Windson, Braz.†.
Potassium iodide (p.1598·1); menthol (p.1711·3).
*Respiratory-tract congestion.*

**Atazid** AstraZeneca, Denm.
Candesartan cilexetil (p.878·3); hydrochlorothiazide (p.933·2).
*Hypertension.*

**Atd** Biolab, Thai.
Fluoxetine hydrochloride (p.292·1).
*Depression.*

**Ate** ABZ, Ger.
Atenolol (p.865·2).
*Angina pectoris; arrhythmias; hypertension.*

**Ate Lich** Lichtenstein, Ger.
Atenolol (p.865·2).
*Angina pectoris; arrhythmias; hypertension; myocardial infarction.*

**Ate Lich comp** Lichtenstein, Ger.
Atenolol (p.865·2); chlortalidone (p.882·3).
*Hypertension.*

**Atebemyxine** Chauvin, Fr.
Neomycin sulfate (p.235·1); polymyxin B sulfate (p.245·1).
*Bacterial eye infections.*

**Ateben** Pharmacia, Arg.
Nortriptyline hydrochloride (p.310·2).
*Depression.*

**Atebeta** Betapharm, Ger.
Atenolol (p.865·2).
*Angina pectoris; arrhythmias; hypertension.*

**Atecard**
Cazi, Braz.; Dabur, India.
Atenolol (p.865·2).
*Angina pectoris; arrhythmias; hypertension.*

**Atecard-D** Dabur, India.
Atenolol (p.865·2); chlortalidone (p.882·3).
*Hypertension.*

**Atecor** Rowex, Irl.
Atenolol (p.865·2).
*Angina pectoris; arrhythmias; hypertension; myocardial infarction.*

**Atedurex** Ecosol, Switz.
Atenolol (p.865·2); chlortalidone (p.882·3).
*Hypertension.*

**Atege** Fresenius Kabi, Spain.
Antithymocyte immunoglobulin (rabbit) (p.1348·3).
*Transplant rejection.*

**Atehexal**
Hexal, Austral.; Hexal, Austria; Hexal, Ger.
Atenolol (p.865·2).
*Angina pectoris; arrhythmias; hypertension; myocardial infarction.*

**Atehexal comp** Hexal, Ger.
Atenolol (p.865·2); chlortalidone (p.882·3).
*Hypertension.*

**Atel**
Note. This name is used for preparations of different composition.
Hexal, Arg.
Atenolol (p.865·2).
*Angina pectoris; arrhythmias; heart failure; hypertension; myocardial infarction.*

Betapharm, Ger.
Atenolol (p.865·2); chlortalidone (p.882·3).
*Hypertension.*

**Atel C** Hexal, Arg.
Atenolol (p.865·2); chlortalidone (p.882·3).
*Hypertension.*

**Atel N** Hexal, Arg.
Atenolol (p.865·2); nifedipine (p.966·2).
*Angina pectoris; hypertension.*

**Atelec** Mochida, Jpn.
Cilnidipine (p.884·1).
*Hypertension.*

**Atem** Promedica, Ital.
Ipratropium bromide (p.787·1).
*Obstructive airways disease.*

**Atemaron N R30** Reckeweg, Ger.
Homoeopathic preparation.

**Atemperator**
Note. This name is used for preparations of different composition.
Armstrong, Arg.
Bromazepam (p.671·3).
*Anxiety.*

Drugtech, Chile; Armstrong, Mex.
Magnesium valproate (p.382·2) or sodium valproate (p.380·1).
*Epilepsy; migraine.*

**Atemur** GlaxoSmithKline, Ger.
Fluticasone propionate (p.1102·3).
*Asthma.*

**Atenase** UCI, Braz.
Niclosamide (p.110·1).
*Cestode infections.*

**Atenativ**
Pharmacia, Austria; Biovitrum, Denm.; Pharmacia, Fin.; Pharmacia, Ger.; Pharmacia Upjohn, Ital.; Pharmacia, Neth.; Biovitrum, Norw.; Pharmacia, Spain; Biovitrum, Swed.; ZLB, Switz.
Antithrombin III (p.742·2).
*Antithrombin III deficiency.*

**Atenblock** Pharmacia, Fin.
Atenolol (p.865·2).
*Angina pectoris; arrhythmias; hypertension; hyperthyroidism; myocardial infarction.*

**Atendol** Pohl, Ger.
Atenolol (p.865·2).
*Arrhythmias; hypertension; ischaemic heart disease; myocardial infarction.*

**Ateneo** Neo Quimica, Braz.
Atenolol (p.865·2).
*Arrhythmias; hypertension.*

**Atenet** Nettopharma, Denm.
Atenolol (p.865·2).
*Angina pectoris; arrhythmias; hypertension; myocardial infarction.*

**Atenetic** Gerard, Irl.
Atenolol (p.865·2); chlortalidone (p.882·3).
*Hypertension.*

**Atenfar** Medipharm, Chile.
Atorvastatin calcium (p.866·1).
*Hypercholesterolaemia.*

**Ateni** Gerard, Irl.
Atenolol (p.865·2).
*Angina pectoris; arrhythmias; hypertension; myocardial infarction.*

**AteNif beta** Betapharm, Ger.
Atenolol (p.865·2); nifedipine (p.966·2).
*Hypertension.*

**Ate-Nife** Rowex, Irl.†.
Atenolol (p.865·2); nifedipine (p.966·2).
*Angina pectoris; hypertension.*

**Atenigron** Mitim, Ital.
Atenolol (p.865·2); chlortalidone (p.882·3).
*Hypertension.*

**Atenil** Ecosol, Switz.
Atenolol (p.865·2).
*Angina pectoris; arrhythmias; hypertension; myocardial infarction.*

**Atenix**
Note. This name is used for preparations of different composition.
Raffo, Arg.
Sertraline (p.317·3).
*Depression.*

Tecnofarma, Chile.
Sibutramine hydrochloride (p.1593·1).
*Obesity.*

Ashbourne, UK.
Atenolol (p.865·2).
*Angina pectoris; arrhythmias; hypertension.*

**AtenixCo** Ashbourne, UK.
Atenolol (p.865·2); chlortalidone (p.882·3).
These ingredients can be described by the British Approved Name Co-tenidone.
*Hypertension.*

**Ateno**
Alpharma-Isis, Ger.; Jean-Marie, Hong Kong.
Atenolol (p.865·2).
*Alcohol withdrawal syndrome; angina pectoris; arrhythmias; hypertension; hyperthyroidism; migraine; myocardial infarction.*

**Ateno comp** Alpharma-Isis, Ger.
Atenolol (p.865·2); chlortalidone (p.882·3).
*Hypertension.*

**ateno-basan** Schonenberger, Switz.
Atenolol (p.865·2).
*Angina pectoris; arrhythmias; hypertension; myocardial infarction.*

**ateno-basan comp.** Schonenberger, Switz.
Atenolol (p.865·2); chlortalidone (p.882·3).
*Hypertension.*

**Atenobene** Ratiopharm, Austria.
Atenolol (p.865·2).
*Angina pectoris; arrhythmias; hypertension; myocardial infarction.*

**Atenobene comp** Ratiopharm, Austria.
Atenolol (p.865·2); chlortalidone (p.882·3).
*Hypertension.*

**Atenoblock** Klonal, Arg.
Atenolol (p.865·2).
*Hypertension.*

**Atenoblok** Triomed, S.Afr.
Atenolol (p.865·2).
*Angina pectoris; hypertension; myocardial infarction.*

**Atenoblok Co** Triomed, S.Afr.
Atenolol (p.865·2); chlortalidone (p.882·3).
*Hypertension.*

**Atenodan** Pharmacodane, Denm.
Atenolol (p.865·2).
*Angina pectoris; arrhythmias; hypertension; myocardial infarction.*

**Atenogamma** Worwag, Ger.
Atenolol (p.865·2).
*Angina pectoris; arrhythmias; hypertension.*

**Atenogamma comp** Worwag, Ger.
Atenolol (p.865·2); chlortalidone (p.882·3).
*Hypertension.*

**Atenogen** Antigen, Irl.
Atenolol (p.865·2).
*Angina pectoris; arrhythmias; hypertension; myocardial infarction.*

**Atenol**
AstraZeneca, Braz.; Pharmacia, Fin.; CT, Ital.; TO-Chemicals, Thai.
Atenolol (p.865·2).
*Angina pectoris; arrhythmias; hypertension; hyperthyroidism; migraine; myocardial infarction.*

**Atenolan** Lannacher, Austria.
Atenolol (p.865·2).
*Angina pectoris; arrhythmias; hypertension; myocardial infarction.*

**Atenolan comp** Lannacher, Austria.
Atenolol (p.865·2); chlortalidone (p.882·3).
*Hypertension.*

**Atenolol AL comp** Aliud, Ger.
Atenolol (p.865·2); chlortalidone (p.882·3).
*Hypertension.*

**Atenolol comp**
Genericon, Austria; Ratiopharm, Ger.; CT, Ger.; Heumann, Ger.; Stada, Ger.
Atenolol (p.865·2); chlortalidone (p.882·3).
*Hypertension.*

**Atenomel** Clonmel, Irl.
Atenolol (p.865·2).
*Angina pectoris; arrhythmias; hypertension; myocardial infarction.*

**Atenomerck** Merck, Ger.†.
Atenolol (p.865·2).
*Angina pectoris; arrhythmias; hypertension.*

**Atenomerck comp** Merck, Ger.†.
Atenolol (p.865·2); chlortalidone (p.882·3).
*Hypertension.*

**Atenopress** Hexal, Braz.
Atenolol (p.865·2).
*Hypertension.*

**Atenor** Durascan, Denm.
Atenolol (p.865·2).
*Angina pectoris; arrhythmias; hypertension; myocardial infarction.*

**Atenoric** Neo Quimica, Braz.
Atenolol (p.865·2); chlortalidone (p.882·3).
*Hypertension.*

**Atenos**
Note. This name is used for preparations of different composition.
UCB, Austria.
Pentoxyverine (p.1126·2), pentoxyverine citrate (p.1126·2), or pentoxyverine hydrochloride (p.1126·3).
*Coughs.*

UCB, Ger.; UCB, Port.
Tulobuterol hydrochloride (p.806·3).
*Obstructive airways disease.*

**Atenotyrol** Tyrol, Austria.
Atenolol (p.865·2).
*Angina pectoris; arrhythmias; hypertension; myocardial infarction.*

**Atenotyrol comp** Tyrol, Austria.
Atenolol (p.865·2); chlortalidone (p.882·3).
*Hypertension.*

**Atens** Farmasa, Braz.
Enalapril maleate (p.909·2).
*Heart failure; hypertension.*

**Atens H** Farmasa, Braz.
Enalapril maleate (p.909·2); hydrochlorothiazide (p.933·2).
*Hypertension.*

**Atenses** Novag, Mex.
Nifedipine (p.966·2).
*Angina pectoris; hypertension.*

**Atensin** Medochemie, Thai.
Propranolol hydrochloride (p.989·3).
*Angina pectoris; arrhythmias; hypertension.*

**Atensina** Boehringer de Angeli, Braz.
Clonidine hydrochloride (p.885·2).
*Diagnosis of phaeochromocytoma; dysmenorrhoea; hypertension; menopausal disorders; migraine; opioid withdrawal syndrome; Tourette's syndrome.*

**Atenual** Tecnofarma, Chile.
Clomipramine (p.290·1).
*Depression; narcoleptic syndrome; nocturnal enuresis; obsessive-compulsive disorder; pain.*

**Atepadene**
Sidus, Arg.; Mayoly-Spindler, Fr.
Adenosine triphosphate disodium (p.1648·1).
*Fibromyalgia; fibromyositis.*

**Atepodin** Medix, Spain.
Adenosine triphosphate sodium (p.1648·1).
*Arrhythmias; muscular dystrophies; prevention of anoxia.*

**Ateran** Eurofarmaco, Ital.
A heparinoid (p.931·1).
*Thrombosis prophylaxis.*

**Aterax** UCB, S.Afr.
Hydroxyzine hydrochloride (p.434·3).
*Anxiety; hypersensitivity reactions; premedication.*

**Atereal** Realpharma, Ger.†.
Atenolol (p.865·2).
*Angina pectoris; arrhythmias; hypertension; myocardial infarction.*

**Aterina**
Eurofarma, Braz.†; Tedec Meiji, Spain.
Sulodexide (p.1009·2).
*Arteriosclerosis; atherosclerosis; thromboembolic disorders.*

**Ateriosan** Microsules Bernabo, Arg.
Amlodipine besilate (p.862·1).
*Angina pectoris; hypertension.*

**Aterkey** Inkeysa, Spain.
Lovastatin (p.949·1).
*Hypercholesterolaemia.*

**Atermin** Magis, Ital.
Atenolol (p.865·2).
*Angina pectoris; arrhythmias; hypertension; myocardial infarction.*

**Ateroclar**
Note. This name is used for preparations of different composition.
Beta, Arg.
Atorvastatin calcium (p.866·1).
*Hypercholesterolaemia.*

Drugtech, Chile.
Ticlopidine hydrochloride (p.1011·2).
*Thromboembolic disorders.*

Medibase, Ital.
Heparin sodium (p.928·1).
*Thromboembolic disorders.*

**Ateroid** Crinos, Ital.
A heparinoid (p.931·1).
Lidocaine hydrochloride (p.1377·3) is included in the intramuscular injection to alleviate the pain of injection.
*Thrombosis prophylaxis.*

**Ateroide** Breves, Braz.†.
*Ointment:* A heparinoid (p.931·1); methyl nicotinate (p.59·2).
*Inflammation.*
*Tablets:* A heparinoid (p.931·1).
*Hyperlipidaemias.*

**Ateroxide** Ripari-Gero, Ital.
A heparinoid (p.931·1).
*Thrombosis prophylaxis.*

**Atesifar** Siphar, Switz.
Atenolol (p.865·2).
*Angina pectoris; arrhythmias; hypertension.*

**At-Eze** Douglas, NZ.
Oxymetazoline hydrochloride (p.1126·1).
*Nasal congestion.*

**ATG**
Aventis, Belg.†; Fresenius, Hong Kong; Fresenius Hemocare, Singapore; Fresenius Medical, Switz.; Fresenius Kabi, Thai.
Antithymocyte immunoglobulin (rabbit) (p.1348·3).
*Graft-versus-host disease; transplant rejection.*

**Atgam**
Pharmacia, Austral.; Pharmacia Upjohn, Belg.†; Pharmacia, Canad.; Pharmacia, Hong Kong; Pharmacia Upjohn, Israel†; Pharmacia, Malaysia; Pharmacia Upjohn, Mex.; Pharmacia, NZ; Pharmacia, S.Afr.; Pharmacia, Singapore; Pharmacia, Spain; Pharmacia, Switz.; Upjohn, USA.
Antithymocyte immunoglobulin (horse) (p.1348·3).
*Aplastic anaemia; renal transplant rejection.*

**ATG-S** Fresenius, Israel.
Antithymocyte immunoglobulin (rabbit) (p.1348·3).
*Transplant rejection.*

**Athelmin** Apsen, Braz.†.
Mebendazole (p.108·2).
*Worm infections.*

**Athenol** *SMB, Belg.*
Atenolol (p.865·2).
*Angina pectoris; arrhythmias; hypertension; myocardial infarction.*

**Athera** *Lane, UK.*
Parsley (p.1728·3); vervain (p.1764·1); senna leaf (p.1288·2); clivers (p.1673·2).
*Menopausal symptoms.*

**Athero** *Ono, Hong Kong†.*
Choline bitartrate (p.1424·3); carbazochrome; rutoside; linoleic acid; vitamin A; vitamin $B_6$; vitamin E.
*Hyperlipidaemias.*

**Athimbin P** *Centeon, Austria†.*
Antithrombin III (p.742·2).
*Antithrombin III deficiency.*

**Athimil** *Organon, Chile.*
Mianserin hydrochloride (p.306·3).
*Depression.*

**Athletes Foot**
*Schering, Arg.; Scholl, Israel.*
Tolnaftate (p.410·1).
*Tinea pedis.*

**Athletes Foot Antifungal** *Pedi-Pak, Canad.†.*
Aluminium chlorohydrate (p.1142·1); undecenoic acid (p.410·3); zinc undecenoate (p.411·1).
*Tinea pedis.*

**Athletes Foot Cream** *Wallis, UK†.*
Clotrimazole (p.396·2).
*Tinea pedis.*

**Athos**
*Note. This name is used for preparations of different composition.*
*Roemmers, Arg.*
Hedera helix.
*Respiratory-tract disorders.*

*Medix, Mex.*
Dextromethorphan hydrobromide (p.1117·3).
*Coughs.*

**Athrofen** *Amino, Switz.*
Diclofenac sodium (p.32·1).
*Inflammation; musculoskeletal and joint disorders; pain.*

**Athru-Derm** *Meyer Zall, S.Afr.*
Diclofenac sodium (p.32·1).
*Inflammation; pain.*

**Athymil** *Organon, Fr.*
Mianserin hydrochloride (p.306·3).
*Depression.*

**Atiflan** *Ederka, Mex.†.*
Naproxen (p.65·1).

**Atilan** *Zambon, Braz.†.*
Fentiazac (p.43·1).
*Musculoskeletal and joint disorders.*

**Atinac** *Diffucap, Braz.*
Loratadine (p.436·1).
*Hypersensitivity reactions.*

**A-Tinic** *Polipharm, Thai.*
Tretinoin (p.1161·1).
*Sun-induced skin damage.*

**Atinorm** *Bioprogress, Ital.*
Atenolol (p.865·2); indapamide (p.938·2).
*Hypertension.*

**Atiramin** *Juste, Spain.*
Azatadine maleate (p.425·1); pseudoephedrine sulfate (p.1129·2).
*Allergic rhinitis.*

**Atirosin** *Piam, Ital.†.*
Infant feed (p.1417·1).
*Tyrosinaemia.*

**Atisuril** *Byk Gulden, Mex.*
Allopurinol (p.412·2).
*Gout; hyperuricaemia; renal calculi.*

**Atiten** *Bayer, Ital.*
Dihydrotachysterol (p.1461·3).
*Hypoparathyroidism; pseudohypoparathyroidism.*

**Ativan**
*Sigma, Austral.; Wyeth-Ayerst, Canad.; Wyeth, Hong Kong; John Wyeth, India; Wyeth, Irl.; Wyeth, Malaysia; Wyeth, Mex.; Wyeth, NZ†; Akromed, S.Afr.; Wyeth, Singapore; Wyeth-Ayerst, Thai.; Wyeth, UK; Biovail, USA.*
Lorazepam (p.704·1).
*Anxiety; insomnia; mania; nausea and vomiting; premedication; status epilepticus.*

**Ativit** *Heralds, Braz.†.*
Cyproheptadine (p.430·2); vitamins and minerals (p.1417·1).
*Reduced appetite; tonic.*

**Atizor** *Medipharm, Chile.*
Azithromycin (p.159·1).
*Bacterial infections.*

**Atkinson & Barker's Gripe Mixture** *Torbet Laboratories, UK.*
Sodium bicarbonate (p.1223·2); caraway oil (p.1667·3); dill oil (p.1680·2).
Formerly contained light magnesium carbonate, sodium bicarbonate, fennel oil, and dill oil.
*Infant colic.*

**Atlansil**
*Roemmers, Arg.; Sanofi Synthelabo, Braz.; Pharma Investi, Chile.*
Amiodarone hydrochloride (p.859·2).
*Arrhythmias.*

**Atma** *Bittner, Austria.*
Homoeopathic preparation.

**Atmadisc** *Sanol, Ger.; Schwarz, Ger.*
Salmeterol xinafoate (p.795·1); fluticasone propionate (p.1102·3).
*Obstructive airways disease.*

**Atmocol** *Adams, UK.*
A deodorant spray for use with colostomies and ileostomies.

**Atmos**
*AstraZeneca, Fin.; AstraZeneca, Norw.; Astra, Swed.*
Testosterone (p.1569·3).
*Erectile dysfunction; hypogonadism; osteoporosis.*

**Atoactive** *Bioethical, Ital.*
Fluocinolone acetonide (p.1101·2).
*Skin disorders.*

**Atock** *Yamanouchi, Jpn.*
Formoterol fumarate (p.786·1).
*Obstructive airways disease.*

**Atodel**
*Remedica, Malaysia; Remedica, Thai.*
Prazosin hydrochloride (p.985·1).
*Heart failure; hypertension; Raynaud's syndrome.*

**Atoderm**
*Note. This name is used for preparations of different composition.*
*Sanofi Synthelabo, Arg.*
Dimeticone (p.1482·1).
*Barrier preparation.*

*Bioderma, Ital.*
Emollient.
*Dry skin disorders.*

**Atolant** *SS, Jpn.*
Neticonazole hydrochloride (p.406·3).
*Fungal skin infections.*

**Atolone** *Major, USA.*
Triamcinolone (p.1110·2).
*Corticosteroid.*

**Atomase**
*Douglas, Hong Kong†; Douglas, Malaysia; Douglas, NZ; Douglas, Singapore; Douglas, Thai.; TTN, Thai.*
Beclometasone dipropionate (p.1091·1).
*Nasal polyps; rhinitis.*

**Atomic Enema** *Health Chemical, Hong Kong.*
Sodium chloride (p.1233·3).
*Constipation.*

**Atomide** *Douglas, NZ†.*
Beclometasone dipropionate (p.1091·1).
*Obstructive airways disease.*

**Atomo Desinflamante C** *Imvi, Arg.*
Amyl salicylate (p.14·3); camphor (p.1665·3); turpentine oil (p.1760·1); salicylic acid (p.1157·1); capsaicin (p.24·2).
*Musculoskeletal and joint disorders; neuralgia.*

**Atomo Desinflamante Depor** *Imvi, Arg.*
Methyl salicylate (p.59·3); menthol (p.1711·3).
*Musculoskeletal, joint, peri-articular, and soft-tissue disorders.*

**Atomo Desinflamante Familiar** *Imvi, Arg.*
Camphor (p.1665·3); menthol (p.1711·3); amyl salicylate (p.14·3); cineole (p.1672·1); terpineol (p.1752·2); guaiacol (p.1122·1).
*Musculoskeletal, joint, and soft-tissue disorders.*

**Atomo Desinflamante G** *Imvi, Arg.*
Methyl salicylate (p.59·3); menthol (p.1711·3); cineole (p.1672·1); terpineol (p.1752·2).
*Musculoskeletal, joint, peri-articular, and soft-tissue disorders; neuralgia.*

**Atomo Desinflamante Geldic** *Imvi, Arg.*
Diclofenac diethylamine (p.32·1).
*Musculoskeletal, joint, and peri-articular disorders; oedema.*

**Atomoderma A** *Imvi, Arg.*
Vitamin A (p.1451·2).
*Skin disorders.*

**Atomoderma A-D** *Imvi, Arg.*
Vitamin A (p.1451·2); vitamin D (p.1461·2); cod-liver oil (p.1425·2).
*Skin disorders.*

**Atomoderma A-E** *Imvi, Arg.*
Vitamin A palmitate (p.1453·1); tocoferil acetate (p.1465·1); allantoin (p.1141·3).
*Skin disorders.*

**Atomoderma Plus** *Imvi, Arg.*
Hydrocortisone (p.1103·3); fish-liver oil; cod-liver oil (p.1425·2); zinc oxide (p.1163·2).
*Anorectal disorders; skin disorders.*

**Atopic** *Dermoteca, Port.*
*Bath gel:* Lactic acid (p.1704·1).
*Cream; topical emulsion:* Evening primrose oil (p.1686·3); lactic acid (p.1704·1).
*Dry skin disorders.*

**Atopil** *IDI, Ital.*
Borage oil; vitamins; selenium (p.1417·1).
*Nutritional supplement.*

**Atorva** *Zydus, India.*
Atorvastatin calcium (p.866·1).
*Hyperlipidaemias.*

**Atorvastan** *Biotenk, Arg.*
Atorvastatin (p.866·2).
*Hypercholesterolaemia.*

**Atosil** *Bayer, Ger.*
Promethazine hydrochloride (p.439·1).
*Agitation; hypersensitivity reactions; insomnia; nausea and vomiting; restlessness.*

**Atossion** *Elofar, Braz.*
Dropropizine (p.1119·3).
*Coughs.*

**Atossisclerol Kreussler** *Also, Ital.*
Lauromacrogol 400 (p.1412·3).
*Sclerotherapy of varices.*

**Atoxecar** *Beta, Arg.*
Oxcarbazepine (p.366·3).
*Epilepsy.*

**ATP** *Hebron, Braz.*
Amino-acid preparation (p.1417·1).

**Atractil**
*Trenker, Belg.†; Trenker, Thai.*
Diethylpropion (p.1587·1).
*Obesity.*

**Atracur** *Libra, Braz.†.*
Atracurium besilate (p.1399·1).
*Competitive neuromuscular blocker.*

**Atralcilina** *Atral, Port.†.*
Benzylpenicillin potassium (p.163·2); procaine benzylpenicillin (p.246·1).
*Bacterial infections.*

**Atralidon** *Atral, Port.*
Paracetamol (p.76·2).
*Fever; pain.*

**Atralmicina** *Atral, Port.*
Benethamine penicillin (p.162·3); benzylpenicillin sodium (p.163·2).
*Bacterial infections.*

**Atretol** *Athena Neurosciences, USA†.*
Carbamazepine (p.353·3).
*Epilepsy; trigeminal neuralgia.*

**Atrican** *Innotech, Fr.*
Tenonitrozole (p.616·3).
*Urogenital trichomoniasis.*

**Atridox**
*Meda, Fin.; Meda, Swed.; Atrix, UK†; CollaGenex, USA.*
Doxycycline hyclate (p.206·2).
*Bacterial mouth infections.*

**Atrilon** *Byk, Port.*
Lonazolac calcium (p.54·2).
*Musculoskeletal, joint, and peri-articular disorders; pain.*

**Atrimon** *Elvetium, Arg.*
Algestone acetophenide (p.1541·3); estradiol enantate (p.1550·1).
*Combined oral contraceptive.*

**Atriscal** *Lacer, Spain.*
Dexibuprofen (p.46·1).
*Dysmenorrhoea; osteoarthritis; pain.*

**Atrisol** *Quimica y Farmacia, Mex.*
Captopril (p.879·2).
*Hypertension.*

**Atrisolon** *Andre, India.*
Atropine sulfate (p.477·1); prednisolone (p.1108·1).
*Inflammatory eye disorders.*

**Atrium**
*Riom, Fr.†.*
Febarbamate (p.698·2); difebarbamate (p.697·2); phenobarbital (p.367·3).
*Alcohol withdrawal syndrome.*

*Roche, Switz.†.*
Tetrabamate, a complex of febarbamate (p.698·2), difebarbamate (p.697·2), and phenobarbital (p.367·3).
*Anxiety disorders; tremor.*

**Atrival** *Careiatrics, Arg.*
Amoxicillin (p.155·3).
*Bacterial infections.*

**Atro Grin** *Grin, Mex.*
Atropine sulfate (p.477·1).
*Production of mydriasis.*

**Atrobel** *Fawns & McAllan, Austral.*
Belladonna herb (p.479·1).
*Peptic ulcer; reduction of secretions; smooth muscle spasm.*

**Atrodual** *Boehringer Ingelheim, Fin.*
Ipratropium bromide (p.787·1); salbutamol sulfate (p.791·3).
*Obstructive airways disease.*

**Atrohist Pediatric** *Medeva, USA†.*
*Capsules:* Pseudoephedrine hydrochloride (p.1129·2); chlorphenamine maleate (p.427·3).
Formerly contained brompheniramine maleate, phenyltoloxamine citrate and phenylephrine hydrochloride.
*Allergic rhinitis; cold symptoms; sinusitis.*
*Oral suspension:* Chlorphenamine tannate (p.428·1); phenylephrine tannate (p.1127·2); mepyramine tannate (p.437·1).
*Cold symptoms; nasal congestion.*

**Atrohist Plus** *Medeva, USA†.*
Phenylpropanolamine hydrochloride (p.1127·3); phenylephrine hydrochloride (p.1126·3); chlorphenamine maleate (p.427·3); hyoscyamine sulfate (p.485·1); atropine sulfate (p.477·1); hyoscine hydrobromide (p.483·3).
*Upper respiratory-tract symptoms.*

**Atrombin** *Leiras, Fin.*
Dipyridamole (p.903·1).
*Thromboembolic disorders.*

**Atromicin** *Teuto, Braz.*
Azithromycin (p.159·1).
*Bacterial infections.*

**Atromidin**
*Zeneca, Belg.†; Zeneca, Denm.†; Zeneca, Swed.†.*
Clofibrate (p.884·3).
*Hyperlipidaemias; prophylaxis of ischaemic heart disease in high-risk patients.*

**Atromid-S**
*Wyeth-Ayerst, Canad.†; Zeneca, Hong Kong†; Zeneca, Irl.†; Zeneca, Mex.†; AstraZeneca, NZ†; Zeneca, Port.; Zeneca, S.Afr.†; AstraZeneca, UK†; Wyeth-Ayerst, USA†.*
Clofibrate (p.884·3).
*Diabetic retinopathy; hyperlipidaemias.*

**Atronase**
*Boehringer Ingelheim, Austria†; Boehringer Ingelheim, Belg.*
Ipratropium bromide (p.787·1).
*Rhinitis.*

**Atrop** *Upha, Malaysia.*
Atropine sulfate (p.477·1).
*Production of mydriasis and cycloplegia.*

**AtroPen** *Survival Technology, USA.*
Atropine sulfate (p.477·1).
*Organophosphorus or carbamate pesticide poisoning.*

**Atropine and Demerol** *Sanofi Winthrop, USA†.*
Atropine sulfate (p.477·1); pethidine hydrochloride (p.80·2).
*Sedative.*

**Atropinol** *Winzer, Ger.*
Atropine (p.476·3).
*Production of mydriasis.*

**Atropion** *Ariston, Braz.*
Atropine sulfate (p.477·1).
*Arrhythmias.*

**Atropisol**
*Novartis Ophthalmics, Canad.; Novartis Ophthalmics, USA†.*
Atropine sulfate (p.477·1).
*Production of mydriasis and cycloplegia.*

**Atropocil** *Edol, Port.*
Atropine sulfate (p.477·1).
*Production of mydriasis and cycloplegia.*

**Atropt**
*Sigma, Austral.; Sigma, NZ.*
Atropine sulfate (p.477·1).
*Production of cycloplegia and mydriasis.*

**Atrosept** *Geneva, USA.*
Methenamine (p.230·1); salol (p.88·1); atropine sulfate (p.477·1); hyoscyamine sulfate (p.485·1); benzoic acid (p.1169·3); methylthioninium chloride (p.1042·2).
*Urinary-tract infections.*

**Atrospan** *Fischer, Israel.*
Atropine sulfate (p.477·1).
*Production of cycloplegia and mydriasis.*

**Atrotil** *Raza, Malaysia; Pharmaniaga, Malaysia.*
Diphenoxylate hydrochloride (p.1261·3).
Atropine sulfate (p.477·1) is included in this preparation to discourage abuse.
*Diarrhoea.*

**Atrovent**
*Boehringer Ingelheim, Arg.; Boehringer Ingelheim, Austral.; Boehringer Ingelheim, Austria; Boehringer Ingelheim, Belg.; Boehringer de Angeli, Braz.; Boehringer Ingelheim, Canad.; Boehringer Ingelheim, Chile; Boehringer Ingelheim, Denm.; Boehringer Ingelheim, Fin.; Boehringer Ingelheim, Fr.; Boehringer Ingelheim, Ger.; Boehringer Ingelheim, Gr.; Boehringer Ingelheim, Hong Kong; Boehringer Ingelheim, Irl.; Boehringer Ingelheim, Ital.†; Teijin, Jpn; Boehringer Ingelheim, Malaysia; Boehringer Ingelheim, Mex.; Boehringer Ingelheim, Neth.; Boehringer Ingelheim, Norw.; Boehringer Ingelheim, NZ; Boehringer Ingelheim, Port.; Boehringer Ingelheim, S.Afr.; Boehringer Ingelheim, Singapore; Boehringer Ingelheim, Spain; Boehringer Ingelheim, Swed.; Boehringer Ingelheim, Switz.; Boehringer Ingelheim, Thai.; Boehringer Ingelheim, UK; Boehringer Ingelheim, USA.*
Ipratropium bromide (p.787·1).
*Obstructive airways disease; rhinitis.*

**Atrovent Beta** *Boehringer Ingelheim, S.Afr.*
Ipratropium bromide (p.787·1); fenoterol hydrobromide (p.785·2).
*Obstructive airways disease.*

**Atrovent Comp** *Boehringer Ingelheim, Fin.*
Ipratropium bromide (p.787·1); fenoterol hydrobromide (p.785·2).
*Obstructive airways disease.*

**Atroveran** *Virtus, Braz.†.*
*Oral solution:* Papaverine hydrochloride (p.1728·1); belladonna (p.479·1); star anise; hyoscyamus (p.485·2); boldo (p.1661·2).
*Smooth muscle spasm.*
*Tablets:* Papaverine hydrochloride (p.1728·1); aspirin (p.15·1); belladonna (p.479·1).
*Pain; smooth muscle spasm.*

**Atrovex** *Medquimica, Braz.†.*
Papaverine (p.1728·1); belladonna (p.479·1); star anise; hyoscyamus (p.485·2); boldo (p.1661·2).
*Smooth muscle spasm.*

**ATS** *Hoechst Marion Roussel, USA.*
Erythromycin (p.208·1).
*Acne.*

**Atse** *IA, Ger.*
Acetylcysteine (p.1112·3).
*Respiratory-tract disorders with excess and viscous mucus.*

**Atta** *Ranbaxy, Thai.†.*
Activated attapulgite (p.1251·1).
*Diarrhoea.*

**Attafur** *Ranbaxy, Thai.†.*
Activated attapulgite (p.1251·1); furazolidone (p.605·2).
*Diarrhoea.*

**Attain** *Sherwood, USA.*
Lactose-free preparation for enteral nutrition (p.1417·1).

**Attenta** *Alphapharm, Austral.*
Methylphenidate hydrochloride (p.1590·2).
*Attention-deficit hyperactivity disorder; narcoleptic syndrome.*

**Attenuvax**
Prodome, Braz.†; Aventis Pasteur, Denm.; Pasteur Merieux, Ital.†; Pro Vaccine, Switz.; Merck, USA.
A live measles vaccine (more attenuated Enders' Edmonston strain) (p.1623·1).
*Active immunisation.*

**Aturgyl**
Note. This name is used for preparations of different composition.
GlaxoSmithKline, Braz.
Fenoxazoline hydrochloride (p.1121·3).
*Nasal congestion.*
Sanofi Synthelabo, Fr.
Oxymetazoline hydrochloride (p.1126·1).
*Rhinopharyngeal congestion.*

**Atus** Metapharma, Ital.
Ambroxol hydrochloride (p.1114·3).
*Respiratory-tract disorders.*

**Atusil** Recalcine, Chile.
Promolate (p.1129·2).
*Coughs.*

**Atuss DM** Atley, USA.
Dextromethorphan hydrobromide (p.1117·3); phenylephrine hydrochloride (p.1126·3); chlorphenamine maleate (p.427·3).
*Coughs and associated respiratory-tract disorders.*

**Atuss-12 DM** Atley, USA.
Pseudoephedrine polistirex (p.1130·1); chlorphenamine polistirex (p.428·1); dextromethorphan polistirex (p.1118·1).
*Upper respiratory-tract disorders.*

**Atuss-12 DX** Atley, USA.
Dextromethorphan polistirex (p.1118·1); guaifenesin (p.1122·1).
*Coughs.*

**Atuss EX** Atley, USA.
Hydrocodone tartrate (p.45·1); guaifenesin (p.1122·1).
*Coughs and associated respiratory-tract disorders.*

**Atuss G** Atley, USA.
Hydrocodone tartrate (p.45·1); phenylephrine hydrochloride (p.1126·3); guaifenesin (p.1122·1).
*Coughs and associated respiratory-tract disorders.*

**Atuss HD** Atley, USA.
Hydrocodone tartrate (p.45·1); phenylephrine hydrochloride (p.1126·3); chlorphenamine maleate (p.427·3).

**Atuxane** Monot, Fr.†.
Dextromethorphan hydrobromide (p.1117·3).
*Coughs.*

**AT-V** Offenbach, Mex.
Diazepam (p.690·1).

**AU 4 Regeneresen** Dyckerhoff, Ger.
Ribonucleic acid (p.1738·2).
*Ear disorders.*

**Aubeline** Arkopharma, Fr.
Crataegus (p.1677·1).
*Cardiac disorders; nervous disorders.*

**Aubril** Novartis, India.
Trimethoprim (p.272·2); sulfadiazine (p.258·2).
*Bacterial infections.*

**Aucusik** Andromaco, Chile.
Benzocaine (p.1370·3); benzethonium chloride (p.1169·2); benzyl alcohol (p.1170·2); menthol (p.1711·3).
*Pruritus.*

**Audax**
Mundipharma, Ger.; SSL, Irl.; SSL, UK.
Choline salicylate (p.26·2).
*Ear wax removal; earache.*

**Audazol** Lesvi, Spain.
Omeprazole (p.1278·2).
*Gastro-oesophageal reflux; peptic ulcer; Zollinger-Ellison syndrome.*

**Audicort**
Wyeth, Irl.; Goldshield, UK.
Neomycin undecylenate (p.235·2); triamcinolone acetonide (p.1110·2).
Formerly contained benzocaine, triamcinolone acetonide, and neomycin undecenoate in the *UK*.
*Inflammatory ear disorders with bacterial infection.*

**Audifluor** Diba, Mex.
Sodium fluoride (p.1444·3).
*Otosclerosis.*

**Audione** Serra Pamies, Spain.
Vitamins (p.1417·1); potassium iodide (p.1598·1).
*Ear disorders; eye disorders.*

**Audispray** Diepharmex, Fr.
Sea water.
*External ear hygiene.*

**Auditol** Sanofi Synthelabo, Braz.†.
Phenazone (p.82·3); procaine (p.1383·2).
*Inflammatory ear disorders.*

**Augelit** Catarinense, Braz.
Diclofenac sodium (p.32·1).
*Inflammation; pain.*

**Augenkraft** Twardy, Ger.†.
Vitamin A (p.1451·2).
*Night-blindness.*

**Augentonicum** Vifor, Switz.
Digitalis (p.894·2); digitoxin (p.894·3); esculoside (p.1648·2).
*Eye disorders.*

**Augentonikum N** Stulln, Ger.
Digitalin (p.1680·1).
Formerly contained digitalin and vitamin A palmitate.
*Eyestrain.*

**Augentropfen Mucokehl D5** Sanum-Kehlbeck, Ger.
Homoeopathic preparation.

**Augentropfen Stulln** Sanova, Austria.
Digitalis (p.894·2); esculoside (p.1648·2).

**Augentropfen Stulln Mono** Stulln, Ger.
Digitalis leaf (p.894·2); esculoside (p.1648·2).
*Eyestrain.*

**Augmaxil** Triomed, S.Afr.
Amoxicillin (p.155·3); clavulanic acid (p.193·3).
*Bacterial infections.*

**Augmentan** GlaxoSmithKline, Ger.
Amoxicillin sodium (p.155·3) or amoxicillin trihydrate (p.155·3); potassium clavulanate (p.193·3).
*Bacterial infections.*

**Augmentin**
GlaxoSmithKline, Austral.; GlaxoSmithKline, Austria; GlaxoSmithKline, Belg.; SmithKline Beecham, Braz.†; GlaxoSmithKline, Chile; GlaxoSmithKline, Fin.; GlaxoSmithKline, Fr.; SmithKline Beecham, Gr.; GlaxoSmithKline, Hong Kong; GlaxoSmithKline, India; GlaxoSmithKline, Irl.; SmithKline Beecham, Israel; GlaxoSmithKline, Ital.; GlaxoSmithKline, Malaysia; SmithKline Beecham, Mex.; GlaxoSmithKline, Neth.; GlaxoSmithKline, NZ; Beecham, Port.; GlaxoSmithKline, S.Afr.; GlaxoSmithKline, Singapore; SmithKline Beecham, Switz.; GlaxoSmithKline, Thai.; GlaxoSmithKline, UK; GlaxoSmithKline, USA.
Amoxicillin sodium (p.155·3) or amoxicillin trihydrate (p.155·3); potassium clavulanate (p.193·3).
These ingredients can be described by the British Approved Name Co-amoxiclav.
*Bacterial infections.*

**Augmentin Bid** GlaxoSmithKline, Chile.
Amoxicillin trihydrate (p.155·3); potassium clavulanate (p.193·3).
*Bacterial infections.*

**Augmentin-Duo** GlaxoSmithKline, UK.
Amoxicillin trihydrate (p.155·3); potassium clavulanate (p.193·3).
These ingredients can be described by the British Approved Name Co-amoxiclav.
*Bacterial infections.*

**Augmentine** GlaxoSmithKline, Spain.
Amoxicillin sodium (p.155·3) or amoxicillin trihydrate (p.155·3); potassium clavulanate (p.193·3).
*Bacterial infections.*

**Aulcer** Alacan, Spain.
Omeprazole (p.1278·2).
*Gastro-oesophageal reflux; peptic ulcer; Zollinger-Ellison syndrome.*

**Aulin**
Grunenthal, Arg.; CSC, Austria; Essex, Chile; Helsinn Birex, Irl.; Roche, Ital.; Helsinn, Port.; Roche, Switz.
Nimesulide (p.67·1).
*Fever; inflammation; musculoskeletal, joint, and periarticular disorders; pain.*

**Aulo Gelio Pie** Aulo Gelio, Arg.
Camphor (p.1665·3); vitamin A (p.1451·2).
*Foot disorders.*

**Aulo Gelio Repelente** Aulo Gelio, Arg.
Citronella oil (p.1673·2).
*Insect repellent.*

**Aunativ**
Pharmacia, Austria; Biovitrum, Denm.; Pharmacia Upjohn, Ger.†; Biovitrum, Norw.; Biovitrum, Swed.
A hepatitis B immunoglobulin (p.1617·2).
*Passive immunisation.*

**Aunativ S.D.** Pharmacia-Upjohn, Gr.
A hepatitis B immunoglobulin (p.1617·2).
*Passive immunisation.*

**Auralgan**
Note. This name is used for preparations of different composition.
Whitehall Consumer, Austral.; Whitehall-Robins, Canad.; Whitehall, NZ.; Wyeth-Ayerst, USA.
Benzocaine (p.1370·3); phenazone (p.82·3); glycerol (p.1694·3).
*Acute otitis media; ear wax removal.*
Wyeth-Ayerst, Thai.
Benzocaine (p.1370·3); phenazone (p.82·3).
*Ear wax removal; otitis media.*

**Auralgicin** Roche, S.Afr.†.
Ephedrine hydrochloride (p.1120·1); phenazone (p.82·3); benzocaine (p.1370·3); potassium hydroxyquinoline sulfate (p.1734·2).
*Otitis media.*

**Auralyt** Wyeth, Mex.
Benzocaine (p.1370·3).

**Auram** Ache, Braz.
Oxcarbazepine (p.366·3).
*Epilepsy.*

**Auramin** Solco, Austria.
Minocycline hydrochloride (p.231·3).
*Bacterial infections.*

**Aurantin** Parke, Davis, Ital.
Phenytoin sodium (p.370·2).
*Arrhythmias; epilepsy.*

**Auraphene-B** Reese, USA.
Urea hydrogen peroxide (p.1195·3).

**Aurasept** Rolab, S.Afr.
Benzocaine (p.1370·3); phenazone (p.82·3).
*Otitis.*

**Auratek hCG** Bio Merieux, UK.
Pregnancy test (p.1734·3).

**Aureciclina** Sanval, Braz.
Tetracycline hydrochloride (p.266·2).
*Bacterial infections.*

**Aurecil** Edol, Port.
Chlortetracycline hydrochloride (p.187·3).
*Bacterial eye infections.*

**Aurene** Armstrong, Arg.
Oxcarbazepine (p.366·3).
*Epilepsy; trigeminal neuralgia.*

**Aureocort**
Wyeth Lederle, Austria; Wyeth Lederle, Fin.†; Wyeth, Irl.†; Teofarma, Ital.; Goldshield, UK.
Chlortetracycline hydrochloride (p.187·3); triamcinolone acetonide (p.1110·2).
*Infected skin disorders.*

**Aureocrem** Puebla, Arg.
Polysaccharides of *Pseudomonas aeruginosa*.

**Aureodelf** Lederle, Ger.
Chlortetracycline hydrochloride (p.187·3); triamcinolone acetonide (p.1110·2).
*Infected skin disorders.*

**Aureodermil** Edol, Port.
Chlortetracycline hydrochloride (p.187·3).
*Bacterial skin infections.*

**Aureomicina**
Wyeth Lederle, Ital.; Wyeth, Mex.†; Alcon, Port.†; Alcon Cusi, Spain; Novartis, Spain.
Chlortetracycline hydrochloride (p.187·3).
*Bacterial infections.*

**Aureomix** SIT, Ital.
Chlortetracycline hydrochloride (p.187·3); sulfacetamide sodium (p.257·3).
*Ear, nose, mouth, throat, and eye infections.*

**Aureomycin**
Wyeth, Austral.†; Wyeth Lederle, Austria; Wyeth Lederle, Belg.; Wyeth-Ayerst, Canad.†; Wyeth Lederle, Denm.†; Wyeth Lederle, Fin.†; Lederle, Ger.; Wyeth, Hong Kong; Wyeth, Irl.†; Lederle, Israel†; Lederle, Neth.†; Wyeth Lederle, Norw.; Wyeth, NZ†; Wyeth, S.Afr.†; Wyeth Lederle, Swed.†; Wyeth-Ayerst, Thai.; Wyeth, UK†.
Chlortetracycline hydrochloride (p.187·3).
*Bacterial infections.*

**Aureomycin N** Wyeth, Ger.
Chlortetracycline hydrochloride (p.187·3); nystatin (p.406·3).
*Vaginal infections.*

**Aureomycine**
Viatris, Belg.; Celltech, Fr.; Lederle, Switz.†.
Chlortetracycline hydrochloride (p.187·3).
*Bacterial infections.*

**Aureotan** Tosse, Ger.†.
Aurothioglucose (p.19·3).
*Chronic polyarthritis; psoriatic arthritis.*

**Auricid** Day, Ital.
Cefonicid sodium (p.174·2).
Lidocaine hydrochloride (p.1377·3) is included in this preparation to alleviate the pain of injection.
*Bacterial infections.*

**Auricularum**
Grimberg, Fr.; Serolam, Israel.
Oxytetracycline hydrochloride (p.241·1); polymyxin B sulfate (p.245·1); dexamethasone sodium phosphate (p.1097·2); nystatin (p.406·3).
*Otitis.*

**Auricum** Dolisos, Canad.
Homoeopathic preparation.

**Auriderm Corps** Finn Vita, Chile.
Vitamin K (p.1466·3).
*Skin discoloration.*

**Auridonal** Ducto, Braz.
Chloramphenicol (p.185·1).
*Bacterial ear infections.*

**Aurigen** Mavi, Mex.
Allopurinol (p.412·2).
*Hyperuricaemia.*

**Aurigoutte** Merck Medication Familiale, Fr.
Hexamidine isetionate (p.1181·3); lidocaine hydrochloride (p.1377·3).
*Ear disorders.*

**Aurisan** Nadeau, Canad.†.
Benzocaine (p.1370·3); camphor (p.1665·3); chlorobutanol (p.1176·3).
*Ear ache.*

**Auristan** Monin, Fr.
Phenylephrine hydrochloride (p.1126·3).
*Otitis externa.*

**Aurita-Bronchialtee** Bittner, Austria.
Althaea (p.1651·3); plantago lanceolata (p.1738·2); thyme (p.1755·2); aniseed (p.1655·2).
*Coughs and cold symptoms.*

**Aurita-Erkaltungstee** Bittner, Austria.
Sambucus (p.1741·3); tilia (p.1756·2); chamomile (p.1669·3); althaea (p.1651·3).
*Cold symptoms.*

**Aurita-Leber-Galletee** Bittner, Austria.
Taraxacum (p.1751·3); peppermint leaf (p.1283·2); achillea (p.1646·2); chamomile (p.1669·3).
*Liver and biliary-tract disorders.*

**Aurita-Nerventee** Bittner, Austria.
Melissa (p.1711·1); bitter-orange peel (p.1723·3); chamomile (p.1669·3); valerian (p.1762·2).
*Nervous disorders.*

**Aurita-Nieren-Blasentee** Bittner, Austria.
Ononis (p.1723·3); equisetum (p.1684·1); viola tricolor; juniper berry (p.1703·1).
*Kidney and bladder disorders.*

**Aurita-Verdauungstee** Bittner, Austria.
Chamomile (p.1669·3); peppermint leaf (p.1283·2); calamus (p.1664·1); fennel (p.1687·2).
*Digestive disorders.*

**Auritricin** Delta, Braz.
Tyrothricin (p.275·1); ethyl metaborate; chlorobutanol (p.1176·3).
*Ear infections.*

**Auro** Del, USA.
Urea hydrogen peroxide (p.1195·3).
*Ear wax removal.*

**Auroanalin N** Hevert, Ger.
Glycol salicylate (p.44·3).
Auroanalin formerly contained glycol salicylate and benzyl nicotinate.
*Inflammation; rheumatism.*

**Aurochobet** Chobet, Arg.
Calcium gold keratinate (p.45·1).
*Musculoskeletal and joint disorders.*

**Auroclim** Juste, Spain.
16 Tablets, estradiol valerate (p.1550·2); 12 tablets, estradiol valerate; levonorgestrel (p.1563·2).
*Menopausal disorders; osteoporosis.*

**Auro-Dri**
Del, Canad.; Del, USA.
Isopropyl alcohol (p.1184·3).
*Ear disorders.*

**Auroguard Otic** SDA, USA.
Benzocaine (p.1370·3); phenazone (p.82·3); hydroxyquinoline sulfate (p.1700·1).
*Ear disorders.*

**Auroken** Kendrick, Mex.
Fluoxetine hydrochloride (p.292·1).
*Depression; mixed anxiety depressive disorders.*

**Aurolate** Pasadena, USA.
Sodium aurothiomalate (p.88·2).

**Auromyose** Nourypharma, Neth.
Aurothioglucose (p.19·3).
*Rheumatoid arthritis.*

**Aurone** Aspen, S.Afr.
Phenazone (p.82·3).
*Earache.*

**Aurone Forte** Aspen Consumer, S.Afr.
Phenazone (p.82·3); benzocaine (p.1370·3).
*Earache.*

**Auroplatin** Steigerwald, Ger.
Homoeopathic preparation.

**Aurorex** Roche, Mex.
Moclobemide (p.308·2).
*Depression; phobias.*

**Aurorix**
Roche, Arg.; Roche, Austral.; Roche, Austria; Roche, Belg.; Roche, Braz.; Roche, Chile; Roche, Denm.; Roche, Fin.; Roche, Ger.; Roche, Gr.; Roche, Hong Kong; Roche, Ital.†; Roche, Neth.; Roche, Norw.; Roche, NZ; Roche, Port.; Roche, S.Afr.; Roche, Singapore; Roche, Swed.; Roche, Switz.; Roche, Thai.
Moclobemide (p.308·2).
*Depression; social phobia.*

**Aurosulfo** Geymonat, Ital.†.
Colloidal gold sulfide.
*Rheumatoid arthritis.*

**Aurosyx N** Syxyl, Ger.
Homoeopathic preparation.

**Auroto** Barre-National, USA.
Benzocaine (p.1370·3); phenazone (p.82·3).
*Earache.*

**Aurum-Gastreu S R2** Reckeweg, Ger.
Homoeopathic preparation.

**Aurumheel** Peithner, Austria.
Homoeopathic preparation.

**Auscap** Sigma, Austral.
Fluoxetine hydrochloride (p.292·1).
*Depression; obsessive-compulsive disorder.*

**Auscard** Sigma, Austral.
Diltiazem hydrochloride (p.900·1).
*Angina pectoris.*

**Ausclav** Sigma, Austral.
Amoxicillin trihydrate (p.155·3); potassium clavulanate (p.193·3).
*Bacterial infections.*

**Ausentron** Laboratorios Chile, Chile.
Clomipramine (p.290·1).
*Depression; nocturnal enuresis; obsessive-compulsive disorder; premature ejaculation.*

**Ausgem** Sigma, Austral.
Gemfibrozil (p.923·1).
*Hyperlipidaemias.*

**Ausobronc** Biotekfarma, Ital.†.
Mesna (p.1041·2).
*Respiratory-tract disorders.*

**Ausomina** Biotekfarma, Ital.†.
Vincamine (p.1764·2).
*Cerebrovascular disorders.*

**Auspril** Sigma, Austral.
Enalapril maleate (p.909·2).
*Heart failure; hypertension.*

**Ausran** Sigma, Austral.
Ranitidine hydrochloride (p.1285·2).
*Gastro-oesophageal reflux; peptic ulcer; Zollinger-Ellison syndrome.*

**Aussie Tan** Or-Dov, Austral.†.
*SPF 4:* Octinoxate (p.1154·3); avobenzone (p.1142·3).
*SPF 7:* Octinoxate (p.1154·3); avobenzone (p.1142·3); oxybenzone (p.1154·3).
*SPF 15 Lotion:* Octinoxate (p.1154·3); avobenzone (p.1142·3); oxybenzone (p.1154·3).
*SPF 15 Topical gel:* Octinoxate (p.1154·3); avobenzone (p.1142·3).
*Sunscreen.*

**Aussie Tan Pre-Tan** Or-Dov, Austral.†.
Tyrosine (p.1451·1); tyrosinase.
*To accelerate tanning.*

**Aussie Tan Skin Moisturiser** *Or-Dov, Austral.†.*
Urea (p.1162·2); lactic acid (p.1704·1).

**Aussie Tan Sunstick** *Or-Dov, Austral.†.*
Salol (p.88·1).
*Sunscreen.*

**Austral-Balm** *Nutri-Pharm, Austral.†.*
Melaleuca oil (p.1710·2); eucalyptus oil (p.1686·2); sweet birch oil (p.60·1); emu oil; lemon oil (p.1706·2); peppermint oil (p.1283·2).
*Musculoskeletal and joint pain.*

**Austrapen** *CSL, Austral.*
Ampicillin sodium (p.157·1).
*Bacterial infections.*

**Austrialens** *Austroflex, Austria†.*
Cleaning, wetting, and storage solutions for hard and gas-permeable contact lenses (p.1164·2).

**Austroflex** *Austroflex, Austria†.*
Range of contact lens solutions (p.1164·2).

**Austrophyllin** *Petrasch, Austria.*
Diprophylline (p.784·3).

**Austrorinse** *Austroflex, Austria†.*
Rinsing solution for contact lenses (p.1164·2).

**Austrosept** *Austroflex, Austria†.*
Hydrogen peroxide (p.1182·2) (p.1164·2).
*Disinfecting solution for soft contact lenses.*

**Austyn**
*Faulding, Austral.†; Faulding, Singapore†.*
Theophylline (p.798·3).
*Obstructive airways disease.*

**Aut** *Elea, Arg.*
Pyrantel embonate (p.113·2).
*Gastrointestinal worm infections.*

**Autan** *Bayer, Ger.†.*
Diethyltoluamide (p.1503·3).
*Insect repellent.*

**Autdol** *Laboratorios Chile, Chile.*
Diclofenac sodium (p.32·1).
*Fever; gout; inflammation; musculoskeletal and joint disorders; pain.*

**Aution Sticks 10EA** *Menarini Diagnostics, Port.*
Test for glucose, protein, bilirubin, urobilinogen, pH, specific gravity, blood, ketones, nitrites, and leucocytes in urine.

**Autohaler** *Cipla, India.*
Isoprenaline sulfate (p.940·2).
*Obstructive airways disease.*

**Autohelios** *Roche-Posay, Arg.*
Dihydroxyacetone (p.1145·2).
*Sunscreen adjunct.*

**Autonic** *Acusan, Ger.†.*
Caffeine (p.782·1).
*Fatigue.*

**Autoplasme Vaillant** *Chefaro Ardeval, Fr.*
Black mustard (p.1718·2).
*Respiratory-tract congestion.*

**Autoplex**
*Baxter, Ger.; Baxter, Swed.; Travenol, UK†.*
A factor VIII inhibitor bypassing fraction (p.752·2).
*Haemorrhage in patients with inhibitors to factor VIII.*

**Autoplex T**
*Baxter, Belg.†.; Baxter, Malaysia; Baxter, Singapore†; Baxter, Spain†; Nabi, USA.*
A factor VIII inhibitor bypassing fraction (p.752·2).
*Haemorrhage in patients with inhibitor to factor VIII.*

**Autosterile** *Allergan, Austria†.*
Contact lens cleaner (p.1164·2).

**Autrin**
*Note. This name is used for preparations of different composition.*
*Wyeth Lederle, India.*
Ferrous fumarate (p.1427·3); folic acid; vitamin $B_{12}$ (p.1417·1).
Vitamin C (p.1460·2) is included in this preparation to increase the absorption and availability of the iron.
*Anaemias.*

*Wyeth, Mex.*
Ferrous fumarate (p.1427·3); folic acid; vitamin $B_{12}$; vitamin E (p.1417·1).
Vitamin C (p.1460·2) is included in this preparation to increase the absorption and availability of iron.
*Anaemias.*

*Wyeth, S.Afr.*
Ferrous fumarate (p.1427·3); folic acid; vitamin $B_{12}$; intrinsic factor (p.1417·1).
Vitamin C (p.1460·2) is included in this preparation to increase the absorption and availability of iron.
*Anaemias.*

**Autrinic Compuesto** *Wyeth, Arg.*
Ferrous fumarate (p.1427·3); ascorbic acid; vitamin $B_{12}$; intrinsic factor; folic acid (p.1417·1).
*Anaemias.*

**Autritis** *Fariberica, Port.*
Indometacin (p.47·3).

**Auxergyl $D_3$** *Aventis, Fr.†.*
Vitamin A (p.1451·2); colecalciferol (p.1461·3).
*Vitamin A and D deficiency.*

**Auxergyl D3** *Roussel, Port.†.*
Vitamin A; vitamin D (p.1417·1).

**Auxiloson** *Boehringer Ingelheim, Ger.*
Dexamethasone isonicotinate (p.1097·2).
*Respiratory-tract disorders.*

**Auxina A + E** *Alcala, Spain.*
Vitamin A palmitate (p.1453·1); tocoferil acetate (p.1465·1).
*Deficiency of vitamins A and E; eye disorders; infertility; recurrent miscarriage; skin disorders.*

**Auxina A Masiva** *Alcala, Spain.*
Vitamin A palmitate (p.1453·1).
*Vitamin A deficiency.*

**Auxina Complejo B** *Alcala, Spain†.*
Vitamin B substances (p.1417·1).

**Auxina E** *Alcala, Spain.*
Tocoferil acetate (p.1465·1).
*Biliary-tract disorders; cystic fibrosis; hypoproteinaemia; prevention of intraventricular haemorrhage in premature neonates; vitamin E deficiency.*

**Auxitrans** *Alpharma, Fr.*
Pentaerythritol (p.1283·2).
*Constipation.*

**Auxofer** *Magis, Ital.*
Ferrous gluconate (p.1428·1).
Ascorbic acid (p.1460·2) is included in this preparation to increase the absorption and availability of iron.
*Iron-deficiency anaemia.*

**Auxxil** *Laboratorios Chile, Chile.*
Levofloxacin (p.225·3).
*Bacterial infections.*

**Avadene** *Schering, Fr.*
16 Tablets, estradiol (p.1550·1); 12 tablets, estradiol; gestodene (p.1556·1).
*Menopausal disorders; osteoporosis.*

**Avafontan** *Alpharma, Mex.*
Dipyrone (p.35·3).
*Fever; pain.*

**Avafortan** *Therabel, Fr.*
Camylofin hydrochloride (p.1666·1) or camylofin noramidopyrine mesilate (p.1666·1); dipyrone (p.35·3).
*Pain; smooth muscle spasm.*

**Avage** *Allergan, USA.*
Tazarotene (p.1160·2).
*Facial wrinkles; skin pigmentation disorders.*

**Avail** *Menley & James, USA.*
Multivitamin and mineral preparation with iron and folic acid (p.1417·1).

**Avala** *Schwabe, Spain.*
Cimicifuga (p.1671·3).
*Menopausal disorders.*

**Avaldrian** *Alpharma, Mex.*
Dipyrone (p.35·3).
*Fever; pain.*

**Avalide**
*Bristol-Myers Squibb, Canad.; Sanofi Synthelabo, Canad.; Bristol-Myers Squibb, USA.*
Irbesartan (p.940·1); hydrochlorothiazide (p.933·2).
*Hypertension.*

**Avalin** *Piam, Ital.†.*
Infant feed (p.1417·1).
*Maple syrup urine disease.*

**Avallone** *Novartis, Austria.*
Ibuprofen (p.45·3).
*Inflammation; musculoskeletal and joint disorders; pain.*

**Avalon** *Difa, Ital.*
Avena (p.1658·2).
*Emollient skin cleanser.*

**Avalox**
*Bayer, Braz.; Bayer, Ger.; Bayer, Ital.; Bayer, Switz.*
Moxifloxacin hydrochloride (p.233·1).
*Bacterial infections.*

**Avamigran**
*Note. This name is used for preparations of different composition.*
*Asta Medica, Austria.*
Ergotamine tartrate (p.467·2); mecloxamine citrate (p.485·3); camylofin hydrochloride (p.1666·1); caffeine (p.782·1); propyphenazone (p.85·3).
*Cluster headache; migraine.*

*Viatris, Port.*
Ergotamine tartrate (p.467·2); propyphenazone (p.85·3).
Formerly contained ergotamine tartrate, propyphenazone, caffeine, camylofin hydrochloride, and mecloxamine citrate.
*Cluster headache; vascular headache.*

*Asta Medica, Thai.*
Ergotamine tartrate (p.467·2); caffeine (p.782·1).
*Migraine and related vascular headaches.*

**Avamigran N** *AWD, Ger.*
Ergotamine tartrate (p.467·2); propyphenazone (p.85·3).
*Cluster headache; migraine.*

**Avance** *SSL, UK.*
Hydropolymer wound dressing containing silver (p.1746·1).
*Exudating wounds.*

**Avancel** *Bago, Chile.*
Tenoxicam (p.93·1).
*Gout; musculoskeletal, joint, and peri-articular disorders.*

**Avancort** *Polifarma, Ital.*
Methylprednisolone aceponate (p.1106·3).
*Skin disorders.*

**Avandamet**
*GlaxoSmithKline, UK; GlaxoSmithKline, USA.*
Rosiglitazone maleate (p.345·2); metformin hydrochloride (p.342·3).
*Diabetes mellitus.*

**Avandia**
*GlaxoSmithKline, Arg.; GlaxoSmithKline, Austral.; GlaxoSmithKline, Belg.; GlaxoSmithKline, Braz.; GlaxoSmithKline, Canad.; GlaxoSmithKline, Chile; GlaxoSmithKline, Denm.; GlaxoSmithKline, Fin.; GlaxoSmithKline, Fr.; GlaxoSmithKline, Ger.; SmithKline Beecham, Gr.; GlaxoSmithKline, Hong Kong; GlaxoSmithKline, Irl.; SmithKline Beecham, Israel; GlaxoSmithKline, Ital.; GlaxoSmithKline, Malaysia; SmithKline Beecham, Mex.; GlaxoSmithKline, Neth.; GlaxoSmithKline, Norw.; GlaxoSmithKline, NZ; Smith Kline & French, Port.; GlaxoSmithKline, S.Afr.; GlaxoSmithKline, Singapore; GlaxoSmithKline, Spain; GlaxoSmithKline, Swed.; SmithKline Beecham, Switz.; GlaxoSmithKline, Thai.; GlaxoSmithKline, UK; SmithKline Beecham, USA.*
Rosiglitazone maleate (p.345·2).
*Diabetes mellitus.*

**Avant** *Medochemie, Malaysia.*
Haloperidol (p.701·2).
*Behavioural disorders; hiccups; movement disorders; psychomotor agitation; stuttering; tics; vomiting.*

**Avant Garde Shampoo** *Avant Garde, Canad.†.*
Pyrithione zinc (p.1156·2).

**Avantrin** *UCB, Ital.*
Trapidil (p.1016·2).
*Ischaemic heart disease.*

**Avanza** *British Pharmaceuticals, Austral.*
Mirtazapine (p.307·3).
*Depression.*

**Avapena** *Novartis, Mex.*
Chloropyramine hydrochloride (p.427·3).
*Hypersensitivity.*

**Avapro**
*Bristol-Myers Squibb, Arg.; Bristol-Myers Squibb, Austral.; Bristol-Myers Squibb, Braz.; Bristol-Myers Squibb, Canad.; Sanofi Synthelabo, Canad.; Bristol-Myers Squibb, Mex.; Sanofi Winthrop, USA; Bristol-Myers Squibb, USA.*
Irbesartan (p.940·1).
*Diabetic nephropathy; hypertension.*

**Avapro HCT**
*Bristol-Myers Squibb, Arg.; Bristol-Myers Squibb, Austral.*
Irbesartan (p.940·1); hydrochlorothiazide (p.933·2).
*Hypertension.*

**Avar** *Sirius, USA.*
Sulfur (p.1158·2); sulfacetamide sodium (p.257·3).
*Acne.*

**Avastin** *Genentech, USA.*
Bevacizumab (p.529·3).
*Colorectal cancer.*

**Avaxim**
*Aventis Pasteur, Arg.; Aventis Pasteur, Austral.; Pasteur Merieux, Austria†; Aventis Pasteur, Braz.; Aventis Pasteur, Canad.; Aventis Pasteur, Chile; Pasteur Merieux, Denm.†; Pasteur Vaccins, Fr.; Aventis Pasteur, Hong Kong; Aventis Pasteur, Irl.; Pasteur Merieux, Israel; Pasteur Merieux, Ital.†; Aventis Pasteur, Malaysia; Pasteur Merieux, Neth.; CSL, NZ; Aventis, S.Afr.; Aventis Pasteur, Singapore; Aventis Pasteur, Spain; Pasteur Merieux, Swed.†; Aventis Pasteur, Thai.; Aventis Pasteur, UK.*
An inactivated hepatitis A vaccine (GBM strain) (p.1617·1).
*Active immunisation.*

**Avazinc** *Rekah, Israel.*
Zinc sulfate (p.1469·3).
*Zinc deficiency.*

**AVC**
*Theramed, Canad.; Hoechst Marion Roussel, USA†.*
Sulfanilamide (p.263·2).
*Vulvovaginal candidiasis.*

**Avecyde**
*3M, Austral.†; 3M, Malaysia; Galderma, Mex.; 3M, Singapore.*
Lactic acid (p.1704·1).
*Skin irritation; soap substitute.*

**Avedorm** *Eberth, Ger.†.*
Valerian (p.1762·2); melissa (p.1711·1); passion flower (p.1729·1).
*Agitation; sleep disorders.*

**Avedorm duo** *Eberth, Ger.*
Valerian (p.1762·2); lupulus (p.1708·1).
*Agitation; sleep disorders.*

**Avedorm N** *Eberth, Ger.†.*
Lupulus (p.1708·1); passiflora; zinc valerianic.
*Nervous disorders.*

**Aveendix** *Glaxo Wellcome, Mex.*
Avena (p.1658·2); borage (p.1661·3); lactyl glutamate; vitamin E acetate (p.1465·1); levomenol (p.1707·1).
*Dry skin; skin irritation.*

**Aveeno**
*Note. This name is used for preparations of different composition.*
*Bioglan, Irl.†.*
Avena (p.1658·2).
*Dry skin.*

*Rydelle, USA.*
Soap-free skin cleanser; emollient and moisturiser.

**Aveeno Acne Treatment** *Johnson & Johnson, Canad.*
Avena (p.1658·2); salicylic acid (p.1157·1).
Formerly known as Aveeno Acne Bar.
*Acne.*

**Aveeno Anti-Itch**
*Note. This name is used for preparations of different composition.*
*Johnson & Johnson, Canad.*
Calamine (p.1144·1); pramocaine hydrochloride (p.1382·2).
Aveeno Anti-Itch cream formerly contained calamine, pramocaine hydrochloride, and camphor.
*Skin disorders.*

*Rydelle, USA†.*
Calamine (p.1144·1); pramocaine hydrochloride (p.1382·2); camphor (p.1665·3).
*Minor skin irritation.*

**Aveeno Cleansing Bar** *Rydelle, USA.*
Sulfur (p.1158·2); salicylic acid (p.1157·1); colloidal oatmeal (p.1658·2).
*Acne.*

**Aveeno Diaper Rash** *Johnson & Johnson, Canad.*
Zinc oxide (p.1163·2).
*Nappy rash.*

**Aveeno Preparations**
*Johnson & Johnson, Canad.; Rydelle, Fr.†; Johnson & Johnson, Ital.; Dermoteca, Port.†; Johnson & Johnson, UK.*
A range of preparations containing avena (p.1658·2).
*Dry skin disorders; skin care.*

**Aveenocream** *Dermoteca, Port.†.*
Avena (p.1658·2); allantoin (p.1141·3).
*Dry skin disorders.*

**Aveenoderm**
*Rydelle, Fr.†; Dermoteca, Port.†.*
Avena (p.1658·2); zinc oxide (p.1163·2); allantoin (p.1141·3).
*Barrier cream; skin disorders.*

**Avelon** *Bayer, S.Afr.*
Moxifloxacin hydrochloride (p.233·1).
*Bacterial infections.*

**Avelox**
*Bayer, Arg.; Bayer, Austral.; Bayer, Austria; Bayer, Belg.; Bayer, Canad.; Bayer, Chile; Bayer, Denm.; Bayer, Fin.; Bayer, Gr.; Bayer, Hong Kong; Bayer, Irl.; Bayer, Malaysia; Bayer, Mex.; Bayer, NZ; Bayer, Port.; Bayer, Singapore; Bayer, Swed.; Bayer, Thai.; Bayer, UK; Bayer, USA.*
Moxifloxacin hydrochloride (p.233·1).
*Bacterial infections.*

**Avena Complex** *Blackmores, Austral.†.*
Rosemary (p.1740·2); avena (p.1658·2); vervain (p.1764·1); kola (p.1765·3); vitamin B substances (p.1417·1).
*Tonic.*

**Avena Med Complex** *Dynamit, Austria.*
Homoeopathic preparation.

**Avena Rihom Komplex** *Richter, Austria.*
Homoeopathic preparation.

**Avena Sativa Comp** *Weleda, UK.*
Avena (p.1658·2); lupulus (p.1708·1); passion flower (p.1729·1); valerian root (p.1762·2); coffea tosta.
*To aid relaxation.*

**Avenaforce** *Bioforce, Switz.*
Avena (p.1658·2).
*Insomnia; nervousness.*

**Avene Antirougeurs** *Avene, Fr.*
Ruscus aculeatus; dextran sulfate (p.1679·2); melilotus.
*Skin redness.*

**Avene Creme Protectrice and Lait Protecteur** *Avene, Fr.*
*SPF 12B 12A:* Cinnamate.
*Sunscreen.*

**Avene Ecran** *Avene, Fr.†.*
*SPF 12; cream SPF 20; SPF 60:* Cinnamate; titanium dioxide (p.1160·3); zinc oxide (p.1163·2).
*SPF 20; SPF 60:* Cinnamate; titanium dioxide (p.1160·3).
*SPF 25; SPF 50:* Titanium dioxide (p.1160·3); zinc oxide (p.1163·2).
*Sunscreen.*

**Avene Ecran Extreme** *Avene, Fr.*
*SPF 50B 15A:* Zinc oxide (p.1163·2); titanium dioxide (p.1160·3).
*SPF 60B 60A:* Cinnamate.
*Sunscreen.*

**Avene Ecran Jour** *Avene, Fr.*
*SPF 15:* Zinc oxide (p.1163·2); titanium dioxide (p.1160·3); cinnamate.
*Sunscreen.*

**Avene Ecran Tres Haute Protection** *Avene, Fr.*
*Cream SPF 20B 20A:* Cinnamate.
*SPF 20B 15A:* Titanium dioxide (p.1160·3); zinc oxide (p.1163·2).
*Stick SPF 20B 20A:* Cinnamate; titanium dioxide (p.1160·3).
*Sunscreen.*

**Avene 50 Proteccion Extrema** *Silesia, Chile.*
*SPF 50:* Titanium dioxide (p.1160·3); zinc oxide (p.1163·2).
*Sunscreen.*

**Avene 20 Proteccion Total** *Silesia, Chile.*
*Cream SPF 20:* Titanium dioxide (p.1160·3); zinc oxide (p.1163·2); cinnamate.
*Stick SPF 20:* Titanium dioxide (p.1160·3); cinnamate.
*Sunscreen.*

**Aveno**
*Note. This name is used for preparations of different composition.*
*Szama, Arg.*
Avena (p.1658·2); melaleuca oil (p.1710·2).
*Skin disorders.*

*Galderma, Braz.*
Barrier preparation; skin cleanser.

**Avenoc**
*Note. This name is used for preparations of different composition.*
*Boiron, Canad.; Boiron, Port.*
Homoeopathic preparation.

*Boiron, Fr.†.*
*Ointment:* Pilewort (p.1732·1); paeonia officinalis; adrenaline; amylocaine hydrochloride (p.1370·2).
*Anorectal disorders; haemorrhoids.*
*Suppositories:* Homoeopathic preparation.

**Aventyl**
*Lilly, Canad.; Lilly, Irl.†; Aspen, S.Afr.†; Lilly, USA.*
Nortriptyline hydrochloride (p.310·2).
*Depression; nocturnal enuresis.*

**Averpan** *Natus, Braz.†.*
Mebendazole (p.108·2).
*Worm infections.*

**Avertex** *Beta, Arg.*
Finasteride (p.1554·2).
*Benign prostatic hyperplasia.*

**Averuk Bruciaporri** *Marco Viti, Ital.†.*
Trichloroacetic acid (p.1162·1).
*Verrucas; warts.*

**Avesoap** *ICN, Arg.*
Soap substitute for sensitive skin.

**Aviane** *Duramed, USA.*
21 Tablets, levonorgestrel (p.1563·2); ethinylestradiol (p.1553·2); 7 tablets, inert.
*Combined oral contraceptive.*

**Avibon** *Theraplix, Fr.*
Vitamin A (p.1451·2) or vitamin A palmitate (p.1453·1).
*Skin disorders; vitamin A deficiency.*

**A-Vicon** *Collins, Mex.*
Vitamin A (p.1451·2).

**A-Vicotrat** *Heyl, Ger.*
Vitamin A palmitate (p.1453·1).
*Vitamin A deficiency.*

**Avigilen**
*Note. This name is used for preparations of different composition.*
*Sanova, Austria.*
Alpha tocoferil acetate (p.1465·1).
*Intermittent claudication; muscle and connective tissue disorders.*

*Riemser, Ger.*
Piracetam (p.1732·1).
*Mental function disorders.*

**Avil**
*Aventis, Austral.; Aventis, Austria; Hexal, Austria; Hoechst Marion Roussel, Ger.†; Aventis, India; Aventis, NZ.*
Pheniramine maleate (p.438·3).
*Hypersensitivity reactions; motion sickness; pruritus; rhinitis; vestibular disorders.*

**Avil Decongestant** *Aventis, Austral.*
Pheniramine maleate (p.438·3); ammonium chloride (p.1115·2); menthol (p.1711·3).
*Bronchial and nasal congestion; coughs.*

**Avil Expectorant** *Aventis, India.*
Pheniramine maleate (p.438·3); ammonium chloride (p.1115·2); menthol (p.1711·3).
*Bronchitis; coughs; respiratory-tract hypersensitivity.*

**Avilac** *Agis, Israel.*
Lactulose (p.1269·1).
*Constipation; hepatic coma.*

**Avinal-Ex** *Sons, Mex.†.*
Vitamin A (p.1451·2).
*Vitamin A deficiency.*

**Avintac** *Mavi, Mex.*
Ranitidine (p.1285·2).

**Avinza** *Elan, USA.*
Morphine sulfate (p.60·2).
*Pain.*

**Avipur** *Taro, Israel.*
Vitamin A (p.1451·2).
*Vitamin A deficiency.*

**Aviral**
*Medley, Braz.; Mepha, Switz.*
Aciclovir (p.626·1).
*Herpesvirus infections.*

**Avirase** *Lampugnani, Ital.*
Aciclovir (p.626·1).
*Herpesvirus infections.*

**Avirax** *Fabrigen, Canad.*
Aciclovir (p.626·1).
*Herpesvirus infections.*

**Avirex-T** *Tecnofarma, Mex.*
Aciclovir (p.626·1).
*Herpesvirus infections.*

**Avirin**
*Note. This name is used for preparations of different composition.*
*Royal, Chile.*
Amlodipine (p.862·2).
*Hypertension; ischaemic heart disease.*

*Eurofarmaco, Ital.*
Inosine pranobex (p.640·2).
*Viral infections.*

**Avirostat** *Cassara, Arg.*
Interferon alfa-2a (p.640·3).
*Anogenital warts; hepatitis; malignant neoplasms.*

**Avirox** *Durascan, Denm.*
Aciclovir (p.626·1).
*Herpesvirus infections of the skin and mucous membranes.*

**Avishot** *Kanebo, Jpn.*
Naftopidil (p.964·1).

**A-Vita**
*Note. A similar name is used for preparations of different composition (see below).*
*Leiras, Fin.*
Vitamin A palmitate (p.1453·1); menthol (p.1711·3).
*Nasal dryness.*

**Avita**
*Note. A similar name is used for preparations of different composition (see above).*
*Penederm, USA.*
Tretinoin (p.1161·1).
*Acne.*

**A-Vitamiini** *Leiras, Fin.*
Vitamin A (p.1451·2).
*Scalp and skin disorders.*

**A-vitamin** *Medic, Denm.*
Vitamin A (p.1451·2).
*Vitamin A deficiency.*

**Avitcid** *Orion, Fin.*
Tretinoin (p.1161·1).
*Acne; keratinisation disorders.*

**A-Vite** *Neves, Port.*
Vitamin A (p.1451·2).
*Vitamin A deficiency.*

**A-Vitel** *Medipharma, Arg.*
Vitamin A palmitate (p.1453·1).
*Skin disorders.*

**A-Vitel E** *Medipharma, Arg.*
Vitamin A (p.1451·2); alpha tocopherol (p.1464·3).
*Skin disorders.*

**Avitene**
*Agepha, Austria†; Bard, Hong Kong; Shionogi, USA.*
Collagen (p.1674·3).
*Haemostasis in surgery.*

**A-Vitex** *Sophia, Mex.†.*
Vitamin A (p.1451·2).

**Avitol** *Lannacher, Austria.*
Vitamin A acetate (p.1453·1).
*Vitamin A deficiency.*

**Avitracid** *Adroka, Switz.*
Isopropyl alcohol (p.1184·3).
*Hand disinfection.*

**Avix** *Ibirn, Ital.*
Aciclovir (p.626·1).
*Herpesvirus infections.*

**Avixis** *Galderma, Arg.*
Alfatradiol.
*Alopecia androgenetica.*

**Avlocardyl** *AstraZeneca, Fr.*
Propranolol hydrochloride (p.989·3).
*Angina pectoris; arrhythmias; hypertension; hyperthyroidism; migraine; myocardial infarction; obstructive cardiomyopathy; oesophageal varices; tremor.*

**Avloclor**
*AstraZeneca, Irl.; Zeneca, Israel; AstraZeneca, Singapore†; AstraZeneca, UK.*
Chloroquine phosphate (p.448·2).
*Hepatic amoebiasis; lupus erythematosus; malaria; rheumatoid arthritis.*

**Avlosulfon**
*Wyeth-Ayerst, Canad.†; Wyeth-Ayerst, Israel.*
Dapsone (p.202·2).
*Actinomycotic mycetoma; dermatitis herpetiformis; leprosy.*

**Avoca** *Bray, UK.*
Silver nitrate (p.1746·1); potassium nitrate (p.1190·1).
*Verrucas; warts.*

**Avoca Menthol Cone** *Bray, UK†.*
Menthol (p.1711·3).
*Headache.*

**Avocin** *Wyeth Lederle, Ital.*
Piperacillin sodium (p.243·1).
Lidocaine hydrochloride (p.1377·3) is included in this preparation to alleviate the pain of injection.
*Bacterial infections.*

**Avodart**
*GlaxoSmithKline, Fr.; GlaxoSmithKline, UK; GlaxoSmithKline, USA.*
Dutasteride (p.1549·2).
*Benign prostatic hyperplasia.*

**Avomine**
*Aventis, Austral.; Rhone-Poulenc Rorer, Hong Kong†; Nicholas Piramal, India; Aventis, NZ; Aspen, S.Afr.; Manx, UK.*
Promethazine teoclate (p.439·2).
*Motion sickness; nausea and vomiting.*

**Avon Footworks** *Avon, Canad.†.*
Tolnaftate (p.410·1).
*Fungal skin infections.*

**Avon Techniques Anti-Dandruff** *Avon, Canad.†.*
Pyrithione zinc (p.1156·2).
*Dandruff.*

**Avonex**
*Abbott, Arg.; Biogen, Austral.; Biogen, Austria; Biogen, Belg.; Abbott, Braz.; Biogen, Canad.; Abbott, Chile; Biogen, Denm.; Biogen, Fin.; Biogen, Fr.; Biogen, Ger.; Biogen, Gr.; Biogen, Irl.; Biogen, Israel; Dompe Biotec, Ital.; Abbott, Mex.; Biogen, Neth.; Biogen, Norw.; Biogen, NZ; CSL, NZ; Schering-Plough, Port.†; Pharmaplan, S.Afr.; Schering-Plough, Spain; Biogen, Swed.; Dompe Biogen, Switz.; Biogen, UK; Biogen, USA.*
Interferon beta-1a (p.645·3).
*Multiple sclerosis.*

**Avorax**
*Xepa-Soul Pattinson, Hong Kong; Xepa-Soul Pattinson, Malaysia; Xepa-Soul Pattinson, Singapore.*
Aciclovir (p.626·1).
*Herpesvirus infections.*

**Avril** *Teofarma, Spain.*
Cod-liver oil (p.1425·2); aluminium acetotartrate (p.1652·3); benzalkonium chloride (p.1168·3); zinc oxide (p.1163·2).
*Burns; wounds.*

**Avural** *Kampel Martian, Arg.*
Indinavir (p.640·1).
*HIV infection.*

**Avyclor** *Uno, Ital.*
Aciclovir (p.626·1).
*Herpesvirus infections.*

**Avyplus** *Epifarma, Ital.*
Aciclovir (p.626·1).
*Herpesvirus infections.*

**Avysal** *Selvi, Ital.*
Aciclovir (p.626·1).
*Herpesvirus infections.*

**Awesome Animals** *New Vision, Canad.*
Multivitamin and mineral preparation (p.1417·1).

**Axacef**
*Durascan, Denm.†; Tika, Swed.†.*
Cefuroxime sodium (p.184·1).
*Bacterial infections.*

**Axagon** *Simesa, Ital.*
Esomeprazole magnesium (p.1265·1).
*Gastro-oesophageal reflux; peptic ulcer.*

**Axal** *Randall, Mex.†.*
Aspirin (p.15·1).

**Axasol** *Silesia, Chile.*
Clotrimazole (p.396·2).
*Balanitis; fungal vaginal infections.*

**Axcil** *Ofimex, Mex.†.*
Amoxicillin (p.155·3).
*Bacterial infections.*

**Axelorax** *Proel, Gr.*
Propylene glycol cefatrizine (p.170·3).
*Bacterial infections.*

**Axelvin** *Proel, Gr.*
Lisinopril (p.946·3).
*Heart failure; hypertension; myocardial infarction.*

**Axepim** *Bristol-Myers Squibb, Fr.*
Cefepime hydrochloride (p.172·1).
*Bacterial infections.*

**Axer** *Wassermann, Ital.*
Naproxen sodium (p.65·1).
*Musculoskeletal and joint disorders; pain.*

**Axert** *Ortho McNeil, USA.*
Almotriptan malate (p.465·2).
*Migraine.*

**Axetine**
*Medochemie, Hong Kong; Medochemie, Thai.*
Cefuroxime sodium (p.184·1).
*Bacterial infections.*

**Axiago** *Ferrer, Spain.*
Esomeprazole magnesium (p.1265·1).
*Gastro-oesophageal reflux; peptic ulcer.*

**Axid**
*Farmoquimica, Braz.; Lilly, Canad.; Pharmaserve Lilly (Φαρμασερβ Λιλλυ), Gr.; Lilly, Hong Kong; Lilly, Irl.; Lilly, Malaysia; Lilly, Mex.; Norgine, Neth.; Lilly, Neth.; Lilly, S.Afr.†; Lilly, Thai.; Lilly, UK; Lilly, USA; Whitehall-Robins, USA.*
Nizatidine (p.1277·2).
*Dyspepsia; gastro-oesophageal reflux; heartburn; peptic ulcer.*

**Axilin** *Fustery, Mex.*
Flunarizine (p.434·2).
*Migraine.*

**Aximad** *Zeus, Ital.*
Cefotaxime sodium (p.175·3).
Lidocaine hydrochloride (p.1377·3) is included in this preparation to alleviate the pain of injection.
*Gram-negative bacterial infections.*

**Axion** *Apsen, Braz.†.*
Citicoline (p.1672·3).

**Axis** *Labinca, Arg.*
Piroxicam (p.84·2).

**Axistal** *Asian Pharm, Thai.*
Bromhexine hydrochloride (p.1115·3).
*Respiratory-tract disorders associated with increased or viscous mucus.*

**Axocet** *Savage, USA†.*
Butalbital (p.673·3); paracetamol (p.76·2).
*Pain.*

**Axocillin** *Malayan, Singapore.*
Cloxacillin sodium (p.198·2).
*Gram-positive bacterial infections.*

**Axofor** *Aventis, Mex.*
Hydroxocobalamin acetate (p.1458·2).
*Anaemias; neuralgias; neuritis; neuropathies; vitamin $B_{12}$ deficiency.*

**Axol**
*Note. This name is used for preparations of different composition.*
*Veritas, Braz.†.*
Iodine (p.1598·1); phenol (p.1188·1); thymol (p.1194·2); menthol (p.1711·3); methyl salicylate (p.59·3); guaiacol (p.1122·1); procaine (p.1383·2); cineole (p.1672·1); cinnamon oil (p.1672·2); aconite (p.1646·3); cariniana brasiliensis; sumatra benzoin (p.1751·1); eucalyptus (p.1686·1).
*Mouth disorders.*

*YSP, Malaysia; Yung Shin, Singapore.*
Ambroxol hydrochloride (p.1114·3).
*Respiratory-tract disorders associated with viscous mucus.*

**Axonyl** *Pfizer, Fr.*
Piracetam (p.1732·1).
*Cerebrovascular insufficiency; mental function disorders; vertigo.*

**Axoren** *GlaxoSmithKline, Ital.*
Buspirone hydrochloride (p.672·2).
*Anxiety.*

**Axotide** *GlaxoSmithKline, Switz.*
Fluticasone propionate (p.1102·3).
*Asthma.*

**Axsain**
*GenDerm, Canad.†; Elan, Irl.; Elan, UK.*
Capsaicin (p.24·2).
*Diabetic neuropathy; neuralgia.*

**Axtin** *Mavi, Mex.*
Fluoxetine (p.296·3).
*Depression.*

**Axura** *Merz, Ger.*
Memantine hydrochloride (p.1711·2).
Formerly known as Akatinol.
*Alzheimer's disease.*

**Axyol** *Richard, Fr.†.*
Iodine (p.1598·1).
*Burns; leg ulcers; wounds.*

**Aydolid** *Farma Lepori, Spain.*
Fosfosal (p.44·2).
*Fever; musculoskeletal, joint, peri-articular, and soft-tissue disorders; pain.*

**Aydolid Codeina** *Farma Lepori, Spain.*
Codeine phosphate (p.27·1); fosfosal (p.44·2).
*Pain.*

**Ayercillin** *Wyeth-Ayerst, Canad.†.*
Procaine benzylpenicillin (p.246·1).
*Bacterial infections.*

**Aygestin** *Barr, USA.*
Norethisterone acetate (p.1562·2).
*Abnormal uterine bleeding; endometriosis; secondary amenorrhoea.*

**Ayoral** *Rayere, Mex.*
Dipyrone (p.35·3); papaverine (p.1728·1).
*Fever; muscle spasm; pain.*

**Ayoral Simple** *Rayere, Mex.*
Dipyrone (p.35·3).
Formerly known as Ayoral F.
*Fever; pain.*

**Ayr-5** *SMB, Chile.*
Urea (p.1162·2).
*Skin disorders.*

**Ayr Saline** *Ascher, USA.*
Sodium chloride (p.1233·3).
*Nasal irritation.*

**Ayrementol** *SMB, Chile.*
Menthol (p.1711·3); camphor (p.1665·3).
*Dry skin; skin irritation.*

**Ayrton's Antiseptic** *McGloin, Austral.†.*
Zinc oxide (p.1163·2); dichlorobenzyl alcohol (p.1178·3).
*Superficial skin infections.*

**Ayrton's Chilblain** *McGloin, Austral.†.*
Camphor (p.1665·3); benzocaine (p.1370·3); peru balsam (p.1730·2); phenol (p.1188·1).
*Chilblains.*

**Ayton** *Maigal, Arg.*
Vegetable oils; soya lecithin (p.1706·1).
*Skin disorders.*

**Aywet** *Willvonseder, Austria†.*
Wetting solution for hard and soft contact lenses (p.1164·2).

**Az** *Sophia, Mex.*
Azelastine hydrochloride (p.425·2).
*Allergic conjunctivitis.*

**AZ 15** *Procter & Gamble, Ital.*
Sodium chloride (p.1233·3); benzalkonium chloride (p.1168·3); azulene (p.1658·3).
*Gum protection; oral hygiene.*

**AZ Junior** *Procter & Gamble, Ital.†.*
Sodium fluoride (p.1444·3); mica-titanium dioxide complex.
*Dental caries prophylaxis.*

**Az Ofteno** *SMB, Chile.*
Azelastine hydrochloride (p.425·2).
*Allergic conjunctivitis.*

**AZ Protezione Completa** *Procter & Gamble, Ital.†.*
Triclosan (p.1195·2); sodium fluoride (p.1444·3).
*Dental caries prophylaxis.*

**AZ Protezione Gengive** *Procter & Gamble, Ital.*
Triclosan (p.1195·2); pyrophosphate; sodium fluoride (p.1444·3).
*Gum disorders.*

**AZ Tartar Control** *Procter & Gamble, Ital.*
Sodium fluoride (p.1444·3); potassium and sodium pyrophosphates.
*Dental caries prophylaxis; dental tartar.*

**AZ Verde** *Procter & Gamble, Ital.*
Sodium fluoride (p.1444·3).
*Dental caries prophylaxis.*

**Azacortid**
*Aventis, Arg.; Aventis, Chile.*
Deflazacort (p.1096·2).
*Corticosteroid.*

**Azactam**
*Bristol-Myers Squibb, Arg.; Bristol-Myers Squibb, Austral.; Bristol-Myers Squibb, Austria; Bristol-Myers Squibb, Belg.; Bristol-Myers Squibb, Braz.; Bristol-Myers Squibb, Chile; Bristol-Myers Squibb, Denm.; Bristol-Myers Squibb, Fin.; Sanofi Synthelabo, Fr.; Bristol-Myers Squibb, Ger.; Bristol-Myers Squibb, Gr.; Bristol-Myers Squibb, Hong Kong; Bristol-Myers Squibb, Irl.; Bristol-Myers Squibb, Israel; Bristol-Myers Squibb, Ital.; Bristol-Myers Squibb, Neth.†; Bristol-Myers Squibb, Norw.; Bristol-Myers Squibb, NZ; Bristol-Myers Squibb, Port.; Bristol-Myers Squibb, S.Afr.; Bristol-Myers Squibb, Singapore; Squibb, Spain; Bristol-Myers Squibb, Swed.; Bristol-Myers Squibb, Switz.; Bristol-Myers Squibb, Thai.†; Bristol-Myers Squibb, UK; Bristol-Myers Squibb, USA.*
Aztreonam (p.160·3).
*Gram-negative bacterial infections.*

**Azadose** *Pfizer, Fr.*
Azithromycin (p.159·1).
*Opportunistic mycobacterial infections.*

**Azafalk** EciFarma, Chile; Falk, Ger.
Azathioprine (p.1349·1).
*Auto-immune disorders; rheumatoid arthritis; transplant rejection.*

**Azahexal** Hexal, Austral.
Azathioprine (p.1349·1).

**Azamedac** Medac, Ger.
Azathioprine (p.1349·1).
*Auto-immune disorders; transplant rejection.*

**Azameno** Wyeth, Switz.†.
Omoconazole nitrate (p.407·2).
*Fungal skin and vulvovaginal infections.*

**Azamun**
Douglas, Austral.; Leiras, Fin.; Douglas, Hong Kong; Douglas, NZ.
Azathioprine (p.1349·1).
*Auto-immune disorders; transplant rejection.*

**Azanplus** Glaxo Wellcome, Mex.
Ranitidine bismuth citrate (p.1287·2).
*Peptic ulcer.*

**Azantac**
GlaxoSmithKline, Fr.; Glaxo Wellcome, Mex.
Ranitidine hydrochloride (p.1285·2).
*Acid aspiration; dyspepsia; gastritis; gastro-oesophageal reflux; gastrointestinal haemorrhage; peptic ulcer; Zollinger-Ellison syndrome.*

**Azapress** Bodene, S.Afr.
Azathioprine (p.1349·1).
*Transplant rejection.*

**Azaron**
Note. This name is used for preparations of different composition.
Sanova, Austria; Chefaro, Ger.; Chefaro, Neth.†; Chefaro, Spain.
Tripelennamine hydrochloride (p.442·3).
*Bites and stings; urticaria.*

Chefaro, Belg.
Diphenhydramine hydrochloride (p.431·3).
*Pruritus; skin irritation.*

**Azasan** Salix, USA.
Azathioprine (p.1349·1).
*Rheumatoid arthritis; transplant rejection.*

**Azathiodura** Merck dura, Ger.
Azathioprine (p.1349·1).
*Auto-immune disorders; transplant rejection.*

**Azatrilem** Lemery, Mex.
Azathioprine (p.1349·1).
*Immunosuppressant.*

**Azatyl** Remedina, Gr.
Ceftriaxone sodium (p.182·3).
*Bacterial infections.*

**Azectol** Help, Gr.
Atenolol (p.865·2).
*Angina; arrythmias; hypertension.*

**Azedavit** Whitehall, Fr.†.
Multivitamin and mineral preparation (p.1417·1).

**Azelan** Schering, Braz.
Azelaic acid (p.1142·3).
*Acne.*

**Azelast** Sigma, Braz.
Azelastine hydrochloride (p.425·2).
*Hypersensitivity reactions.*

**Azelcream** Crinos, Ital.†.
Azelaic acid (p.1142·3).
*Acne.*

**Azelderm** Kleva, Gr.
Azelaic acid (p.1142·3).
*Acne.*

**Azelex** Allergan, USA.
Azelaic acid (p.1142·3).
*Acne.*

**Azenil** Pfizer, Israel.
Azithromycin (p.159·1).
*Bacterial infections.*

**Azep**
Sigma, Austral.; Asta Medica, Hong Kong; German Remedies, India; Asta Medica, Malaysia; Probios, Port.; Asta Medica, Singapore; Asta Medica, Thai.
Azelastine hydrochloride (p.425·2).
*Allergic rhinitis.*

**Azepam** Macrophar, Thai.
Diazepam (p.690·1).
*Anxiety; muscle spasm.*

**Azerodol** Edmond Pharma, Ital.†.
Salicylamide (p.87·3); propyphenazone (p.85·3); caffeine (p.782·1).
*Pain.*

**Azerty** AstraZeneca, Fr.†.
Nalbuphine hydrochloride (p.64·2).
*Pain.*

**Azetavir** Tecnofarma, Mex.
Zidovudine (p.658·2).
*Viral infections.*

**Azi** Sigma, Braz.
Azithromycin (p.159·1).
*Bacterial infections.*

**Aziac** Infabra, Braz.†.
Aluminium hydroxide (p.1249·2); magnesium hydroxide (p.1272·2).
*Gastrointestinal hyperacidity.*

**Aziclav** Spirig, Switz.
Amoxicillin trihydrate (p.155·3); potassium clavulanate (p.193·3).
*Bacterial infections.*

**Aziliv** Delta, Braz.
Ranitidine hydrochloride (p.1285·2).
*Peptic ulcer.*

**Azilline** Spirig, Switz.
Amoxicillin trihydrate (p.155·3).
*Bacterial infections.*

**Azimax**
Note. This name is used for preparations of different composition.
EMS, Braz.†.
Azithromycin (p.159·1).
*Bacterial infections.*

Almirall, Spain†.
Zafirlukast (p.807·1).
*Asthma.*

**Azime** Sedabel, Braz.
Pancreatin (p.1725·3); dimeticone (p.1289·2).
*Digestive disorders; flatulence.*

**Azimix** Ativus, Braz.
Azithromycin (p.159·1).
*Bacterial infections.*

**Azinc**
Arkopharma, Fr.; Arkochim, Spain; Arkopharma, UK.
A range of vitamin and mineral preparations (p.1417·1).

**Aziram** Uniao Quimica, Braz.
Aluminium hydroxide (p.1249·2).
*Antacid.*

**Azithral** Alembic, India.
Azithromycin (p.159·1).
*Bacterial infections.*

**Azitrax** Farmoquimica, Braz.
Azithromycin (p.159·1).
*Bacterial infections.*

**Azitrix** Tecnimede, Port.
Azithromycin (p.159·1).
*Bacterial infections.*

**Azitrocin**
Cibran, Braz.†; Bioindustria, Ital.; Pfizer, Mex.
Azithromycin (p.159·1).
*Bacterial infections.*

**Azitrom** Laboratorios Chile, Chile.
Azithromycin (p.159·1).
*Bacterial infections.*

**Azitromax**
Pfizer, Norw.; Pfizer, Swed.
Azithromycin (p.159·1).
*Bacterial infections.*

**Azitromin** Farmasa, Braz.
Azithromycin (p.159·1).
*Bacterial infections.*

**Azitron** Cifarma, Braz.†.
Azithromycin (p.159·1).
*Bacterial infections.*

**Azitronal** Klonal, Arg.
Azithromycin (p.159·1).
*Bacterial infections.*

**Azitroxil** De Mayo, Braz.
Azithromycin (p.159·1).
*Bacterial infections.*

**Aziwok** Wockhardt, India.
Azithromycin (p.159·1).
*Bacterial infections.*

**Azmacort**
Aventis, Braz.; Rhone-Poulenc Rorer, Canad.†; Rhone-Poulenc Rorer, USA.
Triamcinolone acetonide (p.1110·2).
*Asthma.*

**Azmasol** Beximco, Singapore.
Salbutamol (p.791·3).
*Obstructive airways disease.*

**Azoazol** Gador, Arg.
Zidovudine (p.658·2).
*HIV infection.*

**Azoflune** Decomed, Port.
Fluconazole (p.398·1).
*Fungal infections.*

**Azo-Gen** Berman, Mex.
Phenazopyridine (p.83·2); nalidixic acid (p.234·1).
*Bacterial infections of the urinary tract.*

**Azol**
Note. This name is used for preparations of different composition.
Alphapharm, Austral.; Alphapharm, Malaysia; Merck, Malaysia; Alphapharm, Singapore; Merck, Singapore.
Danazol (p.1545·2).
*Benign breast disorders; endometriosis; gynaecomastia; hereditary angioedema; menorrhagia.*

Kern, Spain.
Sulfanilamide (p.263·2).
*Skin infections.*

**Azolin** Biochem, India.
Cefazolin sodium (p.170·3).
*Bacterial infections.*

**Azoline** Fischer, Israel.
Tetryzoline hydrochloride (p.1131·2).
*Allergic conjunctivitis; eye irritation.*

**Azolmen** Menarini, Ital.
Bifonazole (p.395·1).
*Fungal skin infections.*

**Azomid** Propan, S.Afr.
Acetazolamide (p.849·1).
*Glaucoma.*

**Azomycin** Julphar, UAE.
Azithromycin (p.159·1).
*Bacterial infections.*

**Azomyr**
Kirby, Arg.; Essex, Ital.; Ferraz, Lynce, Port.
Desloratadine (p.431·1).
*Allergic rhinitis; urticaria.*

**Azona**
Note. This name is used for preparations of different composition.
Orion, Fin.
Trazodone hydrochloride (p.319·1).
*Depression; insomnia; psychoses.*

Keton, Mex.†.
Dexamethasone (p.1097·1).
*Corticosteroid.*

**Azonutril**
Pharmacia Upjohn, Fr.†; Rhone-Poulenc Rorer, Spain†.
Amino-acid infusion (p.1417·1).
*Parenteral nutrition.*

**Azopi** Generics, Israel.
Azathioprine (p.1349·1).
*Auto-immune disorders; rheumatoid arthritis; transplant rejection.*

**Azopine** Pinewood, Irl.†.
Azathioprine (p.1349·1).
*Auto-immune disorders; organ transplant rejection.*

**Azopt**
Alcon, Arg.; Alcon, Austral.; Alcon, Austria; Alcon, Belg.; Alcon, Braz.; Alcon, Canad.; Alcon, Chile; Alcon, Denm.; Alcon, Fin.; Alcon, Fr.; Alcon, Ger.; Alkon (Αλκον), Gr.; Alcon, Hong Kong; Alcon, Irl.; Alcon, Israel; Alcon, Ital.; Alcon, Mex.; Alcon, Norw.; Alcon, Port.; Alcon, Singapore; Alcon Cusi, Spain; Alcon, Swed.; Alcon, Switz.; Alcon, Thai.; Alcon, UK; Alcon, USA.
Brinzolamide (p.877·1).
*Glaucoma; ocular hypertension.*

**Azor** Aspen, S.Afr.
Alprazolam (p.668·3).
*Anxiety; mixed anxiety depressive states.*

**Azoran**
Note. This name is used for preparations of different composition.
RPG, India.
Azathioprine (p.1349·1).
*Auto-immune disorders; organ transplantation.*

Columbia, Mex.
Omeprazole (p.1278·2).
*Gastritis; gastro-oesophageal reflux; peptic ulcer.*

**Azo-Standard** PolyMedica, USA.
Phenazopyridine hydrochloride (p.83·1).
*Urinary-tract pain.*

**Azostix**
Bayer, Austral.; Miles, Canad.†; Bayer Diagnostics, Irl.†; Bayer, NZ; Bayer Diagnostics, UK; Bayer, USA.
Test for urea in blood.

**Azotine** Elvetium, Arg.
Zidovudine (p.658·2).
*HIV infection.*

**Azo-Wintomylon**
Sanofi Winthrop, Braz.†; Sanofi Synthelabo, Mex.
Nalidixic acid (p.234·1); phenazopyridine hydrochloride (p.83·1).
*Urinary-tract infections.*

**Aztemin** Protein, Mex.†.
Astemizole (p.424·2).

**Aztil** Offenbach, Mex.
Astemizole (p.424·2).
*Hypersensitivity.*

**Azuben** Ipsen, Spain.
Pefloxacin mesilate (p.241·3).
*Bacterial infections.*

**Azubronchin** Azupharma, Ger.
Acetylcysteine (p.1112·3).
*Respiratory-tract disorders associated with increased or viscous mucus.*

**Azucalcit** Azupharma, Ger.
Calcitonin (salmon) (p.768·2).
*Hypercalcaemia; osteoporosis; Paget's disease of bone; reflex sympathetic dystrophy.*

**Azucaps** Medix, Mex.
Phenformin (p.344·1).
*Diabetes mellitus.*

**Azucimet** Azupharma, Ger.
Cimetidine (p.1255·3).
*Acid aspiration; gastro-oesophageal reflux; gastrointestinal haemorrhage; peptic ulcer; Zollinger-Ellison syndrome.*

**Azuder** Remexa, Mex.†.
Sulfur (p.1158·2).

**Azudoxat** Azupharma, Ger.
Doxycycline hyclate (p.206·2).
*Bacterial infections.*

**Azudoxat comp** Azupharma, Ger.
Doxycycline hyclate (p.206·2); ambroxol hydrochloride (p.1114·3).
*Respiratory-tract infections.*

**Azufibrat**
Azupharma, Ger.; Azupharma, Hong Kong†.
Bezafibrate (p.873·2).
*Hyperlipidaemias.*

**Azufracid** Bajer, Arg.
Sulfur (p.1158·2); iodine (p.1598·1).
*Skin cleanser.*

**Azuglucon** Azupharma, Ger.
Glibenclamide (p.331·2).
*Diabetes mellitus.*

**Azul Metile** Ciba Vision, Spain†.
Methylthioninium chloride (p.1042·2).
*Ophthalmic diagnostic agent.*

**Azulen** Provita, Austria.
Guaiazulene (p.1696·2).
*Hypersensitivity and inflammatory disorders.*

**Azulenal** Agepha, Austria.
Guaiazulene (p.1696·2).
*Hypersensitivity disorders; mucus membrane inflammation; skin disorders.*

**Azulene** Thea, Fr.
Guaiazulene (p.1696·2).
*Conjunctival irritation.*

**Azulfidine**
Pharmacia, Arg.; Pharmacia, Chile; Pharmacia, Ger.; Pharmacia Upjohn, USA.
Sulfasalazine (p.1291·1).
*Inflammatory bowel disease; rheumatoid arthritis.*

**Azulfin** Apsen, Braz.
Sulfasalazine (p.1291·1).
*Rheumatoid arthritis; ulcerative colitis.*

**Azulina** Llorens, Spain.
Tetryzoline hydrochloride (p.1131·2).
Formerly contained methylthioninium chloride and tetryzoline hydrochloride.
*Eye disorders.*

**Azulipont** Azupharma, Ger.
Thioctic acid (p.1754·3).
*Diabetic polyneuropathy.*

**Azulon**
Note. This name is used for preparations of different composition.
Szama, Arg.
Guaiazulene (p.1696·2).
*Hypersensitivity reactions; inflammation.*

Baxter, Ger.
Chamomile (p.1669·3).
*Skin disorders.*

**Azumetop** Azupharma, Ger.
Metoprolol tartrate (p.957·1).
*Angina pectoris; arrhythmias; hypertension; migraine; myocardial infarction.*

**Azumetop HCT** Azupharma, Ger.
Metoprolol tartrate (p.957·1); hydrochlorothiazide (p.933·2).
*Hypertension.*

**Azunaftil** Azupharma, Ger.
Naftidrofuryl oxalate (p.964·1).
*Peripheral vascular disorders.*

**Azunol** Shinyaku, Hong Kong.
Azulene sodium sulfonate (p.1658·3).
*Gastric ulcer; gastritis; mouth and throat disorders.*

**Azupamil** Azupharma, Ger.
Verapamil hydrochloride (p.1019·1).
*Angina pectoris; arrhythmias; hypertension.*

**Azupanthenol** Parke, Davis, Ger.
Guaiazulene (p.1696·2); sodium pantothenate (p.1443·1).
*Gastrointestinal disorders.*

**Azupentat** Azupharma, Ger.
Pentoxifylline (p.979·3).
*Peripheral vascular disorders.*

**Azuperamid** Azupharma, Ger.
Loperamide hydrochloride (p.1271·1).
*Diarrhoea.*

**Azuprostat** Azupharma, Ger.
Sitosterol (p.982·3).
*Benign prostatic hyperplasia.*

**Azuprostat Sabal** Azupharma, Ger.
Saw palmetto (p.1569·1).
*Benign prostatic hyperplasia.*

**Azuprostat Urtica** Azupharma, Ger.
Urtica (p.1762·1).
*Benign prostatic hyperplasia.*

**Azur** Steiner, Ger.
Paracetamol (p.76·2); caffeine (p.782·1).
*Pain.*

**Azur compositum** Steiner, Ger.
Paracetamol (p.76·2); caffeine (p.782·1); codeine phosphate (p.27·1).
*Pain.*

**Azur compositum SC** Steiner, Ger.
Paracetamol (p.76·2); codeine phosphate (p.27·1).
*Pain.*

**Azuranit** Azupharma, Ger.
Ranitidine hydrochloride (p.1285·2).
*Acid aspiration; gastro-oesophageal reflux; gastrointestinal haemorrhage; peptic ulcer; Zollinger-Ellison syndrome.*

**Azuril** Pharmanel, Gr.
Roxithromycin (p.254·2).
*Bacterial infections.*

**Azutranquil** Azupharma, Ger.
Oxazepam (p.712·2).
*Anxiety; insomnia.*

**Azutrimazol** Azupharma, Ger.
Clotrimazole (p.396·2).
*Fungal skin and genito-urinary tract infections.*

**Azym** Zambon, Fr.†.
Magnesium hydroxide (p.1272·2); magnesium carbonate (p.1272·1); anhydrous sodium sulfate (p.1290·1); dibasic sodium phosphate (p.1231·1); calcium carbonate (p.1254·2); sodium bicarbonate (p.1223·2).
*Gastrointestinal disorders.*

**B1-12-15** Italmex, Mex.
Pangamic acid (p.1727·2); cyanocobalamin (p.1458·2); thiamine hydrochloride (p.1455·1).
*Anaemias; neuralgia; neuritis.*

**3B**
*Atlantic, Hong Kong; Atlantic, Malaysia; Atlantic, Singapore†; Atlantic, Thai.*
Vitamin $B_1$ (p.1455·2); vitamin $B_6$ (p.1457·2); vitamin $B_{12}$ (p.1458·2).
*Anaemias; neural disorders.*

**B-6** *Pharmasant, Thai.*
Pyridoxine hydrochloride (p.1456·3).
*Vitamin $B_6$ deficiency.*

**B15** *Natural Life, Arg.*
Pangamic acid (p.1727·2).
*Vitamin B supplement.*

**$B_{12}$ Ankermann** *Worwag, Ger.*
Cyanocobalamin (p.1458·2).
*Vitamin $B_{12}$ deficiency.*

**B Chabre** *Expanpharm, Fr.*
Vitamin B substances (p.1417·1).

**B Complex**
*Jamieson, Canad.; Sante Naturelle, Canad.; Vita Pharm, Canad.; CTI, Israel; Upha, Malaysia.*
Vitamin B substances (p.1417·1).

*Phillips Yeast, UK†.*
Yeast (p.1469·1); vitamin B substances (p.1417·1).

**B-100 Complex** *TP, Thai.*
Vitamin B substances (p.1417·1).

**B Complex 500** *Nobel, Canad.†.*
Vitamin B substances and vitamin C (p.1417·1).

**B Complex with C** *Everest, Canad.†.*
Vitamin B substances and vitamin C (p.1417·1).

**B Complex C 550** *Adams, Canad.*
Vitamin B substances and vitamin C (p.1417·1).

**B Complex Fosforilado** *Alter, Spain†.*
Vitamin B substances (p.1417·1).

**B Complex plus C** *Jamieson, Canad.*
Vitamin B substances and vitamin C (p.1417·1).

**$B_{12}$ Compositum** *Helvepharm, Switz.*
Cyanocobalamin; iron sucrose; calcium glycerophosphate (p.1417·1).
*Tonic.*

**B Compound** *Swiss Herbal, Canad.*
Vitamin B substances (p.1417·1).

**$B_{12}$ Depot-Hevert** *Hevert, Ger.*
Hydroxocobalamin acetate (p.1458·2).
*Vitamin $B_{12}$ deficiency.*

**B12 Depot-Rotexmedica** *Rotexmedica, Ger.*
Hydroxocobalamin acetate (p.1458·2).
*Vitamin $B_{12}$ deficiency.*

**$B_{12}$ Depot-Vicotrat** *Heyl, Ger.†.*
Hydroxocobalamin (p.1458·2).
*Vitamin $B_{12}$ deficiency.*

**$B_{1/6}$ Effekton** *Brenner-Efeka, Ger.†.*
Thiamine hydrochloride (p.1455·1); pyridoxine hydrochloride (p.1456·3).
*Neurological disorders.*

**B12 Ehrl** *Hormosan, Ger.†.*
Cyanocobalamin (p.1458·2).
*Vitamin $B_{12}$ deficiency.*

**$B_{12}$ Fol-Vicotrat** *Heyl, Ger.*
Cyanocobalamin (p.1458·2); folic acid (p.1429·1).
*Vitamin $B_{12}$ and folic acid deficiency.*

**B Forte** *Bio-Health, UK†.*
Vitamin B preparation (p.1417·1).

**B 12-L 90** *Loges, Ger.*
Cyanocobalamin (p.1458·2).
*Anaemias; tonic; vitamin B deficiency.*

**B & O Supprettes No. 15A** *PolyMedica, USA.*
Prepared opium (p.74·2); powdered belladonna extract (p.479·1).
*Ureteral spasm pain.*

**B & O Supprettes No. 16A** *PolyMedica, USA.*
Prepared opium (p.74·2); powdered belladonna extract (p.479·1).
*Ureteral spasm pain.*

**B plus C** *Novopharm, Canad.*
Vitamin B substances and vitamin C (p.1417·1).

**B12 Rotexmedica** *Rotexmedica, Ger.*
Cyanocobalamin (p.1458·2).
*Vitamin $B_{12}$ deficiency.*

**B Six** *Sam-On, Israel.*
Vitamin $B_6$ (p.1456·3).
*Vitamin $B_6$ deficiency.*

**B12 Steigerwald** *Steigerwald, Ger.*
Cyanocobalamin (p.1458·2).
*Vitamin $B_{12}$ deficiency.*

**B Stress C plus Iron & Vitamins** *Stanley, Canad.*
Vitamin preparation with iron (p.1417·1).

**B Stress Select** *Sisu, Canad.*
Vitamin B substances (p.1417·1).

**B Totum** *Desbergers, Canad.†.*
Vitamin B substances and vitamin C (p.1417·1).

**$B_1$ Vicotrat** *Heyl, Ger.*
Thiamine nitrate (p.1455·1).
*Vitamin $B_1$ deficiency.*

**$B_6$ Vicotrat** *Heyl, Ger.*
Pyridoxine hydrochloride (p.1456·3).
*Vitamin $B_6$ deficiency.*

**$B_{12}$ Vicotrat** *Heyl, Ger.*
Cyanocobalamin (p.1458·2).
*Vitamin $B_{12}$ deficiency.*

**B Virol** *Rolmex, Canad.*
Multivitamin preparation (p.1417·1).

**Babcon** *Eisai, Thai.; Toho, Thai.*
Dimethicone (p.1289·2).
*Excess gastrointestinal gas; preparation for gastrointestinal examinations.*

**Babee** *Pfeiffer, USA.*
Benzocaine (p.1370·3); cetalkonium chloride (p.1172·1); camphor (p.1665·3); menthol (p.1711·3); cineole (p.1672·1).
*Oral lesions.*

**Babefen Sus** *Polipharm, Thai.*
Ibuprofen (p.45·3).
*Inflammation; pain.*

**Babic** *Abic, Israel.*
Sodium bicarbonate (p.1223·2).
*Infant colic.*

**Babiforton** *Sanofi Synthelabo, Ger.*
Eucalyptus oil (p.1686·2); pine needle oil; peppermint oil (p.1283·2).
*Nasal congestion.*

**Babigoz Crema Protettiva** *Guigoz, Ital.*
Zinc oxide (p.1163·2); magnesium silicate (p.1580·2); wheat-germ oil.
*Nappy rash.*

**Babix**
*Note. This name is used for preparations of different composition.*
*Stiefel, Arg.*
Liquid paraffin (p.1479·1).
*Skin cleansing.*

*Madaus, Austria.*
Cajuput oil (p.1664·1); pumilio pine oil (p.1737·1); eucalyptus oil (p.1686·2).
*Respiratory-tract disorders.*

*Stiefel, Braz.†.*
Triclosan (p.1195·2).
*Skin disinfection.*

**Babix-Inhalat N** *Mickan, Ger.*
Eucalyptus oil (p.1686·2); Norway spruce oil.
*Respiratory-tract disorders.*

**Babix-Wundsalbe N** *Mickan, Ger.*
Zinc oxide (p.1163·2); lemon oil (p.1706·2); chamomile oil (p.1669·3).
*Skin disorders.*

**Baby AF** *Sam-On, Israel.*
Sodium chloride (p.1233·3).
*Nasal congestion.*

**Baby Agisten** *Agis, Israel.*
Clotrimazole (p.396·2).
*Fungal skin infections.*

**Baby Anbesol** *Whitehall, USA.*
Benzocaine (p.1370·3).
*Teething pain.*

**Baby Block** *Estee Lauder, Canad.*
*SPF 25:* Titanium dioxide (p.1160·3).
*Sunscreen.*

**Baby Cough** *Greater Pharma, Thai.*
Ammonium chloride (p.1115·2); sodium citrate (p.1223·2).
*Coughs.*

**Baby Cough with Antihistamine**
*Atlantic, Hong Kong; Atlantic, Thai.*
Acetic acid (p.1645·2); ammonium chloride (p.1115·2); sodium citrate (p.1223·2); glycerol (p.1694·3); tolu syrup (p.1131·3); chlorphenamine maleate (p.427·3).
*Coughs.*

**Baby Cough Syrup** *Atlantic, Thai.*
Acetic acid (p.1645·2); ammonium chloride (p.1115·2); glycerol (p.1694·3); sodium citrate (p.1223·2); tolu syrup (p.1131·3).
*Coughs.*

**Baby Fact B** *Gemepe, Arg.*
Pulmonary surfactant (p.1736·1).
*Neonatal respiratory distress syndrome.*

**Baby Gel** *Medibrands, Israel.*
Benzocaine (p.1370·3).
*Teething pain.*

**Baby Gripe** *TO-Chemicals, Thai.*
Dill oil (p.1680·2); sodium bicarbonate (p.1223·2).
*Flatulence; infant bloating.*

**Baby Liberol** *Galactina, Switz.†.*
Hyoscyamus oil (p.485·2); eucalyptus oil (p.1686·2); pumilio pine oil (p.1737·1); star anise oil; juniper oil (p.1703·1); methyl salicylate (p.59·3).
*Cold symptoms.*

**Baby Luuf** *Apomedica, Austria.*
Camphor (p.1665·3); eucalyptus oil (p.1686·2); turpentine oil (p.1760·1); majoram oil.
*Respiratory-tract disorders.*

**Baby Orajel**
*Del, Canad.; Instituto Sanitas, Chile; Del, USA.*
Benzocaine (p.1370·3).
*Teething pain.*

**Baby Orajel Tooth and Gum Cleanser** *Del, USA.*
Poloxamer 407 (p.1414·2); simeticone (p.1289·2).
*Dental hygiene.*

**Baby Paste** *Vitamed, Israel.*
Zinc oxide (p.1163·2); starch (p.1449·1).
*Nappy rash; skin irritation.*

**Baby Paste + Chamomile** *Vitamed, Israel.*
Chamomile (p.1669·3); sage (p.1741·2); calamine (p.1144·1); zinc oxide (p.1163·2).
*Skin disorders.*

**Baby Sebamed** *Sebapharma, Thai.*
A range of skin cleansers and emollients.

**Baby Shield**
*Hoe, Malaysia; Hoe, Singapore.*
Barrier preparation.
*Nappy rash; skin irritation.*

**BabyBIG** *California Department of Health, USA.*
Botulism immunoglobulin (p.1610·3).
*Botulism in infants.*

**Babycare** *Trima, Israel†.*
Barrier preparation.

**Babycheck-Plus** *Veda, Fr.*
Pregnancy test (p.1734·3).

**Baby-Drax** *Uniao Quimica, Braz.*
Glucose; sodium chloride; potassium chloride; sodium citrate (p.1222·2).
*Diarrhoea; oral rehydration.*

**Babyfort** *QIF, Braz.†.*
Multivitamin preparation (p.1417·1).

**Babygella**
*Note. This name is used for preparations of different composition.*
*Rottapharm, Fr.*
Zinc oxide (p.1163·2).
*Skin irritation.*

*Rottapharm, Ital.*
*Cream:* Calendula (p.1665·2); chamomile (p.1669·3); zinc oxide (p.1163·2).
*Topical paste:* Squalane; sweet almond oil; lactic acid; zinc oxide (p.1163·2).
*Barrier preparation.*

**Babygencal** *Qualiphar, Belg.†.*
Amylocaine hydrochloride (p.1370·2); potassium bromide (p.1663·1); cloral hydrate (p.684·1).
*Teething pain.*

**Babyglos** *Hertz, Braz.†.*
Allantoin (p.1141·3); panthenol (p.1727·2); triclosan (p.1195·2); zinc (p.1469·2).
*Barrier preparation.*

**Babylax**
*Mann, Ger.†; Mann, Irl.*
Glycerol (p.1694·3).
*Bowel evacuation; constipation.*

**Baby-Line** *Cesam, Port.†.*
Barrier preparation.

**Babypasmil** *Lacefa, Arg.*
Dicycloverine (p.481·2).

**Babypiril** *Zambon, Spain.*
Ibuprofen arginine (p.46·3).
*Fever; pain.*

**Baby-Rinolo** *Bruno, Ital.*
Phenylpropanolamine hydrochloride (p.1127·3); chlorphenamine maleate (p.427·3); paracetamol (p.76·2).
*Respiratory-tract disorders.*

**Babys Own Gripe Water** *Block, Canad.†.*
Anise oil (p.1655·2); dill oil (p.1680·2); fennel oil (p.1687·3); sodium bicarbonate (p.1223·2).
*Gastrointestinal disorders.*

**Babys Own Infant Drops** *Block, Canad.†.*
Simeticone (p.1289·2).
*Infant colic, bloating, and flatulence.*

**Babys Own Ointment** *Block, Canad.*
Zinc oxide (p.1163·2).
*Nappy rash.*

**Babys Own Teething Gel** *Block, Canad.*
Benzyl alcohol (p.1170·2).
*Teething pain.*

**Babysan** *Szama, Arg.*
Alcloxa (p.1141·2).
*Hyperhidrosis; skin disorders.*

**Babysiton** *Faes, Spain.*
Cetylpyridinium chloride (p.1173·1); zinc oxide (p.1163·2).
*Skin disorders.*

**Babysteril** *Eurospital, Ital.*
Zinc oxide (p.1163·2); almond oil (p.1651·1); wheat-germ oil; vitamin A (p.1451·2); vitamin E (p.1464·3).
*Napkin rash.*

**Baby-Transpulmin** *Asta Medica, Ger.†.*
Eucalyptus oil (p.1686·2); pine needle oil.
*Cold symptoms.*

**Babyzim** *Sam-On, Israel.*
Pepsin (p.1729·3); lactic acid (p.1704·1); sodium glycerophosphate (p.1695·2); nicotinic acid (p.1441·1).
*Gastrointestinal disorders.*

**B-A-C** *Mayrand, USA†.*
Butalbital (p.673·3); aspirin (p.15·1); caffeine (p.782·1).
*Tension headache.*

**Bac Resistente** *Sanus, Braz.†.*
*Lactobacillus acidophilus* (p.1704·2).
*Diarrhoea; restoration of gastrointestinal flora.*

**Bac Septin** *Gilton, Braz.†.*
Co-trimoxazole (p.199·3).
*Bacterial infections; Pneumocystis carinii pneumonia; protozoal infections.*

**Bac Septin Balsamico** *Gilton, Braz.†.*
Co-trimoxazole (p.199·3); guaiacol (p.1122·1).
*Respiratory-tract infections.*

**Bacacil** *Pfizer, Ital.*
Bacampicillin hydrochloride (p.161·2).
*Bacterial infections.*

**Bacagen** *Boniscontro & Gazzone, Ital.*
Bacampicillin hydrochloride (p.161·2).
*Bacterial infections.*

**Bacampicin**
*Pharmacia, Belg.; Pharmacia Upjohn, Port.; Pharmacia Upjohn, Switz.†.*
Bacampicillin hydrochloride (p.161·2).
*Bacterial infections.*

**Bacampicine** *Pharmacia, Fr.*
Bacampicillin hydrochloride (p.161·2).
*Bacterial infections.*

**Bacard** *Chew, Thai.*
Chlorhexidine gluconate (p.1173·2); cetrimide (p.1172·1).
*Skin, wound, and instrument disinfection.*

**Bacard Antiseptic** *Chew, Thai.*
Chlorhexidine gluconate (p.1173·2).
*Skin, hand, and wound disinfection.*

**Bacasint** *Piam, Ital.*
Bacampicillin hydrochloride (p.161·2).
*Bacterial infections.*

**Bacattiv** *Uno, Ital.*
Bacampicillin hydrochloride (p.161·2).
*Bacterial infections.*

**Baccalin** *Bode, Ger.*
Benzalkonium chloride (p.1168·3); didecyldimethylammonium chloride (p.1178·3).
*Disinfection.*

**Baccidal**
*Kyorin, Jpn; Abbott, Spain.*
Norfloxacin (p.238·3).
*Bacterial infections.*

**Bacfar** *Elofar, Braz.*
Co-trimoxazole (p.199·3).
*Bacterial infections; Pneumocystis carinii pneumonia; protozoal infections.*

**Bacfar Balsamico** *Elofar, Braz.†.*
Co-trimoxazole (p.199·3); guaifenesin (p.1122·1); ammonium chloride (p.1115·2).
*Bacterial infections.*

**Bacferol** *Grisi, Mex.*
Vitamin E (p.1464·3).
*Vitamin E supplement.*

**Bacgen** *Uniao Quimica, Braz.†.*
Co-trimoxazole (p.199·3).
*Bacterial infections; Pneumocystis carinii pneumonia; protozoal infections.*

**Bacgen Balsamico** *Uniao Quimica, Braz.†.*
Co-trimoxazole (p.199·3); guaifenesin (p.1122·1); ammonium chloride (p.1115·2).
*Bacterial infections.*

**Bach Rescue Remedy** *Bach, UK.*
Homoeopathic preparation.

**Bacibact** *Orion, Fin.*
Bacitracin (p.161·3); neomycin sulfate (p.235·1).
*Infected skin disorders.*

**Bacicoline** *Merck Sharp & Dohme-Chibret, Fr.*
Bacitracin (p.161·3); colistimethate sodium (p.199·1); hydrocortisone acetate (p.1103·3).
*Eye infections.*

**Bacicoline-B** *Merck Sharp & Dohme, Neth.*
Colistimethate sodium (p.199·1); bacitracin (p.161·3); hydrocortisone acetate (p.1103·3).
*Inflammatory ear infections.*

**Bacid**
*Note. This name is used for preparations of different composition.*
*Aventis, Canad.; Ciba, USA.*
*Lactobacillus acidophilus* (p.1704·2).
*Diarrhoea; dietary supplement; stomatitis.*

*Uno, Ital.*
Cefonicid sodium (p.174·2).
Lidocaine hydrochloride (p.1377·3) is included in this preparation to alleviate the pain of injection.
*Bacterial infections.*

**Baciderma** *Confar, Port.*
Bacitracin (p.161·3); neomycin (p.235·1).

**Bacifim** *Medipharma, Arg.*
Rifampicin (p.250·2); isoniazid (p.222·2).
*Tuberculosis.*

**Bacifurane** *Melisana, Belg.*
Nifuroxazide (p.237·2).
*Diarrhoea.*

**Bacigen** *Cazi, Braz.*
Neomycin sulfate (p.235·1); bacitracin zinc (p.161·3).
*Skin infections.*

**Baciguent**
*Johnson & Johnson, Canad.; Upjohn, USA†.*
Bacitracin (p.161·3).
*Bacterial skin infections.*

**Baciguent Plus Pain Reliever** *McNeil Consumer, Canad.†.*
Bacitracin (p.161·3); lidocaine (p.1377·3).
*Pain and infection in burns and wounds.*

**Baci-IM** *Pharma Tek, USA.*
Bacitracin (p.161·3).
*Bacterial infections.*

**Bacillin** *Lafare, Ital.*
Bacampicillin hydrochloride (p.161·2).
*Bacterial infections.*

**Bacillocid rasant** *Bode, Ger.*
Glutaral (p.1180·3); benzalkonium chloride (p.1168·3); didecyldimethylammonium chloride (p.1178·3).
*Surface disinfection.*

**Bacillocid Spezial** *Bode, Ger.†.*
1,6-Dihydroxy-2,5-dioxahexan; glutaral (p.1180·3); benzalkonium chloride (p.1168·3); cocosguanidinium chloride.
*Surface disinfection.*

**Bacillol** *Bode, Ger.*
Propyl alcohol (p.1191·2); isopropyl alcohol (p.1184·3); alcohol (p.1166·1); 1,6-dihydroxy-2,5-dioxahexan; mecetronium etilsulfate (p.1185·2).
*Surface disinfection.*

**Bacillol AF** *Bode, Ger.*
Propyl alcohol (p.1191·2); isopropyl alcohol (p.1184·3); alcohol (p.1166·1).
*Surface disinfection.*

**Bacillol plus** *Bode, Ger.*
Propyl alcohol (p.1191·2); isopropyl alcohol (p.1184·3); glutaral (p.1180·3).
*Surface disinfection.*

**Bacillotox** *Bode, Ger.†.*
Chlorocresol (p.1177·1); orthophenylphenol (p.1187·2); chloroxylenol (p.1177·2); clorophene (p.1177·3).
*Disinfection.*

**Bacilor** *Lyocentre, Fr.*
*Lactobacillus casei* var *rhamnosus* (p.1704·2).
Formerly known as Antibiophilus.
*Diarrhoea.*

**Bacimex** *Alter, Spain†.*
*Injection:* Ampicillin sodium (p.157·1); sulbactam sodium (p.257·2).
Lidocaine hydrochloride (p.1377·3) is included in the intramuscular injection to alleviate the pain of injection.
*Tablets; oral suspension:* Sultamicillin tosilate (p.264·2).
*Bacterial infections.*

**Bacimycin**
*Note. This name is used for preparations of different composition.*
*Grossmann, Hong Kong.*
Bacitracin (p.161·3); neomycin (p.235·1).
*Burns; infected skin disorders; wounds.*
*Alpharma, Norw.*
Bacitracin zinc (p.161·3); chlorhexidine acetate (p.1173·2).
*Bacterial infections of the skin.*
*Grossmann, Switz.*
Bacitracin (p.161·3); neomycin sulfate (p.235·1).
*Infected skin disorders.*

**Bacimyxin** *Pharmascience, Canad.*
Polymyxin B sulfate (p.245·1); bacitracin (p.161·3).
*Bacterial infections.*

**Bacin**
*Atlantic, Hong Kong†; Atlantic, Malaysia; Atlantic, Singapore; Atlantic, Thai.*
Co-trimoxazole (p.199·3).
*Bacterial infections.*

**Bacineo** *Luper, Braz.*
Neomycin sulfate (p.235·1); bacitracin (p.161·3).
*Bacterial skin infections.*

**Bacisporin** *Alcala, Spain.*
Bacitracin zinc (p.161·3); hydrocortisone (p.1103·3); neomycin sulfate (p.235·1); polymyxin B sulfate (p.245·1).
*Infected skin disorders.*

**Bacitin**
*Pharmascience, Canad.; Pharmascience, Hong Kong†.*
Bacitracin (p.161·3).
*Bacterial infections of the skin; burns; wounds.*

**Bacitopic** *Laboratorios Chile, Chile.*
Bacitracin zinc (p.161·3); neomycin sulfate (p.235·1); zinc oxide (p.1163·2).
*Bacterial skin infections; infected burns and wounds.*

**Bacitopic Compuesto** *Laboratorios Chile, Chile.*
Bacitracin zinc (p.161·3); neomycin sulfate (p.235·1); antazoline phosphate (p.424·2); xylometazoline hydrochloride (p.1132·2).
*Cold symptoms; rhinitis; sinusitis.*

**Bacitracina-Neo** *Zimaia, Port.*
Bacitracin (p.161·3); neomycin (p.235·1).

**Backache** *Potter's, UK.*
*Oral mixture:* Bearberry (p.1659·2); juniper (p.1703·1); clivers (p.1673·2); taraxacum (p.1751·3); lappa (p.1704·3).
*Tablets:* Gravel root (p.1695·3); hydrangea root (p.1698·3); buchu (p.1663·1); bearberry (p.1659·2).
*Backache.*

**Backache with Arnica** *Hylands, Canad.*
Homoeopathic preparation.

**Backache Ledum** *Homeocan, Canad.*
Homoeopathic preparation.

**Backache Maximum Strength Relief** *Bristol-Myers Squibb, USA.*
Magnesium salicylate (p.55·1).

**Backache Relief** *Herbal Concepts, UK.*
Buchu (p.1663·1); bearberry (p.1659·2); parsley piert (p.1729·1).
*Backache.*

**Back-Aid** *Technilab, Canad.*
Paracetamol (p.76·2); chlorzoxazone (p.1392·3).

**Back-Ese M** *Dannorth, Canad.†.*
Magnesium salicylate (p.55·1).

**BackOsamine** *Health Perception, UK.*
Glucosamine (p.1694·1); chondroitin; bromelains (p.1662·2); turmeric (p.1058·3).
*Back disorders.*

**Baclo** *Douglas, Austral.*
Baclofen (p.1386·3).
*Skeletal muscle spasm.*

**Baclohexal** *Hexal, Austral.*
Baclofen (p.1386·3).
*Skeletal muscle spasm.*

**Baclon** *Leiras, Fin.*
Baclofen (p.1386·3).
*Spasticity.*

**Baclopar**
*Pharmacia, Fin.; Gerard, Irl.*
Baclofen (p.1386·3).
*Spasticity.*

**Baclosal**
*Unipharm, Israel; M & H, Thai.*
Baclofen (p.1386·3).
*Spasticity.*

**Baclospas** *Ashbourne, UK.*
Baclofen (p.1386·3).
*Skeletal muscle spasm or spasticity.*

**Bacmin** *Marnel, USA.*
Multivitamin and mineral preparation with iron and folic acid (p.1417·1).

**Bacnutri** *Grisi, Mex.*
Vitamins A and D (p.1417·1).
*Vitamin supplement.*

**Bacocil** *Pfizer, Belg.†.*
Bacampicillin hydrochloride (p.161·2).
*Bacterial infections.*

**Bacotan** *TO-Chemicals, Thai.*
Hyoscine butylbromide (p.483·3).
*Smooth muscle spasm.*

**Bacpiryl** *Parggon, Mex.*
Co-trimoxazole (p.199·3).
*Bacterial infections.*

**Bacprotin** *Prodotti, Braz.*
Co-trimoxazole (p.199·3).
*Bacterial infections.*

**Bacris** *Cristalia, Braz.*
Co-trimoxazole (p.199·3).
*Bacterial infections; Pneumocystis carinii pneumonia; protozoal infections.*

**Bacrocin** *ICN, Braz.*
Mupirocin (p.233·1).
*Bacterial skin infections.*

**Bac-Sulfitrin** *Ducto, Braz.*
Co-trimoxazole (p.199·3).
*Bacterial infections.*

**Bacta** *Masa, Thai.*
Co-trimoxazole (p.199·3).
*Bacterial infections.*

**Bactacin** *Osoth, Thai.*
Nitrofurazone (p.238·2).
*Burns; skin ulcers; wounds.*

**Bactedene** *Macrophar, Thai.*
Povidone-iodine (p.1190·3).
*Disinfection of skin, wounds, and burns.*

**Bactelan** *Quimica y Farmacia, Mex.*
Co-trimoxazole (p.199·3).
*Bacterial infections.*

**Bacteomycine** *Merck Medication Familiale, Fr.*
Neomycin sulfate (p.235·1).
Formerly contained bacitracin and neomycin sulfate.
*Infected skin disorders.*

**Bacteracin** *Teuto, Braz.*
Co-trimoxazole (p.199·3).
*Bacterial infections; Pneumocystis carinii pneumonia; protozoal infections.*

**Bacteracin Balsamico** *Teuto, Braz.†.*
Co-trimoxazole (p.199·3); guaifenesin (p.1122·1); ammonium chloride (p.1115·2).
*Bacterial infections.*

**Bacterial** *CT, Ital.†.*
Co-trimoxazole (p.199·3).
*Bacterial infections.*

**Bacterian** *Musa, Braz.*
Benzalkonium chloride (p.1168·3).
Formerly contained thiomersal.
*Disinfection.*

**Bacterianos D** *Anios, Fr.*
Formaldehyde (p.1179·3); glyoxal (p.1181·1); glutaral (p.1180·3); didecyldimethylammonium chloride (p.1178·3).
*Disinfection of surfaces.*

**Bacterinil** *Luper, Braz.*
Ampicillin (p.157·1).
*Bacterial infections.*

**Bacterion** *Opofarm, Braz.†.*
Ampicillin (p.157·1).
*Bacterial infections.*

**Bacterix** *Gifrer Barbezat, Fr.*
Nifuroxazide (p.237·2).

**Bacternil** *Maffioli, Ital.*
Sulfadiazine silver (p.259·1).
*Infected burns and ulcers; infected skin disorders.*

**Bacterol** *Recalcine, Chile.*
Co-trimoxazole (p.199·3).
*Bacterial infections.*

**Bacteroskin** *Stiefel, Arg.*
Coco fatty acids; undecenoic acid (p.410·3); triclocarban (p.1195·1).
*Feminine hygiene; soap substitute.*

**Bacticef** *Mitim, Ital.*
Cefaclor (p.167·1).
*Bacterial infections.*

**Bacticel** *Bago, Arg.*
Co-trimoxazole (p.199·3).
*Bacterial infections.*

**Bacticil** *Continentales, Mex.†.*
Ampicillin (p.157·1).
*Bacterial infections.*

**Bacti-Cleanse** *Pedinol, USA.*
Benzalkonium chloride (p.1168·3).
*Skin cleanser.*

**Bacticlor** *Ranbaxy, UK.*
Cefaclor (p.167·1).
*Bacterial infections.*

**Bacticort** *Montpellier, Arg.*
Betamethasone valerate (p.1093·2); gentamicin sulfate (p.217·1).
*Burns; infected skin disorders; ulcers; wounds.*

**Bacticort Complex** *Montpellier, Arg.*
Betamethasone valerate (p.1093·2); gentamicin sulfate (p.217·1); tolnaftate (p.410·1); nystatin (p.406·3).
*Infected burns; infected skin disorders.*

**Bactidan** *Pierre Fabre, Ital.*
Enoxacin (p.207·2).
*Urinary-tract and respiratory-tract infections.*

**Bactide** *Collins, Mex.*
Co-trimoxazole (p.199·3).
*Bacterial infections.*

**Bactident** *Oberlin, Fr.*
Sodium perborate (p.1192·2); sodium carbonate (p.1747·1); sodium phosphate (p.1231·1); sodium laurilsulfate (p.1574·2).
*False teeth hygiene.*

**Bactidol**
*Pfizer, Hong Kong; Pfizer, Malaysia; Pfizer Consumer, Singapore.*
Hexetidine (p.1182·1).
*Mouth and throat disorders.*

**Bactidox** *TAD, Ger.†.*
Doxycycline (p.206·2).
*Bacterial infections.*

**Bactidron** *Aventis, S.Afr.*
Enoxacin (p.207·2).
*Cystitis; gonorrhoea.*

**Bactifor** *Andromaco, Spain†.*
Co-trimoxazole (p.199·3).
*Bacterial infections; Pneumocystis carinii pneumonia.*

**Bactigras**
*Smith & Nephew, Austral.; Smith & Nephew, Canad.; Braun, Ger.; Smith & Nephew, Hong Kong; Smith & Nephew, S.Afr.; Smith & Nephew, Thai.; Smith & Nephew, UK.*
Chlorhexidine acetate (p.1173·2).
*Burns; skin infections; ulcers; wounds.*

**Bactil** *CEPA, Spain.*
Ebastine (p.433·1).
*Hypersensitivity reactions.*

**Bactilen** *Cryopharma, Mex.*
Co-trimoxazole (p.199·3).
*Bacterial infections.*

**Bactilina** *Richmond, Arg.*
Ampicillin (p.157·1).
*Bacterial infections.*

**Bactine**
*Note. This name is used for preparations of different composition.*
*Bayer Consumer, Canad.*
Benzalkonium chloride (p.1168·3); lidocaine hydrochloride (p.1377·3).
*Skin disorders; wound cleansing.*
*Miles, USA.*
Hydrocortisone (p.1103·3).
*Skin disorders.*

**Bactine Antiseptic** *Miles, USA.*
Lidocaine (p.1377·3); benzalkonium chloride (p.1168·3).
*Skin disorders.*

**Bactine First Aid Antibiotic Plus Anesthetic**
*Miles Laboratories, USA†.*
Polymyxin B sulfate (p.245·1); bacitracin (p.161·3); neomycin sulfate (p.235·1); diperodon hydrochloride (p.1376·2).
*Bacterial skin infections.*

**Bactine Pain Relieving Cleansing** *Bayer, USA.*
*Topical spray:* Lidocaine (p.1377·3); benzalkonium chloride (p.1168·3).
*Topical wipes:* Pramocaine hydrochloride (p.1382·2); benzalkonium chloride (p.1168·3).

**Bactio Rhin** *Byk, Arg.*
Naphazoline hydrochloride (p.1124·3).
*Rhinitis.*

**Bactio Rhin Prednisolona** *Byk, Arg.*
Naphazoline hydrochloride (p.1124·3); prednisolone (p.1108·1).
*Allergic rhinitis.*

**Bactisubtil**
*Sanofi Synthelabo, Belg.; Aventis, Fr.†; Cassella-med, Ger.; Aventis, Port.*
*Bacillus cereus* IP 5832.
*Diarrhoea; restoration of the gastrointestinal flora..*

**Bacti-Uril** *Bago, Arg.*
Co-trimoxazole (p.199·3); phenazopyridine hydrochloride (p.83·1).
*Urinary-tract infections.*

**Bactiver** *Maver, Mex.*
Co-trimoxazole (p.199·3).
*Bacterial infections.*

**Bactocef** *Aspen, S.Afr.†.*
Cefradine (p.179·3).
*Bacterial infections.*

**Bactocill** *SmithKline Beecham, USA†.*
Oxacillin sodium (p.240·2).
*Bacterial infections.*

**Bactocin**
*Note. This name is used for preparations of different composition.*
*Scharper, Ital.*
*Lactobacillus plantarum.*
*Vulvovaginitis.*
*Hormona, Mex.*
Ofloxacin (p.239·3).
*Bacterial infections.*

**Bactoderm** *Agis, Israel.*
Mupirocin (p.233·1).
*Bacterial skin infections.*

**Bactofen** *Rusch, Ital.*
Benzoxonium chloride (p.1170·2).
*Disinfection of skin, mucous membranes, and instruments.*

**Bactoflox**
*Note. This name is used for preparations of different composition.*
*Aurantis, Braz.; Biochimico, Braz.*
Ciprofloxacin hydrochloride (p.188·2).
*Bacterial infections.*
*Probios, Port.*
Ofloxacin (p.239·3).
*Bacterial infections.*

**Bactomicin** *Sigma, Braz.*
Amikacin sulfate (p.154·1).
*Bacterial infections.*

**Bactopumon** *Cinfa, Spain.*
Tolu balsam (p.1131·3); bromhexine hydrochloride (p.1115·3); co-trimoxazole (p.199·3).
*Respiratory-tract infections.*

**Bactoreduct** *Azupharma, Ger.*
Co-trimoxazole (p.199·3).
*Bacterial infections; Pneumocystis carinii pneumonia.*

**Bactoscrub** *Vitamed, Israel.*
Chlorhexidine gluconate (p.1173·2).
*Skin cleansing; skin disinfection.*

**Bactosept** *Vitamed, Israel.*
Chlorhexidine gluconate (p.1173·2).
*Burns; disinfection of instruments and skin; skin cleansing; wounds.*

**BactoShield** *Amsco, USA.*
Chlorhexidine gluconate (p.1173·2); isopropyl alcohol (p.1184·3).
*Skin disinfection.*

**Bactosone Retard** *Belmac, Spain†.*
Ampicillin sodium (p.157·1).
Lidocaine hydrochloride (p.1377·3) is included in this preparation to alleviate the pain of injection.
Formerly contained ampicillin sodium, ampicillin benzathine, bromhexine hydrochloride, and guaifenesin.
*Respiratory-tract infections.*

**Bactox**
*Note. This name is used for preparations of different composition.*
*Windson, Braz.†.*
Co-trimoxazole (p.199·3).
*Bacterial infections; Pneumocystis carinii pneumonia; protozoal infections.*
*Innotech, Fr.*
Amoxicillin sodium (p.155·3) or amoxicillin trihydrate (p.155·3).
*Bacterial infections.*

**Bactox Balsamico** *Windson, Braz.†.*
Co-trimoxazole (p.199·3); guaifenesin (p.1122·1).
*Bacterial infections.*

**Bactracid** *Apogepha, Ger.*
Norfloxacin (p.238·3).
*Urinary-tract infections.*

**Bactrazine** *Smith & Nephew, S.Afr.†.*
Sulfadiazine silver (p.259·1).
*Infected ulcers and burns.*

**Bactren** *Sanval, Braz.†.*
Co-trimoxazole (p.199·3).
*Bacterial infections; Pneumocystis carinii pneumonia; protozoal infections.*

**Bactrex** *Sintofarma, Braz.†.*
Co-trimoxazole (p.199·3); guaifenesin (p.1122·1); ammonium chloride (p.1115·2).
*Bacterial infections.*

**Bactrian** *Loveridge, UK†.*
Cetrimide (p.1172·1).
*Skin infections.*

**Bactricin** *Marjan, Braz.†.*
Co-trimoxazole (p.199·3).
*Bacterial infections; Pneumocystis carinii pneumonia; protozoal infections.*

**Bactricin Balsamico** *Marjan, Braz.†.*
Co-trimoxazole (p.199·3); guaifenesin (p.1122·1); ammonium chloride (p.1115·2).
*Bacterial infections.*

**Bactrim**
*Roche, Arg.; Roche, Austral.; Roche, Austria; Roche, Belg.; Roche, Braz.; Roche, Canad.†; Roche, Denm.†; Roche, Fr.; Roche, Ger.†; Piramal, India; Roche, Irl.†; Roche, Ital.; Roche, Mex.; Roche, Norw.; Roche, NZ†; Roche, Port.; Roche, S.Afr.; Roche, Singapore†; Roche, Swed.; Roche, Switz.; Roche, Thai.; Roche, USA.*
Co-trimoxazole (p.199·3).
*Bacterial infections; Pneumocystis carinii pneumonia; toxoplasmosis.*

**Bactrim Balsamico** *Roche, Arg.*
Co-trimoxazole (p.199·3); guaifenesin (p.1122·1).
*Respiratory-tract infections.*

**Bactrim Compositum** *Roche, Mex.*
Co-trimoxazole (p.199·3); guaifenesin (p.1122·1).
*Respiratory-tract infections.*

**Bactrimel**
Roche, Chile; Roche, Gr.; Roche, Neth.
Co-trimoxazole (p.199·3).
*Bacterial infections; Pneumocystis carinii pneumonia; toxoplasmosis.*

**Bactrisan** Sanval, Braz.
Co-trimoxazole (p.199·3).
*Bacterial infections; Pneumocystis carinii pneumonia; protozoal infections.*

**Bactrisan Balsamico** Sanval, Braz.†.
Co-trimoxazole (p.199·3); guaifenesin (p.1122·1); ammonium chloride (p.1115·2).
*Bacterial infections.*

**Bactrizol** IMA, Braz.
Co-trimoxazole (p.199·3).
*Bacterial infections.*

**Bactroban**
GlaxoSmithKline, Arg.; GlaxoSmithKline, Austral.; GlaxoSmithKline, Austria; GlaxoSmithKline, Belg.; GlaxoSmithKline, Braz.; GlaxoSmithKline, Canad.; GlaxoSmithKline, Chile; GlaxoSmithKline, Denm.; GlaxoSmithKline, Fin.; GlaxoSmithKline, Fr.; SmithKline Beecham, Gr.; GlaxoSmithKline, Hong Kong; GlaxoSmithKline, India; GlaxoSmithKline, Irl.; SmithKline Beecham, Israel; GlaxoSmithKline, Ital.; SmithKline Beecham, Jpn; GlaxoSmithKline, Malaysia; SmithKline Beecham, Mex.; GlaxoSmithKline, Neth.; GlaxoSmithKline, NZ; Beecham, Port.; GlaxoSmithKline, S.Afr.; GlaxoSmithKline, Singapore; GlaxoSmithKline, Spain; GlaxoSmithKline, Swed.; SmithKline Beecham, Switz.; GlaxoSmithKline, Thai.; GlaxoSmithKline, UK; SmithKline Beecham, USA.
Mupirocin (p.233·1) or mupirocin calcium (p.233·2).
*Bacterial skin infections; elimination of nasal staphylococci.*

**Bactroneo** Neo Quimica, Braz.
Mupirocin (p.233·1).
*Bacterial skin infections.*

**Bactropin**
Cimed, Braz.; Sons, Mex.
Co-trimoxazole (p.199·3).
*Bacterial infections; Pneumocystis carinii pneumonia; protozoal infections.*

**Bactropin Balsamico** Cimed, Braz.†.
Co-trimoxazole (p.199·3); guaifenesin (p.1122·1); ammonium chloride (p.1115·2).
*Bacterial infections.*

**Bactyl** Europhta, Mon.
Cethexonium bromide (p.1172·1).
*Eye infections.*

**Bactylisine** Peters, Fr.
Mixed quaternary ammonium salts; polyalkylamine.
*Surface disinfection.*

**Bac-Xolid** Ofimex, Mex.†.
Ceftriaxone (p.183·3).
*Bacterial infections.*

**Bac-Zidim** Ofimex, Mex.†.
Ceftazidime (p.180·2).
*Bacterial infections.*

**Baczole** Nakornpatana, Thai.
Co-trimoxazole (p.199·3).
*Bacterial infections.*

**Badeol** Agepha, Austria.
Sulfur (p.1158·2); soya oil (p.1447·2).
*Skin disorders.*

**Badyket** Tecefarma, Spain.
Dexketoprofen trometamol (p.51·2).
*Inflammation; pain.*

**Bafucin**
Pharmacia, Fin.; Pharmacia, Swed.
Benzocaine (p.1370·3); gramicidin (p.220·2); cetylpyridinium chloride (p.1173·1); dichlorobenzyl alcohol (p.1178·3).
*Mouth and throat disorders.*

**Bagnisan med Heilbad** Klemenz, Ger.†.
Echinacea purpurea (p.1683·2); hamamelis (p.1696·3); chlorophyllin (p.1057·1).
*Bath additive; circulatory disorders; deodorant; nervous disorders; neuralgia; neuritis; skin disorders.*

**Bagno Oculare** Ogna, Ital.; AFOM, Ital.
Zinc sulfate (p.1469·3); boric acid (p.1662·1); borax (p.1661·3).
*Eye irritation.*

**Bagobutam** Bago, Chile.
Dobutamine hydrochloride (p.905·3).
*Heart failure.*

**Bagociletas con Anestesia** Bago, Arg.
Nitrofurantoin (p.237·2); tetracaine dibudinate.
*Mouth and throat disorders.*

**Bagociletas sin Anestesia** Bago, Arg.
Nitrofurantoin (p.237·2); cetrimonium bromide (p.1173·1); hexylresorcinol (p.1182·1).
*Mouth and throat disorders.*

**Bagoderm** Bago, Arg.
Sodium acexamate (p.1646·2); cetrimonium bromide (p.1173·1).
*Burns; cracked nipples; nappy rash; wounds.*

**Bagohepat** Bago, Arg.
Cynara (p.1678·3); dehydrocholic acid (p.1679·2).
*Liver disorders.*

**Bagomicina** Bago, Chile.
Minocycline (p.231·3).
*Bacterial infections.*

**Bagovit A** Bago, Arg.
Vitamin A (p.1451·2).
*Skin disorders.*

**Bagovit A Plus** Bago, Arg.
Vitamin A palmitate (p.1453·1); triamcinolone acetonide (p.1110·2).
*Skin disorders.*

**Bagovit Avant Piel** Bago, Arg.
Vitamin A (p.1451·2); methylsilanol manuronate; dimethylsilanol hyaluronate.
*Skin disorders.*

**Bagovit-A** Bago, Chile.
Vitamin A palmitate (p.1453·1).
*Skin disorders.*

**Bagren** Serono, Braz.
Bromocriptine mesilate (p.1200·3).
*Acromegaly; hyperprolactinaemia; lactation inhibition; male infertility; neuroleptic malignant syndrome; parkinsonism.*

**Baicurina** Regius, Braz.†.
Paracetamol (p.76·2).
*Dysmenorrhoea.*

**Bain antirhumatismal** Kneipp, Switz.
Juniper oil (p.1703·1); sweet birch oil (p.60·1).
*Bath additive; musculoskeletal and joint disorders.*

**Bain contre les refroidissements** Kneipp, Switz.
Eucalyptus oil (p.1686·2); camphor (p.1665·3).
*Bath additive; coughs and colds.*

**Bain de Bouche Lipha** Merck Medication Familiale, Fr.
Veratrol; menthol (p.1711·3); resorcinol (p.1156·3) cloral hydrate (p.684·1).
*Mouthwash.*

**Bain de Soleil**
Note. This name is used for preparations of different composition.
Canderm, Canad.
*SPF 4 lotion*†; *SPF 8*†: Octocrilene (p.1154·3); octinoxate (p.1154·3); titanium dioxide (p.1160·3).
*SPF 15*†; *SPF 30*†: Octocrilene (p.1154·3); octinoxate (p.1154·3); oxybenzone (p.1154·3); titanium dioxide (p.1160·3).
*Sunscreen.*

Schering-Plough, Canad.
*SPF 4 gel:* Octinoxate (p.1154·3); octisalate (p.1154·3).
*Sunscreen.*

Procter & Gamble, USA.
*SPF 4:* Octinoxate (p.1154·3); octisalate (p.1154·3).
*Sunscreen.*

**Bain de Soleil All Day** Procter & Gamble, USA.
*SPF 4; SPF 8:* Octinoxate (p.1154·3); octocrilene (p.1154·3); titanium dioxide (p.1160·3).
*SPF 15; SPF 30:* Octinoxate (p.1154·3); octocrilene (p.1154·3); oxybenzone (p.1154·3); titanium dioxide (p.1160·3).
*Sunscreen.*

**Bain de Soleil Color** Procter & Gamble, USA.
*SPF 8+:* Octinoxate (p.1154·3); octocrilene (p.1154·3).
*SPF 15+; SPF 30+:* Octinoxate (p.1154·3); octocrilene (p.1154·3); oxybenzone (p.1154·3).
*Sunscreen.*

**Bain de Soleil Luminessence** Schering-Plough, Canad.
*SPF 4; SPF 8:* Octinoxate (p.1154·3); oxybenzone (p.1154·3).
*Sunscreen.*

**Bain de Soleil Mega Tanning** Canderm, Canad.†.
*SPF 30:* Octocrilene (p.1154·3); octinoxate (p.1154·3); oxybenzone (p.1154·3).
*Sunscreen.*

**Bain de Soleil Oil Free Faces** Schering-Plough, Canad.
*SPF 15:* Octinoxate (p.1154·3); oxybenzone (p.1154·3).
*Sunscreen.*

**Bain de Soleil Orange** Schering-Plough, Canad.
*SPF 8:* Octinoxate (p.1154·3); octocrilene (p.1154·3); octisalate (p.1154·3); oxybenzone (p.1154·3).
*Sunscreen.*

**Bain de Soleil Protection** Canderm, Canad.†.
*SPF 15:* Avobenzone (p.1142·3); enzacamene (p.1147·1); octisalate (p.1154·3); titanium dioxide (p.1160·3).
*SPF 25:* Titanium dioxide (p.1160·3); zinc oxide (p.1163·2).
*Sunscreen.*

**Bain de Soleil Sport** Canderm, Canad.†.
*SPF 8:* Octocrilene (p.1154·3); octinoxate (p.1154·3); titanium dioxide (p.1160·3).
*SPF 15:* Octocrilene (p.1154·3); octinoxate (p.1154·3); oxybenzone (p.1154·3); titanium dioxide (p.1160·3).
*Sunscreen.*

**Bain de Soleil Tanning Mist** Schering-Plough, Canad.
*SPF 4:* Octocrilene (p.1154·3); octinoxate (p.1154·3).
Formerly known as Bain de Soleil Mega Tan.
*SPF 8:* Octocrilene (p.1154·3); octinoxate (p.1154·3); oxybenzone (p.1154·3).
*Sunscreen.*

**Bain de Soleil Tropical** Schering-Plough, Canad.
*SPF 4:* Octinoxate (p.1154·3); octisalate (p.1154·3); zinc oxide (p.1163·2).
*Sunscreen.*

**Bain extra-doux dermatologique** Widmer, Switz.†.
Coal tar (p.1159·2); chamomile (p.1669·3).
*Skin disorders.*

**Bain extra-doux dermatologique Nouvelle Formule** Widmer, Switz.
Ichthammol (p.1148·2); chamomile (p.1669·3); guaiazulene (p.1696·2).
*Skin disorders.*

**Bains Romains** Couzian, Fr.
Hypericum oil (p.299·2).
*Bath additive; dry skin; skin irritation.*

**Bainto** TP, Thai.
Gamma-aminobutyric acid (p.1690·2).
*Amnesia; hypertension; mental function impairment; palsy; speech disorders.*

**Bajaten**
Note. This name is used for preparations of different composition.
Merck, Arg.
Indapamide (p.938·2).
*Hypertension.*

Instituto Sanitas, Chile.
Enalapril maleate (p.909·2).
*Heart failure; hypertension.*

**Bajaten D** Instituto Sanitas, Chile.
Enalapril maleate (p.909·2); hydrochlorothiazide (p.933·2).
*Heart failure; hypertension.*

**Bajumol** Poen, Arg.
Mepyramine maleate (p.437·1); phenylephrine hydrochloride (p.1126·3); phenazone (p.82·3).
*Eye inflammation and irritation.*

**Bakam** De Salute, Ital.
Bacampicillin hydrochloride (p.161·2).
*Bacterial infections.*

**Bakanasan Einschlaf** Bregenzer, Austria.
Valerian (p.1762·2); lupulus (p.1708·1).
*Anxiety; sleep disorders.*

**Bakanasan Entwasserungs** Bregenzer, Austria.
Birch leaf (p.1660·3).
*Urinary-tract disorders.*

**Bakanasan Leber-Galle** Bregenzer, Austria.
Silybum marianum (p.1043·3); turmeric (p.1058·3).
*Gastrointestinal disorders; liver and gallbladder disorders.*

**Baklinger** Klinger, Braz.†.
Co-trimoxazole (p.199·3).
*Bacterial infections.*

**Baknyl** Ariston, Braz.†.
Erythromycin (p.208·1); bromhexine hydrochloride (p.1115·3).
*Bacterial infections.*

**Bakteriostat "Herbrand"** Herbrand, Ger.†.
Dequalinium chloride (p.1178·1); ascorbic acid (p.1460·2).
*Mouth and throat disorders.*

**Baktobod** Bode, Ger.†.
Glutaral (p.1180·3); glyoxal (p.1181·1); benzalkonium chloride (p.1168·3).
*Surface disinfection.*

**Baktobod N** Bode, Ger.†.
Glyoxal (p.1181·1); benzalkonium chloride (p.1168·3).
*Surface disinfection.*

**Baktonium** Bode, Ger.
Benzalkonium chloride (p.1168·3).
*Hand and skin disinfection.*

**BAL** IFET (IΦET), Gr.
Dimercaprol (p.1037·1).
*Heavy metal poisoning.*

**Bal Tar** Euroderm, Ital.†.
Castor oil (p.1668·2); ichthammol (p.1148·2).
*Seborrhoeic dermatitis.*

**Balad** Korean Drug, Singapore.
Sodium fusidate (p.215·2).
*Bacterial skin infections; infected wounds and burns.*

**Balance ACE** Pharmavite, Canad.
Betacarotene; vitamin C; vitamin E; minerals (p.1417·1).

**Balance Elastin E** Bio-Pharmaceuticals, Malaysia.
Elastin; vitamin E (p.1464·3).
*Dry skin disorders.*

**Balanced B** Adams, Canad.; Hall, Canad.; Pharmavite, Canad.; Stanley, Canad.; General Nutrition, Canad.
Vitamin B substances (p.1417·1).

**Balanced B Complex plus Vitamins C & E** Pharmavite, Canad.
Vitamin B substances, vitamin C, and Vitamin E (p.1417·1).

**Balanced C Complex** Jamieson, Canad.
Ascorbic acid (p.1460·2).

**Balanced E** Jamieson, Canad.†.
Vitamin C, vitamin E, and selenium (p.1417·1).

**Balanced Irrigating Salt Solution** Teva, Israel.
Electrolyte solution (p.1217·1).
*Irrigation of eyes, ears, nose, and throat.*

**Balanced Ratio Cal-Mag** Quest, UK.
Calcium, magnesium, and vitamin D preparation (p.1417·1).

**Balanced Salt Solution**
Alcon, Denm.†; Alcon, NZ; Alcon, UK; Pharmacia, UK; Abbott, USA; Bausch & Lomb, USA; Akorn, USA.
Electrolyte solution (p.1217·1).
*Eye irrigation.*

**Balancid** AstraZeneca, Norw.†.
Magnesium carbonate (p.1272·1); aluminium hydroxide (p.1249·2).
*Gastrointestinal disorders associated with hyperacidity.*

**Balancid Novum**
AstraZeneca, Denm.; AstraZeneca, Fin.
Calcium carbonate (p.1254·2); magnesium hydroxide (p.1272·2).
*Gastritis; gastro-oesophageal reflux; peptic ulcer.*

**Balans** Labomed, Chile.
Betacarotene; alpha tocopherol; ascorbic acid (p.1417·1).
*Vitamin supplement.*

**Balbek** Provit, Mex.
Dextromethorphan (p.1117·3).
*Coughs.*

**B-Alcerin** Medicus, Gr.
Ranitidine hydrochloride (p.1285·2).
*Conditions where gastric acid reduction is beneficial; gastric hypersecretion including Zollinger-Ellison syndrome; peptic ulcer.*

**Balcor**
Baldacci, Braz.; Baldacci, Port.
Diltiazem hydrochloride (p.900·1).
*Angina pectoris; arrhythmias; hypertension.*

**Balcoran** Whitehall-Robins, Mex.†.
Vancomycin (p.275·2).

**Baldin-CE** Neckerman, Braz.†.
Dipyrone (p.35·3); sodium camsilate; ascorbic acid (p.1460·2); guaifenesin (p.1122·1); cineole (p.1672·1); niaouli oil (p.1719·3).
*Cold and influenza symptoms.*

**Baldmin** Mintlab, Chile.
Pipenzolate bromide (p.487·3); phenobarbital (p.367·3).

**Baldracin** Austroplant, Austria.
Valerian (p.1762·2); peppermint leaf (p.1283·2); melissa (p.1711·1); lupulus (p.1708·1).
*Nervous disorders; sleep disorders.*

**Baldrian** Solvay, Spain†.
Passion flower (p.1729·1); valerian (p.1762·2).
*Insomnia; nervous disorders.*

**Baldrian AMA** Kwizda, Austria.
Valerian (p.1762·2); lupulus (p.1708·1).
*Nervous disorders; sleep disorders.*

**Baldrian Dispert Compositum** Solvay, Austria.
Valerian (p.1762·2); lupulus (p.1708·1).
*Nervous disorders; sleep disorders.*

**Baldrian-Dispert** Solvay, Swed.
Valerian (p.1762·2).
*Anxiety; sleep disorders.*

**Baldrian-Dispert Nacht** Solvay, Ger.
Valerian (p.1762·2); lupulus (p.1708·1).
*Insomnia.*

**Baldrian-Elixier** Ehrmann, Austria.
Valerian (p.1762·2); lupulus (p.1708·1); melissa (p.1711·1).
*Nervous disorders; sleep disorders.*

**Baldrian-Krautertonikum** Bioflora, Austria.
Melissa (p.1711·1); valerian (p.1762·2); lupulus (p.1708·1); orange flowers (p.1723·3); lavender flowers (p.1705·1).
*Nervous disorders; sleep disorders.*

**Baldrianox S** Hermes, Ger.†.
Valerian (p.1762·2); lupulus (p.1708·1).
*Nervous and sleep disorders.*

**Baldrinetten** Solvay, Austria.
Valerian (p.1762·2).
*Sedative.*

**Baldriparan** Whitehall-Robins, Switz.
Valerian (p.1762·2); melissa (p.1711·1); lupulus (p.1708·1).
*Nervous disorders.*

**Baldriparan Beruhigungs** Sanova, Austria; Wyeth Lederle, Austria.
Valerian (p.1762·2); lupulus (p.1708·1); melissa (p.1711·1).
*Nervous disorders; sleep disorders.*

**Baldriparan N** Whitehall-Much, Ger.†.
Valerian (p.1762·2); lupulus (p.1708·1).
*Nervous disorders; sleep disorders.*

**Baldriparan N Stark** Whitehall-Much, Ger.
Valerian (p.1762·2); lupulus (p.1708·1); melissa (p.1711·1).
*Nervous disorders; sleep disorders.*

**Baldriparan pour la nuit** Whitehall-Robins, Switz.
Valerian (p.1762·2).
*Sleep disorders.*

**Baldriparan Stark** Whitehall-Much, Ger.
Valerian (p.1762·2).
*Sleep disorders.*

**Baldrisedon** Wild, Switz.
Valerian (p.1762·2).
*Anxiety; sleep disorders.*

**Baldrisedon Mono** Much, Ger.†.
Valerian (p.1762·2).
*Nervous disorders; sleep disorders.*

**Baldurat** Pohl, Ger.
Valerian (p.1762·2).
*Nervous tension; sleep disorders.*

**Balepton** Leovan, Gr.
Ciprofloxacin hydrochloride (p.188·2).
*Bacterial infections.*

**Balgifen** Berk, UK†.
Baclofen (p.1386·3).
*Skeletal muscle spasm or spasticity.*

**Baliartrin** Baliarda, Arg.
Glucosamine sulfate (p.1694·1).
*Musculoskeletal and joint disorders.*

**Balidon** Recalcine, Chile.
Triazolam (p.725·3).
*Sleep disorders.*

**Balin**
Atlantic, Malaysia; Atlantic, Singapore; Atlantic, Thai.†.
Sulfadiazine (p.258·2); trimethoprim (p.272·2).
*Bacterial infections.*

**Balisa** Bioglan, Ger.
Urea (p.1162·2).
*Keratinisation disorders.*

**Balisa VAS** Bioglan, Ger.
Urea (p.1162·2); tretinoin (p.1161·1).
*Keratinisation disorders.*

**Balkis** Dolorgiet, Ger.
*Capsules:* Phenylephrine hydrochloride (p.1126·3); chlorphenamine maleate (p.427·3).
Formerly contained etilefrine polistirex and chlorphenamine polistirex.
*Colds; hay fever.*
*Nasal drops; nasal spray:* Xylometazoline hydrochloride (p.1132·2).
*Nasal congestion.*

**Balkis Spezial** Dolorgiet, Ger.†.
Terfenadine (p.441·1).
*Allergic rhinitis.*

**Balm of Gilead**
Note. This name is used for preparations of different composition.
Healthcrafts, UK†.
*Pastilles:* Balm of Gilead (p.1733·3); squill (p.1130·3); lobelia (p.1589·1).
*Catarrh; coughs.*
Potter's, UK.
*Oral mixture:* Balm of Gilead (p.1733·3); squill (p.1130·3); lobelia (p.1589·1); lungwort.
*Coughs.*

**Balmandol** Spirig, Switz.
Almond oil (p.1651·1); light liquid paraffin (p.1479·1).
*Skin disorders.*

**Balmex**
Note. This name is used for preparations of different composition.
GlaxoSmithKline, Arg.
Zinc oxide (p.1163·2).
*Nappy rash.*
GlaxoSmithKline, Braz.
Zinc oxide (p.1163·2); liquid paraffin (p.1479·1); beeswax (p.1480·1); silicone (p.1482·1); peru balsam (p.1730·2).
*Skin disorders.*
Stafford-Miller, Fr.†.
Zinc oxide (p.1163·2); liquid paraffin (p.1479·1); beeswax (p.1480·1); silicone (p.1482·1).
*Nappy rash.*
GlaxoSmithKline, Port.†.
Zinc oxide (p.1163·2); liquid paraffin (p.1479·1); beeswax (p.1480·1); dimeticone (p.1482·1).
*Nappy rash.*

**Balmex Baby** Macsil, USA.
Zinc oxide (p.1163·2); peru balsam (p.1730·2); corn starch (p.1449·1); calcium carbonate (p.1254·2).
*Nappy rash.*

**Balmex Emollient** Block, USA.
Emollient and moisturiser.

**Balminil** Elfar, Spain.
Nitrendipine (p.973·3).
*Hypertension.*

**Balminil Camphorub** Rougier, Canad.
Camphor (p.1665·3); menthol (p.1711·3); cineole (p.1672·1).
*Pain.*

**Balminil Cough & Flu** Technilab, Canad.
Dextromethorphan hydrobromide (p.1117·3); pseudoephedrine hydrochloride (p.1129·2); guaifenesin (p.1122·1); paracetamol (p.76·2).
*Congestion; coughs.*

**Balminil Decongestant**
Rougier, Canad.†; Rougier, Hong Kong†.
Pseudoephedrine hydrochloride (p.1129·2).
*Nasal and sinus congestion.*

**Balminil DM**
Technilab, Canad.; Rougier, Hong Kong.
Dextromethorphan hydrobromide (p.1117·3).
*Coughs.*

**Balminil DM+Decongestant** Technilab, Canad.
Pseudoephedrine hydrochloride (p.1129·2); dextromethorphan hydrobromide (p.1117·3).
Formerly known as Balminil DM D.
*Congestion; coughs.*

**Balminil DM+Decongestant+Expectorant**
Technilab, Canad.
Dextromethorphan hydrobromide (p.1117·3); pseudoephedrine hydrochloride (p.1129·2); guaifenesin (p.1122·1).
Formerly known as Balminil DM D E.
*Congestion; cough.*

**Balminil DM+Expectorant** Technilab, Canad.
Dextromethorphan hydrobromide (p.1117·3); guaifenesin (p.1122·1).
Formerly known as Balminil DM E.
*Coughs.*

**Balminil Expectorant** Technilab, Canad.
Guaifenesin (p.1122·1).
*Coughs.*

**Balminil Lozenges** Rougier, Canad.†.
Cetylpyridinium chloride (p.1173·1); benzocaine (p.1370·3).
*Mouth and throat disorders.*

**Balminil Nasal Ointment** Rougier, Canad.
Camphor (p.1665·3); menthol (p.1711·3); cineole (p.1672·1); chlorobutanol (p.1176·3); ephedrine hydrochloride (p.1120·1).
*Nasal congestion.*

**Balminil Night-Time** Technilab, Canad.
Dextromethorphan hydrobromide (p.1117·3); diphenhydramine hydrochloride (p.431·3); ammonium chloride (p.1115·2).
*Congestion; coughs.*

**Balminil Suppositories** Technilab, Canad.
Eucalyptus oil (p.1686·2); niaouli oil (p.1719·3); menthol (p.1711·3); sodium dibunate (p.1130·2).
*Coughs.*

**Balmosa** Forest Laboratories, UK.
Methyl salicylate (p.59·3); menthol (p.1711·3); camphor (p.1665·3); capsicum oleoresin (p.1667·1).
*Musculoskeletal, joint, and soft-tissue pain.*

**Balmox**
Yamanouchi, Port.; SmithKline Beecham, Switz.
Nabumetone (p.63·3).
*Musculoskeletal, joint, peri-articular, and soft-tissue disorders.*

**Balneoconzen N** S & K, Ger.
Soya oil (p.1447·2).
*Skin disorders.*

**Balneogel** Boots Healthcare, Spain†.
Allantoin (p.1141·3); chlorophyllin (p.1057·1); guaiazulene (p.1696·2); lauril polyoxyethylene sulfate; riboflavin sodium phosphate (p.1456·1).
*Skin disorders; soap substitute.*

**Balneol** Solvay, USA.
Skin cleanser.

**Balneovit** Mavena, Ger.
Soya oil (p.1447·2).
*Bath additive; skin disorders.*

**Balnetar**
Westwood-Squibb, Canad.; Westwood-Squibb, USA.
Coal tar (p.1159·2).
*Dermatitis; psoriasis.*

**Balneum**
Note. This name is used for preparations of different composition.
Hermal, Austria; Hermal, Ger.; Boots Healthcare, Irl.; Hermal, Israel; Hermal, Port.†; Crookes Healthcare, UK.
Soya oil (p.1447·2).
*Dry skin disorders.*
Hermal, Malaysia; Hermal, Singapore; Boots, Thai.; Hermal, Thai.
*Bath oil:* Light liquid paraffin (p.1479·1).
*Bath additive; dry skin disorders.*
Hermal, Malaysia; Hermal, Singapore; Boots, Thai.; Hermal, Thai.
*Cream; lotion:* White soft paraffin (p.1479·3); light liquid paraffin (p.1479·1); wool fat (p.1483·1).
*Dry skin disorders.*

**Balneum F**
Hermal, Austria; Hermal, Ger.; Hermal, Israel.
Arachis oil (p.1656·1); light liquid paraffin (p.1479·1).
*Bath additive; skin disorders.*

**Balneum Hermal**
Note. This name is used for preparations of different composition.
Hermal, Hong Kong.
White soft paraffin (p.1479·3); wool fat (p.1483·1); light liquid paraffin (p.1479·1).
Formerly contained soya oil.
*Skin disorders.*
Boots Healthcare, Ital.; Boots Healthcare, Switz.
Soya oil (p.1447·2).
*Bath additive; skin disorders.*

**Balneum Hermal F** Boots Healthcare, Switz.
Arachis oil (p.1656·1); liquid paraffin (p.1479·1).
*Skin disorders.*

**Balneum Hermal Forte** Boots Healthcare, Ital.
Liquid paraffin (p.1479·1); arachis oil (p.1656·1).
*Bath additive; skin disorders.*

**Balneum Hermal Plus** Boots Healthcare, Switz.
Soya oil (p.1447·2); macrogol lauril ethers (p.1412·3).
*Skin disorders.*

**Balneum Intensiv**
Note. This name is used for preparations of different composition.
Hermal, Hong Kong.
Ceramide; urea (p.1162·2); lipids.
*Skin disorders.*
Hermal, Malaysia.
Urea (p.1162·2).
*Dry skin disorders.*
Hermal, Singapore; Boots, Thai.; Hermal, Thai.
*Cream; lotion; wash:* Urea (p.1162·2).
*Dry skin disorders.*
Hermal, Singapore; Boots, Thai.; Hermal, Thai.
*Shower gel:* Soap substitute.
*Emollient; moisturiser.*

**Balneum Intensiv Plus**
Hermal, Hong Kong; Hermal, Malaysia; Hermal, Singapore; Boots, Thai.; Hermal, Thai.
Lauromacrogol 400 (p.1412·3); urea (p.1162·2).
*Dry skin disorders.*

**Balneum mit Teer** Hermal, Austria.
Soya oil (p.1447·2); coal tar (p.1159·2).
*Skin disorders.*

**Balneum Plus**
Note. This name is used for preparations of different composition.
Hermal, Austria; Hermal, Ger.; Boots Healthcare, Irl.; Hermal, Israel; Crookes Healthcare, UK.
*Bath additive:* Soya oil (p.1447·2); lauromacrogol 400 (p.1412·3).
*Dry skin; pruritus.*
Crookes Healthcare, UK.
*Cream:* Macrogol lauril ethers (p.1412·3); urea (p.1162·2).
*Skin disorders.*

**Balneum surgras** Merck-Clevenot, Fr.†.
Arachis oil (p.1656·1); liquid paraffin (p.1479·1).
*Bath additive; skin disorders.*

**Balneum with Tar** E. Merck, Irl.†.
Soya oil (p.1447·2); coal tar (p.1159·2).
*Bath additive; skin disorders.*

**Balnostim Bad N** Hoernecke, Ger.†.
Pine needle oil; rosemary oil (p.1740·2).
*Musculoskeletal, joint, and soft-tissue disorders.*

**Balodin** Ferrer, Spain†.
Dirithromycin (p.206·1).
*Bacterial infections.*

**Balpril** Baldacci, Port.
Enalapril maleate (p.909·2).
*Heart failure; hypertension.*

**Balsabit** Pensa, Spain.
Pramocaine hydrochloride (p.1382·2).
*Burns; insect bites; pruritus.*

**Balsamico (Unguento)** AFOM, Ital.; NewFaDem, Ital.; Sella, Ital.
Cineole (p.1672·1); menthol (p.1711·3); camphor (p.1665·3).
*Cold symptoms.*

**Balsamicum** Weleda, UK.
Homoeopathic preparation.

**Balsamin** Ahimsa, Arg.
Hexylresorcinol (p.1182·1); benzocaine (p.1370·3).
*Mouth and throat disorders.*

**Balsamina Kroner** Ceccarelli, Ital.
Sulfogaiacol (p.1131·1); mepyramine maleate (p.437·1).
*Catarrh; coughs.*

**Balsamo Analgesic Karmel** Agua del Carmen, Spain†.
Camphor (p.1665·3); beleo; stramonium (p.489·2); amyl salicylate (p.14·3); menthol (p.1711·3).
Formerly known as Karmel Balsamo.
*Rheumatic and muscle pain.*

**Balsamo Analgesico**
Note. This name is used for preparations of different composition.
Basi, Port.; Upsifarma, Port.
Salicylic acid (p.1157·1); menthol (p.1711·3); methyl salicylate (p.59·3).
Medical, Port.
Salicylic acid (p.1157·1); capsicum (p.1667·1); menthol (p.1711·3).

**Balsamo Analgesico con Fenilbutazona** Instituto Sanitas, Chile.
Phenylbutazone (p.83·2); dimeticones (p.1482·1); methyl salicylate (p.59·3); menthol (p.1711·3).
*Musculoskeletal, joint, and peri-articular pain.*

**Balsamo Analgesico Labesfal** Labesfal, Port.
Methyl salicylate (p.59·3).
Formerly contained salicylic acid, menthol, methyl salicylate, belladonna, and capsicum.

**Balsamo Analgesico Sanitas** Upsifarma, Port.
Methyl salicylate (p.59·3); salicylic acid (p.1157·1); menthol (p.1711·3); capsicum (p.1667·1).
Formerly contained methyl salicylate, salicylic acid, menthol, belladonna, and capsicum.
*Musculoskeletal and joint pain.*

**Balsamo Bengue** Novamed, Braz.
Menthol (p.1711·3); methyl salicylate (p.59·3).
*Musculoskeletal and joint disorders.*

**Balsamo Branco** Catarinense, Braz.†.
Lavender (p.1705·1); melissa (p.1711·1); caraway (p.1667·2); aniseed (p.1655·2); cinnamon (p.1672·2); clove (p.1673·2); lemon (p.1706·2).
*Dyspepsia.*

**Balsamo Ifusa** Ifusa, Mex.
Methyl salicylate (p.59·3); pine oil; peppermint oil (p.1283·2).
*Musculoskeletal and joint pain.*

**Balsamo Italstadium** Falqui, Ital.
Methyl salicylate (p.59·3); menthol (p.1711·3); camphor (p.1665·3).
*Musculoskeletal and joint pain.*

**Balsamo Kneipp** Fher, Spain.
Camphor (p.1665·3); Peru balsam (p.1730·2); cineole (p.1672·1); oleum pini sylvestris; thymol (p.1194·2); menthol (p.1711·3).
*Respiratory-tract disorders.*

**Balsamo Leon** Beiersdorf, Chile.
Menthol (p.1711·3); camphor (p.1665·3); thymol (p.1194·2); pine oil; turpentine oil (p.1760·1); eucalyptus oil (p.1686·2); anfocerina K.
*Coughs and cold symptoms.*

**Balsamo Midalgan** Sanofi Synthelabo, Spain†.
Capsicum (p.1667·1); methyl nicotinate (p.59·2); methyl salicylate (p.59·3).
*Rheumatic and muscle pain.*

**Balsamo Nostrum** Nostrum, Port.
Camphor (p.1665·3); menthol (p.1711·3); methyl salicylate (p.59·3); turpentine oil (p.1760·1).

**Balsamo Primi Denti** Sanofi Synthelabo OTC, Ital.
Milk serum.
*Teething pain.*

**Balsamo Sifcamina** Teofarma, Ital.
Methyl nicotinate (p.59·2); glycol salicylate (p.44·3).
*Musculoskeletal disorders.*

**Balsamorhinol** Etris, Fr.†.
Chlorobutanol (p.1176·3); menthol (p.1711·3).
*Nose and throat infections.*

**Balsan** Labinca, Arg.
Sodium chloride; polysorbate 80 (p.1415·2); benzalkonium chloride.
*Snoring.*

**Balsandin** Dinafarma, Braz.†.
Co-trimoxazole (p.199·3).
*Bacterial infections; Pneumocystis carinii pneumonia; protozoal infections.*

**Balsasulf** Fabra, Arg.
Bromhexine (p.1115·3).
*Respiratory-tract congestion.*

**Balsatux** Edmond Pharma, Ital.
Sulfogaiacol (p.1131·1); dextromethorphan hydrobromide (p.1117·3).
*Coughs.*

**Balsedrina** IQFA, Mex.
Dextromethorphan (p.1117·3).
*Coughs.*

**Balseptol** Hearst, Braz.†.
Thymol (p.1194·2).
*Antiseptic.*

**Balsibron** Liferpal, Mex.
Ambroxol (p.1114·3).
*Respiratory-tract congestion.*

**Balsibron-C** Liferpal, Mex.
Ambroxol hydrochloride (p.1114·3); clenbuterol hydrochloride (p.784·2).
*Respiratory-tract disorders with viscous mucus.*

**Balsiprin** Eurofarma, Braz.†.
Co-trimoxazole (p.199·3); guaifenesin (p.1122·1); ammonium chloride (p.1115·2).
*Bacterial infections.*

**Balsoclase**
Note. This name is used for preparations of different composition.
Bios, Belg.†.
*Oral solution:* Pentoxyverine citrate (p.1126·2); terpin hydrate (p.1131·1).
*Syrup:* Pentoxyverine citrate (p.1126·2); cineole (p.1672·1); terpin hydrate (p.1131·1); thyme (p.1755·2).
*Oral drops:* Pentoxyverine citrate (p.1126·2); guaifenesin (p.1122·1); cineole (p.1672·1); terpin hydrate (p.1131·1); thymol (p.1194·2).
*Coughs.*
UCB, Neth.
Pentoxyverine citrate (p.1126·2).
*Coughs.*

**Balsoclase Antitussivum** UCB, Belg.
Pentoxyverine citrate (p.1126·2).
*Coughs.*

**Balsoclase Compositum** UCB, Neth.†.
Pentoxyverine citrate (p.1126·2); cineole (p.1672·1); sodium citrate (p.1223·2); terpin hydrate (p.1131·1); thyme (p.1755·2).
*Coughs.*

**Balsoclase Expectorans** UCB, Belg.
*Oral solution; syrup:* Pentoxyverine citrate (p.1126·2); guaifenesin (p.1122·1).
*Suppositories:* Pentoxyverine (p.1126·2); guaifenesin (p.1122·1); cineole (p.1672·1).
Balsoclase suppositories formerly contained pentoxyverine, guaifenesin, cineole, terpineol, and terpin hydrate.
*Coughs.*

**Balsoclase-E** UCB, Neth.
Pentoxyverine (p.1126·2); cineole (p.1672·1).
*Coughs.*

**Balsofumine** Sanofi Synthelabo OTC, Fr.
Peru balsam (p.1730·2); sumatra benzoin (p.1751·1); eucalyptus (p.1686·1); lavender oil (p.1705·2); thyme oil (p.1755·3).
*Respiratory-tract congestion.*

**Balsofumine Mentholee** Sanofi Synthelabo OTC, Fr.
Peru balsam (p.1730·2); sumatra benzoin (p.1751·1); eucalyptus (p.1686·1); lavender oil (p.1705·2); thyme oil (p.1755·3); menthol (p.1711·3).
*Respiratory-tract congestion.*

**Balsolene** Cooperation Pharmaceutique, Fr.
Eucalyptus oil (p.1686·2); niaouli oil (p.1719·3); menthol (p.1711·3); siam benzoin (p.1744·1).
*Respiratory-tract congestion.*

**Balsoprim** Juste, Spain.
Bromhexine hydrochloride (p.1115·3); co-trimoxazole (p.199·3).
*Respiratory-tract infections.*

**Balta Intimo** Boots Healthcare, Ital.
Menthol (p.1711·3); cineole (p.1672·1); Iceland moss; undecenoic acid (p.410·3).
*Personal hygiene.*

**Balta-Crin Tar** Boots Healthcare, Ital.
Tar (p.1159·3); allantoin (p.1141·3).
*Seborrhoeic dermatitis.*

**Baltar** E. Merck, Irl.†.
Coal tar (p.1159·2).
*Scalp disorders.*

**Balto Foot Balm** Lane, UK.
Camphor (p.1665·3); menthol (p.1711·3); zinc oxide (p.1163·2); precipitated sulfur (p.1158·2).
*Aching feet; excessive perspiration; hard skin.*

**Balurol** Baldacci, Braz.
Pipemidic acid (p.243·1).
*Urinary-tract infections.*

**Balzide** Malesci, Ital.
Balsalazide sodium (p.1251·2).
*Ulcerative colitis.*

**Bamalite** Tecnobio, Spain.
Lansoprazole (p.1269·3).
*Gastro-oesophageal reflux; peptic ulcer.*

**Bambec**
AstraZeneca, Austria; AstraZeneca, Braz.†; AstraZeneca, Denm.;

Stern, Ger.; AstraZeneca, Ger.; AstraZeneca, Hong Kong; AstraZeneca, Ital.; AstraZeneca, Malaysia; AstraZeneca, Norw.; AstraZeneca, NZ; AstraZeneca, Singapore; Epsilon, Spain; Draco, Swed.; Astra, Switz.†; AstraZeneca, Thai.; AstraZeneca, UK.
Bambuterol hydrochloride (p.781·2).
*Obstructive airways disease.*

**Bambudil** Cipla, India.
Bambuterol hydrochloride (p.781·2).
*Obstructive airways disease.*

**Bamifix**
Farmalab, Braz.; Chiesi, Ital.
Bamifylline hydrochloride (p.781·3).
*Obstructive airways disease.*

**Bamixol** Pulitzer, Ital.
Bamifylline hydrochloride (p.781·3).
*Asthma; bronchospasm.*

**Bamycor**
AstraZeneca, Norw.†; Hassle, Swed.
Aspirin (p.15·1).
*Cardiovascular and cerebrovascular disorders.*

**Bamyl** Hassle, Swed.
Aspirin (p.15·1).
*Fever; inflammation; pain.*

**Bamyl koffein** Hassle, Swed.
Aspirin (p.15·1); caffeine (p.782·1).
*Fever; pain.*

**Bamyl S** Hassle, Swed.
Aspirin (p.15·1).
*Fever; pain.*

**Bamyl S koffein** Hassle, Swed.
Aspirin (p.15·1); caffeine (p.782·1).
*Fever; pain.*

**Bamyxin** Rekah, Israel.
Bacitracin (p.161·3); neomycin sulfate (p.235·1); polymyxin B sulfate (p.245·1).
*Bacterial eye infections.*

**Ban Pain** Triomed, S.Afr.
*Syrup:* Paracetamol (p.76·2); codeine phosphate (p.27·1); promethazine hydrochloride (p.439·1).
*Fever; pain.*
*Tablets:* Paracetamol (p.76·2); codeine phosphate (p.27·1); caffeine (p.782·1); meprobamate (p.706·2).
*Pain with tension.*

**Banadroxin** Pharmanik (Φαρμανικ), Gr.
Propylene glycol cefatrizine (p.170·3).
*Bacterial infections.*

**Banadyne-3** Norstar, USA.
Lidocaine (p.1377·3); menthol (p.1711·3); alcohol (p.1166·1).
*Herpes labialis.*

**Banalg** Forest Pharmaceuticals, USA.
Methyl salicylate (p.59·3); camphor (p.1665·3); menthol (p.1711·3).
*Muscle, joint, and soft-tissue pain; neuralgia.*

**Banan**
Sankyo, Hong Kong; Sankyo, Jpn; Sankyo, Thai.
Cefpodoxime proxetil (p.178·3).
*Bacterial infections.*

**Banana Boat Active Kids** Banana Boat, Canad.
*SPF 30:* Octinoxate (p.1154·3); octisalate (p.1154·3); oxybenzone (p.1154·3); titanium dioxide (p.1160·3).
*SPF 50:* Octocrilene (p.1154·3); octinoxate (p.1154·3); octisalate (p.1154·3); oxybenzone (p.1154·3).
*Sunscreen.*

**Banana Boat Active Sport** Banana Boat, Canad.
*SPF 25:* Homosalate (p.1148·1); octinoxate (p.1154·3); octisalate (p.1154·3); oxybenzone (p.1154·3).
Formerly known as Banana Boat Action Sport.
*Sunscreen.*

**Banana Boat Aloe Vera Lip Balm Sunblock**
Banana Boat, Canad.
*SPF 30†:* Padimate O (p.1155·1); octinoxate (p.1154·3); oxybenzone (p.1154·3).
*SPF 30:* Padimate O (p.1155·1); octinoxate (p.1154·3); oxybenzone (p.1154·3); homosalate (p.1148·1).
*Sunscreen.*

**Banana Boat Baby Sunblock** Banana Boat, Canad.
*SPF 50:* Octinoxate (p.1154·3); octisalate (p.1154·3); oxybenzone (p.1154·3); titanium dioxide (p.1160·3).
Formerly contained octocrilene, octinoxate, octisalate, and oxybenzone.
*Sunscreen.*

**Banana Boat Bite Block** Banana Boat, Canad.†
*SPF 15:* Octinoxate (p.1154·3); oxybenzone (p.1154·3).
*SPF 30:* Homosalate (p.1148·1); octinoxate (p.1154·3); octisalate (p.1154·3); oxybenzone (p.1154·3).
*Sunscreen.*

**Banana Boat Cool Coloring** Banana Boat, Canad.
*SPF 30:* Homosalate (p.1148·1); octinoxate (p.1154·3); octisalate (p.1154·3); oxybenzone (p.1154·3); titanium dioxide (p.1160·3).
*Sunscreen.*

**Banana Boat Cool Colorz** Banana Boat, Canad.
*SPF 30 spray:* Homosalate (p.1148·1); octinoxate (p.1154·3); octisalate (p.1154·3); oxybenzone (p.1154·3); titanium dioxide (p.1160·3).
*Sunscreen.*

**Banana Boat Dark Tanning** Banana Boat, Canad.
*Lotion SPF 4:* Padimate O (p.1155·1).
*Oil SPF 4; oil SPF 8:* Padimate O (p.1155·1); octinoxate (p.1154·3).
*Sunscreen.*

**Banana Boat Faces Plus** Banana Boat, Canad.
*SPF 23:* Octinoxate (p.1154·3); octisalate (p.1154·3); oxybenzone (p.1154·3).
Formerly contained octinoxate, octisalate, oxybenzone, homosalate, titanium dioxide.
*SPF 31†:* Octinoxate (p.1154·3); octisalate (p.1154·3); oxybenzone (p.1154·3); titanium dioxide (p.1160·3).
*Sunscreen.*

**Banana Boat Funky Fruit Lip Balm** Banana Boat, Canad.
*SPF 15:* Padimate O (p.1155·1); homosalate (p.1148·1); octinoxate (p.1154·3); oxybenzone (p.1154·3).
*Sunscreen.*

**Banana Boat Kids Sunblock** Banana Boat, Canad.
*SPF 30:* Homosalate (p.1148·1); octocrilene (p.1154·3); octinoxate (p.1154·3); octisalate (p.1154·3); oxybenzone (p.1154·3).
*Sunscreen.*

**Banana Boat Oil Free** Banana Boat, Canad.†
*SPF 30:* Octinoxate (p.1154·3); octisalate (p.1154·3); oxybenzone (p.1154·3); homosalate (p.1148·1); titanium dioxide (p.1160·3).
Formerly contained octinoxate, octisalate, and oxybenzone.
*Sunscreen.*

**Banana Boat Quik Blok** Banana Boat, Canad.
*SPF 15; SPF 25:* Homosalate (p.1148·1); octinoxate (p.1154·3); octisalate (p.1154·3); oxybenzone (p.1154·3); titanium dioxide (p.1160·3).
*Sunscreen.*

**Banana Boat Sooth-A-Caine** Banana Boat, Canad.
Menthol (p.1711·3); lidocaine (p.1377·3).

**Banana Boat Sport** Banana Boat, Canad.
*SPF 15:* Octinoxate (p.1154·3); octisalate (p.1154·3); oxybenzone (p.1154·3).
*SPF 30:* Octinoxate (p.1154·3); octisalate (p.1154·3); oxybenzone (p.1154·3); titanium dioxide (p.1160·3).
*SPF 50†:* Octinoxate (p.1154·3); octisalate (p.1154·3); oxybenzone (p.1154·3); octocrilene (p.1154·3).
*Sunscreen.*

**Banana Boat Sunblock** Banana Boat, Canad.†
*SPF 15:* Octinoxate (p.1154·3); octisalate (p.1154·3); oxybenzone (p.1154·3).
*Sunscreen.*

**Banana Boat Sunless Tanning** Banana Boat, Canad.†
*SPF 8:* Octinoxate (p.1154·3); oxybenzone (p.1154·3).
*Sunscreen.*

**Banana Boat Sunscreen** Banana Boat, Canad.
*SPF 8:* Padimate O (p.1155·1); oxybenzone (p.1154·3).
*Sunscreen.*

**Banana Boat Ultra** Banana Boat, Canad.
*SPF 30:* Octinoxate (p.1154·3); octisalate (p.1154·3); oxybenzone (p.1154·3); titanium dioxide (p.1160·3).
*Sunscreen.*

**Banana Boat Ultra Plus** Banana Boat, Canad.
*SPF 50:* Octinoxate (p.1154·3); octisalate (p.1154·3); oxybenzone (p.1154·3); octocrilene (p.1154·3).
*Sunscreen.*

**Banana Boat Vitamin E Lip Balm Sunblock**
Banana Boat, Canad.
*SPF 30:* Octinoxate (p.1154·3); homosalate (p.1148·1); oxybenzone (p.1154·3); padimate O (p.1155·1).
Formerly contained octinoxate, octocrilene, oxybenzone, and padimate O.
*Sunscreen.*

**Banatin** Remedina, Gr.
Famotidine (p.1265·2).
*Conditions where gastric acid reduction is beneficial; gastric hypersecretion including Zollinger-Ellison syndrome; peptic ulcer.*

**Bancap HC** Forest Pharmaceuticals, USA.
Hydrocodone tartrate (p.45·1); paracetamol (p.76·2).
*Pain.*

**Band Aid Spruhpflaster** Johnson & Johnson, Ger.
Cellaburat; octyldiphenylphosphate.
*Skin ulcers; wounds.*

**Band-Aid Antibiotic** Johnson & Johnson, Canad.
Bacitracin zinc (p.161·3); polymyxin B sulfate (p.245·1).

**Band-Aid Corn Remover** Johnson & Johnson, Canad.
Salicylic acid (p.1157·1).
*Corns.*

**Bandol** Pharmacia, Spain.
Paracetamol (p.76·2).
*Fever; pain.*

**Bandotan** Teva Tuteur, Arg.
Didanosine (p.630·3).
*HIV infection.*

**Bandrobon** Dupomar, Arg.
Sodium ibandronate (p.772·3).
*Hypercalaemia of malignancy.*

**Banedif**
Note. This name is used for preparations of different composition.
Bago, Chile.
*Ointment:* Bacitracin zinc (p.161·3); neomycin sulfate (p.235·1); zinc oxide (p.1163·2).
*Topical powder:* Bacitracin zinc (p.161·3); neomycin sulfate (p.235·1); aluminium hydroxide (p.1249·2).
*Bacterial skin infections.*
Maxfarma, Spain.
Bacitracin (p.161·3); neomycin sulfate (p.235·1); zinc oxide (p.1163·2).
*Infected skin disorders.*

**Banedif Oftalmico** Bago, Chile.
Bacitracin zinc (p.161·3); neomycin sulfate (p.235·1).
*Bacterial eye infections.*

**Banedif Oftalmico con Prednisolona** Bago, Chile.
Bacitracin zinc (p.161·3); neomycin sulfate (p.235·1); prednisolone (p.1108·1).
*Infected eye disorders with inflammation.*

**Baneocin**
Biochemie, Austria; Biochemie, Malaysia; Biochemie, Singapore.
Bacitracin (p.161·3) or bacitracin zinc (p.161·3); neomycin sulfate (p.235·1).
*Bacterial skin infections.*

**Baneopol** Streuli, Switz.
Bacitracin (p.161·3); polymyxin B sulfate (p.245·1); neomycin sulfate (p.235·1).
*Infected eye and skin disorders.*

**Banflex** Forest Pharmaceuticals, USA.
Orphenadrine citrate (p.486·1).
*Musculoskeletal pain.*

**Banholeum** Sofex, Port.
Soya oil (p.1447·2).
*Skin disorders.*

**Banholeum Composto** Sofex, Port.
Soya oil (p.1447·2); ichthammol (p.1148·2).
*Skin disorders.*

**Banholeum Gel** Sofex, Port.
Soya oil (p.1447·2); liquid paraffin (p.1479·1).
*Skin disorders.*

**Banidor** Hertz, Braz.†
Caffeine (p.782·1); dipyrone (p.35·3); orphenadrine (p.486·2).

**Banimax** SmithKline Beecham, UK†.
Aspirin (p.15·1); paracetamol (p.76·2).

**Banish II** Smith & Nephew, Austral.
Zinc ricinoleate; dipropylene glycol.
*Colostomy and ileostomy odour.*

**Banishing Cream** Avon, Canad.
Hydroquinone (p.1148·1).

**Banlice** Pfizer Consumer, Austral.
Pyrethrins (p.1509·3); piperonyl butoxide (p.1509·2).
*Pediculosis.*

**Banner Protein** Osotspa, Thai.
A preparation for enteral nutrition (p.1417·1).

**Bano Liquido con Eucalipto** Johnson & Johnson, Arg.
Menthol (p.1711·3); cineole (p.1672·1); rosemary oil (p.1740·2).

**Bano Ocular** Poen, Arg.
Tetryzoline hydrochloride (p.1131·2).
*Eye irritation.*

**Banocide** GlaxoSmithKline, India.
Diethylcarbamazine citrate (p.104·1).
*Worm infections.*

**Banocin** Nakornpatana, Thai.
*Ointment:* Neomycin sulfate (p.235·1); polymyxin B sulfate (p.245·1); bacitracin zinc (p.161·3).
*Topical powder:* Clioquinol (p.196·3); bacitracin (p.161·3); neomycin sulfate (p.235·1); zinc stearate (p.1575·3).
*Burns; ulcers; wounds.*

**Banoclus** Frasca, Arg.
Diclofenac (p.32·1).
*Fever; inflammation; pain.*

**Banoftal**
Alcon, Arg.; Alcon Cusi, Spain.
Boric acid (p.1662·1); calendula (p.1665·2); hamamelis (p.1696·3); borax (p.1661·3).
*Eye disorders.*

**Banophen Allergy** Major, USA.
Diphenhydramine hydrochloride (p.431·3).
*Hypersensitivity reactions; insomnia; motion sickness.*

**Banophen Decongestant** Major, USA.
Diphenhydramine hydrochloride (p.431·3); pseudoephedrine hydrochloride (p.1129·2).
*Hypersensitivity reactions; insomnia; motion sickness.*

**Ban-Sol** Remexa, Mex.
*SPF 15; SPF 30:* Avobenzone (p.1142·3); octinoxate (p.1154·3).
*Sunscreen.*

**Bansor** Thornton & Ross, UK.
Cetrimide (p.1172·1).
*Sore gums.*

**Bantel** Nakorn, Thai.
Pyrantel embonate (p.113·2).
*Worm infections.*

**Bantenol** Abello, Spain.
Mebendazole (p.108·2).
*Worm infections.*

**Banthine** Schiapparelli Searle, USA†.
Methantheliniurn bromide (p.485·3).
*Adjunct in peptic ulcer; neurogenic bladder.*

**Baralgin** Hoechst Marion Roussel, Ger.†
Dipyrone (p.35·3).
*Colic; pain.*

**Baralgin M** GlaxoSmithKline, Braz.
Dipyrone (p.35·3).
*Fever; pain.*

**Baralgina M** Aventis, Chile.
Dipyrone (p.35·3).
*Fever; pain.*

**Baran-mild N** Mickan, Ger.†
Benzocaine (p.1370·3); olive oil (p.1723·2); zinc oil (p.1469·2).
*Skin ulcers; wounds.*

**Baratol**
Shire, Irl.; Aspen, S.Afr.†; Shire, UK.
Indoramin hydrochloride (p.939·2).
*Hypertension.*

**Barazan** Dieckmann, Ger.
Norfloxacin (p.238·3).
*Bacterial infections of the urinary tract.*

**Barbamin** Streuli, Switz.
Propyphenazone (p.85·3); diphenhydramine hydrochloride (p.431·3).
*Fever; pain.*

**Barbidonna** Wallace, USA.
Atropine sulfate (p.477·1); hyoscine hydrobromide (p.483·3); hyoscyamine hydrobromide (p.485·1) or hyoscyamine sulfate (p.485·1); phenobarbital (p.367·3).
*Gastrointestinal disorders.*

**Barbitron** Sanval, Braz.
Phenobarbital (p.367·3).
*Convulsions.*

**Barbloc** Alphapharm, Austral.
Pindolol (p.983·2).
*Angina pectoris; arrhythmias; hypertension.*

**Barc** Del, USA†.
Pyrethrins (p.1509·3); piperonyl butoxide (p.1509·2).
*Pediculosis.*

**Barcan**
UCB, Denm.; UCB, Fin.; UCB, Norw.; UCB, Swed.
Aceclofenac (p.11·2).
*Inflammation; musculoskeletal and joint disorders.*

**Barex** Dominguez, Arg.
Macrogol 3350 (p.1709·1); electrolytes (p.1217·1).
*Bowel evacuation; constipation.*

**Barexal** Ipsen, Belg.
Smectite; aluminium hydroxide-magnesium carbonate co-dried gel (p.1250·1).
*Diarrhoea.*

**Baricon** Lafayette, USA.
Barium sulfate (p.1061·1).
*Contrast medium for gastrointestinal radiography.*

**Baridium** Pfeiffer, USA.
Phenazopyridine hydrochloride (p.83·1).
*Irritation of the lower urinary tract.*

**Barigraf**
Justesa Imagen, Arg.; Schering, Chile; Juste, Spain.
Barium sulfate (p.1061·1).
*Contrast medium for gastrointestinal radiography.*

**Barigraf Tac** Juste, Spain†.
Barium sulfate (p.1061·1).
Simeticone (p.1289·2) is included in this preparation to eliminate gas from the gastrointestinal tract before tomography.
*Contrast medium for gastrointestinal computerised axial tomography.*

**Barilux**
Waldheim, Austria; Goldham, Ger.
Barium sulfate (p.1061·1).
Formerly known as Falibaryt and Unibaryt in *Ger.*
*Contrast medium for gastrointestinal radiography.*

**Barilux Brausetabletten** Goldham, Ger.
Sodium bicarbonate (p.1223·2); citric acid (p.1673·1); dimethicone (p.1289·2).
*Adjunct in gastrointestinal radiography.*

**Bario Dif** Rovi, Spain.
Barium sulfate (p.1061·1).
Dimethicone (p.1289·2) is included in this preparation to eliminate gas from the gastrointestinal tract before radiography.
*Contrast medium for gastrointestinal radiography.*

**Bario Llorente** Llorente, Spain.
Barium sulfate (p.1061·1).
*Contrast medium for gastrointestinal radiography.*

**Bariofarma** Varifarma, Arg.
Barium sulfate (p.1061·1).
*Radiographic contrast medium.*

**Bariogel** Cristalia, Braz.†
Barium sulfate (p.1061·1).
*Contrast medium for gastrointestinal radiography.*

**Bariopacin** Serra Pamies, Spain†.
Barium sulfate (p.1061·1).
*Contrast medium for gastrointestinal radiography.*

**Bariotest** Schering, Braz.†
Barium sulfate (p.1061·1).
*Contrast medium for gastrointestinal radiography.*

**Baripril** Lesvi, Spain.
Enalapril maleate (p.909·2).
*Heart failure; hypertension.*

**Baripril Diu** Lesvi, Spain.
Enalapril maleate (p.909·2); hydrochlorothiazide (p.933·2).
*Hypertension.*

**Baritop** Sanochemia, UK.
Barium sulfate (p.1061·1).
*Contrast medium for gastrointestinal tract radiography.*

**Barium Med Complex** Dynamit, Austria.
Homoeopathic preparation.

**Barmicil** Sons, Mex.
Gentamicin sulfate (p.217·1).
*Bacterial infections.*

**Barnetil**
Sanofi Synthelabo, Belg.; Sanofi Synthelabo, Fr.; Synthelabo, Port.
Sultopride hydrochloride (p.723·1).
*Psychoses.*

**Barnotil** Sanofi Synthelabo, Ital.
Sultopride hydrochloride (p.723·1).
*Psychoses.*

**Baro-cat** *Lafayette, USA.*
Barium sulfate (p.1061·1).
*Contrast medium for gastrointestinal radiography.*

**Barokaton** *Sanova, Austria.*
*Injection:* 1-(β-Diethylaminoethyl)-theobromin-ethylbromide; 2-diethylaminoethanol hydrochloride (p.1587·1).
*Tablets:* 1-(β-Diethylaminoethyl)-theobromin-ethylbromide.
*Asthma; cardiovascular disorders.*

**Baropac** *Darrow, Braz.†.*
Barium sulfate (p.1061·1).
*Contrast medium for gastrointestinal radiography.*

**Baros** *Lafayette, USA†.*
Sodium bicarbonate (p.1223·2); tartaric acid (p.1752·1); simeticone (p.1289·2).
*Adjunct in gastrointestinal radiography.*

**Barosperse**
*Mallinckrodt, Arg.; Lafayette, USA.*
Barium sulfate (p.1061·1).
*Contrast medium for gastrointestinal radiography.*

**Barotonal** *Alpharma-Isis, Ger.*
Hydrochlorothiazide (p.933·2); reserpine (p.995·1).
*Hypertension.*

**Baroxal** *Remek, Gr.*
Ranitidine hydrochloride (p.1285·2).
*Conditions where gastric acid reduction is beneficial; gastric hypersecretion including Zollinger-Ellison syndrome; peptic ulcer.*

**Barpil** *Biolab, Thai.†.*
Buspirone hydrochloride (p.672·2).
*Anxiety.*

**Barrier Cream** *National Care, Canad.*
Dimethicone (p.1482·1).
*Skin disorders.*

**Barriere** *Wellspring, Canad.*
Dimethicone (p.1482·1).
*Skin disorders.*

**Barriere-HC** *Shire, Canad.*
Hydrocortisone (p.1103·3).
*Skin disorders.*

**Barrycidal** *Barry, Ital.*
Alkylbenzyldimethylammonium chloride (p.1168·3); benzethonium chloride (p.1169·2); diisobutylcresoxyethoxyethylbenzyldimethylammonium chloride.
*Instrument disinfection.*

**Bartelin N** *OTW, Ger.†.*
Diethylamine salicylate (p.34·1); camphor (p.1665·3); turpentine oil (p.1760·1).
*Musculoskeletal and joint disorders; neuralgia; neuritis.*

**Bartelin nico** *OTW, Ger.†.*
Diethylamine salicylate (p.34·1); benzyl nicotinate (p.21·2); oleum pini sylvestris.
*Musculoskeletal and joint disorders; neuralgia; neuritis.*

**Barytgen** *Fuji, Swed.†.*
Barium sulfate (p.1061·1).
*Contrast medium for gastrointestinal radiography.*

**Basab** *BA Farma, Port.*
Lomefloxacin (p.227·3).

**Basal-H-Insulin** *Hoechst, Ger.†.*
Isophane insulin (human) (p.333·3).
*Diabetes mellitus.*

**Basaljel**
*Note. This name is used for preparations of different composition.*
*Axcan, Canad.*
Aluminium hydroxide (p.1249·2).
*Hyperphosphataemia.*

*Wyeth-Ayerst, USA†.*
Dried basic aluminium carbonate gel (p.1249·1).
*Hyperacidity; hyperphosphataemia.*

**Basan** *Leiras, Fin.*
Basis for topical preparations.

**Bascardial** *Bastian, Ger.*
Potassium aspartate (p.1233·1); magnesium aspartate (p.1227·3).
*Coronary circulation disorders with magnesium and potassium deficiency.*

**Basdene** *Bouchara-Recordati, Fr.*
Benzylthiouracil (p.1596·1).
*Hyperthyroidism.*

**Bas-Dextrano** *Braun, Port.*
Dextran 40 (p.745·3) in glucose or sodium chloride.
*Plasma volume expansion; thromboembolic disorders.*

**Baseler Haussalbe** *Sanico, Belg.†.*
Zinc oxide (p.1163·2); zinc stearate (p.1575·3); bismuth subnitrate (p.1252·2); titanium dioxide (p.1160·3); borax (p.1661·3); sodium salicylate (p.90·1); purified talc (p.1159·1).
*Barrier cream; skin disorders.*

**Basen**
*Takeda, Jpn; Takeda, Thai.*
Voglibose (p.348·3).
*Diabetes mellitus.*

**Baserin** *Raza, Malaysia; Pharmaniaga, Malaysia.*
Co-trimoxazole (p.199·3).
*Bacterial infections.*

**Basicaina** *Senese, Ital.*
Lidocaine hydrochloride (p.1377·3).
*Local anaesthesia.*

**Basilan** *Baldacci, Braz.†.*
Arginine; calcium inositol hexaphosphate; magnesium inositol hexaphosphate; pyridoxine (p.1417·1).
*Nutritional supplement.*

**Basilicao** *Simoes, Braz.*
Colophony (p.1675·1); turpentine.
*Acne.*

**Basinal** *Basi, Port.*
Naltrexone hydrochloride (p.1046·1).
*Opioid withdrawal syndrome.*

**Basireuma** *Basi, Port.*
Phenylbutazone (p.83·2).

**Basiron**
*Galderma, Denm.†; Galderma, Fin.; Galderma, Norw.; Galderma, Swed.; Galderma, Switz.*
Benzoyl peroxide (p.1143·2).
*Acne.*

**Basiter** *Galderma, Ger.*
Coal tar (p.1159·2).
*Eczema; psoriasis.*

**Basiton** *Sarabhai Piramal, India.*
Vitamin B substances; vitamin C; folic acid (p.1417·1).
*Vitamin B and C deficiency.*

**B1-ASmedic** *Dyckerhoff, Ger.*
Thiamine nitrate (p.1455·1).
*Vitamin $B_1$ deficiency.*

**B2-ASmedic** *Dyckerhoff, Ger.*
Riboflavin (p.1456·1).
*Riboflavin deficiency.*

**B6-ASmedic** *Dyckerhoff, Ger.*
Pyridoxine hydrochloride (p.1456·3).
*Vitamin $B_6$ deficiency.*

**$B_{12}$-ASmedic** *Dyckerhoff, Ger.*
Cyanocobalamin (p.1458·2).
*Vitamin $B_{12}$ deficiency.*

**Basocef** *Curasan, Ger.*
Cefazolin sodium (p.170·3).
*Bacterial infections.*

**Basocin** *Galderma, Ger.*
Clindamycin phosphate (p.194·2).
*Acne.*

**Basodexan**
*Procter & Gamble, Austria†; Hermal, Ger.*
Urea (p.1162·2).
*Skin disorders.*

**Basofortina** *Novartis, Arg.*
Methylergometrine maleate (p.1714·2).

**Basoplex** *Riemser, Ger.*
Paracetamol (p.76·2); phenylpropanolamine hydrochloride (p.1127·3); dextromethorphan hydrobromide (p.1117·3).
*Coughs and cold symptoms.*

**Basoquin** *Parke, Davis, India.*
Amodiaquine (p.446·3).
*Malaria.*

**Basotar** *Galderma, Denm.*
Coal tar (p.1159·2).
*Psoriasis; seborrhoeic dermatitis.*

**Bassado** *Monsanto, Ital.*
Doxycycline hyclate (p.206·2).
*Bacterial infections.*

**Basti-Cal** *Bastian, Ger.*
Calcium carbonate (p.1254·2).
*Calcium deficiency; osteoporosis.*

**Basticrat** *Bastian, Ger.*
Crataegus (p.1677·1).
*Cardiac disorders.*

**Bastilong** *Merck, Braz.†.*
Ebastine (p.433·1).
*Hypersensitivity reactions.*

**Basti-Mag** *Bastian, Ger.*
Magnesium aspartate (p.1227·3).
*Magnesium deficiency.*

**Bastiverit** *Bastian, Ger.*
Glibenclamide (p.331·2).
*Diabetes mellitus.*

**Bastoncino** *Whitehall, Ital.†.*
Eugenol (p.1686·2).
*Oral hygiene; temporary dental filling.*

**Bat** *Zeta, Ital.*
Cetylpyridinium chloride (p.1173·1).
*Disinfection of wounds and burns.*

**Bateral** *Allen, Mex.*
Co-trimoxazole (p.199·3).
*Bacterial infections.*

**Bath E45** *Crookes Healthcare, UK.*
Bath additive.
*Dry skin.*

**Batinel** *Teva Tuteur, Arg.*
Mitoxantrone (p.576·1).
*Malignant neoplasms.*

**Batistol** *Serch, Arg.*
Pentane; butane (p.1235·1).
*Local anaesthesia.*

**Batixim** *SoSe, Ital.*
Cefotaxime sodium (p.175·3).
Lidocaine hydrochloride (p.1377·3) is included in this preparation to alleviate the pain of injection.
*Gram-negative bacterial infections.*

**Batmen** *Menarini, Spain.*
Prednicarbate (p.1107·3).
*Skin disorders.*

**Batrafen**
*Aventis, Austria; Aventis, Chile; Aventis, Ger.; Aventis, Hong Kong; Aventis, Irl.; Aventis, Israel; Aventis, Ital.; Aventis, NZ; Aventis, Spain; Knoll, Switz.*
Ciclopirox (p.396·1) or ciclopirox olamine (p.396·1).
*Fungal skin, nail, and vulvovaginal infections.*

**Batramycin** *Geistlich, Singapore.*
Bacitracin (p.161·3); neomycin sulfate (p.235·1).
*Bacterial skin infections.*

**Batramycine** *Geistlich, Switz.*
*Nasal ointment:* Bacitracin (p.161·3); neomycin sulfate (p.235·1); octacaine hydrochloride (p.1382·1).
*Bacterial nasal infections.*
*Ointment; topical powder:* Bacitracin (p.161·3); neomycin sulfate (p.235·1).
*Infected wounds or burns.*

**Batrax** *Gewo, Ger.†.*
*Nasal ointment:* Bacitracin (p.161·3); neomycin sulfate (p.235·1); octacaine hydrochloride (p.1382·1).
*Nasal infections.*
*Ointment; topical powder:* Bacitracin (p.161·3); neomycin sulfate (p.235·1).
*Bacterial skin infections.*

**Batrevac** *SBL, Swed.*
An inactivated influenza vaccine (p.1620·2).
*Active immunisation.*

**Batrizol** *Medimport, Mex.*
Co-trimoxazole (p.199·3).
*Bacterial infections.*

**Baudry** *Boiron, Canad.*
Homoeopathic preparation.

**Baume** *Zeller, Switz.*
Achillea (p.1646·2); absinthium (p.1645·1); poppy flowers (p.1058·1); guaiacum wood; tormentil root (p.1757·2); cinnamon bark (p.1672·2); benzoin (p.1751·1); myrrh (p.1718·3); tolu balsam (p.1131·3).
*Gastrointestinal disorders.*

**Baume Analgesique** *Multi-Pro, Canad.*
Methyl salicylate (p.59·3); camphor (p.1665·3).

**Baume Analgesique Medicamente** *Prodemdis, Canad.*
Methyl salicylate (p.59·3); camphor (p.1665·3); menthol (p.1711·3); eucalyptus oil (p.1686·2).

**Baume Aroma** *Mayoly-Spindler, Fr.*
Clove oil (p.1673·3); capsicum oil; methyl salicylate (p.59·3).
*Muscle and joint pain.*

**Baume Bengue** *URPAC, Fr.*
Methyl salicylate (p.59·3); menthol (p.1711·3).
*Muscle and joint pain.*

**Baume Dalet**
*Note. This name is used for preparations of different composition.*
*COB, Belg.†.*
Menthol (p.1711·3); guaiacol (p.1122·1); chloroform (p.1296·3); methyl salicylate (p.59·3); belladonna (p.479·1).
*Bunions.*

*Phygiene, Fr.†.*
Hyoscyamus oil (p.485·2); amyl salicylate (p.14·3); guaiacol (p.1122·1); menthol (p.1711·3); chloroform (p.1296·3).
*Calluses; corns.*

**Baume de Chine Temple of Heaven blanc** *Panax, Switz.*
Menthol (p.1711·3); camphor (p.1665·3); peppermint oil (p.1283·2); eucalyptus oil (p.1686·2); clove oil (p.1673·3); cinnamon oil (p.1672·2).
*Musculoskeletal and joint disorders; soft-tissue injury.*

**Baume du Chalet** *Plan, Switz.*
Lavender oil (p.1705·2); melissa oil (p.1711·2); spike lavender oil (p.1749·2); terebinthin (p.1760·1).
*Skin disorders; wounds.*

**Baume Esco** *Streuli, Switz.*
Salicylic acid (p.1157·1); menthol (p.1711·3); methyl salicylate (p.59·3).
*Musculoskeletal and joint pain.*

**Baume Esco Forte** *Streuli, Switz.*
Salicylic acid (p.1157·1); menthol (p.1711·3); methyl salicylate (p.59·3); ethyl nicotinate (p.37·2).
*Musculoskeletal and joint pain.*

**Baume Saint-Bernard** *Monot, Fr.†.*
Salicylic acid (p.1157·1); menthol (p.1711·3); camphor (p.1665·3); amyl salicylate (p.14·3); capsicum (p.1667·1); benzylidene acetone.
*Muscle and joint pain.*

**Bausch & Lomb Computer Eye Drops** *Bausch & Lomb, Austral.†.*
Glycerol (p.1694·3).
*Dry eyes; eye irritation.*

**Bausch & Lomb Concentrated Cleaner** *Bausch & Lomb, Austral.†.*
Cleansing solution for gas permeable and hard contact lenses (p.1164·2).

**Bausch & Lomb Conditioning Solution** *Bausch & Lomb, Austral.†.*
Disinfecting and storage solution for gas permeable and hard contact lenses (p.1164·2).

**Bausch & Lomb ReNu** *Bausch & Lomb, Austral.†.*
A range of solutions for soft contact lens care (p.1164·2).

**Bausch & Lomb Saline Plus** *Bausch & Lomb, Austral.†.*
Sodium chloride (p.1233·3) (p.1164·2).
*Solution for soft contact lenses.*

**Bausch & Lomb Sensitive Eyes Daily Cleaner** *Bausch & Lomb, Austral.†.*
Cleansing solution for soft contact lenses (p.1164·2).

**Bausch & Lomb Sensitive Eyes Lens Lubricant** *Bausch & Lomb, Austral.†.*
Povidone (p.1581·2); hypromellose (p.1579·3)(p.1164·2).
*Wetting solution for contact lenses.*

**Bausch & Lomb Sensitive Eyes Protein Removal** *Bausch & Lomb, Austral.†.*
Proteolytic enzyme (p.1164·2).
*Cleanser for soft contact lenses.*

**Bausch & Lomb Sensitive Eyes Saline** *Bausch & Lomb, Austral.†.*
Sodium chloride (p.1233·3) (p.1164·2).
*Saline solution for soft contact lenses.*

**Bauxol** *Mintlab, Chile.*
Bromhexine (p.1115·3); clofedanol (p.1117·1).
*Coughs.*

**Baxan** *Bristol-Myers Squibb, UK.*
Cefadroxil (p.167·2).
*Bacterial infections.*

**Baxapril** *Brasmedica, Braz.†.*
Co-trimoxazole (p.199·3).
*Bacterial infections; Pneumocystis carinii pneumonia; protozoal infections.*

**Baxedin** *Omega, Canad.*
Chlorhexidine gluconate (p.1173·2).
*Disinfection and antisepsis.*

**Baxidin** *Pierrel, Ital.*
Cetrimide (p.1172·1); chlorhexidine gluconate (p.1173·2).
*Disinfection of wounds and burns.*

**Baxi-K** *Baxter, Mex.*
Amikacin sulfate (p.154·1).

**Baxil** *Erfa, Belg.*
Chlorhexidine gluconate (p.1173·2).
*Mouth and throat disorders.*

**Baxo** *Toyama, Jpn.*
Piroxicam (p.84·2).
*Inflammation; musculoskeletal, joint, and peri-articular disorders; pain.*

**Bayaspirina** *Bayer, Arg.*
Aspirin (p.15·1).
*Fever; inflammation; pain; thromboembolism prophylaxis.*

**Bayaspirina C** *Bayer, Arg.*
Aspirin (p.15·1); ascorbic acid (p.1460·2).
*Cold symptoms; fever; pain.*

**Baycaron**
*Bayer, Denm.†; Bayer, Irl.†; Bayer, Neth.; Bayer, Norw.†; Bayer Consumer, UK†.*
Mefruside (p.951·3).
*Diabetes insipidus; hypertension; oedema.*

**Baycidal** *Bayer, Ital.*
Triflumuron (p.1510·3).
*Insecticide.*

**Baycillin** *Bayer, Ger.*
Propicillin potassium (p.246·3).
*Bacterial infections.*

**Baycip**
*Bayer, Chile; Bayer, Spain.*
Ciprofloxacin (p.188·2), ciprofloxacin hydrochloride (p.188·2), or ciprofloxacin lactate (p.188·3).
*Bacterial infections.*

**Baycol**
*Bayer, Canad.†; Bayer, Mex.; Bayer, S.Afr.†; Bayer, USA†.*
Cerivastatin sodium (p.881·3).
*Hypercholesterolaemia.*

**Baycuten**
*Note. This name is used for preparations of different composition.*
*Bayer, Braz.; Bayer, Port.*
Clotrimazole (p.396·2); dexamethasone (p.1097·1).
*Infected skin disorders.*

*Bayer, Chile; Bayer, Ger.*
Clotrimazole (p.396·2); dexamethasone acetate (p.1097·1).
*Infected skin disorders.*

*Bayer, Mex.*
Clotrimazole (p.396·2).
*Fungal skin infections.*

**Baycuten N**
*Note. This name is used for preparations of different composition.*
*Bayer, Malaysia.*
Clotrimazole (p.396·2); dexamethasone acetate (p.1097·1).
*Fungal skin infections.*

*Bayer, Mex.*
Clotrimazole (p.396·2); dexamethasone acetate (p.1097·1); neomycin sulfate (p.235·1).
*Infected skin disorders.*

**Bayer Extra Strength Back & Body Pain** *Bayer, USA.*
Aspirin (p.15·1); caffeine (p.782·1).
*Pain.*

**Bayer Low Adult Strength** *Sterling Health, USA.*
Aspirin (p.15·1).

**Bayer Select Chest Cold** *Sterling Health, USA.*
Dextromethorphan hydrobromide (p.1117·3); paracetamol (p.76·2).

**Bayer Select Flu Relief** *Sterling Health, USA.*
Paracetamol (p.76·2); pseudoephedrine hydrochloride (p.1129·2); dextromethorphan hydrobromide (p.1117·3); chlorphenamine maleate (p.427·3).

**Bayer Select Head Cold** *Sterling Health, USA.*
Pseudoephedrine hydrochloride (p.1129·2); paracetamol (p.76·2).

**Bayer Select Maximum Strength Backache** *Sterling Health, USA.*
Magnesium salicylate (p.55·1).

**Bayer Select Maximum Strength Headache** *Sterling Health, USA†.*
Paracetamol (p.76·2); caffeine (p.782·1).

**Bayer Select Maximum Strength Menstrual** *Sterling Health, USA†.*
Paracetamol (p.76·2); pamabrom (p.978·2).

**Bayer Select Maximum Strength Night Time Pain Relief** *Sterling Health, USA.*
Paracetamol (p.76·2); diphenhydramine hydrochloride (p.431·3).
*Insomnia; pain.*

**Bayer Select Maximum Strength Sinus Pain Relief** *Sterling Health, USA.*
Paracetamol (p.76·2); pseudoephedrine hydrochloride (p.1129·2).
*Nasal congestion; pain.*

**Bayer Select Night Time Cold** *Sterling Health, USA.*
Paracetamol (p.76·2); pseudoephedrine hydrochloride (p.1129·2); dextromethorphan hydrobromide (p.1117·3); triprolidine hydrochloride (p.442·3).

**Bayer Select Pain Relief Formula** *Sterling Health, USA†.*
Ibuprofen (p.45·3).

**Bayer Womens Aspirin Plus Calcium** *Bayer, USA.*
Aspirin (p.15·1); calcium (p.1225·1).
*Pain.*

**Bayers Tonic** *Bayer, India.*
Liver extract; sodium acid phosphate; yeast extract; alcohol (p.1417·1).
*Tonic.*

**Baygam** *Bayer, Canad.*
A normal immunoglobulin (p.1627·2).
*Passive immunisation.*

**Baygon** *Bayer, Ital.*
Propoxur (p.1509·2); tetramethrin (p.1510·2); piperonyl butoxide (p.1509·2).
*Insecticide.*

**BayHep** *Bayer, Israel.*
A hepatitis B immunoglobulin (p.1617·2).
*Passive immunisation.*

**BayHep B**
*Bayer, Canad.; Bayer Biological, Hong Kong; Bayer, Singapore; Bayer, USA.*
A hepatitis B immunoglobulin (p.1617·2).
Formerly known as HyperHep in the *USA*.
*Passive immunisation.*

**Baylotensin** *Mitsubishi, Jpn.*
Nitrendipine (p.973·3).
*Angina pectoris; hypertension.*

**Baymycard** *Bayer, Ger.; Zeneca, Ger.*
Nisoldipine (p.973·2).
*Angina pectoris; hypertension.*

**Bayolin** *Bayer, Austria.*
A heparinoid (p.931·1); glycol salicylate (p.44·3); benzyl nicotinate (p.21·2).
*Bruises; haematomas; musculoskeletal and joint disorders; neuralgia.*

**Bayotensin** *Bayer, Ger.*
Nitrendipine (p.973·3).
*Hypertension.*

**Baypen**
*Bayer, Austria; Bayer, Fr.; Bayer, Ger.; Bayer, Israel; Bayer, Ital.; Bayer, Spain†.*
Mezlocillin sodium (p.231·1).
*Bacterial infections.*

**Baypresol** *Prevision, Spain.*
Nitrendipine (p.973·3).
*Angina pectoris; hypertension; Raynaud's syndrome.*

**Baypress**
*Bayer, Austria; Bayer, Belg.; Bayer, Denm.; Bayer, Fr.; Bayer, Gr.; Bayer, Hong Kong; Bayer, Ital.; Bayer, Mex.; Bayer, Neth.; Bayer, Switz.; Bayer, Thai.*
Nitrendipine (p.973·3).
*Hypertension.*

**BayRab**
*Bayer, Canad.; Bayer Biological, Hong Kong; Probifasa, Mex.; Bayer, Singapore; Bayer, USA.*
A rabies immunoglobulin (p.1635·3).
Formerly known as HyperRab in the *USA*.
*Passive immunisation.*

**BayRho-D**
*Gador, Arg.; Sintofarma, Braz.†; Bayer, Canad.; Bayer, Chile; Bayer Biological, Hong Kong; Bayer, Israel; Probifasa, Mex.; Bayer, Singapore; Bayer, USA.*
An anti-D immunoglobulin (p.1608·1).
Formerly known as HypRho-D in the *USA*.
*Prevention of rhesus sensitisation.*

**Bayro**
*Bayer, Braz.; Bayer, Chile; Bayer, Ital.; Bayer, Mex.; Bayer, Spain†.*
Etofenamate (p.38·1).
*Gout; musculoskeletal, joint, peri-articular, and soft-tissue disorders; pain.*

**Bayro Termo** *Bayer, Mex.*
Etofenamate (p.38·1); benzyl nicotinate (p.21·2).
*Musculoskeletal, joint, and peri-articular disorders.*

**Bayrogel** *Bayer, Arg.*
Etofenamate (p.38·1).
*Musculoskeletal, joint, peri-articular, and soft-tissue disorders.*

**Bayro-Therm** *Bayer, Chile.*
Etofenamate (p.38·1); benzyl nicotinate (p.21·2).
*Musculoskeletal, joint, peri-articular, and soft-tissue disorders.*

**BayTet**
*Bayer, Canad.; Bayer Biological, Hong Kong; Bayer, Israel; Probifasa, Mex.; Bayer, Singapore; Bayer, USA.*
A tetanus immunoglobulin (p.1640·3).
Formerly known as Hyper-Tet in the *USA*.
*Passive immunisation.*

**Baythion EC** *Bayer, Ital.*
Phoxim (p.1509·1).
*Insecticide.*

**Bazalin** *Yamanouchi, Spain.*
Coal tar (p.1159·2); fluocinolone acetonide (p.1101·2); salicylic acid (p.1157·1).
*Keratinisation disorders; psoriasis.*

**Bazoton**
*Schering-Plough, Braz.†; Abbott, Ger.*
Urtica root (p.1762·1).
*Benign prostatic hyperplasia.*

**Bazuctril** *Chrispa (Χρισπα), Gr.*
Roxithromycin (p.254·2).
*Bacterial infections.*

**Bazuka** *Dendron, UK.*
Salicylic acid (p.1157·1); lactic acid (p.1704·1).
*Calluses; corns; verrucas; warts.*

**BB Fleet** *Pisa, Mex.†.*
Glycerol (p.1694·3).

**BB Test** *Innotech, Fr.*
Pregnancy test (p.1734·3).

**BBdent Gel Topico** *Maver, Chile.*
Benzocaine (p.1370·3).

**BB-K8** *Bristol-Myers Squibb, Ital.*
Amikacin sulfate (p.154·1).
*Bacterial infections.*

**BC** *Block, USA.*
Aspirin (p.15·1); salicylamide (p.87·3); caffeine (p.782·1).
*Pain.*

**BC 500** *Whitehall, Irl.†.*
Vitamin B substances and vitamin C (p.1417·1).
*Vitamin supplement.*

**BC Cold-Sinus** *Block, USA†.*
Phenylpropanolamine hydrochloride (p.1127·3); aspirin (p.15·1).
*Upper respiratory-tract symptoms.*

**BC 500 with Iron** *Whitehall, Irl.†.*
Ferrous fumarate (p.1427·3); vitamin B and C substances (p.1417·1).
*Dietary supplement; vitamin B and C and iron deficiencies.*

**BC Multi Symptom Cold Powder** *Block, USA†.*
Phenylpropanolamine hydrochloride (p.1127·3); chlorphenamine maleate (p.427·3); aspirin (p.15·1).
*Upper respiratory-tract symptoms.*

**BCAD 2** *Mead Johnson Nutritionals, USA.*
Food for special diets (p.1417·1).
*Maple syrup urine disease.*

**B-Caroteno** *AM, Arg.*
Betacarotene (p.1422·3).
*Skin pigmentation.*

**B-C-Bid** *Roberts, USA.*
Vitamin B complex with vitamin C (p.1417·1).

**BCM** *Pfizer, Austral.†.*
Vitamin B substances; minerals (p.1417·1).
*Tonic.*

**B-Combin** *Nycomed, Denm.†.*
Vitamin B substances (p.1417·1).

**B-Complex** *Bristol-Myers Squibb, Thai.*
Vitamin B substances (p.1417·1).

**B-Complex Threshold** *GNLD, Austral.†.*
Vitamin B substances (p.1417·1); rutoside (p.1688·2).
*Vitamin B deficiencies.*

**B-Cool** *Julphar, UAE.*
Oxybuprocaine hydrochloride (p.1382·1); cetylpyridinium chloride (p.1173·1); tyrothricin (p.275·1).
*Throat disorders.*

**B-Dol** *Be-Tabs, S.Afr.*
Paracetamol (p.76·2); doxylamine succinate (p.432·3); caffeine (p.782·1); codeine phosphate (p.27·1).
*Pain with tension.*

**Beacolux** *Upha, Malaysia.*
Bisacodyl (p.1251·3).
*Bowel evacuation; constipation.*

**Beacolytic** *Upha, Malaysia.*
Bromhexine hydrochloride (p.1115·3).
*Respiratory-tract disorders associated with viscous mucus.*

**Beacon K** *Upha, Malaysia.*
Potassium chloride (p.1232·2).
*Hypokalaemia.*

**Beacons** *Beacons, Singapore.*
Paracetamol (p.76·2); caffeine (p.782·1); phenylephrine hydrochloride (p.1126·3).
*Cold symptoms.*

**Beactafed** *Beacons, Singapore.*
Codeine phosphate (p.27·1); pseudoephedrine hydrochloride (p.1129·2); triprolidine (p.443·2).
*Allergic rhinitis; cold symptoms; nasal congestion; respiratory-tract congestion; sinusitis.*

**Beafemic**
*Upha, Malaysia; Beacons, Singapore.*
Mefenamic acid (p.55·2).
*Fever; musculoskeletal, joint, and peri-articular disorders; pain.*

**Beaflu-Plus** *Beacons, Singapore.*
Chlorphenamine maleate (p.427·3); paracetamol (p.76·2); pseudoephedrine hydrochloride (p.1129·2).
Formerly known as Beaflu and contained chlorphenamine maleate, paracetamol, and phenylpropanolamine hydrochloride.
*Fever; hypersensitivity reactions; pain.*

**Beagenco** *Beacons, Singapore.*
Paracetamol (p.76·2); pseudoephedrine hydrochloride (p.1129·2); dexchlorpheniramine maleate (p.427·3).
*Fever; hypersensitivity reactions; pain.*

**Beagenta** *Upha, Malaysia.*
Gentamicin sulfate (p.217·1).
*Bacterial skin, eye, and ear infections.*

**Beaglobe** *Upha, Malaysia.*
Sulfadiazine (p.258·2); trimethoprim (p.272·2).
*Bacterial infections.*

**Beagocrine** *Upha, Malaysia.*
Co-dergocrine mesilate (p.1674·1).
*Mental function impairment in the elderly.*

**Beagyne** *Effik, Fr.*
Fluconazole (p.398·1).
*Vaginal and perineal candidiasis.*

**Beahexol** *Beacons, Singapore.*
Trihexyphenidyl hydrochloride (p.490·2).
*Drug-induced extrapyramidal disorders; parkinsonism.*

**Beakopectin** *Upha, Malaysia.*
Kaolin (p.1268·3); pectin (p.1580·3).
*Diarrhoea.*

**Beamat** *Italmex, Mex.†.*
Cimetidine (p.1255·3).
*Peptic ulcer.*

**Beamodium** *Upha, Malaysia.*
Loperamide hydrochloride (p.1271·1).
*Diarrhoea.*

**Beamoken A** *Kendrick, Mex.†.*
Dexamethasone (p.1097·1).
*Corticosteroid.*

**Beamotil** *Upha, Malaysia.*
Diphenoxylate hydrochloride (p.1261·3).
Atropine sulfate (p.477·1) is included in this preparation to discourage abuse.
*Diarrhoea.*

**Beamoxy** *Upha, Malaysia.*
Amoxicillin trihydrate (p.155·3).
*Bacterial infections.*

**Be-Ampicil** *Be-Tabs, S.Afr.*
Ampicillin trihydrate (p.157·2).
*Bacterial infections.*

**Beano**
*Block, Canad.; Stafford-Miller, UK; AkPharma, USA.*
Alpha galactosidase A (p.1651·1).
*Gas/bloating from ingestion of raffinose, stachyose, or verbascose.*

**Beapen** *Upha, Malaysia.*
Phenoxymethylpenicillin potassium (p.242·1).
*Bacterial infections.*

**Beaphenicol**
*Upha, Malaysia; Beacons, Singapore†.*
Chloramphenicol (p.185·1).
*Bacterial infections.*

**Beapizide** *Beacons, Singapore.*
Glipizide (p.332·2).
*Diabetes mellitus.*

**Bear Essentials** *Hall, Canad.†.*
Multivitamin preparation with glucose (p.1417·1).

**Bearax** *Beacons, Singapore.*
Aciclovir (p.626·1).
*Herpesvirus infections.*

**Beatacycline**
*Upha, Malaysia.*
Tetracycline (p.266·2).
*Bacterial infections.*

*Beacons, Singapore.*
Tetracycline hydrochloride (p.266·2).
*Bacterial infections.*

**Beatafed** *Upha, Malaysia.*
Pseudoephedrine hydrochloride (p.1129·2); triprolidine hydrochloride (p.442·3).
*Allergic rhinitis; sinusitis; upper respiratory-tract congestion.*

**Beatafed Compound** *Upha, Malaysia.*
Codeine phosphate (p.27·1); triprolidine hydrochloride (p.442·3).
*Coughs.*

**Beathricin** *Beacons, Singapore.*
Lidocaine hydrochloride (p.1377·3); tyrothricin (p.275·1).
*Mouth and throat infections.*

**Beatifen** *Beacons, Singapore.*
Ketotifen fumarate (p.788·1).
*Allergic conjunctivitis; allergic rhinitis; asthma.*

**Beatizem** *Beacons, Singapore.*
Diltiazem hydrochloride (p.900·1).
*Antina pectoris; hypertension.*

**Beatoconazole** *Beacons, Singapore.*
Ketoconazole (p.403·3).
*Fungal skin infections.*

**Beatolin** *Upha, Malaysia.*
Salbutamol (p.791·3).
*Obstructive airways disease.*

**Beatolin Expectorant** *Upha, Malaysia.*
Guaifenesin (p.1122·1); salbutamol sulfate (p.791·3).
*Coughs.*

**Beatrolol** *Upha, Malaysia.*
Metoprolol tartrate (p.957·1).
*Angina pectoris; arrhythmias; hypertension; hyperthyroidism.*

**Beavate** *Upha, Malaysia.*
Betamethasone valerate (p.1093·2).
*Skin disorders.*

**Beavate N** *Upha, Malaysia.*
Betamethasone valerate (p.1093·2); neomycin sulfate (p.235·1).
*Infected skin disorders.*

**Beazyme** *Upha, Malaysia.*
Papain (p.1727·3).
*Inflammatory disorders; oedema.*

**Bebedermis** *Abbott, Ital.†.*
Glycerol; wool fat; vegetable oil; zinc oxide (p.1163·2).
*Barrier cream.*

**Bebegel**
*Sarget, Fr.; Viatris, Port.*
Glycerol (p.1694·3).
*Bowel evacuation; constipation.*

**Bebelac EC** *Nutricia, Malaysia.*
Infant feed (p.1417·1).
*Gastrointestinal disorders.*

**Bebelac FL** *Nutricia, Malaysia.*
Infant feed (p.1417·1).
*Lactose intolerance.*

**Beben**
*Parke, Davis, Canad.†; Pfizer Consumer, Ital.*
Betamethasone benzoate (p.1093·1).
*Skin disorders.*

**Beben Clorossina** *Pfizer Consumer, Ital.*
Betamethasone benzoate (p.1093·1); chloroxine (p.220·3).
*Infected skin disorders.*

**Bebesales** *Pharmacia, Spain.*
Calcium lactate pentahydrate; citric acid monohydrate; magnesium sulfate; potassium chloride; sodium bicarbonate; sodium chloride; glucose (p.1222·2).
*Oral rehydration therapy.*

**Bebia** *Stiefel, Canad.†.*
Zinc oxide (p.1163·2); kaolin (p.1268·3); talc (p.1159·1).
*Skin disorders.*

**Bebidol** *Nakorn, Thai.*
Dill oil (p.1680·2); sodium bicarbonate (p.1223·2).
*Flatulence; infant bloating.*

**Bebimix** *Sella, Ital.*
Honey (p.1434·2); royal jelly (p.1740·3); myrtillus (p.1718·3).
*Nutritional supplement.*

**Bebulin** *Immuno, Braz.†.*
A factor IX preparation (p.752·2).
*Haemorrhagic disorders.*

**Bebulin TIM 3** *Immuno, Ital.†.*
Factor IX (p.752·2).
*Factor IX deficiency; haemophilia B.*

**Bebulin TIM 4** *Baxter, Spain†.*
Factor IX (p.752·2).
*Factor IX deficiency.*

**Bebulin VH** *Immuno, USA.*
A factor IX preparation (p.752·2).
*Haemophilia B.*

**Bebyderm** *QIF, Braz.†.*
Betamethasone (p.1093·1).
*Skin disorders.*

**Bec** *Maruko, Jpn.*
Aranidipine (p.864·2).
*Hypertension.*

**Becacort** *Upha, Malaysia.*
Hydrocortisone (p.1103·3); miconazole nitrate (p.405·3).
*Infected skin disorders.*

**Becadexamin** *GlaxoSmithKline, India.*
Multivitamin and mineral preparation (p.1417·1).

**Becaltrin** *Natus, Braz.†.*
Co-trimoxazole (p.199·3).
*Bacterial infections; Pneumocystis carinii pneumonia; protozoal infections.*

**Became**
*YSP, Malaysia; Yung Shin, Singapore.*
Carbinoxamine maleate (p.426·3); pseudoephedrine hydrochloride (p.1129·2).
*Rhinitis.*

**Becantex**
*Note. This name is used for preparations of different composition.*
*SmithKline Beecham, Belg.†.*
Sodium dibunate (p.1130·2); guaifenesin (p.1122·1).
*Coughs.*

*CPH, Port.†; Sanofi Synthelabo, Thai.*
Sodium dibunate (p.1130·2).
*Coughs.*

**Becantosse** *Dinafarma, Braz.†.*
Sodium dibunate (p.1130·2); potassium iodide (p.1598·1).
*Coughs.*

**Becaps** *Sigma, Braz.†.*
Thiamine nitrate (p.1455·1).
*Vitamin $B_1$ supplement.*

**Becardin** *Remedica, Hong Kong.*
Propranolol hydrochloride (p.989·3).
*Angina pectoris; arrhythmias; hypertension; hyperthyroidism; migraine; myocardial infarction; obstructive cardiomyopathy; phaeochromocytoma; tremor; variceal haemorrhage.*

**Becarin** *Upha, Malaysia.*
Miconazole nitrate (p.405·3).
*Fungal skin and nail infections.*

**Because** *Schering, USA†.*
Nonoxinol 9 (p.1413·3).
*Contraceptive.*

**Bece** *Codilab, Port.*
Vitamin B substances; vitamin C (p.1417·1).
*Vitamin supplement.*

**Becede** *Vannier, Arg.*
Alprazolam (p.668·3).
*Anxiety.*

**Becenun**
*Bristol-Myers Squibb, Braz.; Bristol-Myers Squibb, Denm.†; Bristol-Myers Squibb, Norw.†; Bristol-Myers Squibb, Swed.†.*
Carmustine (p.535·1).
*Malignant neoplasms.*

**Becetamol**
*Gebro, Austria; Gebro, Switz.*
Paracetamol (p.76·2).
*Fever; pain.*

**Beceze**
*Norton, S.Afr.; Ivax, UK.*
Beclometasone dipropionate (p.1091·1).
*Allergic rhinitis; asthma.*

**Bechilar** *Montefarmaco, Ital.*
Dextromethorphan hydrobromide (p.1117·3).
*Coughs.*

**Bechlomin** *Jean-Marie, Hong Kong.*
Betamethasone (p.1093·1); dexchlorpheniramine maleate (p.427·3).
*Hypersensitivity reactions; inflammatory eye disorders.*

**Becilan** *DB, Fr.*
Pyridoxine hydrochloride (p.1456·3).
*Vitamin $B_6$ deficiency.*

**Beclase** *De Mayo, Braz.†.*
Sodium dibunate (p.1130·2); mepyramine maleate (p.437·1); ephedrine hydrochloride (p.1120·1).
*Coughs.*

**Beclasma**
*Raffo, Arg.; Raffo, Chile.*
Beclometasone dipropionate (p.1091·1); salbutamol (p.791·3).
*Obstructive airways disease.*

**Beclate**
*Cipla, India; Cipla-Medpro, S.Afr.*
Beclometasone dipropionate (p.1091·1).
*Asthma; nasal polyps; rhinitis; skin disorders.*

**Beclate-C** *Cipla, India.*
Beclometasone dipropionate (p.1091·1); clioquinol (p.196·3).
*Infected skin disorders.*

**Beclate-N** *Cipla, India.*
Beclometasone dipropionate (p.1091·1); neomycin sulfate (p.235·1).
*Infected skin disorders.*

**Beclazone**
*Ivax, Hong Kong; Norton Waterford, Irl.; Airflow, NZ; Ivax, Singapore; Norton Healthcare, Singapore; Ivax, UK.*
Beclometasone dipropionate (p.1091·1).
*Asthma.*

**Beclo Aqua** *Galen, UK†.*
Beclometasone dipropionate (p.1091·1).
*Rhinitis.*

**Beclo Asma**
*Aldo-Union, Hong Kong; Aldo-Union, Singapore; Aldo, Spain.*
Beclometasone dipropionate (p.1091·1).
*Asthma.*

**Beclo Rino** *Estedi, Spain.*
Beclometasone dipropionate (p.1091·1).
*Nasal polyps; rhinitis.*

**Beclo Siozwo** *Febena, Ger.*
Beclometasone dipropionate (p.1091·1).
*Allergic rhinitis.*

**Beclodisk** *Glaxo Wellcome, Canad.†.*
Beclometasone dipropionate (p.1091·1).
*Asthma.*

**Becloforte**
*Glaxo Wellcome, Austral.; Glaxo Wellcome, Canad.†; Glaxo Wellcome, Denm.†; GlaxoSmithKline, Hong Kong; GlaxoSmithKline, Israel; GlaxoSmithKline, Malaysia; GlaxoSmithKline, Neth.; GlaxoSmithKline, NZ†; GlaxoSmithKline, S.Afr.; GlaxoSmithKline, Singapore; GlaxoSmithKline, Spain; GlaxoSmithKline, Switz.; GlaxoSmithKline, Thai.; Allen & Hanburys, UK.*
Beclometasone dipropionate (p.1091·1).
*Asthma.*

**Beclogen** *Generics, UK.*
Beclometasone dipropionate (p.1091·1).
*Rhinitis.*

**Beclohale** *Julphar, UAE.*
Beclometasone dipropionate (p.1091·1).
*Asthma.*

**Beclojet** *Chiesi, Fr.*
Beclometasone dipropionate (p.1091·1).
*Asthma.*

**Beclomet**
*Lannacher, Austria; Orion, Denm.; Orion, Fin.; Orion, Ger.; Orion, Malaysia; Orion, Norw.; Orion, Singapore; Ferrer, Spain; Orion, Swed.; Orion, Switz.; Orion, Thai.*
Beclometasone dipropionate (p.1091·1).
*Asthma; nasal polyps; rhinitis.*

**Beclomin** *Jean-Marie, Hong Kong.*
Betamethasone (p.1093·1); dexchlorpheniramine maleate (p.427·3).
*Hypersensitivity reactions; inflammatory eye disorders.*

**Beclonarin** *Rappai, Switz.*
Beclometasone dipropionate (p.1091·1); chamomile (p.1669·3).
*Allergic rhinitis; polyps.*

**Beclonasal** *Orion, Fin.*
Beclometasone dipropionate (p.1091·1).
*Nasal polyps; rhinitis.*

**Beclonato** *Ducto, Braz.*
Betamethasone dipropionate (p.1093·1); betamethasone sodium phosphate (p.1093·1).
*Corticosteroid.*

**Beclone** *Leurquin, Fr.*
Beclometasone dipropionate (p.1091·1).
*Asthma.*

**Beclophar** *Novartis, Belg.*
Beclometasone dipropionate (p.1091·1).
*Asthma.*

**Beclo-Rhino**
*Viatris, Fr.; Goldshield, Irl.*
Beclometasone dipropionate (p.1091·1).
*Allergic rhinitis.*

**Beclorhinol** *Asche Chiesi, Ger.*
Beclometasone dipropionate (p.1091·1).
*Allergic rhinitis; nasal polyps.*

**Beclosema** *Etex, Chile.*
Beclometasone dipropionate (p.1091·1).
*Asthma.*

**Beclosol** *GlaxoSmithKline, Braz.*
Beclometasone dipropionate (p.1091·1).
*Asthma; nasal polyps; rhinitis.*

**Beclosona** *Spyfarma, Spain.*
Beclometasone dipropionate (p.1091·1).
*Skin disorders.*

**Beclotaide** *Glaxo Wellcome, Port.*
Beclometasone dipropionate (p.1091·1).
*Asthma.*

**Beclotamol** *Zambon, Braz.†.*
Beclometasone dipropionate (p.1091·1); salbutamol (p.791·3).
*Asthma.*

**Becloturmant** *Asche Chiesi, Ger.*
Beclometasone dipropionate (p.1091·1).
*Obstructive airways disease.*

**Beclovent**
*Glaxo Wellcome, Canad.†; GlaxoSmithKline, Chile; Glaxo Wellcome, USA.*
Beclometasone dipropionate (p.1091·1).
*Asthma.*

**Beco** *Mepha, Switz.*
Vitamin B substances (p.1417·1).
*Alcoholism; liver disorders; neuropathies; vitamin B deficiency.*

**Becocent** *Glaxo Wellcome, Denm.†.*
Beclometasone dipropionate (p.1091·1).
*Asthma.*

**Becodisk**
*GlaxoSmithKline, NZ†; GlaxoSmithKline, Switz.; GlaxoSmithKline, Thai.*
Beclometasone dipropionate (p.1091·1).
*Asthma.*

**Becodisks**
*GlaxoSmithKline, Hong Kong; Allen & Hanburys, Irl.; GlaxoSmithKline, S.Afr.; Allen & Hanburys, UK.*
Beclometasone dipropionate (p.1091·1).
*Asthma.*

**Becof** *Compu, S.Afr.†.*
Diphenhydramine hydrochloride (p.431·3); ammonium chloride (p.1115·2); sodium citrate (p.1223·2).
*Coughs.*

**Becolim**
*Atlantic, Hong Kong; Atlantic, Malaysia; Atlantic, Singapore; Atlantic, Thai.*
Vitamin B substances (p.1417·1).
*Vitamin B deficiency.*

**Becoloxin** *Upha, Malaysia.*
Meclozine hydrochloride (p.436·3); pyridoxine hydrochloride (p.1456·3).
*Motion sickness; nausea and vomiting.*

**Becombion**
*Merck, Malaysia; Merck, Singapore.*
Vitamin B substances (p.1417·1).
*Vitamin B deficiency.*

**Becomplex**
*Alpharma, Malaysia; Alpharma, Singapore.*
Vitamin B substances (p.1417·1).
*Vitamin B deficiency.*

**Becomplina Fuerte** *Labomed, Chile.*
Thiamine; riboflavine; pyridoxine; cyanocobalamin; nicotinamide; calcium pantothenate (p.1417·1).
*Vitamin B supplement.*

**Beconase**
*GlaxoSmithKline Consumer, Austral.; GlaxoSmithKline, Austria; GlaxoSmithKline, Belg.; Glaxo Wellcome, Canad.†; GlaxoSmithKline, Chile; GlaxoSmithKline, Denm.; GlaxoSmithKline, Fin.; GlaxoSmithKline, Fr.; GlaxoSmithKline, Hong Kong; Allen & Hanburys, Irl.; GlaxoSmithKline, Israel; GlaxoSmithKline, Malaysia; Glaxo Wellcome, Mex.; GlaxoSmithKline, Neth.; Glaxo Wellcome, Port.; GlaxoSmithKline, S.Afr.; Glaxo Wellcome, Singapore†; Allen, Spain; GlaxoSmithKline, Switz.; GlaxoSmithKline, Thai.; GlaxoSmithKline Consumer, UK; Glaxo Wellcome, USA.*
Beclometasone dipropionate (p.1091·1).
*Nasal polyps; rhinitis.*

**Beconase Allergy** *GlaxoSmithKline Consumer, Austral.*
Fluticasone propionate (p.1102·3).
*Allergic rhinitis.*

**Beconase Aquosum** *GlaxoSmithKline, Ger.*
Beclometasone dipropionate (p.1091·1).
*Allergic rhinitis; nasal polyps.*

**Beconase Hayfever** *GlaxoSmithKline, NZ.*
Beclometasone dipropionate (p.1091·1).
*Allergic rhinitis.*

**Beconasol** *GlaxoSmithKline, Switz.*
Beclometasone dipropionate (p.1091·1).
*Nasal polyps; rhinitis.*

**Becoplex Ido** *Novo Nordisk, S.Afr.*
Vitamin B substances (p.1417·1).

**Becortin** *Purissimus, Arg.*
Betamethasone dipropionate (p.1093·1); gentamicin embonate (p.219·1); clotrimazole (p.396·2).
*Infected skin and nail disorders.*

**Becosol** *GHP, Thai.*
Vitamin B substances, glucose, and sodium chloride infusion (p.1417·1).
*Parenteral nutrition.*

**Becosules** *Omni-Protech, India.*
Vitamin B substances; vitamin C (p.1417·1).
*Vitamin B and C deficiency.*

**Becosym**
*Roche Consumer, Irl.; Roche Consumer, UK†.*
Vitamin B substances (p.1417·1).
*Vitamin B deficiency.*

**Becotal** *Streuli, Switz.*
Vitamin B substances (p.1417·1).
*Neuropathies; vitamin B deficiency.*

**Becotide**
*Glaxo Wellcome, Austral.; GlaxoSmithKline, Austria; GlaxoSmithKline, Belg.; Glaxo Wellcome, Denm.†; GlaxoSmithKline, Fin.; GlaxoSmithKline, Fr.; Glaxo Wellcome, Gr.; GlaxoSmithKline, Hong Kong; Allen & Hanburys, Irl.; GlaxoSmithKline, Israel; GlaxoSmithKline, Ital.; GlaxoSmithKline, Malaysia; Glaxo Wellcome, Mex.; GlaxoSmithKline, Neth.; GlaxoSmithKline, Norw.; GlaxoSmithKline, NZ†; GlaxoSmithKline, S.Afr.; GlaxoSmithKline, Singapore; GlaxoSmithKline, Spain; GlaxoSmithKline, Swed.; GlaxoSmithKline, Switz.; GlaxoSmithKline, Thai.; Allen & Hanburys, UK.*
Beclometasone dipropionate (p.1091·1).
*Asthma.*

**Becotide A** *GlaxoSmithKline, Ital.*
Beclometasone dipropionate (p.1091·1).
Formerly known as Inalone A.
*Nose, sinus, and throat disorders; obstructive airways disease.*

**Becovit** *Julphar, UAE.*
Vitamin B substances (p.1417·1).
*Vitamin B deficiency; vitamin B supplement.*

**Becovitan** *Janssen-Cilag, Belg.†.*
Vitamin B substances (p.1417·1).
*Dietary supplementation; digestive disorders; nervous disorders; skin disorders; vitamin B deficiency.*

**Becozym**
*Roche, Austria†; Roche, Israel; Roche, Ital.; Roche, Swed.*
Vitamin B substances (p.1417·1).
*Alcoholism; neuropathies; vitamin B deficiency.*

**Becozym NF** *Roche, Arg.*
Vitamin B substances (p.1417·1).

**Becozym-C** *Roche, Arg.*
Vitamin B substances; vitamin C (p.1417·1).

**Becozyme**
*Roche, Belg.; Roche Nicholas, Fr.; Roche, Port.; Roche, Spain†; Roche, Switz.*
Vitamin B substances (p.1417·1).
*Alcoholism; liver disorders; nausea and vomiting in pregnancy; neuritis; neuropathies; vitamin B deficiency.*

**Becozyme C** *Roche, Port.*
Vitamin B substances; vitamin C (p.1417·1).
*Vitamin B and C deficiency.*

**Becozyme C Forte**
*Piramal, India; Roche, Spain.*
Vitamin B substances; vitamin C (p.1417·1).
*Vitamin B and C deficiency.*

**Becozyme-S** *Roche, Gr.; IFET (ΙΦΕΤ), Gr.*
Multivitamin preparation (p.1417·1).
*Vitamin B deficiency.*

**Bectam** *Labomed, Chile.*
Paroxetine hydrochloride (p.311·2).
*Depression.*

**Bed Wetting** *Hylands, Canad.*
Homoeopathic preparation.

**Bed Wetting Relief** *Brauer, Austral.†.*
Homoeopathic preparation.

**Bedelix** *Beaufour, Fr.*
Montmorillonite beidellitique.
*Gastrointestinal disorders.*

**Bediatil** *Pasteur, Chile.*
Ibuprofen (p.45·3).
*Fever; pain.*

**Bedin** *Pharmasant, Thai.*
Dihydroergocristine mesilate (p.1680·1); clopamide (p.888·2); reserpine (p.995·1).
*Hypertension.*

**Bedix** *Microsules Bernabo, Arg.*
Loratadine (p.436·1).
*Allergic rhinitis; allergic skin disorders.*

**Bedix-D** *Microsules Bernabo, Arg.*
Loratadine (p.436·1); pseudoephedrine sulfate (p.1129·2).
*Allergic rhinitis.*

**Bedocil** *Allen, Mex.*
Cyanocobalamin (p.1458·2); thiamine hydrochloride (p.1455·1).
*Anaemias; neuritis.*

**Bedodeka** *Biogal, Israel.*
Vitamin $B_{12}$ (p.1458·2).
*Anaemias; vitamin $B_{12}$ deficiency.*

**Bedodeka Antineuralgica** *Biogal, Israel.*
Procaine hydrochloride (p.1383·2); vitamin B substances (p.1417·1).
*Arthralgia; neuralgia.*

**Bedorma** *Singer, Switz.*
Diphenhydramine hydrochloride (p.431·3).
*Sleep disorders.*

**Bedovit Pharmaton** *Boehringer Ingelheim, Chile.*
Ginseng; deanol tartrate; vitamins; rutina; minerals; choline; inositol; linoleic acid; linolenic acid; soya lecithin (p.1417·1).
*Tonic.*

**Bedoxine** *Meuse, Belg.*
Pyridoxine hydrochloride (p.1456·3).
*Vitamin $B_6$ deficiency.*

**Bedoyecta** *Grossman, Mex.*
Calcium ascorbate; vitamin B substances; inositol; rutoside (p.1417·1).

**Bedoyecta Tri** *Grossman, Mex.*
Vitamin B substances (p.1417·1).

**Bedoz** *Nadeau, Canad.*
Cyanocobalamin (p.1458·2).

**Bedoze** *Merck, Port.*
Cyanocobalamin (p.1458·2).
*Megaloblastic anaemia; neuralgias; neuritis.*

**Bedozil** *Bunker, Braz.*
Cyanocobalamin (p.1458·2).
*Megaloblastic anaemia; vitamin $B_{12}$ supplement.*

**Bedranol** *Sandoz, UK.*
Propranolol hydrochloride (p.989·3).
*Angina pectoris; hypertension.*

**Beech Nut Cough Drops** *Beta, Canad.*
*Black:* Menthol (p.1711·3); anise oil (p.1655·2).
*Honey-Lemon; wild cherry:* Menthol (p.1711·3); eucalyptus (p.1686·1).
*Menthol:* Menthol (p.1711·3); anethole (p.1654·3); eucalyptus oil (p.1686·2).

**Beecham Lemon** *SmithKline Beecham, Spain.*
Ascorbic acid (p.1460·2); phenylephrine hydrochloride (p.1126·3); paracetamol (p.76·2).
*Cold symptoms.*

**Beecham Lemon Miel** *SmithKline Beecham, Spain†.*
Paracetamol (p.76·2); caffeine (p.782·1); ascorbic acid (p.1460·2).
*Cold symptoms; fever; pain.*

**Beechams All-In-One** *GlaxoSmithKline Consumer, UK.*
Paracetamol (p.76·2); guaifenesin (p.1122·1); phenylephrine hydrochloride (p.1126·3).
*Cold and influenza symptoms.*

**Beechams Cold & Flu** *GlaxoSmithKline Consumer, UK.*
Paracetamol (p.76·2); phenylephrine hydrochloride (p.1126·3); ascorbic acid (p.1460·2).
*Cold and influenza symptoms.*

**Beechams Cold Relief** *SmithKline Beecham Consumer, Irl.†.*
Paracetamol (p.76·2); caffeine (p.782·1); phenylephrine hydrochloride (p.1126·3).
*Cold symptoms.*

**Beechams Decongestant Plus with Paracetamol** *GlaxoSmithKline Consumer, UK.*
Paracetamol (p.76·2); caffeine (p.782·1); phenylephrine hydrochloride (p.1126·3).
*Cold symptoms.*

**Beechams Flu Plus** *SmithKline Beecham Consumer, Irl.*
Paracetamol (p.76·2); ascorbic acid (p.1460·2); caffeine (p.782·1); phenylephrine hydrochloride (p.1126·3).
*Cold and influenza symptoms.*

**Beechams Flu-Plus** *GlaxoSmithKline Consumer, UK.*
*Oral liquid:* Paracetamol (p.76·2); phenylephrine hydrochloride (p.1126·3); vitamin C (p.1460·2).
*Tablets:* Paracetamol (p.76·2); phenylephrine hydrochloride (p.1126·3); caffeine (p.782·1).
*Cold and influenza symptoms.*

**Beechams Hot Lemon** *GlaxoSmithKline, Hong Kong.*
Paracetamol (p.76·2); ascorbic acid (p.1460·2); phenylephrine hydrochloride (p.1126·3).
*Cold and influenza symptoms.*

**Beechams Hot Lemon Decongestant** *SmithKline Beecham Consumer, Irl.*
Paracetamol (p.76·2); ascorbic acid (p.1460·2); phenylephrine hydrochloride (p.1126·3).
*Cold symptoms.*

**Beechams Hot Remedies** *SmithKline Beecham Consumer, Irl.*
Paracetamol (p.76·2); ascorbic acid (p.1460·2).
*Cold symptoms.*

**Beechams Lemon Tablets** *SmithKline Beecham Consumer, UK†.*
Aspirin (p.15·1).
Glycine (p.1433·3) is included in this preparation in an attempt to limit adverse effects on the gastrointestinal mucosa.
*Cold and influenza symptoms; pain.*

**Beechams Max Strength Sore Throat Relief** *GlaxoSmithKline Consumer, UK.*
Hexylresorcinol (p.1182·1); benzalkonium chloride (p.1168·3).
*Sore throat.*

**Beechams for Natural Defence** *GlaxoSmithKline Consumer, UK.*
Ascorbic acid (p.1460·2) with zinc.

**Beechams for Natural Relief** *SmithKline Beecham Consumer, UK†.*
Echinacea (p.1683·2); garlic (p.1691·1).
*Catarrh; cold and influenza symptoms; coughs; rhinitis.*

**Beechams Powders** *GlaxoSmithKline Consumer, UK.*
Aspirin (p.15·1); caffeine (p.782·1).
*Cold and influenza symptoms; pain.*

**Beechams Powders Capsules** *GlaxoSmithKline Consumer, UK.*
Paracetamol (p.76·2); caffeine (p.782·1); phenylephrine hydrochloride (p.1126·3).
*Cold and influenza symptoms.*

**Beechams Remedy** *SmithKline Beecham, Israel†.*
Paracetamol (p.76·2); ascorbic acid (p.1460·2).
*Fever; pain.*

**Beechams Throat-Plus** *GlaxoSmithKline Consumer, UK.*
Benzalkonium chloride (p.1168·3); hexylresorcinol (p.1182·1).
*Sore throat.*

**Beefolic** *Sriprasit, Thai.*
Vitamin B substances with folic acid (p.1417·1).

**Beehive Balsam** *Ayrton, UK.*
Purified honey (p.1434·2); glycerol (p.1694·3); ipecacuanha (p.1122·3).
*Coughs.*

**Beeline** *Lifeplan, UK†.*
Propolis (p.1735·2); pollen; royal jelly (p.1740·3).
*Nutritional supplement.*

**Beelith** *Beach, USA.*
Pyridoxine hydrochloride (p.1456·3); magnesium oxide (p.1272·3).
*Dietary supplement.*

**Beepen-VK** *SmithKline Beecham, USA†.*
Phenoxymethylpenicillin potassium (p.242·1).
*Bacterial infections.*

**Beespan** *Garec, S.Afr.*
Vitamin B substances (p.1417·1).
*Vitamin B deficiencies.*

**Beetrion** *Franco-Indian, India.*
Multivitamin and mineral preparation (p.1417·1).

**Bee-Zee** *Rugby, USA.*
Multivitamin and mineral preparation (p.1417·1).

**Befact** *SMB, Belg.*
Vitamin B substances (p.1417·1).
*Alcoholism; neuritis; vitamin B deficiency.*

**Befelka-Oel** *Befelka, Ger.*
Hypericum oil (p.299·2); calendula oil (p.1665·2); chamomile oil (p.1669·3); olive oil (p.1723·2); viola tricoloris oil; liquid paraffin (p.1479·1).
*Skin disorders.*

**Befelka-Tinktur** *Befelka, Ger.†.*
Aloes (p.1248·2); achillea (p.1646·2); melissa (p.1711·1); juniper fruit (p.1703·1); ononis (p.1723·3); betula (p.1660·3); urtica (p.1762·1); chamomile (p.1669·3); arnica (p.1656·3); pimpinella; turiones pini; liquorice (p.1270·2).
*Circulatory disorders; metabolic disorders; skin disorders.*

**Beferon** *Cristalia, Braz.*
Interferon alfa (p.640·3).

**Befibrat** *Hennig, Ger.*
Bezafibrate (p.873·2).
*Hyperlipidaemias.*

**Befimat** *Biomedica-Chemica, Gr.*
Nimodipine (p.972·3).
*Neurological deficit following subarachnoid haemorrhage.*

**Befizal** *Roche, Fr.*
Bezafibrate (p.873·2).
*Hyperlipidaemias.*

**Beflavine** *Roche Nicholas, Fr.*
Riboflavin (p.1456·1).
*Vitamin B deficiency.*

**Befol** *Biotenk, Arg.*
Rofecoxib (p.86·3).
*Osteoarthritis; pain.*

**Beforplex** *Bournonville, Belg.†.*
Vitamin B substances (p.1417·1).
*Digestive disorders; neuritis; skin disorders; vitamin B deficiency.*

**Befort** *Collins, Mex.*
Multivitamin preparation (p.1417·1).

**Begadon** *Berman, Mex.*
Vitamin B substances (p.1417·1).

**Begalin** *Pfizer, Gr.*
Sultamicillin (p.264·2) or sultamicillin tosilate (p.264·2).
*Bacterial infections.*

**Begalin-P** *Pfizer, Gr.*
Ampicillin sodium (p.157·1); sulbactam sodium (p.257·2).
*Bacterial infections.*

**Begesic**
*Note. This name is used for preparations of different composition.*
*Berlin Pharm, Singapore.*
Methyl salicylate (p.59·3); menthol (p.1711·3); eugenol (p.1686·2); cajuput oil (p.1664·1).
*Muscle pain; musculoskeletal and joint disorders.*

*Berlin Pharm, Thai.*
Methyl salicylate (p.59·3); menthol (p.1711·3); eugenol (p.1686·2).
Formerly contained methyl salicylate, menthol, eugenol, and cajuput oil.
*Lumbago; rheumatic disorders; sciatica.*

**Beglan** *Faes, Spain.*
Salmeterol xinafoate (p.795·1).
*Asthma; bronchitis.*

**Beglunina** *Llorens, Spain†.*
Pyridoxine (p.1457·2).
*Alcohol intoxication; vitamin $B_6$ deficiency.*

**Begrivac**
*Grunenthal, Austria; Chiron, Denm.†; Chiron Behring, Fin.; Chiron Behring, Ger.; Wyeth, Irl.; Chiron, Ital.; Chiron Behring, Norw.; Multichem, NZ; Meda, Swed.; Wyeth, UK.*
An inactivated influenza vaccine (split virion) (p.1620·2).
*Active immunisation.*

**Begrocit** *Grossmann, Switz.*
Vitamin and mineral preparation (p.1417·1).

**Behepan**
*Pharmacia Upjohn, Denm.†.*
Cyanocobalamin (p.1458·2).
*Megaloblastic anaemia.*

*Pharmacia, Swed.*
*Injection:* Hydroxocobalamin acetate (p.1458·2).
*Megaloblastic anaemia; Schilling test; sprue; vitamin $B_{12}$ deficiency.*
*Tablets:* Cyanocobalamin (p.1458·2).
*Megaloblastic anaemia; sprue; vitamin $B_{12}$ deficiency.*

**Behexine** *Osotspa, Thai.*
Bromhexine hydrochloride (p.1115·3).
*Respiratory-tract disorders associated with increased or viscous mucus.*

**Beiklin** *Scherer, Singapore†.*
Multivitamin and mineral preparation (p.1417·1).

**Bekfan** *Arlex, Mex.†.*
Dextromethorphan (p.1117·3).
*Coughs.*

**Bekidiba** *Diba, Mex.*
Dextromethorphan hydrobromide (p.1117·3); guaifenesin (p.1122·1).
*Coughs.*

**Bekidiba Dex** *Diba, Mex.*
Dextromethorphan hydrobromide (p.1117·3).
*Coughs.*

**Beknol** *Kener, Mex.†.*
Benzonatate (p.1115·3).

**Beko** *Orion, Fin.*
Vitamin B substances (p.1417·1).
*Vitamin B deficiency; vitamin B supplement.*

**Bekunis**
*Note. This name is used for preparations of different composition.*
*Schulke & Mayr, Austria; Lavipharm, Gr.; Roha, Irl.†; Roha, Israel; Roha, Port.†; Roha, Switz.*
Senna (p.1288·2).
Formerly contained senna and bisacodyl in *Switz.*
*Bowel evacuation; constipation.*

*Roha, Port.†.*
*Tablets:* Senna (p.1288·2); bisacodyl (p.1251·3).
*Constipation.*

**Bekunis Bisacodyl** *Roha, Ger.*
Bisacodyl (p.1251·3).
*Constipation.*

**Bekunis Complex** *Diafarm, Spain.*
Bisacodyl (p.1251·3); senna (p.1288·2).
*Constipation.*

**Bekunis Dragees** *Roha, Switz.*
Bisacodyl (p.1251·3).
*Constipation.*

**Bekunis Fibra** *Roha, Port.†.*
Ispaghula (p.1268·1).
*Constipation.*

**Bekunis Herbal Tea** *Polcopharma, Austral.†.*
Senna (p.1288·2).
*Constipation.*

**Bekunis Instant**
*Polcopharma, Austral.†; Roha, Ger.*
Senna (p.1288·2).
*Constipation.*

**Bekunis Leicht** *Roha, Ger.†.*
Ispaghula (p.1268·1).
*Constipation.*

**Bekunis Plantago Granule** *Roha, Switz.†.*
Ispaghula (p.1268·1).
*Constipation; diarrhoea; irritable bowel; obesity; stool softener.*

**Bekunis-Krautertee N** *Roha, Ger.*
Senna (p.1288·2).
*Constipation.*

**Belacid** *Nakornpatana, Thai.*
Charcoal (p.1030·2); magnesium hydroxide (p.1272·2); belladonna (p.479·1); peppermint oil (p.1283·2).
*Gastric hyperacidity.*

**Belacodid** *Climax, Braz.*
*Injection:* Codeine phosphate (p.27·1); sparteine sulfate (p.1749·1); homatropine methonitrate (p.483·2).
*Smooth muscle spasm.*
*Oral drops:* Codeine (p.27·1); phenethylamine citrate; pentetrazol (p.1592·1); homatropine methonitrate (p.483·2).
*Coughs.*
*Syrup:* Codeine phosphate (p.27·1); phenethylamine citrate; trolamine thymolsulphonate; pentetrazol (p.1592·1); homatropine methonitrate (p.483·2).
*Coughs.*

**Belagin** *IMA, Braz.*
Copper sulfate (p.1426·1); zinc sulfate (p.1469·3); aluminium (p.1652·2); menthol (p.1711·3); benzalkonium chloride (p.1168·3).
*Gynaecological infections.*

**Belara**
*Grunenthal, Chile; Grunenthal, Ger.; Grunenthal, Switz.*
Ethinylestradiol (p.1553·2); chlormadinone acetate (p.1542·1).
*Androgenisation in women; combined oral contraceptive.*

**Be-Lax** *Be-Tabs, S.Afr.*
Magnesium sulfate (p.1228·2); magnesium carbonate (p.1272·1).
*Constipation.*

**Belbar** *Luar, Arg.*
Neomycin (p.235·1); polymyxin B (p.245·2); dexamethasone (p.1097·1).
*Infected eye disorders.*

**Belcetin** *Sedabel, Braz.*
Bacitracin (p.161·3); neomycin (p.235·1).
*Bacterial skin infections.*

**Belcid**
*Biolab, Malaysia; Biolab, Thai.*
Aluminium oxide (p.1140·1); magnesium hydroxide (p.1272·2); simeticone (p.1289·2).
*Dyspepsia; flatulence; gastric hyperacidity; peptic ulcer.*

**Belcomycine** *Aventis, Neth.*
Colistin sulfate (p.198·3).
*Bacterial infections.*

**Belep** *Lepori, Port.†.*
Ibuprofen guaiacol (p.46·3).
*Fever; pain.*

**Belestar** *Biol, Arg.*
Conjugated oestrogens (p.1543·2).
*Menopausal disorders; osteoporosis.*

**Belexa** *Farmasa, Braz.*
Vitamin B substances (p.1417·1).

**Belfactrin** *Belfar, Braz.†.*
Co-trimoxazole (p.199·3).
*Bacterial infections.*

**Bel-Gel** *Sedabel, Braz.*
Diclofenac diethylamine (p.32·1).

**Belglos** *Belfar, Braz.†.*
Neomycin sulfate (p.235·1); benzalkonium chloride (p.1168·3); ergocalciferol (p.1462·1); vitamin A palmitate (p.1453·1).
*Skin infections.*

**Beliam** *Abbott, Arg.*
Cefalexin (p.168·1).
*Bacterial infections.*

**Belidral** *Almirall, Belg.*
Amiloride hydrochloride (p.858·2); hydrochlorothiazide (p.933·2).
*Ascites; heart failure; hypertension; oedema.*

**Belifax** *Pharmaten (Φαρματεν), Gr.*
Omeprazole (p.1278·2).
*Acid aspiration; eradication of Helicobacter pylori in combination with antimicrobials; peptic ulcer; reflux oesophagitis; Zollinger-Ellison syndrome.*

**Belisina** *CPH, Port.*
Lysine hydrochloride; vitamin B substances (p.1417·1).
*Tonic.*

**Belisir** *Bittner, Austria.*
Crataegus (p.1677·1); lupulus (p.1708·1); melissa (p.1711·1).
*Cardiovascular disorders; sleep disorders.*

**Belivon**
*Organon, Austria; Organon, Ital.*
Risperidone (p.719·2).
*Psychoses.*

**Bell Diono Resolvent** *Bell, India.*
Ethylmorphine (p.37·3); allylthiourea; hydrocortisone (p.1103·3); yellow mercuric oxide (p.1712·3).
*Corneal scars, ulcers, and opacities.*

**Bell Pentolate** *Bell, India.*
Cyclopentolate hydrochloride (p.480·3).
*Production of mydriasis and cycloplegia.*

**Bell Pino-Atrin** *Bell, India.*
Atropine sulfate (p.477·1).
*Production of mydriasis and cycloplegia; uveitis.*

**Bell Resolvent** *Bell, India.*
Ethylmorphine (p.37·3); allylthiourea; hydrocortisone (p.1103·3); yellow mercuric oxide (p.1712·3).
*Corneal scars, ulcers, and opacities.*

**Bellacane** *Treiner, USA.*
Hyoscyamine sulfate (p.485·1); phenobarbital (p.367·3).
*Gastrointestinal disorders.*

**BellaCarotin mono** *3M, Ger.†.*
Betacarotene (p.1422·3).
*Sunburn.*

**Belladol** *Dolisos, Canad.†.*
Homoeopathic preparation.

**Belladonna Med Complex** *Dynamit, Austria.*
Homoeopathic preparation.

**Belladonna-Homaccord** *Peithner, Austria.*
Homoeopathic preparation.

**Belladonnysat Burger** *Ysatfabrik, Ger.*
Belladonna (p.479·1).
*Smooth muscle spasm.*

**Bellafit N** *Streuli, Switz.*
Atropine sulfate (p.477·1).
*Colic; hyperhidrosis; sialorrhoea.*

**Bellagotin** *Streuli, Switz.*
Belladonna (p.479·1); diphenhydramine hydrochloride (p.431·3); ergotamine tartrate (p.467·2).
*Nervous disorders.*

**Bellahist-D** *Cypress, USA.*
Phenylephrine hydrochloride (p.1126·3); hyoscyamine sulfate (p.485·1); hyoscine hydrobromide (p.483·3); chlorphenamine maleate (p.427·3); atropine sulfate (p.477·1).
*Upper respiratory-tract disorders.*

**Bellamine** *Major, USA.*
Levorotatory alkaloids of belladonna (p.479·1); phenobarbital (p.367·3); ergotamine tartrate (p.467·2).
*Gastrointestinal disorders.*

**Bellanorm** *Rosch & Handel, Austria.*
Belladonna (p.479·1).
*Bronchospasm; gastrointestinal disorders; motion sickness; night sweats.*

**Bellanox** *Bios, Belg.†.*
Brallobarbital (p.671·3); amobarbital (p.670·1); secobarbital (p.721·2).
*Insomnia.*

**Bellatal** *Richwood, USA.*
Phenobarbital (p.367·3); hyoscyamine sulfate (p.485·1); atropine sulfate (p.477·1); hyoscine hydrobromide (p.483·3).
*Hypnotic; sedative.*

**Bellatard** *Propan, S.Afr.†.*
Phenobarbital (p.367·3); atropine sulfate (p.477·1); hyoscine hydrobromide (p.483·3); hyoscyamine sulfate (p.485·1).
*Smooth muscle spasm.*

**Bellatotal** *Cetus, Arg.*
Homatropine (p.483·2); dipyrone (p.35·3).
*Pain; smooth muscle spasm.*

**Belle Cream** *Bell, India.*
Zinc oxide (p.1163·2).
*Photodermatoses; sunscreen.*

**Bellergal**
*Novartis, Canad.; Novartis, S.Afr.†; Novartis, Switz.†; Novartis, Thai.*
Belladonna alkaloids (p.479·1); ergotamine tartrate (p.467·2); phenobarbital (p.367·3).
*Cardiovascular disorders; gastrointestinal disorders; menopausal disorders; nervous system disorders; premenstrual syndrome.*

**Bellergal Retardado** *Novartis, Chile.*
Total belladonna alkaloids (p.479·1); ergotamine tartrate (p.467·2); phenobarbital (p.367·3).
*Circulatory disorders; endocrine disorders; gastrointestinal disorders; nervous disorders.*

**Bellergal-S** *Novartis, USA.*
Laevorotatory alkaloids of belladonna (Bellafoline) (p.479·1); ergotamine tartrate (p.467·2); phenobarbital (p.367·3).
*Cardiovascular disorders; gastrointestinal disorders; menopausal disorders; recurrent throbbing headache.*

**Bellergil** *Sandoz, Ital.†.*
Belladonna alkaloids (p.479·1); ergotamine tartrate (p.467·2); phenobarbital (p.367·3).
*Dystonias.*

**Belloform nouvelle formule** *Tentan, Switz.*
Cathine hydrochloride (p.1585·2).
*Obesity.*

**Belloid** *Gedeon Richter, Thai.†.*
Hyoscyamine sulfate (p.485·1); ergotoxine (p.1685·2); butobarbital (p.673·3).
*Central vegetative disorder; dystonias; migraine.*

**Bells Muscle Rub** *Bell, UK.*
Sweet birch oil (p.60·1); cajuput oil (p.1664·1); eucalyptus oil (p.1686·2); methyl salicylate (p.59·3); menthol (p.1711·3).
*Musculoskeletal disorders.*

**Belmacina** *Pliva, Spain.*
Ciprofloxacin hydrochloride (p.188·2).
*Bacterial infections.*

**Belmalax** *Belmac, Spain.*
Lactulose (p.1269·1).
*Constipation; hepatic encephalopathy.*

**Belmalen** *Cetus, Arg.*
Diclofenac (p.32·1); orphenadrine (p.486·2).
*Inflammation; pain.*

**Belmalen Plus** *Cetus, Arg.*
Glucosamine (p.1694·1).
*Musculoskeletal and joint disorders.*

**Belmalip** *Belmac, Spain.*
Simvastatin (p.997·1).
*Hyperlipidaemias; secondary prophylaxis of ischaemic heart disease.*

**Belmazol**
*Daquimed, Port.; Belmac, Spain.*
Omeprazole (p.1278·2).
*Dyspepsia; gastro-oesophageal reflux; peptic ulcer; Zollinger-Ellison syndrome.*

**Belmirax** *Belfar, Braz.†.*
Mebendazole (p.108·2).
*Worm infections.*

**Belnif** *Promed, Ger.; AstraZeneca, Ger.*
Metoprolol tartrate (p.957·1); nifedipine (p.966·2).
*Angina pectoris; hypertension.*

**Beloc**
*Note. This name is used for preparations of different composition.*
*AstraZeneca, Arg.; AstraZeneca, Austria; AstraZeneca, Ger.; Promed, Ger.*
Metoprolol tartrate (p.957·1).
*Angina pectoris; arrhythmias; heart failure; hypertension; hyperthyroidism; migraine; myocardial infarction.*

*Recalcine, Chile.*
Acebutolol (p.848·1).
*Angina pectoris; arrhythmias; hypertension.*

**Beloc comp** *Sanova, Austria; Astra, Ger.†.*
Metoprolol tartrate (p.957·1); hydrochlorothiazide (p.933·2).
*Hypertension.*

**Beloc COR** *AstraZeneca, Switz.*
Metoprolol tartrate (p.957·1).
*Heart failure.*

**Beloc-Zok** *AstraZeneca, Ger.; Promed, Ger.; AstraZeneca, Switz.*
Metoprolol succinate (p.957·1).
*Angina pectoris; arrhythmias; hypertension; ischaemic heart disease; migraine; myocardial infarction.*

**Beloc-Zok comp** *Pharmacia, Ger.*
Metoprolol succinate (p.957·1); hydrochlorothiazide (p.933·2).
*Hypertension.*

**Beloken** *AstraZeneca, Spain.*
Metoprolol succinate (p.957·1) or metoprolol tartrate (p.957·1).
*Angina pectoris; arrhythmias; hypertension; hyperthyroidism; migraine; myocardial infarction.*

**Belomet** *Recalcine, Chile.*
Salbutamol (p.791·3); beclometasone (p.1092·1).
*Asthma.*

**Belpen** *Dermopen, Braz.†.*
Cyclamic acid (p.1426·2); saccharin (p.1443·2).
*Sugar substitute.*

**Bel-Phen-Ergot S** *Goldline, USA.*
Phenobarbital (p.367·3); ergotamine tartrate (p.467·2); belladonna (p.479·1).

**Beltrax Uno** *Baliarda, Arg.*
Saw palmetto (p.1569·1).

**Belupan** *Grunenthal, Chile.*
Papaverine (p.1728·1); phenobarbital (p.367·3); belladonna liquid extract (p.479·1).
*Colic.*

**Belustine**
*Bellon, Fr.†; Rhone-Poulenc Rorer, Hong Kong†; Rhone-Poulenc Rorer, Ital.†; Rhone-Poulenc Rorer, Spain†.*
Lomustine (p.565·2).
*Malignant neoplasms.*

**Bemaz** *Laboratorios Chile, Chile.*
Betaxolol hydrochloride (p.873·1).
*Glaucoma; ocular hypertension.*

**Bemedrex** *Orion, Fr.*
Beclometasone dipropionate (p.1091·1).
*Asthma.*

**Bemetrazole** *Be-Tabs, S.Afr.*
Metronidazole (p.607·2).
*Anaerobic bacterial infections; protozoal infections.*

**Bemetson** *Orion, Fin.*
Betamethasone valerate (p.1093·2).
*Skin disorders.*

**Bemicin** *Northia, Arg.*
Pancuronium bromide (p.1404·3).
*Competitive neuromuscular blocker.*

**Beminal**
*Eurofarma, Braz.; Whitehall-Robins, Canad.†; Whitehall, USA.*
Vitamin B substances with vitamin C (p.1417·1).

**Beminal C Fortis** *Whitehall-Robins, Canad.†.*
Vitamin B substances with ascorbic acid (p.1417·1).

**Beminal Fortis** *Whitehall-Robins, Canad.†.*
Vitamin B substances (p.1417·1).

**Beminal with Iron and Liver** *Whitehall-Robins, Canad.†.*
Vitamin B substances with ferrous sulfate and liver (p.1417·1).

**Beminal Plus** *Eurofarma, Braz.*
Vitamin B substances; vitamin C; vitamin E; minerals (p.1417·1).

**Beminal Z** *Whitehall-Robins, Canad.†.*
Multivitamins (p.1417·1); zinc sulfate (p.1469·3).

**Bemofil** *Veripalvelu, Fin.*
A factor IX preparation (p.752·2).

**Bemolan** *Altana, Spain.*
Magaldrate (p.1271·3).
*Dyspepsia; gastro-oesophageal reflux; gastrointestinal hyperacidity.*

**Bemon** *Bioglan, Ger.*
Betamethasone valerate (p.1093·2).
*Skin disorders.*

**Bemonalcool** *Pierrel, Ital.*
Benzalkonium chloride (p.1168·3); alcohol (p.1166·1).
*Disinfection of skin and wounds.*

**Bemplas** *Casasco, Arg.*
Clonidine hydrochloride (p.885·2); chlortalidone (p.882·3).
*Hypertension.*

**Bena** *Xepa-Soul Pattinson, Malaysia.*
Ammonium chloride (p.1115·2); diphenhydramine hydrochloride (p.431·3); sodium citrate (p.1223·2).
*Coughs; upper respiratory-tract congestion.*

**Benace** *Novartis, India.*
Benazepril hydrochloride (p.867·2).
*Heart failure; hypertension.*

**Benacilina** *Fustery, Mex.*
Benzylpenicillin (p.163·2).
*Bacterial infections.*

**Benacne** *Wyeth Consumer, Port.*
Benzoyl peroxide (p.1143·2).
*Acne.*

**Benactiv** *Boots Healthcare, Ital.*
Flurbiprofen (p.43·3).
*Mouth and throat pain and inflammation.*

**Benaday** *Pfizer, Denm.*
Cetirizine hydrochloride (p.427·1).
*Allergic rhinitis; hay fever; urticaria.*

**Benaderma** *Confar, Port.*
Diphenhydramine hydrochloride (p.431·3).
Formerly contained ammonium chloride, diphenhydramine, and menthol.
*Skin disorders.*

**Benaderma com Calamina** *Confar, Port.*
Calamine (p.1144·1); camphor (p.1665·3); diphenhydramine hydrochloride (p.431·3).
*Skin disorders.*

**Benadon**
*Roche, Arg.; Roche, Austria†; Roche Consumer, Irl.†; Roche, Ital.; Roche, Mex.†; Roche, Port.; Roche, Spain; Roche, Swed.; Roche, Switz.*
Pyridoxine hydrochloride (p.1456·3).
*Alcoholism; blood dyscrasias; nausea and vomiting; neuritis; vitamin $B_6$ deficiency.*

**Benadryl**
*Note. This name is used for preparations of different composition.*
*Parke, Davis, Arg.; Pfizer Consumer, Canad.; Pfizer, Gr.; Pfizer, Hong Kong; Parke, Davis, India; Warner-Lambert, Ital.†; Pfizer Lambert, Spain; Pfizer, Thai.; Warner-Lambert, USA; Parke, Davis, USA.*
Diphenhydramine (p.431·3) or diphenhydramine hydrochloride (p.431·3).
*Hypersensitivity reactions; insomnia; minor skin irritation; motion sickness; parkinsonism.*

*Pfizer, Austria; Pfizer, Braz.; Warner-Lambert, Ital.*
*Oral liquid; oral drops:* Diphenhydramine hydrochloride (p.431·3); ammonium chloride (p.1115·2); sodium citrate (p.1223·2); menthol (p.1711·3).
*Cold and influenza symptoms; coughs.*

*Pfizer, Denm.*
Acrivastine (p.423·3).
*Hypersensitivity reactions.*

**Benadryl Allergy Oral Solution** *Pfizer Consumer, UK.*
Cetirizine hydrochloride (p.427·1).
*Allergic rhinitis; urticaria.*

**Benadryl Allergy Relief** *Pfizer Consumer, UK.*
Acrivastine (p.423·3).
*Allergic rhinitis; urticaria.*

**Benadryl Allergy/Cold** *Warner-Lambert, USA.*
Diphenhydramine hydrochloride (p.431·3); pseudoephedrine hydrochloride (p.1129·2); paracetamol (p.76·2).

**Benadryl Allergy/Congestion** *Warner-Lambert, USA.*
Diphenhydramine hydrochloride (p.431·3); pseudoephedrine hydrochloride (p.1129·2).

**Benadryl Allergy/Sinus Headache**
*Pfizer Consumer, Canad.; Warner-Lambert, USA.*
Diphenhydramine hydrochloride (p.431·3); pseudoephedrine hydrochloride (p.1129·2); paracetamol (p.76·2).
*Eye irritation; headache; upper respiratory-tract disorders.*

**Benadryl Antialergico** *Parke, Davis, Arg.*
Diphenhydramine hydrochloride (p.431·3).
*Hypersensitivity reactions; motion sickness; parkinsonism.*

**Benadryl Antitusivo** *Parke, Davis, Arg.*
Diphenhydramine hydrochloride (p.431·3); ammonium chloride (p.1115·2); menthol (p.1711·3); sodium citrate (p.1223·2).
*Coughs.*

**Benadryl CD**
*Note. This name is used for preparations of different composition.*
*Pfizer, Malaysia; Pfizer, Singapore.*
Diphenhydramine hydrochloride (p.431·3); codeine phosphate (p.27·1); ammonium chloride (p.1115·2).
*Cold symptoms; coughs.*

*Pfizer, Thai.*
Diphenhydramine hydrochloride (p.431·3); codeine phosphate (p.27·1); ammonium chloride (p.1115·2); sodium citrate (p.1223·2); menthol (p.1711·3).
*Coughs.*

**Benadryl Chesty Cough and Nasal Congestion** *Pfizer, NZ.*
Guaifenesin (p.1122·1); pseudoephedrine hydrochloride (p.1129·2).
Formerly known as Benadryl Chesty Cough.
*Coughs; nasal congestion.*

**Benadryl Chesty Forte** *Pfizer, NZ.*
Bromhexine (p.1115·3); guaifenesin (p.1122·1).
*Coughs.*

**Benadryl Childrens Allergy** *Pfizer, USA.*
Diphenhydramine citrate (p.431·3).
*Hypersensitivity reactions.*

**Benadryl Cold Nighttime Formula** *Parke, Davis, USA.*
Pseudoephedrine hydrochloride (p.1129·2); diphenhydramine hydrochloride (p.431·3); paracetamol (p.76·2).
*Upper respiratory-tract symptoms.*

**Benadryl Complex** *Warner-Lambert, Ital.*
Diphenhydramine hydrochloride (p.431·3); dextromethorphan hydrobromide (p.1117·3); pseudoephedrine hydrochloride (p.1129·2); ammonium chloride (p.1115·2); sodium citrate (p.1223·2); menthol (p.1711·3).
*Coughs.*

**Benadryl Cough**
*Note. This name is used for preparations of different composition.*
*Parke, Davis, India; Pfizer, Thai.*
Diphenhydramine hydrochloride (p.431·3); ammonium chloride (p.1115·2); sodium citrate (p.1223·2); menthol (p.1711·3).
*Cold symptoms; coughs; nasal congestion.*

*Pfizer, Malaysia.*
Diphenhydramine hydrochloride (p.431·3); ammonium chloride (p.1115·2).
*Coughs and cold symptoms; rhinitis.*

*Pfizer, Singapore.*
Diphenhydramine hydrochloride (p.431·3); ammonium chloride (p.1115·2); menthol (p.1711·3).
*Cold symptoms; coughs.*

**Benadryl Day & Night**
*Note. This name is used for preparations of different composition.*
*Parke, Davis, Arg.*
Day tablets, paracetamol (p.76·2); phenylpropanolamine hydrochloride (p.1127·3); night tablets, paracetamol; diphenhydramine hydrochloride (p.431·3).
*Cold and influenza symptoms.*

*Warner-Lambert, NZ†.*
Day formula, dextromethorphan hydrobromide (p.1117·3); pseudoephedrine hydrochloride (p.1129·2); night formula, dextromethorphan hydrobromide; pseudoephedrine hydrochloride; diphenhydramine hydrochloride (p.431·3).
*Coughs and cold symptoms.*

**Benadryl Decongestant**
*Warner-Lambert, Canad.†; Pfizer, Thai.; Parke, Davis, USA.*
Diphenhydramine hydrochloride (p.431·3); pseudoephedrine hydrochloride (p.1129·2).
*Coughs; nasal congestion.*

**Benadryl Descongestivo** *Parke, Davis, Arg.*
Diphenhydramine hydrochloride (p.431·3); pseudoephedrine hydrochloride (p.1129·2).

**Benadryl DM Compuesto** *Parke, Davis, Arg.*
Diphenhydramine hydrochloride (p.431·3); dextromethorphan hydrobromide (p.1117·3); phenylephrine hydrochloride (p.1126·3); ammonium chloride (p.1115·2).
*Coughs.*

**Benadryl DMP** *Pfizer, Thai.*
Diphenhydramine hydrochloride (p.431·3); dextromethorphan hydrobromide (p.1117·3); phenylephrine hydrochloride (p.1126·3); ammonium chloride (p.1115·2); sodium citrate (p.1223·2).
*Coughs; respiratory-tract congestion.*

**Benadryl Dry Cough and Nasal Congestion**
*Pfizer, NZ.*
Dextromethorphan hydrobromide (p.1117·3); pseudoephedrine hydrochloride (p.1129·2).
Formerly known as Benadryl Dry Cough and contained dextromethorphan hydrobromide, pseudoephedrine hydrochloride, and diphenhydramine hydrochloride.
*Coughs; nasal congestion.*

**Benadryl Dry Forte** *Pfizer, NZ.*
Dextromethorphan hydrobromide (p.1117·3).
*Coughs.*

**Benadryl Expectorante** *Warner-Lambert, Spain†.*
Ammonium chloride (p.1115·2); diphenhydramine hydrochloride (p.431·3); sodium citrate (p.1223·2); menthol (p.1711·3).
*Respiratory-tract disorders.*

**Benadryl for the Family Chesty Cough & Nasal Congestion** *Pfizer Consumer, Austral.*
Guaifenesin (p.1122·1); pseudoephedrine hydrochloride (p.1129·2).
*Coughs.*

**Benadryl for the Family Chesty Forte** *Pfizer Consumer, Austral.*
Bromhexine hydrochloride (p.1115·3); guaifenesin (p.1122·1).
*Coughs.*

**Benadryl for the Family - Dry** *Pfizer Consumer, Austral.*
Dextromethorphan hydrobromide (p.1117·3); pseudoephedrine hydrochloride (p.1129·2); diphenhydramine hydrochloride (p.431·3).
*Coughs and cold symptoms.*

**Benadryl for the Family Dry Forte** *Pfizer Consumer, Austral.*
Dextromethorphan hydrobromide (p.1117·3).
*Coughs.*

**Benadryl for the Family Original** *Pfizer Consumer, Austral.*
Diphenhydramine hydrochloride (p.431·3); ammonium chloride (p.1115·2); sodium citrate (p.1223·2).
*Allergic rhinitis; cough and cold symptoms.*

**Benadryl Itch** *Warner-Lambert, USA.*
*Cream; topical spray; topical stick:* Diphenhydramine hydrochloride (p.431·3); zinc acetate (p.1469·2).
*Hypersensitivity reactions.*
*Topical gel:* Diphenhydramine hydrochloride (p.431·3).
*Pruritus.*

**Benadryl mit Codein** *Parke, Davis, Austria†.*
Codeine phosphate (p.27·1); diphenhydramine hydrochloride (p.431·3); ammonium chloride (p.1115·2); menthol (p.1711·3); sodium citrate (p.1223·2).
*Coughs.*

**Benadryl N** *Pfizer Consumer, Ger.*
Diphenhydramine hydrochloride (p.431·3).
*Coughs, colds and associated respiratory-tract disorders.*

**Benadryl Nightime** *Pfizer, NZ.*
Dextromethorphan hydrobromide (p.1117·3); diphenhydramine hydrochloride (p.431·3).
*Coughs and cold symptoms.*

**Benadryl One A Day** *Pfizer Consumer, UK.*
Cetirizine hydrochloride (p.427·1).
*Allergic rhinitis; urticaria.*

**Benadryl Original** *Pfizer, NZ.*
Diphenhydramine hydrochloride (p.431·3); ammonium chloride (p.1115·2); sodium citrate (p.1223·2).
*Coughs.*

**Benadryl Plus** *Pfizer Consumer, UK.*
Acrivastine (p.423·3); pseudoephedrine hydrochloride (p.1129·2).
*Allergic rhinitis.*

**Benadryl Skin Allergy Relief**
*Warner-Lambert, Irl.; Pfizer Consumer, UK.*
Diphenhydramine hydrochloride (p.431·3); camphor (p.1665·3); zinc oxide (p.1163·2).
*Allergic skin disorders; skin irritation.*

**Benagol** *Boots Healthcare, Ital.*
Dichlorobenzyl alcohol (p.1178·3); amylmetacresol (p.1168·2).
*Oral hygiene.*

**Benagol Collutorio** *Boots Healthcare, Ital.†.*
Amylmetacresol (p.1168·2).
*Oral hygiene.*

**Benagol Mentolo-Eucaliptolo** *Boots Healthcare, Ital.*
Dichlorobenzyl alcohol (p.1178·3); amylmetacresol (p.1168·2); menthol (p.1711·3).
*Oral hygiene.*

**Benagol Vitamina C** *Boots Healthcare, Ital.*
Dichlorobenzyl alcohol (p.1178·3); amylmetacresol (p.1168·2); sodium ascorbate (p.1460·2); ascorbic acid (p.1460·2).
*Adjunct in cold symptoms; oral hygiene.*

**Benal** *Berman, Mex.*
Vitamin $B_1$ (p.1454·3).

**Benalapril** *Berlin-Chemie, Ger.*
Enalapril maleate (p.909·2).
*Heart failure; hypertension.*

**Benalcon** *Pierrel, Ital.*
Benzalkonium chloride (p.1168·3).
*Disinfection of wounds.*

**Benalet** *Ache, Braz.*
Diphenhydramine hydrochloride (p.431·3); ammonium chloride (p.1115·2); sodium citrate (p.1223·2).

**Benalgis** *Franco-Indian, India.*
Vitamin $B_1$ (p.1454·3).
*Beri-beri; neuritis.*

**Benalix** *Raza, Malaysia; Pharmaniaga, Malaysia.*
Diphenhydramine hydrochloride (p.431·3); ammonium chloride (p.1115·2).
*Coughs; respiratory-tract congestion.*

**Benapen** *Biolab Sanus, Braz.*
Procaine benzylpenicillin (p.246·1); benzylpenicillin potassium (p.163·2).
*Bacterial infections.*

**Benaprost** *Bago, Arg.*
Terazosin hydrochloride (p.1010·3).
*Benign prostatic hyperplasia.*

**Benatoss** *Herus, Braz.†.*
Ambroxol hydrochloride (p.1114·3).
*Respiratory-tract congestion.*

**Benaxima** *Fustery, Mex.*
Cefotaxime sodium (p.175·3).
*Bacterial infections.*

**Benaxona** *Fustery, Mex.*
Ceftriaxone sodium (p.182·3).
*Bacterial infections.*

**Bencard Skin Testing Solutions** *Allergy Therapeutics, UK†.*
Allergen extracts (single and mixed) (p.1650·1).
*Diagnosis of hypersensitivity.*

**Bencelin** *Antibioticos, Mex.*
Benzathine benzylpenicillin (p.162·3).
*Bacterial infections.*

**Bencelin Combinado** *Antibioticos, Mex.*
Benzathine benzylpenicillin (p.162·3); procaine benzylpenicillin (p.246·1); benzylpenicillin (p.163·2).
*Bacterial infections.*

**Bencid**
*Geno, India; Pharmaland, Thai.*
Probenecid (p.416·3).
*Gout; gouty arthritis; hyperuricaemia.*

**Benclamin**
*Cazi, Braz.; Polipharm, Thai.*
Glibenclamide (p.331·2).
*Diabetes mellitus.*

**Bencole** *Propan, S.Afr.*
Co-trimoxazole (p.199·3).
*Bacterial infections.*

**Benda** *Nakorn, Thai.*
Mebendazole (p.108·2).
*Worm infections.*

**Bendalina**
*Angelini, Ital.; Lepori, Port.*
Bendazac lysine (p.20·3).
*Cataracts.*

**Bendapar** *Fustery, Mex.*
Albendazole (p.101·2).
*Worm infections.*

**Bendex** *Ciplo-Medpro, S.Afr.*
Albendazole (p.101·2).
*Giardiasis; worm infections.*

**Bendigon N** *Gepepharm, Ger.*
Mefruside (p.951·3); reserpine (p.995·1).
*Hypertension.*

**Bendracol** Synco, Hong Kong.
Diphenhydramine hydrochloride (p.431·3); ammonium chloride (p.1115·2); sulfogaiacol (p.1131·1); sodium citrate (p.1223·2); terpin hydrate (p.1131·1); menthol (p.1711·3).
*Coughs; respiratory-tract congestion.*

**Bendrax** Haller, Braz.
Mebendazole (p.108·2).
*Worm infections.*

**Bendzon** Dzwon, India.
Oxybuprocaine hydrochloride (p.1382·1).
*Local anaesthesia.*

**Benecid** Valdecasas, Mex.
Probenecid (p.416·3).
*Adjunct to beta-lactam antibacterials; gout.*

**Benectrin** Legrand, Braz.
Co-trimoxazole (p.199·3).
*Bacterial infections; Pneumocystis carinii pneumonia; protozoal infections.*

**Benectrin Balsamico** Legrand, Braz.
Co-trimoxazole (p.199·3); guaifenesin (p.1122·1); ammonium chloride (p.1115·2).
*Bacterial infections.*

**Benecut** Sanova, Austria.
Naftifine hydrochloride (p.406·2).
*Fungal skin infections.*

**Benedaxol** Liomont, Mex.†.
Mebendazole (p.108·2).

**Benedorm**
Note. This name is used for preparations of different composition.
Ariston, Arg.
Bromazepam (p.671·3).
*Alcohol withdrawal syndrome; anxiety.*
Dresden, Ger.†.
Valerian (p.1762·2).
*Anxiety disorders; insomnia.*
ICN, Mex.
Melatonin (p.1710·2).
*Sleep disorders.*

**Benefiber**
Novartis Consumer, Austral.; Novartis, Braz.; Novartis Nutrition, USA.
Guar gum (p.333·2).
*Constipation; diarrhoea; dietary fibre supplement.*

**Benefix**
Wyeth, Arg.; Wyeth, Austral.; Genetics Institute, Austria; Baxter, Belg.†; Wyeth, Braz.; Whitehall, Braz.; Wyeth, Chile; Genetics Institute, Denm.; Baxter, Fr.; Baxter, Ger.; Genetics, Gr.; Baxter, Ital.; Wyeth, Mex.; Baxter, Spain; Baxter, Swed.; Baxter, Switz.; Baxter BioScience, UK; Genetics Institute, USA.
Nonacog alfa (p.752·3).
*Factor IX deficiency.*

**Beneflora** Cedar Health, UK.
*Lactobacillus acidophilus* (p.1704·2); *Bifidobacterium* spp; *Streptococcus thermophilus* (p.1704·2); *Lactobacillus casei*; *Lactobacillus bulgaricus* (p.1704·2); *Bifidobacterium longum*; fructo oligosaccharides; pea fibres.
*Maintenance of normal gastrointestinal flora.*

**Beneflur** Schering, Spain.
Fludarabine phosphate (p.553·2).
*Chronic lymphocytic leukaemia.*

**Benegel** Legrand, Braz.†.
Methyl salicylate (p.59·3); camphor (p.1665·3); menthol (p.1711·3); rosemary oil (p.1740·2); lavender oil (p.1705·2); turpentine oil (p.1760·1); mustard oil (p.1718·2).
*Musculoskeletal and joint disorders.*

**Benegrip** DM, Braz.†.
Salicylamide (p.87·3); chlorphenamine (p.428·1); caffeine (p.782·1); vitamin C (p.1460·2).
*Cold and influenza symptoms.*

**Benemid**
Merck Sharp & Dohme, Austral.†; Merck Frosst, Canad.†; Merck Sharp & Dohme, Irl.†; Merck Sharp & Dohme, NZ†; Merck Sharp & Dohme, S.Afr.†; Merck Sharp & Dohme, Switz.†; Merck Sharp & Dohme, Thai.; Merck Sharp & Dohme, UK†; Merck, USA.
Probenecid (p.416·3).
*Adjunct to beta-lactam antibacterials; gout; hyperuricaemia.*

**Benemide** Doms-Adrian, Fr.
Probenecid (p.416·3).
*Adjunct to beta-lactam antibacterials; gout; hyperuricaemia.*

**Benera** TO-Chemicals, Thai.
Belladonna alkaloids (p.479·1); ergotamine tartrate (p.467·2); phenobarbital (p.367·3).
*Menopausal disorders; migraine; neurocirculatory asthenia; psychosomatic disorders.*

**Beneroc** Roche, Austria†.
Multivitamin and mineral preparation (p.1417·1).

**Benerva**
Roche, Belg.; Roche, Braz.; Roche Nicholas, Fr.; IFET (ΙΦΕΤ), Gr.; Roche Consumer, Irl.; Roche, Ital.; Roche, Mex.; Roche, Spain; Roche, Swed.; Roche, Switz.; Roche Consumer, UK.
Thiamine hydrochloride (p.1455·1).
*Alcoholism; beri beri; neuritis; neuropathies; vitamin $B_1$ deficiency; Wernicke's encephalopathy.*

**Benestan**
Vita, Ital.†; Sanofi Synthelabo, Port.; Sanofi Synthelabo, Spain.
Alfuzosin hydrochloride (p.856·2).
*Benign prostatic hyperplasia.*

**Benetoss** Heralds, Braz.†.
Ambroxol (p.1114·3).
*Respiratory-tract congestion.*

**Benetussin** Janssen-Cilag, Port.
Ammonium chloride (p.1115·2); diphenhydramine (p.431·3); menthol (p.1711·3).
*Coughs.*

**Beneuran** Nycomed, Austria.
Thiamine hydrochloride (p.1455·1).
*Vitamin $B_1$ deficiency.*

**Beneuran compositum** Nycomed, Austria.
Thiamine hydrochloride (p.1455·1); pyridoxine hydrochloride (p.1456·3); folic acid (p.1429·1); cyanocobalamin (p.1458·2).
*Cervical syndrome; funicular myelosis; herpes zoster infection; nervous exhaustion; neuralgia; neuritis; pregnancy induced vomiting.*

**Beneuran Vit B-Komplex** Nycomed, Austria.
Riboflavin sodium phosphate (p.1456·1); pyridoxine hydrochloride (p.1456·3); dexpanthenol (p.1727·2); thiamine hydrochloride (p.1455·1); nicotinamide (p.1441·2).
*Eye disorders; gastrointestinal disorders; liver disorders; mouth and throat disorders; neurological disorders; obstetric disorders; skin disorders; vitamin deficiency.*

**Beneurol** Meuse, Belg.
Thiamine hydrochloride (p.1455·1).
*Beri-beri; dietary supplementation; digestive disorders; neuritis.*

**Beneuron Forte** Franco-Indian, India.
Vitamin B substances; vitamin C (p.1417·1).
*Vitamin B and C deficiency.*

**Benevat** Teuto, Braz.
Betamethasone valerate (p.1093·2).
*Skin disorders.*

**Benevolus** Schwabe, Arg.
Silymarin (p.1043·3).
*Liver disorders.*

**Benevran** Legrand, Braz.
Diclofenac potassium (p.32·1).
*Gout; inflammation; musculoskeletal, joint, and periarticular disorders; pain.*

**Benexol** Roche, Switz.
Vitamin B substances (p.1417·1).
*Alcoholism; neuropathies; vitamin B deficiency.*

**Benexol B12**
Note. This name is used for preparations of different composition.
Roche, Ital.
*Injection:* Cocarboxylase (p.1455·2); pyridoxine hydrochloride (p.1456·3); hydroxocobalamin (p.1458·2).
*Tablets:* Thiamine hydrochloride (p.1455·1); pyridoxine hydrochloride (p.1456·3); cyanocobalamin (p.1458·2).
*Neuropathies; vitamin $B_1$, $B_6$, and $B_{12}$ deficiency; vomiting.*
Roche, Mex.
Thiamine hydrochloride (p.1455·1); pyridoxine hydrochloride (p.1456·3); cyanocobalamin (p.1458·2).
*Megaloblastic and sideroblastic anaemias; neuritis; vitamin B deficiencies.*

**Benexol B1 B6 B12** Roche, Spain.
Cyanocobalamin (p.1458·2); pyridoxine hydrochloride (p.1456·3); thiamine hydrochloride (p.1455·1).
*Vitamin B deficiency.*

**Benfast** Novel, Ital.†.
Ibuprofen sodium (p.46·3).
*Fever; pain.*

**Benflogin**
Note. This name is used for preparations of different composition.
Asta Medica, Braz.
Benzydamine hydrochloride (p.21·1).
*Fever; inflammation; pain.*
Angelini, Ital.
Ibuprofen guaiacol ester (p.46·3).
*Fever; inflammation; pain.*

**Benflorene** Farmalight, Port.†.
Lactic-acid-producing organisms (p.1704·2); dried yeast; vitamin B substances (p.1417·1).
*Dietary supplement.*

**Benflux** Atral, Port.
Ambroxol hydrochloride (p.1114·3).
*Respiratory-tract congestion.*

**Benfofen** Sanofi Synthelabo, Ger.
Diclofenac sodium (p.32·1).
*Gout; inflammation; musculoskeletal, joint, and soft-tissue disorders; pain.*

**Ben-Gay**
Pfizer, Hong Kong; Pfizer, Israel; Pfizer Consumer, Singapore; Pfizer, USA.
Methyl salicylate (p.59·3); menthol (p.1711·3).
*Muscle, joint, and soft-tissue pain; neuralgia.*

**Ben-Gay Ice** Pfizer Consumer, Canad.
Menthol (p.1711·3).
*Muscle and joint pain.*

**Ben-Gay No Odor** Pfizer Consumer, Canad.
Trolamine salicylate (p.95·3).
*Muscle and joint pain.*

**Ben-Gay Original, Ben-Gay Extra Strength**
Pfizer Consumer, Canad.
Methyl salicylate (p.59·3); menthol (p.1711·3).
*Muscle and joint pain.*

**Ben-Gay Patch** Pfizer, USA.
Menthol (p.1711·3).
*Muscle, joint, and soft-tissue pain; neuralgia.*

**Ben-Gay Ultra**
Pfizer Consumer, Canad.; Pfizer, Hong Kong; Pfizer, Israel; Pfizer Consumer, Singapore; Pfizer, USA.
Methyl salicylate (p.59·3); menthol (p.1711·3); camphor (p.1665·3).
*Muscle, joint, and soft-tissue pain; neuralgia.*

**Ben-Gay Vanishing** Pfizer, USA.
Menthol (p.1711·3).
*Muscle, joint, and soft-tissue pain; neuralgia.*

**Benglau** CSC, Austria.
Dapiprazole hydrochloride (p.1679·1).
*Reversal of mydriasis.*

**Bengue's Balsam** Bengue, Irl.†.
Menthol (p.1711·3); methyl salicylate (p.59·3).
*Chilblains; musculoskeletal pain; respiratory-tract congestion.*

**Benhex** PSM, NZ.
Lindane (p.1506·3).
*Scabies.*

**Benical** Roche, Switz.
Dextromethorphan hydrobromide (p.1117·3); pseudoephedrine hydrochloride (p.1129·2); chlorphenamine maleate (p.427·3).
*Coughs.*

**Benicar** Sankyo, USA.
Olmesartan medoxomil (p.975·3).
*Hypertension.*

**Benicar HCT** Sankyo, USA.
Olmesartan medoxomil (p.975·3); hydrochlorothiazide (p.933·2).
*Hypertension.*

**Beni-cur** Biocur, Ger.†.
Garlic (p.1691·1).
*Vascular disorders.*

**Benisan** Fabra, Arg.
Piroxicam (p.84·2).
*Inflammation; pain.*

**Benistina** Ortoquimica, Braz.†.
Mepyramine maleate (p.437·1); pyridoxine (p.1457·2).
*Hypersensitivity reactions.*

**Benium**
Ratiopharm, Austria; Merckle, Ger.†.
Anise oil (p.1655·2); fennel oil (p.1687·3); caraway oil (p.1667·3).
*Gastrointestinal disorders.*

**Benn** Silom, Thai.†.
Betamethasone valerate (p.1093·2); neomycin (p.235·1).
*Bacterial skin infections.*

**Bennasone** Silom, Thai.
Betamethasone valerate (p.1093·2).
*Skin disorders.*

**Bennatuss** Hoe, Singapore.
Diphenhydramine hydrochloride (p.431·3); ammonium chloride (p.1115·2); sodium citrate (p.1223·2).
*Coughs; nasal congestion.*

**Benocten**
Medinova, Singapore; Medinova, Switz.
Diphenhydramine hydrochloride (p.431·3).
*Sleep disorders.*

**Benodent** IMS, Ital.
Sodium fluoride (p.1444·3); chlorhexidine (p.1173·2).
*Dental caries prophylaxis; dental hygiene.*

**Benodent CLX** IMS, Ital.
Chlorhexidine gluconate (p.1173·2).
*Dental disorders.*

**Benodent Gel Gengivale** IMS, Ital.
Chlorhexidine (p.1173·2); potassium nitrate (p.1190·1); potassium glycyrrhetinate.
*Gum disorders.*

**Benoquin**
ICN, Canad.; Mac, India; ICN, USA†.
Monobenzone (p.1154·2).
*Skin hyperpigmentation.*

**Benoral**
Note. This name is used for preparations of different composition.
Sanofi Synthelabo, Irl.; Sanofi Synthelabo, UK†.
Benorilate (p.20·3).
*Fever; inflammation; musculoskeletal and joint disorders; pain.*
Reig Jofre, Spain.
Benzathine phenoxymethylpenicillin (p.163·2).
*Bacterial infections.*

**Benormal** Cristalia, Braz.
Vitamin B substances with calcium (p.1417·1).
*Nutritional supplement.*

**Benosid** Farmasan, Ger.
Budesonide (p.1094·2).
*Obstructive airways disease.*

**Benotrin** EMS, Braz.†.
Ibuprofen (p.45·3).
*Inflammation; pain.*

**Benovate** GlaxoSmithKline, India.
Betamethasone valerate (p.1093·2).
*Skin and scalp disorders.*

**Benoxid** Yamanouchi, Ital.
Benzoyl peroxide (p.1143·2).
*Acne; skin disinfection.*

**Benoxinat SE** Alcon, Ger.
Oxybuprocaine hydrochloride (p.1382·1).
*Local anaesthesia.*

**Benoxinate** Alcon, Hong Kong.
Oxybuprocaine hydrochloride (p.1382·1).
*Local anaesthesia.*

**Benoxinato** Cusi, Spain†.
Oxybuprocaine hydrochloride (p.1382·1).
*Local anaesthesia.*

**Benoxygel**
Stiefel, Port.; Stiefel, Spain.
Benzoyl peroxide (p.1143·2).
*Acne.*

**Benoxyl**
Stiefel, Canad.; Stiefel, Irl.†; Stiefel, Mex.; Stiefel, NZ†; Stiefel, S.Afr.; Stiefel, UK†; Stiefel, USA†.
Benzoyl peroxide (p.1143·2).
*Acne.*

**Benpen**
CSL, Austral.; CSL, NZ.
Benzylpenicillin sodium (p.163·2).
*Bacterial infections.*

**Benpine**
Atlantic, Malaysia; Atlantic, Singapore; Atlantic, Thai.
Chlordiazepoxide hydrochloride (p.674·2).
*Alcohol withdrawal syndrome; anxiety; skeletal muscle spasm.*

**Benquil** Hansam, UK.
Benperidol (p.671·2).
*Deviant sexual behaviour.*

**Bens** Ardern, UK.
Diethyltoluamide (p.1503·3).
*Insect repellent.*

**Bensal HP** 7 Oaks, USA.
Benzoic acid (p.1169·3); salicylic acid (p.1157·1).
*Fungal skin infections.*

**Bensolmin** Continentales, Mex.†.
Mebendazole (p.108·2).

**Bensulf** Fada, Arg.
Thiopental (p.1310·1).

**Bensulfoid** ECR, USA.
Colloidal sulfur (p.1158·2); resorcinol (p.1156·3).
*Acne.*

**Bentasil** Carter Horner, Canad.
*Green lozenges*†: Anethole (p.1654·3); cineole (p.1672·1); menthol (p.1711·3).
*Nasal congestion.*
*Red lozenges; yellow lozenges:* Anethole (p.1654·3); menthol (p.1711·3).
*Coughs; sore throats.*

**Bentasil Black Currant** Carter Horner, Canad.
Menthol (p.1711·3).
*Sore throat.*

**Bentasil Eucalyptus** Carter Horner, Canad.
Eucalyptus oil (p.1686·2); menthol (p.1711·3).
*Coughs; nasal congestion; sore throat.*

**Bentasil Licorice with Echinacea** Carter Horner, Canad.
Ammonium chloride (p.1115·2); anethole (p.1654·3); echinacea (p.1683·2); liquorice (p.1270·2); eucalyptus oil (p.1686·2); menthol (p.1711·3).
*Sore throat.*

**Bentasil Menthol** Carter Horner, Canad.
Eucalyptus oil (p.1686·2); menthol (p.1711·3).
*Coughs; nasal congestion; sore throat.*

**Bentelan** Biofutura, Ital.
Betamethasone disodium phosphate (p.1093·1).
*Corticosteroid.*

**Bentiamin** Haller, Braz.
Albendazole (p.101·2).
*Worm infections.*

**Bentonine** IFET (ΙΦΕΤ), Gr.
Bentonite (p.1577·2).
*Paraquat poisoning.*

**Bentophyto** Panalab, Arg.
Undecenoic acid diethanolamide.
*Fungal skin infections.*

**Bentos**
Novartis Ophthalmics, Fr.; Kaken, Hong Kong†; Kaken, Jpn.
Befunolol hydrochloride (p.867·1).
*Glaucoma; ocular hypertension.*

**Bentyl**
Medley, Braz.; Aventis, Mex.; Axcan, USA.
Dicycloverine hydrochloride (p.481·2).
*Smooth muscle spasm.*

**Bentylol** Aventis, Canad.
Dicycloverine hydrochloride (p.481·2).
*Gastrointestinal spasm.*

**Benur** Bioindustria, Ital.
Doxazosin mesilate (p.908·3).
*Benign prostatic hyperplasia.*

**Ben-u-ron**
Sigmapharm, Austria; Bene, Ger.; Novartis Consumer, Ger.; Bene-Chemie, Hong Kong; Neo-Farmaceutica, Port.; Milupa, Switz.
Paracetamol (p.76·2).
*Fever; pain.*

**Benursil** Benedetti, Ital.
Ursodeoxycholic acid (p.1760·3).
*Biliary disorders; cholesterol gallstones.*

**Benuryl** ICN, Canad.
Probenecid (p.416·3).
*Hyperuricaemia.*

**Benutrex 1000** Organon, Chile.
Thiamine hydrochloride; riboflavine; pyridoxine hydrochloride; nicotinamide; dexpanthenol; cyanocobalamin; hydroxocobalamin (p.1417·1).
*Neuralgia; neuritis; vitamin B deficiency.*

**Benylan**
Note. This name is used for preparations of different composition.
Pfizer, Denm.
Diphenhydramine hydrochloride (p.431·3); ammonium chloride (p.1115·2); menthol (p.1711·3).
*Coughs; hypersensitivity.*
Parke, Davis, Fin.†; Parke, Davis, Swed.†.
Diphenhydramine hydrochloride (p.431·3).
*Hypersensitivity reactions.*

**Benylin**
*Note. This name is used for preparations of different composition.*
*Parke, Davis, Chile.*
Diphenhydramine hydrochloride (p.431·3); ammonium chloride (p.1115·2); sodium citrate (p.1223·2); menthol (p.1711·3).
*Coughs.*

*Pfizer Consumer, Irl.; Pfizer Consumer, Port.*
Diphenhydramine hydrochloride (p.431·3); menthol (p.1711·3).
Formerly contained diphenhydramine hydrochloride, ammonium chloride, and menthol in *Port.*
*Coughs.*

*Pfizer Consumer, S.Afr.; Pfizer, Switz.*
Diphenhydramine hydrochloride (p.431·3); ammonium chloride (p.1115·2).
*Coughs.*

**Benylin a la codeine** *Pfizer, Switz.*
Diphenhydramine hydrochloride (p.431·3); codeine phosphate (p.27·1); ammonium chloride (p.1115·2).
*Coughs.*

**Benylin Active Response** *Pfizer Consumer, UK.*
Echinacea purpurea (p.1683·2).
*Upper respiratory-tract infections.*

**Benylin Adult** *Warner-Lambert, USA.*
Dextromethorphan hydrobromide (p.1117·3).
Formerly called Benylin Cough Syrup and contained diphenhydramine hydrochloride.
*Coughs.*

**Benylin Antihistaminicum** *Pfizer Consumer, Belg.*
Diphenhydramine hydrochloride (p.431·3).
*Hypersensitivity reactions.*

**Benylin Antitusivo** *Pfizer Lambert, Spain.*
Dextromethorphan hydrobromide (p.1117·3).
*Coughs.*

**Benylin Antitussivum** *Warner-Lambert Consumer, Belg.†.*
Dextromethorphan hydrobromide (p.1117·3).
*Coughs.*

**Benylin CD** *Pfizer, Hong Kong.*
Diphenhydramine hydrochloride (p.431·3); codeine phosphate (p.27·1); ammonium chloride (p.1115·2); sodium citrate (p.1223·2); menthol (p.1711·3).
*Coughs.*

**Benylin Chesty** *Pfizer Consumer, S.Afr.*
Orciprenaline sulfate (p.790·2); bromhexine hydrochloride (p.1115·3).
*Coughs.*

**Benylin Chesty Cough Original** *Pfizer Consumer, UK.*
Diphenhydramine hydrochloride (p.431·3); menthol (p.1711·3).
*Coughs.*

**Benylin Chesty Coughs Non-Drowsy** *Pfizer Consumer, UK.*
Guaifenesin (p.1122·1); menthol (p.1711·3).
*Coughs.*

**Benylin Childrens Chesty Coughs**
*Pfizer Consumer, Irl.; Pfizer Consumer, UK.*
Guaifenesin (p.1122·1).
*Coughs.*

**Benylin Childrens Cough** *Pfizer Consumer, Irl.*
Diphenhydramine hydrochloride (p.431·3); sodium citrate (p.1223·2); menthol (p.1711·3).
*Coughs.*

**Benylin Childrens Cough and Cold** *Pfizer Consumer, Irl.*
Dextromethorphan hydrobromide (p.1117·3); triprolidine hydrochloride (p.442·3).
*Coughs and cold symptoms.*

**Benylin Childrens Coughs & Colds** *Pfizer Consumer, UK.*
Dextromethorphan hydrobromide (p.1117·3); triprolidine hydrochloride (p.442·3).
*Coughs and cold symptoms.*

**Benylin Childrens Dry Coughs** *Pfizer Consumer, UK.*
Pholcodine (p.1128·3).
*Coughs.*

**Benylin Childrens Night Coughs** *Pfizer Consumer, UK.*
Diphenhydramine hydrochloride (p.431·3); menthol (p.1711·3).
*Coughs; hypersensitivity symptoms of the respiratory tract.*

**Benylin with Codeine**
*Note. This name is used for preparations of different composition.*
*Pfizer Consumer, Irl.; Pfizer Consumer, UK.*
Diphenhydramine hydrochloride (p.431·3); codeine phosphate (p.27·1); menthol (p.1711·3).
*Coughs.*

*Parke, Davis, Israel†.*
Diphenhydramine hydrochloride (p.431·3); codeine phosphate (p.27·1); sodium citrate (p.1223·2); menthol (p.1711·3).
*Coughs.*

*Pfizer Consumer, S.Afr.*
Diphenhydramine hydrochloride (p.431·3); codeine phosphate (p.27·1); ammonium chloride (p.1115·2).
*Coughs.*

**Benylin Codeine D-E** *Pfizer Consumer, Canad.*
Codeine phosphate (p.27·1); pseudoephedrine hydrochloride (p.1129·2); guaifenesin (p.1122·1).
Formerly known as Benylin Codeine.
*Coughs; nasal congestion.*

**Benylin Cold** *Warner-Lambert, NZ†.*
Paracetamol (p.76·2); pseudoephedrine hydrochloride (p.1129·2); dextromethorphan hydrobromide (p.1117·3).
*Coughs and cold symptoms.*

**Benylin Cough** *Pfizer, Hong Kong.*
Diphenhydramine hydrochloride (p.431·3); ammonium chloride (p.1115·2); sodium citrate (p.1223·2); menthol (p.1711·3).
*Cold symptoms; coughs.*

**Benylin Cough & Congestion** *Pfizer Consumer, UK.*
Diphenhydramine hydrochloride (p.431·3); menthol (p.1711·3); dextromethorphan hydrobromide (p.1117·3); pseudoephedrine hydrochloride (p.1129·2).
*Coughs and cold symptoms.*

**Benylin Day & Night**
*Note. This name is used for preparations of different composition.*
*Pfizer Consumer, Irl.; Warner-Lambert, Ital.†; Parke, Davis, S.Afr.†.*
Day tablets, paracetamol (p.76·2); phenylpropanolamine hydrochloride (p.1127·3); night tablets, paracetamol; diphenhydramine hydrochloride (p.431·3).
*Cold and influenza symptoms; upper respiratory-tract congestion.*

*Pfizer Consumer, UK.*
Daytime tablets, paracetamol (p.76·2); pseudoephedrine hydrochloride (p.1129·2); night-time tablets, diphenhydramine hydrochloride (p.431·3); paracetamol.
The daytime tablets formerly contained paracetamol and phenylpropanolamine hydrochloride.
*Cold and influenza symptoms.*

**Benylin Descongestivo** *Pfizer Lambert, Spain.*
Dextromethorphan hydrobromide (p.1117·3); pseudoephedrine hydrochloride (p.1129·2).
*Coughs; nasal congestion.*

**Benylin DM**
*Pfizer Consumer, Canad.; Parke, Davis, USA†.*
Dextromethorphan hydrobromide (p.1117·3).
*Coughs.*

**Benylin DM-D**
*Pfizer Consumer, Canad.; Pfizer Consumer, S.Afr.*
Dextromethorphan hydrobromide (p.1117·3); pseudoephedrine hydrochloride (p.1129·2).
*Coughs; nasal congestion.*

**Benylin DM-D-E** *Pfizer Consumer, Canad.*
Dextromethorphan hydrobromide (p.1117·3); pseudoephedrine hydrochloride (p.1129·2); guaifenesin (p.1122·1).
*Coughs; nasal congestion.*

**Benylin DM-E** *Pfizer Consumer, Canad.*
Dextromethorphan hydrobromide (p.1117·3); guaifenesin (p.1122·1).
*Coughs.*

**Benylin Dry Cough**
*Note. This name is used for preparations of different composition.*
*Pfizer Consumer, Irl.*
Diphenhydramine hydrochloride (p.431·3); dextromethorphan hydrobromide (p.1117·3); sodium citrate (p.1223·2); menthol (p.1711·3).
*Coughs.*

*Pfizer Consumer, S.Afr.*
Dextromethorphan hydrobromide (p.1117·3).
Formerly known as Benylin DM.
*Coughs.*

**Benylin Dry Coughs Non-Drowsy** *Pfizer Consumer, UK.*
Dextromethorphan hydrobromide (p.1117·3).
*Coughs.*

**Benylin Dry Coughs Original** *Pfizer Consumer, UK.*
Diphenhydramine hydrochloride (p.431·3); dextromethorphan hydrobromide (p.1117·3); menthol (p.1711·3).
*Coughs.*

**Benylin Expectorant** *Warner-Lambert, USA.*
Dextromethorphan hydrobromide (p.1117·3); guaifenesin (p.1122·1).
*Coughs.*

**Benylin First Defense** *Pfizer Consumer, Canad.*
Echinacea (p.1683·2); menthol (p.1711·3).
*Cough and cold symptoms.*

**Benylin 4 Flu**
*Note. This name is used for preparations of different composition.*
*Pfizer Consumer, Canad.*
Dextromethorphan hydrobromide (p.1117·3); pseudoephedrine hydrochloride (p.1129·2); guaifenesin (p.1122·1); paracetamol (p.76·2).
*Coughs and cold symptoms.*

*Pfizer Consumer, Irl.*
Diphenhydramine hydrochloride (p.431·3); paracetamol (p.76·2); pseudoephedrine hydrochloride (p.1129·2).
*Cold and influenza symptoms.*

*Pfizer Consumer, UK.*
*Hot drink†:* Diphenhydramine hydrochloride (p.431·3); paracetamol (p.76·2); phenylephrine hydrochloride (p.1126·3).
*Oral liquid; tablets:* Diphenhydramine hydrochloride (p.431·3); paracetamol (p.76·2); pseudoephedrine hydrochloride (p.1129·2).
*Cold and influenza symptoms.*

**Benylin Multi-Symptom** *Warner-Lambert, USA.*
Dextromethorphan hydrobromide (p.1117·3); pseudoephedrine hydrochloride (p.1129·2); guaifenesin (p.1122·1).
*Cough and cold symptoms.*

**Benylin Non-Drowsy Chesty Cough** *Pfizer Consumer, Irl.*
Guaifenesin (p.1122·1); menthol (p.1711·3).
*Coughs.*

**Benylin Non-Drowsy Dry Cough** *Pfizer Consumer, Irl.*
Dextromethorphan hydrobromide (p.1117·3).
*Coughs.*

**Benylin Paediatric** *Parke, Davis, Israel†.*
*Sugar/colour-free syrup:* Diphenhydramine hydrochloride (p.431·3); menthol (p.1711·3).
*Syrup:* Diphenhydramine hydrochloride (p.431·3); sodium citrate (p.1223·2); menthol (p.1711·3).
*Coughs.*

**Benylin Pediatric** *Warner-Lambert, USA.*
Dextromethorphan hydrobromide (p.1117·3).
*Coughs.*

**Benylin Solid** *Parke, Davis, S.Afr.†.*
Dextromethorphan hydrobromide (p.1117·3).
*Coughs.*

**Benylin Sore Throat Lozenge** *Pfizer Consumer, UK.*
Hexylresorcinol (p.1182·1).
*Sore throat.*

**Benylin Tickly Coughs** *Boots, UK.*
Glycerol (p.1694·3).
*Coughs.*

**Benylin-E** *Pfizer Consumer, Canad.*
Guaifenesin (p.1122·1).
*Coughs.*

**Benza** *Century, USA.*
Benzalkonium chloride (p.1168·3).
*Eye, bladder, urethra, and body cavity irrigation; skin, mucous membrane, and wound disinfection; vaginal douching.*

**Benzac**
*Galderma, Austral.; Galderma, Belg.; Galderma, Braz.†; Galderma, Canad.; Galderma, Chile; Galderma, Ital.; Galderma, Mex.; Galderma, Neth.; Galderma, NZ; Galderma, Port.; Galderma, Singapore; Galderma, Switz.; Galderma, Thai.; Galderma, USA.*
Benzoyl peroxide (p.1143·2).
*Acne.*

**Benzac Eritromicina** *Galderma, Braz.*
Erythromycin (p.208·1); benzoyl peroxide (p.1143·2).
*Acne.*

**Benzac-AC**
*Galderma, Braz.; Galderma, Hong Kong; Galderma, Israel; Galderma, Malaysia; Galderma, S.Afr.*
Benzoyl peroxide (p.1143·2).
*Acne.*

**BenzaClin** *Dermik, USA.*
Clindamycin (p.194·2); benzoyl peroxide (p.1143·2).
*Acne.*

**Benzac-W** *Lavipharm, Gr.*
Benzoyl peroxide (p.1143·2).
*Acne.*

**Benzaderm** *Remexa, Mex.*
Soap.
*Skin cleansing.*
*Topical gel:* Benzoyl peroxide (p.1143·2).
*Acne.*

**Benzagel**
*Galderma, Braz.†; Novartis Consumer, Canad.; Dermik, Canad.; Dermik, USA†.*
Benzoyl peroxide (p.1143·2).
*Acne.*

**Benzaknen**
*AB-Consult, Austria; Galderma, Ger.*
Benzoyl peroxide (p.1143·2).
*Acne.*

**Benzalc** *Asens, Spain†.*
Benzalkonium chloride (p.1168·3).
*Skin and mucous membrane disinfection.*

**Benzalcream** *Argenfarma, Arg.*
Benzalkonium chloride (p.1168·3).
*Mucous membrane disinfection.*

**Benzamycin**
*Ingens, Arg.; Trenker, Belg.; Dermik, Canad.; Finn Vita, Chile; Dermik, Hong Kong; Bioglan, Irl.; Dermik, Israel; Darier, Mex.; Dermik, Singapore; Schwarz, UK; Dermik, USA.*
Benzoyl peroxide (p.1143·2); erythromycin (p.208·1).
*Acne.*

**Benzamycine** *UCB, S.Afr.*
Benzoyl peroxide (p.1143·2); erythromycin (p.208·1).
*Acne.*

**Benzanil Compuesto** *Lakeside, Mex.*
Benzathine benzylpenicillin (p.162·3); procaine benzylpenicillin (p.246·1); benzylpenicillin sodium (p.163·2).
*Bacterial infections.*

**Benzanil Simple** *Lakeside, Mex.*
Benzathine benzylpenicillin (p.162·3).
*Bacterial infections.*

**Benzantine H** *Rekah, Israel.*
Diphenhydramine hydrochloride (p.431·3); hydrocortisone (p.1103·3).
*Skin disorders; skin irritation.*

**Benzapen G** *Teuto, Braz.*
Procaine benzylpenicillin (p.246·1); benzylpenicillin potassium (p.163·2).
*Bacterial infections.*

**Benzashave** *Medicis, USA†.*
Benzoyl peroxide (p.1143·2).
*Acne.*

**Benzatec** *Caps, S.Afr.*
Benzylpenicillin sodium (p.163·2).
*Bacterial infections.*

**Benzatron** *Ariston, Braz.*
Benzathine benzylpenicillin (p.162·3).
*Bacterial infections.*

**Benzecilin** *Teuto, Braz.*
Benzylpenicillin potassium (p.163·2).
*Bacterial infections.*

**Benzedrex** *Ascher, USA.*
Propylhexedrine (p.1592·3).
*Nasal congestion.*

**Benzemul** *McGloin, Austral.*
Benzyl benzoate (p.1500·2).
*Pediculosis; scabies.*

**Benzet** *Rolab, S.Afr.*
Cetrimide (p.1172·1); benzocaine (p.1370·3).
*Mouth and throat disorders.*

**Benzetacil**
*Wyeth, Arg.; Eurofarma, Braz.; Wyeth, Mex.; Antibioticos, Spain.*
Benzathine benzylpenicillin (p.162·3).
*Bacterial infections.*

**Benzetacil Combinado** *Wyeth, Mex.*
Benzathine benzylpenicillin (p.162·3); benzylpenicillin potassium (p.163·2); procaine benzylpenicillin (p.246·1).
*Bacterial infections.*

**Benzetacil Compuesta** *Antibioticos, Spain.*
Benzylpenicillin potassium (p.163·2); procaine benzylpenicillin (p.246·1); benzathine benzylpenicillin (p.162·3).
*Bacterial infections.*

**Benzevit** *Elofar, Braz.*
Nystatin (p.406·3); zinc oxide (p.1163·2).
*Skin infections.*

**Benzibel** *Luper, Braz.*
Benzyl benzoate (p.1500·2).
*Pediculosis; scabies.*

**Benziflex** *EMS, Braz.†.*
Benzydamine hydrochloride (p.21·1).
*Fever; inflammation; pain.*

**Benzihex** *Galderma, Arg.*
Benzoyl peroxide (p.1143·2).
*Acne.*

**Benzilol** *Bunker, Braz.†.*
Benzyl benzoate (p.1500·2); trolamine (p.1758·2).
*Pediculosis; scabies.*

**Benzirin** *Fater, Ital.*
Benzydamine hydrochloride (p.21·1).
*Inflammatory mouth and throat disorders.*

**Benzitrat** *Biolab Sanus, Braz.*
Benzydamine hydrochloride (p.21·1).
*Fever; inflammation; pain.*

**Benzoax** *Ducto, Braz.*
Benzyl benzoate (p.1500·2).
*Pediculosis; scabies.*

**Benzoben** *Osorio de Moraes, Braz.*
Benzyl benzoate (p.1500·2).
*Pediculosis; scabies.*

**Benzocaine PD** *Produits Dentaires, Switz.*
Benzocaine (p.1370·3); hydroxyquinoline sulfate (p.1700·1); eugenol (p.1686·2).
*Dental pain.*

**Benzocan** *Teuto, Braz.*
Benzyl benzoate (p.1500·2).
*Pediculosis; scabies.*

**Benzodent** *Procter & Gamble, USA.*
Benzocaine (p.1370·3).
*Oral lesions.*

**Benzoderm Myco** *Athenstaedt, Ger.*
Clotrimazole (p.396·2).
*Fungal skin infections.*

**Benzogen Ferri** *Cos Farma, Ital.†.*
Benzalkonium chloride (p.1168·3); sodium nitrite (p.1052·3); acetone.
*Instrument disinfection.*

**Benzo-Ginestryl** *Aventis, Mex.*
Estradiol benzoate (p.1550·1).
*Menopausal disorders; menstrual disorders; osteoporosis.*

**Benzo-Ginoestril** *Aventis, Braz.*
Estradiol hexahydrobenzoate (p.1550·1).
*Menopausal disorders; osteoporosis.*

**Benzo-Gynoestryl** *Roussel, Fr.†.*
Estradiol benzoate (p.1550·1) or estradiol hexahydrobenzoate (p.1550·1).
*Oestrogen deficiency.*

**Benzol** *Teuto, Braz.*
Tiabendazole (p.114·2).
*Worm infections.*

**Benzomel** *Granado, Braz.*
Sodium benzoate (p.1169·3); mepyramine maleate (p.437·1); sulfogaiacol (p.1131·1); belladonna (p.479·1); passion flower (p.1729·1).
*Coughs.*

**Benzomix** *Savoma, Ital.†.*
Benzoyl peroxide (p.1143·2).
*Acne; skin disinfection.*

**Benzonal** *Cryopharma, Mex.*
Benzonatate (p.1115·3).
*Coughs.*

**Benzopin** *Alliance, S.Afr.†.*
Diazepam (p.690·1).
*Alcohol withdrawal syndrome; anxiety; premedication.*

**Benzoral** *Billiet, Arg.*
Cyanocobalamin (p.1458·2).
*Anaemias.*

**Benzotal** *Cifarma, Braz.†.*
Ampicillin benzathine (p.158·1); ampicillin sodium (p.157·1).
*Bacterial infections.*

**Benzotal Balsamico** Biosintetica, Braz.†.
Ampicillin benzathine (p.158·1); ampicillin sodium (p.157·1); guaifenesin (p.1122·1); niaouli oil (p.1719·3); cineole (p.1672·1).
*Bacterial infections.*

**Benzotizan** Sanval, Braz.
Benzyl benzoate (p.1500·2).
*Scabies.*

**Benzotran** Pacific, NZ†.
Oxazepam (p.712·2).
*Anxiety.*

**Benzoyt** Bioglan, Ger.
Benzoyl peroxide (p.1143·2).
*Acne.*

**Benzperox** Medphano, Ger.
Benzoyl peroxide (p.1143·2).
*Acne.*

**Benztrop** Pharmalab, Austral.
Benzatropine mesilate (p.479·2).
*Drug-induced extrapyramidal disorders; parkinsonism.*

**Benzum** Lepori, Port.†.
Bendazac (p.20·3).
*Skin disorders.*

**Benzyme** Collins, Mex.†.
Diazepam (p.690·1).

**Beocid Puroptal** Metochem, Austria†.
Sulfacetamide sodium (p.257·3).
*Bacterial eye infections.*

**Beof** Saval, Chile.
Betaxolol hydrochloride (p.873·1).
*Glaucoma; ocular hypertension.*

**Beofenac**
UCB, Austria; UCB, Ger.
Aceclofenac (p.11·2).
*Musculoskeletal and joint disorders.*

**Beofta** Columbia, Mex.
Betaxolol (p.873·1).

**Be-Oxytet** Be-Tabs, S.Afr.
Oxytetracycline hydrochloride (p.241·1).
*Bacterial infections.*

**Bepanten** Roche, Ital.
Dexpanthenol (p.1727·2).
*Intestinal atony.*

**Bepanthen**
Note. This name is used for preparations of different composition.
Roche Consumer, Austral.
Benzalkonium chloride (p.1168·3).
Formerly contained panthenol.
*Minor skin lesions; skin irritation.*

Roche, Austria.
*Cream; ointment:* Dexpanthenol (p.1727·2).
*Skin damage; wounds.*

*Solution:* Dexpanthenol (p.1727·2); domiphen bromide (p.1179·1).
*Gastrointestinal disorders; mouth and throat disorders; nasal disorders; respiratory-tract disorders; skin damage.*

Roche, Fin.; Roche Nicholas, Fr.; Roche Nicholas, Ger.; Roche, Israel; Roche, UK†.
Dexpanthenol (p.1727·2).
*Conjunctivitis; dexpanthenol deficiency disorders; gastrointestinal disorders; mouth and throat disorders; nasal disorders; skin disorders; wounds.*

Roche, NZ.
Panthenol (p.1727·2).
*Burns; skin irritation; skin lesions.*

**Bepanthen Plus**
Roche, Austria; Roche, Israel.
Dexpanthenol (p.1727·2); chlorhexidine hydrochloride (p.1173·3).
*Dry skin; wounds.*

**Bepanthene**
Note. This name is used for preparations of different composition.
Roche, Belg.†.
Panthenol (p.1727·2).
*Hepatitis; intestinal atony; muscular cramps; respiratory-tract disorders; skin disorders.*

Roche, Port.
*Cream; ointment:* Dexpanthenol (p.1727·2).

*Lotion:* Dexpanthenol (p.1727·2); chlorhexidine hydrochloride (p.1173·3).
*Skin disorders; wounds.*

Roche, Spain; Roche, Switz.
Dexpanthenol (p.1727·2).
*Gastrointestinal disorders; mouth and throat disorders; nasal disorders; respiratory-tract disorders; skin disorders.*

**Bepanthene Plus**
Roche, Port.; Roche, Switz.
Dexpanthenol (p.1727·2); chlorhexidine hydrochloride (p.1173·3).
*Skin disorders; wounds.*

**Bepantol**
Roche, Braz.; Roche, Chile; Roche Consumer, S.Afr.
Dexpanthenol (p.1727·2).
*Burns; skin disorders; wounds.*

**Beparine** Biological E, India.
*Cream:* Heparin sodium (p.928·1); benzyl nicotinate (p.21·2).
*Superficial thrombophlebitis.*

*Injection:* Heparin sodium (p.928·1).
*Thromboembolic disorders.*

**Bepeben** Teuto, Braz.
Benzathine benzylpenicillin (p.162·3).
*Bacterial infections.*

**Bepeno** Milano, Thai.
Phenylephrine hydrochloride (p.1126·3); brompheniramine maleate (p.426·1).
*Nasal congestion; respiratory-tract disorders.*

**Bepeno-G** Milano, Thai.
Phenylephrine hydrochloride (p.1126·3); brompheniramine maleate (p.426·1); guaifenesin (p.1122·1).
Formerly contained phenylpropanolamine hydrochloride, phenylephrine hydrochloride, brompheniramine maleate, and guaifenesin.
*Coughs; respiratory-tract congestion.*

**Bepep** Nutrition Care, Austral.†.
Betaine hydrochloride (p.1660·2); pepsin (p.1729·3).
*Digestive disorders.*

**Bephen** Thilo, Hong Kong†.
Trifluridine (p.655·3).
*Herpes simplex eye infections.*

**Beplex** Anglo-French Drugs, India.
Vitamin B substances with or without vitamin C (p.1417·1).
*Vitamin B deficiency.*

**Beplexaron** Ariston, Braz.
Vitamin B substances (p.1417·1).

**Beplex-Zee**
Anglo-French Drugs, India; Anglo-French Drugs, Thai.
Multivitamin preparation with zinc (p.1417·1).

**Beplus** Cazi, Braz.
Vitamin B substances (p.1417·1).

**Beprogel**
Hoe, Malaysia; Hoe, Singapore.
Betamethasone dipropionate (p.1093·1).
*Skin disorders.*

**Beprogent**
Hoe, Malaysia; Hoe, Singapore.
Betamethasone dipropionate (p.1093·1) gentamicin sulfate (p.217·1).
*Infected skin disorders.*

**Beprogenta** Chew, Thai.
Betamethasone dipropionate (p.1093·1); gentamicin sulfate (p.217·1).
*Infected inflammatory skin disorders.*

**Beprosalic**
Hoe, Malaysia; Hoe, Singapore.
Betamethasone dipropionate (p.1093·1); salicylic acid (p.1157·1).
*Skin disorders.*

**Beprosone**
Hoe, Malaysia; Hoe, Singapore; Chew, Thai.
Betamethasone dipropionate (p.1093·1).
*Skin disorders.*

**Beptazine** MM, India.
Propranolol hydrochloride (p.989·3); dihydralazine sulfate (p.899·3).
*Hypertension.*

**Beptazine-H** MM, India.
Propranolol hydrochloride (p.989·3); dihydralazine sulfate (p.899·3); hydrochlorothiazide (p.933·2).
*Hypertension.*

**Bequidril** Teuto, Braz.
Diphenhydramine hydrochloride (p.431·3); ammonium chloride (p.1115·2); sodium citrate (p.1223·2).
*Coughs.*

**Bequipecto** Llorens, Spain†.
Bromelains (p.1662·2); bromhexine (p.1115·3); oxolamine citrate (p.1126·1).
*Respiratory-tract disorders.*

**Bequium** Saval, Chile.
Chlorphenamine maleate (p.427·3); pseudoephedrine hydrochloride (p.1129·2); codeine (p.27·1).
*Coughs; nasal congestion.*

**Beramicina** Berman, Mex.
Gentamicin sulfate (p.217·1).
*Bacterial infections.*

**Beramikin** Berman, Mex.
Amikacin sulfate (p.154·1).
*Bacterial infections.*

**Beramin** Hoechst Marion Roussel, S.Afr.†.
Diphenhydramine hydrochloride (p.431·3); ammonium chloride (p.1115·2).
*Coughs.*

**Berazole** Hoechst Marion Roussel, S.Afr.†.
Metronidazole (p.607·2).
*Anaerobic bacterial infections; protozoal infections.*

**Berberell** Sanorell, Ger.
Homoeopathic preparation.

**Berberil Dry Eye** Mann, Ger.
Hypromellose (p.1579·3).
*Dry eyes.*

**Berberil N** Mann, Ger.
Tetryzoline hydrochloride (p.1131·2).
*Eye disorders.*

**Berberis Complex** Blackmores, Austral.†.
Berberis vulgaris; taraxacum (p.1751·3); greater celandine (p.1695·3); boldo (p.1661·2); lecithin (p.1706·1); methionine (p.1042·1); thiamine hydrochloride (p.1455·1).
*Constipation; dyspepsia; liver disorders.*

**Berberis Cosmoplex** Peithner, Austria.
Homoeopathic preparation.

**Berberis Med Complex** Dynamit, Austria.
Homoeopathic preparation.

**Berberis Oligoplex** Madaus, Ger.
Homoeopathic preparation.

**Bercetina** Microsules Bernabo, Arg.
Flunarizine (p.434·2).

**Berciclina** Berman, Mex.
Tetracycline hydrochloride (p.266·2).
*Bacterial infections.*

**Berciclina Enzimatica** Berman, Mex.
Tetracycline (p.266·2) with enzymes.
*Bacterial infections.*

**Berclomine** Polipharm, Thai.
Dicycloverine hydrochloride (p.481·2); simeticone (p.1289·2).
*Gastrointestinal colic and spasm.*

**Berex** Leiras, Fin.
Vitamin B substances (p.1417·1).
*Vitamin B deficiency; vitamin B supplement.*

**Bergagyn** Bergamon, Ital.
Benzalkonium chloride (p.1168·3).
*Vaginal disinfection.*

**Bergamol** Medichrom, Gr.
Buspirone hydrochloride (p.672·2).
*Generalised anxiety.*

**Bergamon Sapone** Bergamon, Ital.
Tribromsalan (p.1171·2).
*Skin cleansing.*

**Berggeist** Kur und Stadtapotheke, Austria.
Arnica tincture (p.1656·3); urtica tincture (p.1762·1); formic acid (p.1689·3); menthol (p.1711·3); methyl nicotinate (p.59·2); juniper oil (p.1703·1); lavender oil (p.1705·2); eucalyptus oil (p.1686·2); rosemary oil (p.1740·2); pumilio pine oil (p.1737·1).
*Bruising; musculoskeletal and joint disorders; neuralgia.*

**Bergon** MC, Ital.
Orthophenylphenol (p.1187·2); glutaral (p.1180·3); isopropyl alcohol (p.1184·3).
*Disinfection of endoscopes.*

**Beriate** Aventis, Austria.
A factor VIII preparation (p.751·1).
*Factor VIII deficiency.*

**Beriate P**
Aventis Behring, Braz.; Aventis Behring, Ger.; Aventis Behring, Ital.; Aventis Behring, Spain; Aventis Behring, Swed.; Aventis Behring, Switz.; Aventis Behring, UK.
A factor VIII preparation (p.751·1).
*Haemorrhagic disorders.*

**Beribumin** Aventis Behring, Braz.
Albumin (p.740·3).
*Plasma volume expansion.*

**Bericard** Provita, Austria.
Crataegus (p.1677·1).
*Cardiovascular disorders.*

**Beriglobin**
Aventis, Austria; Aventis Behring, Denm.; Aventis Behring, Ger.; Mirren, S.Afr.; Aventis Behring, Swed.
A normal immunoglobulin (p.1627·2).
*Hypogammaglobulinaemia; passive immunisation.*

**Beriglobin P** Aventis Behring, Israel.
A normal immunoglobulin (p.1627·2).
*Hypogammaglobulinaemia; passive immunisation.*

**Beriglobina** Aventis Behring, Braz.
A normal immunoglobulin (p.1627·2).
*Passive immunisation.*

**Beriglobina Anti D-P** Centeon, Spain†.
An anti-D immunoglobulin (p.1608·1).
*Prevention of rhesus sensitisation.*

**Beriglobina P**
Aventis Pasteur, Chile; Centeon, Mex.†; Aventis Behring, Spain.
A normal immunoglobulin (p.1627·2).
*Hypogammaglobulinaemia; passive immunisation.*

**Berigripina** Elea, Arg.
An influenza vaccine (p.1620·2).
*Active immunisation.*

**Berinert**
Aventis, Austria; Aventis Behring, Ger.
Complement C1 esterase inhibitor (p.1675·2).
*Hereditary angioedema.*

**Berinert HS** Aventis Behring, Switz.
Complement C1 esterase inhibitor (p.1675·2).
*Hereditary angioedema.*

**Berinert P** Centeon, UK†.
Complement C1 esterase inhibitor (p.1675·2).
*Hereditary angioedema.*

**Berinin**
Aventis Behring, Braz.; Aventis Behring, Ger.
A factor IX preparation (p.752·2).
*Factor IX deficiency; haemophilia B.*

**Berinin HS** Aventis Behring, Switz.
A factor IX preparation (p.752·2).
*Haemophilia B.*

**Berinin P** Centeon, Mex.†.
A factor IX preparation (p.752·2).
*Factor IX deficiency; haemophilia B.*

**Beriplast**
Aventis, Austria; Centeon, Fin.†; Aventis Behring, Fr.; Aventis Behring, Ger.
1 ampoule, fibrinogen (p.753·2); factor XIII (p.753·1); 1 ampoule, aprotinin (p.742·3); 1 ampoule, thrombin (p.760·1); 1 ampoule, calcium chloride (p.1225·1).
On mixing this forms a fibrin glue (p.753·1).
*Surgical bleeding; wounds.*

**Beriplast P**
Aventis Behring, Braz.; Aventis Pasteur, Chile; Aventis Behring, Hong Kong; Centeon, Israel; Centeon, Mex.†; Aventis Behring, Switz.
1 Ampoule: fibrinogen (p.753·2); factor XIII (p.753·1); 1 ampoule: aprotinin (p.742·3); 1 ampoule: thrombin (p.760·1); 1 ampoule: calcium chloride (p.1225·1).
On mixing this forms a fibrin glue (p.753·1).
*Haemorrhage; wounds.*

**Beriplex** Aventis, Austria.
A factor IX preparation (p.752·2).
*Factor II, VII, IX, and X deficiency; haemorrhagic disorders.*

**Beriplex PN**
Aventis Behring, Braz.; Aventis Behring, Ger.; Centeon, UK†.
A factor IX preparation (p.752·2).
*Anticoagulant overdose; haemorrhagic disorders.*

**Berirab**
Aventis, Austria; Aventis Behring, Ger.; Aventis Behring, Israel.
A rabies immunoglobulin (p.1635·3).
*Passive immunisation.*

**Berirab-P** Zydus, India.
A rabies immunoglobulin (p.1635·3).
*Passive immunisation.*

**Berivine** Meuse, Belg.
Riboflavin (p.1456·1).
*Dietary supplement; nocturnal cramps; vitamin $B_2$ deficiency.*

**Berkamil** Berk, UK†.
Amiloride (p.858·3).
*Heart failure; hepatic cirrhosis with ascites; hypertension.*

**Berkolol** Rhone-Poulenc Rorer, Hong Kong†.
Propranolol hydrochloride (p.989·3).
*Angina pectoris; hypertension.*

**Berlactone** Berlin Pharm, Thai.
Spironolactone (p.1003·1).
*Hypertension; oedema and ascites of heart failure; primary aldosteronism.*

**Berlex** Duncan, Arg.
Alendronate sodium (p.765·3).
*Osteoporosis.*

**Berlicetin**
Chauvin ankerpharm, Ger.
*Eye drops:* Azidamfenicol (p.159·1).
*Bacterial eye infections.*

Wernigerode, Ger.
*Ear drops:* Chloramphenicol (p.185·1); prednisolone (p.1108·1).
*Bacterial ear infections with inflammation.*

**Berlicort** Berlin-Chemie, Ger.
Triamcinolone (p.1110·2) or triamcinolone acetonide (p.1110·2).
*Corticosteroid.*

**Berlinsulin H 20/80, 30/70** Berlin-Chemie, Ger.
Mixtures of insulin injection (human, prb) and isophane insulin injection (human, prb) respectively in the proportions indicated (p.333·3).
*Diabetes mellitus.*

**Berlinsulin H Basal** Berlin-Chemie, Ger.
Isophane insulin injection (human, prb) (p.333·3).
*Diabetes mellitus.*

**Berlinsulin H Normal** Berlin-Chemie, Ger.
Insulin injection (human, prb) (p.333·3).
*Diabetes mellitus.*

**Berlison** Schering, Braz.
Hydrocortisone acetate (p.1103·3).
*Skin disorders.*

**Berlithion** Berlin-Chemie, Ger.†.
Thioctic acid (p.1754·3) or ethylenediamine thioctate (p.1754·3).
*Diabetic polyneuropathy.*

**Berlocid** Berlin-Chemie, Ger.
Co-trimoxazole (p.199·3).
*Bacterial infections; Pneumocystis carinii pneumonia.*

**Berlocombin** Berlin-Chemie, Ger.
Trimethoprim (p.272·2); sulfamerazine (p.260·3).
*Bacterial infections.*

**Berlofen** Elea, Arg.
Aceclofenac (p.11·2).
*Musculoskeletal, joint, and peri-articular disorders; pain.*

**Berlosin** Berlin-Chemie, Ger.
Dipyrone (p.35·3).
*Fever; pain.*

**Berlthyrox** Berlin-Chemie, Ger.
Levothyroxine sodium (p.1600·1).
*Hypothyroidism.*

**Bermacia** CIF, Braz.
Theophylline (p.798·3).
*Obstructive airways disease.*

**Bernadine** Shiwa, Thai.
Povidone-iodine (p.1190·3).
*Disinfection of skin, wounds, burns, and mucous membranes; mouth and throat inflammation.*

**Berniter** Galderma, Ger.
Coal tar (p.1159·2).
*Scalp disorders.*

**Berocca**
Roche Consumer, Austral.; Roche Nicholas, Fr.; Roche, Hong Kong; Roche, Mex.†; Roche Consumer, Singapore; Roche, Swed.; Roche, Thai.; Roche Consumer, UK.
Vitamin B substances; vitamin C; calcium; magnesium (p.1417·1).

Roche, Ital.
Vitamin B substances with vitamin C (p.1417·1).
*Vitamin B and C deficiency.*

Roche, NZ.
Vitamin B substances with vitamin C, and calcium (p.1417·1).
*Nutritional supplement.*

Roche, USA.
Vitamin B substances with vitamin C and folic acid (p.1417·1).

**Berocca Calcio e Magnesio** *Roche, Port.*
Vitamin B substances; vitamin C; calcium; magnesium (p.1417·1).
*Alcoholism; vitamin deficiency.*

**Berocca Calcio y Magnesio** *Roche, Arg.*
Vitamin B substances; vitamin C; calcium; magnesium (p.1417·1).

**Berocca Calcium**
*Roche, Austria†; Roche, S.Afr.†.*
Vitamin B substances with vitamin C and calcium (p.1417·1).

**Berocca Calcium and Magnesium** *Roche, Israel.*
Vitamin B substances with vitamin C, calcium, and magnesium (p.1417·1).
*Nutritional supplement.*

**Berocca calcium, magnesium + zinc** *Roche, Switz.*
Vitamin B substances; vitamin C; calcium; magnesium; zinc (p.1417·1).
*Alcoholism; vitamin deficiency.*

**Berocca Calmag** *Roche, S.Afr.†.*
Vitamin B substances; vitamin C; calcium; magnesium (p.1417·1).

**Berocca Plus**
*Note. This name is used for preparations of different composition.*
*Roche, Arg.; Roche, Austria; Roche, Chile; Roche, Fin.*
Vitamin B substances; vitamin C; minerals (p.1417·1).

*Roche, USA.*
Ferrous fumarate (p.1427·3); folic acid (p.1429·1); multivitamins and minerals (p.1417·1).
*Iron-deficiency anaemias.*

**Beroccal** *Roche, Braz.*
Vitamin B substances; vitamin C; calcium; magnesium (p.1417·1).

**Berodual**
*Boehringer Ingelheim, Arg.; Boehringer Ingelheim, Austria; Boehringer Ingelheim, Chile; Boehringer Ingelheim, Denm.; Boehringer Ingelheim, Ger.; Boehringer Ingelheim, Gr.; Boehringer Ingelheim, Hong Kong; Boehringer Ingelheim, Malaysia; Boehringer Ingelheim, Mex.; Boehringer Ingelheim, Neth.; Boehringer Ingelheim, Port.; Boehringer Ingelheim, Singapore; Boehringer Ingelheim, Spain; Boehringer Ingelheim, Switz.; Boehringer Ingelheim, Thai.*
Fenoterol hydrobromide (p.785·2); ipratropium bromide (p.787·1).
*Obstructive airways disease.*

**Berodualin** *Boehringer Ingelheim, Austria.*
Fenoterol hydrobromide (p.785·2); ipratropium bromide (p.787·1).
*Obstructive airways disease.*

**Berofin** *Sanofi Synthelabo, Arg.*
Biperiden hydrochloride (p.479·3).
*Drug-induced extrapyramidal disorders; parkinsonism.*

**Berofor** *Boehringer Ingelheim, Austria†.*
Interferon alfa-2c (p.640·3).
*Anogenital warts; chronic active hepatitis; herpes infections; malignant neoplasms.*

**Beromin** *Condrugs, Thai.*
Vitamin B$_1$ (p.1455·2); vitamin B$_6$ (p.1457·2); vitamin B$_{12}$ (p.1458·2).
*Neuritis; vitamin B deficiency.*

**Beromun**
*Boehringer Ingelheim, Belg.; Boehringer Ingelheim, Gr.; Boehringer Ingelheim, Ital.; Boehringer Ingelheim, Neth.†; Boehringer Ingelheim, Spain; Boehringer Ingelheim, Swed.*
Tasonermin (p.590·2).
*Soft-tissue sarcoma.*

**Berotec**
*Boehringer Ingelheim, Arg.; Boehringer Ingelheim, Austral.; Boehringer Ingelheim, Austria; Boehringer Ingelheim, Belg.; Boehringer de Angeli, Braz.; Boehringer Ingelheim, Canad.; Boehringer Ingelheim, Chile; Boehringer Ingelheim, Denm.; Boehringer Ingelheim, Fin.; Boehringer Ingelheim, Fr.†; Boehringer Ingelheim, Ger.; Boehringer Ingelheim, Hong Kong; Boehringer Ingelheim, Irl.†; Boehringer Ingelheim, Malaysia; Boehringer Ingelheim, Mex.; Boehringer Ingelheim, Neth.; Boehringer Ingelheim, Norw.; Boehringer Ingelheim, NZ†; Boehringer Ingelheim, Port.; Boehringer Ingelheim, S.Afr.; Boehringer Ingelheim, Singapore; Boehringer Ingelheim, Spain; Boehringer Ingelheim, Swed.; Boehringer Ingelheim, Switz.; Boehringer Ingelheim, Thai.; Boehringer Ingelheim, UK†.*
Fenoterol (p.785·2) or fenoterol hydrobromide (p.785·2).
*Obstructive airways disease; premature labour; uterine hypertonia.*

**Berotec solvens** *Boehringer Ingelheim, Ger.†.*
Fenoterol hydrobromide (p.785·2); bromhexine hydrochloride (p.1115·3).
*Bronchiectasis; bronchitis; emphysema; interstitial lung disease.*

**Berovent** *Boehringer Ingelheim, Gr.*
Salbutamol sulfate (p.791·3); ipratropium bromide (p.787·1).
*Asthma; chronic obstructive pulmonary disease.*

**Berplex** *Schein, USA†.*
Ferrous fumarate (p.1427·3); folic acid (p.1429·1); multivitamins and minerals (p.1417·1).
*Iron-deficiency anaemias.*

**Bersen** *Pasteur, Chile.*
Prednisone (p.1109·3).
*Corticosteroid.*

**Bertocil** *Edol, Port.*
Betaxolol hydrochloride (p.873·1).
*Glaucoma; ocular hypertension.*

**Berubi** *Redel, Ger.†.*
Echinacea (p.1683·2).
Formerly contained cyanocobalamin.
*Cold and influenza symptoms.*

**Besaprin** *Sanofi Winthrop, Braz.†.*
Chlormezanone (p.675·1); aspirin (p.15·1).
*Muscle spasm.*

**Besedan** *Wyeth, Braz.*
Butamirate citrate (p.1116·2).
*Coughs.*

**Besemax** *Covan, S.Afr.*
Orphenadrine citrate (p.486·1); paracetamol (p.76·2).
*Musculoskeletal spasm; pain.*

**Besenol**
*Note. This name is used for preparations of different composition.*
*Adcock Ingram, S.Afr.*
Paracetamol (p.76·2); orphenadrine citrate (p.486·1).
*Musculoskeletal spasm; pain.*

*Covan, S.Afr.†.*
Paracetamol (p.76·2); chlormezanone (p.675·1).
*Fever; pain; skeletal muscle spasm.*

**Beserol** *Sanofi Synthelabo, Braz.*
Diclofenac sodium (p.32·1); carisoprodol (p.1392·1); paracetamol (p.76·2); caffeine (p.782·1).
Formerly contained chlormezanone and dipyrone.
*Muscle spasm; pain.*

**Beserol-S** *Sanofi Synthelabo, Chile.*
Paracetamol (p.76·2); chlorzoxazone (p.1392·3).
*Musculoskeletal spasm; pain.*

**Besidin** *Coup, Gr.*
Cimetidine (p.1255·3).
*Conditions where gastric acid reduction is beneficial; gastric hypersecretion including Zollinger-Ellison syndrome; peptic ulcer.*

**Besitran** *Pfizer, Spain.*
Sertraline hydrochloride (p.317·2).
*Depression; obsessive-compulsive disorder; panic disorder.*

**Besix** *Cooper (Κοπερ), Gr.*
Pyridoxine hydrochloride (p.1456·3).
*Hyperoxaluria; sideroplastic anaemia; vitamin B6 deficiency.*

**Besone**
*Atlantic, Malaysia; Atlantic, Singapore; Atlantic, Thai.*
Betamethasone valerate (p.1093·2).
*Skin disorders.*

**Besone-N**
*Atlantic, Malaysia; Atlantic, Singapore; Atlantic, Thai.*
Betamethasone valerate (p.1093·2); neomycin sulfate (p.235·1).
*Infected skin disorders.*

**Besopartin** *Boehringer Ingelheim, Austria.*
Alteplase (p.857·1).
*Myocardial infarction; peripheral arterial thromboembolism; pulmonary embolism.*

**Bespar**
*Bristol-Myers Squibb, Ger.; Hormosan, Ger.; Mead Johnson, Gr.*
Buspirone hydrochloride (p.672·2).
*Anxiety.*

**Bessasone** *Pharmaland, Thai.*
Betamethasone valerate (p.1093·2).
*Skin disorders.*

**Best EPA** *Contassium Co., UK†.*
Fish oil (eicosapentaenoic acid, and docosahexaenoic acid) (p.976·2).

**Bestafen** *Best, Mex.*
Ibuprofen (p.45·3).
*Inflammation; musculoskeletal, joint, peri-articular, and soft-tissue disorders; pain.*

**Bestatin** *Berlin Pharm, Thai.*
Simvastatin (p.997·1).
*Hypercholesterolaemia.*

**Bestcall** *Takeda, Jpn.*
Cefmenoxime hydrochloride (p.173·2).
Mepivacaine hydrochloride (p.1381·2) is included in the intramuscular injection to alleviate the pain of injection.
*Bacterial infections.*

**Bestelar** *Best, Mex.*
Mebendazole (p.108·2).
*Worm infections.*

**Bester Complex** *Salvat, Spain.*
Thiamine hydrochloride (p.1455·1); hydroxocobalamin acetate (p.1458·2); pyridoxine hydrochloride (p.1456·3).
*Vitamin B deficiency.*

**Bestocin** *Best, Mex.*
Erythromycin estolate (p.208·1).
*Bacterial infections.*

**Bestozyme** *Biological E, India.*
*Capsules:* Amylase (p.1654·2); papain (p.1727·3) simeticone (p.1289·2).
*Paediatric Syrup:* Amylase (p.1654·2); papain (p.1727·3); anise oil (p.1655·2); caraway oil (p.1667·3); cinnamon oil (p.1672·2); dill oil (p.1680·2).
*Syrup:* Amylase (p.1654·2); papain (p.1727·3).
*Dyspepsia.*

**Bestrol** *Cetus, Arg.*
Alprazolam (p.668·3).
*Anxiety; depression.*

**Bestron** *Senju, Jpn.*
Cefmenoxime hydrochloride (p.173·2).
*Bacterial eye infections.*

**Be-Supra** *Irex, Port.*
Vitamin B substances and vitamin C (p.1417·1).

**Beta**
*Note. This name is used for preparations of different composition.*
*Stadmed, India.*
Atenolol (p.865·2).
*Angina pectoris; arrhythmias; hypertension.*

*Upha, Malaysia.*
Betamethasone sodium phosphate (p.1093·1).
*Inflammatory eye and ear disorders.*

*Pacific, NZ; Chew, Thai.*
Betamethasone valerate (p.1093·2).
*Skin disorders.*

**Beta 21** *IDI, Ital.*
Betamethasone valero-acetate (p.1093·2).
*Skin disorders.*

**Beta A-C** *Eagle, Austral.†.*
*Oral powder:* Ascorbic acid (p.1460·2); sodium ascorbate (p.1460·2); calcium ascorbate (p.1460·2); *dl*-alpha-tocoferil acetate (p.1465·1); rutoside (p.1688·2); zinc amino acid chelate (p.1469·3); betacarotene (p.1422·3).
*Tablets:* Ascorbic acid (p.1460·2); sodium ascorbate (p.1460·2); calcium ascorbate (p.1460·2); *dl*-alpha-tocoferil acetate (p.1465·1); rutoside (p.1688·2); zinc amino acid chelate (p.1469·3); betacarotene (p.1422·3); bioflavonoids (p.1688·2).
*Vitamin supplement.*

**Beta Adenil** *Adesil, Arg.*
Betamethasone dipropionate (p.1093·1).
*Skin disorders.*

**Beta Alcanforado** *Betamadrileno, Spain.*
Camphor (p.1665·3); alcohol (p.1166·1).
*Musculoskeletal, joint, and soft-tissue pain.*

**Beta C E with Selenium** *Stanley, Canad.*
Betacarotene, selenium, vitamin C, and vitamin E (p.1417·1).

**Beta Long** *Uniao Quimica, Braz.†.*
Betamethasone acetate (p.1093·1); betamethasone sodium phosphate (p.1093·1).
*Skin disorders.*

**Beta Micoter** *Farmacusi, Spain.*
Betamethasone dipropionate (p.1093·1); clotrimazole (p.396·2).
*Fungal skin infections.*

**Beta Nicardia** *Unique, India.*
Atenolol (p.865·2); nifedipine (p.966·2).
*Angina pectoris; hypertension.*

**Beta Ophtiole** *Kite (Κιτε), Gr.*
Metipranolol hydrochloride (p.956·1); benzalkonium chloride (p.1168·3).
*Glaucoma.*

**Beta plus Vitamins C, E & Selenium** *Quest, Canad.*
Betacarotene, selenium, vitamin C, and vitamin E (p.1417·1).

**Beta Prostate** *Young Again Products, USA.*
Sitosterol (p.982·3); zinc citrate; selenium chelate (p.1444·1).
Formerly contained sitosterol and zinc citrate.
*Dietary supplement.*

**Beta Romero** *Betamadrileno, Spain.*
Alcohol (p.1166·1); rosemary oil (p.1740·2).
*Musculoskeletal pain and fatigue.*

**Beta-Ace Tablets** *Vitaglow, Austral.†.*
Betacarotene (p.1422·3); ascorbic acid (p.1460·2); *d*-alpha tocoferil acid succinate (p.1465·1); zinc amino acid chelate (p.1469·3).
*Dietary supplement.*

**Beta-Adalat**
*Bayer, Austria; Bayer, Belg.; Bayer, Fin.†; Bayer, Irl.; Bayer, Switz.; Bayer, UK.*
Atenolol (p.865·2); nifedipine (p.966·2).
*Angina pectoris; hypertension.*

**Beta-Adalate** *Bayer, Fr.*
Atenolol (p.865·2); nifedipine (p.966·2).
*Hypertension.*

**Betabactyl** *SmithKline Beecham, Ger.†.*
Ticarcillin sodium (p.270·2); potassium clavulanate (p.193·3).
*Bacterial infections.*

**Betabion**
*Merck, Ger.; Bracco, Ital.†; Merck, Swed.*
Thiamine hydrochloride (p.1455·1).
*Vitamin B$_1$ deficiency.*

**Betabioptal** *Farmila, Ital.*
Betamethasone (p.1093·1) or betamethasone sodium phosphate (p.1093·1); chloramphenicol (p.185·1).
*Infected eye disorders.*

**Betabiotic** *Esseti, Ital.*
Flucloxacillin sodium (p.213·3).
Lidocaine hydrochloride (p.1377·3) is included in the intramuscular injection to alleviate the pain of injection.
*Bacterial infections.*

**Betabloc** *USV, India.*
Propranolol hydrochloride (p.989·3).
*Angina pectoris; arrhythmias; hypertension.*

**Be-Tabs Antacid** *Be-Tabs, S.Afr.*
Magnesium trisilicate (p.1272·3); light magnesium carbonate (p.1272·1); sodium bicarbonate (p.1223·2).
*Gastrointestinal disorders associated with hyperacidity.*

**Beta-C** *Chew, Thai.*
Betamethasone valerate (p.1093·2); clioquinol (p.196·3).
*Infected skin disorders.*

**Betacap**
*Dermal Laboratories, Irl.; Dermal Laboratories, UK.*
Betamethasone valerate (p.1093·2).
*Scalp disorders.*

**Betacar** *Sanofi Synthelabo, Chile.*
Atenolol (p.865·2).
*Hypertension.*

**Beta-Cardone** *Celltech, UK.*
Sotalol hydrochloride (p.1001·3).
*Arrhythmias.*

**Betacarpin** *Riel, Austria.*
Pilocarpine hydrochloride (p.1495·1); metipranolol hydrochloride (p.956·1).
*Glaucoma.*

**Betacef**
*Note. This name is used for preparations of different composition.*
*Biochimico, Braz.; Be-Tabs, S.Afr.†.*
Cefalexin (p.168·1).
*Bacterial infections.*

*FIRMA, Ital.†.*
Cefoxitin sodium (p.177·2).
*Bacterial infections.*

**Betacept** *Wampole, Canad.*
Vitamin C, vitamin E, and betacarotene (p.1417·1).

**Betachek** *National Diagnostic, Austral.*
Test for glucose in blood (p.1694·2).

**Betacin**
*Note. This name is used for preparations of different composition.*
*Upha, Malaysia.*
Betamethasone sodium phosphate (p.1093·1); neomycin sulfate (p.235·1).
*Infected eye and ear disorders.*

*Adcock Ingram, S.Afr.*
Indometacin (p.47·3).
Formerly known as Famethacin.
*Gout; musculoskeletal and joint disorders.*

**Betaclar** *Angelini, Ital.*
Befunolol hydrochloride (p.867·1).
*Glaucoma.*

**Betaclomin** *Be-Tabs, S.Afr.*
Dicycloverine hydrochloride (p.481·2); dried aluminium hydroxide gel (p.1249·2); light magnesium oxide (p.1272·3).
*Gastrointestinal hyperacidity.*

**Betaclopramide** *Be-Tabs, S.Afr.*
Metoclopramide hydrochloride (p.1274·3).
*Gastrointestinal disorders.*

**Betacomplesso** *Medosan, Ital.*
Vitamin B substances (p.1417·1).
*Tonic; vitamin B deficiency.*

**Betacort**
*Cassara, Arg.*
*Cream; lotion:* Betamethasone dipropionate (p.1093·1).
*Skin disorders.*
*Injection:* Betamethasone acetate (p.1093·1); betamethasone sodium phosphate (p.1093·1).
*Corticosteroid.*

*ICN, Canad.†.*
Betamethasone valerate (p.1093·2).
*Scalp disorders.*

**Betacorten**
*Trima, Israel; Trima, Singapore; Unipharm, Singapore.*
Betamethasone valerate (p.1093·2).
*Scalp disorders.*

**Betacorten-G** *Trima, Israel.*
Betamethasone valerate (p.1093·2); gentamicin sulfate (p.217·1).
*Infected skin disorders.*

**Betacortone** *Spirig, Switz.*
*Cream:* Halcinonide (p.1103·2); urea (p.1162·2).
*Topical solution:* Halcinonide (p.1103·2).
*Skin disorders.*

**Betacortone S** *Spirig, Switz.*
Halcinonide (p.1103·2); salicylic acid (p.1157·1).
*Skin disorders.*

**BetaCreme** *Lichtenstein, Ger.*
Betamethasone valerate (p.1093·2).
*Skin disorders.*

**Betaderm**
*Note. This name is used for preparations of different composition.*
*Stiefel, Braz.; Taro, Canad.*
Betamethasone valerate (p.1093·2).
*Scalp disorders; skin disorders.*

*Beta, Ital.*
Salicylic acid (p.1157·1); aluminium acetate (p.1652·3); zinc oxide (p.1163·2).
*Skin disinfection.*

**Betaderma** *Safire, Hong Kong.*
Betamethasone valerate (p.1093·2).
*Skin disorders.*

**Betadermic** *Bioglan, Ger.*
Betamethasone dipropionate (p.1093·1); salicylic acid (p.1157·1).
*Skin disorders.*

**Betades** *Farmades, Ital.†.*
Sotalol hydrochloride (p.1001·3).
*Angina pectoris; arrhythmias; hypertension.*

**Betadine**
*Faulding, Austral.; Purdue, Canad.; Leiras, Fin.; Viatris, Fr.; Lavipharm, Gr.; Mundipharma, Hong Kong; Win-Medicare, India; SSL, Irl.; Rafa, Israel†; Asta Medica, Ital.; Mahakam Beta, Malaysia; Viatris, Neth.; Baxter, NZ; Viatris, Port.; Adcock Ingram, S.Afr.; Restan, S.Afr.; Mun-*

*dipharma, Singapore; Viatris, Spain; Mundipharma, Switz.; Mundipharma, Thai.; SSL, UK; Purdue Frederick, USA.*
Povidone-iodine (p.1190·3).
*Burns; infections of the skin, oropharynx, wounds, and vagina; skin, mucous membrane, and wound disinfection.*

**Betadine First Aid Antibiotics + Moisturizer** *Purdue Frederick, USA†.*
Polymyxin B sulfate (p.245·1); bacitracin zinc (p.161·3).
*Minor cuts and burns.*

**Betadine Plus First Aid Antibiotics & Pain Reliever** *Purdue Frederick, USA.*
Polymyxin B sulfate (p.245·1); bacitracin zinc (p.161·3); pramocaine hydrochloride (p.1382·2).
*Minor cuts and burns.*

**Betadine-AD** *Win-Medicare, India.*
Povidone-iodine (p.1190·3).
*Scalp disorders.*

**Beta-Dipo** *Nakorn, Thai.*
Betamethasone dipropionate (p.1093·1); neomycin sulfate (p.235·1).
*Skin disorders.*

**Betadipresan** *Fides Ecopharma, Spain.*
Hydralazine hydrochloride (p.931·2); propranolol hydrochloride (p.989·3).
*Hypertension.*

**Betadipresan Diu** *Fides Ecopharma, Spain.*
Bendroflumethiazide (p.867·3); hydralazine hydrochloride (p.931·2); propranolol hydrochloride (p.989·3).
*Hypertension.*

**Betadiur** *Siphar, Switz.*
Amiloride hydrochloride (p.858·2); hydrochlorothiazide (p.933·2).
*Hypertension; liver failure with ascites; oedema.*

**Betadona** *Mundipharma, Austria.*
Povidone-iodine (p.1190·3).
*Infected wounds and burns.*

**Betadorm-A** *Woelm, Ger.*
Diphenhydramine hydrochloride (p.431·3); 8-chlorotheophylline.
*Sleep disorders.*

**Betadrenol** *Desma, Ger.*
Bupranolol hydrochloride (p.878·1).
*Hypertension; ischaemic heart disease; myocardial infarction.*

**Betadur CR** *Monmouth, UK†.*
Propranolol hydrochloride (p.989·3).
*Angina pectoris; anxiety; essential tremor; hypertension; migraine; variceal haemorrhage.*

**Betaeffe Complex** *Mavi, Ital.*
Carotenoids; vitamin E; vitamin C; vitis vinifera (p.1417·1).
*Nutritional supplement.*

**Betaeffe Plus** *Mavi, Ital.*
Betacarotene, vitamin E, and selenium preparation (p.1417·1).
*Nutritional supplement.*

**Betafact**
*Lab Francais du Fractionnement, Fr.; Vianex (Βιανεξ), Gr.; Omrix, Israel.*
A factor IX preparation (p.752·2).
*Haemorrhagic disorders.*

**Betafed** *Be-Tabs, S.Afr.*
Triprolidine hydrochloride (p.442·3); pseudoephedrine hydrochloride (p.1129·2).
*Nasal congestion.*

**Betaferon**
*Schering, Arg.; Schering, Austral.; Schering, Austria; Schering, Belg.; Schering, Braz.; Schering, Denm.; Schering, Fin.; Schering, Fr.; Schering, Ger.; Schering-Plough, Gr.; Schering, Irl.; Schering, Israel; Schering, Ital.; Schering, Malaysia; Schering, Mex.; Schering, Neth.; Schering, Norw.; Schering, NZ; Schering, Port.; Schering, S.Afr.; Schering, Singapore; Schering, Spain; Schering, Swed.; Schering, Switz.; Schering, UK.*
Interferon beta-1b (p.645·3).
*Multiple sclerosis.*

**Betaflex** *Mer-National, S.Afr.†.*
Paracetamol (p.76·2); chlormezanone (p.675·1).
*Pain and associated tension.*

**Betafloroto** *INTES, Ital.*
Betamethasone sodium phosphate (p.1093·1); tetracycline hydrochloride (p.266·2).
*Ear infections; rhinitis.*

**Betaform Habitat** *Cos Farma, Ital.†.*
Benzalkonium chloride (p.1168·3); a nonoxinol (p.1413·2).
*Surface and room disinfection.*

**Betagalen** *Pharmagalen, Ger.*
Betamethasone valerate (p.1093·2).
*Skin disorders.*

**Betagan**
*Allergan, Arg.; Allergan, Austral.; Allergan, Belg.; Allergan, Braz.; Allergan, Canad.; Allergan, Denm.; Allergan, Fr.; Allergan, Hong Kong; Allergan, Irl.; Allergan, Israel; Allergan, Malaysia; Allergan, Mex.; Allergan, NZ; Allergan, Port.; Allergan, S.Afr.; Allergan, Singapore; Allergan, Spain; Allergan, Swed.†; Allergan, Thai.; Allergan, UK; Allergan, USA.*
Levobunolol hydrochloride (p.946·2).
*Glaucoma; ocular hypertension.*

**Betagard** *GNLD, Austral.†.*
Vitamin, mineral, and amino-acid preparation (p.1417·1).

**Betagen**
*Note. This name is used for preparations of different composition.*
*Allergan, Chile.*
Levobunolol hydrochloride (p.946·2).
*Glaucoma; ocular hypertension.*

*Upha, Malaysia.*
Betamethasone sodium phosphate (p.1093·1); gentamicin sulfate (p.217·1).
*Infected eye and ear disorders.*

**Betagentam** *Winzer, Ger.*
Betamethasone sodium phosphate (p.1093·1); gentamicin sulfate (p.217·1).
*Infected eye disorders.*

**Betagesic** *Restan, S.Afr.*
Ibuprofen (p.45·3).
*Fever; musculoskeletal and joint disorders; pain.*

**Betagon** *Schering, Ital.†.*
Mepindolol sulfate (p.952·2).
*Angina pectoris; cardiac hyperkinesis; hypertension.*

**Betaimune** *Pharmadass, UK.*
Vitamins A, C, and E; selenium; zinc (p.1417·1).
*Antioxidant preparation.*

**Betaine Digestive Aid** *GNLD, Austral.†.*
Betaine hydrochloride (p.1660·2); pepsin (p.1729·3); papain (p.1727·3); pectin (p.1580·3); natural dried beet; rhubarb (p.1287·3); liquorice (p.1270·2).
*Digestive disorders.*

**Betaisodona**
*Mundipharma, Austria; Mundipharma, Ger.*
Povidone-iodine (p.1190·3).
*Burns; mouth and throat infections; skin and mucous membrane disinfection; skin infections; skin ulcers; vaginal infections; wounds.*

**Beta-Isoket** *Gebro, Austria†.*
Bupranolol hydrochloride (p.878·1); isosorbide dinitrate (p.941·1).
*Angina pectoris; myocardial infarction.*

**Betaject** *Sabex, Canad.*
Betamethasone sodium phosphate (p.1093·1); betamethasone acetate (p.1093·1).
*Corticosteroid.*

**Betalevedim** *Libbs, Braz.†.*
Propranolol (p.990·1).
*Hypertension.*

**Betalgil** *Whitehall, Port.†.*
Aluminium hydroxide (p.1249·2); magnesium hydroxide (p.1272·2); oxetacaine (p.1382·1).
*Gastrointestinal disorders.*

**Betalin** *Be-Tabs, S.Afr.*
Diphenhydramine hydrochloride (p.431·3); ammonium chloride (p.1115·2); sodium citrate (p.1223·2); menthol (p.1711·3).
*Coughs.*

**Betaliver** *Luper, Braz.*
Methionine (p.1042·1); adenosine (p.851·2); betaine hydrochloride (p.1660·2); pyridoxine hydrochloride (p.1456·3); choline citrate (p.1424·3).
*Liver disorders.*

**Betalix** *Be-Tabs, S.Afr.†.*
Chlorphenamine maleate (p.427·3); phenylpropanolamine hydrochloride (p.1127·3); phenylephrine hydrochloride (p.1126·3).
*Nasal congestion.*

**Betaloc**
*AstraZeneca, Austral.; AstraZeneca, Canad.; AstraZeneca, Hong Kong; AstraZeneca, India; AstraZeneca, Irl.; AstraZeneca, Malaysia; AstraZeneca, NZ; AstraZeneca, Singapore; AstraZeneca, Thai.; AstraZeneca, UK.*
Metoprolol succinate (p.957·1) or metoprolol tartrate (p.957·1).
*Angina pectoris; arrhythmias; heart failure; hypertension; hyperthyroidism; migraine; myocardial infarction.*

**Betaloc Comp** *AstraZeneca, Hong Kong.*
Metoprolol tartrate (p.957·1); hydrochlorothiazide (p.933·2).
*Hypertension.*

**Betalol** *Berlin Pharm, Thai.*
Propranolol hydrochloride (p.989·3).
*Angina pectoris; anxiety disorders; arrhythmias; hypertension; tremor.*

**Betama-EN** *Samakeephaesaj, Thai.*
Betamethasone valerate (p.1093·2); neomycin sulfate (p.235·1).
*Infected skin disorders.*

**Betamann** *Mann, Ger.*
Metipranolol hydrochloride (p.956·1).
*Glaucoma; ocular hypertension.*

**Betamatil** *Inibsa, Spain†.*
Betamethasone valerate (p.1093·2).
*Skin disorders.*

**Betamatil con Neomicina** *Inibsa, Spain†.*
Betamethasone valerate (p.1093·2); neomycin sulfate (p.235·1).
*Infected skin disorders.*

**Betamaze** *Pfizer, Fr.†.*
Sulbactam sodium (p.257·2).
*Bacterial infections.*

**Betamed** *Kwizda, Austria.*
Bupranolol hydrochloride (p.878·1); diazepam (p.690·1).
*Anxiety disorders.*

**Betamesol** *Proge, Ital.*
Betamethasone dipropionate (p.1093·1).
*Skin disorders.*

**Betametagen** *Kinder, Braz.*
Betamethasone valerate (p.1093·2).
*Skin disorders.*

**Betameth** *Osoth, Thai.*
Betamethasone valerate (p.1093·2).
*Skin disorders.*

**Betamethason Plus** *Heumann, Ger.*
Betamethasone dipropionate (p.1093·1); salicylic acid (p.1157·1).
*Skin disorders.*

**Betameth-N** *Osoth, Thai.*
Betamethasone valerate (p.1093·2); neomycin sulfate (p.235·1).
*Infected skin disorders.*

**Betamican** *Alter, Spain.*
Salmeterol xinafoate (p.795·1).
*Obstructive airways disease.*

**Betamida** *Alcon Cusi, Spain.*
Betamethasone sodium phosphate (p.1093·1); sulfacetamide sodium (p.257·3).
*Eye disorders.*

**Betamil-M** *Merck, India.*
Betamethasone dipropionate (p.1093·1); miconazole nitrate (p.405·3).
*Infected skin disorders.*

**Betamin**
*Aventis, Austral.; Instituto Sanitas, Chile.*
Thiamine hydrochloride (p.1455·1).
*Neuralgia; neuritis; vitamin $B_1$ deficiency.*

**Betamine** *Wolfs, Belg.*
Thiamine hydrochloride (p.1455·1).
*Alcoholic polyneuropathy; beri-beri; neuralgia.*

**Betam-Ophtal** *Winzer, Ger.*
Betamethasone sodium phosphate (p.1093·1).
*Eye disorders.*

**Betamox**
*Note. This name is used for preparations of different composition.*
*Duopharma, Hong Kong; Be-Tabs, S.Afr.*
Amoxicillin trihydrate (p.155·3).
*Bacterial infections.*

*Cipan, Port.*
Amoxicillin trihydrate (p.155·3); potassium clavulanate (p.193·3).
*Bacterial infections.*

**Betamycin** *Be-Tabs, S.Afr.*
Erythromycin estolate (p.208·1).
*Bacterial infections.*

**Beta-N** *Chew, Thai.*
Betamethasone valerate (p.1093·2); neomycin sulfate (p.235·1).
*Infected skin disorders.*

**Betanoid** *Aspen, S.Afr.*
Betamethasone (p.1093·1).
*Corticosteroid.*

**Betanoid N** *Aspen, S.Afr.*
Betamethasone valerate (p.1093·2); neomycin sulfate (p.235·1).
*Infected skin disorders.*

**Betanol** *Europhta, Mon.*
Metipranolol (p.955·3).
*Glaucoma; ocular hypertension.*

**Beta-Ophtiole**
*Riel, Austria; Tramedico, Belg.; Mann, Malaysia; Tramedico, Neth.; Lepori, Port.; Bausch & Lomb, S.Afr.; Mann, Singapore; Bausch & Lomb, Thai.; Mann, Thai.*
Metipranolol hydrochloride (p.956·1).
*Glaucoma; ocular hypertension.*

**Betapace** *Berlex, USA.*
Sotalol hydrochloride (p.1001·3).
*Arrhythmias.*

**Betapam** *Be-Tabs, S.Afr.*
Diazepam (p.690·1).
*Alcohol withdrawal syndrome; anxiety; premedication.*

**Betapect** *Be-Tabs, S.Afr.*
Light kaolin (p.1268·3); apple pectin (p.1580·3).
Formerly known as Pectikon.
*Diarrhoea.*

**Betapen** *Be-Tabs, S.Afr.*
Phenoxymethylpenicillin potassium (p.242·1).
*Bacterial infections.*

**Betaperamide** *Restan, S.Afr.*
Loperamide hydrochloride (p.1271·1).
*Diarrhoea.*

**Betaphlem** *Be-Tabs, S.Afr.*
Carbocisteine (p.1116·2).
*Respiratory-tract disorders with increased mucous.*

**Betapindol** *Helvepharm, Switz.†.*
Pindolol (p.983·2).
Now known as Pindolol Helvepharm.
*Angina pectoris; arrhythmias; hypertension.*

**Betaplex** *Drugtech, Chile.*
Carvedilol (p.881·1).
*Hypertension.*

**Betapred**
*Orphan, Fin.; Swedish Orphan, Swed.*
Betamethasone sodium phosphate (p.1093·1).
*Corticosteroid.*

**Betapresin** *Hoechst Marion Roussel, Mex.†.*
Penbutolol sulfate (p.979·1).

**Betapress** *Polipharm, Thai.*
Propranolol hydrochloride (p.989·3).
*Angina pectoris; arrhythmias; hypertension; tremor.*

**Betapressin** *Wolff, Ger.*
Penbutolol sulfate (p.979·1).
*Arrhythmias; hypertension; ischaemic heart disease; myocardial infarction.*

**Betapressine** *Roussel Diamant, Fr.†.*
Penbutolol sulfate (p.979·1).
*Angina pectoris; hypertension.*

**Betaprofen** *Be-Tabs, S.Afr.*
Ibuprofen (p.45·3).
*Musculoskeletal and joint disorders.*

**Beta-Prograne** *Tillomed, UK.*
Propranolol hydrochloride (p.989·3).
*Angina pectoris; anxiety; essential tremor; hypertension; hyperthyroidism; migraine; prophylaxis of upper gastrointestinal bleeding.*

**Betaprol** *Helvepharm, Switz.†.*
Propranolol hydrochloride (p.989·3).
Now known as Propranolol Helvepharm.
*Angina pectoris; arrhythmias; hypertension; migraine; phaeochromocytoma.*

**Betaprospan** *Uniao Quimica, Braz.*
Betamethasone dipropionate (p.1093·1); betamethasone sodium phosphate (p.1093·1).
*Corticosteroid.*

**Betapyn** *Restan, S.Afr.*
Paracetamol (p.76·2); codeine phosphate (p.27·1); doxylamine succinate (p.432·3); caffeine (p.782·1).
*Fever; muscular tension; pain.*

**Betapyr** *Wolfs, Belg.*
Thiamine hydrochloride (p.1455·1); pyridoxine hydrochloride (p.1456·3).
*Alcoholic polyneuritis; prophylaxis during isoniazid therapy; vitamin $B_1$ and/or $B_6$ deficiency.*

**Betarelix** *Wolff, Ger.*
Penbutolol sulfate (p.979·1); piretanide (p.983·3).
*Hypertension.*

**Betaren** *Dexxon, Israel.*
Diclofenac sodium (p.32·1).
*Inflammation; musculoskeletal and joint disorders; pain.*

**Betaretic** *Be-Tabs, S.Afr.*
Amiloride hydrochloride (p.858·2); hydrochlorothiazide (p.933·2).
*Hypertension; oedema.*

**Betartrinovo** *Llorens, Spain†.*
Betamethasone phosphate (p.1093·2); indometacin (p.47·3).
*Musculoskeletal and joint disorders; peri-articular disorders.*

**Beta-S** *Chew, Thai.*
Betamethasone valerate (p.1093·2); salicylic acid (p.1157·1).
*Skin disorders.*

**BetaSalbe** *Lichtenstein, Ger.*
Betamethasone valerate (p.1093·2).
*Skin disorders.*

**Betasan** *Mundipharma, Austria.*
Povidone-iodine (p.1190·3).
*Infected burns and wounds.*

**Betascor B12** *Manetti Roberts, Ital.†.*
Betaine ascorbate (p.1660·2); cyanocobalamin (p.1458·2).
*Vitamin C deficiency.*

**Betasedar** *Sedar, Braz.†.*
Vitamin B substances (p.1417·1).
*Vitamin supplement.*

**Betasel** *Alcon, Arg.*
Betaxolol hydrochloride (p.873·1).

**Betaselen** *Arkopharma, Fr.*
Multivitamin and mineral preparation (p.1417·1).
*Tonic.*

**Betasemid** *Wolff, Ger.*
Penbutolol sulfate (p.979·1); furosemide (p.919·3).
*Hypertension.*

**Betasept** *Purdue Frederick, USA.*
Chlorhexidine gluconate (p.1173·2).
*Skin and wound disinfection.*

**Betaseptic**
*Note. This name is used for preparations of different composition.*
*Mundipharma, Austria; Asta Medica, Ital.*
Povidone-iodine (p.1190·3).
*Medicated dressing; skin disinfection.*

*Mundipharma, Ger.; Mundipharma, Switz.*
Povidone-iodine (p.1190·3); isopropyl alcohol (p.1184·3); alcohol (p.1166·1).
*Skin and hand disinfection.*

**Betaserc**
*Solvay, Austria; Solvay, Belg.; Sintofarma, Braz.; Solvay, Denm.; Solvay, Fin.; Solvay, Fr.; Solvay, Gr.; Solvay, Hong Kong; Solvay, Malaysia; Solvay, Neth.; Solvay, Port.; Solvay, Singapore; Solvay, Switz.*
Betahistine hydrochloride (p.1660·1).
*Ménière's disease; vestibular disorders.*

**Betaseron**
*Berlex, Canad.; Berlex, USA.*
Interferon beta-1b (p.645·3).
*Multiple sclerosis.*

**Betasit Plus** *Ferrer, Spain†.*
Chlortalidone (p.882·3); atenolol (p.865·2).
*Hypertension.*

**Betasleep** *Restan, S.Afr.*
Diphenhydramine hydrochloride (p.431·3).
*Insomnia.*

**Betasoda** *Restan, S.Afr.*
Citric acid (p.1673·1); sodium bicarbonate (p.1223·2).
*Urinary alkalinisation.*

**Beta-Sol**
*Note. A similar name is used for preparations of different composition (see below).*
*Fawns & McAllan, Austral.*
Thiamine hydrochloride (p.1455·1).
*Vitamin $B_1$ deficiency.*

**Betasol**
*Note. A similar name is used for preparations of different composition*

(see above).
Upha, Malaysia; Chew, Thai.
Clobetasol propionate (p.1095·2).
*Skin disorders.*

**Betasone**
DHA, Hong Kong; Vida, Hong Kong; DHA, Malaysia; DHA, Singapore; Julphar, UAE.
Betamethasone valerate (p.1093·2).
*Skin disorders.*

Julphar, UAE.
*Tablets:* Betamethasone (p.1093·1).
*Corticosteroid.*

**Betasone-G** Klonal, Arg.
Betamethasone (p.1093·1).
*Corticosteroid.*

**Betasone-G 12 Horas** Klonal, Arg.
Betamethasone acetate (p.1093·1); betamethasone sodium phosphate (p.1093·1).
*Corticosteroid.*

**Betaspan**
Note. This name is used for preparations of different composition.
Delta, Braz.
Betamethasone dipropionate (p.1093·1); betamethasone sodium phosphate (p.1093·1).
*Corticosteroid.*

GlaxoSmithKline, India.
Propranolol hydrochloride (p.989·3).
*Angina pectoris; anxiety; hypertension; hyperthyroidism; migraine; tremor.*

**Beta-Stulln** Stulln, Ger.
Betamethasone sodium phosphate (p.1093·1).
*Inflammatory eye disorders.*

**Betasyn** Jacoby, Austria.
Atenolol (p.865·2).
*Angina pectoris; arrhythmias; hypertension; myocardial infarction.*

**Betatab** Raza, Malaysia; Pharmaniaga, Malaysia.
Metoprolol tartrate (p.957·1).
*Angina pectoris; hypertension; hyperthyroidism.*

**Beta-Tablinen** Lichtenstein, Ger.
Propranolol hydrochloride (p.989·3).
*Angina pectoris; anxiety; arrhythmias; essential tremor; hypertension; hyperthyroidism; migraine.*

**Betatene** Swiss Herbal, Canad.
Betacarotene (p.1422·3).

**Betathiazid** Henning, Ger.†.
Propranolol hydrochloride (p.989·3); triamterene (p.1016·2); hydrochlorothiazide (p.933·2).
*Hypertension.*

**Betathiazid A** Henning, Ger.†.
Propranolol hydrochloride (p.989·3); hydrochlorothiazide (p.933·2).
*Hypertension.*

**Beta-Tim** Ciba Vision, Canad.†.
Timolol maleate (p.1012·2).
*Glaucoma.*

**Betaton** Hovid, Malaysia.
Multivitamin and mineral preparation with lecithin (p.1417·1).

**Betaton with Ginseng** Hovid, Malaysia.
Multivitamin and mineral preparation with rutoside, lecithin, and ginseng (p.1417·1).

**Betatop** IPRAD, Fr.
Atenolol (p.865·2).
*Angina pectoris; arrhythmias; hypertension; myocardial infarction.*

**Betatrex** Savage, USA†.
Betamethasone valerate (p.1093·2).
*Skin disorders.*

**Betatul** Viatris, Spain.
Povidone-iodine (p.1190·3).
*Infected skin disorders; skin disinfection.*

**Beta-Turfa** Worwag, Ger.
Propranolol hydrochloride (p.989·3); triamterene (p.1016·2); hydrochlorothiazide (p.933·2).
*Hypertension.*

**Beta-Val** Lemmon, USA.
Betamethasone valerate (p.1093·2).
*Skin disorders.*

**Betavert** Hennig, Ger.
Betahistine mesilate (p.1660·1).
*Vertigo.*

**Betavite** Nicholas Piramal, India.
Vitamin B substances; vitamin C (p.1417·1).
*Vitamin B and C deficiency.*

**Betavix** Genepharm, Gr.
Butamirate citrate (p.1116·2).
*Cough.*

**Beta-Wolff** Wolff, Ger.
Betamethasone valerate (p.1093·2).
*Skin disorders.*

**Betaxin** Abbott, Canad.
Thiamine hydrochloride (p.1455·1).

**Betaxina** Terapeutico, Ital.
Nalidixic acid (p.234·1).
*Gram-negative genito-urinary tract infections.*

**Betaxon** Alcon, USA.
Levobetaxolol hydrochloride (p.946·1).
*Glaucoma; ocular hypertension.*

**Betazim** Sam-On, Israel.
Betaine hydrochloride (p.1660·2); pepsin (p.1729·3).
*Anorexia; diarrhoea; gastritis; gastrointestinal hypoacidity.*

**Betazok** Astra, Irl.†.
Metoprolol succinate (p.957·1).
*Angina pectoris; hypertension.*

**Betazol Cort** Delta, Braz.
Ketoconazole (p.403·3); betamethasone dipropionate (p.1093·1); neomycin sulfate (p.235·1).
*Infected skin disorders.*

**Betazon** Bergamo, Braz.†.
Betamethasone (p.1093·1); phenylbutazone (p.83·2); aluminium glycinate (p.1249·1).

**Betazone** Merck, Hong Kong.
Betamethasone dipropionate (p.1093·1).
*Skin disorders.*

**BETE** Laevosan, Austria†.
Benzatropine hydrochloride (p.479·3).
*Pain with spasmodic disorders.*

**Bethacil** Bioindustria, Ital.
*Injection:* Sulbactam sodium (p.257·2); ampicillin sodium (p.157·1).
Lidocaine hydrochloride (p.1377·3) is included in the intramuscular injection to alleviate the pain of injection.
*Oral suspension*†: Sultamicillin (p.264·2).
*Tablets*†: Sultamicillin tosilate (p.264·2).
*Bacterial infections.*

**Bethasone** Greater Pharma, Thai.
Betamethasone (p.1093·1).
*Skin disorders.*

**Bethasone-N** Greater Pharma, Thai.
Betamethasone (p.1093·1); neomycin sulfate (p.235·1).
*Infected skin disorders.*

**Betim**
Leo, Norw.†; ICN, UK.
Timolol maleate (p.1012·2).
*Angina pectoris; hypertension; hyperthyroidism; migraine; myocardial infarction.*

**Betimol** Novartis Ophthalmics, USA.
Timolol (p.1012·3).
*Glaucoma; ocular hypertension.*

**Betinex** Berk, UK†.
Bumetanide (p.877·2).
*Oedema.*

**Betinjectol** INQ, Braz.†.
Cyanocobalamin (p.1458·2); thiamine (p.1455·2); pyridoxine (p.1457·2).
*Anaemias; vitamin B deficiency.*

**Betiral** Roche, Gr.
Ornidazole (p.612·2).
*Anaerobic bacterial infections; protozoal infections.*

**Betistine** Rafa, Israel.
Betahistine hydrochloride (p.1660·1).
*Vestibular disorders.*

**Betitotal** Propan, S.Afr.
Multivitamin and mineral preparation (p.1417·1).

**Betlife** Euro-Labor, Port.; Grunenthal, Port.
Ticlopidine hydrochloride (p.1011·2).
*Thromboembolic disorders.*

**Betnasol** Glaxo Wellcome, Port.
Betamethasone (p.1093·1).
*Corticosteroid.*

**Betnelan**
Zest, Braz.; GlaxoSmithKline, India; Celltech, Irl.; Celltech, UK.
Betamethasone (p.1093·1).
*Corticosteroid.*

GlaxoSmithKline, Neth.
Betamethasone valerate (p.1093·2).
*Skin disorders.*

**Betnelan-V** GlaxoSmithKline, Belg.
Betamethasone valerate (p.1093·2).
*Skin disorders.*

**Betnelan-VC** GlaxoSmithKline, Belg.
Betamethasone valerate (p.1093·2); clioquinol (p.196·3).
*Infected skin disorders.*

**Betnelan-VN** Glaxo Wellcome, Belg.†.
Betamethasone valerate (p.1093·2); neomycin sulfate (p.235·1).
*Infected skin disorders.*

**Betnesalic**
GlaxoSmithKline, Fr.; GlaxoSmithKline, Ger.†; Cascan, Ger.†; GlaxoSmithKline, Hong Kong; GlaxoSmithKline, Switz.; GlaxoSmithKline, Thai.
Betamethasone valerate (p.1093·2); salicylic acid (p.1157·1).
*Skin disorders.*

**Betnesol**
GlaxoSmithKline, Austria; Glaxo Wellcome, Belg.†; Shire, Canad.; Sigma-Tau, Fr.; Sigma-Tau, Ger.; GlaxoSmithKline, India; Celltech, Irl.; Devries, Israel; GlaxoSmithKline, Malaysia; Defiante, Neth.; GlaxoSmithKline, NZ†; GlaxoSmithKline, S.Afr.; Sigma-Tau, Switz.; Celltech, UK.
Betamethasone sodium phosphate (p.1093·1).
*Corticosteroid; inflammatory disorders of the eye, ear, or nose.*

**Betnesol Aqueous** GlaxoSmithKline, NZ.
Betamethasone sodium phosphate (p.1093·1); naphazoline nitrate (p.1124·3).
*Nasal congestion and inflammation.*

**Betnesol-N**
GlaxoSmithKline, Austria; GlaxoSmithKline, India; Celltech, Irl.; Devries, Israel; GlaxoSmithKline, Malaysia; GlaxoSmithKline, NZ†; GlaxoSmithKline, S.Afr.; Celltech, UK.
Betamethasone sodium phosphate (p.1093·1); neomycin sulfate (p.235·1).
*Infected eye, ear or nose disorders.*

**Betnesol-N Nasal** GlaxoSmithKline, India.
Betamethasone sodium phosphate (p.1093·1); naphazoline nitrate (p.1124·3); neomycin sulfate (p.235·1).
*Nasal disorders.*

**Betnesol-V** GlaxoSmithKline, Ger.
Betamethasone valerate (p.1093·2).
*Scalp disorders; skin disorders.*

**Betneval** GlaxoSmithKline, Fr.
Betamethasone valerate (p.1093·2).
*Mouth disorders; skin disorders.*

**Betneval-Neomycine** GlaxoSmithKline, Fr.
Betamethasone valerate (p.1093·2); neomycin sulfate (p.235·1).
*Infected skin disorders.*

**Betnor** Indoco, India.
Betamethasone sodium phosphate (p.1093·1); neomycin sulfate (p.235·1).
*Inflammatory eye and ear disorders.*

**Betnovat**
GlaxoSmithKline, Denm.; GlaxoSmithKline, Fin.; GlaxoSmithKline, Norw.; GlaxoSmithKline, Swed.
Betamethasone valerate (p.1093·2).
*Otitis externa; skin disorders.*

**Betnovat Comp** GlaxoSmithKline, Fin.
Betamethasone valerate (p.1093·2); phenylephrine hydrochloride (p.1126·3); lidocaine hydrochloride (p.1377·3).
*Anorectal disorders.*

**Betnovat med Chinoform**
GlaxoSmithKline, Denm.; GlaxoSmithKline, Norw.; GlaxoSmithKline, Swed.
Betamethasone valerate (p.1093·2); clioquinol (p.196·3).
*Infected skin disorders.*

**Betnovat med Neomycin** GlaxoSmithKline, Swed.
Betamethasone valerate (p.1093·2); neomycin sulfate (p.235·1).
*Infected skin disorders.*

**Betnovat Rektal** Meda, Denm.
Betamethasone valerate (p.1093·2); lidocaine hydrochloride (p.1377·3); phenylephrine hydrochloride (p.1126·3).
*Anorectal disorders.*

**Betnovat-C** GlaxoSmithKline, Fin.
Betamethasone valerate (p.1093·2); clioquinol (p.196·3).
*Infected skin disorders.*

**Betnovate**
GlaxoSmithKline, Arg.; Sigma, Austral.; GlaxoSmithKline, Austria; GlaxoSmithKline, Braz.; Roberts, Canad.†; GlaxoSmithKline, Chile; Allen, Gr.; GlaxoSmithKline, Hong Kong; GlaxoSmithKline, Irl.; GlaxoSmithKline, Israel; GlaxoSmithKline, Malaysia; Glaxo Wellcome, Mex.; GlaxoSmithKline, NZ; Glaxo Wellcome, Port.; GlaxoSmithKline, S.Afr.; GlaxoSmithKline, Singapore; Celltech, Spain; GlaxoSmithKline, Switz.; GlaxoSmithKline, Thai.; GlaxoSmithKline, UK.
Betamethasone valerate (p.1093·2).
*Skin and scalp disorders.*

**Betnovate Antihemorroidal** GlaxoSmithKline, Arg.
Betamethasone valerate (p.1093·2); phenylephrine hydrochloride (p.1126·3); lidocaine hydrochloride (p.1377·3).
*Anorectal disorders.*

**Betnovate RD (Ready Diluted)** GlaxoSmithKline, UK.
Betamethasone valerate (p.1093·2).
*Skin disorders.*

**Betnovate Rectal Ointment** GlaxoSmithKline, UK†.
Betamethasone valerate (p.1093·2); lidocaine hydrochloride (p.1377·3); phenylephrine hydrochloride (p.1126·3).
*Anorectal disorders.*

**Betnovate-C**
GlaxoSmithKline, Arg.; GlaxoSmithKline, Austria; GlaxoSmithKline, Hong Kong; GlaxoSmithKline, India; GlaxoSmithKline, Irl.; GlaxoSmithKline, Israel; GlaxoSmithKline, NZ; Glaxo Wellcome, Port.; GlaxoSmithKline, S.Afr.; Glaxo Wellcome, Singapore†; GlaxoSmithKline, Switz.; GlaxoSmithKline, Thai.; GlaxoSmithKline, UK.
Betamethasone valerate (p.1093·2); clioquinol (p.196·3).
*Infected skin disorders.*

**Betnovate-GM**
GlaxoSmithKline, India; Glaxo Wellcome, Singapore†.
Betamethasone valerate (p.1093·2); miconazole nitrate (p.405·3); gentamicin sulfate (p.217·1).
*Infected skin disorders.*

**Betnovate-M**
GlaxoSmithKline, India; Glaxo Wellcome, Singapore†.
Betamethasone valerate (p.1093·2); miconazole nitrate (p.405·3).
*Infected skin disorders.*

**Betnovate-N**
GlaxoSmithKline, Arg.; GlaxoSmithKline, Austria; GlaxoSmithKline, Braz.; GlaxoSmithKline, Chile; GlaxoSmithKline, Hong Kong; GlaxoSmithKline, India; GlaxoSmithKline, Irl.; GlaxoSmithKline, Israel; GlaxoSmithKline, Malaysia; Glaxo Wellcome, Port.; GlaxoSmithKline, S.Afr.; Glaxo Wellcome, Singapore†; GlaxoSmithKline, Switz.; GlaxoSmithKline, Thai.; GlaxoSmithKline, UK.
Betamethasone valerate (p.1093·2); neomycin sulfate (p.235·1).
*Infected skin disorders.*

**Betnovate-Q** GlaxoSmithKline, Braz.
Betamethasone valerate (p.1093·2); clioquinol (p.196·3).
*Infected skin disorders.*

**Betnovate-S** GlaxoSmithKline, India.
Betamethasone valerate (p.1093·2); salicylic acid (p.1157·1).
*Skin disorders.*

**Betoid**
Yamanouchi, Denm.†; Yamanouchi, Norw.†; Yamanouchi, Swed.†.
Betamethasone valerate (p.1093·2).
*Skin disorders.*

**Betolvex**
Alpharma, Denm.; Alpharma, Fin.; Alpharma, Norw.; Lagamed, S.Afr.†; Alpharma, Swed.; Alpharma, Switz.
Cyanocobalamin (p.1458·2) or cyanocobalamin tannate (p.1459·1).
*Megaloblastic anaemia; vitamin $B_{12}$ deficiency.*

**Betolvidon** Abigo, Swed.
Cyanocobalamin (p.1458·2).
*Vitamin $B_{12}$ deficiency.*

**Betonin** Knoll, India.
Vitamin B substances (p.1417·1).
*Vitamin B deficiency.*

**Betonvit** Recalcine, Chile.
Thiamine hydrochloride (p.1455·1); pyridoxine hydrochloride (p.1456·3); cyanocobalamin (p.1458·2); procaine hydrochloride (p.1383·2).
*Neuralgia; neuritis; neuropathy; tonic.*

**Betoptic**
Alcon, Austral.; Alcon, Austria; Alcon, Belg.; Alcon, Braz.; Alcon, Canad.; Alcon, Chile; Alcon, Denm.; Alcon, Fin.; Alcon, Fr.; Alkon (Αλκον), Gr.; Alcon, Hong Kong; Alcon, Irl.; Alcon, Israel; Alcon, Ital.; Alcon, Malaysia; Alcon, Mex.; Alcon, Norw.; Alcon, NZ; Alcon, Port.; Alcon, S.Afr.; Alcon, Singapore; Alcon Cusi, Spain; Alcon, Swed.; Alcon, Thai.; Alcon, UK; Alcon, USA.
Betaxolol hydrochloride (p.873·1).
*Glaucoma; ocular hypertension.*

**Betoptic S**
Alkon (Αλκον), Gr.; Alcon, Switz.
Betaxolol hydrochloride (p.873·1).
*Glaucoma; ocular hypertension.*

**Betoptima** Alcon, Ger.
Betaxolol hydrochloride (p.873·1).
*Glaucoma; ocular hypertension.*

**Betoquin** Ioquin, Austral.
Betaxolol hydrochloride (p.873·1).
*Glaucoma; ocular hypertension.*

**Betosalic** TO-Chemicals, Thai.
Betamethasone valerate (p.1093·2); salicylic acid (p.1157·1).
*Skin disorders.*

**Betosone** TO-Chemicals, Thai.
Betamethasone valerate (p.1093·2).
*Skin disorders.*

**Betosone-CE** TO-Chemicals, Thai.
Betamethasone valerate (p.1093·2); clioquinol (p.196·3).
*Infected skin disorders.*

**Be-Total** Carlo Erba OTC, Ital.
Vitamin B substances (p.1417·1).
*Vitamin B deficiency.*

**Betozone** De Mayo, Braz.
*Capsules:* Ferrous fumarate (p.1427·3); folic acid (p.1429·1); ascorbic acid; vitamin B substances (p.1417·1).
*Anaemias.*
*Injection*†: Vitamin B substances (p.1417·1); liver extract.
*Anaemias; vitamin deficiency.*
*Oral liquid:* Ferrous sulfate (p.1428·2); vitamin B substances; lysine hydrochloride (p.1417·1).
*Anaemias.*

**Betrat B** Ativus, Braz.
Betamethasone valerate (p.1093·2).
*Skin disorders.*

**Betres AP** Offenbach, Mex.
Vitamin B substances (p.1417·1).

**Betriphos-C** Schwarz, Fr.†.
Adenosine triphosphate sodium (p.1648·1); vitamin B substances (p.1417·1); ascorbic acid.
*Tonic.*

**Betrivit** Biogal, Israel†.
Hydroxocobalamin (p.1458·2); pyridoxine hydrochloride (p.1456·3); thiamine nitrate (p.1455·1).
Lidocaine hydrochloride (p.1377·3) is included in this preparation to alleviate the pain of injection.
*Metabolic disorders; neuropathies.*

**Betron R** Italfarmaco, Ital.
Interferon beta (human, recombinant) (p.645·3).
*Malignant neoplasms; viral infections.*

**Betsol Z** Zafiro, Mex.
Sodium bicarbonate (p.1223·2).
*Metabolic acidosis.*

**Betsona** Neo Quimica, Braz.
Betamethasone valerate (p.1093·2).
*Skin disorders.*

**Betsuril** Almirall, Spain.
Beclometasone dipropionate (p.1091·1).
*Asthma.*

**Bettamousse**
Vitaflo, Denm.; Vitaflo, Fin.†; Celltech, Irl.; Evans Medical, Israel; Mipharm, Ital.; Vitaflo, Norw.; Celltech, Spain; Vitaflo, Swed.; Celltech, UK.
Betamethasone valerate (p.1093·2).
*Scalp disorders.*

**Better Cholesterol** Young Again Products, USA.
Sitosterol (p.982·3); guggul sterones.

**Better Prostate** Young Again Products, USA.
Sitosterol (p.982·3); zinc citrate.
*Dietary supplement.*

**Betulac** Meda, Swed.†.
Lactulose (p.1269·1).
*Constipation; hepatic encephalopathy.*

**Betuline** *Ferndale, USA.*
Methyl salicylate (p.59·3); camphor (p.1665·3); menthol (p.1711·3).
*Muscle, joint, and soft-tissue pain; neuralgia.*

**Betulla (Specie Composta)** *Dynacren, Ital.*
Birch leaf (p.1660·3); couch-grass (p.1676·2).
*Herbal tea; water retention.*

**Be-Uric** *Be-Tabs, S.Afr.†.*
Allopurinol (p.412·2).
*Gout; hyperuricaemia.*

**Beurises** *Be-Tabs, S.Afr.*
Furosemide (p.919·3).
*Hypertension; oedema.*

**Bevicomplex** *INQ, Braz.†.*
Vitamin B substances (p.1417·1).
*Vitamin supplement.*

**Beviplex** *Meuse, Belg.*
Vitamin B substances (p.1417·1).
*Neuritis; vitamin B deficiency.*

**Beviplex forte** *Abigo, Swed.*
Vitamin B substances (p.1417·1).
*Alcoholism; neuropathies; vitamin B deficiency.*

**Bevispas** *Aspen, S.Afr.*
Mebeverine hydrochloride (p.1273·1).
*Irritable bowel syndrome.*

**Bevit Forte** *Biocur, Ger.*
Thiamine hydrochloride (p.1455·1); pyridoxine hydrochloride (p.1456·3).
*Nervous system disorders.*

**Bevitamel** *Westlake, USA.*
Melatonin (p.1710·2); vitamin $B_{12}$ (p.1458·2); folic acid (p.1429·1).
*Aid in homocysteine metabolism; sleep disorders.*

**Bevitin** *Abbott, Ital.*
Vitamin B substances (p.1417·1).
*Vitamin B deficiency.*

**Bevitine** *DB, Fr.*
Thiamine hydrochloride (p.1455·1).
*Beri beri; neuritis; vitamin B deficiency.*

**Bevitol** *Lannacher, Austria.*
Thiamine hydrochloride (p.1455·1).
*Vitamin $B_1$ deficiency.*

**Bevitotal comp** *Astra, Swed.*
Vitamin B substances with vitamin C (p.1417·1).
*Alcoholism; neuropathies; vitamin B and C deficiency.*

**Bevoren** *Almirall, Belg.*
Glibenclamide (p.331·2).
*Diabetes mellitus.*

**Bewon** *Charton, Canad.†.*
Thiamine hydrochloride (p.1455·1).

**Bex**
*Note. This name is used for preparations of different composition.*
*Roche Consumer, Austral.*
Aspirin (p.15·1).
*Fever; pain.*
*Lalco, Canad.†.*
Vitamin B substances and vitamin C (p.1417·1).

**Bex-Hepar** *Reuffer, Mex.†.*
Betaxolol (p.873·1).

**Bexicortil** *Isdin, Spain.*
Fluorometholone (p.1102·2); miconazole nitrate (p.405·3); neomycin sulfate (p.235·1).
*Infected skin disorders.*

**Bexid** *ACO Hud, Swed.*
Benzoyl peroxide (p.1143·2).
*Acne.*

**Bexident** *Isdin, Port.*
*Dental gel; dental spray; mouthwash:* Chlorhexidine (p.1173·2).
*Gingivitis.*
*Paediatric dental gel:* Potassium glycyrrhizinate; dexpanthenol (p.1727·2).
*Gum protection.*
*Toothpaste:* Triclosan (p.1195·2); sodium fluoride (p.1444·3).
*Gingivitis.*

**Bexidermil** *Isdin, Spain.*
Trolamine salicylate (p.95·3).
*Peri-articular disorders; soft-tissue disorders.*

**Bexine**
*Note. This name is used for preparations of different composition.*
*Collins, Mex.*
Dexamethasone (p.1097·1).
*Corticosteroid.*
*Spirig, Switz.*
Dextromethorphan hydrobromide (p.1117·3).
*Coughs.*

**Bexinor** *Beacons, Singapore.*
Norfloxacin (p.238·3).
*Bacterial infections.*

**Bexon** *Gobbi, Arg.*
*Pessaries:* Metronidazole (p.607·2); nystatin (p.406·3); hydrocortisone (p.1103·3).
*Vaginal infections.*
*Tablets:* Metronidazole (p.607·2).
*Anaerobic bacterial infections; protozoal infections.*

**Bextra**
*Pharmacia, Chile; Pharmacia, Switz.; Pfizer, UK; Pharmacia, USA; Pfizer, USA.*
Valdecoxib (p.96·1).
*Dysmenorrhoea; osteoarthritis; rheumatoid arthritis.*

**Bexxar** *Corixa, USA; GlaxoSmithKline, USA.*
Iodine-131 tositumomab (p.1524·2) (see also Tositumomab (p.589·3)).
*Non-Hodgkin's lymphoma.*

**Beza** *CT, Ger.; ABZ, Ger.; 1A, Ger.*
Bezafibrate (p.873·2).
*Hyperlipidaemias.*

**Bezabeta** *Betapharm, Ger.*
Bezafibrate (p.873·2).
*Hyperlipidaemias.*

**Bezacur**
*Hexal, Arg.; Hexal, Austria; Hexal, Ger.*
Bezafibrate (p.873·2).
*Hyperlipidaemias.*

**Bezadoc** *Docpharm, Ger.*
Bezafibrate (p.873·2).
*Hyperlipidaemias.*

**Bezafisal** *Cryopharma, Mex.*
Bezafibrate (p.873·2).
*Hyperlipidaemias.*

**Bezagamma** *Worwag, Ger.*
Bezafibrate (p.873·2).
*Hyperlipidaemias.*

**Bezagen** *Generics, UK.*
Bezafibrate (p.873·2).
*Hyperlipidaemias.*

**Beza-Lande** *Sanofi Synthelabo, Ger.†.*
Bezafibrate (p.873·2).
*Hyperlipidaemias.*

**Bezalex** *Pharmacos Abug, Mex.*
Bezafibrate (p.873·2).
*Hyperlipidaemias.*

**Bezalip**
*Roche, Arg.; Roche, Austria; Roche, Canad.; Roche, Denm.†; Roche, Fin.; Roche, Gr.; Roche, Hong Kong; Nicholas Piramal, India; Abic, Israel; Roche Diagnostics, Israel; Roche, Ital.; Roche, Jpn; Roche, Mex.; Roche, Neth.; Roche, NZ; Roche, Port.; Roche, S.Afr.; Roche, Singapore; Roche, Swed.; Roche, Thai.; Roche, UK.*
Bezafibrate (p.873·2).
*Hyperlipidaemias.*

**Bezalip Mono** *Roche, UK.*
Bezafibrate (p.873·2).
*Hyperlipidaemias.*

**Bezamerck** *Merck dura, Ger.*
Bezafibrate (p.873·2).
*Hyperlipidaemias.*

**Bezamil** *Milano, Thai.*
Bezafibrate (p.873·2).
*Hyperlipidaemias.*

**Bezapham** *Phamos, Ger.*
Bezafibrate (p.873·2).
*Hyperlipidaemias.*

**Beza-Puren** *Alpharma-Isis, Ger.*
Bezafibrate (p.873·2).
*Hyperlipidaemias.*

**Bezastad** *Stada, Austria.*
Bezafibrate (p.873·2).
*Hyperlipidaemias.*

**B-Feron** *Greater Pharma, Thai.*
Multivitamin and mineral preparation (p.1417·1).

**BFI**
*Note. This name is used for preparations of different composition.*
*SmithKline Beecham Consumer, Austral.†.*
Bismuth-formic-iodide (p.1253·1); zinc *p*-phenolsulfonate (p.1163·3); alum (p.1652·1); bismuth subgallate (p.1252·2); menthol (p.1711·3); cineole (p.1672·1); thymol (p.1194·2); magnesium carbonate (p.1272·1); pentyloxyphenol.
*Damaged skin; pruritus.*
*Menley & James, USA.*
Bismuth-formic-iodide (p.1253·1); zinc phenolsulfonate (p.1163·3); alum (p.1652·1); bismuth subgallate (p.1252·2); boric acid (p.1662·1); menthol (p.1711·3); cineole (p.1672·1); thymol (p.1194·2).
*Antiseptic.*

**B-G Prot** *Merind, India.*
Vitamin B substances (p.1417·1).
*Vitamin B deficiency.*

**BGB Norflox** *Pond's, Thai.*
Norfloxacin (p.238·3).
*Bacterial infections.*

**Bgramin** *Douglas, Austral.*
Amoxicillin trihydrate (p.155·3).
*Bacterial infections.*

**B-Hex** *Xepa-Soul Pattinson, Singapore†.*
Trihexyphenidyl hydrochloride (p.490·2).
*Drug-induced extrapyramidal disorders; parkinsonism.*

**B12-Horfervit** *Arteva, Ger.†.*
Cyanocobalamin (p.1458·2).
*Vitamin $B_{12}$ deficiency.*

**Biactol Antibacterial Facewash** *Procter & Gamble, Irl.†.*
Phenoxypropanol (p.1189·1).
*Acne.*

**Biactol Liquid** *Crookes Healthcare, UK.*
Phenoxypropanol (p.1189·1).
*Acne.*

**Biaferone** *Kedrion, Ital.*
Interferon alfa (p.640·3).
*Anogenital warts; hepatitis; malignant neoplasms.*

**Biafine**
*Craveri, Arg.; Finn Vita, Chile; Medix, Fr.; Medix, Israel; Upsifarma, Port.; Galephar, Switz.*
Trolamine (p.1758·2).
*Burns; erythema; wounds.*

**Biaflu** *Biagini, Ital.†.*
An adsorbed inactivated influenza vaccine (p.1620·2).
*Active immunisation.*

**Biaflu-Zonale SU** *Biagini, Ital.†.*
An influenza vaccine (p.1620·2).
*Active immunisation.*

**Bi-Aglut**
*Distriborg, Fr.†; Novartis Consumer, UK.*
Gluten-free foods (p.1417·1).
*Gluten intolerance.*
*Plasmon, Ital.*
A range of gluten-free and lactose-reduced foods (p.1417·1).
*Gluten and lactose intolerance.*

**Bialcol**
*Novartis, Chile; Novartis Consumer, Ital.*
Benzoxonium chloride (p.1170·2).
*Disinfection of instruments, skin, and wounds.*

**Bialerge** *Elofar, Braz.*
Phenylephrine hydrochloride (p.1126·3); brompheniramine maleate (p.426·1).
*Nasal congestion.*

**Bialminal** *Bial, Port.*
Phenobarbital (p.367·3).
*Epilepsy; sedative.*

**Bialzepam** *Medibial, Port.*
Diazepam (p.690·1).
*Alcohol withdrawal syndrome; anxiety; epilepsy; insomnia; premedication; skeletal muscle spasm.*

**Biamotil** *Allergan, Braz.*
Ciprofloxacin hydrochloride (p.188·2).
*Bacterial eye and ear infections.*

**Biamotil-D** *Allergan-Frumtost, Braz.*
Ciprofloxacin hydrochloride (p.188·2); dexamethasone (p.1097·1).
*Infected eye disorders.*

**Bianco Val** *Edmond Pharma, Ital.*
Valerian (p.1762·2); crataegus (p.1677·1).
*Hyperexcitability; insomnia.*

**Biartac** *Merck Sharp & Dohme, Belg.*
Diflunisal (p.34·1).
*Arthrosis; polyarthritis.*

**Biatos** *Cimed, Braz.*
Ketotifen (p.788·2).
*Asthma.*

**Biavax II** *Merck Sharp & Dohme, USA.*
A rubella and mumps vaccine (Wistar RA 27/3 and Jeryl Lynn (B level) strains respectively) (p.1638·2).
*Active immunisation.*

**Biaven** *Kedrion, Ital.*
A normal immunoglobulin (p.1627·2).
*Hypogammaglobulinaemia; idiopathic thrombocytopenic purpura; immunodeficiency.*

**Biaxin**
*Abbott, Canad.; Abbott, Ger.; Abbott, USA.*
Clarithromycin (p.192·2).
*Bacterial infections; Helicobacter pylori infections.*

**Biaxsig** *Aventis, Austral.*
Roxithromycin (p.254·2).
*Bacterial infections.*

**Biazolina** *Fermenti, Ital.†.*
Cefazolin sodium (p.170·3).
*Bacterial infections.*

**Bibivit Light** *Lampugnani, Ital.*
Multivitamin and carbohydrate preparation with fruit and plant extracts (p.1417·1).
*Nutritional supplement.*

**Bibol Leloup** *Hexa-Medinova, Arg.*
Silymarin (p.1043·3); dehydrocholic acid (p.1679·2); pancreatin (p.1725·3); bile salts (p.1660·3); homatropine methylbromide (p.483·2).
*Liver disorders.*

**Bica** *Finadiet, Arg.*
Calcium carbonate (p.1254·2).
*Antacid.*

**Bicaflac** *Edwards, Spain.*
Range of electrolyte solutions for haemofiltration (p.1221·1).

**Bicain** *Orion, Fin.*
Bupivacaine hydrochloride (p.1371·1).
*Local anaesthesia.*

**Bicam** *Biolab, Thai.*
Piroxicam (p.84·2).
*Musculoskeletal and joint disorders.*

**Bicaprost** *Pharmacia, Arg.*
Bicalutamide (p.530·1).
*Prostatic cancer.*

**Bicarnat** *Pisa, Mex.*
Sodium bicarbonate (p.1223·2).

**BiCart** *Gambro, Swed.†.*
*Concentrates for haemodialysis solutions:* Sodium chloride; potassium chloride; magnesium chloride; calcium chloride glacial acetic acid (p.1221·1).
To be used with BiCart powder.
*Powder for haemodialysis solutions:* Sodium bicarbonate (p.1221·1).
To be used with BiCart concentrates.

**Bicavine** *Cazi, Braz.*
Dipyrone (p.35·3); vitamin B substances (p.1417·1).
*Neuritis; pain.*

**Bicbag**
*Fresenius Medical, Denm.†; Dicamed, Swed.†.*
Sodium bicarbonate (p.1221·1).
*Haemodialysis.*

**Bicetil** *Menarini, Spain.*
Quinapril hydrochloride (p.991·1); hydrochlorothiazide (p.933·2).
*Hypertension.*

**Bicholate** *Sabex, Canad.*
Bile salts (p.1660·3); cascara (p.1255·1); aloin (p.1248·3); bisacodyl (p.1251·3).
Formerly contained bile salts, cascara, phenolphthalein, aloin.
*Constipation.*

**Bicidal Plus** *Kee, India.*
Amoxicillin trihydrate (p.155·3); cloxacillin sodium (p.198·2); *Lactobacillus sporogenes* (p.1704·2).
*Bacterial infections.*

**Bicide** *Fischer, Israel.*
Lindane (p.1506·3).
*Scabies.*

**Bicillin** *Yamanouchi, UK†.*
Procaine benzylpenicillin (p.246·1); benzylpenicillin sodium (p.163·2).
*Bacterial infections.*

**Bicillin A-P** *Wyeth-Ayerst, Canad.†.*
Benzathine benzylpenicillin (p.162·3); procaine benzylpenicillin (p.246·1); benzylpenicillin potassium (p.163·2).
*Bacterial infections.*

**Bicillin C-R** *Monarch, USA.*
Benzathine benzylpenicillin (p.162·3); procaine benzylpenicillin (p.246·1).
*Bacterial infections.*

**Bicillin L-A**
*Wyeth, Austral.; Wyeth-Ayerst, Canad.†; Wyeth, NZ; Akromed, S.Afr.†; Monarch, USA.*
Benzathine benzylpenicillin (p.162·3).
*Bacterial infections.*

**Biciron** *Alcon, Ger.*
Tramazoline hydrochloride (p.1131·3).
*Eye disorders.*

**Bicitra** *Alza, USA.*
Sodium citrate (p.1223·2); citric acid monohydrate (p.1673·1).
*Chronic metabolic acidosis; urine alkalinising agent.*

**Bi-Citrol**
*Pharmethic, Belg.†; Diepharmex, Fr.*
Monosodium citrate (p.1224·1); sodium citrate (p.1223·2).
*Dyspepsia.*

**Biclar** *Abbott, Belg.*
Clarithromycin (p.192·2).
*Bacterial infections.*

**Biclin**
*Bristol-Myers Squibb, Mex.; Bristol-Myers Squibb, Port.; Bristol-Myers, Spain.*
Amikacin sulfate (p.154·1).
*Bacterial infections.*

**Biclinocilline** *Sanofi Synthelabo, Fr.*
Benethamine penicillin (p.162·3); benzylpenicillin sodium (p.163·2).
*Bacterial infections.*

**Biclopan** *Pharbita, Singapore†.*
Diclofenac sodium (p.32·1).
*Gout; inflammation; musculoskeletal, joint, peri-articular, and soft-tissue disorders; pain.*

**BiCNU**
*Bristol-Myers Squibb, Arg.; Bristol-Myers Squibb, Austral.; Bristol, Canad.; Bristol-Myers Squibb, Chile; Bristol-Myers Squibb, Fr.; Bristol-Myers Squibb, Hong Kong; Bristol-Myers Squibb, Irl.; Bristol-Myers Squibb, Israel; Bristol-Myers Squibb, Malaysia; Bristol-Myers Squibb, Mex.; Bristol-Myers Squibb, NZ; Bristol-Myers Squibb, S.Afr.; Bristol-Myers Squibb, Singapore; Bristol-Myers Squibb, Thai.†; Bristol-Myers Squibb, UK; Bristol-Myers Squibb Oncology, USA.*
Carmustine (p.535·1).
*Malignant neoplasms.*

**Bicobon** *PP Lab, Thai.*
Sodium bicarbonate (p.1223·2); activated charcoal (p.1030·2); peppermint oil (p.1283·2).
*Diarrhoea; flatulence; gastrointestinal disorders.*

**Bicofen** *Vilco, Gr.*
Roxithromycin (p.254·2).
*Bacterial infections.*

**Bicold** *Labima, Belg.*
Diphenylpyraline hydrochloride (p.432·3); phenylephrine hydrochloride (p.1126·3).
*Upper respiratory-tract congestion.*

**Bicomplex** *ABC, Ital.*
Vitamin B substances (p.1417·1).
*Vitamin B deficiency.*

**Biconcor**
*Merck, Braz.; Merck, Mex.*
Bisoprolol fumarate (p.875·1); hydrochlorothiazide (p.933·2).
*Hypertension.*

**Bicor** *Alphapharm, Austral.*
Bisoprolol fumarate (p.875·1).
*Heart failure.*

**Bicozene** *Novartis, USA.*
Benzocaine (p.1370·3); resorcinol (p.1156·3).
*Local anaesthesia.*

**Bicromil** *Cetus, Arg.*
Sertraline (p.317·3).
*Depression.*

**Bidanzen** *GlaxoSmithKline, India.*
Serrapeptase (p.1743·2).
*Hyphaema; inflammation; pain; respiratory-tract congestion.*

**Bidiabe** *Sanofi Synthelabo, Ital.*
Chlorpropamide (p.330·3); phenformin hydrochloride (p.344·1).
*Diabetes mellitus.*

**Bidien** *IDI, Ital.*
Budesonide (p.1094·2).
*Skin disorders.*

**Bidor** *Weleda, UK.*
Homoeopathic preparation.

**Bidrolar** *Spyfarma, Spain.*
Pygeum africanum (p.1568·2).
*Benign prostatic hyperplasia.*

**Bidrostat** *Gautier, Arg.*
Bicalutamide (p.530·1).
*Prostatic cancer.*

**Biduret** *GlaxoSmithKline, India.*
Amiloride hydrochloride (p.858·2); hydrochlorothiazide (p.933·2).
*Hepatic cirrhosis with ascites; hypertension; oedema.*

**Bienfait Total** *Lancome, Canad.†.*
*SPF 15:* Octinoxate (p.1154·3); ensulizole (p.1147·1).
*Sunscreen.*

**Bienterico** *Caldeira & Marques, Port.*
Streptomycin sulfate (p.256·2); neomycin sulfate (p.235·1).
*Bowel sterilisation; diarrhoea; hepatic coma.*

**Bi-Euglucon** *Roche, Ital.*
Glibenclamide (p.331·2); phenformin hydrochloride (p.344·1).
*Diabetes mellitus.*

**Bi-Euglucon M**
*Roche, Chile; Roche, Ital.; Roche, Mex.*
Glibenclamide (p.331·2); metformin hydrochloride (p.342·3).
*Diabetes mellitus.*

**Bifardol S** *Liferpal, Mex.*
Naproxen sodium (p.65·1); paracetamol (p.76·2).
*Fever; pain.*

**Bifazol** *Bayer, Ital.*
Bifonazole (p.395·1).
*Fungal skin infections.*

**Bifebral** *Aventis, Mex.*
Ketoprofen sodium (p.51·3); paracetamol (p.76·2).
*Fever; pain.*

**Bifen**
*DHA, Hong Kong; DHA, Malaysia; DHA, Singapore.*
Ibuprofen (p.45·3).
*Fever; musculoskeletal and joint disorders; pain.*

**Bifena** *Panalab, Arg.*
Lotion 1, salicylic acid (p.1157·1); lotion 2, pantothenic acid (p.1442·3).
*Hair disorders.*

**Bifenac** *Pharmacia Upjohn, Mex.*
Tolfenamic acid (p.94·2).
*Fever; gout; inflammation; musculoskeletal, joint and peri-articular disorders; pain.*

**Bifidosa** *Nutricia-Bago, Arg.*
Lactulose (p.1269·1); ferrous sulfate; vitamin B substances (p.1417·1).
*Restoration of normal gastrointestinal flora.*

**Bifilact** *Fidia, Ital.*
*Lactobacillus acidophilus* (p.1704·2); *Lactobacillus lactis* (p.1704·2); *Lactobacillus bulgaricus* (p.1704·2); *Streptococcus thermophilus* (p.1704·2); *Bifidobacterium bifidum* (p.1704·2); *Lactobacillus sporogenes* (p.1704·2); vitamin B substances; brewers yeast (p.1469·1).
*Maintenance of normal gastrointestinal flora.*

**Bifinorma** *Merckle, Ger.*
Lactulose (p.1269·1).
*Constipation; hepatic encephalopathy.*

**Bifiteral**
*Solvay, Austria; Solvay, Belg.; Solvay, Ger.*
Lactulose (p.1269·1).
*Constipation; hepatic encephalopathy.*

**Bifix** *Roche Nicholas, Fr.*
Nifuroxazide (p.237·2).
*Diarrhoea.*

**Bifized** *Iasis, Gr.*
Bifonazole (p.395·1).
*Fungal skin infections.*

**Bifluorid**
*Voco, Denm.; New Ulros, Ital.; Meda, Swed.*
Calcium fluoride (p.1423·3); sodium fluoride (p.1444·3).
*Dental caries prophylaxis; sensitive gums.*

**Bifokey** *Inkeysa, Spain.*
Bifonazole (p.395·1).
*Fungal skin infections.*

**Bifomyk** *Bioglan, Ger.*
Bifonazole (p.395·1).
*Fungal skin infections.*

**Bifon**
*Dermapharm, Ger.; Genepharm, Gr.*
Bifonazole (p.395·1).
*Fungal skin infections.*

**Bifonal** *Fortbenton, Arg.*
Bifonazole (p.395·1).
*Fungal skin infections.*

**Bifort**
*Note. This name is used for preparations of different composition.*
*Finadiet, Arg.*
Sildenafil citrate (p.1744·2).
*Erectile dysfunction.*

*Merck, Spain.*
Cafedrine hydrochloride (p.878·2); theodrenaline hydrochloride (p.1754·3).
*Hypotension.*

**Bifosa** *Troikaa, India.*
Alendronate sodium (p.765·3).
*Osteoporosis.*

**Bifril**
*Lusofarmaco, Ital.; Menarini, Swed.*
Zofenopril calcium (p.1029·3).
*Hypertension; myocardial infarction.*

**Big V** *Tanning Research, Canad.†.*
*SPF 15:* Octinoxate (p.1154·3); oxybenzone (p.1154·3).
*SPF 30:* Homosalate (p.1148·1); octinoxate (p.1154·3); octisalate (p.1154·3); oxybenzone (p.1154·3).
*Sunscreen.*

**Big V Baby** *Tanning Research, Canad.†.*
*SPF 30:* Homosalate (p.1148·1); octinoxate (p.1154·3); octisalate (p.1154·3); oxybenzone (p.1154·3).
*Sunscreen.*

**Big V Cough Lozenge** *Sutton, Canad.†.*
Menthol (p.1711·3).

**Big V Kids** *Tanning Research, Canad.†.*
Octinoxate (p.1154·3); octocrilene (p.1154·3); octisalate (p.1154·3); oxybenzone (p.1154·3).
*Sunscreen.*

**Bigasan** *Phyteia, Switz.†.*
Aluminium hydroxide (p.1249·2); magnesium hydroxide (p.1272·2); magnesium oxide (p.1272·3); magnesium silicate (p.1580·2); mannitol (p.950·2).
*Gastric hyperacidity.*

**Bigenol** *Grisi, Mex.*
Methyltestosterone (p.1559·3); calcium glycerophosphate; calcium anhydroxymethylenediphosphate; magnesium anhydroxymethylenediphosphate; glutamic acid; thiamine hydrochloride; nux vomica (p.1722·3).
*Anabolic.*

**Bigetric** *Casasco, Arg.*
Domperidone (p.1263·2); simeticone (p.1289·2).
*Dyspepsia; flatulence; nausea and vomiting.*

**Bigonist** *Aventis, Fr.*
Buserelin acetate (p.1319·2).
*Prostatic cancer.*

**Bigpen** *GlaxoSmithKline, Spain.*
Amoxicillin trihydrate (p.155·3); potassium clavulanate (p.193·3).
*Bacterial infections.*

**Bikalm** *Byk Gulden, Ger.*
Zolpidem tartrate (p.728·3).
*Sleep disorders.*

**Biklin**
*Bristol-Myers Squibb, Arg.; Bristol-Myers Squibb, Austria; Bristol-Myers Squibb, Denm.†; Bristol-Myers Squibb, Fin.; Bristol-Myers Squibb, Ger.; Bristol-Myers Squibb, Swed.*
Amikacin sulfate (p.154·1).
*Bacterial infections.*

**Bil 13** *Bago, Arg.*
Choline orotate (p.1724·3); dehydrocholic acid (p.1679·2); deoxycholic acid (p.1660·3); casanthranol (p.1255·1); boldine (p.1661·2).
*Constipation; liver and biliary-tract disorders.*

**Bil 13 Enzimatico** *Bago, Arg.*
Metoclopramide hydrochloride (p.1274·3); dehydrocholic acid (p.1679·2); pancreatin (p.1725·3); simeticone (p.1289·2).
*Digestive disorders; flatulence.*

**Bilagit Mono** *Temmler, Ger.*
Javanese turmeric (p.1759·3).
*Dyspepsia.*

**Bilagol**
*Note. This name is used for preparations of different composition.*
*Lazar, Arg.*
Bile salts (p.1660·3); dehydrocholic acid (p.1679·2); domperidone (p.1263·2); simeticone (p.1289·2).
*Digestive disorders; dyspepsia.*

*Janssen-Cilag, Belg.†.*
Diisopromine hydrochloride (p.1261·2); sorbitol (p.1446·3).
*Constipation; hepatobiliary disorders.*

**Bilamide** *Ethnor, India.*
Hydroxymethylnicotinamide (p.1700·1).
*Anorexia; constipation; dyspepsia; flatulence.*

**Bilan** *Biocur, Ger.†.*
Haronga.
*Digestive disorders.*

**Bilaten** *Medipharm, Chile.*
Candesartan (p.878·3).
*Hypertension.*

**Bilatin** *Stada, Austria.*
Lecithin (p.1706·1); liver extract.
*Tonic.*

**Bilatin Fischol** *Stada, Ger.†.*
Marine triglycerides (p.976·2).
*Hyperlipidaemias.*

**Bilaxil** *Roche, Chile.*
Ispaghula husk (p.1268·1); senna (p.1288·2).
*Bowel evacuation; constipation.*

**Bilberry Formula** *Quest, Canad.*
Myrtillus; carrot; citrus bioflavonoids; hesperidin (p.1417·1).

**Bilberry Plus** *Eagle, Austral.†.*
Myrtillus (p.1718·3); euphrasia (p.1686·3); fenugreek (p.1688·1); hydrastis (p.1698·3).
*Eye fatigue.*

**Bilberry Plus Eye Health** *Cenovis, Austral.†.*
Myrtillus (p.1718·3); ginkgo biloba (p.1692·3); tagetes erecta; riboflavin; *dl*-alpha tocoferil acetate; ascorbic acid; zinc gluconate; betacarotene (p.1417·1).
*Eye fatigue; eye irritation.*

**Bilduretic** *Bangkok Lab & Cosmetic, Thai.*
Amiloride hydrochloride (p.858·2); hydrochlorothiazide (p.933·2).
*Hepatic cirrhosis with ascites; hypertension; oedema.*

**Bileco** *Elvetium, Arg.*
Bleomycin sulfate (p.530·2).
*Malignant neoplasms.*

**Bilem** *Lemery, Mex.*
Tamoxifen (p.585·3).

**Bilenor** *Schwarz, Ital.*
Magnesium trihydrate salt of chenodeoxycholic and ursodeoxycholic acids (p.1670·1) (p.1760·3).
*Biliary dyspepsia; gallstones.*

**Bilenzima** *Elofar, Braz.†.*
Bromopride (p.1254·1).
*Gastrointestinal disorders.*

**Biletan** *Gador, Arg.*
Thioctic acid (p.1754·3).
*Diabetic neuropathy; liver disorders.*

**Biletan Enzimatico** *Gador, Arg.*
Thioctic acid (p.1754·3); pancreatin (p.1725·3); cellulase (p.1669·1); simeticone (p.1289·2).
*Digestive disorders.*

**Bilgast echinac** *Bilgast, Ger.†.*
Echinacea purpurea (p.1683·2).
*Respiratory- and urinary-tract infections.*

**Bilicanta** *Roche, Spain.*
Hymecromone (p.1700·1).
*Biliary-tract disorders.*

**Bilicante** *Monot, Fr.†.*
Hymecromone (p.1700·1).

**Bilicura Forte** *Muller Goppingen, Ger.†.*
Kava (p.1703·2); cynara (p.1678·3).
*Biliary disorders; dyspepsia.*

**Bilidren** *Lafage, Arg.*
Cascara (p.1255·1); cynara (p.1678·3); bile salts (p.1660·3).
*Biliary-tract disorders.*

**Biliepar** *Ibirn, Ital.*
Ursodeoxycholic acid (p.1760·3).
*Biliary dyspepsia; gallstones.*

**Bilifel** *Neckerman, Braz.†.*
Cascara (p.1255·1); boldo (p.1661·2); rhubarb (p.1287·3); fig (p.1266·3).
*Constipation.*

**Bilifluine** *Promedica, Fr.†.*
Depigmented and decholesterolised ox bile (p.1660·3); sodium oleate (p.1574·3).
*Constipation; dyspepsia.*

**Biliflux** *Eurofarma, Braz.*
Diisopromine hydrochloride (p.1261·2); sorbitol (p.1446·3).
*Liver disorders.*

**Bilifuge** *Plan, Switz.*
Cynara (p.1678·3); berberis vulgaris; java tea (p.1702·3); kinkeliba (p.1703·3).
*Digestive disorders.*

**Biligrama** *Schering, Braz.†.*
Meglumine ioglicate (p.1064·1).
*Contrast medium for biliary-tract radiography.*

**Bili-Labstix**
*Bayer Diagnostics, Irl.†; Bayer Diagnostici, Ital.; Bayer Diagnostics, UK†; Bayer, USA.*
Test for pH, protein, glucose, ketones, bilirubin, and blood in urine.

**Bilina** *Esteve, Spain.*
Levocabastine hydrochloride (p.435·2).
*Allergic conjunctivitis; allergic rhinitis.*

**Biliosan Compuesto** *Hexa-Medinova, Arg.*
Carqueja; boldo (p.1661·2); cynara (p.1678·3); bile salts (p.1660·3); homatropine methylbromide (p.483·2); peppermint oil (p.1283·2).
*Biliary-tract disorders; digestive disorders.*

**Bilipax** *Taphlan, Switz.*
Naphthylacetic acid (p.1719·1); methylphenylethyl nicotinate.
*Adjuvant in cholangiography; digestive disorders.*

**Bilipeptal Mono** *Evisco, Ger.*
Pancreatin (p.1725·3).
*Pancreatic insufficiency.*

**Biliranin** *Pharmaten (Φαρματεν), Gr.*
Loratadine (p.436·1).
*Allergic rhinitis; pruritus.*

**Bilisan C3** *Repha, Ger.†.*
Silybum marianum (p.1043·3); greater celandine (p.1695·3); Javanese turmeric (p.1759·3).
*Biliary disorders; gallstones; liver disorders.*

**Bilisan Duo** *Repha, Ger.*
Silybum marianum (p.1043·3); Javanese turmeric (p.1759·3).
*Biliary-tract disorders; dyspepsia; liver disorders.*

**Biliscopin**
*Schering, Austral.; Schering, Austria; Schering, Braz.†; Schering, Ger.; Schering, NZ; Schering, Swed.; Schering, Switz.; Schering, UK.*
Meglumine iotroxate (p.1066·1).
*Contrast medium for biliary-tract radiography.*

**Bilisegrol** *Schering, Spain.*
Meglumine iotroxate (p.1066·1).
*Contrast medium for biliary-tract radiography.*

**Bilkaby** *Bailly, Fr.†.*
Menadione (p.1466·3); bile salts (p.1660·3).
*Haemorrhagic disorders due to vitamin K deficiency.*

**Billerol** *Lehning, Fr.*
Homoeopathic preparation.

**Biloban** *Cipan, Port.*
Ginkgo biloba (p.1692·3).
*Vascular disorders.*

**Bilobene**
*Ratiopharm, Austria; Merckle, Ger.*
Fumitory (p.1690·1).
*Biliary-tract disorders.*

**Biloina** *Andromaco, Arg.*
Loratadine (p.436·1).
*Hypersensitivity reactions.*

**Bilol** *Ecosol, Switz.*
Bisoprolol fumarate (p.875·1).
*Angina pectoris; hyperkinetic heart syndrome; hypertension.*

**Bilopaque** *Nycomed, USA†.*
Sodium tyropanoate (p.1067·3).
*Radiographic contrast medium for cholecystography.*

**Biloptin**
*Schering, Austria†; Schering, Ger.†; Schering, Port.†; Schering, S.Afr.†; Schering, Switz.†; Schering, UK.*
Sodium iopodate (p.1065·2).
*Contrast medium for biliary-tract radiography.*

**Bilron** *Aspen, S.Afr.*
Iron bile salts (p.1660·3).
*Bile salt deficiency; biliary-tract disorders.*

**Bilsan** *Abbott, Hong Kong.*
Choline bicitrate (p.1424·3); inositol (p.1701·2); methionine (p.1042·1); vitamin B substances (p.1417·1); dehydrocholic acid (p.1679·2); ox bile (p.1660·3).
*Biliary disorders; liver disorders.*

**Biltricide**
*Bayer, Austral.; Bayer, Canad.; Bayer, Fr.; Bayer, Ger.; IFET (ΙΦΕΤ), Gr.; Bayer, Hong Kong; Bayer, Israel; Bayer, Neth.; Bayer, S.Afr.; Bayer, Thai.†; Bayer, USA.*
Praziquantel (p.112·2).
*Worm infections.*

**Biluen Enzimatico** *Byk, Arg.*
Azintamide (p.1658·3); pancreatin (p.1725·3); cellulase (p.1669·1); simeticone (p.1289·2).
*Liver and biliary-tract disorders.*

**Bilugen**
*Roche Diagnostics, Austral.; Boehringer Mannheim Diagnostics, Irl.†; Roche Diagnostics, UK†.*
Test for urobilinogen and bilirubin in urine.

**Bim** *Elvetium, Arg.*
Bacteria; muramidase hydrochloride (p.1717·2).
*Respiratory-tract infections.*

**Bimicot** *Euroderm, Arg.*
Bifonazole (p.395·1).
*Fungal skin infections.*

**Bi-Miotic** *Bell, India.*
Pilocarpine nitrate (p.1495·1); physostigmine salicylate (p.1494·1).
*Glaucoma.*

**Bimixin** *Sanofi Synthelabo, Ital.*
Bacitracin (p.161·3); neomycin sulfate (p.235·1).
*Enteric infections.*

**Bimolin** *Drugtech, Chile.*
Pemoline (p.1591·2).

**Binaldan** *Vifor, Switz.*
Loperamide hydrochloride (p.1271·1).
*Diarrhoea.*

**Bindazac** *Norma (Νορμα), Gr.*
Ranitidine hydrochloride (p.1285·2).
*Conditions where gastric acid reduction is beneficial; gastric hypersecretion including Zollinger-Ellison syndrome; peptic ulcer.*

**Bi-Nerisona**
*Schering, Braz.; Schering, Chile; Schering, Mex.*
Diflucortolone valerate (p.1099·3); chlorquinaldol (p.187·3).
*Infected skin disorders.*

**Biniwas** *Chiesi, Spain.*
Binifibrate (p.875·1).
*Hyperlipidaemias.*

**Binoctrin** *Cazi, Braz.*
Co-trimoxazole (p.199·3).
*Bacterial infections; Pneumocystis carinii pneumonia; protozoal infections.*

**Binodian** *Schering, Mex.*
Estradiol valerate (p.1550·2); prasterone enantate (p.1565·3).
*Menopausal disorders.*

**Binopen** *Cazi, Braz.†.*
Ampicillin (p.157·1).
*Bacterial infections.*

**Binordiol**
*Wyeth Lederle, Belg.; Wyeth, Neth.†; Wyeth, Switz.*
Levonorgestrel (p.1563·2); ethinylestradiol (p.1553·2).
*Biphasic oral contraceptive; menstrual disorders.*

**Binospan Composto** *Cazi, Braz.*
Hyoscine butylbromide (p.483·3); dipyrone (p.35·3).

**Binotal**
*Bayer, Braz.; Grunenthal, Ger.; Bayer, Mex.*
Ampicillin sodium (p.157·1) or ampicillin trihydrate (p.157·2).
*Bacterial infections.*

**Binotine** *Farmalab, Braz.†.*
Ampicillin benzathine (p.158·1); ampicillin sodium (p.157·1).
*Bacterial infections.*

**Binotine Balsamico** *Farmalab, Braz.†.*
Ampicillin benzathine (p.158·1); sodium camsilate; guaifenesin (p.1122·1); cineole (p.1672·1); niaouli oil (p.1719·3).
*Bacterial infections.*

**Binovum**
*Janssen-Cilag, Irl.†; Janssen-Cilag, UK.*
Norethisterone (p.1562·2); ethinylestradiol (p.1553·2).
*Biphasic oral contraceptive.*

**B-Insulin** *Berlin-Chemie, Ger.†.*
Insulin injection (pork) (p.333·3).
*Diabetes mellitus.*

**Binvex** *Armstrong, Arg.*
Pargeverine hydrochloride (p.487·3); dihydroxydibutylether (p.1680·2).
*Liver and biliary-tract disorders.*

**Bio²** *Bio2, Fr.†.*
Protein, fibre, and vitamin preparation (p.1417·1).
*Low body weight.*

**Bio-200** *Dermofarma, Ital.*
Royal jelly (p.1740·3); pollen.
*Nutritional supplement.*

**Bio Ace** *Blackmores, Austral.†.*
Betacarotene; ascorbic acid; *d*-alpha tocoferil acid succinate; vitamin $B_1$; calcium pantothenate; vitamin $B_6$; vitamin $K_3$; zinc; ginseng; garlic (p.1417·1).
*Tonic.*

**Bio Ace Excell** *Blackmores, Austral.†.*
Vitis vinifera; silybum marianum; betacarotene; vitamin C; *d*-alpha tocopherol; calcium pantothenate; vitamin $B_6$; zinc; vitamin $B_{12}$; folic acid; thiamine nitrate (p.1417·1).
*Tonic.*

**Bio Acidophilus** *Bioceuticals, UK.*
*Lactobacillus acidophilus* (p.1704·2).

**Bio C** *Blackmores, Austral.†.*
Ascorbic acid (p.1460·2); sodium ascorbate (p.1460·2); calcium ascorbate (p.1460·2); bioflavonoids (p.1688·2); rutoside (p.1688·2); hesperidin (p.1688·2); rose fruit (p.1740·1); acerola.
*Vitamin C supplement.*

**Bio Cabal** *Dallas, Arg.*
Dexamethasone (p.1097·1); astemizole (p.424·2).
*Hypersensitivity reactions.*

**Bio E**
*Blackmores, Austral.†; Bio-Health, UK†.*
Vitamin E (p.1464·3).

**Bio Enhaced Natural E** *Nutrition Care, Austral.†.*
*d*-Alpha tocopherol (p.1464·3).
*Vitamin E deficiency.*

**Bio Equisan** *Hexal, Austria.*
Equisetum (p.1684·1).
*Diuretic.*

**Bio Espectrum** *Centrum, Spain†.*
Ampicillin sodium (p.157·1); ampicillin benzathine (p.158·1); bromhexine (p.1115·3).
Lidocaine hydrochloride (p.1377·3) is included in this preparation to alleviate the pain of injection.
*Respiratory-tract infections.*

**Bio Eutrical** *Crinos, Ital.†.*
An amino-acid preparation with vitamins and minerals (p.1417·1).
*Nutritional supplement.*

**Bio Flora** *DermoDuemila, Ital.*
Lactic-acid-producing organisms (p.1704·2); vitamins; minerals (p.1417·1).
*Gastrointestinal disorders.*

**Bio Gelin** *Northia, Arg.*
Chloramphenicol (p.185·1).
*Bacterial infections.*

**Bio Grip C** *Gramon, Arg.*
Aspirin (p.15·1); ascorbic acid (p.1460·2).
*Cold symptoms.*

**Bio Grip Plus** *Gramon, Arg.*
Paracetamol (p.76·2); phenylephrine hydrochloride (p.1126·3); pentoxyverine citrate (p.1126·2); ascorbic acid (p.1460·2); vitamin $B_1$.
*Cold and influenza symptoms.*

**Bio Magnesium** *Blackmores, Austral.†.*
Magnesium (p.1227·3); calcium ascorbate (p.1460·2); vitamin $B_6$ (p.1456·3); colecalciferol (p.1461·3); manganese (p.1440·1).
*Muscle cramps.*

**Bio Slim Silueta** *Natrahealth, UK.*
Poliglusam.
*Slimming aid.*

**Bio Star** *Novag, Spain.*
Ginseng (p.1693·1).
*Tonic.*

**Bio Tarbun** *Duncan, Arg.*
Norfloxacin (p.238·3).
*Bacterial infections.*

**Bio Tears** *Maurino, Arg.*
Polyvinyl alcohol (p.1581·1).
*Dry eyes.*

**Bio Zinc** *Blackmores, Austral.†.*
Multivitamin and mineral preparation (p.1417·1).
*Skin disorders; wounds.*

**Bio-Acerola C Complex** *Solgar, UK†.*
Vitamin C with bioflavonoids (p.1417·1).

**Bioact-D** *Lafepe, Braz.†.*
Dactinomycin (p.545·1).
*Malignant neoplasms.*

**Bioactiv** *Knop, Chile.*
A range of homoeopathic preparations.

**Bioagil** *Merck, Austria†.*
Ascorbic acid (p.1460·2).
*Vitamin C deficiency.*

**Bioaler** *Giscard, Arg.*
Loratadine (p.436·1).
*Hypersensitivity reactions.*

**Bio-Amoksiclav** *Biotech, S.Afr.*
Amoxicillin (p.155·3); clavulanic acid (p.193·3).
*Bacterial infections.*

**Bio-Antioxydant** *Pharma Nord, Fr.*
Vitamin and mineral preparation (p.1417·1).
*Antoxidant.*

**Bioarginina** *Damor, Ital.*
Arginine hydrochloride (p.1421·1).
*Asthenia; hyperammonaemia.*

**Bio-Arscolloid** *SIT, Ital.*
Dichlorobenzyl alcohol (p.1178·3); silver protein (p.1746·2); tyrothricin (p.275·1).
*Bacterial mouth infections.*

**Bio-Ascorbate** *Solgar, UK†.*
Vitamin C with bioflavonoids (p.1417·1).

**Biobalm** *Modern Health Products, UK†.*
Slippery elm bark (p.1747·1); althaea root (p.1651·3); chondrus (p.1578·2).
*Gastrointestinal disorders.*

**Bioband** *Corbridge, Austral.†.*
Triclosan (p.1195·2).
*Medicated bandage; ulcers; wounds.*

**Biobase** *Odan, Canad.*
Alcohol (p.1166·1); (+)-cetyl steryl ethylene oxide.
*Antiseptic vehicle for topical preparations.*

**Biobase-G** *Odan, Canad.*
Alcohol (p.1166·1); glycolic acid (p.1147·3).
*Antiseptic vehicle for topical preparations.*

**Biobees** *Bioceuticals, UK.*
A range of preparations containing royal jelly (p.1740·3).

**Bio-Biol** *Searle, Ital.†.*
Vitamin B substances (p.1417·1); coenzyme A (p.1674·3).
*Vitamin deficiency.*

**Bio-C**
*Pharma Nord, Norw.; Pharma Nord, Thai.*
Calcium ascorbate (p.1460·2).
*Vitamin C deficiency.*

**Bio-C A Vogel** *Bioforce, Switz.†.*
Vitamin C preparation (p.1417·1).

**Bio-C Complex** *Blackmores, Austral.†.*
Ascorbic acid (p.1460·2); sodium ascorbate (p.1460·2); calcium ascorbate (p.1460·2); lemon bioflavonoids (p.1688·2); rutoside (p.1688·2); hesperidin (p.1688·2); acerola.
*Vitamin C preparation.*

**Biocadmio** *Uriach, Spain.*
Cadmium sulfide (p.1663·3).
*Skin and scalp disorders.*

**Biocalcin** *Esseti, Ital.*
Calcitonin (salmon) (p.768·2).
*Hypercalcaemia; osteoporosis; Paget's disease of bone; sympathetic pain syndrome.*

**Biocalcio** *Sedabel, Braz.*
Calcium phosphate; cyanocobalamin; ergocalciferol; sodium fluoride; sodium iodide (p.1417·1).
*Vitamin and mineral supplement.*

**Biocalcium** *Bioprogress, Ital.*
Calcium carbonate (p.1254·2).
*Calcium deficiency.*

**Bio-Calcium + $D_3$** *Pharma Nord, Irl.*
Calcium (p.1225·1); magnesium (p.1227·3); colecalciferol (p.1461·3).
*Calcium deficiency.*

**Bio-Calcium + $D_3$ + K** *Pharma Nord, Irl.*
Calcium (p.1225·1); colecalciferol (p.1461·3); vitamin K (p.1466·3).

**Biocalm**
*Note. This name is used for preparations of different composition.*
*Lizofarm, Ital.*
Valerian (p.1762·2); passion flower (p.1729·1); peppermint leaf (p.1283·2).
*Insomnia.*

*Biolab, Thai.*
Tolperisone hydrochloride (p.1396·3).
*Obliterative vascular diseases; parkinsonism; skeletal muscle spasticity and spasm.*

**Biocalron** *Biomedis, Thai.; Great Eastern, Thai.*
Calcium lactate (p.1225·3); ferrous fumarate (p.1427·3); vitamin C (p.1460·2); rutoside (p.1688·2).

**Biocalyptol**
*Note. This name is used for preparations of different composition.*
*Zambon, Fr.*
Pholcodine (p.1128·3).
Formerly contained pholcodine, cineole, and guaiacol.
*Coughs.*

*Laphal, Hong Kong.*
Pholcodine (p.1128·3); cineole (p.1672·1); guaiacol (p.1122·1).
*Coughs.*

**Bio-Caps**
*Infabra, Braz.†; Bio-Health, UK.*
Multivitamin and mineral preparation (p.1417·1).

**Biocarbo** *Biosintetica, Braz.*
Carboplatin (p.533·3).
*Malignant neoplasms.*

**Biocarbon** *Trenka, Austria.*
Activated charcoal (p.1030·2).
*Diarrhoea; flatulence.*

**Biocarde** *Lehning, Fr.*
Crataegus (p.1677·1); passion flower (p.1729·1); avena (p.1658·2); valerian (p.1762·2); melissa (p.1711·1); motherwort (p.1717·1).
*Insomnia; nervous disorders.*

**Biocarn** *Medice, Ger.*
Levocarnitine (p.1423·3).
*Carnitine deficiency.*

**Biocarnil** *Abiogen, Ital.*
Carnitine hydrochloride (p.1424·1); L-lysine hydrochloride (p.1439·2).
*Carnitine deficiency.*

**Biocarotine** *Bioceuticals, UK.*
Betacarotene (p.1422·3).

**Biocatalase** *Fournier SA, Spain.*
Catalase (p.1668·3).
*Burns; skin disorders; ulcers; wounds.*

**Bioceanat** *Plantes Tropicales, Fr.†.*
Sea water; copper gluconate (p.1425·3).
*Nasal irrigation.*

**Biocebe** *Nutergia, Fr.*
Vitamin, bioflavonoid, and zinc preparation (p.1417·1).
*Nutritional supplement.*

**Biocef**
*Note. This name is used for preparations of different composition.*
*Biochemie, Austria.*
Cefpodoxime proxetil (p.178·3).
*Bacterial infections.*

*Zambon, Spain.*
Ceftibuten (p.182·1).
*Bacterial infections.*

*International Ethical, USA.*
Cefalexin (p.168·1).
*Bacterial infections.*

**Bio-Cest** *Bioresearch, Mex.*
Praziquantel (p.112·2).
*Cysticercosis.*

**Biochetasi** *Sigma-Tau, Ital.*
*Injection; suppositories; effervescent tablets:* Vitamin B substances and electrolytes (p.1417·1).
*Oral granules:* Vitamin B substances, electrolytes, and carbohydrate (p.1417·1).
*Fluid and electrolyte disorders; liver disorders.*

**Biochin** *Biolab, Thai.*
Neomycin sulfate (p.235·1); bacitracin zinc (p.161·3); amylocaine hydrochloride (p.1370·2).
*Mouth and throat disorders.*

**Bio-Chrome**
*Note. This name is used for preparations of different composition.*
*Sante Naturelle, Canad.*
Chromium (p.1425·1).

*Herbaxt, Fr.†.*
Chromium (p.1425·1) from *Saccharomyces cerevisiae*; nicotinamide (p.1441·2).
*Nutritional supplement.*

**Bio-Chromium** *Blackmores, Austral.†.*
Dried yeast (p.1469·1); chromium amino acid chelate (p.1425·1); manganese amino acid chelate (p.1440·2); nicotinamide (p.1441·2); magnesium phosphate (p.1228·1); dibasic potassium phosphate (p.1230·3); zinc amino acid chelate (p.1469·3).
*Alcoholism; hyperglycaemia; hypoglycaemia; sugar cravings.*

**Bio-Ci** *Ceccarelli, Ital.*
Ascorbic acid (p.1460·2).
*Vitamin C deficiency.*

**Biociclin** *Francia, Ital.*
Cefuroxime sodium (p.184·1).
*Bacterial infections.*

**Biocid** *Biochem, India.*
Omeprazole (p.1278·2).
*Gastro-oesophageal reflux; peptic ulcer; Zollinger-Ellison syndrome.*

**Biocidan** *Menarini, Fr.*
*Eye drops:* Cethexonium bromide (p.1172·1).
*Minor eye infections.*
*Nasal spray:* Cethexonium bromide (p.1172·1); phenyltoloxamine citrate (p.439·1).
*Nose and throat disorders.*

**Biocil**
*Note. This name is used for preparations of different composition.*
*Ibirn, Ital.*
Cefonicid sodium (p.174·2).
Lidocaine hydrochloride (p.1377·3) is included in this preparation to alleviate the pain of injection.
*Bacterial infections.*

*Raza, Malaysia; Pharmaniaga, Malaysia.*
Ampicillin trihydrate (p.157·2).
*Bacterial infections.*

*Formula, NZ.*
Povidone-iodine (p.1190·3).
*Herpes labialis; minor cuts and burns; skin disinfection.*

**Biocilin** *Biochem, India.*
Ampicillin (p.157·1) or ampicillin trihydrate (p.157·2).
*Bacterial infections.*

**Biocin**
*Note. This name is used for preparations of different composition.*
*Ibirn, Ital.†.*
Fosfomycin calcium (p.214·2).
*Bacterial infections.*

*Atral, Port.*
Doxycycline (p.206·2).
*Bacterial infections.*

**Biocine Test** *Biovac, S.Afr.*
Tuberculin (p.1759·1).
*Diagnosis of tuberculosis.*

**Biocine Test PPD** *Chiron Vaccines, Ital.*
Tuberculin purified protein derivative (p.1759·1).
*Test for hypersensitivity to tubercle bacillus.*

**Biocitronil** *SMB, Chile.*
Bifonazole (p.395·1).
*Fungal skin infections.*

**Bioclaril** *GNR, Ital.*
Heparin calcium (p.927·3).
*Thromboembolic disorders.*

**Bioclate**
*Centeon, Denm.†; Centeon, Ger.†; Centeon, Spain†; Centeon, UK†; Armour, USA.*
A factor VIII preparation (p.751·1).
*Haemophilia A.*

**Bioclavid**
*Biochemie, Denm.; Biochemie, Fin.; Novartis, Gr.*
Amoxicillin trihydrate (p.155·3); potassium clavulanate (p.193·3).
*Bacterial infections.*

**Bioclin Kera** *Dermoteca, Port.*
Borage; cystine; glycine; zinc gluconate; methionine; arginine; cucurbita; vitis vinifera; calcium pantothenate; biotin; copper gluconate (p.1417·1).
*Hair and nail disorders.*

**Bioclin Sebo Care** *Dermoteca, Port.*
*Capsules:* Borage oil (p.1661·3); Iceland moss; zinc (p.1469·2); cucurbita oil (p.1677·3).
*Seborrhoea.*
*Topical gel:* Glycolic acid (p.1147·3); piroctone olamine (p.1155·2); salicylic acid (p.1157·1); lactic acid (p.1704·1).
*Acne.*

**Bioclox** *Biochem, India.*
Cloxacillin sodium (p.198·2).
*Gram-positive bacterial infections.*

**Biocobal** *Lemery, Mex.*
Hydroxocobalamin (p.1458·2).
*Anaemias; neuritis.*

**Biocodone** *UCB, Belg.*
Hydrocodone bitartrate (p.45·1).
*Coughs.*

**Biocol** *Bio-Transfusion, Fr.†.*
1 Vial, fibrinogen (p.753·2); fibronectin (p.1688·1); factor XIII (p.753·1); 1 syringe, aprotinin (p.742·3); 1 vial, thrombin (p.760·1); calcium chloride (p.1225·1). On mixing this forms a fibrin glue (p.753·1).
*Haemorrhage.*

**Bioconseils** *Yves Ponroy, Fr.†.*
A range of herbal preparations.

**Biocord**
*Note. This name is used for preparations of different composition.*
*Biosintetica, Braz.†.*
Nifedipine (p.966·2).
*Angina pectoris; hypertension; Raynaud's syndrome.*

*Medipharm, Chile.*
Vitamins; minerals; ginseng; soya lecithin; procaine hydrochloride; rutin (p.1417·1).
*Tonic.*

**Biocort** *Salters, S.Afr.†.*
Hydrocortisone acetate (p.1103·3).
*Skin disorders.*

**Biocortin** *Eczane, Arg.*
Hydrocortisone (p.1103·3); neomycin (p.235·1); tetryzoline (p.1131·2).
*Eye disorders.*

**Biocoryl** *Uriach, Spain.*
Procainamide hydrochloride (p.987·1).
*Arrhythmias.*

**Biocos** *APS, Ger.*
Metformin hydrochloride (p.342·3).
*Diabetes mellitus.*

**BioCox** *Iatric, USA†.*
Coccidioidin (p.1674·1).
*Skin test for coccidioidomycosis.*

**Biocream** *BritHealth, UK†.*
Tissue salts; terpineol (p.1752·2); germall.
*Skin disorders.*

**Biocrinal** *Sofex, Port.*
Minoxidil (p.960·1).
*Alopecia androgenetica.*

**Biocrist** *Biosintetica, Braz.*
Vincristine sulfate (p.592·2).
*Malignant neoplasms.*

**Bio-Cuivre** *Herbaxt, Fr.*
Copper pidolate; manganese pidolate (p.1417·1).
*Nutritional supplement.*

**Bio-C-Vitamin** *Pharma Nord, Fin.*
Calcium ascorbate (p.1460·2).
*Vitamin C deficiency; vitamin C supplement.*

**Biocyclin** *Biochemie, Austria.*
Doxycycline hyclate (p.206·2).
*Bacterial and protozoal infections.*

**BioCyst** *CytoChemia, Ger.*
Birch leaf (p.1660·3); solidago virgaurea (p.1748·3); java tea (p.1702·3).
*Urinary-tract disorders.*

**Bio-Dac** *Bioresearch, Mex.*
Sulindac (p.91·2).
*Inflammation.*

**Biodalgic** *Biocodex, Fr.*
Tramadol hydrochloride (p.94·3).
*Pain.*

**Biodan**
*Note. This name is used for preparations of different composition.*
*Bioresearch, Mex.*
Phenytoin sodium (p.370·2).
*Epilepsy.*

*Biomedis, Thai.; Great Eastern, Thai.*
Sulfaguanidine (p.260·3); activated charcoal (p.1030·2); bismuth subcarbonate (p.1252·1); pectin (p.1580·3); dicycloverine hydrochloride (p.481·2).
*Diarrhoea.*

**Bioday** *Biocur, Ger.†.*
Guarana (p.1765·3).
*Fatigue.*

**Bio-Delta Cortilen** *SIFI, Ital.*
Prednisolone acetate (p.1108·1); neomycin sulfate (p.235·1).
*Eye infections.*

**Bioderm** *Odan, Canad.*
Polymyxin B sulfate (p.245·1); bacitracin (p.161·3).
*Bacterial infections.*

**Biodermatin** *Lafare, Ital.*
Biotin (p.1423·2).
*Skin disorders.*

**Biodexan** *Sophia, Mex.*
Dexamethasone sodium phosphate (p.1097·2); neomycin sulfate (p.235·1); polymyxin B sulfate (p.245·1); phenylephrine hydrochloride (p.1126·3).
*Eye disorders.*

**Biodexin** *Silesia, Chile.*
Bacitracin (p.161·3); neomycin sulfate (p.235·1); zinc oxide (p.1163·2).
*Infected burns, ulcers, and wounds; skin infections.*

**Biodezil** *Bioresearch, Mex.*
Captopril (p.879·2).
*Hypertension.*

**Biodif** *Bago, Chile.*
Betacarotene; vitamin E; vitamin C; minerals (p.1417·1).

**Biodinam** *Roux-Ocefa, Arg.*
Vitamin and trace element preparation (p.1417·1).

**Biodine** *Major, USA.*
Povidone-iodine (p.1190·3).
*Skin disinfection.*

**Bio-Disc** *Blackmores, Austral.†.*
Minerals; vitamins (p.1417·1); silicon dioxide (p.1581·3); bromelains (p.1662·2); papain (p.1727·3).
*Delayed bone healing; muscular and joint pain.*

**Biodone** *McGaw Biomed, NZ.*
Methadone hydrochloride (p.57·2).
*Opioid withdrawal syndrome.*

**Biodone Forte** *Biomed, Austral.*
Methadone hydrochloride (p.57·2).
*Opioid dependence.*

**Biodophilus** *Bioceuticals, UK.*
*Lactobacillus acidophilus* (p.1704·2).

**Biodoxi** *Biochem, India.*
Doxycycline (p.206·2).
*Bacterial infections.*

**Biodramina** *Uriach, Spain.*
Dimenhydrinate (p.431·1).
*Motion sickness.*

**Biodramina Cafeina** *Uriach, Spain.*
Caffeine (p.782·1); dimenhydrinate (p.431·1); pyridoxine hydrochloride (p.1456·3).
*Motion sickness; vertigo.*

**Biodrop** *Sidus, Arg.*
Dorzolamide hydrochloride (p.908·3).
*Glaucoma; ocular hypertension.*

**Biodroxil**
*Biochemie, Austria; Novartis, Chile; Biochemie, Hong Kong; Biochemie, Israel; Biochemie, Singapore†.*
Cefadroxil (p.167·2).
*Bacterial infections.*

**Bio-E** *Pharma Nord, Thai.*
*d*-Alpha tocoferil acetate (p.1465·1).
*Vitamin E deficiency.*

**Bio-Energol Plus** *Yabrofarma, Port.*
Arginine aspartate (p.1421·1).
*Tonic.*

**Bioenterine** *DB, Fr.*
Nutritional supplement (p.1417·1).
*Maintenance of gastrointestinal flora.*

**Bioequiseto** *Cabassi, Ital.*
Equisetum (p.1684·1).
*Nutritional supplement.*

**Bioesse Plus** *Mavi, Ital.*
Amino acids; biotin; selenium; saw palmetto (p.1417·1).
*Nutritional supplement.*

**Bio-E-Vitamin**
*Pharma Nord, Fin.; Pharma Nord, Norw.*
*d*-Alpha tocopherol (p.1464·3).
*Vitamin E deficiency.*

**Biofanal** *Pfleger, Ger.*
Nystatin (p.406·3).
*Candidiasis.*

**Biofax** *Maver, Chile.*
Vitamin E; betacarotene; vitamin C; selenium; zinc gluconate (p.1417·1).

**Biofaxil** *Lepori, Port.*
Cefadroxil (p.167·2).
*Bacterial infections.*

**Biofem**
*Note. This name is used for preparations of different composition.*
*Biotenk, Arg.*
Raloxifene (p.1568·3).
*Osteoporosis.*

*Biocur, Ger.*
Vitex agnus castus (p.1649·1).
*Mastalgia; menstrual disorders.*

**Biofenac**
*Note. This name is used for preparations of different composition.*
*UCB, Belg.; UCB, Gr.; Almirall, Neth.; UCB, Port.*
Aceclofenac (p.11·2).
*Inflammation; musculoskeletal, joint, and peri-articular disorders; pain.*

*Ache, Braz.*
Diclofenac diethylamine (p.32·1), diclofenac resinate (p.33·1), or diclofenac sodium (p.32·1).
*Gout; inflammation; musculoskeletal, joint, and peri-articular disorders; pain.*

**Bio-Fer** *Herbaxt, Fr.*
Iron pidolate; folic acid; ascorbic acid (p.1417·1).
*Nutritional supplement.*

**Bioferal** *Bioprogress, Ital.*
Ferrous gluconate (p.1428·1).
Ascorbic acid (p.1460·2) is included in this preparation to increase the absorption and availability of iron.
*Iron-deficiency anaemia.*

**Bioferina** *Bioresearch, Mex.*
Phenazopyridine (p.83·2).
*Urinary-tract infections.*

**Bioferon**
*Sidus, Arg.; Bio Sidus, Thai.*
Interferon alfa-2b (p.640·3).
*Anogenital warts; hepatitis; malignant neoplasms.*

**Bioferon Hepakit** *Sidus, Arg.*
Capsules, ribavirin (p.652·1); injection, interferon alfa-2b (recombinant) (p.640·3).
*Chronic hepatitis C.*

**Bioferro** *Prospa, Port.*
Ferrous gluconate (p.1428·1).
*Iron-deficiency anaemia.*

**Biofiber** *Enila, Braz.*
Guar gum (p.333·2).

**Biofibra** *Pfizer Consumer, Spain†.*
Wheat bran; pectins; oligo-fructose (p.1417·1).
*Dietary fibre supplement.*

**Biofigado** *Simoes, Braz.†.*
Adenosine (p.851·2); methionine (p.1042·1); betaine sodium (p.1660·2); choline citrate (p.1424·3); pyridoxine hydrochloride (p.1456·3); sorbitol (p.1446·3).
*Liver disorders.*

**Biofilm** *Braun, UK.*
Hydrocolloid dressing.
*Ulcers; wounds.*

**Biofim** *Uniao Quimica, Braz.†.*
14 Tablets, mestranol (p.1559·2); 7 tablets, norethisterone (p.1562·2); mestranol; 7 tablets, inert.
*Biphasic oral contraceptive.*

**Bioflac** *Cristalia, Braz.*
Meloxicam (p.56·1).
*Osteoarthritis; rheumatoid arthritis.*

**Bioflam** *Rider, Chile.*
Tenoxicam (p.93·1).
*Gout; musculoskeletal, joint, peri-articular, and soft-tissue disorders.*

**Bioflex** *Rottapharm, Chile.*
Glucosamine sulfate (p.1694·1).
Lidocaine hydrochloride (p.1377·3) is included in the injection to alleviate the pain of injection.
*Degenerative joint disorders.*

**Bioflogil** *Spedrog, Arg.*
Chondroitin sulfate sodium (p.1670·2).
*Osteoarthritis.*

**Bioflor** *Biocodex, Hong Kong.*
*Saccharomyces boulardii* (p.1704·2).
*Diarrhoea; irritable bowel syndrome.*

**Bio-Flora** *Maver, Chile.*
Saccharomyces boulardii (p.1704·2).
*Diarrhoea.*

**Bioflorin**
*Note. This name is used for preparations of different composition.*
*Sanova, Austria.*
Live *Enterococcus faecium* (p.1704·2).
*Gastrointestinal disorders.*

*Hebron, Braz.*
*Saccharomyces cerevisiae* (p.1469·1).
*Diarrhoea; restoration of gastrointestinal flora.*

*Sanofi Synthelabo, Ital.; Sanofi Synthelabo, Switz.*
Lactic-acid-producing enterococci (p.1704·2).
*Gastrointestinal disorders.*

**Bioflox** *Bioresearch, Mex.*
Ciprofloxacin (p.188·2).
*Bacterial infections.*

**Biofloxin** *Biochem, India.*
Norfloxacin (p.238·3).
*Bacterial diarrhoea; gonorrhoea; urinary-tract infections.*

**Biofluor** *Distrifarma, Port.*
Chlorhexidine gluconate (p.1173·2); sodium fluoride (p.1444·3).
*Oral hygiene.*

**Biofluor Sensitive** *Distrifarma, Port.*
Potassium nitrate (p.1190·1); cetylpyridinium chloride (p.1173·1); sodium fluoride (p.1444·3).
*Gingivitis; sensitive teeth.*

**Bioflusin** *Bioresearch, Mex.*
Paracetamol (p.76·2); caffeine (p.782·1); phenylephrine hydrochloride (p.1126·3); chlorphenamine maleate (p.427·3).
Formerly contained chlorphenamine.
*Hay fever.*

**Bioflutin-N** *Sudmedica, Ger.*
Etilefrine hydrochloride (p.914·1).
*Hypotension.*

**Biofolic** *Esseti, Ital.*
Calcium methyltetrahydrofolate (p.1431·2).
*Antidote to folic acid antagonists; folic acid deficiency; reduction of aminopterin and methotrexate toxicity.*

**Bioform** *Salters, S.Afr.†.*
Clioquinol (p.196·3).
*Fungal and bacterial skin infections.*

**Biofreeze** *Lane, UK.*
Menthol (p.1711·3); maté (p.1765·3).
*Musculoskeletal and joint pain.*

**Biofructose** *Bunker, Braz.*
Vitamin B substances, ascorbic acid, and fructose (p.1417·1).

**Biofurex** *KBR, Ital.*
Cefuroxime sodium (p.184·1).
*Bacterial infections.*

**Biofurin** *Bioresearch, Mex.*
Nitrofurantoin (p.237·2).
*Urinary-tract infections.*

**Biofuroso** *Bioresearch, Mex.*
Ferrous fumarate (p.1427·3).
*Iron deficiency anaemia.*

**Biogam** *Biogam, Switz.*
Trace element preparations (p.1417·1).

**Biogaracin** *Biochem, India.*
Gentamicin sulfate (p.217·1).
*Bacterial infections.*

**Biogardol** *Biophytarom, Fr.†.*
Vitamin E; betacarotene; vitamin C (p.1417·1).

**Bio-Garten Entschlackungstee** *Bio-Garten, Austria.*
Birch leaf (p.1660·3); taraxacum leaf (p.1751·3); prunus spinosa; rose fruit (p.1740·1); sambucus (p.1741·3); calendula (p.1665·2).
*Herbal preparation.*

**Bio-Garten Tee fur den Magen** *Bio-Garten, Austria.*
Chamomile (p.1669·3); peppermint leaf (p.1283·2); caraway (p.1667·2); valerian (p.1762·2).
*Gastrointestinal disorders.*

**Bio-Garten Tee fur Leber und Galle** *Bio-Garten, Austria.*
Absinthium (p.1645·1); calamus (p.1664·1); angelica (p.1655·1); peppermint leaf (p.1283·2); bitter-orange leaf (p.1723·3).
*Liver and gallbladder disorders.*

**Bio-Garten Tee fur Niere und Blase** *Bio-Garten, Austria.*
Bearberry (p.1659·2); equisetum (p.1684·1); birch leaf (p.1660·3).
*Kidney and bladder disorders.*

**Bio-Garten Tee gegen Blahungen** *Bio-Garten, Austria.*
Fennel (p.1687·2); chamomile (p.1669·3); caraway (p.1667·2); achillea (p.1646·2); peppermint leaf (p.1283·2).
*Flatulence.*

**Bio-Garten Tee gegen Durchfall** *Bio-Garten, Austria.*
Tormentil (p.1757·2); chamomile (p.1669·3); strawberry leaf; blackberry leaf; raspberry leaf (p.1737·3).
*Diarrhoea.*

**Bio-Garten Tee gegen Erkaltung** *Bio-Garten, Austria.*
Thyme (p.1755·2); althaea (p.1651·3); verbascum flowers (p.1764·1); plantago lanceolata leaf (p.1738·2).
*Catarrh; cold symptoms.*

**Bio-Garten Tee gegen Verstopfung** *Bio-Garten, Austria.*
Prunus spinosa; peppermint leaf (p.1283·2); chamomile (p.1669·3); fennel (p.1687·2).
*Constipation.*

**Bio-Garten Tee zur Beruhigung** *Bio-Garten, Austria.*
Valerian (p.1762·2); melissa (p.1711·1); lupulus (p.1708·1); lavender flowers (p.1705·1); orange flowers (p.1723·3).
*Anxiety; insomnia.*

**Bio-Garten Tee zur Erhohung der Harnmenge** *Bio-Garten, Austria.*
Urtica (p.1762·1); birch leaf (p.1660·3); taraxacum leaf (p.1751·3); prunus spinosa; ononis (p.1723·3).
*Diuretic.*

**Bio-Garten Tee zur Starkung und Kraftigung** *Bio-Garten, Austria.*
Achillea (p.1646·2); bitter-orange peel (p.1723·3); gentian (p.1692·2); rosemary leaf (p.1740·2); rose fruit (p.1740·1).
*Tonic.*

**Bio-Garten Tropfen fur Galle und Leber** *Bio-Garten, Austria.*
Absinthium (p.1645·1); achillea (p.1646·2); taraxacum (p.1751·3).
*Liver and gallbladder disorders.*

**Bio-Garten Tropfen fur Magen und Darm** *Bio-Garten, Austria.*
Peppermint (p.1283·2); valerian (p.1762·2); chamomile (p.1669·3).
*Gastrointestinal disorders.*

**Bio-Garten Tropfen fur Niere und Blase** *Bio-Garten, Austria.*
Birch leaf (p.1660·3); equisetum (p.1684·1).
*Kidney and bladder disorders.*

**Bio-Garten Tropfen gegen Blahungen** *Bio-Garten, Austria.*
Caraway (p.1667·2); coriander (p.1676·1); peppermint (p.1283·2).
*Flatulence.*

**Bio-Garten Tropfen gegen Husten** *Bio-Garten, Austria.*
Thyme (p.1755·2); plantago lanceolata (p.1738·2).
*Catarrh; coughs.*

**Bio-Garten Tropfen zur Beruhigung** *Bio-Garten, Austria.*
Lupulus (p.1708·1); melissa (p.1711·1).
*Nervous disorders.*

**Biogaze** *Zambon, Fr.*
Niaouli oil (p.1719·3); thyme oil (p.1755·3).
*Burns.*

**Biogel**
*Note. This name is used for preparations of different composition.*
*Prater, Chile.*
Ketoconazole (p.403·3).
*Fungal scalp infections.*

*Ghimas, Ital.*
Royal jelly (p.1740·3).

**Biogelat Erkaltungs & Grippe** *Metochem, Austria†.*
Salix (p.87·3).
*Cold and flu symptoms; pain.*

**Biogelat Herzstarkungs** *Metochem, Austria.*
Crataegus (p.1677·1).
*Cardiovascular disorders.*

**Biogelat Leberschutz** *Metochem, Austria.*
Silybum marianum (p.1043·3).
*Liver disorders.*

**Biogelat Schlaf** *Metochem, Austria.*
Valerian (p.1762·2); lupulus (p.1708·1).
*Sleep disorders.*

**Biogena Dermo** *Biogena, Ital.*
Soap substitute.

**Biogenis** *Bayer, Ger.†.*
*dl*-Alpha tocoferil acetate (p.1465·1); magnesium oxide (p.1272·3).
*Vitamin E or magnesium deficiency.*

**Biogenis One-a-Day** *Bayer, Ger.†.*
*d*-Alpha tocoferol (p.1464·3).
*Vitamin E deficiency.*

**Biogenol** *Chemopharma, Chile.*
Vitamin A palmitate; calcium ascorbate; alpha tocoferil acetato; selenium yeast; zinc gluconate; copper gluconate (p.1417·1).
*Nutritional supplement.*

**Biogesic**
*Biomedis, Hong Kong; Biomedis, Malaysia; Biomedis, Singapore; Biomedis, Thai.; Great Eastern, Thai.*
Paracetamol (p.76·2).
*Fever; pain.*

**Bioget** *Michallik, Ger.*
Tannic acid (p.1751·2); cetylpyridinium chloride (p.1173·1).
*Burns; wounds.*

**BioGinkgo** *Pharmanex, USA.*
Ginkgo biloba (p.1692·3).
*Nutritional supplement.*

**Bioglan Acidophilus** *Bioglan, Austral.†.*
*Lactobacillus acidophilus* (p.1704·2).
*Diarrhoea; restoration of gastrointestinal flora.*

**Bioglan Arthri Plus** *Bioglan, Austral.†.*
Celery seed oil (p.1669·1); evening primrose oil (p.1686·3); fish oil (p.976·2); devil's claw root (p.28·2); salix (p.87·3).
*Arthritis; rheumatism; sports injuries.*

**Bioglan 3B Beer Belly Buster** *Bioglan, Austral.†.*
Garcinia; chromium trichloride (p.1425·1); pectin (p.1580·3); methylcellulose (p.1580·2); guarana (p.1765·3); hypericum (p.299·1).
*Obesity.*

**Bioglan Bioage Peripheral** *Bioglan, Austral.†.*
Viola tricolor; crataegus (p.1677·1); olive; magnesium orotate (p.1724·3); *d*-alpha tocoferil acid succinate (p.1465·1).
*Peripheral circulatory disorders.*

**Bioglan The Blue One** *Bioglan, Austral.†.*
Avena (p.1658·2); gokhru; damiana (p.1679·1); capsicum (p.1667·1); eschscholtzia californica; zinc amino acid chelate (p.1469·3); rutoside (p.1688·2).
*Tonic for males.*

**Bioglan Cal C** *Bioglan, Austral.†.*
Calcium ascorbate (p.1460·2).
*Vitamin C supplement.*

**Bioglan Cirflo** *Bioglan, Austral.†.*
Rutoside (p.1688·2); bioflavonoids (p.1688·2); nicotinic acid (p.1441·1); calcium ascorbate (p.1460·2); calcium gluconate (p.1225·2); aesculus (p.1648·2); hamamelis (p.1696·3); pulsatilla (p.1737·1); ruscus aculeatus.
*Peripheral circulatory disorders.*

**Bioglan Cranbiotic Super** *Bioglan, Austral.†.*
Cranberry (p.1676·3); taraxacum (p.1751·3); bearberry (p.1659·2); buchu (p.1663·1); solidago virgaurea (p.1748·3).
*Cystitis.*

**Bioglan Daily Plus** *Bioglan, Austral.*
Vitamin and mineral preparation (p.1417·1).

**Bioglan Daily Plus Max** Bioglan, Austral.†.
Ginseng; garlic; silybum marianum; bladderwrack (p.1742·3); lecithin; vitamins; minerals (p.1417·1).
*Tonic.*

**Bioglan Digestive Zyme** Bioglan, Austral.†.
Betaine hydrochloride (p.1660·2); glutamic acid (p.1433·2); pepsin (p.1729·3).
*Achlorhydria; hypochlorhydria.*

**Bioglan Discone** Bioglan, Austral.†.
Vitamin and mineral preparation (p.1417·1) with bromelain (p.1662·2) and papain (p.1727·3).
*Arthritis; rheumatism; sports injuries.*

**Bioglan Easy Bronz** Bioglan, Austral.†.
Lycopersicon esculatum.
*Skin tanning.*

**Bioglan Fingers & Toes** Bioglan, Austral.†.
Calcium ascorbate (p.1460·2); *d*-alpha tocoferil acid succinate (p.1465·1); rutoside (p.1688·2); bioflavonoids (p.1688·2); nicotinic acid (p.1441·1); aesculus (p.1648·2); hamamelis (p.1696·3); ginkgo biloba (p.1692·3); rosemary oil (p.1740·2).
*Peripheral vascular disorders.*

**Bioglan Formula Four** Bioglan, Austral.†.
Vitamin and mineral preparation (p.1417·1).

**Bioglan Ginger-Vite Forte** Bioglan, Austral.†.
Ginger oil (p.1267·1); ginger (p.1267·1); evening primrose oil (p.1686·3).
*Arthritis; rheumatism; sports injuries.*

**Bioglan Ginsynergy** Bioglan, Austral.†.
Ginseng (p.1693·1); eleutherococcus senticosis root (p.1744·1); withania somnifera; panax quinquefolium.
*Tonic.*

**Bioglan Hemofactor** Bioglan, Austral.
Vitamin preparation with iron and folic acid (p.1417·1).
*Anaemia.*

**Bioglan Joint Mobility** Bioglan, Austral.†.
Glucosamine sulfate (p.1694·1); turmeric (p.1058·3); boswellia serrata (p.1690·1); capsicum (p.1667·1); zinc gluconate (p.1469·2); manganese amino acid chelate (p.1440·2).
*Musculoskeletal and joint disorders.*

**Bioglan Liver-Vite** Bioglan, Austral.†.
Silybum marianum (p.1043·3).
*Liver disorders.*

**Bioglan Maxepa** Bioglan, Austral.†.
Fish oil (p.976·2); *d*-alpha tocoferil acetate (p.1465·1).
*Atherosclerosis; hypertriglyceridaemia.*

**Bioglan Mega C** Bioglan, Austral.†.
Ascorbic acid (p.1460·2); rose fruit (p.1740·1); hesperidin (p.1688·2).
*Vitamin C supplement.*

**Bioglan Mens Super Soy/Clover** Bioglan, Austral.†.
Red clover (p.1737·3); soya bean (p.1447·2); saw palmetto (p.1569·1); damiana (p.1679·1); calcium hydrogen phosphate (p.1225·2).
*Male menopausal disorders.*

**Bioglan Micelle A plus E** Bioglan, Austral.†.
Vitamin A (p.1451·2); *d*-alpha tocoferil acetate (p.1465·1).
*Fat malabsorption syndromes; vitamin A and E supplement.*

**Bioglan Micelle E** Bioglan, Austral.†.
*d*-Alpha tocoferil acetate (p.1465·1).
*Vitamin E supplement.*

**Bioglan Natural E** Bioglan, Austral.†.
*d*-Alpha tocopherol (p.1464·3).
*Vitamin E deficiency; vitamin E supplement.*

**Bioglan Neo Stress** Bioglan, Austral.†.
Multivitamin, mineral, and amino-acid preparation (p.1417·1).

**Bioglan Organic Mineral** Bioglan, Austral.†.
Mineral supplement (p.1417·1).

**Bioglan Panazyme** Bioglan, Austral.†.
Pancreatin (p.1725·3).
*Digestive enzyme supplement.*

**Bioglan PMT-Eze** Bioglan, Austral.†.
Multivitamin and mineral preparation with herbs (bladderwrack, juniper, alchemilla, bearberry, viburnum opulus, vitex agnus castus) (p.1417·1).
*Menstrual disorders.*

**Bioglan Primrose Micelle** Bioglan, Austral.†.
Evening primrose oil (p.1686·3).
*Eczema; mastalgia.*

**Bioglan Primrose-E** Bioglan, Austral.†.
Evening primrose oil (p.1686·3); *d*-alpha tocopherol (p.1464·3).
*Premenstrual syndrome.*

**Bioglan Pro-Guard** Bioglan, Austral.†.
Saw palmetto (p.1569·1).
*Benign prostatic hyperplasia.*

**Bioglan Psylli-Mucil Plus** Bioglan, Austral.†.
Ispaghula (p.1268·1); slippery elm (p.1747·1); peppermint leaf (p.1283·2); ginger (p.1267·1); pectin (p.1580·3).
*Bowel cleanser.*

**Bioglan Pygno-Vite** Bioglan, Austral.†.
Vitis vinifera; myrtillus (p.1718·3).
*Peripheral circulatory disorders.*

**Bioglan Silica-Vite** Bioglan, Austral.†.
Equisetum (p.1684·1).
*Skin disorders; wounds.*

**Bioglan Soy Power Plus** Bioglan, Austral.†.
Red clover (p.1737·3); isoflavones; soya bean (p.1447·2); dioscorea villosa; calcium hydrogen phosphate (p.1225·2).
*Isoflavone and calcium supplement.*

**Bioglan Stress-Relax** Bioglan, Austral.†.
Hypericum (p.299·1).
*Anxiety; nervous disorders.*

**Bioglan Sucro** Bioglan, Austral.†.
Vitamin and mineral preparation (p.1417·1).

**Bioglan Super Cal C** Bioglan, Austral.†.
Calcium ascorbate (p.1460·2); citrus bioflavonoids (p.1688·2); hesperidin (p.1688·2); rutoside (p.1688·2); rose fruit (p.1740·1).
*Vitamin C supplement.*

**Bioglan Supercarotene C&E** Bioglan, Austral.†.
Betacarotene; *d*-alpha tocoferil acid succinate; ascorbic acid (p.1417·1).
*Tonic.*

**Bioglan Superdophilus** Bioglan, Austral.†.
*Lactobacillus acidophilus* (p.1704·2).
*Diarrhoea; restoration of gastrointestinal flora.*

**Bioglan Synergy B** Bioglan, Austral.†.
Vitamin B substances with vitamin C and magnesium (p.1417·1).

**Bioglan Vision-Eze** Bioglan, Austral.†.
Myrtillus (p.1718·3); ginkgo biloba (p.1692·3).
*Eye fatigue; peripheral circulatory disorders; poor night vision.*

**Bioglan Water Soluble E** Bioglan, Austral.†.
*d*-Alpha tocopherol (p.1464·3).
*Vitamin E supplement.*

**Bioglan Zellulean with Escin** Bioglan, Austral.†.
Aesculus (p.1648·2); ginkgo biloba (p.1692·3); vitis vinifera; bladderwrack (p.1742·3); bioflavonoids (p.1688·2); lecithin (p.1706·1); pectin (p.1580·3); tyrosine (p.1451·1); evening primrose oil (p.1686·3); omega-3 marine triglycerides (p.976·2); yellow sweet clover.
*Aid to skin tissue repair; obesity.*

**Bioglan Zinc Chelate** Bioglan, Austral.†.
Zinc amino acid chelate (p.1469·3).
*Zinc deficiency.*

**Bioglan Zn-A-C** Bioglan, Austral.†.
Ascorbic acid (p.1460·2); vitamin A (p.1451·2); zinc amino acid chelate (p.1469·3); calcium pantothenate (p.1442·3); rutoside (p.1688·2).
*Vitamin and mineral supplement.*

**Bioglufer** Euro-Pharma, Ital.
Ferrous gluconate (p.1428·1).
Ascorbic acid (p.1460·2) is included in this preparation to increase the absorption and availability of iron.
*Iron-deficiency anaemia.*

**Bioglusil** Bioresearch, Mex.
Tolbutamide (p.348·1).
*Diabetes mellitus.*

**Biogreen** Euro-Pharma, Ital.
Sodium monofluorophosphate (p.1446·2); propolis (p.1735·2); tabebuia; plant extracts.
*Mouth disorders.*

**Biogrip Forte** Instituto Sanitas, Chile.
Paracetamol (p.76·2); pseudoephedrine sulfate (p.1129·2); chlorphenamine maleate (p.427·3).
*Cold and influenza symptoms.*

**Biogyl** Biolab, Thai.
Metronidazole (p.607·2).
*Anaerobic bacterial infections.*

**Biohepax** Ducto, Braz.
Adenosine (p.851·2); methionine (p.1042·1); betaine (p.1660·1); choline citrate (p.1424·3); pyridoxine hydrochloride (p.1456·3).
*Biliary-tract disorders.*

**Bio-Hep-B** Biotechnology, Israel.
A hepatitis B vaccine (recombinant) (p.1618·1).
*Active immunisation.*

**Biohisdex DM** Everest, Canad.†.
Dextromethorphan hydrobromide (p.1117·3); phenylephrine hydrochloride (p.1126·3); diphenylpyraline hydrochloride (p.432·3).
*Coughs; respiratory congestion.*

**Biohisdine DM** Everest, Canad.†.
Dextromethorphan hydrobromide (p.1117·3); phenylephrine hydrochloride (p.1126·3); diphenylpyraline hydrochloride (p.432·3).
*Coughs; respiratory congestion.*

**Biohist** Propan, S.Afr.
Diphenhydramine hydrochloride (p.431·3); zinc oxide (p.1163·2); calamine (p.1144·1); phenol (p.1188·1).
*Skin disorders.*

**Biohist-LA** Ivax, USA.
Chlorphenamine maleate (p.427·3); pseudoephedrine hydrochloride (p.1129·2).
Formerly contained carbinoxamine maleate and pseudoephedrine hydrochloride.
*Cold symptoms.*

**Bio-H-Tin**
e+b, Austria; e+b, Ger.; Gebro, Switz.
Biotin (p.1423·2).
*Biotin deficiency.*

**Biohulin 70/30, 80/20, and 90/10** Biobras, Braz.
A mixture of isophane insulin injection(human, monocomponent) and insulin injection (human, monocomponent) (p.333·3) in the proportions indicated.
*Diabetes mellitus.*

**Biohulin Humana** Elvetium, Arg.
Insulin zinc suspension (human) (p.333·3).
*Diabetes mellitus.*

**Biohulin L** Biobras, Braz.
Insulin zinc suspension (human, monocomponent) (p.333·3).
*Diabetes mellitus.*

**Biohulin NPH** Biobras, Braz.
Isophane insulin injection (human, monocomponent) (p.333·3).
*Diabetes mellitus.*

**Biohulin R** Biobras, Braz.
Insulin injection (human, monocomponent) (p.333·3).
*Diabetes mellitus.*

**Biohulin Ultralenta** Biobras, Braz.
Insulin zinc suspension (crystalline) (human, monocomponent) (p.333·3).
*Diabetes mellitus.*

**Bio-Insulin I** Guidotti, Ital.
Isophane insulin (human, biosynthetic) (p.333·3).
*Diabetes mellitus.*

**Bio-Insulin 30/70 and 50/50** Guidotti, Ital.
Mixtures of insulin injection (human, biosynthetic) and isophane insulin injection (human, biosynthetic) respectively in the proportions indicated (p.333·3).
*Diabetes mellitus.*

**Bio-Insulin L** Guidotti, Ital.
Insulin zinc suspension (human, biosynthetic) (p.333·3).
*Diabetes mellitus.*

**Bio-Insulin R** Guidotti, Ital.
Insulin (human, biosynthetic) (p.333·3).
*Diabetes mellitus.*

**Bio-Insulin U** Guidotti, Ital.
Insulin zinc suspension (crystalline) (human, biosynthetic) (p.333·3).
*Diabetes mellitus.*

**Bioiodine** Bioceuticals, UK.
Potassium iodate (p.1598·1).

**Biojad** Roche, Austria†.
Multivitamin and iron preparation (p.1417·1).
*Tonic.*

**Biokacin** Rayere, Mex.
Amikacin (p.154·1).
*Bacterial infections.*

**Biokids** Biotherm, Canad.
*SPF 35:* Avobenzone (p.1142·3); enzacamene (p.1147·1); octocrilene (p.1154·3); ecamsule (p.1146·3); titanium dioxide (p.1160·3).
*Sunscreen.*

**Bioklysm** Zekides, Gr.
Dibasic sodium phosphate (p.1231·1); monobasic sodium phosphate (p.1230·3).
*Bowel evacuation; constipation.*

**Biokosma Embrocation** Synpharma, Austria.
Menthol (p.1711·3); peppermint oil (p.1283·2); methyl salicylate (p.59·3); eucalyptus oil (p.1686·2); rosemary oil (p.1740·2); anise oil (p.1655·2); citronella oil (p.1673·2); arnica (p.1656·3).
*Musculoskeletal and joint disorders.*

**Biokosma Medizinalbad** Synpharma, Austria.
Camphor (p.1665·3); anise oil (p.1655·2); eucalyptus oil (p.1686·2); methyl salicylate (p.59·3); niaouli oil (p.1719·3); citronella oil (p.1673·2); peppermint oil (p.1283·2); rosemary oil (p.1740·2); thyme oil (p.1755·3).
*Bath additive; musculoskeletal and joint disorders.*

**Biokosma Red Point-Massagecreme** Synpharma, Austria.
Camphor (p.1665·3); citral; anise oil (p.1655·2); eucalyptus oil (p.1686·2); methyl salicylate (p.59·3); citronella oil (p.1673·2); niaouli oil (p.1719·3); rosemary oil (p.1740·2); thyme oil (p.1755·3); peppermint oil (p.1283·2); cayenne pepper (p.1667·1); mustard oil (p.1718·2); arnica (p.1656·3).
*Musculoskeletal and joint disorders; sports injuries.*

**Biokur** Biocur, Ger.
Biotin (p.1423·2).
*Biotin deficiency.*

**Biol Preo** Biol, Arg.
*Escherichia coli*; *Staphylococcus aureus*; alpha haemolytic streptococcus; *Streptococcus pyogenes*; non-haemolytic streptococcus; *Enterococcus faecalis* (p.1704·2); *Streptococcus pnuemoniae*; *Klebsiella pneumoniae*; *Moraxella catarrhalis*; *Pseudomonas aeruginosa*.
*Respiratory-tract infections.*

**Biolac** Angelini, Ital.
Lactulose (p.1269·1).
*Constipation; hepatic cirrhosis; hepatic encephalopathy.*

**Biolactine** Sella, Ital.
Vitamin B substances (p.1417·1), lactic-acid-producing organisms (p.1704·2); myrtillus (p.1718·3).
*Nutritional supplement.*

**Biolactona** Bioresearch, Mex.
Spironolactone (p.1003·1).
*Hypertension; oedema.*

**Biolactus** Rider, Chile.
*Lactobacillus rhamnosus (p.1704·2).*
*Diarrhoea.*

**Biolactyl** DB, Fr.
*Lactobacillus acidophilus* (p.1704·2); *Lactobacillus casei* var *rhamnosus* (p.1704·2).
*Maintenance of gastrointestinal flora.*

**Biolan Tar** Biopha, Fr.†.
Coal tar (p.1159·2); piroctone olamine (p.1155·2); salicylic acid (p.1157·1).
*Seborrhoeic dermatitis.*

**Biolane** Prater, Chile.
Zinc (p.1469·2).
*Dandruff.*

**Biolau** Luchon, Fr.
Linalol; geraniol; neroli; d-borneol; cinol; cineole (p.1672·1); sodium chloride (p.1233·3).
*Nasal and oral hygiene.*

**Biolavan** Pharmaton, Ger.†.
Equisetum (p.1684·1).
*Oedema; urinary-tract disorders.*

**Biolax** Chatfield Laboratories, UK.
Bisacodyl (p.1251·3).
*Constipation.*

**Biolecit H3** Roche, Austria†.
Procaine hydrochloride (p.1383·2); essential phospholipids; *dl*-alpha tocoferil acetate (p.1417·1).
*Tonic.*

**Biolectra Calcium** Hermes, Ger.
Calcium carbonate (p.1254·2).
*Calcium deficiency; osteoporosis.*

**Biolectra Magnesium** Hermes, Ger.
Magnesium oxide (p.1272·3).
*Muscular disorders associated with magnesium deficiency.*

**Biolectra Zink** Hermes, Ger.
Zinc sulfate (p.1469·3).
*Zinc deficiency.*

**Bioleine** Nutergia, Fr.
Evening primrose oil (p.1686·3).
*Nutritional supplement.*

**Biolid**
Note. This name is used for preparations of different composition.
Bioresearch, Mex.
Loperamide (p.1271·2).
*Diarrhoea.*

Belmac, Spain.
Ispaghula (p.1268·1).
*Constipation; diarrhoea.*

**Biolina** Bioceuticals, UK.
Spirulina (p.1749·2).

**Biolix** Bioresearch, Mex.
Domperidone (p.1263·2).
*Dyspepsia.*

**Bio-Logos** Sigma-Tau, Switz.
Hydroxocobalamin; amino acids (p.1417·1).
*Tonic.*

**Biolon**
BPL-Meizler, Braz.†; Ophtapharma, Canad.; Stulin, Ger.; Biotechnology, Israel; SIFI, Ital.†; Cryopharma, Mex.; Chauvin Novopharma, Switz.†.
Sodium hyaluronate (p.1697·3).
*Aid in ophthalmic surgery.*

**Biolone** Pharmafrica, S.Afr.
Sodium hyaluronate (p.1697·3).
*Aid in eye surgery.*

**Biolucchini** Geymonat, Ital.†.
Proteins (mol. wt 30-300 kD).
*Tissue repair.*

**Biomag**
Note. This name is used for preparations of different composition.
Baliarda, Arg.
Magnesium pidolate (p.1228·2).
*Magnesium supplement.*

Homeocan, Canad.; Lehning, Fr.
Homoeopathic preparation.

Pulitzer, Ital.
Cimetidine (p.1255·3).
*Gastrointestinal hyperacidity; oesophagitis; peptic ulcer; Zollinger-Ellison syndrome.*

**Biomag Vital** Baliarda, Arg.
Levocarnitine; magnesium pidolate; vitamin B substances; vitamin C (p.1417·1).
*Tonic.*

**Biomagnesin** Madaus, Ger.
Dibasic magnesium phosphate (p.1229·1); dibasic magnesium citrate.
*Magnesium deficiency.*

**Bio-Magnesium** Phytomed, Switz.
Homoeopathic preparation.

**Bio-Marine Plus** Pharma Nord, Fr.
Omega-3 marine triglycerides (p.976·2); folic acid; vitamin $B_{12}$ (p.1417·1).
*Nutritional supplement.*

**Biomega-3** Usana, Hong Kong.
Eicosapentaenoic acid (p.976·2); docosahexaenoic acid (p.976·1); omega-3 triglycerides (p.976·1).
*Fatty acid supplement.*

**Biometalle II-Heyl** Heyl, Ger.†.
Mineral preparation (p.1417·1).
*Correction of metal balance following penicillamine therapy.*

**Biometalle III-Heyl** Heyl, Ger.†.
Mineral preparation (p.1417·1).
*Correction of metal balance following penicillamine therapy.*

**Biometrox** Biosintetica, Braz.
Methotrexate sodium (p.568·3).
*Malignant neoplasms.*

**Biomida** Biosintetica, Braz.
Flutamide (p.556·2).

**Biomina** Precimex, Mex.†.
Albumin (human) (p.740·3).

**Biomineral** Biochimici, Ital.
Mineral preparation with cystine (p.1417·1).
*Nutritional supplement.*

**Biomineral 5-Alfa** *Biochimici, Ital.*
Cucurbita oil; soya oil; evening primrose oil; zinc-rich yeast; green tea; biotin (p.1417·1).
*Nutritional supplement; seborrhoea; thinning hair.*

**Bio-Mineral Formula** *Blackmores, Austral.†.*
Mineral preparation (p.1417·1).

**Biomineral One** *Biochimici, Ital.*
Vitamin and mineral preparation with cystine and methionine (p.1417·1).

**Biomineral Plus** *Biochimici, Ital.*
Multivitamin and mineral preparation with cystine and methionine (p.1417·1).
*Nutritional supplement.*

**Biomineral Unghie** *Biochimici, Ital.*
Amino-acid preparation with vitamins and minerals (p.1417·1).
*Nail disorders.*

**Biominol A** *Alter, Spain.*
Vitamin A palmitate (p.1453·1).
*Vitamin A deficiency.*

**Biominol A D** *Alter, Spain.*
Vitamin A palmitate (p.1453·1); ergocalciferol (p.1462·1).
*Deficiency of vitamins A and D.*

**Biomisen** *Bioresearch, Mex.*
Furosemide (p.919·3).

**Biomitin** *Bioresearch, Mex.*
Difenidol (p.1261·1).
*Nausea and vomiting; vertigo.*

**Biomo-lipon** *Biomo, Ger.*
Thioctic acid (p.1754·3).
*Diabetic polyneuropathy.*

**Biomona** *Bioresearch, Mex.*
Metronidazole (p.607·2).
*Vaginitis.*

**Biomont** *Pharmonta, Austria.*
Multivitamin preparation (p.1417·1).

**Biomox** *Biolab, Thai.†.*
Amoxicillin (p.155·3).
*Bacterial infections.*

**Biomoxil** *Biochem, India.*
Amoxicillin (p.155·3) or amoxicillin trihydrate (p.155·3).
*Bacterial infections.*

**Biomunil** *Lusofarmaco, Ital.*
*Klebsiella pneumoniae* ribosomes and membrane fraction; *Streptococcus pneumoniae* ribosomes; *Streptococcus pyogenes* ribosomes; *Haemophilus influenzae* ribosomes.
*Immunostimulant.*

**Bion Tears**
*Alcon, Austral.†; Alcon, Canad.; Alcon, Hong Kong; Alcon, Singapore; Alcon, Swed.; Alcon, Thai.; Alcon, USA.*
Dextran 70 (p.746·2); hypromellose (p.1579·3).
*Dry eyes.*

**Bionafil** *Bioresearch, Mex.*
Enalapril (p.909·2).
*Hypertension.*

**Bionagre plus E** *Bio-Sante, Canad.*
Linoleic acid (p.1690·2); linolenic acid; vitamin E (p.1464·3).

**Bionagrol** *Biophytarom, Fr.*
Evening primrose oil (p.1686·3).
*Nutritional supplement.*

**Bionagrol Plus** *Biophytarom, Fr.*
Evening primrose oil (p.1686·3); omega-3 fatty acids (p.976·1).
*Nutritional supplement.*

**Bionaril** *Bioresearch, Mex.*
Diphenhydramine (p.431·3).
*Hypersensitivity.*

**Bionet** *Carter Horner, Canad.*
Benzocaine (p.1370·3); cetalkonium chloride (p.1172·1).
*Mouth disorders.*

**Bioneural B12** *Labinca, Arg.*
Ibuprofen (p.45·3); hydroxocobalamin (p.1458·2).
*Pain.*

**Bioneuryl** *Bioresearch, Mex.*
Carbamazepine (p.353·3).
*Epilepsy.*

**Bionicard** *Rottapharm, Ital.*
Nicardipine hydrochloride (p.965·1).
*Angina pectoris; hypertension.*

**Bionif** *Bioprogress, Ital.*
Nifedipine (p.966·2).
*Angina pectoris; hypertension.*

**Bionobal** *Bioresearch, Mex.*
Hydralazine (p.933·1).
*Hypertension; oedema.*

**Bionocalcin**
*Delta, Port.†; Ipsen, Spain†.*
Calcitonin (salmon) (p.768·2).
*Hypercalcaemia; metastatic bone pain; osteoporosis; Paget's disease of bone.*

**Bionolip** *Bioresearch, Mex.*
Bezafibrate (p.873·2).
*Hyperlipidaemias.*

**Bionorm** *Merck, Braz.†.*
Amino acids and vitamin B substances (p.1417·1).
*Nutritional supplement.*

**Bionoxol** *Bioresearch, Mex.*
Ambroxol (p.1114·3).
*Respiratory-tract disorders.*

**Bionutrin** *Biomedis, Thai.; Great Eastern, Thai.*
Multivitamin and mineral preparation (p.1417·1).

**Biopasal Fibra** *Synthelabo, Spain†.*
Ispaghula (p.1268·1).
*Constipation.*

**Biopause** *Monin, Fr.*
Soya bean (p.1447·2); magnesium lactate (p.1228·1); yam.
*Menopausal disorders.*

**Biopaxel** *Biosintetica, Braz.*
Paclitaxel (p.577·3).
*Malignant neoplasms.*

**Biopental** *OM, Port.*
Lysates of *Streptococcus pneumoniae*; *Neisseria catarrhalis*; *Staphylococcus aureus*; *Klebsiella pneumoniae*; *Haemophilus influenzae*; *Streptococcus pyogenes*.
*Respiratory-tract infections.*

**Bioperazone** *Biopharma, Ital.*
Cefoperazone sodium (p.174·3).
*Bacterial infections.*

**Bioperidolo** *FIRMA, Ital.†.*
Haloperidol (p.701·2).
*Psychoses.*

**Biophil** *Kemiprogress, Ital.†.*
Vitamin B substances (p.1417·1); myrtillus (p.1718·3).
*Disturbances of the gastrointestinal flora.*

**Biophylin** *Gerard House, UK†.*
Valerian (p.1762·2); skullcap (p.1746·3); Jamaica dogwood (p.1702·3); cimicifuga (p.1671·3).
*Tenseness, restlessness, nervous irritability.*

**Biopim** *Kemyos, Ital.†.*
Pipemidic acid (p.243·1).
*Urinary-tract infections.*

**Biopiper** *Bioprogress, Ital.*
Piperacillin sodium (p.243·1).
Lidocaine hydrochloride (p.1377·3) is included in the intramuscular injection to alleviate the pain of injection.
*Bacterial infections.*

**Bioplak** *Ern, Spain.*
Aspirin (p.15·1).
*Thromboembolism prophylaxis.*

**bioplant-Kamillenfluid** *Serum-Werk Bernburg, Ger.*
Chamomile (p.1669·3); calendula (p.1665·2).
*Bedsores; mouth inflammation; skin inflammation.*

**Bioplasma FDP** *NBI, S.Afr.*
Plasma protein fraction (p.758·2).
*Fluid depletion; haemorrhagic disorders.*

**Bioplatino** *Biosintetica, Braz.*
Cisplatin (p.538·1).
*Malignant neoplasms.*

**Bioplex**
*Note. This name is used for preparations of different composition.*
*Sante Naturelle, Canad.*
Vitamin B substances (p.1417·1).

*Fresenius Kabi, Ital.*
A range of amino-acid infusions (p.1417·1).
*Parenteral nutrition.*

*Biorex, UK.*
Carbenoxolone sodium (p.1254·3).
*Mouth ulcers.*

**Bioplus** *Covan, S.Afr.*
Caffeine; vitamin B substances; calcium citrate; calcium gluconate (p.1417·1).
*Tonic.*

**Biopram** *Bioresearch, Mex.*
Metoclopramide (p.1274·3).
*Nausea and vomiting.*

**Bioprim**
*Norma (Νορμα), Gr.; Bioresearch, Mex.*
Co-trimoxazole (p.199·3).
*Bacterial infections; Pneumocystis carinii pneumonia; toxoplasmosis.*

**Bioprofol** *Biosintetica, Braz.*
Propofol (p.1305·3).
*General anaesthesia.*

**Bioprol** *Bioresearch, Mex.*
Metoprolol (p.956·3).
*Hypertension.*

**Bioprotus** *Carrare, Fr.*
Lactic-acid-producing organisms (p.1704·2).
*Maintenance of gastrointestinal flora.*

**Bioptic** *Biocumed, Arg.*
Tobramycin (p.271·2).
*Bacterial eye infections.*

**Bioptic DX** *Biocumed, Arg.*
Tobramycin (p.271·2); dexamethasone (p.1097·1).
*Infected eye disorders.*

**Bioptimum** *Boiron, Port.†.*
A range of amino-acid, vitamin and mineral preparations (p.1417·1).

**Biopto-E** *Jenapharm, Ger.*
*d*-Alpha tocopherol (p.1464·3).
*Vitamin E deficiency.*

**Biopulmin** *Grunenthal, Chile.*
Erdosteine (p.1121·1).
*Respiratory-tract congestion.*

**Biopyr** *Madaus, Ger.†.*
Homoeopathic preparation.

**Bioquidan** *Bioresearch, Mex.*
Dextromethorphan (p.1117·3).
*Coughs.*

**Bioquil** *Atral, Port.*
Ofloxacin (p.239·3).
*Bacterial infections.*

**Bioquin** *Lafi, Chile.*
Erythromycin ethyl succinate (p.208·1); sulfafurazole (p.260·1).
*Bacterial infections.*

**Bio-Quinon Q10 Super** *Pharma Nord, Fr.*
Ubidecarenone (p.1760·2).
*Nutritional supplement.*

**Bio-Quinone**
*Pharma Nord, Malaysia; Pharma Nord, Thai.*
Ubidecarenone (p.1760·2).

**Bioral**
*Smith & Nephew, Austral.; Merck Consumer, UK.*
Carbenoxolone sodium (p.1254·3).
*Mouth ulcers.*

**Bioralin** *Bioresearch, Mex.*
Chlortalidone (p.882·3).
*Heart failure; hypertension.*

**Bioran** *Bioresearch, Mex.*
Methenamine (p.230·1).
*Urinary-tract infections.*

**Biordin** *Bioresearch, Mex.*
Isosorbide (p.941·1).

**Bio-Real** *Farmetrusca, Ital.†.*
Royal jelly (p.1740·3); yeast (p.1469·1).

**Bio-Real Complex** *Farmetrusca, Ital.†.*
Royal jelly (p.1740·3); ginseng (p.1693·1).

**Bio-Real Plus** *Farmetrusca, Ital.†.*
Royal jelly (p.1740·3); ginseng (p.1693·1).

**Bioreform-Beruhigungstee** *Sanova, Austria.*
Valerian (p.1762·2); melissa (p.1711·1); lupulus (p.1708·1); lavender flower (p.1705·1); orange flower (p.1723·3).
*Anxiety; sleep disturbances.*

**Bioreform-Blasen- und Nierentee** *Sanova, Austria.*
Bearberry (p.1659·2); equisetum (p.1684·1); birch leaf (p.1660·3).
*Kidney and bladder disorders.*

**Bioreform-Entschlackungstee** *Sanova, Austria.*
Birch leaf (p.1660·3); taraxacum (p.1751·3); prunus spinosa; rose fruit (p.1740·1).
*Herbal preparation.*

**Bioreform-Erkaltungstee** *Sanova, Austria.*
Thyme leaf (p.1755·2); althaea (p.1651·3); verbascum flowers (p.1764·1); plantago lanceolata leaf (p.1738·2).
*Mouth and throat disorders; respiratory-tract disorders.*

**Bioreform-Harntreibender Tee** *Sanova, Austria.*
Urtica (p.1762·1); silver birch (p.1660·3); taraxacum (p.1751·3); prunus spinosa; ononis (p.1723·3).
*Diuretic.*

**Bioreform-Leber- und Galletee** *Sanova, Austria.*
Absinthium (p.1645·1); calamus (p.1664·1); angelica (p.1655·1); peppermint leaf (p.1283·2); bitter-orange leaf (p.1723·3).
*Liver and biliary disorders.*

**Bioreform-Magentee** *Sanova, Austria.*
Chamomile (p.1669·3); peppermint leaf (p.1283·2); caraway (p.1667·2); valerian (p.1762·2).
*Gastrointestinal disorders.*

**Bioreform-Starkungs- und Kraftigungstee**
*Sanova, Austria.*
Achillea bitter orange peel; gentian; rosemary leaf; rose fruit.
*Tonic.*

**Bioreform-Tee gegen Durchfall** *Sanova, Austria.*
Tormentil root (p.1757·2); chamomile flower (p.1669·3); fragaria vesca; rubus fruticosus; raspberry leaf (p.1737·3).
*Diarrhoea.*

**Bioreform-Windtreibender Tee** *Sanova, Austria.*
Fennel (p.1687·2); chamomile flower (p.1669·3); caraway (p.1667·2); achillea (p.1646·2); peppermint leaf (p.1283·2).
*Flatulence.*

**Bio-Regenerat S 3** *Dibropharm, Ger.†.*
Adenosine phosphate disodium (p.1647·3).
*Psoriasis.*

**Bioregime** *Azevedos, Port.*
Glucomannan (p.1693·3).
*Obesity.*

**Bioregime Fort** *Azevedos, Port.*
Glucomannan (p.1693·3); yeast (p.1469·1).
*Obesity.*

**Bioregime SlimKit** *Azevedos, Port.*
*Capsules:* Glucomannan (p.1693·3); bromelains (p.1662·2).
*Topical gel:* Caffeine (p.782·1).
*Obesity.*

**Biorenal** *Pharmalink, Swed.†.*
Anhydrous glucose; sodium chloride; sodium lactate; calcium chloride; magnesium chloride (p.1221·1).
*Peritoneal dialysis.*

**Biorenyn** *Bioresearch, Mex.*
Salbutamol (p.791·3).

**Bioreucam** *Helfarma, Port.*
Tenoxicam (p.93·1).
*Gout; musculoskeletal, joint, and peri-articular disorders.*

**Bioreunil** *Bioresearch, Mex.*
Carbamazepine (p.353·3).
*Epilepsy.*

**Biorevit Solar 15** *DNR, Arg.*
Titanium dioxide (p.1160·3); aminobenzoic acid (p.1142·2).
*Sunscreen.*

**Biorganic Geri** *Gisand, Switz.†.*
Vitamin, mineral, and amino-acid preparation (p.1417·1) with ginseng (p.1693·1).
*Dietary supplement; tonic.*

**Biorgasept** *Biorga, Fr.*
Chlorhexidine (p.1173·2).
*Disinfection of skin and wounds; skin infections.*

**Biorinil** *Farmila, Ital.*
Betamethasone (p.1093·1); tetryzoline hydrochloride (p.1131·2).
*Rhinitis; rhinopharyngitis; sinusitis.*

**Bio-Ritmo** *Medinfar, Port.*
Arginine aspartate; pyridoxine; calcium pangamate (p.1417·1).
*Tonic.*

**Biormon** *Amsa, Ital.*
Estradiol benzoate (p.1550·1); progesterone (p.1566·2).
*Amenorrhoea; oligomenorrhoea.*

**Biorphen** *Alliance, UK.*
Orphenadrine hydrochloride (p.486·1).
*Drug-induced extrapyramidal disorders; parkinsonism.*

**Biorrub** *Biosintetica, Braz.*
Doxorubicin hydrochloride (p.547·3).
*Malignant neoplasms.*

**Biortho** *Nutergia, Fr.*
Vitamin and mineral preparation (p.1417·1).
*Nutritional supplement.*

**Biosal**
*Note. This name is used for preparations of different composition.*
*Yauyip, Austral.*
Methyl salicylate (p.59·3); menthol (p.1711·3); camphor (p.1665·3); eucalyptus oil (p.1686·2); pumilio pine oil (p.1737·1).
*Arthritis pain.*

*Bioprogress, Ital.*
Nimesulide (p.67·1).
*Fever; inflammation; pain.*

**Biosan E** *Biocur, Ger.*
*dl*-Alpha tocoferil acetate (p.1465·1).
*Vitamin E deficiency.*

**Biosan Zink** *Biocur, Ger.*
Zinc sulfate (p.1469·3).
*Zinc deficiency.*

**Bioscalin** *Giuliani, Ital.*
Multivitamin and mineral preparation with methionine (p.1417·1).
*Hair and nail disorders.*

**Bioscefal** *Unibios, Spain.*
Cefalexin (p.168·1).
*Bacterial infections.*

**Bioscina** *Biochimico, Braz.†.*
Dipyrone (p.35·3).
*Fever; pain.*

**Bioscina Composta** *Biochimico, Braz.*
Hyoscine butylbromide (p.483·3); dipyrone (p.35·3).
*Smooth muscle spasm.*

**Biosedon S** *Biocur, Ger.†.*
Valerian (p.1762·2); passion flower (p.1729·1); lupulus (p.1708·1).
*Anxiety disorders; insomnia.*

**Bio-Sel** *Ache, Braz.*
Betacarotene; selenium; alpha tocoferol; ascorbic acid (p.1417·1).

**Bio-Selenium** *Herbaxt, Fr.*
Selenium (p.1444·1) from *Saccharomyces cerevisiae*; alpha tocoferil acetate (p.1465·1); wheat-germ oil.
*Muscular disorders; skin disorders.*

**Bioselenium** *Uriach, Spain.*
Selenium sulfide (p.1157·3).
*Skin disorders.*

**Biosern** *Bioprogress, Ital.*
Saw palmetto (p.1569·1).
*Benign prostatic hyperplasia.*

**Biosil** *Enzpharma, NZ.*
Orthosilicic acid (p.1581·3).
*Nutritional supplement.*

**Biosint** *Liomont, Mex.*
Cefotaxime sodium (p.175·3).
*Bacterial infections.*

**Biosol A** *Pharmalink, Swed.†.*
Sodium chloride; potassium chloride; magnesium chloride; calcium chloride; acetic acid; with or without glucose (p.1221·1).
*Haemodialysis.*

**Biosol B** *Pharmalink, Swed.†.*
Sodium bicarbonate (p.1221·1).
*Haemodialysis.*

**Biosonide** *Medicus, Gr.*
Budesonide (p.1094·2).
*Allergic rhinitis.*

**Biosorb** *Nutricia, Port.†.*
Preparation for enteral nutrition (p.1417·1).

**Biosorbin MCT** *Nutricia, Fin.†.*
Preparation for enteral nutrition (p.1417·1).

**Biosor-C** *Hamilton, Austral.†.*
Hesperidin methyl chalcone (p.1688·3); hesperidin (p.1688·2); ascorbic acid (p.1460·2).
*Gingivitis; herpes labialis.*

**Biosoviran** *Bioprogress, Ital.*
Pipemidic acid (p.243·1).
*Urinary-tract infections.*

**Bio-Sport** *Pharma Nord, Fr.*
Capsules, fish oil; borage oil; tablets, betacarotene; vitamins; minerals (p.1417·1).
*Nutritional supplement.*

**Biostan** *Bioresearch, Mex.*
Astemizole (p.424·2).

**Biostatine** *UCB, Spain†.*
Somatostatin acetate (p.1339·3).
*Pancreatic fistulae; variceal haemorrhage.*

**Biostim**
*Aventis, Braz.†; Aventis, Fr.; Aventis, Ital.; Aventis, Mex.; Aventis, Port.*
*Klebsiella pneumoniae* glycoprotein (p.1703·3).
*Prophylaxis of respiratory-tract infections.*

**Biostin** *Bioresearch, Mex.*
Glibenclamide (p.331·2).
*Diabetes mellitus.*

**Biostop** *Vezedes, Fr.*
Copra oil; fruit acids.
*Insect repellent.*

**Bio-Strath**
*Note. This name is used for preparations of different composition.*
*Lizofarm, Ital.†.*
Valerian (p.1762·2); passion flower (p.1729·1); peppermint leaf (p.1283·2).
*Insomnia; sedative.*

*Crefar, Port.*
Amino-acid, vitamin, and mineral preparation (p.1417·1).
*Tonic.*

*Cedar Health, UK.*
*Saccharomyces cerevisiae* (p.1469·1).

**Bio-Strath Artichoke Formula** *Cedar Health, UK.*
Cynara (p.1678·3); thistle seeds (p.1673·3); peppermint leaf (p.1283·2); yeast plasmolysate (p.1469·1).
*Dyspepsia.*

**Bio-Strath Husten** *Parapharm, Austria.*
Thyme (p.1755·2); cowslip (p.1735·1).
*Coughs.*

**Bio-Strath Leber-Galle** *Parapharm, Austria.*
Silybum marianum (p.1043·3); cynara (p.1678·3); peppermint leaf (p.1283·2).
*Digestive disorders; flatulence.*

**Bio-Strath Nieren-Blasen** *Parapharm, Austria.*
Bearberry (p.1659·2); taraxacum (p.1751·3).
*Kidney and bladder disorders.*

**Bio-Strath No 1** *Crefar, Port.†.*
Aesculus (p.1648·2); primula root (p.1735·1).
*Peripheral vascular disorders; venous disorders.*

**Bio-Strath No 5** *Crefar, Port.†.*
Salix (p.87·3); primula root (p.1735·1).
*Musculoskeletal and joint disorders.*

**Bio-Strath No 8** *Crefar, Port.†.*
Valerian (p.1762·2); passion flower (p.1729·1); peppermint leaf (p.1283·2).
*Anxiety; insomnia.*

**Bio-Strath Schleimhaut** *Parapharm, Austria.*
Sage (p.1741·2); chamomile (p.1669·3).
*Catarrh; sore throat.*

**Bio-Strath Valerian Formula** *Cedar Health, UK.*
Valerian (p.1762·2); passion flower (p.1729·1); peppermint leaf (p.1283·2); yeast plasmolysate (p.1469·1).
*Insomnia; irritability; tension.*

**Bio-Strath Willow Formula** *Cedar Health, UK.*
Salix (p.87·3); primula root (p.1735·1); yeast plasmolysate (p.1469·1).
*Musculoskeletal and joint pain.*

**Biosun** *Banana Boat, Canad.†.*
*SPF 45:* Octinoxate (p.1154·3); octisalate (p.1154·3); oxybenzone (p.1154·3); octocrilene (p.1154·3).
*SPF 25; SPF 30:* Octinoxate (p.1154·3); octisalate (p.1154·3); oxybenzone (p.1154·3); titanium dioxide (p.1160·3).
*Sunscreen.*

**Bio-Tab** *International Ethical, USA†.*
Doxycycline hyclate (p.206·2).

**Biotaer** *Disprovent, Arg.*
Bacitracin (p.161·3); neomycin (p.235·1); tyrothricin (p.275·1).
*Mouth and throat infections.*

**Biotaer Gamma** *Disprovent, Arg.*
Immunoglobulin (p.1627·2); neomycin (p.235·1); bacitracin (p.161·3); tyrothricin (p.275·1); phenylephrine (p.1126·3).

**Biotaer Nasal** *Disprovent, Arg.*
Framycetin sulfate (p.215·1); gramicidin (p.220·2); triamcinolone hexacetonide (p.1110·2); chlorphenamine maleate (p.427·3); phenylephrine hydrochloride (p.1126·3); naphazoline nitrate (p.1124·3).
*Nasal congestion.*

**Biotaer Nebulizable** *Disprovent, Arg.*
Nystatin (p.406·3); beclometasone (p.1092·1); neomycin (p.235·1); bacitracin (p.161·3); tyrothricin (p.275·1); phenylephrine (p.1126·3).

**Biotaer Ultrason Nebulizable** *Disprovent, Arg.*
Neomycin (p.235·1); bacitracin (p.161·3); tyrothricin (p.275·1); dexamethasone (p.1097·1); phenylephrine hydrochloride (p.1126·3).

**Biotamoxal** *Hexa-Medinova, Arg.*
Amoxicillin trihydrate (p.155·3).
*Bacterial infections.*

**Biotanica Feminine** *Medikem, Fr.*
Soya bean; lupulus; borage oil; spinach leaf; vitamin E; grape extract; vitamin $B_6$; folic acid (p.1417·1).
*Nutritional supplement.*

**Biotanica Ginsemag** *Medikem, Fr.*
Magnesium glycerophosphate; magnesium lactate; magnesium oxide; ginseng; vitamin $B_6$ (p.1417·1).
*Nutritional supplement.*

**Biotanica Nocturn** *Medikem, Fr.*
Melissa; valerian; lupulus; wheat-germ; spinach leaf; orange leaf; vitamin $B_6$ (p.1417·1).
*Nutritional supplement; sleep disorders.*

**Biotanica Pro Energy** *Medikem, Fr.*
Dried yeast; ginseng; kola; shiitake mushrooms; camelia sinensis; vitamin C; royal jelly; grape extract; B vitamins (p.1417·1).
*Nutritional supplement.*

**Biotanica Regenerance** *Medikem, Fr.*
Marine carotenoids; omega-3 triglycerides; pumpkin seed; grape extract; selenium; vitamin C; zinc sulfate; camelia sinensis; vitamin E; pantothenic acid; folic acid (p.1417·1).
*Nutritional supplement.*

**Biotanica Uricalm** *Medikem, Fr.*
Heather flower; meadowsweet; melissa; lithothamme; zinc sulfate; pumpkin seed (p.1417·1).
*Micturition disorders; nutritional supplement.*

**Biotarson N** *Ifusa, Mex.*
Hydrocortisone acetate (p.1103·3); gramicidin (p.220·2); neomycin (p.235·1).
*Bacterial nose infections.*

**Biotarson O** *Ifusa, Mex.*
Naphazoline (p.1124·3); gramicidin (p.220·2); neomycin (p.235·1).
*Bacterial eye infections.*

**Biotase**
*YSP, Malaysia.*
Amylase (p.1654·2); lipase; newlase.
*Gastrointestinal disorders.*

*Yung Shin, Singapore.*
Biodiastase; lipase; newlase.
*Digestive disorders.*

**Biotassina** *Teofarma, Ital.*
Amino acids; vitamin B substances (p.1417·1); calcium gluconate (p.1225·2).
Lidocaine hydrochloride (p.1377·3) is included in the intramuscular injection to alleviate the pain of injection.
*Asthenia.*

**Biotax**
*Note. This name is used for preparations of different composition.*
*Biochem, India.*
Cefotaxime sodium (p.175·3).
*Bacterial infections.*

*Faulding, Israel.*
Paclitaxel (p.577·3).
*Breast cancer; Kaposi's sarcoma; non-small-cell lung cancer; ovarian cancer.*

**Biotaxime** *Biolab, Thai.*
Cefotaxime sodium (p.175·3).
*Bacterial infections.*

**Biotazol** *Bioresearch, Mex.*
Metronidazole (p.607·2).
*Amoebiasis; giardiasis; trichomoniasis.*

**Biotecan** *Biotenk, Arg.*
Irinotecan hydrochloride (p.564·1).
*Colorectal cancer.*

**Biotel kidney** *Biotel, USA.*
Test for haemoglobin, red blood cells, and albumin in urine.

**Biotene** *Laclede, Singapore.*
Glucose oxidase (p.1694·2); lactoperoxidase; muramidase (p.1717·2); lactoferrin.
*Mouth disorders.*

**Biotene Dry Mouth** *Anglian, UK.*
Lactoperoxidase; glucose oxidase (p.1694·2); lactoferrin; muramidase (p.1717·2).
*Dry mouth.*

**Biotene Oralbalance** *Anglian, UK.*
Lactoperoxidase; glucose oxidase (p.1694·2); xylitol (p.1469·1).
*Dry mouth.*

**Biotens** *Kemyos, Ital.†.*
Labetalol hydrochloride (p.943·3); chlortalidone (p.882·3).
*Hypertension.*

**Biotenzol** *Bioresearch, Mex.*
Methyldopa (p.953·2).
*Hypertension.*

**Bioteral** *Northia, Arg.*
Ceftriaxone (p.183·3).
*Bacterial infections.*

**Bioterona** *Biosintetica, Braz.*
Cyproterone acetate (p.1544·1).

**Biotherm** *Biotherm, Canad.*
*SPF 15; SPF 25; SPF 30:* Avobenzone (p.1142·3); enzacamene (p.1147·1); ecamsule (p.1146·3); titanium dioxide (p.1160·3).
*Sunscreen.*

**Biotherm Gelee Bronzante** *Biotherm, Canad.†.*
*SPF 8:* Octinoxate (p.1154·3); octisalate (p.1154·3); oxybenzone (p.1154·3).
*Sunscreen.*

**Biotherm Gelee Fraiche** *Biotherm, Canad.*
*SPF 8:* Octinoxate (p.1154·3); enzacamene (p.1147·1); ecamsule (p.1146·3); titanium dioxide (p.1160·3).
*Sunscreen.*

**Biotherm Gelee Fraiche Hydrantante** *Biotherm, Canad.*
*SPF 10; SPF 15:* Avobenzone (p.1142·3); octocrilene (p.1154·3); ecamsule (p.1146·3); titanium dioxide (p.1160·3).
*Sunscreen.*

**Biotherm Lait Bronzant** *Biotherm, Canad.*
*SPF 8:* Octinoxate (p.1154·3); ecamsule (p.1146·3); titanium dioxide (p.1160·3).
*Sunscreen.*

**Biotherm Lait Protecteur** *Biotherm, Canad.*
*SPF 15:* Octinoxate (p.1154·3); ecamsule (p.1146·3); titanium dioxide (p.1160·3).
*Sunscreen.*

**Biotherm Soin des Levres** *Biotherm, Canad.*
*SPF 8:* Octinoxate (p.1154·3).
*Sunscreen.*

**Biotherm Soin Solaire** *Biotherm, Canad.*
*SPF 8:* Octinoxate (p.1154·3); ecamsule (p.1146·3); titanium dioxide (p.1160·3).
*Sunscreen.*

**Biotherm Soin Solaire Autobronzant** *Biotherm, Canad.*
*SPF 8:* Avobenzone (p.1142·3); enzacamene (p.1147·1); ecamsule (p.1146·3).
*Sunscreen.*

**Biotherm Stick Ecran** *Biotherm, Canad.†.*
*SPF 20:* Avobenzone (p.1142·3); octocrilene (p.1154·3); titanium dioxide (p.1160·3).
*Sunscreen.*

**Biotherm UV Protectant** *Biotherm, Canad.*
*SPF 25:* Octinoxate (p.1154·3); oxybenzone (p.1154·3); titanium dioxide (p.1160·3).
*Sunscreen.*

**Biothymus** *Biochimici, Ital.†.*
Thymus gland extract (p.1756·1).
*Prevention of hair loss.*

**Biothymus DS** *Biochimici, Ital.*
*Face wash:* Levomenol (p.1707·1); enoxolone (p.36·2); piroctone olamine (p.1155·2); salix (p.87·3).
*Scalp lotion:* Piroctone olamine (p.1155·2); urtica (p.1762·1); salix (p.87·3); salicylic acid (p.1157·1); menthol (p.1711·3).
*Shampoo:* Pyrithione zinc (p.1156·2); potassium glycyrrhizinate.
*Seborrhoeic dermatitis.*

**Biothymus F Urto** *Biochimici, Ital.*
Thymus gland extract (p.1756·1); paeonia suffruticosa.
*Prevention of hair loss.*

**Biothymus M Urto** *Biochimici, Ital.*
Thymus gland extract (p.1756·1); paeonia suffruticosa; saw palmetto (p.1569·1).
*Prevention of hair loss.*

**Biotic** *TRB, Arg.*
Ciprofloxacin hydrochloride (p.188·2).
*Bacterial infections.*

**Bioticaps** *Richet, Arg.*
Chloramphenicol (p.185·1).
*Bacterial infections.*

**Bioticic** *PS, Ital.*
Cefonicid sodium (p.174·2).
Lidocaine hydrochloride (p.1377·3) is included in this preparation to alleviate the pain of injection.
*Gram-negative bacterial infections.*

**Biotin-Asmedic** *Dyckerhoff, Ger.*
Biotin (p.1423·2).
*Biotin deficiency.*

**Bioton** *Sella, Ital.*
Honey (p.1434·2); ginseng (p.1693·1); royal jelly (p.1740·3).
*Nutritional supplement.*

**Biotone** *Laphal, Fr.*
Kola (p.1765·3); phosphoric acid (p.1731·2); manganese glycerophosphate (p.1695·2).
*Tonic.*

**Biotonico Fontoura** *DM, Braz.†.*
Ferrous sulfate (p.1428·2); phosphoric acid (p.1731·2); plant extracts.
*Anaemias.*

**Biotonus** *Gynopharm, Chile.*
Betacarotene; vitamin E; ascorbic acid; minerals (p.1417·1).

**Biototal** *Kanda, Braz.†.*
Dried yeast; malt; honey (p.1417·1).
*Nutritional supplement.*

**Biotrefon L** *Italmex, Mex.*
Cobamamide (p.1459·1).
*Tonic.*

**Biotrefon Plus** *Whitehall, Ital.*
Pollen; royal jelly (p.1740·3); liver extract.

**Biotrexate** *Biochem, India.*
Methotrexate (p.568·2).
*Malignant neoplasms; psoriasis; rheumatoid arthritis.*

**Biotricina** *Bioresearch, Mex.*
Tetracycline (p.266·2).
*Bacterial infections.*

**Biotril** *Bioresearch, Mex.*
Erythromycin (p.208·1).
*Bacterial infections.*

**Biotrivin** *Bioresearch, Mex.*
Vitamin B substances (p.1417·1).
*Neuritis; vitamin B supplement.*

**Biotrixina** *Benedetti, Ital.*
Cefatrizine (p.170·3).
*Bacterial infections.*

**Biotron** *Covan, S.Afr.*
Multivitamin and mineral preparation (p.1417·1).

**Biotropic** *Madaus, Spain†.*
Guar gum (p.333·2).
*Diabetes mellitus.*

**Biotropin**
*Elvetium, Arg.; Enila, Braz.*
Somatropin (p.1327·2).
*Growth hormone deficiency; Turner's syndrome.*

**Bio-Tropin**
*Biotechnology, Israel; Cryopharma, Mex.†.*
Somatropin (p.1327·2).
*Growth disorders in renal failure; growth hormone deficiency; Turner's syndrome.*

**Biotuss** *Spitzner, Ger.*
Thyme (p.1755·2).
Formerly contained thyme, althaea, and drosera.
*Catarrh; coughs.*

**Biotyage** *Bionatec, Fr.†.*
Nutritional supplement (p.1417·1).

**Biovac HB** *Elea, Arg.*
A hepatitis B vaccine (p.1618·1).
*Active immunisation.*

**Bio-Vagin** *Elofar, Braz.*
Metronidazole (p.607·2); nystatin (p.406·3).
*Gynaecological infections.*

**Biovancomin** *Biosintetica, Braz.*
Vancomycin hydrochloride (p.275·2).
*Bacterial infections.*

**Biovelbin** *Biogalenica, Spain†.*
Vinorelbine tartrate (p.594·1).
*Breast cancer; lung cancer.*

**Biovent** *Biomedis, Thai.; Great Eastern, Thai.*
Salbutamol (p.791·3); guaifenesin (p.1122·1).
*Coughs; obstructive airways disease.*

**Biovicerin** *Geyer, Braz.*
*Bacillus cereus.*
*Diarrhoea.*

**Biovigor**
*Note. This name is used for preparations of different composition.*
*Biotrading, Ital.†.*
Royal jelly (p.1740·3); honey (p.1434·2).
*Nutritional supplement.*

*IBSA, Switz.*
Hydroxocobalamin chloride; amino acids (p.1417·1).
*Tonic.*

**Biovir** *GlaxoSmithKline, Braz.*
Lamivudine (p.648·2); zidovudine (p.658·2).
*HIV infection.*

**Biovit** *Roche, Austria.*
Multivitamin preparation with iron (p.1417·1).

**Biovit-A** *Bioceuticals, UK.*
Vitamin A (p.1451·2).

**Biovital**
*Note. This name is used for preparations of different composition.*
*EMS, Braz.*
Multivitamin and mineral preparation (p.1417·1).

*Roche Consumer, Irl.; Roche Consumer, UK†.*
Vitamin B substances; vitamin C; iron; manganese (p.1417·1).

*Lampugnani, Ital.*
Royal jelly (p.1740·3).
*Nutritional supplement.*

**Biovital Aktiv** *Schieffer, Ger.*
*Oral liquid:* Crataegus (p.1677·1); caffeine citrate (p.782·1); ferrous gluconate (p.1428·1); vitamins.
Formerly known as Biovital Forte N.
*Tablets:* Crataegus (p.1677·1); motherwort (p.1717·1); ferrous sulfate (p.1428·2); vitamins (p.1417·1).
*Tonic.*

**Biovital Classic** *Schieffer, Ger.*
Crataegus (p.1677·1); motherwort (p.1717·1); ferric sodium citrate (p.1436·1); vitamins.
Formerly known as Biovital N.
*Tonic.*

**Biovital Ginseng** *Roche, Switz.*
Ginseng (p.1693·1); caffeine (p.782·1); lecithin (p.1706·1); vitamins and minerals (p.1417·1).
*Tonic.*

**Biovital N** *Schieffer, Ger.†.*
Crataegus (p.1677·1); motherwort (p.1717·1); ferrous sulfate (p.1428·2); ferric sodium citrate (p.1436·1); vitamins.
*Tonic.*

**Biovital Weissdorn** *Roche, Austria.*
Crataegus (p.1677·1); magnesium citrate (p.1272·1); ascorbic acid (p.1460·2).
*Tonic.*

**Biovital Weissdorn Tonikum** *Schieffer, Ger.†.*
Crataegus (p.1677·1); motherwort (p.1717·1); vitamins.
*Nervous disorders.*

**Bio-Vitas** *Kyorin, Thai.*
Chlorphenamine maleate (p.427·3); DL-methionine (p.1042·1); vitamin B substances (p.1417·1).
*Skin disorders.*

**Bioxan** *Bioresearch, Mex.*
Naproxen (p.65·1).
*Inflammation; musculoskeletal and joint disorders.*

**Bioxel** *Bioresearch, Mex.*
Fluconazole (p.398·1).
*Fungal infections.*

**Bioxifeno** *Biosintetica, Braz.*
Tamoxifen citrate (p.584·1).
*Malignant neoplasms.*

**Bioxilina** *Northia, Arg.*
Amoxicillin (p.155·3).
*Bacterial infections.*

**Bioxilina Plus** *Northia, Arg.*
Amoxicillin (p.155·3); clavulanic acid (p.193·3).
*Bacterial infections.*

**Bioxima** *Kemyos, Ital.†.*
Cefuroxime sodium (p.184·1).
*Bacterial infections.*

**Bioximicina** *Bioresearch, Mex.*
Doxycycline (p.206·2).
*Bacterial infections.*

**Bioximil** *Bioresearch, Mex.*
Piroxicam (p.84·2).
*Inflammation; musculoskeletal and joint disorders.*

**BioXtra** *Molar, UK.*
Lactoperoxidase; lactoferrin; muramidase (p.1717·2); whey colostrum (p.1611·1); xylitol (p.1469·1).
*Dry mouth; oral hygiene; xerostomia.*

**BioXtra Programme** *Pamex, Irl.*
Artificial saliva, toothpaste, and mouthrinse.
*Dry mouth.*

**Bioxyol** *Richard, Fr.*
Zinc oxide (p.1163·2); zinc peroxide (p.1195·3); titanium dioxide (p.1160·3).
*Ulcers.*

**Bioyetin** *Probiomed, Mex.*
Erythropoietin (p.747·1).
*Anaemias.*

**Biozac** *Niche, Irl.*
Fluoxetine hydrochloride (p.292·1).
*Depression.*

**Bio-Zinc** *Herbaxt, Fr.*
Zinc pidolate; vitamin A; vitamin $B_6$ (p.1417·1).
*Nutritional supplement.*

**Biozole** *Biolab, Thai.*
Fluconazole (p.398·1).
*Fungal infections.*

**Biozolene** *Bioindustria, Ital.*
Fluconazole (p.398·1).
*Fungal infections.*

**Biozolin** *Novartis, Gr.*
Cefazolin sodium (p.170·3).
*Bacterial infections.*

**Biozoral** *Bioresearch, Mex.*
Ketoconazole (p.403·3).
*Fungal infections.*

**Bipasmin**
*Boehringer de Angeli, Braz.†; Promeco, Mex.*
Pargeverine hydrochloride (p.487·3).
*Smooth muscle spasm.*

**Bipasmin Composto** *Boehringer de Angeli, Braz.†.*
Pargeverine hydrochloride (p.487·3); metamizole magnesium (p.36·1).
*Smooth muscle spasm.*

**Bipasmin Compuesto** *Promeco, Mex.*
Pargeverine hydrochloride (p.487·3); metamizole magnesium (p.36·1).
*Smooth muscle pain and spasm.*

**Bipasmin Compuesto NF** *Promeco, Mex.*
Hyoscine butylbromide (p.483·3); ibuprofen (p.45·3).
*Smooth muscle pain and spasm.*

**Bipectinol** *Propan, S.Afr.*
Kaolin (p.1268·3); pectin (p.1580·3); electrolytes (p.1217·1).
*Diarrhoea.*

**Bipencil** *Biochimico, Braz.*
Ampicillin (p.157·1).
*Bacterial infections.*

**Bipensaar** *Rosen, Ger.*
Benzylpenicillin sodium (p.163·2); procaine benzylpenicillin (p.246·1).
Lidocaine hydrochloride (p.1377·3) is included in this preparation to alleviate the pain of injection.
*Bacterial infections.*

**Biphasil**
*Wyeth, Austral.; Wyeth, NZ†; Akromed, S.Afr.*
Levonorgestrel (p.1563·2); ethinylestradiol (p.1553·2).
28-Day packs also contain 7 inert tablets.
*Biphasic oral contraceptive; menstrual disorders.*

**Biphaston** *Agis, Israel.*
Dydrogesterone (p.1549·2).
*Infertility; menorrhagia; menstrual disorders.*

**Biplatrix** *Smith & Nephew, Fr.*
Dried calcium sulfate (p.1665·1).
*External splinting.*

**Bipodial** *Pisa, Mex.*
Sodium bicarbonate; sodium chloride (p.1221·1).
*Haemodialysis.*

**Bipranix** *Ashbourne, UK.*
Bisoprolol fumarate (p.875·1).
*Angina pectoris; hypertension.*

**Bipreterax** *Therval, Fr.*
Perindopril erbumine (p.980·2); indapamide (p.938·2).
*Hypertension.*

**Bipro** *Kenyaku, Thai.*
Betamethasone valerate (p.1093·2).
*Skin disorders.*

**Bi-Profenid**
*Aventis, Braz.; Aventis, Fr.*
Ketoprofen (p.51·2).
*Inflammation; migraine; musculoskeletal, joint and peri-articular disorders.*

**Bipronyl** *Pharmachemie, Singapore.*
Naproxen (p.65·1).
*Gout; musculoskeletal, joint, peri-articular, and soft-tissue disorders.*

**Biquin** *AstraZeneca, Canad.*
Quinidine bisulfate (p.991·3).
*Arrhythmias.*

**Biquinate** *Aventis, Austral.*
Quinine bisulfate (p.460·1).
*Diagnosis of myasthenia gravis; malaria; muscle cramps; myotonia congenita.*

**Bi-Qui-Nol** *Monot, Fr.†.*
Cineole (p.1672·1); guaiacol (p.1122·1); camphor (p.1665·3); bismuth succinate (p.1253·1).
Formerly contained cineole, guaiacol, camphor, bismuth succinate, and quinine sulfate.
*Mouth and throat disorders.*

**Birac** *Pharmacia, Arg.*
Stavudine (p.654·2).
*HIV infection.*

**Biral**
*Madaus, Ger.†; Byk Madaus, S.Afr.*
Valerian (p.1762·2); passion flower (p.1729·1).
*Anxiety; minor nervous disorders.*

**Birley's** *Torbet Laboratories, UK.*
Dried aluminium hydroxide (p.1249·2); magnesium trisilicate (p.1272·3); light magnesium carbonate (p.1272·1).
*Dyspepsia; flatulence; gastric hyperacidity; heartburn.*

**Birobin** *Novartis, Austria†.*
Metolazone (p.956·2).
*Hypertension; oedema.*

**Birodogyl** *Aventis, Fr.*
Spiramycin (p.255·3); metronidazole (p.607·2).
*Bacterial mouth infections.*

**Birofenid** *Aventis, Belg.*
Ketoprofen (p.51·2).
*Inflammation; musculoskeletal, joint, and peri-articular disorders; oedema; pain.*

**Biron** *Douglas, NZ.*
Buspirone hydrochloride (p.672·2).
*Anxiety.*

**Biroxol** *Salus, Ital.*
Ciclopirox olamine (p.396·1).
*Fungal infections.*

**Birvac** *Pharmacia, Arg.*
Lamivudine (p.648·2).
*HIV infection.*

**Bisacolax** *ICN, Canad.*
Bisacodyl (p.1251·3).
*Constipation.*

**Bisalax** *Aspen, Austral.*
Bisacodyl (p.1251·3).
*Bowel evacuation; constipation.*

**Bisa-Lax** *Bergen Brunswig, USA.*
Bisacodyl (p.1251·3).
*Constipation.*

**Biscasil** *Weimer, Hong Kong†.*
Bismuth aluminate (p.1252·1); bismuth subgallate (p.1252·2); bismuth subnitrate (p.1252·2); calcium carbonate (p.1254·2); sodium bicarbonate (p.1223·2); peppermint oil (p.1283·2); silver nitrate (p.1746·1); charcoal (p.1030·2); magnesium phosphate (p.1228·1); silica (p.1581·3).
*Gastrointestinal disorders.*

**Biscotto Plasmon** *Plasmon, Ital.*
Protein, carbohydrate, and lipid preparation with minerals and vitamins (p.1417·1).
*Nutritional supplement.*

**Bisco-Zitron** *Biscova, Ger.*
Bisacodyl (p.1251·3).
*Constipation.*

**Biseko**
*Biotest, Austria; Biotest, Ger.; Biotest, Thai.*
A plasma protein fraction (p.758·2).
*Haemodilution; hypoalbuminaemia; hypogammaglobulinaemia; hypoproteinaemia; hypovolaemia; passive immunisation.*

*Biotest, Hong Kong.*
Albumin (p.740·3).
*Hypoalbuminaemia; hypogammaglobulinaemia; hypoproteinaemia; passive immunisation.*

**Biselic** *ICN, Mex.*
Tripotassium dicitratobismuthate (p.1252·2).
*Dyspepsia; gastritis; gastro-oesophageal reflux; peptic ulcer.*

**Biseptine** *Roche Nicholas, Fr.*
Chlorhexidine gluconate (p.1173·2); benzalkonium chloride (p.1168·3); benzyl alcohol (p.1170·2).
*Bacterial skin infections; skin and wound disinfection.*

**Biserirte Magnesia** *Whitehall, Norw.†.*
Magnesium subcarbonate (p.1272·1); sodium bicarbonate (p.1223·2); bismuth subcarbonate (p.1252·1).
*Gastrointestinal disorders associated with hyperacidity.*

**Biserol-Potassium** *Bichsel, Switz.*
Electrolyte infusion with glucose (p.1217·1).
*Fluid and electrolyte disorders.*

**Bisil** *Sriprasit, Thai.*
Gemfibrozil (p.923·1).
*Hyperlipidaemias.*

**Biskapect** *Propan, S.Afr.*
Light kaolin (p.1268·3); apple pectin (p.1580·3); bismuth subcarbonate (p.1252·1).
*Diarrhoea.*

**Bislan**
*YSP, Malaysia; Yung Shin, Singapore; Yung Shin, Thai.†.*
Bromhexine hydrochloride (p.1115·3).
*Respiratory-tract disorders associated with increased or viscous mucus.*

**Bisma Rex** *Novartis Consumer, S.Afr.*
Bismuth aluminate (p.1252·1); aluminium hydroxide (p.1249·2); magnesium trisilicate (p.1272·3); calcium carbonate (p.1254·2); sodium bicarbonate (p.1223·2); magnesium carbonate (p.1272·1).

**Bismag** *Wyeth Consumer, Singapore.*
Heavy magnesium carbonate (p.1272·1); light magnesium carbonate; sodium bicarbonate (p.1223·2).
*Dyspepsia; gastric hyperacidity.*

**Bisma-Rex** *3M, UK.*
Bismuth subcarbonate (p.1252·1); calcium carbonate (p.1254·2); magnesium trisilicate (p.1272·3); magnesium carbonate (p.1272·1); peppermint oil (p.1283·2).
*Dyspepsia; flatulence.*

**Bismatrol** *Major, USA.*
Bismuth salicylate (p.1252·1).
*Diarrhoea; dyspepsia; nausea.*

**Bismed** *Technilab, Canad.*
*Oral liquid:* Bismuth salicylate (p.1252·1).
*Tablets†:* Bismuth salicylate (p.1252·1); calcium carbonate (p.1254·2).
*Diarrhoea; dyspepsia.*

**Bismofalk**
*Falk, Ger.†; Falk, Hong Kong†.*
Bismuth subgallate (p.1252·2); bismuth subnitrate (p.1252·2).
*Gastrointestinal disorders.*

**Bismofarma** *Farmasa, Mex.*
Tripotassium dicitratobismuthate (p.1252·2).
*Peptic ulcer.*

**Bismolan** *Bittermedizin, Ger.*
Bismuth subnitrate (p.1252·2); butoxycaine hydrochloride (p.1373·1); zinc oxide (p.1163·2).
*Anorectal disorders.*

**Bismolan H Corti** *Bittermedizin, Ger.*
Prednisolone acetate (p.1108·1); bismuth oxychloride (p.1253·1); zinc oxide (p.1163·2).
*Anorectal disorders.*

**Bismolan N** *Bittermedizin, Ger.*
Procaine hydrochloride (p.1383·2); bismuth oxychloride (p.1253·1); zinc oxide (p.1163·2).
*Anorectal disorders.*

**Bismopepsin** *Wiener, Mex.†.*
Tripotassium dicitratobismuthate (p.1252·2).

**Bismorectal** *Vifor, Switz.*
Bismuth succinate (p.1253·1); bismuth hydroxyquinoline (p.1253·1); eucalyptus oil (p.1686·2); sage oil (p.1741·2).
*Mouth and throat disorders.*

**Bismubell** *Sanval, Braz.†.*
Magnesium (p.1227·3); sodium bicarbonate (p.1223·2); acetylmethionine; belladonna (p.479·1).
*Gastrointestinal hyperacidity.*

**Bismu-Jet** *Legrand, Braz.*
Neomycin sulfate (p.235·1); bismuth sodium tartrate; menthol (p.1711·3); procaine hydrochloride (p.1383·2).
*Mouth and throat disorders.*

**Bismultin** *Rafarm, Gr.*
Econazole nitrate (p.397·2).
*Fungal skin and vaginal infections.*

**Bismurectol** *Knoll, Fr.†.*
Bismuth succinate (p.1253·1); cineole (p.1672·1); camphor (p.1665·3).
*Upper respiratory-tract congestion.*

**Bismutal** *Technilab, Canad.*
Bismuth camphocarbonate (p.1253·1); guaifenesin (p.1122·1).
*Sore throat.*

**Bismuth Tulasne** *Rhone-Poulenc Rorer, Switz.†.*
Bismuth subnitrate (p.1252·2).
*Dyspepsia; peptic ulcer.*

**Bismylate** *Stanley, Canad.†.*
Bismuth salicylate (p.1252·1).

**Biso** *1A, Ger.; ABZ, Ger.; Hennig, Ger.*
Bisoprolol fumarate (p.875·1).
*Angina pectoris; hypertension.*

**Biso Lich** *Lichtenstein, Ger.*
Bisoprolol fumarate (p.875·1).
*Angina pectoris; hypertension.*

**Bisobeta** *Betapharm, Ger.*
Bisoprolol fumarate (p.875·1).
*Angina pectoris; hypertension.*

**Bisobloc**
*Azupharma, Ger.; Lederle, Neth.†.*
Bisoprolol fumarate (p.875·1).
*Angina pectoris; hypertension.*

**Bisocor**
*Kwizda, Austria; United Nordic, Denm.; Niche, Irl.*
Bisoprolol fumarate (p.875·1).
*Angina pectoris; hypertension.*

**Bisodol**
*Note. This name is used for preparations of different composition.*
*Wyeth, Irl.; Forest Laboratories, UK.*
*Oral powder:* Heavy magnesium carbonate (p.1272·1); light magnesium carbonate; sodium bicarbonate (p.1223·2).
*Dyspepsia; flatulence; gastric hyperacidity; heartburn.*

*Wyeth, Irl.; Forest Laboratories, UK.*
*Tablets:* Calcium carbonate (p.1254·2); light magnesium carbonate (p.1272·1); sodium bicarbonate (p.1223·2).
*Dyspepsia; flatulence; gastric hyperacidity; heartburn.*

*Wyeth Consumer, Port.*
Calcium carbonate (p.1254·2); magnesium carbonate (p.1272·1); sodium bicarbonate (p.1223·2).
*Dyspepsia; flatulence.*

**Bisodol Extra Strong Mint Tablets** *Whitehall, Irl.*
Calcium carbonate (p.1254·2); magnesium carbonate (p.1272·1); sodium bicarbonate (p.1223·2).
*Dyspepsia; flatulence; heartburn.*

**Bisodol Heartburn Relief** *Forest Laboratories, UK.*
Alginic acid (p.1576·3); magaldrate (p.1271·3); sodium bicarbonate (p.1223·2).
*Dyspepsia; heartburn.*

**Bisodol Wind Relief** *Forest Laboratories, UK.*
Calcium carbonate (p.1254·2); light magnesium carbonate (p.1272·1); sodium bicarbonate (p.1223·2); simeticone (p.1289·2).
Formerly known as Bisodol Extra.
*Dyspepsia; flatulence; gastric hyperacidity; heartburn.*

**Bisogamma** *Worwag, Ger.*
Bisoprolol fumarate (p.875·1).
*Angina pectoris; hypertension.*

**Bisohexal** *Hexal, Ger.*
Bisoprolol fumarate (p.875·1).
*Angina pectoris; hypertension.*

**Bisolapid** *Boehringer Ingelheim, Switz.*
Acetylcysteine (p.1112·3).
*Excess respiratory mucus.*

**Bisolax** *Seng, Thai.*
Bisacodyl (p.1251·3); docusate sodium (p.1262·2); carmellose sodium (p.1577·3).
*Constipation.*

**Bisolbruis** *Boehringer Ingelheim, Neth.*
Acetylcysteine (p.1112·3).
*Respiratory-tract disorders associated with increased mucus.*

**Bisolgrip** *Fher, Spain.*
Chlorphenamine maleate (p.427·3); phenylephrine hydrochloride (p.1126·3); paracetamol (p.76·2).
*Catarrh; cold symptoms.*

**Bisolgrip T** *Boehringer Ingelheim, Port.*
Aspirin (p.15·1); paracetamol (p.76·2); caffeine (p.782·1).
*Fever; inflammation; pain.*

**Bisolnasal** *Boehringer Ingelheim, Neth.*
Tramazoline hydrochloride (p.1131·3).
*Nasal congestion.*

**Bisolol** *Rafa, Israel.*
Bisoprolol fumarate (p.875·1).
*Angina pectoris; hypertension.*

**Bisolrapid** *Boehringer Ingelheim, Austria.*
Acetylcysteine (p.1112·3).
*Respiratory-tract disorders with viscous mucus.*

**Bisolspray** *Boehringer Ingelheim, Port.*
Oxymetazoline hydrochloride (p.1126·1).
Formerly contained fenoxazoline hydrochloride.
*Upper respiratory-tract congestion and inflammation.*

**Bisoltab** *Macrophar, Thai.*
Bromhexine hydrochloride (p.1115·3).
*Coughs.*

**Bisoltus** *Boehringer Ingelheim, Spain.*
Codeine hydrochloride (p.27·1).
*Cough; diarrhoea; pain.*

**Bisolvex** *Boehringer Ingelheim, Switz.†.*
Cineole (p.1672·1); camphor (p.1665·3); niaouli oil (p.1719·3).
*Cold symptoms.*

**Bisolvomycin**
*Boehringer Ingelheim, Ger.†; Boehringer Ingelheim, S.Afr.†.*
Bromhexine hydrochloride (p.1115·3); oxytetracycline hydrochloride (p.241·1).
*Bacterial infections of the respiratory tract.*

**Bisolvon**
*Boehringer Ingelheim, Arg.; Boehringer Ingelheim, Austria; Boehringer Ingelheim, Belg.; Boehringer de Angeli, Braz.; Boehringer Ingelheim, Chile; Boehringer Ingelheim, Denm.; Boehringer Ingelheim, Fin.; Boehringer Ingelheim, Fr.; Boehringer Ingelheim, Ger.; Boehringer Ingelheim, Gr.; Boehringer Ingelheim, Hong Kong; Boehringer Ingelheim, Irl.; Boehringer Ingelheim, Ital.; Boehringer Ingelheim, Malaysia; Boehringer Ingelheim Promeco, Mex.; Boehringer Ingelheim, Neth.; Boehringer Ingelheim, Norw.; Boehringer Ingelheim, Port.; Boehringer Ingelheim, S.Afr.; Boehringer Ingelheim, Singapore; Boehringer Ingelheim, Spain; Boehringer Ingelheim, Swed.; Boehringer Ingelheim, Switz.; Boehringer Ingelheim, Thai.*
Bromhexine hydrochloride (p.1115·3).
*Respiratory-tract disorders associated with increased or viscous mucus.*

**Bisolvon AM** *Thomae, Ger.†.*
Ambroxol hydrochloride (p.1114·3).
*Respiratory-tract disorders associated with increased or viscous mucus.*

**Bisolvon Amoxycilina** *Fher, Spain†.*
Amoxicillin trihydrate (p.155·3); bromhexine hydrochloride (p.1115·3).
*Respiratory-tract infections.*

**Bisolvon Chesty**
*Boehringer Ingelheim, Austral.; Boehringer Ingelheim, NZ.*
Bromhexine hydrochloride (p.1115·3).
*Otitis media; respiratory-tract congestion.*

**Bisolvon Complex** *Boehringer de Angeli, Braz.†.*
Bromhexine hydrochloride (p.1115·3); orciprenaline sulfate (p.790·2); doxylamine succinate (p.432·3).
*Respiratory-tract disorders.*

**Bisolvon Compositum** *Fher, Spain.*
Bromhexine hydrochloride (p.1115·3); codeine hydrochloride (p.27·1); diphenhydramine hydrochloride (p.431·3); ephedrine hydrochloride (p.1120·1).
*Respiratory-tract disorders.*

**Bisolvon Compositum NF** *Boehringer Ingelheim, Arg.*
Bromhexine hydrochloride (p.1115·3); codeine hydrochloride (p.27·1); diphenhydramine hydrochloride (p.431·3); ephedrine hydrochloride (p.1120·1).
*Respiratory-tract disorders.*

**Bisolvon Dry** *Boehringer Ingelheim, Austral.*
Dextromethorphan hydrobromide (p.1117·3).
*Coughs.*

**Bisolvon EX** *Boehringer Ingelheim, Thai.*
Bromhexine hydrochloride (p.1115·3); sulfogaiacol (p.1131·1).
*Respiratory-tract disorders associated with increased or viscous mucus.*

**Bisolvon Linctus** *Boehringer Ingelheim, Switz.*
Bromhexine hydrochloride (p.1115·3); ammonium chloride (p.1115·2).
*Respiratory-tract disorders.*

**Bisolvon Linctus DA** *Boehringer Ingelheim, S.Afr.*
Bromhexine hydrochloride (p.1115·3); orciprenaline sulfate (p.790·2).
*Cough associated with wheeziness.*

**Bisolvon NAC** *Thomae, Ger.†.*
Acetylcysteine (p.1112·3).
*Bronchitis.*

**Bisolvon Sinus**
*Boehringer Ingelheim, Austral.; Boehringer Ingelheim, NZ.*
Bromhexine hydrochloride (p.1115·3); pseudoephedrine hydrochloride (p.1129·2).
*Respiratory-tract congestion.*

**Bisolvonat** *Boehringer Ingelheim, Ger.†.*
Bromhexine hydrochloride (p.1115·3); erythromycin ethyl succinate (p.208·1).
*Bacterial respiratory-tract infections.*

**Bisolvonat Mono** *Thomae, Ger.†.*
Erythromycin (p.208·1) or erythromycin ethyl succinate (p.208·1).
*Bacterial infections.*

**Bisomerck** *Merck dura, Ger.*
Bisoprolol fumarate (p.875·1).
*Angina pectoris; hypertension.*

**Bisomerck Plus** *Merck dura, Ger.*
Bisoprolol fumarate (p.875·1); hydrochlorothiazide (p.933·2).
*Hypertension.*

**Bisopine** *Pinewood, Irl.*
Bisoprolol fumarate (p.875·1).
*Angina pectoris; hypertension.*

**Bisopral** *Alpharma, Fin.*
Bisoprolol fumarate (p.875·1).
*Angina pectoris; hypertension.*

**Bisoprolol-HCT** *Arcana, Austria; Ratiopharm, Austria.*
Bisoprolol fumarate (p.875·1); hydrochlorothiazide (p.933·2).
*Hypertension.*

**Biso-Puren** *Alpharma-Isis, Ger.*
Bisoprolol fumarate (p.875·1).
*Angina pectoris; hypertension.*

**Bisotyrol** *Tyrol, Austria.*
Bisoprolol fumarate (p.875·1).
*Angina pectoris; hypertension.*

**Bispan** *Chinoin, Hung.*
Isopropamide iodide (p.485·2); drotaverine hydrochloride (p.1683·1).
*Peptic ulcer; smooth muscle spasm.*

**Bis-Pectin** *Biotech, Austral.*
Codeine phosphate (p.27·1); kaolin (p.1268·3); aluminium hydroxide (p.1249·2); pectin (p.1580·3).
*Diarrhoea.*

**Bisphonal** *Yamanouchi, Jpn.*
Disodium incadronate (p.773·1).
*Hypercalcaemia of malignancy.*

**Bistatin V** *Bioresearch, Mex.*
Nystatin (p.406·3).
*Fungal vaginal infections.*

**Bisteron** *Jenapharm, Hong Kong†.*
Estradiol valerate (p.1550·2).
*Menopausal disorders; osteoporosis.*

**Bistrepen** *Alembic, India.*
Procaine benzylpenicillin (p.246·1); benzylpenicillin sodium (p.163·2).
*Bacterial infections.*

**Bistryl** *Roux-Ocefa, Arg.*
Ibuprofen (p.45·3).
*Fever; pain.*

**Bisuisan** *DM, Braz.*
Sodium bicarbonate (p.1223·2); calcium carbonate (p.1254·2); magnesium carbonate (p.1272·1); bismuth subcarbonate (p.1252·1); belladonna (p.479·1); rhubarb (p.1287·3); menthol (p.1711·3).
*Gastrointestinal hyperacidity.*

**Bisval** *Valdecasas, Mex.*
Bismuth salicylate (p.1252·1).
*Diarrhoea; gastrointestinal hyperacidity.*

**Bite & Itch Lotion** *Reese, USA.*
Diphenhydramine hydrochloride (p.431·3); pramocaine hydrochloride (p.1382·2).

**Bite Rx** *International Lab Tech, USA.*
Aluminium acetate (p.1652·3).
*Insect bites.*

**Bitecain AA** *Cetus, Arg.*
Aluminium hydroxide (p.1249·2); magnesium hydroxide (p.1272·2); metoclopramide (p.1274·3).
*Gastrointestinal disorders.*

**Bitensil** *UCB, Spain.*
Enalapril maleate (p.909·2).
*Heart failure; hypertension.*

**Bitensil Diu** *UCB, Spain.*
Enalapril maleate (p.909·2); hydrochlorothiazide (p.933·2).
*Hypertension.*

**Bi-Tildiem** *Sanofi Synthelabo, Fr.*
Diltiazem hydrochloride (p.900·1).
*Angina pectoris.*

**Bitteridina** *AFOM, Ital.†.*
Cinchona calisaya (p.1671·3); calumba (p.1665·2); angelica (p.1655·1); cascara (p.1255·1); valerian (p.1762·2).
*Constipation.*

**Bituelve** *Opofarm, Braz.†.*
Cyanocobalamin (p.1458·2); thiamine hydrochloride (p.1455·1).
*Anaemias; vitamin $B_1$ and $B_{12}$ deficiency.*

**Bivacyn**
*Medphano, Ger.; Lek, Hong Kong.*
Neomycin sulfate (p.235·1); bacitracin (p.161·3).
*Burns; ear inflammation; eye disorders; skin disorders; urinary-tract infections; wounds.*

**Bivalem** *Bergamo, Braz.†.*
Mebendazole (p.108·2).
*Worm infections.*

**Bi-Vaspit** *Asche, Ger.*
Fluocortin butyl (p.1102·1); isoconazole nitrate (p.401·3).
*Nappy rash.*

**Bivate** *Douglas, NZ.*
Betamethasone valerate (p.1093·2).
*Skin disorders.*

**Biviol** *Nourypharma, Ger.*
Desogestrel (p.1547·2); ethinylestradiol (p.1553·2).
*Biphasic oral contraceptive.*

**Biviraten**
*Swisspharm, S.Afr.†; Berna, Switz.†.*
A measles and mumps vaccine (p.1624·3).
*Active immunisation.*

**Bivitasi** *Kedrion, Ital.*
Cocarboxylase hydrochloride (p.1455·2).
*Vitamin $B_1$ deficiency.*

**Bivitox** *Terapeutica, Ital.*
Cogalactoisomerase disodium (p.1674·3).
*Liver disorders.*

**Bivorilan** *Medinova (Μεντινοβα), Gr.*
Ciprofloxacin hydrochloride (p.188·2).
*Bacterial infections.*

**B-Ject** *Hyrex, USA.*
Vitamin B substances (p.1417·1).
*Parenteral nutrition.*

**BK** *3M, NZ.*
*Bath oil; lotion:* Liquid paraffin (p.1479·1); oil-soluble dewaxed lanolin fraction (p.1483·1).
*Dry skin disorders; pruritus.*

*Liquid soap:* Lactic acid (p.1704·1).
*Soap substitute in skin disorders.*

**BK HC** *3M, NZ†.*
Hydrocortisone (p.1103·3).
*Skin disorders.*

**B-kombin**
*Leiras, Fin.; ACO, Swed.*
Vitamin B substances (p.1417·1).
*Vitamin B deficiency.*

**B-Laboterol** *Labomed, Chile.*
Betamethasone dipropionate (p.1093·1); clotrimazole (p.396·2).
*Fungal skin infections with inflammation.*

**Black Forest Herbal Tea** *Novartis Consumer, S.Afr.*
Senna (p.1288·2).

**Black Seed** *Be-Tabs, S.Afr.*
Nutritional supplement (p.1417·1).

**Black-Draught** *Chattem, USA.*
*Syrup†:* Casanthranol (p.1255·1); senna (p.1288·2); rhubarb (p.1287·3).

*Tablets; oral granules:* Senna (p.1288·2).

*Constipation.*

**Blackmores B Plus C** *Blackmores, Thai.*
Vitamin B substances; vitamin C (p.1417·1).

**Blackmores Bio** *Blackmores, Thai.*
A range of vitamin preparations with or without minerals (p.1417·1).

**Blackmores Exec B's** *Blackmores, Thai.*
Multivitamin and mineral preparation (p.1417·1).

**Blackmores Naturetime** *Blackmores, Thai.*
A range of vitamin preparations with or without minerals (p.1417·1).

**Blackmores Pregnancy & Breastfeeding Formula** *Blackmores, Austral.†.*
Omega-3 marine triglycerides; dunaliella salina; minerals; vitamins (p.1417·1).
*Dietary supplement.*

**Blackmores for Women Bio Iron** *Blackmores, Austral.†.*
Ferrous fumarate (p.1427·3); folic acid; vitamin C; vitamin $B_{12}$; urtica (p.1417·1).
*Iron deficiency.*

**Blackmores for Women PMT** *Blackmores, Austral.†.*
Vitamins; minerals; viburnum; ginseng; bladderwrack (p.1417·1).
*Premenstrual syndrome.*

**Blackmores for Women Total Calcium** *Blackmores, Austral.†.*
Calcium citrate (p.1225·1); calcium phosphate (p.1225·3); calcium amino acid chelate; minerals; vitamins (p.1417·1).
*Calcium deficiency.*

**Blackoids du Docteur Meur** *SERP, Mon.*
Menthol (p.1711·3); liquorice (p.1270·2).
*Sore throat.*

**Blacor** *Kampel Martian, Arg.*
Betamethasone (p.1093·1).
*Skin disorders.*

**Bladder Irritation** *Hylands, Canad.*
Homoeopathic preparation.

**Bladderon** *Shinyaku, Jpn.*
Flavoxate hydrochloride (p.482·2).
*Pollakisuria.*

**Blader** *Fada, Arg.*
Ciprofloxacin (p.188·2).
*Bacterial infections.*

**Bladex** *Pharma Investi, Chile.*
Ibuprofen (p.45·3).
*Fever.*

**Bladuril**
*Casasco, Arg.; Tecnofarma, Chile; Aventis, Mex.*
Flavoxate hydrochloride (p.482·2).
*Urinary-tract disorders.*

**Blairex Lens Lubricant** *Blairex, USA.*
Range of solutions for soft contact lenses (p.1164·2).

**Blancaler** *Galderma, Mex.*
*Cream:* Titanium dioxide (p.1160·3).

*Topical gel:* Achillea (p.1646·2).

*Skin hyperpigmentation.*

**Blandonal** *Falqui, Ital.†.*
Passion flower (p.1729·1); crataegus (p.1677·1).
*Insomnia.*

**Blanel** *Pfleger, Ger.*
Potassium sodium hydrogen citrate (p.1224·1).
*Renal calculi.*

**Blanoxan** *Bristol-Myers Squibb, Mex.*
Bleomycin sulfate (p.530·2).
*Malignant neoplasms.*

**Blasen- und Nierentee** *Sanova, Austria.*
Bearberry (p.1659·2); equisetum (p.1684·1); birch leaf (p.1660·3); java tea (p.1702·3); maté leaf (p.1765·3).
*Kidney and bladder disorders.*

**Blasen-Nieren-Tee Stada** *Stada, Ger.†.*
Couch-grass (p.1676·2); ononis (p.1723·3); solidago virgaurea (p.1748·3); liquorice (p.1270·2); betulae (p.1660·3).
*Urinary-tract infections.*

**Blasen-Tee** *Mayrhofer, Austria†.*
Bearberry (p.1659·2); herniaria (p.1697·1); juniper (p.1703·1); ononis (p.1723·3); parsley root (p.1728·3); peppermint leaf (p.1283·2).
*Kidney and bladder disorders.*

**Blasentee EF-EM-ES** *Smetana, Austria.*
Birch leaf (p.1660·3); herniaria (p.1697·1); equisetum (p.1684·1); calluna vulgaris.
*Kidney and bladder disorders.*

**Blastocarb**
*Laboratorios Chile, Chile; Lemery, Mex.*
Carboplatin (p.533·3).
*Malignant neoplasms.*

**Blastoestimulina** *Almirall, Spain.*
*Eye drops:* Centella (p.1144·3).
*Eye disorders.*

*Ointment; medicated dressing:* Centella (p.1144·3); neomycin sulfate (p.235·1).
*Burns; skin infections; ulcers; wounds.*

*Pessaries:* Centella (p.1144·3); miconazole nitrate (p.405·3); metronidazole (p.607·2); neomycin sulfate (p.235·1); polymyxin B sulfate (p.245·1).
Formerly contained centella, clodantoin, metronidazole, neomycin sulfate, and polymyxin B sulfate.
*Vulvovaginal infections.*

*Topical aerosol:* Centella (p.1144·3); tetracaine (p.1385·1).
*Burns; ulcers; wounds.*

**Blastolem**
*Laboratorios Chile, Chile; Lemery, Mex.*
Cisplatin (p.538·1).
*Malignant neoplasms.*

**Blaston** *Lacer, Spain.*
Cinitapride acid tartrate (p.1259·2).
*Gastro-oesophageal reflux; gastroparesis.*

**Blastop** *TRB, Arg.*
Folic acid (p.1429·1); vitamin $B_6$ (p.1456·3); vitamin $B_{12}$ (p.1458·2).
*Atherosclerosis; cerebrovascular disorders; dietary supplement; hyperhomocysteinaemia.*

**Blastovin**
*Teva Tuteur, Arg.; Teva, Israel.*
Vinblastine sulfate (p.591·2).
*Malignant neoplasms.*

**Blaubimax** *Blausiegel, Braz.*
Albumin (p.740·3).
*Plasma volume expansion.*

**Blaubumin** *Blausiegel, Braz.*
Albumin (p.740·3).
*Plasma volume expansion.*

**Blauferon** *Blausiegel, Braz.*
Interferon alfa (p.640·3).

**Blauinfuion** *Blausiegel, Braz.†.*
Albumin (p.740·3).
*Plasma volume expansion.*

**Blavin** *Baliarda, Arg.*
Terazosin (p.1011·1).
*Benign prostatic hyperplasia.*

**Bledilait** *Bledina, Fr.*
A range of infant feeds (p.1417·1).
*Allergic disorders; diarrhoea; regurgitation.*

**Bleduran** *Anpharm (Ανφαρμ), Gr.*
Piroxicam (p.84·2).
*Dysmenorrhoea; gout; inflammation; musculoskeletal and joint disorders; pain.*

**Blef-10** *Allergan, Mex.*
Sulfacetamide sodium (p.257·3).
*Eye infections.*

**Blefamide**
*Note. This name is used for preparations of different composition.*
*Allergan, Arg.*
Sulfacetamide sodium (p.257·3); prednisolone acetate (p.1108·1); phenylephrine hydrochloride (p.1126·3).
*Infected eye disorders.*

*Allergan, Chile.*
*Eye drops:* Sulfacetamide sodium (p.257·3); prednisolone acetate (p.1108·1); phenylephrine hydrochloride (p.1126·3).

*Eye ointment:* Sulfacetamide sodium (p.257·3); prednisolone acetate (p.1108·1).

*Eye disorders.*

**Blefamide SF** *Allergan, Mex.*
Sulfacetamide sodium (p.257·3); prednisolone acetate (p.1108·1).
*Eye disorders.*

**Blefamide SOP** *Allergan, Mex.*
Sulfacetamide sodium (p.257·3); prednisolone acetate (p.1108·1).
*Eye disorders.*

**Blefarida**
*Alcon, Port.†.*
Chloramphenicol (p.185·1); cortisone.

*Alcon Cusi, Spain.*
Chloramphenicol (p.185·1); cortisone acetate (p.1096·1).
*Infected eye disorders.*

**Blefarolin** *Bruschettini, Ital.*
Tannic acid (p.1751·2); resorcinol (p.1156·3); menthol (p.1711·3).
*Eye disorders.*

**Blefarosan** *Lersan, Arg.*
Sulfathiazole sodium (p.264·1).
*Bacterial eye infections.*

**Blefcon**
*Note. This name is used for preparations of different composition.*
*Alcon, Ger.†.*
Sulfacetamide sodium (p.257·3); prednisolone acetate (p.1108·1).
*Allergic and inflammatory disorders of the eye.*

*Allergan, Swed.†.*
Sulfacetamide sodium (p.257·3); prednisolone acetate (p.1108·1); phenylephrine hydrochloride (p.1126·3).
*Blepharitis.*

**Blemaren N** *Esparma, Ger.*
Citric acid (p.1673·1); anhydrous sodium citrate (p.1223·2); potassium bicarbonate (p.1223·1).
*Hyperuricaemia; porphyria cutanea tarda; renal calculi.*

**Blemerase** *Young, USA†.*
Benzoyl peroxide (p.1143·2).
*Acne.*

**Bleminol** *Gepepharm, Ger.*
Allopurinol (p.412·2).
*Gout; hyperuricaemia; renal calculi.*

**Blemish Control** *Kay, Canad.*
Salicylic acid (p.1157·1).
*Acne.*

**Blemix** *Ashbourne, UK.*
Minocycline hydrochloride (p.231·3).
*Bacterial infections.*

**Blenamax** *Shinnick, Austral.*
Bleomycin sulfate (p.530·2).
*Malignant neoplasms.*

**Blend-a-Med Periochip** *Procter & Gamble, Austria.*
Chlorhexidine gluconate (p.1173·2).
*Periodontal infections.*

**Blendera** *Otsuka, Thai.*
Preparation for enteral nutrition (p.1417·1).

**Blendox** *Berman, Mex.*
Chlorphenamine (p.428·1).

**Blenox** *Antibioticos, Spain.*
Amoxicillin (p.155·3).
Probenecid (p.416·3) is included in this preparation to reduce renal tubular excretion of amoxicillin.
*Bacterial infections.*

**Blenoxane**
Bristol-Myers Squibb, Austral.; Bristol-Myers Squibb, Braz.; Bristol, Canad.; Bristol-Myers Squibb, NZ; Bristol-Myers Squibb, S.Afr.; Bristol-Myers Squibb Oncology, USA.
Bleomycin sulfate (p.530·2).
*Malignant neoplasms.*

**Bleo** Kyowa, UK.
Bleomycin sulfate (p.530·2).
*Malignant neoplasms.*

**Bleo-cell** Cell Pharm, Ger.
Bleomycin sulfate (p.530·2).
*Malignant neoplasms.*

**Bleocin**
Vianex (Βιανεξ), Gr.; Khandelwal, India; Kayaku, Jpn.
Bleomycin hydrochloride (p.531·2).
*Malignant neoplasms.*

**Bleocris** Kampel Martian, Arg.
Bleomycin (p.531·2).
*Malignant neoplasms.*

**Bleolem**
Lemery, Mex.; Lemery, Thai.
Bleomycin sulfate (p.530·2).
*Malignant neoplasms.*

**Bleo-S** Kayaku, Jpn.
Bleomycin sulfate (p.530·2).
*Skin cancer.*

**Bleph-10**
Allergan, Austral.; Allergan, Canad.†; Allergan, Hong Kong; Allergan, NZ; Allergan, S.Afr.†; Allergan, Thai.; Allergan, USA.
Sulfacetamide sodium (p.257·3).
*Eye infections.*

**Blephagel**
Allergan, Braz.; Thea, Fr.; Pharmacia, Singapore.
Eyelid cleanser.

**Blephamide**
Note. This name is used for preparations of different composition.
Allergan, Austral.†; Allergan, Austria†; Allergan, Hong Kong; Allergan, Malaysia; Allergan, S.Afr.†; Allergan, Singapore.
Sulfacetamide sodium (p.257·3); prednisolone acetate (p.1108·1); phenylephrine hydrochloride (p.1126·3).
*Blepharitis; conjunctivitis.*

Allergan, Canad.; Allergan, Ger.; Allergan, Switz.; Allergan, USA.
Sulfacetamide sodium (p.257·3); prednisolone acetate (p.1108·1).
Formerly contained sulfacetamide sodium, phenazone, sodium thiosulfate, prednisolone acetate, and phenylephrine hydrochloride in *Switz.*
*Blepharitis; conjunctivitis.*

Allergan, Israel; Allergan, NZ.
*Eye drops:* Sulfacetamide sodium (p.257·3); prednisolone acetate (p.1108·1); phenylephrine hydrochloride (p.1126·3).
*Blepharitis; conjunctivitis.*

*Eye ointment:* Sulfacetamide sodium (p.257·3); prednisolone acetate (p.1108·1).
*Inflammatory eye disorders.*

**Blephasol** Pharmacia, Singapore.
Eyelid cleanser.

**Blexit** Laboratorios Chile, Chile.
Bleomycin (p.531·2).
*Malignant neopalsms.*

**Blezamont** Antor, Gr.
Cetirizine hydrochloride (p.427·1).
*Allergic conjunctivitis; allergic rhinitis; pruritus.*

**Blifamol** Allergan, Port.†.
Sulfacetamide sodium (p.257·3); prednisolone acetate (p.1108·1); phenylephrine hydrochloride (p.1126·3).
*Infected eye disorders.*

**Blink** Advanced Medical Optics, UK.
Polyvinyl alcohol (p.1581·1); sodium chloride (p.1233·3) (p.1164·2).
*Dry eyes in contact lens wearers.*

**Blinkene** Allergan-Frumtost, Braz.†.
Polyoxyl 40; macrogol 300 (p.1709·1) (p.1164·2).
*Cleansing solution for contact lens.*

**Blinx** Pilkington Barnes-Hind, USA.
Electrolytes (p.1217·1).
*Eye irrigation.*

**Blio** Faulding, Port.
Bleomycin sulfate (p.530·2).

**Blis K12 Throat Guard** Blis, NZ.
*Streptococcus thermophilus* (p.1704·2).
*Restoration of normal throat bacterial flora.*

**Blisprotex** Rider, Chile.
Zinc oxide (p.1163·2); dimeticone (p.1482·1).
*Nappy rash.*

**BlisterGard** Medtech, USA.
Topical barrier preparation.

**Blistex**
Note. This name is used for preparations of different composition.
Rider, Chile.
Phenol (p.1188·1); camphor (p.1665·3).
*Chapped lips.*

Blistex, USA.
Camphor (p.1665·3); phenol (p.1188·1); allantoin (p.1141·3).
*Oral lesions.*

**Blistex Complete Moisture** Blistex, Canad.
*SPF 15:* Octinoxate (p.1154·3); oxybenzone (p.1154·3).
*Sunscreen.*

**Blistex DCT Lip Balm** Blistex, Canad.
*SPF 15:* Octinoxate (p.1154·3); oxybenzone (p.1154·3); menthol (p.1711·3); phenol (p.1188·1); camphor (p.1665·3).
Formerly contained padimate O, oxybenzone, menthol, phenol, and camphor.
*Chapped lips; sunscreen.*

**Blistex Fruit Smoothies** Rider, Chile.
*SPF 15:* Octinoxate (p.1154·3); oxybenzone (p.1154·3).
*Sunscreen.*

**Blistex Herbal Answer** Blistex, Canad.
*SPF 15:* Octinoxate (p.1154·3); oxybenzone (p.1154·3).
*Sunscreen.*

**Blistex Lip Balm**
Note. This name is used for preparations of different composition.
Blistex, Canad.
*SPF 10:* Padimate O (p.1155·1); oxybenzone (p.1154·3); dimethicone (p.1482·1).
*Chapped lips; sunscreen.*

Blistex, USA.
*SPF 10:* Camphor (p.1665·3); phenol (p.1188·1); allantoin (p.1141·3); dimethicone (p.1482·1); padimate O (p.1155·1); oxybenzone (p.1154·3).
*Chapped lips; sunscreen.*

**Blistex Lip Medex** Blistex, Canad.
Menthol (p.1711·3); camphor (p.1665·3); phenol (p.1188·1).
*Chapped lips; cold sores.*

**Blistex Lip Ointment**
Note. This name is used for preparations of different composition.
Blistex, Canad.
Allantoin (p.1141·3); camphor (p.1665·3); phenol (p.1188·1).
*Chapped lips; herpes labialis.*

Blistex, Hong Kong.
Allantoin (p.1141·3); camphor (p.1665·3); phenol (p.1188·1); menthol (p.1711·3).
*Chapped lips; herpes labialis.*

**Blistex Lip Revitalizer** Key, Austral.†.
*SPF 15:* Octinoxate (p.1154·3); oxybenzone (p.1154·3).
*Dry lips; sunscreen.*

**Blistex Lip Tone**
Note. This name is used for preparations of different composition.
Key, Austral.†.
*SPF 18:* Octinoxate (p.1154·3); oxybenzone (p.1154·3).
*Dry lips; sunscreen.*

Blistex, Canad.
*SPF 15:* Padimate O (p.1155·1); meradimate (p.1151·3); dimethicone (p.1482·1).
*Chapped lips; sunscreen.*

**Blistex Medicated Lip Balm** Key, Austral.†.
*SPF 16:* Padimate O (p.1155·1); oxybenzone (p.1154·3).
*Dry lips; sunscreen.*

**Blistex Medicated Lip Conditioner** Key, Austral.†.
*SPF 15+:* Yellow soft paraffin (p.1479·3); padimate O (p.1155·1); oxybenzone (p.1154·3).
*SPF 20:* Octinoxate (p.1154·3); oxybenzone (p.1154·3).
*Dry lips; sunscreen.*

**Blistex Medicated Lip Conditioner Jar** Blistex, Canad.
*SPF 15:* Camphor (p.1665·3); menthol (p.1711·3); meradimate (p.1151·3); octinoxate (p.1154·3); phenol (p.1188·1).
Formerly contained camphor, menthol, meradimate, padimate O and phenol.
*Chapped lips; herpes labialis.*

**Blistex Medicated Lip Conditioner Tube** Blistex, Canad.†.
*SPF 15:* Padimate O (p.1155·1); oxybenzone (p.1154·3); camphor (p.1665·3).
*Sunscreen.*

**Blistex Medicated Lip Ointment** Key, Austral.†.
*SPF 15:* Padimate O (p.1155·1); oxybenzone (p.1154·3); allantoin (p.1141·3); camphor (p.1665·3).
*Dry lips; sunscreen.*

**Blistex Relief Cream** DDD, UK.
Strong ammonia solution (p.1653·3); ammonia solution aromatic; phenol (p.1188·1).
Formerly known as Blisteze.
*Chapped and cracked lips; herpes labialis.*

**Blistex Ultra** Blistex, USA.
*SPF 30:* Octinoxate (p.1154·3); oxybenzone (p.1154·3); octisalate (p.1154·3); methyl anthranilate (p.1154·1); homosalate (p.1148·1).
*Sunscreen.*

**Blistex Ultra Lip Balm**
Key, Austral.†; Blistex, Canad.
*SPF 30:* Octinoxate (p.1154·3); oxybenzone (p.1154·3); octisalate (p.1154·3); meradimate (p.1151·3); homosalate (p.1148·1).
*Chapped lips; sunscreen.*

**Blistik** Rider, Chile.
*SPF 15:* Padimate o (p.1155·1); oxybenzone (p.1154·3).
*Sunscreen.*

**Blis-To-Sol** Chattem, USA.
*Topical liquid:* Tolnaftate (p.410·1).
*Topical powder:* Zinc undecenoate (p.411·1).
Formerly contained benzoic acid and salicylic acid.
*Fungal skin infections.*

**Bliz** Grisi, Mex.
Boldo (p.1661·2).
*Constipation.*

**Blizer** Ibirn, Ital.
Ferrous gluconate (p.1428·1).
Ascorbic acid (p.1460·2) is included in this preparation to increase the absorption and availability of iron.
*Iron-deficiency anaemia.*

**Blocacid**
Note. This name is used for preparations of different composition.
Ipca, India; IPCA, Singapore.
Famotidine (p.1265·2).
*Gastro-oesophageal reflux; peptic ulcer; Zollinger-Ellison syndrome.*

Collins, Mex.
Naproxen (p.65·1); carisoprodol (p.1392·1).
*Inflammation; pain.*

**Blocadren**
Frosst, Austral.†; Merck Sharp & Dohme, Austria; Merck Sharp & Dohme, Belg.; Merck Frosst, Canad.†; Merck Sharp & Dohme, Hong Kong†; SIT, Ital.; Merck Sharp & Dohme, Mex.†; Merck Sharp & Dohme, Neth.†; Merck Sharp & Dohme, Norw.; Merck Sharp & Dohme, Port.; Merck Sharp & Dohme, S.Afr.†; Merck Sharp & Dohme, Swed.; Merck Sharp & Dohme, Switz.†; Merck Sharp & Dohme, UK†; Merck, USA.
Timolol maleate (p.1012·2).
*Angina pectoris; arrhythmias; glaucoma; hypertension; migraine; myocardial infarction; ocular hypertension.*

**Blocamicina** Gador, Arg.
Bleomycin hydrochloride (p.531·2).
*Malignant neoplasms.*

**Blocan** Grossman, Mex.†.
Cimetidine (p.1255·3).

**Blocanol** Merck Sharp & Dohme, Fin.
Timolol maleate (p.1012·2).
*Angina pectoris; glaucoma; hypertension; migraine; myocardial infarction; ocular hypertension.*

**Blocar** Bago, Chile.
Carvedilol (p.881·1).
*Heart failure; hypertension.*

**Blocatril** Tecnofarma, Mex.
Enalapril (p.909·2).
*Hypertension.*

**Blocotenol**
Azupharma, Ger.; Novartis, Gr.
Atenolol (p.865·2).
*Angina pectoris; arrhythmias; hypertension.*

**Blocotenol comp** Azupharma, Ger.
Atenolol (p.865·2); chlortalidone (p.882·3).
*Hypertension.*

**Blodex** Estedi, Spain.
Vegetable oil (p.1763·3).
*Adjunct in cholecystography and cholangiography.*

**Bloken** Berman, Mex.
Phenylbutazone (p.83·2).
*Inflammation; pain.*

**Blokium**
Note. This name is used for preparations of different composition.
Casasco, Arg.
Diclofenac diethylamine (p.32·1) or diclofenac sodium (p.32·1).
*Gout; inflammation; musculoskeletal, joint, and periarticular disorders; pain.*

Sintesa, Belg.†; Probios, Port.; Almirall, Spain.
Atenolol (p.865·2).
*Angina pectoris; arrhythmias; hypertension; myocardial infarction.*

**Blokium B12** Casasco, Arg.
Diclofenac potassium (p.32·1); betamethasone (p.1093·1) or betamethasone sodium phosphate (p.1093·1); cyanocobalamin (p.1458·2) or hydroxocobalamin (p.1458·2).
*Musculoskeletal and joint disorders.*

**Blokium Cox** Casasco, Arg.
Rofecoxib (p.86·3).
*Osteoarthritis; pain.*

**Blokium Diu**
Probios, Port.; Almirall, Spain.
Atenolol (p.865·2); chlortalidone (p.882·3).
*Hypertension.*

**Blokium Flex** Casasco, Arg.
Diclofenac sodium (p.32·1); pridinol mesilate (p.1395·2).
*Musculoskeletal and joint disorders.*

**Blokium Gesic** Casasco, Arg.
Diclofenac potassium (p.32·1); paracetamol (p.76·2).
*Inflammation; pain.*

**Bloktus** Pisa, Mex.†.
Benzonatate (p.1115·3).

**Blonax** Mintlab, Chile.
Clonixin lysine (p.26·3).
*Pain.*

**Blootec** Ibfarma, Braz.†.
Enalapril maleate (p.909·2).
*Hypertension.*

**Blopresid** Takeda, Ital.
Candesartan cilexetil (p.878·3); hydrochlorothiazide (p.933·2).
*Hypertension.*

**Blopress**
Takeda, Austria; Abbott, Braz.; Abbott, Chile; Takeda, Ger.; Takeda, Hong Kong; Takeda, Ital.; Takeda, Jpn; Takeda, Malaysia; Abbott, Mex.; Seber, Port.; Takeda, Switz.; Takeda, Thai.
Candesartan cilexetil (p.878·3).
*Hypertension.*

**Blopress D** Abbott, Chile.
Candesartan cilexetil (p.878·3); hydrochlorothiazide (p.933·2).
*Hypertension.*

**Blopress 16 mg + 12,5 mg** Seber, Port.
Candesartan cilexetil (p.878·3); hydrochlorothiazide (p.933·2).
*Hypertension.*

**Blopress Plus**
Takeda, Austria; Takeda, Ger.; Takeda, Switz.; Takeda, Thai.
Candesartan cilexetil (p.878·3); hydrochlorothiazide (p.933·2).
*Hypertension.*

**Blosyn** Gufic, India.
Haemoglobin (p.755·2); ferric ammonium citrate (p.1427·2); vitamin $B_{12}$ (p.1458·2); vitamin $B_6$ (p.1457·2) folic acid (p.1429·1).
*Anaemias.*

**Blotex** Novartis, Mex.
Atenolol (p.865·2).
*Angina pectoris; hypertension; myocardial infarction.*

**Blox** Saval, Chile.
Candesartan cilexetil (p.878·3).
*Hypertension.*

**Bloxang** Chauvin, Fr.
Gelatin (porcine) (p.754·3).
*Haemostatic.*

**Blox-D** Saval, Chile.
Candesartan cilexetil (p.878·3); hydrochlorothiazide (p.933·2).
*Hypertension.*

**Bluboro** Allergan Herbert, USA.
Aluminium sulfate (p.1653·1); calcium acetate (p.1225·1).
*Bruises; skin inflammation.*

**Bluco** Hua, Thai.
Codeine phosphate (p.27·1); brompheniramine maleate (p.426·1); pseudoephedrine hydrochloride (p.1129·2).
*Coughs.*

**Bluderm** Quimioterapica, Braz.
Boric acid (p.1662·1); glycerol (p.1694·3); quillaia (p.1416·1).
*Skin disinfection.*

**Blue** Ambix, USA; Moore, USA.
Pyrethrins (p.1509·3); piperonyl butoxide (p.1509·2).
*Pediculosis.*

**Blue Collyrium** Sabex, Canad.†.
Methylthioninium chloride (p.1042·2); naphazoline hydrochloride (p.1124·3).
*Eye irritation.*

**Blue Flag Root Compound** Gerard House, UK†.
Blue flag root (p.1702·1); lappa (p.1704·3); sarsaparilla (p.1742·1).
*Minor skin disorders.*

**Bluesteril** IMS, Ital.
Benzalkonium chloride (p.1168·3).
*Instrument disinfection.*

**Bluetest**
Delta, Fr.; Farmatrading, Port.†.
Pregnancy or fertility test (p.1734·3).

**Blum** Ahimsa, Arg.
Permethrin (p.1508·3).
*Pediculosis.*

**Blumel** Luper, Braz.†.
Honey (p.1434·2); rorippa nasturtium aquaticum.
*Coughs.*

**Blumen** Luper, Braz.
Cod-liver oil (p.1425·2); zinc oxide (p.1163·2).
*Barrier preparation; skin disorders.*

**Blumol** Medinova (Μεντνοβα), Gr.
Ranitidine hydrochloride (p.1285·2).
*Conditions where gastric acid reduction is beneficial; gastric hypersecretion including Zollinger-Ellison syndrome; peptic ulcer.*

**Blunorm** Pharma-Natura, Ital.†.
Hesperidin (p.1688·2); diosmin (p.1688·2); vitamin C (p.1460·2).
*Nutritional supplement in vascular disorders.*

**Blustark** Savio, Ital.
Ferrous gluconate (p.1428·1).
Ascorbic acid (p.1460·2) is included in this preparation to increase the absorption and availability of iron.
*Iron-deficiency anaemia.*

**Blutquick Forte** Duopharm, Ger.†.
Ferrous gluconate (p.1428·1); vitamin B substances (p.1417·1).
*Iron deficiency; tonic.*

**Blutquick Forte S** Duopharm, Ger.†.
Ferrous fumarate (p.1427·3); ferric sodium citrate (p.1436·1); ferrous gluconate (p.1428·1).
*Iron-deficiency anaemia.*

**BM-Accutest**
Roche Diagnostics, Irl.; Roche Diagnostics, UK.
Test for glucose in blood (p.1694·2).
For use with Accutrend blood glucose meters.

**BM-Hopitest** Roche Diagnostics, UK†.
Test for protein, glucose, ketones, and blood in urine.

**BM-Test 1-44**
Roche Diagnostics, Irl.; Roche Diagnostics, NZ; Roche Diagnostics, UK.
Test for glucose in blood (p.1694·2).
Formerly known as BM-Test Glycemie 1-44 in the *UK.*

**BM-Test 3**
Boehringer Mannheim Diagnostics, Irl.†; Roche Diagnostics, UK†.
Test for pH, protein, and glucose in urine.

**BM-Test 4**
Boehringer Mannheim Diagnostics, Irl.†; Roche Diagnostics, UK†.
Test for pH, protein, glucose, and nitrite in urine.

**BM-Test 7** *Boehringer Mannheim Diagnostics, Irl.†; Roche Diagnostics, UK†.*
Test for pH, protein, glucose, ketones, urobilinogen, bilirubin, and blood in urine.

**BM-Test 8** *Boehringer Mannheim Diagnostics, Irl.†; Roche Diagnostics, UK†.*
Test for nitrite, pH, protein, glucose, ketones, urobilinogen, bilirubin, and blood in urine.

**BM-Test BG** *Roche Diagnostics, Austral.; Roche Diagnostics, Ital.†; Roche Diagnostics, UK†.*
Test for glucose in blood (p.1694·2).

**BM-Test Glycemie** *Roche Diagnostics, Fr.*
Test for glucose in blood (p.1694·2).

**BM-Test Glycemie 20-800** *Roche Diagnostics, Austral.*
Test for glucose in blood (p.1694·2).

**BM-Test GP** *Roche Diagnostics, Austral.; Roche Diagnostics, UK†.*
Test for glucose and protein in urine.

**BM-Test 5L** *Boehringer Mannheim Diagnostics, Irl.†; Roche Diagnostics, UK†.*
Test for pH, protein, glucose, ketones, and blood in urine.

**BM-Test LN** *Roche Diagnostics, Fr.†.*
Test for leucocytes and nitrites in urine.

**BM-Test Meconium** *Roche Diagnostics, UK†.*
Test for cystic fibrosis by detection of albumin in the meconium.

**BN** *3M, UK†.*
Turpentine oil (p.1760·1); strong ammonia (p.1653·3); ammonium chloride (p.1115·2).
*Musculoskeletal and joint disorders; pain.*

**BN 53** *Staufen, Ger.*
Homoeopathic preparation.

**BNIL** *Masa, Thai.*
Glibenclamide (p.331·2).
*Diabetes mellitus.*

**Bo-Cal** *Fibertone, USA.*
Calcium with vitamins B and D, and magnesium (p.1417·1).

**Bocasan** *Oral-B, Irl.†; Oral-B, UK†.*
Sodium perborate (p.1192·2).
*Gingivitis; oral hygiene; stomatitis.*

**Bocatriol** *Leo, Austria; Leo, Ger.; Leo, Switz.*
Calcitriol (p.1461·2).
*Hypoparathyroidism; osteoporosis; renal osteodystrophy; rickets.*

**Bocytin** *Asian Pharm, Thai.*
Carbocisteine (p.1116·2).
*Respiratory-tract disorders.*

**Bodaril** *Byk Elmu, Spain†.*
Inosine pranobex (p.640·2).
*Viral infections.*

**Bodigarde** *Lifeplan, UK†.*
Vitamins, fish oils, borage oil, and garlic oil (p.1417·1).
*Nutritional supplement.*

**Bodisan** *Medinfar, Port.*
Amoxicillin trihydrate (p.155·3).
*Bacterial infections.*

**Bodivitin** *Hua, Thai.*
Multivitamin preparation with calcium (p.1417·1).

**Body** *Progest, Ital.†.*
Barrier gel.

**Body Rox** *Usana, Hong Kong.*
A multivitamin and mineral preparation with bioflavonoids (p.1417·1).

**Body Smarts** *Adams, Canad.*
Vitamin or mineral preparations (p.1417·1).

**Body Wash** *Hamilton, Hong Kong.*
Light liquid paraffin (p.1479·1).
*Skin disorders.*

**Bodyguard** *Sanitalia, Ital.*
Echinacea (p.1683·2); salix (p.87·3); devil's claw root (p.28·2); propolis (p.1735·2).
*Nutritional supplement.*

**Boestrol** *Antigen, Irl.*
Diethylstilbestrol (p.1548·1).
*Breast cancer; prostatic cancer.*

**Boflavin** *Milano, Thai.*
Riboflavin (p.1456·1).
*Vitamin $B_2$ deficiency.*

**Bogil** *Llorente, Spain†.*
Aminohydroxybutyric acid (p.353·2).
*Behaviour disorders; emotional disorders; epilepsy.*

**Bo-Gum** *Solvay, Ital.†.*
Cetylpyridinium chloride (p.1173·1); sorbic acid (p.1192·3); bioflavonoids (p.1688·2).
*Oral hygiene.*

**Bogumil-tassenfertiger milder Abfurtee** *Enzypharm, Austria.*
Sambucus (p.1741·3); equisetum (p.1684·1); urtica (p.1762·1); chamomile (p.1669·3); tilia (p.1756·2).
*Constipation; dyspepsia; flatulence.*

**Boi K** *BOI, Spain.*
Potassium ascorbate (p.1233·1).
*Potassium depletion.*

**Boi K Aspartico** *BOI, Spain.*
Potassium ascorbate (p.1233·1).
*Potassium depletion.*

**Boil Ease**
*Note. This name is used for preparations of different composition.*
*Del, Canad.*
Benzocaine (p.1370·3); ichthammol (p.1148·2); sulfur (p.1158·2); cade oil (p.1159·2); camphor (p.1665·3); phenol (p.1188·1); zinc oxide (p.1163·2); thymol (p.1194·2).
*Del, USA; Commerce, USA.*
Benzocaine (p.1370·3); ichthammol (p.1148·2); sulfur (p.1158·2); cade oil (p.1159·2); camphor (p.1665·3); phenol (p.1188·1); zinc oxide (p.1163·2); thymol (p.1194·2); menthol (p.1711·3); eucalyptus oil (p.1686·2).
*Boils.*

**Bokey EMC** *Yung Shin, Singapore.*
Aspirin (p.15·1).
*Thrombosis prophylaxis.*

**Bolchipen** *Cruz, Spain.*
Amoxicillin trihydrate (p.155·3).
*Bacterial infections.*

**Bolcitol** *Lesourd, Fr.*
Fumitory (p.1690·1); boldo (p.1661·2); sage (p.1741·2); fennel (p.1687·2).
*Biliary disorders; gastrointestinal disorders; kidney disorders.*

**Boldex** *Potter's, UK.*
Taraxacum (p.1751·3); butternut bark; boldo (p.1661·2); bladderwrack (p.1742·3).
*Slimming aid.*

**Boldigan** *UCI, Braz.†.*
Acetylmethionine; cynara (p.1678·3); solanum paniculatum; boldo (p.1661·2); liver extract.
*Liver disorders.*

**Boldina He** *Teofarma, Ital.*
Boldine (p.1661·2); aloin (p.1248·3).
*Constipation.*

**Boldo** *Larkhall Laboratories, UK†.*
Boldo (p.1661·2); clivers (p.1673·2); bearberry (p.1659·2); bladderwrack (p.1742·3); taraxacum (p.1751·3).

**Boldo Jurubeba** *Prima, Braz.†.*
Boldo (p.1661·2); solanum paniculatum.
*Liver disorders.*

**Boldo N "Hanosan"** *Hanosan, Ger.†.*
Homoeopathic preparation.

**Boldobeba** *Medquimica, Braz.†.*
Cascara (p.1255·1); boldo (p.1661·2); solanum paniculatum; choline (p.1424·3); vitamin $B_1$ (p.1455·2).
*Liver disorders.*

**Boldocynara** *Bioforce, Switz.*
Cynara (p.1678·3); silybum marianum (p.1043·3); taraxacum (p.1751·3); boldo (p.1661·2); peppermint leaf (p.1283·2).
*Digestive disorders.*

**Boldoflorine**
*Note. This name is used for preparations of different composition.*
*Exflora, Fr.†.*
Boldine (p.1661·2); senna (p.1288·2); frangula bark (p.1266·3); rosemary (p.1740·2).
*Constipation.*
*Exflora, Switz.†.*
*Herbal tea:* Senna (p.1288·2); boldo (p.1661·2); rosemary (p.1740·2); peppermint leaf (p.1283·2); fraxinus excelsior; corylus avellana leaf; castanea vulgaris; frangula bark (p.1266·3); apple; coriander (p.1676·1); elecampane (p.1119·3); liquorice (p.1270·2).
*Tablets:* Boldine (p.1661·2); senna (p.1288·2); frangula bark (p.1266·3); rosemary (p.1740·2).
*Constipation.*

**Boldolaxin** *Diviser Aquilea, Spain.*
Belladonna (p.479·1); bisacodyl (p.1251·3); boldo leaves (p.1661·2); calcium phosphate (p.1225·3); docusate sodium (p.1262·2).
*Bowel evacuation; constipation.*

**Boldopeptan** *Neo Quimica, Braz.*
Cascara (p.1255·1); boldo (p.1661·2); rhubarb (p.1287·3); liver extract.
*Liver disorders.*

**Boldosal** *Ern, Spain†.*
Boldine (p.1661·2); inosine (p.1701·2); magnesium sulfate (p.1228·2); sodium bicarbonate (p.1223·2); dibasic sodium phosphate (p.1231·1); sodium sulfate (p.1290·1).
*Constipation; hepatobiliary disorders.*

**Bolinan** *Roche Nicholas, Fr.*
Povidone (p.1581·2).
*Gastrointestinal disorders.*

**Bolisegna** *Rafarm, Gr.*
Bromhexine hydrochloride (p.1115·3).
*Respiratory disorders associated with viscous mucus.*

**Boljuprima** *Prima, Braz.*
Boldo (p.1661·2); solanum paniculatum.
*Biliary-tract disorders.*

**Bollinol** *Viofar, Gr.*
Loratadine (p.436·1).
*Allergic rhinitis; pruritus.*

**Bolo** *Eagle, Austral.†.*
Vitamin, mineral and amino-acid preparation with eleutherococcus senticosis (p.1417·1).
*Tonic.*

**Boltin** *Organon, Spain.*
Tibolone (p.1572·3).
*Menopausal disorders.*

**Bolus Eucalypti Comp** *Weleda, Austria; Weleda, UK.*
Homoeopathic preparation.

**Bolutol** *Farmasierra, Spain.*
Gemfibrozil (p.923·1).
*Hyperlipidaemias.*

**Bolvidon** *Organon, Israel†.*
Mianserin hydrochloride (p.306·3).
*Depression.*

**B-OM** *OM, Switz.†.*
Cyanocobalamin; sorbitol; yeast (p.1417·1).
*Tonic.*

**B-OM Forte** *OM, Switz.†.*
Cyanocobalamin; nicotinamide; sorbitol; yeast (p.1417·1).
*Tonic.*

**Boma** *Ogna, Ital.*
Borax (p.1661·3); benzocaine (p.1370·3).
*Nausea; oral hygiene.*

**Bomacorin** *Hevert, Ger.*
Crataegus (p.1677·1).
*Heart failure.*

**Bomagall forte S** *Hevert, Ger.†.*
Ammi visnaga; atropin sulf.; carduus marianus; taraxacum; shepherd's purse (p.1744·1); cnicus benedictus (p.1673·3); herb. chelidonii; echinacea; echinaceae pallidae (p.1683·2).
*Painful and spastic biliary disorders.*

**Bomagall mono** *Hevert, Ger.*
Fumitory (p.1690·1).
*Biliary-tract spasm; gastrointestinal spasm.*

**Bomaklim** *Hevert, Ger.*
Homoeopathic preparation.

**Bomapect** *Hevert, Ger.*
Homoeopathic preparation.

**Bomex** *YSP, Malaysia; Yung Shin, Singapore.*
Brompheniramine maleate (p.426·1).
*Hypersensitivity reactions.*

**Bomexin** *Pond's, Thai.*
Bromhexine hydrochloride (p.1115·3).
*Respiratory-tract disorders associated with increased or viscous mucus.*

**Bomix** *Bode, Ger.*
Clorophene (p.1177·3); orthophenylphenol (p.1187·2); chlorocresol (p.1177·1).
*Instrument disinfection.*

**Bonactin** *Almed, Switz.†.*
Zinc sulfate (p.1469·3); heparin sodium (p.928·1).
*Herpesvirus infections.*

**Bonadoxina** *Pfizer, Mex.*
Meclozine hydrochloride (p.436·3); pyridoxine hydrochloride (p.1456·3).
*Nausea and vomiting; vertigo.*

**Bonalen** *Biolab Sanus, Braz.*
Alendronate sodium (p.765·3).
*Osteoporosis.*

**Bonalfa** *White, Arg.; Schering-Plough, Chile; Teijin, Jpn; Schering-Plough, Mex.; Isdin, Port.; Isdin, Spain.*
Tacalcitol (p.1158·3).
*Psoriasis.*

**Bonamina** *Pfizer, Chile.*
Meclozine hydrochloride (p.436·3).
*Nausea and vomiting; vertigo.*

**Bonamine** *Pfizer Consumer, Canad.; Pfizer, Ger.†; Pfizer, Thai.†.*
Meclozine hydrochloride (p.436·3).
*Motion sickness; nausea and vomiting; vestibular disorders.*

**Bonapetit** *Sinterapico, Braz.†.*
Cyproheptadine hydrochloride (p.430·1); vitamins (p.1417·1).
*Reduced appetite.*

**Bonar** *Biosintetica, Braz.*
Bleomycin sulfate (p.530·2).
*Malignant neoplasms.*

**Bonasanit** *Biokanol, Ger.*
Pyridoxine hydrochloride (p.1456·3).
*Vitamin $B_6$ deficiency.*

**Bonased-L** *Dolorgiet, Ger.†.*
Lupulus (p.1708·1).
*Nervous disorders; sleep disorders.*

**Bonatol-R** *Coup, Gr.*
Flurbiprofen (p.43·3).
*Inflammation; musculoskeletal and joint disorders; pain.*

**Bonavit** *QIF, Braz.†.*
Multivitamin and mineral preparation (p.1417·1).

**Bonazin** *Collins, Mex.*
Pyridoxine (p.1457·2); meclozine (p.436·3).
*Nausea and vomiting.*

**Boncordin** *Labinca, Arg.*
Benazepril hydrochloride (p.867·2).
*Hypertension.*

**Bondil** *Vivus, Norw.; Meda, Swed.*
Alprostadil (p.1512·3).
*Erectile dysfunction.*

**Bondiol** *Gry, Ger.*
Alfacalcidol (p.1461·2).
*Hypoparathyroidism; osteomalacia; osteoporosis; renal osteodystrophy; rickets.*

**Bondormin** *Rafa, Israel.*
Brotizolam (p.672·1).
*Insomnia.*

**Bondronat** *Roche, Austria; Roche, Denm.; Roche, Fin.†; Roche, Fr.; Roche, Ger.; Roche, Gr.; Roche, S.Afr.; Roche, Singapore; Kern, Spain; Roche, Swed.; Roche, Switz.; Roche, Thai.; Roche, UK.*
Sodium ibandronate (p.772·3).
*Hypercalcaemia of malignancy; osteolytic bone metastases.*

**Bone Plus** *Tishcon, Hong Kong†.*
Calcium carbonate (p.1254·2); ergocalciferol (p.1462·1).
*Calcium supplement.*

**Bo-Ne-Ca** *ST, Thai.*
Calcium carbonate (p.1254·2).
*Calcium deficiency.*

**Bonefos** *Aventis, Austral.; Calea, Austria; Schering, Belg.; Schering, Braz.; Aventis, Canad.; Schering, Denm.; Leiras, Fin.; AstraZeneca, Ger.; Medac, Ger.; Schering, Hong Kong; Boehringer Ingelheim, Irl.; Leiras, Israel; Schering, Malaysia; Schering, Neth.; Schering, Norw.; Schering, Port.; Schering, Singapore; Schering, Spain; AstraZeneca, Swed.†; Astra, Switz.†; Schering, Thai.; Boehringer Ingelheim, UK.*
Disodium clodronate (p.770·2).
*Hypercalcaemia of malignancy; osteolysis of malignancy.*

**Bonemass** *Apsen, Braz.†.*
Disodium etidronate (p.771·2).
*Osteoporosis.*

**Bongreen** *Welfide, Singapore.*
Alfacalcidol (p.1461·2).
*Osteoporosis; vitamin D metabolic disorders.*

**Boniderma** *Bioethical, Ital.†.*
Fluocinolone acetonide (p.1101·2).
*Skin disorders.*

**Bonidon**
*Mepha, Singapore†.*
Indometacin (p.47·3).
*Gout; inflammation; musculoskeletal, joint, and periarticular disorders; pain.*
*Mepha, Switz.*
Indometacin (p.47·3).
Aluminium glycinate (p.1249·1) is included in the tablets in an attempt to limit adverse effects on the gastrointestinal mucosa.
*Inflammation; pain.*

**Bonifen** *Merck, Mex.; Merck, Port.*
Pyritinol hydrochloride (p.1737·2).
*Cerebrovascular disorders; mental function disorders.*

**Bonine** *Pfizer Consumer, USA.*
Meclozine hydrochloride (p.436·3).
*Motion sickness; vertigo.*

**Boniva** *Roche, USA.*
Sodium ibandronate (p.772·3).
*Osteoporosis.*

**Bonjela** *Reckitt Benckiser, Austral.; Reckitt & Colman, Hong Kong; Reckitt Benckiser, Irl.; Reckitt & Colman, Israel; Reckitt Benckiser, Malaysia; Reckitt Benckiser, NZ; Reckitt Benckiser, S.Afr.; Reckitt Benckiser, Singapore; Reckitt Benckiser, Thai.; Reckitt Benckiser, UK.*
Choline salicylate (p.26·2); cetalkonium chloride (p.1172·1).
*Herpes labialis; oral pain and irritation.*

**Bonjela Teething Gel** *Reckitt Benckiser, UK.*
Lidocaine (p.1377·3); cetalkonium chloride (p.1172·1).
*Infant teething.*

**Bon-Ker** *Baxter, Mex.*
Calcium gluconate (p.1225·2).

**Bonlax** *Synthelabo, Ital.†.*
Cascara (p.1255·1).
*Constipation.*

**Bonmax** *Zydus, India.*
Raloxifene hydrochloride (p.1568·3).
*Osteoporosis.*

**Bonningtons Irish Moss**
*Note. This name is used for preparations of different composition.*
*SmithKline Beecham Consumer, Austral.†.*
Carrageenan (p.1578·2); camphor (p.1665·3); menthol (p.1711·3).
*Coughs; sore throat.*
*GlaxoSmithKline, NZ.*
Menthol (p.1711·3); camphor (p.1665·3); liquorice (p.1270·2); carrageenan (p.1578·2).
*Coughs.*

**Bonocef** *Baldacci, Port.*
Cefixime (p.172·3).
*Bacterial infections.*

**Bonomint** *Intercare, UK†.*
Yellow phenolphthalein (p.1284·1).
*Constipation.*

**Bon-One** *Teijin, Singapore; Teijin, Thai.*
Alfacalcidol (p.1461·2).
*Chronic renal failure; hypoparathyroidism; osteomalacia; osteoporosis; rickets.*

**Bonserin** *Rafa, Israel.*
Mianserin hydrochloride (p.306·3).
*Depression.*

**Bontoss** *Neo Quimica, Braz.*
Guaifenesin (p.1122·1); potassium iodide (p.1598·1).
*Coughs.*

**Bontril** *Carnrick, USA.*
Phendimetrazine tartrate (p.1592·1).
*Obesity.*

**Bonyl** *Orion, Denm.*
Naproxen (p.65·1).
*Inflammation; musculoskeletal and joint disorders; pain.*

**Boost**
*Note. This name is used for preparations of different composition.*
*Mead Johnson Nutritionals, Canad.; Mead Johnson Nutritionals, USA.*
A range of preparations for enteral nutrition (p.1417·1).

*Seven Seas, UK.*
Caffeine (p.782·1); glucose; vitamin B substances; taurine (p.1417·1).
*Fatigue.*

**Boostrix**
*GlaxoSmithKline, Austral.; GlaxoSmithKline, Austria; GlaxoSmithKline, Belg.; GlaxoSmithKline, Fin.; GlaxoSmithKline, Ger.; SmithKline Beecham, Israel; GlaxoSmithKline, Ital.; GlaxoSmithKline, Norw.; GlaxoSmithKline, NZ; GlaxoSmithKline, Spain; SmithKline Beecham, Switz.*
An adsorbed diphtheria, tetanus, and pertussis vaccine (p.1613·3).
*Active immunisation.*

**Boots Antenatal Massage Cream** *Boots Healthcare, Malaysia.*
Aloe vera (p.1141·3); vitamin E (p.1464·3).
*Stretch marks.*

**Boots Chesty Cough Syrup 1 Year Plus** *Boots, UK.*
Guaifenesin (p.1122·1).
*Coughs.*

**Boots Cold & Flu Relief** *Boots, UK.*
Paracetamol (p.76·2); phenylephrine hydrochloride (p.1126·3) caffeine (p.782·1); ascorbic acid (p.1460·2).
*Cold and influenza symptoms.*

**Boots Cold & Flu Relief Hot Lemon** *Boots, UK.*
Paracetamol (p.76·2); vitamin C (p.1460·2).
*Cold and influenza symptoms.*

**Boots Cough & Decongestant Syrup 2 Years Plus** *Boots, UK.*
Guaifenesin (p.1122·1); pseudoephedrine hydrochloride (p.1129·2).
*Coughs.*

**Boots Cough Syrup 3 Months Plus** *Boots, UK.*
Glycerol (p.1694·3).
*Coughs.*

**Boots Covering Cream** *Boots, UK†.*
A covering cream.
*Concealment of birth marks, scars, and disfiguring skin disease.*

**Boots Decongestant Capsules** *Boots, UK.*
Phenylephrine hydrochloride (p.1126·3).
*Cold symptoms.*

**Boots Decongestant Tablets** *Boots, UK.*
Paracetamol (p.76·2); pseudoephedrine hydrochloride (p.1129·2).
*Cold symptoms.*

**Boots Dental Pain Relief** *Boots, UK†.*
Paracetamol (p.76·2); dihydrocodeine tartrate (p.34·3).
*Dental pain.*

**Boots Dry Cough Syrup 1 Year Plus** *Boots, UK.*
Pholcodine (p.1128·3).
*Coughs.*

**Boots Gripe Mixture 1 Month Plus** *Boots, UK.*
Sodium bicarbonate (p.1223·2).
*Dyspepsia.*

**Boots Hayfever Relief Antihistamine** *Boots, UK†.*
Terfenadine (p.441·1).
Formerly known as One-a-Day Antihistamine.
*Hypersensitivity reactions.*

**Boots Maximum Strength Cold & Flu Relief** *Boots, UK.*
Paracetamol (p.76·2); phenylephrine hydrochloride (p.1126·3).
*Cold and influenza symptoms.*

**Boots Medicated Pain Relief Plaster** *Boots, UK†.*
Camphor (p.1665·3); methyl salicylate (p.59·3); menthol (p.1711·3).
*Muscle and soft-tissue pain.*

**Boots Nightime Cough Syrup 1 Year Plus** *Boots, UK.*
Diphenhydramine hydrochloride (p.431·3); pholcodine (p.1128·3).
*Coughs.*

**Boots Pain Relief Suspension 6 Years Plus** *Boots, UK.*
Paracetamol (p.76·2).
*Fever; pain.*

**Boots Tension Headache Relief** *Boots, UK†.*
Paracetamol (p.76·2); doxylamine succinate (p.432·3); caffeine (p.782·1); codeine phosphate (p.27·1).
*Tension headache.*

**Boots Threadworm Tablets 2 Years Plus** *Boots, UK.*
Mebendazole (p.108·2).
*Threadworm.*

**Boots Vapour Rub** *Boots, UK†.*
Eucalyptus oil (p.1686·2); camphor (p.1665·3); turpentine oil (p.1760·1); menthol (p.1711·3); thymol (p.1194·2); pumilio pine oil (p.1737·1).

**Boots Wind Relief** *Boots, UK.*
Aluminium hydroxide (p.1249·2); magnesium hydroxide (p.1272·2); simeticone (p.1289·2).
*Dyspepsia.*

**B.O.P.** *Pautrat, Fr.*
Olive leaf; birch leaf (p.1660·3).
*Oedema.*

**Boplatex** *Pisa, Mex.*
Carboplatin (p.533·3).
*Malignant neoplasms.*

**Boracap** *Sriprasit, Thai.*
Multivitamin preparation with iron and folic acid (p.1417·1).

**Boracelle**
*Swiss Herbal, Canad.†; Bio-Oil Research, UK†.*
Borage oil (p.1661·3).
*Dietary supplement.*

**Boracough** *Sriprasit, Thai.*
Dextromethorphan hydrobromide (p.1117·3); chlorphenamine maleate (p.427·3).
*Coughs.*

**Boradren** *Novartis, Spain†.*
Boric acid (p.1662·1); phenylephrine hydrochloride (p.1126·3); borax (p.1661·3).
*Eye irritation.*

**Boradrine**
*Note. This name is used for preparations of different composition.*
*Bournonville, Belg.†.*
Borax (p.1661·3); boric acid (p.1662·1); phenylephrine hydrochloride (p.1126·3).
*Eye irritation.*

*Bournonville, Neth.†.*
Phenylephrine hydrochloride (p.1126·3).
*Congestion.*

**Borafen** *Sriprasit, Thai.*
Ibuprofen (p.45·3).
*Fever; pain.*

**Borakid** *Sriprasit, Thai.*
Ibuprofen (p.45·3).
*Fever; pain.*

**Boralina** *Veritas, Braz.†.*
Tannic acid (p.1751·2); iodine (p.1598·1); thymol (p.1194·2); salicylic acid (p.1157·1); borax (p.1661·3); boric acid (p.1662·1).
*Skin disorders.*

**Boraline** *Abello, Spain.*
Phenylephrine hydrochloride (p.1126·3).
*Eye irritation.*

**Boramycin** *Sriprasit, Thai.*
Tetracycline phosphate complex (p.266·2).
*Bacterial infections.*

**Borato de Sodio** *Eurofarma, Braz.†.*
Zinc sulfate (p.1469·3); boric acid (p.1662·1); naphazoline hydrochloride (p.1124·3).
*Ocular congestion.*

**Borbalan** *Spyfarma, Spain.*
Amoxicillin trihydrate (p.155·3).
*Bacterial infections.*

**Borea** *Madaus, Spain.*
Megestrol acetate (p.1558·2).
*Breast cancer; endometrial cancer.*

**Born** *Lichtwer, Ger.†.*
Crataegus (p.1677·1).
*Cardiac disorders.*

**Bornilene** *Euphar, Ital.*
Xibornol (p.277·3).
*Mouth and throat infections.*

**Bornosan-Entwasserungsdragees** *Bregenzer, Austria.*
Birch leaf (p.1660·3).
*Diuretic.*

**Bornosan-Leberschutz** *Bregenzer, Austria.*
Silybum marianum (p.1043·3).
*Liver and biliary-tract disorders.*

**Borocaina** *Wassermann, Ital.*
Benzyl alcohol (p.1170·2); sodium benzoate (p.1169·3).
*Mouth and throat disinfection.*

**Borocaina Gola** *Wassermann, Ital.*
Cetylpyridinium chloride (p.1173·1).
*Mouth and throat disinfection.*

**Borocarpin-S** *Winzer, Ger.*
Pilocarpine hydrochloride (p.1495·1).
*Glaucoma; production of miosis.*

**Borocell** *Neutron Technology, USA.*
Sodium monomercaptoundecahydro-closo-dodecaborate.
*Glioblastoma multiforme.*

**Boroclarine** *Novartis Ophthalmics, Fr.*
Borax (p.1661·3); boric acid (p.1662·1); phenylephrine hydrochloride (p.1126·3).
*Conjunctivitis.*

**Borofair Otic** *Major, USA.*
Acetic acid (p.1645·2); aluminium acetate (p.1652·3).

**Borofax** *Warner-Wellcome, USA.*
Zinc oxide (p.1163·2).
Formerly contained boric acid.
*Skin irritation.*

**Boronex** *Remedina, Gr.*
Buspirone hydrochloride (p.672·2).
*Generalised anxiety.*

**Boropak** *Glenwood, USA.*
Aluminium sulfate (p.1653·1); calcium acetate (p.1225·1).
*Inflammatory skin disorders.*

**Boro-Scopol** *Winzer, Ger.*
Hyoscine hydrobromide (p.483·3).
*Eye disorders; production of mydriasis and cycloplegia.*

**Borossigeno Plus Stomatologico** *Warner-Lambert, Ital.†.*
Sodium perborate (p.1192·2); benzethonium chloride (p.1169·2); borax (p.1661·3); boric acid (p.1662·1).
*Oral hygiene.*

**Borostyrol**
*Note. This name is used for preparations of different composition.*
*ACP, Belg.†.*
*Ointment:* Thymol (p.1194·2); benzophenol salicylate; menthol (p.1711·3); boric acid (p.1662·1).
*Burns; skin disorders; wounds.*
*Topical solution:* Thymol (p.1194·2); benzophenol salicylate; menthol (p.1711·3); boric acid (p.1662·1); benzoin (p.1751·1).
*Mouth disorders.*

*Mayoly-Spindler, Fr.*
*Cream:* Thymol (p.1194·2); salol (p.88·1); menthol (p.1711·3).
*Minor burns.*
*Topical solution:* Thymol (p.1194·2); salol (p.88·1); menthol (p.1711·3); boric acid (p.1662·1); siam benzoin (p.1744·1).
*Insect stings; minor skin and mouth disorders.*

**Borostyrol N** *Uhlmann-Eyraud, Switz.*
Thymol (p.1194·2); salol (p.88·1); menthol (p.1711·3); Siam benzoin (p.1744·1).
*Mouth disorders.*

**Borraginol-N** *Takeda, Hong Kong.*
Benzocaine (p.1370·3); cinchocaine hydrochloride (p.1373·2); diphenhydramine hydrochloride (p.431·3); cetrimide (p.1172·1); lithiospermi radix.
*Anorectal disorders.*

**Borymycin**
*YSP, Malaysia; Yung Shin, Singapore.*
Minocycline hydrochloride (p.231·3).
*Bacterial infections.*

**Bosconar** *Teva Tuteur, Arg.*
Bicalutamide (p.530·1).
*Malignant neoplasms.*

**Bosisto's Eucalyptus Inhalant** *Felton, Austral.†.*
Eucalyptus oil (p.1686·2); menthol (p.1711·3).
*Cold symptoms.*

**Bosisto's Eucalyptus Rub** *Felton, Austral.†.*
Eucalyptus oil (p.1686·2); menthol (p.1711·3); methyl salicylate (p.59·3).
*Muscular aches and pains.*

**Bosisto's Eucalyptus Spray** *Felton, Austral.†.*
Eucalyptus oil (p.1686·2).
*Muscular aches and pains.*

**Bosporon** *Tedec Meiji, Spain.*
Lornoxicam (p.54·2).
*Musculoskeletal and joint disorders; pain.*

**Boston**
*Bausch & Lomb, Braz.; Polymer Technology, Canad.; Bausch & Lomb, Fr.†; Polymer Technology, USA.*
Range of solutions for contact lenses (p.1164·2).

**Boston Advance** *Essilor, Austria†.*
Storage solution for hard and gas permeable contact lens (p.1164·2).

**Botaderm** *Zekides, Gr.*
Ketoconazole (p.403·3).
*Fungal scalp infections.*

**Botamycin-N** *Zekides, Gr.*
Clindamycin phosphate (p.194·2).
*Acne.*

**Botanica Hayfever** *Pacific, NZ.*
Chamomile (p.1669·3); lavender (p.1705·1); melissa (p.1711·1); quercetin (p.1688·2); vitamin C (p.1460·2).
*Prevention of minor allergic reactions in the upper respiratory tract.*

**Botastin** *Zekides, Gr.*
Sodium cromoglicate (p.795·3).
*Allergic conjunctivitis; allergic rhinitis.*

**Botox**
*Allergan, Arg.; Allergan, Austral.; Allergan, Austria; Allergan, Belg.; Allergan, Braz.; Allergan, Canad.; Allergan, Denm.; Allergan, Fin.; Allergan, Fr.; Merz, Ger.; Allergan, Gr.; Allergan, Hong Kong; Allergan, Irl.; Allergan, Israel; Allergan, Ital.; Allergan, Jpn; Allergan, Malaysia; Allergan, Mex.; Allergan, Norw.; Allergan, NZ; Allergan, Port.; Allergan, S.Afr.; Allergan, Singapore; Allergan, Spain; Allergan, Swed.; Allergan, Switz.; Allergan, Thai.; Allergan, UK; Allergan, USA.*
Botulinum A toxin (p.1388·3).
*Blepharospasm; cervical dystonia; foot spasticity associated with paediatric cerebral palsy; glabellar lines; hemifacial spasm; hyperhidrosis; spasmodic torticollis; strabismus.*

**Botropase** *Abbott, Ital.*
Batroxobin (p.743·3).
*Haemorrhagic disorders.*

**Bottom Better** *InnoVisions, USA.*
Yellow soft paraffin (p.1479·3); wool fat (p.1483·1).
*Nappy rash.*

**Boucren** *Bouzen, Arg.*
Cetrimide (p.1172·1).
*Skin infections.*

**Bouillet** *Dietetique et Sante, Fr.†.*
Potassium chloride; calcium glutamate; adipic acid; glutamic acid; magnesium carbonate (p.1417·1).
*Dietary salt substitute.*

**Bounty Bears** *Nature's Bounty, USA.*
A range of vitamin preparations (p.1417·1).

**Bourget** *Medipharma, Ger.†.*
Sodium citrate (p.1223·2); sodium bicarbonate (p.1223·2); tartaric acid (p.1752·1).
*Gastrointestinal tract disorders.*

**Bovisan** *Sanum-Kehlbeck, Ger.*
Homoeopathic preparation.

**Bowa** *Nakorn, Thai.*
Aluminium hydroxide gel (p.1249·2); magnesium hydroxide (p.1272·2); simeticone (p.1289·2).
*Flatulence; gastric hyperacidity; peptic ulcer.*

**Boxazin plus C** *Boehringer Ingelheim, Ger.*
Aspirin (p.15·1); ascorbic acid (p.1460·2).
*Fever; pain.*

**Boxocalm** *Cheplapharm, Ger.*
Valerian (p.1762·2); lupulus (p.1708·1).
*Anxiety; insomnia.*

**Boxol** *Pharmacia, Spain.*
Dalteparin sodium (p.891·1).
*Deep-vein thrombosis; myocardial infarction; thrombosis prophylaxis; unstable angina pectoris.*

**Boxolip** *Cheplapharm, Ger.*
Loperamide hydrochloride (p.1271·1).
*Diarrhoea.*

**Boyol Salve** *Pfeiffer, USA.*
Ichthammol (p.1148·2); benzocaine (p.1370·3).
*Skin disorders.*

**Bozaktral** *Chrispa (Χρισπα), Gr.*
Cisapride (p.1259·2).
*Diabetic gastroparesis resistant to other therapy.*

**B-Platin** *Blausiegel, Braz.*
Carboplatin (p.533·3).
*Malignant neoplasms.*

**B-Plex** *Stanley, Canad.*
Vitamin B substances (p.1417·1).

**B-Plex C** *Stanley, Canad.*
Vitamin B substances and vitamin C (p.1417·1).

**B-Plus**
*Volchem, Ital.†.*
Multivitamin preparation (p.1417·1).
*Nutritional supplement.*

*Biolab, Thai.*
Vitamin B substances (p.1417·1).

**BQL** *Cadila, India.*
Enalapril maleate (p.909·2).
*Heart failure; hypertension; myocardial infarction.*

**Braccopiral** *Rhone-Poulenc Rorer, Mex.†.*
Pyrazinamide (p.246·3).

**Brachiapas S** *Pascoe, Ger.†.*
Homoeopathic preparation.

**Brachont** *Azupharma, Ger.†.*
Glycol salicylate (p.44·3); benzyl nicotinate (p.21·2).
*Bruising; muscle and joint disorders.*

**Bradelmin** *Berman, Mex.*
Albendazole (p.101·2).
*Worm infections.*

**Bradimox** *Yamanouchi, Ital.*
Amoxicillin trihydrate (p.155·3).
*Bacterial infections.*

**Bradoral** *Novartis Consumer, Ital.*
Domiphen bromide (p.1179·1).
*Mouth and throat disinfection.*

**Bradosol**
*Note. This name is used for preparations of different composition.*
*Novartis Consumer, Austria.*
Domiphen bromide (p.1179·1); peppermint oil (p.1283·2); eucalyptus oil (p.1686·2); anise oil (p.1655·2).
*Sore throat.*

*Novartis Consumer, Canad.*
Hexylresorcinol (p.1182·1).
*Sore throat.*

*Novartis Consumer, UK.*
Benzalkonium chloride (p.1168·3).
*Sore throat.*

**Bradosol Plus** *Novartis Consumer, UK†.*
Domiphen bromide (p.1179·1); lidocaine hydrochloride (p.1377·3).
*Sore throat.*

**Bradyl** *Lafon, Fr.†.*
Nadoxolol hydrochloride (p.963·3).
*Arrhythmias.*

**Brady's-Magentropfen** *Brady, Austria.*
Cinchona bark (p.1671·3); cinnamon (p.1672·2); aniseed (p.1655·2); coriander (p.1676·1); fennel (p.1687·2); myrrh (p.1718·3); santalum album; gentian (p.1692·2); zedoary.
*Gastrointestinal disorders.*

**Bragg's Medicinal Charcoal** *Bragg, UK.*
Activated charcoal (p.1030·2).
*Dyspepsia; flatulence; heartburn.*

**Brainal**
*Grunenthal, Chile; Andromaco, Spain.*
Nimodipine (p.972·3).
*Mental function impairment; neurological deficit following subarachnoid haemorrhage.*

**Brainox** *Euro-Labor, Port.; Grunenthal, Port.*
Nimodipine (p.972·3).
*Cerebral ischaemia after subarachnoid haemorrhage.*

**Braintop** *Exel, Belg.*
Piracetam (p.1732·1).
*Alcohol withdrawal syndrome; mental function disorders.*

**Bralix** *Remedica, Hong Kong.*
Chlordiazepoxide (p.674·2); clidinium bromide (p.480·2).
*Dysmenorrhoea; gastrointestinal disorders; nocturnal enuresis; ureteral spasm.*

**Bramedil** *Grunenthal, Chile.*
Pargeverine (p.487·3).
*Smooth muscle spasm.*

**Bramedil Compuesto** *Grunenthal, Chile.*
Pargeverine (p.487·3); metamizole magnesium (p.36·1).
*Colic; dysmenorrhoea.*

**Bramin-hepa** *Merz, Ger.*
Isoleucine (p.1438·2); leucine (p.1439·1); valine (p.1451·2); pyridoxine hydrochloride (p.1456·3).
*Hepatic encephalopathy.*

**BranchAmin** *Clintec, USA.*
Amino-acid infusion (p.1417·1).
*Parenteral nutrition in hepatic encephalopathy.*

**Brand- u. Wundgel-Medice N** *Medice, Ger.*
Benzethonium chloride (p.1169·2); lauromacrogol 400 (p.1412·3); urea (p.1162·2).
*Burns; insect stings; skin disorders; wounds.*

**Brand- und Wund-Gel Eu Rho** *Eu Rho, Ger.*
Lidocaine hydrochloride (p.1377·3); allantoin (p.1141·3); cetylpyridinium chloride (p.1173·1); dexpanthenol (p.1727·2).
*Burns; insect stings; skin disorders; wounds.*

**Brandiazin** *Medphano, Ger.*
Sulfadiazine silver (p.259·1).
*Burns.*

**Branigen** *GlaxoSmithKline, Ital.*
Acetylcarnitine hydrochloride (p.1646·1).
*Cerebrovascular disorders; diabetic neuropathy; peripheral nerve disorders.*

**Branitil** *OFF, Ital.*
Acetylcarnitine hydrochloride (p.1646·1).
*Carnitine deficiency.*

**Branolind N** *Hartmann, Ger.†.*
Peru balsam (p.1730·2).
*Burns; skin disorders; wounds.*

**Brasivil** *Stiefel, Ger.†.*
Aluminium oxide (p.1140·1).
*Acne.*

**Brasivol**
*Stiefel, Austral.†; Stiefel, Canad.†; Stiefel, Fr.; Stiefel, Hong Kong; Stiefel, Irl.; Stiefel, UK.*
Aluminium oxide (p.1140·1).
*Acne.*

**Brassel** *Monsanto, Ital.*
Citicoline sodium (p.1672·3).
*Cerebrovascular disorders; parkinsonism.*

**Bratenol** *Byk Elmu, Spain†.*
Pirifibrate (p.984·1).
*Arteriosclerosis; hyperlipidaemias.*

**Braudeide** *Braun, Braz.†.*
Glutaral (p.1180·3).
*Instrument disinfection.*

**Braunoderm**
*Note. This name is used for preparations of different composition.*
*Braun, Austria; Braun, Belg.†; Braun, Ger.; Braun, Irl.†; Braun, Ital.; Braun, Switz.*
Povidone-iodine (p.1190·3); isopropyl alcohol (p.1184·3).
*Skin disinfection; wounds.*

*Braun, Braz.†; Braun, Spain†.*
Povidone-iodine (p.1190·3).
*Skin and mucous membrane disinfection; wounds.*

**Braunol**
*Braun, Austria; Braun, Belg.; Braun, Braz.†; Braun, Ger.; Braun, Irl.†; Braun, Ital.; Braun, Spain†; Braun, Switz.*
Povidone-iodine (p.1190·3).
*Skin and mucous membrane disinfection; wounds.*

**Braunosan**
*Braun, Irl.†; Braun, Switz.*
Povidone-iodine (p.1190·3).
*Hand and wound disinfection.*

**Braunosan H Plus** *Braun, Switz.*
Povidone-iodine (p.1190·3).
*Hand and skin disinfection.*

**Braunovidon**
*Sanova, Austria; Braun, Ger.; Braun, Irl.†; Braun, Switz.*
Povidone-iodine (p.1190·3).
*Burns; infected skin disorders; skin ulcers; vaginal infections; wounds.*

**Bravelle** *Ferring, USA.*
Urofollitropin (p.1342·1).
*Female infertility.*

**Braxan** *Armstrong, Mex.*
Amiodarone hydrochloride (p.859·2).
*Angina pectoris; arrhythmias.*

**Brazepam** *Aspen, S.Afr.*
Bromazepam (p.671·3).
*Anxiety.*

**Breacol**
*ICN, Hong Kong; ICN, Singapore.*
Guaifenesin (p.1122·1).
*Coughs.*

**Breacol Decongestant & Cough Suppressant** *ICN, Malaysia.*
Codeine phosphate (p.27·1); phenylephrine hydrochloride (p.1126·3).
*Coughs; upper respiratory-tract congestion.*

**Breathe Eazy Chest Rub** *Breathe Eazy, Austral.†.*
*Adult formula:* Grindelia (p.1696·1); cajuput oil (p.1664·1); thyme oil (p.1755·3); peppermint oil (p.1283·2); eucalyptus oil (p.1686·2).
*Childrens formula:* Grindelia (p.1696·1); cajuput oil (p.1664·1); thyme oil (p.1755·3); peppermint oil (p.1283·2).
*Respiratory-tract congestion.*

**Breathe Free** *Thompson, USA.*
Sodium chloride (p.1233·3).
*Inflammation and dryness of nasal membranes.*

**Breathe More** *Homeocan, Canad.*
Homoeopathic preparation.

**Breatheze** *Rolab, S.Afr.*
Salbutamol (p.791·3).
*Bronchospasm.*

**Breathquality-UBT** *AB, Ital.*
Carbon-13 labelled urea (p.1667·3).
*Test for gastroduodenal Helicobacter pylori infection.*

**Bredon** *Organon, Mex.*
Oxolamine citrate (p.1126·1).
*Coughs.*

**Breezee Mist Antifungal**
*Note. This name is used for preparations of different composition.*
*Pedinol, USA.*
*Topical powder:* Miconazole nitrate (p.405·3).
*Fungal skin infections.*

*Pedinol, USA.*
*Powder aerosol:* Aluminium chlorohydrate (p.1142·1); menthol (p.1711·3); undecenoic acid (p.410·3).
Formerly contained tolnaftate.
*Fungal skin infections.*

**Brefar** *Farcoral, Mex.*
Paracetamol (p.76·2); phenylephrine hydrochloride (p.1126·3); chlorphenamine maleate (p.427·3).
*Cold symptoms.*

**Brefus** *Hebron, Braz.*
Liquorice (p.1270·2).
*Coughs.*

**Brek** *TRB, Arg.*
Alendronate sodium (p.765·3).
*Osteoporosis.*

**Brelomax** *Abbott, Ger.*
Tulobuterol hydrochloride (p.806·3).
*Obstructive airways disease.*

**Bremagan Flu** *Boehringer Ingelheim Promeco, Mex.*
Guaifenesin (p.1122·1); phenylephrine hydrochloride (p.1126·3); chlorphenamine maleate (p.427·3); paracetamol (p.76·2).
*Allergic rhinitis; hay fever.*

**Bremax**
*Abbott, Austria; Abbott, Mex.†.*
Tulobuterol hydrochloride (p.806·3).
*Obstructive airways disease.*

**Bremicina** *Collins, Mex.*
Ampicillin (p.157·1).
*Bacterial infections.*

**Bremide** *AstraZeneca, Norw.*
Amoxicillin trihydrate (p.155·3); potassium clavulanate (p.193·3).
*Otitis media.*

**Breminal** *Gobbi, Arg.*
Tolterodine (p.490·1).
*Bladder instability.*

**Bremon** *Pensa, Spain.*
Clarithromycin (p.192·2).
*Bacterial infections.*

**Brenazol** *Durascan, Denm.*
Miconazole nitrate (p.405·3).
*Fungal infections.*

**Brenda-35 ED** *Alphapharm, Austral.*
21 Tablets, cyproterone acetate (p.1544·1); ethinylestradiol (p.1553·2); 7 inert tablets.
*Androgenisation in females; combined oral contraceptive.*

**Brennesseltonikum** *Bioflora, Austria.*
Urtica (p.1762·1); taraxacum (p.1751·3); birch leaf (p.1660·3).
*Diuretic.*

**Brenoxil** *Tecnofarma, Mex.*
Amoxicillin (p.155·3).
*Bacterial infections.*

**Brentacort** *Janssen-Cilag, Denm.*
Hydrocortisone (p.1103·3); miconazole nitrate (p.405·3).
*Skin disorders with fungal infection.*

**Brentan**
*Note. This name is used for preparations of different composition.*
*Janssen-Cilag, Denm.*
Miconazole (p.405·2) or miconazole nitrate (p.405·3).
*Fungal infections.*

*Esteve, Spain.*
Hydrocortisone (p.1103·3); miconazole nitrate (p.405·3).
*Fungal infections with inflammation.*

**Breonesin** *Sanofi Winthrop, USA†.*
Guaifenesin (p.1122·1).
*Coughs.*

**Bres** *Farmacologico Milanese, Ital.*
Bromelains (p.1662·2); aescin (p.1648·2).
*Peripheral vascular disorders.*

**Bresal** *Berman, Mex.*
Phenylbutazone (p.83·2).
*Inflammation; musculoskeletal and joint disorders.*

**Bresben** *Azupharma, Ger.*
Atenolol (p.865·2); nifedipine (p.966·2).
*Hypertension.*

**Bresec** *Vocate, Gr.*
Ceftriaxone sodium (p.182·3).
*Bacterial infections.*

**Breston** *Bittner, Austria.*
Senega (p.1130·2); plantago lanceolata (p.1738·2); thyme (p.1755·2); anise oil (p.1655·2).
*Catarrh; coughs.*

**Brethaire** *Novartis, USA†.*
Terbutaline sulfate (p.797·2).
*Asthma; bronchospasm.*

**Brethine** *Novartis, USA.*
Terbutaline sulfate (p.797·2).
*Obstructive airways disease.*

**Bretylate**
*Glaxo Wellcome, Belg.†; Glaxo Wellcome, Canad.†; Wellcome, Irl.†; GlaxoSmithKline, Israel; Glaxo Wellcome, UK†.*
Bretylium tosilate (p.876·2).
*Ventricular arrhythmias.*

**Bretylol** *Sanofi Omnimed, S.Afr.*
Bretylium tosilate (p.876·2).
*Ventricular arrhythmias.*

**Breva** *Valeas, Ital.*
Salbutamol (p.791·3); ipratropium bromide (p.787·1).
*Obstructive airways disease.*

**Brevafen** *Janssen-Cilag, Arg.*
Alfentanil hydrochloride (p.12·2).
*Analgesia in anaesthesia.*

**Brevex** *Bago, Chile.*
Paracetamol (p.76·2); chlorzoxazone (p.1392·3).
*Muscle spasm; pain.*

**Brevibloc**
*Sidus, Arg.; Boots Healthcare, Austral.; Torrex, Austria; Baxter, Belg.†; Cristalia, Braz.; Baxter, Canad.; Baxter, Denm.; Leiras, Fin.; Baxter, Fr.; Baxter, Ger.; Baxter, Gr.; Du Pont, Hong Kong; Boots, Hong Kong; Baxter, Irl.; Du Pont, Israel; Baxter, Ital.; Bristol-Myers Squibb, Malaysia; Aventis, Mex.; Boots Healthcare, NZ; Probios, Port.; Sanofi Synthelabo, S.Afr.; Bristol-Myers Squibb, Singapore; Prasfarma, Spain; Schering, Swed.; Baxter Healthcare, Switz.; Baxter, UK; Baxter, USA.*
Esmolol hydrochloride (p.913·1).
*Hypertension; tachycardia.*

**Brevicon**
*Pharmacia, Canad.; Searle, USA.*
Norethisterone (p.1562·2); ethinylestradiol (p.1553·2).
28-Day packs also contain 7 inert tablets.
*Combined oral contraceptive.*

**Brevilon** *Roche Nicholas, Spain†.*
Passion flower (p.1729·1); valerian (p.1762·2).
*Sedative.*

**Brevimytal** *Lilly, Ger.*
Methohexital sodium (p.1303·2).
*General anaesthesia.*

**Brevinaze** *Intramed, S.Afr.†.*
Ketamine hydrochloride (p.1302·1).
*General anaesthesia.*

**Brevinor**
*Pharmacia, Austral.; Pharmacia, Hong Kong; Pharmacia, Irl.; Pharmacia, NZ; Searle, S.Afr.†; Pharmacia, UK.*
Norethisterone (p.1562·2); ethinylestradiol (p.1553·2).
28-Day packs also contain 7 inert tablets.
*Combined oral contraceptive.*

**Brevital** *Lilly, USA.*
Methohexital sodium (p.1303·2).
*General anaesthesia.*

**Brevoxyl**
*Stiefel, Austral.; Sanova, Austria; Stiefel, Fin.; Stiefel, Fr.; Stiefel, Ger.; Stiefel, Gr.; Stiefel, Hong Kong; Stiefel, Irl.; Stiefel, Malaysia; Stiefel, Norw.; Stiefel, NZ; Stiefel, Singapore; Sylak, Swed.; Stiefel, Thai.; Stiefel, UK; Stiefel, USA.*
Benzoyl peroxide (p.1143·2).
*Acne.*

**Brewers Yeast**
*Jamieson, Canad.†; Nature's Bounty, USA.*
Vitamin B substances (p.1417·1).

*Greater Pharma, Thai.*
Dried yeast (p.1469·1).
*Vitamin B deficiency.*

*Seven Seas, UK.*
Yeast (p.1469·1); vitamin B substances (p.1417·1).

**Brewers Yeast with Garlic** *Phillips Yeast, UK†.*
Yeast (p.1469·1); garlic (p.1691·1); vitamin B substances (p.1417·1).

**Brexecam** *Covan, S.Afr.*
Piroxicam betadex (p.84·2).
*Gout; musculoskeletal and joint disorders.*

**Brexicam** *Pharmacia Upjohn, Mex.*
Piroxicam betadex (p.84·2).
*Gout; inflammation; musculoskeletal, joint, and periarticular disorders; pain.*

**Brexic-DT** *Wockhardt, India.*
Piroxicam (p.84·2).
*Musculoskeletal and joint disorders.*

**Brexidol**
*Biovail, Canad.; Nycomed, Denm.; Nycomed, Fin.; Pharmacia, Ger.; Nycomed, Norw.; Nycomed, Swed.; Chiesi, Switz.; Trinity, UK.*
Piroxicam betadex (p.84·2).
*Gout; inflammation; musculoskeletal, joint, and periarticular disorders; pain.*

**Brexin**
*Note. A similar name is used for preparations of different composition (see below).*
*Pharmacia, Austria; Gross, Braz.; Robapharm, Fr.; Chiesi, Gr.; Chiesi, Hong Kong†; Promedica, Ital.; Chiesi, Malaysia; Germax, Malaysia; Grunenthal, Port.; Chiesi, Singapore; Chiesi, Thai.*
Piroxicam betadex (p.84·2).
*Gout; inflammation; musculoskeletal, joint, and periarticular disorders; pain.*

**Brexin LA**
*Note. A similar name is used for preparations of different composition (see above).*
*Savage, USA†.*
Chlorphenamine maleate (p.427·3); pseudoephedrine hydrochloride (p.1129·2).
*Cold symptoms.*

**Brexine**
*Christiaens, Belg.; Christiaens, Neth.*
Piroxicam betadex (p.84·2).
*Gout; musculoskeletal, joint, and peri-articular disorders; pain.*

**Brexinil** *Grunenthal, Spain.*
Piroxicam betadex (p.84·2).
*Gout; musculoskeletal, joint, and peri-articular disorders; pain.*

**Brexivel** *Promedica, Ital.*
Piroxicam (p.84·2).
*Musculoskeletal and joint disorders.*

**Brexodin** *Quimica y Farmacia, Mex.*
Piroxicam (p.84·2).
*Gout; inflammation; musculoskeletal, joint, periarticular, and soft-tissue disorders; pain.*

**Brexon** *Essex, Chile.*
Vitamin A (p.1451·2); vitamin D (p.1461·2).
*Burns; skin disorders; wounds.*

**Brexonase** *Etex, Chile.*
Fluticasone propionate (p.1102·3).
*Allergic rhinitis.*

**Brexotide** *Etex, Chile.*
Salmeterol xinafoate (p.795·1); fluticasone propionate (p.1102·3).
*Obstructive airways disease.*

**Brexovent** *Etex, Chile.*
Fluticasone propionate (p.1102·3).
*Asthma.*

**Brezal** *Novartis, Ital.*
Choline alfoscerate (p.1488·3).
*Mental function impairment in the elderly.*

**Briazide** *Pierre Fabre, Fr.*
Benazepril hydrochloride (p.867·2); hydrochlorothiazide (p.933·2).
*Hypertension.*

**Bricalin** *Teva, Israel.*
Terbutaline sulfate (p.797·2).
*Obstructive airways disease.*

**Bricanyl**
*AstraZeneca, Arg.; AstraZeneca, Austral.; AstraZeneca, Austria; AstraZeneca, Belg.; AstraZeneca, Braz.; AstraZeneca, Canad.; AstraZeneca, Chile; AstraZeneca, Denm.; AstraZeneca, Fin.; AstraZeneca, Fr.; Stern, Ger.; AstraZeneca, Ger.; AstraZeneca, Hong Kong; AstraZeneca, India; AstraZeneca, Irl.; AstraZeneca, Ital.; AstraZeneca, Malaysia; Astra, Mex.; AstraZeneca, Neth.; AstraZeneca, Norw.; AstraZeneca, NZ; AstraZeneca, Port.; Astra, S.Afr.; AstraZeneca, Singapore; Draco, Swed.; AstraZeneca, Switz.; AstraZeneca, Thai.; AstraZeneca, UK; Hoechst Marion Roussel, USA.*
Terbutaline sulfate (p.797·2).
*Obstructive airways disease; premature labour.*

**Bricanyl comp**
*AstraZeneca, Austria; AstraZeneca, Ger.; Stern, Ger.*
Terbutaline sulfate (p.797·2); guaifenesin (p.1122·1).
*Obstructive airways disease.*

**Bricanyl Composto** *AstraZeneca, Braz.*
Terbutaline sulfate (p.797·2); guaifenesin (p.1122·1).
*Obstructive airways disease.*

**Bricanyl EX** *Astra, Mex.*
Terbutaline sulfate (p.797·2); guaifenesin (p.1122·1).
*Obstructive airways disease.*

**Bricanyl Expectorant**
*AstraZeneca, Hong Kong; AstraZeneca, Irl.; AstraZeneca, Thai.*
Terbutaline sulfate (p.797·2); guaifenesin (p.1122·1).
*Obstructive airways disease.*

**Bricarex** *AstraZeneca, India.*
Terbutaline sulfate (p.797·2); guaifenesin (p.1122·1).
*Asthma; coughs.*

**Bridotrim** *Quimifar, Spain†.*
Co-trimoxazole (p.199·3).
*Bacterial infections; Pneumocystis carinii pneumonia.*

**Briem** *Pierre Fabre, Fr.*
Benazepril hydrochloride (p.867·2).
*Hypertension.*

**Brietal**
*Lilly, Austral.; Lilly, Austria; Lilly, Canad.†; Lilly, Denm.†; Lilly, Irl.†; Lilly, Israel; Lilly, Neth.; Lilly, Norw.†; Lilly, NZ†; Aspen, S.Afr.†; Lilly, Singapore†; Lilly, Swed.†; Lilly, Switz.†.*
Methohexital sodium (p.1303·2).
*General anaesthesia; hypnotic.*

**Briklin** *Bristol-Myers Squibb, Gr.*
Amikacin (p.154·1).
*Bacterial infections.*

**Brimopress**
*Poen, Arg.; Pharma Investi, Chile.*
Brimonidine tartrate (p.876·3).
*Glaucoma; ocular hypertension.*

**Brinaldix**
*Novartis, Ger.; Novartis, India.*
Clopamide (p.888·2).
*Hypertension; oedema.*

**Brinerdin**
*Novartis, Austria; Novartis, S.Afr.; Novartis, Thai.*
Clopamide (p.888·2); dihydroergocristine mesilate (p.1680·1); reserpine (p.995·1).
*Hypertension.*

**Brinerdina**
*Novartis, Ital.; Novartis, Spain.*
Clopamide (p.888·2); dihydroergocristine mesilate (p.1680·1); reserpine (p.995·1).
*Hypertension.*

**Brinerdine**
*Novartis, Port.; Novartis, Switz.*
Clopamide (p.888·2); dihydroergocristine mesilate (p.1680·1); reserpine (p.995·1).
*Hypertension.*

**Brintenal** *Beta, Arg.*
Selegiline hydrochloride (p.1214·1).
*Parkinsonism.*

**Brintoverilte** *Nycomed, Denm.*
Hydrogen peroxide (p.1182·2).
*Mouth infections; oral disinfection.*

**Briocor** *Upsamedica, Ital.†.*
Carnitine (p.1423·3).
*Carnitine deficiency; myocardial ischaemia.*

**Briofil** *Teofarma, Ital.*
Bamifylline hydrochloride (p.781·3).
*Obstructive airways disease.*

**Briogen** *ABC, Ital.*
Glutamine (p.1433·2); DL-phosphoserine; cyanocobalamin (p.1458·2).
*Tonic.*

**Brionil** *Vita, Spain.*
Nedocromil sodium (p.789·3).
*Asthma.*

**Brionot** *Casasco, Arg.*
Piroxicam (p.84·2).
*Gout; musculoskeletal and joint disorders.*

**Brioschi** *Brioschi, Canad.*
Sodium bicarbonate (p.1223·2).

**Briovitan** *Montefarmaco, Ital.*
Multivitamin and mineral preparation with flavonoids (p.1417·1).
*Nutritional supplement.*

**Briovitase** *Montefarmaco, Ital.*
Magnesium aspartate (p.1227·3); potassium aspartate (p.1233·1).
*Magnesium and potassium deficiency.*

**Briscocough** *Quatromed, S.Afr.†.*
Diphenhydramine hydrochloride (p.431·3); ammonium chloride (p.1115·2); sodium citrate (p.1223·2).
*Coughs.*

**Briscopyn** *Quatromed, S.Afr.†.*
Paracetamol (p.76·2); caffeine (p.782·1); meprobamate (p.706·2); codeine phosphate (p.27·1).
Formerly contained paracetamol, caffeine, and meprobamate.
*Pain with tension.*

**Briserin N** *Novartis, Ger.*
Clopamide (p.888·2); reserpine (p.995·1).
*Hypertension.*

**Brisfirina** *Bristol-Myers, Spain.*
Cefapirin sodium (p.170·2).
Lidocaine (p.1377·3) is included in the intramuscular injection to alleviate the pain of injection.
*Bacterial infections.*

**Brisfirina Balsamica** *Bristol-Myers, Spain†.*
Cefapirin (p.170·2); niaouli oil (p.1719·3); guaifenesin (p.1122·1).
*Respiratory-tract infections.*

**Brismucol**
*Bristol-Myers Squibb, Braz.; Bristol-Myers Squibb, Mex.*
Ambroxol acefyllinate (p.1114·3).
*Respiratory-tract disorders.*

**Brisomax** *Bialfar, Port.*
Salmeterol xinafoate (p.795·1); fluticasone propionate (p.1102·3).
*Asthma.*

**Brisoral** *Bristol-Myers, Spain.*
Cefprozil (p.179·2).
*Bacterial infections.*

**Brisovent** *Bialfar, Port.*
Fluticasone propionate (p.1102·3).
*Asthma.*

**Brispen** *Bristol-Myers Squibb, Mex.*
Dicloxacillin (p.205·2).
*Bacterial infections.*

**Bristaciclina** *Pharmacia Upjohn, Spain†.*
Tetracycline hydrochloride (p.266·2).
*Bacterial infections.*

**Bristaciclina Dental** *Pharmacia, Spain.*
Benzydamine hydrochloride (p.21·1); chymotrypsin (p.1671·2); tetracycline hydrochloride (p.266·2); trypsin (p.1758·3).
*Mouth and upper respiratory-tract infections.*

**Bristacol** *Juste, Spain.*
Pravastatin sodium (p.984·3).
*Hypercholesterolaemia; myocardial infarction.*

**Bristaflam**
*Bristol-Myers Squibb, Arg.; Bristol-Myers Squibb, Chile; Bristol-Myers Squibb, Mex.*
Aceclofenac (p.11·2).
*Inflammation; musculoskeletal, joint and peri-articular disorders; pain.*

**Bristamox**
*Bristol-Myers Squibb, Fr.*
Amoxicillin trihydrate (p.155·3).
*Bacterial infections.*

*Bristol-Myers Squibb, Swed.†.*
Amoxicillin (p.155·3).
*Bacterial infections.*

**BrisTaxol** *Bristol-Myers Squibb, Mex.*
Paclitaxel (p.577·3).
*Malignant neoplasms.*

**Bristopen** *Bristol-Myers Squibb, Fr.*
Oxacillin sodium (p.240·2).
*Bacterial infections.*

**Britacil** *Wyeth Lederle, Port.†.*
Ampicillin (p.157·1).
*Bacterial infections.*

**Britaject**
*Lilly, Neth.†; Britannia Pharmaceuticals, UK†.*
Apomorphine hydrochloride (p.1199·1).
*Parkinsonism.*

**Britamox** *Reig Jofre, Spain.*
Amoxicillin trihydrate (p.155·3).
Formerly known as Halitol.
*Respiratory-tract infections.*

**Britane** *Martin, Fr.†.*
Miconazole nitrate (p.405·3).
*Fungal infections.*

**Britapen** *Reig Jofre, Spain.*
Ampicillin sodium (p.157·1) or ampicillin trihydrate (p.157·2).
*Bacterial infections.*

**Britaxol** *Bristol-Myers Squibb, Chile.*
Paclitaxel (p.577·3).
*Kaposi's sarcoma; ovarian cancer.*

**British Army Foot Powder** *Regal, Canad.*
Boric acid (p.1662·1); formaldehyde (p.1179·3); salicylic acid (p.1157·1); zinc oxide (p.1163·2).
*Tinea pedis.*

**Britlofex** *Britannia Pharmaceuticals, UK.*
Lofexidine hydrochloride (p.1041·2).
*Opioid withdrawal symptoms.*

**Brixia**
*Poen, Arg.; Pharma Investi, Chile.*
Azelastine hydrochloride (p.425·2).
*Allergic eye disorders.*

**Brixoral** *Zekides, Gr.*
Ranitidine hydrochloride (p.1285·2).
*Conditions where gastric acid reduction is beneficial; gastric hypersecretion including Zollinger-Ellison syndrome; peptic ulcer.*

**Brizolina** *Bristol-Myers, Spain.*
Cefazolin sodium (p.170·3).
Lidocaine (p.1377·3) is included in the intramuscular injection to alleviate the pain of injection.
*Bacterial infections.*

**Broad Spectrum Sunblock** *Avon, Canad.*
*SPF 15:* Avobenzone (p.1142·3); octinoxate (p.1154·3); oxybenzone (p.1154·3).
*Sunscreen.*

**Brocil** *Berman, Mex.*
Chloramphenicol succinate (p.186·3).
*Bacterial infections.*

**Brocolan** *Berman, Mex.*
Dextromethorphan (p.1117·3).

**Brodifac** *Mintlab, Chile.*
Ketorolac (p.52·3).
*Inflammation; pain.*

**Brodil** *Ofimex, Mex.†.*
Salbutamol (p.791·3).

**Brofed** *Marnel, USA.*
Pseudoephedrine hydrochloride (p.1129·2); brompheniramine maleate (p.426·1).
*Upper respiratory-tract symptoms.*

**Broflex** *Alliance, UK.*
Trihexyphenidyl hydrochloride (p.490·2).
*Drug-induced extrapyramidal disorders; parkinsonism.*

**Brogal** *Rayere, Mex.*
Ambroxol hydrochloride (p.1114·3).
*Respiratory-tract disorders.*

**Brogal Compositum** *Rayere, Mex.*
Ambroxol hydrochloride (p.1114·3); clenbuterol hydrochloride (p.784·2).
*Respiratory-tract disorders.*

**Brogal-T** *Rayere, Mex.*
Ambroxol hydrochloride (p.1114·3); dextromethorphan hydrobromide (p.1117·3).
*Coughs.*

**Brolamina** *Fustery, Mex.*
Hyoscine butylbromide (p.483·3).
*Smooth muscle spasm.*

**Brolene**
*Aventis, Austral.; Aventis, Irl.; Aventis, NZ; Genop, S.Afr.; Aventis, UK.*
Dibrompropamidine isetionate (p.1178·2) or propamidine isetionate (p.1191·2).
*Eye infections.*

**Brolene Cool Eyes** *Aventis, UK.*
Hypromellose (p.1579·3).
*Dry eyes; eye irritation.*

**Brol-eze** *Rhone-Poulenc Rorer, UK†.*
Sodium cromoglicate (p.795·3).
*Allergic conjunctivitis.*

**Brolin**
*Note. This name is used for preparations of different composition.*
*Finn Vita, Chile.*
Cysteine; zinc; pyridoxine; biotin (p.1417·1).
*Hair and nail disorders.*

*Vedim, Spain.*
Famotidine (p.1265·2).
*Gastro-oesophageal reflux; peptic ulcer; Zollinger-Ellison syndrome.*

**Broluidan** *Kenfarma, Spain.*
Letosteine (p.1123·3).
*Respiratory-tract disorders.*

**Bromadine-DM** *Cypress, USA.*
Brompheniramine maleate (p.426·1); dextromethorphan hydrobromide (p.1117·3).
*Coughs.*

**Bromalex** *Vitoria, Port.*
Bromazepam (p.671·3).
*Anxiety.*

**Bromalgina** *Climax, Braz.*
Codeine diethylbarbiturate (p.27·3); dipyrone (p.35·3); methylhomatropine.
*Painful muscle spasm.*

**Bromaline** *Rugby, USA†.*
Phenylpropanolamine hydrochloride (p.1127·3); brompheniramine maleate (p.426·1).
*Upper respiratory-tract symptoms.*

**Bromaline Plus** *Rugby, USA†.*
Phenylpropanolamine hydrochloride (p.1127·3); brompheniramine maleate (p.426·1); paracetamol (p.76·2).
*Upper respiratory-tract symptoms.*

**Bromam** *Durascan, Denm.*
Bromazepam (p.671·3).
*Anxiety.*

**Broman** *Merck, Austria†.*
Bromocriptine mesilate (p.1200·3).
*Parkinsonism.*

**Bromanate**
*Alpharma, Singapore†; Barre-National, USA†.*
Phenylpropanolamine hydrochloride (p.1127·3); brompheniramine maleate (p.426·1).
*Upper respiratory-tract symptoms.*

**Bromarest DX** *Warner Chilcott, USA.*
Brompheniramine maleate (p.426·1); pseudoephedrine hydrochloride (p.1129·2); dextromethorphan hydrobromide (p.1117·3).
*Coughs and cold symptoms.*

**Bromatane DX** *Goldline, USA.*
Pseudoephedrine hydrochloride (p.1129·2); brompheniramine maleate (p.426·1); dextromethorphan hydrobromide (p.1117·3).
*Coughs.*

**Bromatanil** *Hexal, Arg.*
Bromazepam (p.671·3).
*Anxiety.*

**Bromatapp** *Copley, USA†.*
Phenylpropanolamine hydrochloride (p.1127·3); brompheniramine maleate (p.426·1).
*Upper respiratory-tract symptoms.*

**Bromavon** *Hua, Thai.†.*
Brompheniramine maleate (p.426·1); phenylephrine hydrochloride (p.1126·3); phenylpropanolamine hydrochloride (p.1127·3).
*Nasal congestion.*

**Bromax** *Helfarma, Port.*
Ambroxol hydrochloride (p.1114·3).
*Respiratory-tract congestion.*

**Bromaz** *1A, Ger.*
Bromazepam (p.671·3).
*Anxiety; insomnia.*

**Bromazanil** *Hexal, Ger.*
Bromazepam (p.671·3).
*Anxiety; tension.*

**Bromaze** *Hexal, S.Afr.*
Bromazepam (p.671·3).
*Anxiety.*

**Bromazep** *CT, Ger.*
Bromazepam (p.671·3).
*Anxiety; insomnia.*

**Bromazepan** *Dovalle, Braz.*
Bromazepam (p.671·3).
*Anxiety.*

**Bromazolo** *Baldacci, Ital.*
Thiamazole (p.1603·3); dibromotyrosine (p.1597·3).
*Hyperthyroidism.*

**Bromed** *Kolassa, Austria.*
Bromocriptine mesilate (p.1200·3).
*Acromegaly; galactorrhoea; lactation inhibition; menstrual disorders; parkinsonism; prolactinoma.*

**Bromelin** *Hebron, Braz.*
Bromelains (p.1662·2); invertase; glucose oxidase (p.1694·2); ribonuclease (p.1738·1); amylase (p.1654·2).
*Coughs.*

**Bromergon**
*2K, Denm.; Lek, Thai.*
Bromocriptine mesilate (p.1200·3).
*Acromegaly; galactorrhoea; hypogonadism; lactation inhibition; mastalgia; menstrual disorders; parkinsonism; prolactinoma.*

**Bromesep Elixir** *Siam Bheasach, Thai.†.*
Brompheniramine maleate (p.426·1); phenylephrine hydrochloride (p.1126·3); phenylpropanolamine hydrochloride (p.1127·3).
*Hypersensitivity reactions of the respiratory tract.*

**Bromesep Expectorant** *Siam Bheasach, Thai.†.*
Brompheniramine maleate (p.426·1); phenylephrine hydrochloride (p.1126·3); phenylpropanolamine hydrochloride (p.1127·3); guaifenesin (p.1122·1).
*Coughs; hypersensitivity reactions of the respiratory tract.*

**Bromex**
*Qualiphar, Belg.; PP Lab, Thai.*
Bromhexine hydrochloride (p.1115·3).
*Respiratory-tract disorders associated with increased or viscous mucus.*

**Bromexidryl** *Klonal, Arg.*
Bromhexine (p.1115·3).
*Respiratory-tract congestion.*

**Bromfed** *Verum, USA.*
Brompheniramine maleate (p.426·1); phenylephrine hydrochloride (p.1126·3).
Formerly contained brompheniramine maleate and pseudoephedrine hydrochloride.
*Allergic rhinitis; nasal congestion.*

**Bromfed-DM** *Verum, USA.*
Brompheniramine maleate (p.426·1); pseudoephedrine hydrochloride (p.1129·2); dextromethorphan hydrobromide (p.1117·3).
*Allergic rhinitis; coughs; vasomotor rhinitis.*

**Bromfed-PD** *Verum, USA.*
Brompheniramine maleate (p.426·1); phenylephrine hydrochloride (p.1126·3).
Formerly contained brompheniramine maleate and pseudoephedrine hydrochloride.
*Allergic rhinitis; nasal congestion.*

**Bromfenex** *Ethex, USA.*
Brompheniramine maleate (p.426·1); pseudoephedrine hydrochloride (p.1129·2).
*Respiratory-tract disorders.*

**Bromhexine Compound** *Vida, Hong Kong.*
Codeine phosphate (p.27·1); bromhexine hydrochloride (p.1115·3); ephedrine hydrochloride (p.1120·1); brompheniramine maleate (p.426·1); papaverine hydrochloride (p.1728·1).
*Catarrh; coughs; nasal congestion.*

**Bromhist** *Cypress, USA.*
Brompheniramine maleate (p.426·1); pseudoephedrine hydrochloride (p.1129·2).
*Upper respiratory-tract disorders.*

**Bromhist-DM** *Cypress, USA.*
*Oral drops:* Brompheniramine maleate (p.426·1); pseudoephedrine hydrochloride (p.1129·2); dextromethorphan hydrobromide (p.1117·3).
*Coughs; upper respiratory-tract congestion.*
*Syrup:* Brompheniramine maleate (p.426·1); dextromethorphan hydrobromide (p.1117·3); guaifenesin (p.1122·1); pseudoephedrine hydrochloride (p.1129·2).
*Coughs; nasal congestion.*

**Bromhistop** *Neo Dermos, Arg.*
Aluminium chlorohydrate (p.1142·1).
*Hyperhidrosis.*

**Bromidem** *Sandipro, Belg.*
Bromazepam (p.671·3).
*Anxiety; insomnia.*

**Bromidol** *Janssen-Cilag, Denm.†.*
Bromperidol (p.672·1).
*Psychoses.*

**Bromidrastina** *Ibefar, Braz.†.*
Sodium bromide (p.1663·1); hydrastis (p.1698·3); hamamelis (p.1696·3); viburnum prunifolium; gossypium herbaceum.
*Menstrual disorders.*

**Bromifen** *Neo Quimica, Braz.*
Fenoterol hydrobromide (p.785·2).
*Obstructive airways disease.*

**Bromil** *Novamed, Braz.*
*Pastilles:* Menthol (p.1711·3); terpineol (p.1752·2); cineole (p.1672·1); ascorbic acid (p.1460·2); benzocaine (p.1370·3).
*Mouth and throat disorders.*
*Syrup:* Cineole (p.1672·1); terpineol (p.1752·2); menthol (p.1711·3).
*Coughs.*

**Bromi-Lotion** *Gordon, USA.*
Aluminium chlorohydrate (p.1142·1).
*Bromhidrosis; hyperhidrosis.*

**Bromiramin** *Norma (Νορμα), Gr.*
Bromhexine hydrochloride (p.1115·3).
*Respiratory disorders associated with viscous mucus.*

**Bromixen** *Maver, Mex.*
Amoxicillin trihydrate (p.155·3); bromhexine hydrochloride (p.1115·3).
*Respiratory-tract infections.*

**Bromo Madelon** *St Laurent, Canad.*
Sodium bicarbonate (p.1223·2); citric acid (p.1673·1).

**Bromo Seltzer**
*Note. This name is used for preparations of different composition.*
*Numark, Canad.*
Sodium citrate (p.1223·2).
*Dyspepsia; gastric hyperacidity.*

*Warner-Lambert, USA.*
Paracetamol (p.76·2).
*Fever; pain.*

**Bromo Seltzer Effervescent Granules** *Warner-Lambert, USA.*
Sodium bicarbonate (p.1223·2); paracetamol (p.76·2); citric acid (p.1673·1).
*Hyperacidity.*

**Bromocal** *Profarb, Braz.†.*
Calcium lactate (p.1225·3).
*Calcium supplement.*

**Bromocalcio** *Pasteur, Chile.*
Calcium bromolactobionate (p.674·1).
*Insomnia; nervous disorders.*

**Bromocod N** *Streuli, Switz.*
Codeine phosphate (p.27·1); belladonna (p.479·1); drosera (p.1683·1); ipecacuanha (p.1122·3); opium (p.74·2); terpin hydrate (p.1131·1).
*Coughs.*

**Bromocrel** *Hexal, Ger.*
Bromocriptine mesilate (p.1200·3).
*Acromegaly; hyperprolactinaemia; lactation inhibition; parkinsonism.*

**Bromodol** *Janssen-Cilag, Arg.*
Bromperidol (p.672·1) or bromperidol decanoate (p.672·1).
*Behaviour disorders in children; psychoses.*

**Bromohexal** *Hexal, Austral.*
Bromocriptine mesilate (p.1200·3).
*Acromegaly; hyperprolactinaemia; lactation inhibition; parkinsonism.*

**Bromo-Kin** *Irex, Fr.*
Bromocriptine mesilate (p.1200·3).
*Hyperprolactinaemia; lactation inhibition; parkinsonism; prolactinomas.*

**Bromolactin** *Sigma, Austral.*
Bromocriptine mesilate (p.1200·3).
*Acromegaly; hyperprolactinaemia; lactation inhibition; parkinsonism.*

**Bromopar** *Merck, Denm.†.*
Bromocriptine mesilate (p.1200·3).
*Acromegaly; galactorrhoea; hypogonadism; lactation inhibition; mastalgia; menstrual disorders; parkinsonism; prolactinoma.*

**Bromophar** *Qualiphar, Belg.*
Codeine phosphate (p.27·1).
*Coughs.*

**Bromophen TD** *Rugby, USA†.*
Phenylpropanolamine hydrochloride (p.1127·3); phenylephrine hydrochloride (p.1126·3); brompheniramine maleate (p.426·1).
*Upper respiratory-tract symptoms.*

**Bromopirin** *Sigma, Braz.*
Bromazepam (p.671·3); sulpiride (p.722·2).
*Psychoses.*

**Bromoprid** *Teuto, Braz.*
Bromopride (p.1254·1).
*Nausea and vomiting.*

**Bromosedan** *Dovalle, Braz.†.*
Calcium bromide (p.1663·1); sodium bromide (p.1663·1); sparteine sulfate (p.1749·1); phenobarbital (p.367·3); belladonna (p.479·1).
*Sedative.*

**Bromoson**
*Unison, Hong Kong; Unison, Thai.*
Bromhexine hydrochloride (p.1115·3).
*Respiratory-tract disorders associated with increased or viscous mucus.*

**Bromotec** *Teuto, Braz.†.*
Fenoterol hydrobromide (p.785·2).
*Obstructive airways disease.*

**Bromotiren** *Baldacci, Ital.*
Dibromotyrosine (p.1597·3).
*Hyperthyroidism.*

**Bromotuss with Codeine** *Rugby, USA.*
Bromazine hydrochloride (p.425·3); codeine phosphate (p.27·1).
*Coughs and cold symptoms.*

**Bromoxon** *Sanval, Braz.*
Bromazepam (p.671·3).
*Anxiety.*

**Bromped** *Hua, Thai.†.*
Brompheniramine maleate (p.426·1); phenylephrine hydrochloride (p.1126·3); phenylpropanolamine hydrochloride (p.1127·3).
*Nasal congestion.*

**Bromphen DX Cough** *Muro, USA.*
Pseudoephedrine hydrochloride (p.1129·2); brompheniramine maleate (p.426·1); dextromethorphan hydrobromide (p.1117·3).
*Coughs and cold symptoms.*

**Bromphenex** *Ethex, Hong Kong.*
Brompheniramine maleate (p.426·1); pseudoephedrine hydrochloride (p.1129·2).
*Rhinitis.*

**Brompheniramine Cough** *Geneva, USA.*
Pseudoephedrine hydrochloride (p.1129·2); brompheniramine maleate (p.426·1); dextromethorphan hydrobromide (p.1117·3).
*Coughs and cold symptoms.*

**Brompheniramine DC Cough** *Geneva, USA†.*
Phenylpropanolamine hydrochloride (p.1127·3); codeine phosphate (p.27·1); brompheniramine maleate (p.426·1).
*Coughs and cold symptoms.*

**Brom-PP** *Jean-Marie, Hong Kong.*
Brompheniramine maleate (p.426·1); phenylephrine hydrochloride (p.1126·3); phenylpropanolamine hydrochloride (p.1127·3).
*Respiratory-tract disorders.*

**Brom-Ramine Compound** *Universal, Hong Kong.*
Brompheniramine maleate (p.426·1); phenylephrine hydrochloride (p.1126·3); phenylpropanolamine hydrochloride (p.1127·3).
*Respiratory-tract disorders.*

**Bromselon** *Tecnobio, Spain†.*
Ebastine (p.433·1).
*Hypersensitivity reactions.*

**Bromso** *TO-Chemicals, Thai.*
Bromhexine hydrochloride (p.1115·3).
*Respiratory-tract disorders associated with increased or viscous mucus.*

**Bromso-Ex** *TO-Chemicals, Thai.*
Bromhexine hydrochloride (p.1115·3); sulfogaiacol (p.1131·1).
*Respiratory-tract disorders associated with increased or viscous mucus.*

**Bromtine** *Duopharma, Hong Kong.*
Bromocriptine (p.1202·3).
*Acromegaly; hyperprolactinaemia; parkinsonism.*

**Bromtussia** *Asian Pharm, Thai.*
Guaifenesin (p.1122·1); brompheniramine maleate (p.426·1); phenylephrine hydrochloride (p.1126·3).
Formerly contained guaifenesin, brompheniramine maleate, and phenylpropanolamine hydrochloride.
*Nasal congestion.*

**Bromtussia DC** *Asian Pharm, Thai.*
Guaifenesin (p.1122·1); brompheniramine maleate (p.426·1); phenylephrine hydrochloride (p.1126·3); codeine phosphate (p.27·1).
*Coughs; nasal congestion.*

**Bromtussin** *Shiwa, Thai.†.*
Brompheniramine maleate (p.426·1); phenylephrine hydrochloride (p.1126·3); phenylpropanolamine hydrochloride (p.1127·3).
*Cold symptoms.*

**Bromuc**
*Ariston, Braz.; Fujisawa, Ger.*
Acetylcysteine (p.1112·3).
*Respiratory-tract disorders associated with increased or viscous mucus.*

**Bromurex** *Pisa, Mex.*
Pancuronium bromide (p.1404·3).
*Competitive neuromuscular blocker.*

**Bromxin** *Masa, Thai.*
Bromhexine hydrochloride (p.1115·3).
*Respiratory-tract disorders.*

**Bromxine**
*Atlantic, Hong Kong; Atlantic, Malaysia; Atlantic, Singapore; Atlantic, Thai.; General Drugs, Thai.*
Bromhexine hydrochloride (p.1115·3).
*Respiratory-tract disorders associated with increased or viscous mucus.*

**Bron 6** *Capo Sole, Ital.*
Chestnut honey; propolis; althaea; erisimo; thyme; wild rose; niaouli oil (p.1417·1).
*Food supplement; tonic.*

**Bronalide**
*Boehringer Ingelheim, Canad.†; Boehringer Ingelheim, Gr.*
Flunisolide (p.1101·1).
*Asthma.*

**Bronalin Decongestant** *SSL, UK†.*
Pseudoephedrine hydrochloride (p.1129·2).
*Nasal and sinus congestion.*

**Bronalin Dry Cough** *SSL, UK†.*
Dextromethorphan hydrobromide (p.1117·3); pseudoephedrine hydrochloride (p.1129·2).
*Coughs.*

**Bronalin Expectorant** *SSL, UK†.*
Diphenhydramine hydrochloride (p.431·3); sodium citrate (p.1223·2); ammonium chloride (p.1115·2).
*Coughs.*

**Bronalin Junior** *SSL, UK†.*
Diphenhydramine hydrochloride (p.431·3); sodium citrate (p.1223·2).
*Coughs.*

**Broncal**
*Note. This name is used for preparations of different composition.*
*Pharmacobel, Belg.†.*
Pholcodine (p.1128·3); ephedrine hydrochloride (p.1120·1); chlorphenamine maleate (p.427·3); sulfogaiacol (p.1131·1).
*Coughs.*

*Novel, Ital.*
Dextromethorphan hydrobromide (p.1117·3); sulfogaiacol (p.1131·1).
*Coughs.*

**Broncalene** *Martin, Fr.*
Pholcodine (p.1128·3); chlorphenamine maleate (p.427·3); sodium benzoate (p.1169·3).
*Coughs.*

**Broncalene Nourisson** *Martin, Fr.*
Chlorphenamine maleate (p.427·3); sodium benzoate (p.1169·3); tolu balsam (p.1131·3).
*Coughs.*

**Broncard** *Labomed, Chile.*
Levodropropizine (p.1119·3).
*Coughs.*

**Broncasma**
*Berna, Belg.†.; Berna, Hong Kong†; Berna, Switz.†; Berna, Thai.†.*
*Pneumococcus* I, II, III; *Streptococcus*; *Staphylococcus*; *Moraxella catarrhalis*; *Gaffkya tetragena*; *Pseudomonas aeruginosa*; *Klebsiella pneumoniae* (Friedlander); *Haemophilus influenzae*.
*Chronic bronchitis; respiratory-tract infections.*

*Berna, Port.*
An inactivated bacterial vaccine containing lysates of *Haemophilus influenzae*; *Klebsiella pneumoniae*; *Moraxella catarrhalis*; *Neisseria t.*; pneumococcus; staphylococcus; *Streptococcus haemolyticus*; *Streptococcus viridans*.

**Broncasmin Composto** *Opofarm, Braz.†.*
Terbutaline sulfate (p.797·2); guaifenesin (p.1122·1).
*Obstructive airways disease.*

**Broncatar**
*Note. This name is used for preparations of different composition.*
*Cazi, Braz.*
Bromhexine hydrochloride (p.1115·3); thiocol.
*Respiratory-tract congestion.*

*Kramer, Switz.†.*
Carbocisteine (p.1116·2); promethazine hydrochloride (p.439·1).
*Coughs; respiratory-tract congestion.*

**Broncelix** *Pfizer, NZ.*
Choline theophyllinate (p.784·2); guaifenesin (p.1122·1).
*Coughs.*

**Bronch Eze** *Pharmavite, Canad.†.*
Ephedrine hydrochloride (p.1120·1); ammonium chloride (p.1115·2).

**Bronchalene**
*Aventis, Belg.†.*
*Syrup for adults and children:* Pholcodine (p.1128·3); chlorphenamine maleate (p.427·3).
*Coughs.*

*Rhone-Poulenc Rorer, Belg.†.*
*Syrup for infants:* Chlorphenamine maleate (p.427·3).
*Coughs.*

**Bronchalin** *Gubler, Switz.†.*
Ephedrine hydrochloride (p.1120·1); guaifenesin (p.1122·1); hyoscyamine sulfate (p.485·1); castanea vulgaris; drosera (p.1683·1); liquorice (p.1270·2); psyllium seed (p.1268·1); thyme (p.1755·2); belladonna (p.479·1); ipecacuanha (p.1122·3); sodium benzoate (p.1169·3).
*Respiratory-tract disorders.*

**Bronchalis-Heel** *Peithner, Austria.*
Homoeopathic preparation.

**Bronchathiol**
*Aventis, Belg.; Martin, Fr.*
Carbocisteine (p.1116·2).
*Respiratory-tract disorders.*

**Bronchenolo** *GlaxoSmithKline Consumer, Ital.*
*Pastilles:* Cetylpyridinium chloride (p.1173·1).
*Mouth and throat disinfection.*

*Syrup:* Dextromethorphan hydrobromide (p.1117·3); sulfogaiacol (p.1131·1); ammonium acetate (p.1115·1).
*Coughs.*

*Tablets:* Dextromethorphan hydrobromide (adsorbed onto magnesium trisilicate) (p.1117·3).
*Coughs.*

**Bronchenolo Antiflu** *GlaxoSmithKline, Ital.*
Paracetamol (p.76·2); ascorbic acid (p.1460·2).
*Fever; pain.*

**Bronchette** *Aspen, S.Afr.*
Carbocisteine (p.1116·2).
*Respiratory-tract disorders with excess and viscous mucus.*

**Bronchex** *Hilarys, Canad.*
Ammonium chloride (p.1115·2); ammonia (p.1653·3); ammonium carbonate (p.1115·1); glycerol (p.1694·3); liquorice (p.1270·2); menthol (p.1711·3); siberian fir oil; white pine compound.

**Bronchial** *Theralab, Canad.*
Ammonium chloride (p.1115·2); senega (p.1130·2); white pine compound.

**Bronchial Cough** *Hylands, Canad.*
Homoeopathic preparation.

**Bronchial Mixture** *Torbet Laboratories, UK†.*
Squill (p.1130·3); ipecacuanha tincture (p.1122·3); ammonium bicarbonate (p.1115·1).
*Coughs.*

**Bronchialbalsam** *Ratiopharm, Ger.*
Pine needle oil; eucalyptus oil (p.1686·2).
*Catarrh.*

**Bronchialtee N** *TAD, Ger.†.*
Thyme (p.1755·2); hedera helix.
*Bronchitis; catarrh.*

**Bronchiase** *Lafare, Ital.*
Dextromethorphan hydrobromide (p.1117·3); sulfogaiacol (p.1131·1).
*Coughs.*

**Bronchicough** *Aventis, S.Afr.*
Cimicifuga (p.1671·3); grindelia (p.1696·1); pimpinella; cowslip (p.1735·1); quebracho; thyme (p.1755·2); ephedrine hydrochloride (p.1120·1); menthol (p.1711·3); eucalyptus oil (p.1686·2); saponin.
*Coughs.*

**Bronchicum**
*Note. This name is used for preparations of different composition.*
*Aventis, Neth.*
Thyme (p.1755·2); primula root (p.1735·1); grindelia (p.1696·1); pimpinella root; anise oil (p.1655·2); eucalyptus oil (p.1686·2); menthol (p.1711·3); saponin.
*Coughs.*

*Aventis, S.Afr.*
Cimicifuga (p.1671·3); grindelia (p.1696·1); pimpinella; cowslip (p.1735·1); quebracho; thyme (p.1755·2); ephedrine hydrochloride (p.1120·1); menthol (p.1711·3); sodium bromide (p.1663·1); eucalyptus oil (p.1686·2); saponin.
*Bronchitis.*

**Bronchicum Balsam mit Eukalyptusol** *Nattermann, Ger.*
Eucalyptus oil (p.1686·2); camphor (p.1665·3); oleum pini sylvestris.
*Catarrh; cold symptoms.*

**Bronchicum Elixir N** *Nattermann, Ger.*
Grindelia (p.1696·1); pimpinella; primula root (p.1735·1); quebracho; thyme (p.1755·2).
*Bronchial congestion; coughs.*

**Bronchicum Elixir Plus** *Nattermann, Ger.*
Thyme (p.1755·2); plantago lanceolata (p.1738·2); primula root (p.1735·1).
*Bronchial congestion; coughs.*

**Bronchicum Extra Sterk** *Aventis, Neth.*
Ephedrine hydrochloride (p.1120·1); codeine phosphate (p.27·1); vegetable extracts.
*Coughs.*

**Bronchicum Hustentee** *Nattermann, Ger.†.*
Thyme (p.1755·2); fennel oil (p.1687·3); anise oil (p.1655·2); saponaria; liquorice (p.1270·2).
*Coughs and cold symptoms; sore throat.*

**Bronchicum Medizinal-Bad** *Nattermann, Ger.*
Thyme oil (p.1755·3).
*Bath additive; respiratory-tract disorders.*

**Bronchicum Mono Codein** *Nattermann, Ger.*
Codeine phosphate (p.27·1).
*Coughs.*

**Bronchicum Pastillen** *Nattermann, Ger.*
Thyme (p.1755·2).
*Coughs; sore throat.*

**Bronchicum Pflanzlicher** *Nattermann, Ger.*
Thyme (p.1755·2); drosera (p.1683·1).
*Cold symptoms; coughs.*

**Bronchicum Sekret-Loser** *Nattermann, Ger.*
Eucalyptus oil (p.1686·2); primula root (p.1735·1); thyme (p.1755·2).
*Upper respiratory-tract disorders with viscous mucus.*

**Bronchicum Thymian** *Nattermann, Ger.*
Primula root (p.1735·1); thyme (p.1755·2).
*Bronchitis; coughs.*

**Bronchicum Tropfen N** *Nattermann, Ger.*
Quebracho; saponaria; thyme (p.1755·2).
*Bronchitis.*

**Bronchi-Do** *Grasler, Ger.*
Homoeopathic preparation.

**Bronchiflu** *Aventis, S.Afr.*
Mepyramine maleate (p.437·1); menthol (p.1711·3); ammonium chloride (p.1115·2); paracetamol (p.76·2); phenylpropanolamine hydrochloride (p.1127·3).
*Cold symptoms; coughs.*

**Bronchil** *Siam Bheasach, Thai.*
Guaifenesin (p.1122·1); theophylline (p.798·3).
*Obstructive airways disease.*

**Bronchilet** *Nicholas Piramal, India.*
Salbutamol sulfate (p.791·3); etofylline (p.785·1).
*Obstructive airways disease.*

**Bronchilin** *Flordis, Austral.*
Primrose; thyme (p.1755·2).
*Coughs.*

**Bronchilon** *Cesra, Ger.*
Hedera helix.
*Respiratory-tract disorders.*

**Bronchi-Pertu** *Pekana, Ger.*
Homoeopathic preparation.

**Bronchiplant**
*Note. This name is used for preparations of different composition.*
*Apotheke Heiligen Josef, Austria.*
*Balsam:* Eucalyptus oil (p.1686·2); rosemary oil (p.1740·2); camphor (p.1665·3).
*Coughs and cold symptoms.*

*Rosch & Handel, Austria.*
*Oral liquid:* Thyme (p.1755·2); iceland moss; senega root (p.1130·2); bitter-orange peel (p.1723·3).
*Catarrh; coughs.*

**Bronchiplant light** *Rosch & Handel, Austria.*
Iceland moss; senega root (p.1130·2); thyme (p.1755·2); bitter-orange peel (p.1723·3).
*Catarrh; coughs.*

**Bronchipret**
*Note. This name is used for preparations of different composition.*
*Austroplant, Austria.*
Thyme (p.1755·2); hedera helix leaf.
*Bronchitis.*

*Bionorica, Ger.*
*Oral drops; oral liquid:* Thyme (p.1755·2); hedera helix.
*Bronchitis.*

*Pastilles:* Thyme (p.1755·2).
*Bronchitis; cold symptoms; coughs.*

*Tablets:* Primula root (p.1735·1); thyme (p.1755·2).
*Bronchitis.*

**Bronchisaft** *Hilarys, Canad.†.*
Ammonia (p.1653·3); glycerol (p.1694·3); ipecacuanha (p.1122·3); menthol (p.1711·3); sodium citrate (p.1223·2).

**Bronchisan** *Dispergo, Austria†.*
Theophylline (p.798·3); ephedrine hydrochloride (p.1120·1).
*Obstructive airways disease.*

**Bronchiselect** *Dreluso, Ger.*
Homoeopathic preparation.

**Bronchithym** *Austroplant, Austria.*
Thyme (p.1755·2); cowslip (p.1735·1).
*Bronchitis.*

**Bronchitten** *Medopharm, Ger.†.*
Thyme (p.1755·2).
*Bronchial catarrh; bronchitis; coughs.*

**Bronchitten forte K** *Medopharm, Ger.†.*
Thyme (p.1755·2); primula root (p.1735·1).
*Upper respiratory-tract disorders with thickened secretions.*

**Broncho D** *Sam-On, Israel.*
Diphenhydramine hydrochloride (p.431·3); ammonium chloride (p.1115·2).
*Coughs; respiratory-tract congestion.*

**Broncho Fertiginhalat** *Fujisawa, Ger.*
Salbutamol sulfate (p.791·3).
*Obstructive airways disease.*

**Broncho Inhalat** *Fujisawa, Ger.*
Salbutamol sulfate (p.791·3).
*Obstructive airways disease.*

**Broncho Munal**
*Medice, Ger.; Abiogen, Ital.*
Lysates of *Haemophilus influenzae*; *Streptococcus pneumoniae*; *Klebsiella pneumoniae*; *Klebsiella ozaenae*; *Staphylococcus aureus*; *Streptococcus pyogenese*; *Streptococcus viridans*; *Moraxella catarrhalis*.
*Respiratory-tract infections.*

**Broncho Rub** *Mathieu, Canad.†.*
Camphor (p.1665·3); menthol (p.1711·3); cajuput oil (p.1664·1); turpentine.

**Broncho Saline** *Blairex, USA.*
Sodium chloride (p.1233·3).
*Diluent for bronchodilator solutions for inhalation.*

**Bronchobactan** *Klinge, Ger.†.*
Lysate of: *Staphylococcus aureus*; *Streptococcus mitis*; *Streptococcus pyogenes*; *Streptococcus pneumoniae*; *Klebsiella pneumoniae*; *Moraxella catarrhalis*; *Haemophilus influenzae*.
*Respiratory-tract infections.*

**Bronchobel** *Pharmethic, Belg.†.*
Codeine (p.27·1); ephedrine hydrochloride (p.1120·1); sulfogaiacol (p.1131·1); sodium benzoate (p.1169·3).
*Coughs.*

**Bronchobest** *CT, Ger.*
Spike lavender oil (p.1749·2).
*Bronchitis.*

**Bronchocal** *Sam-On, Israel†.*
Guaifenesin (p.1122·1).
*Coughs.*

**Bronchocedin N** *Strathmann, Ger.†.*
Anise oil (p.1655·2); eucalyptus oil (p.1686·2); peppermint oil (p.1283·2).
*Catarrh.*

**Bronchocort** *Fujisawa, Ger.*
Beclometasone dipropionate (p.1091·1).
*Asthma.*

**Bronchocux** *TAD, Ger.†.*
Budesonide (p.1094·2).
*Asthma; bronchitis.*

**Bronchocyst** *SmithKline Beecham, Fr.†.*
Carbocisteine (p.1116·2).
*Respiratory-tract disorders associated with increased or viscous mucus.*

**Bronchodermine** *SERP, Mon.*
*Ointment:* Cineole (p.1672·1); guaiacol (p.1122·1); pine oil.
*Suppositories:* Amylocaine hydrochloride (p.1370·2); cineole (p.1672·1); guaiacol (p.1122·1); pine oil.
*Respiratory disorders.*

**Bronchodex D** *Prodemdis, Canad.†.*
Phenylpropanolamine hydrochloride (p.1127·3); chlorphenamine maleate (p.427·3); pheniramine maleate (p.438·3).

**Bronchodex DM** *Prodemdis, Canad.†.*
Mepyramine maleate (p.437·1); dextromethorphan hydrobromide (p.1117·3); ammonium chloride (p.1115·2); menthol (p.1711·3); sodium citrate (p.1223·2).

**Bronchodex Pastilles** *Prodemdis, Canad.*
Domiphen bromide (p.1179·1).

**Bronchodex Pastilles Antiseptiques** *Prodemdis, Canad.*
Hexylresorcinol (p.1182·1).

**Bronchodex Pediatrique** *Therapex, Canad.†.*
Pseudoephedrine hydrochloride (p.1129·2); pheniramine maleate (p.438·3); dextromethorphan hydrobromide (p.1117·3); guaifenesin (p.1122·1).

**Bronchodex Vapo** *Theralab, Canad.*
Camphor (p.1665·3); eucalyptus oil (p.1686·2); menthol (p.1711·3).

**Bronchodil** *Asta Medica, UK†.*
Reproterol hydrochloride (p.791·2).
*Bronchospasm.*

**Bronchodine** *Pharmethic, Belg.†.*
Codeine phosphate (p.27·1).
*Coughs.*

**Bronchodual** *Boehringer Ingelheim, Fr.*
Fenoterol hydrobromide (p.785·2); ipratropium bromide (p.787·1).
*Obstructive airways disease.*

**Bronchodurat Eucalyptusol** *Pohl, Ger.†.*
Eucalyptus oil (p.1686·2).
*Bronchitis; cold symptoms.*

**Bronchodurat N** *Pohl, Ger.*
Eucalyptus oil (p.1686·2); menthol (p.1711·3).
*Bronchitis; cold symptoms.*

**Broncho-Euphyllin** *Byk Gulden, Ger.*
Theophylline (p.798·3); ambroxol hydrochloride (p.1114·3).
*Obstructive airways disease.*

**Broncho-Fips** *Lichtenstein, Ger.†.*
Acetylcysteine (p.1112·3).
*Respiratory-tract disorders with viscous mucus.*

**Bronchofluid** *DP-Medica, Switz.†.*
*Baby:* Codeine phosphate (p.27·1); ephedrine hydrochloride (p.1120·1); guaifenesin (p.1122·1); belladonna (p.479·1); drosera (p.1683·1); hedera helix; plantago lanceolata (p.1738·2); senega root (p.1130·2); thyme (p.1755·2).
*Infant; Adult:* Codeine phosphate (p.27·1); ephedrine hydrochloride (p.1120·1); guaifenesin (p.1122·1); belladonna (p.479·1); ipecacuanha (p.1122·3); drosera (p.1683·1); hedera helix; plantago lanceolata (p.1738·2); senega root (p.1130·2); thyme (p.1755·2); cherry-laurel.
*Coughs; laryngitis; sore throat.*

**Bronchofluid N** *DP-Medica, Switz.*
Guaifenesin (p.1122·1); drosera (p.1683·1); hedera helix; plantago lanceolata (p.1738·2); senega (p.1130·2); thyme (p.1755·2); anise oil (p.1655·2).
*Coughs with excessive mucus.*

**Bronchoforton**
*Note. This name is used for preparations of different composition.*
*Sanofi Winthrop, Austria†.*
Eucalyptus oil (p.1686·2); oleum pini sylvestris; peppermint oil (p.1283·2).
*Cold and influenza symptoms.*

*Sanofi Synthelabo, Ger.*
*Capsules:* Eucalyptus oil (p.1686·2); anise oil (p.1655·2); peppermint oil (p.1283·2).
*Catarrh.*
*Ointment:* Eucalyptus oil (p.1686·2); Norway spruce oil; peppermint oil (p.1283·2).
*Catarrh; cold symptoms.*
*Oral liquid; oral drops:* Hedera helix.
*Bronchitis; catarrh.*

*Sodip, Switz.†.*
Eucalyptus oil (p.1686·2); pine oil; peppermint oil (p.1283·2).
*Respiratory-tract disorders.*

**Bronchoforton Kinderbalsam** *Sanofi Synthelabo, Ger.*
Eucalyptus oil (p.1686·2); pine needle oil.
*Coughs; respiratory-tract congestion.*

**Bronchoforton-Solinat** *Sanofi Synthelabo, Ger.†.*
Cations: sodium, potassium, magnesium, calcium; anions: chloride, sulfate, bicarbonate.
*Respiratory-tract disorders.*

**Broncho-Grippol-DM** *Technilab, Canad.*
Dextromethorphan hydrobromide (p.1117·3).
*Coughs.*

**Bronchohexal** *Hexal, Austria.*
Acetylcysteine (p.1112·3).
*Respiratory-tract disorders with viscous mucus.*

**Broncho-Kid** *Sam-On, Israel.*
Diphenhydramine hydrochloride (p.431·3); pseudoephedrine hydrochloride (p.1129·2).
*Upper respiratory-tract disorders.*

**Bronchokod** *Aventis, Fr.*
Carbocisteine (p.1116·2).
*Respiratory-tract disorders associated with increased or viscous mucus.*

**Bronchol** *Streuli, Switz.*
Guaifenesin (p.1122·1).
*Upper respiratory-tract disorders.*

**Bronchol N** *DP-Medica, Switz.†.*
Guaifenesin (p.1122·1); ephedrine hydrochloride (p.1120·1); codeine phosphate (p.27·1); camphor (p.1665·3); cineole (p.1672·1); anise oil (p.1655·2).
*Coughs.*

**Broncholate**
*Note. This name is used for preparations of different composition.*
*Sam-On, Israel.*
Diphenhydramine hydrochloride (p.431·3); pseudoephedrine hydrochloride (p.1129·2).
Formerly contained diphenhydramine hydrochloride and phenylpropanolamine hydrochloride.
*Respiratory-tract disorders.*

*Sanofi Winthrop, USA.*
Ephedrine hydrochloride (p.1120·1); guaifenesin (p.1122·1).
*Coughs.*

**Broncholate Forte** *Sam-On, Israel.*
Diphenhydramine hydrochloride (p.431·3); pseudoephedrine hydrochloride (p.1129·2); codeine phosphate (p.27·1).
Formerly contained diphenhydramine hydrochloride, phenylpropanolamine hydrochloride, and codeine phosphate.
*Respiratory-tract disorders.*

**Broncholate Plus** *Sam-On, Israel†.*
Diphenhydramine hydrochloride (p.431·3); phenylpropanolamine hydrochloride (p.1127·3); paracetamol (p.76·2).
*Cold and influenza symptoms; rhinitis; sinusitis.*

**Broncholine** *TO-Chemicals, Thai.*
Terbutaline sulfate (p.797·2).
*Obstructive airways disease.*

**Bronchomed** *Pohl, Ger.†.*
Eucalyptus oil (p.1686·2).
*Bronchitis; cold symptoms.*

**Bronchopan DM** *Atlas, Canad.*
Dextromethorphan hydrobromide (p.1117·3).

**Bronchoparat** *Fujisawa, Ger.*
Theophylline sodium glycinate (p.804·3).
*Obstructive airways disease.*

**Broncho-pectoralis** *Medgenix, Belg.*
Pholcodine (p.1128·3); sulfogaiacol (p.1131·1); red-poppy petal fluidextract.
Formerly contained pholcodine, diphenhydramine hydrochloride, ephedrine sulfate, sulfogaiacol, Desessartz fluidextract, and red-poppy petal fluidextract.
*Coughs and nasal congestion.*

**Bronchoped** *Adcock Ingram, S.Afr.*
Terbutaline sulfate (p.797·2); ammonium chloride (p.1115·2); sodium citrate (p.1223·2).
*Coughs with bronchospasm.*

**Bronchophylline** *Sam-On, Israel†.*
Theophylline (p.798·3); guaifenesin (p.1122·1).
*Respiratory-tract disorders.*

**Bronchoplus** *Nycomed, Austria.*
Acetylcysteine (p.1112·3).
*Respiratory-tract disorders with viscous mucus.*

**Bronchoprex** *Kenyaku, Thai.*
Diphenhydramine hydrochloride (p.431·3); sodium citrate (p.1223·2); dextromethorphan hydrobromide (p.1117·3).
*Respiratory-tract disorders.*

**Bronchoprex Expectorant** *Kenyaku, Thai.*
Diphenhydramine hydrochloride (p.431·3); guaifenesin (p.1122·1); bromhexine hydrochloride (p.1115·3).
*Coughs.*

**Bronchopront**
*Grunenthal, Chile; Mack, Illert., Ger.; Mack, Hong Kong; Ferraz, Lynce, Port.; Mack, Singapore; Mack, Thai.*
Ambroxol hydrochloride (p.1114·3).
*Respiratory-tract disorders associated with increased or viscous mucus.*

**Bronchorectine au Citral** *Mayoly-Spindler, Fr.*
Citral; guaiacol (p.1122·1); terpin hydrate (p.1131·1); oleum pini sylvestris; wild thyme oil.
*Respiratory disorders.*

**Bronchoretard** *Fujisawa, Ger.*
Theophylline (p.798·3).
*Obstructive airways disease.*

**Broncho-Rivo** *Rivopharm, Switz.*
*Adult:* Diphenhydramine hydrochloride (p.431·3); ammonium chloride (p.1115·2); sodium citrate (p.1223·2); menthol (p.1711·3).
*Paediatric:* Diphenhydramine hydrochloride (p.431·3); sodium citrate (p.1223·2); menthol (p.1711·3).
*Coughs.*

**Bronchosan** *Vitasan, Austria.*
Quebracho; saponaria; thyme (p.1755·2).
*Bronchitis.*

**Bronchosan Nouvelle formule** *Bioforce, Switz.*
Hedera helix; thyme (p.1755·2); liquorice (p.1270·2).
Bronchosan formerly contained hedera helix, thyme, pimpinella sax., horehound, and liquorice.
*Coughs.*

**Bronchosedal** *Janssen-Cilag, Belg.*
*Oral liquid:* Dextromethorphan hydrobromide (p.1117·3).
*Syrup:* Codeine phosphate (p.27·1).
Formerly contained cherry-laurel water, aconite tincture, codeine phosphate, and sodium benzoate.
*Coughs.*

**Broncho-Sern** *Truw, Ger.*
Plantago lanceolata (p.1738·2).
*Coughs; inflammation of mouth and throat; respiratory catarrh.*

**Bronchosirum** *Bronchosirum, Canad.†.*
Phenylpropanolamine hydrochloride (p.1127·3); pheniramine maleate (p.438·3); mepyramine maleate (p.437·1); dextromethorphan hydrobromide (p.1117·3).

**Bronchosolvin** *Ipca, India.*
Bromhexine hydrochloride (p.1115·3); terbutaline sulfate (p.797·2); guaifenesin (p.1122·1).
*Coughs.*

**Bronchospasmin**
*Asta Medica, Austria; Viatris, Ger.*
Reproterol hydrochloride (p.791·2).
*Obstructive airways disease.*

**Bronchospasmine** *Asta Medica, Switz.†.*
Reproterol hydrochloride (p.791·2).
*Obstructive airways disease.*

**Bronchospect** *Pfizer Consumer, S.Afr.*
Terbutaline sulfate (p.797·2); guaifenesin (p.1122·1).
*Coughs.*

**Bronchospray**
*Note. This name is used for preparations of different composition.*
*Tissot, Fr.†.*
Guethol nicotinate (p.1122·2); guaifenesin (p.1122·1); cineole (p.1672·1); pine oil; lavender oil (p.1705·2).
Formerly contained guethol nicotinate, guaifenesin, terpineol, cineole, pine oil, and lavender oil.
*Respiratory disorders.*

*Fujisawa, Ger.; Parke-Med, S.Afr.†.*
Salbutamol (p.791·3) or salbutamol sulfate (p.791·3).
*Obstructive airways disease.*

**Bronchostad Hustenloser** *Stada, Ger.*
Hedera helix.
*Cold symptoms.*

**Bronchostop** *Metochem, Austria.*
*Capsules:* Mentholum valerianicum; guaifenesin (p.1122·1); eucalyptus oil (p.1686·2); camphor (p.1665·3).
Formerly known as Nicogelat.
*Coughs.*
*Ointment:* Camphor (p.1665·3); menthol (p.1711·3); eucalyptus oil (p.1686·2); turpentine oil (p.1760·1); pumilio pine oil (p.1737·1); thyme oil (p.1755·3).
*Catarrh; colds; cough; sore throat.*
*Oral drops:* Guaifenesin (p.1122·1); thyme (p.1755·2); chamomile (p.1669·3); anise oil (p.1655·2).
*Coughs.*
*Oral liquid:* Ascorbic acid (p.1460·2); thyme (p.1755·2); althaea syrup (p.1651·3).
*Catarrh; colds; cough; sore throat.*
*Spray:* Sage tincture (p.1741·2); thyme tincture (p.1755·2); peppermint leaf tincture (p.1283·2).
*Mouth and throat inflammation.*

**Bronchostop sine** *Metochem, Austria.*
Thyme (p.1755·2); althaea (p.1651·3).
*Coughs.*

**Bronchosyl** *Pharmalab, Canad.†.*
Ammonium chloride (p.1115·2); cocillana (p.1117·2).

**Bronchosyx N** *Syxyl, Ger.*
Liquorice (p.1270·2); thyme (p.1755·2).
*Cold symptoms.*

**Broncho-Tulisan Eucalyptol** *Logeais, Fr.†.*
Noscapine camsilate (p.1125·3); aspirin (p.15·1); cineole (p.1672·1).
*Coughs.*

**Bronchotussine**
*Note. This name is used for preparations of different composition.*
*Adelco, Gr.*
Bromhexine hydrochloride (p.1115·3).
*Respiratory disorders associated with viscous mucus.*

*Medichemie, Switz.*
Butetamate citrate (p.1116·2); codeine phosphate (p.27·1).
*Coughs.*

**Broncho-Tyrosolvetten** *Roland, Ger.; Byk Gulden, Ger.*
Cetylpyridinium chloride (p.1173·1); ammonium chloride (p.1115·2); liquorice (p.1270·2).
*Mouth and throat infections; respiratory-tract catarrh.*

**Broncho-Vaxom**
*Byk, Austria; Fournier, Belg.; Altana, Braz.; Andromaco, Chile; Byk Gulden, Ger.; OM, Hong Kong; Byk Gulden, Ital.; Knoll, Mex.; OM, Port.; OM, Switz.*
Lysate of: *Haemophilus influenzae*; *Streptococcus pneumoniae*; *Klebsiella pneumoniae*; *Klebsiella ozaenae*; *Staphylococcus aureus*; *Streptococcus pyogenes*; *Streptococcus viridans*; *Moraxella catarrhalis*.
*Respiratory-tract infections.*

**Bronchowern** *Wernigerode, Ger.*
Ambroxol hydrochloride (p.1114·3).
*Respiratory-tract disorders with viscous mucus.*

**Bronchozone** *DC Labs, Canad.*
Ammonium chloride (p.1115·2); ammonium carbonate (p.1115·1); liquorice (p.1270·2); menthol (p.1711·3); senega (p.1130·2).

**Bronchyteine** *Knoll, Fr.†.*
Carbocisteine (p.1116·2).

**Bronchytuc** *Knoll, Fr.†.*
Dextromethorphan hydrobromide (p.1117·3).
Formerly known as Bronchydex.
*Coughs.*

**Broncimucil** *Uriach, Spain.*
Brovanexine hydrochloride (p.1116·1).
*Respiratory-tract disorders associated with increased mucus.*

**Broncivent** *Boehringer Ingelheim, Spain.*
Beclometasone dipropionate (p.1091·1).
*Asthma.*

**Bronclear** *Polipharm, Thai.*
Bromhexine hydrochloride (p.1115·3).
*Respiratory-tract disorders associated with increased or viscous mucus.*

**Broncleer** *Adcock Ingram, S.Afr.*
Diphenhydramine hydrochloride (p.431·3); ammonium chloride (p.1115·2); sodium citrate (p.1223·2).
*Coughs.*

**Broncleer with Codeine** *Adcock Ingram, S.Afr.; Propan, S.Afr.*
Codeine phosphate (p.27·1); diphenhydramine hydrochloride (p.431·3); ammonium chloride (p.1115·2); sodium citrate (p.1223·2).
*Coughs.*

**Broncmel** *La-Sante, Braz.†.*
Grindelia (p.1696·1); aniseed (p.1655·2); senega (p.1130·2); rosa gallica (p.1058·1); thyme (p.1755·2); honey (p.1434·2).
*Coughs.*

**Bronco Aseptilex** *Wasserman, Spain†.*
Sulfadiazine (p.258·2); guaiacol cinnamate (p.1122·1).
*Respiratory-tract infections.*

**Bronco Aseptilex Fuerte** *Chiesi, Spain.*
Bromhexine hydrochloride (p.1115·3); co-trimoxazole (p.199·3); guaiacol cinnamate (p.1122·1).
*Respiratory-tract infections.*

**Bronco Asmo** *Pond's, Thai.*
Terbutaline sulfate (p.797·2).
*Obstructive airways disease.*

**Bronco Asmol** *Herbes Universelles, Canad.*
Ammonium bicarbonate (p.1115·1); anethole (p.1654·3); tolu balsam (p.1131·3); camphor (p.1665·3); squill (p.1130·3).

**Bronco Bactifor** *Andromaco, Spain†.*
Bromhexine (p.1115·3); co-trimoxazole (p.199·3).
*Respiratory-tract infections.*

**Bronco Biotaer** *Disprovent, Arg.*
Ambroxol hydrochloride (p.1114·3); clofedanol hydrochloride (p.1117·1); pseudoephedrine sulfate (p.1129·2); astemizole (p.424·2).

**Bronco Cilimox** *Baldassari, Braz.†.*
Amoxicillin (p.155·3); bromhexine hydrochloride (p.1115·3).
*Bacterial infections.*

**Bronco Etersan** *Dallas, Arg.*
Terpineol (p.1752·2); cineole (p.1672·1); oleum pini sylvestris; turpentine oil (p.1760·1).
*Respiratory-tract disorders.*

**Bronco Lizom** *Pensa, Spain†.*
*Haemophilus influenzae*; *Klebsiella pneumoniae*; *Staphylococcus aureus*; *Streptococcus pyogenes*; *Streptococcus pneumoniae*; *Moraxella catarrhalis*.
*Respiratory-tract infections.*

**Bronco Medical** *Medical, Spain.*
Sulfogaiacol (p.1131·1); dextromethorphan hydrobromide (p.1117·3).
*Coughs.*

**Bronco Pensusan** *Wasserman, Spain†.*
Ampicillin sodium (p.157·1); ampicillin benzathine (p.158·1); bromhexine hydrochloride (p.1115·3).

Lidocaine hydrochloride (p.1377·3) is included in this preparation to alleviate the pain of injection.
*Respiratory-tract infections.*

**Bronco Sergo** Inexfa, Spain†.
Tolu balsam (p.1131·3); bromhexine hydrochloride (p.1115·3); sodium benzoate (p.1169·3); co-trimoxazole (p.199·3).
*Respiratory-tract infections.*

**Bronco Tonic** Vir, Spain.
Amoxicillin trihydrate (p.155·3); bromhexine hydrochloride (p.1115·3).
*Respiratory-tract infections.*

**Bronco-Amoxil** GlaxoSmithKline, Braz.
Amoxicillin (p.155·3); bromhexine hydrochloride (p.1115·3).
*Bacterial infections.*

**Broncocalmine** Oriental, Arg.
Bromhexine (p.1115·3).
*Respiratory-tract congestion.*

**Broncoclar** Oberlin, Fr.
*Granules for oral solution:* Acetylcysteine (p.1112·3).
*Syrup:* Carbocisteine (p.1116·2).
*Respiratory-tract disorders associated with increased or viscous mucus.*

**Broncodeina** Pasteur, Chile.
Codeine phosphate (p.27·1); ephedrine hydrochloride (p.1120·1); belladonna liquid extract (p.479·1); menthol (p.1711·3); sodium benzoate (p.1169·3); terpin hydrate (p.1131·1).
*Coughs.*

**Bronco-Dex** Pastor Farina, Ital.†.
Dextromethorphan hydrobromide (p.1117·3); sulfogaiacol (p.1131·1).
*Coughs.*

**Broncodiazina** Vitoria, Port.
Ammonia solution (p.1653·3); pentetrazol (p.1592·1); sodium benzoate (p.1169·3); sulfadiazine (p.258·2).
*Respiratory-tract disorders.*

**Broncodil**
Note. This name is used for preparations of different composition.
Infabra, Braz.†.
Salbutamol sulfate (p.791·3).
*Obstructive airways disease.*

Epifarma, Ital.†.
Clenbuterol hydrochloride (p.784·2).
*Asthma.*

**Broncodual** Laboratorios Chile, Chile.
Clobutinol (p.1117·1).
*Coughs.*

**Broncodual Compuesto** Laboratorios Chile, Chile.
Clobutinol hydrochloride (p.1117·1); orciprenaline sulfate (p.790·2); ammonium chloride (p.1115·2).
*Coughs; obstructive airways disease.*

**Broncofenil** Zurita, Braz.
Guaifenesin (p.1122·1); lobelia (p.1589·1); aconite (p.1646·3).
*Coughs.*

**Broncofisin** Luper, Braz.
Tolu balsam (p.1131·3); potassium iodide (p.1598·1); sulfogaiacol (p.1131·1).
*Coughs.*

**Broncofluid** Recofarma, Ital.
Prenoxdiazine hibenzate (p.1129·1); carbocisteine (p.1116·2).
*Coughs.*

**Broncoflux** Farmasa, Braz.
Ambroxol hydrochloride (p.1114·3).
*Respiratory-tract congestion.*

**Broncoformo Muco Dexa** Edigen, Spain.
Dexamethasone (p.1097·1); dextromethorphan hydrobromide (p.1117·3); guaifenesin (p.1122·1); sodium benzoate (p.1169·3).
*Respiratory-tract disorders.*

**Broncokin** Geymonat, Ital.
Bromhexine hydrochloride (p.1115·3).
*Respiratory-tract disorders.*

**Broncol**
Note. This name is used for preparations of different composition.
Delta, Braz.
Eucalyptus (p.1686·1); ginger (p.1267·1); siparuna apiosyce; lantana camara; mikania glomerata; belladonna (p.479·1); jaborandi.
*Coughs.*

Crown, S.Afr.
Dextromethorphan hydrobromide (p.1117·3); ammonium chloride (p.1115·2); panthenol (p.1727·2).
*Coughs.*

Pharmaland, Thai.
Ambroxol hydrochloride (p.1114·3).
*Respiratory-tract disorders associated with increased or viscous mucus.*

**Broncolex** Legrand, Braz.
Guaifenesin (p.1122·1); etafedrine hydrochloride (p.1121·2); bufylline (p.781·3); doxylamine succinate (p.432·3).
*Coughs.*

**Broncoliber** Tecnimede, Port.
Ambroxol hydrochloride (p.1114·3).
*Respiratory-tract disorders.*

**Broncolin** Heralds, Braz.†.
Salbutamol sulfate (p.791·3).
*Obstructive airways disease.*

**Broncomed** Liomont, Mex.†.
Dextromethorphan (p.1117·3); guaifenesin (p.1122·1).
*Coughs.*

**Broncomega** Almirall, Spain.
Co-trimoxazole (p.199·3).
*Bacterial infections.*

**Broncomicin Bals** Edigen, Spain†.
Tolu balsam (p.1131·3); sodium benzoate (p.1169·3); ammoniacal aniseed (p.1655·2); sulfadiazine (p.258·2).
*Respiratory-tract infections.*

**Broncomnes** Bracco, Ital.
Ambroxol acefyllinate (p.1114·3).
*Bronchospasm.*

**Broncomucil** GlaxoSmithKline, Ital.
Carbocisteine (p.1116·2).
*Respiratory-tract disorders associated with excess or viscous mucus.*

**Bronconait** GlaxoSmithKline, Ital.
Paracetamol (p.76·2); promethazine hydrochloride (p.439·1); dextromethorphan hydrobromide (p.1117·3).
*Coughs and cold symptoms.*

**Bronconovag** Novag, Spain†.
Amoxicillin trihydrate (p.155·3); bromhexine hydrochloride (p.1115·3).
*Respiratory-tract infections.*

**Bronco-Ped** Stiefel, Braz.†.
Etafedrine hydrochloride (p.1121·2); bufylline (p.781·3); doxylamine succinate (p.432·3); guaifenesin (p.1122·1).
*Coughs.*

**Broncopinol** Luper, Braz.
1 Ampoule, dipyrone (p.35·3); sodium camsilate; guaifenesin (p.1122·1); myrtol; suprarenal cortex (p.1110·1); chlorophyllin copper complex potassium (p.1057·1); cineole (p.1672·1); 1 ampoule, chlorphenamine maleate (p.427·3); vitamin C (p.1460·2).
*Cold and influenza symptoms.*

**Broncoplus** Sigma-Tau, Ital.†.
Stepronin sodium (p.1130·3).
*Respiratory-tract disorders.*

**Bronco-Polimoxil** Legrand, Braz.
Amoxicillin trihydrate (p.155·3); bromhexine hydrochloride (p.1115·3).
*Bacterial infections.*

**Broncopulmin** Ecobi, Ital.†.
Camphor (p.1665·3); niaouli oil (p.1719·3); cineole (p.1672·1); menthol (p.1711·3).
*Respiratory-tract disorders.*

**Broncopulmo** Merck, Port.
Sobrerol (p.1130·2).
*Coughs.*

**Broncoral** Ferrer, Spain.
Formoterol fumarate (p.786·1).
*Obstructive airways disease.*

**Broncorema** Septa, Spain†.
Guaifenesin (p.1122·1); co-trimoxazole (p.199·3).
*Respiratory-tract infections.*

**Broncorinol etats grippaux** Roche Nicholas, Fr.†.
Paracetamol (p.76·2); pseudoephedrine hydrochloride (p.1129·2); chlorphenamine maleate (p.427·3).
*Cold symptoms.*

**Broncorinol Expectorant** Roche Nicholas, Fr.
Carbocisteine (p.1116·2).
*Viscous bronchial secretions.*

**Broncorinol maux de gorge** Roche Nicholas, Fr.
Cetylpyridinium chloride (p.1173·1); tetracaine hydrochloride (p.1385·1); ascorbic acid (p.1460·2).
*Sore throat.*

**Broncorinol rhinites** Roche Nicholas, Fr.
Cetrimide (p.1172·1); tyrothricin (p.275·1).
*Upper respiratory-tract infections.*

**Broncorinol rhume** Roche Nicholas, Fr.
Paracetamol (p.76·2); pseudoephedrine hydrochloride (p.1129·2).
*Cold symptoms.*

**Broncorinol toux seche** Roche Nicholas, Fr.
Pholcodine (p.1128·3); sodium benzoate; senega; eucalyptus.
Formerly contained pholcodine, sodium benzoate, aconite, hyoscyamus, lobelia, senega, and eucalyptus.
*Coughs.*

**Broncort**
Boehringer Ingelheim, Belg.†; Boehringer Ingelheim, Switz.
Flunisolide (p.1101·1).
*Obstructive airways disease.*

**Broncosedina** FAMA, Ital.
Cocillana (p.1117·2); eriodictyon (p.1121·2); marrubium (p.1124·1); grindelia (p.1696·1); juniper (p.1703·1); compound thyme (p.1755·2); pumilio pine oil (p.1737·1); mint oil (p.1715·2).
*Respiratory-tract disorders.*

**Broncosedol** QIF, Braz.†.
Salbutamol sulfate (p.791·3).
*Obstructive airways disease.*

**Broncoserum** Ifusa, Mex.
Sulfogaiacol (p.1131·1).
*Coughs.*

**Broncosil** Basi, Port.
Camphor (p.1665·3); quinine (p.460·1).

**Broncospasmin** Merck, Spain†.
Reproterol hydrochloride (p.791·2).
*Obstructive airways disease.*

**Broncospasmine** Asta Medica, Ital.
Reproterol hydrochloride (p.791·2).
*Asthma.*

**Broncosyl** Homberger, Switz.†.
Homoeopathic preparation.

**Broncot** Recalcine, Chile.
Ambroxol hydrochloride (p.1114·3).
*Respiratory-tract disorders.*

**Broncoten** Farmion, Braz.
Ketotifen fumarate (p.788·1).
*Allergic conjunctivitis; allergic rhinitis; asthma; urticaria.*

**Broncoterol**
Note. This name is used for preparations of different composition.
Bago, Chile.
Salbutamol (p.791·3).
*Obstructive airways disease.*

Quimedical, Port.
Clenbuterol hydrochloride (p.784·2).
*Obstructive airways disease.*

**Broncoterol-B** Bago, Chile.
Salbutamol (p.791·3); beclometasone dipropionate (p.1091·1).
*Obstructive airways disease.*

**Broncotosil** Bago, Chile.
Clenbuterol hydrochloride (p.784·2).
*Obstructive airways disease.*

**Bronco-Turbinal** Valeas, Ital.
Beclometasone dipropionate (p.1091·1).
*Obstructive airways disease.*

**Broncotussan** INQ, Braz.†.
Noscapine (p.1125·3); ammonium benzoate; sulfogaiacol (p.1131·1); bromoform (p.1663·1); lobelia (p.1589·1); drosera (p.1683·1); grindelia (p.1696·1); aconite (p.1646·3).
*Coughs.*

**Broncovaleas** Valeas, Ital.
Salbutamol (p.791·3).
*Obstructive airways disease.*

**Broncovanil** Scalls, Ital.
Guaifenesin (p.1122·1).
*Respiratory-tract disorders.*

**Broncovir** Vir, Spain.
Co-trimoxazole (p.199·3); sulfogaiacol (p.1131·1).
*Respiratory-tract infections.*

**Broncovital**
Note. This name is used for preparations of different composition.
Ifusa, Mex.
Chlorphenamine (p.428·1); guaifenesin (p.1122·1).
*Respiratory-tract disorders.*

Puerto Galiano, Spain.
Cineole (p.1672·1); codeine phosphate (p.27·1); ephedrine hydrochloride (p.1120·1); niaouli oil (p.1719·3); sodium benzoate (p.1169·3); sulfogaiacol (p.1131·1); belladonna (p.479·1); drosera (p.1683·1); quebracho; senega (p.1130·2).
*Respiratory-tract disorders.*

**Brondal** Upha, Malaysia.
Guaifenesin (p.1122·1); theophylline (p.798·3).
*Obstructive airways disease.*

**Brondecon** Pfizer, NZ†.
Choline theophyllinate (p.784·2); guaifenesin (p.1122·1).
*Obstructive airways disease.*

**Brondecon Elixir** Pfizer Consumer, Austral.
Choline theophyllinate (p.784·2).
*Obstructive airways disease.*

**Brondecon Expectorant** Pfizer Consumer, Austral.
Choline theophyllinate (p.784·2); guaifenesin (p.1122·1).
*Obstructive airways disease.*

**Brondil** Great Eastern, Thai.; Therapharma, Thai.
Etafedrine hydrochloride (p.1121·2); theophylline (p.798·3); guaifenesin (p.1122·1).
Formerly contained ephedrine hydrochloride, theophylline, and guaifenesin.
*Obstructive airways disease.*

**Brondilat** Ache, Braz.
Ambroxol acefyllinate (p.1114·3).
*Obstructive airways disease.*

**Brondix** Pentafarm, Spain.
Amoxicillin trihydrate (p.155·3).
*Bacterial infections.*

**Brongenit** Elfar, Spain†.
Co-trimoxazole (p.199·3).
*Bacterial infections; Pneumocystis carinii pneumonia.*

**Bronica** Takeda, Jpn.
Seratrodast (p.795·3).
*Asthma.*

**Bronilide** Aventis, Fr.†.
Flunisolide (p.1101·1).
*Asthma.*

**Bronkaid** Sanofi Synthelabo, Canad.†.
Adrenaline (p.852·2).
*Asthma.*

**Bronkaid Dual Action** Sterling, USA.
Ephedrine sulfate (p.1120·1); guaifenesin (p.1122·1).

**Bronkasma** Sanofi Synthelabo, Arg.
Theophylline (p.798·3); ephedrine sulfate (p.1120·1).
*Asthma.*

**Bronkese** Aspen, S.Afr.
Bromhexine hydrochloride (p.1115·3).
*Respiratory-tract disorders with viscous mucus.*

**Bronkese Compound** Aspen, S.Afr.
Bromhexine hydrochloride (p.1115·3); orciprenaline sulfate (p.790·2).
*Coughs.*

**Bronkirex** Irex, Fr.
Carbocisteine (p.1116·2).
*Respiratory-tract disorders.*

**Bronkotrat** Hexal, Braz.
Bromhexine hydrochloride (p.1115·3); sulfogaiacol (p.1131·1).
Formerly contained ammonium chloride and sulfogaiacol.
*Respiratory-tract congestion.*

**Bronkotuss Expectorant** Hyrex, USA.
Ephedrine sulfate (p.1120·1); chlorphenamine maleate (p.427·3); guaifenesin (p.1122·1).
*Coughs.*

**Bronkyl** Weifa, Norw.
Acetylcysteine (p.1112·3).
*Chronic bronchitis; cystic fibrosis.*

**Bronmycin**
Biolab, Malaysia; Biolab, Singapore; Biolab, Thai.
Doxycycline hyclate (p.206·2).
*Bacterial infections.*

**Bronolban** Sons, Mex.
Ambroxol (p.1114·3).
*Respiratory-tract congestion.*

**Bronpax** Biocodex, Fr.†.
*Paediatric syrup:* Sulfogaiacol (p.1131·1); sodium benzoate (p.1169·3); piscidia (p.1702·3); aconite (p.1646·3); belladonna (p.479·1); pine buds; frangula (p.1266·3); tolu balsam (p.1131·3); terpin hydrate (p.1131·1); liquorice (p.1270·2).
*Respiratory disorders.*

*Pastilles:* Tyrothricin (p.275·1); ethylmorphine hydrochloride (p.37·3); sodium benzoate (p.1169·3); menthol (p.1711·3); glycyrrhizinic acid; sulfogaiacol (p.1131·1); terpin hydrate (p.1131·1).
*Coughs.*

*Syrup:* Codeine (p.27·1); sulfogaiacol (p.1131·1); sodium benzoate (p.1169·3); piscidia (p.1702·3); aconite (p.1646·3); belladonna (p.479·1); pine buds; Desessartz syrup; tolu balsam (p.1131·3); terpin hydrate (p.1131·1); liquorice (p.1270·2).
*Coughs.*

**Bronpect** Kenyaku, Thai.†.
Codeine phosphate (p.27·1); guaifenesin (p.1122·1); phenylpropanolamine hydrochloride (p.1127·3).
*Coughs; nasal congestion.*

**Bronpect-D** Kenyaku, Thai.
Dextromethorphan hydrobromide (p.1117·3); guaifenesin (p.1122·1).
*Coughs.*

**Bronpul** Soria Natural, Spain.
Eucalyptus (p.1686·1); verbascum flower (p.1764·1); althaea (p.1651·3); elecampane (p.1119·3); liquorice (p.1270·2).
*Lower respiratory-tract infections.*

**Bronq-C** Microsules Bernabo, Arg.
Clenbuterol (p.784·2) or clenbuterol hydrochloride (p.784·2).

**Bronquial** OM, Port.
Carbocisteine (p.1116·2); sobrerol (p.1130·2).
*Respiratory-tract congestion.*

**Bronquiasma** Heralds, Braz.†.
Theophylline (p.798·3).
*Obstructive airways disease.*

**Bronquiasmol** Confar, Port.
Ephedrine (p.1120·1); ethylmorphine (p.37·3); sodium benzoate (p.1169·3).
*Coughs.*

**Bronquicisteina** Iquinosa, Spain.
Carbocisteine (p.1116·2); co-trimoxazole (p.199·3).
*Respiratory-tract infections.*

**Bronquico** Zimaia, Port.†.
Camphor (p.1665·3); quinine (p.460·1).

**Bronquidex** Farmalab, Braz.
Potassium iodide (p.1598·1); guaifenesin (p.1122·1); diphenhydramine hydrochloride (p.431·3); sodium benzoate (p.1169·3); ammonium chloride (p.1115·2); belladonna (p.479·1); lobelia (p.1589·1).
*Respiratory-tract congestion.*

**Bronquidiazina CR** Faes, Spain.
Tolu balsam (p.1131·3); bromhexine (p.1115·3); sodium benzoate (p.1169·3); co-trimoxazole (p.199·3).
*Respiratory-tract infections.*

**Bronquimar** Cruz, Spain.
*Oral suspension:* Guaifenesin (p.1122·1); sodium benzoate (p.1169·3); co-trimoxazole (p.199·3).
*Respiratory-tract infections.*

*Suppositories†:* Camphor (p.1665·3); cineole (p.1672·1); niaouli oil (p.1719·3); guaiacol (p.1122·1); propyphenazone (p.85·3); menthol (p.1711·3).
*Upper-respiratory-tract disorders.*

**Bronquimar Vit A** Cruz, Spain†.
Camphor (p.1665·3); cineole (p.1672·1); niaouli oil (p.1719·3); guaiacol (p.1122·1); vitamin A (p.1451·2); menthol (p.1711·3).
*Respiratory-tract disorders.*

**Bronquimucil**
Note. This name is used for preparations of different composition.
Dansk-Flama, Braz.; Prospa, Port.
Brovanexine hydrochloride (p.1116·1).
*Respiratory-tract disorders.*

Uriach, Spain.
Brovanexine hydrochloride (p.1116·1); co-trimoxazole (p.199·3).
*Respiratory-tract infections.*

**Bronquiogem** Prodotti, Braz.
Yucca (p.1766·2); rorippa nasturtium aquaticum; mikania glomerata; lantana camara; passion flower (p.1729·1); erva silvina; oleo vermelho; sodium benzoate (p.1169·3).
*Respiratory-tract disorders.*

**Bronquisedan** *Gramon, Arg.*
Theophylline glycinate (p.804·3); clobutinol hydrochloride (p.1117·1); ambroxol hydrochloride (p.1114·3).
*Bronchtis; coughs.*

**Bronquisedan Elixir** *Gramon, Arg.*
Bromhexine hydrochloride (p.1115·3).
*Catarrh.*

**Bronquisedan Mucolitico** *Gramon, Arg.*
Ambroxol hydrochloride (p.1114·3); clobutinol hydrochloride (p.1117·1).
*Coughs.*

**Bronquitos** *Legrand, Braz.*
Diphenhydramine hydrochloride (p.431·3); guaifenesin (p.1122·1); theophylline (p.798·3); vitamin $B_6$ (p.1456·3).
*Obstructive airways disease.*

**Bronquium** *Ferrer, Spain†.*
Bromhexine hydrochloride (p.1115·3); co-trimoxazole (p.199·3).
*Respiratory-tract infections.*

**Bronquium Amoxicilina** *Ferrer, Spain†.*
Amoxicillin trihydrate (p.155·3); bromhexine hydrochloride (p.1115·3).
*Respiratory-tract infections.*

**Bronsal** *Vedim, Spain.*
Betamethasone sodium phosphate (p.1093·1); diprophylline (p.784·3); guaifenesin (p.1122·1).
*Respiratory-tract disorders.*

**Bronsema** *Leti, Spain.*
Erythromycin ethyl succinate (p.208·1).
*Bacterial infections.*

**Bronsema Expectorante** *Leti, Spain.*
Erythromycin ethyl succinate (p.208·1); guaifenesin (p.1122·1).
*Respiratory-tract infections.*

**Bronsul** *Del Bel, Arg.*
Canthaxanthin (p.1056·3); betacarotene (p.1422·3).
*Suntanning aid.*

**Brontal** *Instituto Sanitas, Chile.*
Bromhexine hydrochloride (p.1115·3); clofedanol hydrochloride (p.1117·1).
*Coughs; respiratory-tract congestion.*

**Bronteril** *Manetti Roberts, Ital.†.*
Guaimesal (p.1122·2).
*Respiratory-tract disorders.*

**Brontex** *Procter & Gamble, USA.*
Codeine phosphate (p.27·1); guaifenesin (p.1122·1).
*Coughs.*

**Brontonyl** *Rhone-Poulenc Rorer, Mex.†.*
Paracetamol (p.76·2).
*Fever; pain.*

**Brontoss** *Teuto, Braz.*
Potassium iodide (p.1598·1); belladonna (p.479·1); lobelia (p.1589·1); diphenhydramine hydrochloride (p.431·3).
*Coughs.*

**Bronuck** *Senju, Jpn.*
Bromfenac sodium (p.21·3).
*Inflammatory eye disorders.*

**Bronx** *Lisapharma, Ital.*
Carbocisteine (p.1116·2).
*Respiratory-tract disorders.*

**Bronze 8882** *Juvex, Fr.†.*
Octinoxate (p.1154·3); oxybenzone (p.1154·3); avobenzone (p.1142·3); mica-titanium dioxide complex (p.1160·3).
*Sunscreen.*

**Bronzearte** *Gramon, Arg.*
Canthaxanthin (p.1056·3).
*Suntanning aid.*

**Brooklax** *Intercare, UK†.*
Yellow phenolphthalein (p.1284·1).
*Constipation.*

**Bropamil** *Offenbach, Mex.*
Bromazepam (p.671·3).
*Anxiety.*

**Bropantil** *Mavi, Mex.†.*
Propantheline (p.489·1).

**Broptin** *IQFA, Mex.*
Bromocriptine (p.1202·3).

**Bros**
*TRB, Arg.*
Cerebral phospholipids (porcine) (p.1709·3).
*Mental function impairment; tonic.*

*TRB, Braz.*
Phosphatidyl serine (p.1731·2).
*Cerebrovascular disorders.*

**Brosol** *Mepha, Switz.†.*
Codeine phosphate (p.27·1); diprophylline (p.784·3); atropine methobromide (p.476·3); thyme oil (p.1755·3).
*Coughs.*

**Brosolan** *Collins, Mex.*
Ambroxol (p.1114·3).
*Respiratory-tract disorders.*

**Brosolan-C** *Collins, Mex.*
Ambroxol (p.1114·3); clenbuterol (p.784·2).
*Coughs.*

**Brosoline-Rectocaps** *Mepha, Switz.*
Noscapine hydrochloride (p.1125·3); guaifenesin (p.1122·1).
*Bronchial disorders.*

**Brostalin** *Synpharma, Austria.*
Urtica root and leaves (p.1762·1); couch-grass (p.1676·2).
*Urinary-tract disorders.*

**Brota Rectal Bals** *Escaned, Spain.*
Camphor (p.1665·3); cineole (p.1672·1); ephedrine hydrochloride (p.1120·1); niaouli oil (p.1719·3); quinine sulfate (p.460·2); sulfogaiacol (p.1131·1).
*Respiratory-tract disorders.*

**Brotazona** *Escaned, Spain.*
Feprazone (p.43·1).
*Gout; musculoskeletal and joint disorders.*

**Brovon**
*GlaxoSmithKline, India; Torbet Laboratories, UK.*
Adrenaline (p.852·2) atropine methonitrate (p.477·1); papaverine hydrochloride (p.1728·1).
*Bronchoconstriction.*

**Brown Mixture** *British Dispensary, Thai.*
Liquorice fluid extract (p.1270·2); antimony potassium tartrate (p.103·1); camphorated opium tincture.
*Coughs.*

**Broxil** *GlaxoSmithKline, Neth.*
Pheneticillin potassium (p.242·1).
*Bacterial infections.*

**Broxine** *Malayan, Singapore.*
Bromhexine hydrochloride (p.1115·3).
*Respiratory-tract disorders associated with increased or viscous mucus.*

**Broxo al Fluoro** *SIT, Ital.*
Levomenol (p.1707·1); sodium fluoride (p.1444·3); sodium monofluorophosphate (p.1446·2).
*Gum disorders; halitosis.*

**Broxodin** *SIT, Ital.*
Sodium fluoride (p.1444·3); sodium monofluorophosphate (p.1446·2).
*Dental caries prophylaxis.*
*Oral drops; oral gel:* Chlorhexidine gluconate (p.1173·2).
*Oral hygiene.*

**Broxofar** *Farcoral, Mex.*
Ambroxol hydrochloride (p.1114·3).

**Broxofar Compuesto** *Farcoral, Mex.*
Ambroxol hydrochloride (p.1114·3); clenbuterol hydrochloride (p.784·2).
*Respiratory-tract disorders with viscous mucus.*

**Broxol**
*Mundipharma, Austria; Pulitzer, Ital.; Carnot, Mex.; Masa, Thai.*
Ambroxol hydrochloride (p.1114·3).
*Respiratory-tract disorders associated with increased or viscous mucus.*

**Broxol Plus** *Carnot, Mex.*
Ambroxol hydrochloride (p.1114·3); clenbuterol hydrochloride (p.784·2).
*Respiratory-tract disorders with viscous mucus.*

**Broxolan** *Collins, Mex.†.*
Ambroxol (p.1114·3).

**Broxsa** *Silom, Thai.*
Ambroxol hydrochloride (p.1114·3).
*Respiratory-tract disorders associated with increased or viscous mucus.*

**Bro-Zedex** *Wockhardt, India.*
Terbutaline sulfate (p.797·2); bromhexine hydrochloride (p.1115·3); guaifenesin (p.1122·1); menthol (p.1711·3).
*Coughs.*

**Brozepax** *Biosintetica, Braz.*
Bromazepam (p.671·3).
*Anxiety.*

**Brozil**
*YSP, Malaysia; Yung Shin, Singapore.*
Gemfibrozil (p.923·1).
*Hyperlipidaemia.*

**Bruciaporri** *Giovanardi, Ital.*
Salicylic acid (p.1157·1); lactic acid (p.1704·1).
*Verrucas; warts.*

**Brufen**
*Abbott, Austral.; Ebewe, Austria; Knoll, Belg.; Abbott, Denm.; Abbott, Fin.; Knoll, Fr.; Kanoldt, Ger.†; Vianex (Βιανεξ), Gr.; Abbott, Hong Kong; Knoll, India; Abbott, Irl.; Abbott, Ital.; Knoll, Neth.; Abbott, Norw.; Abbott, NZ; Abbott, Port.; Knoll, S.Afr.; Knoll, Singapore†; Abbott, Swed.; Knoll, Switz.; Abbott, Thai.; Abbott, UK.*
Ibuprofen (p.45·3) or ibuprofen sodium (p.46·3).
*Fever; gout; inflammation; musculoskeletal, joint, peri-articular, and soft-tissue disorders; pain.*

**Brufort** *Lampugnani, Ital.†.*
Ibuprofen (p.45·3).
*Inflammation; musculoskeletal and joint disorders; pain.*

**Brugesic**
*Raza, Malaysia; Pharmaniaga, Malaysia; Garec, S.Afr.*
Ibuprofen (p.45·3).
*Fever; musculoskeletal and joint disorders; pain.*

**Bruise Cream** *Medipharma, Hong Kong.*
A heparinoid (p.931·1).
*Bruising.*

**Bruiseze** *Bayer Consumer, UK.*
A heparinoid (p.931·1).
*Soft-tissue injury.*

**Brulamycin**
*Torrex, Austria; Medphano, Ger.*
Tobramycin sulfate (p.271·3).
*Bacterial infections.*

**Brulex** *Bailly, Fr.*
Phenazone (p.82·3); zinc oxide (p.1163·2); peru balsam (p.1730·2); phenol (p.1188·1); sodium salicylate (p.90·1).
*Burns; sunburn.*

**Brulidine**
*Aventis, Austral.†; Rhone-Poulenc Rorer, Hong Kong†; Rhone-Poulenc Rorer, Irl.†; Aventis, Norw.; Aventis, NZ†; Manx, UK.*
Dibrompropamidine isetionate (p.1178·2).
*Burns; napkin rash; skin abrasions; skin infections; wounds.*

**Brulstop** *Agepharm, Fr.*
Hydrocolloid dressing.
*Burns.*

**Brumed** *LSP, Thai.*
Ibuprofen (p.45·3).
*Fever; pain.*

**Brumetidina** *Bruschettini, Ital.*
Cimetidine (p.1255·3).
*Gastro-oesophageal reflux; gastrointestinal hyperacidity; peptic ulcer; Zollinger-Ellison syndrome.*

**Brumeton Colloidale S** *Bruschettini, Ital.*
Betamethasone (p.1093·1); sulfacetamide sodium (p.257·3).
*Eye and ear disorders.*

**Brumixol** *Bruschettini, Ital.*
Ciclopirox olamine (p.396·1).
*Fungal skin and vulvovaginal infections.*

**Brunac** *Bruschettini, Ital.*
Acetylcysteine (p.1112·3).
*Eye disorders.*

**Brunacod** *Brunel, S.Afr.*
Promethazine hydrochloride (p.439·1); ephedrine hydrochloride (p.1120·1); codeine phosphate (p.27·1).
*Coughs.*

**Brunal** *Fada, Arg.*
Ibuprofen (p.45·3).
*Inflammation; pain.*

**Brunavera** *Euroderm, Arg.*
Aloe vera (p.1141·3); calendula (p.1665·2); alpha tocopherol (p.1464·3).
*Dry skin.*

**Brunazine** *Brunel, S.Afr.*
Promethazine hydrochloride (p.439·1).
*Hypersensitivity reactions; motion sickness; nausea; vomiting.*

**Brunocillin** *Mepha, Switz.*
Phenoxymethylpenicillin potassium (p.242·1).
*Bacterial infections.*

**Brunomol** *Brunel, S.Afr.*
Paracetamol (p.76·2).
*Fever; pain.*

**Bruprin** *Condrugs, Thai.*
Ibuprofen (p.45·3).
*Musculoskeletal and joint disorders.*

**Brush Off** *SSL, UK†.*
Povidone-iodine (p.1190·3).
*Herpes labialis.*

**Brushtox** *Dentox, UK†.*
Denatured alcohol (p.1166·1); hydroxybenzoate esters (p.1183·2); zinc chloride (p.1469·2).
*Disinfection of toothbrushes.*

**Brusil** *Silom, Thai.*
Ibuprofen (p.45·3).
*Fever; musculoskeletal and joint disorders; pain.*

**Brust- und Hustentee** *Bad Heilbrunner, Ger.*
Thyme (p.1755·2); primula root (p.1735·1).
*Respiratory-tract disorders with viscous mucus.*

**Brust- und Hustentee EF-EM-ES** *Smetana, Austria.*
Castanea vulgaris; plantago lanceolata (p.1738·2); verbascum leaf (p.1764·1); thyme (p.1755·2); rad. enulae.
*Respiratory-tract disorders.*

**Brust- und Husten-Tee Stada N** *Stada, Ger.†.*
Plantago lanceolata (p.1738·2); thyme (p.1755·2); fennel (p.1687·2); liquorice (p.1270·2).
*Bronchitis; tracheitis.*

**Brustan** *Ranbaxy, Thai.*
Ibuprofen (p.45·3); paracetamol (p.76·2).
*Musculoskeletal, joint, peri-articular, and soft-tissue disorders.*

**Brustol** *Vifor, Switz.†.*
Dextromethorphan hydrobromide (p.1117·3); phenylephrine hydrochloride (p.1126·3); chlorphenamine maleate (p.427·3).
*Coughs.*

**Bruvac** *Nikkho, Braz.†.*
A brucellosis vaccine (p.1611·1).
*Active immunisation.*

**Bruxel** *Armstrong, Arg.*
Proglumetacin maleate (p.85·2).
*Gout; musculoskeletal, joint, and peri-articular disorders.*

**Bruxicam** *Bruschettini, Ital.*
Piroxicam (p.84·2).
*Musculoskeletal, joint, peri-articular, and soft-tissue disorders.*

**Brylcreem Anti-Dandruff** *GlaxoSmithKline Consumer, Canad.*
Pyrithione zinc (p.1156·2).
*Dandruff.*

**Bryonon B-Komplex** *Protina, Ger.†.*
Vitamin B substances (p.1417·1).
*Vitamin B deficiency.*

**Bryonon N** *Protina, Ger.†.*
Vitamin B substances (p.1417·1).
*Vitamin B deficiency.*

**Bryorheum** *DHU, Ger.*
Homoeopathic preparation.

**BS**
*Xepa-Soul Pattinson, Hong Kong†; Xepa-Soul Pattinson, Singapore.*
Co-trimoxazole (p.199·3).
*Bacterial infections.*

**B-Salt Forte** *Akorn, USA†.*
Electrolytes (p.1217·1); glucose (p.1432·2); oxiglutatione (p.1040·3).
*Eye irrigation.*

**BS-ratiopharm** *Ratiopharm, Ger.*
Hyoscine butylbromide (p.483·3).
*Smooth muscle spasm.*

**BSS**
*Alcon, Austral.; Alcon, Austria†; Alcon, Belg.†; Alcon, Braz.†; Alcon, Canad.; Alcon, Fr.; Alcon, Ger.; Pharmacia, Ger.; Serag-Wiessner, Ger.; Alkon (Αλκον), Gr.; Alcon, Hong Kong; Alcon, Irl.; Alcon, Israel; Alcon, Malaysia; Alcon, S.Afr.; Alcon, Singapore; Alcon Cusi, Spain†; Alcon, Switz.†; Alcon, Thai.; Alcon, USA.*
Electrolyte solution (p.1217·1).
*Eye irrigation; irrigation of ear, nose, and throat.*

**BSS Compose** *Alcon, Fr.*
Electrolytes (p.1217·1); glucose (p.1432·2); oxiglutatione (p.1040·3).
*Eye irrigation.*

**BSS Plus**
*Alcon, Austral.; Alcon, Austria; Alcon, Belg.†; Alcon, Canad.; Alcon, Ger.; Alkon (Αλκον), Gr.; Alcon, Hong Kong; Alcon, Israel; Alcon, Malaysia; Alcon, Singapore; Alcon, Switz.; Alcon, Thai.; Alcon, UK†; Alcon, USA.*
Electrolytes (p.1217·1); glucose (p.1432·2); oxiglutatione (p.1040·3).
*Eye irrigation.*

**B-Tasone-G** *Beacons, Singapore.*
Betamethasone valerate (p.1093·2); gentamicin sulfate (p.217·1).
*Infected skin disorders.*

**B-Tene** *Vitaglow, Austral.†.*
Betacarotene (p.1422·3).
*Photosensitivity reactions in patients with erythropoietic protoporphyria.*

**B-Tonin** *Nycomed, Norw.†.*
Vitamin B substances (p.1417·1); caffeine (p.782·1).
*Tonic; vitamin B deficiency.*

**BU Pangramin SLIT** *Alk-Scherax, Ger.*
Allergen extracts (p.1650·1).
*Allergen immunotherapy.*

**Buateron** *Pharmedia (Φαρμεντια), Gr.*
Calcium folinate (p.1431·1).
*Antidote to folic acid antagonists; megaloblastic anaemia.*

**Bucagel** *Asta Medica, Port.*
Choline salicylate (p.26·2); cetalkonium chloride (p.1172·1).
*Mouth disorders.*

**Bucain**
*Curasan, Austria; Curasan, Ger.*
Bupivacaine hydrochloride (p.1371·1).
*Local anaesthesia.*

**Bucanil**
*YSP, Malaysia; Yung Shin, Singapore.*
Terbutaline sulfate (p.797·2).
*Obstructive airways disease.*

**Bucaril** *Pharmaland, Thai.*
Terbutaline sulfate (p.797·2).
*Obstructive airways disease.*

**Bucasept** *Aerocid, Fr.†.*
Chlorhexidine gluconate (p.1173·2).
*Mouth and throat disorders.*

**Buccalin**
*Note. This name is used for preparations of different composition.*
*Kwizda, Austria.*
*Haemophilus influenzae*; pneumococci; streptococci; staphylococcus aureus; ox bile extract (p.1660·3).
*Prophylaxis of bacterial infections in patients with colds.*

*SIT, Ital.*
*Streptococcus pneumoniae* I, II, and III; *Streptococcus haemolyticus*; *Staphylococcus aureus*; *Haemophilus influenzae*.
*Prophylaxis of bacterial infections in patients with influenza.*

**Buccalin Complet** *Berna, Spain†.*
Pneumococcus; streptococcus; staphylococcus; *Haemophilus influenzae*.
*Respiratory-tract infections.*

**Buccaline**
*Note. This name is used for preparations of different composition.*
*Berna, Belg.; Berna, Hong Kong; Berna, Switz.; Berna, Thai.*
Pneumococcus I, II, III; streptococcus; staphylococcus; *Haemophilus influenzae*; ox bile (p.1660·3).
*Prophylaxis of colds.*

*Pharmabroker, NZ.*
Pneumococcus; streptococcus; staphylococcus; *Haemophilus influenzae*.
*Common cold prophylaxis.*

**Buccalsone**
*Will-Pharma, Belg.; Will-Pharma, Neth.*
Hydrocortisone sodium succinate (p.1104·1).
*Aphthous stomatitis.*

**Buccapol**
*Berna, Hong Kong†; Berna, Singapore†.*
An oral poliomyelitis vaccine (p.1633·3).
*Active immunisation.*

**Buccard** *AstraZeneca, Denm.*
Glyceryl trinitrate (p.923·2).
*Angina pectoris; heart failure.*

The symbol † denotes a preparation no longer actively marketed

**Buccastem**
Reckitt Benckiser, Irl.; Reckitt Benckiser, NZ; Reckitt Benckiser, UK.
Prochlorperazine maleate (p.716·3).
*Migraine; nausea; vertigo; vomiting.*

**Buccawalter** SmithKline Beecham, Fr.†.
Lidocaine hydrochloride (p.1377·3); cetrimide (p.1172·1); sodium salicylate (p.90·1); phenol (p.1188·1).
Formerly contained amylocaine hydrochloride, cloral hydrate, phenosalyl, and borax.
*Mouth and throat disorders.*

**Buccosan** Pfizer Consumer, Belg.
Dequalinium chloride (p.1178·1); lidocaine hydrochloride (p.1377·3).
*Mouth and throat disorders.*

**Bucco-Spray** Warner-Lambert Consumer, Belg.†.
Dequalinium chloride (p.1178·1); lidocaine hydrochloride (p.1377·3).
*Mouth and throat disorders.*

**Bucco-Tantum** Roche, Switz.
Benzydamine hydrochloride (p.21·1).
*Mouth and throat inflammation.*

**Buchex** Microsules Bernabo, Arg.
Hexetidine (p.1182·1); benzydamine hydrochloride (p.21·1).
*Mouth disorders.*

**Buchol** Palmicol, Ger.†.
Sage oil (p.1741·2).
*Hyperhidrosis.*

**Buchzine** Upha, Malaysia.
Buclizine hydrochloride (p.426·3).
*Appetite loss; hypersensitivity reactions.*

**Bucin** Masa, Thai.
Indometacin (p.47·3).
*Musculoskeletal, joint, and peri-articular disorders.*

**Buckley's Bedtime** Buckley, Canad.
Diphenhydramine hydrochloride (p.431·3); menthol (p.1711·3).
*Cold symptoms; coughs.*

**Buckley's Cough, Cold & Flu Daytime Relief** Buckley, Canad.
Pseudoephedrine hydrochloride (p.1129·2); dextromethorphan hydrobromide (p.1117·3); paracetamol (p.76·2).
*Cold and influenza symptoms; coughs.*

**Buckley's Cough, Cold & Flu Nighttime Relief** Buckley, Canad.
Pseudoephedrine hydrochloride (p.1129·2); dextromethorphan hydrobromide (p.1117·3); paracetamol (p.76·2); chlorphenamine maleate (p.427·3).
*Cold and influenza symptoms; coughs.*

**Buckley's DM** Buckley, Canad.
Dextromethorphan hydrobromide (p.1117·3).
*Dry cough.*

**Buckley's DM Decongestant** Buckley, Canad.
Pseudoephedrine hydrochloride (p.1129·2); dextromethorphan hydrobromide (p.1117·3).
*Coughs and cold symptoms.*

**Buckley's Mixture** Buckley, Canad.
Ammonium carbonate (p.1115·1); potassium bicarbonate (p.1223·1); menthol (p.1711·3); camphor (p.1665·3).
*Cough.*

**Buckleys Pain Relief** Buckley, Canad.
Methyl salicylate (p.59·3); menthol (p.1711·3).
*Muscle and joint pain.*

**Buckley's White Rub** Buckley, Canad.
Menthol (p.1711·3); camphor (p.1665·3); methyl salicylate (p.59·3); thymol (p.1194·2).
*Cold symptoms; muscle and joint pain.*

**Bucladin-S Softab** Stuart, USA.
Buclizine hydrochloride (p.426·3).
*Motion sickness.*

**Buclamin** Teuto, Braz.
Buclizine hydrochloride (p.426·3); tryptophan; lysine hydrochloride; pyridoxine; cyanocobalamin (p.1417·1).
*Reduced appetite; tonic.*

**Bucliamin** Baldassari, Braz.†.
Buclizine hydrochloride (p.426·3); tryptophan hydrochloride; carnitine hydrochloride; lysine hydrochloride; vitamin $B_6$; vitamin $B_{12}$ (p.1417·1).
*Reduced appetite; tonic.*

**Buclifen-Vit** Profarb, Braz.†.
Buclizine hydrochloride (p.426·3); lysine; vitamin $B_{12}$ (p.1417·1).
*Reduced appetite; tonic.*

**Buclina**
Sanofi Synthelabo, Braz.
Buclizine hydrochloride (p.426·3).
*Motion sickness; reduced appetite.*

Vedim, Port.
Buclizine (p.426·3).

**Bucliplex** Dovalle, Braz.
Buclizine hydrochloride (p.426·3); vitamin B substances (p.1417·1).
*Reduced appetite; tonic.*

**Buclitina** Heralds, Braz.†.
Buclizine (p.426·3); carnitine; gamma-aminobutyric acid; lysine; vitamin B substances (p.1417·1).
*Reduced appetite; tonic.*

**Buco Regis** Ramon Sala, Spain.
Ipecacuanha (p.1122·3); methyl salicylate (p.59·3); myrrh (p.1718·3); sulfanilamide (p.263·2); zinc chloride (p.1469·2); menthol (p.1711·3).
*Mouth and throat inflammation; pyorrhoea.*

**Bucodrin** Fardi, Spain.
Chlorhexidine hydrochloride (p.1173·3); benzocaine (p.1370·3).
Formerly contained ephedrine ricinoleate, ethacridine lactate, and sulfathiazole.
*Mouth and throat disorders.*

**Bucometasana** Solvay, Spain.
Chlorhexidine hydrochloride (p.1173·3); benzocaine (p.1370·3); tyrothricin (p.275·1).
*Mouth and throat disorders.*

**Buconif** Nycomed, Austria.
Nifedipine (p.966·2).
*Hypertension; ischaemic heart disease; Raynaud's syndrome.*

**Bucort** Orion, Fin.
Hydrocortisone butyrate (p.1104·1).
*Skin disorders.*

**Bucoseptil** Instituto Sanitas, Chile.
Chlorhexidine gluconate (p.1173·2).
*Mouth and throat disorders; oral hygiene.*

**Bucospray** Teofarma, Spain.
Chlorhexidine gluconate (p.1173·2); benzocaine (p.1370·3).
*Mouth and throat disorders.*

**Bucotricin** Monserrat, Arg.
Tyrothricin (p.275·1); benzocaine (p.1370·3).
*Mouth and throat disorders.*

**Bucovacuna** Nezel, Spain†.
*Streptococcus pneumoniae; Micrococcus pyogenes; Haemophilus influenzae*(p.0·0); *Gaffkya tetragena; Moraxella catarrhalis; Klebsiella pneumoniae; Moraxella.*
*Prophylaxis of respiratory-tract infections.*

**Budamax** PMC, Austral.
Budesonide (p.1094·2).
*Allergic rhinitis; nasal polyps.*

**Budapp** Dermapharm, Ger.
Budesonide (p.1094·2).
*Obstructive airways disease.*

**Budecol** Astra-Zeneca, Gr.
Budesonide (p.1094·2).
*Inflammatory bowel disease.*

**Budecort**
AstraZeneca, Braz.; Fujisawa, Ger.; Cipla, Thai.
Budesonide (p.1094·2).
*Asthma; nasal polyps; rhinitis.*

**Budefarma** ICN, Arg.
Budesonide (p.1094·2).
*Skin disorders.*

**Budefat** Fatol, Ger.
Budesonide (p.1094·2).
*Obstructive airways disease.*

**Budeflam** Cipla-Medpro, S.Afr.
Budesonide (p.1094·2).
*Allergic rhinitis; asthma.*

**Budenofalk**
Codali, Belg.; EciFarma, Chile; Falk, Ger.; Galenica, Gr.; Falk, Hong Kong; Medichemie, Switz.; Provalis, UK.
Budesonide (p.1094·2).
*Inflammatory bowel disease.*

**Budepur E** BASF, Ger.†.
Budesonide (p.1094·2).
*Obstructive airways disease.*

**Budes** Hexal, Ger.
Budesonide (p.1094·2).
*Obstructive airways disease.*

**Budesan** Zekides, Gr.
Budesonide (p.1094·2).
*Allergic rhinitis; topical corticosteroid.*

**Budeson**
Danes, Arg.; Rafa, Israel.
Budesonide (p.1094·2).
*Asthma; Crohn's disease; nasal polyps; rhinitis.*

**Budicort** Teva, Israel.
Budesonide (p.1094·2).
*Asthma.*

**Budon** Lindopharm, Ger.
Budesonide (p.1094·2).
*Obstructive airways disease.*

**Budo-san** Merck, Austria.
Budesonide (p.1094·2).
*Crohn's disease.*

**Buenas Noches** ISA, Arg.
Melatonin (p.1710·2).
*Sleep disorders.*

**Buenoson N** Zilly, Ger.
Hypericum oil; wheat-germ oil; avocado oil; birch tar oil; thiamine hydrochloride; dilute formic acid; garlic juice; birch leaf; juniper berry; gentian root; lupulus; clove; male fern leaf.
*Herbal preparation.*

**Buer Vitamin E + Magnesium** Roland, Ger.†.
α-Tocoferil acetate (p.1465·1); magnesium oxide (p.1272·3).
*Muscle weakness.*

**Buerlecithin**
Note. This name is used for preparations of different composition.
Polcopharma, Austral.†; Altana, Ger.
Lecithin (p.1706·1).
*Tonic.*

Byk, Austria.
Lecithin (p.1706·1) with or without vitamins (p.1417·1).
*Tonic.*

**Buerlecithin Compact**
Byk, Austria; Altana, Switz.
Lecithin (p.1706·1).
*Tonic.*

**Bufacyl** Medipharm, Chile.
Octatropine methylbromide (p.486·1); phenobarbital (p.367·3).
*Colic; dysmenorrhoea; vomiting in infants.*

**Bufederm** Galen, Ger.
Bufexamac (p.21·3).
*Skin disorders.*

**Bufedil**
Abbott, Braz.; Abbott, Ger.
Buflomedil hydrochloride (p.877·2).
*Peripheral vascular disorders.*

**Bufedon** Byk, Belg.†.
Ibuprofen (p.45·3).
*Gout; musculoskeletal, joint, and peri-articular disorders; pain.*

**Bufencon**
YSP, Malaysia; Yung Shin, Singapore.
Betamethasone dipropionate (p.1093·1); betamethasone sodium phosphate (p.1093·1).
*Corticosteroid.*

**Bufene** Ist. Chim. Inter., Ital.†.
Buflomedil hydrochloride (p.877·2).
*Vascular disorders.*

**Bufeno** Helvepharm, Switz.†.
Ibuprofen (p.45·3).
*Musculoskeletal and joint disorders.*

**Bufeproct** Hexal, Ger.†.
Bufexamac (p.21·3); lidocaine hydrochloride (p.1377·3); bismuth subgallate (p.1252·2); titanium dioxide (p.1160·3).
*Haemorrhoids.*

**Bufex** Wyeth Lederle, Austria.
Bufexamac (p.21·3).
*Skin disorders.*

**Bufexan**
Note. This name is used for preparations of different composition.
Labinca, Arg.
Mesalazine (p.1273·2).
*Inflammatory bowel disease.*

Lannacher, Austria.
Bufexamac (p.21·3).
*Inflammatory skin disorders.*

**Bufexine** Continental Pharma, Belg.
Bufexamac (p.21·3).
*Arthritis; peri-articular inflammation.*

**Buffelin** Opto-Pharm, Singapore†.
Boric acid (p.1662·1); sodium chloride (p.1233·3).
*Eye irritation.*

**Buffered C** Quest, UK.
Calcium ascorbate (p.1460·2).

**Buffered C 500** Bio-Health, UK.
Calcium ascorbate (p.1460·2).

**Bufferin**
Bristol-Myers Squibb, Arg.; Bristol-Myers Squibb, Braz.; Bristol-Myers Squibb, Canad.; Bristol-Myers Squibb, Ital.; Bristol-Myers Products, USA.
Aspirin (p.15·1).
Calcium carbonate (p.1254·2), magnesium carbonate (p.1272·1), and magnesium oxide (p.1272·3) are included in this preparation in an attempt to limit adverse effects on the gastrointestinal mucosa.
*Fever; inflammation; myocardial infarction; pain; transient ischaemic attacks.*

Bristol-Myers Squibb, Singapore.
Aspirin (p.15·1).
*Thrombosis prophylaxis.*

**Bufferin AF Nite Time** Bristol-Myers Squibb, USA.
Diphenhydramine citrate (p.431·3); paracetamol (p.76·2).
*Insomnia.*

**Bufferin Low Dose** Bristol-Myers Squibb, Malaysia.
Aspirin (p.15·1).
*Thromboembolic disorders.*

**Buffets II** JMI, USA†.
Paracetamol (p.76·2); aspirin (p.15·1); caffeine (p.782·1).
Aluminium hydroxide (p.1249·2) is included in this preparation in an attempt to limit adverse effects on the gastrointestinal mucosa.
*Pain.*

**Buffex** Roberts, USA.
Aspirin (p.15·1).
Aluminium glycinate (p.1249·1) and magnesium carbonate (p.1272·1) are included in this preparation in an attempt to limit adverse effects on the gastrointestinal mucosa.
*Fever; inflammation; myocardial infarction; pain; transient ischaemic attacks.*

**Bufigen**
Note. This name is used for preparations of different composition.
Antigen, Irl.
Ibuprofen (p.45·3).
*Musculoskeletal, joint, and peri-articular disorders; pain; soft-tissue injuries.*

Pisa, Mex.
Nalbuphine hydrochloride (p.64·2).
*Pain.*

**Bufilem** Lemery, Mex.
Nalbuphine (p.64·3).
*Pain.*

**Buflan** Fournier, Ital.
Buflomedil hydrochloride (p.877·2).
*Vascular disorders.*

**Buflo** ABZ, Ger.; 1A, Ger.
Buflomedil hydrochloride (p.877·2).
*Peripheral vascular disorders.*

**Buflocit** CT, Ital.
Buflomedil hydrochloride (p.877·2).
*Cerebral and peripheral vascular disorders.*

**Buflofar** Upsamedica, Ital.
Buflomedil hydrochloride (p.877·2).
*Cerebral and peripheral vascular disorders.*

**Buflohexal**
Hexal, Austria; Hexal, Ger.
Buflomedil hydrochloride (p.877·2).
*Peripheral vascular disorders.*

**Buflomed**
Scott-Cassara, Arg.
Buflomedil (p.877·2).
*Cerebral and peripheral vascular disorders.*

Genericon, Austria.
Buflomedil hydrochloride (p.877·2).
*Peripheral vascular disorders.*

**Buflo-POS** Ursapharm, Ger.
Buflomedil hydrochloride (p.877·2).
*Peripheral vascular disorders.*

**Buflo-Puren** Alpharma-Isis, Ger.
Buflomedil hydrochloride (p.877·2).
*Peripheral vascular disorders.*

**Buflo-Reu** Reusch, Ger.†.
Buflomedil hydrochloride (p.877·2).
*Peripheral vascular disorders.*

**Bufoxin** Fulton, Ital.†.
Buflomedil pyridoxal phosphate compound (p.877·2).
*Cerebral and peripheral vascular disorders.*

**Buftyl** Hexal, Austria.
Buflomedil hydrochloride (p.877·2).
*Peripheral vascular disorders.*

**Bug Guards** Go Travel, UK†.
Diethyltoluamide (p.1503·3).
*Insect repellent.*

**Bug Proof** Nomad, UK†.
Permethrin (p.1508·3).
*Insect repellent for clothing.*

**Bugazon** Pharmacos Abug, Mex.
Captopril (p.879·2).
*Hypertension.*

**Bugesic** Cipla, Austral.
Ibuprofen (p.45·3).

**Bugs Bunny**
Bayer Consumer, Canad.; Bayer Consumer, Singapore; Miles, USA.
Multivitamins or multivitamins with minerals (p.1417·1).

**Bulboid** Melisana, Switz.
Glycerol (p.1694·3).
*Bowel evacuation; constipation.*

**Bulboshap** Farmagan, Ital.
Shampoo containing achillea, chamomile, cinchona, cornflower, gentian, lilly, and almond.
*Seborrhoeic dermatitis.*

**Bulgarolax** Laboratorios Chile, Chile.
Phenolphthalein (p.1284·1); cascara (p.1255·1); aloes (p.1248·2).
*Constipation.*

**Bulk** Agepha, Austria.
Methylcellulose (p.1580·2).
*Constipation.*

**Bullfrog** Chattem, USA.
*Gel SPF 18:* Oxybenzone (p.1154·3); octocrilene (p.1154·3); octinoxate (p.1154·3).
*SPF 36:* Oxybenzone (p.1154·3); octocrilene (p.1154·3); octinoxate (p.1154·3).
*Stick SPF 18:* Oxybenzone (p.1154·3); octinoxate (p.1154·3).
*Sunscreen.*

**Bullfrog for Kids** Chattem, USA.
*SPF 18:* Octocrilene (p.1154·3); octinoxate (p.1154·3) octisalate (p.1154·3).
*Sunscreen.*

**Bullfrog Sport** Chattem, USA.
*SPF 18:* Oxybenzone (p.1154·3); octocrilene (p.1154·3); octinoxate (p.1154·3) octisalate (p.1154·3); titanium dioxide (p.1160·3).
*Sunscreen.*

**Bullrich Salz** Mundipharma, Austria.
Sodium bicarbonate (p.1223·2).
*Dyspepsia.*

**Bumaflex N** Byk, Arg.
Naproxen (p.65·1).
*Inflammation.*

**Bumed** Medifive, Thai.
Ibuprofen (p.45·3).
*Inflammation; musculoskeletal and joint disorders; pain.*

**Bumedyl** Atlantis, Mex.
Bumetanide (p.877·2).
*Cirrhosis with ascites; heart failure; hypertension; oedema.*

**Bumex** Roche, USA.
Bumetanide (p.877·2).
*Oedema.*

**Buminate**
Baxter-Hyland, Hong Kong; Baxter, Malaysia; Baxter, Singapore†; Baxter, Thai.; Baxter, USA.
Albumin (p.740·3).
*Adult respiratory distress syndrome; burns; cardiopulmonary bypass surgery; hypoalbuminaemia; hypovolaemia; neonatal hyperbilirubinaemia; nephrosis.*

**Bumps and Bruises** *Hylands, Canad.*
Homoeopathic preparation.

**Bumps 'n Falls** *Dermamend, UK†.*
Benzalkonium chloride (p.1168·3); oxyesterified triglycerides.
*Cuts; soft-tissue injury.*

**Bunafon** *Unipharma, Gr.*
Ambroxol hydrochloride (p.1114·3).
*Respiratory disorders associated with viscous mucus.*

**Bunil** *Lundbeck, Port.*
Melperone (p.706·1).
*Agitation; alcohol withdrawal syndrome; confusion; insomnia; psychoses.*

**Bunion Salve** *Cress, Canad.†.*
Camphor (p.1665·3); menthol (p.1711·3); phenol (p.1188·1); tannic acid (p.1751·2).

**Bupafen** *Biomed, NZ.*
Bupivacaine hydrochloride (p.1371·1); fentanyl citrate (p.40·1).
*Epidural analgesia.*

**Bupap** *ECR, USA.*
Butalbital (p.673·3); paracetamol (p.76·2).
*Pain.*

**Buphenyl** *Ucyclyd, USA.*
Sodium phenylbutyrate (p.1748·2).
*Urea cycle disorders.*

**Bupiabbott** *Abbott, Braz.*
Bupivacaine hydrochloride (p.1371·1).
*Local anaesthesia.*

**Bupiabbott Plus** *Abbott, Braz.*
Bupivacaine hydrochloride (p.1371·1).
Adrenaline (p.852·2) is included in this preparation as a vasoconstrictor to diminish absorption and localise the effect of the local anaesthetic.
*Local anaesthesia.*

**Bupibil** *Biologici Italia, Ital.*
Bupivacaine hydrochloride (p.1371·1).
*Local anaesthesia.*

**Bupicain** *Monico, Ital.*
Bupivacaine hydrochloride (p.1371·1).
Adrenaline acid tartrate (p.852·2) is included in some injections as a vasoconstrictor to diminish absorption and localise the effect of the local anaesthetic.
*Local anaesthesia.*

**Bupicaina** *Scott-Cassara, Arg.*
Bupivacaine (p.1372·1).
*Local anaesthesia.*

**Bupiforan** *Baxter, Ital.*
Bupivacaine hydrochloride (p.1371·1).
Adrenaline acid tartrate (p.852·2) is included in some injections as a vasoconstrictor to diminish absorption and localise the effect of the local anaesthetic.
*Local anaesthesia.*

**Bupinex** *Richmond, Arg.*
Bupivacaine (p.1372·1).
*Local anaesthesia.*

**Bupinostrum Adrenalina** *Nostrum, Port.*
Bupivacaine hydrochloride (p.1371·1).
Adrenaline (p.852·2) is included in this preparation as a vasoconstrictor to diminish absorption and localise the effect of the local anaesthetic.
*Local anaesthesia.*

**Bupisen** *Senese, Ital.*
Bupivacaine hydrochloride (p.1371·1).
Adrenaline acid tartrate (p.852·2) is included in some injections as a vasoconstrictor to diminish absorption and localise the effect of the local anaesthetic.
*Local anaesthesia.*

**Bupisolver** *Solver, Ital.*
Bupivacaine hydrochloride (p.1371·1).
Adrenaline acid tartrate (p.852·2) is included in some injections as a vasoconstrictor to diminish absorption and localise the effect of the local anaesthetic.
*Local anaesthesia.*

**Bupixamol** *Molteni, Ital.*
Bupivacaine hydrochloride (p.1371·1).
Adrenaline acid tartrate (p.852·2) is included in some injections as a vasoconstrictor to diminish absorption and localise the effect of the local anaesthetic.
*Local anaesthesia.*

**Bupogesic** *Merck, Hong Kong.*
Ibuprofen (p.45·3).
*Musculoskeletal, joint, and peri-articular disorders.*

**Buprenex** *Reckitt & Colman, USA.*
Buprenorphine hydrochloride (p.21·3).
*Pain.*

**Buprex**
*Schering-Plough, Port.; Schering-Plough, Spain.*
Buprenorphine hydrochloride (p.21·3).
*Pain.*

**Buprine** *Siam Bheasach, Thai.*
Buprenorphine hydrochloride (p.21·3).
*Pain.*

**Bupyl** *Molteni, Ital.†.*
Bupivacaine hydrochloride (p.1371·1).
Adrenaline acid tartrate (p.852·2) is included in some injections as a vasoconstrictor to diminish absorption and localise the effect of the local anaesthetic.
*Local anaesthesia.*

**Buram**
*Leo, Denm.; Leo, Irl.*
Amiloride hydrochloride (p.858·2); bumetanide (p.877·2).
*Oedema.*

The symbol † denotes a preparation no longer actively marketed

**Burana** *Orion, Fin.*
Ibuprofen (p.45·3).
*Gout; inflammation; musculoskeletal, joint, and peri-articular disorders; pain.*

**Burana-C** *Orion, Fin.*
Ibuprofen (p.45·3); ascorbic acid (p.1460·2).
*Influenza symptoms.*

**Buraton 10 F** *Schulke & Mayr, Ger.†.*
Glyoxal (p.1181·1); formaldehyde (p.1179·3); glutaral (p.1180·3); ethylhexanal.
*Surface disinfection.*

**Burgerstein Geriatrikum** *Antistress, Switz.*
Multivitamin and mineral preparation (p.1417·1).
*Tonic.*

**Burgerstein S** *Antistress, Switz.*
Vitamin and mineral preparation (p.1417·1).
*Liver disorders.*

**Burgerstein TopVital** *Antistress, Switz.*
Multivitamin and mineral preparation with ginseng (p.1417·1)(p.1693·1).
*Tonic.*

**Burgodin** *Janssen-Cilag, Belg.†.*
Bezitramide (p.21·2).
*Pain.*

**Burinax** *Sintofarma, Braz.*
Bumetanide (p.877·2).
*Hypercalcaemia; hypertension; oedema.*

**Burinex**
*CSL, Austral.; Leo, Austria; Leo, Belg.; Leo, Canad.; Leo, Denm.; Leo, Fin.†; Leo, Fr.; Leo, Ger.; IFET (ΙΦΕΤ), Gr.; Leo, Hong Kong†; Leo, Irl.; Leo, Malaysia; Leo, Neth.; Leo, Norw.; CSL, NZ; Leo, NZ; Adcock Ingram, S.Afr.; Leo, Singapore; Leo, Swed.; Leo, Switz.; Leo, Thai.; Leo, UK.*
Bumetanide (p.877·2).
*Forced diuresis; hypertension; oedema; renal failure.*

**Burinex A** *Leo, UK.*
Bumetanide (p.877·2); amiloride hydrochloride (p.858·2).
*Oedema.*

**Burinex K**
*Leo, Hong Kong†; Leo, Irl.; Leo, Malaysia; Leo, Norw.; Adcock Ingram, S.Afr.; Leo, Singapore; Leo, UK.*
Bumetanide (p.877·2); potassium chloride (p.1232·2).
*Oedema.*

**Burinex med kaliumklorid** *Leo, Denm.*
Bumetanide (p.877·2); potassium chloride (p.1232·2).
*Hypertension; oedema.*

**Burmicin** *I Farmacologia, Spain.*
Amoxicillin trihydrate (p.155·3); potassium clavulanate (p.193·3).
*Bacterial infections.*

**Burn Cream** *Medipharma, Hong Kong.*
Aminoacridine hydrochloride (p.1165·3); thymol (p.1194·2); allantoin (p.1141·3); lidocaine hydrochloride (p.1377·3).
*Burns.*

**Burn Healing Cream** *Brauer, Austral.†.*
Homoeopathic preparation.

**Burnaid** *Rye, Singapore.*
Melaleuca oil (p.1710·2); triclosan (p.1195·2).
*Burns; scalds.*

**Burnaid First Aid Burn Gel** *Rye, Austral.†.*
Melaleuca oil (p.1710·2); triclosan (p.1195·2).
*Burns.*

**Burn-A-Sept** *Salters, S.Afr.†.*
Tannic acid (p.1751·2); phenol (p.1188·1).
*Burns.*

**Burneze** *SSL, UK.*
Benzocaine (p.1370·3).
*Burns; scalds.*

**Burnocaine** *Salters, S.Afr.†.*
Benzocaine (p.1370·3); chlorhexidine acetate (p.1173·2); cetrimide (p.1172·1); benzyl alcohol; vitamin A palmitate; castor oil.
*Burns.*

**Burnol Plus**
*Boots Healthcare, Malaysia; Boots, Singapore; Boots, Thai.*
Aminoacridine hydrochloride (p.1165·3); cetrimide (p.1172·1); thymol (p.1194·2).
*Burns; insect bites; skin rashes; wounds.*

**Burns Cream** *Nelson, UK.*
Homoeopathic preparation.

**Burnshield Gel** *Travel-Safe, UK.*
Melaleuca oil (p.1710·2).
*Burns; scalds.*

**Buro Derm** *Trans Canaderm, Canad.†.*
Aluminium acetate (p.1652·3); benzethonium chloride (p.1169·2).

**Buronil**
*Lundbeck, Austria; Lundbeck, Belg.; Lundbeck, Denm.; Lundbeck, Fin.; Lundbeck, Norw.†; Lundbeck, Swed.*
Melperone hydrochloride (p.706·1).
*Anxiety disorders; dementia; drug and alcohol withdrawal syndromes; pain; psychoses; sleep disorders.*

**Buro-Sol**
*Trans Canaderm, Canad.; Doak, USA.*
Aluminium acetate (p.1652·3).
*Skin inflammation.*

**Burow's** *Rugby, USA.*
Acetic acid (p.1645·2); aluminium acetate (p.1652·3).
*Ear infections.*

**Burten** *Laboratorios Chile, Chile.*
Ketorolac trometamol (p.52·1).
*Pain.*

**Busala** *Selz, Ger.†.*
Dimethicone (p.1289·2).
*Gastrointestinal disorders.*

**Busansil** *Lepori, Port.*
Buspirone hydrochloride (p.672·2).
*Anxiety.*

**Buscalm** *Wockhardt, India.*
Buspirone hydrochloride (p.672·2).
*Anxiety.*

**Buscalma** *Euro-Labor, Port.; Grunenthal, Port.*
Buspirone hydrochloride (p.672·2).
*Anxiety.*

**Buscapina**
*Boehringer Ingelheim, Arg.; Boehringer Ingelheim, Chile; Boehringer Ingelheim, Mex.; Boehringer Ingelheim, Spain.*
Hyoscine butylbromide (p.483·3).
*Adjuvant in gastrointestinal radiography; smooth muscle spasm.*

**Buscapina Compositum**
*Boehringer Ingelheim, Arg.; Boehringer Ingelheim, Chile; Boehringer Ingelheim, Mex.; Boehringer Ingelheim, Spain.*
Hyoscine butylbromide (p.483·3); dipyrone (p.35·3).
*Painful smooth muscle spasm.*

**Buscapina Compositum N**
*Boehringer Ingelheim, Arg.; Boehringer Ingelheim, Mex.*
Hyoscine butylbromide (p.483·3); paracetamol (p.76·2).
*Painful smooth muscle spasm.*

**Buscofen** *Boehringer Ingelheim, Ital.*
Ibuprofen (p.45·3).
*Pain.*

**Buscolysin** *Medphano, Ger.*
Hyoscine butylbromide (p.483·3).
*Smooth muscle spasm.*

**Busconet** *Sons, Mex.*
Hyoscine butylbromide (p.483·3); dipyrone (p.35·3).
*Painful smooth muscle spasm.*

**Buscono** *Milano, Thai.*
Hyoscine butylbromide (p.483·3).
*Smooth muscle spasm.*

**Buscopamol** *Boehringer Ingelheim, Austria.*
Hyoscine butylbromide (p.483·3); paracetamol (p.76·2).
*Pain; smooth muscle spasm.*

**Buscopan**
*Boehringer Ingelheim, Austral.; Boehringer Ingelheim, Austria; Boehringer Ingelheim, Belg.; Boehringer de Angeli, Braz.; Boehringer Ingelheim, Canad.; Boehringer Ingelheim, Denm.; Boehringer Ingelheim, Fin.; Boehringer Ingelheim, Ger.; Boehringer Ingelheim, Gr.; Boehringer Ingelheim, Hong Kong; German Remedies, India; Boehringer Ingelheim, Irl.; Boehringer Ingelheim, Ital.; Boehringer Ingelheim, Malaysia; Boehringer Ingelheim, Neth.; Boehringer Ingelheim, Norw.; Boehringer Ingelheim, NZ; Boehringer Ingelheim, Port.; Boehringer Ingelheim, S.Afr.; Boehringer Ingelheim, Singapore; Boehringer Ingelheim, Swed.; Boehringer Ingelheim, Switz.; Boehringer Ingelheim, Thai.; Boehringer Ingelheim, UK.*
Hyoscine butylbromide (p.483·3).
*Diagnostic aid in radiology or endoscopy; smooth muscle spasm.*

**Buscopan Compositum**
*Note. This name is used for preparations of different composition.*
*Boehringer Ingelheim, Austria; Boehringer Ingelheim, Belg.; Boehringer Ingelheim, S.Afr.*
Hyoscine butylbromide (p.483·3); dipyrone (p.35·3).
*Smooth muscle spasm and pain.*

*Boehringer Ingelheim, Ital.*
Hyoscine butylbromide (p.483·3); paracetamol (p.76·2).
Formerly contained hyoscine butylbromide and dipyrone.
*Smooth muscle spasm.*

**Buscopan Compositum N** *Boehringer Ingelheim, Port.*
Hyoscine butylbromide (p.483·3); paracetamol (p.76·2).
*Smooth muscle spasm.*

**Buscopan Composto** *Boehringer de Angeli, Braz.*
Hyoscine butylbromide (p.483·3); dipyrone (p.35·3).
*Smooth muscle spasm.*

**Buscopan Plus**
*Boehringer de Angeli, Braz.; Boehringer Ingelheim, Ger.; Boehringer Ingelheim, Thai.*
Hyoscine butylbromide (p.483·3); paracetamol (p.76·2).
*Smooth muscle spasm.*

**Buscoveran Composto** *Bunker, Braz.*
Hyoscine butylbromide (p.483·3); dipyrone (p.35·3).
*Smooth muscle spasm.*

**Busepan** *Offenbach, Mex.*
Hyoscine butylbromide (p.483·3); dipyrone (p.35·3).
*Smooth muscle spasm.*

**Bush Formula** *Or-Dov, Austral.†.*
Chlorhexidine gluconate (p.1173·2).
*Acne; skin rashes.*

**Bushi** *Andromaco, Arg.*
Calendula (p.1665·2); allantoin (p.1141·3).
*Nipple care.*

**Busidril** *Omega, Spain.*
Ebastine (p.433·1).
*Hypersensitivity reactions.*

**Busilvex** *Pierre Fabre, UK.*
Busulfan (p.532·2).
*Malignant neoplasms.*

**Busina** *Jofrain, Mex.†.*
Hyoscine butylbromide (p.483·3).

**Busonid** *Biosintetica, Braz.*
Budesonide (p.1094·2).
*Corticosteroid.*

**Busopin** *Jean-Marie, Hong Kong.*
Hyoscine butylbromide (p.483·3).
*Smooth muscle spasm.*

**Busp** *Hexal, Ger.*
Buspirone hydrochloride (p.672·2).
*Anxiety disorders.*

**Buspanil** *Novartis, Braz.*
Buspirone hydrochloride (p.672·2).
*Anxiety.*

**Buspar**
*Bristol-Myers Squibb, Austral.; Bristol-Myers Squibb, Austria; Bristol-Myers Squibb, Belg.; Bristol-Myers Squibb, Braz.; Bristol, Canad.; Bristol-Myers Squibb, Denm.; Orion, Fin.; Bristol-Myers Squibb, Fin.; UPSA, Fr.; Bristol-Myers Squibb, Hong Kong; Bristol-Myers Squibb, Irl.; Bristol-Myers Squibb, Ital.; Bristol-Myers Squibb, Mex.; Bristol-Myers Squibb, Neth.; Bristol-Myers Squibb, Norw.; Bristol-Myers Squibb, NZ; Bristol-Myers Squibb, Port.; Bristol-Myers Squibb, S.Afr.; Bristol-Myers Squibb, Singapore†; Bristol-Myers, Spain; Bristol-Myers Squibb, Swed.; Bristol-Myers Squibb, Switz.; IXL, UK; Bristol-Myers Squibb, USA.*
Buspirone hydrochloride (p.672·2).
*Anxiety.*

**Buspimen** *Menarini, Ital.*
Buspirone hydrochloride (p.672·2).
*Anxiety.*

**Buspirex** *Technilab, Canad.*
Buspirone hydrochloride (p.672·2).
*Anxiety.*

**Buspirol** *Bristol-Myers Squibb, Israel.*
Buspirone hydrochloride (p.672·2).
*Anxiety.*

**Buspisal** *Lesvi, Spain†.*
Buspirone hydrochloride (p.672·2).
*Anxiety.*

**Buspril** *Sintofarma, Braz.†.*
Buspirone hydrochloride (p.672·2).
*Anxiety.*

**Busprina** *Farcoral, Mex.*
Hyoscine butylbromide (p.483·3); dipyrone (p.35·3).
*Smooth muscle spasm and pain.*

**Busprina-S** *Farcoral, Mex.*
Hyoscine butylbromide (p.483·3).
*Smooth muscle spasm.*

**Bustab** *ICN, Canad.†.*
Buspirone hydrochloride (p.672·2).
*Anxiety.*

**Bustrix** *GlaxoSmithKline, Arg.*
A diphtheria, tetanus, and pertussis vaccine (p.1613·3).
*Active immunisation.*

**Busulfex**
*Orphan Medical, Canad.; Orphan Medical, Israel; Orphan Medical, USA.*
Busulfan (p.532·2).
*Malignant neoplasms.*

**Buta** *PD, Thai.*
Phenylbutazone sodium (p.84·1).
Lidocaine hydrochloride (p.1377·3) is included in this preparation to alleviate the pain of injection.
*Gout; musculoskeletal and joint disorders.*

**Buta Pee Dee** *PD, Thai.*
Phenylbutazone (p.83·2); methyl salicylate (p.59·3).
*Musculoskeletal and joint disorders.*

**Buta Rut B12** *Fabra, Arg.*
Cyanocobalamin (p.1458·2); piroxicam (p.84·2).
*Inflammation; pain.*

**Butacort** *Pacific, NZ.*
Budesonide (p.1094·2).
*Nasal polyps; rhinitis.*

**Butacortelone** *Riker, Mex.†.*
Ibuprofen (p.45·3).
*Inflammation; musculoskeletal and joint disorders; pain.*

**Butacote** *Novartis, UK†.*
Phenylbutazone (p.83·2).
*Ankylosing spondylitis.*

**Butadion** *Streuli, Switz.*
Phenylbutazone (p.83·2) or phenylbutazone sodium (p.84·1).
Lidocaine hydrochloride (p.1377·3) is included in the intramuscular injection to alleviate the pain of injection.
*Gout; musculoskeletal and joint disorders; phlebitis; soft-tissue disorders.*

**Butafen** *Tocogino, Mex.†.*
Oxyphenbutazone (p.76·1).

**Butahale** *Reddy, Singapore.*
Salbutamol sulfate (p.791·3).
*Obstructive airways disease.*

**Butalen** *Allen, Mex.*
Phenylbutazone (p.83·2).
*Musculoskeletal and joint disorders.*

**Butalin** *Julphar, UAE.*
Salbutamol sulfate (p.791·3).
*Obstructive airways disease; premature labour.*

**Butaline** *Upha, Malaysia.*
Terbutaline sulfate (p.797·2).
*Obstructive airways disease.*

**Butaliret** *Fatol, Ger.*
Terbutaline sulfate (p.797·2).
*Obstructive airways disease.*

**Butalitab** *Fatol, Ger.*
Terbutaline sulfate (p.797·2).
*Obstructive airways disease.*

**Butamine** *Taro, Israel.*
Dobutamine hydrochloride (p.905·3).
*Heart failure.*

**Butamir** *Pharmanel, Gr.*
Butamirate citrate (p.1116·2).
*Cough.*

**Butamol** *Pharmaland, Thai.*
Salbutamol sulfate (p.791·3).
*Obstructive airways disease; premature labour.*

**Butanil** *Raza, Malaysia; Pharmaniaga, Malaysia.*
Terbutaline sulfate (p.797·2).
*Asthma.*

**Butaparin** *Streuli, Switz.*
Heparin sodium (p.928·1); phenylbutazone (p.83·2); thymol (p.1194·2).
*Peripheral vascular disorders.*

**Butapirin** *IQB, Braz.†.*
Phenylbutazone calcium (p.84·1); paracetamol (p.76·2).
*Fever; inflammation; pain.*

**Buta-Proxyvon** *Wockhardt, India.*
*Capsules:* Diclofenac sodium (p.32·1); dextropropoxyphene hydrochloride (p.28·3); paracetamol (p.76·2).
*Inflammation; musculoskeletal and joint disorders.*
*Topical gel:* Diclofenac diethylamine (p.32·1); linseed oil (p.1707·2); methyl salicylate (p.59·3); menthol (p.1711·3).
*Musculoskeletal, joint, and soft-tissue disorders.*

**Butarion** *Chew, Thai.*
Phenylbutazone (p.83·2); dipyrone (p.35·3).
*Gout; musculoskeletal and joint disorders.*

**Butartrol** *Instituto Sanitas, Chile.*
Ibuprofen (p.45·3); meprobamate (p.706·2).
*Gout; musculoskeletal, joint, and peri-articular disorders.*

**Butasona** *Fabra, Arg.*
Betamethasone (p.1093·1).
*Corticosteroid.*

**Butasona RL** *Fabra, Arg.*
Betamethasone acetate (p.1093·1); betamethasone sodium phosphate (p.1093·1).
*Corticosteroid.*

**Butavate** *Allen, Gr.*
Clobetasol propionate (p.1095·2).
*Topical corticosteroid.*

**Butayonacol** *Ifusa, Mex.*
Salicylamide (p.87·3); phenylbutazone (p.83·2); colchicine (p.415·1).
*Inflammation; musculoskeletal and joint disorders.*

**Butazil** *Neo Quimica, Braz.*
Phenylbutazone (p.83·2); paracetamol (p.76·2).
*Fever; inflammation; pain.*

**Butazolidin**
*Novartis, Austral.†; Novartis, Austria; Novartis, Belg.; Novartis, Ger.†; Novartis, Neth.*
Phenylbutazone (p.83·2) or phenylbutazone sodium (p.84·1).
Cinchocaine (p.1373·2) is included in the injection to alleviate the pain of injection.
*Ankylosing spondylitis; gouty arthritis; osteoarthritis; rheumatoid arthritis.*

**Butazolidina**
*Novartis, Braz.; Novartis, Mex.; Novartis, Spain.*
Phenylbutazone (p.83·2).
Lidocaine (p.1377·3) may be included in the intramuscular injection to alleviate the pain of injection.
*Ankylosing spondylitis; arthrosis; gout; rheumatoid arthritis.*

**Butazolidine**
*Novartis, Fr.; Geigy, Switz.†.*
Phenylbutazone (p.83·2) or phenylbutazone sodium (p.84·1).
Cinchocaine (p.1373·2) may be included in the intramuscular injection to alleviate the pain of injection.
*Ankylosing spondylitis; arthrosis; gout; rheumatoid arthritis.*

**Butazolon** *Dovalle, Braz.*
Phenylbutazone (p.83·2).
Aluminium hydroxide (p.1249·2) is included in this preparation in an attempt to limit adverse effects on the gastrointestinal tract.
*Gout; musculoskeletal, joint, and peri-articular disorders.*

**Butazona** *Boehringer de Angeli, Braz.*
Phenylbutazone calcium (p.84·1).
*Gout; musculoskeletal, joint, and peri-articular disorders.*

**Butazone** *DDSA Pharmaceuticals, UK†.*
Phenylbutazone (p.83·2).

**Butazonil** *Teuto, Braz.*
Phenylbutazone (p.83·2).
*Gout; musculoskeletal, joint, and peri-articular disorders.*

**Buteridol** *Lundbeck, Ger.†.*
Haloperidol (p.701·2).
*Anxiety; behaviour disorders; movement disorders; pain; psychoses; stuttering; vomiting.*

**Butesin Picrate**
*Note. This name is used for preparations of different composition.*
*Abbott, Austral.*
Butyl aminobenzoate picrate (p.1373·1); nitromersol (p.1186·3).
*Burns; skin abrasions.*
*Abbott, USA†.*
Butyl aminobenzoate picrate (p.1373·1).
*Burns.*

**Butex** *Athlon, USA.*
Paracetamol (p.76·2); butalbital (p.673·3).
*Pain.*

**Butibel** *Wallace, USA.*
Belladonna (p.479·1); secbutabarbital sodium (p.721·2).
*Gastrointestinal disorders.*

**Buticina** *Rudefsa, Mex.†.*
Hyoscine butylbromide (p.483·3).

**Buticrem** *Raffo, Arg.*
Butenafine hydrochloride (p.395·2).
*Fungal skin infections.*

**Butidiona** *Roux-Ocefa, Arg.*
*Cream:* Ibuprofen (p.45·3); benzyl nicotinate (p.21·2).
*Tablets:* Ibuprofen (p.45·3).
*Inflammation.*

**Butilamin** *Sanval, Braz.†.*
Dipyrone (p.35·3); hyoscine (p.483·3).
*Smooth muscle spasm.*

**Butimerin** *Ariston, Arg.*
*Paste:* Benzethonium chloride (p.1169·2) butimerin; titanium dioxide (p.1160·3).
*Cracked nipples; infected skin disorders; nappy rash.*
*Topical powder:* Bacitracin (p.161·3); neomycin sulfate (p.235·1); papain (p.1727·3); butimerin.
*Burns; skin infections; ulcers; wounds.*

**Butin**
*YSP, Malaysia; Yung Shin, Singapore.*
Bromocriptine mesilate (p.1200·3).
*Acromegaly; hyperprolactinaemia; lactation inhibition; parkinsonism.*

**Butinat** *Sanofi Synthelabo, Arg.*
Bumetanide (p.877·2).
*Heart failure; hepatic cirrhosis; hypertension; oedema.*

**Butiral** *Rayere, Mex.*
Hyoscine butylbromide (p.483·3).
*Muscle spasm.*

**Butiran** *Ecobi, Ital.*
Butamirate citrate (p.1116·2).
*Coughs.*

**Butisol**
*Carter Horner, Canad.†; Wallace, USA.*
Secbutabarbital sodium (p.721·2).
*Insomnia; sedative.*

**Buti-Spirobene** *Ratiopharm, Austria.*
Butizide (p.878·2); spironolactone (p.1003·1).
*Aldosteronism; oedema.*

**Butix** *Pierre Fabre, Fr.*
*Tablets†:* Mequitazine (p.437·2).
*Hypersensitivity disorders; skin disorders.*
*Topical gel:* Diphenhydramine hydrochloride (p.431·3).
*Insect stings; pruritus; urticaria.*

**Buto Asma**
*Aldo-Union, Hong Kong; Aldo, Spain; Aldo-Union, Thai.*
Salbutamol (p.791·3) or salbutamol sulfate (p.791·3).
*Obstructive airways disease.*

**Butohaler** *Chiesi, Switz.†.*
Salbutamol (p.791·3).
*Bronchospasm.*

**Buton** *Mintlab, Chile.*
Papaverine hydrochloride (p.1728·1); atropine sulfate (p.477·1).
*Muscle spasm.*

**Butosali** *Valdecasas, Mex.*
Furosemide (p.919·3).
*Diuretic.*

**Butosol** *Aldo, Spain.*
Beclometasone dipropionate (p.1091·1); salbutamol (p.791·3).
*Obstructive airways disease.*

**Butotal**
*Grunenthal, Chile; Kener, Mex.†.*
Salbutamol (p.791·3).
*Obstructive airways disease.*

**Butotal B** *Grunenthal, Chile.*
Salbutamol (p.791·3); beclometasone dipropionate (p.1091·1).
*Obstructive airways disease.*

**Butovent**
*Siphar, Switz.†; Chiesi, Thai.*
Salbutamol (p.791·3).
*Obstructive airways disease.*

**Buttercup Infant Cough Syrup** *Pfizer Consumer, UK.*
Ipecacuanha (p.1122·3); glucose (p.1432·2); menthol (p.1711·3).
*Coughs; sore throat.*

**Buttercup Lozenges** *LRC Products, UK†.*
Bee propolis (p.1735·2).
*Coughs.*

**Buttercup Pol'N'Count** *LRC Products, UK†.*
Echinacea (p.1683·2); garlic (p.1691·1).
*Hay fever.*

**Buttercup Syrup** *Pfizer Consumer, UK.*
Squill liquid extract (p.1130·3); capsicum tincture (p.1667·1).
*Coughs.*

**Buttercup Syrup (Blackcurrant flavour)** *Pfizer Consumer, UK†.*
Ipecacuanha (p.1122·3); glucose (p.1432·2); menthol (p.1711·3).
*Coughs.*

**Buttercup Syrup (Honey and Lemon flavour)** *Pfizer Consumer, UK.*
Ipecacuanha (p.1122·3); glucose (p.1432·2); menthol (p.1711·3); honey (p.1434·2).
*Coughs.*

**Butt-Out** *Paradise, Canad.*
Lobelia (p.1589·1).
*Aid to smoking withdrawal.*

**Butyl** *Masa, Thai.*
Hyoscine butylbromide (p.483·3).
*Smooth muscle spasm.*

**Butylin** *Hovid, Singapore†.*
Terbutaline sulfate (p.797·2).
*Obstructive airways disease.*

**Buvacaina** *Pisa, Mex.*
Bupivacaine hydrochloride (p.1371·1).
Adrenaline acid tartrate (p.852·2) is included in some injections as a vasoconstrictor to diminish absorption and localise the effect of the local anaesthetic.
*Local anaesthesia.*

**Buventol**
*Lannacher, Austria; Orion, Denm.; Orion, Fin.; Orion, Fr.; Orion, Malaysia; Orion, Norw.; Orion, Singapore; Orion, Swed.; Orion, Switz.; Orion, Thai.*
Salbutamol (p.791·3) or salbutamol sulfate (p.791·3).
*Obstructive airways disease.*

**Buxon** *Saval, Chile.*
Bupropion hydrochloride (p.287·2).
*Aid to smoking withdrawal; depression.*

**Buzpel** *Torbet Laboratories, UK†.*
Pyrethrins (p.1509·3); piperonyl butoxide (p.1509·2).
*Insect repellent.*

**B-Vasc** *Garec, S.Afr.*
Atenolol (p.865·2).
*Angina pectoris; hypertension.*

**B-Vesil** *Daudt, Braz.*
*Oral solution:* Dehydrocholic acid (p.1679·2); glycine (p.1433·3); choline chloride (p.1424·3).
*Tablets:* Dehydrocholic acid (p.1679·2); bovine bile extract (p.1660·3).
*Digestive disorders.*

**BVK Roche plus C** *Roche Nicholas, Ger.*
Vitamin B substances with ascorbic acid (p.1417·1).
*Vitamin B and C deficiency.*

**Byclomine** *Major, USA.*
Dicycloverine hydrochloride (p.481·2).
*Functional bowel/irritable bowel syndrome.*

**Bye Bye Bite** *Daniels, Canad.†.*
Diphenhydramine hydrochloride (p.431·3); menthol (p.1711·3); benzocaine (p.1370·3).
*Bites and stings.*

**Bye Bye Burn** *Daniels, Canad.†.*
Benzocaine (p.1370·3); cetrimonium bromide (p.1173·1); allantoin (p.1141·3); vitamin E (p.1464·3).
*Burns.*

**Bykomycin**
*Byk, Austria; Byk Gulden, Ger.*
Neomycin sulfate (p.235·1).
*Hepatic coma.*

**Byl** *Medical, Port.*
Agar (p.1576·3); ox bile (p.1660·3); phenolphthalein (p.1284·1).
*Gastrointestinal disorders; liver disorders.*

**By-Madol** *Ergha, Irl.*
Tramadol hydrochloride (p.94·3).
*Pain.*

**Bymeniere** *Toho, Hong Kong.*
Betahistine mesilate (p.1660·1).
*Ménière's disease.*

**By-Mycin** *Ergha, Irl.*
Doxycycline hyclate (p.206·2).
*Bacterial infections.*

**Byodin** *Lucchini, Ital.†.*
Proteins (mol. wt 30-300 kD).
*Tissue repair.*

**Byodinoral** *MDM, Ital.*
Multivitamin preparation with thioctic acid (p.1754·3) (p.1417·1).
*Neuropathies.*

**By-Vertin** *Ergha, Irl.*
Betahistine hydrochloride (p.1660·1).
*Ménière's disease; tinnitus; vertigo.*

**C-20** *Osoth, Thai.*
Chlorhexidine gluconate (p.1173·2).
*Mouth infections.*

**C-86** *LDA, Arg.*
Ketoconazole (p.403·3).
*Scalp disorders.*

**C500** *Rekah, Israel.*
Vitamin C (p.1460·2).
*Vitamin C deficiency; vitamin C supplement.*

**C-1000**
*Seroyal, Canad.†; Richlife, Hong Kong†.*
Vitamin C (p.1460·2).

**C-3000** *Seroyal, Canad.†.*
Ascorbic acid (p.1460·2).

**C Calcio** *EMS, Braz.*
Vitamins C, D, and $B_6$ with calcium carbonate (p.1417·1).
*Nutritional supplement.*

**C2 with Codeine** *Wampole, Canad.*
Aspirin (p.15·1); caffeine (p.782·1); codeine phosphate (p.27·1).
Aluminium hydroxide (p.1249·2) and magnesium hydroxide (p.1272·2) are included in this preparation in an attempt to limit adverse effects on the gastrointestinal mucosa.
*Cardiovascular disorders; fever; inflammation; pain.*

**C Factors "1000" Plus** *Solgar, USA.*
Vitamin C (p.1460·2); rose hips (p.1740·1); citrus bioflavonoids complex (p.1688·2); rutoside (p.1688·2); hesperidin (p.1688·2).
*Capillary bleeding.*

**C Forte** *Frega, Canad.†.*
Ascorbic acid (p.1460·2).

**C1 Inattivatore Umano** *Baxter, Ital.*
Complement C1 esterase inhibitor (p.1675·2).
*Hereditary angioedema.*

**C Mon** *PP Lab, Thai.*
Ascorbic acid (p.1460·2).
*Scurvy.*

**C Monovit** *Esseti, Ital.*
Sodium ascorbate (p.1460·2).
*Vitamin C deficiency.*

**C Pal** *Eagle, Austral.†.*
Vitamin and mineral preparation with lysine (p.1417·1).

**C Plus E Natural** *Larkhall Laboratories, UK†.*
Vitamin C and E preparation (p.1417·1).

**C Rose Hips** *Richlife, Hong Kong†.*
Vitamin C (p.1460·2).

**C Supa + Bioflavonoids** *Vitaplex, Austral.†.*
Calcium ascorbate (p.1460·2); citrus bioflavonoids (p.1688·2); hesperidin (p.1688·2); rutoside (p.1688·2); rose fruit (p.1740·1).
*Vitamin C deficiency.*

**Ca Lac** *Raza, Malaysia; Pharmaniaga, Malaysia.*
Calcium lactate (p.1225·3).
*Calcium deficiency.*

**Caas** *EMS, Braz.*
Aspirin (p.15·1).
*Fever; inflammation; pain; thromboembolism prophylaxis.*

**Cabal** *Dallas, Arg.*
Cetirizine hydrochloride (p.427·1).
*Hypersensitivity reactions.*

**Cabaser**
*Pharmacia, Arg.; Pharmacia, Austral.; Pharmacia, Denm.; Pharmacia, Fin.; Pharmacia, Irl.; Pharmacia, Israel; Pharmacia Upjohn, Ital.; Pharmacia, Norw.; Pharmacia, Swed.; Pharmacia, Switz.; Pharmacia, UK.*
Cabergoline (p.1203·3).
*Parkinsonism.*

**Cabaseril**
*Pharmacia, Austria; Pharmacia, Ger.*
Cabergoline (p.1203·3).
*Parkinsonism.*

**Cabdrivers Sugar-Free Linctus** *Seven Seas, UK†.*
Ephedrine hydrochloride (p.1120·1); dextromethorphan hydrobromide (p.1117·3).
*Coughs.*

**Ca-C**
*Novartis Sante, Fr.*
Ascorbic acid (p.1460·2); calcium lactate gluconate (p.1225·3).
*Asthenia.*
*Novartis, Hong Kong; Novartis Consumer, Port.; Novartis Consumer, S.Afr.†; Novartis Nutrition, Singapore; Novartis Consumer, Switz.; Novartis, Thai.*
Ascorbic acid (p.1460·2); calcium carbonate (p.1254·2); calcium lactate gluconate (p.1225·3).
*Adjunct in colds and influenza; calcium deficiency; vitamin C deficiency.*

**Caceff** *Lupin, India.*
Cefalexin (p.168·1); carbocisteine (p.1116·2).
*Otitis media; respiratory-tract infections.*

**Cachexon** *Telluride, USA.*
Glutathione (p.1040·3).
*AIDS-associated cachexia.*

**Cacit**
*Procter & Gamble, Belg.; Procter & Gamble, Fr.; Procter & Gamble, Irl.; Procter & Gamble, Ital.; Procter & Gamble, Neth.; Procter & Gamble, UK.*
Calcium carbonate (p.1254·2).
*Calcium deficiency; osteoporosis.*

**Cacit D3** *Procter & Gamble, UK.*
Calcium carbonate (p.1254·2); colecalciferol (p.1461·3).
*Calcium and vitamin D deficiency; osteoporosis.*

**Cacit mit Vitamin $D_3$** *Asta Medica, Austria.*
Calcium carbonate (p.1254·2); colecalciferol (p.1461·3).
*Calcium and vitamin D deficiency; osteoporosis.*

**Cacit Vitamina D3** *Procter & Gamble, Ital.*
Calcium carbonate (p.1254·2); colecalciferol (p.1461·3).
*Calcium and vitamin D deficiency; osteoporosis.*

**Cacit Vitamine $D_3$**
*Procter & Gamble, Belg.; Procter & Gamble, Fr.*
Calcium carbonate (p.1254·2); colecalciferol (p.1461·3).
*Calcium and vitamin D deficiency; osteoporosis.*

**Cacital** *Parke, Davis, Spain†.*
Papain (p.1727·3).
*Hypersensitivity reactions; tissue injury.*

**Cactus compositum** *Peithner, Austria.*
Homoeopathic preparation.

**CaD** *Will-Pharma, Neth.*
Calcium carbonate (p.1254·2); colecalciferol (p.1461·3).
*Calcium and vitamin D deficiency; osteoporosis.*

**Cadencial Plus** *Poen, Arg.*
Cinnarizine (p.428·3); gamma-aminobutyric acid (p.1690·2); vitamin $B_6$ (p.1456·3).
*Cerebrovascular disorders; vascular eye disorders; vestibular disorders.*

**Cadens** *Zambon, Fr.*
Calcitonin (salmon) (p.768·2).
*Hypercalcaemia; hyperphosphataemia; osteoporosis; Paget's disease of bone; reflex sympathetic dystrophy.*

**Cadevit** *Gynopharm.*
Calcium carbonate (p.1254·2); colecalciferol (p.1461·3).
*Calcium and vitamin D supplement.*

**Cadex** *Dexcel, Israel.*
Doxazosin mesilate (p.908·3).
*Benign prostatic hyperplasia; hypertension.*

**Cadexcin-N** *Nakorn, Thai.*
Dexamethasone phosphate (p.1097·2); neomycin sulfate (p.235·1).
*Bacterial eye and ear infections.*

**Cadicon** *Pharmasant, Thai.*
Gliclazide (p.332·1).
*Diabetes mellitus.*

**Cadifen** *CaDiGroup, Ital.*
Fennel (p.1687·2); aniseed (p.1655·2); chamomile (p.1669·3); liquorice (p.1270·2); caraway (p.1667·2); coriander (p.1676·1).
*Bloating; digestive disorders.*

**Cadimasol** *Asta Medica, Ital.*
Vitamin D and mineral preparation (p.1417·1).

**Cadimint** *CaDiGroup, Ital.*
Peppermint (p.1283·2); fennel (p.1687·2); aniseed (p.1655·2); chamomile (p.1669·3); liquorice (p.1270·2); caraway (p.1667·2); coriander (p.1676·1).
*Gastrointestinal bloating.*

**Cadinol** *Andromaco, Chile.*
Dimeticone (p.1482·1).
*Flatulence.*

**Cadinyl** *Medifive, Thai.*
Diphenhydramine hydrochloride (p.431·3); calamine (p.1144·1); zinc oxide (p.1163·2).
*Skin irritation.*

**Cadiphylate** *Zydus, India.*
Acefylline piperazine (p.780·1); ephedrine hydrochloride (p.1120·1); phenobarbital (p.367·3); guaifenesin (p.1122·1).
*Obstructive airways disease.*

**Cadisper C** *Cadila, India.*
Methyl hesperidin; rutoside (p.1688·2); vitamin C (p.1460·2); carbazochrome (p.745·1); menadione sodium bisulfite (p.1466·3); calcium hydrogen phosphate (p.1225·2).
*Haemorrhage.*

**Caditar** *IPRAD, Fr.*
Cade oil (p.1159·2).
*Psoriasis; seborrhoeic dermatitis.*

**Cadolac** *Cadila, India.*
Ketorolac trometamol (p.52·1).
*Pain.*

**Cadramine** *Vana, Thai.*
Calamine (p.1144·1); zinc oxide (p.1163·2); diphenhydramine hydrochloride (p.431·3); camphor (p.1665·3); menthol (p.1711·3).
*Skin irritation.*

**Cadramine-V** *Atlantic, Hong Kong.*
Calamine (p.1144·1); zinc oxide (p.1163·2); diphenhydramine hydrochloride (p.431·3); camphor (p.1665·3); menthol (p.1711·3).
*Skin disorders.*

**Cadraten** *GlaxoSmithKline, Ital.*
Cadralazine (p.878·2).
*Hypertension.*

**Cadrilan** *Ciba, Ital.†.*
Cadralazine (p.878·2).
*Hypertension.*

**Cadrox** *Dinafarma, Braz.†.*
Calcium carbonate (p.1254·2); aluminium hydroxide (p.1249·2).
*Gastrointestinal hyperacidity.*

**Caduet** *Pfizer, USA.*
Amlodipine besilate (p.862·1); atorvastatin calcium (p.866·1).
*Hypercholesterolaemia; hypertension.*

**Cadvion** *Merck, India.*
Eicosapentaenoic acid (p.976·2); docosahexaenoic acid (p.976·1); vitamin E (p.1464·3).
*Hyperlipidaemias.*

**Cadyoil** *Cody, Ital.†.*
Emollient.

**C-A-E** *Seroyal, Canad.†.*
Vitamins A, C, and E (p.1417·1).

**Caedax**
*Aesca, Austria; Schering-Plough, Gr.; Schering-Plough, Port.*
Ceftibuten (p.182·1).
*Bacterial infections.*

**Caelyx**
*Essex, Arg.; Schering-Plough, Austral.; Sequus, Austria; Schering-Plough, Belg.; Schering-Plough, Braz.†; Schering, Canad.; Schering-Plough, Chile; Schering-Plough, Denm.; Schering-Plough, Fin.; Schering-Plough, Fr.; Essex, Ger.; Schering-Plough, Gr.; Schering-Plough, Hong Kong; Schering-Plough, Irl.; Sequus, Israel; Schering-Plough, Ital.; Schering-Plough, Malaysia; Schering-Plough, Mex.; Schering-Plough, Neth.; Schering-Plough, Norw.; Schering-Plough, Port.†; Schering-Plough, S.Afr.; Schering-Plough, Singapore; Schering-Plough, Spain; Schering-Plough, Swed.; Essex, Switz.; Schering-Plough, Thai.; Schering-Plough, UK.*
Liposomal doxorubicin hydrochloride (p.547·3) (p.547·3).
*Kaposi's sarcoma; ovarian cancer.*

**Caext** *Dallas, Arg.*
Benzocaine (p.1370·3); neomycin sulfate (p.235·1); gramicidin (p.220·2).
*Mouth and throat disorders.*

**Cafadol** *Typharm, UK†.*
Paracetamol (p.76·2); caffeine (p.782·1).
*Fever; pain.*

**Cafalena** *Dinafarma, Braz.†.*
Dipyrone (p.35·3); sodium camsilate.
*Cold and influenza symptoms.*

**Cafatine** *Major, USA.*
Ergotamine tartrate (p.467·2); caffeine (p.782·1).
*Migraine.*

**Cafatine-PB** *Major, USA.*
Ergotamine tartrate (p.467·2); caffeine (p.782·1); belladonna (p.479·1); pentobarbital sodium (p.713·3).
*Migraine.*

**Cafcit**
*IFET (ΙΦΕΤ), Gr.; Mead Johnson Nutritionals, USA.*
Caffeine citrate (p.782·1).
*Acute alcohol intoxication; apnoea of prematurity; lumbar puncture headache.*

**Cafergot**
*Note. This name is used for preparations of different composition.*
*Novartis, Arg.; Novartis, Austral.; Novartis, Austria; Novartis, Belg.; Novartis, Braz.†; Novartis, Canad.; Novartis, Gr.; Novartis, Hong Kong; Novartis, Irl.†; Novartis, Israel; Novartis, Ital.; Novartis, Malaysia; Novartis, Mex.; Novartis, Neth.; Novartis, NZ; Novartis, S.Afr.; Novartis, Singapore; Novartis, Spain; Novartis, Swed.; Novartis, Switz.; Novartis, Thai.; Alliance, UK; Novartis, USA.*
Ergotamine tartrate (p.467·2); caffeine (p.782·1).
*Migraine and related vascular headache.*

**Cafergot N** *Novartis, Ger.*
Ergotamine tartrate (p.467·2); caffeine (p.782·1).
*Headache including migraine.*

**Cafergot-PB**
*Note. This name is used for preparations of different composition.*
*Novartis, Canad.*
Ergotamine tartrate (p.467·2); caffeine (p.782·1); laevorotatory alkaloids of belladonna (p.479·1); pentobarbital (p.713·2).
*Migraine and related vascular headache.*

*Novartis, Chile; Novartis, S.Afr.; Novartis, Spain; Novartis, Switz.*
Ergotamine tartrate (p.467·2); caffeine (p.782·1); total belladonna alkaloids (p.479·1); butalbital (p.673·3).
*Migraine.*

**Cafetrate** *Schein, USA†.*
Ergotamine tartrate (p.467·2); caffeine (p.782·1).
*Migraine.*

**Caffalgina** *Whitehall, Ital.†.*
Propyphenazone (p.85·3); caffeine (p.782·1).
*Pain.*

**Caffedrine** *Thompson, USA.*
Caffeine (p.782·1).
*Fatigue.*

**Caffeine Withdrawal Support** *Homeocan, Canad.*
Homoeopathic preparation.

**Cafiaspirina**
*Bayer, Arg.; Bayer, Braz.; Bayer, Chile; Bayer, Ital.†; Bayer, Port.; Bayer, Spain.*
Aspirin (p.15·1); caffeine (p.782·1).
*Fever; pain.*

**Cafinitrina** *Almirall, Spain.*
Caffeine citrate (p.782·1); glyceryl trinitrate (p.923·2).
*Angina pectoris; biliary-tract spasm; vasospasm.*

**Caginal** *Pond's, Thai.*
Clotrimazole (p.396·2).
*Trichomoniasis; vaginal candidiasis.*

**Caina G** *Gray, Arg.*
Bupivacaine hydrochloride (p.1371·1).
Adrenaline (p.852·2) is included in some injections as a vasoconstrictor to diminish absorption and localise the effect of the local anaesthetic.
*Local anaesthesia.*

**Cal-500** *Pro Doc, Canad.*
Calcium carbonate (p.1254·2).

**Cal Alkyline** *Eagle, Austral.†.*
Calcium carbonate (p.1254·2); slippery elm (p.1747·1); glycine (p.1433·3); equisetum (p.1684·1); dibasic sodium phosphate (p.1231·1); spirulina (p.1749·2); magnesium carbonate (p.1272·1); ginger (p.1267·1).
*Gastric hyperacidity.*

**Cal D** *Pro Doc, Canad.*
Calcium carbonate (p.1254·2); vitamin D (p.1461·2).

**Cal Gel** *Lalco, Canad.†.*
Calcium phosphate (p.1225·3).

**Cal Mag plus Vitamin D** *Quest, Canad.*
Calcium, magnesium, and vitamin D (p.1417·1).

**Cal Mo Dol** *Herbes Universelles, Canad.*
Methyl salicylate (p.59·3); camphor (p.1665·3); menthol (p.1711·3); cineole (p.1672·1); turpentine oil (p.1760·1); peppermint oil (p.1283·2).

**CAL Ocean** *Proceane, Fr.*
Calcium (from oyster shells) (p.1225·1).
*Calcium supplement.*

**Calaband**
*SSL, Austral.; SSL, UK.*
Calamine (p.1144·1); zinc oxide (p.1163·2).
*Medicated bandage.*

**Calabren**
*Teva, Hong Kong; Berk, UK†.*
Glibenclamide (p.331·2).
*Diabetes mellitus.*

**Caladaryl Panal** *Parke, Davis, Arg.*
Zinc oxide (p.1163·2).
*Nappy rash.*

**Caladerm**
*Note. This name is used for preparations of different composition.*
*Klinger, Braz.*
Diphenhydramine (p.431·3) or diphenhydramine hydrochloride (p.431·3); calamine (p.1144·1); camphor (p.1665·3).
*Pruritus; skin irritation.*

*Macrophar, Thai.*
Diphenhydramine hydrochloride (p.431·3); calamine (p.1144·1).
*Pruritus; skin irritation.*

**Caladryl**
*Note. This name is used for preparations of different composition.*
*Parke, Davis, Arg.; Pfizer Consumer, Canad.; Warner-Lambert, Neth.; Pfizer Consumer, S.Afr.*
Diphenhydramine hydrochloride (p.431·3); calamine (p.1144·1).
*Pruritus; skin irritation.*

*Warner-Lambert, Austral.†.*
Lidocaine (p.1377·3) or lidocaine hydrochloride (p.1377·3); calamine (p.1144·1); camphor (p.1665·3).
*Pruritus; skin irritation.*

*Ache, Braz.; Pfizer, Hong Kong; Parke, Davis, India; Warner-Lambert, Irl.†; Pfizer Consumer, Port.; Pfizer, Thai.*
Diphenhydramine hydrochloride (p.431·3); calamine (p.1144·1); camphor (p.1665·3).
*Pruritus; skin irritation.*

*Pfizer Lambert, Spain.*
*Cream:* Diphenhydramine hydrochloride (p.431·3); calamine (p.1144·1).
Formerly contained diphenhydramine hydrochloride, calamine, and camphor.
*Topical solution:* Diphenhydramine (p.431·3); camphor (p.1665·3); zinc oxide (p.1163·2).
*Pruritus; skin irritation.*

*Warner-Lambert Consumer, Switz.†; Warner-Lambert, UK†.*
Diphenhydramine hydrochloride (p.431·3); zinc oxide (p.1163·2); camphor (p.1665·3).
Formerly contained diphenhydramine hydrochloride, calamine, and camphor in the *UK*.
*Skin irritation; urticaria.*

*Warner-Lambert, USA.*
Pramocaine hydrochloride (p.1382·2); calamine (p.1144·1).

**Caladryl Clear**
*Note. This name is used for preparations of different composition.*
*Parke, Davis, Chile.*
Pramocaine hydrochloride (p.1382·2); camphor (p.1665·3); zinc acetate (p.1469·2).
*Skin irritation; urticaria.*

*Warner-Lambert, USA.*
Pramocaine hydrochloride (p.1382·2); zinc acetate (p.1469·2).

**Caladryl Incoloro** *Parke, Davis, Arg.*
Diphenhydramine hydrochloride (p.431·3); zinc acetate (p.1469·2) or zinc oxide (p.1163·2).
*Skin irritation.*

**Cala-gen** *Goldline, USA†.*
Diphenhydramine hydrochloride (p.431·3); camphor (p.1665·3).
*Pruritus.*

**Cal-Aid** *Indoco, India.*
Calcium carbonate (p.1254·2); colecalciferol (p.1461·3).
*Calcium supplement.*

**Calais** *Mead Johnson Nutritionals, Canad.†.*
Calcium glycerophosphate hydroxide (p.1225·2).

**Calamatum** *Blair, USA†.*
Calamine (p.1144·1); zinc oxide (p.1163·2); menthol (p.1711·3); camphor (p.1665·3); benzocaine (p.1370·3).
*Minor skin irritation.*

**Calamina** *Bunker, Braz.; Delta, Braz.; Prodotti, Braz.; Sedabel, Braz.*
Diphenhydramine (p.431·3) or diphenhydramine hydrochloride (p.431·3); calamine (p.1144·1); camphor (p.1665·3).
*Pruritus; skin irritation.*

**Calamina Composta**
*Note. This name is used for preparations of different composition.*
*Neo Quimica, Braz.; Prodotti, Braz.*
Calamine (p.1144·1); diphenhydramine (p.431·3) or diphenhydramine hydrochloride (p.431·3); camphor (p.1665·3).
Also known as Calamyn.
*Pruritus; skin irritation.*

*QIF, Braz.†.*
Calamine (p.1144·1); diphenhydramine hydrochloride (p.431·3).
*Pruritus; skin irritation.*

**Calamine Antihistamine** *Stanley, Canad.*
Calamine (p.1144·1); diphenhydramine hydrochloride (p.431·3).
*Pruritus.*

**Calamine Lotion**
*Note. This name is used for preparations of different composition.*
*McGloin, Austral.†.*
Calamine (p.1144·1); zinc oxide (p.1163·2); phenol (p.1188·1).
*Insect bites; skin irritation; sunburn.*

*Floris, Israel; Sam-On, Israel; Vitamed, Israel.*
Calamine (p.1144·1); zinc oxide (p.1163·2).
*Pruritus.*

**Calamine-D** *Medipharma, Hong Kong.*
Calamine (p.1144·1); zinc oxide (p.1163·2); kaolin (p.1268·3); diphenhydramine hydrochloride (p.431·3).
*Pruritus.*

**Calamox** *Hauck, USA†.*
Calamine (p.1144·1).
*Minor skin irritation.*

**Calamycin** *Pfeiffer, USA.*
Zinc oxide (p.1163·2); calamine (p.1144·1); benzocaine (p.1370·3); chloroxylenol (p.1177·2); mepyramine maleate (p.437·1).
*Pruritus.*

**Calan**
*Note. This name is used for preparations of different composition.*
*Takeda, Jpn†.*
Vinpocetine (p.1764·2).
*Cerebrovascular disorders.*

*Searle, USA.*
Verapamil hydrochloride (p.1019·1).
*Angina pectoris; arrhythmias; hypertension.*

**Calanda** *Atlantis, Mex.*
Multivitamin and mineral preparation (p.1417·1).

**Calanif** *Berk, UK†.*
Nifedipine (p.966·2).
*Angina pectoris; hypertension; Raynaud's syndrome.*

**Calanol** *Nakornpatana, Thai.*
Diphenhydramine hydrochloride (p.431·3); calamine (p.1144·1).
*Skin irritation.*

**Cal-Antagon** *Ferring, Port.*
Diltiazem hydrochloride (p.900·1).
*Angina pectoris; arrhythmias; hypertension.*

**Calapro** *Progress, Thai.*
Calamine (p.1144·1); diphenhydramine hydrochloride (p.431·3).
*Skin irritation.*

**Calaptin** *Nicholas Piramal, India.*
Verapamil hydrochloride (p.1019·1).
*Angina pectoris; arrhythmias; hypertension.*

**Calasthetic** *Restan, S.Afr.*
Calamine (p.1144·1); benzocaine (p.1370·3); pheniramine maleate (p.438·3); phenol (p.1188·1).
*Skin disorders.*

**Calatrim** *Trima, Israel.*
Calamine (p.1144·1); zinc oxide (p.1163·2).
*Sunburn; urticaria.*

**Calatrim cum Sulphur** *Trima, Israel.*
Calamine (p.1144·1); zinc oxide (p.1163·2); sulfur (p.1158·2).
*Pruritus.*

**Calax** *Odan, Canad.*
Docusate calcium (p.1262·1).
*Constipation.*

**Calbion** *Merck, Spain†.*
Calcium pidolate (p.1226·1).
*Hypocalcaemia; osteoporosis.*

**Calbisan** *Pontafarm, Ital.*
Calcium carbonate (p.1254·2).
*Calcium deficiency; calcium supplement.*

**Calburst** *Pharmavite, Canad.*
Vitamin D (p.1461·2); calcium carbonate (p.1254·2).

**Calcanate** *ST, Thai.*
Calcium carbonate (p.1254·2).
*Calcium deficiency.*

**Cal-Car** *Selvi, Ital.*
Calcium carbonate (p.1254·2).
*Calcium deficiency; calcium supplement.*

**Calcarb with Vitamin D** *Ivax, USA.*
Calcium carbonate (p.1254·2); vitamin D (p.1461·2).

**Calcascorbin** *Pharmonta, Austria.*
Calcium ascorbate (p.1460·2).
*Vitamin C deficiency.*

**Calcedon** *Worwag, Ger.†.*
*Tablets:* Calcium carbonate (p.1254·2).
*Calcium deficiency.*

**Calcefor** *Laboratorios Chile, Chile.*
Calcium carbonate (p.1254·2).
*Calcium deficiency; osteoporosis.*

**Calcefor Cap** *Laboratorios Chile, Chile.*
Calcium carbonate (p.1254·2).
*Calcium deficiency; osteoporosis.*

**Calcefor D** *Laboratorios Chile, Chile.*
Calcium carbonate (p.1254·2); colecalciferol (p.1461·3).
*Calcium and vitamin D deficiency; osteoporosis.*

**Calceos** *Provalis, UK.*
Calcium carbonate (p.1254·2); colecalciferol (p.1461·3).
*Calcium and vitamin D deficiency; osteoporosis.*

**Calcet** *Mission Pharmacal, USA.*
Calcium lactate (p.1225·3); calcium gluconate (p.1225·2); calcium carbonate (p.1254·2); vitamin D (p.1461·2).
*Calcium supplement.*

**Calcet Plus** *Mission Pharmacal, USA.*
Multivitamin and mineral preparation with iron and folic acid (p.1417·1).
*Low-calcium leg cramping; nursing mothers; osteoporosis; patients with milk allergies; pre- and postoperative patients.*

**Calcetat** *Giovanardi, Ital.*
Calcium acetate (p.1225·1).
*Calcium supplement.*

**Calcette** *Ashbourne, UK†.*
Calcium carbonate (p.1254·2).
*Calcium supplement; hyperphosphataemia; osteoporosis.*

**Calcevita**
*Roche Consumer, Neth.; Roche, Swed.*
Multivitamin preparation with calcium (p.1417·1).
*Calcium and vitamin deficiency.*

**Calchan** *Ranbaxy, UK.*
Nifedipine (p.966·2).
*Angina pectoris; hypertension.*

**Calchek** *Ipca, India.*
Amlodipine besilate (p.862·1).
*Angina pectoris; hypertension.*

**Calchew** *Ranbaxy, Thai.*
Calcium carbonate (p.1254·2); calcium gluconate (p.1225·2).
*Calcium supplement; hypocalcaemia.*

**Calci** *Hexal, Ger.*
Calcitonin (salmon) (p.768·2).
*Hypercalcaemia; osteolysis; osteoporosis; Paget's disease of bone; reflex sympathetic dystrophy.*

**Calcia** *Peter Black, UK.*
Calcium carbonate (p.1254·2) with vitamins and iron (p.1417·1).

**Calciben** *FIRMA, Ital.*
Calcitonin (salmon) (p.768·2).
*Hypercalcaemia; osteoporosis; Paget's disease of bone; prevention of fracture in osteoporosis; reflex sympathetic dystrophy.*

**Calcibind** *Mission Pharmacal, USA.*
Sodium cellulose phosphate (p.1052·1).
*Ion exchange resin binding calcium.*

**Calcibon** *Masa, Thai.*
Calcium citrate (p.1225·1).
*Calcium deficiency.*

**Calcibronat**
*Novartis, Fr.; Novartis, Ital.; Novartis, Mex.*
Calcium bromolactobionate (p.674·1).
*Nervous disorders; sedative; sleep disorders.*

**CalciCaps** *Nion, USA.*
Calcium with vitamin D and phosphorus (p.1417·1).
*Calcium deficiency; dietary supplement.*

**CalciCaps with iron** *Nion, USA.*
Calcium with vitamin D, phosphorus, and iron (p.1417·1).
*Calcium deficiency; dietary supplement.*

**CalciCaps M-Z** *Nion, USA.*
Calcium with vitamins A and D, and minerals (p.1417·1).

**Calcicard**
*Note. This name is used for preparations of different composition.*
*Pharma Dynamics, S.Afr.*
Verapamil hydrochloride (p.1019·1).
*Angina pectoris; arrhythmias; hypertension.*

*Ivax, UK.*
Diltiazem hydrochloride (p.900·1).
*Angina pectoris; hypertension.*

**Calcichell** *Ativus, Braz.*
Calcium amino-acid chelate.
*Calcium supplement.*

**Calci-Chew**
*Piette, Belg.†; Christiaens, Neth.; R&D, USA.*
Calcium carbonate (p.1254·2).
*Calcium deficiency; calcium supplement; hyperphosphataemia; osteoporosis.*

**Calcichew**
*Nycomed, Fin.; Nycomed, Hong Kong; Shire, Irl.; Shire, UK.*
Calcium carbonate (p.1254·2).
*Calcium deficiency; hyperphosphataemia; osteoporosis.*

**Calcichew $D_3$**
*Nycomed, Denm.; Nycomed, Fin.; Nycomed, Hong Kong; Shire, Irl.; Nycomed, Swed.; Shire, UK.*
Calcium carbonate (p.1254·2); colecalciferol (p.1461·3).
*Calcium and vitamin D deficiency; osteomalacia; osteoporosis.*

**Calciday** *Nature's Bounty, USA†.*
Calcium carbonate (p.1254·2).
*Calcium deficiency; dietary supplement.*

**Calcidia** *Roche Nicholas, Fr.*
Calcium carbonate (p.1254·2).
*Hypocalcaemia and hyperphosphoraemia related to kidney disorders; renal osteodystrophy.*

**Calcidon** *Roche, Ital.*
Calcium carbonate (p.1254·2); colecalciferol (p.1461·3).
*Calcium and vitamin D deficiency.*

**Calcidose** *Opocalcium, Fr.*
Calcium carbonate (p.1254·2).
*Calcium deficiency; osteoporosis.*

**Calcidose Vitamine D** *Opocalcium, Fr.*
Calcium carbonate (p.1254·2); colecalciferol (p.1461·3).
*Calcium and vitamin D deficiency; osteoporosis.*

**Calcidrine** *Abbott, USA.*
Codeine (p.27·1); calcium iodide (p.1116·2).
*Coughs.*

**Calcidrink** *Shire, UK†.*
Calcium carbonate (p.1254·2).
*Calcium deficiency; osteoporosis.*

**Calcifar** *Farcoral, Mex.*
Calcium carbonate (p.1254·2).

**Calciferol**
*Note. This name is used for preparations of different composition.*
*Heralds, Braz.†.*
Ergocalciferol; calcium phosphate; cyanocobalamin; sodium fluoride (p.1417·1).
*Vitamin and mineral supplement.*

*Schwarz, USA.*
Ergocalciferol (p.1462·1).
*Familial hypophosphataemia; gastrointestinal, liver, or biliary disease associated with malabsorption of vitamin D; hypoparathyroidism; refractory rickets.*

**Calciferol B12**
*EMS, Braz.*
Ergocalciferol; vitamin $B_{12}$; calcium chloride; calcium phosphate; sodium fluoride (p.1417·1).
*Vitamin and mineral supplement.*

*Medquimica, Braz.†.*
Ergocalciferol; vitamin $B_{12}$; calcium phosphate; sodium fluoride (p.1417·1).
*Vitamin and mineral supplement.*

**Calciferol Composto** *Delta, Braz.*
Ergocalciferol; vitamin $B_{12}$; calcium gluconate; calcium phosphate; sodium fluoride (p.1417·1).
Also known as Calferon.
*Vitamin and mineral supplement.*

**Calcifluol** *Cimed, Braz.*
Calcium chloride; ergocalciferol; sodium fluoride; sodium phosphate; lysine (p.1417·1).
*Nutritional supplement.*

**Calcifluor** *Crinex, Fr.*
Calcium fluoride (p.1423·3).
*Dental caries prophylaxis.*

**Calcifolin**
*Kleva, Gr.; Ibirn, Ital.*
Calcium folinate (p.1431·1).
*Antidote to folic acid antagonists; folic acid deficiency; megaloblastic anaemia.*

**Calcifort** *Labinca, Arg.*
Disodium calcium edetate; ergocalciferol; cyanocobalamin (p.1417·1).
*Calcium and vitamin supplement.*

**Calciforte** *Grimberg, Fr.*
*Oral liquid:* Calcium gluconate (p.1225·2); calcium lactate (p.1225·3); calcium gluceptate (p.1225·2); calcium chloride (p.1225·1); yeast (*Saccharomyces cerevisiae*) (p.1469·1).
*Powder for oral solution:* Calcium gluconate (p.1225·2); calcium lactate (p.1225·3); calcium gluceptate (p.1225·2); calcium chloride (p.1225·1); calcium carbonate (p.1254·2); yeast (*Saccharomyces cerevisiae*) (p.1469·1).
*Calcium deficiency; osteoporosis.*

**Calcigamma** *Worwag, Ger.*
Calcium carbonate (p.1254·2).
*Calcium deficiency; osteoporosis.*

**Calcigard**
*Torrent, India; Torrent, Thai.*
Nifedipine (p.966·2).
*Angina pectoris; heart failure; hypertension; myocardial infarction.*

**Calcigen D** *Opfermann, Ger.*
Calcium carbonate (p.1254·2); colecalciferol (p.1461·3).
*Calcium and vitamin D deficiency; osteoporosis.*

**Calcigenol** *Korangi, Port.*
Calcium phosphate (p.1225·3); ergocalciferol (p.1462·1).
Formerly contained calcium phosphate.
*Calcium and vitamin D supplement; osteoporosis; rickets; tetany.*

**Calcigenol B12**
*Note. This name is used for preparations of different composition.*
*GlaxoSmithKline, Arg.*
Calcium phosphate; calciferol; vitamin $B_{12}$ (p.1417·1).
*Vitamin and calcium supplement.*

*Aventis, Braz.†.*
Calcium phosphate; vitamin $B_{12}$; vitamin D; sodium fluoride (p.1417·1).
*Vitamin and mineral supplement.*

**Calcigenol Irradiado** *Aventis, Braz.†.*
Calcium phosphate (p.1225·3); sodium fluoride (p.1444·3).
*Calcium and sodium deficiencies.*

**Calcigran**
*Note. This name is used for preparations of different composition.*
*Labomed, Chile.*
Calcium carbonate (p.1254·2); calcium hydrogen phosphate (p.1225·2); ascorbic acid (p.1460·2); ergocalciferol (p.1462·1).
*Calcium and vitamin D deficiency; osteoporosis.*

*Nycomed, Norw.*
*Chewable tablets:* Calcium carbonate (p.1254·2); colecalciferol (p.1461·3).
*Oral granules†:* Calcium carbonate (p.1254·2); ascorbic acid (p.1460·2); colecalciferol (p.1461·3).
*Calcium supplement; osteoporosis.*

**Calci-Gry** *Gry, Ger.*
Calcium carbonate (p.1254·2).
*Calcium deficiency; osteoporosis.*

**Calcihep** *Aventis, Austral.*
Heparin calcium (p.927·3).
*Thromboembolic disorders.*

**Calcihexal** *Hexal, Austria.*
Calcium carbonate (p.1254·2).
*Calcium deficiency.*

**Calciject** *Omega, Canad.*
Calcium chloride (p.1225·1).
*Calcium supplement.*

**Calcijex**
*Abbott, Austral.; Abbott, Austria; Abbott, Braz.; Abbott, Canad.†; Abbott, Fin.; Abbott, Hong Kong; Abbott, Irl.; Abbott, Israel; Abbott, Ital.; Abbott, Mex.†; Abbott, Norw.; Abbott, Singapore; Abbott, Spain; Abbott, Swed.; Abbott, Switz.; Abbott, UK; Abbott, USA.*
Calcitriol (p.1461·2).
*Hyperparathyroidism; hypocalcaemia in chronic renal dialysis.*

**Calcilac KT** *Jenapharm, Ger.*
Calcium carbonate (p.1254·2); colecalciferol (p.1461·3).
*Calcium and vitamin D deficiency; osteoporosis.*

**Calcilat** *Eastern Pharmaceuticals, UK†.*
Nifedipine (p.966·2).
*Angina pectoris; hypertension; Raynaud's syndrome.*

**Calcilean** *Organon Teknika, Canad.†.*
Heparin calcium (p.927·3).
*Thromboembolic disorders; thrombosis prophylaxis.*

**Calciless** *Sam-On, Israel.*
Dibasic sodium phosphate (p.1231·1); monobasic potassium phosphate (p.1230·3).
*Calcium oxalate renal calculi.*

**Calcilin** *Laevosan, Austria†.*
Calcium levulinate (p.1225·3).
*Allergic and anaphylactic conditions; calcium deficiency; haemorrhage; inflammation.*

**Calcilin compositum** *Laevosan, Austria†.*
Chlorphenoxamine hydrochloride (p.428·3); calcium levulinate (p.1225·3); calcium gluconate (p.1225·2).
*Allergic disorders.*

**Calcilo XD** *Ross, USA.*
Low calcium, vitamin D-free infant feed (p.1417·1).
*Hypercalcaemia; osteopetrosis.*

**Calcilos** *TAD, Ger.†.*
Calcium carbonate (p.1254·2).
*Calcium deficiency.*

**Calcimagon** *Orion, Ger.*
Calcium carbonate (p.1254·2).
*Calcium deficiency; osteoporosis.*

**Calcimagon-D3**
*Orion, Ger.; Nycomed, Switz.*
Calcium carbonate (p.1254·2); colecalciferol (p.1461·3).
*Calcium and vitamin D deficiency; osteoporosis.*

**Calcimar**
*Aventis, Canad.; Rhone-Poulenc Rorer, USA.*
Calcitonin (salmon) (p.768·2).
*Hypercalcaemia; osteoporosis; Paget's disease of bone.*

**Calcimax**
*Note. This name is used for preparations of different composition.*
*Gador, Arg.*
Calcium citrate (p.1225·1).
*Calcium supplement; hyperparathyroidism; osteoporosis.*

*Carmaran, Canad.†.*
Calcium lactate (p.1225·3).

*Wallace Mfg Chem., UK.*
Calcium levulinate (p.1225·3); calcium chloride (p.1225·1); vitamins (p.1417·1).

**Calcimax D3** *Gador, Arg.*
Calcium citrate (p.1225·1); colecalciferol (p.1461·3).
*Calcium and vitamin D supplement; osteopenia; osteoporosis.*

**Calcimed** *Hermes, Ger.*
Calcium carbonate (p.1254·2).
*Calcium deficiency; osteoporosis.*

**Calcimed $D_3$** *Hermes, Ger.*
Calcium carbonate (p.1254·2); colecalciferol (p.1461·3).
*Calcium and vitamin D deficiency; osteoporosis.*

**Calcimega** *Larkhall Laboratories, UK†.*
Calcium with vitamins and minerals (p.1417·1).

**Calcimex** *Dutch Lady, Malaysia.*
Preparation for enteral nutrition (p.1417·1).

**Calci-Mix** *R&D, USA.*
Calcium carbonate (p.1254·2).
*Calcium deficiency; dietary supplement.*

**Calcimon** *Byk, Port.*
Calcitonin (salmon) (p.768·2).
*Hypercalcaemia; osteolytic bone pain; osteoporosis; Paget's disease of bone.*

**Calcimonta** *Byk Tosse, Ger.†; Byk Gulden, Ger.†.*
Calcitonin (salmon) (p.768·2).
*Hypercalcaemia; osteolysis; osteoporosis; Paget's disease of bone; reflex sympathetic dystrophy.*

**Calcimore** *Taro, Israel.*
Calcium carbonate (p.1254·2).
*Calcium supplement; gastritis; gastrointestinal hyperacidity; heartburn; peptic ulcer.*

**Calcinatal** *Pfizer Lambert, Spain.*
Multivitamin and mineral preparation (p.1417·1).

**Calcinil** *Sclavo, Ital.†.*
Elcatonin (p.768·3).
*Hypercalcaemia; osteoporosis; Paget's disease of bone; reflex sympathetic dystrophy.*

**Calcinol** *Raptakos, India.*
*Oral powder:* Calcium carbonate (p.1254·2); colecalciferol (p.1461·3).
*Syrup:* Calcium lactate (p.1225·3); calcium gluconate (p.1225·2); colecalciferol (p.1461·3); vitamin $B_{12}$ (p.1458·2); magnesium chloride (p.1228·1).
*Tablets:* Calcium carbonate (p.1254·2); calcium phosphate (p.1225·3); calcium fluoride (p.1423·3); magnesium hydroxide (p.1272·2); colecalciferol (p.1461·3).
*Calcium deficiency; calcium supplement.*

**Calcio 20** *Madariaga, Spain.*
Calcium carbonate (p.1254·2).
*Calcium deficiency; osteoporosis.*

**Calcio 520** *Knop, Chile.*
Calcium phosphate (p.1225·3); calcium gluconate (p.1225·2); calcium carbonate (p.1254·2); magnesium oxide (p.1272·3); alfalfa (p.1649·1) rose fruit (p.1740·1).
*Calcium supplement; osteoporosis.*

**Calcio Cit** *TRB, Arg.*
Calcium citrate (p.1225·1); colecalciferol (p.1461·3).
*Calcium supplement; osteoporosis; renal calculi; renal osteodystrophy.*

**Calcio Cit Simple** *TRB, Arg.*
Calcium citrate (p.1225·1).
*Calcium supplement; osteoporosis; renal calculi; renal osteodystrophy.*

**Calcio Cm** *Labomed, Chile.*
Calcium carbonate (p.1254·2); calcium phosphate (p.1225·3); magnesium sulfate; vitamin C (p.1417·1).
*Calcium supplement; osteoporosis.*

**Calcio 20 Complex** *Madariaga, Spain.*
Ascorbic acid (p.1460·2); calcium phosphate (p.1225·3); calcium pantothenate (p.1442·3); cyanocobalamin (p.1458·2); colecalciferol (p.1461·3); vitamin A palmitate (p.1453·1).
*Calcium deficiency; osteoporosis.*

**Calcio Day D**
*Sintofarma, Braz.†; Silesia, Chile.*
Calcium carbonate (p.1254·2); magnesium oxide (p.1272·3); vitamin D (p.1461·2).
*Calcium, magnesium, and vitamin D supplement; osteoporosis.*

**Calcio Dobetin** *Angelini, Ital.*
Cyanocobalamin (p.1458·2); calcium gluconate (p.1225·2); calcium gluceptate (p.1225·2).
*Calcium and vitamin $B_{12}$ deficiency.*

**Calcio 20 Emulsion** *Madariaga, Spain.*
Calcium phosphate (p.1225·3).
*Calcium deficiency; osteomalacia; osteoporosis.*

**Calcio 20 Fuerte** *Madariaga, Spain.*
Calcium phosphate (p.1225·3); colecalciferol (p.1461·3).
*Calcium deficiency; osteoporosis.*

**Calcio Geve D y C** *Reig Jofre, Spain†.*
Ascorbic acid (p.1460·2); calcium carbonate (p.1254·2); calcium fluoride (p.1423·3); calcium phosphate (p.1225·3); colecalciferol (p.1461·3).
Formerly contained ascorbic acid, calcium gluceptate, calcium hypophosphite, and calcium laevulinolactogluconate.
*Calcium deficiency; vitamin C and D deficiency.*

**Calcio Masticable** *AM, Arg.*
Calcium carbonate (p.1254·2); vitamin D (p.1461·2).
*Calcium supplement.*

**Calcio Nil** *Andromaco, Chile.*
Calcium phosphate (p.1225·3); calcium lactate (p.1225·3); sodium chloride; magnesium oxide; calciferol (p.1417·1).
*Calcium deficiency.*

**Calcio Nil Forte** *Andromaco, Chile.*
Calcium carbonate (p.1254·2); calcium citrate (p.1225·1); calcium lactate (p.1225·3); calcium phosphate (p.1225·3); ergocalciferol (p.1462·1); magnesium oxide (p.1272·3).
*Calcium deficiency; osteomalacia; osteoporosis.*

**Calcio Vitam D3** *Berenguer Infale, Spain†.*
Calcium hydrogen phosphate (p.1225·2); colecalciferol (p.1461·3).
*Bone and dental disorders; calcium deficiency; osteomalacia.*

**Calcio Vitaminado** *Bunker, Braz.†.*
Calcium phosphate; vitamin $B_{12}$; ergocalciferol; sodium fluoride; gastric mucosa extract (p.1417·1).
*Nutritional supplement.*

**Calcio Vitaminado B12** *Neo Quimica, Braz.†.*
Calcium phosphate; calcium glycerophosphate; vitamin A; vitamin $B_{12}$; ergocalciferol (p.1417·1).
*Calcium and vitamin supplement.*

**Calciobion** *Ibefar, Braz.†.*
Calcium phosphate; ergocalciferol; vitamin $B_{12}$; sodium fluoride (p.1417·1).
*Nutritional supplement.*

**Calcioday-D**
*Eurodrug, Hong Kong; Eurodrug, Malaysia; Eurodrug, Singapore; Eurodrug, Thai.*
Calcium (p.1225·1); colecalciferol (p.1461·3); magnesium (p.1227·3).
*Calcium, magnesium and vitamin D supplement.*

**Calciodie** *Epifarma, Ital.*
Calcium carbonate (p.1254·2).
*Calcium deficiency; calcium supplement.*

**Calciofix** *Damor, Ital.*
L-Arginine (p.1421·1); L-lysine (p.1439·1); glycerophosphoric acid (p.1695·2).
*Bone and dental disorders; tonic.*

**Calciokatabios** *SIT, Ital.*
Calcium and vitamin preparation (p.1417·1).
*Nutritional supplement.*

**Calcional** *Spedrog, Arg.*
Calcium carbonate (p.1254·2).
*Calcium supplement.*

**Calciopen** Astra, Swed.†.
Phenoxymethylpenicillin potassium (p.242·1).
*Bacterial infections.*

**Calciopiu** Lafare, Ital.
Calcium carbonate (p.1254·2).
*Calcium deficiency; calcium supplement.*

**Calcior** Delta, Port.
Calcium carbonate (p.1254·2).

**Calcioral**
Nycomed, Gr.; Novartis Consumer, Port.
Calcium carbonate (p.1254·2).
*Prevention and treatment of calcium deficiency.*

**Calcioral D3** Nycomed, Gr.
Calcium carbonate (p.1254·2); colecalciferol (p.1461·3).
*Prevention and treatment of calcium deficiency.*

**Calcioretard** Farmapros, Spain†.
Calcium ascorbate (p.1460·2); lysine hydrochloride (p.1439·2); tryptophan (p.320·3).
*Bone and dental disorders; calcium deficiency; osteomalacia; rickets.*

**Calciosan** Provita, Ital.†.
Multivitamin and mineral preparation (p.1417·1).

**Calciosint** Pulitzer, Ital.
Calcitonin (salmon) (p.768·2).
*Hypercalcaemia; osteoporosis; Paget's disease of bone; reflex sympathetic dystrophy.*

**Calcioton** San Carlo, Ital.
Calcitonin (salmon) (p.768·2).
*Hypercalcaemia; osteoporosis; Paget's disease of bone; reflex sympathetic dystrophy.*

**Calciovit Puro** Laboratorios Chile, Chile.
Vitamin D (p.1461·2); calcium hydrogen phosphate (p.1225·2).
*Hypocalcaemia; osteomalacia; rickets.*

**Calciovit Urto** Lafare, Ital.†.
Calcium oleate; ergocalciferol (p.1462·1).
*Vitamin deficiency.*

**Calciovital Irradiado** Heralds, Braz.†.
Calcium phosphate; vitamin A palmitate; ergocalciferol; cyanocobalamin (p.1417·1).
*Calcium and vitamin supplement.*

**Calciozim** Monsanto, Ital.
Colecalciferol (p.1461·3); calcium gluconate (p.1225·2); calcium gluceptate (p.1225·2).
*Bone metabolic disorders; calcium deficiency.*

**Calciparin**
Sanofi Synthelabo, Austria; Sanofi Synthelabo, Ger.; Choay, Israel.
Heparin calcium (p.927·3).
*Thromboembolic disorders.*

**Calciparina**
Italfarmaco, Ital.; Sanofi Synthelabo, Port.; Sanofi Synthelabo, Spain.
Heparin calcium (p.927·3).
*Thromboembolic disorders.*

**Calciparine**
Sanofi Synthelabo, Arg.; Sanofi Synthelabo, Austral.; Sanofi Synthelabo, Fr.; Sanofi Synthelabo, Irl.; Mer-National, S.Afr.; Sanofi Synthelabo, Switz.; Sanofi Synthelabo, UK.
Heparin calcium (p.927·3).
*Thromboembolic disorders.*

**Calci-Ped** Stiefel, Braz.
Multivitamin and mineral preparation (p.1417·1).

**Calcipen**
Leo, Denm.; Leo, Norw.
Phenoxymethylpenicillin calcium (p.242·1).
*Bacterial infections.*

**Calciplex** Vitaplex, Austral.†.
Mineral and vitamin D preparation (p.1417·1).
*Calcium deficiency; osteoporosis.*

**Calciplus**
Note. This name is used for preparations of different composition.
Alvia (Αλβια), Gr.
Calcitonin (p.768·2).
*Osteoporosis.*

Chemedica, Switz.†.
Calcium carbonate (p.1254·2); colecalciferol (p.1461·3).
*Calcium deficiency.*

**Calcipor** Ibirn, Ital.†.
Heparin calcium (p.927·3).
*Thromboembolic disorders.*

**Calcipot** 3M, Ger.
*Effervescent tablets*†: Calcium gluconate (p.1225·2).
*Tablets:* Calcium citrate (p.1225·1); calcium hydrogen phosphate (p.1225·2).
*Calcium deficiency.*

**Calcipot C** Kolassa, Austria.
Vitamin C (p.1460·2); rutoside (p.1688·2); calcium citrate (p.1225·1); calcium glycerophosphate (p.1225·2).
*Calcium and vitamin C deficiency.*

**Calcipot D$_3$** Kolassa, Austria.
Colecalciferol (p.1461·3); calcium citrate (p.1225·1); calcium glycerophosphate (p.1225·2).
*Calcium and vitamin D deficiency.*

**Calciprat** IPRAD, Fr.
Calcium carbonate (p.1254·2).
*Calcium deficiency; osteoporosis.*

**Calciprat D$_3$** IPRAD, Fr.
Calcium carbonate (p.1254·2); colecalciferol (p.1461·3).
*Calcium and vitamin D deficiency; osteoporosis.*

**Calcipulpe** Septodont, Switz.†.
Barium sulfate (p.1061·1); calcium hydroxide (p.1664·3).
*Covering for dental pulp.*

**Calci-Rav** Asta Medica, Israel.
Calcium carbonate (p.1254·2).
*Calcium supplement.*

**Calciretard** Kohler-Pharma, Ger.
Calcium aspartate (p.1226·1).
*Hypocalcaemia.*

**Calcirol** Cadila, India.
Colecalciferol (p.1461·3).
*Osteomalacia; rickets.*

**Calcisan** Petrasch, Austria.
Calcium hydrogen phosphate (p.1225·2); calcium carbonate (p.1254·2).
*Calcium deficiency; osteoporosis.*

**Calcisan B + C** Petrasch, Austria.
Calcium hydrogen phosphate (p.1225·2); calcium carbonate (p.1254·2); ascorbic acid (p.1460·2); thiamine hydrochloride (p.1455·1).
*Calcium, vitamin B$_1$, and vitamin C deficiency; osteoporosis.*

**Calcisan C** Petrasch, Austria.
Calcium hydrogen phosphate (p.1225·2); calcium carbonate (p.1254·2); ascorbic acid (p.1460·2).
*Calcium and vitamin C deficiency.*

**Calcisan D** Petrasch, Austria.
Calcium hydrogen phosphate (p.1225·2); calcium carbonate (p.1254·2); ergocalciferol (p.1462·1).
*Calcium and vitamin D deficiency; osteoporosis.*

**Calcisorb**
3M, Austral.†; 3M, Belg.†; 3M, Israel; 3M, Neth.; 3M, NZ†; 3M, UK†.
Sodium cellulose phosphate (p.1052·1).
*Hypercalcaemia; hypercalciuria; osteopetrosis; renal calculi; vitamin D intoxication.*

**Calcitab** ITF, Port.
Calcium carbonate (p.1254·2).
*Calcium deficiency; calcium supplement; osteoporosis.*

**Calcitab D** ITF, Port.
Calcium carbonate (p.1254·2); colecalciferol (p.1461·3).
*Calcium deficiency; osteoporosis.*

**Calcitar**
Specia, Fr.†; Rhone-Poulenc Rorer, Ital.†.
Calcitonin (pork) (p.768·2).
*Algodystrophies; hypercalcaemia; hyperphosphatasia; osteoporosis; Paget's disease of bone.*

**Calcitare** Rhone-Poulenc Rorer, Austral.†.
Calcitonin (pork) (p.768·2).
*Hypercalcaemia; Paget's disease of bone.*

**Calcite** Riva, Canad.
Calcium carbonate (p.1254·2).
*Calcium supplement.*

**Calcite D** Riva, Canad.
Calcium carbonate (p.1254·2); vitamin D (p.1461·2).
*Dietary supplement.*

**Calcitol** Frega, Canad.†.
Vitamin A, vitamin D, and calcium (p.1417·1).

**Calcitonin** Novartis, Austria.
Calcitonin (salmon) (p.768·2).
*Bone pain and osteolysis in malignancy; hypercalcaemia; osteoporosis; Paget's disease of bone; reflex sympathetic dystrophy.*

**Calcitonina** Novartis, Ital.; Aventis, Ital.
Calcitonin (salmon) (p.768·2).
*Hypercalcaemia; osteoporosis; Paget's disease of bone; reflex sympathetic dystrophy.*

**Calcitoran** Teikoku, Jpn.
Calcitonin (salmon) (p.768·2).
*Osteoporosis.*

**Calcitran B12** Eversil, Braz.
Cyanocobalamin; ergocalciferol; calcium phosphate; calcium glycerophosphate; sodium fluoride (p.1417·1).
*Vitamin and mineral supplement.*

**Calcitrans** Fresenius-Praxis, Ger.†.
Calcium gluconate (p.1225·2); calcium gluceptate (p.1225·2); calcium saccharate (p.1665·1).
*Calcium deficiency.*

**Calcitrat** Merckle, Ger.
Calcium citrate (p.1225·1).
*Calcium deficiency; osteoporosis.*

**Cal-Citrate** Bio-Tech, USA.
Calcium citrate (p.1225·1).
*Calcium supplement.*

**Calcitridin**
Note. This name is used for preparations of different composition.
Opfermann, Ger.
Calcium carbonate (p.1254·2).
*Calcium deficiency; osteoporosis.*

Rottapharm, Ital.
Sodium monofluorophosphate (p.1446·2); calcium carbonate (p.1254·2).
*Osteoporosis.*

**Calcitugg** Nycomed, Swed.
Calcium carbonate (p.1254·2).
*Calcium deficiency; hyperphosphataemia; osteoporosis.*

**Calcium 600**
Wyeth Lederle, Port.
Calcium phosphate (p.1225·3); colecalciferol (p.1461·3).

Solgar, USA.
Calcium carbonate (p.1254·2); vitamin D (p.1461·2).

**Calcium AL** Aliud, Ger.
Calcium carbonate (p.1254·2).
*Calcium supplement.*

**Calcium beta** Betapharm, Ger.
Calcium carbonate (p.1254·2).
*Calcium supplement; osteoporosis.*

**Calcium Braun** Braun, Ger.
Calcium gluconate (p.1225·2); calcium saccharate (p.1665·1).
*Calcium deficiency.*

**Calcium C** Labinca, Arg.
Sodium calcium edetate (p.1051·3); ascorbic acid (p.1460·2).

**Calcium Chewable** Richlife, Hong Kong†.
Calcium; phosphorus; magnesium; vitamin D (p.1417·1).
*Dietary supplement.*

**Calcium Clear** Nutraceuticals, UK.
Calcium lactate (p.1225·3); magnesium carbonate (p.1272·1).
*Calcium supplement.*

**Calcium Corbiere** Sanofi Winthrop, Fr.†.
Calcium glucoheptogluconate (p.1225·2).
*Hypocalcaemia.*

**Calcium Corbiere vitamine CDPP** Sanofi Winthrop, Fr.†.
Anhydrous calcium gluceptate (p.1225·2) or calcium glucoheptogluconate with vitamins (p.1417·1).
*Asthenia.*

**Calcium D**
Novartis, Arg.
Calcium lactate gluconate (p.1225·3); calcium carbonate (p.1254·2); colecalciferol (p.1461·3).
*Calcium and vitamin D supplement.*

Trianon, Canad.
Calcium carbonate (p.1254·2); vitamin D (p.1461·2).
*Calcium and vitamin D supplement.*

**Calcium D$_3$** Aliud, Ger.; Betapharm, Ger.; Ratiopharm, Ger.; Stada, Ger.
Calcium carbonate (p.1254·2); colecalciferol (p.1461·3).
*Calcium and vitamin D deficiency; osteoporosis.*

**Calcium D Sauter** Roche, Switz.
Calcium hydrogen phosphate (p.1225·2); calcium gluconate (p.1225·2); calcium lactate (p.1225·3); ergocalciferol (p.1462·1); ascorbic acid (p.1460·2).
*Calcium supplement; disorders of calcium and phosphorus metabolism; vitamin C and D deficiencies.*

**Calcium Dago** Steiner, Ger.
Calcium carbonate (p.1254·2).
*Calcium deficiency; osteoporosis.*

**Calcium Docuphen** Pharmascience, Canad.†.
Docusate calcium (p.1262·1); yellow phenolphthalein (p.1284·1).
*Constipation.*

**Calcium Eifelfango** Eifelfango, Ger.
Calcium gluconate (p.1225·2); calcium levulinate (p.1225·3).
Formerly known as Calcium gluconicum.
*Calcium deficiency.*

**Calcium and Ergocalciferol Tablets** Cox, UK.
Calcium lactate 300 mg (p.1225·3); calcium phosphate 150 mg (p.1225·3); ergocalciferol 10 µg (p.1462·1).
Each tablet contains 400 units of vitamin-D activity. They should be crushed or chewed before administration.
Distinguish from Calcium with Vitamin D Tablets (BPC 1973).

**Calcium Factor** Novartis, Chile.
Calcium carbonate (p.1254·2).
*Calcium supplement; osteomalacia; osteoporosis, rickets.*

**Calcium Forte D** Novartis, Chile.
Calcium lactogluconate; calcium carbonate (p.1254·2); colecalciferol (p.1461·3).
*Hypocalcaemia; osteoporosis.*

**Calcium Fresenius**
Fresenius Kabi, Austria.
Calcium gluconate (p.1225·2); calcium saccharate (p.1665·1).
*Hypocalcaemia; osteoporosis.*

Fresenius Kabi, Ger.
Calcium gluconate (p.1225·2); calcium gluceptate (p.1225·2); calcium saccharate (p.1665·1).
*Calcium deficiency.*

**Calcium Heumann** Heumann, Ger.
Calcium carbonate (p.1254·2).
*Calcium deficiency; osteoporosis.*

**Calcium Hexal** Hexal, Ger.
Calcium carbonate (p.1254·2).
*Calcium deficiency; osteoporosis.*

**Calcium Magnesium Plus** Shaklee, Canad.
Vitamin D (p.1461·2); calcium phosphate (p.1225·3); magnesium carbonate (p.1272·1).

**Calcium 600mg** Pharmadass, UK†.
Calcium carbonate (p.1254·2); vitamins A and D (p.1417·1).

**Calcium Novartis** Novartis Consumer, Austria.
Calcium carbonate (p.1254·2); calcium lactate gluconate (p.1225·3).
*Calcium deficiency; osteoporosis.*

**Calcium Oyster Shell** Novopharm, Canad.
Calcium carbonate (p.1254·2).
*Calcium supplement.*

**Calcium Plus** General Nutrition, Canad.
Multivitamin and mineral preparation (p.1417·1).

**Calcium Resonium**
Sanofi Synthelabo, Austral.; Sanofi Synthelabo, Ger.; Sanofi Synthelabo, Gr.; Sanofi Synthelabo, Hong Kong; Sanofi Synthelabo, Irl.; Sanofi Synthelabo, NZ; Sanofi Synthelabo, UK.
Calcium polystyrene sulfonate (p.1032·3).
*Hyperkalaemia.*

**Calcium Rich Rolaids** Warner-Lambert, USA.
Magnesium hydroxide (p.1272·2); calcium carbonate (p.1254·2).
*Hyperacidity.*

**Calcium Stada** Stada, Ger.
Calcium carbonate (p.1254·2).
*Calcium deficiency; osteoporosis.*

**Calcium Stanley** Stanley, Canad.
Calcium gluceptate (p.1225·2); calcium gluconate (p.1225·2).
*Calcium deficiency; calcium supplement.*

**Calcium Truw** Truw, Ger.†.
Calcium gluconate (p.1225·2); calcium saccharate (p.1665·1).
*Calcium deficiency.*

**Calcium Unison**
Unison, Hong Kong; Unison, Thai.
Calcium lactate (p.1225·3).
*Calcium deficiency; calcium supplement.*

**Calcium Verla** Verla, Ger.
*Coated tablets; effervescent tablets:* Calcium carbonate (p.1254·2).
*Calcium deficiency; osteoporosis.*
*Injection*†: Calcium gluconate (p.1225·2); calcium saccharate (p.1665·1).
*Allergic disorders; calcium deficiency; lead poisoning; tetany.*
*Tablets*†: Calcium phosphate (p.1225·3); calcium citrate (p.1225·1).
*Allergic reactions; calcium deficiency; osteomalacia; osteoporosis; tetany.*

**Calcium Verla D** Verla, Ger.
Calcium carbonate (p.1254·2); colecalciferol (p.1461·3).
*Calcium and vitamin D$_3$ deficiency; osteoporosis.*

**Calcium Vitis** Neopharma, Ger.
Sodium calcium edetate (p.1051·3).
*Heavy-metal poisoning.*

**Calcium von CT** CT, Ger.
Calcium carbonate (p.1254·2).
*Calcium deficiency; osteoporosis.*

**Calcium-D-Redoxon**
Roche, Hong Kong; Roche Consumer, Singapore; Roche, Thai.
Calcium; vitamin C; vitamin B$_6$; vitamin D (p.1417·1).
*Calcium and vitamin deficiency.*

**Calcium-D-Sandoz**
Novartis Consumer, Austria; Novartis Consumer, Ger.; Novartis Consumer, Port.
Calcium carbonate (p.1254·2); colecalciferol (p.1461·3).
*Calcium and vitamin D deficiency; osteoporosis.*

**Calcium-D3-Sandoz** Novartis Consumer, Ital.
Calcium carbonate (p.1254·2); colecalciferol (p.1461·3).
*Calcium and vitamin D deficiency; calcium and vitamin D supplement; osteoporosis.*

**Calcium-dura** Merck dura, Ger.
Calcium carbonate (p.1254·2).
*Osteoporosis.*

**Calcium-dura Vit D$_3$** Merck dura, Ger.
Calcium carbonate (p.1254·2) or calcium phosphate (p.1225·3); colecalciferol (p.1461·3).
*Calcium and vitamin D deficiency.*

**Calcium-EAP** Kohler-Pharma, Ger.
Phosphorylcolamine calcium.
*Multiple sclerosis.*

**Calcium-Rougier** Rougier, Canad.
Calcium gluceptate (p.1225·2); calcium gluconate (p.1225·2).
*Calcium supplement.*

**Calcium-Rutinion** Biomo, Ger.
Rutoside (p.1688·2); calcium gluconate (p.1225·2).
*Capillary disorders; hypersensitivity reactions.*

**Calcium-Sandoz**
Note. This name is used for preparations of different composition.
Novartis, Arg.
Calcium lactate gluconate (p.1225·3); calcium carbonate (p.1254·2).
*Calcium supplement; osteomalacia; osteoporosis; rickets; tetany.*

Novartis Consumer, Austria; Novartis Consumer, Canad.; Novartis, Denm.; Novartis, Fin.; Novartis, Fr.; Novartis Consumer, Ger.; Novartis, Israel; Novartis Consumer, Neth.; Novartis, Norw.; Novartis Consumer, S.Afr.; Novartis, Swed.; Novartis, Switz.
*Effervescent tablets; powder for oral solution:* Calcium lactate gluconate (p.1225·3); calcium carbonate (p.1254·2).
*Calcium deficiency; calcium supplement; osteoporosis.*

Novartis Consumer, Austria; Novartis, Denm.; Novartis, Fin.; Novartis, Israel; Novartis Consumer, Neth.; Novartis, S.Afr.; Novartis, Swed.; Novartis, Switz.
*Injection:* Calcium glubionate (p.1225·1).
*Hyperkalaemia; hypocalcaemia; lead and fluoride poisoning; osteomalacia; osteoporosis; rickets; tetanus.*

Novartis, Braz.
Calcium gluconate (p.1225·2); calcium lactobionate (p.1225·3).
*Calcium deficiency.*

Novartis Consumer, Canad.†; Novartis, Irl.; Alliance, UK.
*Syrup:* Calcium glubionate (p.1225·1); calcium lactobionate (p.1225·3).
*Calcium deficiency; osteoporosis.*

Novartis, Chile.
Calcium lactogluconate; calcium carbonate (p.1254·2).
*Calcium supplement; osteomalacia; osteoporosis; rickets.*

Sandoz, Fr.†.
*Syrup:* Calcium gluconate (p.1225·2); calcium lactobionate (p.1225·3).
*Calcium deficiency; normocalcaemic tetany; prevention of bone loss in immobilisation; rickets.*

Novartis Consumer, Ger.
*Injection:* Calcium gluconate (p.1225·2); calcium lactobionate (p.1225·3).
*Calcium deficiency.*

Novartis, Hong Kong.
Calcium lactate gluconate (p.1225·3); calcium carbonate (p.1254·2).
*Calcium deficiency; osteomalacia; osteoporosis; rickets; tetany.*

Novartis, India.
Calcium carbonate (p.1254·2) or calcium glubionate (p.1225·1).
*Calcium deficiency.*

Novartis Consumer, Ital.
Calcium lactate gluconate (p.1225·3); calcium carbonate (p.1254·2).
*Calcium deficiency; osteomalacia; osteoporosis.*

Novartis, Mex.
Calcium lactate gluconate (p.1225·3); calcium carbonate (p.1254·2).
*Calcium supplement; osteomalacia; osteoporosis; rickets; tetany.*

Novartis, NZ.
Calcium lactate gluconate (p.1225·3); calcium carbonate (p.1254·2).
*Calcium supplement.*

Novartis Consumer, Port.
Calcium carbonate (p.1254·2); calcium lactate gluconate (p.1225·3).

Novartis Nutrition, Singapore.
Calcium lactate gluconate (p.1225·3); calcium carbonate (p.1254·2).
*Calcium deficiency; osteoporosis.*

Novartis Consumer, Spain.
Calcium glubionate (p.1225·1).
*Calcium deficiency.*

Novartis, Thai.
Calcium lactate gluconate (p.1225·3); calcium carbonate (p.1254·2).
*Bone demineralisation; calcium supplement; osteomalacia; osteoporosis; rickets; tetany.*

**Calcium-Sandoz C** Novartis, Spain†.
Ascorbic acid (p.1460·2); calcium glubionate (p.1225·1).
*Calcium deficiency; vitamin C deficiency.*

**Calcium-Sandoz F** Novartis, Braz.
Calcium lactate gluconate (p.1225·3); calcium carbonate (p.1254·2).
*Calcium deficiency.*

**Calcium-Sandoz Forte**
Novartis, Malaysia.
Calcium carbonate (p.1254·2); calcium lactate gluconate (p.1225·3).
*Calcium deficiency; osteomalacia; osteoporosis; rickets.*

Novartis Consumer, Spain.
Calcium carbonate (p.1254·2); calcium glubionate (p.1225·1).
*Calcium deficiency; hypoparathyroidism; osteomalacia; osteoporosis; rickets.*

**Calcium-Sandoz Forte D**
Novartis, Chile.
Calcium carbonate (p.1254·2); calcium lactobionate (p.1225·3); vitamin D (p.1461·2).
*Hypocalcaemia; osteoporosis.*

Novartis Consumer, Spain.
Calcium gluceptate (p.1225·2); colecalciferol(p.1461·3); calcium carbonate (p.1254·2).
*Deficiencies of calcium and vitamin D; osteoporosis.*

**Calcium-Sandoz + Vit C** Novartis, Israel.
Calcium gluconate (p.1225·2); calcium lactate (p.1225·3); calcium carbonate (p.1254·2); vitamin C (p.1460·2).
*Calcium and vitamin C supplement.*

**Calcium-Sandoz + Vitamin C** Novartis, Malaysia.
Ascorbic acid (p.1460·2); calcium carbonate (p.1254·2); calcium lactate gluconate (p.1225·3).
*Calcium and vitamin C supplement.*

**Calcium-Sandoz + Vitamina C** Novartis, Braz.
Calcium carbonate (p.1254·2); calcium lactobionate (p.1225·3); ascorbic acid (p.1460·2).
*Calcium and vitamin C supplement.*

**Calcium-Sorbisterit** Fresenius, Fr.†.
Calcium polystyrene sulfonate (p.1032·3).
*Hyperkalaemia related to renal insufficiency.*

**Calciumvit** Viternat, Braz.
Calcium carbonate (p.1254·2).
*Calcium deficiency.*

**Calciumvit Infantil** Viternat, Braz.
Calcium carbonate (p.1254·2); cod-liver oil (p.1425·2).
*Nutritional supplement.*

**Calcival** Valdecasas, Mex.
Calcium citrate (p.1225·1).
*Calcium deficiency; calcium supplement; osteomalacia, rickets; osteoporosis.*

**Calcivit** UB Interpharm, Switz.
Calcium hydrogen phosphate (p.1225·2); colecalciferol (p.1461·3).
*Hypocalcaemia.*

**Calcivit D** Hexal, Ger.
Calcium carbonate (p.1254·2); colecalciferol (p.1461·3).
*Calcium and vitamin $D_3$ deficiency; osteoporosis.*

**Calcivit F** Hexal, Ger.
Calcium carbonate (p.1254·2); sodium fluorophosphate (p.1446·2).
*Osteoporosis.*

**calcivitase** Biosyn, Ger.
Calcium citrate (p.1225·1); calcium gluconate (p.1225·2); calcium glycerophosphate (p.1225·2); calcium silicate (p.1226·1); colecalciferol (p.1461·3).
*Calcium deficiency.*

**Calcivorin** Mintlab, Chile.
Calcium carbonate (p.1254·2).
*Calcium supplement.*

**Calcivorin D** Mintlab, Chile.
Calcium carbonate (p.1254·2); vitamin D (p.1461·2).
*Calcium and vitamin D supplement.*

**Calco**
Kwizda, Austria; Iasis, Gr.; Lisapharma, Ital.; Lisapharma, Singapore; Lisapharma, Thai.
Calcitonin (salmon) (p.768·2).
*Hypercalcaemia; osteoporosis; Paget's disease of bone; reflex sympathetic dystrophy.*

**Calcort**
Aventis, Braz.; Galen, Ger.; Shire, Irl.; Aventis, Mex.; Aventis, Switz.; Shire, UK.
Deflazacort (p.1096·2).
*Corticosteroid.*

**Calcos Vitamine $D_3$** Arkomedika, Fr.
Calcium carbonate (p.1254·2); colecalciferol (p.1461·3).
*Calcium and vitamin D deficiency; osteoporosis.*

**Cal-C-Tose** Roche, Mex.†.
Multivitamin and mineral preparation (p.1417·1).

**Calcufel Aqua** Hevert, Ger.
Solidago virgaurea (p.1748·3).
*Renal calculi; urinary-tract disorders.*

**Calculi H** Pfluger, Ger.
Homoeopathic preparation.

**Calculina** Ferro, Arg.
No 1, podophyllum (p.1155·2); no 2, cascara (p.1255·1); rhubarb (p.1287·3); senna (p.1288·2); no 3, olive oil (p.1723·2); no 4, castor oil (p.1668·2); no 5, methenamine (p.230·1).
*Biliary-tract disorders.*

**Calcusan** Monserrat, Arg.
Calamine (p.1144·1); diphenhydramine (p.431·3).
*Allergic skin reactions; skin irritation.*

**Cal-C-Vita**
Roche, Arg.; Roche, Austria; Roche, Israel; Roche, Mex.†; Roche Consumer, S.Afr.; Roche, Switz.
Calcium carbonate (p.1254·2); vitamins (p.1417·1).
*Calcium supplement; tonic.*

**Cal-C-Vita Fluor** Roche, Arg.
Calcium carbonate (p.1254·2); sodium fluoride (p.1444·3); vitamins (p.1417·1).
*Calcium and fluoride supplement.*

**Cal-D3** Cotek, Singapore.
Calcium carbonate (p.1254·2); colecalciferol (p.1461·3).
*Calcium supplement.*

**Caldar-D** Medipharm, Chile.
Calcium carbonate (p.1254·2); vitamin D (p.1461·2).
*Calcium deficiency; osteoporosis.*

**Cal-De**
Asta Medica, Austria; Novartis, Switz.
Calcium carbonate (p.1254·2); colecalciferol (p.1461·3).
*Vitamin D and calcium deficiency.*

**Caldease** Roche Consumer, Irl.
Zinc oxide (p.1163·2); cod-liver oil (p.1425·2).
*Burns; nappy rash; skin irritation; wounds.*

**CaldeCort** Novartis Consumer, USA.
Hydrocortisone (p.1103·3) or hydrocortisone acetate (p.1103·3).
*Skin disorders.*

**Calderol** Organon, USA.
Calcifediol (p.1461·2).
*Hypocalcaemia associated with renal dialysis; metabolic bone disease.*

**Caldesene**
Note. This name is used for preparations of different composition.
Novartis Consumer, Canad.†; Fisons, USA.
*Ointment:* Cod-liver oil (p.1425·2); zinc oxide (p.1163·2).
*Skin disorders.*

Novartis Consumer, Canad.†; Fisons, USA.
*Topical powder:* Calcium undecenoate (p.410·3).
*Bromhidrosis; fungal skin infections; hyperhidrosis; minor skin irritation; nappy rash.*

Roche Consumer, Irl.
Calcium undecenoate (p.410·3).
*Nappy rash; skin irritation.*

**Caldeval** Saval, Chile.
Calcium (p.1225·1); vitamin D (p.1461·2).
*Calcium and vitamin D deficiency; osteomalacia; osteoporosis; rickets.*

**Caldine** Boehringer Ingelheim, Fr.
Lacidipine (p.944·2).
*Hypertension.*

**Caldomine-DH** Technilab, Canad.†.
Hydrocodone tartrate (p.45·1); phenylpropanolamine hydrochloride (p.1127·3); mepyramine maleate (p.437·1); pheniramine maleate (p.438·3).
*Coughs.*

**Cal-D-or** Nycomed, Austria.
Calcium carbonate (p.1254·2); colecalciferol (p.1461·3).
*Calcium and vitamin D deficiency; osteoporosis.*

**Caldramine** Silom, Thai.†.
Calamine (p.1144·1); diphenhydramine hydrochloride (p.431·3); camphor (p.1665·3).
*Skin irritation.*

**Cal-D-Vita**
Roche, Austria; Roche, Swed.; Roche, Thai.
Calcium carbonate (p.1254·2); colecalciferol (p.1461·3).
*Calcium and vitamin D deficiency; osteoporosis.*

**Calel-D** Rhone-Poulenc Rorer, USA.
Calcium carbonate (p.1254·2); colecalciferol (p.1461·3).
*Nutritional supplement.*

**Calendaderm** Knop, Chile.
Homoeopathic preparation.

**Calendolon** Weleda, UK.
Calendula (p.1665·2).
*Minor wounds and abrasions.*

**Calendula +** Homeocan, Canad.
Homoeopathic preparation.

**Calendula Concreta** Simoes, Braz.
Calendula (p.1665·2); zinc oxide (p.1163·2).
*Skin disorders.*

**Calendula Echinacea Comp** Knop, Chile.
Homoeopathic preparation.

**Calendula Nappy Change Cream** Weleda, UK.
Calendula (p.1665·2); chamomile (p.1669·3); almond oil (p.1651·1).
*Nappy rash.*

**Calendulene** Thea, Fr.
Calendula (p.1665·2).
*Eye hygiene.*

**Calendumed**
Peithner, Austria; DHU, Ger.
Homoeopathic preparation.

**Calfate** Helsinn, Port.
Sucralfate (p.1290·2).
*Duodenitis; gastritis; gastro-oesophageal reflux; peptic ulcer.*

**Calfolex** Crinos, Ital.
Calcium folinate (p.1431·1).
*Antidote to folic acid antagonists; folic acid deficiency; reduction of aminopterin and methotrexate toxicity.*

**Calfolin** Eurofarma, Braz.†.
Calcium folinate (p.1431·1).
*Adjunct to antineoplastic therapy; anaemias; antidote to folic acid antagonists.*

**Calfosina** Grunenthal, Chile.
Calcitonin (salmon) (p.768·2).
*Hypercalcaemia; osteoporosis; Paget's disease of bone.*

**Calfovit D3** Trinity, UK.
Calcium phosphate (p.1225·3); colecalciferol (p.1461·3).
*Calcium and vitamin D deficiency; osteoporosis.*

**Calgayan** Grossman, Mex.
Paracetamol (p.76·2); chlorphenamine maleate (p.427·3); phenylpropanolamine hydrochloride (p.1127·3).
*Upper respiratory-tract disorders.*

**Calgel** Pfizer Consumer, UK.
Lidocaine hydrochloride (p.1377·3); cetylpyridinium chloride (p.1173·1).
*Teething pain.*

**Calibral** Solvay, Port.
Tenoxicam (p.93·1).
*Gout; musculoskeletal, joint, and peri-articular disorders.*

**Calicida Indiano** Medical, Port.
*Ointment:* Acetic acid (p.1645·2); salicylic acid (p.1157·1).
*Topical solution:* Lactic acid (p.1704·1); salicylic acid (p.1157·1).

**Caliderm** Darier, Mex.
Calcium hydroxide (p.1664·3); almond oil (p.1651·1).
*Skin disorders.*

**Califig** Merck Consumer, UK.
*Chewable bar:* Senna (p.1288·2); fig (p.1266·3); dietary fibre (p.1417·1).
*Constipation.*
*Effervescent tablets†:* Dietary fibre supplement (p.1417·1).
*Oral liquid:* Senna (p.1288·2); fig (p.1266·3).
*Constipation.*
*Tablets†:* Taraxacum (p.1751·3); peppermint oil (p.1283·2); senna (p.1288·2).
*Constipation.*

**Calimal** Sussex, UK.
Chlorphenamine maleate (p.427·3).
*Hypersensitivity reactions.*

**Calinat** Aesculapius, Ital.
Calcium folinate (p.1431·1).
*Folate deficiency; reduction of aminopterin and methotrexate toxicity.*

**Calinofen** Medimport, Mex.
Paracetamol (p.76·2).
*Fever; pain.*

**Calista** Ecobrands, UK.
Fertility test (p.1734·3).

**Calisvit** Menarini, Ital.
Colecalciferol (p.1461·3); tribasic calcium phosphate (p.1225·3).
*Calcium and vitamin D deficiency.*

**Cal-Lac** Bio-Tech, USA.
Calcium lactate (p.1225·3).
*Calcium supplement.*

**Callicida**
Note. This name is used for preparations of different composition.
Asofarma, Arg.; Gezzi, Arg.
Salicylic acid (p.1157·1).
*Callus removal.*

Cabuchi, Arg.
Salicylic acid (p.1157·1); lactic acid (p.1704·1); phenol (p.1188·1); acetic acid (p.1645·2); benzocaine (p.1370·3); collodion.
*Callus removal.*

Eczane, Arg.; Lauria, Arg.
Salicylic acid (p.1157·1); resorcinol (p.1156·3); lactic acid (p.1704·1).
*Callus removal.*

El Monje, Arg.
*Ointment:* Salicylic acid (p.1157·1).
*Topical solution:* Salicylic acid (p.1157·1); lactic acid (p.1704·1); zinc chloride (p.1469·2).
*Callus removal.*

**Callicida 2** Schering-Plough, Arg.
Salicylic acid (p.1157·1); Canada balsam; acetone; collodion.
*Callus removal.*

**Callicida Brujo** Perez Gimenez, Spain†.
Flexible collodion; lactic acid (p.1704·1); salicylic acid (p.1157·1).
*Callosities.*

**Callicida Brum** Brum, Spain.
Flexible collodion; salicylic acid (p.1157·1); trichloroacetic acid (p.1162·1).
*Callosities.*

**Callicida Cor Pik** Quimifar, Spain.
Acetic acid (p.1645·2); flexible collodion; lactic acid (p.1704·1); castor oil; salicylic acid (p.1157·1).
*Callosities.*

**Callicida Durcall** Llorens, Spain†.
Acetic acid (p.1645·2); flexible collodion; lactic acid (p.1704·1); salicylic acid (p.1157·1).
*Callosities.*

**Callicida Globodermis** Weinco, Spain†.
Salicylic acid (p.1157·1).
*Callosities.*

**Callicida Gras** Quimifar, Spain.
Salicylic acid (p.1157·1).
*Callosities.*

**Callicida Rojo** Escaned, Spain.
Acetic acid (p.1645·2); flexible collodion; benzocaine (p.1370·3); salicylic acid (p.1157·1); iodine tincture (p.1598·1).
*Callosities.*

**Callicida Salve** Cederroth, Spain.
Salicylic acid (p.1157·1).
*Callosities.*

**Callimon**
Grossmann, Hong Kong.
Calcium (p.1225·1); vitamin C (p.1460·2).
*Calcium and vitamin C supplement.*

Grossmann, Switz.
Calcium carbonate (p.1254·2); calcium lactate (p.1225·3); ascorbic acid (p.1460·2).
*Vitamin C and calcium deficiency.*

**Callivoro Marthand** Martinez Llenas, Spain.
Salicylic acid (p.1157·1); benzocaine (p.1370·3).
*Callosities.*

**Callix** Perez Gimenez, Spain.
Flexible collodion; benzocaine (p.1370·3); lactic acid (p.1704·1); salicylic acid (p.1157·1).
*Callosities.*

**Callofin** Alcor, Spain.
Salicylic acid (p.1157·1).
*Callosities.*

**Callus Salve** Cress, Canad.†.
Salicylic acid (p.1157·1).

**Calma** Uno, Ital.
Calcium carbonate (p.1254·2).
*Calcium deficiency; calcium supplement.*

**Calmaben** Montavit, Austria.
Diphenhydramine hydrochloride (p.431·3).
*Hypersensitivity reactions; sedative.*

**Calmaderm** Whitehall, Fr.†.
Bufexamac (p.21·3).
*Pruritus.*

**Calmador** Finadiet, Arg.
Tramadol hydrochloride (p.94·3).
*Pain.*

**Cal-Mag**
Note. This name is used for preparations of different composition.
Seroyal, Canad.†.
Calcium carbonate (p.1254·2); magnesium oxide (p.1272·3).

Swiss Herbal, Canad.
Calcium, magnesium, zinc, vitamin C and vitamin D (p.1417·1).
Formerly contained calcium carbonate and magnesium carbonate.

Quest, UK.
Calcium, magnesium, and vitamin D (p.1417·1).

**Cal-Mag Citrate with Vitamin D & Zinc** *Swiss Herbal, Canad.*
Calcium, magnesium, zinc, and vitamin D (p.1417·1).

**Calmag D** *Gerbex, Canad.*
Calcium, magnesium, and vitamin D (p.1417·1).

**CalMag Plus**
*Usana, Hong Kong; USANA, USA.*
Calcium citrate; magnesium amino acid chelate; silicon amino acid chelate; boron amino acid chelate; vitamin D (p.1417·1).
*Nutritional supplement.*

**Cal-Mag plus Vitamin D** *Quest, Canad.*
Calcium, magnesium, and vitamin D (p.1417·1).

**Cal-Mag Vitamin C & Zinc** *Swiss Herbal, Canad.*
Calcium, magnesium, zinc, and vitamin C (p.1417·1).

**Cal-Mag with Vitamin D & Zinc** *Swiss Herbal, Canad.*
Calcium, magnesium, zinc, and vitamin D (p.1417·1).

**Cal-Mag & Vitamins C & D** *Swiss Herbal, Canad.*
Calcium and magnesium with vitamins C and D (p.1417·1).

**Calmag Zn** *Vita Health, Singapore†.*
Calcium, magnesium, and zinc (p.1417·1).
*Calcium deficiency; osteoporosis.*

**Calman** *Ativus, Braz.*
Passion flower (p.1729·1); crataegus (p.1677·1); salix (p.87·3).
*Sedative.*

**Calmanervin** *Sam-On, Israel.*
*Elixir:* Passion flower (p.1729·1); valerian (p.1762·2).
*Tablets:* Passion flower (p.1729·1); valerian (p.1762·2); thiamine hydrochloride (p.1455·1); pyridoxine hydrochloride (p.1456·3).
*Anxiety; insomnia.*

**Calmant Martou** *Sanico, Belg.†.*
Belladonna extract (p.479·1); mint oil (p.1715·2); cinnamon oil (p.1672·2); orange-peel oil (p.1723·3); melissa oil (p.1711·2); eugenol (p.1686·2); anethole (p.1654·3); saffron (p.1058·2).
*Gastrointestinal disorders.*

**Calmante Creosotado** *Phos-Kola, Braz.†.*
Eucalyptus (p.1686·1); hypophosphite; Desessartz syrup; laurana camara; tolu balsam (p.1131·3); creosote (p.1117·2).
*Coughs.*

**Calmante De Aftas** *Drag, Chile.*
Lidocaine (p.1377·3); methylrosanilinium chloride (p.1186·1).

**Calmante De Denticion** *Drag, Chile.*
Lidocaine (p.1377·3).

**Calmante Vitaminado P G** *Perez Gimenez, Spain.*
Aspirin (p.15·1); caffeine (p.782·1); thiamine (p.1455·2).
*Fever; pain.*

**Calmante Vitaminado PG Efervescente** *Perez Gimenez, Spain.*
Aspirin (p.15·1); caffeine (p.782·1); thiamine nitrate (p.1455·1); ascorbic acid (p.1460·2).
*Fever; pain.*

**Calmante Vitaminado Rinver** *Monik, Spain.*
Aspirin (p.15·1); thiamine (p.1455·2).
*Fever; inflammation; pain.*

**Calmanticold** *Perez Gimenez, Spain.*
Paracetamol (p.76·2).
*Fever; pain.*

**Calmanticold Vit C** *Calmante Vitaminado, Spain†.*
Ascorbic acid (p.1460·2); paracetamol (p.76·2).
*Fever; pain.*

**Calmantina** *Inexfa, Spain†.*
Aspirin (p.15·1).
*Fever; inflammation; pain; thromboembolism prophylaxis.*

**Calmapax** *Delta, Braz.*
Chamomile (p.1669·3); erythrina mulungu (p.1717·2); melissa (p.1711·1); passion flower (p.1729·1).
*Sedative.*

**Calmapele** *Luper, Braz.†.*
Calamine (p.1144·1); zinc oxide (p.1163·2); diphenhydramine hydrochloride (p.431·3); camphor (p.1665·3).
*Pruritus; skin irritation.*

**Calmapica** *Perez Gimenez, Spain.*
Ammonia (p.1653·3).
*Insect bites; stings.*

**Calmapir** *Elvetium, Arg.*
Piroxicam (p.84·2).
*Inflammation; osteoarthritis; pain; rheumatoid arthritis; tendinitis.*

**Calmapir-P** *Elvetium, Arg.*
Piroxicam (p.84·2); paracetamol (p.76·2).
*Inflammation; osteoarthritis; pain; rheumatoid arthritis.*

**Calmaril** *Siam Bheasach, Thai.*
Thioridazine hydrochloride (p.724·2).
*Anxiety; behaviour disorders; mania; schizophrenia.*

**Calmarum** *Medical, Port.*
Sulfogaiacol (p.1131·1); ephedrine hydrochloride (p.1120·1); ethylmorphine (dionina) (p.37·3); sodium benzoate (p.1169·3); aconite (p.1646·3); thyme (p.1755·2); senega (p.1130·2).
*Coughs.*

**Calmatel** *Almirall, Spain.*
Piketoprofen (p.84·1) or piketoprofen hydrochloride (p.84·1).
*Peri-articular and soft-tissue disorders.*

**Calmatoss** *Herbarium, Braz.*
Grindelia (p.1696·1); guaco; tolu balsam (p.1131·3); propolis (p.1735·2); copaiba; nasturtium; honey (p.1434·2).
*Coughs.*

**Calmaven** *Alter, Spain†.*
Diazepam (p.690·1).
*Alcohol withdrawal syndrome; anxiety; epilepsy; febrile convulsions; insomnia; premedication; skeletal muscle spasm.*

**Calmaverine** *Taphlan, Switz.*
Caroverine (p.1668·1) or caroverine hydrochloride (p.1668·1).
*Smooth muscle spasm.*

**Calmax** *Ergha, Irl.*
Alprazolam (p.668·3).
*Anxiety.*

**Calmaxid** *Norgine, Switz.*
Nizatidine (p.1277·2).
*Gastric hyperacidity; gastro-oesophageal reflux; peptic ulcer.*

**Calmazin** *Ibefar, Braz.†.*
Papaverine hydrochloride (p.1728·1); homatropine methylbromide (p.483·2); passion flower (p.1729·1); adonis vernalis (p.1648·1); crataegus (p.1677·1).
*Sedative.*

**Calmday**
*Will-Pharma, Belg.; Will-Pharma, Neth.*
Nordazepam (p.710·3).
*Anxiety.*

**Calmerphan** *Doetsch, Grether, Switz.†.*
Dextromethorphan hydrobromide (p.1117·3).
*Coughs.*

**Calmerphan-L** *Doetsch, Grether, Switz.*
Dextromethorphan resin (p.1117·3).
*Bronchitis; coughs.*

**Calmese** *Themis Chemicals, India.*
Lorazepam (p.704·1).
*Premedication.*

**Calmesine** *Mepha, Switz.*
Dextromethorphan resin (p.1118·1).
*Coughs.*

**Calmettes** *Aventis, S.Afr.*
Valerian (p.1762·2).
*Anxiety; nervous disorders.*

**Calmex**
*Note. This name is used for preparations of different composition.*
*Heralds, Braz.†.*
Bromazepam (p.671·3).
*Anxiety.*

*Novopharm, Canad.*
Diphenhydramine hydrochloride (p.431·3).
*Insomnia.*

*Roerig, Chile.*
Doxylamine succinate (p.432·3).
*Insomnia.*

**Calmine** *Bouty, Ital.*
Ibuprofen (p.45·3).
*Pain.*

**Calminex Atleta** *Schering-Plough, Braz.*
Methyl salicylate (p.59·3); belladonna (p.479·1); camphor (p.1665·3).
*Musculoskeletal and joint disorders.*

**Calminex H** *Schering-Plough, Braz.*
Methyl salicylate (p.59·3); zinc oxide (p.1163·2); belladonna (p.479·1); peru balsam (p.1730·2); camphor (p.1665·3).
*Musculoskeletal and joint disorders.*

**Calmiphase** *Arkomedika, Fr.*
Chamomile (p.1669·3); centella (p.1144·3).
*Skin disorders.*

**Calmiplan** *Bunker, Braz.*
Passion flower (p.1729·1); crataegus (p.1677·1); salix (p.87·3).

**Calmiton** *Bunker, Braz.*
Kava (p.1703·2).
*Anxiety.*

**Calmixene** *Novartis, Fr.*
Pimethixene (p.439·1).
*Coughs.*

**Calmo**
*Note. This name is used for preparations of different composition.*
*Eagle, Austral.†.*
Mistletoe (p.1715·3); valerian (p.1762·2); vervain (p.1764·1); gentian (p.1692·2); avena (p.1658·2); passion flower (p.1729·1); skullcap (p.1746·3); tansy (p.1751·3); pulsatilla (p.1737·1).
*Hypnotic; tension; tension headache.*

*Lab, Port.†.*
Anemone; belladonna (p.479·1); passion flower (p.1729·1); crataegus (p.1677·1).

**Calmobrul** *SVR, Fr.*
Hypericum oil; wheatgerm oil; allantoin; vitamin E; niaouli oil; rosemary oil.
*Sunburn.*

**Calmociteno** *Medley, Braz.*
Diazepam (p.690·1).
*Alcohol withdrawal syndrome; anxiety; epilepsy; insomnia; premedication; sedative; skeletal muscle spasm.*

**Calmoflorine** *Coup, Gr.*
Sulpiride (p.722·2).
*Psychoses.*

**Calmogel** *Aventis, Ital.*
Isothipendyl hydrochloride (p.435·2).
*Insect bites; pruritus; sunburn.*

**Calmogenol** *Brasmedica, Braz.†.*
Lorazepam (p.704·1).
*Alcohol withdrawal syndrome; anxiety; epilepsy; insomnia; nausea and vomiting; premedication; sedative.*

**Calmol** *Mentholatum, USA.*
Zinc oxide (p.1163·2); bismuth subgallate (p.1252·2).
*Anorectal disorders.*

**Calmomusc** *Cardinaux, Canad.†.*
Methyl salicylate (p.59·3); menthol (p.1711·3); cineole (p.1672·1).

**Calmonex** *Delta, Braz.*
Kava (p.1703·2).
*Anxiety.*

**Calmophytum** *Holistica, Fr.*
Tilia (p.1756·2); orange buds (p.1723·3); chamomile (p.1669·3); vervain (p.1764·1); hibiscus.
*Insomnia.*

**Calmopirin** *Fada, Arg.*
Dextropropoxyphene (p.28·3); dipyrone (p.35·3).
*Fever; pain.*

**Calmoplex** *Teofarma, Spain.*
Codeine phosphate (p.27·1); hydroxyzine hydrochloride (p.434·3); propyphenazone (p.85·3).
*Coughs; fever; pain.*

**Calmoroide** *Warner-Lambert, Fr.†.*
Ruscogenin (p.1741·1); vitamin A palmitate (p.1453·1).
*Haemorrhoids.*

**Calmose** *Welt, Arg.*
Aluminium hydroxide (p.1249·2); magnesium hydroxide (p.1272·2); magnesium carbonate (p.1272·1).
*Antacid.*

**Calmosedan** *Recalcine, Chile.*
Chlormezanone (p.675·1); diazepam (p.690·1).
*Anxiety; muscle spasm.*

**Calmosine** *Legras, Fr.*
Dill seed (p.1680·2); sodium bicarbonate (p.1223·2).
*Infant colic.*

**Calmovarin** *Faria, Braz.†.*
Diethylstilbestrol (p.1548·1); papaverine (p.1728·1); calcium gluconate (p.1225·2); viburnum; berberis.
*Smooth muscle spasm.*

**Calmpose**
*Ranbaxy, India; Ranbaxy, S.Afr.*
Diazepam (p.690·1).
*Alcohol withdrawal syndrome; anxiety; premedication; skeletal muscle spasm; status epilepticus; tetanus.*

**Calms** *Hylands, Canad.*
Homoeopathic preparation.

**Calms Forte** *Hylands, Canad.*
Homoeopathic preparation.

**Calmtabs** *Natural Life, Arg.*
Valerian (p.1762·2); passion flower (p.1729·1); celery (p.1669·1); cataria; lupulus (p.1708·1); dried orange peel (p.1723·3).
*Sedative.*

**Calm-U** *Wilson, NZ.*
Diphenhydramine hydrochloride (p.431·3); salicylamide (p.87·3).
*Anxiety; insomnia.*

**Calmurid**
*Note. This name is used for preparations of different composition.*
*Galderma, Austral.; AB-Consult, Austria; Galderma, Belg.; Galderma, Canad.†; Galderma, Ger.; Galderma, Irl.; Galpharma, Israel; Galderma, Neth.; Galderma, NZ; Jaba, Port.; Galderma, Switz.; Galderma, UK.*
Urea (p.1162·2); lactic acid (p.1704·1).
*Dry skin; hyperkeratosis.*

*Grunenthal, Chile.*
Hydrocortisone (p.1103·3).
*Skin disorders.*

**Calmurid comp** *AB-Consult, Austria.*
Urea (p.1162·2); sodium chloride (p.1233·3).
*Psoriasis.*

**Calmurid HC**
*Note. This name is used for preparations of different composition.*
*AB-Consult, Austria; Galderma, Canad.†; Galderma, Ger.†; Galderma, Irl.; Galderma, Israel; Galderma, Switz.; Galderma, UK.*
Urea (p.1162·2); lactic acid (p.1704·1); hydrocortisone (p.1103·3).
*Skin disorders.*

*Galderma, Neth.; Galderma, S.Afr.*
Urea (p.1162·2); hydrocortisone (p.1103·3).
*Skin disorders.*

**Calmuril**
*Pharmacia, Fin.; Pharmacia, Swed.*
Urea (p.1162·2); lactic acid (p.1704·1).
*Dry skin; eczema; keratinisation disorders.*

**Calmuril-Hydrokortison** *Pharmacia Upjohn, Swed.†.*
Urea (p.1162·2); hydrocortisone (p.1103·3).
*Skin disorders.*

**Calm-X** *Republic, USA.*
Dimenhydrinate (p.431·1).
*Motion sickness.*

**Calmydone** *Technilab, Canad.*
Hydrocodone tartrate (p.45·1); etafedrine hydrochloride (p.1121·2); doxylamine succinate (p.432·3).
*Coughs.*

**Calmylin #1** *Technilab, Canad.*
Dextromethorphan hydrobromide (p.1117·3).
*Coughs.*

**Calmylin #2** *Technilab, Canad.*
Dextromethorphan hydrobromide (p.1117·3); pseudoephedrine hydrochloride (p.1129·2).
Formerly known as Calmylin-DM-D.
*Coughs.*

**Calmylin #3** *Technilab, Canad.*
Dextromethorphan hydrobromide (p.1117·3); pseudoephedrine hydrochloride (p.1129·2); guaifenesin (p.1122·1).
Formerly known as Calmylin-DM-D-E.
*Coughs.*

**Calmylin #4** *Technilab, Canad.*
Diphenhydramine hydrochloride (p.431·3); ammonium chloride (p.1115·2); dextromethorphan hydrobromide (p.1117·3).
Formerly known as Calmylin-DM.
*Coughs.*

**Calmylin Ace** *Technilab, Canad.*
Guaifenesin (p.1122·1); pheniramine maleate (p.438·3); codeine phosphate (p.27·1).
*Coughs.*

**Calmylin with Codeine** *Technilab, Canad.*
Pseudoephedrine hydrochloride (p.1129·2); codeine phosphate (p.27·1); guaifenesin (p.1122·1).
Formerly known as Calmylin Codeine D-E.

**Calmylin Cough & Flu** *Technilab, Canad.*
Dextromethorphan hydrobromide (p.1117·3); pseudoephedrine hydrochloride (p.1129·2); guaifenesin (p.1122·1); paracetamol (p.76·2).
*Coughs and cold symptoms.*

**Calmylin Expectorant** *Technilab, Canad.*
Guaifenesin (p.1122·1).
*Coughs.*

**Calmylin Original with Codeine** *Technilab, Canad.*
Diphenhydramine hydrochloride (p.431·3); ammonium chloride (p.1115·2); codeine phosphate (p.27·1).
*Coughs.*

**Calmylin Pediatric** *Technilab, Canad.*
Dextromethorphan hydrobromide (p.1117·3); pseudoephedrine hydrochloride (p.1129·2).
*Coughs and cold symptoms.*

**Cal-Nate** *Ethex, USA.*
Vitamin and mineral preparation (p.1417·1).

**Calner** *Medipharm, Chile.*
Dipotassium clorazepate (p.685·1).
*Anxiety.*

**Calnisan** *Osteolab, Chile.*
Calcitonin (salmon) (p.768·2).
*Osteoporosis.*

**Calnit** *Elan, Spain.*
Nimodipine (p.972·3).
*Mental function impairment; neurological deficit following subarachnoid haemorrhage.*

**Calociclina** *ISI, Ital.†.*
Tetracycline hydrochloride (p.266·2).
*Bacterial infections.*

**Calogen**
*Note. This name is used for preparations of different composition.*
*Scientific Hospital Supplies, Austral.; Nutricia, Fin.; Scientific Hospital Supplies, Irl.; Nutricia, Ital.; Scientific Hospital Supplies, NZ; Nutricia, NZ; Scientific Hospital Supplies, UK.*
Arachis oil (p.1656·1).
*Carbohydrate malabsorption; dietary supplement; disorders of amino acid metabolism; ketogenic diet in epilepsy.*

*Probios, Port.; Almirall, Spain.*
Calcitonin (salmon) (p.768·2).
*Hypercalcaemia; metastatic bone pain; osteoporosis; Paget's disease of bone.*

*SHS, Singapore†.*
Dietary fat supplement (p.1417·1).

**Calonat** *Democal, Switz.†.*
Carbasalate calcium (p.25·1); ascorbic acid (p.1460·2).
*Fever; pain.*

**Calope** *Simoes, Braz.*
Phenylacetic acid; lactic acid (p.1704·1); thuja (p.1755·1).
*Keratinisation disorders.*

**Caloreen**
*Nestle, Fr.; IFET (ΙΦΕΤ), Gr.; Clintec, Irl.†; Roussel, S.Afr.†; Nestle, UK.*
Dextrin (p.1427·1).
*Food for special diets.*

**Calotrat** *Galenogal, Braz.†.*
Lactic acid (p.1704·1); salicylic acid (p.1157·1).
*Hyperkeratosis.*

**Calox**
*Note. This name is used for preparations of different composition.*
*Qualiphar, Belg.†.*
Sterculia (p.1290·2).
Formerly known as Fixobel.
*Denture fixative.*

*Medipharma, Hong Kong.*
Diphenhydramine hydrochloride (p.431·3).
*Pruritus.*

**Calpan** *ICN, Canad.†.*
Calcium pantothenate (p.1442·3).

**Calparine**
*Sanofi Synthelabo, Belg.; Sanofi Synthelabo, Neth.†.*
Heparin calcium (p.927·3).
*Thrombosis prophylaxis.*

**Calperos**
*Bouchara-Recordati, Fr.; Robapharm, Switz.*
Calcium carbonate (p.1254·2).
*Calcium deficiency; osteoporosis.*

**Calperos $D_3$** *Bouchara-Recordati, Fr.; Bouchara-Recordati, Hong Kong; Robapharm, Switz.*
Calcium carbonate (p.1254·2); colecalciferol (p.1461·3).
*Calcium and vitamin D deficiency; osteoporosis.*

**Calphosan** *Glenwood, USA.*
Calcium glycerophosphate (p.1225·2); calcium lactate (p.1225·3).
*Calcium deficiency.*

**Calphron** *Nephro-Tech, USA†.*
Calcium acetate (p.1225·1).
*Hyperphosphataemia.*

**Calpix** *Euro-Labor, Port.; Grunenthal, Port.*
Captopril (p.879·2).
*Heart failure; hypertension.*

**Cal-Plus** *Geriatric Pharm. Corp., USA†.*
Calcium carbonate (p.1254·2).
*High-potency calcium supplement.*

**CalplusD3** *Guidotti, Ital.*
Tribasic calcium phosphate (p.1225·3); colecalciferol (p.1461·3).
*Calcium and vitamin deficiency; osteoporosis.*

**Calpol** *Glaxo Wellcome, Braz.†; GlaxoSmithKline, Hong Kong; GlaxoSmithKline, India; Warner-Lambert, Irl.; Glaxo Wellcome, Mex.†; GlaxoSmithKline, S.Afr.; GlaxoSmithKline, Singapore; GlaxoSmithKline, Thai.; Pfizer Consumer, UK.*
Paracetamol (p.76·2).
*Fever; pain.*

**Calpol Extra** *Warner-Lambert, UK†.*
Paracetamol (p.76·2); codeine phosphate (p.27·1); caffeine (p.782·1).
*Fever; pain.*

**Calporo** *Eagle, Austral.†.*
Vitamin and mineral supplement with rose fruit, irish moss, echinacea, equisetum, lysine, and bone powder (p.1417·1).
*Bone disorders; mineral supplement.*

**Calpred** *Grossmann, Switz.*
Prednisolone acetate (p.1108·1); mepyramine maleate (p.437·1); calcium levulinate (p.1225·3).
*Skin disorders.*

**Calpres** *Temis, Arg.*
Amlodipine besilate (p.862·1).
*Angina pectoris; hypertension.*

**Calprimum** *Iderne, Fr.*
Calcium carbonate (p.1254·2).
*Calcium deficiency; osteoporosis.*

**Calprofen** *Pfizer Consumer, UK.*
Ibuprofen (p.45·3).
*Fever; pain.*

**Calron** *East India Pharma, India.*
Multivitamin and mineral preparation (p.1417·1).

**Calrub** *Pfizer Consumer, UK.*
Eucalyptus (p.1686·1); menthol (p.1711·3).
*Respiratory-tract congestion.*

**Cal-Rutina** *ICN, Mex.*
Rutoside (p.1688·2); vitamin C (p.1460·2).
*Capillary fragility.*

**Calsalettes** *Torbet Laboratories, UK.*
Aloin (p.1248·3).
*Constipation.*

**Calsan** *Novartis, Braz.; Novartis Consumer, Canad.; Novartis, Mex.; Novartis, Switz.†.*
Calcium carbonate (p.1254·2).
*Calcium supplement; osteoporosis.*

**Calsein** *Manuell, Mex.*
Calcium caseinate.

**Calshake** *Fresenius Kabi, Irl.; Fresenius Kabi, UK.*
Preparation for enteral nutrition (p.1417·1).

**Calsip** *Rowa, Irl.†.*
Food for special diets (p.1417·1).

**Calslot** *Takeda, Jpn.*
Manidipine hydrochloride (p.950·2).
*Hypertension.*

**Calsorp** *Thaipharmed, Thai.*
Calcium citrate (p.1225·1).
*Calcium deficiency.*

**Calsum Forte** *Sriprasit, Thai.*
Calcium carbonate (p.1254·2).
*Calcium deficiency; osteomalacia; osteoporosis; rickets.*

**Cal-Sup** *3M, Austral.; 3M, Malaysia; 3M, NZ†; 3M, Singapore.*
Calcium carbonate (p.1254·2).
*Calcium deficiency; calcium supplement.*

**Calsyn** *Aventis, Fr.; Aventis, Port.*
Calcitonin (salmon) (p.768·2).
*Algodystrophies; hypercalcaemia; hyperphosphatasia; osteoporosis; Paget's disease of bone; prevention of bone loss in immobilisation.*

**Calsynar** *Aventis, Arg.; Rhone-Poulenc Rorer, Austral.†; Aventis, Belg.; Aventis, Braz.; Aventis, Ger.; Aventis, Gr.; Rhone-Poulenc Rorer, Hong Kong†; Rhone-Poulenc Rorer, Irl.†; Rhone-Poulenc Rorer, Israel†; Aventis, Spain; Aventis, UK†.*
Calcitonin (salmon) (p.768·2) or calcitonin (salmon) acetate (p.769·2).
*Bone pain in malignancy; hypercalcaemia; osteoporosis; Paget's disease of bone; reflex sympathetic dystrophy.*

**Calsynar Lyo** *Rhone-Poulenc Rorer, Ger.†.*
Calcitonin (salmon) (p.768·2).
*Bone pain in malignancy; hypercalcaemia; osteoporosis; Paget's disease of bone; reflex sympathetic dystrophy.*

**Caltab** *Masa, Thai.*
Calcium carbonate (p.1254·2).
*Calcium deficiency; calcium supplement.*

**Caltabs** *Lifeplan, UK†.*
Vitamin and mineral preparation (p.1417·1).

**Caltheon** *Chephasaar, Ger.*
Tetryzoline hydrochloride (p.1131·2).
*Nasal congestion.*

**Caltine** *Ferring, Canad.*
Calcitonin (salmon) (p.768·2).
*Hypercalcaemia; Paget's disease of bone.*

**Caltoson Balsamico** *Rottapharm, Spain.*
Cineole (p.1672·1); benzocaine (p.1370·3); pholcodine (p.1128·3); cherry-laurel; terpineol (p.1752·2); menthol (p.1711·3).
*Respiratory-tract disorders.*

**Caltrate**
*Note. This name is used for preparations of different composition.*
*Whitehall Consumer, Austral.; Whitehall-Robins, Canad.; Whitehall, Fr.; Wyeth, Hong Kong; Lederle, Israel; Wyeth Consumer, Malaysia; Wyeth, Mex.; Whitehall, NZ; Whitehall, S.Afr.; Wyeth Consumer, Singapore; Whitehall, Thai.; Lederle, USA.*
Calcium carbonate (p.1254·2).
*Calcium deficiency; calcium supplement; osteomalacia; osteoporosis.*

*Whitehall, Ital.; Whitehall, UK†.*
Calcium (p.1225·1); vitamin D (p.1461·2).
*Calcium deficiency.*

**Caltrate with D** *Whitehall-Robins, Canad.*
Calcium carbonate (p.1254·2); vitamin D (p.1461·2).
*Calcium supplement.*

**Caltrate + D** *Wyeth-Whitehall, Arg.; Whitehall, Braz.; Wyeth, Hong Kong; Wyeth Consumer, Malaysia; Wyeth, Mex.; Whitehall, Thai.*
Calcium (p.1225·1); vitamin D (p.1461·2).
*Calcium and vitamin D supplement; osteomalacia; osteoporosis; rickets; tetany.*

**Caltrate + Iron & Vitamin D** *Whitehall-Robins, Canad.†; Lederle, USA.*
Calcium carbonate (p.1254·2); ferrous fumarate (p.1427·3); vitamin D (p.1461·2).
*Calcium and iron deficiency.*

**Caltrate Jr** *Lederle, USA†.*
Calcium carbonate (p.1254·2).
Formerly contained calcium carbonate and vitamin D.
*Calcium deficiency.*

**Caltrate + M** *Whitehall, Braz.*
Calcium carbonate (p.1254·2); vitamin D (p.1461·2); minerals.

**Caltrate Plus**
*Note. This name is used for preparations of different composition.*
*Whitehall Consumer, Austral.; Whitehall-Robins, Canad.*
Calcium carbonate (p.1254·2); vitamin D (p.1461·2); copper oxide; magnesium oxide; manganese sulfate; zinc oxide (p.1417·1).
*Calcium deficiency; calcium supplement; osteomalacia; osteoporosis.*

*Wyeth, Hong Kong; Wyeth Consumer, Irl.; Whitehall, Israel; Wyeth Consumer, Port.; Wyeth Consumer, Singapore; Whitehall, Thai.; Wyeth Consumer, UK; Lederle, USA.*
Calcium (p.1225·1); colecalciferol (p.1461·3); boron; copper; magnesium; manganese; zinc (p.1417·1).
*Calcium deficiency; calcium supplement; osteomalacia; osteoporosis.*

**Caltrate Plus Mastigavel** *Wyeth Consumer, Port.*
Calcium carbonate (p.1254·2); colecalciferol (p.1461·3); magnesium; zinc; copper; manganese; boron (p.1417·1).
*Osteoporosis.*

**Caltrate + Vit D** *Lederle, Israel; Wyeth Consumer, Singapore.*
Calcium carbonate (p.1254·2); vitamin D (p.1461·2).
*Calcium and vitamin D deficiency.*

**Caltrate + Vitamin D** *Whitehall Consumer, Austral.; Lederle, USA.*
Calcium carbonate (p.1254·2); vitamin D (p.1461·2).
*Calcium and vitamin D deficiency; calcium supplement; osteomalacia; osteoporosis.*

**Caltrate Vitamine $D_3$** *Whitehall, Fr.*
Calcium carbonate (p.1254·2); colecalciferol (p.1461·3).
*Calcium and vitamin D deficiency; osteoporosis.*

**Caltrec** *Columbia, Mex.*
Calcium (p.1225·1); colecalciferol (p.1461·3).
*Calcium supplement.*

**Caltren** *Libbs, Braz.*
Nitrendipine (p.973·3).
*Angina pectoris; heart failure; hypertension; myocardial infarction.*

**Caltro** *Geneva, USA.*
Calcium with vitamin D (p.1417·1).
*Calcium deficiency; dietary supplement.*

**Caltusine** *Rudefsa, Mex.*
Carbocisteine (p.1116·2); oxolamine citrate (p.1126·1).
*Respiratory-tract disorders.*

**Calvakehl** *Sanum-Kehlbeck, Ger.*
Homoeopathic preparation.

**Calvepen** *Leo, Irl.*
Phenoxymethylpenicillin calcium (p.242·1).
*Bacterial infections.*

**Calvidin** *Ergha, Irl.*
Calcium carbonate (p.1254·2); colecalciferol (p.1461·3).
*Calcium and vitamin D deficiency; osteoporosis.*

**Calvita** *Roche Consumer, Austral.†.*
Calcium phosphate (p.1225·3); vitamins and iron (p.1417·1).
*Calcium supplement; dietary supplement.*

**Calvita B12** *De Mayo, Braz.*
Calcium lactate; calcium phosphate; sodium fluoride; colecalciferol; vitamin $B_{12}$ (p.1417·1).

**Calypsol** *Gedeon Richter, Malaysia; Gedeon Richter, Thai.*
Ketamine hydrochloride (p.1302·1).
*General anaesthesia.*

**Calyptol** *Aventis, Ital.*
Cineole (p.1672·1); terpineol (p.1752·2); pine oil; thyme oil (p.1755·3); rosemary oil (p.1740·2).
*Respiratory-tract congestion.*

*Techni-Pharma, Mon.*
Cineole (p.1672·1); terpineol (p.1752·2); oleum pini sylvestris thyme oil (p.1755·3); rosemary oil (p.1740·2).
*Respiratory-tract congestion.*

**Calyptol Inhalante** *Aventis, Spain†.*
Oleum pini sylvestris; rosemary oil (p.1740·2); terpineol (p.1752·2); thyme oil (p.1755·3); eucalyptus (p.1686·1).
*Respiratory-tract congestion.*

**CAM**
*Note. A similar name is used for preparations of different composition (see below).*
*Eversil, Braz.†.*
Theophylline calcium salicylate (p.804·3); potassium iodide (p.1598·1).
*Obstructive airways disease.*

*Rybar, Irl.†.*
Butetamate citrate (p.1116·2).
*Bronchospasm.*

*Cambridge Healthcare, UK.*
Ephedrine hydrochloride (p.1120·1).
*Bronchospasm; cough.*

**Cam**
*Note. A similar name is used for preparations of different composition (see above).*
*Laboratorios Chile, Chile.*
Dexchlorpheniramine maleate (p.427·3); betamethasone (p.1093·1).
*Hypersensitivity reactions.*

**Cama Arthritis Pain Reliever** *Novartis, USA.*
Aspirin (p.15·1).
Aluminium hydroxide (p.1249·2) and magnesium oxide (p.1272·3) are included in this preparation in an attempt to limit adverse effects on the gastrointestinal mucosa.
*Arthritis; pain.*

**Camalox** *Rhone-Poulenc Rorer, Swed.†.*
Aluminium hydroxide (p.1249·2); magnesium hydroxide (p.1272·2); calcium carbonate (p.1254·2).
*Heartburn; peptic ulcer.*

**Camazol** *Xepa-Soul Pattinson, Malaysia; Xepa-Soul Pattinson, Singapore.*
Carbimazole (p.1596·2).
*Hyperthyroidism.*

**Cambem** *UCI, Braz.*
Cambendazole (p.103·3).
*Strongyloidiasis.*

**Camboacy** *Farmavy, Braz.†.*
*Lactobacillus acidophilus* (p.1704·2).
*Diarrhoea; restoration of gastrointestinal flora.*

**Camcolit** *Norgine, Belg.; Norgine, Hong Kong; Norgine, Irl.; Norgine, S.Afr.; Norgine, Singapore; Norgine, UK.*
Lithium carbonate (p.301·1).
*Bipolar disorder; depression; disturbed behaviour; mania.*

**Camegel** *Bonomelli, Ital.†.*
Vitamin and fibre preparation (p.1417·1).
*Diarrhoea.*

**Cameo** *Medco, USA.*
Emollient.

**Camil** *Martin, Spain.*
Cefazolin sodium (p.170·3).
*Bacterial infections.*

**Camilia** *Boiron, Canad.*
Homoeopathic preparation.

**Camiline** *Arkopharma, Fr.*
Camelia sinensis (p.1765·3).
*Asthenia; slimming aid.*

**Caminol** *Geminis, Arg.*
Salicylic acid (p.1157·1); lactic acid (p.1704·1).
*Callus removal.*

**Camoderm**
*Note. This name is used for preparations of different composition.*
*Link, Austral.†.*
Chamomile (p.1669·3); chamomile oil (p.1669·3).
*Nappy rash; skin irritation; sore nipples.*

*Norgine, Hong Kong†.*
Chamomile (p.1669·3); levomenol (p.1707·1).
*Skin irritation.*

**Camomila** *Catarinense, Braz.†.*
Aloes (p.1248·2); paregoric (p.74·2); aniseed (p.1655·2); peppermint leaf (p.1283·2); melissa (p.1711·1); chamomile (p.1669·3); centaury (p.1669·2); condurango (p.1675·3); Fuller's earth (p.1039·3); gentian (p.1692·2); absinthium (p.1645·1); quassia (p.1737·2); rhubarb (p.1287·3); bixa orellana.
*Digestive disorders.*

**Camomilina C** *Igefarma, Braz.†.*
Chamomile (p.1669·3); liquorice (p.1270·2); colecalciferol; vitamin C; calcium phosphate (p.1417·1).
*Nutritional supplement.*

**Camomilla (Specie Composta)** *Dynacren, Ital.*
Valerian (p.1762·2); chamomile (p.1669·3); caraway (p.1667·2); peppermint leaf (p.1283·2).
*Herbal tea; sedative.*

**Camoquin** *Parke, Davis, India.*
Amodiaquine hydrochloride (p.446·3).
*Malaria.*

**Camoxin** *Klinger, Braz.*
Amoxicillin (p.155·3).
*Bacterial infections.*

**Campanyl** *Temmler, Ger.†.*
Potassium polystyrene sulfonate (p.1050·1).
*Hypercalciuria.*

**Campath** *Berlex, USA.*
Alemtuzumab (p.526·1).
*Chronic lymphocytic leukaemia.*

**Campel** *Chiesi, Fr.*
Chromocarb diethylamine (p.1670·3).
*Circulatory disorders; haemorrhoids.*

**Camphoderm N** *Li-il, Ger.*
Camphor (p.1665·3).
*Catarrh; musculoskeletal, joint, and soft-tissue disorders.*

**Camphodionyl** *Distri B3, Fr.*
Sulfogaiacol (p.1131·1); codeine (p.27·1).
*Coughs.*

**Campho-Phenique** *Winthrop Consumer, USA; Sterling, USA.*
Phenol (p.1188·1); camphor (p.1665·3).
*Burns; cuts; herpes labialis; infections; insect bites; pain.*

**Campho-Phenique Antibiotic Plus Pain Reliever Ointment** *Winthrop Consumer, USA†.*
Bacitracin (p.161·3); neomycin sulfate (p.235·1); polymyxin B sulfate (p.245·1); lidocaine (p.1377·3).
Formerly contained diperodon hydrochloride in place of lidocaine.
*Infection prophylaxis and pain relief in minor skin lesions.*

**Camphopin** *Schoning-Berlin, Ger.*
Methyl salicylate (p.59·3); benzyl nicotinate (p.21·2); camphor (p.1665·3).
*Frostbite; neuralgia; rheumatic disorders; sciatica; tendinitis.*

**Campho-Pneumine** *Marion Merrell, Fr.†.*
*Adult suppositories:* Camphor (p.1665·3); guaiacol (p.1122·1); cineole (p.1672·1); guaifenesin (p.1122·1); amylocaine hydrochloride (p.1370·2).
*Suppositories child:* Camphor (p.1665·3); guaiacol (p.1122·1); cineole (p.1672·1); guaifenesin (p.1122·1).
*Suppositories infant:* Cineole (p.1672·1); guaifenesin (p.1122·1).
*Respiratory-tract disorders.*

**Camphor Linctus Compound** *McGloin, Austral.†.*
Camphor (p.1665·3); tolu balsam (p.1131·3).
*Coughs.*

**Camphre Compose** *Valmo, Canad.†.*
Camphor (p.1665·3); menthol (p.1711·3); cineole (p.1672·1).

**Camphrice Du Canada** *Homme de Fer, Fr.*
Camphor (p.1665·3).
*Skin disorders.*

**Campicilin** *Cadila, India.*
Ampicillin (p.157·1).
*Bacterial infections.*

**Campral** *Merck, Arg.; Alphapharm, Austral.; Merck, Austria; Merck, Belg.; Merck, Braz.; Merck, Chile; Lipha, Denm.; Merck, Ger.; Merck-Lipha, Hong Kong; Lipha, Irl.; Merck, Mex.; Merck, Neth.; Lipha, Norw.; Merck, Port.; Merck, Singapore; Merck-Lipha, Singapore; Merck, Spain; Merck, Swed.; Lipha, Switz.; Merck, UK.*
Acamprosate calcium (p.668·1).
*Alcoholism.*

**Campto** *Aventis, Austria; Aventis, Belg.; Aventis, Denm.; Aventis, Fin.; Aventis, Fr.; Aventis, Ger.; Rhone-Poulenc Rorer, Gr.; Aventis, Hong Kong; Aventis, Irl.; Aventis, Israel; Aventis, Ital.; Aventis, Malaysia; Aventis, Neth.; Aventis, Norw.; Aventis, Port.; Aventis, S.Afr.; Aventis, Singapore; Pras, Spain; Aventis, Swed.; Aventis, Switz.; Aventis, Thai.; Aventis, UK.*
Irinotecan hydrochloride (p.564·1).
*Colorectal cancer.*

**Camptosar** *Pharmacia, Arg.; Pharmacia, Austral.; Pharmacia, Braz.; Pharmacia, Canad.; Pharmacia, Chile; Pharmacia Upjohn, Mex.; Pharmacia, NZ; Pharmacia, USA.*
Irinotecan hydrochloride (p.564·1).
*Colorectal cancer.*

**Canadine** *Nakorn, Thai.*
Clotrimazole (p.396·2).
*Fungal skin infections.*

**Canadiol** *Esteve, Spain.*
Itraconazole (p.401·3).
*Fungal infections.*

**Canalba** *Aspen, S.Afr.*
Clotrimazole (p.396·2).
*Fungal skin and vulvovaginal infections.*

**Canasa** *Axcan, USA.*
Mesalazine (p.1273·2).
*Inflammatory bowel disease.*

**Canasone** *Nakorn, Thai.*
Clotrimazole (p.396·2); betamethasone dipropionate (p.1093·1).
*Fungal skin infections.*

**Canazol**
*Durascan, Denm.†; TO-Chemicals, Thai.*
Clotrimazole (p.396·2).
*Fungal skin, oropharyngeal, and vaginal infections; trichomoniasis.*

**Canazol-BE** *TO-Chemicals, Thai.*
Clotrimazole (p.396·2); betamethasone valerate (p.1093·2).
*Fungal skin infections.*

**Cancidas**
*Merck Sharp & Dohme, Arg.; Merck Sharp & Dohme, Austral.; Merck Sharp & Dohme, Chile; Merck Sharp & Dohme, Hong Kong; Merck Sharp & Dohme, NZ; Merck Sharp & Dohme, Singapore; Merck Sharp & Dohme, UK; Merck, USA.*
Caspofungin acetate (p.395·3).
*Aspergillosis.*

**Candacide** *Be-Tabs, S.Afr.*
Nystatin (p.406·3).
*Oral candidiasis.*

**Candacort** *Hoe, Malaysia.*
Clotrimazole (p.396·2); hydrocortisone (p.1103·3).
*Fungal skin infections.*

**Candalba** *Brauer, Austral.†.*
Homoeopathic preparation.

**Candaspor** *Be-Tabs, S.Afr.*
Clotrimazole (p.396·2).
*Fungal skin and vulvovaginal infections.*

**Candazol** *Apogepha, Ger.*
Clotrimazole (p.396·2).
*Fungal and bacterial vaginal infections; trichomoniasis.*

**Candazole**
*Hoe, Malaysia; Hoe, Singapore.*
Clotrimazole (p.396·2).
*Fungal skin infections.*

**Canderel**
*Searle, Mex.†; Monsanto, Port.†.*
Aspartame (p.1422·1).
*Sugar substitute.*

**Canderme** *Legrand, Braz.*
Metronidazole (p.607·2) or metronidazole benzoate (p.607·2).

**Candermil** *Kampel Martian, Arg.*
Nystatin (p.406·3).
*Fungal infections.*

**Candermyl** *Galderma, Austral.†.*
Emollient.

**Candesar** *Stancare, India.*
Candesartan (p.878·3).
*Hypertension.*

**Candibene** *Ratiopharm, Austria.*
Clotrimazole (p.396·2).
*Fungal infections; trichomoniasis.*

**Candicort** *Ache, Braz.*
Ketoconazole (p.403·3); betamethasone (p.1093·1).
*Infected skin disorders.*

**Candid**
*Neves, Port.; Glenmark, Thai.*
Clotrimazole (p.396·2).
*Fungal ear, mouth, skin, and vaginal infections; trichomoniasis.*

**Candida Yeast** *Homeocan, Canad.*
Homoeopathic preparation.

**Candiden** *Akita, UK.*
Clotrimazole (p.396·2).
*Fungal infections.*

**Candiderm** *Ache, Braz.*
Ketoconazole (p.403·3).
*Fungal skin infections.*

**Candidine** *Stallergenes, Fr.†.*
Candida albicans antigen (p.1650·1).
*Allergen immunotherapy of Candida albicans; diagnosis of hypersensitivity to Candida albicans.*

**Candimon** *Andromaco, Mex.*
Clotrimazole (p.396·2).
*Fungal skin and vaginal infections.*

**Candimyc** *Viofar, Gr.*
Ciclopirox olamine (p.396·1).
*Fungal skin infections.*

**Candinox** *Charoen, Thai.*
Clotrimazole (p.396·2).
*Fungal mouth, throat, and vaginal infections; trichomoniasis.*

**Candio**
*Hermal, Austria; Hermal, Ger.; Boots Healthcare, Switz.†.*
Nystatin (p.406·3).
*Fungal infections.*

**Candio-Hermal Plus** *Hermal, Ger.*
Nystatin (p.406·3); fluprednidene acetate (p.1102·2).
Formerly known as Candio E comp N.
*Inflammatory skin disorders with fungal infection.*

**Candiplas**
*Medochemie, Singapore†; Medochemie, Thai.†.*
Miconazole nitrate (p.405·3).
*Fungal and Gram-positive bacterial infections.*

**Candipres** *Precimex, Mex.†.*
Amphotericin B (p.391·2).
*Fungal infections.*

**Candistat** *Merck, India.*
Itraconazole (p.401·3).
*Fungal infections.*

**Candistatin**
*Cristalia, Braz.; Teuto, Braz.; Westwood-Squibb, Canad.*
Nystatin (p.406·3).
*Fungal infections.*

**Canditral** *Glenmark, Singapore.*
Itraconazole (p.401·3).
*Fungal infections.*

**Candizol**
*Ache, Braz.; Fustery, Mex.*
Fluconazole (p.398·1).
*Fungal infections.*

**Candizole** *Aspen, S.Afr.*
Clotrimazole (p.396·2).
*Fungal skin and vulvovaginal infections.*

**Candizole-T** *Unichem, India.*
Tinidazole (p.617·1); miconazole nitrate (p.405·3); neomycin sulfate (p.235·1).
*Vaginal candidiasis.*

**Candoral** *Ache, Braz.*
Ketoconazole (p.403·3).
*Fungal infections.*

**Candyl**
*Douglas, Austral.; Douglas, Thai.†; TTN, Thai.†.*
Piroxicam (p.84·2).
*Musculoskeletal and joint disorders.*

**Candyl-D** *Douglas, NZ.*
Piroxicam (p.84·2).
*Dysmenorrhoea; gout; musculoskeletal and joint disorders.*

**Canef**
*AstraZeneca, Denm.; AstraZeneca, Fin.; Astra, Mex.; AstraZeneca, Neth.; AstraZeneca, Norw.†; AstraZeneca, Port.; Hassle, Swed.*
Fluvastatin sodium (p.918·2).
*Atherosclerosis; hypercholesterolaemia.*

**Canephron** *Bionorica, Ger.*
Centaury (p.1669·2); lovage (p.1708·1); rosemary (p.1740·2).
*Renal calculi; urinary-tract disorders.*

**Canephron N** *Bionorica, Hong Kong†.*
Centaury (p.1669·2); lovage (p.1708·1); rosemary (p.1740·2).
*Urinary-tract disorders.*

**Canephron novo** *Bionorica, Ger.*
Birch leaf (p.1660·3); java tea (p.1702·3); solidago virgaurea (p.1748·3).
*Renal calculi; urinary-tract disorders.*

**Canephron S** *Bionorica, Ger.*
Solidago virgaurea (p.1748·3).
*Renal calculi; urinary-tract disorders.*

**Canesten**
*Bayer, Austral.; Bayer, Austria; Bayer, Braz.; Bayer Consumer, Canad.; Bayer, Chile; Bayer, Denm.; Bayer, Fin.; Bayer, Ger.; Bayer, Gr.; Bayer, Hong Kong; Bayer, Irl.; Bayer, Ital.; Bayer Consumer, Malaysia; Bayer Consumer, Mex.†; Bayer, Neth.; Bayer, Norw.; Bayer, NZ; Bayer, Port.; Bayer, S.Afr.; Bayer Consumer, Singapore; Bayer, Spain; Bayer, Swed.; Bayer, Thai.; Bayer Consumer, UK.*
Clotrimazole (p.396·2).
*Fungal and bacterial infections; trichomoniasis.*

**Canesten AF Once Daily** *Bayer Consumer, UK.*
Bifonazole (p.395·1).
*Athlete's foot.*

**Canesten Combi** *Bayer Consumer, UK.*
*Combination pack containing Canesten Cream and Canesten 1 pessary:* Clotrimazole (p.396·2).
*Vulvovaginal candidiasis.*

**Canesten Extra** *Bayer, Ger.*
Bifonazole (p.395·1).
*Fungal skin infections.*

**Canesten HC**
*Bayer, Ger.; Bayer, Hong Kong; Bayer, Irl.; Bayer Consumer, Singapore; Bayer Consumer, UK.*
Clotrimazole (p.396·2); hydrocortisone (p.1103·3).
*Fungal skin infections with inflammation.*

**Canesten Oasis** *Bayer Consumer, UK.*
Sodium citrate (p.1223·2).
*Cystitis.*

**Canesten Once Daily** *Bayer, Austral.*
Bifonazole (p.395·1).
*Fungal skin infections.*

**Canesten Oral** *Bayer, UK.*
Fluconazole (p.398·1).
*Candidal balanitis; vaginal candidiasis.*

**Canestene**
*Bayer, Belg.; Bayer, Switz.*
Clotrimazole (p.396·2).
*Fungal and bacterial infections; trichomoniasis.*

**Canex** *Alliance, S.Afr.*
Clotrimazole (p.396·2).
*Fungal skin and vulvovaginal infections.*

**Canfomenol** *Brasmedica, Braz.†.*
Niaouli oil (p.1719·3); camphor (p.1665·3); cineole (p.1672·1); guaiacol (p.1122·1); menthol (p.1711·3); ephedrine (p.1120·1).
*Respiratory-tract congestion.*

**Canfosalicilica** *Farmatre, Ital.; Ogna, Ital.; Sella, Ital.*
Camphor (p.1665·3); methyl salicylate (p.59·3).
*Muscle and joint pain.*

**Canifug** *Wolff, Ger.*
Clotrimazole (p.396·2).
*Fungal and bacterial infections; trichomoniasis.*

**Cankerol** *Coradol, Ger.*
Homoeopathic preparation.

**Canoderm** *ACO Hud, Swed.*
Urea (p.1162·2).
*Dry skin.*

**Canol** *Jolly-Jatel, Fr.*
Cynara (p.1678·3); chimaphylla; aphloia.
*Dyspepsia.*

**Canovex** *Microsules, Arg.*
Dipyrone (p.35·3); dextropropoxyphene napsilate (p.28·3) or dextropropoxyphene hydrochloride (p.28·3).
*Fever; pain.*

**Canrenol** *Grunenthal, Belg.*
Potassium canrenoate (p.984·2).
*Cirrhosis; electrolyte disturbances; heart failure; hyperaldosteronism; hypertension; nephrotic syndrome.*

**Canscreen** *Draxis, Canad.*
Avobenzone (p.1142·3); octinoxate (p.1154·3); oxybenzone (p.1154·3).
*Sunscreen.*

**Canstat** *Wyeth, S.Afr.†.*
Nystatin (p.406·3).
*Candidiasis.*

**Cantabilin** *Formenti, Ital.*
Hymecromone (p.1700·1).
*Biliary-tract disorders; liver disorders.*

**Cantabiline**
*Merck, Belg.; Lipha Sante, Fr.*
Hymecromone (p.1700·1).
*Biliary-tract disorders; dyspepsia.*

**Cantadrill** *Pierre Fabre Sante, Fr.*
Erysimum.
*Mouth and throat disorders.*

**Cantalene** *Cooperation Pharmaceutique, Fr.*
Muramidase hydrochloride (p.1717·2); chlorhexidine acetate (p.1173·2); tetracaine hydrochloride (p.1385·1).
*Mouth and throat disorders.*

**Cantamac** *Cantassium Co., UK†.*
Multivitamin and mineral preparation (p.1417·1).

**Cantamega** *Larkhall Laboratories, UK†.*
Multivitamin and mineral preparation (p.1417·1).

**Cantapollen** *Cantassium Co., UK†.*
Dolomite; bee pollen.

**Cantassium Discs** *Cantassium Co., UK†.*
Mineral preparation (p.1417·1).

**Cantavite with FF** *Cantassium Co., UK†.*
Multivitamin and mineral preparation (p.1417·1).

**Canthacur**
*Paladin, Canad.; Pharmascience, Singapore†.*
Cantharidin (p.1667·1).
*Molluscum contagiosum; warts.*

**Canthacur-PS** *Paladin, Canad.*
Cantharidin (p.1667·1); podophyllum resin (p.1155·2); salicylic acid (p.1157·1).
*Molluscum contagiosum; warts.*

**Cantharis Med Complex** *Dynamit, Austria.*
Homoeopathic preparation.

**Cantharone** *Dormer, Canad.*
Cantharidin (p.1667·1).
*Molluscum contagiosum; warts.*

**Cantharone Plus** *Dormer, Canad.*
Cantharidin (p.1667·1); podophyllum resin (p.1155·2); salicylic acid (p.1157·1).
*Warts.*

**Cantil**
*Tika, Swed.; Hoechst Marion Roussel, USA.*
Mepenzolate bromide (p.485·3).
*Adjunctive therapy in peptic ulcer; spasmodic disorders of the colon.*

**Cantipal** *Loren, Mex.*
Paracetamol (p.76·2); caffeine (p.782·1); chlorphenamine (p.428·1); phenylephrine (p.1126·3).
*Cold symptoms.*

**Cantopal** *Larkhall Laboratories, UK†.*
Calcium pantothenate (p.1442·3).

**Cantril** *Talcris, Arg.*
Clobetasol (p.1095·3).
*Skin disorders.*

**Canusal** *CP Pharmaceuticals, UK.*
Heparin sodium (p.928·1).
*To maintain patency of in-dwelling intravascular lines.*

**Caolax** *Labima, Belg.†.*
Phenolphthalein (p.1284·1).
*Bowel evacuation; constipation.*

**Caomet** *AstraZeneca, Ital.†.*
Ubidecarenone (p.1760·2).
*Cardiac disorders.*

**Caopecfar** *Alpharma, Mex.*
Furazolidone (p.605·2); pectin (p.1580·3); kaolin (p.1268·3).
*Diarrhoea.*

**Caosina** *Ern, Spain.*
Calcium carbonate (p.1254·2).
*Calcium deficiency; calcium supplement; osteoporosis.*

**Caosina D** *Ern, Spain.*
Calcium carbonate (p.1254·2); colecalciferol (p.1461·3).
*Calcium and vitamin D deficiency.*

**Capace**
*Amrad, Austral.†; Hexal, Austria; Garec, S.Afr.*
Captopril (p.879·2).
*Diabetic nephropathy; heart failure; hypertension; myocardial infarction.*

**Capadex**
*Fawns & McAllan, Austral.; Sigma, NZ.*
Dextropropoxyphene hydrochloride (p.28·3); paracetamol (p.76·2).
*Fever; pain.*

**Caparin** *Osotspa, Thai.*
Aspirin (p.15·1).
Glycine (p.1433·3) is included in this preparation in an attempt to limit adverse effects on the gastrointestinal mucosa.
*Thromboembolism prophylaxis.*

**Capasal**
*Dermal Laboratories, Irl.; Dermal, Israel; Dermal Laboratories, UK.*
Salicylic acid (p.1157·1); coal tar (p.1159·2).
*Scalp disorders.*

**Capastat**
*Lilly, Austral.; Lilly, Austria; Lilly, Canad.†; IFET (ΙΦΕΤ), Gr.; Dista, Spain; King, UK; Dura, USA.*
Capreomycin sulfate (p.166·1).
*Pulmonary tuberculosis.*

**CAPD**
*Fresenius, Israel; Fresenius Medical, Spain.*
A range of electrolyte solutions with glucose (p.1221·1).
*Peritoneal dialysis.*

**CAPD/DPCA**
*Fresenius Medical, Denm.; Fresenius Medical, Spain; Dicamed, Swed.*
Anhydrous glucose; sodium chloride; sodium lactate; calcium chloride; magnesium chloride (p.1221·1).
Formerly known as Lockolys in *Swed.*
*Peritoneal dialysis.*

**Capel** *Ache, Braz.*
Ketoconazole (p.403·3); panthenol (p.1727·2).
*Seborrhoeic dermatitis.*

**Capent** *Andromaco, Chile.*
Loperamide (p.1271·2).
*Diarrhoea.*

**Capergyl** *Bailleul, Fr.*
Co-dergocrine mesilate (p.1674·1).
*Mental function disorders.*

**Capex**
*Galderma, Canad.; Galderma, USA.*
Fluocinolone acetonide (p.1101·2).
Formerly known as FS in the *USA.*
*Scalp disorders.*

**Capginvit**
*Atlantic, Hong Kong; Atlantic, Thai.*
Multivitamin preparation (p.1417·1).

**Capibaryne** *Osorio de Moraes, Braz.†.*
Vitamin B substances with minerals (p.1417·1).

**Capilarema**
*Baldacci, Braz.; Baldacci, Port.; Zambon, Spain.*
Aminaphthone (p.741·3).
*Capillary disorders; haemorrhage.*

**Capill** *Pharma Italia, Ital.*
Centella (p.1144·3); aesculus (p.1648·2); red vine; myrtillus (p.1718·3); vitamin C (p.1460·2); vitamin E (p.1464·3).
*Capillary disorders; oedema.*

**Capillarema** *Baldacci, Ital.*
Aminaphthone (p.741·3).
*Capillary disorders.*

**Capillaron** *Madaus, Ger.*
Homoeopathic preparation.

**Capillon** *Gramse, Israel†.*
Cetrimide (p.1172·1).
*Seborrhoeic dermatitis of the scalp.*

**Capiloton** *Virtus, Braz.†.*
Jaborandi; sweet birch oil (p.60·1).
*Alopecia.*

**Capistan** *Sanofi Winthrop, Fr.†.*
Saw palmetto (p.1569·1).
*Benign prostatic hyperplasia.*

**Capital with Codeine** *Carnrick, USA.*
Paracetamol (p.76·2); codeine phosphate (p.27·1).
*Pain.*

**Capitis** *Fecofar, Arg.*
*Cream:* Permethrin (p.1508·3).
*Lotion:* Deltamethrin (p.1503·1); piperonyl butoxide (p.1509·2).
*Pediculosis.*

**Capitrol** *Westwood-Squibb, USA.*
Chloroxine (p.220·3).
*Seborrhoeic dermatitis.*

**Capiven** *Servier, Denm.*
Diosmin (p.1688·2); hesperidin (p.1688·2).
*Haemorrhoids; venous insufficiency.*

**Caplenal**
*Rhone-Poulenc Rorer, Hong Kong†; Berk, Irl.†; Berk, UK.*
Allopurinol (p.412·2).
*Gout; hyperuricaemia; renal calculi.*

**Capocard** *Dar Al Dawa, Hong Kong.*
Captopril (p.879·2).
*Heart failure; hypertension.*

**Caposan** *Adler, Switz.*
Propyphenazone (p.85·3); paracetamol (p.76·2); caffeine (p.782·1).
*Fever; pain.*

**Caposten** *Chinoin, Mex.*
Hydroxyprogesterone (p.1556·3).

**Capoten**
*Bristol-Myers Squibb, Austral.; Bristol-Myers Squibb, Belg.; Bristol-Myers Squibb, Braz.; Squibb, Canad.; Bristol-Myers Squibb, Chile; Bristol-Myers Squibb, Denm.; Bristol-Myers Squibb, Fin.; Bristol-Myers Squibb, Gr.; Bristol-Myers Squibb, Hong Kong; Bristol-Myers Squibb, Irl.; Bristol-Myers Squibb, Ital.; Bristol-Myers Squibb, Malaysia; Bristol-Myers Squibb, Neth.; Bristol-Myers Squibb, Norw.; Bristol-Myers Squibb, NZ; Bristol-Myers Squibb, Port.; Bristol-Myers Squibb, S.Afr.; Bristol-Myers Squibb, Singapore; Squibb, Spain; Bristol-Myers Squibb,*

Swed.; Bristol-Myers Squibb, Thai.; Bristol-Myers Squibb, UK; Bristol-Myers Squibb, USA.
Captopril (p.879·2).
*Diabetic nephropathy; heart failure; hypertension; myocardial infarction.*

**Capotena** Bristol-Myers Squibb, Mex.
Captopril (p.879·2).
*Heart failure; hypertension; myocardial infarction.*

**Capotril** Neo Quimica, Braz.
Captopril (p.879·2).
*Hypertension.*

**Capozid**
Bristol-Myers Squibb, Denm.; Bristol-Myers Squibb, Swed.†.
Captopril (p.879·2); hydrochlorothiazide (p.933·2).
*Hypertension.*

**Capozide**
Bristol-Myers Squibb, Austria; Bristol-Myers Squibb, Ger.; Bristol-Myers Squibb, Irl.; Bristol-Myers Squibb, Mex.; Bristol-Myers Squibb, Neth.; Bristol-Myers Squibb, NZ†; Bristol-Myers Squibb, S.Afr.; Bristol-Myers Squibb, Switz.; Bristol-Myers Squibb, UK; Bristol-Myers Squibb, USA.
Captopril (p.879·2); hydrochlorothiazide (p.933·2).
These ingredients can be described by the British Approved Name Co-zidocapt.
*Hypertension.*

**Capramin** Glaxo Wellcome, Austria†.
Aspirin (p.15·1); carbinoxamine maleate (p.426·3); phenylephrine hydrochloride (p.1126·3); caffeine (p.782·1).
*Cold and influenza symptoms.*

**Capricin** Sisu, Canad.†.
Octanoic acid (p.1723·1).
*Elimination of intestinal Candida albicans.*

**Capril**
Teuto, Braz.; Merck, Hong Kong.
Captopril (p.879·2).
*Diabetic nephropathy; heart failure; hypertension; myocardial infarction.*

**Caprilate** Eagle, Austral.†.
Sodium octanoate (p.1723·1); berberis vulgaris; magnesium chloride (p.1228·1); zinc gluconate (p.1469·2); lithium chloride (p.305·1); sorbic acid (p.1192·3).
*Inhibition of gastrointestinal yeast growth.*

**Caprilon**
Note. This name is used for preparations of different composition.
Scientific Hospital Supplies, Austral.; Scientific Hospital Supplies, Irl.; Nutricia, Ital.; Scientific Hospital Supplies, UK.
Preparation for enteral nutrition containing medium-chain triglycerides (p.1440·3).
*Disorders of fat metabolism.*

Leiras, Fin.
Tranexamic acid (p.760·3).
*Fibrinolysis; hereditary angioedema.*

**Caprimida** Osteolab, Chile.
Calcium carbonate (p.1254·2).
*Calcium supplement.*

**Caprimida D** Osteolab, Chile.
Calcium carbonate (p.1254·2); colecalciferol (p.1461·3).
*Calcium and vitamin D supplement.*

**Caprin**
Sinclair, Irl.; Sinclair, UK.
Aspirin (p.15·1).
*Fever; inflammation; pain; thrombosis prophylaxis.*

**Caprisana** Sidroga, Switz.†.
Camphor (p.1665·3); juniper oil (p.1703·1); rosemary oil (p.1740·2); turpentine oil (p.1760·1); thyme oil (p.1755·3); larch oil.
*Musculoskeletal and joint pain.*

**Caprisset** Solfran, Mex.
Multivitamin and mineral preparation (p.1417·1).

**Caproamin** Fides Ecopharma, Spain.
Aminocaproic acid (p.741·3).
*Haemorrhage.*

**Caprofides Hemostatico** Fides Ecopharma, Spain.
Aminocaproic acid (p.741·3); esculoside (p.1648·2); hesperidin methyl chalcone (p.1688·3); menadione (p.1466·3); creatinine sulfate.
*Haemorrhage.*

**Caprolisin** Malesci, Ital.
Aminocaproic acid (p.741·3).
*Haemorrhagic disorders.*

**Capros** Medac, Ger.
Morphine sulfate (p.60·2).
*Pain.*

**Caprysin** Leiras, Fin.†.
Clonidine hydrochloride (p.885·2).
*Hypertension; opioid and alcohol withdrawal syndromes.*

**Capsamol** Worwag, Ger.
*Ointment:* Capsicum (p.1667·1).
*Musculoskeletal and joint pain.*

*Topical application:* Benzyl nicotinate (p.21·2); capsaicin (p.24·2).
*Rheumatic disorders.*

**Capsic** Pierre Fabre Sante, Fr.†.
*Dressing:* Capsicum (p.1667·1); methyl salicylate (p.59·3); camphor (p.1665·3).
*Ointment:* Capsaicin (p.24·2); methyl nicotinate (p.59·2).
*Muscle cramp.*

**Capsicin** Vinas, Spain.
Capsaicin (p.24·2).
*Diabetic neuropathy.*

**Capsicof** Pharmacaps, Mex.†.
Benzonatate (p.1115·3).
*Coughs.*

**Capsicum + Arthri-Cream** Homeocan, Canad.
Homoeopathic preparation.

**Capsicum Farmaya** Alacan, Spain.
Capsaicin (p.24·2).
*Diabetic neuropathy.*

**Capsidol**
Janssen, Mex.; Vinas, Spain.
Capsaicin (p.24·2).
*Diabetic neuropathy; musculoskeletal and joint disorders.*

**Capsin** Fleming, USA.
Capsaicin (p.24·2).
*Neuralgia; pain.*

**Capsina** Bioglan, Swed.
Capsaicin (p.24·2).
*Postherpetic neuralgia.*

**Capsiplast** Beiersdorf, Austria†.
Capsicum (p.1667·1).
*Musculoskeletal and joint disorders.*

**Capso** RDC, Ital.
Capsicum oleoresin (p.1667·1); aloe vera (p.1141·3).
*Skin disorders.*

**Capsoid** Caps, S.Afr.
Prednisolone (p.1108·1).
*Corticosteroid.*

**Capsolin**
Note. This name is used for preparations of different composition.
Parke, Davis, Austral.†.
Capsicum oleoresin (p.1667·1); camphor (p.1665·3); turpentine oil (p.1760·1); cajuput oil (p.1664·1).
*Joint and muscle pain.*

Warner-Lambert, Ital.; Parke, Davis, Switz.†.
Capsicum oleoresin (p.1667·1); camphor (p.1665·3); turpentine oil (p.1760·1); eucalyptus oil (p.1686·2).
*Joint and muscle pain; soft-tissue disorders.*

**Capson** Pharmatrix, Arg.
Aloe vera (p.1141·3).
*Skin disorders.*

**Capsulas Handel** Casasco, Arg.
Castor oil (p.1668·2).
*Constipation.*

**Capsules laxatives Nattermann Nr. 13** Piraud, Switz.†.
Senna (p.1288·2); caraway oil (p.1667·3); anise oil (p.1655·2).
*Bowel evacuation; constipation.*

**Capsules-vital** Biomed, Switz.
Ginkgo biloba (p.1692·3); glutamic acid; magnesium glycerophosphate; magnesium orotate (p.1417·1).
*Tonic.*

**Capsuvac** Galen, UK.
Dantron (p.1261·1); docusate sodium (p.1262·2).
These ingredients can be described by the British Approved Name Co-danthrusate.
*Constipation.*

**Capsyl** Sandoz, Fr.†.
Dextromethorphan hydrobromide (p.1117·3).
*Coughs.*

**Captagon**
Viatris, Belg.; Viatris, Ger.
Fenetylline hydrochloride (p.1588·2).
*Hyperactivity disorders; tonic.*

**Captaton** Biotenk, Arg.
Fluoxetine hydrochloride (p.292·1).
*Depression.*

**Captea** Aventis, Fr.
Captopril (p.879·2); hydrochlorothiazide (p.933·2).
*Hypertension.*

**Capti** Genpharm, Israel.
Captopril (p.879·2).
*Diabetic nephropathy; heart failure; hypertension; myocardial infarction.*

**Captil** Hebron, Braz.
Captopril (p.879·2).
*Hypertension.*

**Captimer** MIT, Ger.
Tiopronin (p.1054·3).
*Cystinuria; heavy metal poisoning; liver disorders.*

**Captin** Krewel, Ger.
Paracetamol (p.76·2).
*Fever; pain.*

**Captirex** Irex, Fr.†.
Captopril (p.879·2).
*Heart failure; hypertension.*

**Capto** CT, Ger.; ABZ, Ger.; corax, Ger.; Eu Rho, Ger.; Alpharma-Isis, Ger.; Lichtenstein, Ger.; 1A, Ger.
Captopril (p.879·2).
*Heart failure; hypertension.*

**Capto Comp** 1A, Ger.; CT, Ger.; corax, Ger.; Lichtenstein, Ger.
Captopril (p.879·2); hydrochlorothiazide (p.933·2).
*Hypertension.*

**Capto Plus** Isis Puren, Ger.
Captopril (p.879·2); hydrochlorothiazide (p.933·2).
*Hypertension.*

**capto-basan** Schonenberger, Switz.
Captopril (p.879·2).
*Diabetic nephropathy; heart failure; hypertension; left ventricular dysfunction following myocardial infarction.*

**Captobeta** Betapharm, Ger.
Captopril (p.879·2).
*Heart failure; hypertension.*

**Captobeta Comp** Betapharm, Ger.
Captopril (p.879·2); hydrochlorothiazide (p.933·2).
*Hypertension.*

**Capto-Co** Ivax, UK.
Captopril (p.879·2); hydrochlorothiazide (p.933·2).
These ingredients can be described by the British Approved Name Co-zidocapt.
*Hypertension.*

**Captocomp** Ebewe, Austria.
Verapamil hydrochloride (p.1019·1); captopril (p.879·2).
*Hypertension.*

**Captodan** Pharmacodane, Denm.
Captopril (p.879·2).
*Heart failure; hypertension.*

**Captodoc** Docpharm, Ger.
Captopril (p.879·2).
*Heart failure; hypertension.*

**Captodoc Comp** Docpharm, Ger.
Captopril (p.879·2); hydrochlorothiazide (p.933·2).
*Hypertension.*

**Capto-dura Cor** Durachemie, Ger.†.
Captopril (p.879·2).
*Heart failure; hypertension.*

**Capto-dura M** Merck dura, Ger.
Captopril (p.879·2).
*Heart failure; hypertension.*

**Captoflux** Hennig, Ger.
Captopril (p.879·2).
*Heart failure; hypertension.*

**Captogamma** Worwag, Ger.
Captopril (p.879·2).
*Heart failure; hypertension.*

**Captogamma HCT** Worwag, Ger.
Captopril (p.879·2); hydrochlorothiazide (p.933·2).
*Hypertension.*

**Captohexal**
Hexal, Austral.; Hexal, Ger.; Hexal, NZ; Hexal, S.Afr.
Captopril (p.879·2).
*Diabetic nephropathy; heart failure; hypertension; myocardial infarction.*

**Captohexal Comp** Hexal, Ger.
Captopril (p.879·2); hydrochlorothiazide (p.933·2).
*Hypertension.*

**Captol**
Note. This name is used for preparations of different composition.
Durascan, Denm.
Captopril (p.879·2).
*Diabetic nephropathy; heart failure; hypertension; myocardial infarction.*

Pacific, NZ.
Oxprenolol hydrochloride (p.978·1).
*Angina pectoris; arrhythmias; hypertension.*

**Captolane** Aventis, Fr.
Captopril (p.879·2).
*Diabetic nephropathy; heart failure; hypertension; myocardial infarction.*

**Captomax** Parke-Med, S.Afr.
Captopril (p.879·2).
*Heart failure; hypertension; myocardial infarction.*

**Captomed**
Ebewe, Austria; Cimed, Braz.
Captopril (p.879·2).
*Diabetic nephropathy; heart failure; hypertension; myocardial infarction.*

**Captomerck** Merck dura, Ger.
Captopril (p.879·2).
*Heart failure; hypertension.*

**Captomin** Ratiopharm, Fin.
Captopril (p.879·2).
*Diabetic nephropathy; heart failure; hypertension; myocardial infarction.*

**Capton** Royton, Braz.
Captopril (p.879·2).
*Hypertension.*

**Capton Diet** Dexo, Switz.†.
Phenylpropanolamine hydrochloride (p.1127·3).
*Obesity.*

**Captopiril** Bunker, Braz.
Captopril (p.879·2).
*Hypertension.*

**Captoplus** Ratiopharm, Austria.
Captopril (p.879·2); hydrochlorothiazide (p.933·2).
*Hypertension.*

**Captopril Comp** Heumann, Ger.; Basics, Ger.
Captopril (p.879·2); hydrochlorothiazide (p.933·2).
*Hypertension.*

**Captopril Compositum** Faromed, Austria; Mayrhofer, Austria.
Captopril (p.879·2); hydrochlorothiazide (p.933·2).
*Hypertension.*

**Captopril HCT** Acis, Ger.; Aliud, Ger.; Stada, Ger.
Captopril (p.879·2); hydrochlorothiazide (p.933·2).
*Hypertension.*

**Captopril Plus** Verla, Ger.
Captopril (p.879·2); hydrochlorothiazide (p.933·2).
*Hypertension.*

**Captor**
Hexal, Austria; Rowex, Irl.
Captopril (p.879·2).
*Diabetic nephropathy; heart failure; hypertension; myocardial infarction.*

**Captoreal** Realpharma, Ger.†.
Captopril (p.879·2).
*Heart failure; hypertension.*

**Captoretic** Hexal, S.Afr.
Captopril (p.879·2); hydrochlorothiazide (p.933·2).
*Hypertension.*

**Captor-HCT** Rowex, Irl.
Captopril (p.879·2); hydrochlorothiazide (p.933·2).
*Hypertension.*

**Captoser** Serral, Mex.
Captopril (p.879·2).
*Hypertension.*

**Captosina** Ciclum, Spain.
Captopril (p.879·2).
*Diabetic nephropathy; heart failure; hypertension; myocardial infarction.*

**Captosol** Ecosol, Switz.
Captopril (p.879·2).
*Diabetic nephropathy; heart failure; hypertension; left ventricular dysfunction following myocardial infarction.*

**Captosol comp** Ecosol, Switz.
Captopril (p.879·2); hydrochlorothiazide (p.933·2).
*Heart failure; hypertension.*

**Captostad** Berner, Fin.
Captopril (p.879·2).
*Heart failure; hypertension.*

**Captotec** Hexal, Braz.
Captopril (p.879·2).
*Hypertension.*

**Captotec + HCT** Hexal, Braz.
Captopril (p.879·2); hydrochlorothiazide (p.933·2).
*Hypertension.*

**Captotyrol** Tyrol, Austria.
Captopril (p.879·2).
*Diabetic nephropathy; heart failure; hypertension; myocardial infarction.*

**Captral** Silanes, Mex.
Captopril (p.879·2).
*Heart failure; hypertension; myocardial infarction.*

**Captril** Technilab, Canad.†.
Captopril (p.879·2).

**Captrizin** Prodotti, Braz.
Captopril (p.879·2).
*Hypertension.*

**Captus** Laboratorios Chile, Chile.
Pseudoephedrine hydrochloride (p.1129·2); paracetamol (p.76·2); noscapine (p.1125·3); ascorbic acid (p.1460·2).
*Cold and influenza symptoms.*

**Capurate** Sigma, Austral.
Allopurinol (p.412·2).
*Gout; hyperuricaemia; renal calculi.*

**Capval** Dreluso, Ger.
Noscapine resinate or noscapine hydrochloride (p.1125·3).
*Coughs and associated respiratory-tract disorders.*

**Capxidin** Malayan, Singapore.
Piroxicam (p.84·2).
*Gout; musculoskeletal and joint disorders; pain.*

**Capzasin-P**
Stella, Canad.†; Thompson, USA.
Capsaicin (p.24·2).
*Pain.*

**Car Ti Buron** Lafarmen, Arg.
Cartilage (shark).
*Musculoskeletal and joint disorders.*

**Carac** Dermik, USA.
Fluorouracil (p.554·2).
*Actinic keratoses; solar keratoses.*

**Carace**
Du Pont, Irl.; Bristol-Myers Squibb, UK.
Lisinopril (p.946·3).
*Heart failure; hypertension; myocardial infarction.*

**Carace Plus**
Du Pont, Irl.; Bristol-Myers Squibb, UK.
Lisinopril (p.946·3); hydrochlorothiazide (p.933·2).
*Hypertension.*

**Caradrin** Fresenius Kabi, Austria†.
Proscillaridin (p.990·3).
*Cardiac disorders.*

**Carafate**
Aspen, Austral.; Aventis, NZ; Axcan, USA.
Sucralfate (p.1290·2).
*Peptic ulcer.*

**Caramelle alle Erbe Digestive** Giuliani, Ital.
Gentian (p.1692·2); rhubarb (p.1287·3); boldo (p.1661·2).
*Aid to digestion.*

**Caramelos Agua del Carmen** Fardi, Spain.
Cineole (p.1672·1); melissa (p.1711·1); menthol (p.1711·3).
*Nasal congestion.*

**Caramelos Antibioticos**
Note. This name is used for preparations of different composition.
Fecofar, Arg.; Richet, Arg.
Benzocaine (p.1370·3); tyrothricin (p.275·1).
*Mouth and throat disorders.*

Raymos, Arg.
Hexylresorcinol (p.1182·1); benzocaine (p.1370·3); tyrothricin (p.275·1).
*Mouth and throat disorders.*

**Caramelos Antibioticos Bucoangin** Northia, Arg.
Hexylresorcinol (p.1182·1); neomycin (p.235·1); tyrothricin (p.275·1).
*Mouth and throat disorders.*

**Caramelos Balsam** Alcala, Spain†.
Cineole (p.1672·1); oleum pini sylvestris; menthol (p.1711·3).
*Throat irritation.*

**Caramelos Oriental** Oriental, Arg.
Hexylresorcinol (p.1182·1); benzocaine (p.1370·3).
*Mouth and throat disorders.*

**Caramelos Vit C** Alcala, Spain†.
Ascorbic acid (p.1460·2).
*Deficiency of vitamin C.*

**Carasel** Almirall, Spain.
Ramipril (p.994·1).
*Diabetic nephropathy; heart failure; hypertension; myocardial infarction.*

**Carba** ABZ, Ger.; CT, Ger.
Carbamazepine (p.353·3).
*Alcohol withdrawal syndrome; bipolar disorder; diabetic neuropathy; epilepsy; multiple sclerosis; neuralgias.*

**Carbabeta** Betapharm, Ger.
Carbamazepine (p.353·3).
*Alcohol withdrawal syndrome; bipolar disorder; diabetic neuropathy; epilepsy; multiple sclerosis; neuralgias.*

**Carbac** Syntex, Mex.
Loracarbef (p.228·1).
*Bacterial infections.*

**Carbacide** Fischer, Israel†.
Carbaryl (p.1501·2).
*Pediculosis.*

**Carbactive** Cooperation Pharmaceutique, Fr.
Activated charcoal (p.1030·2).
*Gastrointestinal disorders.*

**Carbactol Retard** Laboratorios Chile, Chile.
Carbamazepine (p.353·3).
*Diabetes insipidus; epilepsy; neuralgia.*

**Carbaderme** Lepori, Port.
Emollient.

**Carbadura** Merck dura, Ger.
Carbamazepine (p.353·3).
*Alcohol withdrawal syndrome; bipolar disorder; diabetic neuropathy; epilepsy; multiple sclerosis; neuralgia.*

**Carbaflux** Hennig, Ger.
Carbamazepine (p.353·3).
*Alcohol withdrawal syndrome; bipolar disorder; diabetic neuropathy; epilepsy; multiple sclerosis; neuralgias.*

**Carbagamma** Worwag, Ger.
Carbamazepine (p.353·3).
*Alcohol withdrawal syndrome; diabetic neuropathy; epilepsy; multiple sclerosis; neuralgias.*

**Carbagen** Generics, UK.
Carbamazepine (p.353·3).
*Epilepsy.*

**Carbager-Plus** Streger, Mex.
Methocarbamol (p.1395·1); ibuprofen (p.45·3).
*Gout; inflammation; musculoskeletal, joint and periarticular disorders; pain.*

**Carbaglu**
Orphan, Austria; Orphan, Denm.; Orphan, Fr.; Orphan, UK.
Carglumic acid (p.1668·1).
*Hyperammonaemia.*

**Carbagramon** Gramon, Arg.
Carbamazepine (p.353·3).
*Epilepsy; neuralgia.*

**Carbaica** Pharmafar, Ital.
Urazamide (p.1760·3).
*Liver disorders.*

**Carbalan** Quimica y Farmacia, Mex.
Carbamazepine (p.353·3).
*Epilepsy.*

**Carbalax** Forest Laboratories, UK.
Monobasic sodium phosphate (p.1230·3); sodium bicarbonate (p.1223·2).
*Bowel evacuation; constipation.*

**Carbamann** Mann, Ger.
Carbachol (p.1488·1).
*Glaucoma.*

**Carbamat** Pharmacia, Arg.
Carbamazepine (p.353·3).
*Alcohol withdrawal syndrome; deafferenation pain; diabetes insipidus; diabetic neuropathy; epilepsy; trigeminal neuralgia.*

**Carbamid + VAS** Widmer, Ger.
Tretinoin (p.1161·1); urea (p.1162·2).
*Skin disorders.*

**Carbamide Creme** Widmer, Switz.
Urea (p.1162·2); vitamin A palmitate (p.1453·1); dexpanthenol (p.1727·2).
*Skin disorders.*

**Carbamide + VAS** Widmer, Switz.
Tretinoin (p.1161·1); urea (p.1162·2); dexpanthenol (p.1727·2).
*Skin disorders.*

**Carbamox** Offenbach, Mex.
Methocarbamol (p.1395·1); aspirin (p.15·1).
*Fever; muscle spasm; pain.*

**Carbastat**
Novartis Ophthalmics, Canad.; Novartis Ophthalmics, USA.
Carbachol (p.1488·1).
*Production of miosis.*

**Carbatil** Loren, Mex.
Mebendazole (p.108·2).
*Worm infections.*

**Carbatrol** Shire Richwood, USA.
Carbamazepine (p.353·3).
*Epilepsy; trigeminal neuralgia.*

**Carbaval** Valdecasas, Mex.
Carbamazepine (p.353·3).
*Epilepsy; neuralgia.*

**Carbazene** Medifive, Thai.
Carbamazepine (p.353·3).
*Epilepsy; trigeminal neuralgia.*

**Carbazep** Cryopharma, Mex.
Carbamazepine (p.353·3).
*Diabetic neuropathy; epilepsy; neuralgias.*

**Carbazina** Psicofarma, Mex.
Carbamazepine (p.353·3).
*Epilepsy; neuralgias.*

**Carbecin** Sanfer, Mex.
Carbenicillin sodium (p.166·2).
*Bacterial infections.*

**Carbellon** Torbet Laboratories, UK.
Activated charcoal (p.1030·2); magnesium hydroxide (p.1272·2); peppermint oil (p.1283·2).
*Dyspepsia; flatulence; gastric hyperacidity.*

**Carbem** Lilly, Ital.†.
Loracarbef (p.228·1).
*Bacterial infections.*

**Carbenin** Sankyo, Jpn.
Panipenem (p.241·3); betamipron (p.165·3).
*Bacterial infections.*

**Carbex**
Note. This name is used for preparations of different composition.
Ferring, Irl.; Nordic, UK.
Oral granules, sodium bicarbonate (p.1223·2); simeticone (p.1289·2); solution, anhydrous citric acid (p.1673·1).
*Adjunct to contrast media for gastrointestinal radiography.*

Endo, USA.
Selegiline hydrochloride (p.1214·1).
*Parkinsonism.*

**Carbi** Gerard, Israel.
Carbamazepine (p.353·3).
*Bipolar disorder; diabetes insipidus; epilepsy; mania; trigeminal neuralgia.*

**Carbicalcin**
Procter & Gamble, Ital.; Alcala, Spain.
Elcatonin (p.768·3).
*Hypercalcaemia; osteoporosis; Paget's disease of bone; reflex sympathetic dystrophy.*

**Carbidol** Teuto, Braz.
Carbidopa (p.1204·3); levodopa (p.1205·2).
*Parkinsonism.*

**Carbilev** Aspen, S.Afr.
Levodopa (p.1205·2); carbidopa (p.1204·3).
*Parkinsonism.*

**Carbinib** Edol, Port.
Acetazolamide (p.849·1).
*Glaucoma.*

**Carbinoxamine Compound** Morton Grove, USA.
Carbinoxamine maleate (p.426·3); pseudoephedrine hydrochloride (p.1129·2); dextromethorphan hydrobromide (p.1117·3).
*Coughs and cold symptoms.*

**Carbiset** Nutripharm, USA.
Pseudoephedrine hydrochloride (p.1129·2); carbinoxamine maleate (p.426·3).
*Upper respiratory-tract symptoms.*

**Carbistad** Stada, Austria.
Carbimazole (p.1596·2).
*Hyperthyroidism.*

**Carbium**
Hexal, Austral.†; Hexal, Ger.
Carbamazepine (p.353·3).
*Alcohol withdrawal syndrome; bipolar disorder; diabetic neuropathy; epilepsy; multiple sclerosis; neuralgias.*

**Carbloc** Labomed, Chile.
Nifedipine (p.966·2).
*Hypertension.*

**Carbo** Max Farma, Ital.
Calcium carbonate (p.1254·2).
*Calcium deficiency; calcium supplement.*

**Carbo Konigsfeld** Muller Goppingen, Ger.
Carbo coffea (p.1765·3).
*Diarrhoea.*

**Carbo Veg** Brauer, Austral.†.
Homoeopathic preparation.

**Carbobel** Medgenix, Belg.
Activated charcoal (p.1030·2); methenamine (p.230·1); magnesium citrate (p.1272·1).
*Diarrhoea; dyspepsia; poisoning.*

**Carbocain**
AstraZeneca, Denm.; AstraZeneca, Norw.; AstraZeneca, Swed.
Mepivacaine hydrochloride (p.1381·2).
Adrenaline acid tartrate (p.852·2) is included in some injections as a vasoconstrictor to diminish absorption and localise the effect of the local anaesthetic.
*Local anaesthesia.*

**Carbocaina**
Note. This name is used for preparations of different composition.
AstraZeneca, Ital.
Mepivacaine hydrochloride (p.1381·2).
Adrenaline acid tartrate (p.852·2) is included in some injections as a vasoconstrictor to diminish absorption and localise the effect of the local anaesthetic.
*Local anaesthesia.*

Bucca, Spain.
Phenol (p.1188·1); methyl salicylate (p.59·3); tetracaine hydrochloride (p.1385·1).
*Local anaesthesia.*

**Carbocaine**
AstraZeneca, Austral.; Abbott, Canad.; AstraZeneca, Fr.; Adcock Ingram, S.Afr.; Sanofi Winthrop, USA; Cook-Waite, USA.
Mepivacaine hydrochloride (p.1381·2).
Corbadrine (p.1675·3) is included in some injections as a vasoconstrictor to diminish absorption and localise the effect of the local anaesthetic.
*Local anaesthesia.*

**Carbocaine with Neo-Cobefrin** Cook-Waite, USA.
Mepivacaine hydrochloride (p.1381·2).
Corbadrine (p.1675·3) is included in this preparation as a vasoconstrictor to diminish absorption and localise the effect of the local anaesthetic.
*Local anaesthesia.*

**Carbocal** Madariaga, Spain†.
Calcium carbonate (p.1254·2).
*Hypocalcaemia; osteoporosis.*

**Carbocal D** Madariaga, Spain.
Calcium carbonate (p.1254·2); colecalciferol (p.1461·3).
*Calcium and vitamin D deficiency; osteoporosis.*

**Carbocin** Cimed, Braz.
Carbocisteine (p.1116·2).
*Respiratory-tract congestion.*

**Carbocit** CT, Ital.
Carbocisteine (p.1116·2).
*Respiratory-tract disorders.*

**Carbodec** Rugby, USA.
Carbinoxamine maleate (p.426·3); pseudoephedrine hydrochloride (p.1129·2).
*Allergic rhinitis; nasal congestion.*

**Carbodec DM** Rugby, USA.
Pseudoephedrine hydrochloride (p.1129·2); dextromethorphan hydrobromide (p.1117·3); carbinoxamine maleate (p.426·3).
*Coughs and cold symptoms.*

**Carbodex DM** Tri-Med, USA.
*Oral drops:* Dextromethorphan hydrobromide (p.1117·3); carbinoxamine maleate (p.426·3); pseudoephedrine hydrochloride (p.1129·2).
*Syrup:* Dextromethorphan hydrobromide (p.1117·3); brompheniramine maleate (p.426·1); pseudoephedrine hydrochloride (p.1129·2).
*Upper respiratory-tract disorders.*

**Carbo-Dome** Sandoz, UK.
Coal tar (p.1159·2).
*Psoriasis.*

**Carbofan** Bunker, Braz.
Carbocisteine (p.1116·2).
*Respiratory-tract congestion.*

**Carboflex**
Note. This name is used for preparations of different composition.
Convatec, Austral.; Convatec, Fr.
Activated charcoal (p.1030·2); alginate.
*Wounds.*

Convatec, Port.
Activated charcoal (p.1030·2); calcium-sodium alginate (p.745·1) (p.1577·1); carmellose sodium (p.1577·3).
*Ulcers; wounds.*

**Carbogasol** Montpellier, Arg.
*Oral drops:* Simeticone (p.1289·2).
*Meteorism; preparation for radiography.*
*Tablets:* Simeticone (p.1289·2); charcoal (p.1030·2); homatropine methylbromide (p.483·2).
*Dyspepsia; meteorism.*

**Carbogasol Antiacido** Montpellier, Arg.
Magaldrate (p.1271·3); simeticone (p.1289·2).
*Dyspepsia; gastritis; gastro-oesophageal reflux; hiatus hernia; peptic ulcer.*

**Carbogasol Digestivo** Montpellier, Arg.
Pancreatin (p.1725·3); simeticone (p.1289·2); thioctic acid (p.1754·3); deoxycholic acid (p.1660·3); dehydrocholic acid (p.1679·2).
*Dyspepsia.*

**Carbogasol Forte** Montpellier, Arg.
Simeticone (p.1289·2).
*Dyspepsia; meteorism; preparation for radiography.*

**Carbohydrate-Free Mixture** Scientific Hospital Supplies, Austral.
Food for special diets (p.1417·1).

**Carbo-Levedo** Itaca, Braz.†.
Vegetable charcoal (p.1030·3); yeast (p.1469·1).
*Diarrhoea.*

**Carbolevure**
Vedim, Fr.
*Saccharomyces cerevisiae* (p.1469·1); activated charcoal (p.1030·2).
*Gastrointestinal disorders.*

UCB, Switz.
Dried yeast (p.1469·1); activated charcoal (p.1030·2).
*Gastrointestinal disorders.*

**Carbolim** Dansk-Flama, Braz.
Lithium carbonate (p.301·1).
*Bipolar disorder; depression; migraine and vascular headaches; neutropenia; schizophrenia.*

**Carbolit**
Raffo, Chile; Psicofarma, Mex.
Lithium carbonate (p.301·1).
*Bipolar disorder; migraine; psychoses.*

**Carbolith** ICN, Canad.
Lithium carbonate (p.301·1).
*Bipolar disorder.*

**Carbolithium** Elan, Ital.
Lithium carbonate (p.301·1).
*Adjunct in drug-induced leucopenia; cluster headache; psychiatric disorders.*

**Carbolitium** Eurofarma, Braz.
Lithium carbonate (p.301·1).
*Bipolar disorder; depression; migraine and vascular headaches; neutropenia; schizophrenia.*

**Carbomix**
Leiras, Fin.; Pharmygiene, Fr.; IFET (ΙΦΕΤ), Gr.; Penn, Irl.; Vaillant, Ital.; Selena, Swed.; Meadow, UK.
Activated charcoal (p.1030·2).
*Acute poisoning; diarrhoea.*

**Carbomox** Win-Medicare, India.
Amoxicillin (p.155·3) or amoxicillin trihydrate (p.155·3); carbocisteine (p.1116·2).
*Otitis media; respiratory-tract infections.*

**Ca-R-Bon** Greater Pharma, Thai.
Activated charcoal (p.1030·2).
*Abdominal distension; diarrhoea; poisoning.*

**Carbon Tabs** Hexa-Medinova, Arg.
Activated charcoal (p.1030·2); phthalylsulfathiazole (p.242·3); homatropine methylbromide (p.483·2).
*Gastrointestinal disorders.*

**Carbondifer** Trenka Difer, Ital.†.
Senna (p.1288·2); rhubarb (p.1287·3); vegetable charcoal (p.1030·3); sublimed sulfur (p.1158·2).
Formerly known as Eucarbon.
*Constipation.*

**Carbone Composto** AFOM, Ital.; Dynacren, Ital.; Ottolenghi, Ital.; Zeta, Ital.
Vegetable charcoal (p.1030·3); magnesium hydroxide (p.1272·2); calcium carbonate (p.1254·2).
*Gastrointestinal disorders.*

**Carbonesia** Geymonat, Ital.
Activated charcoal (p.1030·2); magnesium oxide (p.1272·3); calcium carbonate (p.1254·2); magnesium peroxide (p.1185·2).
*Gastrointestinal disorders.*

**Carbonet**
Smith & Nephew, Fr.; Smith & Nephew, Irl.; Smith & Nephew, UK.
Activated charcoal (p.1030·2).
*Malodorous wounds.*

**Carbonex** Richelet, Fr.
Magnesium hydroxide (p.1272·2).
Formerly contained sublimed sulfur and magnesium hydroxide.
*Constipation.*

**Carbonpectate** Chew, Thai.
Activated charcoal (p.1030·2); magnesium carbonate (p.1272·1); pectin (p.1580·3).
*Diarrhoea; flatulence.*

**Carbophagix** UCB, Fr.†.
Activated charcoal (p.1030·2); *Saccharomyces cerevisiae* (p.1469·1).
*Gastrointestinal disorders.*

**Carbophos** UPSA, Fr.
Vegetable charcoal (p.1030·3); calcium carbonate (p.1254·2); calcium phosphate (p.1225·3).
*Gastrointestinal disorders.*

**Carboplat**
Pharmacia, Arg.; Bristol-Myers Squibb, Ger.; Asofarma, Mex.
Carboplatin (p.533·3).
*Malignant neoplasms.*

**Carboron** Royal, Chile.
Lithium carbonate (p.301·1).
*Alcohol withdrawal; bipolar disorder; migraine; obsessive-compulsive disorder; schizophrenia.*

**Carbosan** Rowa, Irl.
Carbenoxolone sodium (p.1254·3).
*Aphthous stomatitis; herpes labialis; lip sores.*

**Carbosen** Senese, Ital.
Mepivacaine hydrochloride (p.1381·2).
Adrenaline acid tartrate (p.852·2) is included in some injections as a vasoconstrictor to diminish absorption and localise the effect of the local anaesthetic.
*Local anaesthesia.*

**Carboseptol** Herbes Universelles, Canad.
Menthol (p.1711·3); cineole (p.1672·1); methyl salicylate (p.59·3); thymol (p.1194·2); zinc oxide (p.1163·2).

**Carbosin**
Nettopharma, Denm.†; Nycomed, Fin.; Chemipharma, Gr.; Nycomed, Norw.; Asta Medica, NZ; NZ Medical & Scientific, NZ; Pharmachemie, S.Afr.; Pharmachemie, Thai.; Teva, Thai.
Carboplatin (p.533·3).
*Malignant neoplasms.*

**Carbosint** Boniscontro & Gazzone, Ital.
Calcium carbonate (p.1254·2).
*Calcium deficiency; calcium supplement.*

**Carbosol** Sanova, Austria.
Carboplatin (p.533·3).
*Malignant neoplasms.*

**Carbosorb**
Pharmacia, Austral.; Pharmacia, NZ.
Activated charcoal (p.1030·2).
*Drug overdose; poisoning.*

**Carbosorb S**
Pharmacia, Austral.; Pharmacia, NZ.
Activated charcoal (p.1030·2); sorbitol (p.1446·3).
*Drug overdose; poisoning.*

**Carbospare** Abbott, Fin.
Preparation for enteral nutrition (p.1417·1).

**Carbospect** Mer-National, S.Afr.†.
Carbocisteine (p.1116·2).
*Respiratory-tract disorders.*

**Carbostesin**
*Note. This name is used for preparations of different composition.*
AstraZeneca, Austria; AstraZeneca, Ger.; AstraZeneca, Switz.
Bupivacaine hydrochloride (p.1371·1).
Adrenaline acid tartrate (p.852·2) is included in some injections as a vasoconstrictor to diminish absorption and localise the effect of the local anaesthetic.
*Local anaesthesia.*

Asta Medica, Braz.†.
Articaine hydrochloride (p.1370·3).
Adrenaline acid tartrate (p.852·2) is included in this preparation as a vasoconstrictor to diminish absorption and localise the effect of the local anaesthetic.
*Local anaesthesia.*

**Carbosylane** Grimberg, Fr.; Trima, Israel.
Activated charcoal (p.1030·2); simeticone (p.1289·2).
*Dyspepsia; flatulence; meteorism.*

**Carbosymag** Grimberg, Fr.
Charcoal (p.1030·2); simeticone (p.1289·2); magnesium oxide (p.1272·3).
*Dyspepsia; meteorism.*

**Carbotec** Columbia, Mex.†.
Carboplatin (p.533·3).
*Malignant neoplasms.*

**Carboticon** Interdelta, Switz.
Activated charcoal (p.1030·2); simeticone (p.1289·2).
*Digestive disorders; flatulence.*

**Carbotiol** Bouty, Ital.†.
Killed bacteria: *Escherichia coli*; *Streptococcus ovalis*; *Micrococcus pyogenes* var. *aureus*; *Proteus vulgaris*; vegetable charcoal (p.1030·3); kaolin (p.1268·3); sodium sulfate (p.1290·1); sodium bicarbonate (p.1223·2).
*Gastrointestinal disorders.*

**Carbotop** Pulitzer, Ital.
Calcium carbonate (p.1254·2).
*Calcium deficiency; calcium supplement.*

**Carboxine** Cypress, USA.
Carbinoxamine maleate (p.426·3).
*Rhinitis.*

**Carboxine-PSE** Cypress, USA.
Carbinoxamine maleate (p.426·3); pseudoephedrine hydrochloride (p.1129·2).
*Rhinitis.*

**Carboxtie** Gautier, Arg.
Carboplatin (p.533·3).
*Malignant neoplasms.*

**Carboyoghurt** SIT, Ital.
Vegetable charcoal (p.1030·3); simeticone (p.1289·2).
*Gastrointestinal disorders.*

**Carcinil** Abbott, Ger.†.
Leuprorelin acetate (p.1331·1).
*Prostatic cancer.*

**Cardace**
Aventis, Fin.; Aventis, India.
Ramipril (p.994·1).
*Diabetic nephropathy; heart failure; hypertension; myocardial infarction.*

**Cardace Comp** Aventis, Fin.
Ramipril (p.994·1); hydrochlorothiazide (p.933·2).
*Hypertension.*

**Cardactona** Pasteur, Chile.
Spironolactone (p.1003·1).
*Heart failure; hyperaldosteronism; hypertension; oedema.*

**Cardalept** Synpharma, Austria.
Crataegus (p.1677·1); melissa (p.1711·1); rosemary (p.1740·2).
*Cardiac disorders.*

**Cardalin** Sintofarma, Braz.
Nifedipine (p.966·2).
*Angina pectoris; hypertension; Raynaud's syndrome.*

**Cardanat** Temmler, Ger.
Etilefrine hydrochloride (p.914·1).
*Hypotension.*

**Cardaxen** Spirig, Switz.
Atenolol (p.865·2).
*Angina pectoris; arrhythmias; hypertension; myocardial infarction.*

**Cardaxen plus** Spirig, Switz.
Atenolol (p.865·2); chlortalidone (p.882·3).
*Hypertension.*

**Cardcal** Amrad, Austral.†.
Diltiazem hydrochloride (p.900·1).
*Angina pectoris.*

**Cardcor** Teuto, Braz.
Digoxin (p.895·2).
*Arrhythmias.*

**Cardec** Dermopen, Braz.†.
Methyl salicylate (p.59·3); menthol (p.1711·3); camphor (p.1665·3).
*Musculoskeletal and joint disorders.*

**Cardec DM** Alpharma, USA†.
Pseudoephedrine hydrochloride (p.1129·2); dextromethorphan hydrobromide (p.1117·3); carbinoxamine maleate (p.426·3).
*Coughs and cold symptoms.*

**Cardec-S** Alpharma, USA†.
Pseudoephedrine hydrochloride (p.1129·2); carbinoxamine maleate (p.426·3).
*Upper respiratory-tract symptoms.*

**Cardegic**
Sanofi Synthelabo, Belg.; Sanofi Synthelabo, Neth.
Lysine aspirin (p.54·3).
*Thromboembolic disorders.*

**Cardeloc** TO-Chemicals, Thai.
Metoprolol tartrate (p.957·1).
*Angina pectoris; arrhythmias; hypertension; hyperthyroidism; myocardial infarction.*

**Cardem** Aventis, Spain.
Celiprolol hydrochloride (p.881·3).
*Angina pectoris; hypertension.*

**Cardenalin** Pfizer, Jpn.
Doxazosin mesilate (p.908·3).
*Hypertension.*

**Cardene**
Roche, Canad.†; Yamanouchi, Irl.; Yamanouchi, Neth.; Yamanouchi, UK; Wyeth-Ayerst, USA.
Nicardipine hydrochloride (p.965·1).
*Angina pectoris; hypertension.*

**Cardenol** TO-Chemicals, Thai.
Propranolol hydrochloride (p.989·3).
*Angina pectoris; arrhythmias; hypertension; tremor.*

**Cardensiel** Lipha Sante, Fr.
Bisoprolol fumarate (p.875·1).
*Heart failure.*

**Cardepine**
Imperial, Malaysia; Westmont, Thai.; Great Eastern, Thai.
Nicardipine hydrochloride (p.965·1).
*Angina pectoris; cerebrovascular disorders; heart failure; hypertension.*

**Cardeymin** Cantassium Co., UK†.
Magnesium orotate (p.1724·3); bromelain (p.1662·2); potassium orotate (p.1724·3).

**Card-Floe II** Sisu, Canad.
Multivitamin and mineral preparation (p.1417·1).

**Cardiace** Triomed, S.Afr.
Captopril (p.879·2).
*Diabetic nephropathy; heart failure; hypertension.*

**Cardiacton** Byk, Austria†.
Diltiazem hydrochloride (p.900·1).
*Angina pectoris; hypertension.*

**Cardiacum PMD** Plantamed, Ger.†.
Homoeopathic preparation.

**Cardiaforce** Bioforce, Switz.
Crataegus (p.1677·1); melissa (p.1711·1); wine.
*Sleep disorders; tachycardia.*

**Cardiagen** APS, Ger.
Captopril (p.879·2).
Formerly contained crataegus and camphor.
*Heart failure; hypertension.*

**Cardiagen HCT** APS, Ger.
Captopril (p.879·2); hydrochlorothiazide (p.933·2).
*Hypertension.*

**Cardialgine** MIP, Ger.
Etilefrine hydrochloride (p.914·1).
*Hypotension.*

**Cardiavis N** Truw, Ger.
Homoeopathic preparation.

**Cardiax** Sidus, Arg.
Aspirin (p.15·1); vitamin C (p.1460·2); vitamin E (p.1464·3).
*Thrombosis prophylaxis.*

**Cardiazem** Instituto Sanitas, Chile.
Nitrendipine (p.973·3).
*Hypertension.*

**Cardiazidine** Pharmacia Upjohn, Fr.†.
Trimetazidine hydrochloride (p.1018·1).
*Angina pectoris; vascular eye disorders; vestibular disorders.*

**Cardiazol-Dicodid** Nicholas Piramal, India.
Pentetrazol (p.1592·1); hydrocodone hydrochloride (p.45·1).
*Coughs.*

**Cardiazol-Paracodina** Abbott, Ital.
Pentetrazol (p.1592·1); dihydrocodeine thiocyanate (p.35·2).
*Coughs.*

**Cardibisana** Riemser, Ger.
Crataegus (p.1677·1); cinchona bark (p.1671·3); kola (p.1765·3); convallaria (p.1675·3); cereus (p.1669·2); ephedra (p.1119·3); ginseng (p.1693·1); camphora; thiamine hydrochloride; veratrum; strophanthus; phosphor; glonoinum; ars. alb.
*Cardiovascular disorders.*

**Cardibloc** Imperial, Singapore.
Nicardipine hydrochloride (p.965·1).
*Angina pectoris; hypertension.*

**Cardiblok** Xixia, S.Afr.†.
Propranolol hydrochloride (p.989·3).
*Angina pectoris; arrhythmias; hypertension; hyperthyroidism; phaeochromocytoma; tachycardia; tremor.*

**Cardicon** Labomed, Chile.
Nifedipine (p.966·2).
*Angina pectoris; hypertension; myocardial infarction.*

**Cardicor**
Merck, Denm.; Merck, Irl.; Merck, UK.
Bisoprolol fumarate (p.875·1).
*Heart failure.*

**Cardif Beta** Concept, India.
Nitrendipine (p.973·3); atenolol (p.865·2).
*Hypertension.*

**Cardifen** Aspen, S.Afr.
Nifedipine (p.966·2).
*Angina pectoris.*

**Cardiject** Sun, Thai.
Dobutamine hydrochloride (p.905·3).
*Heart failure.*

**Cardil**
Orion, Denm.; Gerolimatos (Γερολυματος), Gr.; Orion, Malaysia; Orion, Singapore; Orion, Thai.
Diltiazem hydrochloride (p.900·1).
*Angina pectoris; hypertension.*

**Cardilat** Triomed, S.Afr.
Nifedipine (p.966·2).
*Angina pectoris; hypertension.*

**Cardilate**
*Note. A similar name is used for preparations of different composition (see below).*
Glaxo Wellcome, Ital.†.
Eritrityl tetranitrate (p.913·1).
*Angina pectoris.*

**Cardilate MR**
*Note. A similar name is used for preparations of different composition (see above).*
Ivax, Hong Kong; Ivax, UK.
Nifedipine (p.966·2).
*Angina pectoris; hypertension.*

**Cardiloc** Unipharm, Israel.
Bisoprolol fumarate (p.875·1).
*Angina pectoris; hypertension.*

**Cardilol**
*Note. This name is used for preparations of different composition.*
Libbs, Braz.
Carvedilol (p.881·1).
*Angina pectoris; heart failure; hypertension.*

Julphar, UAE.
Propranolol hydrochloride (p.989·3).
*Angina pectoris; anxiety; arrhythmias; hypertension; hyperthyroidism; migraine; myocardial infarction; phaeochromocytoma; tremor; variceal haemorrhage.*

**Cardimet** Errekappa, Ital.†.
Carnitine (p.1423·3).
*Carnitine deficiency; myocardial ischaemia.*

**Cardin** Farmoquimica, Braz.†.
Methyldopa (p.953·2).
*Hypertension.*

**Cardinit** Knoll, Mex.
Glyceryl trinitrate (p.923·2).
*Angina pectoris; heart failure.*

**Cardinol**
Pacific, NZ; CP Pharmaceuticals, UK†.
Propranolol hydrochloride (p.989·3).
*Angina pectoris; anxiety; arrhythmias; hypertension; hyperthyroidism; hypertrophic obstructive cardiomyopathy; migraine; myocardial infarction; phaeochromocytoma; thyrotoxicosis; tremor.*

**Cardinorm**
*Note. This name is used for preparations of different composition.*
Hexal, Austral.
Amiodarone hydrochloride (p.859·2).
*Arrhythmias.*

Benedetti, Ital.
Verapamil hydrochloride (p.1019·1).
*Angina pectoris; arrhythmias; hypertension; myocardial infarction.*

**Cardinorma** Pekana, Ger.
Homoeopathic preparation.

**Cardioace** Vitabiotics, UK.
Omega-3 fish oil; garlic; lecithin; vitamins; minerals (p.1417·1).

**Cardioaspirin** Bayer, Ital.
Aspirin (p.15·1).
*Thromboembolic disorders.*

**Cardioaspirina**
Bayer, Arg.; Bayer, Chile.
Aspirin (p.15·1).
*Thrombosis prophylaxis.*

**Cardioaspirine** Bayer, Belg.
Aspirin (p.15·1).
*Thromboembolic disorders.*

**Cardiobil** Biologici Italia, Ital.
Levocarnitine (p.1423·3).
*Carnitine deficiency.*

**Cardiobron** Fada, Arg.
Alprostadil (p.1512·3).

**Cardiocalm** Pharmastra, Fr.
Crataegus (p.1677·1).
Formerly contained crataegus and phenobarbital.
*Insomnia; nervous disorders.*

**Cardiocap** Miba, Ital.†.
Carbocromen hydrochloride (p.880·2).
*Ischaemic heart disease.*

**Cardiocor**
Merck, Austria; Wyeth Lederle, Fr.
Bisoprolol fumarate (p.875·1).
*Heart failure.*

**Cardiodisco** Juste, Spain†.
Glyceryl trinitrate (p.923·2).
*Angina pectoris.*

**Cardiodopa** Royton, Braz.
Methyldopa (p.953·2).
*Hypertension.*

**Cardiodoron**
Weleda, Austria; Weleda, Ger.
Hyoscyamus niger; onopordon acanthium; cowslip flower (p.1735·1).
*Cardiac disorders; sleep disorders.*

**Cardiofort** Kwizda, Austria.
Crataegus (p.1677·1).
*Cardiovascular disorders.*

**Cardiofrik** Fresenius Kabi, Austria†.
Convallaria (p.1675·3); crataegus (p.1677·1); valerian (p.1762·2).
*Cardiac disorders.*

**Cardiogen** UCB, Ital.
Levocarnitine (p.1423·3).
*Carnitine deficiency.*

**Cardiogoxin** Medipharma, Arg.
Digoxin (p.895·2).

**Cardio-Green**
Paesel, Ger.†; Becton Dickinson, USA.
Indocyanine green (p.1701·1).
*Diagnostic aid.*

**Cardioguard** Clonmel, Irl.
Folic acid (p.1429·1).
*Hyperhomocysteinaemia.*

**Cardiol**
*Note. This name is used for preparations of different composition.*
Roche, Fin.
Carvedilol (p.881·1).
*Angina pectoris; heart failure; hypertension.*

Bial, Port.
Fluvastatin sodium (p.918·2).
*Hypercholesterolaemia.*

**Cardiolan** Tosi, Ital.†.
Metildigoxin (p.955·2).
*Heart failure.*

**Cardiolen** Instituto Sanitas, Chile.
Verapamil hydrochloride (p.1019·1).
*Angina pectoris; arrhythmias; hypertension.*

**Cardiolite**
New England Nuclear, Austria; Bristol-Myers Squibb, Belg.; Du Pont, Fr.; Du Pont, Irl.; Bristol-Myers, Spain; Bristol-Myers Squibb, UK; Du Pont, USA.
Technetium-99m sestamibi (p.1525·2).
*Diagnosis and location of myocardial infarction; diagnosis of breast cancer; diagnosis of hyperparathyroidism; diagnosis of myocardial ischaemia and ventricular dysfunction.*

**Cardio-Longoral** Artesan, Ger.; Cassella-med, Ger.
Potassium aspartate (p.1233·1); magnesium aspartate (p.1227·3); crataegus (p.1677·1).
*Cardiac disorders.*

**Cardi-Omega 3** Thompson, USA.
Omega-3 marine triglycerides (p.976·2).
*Dietary supplement.*

**Cardiomin** Andromaco, Chile.
Aminophylline (p.780·2).
*Obstructive airways disease; status asthmaticus.*

**Cardionil**
Ducto, Braz.; CEPA, Spain.
Isosorbide mononitrate (p.942·1).
*Angina pectoris.*

**Cardionorm** Knoll, Braz.†.
Sotalol hydrochloride (p.1001·3).
*Arrhythmias; hypertension.*

**Cardionox** Alter, Port.
Amlodipine besilate (p.862·1).
*Angina pectoris.*

**Cardiopina** Farmion, Braz.†.
Nifedipine (p.966·2).
*Angina pectoris; hypertension.*

**Cardiopine** Julphar, UAE.
Nifedipine (p.966·2).
*Angina pectoris; hypertension.*

**Cardio-Plantina** Plantina, Ger.†.
Homoeopathic preparation.

**Cardioplegia**
Mayne, Hong Kong; Faulding, Malaysia; Bull, Singapore; DBL, Thai.; Faulding, Thai.
Magnesium chloride (p.1228·1); potassium chloride (p.1232·2); procaine hydrochloride (p.1383·2).
*Induction of cardioplegic arrest in open-heart surgery.*

**Cardioplegia A** Baxter, Austral.
Sodium chloride (p.1233·3); potassium chloride (p.1232·2); magnesium chloride (p.1228·1); calcium chloride (p.1225·1).
*Induction of cardiac arrest during heart surgery.*

**Cardioplegia Concentrate** Mayne, Austral.
Magnesium chloride (p.1228·1); potassium chloride (p.1232·2); procaine hydrochloride (p.1383·2).

**Cardioplegin N** Kohler, Ger.
Magnesium aspartate (p.1227·3); procaine hydrochloride (p.1383·2); xylitol (p.1469·1).
*Cardioplegia in open-heart surgery.*

**Cardiopril** Pharmacia, Switz.
Spirapril hydrochloride (p.1003·1).
*Hypertension.*

**Cardioprotect** BASF, Ger.†.
Verapamil hydrochloride (p.1019·1).
*Arrhythmias; hypertension; ischaemic heart disease.*

**Cardioquin**
Purdue Frederick, Canad.†; Viatris, Neth.; Purdue Frederick, USA†.
Quinidine polygalacturonate (p.991·3).
*Arrhythmias.*

**Cardioquine**
Asta Medica, Fr.†; Almirall, Spain†.
Quinidine polygalacturonate (p.991·3).
*Arrhythmias.*

**Cardioreg** Rhone-Poulenc Rorer, Ital.
β-Acetyldigoxin (p.851·1).
*Heart failure.*

**Cardioregis** Zambon, Braz.†.
Convallatoxin; nikethamide (p.1591·2).
*Respiratory insufficiency.*

**Cardiorex** *Bago, Arg.*
Amlodipine (p.862·2).
*Angina pectoris; heart failure; hypertension.*

**Cardiorona** *Columbia, Mex.†.*
Amiodarone (p.859·2).

**Cardiosedantol** *Recalcine, Chile.*
Pentaerithrityl tetranitrate (p.979·1); diazepam (p.690·1); chlormezanone (p.675·1).
*Anxiety.*

**Cardioselect N** *Dreluso, Ger.*
Homoeopathic preparation.

**Cardiosolupsan** *Bristol-Myers Squibb, Fr.*
Carbasalate calcium (p.25·1).
*Thromboembolism prophylaxis.*

**Cardiostenol** *Molteni, Ital.*
Morphine hydrochloride (p.60·1); atropine sulfate (p.477·1).
*Adjuvant in anaesthesia; pain.*

**Cardioten** *OFF, Ital.*
Nicardipine hydrochloride (p.965·1).
*Angina pectoris; heart failure; hypertension.*

**Cardioton** *NCSN, Ital.†.*
Ubidecarenone (p.1760·2).
*Cardiopathy; coenzyme Q10 deficiency.*

**Cardiotone** *VHB, India.*
Amrinone lactate (p.862·3).
*Heart failure.*

**Cardiotonicum (Rowo-15)** *Pharmakon, Ger.†.*
Homoeopathic preparation.
Lidocaine hydrochloride (p.1377·3) is included in this preparation to alleviate the pain of injection.

**Cardiovas** *Abbott, Spain.*
Isosorbide mononitrate (p.942·1).
*Angina pectoris; heart failure.*

**Cardiovasc** *Rottapharm, Ital.*
Lercanidipine hydrochloride (p.946·1).
*Hypertension.*

**Cardioxane**
*CSC, Austria; Zodiac, Braz.; Tecnofarma, Chile; Chiron, Denm.; Chiron, Fr.; Chiron, Israel; Chiron, Ital.; Asofarma, Mex.*
Dexrazoxane hydrochloride (p.1036·2).
*Prevention of doxorubicin cardiotoxicity.*

**Cardioxin** *Novartis, India.*
Digoxin (p.895·2).
*Arrhythmias; heart failure.*

**Cardip** *Francia, Ital.*
Nicardipine hydrochloride (p.965·1).
*Angina pectoris; heart failure; hypertension.*

**Cardiphyt** *Austroplant, Austria.*
Crataegus (p.1677·1).
*Cardiac disorders.*

**Cardipin** *Spirig, Switz.*
Nifedipine (p.966·2).
*Angina pectoris; hypertension; myocardial infarction.*

**Cardiplant** *Schwabe, Switz.*
Crataegus (p.1677·1).
*Cardiac disorders.*

**Cardipril**
*Note. This name is used for preparations of different composition.*
*Liomont, Mex.*
Captopril (p.879·2).
*Diabetic nephropathy; heart failure; hypertension; myocardial infarction.*

*Bial, Port.*
Imidapril hydrochloride (p.938·2).
*Hypertension.*

**Cardiprin**
*Reckitt Benckiser, Austral.; Reckitt Benckiser, Hong Kong; Reckitt Benckiser, Malaysia; Reckitt Benckiser, NZ; Reckitt Benckiser, Singapore; Reckitt Benckiser, Thai.*
Aspirin (p.15·1).
Glycine (p.1433·3) is included in this preparation in an attempt to limit adverse effects on the gastrointestinal mucosa.
*Thromboembolism prophylaxis.*

**Cardirenal** *Lafage, Arg.*
Aminophylline (p.780·2).
*Obstructive airways disease.*

**Cardirene** *Sanofi Synthelabo, Ital.*
Lysine aspirin (p.54·3).
*Thrombosis prophylaxis.*

**Cardiser** *Merck, Spain.*
Diltiazem hydrochloride (p.900·1).
*Angina pectoris; hypertension.*

**Cardispan** *Grossman, Mex.*
Levocarnitine (p.1423·3).
*Carnitine deficiency.*

**Cardium**
*DHA, Hong Kong; DHA, Singapore.*
Diltiazem hydrochloride (p.900·1).
*Angina pectoris; hypertension.*

**Cardizem**
*Aventis, Austral.; Boehringer de Angeli, Braz.; Biovail, Canad.; Novo Nordisk, Denm.; Pharmacia, Fin.; Pharmacia, Norw.; Aventis, NZ; Pharmacia, Swed.; Biovail, USA.*
Diltiazem hydrochloride (p.900·1).
*Angina pectoris; arrhythmias; hypertension.*

**Cardol** *Alphapharm, Austral.*
Sotalol hydrochloride (p.1001·3).
*Arrhythmias.*

**Cardopar** *DHA, Singapore.*
Levodopa (p.1205·2); carbidopa (p.1204·3).
*Parkinsonism.*

**Cardopax** *Orion, Denm.*
Isosorbide dinitrate (p.941·1).
*Angina pectoris; heart failure.*

**Cardoral** *Pfizer, Israel.*
Doxazosin mesilate (p.908·3).
*Benign prostatic hyperplasia; hypertension.*

**Cardoxan** *Douglas, NZ.*
Doxazosin mesilate (p.908·3).
*Benign prostatic hyperplasia; hypertension.*

**Cardoxin** *Rafa, Israel.*
Dipyridamole (p.903·1).
*Adjunct to cardiac imaging; nephrotic syndrome; pre-eclampsia; thrombosis prophylaxis.*

**Cardoxone** *Remedica, Thai.*
Metoprolol tartrate (p.957·1).
*Angina pectoris; hypertension; migraine.*

**Cards HCG-Urine** *Point of Care Diagnostics, NZ.*
Pregnancy test (p.1734·3).

**Carduben** *Madaus, Ger.†.*
Ammi visnaga fruit (p.1653·3).
*Cardiac disorders.*

**Cardular** *Pfizer, Ger.*
Doxazosin mesilate (p.908·3).
*Benign prostatic hyperplasia; hypertension.*

**Cardules** *Nicholas Piramal, India.*
Nifedipine (p.966·2).
*Angina pectoris; hypertension.*

**Cardules Plus** *Nicholas Piramal, India.*
Atenolol (p.865·2); nifedipine (p.966·2).
*Angina pectoris; hypertension.*

**Carduokatt N** *Kattwiga, Ger.*
Homoeopathic preparation.

**Cardura**
*Pfizer, Arg.; AstraZeneca, Canad.; Roerig, Chile; Pfizer, Gr.; Pfizer, Hong Kong; Pfizer, Irl.; Pfizer, Ital.; Pfizer, Malaysia; Pfizer, Mex.; Pfizer, Neth.; Pfizer, S.Afr.; Pfizer, Singapore; Pfizer, Switz.; Pfizer, Thai.; Pfizer, UK; Pfizer, USA.*
Doxazosin mesilate (p.908·3).
*Benign prostatic hyperplasia; hypertension.*

**Carduran**
*Pfizer, Austral.†; Pfizer, Braz.; Pfizer, Denm.; Pfizer, Norw.; Pfizer, Spain.*
Doxazosin mesilate (p.908·3).
*Benign prostatic hyperplasia; hypertension.*

**Carduus-monoplant** *Weber & Weber, Ger.†.*
Silybum marianum (p.1043·3).
*Liver disorders.*

**Cardyl** *Pfizer, Spain.*
Atorvastatin calcium (p.866·1).
*Hyperlipidaemias.*

**Care 55+ Multi** *Blackmores, Austral.†.*
Multivitamin, mineral and ginkgo biloba preparation (p.1417·1).

**Careflu** *Uno, Ital.*
Flunisolide (p.1101·1).
*Allergic disorders of the respiratory tract.*

**Carencil** *Jaba, Port.*
Captopril (p.879·2).
*Heart failure; hypertension.*

**Carencyl** *Lyocentre, Fr.*
Multivitamin, amino-acid, and mineral preparation (p.1417·1).
*Tonic.*

**Carentil** *Wyeth, Spain†.*
Conjugated oestrogens (p.1543·2).
*Female hypogonadism; menopausal disorders; osteoporosis.*

**Caresel** *Wassen, Ital.*
Vitamin C; vitamin E; selenium; zinc; betacarotene; astaxanthin (p.1417·1).
*Nutritional supplement.*

**Caress** *Schering-Plough, Swed.*
Urea (p.1162·2).
*Dry skin.*

**Carexan** *Pisa, Mex.*
Itraconazole (p.401·3).
*Fungal infections.*

**Careza** *Silesia, Chile.*
24 Tablets, ethinylestradiol (p.1553·2); gestodene (p.1556·1); 4 tablets, inert.
*Combined oral contraceptive.*

**Carfosid** *Palmares, Ital.*
Iron-rich yeast (p.1434·3); levocarnitine (p.1423·3); calcium folinate (p.1431·1).
*Anaemias.*

**Carginine** *Coraltis, Israel.*
L-Arginine (p.1421·1).
*Amino-acid deficiency.*

**Cargosil** *Genepharm, Gr.*
Aciclovir (p.626·1).
*Herpes simplex infections.*

**Cariamyl** *Prater, Chile.*
Menthol (p.1711·3); camphor (p.1665·3); triclosan (p.1195·2); benzocaine (p.1370·3).
*Skin irritation.*

**Cariban** *Inibsa, Spain.*
Doxylamine succinate (p.432·3); pyridoxine hydrochloride (p.1456·3).
*Nausea; vomiting.*

**Caricef** *Antibioticos, Spain.*
Cefazolin sodium (p.170·3).
Lidocaine hydrochloride (p.1377·3) is included in the intramuscular injection to alleviate the pain of injection.
*Bacterial infections.*

**Caril** *Nutricia, Fr.*
Carrots, rice, dextrin-maltose, glucose, and electrolytes (p.1222·2).
*Diarrhoea.*

**Carilax** *Strallhofer, Austria.*
Fig (p.1266·3); senna (p.1288·2).
*Bowel evacuation; constipation.*

**Carin** *CCM, Malaysia.*
Loratadine (p.436·1).
*Allergic rhinitis; allergic skin disorders; eye irritation.*

**Carinose** *Community Pharmacy, Thai.*
Loratadine (p.436·1).
*Allergic rhinitis; allergic skin disorders; hay fever.*

**Cariomix** *INTES, Ital.†.*
Xanthopterin; human placenta extract.
*Corneal ulcers, burns, and wounds; herpetic keratitis.*

**Carisano** *Truw, Ger.*
Garlic (p.1691·1).
*Lipid disorders.*

**Cariso-Co** *PP Lab, Thai.*
Paracetamol (p.76·2); carisoprodol (p.1392·1).
*Musculoskeletal disorders.*

**Carisoma**
*Wallace, India; Forest Laboratories, UK.*
Carisoprodol (p.1392·1).
*Skeletal muscle spasm.*

**Carisoma Compound**
*Note. This name is used for preparations of different composition.*
*Wallace, India.*
Carisoprodol (p.1392·1); paracetamol (p.76·2); caffeine (p.782·1).
*Musculoskeletal pain.*

*Carter Horner, Thai.*
Carisoprodol (p.1392·1); paracetamol (p.76·2).
*Musculoskeletal and joint disorders.*

**Caristop** *Maver, Chile.*
*Mouthwash:* Sodium fluoride (p.1444·3).
*Toothpaste:* Sodium monofluorophosphate (p.1446·2); sodium fluoride (p.1444·3); sodium benzoate (p.1169·3).
*Dental caries prophylaxis.*

**Caritasone** *Chinta, Thai.*
Carisoprodol (p.1392·1); paracetamol (p.76·2).
*Musculoskeletal and joint disorders.*

**Caritec** *Stancare, India.*
Benidipine hydrochloride (p.868·2).
*Angina pectoris; hypertension.*

**Carito mono**
*Europharm, Austria; Hoyer, Ger.*
Java tea (p.1702·3).
*Urinary-tract disorders.*

**Carl Baders Divinal** *Apotheke Heiligen Rupertus, Austria.*
Camphor and camphor spirit (p.1665·3); methyl salicylate (p.59·3); salicylic acid (p.1157·1); salol (p.88·1); turpentine oil (p.1760·1); rosemary oil (p.1740·2); menthol (p.1711·3).
*Musculoskeletal and joint disorders.*

**Carli** *Boncour, Fr.†.*
Magnesium aspartate; potassium aspartate; arnica (p.1656·3).
*Musculoskeletal and soft-tissue disorders.*

**Carloc**
*Cipla, India; Cipla-Medpro, S.Afr.*
Carvedilol (p.881·1).
*Heart failure; hypertension.*

**Carloxan** *Orion, Denm.*
Cyclophosphamide (p.540·2).
*Malignant neoplasms.*

**Carlytene** *Viatris, Fr.*
Moxisylyte hydrochloride (p.962·2).
*Circulatory disorders.*

**Carmapine** *Pharmasant, Thai.*
Carbamazepine (p.353·3).
*Alcohol withdrawal syndrome; diabetic neuropathy; epilepsy; glossopharyngeal neuralgia; trigeminal neuralgia.*

**Carmatis** *Carmaran, Canad.†.*
Methyl salicylate (p.59·3); camphor (p.1665·3); menthol (p.1711·3).

**Carmazin** *Teuto, Braz.*
Carbamazepine (p.353·3).
*Epilepsy.*

**Carmen** *Berlin-Chemie, Ger.*
Lercanidipine hydrochloride (p.946·1).
*Hypertension.*

**Carmian** *Teofarma, Ital.*
Atenolol (p.865·2); chlortalidone (p.882·3).
*Hypertension.*

**Carmicide**
*Indoco, India; Indoco, Thai.*
Sodium citrate (p.1223·2); citric acid (p.1673·1); ginger tincture (p.1267·1); aromatic cardamom tincture (p.1667·3); cinnamon tincture (p.1672·2).
*Colic; flatulence.*

**Carmicina** *Irex, Port.*
Ciprofloxacin hydrochloride (p.188·2).
*Bacterial infections.*

**Carminagal N** *Galenika, Ger.*
Cynara (p.1678·3).
Formerly contained cynara, pancreatin, and dimethicone.
*Dyspepsia.*

**Carminative** *Sanova, Austria.*
Caraway tincture (p.1667·2); coriander tincture (p.1676·1); spearmint tincture (p.1749·1).
*Flatulence.*

**Carminative Tea** *Weleda, UK†.*
Fennel seed (p.1687·2); aniseed (p.1655·2); caraway seed (p.1667·2); achillea (p.1646·2); chamomile flowers (p.1669·3).
*Flatulence.*

**Carminativo Ibys** *Pharmacia, Spain.*
Anise oil (p.1655·2); sodium bicarbonate (p.1223·2).
*Aerophagia.*

**Carminativo Juventus** *Juventus, Spain.*
Anise oil (p.1655·2); belladonna tincture (p.479·1); sodium bicarbonate (p.1223·2).
*Aerophagia; meteorism; vomiting.*

**Carminativum Babynos**
*Byk, Austria; Dentinox, Ger.*
Fennel (p.1687·2); coriander (p.1676·1); chamomile (p.1669·3).
*Gastrointestinal disorders.*

**Carminativum-Hetterich N** *Galenika, Ger.*
Chamomile (p.1669·3); peppermint leaf (p.1283·2); caraway (p.1667·2); fennel (p.1687·2); dried bitter-orange peel (p.1723·3).
*Gastrointestinal disorders.*

**Carminativum-Pascoe** *Pascoe, Ger.*
Peppermint leaf (p.1283·2); chamomile (p.1669·3); caraway (p.1667·2).
*Dyspepsia.*

**Carminetum** *Galenika, Ger.†.*
Peppermint oil (p.1283·2).
*Gastrointestinal disorders; muscle and nerve pain; respiratory-tract catarrh.*

**Carminex** *Propan, S.Afr.*
Magnesium carbonate (p.1272·1); sodium bicarbonate (p.1223·2); sodium citrate (p.1223·2).
*Hyperacidity.*

**Carmint** *Sofar, Ital.*
Peppermint oil (p.1283·2).
*Gastrointestinal disorders.*

**Carmitol** *Medinfar, Port.*
Urea (p.1162·2); panthenol (p.1727·2).
*Dry skin; pruritus.*

**Carmol**
*Note. This name is used for preparations of different composition.*
*Schmidgall, Austria.*
Dementholised mint oil (p.1715·2).
*Gastrointestinal disorders; headache; migraine; musculoskeletal, joint, and soft-tissue disorders; respiratory-tract disorders.*

*Doak, Hong Kong; Doak, USA.*
Urea (p.1162·2).
*Dry skin; hyperkeratosis.*

**Carmol HC** *Doak, USA.*
Hydrocortisone acetate (p.1103·3).
*Corticosteroid.*

**Carmol Magen-Galle-Darm** *Omegin, Ger.*
Taraxacum (p.1751·3); peppermint leaf (p.1283·2); cynara (p.1678·3).
*Biliary-tract disorders.*

**Carmubris**
*Bristol-Myers Squibb, Austria; Bristol-Myers Squibb, Ger.*
Carmustine (p.535·1).
*Malignant neoplasms.*

**Carnabol** *Ache, Braz.*
Buclizine (p.426·3); caffeine (p.782·1); lysine; vitamin B substances (p.1417·1).
*Reduced appetite; tonic.*

**Carnation**
*Note. This name is used for preparations of different composition.*
*Clintec, Canad.†.*
A range of preparations for enteral nutrition (p.1417·1).

*Cuxson, Gerrard, Canad.; Cuxson, Gerrard, UK.*
Salicylic acid (p.1157·1).
*Calluses; corns; verrucas.*

**Carneferrol** *INQ, Braz.†.*
Ferric ammonium citrate (p.1427·2); sodium methylarsinate (p.1748·1); tissue extracts.
*Anaemias.*

**Carnicor**
*Labomed, Chile; Max Farma, Ital.†.*
Levocarnitine (p.1423·3).
*Carnitine deficiency; myocardial ischaemia.*

*Sigma-Tau, Spain.*
Carnitine (p.1423·3).
*Carnitine deficiency.*

**Carnigen**
*Aventis, Austria; Aventis, Ger.*
Oxilofrine hydrochloride (p.977·3).
*Circulatory disorders; orthostatic hypotension.*

**Carnitene**
*Sigma-Tau, Hong Kong; Sigma-Tau, Ital.*
Levocarnitine (p.1423·3).
*Carnitine deficiency; myocardial ischaemia.*

**Carnitolo** *Recofarma, Ital.*
Levocarnitine hydrochloride (p.1424·1).
*Carnitine deficiency.*

**Carnitop** *Infosint, Ital.*
Levocarnitine (p.1423·3).
*Carnitine deficiency.*

**Carnitor**
*Sigma-Tau, Canad.; Sigma-Tau, Hong Kong; Shire, UK; Sigma-Tau, USA.*
Levocarnitine (p.1423·3).
*Carnitine deficiency.*

**Carnivora VF** *Carnivora, Ger.†.*
Dionaea muscipula.
*Malignant neoplasms.*

**Carnizin** *Bergamo, Braz.†.*
Buclizine (p.426·3); carnitine; lysine; vitamin B substances (p.1417·1).
*Reduced appetite; tonic.*

**Carnot Colutorio** *Esme, Arg.*
Bacitracin (p.161·3); gramicidin (p.220·2); benzocaine (p.1370·3); lidocaine (p.1377·3).
*Mouth disorders.*

**Carnot Topico** *Esme, Arg.*
Aluminium chloride (p.1142·1); acriflavinium chloride (p.1165·3); lidocaine hydrochloride (p.1377·3).
*Mouth disorders.*

**Carnotprim** *Carnot, Mex.*
Metoclopramide hydrochloride (p.1274·3).
*Gastrointestinal disorders; migraine; nausea and vomiting.*

**Carnovis** *Glaxo Allen, Ital.*
Levocarnitine (p.1423·3).
*Carnitine deficiency; myocardial ischaemia.*

**Carnum** *FIRMA, Ital.*
Levocarnitine (p.1423·3).
*Carnitine deficiency.*

**Carobel**
*Cow & Gate, Irl.; Cow & Gate, UK.*
Carob seed flour (p.1579·1).
*Feed thickener to control vomiting.*

**Carofril** *Arlex, Mex.†.*
Paracetamol (p.76·2).
*Fever; pain.*

**Carogil** *Novartis Nutrition, Fr.*
Carrots, rice, dextrin-maltose, and electrolytes (p.1222·2).
*Diarrhoea.*

**Caroid**
*Note. This name is used for preparations of different composition.*
*Mentholatum, Canad.†.*
Cascara (p.1255·1); phenolphthalein (p.1284·1); ox bile (p.1660·3).

*Lepori, Port.*
Capsicum (p.1667·1); cascara (p.1255·1); phenolphthalein (p.1284·1); papain (p.1727·3); bile salts (p.1660·3).
*Constipation.*

**Carominthe** *Lehning, Fr.*
Homoeopathic preparation.

**Carotaben**
*Merck, Austria; Hermal, Ger.; Boots Healthcare, Neth.†; Boots Healthcare, Switz.*
Betacarotene (p.1422·3).
*Erythropoietic protoporphyria; photodermatoses; skin pigmentation disorders.*

**Carotenoplos** *Laboratorios Chile, Chile.*
Betacarotene; *dl*-alpha tocoferil acetate; calcium ascorbate; zinc sulfate; selenium yeast (p.1417·1).
*Nutritional supplement.*

**Carotenos** *Natufarma, Arg.*
Ascorbic acid; betacarotene; alfa tocopherol (p.1417·1).
*Vitamin supplement.*

**Carotin** *Twardy, Ger.*
Betacarotene (p.1422·3); biotin (p.1423·2); calcium pantothenate (p.1442·3).
*Suntanning aid.*

**Carovit** *Biochimici, Ital.*
Betacarotene with vitamins C and E (p.1417·1).
*Nutritional supplement.*

**Carovit Forte** *Biochimici, Ital.*
Betacarotene with vitamins E and C (p.1417·1).
*Nutritional supplement.*

**Carovit Melanin** *Biochimici, Ital.*
Amino-acid preparation with vitamins and minerals (p.1417·1).
*Nutritional supplement.*

**Carovit Repair** *Biochimici, Ital.*
Evening primrose oil; fish oil; zinc-rich yeast; vitamin E; dried yeast; betacarotene (p.1417·1).
*Nutritional supplement.*

**Carpantin** *Sanofi Synthelabo, Ital.*
Pantethine (p.978·3); carnitine chloride (p.1424·1); cyproheptadine hydrochloride (p.430·1).
*Anorexia; insufficient body weight.*

**Carpilo** *Chauvin, Fr.*
Pilocarpine hydrochloride (p.1495·1); carteolol hydrochloride (p.880·3).
*Glaucoma; ocular hypertension.*

**Carpin** *Novag, Mex.*
Carbamazepine (p.353·3).
*Epilepsy.*

**Carpine** *Atlantic, Thai.*
Carbamazepine (p.353·3).
*Bipolar disorder; epilepsy; trigeminal neuralgia.*

**Carpo-Miotic** *Bell, India.*
Pilocarpine nitrate (p.1495·1).
*Glaucoma.*

**Carrasyn** *Carrington, USA.*
Acemannan (p.1645·2).
*Wounds.*

**Carreldon** *Bama, Spain.*
Diltiazem hydrochloride (p.900·1).
*Angina pectoris; hypertension.*

**Carrier** *Chiesi, Ital.*
Levocarnitine (p.1423·3).
*Carnitine deficiency.*

**Carsuquin** *Berman, Mex.*
Diiodohydroxyquinoline (p.603·3).
*Amoebiasis; trichomoniasis.*

**Cartan** *Quesada, Arg.*
Losartan (p.948·2).
*Hypertension.*

**Carteabak** *Thea, Fr.*
Carteolol hydrochloride (p.880·3).
*Glaucoma; ocular hypertension.*

**Carteol**
*Viatris, Belg.; Chauvin, Fr.; SIFI, Ital.*
Carteolol hydrochloride (p.880·3).
*Ocular hypertension; open-angle glaucoma.*

**Carteopil** *Viatris, Belg.*
Pilocarpine hydrochloride (p.1495·1); carteolol hydrochloride (p.880·3).
*Glaucoma; ocular hypertension.*

**Carter Petites Pilules** *Carter-Wallace, Switz.†.*
Aloin (p.1248·3); phenolphthalein (p.1284·1); liquorice (p.1270·2).
*Constipation.*

**Carters** *Therabel, Belg.*
Bisacodyl (p.1251·3).
Formerly contained aloes, and podophyllum resin.
*Constipation.*

**Carters Little Pills** *Carter Horner, Canad.*
Bisacodyl (p.1251·3).
Formerly contained aloin and phenolphthalein.
*Constipation.*

**Carthamex** *Rolmex, Canad.*
Vitamin $B_6$ (p.1457·2) in safflower oil.

**Cartia**
*Note. This name is used for preparations of different composition.*
*GlaxoSmithKline, Austral.; GlaxoSmithKline, Hong Kong; SmithKline Beecham, Israel; GlaxoSmithKline, NZ; Lusofarmaco, Port.*
Aspirin (p.15·1).
*Thromboembolism prophylaxis.*

*Andrx, USA.*
Diltiazem hydrochloride (p.900·1).
*Angina pectoris; hypertension.*

**Cartidont** *Curaden, Ital.*
Articaine hydrochloride (p.1370·3).
Adrenaline acid tartrate (p.852·2) is included in this preparation as a vasoconstrictor to diminish absorption and localise the effect of the local anaesthetic.
*Local anaesthesia.*

**Cartilade** *Cartilade, Arg.*
Cartilage (shark).
*Dietary supplement.*

**Cartilag** *Eagle, Austral.†.*
Cartilage (bovine).
*Dietary supplement.*

**Cartilago Compuesto** *Hochstetter, Chile.*
Cartillage; potassium dichromate.
*Arthritis.*

**Cartisorb** *Bioiberica, Spain.*
Glucosamine sulfate (p.1694·1).
*Osteoarthritis.*

**Cartivix** *Jaba, Port.*
Diacerein (p.30·1).
*Osteoarthritis.*

**Cartrax** *Pfizer, Braz.*
Tioconazole (p.409·3); tinidazole (p.617·1).
*Vulvovaginal infections.*

**Cartrol** *Abbott, USA.*
Carteolol hydrochloride (p.880·3).
*Hypertension.*

**Carudol**
*Note. This name is used for preparations of different composition.*
*Boehringer Ingelheim, Fr.†; Fher, Spain†.*
Phenylbutazone piperazine (p.84·1).
Formerly contained phenylbutazone piperazine, methyl nicotinate, and piperazine hydrate in *Fr.*
*Gout; musculoskeletal and joint disorders.*

*Wild, Switz.†.*
Phenylbutazone piperazine (p.84·1); piperazine hydrate (p.111·2).
*Musculoskeletal, joint, and peri-articular pain; soft-tissue disorders.*

**Carvasin**
*Teofarma, Ital.; Wyeth, NZ†.*
Isosorbide dinitrate (p.941·1).
*Angina pectoris; heart failure.*

**Carvicum** *Duopharm, Ger.*
Taraxacum (p.1751·3).
*Appetite loss; biliary disorders; digestive disorders; diuretic.*

**Carvil** *Zydus, India.*
Carvedilol (p.881·1).
*Hypertension.*

**Carvipress** *Gentili, Ital.*
Carvedilol (p.881·1).
*Angina pectoris; hypertension.*

**Carvis** *Volchem, Ital.†.*
Carnitine (p.1423·3).
*Tonic.*

**Carvit** *AGIPS, Ital.†.*
Carnitine (p.1423·3).
*Carnitine deficiency; myocardial ischaemia.*

**Carvomin** *Wernigerode, Ger.*
Angelica (p.1655·1); cnicus benedictus (p.1673·3); peppermint leaf (p.1283·2).
*Gastrointestinal disorders.*

**Carvomin Magentropfen mit Pomeranze**
*Madaus, Ger.*
Bitter-orange peel (p.1723·3).
*Dyspepsia.*

**Carylderm**
*Seton, Irl.†; SSL, UK.*
Carbaryl (p.1501·2).
Carylderm Liquid was formerly known as Derbac-C in the *UK.*
*Pediculosis.*

**Caryolysine**
*Genopharm, Fr.†; IFET (ΙΦΕΤ), Gr.*
Chlormethine hydrochloride (p.537·1).
*Malignant effusions; malignant neoplasms; psoriasis.*

**Carzem** *Rottapharm, Ital.†.*
Diltiazem hydrochloride (p.900·1).
*Hypertension; ischaemic heart disease.*

**Carzepine** *Condrugs, Thai.*
Carbamazepine (p.353·3).
*Alcohol withdrawal syndrome; diabetic neuropathy; epilepsy; trigeminal neuralgia.*

**Carzilasa** *Manuell, Mex.*
Cocarboxylase (p.1455·2).
*Cardiovascular, cerebrovascular, and metabolic disorders.*

**Carzodelan** *Gaschler, Ger.*
Pancreatin (p.1725·3).
*Inflammatory disorders.*

**Casacol** *Helsinn Birex, Irl.*
Methoxyphenamine hydrochloride (p.1124·2); guaifenesin (p.1122·1); sodium citrate (p.1223·2).
*Coughs.*

**Casalm**
*Pharmacia, Austria; Pharmacia, Ger.*
Calcitonin (salmon) (p.768·2).
*Hypercalcaemia and osteolysis in malignancy; osteoporosis; Paget's disease of bone; pancreatic transplantation; reflex sympathetic dystrophy.*

**Casbol** *Fournier SA, Spain.*
Paroxetine hydrochloride (p.311·2).
*Anxiety disorders; depression; obsessive-compulsive disorder; social phobia.*

**Cascade** *Lane, UK.*
Bearberry (p.1659·2); clivers (p.1673·2); lappa root (p.1704·3).
*Water retention.*

**Cascalax** *Will-Pharma, Belg.*
Casanthranol (p.1255·1).
*Constipation.*

**Cascapride** *Merck, Ger.†.*
Bromopride (p.1254·1).
*Gastrointestinal motility disorders; nausea; vomiting.*

**Cascara Sagrada Puler** *Serch, Arg.*
Cascara (p.1255·1); phenolphthalein (p.1284·1).
*Constipation.*

**Cascara Sagrada Sanaplex** *Bouzen, Arg.*
Cascara (p.1255·1); belladonna (p.479·1); bile salts (p.1660·3); phenolphthalein (p.1284·1).
*Constipation.*

**Cascara-Salax**
*Ferring, Austria; Ferring, Ger.†; Ferring, Switz.†.*
Powder for oral solution, dried magnesium sulfate (p.1229·1); tablets, cascara (p.1255·1).
*Bowel evacuation.*

**Cascor**
*Ranbaxy, Malaysia; Ranbaxy, Thai.*
Diltiazem hydrochloride (p.900·1).
*Angina pectoris; hypertension.*

**Casec**
*Mead Johnson, Austral.†.*
Dietary protein supplement (p.1417·1).

*Mead Johnson Nutritionals, Canad.; Mead Johnson, Israel; Mead Johnson Nutritionals, USA.*
Calcium caseinate.
*Protein supplement.*

**Caseical** *Support, Braz.*
Preparation for enteral nutrition (p.1417·1).

**Caseincal** *Novag, Mex.*
Calcium caseinate.
*Dietary supplement.*

**Casenfilus** *Casen Fleet, Spain.*
*Lactobacillus acidophilus* (p.1704·2).
*Restoration of gastrointestinal flora.*

**Casfen** *Menarini, Port.*
*Infant suppositories†:* Aspirin (p.15·1); paracetamol (p.76·2); codeine phosphate (p.27·1).
*Tablets:* Aspirin (p.15·1); paracetamol (p.76·2); codeine phosphate (p.27·1); caffeine (p.782·1).
*Fever; pain.*

**Casilan** *Glaxo Wellcome, Mex.*
Protein supplement (p.1417·1).

**Casodex**
*AstraZeneca, Arg.; AstraZeneca, Austria; AstraZeneca, Belg.; AstraZeneca, Braz.; AstraZeneca, Canad.; AstraZeneca, Chile; AstraZeneca, Denm.; AstraZeneca, Fin.; AstraZeneca, Fr.; AstraZeneca, Ger.; Astra-Zeneca, Gr.; AstraZeneca, Hong Kong; AstraZeneca, Irl.; AstraZeneca, Israel; AstraZeneca, Ital.; AstraZeneca, Malaysia; AstraZeneca, Mex.; AstraZeneca, Neth.; AstraZeneca, Norw.; AstraZeneca, Port.; Zeneca, S.Afr.; AstraZeneca, Singapore; AstraZeneca, Spain; AstraZeneca, Swed.; AstraZeneca, Switz.; AstraZeneca, Thai.; AstraZeneca, UK; Zeneca, USA.*
Bicalutamide (p.530·1).
*Prostatic cancer.*

**Caspacil** *Cazi, Braz.*
Selenium sulfide (p.1157·3).
*Dandruff.*

**Caspiselenio** *Diafarm, Spain.*
Selenium sulfide (p.1157·3).
*Scalp disorders.*

**Casprin** *YSP, Malaysia.*
Aspirin (p.15·1).
*Thromboembolism prophylaxis.*

**Cassadan** *Temmler, Ger.*
Alprazolam (p.668·3).
*Anxiety.*

**Castaderm** *Lannett, USA.*
Resorcinol (p.1156·3); boric acid (p.1662·1); phenol (p.1188·1).
*Fungal skin infections.*

**Castanha de India Composta** *Infabra, Braz.†.*
Aesculus (p.1648·2); rutoside (p.1688·2); vitamin C (p.1460·2).
*Venous insufficiency.*

**Castel** *Syosset, USA.*
Resorcinol (p.1156·3).
*Fungal skin infections.*

**Castellani mit Miconazol** *Hollborn, Ger.*
Miconazole (p.405·2).
*Fungal and bacterial skin infections.*

**Castilium** *Aventis, Port.*
Clobazam (p.358·2).
*Anxiety disorders; epilepsy.*

**Castindia** *IMO, Ital.†.*
Aesculus (p.1648·2); silybum marianum (p.1043·3); hamamelis (p.1696·3).
*Peripheral vascular disorders.*

**Castoria** *Mentholatum, Canad.†.*
Sennoside A and B (p.1288·2).

**Castufemin** *Ardeypharm, Ger.*
Agnus castus (p.1649·1).
*Mastalgia; menstrual disorders.*

**Catabex** *UCB, Belg.*
Dropropizine (p.1119·3).
*Coughs.*

**Catabex Expectorans** *UCB, Belg.*
Dropropizine (p.1119·3); guaifenesin (p.1122·1).
*Coughs.*

**Catabina** *Tecnifar, Port.*
Dropropizine (p.1119·3).
*Coughs.*

**Catabina Expectorante** *Tecnifar, Port.*
Dropropizine (p.1119·3); guaifenesin (p.1122·1).
*Coughs.*

**Cataclot** *Ono, Jpn.*
Ozagrel sodium (p.1725·2).
*Cerebrovascular disorders.*

**Catacol**
*Alcon, Fr.*
Disodium inosinate phosphate.
*Lens opacities.*

*Alcon, Switz.†.*
Disodium inosinate (p.1681·3).
*Eye disorders.*

**Cataflam**
*Novartis, Arg.; Novartis, Belg.; Novartis, Braz.; Novartis, Chile; Novartis, Gr.; Novartis, Hong Kong; Novartis, Irl.; Novartis, Israel; Ciba, Ital.†; Novartis, Malaysia; Novartis, Mex.; Novartis, Neth.; Novartis, Norw.; Novartis, NZ; Bykomed, Port.; Novartis, S.Afr.; Novartis, Singapore; Novartis, Thai.; Novartis, USA.*
Diclofenac (p.32·1), diclofenac diethylamine (p.32·1), diclofenac potassium (p.32·1), diclofenac resinate (p.33·1), or diclofenac sodium (p.32·1).
*Gout; inflammation; musculoskeletal, joint, and peri-articular disorders; pain.*

**Catalgem** *Ibfarma, Braz.†.*
Diclofenac potassium (p.32·1).

**Catalgine** *Lipha Sante, Fr.†.*
Sodium aspirin (p.17·3).
*Fever; musculoskeletal and joint disorders; myocardial infarction; pain.*

**Catalgix** *Rhone-Poulenc Rorer, Belg.†.*
Aspirin (p.15·1).
*Fever; migraine; rheumatic disorders.*

**Catalgix C** *Rhone-Poulenc Rorer, Belg.†.*
Aspirin (p.15·1); ascorbic acid (p.1460·2).
*Fever; migraine; rheumatic disorders.*

**Catalin**
*Allergan, Arg.; Takeda, Hong Kong; Allergan, India; Senju, Jpn; Takeda, Malaysia; Takeda, Singapore; Takeda, Thai.*
Pirenoxine (p.1732·2) or pirenoxine sodium (p.1732·2).
*Cataract.*

**Catalip** *Fournier, Port.*
Fenofibrate (p.915·2).
*Hyperlipidaemias.*

**Catamin** *Riedel-Zabinka, Braz.†.*
Sulfur (p.1158·2); zinc oxide (p.1163·2).
*Acne.*

**Catanac** *Pharmasant, Thai.*
Diclofenac potassium (p.32·1).
*Inflammation; pain.*

**Catapres**
*Boehringer Ingelheim, Austral.; Boehringer Ingelheim, Canad.; Boehringer Ingelheim, Hong Kong; German Remedies, India; Boehringer Ingelheim, Irl.; Boehringer Ingelheim, NZ; Boehringer Ingelheim, S.Afr.†; Boehringer Ingelheim, Thai.; Boehringer Ingelheim, UK; Boehringer Ingelheim, USA.*
Clonidine (p.885·2) or clonidine hydrochloride (p.885·2).
*Hypertension; menopausal flushing; migraine and vascular headache.*

**Catapres Diu** *German Remedies, India.*
Clonidine hydrochloride (p.885·2); chlortalidone (p.882·3).
*Hypertension.*

**Catapresan**
*Boehringer Ingelheim, Austria; Boehringer Ingelheim, Chile; Boehringer Ingelheim, Denm.; Boehringer Ingelheim, Fin.; Boehringer Ingelheim, Ger.; Boehringer Ingelheim, Gr.; Boehringer Ingelheim, Ital.; Boehringer Ingelheim, Mex.; Boehringer Ingelheim, Neth.; Boehringer Ingelheim, Norw.; Boehringer Ingelheim, Port.; Boehringer Ingelheim, Spain; Boehringer Ingelheim, Swed.; Boehringer Ingelheim, Switz.*
Clonidine (p.885·2) or clonidine hydrochloride (p.885·2).
*Hypertension; menopausal disorders; migraine; opioid withdrawal syndrome.*

**Catapressan**
*Boehringer Ingelheim, Belg.; Boehringer Ingelheim, Fr.*
Clonidine hydrochloride (p.885·2).
*Hypertension.*

**Cataren** *INQ, Braz.†.*
Diclofenac potassium (p.32·1).
*Gout; inflammation; musculoskeletal, joint, and periarticular disorders; pain.*

**Cataridol** *Novartis Ophthalmics, Fr.*
Calcium chloride (p.1225·1); magnesium chloride (p.1228·1); sodium chloride (p.1233·3).
Formerly contained sodium iodide and calcium chloride.
*Lens opacities.*

**Catarrh** *Larkhall Laboratories, UK†.*
Achillea (p.1646·2); vervain (p.1764·1); horehound (p.1124·1); salvia (p.1741·2).

**Catarrh Cream** *Weleda, UK.*
Homoeopathic preparation.

**Catarrh Mixture** *Potter's, UK.*
Boneset (p.1661·3); blue flag (p.1702·1); lapp root (p.1704·3); hyssop; capsicum (p.1667·1).
*Catarrh.*

**Catarrh Pastilles**
*Note. This name is used for preparations of different composition.*
*Healthcrafts, UK†.*
Squill vinegar (p.1130·3); menthol (p.1711·3); pumilio pine oil (p.1737·1); eucalyptus oil (p.1686·2).
*Cough and cold symptoms.*

*Unichem, UK†.*
Menthol (p.1711·3); siberian fir oil; oleum pini sylvestris; creosote (p.1117·2).
*Catarrh; coughs.*

**Catarrh Tablets** *Healthcrafts, UK†.*
Horehound (p.1124·1); squill (p.1130·3).
*Catarrh; coughs.*

**Catarrh-eeze** *Chefaro, UK.*
Marrubium (p.1124·1); achillea (p.1646·2); elecampane (p.1119·3).
*Catarrh.*

**Catarrh-Ex** *Thompson, UK.*
Phenylephrine hydrochloride (p.1126·3); paracetamol (p.76·2); caffeine (p.782·1).
*Cold symptoms.*

**Catarrosan** *Tentan, Switz.*
Homoeopathic preparation.

**Catarrosine** *Fecofar, Arg.*
Bromhexine (p.1115·3).
*Respiratory-tract congestion.*

**Catarstat**
*Chauvin, Fr.; Bausch & Lomb, Switz.*
Pyridoxine hydrochloride (p.1456·3); amino acids.
*Cataracts.*

**Catazyme-P** *Stadmed, India.*
*Oral drops:* Amylase (p.1654·2); cinnamon oil (p.1672·2); caraway oil (p.1667·3); cardamom oil (p.1668·1).
*Syrup:* Amylase (p.1654·2); papain (p.1727·3).
*Dyspepsia; flatulence.*

**CAT-Barium (E-Z-CAT)** *Bracco, Switz.*
Barium sulfate (p.1061·1).
*Contrast medium for gastrointestinal radiography.*

**Caterol** *Pharmasant, Thai.*
Procaterol hydrochloride (p.791·1).
*Obstructive airways disease.*

**Catex** *Cantabria, Spain.*
Ciprofloxacin hydrochloride (p.188·2).
*Bacterial infections.*

**Cathejell**
*Montavit, Austria; Pfleger, Ger.†; Montavit, Israel.*
Diphenhydramine hydrochloride (p.431·3); chlorhexidine hydrochloride (p.1173·3).
*Cystoscopy; endoscopy; lubrication for catheter insertion.*

**Cathejell with Lidocaine**
*Montavit, Thai.; Mediplus, UK.*
Chlorhexidine hydrochloride (p.1173·3); lidocaine hydrochloride (p.1377·3).
*Catheter insertion; instrument insertion.*

**Cathejell mit Lidocain**
*Montavit, Austria; Pfleger, Ger.*
Chlorhexidine hydrochloride (p.1173·3); lidocaine hydrochloride (p.1377·3).
*Catheterisation; instrument insertion.*

**Cathejell N** *Geistlich, Switz.†.*
Chlorhexidine hydrochloride (p.1173·3); lidocaine hydrochloride (p.1377·3).
*Catheterisation.*

**Cathejell S** *Pfleger, Ger.*
Chlorhexidine hydrochloride (p.1173·3).
*Catheterisation.*

**Catheter Preparation** *Pharmacia Upjohn, Austral.*
Chlorhexidine gluconate (p.1173·2).
*Genital disinfection before bladder catheterisation.*

**Catiz Plus** *Merck, Arg.*
Saw palmetto (p.1569·1); pygeum africanum (p.1568·2).
*Benign prostatic hyperplasia.*

**Catlep** *Sumitomo, Jpn; Teikoku Seiyaku, Jpn.*
Indometacin (p.47·3).
*Inflammation; musculoskeletal, joint, and periarticular disorders; pain.*

**Cato-Bell** *Bell, India.*
Potassium iodide (p.1598·1); sodium chloride (p.1233·3); calcium chloride (p.1225·1).
*Cataract; lens opacities.*

**Catona** *Mavi, Mex.*
Captopril (p.879·2).
*Hypertension.*

**Catonet** *Nettopharma, Denm.*
Captopril (p.879·2).
*Heart failure; hypertension.*

**Catonin** *Magis, Ital.*
Calcitonin (salmon) (p.768·2).
*Hypercalcaemia; osteoporosis; Paget's disease of bone; reflex sympathetic dystrophy.*

**Catoplin** *Beacons, Singapore.*
Captopril (p.879·2).
*Heart failure; hypertension.*

**Catoprol** *Medley, Braz.*
Captopril (p.879·2).
*Diabetic nephropathy; heart failure; hypertension; myocardial infarction.*

**Catorid** *Boehringer Ingelheim, Belg.†.*
Prolintane hydrochloride (p.1592·3).
*Narcoleptic syndrome.*

**Catovit** *Boehringer Ingelheim, S.Afr.†.*
Prolintane hydrochloride (p.1592·3); multivitamins (p.1417·1).
*Tonic.*

**Catovit N** *Boehringer Ingelheim, S.Afr.†.*
Prolintane hydrochloride (p.1592·3).
*Tonic.*

**Catrix**
*Note. This name is used for preparations of different composition.*
*ICN, Port.*
Collagen (p.1674·3).
*Skin ulcers.*

*Donell DerMedex, USA.*
Emollient and moisturiser.

**Catrix Correction** *Donell DerMedex, USA.*
*SPF 15:* Octinoxate (p.1154·3); methyl anthranilate (p.1154·1); oxybenzone (p.1154·3); titanium dioxide (p.1160·3).
*Sunscreen.*

**Catrix Lip** *Donell DerMedex, USA.*
*SPF 15:* Octinoxate (p.1154·3); oxybenzone (p.1154·3).
*Sunscreen.*

**Catuaba** *Cazi, Braz.†.*
Erythroxylon catuaba; guarana (p.1765·3); liriosma ovata; ginger (p.1267·1); bitter orange (p.1723·3).
*Tonic.*

**Catuama** *Catarinense, Braz.†.*
Erythroxylon catuaba; guarana (p.1765·3); liriosma ovata; ginger (p.1267·1).

**Caulophyllum Complex** *Dolisos, Canad.*
Homoeopathic preparation.

**Causalon** *Phoenix, Arg.*
Paracetamol (p.76·2).
*Fever; pain.*

**Causalon Bronquial** *Phoenix, Arg.*
Clofedanol hydrochloride (p.1117·1); guaifenesin (p.1122·1); oxatomide (p.438·1).
*Coughs.*

**Causalon Gesic** *Phoenix, Arg.*
Paracetamol (p.76·2); ibuprofen (p.45·3).
*Fever; inflammation; pain.*

**Causalon Grip** *Phoenix, Arg.*
Paracetamol (p.76·2); oxatomide (p.438·1); phenylephrine hydrochloride (p.1126·3).
*Respiratory-tract disorders.*

**Causalon Pro** *Phoenix, Arg.*
Naproxen (p.65·1) or naproxen sodium (p.65·1).
*Fever; pain.*

**Causat** *Sanofi Synthelabo, Austria.*
Procaine hydrochloride (p.1383·2); atropine sulfate (p.477·1).
*Migraine; neuralgia; neuritis.*

**Causat B12 N** *Sanofi Synthelabo, Ger.†.*
Procaine hydrochloride (p.1383·2); atropine sulfate (p.477·1); hydroxocobalamin hydrochloride (p.1459·1).
*Arthrosis; migraine; neuralgia; neuritis.*

**Causat N** *Sanofi Synthelabo, Ger.†.*
Procaine hydrochloride (p.1383·2); atropine sulfate (p.477·1).
*Migraine; neuralgia; neuritis; postherpetic neuralgia; trigeminal neuralgia.*

**Caustinerf forte** *Septodont, Switz.*
Lidocaine (p.1377·3); phenol (p.1188·1); paraformaldehyde (p.1187·3).
*Dental pain.*

**Cauterex** *Ache, Braz.*
Fibrinolysin (p.916·2); dornase alfa (p.1119·1); gentamicin (p.219·1).
*Wounds.*

**Cauteridol** *Ederka, Mex.†.*
Ranitidine (p.1285·2).

**Caved-S**
*Note. This name is used for preparations of different composition.*
*Casen Fleet, Spain†.*
Deglycyrrhizinised liquorice (p.1270·2); colloidal aluminium hydroxide (p.1249·2); magnesium carbonate (p.1272·1); sodium bicarbonate (p.1223·2); calamus (p.1664·1); frangula bark (p.1266·3).
*Gastrointestinal hyperacidity.*

*Pharmakon, Switz.†.*
Deglycyrrhizinised liquorice (p.1270·2); dried aluminium hydroxide gel (p.1249·2); magnesium carbonate (p.1272·1); sodium bicarbonate (p.1223·2); frangula (p.1266·3); calamus (p.1664·1); fennel (p.1687·2).
*Gastrointestinal disorders.*

**Caveril** *Remedica, Thai.*
Verapamil hydrochloride (p.1019·1).
*Angina pectoris; arrhythmias; hypertension.*

**Caverject**
*Pharmacia, Arg.; Pharmacia, Austral.; Pharmacia, Austria; Pharmacia, Belg.; Pharmacia, Braz.; Pharmacia, Canad.; Pharmacia, Chile; Pharmacia, Denm.; Pharmacia, Fin.; Pharmacia, Fr.; Pharmacia, Ger.; Pharmacia-Upjohn, Gr.; Pharmacia, Hong Kong; Pharmacia, Irl.; Pharmacia Upjohn, Israel; Pharmacia Upjohn, Ital.; Pharmacia, Malaysia; Pharmacia Upjohn, Mex.; Pharmacia, Neth.; Pharmacia, Norw.; Pharmacia, NZ; Pharmacia, Port.; Pharmacia, S.Afr.; Pharmacia, Singapore; Pharmacia, Spain; Pharmacia, Swed.; Pharmacia, Switz.; Pharmacia, Thai.; Pharmacia, UK; Pharmacia, USA.*
Alprostadil (p.1512·3) or alprostadil alfadex (p.1512·3).
*Erectile dysfunction.*

**Caverta** *Ranbaxy, India.*
Sildenafil citrate (p.1744·2).
*Erectile dysfunction.*

**Caviamina** *De Mayo, Braz.*
Vitamin B substances; vitamin C; fructose (p.1417·1).

**CaviD** *Nycomed, Denm.*
Calcium carbonate (p.1254·2); colecalciferol (p.1461·3).
*Calcium and vitamin D deficiency; osteoporosis.*

**Cavilon**
*3M, Arg.; 3M, Fr.; 3M, UK.*
A range of barrier preparations.

**Cavinton**
*Bago, Arg.; Thiemann, Ger.; Armstrong, Mex.†; Biosaude, Port.; Gedeon Richter, Singapore; Gedeon Richter, Thai.*
Vinpocetine (p.1764·2).
*Cerebrovascular disorders; vascular eye disorders.*

**Cavirox** *Roux-Ocefa, Arg.*
Calcium carbonate (p.1254·2); colecalciferol (p.1461·3).
*Calcium supplement; osteoporosis.*

**Cavirox Junior** *Roux-Ocefa, Arg.*
Calcium carbonate (p.1254·2).
*Calcium supplement.*

**Cavit-D3** *Merck, Singapore.*
Calcium hydrogen phosphate (p.1225·2); colecalciferol (p.1461·3).
*Calcium and vitamin D deficiency; calcium and vitamin D supplement; osteoporosis.*

**Cavodan** *Lacefa, Arg.*
Hyoscine (p.483·3); nitrazepam (p.710·1); oxazepam (p.712·2).
*Sedative.*

**Cavodine** *Biolab, Thai.*
Povidone-iodine (p.1190·3).
*Skin, burn, and wound disinfection.*

**Cavumox** *Siam Bheasach, Thai.*
Amoxicillin trihydrate (p.155·3); potassium clavulanate (p.193·3).
*Bacterial infections.*

**Caye Balsam** *Medopharm, Ger.*
Glycol salicylate (p.44·3); sodium salamidacetate (p.87·3); benzyl nicotinate (p.21·2); capsicum (p.1667·1); coumarin (p.1676·2).
*Musculoskeletal, joint, and soft-tissue disorders.*

**Cayenne Plus** *Nutrovite, Canad.*
Cayenne (p.1667·1); ginger root (p.1267·1).

**Caziderm** *Cazi, Braz.*
Nitrofurazone (p.238·2).
*Burns; skin infections.*

**Cazigeran** *Cazi, Braz.*
Vitamin B substances; vitamin E; magnesium; potassium (p.1417·1).

**Cazmar** *Fucus, Arg.*
Vitamin A (p.1451·2).
*Skin disorders.*

**Cazole**
*Malpharm, Hong Kong; Malaysia Chemist, Singapore.*
Carbimazole (p.1596·2).
*Hyperthyroidism.*

**C-1000-C**
*Novartis, Chile.*
Ascorbic acid (p.1460·2); calcium lactobionate (p.1225·3); calcium carbonate (p.1254·2).
*Calcium and vitamin C supplement.*

*Novartis, Mex.*
Ascorbic acid (p.1460·2); calcium lactate gluconate (p.1225·3).
*Calcium and vitamin C supplement.*

**C-Calcium** *Streuli, Switz.*
Calcium gluconate (p.1225·2); ascorbic acid (p.1460·2); calcium saccharate (p.1665·1).
*Vitamin C and calcium deficiency.*

**CCK** *Sanitas, Arg.*
Co-dergocrine mesilate (p.1674·1).
*Cerebrovascular disorders.*

**CCK Flunarizina** *Sanitas, Arg.*
Co-dergocrine mesilate (p.1674·1); flunarizine hydrochloride (p.434·1).
*Cerebral and peripheral vascular disorders; vestibular disorders.*

**CC-Nefro** *Medice, Ger.*
Calcium carbonate (p.1254·2).
*Hyperphosphataemia.*

**CCNU** *Medac, UK.*
Lomustine (p.565·2).
*Malignant neoplasms.*

**C-Destrosio** *Amsa, Ital.†.*
Ascorbic acid (p.1460·2); glucose (p.1432·2).
*Vitamin C deficiency.*

**C-Dose** *Medgenix, Belg.*
Ascorbic acid (p.1460·2).
*Scurvy; vitamin C deficiency.*

**CDT**
*CSL, Austral.; CSL, NZ†.*
An adsorbed diphtheria and tetanus vaccine (p.1613·1).
*Active immunisation of infants and young children.*

**Ceanel**
*Quinoderm, Irl.; Hoechst Marion Roussel, S.Afr.†; Ferndale, UK.*
Cetrimide (p.1172·1); undecenoic acid (p.410·3); phenethyl alcohol (p.1188·1).
*Dandruff; psoriasis; seborrhoeic dermatitis.*

**CEA-Scan**
*Byk Gulden, Ital.; Nuclear, Spain; Immunomedics, UK; Immunomedics, USA.*
Technetium-99m arcitumomab (p.1525·2).
*Detection of colorectal cancer.*

**Cebedex** *Chauvin, Fr.†.*
Dexamethasone sodium phosphate (p.1097·2).
*Eye disorders.*

**Cebedexacol** *Chauvin, Fr.*
Chloramphenicol (p.185·1); dexamethasone sodium phosphate (p.1097·2).
*Eye infections.*

**Cebemyxine**
*Chauvin, Fr.; Chauvin, Hong Kong.*
Neomycin sulfate (p.235·1); polymyxin B sulfate (p.245·1).
*Bacterial eye infections.*

**Cebenicol** *Chauvin, Fr.*
Chloramphenicol (p.185·1).
*Eye infections.*

**Cebera** *Irex, Fr.*
Alibendol (p.1649·3).
*Dyspepsia.*

**Cebesine** *Chauvin, Fr.*
Oxybuprocaine hydrochloride (p.1382·1).
*Local anaesthesia.*

**Cebexin** *Indian Drugs, India.*
Vitamin B substances; vitamin C (p.1417·1).
*Vitamin B and C deficiency.*

**Cebid** *Hauck, USA†.*
Ascorbic acid (p.1460·2).
*Scurvy; vitamin C deficiency.*

**Cebiolon** *Merck, Port.*
Ascorbic acid (p.1460·2).
*Vitamin C supplement.*

**Cebion**
*Merck, Arg.; Merck, Austria; Merck, Braz.; Merck, Chile; Merck, Ger.; Galenica, Gr.; Bracco, Ital.; Merck, Port.†; Merck, Spain.*
Ascorbic acid (p.1460·2).
*Vitamin C deficiency.*

**Cebion Calcico** *Merck, Chile.*
Vitamin C; calcium carbonate; rutin; colecalciferol (p.1417·1).
*Calcium supplement; tonic.*

**Cebion Calcio** *Merck, Braz.*
Ascorbic acid (p.1460·2); calcium carbonate (p.1254·2).
*Calcium and vitamin C supplement.*

**Cebion Erkaltungs** *Merck, Ger.*
Aspirin (p.15·1); ascorbic acid (p.1460·2).
*Cold symptoms; fever; pain.*

**Cebion Glicose** *Merck, Braz.†.*
Ascorbic acid (p.1460·2); glucose (p.1432·2).
*Glucose and vitamin C supplement.*

**Cebion Multi** *Merck, Port.†.*
Multivitamin and mineral preparation (p.1417·1).

**Cebion N** *Merck, Ger.*
Sodium ascorbate (p.1460·2).
*Methaemoglobinaemia; vitamin C deficiency.*

**Cebion Plus Calcio** *Merck, Port.†.*
Ascorbic acid (p.1460·2); calcium carbonate (p.1254·2).
*Nutritional supplement.*

**Cebion Plus Com Minerais** *Merck, Braz.*
Ascorbic acid (p.1460·2); minerals.
*Nutritional supplement.*

**Cebion Plus Magnesio**
*Merck, Braz.; Merck, Port.†.*
Ascorbic acid (p.1460·2); magnesium carbonate (p.1272·1).
*Nutritional supplement.*

**Cebion Plus Minerals** *Merck, Port.†.*
Ascorbic acid and minerals (p.1417·1).
*Nutritional supplement.*

**Cebion-Calcium N** *Merck, S.Afr.†.*
Calcium carbonate (p.1254·2); ascorbic acid (p.1460·2).
*Calcium and vitamin C supplement.*

**Cebiopirina** *Brocco, Ital.†.*
Ascorbic acid (p.1460·2); aspirin (p.15·1).
*Cold symptoms; pain.*

**Cebralat** *Libbs, Braz.†.*
Cilostazol (p.884·1).
*Thromboembolic disorders.*

**Cebran** *Garant, Ital.*
Nicergoline (p.1719·3).
*Cerebral and peripheral vascular disorders; headache; hypertension.*

**Cebrilin** *Libbs, Braz.*
Paroxetine hydrochloride (p.311·2).
*Depression.*

**Cebrocal** *Lafi, Chile.*
Gamma-aminobutyric acid; gamma-amino beta-hidroxybutyric acid; acetylglutamin; vitamin B (p.1417·1).

**Cebrofort** *Baliarda, Arg.*
Nimodipine (p.972·3).
*Cerebrovascular disorders.*

**Cebrotex** *Janssen-Cilag, Port.*
Glutamine (p.1433·2).

**Cebroton** *Tubilux, Ital.*
Citicoline sodium (p.1672·3).
*Cerebrovascular disorders; mental function impairment; parkinsonism.*

**Cebrotonin**
*Ritter, Malaysia; Ritter, Singapore.*
Piracetam (p.1732·1).
*Mental function impairment in the elderly.*

**Cebutid** *Shire, Fr.*
Flurbiprofen (p.43·3).
*Inflammation; musculoskeletal, joint, and peri-articular disorders; pain.*

**Cec**
*Hexal, Arg.; Hexal, Austria; Hexal, Ger.; Hexal, S.Afr.*
Cefaclor (p.167·1).
*Bacterial infections.*

**Cecap**
*Atlantic, Hong Kong; Atlantic, Malaysia.*
Ascorbic acid (p.1460·2).
*Tonic; vitamin C deficiency.*

**Cecenu**
*Rhone-Poulenc Rorer, Belg.†; Medac, Ger.*
Lomustine (p.565·2).
*Malignant neoplasms.*

**Ceclor**
*Lilly, Austral.; Lilly, Austria; Lilly, Belg.; Lilly, Braz.; Lilly, Canad.; Pharmaserve Lilly (Φαρμασερβ Λιλλυ), Gr.; Lilly, Hong Kong; Lilly, Israel; Lilly, Mex.; Lilly, Neth.; Lilly, NZ†; Medinfar, Port.; Lilly, S.Afr.; Spaly, Spain; Lilly, Switz.; Dura, USA; Lilly, USA.*
Cefaclor (p.167·1).
*Bacterial infections.*

**Ceclorbeta** *Betapharm, Ger.*
Cefaclor (p.167·1).
*Bacterial infections.*

**Cecon**
*Abbott, Austral.†; Abbott, India; Abbott, Ital.†; Abbott, USA.*
Ascorbic acid (p.1460·2).
*Scurvy; vitamin C deficiency.*

*Abbott, Ital.†.*
*Tablets:* Sodium ascorbate (p.1460·2); ascorbic acid (p.1460·2).
*Vitamin C deficiency.*

**Cecrisina** *Janssen-Cilag, Port.*
Ascorbic acid (p.1460·2).
*Vitamin C supplement.*

**Ced Compl** *Sigma, Braz.†.*
Multivitamin preparation (p.1417·1).

**Cedax**
*White, Arg.; Schering-Plough, Fin.†; Schering-Plough, Hong Kong; Schering-Plough, Irl.†; Schering-Plough, Israel†; Schering-Plough, Ital.; Schering-Plough, Malaysia; Schering-Plough, Mex.; Schering-Plough, Neth.; Schering-Plough, S.Afr.; Schering-Plough, Singapore; Schering-Plough, Spain; Schering-Plough, Swed.; Essex, Switz.; Schering-Plough, Thai.; Schering, USA.*
Ceftibuten (p.182·1).
*Bacterial infections.*

**Cedelate** *Nakorn, Thai.*
Flunarizine (p.434·2).
*Migraine; vestibular disorders.*

**Cedilanid** *Novartis, Austria†.*
*Injection:* Deslanoside (p.893·1).
*Tablets:* Lanatoside C (p.945·1).
*Arrhythmias; heart failure.*

**Cedilanide**
*Novartis, Braz.; Novartis, Fr.†.*
Deslanoside (p.893·1).
*Heart failure; pulmonary oedema; supraventricular arrhythmias.*

**Cedine** *Rowex, Irl.*
Cimetidine (p.1255·3).
*Gastric hyperacidity; peptic ulcer; Zollinger-Ellison syndrome.*

**Cedium** *Qualiphar, Belg.*
Benzalkonium chloride (p.1168·3).
*Disinfection of the skin, wounds, and hands.*

**Cedixen** *Aventis, Austria.*
Cefpirome sulfate (p.178·2).
*Bacterial infections.*

**Cedocard**
*Byk, Austria; Byk, Belg.; Paladin, Canad.; Pharmacia Upjohn, Irl.†; Byk, Neth.; Pacific, Thai.†; Pharmacia, UK.*
Isosorbide dinitrate (p.941·1).
*Angina pectoris; heart failure; myocardial infarction; pulmonary hypertension.*

**Cedol** *Eurofarmaco, Ital.†.*
Cefamandole nafate (p.169·3).
*Bacterial infections.*

**Cedozelin** *Sigma, Braz.*
Vitamin B substances; fructose; vitamin C (p.1417·1).
*Anaemias.*

**Cedril** *MC, Ital.†.*
Benzalkonium chloride (p.1168·3); benzethonium chloride (p.1169·2); didecyldimethylammonium chloride (p.1178·3).
*Disinfection of ulcers, burns, and wounds.*

**Cedril Strumenti** *MC, Ital.†.*
Benzalkonium chloride (p.1168·3); benzethonium chloride (p.1169·2); didecyldimethylammonium chloride (p.1178·3); alcohol (p.1166·1).
*Instrument disinfection.*

**Cedrin** *Schering-Plough, Braz.*
Pseudoephedrine sulfate (p.1129·2); azatadine maleate (p.425·1).
*Nasal congestion.*

**Cedrol** *Astra, Spain†.*
Zolpidem tartrate (p.728·3).
*Insomnia.*

**Cedrox** *Hexal, Ger.*
Cefadroxil (p.167·2).
*Bacterial infections.*

**Cedur**
*Roche, Belg.; Roche, Braz.; Roche, Ger.; Roche, Switz.*
Bezafibrate (p.873·2).
*Hyperlipidaemias.*

**Ceelin** *Pediatrica, Malaysia.*
Ascorbic acid (p.1460·2).
*Vitamin C deficiency; vitamin C supplement.*

**CeeNU**
*Bristol-Myers Squibb, Arg.; Bristol-Myers Squibb, Austral.; Bristol, Canad.; Bristol-Myers Squibb, Chile; Bristol-Myers Squibb, Hong Kong; Bristol-Myers Squibb, Israel; Bristol-Myers Squibb, Malaysia; Bristol-Myers Squibb, Mex.; Bristol-Myers Squibb, NZ; Bristol-Myers Squibb, S.Afr.†; Bristol-Myers Squibb, Singapore; Bristol-Myers Squibb, Thai.†; Bristol-Myers Squibb Oncology, USA.*
Lomustine (p.565·2).
*Malignant neoplasms.*

**Ceerexin** *Leiras, Fin.*
Ascorbic acid (p.1460·2).
*Vitamin C deficiency.*

**Ceezinc** *Lifeplan, UK†.*
Zinc (p.1469·2); vitamin C (p.1460·2).

**CEF-3** *Siam Bheasach, Thai.*
Ceftriaxone sodium (p.182·3).
*Bacterial infections.*

**CEF-4** *Siam Bheasach, Thai.*
Ceftazidime (p.180·2).
*Bacterial infections.*

**Cefa Resan** *Alacan, Spain.*
Cefazolin sodium (p.170·3).
Lidocaine hydrochloride (p.1377·3) is included in this preparation to alleviate the pain of injection.
*Bacterial infections.*

**Cefaben** *Cazi, Braz.*
Cefalexin (p.168·1).
*Bacterial infections.*

**Cefabene** *Cefak, Ger.*
Stipites dulcamarae (p.1683·1).
*Eczema.*

**Cefabiot** *Hexal, Arg.*
Cefadroxil (p.167·2).
*Bacterial infections.*

**Cefabiozim** *IPA, Ital.*
Cefazolin sodium (p.170·3).
Lidocaine hydrochloride (p.1377·3) is included in this preparation to alleviate the pain of injection.
*Bacterial infections.*

**Cefabol**
*Note. This name is used for preparations of different composition.*
*Cefak, Ger.†.*
Boldo (p.1661·2).
*Dyspepsia; gastrointestinal spasm.*

*Robert, Spain.*
Sodium cytidine monophosphate; gamma-aminobutyric acid (p.1690·2); aminohydroxybutyric acid (p.353·2); magnesium glutamate hydrobromide (p.1709·2); trisodium uridine triphosphate (p.1760·3); pyridoxine hydrochloride (p.1456·3).
*Mental function disorders; tonic.*

**Cefabrina** *Neo Quimica, Braz.*
Paracetamol (p.76·2).
*Fever; pain.*

**Cefabronchin** *Cefak, Ger.†.*
Thyme (p.1755·2); Iceland moss; saponaria; pimpinella; eucalyptus (p.1686·1); fennel (p.1687·2); star anise.
*Respiratory-tract inflammation.*

**Cefacar** *Bristol-Myers Squibb, Arg.*
Cefadroxil (p.167·2).
*Bacterial infections.*

**Cefacar Mucolitico** *Bristol-Myers Squibb, Arg.*
Cefadroxil (p.167·2); ambroxol hydrochloride (p.1114·3).
*Respiratory-tract infections.*

**Cefacene** *Centrum, Spain.*
Cefazolin sodium (p.170·3).
Lidocaine (p.1377·3) is included in this preparation to alleviate the pain of injection.
*Bacterial infections.*

**Cefacet** *Norgine, Fr.*
Cefalexin (p.168·1).
*Bacterial infections.*

**Cefachol** *Cefak, Ger.†.*
Greater celandine (p.1695·3); taraxacum (p.1751·3); silybum marianum (p.1043·3).
*Biliary disorders; liver disorders.*

**Cefacidal**
*Bristol-Myers Squibb, Belg.; Bristol-Myers Squibb, Fr.; Bristol-Myers Squibb, Mex.†; Bristol-Myers Squibb, Neth.; Bristol-Myers Squibb, S.Afr.; Bristol-Myers Squibb, Thai.†.*
Cefazolin sodium (p.170·3).
Lidocaine (p.1377·3) my be included in the intramuscular injection to alleviate the pain of injection.
*Bacterial infections.*

**Cefacile** *Bristol-Myers Squibb, Port.*
Cefadroxil (p.167·2).
*Bacterial infections.*

**Cefacilina** *Montpellier, Arg.*
Cefadroxil (p.167·2).
*Bacterial infections.*

**Cefacilina Bronquial** *Montpellier, Arg.*
Cefadroxil (p.167·2); ambroxol hydrochloride (p.1114·3).
*Respiratory-tract infections.*

**Cefacin-M** *Bright Future, Hong Kong.*
Cefalexin (p.168·1).
*Bacterial infections.*

**Cefacolin** *Northia, Arg.*
Cefotaxime (p.176·3).
*Bacterial infections.*

**Cefacor** *Cefak, Ger.†.*
Scoparium (p.1742·2).
*Cardiac disorders.*

**Cefacure** *Orchid, Hong Kong.*
Cefalexin (p.168·1).
*Bacterial infections.*

**Cefacynar** *Cefak, Ger.*
Cynara (p.1678·3).
*Biliary-tract disorders.*

**Cefade** *Klonal, Arg.*
Cefalotin (p.168·3).
*Bacterial infections.*

**Cefadel** *Francia, Ital.†.*
Cefmetazole sodium (p.173·3).
Lidocaine hydrochloride (p.1377·3) is included in this preparation to alleviate the pain of injection.
*Bacterial infections.*

**Cefadian** *Cefak, Ger.*
Potentilla anserina.
*Dysmenorrhoea.*

**Cefadin**
*Atlantic, Singapore; Vana, Thai.*
Cefalotin sodium (p.168·3).
*Bacterial infections.*

**Cefadol** *Atlantic, Thai.*
Cefamandole nafate (p.169·3).
*Bacterial infections.*

**Cefadolor** *Cefak, Ger.*
Guaiacum wood.
*Rheumatic disorders.*

**Cefadolor H** *Cefak, Ger.*
Homoeopathic preparation.

**Cefadrex** *Vir, Spain.*
Cefazolin sodium (p.170·3).
Lidocaine (p.1377·3) is included in the injection to alleviate the pain of injection.
*Bacterial infections.*

**Cefadril**
*AGIPS, Ital.; LSP, Thai.*
Cefadroxil (p.167·2).
*Bacterial infections.*

**Cefadrin** *Cefak, Ger.*
Ephedra (p.1119·3); thyme (p.1755·2); ammi visnaga (p.1653·3).
Formerly known as Cefedrin N.
*Asthma; coughs.*

**Cefadrox** *Mer-National, S.Afr.†.*
Cefadroxil (p.167·2).
*Bacterial infections.*

**Cefadroxon** *Sanval, Braz.*
Cefadroxil (p.167·2).
*Bacterial infections.*

**Cefadyn** *Cefak, Ger.†.*
Ruscus aculeatus.
*Chronic venous insufficiency.*

**Cefadysbasin** *Cefak, Ger.†.*
Secale corn.; aesculus (p.1648·2); potentilla anserina.
*Peripheral, coronary, and central circulatory disorders.*

**Cefafloria** *Cefak, Ger.*
Ethyl linoleate.
Formerly known as Floriabene.
*Skin disorders.*

**Cefagastrin** *Cefak, Ger.†.*
Chamomile (p.1669·3); calendula (p.1665·2); peppermint leaf (p.1283·2); centaury (p.1669·2); absinthium (p.1645·1); arnica (p.1656·3); fennel (p.1687·2).
*Gastrointestinal disorders.*

**Cefager** *Gerard, Irl.*
Cefaclor (p.167·1).
*Bacterial infections.*

**Cefagil** *Cefak, Ger.*
Homoeopathic preparation.

**Cefagon** *Ibfarma, Braz.†.*
Cefalexin (p.168·1).
*Bacterial infections.*

**Cefagran** *Legrand, Braz.*
Cefalexin (p.168·1).
*Bacterial infections.*

**Cefakava** *Cefak, Ger.†.*
Kava (p.1703·2).
*Anxiety; nervousness; tension.*

**Cefakes** *Inexfa, Spain†.*
Cefazolin sodium (p.170·3).
*Bacterial infections.*

**Cefakliman** *Cefak, Ger.*
Homoeopathic preparation.

**Cefakliman mono** *Cefak, Ger.*
Cimicifuga (p.1671·3).
*Menopausal disorders.*

**Cefakliman N** *Cefak, Ger.†.*
Homoeopathic preparation.

**Cefaktivon** *Cefak, Ger.†.*
Cerium (III)-chloride; echinacea (p.1683·2); hypericum (p.299·1); menyanthes (p.1712·1); calendula (p.1665·2).
*Tonic.*

**Cefalan** *Merck, Mex.*
Cefaclor (p.167·1).
*Bacterial infections.*

**Cefaldina** *IMA, Braz.*
Isometheptene mucate (p.1702·1); dipyrone (p.35·3); caffeine (p.782·1).
*Migraine.*

**Cefalektin** *Cefak, Ger.*
Mistletoe (p.1715·3).
*Malignant neoplasms.*

**Cefalen** *Byk, Braz.†.*
Cefalexin (p.168·1).
*Bacterial infections.*

**Cefalex** *Bago, Arg.*
Ergotamine tartrate (p.467·2); caffeine (p.782·1); chlorphenamine maleate (p.427·3); paracetamol (p.76·2).
*Migraine.*

**Cefalexan** *Sanval, Braz.*
Cefalexin (p.168·1).
*Bacterial infections.*

**Cefalexgobens** *Normon, Spain.*
Cefalexin (p.168·1).
*Bacterial infections.*

**Cefalexi** *Arion, Arg.*
Cefalexin (p.168·1).
*Bacterial infections.*

**Cefalin**
*Note. This name is used for preparations of different composition.*
*Generics, Israel.*
Cefalexin (p.168·1).
*Bacterial infections.*

*Vana, Thai.*
Cefazolin sodium (p.170·3).
*Bacterial infections.*

**Cefaline Hauth** *Homme de Fer, Fr.*
Paracetamol (p.76·2); caffeine (p.782·1).
*Fever; pain.*

**Cefaline-Pyrazole** *Homme de Fer, Fr.*
Dipyrone (p.35·3); caffeine (p.782·1).
*Pain.*

**Cefalium** *Ache, Braz.*
Paracetamol (p.76·2); dihydroergotamine mesilate (p.465·3); metoclopramide hydrochloride (p.1274·3); caffeine (p.782·1).
*Migraine.*

**Cefaliv** *Ache, Braz.*
Dihydroergotamine mesilate (p.465·3); dipyrone (p.35·3); caffeine (p.782·1).
*Migraine.*

**Cefallone** *Azupharma, Ger.†.*
Cefaclor (p.167·1).
*Bacterial infections.*

**Cefalmin** *Instituto Sanitas, Chile.*
Ergotamine tartrate (p.467·2); dipyrone (p.35·3); chlorphenamine maleate (p.427·3); caffeine (p.782·1).
*Migraine and other vascular headache.*

**Cefaloject** *Bristol-Myers Squibb, Fr.*
Cefapirin sodium (p.170·2).
Lidocaine hydrochloride (p.1377·3) is included in the intramuscular injection to alleviate the pain of injection.
*Bacterial infections.*

**Cefalom** *Help, Gr.*
Cefadroxil (p.167·2).
*Bacterial infections.*

**Cefalomicina** *Bago, Arg.*
Cefazolin (p.170·3).
Lidocaine hydrochloride (p.1377·3) is included in some injections to alleviate the pain of injection.
*Bacterial infections.*

**Cefalor**
*Merck, Hong Kong; Vitamed, Israel.*
Cefaclor (p.167·1).
*Bacterial infections.*

**Cefalot** *Teuto, Braz.*
Cefalotin sodium (p.168·3).
*Bacterial infections.*

**Cefaluffa** *Cefak, Ger.†.*
Homoeopathic preparation.

**Cefalver** *Maver, Mex.*
Cefalexin (p.168·1).
*Bacterial infections.*

**Cefalymphat** *Cefak, Ger.†.*
Homoeopathic preparation.

**Cefam** Magis, Ital.
Cefamandole nafate (p.169·3).
Lidocaine hydrochloride (p.1377·3) is included in this preparation to alleviate the pain of injection.
*Bacterial infections.*

**Cefamadar** Cefak, Ger.
Homoeopathic preparation.

**Cefamar**
Note. This name is used for preparations of different composition.
Mar, Arg.
Cefadroxil (p.167·2).
*Bacterial infections.*

FIRMA, Ital.†; Menarini, Thai.
Cefuroxime sodium (p.184·1).
*Bacterial infections.*

**Cefamezin**
Gador, Arg.; Sigma, Austral.†; Hoechst Marion Roussel, Braz.†; Fujisawa, Hong Kong; Teva, Israel; Pharmacia Upjohn, Ital.; Fujisawa, Jpn; Hikma, Port.; Knoll, Spain†; Fujisawa, Thai.
Cefazolin sodium (p.170·3).
Lidocaine (p.1377·3) or lidocaine hydrochloride (p.1377·3) may be included in the intramuscular injection to alleviate the pain of injection.
*Bacterial infections.*

**Cefamig** Richelet, Fr.
Chamomile (p.1669·3).
*Headache.*

**Cefamiso** Inexfa, Spain†.
Cefalexin (p.168·1).
*Bacterial infections.*

**Cefamox**
Bristol-Myers Squibb, Braz.; Bristol-Myers Squibb, Chile; Bristol-Myers Squibb, Mex.; Bristol-Myers Squibb, Swed.
Cefadroxil (p.167·2).
*Bacterial infections.*

**Cefamusel** Cruz, Spain†.
Cefazolin sodium (p.170·3).
Lidocaine (p.1377·3) is included in the intramuscular injection to alleviate the pain of injection.
*Bacterial infections.*

**Cefanal** Bunker, Braz.
Cefalexin (p.168·1).
*Bacterial infections.*

**Cefanalgin** Cefak, Ger.†.
Homoeopathic preparation.

**Cefanephrin** Cefak, Ger.†.
Solidago virgaurea (p.1748·3); bearberry (p.1659·2).
*Urinary-tract disorders.*

**Cefanex** Apothecon, USA.
Cefalexin (p.168·1).
*Bacterial infections.*

**Cefangipect** Cefak, Ger.†.
Homoeopathic preparation.

**Cefanorm** Cefak, Ger.
Agnus castus (p.1649·1).
*Mastalgia; menstrual disorders.*

**Cefaperos**
Bristol-Myers Squibb, Belg.; Bristol-Myers Squibb, Fr.
Cefatrizine (p.170·3) or propylene glycol cefatrizine (p.170·3).
*Bacterial infections.*

**Cefaporex** Haller, Braz.†.
Cefalexin (p.168·1).
*Bacterial infections.*

**Cefapoten** Del Bel, Arg.
Cefalexin (p.168·1).
*Bacterial infections.*

**Cefapulmon mono** Cefak, Ger.
Hedera helix.
*Bronchial catarrh.*

**Cefarheumin N** Cefak, Ger.†.
Pumilio pine oil (p.1737·1); rosemary oil (p.1740·2); camphor (p.1665·3).
*Muscle, joint, and nerve pain; neuritis.*

**Cefarheumin S** Cefak, Ger.†.
Homoeopathic preparation.

**Cefariston** Ariston, Braz.
Cefalotin (p.169·2).
*Bacterial infections.*

**Cefasabal** Cefak, Ger.
Saw palmetto (p.1569·1); solidago virgaurea (p.1748·3); aesculus (p.1648·2).
*Prostatic disorders.*

**Cefascillan** Cefak, Ger.†.
Squill (p.1130·3); convallaria (p.1675·3).
*Cardiac disorders; oedema.*

**Cefasedativ** Cefak, Ger.
Valerian (p.1762·2); lupulus (p.1708·1).
Formerly contained valerian, lupulus, and crataegus.
*Anxiety disorders; insomnia.*

**Cefasel**
Cefak, Ger.
Sodium selenite (p.1444·1).
*Selenium deficiency.*

Cefak, Ger.†.
Homoeopathic preparation.

**Cefasept** Cefak, Ger.
*Injection; oral drops:* Homoeopathic preparation.
*Tablets:* Echinacea angustifolia (p.1683·2).
*Infections.*

**Cefasept mono** Cefak, Ger.†.
Echinacea purpura (p.1683·2).
*Immunostimulant in respiratory-tract infections.*

**Cefasin** Sintesina, Arg.
Cefadroxil (p.167·2).
*Bacterial infections.*

**Cefasliymarin** Cefak, Ger.
Silybum marianum (p.1043·3).
*Liver disorders.*

**Cefaspasmon N** Cefak, Ger.†.
Homoeopathic preparation.

**Cefasporina** Oriental, Arg.
Cefalexin (p.168·1).
*Bacterial infections.*

**Cefassin** Cefak, Ger.
Symphoricarpus; euphorbium cypariss.; gold in form of tetrachlorogold acid (p.1695·3).
Formerly known as Cefossin H.
*Joint disorders.*

**Cefastad** Stada, Austria.
Cefaclor (p.167·1).
*Bacterial infections.*

**Cefasulfon N** Cefak, Ger.†.
Homoeopathic preparation.

**Cefatec** Cefak, Ger.
Devil's claw root (p.28·2).
*Musculoskeletal and joint disorders.*

**Cefatenk** Biotenk, Arg.
Cefadroxil (p.167·2).
*Bacterial infections.*

**Cefatox** Cefak, Ger.
Echinacea purpurea (p.1683·2).
*Respiratory-tract infections.*

**Cefatrex** Bristol-Myers Squibb, Gr.
Cefapirin sodium (p.170·2).
*Bacterial infections.*

**Cefatrix** Levofarma, Ital.
Propylene glycol cefatrizine (p.170·3).
*Bacterial infections.*

**Cefavale** Cefak, Ger.†.
Lycopus europaeus.
*Thyroid disorders.*

**Cefavora** Cefak, Ger.
Homoeopathic preparation.

**Cefawell** Cefak, Ger.
Calendula (p.1665·2); arnica (p.1656·3).
*Skin disorders; wounds.*

**Cefa-Wolff** Wolff, Ger.
Cefaclor (p.167·1).
*Bacterial infections.*

**Cefax**
Note. This name is used for preparations of different composition.
Hexal, Austria.
Cefaclor (p.167·1).
*Bacterial infections.*

Inga, Malaysia.
Cefalexin (p.168·1).
*Bacterial infections.*

**Cefaxicina** CEPA, Spain†.
Cefoxitin sodium (p.177·2).
Lidocaine hydrochloride (p.1377·3) is included in the intramuscular injection to alleviate the pain of injection.
*Bacterial infections.*

**Cefaxim** Ofimex, Mex.†.
Cefotaxime (p.176·3).
*Bacterial infections.*

**Cefaxon** Ariston, Braz.
Cefalexin (p.168·1).
*Bacterial infections.*

**Cefaxona** Pisa, Mex.
Ceftriaxone sodium (p.182·3).
Lidocaine hydrochloride (p.1377·3) is included in the intramuscular injection to alleviate the pain of injection.
*Bacterial infections.*

**Cefaxone** Shin Poong, Singapore.
Ceftriaxone sodium (p.182·3).
*Bacterial infections.*

**Cefazil** Italfarmaco, Ital.
Cefazolin sodium (p.170·3).
Lidocaine hydrochloride (p.1377·3) is included in this preparation to alleviate the pain of injection.
*Bacterial infections.*

**Cefazillin** TP, Thai.
Cefazolin sodium (p.170·3).
*Bacterial infections.*

**Cefazima** Biochimico, Braz.
Ceftazidime (p.180·2).
*Bacterial infections.*

**Cefazink** Cefak, Ger.
Zinc gluconate (p.1469·2).
*Zinc deficiency.*

**Cefazol** General Drugs, Thai.
Cefazolin sodium (p.170·3).
*Bacterial infections.*

**Cefazone**
Teuto, Braz.; Locatelli, Ital.†.
Cefoperazone sodium (p.174·3).
Lidocaine hydrochloride (p.1377·3) is included in this preparation to alleviate the pain of injection.
*Bacterial infections.*

**Cef-Diolan** Brahms, Ger.
Cefaclor (p.167·1).
*Bacterial infections.*

**Cefec** Tecnifar, Port.
Cefetamet pivoxil hydrochloride (p.172·3).
*Bacterial infections.*

**Cefen** Pharmasant, Thai.
Ibuprofen (p.45·3).
*Fever; inflammation; musculoskeletal, joint, and soft-tissue disorders; pain.*

**Ceferro** Teofarma, Ger.
Ferrous sulfate (p.1428·2).
*Iron-deficiency; iron-deficiency anaemias.*

**Cefexin** Unison, Thai.
Cefalexin (p.168·1).
*Bacterial infections.*

**Cefimix** Faribérica, Port.
Cefixime (p.172·3).
*Bacterial infections.*

**Cefin** Korea United, Singapore.
Ceftriaxone sodium (p.182·3).
*Bacterial infections.*

**Cefine** Nakorn, Thai.
Ceftriaxone sodium (p.182·3).
*Bacterial infections.*

**Cefiran** Searle, Ital.†.
Cefamandole nafate (p.169·3).
Lidocaine hydrochloride (p.1377·3) is included in this preparation to alleviate the pain of injection.
*Bacterial infections.*

**Cefirex** Irex, Fr.†.
Cefradine (p.179·3).
*Bacterial infections.*

**Cefiton** Clintex, Port.
Cefixime (p.172·3).
*Bacterial infections.*

**Cefixoral** Menarini, Ital.
Cefixime (p.172·3).
*Bacterial infections.*

**Cefizox**
Roche, Austria†; GlaxoSmithKline, Canad.; Aventis, Fr.; GlaxoSmithKline, India; Wellcome, Irl.†; Promeco, Mex.; Yamanouchi, Neth.; Hikma, Port.; SmithKline, Spain†; Fujisawa, USA.
Ceftizoxime sodium (p.182·2).
Lidocaine hydrochloride (p.1377·3) may be included in the intramuscular injection to alleviate the pain of injection.
*Bacterial infections.*

**Cefkor** Douglas, Austral.
Cefaclor (p.167·1).
*Bacterial infections.*

**Ceflacid** Collins, Mex.
Cefaclor (p.167·1).
*Bacterial infections.*

**Ceflax** Hikma, Port.
Cefalexin (p.168·1).
*Bacterial infections.*

**Ceflexin** Luper, Braz.
Cefalexin (p.168·1).
*Bacterial infections.*

**Ceflin** Hexal, Austral.†.
Cefalexin (p.168·1).
*Bacterial infections.*

**Ceflour** YSP, Malaysia.
Cefuroxime sodium (p.184·1).
*Bacterial infections.*

**Ceflux** Ahimsa, Arg.
Cefuroxime (p.184·1).
*Bacterial infections.*

**Cefmandol** General Drugs, Thai.
Cefamandole (p.169·3).
*Bacterial infections.*

**Cefmetazon**
Sankyo, Hong Kong; Sankyo, Jpn; Sankyo, Thai.†.
Cefmetazole sodium (p.173·3).
*Bacterial infections.*

**Cefnax** Teuto, Braz.
Cefixime (p.172·3).
*Bacterial infections.*

**Cefobacter** AGIPS, Ital.
Cefonicid sodium (p.174·2).
Lidocaine hydrochloride (p.1377·3) is included in this preparation to alleviate the pain of injection.
*Gram-negative bacterial infections.*

**Cefobid**
Pfizer, Arg.; Pfizer, Austria; Pfizer, Braz.†; Pfizer, Hong Kong; Pfizer, Jpn; Pfizer, Malaysia; Pfizer, Singapore; Farmasierra, Spain; Pfizer, Thai.; Pfizer, USA.
Cefoperazone sodium (p.174·3).
*Bacterial infections.*

**Cefobis**
Pfizer, Fr.†; Pfizer, Ger.†.
Cefoperazone sodium (p.174·3).
*Bacterial infections.*

**Cefociclin** Francia, Ital.
Cefoxitin sodium (p.177·2).
Lidocaine hydrochloride (p.1377·3) is included in this preparation to alleviate the pain of injection.
*Gram-negative bacterial infections.*

**Cefoclin** Wayne, Mex.†.
Cefotaxime (p.176·3).
*Bacterial infections.*

**Cefodie** GlaxoSmithKline, Ital.
Cefonicid sodium (p.174·2).
Lidocaine hydrochloride (p.1377·3) is included in the intramuscular injections to alleviate the pain of injection.
*Bacterial infections.*

**Cefodime** LBS, Thai.
Ceftazidime (p.180·2).
*Bacterial infections.*

**Cefodox**
Aventis, Irl.; Scharper, Ital.
Cefpodoxime proxetil (p.178·3).
*Bacterial infections.*

**Cefofix** Hikma, Port.
Cefuroxime sodium (p.184·1).
*Bacterial infections.*

**Cefogen** Cadila, Thai.
Cefuroxime sodium (p.184·1).
*Bacterial infections.*

**Cefoger** De Salute, Ital.
Cefonicid sodium (p.174·2).
Lidocaine hydrochloride (p.1377·3) is included in this preparation to alleviate the pain of injection.
*Gram-negative bacterial infections.*

**Cefogram**
Note. This name is used for preparations of different composition.
Richmond, Arg.
Cefuroxime (p.184·1).
*Bacterial infections.*

Metapharma, Ital.†.
Cefoperazone sodium (p.174·3).
Lidocaine hydrochloride (p.1377·3) is included in this preparation to alleviate the pain of injection.
*Bacterial infections.*

**Cefok** KBR, Ital.
Cefonicid sodium (p.174·2).
Lidocaine hydrochloride (p.1377·3) is included in this preparation to alleviate the pain of injection.
*Gram-negative bacterial infections.*

**Cefol**
Abbott, Hong Kong; Abbott, USA.
Multivitamin preparation (p.1417·1).

**Cefomic** LBS, Thai.
Cefotaxime sodium (p.175·3).
*Bacterial infections.*

**Cefomycin** Cadila, India.
Cefoperazone sodium (p.174·3).
*Bacterial infections.*

**Cefoneg** Tosi, Ital.
Cefoperazone sodium (p.174·3).
Lidocaine hydrochloride (p.1377·3) is included in the intramuscular injection to alleviate the pain of injection.
*Gram-negative bacterial infections.*

**Cefoper** Menarini, Ital.
Cefoperazone sodium (p.174·3).
Lidocaine hydrochloride (p.1377·3) is included in the intramuscular injection to alleviate the pain of injection.
*Gram-negative bacterial infections.*

**Cefoplus** Aesculapius, Ital.
Cefonicid sodium (p.174·2).
Lidocaine hydrochloride (p.1377·3) is included in this preparation to alleviate the pain of injection.
*Gram-negative bacterial infections.*

**Cefoprim** Esseti, Ital.
Cefuroxime sodium (p.184·1).
Lidocaine hydrochloride (p.1377·3) is included in this preparation to alleviate the pain of injection.
*Gram-negative bacterial infections.*

**Ceforal**
Note. This name is used for preparations of different composition.
Teva, Israel.
Cefalexin (p.168·1).
*Bacterial infections.*

Euro-Labor, Port.; Grunenthal, Port.
Cefadroxil (p.167·2).
*Bacterial infections.*

**Ceforan**
Uniao Quimica, Braz.; General Drugs, Thai.
Cefotaxime sodium (p.175·3).
*Bacterial infections.*

**Cefortam** Glaxo Wellcome, Port.
Ceftazidime sodium (p.181·2).
*Bacterial infections.*

**Cefosint** Crosara, Ital.†.
Cefoperazone sodium (p.174·3).
Lidocaine hydrochloride (p.1377·3) is included in this preparation to alleviate the pain of injection.
*Bacterial infections.*

**Cefosporen** TRB, Arg.
Cefalexin (p.168·1).
*Bacterial infections.*

**Cefosporin** Esseti, Ital.
Cefonicid sodium (p.174·2).
Lidocaine hydrochloride (p.1377·3) is included in the intramuscular injection to alleviate the pain of injection.
*Gram-negative bacterial infections.*

**Cefossin** Cefak, Ger.†.
Homoeopathic preparation.

**Cefotan**
Wyeth-Ayerst, Canad.; Zeneca, USA.
Cefotetan disodium (p.177·1).
*Bacterial infections.*

**Cefotax**
Eurofarma, Braz.†; Vana, Thai.
Cefotaxime sodium (p.175·3).
*Bacterial infections.*

**Cefotex** Precimex, Mex.†.
Cefotaxime (p.176·3).
*Bacterial infections.*

**Cefotrizin** FIRMA, Ital.†.
Propylene glycol cefatrizine (p.170·3).
*Bacterial infections.*

**Cefovis** *Ripari-Gero, Ital.†.*
Cefonicid sodium (p.174·2).
Lidocaine hydrochloride (p.1377·3) is included in this preparation to alleviate the pain of injection.
*Gram-negative bacterial infections.*

**Cefovit** *Vitamed, Israel.*
Cefalexin (p.168·1).
*Bacterial infections.*

**Cefoxan** *Royton, Braz.*
Cefoxitin (p.178·1).
*Bacterial infections.*

**Cefoxin**
*Royton, Braz.; Merck Sharp & Dohme, Thai.*
Cefoxitin sodium (p.177·2).
Lidocaine hydrochloride (p.1377·3) may be included in the intramuscular injection to alleviate the pain of injection.
*Bacterial infections.*

**Cefozone**
*Atlantic, Hong Kong†; Atlantic, Singapore; Vana, Thai.*
Cefoperazone sodium (p.174·3).
*Bacterial infections.*

**Cefra** *OM, Port.*
Cefadroxil (p.167·2).
*Bacterial infections.*

**Cefrabiotic** *Prospa, Ital.*
Cefradine (p.179·3).
*Bacterial infections.*

**Cefraden** *Merck, Mex.†.*
Ceftriaxone sodium (p.182·3).
*Bacterial infections.*

**Cefradil** *Merck, Mex.†.*
Cefotaxime sodium (p.175·3).
*Bacterial infections.*

**Cefradur** *Atral-Vida, Port.*
Cefradine (p.179·3).
*Bacterial infections.*

**Cefral** *Lilly, Arg.*
Cefaclor (p.167·1).
*Bacterial infections.*

**Cefril** *Bristol-Myers Squibb, S.Afr.*
Cefradine (p.179·3).
*Bacterial infections.*

**Cefrin** *Julphar, UAE.*
Cefalexin (p.168·1).
*Bacterial infections.*

**Cefrom**
*Aventis, Austral.; Aventis, Austria; Aventis, Belg.; Hoechst Marion Roussel, Denm.†; Hoechst Marion Roussel, Fin.†; Aventis, Fr.; Hoechst Marion Roussel, Hong Kong†; Aventis, India; Aventis, Irl.; Aventis, Mex.; Aventis, Neth.; Aventis, NZ; Aventis, S.Afr.; Hoechst Marion Roussel, Singapore†; Hoechst Marion Roussel, Swed.†; Hoechst Marion Roussel, Switz.†; Aventis, Thai.; Aventis, UK.*
Cefpirome sulfate (p.178·2).
*Bacterial infections.*

**Cefron** *Aventis, Braz.†.*
Cefpirome sulfate (p.178·2).
*Bacterial infections.*

**Cefspan**
*Grunenthal, Chile; Fujisawa, Jpn; Fujisawa, Thai.*
Cefixime (p.172·3).
*Bacterial infections.*

**Ceft** *Sanval, Braz.*
Ceftriaxone sodium (p.182·3).
*Bacterial infections.*

**Ceftaran** *Nakorn, Thai.*
Cefotaxime sodium (p.175·3).
*Bacterial infections.*

**Ceftazidon** *Ariston, Braz.*
Ceftazidime (p.180·2).
*Bacterial infections.*

**Ceftazin** *Remedina, Gr.*
Propylene glycol cefatrizine (p.170·3).
*Bacterial infections.*

**Ceften** *Teuto, Braz.*
Ceftazidime (p.180·2).
*Bacterial infections.*

**Ceftidin** *Lyka, India.*
Ceftazidime (p.180·2).
*Bacterial infections.*

**Ceftim** *Glaxo Allen, Ital.*
Ceftazidime (p.180·2).
*Gram-negative bacterial infections.*

**Ceftin**
*GlaxoSmithKline, Canad.; GlaxoSmithKline, USA.*
Cefuroxime axetil (p.184·1).
*Bacterial infections.*

**Ceftina** *Galen, Mex.*
Cefalotin sodium (p.168·3).
*Bacterial infections.*

**Ceftix**
*Gador, Arg.*
Ceftizoxime (p.182·3).
*Bacterial infections.*

*Boehringer Mannheim, Ger.†.*
Ceftizoxime sodium (p.182·2).
*Bacterial infections.*

**Ceftizon** *Bago, Arg.*
Ceftizoxime sodium (p.182·2).
*Bacterial infections.*

**Cefton** *Ariston, Braz.*
Cefoxitin (p.178·1).
*Bacterial infections.*

**Ceftoral** *Vianex (Βιανεξ), Gr.*
Cefixime (p.172·3).
*Bacterial infections.*

**Ceftrat** *Uniao Quimica, Braz.†.*
Cefazolin sodium (p.170·3).
*Bacterial infections.*

**Ceftrex**
*Biolab, Malaysia; Columbia, Mex.; Biolab, Thai.*
Ceftriaxone sodium (p.182·3).
Lidocaine (p.1377·3) may be included in the intramuscular injection to alleviate the pain of injection.
*Bacterial infections.*

**Ceftriax** *Sigma, Braz.*
Ceftriaxone (p.183·3).
Lidocaine (p.1377·3) is included in the intramuscular injection to alleviate the pain of injection.
*Bacterial infections.*

**Ceftriaz** *Klonal, Arg.*
Ceftriaxone (p.183·3).
*Bacterial infections.*

**Ceftrilem** *Lemery, Mex.*
Ceftriaxone sodium (p.182·3).
Lidocaine (p.1377·3) is included in the intramuscular injection to alleviate the pain of injection.
*Bacterial infections.*

**Ceftrinal** *Pharmedia (Φαρμεντια), Gr.*
Ranitidine hydrochloride (p.1285·2).
*Conditions where gastric acid reduction is beneficial; gastric hypersecretion including Zollinger-Ellison syndrome; peptic ulcer.*

**Ceftriphin** *General Drugs, Thai.*
Ceftriaxone sodium (p.182·3).
*Bacterial infections.*

**Cefudura** *Merck dura, Ger.*
Cefuroxime axetil (p.184·1).
*Bacterial infections.*

**Cefuhexal** *Hexal, Ger.*
Cefuroxime axetil (p.184·1).
*Bacterial infections.*

**Cefulton** *Fulton, Ital.*
Cefaclor (p.167·1).
*Bacterial infections.*

**Cefumax** *SoSe, Ital.*
Cefuroxime sodium (p.184·1).
Lidocaine hydrochloride (p.1377·3) is included in this preparation to alleviate the pain of injection.
*Gram-negative bacterial infections.*

**Cefunk** *Apsen, Braz.†.*
Mepyramine maleate (p.437·1); aspirin (p.15·1); caffeine (p.782·1); ascorbic acid (p.1460·2).
Aluminium hydroxide (p.1249·2) is included in this preparation in an attempt to limit adverse effects on the gastrointestinal mucosa.
*Cold and influenza symptoms.*

**Cefur** *Eurofarmaco, Ital.*
Cefuroxime sodium (p.184·1).
*Gram-negative bacterial infections.*

**Cefuracet** *Columbia, Mex.*
Cefuroxime axetil (p.184·1).
*Bacterial infections.*

**Cefurax** *Lindopharm, Ger.*
Cefuroxime axetil (p.184·1).
*Bacterial infections.*

**Cefurex** *Salus, Ital.*
Cefuroxime sodium (p.184·1).
*Gram-negative bacterial infections.*

**Cefurim** *General Drugs, Thai.*
Cefuroxime (p.184·1).
*Bacterial infections.*

**Cefurin** *Magis, Ital.*
Cefuroxime sodium (p.184·1).
*Gram-negative bacterial infections.*

**Cefuro-Puren** *Alpharma-Isis, Ger.*
Cefuroxime axetil (p.184·1).
*Bacterial infections.*

**Cefurox** *GlaxoSmithKline, Arg.*
Cefuroxime (p.184·1) or cefuroxime axetil (p.184·1).
*Bacterial infections.*

**Cefurox-Reu** *Reusch, Ger.†.*
Cefuroxime sodium (p.184·1).
*Bacterial infections.*

**Cefurox-Wolff** *Wolff, Ger.*
Cefuroxime axetil (p.184·1).
*Bacterial infections.*

**Cefuzime** *Julphar, UAE.*
Cefuroxime axetil (p.184·1).
*Bacterial infections.*

**Cefxin** *Community Pharmacy, Thai.*
Cefalexin (p.168·1).
*Bacterial infections.*

**Cefxitin** *Siam Bheasach, Thai.*
Cefoxitin sodium (p.177·2).
*Bacterial infections.*

**Cefzil**
*Bristol-Myers Squibb, Braz.; Bristol-Myers Squibb, Canad.; Bristol-Myers Squibb, UK; Bristol-Myers Squibb, USA.*
Cefprozil (p.179·2).
*Bacterial infections.*

**Cefzon** *Fujisawa, Jpn.*
Cefdinir (p.171·3).
*Bacterial infections.*

**Ceglution** *Ariston, Arg.*
Lithium carbonate (p.301·1).
*Bipolar disorder.*

**Cegripe** *Janssen-Cilag, Port.*
Chlorphenamine maleate (p.427·3); paracetamol (p.76·2); hesperidin (p.1688·2); vitamin C (p.1460·2).
*Cold symptoms.*

**Cegrovit**
*Grossmann, Hong Kong; Grossmann, Switz.*
Ascorbic acid (p.1460·2).
*Vitamin C deficiency.*

**Cehafolin** *Sanova, Austria†.*
Calcium folinate (p.1431·1).
*Enhancement of fluorouracil activity; methotrexate toxicity.*

**Cehapark** *Sanova, Austria.*
Bromocriptine mesilate (p.1200·3).
*Acromegaly; parkinsonism.*

**Cehasol** *Sanova, Austria.*
*Bath additive:* Eucalyptus oil (p.1686·2); camphor (p.1665·3); menthol (p.1711·3).
*Cold symptoms.*
*Ointment:* Sulfur-rich shale oil (Cehasol); vitamin F-glycerinester.
*Skin disorders.*

**Ceklin** *Klinger, Braz.*
Ascorbic acid (p.1460·2).
*Vitamin C supplement.*

**Celamine** *Pharmasant, Thai.*
Imipramine hydrochloride (p.300·1).
*Depression; nocturnal enuresis; pain; panic attacks; parkinsonism.*

**Celance**
*Pharmacia, Arg.; Lilly, Braz.; Lilly, Chile; Lilly, Fr.; Pharmaserve Lilly (Φαρμασερβ Λιλλυ), Gr.; Lilly, Hong Kong; Lilly, Irl.; Lilly, Singapore†; Lilly, Thai.; Lilly, UK.*
Pergolide mesilate (p.1211·2).
*Parkinsonism.*

**Celapram** *Alphapharm, Austral.*
Citalopram hydrobromide (p.289·1).
*Depression.*

**Celco** *Unison, Thai.*
Cefaclor (p.167·1).
*Bacterial infections.*

**Celcox** *Trima, Israel.*
Celecoxib (p.25·2).
*Osteoarthritis; rheumatoid arthritis.*

**Celebra**
*Pharmacia, Braz.; Pfizer, Chile; Pharmacia, Denm.; Pfizer, Fin.; Pharmacia, Fin.; Searle, Israel; Pfizer, Norw.; Pharmacia, Norw.; Pfizer, Swed.; Pharmacia, Swed.*
Celecoxib (p.25·2).
*Familial adenomatous polyposis; osteoarthritis; pain; rheumatoid arthritis.*

**Celebrex**
*Pharmacia, Arg.; Pharmacia, Austral.; Pharmacia, Austria; Pharmacia, Belg.; Pharmacia, Canad.; Pharmacia, Fr.; Pharmacia, Ger.; Pharmacia, Hong Kong; Pfizer, Hong Kong; Pharmacia, Irl.; Monsanto, Ital.; Pharmacia, Malaysia; Pfizer, Malaysia; Searle, Mex.; Pharmacia, Neth.; Pharmacia, NZ; Pharmacia, Port.; Pharmacia, S.Afr.; Pfizer, Singapore; Pharmacia, Singapore; Pharmacia, Spain; Pharmacia, Switz.; Pfizer, Thai.; Pharmacia, Thai.; Pharmacia, UK; Searle, USA.*
Celecoxib (p.25·2).
*Familial adenomatous polyposis; osteoarthritis; pain; rheumatoid arthritis.*

**Celectol**
*Aventis, Fr.; Pantheon, UK.*
Celiprolol hydrochloride (p.881·3).
*Angina pectoris; hypertension.*

**Celemax** *Elvetium, Arg.*
Celecoxib (p.25·2).
*Osteoarthritis; rheumatoid arthritis.*

**Celemin** *Galen, Mex.*
Quinfamide (p.615·2).
*Amoebiasis.*

**Celen** *Ranbaxy, Braz.*
Cefalexin (p.168·1).
*Bacterial infections.*

**Celenid**
*Biopharm, Hong Kong; Biolab, Malaysia; Biolab, Singapore; Biolab, Thai.*
Cinnarizine (p.428·3).
*Cerebrovascular disorders; migraine; motion sickness; peripheral vascular disease; vestibular disorders.*

**Celesdepot** *Schering-Plough, Port.*
Betamethasone sodium phosphate (p.1093·1); betamethasone acetate (p.1093·1).
*Corticosteroid.*

**Celesemine** *Schering-Plough, Spain.*
Betamethasone (p.1093·1); dexchlorpheniramine maleate (p.427·3).
*Hypersensitivity reactions.*

**Celestamil** *Teuto, Braz.*
Betamethasone (p.1093·1); dexchlorpheniramine maleate (p.427·3).
*Hypersensitivity reactions.*

**Celestamin** *Aesca, Austria.*
Betamethasone (p.1093·1); dexchlorpheniramine maleate (p.427·3).
*Hypersensitivity disorders.*

**Celestamine**
*Key, Arg.; Schering-Plough, Braz.; Schering-Plough, Chile; Schering-Plough, Fr.; Essex, Ger.; Schering-Plough, Hong Kong; Schering-Plough, Mex.; Schering-Plough, S.Afr.; Essex, Switz.*
Betamethasone (p.1093·1); dexchlorpheniramine maleate (p.427·3).
*Hypersensitivity reactions.*

**Celestamine N** *Essex, Ger.*
Betamethasone (p.1093·1).
*Corticosteroid.*

**Celestamine NS** *Schering-Plough, Mex.*
Betamethasone (p.1093·1); loratadine (p.436·1).
*Hypersensitivity.*

**Celestamine-F** *Schering-Plough, Mex.*
Betamethasone (p.1093·1); dexchlorpheniramine maleate (p.427·3).
*Hypersensitivity.*

**Celestamine-L** *Key, Arg.*
Betamethasone (p.1093·1); loratadine (p.436·1).
*Hypersensitivity reactions.*

**Celestan**
*Aesca, Austria.*
Betamethasone (p.1093·1) or betamethasone sodium phosphate (p.1093·1) and betamethasone acetate (p.1093·1).
*Corticosteroid.*

*Teuto, Braz.*
Betamethasone sodium phosphate (p.1093·1).
*Corticosteroid.*

**Celestan Depot** *Essex, Ger.*
Betamethasone sodium phosphate (p.1093·1); betamethasone acetate (p.1093·1).
*Corticosteroid.*

**Celestan solubile** *Essex, Ger.*
Betamethasone sodium phosphate (p.1093·1).
*Corticosteroid.*

**Celestan-V** *Essex, Ger.*
Betamethasone valerate (p.1093·2).
*Scalp disorders; skin disorders.*

**Celestene**
*Schering-Plough, Fr.; IFET (ΙΦΕΤ), Gr.*
Betamethasone (p.1093·1) or betamethasone sodium phosphate (p.1093·1).
*Corticosteroid.*

**Celestene Chronodose** *Schering-Plough, Fr.*
Betamethasone sodium phosphate (p.1093·1); betamethasone acetate (p.1093·1).
*Corticosteroid.*

**Celestial Seasonings** *Warner-Lambert, Canad.†.*
Menthol (p.1711·3).

**Celestoderm**
*Schering, Canad.; Schering-Plough, Fin.; Schering-Plough, Fr.; Schering-Plough, Neth.; Schering-Plough, Spain.*
Betamethasone valerate (p.1093·2).
*Scalp disorders.*

**Celestoderm cum Chinoform** *Schering-Plough, Fin.*
Betamethasone valerate (p.1093·2); clioquinol (p.196·3).
*Infected skin disorders.*

**Celestoderm cum Garamycin** *Schering-Plough, Fin.*
Betamethasone valerate (p.1093·2); gentamicin sulfate (p.217·1).
*Infected skin disorders.*

**Celestoderm Gentamicina** *Schering-Plough, Spain.*
Betamethasone valerate (p.1093·2); gentamicin sulfate (p.217·1).
*Infected skin disorders.*

**Celestoderm met Neomycine** *Schering-Plough, Neth.*
Betamethasone valerate (p.1093·2); neomycin sulfate (p.235·1).
*Infected skin disorders.*

**Celestoderm-V**
*Schering-Plough, Gr.; Schering-Plough, Hong Kong; Schering-Plough, Israel†; Schering-Plough, Ital.; Schering-Plough, Malaysia; Schering-Plough, Mex.; Schering-Plough, S.Afr.; Schering-Plough, Singapore; Schering-Plough, Spain; Essex, Switz.; Schering-Plough, Thai.†.*
Betamethasone valerate (p.1093·2).
*Skin disorders.*

**Celestoderm-V with Garamycin**
*Schering-Plough, Hong Kong; Schering-Plough, Israel†; Schering-Plough, Malaysia; Schering-Plough, S.Afr.; Schering-Plough, Singapore.*
Betamethasone valerate (p.1093·2); gentamicin sulfate (p.217·1).
*Infected skin disorders.*

**Celestoderm-V with Neomycin**
*Schering-Plough, Hong Kong†; Schering-Plough, Singapore; Schering-Plough, Thai.†.*
Betamethasone valerate (p.1093·2); neomycin sulfate (p.235·1).
*Infected skin disorders.*

**Celestoform** *Schering-Plough, Neth.*
Betamethasone valerate (p.1093·2); clioquinol (p.196·3).
*Infected skin disorders.*

**Celeston**
*Schering-Plough, Denm.*
*Cream; liniment; ointment; topical solution:* Betamethasone valerate (p.1093·2).
*Skin disorders.*

*Schering-Plough, Denm.; Schering-Plough, Norw.*
*Injection:* Betamethasone acetate (p.1093·1); betamethasone sodium phosphate (p.1093·1).
*Corticosteroid.*

*Schering-Plough, Denm.†.*
*Tablets:* Betamethasone (p.1093·1).
*Corticosteroid.*

*Schering-Plough, Swed.*
*Injection:* Betamethasone sodium phosphate (p.1093·1).
*Corticosteroid.*

**Celeston bifas** *Schering-Plough, Swed.*
Betamethasone acetate (p.1093·1); betamethasone sodium phosphate (p.1093·1).
*Corticosteroid.*

**Celeston Chronodose** *Schering-Plough, Fin.*
Betamethasone acetate (p.1093·1); betamethasone sodium phosphate (p.1093·1).
*Corticosteroid.*

**Celeston med Chinoform** *Schering-Plough, Denm.*
Betamethasone valerate (p.1093·2); clioquinol (p.196·3).
*Infected skin disorders.*

**Celeston valerat** *Schering-Plough, Swed.*
Betamethasone valerate (p.1093·2).
*Otitis externa; skin disorders.*

**Celeston valerat comp** *Schering-Plough, Swed.*
Betamethasone valerate (p.1093·2); neomycin sulfate (p.235·1).
*Infected skin disorders.*

**Celeston valerat med chinoform** *Schering-Plough, Swed.*
Betamethasone valerate (p.1093·2); clioquinol (p.196·3).
*Infected skin disorders; otitis externa.*

**Celeston valerat med gentamicin** *Schering-Plough, Swed.*
Betamethasone valerate (p.1093·2); gentamicin sulfate (p.217·1).
*Infected skin disorders.*

**Celestone**
*Kirby, Arg.; Schering-Plough, Belg.; Schering-Plough, Braz.; Schering, Canad.†; Schering-Plough, Hong Kong; Schering-Plough, Ital.; Schering-Plough, Malaysia; Schering-Plough, Mex.; Schering-Plough, Neth.; Schering-Plough, Port.; Schering-Plough, S.Afr.; Schering-Plough, Singapore†; Schering-Plough, Spain; Essex, Switz.; Schering-Plough, Thai.†; Schering, USA.*
Betamethasone (p.1093·1) or betamethasone sodium phosphate (p.1093·1).
*Corticosteroid.*

**Celestone V** *Schering-Plough, Austral.*
Betamethasone valerate (p.1093·2).
*Skin disorders.*

**Celestone Chronodose**
*Schering-Plough, Austral.; Schering-Plough, Belg.; Schering-Plough, Gr.; Schering-Plough, Israel; Schering-Plough, Neth.; Schering-Plough, NZ; Essex, Switz.*
Betamethasone sodium phosphate (p.1093·1); betamethasone acetate (p.1093·1).
*Corticosteroid.*

**Celestone Cronodose**
*Kirby, Arg.; Schering-Plough, Ital.; Schering-Plough, Spain.*
Betamethasone acetate (p.1093·1); betamethasone sodium phosphate (p.1093·1).
*Corticosteroid.*

**Celestone M** *Schering-Plough, Austral.*
Betamethasone valerate (p.1093·2).
*Skin disorders.*

**Celestone S** *Schering-Plough, Spain.*
Betamethasone (p.1093·1); sulfacetamide sodium (p.257·3).
*Infected eye disorders.*

**Celestone Soluspan**
*Schering-Plough, Braz.; Schering, Canad.; Schering-Plough, Mex.; Schering-Plough, S.Afr.; Schering, USA.*
Betamethasone acetate (p.1093·1); betamethasone sodium phosphate (p.1093·1).
*Corticosteroid.*

**Celestone VG** *Schering-Plough, Austral.*
Betamethasone valerate (p.1093·2); gentamicin sulfate (p.217·1).
*Infected skin disorders.*

**Celevac**
*Shire, Irl.; Monmouth, UK.*
Methylcellulose (p.1580·2).
*Constipation; diarrhoea; diverticular disease; obesity; ostomy management; ulcerative colitis.*

**Celex** *Masa, Thai.*
Cefalexin (p.168·1).
*Bacterial infections.*

**Celexa**
*Lundbeck, Canad.; Forest Pharmaceuticals, USA.*
Citalopram hydrobromide (p.289·1).
*Depression.*

**Celexin**
*Schering-Plough, Braz.; Hovid, Malaysia; Hovid, Singapore; Vana, Thai.*
Cefalexin (p.168·1).
*Bacterial infections.*

**Celfax** *Degorts, Mex.*
Ketorolac trometamol (p.52·1).
*Pain.*

**Celib** *Unichem, India.*
Celecoxib (p.25·2).
*Osteoarthritis; rheumatoid arthritis.*

**Ce-Limo** *Asta Medica, Austria.*
Ascorbic acid (p.1460·2).
*Vitamin C deficiency.*

**Ce-Limo plus 10 Vitamine** *Asta Medica, Austria.*
Multivitamin preparation (p.1417·1).

**Ce-Limo-Calcium** *Asta Medica, Austria.*
Ascorbic acid (p.1460·2); calcium carbonate (p.1254·2).
*Calcium and vitamin C deficiency.*

**Celin**
*GlaxoSmithKline, Hong Kong; GlaxoSmithKline, India.*
Vitamin C (p.1460·2).
*Vitamin C supplement.*

**Celipro** *Lichtenstein, Ger.*
Celiprolol hydrochloride (p.881·3).
*Angina pectoris; hypertension.*

**Celit** *Fada, Arg.*
Metoclopramide (p.1274·3).
*Nausea and vomiting.*

**Celkalm** *Aerocid, Fr.†.*
Loperamide hydrochloride (p.1271·1).
*Diarrhoea.*

**Cellasene** *Cinetic, Arg.*
Bearberry; melilotus; ginkgo biloba; bladderwrack (p.1742·3); centella; fish oil; borage oil; soya lecithin; fatty acids (p.1417·1).
*Antioxidant; cellulitis.*

**Cellavie** *Ferrosan, Fin.*
*d*-Alpha tocoferil acetate (p.1465·1); ascorbic acid (p.1460·2).
*Vitamin E and vitamin C deficiency.*

**Cellblastin** *Cell Pharm, Ger.*
Vinblastine sulfate (p.591·2).
*Malignant neoplasms.*

**CellCept**
*Roche, Arg.; Roche, Austral.; Roche, Austria; Roche, Belg.; Roche, Braz.; Roche, Canad.; Roche, Chile; Roche, Denm.; Roche, Fin.; Roche, Fr.; Roche, Ger.; Roche, Gr.; Roche, Hong Kong; Roche, Irl.; Roche, Israel; Roche, Ital.; Chugai, Jpn; Roche, Mex.; Roche, Neth.; Roche, Norw.; Roche, NZ; Roche, Port.; Roche, S.Afr.; Roche, Singapore; Roche, Spain; Roche, Swed.; Roche, Switz.; Roche, Thai.; Roche, UK; Roche, USA.*
Mycophenolate mofetil (p.1361·2) or mycophenolate mofetil hydrochloride (p.1362·2).
*Cardiac, renal, or hepatic transplant rejection.*

**Cellcristin** *Cell Pharm, Ger.*
Vincristine sulfate (p.592·2).
*Malignant neoplasms.*

**Cellferon** *Cell Pharm, Ger.†.*
Interferon alpha-1 (p.640·3).
*Hairy-cell leukaemia.*

**Cellidrin** *Hennig, Ger.*
Allopurinol (p.412·2).
*Gout; hyperuricaemia; renal calculi.*

**Cellidrine** *Sanofi, Switz.*
Allopurinol (p.412·2).
*Hyperuricaemia.*

**cellmustin** *Cell Pharm, Ger.*
Estramustine sodium phosphate (p.551·1).
*Prostatic cancer.*

**Cellobexon** *Agepha, Austria.*
Methylcellulose (p.1580·2); thiamine hydrochloride (p.1455·1); vitamin C (p.1460·2).
*Constipation; obesity.*

**Celloid Compounds Magcal Plus** *Blackmores, Austral.†.*
Dibasic sodium phosphate (p.1231·1); magnesium phosphate (p.1228·1); calcium phosphate (p.1225·3); dibasic potassium phosphate (p.1230·3); iron phosphate.

**Celloid Compounds Sodical Plus** *Blackmores, Austral.†.*
Dibasic sodium phosphate (p.1231·1); calcium phosphate (p.1225·3); iron phosphate.

**Celloids CF 43** *Blackmores, Austral.†.*
Homoeopathic preparation.

**Celloids CP 57** *Blackmores, Austral.†.*
Calcium phosphate (p.1225·3).

**Celloids CS 36** *Blackmores, Austral.†.*
Calcium sulfate (p.1665·1).

**Celloids IP 82** *Blackmores, Austral.†.*
Iron phosphate.

**Celloids MP 65** *Blackmores, Austral.†.*
Magnesium phosphate (p.1228·1).

**Celloids PC 73** *Blackmores, Austral.†.*
Potassium chloride (p.1232·2).

**Celloids PP 85** *Blackmores, Austral.†.*
Potassium phosphate (p.1230·3).

**Celloids PS 29** *Blackmores, Austral.†.*
Potassium sulfate (p.1232·2).

**Celloids S 79** *Blackmores, Austral.†.*
Silicon dioxide (p.1581·3).

**Celloids SP 96** *Blackmores, Austral.†.*
Dibasic sodium phosphate (p.1231·1).

**Celloids SS 69** *Blackmores, Austral.†.*
Anhydrous sodium sulfate (p.1290·1).

**Celltop** *Baxter Oncology, Fr.*
Etoposide (p.551·3).
*Malignant neoplasms.*

**Cellufresh**
*Allergan, Arg.; Allergan, Austral.; Allergan, Braz.; Allergan, Canad.†; Allergan, Ital.; Allergan, NZ; Allergan, S.Afr.; Allergan, Singapore†; Allergan, Spain; Allergan, Thai.*
Carmellose sodium (p.1577·3) (p.1164·2).
*Dry eyes; eye irritation; lubricating solution for contact lens.*

**Cellugel** *Alcon, Ger.*
Hypromellose (p.1579·3).
*Adjunct in ophthalmic surgery.*

**Cellular Formula** *General Nutrition, Canad.*
Multivitamin and trace element preparation (p.1417·1).

**Cellulin Retinale** *INTES, Ital.*
Retina extract.
*Eye disorders.*

**Cellulone** *Alphapharm, Austral.†.*
Methylcellulose (p.1580·2).
*Bowel disorders; constipation; diarrhoea.*

**Celluson** *CS, Fr.†.*
Bran (p.1253·2).
*Dietary fibre supplement.*

**Celluspan** *Fischer, Israel.*
Cellulose derivatives (p.1578·3); electrolytes (p.1217·1).
*Aid in gonioscopy.*

**Celluvisc**
*Allergan, Arg.; Allergan, Austral.; Allergan, Canad.; Allergan, Denm.; Allergan, Fin.; Allergan, Fr.; Allergan, Ger.; Alvia (Αλβια), Gr.; Allergan, Hong Kong†; Allergan, Ital.; Allergan, Mex.; Allergan, NZ; Allergan, Port.; Allergan, S.Afr.; Allergan, Singapore; Allergan, Spain; Allergan, Swed.; Allergan, Switz.; Allergan, Thai.; Allergan, UK; Allergan, USA.*
Carmellose sodium (p.1577·3).
*Dry eyes.*

**Cellvital** *Pharma Investi, Chile.*
Selenium yeast; zinc gluconate; copper gluconate; Vitamins (p.1417·1).
*Dietary supplement.*

**Celnium** *Sanofi Synthelabo, Fr.†.*
Selenium (p.1444·1) from *Saccharomyces cerevisiae*.
*Skin and muscular disorders.*

**Celobar** *Enila, Braz.*
Barium sulfate (p.1061·1).
*Contrast medium for gastrointestinal radiography.*

**Celocurin** *Ipex, Swed.*
Suxamethonium chloride (p.1406·2).
*Depolarising neuromuscular blocker.*

**Celocurine** *Pharmacia, Fr.*
Suxamethonium chloride (p.1406·2).
*Depolarising neuromuscular blocker.*

**Celoftal**
*Alcon, Ger.; Cusi, Singapore†.*
Hypromellose (p.1579·3).
*Aid in eye surgery.*

**Celol** *Pacific, NZ.*
Celiprolol hydrochloride (p.881·3).
*Angina pectoris; hypertension.*

**Celontin**
*Pfizer, Canad.; Parke, Davis, Israel; Parke, Davis, Neth.; Parke, Davis, USA.*
Mesuximide (p.366·2).
*Absence seizures.*

**Celucrem** *ICN, Arg.*
Lactic acid (p.1704·1).
*Skin disorders.*

**Cel-U-Jec** *Hauck, USA.*
Betamethasone sodium phosphate (p.1093·1).
*Corticosteroid.*

**Celulase** *Rider, Chile.*
Centella (p.1144·3).
*Burns; fibrosis; lipodystrophy; ulcers; venous insufficiency; wounds.*

**Celulase Con Neomicina** *Rider, Chile.*
Centella (p.1144·3); neomycin sulfate (p.235·1).
*Burns; skin infections; ulcers; wounds.*

**Celulase Plus** *Rider, Chile.*
Centella (p.1144·3).
*Burns; fibrosis; lipodystrophy; ulcers; wounds.*

**Celulose** *Grin, Mex.*
Hypromellose (p.1579·3).
*Aid in ophthalmic procedures; dry eyes.*

**Celumax** *Sanofi Winthrop, Braz.†.*
Centella (p.1144·3).
*Cellulite.*

**Celupan** *Lacer, Spain.*
Naltrexone hydrochloride (p.1046·1).
*Alcoholism; opioid withdrawal.*

**Celuvital** *Beta, Arg.*
Vitamin A palmitate (p.1453·1); collagen (p.1674·3).
*Barrier cream.*

**Celvista** *Lilly, Thai.*
Raloxifene hydrochloride (p.1568·3).
*Osteoporosis.*

**Cemac B12** *Larkhall Laboratories, UK†.*
Vitamin $B_{12}$ (p.1458·2).

**Cemado** *Francia, Ital.*
Cefamandole nafate (p.169·3).
Lidocaine hydrochloride (p.1377·3) is included in this preparation to alleviate the pain of injection.
*Gram-negative bacterial infections.*

**Cemaflavone** *Bailleul, Fr.*
Citroflavonoids (p.1688·2); magnesium ascorbate (p.1227·3).
*Haemorrhoids; venous insufficiency; visual disorders.*

**Cemalyt** *Saros, Spain.*
Triamcinolone (p.1110·2); centella (p.1144·3).
Formerly contained human placenta extract, triamcinolone acetonide, and calendula officinalis.
*Skin disorders.*

**Cemaquin**
*Cimex, Hong Kong; Cimex, Switz.*
Benzethonium chloride (p.1169·2); ascorbic acid (p.1460·2).
*Mouth and throat infections.*

**Cementin**
*DHA, Hong Kong; DHA, Singapore.*
Cimetidine (p.1255·3).
*Gastro-oesophageal reflux; peptic ulcer; Zollinger-Ellison syndrome.*

**Cemetol** *Pharmacia Upjohn, Spain†.*
Cefmetazole sodium (p.173·3).
Lidocaine hydrochloride (p.1377·3) is included in the intramuscular injection to alleviate the pain of injection.
*Bacterial infections.*

**Cemidin** *Dexxon, Israel.*
Cimetidine (p.1255·3).
*Gastro-oesophageal reflux; peptic ulcer; Zollinger-Ellison syndrome.*

**Cemidon** *Alcala, Spain.*
Isoniazid (p.222·2).
*Opportunistic mycobacterial infections; tuberculosis.*

**Cemidon B6** *Alcala, Spain.*
Isoniazid (p.222·2).
Pyridoxine hydrochloride (p.1456·3) is included in this preparation for the prophylaxis of peripheral neuropathy.
*Opportunistic mycobacterial infections; tuberculosis.*

**Cemina** *Medix, Mex.*
Ascorbic acid (p.1460·2).
*Vitamin supplement.*

**Cemirit** *Bayer, Ital.*
Aspirin (p.15·1).
*Fever; inflammation; influenza symptoms; pain.*

**Cemol** *Pharmasant, Thai.*
Paracetamol (p.76·2).
*Fever; pain.*

**Cenacert** *Phoenix, Arg.*
Oxatomide (p.438·1).
*Hypersensitivity reactions.*

**Cenafed** *Century, USA.*
Pseudoephedrine hydrochloride (p.1129·2).
*Nasal congestion.*

**Cenafed Plus** *Century, USA.*
Pseudoephedrine hydrochloride (p.1129·2); triprolidine hydrochloride (p.442·3).
*Upper respiratory-tract symptoms.*

**Cenai** *The Forty-Two, Thai.*
Cinnarizine (p.428·3).
*Cerebrovascular disorders; migraine; motion sickness; peripheral vascular disease; vestibular disorders.*

**Cena-K** *Century, USA.*
Potassium chloride (p.1232·2).
*Hypokalaemia; potassium depletion.*

**Cenalfan** *Sigma, Braz.*
Vitamins A, C, and E (p.1417·1).

**Cenalfan Plus** *Sigma, Braz.*
Multivitamin and mineral preparation (p.1417·1).

**Cenat** *Madaus, Spain.*
Ispaghula (p.1268·1).
*Constipation; functional diarrhoeas.*

**Cencamet** *Pharmasant, Thai.*
Cimetidine (p.1255·3).
*Gastric hyperacidity; gastro-oesophageal reflux; peptic ulcer.*

**Cencopan** *Pharmasant, Thai.*
Hyoscine butylbromide (p.483·3).
*Smooth muscle spasm.*

**Cendalon** *Teva Tuteur, Arg.*
Letrozole (p.565·1).

**Ceneo** *Pensa, Spain.*
Hydrocortisone butyrate (p.1104·1) or hydrocortisone propionate (p.1104·2).
*Skin disorders.*

**Cenestin** *Duramed, USA.*
Synthetic conjugated oestrogens, A (p.1543·2).
*Menopausal disorders.*

**Cenevit** *Legrand, Braz.*
Ascorbic acid (p.1460·2).
*Vitamin C supplement.*

**Cenilene** *Schering-Plough, Port.*
Fluphenazine hydrochloride (p.699·3).

**Cenlidac** *Pharmasant, Thai.*
Sulindac (p.91·2).
*Musculoskeletal, joint, and peri-articular disorders.*

**Cennlacs** *Westward, Canad.†.*
Senna (p.1288·2); liquorice (p.1270·2).

**Cenogen Ultra** *US Pharmaceutical, USA.*
Vitamin and mineral preparation with iron and folic acid (p.1417·1).

**Cenogen-OB** *US Pharmaceutical, USA.*
Multivitamin and mineral preparation with iron (p.1417·1).

**Cenol** *Solvay, Belg.†.*
Ascorbic acid (p.1460·2).
*Dietary supplement; methaemoglobinaemia; scurvy.*

**Cenolate** *Abbott, USA.*
Sodium ascorbate (p.1460·2).
*Scurvy; vitamin C deficiency.*

**Cenpine** *Pharmasant, Thai.†.*
Nicardipine hydrochloride (p.965·1).
*Angina pectoris; cerebrovascular disorders; hypertension.*

**Centa Vite** *Cypress, USA.*
Vitamin and mineral preparation (p.1417·1).

**Centabel** *Silesia, Chile.*
Centella (p.1144·3).
*Burns; ulcers; venous insufficiency; wounds.*

**Centagin** *Pharmasant, Thai.*
Dipyrone (p.35·3).
*Fever; pain.*

**Centany** *Ortho Dermatological, USA.*
Mupirocin (p.233·1).
*Bacterial skin infections.*

**Centapp** *Pharmasant, Thai.*
Brompheniramine maleate (p.426·1); phenylephrine hydrochloride (p.1126·3).

Formerly contained brompheniramine maleate, phenylephrine hydrochloride, and phenylpropanolamine hydrochloride.
*Cold symptoms; nasal congestion.*

**Centaurea (Specie Composta)** *Dynacren, Ital.*
Centaury (p.1669·2); taraxacum (p.1751·3); gentian (p.1692·2).
*Gastrointestinal disorders; herbal tea.*

**Centella Complex** *Peter, Ital.*
*Tablets:* Centella asiatica (p.1144·3); hamamelis (p.1696·3); aesculus (p.1648·2); pineapple; vitamin C (p.1460·2).
*Circulatory disorders; nutritional supplement.*
*Topical gel:* Centella asiatica (p.1144·3); aesculus (p.1648·2); pineapple; hamamelis (p.1696·3); allantoin (p.1141·3).

**Centella Queen Complex** *Temis, Arg.*
*Cream:* Centella (p.1144·3); marine algae; equisetum (p.1684·1).
*Cellulitis.*
*Tablets:* Bladderwrack (p.1742·3); vitamin E; centella; ginkgo biloba (p.1417·1).
*Dietary supplement.*

**Centella Queen Reductora** *Temis, Arg.*
Centella (p.1144·3); fibre (p.1253·2).
*Slimming aid.*

**Centellase**
*Hoechst, Ital.; Tai Guk, Singapore.*
Centella asiatica (p.1144·3).
*Burns; scars; skin ulcers; venous insufficiency; wounds.*

**Centella-Vit** *Fontovit, Braz.*
Centella (p.1144·3).

**Center-Al** *Center, USA.*
Range of allergen extracts (p.1650·1).
*Allergen immunotherapy.*

**Centerfen** *Pharmasant, Thai.†.*
Terfenadine (p.441·1).
*Allergic rhinitis; urticaria.*

**Centeril H** *Errekappa, Ital.*
*Cream:* Zinc oxide (p.1163·2); centella asiatica (p.1144·3); hamamelis (p.1696·3); aesculus (p.1648·2); peppermint (p.1283·2); menthol (p.1711·3).
*Topical solution:* Centella asiatica (p.1144·3); hamamelis (p.1696·3); aesculus (p.1648·2).
*Anorectal disorders.*

**Centica** *Samjin, Singapore.*
Centella asiatica (p.1144·3).
*Burns; scars; skin ulcers; wounds.*

**Centilux** *Alcon Cusi, Spain.*
Methylthioninium chloride (p.1042·2); naphazoline hydrochloride (p.1124·3).
*Eye disorders.*

**Centra Acid** *Therapex, Canad.†.*
Aluminium hydroxide (p.1249·2); magnesium hydroxide (p.1272·2).

**Centra Acid Plus** *Therapex, Canad.†.*
Aluminium hydroxide (p.1249·2); magnesium hydroxide (p.1272·2); simeticone (p.1289·2).

**Centrac** *Pfizer, Gr.*
Prazepam (p.716·2).
*Anxiety disorders.*

**Centracetam** *UCB, Port.*
Piracetam (p.1732·1); vincamine (p.1764·2).

**Centracol** *Therapex, Canad.†.*
Phenylephrine hydrochloride (p.1126·3); phenylpropanolamine hydrochloride (p.1127·3); brompheniramine maleate (p.426·1).

**Centracol DM** *Prometic, Canad.†.*
Phenylpropanolamine hydrochloride (p.1127·3); pheniramine maleate (p.438·3); mepyramine maleate (p.437·1); dextromethorphan hydrobromide (p.1117·3).

**Centracol Pediatrique** *Prometic, Canad.†.*
Pseudoephedrine hydrochloride (p.1129·2); pheniramine maleate (p.438·3); dextromethorphan hydrobromide (p.1117·3); guaifenesin (p.1122·1).

**Centralgine** *Amino, Switz.†.*
Pethidine hydrochloride (p.80·2).
*Pain; smooth muscle spasm.*

**Centralgol** *Zyma, Fr.†.*
Proxibarbal (p.718·1).
*Anxiety; menopausal symptoms.*

**Centramin** *Rosch & Handel, Austria.*
Glycine (p.1433·3); magnesium chloride (p.1228·1); calcium chloride (p.1225·1); potassium chloride (p.1232·2).
*Pruritus; tetany.*

**Centramina** *Miquel Otsuka, Spain†.*
Amfetamine sulfate (p.1584·3).
*Hyperactivity; narcoleptic syndrome.*

**Centratuss DM** *Therapex, Canad.†.*
Dextromethorphan hydrobromide (p.1117·3).

**Centratuss DM Expectorant** *Therapex, Canad.†.*
Dextromethorphan hydrobromide (p.1117·3); guaifenesin (p.1122·1).

**Centratuss DM-D** *Therapex, Canad.†.*
Dextromethorphan hydrobromide (p.1117·3); pseudoephedrine hydrochloride (p.1129·2).

**Centrax** *Parke, Davis, Irl.*
Prazepam (p.716·2).
*Anxiety disorders.*

**Centromicina** *Boehringer Ingelheim, Arg.*
Clarithromycin (p.192·2).
*Bacterial infections.*

**Centron** *Torrent, India.*
Ormeloxifene (p.1564·3).
*Oral contraceptive.*

**Centrophene** *Alpharma, Fr.*
Trimetazidine hydrochloride (p.1018·1).
*Angina pectoris; vertigo; visual disorders.*

**Centrovite** *Rugby, USA.*
A range of multivitamin and mineral preparations with iron and folic acid (p.1417·1).

**Centrum**
*Note. This name is used for preparations of different composition.*
*Wyeth-Whitehall, Arg.; Whitehall Consumer, Austral.; Wyeth Lederle, Austria; Whitehall, Braz.; Whitehall-Robins, Canad.; Wyeth, Hong Kong; Wyeth, Irl.; Lederle, Israel; Wyeth Consumer, Malaysia; Wyeth, Mex.; Wyeth Consumer, Port.; Wyeth Consumer, Singapore; Whitehall, Thai.; Wyeth Consumer, UK; Wyeth-Ayerst, USA.*
A range of multivitamin and mineral preparations (p.1417·1).

*Polifarma, Ital.*
Cytidine; uridine (p.1760·3).
*Mental function impairment.*

**Centural Gold** *Goldshield, Singapore.*
Multivitamin and mineral preparation (p.1417·1).

**Centurion A–Z** *Mission Pharmacal, USA.*
Iron (p.1434·3); folic acid (p.1429·1); multivitamins and minerals (p.1417·1).
*Iron-deficiency anaemias.*

**Centyl**
*Leo, Denm.; Leo, Irl.; Leo, Norw.*
Bendroflumethiazide (p.867·3).
*Diabetes insipidus; hypertension; oedema; renal calcium stones.*

**Centyl K**
*Leo, Irl.; Leo, UK.*
Bendroflumethiazide (p.867·3); potassium chloride (p.1232·2).
*Hypertension; oedema; renal calculi.*

**Centyl med Kaliumklorid**
*Leo, Denm.; Leo, Norw.*
Bendroflumethiazide (p.867·3); potassium chloride (p.1232·2).
*Diabetes insipidus; hypertension; oedema; renal calcium stones.*

**Ceolat**
*Solvay, Denm.†; Solvay, Fin.†; Rekawan, Ger.; Solvay, Gr.; Vemedia, Neth.; Solvay, Norw.; Solvay Duphar, Swed.†.*
Dimethicone (p.1289·2).
*Flatulence.*

**Ceolat Compositum** *Lannacher, Austria.*
Dimeticone (p.1482·1); metoclopramide (p.1274·3).
*Gastrointestinal disorders.*

**Ceo-Two** *Beutlich, USA.*
Sodium bicarbonate (p.1223·2); potassium acid tartrate (p.1284·3).
*Constipation.*

**Ceoxil** *Magis, Ital.*
Cefadroxil (p.167·2).
*Bacterial infections.*

**Ceoxx**
*Merck Sharp & Dohme, Chile; Merck Sharp & Dohme, Irl.; Merck Sharp & Dohme, Port.; Merck Sharp & Dohme, Spain.*
Rofecoxib (p.86·3).
*Osteoarthritis; pain; rheumatoid arthritis.*

**Cepa Med Complex** *Dynamit, Austria.*
Homoeopathic preparation.

**Cepacaina** *Aventis, Braz.*
Benzocaine (p.1370·3); cetylpyridinium chloride (p.1173·1).
*Antiseptic; local anaesthetic.*

**Cepacaine**
*Note. This name is used for preparations of different composition.*
*Roche Consumer, Austral.; Roche, NZ; Adcock Ingram, S.Afr.*
Benzocaine (p.1370·3); cetylpyridinium chloride (p.1173·1).
*Mouth and throat disorders.*

*Adcock Ingram, S.Afr.*
*Mouthwash:* Benzocaine (p.1370·3); cinchocaine hydrochloride (p.1373·2); cetylpyridinium chloride (p.1173·1).
*Mouth and throat disorders.*

**Cepacilina** *Reig Jofre, Spain.*
Benzathine benzylpenicillin (p.162·3).
*Bacterial infections; rheumatic fever.*

**Cepacilina 633** *Reig Jofre, Spain.*
Benzylpenicillin sodium (p.163·2); procaine benzylpenicillin (p.246·1); benzathine benzylpenicillin (p.162·3).
*Bacterial infections; rheumatic fever.*

**Cepacol**
*Note. This name is used for preparations of different composition.*
*GlaxoSmithKline Consumer, Canad.; Aventis, Hong Kong; Roche, NZ; Restan, S.Afr.; Marion Merrell Dow, Singapore; Aventis, Thai.*
Cetylpyridinium chloride (p.1173·1).
*Mouth and throat disorders.*

*Lepetit, Ital.†.*
Alkylbenzyldimethylammonium saccharinate (p.1169·1); sodium monofluorophosphate (p.1446·2); calcium hydrogen phosphate (p.1225·2).
*Oral disinfection; oral hygiene.*

*Restan, S.Afr.*
*Linctus:* Dextromethorphan hydrobromide (p.1117·3); doxylamine succinate (p.432·3); sodium citrate (p.1223·2); cetylpyridinium chloride (p.1173·1).
*Coughs.*

**Cepacol Anaesthetic** *Roche, NZ.*
Benzocaine (p.1370·3); cetylpyridinium chloride (p.1173·1).
*Mouth and throat disorders.*

**Cepacol Anesthetic** *JB Williams, USA.*
Benzocaine (p.1370·3); cetylpyridinium chloride (p.1173·1).
*Sore throat.*

**Cepacol Antibacterial** *Roche Consumer, Austral.*
*Honey and Lemon; Orange Citrus:* Cetylpyridinium chloride (p.1173·1).
*Menthol and Eucalyptus:* Cetylpyridinium chloride (p.1173·1); eucalyptus oil (p.1686·2); menthol (p.1711·3).
*Mouth and throat disorders.*

**Cepacol Citrus** *GlaxoSmithKline Consumer, Canad.*
Benzocaine (p.1370·3); cetylpyridinium chloride (p.1173·1).
Formerly known as Cepacol Anesthetic.
*Mouth and throat disorders.*

**Cepacol Cough +** *Roche Consumer, Austral.*
Dextromethorphan hydrobromide (p.1117·3); cetylpyridinium chloride (p.1173·1); benzocaine (p.1370·3); menthol (p.1711·3).
Formerly known as Cepacol Cough and Sore Throat.
*Coughs; sore throat.*

**Cepacol Cough Discs**
*Note. This name is used for preparations of different composition.*
*Roche, NZ.*
Dextromethorphan hydrobromide (p.1117·3); cetylpyridinium chloride (p.1173·1); benzocaine (p.1370·3); menthol (p.1711·3).
*Coughs; mouth and throat disorders.*

*Restan, S.Afr.*
Dextromethorphan hydrobromide (p.1117·3); cetylpyridinium chloride (p.1173·1); benzocaine (p.1370·3).
*Coughs; sore throat.*

**Cepacol with Fluoride** *GlaxoSmithKline Consumer, Canad.*
Cetylpyridinium chloride (p.1173·1); sodium fluoride (p.1444·3).

**Cepacol Maximum Strength Sore Throat** *JB Williams, USA.*
*Lozenges:* Benzocaine (p.1370·3); menthol (p.1711·3); cetylpyridinium chloride (p.1173·1).
*Throat spray:* Dyclonine hydrochloride (p.1376·2); cetylpyridinium chloride (p.1173·1).
*Sore throat.*

**Cepacol Mint** *Roche Consumer, Austral.†.*
Cetylpyridinium chloride (p.1173·1).
*Mouth and throat disorders; oral hygiene.*

**Cepacol Mouthwash** *JB Williams, USA.*
Cetylpyridinium chloride (p.1173·1).
*Minor mouth or throat disorders.*

**Cepacol Plus with Anaesthetic** *Roche Consumer, Austral.*
Benzocaine (p.1370·3); cetylpyridinium chloride (p.1173·1).
Formerly known as Cepacol Anaesthetic.
*Mouth and throat disorders.*

**Cepacol Regular** *Roche Consumer, Austral.†.*
Cetylpyridinium chloride (p.1173·1).
*Mouth and throat disorders; oral hygiene.*

**Cepacol Regular Strength** *JB Williams, USA.*
Menthol (p.1711·3); cetylpyridinium chloride (p.1173·1).
*Sore throat.*

**Cepacol Throat** *JB Williams, USA.*
Benzyl alcohol (p.1170·2); cetylpyridinium chloride (p.1173·1).
*Sore throat.*

**Cepacol Viractin** *GlaxoSmithKline Consumer, Canad.*
Tetracaine hydrochloride (p.1385·1).

**Cepacol Viractin Cold Sore Treatment** *JB Williams, USA.*
Tetracaine (p.1385·1) or tetracaine hydrochloride (p.1385·1).
*Topical anaesthesia.*

**Cepadont** *Agis, Israel.*
Cetylpyridinium chloride (p.1173·1); chlorobutanol (p.1176·3).
*Mouth disinfection.*

**Cepadyne** *Infan, Mex.†.*
Cetylpyridinium chloride (p.1173·1).

**Cepal**
*Note. This name is used for preparations of different composition.*
*Demo, Gr.*
Famotidine (p.1265·2).
*Conditions where gastric acid reduction is beneficial; gastric hypersecretion including Zollinger-Ellison syndrome; peptic ulcer.*

*Pharmasant, Thai.*
Fenbufen (p.39·1).
*Musculoskeletal and joint disorders.*

**Cepasium** *Cortunon, Canad.†.*
Magnesium carbonate (p.1272·1).

**Cepastat**
*Note. This name is used for preparations of different composition.*
*GlaxoSmithKline Consumer, Canad.; SmithKline Beecham Consumer, USA.*
Phenol (p.1188·1); menthol (p.1711·3); eucalyptus oil (p.1686·2).
*Mouth and throat disorders.*

*Aventis, Hong Kong; Marion Merrell Dow, Singapore.*
Phenol (p.1188·1); menthol (p.1711·3).
*Mouth and throat disorders.*

**Cepastat Cherry** *SmithKline Beecham Consumer, USA.*
Phenol (p.1188·1); menthol (p.1711·3).
*Sore throat.*

**Cepazine** *Novaxo, Fr.*
Cefuroxime axetil (p.184·1).
*Bacterial infections.*

**Cepevit** *Darci, Fr.†.*
Ascorbic acid (p.1460·2); hesperidin methyl chalcone (p.1688·3); hesperidin (p.1688·2); esculoside (p.1648·2).
*Capillary fragility.*

**Cepexin** *Glaxo Wellcome, Austria.*
Cefalexin (p.168·1).
*Bacterial infections.*

**Cephadol**
*Shinyaku, Hong Kong; Shinyaku, Jpn; Shinyaku, Malaysia; Shinyaku, Singapore; Shinyaku, Thai.*
Difenidol hydrochloride (p.1261·1).
*Dizziness; vertigo.*

**Cephalen** *Beximco, Singapore.*
Cefalexin (p.168·1).
*Bacterial infections.*

**Cephalex** *CT, Ger.*
Cefalexin (p.168·1).
*Bacterial infections.*

**Cephalexyl** *Bangkok Lab & Cosmetic, Thai.*
Cefalexin (p.168·1).
*Bacterial infections.*

**Cephalgan** *UPSA, Fr.*
Carbasalate calcium (p.25·1); metoclopramide hydrochloride (p.1274·3).
*Migraine.*

**Cephalobene** *Ratiopharm, Austria.*
Cefalexin (p.168·1).
*Bacterial infections.*

**Cephalodoc** *Docpharm, Ger.*
Cefaclor (p.167·1).
*Bacterial infections.*

**Cephaloplant** *Infirmarius-Rovit, Ger.*
Homoeopathic preparation.

**Cephanmycin** *Yung Shin, Singapore.*
Cefalexin (p.168·1).
*Bacterial infections.*

**Cephanol** *Riva, Canad.*
Paracetamol (p.76·2).

**Cephaxin** *Biochem, India.*
Cefalexin (p.168·1).
*Bacterial infections.*

**Ceph-Biocin** *Orion, Ger.†.*
Cefaclor (p.167·1).
*Bacterial infections.*

**Cephin** *General Drugs, Thai.*
Cefalexin (p.168·1).
*Bacterial infections.*

**Cephoral**
*Merck, Ger.; Klinge, Switz.*
Cefixime (p.172·3).
*Bacterial infections.*

**Cephos** *CT, Ital.*
Cefadroxil (p.167·2).
*Bacterial infections.*

**Cephulac**
*Hoechst Marion Roussel, Canad.†; Hoechst Marion Roussel, USA.*
Lactulose (p.1269·1).
*Hepatic encephalopathy.*

**Cephyl**
*Note. This name is used for preparations of different composition.*
*Boiron, Fr.*
Aspirin (p.15·1); caffeine (p.782·1); belladonna; iris versicolor; nux vomica; spigelia; gelsemium.
Formerly contained aspirin, ethenzamide, caffeine hydrate, belladonna, iris versicolor, nux vomica, spigelia, and gelsemium.
*Fever; pain.*

*Boiron, Port.*
Aspirin (p.15·1); ethenzamide(p.37·2); caffeine (p.782·1); belladonna; iris versicolor; nux vomica; spigelia; gelsemium.
*Fever; pain.*

**Cepifran** *Juste, Spain.*
Ceftibuten (p.182·1).
*Bacterial infections.*

**Cepim** *Polifarma, Ital.*
Cefepime hydrochloride (p.172·1).
*Bacterial infections.*

**Cepimex** *Upsa, Ital.*
Cefepime hydrochloride (p.172·1).
*Bacterial infections.*

**Ceplac** *Rhone-Poulenc Rorer, UK†.*
Erythrosine (p.1057·2).
*Disclosing agent for plaque.*

**Cepodem** *Stancare, India.*
Cefpodoxime proxetil (p.178·3).
*Bacterial infections.*

**Ceporacin** *Bioniche, Canad.*
Cefalotin sodium (p.168·3).
*Bacterial infections.*

**Ceporan** *Glaxo Wellcome, Mex.†.*
Cefaloridine (p.168·3).
*Bacterial infections.*

**Ceporex**
*GlaxoSmithKline, Belg.; GlaxoSmithKline, Hong Kong; GlaxoSmithKline, Irl.; GlaxoSmithKline, Ital.; GlaxoSmithKline, Malaysia; Glaxo*

Wellcome, Mex.; Glaxo Wellcome, Port.; Glaxo Wellcome, Singapore; GlaxoSmithKline, Thai.; Galen, UK.
Cefalexin (p.168·1).
*Bacterial infections.*

**Ceporexin**
Investi, Arg.; GlaxoSmithKline, Braz.; Aventis, Ger.; GlaxoSmithKline, Ger.
Cefalexin (p.168·1).
*Bacterial infections.*

**Ceporexine** GlaxoSmithKline, Fr.
Cefalexin (p.168·1).
*Bacterial infections.*

**Ceposil** Pisa, Mex.
Potassium acetate (p.1232·1).

**Cepral** Kemyos, Ital.†.
Aluminium sulfate (p.1653·1); cetylpyridinium chloride (p.1173·1).
*Mouth and throat disorders.*

**Ceprandal** Sigma-Tau, Spain.
Omeprazole (p.1278·2).
*Gastro-oesophageal reflux; peptic ulcer; Zollinger-Ellison syndrome.*

**Ceprater** Richmond, Arg.
Cyproterone (p.1544·3).

**Ceprazol** Laboratorios Chile, Chile.
Albendazole (p.101·2).
*Worm infections.*

**Ceprimax** Fides Ecopharma, Spain.
Ciprofloxacin hydrochloride (p.188·2).
*Bacterial infections.*

**Ceprin** Dolisos, Canad.
Homoeopathic preparation.

**Ceprofen** Neo Quimica, Braz.
Ketoprofen (p.51·2).

**Ceprotin**
Baxter, Denm.; Baxter, Fin.; Baxter, Fr.; Baxter, Ger.; Baxter, Ital.; Baxter, Spain; Baxter, Swed.; Baxter BioScience, UK.
Protein C (p.759·2).
*Thromboembolic disorders.*

**Ceprovit** Wider, Ger.†.
Lemon oil (p.1706·2); chamomile oil (p.1669·3); arnica (p.1656·3).
*Healing of amputations.*

**Ceptaz**
GlaxoSmithKline, Canad.; Glaxo Wellcome, USA.
Ceftazidime (p.180·2).
*Bacterial infections.*

**Cepton** Eastern Pharmaceuticals, UK.
Chlorhexidine gluconate (p.1173·2).
*Acne.*

**Cequinyl** GlaxoSmithKline Sante, Fr.
Paracetamol (p.76·2); pseudoephedrine hydrochloride (p.1129·2); ascorbic acid (p.1460·2).
Formerly contained paracetamol, ascorbic acid, and quinine hydrochloride.
*Fever; nasal congestion; pain.*

**Ceractiv** Andromaco, Chile.
Pemoline (p.1591·2).
*Attention-deficit hyperactivity disorder.*

**Ceradolan**
Takeda, Hong Kong†; Takeda, Singapore; Takeda, Thai.
Cefotiam hydrochloride (p.177·2).
*Bacterial infections.*

**Ceralan** Orion, Fin.
Emollient.
*Dry skin.*

**Ceralip**
Roche-Posay, Arg.; Roche-Posay, Braz.; Roche-Posay, Irl.
Emollient.
*Dry lips; mucous membrane damage.*

**Cerasorb** Curasan, Ger.
Calcium phosphate (p.1225·3).
*Artificial bone and dental enamel.*

**Cerat Inalterable** Roche-Posay, Fr.
Titanium dioxide (p.1160·3); aluminium silicate (p.1250·2); white beeswax (p.1480·1); light liquid paraffin (p.1479·1).
*Barrier ointment.*

**Cerax**
Note. This name is used for preparations of different composition.
GlaxoSmithKline, Arg.
Benzocaine (p.1370·3).
*Removal of ear wax.*

Pharmasant, Thai.
Hydroxyzine hydrochloride (p.434·3).
*Hypersensitivity reactions; sedative.*

**Cerazet** Organon, Spain.
Desogestrel (p.1547·2).
*Progestogen-only oral contraceptive.*

**Cerazette**
Organon, Arg.; Organon, Belg.; Organon, Braz.; Organon, Chile; Organon, Denm.; Organon, Fin.; Organon, Fr.; Organon, Ger.; Organon, Ital.; Organon, Mex.; Organon, Neth.; Organon, NZ; Organon, Port.; Organon, Swed.; Organon, Switz.; Organon, UK.
Desogestrel (p.1547·2).
*Progestogen-only oral contraceptive.*

**Cerbon** Confar, Port.
Pyritinol hydrochloride (p.1737·2).
*Cerebrovascular disorders; mental function disorders.*

**Cercon** Lakeside, Mex.†.
Praziquantel (p.112·2).

**Cere** Kolassa, Austria.
Ornithine aspartate (p.1442·3).
*Hepatic encephalopathy.*

**Cerebokan** Austroplant, Austria.
Ginkgo biloba (p.1692·3).
*Cerebral and peripheral vascular disorders.*

**Cerebral-Do** Grasler, Ger.
Homoeopathic preparation.

**Cerebramed** Orion, Ger.†.
Amantadine hydrochloride (p.1197·2).
*Drug-induced extrapyramidal disorders; influenza A; parkinsonism.*

**Cerebrex** Luper, Braz.
Vitamin B substances; glutamic acid; calcium glycerophosphate; calcium phosphate (p.1417·1).
*Nutritional supplement.*

**Cerebrino** Mandri, Spain.
Aspirin (p.15·1); paracetamol (p.76·2); caffeine (p.782·1).
*Influenza symptoms; pain.*

**Cerebroad** Chinta, Thai.
Cinnarizine (p.428·3).
*Cerebrovascular disorders; migraine; peripheral vascular disorders; vestibular disorders.*

**Cerebroforte** Azupharma, Ger.
Piracetam (p.1732·1).
*Mental function disorders.*

**Cerebrol**
Note. This name is used for preparations of different composition.
Boehringer Ingelheim, Fr.†.
Diethylaminoethanol malate (p.1587·1).
*Asthenia.*

Actipharm, Switz.
Codeine phosphate (p.27·1); caffeine (p.782·1); paracetamol (p.76·2); propyphenazone (p.85·3).
*Pain.*

**Cerebrol sans codeine** Actipharm, Switz.
Caffeine (p.782·1); paracetamol (p.76·2).
*Pain.*

**Cerebrolysin**
Ebewe, Austria; Abbott, Ger.; Ebewe, Hong Kong; Ebewe, Thai.
Brain extract (p.1709·3).
*Brain injury; epilepsy; mental function impairment; mental retardation; parkinsonism; senile dementia; stroke.*

**Cerebropan** Kedrion, Ital.
Piracetam (p.1732·1).
*Mental function impairment.*

**Cerebrotonin** Ebewe, Austria.
Porcine brain protein (p.1709·3).
*Cerebral disorders.*

**Cerebroxine** Therabel, Belg.
Vincamine (p.1764·2).
*Cerebrovascular disorders.*

**Cerebryl** Kwizda, Austria.
Piracetam (p.1732·1).
*Cerebral disorders.*

**Cerebyx**
Pfizer, Canad.; Parke, Davis, USA.
Fosphenytoin sodium (p.361·3).
*Epilepsy.*

**Ceredase**
Genzyme, Ger.†; Genzyme, Israel; Genzyme, Jpn; Genzyme, Spain†; Genzyme, USA.
Alglucerase (p.1649·1).
*Gaucher disease.*

**Cereginkgo** Pfluger, Ger.
Homoeopathic preparation.

**Ceregumil** Azevedos, Port.
Preparation for enteral nutrition (p.1417·1).

**Cerekinon**
Tanabe, Hong Kong; Tanabe, Jpn; Tanabe, Malaysia; Tanabe, Singapore; Tanabe, Thai.
Trimebutine maleate (p.1758·1).
*Chronic gastritis; irritable bowel syndrome.*

**Cerelac**
Nestle, Braz.
Preparation for enteral nutrition (p.1417·1).

Nestle, Port.
Range of gluten-free infant feeds (p.1417·1).
*Gluten intolerance.*

**Cerella** Asche, Ger.
Estradiol (p.1550·1).
*Menopausal disorders.*

**Cereloid** Sun, India.
Co-dergocrine mesilate (p.1674·1).
*Dementia.*

**Cereluc** Beta, Arg.
Pioglitazone hydrochloride (p.344·1).
*Diabetes mellitus.*

**Ceremin**
Note. This name is used for preparations of different composition.
Madaus, Austria.
Ginkgo biloba (p.1692·3).
*Cerebral and peripheral vascular disorders.*

Polipharm, Thai.
Cinnarizine (p.428·3).
*Cerebrovascular disorders; migraine; motion sickness; peripheral vascular disorders; vestibular disorders.*

**Cereneu** Pfizer, Spain.
Fosphenytoin sodium (p.361·3).
*Epilepsy.*

**Cereon** Biogal, Israel.
Ascorbic acid (p.1460·2).
*Scurvy.*

**Cerepar** Mepha, Switz.
Cinnarizine (p.428·3).
*Vertigo; vestibular disorders.*

**Cerepar N** Merckle, Ger.
Piracetam (p.1732·1).
*Mental function impairment.*

**Cereron** Raza, Malaysia; Pharmaniaga, Malaysia.
Cinnarizine (p.428·3).
*Cerebrovascular disorders; motion sickness; peripheral vascular disorders; vestibular disorders.*

**Cerestabon** Seber, Port.
Idebenone (p.1700·3).
*Cerebrovascular disorders; mental function disorders.*

**Cerestar** Ranbaxy, Malaysia.
Ginkgo biloba (p.1692·3); ginseng (p.1693·1).
*Tonic.*

**Ceretec**
Amersham, Austral.; Nycomed, Austria; Amersham, Fr.†; Nycomed, Ital.; Amersham, Spain; Nycomed Amersham, UK.
Technetium-99m exametazime (p.1525·2).
*Cerebral blood flow scintigraphy; leucocyte labelling.*

**Cerevon** Wellcome, Canad.†.
Ferrous succinate (p.1428·2).
*Iron-deficiency anaemias.*

**Cerexin** Rolab, S.Afr.†.
Cefalexin (p.168·1).
*Bacterial infections.*

**Cerezyme**
Genzyme, Austral.; Genzyme, Austria; Genzyme, Denm.; Genzyme, Fr.†; Genzyme, Ger.; Genzyme, Hong Kong; Genzyme, Israel; Genzyme, Ital.; Genzyme, Jpn; Medra, NZ; Enzifarma, Port.; Genzyme, Spain; Genzyme, Switz.; Genzyme, UK; Genzyme, USA.
Imiglucerase (p.1649·2).
*Gaucher disease.*

**Cergem** Nourypharma, Ger.
Gemeprost (p.1518·1).
*Cervical dilatation.*

**Cergodun** Duncan, Arg.
Nicergoline (p.1719·3).

**Ceridal**
Stiefel, Fin.; Rhone-Poulenc Rorer, Irl.†.
A range of emollient preparations.
*Dry skin and scalp disorders.*

**Cerina** Wyeth, Switz.
Estradiol (p.1550·1).
*Menopausal disorders; osteoporosis.*

**Ceri-Nutrina** Prospa, Port.
Preparation for enteral nutrition (p.1417·1).

**Ceris** Madaus, Fr.
Trospium chloride (p.491·2).
*Bladder instability.*

**Cerivikehl** Sanum-Kehlbeck, Ger.
Homoeopathic preparation.

**Cermox** Rontag, Arg.
Ciclosporin (p.1351·2).
*Immunosuppressant.*

**Cernevit**
Baxter Immuno, Arg.; Baxter, Austral.; Baxter, Austria; Baxter, Belg.†; Baxter, Braz.†; Baxter, Fr.; Baxter, Ger.; Baxter, Gr.; Clintec, Irl.†; Baxter, Ital.; Baxter, NZ; Baxter, Spain; Baxter, Swed.; Baxter, Switz.; Baxter, UK; Baxter, USA.
A multivitamin preparation (p.1417·1).
*Parenteral nutrition.*

**Cernilton**
Temis, Arg.; Strathmann, Ger.; Fuso, Jpn.
Cernitin pollen extract.
*Benign prostatic hyperplasia; prostatitis.*

**Cerofene** Medicus, Gr.
Cefuroxime sodium (p.184·1).
*Bacterial infections.*

**Cerose DM** Wyeth-Ayerst, USA.
Dextromethorphan hydrobromide (p.1117·3); chlorphenamine maleate (p.427·3); phenylephrine hydrochloride (p.1126·3).
*Coughs and cold symptoms.*

**Cerotto Bertelli Arnikos** Kelemata, Ital.
Capsicum oleoresin (p.1667·1).
*Musculoskeletal disorders.*

**Cerovite** Rugby, USA.
Multivitamin and mineral preparation with iron and folic acid (p.1417·1).

**Cerox** Bouty, Ital.
Benzalkonium chloride (p.1168·3); allantoin (p.1141·3); quaternium-14.
*Skin, wound, and burn disinfection.*

**Ceroxmed Steril** Bouty, Ital.†.
Benzalkonium chloride (p.1168·3).
*Instrument and surface disinfection; skin, wound, and hand disinfection.*

**Cerson** Riemser, Ger.
Flumetasone pivalate (p.1101·1).
*Skin disorders.*

**Certagen** Goldline, USA.
*Oral liquid:* Multivitamin and mineral preparation (p.1417·1).
*Tablets:* Ferrous fumarate (p.1427·3); folic acid (p.1429·1); multivitamins and minerals (p.1417·1).
*Iron-deficiency anaemias.*

**Certagen Senior** Goldline, USA.
Multivitamin and mineral preparation with iron and folic acid (p.1417·1).

**Certalac** Celltech, Belg.
Lactulose (p.1269·1).
*Constipation.*

**Certa-Vite** Major, USA.
Multivitamin and mineral preparation (p.1417·1).

**Certified Decongestant** Prodemdis, Canad.
Xylometazoline hydrochloride (p.1132·2).

**Certified Ice** Prodemdis, Canad.
Menthol (p.1711·3).

**Certified Nasal** Prodemdis, Canad.
Sodium chloride (p.1233·3).

**Certiva** North American Vaccine, USA†.
A diphtheria, tetanus, and acellular pertussis vaccine (p.1613·3).
*Active immunisation.*

**Certobil** Metapharma, Ital.†.
Dehydrocholic acid (p.1679·2); rhubarb (p.1287·3); cascara (p.1255·1); boldo (p.1661·2); manna (p.1273·1).
*Constipation.*

**Certomycin**
Aesca, Austria; Essex, Ger.
Netilmicin sulfate (p.236·3).
*Bacterial infections.*

**Certonal** Riemser, Ger.
Moxaverine hydrochloride (p.1717·2).
*Circulatory disorders.*

**Certovermil** Farmedica, Braz.†.
Mebendazole (p.108·2).
*Worm infections.*

**Certuss** Prodotti, Braz.
Carbocisteine (p.1116·2).
*Respiratory-tract congestion.*

**Ceru Spray** Ghimas, Ital.
Chamomile (p.1669·3).
*Aural hygiene.*

**Cerubidin**
Aventis, Denm.; Aventis, Irl.; Aventis, Norw.; Aventis, S.Afr.; Aventis, Swed.; Rhone-Poulenc Rorer, UK†.
Daunorubicin hydrochloride (p.545·3).
*Leukaemias.*

**Cerubidine**
Aventis, Belg.; Aventis, Canad.; Aventis, Fr.; Aventis, Israel; Aventis, Neth.; Aventis, NZ†; Aventis, Switz.; Bedford, USA.
Daunorubicin hydrochloride (p.545·3).
*Leukaemias and lymphomas.*

**Cerucal** Temmler, Ger.
Metoclopramide hydrochloride (p.1274·3).
*Gastrointestinal disorders.*

**Cerulisina** Bouty, Ital.
Xylene (p.1478·2).
*Ear wax removal.*

**Cerulyse** Chauvin, Fr.
Xylene (p.1478·2).
*Ear wax removal.*

**Cerumenex**
Purdue, Canad.; Asta Medica, Ital.†; Aventis, S.Afr.†; Mundipharma, Switz.; Purdue Frederick, USA.
Trolamine polypeptide oleate-condensate (p.1758·2).
*Ear wax removal.*

**Cerumenex N** Mundipharma, Ger.
Trolamine polypeptide oleate-condensate (p.1758·2).
*Ear wax removal.*

**Cerumenol**
Note. This name is used for preparations of different composition.
Martin, Fr.
Polysorbate 80 (p.1415·2).
*Ear wax removal.*

Berna, Spain.
Potassium hydroxide (p.1734·2).
*Ear wax removal.*

Schonenberger, Switz.
Paradichlorobenzene (p.1728·3); chlorobutanol hemihydrate (p.1176·3); turpentine oil (p.1760·1); orthodichlorobenzene (p.1724·3); methoxybutyl acetate.
*Ear wax removal.*

**Cerumex** Cassara, Arg.
Docusate sodium (p.1262·2).
*Ear wax removal.*

**Cerumin** Alcon, Braz.
Hydroxyquinoline borate (p.1700·1); trolamine (p.1758·2).
*Ear wax removal.*

**Cerumol**
Note. This name is used for preparations of different composition.
Culver, Austral.
Paradichlorobenzene (p.1728·3); chlorobutanol (p.1176·3); orthodichlorobenzene (p.1724·3); arachis oil (p.1656·1).
*Ear wax removal.*

Paladin, Canad.; Laboratories for Applied Biology, Irl.†.
Paradichlorobenzene (p.1728·3); chlorobutanol (p.1176·3); turpentine oil (p.1760·1).

Laboratories for Applied Biology, Hong Kong†; Tamar, Israel; Pharmafrica, S.Afr.; Laboratories for Applied Biology, Singapore; Laboratories for Applied Biology, UK.
Paradichlorobenzene (p.1728·3); chlorobutanol (p.1176·3); arachis oil (p.1656·1).
Formerly contained paradichlorobenzene, chlorobutanol, benzocaine, and turpentine oil in *Israel*.
The name Cerumenol has also been used for this preparation in the *UK*.
*Ear wax removal.*

Laboratories for Applied Biology, Malaysia.
Paradichlorobenzene (p.1728·3); chlorobutanol (p.1176·3).
*Ear wax removal.*

**Cerutil** Alpharma-Isis, Ger.
Meclofenoxate hydrochloride (p.1710·1).
*Cerebrovascular disorders; mental function impairment.*

**Ceruxim** Antor, Gr.
Cefuroxime sodium (p.184·1).
*Bacterial infections.*

**Cervagem**
Aventis, Austral.; Aventis, Denm.; Aventis, Fin.; Aventis, Hong Kong; Aventis, Malaysia; Aventis, Norw.; Aventis, NZ; Aventis, Singapore; Aventis, Swed.
Gemeprost (p.1518·1).
*Cervical dilatation; termination of pregnancy.*

**Cervageme** Aventis, Fr.
Gemeprost (p.1518·1).
*Cervical dilatation prior to uterine procedures; termination of pregnancy.*

**Cervasta** Fournier, Ital.†.
Cerivastatin sodium (p.881·3).
*Hypercholesterolaemia.*

**Cervekanin** Romer, Mex.†.
Brewers' yeast (p.1469·1).

**Cervep** Menarini, Arg.
Heparin sodium (p.928·1).
*Soft-tissue injury; thrombophlebitis.*

**Cervidil**
Note. This name is used for preparations of different composition.
CSL, Austral.; Ferring, Canad.; Forest Pharmaceuticals, USA.
Dinoprostone (p.1515·1).
*Labour induction.*

Serono, Ital.
Gemeprost (p.1518·1).
*Cervical dilatation.*

**Cervilan** Aventis, Mex.
Lomifylline; dihydroergocristine mesilate (p.1680·1).
*Cerebrovascular disorders.*

**Cervilane**
Aventis, Arg.; Aventis, Chile; Cassenne, Fr.†; Roussel, Port.
Lomifylline; dihydroergocristine mesilate (p.1680·1).
*Cerebrovascular disorders; vestibular disorders.*

**Cervinca** Basi, Port.
Vincamine (p.1764·2).
*Cerebrovascular disorders.*

**Cerviprime** AstraZeneca, India.
Dinoprostone (p.1515·1).
*Cervical dilatation.*

**Cerviprost** Nourypharma, Ger.†.
Dinoprostone (p.1515·1).
*Labour induction.*

**Cervitec** DAB, Swed.
Chlorhexidine acetate (p.1173·2).
*Dental hygiene.*

**Cervoxan**
Pharmafarm, Fr.; Decomed, Port.; Mabo, Spain.
Vinburnine (p.1764·2).
*Cerebrovascular disorders.*

**Cervusen** ADP, Hong Kong.
Deer antler cartilage.
*Osteoarthritis; rheumatoid arthritis; systemic lupus erythematosus.*

**CES** ICN, Canad.
Conjugated oestrogens (p.1543·2).
*Menopausal disorders; osteoporosis.*

**Cesamet**
ICN, Canad.; Lilly, Irl.; Cambridge, UK†.
Nabilone (p.1277·1).
Now available as Nabilone Capsules in the *UK*.
*Nausea and vomiting associated with cancer chemotherapy.*

**Cesbron** Sanofi Synthelabo, Port.
Clenbuterol (p.784·2).

**Cesol**
Note. This name is used for preparations of different composition.
Merck, Chile; Merck, Ger.; Merck, Mex.
Praziquantel (p.112·2).
*Cestode infections.*

Cesam, Port.†.
Ketoconazole (p.403·3).
*Pityriasis versicolor; seborrhoeic dermatitis.*

**Cesoline** Pharmasant, Thai.
Hydralazine hydrochloride (p.931·2).
*Hypertension.*

**Cesplon** Esteve, Spain.
Captopril (p.879·2).
*Diabetic nephropathy; heart failure; hypertension; myocardial infarction.*

**Cesplon Plus** Esteve, Spain.
Hydrochlorothiazide (p.933·2); captopril (p.879·2).
*Hypertension.*

**Cesradyston** Cesra, Ger.
Hypericum (p.299·1).
Formerly contained belladonna, phenobarbital, secalia corn., gelsemium, atropine sulfate, and hamamelis.
*Depression.*

**Cesran** Cesra, Ger.†.
Hypericum (p.299·1).
*Depression.*

**Cesrasanol** Cesra, Ger.
Chamomile; hamamelis; calendula; arnica; achillea; centaury.
*Inflammation; spasms.*

**Cessagripe** Neckerman, Braz.†.
Nux vomica (p.1722·3).

**Cessatosse** Regius, Braz.†.
Sodium dibunate (p.1130·2); sulfogaiacol (p.1131·1); belladonna (p.479·1); sodium benzoate (p.1169·3).
*Coughs.*

**Cessaverm** INQ, Braz.†.
Mebendazole (p.108·2).
*Worm infections.*

**Cestop** Drag, Chile.
Clotrimazole (p.396·2).
*Fungal skin infections.*

**Cestop B** Drag, Chile.
Betamethasone (p.1093·1); clotrimazole (p.396·2).
*Infected skin disorders.*

**Cestox** Merck, Braz.
Praziquantel (p.112·2).
*Cestode infections; trematode infections.*

**Ceta** C & M, USA.
Skin cleanser.

**Ceta Plus** Seatrace, USA.
Hydrocodone tartrate (p.45·1); paracetamol (p.76·2).
*Pain.*

**Ceta Sulfa** Grin, Mex.†.
Sulfacetamide sodium (p.257·3).
*Bacterial eye infections.*

**Cetabon** Great Eastern, Thai.; Therapharma, Thai.
Stanozolol (p.1569·2); vitamin B substances (p.1417·1).
*Anabolic.*

**Cetacaine** Cetylite, USA.
Benzocaine (p.1370·3); butyl aminobenzoate (p.1373·1); tetracaine hydrochloride (p.1385·1).
*Local anaesthesia.*

**Cetacort** Healthpoint, USA.
Hydrocortisone (p.1103·3).
*Skin disorders.*

**Cetafeine** Arkomedika, Fr.†.
Paracetamol (p.76·2); caffeine (p.782·1).
*Fever; pain.*

**Cetafrin** Luper, Braz.
Paracetamol (p.76·2).
*Fever; pain.*

**Cetal**
Pfizer, Austria; Parke, Davis, Ger.†; Pfizer, Switz.
Vincamine (p.1764·2).
*Ménière's disease; mental function disorders; metabolic and circulatory disorders of the brain, retina, and ear.*

**Cetam** Yung Shin, Singapore.
Piracetam (p.1732·1).
*Mental function disorders.*

**Cetamide**
Alcon, Canad.; Alcon, USA.
Sulfacetamide sodium (p.257·3).
*Bacterial eye infections.*

**Cetamine**
Note. This name is used for preparations of different composition.
Wolfs, Belg.
Ascorbic acid (p.1460·2).
*Vitamin C deficiency; vitamin C supplement.*

Covan, S.Afr.†.
*Syrup:* Paracetamol (p.76·2); mepyramine maleate (p.437·1); phenylephrine hydrochloride (p.1126·3); caffeine (p.782·1).
*Tablets:* Quinine sulfate (p.460·2); ascorbic acid (p.1460·2); paracetamol (p.76·2); mepyramine maleate (p.437·1); phenylephrine hydrochloride (p.1126·3).
*Cold and influenza symptoms.*

**Cetampril** Clintex, Port.
Enalapril maleate (p.909·2).
*Heart failure; hypertension.*

**Cetan** Pharmasant, Thai.†.
Ibuprofen (p.45·3); paracetamol (p.76·2).
*Musculoskeletal, joint, peri-articular, and soft-tissue disorders.*

**Cetanorm** Norma, UK.
Benzalkonium chloride (p.1168·3); aldioxa (p.1141·2); chlorobutanol (p.1176·3); cetrimide (p.1172·1).
*Nappy rash; wounds.*

**Cetaphil**
Galderma, Austral.; Galderma, Braz.; Galderma, Canad.; Galderma, Chile; Galderma, Hong Kong; Galderma, Malaysia; Galderma, Mex.; Galderma, NZ; Galderma, Port.; Galderma, Singapore; Galderma, Spain; Galderma, Thai.; Galderma, UK; Galderma, USA.
A range of skin cleansers and emollients.

**Cetaphil Daily Facial** Galderma, Canad.
*SPF 15:* Avobenzone (p.1142·3); octocrilene (p.1154·3).
*Sunscreen.*

**Cetapred**
Alcon, Belg.†; Alcon, USA†.
Prednisolone acetate (p.1108·1); sulfacetamide sodium (p.257·3).
*Bacterial eye infections with inflammation.*

**Cetapril** Dainippon, Jpn.
Alacepril (p.856·2).
*Hypertension.*

**Cetasil** Silom, Thai.†.
Sulfacetamide sodium (p.257·3).
*Bacterial eye infections.*

**Cetavlex**
Note. This name is used for preparations of different composition.
Tramedico, Belg.
Cetrimonium bromide (p.1173·1); chlorhexidine gluconate (p.1173·2).
*Disinfection of wounds, skin, and hands; skin disorders.*

Bioglan, Irl.; Bioglan, Malaysia; CS, Port.†; Bioglan, Singapore†; Centrapharm, UK.
Cetrimide (p.1172·1).
*Burns; nappy rash; skin disorders; wounds.*

**Cetavlon**
CS, Fr.; AstraZeneca, Neth.†; Genop, S.Afr.†; AstraZeneca, Spain.
Cetrimide (p.1172·1).
*Burns; disinfection; wounds.*

**Cetaxim** TRB, Arg.
Cefixime (p.172·3).
*Bacterial infections.*

**Cetaz** Uniao Quimica, Braz.
Ceftazidime (p.180·2).
*Bacterial infections.*

**Cetazin** Sigmapharm, Austria.
Sulfacetamide sodium (p.257·3).
*Bacterial eye infections.*

**Cetebe**
SmithKline Beecham, Austria; GlaxoSmithKline Consumer, Ger.; SmithKline Beecham Consumer, Switz.
Ascorbic acid (p.1460·2).
*Vitamin C deficiency; vitamin C supplement.*

**Ceti** TAD, Ger.
Cetirizine hydrochloride (p.427·1).
*Hypersensitivity reactions.*

**Cetidura** Merck dura, Ger.
Cetirizine hydrochloride (p.427·1).
*Allergic rhinitis.*

**Cetihis** Unison, Thai.
Cetirizine hydrochloride (p.427·1).
*Allergic rhinitis; pruritus; urticaria.*

**Cetildrops** Luper, Braz.
Cetylpyridinium chloride (p.1173·1); benzocaine (p.1370·3).
*Mouth and throat disorders.*

**Cetilsan** Sella, Ital.
Cetylpyridinium chloride (p.1173·1).
*Oral hygiene; skin and wound disinfection.*

**Cetimil** Lesvi, Spain.
Nedocromil sodium (p.789·3).
*Asthma.*

**Cetina** Infan, Mex.†.
Chloramphenicol (p.185·1).
*Bacterial infections.*

**Cetiprin**
Pharmacia, Austria; Darrow, Braz.; Pharmacia, Denm.; Pharmacia Upjohn, Irl.†; Pharmacia, Neth.; Pharmacia, Norw.; Pharmacia Upjohn, NZ†; Pharmacia, Swed.; Pharmacia, Switz.†.
Emepronium bromide (p.482·1) or emepronium carrageenate (p.482·1).
*Bladder disorders; pancreatitis; smooth muscle spasm.*

**Cetiprin Novum**
Pharmacia, Fin.; Pharmacia Upjohn, Hong Kong†.
Emepronium carrageenate (p.482·1).
*Tenesmus; urinary frequency; urinary incontinence.*

**Cetiram** Specifar (Σπεσιφαρ), Gr.
Cetirizine hydrochloride (p.427·1).
*Allergic conjunctivitis; allergic rhinitis; pruritus.*

**Cetirlan** Krewel, Ger.
Cetirizine hydrochloride (p.427·1).
*Allergic conjunctivitis; allergic rhinitis; urticaria.*

**Cetirocol** Approved Prescription Services, UK†.
Cetirizine hydrochloride (p.427·1).
*Allergic rhinitis; urticaria.*

**Cetiva AE** Farmasa, Braz.
Vitamins A, C, and E (p.1417·1).

**Cetobeta** Bunker, Braz.
Betamethasone dipropionate (p.1093·1); ketoconazole (p.403·3); neomycin sulfate (p.235·1).
*Infected skin disorders.*

**Cetocort** Teuto, Braz.
Betamethasone dipropionate (p.1093·1); ketoconazole (p.403·3).
*Infected skin disorders.*

**Cetoglutaran** Tradiphar, Fr.
Calcium di-oxoglurate.
*Asthenia.*

**Cetohexal** Hexal, Braz.
Ketoconazole (p.403·3).
*Fungal infections.*

**Cetomed** Cimed, Braz.
Ketoconazole (p.403·3).
*Fungal infections.*

**Cetona Plus** Democal, Switz.†.
Aluminium acetate (p.1652·3); arnica (p.1656·3); spilantes.
Formerly contained aluminium acetate, arnica, chamomile, calendula, hypericum, comfrey, dexpanthenol, and lidocaine hydrochloride.
*Musculoskeletal, joint, peri-articular, and soft-tissue disorders; skin irritation.*

**Cetonax** Janssen-Cilag, Braz.
Ketoconazole (p.403·3).
*Fungal infections.*

**Cetoneo** Neo Quimica, Braz.
Ketoconazole (p.403·3).
*Fungal infections.*

**Cetonil**
Stiefel, Arg.; Stiefel, Braz.
Ketoconazole (p.403·3).
*Fungal infections.*

**Cetoquina Y** Solfran, Mex.
Fluocinolone acetonide (p.1101·2); clioquinol (p.196·3).
*Infected skin disorders.*

**Cetornan** Chiesi, Fr.
Ornithine oxoglurate (p.1442·3).
*Nutritional supplement.*

**Cetoteron** Eurofarma, Braz.
Cyproterone acetate (p.1544·1).

**Cetovinca**
Schering, Mex.†; Byk Elmu, Spain†.
Vincamine oxoglurate (p.1764·2).
*Cerebral trauma; cerebrovascular disorders.*

**Cetoxil** Fustery, Mex.
Cefuroxime axetil (p.184·1) or cefuroxime sodium (p.184·1).
*Bacterial infections.*

**Cetoxol** Aspen Consumer, S.Afr.†.
Benzocaine (p.1370·3); cetylpyridinium chloride (p.1173·1).
*Sore throat.*

**Cetozan** Royton, Braz.
Ketoconazole (p.403·3).
*Fungal infections.*

**Cetozol** Cazi, Braz.
Ketoconazole (p.403·3).
*Fungal infections.*

**Cetozone** De Mayo, Braz.
Ascorbic acid (p.1460·2).
*Vitamin C supplement.*

**Cetraben**
Lyka, India; Sankyo, UK.
White soft paraffin (p.1479·3); liquid paraffin (p.1479·1).
*Dry skin.*

**Cetraben Bath Oil** Sankyo, UK.
Light liquid paraffin (p.1479·1).
*Dry skin.*

**Cetralon** Julphar, UAE.
Cetirizine hydrochloride (p.427·1).
*Hypersensitivity reactions.*

**Cetraria Salbe** Helixor, Ger.†.
Iceland moss; laminaria (p.1704·3).
*Skin disorders; skin ulcers.*

**Cetraxal** Salvat, Spain.
Ciprofloxacin (p.188·2) or ciprofloxacin hydrochloride (p.188·2).
*Bacterial infections.*

**Cetraxal Plus** Salvat, Spain.
Ciprofloxacin (p.188·2); fluocinolone acetonide (p.1101·2).
*Otitis externa.*

**Cetrazil** Infosint, Ital.
Propylene glycol cefatrizine (p.170·3).
*Bacterial infections.*

**Cetrexidin** Vebas, Ital.
Chlorhexidine gluconate (p.1173·2); cetrimide (p.1172·1).
*Mouth disinfection.*

**Cetriderm con Triclosan** Gedis, Ital.
Triclosan (p.1195·2).
*Skin cleansing.*

**Cetrilan** Igefarma, Braz.†.
Cetrimide (p.1172·1); benzalkonium chloride (p.1168·3).
*Skin disinfection.*

**Cetriler** Roux-Ocefa, Arg.
Cetirizine hydrochloride (p.427·1).
*Allergic rhinitis; allergic skin disorders; urticaria.*

**Cetriler D** Roux-Ocefa, Arg.
Cetirizine hydrochloride (p.427·1); pseudoephedrine hydrochloride (p.1129·2).
*Nasal congestion.*

**Cetrimed** Medifive, Thai.
Cetirizine hydrochloride (p.427·1).
*Allergic conjunctivitis; allergic rhinitis; allergic skin disorders; insect bites.*

**Cetrin** Vitamed, Israel.
Cetrimide (p.1172·1); chlorhexidine gluconate (p.1173·2).
*Skin disinfection.*

**Cetrine** Reddy, Thai.
Cetirizine hydrochloride (p.427·1).
*Allergic conjunctivitis; allergic rhinitis; allergic skin disorders; insect bites.*

**Cetrinets**
Westmont, Hong Kong; Westmont, Malaysia; Westmont, Singapore.
Ascorbic acid (p.1460·2).
*Vitamin C deficiency.*

**Cetrinox** Magis, Ital.
Propylene glycol cefatrizine (p.170·3).
*Bacterial infections.*

**Cetrisan** Gedis, Ital.
Chlorhexidine gluconate (p.1173·2); cetrimide (p.1172·1).
*Surface disinfection.*

**Cetriwal** Wallace, India.
Cetirizine hydrochloride (p.427·1).
*Allergic rhinitis; urticaria.*

**Cetrizet**
Sun, India; Sun, Thai.
Cetirizine hydrochloride (p.427·1).
*Allergic skin disorders; rhinitis.*

**Cetrizin**
Note. This name is used for preparations of different composition.
Sintofarma, Braz.; TO-Chemicals, Thai.
Cetirizine hydrochloride (p.427·1).
*Allergic conjunctivitis; allergic rhinitis; allergic skin disorders; insect bites.*

Elpen (Ελπεν), Gr.
Propylene glycol cefatrizine (p.170·3).
*Bacterial infections.*

**Cetrolac** Genom, Braz.
Ketorolac trometamol (p.52·1).
*Eye disorders.*

**Cetron** Raffo, Arg.
Ondansetron (p.1281·1).
*Nausea and vomiting.*

**Cetrotide**
Serono, Arg.; Serono, Austral.; Serono, Austria; Serono, Belg.†; Serono, Denm.; Serono, Fin.; Serono, Fr.; Serono, Ger.; Asta, Gr.; Serono, Hong Kong; Serono, Israel; Serono, Ital.; Serono, Neth.; Serono, Norw.; Douglas, NZ; Serono, Port.; Serono, Singapore; Serono, Spain; Serono, Swed.; Serono, Thai.; Serono, UK; Asta Medica, USA.
Cetrorelix acetate (p.1320·2).
*Controlled ovarian stimulation.*

**Cetylcide II** Cetylite, USA.
Alkyldimethylbenzylammonium chloride (p.1168·3); alkyldimethylethylbenzylammonium chloride.
*Surface disinfection.*

**Cetylcide-G** Cetylite, USA.
Glutaral (p.1180·3).
*Instrument disinfection.*

**Cetylyre** Oberlin, Fr.
Cetylpyridinium chloride (p.1173·1).
*Eye disorders.*

**Cetynol** Brasmedica, Braz.†.
Paracetamol (p.76·2).
*Fever; pain.*

**Cevaderm** Cevallos, Arg.
Betamethasone (p.1093·1); tolnaftate (p.410·1); gentamicin (p.219·1).
*Skin infections.*

**Cevalin** Lilly, Mex.
Ascorbic acid (p.1460·2).
*Vitamin C deficiency.*

**Cevanil** Pharmasant, Thai.
Pirenzepine hydrochloride (p.488·1).
*Peptic ulcer.*

**Cevi-Bid** Geriatric Pharm. Corp., USA.
Ascorbic acid (p.1460·2).
*Vitamin C deficiency.*

**Cevicort** Cevallos, Arg.
Betamethasone (p.1093·1).
*Corticosteroid.*

**Cevi-drops** Centropharm, Belg.
Ascorbic acid (p.1460·2); calcium ascorbate (p.1460·2).
*Vitamin C deficiency; vitamin C supplement.*

**Cevi-Fer** Geriatric Pharm. Corp., USA.
Ferrous fumarate (p.1427·3); folic acid (p.1429·1).
Ascorbic acid (p.1460·2) is included in this preparation to increase the absorption and availability of iron.
*Iron and folic acid deficiency.*

**Cevigen** Bros, Gr.
Azelaic acid (p.1142·3).
*Acne.*

**Cevinolon** Bros, Gr.
Aciclovir (p.626·1).
*Herpes simplex infections.*

**Cevirin** Esseti, Ital.
Aciclovir (p.626·1).
*Herpesvirus infections.*

**Ceviron** Hearst, Braz.†.
Ferrous sulfate (p.1428·2); thiamine (p.1455·2).
*Anaemias.*

**Cevita** Teuto, Braz.
Ascorbic acid (p.1460·2).
*Vitamin C supplement.*

**Cevi-Tabs** Ferrosan, Fin.
Ascorbic acid (p.1460·2).
*Vitamin C deficiency.*

**Cevitol** Lannacher, Austria.
Ascorbic acid (p.1460·2) or sodium ascorbate (p.1460·2).
*Vitamin C deficiency.*

**Ceviton** Ariston, Braz.
Ascorbic acid (p.1460·2).

**Cewin**
Sanofi Synthelabo, Arg.; Sanofi Synthelabo, Braz.
Ascorbic acid (p.1460·2).
*Vitamin C supplement.*

**Cexidal Otico** Salvat, Spain.
Ciprofloxacin (p.188·2); fluocinolone acetonide (p.1101·2).
*Otitis externa.*

**Cezane**
Note. This name is used for preparations of different composition.
Hexa-Medinova, Arg.
Astemizole (p.424·2).
*Allergic rhinitis; urticaria.*

Laborsil, Braz.†.
Acriflavinium chloride (p.1165·3); methenamine mandelate (p.230·2); methylthioninium chloride (p.1042·2).
*Urinary-tract infections.*

**Cezin** UAD, USA.
Multivitamin and mineral preparation (p.1417·1).

**Cezolin**
Note. This name is used for preparations of different composition.
Biochimico, Braz.
Cefazolin (p.170·3).
*Bacterial infections.*

Remedina, Gr.
Ketoconazole (p.403·3).
*Fungal infections.*

**Cezox** Pharmasant, Thai.
Chlorzoxazone (p.1392·3); paracetamol (p.76·2).
*Skeletal muscle pain and spasm.*

**CF Vite** Cypress, USA.
Multivitamin and zinc preparation (p.1417·1).
*Dietary supplement.*

**C-Film**
Geymonat, Ital.†; Lucchini, Switz.
A nonoxinol (p.1413·2).
*Contraceptive.*

Arun, UK†.
Nonoxinol 9 (p.1413·3).
*Contraceptive.*

**C-Flox** Alphapharm, Austral.
Ciprofloxacin hydrochloride (p.188·2).
*Bacterial infections.*

**C-Floxacin** SM, Thai.
Ciprofloxacin hydrochloride (p.188·2).
*Bacterial infections.*

**C-G** ICN, Arg.
Sulfacetamide sodium (p.257·3); sulfur (p.1158·2).
*Acne; rosacea; seborrhoeic dermatitis.*

**CGT** Libbs, Braz.
Multivitamin and mineral preparation (p.1417·1).

**Chalena** Sibras, Braz.†.
Paracetamol (p.76·2).
*Fever; pain.*

**Chamillamont** Pharmonta, Austria.
Chamomile (p.1669·3).
*Gastrointestinal disorders; mouth disorders; respiratory-tract disorders; skin disorders.*

**Chamo S** Ysatfabrik, Ger.
Chamomile flowers (p.1669·3).
*Anorectal disorders; gastrointestinal disorders; mouth and throat inflammation; respiratory-tract disorders; skin disorders; vaginitis; wounds.*

**Chamoca M** Hanosan, Ger.
Homoeopathic preparation.

**Chamomile Blend** Lifeplan, UK.
Valerian; chamomile; lupulus; passion flower (p.1417·1).
*Herbal supplement.*

**Chamomilla Comp** Weleda, Ger.
Homoeopathic preparation.

**Championyl** Sanofi Synthelabo, Ital.
Sulpiride (p.722·2).
*Dysthymia; psychoses.*

**Champuacid** Bajer, Arg.
Zinc undecenoate (p.411·1); salicylic acid (p.1157·1); coal tar (Alcoderm) (p.1159·2).
*Scalp disorders.*

**Chantaline** Altana, Spain.
Theophylline (p.798·3).
*Asthma; bronchospasm; heart failure; paroxysmal dyspnoea.*

**Chap Stick** Whitehall, NZ.
*Lip Balm Classic SPF 4:* Padimate O (p.1155·1).
*Lip Balm SPF 15:* Oxybenzone (p.1154·3); padimate O (p.1155·1).
*Lip Balm Strawberry SPF 15; Flava-Craze Passion Crush SPF 15:* Octinoxate (p.1154·3); oxybenzone (p.1154·3).
*Lip Balm Ultra SPF 30+:* Octinoxate (p.1154·3); octocrilene (p.1154·3); octisalate (p.1154·3); oxybenzone (p.1154·3).
*Lip Conditioner SPF 15:* Aloe vera (p.1141·3) octinoxate (p.1154·3); oxybenzone (p.1154·3); vitamin E (p.1464·3).
*Chapped lips; sunscreen.*

**Chapstick**
Note. This name is used for preparations of different composition.
Whitehall, Austral.†.
Padimate O (p.1155·1).
*SPF 15:* Padimate O (p.1155·1); oxybenzone (p.1154·3).
*Dry or chapped lips; sunscreen for lips.*

Whitehall, Braz.
*Lipbalm:* Padimate O (p.1155·1); camphor (p.1665·3); titanium dioxide (p.1160·3).
*Lipbalm SPF15:* Padimate O (p.1155·1); oxybenzone (p.1154·3); camphor (p.1665·3); titanium dioxide (p.1160·3).
*Dry or chapped lips; sunscreen.*

Whitehall, Port.†.
*SPF 4:* Padimate (p.1155·1).
*Dry or chapped lips; sunscreen.*

Robins, USA.
*Lip balm SPF 15:* Padimate O (p.1155·1); oxybenzone (p.1154·3); titanium dioxide (p.1160·3).
*Ointment SPF 15:* Padimate O (p.1155·1); oxybenzone (p.1154·3).
*Sunscreen.*

**Chapstick Lip Balm** Blistex, Canad.
Padimate O (p.1155·1).
*Sunscreen.*

**Chapstick Lip Moisturizer**
Whitehall-Robins, Canad.; Wyeth Consumer, Chile.
Octinoxate (p.1154·3); oxybenzone (p.1154·3).
*Chapped lips; sunscreen.*

**Chapstick Medicated** Wyeth Consumer, Chile.
White soft paraffin (p.1479·3); camphor (p.1665·3); menthol (p.1711·3); phenol (p.1188·1).
*Chapped lips.*

**Chapstick Medicated Lip Balm**
Whitehall-Robins, Canad.; Robins, USA.
Camphor (p.1665·3); menthol (p.1711·3); soft paraffin (p.1479·3); phenol (p.1188·1).

**Chapstick Mint** Wyeth Consumer, Chile.
Padimate o (p.1155·1).
*Chapped lips; sunscreen.*

**Chapstick Regular** Wyeth Consumer, Chile.
Padimate o (p.1155·1); titanium dioxide (p.1160·3).
*Chapped lips; sunscreen.*

**Chapstick Sun Block** Whitehall, Port.†.
*SPF 15:* Padimate (p.1155·1); oxybenzone (p.1154·3).
*Dry or chapped lips; sunscreen.*

**Chapstick Sunblock** Whitehall-Robins, Canad.
*SPF 15:* Padimate O (p.1155·1); oxybenzone (p.1154·3).
*Sunscreen.*

**Chapstick Ultra** Wyeth Consumer, Chile.
*SPF 30:* Octinoxate (p.1154·3); octocrilene (p.1154·3); octisalate (p.1154·3); oxybenzone (p.1154·3); titanium dioxide (p.1160·3).
*Chapped lips; sunscreen.*

**Charabs** Lane, UK†.
Caffeine (p.782·1); vitamin B substances (p.1417·1).
*Tonic.*

**Charac** Omega, Canad.
Activated charcoal (p.1030·2).
*Poison antidote.*

**Charac Tol** Omega, Canad.
Activated charcoal (p.1030·2); sorbitol (p.1446·3).
*Poison antidote.*

**Charbon de Belloc** Chefaro Ardeval, Fr.
Activated charcoal (p.1030·2).
*Gastrointestinal disorders.*

**Charcoaid** Requa, USA.
Activated charcoal (p.1030·2).
*Emergency treatment of poisoning.*

**Charcoal Plus** Kramer, USA.
Activated charcoal (p.1030·2).
Formerly contained simeticone and activated charcoal.
*Flatulence.*

**Charcocaps**
Key, Austral.†; Requa, USA.
Activated charcoal (p.1030·2).
*Diarrhoea; flatulence; poisoning.*

**Charcodote**
Pharmascience, Canad.; Pharmascience, Hong Kong; Formulex, Israel; Pliva, UK.
Activated charcoal (p.1030·2) with or without sorbitol (p.1446·3).
*Emergency treatment of poisoning.*

**Charcodote Aqueous** Pharmascience, Canad.
Activated charcoal (p.1030·2).
*Poison antidote.*

**Charcotabs** Key, Austral.†.
Activated charcoal (p.1030·2).
*Diarrhoea; drug poisoning; excess gastrointestinal gas.*

**Charlieu Anti-Poux** Mayoly-Spindler, Fr.
Permethrin (p.1508·3); piperonyl butoxide (p.1509·2).
*Lice infestation.*

**Charlieu Topic** Nigy, Fr.
Urea (p.1162·2).
*Dry skin disorders.*

**Charlieu Topicrem** Nigy, Fr.
Urea (p.1162·2); glycerol (p.1694·3).
*Dry skin disorders.*

**Chase Coldsorex** Stella, Canad.
Benzoin (p.1751·1); camphor (p.1665·3); menthol (p.1711·3); myrrh (p.1718·3).

**Chase Kolik Gripe Water** Stella, Canad.
Alcohol (p.1166·1); ginger (p.1267·1); dill oil (p.1680·2); sodium bicarbonate (p.1223·2).

**Chase Kolik Gripe Water Alcohol-Free** Stella, Canad.
Fennel oil (p.1687·3); sodium bicarbonate (p.1223·2).

**Chebil** Basi, Port.
Chenodeoxycholic acid (p.1670·1).

**Check-Mate** BHR, UK.
Pregnancy test (p.1734·3).

**Chefarine 4** Chefaro, Neth.†.
Aspirin (p.15·1); paracetamol (p.76·2).
*Fever; pain.*

**Chefir** Drug Research, Ital.
Cefonicid sodium (p.174·2).
Lidocaine hydrochloride (p.1377·3) is included in this preparation to alleviate the pain of injection.
*Gram-negative bacterial infections.*

**Cheiranthol** Klein, Ger.
Cheiranthus cheiri; silybum marianum (p.1043·3); cnicus benedictus (p.1673·3); achillea (p.1646·2); hypericum (p.299·1).
*Liver disorders.*

**Chek-Stix** Bayer, Austral.
Positive and negative controls for tests for glucose, bilirubin, ketones, specific gravity, blood, pH, protein, urobilinogen, nitrite, and leucocytes in urine.

**Chelated Bone Meal** Swiss Herbal, Canad.
Calcium; phosphorus (p.1417·1).

**Chelated Cal-Mag** GNLD, Austral.†.
Calcium glycinate (p.1226·3); magnesium glycinate (p.1229·1); fish-liver oil.
*Calcium and magnesium deficiency.*

**Chelated Cal-Mag plus Vitamin** Swiss Herbal, Canad.
Calcium; magnesium; vitamin C; vitamin D (p.1417·1).

**Chelated Dol Mite** Swiss Herbal, Canad.
Calcium; magnesium (p.1417·1).

**Chelated Dolomite** Jamieson, Canad.†.
Calcium; magnesium (p.1417·1).

**Chelated Solamins** Solgar, UK.
Minerals as amino-acid chelates (p.1417·1).

**Chelated Zinc** Richlife, Hong Kong†.
Zinc gluconate (p.1469·2); zinc proteinate (p.1469·3).
*Mineral supplement.*

**Chelatran** SERB, Fr.
Disodium edetate (p.1037·3).
*Digitalis intoxication.*

**Chelidonium Compose** Boiron, Fr.
Homoeopathic preparation.

**Chelidophyt** Galenika, Ger.†.
Greater celandine (p.1695·3).
Formerly contained greater celandine, achillea, peppermint leaf, and scopolia root.
*Biliary and gastrointestinal spasm.*

**Chelintox** Braun, Switz.
Sodium calcium edetate (p.1051·3).
*Heavy-metal poisoning.*

**Chemacin** CT, Ital.
Amikacin sulfate (p.154·1).
*Bacterial infections.*

**Chemcard** Marco, Austral.
Test for cholesterol in blood.

**Chemet**
Janssen-Cilag, Austria†; Ovation, USA.
Succimer (p.1054·2).
*Lead poisoning.*

**Chemicetina**
Fournier, Ital.
Chloramphenicol (p.185·1) or chloramphenicol sodium succinate (p.185·1).
*Bacterial infections.*

Tau, Spain.
Chloramphenicol palmitate (p.185·1).
*Bacterial infections.*

**Chemiofurin** Torlan, Spain†.
Nitrofurantoin (p.237·2).
*Urinary-tract infections.*

**Chemionazolo** NCSN, Ital.
Econazole nitrate (p.397·2).
*Fungal and bacterial skin and vulvovaginal infections.*

**Chemisolv** Iasis, Gr.
Butamirate citrate (p.1116·2).
*Cough.*

**Chemists Own Chesty Cough** Herron, Austral.
Bromhexine hydrochloride (p.1115·3); pseudoephedrine hydrochloride (p.1129·2); guaifenesin (p.1122·1).
Formerly known as Chemists Own Mucotuss.
*Coughs and cold symptoms.*

**Chemists Own Chesty Mucus Cough** Herron, Austral.
Bromhexine hydrochloride (p.1115·3); guaifenesin (p.1122·1).
Formerly known as Chemists Own Noesude.
*Coughs and cold symptoms.*

**Chemists Own Clozole** Herron, Austral.
Clotrimazole (p.396·2).
*Vaginal candidiasis.*

**Chemists Own Cold & Allergy** Herron, Austral.
Chlorphenamine maleate (p.427·3); phenylephrine hydrochloride (p.1126·3).
Formerly known as Chemists Own Zaymaz.
*Cold symptoms; hypersensitivity reactions.*

**Chemists Own Cold & Flu Day/Night** Herron, Austral.
Day tablets, Paracetamol (p.76·2); pseudoephedrine hydrochloride (p.1129·2); codeine phosphate (p.27·1); night tablets, paracetamol; pseudoephedrine hydrochloride; chlorphenamine maleate (p.427·3).
Formerly known as Chemists Own Cold & Flu Medication for Day & Night.
*Cold and influenza symptoms.*

**Chemists Own Cold & Flu Relief** Herron, Austral.
Paracetamol (p.76·2); pseudoephedrine hydrochloride (p.1129·2); codeine phosphate (p.27·1).
*Cold and influenza symptoms.*

**Chemists Own Cold Sore** Herron, Austral.
Aciclovir (p.626·1).
*Herpes labialis.*

**Chemists Own Coldeze** Herron, Austral.
Paracetamol (p.76·2); chlorphenamine maleate (p.427·3).
*Cold and influenza symptoms; hay fever.*

**Chemists Own Cough Suppressant** Herron, Austral.
Ammonium chloride (p.1115·2); codeine phosphate (p.27·1); menthol (p.1711·3).
*Coughs.*

**Chemists Own De Worm** Chemists Own, Austral.
Mebendazole (p.108·2).
*Worm infections.*

**Chemists Own Decongestant Nasal Spray** *Herron, Austral.*
Oxymetazoline hydrochloride (p.1126·1).
*Nasal congestion.*

**Chemists Own Diarrhoea Mixture** *Herron, Austral.*
Aluminium hydroxide (p.1249·2); calcium carbonate (p.1254·2); catechu tincture (p.1668·3); codeine phosphate (p.27·1); kaolin (p.1268·3); magnesium trisilicate (p.1272·3).
*Diarrhoea.*

**Chemists Own Diarrhoea Relief** *Herron, Austral.*
Loperamide hydrochloride (p.1271·1).
*Diarrhoea.*

**Chemists Own Difenacol** *Herron, Austral.*
Ammonium chloride (p.1115·2); diphenhydramine hydrochloride (p.431·3); menthol (p.1711·3); sodium citrate (p.1223·2).
*Coughs.*

**Chemists Own Dry Cough** *Herron, Austral.*
Codeine phosphate (p.27·1); pseudoephedrine hydrochloride (p.1129·2).
*Coughs; nasal congestion.*

**Chemists Own Dry Raspy Cough** *Herron, Austral.*
Chlorphenamine maleate (p.427·3); pseudoephedrine hydrochloride (p.1129·2); dextromethorphan hydrobromide (p.1117·3).
Formerly known as Chemists Own Dexolix.
*Coughs and cold symptoms.*

**Chemists Own Expectalix** *Herron, Austral.*
Ammonium chloride (p.1115·2); codeine phosphate (p.27·1); guaifenesin (p.1122·1); phenylephrine hydrochloride (p.1126·3); pseudoephedrine hydrochloride (p.1129·2).
*Coughs; nasal congestion.*

**Chemists Own Hayfever Sinus Relief** *Herron, Austral.*
Chlorphenamine maleate (p.427·3); pseudoephedrine hydrochloride (p.1129·2); paracetamol (p.76·2).
Formerly known as Chemists Own Allergy Hayfever Sinus Relief.
*Hay fever; nasal and sinus congestion.*

**Chemists Own Junior Cough & Cold** *Herron, Austral.*
Chlorphenamine maleate (p.427·3); dextromethorphan hydrobromide (p.1117·3); pseudoephedrine hydrochloride (p.1129·2).
*Cold symptoms; coughs.*

**Chemists Own Kiddicol** *Herron, Austral.*
Ammonium chloride (p.1115·2); chlorphenamine maleate (p.427·3); phenylephrine hydrochloride (p.1126·3); pholcodine (p.1128·3).
*Coughs; nasal congestion.*

**Chemists Own Natural Laxative with Softener** *Herron, Austral.*
Docusate sodium (p.1262·2); senna leaf (p.1288·2); sennosides (p.1288·2).
*Constipation.*

**Chemists Own Pain** *Herron, Austral.*
Paracetamol (p.76·2); codeine phosphate (p.27·1).
*Pain.*

**Chemists Own Pain & Fever** *Chemists Own, Austral.*
Paracetamol (p.76·2).
*Fever; pain.*

**Chemists Own Peetalix** *Herron, Austral.*
Alimemazine tartrate (p.423·3).

**Chemists Own Period Pain Tablets** *Herron, Austral.*
Naproxen sodium (p.65·1).
*Dysmenorrhoea.*

**Chemists Own Phescode** *Hunter, Austral.†.*
Codeine phosphate (p.27·1); pseudoephedrine hydrochloride (p.1129·2).
*Coughs and cold symptoms.*

**Chemists Own Sinus Relief** *Herron, Austral.*
Pseudoephedrine hydrochloride (p.1129·2).
*Nasal congestion.*

**Chemists Own Sinus-Pain Relief** *Herron, Austral.*
Paracetamol (p.76·2); pseudoephedrine hydrochloride (p.1129·2).
*Nasal congestion; sinusitis.*

**Chemists Own Ultra Sun** *Hunter, Austral.†.*
*SPF 30+:* Octinoxate (p.1154·3); oxybenzone (p.1154·3); octocrilene (p.1154·3); zinc oxide (p.1163·2).
*Sunscreen.*

**Chemists Own Zapazole** *Hunter, Austral.†.*
Miconazole (p.405·2).
*Fungal skin infections.*

**Chemisulide** *Iasis, Gr.*
Nimesulide (p.67·1).
*Inflammation; musculoskeletal disorders; pain.*

**Chemitrim**
*Biomedica, Hong Kong; Biomedica, Ital.*
Co-trimoxazole (p.199·3).
*Bacterial infections.*

**Chemix**
*YSP, Malaysia; Yung Shin, Singapore.*
Co-trimoxazole (p.199·3).
*Bacterial infections; Pneumocystis carinii pneumonia.*

**Chemopent** *Diffucap, Braz.*
Pentoxifylline (p.979·3).

**Chemoprim**
*Biolab, Hong Kong; Biolab, Singapore; Biolab, Thai.*
Co-trimoxazole (p.199·3).
*Bacterial infections.*

**Chemotrim** *Rosemont, UK†.*
Co-trimoxazole (p.199·3).
*Bacterial infections.*

**Chemstrip 6** *Boehringer Mannheim, USA.*
Test for glucose, protein, blood, ketones, leukocytes, and pH in urine.

**Chemstrip 7** *Boehringer Mannheim, USA.*
Test for glucose, protein, blood, ketones, bilirubin, leukocytes, and pH in urine.

**Chemstrip 8** *Boehringer Mannheim, USA.*
Test for glucose, protein, blood, ketones, bilirubin, urobilinogen, leukocytes, and pH in urine.

**Chemstrip 9** *Boehringer Mannheim, USA.*
Test for glucose, protein, blood, ketones, bilirubin, urobilinogen, nitrite, leukocytes, and pH in urine.

**Chemstrip bG**
*Boehringer Mannheim, Canad.†; Boehringer Mannheim Diagnostics, USA.*
Test for glucose in blood (p.1694·2).

**Chemstrip 2 GP** *Boehringer Mannheim, USA.*
Test for glucose and protein in urine.

**Chemstrip K**
*Roche Diagnostics, Canad.; Boehringer Mannheim, USA.*
Test for ketones in urine.

**Chemstrip 2 LN** *Boehringer Mannheim, USA.*
Test for nitrite and leukocytes in urine.

**Chemstrip Micral** *Boehringer Mannheim, USA.*
Test for albumin in urine.

**Chemstrip 4 the OB** *Boehringer Mannheim, USA.*
Test for glucose, protein, blood, and leukocytes in urine.

**Chemstrip 10 with SG** *Boehringer Mannheim, USA.*
Test for nitrite, pH, protein, glucose, ketones, urobilinogen, bilirubin, blood, leucocytes, and specific gravity in urine.

**Chemstrip uG**
*Roche Diagnostics, Canad.; Boehringer Mannheim, USA.*
Test for glucose in urine (p.1694·2).

**Chemstrip uG 5000K** *Roche Diagnostics, Canad.*
Test for glucose and ketones in urine.

**Chemstrip uGK** *Boehringer Mannheim, USA.*
Test for glucose and ketones in urine.

**Chemstrip uG/K** *Roche Diagnostics, Canad.*
Test for glucose and ketones in urine.

**Chemydur** *Sovereign, UK.*
Isosorbide mononitrate (p.942·1).
*Angina pectoris.*

**Chemyparin** *SIT, Ital.†.*
Heparin sodium (p.928·1).
*Eye disorders.*

**Chendol** *CP Pharmaceuticals, Irl.†.*
Chenodeoxycholic acid (p.1670·1).
*Cholesterol gallstones.*

**Chenofalk**
*Merck, Austria; Codali, Belg.; Falk, Ger.; Falk, Hong Kong; Antigen, Irl.†; Farmasa, Mex.; Tramedico, Neth.; Phardi, Switz.†.*
Chenodeoxycholic acid (p.1670·1).
*Cholesterol gallstones.*

**Chephapyrin N** *MIP, Ger.*
Aspirin (p.15·1); paracetamol (p.76·2); caffeine (p.782·1).
*Cold symptoms; fever; pain.*

**Cheracap** *Pharmacia, Braz.†.*
Chlorphenamine (p.428·1); aspirin (p.15·1); caffeine (p.782·1); methoxyphenamine (p.1124·2).
*Cold and influenza symptoms.*

**Cheracap S** *Pharmacia, Braz.*
Chlorphenamine maleate (p.427·3); aspirin (p.15·1); caffeine (p.782·1).
*Cold and influenza symptoms.*

**Cheracol**
*Note. This name is used for preparations of different composition.*
*Shire, Canad.*
Codeine phosphate (p.27·1); guaifenesin (p.1122·1); ammonium chloride (p.1115·2).
*Coughs.*

*Pharmacia, Chile; Pharmacia Upjohn, Mex.*
Aspirin (p.15·1); caffeine (p.782·1); chlorphenamine maleate (p.427·3); methoxyphenamine hydrochloride (p.1124·2).
*Cold and influenza symptoms.*

**Cheracol Cough** *Roberts, USA.*
Codeine phosphate (p.27·1); guaifenesin (p.1122·1).
*Coughs.*

**Cheracol D** *Pharmacia Upjohn, Mex.*
Dextromethorphan hydrobromide (p.1117·3); guaifenesin (p.1122·1).
*Coughs.*

**Cheracol D Cough** *Roberts, USA.*
Dextromethorphan hydrobromide (p.1117·3); guaifenesin (p.1122·1).
*Coughs.*

**Cheracol Nasal** *Roberts, USA†.*
Oxymetazoline hydrochloride (p.1126·1).

**Cheracol Plus** *Lee, USA.*
Dextromethorphan hydrobromide (p.1117·3); guaifenesin (p.1122·1).
Formerly contained phenylpropanolamine hydrochloride, chlorphenamine maleate, and dextromethorphan hydrobromide.
*Coughs and cold symptoms.*

**Cheracol Sore Throat** *Roberts, USA.*
Phenol (p.1188·1).
*Sore throat.*

**Cheripex** *Ranbaxy, Thai.†.*
Diphenhydramine hydrochloride (p.431·3); sodium citrate (p.1223·2); ammonium chloride (p.1115·2); menthol (p.1711·3).
*Cough and cold symptoms.*

**Chest Cold Relief** *Brauer, Austral.†.*
Homoeopathic preparation.
Formerly known as Chest Cold Complex.

**Chest Mixture** *Potter's, UK.*
Horehound (p.1124·1); pleurisy root (p.1733·1); senega (p.1130·2); lobelia (p.1589·1); acetum scillae (p.1130·3).
*Catarrh; coughs.*

**Chest Rub** *Mentholatum, Canad.†.*
Camphor (p.1665·3); eucalyptus oil (p.1686·2); menthol (p.1711·3).
Formerly known as Cherry Chest Rub.

**Chesty Cough Relief** *Herbal Concepts, UK.*
Senega (p.1130·2); catechu (p.1668·3); liquorice (p.1270·2); tolu (p.1131·3); coltsfoot (p.1117·2).
*Coughs.*

**Chetofen** *Pulitzer, Ital.*
Ketotifen fumarate (p.788·1).
*Asthma; bronchitis; hay fever.*

**Chetotest** *SPA, Ital.†.*
Test for acetone in urine.

**Chew-E**
*Eagle, Austral.†.*
*d*-Alpha tocoferil acid succinate (p.1465·1).
*Vitamin E supplement.*

*Ranbaxy, Thai.†.*
*dl*-Alpha tocoferil acetate (p.1465·1).
*Vitamin E deficiency.*

**Chewette C** *Hovid, Malaysia.*
Ascorbic acid (p.1460·2).
*Vitamin C supplement.*

**Chewies** *Malayan, Hong Kong†.*
Vitamin C (p.1460·2).
*Vitamin C deficiency; vitamin C supplement.*

**Chewy C** *Be-Tabs, S.Afr.*
Ascorbic acid (p.1460·2).
*Vitamin C supplement.*

**Chiana** *Bio-Diät, Ger.*
Peppermint oil (p.1283·2).
*Irritable bowel syndrome.*

**Chibretico** *Chibret, Port.*
Amiloride hydrochloride (p.858·2); hydrochlorothiazide (p.933·2).
*Hypertension; oedema.*

**Chibro Uvelina** *Merck Sharp & Dohme, Spain†.*
Methylhydroxyquinoline metilsulfate (p.1714·2).
*Eye irritation.*

**Chibro-Amuno 3** *Chibret, Ger.†.*
Indometacin (p.47·3).
*Macular oedema following cataract surgery.*

**Chibro-Atropine** *Merck Sharp & Dohme-Chibret, Fr.†.*
Atropine sulfate (p.477·1).
*Eye disorders; production of cycloplegia.*

**Chibro-Boraline** *Merck Sharp & Dohme, Switz.†.*
Oxedrine tartrate (p.977·3); borax (p.1661·3); boric acid (p.1662·1).
*Eye irritation.*

**Chibro-Cadron**
*Merck Sharp & Dohme-Chibret, Fr.; Chibret, Ger.†.*
Dexamethasone sodium phosphate (p.1097·2); neomycin sulfate (p.235·1).
*Eye disorders.*

**Chibro-Kerakain** *Chibret, Ger.†.*
Proxymetacaine hydrochloride (p.1384·1).
*Local anaesthesia.*

**Chibro-Pilocarpine** *Merck Sharp & Dohme-Chibret, Fr.†.*
Pilocarpine nitrate (p.1495·1).
*Glaucoma; reversal of mydriasis.*

**Chibro-Proscar** *Merck Sharp & Dohme-Chibret, Fr.*
Finasteride (p.1554·2).
*Benign prostatic hyperplasia.*

**Chibro-Timoptol** *Chibret, Ger.*
Timolol maleate (p.1012·2).
*Glaucoma; ocular hypertension.*

**Chibroxin**
*Merck Sharp & Dohme, Arg.; Merck Sharp & Dohme, Braz.; Merck Sharp & Dohme, Chile; Chibret, Ger.; Merck Sharp & Dohme, Hong Kong†; Merck Sharp & Dohme, Israel; Merck Sharp & Dohme, Malaysia; Merck Sharp & Dohme, Singapore; Merck Sharp & Dohme, Spain; Merck, USA†.*
Norfloxacin (p.238·3).
*Bacterial eye infections.*

**Chibroxine** *Merck Sharp & Dohme-Chibret, Fr.*
Norfloxacin (p.238·3).
*Eye infections.*

**Chibroxol**
*Merck Sharp & Dohme, Belg.; Merck Sharp & Dohme, Neth.; Chibret, Port.†; Merck Sharp & Dohme, Switz.*
Norfloxacin (p.238·3).
*Bacterial eye infections.*

**Chiclida** *Torrens, Spain.*
Meclozine hydrochloride (p.436·3).
*Motion sickness.*

**Chicovit Pharmaton** *Boehringer Ingelheim, Chile.*
Lysine hydrochloride; calcium; phosphorus; vitamins (p.1417·1).
*Tonic.*

**Chiggerex** *Scherer, USA.*
Benzocaine (p.1370·3); camphor (p.1665·3); menthol (p.1711·3).
*Skin disorders.*

**Chigger-Tox** *Scherer, USA.*
Benzocaine (p.1370·3).
*Local anaesthesia.*

**Chilblain Formula** *Vitaplex, Austral.†.*
Nicotinamide (p.1441·2); acetomenaphthone (p.1466·3).
*Chilblains; poor peripheral circulation.*

**Chilblains Cream** *Nelson, UK.*
Homoeopathic preparation.

**Child Chesty Cough** *Numark, UK.*
Diphenhydramine (p.431·3).
*Coughs.*

**Child Chew C** *Bullivants, Austral.†.*
Calcium ascorbate (p.1460·2); bioflavonoids (p.1688·2).
*Vitamin C supplement.*

**Child Formula** *Avon, Canad.*
Multivitamin and mineral preparation (p.1417·1).

**Childrens Advil Cold** *Whitehall-Robins, USA.*
Pseudoephedrine hydrochloride (p.1129·2); ibuprofen (p.45·3).
*Upper respiratory-tract disorders.*

**Children's Allerest** *Ciba, USA†.*
Phenylpropanolamine hydrochloride (p.1127·3); chlorphenamine maleate (p.427·3).
*Upper respiratory-tract symptoms.*

**Children's Allergy Formula** *Stanley, Canad.*
Diphenhydramine hydrochloride (p.431·3).

**Childrens Appetite Tonic** *Bullivants, Austral.†.*
Lysine hydrochloride; ferric pyrophosphate; vitamin B substances (p.1417·1).
*Loss of appetite; tonic.*

**Children's Calcium With Minerals** *Cenovis, Austral.†; Vitelle, Austral.†.*
Calcium ascorbate (p.1460·2); colecalciferol (p.1461·3); ferrous fumarate (p.1427·3); folic acid (p.1429·1); zinc amino acid chelate (p.1469·3).
*Dietary supplement.*

**Childrens Cepacol** *JB Williams, USA.*
Paracetamol (p.76·2); pseudoephedrine hydrochloride (p.1129·2).
*Upper respiratory-tract disorders.*

**Childrens Cherry Sucrets** *SmithKline Beecham, Israel.*
Dyclonine hydrochloride (p.1376·2).
*Sore throat.*

**Childrens Chewable**
*Adams, Canad.; DC Labs, Canad.; Hall, Canad.; Jamieson, Canad.; Novopharm, Canad.; Quest, Canad.; Stanley, Canad.*
Multivitamin preparations with or without minerals (p.1417·1).

*Quest, UK†.*
Multivitamin and mineral preparation (p.1417·1).

**Childrens Chewable Vita-Mins** *Seroyal, Canad.†.*
Multivitamin and mineral preparation (p.1417·1).

**Childrens Chewables** *Sisu, Canad.*
Multivitamin and mineral preparation (p.1417·1).

**Children's Choice** *Swiss Herbal, Canad.*
Multivitamin preparation with or without iron (p.1417·1).

**Childrens Coltalin with Vit $B_1$** *Fortune, Hong Kong.*
Paracetamol (p.76·2); chlorphenamine maleate (p.427·3); phenylephrine hydrochloride (p.1126·3); vitamin $B_1$ (p.1455·2).
*Respiratory-tract disorders.*

**Childrens Diarrhoea Mixture** *Unichem, UK.*
Kaolin (p.1268·3).
*Diarrhoea.*

**Childrens Dynafed Jr** *BDI, USA.*
Paracetamol (p.76·2).
*Fever; pain.*

**Childrens Feverhalt** *Wampole, Canad.*
Paracetamol (p.76·2).
*Fever; pain.*

**Children's Formula Cough** *Pharmakon, USA.*
Dextromethorphan hydrobromide (p.1117·3); guaifenesin (p.1122·1).
*Coughs.*

**Children's Kaopectate** *Pharmacia, USA.*
Bismuth salicylate (p.1252·1).
Formerly contained attapulgite.
*Diarrhoea.*

**Childrens Mapap** *Major, USA.*
Paracetamol (p.76·2).
*Fever; pain.*

**Childrens Motion Sickness Liquid** *Tanta, Canad.*
Dimenhydrinate (p.431·1).

**Childrens Motrin Cold** *McNeil Consumer, USA.*
Ibuprofen (p.45·3); pseudoephedrine hydrochloride (p.1129·2).
*Cold and influenza symptoms.*

**Childrens Multi** *Vitaplex, Austral.†.*
Multivitamin and mineral preparation with lysine hydrochloride (p.1417·1).

**Children's Multivitamins** *Cenovis, Austral.†; Vitelle, Austral.†.*
Multivitamin and mineral preparation (p.1417·1).

**Children's Nostril** *Ciba, USA.*
Phenylephrine hydrochloride (p.1126·3).
*Nasal congestion.*

**Childrens Nyquil** *Procter & Gamble, Canad.*
Pseudoephedrine hydrochloride (p.1129·2); chlorphenamine maleate (p.427·3); dextromethorphan hydrobromide (p.1117·3).
*Coughs and cold symptoms.*

**Childrens Panadol** *SmithKline Beecham Consumer, Austral.†.*
Paracetamol (p.76·2).
*Fever; pain.*

**Childrens Panadol Cold & Flu** *GlaxoSmithKline, Singapore.*
Pseudoephedrine hydrochloride (p.1129·2); chlorphenamine maleate (p.427·3); paracetamol (p.76·2).
*Cold and influenza symptoms.*

**Childrens Panadol Cold Relief Elixir** *GlaxoSmithKline Consumer, Austral.*
Paracetamol (p.76·2); pseudoephedrine hydrochloride (p.1129·2); chlorphenamine maleate (p.427·3).
Formerly known as Panadol Childrens Cold.
*Cold symptoms; fever; nasal congestion; pain.*

**Childrens Panadol Drops for Infants** *GlaxoSmithKline, Singapore.*
Paracetamol (p.76·2).
*Fever; pain.*

**Childrens Sudafed Cold & Cough** *Warner-Lambert, USA.*
Pseudoephedrine hydrochloride (p.1129·2); dextromethorphan hydrobromide (p.1117·3).
*Coughs and cold symptoms.*

**Childrens Sudafed Nasal Decongestant** *Warner-Lambert, USA.*
Pseudoephedrine hydrochloride (p.1129·2).
*Nasal congestion.*

**Children's SunKist Multivitamins Complete** *Ciba, USA.*
Multivitamin and mineral preparation (p.1417·1).

**Children's SunKist Multivitamins + Extra C** *Ciba, USA.*
Multivitamin preparation (p.1417·1).

**Children's SunKist Multivitamins + Iron** *Ciba, USA†.*
Multivitamin preparation with iron (p.1417·1).

**Children's Tylenol** *Johnson & Johnson, Hong Kong.*
Paracetamol (p.76·2).
*Fever; pain.*

**Children's Tylenol Cold Multi-Symptom** *McNeil Consumer, USA.*
Pseudoephedrine hydrochloride (p.1129·2); chlorphenamine maleate (p.427·3); paracetamol (p.76·2).
*Upper respiratory-tract symptoms.*

**Children's Tylenol Cold Multi-Symptom Plus Cough** *McNeil Consumer, USA.*
Paracetamol (p.76·2); dextromethorphan hydrobromide (p.1117·3); chlorphenamine maleate (p.427·3); pseudoephedrine hydrochloride (p.1129·2).
*Coughs and cold symptoms.*

**Children's Tylenol Cold Plus Cough** *Johnson & Johnson, Hong Kong.*
Paracetamol (p.76·2); chlorphenamine maleate (p.427·3); dextromethorphan hydrobromide (p.1117·3); pseudoephedrine hydrochloride (p.1129·2).
*Upper respiratory-tract disorders.*

**Childrevit** *Diviser Aquilea, Spain.*
Cyproheptadine hydrochloride (p.430·1); amino acids and vitamins (p.1417·1).
*Tonic.*

**Chilvax** *Proel, Gr.*
Carbocisteine (p.1116·2).
*Respiratory disorders associated with viscous mucus.*

**Chimar** *Menarini, Port.*
Chymotrypsin (p.1671·2); trypsin (p.1758·3).
*Adjunct to antibiotics; inflammation; oedema; respiratory-tract congestion.*

**Chimax** *Chiron, UK.*
Flutamide (p.556·2).
*Prostatic cancer.*

**Chimodil** *Yamanouchi, Ital.*
Aluminium hydroxide (p.1249·2); magnesium hydroxide (p.1272·2).
*Dyspepsia.*

**Chimono** *Lusofarmaco, Ital.*
Lomefloxacin hydrochloride (p.227·2).
*Bacterial infections.*

**China Diarrhea L107** *Homeocan, Canad.*
Homoeopathic preparation.

**China Eisenwein** *Ungar, Austria†.*
Ferrous citrate (p.1436·1); tinct. cinchona comp (p.1671·3).
*Iron deficiency; tonic.*

**China Med Complex** *Dynamit, Austria.*
Homoeopathic preparation.

**China-Balsam**
*Note. This name is used for preparations of different composition.*
*Sanomed, Austria.*
Camphor (p.1665·3); clove oil (p.1673·3); menthol (p.1711·3).
*Musculoskeletal and joint disorders; neuralgia; respiratory-tract disorders.*

*Bio-Diat, Ger.*
Camphor (p.1665·3); clove oil (p.1673·3); eucalyptus oil (p.1686·2); Norway spruce oil; menthol (p.1711·3).
*Catarrh; fatigue; headache; musculoskeletal and joint disorders; toothache.*

**Chinacin-T** *Chinta, Thai.*
Clindamycin (p.194·2).
*Acne.*

**China-Eisenwein** *Mayrhofer, Austria.*
Mace flowers (p.1708·2); gentian (p.1692·2); bitter-orange peel (p.1723·3); centaury (p.1669·2); ceratonia (p.1579·1); cinchona bark (p.1671·3); cinnamon (p.1672·2); ferrous citrate (p.1436·1); ferrous ascorbate (p.1427·3).
*Tonic.*

**China-Homaccord** *Peithner, Austria.*
Homoeopathic preparation.

**China-Oel** *Bio-Diat, Ger.*
Peppermint oil (p.1283·2).
*Cold symptoms; neuromuscular pain; smooth muscle spasm.*

**China-Ol** *Sanomed, Austria.*
Peppermint oil (p.1283·2).
*Gastrointestinal disorders; musculoskeletal pain; respiratory-tract disorders.*

**Chinclonac** *Chinta, Thai.*
Diclofenac diethylamine (p.32·1).
*Musculoskeletal, joint, and peri-articular disorders.*

**Chingazol** *Chinta, Thai.*
Clotrimazole (p.396·2).
*Fungal skin infections; trichomoniasis; vaginal candidiasis.*

**Chinoidina** *Giovanardi, Ital.*
Cinchona calisaya (p.1671·3); gentian (p.1692·2); kola (p.1765·3).
*Dyspepsia.*

**Chinosol** *Chinosolfabrik, Ger.*
Hydroxyquinoline sulfate (p.1700·1); potassium sulfate (p.1232·2).
*Skin disinfection.*

**Chinosol S Vaseline** *Chinosolfabrik, Ger.†.*
Hydroxyquinoline sulfate (p.1700·1); potassium sulfate (p.1232·2).
*Infective skin disorders.*

**Chinta** *Chinta, Thai.†.*
Dextromethorphan hydrobromide (p.1117·3); ammonium chloride (p.1115·2); calcium pantothenate (p.1442·3); liquorice (p.1270·2).
*Coughs.*

**Chintaral** *Chinta, Thai.*
Ketoconazole (p.403·3).
*Scalp disorders.*

**Chinteina** *Lafare, Ital.*
Quinidine sulfate (p.991·3).
*Arrhythmias.*

**Chirocaine**
*Abbott, Austral.; Abbott, Austria; Abbott, Belg.; Abbott, Braz.†; Abbott, Fin.; Abbott, Gr.; Abbott, Irl.; Abbott, Ital.; Abbott, Neth.; Abbott, NZ; Abbott, Swed.; Abbott, UK; Purdue Frederick, USA.*
Levobupivacaine hydrochloride (p.1377·1).
*Local anaesthesia.*

**Chiroflu**
*Esteve, Port.; Esteve, Spain.*
An inactivated influenza vaccine (subunits) (p.1620·2).
*Active immunisation.*

**Chirofossat N** *Dreluso, Ger.*
Homoeopathic preparation.

**Chiromas** *Esteve, Spain.*
An influenza vaccine (p.1620·2).
*Active immunisation.*

**Chiron Barrier Cream** *Portex, UK.*
Aluminium chlorohydrate (p.1142·1).

**Chironair Odour Control Liquid** *Portex, UK.*
A deodorant for use with colostomies and ileostomies.

**Chiroplexan H** *Pflüger, Ger.*
Homoeopathic preparation.

**Chitodine** *IMS, Ital.*
Iodine (p.1598·1).
*Skin and wound disinfection.*

**Chito-Lafarmen** *Lafarmen, Arg.*
Poliglusam.
*Obesity.*

**Chiton** *INTES, Ital.*
Vitamin B substances; methionine; copper; zinc; omega-3 and omega-6 marine triglycerides (p.1417·1).
*Nutritional supplement.*

**Chitosan C** *YSP, Malaysia.*
Vitamin C (p.1460·2); poliglusam.
*Nutritional supplement.*

**Chitosano** *SIRC, Singapore.*
Poliglusam; hydroxycitric acid; chromium; vitamin C; guar gum; zinc sulfate; ferrous gluconate; vanadium pentoxide (p.1417·1).
*Dietary aid in weight reduction.*

**Chlo-Amine** *Hollister-Stier, USA.*
Chlorphenamine maleate (p.427·3).
*Hypersensitivity reactions.*

**Chlobax** *Beacons, Singapore.*
Chlordiazepoxide (p.674·2); clidinium bromide (p.480·2).
*Gastrointestinal disorders.*

**Chloment** *Denk, Hong Kong.*
Chloramphenicol (p.185·1).
*Eye infections.*

**Chlomide** *Malayan, Singapore.*
Chlorpropamide (p.330·3).
*Diabetes insipidus; diabetes mellitus.*

**Chlomy-P** *Sankyo, Hong Kong.*
Chloramphenicol (p.185·1); neomycin sulfate (p.235·1); prednisolone (p.1108·1).
*Infected skin disorders.*

**Chlor-3** *Fleming, USA.*
Sodium chloride (p.1233·3); potassium chloride (p.1232·2); magnesium chloride (p.1228·1).
*Medical condiment; table salt substitute.*

**Chloracil** *Siam Bheasach, Thai.*
Chloramphenicol (p.185·1).
*Bacterial eye or ear infections.*

**Chloractil** *DDSA Pharmaceuticals, UK†.*
Chlorpromazine hydrochloride (p.675·2).
*Anxiety; intractable hiccup; premedication; psychoses; vomiting.*

**Chloraethyl "Dr Henning"** *Henning Walldorf, Ger.*
Ethyl chloride (p.1376·2).
*Local anaesthesia.*

**Chlorafed** *Roberts, USA.*
Chlorphenamine maleate (p.427·3); pseudoephedrine hydrochloride (p.1129·2).
*Cold symptoms.*

**Chloraldurat**
*Sanova, Austria†; Pohl, Ger.; Pohl, Switz.*
Cloral hydrate (p.684·1).
*Insomnia; sedative.*

**Chloram-D**
*Note. This name is used for preparations of different composition.*
*Duopharma, Hong Kong.*
Chloramphenicol (p.185·1); dexamethasone sodium phosphate (p.1097·2).
*Eye inflammation with bacterial infection.*

*Nakornpatana, Thai.†.*
Chloramphenicol palmitate (p.185·1).
*Bacterial infections.*

**Chloramex** *Aspen, S.Afr.*
Chloramphenicol (p.185·1).
*Bacterial eye infections.*

**Chloramine** *Upha, Malaysia.*
Chlorphenamine maleate (p.427·3).
*Hypersensitivity reactions.*

**Chloraminophene** *Techni-Pharma, Mon.*
Chlorambucil (p.536·1).
*Glomerulonephritis; leukaemia; lymphoma.*

**Chlorammonic** *Chiesi, Fr.*
Ammonium chloride (p.1115·2).
*Alkalosis; urinary-tract disorders.*

**Chloramno** *Milano, Thai.*
Chloramphenicol (p.185·1).
*Bacterial infections.*

**Chloramon** *Streuli, Switz.*
Ammonium chloride (p.1115·2).
*Bronchitis; metabolic alkalosis.*

**Chloramsaar N** *Chephasaar, Ger.*
Chloramphenicol (p.185·1).
*Bacterial infections.*

**Chloranic** *Norma (Νορμα), Gr.*
Chloramphenicol sodium succinate (p.185·1).
*Bacterial infections.*

**Chlorasept** *Baxter, UK†.*
Chlorhexidine acetate (p.1173·2).
*Bladder irrigation; skin disinfection.*

**Chloraseptic Lozenges** *Procter & Gamble, Canad.*
Benzocaine (p.1370·3); menthol (p.1711·3).
*Sore throat and mouth.*

**Chloraseptic Sore Throat Spray** *Procter & Gamble, Canad.*
Phenol (p.1188·1).

**Chloraseptine** *Pharmacobel, Belg.*
Tosylchloramide sodium (p.1194·3).
*Disinfection; water purification.*

**Chlorasol**
*Seton, Israel; SSL, UK.*
Sodium hypochlorite (p.1192·1).
*Cleansing of skin ulcers; skin disinfection.*

**Chlorazin** *Streuli, Switz.*
Chlorpromazine hydrochloride (p.675·2).
*Nausea; pain; pruritus; psychoses; vertigo; vomiting.*

**Chlorazol** *Qualiphar, Belg.*
Tosylchloramide sodium (p.1194·3).
*Disinfection.*

**Chlorcol** *Propan, S.Afr.*
Chloramphenicol (p.185·1).
*Bacterial infections.*

**Chlordex GP** *Cypress, USA.*
Dextromethorphan hydrobromide (p.1117·3); chlorphenamine maleate (p.427·3); phenylephrine hydrochloride (p.1126·3); guaifenesin (p.1122·1).
*Coughs; respiratory-tract congestion.*

**Chlordrine** *Rugby, USA.*
Pseudoephedrine hydrochloride (p.1129·2); chlorphenamine maleate (p.427·3).
*Upper respiratory-tract symptoms.*

**Chloresium** *Rystan, USA.*
Chlorophyllin copper complex (p.1057·1).
*Relief of malodour of wounds and ulcers; wound healing.*

**Chlorestrol** *Pond's, Thai.*
Gemfibrozil (p.923·1).
*Hyperlipidaemias.*

**Chlorethyl** *Adroka, Switz.*
Ethyl chloride (p.1376·2).
*Local anaesthesia.*

**Chlorex-A** *Cypress, USA.*
Phenyltoloxamine citrate (p.439·1); phenylephrine hydrochloride (p.1126·3); chlorphenamine maleate (p.427·3).
*Allergic rhinitis.*

**Chlorformin** *Cadila, India.*
Chlorpropamide (p.330·3); phenformin hydrochloride (p.344·1).
*Diabetes mellitus.*

**Chlorgest** *Ranbaxy, Thai.*
Chlorphenamine maleate (p.427·3); phenylephrine hydrochloride (p.1126·3).
*Nasal congestion.*

**Chlorhex** *Polipharm, Thai.*
Chlorhexidine gluconate (p.1173·2).
*Skin disinfection.*

**Chlorhexamed**
*Block, Austria; GlaxoSmithKline Consumer, Ger.; Stafford-Miller, Switz.*
Chlorhexidine gluconate (p.1173·2).
*Mouth infections; oral hygiene.*

**Chlorhex-C** *Polipharm, Thai.*
Chlorhexidine gluconate (p.1173·2); cetrimide (p.1172·1).
*Disinfection.*

**Chlorhexseptic** *Pharmascience, Canad.†.*
Chlorhexidine gluconate (p.1173·2).
*Disinfection.*

**Chlorhist** *Propan, S.Afr.*
Chlorphenamine maleate (p.427·3).
*Hypersensitivity reactions.*

**Chlorhist Baby Cough** *Sriprasit, Thai.*
Diphenhydramine hydrochloride (p.431·3); ammonium chloride (p.1115·2); sodium citrate (p.1223·2).
*Coughs.*

**Chlorhist Cough** *Sriprasit, Thai.*
Diphenhydramine hydrochloride (p.431·3); ammonium chloride (p.1115·2); sodium citrate (p.1223·2); dextromethorphan hydrobromide (p.1117·3); menthol (p.1711·3).
*Coughs.*

**Chlorhistan** *Hua, Thai.*
Chlorphenamine maleate (p.427·3); phenylephrine hydrochloride (p.1126·3); paracetamol (p.76·2).
*Cold symptoms; nasal congestion.*

**Chlorispray** *Anios, Fr.*
Chlorhexidine gluconate (p.1173·2); formaldehyde (p.1179·3); glutaral (p.1180·3); didecyldimethylammonium chloride (p.1178·3); alcohol (p.1166·1).
*Surface disinfection.*

**Chlorleate** *Silom, Thai.*
Chlorphenamine maleate (p.427·3).
*Hypersensitivity reactions.*

**Chlorleate Expectorant** *Silom, Thai.*
Chlorphenamine maleate (p.427·3); ammonium chloride (p.1115·2); sodium citrate (p.1223·2).
*Coughs; nasal congestion.*

**Chlor-Mes D** *Cypress, USA.*
Phenylephrine hydrochloride (p.1126·3); chlorphenamine maleate (p.427·3); hyoscine methonitrate (p.483·3).
*Respiratory-tract congestion; rhinitis; sinusitis.*

**Chlormixin** *Noir, India.*
Polymyxin B sulfate (p.245·1); chloramphenicol (p.185·1).
*Bacterial eye infections.*

**Chlornamol** *Upha, Malaysia.*
Chlorphenamine maleate (p.427·3); paracetamol (p.76·2).
*Cold and influenza symptoms.*

**Chlornicol** *Genpharm, S.Afr.†.*
Chloramphenicol (p.185·1).
*Bacterial eye infections.*

**Chlorochin** *Streuli, Switz.*
Chloroquine phosphate (p.448·2).
*Lupus erythematosus; malaria; polyarthritis.*

**Chlorocort** *Parke, Davis, Austral.†.*
Chloramphenicol (p.185·1); hydrocortisone acetate (p.1103·3).
*Eye infections.*

**Chlorohex**
*Colgate Oral Care, Austral.†; Asta Medica, Port.†; Colgate-Palmolive, UK.*
Chlorhexidine gluconate (p.1173·2).
*Mouth infections; oral hygiene.*

*Geistlich, Singapore.*
Chlorhexidine (p.1173·2).
*Skin and wound disinfection.*

*Geistlich, Switz.*
Chlorhexidine gluconate (p.1173·2) and/or chlorhexidine hydrochloride (p.1173·3).
*Skin and hand disinfection.*

**Chlorohistol** *Julphar, UAE.*
Chlorphenamine maleate (p.427·3).
*Hypersensitivity.*

**Chloro-Magnesion** *Pautrat, Fr.*
Magnesium chloride (p.1228·1); calcium chloride (p.1225·1).
*Magnesium deficiency.*

**Chloromycetin**
*Parke, Davis, Arg.; Pfizer, Austral.; Pfizer, Canad.; Pfizer, Fin.; Parke, Davis, India; Goldshield, Irl.; Parke, Davis, Ital.†; Warner-Lambert, Mex.; Pfizer, NZ; Pfizer, S.Afr.; Pfizer, Spain; Pfizer, Swed.; Parke, Davis, Switz.†; Forley, UK; Monarch, USA.*
Chloramphenicol (p.185·1), chloramphenicol palmitate (p.185·1), chloramphenicol sodium succinate (p.185·1), or chloramphenicol succinate (p.186·3).
*Bacterial infections.*

**Chloromycetin Ear Drops** *Parke, Davis, India.*
Chloramphenicol (p.185·1); benzocaine (p.1370·3).
*Bacterial ear infections.*

**Chloronguent** *Pharmacobel, Belg.*
Tosylchloramide sodium (p.1194·3).
*Wounds.*

**Chloropect** *Covan, S.Afr.*
Kaolin (p.1268·3); pectin (p.1580·3); bismuth subcarbonate (p.1252·1); chloroform and morphine tincture (p.60·1).
*Diarrhoea.*

**Chloroph**
*Seng, Hong Kong; Seng, Thai.*
Chloramphenicol (p.185·1).
*Bacterial eye infections.*

**Chlorophyl liquid "Schuh"** *Coradol, Ger.*
Chlorophyllin (p.1057·1); crataegus (p.1677·1).
*Asthenia; deodorant.*

**Chlorophyll** *Potter's, UK.*
Kola nut (p.1765·3); chlorophyllin (p.1057·1).
*Tonic.*

**Chlorophyllin Salbe "Schuh"** *Coradol, Ger.*
Chlorophyllin (p.1057·1); chamomilla; arnica; hamamelis (p.1696·3).
*Wounds.*

**Chloropotassuril** *Melisana, Belg.*
Potassium chloride (p.1232·2).
*Potassium depletion.*

**Chloroptic**
*Allergan, Canad.†; Allergan, Irl.†; Allergan, Israel; Allergan, NZ†; Allergan, S.Afr.; Allergan, USA.*
Chloramphenicol (p.185·1).
*Bacterial eye infections.*

**Chlorosin** *General Drugs, Thai.*
Chloramphenicol palmitate (p.185·1).
*Bacterial infections.*

**Chlorotracin** *Chew, Thai.*
Chloramphenicol (p.185·1); clioquinol (p.196·3); phthalylsulfathiazole (p.242·3).
*Gastrointestinal infections.*

**Chlorphed-LA** *Roberts, USA; Hauck, USA.*
Oxymetazoline hydrochloride (p.1126·1).
*Nasal congestion.*

**Chlorphedrine SR** *Goldline, USA.*
Pseudoephedrine hydrochloride (p.1129·2); chlorphenamine maleate (p.427·3).
*Upper respiratory-tract symptoms.*

**Chlorphen** *Caps, S.Afr.*
Chloramphenicol (p.185·1).
*Bacterial infections.*

**Chlorpheno** *Milano, Thai.*
Chlorphenamine maleate (p.427·3).
*Hypersensitivity reactions.*

**Chlor-Pro** *Schein, USA.*
Chlorphenamine maleate (p.427·3).
*Hypersensitivity reactions.*

**Chlorpromanyl** *Technilab, Canad.*
Chlorpromazine hydrochloride (p.675·2).
*Nausea and vomiting; psychoses.*

**Chlorpromasit** *Sriprasit, Thai.*
Chlorpromazine (p.675·1).
*Anxiety; nausea and vomiting; psychoses.*

**Chlorpromed** *Medifive, Thai.*
Chlorpromazine hydrochloride (p.675·2).
*Mania; nausea and vomiting; schizophrenia; sedation.*

**Chlorpyramine** *Atlantic, Malaysia.*
Chlorphenamine maleate (p.427·3).
*Hypersensitivity reactions.*

**Chlorpyrimine**
*Atlantic, Hong Kong; Atlantic, Singapore; Atlantic, Thai.*
Chlorphenamine maleate (p.427·3).
*Hypersensitivity reactions.*

**Chlorquin**
*Aspen, Austral.; Fisons, Hong Kong†.*
Chloroquine phosphate (p.448·2).
*Amoebic hepatitis; lupus erythematosus; malaria; rheumatoid arthritis and related collagen disease.*

**Chlor-Rest** *Rugby, USA†.*
Phenylpropanolamine hydrochloride (p.1127·3); chlorphenamine maleate (p.427·3).
*Upper respiratory-tract symptoms.*

**Chlorsig**
*Sigma, Austral.; Sigma, Hong Kong; Sigma, NZ.*
Chloramphenicol (p.185·1).
*Bacterial eye infections.*

**Chlortralim**
*Atlantic, Hong Kong; Atlantic, Malaysia; Atlantic, Singapore; Atlantic, Thai.*
Chlortetracycline hydrochloride (p.187·3).
*Bacterial eye infections.*

**Chlor-Trimeton**
*Schering-Plough, S.Afr.; Schering-Plough, USA.*
Chlorphenamine maleate (p.427·3).
*Hypersensitivity reactions.*

**Chlor-Trimeton Allergy Sinus** *Schering-Plough, USA†.*
Phenylpropanolamine hydrochloride (p.1127·3); chlorphenamine maleate (p.427·3); paracetamol (p.76·2).
*Upper respiratory-tract symptoms.*

**Chlor-Trimeton 4 Hour Relief** *Schering-Plough, USA.*
Pseudoephedrine sulfate (p.1129·2); chlorphenamine maleate (p.427·3).
*Upper respiratory-tract symptoms.*

**Chlor-Trimeton 12 Hour Relief** *Schering-Plough, USA.*
Pseudoephedrine sulfate (p.1129·2); chlorphenamine maleate (p.427·3).
*Upper respiratory-tract symptoms.*

**Chlor-Tripolon** *Schering, Canad.*
Chlorphenamine maleate (p.427·3).
*Hypersensitivity disorders; pruritus.*

**Chlor-Tripolon Decongestant** *Schering, Canad.*
*Syrup†:* Chlorphenamine maleate (p.427·3); phenylpropanolamine hydrochloride (p.1127·3).
*Tablets:* Chlorphenamine maleate (p.427·3); pseudoephedrine sulfate (p.1129·2).
*Respiratory congestion.*

**Chlor-Tripolon ND** *Schering, Canad.*
Loratadine (p.436·1); pseudoephedrine sulfate (p.1129·2).
*Upper respiratory-tract congestion.*

**Chlorumagene**
*SERP, Mon.; Thepenier, Switz.†.*
Magnesium hydroxide (p.1272·2).
*Constipation.*

**Chlorvescent**
*Aspen, Austral.*
Potassium chloride (p.1232·2); potassium bicarbonate (p.1223·1); potassium carbonate.
*Potassium deficiency.*

*Aventis, NZ.*
Potassium chloride (p.1232·2).
*Potassium supplement.*

**Chlorzide** *Malayan, Singapore.*
Chlorothiazide (p.882·1).
*Hypertension; oedema.*

**Chlorzox** *Pharmasant, Thai.*
Chlorzoxazone (p.1392·3).
*Skeletal muscle pain and spasm.*

**Chlotride**
*Amrad, Austral.†; Merck Sharp & Dohme, Denm.†; Merck Sharp & Dohme, Neth.†.*
Chlorothiazide (p.882·1).
*Hypertension; oedema.*

**Choanol N** *Hanosan, Ger.*
Homoeopathic preparation.

**Chocaton** *Mirren, S.Afr.*
Multivitamin preparation (p.1417·1).

**Chocovite**
*Torbet, Irl.; Torbet Laboratories, UK†.*
Calcium gluconate (p.1225·2); ergocalciferol (p.1462·1).
*Calcium deficiency; vitamin D deficiency.*

**Chofabol** *Allen, Mex.*
Magnesium sulfate (p.1228·2); boldo (p.1661·2); cynara (p.1678·3); belladonna (p.479·1); peptone.
*Biliary-tract disorders.*

**Chofitol** *GlaxoSmithKline, Arg.*
Cynara (p.1678·3).
*Biliary-tract disorders; diuretic; hypercholesterolaemia.*

**Chofranina** *De Mayo, Braz.*
Cascara (p.1255·1); cynara (p.1678·3); carmellose (p.1577·3).
*Constipation.*

**Choice DM**
*Mead Johnson Nutritionals, Canad.; Mead Johnson, Hong Kong†; Mead Johnson, Singapore†; Mead Johnson Nutritionals, Thai.; Mead Johnson Nutritionals, USA.*
Preparation for enteral nutrition (p.1417·1).
*Abnormal glucose tolerance.*

**Chol 4000** *Lichtenstein, Ger.†.*
Greater celandine (p.1695·3).
*Biliary and gastrointestinal spasm.*

**Cholac** *Alra, USA.*
Lactulose (p.1269·1).
*Constipation; hepatic encephalopathy.*

**Cholacid** *Madaus, Ger.†.*
Ursodeoxycholic acid (p.1760·3).
*Biliary-tract disorders.*

**Cholagogum F** *Nattermann, Ger.*
Turmeric (p.1058·3); greater celandine (p.1695·3).
*Biliary-tract disorders.*

**Cholagogum N** *Nattermann, Ger.*
Greater celandine (p.1695·3); turmeric (p.1058·3); peppermint oil (p.1283·2).
*Biliary disorders; gallstones.*

**Cholagutt** *Korangi, Port.*
Greater celandine (p.1695·3); silybum marianum (p.1043·3); peppermint leaf (p.1283·2); lavender (p.1705·1); calamus (p.1664·1); podophyllum (p.1155·2).
*Biliary tract disorders.*

**Cholagutt-N** *Biocur, Ger.*
Greater celandine (p.1695·3); spike lavender (p.1749·2); peppermint leaf (p.1283·2).
*Biliary disorders; gallstones.*

**Cholaktol** *Medopharm, Ger.†.*
Peppermint oil (p.1283·2).
*Gastrointestinal and biliary spasm.*

**Cholal Modificado** *Italmex, Mex.*
Liver antitoxin; sodium sulfate; magnesium sulfate; sodium chloride; potassium nitrate (p.1217·1).
*Biliary-tract disorders; liver disorders.*

**Cholan-HMB** *Ciba Consumer, USA.*
Dehydrocholic acid (p.1679·2).
*Biliary stasis; constipation.*

**Cholapret** *Bionorica, Ger.†.*
Boldo (p.1661·2); greater celandine (p.1695·3); Javanese turmeric (p.1759·3).
*Biliary disorders; gastrointestinal disorders; liver disorders.*

**Chol-Arbuz N** *Bittermedizin, Ger.*
Papain (p.1727·3); pancreatin (p.1725·3); turmeric (p.1058·3).
*Biliary-tract disorders; liver disorders.*

**Cholarist** *Steiner, Ger.*
Greater celandine (p.1695·3).
*Smooth muscle spasm.*

**Cholasitrol** *Lifeplan, UK†.*
Sitosterol (p.982·3); vitamins; minerals (p.1417·1).
*Nutritional supplement.*

**Cholasyn** *Rolmex, Canad.*
Cascara (p.1255·1); senna (p.1288·2).
Formerly contained cascara and phenolphthalein.

**Cholasyn II** *Rolmex, Canad.*
Cascara (p.1255·1); senna (p.1288·2); bile salts (p.1660·3).
Formerly contained cascara and senna.

**Cholax** *Maver, Chile.*
Senna (p.1288·2).
*Constipation.*

**Choldestal** *Krugmann, Ger.*
*Capsules:* Turmeric (p.1058·3).
*Dyspepsia.*

**Chol-Do** *Grasler, Ger.*
Homoeopathic preparation.

**Cholebine** *Mitsubishi, Jpn.*
Colestilan (p.889·2).
*Hypercholesterolaemia.*

**Cholebrin** *Nycomed, Swed.†.*
Iocetamic acid (p.1063·2).
*Contrast medium for cholecystography.*

**Cholebrine** *Viatris, Neth.*
Iocetamic acid (p.1063·2).
*Contrast medium for cholecystography.*

**Cholecis** *Schering, UK.*
Technetium-99m mebrofenin (p.1525·2).
*Assessment of liver function; hepatobiliary imaging.*

**Chole-cyl Ho-Len-Complex** *Liebermann, Ger.*
Homoeopathic preparation.

**Cholecysmon** *Riemser, Ger.*
Ox bile extract (p.1660·3).
*Liver, bile, and pancreas disorders.*

**Choledyl**
*Pfizer, Canad.; Galenica, Gr.; Parke, Davis, Irl.†; Parke, Davis, S.Afr.†; Warner Chilcott, USA.*
Choline theophyllinate (p.784·2).
*Obstructive airways disease.*

**Choledyl Expectorant** *Pfizer, Canad.*
Choline theophyllinate (p.784·2); guaifenesin (p.1122·1).
*Obstructive airways disease.*

**Cholegerol** *Holistica, Fr.*
Soya lecithin (p.1706·1); wheat germ; shiitake; herbs (p.1417·1).
*Cholesterol reduction.*

**Choleodoron**
*Note. This name is used for preparations of different composition.*
*Weleda, Austria.*
Greater celandine (p.1695·3); Javanese turmeric (p.1759·3).
*Liver and gallbladder disorders.*

*Weleda, Fr.; Weleda, Ger.; Weleda, UK.*
Homoeopathic preparation.

**Cholesolvin** *Cyanamid, Ital.†.*
Simfibrate (p.997·1).
*Hyperlipidaemias.*

**Cholestabyl** *Fournier, Ger.*
Colestipol hydrochloride (p.889·2).
*Hypercholesterolaemia.*

**Cholesterol Reducing Plan** *Natural Life, Arg.*
Sitosterol (p.982·3); omega-3 fish oil (p.976·2); ispaghula (p.1268·1); lecithin (p.1706·1); avena (p.1658·2); chromium (p.1425·1); vitamins.
*Hypercholesterolaemia.*

**Cholesterol Support** *Reese, USA.*
Sitosterol (p.982·3); zinc citrate.

**Cholestin** *Pharmanex, USA.*
Policosanol (p.984·2).
Formerly contained *Monascus purpureus* Went.
*Nutritional supplement.*

**Cholest-X L112** *Homeocan, Canad.*
Homoeopathic preparation.

**Choletec** *Squibb Diagnostics, Canad.†.*
Technetium-99m mebrofenin (p.1525·2).
*Hepatobiliary imaging.*

**Cholex** *Silanes, Mex.*
Menthol (p.1711·3); pinene; menthone; borneol; camphene; cineole (p.1672·1).
*Biliary-tract disorders.*

**Chol-Grandelat** *Synpharma, Austria.*
Chamomile (p.1669·3); peppermint oil (p.1283·2); achillea (p.1646·2).
*Gallbladder disorders.*

**Cholhepan** *Doctum, Gr.*
Gemfibrozil (p.923·1).
*Hyperlipidaemias.*

**Cholhepan N** *Schuck, Ger.*
Silybum marianum (p.1043·3); greater celandine (p.1695·3); aloes (p.1248·2).
*Constipation.*

**Choliatron** *Seber, Port.*
Trepibutone (p.1757·2).
*Biliary-tract disorders.*

**Cholidase** *Freeda, USA†.*
Vitamin B substances with vitamin E (p.1417·1).

**Cholinogo** *Pasteur, Chile.*
Peptone magnesium sulfate (p.1228·2).
*Biliary-tract and liver disorders.*

**Cholinoid** *Goldline, USA.*
Vitamin B substances with vitamin C (p.1417·1); lemon bioflavonoids (p.1688·2).

**Cholipin** *Boehringer Ingelheim, Port.†.*
Fenipentol (p.1687·2); octibenzonium bromide.
*Biliary-tract disorders.*

**Cholit-Ursan** *Niddapharm, Ger.*
Ursodeoxycholic acid (p.1760·3).
*Cholesterol gallstones.*

**Chol-Kugeletten Neu** *Dolorgiet, Ger.*
Greater celandine (p.1695·3); aloes (p.1248·2).
*Constipation.*

**Chol-Less** *Rafa, Israel.*
Colestyramine (p.889·3).
*Atherosclerosis; hypercholesterolaemia; myocardial infarction; pruritus in partial biliary obstruction.*

**Cholofalk** *Falk, Ger.*
Ursodeoxycholic acid (p.1760·3).
*Primary biliary cirrhosis.*

**Cholografin**
*Squibb Diagnostics, Canad.†; Squibb Diagnostics, USA.*
Meglumine adipiodone (p.1060·1).
*Contrast medium for biliary-tract radiography.*

**Cholonerton** *Sanova, Austria.*
Hymecromone (p.1700·1).
*Liver and gallbladder disorders.*

**Cholosan** *Spreewald, Ger.†.*
Raphanus sativus var nigra.
*Dyspepsia.*

**Cholosom Phyto N** *Hevert, Ger.*
Greater celandine (p.1695·3); turmeric (p.1058·3).
Cholosom Phyto formerly contained greater celandine, turmeric, and taraxacum.
*Liver and bile disorders.*

**Cholosom SL** *Hevert, Ger.*
Greater celandine (p.1695·3); Javanese turmeric (p.1759·3); taraxacum (p.1751·3).
*Liver and bile disorders.*

**Cholosom-Tee** *Hevert, Ger.*
Caraway (p.1667·2); Javanese turmeric (p.1759·3); taraxacum (p.1751·3); silybum marianum (p.1043·3); peppermint leaf (p.1283·2).
*Biliary-tract disorders; gastrointestinal disorders.*

**Choloxin**
*Knoll, Canad.†; Boots-Flint, USA†.*
Dextrothyroxine sodium (p.893·2).
*Hyperlipidaemias.*

**Cholspasmin** *Merck, Ger.*
Hymecromone (p.1700·1) or hymecromone sodium (p.1700·2).
*Biliary-tract disorders.*

**Cholspasmin Phyto** *Merck, Ger.*
Greater celandine (p.1695·3).
*Biliary and gastrointestinal spasm.*

**Cholspasminase N** *Merck, Ger.*
Pancreatin (p.1725·3).
*Pancreatic disorders.*

**Chol-Spasmoletten** *Dolorgiet, Ger.*
Hymecromone (p.1700·1).
*Biliary disorders.*

**Cholstat**
*Fournier, Belg.†.*
Cerivastatin sodium (p.881·3).
*Hypercholesterolaemia.*

*Fournier, Fr.†.*
Cerivastatin (p.881·3).
*Hypercholesterolaemia.*

**Chol-Truw S** *Truw, Ger.†.*
*Oral drops:* Homoeopathic preparation.
*Tablets:* Javanese turmeric (p.1759·3); greater celandine (p.1695·3); acetic acid (p.1645·2); absinthium (p.1645·1).
*Biliary disorders.*

**Chomelanum**
*Brady, Austria; Schur, Ger.*
Choline stearate.
*Burns; insect stings; skin disorders; soft-tissue disorders; wounds.*

**Chondrosteo** *Equilibre Attitude, Fr.*
Glucosamine sulfate; maltodextrin; chondroitin sulfate; harpagophytum; meadowsweet; black currant; bamboo; minerals (p.1417·1).
*Musculoskeletal and joint disorders; nutritional supplement.*

**Chondrosulf** *Genevrier, Fr.*
Chondroitin sulfate sodium (p.1670·2).
*Coxarthrosis; gonococcal arthritis.*

**Chooz** *Schering-Plough, USA.*
Calcium carbonate (p.1254·2).
*Hyperacidity.*

**Chophytol**
*Millet Roux, Braz.; Rosa-Phytopharma, Fr.; Rosa-Phytopharma, Switz.†.*
Cynara scolymus (p.1678·3).
*Dyspepsia; gastrointestinal disorders; kidney disorders.*

**Choragon**
*Ferring, Braz.†; Ferring, Ger.; Ferring, Irl.†; Ferring, UK.*
Chorionic gonadotrophin (p.1320·3).
*Cryptorchidism; delayed puberty; female infertility; oligospermia.*

**Chorex** *Hyrex, USA.*
Chorionic gonadotrophin (p.1320·3).
*Male and female infertility; male hypogonadism; prepubertal cryptorchidism.*

**Chorigon** *Teva, Israel.*
Chorionic gonadotrophin (p.1320·3).
*Cryptorchidism; female infertility; male hypogonadism.*

**Choriomon**
*IBSA, Hong Kong; IBSA, Switz.*
Chorionic gonadotrophin (p.1320·3).
*Cryptorchidism; delayed puberty; female infertility; male hypogonadism.*

**Choron** *Forest Pharmaceuticals, USA.*
Chorionic gonadotrophin (p.1320·3).
*Male and female infertility; male hypogonadism; prepubertal cryptorchidism.*

**Chributan** *Chrispa (Χρισπα), Gr.*
Butamirate citrate (p.1116·2).
*Cough.*

**Chromagen** *Savage, USA.*
Ferrous fumarate (p.1427·3); cyanocobalamin (p.1458·2); intrinsic factor (stomach preparation).
Ascorbic acid (p.1460·2) is included in this preparation to increase the absorption and availability of iron.
*Anaemias.*

**Chromagen FA** *Savage, USA.*
Ferrous fumarate (p.1427·3); cyanocobalamin (p.1458·2); folic acid (p.1429·1).
Ascorbic acid (p.1460·2) is included in this preparation to increase the absorption and availability of iron.
*Anaemias.*

**Chromagen Forte** *Savage, USA.*
Ferrous fumarate (p.1427·3); cyanocobalamin (p.1458·2); folic acid (p.1429·1).
Ascorbic acid (p.1460·2) is included in this preparation to increase the absorption and availability of iron.
*Anaemias.*

**Chromagen OB** *Savage, USA.*
Multivitamin and mineral preparation (p.1417·1).

**Chroma-Pak** *Smith & Nephew SoloPak, USA.*
Chromium trichloride (p.1425·1).
*Additive for intravenous total parenteral nutrition solutions.*

**Chromargon** *Richard, Fr.*
Hydroxyquinoline sulfate (p.1700·1); acriflavinium chloride (p.1165·3).
*Skin infections.*

**Chrome** *Eagle, Austral.†.*
Chromium amino acid chelate (p.1425·1).
*Dietary supplement.*

**Chromelin Complexion Blender** *Summers, USA.*
Dihydroxyacetone (p.1145·2).
*Hypopigmentation; vitiligo.*

**Chronadalate** *Bayer, Fr.*
Nifedipine (p.966·2).
*Angina pectoris; hypertension.*

**Chronexan** *Asta Medica, Fr.†.*
Xipamide (p.1029·2).
*Hypertension; oedema.*

**Chronocard N** *Cesra, Ger.*
Crataegus (p.1677·1).
*Heart failure.*

**Chronocorte** *Streuli, Switz.*
Dexamethasone (p.1097·1); dexamethasone sodium phosphate (p.1097·2).
*Corticosteroid.*

**Chrono-Indocid** *Merck Sharp & Dohme-Chibret, Fr.*
Indometacin (p.47·3).
*Musculoskeletal and joint disorders.*

**Chronophyllin** *Byk Madaus, S.Afr.*
Theophylline (p.798·3).
*Obstructive airways disease.*

**Chronovera**
*Pharmacia, Austria; Pharmacia, Canad.; Searle, Neth.*
Verapamil hydrochloride (p.1019·1).
*Angina pectoris; hypertension.*

**Chronulac**
*Hoechst Marion Roussel, Canad.†; Hoechst Marion Roussel, USA.*
Lactulose (p.1269·1).
*Constipation.*

**Chrysocor** *Sanum-Kehlbeck, Ger.*
Placenta extracts (human).
*Sexual disorders.*

**Chuker** *Merisant, Arg.*
*Oral liquid:* Saccharin sodium (p.1443·3); sodium cyclamate (p.1426·2).
*Tablets:* Saccharin sodium (p.1443·3); sodium cyclamate (p.1426·2); calcium cyclamate (p.1426·2).
*Sugar substitute.*

**CHX Dental Gel** *Dentsply, Ger.*
Chlorhexidine gluconate (p.1173·2).
*Mouth disorders.*

**Chymex** *Adria, USA†.*
Bentiromide (p.1659·2).
*Diagnosis of pancreatic insufficiency.*

**Chymodiactin**
*Link, Austral.; Knoll, Canad.†; Knoll, Irl.†; Eight, Spain; Knoll, UK†; Boots-Flint, USA†.*
Chymopapain (p.1671·1).
*Herniated lumbar intervertebral disc.*

**Chymodiactine** *Knoll, Fr.†.*
Chymopapain (p.1671·1).
*Herniated lumbar intervertebral disc.*

**Chymol** *Anglian, UK.*
Eucalyptus oil (p.1686·2); terpineol (p.1752·2); methyl salicylate (p.59·3); phenol (p.1188·1).
*Bruises; chapped skin; chilblains; sprains.*

**Ciagen** *Craveri, Arg.*
Thioctic acid (p.1754·3).
*Diabetic neuropathy.*

**Cialis**
*Lilly, Austral.; Lilly, Denm.; Lilly, Fr.; Lilly, Ger.; Lilly, Irl.; Lilly, Port.; Lilly, Swed.; Lilly, UK; Lilly, USA.*
Tadalafil (p.1751·1).
*Erectile dysfunction.*

**Cianomin** *Offenbach, Mex.*
Multivitamin and mineral preparation (p.1417·1).

**Cianon B12** *Ducto, Braz.*
Cyanocobalamin (p.1458·2).

**Cianotrat** *Delta, Braz.*
Vitamin B substances (p.1417·1).

**Cianotrat-Dexa** *Delta, Braz.*
Thiamine hydrochloride (p.1455·1); pyridoxine hydrochloride (p.1456·3); cyanocobalamin (p.1458·2); dexamethasone (p.1097·1) or dexamethasone phosphate (p.1097·2).
Procaine hydrochloride (p.1383·2) is included in the injection to alleviate the pain of injection.
*Neuralgia; neuritis.*

**Ciapar** *Fada, Arg.*
Isoprenaline (p.940·2).

**Ciarbiot** *Vir, Spain†.*
Ampicillin trihydrate (p.157·2).
*Bacterial infections.*

**Ciatyl-Z** *Bayer, Ger.*
Zuclopenthixol acetate (p.730·3), zuclopenthixol decanoate (p.730·3), or zuclopenthixol hydrochloride (p.730·3).
Formerly known as Sedanxol.
*Psychoses.*

**Ciba Vision Cleaner For Sensitive Eyes** *Ciba Vision, USA.*
Cleaning solution for soft contact lenses (p.1164·2).

**Cibacalcin**
*Novartis, Austria; Novartis, Ger.; Novartis, Israel†; Novartis, Ital.†; Novartis, Neth.†; Novartis, Swed.†.*
Calcitonin (human) (p.768·2).
*Hypercalcaemia; osteolysis; osteoporosis; Paget's disease of bone; reflex sympathetic dystrophy.*

**Cibacalcina**
*Novartis, Braz.; Novartis, Port.; Novartis, Spain†.*
Calcitonin (human) (p.768·2).
*Hypercalcaemia; metastatic bone pain; osteoporosis; Paget's disease of bone.*

**Cibacalcine**
*Ciba-Geigy, Belg.†; Novartis, Fr.; Ciba, Switz.†.*
Calcitonin (human) (p.768·2).
*Hypercalcaemia; hyperphosphatasia; osteoporosis; Paget's disease of bone; prevention of bone loss in immobilisation; reflex sympathetic dystrophy.*

**Cibace** *Novartis, S.Afr.*
Benazepril hydrochloride (p.867·2).
*Heart failure; hypertension.*

**Cibacen**
*Novartis, Austria†; Novartis, Belg.; Novartis, Denm.; Novartis, Ger.; Novartis, Gr.; Novartis, Irl.; Novartis, Israel; Novartis, Ital.; Novartis, Neth.; Novartis, NZ†; Novartis, Spain; Novartis, Switz.*
Benazepril hydrochloride (p.867·2).
*Heart failure; hypertension; renal failure.*

**Cibacene** *Novartis, Fr.*
Benazepril hydrochloride (p.867·2).
*Hypertension.*

**Cibadrex**
*Novartis, Austria†; Novartis, Denm.†; Novartis, Fr.; Novartis, Ger.; Novartis, Ital.; Novartis, Neth.; Novartis, S.Afr.; Novartis, Switz.*
Benazepril hydrochloride (p.867·2); hydrochlorothiazide (p.933·2).
*Hypertension.*

**Cibaflam** *Novartis Ophthalmics, Ger.*
Fluorometholone (p.1102·2); gentamicin sulfate (p.217·1).
*Inflammatory eye infections.*

**Cibalena A** *Novartis, Braz.*
Aspirin (p.15·1); paracetamol (p.76·2); caffeine (p.782·1).
*Fever; pain.*

**Cibalgin Compositum N** *Novartis, Ger.*
Propyphenazone (p.85·3); codeine phosphate (p.27·1).
*Pain.*

**Cibalgina Due Fast** *Novartis Consumer, Ital.*
Ibuprofen (p.45·3).
*Fever; influenza symptoms; pain.*

**Cibenol** *Fujisawa, Jpn.*
Cibenzoline succinate (p.883·2).
*Tachyarrhythmias.*

**Cibis** *Siam Bheasach, Thai.*
Chlorphenamine maleate (p.427·3); lidocaine hydrochloride (p.1377·3); hexachlorophene (p.1181·2); methyl salicylate (p.59·3); menthol (p.1711·3); camphor (p.1665·3).
*Dermatitis; eczema; insect bites; pruritus; scalds; wounds.*

**Ciblex** *Drugtech, Chile.*
Mirtazapine (p.307·3).
*Depression.*

**Ciblor** *Inava, Fr.*
Amoxicillin trihydrate (p.155·3); potassium clavulanate (p.193·3).
*Bacterial infections.*

**Cibral** *Ranbaxy, UK.*
Isosorbide mononitrate (p.942·1).
*Angina pectoris.*

**Cibramicina**
*Note. This name is used for preparations of different composition.*
*Cibran, Braz.†.*
Benzylpenicillin potassium (p.163·2); procaine benzylpenicillin (p.246·1).
*Bacterial infections.*

*Cibran, Braz.†.*
Amoxicillin (p.155·3).
*Bacterial infections.*

**Cibronal** *Liferpal, Mex.*
Amoxicillin trihydrate (p.155·3); ambroxol hydrochloride (p.1114·3).
*Respiratory-tract infections.*

**Cica-Care**
*Smith & Nephew, Fr.; Smith & Nephew, Ital.; Smith & Nephew Healthcare, UK.*
Silicone (p.1482·1).
*Hypertrophic and keloid scars.*

**Cicaderma**
*Note. This name is used for preparations of different composition.*
*Boiron, Canad.*
Homoeopathic preparation.

*Boiron, Fr.†; Boiron, Port.*
Calendula (p.1665·2); hypericum perforatum (p.299·1); achillea (p.1646·2); ledum palustre; pulsatilla (p.1737·1).
*Minor burns and wounds.*

**Cicafissan** *Uhlmann-Eyraud, Switz.*
Casein hydrolysate; kaolin (p.1268·3); bismuth subnitrate (p.1252·2); zinc oxide (p.1163·2).
*Burns; skin disorders; wounds.*

**Cicalfate** *Avene, Fr.*
Sucralfate (p.1290·2); copper sulfate (p.1426·1); zinc sulfate (p.1469·3); zinc oxide (p.1163·2).
*Skin irritation; wounds.*

**Cicamosa** *Boots Healthcare, Fr.*
Mimosa tenuiflora.
*Skin disorders.*

**Cicapost** *Isdin, Port.*
Dexpanthenol (p.1727·2); rose oil (p.1740·2); glycerol (p.1694·3); nicotinamide; cravagem asiatica triterpenes; alfa tocoferil acetate; dextran sulfate (p.1679·2).
*Cicatrisation.*

**Cicatral** *Diviser Aquilea, Spain.*
Peru balsam (p.1730·2); ergocalciferol (p.1462·1); estrone (p.1553·1); benzocaine (p.1370·3); vitamin A (p.1451·2); tyrothricin (p.275·1).
*Burns; skin disorders; ulcers; wounds.*

**Cicatrene**
*Note. This name is used for preparations of different composition.*
*Zest, Braz.*
Neomycin sulfate (p.235·1); bacitracin zinc (p.161·3); cysteine; glycine; threonine.
*Skin infections.*

*Warner-Lambert, Ital.*
*Cream; topical powder:* Neomycin sulfate (p.235·1); bacitracin zinc (p.161·3).
*Topical spray:* Polymyxin B sulfate (p.245·1); bacitracin zinc (p.161·3).
*Skin infections.*

**Cicatrex**
*GlaxoSmithKline, Arg.; GlaxoSmithKline, Austria; GlaxoSmithKline, Ger.; Pfizer, Switz.*
Bacitracin zinc (p.161·3); neomycin sulfate (p.235·1); cysteine; glycine; DL-threonine.
*Bacterial skin infections; infected wounds and burns.*

**Cicatrin**
*Pfizer Consumer, Austral.; GlaxoSmithKline, Canad.; Glaxo Wellcome, Irl.; Wellcome, Port.†; GlaxoSmithKline, S.Afr.; GlaxoSmithKline, UK.*
Bacitracin zinc (p.161·3); neomycin sulfate (p.235·1); L-cysteine; glycine DL-threonine.
*Bacterial skin infections; burns; wounds.*

**Cicatrina** *Fada, Arg.*
Zinc (p.1469·2); ichthammol (p.1148·2).
*Skin disorders.*

**Cicatrizan** *Johnson & Johnson, Braz.*
Neomycin sulfate (p.235·1); bacitracin zinc (p.161·3); cysteine; glycine; threonine.
*Skin infections.*

**Cicatrol** *Hexa-Medinova, Arg.*
Zinc undecenoate (p.411·1); zinc oxide (p.1163·2); sodium propionate (p.408·1); salicylic acid (p.1157·1); coal tar (p.1159·2).
*Burns; fungal skin infections; ulcers; wounds.*

**Cicatryl** *UCB, Fr.*
Allantoin (p.1141·3); guaiazulene (p.1696·2); chlorocresol (p.1177·1); alpha tocoferil acetate (p.1465·1).
*Superficial burns and wounds.*

**Cicatul** *ICN, Arg.*
Wheat germ; phenoxyethanol (p.1189·1).
*Wounds.*

**Cicladol**
*Farmalab, Braz.; Master Pharma, Ital.*
Piroxicam betadex (p.84·2).
*Gout; musculoskeletal, joint, and peri-articular disorders; pain.*

**Ciclafast** *Master Pharma, Ital.*
Piroxicam pivalate (p.85·1).
*Musculoskeletal, joint, and peri-articular disorders.*

**Ciclamil**
*Note. This name is used for preparations of different composition.*
*Kampel Martian, Arg.*
Cyproterone (p.1544·3).

*Silesia, Chile.*
Cyclobenzaprine hydrochloride (p.1393·1).
*Musculoskeletal spasm.*

**Ciclavix** *Luper, Braz.*
Aciclovir (p.626·1).

**Ciclidon** *Osteolab, Chile.*
Desogestrel (p.1547·2); ethinylestradiol (p.1553·2).
*Combined oral contraceptive.*

**Ciclinalgin** *IMA, Braz.†.*
Benzydamine hydrochloride (p.21·1).
*Fever; inflammation; pain.*

**Ciclisan** *Sanval, Braz.*
Doxycycline hyclate (p.206·2).
*Bacterial infections.*

**Ciclo** *Uniao Quimica, Braz.*
Ethinylestradiol (p.1553·2); levonorgestrel (p.1563·2).
*Combined oral contraceptive.*

**Ciclobiotico** *Atral, Port.*
*Capsules; oral suspension:* Tetracycline hydrochloride (p.266·2).
*Eye ointment; ointment:* Tetracycline hydrochloride (p.266·2); prednisone (p.1109·3).
*Bacterial infections.*

**Ciclochem** *Novag, Spain.*
Ciclopirox olamine (p.396·1).
*Fungal skin and nail infections; vulvovaginal candidiasis.*

**Ciclocris** *Cristalia, Braz.*
Aciclovir (p.626·1).

**Ciclocur** *Schering, Arg.*
White tablets, estradiol valerate (p.1550·2); coloured tablets, estradiol valerate; levonorgestrel (p.1563·2).
*Menopausal disorders; menstrual disorders.*

**Cicloderm**
*Trima, Israel; Trima, Thai.*
Ciclopirox olamine (p.396·1).
*Fungal skin infections.*

**Cicloderm-C** *Trima, Israel.*
Ciclopirox olamine (p.396·1); clobetasone butyrate (p.1095·3); gentamicin sulfate (p.217·1).
*Infected skin disorders.*

**Ciclofalina** *Almirall, Spain.*
Piracetam (p.1732·1).
*Cortical myoclonia; mental function impairment.*

**Cicloferon** *Liomont, Mex.*
Aciclovir (p.626·1).
*Herpesvirus infections.*

**Ciclohexal** *Hexal, S.Afr.*
Ciclosporin (p.1351·2).
*Graft-versus-host disease; psoriasis; transplant rejection.*

**Ciclolux** *Allergan, Ital.*
Cyclopentolate hydrochloride (p.480·3).
*Production of mydriasis and cycloplegia.*

**Ciclomestril** *QIF, Braz.†.*
Ethinylestradiol (p.1553·2); levonorgestrel (p.1563·2).
*Combined oral contraceptive.*

**Ciclomex** *Gynopharm, Chile.*
Gestodene (p.1556·1); ethinylestradiol (p.1553·2).
28-Day packs contain 24 active tablets and 4 inert tablets.
*Combined oral contraceptive.*

**Ciclon** *Haller, Braz.*
Levonorgestrel (p.1563·2); ethinylestradiol (p.1553·2).
*Combined oral contraceptive.*

**Ciclopenal** *Alcon, Arg.*
Cyclopentolate hydrochloride (p.480·3).
*Production of mydriasis and cycloplegia.*

**Cicloplant** *Knoll, Mex.*
Agnus castus (p.1649·1).
*Menstrual disorders.*

**Ciclople** *Llorens, Spain†.*
Cyclopentolate hydrochloride (p.480·3).
*Eye disorders; production of mydriasis.*

**Cicloplegicedol** *Edol, Port.*
Cyclopentolate hydrochloride (p.480·3).
*Production of mydriasis.*

**Cicloplegico** *Allergan, Braz.*
Cyclopentolate hydrochloride (p.480·3).
*Production of mydriasis and cycloplegia.*

**Cicloplejic** *Novartis, Spain†.*
Cyclopentolate hydrochloride (p.480·3).
*Production of mydriasis; uveitis.*

**Cicloplejico** *Alcon Cusi, Spain; Llorens, Spain.*
Cyclopentolate hydrochloride (p.480·3).
*Production of mydriasis; uveitis.*

**Cicloprimogyna** *Schering, Braz.*
White tablets, estradiol valerate (p.1550·2); red tablets, estradiol valerate; levonorgestrel (p.1563·2).
*Menopausal disorders.*

**Ciclor** *Galen, Mex.†.*
Aciclovir (p.626·1).

**Cicloral** *Hexal, Ger.*
Ciclosporin (p.1351·2).
*Atopic eczema; graft-versus-host disease; nephrotic syndrome; psoriasis; rheumatoid arthritis; transplant rejection; uveitis.*

**Ciclosmida** *Eurofarma, Braz.†.*
Cyclophosphamide (p.540·2).
*Malignant neoplasms.*

**Ciclospasmol** *Yamanouchi, Ital.*
Cyclandelate (p.890·3).
*Cerebral and peripheral vascular disorders.*

**Ciclotal** *Lemery, Mex.*
Medroxyprogesterone acetate (p.1557·2).
*Malignant neoplasms; progestogen-only contraceptive.*

**Ciclotetryl** *Fortbenton, Arg.*
Tetracycline (p.266·2).
*Bacterial infections.*

**Ciclotos** *Lafi, Chile.*
Codeine phosphate (p.27·1); ammonium chloride (p.1115·2).
*Coughs.*

**Ciclotran** *Beta, Arg.*
Raloxifene hydrochloride (p.1568·3).
*Osteoporosis.*

**Cicloven** *AGIPS, Ital.*
Pyricarbate (p.1737·1).
*Vascular disorders.*

**Cicloviral** *Medinfar, Port.*
Aciclovir (p.626·1) or aciclovir sodium (p.626·1).
*Herpesvirus infections.*

**Ciclovular** *Biolab Sanus, Braz.†.*
Estradiol enantate (p.1550·1); algestone (p.1541·3).
*Injectable contraceptive.*

**Ciclovulon** *Sanval, Braz.*
Ethinylestradiol (p.1553·2); norethisterone (p.1562·2).
*Combined oral contraceptive.*

**Cicloxal** *Prodes, Spain†.*
Cyclophosphamide (p.540·2).
*Malignant neoplasms.*

**Cicnor** *Sanofi Synthelabo, Port.*
Algestone acetophenide (p.1541·3); estradiol enantate (p.1550·1).

**Ciconazol** *Cimed, Braz.*
Miconazole (p.405·2).
*Fungal infections.*

**Cidalin** *Agis, Israel.*
Mebhydrolin napadisilate (p.436·3).
*Hypersensitivity reactions.*

**Cidegol C** *Hofmann & Sommer, Ger.*
Chlorhexidine gluconate (p.1173·2).
*Mouth and throat disorders.*

**Cideox** *Alpharma, Mex.†.*
Oxolamine (p.1126·1).

**Cidermex**
*Note. This name is used for preparations of different composition.*
*Panalab, Arg.*
Pantothenic acid (p.1442·3).
*Scalp disorders.*
*Celltech, Fr.*
Triamcinolone acetonide (p.1110·2); neomycin sulfate (p.235·1).
*Skin and eye disorders.*

**Cidetox** *Offenbach, Mex.*
Aluminium (p.1652·2); magnesium (p.1227·3); dimeticone (p.1289·2).
*Gastrointestinal hyperacidity.*

**Cidex**
*Johnson & Johnson Medical, Fr.; Johnson & Johnson, Ger.; Ethicon, Ital.†; Johnson & Johnson Medical, UK†; Johnson & Johnson Medical, USA.*
Glutaral (p.1180·3).
*Instrument disinfection.*

**Cidex OPA**
*Johnson & Johnson, Fr.; Advanced Sterilization Products, USA.*
*o*-Phthaldialdehyde (p.1189·3).
*Instrument disinfection.*

**Cidezyme** *Johnson & Johnson, Fr.*
Proteolytic enzymes.
*Instrument disinfection.*

**Cidilin** *Errekappa, Ital.*
Citicoline sodium (p.1672·3).
*Cerebrovascular disorders; parkinsonism.*

**Cidine**
*Note. This name is used for preparations of different composition.*
*Almirall, Spain.*
Cinitapride acid tartrate (p.1259·2).
*Gastro-oesophageal reflux; gastroparesis.*
*Medifive, Thai.*
Cimetidine (p.1255·3).
*Peptic ulcer; Zollinger-Ellison syndrome.*

**Cidomel** *Clonmel, Irl.*
Indometacin (p.47·3).
*Gout; musculoskeletal, joint, and peri-articular disorders.*

**Cidomycin**
*Hoechst Marion Roussel, Canad.†; Aventis, Irl.; Aventis, Israel; Aventis, S.Afr.†; Aventis, UK; Beacon, UK.*
Gentamicin sulfate (p.217·1).
*Bacterial infections.*

**Cidoten** *Schering-Plough, Chile.*
Betamethasone (p.1093·1) or betamethasone sodium phosphate (p.1093·1).
*Corticosteroid.*

**Cidoten V** *Schering-Plough, Chile.*
Betamethasone valerate (p.1093·2).
*Skin disorders.*

**Cidoten Rapilento** *Schering-Plough, Chile.*
Betamethasone sodium phosphate (p.1093·1); betamethasone acetate (p.1093·1).
Lidocaine (p.1377·3) is included in some injections to alleviate the pain of injection.
*Corticosteroid.*

**Cidrin** *Abbott, Chile.*
Metamfetamine hydrochloride (p.1589·2).
*Attention-deficit hyperactivity disorder.*

**Ciella** *Cooperation Pharmaceutique, Fr.*
Salicylic acid (p.1157·1).
Formerly contained chlorobutanol and zinc sulfate.
*Eye disorders.*

**Cif Candioli** *Papaellinas (Παπαελληνας), Gr.*
Tetramethrin (p.1510·2); phenothrin (p.1509·1).
*Head, body, and crab lice.*

**Cifespasmo** *Northia, Arg.*
Hyoscine (p.483·3).
*Muscle spasm.*

**Cifespasmo Compuesto** *Northia, Arg.*
Hyoscine (p.483·3); dipyrone (p.35·3).
*Muscle spasm; pain.*

**Ciflan** *Azevedos, Port.*
Ciprofloxacin hydrochloride (p.188·2).
*Bacterial infections.*

**Cifloc** *Triomed, S.Afr.*
Ciprofloxacin (p.188·2).
*Bacterial infections.*

**Ciflogex** *Cimed, Braz.*
Benzydamine hydrochloride (p.21·1).
*Fever; inflammation; pain.*

**Ciflolan** *Olan-Kemed, Thai.*
Ciprofloxacin (p.188·2).
*Bacterial infections.*

**Ciflox**
*Note. This name is used for preparations of different composition.*
*Medley, Braz.; Bayer, Fr.*
Ciprofloxacin (p.188·2) or ciprofloxacin hydrochloride (p.188·2).
*Bacterial infections.*
*Alcon, Denm.*
Ciprofloxacin hydrochloride (p.188·2); hydrocortisone (p.1103·3).
*Infected ear disorders.*

**Cifloxin**
*Lafi, Chile.*
Ciprofloxacin (p.188·2).
*Bacterial infections.*
*Siam Bheasach, Thai.*
Ciprofloxacin hydrochloride (p.188·2) or ciprofloxacin lactate (p.188·3).
*Bacterial infections.*

**Cifloxtron** *Ariston, Braz.*
Ciprofloxacin (p.188·2).
*Bacterial infections.*

**Cifran**
*Ranbaxy, India; Ranbaxy, Thai.*
Ciprofloxacin hydrochloride (p.188·2) or ciprofloxacin lactate (p.188·3).
*Bacterial infections.*
*Ranbaxy, S.Afr.*
Ciprofloxacin (p.188·2).
*Bacterial infections.*

**Cifrantil** *Heralds, Braz.†.*
Erythromycin (p.208·1); muramidase (p.1717·2).
*Bacterial infections.*

**Cigamet** *General Drugs, Thai.*
Cimetidine (p.1255·3).
*Gastric hyperacidity; peptic ulcer.*

**Ciganclor** *Richmond, Arg.*
Ganciclovir (p.635·3).
*Viral infections.*

**Cig-Ridettes** *Or-Dov, Austral.†.*
Lobeline hydrochloride (p.1589·1).
*Aid to smoking withdrawal.*

**Cikavit** *Knop, Chile.*
Zinc oxide (p.1163·2); cod-liver oil (p.1425·2).
*Skin irritation; wounds.*

**CIL** *Lichtenstein, Ger.*
Fenofibrate (p.915·2).
*Hyperlipidaemias.*

**Cilab** *Biolab, Thai.*
Ciprofloxacin (p.188·2).
*Bacterial infections.*

**Cilamin** *Panacea, India.*
Penicillamine (p.1046·3).
*Cystinuria; rheumatoid arthritis; Wilson's disease.*

**Cilamox** *Sigma, Austral.*
Amoxicillin trihydrate (p.155·3).
*Bacterial infections.*

**Cilatron** *Quesada, Arg.*
Isosorbide mononitrate (p.942·1).
*Angina pectoris.*

**Cilaxoral** *Ferring, Swed.*
Sodium picosulfate (p.1289·3).
*Constipation.*

**Cilclar** *Novartis Ophthalmics, Braz.*
Preparation for eye cleansing.

**Cildox** *Novartis, Spain†.*
Doxycycline hyclate (p.206·2).
*Bacterial infections; malaria.*

**Cilergil** *Janssen-Cilag, Braz.†.*
Astemizole (p.424·2).
*Hypersensitivity reactions.*

**Cilest**
*Janssen-Cilag, Arg.; Janssen-Cilag, Belg.; Janssen-Cilag, Denm.; Janssen-Cilag, Fin.; Janssen-Cilag, Fr.; Janssen-Cilag, Ger.; Janssen-Cilag, Irl.; Cilag, Mex.; Janssen-Cilag, Neth.; Janssen-Cilag, S.Afr.; Janssen-Cilag, Swed.; Janssen-Cilag, Switz.; Janssen-Cilag, UK.*
Norgestimate (p.1563·2); ethinylestradiol (p.1553·2).
*Combined oral contraceptive.*

**Cileste** *Janssen-Cilag, Austria.*
Norgestimate (p.1563·2); ethinylestradiol (p.1553·2).
*Combined oral contraceptive.*

**Cilestoderme** *Schering-Plough, Port.*
Betamethasone valerate (p.1093·2).
*Skin disorders.*

**Cilex** *Douglas, Austral.*
Cefalexin (p.168·1).
*Bacterial infections.*

**Cilfer-12-F** *Duphar-Interfran, Thai.†.*
Colloidal iron (p.1434·3); vitamin $B_{12}$ (p.1458·2); folic acid (p.1429·1).
*Anaemias.*

**Cilferon-A** *Janssen-Cilag, Ital.*
Interferon alfa (p.640·3).
*Anogenital warts; hepatitis; malignant neoplasms.*

**Ciliar** *Crinos, Ital.†.*
Timonacic methyl hydrochloride (p.1756·3).
*Respiratory-tract disorders associated with viscous mucus.*

**Cilicaine** *Sigma, NZ.*
Procaine benzylpenicillin (p.246·1).
*Bacterial infections.*

**Cilicaine V** *Fawns & McAllan, Austral.*
Benzathine phenoxymethylpenicillin (p.163·2).
*Bacterial infections.*

**Cilicaine Syringe** *Sigma, Austral.*
Procaine benzylpenicillin (p.246·1).
*Bacterial infections.*

**Cilicaine VK**
*Fawns & McAllan, Austral; Sigma, NZ.*
Phenoxymethylpenicillin potassium (p.242·1).
*Bacterial infections.*

**Cilinafosal** *Medical, Spain.*
Ephedrine hydrochloride (p.1120·1); sulfanilamide sodium mesilate (p.263·3).
*Nasal congestion and infection.*

**Cilinafosal DHD Estrep** *Medical, Spain.*
Dihydrostreptomycin sulfate (p.205·3); ephedrine hydrochloride (p.1120·1); sulfanilamide sodium mesilate (p.263·3).
*Nasal congestion and infection.*

**Cilinafosal Hidrocort** *Medical, Spain.*
Ephedrine hydrochloride (p.1120·1); hydrocortisone acetate (p.1103·3); neomycin sulfate (p.235·1); sulfanilamide sodium mesilate (p.263·3).
*Nasal congestion and infection.*

**Cilinafosal Neomicina** *Medical, Spain†.*
Ephedrine hydrochloride (p.1120·1); neomycin sulfate (p.235·1).
*Nasal congestion and infection.*

**Cilinase** *Dovalle, Braz.*
Ciclacillin (p.188·1).
*Bacterial infections.*

**Cilinavagin Neomicina** *Medical, Spain†.*
Diethylstilbestrol dipropionate (p.1548·1); neomycin sulfate (p.235·1); sulfanilamide sodium mesilate (p.263·3); zinc sulfate (p.1469·3).
*Vulvovaginal infections.*

**Cilinon** *Ariston, Braz.*
Ampicillin (p.157·1).

**Cilipen** *Elofar, Braz.*
Ampicillin (p.157·1).
*Bacterial infections.*

**Cillimicina** *Normon, Spain.*
Lincomycin hydrochloride (p.226·2).
*Bacterial infections.*

**Cilodex** *Alcon, Braz.*
Ciprofloxacin hydrochloride (p.188·2); dexamethasone (p.1097·1).
*Infected eye disorders.*

**Cilopen VK** *Douglas, Austral.*
Phenoxymethylpenicillin potassium (p.242·1).
*Bacterial infections.*

**Ciloprin**
*Janssen-Cilag, Denm.†; Janssen-Cilag, Swed.†.*
Acediasulfone sodium (p.153·3); oxymethurea (p.1187·2).
*Ear infections.*

**Ciloprin cum Anaesthetico**
*Janssen-Cilag, Austria; Janssen-Cilag, Fin.*
Acediasulfone (p.153·3); cinchocaine (p.1373·2); oxymethurea (p.1187·2).
*Ear disorders.*

**Ciloprine ca** *Janssen-Cilag, Switz.*
Acediasulfone sodium (p.153·3); cinchocaine (p.1373·2); oxymethurea (p.1187·2).
*Otitis.*

**Ciloquin** *Ioquin, Austral.*
Ciprofloxacin hydrochloride (p.188·2).
*Bacterial eye infections.*

**Cilox** *Alcon, Norw.*
Ciprofloxacin hydrochloride (p.188·2).
*Bacterial keratitis.*

**Ciloxacin** *Alcon, Chile.*
Ciprofloxacin hydrochloride (p.188·2).
*Bacterial eye infections.*

**Ciloxan**
*Alcon, Arg.; Alcon, Austral.; Alcon, Austria; Alcon, Belg.; Alcon, Braz.; Alcon, Canad.; Alcon, Denm.; Alcon, Fr.; Alcon, Ger.; Alkon (Αλκον), Gr.; Alcon, Hong Kong; Alcon, Israel; Alcon, Malaysia; Alcon, Mex.; Alcon, NZ; Alcon, S.Afr.; Alcon, Singapore; Alcon, Swed.; Alcon, Switz.; Alcon, Thai.; Alcon, UK; Alcon, USA.*
Ciprofloxacin hydrochloride (p.188·2).
*Bacterial ear infections; bacterial eye infections.*

**Cilpen** *Antibioticos, Mex.*
Dicloxacillin sodium (p.205·2).
*Bacterial infections.*

**Cilpier** *Pierrel, Ital.*
Piperacillin sodium (p.243·1).
Lidocaine hydrochloride (p.1377·3) is included in this preparation to alleviate the pain of injection.
*Bacterial infections.*

**Cilroton** *Janssen-Cilag, Gr.*
Domperidone (p.1263·2).
*Acid aspiration; aid in diagnostic procedures; delayed gastric emptying; gastro-oesophageal reflux disease; nausea and vomiting.*

**Cim** *Decomed, Port.*
Cimetidine (p.1255·3).
*Gastric hyperacidity; gastro-oesophageal reflux; gastrointestinal haemorrhage; peptic ulcer; Zollinger-Ellison syndrome.*

**Cimaas** *Cimed, Braz.*
Aspirin (p.15·1).
*Fever; inflammaion; pain.*

**Cimag** *TP, Thai.†.*
Cimetidine (p.1255·3).
*Gastric hyperacidity; peptic ulcer.*

**Cimagen** *Antigen, Irl.*
Cimetidine (p.1255·3).
*Gastric hyperacidity; peptic ulcer; Zollinger-Ellison syndrome.*

**Cimal**
*Note. This name is used for preparations of different composition.*
*Drugtech, Chile.*
Citalopram hydrobromide (p.289·1).
*Depression.*
*Alpharma, Norw.*
Cimetidine (p.1255·3).
*Aspiration syndrome; gastro-oesophageal reflux; peptic ulcer; Zollinger-Ellison syndrome.*

**Cimascal** *Belmac, Spain.*
Calcium carbonate (p.1254·2).
*Calcium deficiency; osteoporosis.*

**Cimascal D** *Belmac, Spain.*
Calcium carbonate (p.1254·2); colecalciferol (p.1461·3).
*Calcium deficiency; osteoporosis.*

**Cime** *ABZ, Ger.; Eu Rho, Ger.; Alpharma-Isis, Ger.*
Cimetidine (p.1255·3).
*Aspiration syndromes; gastro- oesophageal reflux; gastro-intestinal haemorrhage; peptic ulcer; Zollinger-Ellison syndrome.*

**Cimebec** *Farcoral, Mex.*
Cimetidine (p.1255·3).
*Peptic ulcer.*

**Cimebeta** *Betapharm, Ger.*
Cimetidine (p.1255·3).
*Aspiration syndromes; gastro-oesophageal reflux; gastrointestinal haemorrhage; peptic ulcer; Zollinger-Ellison syndrome.*

**Cimecard** *Cimed, Braz.*
Digoxin (p.895·2).

**Cimecodan** *Pharmacodane, Denm.*
Cimetidine (p.1255·3).
*Acid aspiration; gastro-oesophageal reflux; peptic ulcer; Zollinger-Ellison syndrome.*

**Cimedine** *Dar Al Dawa, Hong Kong.*
Cimetidine (p.1255·3).
*Gastro-oesophageal reflux; peptic ulcer; Zollinger-Ellison syndrome.*

**Cimedul** *Offenbach, Mex.*
Cimetidine (p.1255·3).
*Peptic ulcer.*

**Cimefer** *Cimed, Braz.*
Ferrous sulfate (p.1428·2).
*Iron-deficiency anaemia.*

**Cimegripe** *Cimed, Braz.*
Paracetamol (p.76·2); chlorphenamine (p.428·1); phenylephrine (p.1126·3).
*Unfluenza symptoms.*

**Cimehexal**
*Hexal, Austral.; Hexal, Ger.*
Cimetidine (p.1255·3) or cimetidine hydrochloride (p.1255·3).
*Acid aspiration; gastro-oesophageal reflux; gastrointestinal haemorrhage; peptic ulcer; Zollinger-Ellison syndrome.*

**Cimeldine** *Clonmel, Irl.*
Cimetidine (p.1255·3).
*Gastric hyperacidity; peptic ulcer; Zollinger-Ellison syndrome.*

**Cimelide** *Cimed, Braz.*
Nimesulide (p.67·1).
*Inflammation.*

**Cimelin** *Sanova, Austria.*
Acetylcysteine (p.1112·3).
*Respiratory-tract disorders with viscous mucus.*

**Cimemerck** *Merck, Ger.†.*
Cimetidine (p.1255·3).
*Acid aspiration; gastro-oesophageal reflux; gastrointestinal haemorrhage; peptic ulcer; Zollinger-Ellison syndrome.*

**Cimephil** *Philopharm, Ger.†.*
Cimetidine (p.1255·3).
*Acid aspiration; gastro-oesophageal reflux; peptic ulcer; Zollinger-Ellison syndrome.*

**Cimet** *Thiemann, Ger.*
Cimetidine (p.1255·3).
*Gastro-oesophageal reflux; gastrointestinal haemorrhage; peptic ulcer; Zollinger-Ellison syndrome.*

**Cimeta** *Jean-Marie, Hong Kong.*
Cimetidine (p.1255·3).
*Dyspepsia; peptic ulcer.*

**Cimetag**
GlaxoSmithKline, Austria; Teva, Israel; Julphar, UAE.
Cimetidine (p.1255·3) or cimetidine hydrochloride (p.1255·3).
*Acid aspiration; dyspepsia; gastro-oesophageal reflux; gastrointestinal haemorrhage; pancreatic insufficiency; peptic ulcer; Zollinger-Ellison syndrome.*

**Cimetase** Liomont, Mex.
Cimetidine (p.1255·3).
*Gastro-oesophageal reflux; gastrointestinal haemorrhage; peptic ulcer; Zollinger-Ellison syndrome.*

**Cimetid** Nycomed, Norw.†.
Cimetidine (p.1255·3).
*Acid aspiration; gastro-oesophageal reflux; gastrointestinal haemorrhage; peptic ulcer; Zollinger-Ellison syndrome.*

**Cimetidan** Cimed, Braz.
Cimetidine (p.1255·3).
*Gastro-oesophageal reflux; gastrointestinal haemorrhage; peptic ulcer; Zollinger-Ellison syndrome.*

**Cimetil** Infabra, Braz.†.
Cimetidine (p.1255·3).
*Gastro-oesophageal reflux; gastrointestinal haemorrhage; peptic ulcer; Zollinger-Ellison syndrome.*

**Cimetimax** PMC, Austral.†.
Cimetidine (p.1255·3).
*Gastro-oesophageal reflux; peptic ulcer; scleroderma oesophagus; Zollinger-Ellison syndrome.*

**Cimetin** Cristalia, Braz.
Cimetidine (p.1255·3).
*Acid aspiration; gastro-oesophageal reflux; gastrointestinal haemorrhage; peptic ulcer; Zollinger-Ellison syndrome.*

**Cimetina** Hexal, Braz.
Cimetidine (p.1255·3).
*Peptic ulcer.*

**Cimetinax** Ducto, Braz.
Cimetidine (p.1255·3).
*Peptic ulcer.*

**Cimetine** Sriprasit, Thai.
Cimetidine (p.1255·3).
*Peptic ulcer.*

**Cimetival** Sanval, Braz.
Cimetidine (p.1255·3).
*Peptic ulcer.*

**Cimet-P** PP Lab, Thai.
Cimetidine (p.1255·3).
*Gastric hyperacidity; peptic ulcer.*

**Cimetrin** Cimex, Switz.†.
Erythromycin ethyl succinate (p.208·1) or erythromycin stearate (p.208·2).
*Bacterial infections.*

**Cimex**
Baldacci, Braz.†; Pharmacia Upjohn, Fin.†.
Cimetidine (p.1255·3).
*Gastro-oesophageal reflux; gastrointestinal haemorrhage; peptic ulcer; Zollinger-Ellison syndrome.*

**Cimex Sirop contre la toux** Cimex, Switz.†.
Codeine phosphate (p.27·1); ephedrine hydrochloride (p.1120·1); ipecacuanha (p.1122·3); tolu balsam (p.1131·3); cherry-laurel.
*Coughs.*

**Cimexyl** Sanova, Austria.
Acetylcysteine (p.1112·3).
*Respiratory-tract disorders with viscous mucus.*

**Cimi** Gerard, Israel.
Cimetidine (p.1255·3).
*Gastro-oesophageal reflux; peptic ulcer.*

**Cimicifuga comp** Steigerwald, Ger.
Homoeopathic preparation.
Formerly known as Auroplatin.

**Cimicifuga Med Complex** Dynamit, Austria.
Homoeopathic preparation.

**Cimicifuga Oligoplex** Madaus, Ger.
Homoeopathic preparation.

**Cimidine** Berlin Pharm, Thai.
Cimetidine (p.1255·3).
*Gastro-oesophageal reflux; peptic ulcer; systemic mastocytosis; Zollinger-Ellison syndrome.*

**Cimifemine** Zeller, Switz.
Cimicifuga (p.1671·3).
*Menopausal disorders.*

**Cimipax** IPRAD, Fr.
Cimicifuga (p.1671·3).
*Insomnia; nervous disorders.*

**Cimisan** APS, Ger.
Cimicifuga (p.1671·3).
*Menopausal disorders.*

**CimLich** Lichtenstein, Ger.
Cimetidine (p.1255·3).
*Acid aspiration; gastro-oesophageal reflux; peptic ulcer; Zollinger-Ellison syndrome.*

**Cimlok** Be-Tabs, S.Afr.
Cimetidine (p.1255·3).
*Gastro-oesophageal reflux; peptic ulcer; Zollinger-Ellison syndrome.*

**Cimogal** Galen, Mex.
Ciprofloxacin hydrochloride (p.188·2).
*Bacterial infections.*

**Cimulcer**
Biopharm, Hong Kong; Biolab, Malaysia; Biolab, Singapore; Biolab, Thai.
Cimetidine (p.1255·3).
*Peptic ulcer; Zollinger-Ellison syndrome.*

**Cinabel**
Note. This name is used for preparations of different composition.
Andromaco, Chile.
Ergotamine tartrate (p.467·2); caffeine (p.782·1); dipyrone (p.35·3); chlorphenamine maleate (p.427·3).
*Migraine and other vascular headaches.*

Columbia, Mex.†.
Clotrimazole (p.396·2).

**Cinacris** Elvetium, Arg.
Cinnarizine (p.428·3); dihydroergocristine (p.1680·1).
*Cerebrovascular disorders.*

**Cinactiv** Labomed, Chile.
Erythromycin-zinc complex (p.208·1).
*Acne.*

**Cinadine** Garec, S.Afr.
Cimetidine (p.1255·3).
*Gastro-oesophageal reflux; peptic ulcer; upper gastrointestinal haemorrhage; Zollinger-Ellison syndrome.*

**Cinaflan** Brasterapica, Braz.†.
Diclofenac potassium (p.32·1).

**Cinageron** Cibran, Braz.†.
Cinnarizine (p.428·3).
*Peripheral vascular disorders; vestibular disorders.*

**Cinalong** Fujirebio, Jpn.
Cilnidipine (p.884·1).
*Hypertension.*

**Cinaran** Cazi, Braz.
Cinnarizine (p.428·3).

**Cinarix** Royton, Braz.
Cinnarizine (p.428·3).

**Cinarizina-Cinarin** Igefarma, Braz.†.
Cinnarizine (p.428·3).
*Peripheral vascular disorders; vertigo.*

**Cinaro Bilina** Semar, Spain†.
Cynara scolymus (p.1678·3); aloes (p.1248·2).
*Constipation; hepatobiliary disorders.*

**Cinaryl** Themis, India.
Chlorphenamine maleate (p.427·3); phenylephrine hydrochloride (p.1126·3); paracetamol (p.76·2).
*Allergic rhinitis; cold symptoms; sinusitis.*

**Cinaziere** Ashbourne, UK.
Cinnarizine (p.428·3).

**Cinazon** Sanval, Braz.
Cinnarizine (p.428·3).

**Cinazyn** Italchimici, Ital.
Cinnarizine (p.428·3).
*Cerebral and peripheral vascular disorders; vestibular disorders.*

**Cincain**
Ophtha, Denm.; Ipex, Swed.
Cinchocaine (p.1373·2).
*Eye disorders.*

**Cinclamina** Laborsil, Braz.†.
Nikethamide (p.1591·2).
*Respiratory depression.*

**Cincofarm**
Lepori, Port.; Farma Lepori, Spain.
Oxitriptan (p.311·1).
*Depression; epilepsy; hepatic coma; myoclonus; parkinsonism; phenylketonuria; schizophrenia; sleep disorders; trigeminal neuralgia.*

**Cinco-Fu** Pharmacia, Arg.
Fluorouracil (p.554·2).
*Malignant neoplasms.*

**Cincopal** Wyeth, Spain†.
Fenbufen (p.39·1).
*Gout; musculoskeletal disorders; pain; peri-articular disorders.*

**Cincordil** Sigma, Braz.
Isosorbide mononitrate (p.942·1).
*Angina pectoris.*

**Cincuental** Schwabe, Arg.
Vincamine (p.1764·2).
*Mental function impairment.*

**Cinergil** Labomed, Chile.
Cinnarizine (p.428·3).
*Mental function impairment; peripheral vascular disorders; vertigo.*

**Cinerine** Pharmasant, Thai.
Cinnarizine (p.428·3).
*Cerebrovascular disorders; motion sickness; peripheral vascular disorders; vestibular disorders.*

**Cinet** Medinfar, Port.
Domperidone (p.1263·2).
*Dyspepsia; nausea; vomiting.*

**Cinetic**
Note. This name is used for preparations of different composition.
Biolab Sanus, Braz.†.
Cisapride (p.1259·2).
*Gastrointestinal motility disorders.*

Teofarma, Ital.
Thyroid (p.1604·2).
*Hypothyroidism.*

**Cinetol** Cristalia, Braz.
Biperiden hydrochloride (p.479·3) or biperiden lactate (p.479·3).
*Parkinsonism.*

**Cinfacromin** Cinfa, Spain.
Merbromin (p.1185·3).
*Skin disinfection.*

**Cinfamar** Cinfa, Spain.
Dimenhydrinate (p.431·1).
*Motion sickness; vertigo.*

**Cinfamar Cafeina** Cinfa, Spain.
Caffeine (p.782·1); dimenhydrinate (p.431·1).
*Motion sickness; vertigo.*

**Cinfatos** Cinfa, Spain.
Dextromethorphan hydrobromide (p.1117·3).
*Cough.*

**Cinfatos Complex** Cinfa, Spain.
Dextromethorphan hydrobromide (p.1117·3); paracetamol (p.76·2); pseudoephedrine hydrochloride (p.1129·2).
*Coughs and cold symptoms.*

**Cinfatos Expectorante** Cinfa, Spain†.
Dextromethorphan hydrobromide (p.1117·3); guaifenesin (p.1122·1).
*Coughs and cold symptoms.*

**Cinfloxine** Progress, Thai.
Ciprofloxacin hydrochloride (p.188·2).
*Bacterial infections.*

**Cinifa** Nakorn, Thai.†.
Rifampicin (p.250·2).
*Gonorrhoea; leprosy; tuberculosis.*

**Cinkef-U** Faulding, Port.
Fluorouracil (p.554·2).

**Cinna**
YSP, Malaysia; Yung Shin, Singapore.
Cinnarizine (p.428·3).
*Motion sickness; peripheral vascular disorders; vestibular disorders.*

**Cinnabene** Ratiopharm, Austria.
Cinnarizine (p.428·3).
*Cerebral and peripheral vascular disease; vestibular disorders.*

**Cinnacet** Sanofi Synthelabo, Ger.†.
Cinnarizine (p.428·3).
*Cerebral and peripheral circulatory disorders; vestibular disorders.*

**Cinnageron** Streuli, Switz.
Cinnarizine (p.428·3).
*Cochlear disorders; motion sickness; vestibular disorders.*

**Cinnamed** Medika, Switz.
Cinnarizine (p.428·3).
*Vestibular disorders.*

**Cinnar**
Atlantic, Singapore; Atlantic, Thai.
Cinnarizine (p.428·3).
*Cerebrovascular disorders; migraine; motion sickness; peripheral vascular disorders; vestibular disorders.*

**Cinnaron**
Remedica, Malaysia; Remedica, Singapore.
Cinnarizine (p.428·3).
*Motion sickness; vestibular disorders.*

**Cinnarplus** Gerot, Austria.
Cinnarizine (p.428·3); etamivan (p.1588·1).
*Cerebral and peripheral vascular disease.*

**Cinnaza** Pharmaland, Thai.
Cinnarizine (p.428·3).
*Cerebrovascular disorders; migraine; peripheral vascular disorders; vestibular disorders.*

**Cinnipirine** Artu, Neth.†.
Cinnarizine (p.428·3).
*Hypersensitivity reactions; motion sickness; vertigo; vestibular disorders.*

**Cinobac**
Lilly, Belg.†; Bruno, Ital.; Lilly, UK†; Oclassen, USA.
Cinoxacin (p.188·1).
*Urinary-tract infections.*

**Cinobactin**
Lilly, Ger.†; Pharmaserve Lilly (Φαρμασερβ Λιλλυ), Gr.; Quatromed, S.Afr.†.
Cinoxacin (p.188·1).
*Urinary-tract infections.*

**Cinocil** Uno, Ital.
Cinoxacin (p.188·1).
*Urinary-tract infections.*

**Cinoflax** Ativus, Braz.
Ciprofloxacin hydrochloride (p.188·2).
*Bacterial infections.*

**Cinon** Azevedos, Port.
Cinnarizine (p.428·3).
*Cerebral and peripheral vascular disorders; vestibular disorders.*

**Cinopal**
Wyeth Lederle, Denm.†; Wyeth Lederle, Fr.†; Cyanamid, Ital.†; Wyeth, S.Afr.†; Wyeth-Ayerst, Thai.
Fenbufen (p.39·1).
*Inflammation; musculoskeletal, joint, and peri-articular disorders; pain.*

**Cinotec** Medipharma, Hong Kong.
Fluocinolone acetonide (p.1101·2).
*Skin disorders.*

**Cinoxen** Ibirn, Ital.
Cinoxacin (p.188·1).
*Urinary-tract infections.*

**Cinquerix** GlaxoSmithKline, Ital.
A diphtheria, tetanus, pertussis, poliomyelitis, and haemophilus influenzae vaccine (p.1615·1).
*Active immunisation.*

**Cinrizine** Medifive, Thai.
Cinnarizine (p.428·3).
*Circulatory disorders; migraine; motion sickness; vestibular disorders.*

**Cintigo** Wallace, India.
Cinnarizine (p.428·3).
*Ménière's disease; tinnitus; vertigo.*

**Cintilan** Medley, Braz.
Piracetam (p.1732·1).
*Alcoholism; behaviour disorders in children; cerebrovascular disorders; senile dementia; vertigo.*

**Cinton** Ariston, Braz.
Cimetidine (p.1255·3).
*Peptic ulcer.*

**Ciocar** Mavi, Mex.
Calcium carbonate (p.1254·2).
*Calcium supplement.*

**Cional** Nycomed, Austria.
Aluminium formate; chamomile (p.1669·3); sage (p.1741·2); arnica (p.1656·3).
*Mouth and throat disorders.*

**Cipadur** Cipla-Medpro, S.Afr.
Cefadroxil (p.167·2).
*Bacterial infections.*

**Cipalat** Cipla-Medpro, S.Afr.
Nifedipine (p.966·2).
*Angina pectoris; hypertension.*

**Cipamox** Cipan, Port.
Amoxicillin sodium (p.155·3) or amoxicillin trihydrate (p.155·3).
*Bacterial infections.*

**Cipanfeno** Cipan, Port.
Ketotifen fumarate (p.788·1).
*Allergic conjunctivitis; allergic rhinitis; allergic skin disorders; asthma.*

**Cipasid** Siam Bheasach, Thai.
Cisapride (p.1259·2).
*Constipation; dyspepsia; gastro-oesophageal reflux; gastroparesis; intestinal pseudo-obstruction.*

**Cipex** Cipla-Medpro, S.Afr.
Mebendazole (p.108·2).
*Worm infections.*

**Cipflocin** Asian Pharm, Thai.
Ciprofloxacin (p.188·2).
*Bacterial infections.*

**Cipide** Merck, Hong Kong.
Ciprofloxacin hydrochloride (p.188·2).
*Bacterial infections.*

**Ciplactin** Cipla, India.
Cyproheptadine hydrochloride (p.430·1).
*Hypersensitivity reactions; migraine.*

**Ciplar** Cipla, India.
Propranolol hydrochloride (p.989·3).
*Angina pectoris; arrhythmias; hypertension.*

**Ciplar-H** Cipla, India.
Propranolol hydrochloride (p.989·3); hydrochlorothiazide (p.933·2).
*Hypertension.*

**Ciplatec** Cipla-Medpro, S.Afr.
Enalapril maleate (p.909·2).
*Heart failure; hypertension.*

**Ciplazin** Prater, Chile.
Hypericum (p.299·1).
*Depression.*

**Ciplin** Cipla, India.
Co-trimoxazole (p.199·3).
*Bacterial infections; Pneumocystis carinii pneumonia.*

**Ciplox**
Cipla, India; Cipan, Port.
Ciprofloxacin (p.188·2), ciprofloxacin hydrochloride (p.188·2), or ciprofloxacin lactate (p.188·3).
*Bacterial infections.*

**Cipobacter** Rubio, Spain.
Ciprofloxacin hydrochloride (p.188·2).
*Bacterial infections.*

**Cipofix** Cipla-Medpro, S.Afr.
Cefuroxime sodium (p.184·1).
*Bacterial infections.*

**Ciprain** Maver, Mex.
Ciprofloxacin (p.188·2).
*Bacterial infections.*

**Cipralan**
Pharmacia, Belg.; Bristol-Myers Squibb, Fr.
*Tablets:* Cibenzoline succinate (p.883·2).
*Arrhythmias.*

Bristol-Myers Squibb, Fr.
*Injection:* Cibenzoline succinate (p.883·2); cibenzoline (p.883·1).
*Arrhythmias.*

**Cipralex**
Lundbeck, Norw.; Lundbeck, UK.
Escitalopram oxalate (p.292·1).
*Depression; panic attacks.*

**Cipram**
Lundbeck, Austria; Lundbeck, Hong Kong; Lundbeck, Malaysia; Lundbeck, Singapore; Lundbeck, Thai.
Citalopram hydrobromide (p.289·1) or citalopram hydrochloride (p.289·1).
*Anxiety; depression; obsessive-compulsive disorder; panic attacks.*

**Cipramil**
Lundbeck, Austral.; Lundbeck, Belg.; Schering-Plough, Braz.; Silesia, Chile; Lundbeck, Denm.; Lundbeck, Fin.; Lundbeck, Ger.; Lundbeck, Irl.; Lundbeck, Israel; Lundbeck, Neth.; Lundbeck, Norw.; Lundbeck, NZ; Zuellig, NZ; Lundbeck, S.Afr.; Lundbeck, Swed.; Lundbeck, UK.
Citalopram hydrobromide (p.289·1) or citalopram hydrochloride (p.289·1).
*Anxiety disorders; depression; obsessive-compulsive disorder; panic attacks.*

**Ciprenit Otico** Vita, Spain.
Ciprofloxacin hydrochloride (p.188·2).
*Otitis externa; otitis media.*

**Ciprex** *Sintofarma, Braz.*†.
Ciprofloxacin hydrochloride (p.188·2).
*Bacterial infections.*

**Cipridanol** *Richmond, Arg.*
Methylprednisolone (p.1106·1).
*Corticosteroid.*

**Cipride** *Biolab, Thai.*
Cisapride (p.1259·2).
*Anorexia nervosa; constipation; dyspepsia; gastro-oesophageal reflux; gastroparesis; intestinal pseudo-obstruction.*

**Cipril**
*Note. This name is used for preparations of different composition.*
*Cipla, India.*
Lisinopril (p.946·3).
*Heart failure; hypertension.*

*Italchimici, Ital.*†.
Cisapride (p.1259·2).
*Gastrointestinal disorders.*

**Cipril-H** *Cipla, India.*
Lisinopril (p.946·3); hydrochlorothiazide (p.933·2).
*Hypertension.*

**Ciprin** *Pharmacia, Switz.*
Ciprofloxacin (p.188·2).
*Bacterial infections.*

**Cipro**
*Bayer, Arg.; Bayer, Braz.; Bayer, Canad.; Bayer, USA.*
Ciprofloxacin (p.188·2), ciprofloxacin hydrochloride (p.188·2), or ciprofloxacin lactate (p.188·3).
*Bacterial infections.*

**Cipro HC**
*Bayer, Arg.; Alcon, Braz.; Alcon, Canad.; Alcon, Hong Kong; Bayer, USA.*
Ciprofloxacin hydrochloride (p.188·2); hydrocortisone (p.1103·3).
*Infected ear disorders.*

**Ciprobac** *Pisa, Mex.*
Ciprofloxacin lactate (p.188·3).
*Bacterial infections.*

**Ciprobay**
*Bayer, Ger.; Bayer, Malaysia; Bayer, S.Afr.; Bayer, Singapore; Bayer, Thai.*
Ciprofloxacin (p.188·2), ciprofloxacin hydrochloride (p.188·2), or ciprofloxacin lactate (p.188·3).
*Bacterial infections.*

**Ciprobay HC**
*Alcon, S.Afr.*
Ciprofloxacin hydrochloride (p.188·2); hydrocortisone (p.1103·3).
*Otitis externa.*

*Alcon, Singapore.*
Ciprofloxacin (p.188·2); hydrocortisone (p.1103·3).
*Infected ear disorders.*

**Ciprobeta** *Betapharm, Ger.*
Ciprofloxacin hydrochloride (p.188·2).
*Bacterial infections.*

**Ciprobid**
*Cadila, India.*
Ciprofloxacin hydrochloride (p.188·2) or ciprofloxacin lactate (p.188·3).
*Bacterial infections.*

*Cadila, Thai.*
Ciprofloxacin (p.188·2).
*Bacterial infections.*

**Ciprobiot** *Hexal, Braz.*
Ciprofloxacin hydrochloride (p.188·2).
*Bacterial infections.*

**Ciprobiotic** *Cryopharma, Mex.*
Ciprofloxacin hydrochloride (p.188·2).
*Bacterial infections.*

**Cipro-Cent** *Centaur, India.*
Ciprofloxacin hydrochloride (p.188·2).
*Bacterial eye infections.*

**Ciprocep** *TO-Chemicals, Thai.*
Ciprofloxacin (p.188·2).
*Bacterial infections.*

**Ciprocin** *Eurofarma, Braz.*†.
Ciprofloxacin (p.188·2).
*Bacterial infections.*

**Ciprocina** *Zeus, Braz.*
Ciprofloxacin (p.188·2).
*Bacterial infections.*

**Ciprocort** *Beta, Arg.*
*Cream; topical spray:* Ketoconazole (p.403·3); hydrocortisone acetate (p.1103·3); gentamicin sulfate (p.217·1).
*Burns; skin disorders.*

*Injection:* Dexamethasone sodium phosphate (p.1097·2); cyproheptadine hydrochloride (p.430·1).
*Hypersensitivity reactions.*

*Pessaries:* Miconazole nitrate (p.405·3); hydrocortisone (p.1103·3); metronidazole (p.607·2).
*Vaginal infections.*

**Ciprocort D** *Beta, Arg.*
Loratadine (p.436·1); pseudoephedrine sulfate (p.1129·2).
*Respiratory-tract disorders.*

**Ciprocort L** *Beta, Arg.*
Loratadine (p.436·1); betamethasone (p.1093·1).
*Hypersensitivity reactions.*

**Ciprodex**
*Saval, Chile; Alcon, USA.*
Ciprofloxacin (p.188·2); dexamethasone (p.1097·1).
*Bacterial eye infections with inflammation; infected ear disorders.*

**Ciprodexol** *Collins, Mex.*
Cyproheptadine (p.430·2); vitamins (p.1417·1).
*Appetite loss.*

**Ciprodine** *Sanval, Braz.*
Ciprofloxacin hydrochloride (p.188·2).
*Bacterial infections.*

**Ciprodura** *Merck dura, Ger.*
Ciprofloxacin hydrochloride (p.188·2).
*Bacterial infections.*

**Ciprofar** *Elofar, Braz.*
Ciprofloxacin hydrochloride (p.188·2).
*Bacterial infections.*

**Ciprofarma** *Varifarma, Arg.*
Cyproterone (p.1544·3).

**Ciprofin** *Utopian, Thai.*
Ciprofloxacin (p.188·2).
*Bacterial infections.*

**Ciproflox**
*Hebron, Braz.*
Ciprofloxacin (p.188·2).
*Bacterial infections.*

*CT, Ger.*
Ciprofloxacin hydrochloride (p.188·2).
*Bacterial infections.*

*Senosiain, Mex.*
Ciprofloxacin hydrochloride (p.188·2) or ciprofloxacin lactate (p.188·3).
*Bacterial infections.*

**Ciprofur** *Fustery, Mex.*
Ciprofloxacin hydrochloride (p.188·2).
*Bacterial infections.*

**Ciprogamma** *Worwag, Ger.*
Ciprofloxacin hydrochloride (p.188·2).
*Bacterial infections.*

**Ciprogen** *General Drugs, Thai.*
Ciprofloxacin (p.188·2).
*Bacterial infections.*

**Ciprogis** *Agis, Israel.*
Ciprofloxacin (p.188·2).
*Bacterial infections.*

**Ciproglen** *Glenmark, Thai.*
Ciprofloxacin (p.188·2).
*Bacterial infections.*

**Ciprohexal** *Hexal, Ger.*
Ciprofloxacin (p.188·2) or ciprofloxacin hydrochloride (p.188·2).
*Bacterial infections.*

**Ciprok** *Sanofi Synthelabo, Spain*†.
Ciprofloxacin hydrochloride (p.188·2).
*Bacterial infections.*

**Ciprol** *Arrow, Austral.*
Ciprofloxacin hydrochloride (p.188·2).
*Bacterial infections.*

**Ciprolet** *Reddy, Thai.*
Ciprofloxacin hydrochloride (p.188·2) or ciprofloxacin lactate (p.188·3).
*Bacterial infections.*

**Cipro-Lich** *Lichtenstein, Ger.*
Ciprofloxacin hydrochloride (p.188·2).
*Bacterial infections.*

**Ciprolisina** *AF, Mex.*
Cyproheptadine hydrochloride (p.430·1); cyanocobalamin (p.1458·2).
*Tonic.*

**Ciprom-H** *M & H, Thai.*
Ciprofloxacin lactate (p.188·3).
*Bacterial infections.*

**Cipromycin** *Medichrom, Gr.*
Ciprofloxacin hydrochloride (p.188·2).
*Bacterial infections.*

**Cipronal** *Cazi, Braz.*
Ciprofloxacin hydrochloride (p.188·2).
*Bacterial infections.*

**Cipro-Otico** *Alcon, Arg.*
Ciprofloxacin hydrochloride (p.188·2).
*Bacterial ear infections.*

**Ciproplex** *Teva Tuteur, Arg.*
Cyproterone (p.1544·3).

**Ciproquinol** *Ferring, Port.*
Ciprofloxacin (p.188·2).
*Bacterial infections.*

**Ciproser** *Serral, Mex.*
Ciprofloxacin (p.188·2).
*Bacterial infections.*

**Ciprospes** *Specifar (Σπεσιφαρ), Gr.*
Ciprofloxacin hydrochloride (p.188·2).
*Bacterial infections.*

**Ciprosun** *Sun, Thai.*
Ciprofloxacin (p.188·2).
*Bacterial infections.*

**Ciprotenk** *Biotenk, Arg.*
Ciprofloxacin hydrochloride (p.188·2) or ciprofloxacin lactate (p.188·3).
*Bacterial infections.*

**Ciproval** *Saval, Chile.*
Ciprofloxacin (p.188·2) or ciprofloxacin hydrochloride (p.188·2).
*Bacterial infections.*

**Ciproviron** *Schering, Chile.*
Cyproterone acetate (p.1544·1).
*Androgen-induced acne, alopecia, hirsutism, or seborrhoea in women; prostatic cancer; sexual deviation in men.*

**Ciprovit Calcio** *Beta, Arg.*
Cyproheptadine hydrochloride (p.430·1); calcium phosphate; cyanocobalamin (p.1417·1).
*Tonic.*

**Ciprovit Energizante** *Beta, Arg.*
Cyproheptadine hydrochloride (p.430·1); vitamins; ginkgo biloba; pyritinol hydrochloride (p.1417·1).
*Tonic.*

**Ciprovit Magnesico** *Beta, Arg.*
Cyproheptadine hydrochloride (p.430·1); vitamins; magnesium chloride (p.1417·1).
*Tonic.*

**Ciprowin** *Alembic, India.*
Ciprofloxacin (p.188·2).
*Bacterial infections.*

**Cipro-Wolff** *Wolff, Ger.*
Ciprofloxacin hydrochloride (p.188·2).
*Bacterial infections.*

**Ciproxan**
*Royton, Braz.; Bayer, Jpn; Pond's, Thai.*
Ciprofloxacin (p.188·2) or ciprofloxacin hydrochloride (p.188·2).
*Bacterial infections.*

**Ciproxil** *Haller, Braz.*
Ciprofloxacin hydrochloride (p.188·2).
*Bacterial infections.*

**Ciproxin**
*Bayer, Austral.; Bayer, Austria; Bayer, Denm.; Bayer, Fin.; Bayer, Gr.; Bayer, Hong Kong; Bayer, Irl.; Bayer, Israel; Bayer, Ital.; Bayer, Neth.; Bayer, Norw.; Bayer, NZ; Bayer, Swed.; Bayer, UK.*
Ciprofloxacin (p.188·2), ciprofloxacin hydrochloride (p.188·2), or ciprofloxacin lactate (p.188·3).
*Bacterial infections.*

**Ciproxin HC**
*Alcon, Austral.; Alcon, Austria; Alcon, Israel; Alcon, NZ; Alcon, Switz.*
Ciprofloxacin hydrochloride (p.188·2); hydrocortisone (p.1103·3).
*Infected ear disorders.*

**Ciproxina**
*Note. This name is used for preparations of different composition.*
*Bayer, Mex.; Bayer, Port.*
Ciprofloxacin hydrochloride (p.188·2) or ciprofloxacin lactate (p.188·3).
*Bacterial infections.*

*Alcon Cusi, Spain.*
Ciprofloxacin hydrochloride (p.188·2); hydrocortisone (p.1103·3).
*Otitis externa.*

**Ciproxine**
*Bayer, Belg.; Bayer, Switz.*
Ciprofloxacin (p.188·2), ciprofloxacin hydrochloride (p.188·2), or ciprofloxacin lactate (p.188·3).
*Bacterial infections.*

**Ciproxin-Hydrocortison** *Alcon, Fin.*
Ciprofloxacin hydrochloride (p.188·2); hydrocortisone (p.1103·3).
*Otitis externa.*

**Ciproxino** *Andromaco, Chile.*
Ciprofloxacin (p.188·2).
*Bacterial infections.*

**Ciproxyl** *Farmaline, Thai.*
Ciprofloxacin hydrochloride (p.188·2).
*Bacterial infections.*

**Ciqfadin** *IQFA, Mex.*
Ciprofloxacin (p.188·2).
*Bacterial infections.*

**Circanetten**
*Eversil, Braz.*†; *Evers, Thai.*
Potassium acid tartrate (p.1284·3); senna (p.1288·2); sulfur (p.1158·2).
*Haemorrhoids; varices.*

**Circanol** *3M, Ger.*
Co-dergocrine mesilate (p.1674·1).
*Hypertension; mental function disorders.*

**Circavite-T** *Circle, USA.*
Multivitamin and mineral preparation with iron (p.1417·1).

**Circo-Maren** *Krewel, Ger.*
Nicergoline (p.1719·3).
*Mental function disorders.*

**Circonyl** *TRB, Arg.*
Quinine sulfate (p.460·2).
*Nocturnal leg cramps.*

**Circonyl N** *Medidom, Switz.*†.
Quinine sulfate (p.460·2).
*Nocturnal leg cramps.*

**Circovenil** *Wyeth, Spain*†.
Buphenine hydrochloride (p.1663·2); aescin (p.1648·2); sodium polygalacturonate sulfonate.
*Peripheral vascular disorders.*

**Circovenil Fuerte** *Wyeth, Spain*†.
Buphenine hydrochloride (p.1663·2); aescin (p.1648·2); esculoside (p.1648·2); hesperidin (p.1688·2).
*Circulatory disorders.*

**Circularine** *Lerads, Fr.*†.
Alpha tocoferil acetate (p.1465·1); troxerutin (p.1688·3); esculoside (p.1648·2).
*Peripheral vascular disorders.*

**Circulation** *Homeocan, Canad.*
Homoeopathic preparation.

**Circulatonic** *Phytomedica, Fr.*
Menthol (p.1711·3); camphor (p.1665·3); cypress oil; equisetum (p.1684·1).
*Circulatory disorders.*

**Circumax** *ISA, Arg.*
Ginkgo biloba; centella; selenium; garlic (p.1417·1).
*Dietary supplement.*

**Circupon**
*Kolassa, Austria; Medichemie, Switz.*†.
Etilefrine hydrochloride (p.914·1).
*Hypotension.*

**Circupon RR** *Gepepharm, Ger.*†.
Etilefrine hydrochloride (p.914·1).
*Hypotension.*

**Circuvit** *Ariston, Arg.*
Warfarin sodium (p.1022·2).
*Thromboembolic disorders.*

**Circuvit E** *Wernigerode, Ger.*
Etilefrine hydrochloride (p.914·1).
*Hypotension.*

**Cirflox-G** *Klonal, Arg.*
Ciprofloxacin (p.188·2).
*Bacterial infections.*

**Ciriax** *Roemmers, Arg.*
Ciprofloxacin (p.188·2).
*Bacterial infections.*

**Ciriax Otic** *Roemmers, Arg.*
Ciprofloxacin hydrochloride (p.188·2); hydrocortisone (p.1103·3).
*Otitis externa.*

**Cirkan** *Sinbio, Fr.*
Ruscus aculeatus; ascorbic acid (p.1460·2); hesperidin methyl chalcone (p.1688·3).
Formerly contained pancreatic enzymes (expressed as chymotrypsin and trypsin activities), ruscosides, ascorbic acid, hesperidin methyl chalcone, and metesculetol sodium.
*Haemorrhoids; venous insufficiency.*

**Cirkan a la Prednacinolone** *Sinbio, Fr.*
Desonide (p.1096·3); lidocaine hydrochloride (p.1377·3); vitamin A palmitate (p.1453·1); ruscosides; tocoferil acetate (p.1465·1); heparin sodium (p.928·1).
*Anorectal disorders.*

**Cirku Sed** *Roha, Hong Kong.*
Valerian (p.1762·2).
*Insomnia.*

**Cirkufemal** *Roha, Ger.*†.
Cimicifuga (p.1671·3).
*Menopausal disorders.*

**Cirkulin Baldrian** *Schulke & Mayr, Austria*†.
Valerian (p.1762·2).
*Sedative.*

**Cirkuprostan** *Roha, Ger.*†.
Urtica root (p.1762·1).
*Prostatic hyperplasia.*

**Cirkused** *Diafarm, Spain.*
Valerian (p.1762·2).
*Insomnia; nervous disorders.*

**Cirrus**
*UCB, Austria; UCB, Belg.; UCB, Fin.; UCB, Hong Kong; UCB, Malaysia; UCB, Singapore.*
Cetirizine hydrochloride (p.427·1); pseudoephedrine hydrochloride (p.1129·2).
*Nasal congestion; rhinitis.*

**Cirulan** *Novag, Mex.*
Metoclopramide (p.1274·3).
*Gastrointestinal motility disorders.*

**Cirulaxia** *Byk, Arg.*
*Chewable tablets:* Sodium picosulfate (p.1289·3).
*Syrup:* Prune (p.1285·1); senna (p.1288·2).
*Constipation.*

**Cisaken** *Kendrick, Mex.*
Cinnarizine (p.428·3).
*Cerebrovascular disorders; motion sickness; vestibular disorders.*

**Cisalone** *Sigma, India.*
Cisapride (p.1259·2).
*Delayed gastric emptying; gastro-oesophageal reflux.*

**Cisap** *Dominguez, Arg.*
Cisapride (p.1259·2).
*Gastro-oesophageal reflux; gastrointestinal motility disorders.*

**Cisapan** *UCI, Braz.*†.
Cisapride (p.1259·2).
*Gastrointestinal motility disorders.*

**Cisapin** *LSP, Thai.*
Cisapride (p.1259·2).
*Gastro-oesophageal reflux; gastroparesis.*

**Cisatec** *Ache, Braz.*†.
Cisapride (p.1259·2).
*Gastrointestinal motility disorders.*

**Cisday** *BASF, Ger.*†.
Nifedipine (p.966·2).
*Angina pectoris.*

**Cis-Gry** *Gry, Ger.*
Cisplatin (p.538·1).
*Malignant neoplasms.*

**Cishexal** *Hexal, Austria.*
Cisplatin (p.538·1).
*Malignant neoplasms.*

**Cisordinol**
*Lundbeck, Austria; Silesia, Chile; Lundbeck, Denm.; Lundbeck, Fin.; Lundbeck, Neth.; Lundbeck, Norw.; Lundbeck, Port.; Solvay, Spain; Lundbeck, Swed.*
Zuclopenthixol acetate (p.730·3), zuclopenthixol decanoate (p.730·3), or zuclopenthixol hydrochloride (p.730·3).
*Psychoses.*

**Cisplatex** *Eurofarma, Braz.*
Cisplatin (p.538·1).
*Malignant neoplasms.*

**Cisplatyl**
*Aventis, Braz.†; Aventis, Fr.; Aventis, Gr.; Rhone-Poulenc Rorer, Israel†.*
Cisplatin (p.538·1).
*Malignant neoplasms.*

**Cispride**
*Klonal, Arg.; Sintofarma, Braz.†.*
Cisapride (p.1259·2).
*Gastrointestinal motility disorders.*

**Cistalgan** *Recordati, Ital.*
Flavoxate hydrochloride (p.482·2); propyphenazone (p.85·3).
*Spasm of the female genital tract; urinary-tract disorders.*

**Cistalgina** *Fortbenton, Arg.*
Phenazopyridine (p.83·2).
*Urinary-tract pain.*

**Cistamine** *LBS, Thai.*
Cetirizine hydrochloride (p.427·1).
*Allergic conjunctivitis; allergic skin disorders; rhinitis.*

**Cisticid**
*Merck, Braz.; Merck, Chile; Merck, Mex.*
Praziquantel (p.112·2).
*Cestode infections; trematode infections.*

**Cistidil** *IDI, Ital.*
L-Cystine (p.1426·3).
*Skin disorders.*

**Cistimax** *Fortbenton, Arg.*
*Lotion:* Methionine; pyridoxine; zinc (p.1417·1).
*Hair loss.*
*Oral solution; tablets:* Vitamin and mineral preparation (p.1417·1).

**Cistobil**
*Bracco, Ital.; Bracco, Switz.†.*
Iopanoic acid (p.1065·1).
*Contrast medium for biliary-tract radiography.*

**Cistofuran** *Crosara, Ital.†.*
Nitrofurantoin (p.237·2).
*Urinary-tract infections.*

**Cistomid** *Uno, Ital.*
Pipemidic acid (p.243·1).
*Urinary-tract infections.*

**Cistopax** *Zimaia, Port.*
Oxolinic acid (p.240·3).
*Urinary-tract infections.*

**Cistoquine Plus** *Casasco, Arg.*
Debutil; simeticone (p.1289·2).
*Biliary-tract disorders; flatulence.*

**Cistosan** *Apsen, Braz.†.*
Pentosan.

**Cistus canadensis Oligoplex** *Madaus, Ger.*
Homoeopathic preparation.

**Citab** *Eurofarma, Braz.*
Cytarabine hydrochloride (p.544·1).
*Malignant neoplasms.*

**Citadura** *Merck dura, Ger.*
Citalopram hydrobromide (p.289·1).
*Depression.*

**Citagenin** *Elvetium, Arg.*
Cytarabine (p.543·1).
*Malignant neoplasms.*

**Cital** *Bichsel, Switz.*
Mannitol (p.950·2); sorbitol (p.1446·3).
*Irrigation solution.*

**Citalgan** *Merck, Mex.*
Ibuprofen (p.45·3).
*Inflammation; musculoskeletal, joint and peri-articular disorders; pain.*

**Citalor** *Pfizer, Braz.*
Atorvastatin (p.866·2).
*Hyperlipidaemias.*

**Citaloxan** *Faulding, Port.*
Cytarabine (p.543·1).

**Citanest**
*Note. This name is used for preparations of different composition.*
*AstraZeneca, Austral.; AstraZeneca, Belg.; Dentsply, Braz.; AstraZeneca, Canad.; AstraZeneca, Fin.†; Astra, Irl.†; AstraZeneca, Neth.; AstraZeneca, NZ; Inibsa, Spain; AstraZeneca, Swed.; AstraZeneca, UK; Dentsply, UK; Astra, USA.*
Prilocaine hydrochloride (p.1382·3).
Adrenaline (p.852·2), adrenaline acid tartrate (p.852·2), or felypressin (p.1324·2) may be included in some injections as a vasoconstrictor to diminish absorption and localise the effect of the local anaesthetic.
*Local anaesthesia.*

*AstraZeneca, Fin.†; AstraZeneca, Norw.†.*
*Gel:* Prilocaine hydrochloride (p.1382·3); chlorhexidine gluconate (p.1173·2).
*Cystitis; cystoscopy; local anaesthesia.*

**Citanest con Octapressin** *Dentsply, Ital.*
Prilocaine hydrochloride (p.1382·3).
Felypressin (p.1324·2) is included in this preparation as a vasoconstrictor to diminish absorption and localise the effect of the local anaesthetic.
*Local anaesthesia.*

**Citanest Dental** *Dentsply, Austral.*
Prilocaine hydrochloride (p.1382·3).
Adrenaline (p.852·2) or felypressin (p.1324·2) is included in some injections as a vasoconstrictor to diminish absorption and localise the effect of the local anaesthetic.
*Local anaesthesia.*

**Citanest Octapresin** *Astra, Mex.*
Prilocaine hydrochloride (p.1382·3).
Felypressin (p.1324·2) is included in this preparation as a vasoconstrictor to diminish absorption and localise the effect of the local anaesthetic.
*Local anaesthesia in dentistry.*

**Citanest Octapressin**
*AstraZeneca, Denm.; Dentsply, Fin.; AstraZeneca, Norw.; Astra, Port.†; Inibsa, Spain; AstraZeneca, Swed.*
Prilocaine hydrochloride (p.1382·3).
Felypressin (p.1324·2) is included in this preparation as a vasoconstrictor to diminish absorption and localise the effect of the local anaesthetic.
*Local anaesthesia.*

**Citanest with Octapressin**
*Astra, Irl.†; AstraZeneca, NZ; Dentsply, UK.*
Prilocaine hydrochloride (p.1382·3).
Felypressin (p.1324·2) is included in this preparation as a vasoconstrictor to diminish absorption and localise the effect of the local anaesthetic.
*Local anaesthesia.*

**Citanest Octapressine** *AstraZeneca, Neth.†.*
Prilocaine hydrochloride (p.1382·3).
Felypressin (p.1324·2) is included in this preparation as a vasoconstrictor to diminish absorption and localise the effect of the local anaesthetic.
*Local anaesthesia.*

**Citavi** *Labocor, Port.*
Ascorbic acid (p.1460·2).
*Tonic.*

**Citavir** *Eurofarma, Braz.†.*
Zalcitabine (p.657·1).
*HIV infection.*

**Citax F** *Biogam, Arg.*
A normal immunoglobulin (p.1627·2).
*Passive immunisation.*

**Citemul S** *Medopharm, Ger.*
Mesulphen (p.1152·1).
*Scabies; skin disorders.*

**Citicef** *CT, Ital.†.*
Cefradine (p.179·3).
*Bacterial infections.*

**Citicil** *CT, Ital.†.*
Ampicillin (p.157·1) or ampicillin sodium (p.157·1).
*Bacterial infections.*

**Citiclor** *CT, Ital.*
Cefaclor (p.167·1).
*Bacterial infections.*

**Citidel** *Del Saz & Filippini, Ital.†.*
Citicoline sodium (p.1672·3).
*Cerebrovascular disorders; parkinsonism.*

**Citidine**
*Atlantic, Hong Kong; Atlantic, Singapore; Atlantic, Thai.*
Cimetidine (p.1255·3).
*Gastro-oesophageal reflux; peptic ulcer; Zollinger-Ellison syndrome.*

**Citifar** *Lafare, Ital.*
Citicoline (p.1672·3).
*Cerebrovascular disorders.*

**Citiflux** *CT, Ital.*
Flunisolide (p.1101·1).
*Asthma.*

**Citilat** *CT, Ital.*
Nifedipine (p.966·2).
*Hypertension; ischaemic heart disease.*

**Citimid** *CT, Ital.†.*
Cimetidine (p.1255·3).
*Gastro-oesophageal reflux; gastrointestinal haemorrhage; peptic ulcer; Zollinger-Ellison syndrome.*

**Citinoides** *Serra Pamies, Spain.*
Lithium carbonate (p.301·1); sodium bicarbonate (p.1223·2); tartaric acid (p.1752·1).
*Dyspepsia; gastrointestinal hyperacidity.*

**Citiolase** *Hoechst Marion Roussel, Ital.†.*
Citiolone (p.1672·3).
*Liver disorders.*

**Cition** *Eurofarmaco, Ital.*
Citicoline sodium (p.1672·3).
*Cerebrovascular disorders; parkinsonism.*

**Citireuma** *CT, Ital.†.*
Sulindac (p.91·2).
*Gout; musculoskeletal, joint, and peri-articular disorders.*

**Citivir** *CT, Ital.*
Aciclovir (p.626·1).
*Herpesvirus infections.*

**Citizem** *CT, Ital.*
Diltiazem hydrochloride (p.900·1).
*Angina pectoris; hypertension.*

**Citoburol** *Richter, Austria.*
Calcium acetate (p.1225·1); aluminium sulfate (p.1653·1).
*Bruises; inflammation.*

**Citocaina** *Cristalia, Braz.*
Prilocaine hydrochloride (p.1382·3).
Felypressin (p.1324·2) is included in this preparation as a vasoconstrictor to diminish absorption and localise the effect of the local anaesthetic.
*Local anaesthesia.*

**Citocartin** *Molteni, Ital.*
Articaine hydrochloride (p.1370·3).
Adrenaline acid tartrate (p.852·2) is included in this preparation as a vasoconstrictor to diminish absorption and localise the effect of the local anaesthetic.
*Local anaesthesia in dentistry.*

**Citochol** *Strallhofer, Austria.*
Taraxacum (p.1751·3); achillea (p.1646·2); peppermint oil (p.1283·2).
*Biliary disorders; gastrointestinal disorders.*

**Citodon**
*Durascan, Denm.; Astra, Swed.*
Codeine phosphate (p.27·1); paracetamol (p.76·2).
*Pain.*

**Citodox** *Pharmacia, Arg.*
Etoposide (p.551·3).
*Malignant neoplasms.*

**Citofolin** *Bracco, Ital.*
Calcium folinate (p.1431·1).
*Antidote to folic acid antagonists; folic acid deficiency; reduction of aminopterin and methotrexate toxicity.*

**Citofur** *Lusofarmaco, Ital.*
Tegafur (p.586·2).
*Malignant neoplasms.*

**Citogel**
*Gebro, Austria; Geymonat, Ital.*
Sucralfate (p.1290·2).
*Gastrointestinal disorders associated with hyperacidity.*

**Cito-Guakalin** *Stada, Ger.*
Sodium dibunate (p.1130·2); guaifenesin (p.1122·1); thyme (p.1755·2).
*Coughs and associated respiratory-tract disorders.*

**Citoken T** *Kendrick, Mex.*
Piroxicam (p.84·2).
*Inflammation; musculoskeletal and joint disorders; pain.*

**Citomid**
*Laboratorios Chile, Chile; Lemery, Mex.*
Vincristine sulfate (p.592·2).
*Idiopathic thrombocytopenic purpura; malignant neoplams.*

**Citoneurin** *Merck, Braz.*
Thiamine hydrochloride (p.1455·1); pyridoxine hydrochloride (p.1456·3); cyanocobalamin (p.1458·2).
*Vitamin B deficiency; vitamin B supplement.*

**Citoneuron** *Andromaco, Chile.*
Sodium cytidine monophosphate; trisodium uridine triphosphate (p.1760·3); hydroxocobalamin (p.1458·2).
*Myopathy; neuralgia; neuritis.*

**Citonina** *Pharmacia, Arg.*
Calcitonin (salmon) (p.768·2).
*Hypercalcaemia; metastatic bone pain; osteoporosis; Paget's disease of bone; pancreatitis; sympathetic dystrophy.*

**Citopam** *Sun, India.*
Citalopram (p.289·1).
*Depression; panic disorder.*

**Citoplatino** *Aventis, Ital.*
Cisplatin (p.538·1).
*Malignant neoplasms.*

**Citorsal** *Ern, Spain.*
Calcium lactate; citric acid; magnesium sulfate; potassium chloride; sodium citrate; sodium chloride; tribasic sodium phosphate; glucose (p.1222·2).
*Oral rehydration.*

**Citosin** *Nettopharma, Denm.†.*
Cisplatin (p.538·1).
*Malignant neoplasms.*

**Citostal** *Bristol-Myers Squibb, Braz.*
Lomustine (p.565·2).
*Malignant neoplasms.*

**Citovirax** *Roche, Ital.*
Ganciclovir (p.635·3) or ganciclovir sodium (p.635·3).
*Cytomegalovirus infections.*

**Citra pH** *ValMed, USA.*
Sodium citrate (p.1223·2).
*Hyperacidity.*

**Citracal**
*Note. This name is used for preparations of different composition.*
*Mission, Austral.; Mission Pharmacal, Hong Kong; Mission Pharmacal, Malaysia; Mission Pharmacal, Singapore†; Mission Pharmacal, USA.*
Calcium citrate (p.1225·1).
*Calcium supplement; hyperphosphataemia; osteoporosis.*

*Bruno, Ital.*
Calcium carbonate (p.1254·2).
*Calcium deficiency; calcium supplement.*

**Citracal + D**
*Mission Pharmacal, Hong Kong; Mission Pharmacal, Malaysia.*
Calcium citrate (p.1225·1); colecalciferol (p.1461·3).
*Calcium deficiency; hyperphosphataemia; osteoporosis.*

*Mission Pharmacal, USA.*
Calcium citrate (p.1225·1); ergocalciferol (p.1462·1).

**Citracal Plus with Magnesium** *Mission Pharmacal, USA.*
Calcium (p.1225·1); vitamin D (p.1462·1); pyridoxine; minerals (p.1417·1).

**Citralite** *Aventis, Austral.*
Sodium bicarbonate (p.1223·2); citric acid (p.1673·1); tartaric acid (p.1752·1).
*Urinary alkalinisation.*

**Citralka** *Parke, Davis, India.*
Sodium acid citrate (p.1223·2).
*Acidosis.*

**Citramag** *Sanochemia, UK.*
Magnesium citrate (p.1272·1).
*Bowel evacuation.*

**Citramar** *Dupomar, Arg.*
Calcium citrate (p.1225·1).
*Calcium deficiency; osteoporosis.*

**Citramar D** *Dupomar, Arg.*
Calcium citrate (p.1225·1); colecalciferol (p.1461·3).
*Calcium and vitamin D deficiency; osteopenia; osteoporosis.*

**Citranacea** *Nutravite, Canad.*
Echinacea (p.1683·2).

**Citrarginine** *Laphal, Fr.*
Neutral arginine citrate (p.1421·2); betaine (p.1660·1); betaine hydrochloride (p.1660·2).
*Liver disorders.*

**Citrato Espresso Gabbiani** *Montefarmaco, Ital.*
Magnesium oxide (p.1272·3); magnesium carbonate (p.1272·1).
*Gastrointestinal disorders.*

**Citrato Espresso S. Pellegrino** *Sanofi Synthelabo, Ital.*
Magnesium hydroxide (p.1272·2).
*Constipation.*

**Citravescent**
*Aventis, Austral.; Aventis, Malaysia.*
Sodium bicarbonate (p.1223·2); citric acid (p.1673·1); tartaric acid (p.1752·1).
*Urinary alkalinisation.*

*Pacific, NZ.*
Sodium citrotartrate (p.1224·1).
*Acidosis; gastric hyperacidity; urinary alkalinisation.*

**Citravite**
*Pharmed, India.*
Ascorbic acid (p.1460·2); sodium ascorbate (p.1460·2).
*Adjunct in wounds and infections; scurvy.*

*Boots Healthcare, NZ.*
Ascorbic acid (p.1460·2).
*Vitamin C supplement.*

**Citrec** *Orion, Swed.†.*
Calcium folinate (p.1431·1).
*Methotrexate antagonist.*

**Citredici UBT Kit** *Cortex, Ital.*
Carbon-13 labelled urea (p.1667·3).
*Diagnosis of gastroduodenal Helicobacter pylori infection.*

**Citrex** *Raza, Malaysia; Pharmaniaga, Malaysia.*
Vitamin C (p.1460·2).
*Vitamin C deficiency.*

**Citrex Vitamin E** *Raza, Malaysia.*
Vitamin E (p.1464·3).
*Vitamin E deficiency.*

**Citri Slim+Trim** *Bioglan, Austral.†.*
Garcinia; chromium trichloride (p.1425·1); pectin (p.1580·3); methylcellulose (p.1580·2); magnesium amino acid chelate (p.1229·1).
*Dietary supplement; obesity.*

**Citrihexal** *Hexal, Austral.*
Calcitriol (p.1461·2).
*Hypocalcaemia; hypoparathyroidism; osteoporosis; rickets.*

**Citrimax** *Natural Life, Arg.*
Garcinia cambogia.
*Slimming aid.*

**Citrisource** *Sandoz Nutrition, Canad.†.*
Preparation for enteral nutrition (p.1417·1).

**Citrizan** *IDI, Ital.*
Catalase (equine) (p.1668·3).
*Burns; skin ulceration.*

**Citrizan Antibiotico** *IDI, Ital.*
Catalase (equine) (p.1668·3); gentamicin sulfate (p.217·1).
*Infected burns and skin ulcers.*

**Citro Jod** *Esoform, Ital.*
Povidone-iodine (p.1190·3).
*Skin disinfection.*

**Citrocarbonate**
*Roberts, Canad.†.*
Sodium bicarbonate (p.1223·2); sodium citrate (p.1223·2); anhydrous citric acid (p.1673·1).
*Antacid; urinary alkaliniser.*

*Roberts, USA; Hauck, USA.*
Sodium bicarbonate (p.1223·2); anhydrous sodium citrate (p.1223·2).
*Hyperacidity.*

**Citrocholine** *Bailleul, Fr.*
*Granules for oral solution†:* Sodium citrate (p.1223·2); magnesium citrate (p.1272·1); choline citrate (p.1424·3).
*Oral solution:* Choline citrate (p.1424·3); sodium acid citrate (p.1223·2); citric acid monohydrate (p.1673·1); light magnesium carbonate (p.1272·1).
*Dyspepsia.*

**Citrocil** *Reig Jofre, Spain.*
Dihydrostreptomycin sulfate (p.205·3); sodium citrate (p.1223·2).
*Gastrointestinal infections.*

**Citrocit** *Premier, S.Afr.*
Citric acid (p.1673·1); sodium bicarbonate (p.1223·2).
*Urinary alkalinisation.*

**Citroepatina** *Roche, Ital.*
Betaine monocitrate (p.1660·2); sorbitol (p.1446·3); sodium bicarbonate (p.1223·2); anhydrous citric acid (p.1673·1).
*Digestive disorders.*

**Citro-Flav** *Goldline, USA.*
Citrus bioflavonoids complex (p.1688·2).
*Capillary bleeding.*

**Citroflavona** Almirall, Spain†.
Ascorbic acid (p.1460·2); bioflavonoids (p.1688·2).
*Capillary disorders.*

**Citroflavona Mag** Funk, Spain†.
Ascorbic acid (p.1460·2); bioflavonoids (p.1688·2); hydroxyflavone.
*Capillary disorders.*

**Citroftalmina** SIFI, Ital.†.
Zinc phenolsulfonate (p.1163·3); procaine hydrochloride (p.1383·2).
*Eye irritation and congestion.*

**Citroftalmina VC** SIFI, Ital.†.
Naphazoline nitrate (p.1124·3); zinc phenolsulfonate (p.1163·3); procaine hydrochloride (p.1383·2).
*Eye irritation and congestion.*

**Citrokehl** Sanum-Kehlbeck, Ger.
Homoeopathic preparation.

**Citrolider** Farmalider, Spain†.
Ascorbic acid (p.1460·2).
*Vitamin C deficiency.*

**Citrolith** Beach, USA†.
Anhydrous potassium citrate (p.1223·1); anhydrous sodium citrate (p.1223·2).
*Urinary alkalinising agent.*

**Citro-Mag**
Rougier, Canad.; Rougier, Hong Kong.
Magnesium citrate (p.1272·1).
*Bowel evacuation; constipation.*

**Citromed** Esoform, Ital.
Chlorhexidine gluconate (p.1173·2); isopropyl alcohol (p.1184·3).
*Skin disinfection.*

**Citromed 80 and 85** Esoform, Ital.
Chlorhexidine gluconate (p.1173·2); benzalkonium chloride (p.1168·3); alcohol (p.1166·1).
*Skin disinfection.*

**Citromed Chirurgico** Esoform, Ital.
Benzalkonium chloride (p.1168·3); alcohol (p.1166·1); chlorhexidine gluconate (p.1173·2).
*Skin disinfection.*

**Citromed Chlor** Esoform, Ital.
Tosylchloramide sodium (p.1194·3).
*Surface disinfection.*

**Citromed Soap** Esoform, Ital.
Cetylpyridinium chloride (p.1173·1).
*Skin disinfection.*

**Citromedics Disinfettante** Esoform, Ital.
Sodium *o*-phenylphenol (p.1187·2).
*Surface disinfection.*

**Citromedics Pronto** Esoform, Ital.
Benzalkonium chloride (p.1168·3); chlorhexidine gluconate (p.1173·2).
*Instrument disinfection.*

**Citromel** Knop, Chile.
Melissa (p.1711·1).
*Anxiety; gastrointestinal disorders.*

**Citron** Infabra, Braz.†.
Ascorbic acid (p.1460·2).
*Vitamin C supplement.*

**Citron Chaud** Prodemdis, Canad.†.
Phenylephrine hydrochloride (p.1126·3); pheniramine maleate (p.438·3); paracetamol (p.76·2); ascorbic acid (p.1460·2).

**Citron Chaud DM** Prodemdis, Canad.
Phenylephrine hydrochloride (p.1126·3); pheniramine maleate (p.438·3); dextromethorphan hydrobromide (p.1117·3); ascorbic acid (p.1460·2).

**Citropepsin** Byk Gulden, Ger.
Pepsin (p.1729·3); citric acid (p.1673·1).
*Gastrointestinal disorders.*

**Citropiperazina** Aventis, Ital.
Piperazine citrate (p.111·2).
*Urinary alkalinisation.*

**Citroplex** Neo Quimica, Braz.
Ascorbic acid (p.1460·2).
*Vitamin C supplement.*

**Citroplus**
Medley, Braz.; Whitehall, Ital.
Metoclopramide hydrochloride (p.1274·3).
*Adjunct in gastrointestinal procedures; gastrointestinal motility disorders; nausea and vomiting.*

**Citrosan** Boots Healthcare, Neth.
Paracetamol (p.76·2); ascorbic acid (p.1460·2); sodium citrate (p.1223·2).
*Cold and influenza symptoms; fever; pain.*

**Citrosil**
Note. This name is used for preparations of different composition.
Dolisos, Fr.†.
Thyme oil (p.1755·3); lemon oil (p.1706·2); lavender oil (p.1705·2).
*House dust mite acaricide.*

Manetti Roberts, Ital.
Benzalkonium chloride (p.1168·3).
*Disinfection of skin, burns, and wounds.*

**Citrosil Alcolico Azzuro** Manetti Roberts, Ital.
Benzalkonium chloride (p.1168·3); alcohol (p.1166·1); sodium nitrite (p.1052·3).
*Instrument disinfection.*

**Citrosil Alcolico Bruno** Manetti Roberts, Ital.
Benzalkonium chloride (p.1168·3); alcohol (p.1166·1).
*Skin and wound disinfection.*

**Citrosil Alcolico Incolore** Manetti Roberts, Ital.
Benzalkonium chloride (p.1168·3); alcohol (p.1166·1).
*Skin and wound disinfection.*

**Citrosil Nubesan** Manetti Roberts, Ital.
Benzalkonium chloride (p.1168·3); benzoin resin (p.1751·1).
*Surface disinfection.*

**Citrosil Sapone** Manetti Roberts, Ital.
Triclocarban (p.1195·1).
*Skin cleansing.*

**Citro-Soda** Abbott, S.Afr.
Sodium citrate (p.1223·2); sodium bicarbonate (p.1223·2); tartaric acid (p.1752·1); citric acid (p.1673·1).
*Antacid; urinary alkalinisation.*

**Citrosodina** Roche, Ital.
Sodium citrate (p.1223·2).
*Gastric hyperacidity.*

**Citrosodine** Prima, Braz.
*Oral granules:* Citric acid (p.1673·1); sodium bicarbonate (p.1223·2); sodium citrate (p.1223·2).
*Tablets:* Sodium citrate (p.1223·2).
*Gastrointestinal hyperacidity.*

**Citrosteril** Fresenius, Ger.†.
Citric acid monohydrate (p.1673·1).
*Instrument disinfection.*

**Citrosteril Ambiente** Sanitas, Ital.
Benzalkonium chloride (p.1168·3).
*Linen disinfection.*

**Citrosteril Aspiratori** Sanitas, Ital.
Orthophenylphenol (p.1187·2).
*Disinfection of aspirators.*

**Citrosteril Deterferri** Sanitas, Ital.
Benzalkonium chloride (p.1168·3).
*Instrument disinfection.*

**Citrosteril Impronte** Sanitas, Ital.
Glutaral (p.1180·3); benzalkonium chloride (p.1168·3).
*Disinfection in dentistry.*

**Citrosteril Pronto** Sanitas, Ital.
Benzalkonium chloride (p.1168·3); chlorhexidine (p.1173·2).
*Disinfection in dentistry.*

**Citrosteril Sterilferri** Sanitas, Ital.
Glutaral (p.1180·3).
*Instrument disinfection.*

**Citrosteril Strumenti** Sanitas, Ital.
Benzalkonium chloride (p.1168·3); alcohol (p.1166·1).
*Instrument disinfection.*

**Citrosystem** Antipiol, Ital.
Citronella oil (p.1673·2); basil oil; lavender oil (p.1705·2).
*Insect repellent.*

**Citrotein**
Sandoz Nutrition, Canad.†; Sandoz Nutrition, USA.
Preparation for enteral nutrition (p.1417·1).

**Citrovenot** Bros, Gr.
Ciprofloxacin hydrochloride (p.188·2).
*Bacterial infections.*

**Citrovit**
Aventis, Braz.; Abello, Spain.
Ascorbic acid (p.1460·2).
*Vitamin C deficiency.*

**Citrucel** GlaxoSmithKline, USA.
Methylcellulose (p.1580·2).
*Bowel evacuation; constipation.*

**Citrus C with Acerola** Blackmores, Austral.†.
Ascorbic acid (p.1460·2); sodium ascorbate (p.1460·2).
*Vitamin C deficiency.*

**Citrus-flav C** Fibertone, USA.
Citrus bioflavonoids complex (p.1688·2); vitamin C (p.1460·2); hesperidin (p.1688·2); acerola; rutoside (p.1688·2).
*Capillary bleeding.*

**Citsav** Savio, Ital.†.
Citicoline sodium (p.1672·3).
*Cerebrovascular disorders.*

**Cituridina** Zambon, Ital.†.
Cytidine; uridine (p.1760·3).
*Hepatic encephalopathy.*

**Ciuk** BASF, Ger.†.
Cimetidine (p.1255·3).
*Acid aspiration; gastro-oesophageal reflux; gastrointestinal haemorrhage; peptic ulcer; Zollinger-Ellison syndrome.*

**Civeran** Lesvi, Spain.
Loratadine (p.436·1).
*Hypersensitivity reactions.*

**Civicor**
Douglas, NZ; Douglas, Singapore†; Douglas, Thai.; TTN, Thai.
Verapamil hydrochloride (p.1019·1).
*Angina pectoris; arrhythmias; hypertension.*

**Civigel** Novartis Ophthalmics, Fr.
Carbomer 980 (p.1577·2).
*Dry eyes.*

**Cizoren** Stadmed, India.
Haloperidol (p.701·2).
*Childhood behaviour disorders; psychoses.*

**C-L90** Loges, Ger.
Ascorbic acid (p.1460·2).
*Vitamin C deficiency.*

**CL tre** Nova Argentia, Ital.
Trichloroacetic acid (p.1162·1).
*Warts.*

**Claben** Raza, Malaysia; Pharmaniaga, Malaysia.
Glibenclamide (p.331·2).
*Diabetes mellitus.*

**Clabin**
Note. This name is used for preparations of different composition.
Chefaro, Ger.
Salicylic acid (p.1157·1); lactic acid (p.1704·1).
Formerly contained salicylic acid, lactic acid, and resorcinol.
*Calluses; corns; warts.*

Schonenberger, Switz.
Salicylic acid (p.1157·1); lactic acid (p.1704·1); resorcinol (p.1156·3).
*Calluses; corns; verrucas; warts.*

**Clacef** Dexa, Singapore.
Cefotaxime sodium (p.175·3).
*Bacterial infections.*

**Claforan**
Aventis, Austral.; Aventis, Austria; Aventis, Belg.; Aventis, Braz.†; Aventis, Canad.; Aventis, Denm.; Aventis, Fin.; Roussel Diamant, Fr.; Aventis, Ger.; Hoechst Marion Roussel, Gr.; Aventis, Hong Kong; Aventis, India; Aventis, Irl.; Aventis, Israel; Lepetit, Ital.; Aventis, Malaysia; Aventis, Mex.; Aventis, Neth.; Aventis, Norw.; Aventis, NZ; Aventis, S.Afr.; Aventis, Singapore; Aventis, Spain; Aventis, Swed.; Aventis, Switz.; Aventis, Thai.; Aventis, UK; Hoechst Marion Roussel, USA.
Cefotaxime sodium (p.175·3).
Lidocaine hydrochloride (p.1377·3) may be included in the intramuscular injection to alleviate the pain of injection.
*Bacterial infections.*

**Clafordil** Ariston, Braz.
Cefotaxime (p.176·3).
*Bacterial infections.*

**Claim** Apomedica, Austria.
Curcumae oleosum extract (p.1058·3); *p*,α-dimethylbenzyl alcohol (p.1680·3); peppermint oil (p.1283·2); eucalyptus oil (p.1686·2); camphor (p.1665·3); menthol (p.1711·3).
*Gastrointestinal disorders.*

**Clairo Tea** Weleda, UK†.
Senna leaf (p.1288·2); peppermint leaf (p.1283·2); aniseed (p.1655·2); clove (p.1673·2).
*Constipation.*

**Clairodermyl** BCS, Fr.†.
Mequinol (p.1151·3).
*Hyperpigmentation.*

**Clamarvit** Clariana, Spain.
Ascorbic acid (p.1460·2); vitamin B substances (p.1417·1); ferrous gluconate (p.1428·1); ferrous gluceptate (p.1428·1).
*Anaemias; tonic.*

**Clamentin** Xixia, S.Afr.
Amoxicillin (p.155·3); clavulanic acid (p.193·3).
*Bacterial infections.*

**Clamiben** Teuto, Braz.
Glibenclamide (p.331·2).
*Diabetes mellitus.*

**Clamicin** Medley, Braz.
Clarithromycin (p.192·2).
*Bacterial infections.*

**Clamide**
Hovid, Hong Kong; Hovid, Singapore.
Glibenclamide (p.331·2).
*Diabetes mellitus.*

**Clamist** Wander, India.
Clemastine fumarate (p.429·1).
*Hypersensitivity reactions.*

**Clamonex** Yungjin, Singapore.
Amoxicillin trihydrate (p.155·3); potassium clavulanate (p.193·3).
*Bacterial infections.*

**Clamox** GlaxoSmithKline, Fin.
Amoxicillin trihydrate (p.155·3).
*Bacterial infections.*

**Clamoxin** Maver, Mex.
Amoxicillin trihydrate (p.155·3); clavulanic acid (p.193·3).
*Bacterial infections.*

**Clamoxyl**
Note. This name is used for preparations of different composition.
GlaxoSmithKline, Austral.
Amoxicillin trihydrate (p.155·3); potassium clavulanate (p.193·3).
*Bacterial infections.*

GlaxoSmithKline, Austria; GlaxoSmithKline, Belg.; GlaxoSmithKline, Fr.; GlaxoSmithKline, Ger.; GlaxoSmithKline, Neth.; Beecham, Port.; GlaxoSmithKline, Spain; SmithKline Beecham, Switz.
Amoxicillin sodium (p.155·3) or amoxicillin trihydrate (p.155·3).
*Bacterial infections.*

**Clamoxyl Mucolitico** SmithKline Beecham, Spain.
Amoxicillin trihydrate (p.155·3); bromhexine hydrochloride (p.1115·3).
*Respiratory-tract infections.*

**Clamycin** Julphar, UAE.
Clarithromycin (p.192·2).
*Bacterial infections.*

**Clanzoflat** Wyeth, Spain.
Dimethicone (p.1289·2); clebopride (p.1260·3).
*Gastrointestinal disorders.*

**Clanzol** Orfi, Spain†.
Clebopride malate (p.1260·3).
*Gastrointestinal disorders; nausea and vomiting.*

**Claradol** Roche Nicholas, Fr.
Paracetamol (p.76·2).
*Fever; pain.*

**Claradol Cafeine** Roche Nicholas, Fr.
Paracetamol (p.76·2); caffeine (p.782·1).
*Fever; pain.*

**Claradol Codeine** Roche Nicholas, Fr.
Paracetamol (p.76·2); codeine phosphate (p.27·1).
*Pain.*

**Claragine** Roche Nicholas, Fr.
Aspirin (p.15·1).
*Fever; pain.*

**Claral** Schering, Spain.
Diflucortolone valerate (p.1099·3).
*Skin disorders.*

**Claral Plus** Schering, Spain.
Chlorquinaldol (p.187·3); diflucortolone valerate (p.1099·3).
*Infected skin disorders.*

**Claramax** Schering-Plough, NZ.
Desloratadine (p.431·1).
*Allergic rhinitis.*

**Claramid**
Zambon, Belg.; Pfizer, Fr.
Roxithromycin (p.254·2).
*Bacterial infections.*

**Claratyne**
Schering-Plough, Austral.; Schering-Plough, NZ.
Loratadine (p.436·1).
*Allergic skin disorders; rhinitis; urticaria.*

**Claratyne Decongestant** Schering-Plough, NZ†.
Loratadine (p.436·1); pseudoephedrine sulfate (p.1129·2).
*Upper respiratory-tract congestion.*

**Claravis** Barr, USA.
Isotretinoin (p.1148·3).
*Acne.*

**Claraxim** Siam Bheasach, Thai.
Cefotaxime sodium (p.175·3).
*Bacterial infections.*

**Clarema** Damor, Ital.
Suleparoid (p.1009·1).
*Superficial vascular disorders; thrombosis prophylaxis.*

**Clarens** Schiapparelli, Ital.
Sulodexide (p.1009·2).
*Thrombosis prophylaxis.*

**Claribid** Abbott, India.
Clarithromycin (p.192·2).
*Bacterial infections.*

**Claricort** Undra, Mex.
Betamethasone (p.1093·1); loratadine (p.436·1).
*Hypersensitivity.*

**Clariderm** Stiefel, Braz.†.
Hydroquinone (p.1148·1).
*Skin pigmentation disorders.*

**Claridon** Schering-Plough, Port.
Loratadine (p.436·1); pseudoephedrine (p.1129·2).

**Clariflu**
Schering-Plough, Hong Kong; Schering-Plough, Mex.
Loratadine (p.436·1); pseudoephedrine sulfate (p.1129·2); paracetamol (p.76·2).
*Allergic rhinitis; cold symptoms.*

**Clarifriol**
Key, Arg.; Undra, Mex.
Loratadine (p.436·1); pseudoephedrine sulfate (p.1129·2); paracetamol (p.76·2).
*Allergic rhinitis; cold symptoms.*

**Claril** Alcon, Braz.
Naphazoline hydrochloride (p.1124·3); pheniramine maleate (p.438·3).
*Ocular congestion.*

**Clarilerg** Hexal, Braz.
Loratadine (p.436·1).
*Hypersensitivity reactions.*

**Clarimac** Cadila, India.
Clarithromycin (p.192·2).
*Bacterial infections.*

**Clarimax**
Pharmus, Braz.†; Andromaco, Chile.
Clarithromycin (p.192·2).
*Bacterial infections.*

**Clarimid** Epicaris, Arg.
Clarithromycin (p.192·2).
*Bacterial infections.*

**Clarimir** Andromaco, Chile.
Naphazoline hydrochloride (p.1124·3).
*Eye irritation.*

**Clarimir F** Andromaco, Chile.
Naphazoline hydrochloride (p.1124·3); pheniramine maleate (p.438·3).
*Allergic eye disorders; eye irritation.*

**Clarinase**
Schering-Plough, Austral.; Aesca, Austria; Schering-Plough, Belg.; Essex, Chile; Schering-Plough, Denm.; Schering-Plough, Fin.; Schering-Plough, Fr.; Schering-Plough, Hong Kong; Schering-Plough, Israel; Schering-Plough, Malaysia; Undra, Mex.; Schering-Plough, NZ; Schering-Plough, Singapore; Essex, Spain†; Schering-Plough, Thai.
Loratadine (p.436·1); pseudoephedrine sulfate (p.1129·2).
*Allergic rhinitis; cold symptoms.*

**Clarineo** Neo Quimica, Braz.
Clarithromycin (p.192·2).
*Bacterial infections.*

**Clarinex**
Note. This name is used for preparations of different composition.
Schering-Plough, Denm.†.
Loratadine (p.436·1); pseudoephedrine sulfate (p.1129·2).
*Allergic rhinitis.*

Schering, USA.
Desloratadine (p.431·1).
*Allergic rhinitis; urticaria.*

**Claripel** Stiefel, Arg.; Stiefel, Braz.
Hydroquinone (p.1148·1).
*Skin pigmentation disorders.*

Stiefel, USA.
Hydroquinone (p.1148·1) in a sunblocking basis.
*Hyperpigmented skin disorders.*

**Claripex AL** Sanofi Winthrop, Braz.†.
Aluminium clofibrate (p.884·3).
*Hyperlipidaemias.*

**Clarisco** Schwarz, Ital.
Heparin sodium (p.928·1).
*Soft-tissue injury; superficial vascular disorders; thromboembolic disorders.*

**Claritab** Ache, Braz.†.
Clarithromycin (p.192·2).
*Bacterial infections.*

**Clariteyes** Schering-Plough, UK.
Sodium cromoglicate (p.795·3).
*Allergic conjunctivitis.*

**Claritin**
Schering-Plough, Braz.; Schering, Canad.; Schering-Plough, USA.
Loratadine (p.436·1).
*Allergic conjunctivitis; allergic rhinitis; hypersensitivity reactions of the skin.*

**Claritin Allergic Congestion Relief** Schering, Canad.
Oxymetazoline hydrochloride (p.1126·1).
*Nasal congestion.*

**Claritin Extra** Schering, Canad.
Loratadine (p.436·1); pseudoephedrine sulfate (p.1129·2).
*Upper respiratory-tract congestion.*

**Claritin Eye Allergy Relief** Schering, Canad.
Oxymetazoline hydrochloride (p.1126·1).
*Conjunctivitis.*

**Claritin Skin Itch Relief** Schering, Canad.
Hydrocortisone (p.1103·3).
*Skin disorders.*

**Claritin-D**
Schering-Plough, Braz.; Schering, USA.
Loratadine (p.436·1); pseudoephedrine (p.1129·2) or pseudoephedrine sulfate (p.1129·2).
*Allergic rhinitis; nasal congestion.*

**Claritine**
Schering-Plough, Belg.; Schering-Plough, Neth.; Schering-Plough, Port.; Essex, Switz.
Loratadine (p.436·1).
*Allergic rhinitis; urticaria.*

**Claritone** Fischer, Israel.
Comfort solution for contact lens (p.1164·2).

**Clarityn**
Note. This name is used for preparations of different composition.
Aesca, Austria; Schering-Plough, Denm.; Schering-Plough, Fin.; Schering-Plough, Irl.; Schering-Plough, Ital.; Schering-Plough, Norw.; Schering-Plough, Swed.; Schering-Plough, UK.
Loratadine (p.436·1).
*Allergic conjunctivitis; allergic rhinitis; pruritus; urticaria.*

Schering-Plough, UK.
*Eye drops:* Sodium cromoglicate (p.795·3).
*Allergic conjunctivitis.*

**Clarityne**
Kirby, Arg.; Essex, Chile; Schering-Plough, Fr.; Schering-Plough, Gr.; Schering-Plough, Hong Kong; Schering-Plough, Malaysia; Schering-Plough, Mex.; Schering-Plough, S.Afr.; Schering-Plough, Singapore; Schering-Plough, Spain; Schering-Plough, Thai.
Loratadine (p.436·1).
*Allergic conjunctivitis; allergic rhinitis; allergic skin disorders; urticaria.*

**Clarityne Cort** Kirby, Arg.
Loratadine (p.436·1); betamethasone (p.1093·1).
*Hypersensitivity reactions.*

**Clarityne D**
Kirby, Arg.; Schering-Plough, Mex.; Schering-Plough, S.Afr.
Loratadine (p.436·1); pseudoephedrine sulfate (p.1129·2).
*Upper respiratory-tract disorders.*

**Clarix** Cooperation Pharmaceutique, Fr.
Erysimum; pholcodine (p.1128·3).
*Coughs.*

**Claroft** Alcon, Braz.
Naphazoline hydrochloride (p.1124·3).
*Eye irritation.*

**Claroftal** Poen, Arg.
Sodium cromoglicate (p.795·3).
*Blepharitis; conjunctivitis.*

**Clarograf**
Justesa Imagen, Arg.; Juste, Spain.
Iopromide (p.1065·2).
*Radiographic contrast medium.*

**Clarover** Ciba Vision, Ital.
Povidone (p.1581·2).
*Dry eyes.*

**Clarvisan**
Allergan, Ital.; Hormona, Mex.; Seber, Port.; Alcon Cusi, Spain.
Pirenoxine sodium (p.1732·2).
*Cataracts.*

**Clarvisol** Allergan, Braz.
Pirenoxine sodium (p.1732·2).
Formerly contained pirenoxine and taurine.
*Cataracts.*

**Clarvisor** Alcon, Ger.
Pirenoxine sodium (p.1732·2).
*Cataracts.*

**Clarvix** Beta, Arg.
Ginkgo biloba (p.1692·3).
*Cerebral and peripheral vascular disorders.*

**Clasifel**
Stiefel, Chile; Stiefel, Mex.
Hydroquinone (p.1148·1); padimate O (p.1155·1); dioxybenzone (p.1145·3); oxybenzone (p.1154·3).
*Skin pigmentation disorders.*

**Classic Swiss One** Swiss Herbal, Canad.
Multivitamin and mineral preparation (p.1417·1).

**Clasteon** Abiogen, Ital.
Disodium clodronate (p.770·2).
*Hyperparathyroidism; multiple myeloma; osteolytic tumours; osteoporosis.*

**Clastidin** Nutrifar, Ital.
Cefonicid sodium (p.174·2).
Lidocaine hydrochloride (p.1377·3) is included in this preparation to alleviate the pain of injection.
*Gram-negative bacterial infections.*

**Clastoban** Schering, Fr.
Disodium clodronate (p.770·2).
*Hypercalcaemia of malignancy; osteolysis of malignancy.*

**Clatromicin** Labinca, Arg.
Clarithromycin (p.192·2).
*Bacterial infections.*

**Claudemor**
Sankyo, Braz.
Thromboplastin (p.760·2); benzocaine (p.1370·3); procaine hydrochloride (p.1383·2); zinc oxide (p.1163·2); bismuth subgallate (p.1252·2); peru balsam (p.1730·2).
*Anorectal disorders.*

Sankyo, Port.
Thromboplastin (p.760·2); benzocaine (p.1370·3); procaine (p.1383·2); zinc oxide (p.1163·2); bismuth subgallate (p.1252·2); peru balsam (p.1730·2).
*Anorectal disorders.*

**Claudicat**
Byk Gulden, Ger.; Byk, Port.
Pentoxifylline (p.979·3).
*Cerebral and peripheral vascular disorders.*

**Clauparest** Pekana, Ger.
Homoeopathic preparation.

**Clavamel** Clonmel, Irl.
Amoxicillin trihydrate (p.155·3); potassium clavulanate (p.193·3).
*Bacterial infections.*

**Clavamox**
Tyrol, Austria; Cimex, Israel; Bial, Port.; Grunenthal, Switz.
Amoxicillin sodium (p.155·3) or amoxicillin trihydrate (p.155·3); potassium clavulanate (p.193·3).
*Bacterial infections.*

**Claventin** GlaxoSmithKline, Fr.
Ticarcillin sodium (p.270·2); potassium clavulanate (p.193·3).
*Bacterial infections.*

**Clavepen**
Clintex, Port.; Almirall, Spain.
Amoxicillin trihydrate (p.155·3); potassium clavulanate (p.193·3).
*Bacterial infections.*

**Claversal**
Merck, Austria; Tramedico, Belg.; Merckle, Ger.; GlaxoSmithKline, Ital.; Byk, Port.; GlaxoSmithKline, Spain.
Mesalazine (p.1273·2).
*Inflammatory bowel disease.*

**Clavigrenin** Hormosan, Ger.
Dihydroergotamine mesilate (p.465·3).
*Hypotension; migraine and related vascular headaches.*

**Clavinex** Saval, Chile.
Potassium clavulanate (p.193·3); amoxicillin (p.155·3).
*Bacterial infections.*

**Clavinex Duo** Saval, Chile.
Amoxicillin (p.155·3); clavulanic acid (p.193·3).
*Bacterial infections.*

**Clavoxil** Haller, Braz.
Amoxicillin (p.155·3) or amoxicillin sodium (p.155·3); potassium clavulanate (p.193·3).
*Bacterial infections.*

**Clavoxilina Bid** Recalcine, Chile.
Amoxicillin trihydrate (p.155·3); potassium clavulanate (p.193·3).
*Bacterial infections.*

**Clavucar** Geymonat, Ital.
Ticarcillin sodium (p.270·2); potassium clavulanate (p.193·3).
Lidocaine hydrochloride (p.1377·3) is included in the intramuscular injection to alleviate the pain of injection.
*Bacterial infections.*

**Clavucid**
Yamanouchi, Belg.; Recordati, Spain.
Amoxicillin trihydrate (p.155·3); potassium clavulanate (p.193·3).
*Bacterial infections.*

**Clavulin**
Arrow, Austral.; GlaxoSmithKline, Canad.; Fournier, Ital.; Sanfer, Mex.
Amoxicillin trihydrate (p.155·3); potassium clavulanate (p.193·3).
*Bacterial infections.*

GlaxoSmithKline, Braz.
Amoxicillin (p.155·3); clavulanic acid (p.193·3) or potassium clavulanate (p.193·3).
*Bacterial infections.*

**Clavulox** GlaxoSmithKline, Arg.
Amoxicillin trihydrate (p.155·3); potassium clavulanate (p.193·3).
*Bacterial infections.*

**Clavulox Duo** GlaxoSmithKline, Arg.
Amoxicillin trihydrate (p.155·3); potassium clavulanate (p.193·3).
*Bacterial infections.*

**Clavumox**
Aspen, S.Afr.
Amoxicillin (p.155·3); clavulanic acid (p.193·3).
*Bacterial infections.*

Pharmacia, Spain.
Amoxicillin trihydrate (p.155·3); potassium clavulanate (p.193·3).
*Bacterial infections.*

**Clavurion** Orion, Fin.
Amoxicillin trihydrate (p.155·3); potassium clavulanate (p.193·3).
*Bacterial infections.*

**Cleactor** Eisai, Jpn.
Monteplase (p.961·3).
*Myocardial infarction.*

**Clean & Clear Deep Cleaning Astringent** Johnson & Johnson, Canad.
Salicylic acid (p.1157·1).
*Acne.*

**Clean & Clear Foaming Cleanser** Johnson & Johnson, Canad.
Triclosan (p.1195·2).
*Acne.*

**Clean & Clear Gel Secativo** Johnson & Johnson, Braz.
Salicylic acid (p.1157·1).
*Acne.*

**Clean & Clear Hidratante** Johnson & Johnson, Braz.
Salicylic acid (p.1157·1).
*Acne.*

**Clean & Clear Invsible Blemish** Johnson & Johnson, Canad.
Salicylic acid (p.1157·1).
*Acne.*

**Clean & Clear Locao Adstringente** Johnson & Johnson, Braz.
Salicylic acid (p.1157·1).
*Acne.*

**Clean & Clear Persa** Johnson & Johnson, Canad.
Benzoyl peroxide (p.1143·2).
*Acne.*

**Clean & Clear Sabonete Liquido Facial** Johnson & Johnson, Braz.
Triclosan (p.1195·2).
*Acne.*

**Clean & Clear Sabonete Liquido Refrescante** Johnson & Johnson, Braz.
Salicylic acid (p.1157·1).
*Acne.*

**Clean Hair** Neo Quimica, Braz.
Permethrin (p.1508·3).
*Pediculosis.*

**Clean Skin Anti Acne** Mentholatum, Austral.†.
Melaleuca oil (p.1710·2).
*Acne.*

**Clean Skin Face Wash** Mentholatum, Austral.†.
Melaleuca oil (p.1710·2); benzalkonium chloride (p.1168·3).
*Acne.*

**Clean-AC**
Pierre Fabre Dermo-Cosmetique, Arg.; Silesia, Chile.
Cucurbita (p.1677·3); zinc gluconate (p.1469·2).
*Acne.*

**Clean-AF** Floris, Israel.
Sodium chloride (p.1233·3).
*Nasal congestion.*

**Cleanal** Mitsubishi, Jpn.
Fudosteine (p.1121·3).
*Respiratory-tract congestion.*

**Cleanance**
Note. This name is used for preparations of different composition.
Pierre Fabre Dermo-Cosmetique, Arg.
Cucurbita (p.1677·3); zinc gluconate (p.1469·2).
*Seborrhoea.*

Silesia, Chile.
*Topical emulsion:* Cucurbita (p.1677·3); zinc gluconate (p.1469·2); salicylic acid (p.1157·1).
*Topical gel:* Cucurbita (p.1677·3); zinc gluconate (p.1469·2).
*Seborrhoea.*

**Cleancef** Shin Poong, Singapore.
Cefaclor (p.167·1).
*Bacterial infections.*

**Cleaner No 4** Fischer, Israel†.
Thiomersal (p.1194·1); disodium edetate (p.1037·3)(p.1164·2).
*Cleaning solution for soft contact lenses.*

**Clean-N-Soak**
Allergan, Austral.†.
Hard and gas permeable contact lens cleaning and soaking solution (p.1164·2).

Allergan, Israel†.
Phenylmercuric nitrate (p.1189·2) (p.1164·2).
*Cleaning and soaking solution for hard contact lenses.*

**Cleanomed** Agepha, Austria.
Alcohol (p.1166·1); isopropyl alcohol (p.1184·3).
*Skin disinfection.*

**Cleansing Herbs** Potter's, UK.
Buckthorn (p.1254·1); psyllium (p.1268·1); senna leaves (p.1288·2); sambucus (p.1741·3); fennel seed (p.1687·2); maté (p.1765·3).
Cleansing Herb Tablets formerly contained senna leaves, aloes, cascara, taraxacum, and fennel seed.
*Constipation.*

**Cleanxate** Sam Chun Dang, Singapore.
Flavoxate hydrochloride (p.482·2).
*Urinary-tract disorders.*

**Clear Away**
Schering-Plough, Austral.; Schering-Plough, Canad.†; Schering-Plough, NZ†.
Salicylic acid (p.1157·1).
*Warts.*

**Clear By Design** SmithKline Beecham Consumer, USA†.
Benzoyl peroxide (p.1143·2).
*Acne.*

**Clear Cough** Be-Tabs, S.Afr.
Diphenhydramine hydrochloride (p.431·3); ammonium chloride (p.1115·2); sodium citrate (p.1223·2).
*Coughs.*

**Clear Ear** Co-Pharma, UK.
Docusate sodium (p.1262·2).
*Ear wax removal.*

**Clear Eyes**
Abbott, Austral.; Abbott, Canad.; Abbott, NZ; Ross, USA.
Naphazoline hydrochloride (p.1124·3).
*Eye irritation.*

**Clear Eyes ACR**
Abbott, NZ; Ross, USA.
Naphazoline hydrochloride (p.1124·3); zinc sulfate (p.1469·3).
*Eye irritation.*

**Clear Eyes CLR** Ross, USA.
Sodium chloride (p.1233·3); hypromellose (p.1579·3) (p.1164·2).
*Moistening drops for contact lenses.*

**Clear Pore**
Professional Health, Canad.†; Neutrogena, Fr.†.
Salicylic acid (p.1157·1).
*Acne; seborrhoea.*

**Clear Total Lice Elimination System** Care, USA†.
Shampoo, pyrethrum extract (p.1509·3); piperonyl butoxide (p.1509·2); enzymic lice egg remover; comb.
*Pediculosis.*

**Clear Tussin 30** Goldline, USA.
Guaifenesin (p.1122·1); dextromethorphan hydrobromide (p.1117·3).
*Coughs.*

**ClearAc** Hylands, Canad.
Homoeopathic preparation.

**ClearAc Cleanser** Hylands, Canad.
Homoeopathic preparation.

**Clearamed** Boots Healthcare, Spain†.
Benzoyl peroxide (p.1143·2).
*Acne.*

**Clearasil**
Note. This name is used for preparations of different composition.
Procter & Gamble, Braz.†.
Sulfur (p.1158·2); resorcinol (p.1156·3); triclosan (p.1195·2).
*Acne.*

Boots Healthcare, NZ.
Sulfur (p.1158·2); triclosan (p.1195·2).
*Acne.*

Richardson-Vicks Personal Care, USA.
Benzoyl peroxide (p.1143·2).
*Acne.*

**Clearasil Acne Cream** Procter & Gamble, Canad.
Sulfur (p.1158·2); resorcinol (p.1156·3).
Formerly contained sulfur, resorcinol, and triclosan.
*Acne.*

**Clearasil Acne Treatment Cream** Boots Healthcare, Austral.
Sulfur (p.1158·2); triclosan (p.1195·2).
*Acne.*

**Clearasil Active Treatment Cream** Crookes Healthcare, UK.
Triclosan (p.1195·2); sulfur (p.1158·2).
Formerly known as Clearasil Treatment Cream.
*Acne.*

**Clearasil Antibacterial** Richardson-Vicks Personal Care, USA.
Triclosan (p.1195·2); glycerol (p.1694·3); titanium dioxide (p.1160·3).
*Acne.*

**Clearasil B.P. Plus** Procter & Gamble, Canad.
Benzoyl peroxide (p.1143·2).
*Acne.*

**Clearasil Cleanser** Procter & Gamble, Canad.
*Lotion:* Salicylic acid (p.1157·1).
*Acne.*

**Clearasil Clearstick**
Procter & Gamble, Canad.; Procter & Gamble, USA.
Salicylic acid (p.1157·1).
*Acne.*

**Clearasil Daily Face Wash**
Note. This name is used for preparations of different composition.
Boots Healthcare, Austral.
Phenoxyisopropanol (p.1189·2).
*Acne.*

*Procter & Gamble, USA.*
Triclosan (p.1195·2).

**Clearasil Double Action Pads** *Crookes Healthcare, UK.*
Salicylic acid (p.1157·1).
Formerly known as Clearasil Dual Action Pads.
*Acne.*

**Clearasil Double Clear** *Richardson-Vicks, USA.*
Salicylic acid (p.1157·1); alcohol (p.1166·1); hamamelis (p.1696·3).

**Clearasil Double Textured Pads** *Procter & Gamble, USA.*
Salicylic acid (p.1157·1); alcohol (p.1166·1).

**Clearasil Face Wash** *Procter & Gamble, Canad.*
Triclosan (p.1195·2).
Formerly contained phenoxypropanol.
*Acne.*

**Clearasil Jabon** *Procter & Gamble, Mex.†.*
Triclosan (p.1195·2).

**Clearasil Max 10** *Procter & Gamble (H&B Care), UK†.*
Benzoyl peroxide (p.1143·2).
*Acne.*

**Clearasil Medicated Cleanser** *Procter & Gamble, Canad.†.*
Salicylic acid (p.1157·1); alcohol (p.1166·1).
*Acne.*

**Clearasil Medicated Face Wash** *Procter & Gamble (H&B Care), UK†.*
Phenoxypropanol (p.1189·1).
*Acne.*

**Clearasil Medicated Moisturiser** *Procter & Gamble (H&B Care), UK†.*
Triclosan (p.1195·2).
*Acne.*

**Clearasil Medicated Wipes** *Boots Healthcare, Austral.*
Salicylic acid (p.1157·1).
*Acne.*

**Clearasil Nightclear** *Procter & Gamble (H&B Care), UK†.*
Salicylic acid (p.1157·1).
*Acne.*

**Clearasil Pads**
*Procter & Gamble, Canad.; Procter & Gamble, Mex.†.*
Salicylic acid (p.1157·1).
*Acne.*

**Clearasil Plus** *Procter & Gamble, Mex.†.*
Benzoyl peroxide (p.1143·2).

**Clearasil Pore Cleansing Lotion** *Crookes Healthcare, UK.*
Chlorhexidine gluconate (p.1173·2); alcohol (p.1166·1).
Formerly known as Clearasil Medicated Lotion.
*Acne.*

**Clearasil Sensitive Skin Cleanser** *Procter & Gamble, Canad.†.*
Cetrimonium bromide (p.1173·1); chlorhexidine gluconate (p.1173·2); alcohol (p.1166·1).
*Acne.*

**Clearasil Soap** *Procter & Gamble (H&B Care), UK†.*
Triclosan (p.1195·2).
*Acne.*

**Clearasil Stay Clear** *Procter & Gamble, Canad.*
Salicylic acid (p.1157·1).
*Acne.*

**Clearasil Ultra**
*Boots Healthcare, Austral.; Procter & Gamble, Ital.†; Boots Healthcare, NZ.*
Benzoyl peroxide (p.1143·2).
*Acne.*

**Clearasil Wash Antiseptico** *Procter & Gamble, Mex.†.*
Triclosan (p.1195·2).

**Clearblue**
*Novartis Consumer, Canad.; Polive, Fr.; Unipath, Israel; Farmades, Ital.; Pfizer, NZ; Unipath, UK.*
Pregnancy or fertility test (p.1734·3).

**Clearblue Easy**
*Whitehall, Braz.; Whitehall, USA.*
Pregnancy test (p.1734·3).

**Clearblue One Step** *Pfizer Consumer, Austral.*
Pregnancy test (p.1734·3).

**Clearex** *Medibrands, Israel.*
Salicylic acid (p.1157·1).
*Acne.*

**Clearex Cover Up** *Medibrands, Israel.*
Benzoyl peroxide (p.1143·2).
*Acne.*

**Clear-Flex Formula 13, 15, 55, 62, 91, AA, AB, AC** *Bieffe, Switz.†.*
A range of glucose and electrolyte solutions for peritoneal dialysis (p.1221·1).

**Clearine** *Dominion, India.*
Naphazoline hydrochloride (p.1124·3).
*Eye irritation.*

**Clearon** *Sanofi Synthelabo, Spain†.*
Binifibrate (p.875·1).
*Hyperlipidaemias.*

**Clearplan**
*Novartis Consumer, Canad.; Wyeth Consumer, Chile; Polive, Fr.; Farmades, Ital.; Pfizer, NZ; Whitehall-Robins, Switz.; Unipath, UK†.*
Fertility test (p.1734·3).

**Clearplan Easy** *Whitehall, USA.*
Fertility test (p.1734·3).

**Clearplan One Step** *Pfizer Consumer, Austral.*
Fertility test (p.1734·3).

**Clearsing** *Duncan, Arg.*
Azithromycin (p.159·1).
*Bacterial infections.*

**Clearskin Acne Defense Stick** *Avon, Canad.*
Salicylic acid (p.1157·1).
*Acne.*

**Clearskin Antibacterial** *Avon, Canad.*
*Cream:* Benzethonium chloride (p.1169·2).
*Soap:* Triclosan (p.1195·2).
*Acne.*

**Clearskin Cleansing** *Avon, Canad.*
Salicylic acid (p.1157·1).
*Acne.*

**Clearskin Medicated Cleanser** *Avon, Canad.*
Triclosan (p.1195·2).
*Acne.*

**Clearskin Medicated Wash** *Avon, Canad.*
Salicylic acid (p.1157·1).
*Acne.*

**Clearskin 2 Medicated Wash** *Avon, Canad.†.*
Salicylic acid (p.1157·1).
*Acne.*

**Clearskin Overnight Acne Treatment** *Avon, Canad.*
Salicylic acid (p.1157·1).
*Acne.*

**Clearskin 2 Overnight Acne Treatment** *Avon, Canad.†.*
Salicylic acid (p.1157·1); alcohol (p.1166·1).
*Acne.*

**Clearskin 2 Tinted Blemish** *Avon, Canad.†.*
Sulfur (p.1158·2); resorcinol (p.1156·3).
*Acne.*

**Clearskin 2 Triple Action** *Avon, Canad.†.*
Salicylic acid (p.1157·1).
*Acne.*

**Clearsol** *Coventry, UK†.*
Tar acids (p.1193·3).

**Clearsore** *Pinewood, UK.*
Aciclovir (p.626·1).
*Herpes simplex infections of the lips and face.*

**Clear-View**
*Note. A similar name is used for preparations of different composition (see below).*
*Colgate Oral Care, Austral.†.*
Demisting solution for dental mirrors and spectacles.

**Clearview HCG**
*Note. A similar name is used for preparations of different composition (see above).*
*Pfizer Consumer, Austral.; Searle, Port.†; Unipath, UK; Wampole, USA.*
Pregnancy test (p.1734·3).

**Clebofex** *Quimedical, Port.*
Clebopride malate (p.1260·3).
*Gastrointestinal disorders; neuroses.*

**Cleboril** *Almirall, Spain.*
Clebopride malate (p.1260·3).
*Gastrointestinal disorders; nausea and vomiting.*

**Clebudan** *Grunenthal, Chile.*
Budesonide (p.1094·2).
*Nasal polyps; obstructive airways disease; rhinitis.*

**Clebutec** *Pharmacia, Port.*
Clebopride malate (p.1260·3).
*Gastrointestinal disorders.*

**Cledist** *Jaldes, Fr.*
Selenium; zinc citrate; ascorbic acid; vitamin E (p.1417·1).
*Nutritional supplement.*

**Cleensheen** *Florafaun, Austral.†.*
Malathion (Maldison) (p.1507·1).
*Pediculosis.*

**Clematis III Oligoplex** *Madaus, Arg.*
Hamamelis (p.1696·3); clematis recta; sanguinaria (p.1741·3).
*Inflammation.*

**Clembroxol** *Ferring, Port.†.*
Ambroxol hydrochloride (p.1114·3); clenbuterol hydrochloride (p.784·2).
*Respiratory-tract disorders.*

**Clembumar** *Dupomar, Arg.*
Clenbuterol hydrochloride (p.784·2).
*Obstructive airways disease.*

**Clemental** *Therabel, Fr.*
Tiapride hydrochloride (p.725·1).
*Aggression; agitation; childhood behaviour disorders; choreas; pain; Tourette's syndrome.*

**Clements Iron** *Felton, Austral.†.*
Multivitamin, mineral, and glucose preparation with iron (p.1434·3)(p.1417·1).
*Iron deficiency; nutritional anaemia.*

**Clements Tonic** *Felton, Austral.†.*
Mineral preparation with malt, honey, thiamine, and yeast (p.1417·1).
*Dietary supplement.*

**Clemenzil ST** *Medopharm, Ger.†.*
Melilotus officinalis.
*Chronic venous insufficiency; haemorrhoids; thrombophlebitis.*

**Clenasma**
*Biomedica, Hong Kong; Biomedica, Ital.*
Clenbuterol hydrochloride (p.784·2).
*Obstructive airways disease.*

**Clenia** *Upsher-Smith, USA.*
Sulfacetamide sodium (p.257·3); sulfur (p.1158·2).
*Acne.*

**Cleniderm** *Chiesi, Ital.†.*
Beclometasone dipropionate (p.1091·1).
*Skin disorders.*

**Clenil**
*Note. This name is used for preparations of different composition.*
*Farmalab, Braz.; Chiesi, Hong Kong†; Chiesi, Ital.; Rolab, S.Afr.; Chiesi, Singapore; Chiesi, Thai.*
Beclometasone dipropionate (p.1091·1).
*Nasal polyps; obstructive airways disease; rhinitis; sinusitis.*

*Chiesi, Gr.*
Dexamethasone dipropionate (p.1097·3).
*Allergic rhinitis.*

**Clenil Compositum**
*Farmalab, Braz.; Promedica, Ital.; Chiesi, Singapore; Chiesi, Thai.*
Beclometasone dipropionate (p.1091·1); salbutamol (p.791·3) or salbutamol sulfate (p.791·3).
*Obstructive airways disease.*

**Clenil "Forte Jet"** *Chiesi, Gr.*
Beclometasone dipropionate (p.1091·1).
*Asthma.*

**Clenilexx** *Promedica, Ital.*
Beclometasone dipropionate (p.1091·1).
*Obstructive airways disease.*

**Clen-Zym** *Alcon, UK.*
Pancreatin (p.1725·3) (p.1164·2).
*Soft contact lens cleanser.*

**Cleocin**
*Pharmacia, Austral.; Pharmacia, Austria; Pharmacia Upjohn, Ital.; Pharmacia, USA.*
Clindamycin hydrochloride (p.194·2) or clindamycin phosphate (p.194·2).
*Bacterial infections.*

**Cleocin T** *Pharmacia, USA.*
Clindamycin phosphate (p.194·2).
*Acne.*

**Cleregil** *Monot, Fr.†.*
Deanol aceglumate (p.1585·3).
*Asthenia.*

**Cleridium** *IPRAD, Fr.*
Dipyridamole (p.903·1).
*Thromboembolism prophylaxis.*

**Clerz**
*Ciba Vision, Austral.†; Ciba Vision, Canad.*
Poloxamer 407 (p.1414·2) (p.1164·2).
*Lubricating, cleansing, and hydrating eye drops for contact lenses.*

*Alcon, USA.*
Range of solutions for contact lenses (p.1164·2).

**Clerz Moisturising Drops** *Ciba Vision, Austral.†.*
Povidone (p.1581·2).
Formerly contained hyetellose and poloxamer 407.
*Dry eyes.*

**Clesidren** *FD, Ital.†.*
Epomediol (p.1683·3).
*Liver disorders.*

**Cletonol** *Merck, Arg.*
Nimodipine (p.972·3).
*Neurological deficit following subarachnoid haemorrhage.*

**Clever** *Chiesi, Ital.*
Ebastine (p.433·1).
*Allergic conjunctivitis; allergic rhinitis; urticaria.*

**Cleveral** *Aesculapius, Ital.†.*
Piracetam (p.1732·1).
*Mental function impairment.*

**Cleveron** *TRB, Braz.*
Alendronate sodium (p.765·3).
*Osteoporosis.*

**Clevian** *Aesculapius, Ital.*
Piroxicam (p.84·2).
*Musculoskeletal and joint disorders.*

**Clevosan** *Baliarda, Arg.*
*Ointment:* Centella (p.1144·3); neomycin sulfate (p.235·1).
*Topical powder:* Centella (p.1144·3); neomycin (p.235·1); zinc undecenoate (p.411·1); zinc oxide (p.1163·2).
*Topical spray:* Centella (p.1144·3); tetracaine (p.1385·1).
*Skin disorders.*

**Clexane**
*Aventis, Arg.; Aventis, Austral.; Aventis, Belg.; Aventis, Braz.; Aventis, Chile; Aventis, Ger.; Aventis, Gr.; Aventis, Hong Kong; Aventis, India; Aventis, Irl.; Aventis, Israel; Aventis, Ital.; Aventis, Malaysia; Aventis, Mex.; Aventis, Neth.; Aventis, NZ; Aventis, S.Afr.; Aventis, Singapore; Aventis, Spain; Aventis, Switz.; Aventis, Thai.; Aventis, UK.*
Enoxaparin sodium (p.910·3).
*Deep-vein thrombosis; myocardial infarction; prevention of clotting during haemodialysis; pulmonary embolism; thromboembolism prophylaxis; unstable angina.*

**Cliacil** *Aventis, Austria.*
Phenoxymethylpenicillin potassium (p.242·1).
*Bacterial infections.*

**Cliane**
*Schering, Braz.; Schering, Chile; Schering, Mex.; Schering, NZ.*
Estradiol (p.1550·1); norethisterone acetate (p.1562·2).
*Menopausal disorders; osteoporosis.*

**Clibium** *Klinger, Braz.*
Ginkgo biloba (p.1692·3).
*Vascular disorders.*

**Clidets** *Stiefel, Chile.*
Clindamycin phosphate (p.194·2).
*Acne.*

**Clifemin** *Herbarium, Braz.*
Cimicifuga (p.1671·3).
*Menopausal symptoms.*

**Clifordin** *Knoll, Belg.†.*
Doxycycline (p.206·2) or doxycycline hyclate (p.206·2).
*Bacterial infections.*

**Climabelle** *Schering, Austria.*
16 Tablets, estradiol valerate (p.1550·2); 12 tablets, estradiol valerate; levonorgestrel (p.1563·2).
*Menopausal disorders; osteoporosis.*

**Climacilin** *Climax, Braz.†.*
Benzylpenicillin sodium (p.163·2); procaine benzylpenicillin (p.246·1); streptomycin sulfate (p.256·2).
*Bacterial infections.*

**Climacteron** *Sabex, Canad.*
Testosterone enantate benzilic acid hydrazone (p.1571·2); estradiol dienanthate (p.1550·1); estradiol benzoate (p.1550·1).
*Menopausal disorders; osteoporosis.*

**Climadan** *Dankos, Singapore.*
Clindamycin hydrochloride (p.194·2).
*Bacterial infections.*

**Climaderm**
*Wyeth, Arg.; Wyeth, Braz.; Wyeth, Chile; Wyeth, Mex.*
Estradiol (p.1550·1).
*Menopausal disorders; osteoporosis.*

**Climadil** *Marjan, Braz.*
Red clover (p.1737·3).
*Menopausal symptoms.*

**Climagest** *Novartis, UK.*
16 Tablets, estradiol valerate (p.1550·2); 12 tablets, estradiol valerate; norethisterone (p.1562·2).
*Menopausal disorders.*

**Climara**
*Schering, Austral.; Schering, Austria; Schering, Belg.; Berlex, Canad.; Schering, Denm.; Schering, Fin.; Schering, Fr.; Schering, Irl.; Schering, Israel†; Schering, Ital.; Schering, Neth.; Schering, Norw.; Schering, NZ; Schering, Port.; Schering, S.Afr.; Schering, Swed.; Schering, Switz.; Schering, Thai.; Berlex, USA.*
Estradiol (p.1550·1).
*Menopausal disorders; osteoporosis.*

**Climara Duo**
*Schering, Fin.*
Patch I, estradiol (p.1550·1); patch II, estradiol; levonorgestrel (p.1563·2).
*Hormone replacement therapy.*

*Schering, Port.*
4 Patches, estradiol (p.1550·1); 4 patches, estradiol; levonorgestrel (p.1563·2).
*Menopausal disorders.*

**ClimaraPro** *Berlex, USA.*
Estradiol (p.1550·1); levonorgestrel (p.1563·2).
*Menopausal disorders.*

**Climarest** *Wyeth, Ger.*
Conjugated oestrogens (p.1543·2).
*Menopausal disorders; osteoporosis.*

**Climaston** *Solvay, Fr.*
*Tablets 1mg/5mg:* Estradiol (p.1550·1); dydrogesterone (p.1549·2).
*Tablets, 1mg/10mg; tablets 2mg/10mg:* 14 Tablets, estradiol (p.1550·1); 14 tablets, estradiol; dydrogesterone (p.1549·2).
*Menopausal disorders; osteoporosis.*

**Climatidine** *Climax, Braz.*
Cimetidine (p.1255·3).
*Gastro-oesophageal reflux; gastrointestinal haemorrhage; peptic ulcer; Zollinger-Ellison syndrome.*

**Climatrol E** *Gynopharm, Chile.*
Conjugated oestrogens (p.1543·2).
*Menopausal disorders.*

**Climatrol Ht** *Gynopharm, Chile.*
17 Tablets, conjugated oestrogens (p.1543·2); 13 tablets, conjugated oestrogens; medroxyprogesterone acetate (p.1557·2).
*Menopausal disorders.*

**Climatrol Ht Continuo** *Gynopharm, Chile.*
Conjugated oestrogens (p.1543·2); medroxyprogesterone acetate (p.1557·2).
*Menopausal disorders.*

**Climaval** *Novartis, UK.*
Estradiol valerate (p.1550·2).
*Menopausal disorders.*

**Climaxol** *Lehning, Fr.*
Hamamelis (p.1696·3); viburnum; ruscus aculeatus; hydrastis (p.1698·3); aesculus (p.1648·2).
*Peripheral vascular disorders.*

**Climen**
*Schering, Austral.*
11 Tablets, estradiol valerate (p.1550·2); 10 tablets, cyproterone acetate (p.1544·1); estradiol valerate.
28-Day packs contain 16 and 12 tablets, respectively.
*Menopausal disorders.*

*Schering, Austria; Schering, Belg.; Schering, Denm.; Schering, Ger.; Schering, Hong Kong; Schering, Ital.; Schering, Malaysia; Schering, Norw.; Schering, Port.; Schering, Singapore; Schering, Spain; Schering, Switz.; Schering, Thai.*
11 Tablets, estradiol valerate (p.1550·2); 10 tablets, estradiol valerate; cyproterone acetate (p.1544·1).
*Menopausal disorders; menstrual disorders; osteoporosis.*

Schering, S.Afr.
11 Tablets, estradiol valerate (p.1550·2); 10 tablets, estradiol valerate; cyproterone acetate (p.1544·1); 7 tablets, inert.
*Menopausal disorders; osteoporosis.*

**Climene** Schering, Arg.; Schering, Braz.
White tablets, estradiol valerate (p.1550·2); pink tablets, estradiol valerate; cyproterone acetate (p.1544·1).
*Menopausal disorders; osteoporosis.*

Schering, Chile; Schering, Fr.; Schering, Mex.
11 Tablets, estradiol valerate (p.1550·2); 10 tablets, cyproterone acetate (p.1544·1); estradiol valerate.
*Menopausal disorders; osteoporosis.*

Schering, Neth.
16 Tablets, estradiol valerate (p.1550·2); 12 tablets, cyproterone acetate (p.1544·1); estradiol valerate.
*Menopausal disorders; osteoporosis.*

**Climesse** Novartis, UK.
Estradiol valerate (p.1550·2); norethisterone (p.1562·2).
*Menopausal disorders; osteoporosis.*

**Climil-80** Wassen, Ital.
Soya (p.1447·2); cimicifuga (p.1671·3).

**Climil Complex** Wassen, Ital.
Soya (p.1447·2); cimicifuga (p.1671·3); griffonia simplicifolia (p.1696·1).

**Climil Gel** Wassen, Ital.
Soya isoflavones (p.1447·2); mimosa tenuiflora.

**Climodien** Schering, Denm.; Schering, Ger.; Schering, Norw.; Schering, Port.; Schering, Spain; Schering, Swed.
Estradiol valerate (p.1550·2); dienogest (p.1548·1).
*Menopausal disorders.*

**Climopax** Wyeth, Ger.
Conjugated oestrogens (p.1543·2); medroxyprogesterone acetate (p.1557·2).
*Menopausal disorders; osteoporosis.*

**Climopax Cyclo** Wyeth, Ger.
14 Tablets, conjugated oestrogens (p.1543·2); 14 tablets, conjugated oestrogens; medroxyprogesterone acetate (p.1557·2).
*Menopausal disorders; osteoporosis.*

**Clinac**
Note. This name is used for preparations of different composition.
Pacific, Hong Kong.
Clindamycin (p.194·2).
*Acne.*

Pacific, NZ.
Clindamycin phosphate (p.194·2).
*Acne.*

Edol, Port.
Erythromycin (p.208·1).
*Acne.*

**Clinac BPO** Ferndale, USA.
Benzoyl peroxide (p.1143·2).
*Acne.*

**Clinadil** Grunenthal, Spain.
Cinnarizine (p.428·3); dihydroergocristine mesilate (p.1680·1).
*Cerebrovascular disorders.*

**Clinadil Compositum** Grunenthal, Spain.
Cinnarizine (p.428·3); co-dergocrine mesilate (p.1674·1); heptaminol acefyllinate (p.786·3).
*Cerebrovascular disorders.*

**Clinadol** Gador, Arg.
Flurbiprofen (p.43·3).
*Musculoskeletal, joint, and peri-articular disorders; pain.*

**Clinadryl** Bangkok Lab & Cosmetic, Thai.
Diphenhydramine hydrochloride (p.431·3); ammonium chloride (p.1115·2).
*Bronchitis; cold symptoms; hypersensitivity reactions.*

**Clinagel** Stiefel, Braz.
Clindamycin phosphate (p.194·2).
*Acne.*

**Clinal** Andromaco, Arg.
Sulfanilamide (p.263·2); zinc oxide (p.1163·2); vitamin A; vitamin D.
*Skin disorders.*

**Clinasol** Gambar, Ital.†.
Sodium tetrachloroiodite.
*Infections; water purification.*

**Clinda** 1A, Ger.; Hameln, Ger.; Lichtenstein, Ger.; Wolff, Ger.
Clindamycin hydrochloride (p.194·2), clindamycin palmitate hydrochloride (p.194·2), or clindamycin phosphate (p.194·2).
*Bacterial infections.*

**Clindabeta** Betapharm, Ger.
Clindamycin hydrochloride (p.194·2).
*Bacterial infections.*

**Clindac** Hexal, Austria.
Clindamycin hydrochloride (p.194·2).
*Bacterial infections.*

Intramed, S.Afr.†.
Clindamycin (p.194·2).
*Bacterial infections.*

**Clindacin** Panalab, Arg.
Clindamycin phosphate (p.194·2).
*Acne.*

**Clindacne** Igefarma, Braz.†.
Clindamycin (p.194·2).
*Acne.*

**Clinda-Derm** Paddock, USA†.
Clindamycin phosphate (p.194·2).
*Acne.*

**Clindagel** Galderma, USA.
Clindamycin phosphate (p.194·2).
*Acne.*

**Clindahexal** Hexal, Ger.; Hexal, S.Afr.
Clindamycin hydrochloride (p.194·2) or clindamycin phosphate (p.194·2).
*Bacterial infections.*

**Clindal**
Note. This name is used for preparations of different composition.
Hexal, Austria.
Clindamycin hydrochloride (p.194·2).
*Bacterial infections.*

Merck, Braz.
Azithromycin (p.159·1).
*Bacterial infections.*

**ClindaMax** PharmaDerm, USA.
Clindamycin phosphate (p.194·2).
*Acne.*

**Clindamin C** Teuto, Braz.
Clindamycin hydrochloride (p.194·2).
*Bacterial infections.*

**Clindarix** Ariston, Braz.
Clindamycin (p.194·2).
*Bacterial infections.*

**Clinda-saar** Rosen, Ger.
Clindamycin hydrochloride (p.194·2) or clindamycin phosphate (p.194·2).
*Bacterial infections.*

**Clindastad** Stada, Ger.
Clindamycin hydrochloride (p.194·2).
*Bacterial infections.*

**Clindatech** Dermatech, Austral.; Dermatech, Singapore.
Clindamycin hydrochloride (p.194·2).
*Acne.*

**Clindaz** Merck, Braz.†.
Azithromycin (p.159·1).
*Bacterial infections.*

**Clindazyn** Lemery, Mex.
Clindamycin phosphate (p.194·2).
*Bacterial infections.*

**Clindets** Stiefel, USA.
Clindamycin phosphate (p.194·2).
*Acne.*

**Clindex** Chelsea, USA.
Clidinium bromide (p.480·2); chlordiazepoxide hydrochloride (p.674·2).
*Gastrointestinal disorders.*

**Clindopax** Lagos, Arg.
Clindamycin phosphate (p.194·2).
*Bacterial infections.*

**Clinensol** Allergan, Braz.
Miranol (p.1164·2).
*Cleansing solution for contact lenses.*

**Clinesfar** Essex, Ger.
Erythromycin (p.208·1); tretinoin (p.1161·1).
*Acne.*

**Clinfar** Merck, Braz.
Simvastatin (p.997·1).
*Hyperlipidaemias.*

**Clinic A Retinol Vital Day** Jamieson, Canad.
*SPF 20:* Meradimate (p.1151·3); octinoxate (p.1154·3); octisalate (p.1154·3); oxybenzone (p.1154·3).
*Sunscreen.*

**Clinical Program Thickened Juice** Nutricia, Austral.
Food thickener (p.1417·1).
*Dysphagia.*

**Cliniderm** Wild, Switz.
*Cream:* Polyethylene granules (abrasive) (p.1140·1); salicylic acid (p.1157·1).
*Topical solution:* Triclosan (p.1195·2).
*Acne; seborrhoea.*

**Clinifeed** Clintec, Irl.†; Nestle, UK†.
Preparation for enteral nutrition (p.1417·1).

**Clinigel** Orion, Austral.; Orion, NZ.
Lubricating gel.

**Clinikold** Bangkok Lab & Cosmetic, Thai.
Triprolidine hydrochloride (p.442·3); pseudoephedrine hydrochloride (p.1129·2).
*Allergic rhinitis; cold symptoms; nasal congestion.*

**Clinimet** Bangkok Lab & Cosmetic, Thai.
Cimetidine (p.1255·3).
*Peptic ulcer; Zollinger-Ellison syndrome.*

**Clinimix** Clintec, Austria; Baxter, Belg.†; Clintec, Denm.; Baxter, Fin.; Baxter, Fr.; Baxter, Ger.; Baxter, Gr.; Baxter, Ital.; Baxter, Spain; Baxter, Swed.; Baxter, UK.
A range of amino-acid and carbohydrate infusions with or without electrolytes (p.1417·1).
*Parenteral nutrition.*

**Clinimycin** Galen, Irl.
Oxytetracycline (p.241·1).
*Bacterial infections.*

**Clinique Acne Spot Treatment** Clinique, Canad.
Salicylic acid (p.1157·1).
*Acne.*

**Clinisorb** CliniMed, UK.
Activated charcoal (p.1030·2).
*Malodorous wounds.*

**Clinistix** Bayer, Austral.; Miles, Canad.†; Bayer Diagnostics, Fr.; Bayer Diagnostics, Irl.; Ames, Israel; Bayer Diagnostici, Ital.; Bayer, NZ; Bayer, Port.; Bayer Diagnostics, UK; Bayer, USA.
Test for glucose in urine (p.1694·2).

**Clinit N** Hormosan, Ger.
Sodium salamidacetate (p.87·3).
Lidocaine (p.1377·3) is included in this preparation to alleviate the pain of injection.
Formerly consisted of 2 ampoules: ampoule 1, sodium salamidacetate and ampoule 2, cyanocobalamin.
*Joint disorders; severe pain.*

**Clinitar** Shire, Irl.†; Cambridge Healthcare, UK.
Coal tar (Stantar) (p.1159·2).
*Dandruff; eczema; psoriasis; seborrhoeic dermatitis.*

**Clinitek HCG** Bayer, Austral.
Pregnancy test (p.1734·3).

**Clinitek Microalbumin** Bayer, Austral.
Test for albumin and creatinine in urine.

**Clinitest** Bayer, Austral.; Bayer, Canad.; Bayer Diagnostics, Fr.; Bayer Diagnostics, Irl.; Ames, Israel; Bayer Diagnostici, Ital.; Bayer Diagnostics, Mex.; Bayer, NZ; Bayer Diagnostics, UK; Bayer, USA.
Test for reducing substances in urine (p.1694·2).
In the *UK* these are described in the Drug Tariff as Copper Solution Reagent Tablets.

**Clinium**
Note. This name is used for preparations of different composition.
Instituto Sanitas, Chile.
Fluoxetine hydrochloride (p.292·1).
*Bulimia; depression; obsessive-compulsive disorder.*

Ethnor, India.
Lidoflazine (p.946·3).
*Ischaemic heart disease.*

**Clinoderm** Bangkok Lab & Cosmetic, Thai.
Clobetasol propionate (p.1095·2).
*Skin disorders.*

**Clinofar** SmithKline Beecham, Gr.
Sodium chloride (p.1233·3).
*Nasal congestion.*

**Clinofem** Pharmacia, Ger.
Medroxyprogesterone acetate (p.1557·2).
*Endometriosis; menopausal disorders; menstrual disorders; test of ovarian function.*

**Clinofug D** Wolff, Ger.
Doxycycline hyclate (p.206·2).
*Acne.*

**Clinofug Gel** Wolff, Ger.†.
Erythromycin (p.208·1).
*Acne.*

**Clinogel** Viatris, Fr.
Isopropyl alcohol (p.1184·3); triclosan (p.1195·2).
*Hand disinfection.*

**Clinoleic** Baxter Immuno, Arg.; Clintec, Austria; Baxter, Belg.†; Clintec, Denm.; Baxter, Fin.; Baxter, Fr.; Baxter, Ger.; Clintec, Gr.; Clintec, Israel; Baxter, Ital.; Baxter, Mex.; Baxter, Spain; Baxter, Swed.; Baxter, Switz.; Baxter, UK.
Olive oil (p.1723·2); soya oil (p.1447·2).
May contain egg lecithin or egg phosphatides.
*Lipid infusion for parenteral nutrition.*

**Clinomel** Baxter Immuno, Arg.; Clintec, Austria; Baxter, Belg.†; Baxter, Fin.; Baxter, Fr.; Baxter, Ger.; Clintec, Gr.; Baxter, Ital.; Adcock Ingram Critical Care, S.Afr.; Baxter, Spain; Baxter, Swed.; Baxter, UK†.
Amino-acid, electrolyte, glucose, and lipid (from soya oil (p.1447·2)) infusion (p.1417·1).
May contain egg lecithin or egg phosphatides.
*Parenteral nutrition.*

Baxter, Braz.†.
Amino-acid, glucose, and lipid infusion (p.1417·1).
*Parenteral nutrition.*

**Clinopront** Bangkok Lab & Cosmetic, Thai.
Codeine phosphate (p.27·1); guaifenesin (p.1122·1).
*Coughs.*

**Clinoril** Merck Sharp & Dohme, Austral.; Merck Sharp & Dohme, Austria; Merck Sharp & Dohme, Belg.; Merck Frosst, Canad.†; Merck Sharp & Dohme, Denm.; Merck Sharp & Dohme, Hong Kong; Merck Sharp & Dohme, Irl.; Neopharmed, Ital.; Merck Sharp & Dohme, Malaysia; Merck Sharp & Dohme, Mex.; Merck Sharp & Dohme, Neth.; Merck Sharp & Dohme, Norw.; Merck Sharp & Dohme, NZ; Merck Sharp & Dohme, S.Afr.†; Merck Sharp & Dohme, Swed.; Merck Sharp & Dohme, Switz.; Merck Sharp & Dohme, Thai.; Merck Sharp & Dohme, UK; Merck, USA.
Sulindac (p.91·2).
*Gout; musculoskeletal, joint, and peri-articular disorders.*

**Clinovir**
Note. This name is used for preparations of different composition.
Pharmacia, Ger.
Medroxyprogesterone acetate (p.1557·2).
*Breast cancer; endometrial cancer.*

Bangkok Lab & Cosmetic, Thai.
Aciclovir (p.626·1).
*Herpes simplex infections of the skin and mucous membranes.*

**Clin-Sanorania** Lichtenstein, Ger.
Clindamycin hydrochloride (p.194·2).
*Bacterial infections.*

**Clintopic** ICN, Arg.
Clindamycin hydrochloride (p.194·2).
*Acne.*

**Clinutren** Nestle, Fr.; Nestle Clinical, Irl.; Nestle, Ital.; Nestle, UK.
A range of preparations for enteral nutrition (p.1417·1).

**Clinvit** Plants, Ital.
Royal jelly (p.1740·3).
*Nutritional supplement.*

**Clinwas** Chiesi, Spain.
Clindamycin phosphate (p.194·2).
*Bacterial infections.*

**Clio-Betnovate** Glaxo Wellcome, Mex.
Betamethasone valerate (p.1093·2); clioquinol (p.196·3).
*Infected skin disorders.*

**Cliogan** Juste, Spain.
Estradiol (p.1550·1).
*Menopausal disorders; osteoporosis.*

**Cliovyl** Zarbi (Ζαρμπη), Gr.
Nimesulide (p.67·1).
*Inflammation; musculoskeletal disorders; pain.*

**Clipper** Chiesi, Ital.
Beclometasone dipropionate (p.1091·1).
*Ulcerative colitis.*

**Clipto** Quimifar, Spain.
Enalapril maleate (p.909·2).
*Heart failure; hypertension.*

**Cliptol** Pierre Fabre Sante, Fr.
Ibuprofen (p.45·3); menthol (p.1711·3).
*Soft-tissue disorders.*

**Cliptol Sport** Pierre Fabre Sante, Fr.
Methyl nicotinate (p.59·2); capsaicin (p.24·2).
*Muscle cramps; sports injuries.*

**C-Lisa** Lisapharma, Ital.
Ascorbic acid (p.1460·2).
*Vitamin C deficiency.*

**Clisemina** Juventus, Spain†.
Doxycycline hyclate (p.206·2).
*Bacterial infections.*

**Clisflex** Sella, Ital.
Monobasic sodium phosphate (p.1230·3); dibasic sodium phosphate (p.1231·1).
*Bowel evacuation; constipation.*

**Clisin** Juste, Spain.
11 Tablets, estradiol valerate (p.1550·2); 10 tablets estradiol valerate; cyproterone acetate (p.1544·1).
*Menopausal disorders; osteoporosis.*

**Clisma Bieffe Medital** Bieffe, Spain†.
Monobasic sodium phosphate (p.1230·3); dibasic sodium phosphate (p.1231·1).
*Bowel evacuation; constipation.*

**Clisma Fleet** Bergamon, Ital.
Monobasic sodium phosphate (p.1230·3); dibasic sodium phosphate (p.1231·1).
*Bowel evacuation; constipation.*

**Clisma-Lax** Sofar, Ital.
Monobasic sodium phosphate monohydrate (p.1230·3); hydrated dibasic sodium phosphate (p.1231·1).
*Bowel evacuation; constipation.*

**Clistin**
Note. This name is used for preparations of different composition.
Klinger, Braz.
Loratadine (p.436·1).
*Hypersensitivity reactions.*

Ethnor, India.
Dextromethorphan hydrobromide (p.1117·3); carbinoxamine maleate (p.426·3); ammonium chloride (p.1115·2); sodium citrate (p.1223·2).
*Coughs.*

**Clitaxel** Pharmacia, Arg.
Paclitaxel (p.577·3).
*Breast cancer; Kaposi's sarcoma; non-small cell lung cancer; ovarian cancer.*

**Clivarin** Baxter, Austria; Abbott, Denm.; Knoll, Fin.†; Abbott, Ger.; Knoll, Norw.†; Knoll, Port.; Knoll, Swed.†.
Reviparin sodium (p.995·3).
*Thromboembolism prophylaxis.*

**Clivarina** Schwarz, Ital.
Reviparin sodium (p.995·3).
*Thromboembolic disorders.*

**Clivarine** Knoll, Fr.; Knoll, India; ICN, UK.
Reviparin sodium (p.995·3).
*Thromboembolism prophylaxis.*

**Clivasol** Eczane, Arg.
Povidone-iodine (p.1190·3).
*Disinfection.*

**Clivoten** Italfarmaco, Ital.
Isradipine (p.942·2).
*Hypertension.*

**Clo-5** Danes, Arg.
Sodium cromoglicate (p.795·3).
*Bronchospasm.*

**Clo Zinc** Llorens, Spain†.
Chloramphenicol (p.185·1); naphazoline hydrochloride (p.1124·3); zinc sulfate (p.1469·3).
*Eye disorders; eye infections.*

**Clobasol** Jean-Marie, Hong Kong.
Clobetasol propionate (p.1095·2).
*Skin disorders.*

**Clobasone** Pharmaland, Thai.
Clobetasol propionate (p.1095·2).
*Skin disorders.*

**Clobatos** Bago, Chile.
Clobutinol hydrochloride (p.1117·1).
*Coughs.*

**Clobegalen** Galen, Ger.
Clobetasol propionate (p.1095·2).
*Skin disorders.*

**Clobemix** Douglas, Austral.
Moclobemide (p.308·2).
*Depression.*

**Clobendian** Efarmes, Spain.
Diltiazem hydrochloride (p.900·1).
*Angina pectoris; hypertension.*

**Cloben-G** Indoco, India.
Clotrimazole (p.396·2); beclometasone dipropionate (p.1091·1); gentamicin (p.219·1).
*Allergic skin disorders; fungal skin infections.*

**Clobeplus** Defuen, Arg.
Clobetasol propionate (p.1095·2); ammonium lactate (p.1142·3).
*Skin disorders.*

**Clobesol**
ICN, Arg.; ICN, Braz.; GlaxoSmithKline, Ital.
Clobetasol propionate (p.1095·2).
*Skin disorders.*

**Clobesol LA** ICN, Arg.
Clobetasol propionate (p.1095·2); ammonium lactate (p.1142·3).
*Skin disorders.*

**Clobeson** Dong Kook, Singapore.
Clobetasol propionate (p.1095·2).
*Skin disorders.*

**Clobet**
Angelini, Ital.; Biolab, Malaysia; Biolab, Thai.
Clobetasol propionate (p.1095·2).
*Eye disorders; skin disorders.*

**Clobetate** Polipharm, Thai.
Clobetasol propionate (p.1095·2).
*Skin disorders.*

**Clobex** Galderma, USA.
Clobetasol propionate (p.1095·2).
*Skin disorders.*

**Cloburate** Dominion, UK†.
Clobetasone butyrate (p.1095·3).
Formerly known as Eumovate Eye Drops.
*Eye disorders.*

**Clob-X** Galderma, Braz.
Clobetasol propionate (p.1095·2).
*Skin disorders.*

**Clocim** Cimex, Switz.†.
Clotrimazole (p.396·2).
*Fungal skin and vaginal infections.*

**Clocream** Roberts, USA.
Cod-liver oil (p.1425·2); colecalciferol (p.1461·3); vitamin A palmitate (p.1453·1).
*Skin disorders.*

**Clocreme**
Pacific, Hong Kong; Pacific, NZ.
Clotrimazole (p.396·2).
*Fungal infections.*

**Clodavan** Medipharm, Chile.
Clobetasol propionate (p.1095·2).
*Skin disorders.*

**Cloderm**
Note. This name is used for preparations of different composition.
Dermapharm, Ger.
Clotrimazole (p.396·2).
*Fungal skin infections.*

Hoe, Malaysia; Hoe, Singapore.
Clobetasol propionate (p.1095·2).
*Skin and scalp disorders.*

Healthpoint, USA.
Clocortolone pivalate (p.1096·1).
*Skin disorders.*

**Clodron** Fidia, Ital.
Disodium clodronate (p.770·2).
*Hyperparathyroidism; multiple myeloma; osteolysis of malignancy; osteoporosis.*

**Clody** Promedica, Ital.
Disodium clodronate (p.770·2).
*Hyperparathyroidism; multiple myeloma; osteolysis of malignancy; osteoporosis.*

**Cloel** Aesculapius, Ital.
Cloperastine fendizoate (p.1117·2).
*Coughs.*

**Clo-Far** Farcoral, Mex.
Diclofenac potassium (p.32·1).
*Inflammation; musculoskeletal and joint disorders; pain.*

**Clofaren** Royton, Braz.
Diclofenac diethylamine (p.32·1).
*Musculoskeletal and joint disorders.*

**Clofec**
Atlantic, Hong Kong; Atlantic, Malaysia; Atlantic, Singapore; Vana, Thai.
Diclofenac sodium (p.32·1).
*Inflammation; musculoskeletal, joint, and peri-articular disorders.*

**Clofeme** Hexal, Austral.
Clotrimazole (p.396·2).
*Vaginal candidiasis.*

**Clofen**
Note. This name is used for preparations of different composition.
Alphapharm, Austral.; Alphapharm, Malaysia; Merck, Malaysia.
Baclofen (p.1386·3).
*Skeletal muscle spasm or spasticity.*

Neckerman, Braz.†; Julphar, UAE.
Diclofenac diethylamine (p.32·1), diclofenac potassium (p.32·1), or diclofenac sodium (p.32·1).
*Gout; inflammation; musculoskeletal, joint, peri-articular, and soft-tissue disorders; pain.*

**Clofenac**
Hovid, Hong Kong; Hovid, Malaysia; Hovid, Singapore.
Diclofenac sodium (p.32·1).
*Gout; musculoskeletal and joint disorders; pain.*

**Clofenak** Medley, Braz.
Diclofenac potassium (p.32·1).
*Gout; inflammation; musculoskeletal, joint, and peri-articular disorders; pain.*

**Clofend** Fidia, Ital.
Cloperastine fendizoate (p.1117·2).
*Coughs.*

**Clofert** Sigma, India.
Clomifene citrate (p.1542·2).
*Anovulatory infertility.*

**Clofexan** Bago, Chile.
Betamethasone (p.1093·1); dexchlorpheniramine maleate (p.427·3).
*Hypersensitivity reactions.*

**Clofon** YF Chem, Thai.
Diclofenac sodium (p.32·1).
*Musculoskeletal, joint, and peri-articular disorders.*

**Clofozine** AstraZeneca, India.
Clofazimine (p.197·1).
*Lepra reactions; leprosy.*

**Clofranil** Sun, Thai.
Clomipramine hydrochloride (p.289·3).
*Depression; narcoleptic syndrome; obsessive-compulsive disorder; phobic states.*

**Clogar** Self-Care Products, UK.
Cod-liver oil (p.1425·2); garlic (p.1691·1).

**Clogen** UCI, Braz.†.
Clotrimazole (p.396·2).
*Fungal skin infections.*

**Cloisone** Psicofarma, Mex.
Levodopa (p.1205·2); carbidopa (p.1204·3).
*Parkinsonism.*

**Clo-Kit** Indoco, India.
Chloroquine phosphate (p.448·2).
*Hepatic amoebiasis; lupus erythematosus; malaria; rheumatoid arthritis.*

**Clomaderm** Parke-Med, S.Afr.†.
Clotrimazole (p.396·2).
*Fungal skin infections.*

**Clomazen** Uniao Quimica, Braz.
Clotrimazole (p.396·2).
*Fungal skin infections.*

**Clomhexal**
Hexal, Austral.; Hexal, Ger.
Clomifene citrate (p.1542·2).
*Anovulatory infertility.*

**Clomicin** IQFA, Mex.
Dicloxacillin sodium (p.205·2).
*Bacterial infections.*

**Clomid**
Aventis, Austral.; Hoechst Marion Roussel, Austria†; Aventis, Belg.; Medley, Braz.; Aventis, Canad.; Aventis, Fr.; Aventis, Hong Kong; Aventis, Irl.; Bruno, Ital.; Aventis, Malaysia; Aventis, Neth.; Aventis, NZ†; Mer-National, S.Afr.; Aventis, Singapore; Aventis, Switz.; Aventis, Thai.; Aventis, UK; Hoechst Marion Roussel, USA.
Clomifene citrate (p.1542·2).
*Anovulatory infertility; male infertility.*

**Clomifen** Leiras, Fin.
Clomifene citrate (p.1542·2).
*Anovulatory infertility; male infertility.*

**Clomifeno** Casen Fleet, Spain†.
Clomifene citrate (p.1542·2).
*Anovulatory infertility; male infertility.*

**Clomihexal** Hexal, S.Afr.
Clomifene citrate (p.1542·2).
*Anovulatory infertility.*

**Clomin**
Quatromed, S.Afr.; Ranbaxy, Thai.†.
Dicycloverine hydrochloride (p.481·2).
*Smooth muscle spasm.*

**Clomivid**
AstraZeneca, Denm.†; AstraZeneca, Norw.†; Tika, Swed.†.
Clomifene citrate (p.1542·2).
*Anovulatory infertility.*

**Clomycin**
Note. This name is used for preparations of different composition.
Neo-Pharma, India.
Clotrimazole (p.396·2); gentamicin (p.219·1).
*Skin and nail infections.*

Roberts, USA†.
Bacitracin (p.161·3); neomycin sulfate (p.235·1); polymyxin B sulfate (p.245·1); lidocaine (p.1377·3).
*Skin infections.*

**Clonagin** Baliarda, Arg.
Clonazepam (p.359·1).
*Anxiety; epilepsy; panic attacks.*

**Clonalgin** Chemopharma, Chile.
Clonixin lysine (p.26·3).
*Pain.*

**Clonalgin Compuesto** Chemopharma, Chile.
Clonixin lysine (p.26·3); ergotamine tartrate (p.467·2).
*Migraine and other vascular headaches.*

**Clonalin** Clonmel, Irl.†.
Diphenhydramine hydrochloride (p.431·3); sodium citrate (p.1223·2); ammonium chloride (p.1115·2); menthol (p.1711·3).
*Coughs; respiratory-tract congestion.*

**Clonamox** Clonmel, Irl.
Amoxicillin trihydrate (p.155·3).
*Bacterial infections.*

**Clonamp** Clonmel, Irl.
Ampicillin trihydrate (p.157·2).
*Bacterial infections.*

**Clonapam**
ICN, Canad.; Laboratorios Chile, Chile.
Clonazepam (p.359·1).
*Anxiety; convulsions; epilepsy; panic attacks; sleep disorders.*

**Clonasten** Teuto, Braz.†.
Clotrimazole (p.396·2).
*Fungal infections.*

**Clonax** Beta, Arg.
Clonazepam (p.359·1).
*Epilepsy; panic attacks.*

**Clonazine** Clonmel, Irl.
Chlorpromazine hydrochloride (p.675·2).
*Hypothermia induction; premedication; schizophrenia; sedative; vomiting.*

**Clondepryl** Clonmel, Irl.†.
Selegiline hydrochloride (p.1214·1).
*Parkinsonism.*

**Clonea** Alphapharm, Austral.
Clotrimazole (p.396·2).
*Fungal skin infections.*

**Clonesina** Teuto, Braz.
Clonidine hydrochloride (p.885·2).
*Hypertension.*

**Clonex** Teva, Israel.
Clonazepam (p.359·1).
*Epilepsy.*

**Clonfolic** Clonmel, Irl.
Folic acid (p.1429·1).
*Prevention of fetal neural tube defects.*

**Clonid-Ophtal** Winzer, Ger.
Clonidine hydrochloride (p.885·2).
*Glaucoma; ocular hypertension.*

**Clonidural** Richmond, Arg.
Clonidine (p.885·2).
*Hypertension.*

**Clonilix** Clonmel, Irl.†.
Indapamide (p.938·2).
*Hypertension.*

**Clonistada** Stada, Ger.
Clonidine hydrochloride (p.885·2).
*Hypertension.*

**Clonix** Janssen-Cilag, Port.
Clonixin (p.26·3).
*Pain.*

**Clonixil** Richmond, Arg.
Clonixin lysine (p.26·3).
*Fever; inflammation; pain.*

**Clonnirit** Rafa, Israel.
Clonidine hydrochloride (p.885·2).
*Menopausal flushing; migraine and other vascular headaches.*

**Clonodifen** Tecnofarma, Mex.
Diclofenac sodium (p.32·1).
*Inflammation; pain.*

**Clonofilin** Clonmel, Irl.†.
Aminophylline (p.780·2).
*Obstructive airways disease.*

**Clonorax** Clonmel, Irl.†.
Aciclovir (p.626·1).
*Herpes simplex infections of the lips and face.*

**Clonovate** TO-Chemicals, Thai.
Clobetasol propionate (p.1095·2).
*Skin disorders.*

**Clonoxifen** Clonmel, Irl.†.
Tamoxifen citrate (p.584·1).
*Breast cancer; endometrial cancer.*

**Clont** Bayer, Ger.
Metronidazole (p.607·2).
*Amoebiasis; anaerobic bacterial infections; giardiasis; trichomoniasis.*

**Clonteric** Clonmel, Irl.†.
Aspirin (p.15·1).
*Fever; inflammation; pain; thrombosis prophylaxis.*

**Clonuretic** Clonmel, Irl.†.
Amiloride hydrochloride (p.858·2); hydrochlorothiazide (p.933·2).
*Heart failure; hepatic cirrhosis; hypertension; oedema.*

**Clopamon** Aspen, S.Afr.
Metoclopramide hydrochloride (p.1274·3).
*Gastrointestinal disorders.*

**Clopan** FIRMA, Ital.
Metoclopramide hydrochloride (p.1274·3).
*Gastrointestinal disorders.*

**Clopine**
Mayne, Austral.; Douglas, NZ.
Clozapine (p.685·3).
*Schizophrenia.*

**Clopirim** Quimioterapica, Braz.
Chloroquine phosphate (p.448·2); pyrimethamine (p.458·1).
*Malaria.*

**Clopixol**
Lundbeck, Austral.; Lundbeck, Belg.; Schering-Plough, Braz.; Lundbeck, Canad.; Lundbeck, Fr.; Lundbeck, Gr.; Lundbeck, Hong Kong; Lundbeck, India; Lundbeck, Irl.; Lundbeck, Israel; Lundbeck, Ital.; Lundbeck, Malaysia; Organon, Mex.; Lundbeck, NZ; Lundbeck, S.Afr.; Lundbeck, Singapore; Lundbeck, Spain; Lundbeck, Switz.; Lundbeck, Thai.; Lundbeck, UK.
Zuclopenthixol (p.730·3), zuclopenthixol acetate (p.730·3), zuclopenthixol decanoate (p.730·3), or zuclopenthixol hydrochloride (p.730·3).
*Psychoses.*

**Clopra**
Ortoquimica, Braz.†.
Metoclopramide (p.1274·3).
*Nausea and vomiting.*

Quantum, USA.
Metoclopramide hydrochloride (p.1274·3).
*Nausea and vomiting.*

**Clopram** Douglas, Austral.
Clomipramine hydrochloride (p.289·3).
*Depression; narcoleptic syndrome; obsessive-compulsive disorder.*

**Cloprane** Luitpold, Ital.†.
Ronifibrate (p.996·1).
*Hyperlipidaemias.*

**Clopress**
Alphapharm, Malaysia; Merck, Malaysia; Pacific, NZ.
Clomipramine hydrochloride (p.289·3).
*Depression; narcoleptic syndrome; nocturnal enuresis; obsessive-compulsive disorder; pain; panic attacks; phobias.*

**Clopsine** Psicofarma, Mex.
Clozapine (p.685·3).
*Schizophrenia.*

**Cloptison**
Merck Sharp & Dohme, Norw.; Merck Sharp & Dohme, Switz.†.
Clobetasone butyrate (p.1095·3).
*Eye disorders.*

**Cloptison-N**
Merck Sharp & Dohme, Arg.; Merck Sharp & Dohme, Switz.†.
Clobetasone butyrate (p.1095·3); neomycin sulfate (p.235·1).
*Infected eye disorders.*

**CloraCEF** Ranbaxy, S.Afr.
Cefaclor (p.167·1).
*Bacterial infections.*

**Clorad** ACS Dobfar, Ital.
Cefaclor (p.167·1).
*Bacterial infections.*

**Cloradex** Tubilux, Ital.
Dexamethasone (p.1097·1); chloramphenicol (p.185·1).
*Infected inflammatory eye disorders.*

**Cloradryn** Recordati, Ital.†.
Cloprednol (p.1096·1).
*Corticosteroid.*

**Clorafen** Merck, Mex.
Chloramphenicol (p.185·1) or chloramphenicol palmitate (p.185·1).
*Bacterial infections.*

**Clorafenil** Teuto, Braz.
Chloramphenicol (p.185·1).
*Bacterial infections.*

**Cloram Hemidexa** Llorens, Spain.
Boric acid (p.1662·1); chloramphenicol (p.185·1); dexamethasone phosphate (p.1097·2).
Formerly known as Cloranfe Hemidex.
*Infected eye disorders.*

**Cloram Zinc** Llorens, Spain.
Chloramphenicol (p.185·1); naphazoline hydrochloride (p.1124·3); zinc sulfate (p.1469·3).
Formerly known as Cloranfenic Zinc.
*Bacterial eye infections.*

**Cloramed**
Note. This name is used for preparations of different composition.
Medimport, Mex.
Chloramphenicol (p.185·1).
*Bacterial infections.*

Medifive, Thai.
Dipotassium clorazepate (p.685·1).
*Anxiety; insomnia.*

**Cloramfen** Nuovo ISM, Ital.
Chloramphenicol (p.185·1).
*Bacterial eye infections.*

**Cloramfeni** Sophia, Mex.
Chloramphenicol (p.185·1).
*Bacterial eye infections.*

**Cloramfenil** Pisa, Mex.†.
Chloramphenicol (p.185·1).
*Bacterial infections.*

**Clorampast** Pasteur, Chile.
Chloramphenicol (p.185·1).
*Vulvovaginal infections.*

**Cloran** Grin, Mex.
Chloramphenicol (p.185·1).
*Bacterial eye infections.*

**Cloran Otico** Grin, Mex.
Chloramphenicol (p.185·1); benzocaine (p.1370·3).
*Bacterial ear infections.*

**Clorana** Sanofi Synthelabo, Braz.
Hydrochlorothiazide (p.933·2).
*Diabetes insipidus; hypertension; oedema; renal calculi.*

**Cloranfe** Llorens, Spain†.
Chloramphenicol (p.185·1).
*Bacterial eye infections.*

**Cloranfenic** Laus, Spain.
Chloramphenicol (p.185·1).
*Bacterial eye infections.*

**Cloranfenil** *Sanval, Braz.*
Chloramphenicol (p.185·1).
*Bacterial infections.*

**Cloranpectina** *Basi, Port.*
Chloramphenicol (p.185·1); phthalylsulfathiazole (p.242·3); pectin (p.1580·3).
*Gastrointestinal infections.*

**Cloraseptic**
*Note. This name is used for preparations of different composition.*
*Legrand, Braz.*
Phenol (p.1188·1); sodium phenolate; borax (p.1661·3); thymol (p.1194·2); menthol (p.1711·3).
Formerly contained tyrothricin and benzocaine.
*Mouth and throat disorders.*
*Diviser Aquilea, Spain†.*
Chlorhexidine gluconate (p.1173·2); chlorobutanol (p.1176·3).
*Mouth and throat infections.*

**Cloraxene** *TO-Chemicals, Thai.*
Dipotassium clorazepate (p.685·1).
*Anxiety; insomnia.*

**Clorazin** *Tecnofarma, Mex.*
Chloramphenicol (p.185·1).
*Bacterial infections.*

**Clorcin-Ped** *Stiefel, Braz.*
Cefaclor (p.167·1).
*Bacterial infections.*

**Clorcorticil** *Edol, Port.*
Chloramphenicol (p.185·1); hydrocortisone acetate (p.1103·3).
*Bacterial eye infections with inflammation.*

**Clordil** *Diba, Mex.*
Chloramphenicol (p.185·1).
*Bacterial infections.*

**Clordispenser** *Molteni, Ital.†.*
Halazone (p.1181·2).
*Waste disinfection.*

**Clordox** *Teuto, Braz.*
Doxycycline hyclate (p.206·2).
*Bacterial infections.*

**Cloretilo Chemirosa** *Ern, Spain.*
Ethyl chloride (p.1376·2).
*Local anaesthesia.*

**Clorevan** *Ariston, Braz.†.*
Chlorphenoxamine (p.428·3).
*Hypersensitivity reactions.*

**Clorexan** *IMS, Ital.*
Chlorhexidine gluconate (p.1173·2); isopropyl alcohol (p.1184·3).
*Wound disinfection.*

**Clorexan Ferri** *IMS, Ital.*
Chlorhexidine gluconate (p.1173·2); alcohol (p.1166·1).
*Instrument disinfection.*

**Clorexident** *Warner-Lambert, Ital.†.*
Chlorhexidine gluconate (p.1173·2).
*Mouth disorders; oral disinfection.*

**Clorexident Ortodontico** *Warner-Lambert, Ital.†.*
Chlorhexidine gluconate (p.1173·2); sodium fluoride (p.1444·3).
*Oral disinfection; prophylaxis of dental caries and gingivitis.*

**Clorfenil**
*Allergan-Frumtost, Braz.†; Rayere, Mex.*
Chloramphenicol (p.185·1).
*Bacterial infections.*

**Clorfibrase** *Parke, Davis, Arg.*
Chloramphenicol (p.185·1); fibrinolysin (p.916·2); deoxyribonuclease (p.1119·1).
*Wounds.*

**Clorfriol** *Rayere, Mex.*
Paracetamol (p.76·2); chlorphenamine (p.428·1); ascorbic acid (p.1460·2); moroxydine hydrochloride (p.649·3).
*Cold and influenza symptoms.*

**Clorhexitulle** *Aventis, Austral.*
Chlorhexidine acetate (p.1173·2).
*Burns; infected skin disorders; skin ulcers; wounds.*

**Clorimet-Z** *Zafiro, Mex.*
Metoclopramide hydrochloride (p.1274·3).
*Gastrointestinal motility disorders; nausea and vomiting.*

**Clorina**
*Lysoform, Ger.; Squibb, Spain.*
Tosylchloramide sodium (p.1194·3).
*Antiseptic; hand disinfection; skin and wound disinfection; surface disinfection; water purification.*

**Cloritines** *Torlan, Spain†.*
Halazone (p.1181·2); sodium carbonate (p.1747·1); sodium chloride (p.1233·3).
*Disinfection of drinking water.*

**Clor-K-Zaf** *Zafiro, Mex.*
Potassium chloride (p.1232·2).
*Hypokalaemia; potassium supplement.*

**Cloroboral** *Inexfa, Spain†.*
Alum (p.1652·1); boric acid (p.1662·1); potassium chlorate (p.1734·2); thymol (p.1194·2); menthol (p.1711·3).
*Gingivitis; mouth and throat irritation; pyorrhoea; stomatitis.*

**Clorocil** *Edol, Port.*
Chloramphenicol (p.185·1).
*Bacterial eye infections.*

**Cloromi-T** *Formenti, Ital.†.*
Tosylchloramide sodium (p.1194·3).
*Disinfection of minor wounds.*

**Clorosan** *Lachifarma, Ital.*
Chlorhexidine gluconate (p.1173·2).
*Disinfection of skin, wounds, and burns.*

**Clorotir** *Novartis, NZ; Biochemie, NZ.*
Cefaclor (p.167·1).
*Bacterial infections.*

**Cloro-Trimeton** *Schering-Plough, Mex.*
Chlorphenamine maleate (p.427·3).
*Hypersensitivity.*

**Clorpactin** *Guardian, Canad.†.*
Sodium oxychlorosene (p.1187·2).
*Antiseptic.*

**Clorpactin WCS-90** *Guardian, USA.*
Sodium oxychlorosene (p.1187·2).
*Disinfection; skin infections.*

**Clorpamina** *Andromaco, Mex.*
Dopamine hydrochloride (p.907·1).
*Heart failure; shock.*

**Clorpres** *Bertek, USA.*
Clonidine hydrochloride (p.885·2); chlortalidone (p.882·3).
*Hypertension.*

**Clorprimeton** *Essex, Chile.*
Chlorphenamine maleate (p.427·3).
*Hypersensitivity reactions.*

**Clorpromaz** *Uniao Quimica, Braz.*
Chlorpromazine hydrochloride (p.675·2).
*Psychoses.*

**Clortalil** *Legrand, Braz.*
Chlortalidone (p.882·3).
*Hypertension; oedema; renal calculi.*

**Clortanol** *CT, Ital.*
Atenolol (p.865·2); chlortalidone (p.882·3).
*Hypertension.*

**Clortil** *Teuto, Braz.*
Chlortalidone (p.882·3).
*Hypertension.*

**Clorxil** *Pan Quimica, Spain.*
Chlorhexidine gluconate (p.1173·2).
*Disinfection of skin and wounds.*

**Closcript** *Ranbaxy, S.Afr.*
Clotrimazole (p.396·2).
*Fungal skin and vulvovaginal infections.*

**Closecs** *Eurofarma, Braz.†; Inaf, Braz.†.*
Loperamide (p.1271·2).
*Diarrhoea.*

**Closin** *Combustin, Ger.*
Promethazine hydrochloride (p.439·1).
*Hypersensitivity reactions; motion sickness; psychoses; sleep disorders.*

**Closina** *Lilly, Austral.*
Cycloserine (p.202·1).
*Tuberculosis; urinary-tract infections.*

**Clostedal** *Silanes, Mex.*
Carbamazepine (p.353·3).
*Alcohol and benzodiazepine withdrawal syndromes; bipolar disorder; diabetes insipidus; diabetic neuropathy; epilepsy; neuralgias; polydypsia; polyuria.*

**Clostet** *Chiron Vaccines, UK.*
An adsorbed tetanus vaccine (p.1640·3).
*Active immunisation.*

**Clostilbegyt**
*Medphano, Ger.†; Egis, Hong Kong; Egis, Malaysia; Egis, Singapore.*
Clomifene citrate (p.1542·2).
*Anovulatory infertility; oligospermia.*

**Clotam**
*Sanova, Austria†; Gea, Denm.; Gea, Fin.; Bristol-Myers Squibb, Gr.; Ecosol, Switz.; Provalis, UK.*
Tolfenamic acid (p.94·2).
*Inflammation; musculoskeletal and joint disorders; pain.*

**Clotan** *SmithKline Beecham, Braz.†.*
Tolfenamic acid (p.94·2).
*Musculoskeletal and joint disorders.*

**Clotassio** *Bunker, Braz.*
Potassium chloride (p.1232·2).
*Hypokalaemia.*

**Clotest** *Bripharm, Irl.*
Test for *Helicobacter pylori* from biopsy specimens.

**Cloton** *Nakorn, Thai.*
Chlorphenamine maleate (p.427·3); ammonium chloride (p.1115·2).
*Coughs; nasal congestion; rhinitis.*

**Clotramid** *Molteni, Ital.*
Chlorhexidine gluconate (p.1173·2); cetrimide (p.1172·1).
*Mouth disinfection.*

**Clotrason** *Schering-Plough, Denm.*
Betamethasone dipropionate (p.1093·1); clotrimazole (p.396·2).
*Fungal skin infections.*

**Clotrasone**
*Schering-Plough, Singapore; Schering-Plough, Spain; Schering-Plough, Thai.*
Betamethasone dipropionate (p.1093·1); clotrimazole (p.396·2).
*Fungal skin infections.*

**Clotreme** *Hexal, Austral.*
Clotrimazole (p.396·2).
*Fungal skin infections.*

**Clotren** *Teuto, Braz.*
Clotrimazole (p.396·2).
*Fungal infections.*

**Clotri** *Polipharm, Thai.*
Clotrimazole (p.396·2).
*Vaginal candidiasis.*

**Clotri OPT** *Optimed, Ger.†.*
Clotrimazole (p.396·2).
*Fungal skin infections.*

**Clotricin** *Seng, Thai.*
Clotrimazole (p.396·2).
*Fungal vaginal infections; trichomoniasis.*

**Clotri-Denk** *Denk, Hong Kong.*
Clotrimazole (p.396·2).
*Fungal and bacterial vaginal infections; fungal skin infections; trichomoniasis.*

**Clotrifug** *Wolff, Ger.†.*
Clotrimazole (p.396·2).
*Fungal and bacterial vaginal infections.*

**Clotrigalen** *Galen, Ger.*
Clotrimazole (p.396·2).
*Fungal skin infections.*

**Clotrihexal** *Hexal, NZ.*
Clotrimazole (p.396·2).
*Vaginal candidiasis.*

**Clotrimaderm**
*Taro, Canad.; Taro, Israel; AFT, NZ.*
Clotrimazole (p.396·2).
*Fungal infections; trichomoniasis.*

**Clotrimin** *Medipharm, Chile.*
Clotrimazole (p.396·2).
*Fungal skin and vulvovaginal infections.*

**Clotrimin-B** *Medipharm, Chile.*
Clotrimazole (p.396·2); betamethasone dipropionate (p.1093·1).
*Fungal skin infections with inflammation.*

**Clotrimix** *Eversil, Braz.*
Clotrimazole (p.396·2).
*Fungal skin infections.*

**Clotrinolon** *Jean-Marie, Hong Kong.*
Clotrimazole (p.396·2); triamcinolone acetonide (p.1110·2).
*Fungal skin infections with inflammation.*

**Clotrizan** *Prodotti, Braz.*
Clotrimazole (p.396·2).
*Fungal infections.*

**Cloval** *Saval, Chile.*
Clobutinol hydrochloride (p.1117·1).
*Coughs.*

**Cloval Compuesto** *Saval, Chile.*
Clobutinol hydrochloride (p.1117·1); orciprenaline sulfate (p.790·2).
*Coughs.*

**Clovate** *Celltech, Spain.*
Clobetasol propionate (p.1095·2).
*Skin disorders.*

**Clovin** *Nakornpatana, Thai.*
Aciclovir (p.626·1).
*Herpes simplex infections of the skin and mucous membranes.*

**Clovir** *Cazi, Braz.*
Aciclovir (p.626·1).

**Clovira** *M & H, Thai.*
Aciclovir (p.626·1).
*Herpes simplex infections of the skin and mucous membranes.*

**Clovirax** *Cooper (Κοπερ), Gr.*
Aciclovir (p.626·1).
*Labial and genital herpes simplex infections.*

**Clox** *Caber, Ital.*
Ticlopidine hydrochloride (p.1011·2).
*Thrombosis prophylaxis.*

**Cloxa** *Hua, Thai.; M & H, Thai.*
Cloxacillin sodium (p.198·2).
*Bacterial infections.*

**Cloxacap** *Hovid, Singapore.*
Cloxacillin sodium (p.198·2).
*Gram-positive bacterial infections.*

**Cloxalin** *Siam Bheasach, Thai.*
Cloxacillin sodium (p.198·2).
*Bacterial infections.*

**Cloxam**
*Note. This name is used for preparations of different composition.*
*Bonafarma, Port.*
Cloxazolam (p.685·3).
*Anxiety disorders.*
*Aspen, S.Afr.*
Ampicillin (p.157·1); cloxacillin (p.198·2).
*Bacterial infections.*
*Macrophar, Thai.*
Cloxacillin (p.198·2).
*Bacterial infections.*

**Cloxan** *Orion, Fin.*
Chlorprothixene hydrochloride (p.682·3).
*Psychoses.*

**Cloxanbin** *ANB, Thai.*
Cloxacillin sodium (p.198·2).
*Bacterial infections.*

**Cloxapan** *Nakorn, Thai.†.*
Cloxacillin sodium (p.198·2).
*Bacterial infections.*

**Cloxapen**
*Pasteur, Chile.*
Cloxacillin (p.198·2).
*Bacterial infections.*
*SmithKline Beecham, USA†.*
Cloxacillin sodium (p.198·2).
*Bacterial infections.*

**Cloxasian** *Asian Pharm, Thai.*
Cloxacillin sodium (p.198·2).
*Bacterial infections.*

**Cloxgen** *General Drugs, Thai.*
Cloxacillin (p.198·2) or cloxacillin sodium (p.198·2).
*Bacterial infections.*

**Cloxil**
*Note. This name is used for preparations of different composition.*
*Duopharma, Hong Kong; Ranbaxy, Thai.*
Cloxacillin sodium (p.198·2).
*Bacterial infections.*
*Ofimex, Mex.†.*
Dicloxacillin (p.205·2).
*Bacterial infections.*

**Cloxillin**
*Note. This name is used for preparations of different composition.*
*Ibirn, Ital.*
Flucloxacillin sodium (p.213·3).
*Bacterial infections.*
*British Dispensary, Thai.*
Cloxacillin sodium (p.198·2).
*Bacterial infections.*

**Cloximar Duo** *Dupomar, Arg.*
Amoxicillin trihydrate (p.155·3); potassium clavulanate (p.193·3).
*Bacterial infections.*

**Cloxin** *Aspen, S.Afr.*
Cloxacillin sodium (p.198·2).
*Staphylococcal infections.*

**Cloxipen** *Welfer, Mex.†.*
Dicloxacillin (p.205·2).
*Bacterial infections.*

**Cloxydin** *Biomedis, Thai.; Great Eastern, Thai.*
Dicloxacillin (p.205·2).
*Bacterial infections.*

**Clozal** *Sankyo, Braz.*
Cloxazolam (p.685·3).
*Anxiety.*

**Clozan** *Pfizer, Belg.*
Clotiazepam (p.685·2).
*Anxiety disorders.*

**Clozanil** *Instituto Sanitas, Chile.*
Clonazepam (p.359·1).
*Epilepsy; panic attacks.*

**Clozaril**
*Novartis, Austral.; Novartis, Canad.; Novartis, Hong Kong; Novartis, Irl.; Novartis, Malaysia; Novartis, NZ; Novartis, Singapore; Novartis, Thai.; Novartis, UK; Novartis, USA.*
Clozapine (p.685·3).
*Psychoses associated with parkinsonism; schizophrenia.*

**Clozole**
*Genpharm, Austral.†; Jean-Marie, Hong Kong; Jean-Marie, Singapore†.*
Clotrimazole (p.396·2).
*Fungal skin infections; fungal vulvovaginal infections.*

**Clusivol**
*Whitehall, Braz.; Akromed, S.Afr.*
Multivitamin and mineral preparation (p.1417·1).

**Clusivol Composto** *Whitehall, Braz.*
Vitamin, amino-acid, and mineral preparation (p.1417·1).

**Cluyer** *Fada, Arg.*
Pethidine (p.81·3).
*Pain.*

**Clysmol** *Pharmacia, Austria.*
Monobasic sodium phosphate (p.1230·3); dibasic sodium phosphate (p.1231·1).
*Bowel evacuation; constipation.*

**Clyss-Go**
*Novag, Mex.; Prospa, Port.*
Docusate sodium (p.1262·2); sorbitol (p.1446·3).
*Bowel evacuation; constipation.*

**CMD** *Nakorn, Thai.*
Cimetidine (p.1255·3).
*Gastro-oesophageal reflux; hypersensitivity reactions; peptic ulcer; Zollinger-Ellison syndrome.*

**C-Mox** *Columbia, S.Afr.†.*
Amoxicillin trihydrate (p.155·3).
*Bacterial infections.*

**CMP** *Klonal, Arg.*
Carbamazepine (p.353·3).
*Epilepsy.*

**CMV Immunoglobulin** *CSL, Austral.*
A cytomegalovirus immunoglobulin (human) (p.1612·1).
*Passive immunisation.*

**CMV Iveegam** *Immuno, Canad.†.*
A cytomegalovirus immunoglobulin (p.1612·1).
*Passive immunisation.*

**CMW** *DePuy, Ger.*
Polymethylmethacrylate (p.1714·3).
*Bone cement for orthopaedic surgery.*

**CMW mit Gentamicin** *DePuy, Ger.*
Polymethylmethacrylate (p.1714·3); gentamicin sulfate (p.217·1).
*Bone cement for orthopaedic surgery.*

**C-Mycin** *Hoe, Malaysia.*
Clindamycin phosphate (p.194·2).
*Acne.*

**CN-25** *Masa, Thai.*
Cinnarizine (p.428·3).
*Cerebrovascular disorders; peripheral vascular disorders.*

**C-Naryl** *Homberger, Switz.†.*
Ascorbic acid (p.1460·2).
*Vitamin C supplement.*

**C'Nergil** *Medinfar, Port.*
Ascorbic acid (p.1460·2).
*Vitamin C deficiency.*

**Co Amoxin** *Smaller, Spain.*
Amoxicillin trihydrate (p.155·3).
*Bacterial infections.*

**Co Bucal** *Smaller, Spain.*
Alum (p.1652·1); procaine hydrochloride (p.1383·2); salicylic acid (p.1157·1); sodium chlorate (p.1747·2); thymol (p.1194·2); cherry laurel water; peppermint oil.
*Gingivitis; pyorrhoea; stomatitis.*

**Co Fluocin Fuerte** *Smaller, Spain.*
Fluocinolone acetonide (p.1101·2).
*Skin disorders.*

**$CO_2$ Granulat**
*Sanova, Austria; Guerbet, Ger.*
Betaine hydrochloride (p.1660·2); sodium bicarbonate (p.1223·2); dimeticone (p.1289·2); colloidal silicon dioxide (p.1581·3).
*Adjunct in double contrast radiography.*

**Co Hepa B12** *Smaller, Spain†.*
Vitamin B substances (p.1417·1); liver extract.
*Tonic; vitamin B deficiency.*

**Co-Acetan** *Kwizda, Austria.*
Lisinopril (p.946·3); hydrochlorothiazide (p.933·2).
*Hypertension.*

**CoActifed** *GlaxoSmithKline, Canad.*
*Expectorant:* Triprolidine hydrochloride (p.442·3); pseudoephedrine hydrochloride (p.1129·2); guaifenesin (p.1122·1); codeine phosphate (p.27·1).
*Syrup; tablets:* Triprolidine hydrochloride (p.442·3); pseudoephedrine hydrochloride (p.1129·2); codeine phosphate (p.27·1).
*Coughs.*

**Coalgan** *Brothier, Fr.*
Calcium alginate (p.745·1).
*Haemorrhage.*

**Coalip** *GlaxoSmithKline, Ital.†.*
Coenzyme A (p.1674·3).
*Hypertriglyceridaemia.*

**Coaltar Saponine le Beuf** *Gerda, Fr.†.*
Coal tar (p.1159·2); quillaia (p.1416·1).
*Skin disorders.*

**Co-Amilorid** *Cophar, Switz.*
Amiloride hydrochloride (p.858·2); hydrochlorothiazide (p.933·2).
*Hypertension; oedema.*

**Coamox** *Community Pharmacy, Thai.*
Amoxicillin trihydrate (p.155·3).
*Bacterial infections.*

**Co-Amoxi** *Mepha, Switz.*
Amoxicillin trihydrate (p.155·3); potassium clavulanate (p.193·3).
*Bacterial infections.*

**Co-Apap** *Rugby, USA.*
Chlorphenamine maleate (p.427·3); dextromethorphan hydrobromide (p.1117·3); paracetamol (p.76·2); pseudoephedrine hydrochloride (p.1129·2).
*Coughs and cold symptoms.*

**CoAprovel**
*Sanofi Synthelabo, Arg.; Sanofi Synthelabo, Belg.; Sanofi Synthelabo, Chile; Sanofi Synthelabo, Denm.; Bristol-Myers Squibb, Fr.; Synthelabo, Fr.; Sanofi Synthelabo, Ger.; Bristol-Myers Squibb, Irl.; Sanofi Synthelabo, Irl.; Sanofi Synthelabo, Ital.; Sanofi Synthelabo, Malaysia; Sanofi Winthrop, Neth.; Bristol-Myers Squibb, Neth.; Sanofi Synthelabo, Norw.; Bristol-Myers Squibb, Norw.; Bristol-Myers Squibb, Port.; Sanofi Synthelabo, Port.; Sanofi Synthelabo, S.Afr.; Sanofi Synthelabo, Singapore; Sanofi Synthelabo, Spain; Sanofi Synthelabo, Swed.; Bristol-Myers Squibb, Swed.; Sanofi Synthelabo, Switz.; Bristol-Myers Squibb, Switz.; Bristol-Myers Squibb, UK; Sanofi Synthelabo, UK.*
Irbesartan (p.940·1); hydrochlorothiazide (p.933·2).
*Hypertension.*

**Coarol** *Andromaco, Chile.*
Acenocoumarol (p.848·3).
*Thromboembolic disorders.*

**Coartem**
*Novartis, S.Afr.; Novartis, Thai.*
Artemether (p.447·2); lumefantrine (p.453·3).
*Malaria.*

**Co-Atenolol** *Cophar, Switz.*
Atenolol (p.865·2); chlortalidone (p.882·3).
*Hypertension.*

**Cobactin** *Zambon, Braz.*
Cyproheptadine hydrochloride (p.430·1); cobamamide (p.1459·1).
*Reduced appetite; tonic.*

**Cobadex Forte** *GlaxoSmithKline, India.*
Vitamin B substances; vitamin C (p.1417·1).
*Vitamin B and C deficiency.*

**Cobaforte** *EG, Ital.*
Cobamamide (p.1459·1).
*Vitamin $B_{12}$ deficiency.*

**Cobaglobal** *Legrand, Braz.*
Cobamamide (p.1459·1); cyproheptadine hydrochloride (p.430·1).
*Tonic.*

**Cobalatec** *Cops, S.Afr.*
Cyanocobalamin (p.1458·2).
*Vitamin $B_{12}$ deficiency.*

**Cobaldoze** *Kinder, Braz.*
Ferrous sulfate (p.1428·2); vitamin B substances (p.1417·1).
Ascorbic acid (p.1460·2) is included in this preparation to increase the absorption and availability of iron.

**Cobalin-H** *Link, UK.*
Hydroxocobalamin (p.1458·2).
*Anaemia due to $B_{12}$ deficiency; Leber's atrophy; tobacco amblyopia.*

**Cobalplex** *UCI, Braz.†.*
Ferric ammonium citrate (p.1427·2); folic acid (p.1429·1); vitamin $B_6$; vitamin $B_{12}$; lysine hydrochloride; tryptophan; threonine; liver extract; gastric mucosa extract (p.1417·1).
*Anaemias.*

**Cobalti** *Lepori, Port.*
Ferric ammonium citrate (p.1427·2).
*Anaemias; tonic.*

**Cobamet** *Roussel, Port.*
Mecobalamin (p.1459·1).
*Anaemias.*

**Cobamin** *Santen, Hong Kong.*
Cyanocobalamin (p.1458·2).
*Eye disorders.*

**Cobamol** *Maver, Mex.*
Salbutamol (p.791·3).

**Cobantril** *Pfizer, Switz.*
Pyrantel embonate (p.113·2).
*Nematode infections.*

**Cobanzyme** *SERB, Fr.*
Cobamamide (p.1459·1).
*Megaloblastic anaemia.*

**Cobavital** *Sintofarma, Braz.*
Cobamamide (p.1459·1); cyproheptadine hydrochloride (p.430·1).
*Reduced appetite; tonic.*

**Cobaxid** *Tecnifar, Port.*
Cobamamide (p.1459·1).
*Anaemias; neuralgias; neuritis; tonic.*

**Cobederm-H** *Sarabhai Piramal, India.*
Halcinonide (p.1103·2); econazole nitrate (p.397·2).
*Infected skin disorders.*

**Cobefen** *Instituto Sanitas, Chile.*
Dexchlorpheniramine maleate (p.427·3); betamethasone (p.1093·1).
*Hypersensitivity reactions.*

**Cobenexol Forte** *Roche, Arg.*
Cocarboxylase (p.1455·2); pyridoxine hydrochloride (p.1456·3); cyanocobalamin (p.1458·2).
*Neuritis; radiotherapy-induced vomiting; vitamin B deficiency; vomiting of pregnancy.*

**Cobenexol Fuerte** *Roche, Arg.*
Vitamin $B_1$ (p.1454·3); vitamin $B_6$ (p.1456·3); vitamin $B_{12}$ (p.1458·2).
*Neuralgias; neuritis; vitamin B deficiency.*

**Cobenzil Compuesto** *Abbott, Arg.*
Dextromethorphan hydrobromide (p.1117·3); carbinoxamine maleate (p.426·3); ephedrine hydrochloride (p.1120·1); ipecacuanha (p.1122·3); ammonium chloride (p.1115·2); tolu balsam (p.1131·3).
*Coughs.*

**Co-Betaloc**
*Pharmacia, Irl.; Pharmacia, UK.*
Metoprolol tartrate (p.957·1); hydrochlorothiazide (p.933·2).
*Hypertension.*

**cobidec n** *Pfizer Consumer, Ger.*
Multivitamin and mineral preparation (p.1417·1).

**Cobiona** *Esteve, Spain.*
Oxatomide (p.438·1).
*Hypersensitivity reactions.*

**Cobirolyte** *Allen, Mex.*
Oral rehydration therapy (p.1222·2).

**Cobotiaxina** *Ifusa, Mex.*
Cyanocobalamin (p.1458·2); pyridoxine (p.1457·2); thiamine (p.1455·2).
*Anaemias; neuritis.*

**Co-Captopril** *Genericon, Austria.*
Captopril (p.879·2); hydrochlorothiazide (p.933·2).
*Hypertension.*

**Co-Captral** *Silanes, Mex.*
Captopril (p.879·2); hydrochlorothiazide (p.933·2).
*Hypertension.*

**Co-Carnetina B12** *Sigma-Tau, Ital.*
Cobamamide (p.1459·1); levocarnitine (p.1423·3).
*Tonic.*

**Coccila** *Nakorn, Thai.*
*Syrup:* Furazolidone (p.605·2); neomycin (p.235·1); kaolin (p.1268·3).
*Tablets:* Diiodohydroxyquinoline (p.603·3); neomycin sulfate (p.235·1); phthalylsulfathiazole (p.242·3); light kaolin (p.1268·3); furazolidone (p.605·2).
*Gastrointestinal infections.*

**Cocculine**
*Boiron, Canad.; Boiron, Fr.; Boiron, Port.*
Homoeopathic preparation.

**Cocculus Oligoplex** *Madaus, Ger.*
Homoeopathic preparation.

**Cocculus-Homaccord** *Peithner, Austria.*
Homoeopathic preparation.

**Cocillana** *Orion, Fin.*
Ethylmorphine hydrochloride (p.37·3).
*Coughs.*

**Cocillana Co** *Propan, S.Afr.*
Cocillana (p.1117·2); squill (p.1130·3); menthol (p.1711·3).
*Coughs.*

**Cocillana Compound**
*Note. This name is used for preparations of different composition.*
*Synco, Hong Kong.*
Cocillana (p.1117·2); euphorbia (p.1686·3); senega (p.1130·2); squill (p.1130·3); antimony potassium tartrate (p.103·1); menthol (p.1711·3).
*Coughs; respiratory-tract congestion.*

*Universal, Hong Kong.*
Cocillana (p.1117·2); euphorbia (p.1686·3); squill (p.1130·3); senega (p.1130·2); codeine phosphate (p.27·1).
*Coughs.*

*Vida, Hong Kong.*
Cocillana (p.1117·2); euphorbia (p.1686·3); squill (p.1130·3).
*Cold symptoms; coughs.*

**Cocillana-Etyfin** *Pharmacia, Swed.*
Ethylmorphine hydrochloride (p.37·3); senega (p.1130·2); cocillana (p.1117·2).
*Coughs.*

**Co-Cillin** *Docmed, S.Afr.†.*
Ampicillin trihydrate (p.157·2).
*Bacterial infections.*

**Cocktail Reale** *Sella, Ital.†.*
Honey (p.1434·2); pollen; ginseng (p.1693·1); royal jelly (p.1740·3); propolis (p.1735·2).
*Nutritional supplement.*

**Co-Codamol** *Alpharma, Singapore; Cox, Singapore.*
Codeine phosphate (p.27·1); paracetamol (p.76·2).
*Fever; pain.*

**Cocois**
*Bioglan, Hong Kong; Celltech, Irl.; Bioglan, Malaysia; AFT, NZ; Celltech, UK.*
Coal tar (p.1159·2); salicylic acid (p.1157·1); precipitated sulfur (p.1158·2).
*Scalp conditions.*

**Cocydal** *Xixia, S.Afr.†.*
Co-trimoxazole (p.199·3).
*Bacterial infections.*

**Cocyntal** *Boiron, Canad.*
Homoeopathic preparation.

**Cod Efferalgan** *Upsamedica, Spain.*
Paracetamol (p.76·2); codeine phosphate (p.27·1).
*Pain.*

**COD N 70** *Fresenius Kabi, Ital.*
Amino-acid infusion (p.1417·1).
*Parenteral nutrition.*

**Codabrol** *Rekah, Israel.*
Paracetamol (p.76·2); codeine phosphate (p.27·1).
*Coughs; fever; pain.*

**Cod-Acamol Forte** *Teva, Israel.*
Paracetamol (p.76·2); codeine phosphate (p.27·1).
*Coughs; fever; pain.*

**Codaewon** *Daewon, Hong Kong.*
Dihydrocodeine tartrate (p.34·3); guaifenesin (p.1122·1); methylephedrine hydrochloride (p.1124·2); chlorphenamine maleate (p.427·3).
*Coughs.*

**Co-Dafalgan** *Upsamedica, Switz.*
Paracetamol (p.76·2); codeine phosphate (p.27·1).
*Pain.*

**Codafen Continus**
*Napp, Irl.; Napp, UK.*
Ibuprofen (p.45·3); codeine phosphate (p.27·1).
*Inflammation; musculoskeletal, joint, and peri-articular disorders; pain.*

**Codalax**
*Napp, Irl.; Douglas, NZ; Napp, UK.*
Dantron (p.1261·1); poloxamer 188 (p.1414·2).
These ingredients can be described by the British Approved Name Co-danthramer.
*Constipation.*

**Codal-DH** *Cypress, USA.*
Hydrocodone tartrate (p.45·1); phenylephrine hydrochloride (p.1126·3); mepyramine maleate (p.437·1).
*Allergic rhinitis; coughs and cold symptoms.*

**Codal-DM** *Cypress, USA.*
Dextromethorphan hydrobromide (p.1117·3); phenylephrine hydrochloride (p.1126·3); mepyramine maleate (p.437·1).
*Allergic rhinitis; coughs and cold symptoms.*

**Codalgin**
*Note. This name is used for preparations of different composition.*
*Fawns & McAllan, Austral.*
Paracetamol (p.76·2); codeine phosphate (p.27·1).
*Fever; pain.*

*Nycomed, Norw.†.*
Phenazone (p.82·3); codeine phosphate (p.27·1).
*Pain.*

**Codalgin Plus** *Sigma, Austral.*
Paracetamol (p.76·2); codeine phosphate (p.27·1); doxylamine succinate (p.432·3).
*Fever; pain.*

**Coda-Med** *Brauer, UK†.*
Paracetamol (p.76·2); codeine phosphate (p.27·1); caffeine citrate (p.782·1).

**Codamine** *Barre-National, USA†.*
Phenylpropanolamine hydrochloride (p.1127·3); hydrocodone tartrate (p.45·1).
*Coughs and cold symptoms.*

**Codant** *Antigen, Irl.*
Codeine phosphate (p.27·1).
*Pain.*

**Codapane** *Alphapharm, Austral.*
Paracetamol (p.76·2); codeine phosphate (p.27·1).
*Fever; pain.*

**Codaphed** *Julphar, UAE.*
Ephedrine hydrochloride (p.1120·1); chlorphenamine maleate (p.427·3); codeine phosphate (p.27·1).
*Coughs.*

**Codaphed Plus** *Julphar, UAE.*
Ephedrine hydrochloride (p.1120·1); chlorphenamine maleate (p.427·3); codeine phosphate (p.27·1); ammonium chloride (p.1115·2); menthol (p.1711·3).
*Coughs.*

**Codedrill** *Pierre Fabre Sante, Fr.*
Codeine phosphate (p.27·1).
Formerly known as Pectoral Edulcor.
*Coughs.*

**Codef** *Be-Tabs, S.Afr.*
Codeine phosphate (p.27·1); mepyramine maleate (p.437·1); ephedrine hydrochloride (p.1120·1).
*Coughs.*

**Codegest Expectorant** *Great Southern, USA†.*
Phenylpropanolamine hydrochloride (p.1127·3); codeine phosphate (p.27·1); guaifenesin (p.1122·1).
*Coughs.*

**Codehist DH** *Geneva, USA.*
Pseudoephedrine hydrochloride (p.1129·2); chlorphenamine maleate (p.427·3); codeine phosphate (p.27·1).
*Coughs and cold symptoms.*

**Codeine Contin** *Purdue, Canad.*
Codeine (p.27·1); codeine sulfate (p.27·1).
*Pain.*

**Codeinol** *Saba, Ital.†.*
Codeine hydrochloride (p.27·1); ephedrine hydrochloride (p.1120·1).
*Respiratory-tract symptoms with cough.*

**Codeipar** *Andromaco, Chile.*
Paracetamol (p.76·2); codeine phosphate (p.27·1).
*Pain.*

**Codeisan**
*Note. This name is used for preparations of different composition.*
*Labocor, Port.†.*
*Syrup:* Codeine phosphate (p.27·1); ephedrine hydrochloride (p.1120·1); cowslip (p.1735·1); sodium benzoate (p.1169·3).
*Catarrh; coughs.*
*Tablets:* Codeine phosphate (p.27·1).
*Coughs; pain.*

*Belmac, Spain.*
Codeine phosphate (p.27·1).
*Coughs; diarrhoea; pain.*

**Codelasa**
*Note. This name is used for preparations of different composition.*
*Andromaco, Arg.*
Codeine (p.27·1); guaifenesin (p.1122·1).
*Coughs.*

*Procter & Gamble, Braz.†.*
Codeine (p.27·1); ephedrine hydrochloride (p.1120·1); sodium benzoate (p.1169·3); coal tar (p.1159·2); pine oil; tolu balsam (p.1131·3).
*Coughs.*

*Andromaco, Chile.*
Codeine (p.27·1); ethylmorphine (p.37·3); homatropine methylbromide (p.483·2).
*Coughs.*

**Codella** *Napp, UK†.*
Glycerol (p.1694·3); kaolin (p.1268·3); povidone-iodine (p.1190·3).
*Dry skin.*

**Codelum** *Sanova, Austria.*
Thyme (p.1755·2); codeine phosphate (p.27·1).
*Coughs.*

**Codenfan** *Bouchara-Recordati, Fr.*
Codeine phosphate (p.27·1).
*Pain.*

**Codepect** *Neopharm, Thai.*
Codeine phosphate (p.27·1); guaifenesin (p.1122·1).
Formerly contained codeine phosphate, guaifenesin, and phenylpropanolamine.
*Cold symptoms; coughs; nasal congestion.*

**Codergine** *Shiwa, Thai.*
Co-dergocrine mesilate (p.1674·1).
*Cerebrovascular disorders; peripheral vascular disorders.*

**Coderit** *Chinoin, Mex.*
Codeine (p.27·1); ephedrine (p.1120·1).
*Coughs.*

**Codesan Comp** *Leiras, Fin.*
Codeine phosphate (p.27·1); ephedrine hydrochloride (p.1120·1); diphenhydramine hydrochloride (p.431·3); cocillana (p.1117·2).
*Coughs.*

**Codesan N** *Leiras, Fin.*
Noscapine (p.1125·3); cocillana (p.1117·2).
*Coughs.*

**Codesia** *Asian Pharm, Thai.*
Codeine phosphate (p.27·1); guaifenesin (p.1122·1).
*Coughs.*

**Codesic** *Raza, Malaysia; Pharmaniaga, Malaysia.*
Dihydrocodeine tartrate (p.34·3).
*Pain.*

**Codethyline**
*Erfa, Belg.; Hoechst, Fr.†.*
Ethylmorphine hydrochloride (p.37·3).
*Coughs.*

**Codetilina-Eucaliptolo He** *Teofarma, Ital.†.*
Ethylmorphine hydrochloride (p.37·3); cineole (p.1672·1).
*Coughs.*

**Codetol** *Laboratorios Chile, Chile.*
Codeine phosphate (p.27·1); pseudoephedrine hydrochloride (p.1129·2); chlorphenamine maleate (p.427·3).
*Coughs; respiratory-tract congestion.*

**Codetol PM** *Laboratorios Chile, Chile.*
Codeine phosphate (p.27·1); pseudoephedrine hydrochloride (p.1129·2); chlorphenamine maleate (p.427·3); avocado leaf; eucalyptus leaf (p.1686·1).
*Coughs; nasal congestion.*

**Codetricine** *Byk, Fr.*
Tyrothricin (p.275·1).
*Mouth and throat disorders.*

**Codetricine vitamine C** *Byk, Fr.*
Tyrothricin (p.275·1); tetracaine hydrochloride (p.1385·1); ascorbic acid (p.1460·2).
*Mouth and throat disorders.*

**Codeverin** *Luper, Braz.*
Dipyrone (p.35·3); papaverine hydrochloride (p.1728·1); homatropine methylbromide (p.483·2).
*Muscle spasm; pain.*

**Codex** *Zambon, Ital.*
*Saccharomyces boulardii* (p.1704·2).
*Gastrointestinal disorders.*

**Codexine-R** *Coup, Gr.*
Butamirate citrate (p.1116·2).
*Cough.*

**Cod-Guaiacol** *Vitamed, Israel.*
Sulfogaiacol (p.1131·1); codeine phosphate (p.27·1).
*Coughs.*

**codi OPT** *Optimed, Ger.*
Codeine phosphate (p.27·1).
*Pain.*

**Codical** *Sam-On, Israel.*
Codeine phosphate (p.27·1).
*Coughs.*

**Codicaps** *Thiemann, Ger.*
Codeine (p.27·1); chlorphenamine maleate (p.427·3).
*Catarrh; coughs.*

**Codicaps mono** *Thiemann, Ger.*
Codeine (p.27·1).
*Coughs.*

**Codicaps N** *Thiemann, Ger.*
Codeine (p.27·1).
*Coughs.*

**Codicet** *Hua, Thai.*
Codeine phosphate (p.27·1); paracetamol (p.76·2).
*Pain.*

**Codiclear DH** *Schwarz, USA.*
Hydrocodone tartrate (p.45·1); guaifenesin (p.1122·1).
*Coughs.*

**Codicompren** *GlaxoSmithKline, Ger.*
Codeine phosphate (p.27·1).
*Coughs.*

**Codicontin**
*Viatris, Belg.; Mundipharma, Switz.*
Dihydrocodeine tartrate (p.34·3).
*Pain.*

**Codidol** *Mundipharma, Austria.*
Dihydrocodeine tartrate (p.34·3).
*Pain.*

**Codiforton** *Sanofi Winthrop, Ger.†.*
Codeine phosphate (p.27·1).
*Coughs.*

**Codigesic** *Bangkok Lab & Cosmetic, Thai.*
Codeine phosphate (p.27·1); paracetamol (p.76·2).
*Pain.*

**Co-Dilatrend** *Roche, Austria.*
Carvedilol (p.881·1); hydrochlorothiazide (p.933·2).
*Hypertension.*

**Codilergi** *Codilab, Port.*
Diphenhydramine hydrochloride (p.431·3).

**Codimal DH** *Schwarz, USA.*
Hydrocodone tartrate (p.45·1); phenylephrine hydrochloride (p.1126·3); mepyramine maleate (p.437·1).
*Coughs and cold symptoms.*

**Codimal DM** *Schwarz, USA.*
Dextromethorphan hydrobromide (p.1117·3); phenylephrine hydrochloride (p.1126·3); mepyramine maleate (p.437·1).
*Coughs.*

**Codimal PH** *Schwarz, USA.*
Codeine phosphate (p.27·1); phenylephrine hydrochloride (p.1126·3); mepyramine maleate (p.437·1).
*Coughs and cold symptoms.*

**Codimin** *Biomedica-Chemica, Gr.*
Butamirate citrate (p.1116·2).
*Cough.*

**Codimol** *Raza, Malaysia; Pharmaniaga, Malaysia.*
Dihydrocodeine tartrate (p.34·3); paracetamol (p.76·2).
*Pain.*

**Co-Diovan**
*Novartis, Austria; Novartis, Ger.; Novartis, Hong Kong; Novartis, Irl.; Novartis, Israel; Novartis, Malaysia; Novartis, Mex.; Novartis, Neth.; Novartis, Port.; Novartis, S.Afr.; Novartis, Singapore; Novartis, Spain; Novartis, Switz.; Novartis, Thai.*
Valsartan (p.1018·3); hydrochlorothiazide (p.933·2).
*Hypertension.*

**Co-Diovane** *Novartis, Belg.*
Valsartan (p.1018·3); hydrochlorothiazide (p.933·2).
*Hypertension.*

**Codipar** *Goldshield, UK.*
Paracetamol (p.76·2); codeine phosphate (p.27·1).
These ingredients can be described by the British Approved Name Co-codamol.
*Pain.*

**Codipertussin**
*Klinge, Austria.*
Codeine polistirex (p.27·3).
*Bronchitis; coughs.*

*Tussin, Ger.*
Codeine phosphate (p.27·1).
*Coughs.*

**Codiphen** *Pfizer Consumer, Austral.*
Codeine phosphate (p.27·1); aspirin (p.15·1).
*Fever; pain.*

**Codipront**
*Pfizer, Austria; Grunenthal, Chile; Mack, Illert., Ger.; Mack, Hong Kong; Bracco, Ital.; Ferraz, Lynce, Port.; Mack, Singapore; Pfizer, Spain; Mack, Switz.; Mack, Thai.*
Codeine phosphate (p.27·1) or codeine polistirex (p.27·3); phenyltoloxamine citrate (p.439·1) or phenyltoloxamine polistirex (p.439·1).
*Coughs.*

**Codipront cum Expectorans**
Note. This name is used for preparations of different composition.
*Mack, Hong Kong†.*
Codeine polistirex (p.27·3); phenyltoloxamine polistirex (p.439·1); guaifenesin (p.1122·1).
*Coughs.*

*Mack, Switz.*
*Capsules:* Codeine resinate (p.27·3); phenyltoloxamine resinate (p.439·1); guaifenesin (p.1122·1).
*Syrup:* Codeine resinate (p.27·3); phenyltoloxamine resinate (p.439·1); guaifenesin (p.1122·1); thyme (p.1755·2).
*Coughs.*

**Codipront Mono**
*Pfizer, Austria; Mack, Illert., Ger.*
Codeine polistirex (p.27·3).
*Coughs.*

**Codipront N**
*Galenica, Gr.*
Codeine polistirex (p.27·3); codeine phosphate (p.27·1).
*Cough.*

*Mack, Hong Kong.*
Codeine polistirex (p.27·3).
*Coughs.*

**Codis**
*Reckitt Benckiser, Austral.; Reckitt & Colman, Belg.†; Reckitt Benckiser, Irl.; Reckitt Benckiser, S.Afr.; Reckitt & Colman, Singapore†; Reckitt Benckiser, UK.*
Aspirin (p.15·1); codeine phosphate (p.27·1).
*Fever; pain.*

**Codisal Forte** *Rafa, Israel.*
Paracetamol (p.76·2); codeine phosphate (p.27·1).
*Cold symptoms; coughs; fever; pain.*

**Coditard** *Klinge, Austria.*
Codeine polistirex (p.27·3).
*Coughs.*

**Codivis** *CTI, Israel.*
Codeine (p.27·1); phenyltoloxamine (p.439·1).
*Coughs.*

**Codivite** *Codilab, Port.†.*
Lysine hydrochloride; vitamin B substances (p.1417·1).
*Tonic.*

**Codocalyptol** *Qualiphar, Belg.†.*
Codeine (p.27·1).
*Coughs.*

**Codoforme** *Azevedos, Port.†.*
Codeine (p.27·1); aconite (p.1646·3); belladonna (p.479·1); trimethylamino triaminomethyl bromoform; sodium benzoate (p.1169·3); terpin (p.1131·1).
*Coughs.*

**Codol**
Note. This name is used for preparations of different composition.
*Confar, Port.*
Codeine (p.27·1); vegetable extract.

*Mundipharma, Switz.*
Paracetamol (p.76·2); codeine phosphate (p.27·1).
*Fever; pain.*

**Codoliprane** *Theraplix, Fr.*
Paracetamol (p.76·2); codeine phosphate (p.27·1).
*Pain.*

**Codomex Orange** *Medipharma, Hong Kong.*
Codeine phosphate (p.27·1); papaverine hydrochloride (p.1728·1); chlorphenamine maleate (p.427·3).
*Cold and influenza symptoms.*

**Codomex Purple** *Medipharma, Hong Kong.*
Codeine phosphate (p.27·1); papaverine hydrochloride (p.1728·1); chlorphenamine maleate (p.427·3); guaifenesin (p.1122·1).
*Cold and influenza symptoms.*

**Codomill** *Brunel, S.Afr.*
Mepyramine maleate (p.437·1); codeine phosphate (p.27·1).
Formerly contained mepyramine maleate, codeine phosphate, and ephedrine hydrochloride.
*Coughs.*

**Codoplex** *Jean-Marie, Hong Kong.*
*Injection†:* Codeine phosphate (p.27·1); papaverine hydrochloride (p.1728·1); chlorphenamine maleate (p.427·3); ephedrine hydrochloride (p.1120·1).
*Syrup:* Codeine phosphate (p.27·1); papaverine hydrochloride (p.1728·1); guaifenesin (p.1122·1); chlorphenamine maleate (p.427·3).
*Tablets:* Codeine phosphate (p.27·1); papaverine hydrochloride (p.1728·1); chlorphenamine maleate (p.427·3); terpin hydrate (p.1131·1); caffeine (p.782·1).
Formerly contained codeine phosphate, papaverine hydrochloride, chlorphenamine maleate, terpin hydrate, phenolphthalein, and caffeine.
*Coughs.*

**Codotusil** *Medifarma, Mex.*
Ammonium chloride (p.1115·2); diphenhydramine (p.431·3); ephedrine hydrochloride (p.1120·1).
*Coughs.*

**Codotussyl Expectorant** *Whitehall, Fr.*
*Oral solution:* Acetylcysteine (p.1112·3).
*Syrup:* Carbocisteine (p.1116·2).
*Respiratory-tract congestion.*

**Codotussyl Maux de Gorge** *Whitehall, Fr.*
Lidocaine hydrochloride (p.1377·3); sodium benzoate (p.1169·3); benzyl alcohol (p.1170·2).
*Mouth and throat disorders.*

**Codotussyl Toux Seche** *Whitehall, Fr.*
*Capsules:* Dextromethorphan hydrobromide (p.1117·3).
*Syrup:* Pholcodine (p.1128·3).
Formerly contained pholcodine, sodium benzoate, sulfogaiacol, aconite, belladonna, cherry-laurel water, tolu syrup, and Desessartz syrup.
*Coughs.*

**Codox** *Boots Healthcare, Austral.*
Aspirin (p.15·1); dihydrocodeine tartrate (p.34·3).
*Coughs; fever; pain.*

**Codral Cold & Flu**
*Pfizer Consumer, Austral.; Pfizer, NZ.*
Paracetamol (p.76·2); pseudoephedrine hydrochloride (p.1129·2); codeine phosphate (p.27·1).
*Cold and influenza symptoms.*

**Codral Cough** *Warner-Lambert, NZ†.*
Dextromethorphan hydrobromide (p.1117·3); pseudoephedrine hydrochloride (p.1129·2).
*Coughs.*

**Codral Cough, Cold & Flu Day & Night**
*Pfizer Consumer, Austral.; Pfizer, NZ.*
Day capsules, paracetamol (p.76·2); pseudoephedrine hydrochloride (p.1129·2); dextromethorphan hydrobromide (p.1117·3); night capsules, paracetamol; dextromethorphan hydrobromide; chlorphenamine maleate (p.427·3).
*Cold and influenza symptoms.*

**Codral Daytime/Nightime**
*Pfizer Consumer, Austral.; Pfizer, NZ.*
Day tablets, paracetamol (p.76·2); pseudoephedrine hydrochloride (p.1129·2); codeine phosphate (p.27·1); night tablets, paracetamol; codeine phosphate; triprolidine hydrochloride (p.442·3).
*Cold and influenza symptoms; nasal congestion.*

**Codral Dry Cough** *Pfizer Consumer, Austral.*
Pseudoephedrine hydrochloride (p.1129·2); codeine phosphate (p.27·1).
*Coughs; nasal congestion.*

**Codral Expectorant** *Warner-Lambert, NZ†.*
Guaifenesin (p.1122·1); pseudoephedrine hydrochloride (p.1129·2).
*Coughs.*

**Codral 4 Flu**
*Pfizer Consumer, Austral.; Pfizer, NZ.*
Paracetamol (p.76·2); codeine phosphate (p.27·1); pseudoephedrine hydrochloride (p.1129·2); chlorphenamine maleate (p.427·3).
*Cold and influenza symptoms.*

**Codral Forte** *GlaxoSmithKline, Austral.*
Aspirin (p.15·1); codeine phosphate (p.27·1).
*Coughs; pain.*

**Codral Linctus** *Warner-Lambert, Austral.†.*
Pseudoephedrine hydrochloride (p.1129·2); codeine phosphate (p.27·1).
*Cold symptoms; coughs.*

**Codral Pain Relief**
*Pfizer Consumer, Austral.; Pfizer, NZ.*
Paracetamol (p.76·2); codeine phosphate (p.27·1).
*Fever; pain.*

**Codrinan** *Cimed, Braz.*
Theophylline (p.798·3).
*Obstructive airways disease.*

**Coduretas Gragenil** *Reig Jofre, Spain.*
Codeine phosphate (p.27·1); diphenhydramine hydrochloride (p.431·3); ephedrine hydrochloride (p.1120·1).
Formerly known as Gragenil.
*Cough; respiratory-tract disorders.*

**Codyl** *Leo, Denm.†.*
Aspirin (p.15·1); codeine phosphate (p.27·1).
*Pain.*

**Coease** *Advance, USA.*
Sodium hyaluronate (p.1697·3).
*Aid in eye surgery.*

**Coedieci** *Mitim, Ital.*
Ubidecarenone (p.1760·2).
*Cardiopathy; coenzyme Q10 deficiency.*

**Co-Efferalagan** *Upsa, Ital.*
Paracetamol (p.76·2); codeine phosphate (p.27·1).
*Pain.*

**Co-Enaran** *Kwizda, Austria.*
Enalapril maleate (p.909·2); hydrochlorothiazide (p.933·2).
*Hypertension.*

**Coenrelax** *Centrum, Spain.*
Valerian (p.1762·2).
*Insomnia; nervous disorders.*

**Coergot** *Masa, Thai.†.*
Co-dergocrine mesilate (p.1674·1).
*Cerebrovascular disorders; mental function impairment; peripheral vascular disorders; vascular headaches.*

**Coex** *Farmasa, Braz.*
Ubidecarenone (p.1760·2).

**Cofasol** *UCI, Braz.†.*
Tetramisole hydrochloride (p.114·1).
*Nematode infections.*

**Cofbron** *Macrophar, Thai.*
Terbutaline sulfate (p.797·2); guaifenesin (p.1122·1).
*Coughs; obstructive airways disease.*

**Cofed** *M & H, Thai.*
Triprolidine hydrochloride (p.442·3); pseudoephedrine hydrochloride (p.1129·2).
*Allergic rhinitis; cold symptoms; hay fever.*

**Cofena** *Sanobia, Port.†.*
Aspirin (p.15·1); codeine phosphate (p.27·1); caffeine (p.782·1).
*Fever; pain.*

**Cofendyl** *Aspen, S.Afr.*
Paracetamol (p.76·2); codeine phosphate (p.27·1); pseudoephedrine hydrochloride (p.1129·2).
*Cold and influenza symptoms.*

**Coffalon N** *Stark, Ger.*
Paracetamol (p.76·2); caffeine (p.782·1).
Coffalon formerly contained paracetamol, salicylamide, caffeine, and tiemonium iodide.
*Pain.*

**Coffeemed N** *Passauer, Ger.*
Caffeine (p.782·1); phenazone (p.82·3).
*Pain.*

**Coffekapton** *Strallhofer, Austria.*
Caffeine (p.782·1).
*Fatigue; vascular headache.*

**Coffetylin** *Bristol-Myers Squibb, Ger.†.*
Aspirin (p.15·1); caffeine (p.782·1).
*Fever; pain.*

**Coffo Selt** *Rosch & Handel, Austria.*
Phenazone (p.82·3); caffeine (p.782·1).
*Pain.*

**Coff-Rest** *Garec, S.Afr.*
Triprolidine hydrochloride (p.442·3); pseudoephedrine hydrochloride (p.1129·2); dextromethorphan hydrobromide (p.1117·3).
*Coughs.*

**Coff-Up** *Propan, S.Afr.†.*
Pheniramine maleate (p.438·3); menthol (p.1711·3); ammonium chloride (p.1115·2); sodium citrate (p.1223·2).
*Respiratory-tract congestion.*

**Coficold-Ped** *Stiefel, Braz.†.*
Paracetamol (p.76·2); pentoxyverine citrate (p.1126·2); phenylephrine hydrochloride (p.1126·3); carbinoxamine maleate (p.426·3).
*Influenza symptoms.*

**Cofi-Tabs** *Vitabalans, Fin.*
Caffeine (p.782·1).
*Fatigue.*

**Co-Flem** *Aspen, S.Afr.*
Carbocisteine (p.1116·2).
*Respiratory-tract congestion.*

**Cofrel** *Pfizer, Hong Kong.*
Benproperine (p.1115·2).
*Coughs.*

**Cofron**
*Abbott, Arg.; Abbott, Chile.*
Clofedanol hydrochloride (p.1117·1); bromhexine hydrochloride (p.1115·3).
*Coughs.*

**Cofsed** *Greater Pharma, Thai.*
Diphenhydramine hydrochloride (p.431·3); ammonium chloride (p.1115·2); sodium citrate (p.1223·2).
*Coughs; nasal congestion.*

**Co-Gel** *Aspen, S.Afr.*
Dicycloverine hydrochloride (p.481·2); aluminium hydroxide (p.1249·2); light magnesium oxide (p.1272·3).
*Gastrointestinal disorders.*

**Cogenate** *General Drugs, Thai.*
Chloramphenicol sodium succinate (p.185·1).
*Bacterial infections.*

**Cogentin**
*Merck Sharp & Dohme, Austral.; Merck Sharp & Dohme, Austria; Merck Frosst, Canad.; Merck Sharp & Dohme, Denm.; Merck Sharp & Dohme, Hong Kong; Merck Sharp & Dohme, Irl.; Merck Sharp & Dohme, Norw.; Merck Sharp & Dohme, NZ; Merck Sharp & Dohme, Port.; Merck Sharp & Dohme, Swed.†; Merck Sharp & Dohme, Thai.; Merck Sharp & Dohme, UK; Merck, USA.*
Benzatropine mesilate (p.479·2).
*Drug-induced extrapyramidal disorders; parkinsonism.*

**Cogentinol** *Astra, Ger.†.*
Benzatropine mesilate (p.479·2).
*Parkinsonism.*

**Co-Gesic**
Note. This name is used for preparations of different composition.
*Aspen, S.Afr.*
Paracetamol (p.76·2); codeine phosphate (p.27·1).
*Fever; pain.*

*Schwarz, USA.*
Paracetamol (p.76·2); hydrocodone tartrate (p.45·1).
*Pain.*

**Cogetine** *General Drugs, Thai.*
Chloramphenicol (p.185·1).
*Bacterial eye infections.*

**Cogitum**
*GlaxoSmithKline Sante, Fr.; Korangi, Port.*
Bipotassium acetylaspartate.
*Asthenia.*

**Cognex**
*Pfizer, Austral.†; Parke, Davis, Austria†; Parke, Davis, Belg.†; Parke, Davis, Braz.†; Parke, Davis, Fr.†; Parke, Davis, Ger.†; Genesis, Gr.; Parke, Davis, Hong Kong†; Parke, Davis, Israel†; Parke, Davis, NZ†; Parke, Davis, Port.†; OTL, Spain; Parke, Davis, Swed.†; Parke, Davis, Switz.†; Parke, Davis, USA.*
Tacrine hydrochloride (p.1497·2).
*Alzheimer's disease.*

**Cognitiv**
*Note. This name is used for preparations of different composition.*
*Rontag, Arg.*
Tacrine hydrochloride (p.1497·2).
*Alzheimer's disease.*

*Ebewe, Austria.*
Selegiline hydrochloride (p.1214·1).
*Parkinsonism.*

**Cognito** *Health Perception, UK.*
Phosphatidyl serine (p.1731·2).
*Memory impairment.*

**Cohemin** *Orion, Fin.*
Hydroxocobalamin acetate (p.1458·2).
*Megaloblastic anaemia; neuropathies; vitamin $B_{12}$ deficiency.*

**Co-Hist** *Roberts, USA.*
Pseudoephedrine hydrochloride (p.1129·2); chlorphenamine (p.428·1); paracetamol (p.76·2).
*Upper respiratory-tract symptoms.*

**Cohistan** *Biomedis, Thai.; Great Eastern, Thai.*
Chlorphenamine maleate (p.427·3).
*Hypersensitivity reactions.*

**Cohistan Expectorant** *Biomedis, Thai.; Great Eastern, Thai.*
Guaifenesin (p.1122·1); chlorphenamine maleate (p.427·3).
*Coughs.*

**Cohortan** *Fher, Spain.*
*Cream†:* Benzoxonium chloride (p.1170·2); hydrocortisone acetate (p.1103·3).
*Infected skin disorders.*

*Rectal ointment:* Hydrocortisone (p.1103·3); tyrothricin (p.275·1); isopropyl benzatropine mesilate.
*Anorectal disorders.*

**Cohortan Antibiotico** *Fher, Spain†.*
Hydrocortisone (p.1103·3); tyrothricin (p.275·1); benzoxonium chloride (p.1170·2).
*Infected skin disorders.*

**Co-Hypert** *Pekana, Ger.*
Homoeopathic preparation.

**Co-Inhibace** *Roche, Belg.*
Cilazapril (p.883·3); hydrochlorothiazide (p.933·2).
*Hypertension.*

**Cokenzen** *Takeda, Fr.*
Candesartan cilexetil (p.878·3); hydrochlorothiazide (p.933·2).
*Hypertension.*

**Cola Tonic** *Fiori, Ital.*
Fructose; kola; ginseng; fieno greco; guarana (p.1417·1).
*Nutritional supplement.*

**Colace**
*Wellspring, Canad.; Purdue, USA.*
Docusate sodium (p.1262·2).
*Constipation.*

**Colace Infant/Child** *Purdue, USA.*
Glycerol (p.1694·3).
*Constipation.*

**Colachofra** *EMS, Braz.*
Sorbitol (p.1446·3); betaine hydrochloride (p.1660·2); cynara (p.1678·3); boldo (p.1661·2); solanum paniculatum.
*Liver disorders.*

**Coladren** *Coop. Farm., Ital.*
Cascara (p.1255·1); boldo (p.1661·2).
*Constipation.*

**Colagain** *Metochem, Austria†.*
Kola (p.1765·3); soya lecithin (p.1706·1); vitamin E (p.1464·3).
*Tonic.*

**Colagenan** *Herbarium, Braz.*
Gelatin (p.754·3).

**Colagolen** *EMS, Braz.†.*
Methenamine mandelate (p.230·2); dehydrocholic acid (p.1679·2); bilineurin; sodium glycolate (p.1660·3); cynarine (p.1678·3); sodium citrate (p.1223·2); sodium benzoate (p.1169·3).
*Liver disorders.*

**Colagotil** *Cazi, Braz.†.*
Dehydrocholic acid (p.1679·2); acetylmethionine; choline chloride (p.1424·3); liquorice (p.1270·2); solanum paniculatum.
*Liver disorders.*

**Colambil** *Madaus, Spain†.*
Fumitory (p.1690·1).
*Biliary-tract disorders.*

**Colamin** *Solvay, Ital.†.*
Cascara (p.1255·1).
*Constipation.*

**Colatan** *Allen, Spain.*
Naratriptan hydrochloride (p.470·1).
*Migraine.*

**Colatus** *Nakorn, Thai.*
Paracetamol (p.76·2); phenylephrine hydrochloride (p.1126·3); chlorphenamine maleate (p.427·3); dextromethorphan hydrobromide (p.1117·3).
Formerly contained paracetamol, phenylpropanolamine hydrochloride, phenylephrine hydrochloride, chlorphenamine maleate, and dextromethorphan hydrobromide.
*Cold symptoms.*

**Co-Lav** *Copley, USA†.*
Macrogol 3350 (p.1709·1); electrolytes (p.1217·1).
*Bowel evacuation.*

**Colax** *OFF, Ital.*
Senna (p.1288·2); rhubarb (p.1287·3); cynara (p.1678·3); boldo (p.1661·2).
*Constipation; digestive disorders; loss of appetite.*

**Colax-C** *Metapharma, Canad.†.*
Docusate calcium (p.1262·1).
*Constipation.*

**Colax-S** *Metapharma, Canad.†.*
Docusate sodium (p.1262·2).
*Constipation.*

**Colazal** *Salix, USA.*
Balsalazide sodium (p.1251·2).
*Ulcerative colitis.*

**Colazid**
*Shire, Norw.; Meda, Swed.*
Balsalazide sodium (p.1251·2).
*Ulcerative colitis.*

**Colazide** *Shire, UK.*
Balsalazide sodium (p.1251·2).
*Ulcerative colitis.*

**ColBenemid** *Merck, USA.*
Probenecid (p.416·3); colchicine (p.415·1).
*Chronic gouty arthritis.*

**Colbiocin** *SIFI, Ital.*
*Eye drops:* Rolitetracycline (p.254·1); chloramphenicol (p.185·1); colistimethate sodium (p.199·1).
*Eye ointment:* Tetracycline (p.266·2); chloramphenicol (p.185·1); colistimethate sodium (p.199·1).
*Eye infections.*

**Colbuzer** *Zerboni, Mex.†.*
Probucol (p.986·3).

**Colcaps** *Covan, S.Afr.*
*Capsules:* Phenylpropanolamine hydrochloride (p.1127·3); phenylephrine hydrochloride (p.1126·3); mepyramine maleate (p.437·1); caffeine (p.782·1); salicylamide (p.87·3); chlorphenamine maleate (p.427·3).
*Cold and influenza symptoms; nasal congestion; rhinitis.*
*Effervescent tablets:* Paracetamol (p.76·2); phenylephrine hydrochloride (p.1126·3); vitamin C (p.1460·2).
*Cold and influenza symptoms.*
*Syrup:* Paracetamol (p.76·2); codeine phosphate (p.27·1); promethazine hydrochloride (p.439·1); pseudoephedrine hydrochloride (p.1129·2).
*Cold and influenza symptoms; nasal congestion; rhinitis.*

**Colchicum Med Complex** *Dynamit, Austria.*
Homoeopathic preparation.

**Colchily** *Pharmasant, Thai.*
Colchicine (p.415·1).
*Gout.*

**Colchimax**
*Note. This name is used for preparations of different composition.*
*Aventis, Fr.*
Colchicine (p.415·1); tiemonium metilsulfate (p.489·3); opium powder (p.74·2).
*Gout; inflammatory disorders.*

*Seid, Spain.*
Colchicine (p.415·1); dicycloverine hydrochloride (p.481·2).
*Gout.*

**Colchiquim** *Quimica y Farmacia, Mex.*
Colchicine (p.415·1).
*Gout; hepatic cirrhosis.*

**Colchis** *Apsen, Braz.*
Colchicine (p.415·1).
*Familial Mediterranean fever; gout; psoriasis; sarcoidosis; scleroderma.*

**Colchysat** *Ysatfabrik, Ger.*
Colchicum autumnale (p.416·3).
*Gout.*

**Colcine** *Fascino, Thai.*
Colchicine (p.415·1).
*Gout.*

**Colcleer** *Propan, S.Afr.*
Chlorphenamine maleate (p.427·3); ephedrine hydrochloride (p.1120·1); paracetamol (p.76·2); caffeine (p.782·1).
*Cold and influenza symptoms.*

**Cold & Allergy** *Prometic, Canad.†.*
Phenylpropanolamine hydrochloride (p.1127·3); phenylephrine hydrochloride (p.1126·3); brompheniramine maleate (p.426·1).

**Cold & Allergy Relief** *Stanley, Canad.†.*
Phenylpropanolamine hydrochloride (p.1127·3); phenylephrine hydrochloride (p.1126·3); brompheniramine maleate (p.426·1).

**Cold Control** *Reese, USA.*
Diphenhydramine hydrochloride (p.431·3); pseudoephedrine hydrochloride (p.1129·2); paracetamol (p.76·2).
*Cold symptoms.*

**Cold Cream Avene** *Silesia, Chile.*
White beeswax (p.1480·1); liquid paraffin (p.1479·1).
*Dry skin disorders.*

**Cold Cream Naturel**
*Roche-Posay, Arg.*
Cetyl esters wax (p.1480·3); white beeswax (p.1480·1); light liquid paraffin (p.1479·1).
*Nappy rash; vehicle for dermatological agents.*

*Roche-Posay, Fr.*
Cetyl palmitate; white beeswax (p.1480·1); light liquid paraffin (p.1479·1).
*Skin dryness and irritation.*

**Cold Cream Salicyle** *Roche-Posay, Fr.*
Salicylic acid (p.1157·1); titanium dioxide (p.1160·3).
*Skin disorders.*

**Cold Decongestant** *Novopharm, Canad.†.*
Phenylpropanolamine hydrochloride (p.1127·3); chlorphenamine maleate (p.427·3); pheniramine maleate (p.438·3).

**Cold & Flu (Non-Drowsy) Tablets** *Biotech, Austral.†.*
Codeine phosphate (p.27·1); paracetamol (p.76·2); pseudoephedrine hydrochloride (p.1129·2).
*Cold and influenza symptoms.*

**Cold and Flu Relief** *Brauer, Austral.†.*
Ascorbic acid (p.1460·2); echinacea angustifolia (p.1683·2); zinc gluconate (p.1469·2); apis mel.; arsen. alb.; aurum met.; baptisia tinct.; belladonna; bryonia; ferrum phos.; merc. sol.
*Cold and influenza symptoms.*

**Cold & Flu Tablets**
*Note. This name is used for preparations of different composition.*
*Biotech, Austral.†.*
Codeine phosphate (p.27·1); paracetamol (p.76·2); pseudoephedrine hydrochloride (p.1129·2); chlorphenamine maleate (p.427·3); belladonna (p.479·1).
*Cold and influenza symptoms.*

*Hamilton, Austral.†.*
Paracetamol (p.76·2); pseudoephedrine hydrochloride (p.1129·2); codeine phosphate (p.27·1).
*Cold and influenza symptoms.*

**Cold & Flu Tablets Non Drowsy** *Or-Dov, Austral.†.*
Pseudoephedrine hydrochloride (p.1129·2); paracetamol (p.76·2); phenylephrine hydrochloride (p.1126·3); citrus bioflavonoids (p.1688·2); ascorbic acid (p.1460·2).
*Cold and influenza symptoms; hay fever.*

**Cold Max** *Reese, USA†.*
Chlorphenamine (p.428·1); phenylpropanolamine (p.1127·3).
*Cold symptoms.*

**Cold Medication D** *Prodemdis, Canad.*
Pseudoephedrine hydrochloride (p.1129·2); dextromethorphan hydrobromide (p.1117·3); paracetamol (p.76·2).

**Cold Medication Daytime Relief** *Stanley, Canad.†; WestCan, Canad.†.*
Pseudoephedrine hydrochloride (p.1129·2); dextromethorphan hydrobromide (p.1117·3); paracetamol (p.76·2).

**Cold Medication N** *Prodemdis, Canad.*
Pseudoephedrine hydrochloride (p.1129·2); chlorphenamine maleate (p.427·3); dextromethorphan hydrobromide (p.1117·3); paracetamol (p.76·2).

**Cold Medication Nighttime Relief** *WestCan, Canad.†.*
Pseudoephedrine hydrochloride (p.1129·2); chlorphenamine maleate (p.427·3); dextromethorphan hydrobromide (p.1117·3); paracetamol (p.76·2).

**Cold Relief**
*Note. This name is used for preparations of different composition.*
*Sussex, UK†.*
Paracetamol (p.76·2); caffeine (p.782·1); phenylephrine hydrochloride (p.1126·3).
*Cold symptoms.*

*Unichem, UK.*
*Capsules:* Paracetamol (p.76·2); caffeine (p.782·1); phenylephrine hydrochloride (p.1126·3).
*Oral powders:* Paracetamol (p.76·2); ascorbic acid (p.1460·2).
*Cold and influenza symptoms.*

*Rugby, USA†.*
Chlorphenamine maleate (p.427·3); dextromethorphan hydrobromide (p.1117·3); paracetamol (p.76·2); phenylpropanolamine hydrochloride (p.1127·3).
*Coughs and cold symptoms.*

**Cold Relief Daytime** *Unichem, UK†.*
Paracetamol (p.76·2); pholcodine (p.1128·3); pseudoephedrine hydrochloride (p.1129·2).
*Cold and influenza symptoms.*

**Cold Relief Night-Time** *Unichem, UK†.*
Paracetamol (p.76·2); pholcodine (p.1128·3); pseudoephedrine hydrochloride (p.1129·2); diphenhydramine hydrochloride (p.431·3).
*Cold and influenza symptoms.*

**Cold Sore** *ICN, NZ.*
Menthol (p.1711·3); camphor (p.1665·3); benzoin (p.1751·1).
*Herpes labialis.*

**Cold Sore Balm**
*Abbott, Austral.†; Abbott, NZ†.*
Lidocaine (p.1377·3); nitromersol (p.1186·3).
*Herpes labialis.*

**Cold Sore Lotion**
*Note. This name is used for preparations of different composition.*
*DC Labs, Canad.*
Benzocaine (p.1370·3); benzoin (p.1751·1); camphor (p.1665·3); menthol (p.1711·3); myrrh (p.1718·3).

*Sabex, Canad.†.*
Menthol (p.1711·3); myrrh (p.1718·3); benzoin (p.1751·1) (p.1744·1); camphor (p.1665·3); alcohol (p.1166·1).
*Herpes labialis.*

*Stanley, Canad.; Rougier, Canad.*
Benzoin (p.1751·1); camphor (p.1665·3); menthol (p.1711·3).

**Cold Sore Relief** *Vitaplex, Austral.†.*
Lysine hydrochloride (p.1439·2); ascorbic acid (p.1460·2); zinc amino acid chelate (p.1469·3).
*Herpes labialis.*

**Cold Sore Tablets** *Vitaglow, Austral.†.*
Lysine hydrochloride (p.1439·2); ascorbic acid (p.1460·2); betacarotene (p.1422·3); zinc amino acid chelate (p.1469·3).
*Herpes labialis.*

**Cold Sores, Fever Blisters** *Hylands, Canad.*
Homoeopathic preparation.

**Cold Tablets with Zinc** *Hylands, Canad.*
Homoeopathic preparation.

**Colda** *Sigmapharm, Austria.*
Sage oil (p.1741·2); thuja oil (p.1755·1); pumilio pine oil (p.1737·1); camphor (p.1665·3); oleum pini sylvestris; dexpanthenol (p.1727·2); eucalyptus oil (p.1686·2).
*Respiratory-tract disorders.*

**Coldacrom** *Sigmapharm, Austria.*
Sodium cromoglicate (p.795·3).
*Conjunctivitis.*

**Coldadolin** *Sigmapharm, Austria.*
Ethenzamide (p.37·2); paracetamol (p.76·2); caffeine (p.782·1); butetamate citrate (p.1116·2).
*Smooth muscle spasm and pain.*

**Coldagrippin** *Sigmapharm, Austria.*
Paracetamol (p.76·2); propyphenazone (p.85·3); caffeine (p.782·1).
*Fever; pain.*

**Coldan**
*Sigmapharm, Austria; Kotsopoulos (Κωτσοπουλος), Gr.*
Naphazoline hydrochloride (p.1124·3).
*Adjunct in rhinoscopy; conjunctivitis; hay fever; rhinitis; sinusitis; sore throat.*

**Coldangin** *Sigmapharm, Austria.*
Dichlorobenzyl alcohol (p.1178·3); amylmetacresol (p.1168·2).
*Mouth and throat disorders.*

**Coldargan** *Sigmapharm, Austria.*
Silver protein (p.1746·2); ephedrine levulinate (p.1120·3); calcium levulinate (p.1225·3); sodium levulinate.
*Mouth and throat disorders; rhinitis; sinusitis.*

**Coldastop** *Desitin, Ger.*
Vitamin A palmitate (p.1453·1); alpha tocoferil acetate (p.1465·1).
*Rhinitis.*

**Coldate** *Chew, Thai.†.*
Dextromethorphan hydrobromide (p.1117·3); brompheniramine maleate (p.426·1); phenylpropanolamine hydrochloride (p.1127·3); paracetamol (p.76·2).
*Coughs and cold symptoms.*

**Coldec D** *Breckenridge, USA.*
Pseudoephedrine hydrochloride (p.1129·2); carbinoxamine maleate (p.426·3).
*Upper respiratory-tract disorders.*

**Coldec DM** *Silarx, USA.*
Brompheniramine maleate (p.426·1); pseudoephedrine hydrochloride (p.1129·2); dextromethorphan hydrobromide (p.1117·3).
*Coughs.*

**Cold-eeze** *English Grains, UK†.*
Garlic (p.1691·1); echinacea (p.1683·2).
*Cold symptoms.*

**Coldenza** *Nelson, UK.*
Homoeopathic preparation.

**Colderina** *Wayne, Mex.†.*
Paracetamol (p.76·2).
*Fever; pain.*

**Coldetab** *Chew, Thai.†.*
Paracetamol (p.76·2); chlorphenamine maleate (p.427·3); phenylpropanolamine (p.1127·3).
*Coughs and cold symptoms.*

**Coldex** *Teva, Israel.*
Caffeine (p.782·1); chlorphenamine maleate (p.427·3); phenylephrine hydrochloride (p.1126·3); paracetamol (p.76·2).
*Cold symptoms; sinusitis.*

**Cold-Gard** *Weider, UK†.*
Zinc acetate (p.1469·2).
*Cold symptoms.*

**Coldil** *Dolisos, Canad.†.*
Homoeopathic preparation.

**Coldin** *Aventis, Chile.*
Carbocisteine (p.1116·2).
*Respiratory-tract disorders with viscous mucus.*

**Coldistan** *Sigmapharm, Austria.*
*Eye drops; nasal drops:* Diphenhydramine hydrochloride (p.431·3); naphazoline hydrochloride (p.1124·3).
*Allergic eye disorders; eye irritation; rhinitis; sinusitis.*
*Nasal ointment:* Diphenhydramine hydrochloride (p.431·3); phenylephrine hydrochloride (p.1126·3); calcium levulinate (p.1225·3); cetylpyridinium chloride (p.1173·1); dexpanthenol (p.1727·2); sage oil (p.1741·2).
*Hay fever; rhinitis; sinusitis.*

**Coldistop**
*Sigmapharm, Austria; Sigmapharm, Switz.*
Vitamin A palmitate (p.1453·1); alpha tocoferil acetate (p.1465·1).
*Nasal and sinus disorders.*

**Coldloc** *Fleming, USA†.*
Guaifenesin (p.1122·1); phenylpropanolamine hydrochloride (p.1127·3); phenylephrine hydrochloride (p.1126·3).
*Upper respiratory-tract symptoms.*

**Coldloc-LA** *Fleming, USA†.*
Phenylpropanolamine hydrochloride (p.1127·3); guaifenesin (p.1122·1).
*Upper respiratory-tract symptoms.*

**Coldoff** *Stadmed, India.*
Phenylephrine hydrochloride (p.1126·3); paracetamol (p.76·2); chlorphenamine maleate (p.427·3); caffeine (p.782·1).
*Cold symptoms.*

**Coldophthal** *Sigmapharm, Austria.*
Naphazoline hydrochloride (p.1124·3); mercuric oxycyanide (p.1713·3); boric acid (p.1662·1).
*Conjunctivitis; eye irritation.*

**Coldosian** *Asian Pharm, Thai.*
*Syrup:* Paracetamol (p.76·2); chlorphenamine maleate (p.427·3).
Formerly contained paracetamol, chlorphenamine maleate, and phenylpropanolamine hydrochloride.
*Tablets:* Paracetamol (p.76·2); chlorphenamine maleate (p.427·3).
Formerly contained paracetamol, chlorphenamine maleate, phenylpropanolamine hydrochloride, and caffeine.
*Cold symptoms; sinusitis.*

**Coldrex**
*Note. This name is used for preparations of different composition.*
*GlaxoSmithKline, Fin.*
Aspirin (p.15·1); guaifenesin (p.1122·1); caffeine (p.782·1); ascorbic acid (p.1460·2).
*Cold and influenza symptoms.*
*GlaxoSmithKline, Hong Kong.*
Paracetamol (p.76·2); phenylephrine hydrochloride (p.1126·3); vitamin C (p.1460·2); noscapine (p.1125·3); terpin hydrate (p.1131·1); caffeine (p.782·1).
*Cold and influenza symptoms; sinusitis.*

**Coldrex C** *SmithKline Beecham Consumer, Neth.*
Aspirin (p.15·1); ascorbic acid (p.1460·2).
*Cold and influenza symptoms.*

**Coldrex Day/Night** *GlaxoSmithKline, NZ.*
Day tablets, paracetamol (p.76·2); pseudoephedrine hydrochloride (p.1129·2); night tablets, chlorphenamine maleate (p.427·3); paracetamol; pseudoephedrine hydrochloride.
*Cold and influenza symptoms; nasal congestion.*

**Coldrex Flu** *SmithKline Beecham, NZ†.*
Paracetamol (p.76·2); dextromethorphan hydrobromide (p.1117·3); chlorphenamine maleate (p.427·3); pseudoephedrine hydrochloride (p.1129·2).
*Cold and influenza symptoms.*

**Coldrex Head & Chest Cold** *GlaxoSmithKline, NZ.*
Paracetamol (p.76·2); pseudoephedrine hydrochloride (p.1129·2); dextromethorphan hydrobromide (p.1117·3).
*Cold and influenza symptoms.*

**Coldrex Head Cold** *GlaxoSmithKline, NZ.*
Paracetamol (p.76·2); pseudoephedrine hydrochloride (p.1129·2).
*Sinusitis.*

**Coldrex Night Relief** *SmithKline Beecham, NZ†.*
Paracetamol (p.76·2); promethazine hydrochloride (p.439·1); dextromethorphan hydrobromide (p.1117·3).
*Cold and influenza symptoms.*

**Coldrin**
*Note. This name is used for preparations of different composition.*
*Janssen-Cilag, Braz.*
Cinnarizine (p.428·3); phenylephrine hydrochloride (p.1126·3); pentoxyverine citrate (p.1126·2); paracetamol (p.76·2); ascorbic acid (p.1460·2).
*Influenza symptoms.*
*Shinyaku, Hong Kong; Shinyaku, Singapore.*
Clofedanol hydrochloride (p.1117·1).
*Coughs.*

**Coldrine** *Roberts, USA; Hauck, USA.*
Pseudoephedrine hydrochloride (p.1129·2); paracetamol (p.76·2).
*Upper respiratory-tract symptoms.*

**Coldstat** *Prater, Chile.*
Aspirin (p.15·1); caffeine (p.782·1); chlorphenamine (p.428·1).
*Cold and influenza symptoms.*

**Coldvac** *Byk Madaus, S.Afr.*
Pneumococci; streptococci; staphylococci; *Haemophilus influenzae*(p.0·0).
*Respiratory-tract disorders.*

**Coldy** *The Forty-Two, Thai.†.*
Paracetamol (p.76·2); chlorphenamine (p.428·1) or chlorphenamine maleate (p.427·3); phenylpropanolamine (p.1127·3) or phenylpropanolamine hydrochloride (p.1127·3).
*Allergic rhinitis; cold symptoms; hay fever; sinusitis.*

**Coleb** *Promed, Ger.; AstraZeneca, Ger.*
Isosorbide mononitrate (p.942·1).
*Angina pectoris.*

**Colebrina** *Schering, Braz.†*
Iocetamic acid (p.1063·2).
*Contrast medium for biliary-tract radiography.*

**Coledis** *Sidus, Arg.*
Simvastatin (p.997·1).
*Hypercholesterolaemia.*

**Coledos** *Prospa, Ital.*
Ursodeoxycholic acid (p.1760·3).
*Biliary-tract disorders.*

**Colegraf** *Estedi, Spain.*
Iopanoic acid (p.1065·1).
*Contrast medium for biliary-tract radiography.*

**Colemin** *Biohorm, Spain.*
Simvastatin (p.997·1).
*Hyperlipidaemias.*

**Colenon** *SIRC, Singapore.*
Poliglusam; garcinia cambogia; hydroxycitric acid; chromium; vitamin C (p.1417·1).
*Dietary aid.*

**Colepren** *Randall, Mex.*
Hyoscine butylbromide (p.483·3); dipyrone (p.35·3).
*Smooth muscle spasm.*

**Colerin** *Lab, Port.*
Azintamide (p.1658·3).
*Digestive insufficiency.*

**Colerin-F** *Lab, Port.*
Azintamide (p.1658·3); cellulase (p.1669·1); pancreatin (p.1725·3).
*Digestive insufficiency.*

**Colese** *Alphapharm, Austral.*
Mebeverine hydrochloride (p.1273·1).
*Irritable bowel syndrome.*

**Colesom** *Temis, Arg.*
Iopanoic acid (p.1065·1).
*Contrast medium for cholecystography.*

**Colestase** *Sanofi Synthelabo, Braz.*
Furazolidone (p.605·2); diphenoxylate hydrochloride (p.1261·3).
Atropine sulfate (p.477·1) is included in this preparation to discourage abuse.
Formerly contained furazolidone, diphenoxylate hydrochloride, pectin, aluminium silicate, and magnesium hydroxide.
*Diarrhoea.*

**Colesterinex** *Almirall, Spain†.*
Pyricarbate (p.1737·1).
*Hyperlipidaemias.*

**Colesthexal** *Hexal, Ger.*
Colestyramine (p.889·3).
*Hyperlipidaemias.*

**Colestid**
*Pharmacia, Austral.; Pharmacia, Belg.; Pharmacia, Canad.; Pharmacia, Ger.; Pharmacia, Irl.; Pharmacia Upjohn, Israel; Pharmacia Upjohn, Mex.†; Pharmacia, Neth.; Pharmacia, NZ; Pharmacia, Port.; Pharmacia, Spain; Pharmacia, Switz.; Pharmacia, UK; Pharmacia Upjohn, USA.*
Colestipol hydrochloride (p.889·2).
*Hypercholesterolaemia.*

**Colesto Cero** *Garden House, Arg.*
Commiphora mukul.
*Dietary supplement.*

**Colestyr** *CT, Ger.*
Colestyramine (p.889·3).
*Hyperlipidaemias.*

**Colesvir** *Vir, Spain.*
Lovastatin (p.949·1).
*Atherosclerosis; hypercholesterolaemia.*

**Colevix** *Royal, Chile.*
Lovastatin (p.949·1).
*Hypercholesterolaemia.*

**Colex** *Tramedico, Neth.*
Dibasic sodium phosphate (p.1231·1); monobasic sodium phosphate (p.1230·3).
*Bowel evacuation; constipation.*

**Colfed-A** *Parmed, USA.*
Pseudoephedrine hydrochloride (p.1129·2); chlorphenamine maleate (p.427·3).
*Upper respiratory-tract symptoms.*

**Colfur** *Carter-Wallace, Mex.*
*Oral suspension:* Colistin sulfate (p.198·3); furazolidone (p.605·2); kaolin (p.1268·3); pectin (p.1580·3).
*Tablets:* Colistin sulfate (p.198·3); furazolidone (p.605·2).
*Gastrointestinal infections.*

**Colgen** *Bournonville, Belg.†.*
Collagen (bovine, non-denatured) (p.1674·3).
*Haemorrhage.*

**Colgout**
*Aspen, Austral.; Aspen, Hong Kong.*
Colchicine (p.415·1).
*Gout; polyarthritis associated with sarcoidosis.*

**Colhidrol** *Teva Tuteur, Arg.*
Doxorubicin (p.547·3).
*Malignant neoplasms.*

**Coliacron** *Enzypharm, Neth.†.*
Glutamine synthetase; acetylcoenzyme A kinase; oxidative phosphorylating enzymes.
*Psychosomatic and neurovegetative disorders.*

**Colibiogen** *Laves, Ger.*
Peptide extract from *Escherichia coli.*
*Gastrointestinal disorders; hypersensitivity; musculoskeletal and joint disorders; skin disorders.*

**Colic** *Hylands, Canad.*
Homoeopathic preparation.

**Colic Relief** *Brauer, Austral.†.*
Homoeopathic preparation.

**Colicon** *Reese, USA.*
Simeticone (p.1289·2).

**Colicort** *Merck Sharp & Dohme-Chibret, Fr.†.*
Colistimethate sodium (p.199·1); tetracycline hydrochloride (p.266·2); prednisolone sodium phosphate (p.1108·1).
*Infections of the ear, nose, and throat.*

**Colief**
*Clonmel, Irl.; Britannia Health, UK.*
Tilactase (p.1756·2).
*Colic associated with lactose intolerance.*

**Colifagina S** *ABC, Ital.*
Lysate of *Escherichia coli*; *Bacillus pumilus*; *Morganella morgani*; *Alcaligenes faecalis*; *Shigella flexneri*; *Enterococcus faecalis* (p.1704·2); *Bacillus subtilis*; *Proteus vulgaris.*
*Gastrointestinal infections; genito-urinary infections.*

**Coli-Fagina S** *ABC, Port.*
Lysates of *Escherichia coli*; *Bacillus morgani*; *B. faecalis alcaligenes*; *E. pseudodysenteriae*; *Bacillus subtilis*; *Proteus vulgaris*; *Enterococcus faecalis* (p.1704·2); *B. mesentericus.*
*Gastrointestinal infections; genito-urinary infections.*

**Colifilm** *Merck, Arg.*
Loperamide (p.1271·2).
*Diarrhoea; ileostomy management.*

**Colifoam**
*Stafford-Miller, Austral.; Block, Austria; GlaxoSmithKline Consumer, Belg.†; Meda, Denm.; Meda, Fin.; Trommsdorff, Ger.; GlaxoSmithKline Consumer, Ger.; Kite (Κιτε), Gr.; Stafford-Miller, Irl.; Stafford-Miller, Israel†; Stafford-Miller, Ital.; Schwarz, Norw.; Stafford-Miller, NZ; GlaxoSmithKline, Port.; Omnimed, S.Afr.; Meda, Swed.; Stafford-Miller, Switz.†; Meda, UK.*
Hydrocortisone acetate (p.1103·3).
*Inflammatory bowel disease.*

**Colifossim** *Day, Ital.*
Cefuroxime sodium (p.184·1).
*Bacterial infections.*

**Colimax** *Qualiphar, Belg.*
Ephedrine hydrochloride (p.1120·1); sodium benzoate (p.1169·3); aconite (p.1646·3); belladonna (p.479·1); thyme (p.1755·2); wild thyme; maidenhair fern.
*Coughs.*

**Colimet** *Collins, Mex.*
Cimetidine (p.1255·3).
*Peptic ulcer.*

**Colimex** *Wallace, India.*
*Oral drops:* Dicycloverine hydrochloride (p.481·2); simeticone (p.1289·2).
*Colic; flatulence; gastrointestinal spasm; irritable bowel.*
*Tablets:* Dicycloverine hydrochloride (p.481·2); paracetamol (p.76·2).
*Colic; dysmenorrhoea.*

**Colimicina**
*UCB, Ital.*
*Injection:* Colistimethate sodium (p.199·1).
*Gram-negative bacterial infections.*
*Tablets; oral drops:* Colistin sulfate (p.198·3).
*Gram-negative bacterial infections of the gastrointestinal tract.*
*Quimifar, Spain.*
Colistin sulfate (p.198·3).
*Bacterial infections.*

**Colimil** *Milte, Ital.*
Melissa (p.1711·1); chamomile (p.1669·3); fennel (p.1687·2).
*Infant colic.*

**Colimix**
*Xepa-Soul Pattinson, Hong Kong; Xepa-Soul Pattinson, Malaysia; Xepa-Soul Pattinson, Singapore.*
Dicycloverine hydrochloride (p.481·2); simeticone (p.1289·2).
*Flatulence; gastrointestinal spasm; infant colic.*

**Colimune** *Aventis, Ger.*
Sodium cromoglicate (p.795·3).
*Food hypersensitivity; ulcerative colitis; ulcerative proctitis.*

**Colimycin**
*Lundbeck, Denm.; Lundbeck, Norw.*
Colistimethate sodium (p.199·1).
*Bacterial infections.*

**Colimycine**
*Glaxo Wellcome, Belg.†; Aventis, Fr.; Aventis, Neth.*
Colistin sulfate (p.198·3) or colistimethate sodium (p.199·1).
*Bacterial infections.*

**Colin** *Strand, Malaysia.*
Salbutamol sulfate (p.791·3).
*Obstructive airways disease; status asthmaticus.*

**Colina** *Intersan, Ger.*
Smectite.
*Diarrhoea; gastrointestinal disorders.*

**Colina Spezial** *Intersan, Ger.*
Smectite; aluminium hydroxide-magnesium carbonate gel (p.1250·1).
*Diarrhoea; gastrointestinal disorders.*

**Colinex** *Brasterapica, Braz.†.*
Papaverine hydrochloride (p.1728·1); belladonna (p.479·1); hyoscyamus (p.485·2); boldo (p.1661·2); valerian (p.1762·2).
*Gastrointestinal disorders.*

**Colinsan** *Ferring, Ger.*
Azathioprine (p.1349·1).
*Auto-immune disorders; dermatomyositis; idiopathic thrombocytopenic purpura; inflammatory bowel disease; polyarteritis nodosa; rheumatoid arthritis; transplant rejection.*

**Colinvintol** *Sedar, Braz.†.*
Adenosine (p.851·2); methionine (p.1042·1); betaine hydrochloride (p.1660·2); choline (p.1424·3); pyridoxine (p.1457·2); glucose (p.1432·2).
*Liver disorders.*

**Coli-Om** *OM, Port.*
Lysate of *Escherichia coli.*
*Gastrointestinal infections; urinary-tract infections.*

**Coliopan**
*Eisai, Hong Kong†; Eisai, Jpn; Eisai, Malaysia; Eisai, Singapore.*
Butropium bromide (p.480·1).
*Painful gastrointestinal spasm.*

**Coliper** *Mintlab, Chile.*
Loperamide (p.1271·2).
*Diarrhoea.*

**Coliquifilm**
*Allergan, Ger.; Allergan, Switz.*
White soft paraffin (p.1479·3); wool alcohols (p.1482·3); light liquid paraffin (p.1479·1).
*Eye disorders.*

**Coliracin** *Rafa, Israel.*
Colistimethate sodium (p.199·1).
*Bacterial infections.*

**Colircusi Anestesico** *Alcon, Port.*
Tetracaine (p.1385·1); naphazoline (p.1124·3).
*Eye disorders.*

**Colircusi Cicloplejico** *Alcon Cusi, Malaysia.*
Cyclopentolate hydrochloride (p.480·3).
*Production of mydriasis and cycloplegia.*

**Colircusi Gentadexa** *Cusi, Hong Kong†.*
Gentamicin sulfate (p.217·1); dexamethasone sodium phosphate (p.1097·2); tetryzoline hydrochloride (p.1131·2).
*Infected eye and ear disorders.*

**Colircusi Iodine-Thio-Calcic** *Cusi, Hong Kong†.*
Sodium iodide (p.1598·1); potassium iodide (p.1598·1); calcium (p.1225·1); sodium thiosulfate (p.1053·3).
*Cataract; fungal eye infections.*

**Colirid** *Cadila, India.*
Dicycloverine hydrochloride (p.481·2); paracetamol (p.76·2); simeticone (p.1289·2).
*Colic; dysmenorrhoea; irritable bowel syndrome.*

**Colirio Blumen** *Luper, Braz.†.*
Zinc sulfate (p.1469·3); naphazoline hydrochloride (p.1124·3).
*Ocular congestion.*

**Colirio de Argyrol** *Quimioterapica, Braz.†.*
Silver protein (p.1746·2).
*Bacterial eye infections.*

**Colirio Helios** *Windson, Braz.†.*
Zinc sulfate (p.1469·3); chlorobutanol (p.1176·3).
*Eye disorders.*

**Colirio Legrand** *Legrand, Braz.*
Naphazoline (p.1124·3); zinc sulfate (p.1469·3).
*Ocular congestion.*

**Colirio Moura Brasil** *Aventis, Braz.†.*
Zinc sulfate (p.1469·3); naphazoline (p.1124·3).
*Ocular congestion.*

**Colirio Sulvi** *Grin, Mex.*
Naphazoline (p.1124·3); sulfacetamide (p.257·3).
*Eye disorders.*

**Colirio Teuto** *Teuto, Braz.*
Zinc sulfate (p.1469·3); naphazoline hydrochloride (p.1124·3).
*Ocular congestion.*

**Colirio Vima** *DM, Braz.†.*
Zinc sulfate (p.1469·3); naphazoline (p.1124·3).
*Ocular congestion.*

**Coliriocilina** *Medical, Spain.*
Benzylpenicillin potassium (p.163·2).
*Eye infections.*

**Coliriocilina Adren Astr** *Medical, Spain.*
Boric acid (p.1662·1); adrenaline hydrochloride (p.852·3); naphazoline hydrochloride (p.1124·3); procaine hydrochloride (p.1383·2); zinc sulfate (p.1469·3).
*Eye disorders.*

**Coliriocilina Espectro** *Medical, Spain†.*
Neomycin sulfate (p.235·1); oxytetracycline (p.241·1).
*Bacterial eye infections.*

**Coliriocilina Gentam** *Medical, Spain.*
Gentamicin sulfate (p.217·1).
*Eye infections.*

**Coliriocilina Homatrop** *Medical, Spain†.*
Homatropine hydrobromide (p.483·2).
*Production of mydriasis and cycloplegia; uveitis.*

**Coliriocilina Prednisona** *Medical, Spain.*
Neomycin sulfate (p.235·1); prednisone (p.1109·3).
*Eye disorders.*

**Colistop** *Hexa-Medinova, Arg.*
Phthalylsulfathiazole (p.242·3); bismuth subcarbonate (p.1252·1); homatropine methylbromide (p.483·2).
*Gastro-enteritis.*

**Colistoral** *Bristol-Myers Squibb, Arg.*
Phthalylsulfathiazole (p.242·3); bismuth subgallate (p.1252·2).
*Diarrhoea; gastroenteritis.*

**Colitofalk** *Codali, Belg.*
Mesalazine (p.1273·2).
*Inflammatory bowel disease.*

**Colitromin** *Collins, Mex.*
Erythromycin (p.208·1).
*Bacterial infections.*

**Colix** *Prolabor, Braz.†.*
Sodium hypochlorite (p.1192·1).
*Skin, wound, instrument, and surface disinfection.*

**Colizin** *Sedabel, Braz.*
Phenylephrine hydrochloride (p.1126·3); chlorphenamine maleate (p.427·3).
*Ocular congestion.*

**Colizole** *East India Pharma, India.*
Co-trimoxazole (p.199·3).
*Bacterial infections; Pneumocystis carinii pneumonia; toxoplasmosis.*

**Collafilm** *Immuno, Fr.†.*
Collagen (p.1674·3).
*Ulcers; wounds.*

**Collatamp G** *Schering-Plough, Fr.*
Collagen (bovine) (p.1674·3); gentamicin (p.219·1).
*Haemorrhage.*

**Collaven** *Roche, Austria†.*
Centella (p.1144·3).
*Chronic venous insufficiency.*

**Collazin** *Selmag, Switz.*
Zinc sulfate (p.1469·3).
*Zinc deficiency.*

**Colleofer** *Medo, Fin.†.*
Iron polymaltose (p.1437·3).
*Iron-deficiency anaemia.*

**Colli** *Gricar, Ital.†.*
Benzalkonium chloride (p.1168·3); hamamelis; chamomile.
*Eye disinfection; eye irritation.*

**Collins Elixir** *Collins Elixir, UK.*
Ethylmorphine hydrochloride (p.37·3).
*Coughs.*

**Collins Elixir Decongesant Pasilles** *Collins Elixir, UK.*
Menthol (p.1711·3); eucalyptus (p.1686·1).
*Coughs; nasal congestion.*

**Collins Elixir Pastilles** *Collins Elixir, UK†.*
Citric acid (p.1673·1); lemon oil (p.1706·2); squill vinegar (p.1130·3); glycerol (p.1694·3).
*Coughs; sore throats.*

**Collirio Alfa** *Bracco, Ital.*
Naphazoline nitrate (p.1124·3).
*Eye irritation.*

**Collirio Alfa Antistaminico** *Bracco, Ital.*
Thonzylamine hydrochloride (p.442·2); naphazoline nitrate (p.1124·3).
*Conjunctival disorders.*

**Collirium Geymonat** *Geymonat, Ital.†.*
Benzalkonium chloride (p.1168·3).
*Eye infections.*

**Collis Browne's** *Thornton & Ross, UK.*
*Oral mixture:* Morphine (p.60·1); peppermint oil (p.1283·2).
*Coughs; diarrhoea.*
*Tablets:* Light kaolin (p.1268·3); morphine hydrochloride (p.60·1); heavy calcium carbonate (p.1254·2).
*Diarrhoea.*

**Collodyne** *Universal, S.Afr.†.*
Light kaolin (p.1268·3); pectin (p.1580·3); bismuth subcarbonate (p.1252·1); chloroform and morphine tincture (p.60·1).
*Diarrhoea.*

**Colloidal 75** *Douglas, NZ.*
Mineral (p.1217·1) and trace-element preparation (p.1417·1).
*Nutritional supplement.*

**Colloidine** *Rudefsa, Mex.†.*
Propylhexedrine (p.1592·3).
*Obesity.*

**Collomack**
*Mack, Illert., Ger.; Mack, Hong Kong; Mack, Malaysia; Mack, Singapore; Mack, Thai.*
Salicylic acid (p.1157·1); lactic acid (p.1704·1); lauromacrogol 400 (p.1412·3).
*Calluses; corns; hard skin; warts.*

**Collosol**
*Note. This name is used for preparations of different composition.*
*Amido, Fr.†.*
Soap substitute.
*Solvay, India.*
Iodine (p.1598·1).
*Hyperthyroidism; hypothyroidism.*

**Collubiazol** *GlaxoSmithKline, Arg.*
*Pastilles:* Sulfachrysoidine sodium; benzocaine (p.1370·3); cetylpyridinium chloride (p.1173·1).
*Spray:* Sulfachrysoidine sodium; benzocaine (p.1370·3).
*Mouth and throat disorders.*

**Collu-Blache** *Bausch & Lomb, Switz.*
Chlorhexidine gluconate (p.1173·2); oxybuprocaine hydrochloride (p.1382·1).
*Mouth and throat disorders.*

**Collubleu** *Medeva, Fr.†.*
Methylthioninium chloride (p.1042·2).
*Bacterial mouth and throat infections.*

**Colludol**
*Aventis, Belg.; Cooperation Pharmaceutique, Fr.*
Hexamidine isetionate (p.1181·3); lidocaine hydrochloride (p.1377·3).
*Mouth and throat disorders.*

**Collu-Hextril**
*Pfizer Sante, Fr.; Pfizer Consumer, Port.*
Hexetidine (p.1182·1).
*Mouth and throat disorders.*

**Collunosol-N** *Sanofi, Switz.*
Chlorhexidine gluconate (p.1173·2); lidocaine hydrochloride (p.1377·3).
*Mouth and throat disorders.*

**Collunovar**
*Note. This name is used for preparations of different composition.*
*Dexo, Fr.*
*Mouthwash; throat spray:* Chlorhexidine gluconate (p.1173·2).
*Pastilles:* Bacitracin zinc (p.161·3); tyrothricin (p.275·1).
*Mouth and throat infections.*
*Actipharm, Switz.†.*
Chlorhexidine gluconate (p.1173·2).
*Mouth and throat disorders.*

**Collupressine** *Synthelabo, Fr.†.*
Felypressin (p.1324·2); chlorhexidine gluconate (p.1173·2).
*Mouth and throat disorders.*

**Collustan** *Oberlin, Fr.†.*
Chlorhexidine gluconate (p.1173·2); amylocaine hydrochloride (p.1370·2); menthol.
*Mouth and throat disorders.*

**Collylarm** *Vifor, Switz.*
Povidone (p.1581·2); polyvinyl alcohol (p.1581·1).
*Dry eyes.*

**Collypan** *Vifor, Switz.*
Tetryzoline hydrochloride (p.1131·2); zinc sulfate (p.1469·3); digitalis (p.894·2); hamamelis (p.1696·3); euphrasia (p.1686·3).
*Eye irritation.*

**Collyre Alpha** *Bracco, Switz.*
Naphazoline nitrate (p.1124·3); camphor (p.1665·3).
*Eye irritation.*

**Collyre Bleu**
*Sabex, Canad.*
Methylthioninium chloride (p.1042·2); naphazoline hydrochloride (p.1124·3).
*Leurquin, Fr.*
Methylthioninium chloride (p.1042·2); naphazoline nitrate (p.1124·3).
*Eye irritation.*

**Collyre Bleu Laiter** *Leurquin, Switz.*
Methylthioninium chloride (p.1042·2); naphazoline nitrate (p.1124·3).
*Eye irritation.*

**Collyrex** *SmithKline Beecham Sante, Fr.†.*
Thiomersal (p.1194·1); phenylephrine hydrochloride (p.1126·3); pentosan polysulfate (p.979·2).
*Eye disorders.*

**Collyria** *Nova Argentia, Ital.*
Benzalkonium chloride (p.1168·3); guaiazulene (p.1696·2); polyvinyl alcohol (p.1581·1).
*Eye hygiene; eye irritation.*

**Collyrium** *Charton, Canad.†.*
Tetryzoline hydrochloride (p.1131·2); glycerol (p.1694·3).
*Eye irritation.*

**Collyrium Fresh** *Wyeth-Ayerst, USA.*
Tetryzoline hydrochloride (p.1131·2); glycerol (p.1694·3).
*Eye irritation.*

**Collyrium for Fresh Eyes** *Bausch & Lomb, USA.*
Borax (p.1661·3); boric acid (p.1662·1).
*Eye irrigation.*

**Colmax** *Andromaco, Chile.*
Clonixin lysine (p.26·3).
*Pain.*

**Colme**
*Croma, Austria; Ipsen, Spain.*
Calcium carbimide (p.1664·2).
*Alcoholism.*

**Colobolina** *Fabra, Arg.*
Hyoscine butylbromide (p.483·3).
*Muscle spasm.*

**Colobolina D** *Fabra, Arg.*
Hyoscine butylbromide (p.483·3); dipyrone (p.35·3).
*Muscle spasm; pain.*

**Colocarb** *Expanpharm, Fr.*
Activated charcoal (p.1030·2).
*Gastrointestinal disorders.*

**ColoCare** *Helena, USA.*
Test for occult blood in faeces.

**Colodium**
*Hovid, Hong Kong; Hovid, Singapore.*
Loperamide hydrochloride (p.1271·1).
*Diarrhoea; ileostomy management.*

**Colofac**
*Solvay, Austral.; Solvay, Austria; Solvay, Irl.; Duphar, NZ; Solvay, S.Afr.; Solvay, Thai.; Solvay, UK.*
Mebeverine embonate (p.1273·1) or mebeverine hydrochloride (p.1273·1).
*Gastrointestinal spasm; irritable bowel syndrome.*

**Colofiber** *Madaus, Belg.*
Ispaghula (p.1268·1).
*Colopathy; constipation.*

**Colofoam** *Norgine, Fr.*
Hydrocortisone acetate (p.1103·3).
*Inflammatory bowel disease.*

**Cololyt** *Spirig, Switz.*
Macrogol 4000 (p.1709·1); electrolytes (p.1217·1).
*Bowel evacuation.*

**Colomba spezial** *Mauermann, Ger.*
Homoeopathic preparation.

**Colominte** *Helsinn, Port.*
Peppermint oil (p.1283·2).
*Irritable bowel syndrome.*

**Colominthe** *Arkopharma, Fr.†.*
Peppermint leaf (p.1283·2); fennel (p.1687·2); melissa (p.1711·1).
*Gastrointestinal disorders.*

**Colomycin**
*Pharmax, Irl.; Forest Laboratories, UK.*
Colistin sulfate (p.198·3) or colistimethate sodium (p.199·1).
*Bacterial infections.*

**Colonic Lavage Powder** *Biotech, Austral.*
Macrogol 3350 (p.1709·1); electrolytes (p.1217·1).
*Bowel evacuation.*

**Colonlytely** *Dendy, Austral.*
Macrogol 3350 (p.1709·1); electrolytes (p.1217·1).
*Bowel evacuation; constipation.*

**Colonorm** *Mundipharma, Austria.*
Senna (p.1288·2).
*Anorectal disorders; constipation.*

**Colonorm N** *Mundipharma, Ger.*
Macrogol 3350 (p.1709·1) electrolytes (p.1217·1).
*Bowel evacuation.*

**Colonprep** *Dendy, Austral.*
1 Sachet, macrogol 3350 (p.1709·1); electrolytes (p.1217·1) (Colonlytely); 2 sachets, sodium picosulfate (p.1289·3) (Picolax).
*Bowel evacuation.*

**Colonsteril** *Orion, Fin.*
Electrolytes (p.1217·1); macrogol 4000 (p.1709·1).
*Bowel evacuation; constipation.*

**Colopeg**
*Roche, Belg.; Roche Nicholas, Fr.*
Electrolytes (p.1217·1); macrogol 3350 (p.1709·1).
*Bowel evacuation.*

**Colophos** *Spirig, Switz.*
Monobasic sodium phosphate (p.1230·3); dibasic sodium phosphate (p.1231·1).
*Bowel evacuation.*

**Coloplast OAD (Sween)** *Coloplast, UK.*
A deodorant for stoma care.

**Colo-Pleon**
*Sanofi Synthelabo, Austria; Henning, Ger.*
Sulfasalazine (p.1291·1).
*Inflammatory bowel disease.*

**Colo-Prep** *Anmarate, S.Afr.*
Monobasic sodium phosphate (p.1230·3); dibasic sodium phosphate (p.1231·1).
*Bowel evacuation.*

**Colopriv** *Biotherapie, Fr.*
Mebeverine hydrochloride (p.1273·1).
*Gastrointestinal and biliary-tract disorders.*

**Colopten** *Fournier, Ital.*
Purified antigenic fraction of *Staphylococcus aureus*; *Escherichia coli*; *Klebsiella pneumoniae*; *Proteus vulgaris*.
*Diarrhoea.*

**Colo-Rectal Test** *Roche, Canad.†.*
Test for occult blood in stools.

**Colosan mite** *Medichemie, Switz.*
Sterculia (p.1290·2).
*Constipation; obesity.*

**Colosan plus** *Medichemie, Switz.*
Sterculia (p.1290·2); frangula (p.1266·3).
*Constipation.*

**Coloscreen**
*Biolab, NZ; Helena, USA.*
Test for faecal occult blood.

**Colosina** *Lemery, Mex.†.*
Ciclosporin (p.1351·2).

**Colosoft** *Medichemie, Switz.*
Ispaghula (p.1268·1).
*Constipation.*

**Colo-Sol** *Medichemie, Switz.*
Macrogol 3350 (p.1709·1); electrolytes (p.1217·1).
*Bowel evacuation.*

**Colospa** *Solvay, India.*
Mebeverine hydrochloride (p.1273·1).
*Irritable bowel syndrome.*

**Colospan**
*Hovid, Malaysia; Hovid, Singapore.*
Hyoscine butylbromide (p.483·3).
*Smooth muscle spasm.*

**Colostrum**
*Note. This name is used for preparations of different composition.*
*Eagle, Austral.†.*
Milk extract (p.1417·1).
*Dietary supplement.*
*Nathura, Ital.*
Colostrum (p.1611·1); melaleuca viridiflora; cupressus sempervirens.
*Skin disorders; wounds.*

**Colotal** *Agis, Israel.*
Mebeverine hydrochloride (p.1273·1).
*Gastrointestinal disorders.*

**Coloxyl**
*Note. This name is used for preparations of different composition.*
*Fawns & McAllan, Austral.; Sigma, NZ.*
*Enema; tablets:* Docusate sodium (p.1262·2).
*Bowel evacuation; constipation.*
*Oral drops:* Poloxamer (p.1414·2).
*Constipation.*
*Suppositories:* Docusate sodium (p.1262·2); bisacodyl (p.1251·3).
*Bowel evacuation; constipation.*

**Coloxyl with Senna**
*Fawns & McAllan, Austral.; Sigma, NZ.*
Docusate sodium (p.1262·2); sennosides (p.1288·2).
*Constipation.*

**Colpacid** *Dansk-Flama, Braz.†.*
Tyrothricin (p.275·1); nitrofurazone (p.238·2); lactic acid (p.1704·1); sodium lactate (p.1223·2).
*Vulvovaginal disorders.*

**Colpagex N** *Marjan, Braz.*
Neomycin sulfate (p.235·1); tyrothricin (p.275·1); nystatin (p.406·3); sodium propionate (p.408·1); boric acid (p.1662·1).
*Vulvovaginal infections.*

**Colpanist** *Dansk-Flama, Braz.†.*
Metronidazole (p.607·2); nystatin (p.406·3); benzalkonium chloride (p.1168·3); urea (p.1162·2).
*Vulvovaginal infections.*

**Colpatrin** *Teuto, Braz.*
Metronidazole (p.607·2); nystatin (p.406·3); benzalkonium chloride (p.1168·3).
*Vulvovaginal infections.*

**Colpermin**
*Germania, Austria.; Pharmascience, Canad.†; Tillotts, Hong Kong; Pharmacia, Irl.; Schering-Plough, Mex.; Baxter, NZ†; Tillotts, NZ†; Tillotts, Switz.; Tillotts, Thai.; Pfizer Consumer, UK.*
Peppermint oil (p.1283·2).
*Irritable bowel syndrome.*

**Colphen** *Propan, S.Afr.*
Codeine phosphate (p.27·1); chlorphenamine maleate (p.427·3); sodium salicylate (p.90·1); guaifenesin (p.1122·1); phenylephrine hydrochloride (p.1126·3); caffeine (p.782·1); cetylpyridinium chloride (p.1173·1).
*Coughs.*

**Colpist** *Ativus, Braz.*
Metronidazole benzoate (p.607·2); nystatin (p.406·3); benzalkonium chloride (p.1168·3).
*Vulvovaginal infections.*

**Colpistar** *Farmoquimica, Braz.*
*Vaginal cream:* Metronidazole (p.607·2); nystatin (p.406·3); benzalkonium chloride (p.1168·3); muramidase (p.1717·2).
*Vaginal tablets†:* Metronidazole (p.607·2); nystatin (p.406·3).
*Vulvovaginal infections.*

**Colpistatin** *Ache, Braz.*
Metronidazole benzoate (p.607·2); nystatin (p.406·3); benzalkonium chloride (p.1168·3).
*Vulvovaginal infections.*

**Colpocin-T** *Demo, Gr.*
Metronidazole (p.607·2).
*Anaerobic bacterial infections.*

**Colpogyn** *Angelini, Ital.*
Estriol (p.1552·3).
*Cervical erosion; menopausal disorders.*

**Colpolase** *De Mayo, Braz.*
*Topical solution:* Neomycin sulfate (p.235·1); tyrothricin (p.275·1); hydroxyquinoline sulfate (p.1700·1); lactic acid (p.1704·1); menthol (p.1711·3).
*Vaginal capsules; vaginal cream:* Neomycin sulfate (p.235·1); polymyxin B sulfate (p.245·1); nystatin (p.406·3); tinidazole (p.617·1).
*Vulvovaginal infections.*

**Colposeptine**
*Merck-Theramex, Hong Kong; Theramex, Mon.*
Chlorquinaldol (p.187·3); promestriene (p.1568·2).
*Vaginal atrophy.*

**Colpotrofin** *Grunenthal, Spain.*
Promestriene (p.1568·2).
*Vulvovaginal disorders.*

**Colpotrofine** *Altana, Braz.*
Promestriene (p.1568·2).
*Vulvovaginal disorders.*

**Colpotrophine**
*Temis, Arg.; Merck-Theramex, Hong Kong; Theramex, Ital.; Theramex, Mon.; Merck, Port.; Merck, Singapore; Golaz, Switz.*
Promestriene (p.1568·2).
*Vulvovaginal disorders.*

**Colpovis** *SIT, Ital.†.*
Quinestradol (p.1568·2).
*Vulvovaginal disorders.*

**Colpro**
*Wyeth Lederle, Belg.; Wyeth, Neth.†; Wyeth, S.Afr.; Wyeth, Spain; Wyeth, Switz.*
Medrogestone (p.1557·1).
*Benign breast disorders; endometriosis; infertility; menopausal disorders; menorrhagia; menstrual disorders.*

**Colpron** *Wyeth Lederle, Austria.*
Medrogestone (p.1557·1).
*Hormone replacement therapy; menorrhagia; secondary amenorrhoea.*

**Colprone**
*Wyeth-Ayerst, Canad.†; Wyeth Lederle, Fr.; Wyeth, Hong Kong; Wyeth Lederle, Ital.; Wyeth-Ayerst, Thai.†.*
Medrogestone (p.1557·1).
*Dysfunctional uterine bleeding; endometriosis; fibroids; infertility; menopausal disorders; menstrual disorders; threatened or recurrent miscarriage.*

**Colpuril** *Bristol-Myers Squibb, Arg.*
Allopurinol (p.412·2); colchicine (p.415·1).
*Gout; hyperuricaemia.*

**Colsanac** *Pierre Fabre, Port.*
Lactulose (p.1269·1).
*Constipation; hepatic coma; hepatic encephalopathy.*

**Colser** *Serral, Mex.*
Bezafibrate (p.873·2).
*Hypercholesterolaemia.*

**Colsor**
*Note. This name is used for preparations of different composition.*
*Seng, Thai.*
Aciclovir (p.626·1).
*Herpes simplex infections of the skin and mucous membranes.*

*Pickles, UK.*
Phenol (p.1188·1); menthol (p.1711·3); tannic acid (p.1751·2).
*Herpes labialis.*

**Colsprin** *Reckitt Benckiser, India.*
Aspirin (p.15·1).
*Prophylaxis of cerebrovascular disorders or myocardial infarction after by-pass surgery.*

**Colstat**
*Note. This name is used for preparations of different composition.*
*Fournier, Port.†.*
Cerivastatin sodium (p.881·3).
*Hypercholesterolaemia.*

*Restan, S.Afr.*
Paracetamol (p.76·2); ascorbic acid (p.1460·2); caffeine (p.782·1); phenylephrine hydrochloride (p.1126·3); chlorphenamine maleate (p.427·3); atropine sulfate (p.477·1).
*Cold and influenza symptoms.*

**Coltalin with Vit $B_1$** *Fortune, Hong Kong.*
Paracetamol (p.76·2); caffeine (p.782·1); chlorphenamine maleate (p.427·3); phenylephrine hydrochloride (p.1126·3); vitamin $B_1$ (p.1455·2).
*Respiratory-tract disorders.*

**Coltapaste**
*Note. This name is used for preparations of different composition.*
*Smith & Nephew, Irl.†.*
Zinc oxide (p.1163·2).
*Medicated bandage.*

*Smith & Nephew, UK†.*
Zinc oxide (p.1163·2); coal tar (p.1159·2).
*Medicated bandage.*

**Colther** *Vilco, Gr.*
Tobramycin (p.271·2).
*Eye infections.*

**Coltix** *Medical, Arg.*
Salicylic acid (p.1157·1); resorcinol (p.1156·3); lactic acid (p.1704·1); benzocaine (p.1370·3).
*Calluses.*

**Coltramyl**
*Theraplix, Fr.; Aventis, Port.*
Thiocolchicoside (p.1395·2).
*Muscle spasm.*

**Coltrax** *Aventis, Braz.*
Thiocolchicoside (p.1395·2).
*Painful muscle spasm.*

**Colubiazol** *Aventis, Braz.†.*
Sulfachrysoidine (p.258·1).
*Mouth infections.*

**Colufase** *Columbia, Mex.*
Sodium benzoate (p.1169·3).
*Hyperammonaemia.*

**Columbia Antiseptic Powder** *Sturtevant, USA.*
Zinc oxide (p.1163·2); talc (p.1159·1); phenol (p.1188·1); boric acid (p.1662·1).

**Columina** *Columbia, Mex.†.*
Cimetidine (p.1255·3).

**Colutoide** *Cimed, Braz.*
Prednisolone (p.1108·1); neomycin sulfate (p.235·1); bismuth sodium tartrate; procaine hydrochloride (p.1383·2).
*Mouth and throat disorders.*

**Coly-Mycin M**
*Pfizer, Austral.; Pfizer, Canad.; Pfizer, NZ; Monarch, USA.*
Colistimethate sodium (p.199·1).
*Bacterial infections.*

**Coly-Mycin S Otic**
*Pfizer, NZ†; Parke, Davis, USA.*
Colistin sulfate (p.198·3); neomycin sulfate (p.235·1); hydrocortisone acetate (p.1103·3); tonzonium bromide (p.1757·2).
*Bacterial ear infections.*

**Colyrazul** *Lessel, Braz.†.*
Naphazoline hydrochloride (p.1124·3); methylthioninium chloride (p.1042·2).
*Ocular congestion.*

**CoLyte**
*Reed & Carnrick, Canad.; Schwarz, USA.*
Macrogol 3350 (p.1709·1); electrolytes (p.1217·1).
*Bowel evacuation.*

**Comafusin Hepar** *Baxter, Ger.*
Amino-acid, vitamin, and electrolyte infusion with xylitol (p.1417·1).
*Hepatic coma.*

**Comagis** *Agis, Israel.*
Bifonazole (p.395·1); fluocinonide (p.1101·3).
*Infected skin disorders.*

**Comalose-R** *Rougier, Canad.†.*
Lactulose (p.1269·1).
*Hepatic encephalopathy.*

**Comat** *Milano, Thai.*
Clotrimazole (p.396·2).
*Fungal and bacterial vaginal infections; trichomoniasis.*

**Combacid** *Streuli, Switz.*
Aluminium hydroxide-magnesium carbonate co-dried gel (p.1250·1); simeticone (p.1289·2).
*Gastric hyperacidity.*

**Combactam**
*Pfizer, Austria; Pfizer, Ger.*
Sulbactam sodium (p.257·2).
*Adjunct to beta-lactam antibiotics.*

**Combact-HIB** *Aventis, S.Afr.*
An adsorbed diphtheria, tetanus, pertussis and haemophilus influenzae conjugate vaccine (p.1614·2).
*Active immunisation.*

**Combantrin**
*Pfizer Consumer, Austral.; Pfizer, Austria; Pfizer Consumer, Canad.; Teofarma, Fr.; Pfizer, Gr.; Pfizer, Hong Kong; Pfizer, Israel; Pfizer, Ital.; Pfizer, Mex.; Pfizer, NZ; Pfizer, Port.; Pfizer Consumer, S.Afr.; Pfizer, Thai.†.*
Pyrantel embonate (p.113·2).
*Worm infections.*

**Combantrin-1** *Pfizer, NZ.*
Mebendazole (p.108·2).
*Worm infections.*

**Combantrin-1 with Mebendazole** *Pfizer Consumer, Austral.*
Mebendazole (p.108·2).
*Worm infections.*

**Combaren** *Novartis, Ger.*
Diclofenac sodium (p.32·1); codeine phosphate (p.27·1).
*Pain.*

**Combetasi** *Kedrion, Ital.*
Vitamin B substances (p.1417·1).
*Tonic.*

**Combi-Cal** *Asta Medica, Thai.*
Calcium (p.1225·1); colecalciferol (p.1461·3).
*Calcium and vitamin D deficiency; osteoporosis.*

**Combid** *GlaxoSmithKline, Thai.*
Lamivudine (p.648·2); zidovudine (p.658·2).
*HIV infection.*

**Combiderm**
*Note. This name is used for preparations of different composition.*
*Convatec, Austral.*
Hydrocolloid dressing.
*Skin ulcers; wounds.*

*Convatec, Port.†.*
Carmellose sodium (p.1577·3); pectin (p.1580·3); gelatin (p.754·3).
*Ulcers; wounds.*

*Kalbe, Singapore.*
Betamethasone dipropionate (p.1093·1); clotrimazole (p.396·2); gentamicin sulfate (p.217·1).
*Infected skin disorders.*

**Combiflam** *Aventis, India.*
Ibuprofen (p.45·3); paracetamol (p.76·2).
*Fever; inflammation; pain.*

**Combifusin** *Baxter, Ger.*
Amino-acid, carbohydrate, and electrolyte infusion (p.1417·1).
*Parenteral nutrition.*

**Combilosung** *Agepha, Austria.*
Disinfection and storage solution for contact lens (p.1164·2).

**Combina** *Omega, Irl.*
Test for glucose, ketones, nitrates, pH, specific gravity, bilirubin, urobilinogen, protein, and blood in urine.

**Combina 2** *Omega, Irl.*
Test for glucose and ketones in urine.

**Combina 3** *Omega, Irl.*
Test for glucose, pH, and protein in urine.

**Combina Glucose** *Omega, Irl.*
Test for glucose in urine (p.1694·2).

**Combinacion Pl** *Pisa, Mex.*
Glucose (p.1432·2); electrolytes (p.1217·1).

**Combinacion Rubin-Calcagno** *Pisa, Mex.*
Electrolyte infusion (p.1217·1).

**Combinovita** *Sedabel, Braz.*
Amino-acid, vitamin, and mineral preparation (p.1417·1).
*Tonic.*

**Combinplex** *Hua, Thai.*
Vitamin B substances (p.1417·1).

**Combion-B** *Merck, Thai.†.*
Vitamin B substances (p.1417·1).

**CombiPatch** *Rhone-Poulenc Rorer, USA.*
Estradiol (p.1550·1); norethisterone acetate (p.1562·2).
*Menopausal disorders.*

**Combiplasmal** *Braun, Ger.*
Amino-acid, carbohydrate, and electrolyte infusion (p.1417·1).
*Parenteral nutrition.*

**Combipres**
*Boehringer Ingelheim, Canad.†; Boehringer Ingelheim, USA.*
Clonidine hydrochloride (p.885·2); chlortalidone (p.882·3).
*Hypertension.*

**Combipresan** *Boehringer Ingelheim, Ger.*
Clonidine hydrochloride (p.885·2); chlortalidone (p.882·3).
*Hypertension.*

**Combiron** *Ache, Braz.*
Ferrous sulfate (p.1428·2); vitamin B substances (p.1417·1).
Ascorbic acid (p.1460·2) is included in this preparation to increase the absorption and availability of iron.
*Anaemias.*

**Combisartan** *Menarini, Ital.*
Valsartan (p.1018·3); hydrochlorothiazide (p.933·2).
*Hypertension.*

**Combiseven** *Bracco, Ital.*
Patch 1, estradiol (p.1550·1); patch 2, estradiol; levonorgestrel (p.1563·2).
*Menopausal disorders.*

**Combistix** *Bayer, USA.*
Test for pH, protein, and glucose in urine.

**Combithyrex** *Biochemie, Austria.*
Levothyroxine sodium (p.1600·1); liothyronine sodium (p.1602·2).
*Hypothyroidism.*

**Combitora** *Solvay, Spain†.*
Amoxicillin trihydrate (p.155·3).
*Bacterial infections.*

**Combitorax** *Nezel, Spain†.*
*Capsules:* Amoxicillin trihydrate (p.155·3); bromhexine hydrochloride (p.1115·3).
*Oral suspension:* Amoxicillin trihydrate (p.155·3); bromhexine (p.1115·3); guaifenesin (p.1122·1); senega (p.1130·2); liquorice (p.1270·2).
*Respiratory-tract infections.*

**Combitrex** *Heralds, Braz.†.*
Tetracycline hydrochloride (p.266·2).
*Bacterial infections.*

**Combivax** *SmithKline Beecham, Belg.†.*
An adsorbed diphtheria, tetanus, and pertussis vaccine (p.1613·3).
*Active immunisation.*

**Combivent**
*Boehringer Ingelheim, Arg.; Boehringer Ingelheim, Austral.; Boehringer Ingelheim, Austria; Boehringer Ingelheim, Belg.; Boehringer de Angeli, Braz.; Boehringer Ingelheim, Canad.; Boehringer Ingelheim, Chile; Boehringer Ingelheim, Denm.; Boehringer Ingelheim, Fr.; Boehringer Ingelheim, Hong Kong; Boehringer Ingelheim, Irl.; Boehringer Ingelheim, Malaysia; Boehringer Ingelheim, Mex.; Boehringer Ingelheim, Neth.†; Boehringer Ingelheim, NZ; Boehringer Ingelheim, Port.; Boehringer Ingelheim, S.Afr.; Boehringer Ingelheim, Singapore; Boehringer Ingelheim, Spain; Boehringer Ingelheim, Swed.; Boehringer Ingelheim, Thai.; Boehringer Ingelheim, UK; Boehringer Ingelheim, USA.*
Ipratropium bromide (p.787·1); salbutamol sulfate (p.791·3).
*Obstructive airways disease.*

**Combivir**
*GlaxoSmithKline, Austral.; Glaxo, Austria; GlaxoSmithKline, Belg.; Glaxo Wellcome, Braz.†; GlaxoSmithKline, Canad.; GlaxoSmithKline, Chile; Glaxo Wellcome, Denm.; GlaxoSmithKline, Fin.; GlaxoSmithKline, Fr.; GlaxoSmithKline, Ger.; Glaxo Wellcome, Gr.; GlaxoSmithKline, Hong Kong; Glaxo Wellcome, Irl.; GlaxoSmithKline, Israel; GlaxoSmithKline, Ital.; GlaxoSmithKline, Malaysia; Glaxo Wellcome, Mex.; GlaxoSmithKline, Neth.; GlaxoSmithKline, Norw.; GlaxoSmithKline, NZ; Glaxo Wellcome, Port.; GlaxoSmithKline, S.Afr.; GlaxoSmithKline, Singapore; GlaxoSmithKline, Spain; GlaxoSmithKline, Swed.; GlaxoSmithKline, Switz.; GlaxoSmithKline, UK; Glaxo Wellcome, USA.*
Lamivudine (p.648·2); zidovudine (p.658·2).
*HIV infection.*

**Combivitol** *Lannacher, Austria.*
Multivitamin preparation (p.1417·1).

**Combizym**
*Note. This name is used for preparations of different composition.*
*Sankyo, Austria; Luitpold, Belg.†; Sankyo, Fin.; Sankyo, Ger.; Sankyo, Hong Kong; Sankyo, Ital.; Will-Pharma, Neth.; Sankyo, Norw.; Wilson, NZ; Sankyo, Port.; Selena, Swed.; Sankyo, Switz.; Sankyo, Thai.*
Pancreatin (p.1725·3); enzymes from *Aspergillus oryzae*.
*Digestive disorders; pancreatic insufficiency.*

*Sankyo Luitpold, Braz.†.*
Pancreatin (p.1725·3); enzymes from *Aspergillus oryzae*; ox bile (p.1660·3).
*Digestive disorders.*

*Sanofi Synthelabo, Chile.*
Digestive enzymes; bile salts (p.1660·3).
*Digestive disorders.*

**Combizym Compositum**
*Sankyo, Austria; Sanofi Synthelabo, Chile; Sankyo, Fin.; Sankyo, Ger.; Luitpold, Neth.†; Sankyo, NZ†; Searle, NZ†; Sankyo, Port.; Selena, Swed.; Sankyo, Switz.†; Sankyo, Thai.*
Pancreatin (p.1725·3); enzymes from *Aspergillus oryzae*; ox bile extract (p.1660·3).
*Digestive disorders.*

**Combizym Composto** *Sankyo, Braz.*
Enzymes from *Aspergillus oryzae*; pancreatin (p.1725·3).

**Combudoron**
*Note. This name is used for preparations of different composition.*
*Weleda, Ger.*
Arnica (p.1656·3); urtica (p.1762·1).
*Burns; insect stings.*

*Weleda, UK.*
Homoeopathic preparation.

**Combunex** *Lupin, India.*
Ethambutol (p.212·2); isoniazid (p.222·2).
*Tuberculosis.*

**Combur 3** *Roche Diagnostics, Irl.*
Test for pH, protein, and glucose in urine.

**Combur 8** *Roche Diagnostics, Irl.*
Test for nitrite, pH, protein, glucose, ketones, urobilinogen, bilirubin, and blood in urine.

**Combur 10** *Roche Diagnostics, Irl.*
Test for specific gravity, nitrite, pH, leucocytes, protein, glucose, ketones, urobilirubin, and blood in urine.

**Combur 4 D** *Roche Diagnostics, Irl.*
Test for protein, glucose, ketones, and blood in urine.

**Combur 5 D** *Roche Diagnostics, Irl.*
Test for pH, protein, glucose, ketones, and blood in urine.

**Combur Test** *Roche Diagnostics, Austral.*
Test for pH, protein, and glucose in urine.

**Combur 4 Test** *Roche Diagnostics, Austral.†.*
Test for protein, glucose, leucocytes, and blood in urine.

**Combur 7 Test** *Roche Diagnostics, Austral.*
Test for pH, protein, glucose, ketones, bilirubin, urobilinogen, and blood in urine.

**Combur 8 Test** *Roche Diagnostics, Austral.*
Test for ketones, urobilinogen, bilirubin, blood, nitrite, pH, protein, and glucose in urine.

**Combur 9 Test** *Roche Diagnostics, Austral.*
Test for leucocytes, nitrite, pH, protein, glucose, ketones, urobilinogen, bilirubin, and blood in urine.

**Combur 10 Test**
*Roche Diagnostics, Austral.; Roche Diagnostics, Fr.*
Test for specific gravity, leucocytes, nitrite, pH, protein, glucose, ketones, urobilinogen, bilirubin, and blood in urine.

**Combur 5 Test D** *Roche Diagnostics, Austral.*
Test for pH, protein, glucose, ketones, and blood in urine.

**Combur 3 Test E** *Roche Diagnostics, Austral.*
Test for protein, glucose, and blood in urine.

**Combur 2 Test LN**
*Roche Diagnostics, Austral.†; Roche Diagnostics, Fr.*
Test for leucocytes and nitrite in urine.

**Comburic** *Therabel, Belg.*
Allopurinol (p.412·2); benzbromarone (p.414·3).
*Gout; hyperuricaemia.*

**Combustin Heilsalbe** *Combustin, Ger.*
Bismuth subgallate (p.1252·2); zinc oxide (p.1163·2); benzocaine (p.1370·3).
*Burns; haemorrhoids; skin disorders; skin ulceration; wounds.*

**Combutol** *Lupin, India.*
Ethambutol (p.212·2).
*Tuberculosis.*

**Comenter** *Raffo, Arg.*
Mirtazapine (p.307·3).
*Depression.*

**Co-Mepril** *Kwizda, Austria.*
Enalapril maleate (p.909·2); hydrochlorothiazide (p.933·2).
*Hypertension.*

**Cometon** *Metapharma, Ital.†.*
Vitamin B substances (p.1417·1).
*Vitamin B deficiency.*

**Comfeel**
*Note. This name is used for preparations of different composition.*
*Coloplast, Arg.; Coloplast, Fr.; Coloplast, Switz.†; Coloplast, UK.*
*Medicated dressing:* Carmellose sodium (p.1577·3).
*Burns; ulcers; wounds.*

*Coloplast, UK.*
Barrier cream.
*Peristomal care.*

**Comfeel Plus** *Coloplast, UK.*
Carmellose sodium (p.1577·3); calcium alginate (p.745·1).
*Wounds.*

**Comfeel Purilon** *Coloplast, Arg.*
Calcium alginate (p.745·1); carmellose sodium (p.1577·3).
*Ulcers; wounds.*

**Comfeel Seasorb**
*Coloplast, Arg.; Coloplast, Fr.*
Calcium alginate (p.745·1); sodium alginate (p.1577·1); carmellose sodium (p.1577·3).
*Ulcers; wounds.*

*Coloplast, UK.*
Calcium sodium alginate (p.745·1) (p.1577·1).
*Exudating wounds.*

**Comfort** *Durex, Canad.†.*
Nonoxinol 9 (p.1413·3).
*Contraceptive.*

**Comfort Eye Drops** *Pilkington Barnes-Hind, USA.*
Naphazoline hydrochloride (p.1124·3).
*Minor eye irritation.*

**Comfort Tears** *Pilkington Barnes-Hind, USA.*
Hyetellose (p.1579·2).
*Dry eyes.*

**Comfortcare Dual Action** *Allergan, Canad.*
Subtilisin; poloxamer 228 (p.1164·2).
*Cleanser for gas permeable contact lenses.*

**Comfortcare GP** *Pilkington Barnes-Hind, USA.*
Disinfecting, wetting, and soaking solution for gas permeable contact lenses (p.1164·2).

**Comfortcare Wetting & Soaking** *Allergan, Canad.*
Wetting and soaking solution for gas permeable contact lenses (p.1164·2).

**Comfortine** *Dermik, USA†.*
Vitamin A (p.1451·2); vitamin E (p.1464·3); zinc oxide (p.1163·2); chloroxylenol (p.1177·2).
*Skin disorders.*

**Comfrey Plus** *Herbal, Israel.*
Comfrey (p.1675·2); allantoin (p.1141·3).
*Burns; cuts; insect bites; nappy rash; soft-tissue injury.*

**Comfy** *Polipharm, Thai.*
Dextromethorphan hydrobromide (p.1117·3); chlorphenamine maleate (p.427·3); pseudoephedrine hy-

drochloride (p.1129·2); ammonium chloride (p.1115·2).
*Cold symptoms; coughs; nasal congestion.*

**Comhist LA** *Procter & Gamble, USA.*
Chlorphenamine maleate (p.427·3); phenyltoloxamine citrate (p.439·1); phenylephrine hydrochloride (p.1126·3).
*Nasal congestion; rhinorrhoea.*

**Co-Micardis** *Boehringer Ingelheim, S.Afr.*
Telmisartan (p.1010·1); hydrochlorothiazide (p.933·2).
*Hypertension.*

**Comilorid** *Mepha, Switz.*
Amiloride hydrochloride (p.858·2); hydrochlorothiazide (p.933·2).
*Hypertension; liver cirrhosis with ascites; oedema.*

**Comital L**
*Bayer, Port.†; Bayer, Spain.*
Phenytoin (p.370·2); methylphenobarbital (p.366·3); phenobarbital (p.367·3).
*Epilepsy; Sydenham's chorea.*

**Comizial** *Ogna, Ital.*
Phenobarbital (p.367·3).
*Chorea; epilepsy.*

**Commit** *GlaxoSmithKline, USA.*
Nicotine polacrilex (p.1720·1).
*Aid to smoking withdrawal.*

**Comoprin** *British Dispensary, Thai.*
Aspirin (p.15·1).
*Fever; pain.*

**Compact** *Roche Diagnostics, Irl.*
Test for glucose in blood (p.1694·2).

**Compact Sorb** *Esoform, Ital.*
Sodium polyacrylate.
*Spillage of biological fluids.*

**Compagel** *Sanofi Synthelabo, Spain.*
Aluminium hydroxide (p.1249·2); magnesium hydroxide (p.1272·2); magaldrate (p.1271·3).
*Gastrointestinal hyperacidity.*

**Compagen** *Solfran, Mex.*
Multivitamin and mineral preparation (p.1417·1).

**Companion 2** *Medisense, Canad.†.*
Test for glucose in blood (p.1694·2).

**Compaz** *Cristalia, Braz.*
Diazepam (p.690·1).
*Anxiety.*

**Compazine** *SmithKline Beecham, USA.*
Prochlorperazine (p.716·2), prochlorperazine edisilate (p.716·2), or prochlorperazine maleate (p.716·3).
*Non-psychotic anxiety; psychoses; severe nausea and vomiting.*

**Compendium** *Polifarma, Ital.*
Bromazepam (p.671·3).
*Anxiety disorders; insomnia.*

**Compensal** *Provit, Mex.*
Cyanocobalamin (p.1458·2).

**Compensan** *Lannacher, Austria.*
Morphine hydrochloride (p.60·1).
*Opioid withdrawal syndrome.*

**Compete** *Mission Pharmacal, USA.*
Ferrous gluconate (p.1428·1); folic acid (p.1429·1); multivitamins and minerals (p.1417·1).
*Iron-deficiency anaemias.*

**Complamin**
*SmithKline Beecham, Belg.†; SmithKline Beecham, Canad.†; Riemser, Ger.; Aventis, Ital.; GlaxoSmithKline, Neth.; Tika, Swed.†; Doetsch, Grether, Switz.*
Xantinol nicotinate (p.1029·1).
*Cerebral circulatory and metabolic disorders; hearing disorders; Ménière's disease; peripheral arterial disorders; retinal vascular disorders.*

**Complamin spezial** *Riemser, Ger.*
Xantinol nicotinate (p.1029·1).
*Lipid disorders.*

**Complamina** *German Remedies, India.*
Xantinol nicotinate (p.1029·1).
*Cerebral and peripheral vascular disorders.*

**Complan**
*Boots, Hong Kong†; Glaxo Wellcome, Mex.; Heinz-Wattie, NZ; Heinz, UK.*
Preparation for enteral nutrition (p.1417·1).

**Compleat**
*Novartis, Arg.; Novartis, Braz.; Novartis Nutrition, Canad.†; Sandoz Nutrition, USA.*
A range of preparations for enteral nutrition (p.1417·1).

**Compleat Modified** *Novartis Nutrition, Hong Kong.*
Preparation for enteral nutrition (p.1417·1).

**Complegel Novo** *Boehringer Ingelheim, Arg.*
Citicoline (p.1672·3).
*Cerebrovascular disorders.*

**Complegil** *Diepal, Fr.†.*
Nutritional supplement (p.1417·1).
*Convalescence.*

**Complejo B** *Carnot, Mex.; Collins, Mex.; Medifarma, Mex.*
Vitamin B substances (p.1417·1).

**Complementa** *Carlo Erba OTC, Ital.*
Multivitamin and mineral preparation (p.1417·1).

**Complenatal FF** *Pharmaceutical Enterprises, S.Afr.*
Multivitamin and mineral preparation (p.1417·1).

**Complesso B** *Carlo Erba OTC, Ital.*
Vitamin B substances (p.1417·1).
*Vitamin deficiency.*

**Completax Plus** *Silesia, Chile.*
Pseudoephedrine sulfate (p.1129·2); chlorphenamine maleate (p.427·3); paracetamol (p.76·2).
*Cold and influenza symptoms.*

**Complete**
*Allergan, Ger.†.*
Polihexanide (p.1190·1); tyloxapol (p.1416·3); trometamol (p.1758·2); disodium edetate (p.1037·3)(p.1164·2).
*Disinfectant, storage, and rinsing solution for soft contact lenses.*

*AMO, UK.*
A range of preparations for contact lens care (p.1164·2).

**Complete All-In-One**
*Allergan, Canad.*
A cleansing, rinsing, disinfecting and lubricating solution for soft contact lenses (p.1164·2).

*Allergan, Israel†.*
Polihexanide (p.1190·1); trometamol (p.1758·2); tyloxapol (p.1416·3)(p.1164·2).
*Disinfectant, storage, rinsing, and lubricant solution for soft contact lenses.*

**Complete Comfort Plus**
*Allergan, Braz.; Allergan, NZ.*
Preparation for contact lens care (p.1164·2).

**Complete Multi Pre- and Post-Natal** *Wampole, Canad.*
Multivitamin and mineral preparation (p.1417·1).

**Complete Multi-Adult** *Wampole, Canad.*
Multivitamin and mineral preparation (p.1417·1).

**Complete Protein Remover**
*Allergan, Austral.†; Allergan, Canad.; Allergan, Israel†.*
Substilisin A (p.1164·2).
*Protein remover for soft contact lenses.*

**Complete Solution** *Allergan, Austral.†.*
Cleaning, rinsing, disinfecting, storage, and lubricating solution for soft contact lenses (p.1164·2).

**Compleven**
*Fresenius Kabi, Austria; Fresenius Kabi, Fin.; Fresenius Kabi, Ger.; Fresenius Kabi, Port.; Fresenius Kabi, Swed.; Fresenius Kabi, Switz.; Fresenius Kabi, UK.*
Amino-acid, carbohydrate, electrolyte, and lipid (from soya oil (p.1447·2)) infusion (p.1417·1).
May contain egg lecithin or egg phospholipids.
*Parenteral nutrition.*

**Complevit**
*Note. This name is used for preparations of different composition.*
*EMS, Braz.†.*
Buclizine (p.426·3); gamma-aminobutyric acid (p.1690·2).
*Reduced appetite; tonic.*

*Pharma Investi, Chile.*
Vitamin and mineral preparation (p.1417·1).

**Complevit Pediatrico** *Pharma Investi, Chile.*
Vitamin preparation (p.1417·1).

**Complevitan** *Bunker, Braz.*
Vitamin B substances (p.1417·1).

**Complex 15**
*Schering-Plough, Canad.*
Dimethicone (p.1482·1); lecithin (p.1706·1).
*Emollient.*

*Schering-Plough, USA.*
Emollient and moisturiser.

**Complex 75** *Frega, Canad.†.*
Vitamin B substances (p.1417·1).

**Complex B** *Pharmalab, Canad.†.*
Vitamin B substances (p.1417·1).

**Complexan B** *Upsifarma, Port.†.*
Vitamin B substances (p.1417·1).
*Vitamin B deficiency.*

**Complexe B Compose** *Bio-Sante, Canad.*
Vitamin B substances (p.1417·1).

**Complexe** *Lehning, Fr.*
A range of homoeopathic preparations.

**Complexo B** *Basi, Port.*
Vitamin B substances (p.1417·1).

**Complidermol** *Medea, Spain.*
Multivitamins and amino acids (p.1417·1); inositol (p.1701·2).
*Skin disorders.*

**Comploment Continus**
*SSL, Irl.; Mundipharma, Switz.; SSL, UK†.*
Pyridoxine hydrochloride (p.1456·3).
*Premenstrual syndrome; vitamin $B_6$ deficiency.*

**Complutine** *Novartis Consumer, Spain.*
Diazepam (p.690·1).
Contains pyridoxine hydrochloride.
*Alcohol withdrawal syndrome; anxiety; febrile convulsions; insomnia; skeletal muscle spasm.*

**Comply** *Sherwood, USA.*
Lactose-free preparation for enteral nutrition (p.1417·1).

**Compocillin** *Abbott, NZ†.*
Phenoxymethylpenicillin (p.242·1).
*Bacterial infections.*

**Composto Anticelulitico** *Infabra, Braz.†.*
Ginkgo biloba (p.1692·3); bearberry (p.1659·2); bladderwrack (p.1742·3); centella (p.1144·3).

**Composto Emagrecedor** *Viternat, Braz.*
Cynara (p.1678·3); bladderwrack (p.1742·3); centella (p.1144·3); dried yeast (p.1469·1); passion flower (p.1729·1); cascara (p.1255·1).
*Slimming aid.*

**Compound V** *SSL, UK†.*
Salicylic acid (p.1157·1).
*Verrucas.*

**Compound Inhalation of Menthol** *McGloin, Austral.†.*
Menthol (p.1711·3); siberian fir oil; creosote (p.1117·2).
*Cold symptoms.*

**Compound W**
*Whitehall-Robins, Canad.; SSL, Irl.; SSL, UK; Medtech, USA.*
Salicylic acid (p.1157·1).
*Verrucas; warts.*

**Compound W Plus** *Whitehall-Robins, Canad.*
Salicylic acid (p.1157·1).
*Warts.*

**Compoz Night-time Sleep Aid** *Medtech, USA.*
Diphenhydramine hydrochloride (p.431·3).
*Insomnia.*

**Compralgyl** *Gifrer Barbezat, Fr.*
Aspirin (p.15·1); codeine phosphate (p.27·1).
*Fever; pain.*

**Compralsol** *Gifrer Barbezat, Fr.†.*
Paracetamol (p.76·2).
*Fever; pain.*

**Comprecin** *Warner-Lambert, Mex.†.*
Enoxacin (p.207·2).
*Bacterial infections.*

**Comprimes analgesiques no 534** *Renapharm, Switz.†.*
Paracetamol (p.76·2).
*Fever; pain.*

**Comprimes analgesiques "S"** *Synpharma, Switz.*
Paracetamol (p.76·2); caffeine (p.782·1); propyphenazone (p.85·3).
*Fever; pain.*

**Comprimes contre la toux** *Zeller, Switz.*
Hedera helix.
*Bronchial disorders with viscous mucus.*

**Comprimes Gynecologiques Pharmatex** *Innothera, Fr.†.*
Benzalkonium chloride (p.1168·3).
*Contraceptive.*

**Comprimes pour l'estomac** *Zeller, Switz.*
Calcium carbonate (p.1254·2); magnesium trisilicate (p.1272·3).
*Gastric hyperacidity.*

**Comprimes somniferes formule 533** *Renapharm, Switz.†.*
Diphenhydramine hydrochloride (p.431·3).
*Insomnia.*

**Comprimes somniferes "S"** *Synpharma, Switz.*
Diphenhydramine (p.431·3).
*Agitation; insomnia; nervousness.*

**Compro** *Paddock, USA.*
Prochlorperazine (p.716·2).
*Nausea and vomiting.*

**Compu-Gel** *Docmed, S.Afr.†.*
Aluminium hydroxide (p.1249·2); magnesium oxide (p.1272·3).
*Gastric hyperacidity.*

**Computer Eye Drops** *Bausch & Lomb, USA.*
Glycerol (p.1694·3).
*Eye irritation.*

**Comstrong** *Unison, Thai.*
Vitamin B substances (p.1417·1).

**Comtan**
*Novartis, Arg.; Novartis, Austral.; Novartis, Austria; Novartis, Belg.; Novartis, Braz.; Novartis, Canad.; Novartis, Fr.; Novartis, Gr.; Novartis, Hong Kong; Orion, Israel; Novartis, Ital.; Novartis, Malaysia; Novartis, Mex.; Novartis, Neth.; Novartis, NZ; Novartis, Port.; Novartis, S.Afr.; Novartis, Singapore; Novartis, Spain; Novartis, Switz.; Novartis, Thai.; Novartis, USA.*
Entacapone (p.1205·1).
*Parkinsonism.*

**Comtaplex** *Greater Pharma, Thai.*
Vitamin B substances (p.1417·1).

**Comtess**
*Orion, Denm.; Orion, Fin.; Orion, Ger.; Orion, Irl.; Orion, Norw.; Orion, Swed.; Orion, UK.*
Entacapone (p.1205·1).
*Parkinsonism.*

**Comtrex** *Bristol-Myers Products, USA.*
Paracetamol (p.76·2); pseudoephedrine hydrochloride (p.1129·2); chlorphenamine maleate (p.427·3); dextromethorphan hydrobromide (p.1117·3).
*Coughs and cold symptoms.*

**Comtrex Allergy-Sinus** *Bristol-Myers Products, USA.*
Paracetamol (p.76·2); pseudoephedrine hydrochloride (p.1129·2); chlorphenamine maleate (p.427·3).
*Upper respiratory-tract symptoms.*

**Comtrex Day & Night Maximum Strength**
*Bristol-Myers Products, USA.*
Orange caplets, dextromethorphan hydrobromide (p.1117·3); paracetamol (p.76·2); pseudoephedrine hydrochloride (p.1129·2); blue tablets, dextromethorphan hydrobromide (p.1117·3); paracetamol (p.76·2); pseudoephedrine hydrochloride (p.1129·2); chlorphenamine maleate (p.427·3).
*Coughs and cold symptoms.*

**Comtrex Day & Night Multi-Symptom** *Bristol-Myers Products, USA.*
Orange caplets, dextromethorphan hydrobromide (p.1117·3); paracetamol (p.76·2); pseudoephedrine hydrochloride (p.1129·2); yellow tablets, dextromethorphan hydrobromide (p.1117·3); paracetamol (p.76·2); pseudoephedrine hydrochloride (p.1129·2); chlorphenamine maleate (p.427·3).
*Coughs and cold symptoms.*

**Comtrex Hot Flu Relief** *Bristol-Myers Products, USA.*
Chlorphenamine maleate (p.427·3); dextromethorphan hydrobromide (p.1117·3); paracetamol (p.76·2); pseudoephedrine hydrochloride (p.1129·2).
*Coughs and cold symptoms.*

**Comtrex Liqui-Gels** *Bristol-Myers Products, USA†.*
Chlorphenamine maleate (p.427·3); dextromethorphan hydrobromide (p.1117·3); paracetamol (p.76·2); phenylpropanolamine hydrochloride (p.1127·3).
*Coughs and cold symptoms.*

**Comvax**
*Merck Sharp & Dohme, Austral.; Merck Sharp & Dohme, Mex.; Merck, USA.*
A haemophilus influenzae and hepatitis B vaccine (p.1616·3).
*Active immunisation in infants.*

**Conacid** *Purissimus, Arg.*
Folic acid (p.1429·1).
*Anaemias; prevention of neural tube defects.*

**Conadyl** *TO-Chemicals, Thai.†.*
Codeine phosphate (p.27·1); promethazine hydrochloride (p.439·1).
*Coughs.*

**Conamic** *Pharmasant, Thai.*
Mefenamic acid (p.55·2).
*Inflammation; musculoskeletal and joint disorders; pain.*

**Conan** *Mitsubishi, Jpn.*
Quinapril hydrochloride (p.991·1).
*Hypertension.*

**Conazine** *Condrugs, Thai.*
Perphenazine (p.714·2).
*Anxiety; nausea and vomiting.*

**Conazol** *Liomont, Mex.*
Ketoconazole (p.403·3).
*Fungal infections.*

**Conazole** *DHA, Singapore.*
Betamethasone valerate (p.1093·2); miconazole nitrate (p.405·3); gentamicin sulfate (p.217·1).
*Infected skin disorders.*

**Conbutol** *Continental-Pharm, Thai.*
Ethambutol hydrochloride (p.211·3).
*Tuberculosis.*

**Concatag** *Lafedar, Arg.*
Neomycin sulfate (p.235·1).
*Bacterial eye infections.*

**Concavit** *Wallace Mfg Chem., UK.*
Multivitamin preparation (p.1417·1).

**Conceive** *Pharmascience, Canad.†.*
Fertility test or pregnancy test (p.1734·3).

**Conceive Ovulation Predictor** *Quidel, USA.*
Fertility test (p.1734·3).

**Conceive Pregnancy** *Quidel, USA.*
Pregnancy test (p.1734·3).

**Concentrado Acido** *Reccius, Chile.*
Sodium chloride; calcium chloride; magnesium chloride; potassium chloride; acetic acid; glucose (p.1221·1).
*Haemodialysis.*

**Concentrado Basico** *Reccius, Chile.*
Sodium chloride (p.1233·3); sodium bicarbonate (p.1223·2).
*Haemodialysis.*

**Concentrated Cleaner** *Bausch & Lomb, NZ.*
Cleaning solution for contact lens care (p.1164·2).

**Concentrated Milk of Magnesia-Cascara** *Roxane, USA.*
Magnesium hydroxide (p.1272·2); cascara (p.1255·1).

**Concentrin** *CT, Ger.*
Aesculus (p.1648·2).
*Soft-tissue disorders; venous insufficiency.*

**Conceplan M** *Grunenthal, Ger.*
Ethinylestradiol (p.1553·2); norethisterone (p.1562·2).
*Combined oral contraceptive.*

**Concept** *Sea-Band, UK.*
Pregnancy test (p.1734·3).

**Concerta**
*Janssen-Cilag, Austral.; Janssen-Cilag, Swed.; Janssen-Cilag, UK; McNeil Pharmaceutical, USA.*
Methylphenidate hydrochloride (p.1590·2).
*Attention-deficit hyperactivity disorder.*

**Conchae comp.** *Weleda, UK.*
Homoeopathic preparation.

**Conchivit** *Ghimas, Ital.†.*
Multivitamin preparation (p.1417·1).
*Vitamin supplement.*

**Concor**
*Merck, Arg.; Merck, Austria; Merck, Braz.; Merck, Chile; Merck, Ger.; Merck, Hong Kong; Merck, India; Merck, Israel; Bracco, Ital.; Merck, Malaysia; Merck, Port.; Merck, S.Afr.; Merck, Singapore; Merck, Switz.; Merck, Thai.*
Bisoprolol fumarate (p.875·1).
*Angina pectoris; hypertension.*

**Concor Plus**
*Merck, Austria; Merck, Ger.; Merck, Port.; Merck, Switz.*
Bisoprolol fumarate (p.875·1); hydrochlorothiazide (p.933·2).
*Hypertension.*

**Concordin** Merck Sharp & Dohme, Denm.†; Merck Sharp & Dohme, Irl.†; Merck Sharp & Dohme, Swed.†; Merck Sharp & Dohme, UK†.
Protriptyline hydrochloride (p.316·2).
*Depression.*

**Condelone** Lacer, Spain†.
Podophyllotoxin (p.1155·3).
*Anogenital warts.*

**Condil** Protermex, Mex.†; Selder, Mex.†.
Podophyllum (p.1155·2).

**Conditioning Solution** Bausch & Lomb, NZ.
Chlorhexidine gluconate (p.1173·2); disodium edetate (p.1037·3) (p.1164·2).
*Soaking and wetting of contact lens.*

**Condiuren** Gentili, Ital.
Enalapril maleate (p.909·2); hydrochlorothiazide (p.933·2).
*Hypertension.*

**Condral** SPA, Ital.
A heparinoid (p.931·1).
*Osteoarthritis; pain.*

**Condress** Gentili, Ital.
Collagen (p.1674·3).
*Cicatrisation of wounds and skin ulcers.*

**Condro Sorb** Andromaco, Chile.
Chondroitin sulfate.
*Osteoarthritis; rheumatoid arthritis.*

**Condrofer** UCB, Ital.
Chondroitin sulfate A-iron complex (p.1425·1).
*Iron deficiency; iron deficiency anaemias.*

**Condroitina** Dominguez, Arg.
Chondroitin sulfate sodium (p.1670·2).
*Osteoarthritis.*

**Condrosamina** Andromaco, Chile.
Chondroitin sulfate; glucosamine hydrochloride.
*Osteoarthritis; rheumatoid arthritis.*

**Condrosulf** Pharmacia, Arg.; Sanova, Austria; Labomed, Chile; IBSA, Switz.
Chondroitin sulfate sodium (p.1670·2).
*Joint disorders.*

**Condrotec** Searle, UK†.
Naproxen (p.65·1).
Misoprostol (p.1519·2) is included in this preparation in an attempt to limit adverse effects on the gastrointestinal mucosa.
*Ankylosing spondylitis; osteoarthritis; rheumatoid arthritis.*

**Conducat** Baxter, Mex.
Magnesium sulfate (p.1228·2).

**Conductasa** Teofarma, Spain.
Pyridoxine oxoglurate (p.1457·2).
*Vitamin B6 deficiency.*

**Conducton** Klinge, Austria; Fujisawa, Ger.
Carazolol (p.880·2).
*Angina pectoris; arrhythmias; heart failure; hypertension; myocardial infarction.*

**Condyline** Hamilton, Austral.; Yamanouchi, Belg.†; Canderm, Canad.; Galderma, Denm.; Galderma, Fin.; Yamanouchi, Fr.; Nycomed, Irl.; Yamanouchi, Ital.; Yamanouchi, Neth.; Galderma, Norw.; CSL, NZ; Yamanouchi, NZ; Yamanouchi, Port.†; Galderma, Swed.; Nycomed, Switz.; Ardern, UK.
Podophyllotoxin (p.1155·3).
*Anogenital warts.*

**Condylox** Gerot, Austria; Wolff, Ger.; Agis, Israel; Oclassen, USA.
Podophyllotoxin (p.1155·3).
*Anogenital warts.*

**Conectol** Elvetium, Arg.
Aniracetam (p.1655·1).
*Mental function impairment.*

**Conef** Defuen, Arg.
Finasteride (p.1554·2).
*Alopecia androgenetica.*

**Conevit** Loren, Mex.
Vitamin preparation with lysine and iron (p.1417·1).

**Conex** Forest Pharmaceuticals, USA†.
Phenylpropanolamine hydrochloride (p.1127·3); guaifenesin (p.1122·1).
*Coughs.*

**Conex with Codeine** Forest Pharmaceuticals, USA†.
Phenylpropanolamine hydrochloride (p.1127·3); guaifenesin (p.1122·1); codeine phosphate (p.27·1).
*Coughs.*

**Conexine** Beta, Arg.
Memantine hydrochloride (p.1711·2).
*Mental function impairment; spasticity.*

**Confer** Merck, Chile.
Ferrous fumarate; folic acid; cyanocobalamin (p.1417·1).
Ascorbic acid (p.1460·2) is included in this preparation to increase the absorption and availability of iron.
*Dietary supplement.*

**Conferma 3 Plus** Aventis, Ital.
Pregnancy test (p.1734·3).

**Confetti Lassativi CM** Giuliani, Ital.
Senna (p.1288·2); boldo (p.1661·2); cascara (p.1255·1).
*Constipation.*

**Confetto CM** Falqui, Ital.
Bisacodyl (p.1251·3).
*Constipation.*

**Confiance** Helsinn, Port.; Wassen, UK†.
Multivitamin and mineral preparation (p.1417·1).

**Confiance Donna** Wassen, Ital.
Multivitamin and mineral preparation (p.1417·1).
*Nutritional supplement.*

**Confidelle** Carter Horner, Canad.
Pregnancy test (p.1734·3).

**Confidelle Progress** Bouty, Ital.
Pregnancy test (p.1734·3).

**Confidol** Medopharm, Ger.†.
Etilefrine hydrochloride (p.914·1).
*Circulatory disorders; hypotension.*

**Confirm** Durex, Canad.
Pregnancy test (p.1734·3).

**Confit** Procter & Gamble, Austria.
Verapamil hydrochloride (p.1019·1); triamterene (p.1016·2); hydrochlorothiazide (p.933·2).
*Hypertension.*

**Confludin N** Truw, Ger.
Homoeopathic preparation.

**Confobos** Smaller, Spain.
Famotidine (p.1265·2).
*Gastro-oesophageal reflux; peptic ulcer; Zollinger-Ellison syndrome.*

**Conformal** Elvetium, Arg.
Carbamazepine (p.353·3).
*Alcohol withdrawal syndrome; bipolar disorder; epilepsy; trigeminal neuralgia.*

**Conformil** Milupa, Port.
Infant feed (p.1417·1).
*Milk intolerance.*

**Confor-Tar** ICN, Arg.
Betamethasone valerate (p.1093·2); salicylic acid (p.1157·1); coal tar (p.1159·2).
*Skin disorders.*

**Confortel** Forder, Arg.
Levomenol (p.1707·1); pilewort (p.1732·1).
*Skin disorders.*

**Confortid** Alpharma, Denm.; Alpharma, Fin.; Alpharma-Isis, Ger.; Alpharma, Norw.; Alpharma, Swed.
Indometacin (p.47·3) or indometacin sodium (p.47·3).
*Gout; inflammation; musculoskeletal, joint, and periarticular disorders; pain; renal and biliary colic.*

**Congest** Trianon, Canad.
Conjugated oestrogens (p.1543·2).
*Oestrogen therapy.*

**Congest Aid** Zee, Canad.
Pseudoephedrine hydrochloride (p.1129·2).

**Congestac** Ascher, USA.
Pseudoephedrine hydrochloride (p.1129·2); guaifenesin (p.1122·1).
*Coughs.*

**Congestaid** Zee, USA.
Pseudoephedrine hydrochloride (p.1129·2).
*Nasal congestion.*

**Congestant** Rugby, USA.
Paracetamol (p.76·2); chlorphenamine maleate (p.427·3).
*Upper respiratory-tract symptoms.*

**Congestant D** Rugby, USA†.
Phenylpropanolamine hydrochloride (p.1127·3); chlorphenamine maleate (p.427·3); paracetamol (p.76·2).
*Upper respiratory-tract symptoms.*

**Congestex** Recalcine, Chile.
Paracetamol (p.76·2); pseudoephedrine hydrochloride (p.1129·2); noscapine (p.1125·3); ascorbic acid (p.1460·2).
*Cold and influenza symptoms.*

**Congest-Eze** Stanley, Canad.
Pseudoephedrine hydrochloride (p.1129·2).

**Congestion Relief** Schein, USA†.
Pseudoephedrine hydrochloride (p.1129·2).
*Nasal congestion.*

**Congex** Schwabe, Arg.
Naproxen (p.65·1).
*Dysmenorrhoea; gout; musculoskeletal and joint disorders.*

**Conidrin** Dansk-Flama, Braz.
Naphazoline hydrochloride (p.1124·3); mepyramine maleate (p.437·1).
*Nasal congestion.*

**Coniel** Kyowa, Jpn.
Benidipine hydrochloride (p.868·2).
*Angina pectoris; hypertension.*

**Conjonctyl** Sedifa, Mon.†.
Sodium methylsilanetriol salicylate.
*Arteritis; mastalgia; osteoporosis.*

**Conjugen** Klinge, Austria; Klinge, Ger.†; Ridupharm, Switz.†.
Conjugated oestrogens (p.1543·2).
*Menopausal disorders; osteoporosis.*

**Conjuncain-EDO** Mann, Ger.
Oxybuprocaine hydrochloride (p.1382·1).
*Local anaesthesia.*

**Conjunctilone** Allergan, Port.
Neomycin sulfate (p.235·1); polymyxin B sulfate (p.245·1).
*Bacterial eye infections.*

**Conjunctilone-S** Allergan, Port.
Neomycin sulfate (p.235·1); polymyxin B sulfate (p.245·1); prednisolone acetate (p.1108·1).
*Infected eye disorders.*

**Conjunctisan-A** Vitorgan, Ger.
Homoeopathic preparation.

**Conjunctisan-B** Vitorgan, Ger.
Homoeopathic preparation.

**Conjuntin** Allergan-Frumtost, Braz.†.
Neomycin sulfate (p.235·1); polymyxin B sulfate (p.245·1).
*Bacterial eye infections.*

**Conjunto Soramin Hipercalorico** Darrow, Braz.†.
Amino-acid infusion (p.1417·1).
*Parenteral nutrition.*

**Conjuvac** Stallergenes, Ital.†.
An allergen extract (p.1650·1).
*Allergen immunotherapy.*

**Conludag** Pharmacia, Norw.
Norethisterone (p.1562·2).
*Progestogen-only oral contraceptive.*

**Conmel** Farmasa, Braz.; Recalcine, Chile; Sanofi Synthelabo, Mex; Sanofi Synthelabo, Port.
Dipyrone (p.35·3).
*Fever; pain.*

**Connettivina** Kolassa, Austria; Fidia, Hong Kong; Fidia, Ital.; Fidia, Thai.
Sodium hyaluronate (p.1697·3).
*Burns; ulcers; varices; wounds.*

**Connettivina Plus** Fidia, Ital.
Sodium hyaluronate (p.1697·3); sulfadiazine silver (p.259·1).
*Burns; skin ulceration; wound.*

**Conotrane** Yamanouchi, Irl.; Yamanouchi, UK.
Benzalkonium chloride (p.1168·3); dimeticone (p.1482·1).
Formerly contained hydrargaphen and dimeticone in the *UK*.
*Barrier cream.*

**Conova** Searle, Belg.†; Searle, Denm.†.
Etynodiol diacetate (p.1554·2); ethinylestradiol (p.1553·2).
*Combined oral contraceptive; menstrual disorders.*

**Conpin** TAD, Ger.
Isosorbide mononitrate (p.942·1).
*Angina pectoris.*

**Conpremin** Wyeth, Chile.
Conjugated oestrogens (p.1543·2).
*Menopausal disorders; oestrogen deficiency; osteoporosis.*

**Conpremin Pak** Wyeth, Chile.
White tablets, conjugated oestrogens (p.1543·2); blue tablets, conjugated oestrogens; medroxyprogesterone acetate (p.1557·2).
*Menopausal disorders.*

**Conpremin Pak Plus** Wyeth, Chile.
28 Tablets, conjugated oestrogens (p.1543·2); 14 tablets, medroxyprogesterone acetate (p.1557·2).
*Menopausal disorders.*

**Conprim** Condrugs, Thai.
Co-trimoxazole (p.199·3).
*Bacterial infections.*

**Conrax** Fada, Arg.
Chlorpromazine (p.675·1).

**Conray** Mallinckrodt, Arg.; Humana, Braz.†; Mallinckrodt, Canad.; Bracco, Ital.; Mallinckrodt, UK; Mallinckrodt, USA.
Meglumine iotalamate (p.1065·3) or sodium iotalamate (p.1065·3).
*Radiographic contrast medium.*

**Conray 30** Tyco, Ger.
Meglumine iotalamate (p.1065·3).
*Radiographic contrast medium.*

**Conray 60** Tyco, Ger.
Meglumine iotalamate (p.1065·3).
*Radiographic contrast medium.*

**Conray 70** Mallinckrodt, Ger.†.
Meglumine iotalamate (p.1065·3); sodium iotalamate (p.1065·3).
*Radiographic contrast medium.*

**Conray 280** Mallinckrodt, Austral.
Meglumine iotalamate (p.1065·3).
*Radiographic contrast medium for urography and angiography.*

**Conray 420** Mallinckrodt, Austral.†.
Sodium iotalamate (p.1065·3).
*Contrast medium for urography and angiography.*

**Conray FL** Mallinckrodt, Ger.†.
Meglumine iotalamate (p.1065·3).
*Contrast medium for urography.*

**Consec** Jagson, India.
Ranitidine hydrochloride (p.1285·2).
*Dyspepsia; gastro-oesophageal reflux; gastrointestinal hyperacidity; peptic ulcer; Zollinger-Ellison syndrome.*

**Consept Step 1** Allergan, Canad.†.
Hydrogen peroxide (p.1182·2) (p.1164·2).
*Cleansing and disinfecting solution for soft contact lenses.*

**Consept Step 2** Allergan, Canad.†.
Sodium thiosulfate (p.1053·3) (p.1164·2).
*Wetting and soaking solution for soft contact lenses.*

**Consil** Barnes Hind, Arg.
Polyvinyl alcohol (p.1581·1); chlorhexidine gluconate (p.1173·2) (p.1164·2).
*Disinfecting and wetting solution for gas permeable contact lenses.*

**Consil Clean** Barnes Hind, Arg.
Miranol; norfox (p.1164·2).
*Cleaning of gas permeable contact lenses.*

**Consinut** Continental-Pharm, Thai.
Pseudoephedrine hydrochloride (p.1129·2); chlorphenamine maleate (p.427·3).
*Allergic rhinitis; nasal congestion.*

**Consolin** Dolisos, Canad.
Homoeopathic preparation.

**Constilac** Alra, USA.
Lactulose (p.1269·1).
*Constipation.*

**Constilax** Bros, Gr.
Norfloxacin (p.238·3).
*Urinary tract infections.*

**Constipal** Plough, Port.
Dexbrompheniramine maleate (p.426·1); pseudoephedrine sulfate (p.1129·2).
*Respiratory-tract congestion.*

**Constipation** Lalco, Canad.
Frangula (p.1266·3); senna (p.1288·2).
*Constipation.*

**Constipation L106** Homeocan, Canad.
Homoeopathic preparation.

**Constrilia** Alcon, Fr.
Tetryzoline hydrochloride (p.1131·2).
*Eye disorders.*

**Constulose** Barre-National, USA.
Lactulose (p.1269·1).
*Constipation.*

**Consudine** Condrugs, Thai.
Pseudoephedrine hydrochloride (p.1129·2); triprolidine hydrochloride (p.442·3).
*Cold symptoms; hypersensitivity reactions; nasal congestion; rhinitis.*

**Consupren** Galena, Thai.; SPB, Thai.
Ciclosporin (p.1351·2).
*Auto-immune disorders; graft-versus-host disease; transplant rejection.*

**Contac**
Note. This name is used for preparations of different composition.
SmithKline Beecham Consumer, Austral.†.
Atropine sulfate (p.477·1); hyoscine hydrobromide (p.483·3); hyoscyamine sulfate (p.485·1); pseudoephedrine hydrochloride (p.1129·2).
*Cold symptoms.*
GlaxoSmithKline, Chile; GlaxoSmithKline Consumer, Ger.†; SmithKline Beecham, Singapore†.
Chlorphenamine maleate (p.427·3); phenylpropanolamine hydrochloride (p.1127·3).
*Cold symptoms.*
SmithKline Beecham, Hong Kong†; SmithKline Beecham, Thai.†.
Phenylpropanolamine hydrochloride (p.1127·3); belladonna alkaloids (p.479·1).
*Cold symptoms.*

**Contac Allergy Formula** SmithKline Beecham Consumer, Canad.†.
Terfenadine (p.441·1).
*Hypersensitivity disorders.*

**Contac Cold** SmithKline Beecham Consumer, Canad.†.
Chlorphenamine maleate (p.427·3); phenylpropanolamine hydrochloride (p.1127·3).
Formerly known as Contac C.
*Respiratory congestion.*

**Contac Cold & Fever** GlaxoSmithKline Consumer, Canad.
Pseudoephedrine hydrochloride (p.1129·2); diphenhydramine hydrochloride (p.431·3); paracetamol (p.76·2).

**Contac Cold Nondrowsy** GlaxoSmithKline Consumer, Canad.
Pseudoephedrine hydrochloride (p.1129·2).
Formerly known as Contac C Nondrowsy.

**Contac Cold & Sore Throat** GlaxoSmithKline Consumer, Canad.
Pseudoephedrine hydrochloride (p.1129·2); dextromethorphan hydrobromide (p.1117·3); paracetamol (p.76·2).

**Contac Cough Cold and Flu** SmithKline Beecham Consumer, Canad.†.
Paracetamol (p.76·2); chlorphenamine maleate (p.427·3); dextromethorphan hydrobromide (p.1117·3); phenylpropanolamine hydrochloride (p.1127·3).
Formerly known as Contac C Cold Care Formula.
*Coughs and cold symptoms.*

**Contac Cough Cold and Flu Day & Night** GlaxoSmithKline Consumer, Canad.
Yellow caplets, pseudoephedrine hydrochloride (p.1129·2); dextromethorphan hydrobromide (p.1117·3); paracetamol (p.76·2); blue caplets, diphenhydramine hydrochloride (p.431·3); pseudoephedrine hydrochloride; paracetamol.
Formerly known as Contac Day & Night Cold and Flu.
*Cold symptoms.*

**Contac Cough, Cold & Flu Nighttime** SmithKline Beecham Consumer, Canad.†.
Pseudoephedrine hydrochloride (p.1129·2); diphenhydramine hydrochloride (p.431·3); paracetamol (p.76·2).
Formerly known as Contac C Nighttime.

**Contac Coughcaps** SmithKline Beecham Consumer, UK†.
Dextromethorphan hydrobromide (p.1117·3).
*Coughs.*

**Contac Day** SmithKline Beecham Consumer, Canad.†.
Pseudoephedrine hydrochloride (p.1129·2); dextromethorphan hydrobromide (p.1117·3); paracetamol (p.76·2).

**Contac Day & Night Allergy Sinus** *SmithKline Beecham Consumer, USA.*
Paracetamol (p.76·2); pseudoephedrine hydrochloride (p.1129·2); diphenhydramine hydrochloride (p.431·3).

**Contac Day and Night Cold & Flu Caplets** *SmithKline Beecham Consumer, USA.*
Pseudoephedrine hydrochloride (p.1129·2); dextromethorphan hydrobromide (p.1117·3); paracetamol (p.76·2).
*Coughs and cold symptoms.*

**Contac Day & Night Sinus/Allergy** *SmithKline Beecham Consumer, Canad.†.*
Paracetamol (p.76·2); pseudoephedrine hydrochloride (p.1129·2); diphenhydramine hydrochloride (p.431·3).
*Cold symptoms; coughs.*

**Contac Erkaltungs-Trunk** *GlaxoSmithKline Consumer, Ger.*
Paracetamol (p.76·2).
*Fever; pain.*

**Contac Erkaltungs-Trunk Forte** *GlaxoSmithKline Consumer, Ger.*
Paracetamol (p.76·2); phenylephrine hydrochloride (p.1126·3); dextromethorphan hydrobromide (p.1117·3).
*Cold and influenza symptoms; coughs.*

**Contac H** *SmithKline Beecham OTC, Ger.†.*
Chlorphenamine maleate (p.427·3); dextromethorphan hydrobromide (p.1117·3); phenylpropanolamine hydrochloride (p.1127·3).
*Cold symptoms; coughs.*

**Contac Head & Chest Congestion** *GlaxoSmithKline Consumer, Canad.*
Pseudoephedrine hydrochloride (p.1129·2); guaifenesin (p.1122·1).

**Contac 12 Hour** *SmithKline Beecham Consumer, USA†.*
Chlorphenamine maleate (p.427·3); phenylpropanolamine hydrochloride (p.1127·3).
*Upper respiratory-tract symptoms.*

**Contac 12 Hour Allergy** *SmithKline Beecham Consumer, USA.*
Clemastine fumarate (p.429·1).

**Contac Husten-Trunk** *Fink, Ger.†.*
Ambroxol hydrochloride (p.1114·3).
*Respiratory disorders associated with viscid or excessive mucus.*

**Contac Non Drowsy** *GlaxoSmithKline Consumer, UK.*
Pseudoephedrine hydrochloride (p.1129·2).
Contac 400 formerly contained chlorphenamine maleate and phenylpropanolamine hydrochloride.
*Cold symptoms.*

**Contac Rhume** *SmithKline Beecham Consumer, Switz.*
Chlorphenamine maleate (p.427·3); phenylpropanolamine hydrochloride (p.1127·3).
*Cold symptoms; hay fever.*

**Contac Schnupfen** *SmithKline Beecham, Austria.*
Chlorphenamine maleate (p.427·3); phenylpropanolamine hydrochloride (p.1127·3).
*Allergic rhinitis; cold symptoms.*

**Contac Sinus** *GlaxoSmithKline Consumer, Canad.*
Paracetamol (p.76·2); pseudoephedrine hydrochloride (p.1129·2).
*Sinus pain and congestion.*

**Contac Toux** *SmithKline Beecham Consumer, Switz.*
Chlorphenamine maleate (p.427·3); phenylpropanolamine hydrochloride (p.1127·3); dextromethorphan hydrobromide (p.1117·3).
*Coughs.*

**Contac-CC** *GlaxoSmithKline, India.*
Phenylpropanolamine hydrochloride (p.1127·3); guaifenesin (p.1122·1).
*Coughs; influenza; nasal congestion; sinusitis.*

**Contaclair** *Akripan, Austria†.*
Rinsing, disinfecting and storage solution for contact lens (p.1164·2).

**Contact** *VAAS, Ital.†.*
Chlorhexidine hydrochloride (p.1173·3).
*Skin disinfection; wounds.*

**Contact Eyes** *Abbott, Austral.†.*
Comfort solution for soft contact lenses (p.1164·2).

**Contactol** *Merck Sharp & Dohme-Chibret, Fr.†.*
Hypromellose 4000 (p.1579·3).
*Contact lens and ocular prostheses; dry eye disorders.*

**Contafilm** *Allergan, Ger.†.*
Polyvinyl alcohol (p.1581·1).
*Dry eye disorders.*

**Contalax**
*Chefaro Ardeval, Fr.; Fischer, Israel.*
Bisacodyl (p.1251·3).
*Bowel evacuation; constipation.*

**Conta-Lens Wetting** *Baif, Ital.†.*
Benzalkonium chloride (p.1168·3); edetic acid (p.1038·2); methylcellulose (p.1580·2)(p.1164·2).
*Wetting solution for hard contact lens.*

**Contalgin** *Pharmacia, Denm.*
Morphine sulfate (p.60·2).
*Pain.*

**Contaren** *Almirall, Belg.*
Canrenone (p.879·1).
*Hypertension; oedema.*

**Contefur** *Loren, Mex.*
Furazolidone (p.605·2); clioquinol (p.196·3); homatropine (p.483·2); kaolin (p.1268·3); pectin (p.1580·3).
*Diarrhoea.*

**Contem** *Ahimsa, Arg.*
Loperamide (p.1271·2).
*Diarrhoea.*

**ConTE-PAK** *SoloPak, USA†.*
Trace element preparation (p.1417·1).
*Additive for intravenous total parenteral nutrition solutions.*

**Conthram** *Pacific, NZ.*
Dantron (p.1261·1); poloxamer (p.1414·2).
*Constipation.*

**Contiabe** *Cazi, Braz.*
Vitamin B substances (p.1417·1).

**Contigen** *Bard, UK.*
Bovine dermal collagen (p.1674·3).
*Urinary incontinence.*

**Contilen** *Legrand, Braz.*
Chlorphenamine maleate (p.427·3); phenylpropanolamine hydrochloride (p.1127·3).
*Nasal congestion.*

**Contimit** *Lindopharm, Ger.*
Terbutaline sulfate (p.797·2).
*Obstructive airways disease.*

**Continucor** *Parke, Davis, Austria†.*
Quinapril hydrochloride (p.991·1).
*Heart failure; hypertension.*

**Contiphyllin** *Lindopharm, Ger.*
Theophylline (p.798·3).
*Obstructive airways disease.*

**Contopharma** *Silhouette, Austria†.*
Wetting, disinfecting, and storage solutions for contact lenses (p.1164·2).

**Contra Combustiones** *Vitamed, Israel†.*
Aluminium acetate (p.1652·3); zinc oxide (p.1163·2); peru balsam (p.1730·2); bismuth subcarbonate (p.1252·1).
*Nappy rash; skin irritation.*

**Contracep**
*Sigma, Braz.; Nakorn, Thai.*
Medroxyprogesterone acetate (p.1557·2).
*Progestogen-only injectable contraceptive.*

**Contracid** *Thiemann, Ger.†.*
Cimetidine (p.1255·3).
*Gastro-oesophageal reflux; peptic ulcer; Zollinger-Ellison syndrome.*

**Contracide**
*Norgine, Fr.; Norgine, Ital.*
Aluminium hydroxide (p.1249·2); magnesium trisilicate (p.1272·3); dimeticone (p.1289·2).
*Aerophagia; gastrointestinal hyperacidity; meteorism.*

**Contra-Coff** *Universal, S.Afr.†.*
Pholcodine (p.1128·3); squill (p.1130·3).
*Coughs.*

**Contractubex**
*Grunenthal, Arg.; Merz, Ger.; Merz, Hong Kong; Merz, Switz.*
Onion (p.1723·2); heparin sodium (p.928·1); allantoin (p.1141·3).
*Keloids; scars.*

*Kolassa, Austria.*
Onion (p.1723·2); heparin (p.927·3); allantoin (p.1141·3).
*Contractures; scars.*

**Contradol** *Gemballa, Braz.*
Paracetamol (p.76·2).
*Fever; pain.*

**Contraforte** *Sanochemia, Austria.*
Propyphenazone (p.85·3); dextropropoxyphene (p.28·3); caffeine (p.782·1).
*Pain.*

**Contralgen** *Pietrasanta, Ital.*
Paracetamol (p.76·2); aspirin (p.15·1).
*Cold and influenza symptoms; fever; pain.*

**Contralmor** *Laboratorios Chile, Chile.*
Betamethasone dipropionate (p.1093·1); lidocaine (p.1377·3); zinc oxide (p.1163·2).
*Anorectal disorders.*

**Contralorin** *Sanochemia, Austria.*
Propyphenazone (p.85·3); paracetamol (p.76·2); caffeine (p.782·1).
*Fever; pain.*

**Contralum Ultra**
*Note. This name is used for preparations of different composition.*
*Boots Healthcare, Neth.*
Enzacamene (p.1147·1); avobenzone (p.1142·3); sodium 2-phenyl-1*H*-benzimidazole-5-sulfonate (p.1147·1).
*Photosensitive skin disorders; sunscreen.*

*Boots Healthcare, Switz.†.*
Enzacamene (p.1147·1); avobenzone (p.1142·3); ensulizole (p.1147·1).
*Sunscreen.*

**Contramal**
*Continental Pharma, Belg.; Grunenthal, Fr.; Sarabhai Piramal, India; Formenti, Ital.*
Tramadol hydrochloride (p.94·3).
*Pain.*

**Contramareo** *Torrens, Spain.*
Dimenhydrinate (p.431·1).
*Motion sickness.*

**Contramutan** *Nattermann, Ger.*
Homoeopathic preparation.

**Contraneural** *Pfleger, Ger.*
Ibuprofen (p.45·3).
*Fever; inflammation; musculoskeletal and joint disorders; pain.*

**Contraneural Paracetamol/Codeine** *Pfleger, Ger.*
Paracetamol (p.76·2); codeine phosphate (p.27·1).
Formerly known as Contraneural Forte.
*Pain.*

**Contrasmina** *Falqui, Ital.†.*
Clenbuterol hydrochloride (p.784·2).
*Obstructive airways disease.*

**Contraspasmin** *Viatris, Ger.*
Clenbuterol hydrochloride (p.784·2).
*Obstructive airways disease.*

**Contrasthenyl** *Doms, Switz.†.*
Vitamin $B_6$ preparation with minerals (p.1417·1).
*Asthenia.*

**Contrathion**
*Aventis, Arg.; Aventis, Braz.; SERB, Fr.; Rhone-Poulenc Rorer, Gr.; Aventis, Ital.*
Pralidoxime metilsulfate (p.1050·2).
*Organophosphorus poisoning.*

**Contravert $B_6$** *Sanochemia, Austria.*
Meclozine hydrochloride (p.436·3); pyridoxine hydrochloride (p.1456·3).
*Motion sickness; vertigo; vomiting.*

**Contre-Coups de l'Abbe Perdrigeon** *Pionneau, Fr.*
Aloes (p.1248·2).
*Skin disorders; soft-tissue disorders.*

**Contre-Douleurs** *Wild, Switz.*
Aspirin (p.15·1); paracetamol (p.76·2); caffeine (p.782·1).
Colloidal aluminium hydroxide (p.1249·2) is included in the tablets in an attempt to limit adverse effects on the gastrointestinal mucosa.
*Fever; pain.*

**Contre-Douleurs C** *Wild, Switz.*
Aspirin (p.15·1); paracetamol (p.76·2); caffeine (p.782·1); ascorbic acid (p.1460·2).
*Cold symptoms; fever.*

**Contre-Douleurs P** *Wild, Switz.*
Paracetamol (p.76·2).
*Fever; pain.*

**Contre-Douleurs plus** *Wild, Switz.*
Aspirin (p.15·1); caffeine (p.782·1).
Aluminium hydroxide (p.1249·2) is included in this preparation in an attempt to limit adverse effects on the gastrointestinal mucosa.
*Pain.*

**Contreet** *Coloplast, UK.*
Hydrocolloid hydroactivated silver dressing (p.1746·1).
*Burns; ulcers; wounds.*

**Contrelmin** *UCI, Braz.†.*
Tiabendazole (p.114·2); pyrvinium embonate (p.113·3).
*Nematode infections.*

**Contrheuma** *Spitzner, Ger.†.*
Glycol salicylate (p.44·3); benzyl nicotinate (p.21·2).
*Circulatory disorders; inflammatory disorders; muscle and nerve pain; rheumatism.*

**Contrheuma Bad L** *Spitzner, Ger.†.*
Salicylic acid (p.1157·1); sodium humate.
*Bath additive; neuromuscular, musculoskeletal, and joint disorders.*

**Contrheuma V + T Bad N** *Spitzner, Ger.†.*
Glycol salicylate (p.44·3); diethylamine salicylate (p.34·1); oleum pini sylvestris.
*Bath additive; cold symptoms; musculoskeletal and joint disorders; neuralgia; peripheral circulatory disorders.*

**Contrheuma-Gel forte N** *Spitzner, Ger.†.*
Bornyl salicylate (p.21·2); ethyl salicylate (p.37·3); methyl nicotinate (p.59·2).
*Neuralgia; neuritis; rheumatism; sports injuries.*

**Contrin** *Geneva, USA.*
Ferrous fumarate (p.1427·3); folic acid (p.1429·1); intrinsic factor; vitamin $B_{12}$ substances (p.1458·2).
Vitamin C (p.1460·2) is included in this preparation to increase the absorption and availability of iron.
*Anaemias.*

**Control**
*Note. This name is used for preparations of different composition.*
*Farmasa, Braz.*
Chitosane; fruit oligosaccharides; sodium ascorbate; citric acid.

*Bio-Sante, Canad.*
Cascara (p.1255·1); sennosides A and B (p.1288·2).

*Bayer, Ital.*
Lorazepam (p.704·1).
*Convulsions; nervous disorders; sedative.*

*Thompson, USA†.*
Phenylpropanolamine hydrochloride (p.1127·3).
*Obesity.*

**Control K** *Merck, Arg.*
Potassium chloride (p.1232·2).
*Potassium deficiency.*

**Controlip** *Knoll, Mex.*
Fenofibrate (p.915·2).
*Hyperlipidaemias.*

**Controloc**
*Sanofi Synthelabo, Gr.*
Pantoprazole sodium (p.1283·1).
*Peptic ulcer; reflux oesophagitis.*

*Pharma Clal, Israel; Altana, Malaysia; Bayer, S.Afr.; Byk Gulden, Singapore; Pacific Biosciences, Singapore; Byk Gulden, Thai.; Schering-Plough, Thai.*
Pantoprazole (p.1283·1).
*Gastro-oesophageal reflux; peptic ulcer.*

**ControlRx** *Omnii, USA.*
Sodium fluoride (p.1444·3); dimeticone (p.1482·1); poloxamer 407 (p.1414·2).
*Dental caries prophylaxis.*

**Controlvas** *Shire, Spain.*
Enalapril maleate (p.909·2).
*Heart failure; hypertension.*

**Contromet** *Propan, S.Afr.*
Metoclopramide hydrochloride (p.1274·3).
*Gastrointestinal disorders.*

**Contugesic** *Viatris, Spain.*
Dihydrocodeine tartrate (p.34·3).
*Pain.*

**Contumax** *Casen Fleet, Spain.*
Sodium picosulfate (p.1289·3).
*Constipation.*

**Contusil** *Farmatre, Ital.†.*
Benzalkonium chloride (p.1168·3).
*Skin, wound, and burn disinfection.*

**Contusin**
*Note. This name is used for preparations of different composition.*
*Lacer, Spain.*
Diethylamine salicylate (p.34·1); camphor (p.1665·3); thymol (p.1194·2); menthol (p.1711·3); aesculus (p.1648·2).
*Musculoskeletal, joint, and soft-tissue disorders.*

*Herbamed, Switz.*
Homoeopathic preparation.

**Contuss**
*Note. This name is used for preparations of different composition.*
*SmithKline Beecham, Thai.†.*
Diphenhydramine hydrochloride (p.431·3); dextromethorphan hydrobromide (p.1117·3); ammonium chloride (p.1115·2); sodium citrate (p.1223·2).
*Cold symptoms; coughs.*

*Parmed, USA†.*
Phenylpropanolamine hydrochloride (p.1127·3); guaifenesin (p.1122·1); phenylephrine hydrochloride (p.1126·3).
*Coughs.*

**Contuxin** *Continentales, Mex.†.*
Oxolamine (p.1126·1).

**Convacard** *Cheplapharm, Ger.*
Convallaria glycosides (p.1675·3).
*Heart failure.*

**Conva-cyl Ho-Len-Complex** *Liebermann, Ger.*
Homoeopathic preparation.

**Convallocor** *Hevert, Ger.†.*
Homoeopathic preparation.

**Convallocor-SL** *Hevert, Ger.†.*
Crataegus (p.1677·1); convallaria (p.1675·3).
*Cardiac disorders.*

**Convastabil** *Klein, Ger.*
Convallaria (p.1675·3); crataegus (p.1677·1).
*Cardiac disorders.*

**Convectal** *Vita Elan, Spain†.*
Diltiazem hydrochloride (p.900·1).
*Angina pectoris; hypertension; myocardial infarction.*

**Convertal** *Tecnimede, Port.*
Captopril (p.879·2).

**Converten** *Gentili, Ital.*
Enalapril maleate (p.909·2).
*Heart failure; hypertension; ischaemic heart disease.*

**Convertin** *Merck Sharp & Dohme, Israel.*
Enalapril maleate (p.909·2).
*Heart failure; hypertension.*

**Convifer C/Hierro** *Degorts, Mex.*
Vitamins with iron and lysine (p.1417·1).
*Tonic.*

**Conviron-TR** *Ranbaxy, India.*
Dried ferrous sulfate (p.1428·2); folic acid (p.1429·1); vitamin $B_{12}$ (p.1458·2); vitamin $B_6$ (p.1457·2).
Vitamin C (p.1460·2) is included in this preparation to increase the absorption and availability of iron.
*Iron-deficiency anaemia.*

**Convulex**
*Gerot, Austria; Byk, Belg.; Lundbeck, Ger.; Byk, Neth.; Byk Madaus, S.Afr.; Gerot, Singapore; Gerot, Switz.; Pharmacia, UK.*
Valproic acid (p.380·1) or sodium valproate (p.380·1).
*Epilepsy.*

**Convulsan** *Sanval, Braz.*
Carbamazepine (p.353·3).
*Epilepsy.*

**Convulsofin** *AWD, Ger.*
Calcium valproate (p.382·2) or sodium valproate (p.380·1).
*Epilepsy.*

**Coolips** *Mintlab, Chile.*
Cetirizine hydrochloride (p.427·1).

**Cool-Mint Listerine** *Warner-Lambert, USA.*
Thymol (p.1194·2); cineole (p.1672·1); methyl salicylate (p.59·3); menthol (p.1711·3).

**Cooper AR** *Coopervision, Canad.†.*
Antazoline phosphate (p.424·2); naphazoline hydrochloride (p.1124·3).

**Cooper Tears** *Coopervision, Canad.†.*
Polyvinyl alcohol (p.1581·1).

**Copal**
*Note. This name is used for preparations of different composition.*
*Biomet Merck, Ger.*
Polymethylmethacrylate methylmethacrylate copolymer (p.1714·3); gentamicin sulfate (p.217·1); clindamycin hydrochloride (p.194·2).
*Bone infections.*

*Galen, Mex.*
Sulindac (p.91·2).
*Gout; musculoskeletal, joint and peri-articular disorders.*

**Copaltra** Plantes Tropicales, Fr.†.
Coutarea (p.1676·3); centaury (p.1669·2).
*Diabetes.*

**Copamide** Dey's, India.
Chlorpropamide (p.330·3).
*Diabetes mellitus.*

**Copan** Duopharma, Hong Kong.
Hyoscine butylbromide (p.483·3).
*Smooth muscle spasm.*

**Copastin** YSP, Malaysia.
Cloperastine hydrochloride (p.1117·2).
*Coughs.*

**Copaxone**
Teva Tuteur, Arg.; Aventis, Austral.; Biosintetica, Braz.; Teva, Canad.; Teva, Denm.; Aventis, Fin.; Aventis, Irl.; Teva, Israel; Aventis, Ital.; Aventis, Neth.; Teva, Norw.; Aventis, Port.; Aventis, Spain; Aventis, Swed.; Aventis, Switz.; Aventis, UK; Teva, UK; Teva, USA.
Glatiramer acetate (p.1693·3).
*Multiple sclerosis.*

**Cope** Mentholatum, USA.
Aspirin (p.15·1); caffeine (p.782·1).
Aluminium hydroxide (p.1249·2) and magnesium hydroxide (p.1272·2) are included in this preparation in an attempt to limit adverse effects on the gastrointestinal mucosa.
*Pain.*

**Copegus**
Roche, NZ; Roche, Port.; Roche, UK; Roche, USA.
Ribavirin (p.652·1).
Used in combination with peginterferon alfa-2a.
*Chronic hepatitis C.*

**Copena** Ariston, Braz.†.
Chlorophenothiazinylscopine; vitamin $B_1$ (p.1455·2).
*Nausea and vomiting.*

**Copercilex** Cooper (Κοπερ), Gr.
Ampicillin sodium (p.157·1).
*Eye infections.*

**Cophene No. 2** Dunhall, USA.
Pseudoephedrine hydrochloride (p.1129·2); chlorphenamine maleate (p.427·3).
*Upper respiratory-tract symptoms.*

**Cophene XP** Dunhall, USA.
Pseudoephedrine hydrochloride (p.1129·2); guaifenesin (p.1122·1); hydrocodone tartrate (p.45·1).
*Coughs.*

**Cophene-X** Dunhall, USA†.
Phenylephrine hydrochloride (p.1126·3); phenylpropanolamine hydrochloride (p.1127·3); pentoxyverine citrate (p.1126·2); sulfogaiacol (p.1131·1).
*Coughs.*

**Cophenylcaine** Paedpharm, Austral.
Phenylephrine hydrochloride (p.1126·3); lidocaine hydrochloride (p.1377·3).
*Aid in upper respiratory-tract investigations; epistaxis; preparation of nasal mucosa for surgical procedures.*

**Cophylac** Hoechst Marion Roussel, Canad.†.
*Expectorant:* Normethadone hydrochloride (p.1125·2); oxilofrine hydrochloride (p.977·3); emetine hydrochloride (p.604·3).
*Oral solution:* Normethadone hydrochloride (p.1125·2); oxilofrine hydrochloride (p.977·3).
*Coughs.*

**6 Copin** Ariston, Arg.
*Injection:* Hyoscine methobromide (p.483·3); chlorpromazine hydrochloride (p.675·2); pyridoxine hydrochloride (p.1456·3).
*Oral drops; tablets:* Hyoscine methobromide (p.483·3); chlorpromazine hydrochloride (p.675·2); pyridoxine hydrochloride (p.1456·3); procaine hydrochloride (p.1383·2).
*Vomiting.*

**Copinal** Vinas, Spain.
Zinc acexamate (p.1646·2).
*Peptic ulcer.*

**Copiron** Microsules, Arg.
Ibuprofen (p.45·3).
*Fever; pain.*

**Coplexina** Sanofi Synthelabo, Arg.
Co-dergocrine mesilate (p.1674·1).
*Cerebrovascular disorders.*

**Copovan** Biologici Italia, Ital.
Vancomycin hydrochloride (p.275·2).
*Bacterial infections.*

**Coppertone** Balmar, NZ.
*Lotion SPF 4+:* Octinoxate (p.1154·3); oxybenzone (p.1154·3).
*Lotion SPF 15+:* Avobenzone (p.1142·3); octinoxate (p.1154·3); oxybenzone (p.1154·3).
*Lotion SPF 30+:* Avobenzone (p.1142·3); octinoxate (p.1154·3); octisalate (p.1154·3); oxybenzone (p.1154·3).
*Oil SPF 2:* Homosalate (p.1148·1).
*Sunscreen.*

**Coppertone Bug & Sun Adult** Schering-Plough, USA.
*SPF 15:* Octinoxate (p.1154·3); oxybenzone (p.1154·3); octisalate (p.1154·3); homosalate (p.1148·1).
*Sunscreen.*

**Coppertone Bug & Sun Kids** Schering-Plough, USA.
*SPF 30:* Octinoxate (p.1154·3); oxybenzone (p.1154·3); octocrilene (p.1154·3).
*Sunscreen.*

**Coppertone Bug & Sunblock** Schering-Plough, Canad.
*SPF 15:* Homosalate (p.1148·1); octinoxate (p.1154·3); octisalate (p.1154·3); oxybenzone (p.1154·3).
*SPF 30:* Octocrilene (p.1154·3); octinoxate (p.1154·3); oxybenzone (p.1154·3).
*Insect repellent; sunscreen.*

**Coppertone Kids**
Note. This name is used for preparations of different composition.
Schering-Plough, Canad.
*SPF 30; SPF 40:* Homosalate (p.1148·1); octinoxate (p.1154·3); octisalate (p.1154·3); oxybenzone (p.1154·3).
*Sunscreen.*

Schering-Plough, USA.
*SPF 15:* Octinoxate (p.1154·3); octisalate (p.1154·3); homosalate (p.1148·1); oxybenzone (p.1154·3).
*SPF 30:* Octinoxate (p.1154·3); octisalate (p.1154·3); oxybenzone (p.1154·3); octocrilene (p.1154·3).
*Sunscreen.*

**Coppertone Kids Colorblok** Schering-Plough, Canad.
*SPF 40:* Octocrilene (p.1154·3); octinoxate (p.1154·3); octisalate (p.1154·3); oxybenzone (p.1154·3).
*Sunscreen.*

**Coppertone Kids Sunblock with Parsol 1789**
Schering-Plough, Canad.
*SPF 30:* Avobenzone (p.1142·3); homosalate (p.1148·1); octinoxate (p.1154·3); octisalate (p.1154·3); oxybenzone (p.1154·3).
*Sunscreen.*

**Coppertone Lipkote**
Schering-Plough, Canad.†; Schering-Plough, USA.
*SPF 15:* Octinoxate (p.1154·3); oxybenzone (p.1154·3).
*Sunscreen.*

**Coppertone Mist** Schering-Plough, Canad.
*SPF 4:* Homosalate (p.1148·1); oxybenzone (p.1154·3).
*Sunscreen.*

**Coppertone Moisturizing** Schering-Plough, USA.
*SPF 2:* Homosalate (p.1148·1).
*SPF 45:* Octinoxate (p.1154·3); octisalate (p.1154·3); octocrilene (p.1154·3); oxybenzone (p.1154·3).
*SPF 25; SPF 30:* Octinoxate (p.1154·3); octisalate (p.1154·3); homosalate (p.1148·1); oxybenzone (p.1154·3).
*SPF 4; SPF 6; SPF 8; SPF 15:* Octinoxate (p.1154·3); oxybenzone (p.1154·3).
*Sunscreen.*

**Coppertone Noskote** Schering-Plough, Canad.†.
*SPF 15:* Octinoxate (p.1154·3); octisalate (p.1154·3); oxybenzone (p.1154·3).
*Sunscreen.*

**Coppertone Oil-Free** Schering-Plough, Canad.
*SPF 15:* Octinoxate (p.1154·3); oxybenzone (p.1154·3).
*SPF 30; SPF 45:* Homosalate (p.1148·1); octinoxate (p.1154·3); octisalate (p.1154·3); oxybenzone (p.1154·3).
*Sunscreen.*

**Coppertone Radiance** Schering-Plough, Canad.†.
*SPF 15:* Homosalate (p.1148·1); octinoxate (p.1154·3); octisalate (p.1154·3); oxybenzone (p.1154·3).
*Sunscreen.*

**Coppertone Skin Selects** Schering-Plough, Canad.†.
*SPF 15:* Octinoxate (p.1154·3); oxybenzone (p.1154·3).
*Sunscreen.*

**Coppertone Skin Selects Sensitive** Schering-Plough, Canad.†.
*SPF 15:* Octinoxate (p.1154·3); titanium dioxide (p.1160·3).
*Sunscreen.*

**Coppertone Spectra** Schering-Plough, Canad.†.
*SPF 30:* Avobenzone (p.1142·3); homosalate (p.1148·1); octinoxate (p.1154·3); octisalate (p.1154·3); oxybenzone (p.1154·3).
*Sunscreen.*

**Coppertone Sport**
Note. This name is used for preparations of different composition.
Schering-Plough, Canad.
*SPF 15:* Octinoxate (p.1154·3); octisalate (p.1154·3); oxybenzone (p.1154·3).
*SPF 8†; SPF 15†:* Octinoxate (p.1154·3); oxybenzone (p.1154·3).
*Sunscreen.*

Schering-Plough, USA.
*SPF 30:* Octinoxate (p.1154·3); octisalate (p.1154·3); oxybenzone (p.1154·3).
*SPF 4; SPF 8; SPF 15:* Octinoxate (p.1154·3); oxybenzone (p.1154·3).
*Sunscreen.*

**Coppertone Sport Spray** Schering-Plough, Canad.
*SPF 15; SPF 30:* Homosalate (p.1148·1); octinoxate (p.1154·3); octisalate (p.1154·3); oxybenzone (p.1154·3).
*Sunscreen.*

**Coppertone Spray** Schering-Plough, Canad.
*SPF 15; SPF 30:* Homosalate (p.1148·1); octinoxate (p.1154·3); octisalate (p.1154·3); oxybenzone (p.1154·3).
*Sunscreen.*

**Coppertone Spray'n Play** Schering-Plough, Canad.
*SPF 30:* Homosalate (p.1148·1); octinoxate (p.1154·3); octisalate (p.1154·3); oxybenzone (p.1154·3).
*Sunscreen.*

**Coppertone Sunblock** Schering-Plough, Canad.†.
*SPF 45:* Homosalate (p.1148·1); octinoxate (p.1154·3); octisalate (p.1154·3); oxybenzone (p.1154·3).
*Sunscreen.*

**Coppertone Sunscreen** Schering-Plough, Canad.
*SPF 8:* Octinoxate (p.1154·3); oxybenzone (p.1154·3).
*Sunscreen.*

**Coppertone Sunstick** Cheshire, UK†.
*SPF 15:* Titanium dioxide (p.1160·3).
*Sunscreen.*

**Coppertone Suntan** Schering-Plough, Canad.
*SPF 4:* Octinoxate (p.1154·3); oxybenzone (p.1154·3).
*Sunscreen.*

**Coppertone Supershade** Cheshire, UK†.
*SPF 15:* Oxybenzone (p.1154·3); padimate O (p.1155·1).
*Sunscreen.*

**Coppertone Tan Magnifier** Schering-Plough, USA.
*Gel SPF 4:* Ensulizole (p.1147·1).
*Lotion SPF 4:* Octinoxate (p.1154·3).
*SPF 2:* Trolamine salicylate (p.95·3).
*Sunscreen.*

**Coppertone Ultrashade** Cheshire, UK†.
*SPF 23:* Octinoxate (p.1154·3); oxybenzone (p.1154·3); padimate O (p.1155·1).
*Sunscreen.*

**Coppertone UVGuard** Schering-Plough, Canad.†.
*SPF 15:* Avobenzone (p.1142·3); octinoxate (p.1154·3); oxybenzone (p.1154·3).
*SPF 30:* Avobenzone (p.1142·3); octinoxate (p.1154·3); oxybenzone (p.1154·3); octisalate (p.1154·3).
*Sunscreen.*

**Coppertone Waterbabies**
Schering-Plough, Canad.; Schering-Plough, USA.
*SPF 30; SPF 45:* Homosalate (p.1148·1); octinoxate (p.1154·3); oxybenzone (p.1154·3); octisalate (p.1154·3).
*Sunscreen.*

**Coppertone Waterproof Sunblock** Schering-Plough, Canad.
*SPF 15:* Octinoxate (p.1154·3); oxybenzone (p.1154·3).
*SPF 15; SPF 30:* Avobenzone (p.1142·3); octocrilene (p.1154·3); octisalate (p.1154·3); oxybenzone (p.1154·3).
*SPF 30; SPF 45:* Octinoxate (p.1154·3); homosalate (p.1148·1); octisalate (p.1154·3); oxybenzone (p.1154·3).
*Sunscreen.*

**Co-Pressotec** Teuto, Braz.
Enalapril maleate (p.909·2); hydrochlorothiazide (p.933·2).
*Hypertension.*

**Coptin** Axcan, Canad.
Sulfadiazine (p.258·2); trimethoprim (p.272·2).
*Bacterial infections of the urinary tract.*

**Copyrkal N** Berlin-Chemie, Ger.
Propyphenazone (p.85·3); caffeine (p.782·1).
*Fever; pain.*

**Co-Pyronil**
Lilly, Thai.; Dista, USA†.
Chlorphenamine maleate (p.427·3); pseudoephedrine hydrochloride (p.1129·2).
*Upper respiratory-tract symptoms.*

**Co-Q-10**
Swiss Herbal, Canad.; Larkhall Laboratories, UK; Carlson, USA.
Ubidecarenone (p.1760·2).
*Metabolic disorders.*

**Coquelusedal** Elerte, Fr.
Niaouli oil (p.1719·3); grindelia (p.1696·1); gelsemium (p.1691·3).
Formerly contained niaouli oil, grindelia, gelsemium, and phenobarbital.
*Coughs.*

**Coquelusedal Paracetamol** Elerte, Fr.
Paracetamol (p.76·2); niaouli oil (p.1719·3); grindelia (p.1696·1); gelsemium (p.1691·3).
*Respiratory-tract disorders.*

**Coquevit** Brasmedica, Braz.†.
Sodium dibunate (p.1130·2); ephedrine (p.1120·1); vitamin C (p.1460·2).
*Coughs.*

**CoQuinone**
Usana, Hong Kong; USANA, USA.
Ubidecarenone (p.1760·2).
*Nutritional supplement.*

**Cor Mio** Hexal, Braz.
Amiodarone hydrochloride (p.859·2).
*Arrhythmias.*

**cor tensobon** Schwarz, Ger.
Captopril (p.879·2).
*Diabetic nephropathy; heart failure; hypertension.*

**Coraben** Medic, Braz.
Ferrous sulfate (p.1428·2); folic acid (p.1429·1); vitamin $B_{12}$ (p.1458·2).
Succinic acid is included in this preparation to increase the absorption and availability of iron.
*Anaemias.*

**Coracten**
Vianex (Βιανέξ), Gr.; ICN, Hong Kong; ICN, Thai.; Celltech, UK.
Nifedipine (p.966·2).
*Angina pectoris; hypertension.*

**Coradol** Coradol, Ger.
Homoeopathic preparation.

**Coradur** Glaxo Wellcome, Canad.†.
Isosorbide dinitrate (p.941·1).
*Angina pectoris.*

**Coral** SoSe, Ital.
Nifedipine (p.966·2).
*Angina pectoris; hypertension; Raynaud's syndrome.*

**Coralen** Alter, Spain.
Ranitidine hydrochloride (p.1285·2).
*Acid aspiration; gastro-oesophageal reflux; gastrointestinal haemorrhage; gastrointestinal hyperacidity; peptic ulcer; Zollinger-Ellison syndrome.*

**Coralgesic** Vesta, S.Afr.†.
Paracetamol (p.76·2); codeine phosphate (p.27·1); vitamin B substances (p.1417·1).
*Fever; pain.*

**Coralmyn** Bioclon, Mex.
Snake venom antiserum (p.1639·1).
*Micrurus spp bites.*

**Coralzul** Farcoral, Mex.
Furazolidone (p.605·2); homatropine (p.483·2); kaolin (p.1268·3); pectin (p.1580·3); diiodohydroxyquinoline (p.603·3).
*Gastrointestinal disorders.*

**Coramedan** Medice, Ger.
Digitoxin (p.894·3).
*Arrhythmias; heart failure.*

**Coramil** Sanofi Synthelabo, Swed.
Diltiazem hydrochloride (p.900·1).
*Angina pectoris; hypertension.*

**Coramine Glucose** Novartis Sante, Fr.
Nikethamide (p.1591·2); glucose monohydrate (p.1432·2).
*Asthenia; fainting.*

**Corangin**
Novartis, Austria†; Novartis, Ger.; Novartis, Hong Kong; Novartis, NZ.
Isosorbide mononitrate (p.942·1).
*Angina pectoris; heart failure.*

**Corangin Nitrokapseln and Nitrospray** Novartis, Ger.
Glyceryl trinitrate (p.923·2).
*Angina pectoris; heart failure; myocardial infarction.*

**Corangine** Novartis, Switz.
Isosorbide mononitrate (p.942·1).
*Heart failure; ischaemic heart disease.*

**Coras** Alphapharm, Austral.
Diltiazem hydrochloride (p.900·1).
*Angina pectoris.*

**Corase** Medac, Ger.
Urokinase (p.1018·2).
*Thromboembolic disorders.*

**Coraspir** Armstrong, Mex.
Lysine aspirin (p.54·3).
*Fever; pain; thromboembolism prophylaxis.*

**Corathiem** Ohta, Hong Kong†.
Cinnarizine (p.428·3).
*Cerebrovascular disorders.*

**Coratol** Scan Lab, Thai.
Atenolol (p.865·2).
*Angina pectoris; arrhythmias; hypertension; myocardial infarction.*

**Corazem** Mundipharma, Austria.
Diltiazem hydrochloride (p.900·1).
*Angina pectoris; heart failure; hypertension; myocardial infarction.*

**Corazet** Mundipharma, Ger.
Diltiazem hydrochloride (p.900·1).
*Angina pectoris; hypertension.*

**Corbar** Covan, S.Afr.
Guaifenesin (p.1122·1); ephedrine hydrochloride (p.1120·1); codeine phosphate (p.27·1); chlorphenamine maleate (p.427·3); co. cocillana syrup (p.1117·2).
*Coughs.*

**Corbar M** Covan, S.Afr.†.
Carbocisteine (p.1116·2).
*Respiratory-tract disorders.*

**Corbar S** Covan, S.Afr.†.
Fedrilate (p.1121·2).
*Coughs.*

**Corbeta** Sarabhai Piramal, India.
Propranolol hydrochloride (p.989·3).
*Angina pectoris.*

**Corbetazine** Sarabhai Piramal, India.
Propranolol hydrochloride (p.989·3); hydralazine hydrochloride (p.931·2).
*Hypertension.*

**Corbeton** Alphapharm, Austral.
Oxprenolol hydrochloride (p.978·1).
*Angina pectoris; arrhythmias; hypertension.*

**Corbin** Pharmaland, Thai.
Cloxacillin sodium (p.198·2).
*Gram-positive bacterial infections.*

**Corbionax** Irex, Fr.
Amiodarone hydrochloride (p.859·2).
*Arrhythmias.*

**Corbis** Roemmers, Arg.
Bisoprolol fumarate (p.875·1).
*Angina pectoris; heart failure; hypertension.*

**Corcanfol** Lafage, Arg.
Etilefrine (p.914·1).
*Hypotension.*

**Corciclen** Allergan, Braz.
Chlortetracycline hydrochloride (p.187·3); cortisone acetate (p.1096·1); bismuth loretinate.
*Infected eye disorders.*

**Cordalin** *AWD, Ger.*
Bisoprolol fumarate (p.875·1).
*Angina pectoris; hypertension.*

**Cordanum** *AWD, Ger.*
Talinolol (p.1009·2).
*Arrhythmias; hypertension; ischaemic heart disease; myocardial infarction.*

**Cordapur Novo** *APS, Ger.*
Crataegus (p.1677·1).
*Heart failure.*

**Cordarex**
*Note. This name is used for preparations of different composition.*
*Biosintetica, Braz.*
Amlodipine besilate (p.862·1).
*Hypertension; ischaemic heart disease.*

*Sanofi Synthelabo, Ger.*
Amiodarone hydrochloride (p.859·2).
*Arrhythmias.*

**Cordarone**
*Sanofi Synthelabo, Belg.; Wyeth-Ayerst, Canad.; Sanofi Synthelabo, Chile; Sanofi Winthrop, Denm.; Sanofi Synthelabo, Fin.; Sanofi Synthelabo, Fr.; Sanofi Synthelabo, Hong Kong; Sanofi Torrent, India; Sanofi Synthelabo, Ital.; Sanofi Synthelabo, Malaysia; Sanofi Synthelabo, Mex.; Sanofi Synthelabo, Neth.; Sanofi Synthelabo, Norw.; Sanofi Synthelabo, NZ; Sanofi Synthelabo, Port.; Sanofi Synthelabo, Singapore; Sanofi Synthelabo, Swed.; Sanofi Synthelabo, Switz.; Sanofi Synthelabo, Thai.; Wyeth-Ayerst, USA.*
Amiodarone hydrochloride (p.859·2).
*Arrhythmias.*

**Cordarone X**
*Sanofi Synthelabo, Austral.; Sanofi Synthelabo, Irl.; Sanofi Synthelabo, S.Afr.; Sanofi Synthelabo, UK.*
Amiodarone hydrochloride (p.859·2).
*Arrhythmias.*

**Cordes Beta** *Ichthyol, Ger.*
Betamethasone valerate (p.1093·2).
*Skin disorders.*

**Cordes BPO** *Ichthyol, Ger.*
Benzoyl peroxide (p.1143·2).
*Acne.*

**Cordes Estriol** *APS, Ger.*
Estriol (p.1552·3).
*Vaginal disorders.*

**Cordes Nystatin Soft** *Ichthyol, Ger.†.*
Nystatin (p.406·3).
*Fungal skin infections.*

**Cordes VAS** *Ichthyol, Ger.*
Tretinoin (p.1161·1).
*Acne.*

**Cordesin** *Serag-Wiessner, Ger.*
Potassium aspartate (p.1233·1); magnesium aspartate (p.1227·3).
*Heart failure; myocardial infarction; potassium and magnesium deficiency.*

**Cordiax** *Crinos, Ital.*
Celiprolol hydrochloride (p.881·3).
*Angina pectoris; hypertension.*

**Cordicant** *Mundipharma, Ger.*
Nifedipine (p.966·2).
*Angina pectoris; hypertension.*

**Cordichin** *Abbott, Ger.*
Verapamil hydrochloride (p.1019·1); quinidine (p.991·3).
*Arrhythmias.*

**Cordil** *Dexxon, Israel.*
Isosorbide dinitrate (p.941·1).
*Angina pectoris; heart failure.*

**Cordilan** *Roche, Spain†.*
Nifedipine (p.966·2).
*Angina pectoris; hypertension; Raynaud's syndrome.*

**Cordilat**
*Note. This name is used for preparations of different composition.*
*Cristalia, Braz.*
Verapamil hydrochloride (p.1019·1).

*Tecnofarma, Mex.*
Nifedipine (p.966·2).
*Angina pectoris; hypertension.*

**Cordilox**
*Abbott, Austral.; Ivax, UK.*
Verapamil hydrochloride (p.1019·1).
*Angina pectoris; arrhythmias; hypertension.*

**Cordinal** *Roemmers, Arg.*
Bifemelane hydrochloride (p.1660·2).
*Mental function impairment.*

**Cordiodoron** *Weleda, Ger.*
Homoeopathic preparation.

**Cordipatch** *Schwarz, Fr.*
Glyceryl trinitrate (p.923·2).
*Angina pectoris.*

**Cordipin** *KRKA, Singapore.*
Nifedipine (p.966·2).
*Angina pectoris; hypertension; Raynaud's syndrome.*

**Cordipina**
*Note. This name is used for preparations of different composition.*
*Farmasa, Braz.*
Amlodipine besilate (p.862·1).
*Hypertension.*

*IBP, Ital.†.*
Nicardipine hydrochloride (p.965·1).
*Angina pectoris; heart failure; hypertension.*

**Cordiplast**
*Gebro, Austria; CEPA, Spain.*
Glyceryl trinitrate (p.923·2).
*Angina pectoris.*

**Cordisol** *Bioprogress, Ital.*
Nicardipine hydrochloride (p.965·1).
*Angina pectoris; heart failure; hypertension.*

**Corditrine** *Specia, Fr.†.*
Glyceryl trinitrate (p.923·2).
*Angina pectoris; heart failure.*

**Cordium**
*Aaciphar, Belg.†; Riom, Fr.†.*
Bepridil hydrochloride (p.868·3).
*Angina pectoris.*

**Cordodopa** *Sanofi Synthelabo, Port.*
Dopamine hydrochloride (p.907·1).
*Shock.*

**Cordran** *Oclassen, USA.*
Fludroxycortide (p.1100·3).
*Skin disorders.*

**Cordymax** *Pharmanex, USA.*
*Cordyceps sinensis* mushroom mycelia.
*Fatigue.*

**Coreg**
*Roche, Braz.; GlaxoSmithKline, Canad.; GlaxoSmithKline, USA.*
Carvedilol (p.881·1).
*Angina pectoris; heart failure; hypertension.*

**Corega** *GlaxoSmithKline, Braz.*
Sterculia (p.1290·2).

**Coreine** *Germania, Austria.*
Carrageenan (p.1578·2).
*Constipation.*

**Co-Renitec**
*Merck Sharp & Dohme, Arg.; Merck Sharp & Dohme, Austria; Merck Sharp & Dohme, Belg.; Merck Sharp & Dohme, Braz.; Merck Sharp & Dohme, Denm.; Merck Sharp & Dohme-Chibret, Fr.; Merck Sharp & Dohme, Hong Kong; Merck Sharp & Dohme, Mex.; Merck Sharp & Dohme, Neth.; Merck Sharp & Dohme, NZ; Merck Sharp & Dohme, S.Afr.; Merck Sharp & Dohme, Singapore†; Merck Sharp & Dohme, Spain.*
Enalapril maleate (p.909·2); hydrochlorothiazide (p.933·2).
*Hypertension.*

**Co-Reniten** *Merck Sharp & Dohme, Switz.*
Enalapril maleate (p.909·2); hydrochlorothiazide (p.933·2).
*Hypertension.*

**Corenza C** *Restan, S.Afr.*
Aspirin (p.15·1); ascorbic acid (p.1460·2); chlorphenamine maleate (p.427·3); phenylephrine hydrochloride (p.1126·3); moroxydine hydrochloride (p.649·3).
*Cold and influenza symptoms.*

**Coreptil** *Sanofi Synthelabo, Ital.*
Heptaminol hydrochloride (p.1697·1).
*Adjunct in overdosage with neuroleptics and barbiturates; cardiac disorders.*

**Coretec** *Eisai, Jpn.*
Olprinone hydrochloride (p.976·1).
*Heart failure.*

**Corethium** *Johnson & Johnson Medical, UK†.*
Porcine skin (p.1158·1).
*Skin grafts.*

**Corex** *Pfizer, India.*
Chlorphenamine maleate (p.427·3); codeine phosphate (p.27·1); menthol (p.1711·3).
*Coughs.*

**Corex Dx** *Pfizer, India.*
Chlorphenamine maleate (p.427·3); dextromethorphan hydrobromide (p.1117·3); menthol (p.1711·3).
*Coughs.*

**Corfen-DM** *Cypress, USA.*
Dextromethorphan hydrobromide (p.1117·3); phenylephrine hydrochloride (p.1126·3); chlorphenamine maleate (p.427·3).
*Coughs; respiratory-tract congestion.*

**Corflo** *Wockhardt, India.*
Nicorandil (p.965·3).
*Angina pectoris.*

**Corgard**
*Bristol-Myers Squibb, Arg.; Bristol-Myers Squibb, Belg.; Bristol-Myers Squibb, Braz.; Squibb, Canad.; Bristol-Myers Squibb, Chile; Sanofi Synthelabo, Fr.; Bristol-Myers Squibb, Hong Kong; Bristol-Myers Squibb, Ital.; Bristol-Myers Squibb, Malaysia; Bristol-Myers Squibb, NZ†; Bristol-Myers Squibb, S.Afr.; Squibb, Spain; Bristol-Myers Squibb, Switz.; Sanofi Synthelabo, UK; Monarch, USA.*
Nadolol (p.963·1).
*Angina pectoris; arrhythmias; hypertension; hyperthyroidism; migraine; myocardiol infarction; obstructive cardiomyopathy; tremor.*

**Corgaretic**
*Bristol-Myers Squibb, S.Afr.; Bristol-Myers Squibb, Switz.†; Sanofi Synthelabo, UK†.*
Nadolol (p.963·1); bendroflumethiazide (p.867·3).
*Hypertension.*

**Corguttin N plus** *Roland, Ger.†.*
Adonis vernalis (p.1648·1); convallaria (p.1675·3); crataegus (p.1677·1).
*Cardiovascular disorders.*

**Coric** *Bristol-Myers Squibb, Ger.*
Lisinopril (p.946·3).
*Heart failure; hypertension; myocardial infarction.*

**Coric Plus** *Bristol-Myers Squibb, Ger.*
Lisinopril (p.946·3); hydrochlorothiazide (p.933·2).
*Hypertension.*

**Coricide le Diable** *Sodia, Fr.*
Salicylic acid (p.1157·1).
*Callosities; corns; verrucae.*

**Coricidil-D** *Plough, Port.*
Paracetamol (p.76·2); chlorphenamine maleate (p.427·3); phenylpropanolamine hydrochloride (p.1127·3).
*Cold symptoms; rhinitis; sinusitis.*

**Coricidin**
*Note. This name is used for preparations of different composition.*
*Schering-Plough, Canad.*
Chlorphenamine maleate (p.427·3); aspirin (p.15·1).
Formerly known as Coricidin Cold.
*Cold symptoms.*

*Schering-Plough, Ital.*
Oxymetazoline hydrochloride (p.1126·1).
*Allergic rhinitis; cold symptoms; sinusitis.*

*Schering-Plough, Spain.*
Ascorbic acid (p.1460·2); caffeine (p.782·1); chlorphenamine maleate (p.427·3); salicylamide (p.87·3).
*Fever; nasal congestion; pain.*

*Schering-Plough, USA.*
Paracetamol (p.76·2); chlorphenamine maleate (p.427·3).
*Upper respiratory-tract symptoms.*

**Coricidin D**
*Note. This name is used for preparations of different composition.*
*Schering, Canad.†.*
*Long-acting tablets:* Chlorphenamine maleate (p.427·3); phenylpropanolamine hydrochloride (p.1127·3).
*Tablets:* Chlorphenamine maleate (p.427·3); aspirin (p.15·1); phenylpropanolamine (p.1127·3).
*Cold symptoms; respiratory congestion.*

*Schering-Plough, USA†.*
Phenylpropanolamine hydrochloride (p.1127·3); chlorphenamine maleate (p.427·3); paracetamol (p.76·2).
*Upper respiratory-tract symptoms.*

**Coricidin Expec** *Schering-Plough, Mex.*
Loratadine (p.436·1); ambroxol hydrochloride (p.1114·3).
Formerly contained dextromethorphan hydrobromide, guaifenesin, and phenylpropanolamine hydrochloride.
*Respiratory-tract disorders associated with viscous mucus.*

**Coricidin F** *Schering-Plough, Mex.*
Paracetamol (p.76·2); caffeine (p.782·1); phenylephrine hydrochloride (p.1126·3); chlorphenamine maleate (p.427·3).
Formerly contained paracetamol, phenylpropanolamine hydrochloride, and chlorphenamine maleate.
*Nasal congestion.*

**Coricidin Fuerte** *Schering-Plough, Spain†.*
Chlorphenamine maleate (p.427·3); phenylpropanolamine hydrochloride (p.1127·3); paracetamol (p.76·2).
*Fever; nasal congestion; pain.*

**Coricidin HBP Chest Congestion & Cough** *Schering-Plough, USA.*
Dextromethorphan hydrobromide (p.1117·3); guaifenesin (p.1122·1).
*Upper respiratory-tract disorders.*

**Coricidin Maximum Strength Sinus Headache** *Schering-Plough, USA†.*
Phenylpropanolamine hydrochloride (p.1127·3); chlorphenamine maleate (p.427·3); paracetamol (p.76·2).
*Upper respiratory-tract symptoms.*

**Coricidin Non-Drowsy** *Schering, Canad.†.*
Phenylpropanolamine hydrochloride (p.1127·3); aspirin (p.15·1).
*Sinus pain and congestion.*

**Coricidin Pediatrico NF** *Schering-Plough, Mex.*
Chlorphenamine maleate (p.427·3); paracetamol (p.76·2); phenylpropanolamine hydrochloride (p.1127·3).
Formerly known as Coricidin Pediatrico and contained chlorphenamine maleate and paracetamol.
*Respiratory-tract congestion.*

**Coricidin Sinus Headache** *Schering, Canad.†.*
Paracetamol (p.76·2); phenylpropanolamine hydrochloride (p.1127·3); chlorphenamine maleate (p.427·3).
*Cold symptoms; nasal congestion; sinus headache.*

**Coridil** *Ecosol, Switz.*
Diltiazem hydrochloride (p.900·1).
*Hypertension; ischaemic heart disease.*

**Corifeo** *UCB, Ger.*
Lercanidipine hydrochloride (p.946·1).
*Hypertension.*

**Corifin** *Raza, Malaysia; Pharmaniaga, Malaysia.*
Guaifenesin (p.1122·1); pseudoephedrine hydrochloride (p.1129·2).
*Coughs; respiratory-tract congestion.*

**Corifina** *Farma Lepori, Spain.*
Azelastine hydrochloride (p.425·2).
*Allergic conjunctivitis; allergic rhinitis.*

**Corilax** *Community Pharmacy, Thai.*
Orphenadrine citrate (p.486·1); paracetamol (p.76·2).
*Musculoskeletal pain; neuralgia; tension headache.*

**Corilin F** *Schering-Plough, Mex.*
Paracetamol (p.76·2); caffeine (p.782·1); phenylephrine hydrochloride (p.1126·3); chlorphenamine maleate (p.427·3).
*Nasal congestion.*

**Corilisina** *Pensa, Spain.*
Oxymetazoline hydrochloride (p.1126·1).
*Nasal congestion.*

**Corindocomb** *Schering, Ger.*
Mepindolol sulfate (p.952·2); hydrochlorothiazide (p.933·2).
*Hypertension.*

**Corindolan**
*Schering, Austria†; Schering, Ger.*
Mepindolol sulfate (p.952·2).
*Angina pectoris; cardiac hyperkinetic syndrome; hypertension.*

**Corinfar** *AWD, Ger.*
Nifedipine (p.966·2).
*Angina pectoris; hypertension; Raynaud's syndrome.*

**Coriodal** *Instituto Sanitas, Chile.*
Propranolol hydrochloride (p.989·3).
*Angina pectoris; arrhythmias; hypertension; migraine.*

**Corion** *Win-Medicare, India.*
Chorionic gonadotrophin (p.1320·3).
*Cryptorchidism; delayed puberty; female infertility; habitual miscarriage; male hypogonadism; oligospermia; pituitary dwarfism.*

**Coriosta Vitaltonikum N** *Niedermaier, Ger.*
Ginseng (p.1693·1).
*Tonic.*

**Coriovaccine** *Disprovent, Arg.*
*Staphylococcus*; *Micrococcus*; *Pneumococcus*; *Streptococcus*; *Klebsiella*; *Moraxella catarrhalis*; *Haemophilus influenzae*; vitamin C (p.1460·2).

**Corisol** *Ecosol, Switz.*
Clotrimazole (p.396·2).
*Fungal skin infections.*

**Coristex-DH** *Technilab, Canad.*
Phenylephrine hydrochloride (p.1126·3); hydrocodone tartrate (p.45·1).
*Coughs.*

**Coristina D** *Schering-Plough, Braz.*
Dexchlorpheniramine maleate (p.427·3); phenylephrine hydrochloride (p.1126·3); caffeine (p.782·1); aspirin (p.15·1).
*Cold and influenza symptoms.*

**Coristina R** *Schering-Plough, Braz.*
Salicylamide (p.87·3); dexchlorpheniramine maleate (p.427·3); phenylephrine hydrochloride (p.1126·3); caffeine (p.782·1).
*Influenza symptoms.*

**Coristina Reforcada** *Schering-Plough, Braz.†.*
Dexchlorpheniramine maleate (p.427·3); phenylephrine hydrochloride (p.1126·3); caffeine (p.782·1); salicylamide (p.87·3).
*Bronchodilator.*

**Coristine-DH** *Technilab, Canad.*
Hydrocodone tartrate (p.45·1); phenylephrine hydrochloride (p.1126·3).
*Coughs.*

**Coritab**
*Atlantic, Hong Kong; Atlantic, Singapore†; Atlantic, Thai.†.*
Paracetamol (p.76·2); phenylpropanolamine hydrochloride (p.1127·3); chlorphenamine maleate (p.427·3).
*Cold symptoms; nasal congestion; rhinitis.*

**Coritensil** *Roux-Ocefa, Arg.*
Carvedilol (p.881·1).

**Coritex** *Bago, Chile.*
Betamethasone (p.1093·1).
*Corticosteroid.*

**Coritussal**
*Note. This name is used for preparations of different composition.*
*Mack, Hong Kong.*
Dextromethorphan hydrobromide (p.1117·3); phenylephrine hydrochloride (p.1126·3); carbinoxamine maleate (p.426·3).
*Coughs; rhinitis.*

*Mack, Singapore†.*
Dextromethorphan (p.1117·3); phenylpropanolamine (p.1127·3); carbinoxamine (p.426·3).
*Coughs; rhinitis.*

**Corium** *ICN, Canad.†.*
Chlordiazepoxide hydrochloride (p.674·2); clidinium bromide (p.480·2).
*Gastrointestinal disorders with associated anxiety.*

**Coriver** *Maver, Mex.*
Paracetamol (p.76·2).
*Fever; pain.*

**Corizina**
*Note. A similar name is used for preparations of different composition (see below).*
*Cetus, Arg.*
Ascorbic acid (p.1460·2); paracetamol (p.76·2); diphenhydramine (p.431·3).
*Influenza symptoms.*

**Corizzina**
*Note. A similar name is used for preparations of different composition (see above).*
*SIT, Ital.*
Tetracaine hydrochloride (p.1385·1); naphazoline nitrate (p.1124·3).
*Nasal congestion.*

**cor-L 90 N** *Loges, Ger.*
Homoeopathic preparation.

**Corlan**
*Celltech, Irl.; Celltech, UK.*
Hydrocortisone sodium succinate (p.1104·1).
*Aphthous stomatitis.*

**Cor-loges** *Loges, Ger.*
Squill (p.1130·3); convallaria (p.1675·3).
*Cardiac disorders; oedema.*

**Corlopam**
*Elan, Irl.; Segix, Ital.; Neurex, USA.*
Fenoldopam mesilate (p.915·3).
*Hypertension.*

**Cormagnesin** *Asta Medica, Austria; Worwag, Ger.*
Magnesium sulfate (p.1228·2).
*Arrhythmias; eclampsia; magnesium deficiency; myocardial infarction; premature labour.*

**Cormax** *Oclassen, USA.*
Clobetasol propionate (p.1095·2).
*Skin disorders.*

**Cormelian** *Khandelwal, India; Schering, Ital.†.*
Dilazep hydrochloride (p.900·1).
*Cardiac disorders.*

**Corn Huskers** *Warner-Lambert, USA.*
Emollient and moisturiser.

**Corn Removing Liquid** *Scholl, Israel.*
Salicylic acid (p.1157·1); camphor (p.1665·3).
*Corns.*

**Corn Salve** *Cress, Canad.†.*
Methyl salicylate (p.59·3); salicylic acid (p.1157·1).

**Cornaron** *TAD, Ger.*
Amiodarone hydrochloride (p.859·2).
*Arrhythmias.*

**Cornel** *Almirall, Spain.*
Nisoldipine (p.973·2).
*Angina pectoris; hypertension.*

**Corneregel** *Mann, Ger.*
Dexpanthenol (p.1727·2).
*Eye disorders.*

**Corni Limp** *Sophia, Mex.†.*
Sodium chloride (p.1233·3).

**Cornina**
*Note. This name is used for preparations of different composition.*
*Beiersdorf, Chile.*
Triclosan (p.1195·2); dichlorobenzyl alcohol (p.1178·3).
*Bacterial and fungal foot infections.*

*Beiersdorf, Spain.*
Salicylic acid (p.1157·1).
*Corns.*

**Cornina Hornhaut** *Beiersdorf, Ger.†.*
Salicylic acid (p.1157·1).
*Calluses; corns.*

**Cornina Huhneraugen** *Beiersdorf, Ger.†.*
Salicylic acid (p.1157·1).
*Corns.*

**Cornkil** *Norgine, Austral.*
Benzocaine (p.1370·3); salicylic acid (p.1157·1); lactic acid (p.1704·1).
*Corns.*

**Corocrat** *Biomo, Ger.*
Crataegus (p.1677·1).
*Heart failure.*

**Coroday** *Generics, UK.*
Nifedipine (p.966·2).
*Angina pectoris; hypertension.*

**Corodil** *Gea, Denm.*
Enalapril maleate (p.909·2).
*Heart failure; hypertension.*

**Corodil Comp** *Gea, Denm.*
Enalapril maleate (p.909·2); hydrochlorothiazide (p.933·2).
*Hypertension.*

**Corodin** *Drugtech, Chile.*
Losartan potassium (p.947·2).
*Hypertension.*

**Corodin D** *Drugtech, Chile.*
Losartan potassium (p.947·2); hydrochlorothiazide (p.933·2).
*Hypertension.*

**Corodoc S** *Fides, Ger.*
Homoeopathic preparation.

**Corodyn** *Schmidgall, Austria.*
Crataegus tincture (p.1677·1); camphor (p.1665·3); menthol (p.1711·3).
*Cardiovascular disorders.*

**Corogal** *Galen, Mex.*
Nifedipine (p.966·2).
*Angina pectoris; hypertension.*

**Corolater** *Elan, Spain.*
Diltiazem hydrochloride (p.900·1).
*Angina pectoris; hypertension.*

**Corolin** *Leiras, Fin.*
Simvastatin (p.997·1).
*Coronary artery disease; hypercholesterolaemia.*

**Coromert** *Mertens, Arg.*
Flunarizine (p.434·2).
*Migraine; vertigo.*

**Coronar** *Biolab Sanus, Braz.*
Propatylnitrate (p.989·3).
*Angina pectoris.*

**Coronarine** *Negma, Fr.†.*
Dipyridamole (p.903·1).
*Thromboembolic disorders.*

**Coronator** *Roland, Ger.†.*
Crataegus (p.1677·1).
*Heart failure.*

**Coronex** *Pacific, NZ.*
Isosorbide dinitrate (p.941·1).

**Coro-Nitro**
*3M, Ger.; Roche, UK.*
Glyceryl trinitrate (p.923·2).
*Angina pectoris; heart failure; myocardial infarction.*

**Coronorm** *Wolff, Ger.*
Captopril (p.879·2).
*Heart failure; hypertension.*

**Coronovo**
*Note. This name is used for preparations of different composition.*
*Labinca, Arg.*
Amiodarone hydrochloride (p.859·2).
*Arrhythmias.*

*Recalcine, Chile.*
Nifedipine (p.966·2).
*Angina pectoris; hypertension.*

**Coronur** *Roche, Spain.*
Isosorbide mononitrate (p.942·1).
*Angina pectoris.*

**Coropres** *Roche, Spain.*
Carvedilol (p.881·1).
*Heart failure; hypertension; ischaemic heart disease.*

**Cororell** *Sanorell, Ger.*
Homoeopathic preparation.

**Corosan** *Farmacologico Milanese, Ital.*
Dipyridamole (p.903·1).
*Vascular disorders.*

**Corotal** *Rosch & Handel, Austria.*
β-Acetyldigoxin (p.851·1).
*Arrhythmias; heart failure.*

**Corotenol**
*Mepha, Hong Kong†; Mepha, Malaysia.*
Atenolol (p.865·2).
*Angina pectoris; arrhythmias; hypertension; myocardial infarction.*

**Corotrend**
*BASF, Ger.†; Rhein, Mex.; Medika, Switz.*
Nifedipine (p.966·2).
*Hypertension; ischaemic heart disease; Raynaud's syndrome.*

**Corotrop**
*Sanofi Synthelabo, Austria; Sanofi Synthelabo, Ger.; Sanofi Synthelabo, Switz.*
Milrinone (p.959·2).
*Heart failure.*

*Sanofi Synthelabo, Swed.*
Milrinone lactate (p.959·2).
*Heart failure.*

**Corotrope**
*Sanofi Synthelabo, Arg.; Sanofi Synthelabo, Belg.; Sanofi Synthelabo, Gr.; Sanofi Synthelabo, Spain.*
Milrinone (p.959·2).
*Heart failure.*

*Sanofi Synthelabo, Fr.; Sanofi Synthelabo, Neth.*
Milrinone lactate (p.959·2).
*Heart failure.*

**Coroval** *Labinca, Arg.*
Amlodipine besilate (p.862·1).
*Hypertension.*

**Coroval B** *Labinca, Arg.*
Amlodipine besilate (p.862·1); benazepril hydrochloride (p.867·2).
*Hypertension.*

**Coroverlan** *Verla, Ger.†.*
Magnesium aspartate (p.1227·3); potassium aspartate (p.1233·1); etofylline (p.785·1); crataegus (p.1677·1).
*Cardiac disorders.*

**Corovliss** *Boehringer Mannheim, Ger.†.*
Isosorbide dinitrate (p.941·1).
*Cardiac disorders.*

**Corozell** *Fresenius Kabi, Austria.*
Potassium chloride (p.1232·2); magnesium aspartate (p.1227·3).
*Potassium and magnesium deficiency.*

**Corpamil** *Helvepharm, Switz.*
Verapamil hydrochloride (p.1019·1).
*Angina; arrhythmias; hypertension.*

**Corpea** *Normon, Spain.*
Molsidomine (p.961·3).
*Angina pectoris.*

**Corpendol** *Sanofi Synthelabo, Port.*
Propranolol hydrochloride (p.989·3).
*Angina pectoris; arrhythmias; essential tremor; gastrointestinal haemorrhage; hypertension; migraine; myocardial infarction; obstructive cardiomyopathy; thyrotoxicosis.*

**Corplus** *Bago, Arg.*
Lysine aspirin (p.54·3).
*Thromboembolism prophylaxis.*

**Corpotasin CL** *Armstrong, Mex.*
Potassium bicarbonate (p.1223·1); potassium chloride (p.1232·2); lysine hydrochloride (p.1439·2).
*Digitalis intoxication; potassium and chloride supplement.*

**Corpril** *Ranbaxy, Thai.*
Ramipril (p.994·1).
*Congestive heart failure; hypertension; myocardial infarction.*

**Corprilor**
*Rubio, Singapore; Rubio, Spain.*
Enalapril maleate (p.909·2).
*Heart failure; hypertension.*

**Corque** *Geneva, USA.*
Hydrocortisone (p.1103·3); clioquinol (p.196·3).
*Skin disorders.*

**Correctol**
*Note. This name is used for preparations of different composition.*
*Schering-Plough, Canad.; Schering-Plough, Hong Kong†; Schering-Plough, USA.*
Bisacodyl (p.1251·3).
Formerly contained docusate sodium and phenolphthalein in the *USA*.
*Constipation.*

*Alcon, Fr.*
Disodium inosinate (p.1681·3).
*Visual disturbances.*

*Schering-Plough, Mex.*
Docusate sodium (p.1262·2).
*Constipation.*

*Alcon, Port.†.*
Inosine monophosphate.

**Correctol Stool Softener** *Schering-Plough, Canad.*
Docusate sodium (p.1262·2).
Formerly contained docusate sodium and phenolphthalein.
*Constipation.*

**Corrigast** *Continental, Spain†.*
Misoprostol (p.1519·2).
*Peptic ulcer.*

**Corsalbene** *Ratiopharm, Austria†.*
Aspirin (p.15·1).
*Migraine; myocardial infarction; thrombosis prophylaxis.*

**Cor-Select** *Dreluso, Ger.*
*Ointment:* Crataegus (p.1677·1); valerian (p.1762·2); camphor (p.1665·3); ol. sinapis (p.1718·2); benzyl nicotinate (p.21·2); peppermint oil (p.1283·2); melissa oil (p.1711·2).
*Cardiovascular disorders.*
*Oral drops:* Homoeopathic preparation.

**Corsifar** *Siphar, Switz.*
Molsidomine (p.961·3).
*Ischaemic heart disease.*

**Corsodyl**
*GlaxoSmithKline Consumer, Belg.; GlaxoSmithKline, Fin.; GlaxoSmithKline Sante, Fr.; GlaxoSmithKline Consumer, Ger.†; GlaxoSmithKline, Hong Kong; GlaxoSmithKline, Irl.; SmithKline Beecham, Israel; GlaxoSmithKline, Ital.; SmithKline Beecham Consumer, Neth.; GlaxoSmithKline, Norw.; Sterling, Port.†; GlaxoSmithKline Consumer, Swed.; SmithKline Beecham Consumer, Switz.; GlaxoSmithKline Consumer, UK.*
Chlorhexidine gluconate (p.1173·2).
*Mouth infections; oral hygiene.*

**CorSotalol** *Merck dura, Ger.*
Sotalol hydrochloride (p.1001·3).
*Arrhythmias.*

**Corsym** *Novartis Consumer, Canad.†.*
Phenylpropanolamine polistirex (p.1128·2); chlorphenamine polistirex (p.428·1).
*Nasal congestion.*

**Cortacet** *Whitehall-Robins, Canad.*
Hydrocortisone acetate (p.1103·3).
*Skin disorders.*

**Cortafrin** *Streger, Mex.*
Paracetamol (p.76·2); chlorphenamine maleate (p.427·3); phenylephrine hydrochloride (p.1126·3).
*Fever; nasal congestion; pain.*

**Cortafriol C** *Sanofi Synthelabo, Spain.*
Paracetamol (p.76·2); pseudoephedrine sulfate (p.1129·2); ascorbic acid (p.1460·2).
*Fever; influenza and cold symptoms; pain.*

**Cortafriol Complex** *Sanofi Synthelabo, Spain.*
Paracetamol (p.76·2); pseudoephedrine sulfate (p.1129·2); chlorphenamine maleate (p.427·3).
*Fever; nasal congestion; pain.*

**Cor-Tagrip**
*Note. A similar name is used for preparations of different composition (see below).*
*Benitol, Arg.*
Paracetamol (p.76·2); pseudoephedrine (p.1129·2); astemizole (p.424·2); bromhexine (p.1115·3).
*Influenza symptoms.*

**Cortagrip**
*Note. A similar name is used for preparations of different composition (see above).*
*UCI, Braz.†.*
Dipyrone (p.35·3); sodium camsilate; guaifenesin (p.1122·1); cineole (p.1672·1); niaouli oil (p.1719·3); vitamin C (p.1460·2).
*Cold and influenza symptoms.*

**Cortagrip D** *UCI, Braz.†.*
Dipyrone (p.35·3); chlorphenamine maleate (p.427·3); guaifenesin (p.1122·1); terpin hydrate (p.1131·1); sodium camsilate.
*Cold and influenza symptoms.*

**Cortaid**
*Dermatech, Austral.; Carlo Erba OTC, Ital.; Pharmacia Upjohn, NZ†; Pharmacia Upjohn, USA.*
Hydrocortisone (p.1103·3) or hydrocortisone acetate (p.1103·3).
*Skin disorders.*

**Cortaid with Aloe** *Pharmacia, Singapore.*
Hydrocortisone acetate (p.1103·3); aloe vera (p.1141·3).
*Skin disorders.*

**Cortal** *Organon, Swed.†.*
Cortisone acetate (p.1096·1).
*Corticosteroid.*

**Cortal for Adults** *GlaxoSmithKline, Hong Kong.*
Aspirin (p.15·1); caffeine (p.782·1).
*Fever; pain.*

**Cortal for Children** *GlaxoSmithKline, Hong Kong.*
Paracetamol (p.76·2).
*Fever; pain.*

**Cortalen C** *Ativus, Braz.*
Clobetasol propionate (p.1095·2).
*Skin disorders.*

**Cortaler Novo** *Phoenix, Arg.*
Dexamethasone (p.1097·1); terfenadine (p.441·1).
*Hypersensitivity reactions.*

**Cortamed** *Sabex, Canad.†.*
Hydrocortisone acetate (p.1103·3).
*Eye disorders.*

**Cortamide** *Ottolenghi, Ital.*
Fluocinolone acetonide (p.1101·2).
*Skin disorders.*

**Cortancyl** *Aventis, Fr.*
Prednisone (p.1109·3).
*Corticosteroid.*

**Cortane-B** *Blansett, USA.*
Chloroxylenol (p.1177·2); pramocaine hydrochloride (p.1382·2); hydrocortisone (p.1103·3).

**Cortanest** *Piam, Ital.†.*
Hydrocortamate hydrochloride (p.1103·3); lidocaine hydrochloride (p.1377·3).
*Burns; skin disorders; wounds.*

**Cortanest Plus** *Piam, Ital.*
Fluocinolone acetonide (p.1101·2); lidocaine hydrochloride (p.1377·3).
*Anogenital disorders; burns; skin disorders.*

**Cortapaisyl** *Merck Medication Familiale, Fr.*
Hydrocortisone (p.1103·3).
*Skin disorders.*

**Cortasm** *Zambon, Braz.†.*
Budesonide (p.1094·2).
*Corticosteroid.*

**Cortate**
*Note. This name is used for preparations of different composition.*
*Aspen, Austral.*
Cortisone acetate (p.1096·1).
*Oral corticosteroid.*

*Schering, Canad.; Schering-Plough, Canad.*
Hydrocortisone (p.1103·3).
*Skin disorders.*

**Cortatrigen** *Goldline, USA.*
Hydrocortisone (p.1103·3); neomycin sulfate (p.235·1); polymyxin B (p.245·2).
*Bacterial ear infections.*

**Cortax** *Ativus, Braz.*
Deflazacort (p.1096·2).
*Corticosteroid.*

**Cort-Dome** *Miles, USA.*
Hydrocortisone (p.1103·3) or hydrocortisone acetate (p.1103·3).
*Anorectal disorders; skin disorders.*

**Cortef**
*Dermatech, Austral.*
Hydrocortisone acetate (p.1103·3).
*Skin disorders.*

*Pharmacia, Canad.; McNeil Consumer, Canad.*
Hydrocortisone (p.1103·3).
*Corticosteroid.*

*Upjohn, USA.*
Hydrocortisone (p.1103·3) or hydrocortisone cipionate (p.1104·1).
*Corticosteroid.*

**Cortef Feminine Itch** *Upjohn, USA.*
Hydrocortisone acetate (p.1103·3).
*Pruritus.*

**Cortegripan** *Heralds, Braz.†.*
Dipyrone (p.35·3); guaifenesin (p.1122·1); sodium camsilate; ascorbic acid (p.1460·2); lidocaine (p.1377·3).
*Cold and influenza symptoms.*

**Cortenem** *Pharmacia, Arg.*
Hydrocortisone (p.1103·3).
*Inflammatory bowel disease.*

**Cortenema**
*Note. This name is used for preparations of different composition.*
*Axcan, Canad.; Solvay, USA.*
Hydrocortisone (p.1103·3).
*Inflammatory bowel disease.*

*Casen Fleet, Spain.*
Allantoin (p.1141·3); hydrocortisone hydrogen succinate (p.1104·1); homatropine methylbromide (p.483·2); zinc oxide (p.1163·2).
*Anorectal disorders.*

**Corteroid** *Montpellier, Arg.*
Betamethasone (p.1093·1), betamethasone sodium phosphate (p.1093·1), or betamethasone valerate (p.1093·2).
*Corticosteroid.*

**Corteroid Gesic** *Montpellier, Arg.*
Betamethasone (p.1093·1) or betamethasone sodium phosphate (p.1093·1); diclofenac sodium (p.32·1); cyanocobalamin (p.1458·2) or hydroxocobalamin (p.1458·2).
*Gout; musculoskeletal, joint, and peri-articular disorders; neuritis.*

**Corteroid Retard** *Montpellier, Arg.*
Betamethasone sodium phosphate (p.1093·1); betamethasone acetate (p.1093·1).
*Corticosteroid.*

**Corti Biciron N** *S & K, Ger.*
Dexamethasone isonicotinate (p.1097·2); oxytetracycline hydrochloride (p.241·1).
*Infected eye disorders.*

**Corti Jaikal** *S & K, Ger.*
Hydrocortisone acetate (p.1103·3); sodium thiosulfate (p.1053·3); salicylic acid (p.1157·1).
*Acne.*

**Corti-Arscolloid** *SIT, Ital.*
Dichlorobenzyl alcohol (p.1178·3); silver protein (p.1746·2); dexamethasone sodium phosphate (p.1097·2).
*Stomatitis.*

**Cortibiotique** *Chauvin, Fr.†.*
Hydrocortisone acetate (p.1103·3); framycetin sulfate (p.215·1).
*Infected skin disorders.*

**Cortic**
*Note. This name is used for preparations of different composition.*
*Sigma, Austral.*
Hydrocortisone acetate (p.1103·3).
*Anogenital pruritus; skin disorders.*
*Everett, USA.*
Hydrocortisone (p.1103·3); pramocaine hydrochloride (p.1382·2); chloroxylenol (p.1177·2).
*Inflammatory ear disorders.*

**Corticaine** *Glaxo, USA.*
*Rectal cream:* Hydrocortisone acetate (p.1103·3); cinchocaine (p.1373·2).
*Anorectal disorders.*
*UCB, USA.*
*Cream:* Hydrocortisone acetate (p.1103·3).
*Skin disorders.*

**Cortical** *Caber, Ital.*
Diflucortolone valerate (p.1099·3).
*Skin disorders.*

**Corticel** *Serono, Arg.*
Methylprednisolone sodium succinate (p.1106·2).
*Corticosteroid.*

**Corticetine**
*Chauvin, Fr.; Bausch & Lomb, Switz.*
Framycetin sulfate (p.215·1); dexamethasone sodium phosphate (p.1097·2).
*Otitis.*

**Corticil T** *Edol, Port.*
Oxytetracycline hydrochloride (p.241·1); hydrocortisone (p.1103·3).
*Infected skin disorders.*

**Corticin** *Medipharma, Hong Kong.*
Hydrocortisone (p.1103·3); neomycin sulfate (p.235·1).
*Infected skin disorders.*

**Corti-Clyss** *Braun, Switz.*
Prednisolone metasulfobenzoate sodium (p.1108·1).
*Crohn's disease; ulcerative colitis.*

**Corticoderm**
*Hermal, Denm.†; Hermal, Norw.†; Meda, Swed.*
Fluprednidene acetate (p.1102·2).
*Skin disorders.*

**Corticorten** *Neo Quimica, Braz.*
Prednisone (p.1109·3).
*Corticosteroid.*

**Corticotulle Lumiere**
*Solvay, Fr.; Hefa, Ger.*
Neomycin sulfate (p.235·1); polymyxin B sulfate (p.245·1); triamcinolone acetonide (p.1110·2).
*Burns; wounds.*

**Corticreme**
*Rougier, Canad.†; Rougier, Hong Kong†.*
Hydrocortisone acetate (p.1103·3).
*Skin disorders.*

**Cortidax** *Raza, Malaysia; Pharmaniaga, Malaysia.*
Dexamethasone (p.1097·1).
*Corticosteroid.*

**Cortidene** *Berna, Spain.*
Paramethasone acetate (p.1107·3).
*Corticosteroid.*

**Cortiderma** *Mertens, Arg.*
Betamethasone valerate (p.1093·2).
*Skin disorders.*

**Cortidex** *Rayere, Mex.*
Dexamethasone (p.1097·1).
*Corticosteroid.*

**Cortidexason** *Dermapharm, Ger.*
Dexamethasone (p.1097·1).
*Skin and scalp disorders.*

**Cortidexason comp** *Dermapharm, Ger.*
Dexamethasone (p.1097·1); neomycin sulfate (p.235·1).
*Infected skin disorders.*

**Cortidro** *Sofar, Ital.*
Hydrocortisone acetate (p.1103·3).
*Bites and stings; burns; eczema; pruritus.*

**Corti-Dynexan** *Kreussler, Ger.*
Prednisolone acetate (p.1108·1); lauromacrogol 400 (p.1412·3); dequalinium chloride (p.1178·1).
*Inflammatory disorders of the mouth.*

**Cortiespec** *Centrum, Spain.*
Fluocinolone acetonide (p.1101·2).
*Skin disorders.*

**Cortifenol H** *Novartis, Chile.*
Chloramphenicol (p.185·1); hydrocortisone acetate (p.1103·3).
*Bacterial eye infections with inflammation.*

**Corti-Flexiole** *Mann, Ger.†.*
Hydrocortisone (p.1103·3); chloramphenicol (p.185·1); vitamin A palmitate (p.1453·1).
*Infected skin disorders.*

**Cortifluid N** *Streuli, Switz.*
Calcium pantothenate (p.1442·3); hydrocortisone acetate (p.1103·3); neomycin sulfate (p.235·1).
*Infected skin disorders.*

**Corti-Fluoral** *Schering, Ital.*
Josamycin propionate (p.224·3); diflucortolone valerate (p.1099·3).
*Mouth disorders.*

**Cortifoam**
*Reed & Carnrick, Canad.; Medis, Israel; Schwarz, USA.*
Hydrocortisone acetate (p.1103·3).
*Colitis; ulcerative proctitis.*

**Cortiglanden** *Disperga, Austria†.*
Suprarenal cortex (p.1110·1).
*Adrenocortical insufficiency; congenital adrenal hyperplasia.*

**Cortigrin**
*Note. This name is used for preparations of different composition.*
*Collins, Mex.*
Tetracycline (p.266·2).
*Bacterial infections.*
*Collins, Mex.*
Chlorphenamine (p.428·1); aspirin (p.15·1); moroxydine hydrochloride (p.649·3).
*Cold and influenza symptoms.*

**Cortigrip** *Medipharm, Chile.*
Paracetamol (p.76·2); pseudoephedrine (p.1129·2).
*Cold and influenza symptoms.*

**Cortigrip Dia/Noche** *Medipharm, Chile.*
Day tablets, pseudoephedrine hydrochloride (p.1129·2); paracetamol (p.76·2); night tablets, pseudoephedrine hydrochloride; paracetamol; chlorphenamine maleate (p.427·3).
*Cold and influenza symptoms.*

**Cortigripe** *Zimaia, Port.*
Aspirin (p.15·1); hydrocortisone (p.1103·3).

**Cortilate** *Micro, India.*
Halcinonide (p.1103·2).
*Skin disorders.*

**Cortilona** *Offenbach, Mex.*
Fluocinolone acetonide (p.1101·2).
*Skin disorders.*

**Cortilona Compuesta** *Offenbach, Mex.*
Fluocinolone acetonide (p.1101·2); clioquinol (p.196·3).
*Skin disorders.*

**Cortiment** *Hoechst Marion Roussel, Canad.†.*
Hydrocortisone acetate (p.1103·3).
*Anorectal inflammatory disorders.*

**Cortimycin** *Medical Ophthalmics, USA.*
*Eye drops:* Hydrocortisone (p.1103·3); neomycin (p.235·1); polymyxin B (p.245·2).
*Eye ointment:* Hydrocortisone (p.1103·3); neomycin (p.235·1); bacitracin (p.161·3); polymyxin B (p.245·2).
*Infected eye disorders.*

**Cortimycine** *Drossapharm, Switz.*
*Cream:* Hydrocortisone acetate (p.1103·3); neomycin sulfate (p.235·1); dexpanthenol (p.1727·2).
*Infected skin disorders.*
*Ear drops; nose drops; eye drops; eye ointment; ointment:* Hydrocortisone acetate (p.1103·3); neomycin sulfate (p.235·1).
*Infected inflammatory disorders.*

**Cortimyk** *CCS, Swed.*
Miconazole nitrate (p.405·3); hydrocortisone (p.1103·3).
*Fungal skin infections with inflammation.*

**Cortimyxin** *Sabex, Canad.*
Hydrocortisone (p.1103·3); neomycin sulfate (p.235·1); polymyxin B sulfate (p.245·1).
*Ear disorders.*

**Cort-Inal** *Teofarma, Ital.*
Hydrocortisone acetate (p.1103·3); diprophylline (p.784·3).
*Bronchial catarrh.*

**Cortine Naturelle** *Roche Nicholas, Fr.†.*
Suprarenal cortex (porcine) (p.1110·1).
*Asthenia.*

**Cortinorex** *Spyfarma, Spain†.*
Cyanocobalamin; suprarenal cortex; glutathione; liver extract; inosine (p.1417·1).
*Tonic.*

**Cortiphenol H** *Novartis Ophthalmics, Hong Kong.*
Chloramphenicol (p.185·1); hydrocortisone acetate (p.1103·3).
*Infected eye disorders.*

**Cortiprex** *Laboratorios Chile, Chile.*
Prednisone (p.1109·3).
*Corticosteroid.*

**Cortipyren B** *Gador, Arg.*
Meprednisone (p.1106·1).
*Corticosteroid.*

**Cortirel**
*Note. A similar name is used for preparations of different composition (see below).*
*Curatis, Ger.*
Corticorelin triflutate (p.1321·3).
*Diagnosis of corticotrophic pituitary function.*

**Cortirell**
*Note. A similar name is used for preparations of different composition (see above).*
*Sanorell, Ger.*
Homoeopathic preparation.

**Cortiron**
*Schering, Austria†.; Schering, Ital.*
Desoxycortone acetate (p.1097·1) or desoxycortone enantate (p.1097·1).
*Adrenocortical insufficiency.*

**Cortisal** *Dexo, Fr.*
Dipropylene glycol mono- and disalicylate (p.44·3); prednisolone (p.1108·1).
*Peri-articular and soft-tissue disorders.*

**Cortisdin Urea** *Isdin, Spain.*
Fluorometholone (p.1102·2); urea (p.1162·2).
*Skin disorders.*

**Cortisolona** *Klonal, Arg.*
Methylprednisolone (p.1106·1).
*Corticosteroid.*

**Cortison Chemicet Topica** *Teofarma, Spain.*
Chloramphenicol (p.185·1); hydrocortisone acetate (p.1103·3).
*Infected skin disorders.*

**Cortison Chemicetina** *Fournier, Ital.*
Chloramphenicol (p.185·1); hydrocortisone acetate (p.1103·3).
*Infected eye or skin disorders.*

**Cortison Kemicetin** *Pharmacia, Austria.*
Chloramphenicol (p.185·1); hydrocortisone acetate (p.1103·3).
*Bacterial eye infections; inflammation.*

**Cortison Kemicetine**
*Note. This name is used for preparations of different composition.*
*Pharmacia Upjohn, Hong Kong†.*
*Eye/ear drops:* Chloramphenicol (p.185·1); hydrocortisone caprylate (p.1104·2).
*Infected eye and ear disorders.*
*Ointment:* Chloramphenicol (p.185·1); hydrocortisone acetate (p.1103·3).
*Infected eye disorders; infected skin disorders; periodontitis.*
*Rectal ointment:* Chloramphenicol (p.185·1); prednisolone (p.1108·1); phenylephrine hydrochloride (p.1126·3); lidocaine hydrochloride (p.1377·3); tannic acid (p.1751·2); peru balsam (p.1730·2).
*Anorectal disorders.*
*Mac, India.*
Hydrocortisone acetate (p.1103·3); chloramphenicol (p.185·1).
*Allergic and infected skin disorders.*

**Cortisonal** *Uniao Quimica, Braz.*
Hydrocortisone sodium succinate (p.1104·1).
*Corticosteroid.*

**Cortispec** *Euroderm, Arg.*
Betamethasone dipropionate (p.1093·1); clotrimazole (p.396·2).
*Infected skin disorders.*

**Cortisporin**
*Note. This name is used for preparations of different composition.*
*GlaxoSmithKline, Canad.; Monarch, USA.*
*Eye drops; ear drops:* Polymyxin B sulfate (p.245·1); neomycin sulfate (p.235·1); hydrocortisone (p.1103·3).
*Bacterial infections with inflammation.*
*GlaxoSmithKline, Canad.; Monarch, USA.*
*Ointment; eye ointment:* Polymyxin B sulfate (p.245·1); bacitracin zinc (p.161·3); neomycin sulfate (p.235·1); hydrocortisone (p.1103·3).
*Infected skin and eye disorders.*
*Glaxo Wellcome, Mex.*
Polymyxin B sulfate (p.245·1); neomycin sulfate (p.235·1); hydrocortisone (p.1103·3).
*Otitis externa.*
*Monarch, USA.*
*Cream:* Polymyxin B sulfate (p.245·1); neomycin sulfate (p.235·1); hydrocortisone acetate (p.1103·3).
*Infected skin disorders.*

**Cortisporin-TC** *Monarch, USA.*
Colistin sulfate (p.198·3); neomycin sulfate (p.235·1); hydrocortisone acetate (p.1103·3); tonzonium bromide (p.1757·2).
*Infected ear disorders.*

**Cortistamin L** *Bago, Arg.*
Betamethasone (p.1093·1); loratadine (p.436·1).
*Hypersensitivity reactions.*

**Cortistamin NF** *Bago, Arg.*
Betamethasone (p.1093·1); terfenadine (p.441·1).
*Hypersensitivity reactions.*

**Cortisteron** *Streuli, Switz.*
Desoxycortone acetate (p.1097·1).
Lidocaine hydrochloride (p.1377·3) is included in some injections to alleviate the pain of injection.
*Adrenocortical insufficiency.*

**Cortiston** *Ariston, Braz.*
Hydrocortisone (p.1103·3).
*Corticosteroid.*

**Cortisumman** *Winzer, Ger.*
Dexamethasone (p.1097·1).
*Eye disorders.*

**Cortisyl** *Aventis, UK.*
Cortisone acetate (p.1096·1).
*Corticosteroid.*

**Cortival** *Fawns & McAllan, Austral.*
Betamethasone valerate (p.1093·2).
*Skin disorders.*

**Cortivent** *Leiras, Fin.*
Budesonide (p.1094·2).
*Asthma.*

**Cortizone**
*Pfizer, Israel; Pfizer, USA.*
Hydrocortisone (p.1103·3).
*Skin disorders.*

**Cortizul** *Lersan, Arg.*
*Eye drops:* Prednisolone (p.1108·1); phenylephrine hydrochloride (p.1126·3).
*Eye ointment:* Prednisolone (p.1108·1).
*Inflammatory eye disorders.*

**Cortobion** *Laborsil, Braz.†.*
Desoxycortone (p.1097·1); ascorbic acid (p.1460·2).
*Corticosteroid.*

**Cortoderm**
*Note. This name is used for preparations of different composition.*
*Taro, Canad.*
Hydrocortisone (p.1103·3).
*Skin disorders.*
*Aspen, S.Afr.*
Fluocinolone acetonide (p.1101·2).
*Skin disorders.*

**Cortoftal**
*Alcon Cusi, Malaysia; Alcon Cusi, Spain.*
Clobetasone butyrate (p.1095·3).
*Inflammatory eye disorders.*

**Cortogen** *Schering-Plough, S.Afr.*
Cortisone acetate (p.1096·1).
*Corticosteroid.*

**Cortola-m** *East India Pharma, India.*
Sulfacetamide sodium (p.257·3); hydrocortisone acetate (p.1103·3).
*Infected eye disorders.*

**Cortone**
*Merck Sharp & Dohme, Austria†; Merck Frosst, Canad.; Ist. Chim. Inter., Ital.; Merck Sharp & Dohme, Norw.†; Merck Sharp & Dohme, Swed.†; Merck, USA.*
Cortisone acetate (p.1096·1).
*Corticosteroid.*

**Cortop** *Biologici Italia, Ital.*
Hydrocortisone sodium succinate (p.1104·1).
*Corticosteroid.*

**Cortopic** *Laboratorios Chile, Chile.*
Clobetasol propionate (p.1095·2).
*Skin disorders.*

**Cortopin**
*Pinewood, Irl.; Lexon, UK.*
Hydrocortisone (p.1103·3).
*Skin disorders.*

**Cortoquinol** *East India Pharma, India.*
Clioquinol (p.196·3); hydrocortisone (p.1103·3).
*Fungal skin infections.*

**Cortos** *Raffo, Arg.*
Ambroxol (p.1114·3).
*Respiratory-tract congestion.*

**Corto-Tavegil** *Novartis Consumer, Ger.*
*Tablets:* Clemastine fumarate (p.429·1); dexamethasone (p.1097·1).
*Hypersensitivity reactions.*
*Topical gel:* Clemastine fumarate (p.429·1); clocortolone pivalate (p.1096·1).
*Insect stings; skin disorders; sunburn.*

**Cortril**
*Pfizer, Belg.; Pfizer, Fin.†.*
Hydrocortisone (p.1103·3) or hydrocortisone acetate (p.1103·3).
*Eye disorders; skin disorders.*

**Cortropin** *Pinewood, UK.*
Hydrocortisone (p.1103·3).
*Skin disorders.*

**Cortrosina** *Akzo, Braz.†.*
Tetracosactide (p.1340·2).
*Diagnosis of adrenocortical insufficiency.*

**Cortrosyn**
*Organon, Canad.; Organon (Οργανον), Gr.; Organon, Israel; Organon, Ital.; Amphastar, USA.*
Tetracosactide (p.1340·2).
*Adrenocorticotrophic hormone; diagnosis of adrenocortical insufficiency; infantile spasm; multiple sclerosis.*
*Organon, Hong Kong.*
Tetracosactide hexa-acetate (p.1340·3).
*Adrenocorticotrophic hormone.*

**Cortuss** *Pharmaland, Thai.*
Dextromethorphan hydrobromide (p.1117·3).
*Coughs.*

**Coruno** *Therabel, Belg.*
Molsidomine (p.961·3).
*Angina pectoris; heart failure.*

**Corus** *Biosintetica, Braz.*
Losartan potassium (p.947·2).
*Hypertension.*

**Corus H** *Biosintetica, Braz.*
Losartan potassium (p.947·2); hydrochlorothiazide (p.933·2).
*Hypertension.*

**Coruzol** *Schlatter, Switz.*
Acetic acid (p.1645·2); lactic acid (p.1704·1); salicylic acid (p.1157·1).
*Hard skin.*

**Corvasal** *Aventis, Fr.*
*Injection:* Linsidomine hydrochloride (p.946·3).
*Angina pectoris; cardiac investigations; coronary arterial spasm.*
*Tablets:* Molsidomine (p.961·3).
*Angina pectoris.*

**Corvatard** *Therabel, Belg.*
Molsidomine (p.961·3).
*Angina pectoris; heart failure.*

**Corvaton**
*Therabel, Belg.; Hoechst Marion Roussel, Ger.; Aventis, Switz.*
Molsidomine (p.961·3).
*Angina pectoris; heart failure; myocardial infarction; pulmonary hypertension.*

**Cor-Vel** *Truw, Ger.*
Camphor (p.1665·3); menthol (p.1711·3); Norway spruce oil; rosemary oil (p.1740·2).
*Cardiac disorders.*

**Cor-Vel N** *Truw, Ger.†.*
*Oral drops:* Convallaria (p.1675·3); squill (p.1130·3).
*Tablets:* Convallaria (p.1675·3); crataegus (p.1677·1).
*Heart failure.*

**Corvert**
*Pharmacia, Austria; Pharmacia, Braz.†; Pharmacia, Fin.; Pharmacia, Fr.; Gerolimatos (Γερολυματος), Gr.; Pharmacia Upjohn, Ital.; Pharmacia, Neth.; Pharmacia, Norw.; Pharmacia, Swed.; Pharmacia, Switz.; Pharmacia Upjohn, USA.*
Ibutilide fumarate (p.938·1).
*Arrhythmias.*

**Corvipas** *Pascoe, Ger.†.*
Homoeopathic preparation.

**Corvo** *TAD, Ger.*
Enalapril maleate (p.909·2).
*Heart failure; hypertension.*

**Corwin**
*Zeneca, Belg.†; AstraZeneca, UK†.*
Xamoterol fumarate (p.1029·1).
*Heart failure.*

**Coryaid** *Pfizer, Hong Kong†.*
Salicylamide (p.87·3); caffeine (p.782·1); vitamin C (p.1460·2); chlorphenamine maleate (p.427·3); phenylpropanolamine hydrochloride (p.1127·3).
*Cold symptoms.*

**Coryfin C** *SIT, Ital.*
Menglytate (p.1124·2); ascorbic acid (p.1460·2).
*Coughs; hoarseness.*

**Corymunun** *Fund a Paiva, Braz.†.*
*Corynebacterium parvum* (p.540·2).
*Immunostimulant.*

**Coryphen** *Rougier, Canad.†.*
Aspirin (p.15·1).

**Coryx** *Mirren, S.Afr.*
*Effervescent tablets:* Chlorphenamine maleate (p.427·3); pseudoephedrine hydrochloride (p.1129·2); aspirin (p.15·1); ascorbic acid (p.1460·2).
*Syrup:* Triprolidine hydrochloride (p.442·3); pseudoephedrine hydrochloride (p.1129·2); vitamin C (p.1460·2).
*Cold and influenza symptoms.*

**Coryzalia**
*Boiron, Canad.; Boiron, Fr.; Boiron, Port.*
Homoeopathic preparation.

**Corzide**
*Squibb, Canad.†; Monarch, USA.*
Nadolol (p.963·1); bendroflumethiazide (p.867·3).
*Hypertension.*

**Cosaar**
*Merck Sharp & Dohme, Austria; Merck Sharp & Dohme, Switz.*
Losartan potassium (p.947·2).
*Heart failure; hypertension.*

**Cosaar Plus**
*Merck Sharp & Dohme, Austria; Merck Sharp & Dohme, Switz.*
Losartan potassium (p.947·2); hydrochlorothiazide (p.933·2).
*Hypertension.*

**Cosaldon**
*Note. This name is used for preparations of different composition.*
*Hoechst Marion Roussel, Austria†; Aventis, S.Afr.*
Pentifylline (p.979·2); nicotinic acid (p.1441·1).
*Cerebral and peripheral vascular disorders; vascular eye disorders.*

*Aventis, Ger.*
Pentifylline (p.979·2).
*Cerebrovascular insufficiency; vascular eye disorders; vestibular disorders.*

**Cosaldon A** *Hoechst Marion Roussel, Ger.†.*
Pentifylline (p.979·2); vitamin A palmitate (p.1453·1).
*Vascular eye disorders; vestibular disorders.*

**Cosalgesic**
*Cox, Hong Kong; Cox, Irl.†; Alpharma, UK.*
Dextropropoxyphene hydrochloride (p.28·3); paracetamol (p.76·2).
These ingredients can be described by the British Approved Name Co-proxamol.
*Pain.*

**Co-Salt** *Pharmacia, Arg.*
Potassium chloride (p.1232·2).
*Salt substitute.*

**Cosamin** *Nutramax, USA.*
Glucosamine hydrochloride; sodium chondroitin sulfate; manganese ascorbate (p.1417·1).
*Nutritional supplement.*

**Cosavil** *Aventis, India.*
Pheniramine maleate (p.438·3); paracetamol (p.76·2).
*Cold symptoms.*

**Coscopin** *Biological E, India.*
Noscapine (p.1125·3); citric acid (p.1673·1); sodium citrate (p.1223·2); ammonium chloride (p.1115·2).
*Coughs.*

**Coscopin BR** *Biological E, India.*
Pseudoephedrine (p.1129·2); bromhexine hydrochloride (p.1115·3); menthol (p.1711·3).
*Coughs.*

**Coscopin Plus** *Biological E, India.*
Noscapine (p.1125·3); citric acid (p.1673·1); sodium citrate (p.1223·2); ammonium chloride (p.1115·2).
*Coughs.*

**Cose-Anal** *Will-Pharma, Belg.*
Sodium oleate (p.1574·3); lauromacrogol 400 (p.1412·3).
*Haemorrhoids.*

**Cosig** *Sigma, Austral.*
Co-trimoxazole (p.199·3).
*Bacterial infections; Pneumocystis carinii pneumonia.*

**Coslan** *Pfizer, Spain.*
Mefenamic acid (p.55·2).
*Fever; inflammation; pain.*

**Coslyte** *CFL, India.*
Potassium chloride; sodium chloride; sodium citrate; glucose (p.1222·2).
*Oral rehydration therapy.*

**Cosmaxil** *Cosmofarma, Port.*
Atropine sulfate (p.477·1); papaverine hydrochloride (p.1728·1); ephedrine hydrochloride (p.1120·1); phenobarbital (p.367·3); theophylline (p.798·3).
*Obstructive airways disease.*

**Cosmegen**
*Sidus, Arg.; Merck Sharp & Dohme, Austral.; Merck Sharp & Dohme, Austria; Prodome, Braz.; Merck Frosst, Canad.; Merck Sharp & Dohme, Fin.; IFET (ΙΦΕΤ), Gr.; Merck Sharp & Dohme, Hong Kong; Merck Sharp & Dohme, Irl.; Merck Sharp & Dohme, Ital.; Merck Sharp & Dohme, Malaysia; Merck Sharp & Dohme, Norw.; Merck Sharp & Dohme, NZ; Merck Sharp & Dohme, S.Afr.†; Merck Sharp & Dohme, Swed.; Merck Sharp & Dohme, Switz.; Merck Sharp & Dohme, Thai.; Merck Sharp & Dohme, UK; Merck, USA.*
Dactinomycin (p.545·1).
*Malignant neoplasms.*

**Cosmetar-S** *Promedica, Fr.†.*
Coal tar (Stantar) (p.1159·2).
*Seborrhoeic dermatitis.*

**Cosmiciclina** *INTES, Ital.*
Oxytetracycline hydrochloride (p.241·1); chloramphenicol (p.185·1); sulfacetamide sodium (p.257·3).
*Bacterial infections of the eye or ear.*

**Cosmofer**
*Gry, Ger.; Demo, Gr.; Nebo, Hong Kong; Schwarz, Hong Kong; Vitaline, UK.*
Iron dextran (p.1436·3).
*Iron-deficiency anaemia.*

**Cosmopril** *Cosmopharm, Gr.*
Selegiline hydrochloride (p.1214·1).
*Parkinsonism.*

**Coso** *McGloin, Austral.†.*
Menthol (p.1711·3); camphor (p.1665·3); benzyl alcohol (p.1170·2).
*Herpes labialis.*

**Cosome** *Merck, India.*
Dextromethorphan hydrobromide (p.1117·3); phenylpropanolamine hydrochloride (p.1127·3); chlorphenamine maleate (p.427·3).
*Cold symptoms; coughs; nasal congestion.*

**Cosopt**
*Merck Sharp & Dohme, Arg.; Merck Sharp & Dohme, Austral.; Merck Sharp & Dohme, Austria; Merck Sharp & Dohme, Belg.; Merck Sharp & Dohme, Braz.; Merck Frosst, Canad.; Merck Sharp & Dohme, Chile; Merck Sharp & Dohme, Denm.; Merck Sharp & Dohme, Fin.; Merck Sharp & Dohme-Chibret, Fr.; Chibret, Ger.; Vianex (Βιανεξ), Gr.; Merck Sharp & Dohme, Hong Kong; Merck Sharp & Dohme, Irl.; Merck Sharp & Dohme, Israel; Merck Sharp & Dohme, Ital.; Merck Sharp & Dohme, Mex.; Merck Sharp & Dohme, Neth.; Merck Sharp & Dohme, Norw.; Merck Sharp & Dohme, NZ; Merck Sharp & Dohme, S.Afr.; Merck Sharp & Dohme, Singapore; Merck Sharp & Dohme, Swed.; Merck Sharp & Dohme, Switz.; Merck Sharp & Dohme, Thai.; Merck Sharp & Dohme, UK; Merck, USA.*
Dorzolamide hydrochloride (p.908·3); timolol maleate (p.1012·2).
*Glaucoma; ocular hypertension.*

**Cospanon**
*Eisai, Hong Kong†; Eisai, Jpn.*
Flopropione (p.1689·1).
*Smooth muscle spasm.*

**Cost** *Fada, Arg.*
Ketamine (p.1303·1).
*General anaesthesia.*

**Costi**
*Medochemie, Hong Kong; Medochemie, Thai.†.*
Domperidone (p.1263·2).
*Digestive disorders; dyspepsia; flatulence; gastro-oesophageal reflux; heartburn; nausea and vomiting.*

**Costop** *Standard, Hong Kong†.*
Cloperastine hydrochloride (p.1117·2).
*Coughs.*

**Cosudex**
*AstraZeneca, Austral.; AstraZeneca, NZ.*
Bicalutamide (p.530·1).
*Prostatic cancer.*

**Cosuric** *DDSA Pharmaceuticals, UK.*
Allopurinol (p.412·2).
*Gout; hyperuricaemia.*

**Cosylan**
*Parke, Davis, Denm.†; Pfizer, Norw.; Parke, Davis, Swed.†.*
Ethylmorphine hydrochloride (p.37·3); cascara (p.1255·1); menthol (p.1711·3).
*Coughs; respiratory-tract irritation.*

**Cosyr** *Great Eastern, Thai.; United American, Thai.*
Dextromethorphan hydrobromide (p.1117·3); chlorphenamine maleate (p.427·3); guaifenesin (p.1122·1).
Formerly contained dextromethorphan hydrobromide, chlorphenamine maleate, phenylpropanolamine hydrochloride, and guaifenesin.
*Coughs.*

**Cosyr (Reformulated)** *United American, Hong Kong.*
Dextromethorphan hydrobromide (p.1117·3); chlorphenamine maleate (p.427·3).
Cosyr formerly contained dextromethorphan hydrobromide, chlorphenamine maleate, phenylpropanolamine, and guaifenesin.
*Coughs.*

**Cotamox** *Asian Pharm, Thai.*
Co-trimoxazole (p.199·3).
*Bacterial infections.*

**Cotareg**
*Biosintetica, Braz.; Novartis, Fr.; Novartis, Ital.*
Valsartan (p.1018·3); hydrochlorothiazide (p.933·2).
*Hypertension.*

**Co-Tareg** *Helsinn, Port.*
Valsartan (p.1018·3); hydrochlorothiazide (p.933·2).
*Hypertension.*

**Cotaryl** *FDC, India.*
Urea (p.1162·2); calcium lactate (p.1225·3); lactic acid (p.1704·1); potassium chloride (p.1232·2); magnesium chloride (p.1228·1); glycine (p.1433·3); monobasic sodium phosphate (p.1230·3); ammonium chloride (p.1115·2); sodium chloride (p.1233·3).
*Hyperkeratosis; ichthyosis.*

**Co-Tasian** *Asian Pharm, Thai.*
Co-trimoxazole (p.199·3).
*Bacterial infections.*

**Cotazym**
*Note. This name is used for preparations of different composition.*
*Organon, Braz.; Thiemann, Ger.*
Pancreatin (p.1725·3).
*Pancreatic enzyme deficiency.*

*Organon, Canad.; Organon, NZ; Organon, USA†.*
Pancrelipase (p.1725·3).
*Pancreatic enzyme deficiency.*

**Cotazym S Forte** *Organon, Austral.*
Pancrelipase (p.1725·3).
*Pancreatic enzyme deficiency.*

**Cotenol** *TP, Thai.*
Paracetamol (p.76·2); codeine phosphate (p.27·1).
*Pain.*

**Cotenolol** *Mepha, Switz.*
Atenolol (p.865·2); chlortalidone (p.882·3).
*Hypertension.*

**Cotenomel** *Clonmel, Irl.†.*
Atenolol (p.865·2); chlortalidone (p.882·3).
*Hypertension.*

**Cotesifar** *Siphar, Switz.*
Atenolol (p.865·2); chlortalidone (p.882·3).
*Hypertension.*

**Cotet** *Rolab, S.Afr.*
Oxytetracycline hydrochloride (p.241·1).
*Bacterial infections; protozoal infections.*

**Cothilyne** *Haemacure, Canad.†.*
Centella (p.1144·3).
*Wounds.*

**Cotibin Compuesto** *Andromaco, Chile.*
*Oral suspension:* Paracetamol (p.76·2); pseudoephedrine hydrochloride (p.1129·2).
*Cold and influenza symptoms.*
*Tablets:* Paracetamol (p.76·2).
*Fever; pain.*

**Cotibin Dia y Noche** *Andromaco, Chile.*
Day tablets, pseudoephedrine hydrochloride (p.1129·2); paracetamol (p.76·2); night tablets, pseudoephedrine hydrochloride; paracetamol; chlorphenamine maleate (p.427·3).
*Cold and influenza symptoms.*

**Cotibin Flu** *Andromaco, Chile.*
Paracetamol (p.76·2); noscapine (p.1125·3); caffeine (p.782·1); ascorbic acid (p.1460·2).
*Cold and influenza symptoms.*

**Cotina** *Instituto Sanitas, Chile.*
Nicotinic acid (p.1441·1).
*Chilblains; hyperlipidaemias; peripheral vascular disorders; venous ulcers.*

**Cotinazin** *Pfizer, Gr.*
Tioconazole (p.409·3).
*Fungal skin and vaginal infections.*

**Co-Tioctan** *Purissimus, Arg.*
Cocarboxylase (p.1455·2); thioctic acid (p.1754·3).
*Liver disorders; metabolic disorders; poisoning.*

**Cotofin** *Loren, Mex.*
Paracetamol (p.76·2); chlorphenamine (p.428·1).
*Hypersensitivity.*

**Cotone Emostatico** *Farmatre, Ital.; Nova Argentia, Ital.*
Ferric chloride (p.1688·1).
*Styptic.*

**Cotrane** *Sanofi Synthelabo, Belg.*
Dimethoxanate hydrochloride (p.1119·1).
*Coughs.*

**Cotrazol** *Valomed, Spain.*
Guaifenesin (p.1122·1); co-trimoxazole (p.199·3).
*Respiratory-tract infections.*

**Cotren**
*Biopharm, Hong Kong; Biolab, Malaysia; Biolab, Singapore; Biolab, Thai.*
Clotrimazole (p.396·2).
*Fungal skin and vaginal infections; trichomoniasis.*

**Cotribene** *Ratiopharm, Austria.*
Co-trimoxazole (p.199·3).
*Bacterial infections; Pneumocystis carinii pneumonia.*

**Cotridin** *Technilab, Canad.*
Triprolidine hydrochloride (p.442·3); pseudoephedrine hydrochloride (p.1129·2); codeine phosphate (p.27·1).
*Coughs.*

**Cotridin Expectorant** *Technilab, Canad.*
Triprolidine hydrochloride (p.442·3); pseudoephedrine hydrochloride (p.1129·2); guaifenesin (p.1122·1); codeine phosphate (p.27·1).
*Coughs.*

**Cotrim**
*Ratiopharm, Fin.; 1A, Ger.; Hefa, Ger.; Heumann, Ger.; CT, Ger.; Ratiopharm, Ger.; Medochemie, Malaysia; Ratiopharm, Port.; Spirig, Switz.; Lemmon, USA.*
Co-trimoxazole (p.199·3).
*Bacterial infections; Pneumocystis carinii pneumonia.*

**Cotrimazol** *Lafon, Fr.†.*
Co-trimoxazole (p.199·3).
*Bacterial infections; Pneumocystis carinii pneumonia; toxoplasmosis.*

**Cotrim-Diolan** *Brahms, Ger.*
Co-trimoxazole (p.199·3).
*Bacterial infections; fungal mycetoma; paracoccidioidomycosis.*

**Co-Trimed** *Medifive, Thai.*
Co-trimoxazole (p.199·3).
*Bacterial infections.*

**Cotrimel** *Clonmel, Irl.†.*
Co-trimoxazole (p.199·3).
*Bacterial infections.*

**Cotrimhexal** *Hexal, Ger.*
Co-trimoxazole (p.199·3).
*Bacterial infections.*

**Cotrimox-Wolff** *Wolff, Ger.*
Co-trimoxazole (p.199·3).
*Bacterial infections.*

**Cotrimstada** *Stada, Ger.*
Co-trimoxazole (p.199·3).
*Bacterial infections; Pneumocystis carinii pneumonia.*

**Co-trim-Tablinen** *Sanorania, Ger.†.*
Co-trimoxazole (p.199·3).
*Bacterial infections; fungal mycetoma; paracoccidioidomycosis; Pneumocystis carinii pneumonia.*

**Cotrisan** *Instituto Sanitas, Chile.*
Clotrimazole (p.396·2).
*Fungal skin infections.*

**Cotristad** *Stada, Austria.*
Co-trimoxazole (p.199·3).
*Bacterial infections; Pneumocystis carinii pneumonia.*

**Cotrizol-G** *Klonal, Arg.*
Co-trimoxazole (p.199·3).
*Bacterial infections.*

**Cotron** *Pinewood, Irl.*
Dantron (p.1261·1); poloxamer 188 (p.1414·2).
*Constipation.*

**Co-Tuss V** *Rugby, USA.*
Hydrocodone tartrate (p.45·1); guaifenesin (p.1122·1).
*Coughs.*

**Cotussin** *TP, Thai.*
Diphenhydramine hydrochloride (p.431·3); ammonium chloride (p.1115·2); sodium citrate (p.1223·2).
*Coughs; nasal congestion.*

**Co-Tylenol**
*Note. This name is used for preparations of different composition.*
*Johnson & Johnson, Austria†.*
Paracetamol (p.76·2); carbinoxamine maleate (p.426·3); phenylephrine hydrochloride (p.1126·3).
*Cold symptoms; sinusitis.*

*Cilag, Mex.*
Paracetamol (p.76·2); pseudoephedrine hydrochloride (p.1129·2); chlorphenamine maleate (p.427·3); dextromethorphan hydrobromide (p.1117·3).
*Upper respiratory-tract disorders.*

**Cough & Cold** *Homeocan, Canad.*
Homoeopathic preparation.

**Cough, Cold & Allergy Relief** *Stanley, Canad.†.*
Phenylephrine hydrochloride (p.1126·3); phenylpropanolamine hydrochloride (p.1127·3); brompheniramine maleate (p.426·1); dextromethorphan hydrobromide (p.1117·3).

**Cough & Cold L52** *Homeocan, Canad.*
Homoeopathic preparation.

**Cough Control Sucrets** *SmithKline Beecham, Israel†.*
Dextromethorphan hydrobromide (p.1117·3).
*Coughs.*

**Cough Drops**
*Note. This name is used for preparations of different composition.*
*Zee, Canad.*
Menthol (p.1711·3).

*Weleda, UK.*
Homoeopathic preparation.

**Cough Elixir** *Weleda, UK.*
Homoeopathic preparation.

**Cough & Flu Syrup** *Technilab, Canad.*
Pseudoephedrine hydrochloride (p.1129·2); dextromethorphan hydrobromide (p.1117·3); guaifenesin (p.1122·1); paracetamol (p.76·2).

**Cough Formula Comtrex** *Bristol-Myers Products, USA.*
Paracetamol (p.76·2); pseudoephedrine hydrochloride (p.1129·2); guaifenesin (p.1122·1); dextromethorphan hydrobromide (p.1117·3).
*Coughs and cold symptoms.*

**Cough L64** *Homeocan, Canad.*
Homoeopathic preparation.

**Cough Lozenges** *Sutton, Canad.*
Menthol (p.1711·3).

**Cough N Cold Syrup** *Golden Pride, Canad.†; Rawleigh, Canad.†.*
Ephedrine hydrochloride (p.1120·1); guaifenesin (p.1122·1); sodium citrate (p.1223·2).

**Cough Relief** *Brauer, Austral.†.*
*Oral liquid:* Anise oil (p.1655·2); althaea (p.1651·3); bryonia (p.1663·1); Iceland moss; echinacea (p.1683·2); chamomile (p.1669·3); thyme (p.1755·2); urtica (p.1762·1); aconitum nap.; coccus cacti; corallium rub.; drosera; ipecacuanha; kali bich.; kreosotum; spongia tosta; sticta pulm.
*Coughs.*
*Oral spray:* Homoeopathic preparation.

**Cough Suppressant Syrup DM** *Drug Trading, Canad.†.*
Dextromethorphan hydrobromide (p.1117·3).

**Cough Syrup**
*Note. This name is used for preparations of different composition.*
*Marc-O, Canad.†.*
Dextromethorphan hydrobromide (p.1117·3).
*Stanley, Canad.†.*
Pseudoephedrine hydrochloride (p.1129·2); codeine phosphate (p.27·1); guaifenesin (p.1122·1).
*Technilab, Canad.*
Diphenhydramine hydrochloride (p.431·3); codeine phosphate (p.27·1); ammonium chloride (p.1115·2).
*Goldline, USA.*
Phenylephrine hydrochloride (p.1126·3); dextromethorphan hydrobromide (p.1117·3); guaifenesin (p.1122·1).
*Coughs.*

**Cough Syrup with Codeine** *Stanley, Canad.*
Diphenhydramine hydrochloride (p.431·3); codeine phosphate (p.27·1); ammonium chloride (p.1115·2).

**Cough Syrup DM** *Stanley, Canad.; WestCan, Canad.*
Dextromethorphan hydrobromide (p.1117·3).

**Cough Syrup DM Decongestant** *WestCan, Canad.*
Dextromethorphan hydrobromide (p.1117·3); pseudoephedrine hydrochloride (p.1129·2).

**Cough Syrup DM Decongestant for Children** *Stanley, Canad.*
Dextromethorphan hydrobromide (p.1117·3); pseudoephedrine hydrochloride (p.1129·2).

**Cough Syrup DM Decongestant Expectorant** *Stanley, Canad.*
Dextromethorphan hydrobromide (p.1117·3); pseudoephedrine hydrochloride (p.1129·2); guaifenesin (p.1122·1).

**Cough Syrup DM Expectorant** *Stanley, Canad.*
Dextromethorphan hydrobromide (p.1117·3); guaifenesin (p.1122·1).

**Cough Syrup DM-D-E** *WestCan, Canad.*
Dextromethorphan hydrobromide (p.1117·3); pseudoephedrine hydrochloride (p.1129·2); guaifenesin (p.1122·1).

**Cough Syrup DM-E** *WestCan, Canad.*
Dextromethorphan hydrobromide (p.1117·3); guaifenesin (p.1122·1).

**Cough Syrup Expectorant** *Stanley, Canad.; WestCan, Canad.*
Guaifenesin (p.1122·1).

**Cough Syrup with Guaifenesin & Dextromethorphan** *Tanta, Canad.*
Dextromethorphan hydrobromide (p.1117·3); guaifenesin (p.1122·1).

**Cough Syrup with Honey** *Hylands, Canad.*
Homoeopathic preparation.

**Coughcod** *Aspen, S.Afr.*
Ephedrine hydrochloride (p.1120·1); ammonium chloride (p.1115·2); sodium citrate (p.1223·2); codeine phosphate (p.27·1); mepyramine maleate (p.437·1).
*Coughs.*

**Cough-eeze** *English Grains, UK†.*
Ipecacuanha (p.1122·3); marrubium (p.1124·1); elecampane (p.1119·3).
*Coughs.*

**Cough-EN**
*Xepa-Soul Pattinson, Hong Kong; Xepa-Soul Pattinson, Malaysia; Xepa-Soul Pattinson, Singapore.*
Dextromethorphan hydrobromide (p.1117·3); pseudoephedrine hydrochloride (p.1129·2); triprolidine hydrochloride (p.442·3).
*Coughs; respiratory-tract congestion.*

**Coughlax** *Malaysia Chemist, Singapore.*
Ammonium chloride (p.1115·2); chlorphenamine maleate (p.427·3); codeine phosphate (p.27·1); ephedrine hydrochloride (p.1120·1).
*Coughs; respiratory-tract congestion; sneezing.*

**Coughmin** *Kyorin, Thai.*
Sodium dibunate (p.1130·2); chlorphenamine maleate (p.427·3); *dl*-methylephedrine hydrochloride (p.1124·2).
*Coughs.*

**Coughnadryl** *Condrugs, Thai.*
Diphenhydramine hydrochloride (p.431·3); ammonium chloride (p.1115·2); sodium citrate (p.1223·2); menthol (p.1711·3).
*Coughs; nasal congestion; sneezing.*

**Cough-X** *Ascher, USA.*
Dextromethorphan hydrobromide (p.1117·3); benzocaine (p.1370·3).
*Coughs.*

**Couldina** *Alter, Spain.*
Aspirin (p.15·1); chlorphenamine maleate (p.427·3); phenylephrine hydrochloride (p.1126·3).
*Bronchospasm; fever; nasal congestion; pain.*

**Couldina C** *Alter, Spain.*
Aspirin (p.15·1); ascorbic acid (p.1460·2); chlorphenamine maleate (p.427·3); phenylephrine (p.1126·3).
*Bronchospasm; fever; nasal congestion; pain.*

**Couldina Instant** *Alter, Spain.*
Aspirin (p.15·1); chlorphenamine maleate (p.427·3); phenylephrine hydrochloride (p.1126·3).
Formerly contained aspirin, chlorphenamine maleate, and ascorbic acid.
*Bronchospasm; fever; nasal congestion; pain.*

**Coumadin**
*Sidus, Arg.; Boots Healthcare, Austral.; Du Pont, Canad.; Aventis, Chile; Bristol-Myers Squibb, Ger.; Taro, Israel; Bristol-Myers Squibb, Ital.; Bristol-Myers Squibb, Malaysia; Boots Healthcare, NZ; Sanofi Omnimed, S.Afr.; Bristol-Myers Squibb, Singapore; Bristol-Myers Squibb, USA.*
Warfarin sodium (p.1022·2).
*Thromboembolic disorders.*

**Coumadine** *Bristol-Myers Squibb, Fr.*
Warfarin sodium (p.1022·2).
*Thromboembolic disorders.*

**Counterpain**
*Bristol-Myers Squibb, Hong Kong; Bristol-Myers Squibb, S.Afr.; Bristol-Myers Squibb, Thai.*
Eugenol (p.1686·2); menthol (p.1711·3); methyl salicylate (p.59·3).
*Muscle and joint pain.*

**Counterpain Cool** *Bristol-Myers Squibb, Thai.*
Menthol (p.1711·3).
*Muscle and joint pain.*

**Co-Vals** *Esteve, Spain.*
Valsartan (p.1018·3); hydrochlorothiazide (p.933·2).
*Hypertension.*

**Covamet** *Covan, S.Afr.*
Cyclizine hydrochloride (p.429·3).
*Nausea; vestibular disorders; vomiting.*

**Covan** *Pharmascience, Canad.*
Codeine phosphate (p.27·1); triprolidine hydrochloride (p.442·3); pseudoephedrine hydrochloride (p.1129·2).
*Upper respiratory-tract symptoms.*

**Covancaine** *Covan, S.Afr.*
Phenazone (p.82·3); urea (p.1162·2); sulfacetamide sodium (p.257·3); benzocaine (p.1370·3).
*Otitis externa; otitis media.*

**Covance** *Stancare, India.*
Losartan potassium (p.947·2).
*Hypertension.*

**Covangesic** *Wallace, USA†.*
Phenylpropanolamine hydrochloride (p.1127·3); phenylephrine hydrochloride (p.1126·3); chlorphenamine maleate (p.427·3); mepyramine maleate (p.437·1); paracetamol (p.76·2).
*Upper respiratory-tract symptoms.*

**Covarex** *MZ, S.Afr.*
Miconazole nitrate (p.405·3).
*Fungal skin infections.*

**Covastin** *Xepa-Soul Pattinson, Malaysia.*
Simvastatin (p.997·1).
*Atherosclerosis; hyperlipidaemias.*

**Covatine** *Bailly, Fr.*
Captodiame hydrochloride (p.674·1).
*Anxiety.*

**Covaxis** *Aventis Pasteur, Ger.*
A diphtheria, tetanus, and pertussis vaccine (p.1613·3).
*Active immunisation.*

**Covera** *Searle, USA.*
Verapamil hydrochloride (p.1019·1).
*Angina pectoris; hypertension.*

**Coverene** *Servier, Arg.*
Perindopril erbumine (p.980·2).
*Heart failure; hypertension.*

**Covermark**
*MDM, Fr.; Epiderm, UK.*
A range of covering creams.
*Concealment of birth marks, scars, and disfiguring skin disease.*

**Coversum**
*Servier, Austria; Servier, Ger.; Servier, Switz.*
Perindopril erbumine (p.980·2).
*Heart failure; hypertension.*

**Coversum Combi**
*Servier, Ger.; Servier, Switz.*
Perindopril erbumine (p.980·2); indapamide (p.938·2).
*Hypertension.*

**Coversyl**
*Servier, Austral.; Servier, Belg.; Servier, Braz.; Servier, Canad.; Servier, Chile; Servier, Denm.; Pharmacal, Fin.; Servier, Fr.; Servier, Gr.; Serdia, India; Servier, Irl.; Servier, Ital.; Daiichi, Jpn; Servier, Malaysia; Sanfer, Mex.; Servier, Neth.; Servier, NZ; Servier, Port.; Servier, S.Afr.; Servier, Singapore; Servier, Spain; Servier, Thai.; Servier, UK.*
Perindopril erbumine (p.980·2).
*Heart failure; hypertension.*

**Coversyl Plus**
*Servier, Austral.; Servier, Neth.; Servier, S.Afr.; Servier, UK.*
Perindopril erbumine (p.980·2); indapamide (p.938·2).
*Hypertension.*

**Co-Vibedoze** *Delta, Port.*
Cobamamide (p.1459·1).
*Vitamin B supplement.*

**Covitasa B12** *Seid, Spain.*
Cyproheptadine hydrochloride (p.430·1); cobamamide (p.1459·1).
*Tonic.*

**Covite** *Covan, S.Afr.†.*
Haematoporphyrin; liver extracts; caffeine; yeast (p.1417·1).
*Tonic.*

**Covochol** *Covan, S.Afr.*
Acetylcholine chloride (p.1487·1).
*Production of miosis in eye surgery.*

**Covocort** *Rolab, S.Afr.*
Hydrocortisone (p.1103·3).
*Corticosteroid.*

**Covomycin** *Covan, S.Afr.*
Chloramphenicol (p.185·1); neomycin sulfate (p.235·1); naphazoline hydrochloride (p.1124·3).
*Eye, ear, and nose infections.*

**Covomycin-D** *Covan, S.Afr.*
Chloramphenicol (p.185·1); neomycin sulfate (p.235·1); dexamethasone sodium phosphate (p.1097·2).
*Inflammatory eye and ear infections.*

**Covonia Bronchial Balsam** *Thornton & Ross, UK.*
Dextromethorphan hydrobromide (p.1117·3); menthol (p.1711·3).
*Coughs.*

**Covonia for Children** *Thornton & Ross, UK†.*
Dextromethorphan hydrobromide (p.1117·3).
*Coughs.*

**Covonia Mentholated** *Thornton & Ross, UK.*
Menthol (p.1711·3); squill tincture (p.1130·3); liquorice (p.1270·2).
*Coughs.*

**Covonia Night-Time** *Thornton & Ross, UK.*
Dextromethorphan hydrobromide (p.1117·3); diphenhydramine hydrochloride (p.431·3).
*Coughs.*

**Covonia Throat Spray** *Thornton & Ross, UK.*
Chlorhexidine gluconate (p.1173·2); lidocaine hydrochloride (p.1377·3).
*Sore throat.*

**Covorit** *Laboratorios Chile, Chile.*
Folinic acid (p.1431·1).
*Adjunct to fluorouracil in colorectal cancer; megaloblastic anaemia; reduction of methotrexate toxicity.*

**Covosan** *Covan, S.Afr.*
Naphazoline hydrochloride (p.1124·3); antazoline phosphate (p.424·2); sulfacetamide sodium (p.257·3).
*Conjunctivitis.*

**Covospor** *Covan, S.Afr.*
Clotrimazole (p.396·2).
*Fungal skin and vulvovaginal infections.*

**Covostet** *Covan, S.Afr.*
Tetracaine hydrochloride (p.1385·1).
*Local anaesthesia.*

**Covosulf** *Covan, S.Afr.*
Sulfacetamide sodium (p.257·3).
*Conjunctivitis.*

**Covotop** *Covan, S.Afr.*
Chloramphenicol (p.185·1); benzocaine (p.1370·3).
*Ear infections.*

**Cow & Gate Formula-S** *Nutricia, Hong Kong.*
Infant feed (p.1417·1).
*Lactose intolerance; milk protein allergy.*

**Cow & Gate Pepti-Junior** *Nutricia, Hong Kong.*
Infant feed (p.1417·1).
*Diarrhoea; food hypersensitivity; malabsorption syndromes; malnutrition; short-bowel syndrome.*

**Coxa-cyl Ho-Len-Complex** *Liebermann, Ger.*
Homoeopathic preparation.

**Coxanturenasi** *Teofarma, Ital.*
Pyridoxine hydrochloride (p.1456·3); pyridoxal phosphate (p.1456·3).
Lidocaine hydrochloride (p.1377·3) is included in the intramuscular injection to alleviate the pain of injection.
*Vitamin $B_6$ and its co-enzyme deficiency.*

**Coxel** *Beta, Arg.*
Celecoxib (p.25·2).
*Osteoarthritis; rheumatoid arthritis.*

**Coxflam** *Cipla-Medpro, S.Afr.*
Meloxicam (p.56·1).
*Musculoskeletal and joint disorders.*

**Coxiro** *Dosa, Arg.*
Rofecoxib (p.86·3).
*Inflammation; pain.*

**Coxtenk** *Biotenk, Arg.*
Celecoxib (p.25·2).
*Osteoarthritis; rheumatoid arthritis.*

**Coxxil**
*Merck Sharp & Dohme, Austria; Gentili, Ital.; Ferraz, Lynce, Port.*
Rofecoxib (p.86·3).
*Osteoarthritis; rheumatoid arthritis.*

**Cozaar**
*Merck Sharp & Dohme, Austral.; Merck Sharp & Dohme, Belg.; Merck Sharp & Dohme, Braz.; Merck Frosst, Canad.; Merck Sharp & Dohme, Chile; Merck Sharp & Dohme, Denm.; Merck Sharp & Dohme, Fin.; Merck Sharp & Dohme-Chibret, Fr.; Vianex (Βιανεξ), Gr.; Merck Sharp & Dohme, Hong Kong; Merck Sharp & Dohme, Irl.; Merck Sharp & Dohme, Malaysia; Merck Sharp & Dohme, Mex.; Merck Sharp & Dohme, Neth.; Merck Sharp & Dohme, Norw.; Merck Sharp & Dohme, NZ; Merck Sharp & Dohme, Port.; Merck Sharp & Dohme, S.Afr.; Merck Sharp & Dohme, Singapore; Merck Sharp & Dohme, Spain; Merck Sharp & Dohme, Swed.; Merck Sharp & Dohme, Thai.; Merck Sharp & Dohme, UK; Merck, USA.*
Losartan potassium (p.947·2).
*Diabetic nephropathy; heart failure; hypertension.*

**Cozaar Comp**
*Merck Sharp & Dohme, Denm.; Merck Sharp & Dohme, Fin.; Merck Sharp & Dohme, Irl.; Merck Sharp & Dohme, Norw.; Merck Sharp & Dohme, S.Afr.; Merck Sharp & Dohme, Swed.; Merck Sharp & Dohme, UK.*
Losartan potassium (p.947·2); hydrochlorothiazide (p.933·2).
*Hypertension.*

**Cozaar Plus**
*Merck Sharp & Dohme, Belg.; Merck Sharp & Dohme, Port.; Merck Sharp & Dohme, Spain.*
Losartan potassium (p.947·2); hydrochlorothiazide (p.933·2).
*Hypertension.*

**Cozaarex** *Merck Sharp & Dohme, Arg.*
Losartan potassium (p.947·2).
*Heart failure; hypertension.*

**Cozaarex D** *Merck Sharp & Dohme, Arg.*
Losartan potassium (p.947·2); hydrochlorothiazide (p.933·2).
*Hypertension.*

**Cozole** *Be-Tabs, S.Afr.*
Co-trimoxazole (p.199·3).
*Bacterial infections.*

**CP Tannic** *Cypress, USA.*
Chlorphenamine tannate (p.428·1); pseudoephedrine tannate (p.1130·1).
*Nasal congestion; rhinitis; sinusitis.*

**CPD** *Elvetium, Arg.*
Cyproterone acetate (p.1544·1).
*Androgen-induced acne, alopecia, hirsutism, and seborrhoea in women; male sexual deviation; precocious puberty; prostatic cancer.*

**C-Pela** *Nakorn, Thai.*
Cinnarizine (p.428·3).
*Cerebral and peripheral vascular disorders; motion sickness; nausea and vomiting; vestibular disorders.*

**C-Platin** *Blausiegel, Braz.*
Cisplatin (p.538·1).
*Malignant neoplasms.*

**C-Plus** *Hylands, Canad.*
Homoeopathic preparation.

**CPM PSE MSC** *Cypress, USA.*
Chlorphenamine maleate (p.427·3); pseudoephedrine hydrochloride (p.1129·2); hyoscine methonitrate (p.483·3).
*Rhinitis.*

**CPM/PE/MSC** *Cypress, USA.*
Chlorphenamine maleate (p.427·3); phenylephrine hydrochloride (p.1126·3); hyoscine methonitrate (p.483·3).
*Allergic rhinitis.*

**C-Poretta** *Leiras, Fin.†.*
Ascorbic acid (p.1460·2).
*Dietary supplement; vitamin C deficiency.*

**CPS Pulver**
*Brady, Austria; Gry, Ger.*
Calcium polystyrene sulfonate (p.1032·3).
*Hyperkalaemia.*

**CPT** *Varifarma, Arg.*
Irinotecan (p.564·3).
*Malignant neoplasms.*

**Cracoa B** *Gelos, Spain†.*
Aluminium hydroxide (p.1249·2); calcium carbonate (p.1254·2); magnesium carbonate (p.1272·1); magnesium trisilicate (p.1272·3).
*Gastrointestinal hyperacidity.*

**Cradocap** *Napp, UK†.*
Cetrimide (p.1172·1).
*Cradle cap.*

**Craegium** *Biocur, Ger.*
Crataegus (p.1677·1).
*Heart failure.*

**Crafilm** *Francia, Ital.*
Sucralfate (p.1290·2).
*Gastrointestinal disorders associated with hyperacidity.*

**Cralonin**
*Peithner, Austria; Heel, Ger.*
Homoeopathic preparation.

**Cralsanic** *Hexal, S.Afr.†.*
Sucralfate (p.1290·2).
*Peptic ulcer.*

**Cramigen** *Wayne, Mex.†.*
Amikacin (p.154·1).
*Bacterial infections.*

**Crampex** *Thornton & Ross, UK.*
Calcium gluconate (p.1225·2); nicotinic acid (p.1441·1); colecalciferol (p.1461·3).
*Night cramps.*

**Crampiton** *Orion, Fin.*
Quinine hydrochloride (p.460·2); meprobamate (p.706·2).
*Muscle spasm; restless leg syndrome.*

**Cranberry Complex** *Cenovis, Austral.†.*
Cranberry (p.1676·3); buchu (p.1663·1); bearberry (p.1659·2); ascorbic acid (p.1460·2).
*Cystitis; fluid retention.*

**Cranio-cyl Ho-Len-Complex** *Liebermann, Ger.*
Homoeopathic preparation.

**Cranoc** *Fujisawa, Ger.*
Fluvastatin sodium (p.918·2).
*Hypercholesterolaemia.*

**Crasnitin** *Bayer, Ital.†.*
Asparaginase (p.528·3).
*Leukaemia.*

**Crataegan** *Austroplant, Austria.*
Crataegus (p.1677·1).
*Cardiac disorders.*

**Crataegisan** *Bioforce, Switz.*
Crataegus (p.1677·1).
*Cardiac disorders.*

**Crataegitan** *Amino, Switz.*
Crataegus (p.1677·1).
*Cardiac disorders.*

**Crataegol** *LDM, Fr.†.*
Crataegus (p.1677·1).
*Insomnia; nervous disorders.*

**Crataegus Complex** *Blackmores, Austral.†.*
Tilia platyphyllos (p.1756·2); achillea (p.1646·2); crataegus (p.1677·1); garlic (p.1691·1); ascorbic acid (p.1460·2); hesperidin (p.1688·2); rutoside (p.1688·2).
*Cardiovascular disorders.*

**Crataegus Med Complex** *Dynamit, Austria.*
Homoeopathic preparation.

**Crataegutt**
*Peithner, Austria; Schwabe, Ger.; Schwabe, Neth.†; Schwabe, Spain†.*
Crataegus (p.1677·1).
*Heart failure; hypertension; ischaemic heart disease.*

**Crataegysat F** *Ysatfabrik, Ger.*
Crataegus (p.1677·1).
*Cardiac disorders.*

**Crataelanat** *Schwabe, Ger.†.*
Digoxin (p.895·2); crataegus (p.1677·1).
*Heart failure.*

**Cratae-Loges** *Loges, Ger.*
Crataegus (p.1677·1).
*Heart failure.*

**Crataepas** *Pascoe, Ger.*
Crataegus (p.1677·1).
*Heart failure.*

**Crataezyma** *Zyma, Ger.†.*
Crataegus (p.1677·1).
*Cardiac disorders.*

**Cratecor** *Bionorica, Ger.*
Crataegus (p.1677·1).
*Heart failure.*

**Cratenox** *Knop, Chile.*
Crataegus (p.1677·1).
*Cardiovascular disorders.*

**Cratimon** *Madaus, Spain†.*
Benzydamine aescinate (p.21·1).
*Peri-articular disorders; soft-tissue disorders.*

**Craun** *Fada, Arg.*
Paracetamol (p.76·2); diphenhydramine (p.431·3); dipyrone (p.35·3).

**Craviscum mono** *CPF, Ger.†.*
Crataegus (p.1677·1).
*Cardiac disorders.*

**Cravit**
*Daiichi, Hong Kong; Daiichi, Jpn; Daiichi, Malaysia; Daiichi, Singapore; Daiichi, Thai.*
Levofloxacin (p.225·3).
*Bacterial infections.*

**Cravo-Espin** *Virtus, Braz.†.*
Triclosan (p.1195·2); resorcinol (p.1156·3); sulfur (p.1158·2); bentonite.
*Acne.*

**Creacal** *Diviser Aquilea, Spain.*
Calcium phosphate (p.1225·3); colecalciferol (p.1461·3).
*Calcium and vitamin D deficiency; osteoporosis.*

**Creagin** *Infosint, Ital.*
Multivitamin and mineral preparation with creatine, ginkgo biloba and ginseng (p.1417·1).
*Tonic.*

**Cream E45** *Boots Healthcare, NZ.*
Emollient.
*Dry skin.*

**Creamy Tar** *C & M, USA.*
Coal tar (p.1159·2).
*Scalp disorders.*

**Creanolona** *Bohm, Spain.*
Fluocinolone acetonide (p.1101·2); neomycin (p.235·1); polymyxin B (p.245·2).
*Skin infections with inflammation.*

**Creatile** *New Farma, Ital.*
Creatine (p.1677·2).
*Nutritional supplement.*

**Creatyl** *Volchem, Ital.*
Amino-acid preparation or amino-acid and carbohydrate preparation (p.1417·1).
*Nutritional supplement.*

**Creavit** *Medisint, Ital.*
Carnitine; creatine; minerals; vitamins (p.1417·1).
*Tonic.*

**Crecil** *Vinas, Spain.*
Cystine (p.1426·3).
Formerly known as Vitacrecil.
*Cystine deficiency.*

**Credaxol** *Quimica y Farmacia, Mex.*
Ranitidine (p.1285·2).
*Peptic ulcer.*

**Crelo Blanco** *Yamanouchi, Ital.*
Emollient.
*Dry skin disorders; pharmaceutical base.*

**Crema Axel** *Grisi, Mex.*
Sulfur (p.1158·2); triclosan (p.1195·2); resorcinol (p.1156·3).
*Acne.*

**Crema Blanca** *Bustillos, Mex.*
Hydroquinone (p.1148·1).
*Skin hyperpigmentation disorders.*

**Crema Coloreada de Proteccion Total** *Pierre Fabre Dermo-Cosmetique, Arg.*
Titanium dioxide (p.1160·3); zinc oxide (p.1163·2); cinnamate.
*Sunscreen.*

**Crema Compensadora Avene** *Silesia, Chile.*
Emollient.
*Eczema.*

**Crema Contracepti Lanzas** *Ipsen, Spain.*
Benzalkonium chloride (p.1168·3).
*Contraceptive.*

**Crema de Magnesia** *Cinfa, Spain†.*
Magnesium hydroxide (p.1272·2).
*Constipation; gastrointestinal hyperacidity.*

**Crema de Ordene** *Spineda, Arg.*
Vitamin A (p.1451·2); benzalkonium chloride (p.1168·3); zinc (p.1469·2).
*Skin disorders.*

**Crema de Proteccion Extrema 50B** *Pierre Fabre Dermo-Cosmetique, Arg.*
*SPF 50:* Titanium dioxide (p.1160·3); zinc oxide (p.1163·2).
*Sunscreen.*

**Crema Facial De Dia AHA Formula 405** *Dermaclin, Mex.*
*SPF 15:* Octinoxate (p.1154·3); oxybenzone (p.1154·3).
*Sunscreen.*

**Crema Facial De Noche AHA Formula 405** *Dermaclin, Mex.*
Moisturiser.

**Crema Invisible de Proteccion Total** *Pierre Fabre Dermo-Cosmetique, Arg.*
Titanium dioxide (p.1160·3); zinc oxide (p.1163·2); cinnamate.
*Sunscreen.*

**Crema Para Pieles Intolerantes Avene** *Silesia, Chile.*
Emollient.
*Dry skin.*

**Cremaffin** *Knoll, India.*
Magnesium hydroxide (p.1272·2); liquid paraffin (p.1479·1).
*Constipation.*

**Cremalax** *Knoll, India.*
Sodium picosulfate (p.1289·3).
*Bowel evacuation; constipation.*

**Cremalgin** *Co-Pharma, UK.*
Methyl nicotinate (p.59·2); glycol salicylate (p.44·3); capsicum oleoresin (p.1667·1).
*Musculoskeletal and joint pain.*

**Crema-U** *Jean-Marie, Hong Kong†.*
Propantheline bromide (p.489·1); hyoscine methobromide (p.483·3); dicycloverine hydrochloride (p.481·2); chlorophyllin copper complex sodium (p.1057·1); methiosulfonium chloride (p.1714·1); simeticone (p.1289·2); magnesium hydroxide (p.1272·2); magnesium trisilicate (p.1272·3); dried aluminium hydroxide gel (p.1249·2).
*Flatulence; gastrointestinal hyperacidity; painful gastrointestinal spasm; peptic ulcer.*

**Creme Anti-Rides Auto-Bronzante** *Clarins, Canad.†.*
*SPF 15:* Octinoxate (p.1154·3); oxybenzone (p.1154·3); titanium dioxide (p.1160·3).
*Sunscreen.*

**Creme au Melilot Composee** *Avene, Fr.*
Dextran sulfate (p.1679·2); melilotus; rusculus aculeatus.
*Skin redness.*

**Creme Auto-Bronzant** *Clarins, Canad.†.*
*SPF 15:* Avobenzone (p.1142·3); enzacamene (p.1147·1); oxybenzone (p.1154·3).
*Sunscreen.*

**Creme Autobronzante Visage** *Lancome, Canad.†.*
Avobenzone (p.1142·3); enzacamene (p.1147·1).
*Sunscreen.*

**Creme de base** *Glaxo Wellcome, Switz.†.*
Emollient.
*Skin disorders.*

**Creme des 3 Fleurs d'Orient** *Creme d'Orient, Fr.†.*
*Cream:* Hydroquinone (p.1148·1).
*Ointment:* Mequinol (p.1151·3).
*Hyperpigmentation.*

**Creme Ecran Total** *Lancome, Canad.*
*SPF 40:* Avobenzone (p.1142·3); enzacamene (p.1147·1); ecamsule (p.1146·3); titanium dioxide (p.1160·3).
*Sunscreen.*

**Creme Gordo Barral** *Lepori, Port.*
Emollient.

**Creme Haute Protection** *Lancome, Canad.*
*SPF 15:* Avobenzone (p.1142·3); enzacamene (p.1147·1); ecamsule (p.1146·3); titanium dioxide (p.1160·3).
*Sunscreen.*

**Creme Laser Hidrante** *Dermoteca, Port.*
Squalane (p.1482·2); proline (p.1443·2); urea (p.1162·2); lactic acid (p.1704·1); citric acid (p.1673·1); *dl*-alpha tocopherol (p.1464·3); ruscus aculeatus.
*Dry skin; skin irritation.*

**Creme Protectrice** *Lancome, Canad.†.*
*SPF 15:* Avobenzone (p.1142·3); enzacamene (p.1147·1); ecamsule (p.1146·3); titanium dioxide (p.1160·3).
*Sunscreen.*

**Creme Rap** *IPRAD, Fr.*
Scoparium (p.1742·2); arnica (p.1656·3); aesculus (p.1648·2); hyoscyamus (p.485·2).
*Soft-tissue disorders; venous insufficiency.*

**Creme Solaire Anti-Rides** *Clarins, Canad.†.*
*SPF 10:* Octinoxate (p.1154·3); oxybenzone (p.1154·3); titanium dioxide (p.1160·3).
*Sunscreen.*

**Creme Solaire Bronzage** *Clarins, Canad.†.*
*SPF 15:* Octinoxate (p.1154·3); oxybenzone (p.1154·3); titanium dioxide (p.1160·3).
*Sunscreen.*

**Creme Solaire Bronzage Rapide** *Clarins, Canad.*
*SPF 10:* Avobenzone (p.1142·3); octinoxate (p.1154·3); octisalate (p.1154·3); oxybenzone (p.1154·3).
*Sunscreen.*

**Creme Solaire Bronzage Securite** *Clarins, Canad.*
*SPF 20:* Octinoxate (p.1154·3); octisalate (p.1154·3); oxybenzone (p.1154·3); titanium dioxide (p.1160·3).
*Sunscreen.*

**Creme Solaire Bronzage Securite Special** *Clarins, Canad.*
*SPF 15:* Avobenzone (p.1142·3); enzacamene (p.1147·1); octinoxate (p.1154·3); oxybenzone (p.1154·3).
*Sunscreen.*

**Creme Solaire Ecran Special Visage** *Clarins, Canad.†.*
*SPF 30:* Avobenzone (p.1142·3); enzacamene (p.1147·1); octinoxate (p.1154·3); oxybenzone (p.1154·3); ensulizole (p.1147·1); titanium dioxide (p.1160·3).
*Sunscreen.*

**Creme Solaire Haute Protection** *Clarins, Canad.*
Octocrilene (p.1154·3); octinoxate (p.1154·3); octisalate (p.1154·3); oxybenzone (p.1154·3); ensulizole (p.1147·1); titanium dioxide (p.1160·3).
*Sunscreen.*

**Creme Universal** *Merck, Braz.*
Emollient.

**Cremederme** *Bunker, Braz.*
Betamethasone valerate (p.1093·2); gentamicin sulfate (p.217·1); tolnaftate (p.410·1); clioquinol (p.196·3).
*Infected skin disorders.*

**Cremicort-H** *Chefaro, Belg.*
Hydrocortisone (p.1103·3).
*Skin disorders.*

**Creminem** *Mintlab, Chile.*
Clotrimazole (p.396·2).
*Fungal skin infections.*

**Creminem-B** *Mintlab, Chile.*
Clotrimazole (p.396·2); betamethasone dipropionate (p.1093·1).
*Fungal skin infections.*

**Cremirit** *Mintlab, Chile.*
Betamethasone dipropionate (p.1093·1).
*Skin disorders.*

**Cremisona**
*Note. This name is used for preparations of different composition.*
*ICN, Arg.*
Sodium lactate (p.1223·2); urea (p.1162·2); squalane (p.1482·2); hyaluronic acid (p.1697·3).
*Dry skin disorders.*

*Diba, Mex.*
Fluocinolone (p.1101·2).
*Skin disorders.*

**Cremol-P** *Max Ritter, Switz.†.*
Evening primrose oil (p.1686·3).
*Dry skin.*

**Cremol-Ritter** *Gebro, Switz.*
A range of skin cleansing and emollient preparations.
*Skin disorders.*

**Cremosan** *Quimica y Farmacia, Mex.*
Ketoconazole (p.403·3).
*Fungal skin infections.*

**Cremsol** *Quimifar, Spain.*
Linseed oil; calcium hydroxide (p.1664·3); benzocaine (p.1370·3); sulfathiazole (p.264·1); triamcinolone acetonide (p.1110·2); zinc oxide (p.1163·2).
*Infected skin disorders.*

**Cremsor N** *Kampel Martian, Arg.*
Allantoin (p.1141·3); coal tar (p.1159·2); urea (p.1162·2).
*Skin disorders.*

**Crenodyn** *Francia, Ital.†.*
Cefadroxil (p.167·2).
*Bacterial infections.*

**Creo Grippe** *Marc-O, Canad.†.*
Camphor (p.1665·3); cineole (p.1672·1); guaifenesin (p.1122·1).

**Creodermol** *Medical, Port.†.*
Creosote (p.1117·2); niaouli oil (p.1719·3); thyme oil (p.1755·3); ephedrine hydrochloride (p.1120·1).
*Coughs; respiratory-tract disorders.*

**Creolina** *Pearson, Ital.*
Cresol (p.1177·3).
*Surface disinfection.*

**Creon**
*Byk, Arg.; Solvay, Austral.; Solvay, Belg.; Solvay, Canad.; Grunenthal, Chile; Solvay, Fr.; Solvay, Gr.; Solvay, Hong Kong; Solvay, Irl.; Solvay, Israel; Solvay, Ital.; Solvay, Malaysia; Byk Gulden, Mex.; Solvay, Neth.; Boehringer Ingelheim, NZ; Solvay, S.Afr.; Rotta, Singapore; Solvay, Switz.; Solvay, Thai.; Solvay, UK; Solvay, USA.*
Pancreatin (p.1725·3).
*Pancreatic insufficiency.*

**Creo-Rectal** *Nadeau, Canad.*
Diphenylpyraline hydrochloride (p.432·3); guaiacol carbonate (p.1122·1); camphor (p.1665·3).
*Coughs.*

**Creosedin** *Pharmacia, Arg.*
Bromazepam (p.671·3).
*Alcohol withdrawal syndrome; anxiety.*

**Creosoto Composto** *Ogna, Ital.*
Creosote (p.1117·2); phenol (p.1188·1); lidocaine hydrochloride (p.1377·3); eugenol (p.1686·2).
*Dental pain.*

**Creo-Terpin** *Lee, USA.*
Dextromethorphan hydrobromide (p.1117·3).

**Crescicalcio** *Prodotti, Braz.†.*
Calcium phosphate (p.1225·3); vitamins A, $D_2$, and $B_{12}$ (p.1417·1).
*Calcium and vitamin supplement.*

**Crescom** *Esoform, Ital.*
Sodium *o*-phenylphenol (p.1187·2).
*Instrument disinfection; surface disinfection.*

**Cresolox** *Coventry, UK†.*
Tar acids (p.1193·3).

**Cresophene**
*Note. This name is used for preparations of different composition.*
*Prats, Spain.*
Dexamethasone (p.1097·1); hexachlorophene (p.1181·2); prajmalium bitartrate (p.984·3); parachlorophenol (p.1187·3).
*Dental caries; oral disinfection.*

*Septodont, Switz.*
Dexamethasone acetate (p.1097·1); thymol (p.1194·2); parachlorophenol (p.1187·3); camphor (p.1665·3).
*Root canal infections.*

**Crestanon** *Organon, Mex.†.*
Allylestrenol (p.1541·3).

**Crestor**
*AstraZeneca, UK; AstraZeneca, USA.*
Rosuvastatin calcium (p.996·2).
*Hyperlipidaemias.*

**Cresylate** *Recsei, USA.*
*m*-Cresyl acetate (p.1178·1); isopropyl alcohol (p.1184·3).
*Ear infection.*

**Crevet** *Prater, Chile.*
Ascorbic acid (p.1460·2).
*Vitamin C supplement.*

**CRH**
*Ferring, Austria; Ferring, Ger.; Ferring, Neth.*
Corticorelin triflutate (p.1321·3).
*Diagnosis of adrenal disorders.*

**Criam** *Psicofarma, Mex.*
Magnesium valproate (p.382·2).
*Epilepsy.*

**Crilem** *Lemery, Mex.*
Bromocriptine mesilate (p.1200·3).

**Crima** *Fada, Arg.*
Ceftazidime (p.180·2).
*Bacterial infections.*

**Crimanex** *Drossapharm, Switz.*
Dipyrithione (p.1146·1); undecenoic acid diethanolamide.
*Scalp disorders.*

**Crinalsofex** *Sofex, Port.*
Minoxidil (p.960·1).
*Alopecia androgenetica.*

**Criniton**
*Richter, Austria; Atzinger, Ger.*
Thymol (p.1194·2); salicylic acid (p.1157·1); rosemary oil (p.1740·2).
*Scalp disorders.*

**Crino Cordes** *Ichthyol, Austria.*
Sodium bituminosulphonate (p.1148·3); sodium sulfosuccinated undecenoic acid monoethanolamide (p.411·1).
*Scalp disorders.*

**Crino Cordes N** *Ichthyol, Ger.*
Ictasol (p.1148·3).
*Scalp disorders; skin disorders.*

**Crinohermal fem** *Hermal, Ger.*
Fluprednidene acetate (p.1102·2); estradiol (p.1550·1).
*Female hair loss.*

**Crino-Kaban N** *Asche, Ger.*
Clocortolone pivalate (p.1096·1); salicylic acid (p.1157·1).
*Scalp disorders.*

**Crinone**
*Serono, Arg.; Serono, Braz.; Serono, Canad.; Serono, Fin.; Serono, Ger.; Serono, Gr.; Serono, Hong Kong; Serono, Irl.; Serono, Ital.; Serono, Mex.; Serono, Norw.; Serono, Port.; Serono, Singapore†; Serono, Spain; Serono, Swed.; Serono, Switz.; Serono, UK; Serono, USA.*
Progesterone (p.1566·2).
*Female infertility; menopausal disorders; menstrual disorders.*

**Crinopex** *Schering-Plough, Swed.†.*
Pyrethrin (p.1509·3); piperonyl butoxide (p.1509·2).
*Pediculosis.*

**Crinoren** *Uriach, Spain.*
Enalapril maleate (p.909·2).
*Heart failure; hypertension.*

**Crinoretic** *Uriach, Spain.*
Enalapril maleate (p.909·2); hydrochlorothiazide (p.933·2).
*Hypertension.*

**Crinotar** *Agpharm, Switz.†.*
Pyrithione zinc (p.1156·2); coal tar (p.1159·2).
*Scalp disorders.*

**Criostat SD 2** *Grifols, Spain†.*
Factor VIII (p.751·1).
*Factor VIII deficiency.*

**Criotonal** *Amnol, Ital.*
Aescin; caffeine; ruscus; centella; arnica; hedera; capsicum; ginkgo biloba; menthol.
*Skin disorders.*

**Cripar**
*Taurus, Ger.; Knoll, Ger.; Hormosan, Ger.; Poli, Switz.*
Dihydroergocryptine mesilate (p.1680·1).
*Migraine; parkinsonism.*

**Criptamine** *Raza, Malaysia; Pharmaniaga, Malaysia.*
Bromocriptine mesilate (p.1200·3).
*Acromegaly; benign breast disorders; galactorrhoea; hyperprolactinaemia; hypogonadism; male and female infertility; menstrual disorders; parkinsonism.*

**CRI-regen** *Pekana, Ger.*
Homoeopathic preparation.

**Crisabon** *Teva Tuteur, Arg.*
Epirubicin (p.550·3).
*Malignant neoplasms.*

**Crisacide** *Kampel Martian, Arg.*
Ciprofloxacin (p.188·2).
*Bacterial infections.*

**Crisafeno** *Kampel Martian, Arg.*
Tamoxifen (p.585·3).

**Crisapla** *Kampel Martian, Arg.*
Oxaliplatin (p.577·1).
*Malignant neoplasms.*

**Crisasma** *Sintesina, Arg.*
Theophylline (p.798·3).
*Obstructive airways disease.*

**Crisazet** *Kampel Martian, Arg.*
Zidovudine (p.658·2).
*HIV infection.*

**Crisdazol** *Cristalia, Braz.*
Mebendazole (p.108·2).
*Worm infections.*

**Crislaxo** *Quimifar, Spain.*
Aloes (p.1248·2); aniseed (p.1655·2); cascara (p.1255·1); senna (p.1288·2); fennel (p.1687·2); rhubarb (p.1287·3); sulfur (p.1158·2); belladonna (p.479·1).
*Constipation.*

**Crismol**
*Note. This name is used for preparations of different composition.*
*Royal, Chile.*
Clonazepam (p.359·1).
*Epilepsy; panic attacks.*

*Almirall, Spain†.*
Fenoterol hydrobromide (p.785·2); ipratropium bromide (p.787·1).
*Obstructive airways disease.*

**Crisofimina** *Teva Tuteur, Arg.*
Mitomycin (p.573·3).
*Malignant neoplasms.*

**Crisomet** *Juste, Spain.*
Lamotrigine (p.363·3).
*Epilepsy.*

**Cristaclar** *Beta, Arg.*
Donepezil hydrochloride (p.1489·2).
*Alzheimer's disease.*

**Cristal**
*Note. This name is used for preparations of different composition.*
*Pfizer, Ital.†.*
Multivitamin preparation (p.1417·1).

*Vifor, Switz.†.*
Glycerol (p.1694·3).
*Constipation.*

**Cristalcrom** *Cinfa, Spain.*
Chlorhexidine gluconate (p.1173·2).
*Skin and wound disinfection.*

**Cristalmina** *Salvat, Spain.*
Chlorhexidine gluconate (p.1173·2).
*Skin and wound disinfection.*

**Cristalomicina** *Armstrong, Arg.*
*Ear drops:* Kanamycin sulfate (p.225·1); hydrocortisone (p.1103·3); phenazone (p.82·3); benzocaine (p.1370·3).
*Otitis externa; otitis media.*

*Injection:* Kanamycin sulfate (p.225·1).
*Bacterial infections.*

**Cristalpen** *Biolab Sanus, Braz.*
Benzylpenicillin potassium (p.163·2).
*Bacterial infections.*

**Cristan** *Shin Poong, Singapore.*
Clotrimazole (p.396·2).
*Fungal skin infections; vulvovaginal candidiasis.*

**Cristerona** *Gador, Arg.*
Estradiol (p.1550·1); progesterone (p.1566·2).
*Menstrual disorders.*

**Cristopal** *Alcon, Fr.*
Calcium chloride (p.1225·1); sodium succinate (p.1748·3); magnesium aspartate (p.1227·3); glycine (p.1433·3).
Formerly contained calcium chloride, sodium iodide, and glycine.
*Lens opacities.*

**Criten** *Tecnofarma, Chile.*
Bromocriptine mesilate (p.1200·3).
*Acromegaly; hyperprolactinaemia; parkinsonism.*

**Criticare HN**
*Mead Johnson, Austral.; Mead Johnson Nutritionals, Canad.; Mead Johnson, Hong Kong†; Mead Johnson Nutritionals, USA.*
Preparation for enteral nutrition (p.1417·1).

**Critichol** *Angelini, Ital.*
Fenipentol hemisuccinate (p.1687·2); cascara (p.1255·1); boldo (p.1661·2); rhubarb (p.1287·3).
*Constipation.*

**Crivion** *Vilco, Gr.*
Nitrendipine (p.973·3).
*Hypertension.*

**Crixivan**
*Merck Sharp & Dohme, Arg.; Merck Sharp & Dohme, Austral.; Merck Sharp & Dohme, Austria; Merck Sharp & Dohme, Belg.; Merck Sharp & Dohme, Braz.; Merck Frosst, Canad.; Merck Sharp & Dohme, Chile; Merck Sharp & Dohme, Denm.; Merck Sharp & Dohme, Fin.; Merck Sharp & Dohme-Chibret, Fr.; Merck Sharp & Dohme, Ger.; Merck, Gr.; Merck Sharp & Dohme, Hong Kong; Merck Sharp & Dohme, Irl.; Merck Sharp & Dohme, Israel; Merck Sharp & Dohme, Ital.; Banyu, Jpn; Merck Sharp & Dohme, Malaysia; Merck Sharp & Dohme, Mex.; Merck Sharp & Dohme, Neth.; Merck Sharp & Dohme, Norw.; Merck Sharp & Dohme, NZ; Merck Sharp & Dohme, Port.; Merck Sharp & Dohme, S.Afr.; Merck Sharp & Dohme, Singapore; Merck Sharp & Dohme, Spain; Merck Sharp & Dohme, Swed.; Merck Sharp & Dohme, Switz.; Merck Sharp & Dohme, Thai.; Merck Sharp & Dohme, UK; Merck, USA.*
Indinavir sulfate (p.638·2).
*HIV infection.*

**Cro 50** *Investigaciones Filosoficas y Cientificas, Mex.†.*
Ribonuclease (p.1738·1).

**Croben** *Wassen, Ital.*
Chromium (p.1425·1).
*Nutritional supplement.*

**Crocin** *GlaxoSmithKline, India.*
Paracetamol (p.76·2).
*Fever; pain.*

**CroFab** *Altana, USA.*
Crotalidae polyvalent immune fab (p.1639·2).
*Rattlesnake bites.*

**Croferron** *Degorts, Mex.*
Ferrous fumarate (p.1427·3).
*Iron-deficiency anaemia.*

**Croglina** *Edol, Port.*
Sodium cromoglicate (p.795·3).
*Allergic conjunctivitis.*

**Croix Blanche** *SMB, Belg.*
Paracetamol (p.76·2); caffeine (p.782·1).
*Fever; pain.*

**Crolidin** *Kleva, Gr.*
Sodium cromoglicate (p.795·3).
*Allergic conjunctivitis; allergic rhinitis.*

**Crolix** *Rayere, Mex.*
Roxithromycin (p.254·2).
*Bacterial infections.*

**Crolom** *Dura, USA.*
Sodium cromoglicate (p.795·3).
*Inflammatory disorders of the eye.*

**Crom 80** *Selvi, Ital.*
Ferrous gluconate (p.1428·1).
Ascorbic acid (p.1460·2) is included in this preparation to increase the absorption and availability of iron.
*Iron-deficiency anaemia.*

**Cromabak**
*Allergan-Frumtost, Braz.†; Thea, Fr.; Thea, Hong Kong; Pharmacia, Singapore.*
Sodium cromoglicate (p.795·3).
*Allergic eye disorders.*

**Cromadoses** *Thea, Fr.*
Sodium cromoglicate (p.795·3).
*Allergic eye disorders.*

**Cromal**
*Mundipharma, Austria; Cipla, India; Cipla-Medpro, S.Afr.†.*
Sodium cromoglicate (p.795·3).
*Obstructive airways disease.*

**Cromantal** *Alcon, Ital.*
Sodium cromoglicate (p.795·3).
*Allergic rhinitis.*

**Cro-Man-Zin** *Freeda, USA.*
Chromium, manganese, and zinc preparation (p.1417·1).
*Mineral supplement.*

**Cromatonbic B12** *Menarini, Spain.*
Cyanocobalamin (p.1458·2).
*Vitamin B12 deficiency.*

**Cromatonbic Ferro**
*Menarini, Arg.; Menarini, Spain.*
Ferrous lactate (p.1428·2).
*Iron deficiency; iron-deficiency anaemia.*

**Cromatonbic Folinico**
*Menarini, Arg.; Menarini, Spain.*
Calcium folinate (p.1431·1).
*Folate deficiency; megaloblastic anaemia.*

**Cromatonferro** *Menarini, Ital.*
Ferrous gluconate (p.1428·1).
Ascorbic acid (p.1460·2) is included in the tablets to increase the absorption and availability of iron.
*Anaemias; iron deficiency.*

**Cromedil** *Europhta, Mon.*
Sodium cromoglicate (p.795·3).
Formerly known as Allergodose.
*Allergic eye disorders.*

**Cromer Orto** *Normon, Spain.*
Merbromin (p.1185·3).
*Skin and wound disinfection.*

**Cromese** *Pharmacia, Austral.*
Sodium cromoglicate (p.795·3).
*Asthma.*

**Cromex** *Davi, Port.*
Sodium cromoglicate (p.795·3).
*Allergic conjunctivitis.*

**Cromezin** *SoSe, Ital.*
Cefazolin sodium (p.170·3).
*Bacterial infections.*

**Cromifusin** *Pisa, Mex.*
Chromium trichloride (p.1425·1).

**Cromo** *Ratiopharm, Ger.; CT, Ger.; Stulln, Ger.*
Sodium cromoglicate (p.795·3).
*Allergic conjunctivitis; allergic rhinitis; asthma; hypersensitivity reactions.*

**Cromo Asma** *Aldo, Spain.*
Sodium cromoglicate (p.795·3).
*Asthma; bronchospasm.*

**Cromocato** *Neo Quimica, Braz.*
Sodium cromoglicate (p.795·3).

**Cromocur** *Tipomark, Ital.*
Merbromin (p.1185·3).
*Wound disinfection.*

**Cromodyn** *Rappai, Switz.*
Sodium cromoglicate (p.795·3).
*Allergic rhinitis.*

**Cromoftol** *Merck Sharp & Dohme, Spain†.*
Chlorphenamine maleate (p.427·3); sodium cromoglicate (p.795·3).
*Eye disorders.*

**Cromogen**
*Ivax, Irl.; Norton, Israel; Norton, S.Afr.†; Ivax, UK.*
Sodium cromoglicate (p.795·3).
*Asthma.*

**Cromoglicin** *Heumann, Ger.*
Sodium cromoglicate (p.795·3).
*Allergic conjunctivitis; allergic rhinitis; asthma.*

**Cromoglin** *Ratiopharm, Austria.*
Sodium cromoglicate (p.795·3).
*Allergic eye disorders; obstructive airways disease; rhinitis.*

**Cromohexal**
*Hexal, Ger.; Hexal, S.Afr.*
Sodium cromoglicate (p.795·3).
*Allergic conjunctivitis; allergic rhinitis; asthma.*

**Cromol** *Betapharm, Ger.†.*
Sodium cromoglicate (p.795·3).
*Hay fever.*

**Cromolerg** *Allergan, Braz.*
Sodium cromoglicate (p.795·3).
*Allergic conjunctivitis.*

**Cromolergin UD** *Pharmanel, Gr.*
Sodium cromoglicate (p.795·3).
*Allergic conjunctivitis; allergic rhinitis.*

**Cromolind** *Lindopharm, Ger.*
Sodium cromoglicate (p.795·3).
*Asthma.*

**Cromolyn**
*Pharmascience, Canad.; Fatol, Ger.†; Orion, Ger.†; Genmedix, Israel.*
Sodium cromoglicate (p.795·3).
*Allergic eye disorders; allergic rhinitis; asthma.*

**Cromophtal** *Agepha, Austria.*
Sodium cromoglicate (p.795·3).
*Conjunctivitis.*

**Crom-Ophtal** *Winzer, Ger.*
Sodium cromoglicate (p.795·3).
*Allergic conjunctivitis; allergic rhinitis.*

**Cromopp** *Dermapharm, Ger.*
Sodium cromoglicate (p.795·3).
*Asthma.*

**Cromoptic**
*Chauvin, Fr.; Vitamed, Israel.*
Sodium cromoglicate (p.795·3).
*Allergic eye disorders.*

**Cromosan**
*Note. This name is used for preparations of different composition.*
*Quimioterapica, Braz.†.*
*Injection:* Magnesium chromate; magnesium acetate (p.1227·3).
*Oral gel:* Magnesium bromate; magnesium acetate (p.1227·3); magnesium oxide (p.1272·3); aluminium hydroxide (p.1249·2).
*Gastrointestinal hyperacidity.*

*Medici, Ital.*
Sodium cromoglicate (p.795·3).
*Food hypersensitivity.*

**Cromoseptil Plus** *Azevedos, Port.†.*
Povidone-iodine (p.1190·3).
*Skin and wound disinfection.*

**Cromosoft** *Thea, Fr.*
Sodium cromoglicate (p.795·3).

**Cromosol Ophta** *Ecosol, Switz.*
Sodium cromoglicate (p.795·3).
*Conjunctivitis.*

**Cromosol UD** *Ecosol, Switz.*
Sodium cromoglicate (p.795·3).
*Asthma.*

**Cromotex** *Medix, Mex.*
Chromium dinicotinate (ChromeMate).
*Chromium supplement.*

**Cromovisus** *DMG, Ital.*
Calcium phosphate; bioflavonoids; yeast; vitamins (p.1417·1).
*Nutritional supplement.*

**Cromoxin K** *Rius, Spain.*
Carbazochrome (p.745·1); phytomenadione (p.1467·1).
*Haemorrhage.*

**Cromozil** *Tubilux, Ital.*
Tetryzoline hydrochloride (p.1131·2); sodium cromoglicate (p.795·3).
*Conjunctivitis.*

**Cromunal** *Agis, Israel†.*
Sodium cromoglicate (p.795·3).
*Allergic rhinitis; asthma; bronchitis.*

**Cromycin** *Croma, Austria.*
Tobramycin (p.271·2).
*Bacterial eye infections.*

**Cronacol** *Biotekfarma, Ital.†.*
Sodium cromoglicate (p.795·3).
*Food hypersensitivity.*

**Cronal** *Valdecasas, Mex.*
Chlorphenamine maleate (p.427·3).
*Hypersensitivity.*

**Cronase** *Vitamed, Israel.*
Sodium cromoglicate (p.795·3).
*Allergic rhinitis.*

**Cronasma** *Orion, Ger.*
Theophylline (p.798·3).
*Obstructive airways disease.*

**Cronassial** *Fidia, Thai.†.*
Gangliosides (p.1691·1).
*Peripheral neuropathies; polyneuropathies.*

**Cronavit** *Degorts, Mex.*
Multivitamin preparation with iron (p.1417·1).
*Tonic.*

**Croneparina**
*Armstrong, Arg.; UCB, Ital.*
Heparin calcium (p.927·3).
*Atherosclerosis; thromboembolic disorders.*

**Cronizat** *Caber, Ital.*
Nizatidine (p.1277·2).
*Gastro-oesophageal reflux; peptic ulcer.*

**Cronobe** *Biolab Sanus, Braz.*
Cobamamide (p.1459·1).
*Tonic.*

**Cronocaps** *Medix, Mex.*
Melatonin (p.1710·2).
*Insomnia.*

**Cronocef** *Bristol-Myers Squibb, Ital.*
Cefprozil (p.179·2).
*Bacterial infections.*

**Cronocol** *Schering-Plough, Port.†.*
Gentamicin sulfate (p.217·1).
*Bone infections.*

**Cronocorteroid** *Montpellier, Arg.*
Betamethasone dipropionate (p.1093·1); betamethasone sodium phosphate (p.1093·1).
*Corticosteroid.*

**Cronodine** *Alacan, Spain.*
Diltiazem hydrochloride (p.900·1).
*Angina pectoris; hypertension.*

**Cronoferril** *Grunenthal, Chile.*
Ferrous fumarate (p.1427·3); vitamin $B_{12}$ (p.1458·2); folic acid (p.1429·1).
Vitamin C (p.1460·2) is included in this preparation to increase the absorption and availability of iron.
*Iron and folic acid deficiency; iron-deficiency anaemia.*

**Cronogeron** *Dansk-Flama, Braz.*
Cinnarizine (p.428·3).
*Peripheral vascular disorders; vestibular disorders.*

**Cronol** *Solvay, Spain.*
Famotidine (p.1265·2).
*Gastro-oesophageal reflux; peptic ulcer; Zollinger-Ellison syndrome.*

**Cronolax** *Master, Chile.*
Sodium picosulfate (p.1289·3).
*Constipation.*

**Cronolevel**
*White, Arg.; Essex, Chile; Undra, Mex.*
Betamethasone dipropionate (p.1093·1); betamethasone sodium phosphate (p.1093·1).
Lidocaine (p.1377·3) is included in some injections to alleviate the pain of injection.
*Corticosteroid.*

**Cronomet** *Merck Sharp & Dohme, Braz.*
Carbidopa (p.1204·3); levodopa (p.1205·2).
*Parkinsonism.*

**Cronopen** *Elea, Arg.*
Azithromycin (p.159·1).
*Bacterial infections.*

**Cronopen Balsamico** *Elea, Arg.*
Ampicillin sodium (p.157·1); ampicillin benzathine (p.158·1); dipyrone (p.35·3); guaifenesin (p.1122·1).
*Respiratory-tract infections.*

**Cronoplex** *Delta, Braz.*
Bisacodyl (p.1251·3); sodium picosulfate (p.1289·3).
*Constipation.*

**Cronovera**
*Pharmacia, Braz.; Searle, Mex.*
Verapamil hydrochloride (p.1019·1).
*Angina pectoris; arrhythmias; hypertension.*

**Crotamitex** *Gepepharm, Ger.*
Crotamiton (p.1145·1).
*Scabies.*

**Crotorax** *Sarabhai Piramal, India.*
Crotamiton (p.1145·1).
*Pediculosis; pruritus; scabies.*

**Crotorax-HC** *Sarabhai Piramal, India.*
Crotamiton (p.1145·1); hydrocortisone (p.1103·3).
*Pruritus.*

**Crowne** Master, Chile.
Potassium nitrate (p.1190·1).
*Hypersensitive teeth.*

**Crucial** Nestle, Fr.
Preparation for enteral nutrition (p.1417·1).

**Cruex**
Note. This name is used for preparations of different composition.
Novartis Consumer, Canad.†; Ciba Consumer, USA.
*Aerosol; cream:* Undecenoic acid (p.410·3); zinc undecenoate (p.411·1).
*Bromhidrosis; fungal skin infections; hyperhidrosis; minor skin irritation; nappy rash.*
*Topical powder:* Calcium undecenoate (p.410·3).
*Bromhidrosis; fungal skin infections; hyperhidrosis; minor skin irritation; nappy rash.*
Rhone-Poulenc Rorer, Mex.†.
Calcium undecenoate (p.410·3).

**Cruscasohn** Antonetto, Ital.
Cereal fibre; guar gum (p.333·2); pectin (p.1580·3).
*Constipation.*

**Crusken**
GlaxoSmithKline Consumer, Ital.; Sterling Midy, Ital.†.
A range of dietary fibre supplements (p.1253·2).
*Delayed gastrointestinal transit.*

**Cruzzy** SIT, Ital.
Bioallethrin (p.1500·3); piperonyl butoxide (p.1509·2).
*Pediculosis.*

**Cruzzy Antiparassitario** SIT, Ital.†.
Pyrethrum (p.1509·3); piperonyl butoxide (p.1509·2).
*Pediculosis.*

**Cruzzy Shampoo Potenziato alla Sumitrina**
SIT, Ital.
Phenothrin (p.1509·1).
*Pediculosis.*

**Cryobutol** Cryopharma, Mex.
Dobutamine hydrochloride (p.905·3).

**Cryocriptina** Cryopharma, Mex.
Bromocriptine (p.1202·3).
*Hyperprolactinaemia; lactation inhibition.*

**Cryogenine Plus** Andromaco, Chile.
Paracetamol (p.76·2).
*Fever; pain.*

**Cryogesic** Acorus, UK.
Ethyl chloride (p.1376·2).
*Local anaesthesia; testing of regional blockade; testing of tooth vitality.*

**Cryometasona** Cryopharma, Mex.
Dexamethasone (p.1097·1).
*Corticosteroid.*

**Cryoperacid** Cryopharma, Mex.
Loperamide hydrochloride (p.1271·1).
*Diarrhoea.*

**Cryopina** Cryopharma, Mex.
Hyoscine butylbromide (p.483·3).

**Cryopril** Cryopharma, Mex.
Captopril (p.879·2).
*Heart failure; hypertension.*

**Cryosolona** Cryopharma, Mex.
Methylprednisolone sodium succinate (p.1106·2).
*Corticosteroid.*

**Cryotol** Cryopharma, Mex.
Propofol (p.1305·3).
*General anaesthesia; sedative.*

**Cryo-Tropin** Cryopharma, Mex.
Somatropin (p.1327·2).
*Growth hormone deficiency; Turner's syndrome.*

**Cryoval** Cryopharma, Mex.†.
Valproic acid (p.380·1).
*Epilepsy.*

**Cryovin** Cryopharma, Mex.†.
Ergometrine (p.1684·2).

**Cryoxifeno** Pizzard, Mex.
Tamoxifen (p.585·3).

**Cryozol** Cryopharma, Mex.†.
Metronidazole (p.607·2).

**Cryptocur** Aventis, Neth.
Gonadorelin (p.1325·1).
*Cryptorchidism.*

**Crysanal** Roche, Austral.
Naproxen sodium (p.65·1).
*Inflammation; musculoskeletal and joint disorders; pain.*

**Cryselle** Barr, USA.
21 Tablets, ethinylestradiol (p.1553·2); norgestrel (p.1563·2); 7 tablets, inert.
*Combined oral contraceptive.*

**Crystacide**
Tramedico, Belg.; Bioglan, Ger.; Bioglan, Hong Kong; Bioglan, Irl.; Bioglan, Israel; Mipharm, Ital.; AFT, NZ; Celltech, Spain; Bioglan, UK.
Hydrogen peroxide (p.1182·2).
*Skin infections.*

**Crystacit** Be-Tabs, S.Afr.
Potassium citrate (p.1223·1); citric acid (p.1673·1).
*Urinary alkalinisation.*

**Crystal Clear**
ACS, Austral.; Douglas, NZ.
Pregnancy test (p.1734·3).

**Crystamine** Dunhall, USA.
Cyanocobalamin (p.1458·2).
*Schilling test; vitamin $B_{12}$ deficiency.*

**Crystapen**
Bioniche, Canad.; Britannia Pharmaceuticals, Irl.; Britannia Pharmaceuticals, UK.
Benzylpenicillin sodium (p.163·2).
*Bacterial infections.*

**Crysti 1000** Roberts, USA; Hauck, USA.
Cyanocobalamin (p.1458·2).
*Schilling test; vitamin $B_{12}$ deficiency.*

**Crysticillin** Apothecon, USA.
Procaine benzylpenicillin (p.246·1).
*Bacterial infections.*

**Crystodigin** Lilly, USA.
Digitoxin (p.894·3).
*Atrial flutter and fibrillation; heart failure; supraventricular tachycardia.*

**Crytion** Temis, Arg.
Sodium aurotiosulfate (p.90·1).
*Rheumatoid arthritis.*

**Crytioro** Drag, Chile.
Aurotiosulfate.

**C-Sik** Frankin, Hong Kong.
Cinnarizine (p.428·3); pyridoxine (p.1457·2).
*Motion sickness.*

**C-Soft** Austroflex, Austria.
Rinsing and storage solution for soft contact lenses (p.1164·2).

**C-Solve** Syosset, USA.
Vehicle for topical preparations.

**CST** Pose, Thai.
Clotrimazole (p.396·2).
*Fungal vaginal infections; trichomoniasis.*

**CT Ointment** Life, Israel.
Coal tar (p.1159·2); dead sea minerals.
*Psoriasis; seborrhoeic dermatitis.*

**CT Pommade** Life, Israel.
Coal tar (p.1159·2); salicylic acid (p.1157·1); dead sea minerals.
*Psoriasis of the scalp.*

**CT Shampoo** Life, Israel.
Coal tar (p.1159·2); tar (p.1159·3); cade oil (p.1159·2); dead sea minerals.
*Psoriasis; seborrhoeic dermatitis.*

**C-Tabs** Ferrosan, Fin.
Ascorbic acid (p.1460·2).
*Dietary supplement; vitamin C deficiency.*

**C-Tanna 12D** Prasco, USA.
Pentoxyverine tannate (p.1126·3); mepyramine tannate (p.437·1); phenylephrine tannate (p.1127·2).
*Upper respiratory-tract disorders.*

**C-Tard** Whitehall, Ital.
Ascorbic acid (p.1460·2).
*Adjunct in stomatitis and gingivitis; vitamin C deficiency.*

**C-Tron Calcium** Mavena, Switz.
Vitamin C and D preparation with calcium (p.1417·1).
*Cold symptoms; tonic.*

**C/T/S** Hoechst Marion Roussel, USA†.
Clindamycin phosphate (p.194·2).
*Acne.*

**Cuadel** Cetus, Arg.
Diazepam (p.690·1).
*Anxiety; muscle spasm.*

**Cuait D** Ariston, Arg.
Trifluoperazine hydrochloride (p.726·3); tranylcypromine sulfate (p.318·3).
*Depression.*

**Cuait N** Ariston, Arg.
Trifluoperazine hydrochloride (p.726·3); amobarbital (p.670·1).
*Insomnia.*

**Cuantil** Teva Tuteur, Arg.
Ifosfamide (p.561·1).
*Malignant neoplasms.*

**Cuatroderm** Schering-Plough, Spain.
Betamethasone valerate (p.1093·2); clioquinol (p.196·3); gentamicin sulfate (p.217·1); tolnaftate (p.410·1).
*Infected skin disorders.*

**Cuatroepi** Varifarma, Arg.
Epirubicin (p.550·3).
*Malignant neoplasms.*

**Cuatromin** Grunenthal, Chile.
Vitamin preparation (p.1417·1).

**Cubicin** Cubist, USA.
Daptomycin (p.204·2).
*Bacterial skin and skin structure infections.*

**Cubison**
Nutricia, Austral.; Nutricia, Port.
Preparation for enteral nutrition (p.1417·1).
*Dietary management of chronic wounds.*

**Cubitan**
Nutricia, Austral.; Support, Braz.; Nutricia, Fin.; Nutricia, Fr.† Nutricia, Irl.; Nutricia, Ital.; Nutricia, Port.
Nutritional supplement (p.1417·1).
*Pressure sores.*

**Cucurbita Compuesta** Hochstetter, Chile.
Homoeopathic preparation.

**Cuerpo Amarillo Fuerte** Hormona, Mex.
Progesterone (p.1566·2).

**Cuidaderma** Caldeira & Marques, Port.
Zinc oxide (p.1163·2); almond oil (p.1651·1); starch (p.1449·1); talc (p.1159·1).
*Skin irritation.*

**Culat** Roche, Austria.
Epoetin beta (p.747·2).
*Anaemia of prematurity, chronic renal failure or malignant disease; autologous blood transfusions.*

**Cullens Headache Powders** Cullen & Davison, UK.
Aspirin (p.15·1); caffeine (p.782·1).

**Cultivo BCG** Lemery, Mex.
BCG vaccine (p.1609·2).
*Bladder cancer.*

**Culture Care** Lifeplan, UK.
*Lactobacillus acidophilus* (p.1704·2); *Lactobacillus casei*; *Lactococcus lactis* (p.1704·2); *Bifidobacteria bifidum* (p.1704·2); fructo-oligosaccharides.
*Maintenance of normal gastrointestinal flora.*

**Culturelle LCG** Nordic, UK†.
Lactobacillus GG (p.1704·2).
*Maintenance of healthy gastrointestinal flora.*

**Cumatil L** Bayer, Arg.
Phenytoin (p.370·2); methylphenobarbital (p.366·3); phenobarbital (p.367·3).
*Epilepsy.*

**Cunesin** Recordati, Spain.
Ciprofloxacin hydrochloride (p.188·2).
*Bacterial infections.*

**Cunil** Helsinn Birex, Irl.†.
Ibuprofen (p.45·3).
*Musculoskeletal, joint, and peri-articular disorders; pain; soft-tissue injuries.*

**CuNova T** Leiras, Denm.†.
Copper-wound plastic (p.1425·3) with a silver core (p.1746·1).
*Intra-uterine contraceptive device.*

**Cunticina** Warner-Lambert, Spain†.
Albumin tannate (p.1248·1).
*Diarrhoea.*

**Cupanol** Dermofarm, Spain.
Paracetamol (p.76·2).
*Fever; pain.*

**Cuplaton**
Orion, Fin.; Orion, Malaysia; Orion, Singapore.
Dimeticone (p.1289·2).
*Aid in gastrointestinal radiography and gastroscopy; flatulence; meteorism.*

**Cuplex**
Trans Canaderm, Canad.†; Smith & Nephew, Irl.; Crawford, UK.
Salicylic acid (p.1157·1); lactic acid (p.1704·1).
*Calluses; corns; warts.*

**Cupressin**
Takeda, Malaysia; Takeda, Singapore; Takeda, Thai.
Delapril hydrochloride (p.892·2).
*Hypertension.*

**Cupridium** DHU, Ger.
Homoeopathic preparation.

**Cuprifusin** Pisa, Mex.
Copper sulfate (p.1426·1).

**Cuprimine**
Sidus, Arg.; Prodome, Braz.; Merck Frosst, Canad.; Merck Sharp & Dohme, Hong Kong; Merck Sharp & Dohme, Israel; Merck Sharp & Dohme, Neth.†; Merck Sharp & Dohme, Norw.; Merck Sharp & Dohme, Swed.†; Merck Sharp & Dohme, Thai.; Merck, USA.
Penicillamine (p.1046·3).
*Cystinuria; heavy metal poisoning; rheumatoid arthritis; Wilson's disease.*

**Cupripen**
Omedir, Arg.; Rubio, Spain.
Penicillamine (p.1046·3).
*Cystinuria; heavy-metal poisoning; rheumatoid arthritis; Wilson's disease.*

**Cuprocept CCL** Cuprocept, S.Afr.
Copper-wound plastic (p.1425·3).
*Intra-uterine contraceptive device.*

**Cuprofen** SSL, UK.
Ibuprofen (p.45·3).
*Cold and influenza symptoms; fever; inflammation; pain.*

**Cuprofen Plus** SSL, UK.
Ibuprofen (p.45·3); codeine phosphate (p.27·1).
*Pain.*

**Cuprosodio** Bier, Ital.
Cetrimide (p.1172·1); copper sulfate (p.1426·1); zinc sulfate (p.1469·3).
*Personal hygiene.*

**Cuprosodio Plus** Bier, Ital.
Chlorhexidine gluconate (p.1173·2); copper sulfate (p.1426·1); zinc sulfate (p.1469·3).
*Genital hygiene.*

**Cura** Arnaldi-Uscio, Ital.†.
*Tablets (500 mg):* Aloes (p.1248·2); senna (p.1288·2); althaea (p.1651·3); liquorice (p.1270·2); ferrous sulfate (p.1428·2); vegetable charcoal (p.1030·3).
*Tablets (1 g); oral powder:* Melissa (p.1711·1); cascarilla; quassia (p.1737·2); senna (p.1288·2); ginger (p.1267·1); aloes (p.1248·2); althaea (p.1651·3); laurel; myrtle; bergamot oil (p.1659·3).
*Constipation.*

**Curacid** Finadiet, Arg.
Fatty acid glycerides; fatty acid triglycerides; vitamin A; vitamin D.
*Haemorrhoids; skin disorders; vaginal disorders.*

**Curacit** Nycomed, Norw.
Suxamethonium chloride (p.1406·2).
*Depolarising neuromuscular blocker.*

**Curacleanse** Curacel, Austral.
Cetrimide (p.1172·1); chlorhexidine gluconate (p.1173·2).
*Skin and wound disinfection.*

**Curacne** Pierre Fabre, Fr.
Isotretinoin (p.1148·3).
*Acne.*

**Curadent** Leti, Spain†.
Lidocaine hydrochloride (p.1377·3).
*Local anaesthesia in dentistry.*

**Curaderm** Curacel, Austral.
Salicylic acid (p.1157·1); urea (p.1162·2); melaleuca oil (p.1710·2); linolenic acid; solasodine glycosides.
*Solar keratoses; sunspots.*

**Curadon** Tika, Swed.
Paracetamol (p.76·2).
*Fever; pain.*

**Curadona** Lainco, Spain.
Povidone-iodine (p.1190·3).
*Skin disinfection.*

**Curafil** Betamadrileno, Spain.
Chlorhexidine gluconate (p.1173·2).
*Skin and wound disinfection.*

**Curakalos** Stevia, Braz.†.
Salicylic acid (p.1157·1).
*Keratinisation disorders.*

**Curam**
Biochemie, Austria.
Amoxicillin trihydrate (p.155·3); potassium clavulanate (p.193·3).
*Bacterial infections.*
Biochemie, Hong Kong; Biochemie, Malaysia; Biochemie, Singapore; Biochemie, Thai.; Novartis, Thai.
Amoxicillin (p.155·3); clavulanic acid (p.193·3).
*Bacterial infections.*

**Curandron** Schering, Austria.
Cyproterone acetate (p.1544·1).
*Androgen-induced hirsutism, alopecia, acne, and seborrhoea in females; prostatic cancer.*

**Curantyl N** Berlin-Chemie, Ger.
Dipyridamole (p.903·1).
*Thrombosis prophylaxis.*

**Curapic** Leti, Spain†.
Diphenhydramine hydrochloride (p.431·3); lidocaine hydrochloride (p.1377·3).
*Insect stings; pruritus.*

**Curarina Miro** Palex, Spain†.
Tubocurarine chloride (p.1409·2).
*Competitive neuromuscular blocker.*

**Curarine** Taro, Israel.
Tubocurarine chloride (p.1409·2).
*Competitive neuromuscular blocker.*

**Curash Anti-Rash** Carter-Wallace, Austral.
Zinc oxide (p.1163·2).
*Hyperhidrosis; nappy rash; skin irritation.*

**Curash Baby Wipes** Carter-Wallace, Austral.†.
Vitamin E (p.1464·3); sorbolene.
*Skin cleanser and moisturiser.*

**Curash Babycare** Carter-Wallace, Austral.
*dl*-Alpha tocoferil acetate (p.1465·1); zinc oxide (p.1163·2); almond oil (p.1651·1).
*Nappy rash.*

**Curash Medicated** Carter-Wallace, Austral.†.
Zinc oxide (p.1163·2).
*Skin irritation.*

**Curastatin** Curamed, Austria.
Somatostatin acetate (p.1339·3).
*Gastrointestinal haemorrhage; prevention of postoperative complications following pancreatic surgery.*

**Curasten** Therabel, Fr.
Lysine hydrochloride (p.1439·2); calcium gluceptate (p.1225·2).
*Asthenia.*

**Curatane** Douglas, Israel.
Isotretinoin (p.1148·3).
*Acne.*

**Curatin**
Note. This name is used for preparations of different composition.
Carter-Wallace, Austral.†.
Tolnaftate (p.410·1).
*Fungal skin infections.*
Sanova, Austria.
Biotin (p.1423·2).
*Hair and nail disorders.*

**Curativ** Hexal, Braz.†.
Thiomersal (p.1194·1).
*Skin and wound disinfection; skin disorders.*

**Curatoderm**
Hermal, Austria; Boots Healthcare, Belg.; Hermal, Ger.; Hermal, Israel; Boots Healthcare, Switz.; Crookes Healthcare, UK.
Tacalcitol (p.1158·3).
*Psoriasis.*

**Curaven** Boehringer Ingelheim, Ital.
Aesculus (p.1648·2).
*Peripheral vascular disorders.*

**Curazink** Redino, Ger.
Zinc histidinate (p.1469·3).
*Zinc deficiency.*

**Curban** Rafarm, Gr.
Nimodipine (p.972·3).
*Neurological deficit following subarachnoid haemorrhage.*

**Curcumen** Temmler, Ger.
Javanese turmeric (p.1759·3).
*Dyspepsia.*

**Curcu-Truw** Truw, Ger.
Javanese turmeric (p.1759·3).
*Dyspepsia.*

**Curel** *Jergens, Canad.; Bausch & Lomb, USA.*
Emollient and moisturiser.

**Curethyl** *AJC, Fr.†.*
Alcohol (p.1166·1).
*Alcohol withdrawal syndromes.*

**Curine** *Leti, Spain.*
Benzalkonium chloride (p.1168·3); lidocaine hydrochloride (p.1377·3).
*Pain; pruritus.*

**Curinflam** *Duncan, Arg.*
Diclofenac (p.32·1) or diclofenac diethylamine (p.32·1).
*Inflammation; pain.*

**Curisept** *Excelentia, Arg.*
Piroxoline; hydroxyquinoline (p.1700·1).
*Wounds.*

**Curlem** *Lemery, Mex.*
Vecuronium bromide (p.1409·3).
*Competitive neuromuscular blocker.*

**Curocef**
*GlaxoSmithKline, Austria; GlaxoSmithKline, Chile.*
Cefuroxime axetil (p.184·1) or cefuroxime sodium (p.182·3).
*Bacterial infections.*

**Curol** *Kwizda, Austria.*
Rhatany (p.1738·1); salix bark (p.87·3).
*Mouth and throat disorders.*

**Curon-B** *Intramed, S.Afr.†.*
Pancuronium bromide (p.1404·3).
*Competitive neuromuscular blocker.*

**Curosurf**
*Serono, Austria; Nycomed, Austria; Farmalab, Braz.; Nycomed, Denm.; Nycomed, Fin.; Chiesi, Fr.; Nycomed, Ger.; Serono, Irl.; SLE, Israel; Chiesi, Ital.; Serono, Neth.; Nycomed, Norw.; Serono, Port.†; Safeline, S.Afr.; Chiesi, Spain; Nycomed, Swed.; Nycomed, Switz.; Trinity, UK; Dey, USA.*
Poractant alfa (p.1736·2).
*Neonatal respiratory distress syndrome.*

**Curoveinyl** *Pharmygiene, Fr.†.*
Aesculus (p.1648·2); hamamelis (p.1696·3); hydrastis (p.1698·3); cupressus sempervirens; scoparium (p.1742·2); nux vomica (p.1722·3).
*Peripheral vascular disorders.*

**Curoxim** *GlaxoSmithKline, Ital.*
Cefuroxime sodium (p.184·1).
*Gram-negative bacterial infections.*

**Curoxima** *GlaxoSmithKline, Spain.*
Cefuroxime sodium (p.184·1).
*Bacterial infections.*

**Curoxime** *Glaxo Wellcome, Port.*
Cefuroxime sodium (p.184·1).
*Bacterial infections.*

**Curpol** *Pfizer Consumer, Belg.*
Paracetamol (p.76·2).
*Fever; pain.*

**Curyken** *Kendrick, Mex.*
Loratadine (p.436·1).
*Allergic rhinitis; pruritus; urticaria.*

**Cusate** *Pharmasant, Thai.*
Docusate sodium (p.1262·2).
*Constipation.*

**Cuscutine** *Geymonat, Ital.*
Senna (p.1288·2); aloin (p.1248·3).
*Constipation.*

**Cusicrom**
*Alcon, Hong Kong†; Alcon Cusi, Malaysia; Kener, Mex.†; Alcon, Port.; Cusi, Singapore†; Alcon Cusi, Spain.*
Sodium cromoglicate (p.795·3).
*Allergic eye disorders; allergic rhinitis; hay fever.*

**Cusigel** *Farmacusi, Spain†.*
Fluocinonide (p.1101·3).
*Skin disorders.*

**Cusimolol**
*Alcon, Hong Kong†; Alcon, Ital.; Alcon Cusi, Malaysia; Kener, Mex.†; Alcon, Port.; Alcon Cusi, Spain.*
Timolol maleate (p.1012·2).
*Glaucoma; ocular hypertension.*

**Cusiter** *Cusi, Spain†.*
Lactic acid (p.1704·1); triclocarban (p.1195·1).
*Skin disinfection.*

**Cusiviral**
*Alcon, Hong Kong; Alcon Cusi, Malaysia; Cusi, Singapore; Alcon Cusi, Spain†.*
Aciclovir (p.626·1).
*Herpes simplex keratitis.*

**Custey** *Microsules, Arg.*
Loperamide hydrochloride (p.1271·1).
*Diarrhoea.*

**Custodial** *Schwabe, Arg.*
Paracetamol (p.76·2).
*Fever; pain.*

**Custodiol**
*Kohler, Austria; Tramedico, Belg.; Kohler, Ger.*
Organ perfusion solution (p.1217·1).

**Customed** *Chefaro, Ger.†.*
Bromhexine hydrochloride (p.1115·3); thymol (p.1194·2).
*Coughs; respiratory-tract disorders; sinusitis.*

**Custoplex** *Biogam, Arg.*
Organ perfusion solution (p.1217·1).

**Cutacelan**
*Schering, Arg.; Schering, Mex.*
Azelaic acid (p.1142·3).
*Acne.*

**Cutaclin** *ICN, Mex.*
Clindamycin phosphate (p.194·2).
*Acne; pyodermas.*

**Cutacnyl** *Galderma, Fr.*
Benzoyl peroxide (p.1143·2).
*Acne.*

**Cutaderm** *Schering-Plough, S.Afr.*
Hydrocortisone (p.1103·3).
*Skin disorders.*

**Cutanil** *ITF, Chile.*
Clotrimazole (p.396·2); zinc oxide (p.1163·2).
*Fungal skin infections.*

**Cutaninfant** *Rubiepharm, Ger.*
Zinc oxide (p.1163·2).
*Skin disorders.*

**Cutanit** *Yamanouchi, Spain.*
Fluclorolone acetonide (p.1100·1).
*Skin disorders.*

**Cutanplast** *Mascia Brunelli, Ital.*
Gelatin (p.754·3).
*Haemostasis.*

**Cutanum** *Jenapharm, Ger.*
Estradiol (p.1550·1).
*Menopausal disorders.*

**Cutar** *Summers, USA†.*
Coal tar (p.1159·2).
*Skin disorders.*

**Cutasept**
*Beiersdorf, Austria; Bode, Ger.; Beiersdorf, Switz.*
Isopropyl alcohol (p.1184·3); benzalkonium chloride (p.1168·3).
*Skin disinfection.*

**Cutemol** *Summers, USA.*
Emollient and moisturiser.

**Cutemul** *Medopharm, Ger.†.*
Dexpanthenol (p.1727·2).
*Burns; inflammatory skin disorders; wounds.*

**Cuteral** *Panalab, Arg.*
Budesonide (p.1094·2).
*Skin disorders.*

**Cuterpes**
*Chauvin, Fr.; Chauvin, Hong Kong†.*
Ibacitabine (p.637·3).
*Herpes simplex infections.*

**Cuticura**
*Note. This name is used for preparations of different composition.*
*Novartis Consumer, S.Afr.*
Hydroxyquinoline (p.1700·1); sulfur (p.1158·2); phenol (p.1188·1).

*DEP, USA.*
Triclocarban (p.1195·1).
*Skin cleanser.*

**Cutiderm** *Prodotti, Braz.*
Bacitracin (p.161·3); neomycin sulfate (p.235·1).
*Skin infections.*

**Cutidermin** *Phoenix, Arg.*
Resorcinol (p.1156·3); bismuth salicylate (p.1252·1).
*Skin disorders.*

**Cuti-Do** *Grasler, Ger.*
Homoeopathic preparation.

**Cutifitol** *Llorente, Spain†.*
Progesterone (p.1566·2).
*Hair, scalp, and skin disorders.*

**Cutimian** *Bioharm, Spain†.*
Flutrimazole (p.400·3).
*Tinea pedis.*

**Cutimix** *Metochem, Austria.*
Zinc oxide (p.1163·2); talc (p.1159·1).
*Skin disorders.*

**Cutinova** *Smith & Nephew Healthcare, UK.*
Polyurethane foam dressing.
*Burns; ulcers; wounds.*

**Cutinova Alginate** *Smith & Nephew, Ital.*
Calcium alginate (p.745·1).
*Wounds.*

**Cutiphile** *Braun, Fr.*
Bismuth subgallate (p.1252·2); bismuth subnitrate (p.1252·2); zinc oxide (p.1163·2).
*Skin disorders.*

**Cutisan** *Boots Healthcare, Fr.*
Triclocarban (p.1195·1).
*Skin disorders.*

**Cutisanol** *Millet Roux, Braz.*
*Ointment:* Magnesium silicate (p.1580·2); thymol iodide (p.1194·3); zinc oxide (p.1163·2); bismuth subgallate (p.1252·2).
*Topical gel:* Zinc oxide (p.1163·2); bismuth subgallate (p.1252·2).
*Skin disorders.*

**cutistad**
*Stada, Ger.; Helvepharm, Switz.†.*
Clotrimazole (p.396·2).
*Fungal skin infections.*

**Cutivat** *GlaxoSmithKline, Denm.*
Fluticasone propionate (p.1102·3).
*Skin disorders.*

**Cutivate**
*GlaxoSmithKline, Arg.; GlaxoSmithKline, Austria; GlaxoSmithKline, Belg.; GlaxoSmithKline, Hong Kong; GlaxoSmithKline, Israel; GlaxoSmithKline, Malaysia; Glaxo Wellcome, Mex.; GlaxoSmithKline, Neth.; Glaxo Wellcome, Port.; GlaxoSmithKline, S.Afr.; GlaxoSmithKline, Singapore; Glaxo Wellcome, Spain†; GlaxoSmithKline, Switz.; GlaxoSmithKline, UK; Glaxo Wellcome, USA.*
Fluticasone propionate (p.1102·3).
*Skin disorders.*

**Cuvalit** *Schering, Ger.*
Lisuride maleate (p.1210·3).
*Migraine.*

**Cuvefilm** *Perez Gimenez, Spain.*
Chlorhexidine gluconate (p.1173·2).
*Skin and wound disinfection.*

**Cuxabrain** *TAD, Ger.*
Piracetam (p.1732·1).
*Mental function disorders.*

**Cuxafenon** *TAD, Ger.*
Propafenone hydrochloride (p.988·3).
*Arrhythmias.*

**Cuxanorm** *TAD, Ger.*
Atenolol (p.865·2).
*Arrhythmias; hypertension; ischaemic heart disease.*

**C-vimin**
*AstraZeneca, Fin.; Astra, Swed.*
Ascorbic acid (p.1460·2).
*Vitamin C deficiency.*

**C-Vit** *Novartis Consumer, Austria.*
Ascorbic acid (p.1460·2).
*Vitamin C deficiency.*

**CVP**
*Sterling, India; Rhone-Poulenc Rorer, Ital.†.*
Bioflavonoids (p.1688·2); ascorbic acid (p.1460·2).
*Capillary fragility; gingivitis; stomatitis; vitamin C deficiency.*

**CVP B1 B6 B12** *Phoenix, Arg.*
Vitamin $B_1$ (p.1455·1); vitamin $B_6$ (p.1456·3); vitamin $B_{12}$ (p.1458·2); vitamin C (p.1460·2); bioflavonoids (p.1688·2).
*Capillary disorders; neuralgias; neuritis; vitamin B and C supplement.*

**CVP Duo** *Phoenix, Arg.*
Bioflavonoids (p.1688·2); ascorbic acid (p.1460·2).
*Vascular disorders.*

**CVP Flebo** *Phoenix, Arg.*
Ruscus aculeatus; hesperidin methyl chalcone (p.1688·3); ascorbic acid (p.1460·2).
*Haemorrhoids; varices.*

**CVP Forte** *Phoenix, Arg.*
Ascorbic acid (p.1460·2); bioflavonoids (p.1688·2).
*Arteriopathy; phlebopathy.*

**C-Will**
*Will-Pharma, Belg.; Will-Pharma, Neth.; Willpharma, Thai.; SPB, Thai.*
Ascorbic acid (p.1460·2).
*Vitamin C deficiency.*

**Cx-3** *Cadila, India.*
Rifampicin (p.250·2); isoniazid (p.222·2); vitamin $B_6$ (p.1457·2).
*Tuberculosis.*

**Cx-4** *Cadila, India.*
1 Tablet, rifampicin (p.250·2); isoniazid (p.222·2); vitamin $B_6$ (p.1457·2); 1 tablet ethambutol (p.212·2).
*Tuberculosis.*

**Cx-5** *Cadila, India.*
1 Capsule, rifampicin (p.250·2); 2 tablets, pyrazinamide (p.246·3); 1 tablet, ethambutol (p.212·2); isoniazid (p.222·2); vitamin $B_6$ (p.1457·2).
*Tuberculosis.*

**CX Powder** *Adams, UK.*
Chlorhexidine acetate (p.1173·2).
*Skin disinfection.*

**Cyanide Antidote Package** *Lilly, USA.*
*Combination pack:* 2 Ampoules, sodium nitrite (p.1052·3); 2 ampoules, sodium thiosulfate (p.1053·3); 12 aspirols, amyl nitrite (p.1032·1).
*Cyanide poisoning.*

**Cyanoject** *Mayrand, USA†.*
Cyanocobalamin (p.1458·2).
*Schilling test; vitamin $B_{12}$ deficiency.*

**Cyanokit**
*Lipha Sante, Fr.; Merck-Lipha, Hong Kong.*
Hydroxocobalamin (p.1458·2).
*Cyanide poisoning.*

**Cyater** *Sigma-Tau, Spain.*
Terfenadine (p.441·1).
*Hypersensitivity reactions.*

**Cybutol** *Pharmachemie, S.Afr.; Rolab, S.Afr.*
Salbutamol sulfate (p.791·3).
*Obstructive airways disease.*

**Cycin** *Dong, Singapore.*
Ciprofloxacin hydrochloride (p.188·2).
*Bacterial infections.*

**Cyclabil**
*Schering, Fin.; Schering, Norw.; Schering, Swed.*
11 Tablets, estradiol valerate (p.1550·2); 10 tablets, estradiol valerate; levonorgestrel (p.1563·2).
*Menopausal disorders; menstrual disorders; osteoporosis.*

**Cyclacur**
*Schering, Austria; Shepa, Gr.; Schering, Switz.*
11 Tablets, estradiol valerate (p.1550·2); 10 tablets, estradiol valerate; norgestrel (p.1563·2).
*Menopausal disorders; menstrual disorders.*

**Cycladol**
*Chiesi, Fr.; Chiesi, Spain.*
Piroxicam betadex (p.84·2).
*Gout; musculoskeletal, joint, and peri-articular disorders; pain.*

**Cyclafem** *Dolisos, Canad.†.*
Homoeopathic preparation.

**Cyclan** *BPL-Meizler, Braz.*
Cyclophosphamide (p.540·2).
*Malignant neoplasms.*

**Cycleane** *Organon, Fr.*
Desogestrel (p.1547·2); ethinylestradiol (p.1553·2).
*Combined oral contraceptive.*

**Cyclen** *Janssen-Ortho, Canad.*
Norgestimate (p.1563·2); ethinylestradiol (p.1553·2).
28-Day packs also contain 7 inert tablets.
*Combined oral contraceptive.*

**Cyclergine** *Poirier, Fr.*
Cyclandelate (p.890·3).
*Peripheral vascular disorders.*

**Cyclessa** *Organon, USA.*
21 Tablets, desogestrel (p.1547·2); ethinylestradiol (p.1553·2); 7 tablets, inert.
*Triphasic oral contraceptive.*

**Cyclidox** *Triomed, S.Afr.*
Doxycycline hyclate (p.206·2).
*Bacterial infections.*

**Cyclimorph**
*Calmic, Irl.; GlaxoSmithKline, S.Afr.; CeNeS, UK.*
Morphine tartrate (p.60·3); cyclizine tartrate (p.429·3).
*Pain.*

**Cyclimycin** *Aspen, S.Afr.*
Minocycline (p.231·3).
*Bacterial infections.*

**Cyclinex** *Ross, USA.*
A range of preparations for enteral nutrition including an infant feed (p.1417·1).
*Gyrate atrophy; urea cycle disorder.*

**Cyclivex** *Aspen, S.Afr.*
Aciclovir (p.626·1).
*Herpesvirus infections.*

**Cyclo 3**
*Note. This name is used for preparations of different composition.*
*Casasco, Arg.; Pierre Fabre, Port.*
Ruscus aculeatus; hesperidin methyl chalcone (p.1688·3); ascorbic acid (p.1460·2).
*Haemorrhoids; metrorrhagia; venous insufficiency.*

*Pierre Fabre, Fr.; Pierre Fabre, Singapore.*
Ruscus aculeatus; melilot.
*Circulatory disorders.*

**Cyclo 3 Fort**
*Pierre Fabre, Fr.; Pierre Fabre, Singapore; Pierre Fabre, Thai.*
Ruscus aculeatus; hesperidin methyl chalcone (p.1688·3); vitamin C (p.1460·2).
*Bleeding during oral contraceptive or intra-uterine device use; circulatory disorders; haemorrhoids.*

**Cyclobiol** *Yves Ponroy, Fr.†.*
Nutritional supplement (p.1417·1).
*Premenstrual syndrome.*

**Cycloblastin**
*Pharmacia, Austral.; Pharmacia, NZ; Pharmacia, S.Afr.*
Cyclophosphamide (p.540·2).
*Auto-immune diseases; malignant neoplasms; transplant rejection.*

**Cycloblastine** *Pharmacia Upjohn, Belg.†.*
Cyclophosphamide (p.540·2).
*Malignant neoplasms.*

**Cyclo-cell** *Cell Pharm, Ger.†.*
Cyclophosphamide (p.540·2).
*Malignant neoplasms.*

**Cyclocort**
*Stiefel, Canad.; Fujisawa, USA.*
Amcinonide (p.1091·1).
*Skin disorders.*

**Cyclocur**
*Schering, Belg.; Schering, Neth.*
11 Tablets, estradiol valerate (p.1550·2); 10 tablets, estradiol valerate; norgestrel (p.1563·2).
*Hormone replacement therapy; menopausal disorders; menstrual disorders.*

**Cycloderm** *CSC, Austria.*
Estradiol (p.1550·1).
*Menopausal disorders; osteoporosis.*

**Cyclodox** *Berk, UK†.*
Doxycycline (p.206·2).
*Bacterial infections.*

**Cyclofem** *Master, Chile.*
Medroxyprogesterone acetate (p.1557·2); estradiol cipionate (p.1550·1).
*Combined injectable contraceptive.*

**Cyclofemina**
*Millet Roux, Braz.; Carnot, Mex.*
Estradiol cipionate (p.1550·1); medroxyprogesterone acetate (p.1557·2).
*Injectable contraceptive.*

**Cyclogest**
*Cox, Hong Kong; Aventis, S.Afr.; Alpharma, Singapore; Aventis, Thai.; Alpharma, UK.*
Progesterone (p.1566·2).
*Female infertility; premenstrual syndrome; puerperal depression.*

**Cyclogyl**
*Alcon, Austral.; Alcon, Canad.; Alcon, Chile; Alcon, Denm.; Alkon (Αλκον), Gr.; Alcon, Hong Kong; Andre, India; Alcon, Malaysia; Alcon, NZ; Alcon, S.Afr.; Alcon, Singapore; Alcon, Swed.; Alcon, Switz.; Alcon, Thai.; Alcon, USA.*
Cyclopentolate hydrochloride (p.480·3).
*Production of mydriasis and cycloplegia.*

**Cyclomandol** *Yamanouchi, Swed.*
Cyclandelate (p.890·3).
*Vascular disorders.*

**Cyclomed** *Medibrands, Israel.*
Aciclovir (p.626·1).
*Herpes simplex infections.*

**Cyclo-Meff** *Indoco, India.*
Mefenamic acid (p.55·2); dicycloverine hydrochloride (p.481·2).
*Smooth muscle spasm.*

**Cyclomen** *Sanofi Synthelabo, Canad.*
Danazol (p.1545·2).
*Endometriosis; mastalgia; primary menorrhagia.*

**Cyclo-Menorette** *Wyeth, Ger.*
11 Tablets, estradiol valerate (p.1550·2); estriol (p.1552·3); 10 tablets, estradiol valerate; estriol; levonorgestrel (p.1563·2).
*Menopausal disorders; osteoporosis.*

**Cyclominol** *Noel, India.*
Dicycloverine hydrochloride (p.481·2).
*Colic; gastrointestinal spasm; irritable bowel syndrome; peptic ulcer.*

**Cyclomydril**
*Alcon, Malaysia; Alcon, S.Afr.; Alcon, Singapore; Alcon, USA.*
Cyclopentolate hydrochloride (p.480·3); phenylephrine hydrochloride (p.1126·3).
*Production of mydriasis.*

**CycloOstrogynal** *Asche, Ger.*
11 Tablets, estradiol valerate (p.1550·2); estriol (p.1552·3); 10 tablets, estradiol valerate; estriol; levonorgestrel (p.1563·2).
*Menopausal disorders.*

**Cyclopam** *Indoco, India.*
*Injection:* Dicycloverine hydrochloride (p.481·2).
*Oral suspension; oral drops:* Dicycloverine hydrochloride (p.481·2); dimeticone (p.1289·2).
*Tablets:* Dicycloverine hydrochloride (p.481·2); paracetamol (p.76·2).
*Colic; dysmenorrhoea; irritable bowel syndrome.*

**Cyclopentol** *Viatris, Belg.*
Cyclopentolate hydrochloride (p.480·3).
*Prevention of iridocrystalline adherences; prevention of synechiae; production of mydriasis and cycloplegia.*

**CycloPolar** *Orion, Ger.†.*
White tablets, estradiol valerate (p.1550·2); blue tablets, estradiol valerate; medroxyprogesterone acetate (p.1557·2).

**Cyclo-Premarin-MPA** *Wyeth Lederle, Austria†.*
Redbrown tablets, conjugated oestrogens (p.1543·2); blue tablets, conjugated oestrogens; medroxyprogesterone acetate (p.1557·2).
*Menopausal disorders.*

**Cyclo-Premella** *Wyeth, Switz.†.*
28 Tablets, conjugated oestrogens (p.1543·2); 14 tablets medroxyprogesterone acetate (p.1557·2).
*Menopausal disorders; oestrogen deficiency.*

**Cyclo-Premella ST** *Wyeth, Switz.*
14 Tablets, conjugated oestrogens (p.1543·2); 14 tablets, conjugated oestrogens; medroxyprogesterone acetate (p.1557·2).
*Menopausal disorders; oestrogen deficiency.*

**Cyclo-Progynon** *Schering, Denm.*
11 Tablets, estradiol valerate (p.1550·2); 10 tablets, estradiol valerate; levonorgestrel (p.1563·2).
*Menopausal disorders; osteoporosis.*

**Cyclo-Progynova**
*Schering, Ger.; Schering, Thai.*
11 Tablets, estradiol valerate (p.1550·2); 10 tablets, estradiol valerate; norgestrel (p.1563·2).
*Menopausal disorders; menstrual disorders; osteoporosis.*

**Cyclo-Progynova 1 mg** *Viatris, UK.*
11 Tablets, estradiol valerate (p.1550·2); 10 tablets, estradiol valerate; levonorgestrel (p.1563·2).
*Menopausal disorders.*

**Cyclo-Progynova 2 mg** *Viatris, UK.*
11 Tablets, estradiol valerate (p.1550·2); 10 tablets, estradiol valerate; norgestrel (p.1563·2).
*Menopausal disorders.*

**Cyclorax**
*Atlantic, Hong Kong; Atlantic, Thai.*
Aciclovir (p.626·1).
*Herpes simplex infections of the skin and mucous membranes.*

**Cyclorel** *Alpharma, Fr.*
Naringin sodium.
*Circulatory disorders.*

**Cyclorine** *Lupin, India.*
Cycloserine (p.202·1).
*Tuberculosis.*

**Cyclosa** *Nourypharma, Ger.*
7 Tablets, ethinylestradiol (p.1553·2); 15 tablets, ethinylestradiol; desogestrel (p.1547·2).
*Menstrual disorders.*

**Cycloserine** *King, UK.*
Cycloserine (p.202·1).
*Tuberculosis; urinary-tract infections.*

**Cycloson** *Pharmachemie, S.Afr.; Rolab, S.Afr.*
Beclometasone dipropionate (p.1091·1).
*Asthma.*

**Cyclospasmol**
*Yamanouchi, Belg.; Wyeth-Ayerst, Canad.†; Yamanouchi, Fin.; Yamanouchi, Fr.†; Yamanouchi, Port.*
Cyclandelate (p.890·3).
*Peripheral and cerebral vascular disorders.*

**Cyclostin** *Pharmacia, Ger.*
Cyclophosphamide (p.540·2).
*Malignant neoplasms.*

**Cycloteriam** *Roussel Diamant, Fr.†.*
Triamterene (p.1016·2); cyclothiazide (p.891·1).
*Hypertension; oedema.*

**Cyclovax**
*Remedica, Hong Kong; Raza, Malaysia; Pharmaniaga, Malaysia.*
Aciclovir (p.626·1).
*Herpesvirus infections.*

**Cycloven Forte N** *CT, Ger.*
Aesculus (p.1648·2); esculoside (p.1648·2); rutoside (p.1688·2).
*Peripheral vascular disorders; venous insufficiency.*

**Cyclovir**
*Medichrom, Gr.; Cadila, India.*
Aciclovir (p.626·1).
*Herpesvirus infections.*

**Cycloviran**
*Medichrom, Gr.; Sigma-Tau, Ital.*
Aciclovir (p.626·1).
*Herpesvirus infections.*

**Cycloxan** *Biochem, India.*
Cyclophosphamide (p.540·2).
*Immunosuppressant; malignant neoplasms.*

**Cycofed** *Cypress, USA.*
Codeine phosphate (p.27·1); pseudoephedrine hydrochloride (p.1129·2); guaifenesin (p.1122·1).
*Coughs.*

**Cycrin**
*Wyeth, Arg.; Wyeth, Braz.; Wyeth, Mex.; ESI, USA.*
Medroxyprogesterone acetate (p.1557·2).
*Abnormal uterine bleeding; menopausal disorders; secondary amenorrhoea.*

**Cydec** *Cypress, USA.*
Carbinoxamine maleate (p.426·3); pseudoephedrine hydrochloride (p.1129·2).

**Cydec DM** *Cypress, USA.*
Carbinoxamine maleate (p.426·3); pseudoephedrine hydrochloride (p.1129·2); dextromethorphan hydrobromide (p.1117·3).

**Cydoxmine-B** *PD, Thai.*
Vitamin $B_1$ (p.1455·2); vitamin $B_6$ (p.1457·2); vitamin $B_{12}$ (p.1458·2).
*Megaloblastic anaemia; nausea and vomiting; neuritis; polyneuritis.*

**Cyflox** *Greater Pharma, Thai.*
Ciprofloxacin (p.188·2).
*Bacterial infections.*

**Cy-Gesic** *Cypress, USA.*
Phenylephrine hydrochloride (p.1126·3); phenazone (p.82·3); benzocaine (p.1370·3).
*Earache.*

**Cyheptine** *Greater Pharma, Thai.*
Cyproheptadine (p.430·2).
*Hypersensitivity reactions; pruritus; reduced appetite.*

**Cyklo-F**
*Pharmacia, Austria; Pharmacia, Neth.; Pharmacia, Swed.*
Tranexamic acid (p.760·3).
*Menorrhagia.*

**Cyklokapron**
*Pharmacia, Austral.; Pharmacia, Austria; Pharmacia, Canad.; Pharmacia, Denm.; Pharmacia, Fin.; Pharmacia, Ger.; Pharmacia, Hong Kong; Pharmacia, Irl.; Pharmacia, Neth.; Pharmacia, Norw.; Pharmacia, NZ; Pharmacia, S.Afr.; Pharmacia, Singapore; Pharmacia, Swed.; Pharmacia, Switz.; Pharmacia, UK; Kabivitrum, USA.*
Tranexamic acid (p.760·3).
*Dental extraction in haemophiliacs; fibrinolysis; hereditary angioedema; menorrhagia.*

**Cykrina**
*Wyeth Lederle, Fin.†; Wyeth Lederle, Swed.†.*
Medroxyprogesterone acetate (p.1557·2).
*Endometriosis; menopausal disorders; menstrual disorders.*

**Cylert**
*Abbott, Canad.†; Abbott, Chile; Abbott, Israel; Abbott, USA.*
Pemoline (p.1591·2).
*Attention deficit hyperactivity disorder.*

**Cylex** *Pharmakon, USA.*
Benzocaine (p.1370·3); cetylpyridinium chloride (p.1173·1).
*Sore throat.*

**Cyllind** *Abbott, Ger.*
Clarithromycin (p.192·2).
*Bacterial infections.*

**Cylocide** *Shinyaku, Jpn.*
Cytarabine (p.543·1).
*Acute leukaemias.*

**Cyltabs** *Solvay, India.*
Multivitamin and mineral preparation with liver (p.1417·1).
*Tonic.*

**Cymalon**
*Thornton & Ross, Irl.; Thornton & Ross, UK.*
Sodium citrate (p.1223·2); anhydrous citric acid (p.1673·1); sodium bicarbonate (p.1223·2); sodium carbonate (p.1747·1).
*Cystitis.*

**Cymerin** *Mitsubishi, Jpn.*
Ranimustine (p.582·2).
*Malignant neoplasms; polycythaemia vera; thrombocythaemia.*

**Cymerion** *Azevedos, Port.*
Zolpidem tartrate (p.728·3).
*Insomnia; sedative.*

**Cymevan** *Roche, Fr.*
Ganciclovir (p.635·3) or ganciclovir sodium (p.635·3).
*Cytomegalovirus infections.*

**Cymeven** *Syntex, Ger.; Roche, Ger.*
Ganciclovir (p.635·3) or ganciclovir sodium (p.635·3).
*Cytomegalovirus infections.*

**Cymevene**
*Roche, Arg.; Roche, Austral.; Roche, Austria; Roche, Belg.; Roche, Braz.; Roche, Chile; Roche, Denm.; Roche, Fin.; Roche, Gr.; Roche, Hong Kong; Roche, Irl.; Roche, Israel; Recordati, Ital.; Roche, Mex.; Roche, Neth.; Roche, Norw.; Roche, NZ; Roche, Port.; Roche, S.Afr.; Roche, Singapore; Roche, Spain; Roche, Swed.; Roche, Switz.; Roche, Thai.; Roche, UK.*
Ganciclovir (p.635·3) or ganciclovir sodium (p.635·3).
*Cytomegalovirus infections.*

**Cymex** *De Witt, UK.*
Urea (p.1162·2); dimethicone (p.1482·1); cetrimide (p.1172·1); chlorocresol (p.1177·1).
*Cracked lips; herpes labialis.*

**Cymine** *Pharmasant, Thai.*
Dicycloverine hydrochloride (p.481·2); simeticone (p.1289·2).
*Gastrointestinal colic and spasm.*

**Cyna Bilisan** *Repha, Ger.*
Cynara (p.1678·3).
*Dyspepsia.*

**Cynacur** *Biocur, Ger.*
Cynara (p.1678·3).
*Dyspepsia.*

**Cynafol** *Kanoldt, Ger.†.*
Cynara (p.1678·3).
*Dyspepsia.*

**Cynarex** *Roux-Ocefa, Arg.*
Cynara (p.1678·3).

**Cynarix** *Montavit, Austria.*
Cynara (p.1678·3).
Formerly contained cynara and rhubarb.
*Liver and biliary disorders.*

**Cynarix comp** *Montavit, Austria.*
Cynara (p.1678·3); salverine hydrochloride (p.1741·3).
Formerly contained cynara, rhubarb, and salverine hydrochloride.
*Biliary disorders.*

**Cynarix N** *Sabona, Ger.*
Cynara (p.1678·3).
*Dyspepsia.*

**Cynaro Bilina** *Dermofarm, Spain.*
Cynara (p.1678·3); aloes (p.1248·2).
*Biliary-tract disorders; constipation.*

**Cynarobil** *Uniao Quimica, Braz.†.*
Belladonna (p.479·1); boldo (p.1661·2); cynara (p.1678·3).
*Liver disorders.*

**Cynarol** *Pharmethic, Belg.†.*
Cynara (p.1678·3).
*Biliary disorders; promotion of diuresis.*

**Cynaron** *Enila, Braz.†.*
Cynarine (p.1678·3).
*Liver disorders.*

**Cynarzym N** *Altana, Ger.*
Cynara (p.1678·3); boldo (p.1661·2); greater celandine (p.1695·3).
*Digestive disorders; liver disorders.*

**Cynatrop** *Biologia, Braz.†.*
Betaine hydrochloride (p.1660·2); choline (p.1424·3); liver extract.
*Liver disorders.*

**Cyndal** *Cypress, USA†.*
Codeine phosphate (p.27·1); phenylpropanolamine hydrochloride (p.1127·3); guaifenesin (p.1122·1).
*Coughs; nasal and sinus congestion.*

**Cyndal HD** *Cypress, USA.*
Hydrocodone tartrate (p.45·1); phenylephrine hydrochloride (p.1126·3); chlorphenamine maleate (p.427·3).

**Cyne** *Novartis, Gr.*
Butamirate citrate (p.1116·2).
*Cough.*

**Cynomel**
*Enila, Braz.; Aventis, Fr.; Grossman, Mex.*
Liothyronine sodium (p.1602·2).
*Hypothyroidism.*

**Cynomycin** *Wyeth Lederle, India.*
Minocycline hydrochloride (p.231·3).
*Bacterial infections.*

**Cynoplus** *Grossman, Mex.*
Liothyronine sodium (p.1602·2); levothyroxine sodium (p.1600·1).
*Hypothyroidism.*

**Cynovit** *Julphar, UAE.*
Cyanocobalamin (p.1458·2).
*Megaloblastic anaemia; vitamin $B_{12}$ deficiency; vitamin $B_{12}$ supplement.*

**Cynt**
*Lilly, Braz.; Lilly, Ger.; Pharmaserve Lilly (Φαρμασερβ Λιλλυ), Gr.; Lilly, Spain†.*
Moxonidine (p.962·3).
*Hypertension.*

**Cyntex** *Cypress, USA†.*
Phenylephrine hydrochloride (p.1126·3); phenylpropanolamine hydrochloride (p.1127·3); guaifenesin (p.1122·1).
*Respiratory-tract congestion.*

**Cyomin** *Forest Pharmaceuticals, USA.*
Cyanocobalamin (p.1458·2).
*Schilling test; vitamin $B_{12}$ deficiency.*

**Cyotic** *Cypress, USA.*
Hydrocortisone (p.1103·3); pramocaine hydrochloride (p.1382·2); chloroxylenol (p.1177·2).
*External ear disorders.*

**Cypex** *Cypress, USA.*
Guaifenesin (p.1122·1); sulfogaiacol (p.1131·1).
*Coughs.*

**Cyprid** *Janssen-Cilag, Belg.†.*
Cisapride (p.1259·2).
*Digestive disorders.*

**Cyprogin**
*Atlantic, Hong Kong; Vana, Thai.*
Cyproheptadine hydrochloride (p.430·1).
*Hypersensitivity reactions; migraine; pruritus; reduced appetite.*

**Cypron** *Generics, Israel.*
Cyproterone acetate (p.1544·1).
*Androgenisation; male sexual disorders; prostatic cancer.*

**Cyprone** *Alphapharm, Austral.*
Cyproterone acetate (p.1544·1).
*Androgenisation in females; prostatic cancer; sexual deviation in men.*

**Cyprono** *Milano, Thai.*
Cyproheptadine hydrochloride (p.430·1).
*Hypersensitivity reactions; pruritus; reduced appetite.*

**Cyprosian** *Asian Pharm, Thai.*
Cyproheptadine hydrochloride (p.430·1).
*Hypersensitivity reactions; pruritus; reduced appetite.*

**Cyprostat**
*Schering, Austral.; Schering, UK.*
Cyproterone acetate (p.1544·1).
*Androgen-dependent acne, alopecia, hirsutism, and seborrhoea in females; prostatic cancer; sexual deviation in men.*

**Cyprostol** *Sanova, Austria.*
Misoprostol (p.1519·2).
*Peptic ulcer.*

**Cyral** *Gerot, Austria.*
Primidone (p.376·3).
*Epilepsy.*

**Cyress** *Yamanouchi, Neth.*
Barnidipine hydrochloride (p.866·3).
*Hypertension.*

**Cyriamine** *Pharmasant, Thai.*
Vitamin $B_1$ (p.1455·2); vitamin $B_6$ (p.1457·2); vitamin $B_{12}$ (p.1458·2).
*Vitamin B deficiency.*

**Cyrpon** *Kolassa, Austria.*
Meprobamate (p.706·2).
*Anxiety.*

**Cysporin** *Mayne, Austral.*
Ciclosporin (p.1351·2).
*Atopic dermatitis; nephrotic syndrome; psoriasis; rheumatoid arthritis; transplant rejection.*

**Cystadan** *Orphan Medical, Israel.*
Betaine (p.1660·1).
*Homocystinuria.*

**Cystadane**
*Orphan, Austral.; Orphan Medical, Canad.; Orphan Medical, USA.*
Betaine (p.1660·1).
*Homocystinuria.*

**Cystagon**
*Orphan, Austral.; Orphan, Denm.; Orphan, Fin.; Orphan, Fr.; Orphan, Ger.; Orphan, Ital.; Orphan, Spain; Swedish Orphan, Swed.; Orphan, UK.*
Mercaptamine bitartrate (p.1712·1).
*Nephropathic cystinosis.*

**Cystel Antipelliculaire** *Bailleul, Fr.*
Piroctone olamine (p.1155·2).
Formerly known as Cystelle Antipelliculaire.
*Seborrhoeic dermatitis.*

**Cystel Shampooing Antiseborrheique** *Bailleul, Fr.*
Cade oil (p.1159·2); zinc sulfate (p.1469·3).
Formerly known as Cystelle Shampooing Cheveux Gras.
*Seborrhoea.*

**Cystemme** *Abbott, UK.*
Sodium citrate (p.1223·2).
*Cystitis.*

**Cystex**
*Note. This name is used for preparations of different composition.*
*EMS, Braz.*
Acriflavinium chloride (p.1165·3); methenamine (p.230·1); methylthioninium chloride (p.1042·2); belladonna (p.479·1).
*Urinary-tract infections.*

*Numark, USA.*
Methenamine (p.230·1); sodium salicylate (p.90·1); benzoic acid (p.1169·3).
*Urinary-tract infections.*

**Cystibosin B 48** *Bock, Ger.†.*
Homoeopathic preparation.

**Cystichol** *Bailleul, Fr.†.*
Cystine (p.1426·3); choline bitartrate (p.1424·3).
*Dyspepsia.*

**Cysticide**
*Merck, Ger.; Merck, S.Afr.*
Praziquantel (p.112·2).
*Neurocysticercosis.*

**Cystine $B_6$** *Bailleul, Fr.*
Cystine (p.1426·3); pyridoxine hydrochloride (p.1456·3).
*Eye disorders; nail and hair disorders.*

**Cystinex** *Sofex, Port.*
Gelatin; cystine; pyridoxine hydrochloride; zinc gluconate; vitamin A acetate (p.1417·1).
*Hair loss; nail disorders.*

**Cystinol** *Hoyer, Ger.*
Birch leaf (p.1660·3); equisetum (p.1684·1); solidago virgaurea (p.1748·3); bearberry (p.1659·2).
*Urinary-tract disorders.*

**Cystinol Akut** *Hoyer, Ger.*
Bearberry (p.1659·2).
*Urinary-tract inflammation.*

**Cystinol Long** *Hoyer, Ger.*
Solidago virgaurea (p.1748·3).
*Renal calculi; urinary-tract disorders.*

**Cystiselect N** *Dreluso, Ger.†.*
Homoeopathic preparation.

**Cystistat**
*Paladin, Canad.; Pliva, UK.*
Sodium hyaluronate (p.1697·3).
*Interstitial cystitis.*

**Cystit** *Bristol-Myers Squibb, Ger.†.*
Nitrofurantoin (p.237·2).
*Urinary-tract infections.*

**Cystitis Juniperus** *Homeocan, Canad.*
Homoeopathic preparation.

**Cystitis Relief** *Numark, UK; Thornton & Ross, UK.*
Sodium citrate (p.1223·2).
*Cystitis.*

**Cystium Solidago** *Wernigerode, Ger.*
Solidago virgaurea (p.1748·3).
*Renal calculi; urinary-tract disorders.*

**Cystium-wern** *Wernigerode, Ger.*
Fennel oil (p.1687·3); camphor oil.
*Renal calculi.*

**Cysti-Z** *Bailleul, Fr.*
DL-Methionine (p.1042·1); zinc sulfate (p.1469·3); pyridoxine hydrochloride (p.1456·3).
*Alopecia; seborrhoea.*

**Cysto Fink**
*Kade, Ger.†; SmithKline Beecham OTC, Ger.†.*
*Capsules:* Rhus aromatica (p.1738·1); kava (p.1703·2); lupulus (p.1708·1); bearberry (p.1659·2); cucurbita oil (p.1677·3).
*Urinary-tract disorders.*
*SmithKline Beecham OTC, Ger.†.*
*Tea:* Birch leaf (p.1660·3); solidago (p.1748·3); java tea (p.1702·3); black currant (p.1661·1); bearberry (p.1659·2).
*Urinary-tract disorders.*

**Cysto Fink Mono** *GlaxoSmithKline Consumer, Ger.*
Solidago virgaurea (p.1748·3).
*Urinary-tract disorders.*

**Cystocalm** *Galpharm, UK.*
Sodium citrate (p.1223·2).
*Cystitis.*

**Cysto-Caps Chassot** *Ebi, Switz.†.*
Bearberry (p.1659·2); cucurbita (p.1677·3); kava (p.1703·2); lupulus (p.1708·1); rhus aromatica (p.1738·1).
*Bladder disorders.*

**Cysto-Conray**
*Mallinckrodt, Arg.; Mallinckrodt, Canad.; Mallinckrodt, USA.*
Meglumine iotalamate (p.1065·3).
*Radiographic contrast medium.*

**Cysto-cyl Ho-Len-Complex** *Liebermann, Ger.*
Homoeopathic preparation.

**Cystofem** *Sussex, UK†.*
Sodium citrate (p.1223·2).
*Cystitis.*

**Cysto-Gastreu S R18** *Reckeweg, Ger.*
Homoeopathic preparation.

**Cystografin** *Squibb Diagnostics, USA.*
Meglumine amidotrizoate (p.1060·2).
*Radiographic contrast medium.*

**Cystoleve** *SSL, UK†.*
Sodium citrate (p.1223·2).
*Cystitis.*

**Cysto-Myacyne N** *Schur, Ger.*
Neomycin sulfate (p.235·1).
*Urinary-tract infections.*

**Cystonorm** *Esparma, Ger.*
Oxybutynin (p.487·1).
*Bladder instability; neurogenic bladder.*

**Cystopurin**
*Roche Consumer, Irl.; Roche Consumer, UK.*
Potassium citrate (p.1223·1).
*Cystitis.*

**Cysto-Saar** *MIP, Ger.*
Nitroxoline (p.238·3).
*Urinary-tract infections.*

**Cystosol** *Unimedic, Swed.*
Sorbitol (p.1446·3).
*Bladder irrigation.*

**Cystospaz** *PolyMedica, USA.*
Hyoscyamine (p.485·1).
*Urinary-tract spasm.*

**Cystospaz-M** *PolyMedica, USA†.*
Hyoscyamine sulfate (p.485·1).
*Urinary-tract spasm.*

**Cysto-Urgenin** *Hoyer, Ger.*
Cucurbita oil (p.1677·3).
*Bladder irritability.*

**Cystrin**
*Sanofi Synthelabo, Austria; Sanofi Synthelabo, Fin.; Sanofi Synthelabo, Irl.; Sanofi Synthelabo, UK.*
Oxybutynin hydrochloride (p.486·3).
*Neurogenic bladder disorders; nocturnal enuresis; urinary incontinence.*

**Cytacon**
*Goldshield, Irl.; Goldshield, UK.*
Cyanocobalamin (p.1458·2).
*Megaloblastic anaemia; vitamin $B_{12}$ deficiency.*

**Cytadren**
*Novartis, Austral.; Novartis, NZ; Novartis, USA.*
Aminoglutethimide (p.526·3).
*Breast cancer; Cushing's syndrome; prostatic cancer.*

**Cytagon** *Pharmaland, Thai.*
Glibenclamide (p.331·2).
*Diabetes mellitus.*

**Cytamen**
*Mayne, Austral.; Celltech, Irl.; Celltech, UK.*
Cyanocobalamin (p.1458·2).
*Anaemia due to $B_{12}$ deficiency; Schilling test.*

**Cytarbel** *Bellon, Fr.†.*
Cytarabine (p.543·1).
*Malignant neoplasms.*

**Cytarine**
*Dabur, India; Dabur, Thai.*
Cytarabine (p.543·1).
*Malignant neoplasms.*

**Cyteal**
*Sinbio, Fr.; Pierre Fabre, Port.*
Chlorhexidine gluconate (p.1173·2); chlorocresol (p.1177·1); hexamidine isetionate (p.1181·3).
*Skin and vulvovaginal infections; skin and wound disinfection.*
*Pierre Fabre, Singapore.*
Chlorhexidine gluconate (p.1173·2); chlorocresol (p.1177·1); hexamidine (p.1182·1).
*Skin and vulvovaginal infections; skin and wound disinfection.*

**Cytelium** *Ducray, Fr.*
Avena (p.1658·2); zinc oxide (p.1163·2).
*Skin disorders.*

**Cytine** *Douglas, NZ.*
Cimetidine (p.1255·3).
*Gastro-oesophageal reflux; peptic ulcer; Zollinger-Ellison syndrome.*

**Cyto-Bifidus** *Eagle, Austral.†.*
*Lactobacillus acidophilus; L. bulgaricus; L. rhamnosus; L. casei; L. plantarum; L. salivarius; L. brevis; L. lactis* (p.1704·2).
*Gastrointestinal disorders.*

**Cytobion** *Merck, Ger.*
Cyanocobalamin (p.1458·2).
*Vitamin $B_{12}$ deficiency.*

**Cytoblastin** *Cipla, India.*
Vinblastine sulfate (p.591·2).
*Malignant neoplasms.*

**Cytocristin** *Cipla, India.*
Vincristine sulfate (p.592·2).
*Acute leukaemias.*

**CytoGam**
*Purissimus, Arg.; Medimmune, USA.*
A cytomegalovirus immunoglobulin (p.1612·1).
*Passive immunisation.*

**Cytoglobin**
*Bayer, Austria; Bayer, Ger.*
A cytomegalovirus immunoglobulin (p.1612·1).
*Passive immunisation.*

**Cytolog** *Zydus, India.*
Misoprostol (p.1519·2).
*Peptic ulcer.*

**Cytomel**
*SK-RIT, Belg.†; Theramed, Canad.; SmithKline Beecham, Neth.; Jones, USA.*
Liothyronine sodium (p.1602·2).
*Evaluation of thyroid function; hypothyroidism; nontoxic goitre.*

**Cytophosphan** *Taro, Israel.*
Cyclophosphamide (p.540·2).
*Malignant neoplasms; systemic lupus erythematosus.*

**Cytosar**
*Pharmacia, Austria; Pharmacia, Belg.; Pharmacia, Canad.; Pharmacia, Denm.; Pharmacia, Hong Kong; Pharmacia, Irl.; Pharmacia Upjohn, Israel; Pharmacia, Neth.; Pharmacia, Norw.; Pharmacia, Port.; Pharmacia, S.Afr.; Pharmacia, Singapore; Pharmacia, Swed.; Pharmacia, Switz.; Pharmacia, Thai.; Pharmacia, UK†.*
Cytarabine (p.543·1).
*Leukaemias; non-Hodgkin's lymphoma.*

**Cytosar-U**
*Pharmacia, Austral.†; Pharmacia, Malaysia; Pharmacia Upjohn, NZ†; Gensia, USA.*
Cytarabine (p.543·1).
*Leukaemias; non-Hodgkin's lymphoma.*

**Cytotec**
*Pharmacia, Austral.; Pharmacia, Belg.; Pharmacia, Braz.; Pharmacia, Canad.; Pharmacia, Denm.; Pharmacia, Fin.; Pharmacia, Fr.; Pharmacia, Ger.; Pharmacia-Upjohn, Gr.; Pharmacia, Hong Kong; Pharmacia, Irl.; Searle, Israel; Monsanto, Ital.; Pharmacia, Malaysia; Searle, Mex.; Pharmacia, Neth.; Pharmacia, Norw.; Pharmacia, NZ; Pharmacia, Port.; Pharmacia, S.Afr.; Searle, Singapore†; Pharmacia, Spain; Pharmacia, Swed.; Pharmacia, Switz.; Pharmacia, Thai.; Pharmacia, UK; Searle, USA.*
Misoprostol (p.1519·2).
*Peptic ulcer.*

**Cytotect**
*Biotest, Austria; Pentafarma, Chile; Biotest, Ger.; Biotest, Hong Kong; Biotest, Ital.; Biotest, Switz.*
A cytomegalovirus immunoglobulin (p.1612·1).
*Passive immunisation.*

**Cytovene**
*Rontag, Arg.; Roche, Canad.; Roche, USA.*
Ganciclovir (p.635·3) or ganciclovir sodium (p.635·3).
*Cytomegalovirus infections.*

**Cytoxan**
*Bristol, Canad.; Bristol-Myers Squibb, Israel; Bristol-Myers Squibb, NZ; Bristol-Myers Squibb Oncology, USA.*
Cyclophosphamide (p.540·2).
*Glomerular kidney disease; malignant neoplasms.*

**Cytra-2** *Cypress, USA.*
Citric acid monohydrate (p.1673·1); sodium citrate (p.1223·2).
*Metabolic acidosis; urinary alkalinisation.*

**Cytra-3** *Cypress, USA.*
Citric acid monohydrate (p.1673·1); potassium citrate (p.1223·1); sodium citrate (p.1223·2).
*Metabolic acidosis; urinary alkalinisation.*

**Cytra-K** *Cypress, USA.*
Citric acid monohydrate (p.1673·1); potassium citrate (p.1223·1).
*Metabolic acidosis; urinary alkalinisation.*

**Cytra-LC** *Cypress, USA.*
Citric acid monohydrate (p.1673·1); potassium citrate (p.1223·1); sodium citrate (p.1223·2).
*Metabolic acidosis; urinary alkalinisation.*

**Cytur Test** *Roche Diagnostics, Austral.*
Test for leucocytes in urine.

**Cytuss HC** *Cypress, USA.*
Hydrocodone tartrate (p.45·1); phenylephrine hydrochloride (p.1126·3); chlorphenamine maleate (p.427·3).

**Cyzine** *Pharmasant, Thai.*
Cetirizine hydrochloride (p.427·1).
*Allergic conjunctivitis; allergic skin disorders; rhinitis.*

**D-204** *Gambro, Israel.*
Electrolyte solution (p.1221·1).
*Haemodialysis solution.*

**D-248** *Gambro, Israel.*
Electrolyte solution (p.1221·1).
*Haemodialysis solution.*

**D-300** *Gambro, Israel.*
Electrolyte solution (p.1221·1).
*Haemodialysis solution.*

**D-326** *Gambro, Israel.*
Electrolyte solution (p.1221·1).
*Haemodialysis solution.*

**D 4** *Fouchard, Chile.*
Hydroquinone (p.1148·1); kojic acid (p.1151·2); glycolic acid (p.1147·3).
*Skin pigmentation disorders.*

**d Epifrin** *Allergan, Ger.*
Dipivefrine hydrochloride (p.1681·2).
*Glaucoma.*

**D Sucril** *Pierre Fabre, Fr.†.*
Aspartame (p.1422·1).
*Sugar substitute.*

**$D_3$ Vicotrat** *Heyl, Ger.*
Colecalciferol (p.1461·3).
*Vitamin D deficiency.*

**DA II** *Dura, USA.*
Chlorphenamine maleate (p.427·3); phenylephrine hydrochloride (p.1126·3); hyoscine methonitrate (p.483·3).
*Upper respiratory-tract symptoms.*

**DA Chewable** *Dura, USA.*
Chlorphenamine maleate (p.427·3); phenylephrine hydrochloride (p.1126·3); hyoscine methonitrate (p.483·3).
*Allergic rhinitis; cold symptoms; sinusitis.*

**Daben** *Solfran, Mex.*
Mebendazole (p.108·2).
*Worm infections.*

**Dabenzol**
Note. This name is used for preparations of different composition.
*Filaxis, Arg.*
Oxaliplatin (p.577·1).
*Malignant neoplasms.*
*Tecnofarma, Mex.†.*
Albendazole (p.101·2).

**Dabetil** *Liferpal, Mex.*
Tolbutamide (p.348·1).
*Diabetes mellitus.*

**Dabex** *Merck, Mex.*
Metformin hydrochloride (p.342·3).
*Diabetes mellitus.*

**Dabex G** *Merck, Mex.†.*
Metformin hydrochloride (p.342·3); glibenclamide (p.331·2).
*Diabetes mellitus.*

**Dabonal** *Vita, Spain.*
Enalapril maleate (p.909·2).
*Heart failure; hypertension.*

**Dabonal Plus** *Vita, Spain.*
Hydrochlorothiazide (p.933·2); enalapril maleate (p.909·2).
*Hypertension.*

**Dabroson** *Norma (Νορμα), Gr.*
Gentamicin sulfate (p.217·1).
*Bacterial infections.*

**Dacam** *Laboratorios Chile, Chile.*
Betamethasone sodium phosphate (p.1093·1).
*Corticosteroid.*

**Dacam RL** *Laboratorios Chile, Chile.*
Betamethasone acetate (p.1093·1); betamethasone sodium phosphate (p.1093·1).
*Corticosteroid.*

**Dacarb** *Eurofarma, Braz.*
Dacarbazine (p.544·2).
*Malignant neoplasms.*

**Dacarbaziba** *Libra, Braz.†.*
Dacarbazine (p.544·2).
*Malignant neoplasms.*

**Dacatic** *Orion, Fin.*
Dacarbazine (p.544·2).
*Malignant neoplasms.*

**Dacef** *Aspen, S.Afr.*
Cefadroxil (p.167·2).
*Bacterial infections.*

**Dacin-F** *Farmaline, Thai.*
Clindamycin hydrochloride (p.194·2) or clindamycin phosphate (p.194·2).
*Bacterial infections.*

**Daclin**
Note. This name is used for preparations of different composition.
*Laboratorios Chile, Chile.*
Clindamycin phosphate (p.194·2).
*Bacterial infections.*
*Pacific, NZ.*
Sulindac (p.91·2).
*Musculoskeletal, joint, and peri-articular disorders.*

**Dacmozen** *VHB, India.*
Dactinomycin (p.545·1).
*Malignant neoplasms.*

**Dacoren** *Aventis, Ger.†.*
Co-dergocrine mesilate (p.1674·1).
*Hypertension; mental function disorders.*

**Dacortin** *Merck, Spain.*
Prednisone (p.1109·3).
*Corticosteroid.*

**Dacortin H** *Merck, Spain.*
Prednisolone (p.1108·1).
*Corticosteroid.*

**Dacovo** *Tafir, Spain.*
Cefazolin sodium (p.170·3).
*Bacterial infections.*

**Dacplat** *Pharmacia, Arg.*
Oxaliplatin (p.577·1).
*Colorectal cancer.*

**Dacrin**
*Merck Sharp & Dohme, Austria; Chibret, Ger.†.*
Hydrastinine hydrochloride; oxedrine tartrate (p.977·3).
*Conjunctivitis.*

**Dacrine**
*Chibret, Port.†; Merck Sharp & Dohme, Switz.†.*
Hydrastinine hydrochloride; oxedrine tartrate (p.977·3).
*Eye irritation.*

**Dacrio Gel** *Alkon (Αλκον), Gr.*
Carbomer (p.1577·2).
*Dry eyes.*

**Dacriogel** *Alcon, Ital.*
Carbomer (p.1577·2).
*Dry eyes.*

**Dacriose** *Novartis Ophthalmics, USA.*
Electrolytes (p.1217·1).
*Eye irrigation.*

**Dacriosol**
*Alcon, Denm.; Alcon, Ital.*
Dextran 70 (p.746·2); hypromellose (p.1579·3).
*Dry eyes.*

**Dacrodil** *Teva Tuteur, Arg.*
Hydroxycarbamide (p.559·1).
*Malignant neoplasms.*

**Dacrolux**
*Alcon Cusi, Malaysia; Cusi, Singapore; Alcon Cusi, Spain.*
Dextran 70 (p.746·2); hypromellose (p.1579·3).
*Dry eyes.*

**Dacryne**
*Martin, Fr.*
Oxedrine tartrate (p.977·3); chlorhexidine gluconate (p.1173·2).
Formerly known as Dacryoseptil.
*Eye disorders.*
*Martin, Fr.†.*
Hydrastinine hydrochloride; oxedrine tartrate (p.977·3); chlorhexidine gluconate (p.1173·2).
*Conjunctivitis; eye irritation.*

**Dacryoboraline** *Martin, Fr.*
Oxedrine tartrate (p.977·3); borax (p.1661·3); boric acid (p.1662·1).
*Eye irritation.*

**Dacryolarmes** *Martin, Fr.*
Methylcellulose 4000 (p.1580·2).
*Dry eyes; protection during eye examinations.*

**Dacryoserum** *Martin, Fr.*
Boric acid (p.1662·1); borax (p.1661·3); sodium chloride (p.1233·3).
*Eye irritation.*

**Dacten** *Phoenix, Arg.*
Candesartan cilexetil (p.878·3).
*Hypertension.*

**Dactil OB**
Note. This name is used for preparations of different composition.
Aventis, Braz.
Piperidolate hydrochloride (p.487·3); hesperidin (p.1688·2); ascorbic acid (p.1460·2).
*Smooth muscle spasm.*

Aventis, Mex.
Piperidolate hydrochloride (p.487·3).
*Dysmenorrhoea; premature labour; threatened miscarriage.*

**Dacudoses** Thea, Fr.
Boric acid (p.1662·1); borax (p.1661·3).
*Eye irritation.*

**Daewo** Costec, Arg.
*Soap:* Triclosan (Irgasan DP-300) (p.1195·2).
*Skin and hand disinfection.*
*Topical solution:* Aluminium chlorohydrate (p.1142·1).
*Hyperhidrosis.*

**Dafalgan**
Bristol-Myers Squibb, Belg.; UPSA, Fr.; Bristol-Myers Squibb, Port.; Upsamedica, Spain; Upsamedica, Switz.
Paracetamol (p.76·2).
*Fever; pain.*

**Dafalgan Codeine**
Bristol-Myers Squibb, Belg.; UPSA, Fr.
Paracetamol (p.76·2); codeine phosphate (p.27·1).
*Pain.*

**Daflon**
Servier, Arg.; Servier, Austria; Servier, Belg.; Servier, Hong Kong; Sanfer, Mex.; Servier, Port.; Servier, Thai.
Diosmin (p.1688·2); hesperidin (p.1688·2).
*Haemorrhoids; venous insufficiency.*

Servier, Braz.; Servier, Spain†.
Diosmin (p.1688·2).
*Haemorrhoids; menorrhagia; venous insufficiency.*

Servier, Fr.
Bioflavonoids (p.1688·2).
*Vascular disorders.*

**Daflon 500**
Servier, Chile; Servier, Ital.; Servier, Malaysia; Servier, Singapore; Servier, Spain; Servier, Switz.
Diosmin (p.1688·2); hesperidin (p.1688·2).
*Haemorrhoids; venous insufficiency.*

**Dafloxen** Liomont, Mex.
Naproxen (p.65·1) or naproxen sodium (p.65·1).
*Gout; inflammation; musculoskeletal, joint and peri-articular disorders; pain.*

**Dafloxen F** Liomont, Mex.
Naproxen sodium (p.65·1); paracetamol (p.76·2).
*Fever; inflammation; pain.*

**Dafne** Omega, Arg.
Dicycloverine hydrochloride (p.481·2); diazepam (p.690·1); aluminium glycinate (p.1249·1); magnesium oxide (p.1272·3); lidocaine (p.1377·3); simeticone (p.1289·2).
*Dyspepsia; gastrointestinal motility disorders; peptic ulcer.*

**Dafnegil**
Lepori, Port.; Poli, Switz.†.
Nifuratel (p.611·2); nystatin (p.406·3).
*Balanitis; skin infections; vulvovaginal infections.*

**Dafnegil Neo** Poli, Switz.
Ciclopirox olamine (p.396·1).
*Vulvovaginal candidiasis.*

**Dafnegin** Monsanto, Ital.
Ciclopirox olamine (p.396·1).
*Vulvovaginal and peri-anal candidiasis.*

**Daforin** Sigma, Braz.
Fluoxetine hydrochloride (p.292·1).
*Depression; obsessive-compulsive disorder.*

**Daga** Aventis, Thai.
Paracetamol (p.76·2).
*Fever; pain.*

**Dagan** Tedec Meiji, Spain.
Nicardipine hydrochloride (p.965·1).
*Angina pectoris; cerebrovascular disorders; hypertension.*

**Dagenan** Rhone-Poulenc Rorer, Canad.†.
Sulfapyridine (p.263·3).
*Bacterial infections.*

**Dagol** Cetus, Arg.
Sodium picosulfate (p.1289·3).
*Constipation.*

**Dagotil** Royal, Chile.
Risperidone (p.719·2).
*Schizophrenia.*

**Dagra Fluor** Asta Medica, Neth.†.
Sodium fluoride (p.1444·3).
*Dental caries prophylaxis.*

**Dagracycline** Viatris, Neth.
Doxycycline fosfatex (p.206·2).
*Bacterial infections.*

**Dagragel** Viatris, Port.
Gelatin (p.754·3); glycerol (p.1694·3).
Formerly contained bile and glycerol.
*Bowel evacuation; constipation.*

**Dagramycine** Asta Medica, Belg.†.
Doxycycline polyphosphate sodium (p.206·2).
*Bacterial infections.*

**Dagravit** Viatris, Port.
A range of vitamin preparations with or without minerals (p.1417·1).

**Dagravit A** Asta Medica, Belg.†.
Vitamin A acetate (p.1453·1).
*Vitamin A deficiency.*

**Dagravit A Forte** Viatris, Neth.
Vitamin A acetate (p.1453·1).
*Vitamin A deficiency.*

**Dagravit A-E** Asta Medica, Belg.†.
Vitamin A palmitate (p.1453·1); *dl*-alpha tocoferil acetate (p.1465·1).
*Vitamin A and E deficiency.*

**Dagravit A-E Forte** Viatris, Neth.
Vitamin A palmitate (p.1453·1); *dl*-alpha-tocoferil acetate (p.1465·1).
*Vitamin A and E deficiency.*

**Dagravit B-Complex** Viatris, Belg.†.
Vitamin B substances (p.1417·1).
*Vitamin B deficiency.*

**Dagravit B-Complex Forte** Asta Medica, Neth.†.
Vitamin B substances (p.1417·1); intrinsic factor.
*Vitamin B deficiency.*

**Dagravit Totaal 8** Viatris, Neth.
Multivitamin preparation (p.1417·1).

**Dagravit Total** Asta Medica, Belg.†.
Multivitamin preparation with iron (p.1417·1).

**Dagravit Total 8** Asta Medica, Belg.†.
Multivitamin preparation (p.1417·1).

**Dagrilan** Pharmacypria, Gr.
Fluoxetine hydrochloride (p.292·1).
*Depression; obsessive-compulsive disorder; panic disorder.*

**Dagynil** Viatris, Neth.
Conjugated oestrogens (p.1543·2).
*Menopausal disorders; osteoporosis; prostatic cancer.*

**Dai Natha** Lopes, Braz.†.
Tar (p.1159·3); cade oil (p.1159·2); coal tar (p.1159·2).
*Seborrhoeic dermatitis.*

**Daiet B** Humana, Ital.
Fatty-acid, lipid, and vitamin preparation (p.1417·1).
*Nutritional supplement.*

**Dailat** Pharmasant, Thai.
Serrapeptase (p.1743·2).
*Inflammation; oedema.*

**Daily** Pierre Fabre Sante, Fr.
Ethinylestradiol (p.1553·2); levonorgestrel (p.1563·2).
*Triphasic oral contraceptive.*

**Daily Balance** Pharmavite, Canad.†.
Multivitamin preparation (p.1417·1).

**Daily Benefits** Kay, Canad.
Multivitamin and mineral preparations (p.1417·1).

**Daily Conditioning** Blistex, USA.
*SPF 20:* Octinoxate (p.1154·3); oxybenzone (p.1154·3).
*Sunscreen.*

**Daily Fatigue Relief** Herbal Concepts, UK.
Kola (p.1765·3); damiana (p.1679·1); saw palmetto (p.1569·1).
*Fatigue.*

**Daily Gold Pack** Solgar, UK.
Multivitamin and mineral preparation (p.1417·1).

**Daily Menopause Relief** Herbal Concepts, UK.
Tilia (p.1756·2); motherwort (p.1717·1); pulsatilla (p.1737·1); valerian (p.1762·2).
*Menopausal disorders.*

**Daily Multi** Vitaplex, Austral.†.
Multivitamin, mineral, and amino-acid preparation (p.1417·1).

**Daily Overwork & Mental Fatigue Relief** Herbal Concepts, UK.
Avena (p.1658·2); zanthoxylum (p.1766·3).
*Tonic.*

**Daily Protection Moisturizer** Kay, Canad.
*SPF 15:* Octinoxate (p.1154·3); oxybenzone (p.1154·3).
*Sunscreen.*

**Daily Tension & Strain Relief** Herbal Concepts, UK.
Asafetida (p.1658·1); valerian (p.1762·2); avena (p.1658·2); passion flower (p.1729·1).
*Strain; tension.*

**Daily-Vite** Rugby, USA.
Multivitamin and mineral preparation with iron and folic acid (p.1417·1).

**Daimeton** Drag, Chile.
Paracetamol (p.76·2).
*Fever; pain.*

**Dairy Ease** Blistex, USA.
Tilactase (p.1756·2).
*Lactase insufficiency.*

**Dairyaid** Tanta, Canad.
Tilactase (p.1756·2).
*Lactase insufficiency.*

**Daiv** Fada, Arg.
Diazepam (p.690·1).
*Anxiety.*

**Daivobet**
Leo, Denm.; Leo, Ger.; Leo, Norw.; Farmacusi, Spain; Leo, Swed.
Calcipotriol (p.1144·1); betamethasone dipropionate (p.1093·1).
*Psoriasis.*

**Daivonex**
Andromaco, Arg.; CSL, Austral.; Leo, Belg.; Schering-Plough, Braz.; Andromaco, Chile; Leo, Denm.; Leo, Fin.; Leo, Fr.; Leo, Ger.; Leo, Hong Kong; Leo, Israel; Formenti, Ital.; Leo, Malaysia; Senosiain, Mex.; Leo, Neth.; Leo, Norw.; CSL, NZ; Leo, NZ; Leo, Port.; Leo, Singapore; Farmacusi, Spain; Leo, Swed.; Leo, Switz.; Leo, Thai.
Calcipotriol (p.1144·1).
*Psoriasis.*

**Dakar** Aventis, Belg.
Lansoprazole (p.1269·3).
*Gastro-oesophageal reflux; peptic ulcer; Zollinger-Ellison syndrome.*

**Dakin** Cooperation Pharmaceutique, Fr.
Sodium hypochlorite (p.1192·1).
*Skin, mucous membrane, and wound disinfection.*

**Dakincooper** Melisana, Belg.
Sodium hypochlorite (p.1192·1).
*Skin and mucous membrane disinfection.*

**Daktacort**
Janssen-Cilag, Austria†; Janssen-Cilag, Belg.; Orion, Fin.; Janssen-Cilag, Fr.†; Janssen, Hong Kong; Ethnor, India; Janssen-Cilag, Irl.; Janssen-Cilag, Israel; Janssen-Cilag, Malaysia; Janssen, Mex.; Janssen-Cilag, Neth.; Janssen-Cilag, Norw.; Janssen-Cilag, NZ; Janssen-Cilag, Port.; Janssen-Cilag, S.Afr.; Janssen-Cilag, Singapore; Janssen-Cilag, Swed.; Janssen-Cilag, Switz.; Janssen-Cilag, Thai.; Janssen-Cilag, UK.
Miconazole nitrate (p.405·3); hydrocortisone (p.1103·3).
*Fungal and Gram-positive bacterial skin infections with inflammation.*

**Daktacort HC** Johnson & Johnson MSD Consumer, UK.
Miconazole nitrate (p.405·3); hydrocortisone acetate (p.1103·3).
*Infected skin disorders.*

**Daktagold**
Janssen-Cilag, Austral.; Janssen-Cilag, NZ.
Ketoconazole (p.403·3).
*Fungal skin infections; seborrhoeic dermatitis.*

**Daktar**
Janssen-Cilag, Belg.; Janssen-Cilag, Ger.; Janssen-Cilag, Norw.; Janssen-Cilag, Swed.
Miconazole (p.405·2) or miconazole nitrate (p.405·3).
*Fungal and Gram-positive bacterial infections.*

**Daktarin**
Janssen-Cilag, Arg.; Janssen-Cilag, Austral.; Janssen-Cilag, Austria; Janssen-Cilag, Belg.; Janssen-Cilag, Braz.; Janssen-Cilag, Chile; Orion, Fin.; Janssen-Cilag, Fr.; Janssen-Cilag, Gr.; Janssen, Hong Kong; Ethnor, India; Janssen-Cilag, Irl.; Janssen-Cilag, Israel; Janssen-Cilag, Ital.; Janssen-Cilag, Malaysia; Janssen, Mex.; Janssen-Cilag, Neth.; Janssen-Cilag, NZ; Janssen-Cilag, Port.; Janssen-Cilag, S.Afr.; Janssen-Cilag, Singapore; Esteve, Spain; Janssen-Cilag, Switz.; Janssen-Cilag, Thai.; Janssen-Cilag, UK; Johnson & Johnson MSD Consumer, UK.
Miconazole (p.405·2) or miconazole nitrate (p.405·3).
*Fungal and Gram-positive bacterial infections.*

**Daktarin Gold** Johnson & Johnson MSD Consumer, UK.
Ketoconazole (p.403·3).
*Fungal skin infections.*

**Daktazol** Neo Quimica, Braz.
Miconazole nitrate (p.405·3).
*Fungal infections.*

**Daktodor** Janssen-Cilag, Gr.
Hydrocortisone (p.1103·3); miconazole nitrate (p.405·3).
*Fungal skin infections with inflammation.*

**Daktozin**
Janssen-Cilag, Arg.; Janssen-Cilag, Austral.; Janssen-Cilag, Belg.; Janssen-Cilag, Braz.†; Janssen-Cilag, NZ.
Miconazole nitrate (p.405·3); zinc oxide (p.1163·2).
*Nappy rash with secondary candidiasis.*

**Dal** Osteolab, Chile.
21 Tablets, desogestrel (p.1547·2); ethinylestradiol (p.1553·2); 5 tablets, ethinylestradiol; 2 tablets, placebo.
*Biphasic oral contraceptive.*

**Dalacin**
Pharmacia, Arg.; Pharmacia, Austria; Pharmacia, Chile; Pharmacia, Denm.; Pharmacia, Fin.; Pharmacia Upjohn, India; Pharmacia, Irl.; Pharmacia, Norw.; Pharmacia, NZ; Pharmacia, Spain; Pharmacia, Swed.; Pharmacia, UK.
Clindamycin hydrochloride (p.194·2), clindamycin palmitate hydrochloride (p.194·2), or clindamycin phosphate (p.194·2).
*Bacterial infections.*

**Dalacin V**
Pharmacia, Austral.; Pharmacia, Chile; Pharmacia Upjohn, Hong Kong†; Pharmacia Upjohn, Mex.; Pharmacia, Neth.; Pharmacia Upjohn, NZ†; Pharmacia, Port.; Pharmacia, Switz.
Clindamycin phosphate (p.194·2).
*Bacterial vaginitis.*

Pharmacia, Braz.
Clindamycin hydrochloride (p.194·2).
*Bacterial vaginitis.*

**Dalacin C**
Pharmacia, Arg.; Pharmacia, Austral.; Pharmacia, Belg.; Pharmacia, Braz.; Pharmacia, Canad.; Pharmacia, Chile; Pharmacia-Upjohn, Gr.; Pharmacia, Hong Kong; Pharmacia, Irl.; Pharmacia Upjohn, Israel; Pharmacia Upjohn, Ital.; Pharmacia, Malaysia; Pharmacia Upjohn, Mex.; Pharmacia, Neth.; Pharmacia, Port.; Pharmacia, S.Afr.; Pharmacia, Singapore; Pharmacia, Switz.; Pharmacia, Thai.; Pharmacia, UK.
Clindamycin hydrochloride (p.194·2), clindamycin palmitate hydrochloride (p.194·2) or clindamycin phosphate (p.194·2).
*Bacterial infections.*

**Dalacin ST** Pharmacia, Arg.
Clindamycin phosphate (p.194·2).
*Acne.*

**Dalacin T**
Pharmacia, Austral.; Pharmacia, Braz.; Pharmacia, Canad.; Pharmacia, Chile; Pharmacia, Hong Kong; Pharmacia, Irl.; Pharmacia Upjohn, Ital.; Pharmacia, Malaysia; Pharmacia Upjohn, Mex.; Pharmacia, Neth.; Pharmacia, NZ; Pharmacia, Port.; Pharmacia, S.Afr.; Pharmacia, Singapore; Pharmacia, Switz.; Pharmacia, Thai.; Pharmacia, UK.
Clindamycin phosphate (p.194·2).
*Acne.*

**Dalacin T Prewash** Pharmacia, NZ.
Triclosan (p.1195·2).
*Skin cleansing.*

**Dalacin Topical** Pharmacia, Belg.
Clindamycin phosphate (p.194·2).
Formerly known as Dalacin T.
*Acne.*

**Dalacin Vaginal**
Pharmacia, Belg.; Pharmacia, Canad.; Pharmacia Upjohn, Israel.
Clindamycin phosphate (p.194·2).
*Bacterial vaginitis.*

**Dalacin VC** Pharmacia, S.Afr.
Clindamycin phosphate (p.194·2).
*Bacterial vaginosis.*

**Dalacine** Pharmacia, Fr.
Clindamycin hydrochloride (p.194·2) or clindamycin phosphate (p.194·2).
*Bacterial infections.*

**Dalacine T** Pharmacia, Fr.
Clindamycin phosphate (p.194·2).
*Acne.*

**Dalagis T** Agis, Israel.
Clindamycin phosphate (p.194·2).
*Acne.*

**Dalalgan Codeina** Bristol-Myers Squibb, Port.
Paracetamol (p.76·2); codeine phosphate (p.27·1).
*Pain.*

**Dalalone** Forest Pharmaceuticals, USA.
Dexamethasone acetate (p.1097·1).
*Corticosteroid.*

**Dalam** Richmond, Arg.
Midazolam (p.707·1).
*Sedative.*

**Dalamon** Alter, Spain.
*Capsules†:* Cobamamide (p.1459·1); pyridoxine phosphate (p.1457·2); thiamine phosphate (p.1455·2).
*Neuralgia; neuritis.*
*Injection:* Cyanocobalamin (p.1458·2); dexamethasone sodium diacid phosphate (p.1097·2); pyridoxine hydrochloride (p.1456·3); thiamine hydrochloride (p.1455·1).
Lidocaine hydrochloride (p.1377·3) is included in this preparation to alleviate the pain of injection.
*Myalgia; neuralgia; neuritis; rheumatism.*

**Dalamon Inyectable** Alter, Spain.
Dexamethasone sodium phosphate (p.1097·2).
*Corticosteroid.*

**Dalcap** Unichem, India.
Clindamycin hydrochloride (p.194·2).
*Bacterial infections.*

**Dalcept** Cuprocept, S.Afr.
Copper-wound plastic (p.1425·3).
*Intra-uterine contraceptive device.*

**Dalcipran**
Roche, Arg.; Sanofi Synthelabo, Austria.
Milnacipran hydrochloride (p.307·3).
*Depression.*

**Dal-E** Dal-Vita, Austral.†.
*d*-Alpha tocoferil acetate (p.1465·1).
*Burns; minor wounds; skin irritation.*

**Dalet Med Balsam** Mauermann, Ger.
Guaiacol (p.1122·1); methyl salicylate (p.59·3); belladonna (p.479·1); menthol (p.1711·3).
*Hallux valgus; inflammation of big toe joint.*

**Dalfaz**
Sanofi Synthelabo, Arg.; Synthelabo, Spain†.
Alfuzosin hydrochloride (p.856·2).
*Benign prostatic hyperplasia.*

**Dalgan** Astra, USA†.
Dezocine (p.30·1).
*Pain.*

**Dalgen** Recordati, Spain.
Fepradinol (p.43·1) or fepradinol hydrochloride (p.43·1).
*Peri-articular disorders; soft-tissue disorders.*

**Dalgex** Daudt, Braz.
Orphenadrine citrate (p.486·1); dipyrone (p.35·3); caffeine (p.782·1).
*Pain; skeletal muscle spasm.*

**Dalidome** Serral, Mex.
Copper sulfate (p.1426·1); zinc sulfate (p.1469·3); camphor (p.1665·3).
*Skin disorders.*

**Dalinar** Essex, Spain†.
Netilmicin sulfate (p.236·3).
*Bacterial infections.*

**Dalisol** Lemery, Mex.
Calcium folinate (p.1431·1).
*Adjunct to fluorouracil therapy; antidote to folic acid antagonists; megaloblastic anaemia; reduction of methotrexate toxicity.*

**Dalivit**
Ariston, Braz.
Vitamin B substances; vitamin C; fructose (p.1417·1).

Eastern Pharmaceuticals, UK.
Multivitamin preparation (p.1417·1).

**Dallamizol-D** Dallas, Arg.
Pseudoephedrine sulfate (p.1129·2); astemizole (p.424·2).

**Dallapasmo** Dallas, Arg.
Homatropine methylbromide (p.483·2).
*Muscle spasm.*

**Dallergy** *Laser, USA.*
Chlorphenamine maleate (p.427·3); phenylephrine hydrochloride (p.1126·3); hyoscine methonitrate (p.483·3).
*Upper respiratory-tract symptoms.*

**Dallergy-D** *Laser, USA.*
*Capsules:* Pseudoephedrine hydrochloride (p.1129·2); chlorphenamine maleate (p.427·3).
*Syrup:* Phenylephrine hydrochloride (p.1126·3); chlorphenamine maleate (p.427·3).
*Upper respiratory-tract symptoms.*

**Dallergy-JR** *Laser, USA.*
Phenylephrine hydrochloride (p.1126·3); chlorphenamine maleate (p.427·3).
Formerly contained brompheniramine maleate and pseudoephedrine hydrochloride.
*Allergic rhinitis; nasal congestion.*

**Dalmacol** *Riva, Canad.*
Hydrocodone tartrate (p.45·1); etafedrine hydrochloride (p.1121·2); sodium citrate (p.1223·2); doxylamine succinate (p.432·3).
*Respiratory-tract disorders.*

**Dalmadorm**
*ICN, Braz.; Roche, Hong Kong; ICN, Neth.; ICN, Singapore; ICN, Switz.*
Flurazepam hydrochloride (p.700·3).
*Insomnia.*
*ICN, Ger.; ICN, Ital.; ICN, Port.; Pharmaco, S.Afr.; ICN, Thai.*
Flurazepam monohydrochloride (p.700·3).
*Insomnia.*

**Dalmane**
*ICN, Canad.; ICN, Irl.; Roche, USA.*
Flurazepam dihydrochloride (p.700·3).
*Insomnia.*
*ICN, UK.*
Flurazepam monohydrochloride (p.700·3).
*Insomnia.*

**Dalmasin** *Columbia, Mex.†.*
Dipyrone (p.35·3).
*Fever; pain.*

**Dalminette** *Norma (Νορμα), Gr.*
Paracetamol (p.76·2).
*Fever; pain.*

**Dalparan** *Farma Lepori, Spain.*
Zolpidem tartrate (p.728·3).
*Insomnia.*

**Dalsin** *Offenbach, Mex.*
Dipyrone (p.35·3).
*Fever; muscle spasm; pain.*

**Dalsy**
*Abbott, Braz.; Abbott, Spain.*
Ibuprofen (p.45·3).
*Fever; musculoskeletal, joint, and peri-articular disorders; pain.*

**Daltroid** *Lemery, Mex.*
Levothyroxine sodium (p.1600·1).

**Dalun** *Medipharm, Chile.*
Hydroxyzine hydrochloride (p.434·3).
*Agitation; anxiety; hypersensitivity reactions.*

**Dalys** *Dosa, Arg.*
Paclitaxel (p.577·3).
*Malignant neoplasms.*

**Dalzolston** *Ariston, Braz.*
Metronidazole (p.607·2).

**Dam** *Terapeutico, Ital.*
Damiana (p.1679·1); muira puama; santoreggia; kola (p.1765·3); cinnamon (p.1672·2).
*Erectile dysfunction.*

**Dama-Lax** *Schering-Plough, Spain†.*
Docusate sodium (p.1262·2).
Formerly contained docusate sodium and phenolphthalein.
*Constipation.*

**Damason-P** *Mason, USA.*
Hydrocodone tartrate (p.45·1); aspirin (p.15·1).
*Pain.*

**Damax** *Offenbach, Mex.*
Estradiol benzoate (p.1550·1); progesterone (p.1566·2).

**Damiana and Kola Tablets** *Dorwest, UK.*
Kola (p.1765·3); damiana (p.1679·1); saw palmetto (p.1569·1).
*Tonic.*

**Damiana-Sarsaparilla Formula** *Quest, Canad.*
Damiana leaf (p.1679·1); kelp (p.1742·3); liquorice root (p.1270·2); sarsaparilla root (p.1742·1); saw palmetto berry (p.1569·1); ginseng root (p.1693·1).

**Damiclin** *Fustery, Mex.*
Clindamycin (p.194·2).
*Bacterial infections.*

**Damide** *Benedetti, Ital.*
Indapamide (p.938·2).
*Hypertension.*

**Daminate** *Sriprasit, Thai.*
Brompheniramine maleate (p.426·1); phenylephrine hydrochloride (p.1126·3); guaifenesin (p.1122·1).
*Nasal congestion.*

**Damira** *Wander Health Care, Switz.*
Preparation for enteral nutrition (p.1417·1).
*Cow's milk intolerance.*

**Damixa** *Merck, Arg.*
Diclofenac (p.32·1), diclofenac diethylamine (p.32·1), diclofenac potassium (p.32·1), diclofenac resinate (p.33·1), or diclofenac sodium (p.32·1).
*Gout; musculoskeletal, joint, peri-articular, and soft-tissue disorders; pain; renal colic.*

**Damosal** *Salus, Mex.†.*
Dipyridamole (p.903·1).

**Damoxicil** *Byk Elmu, Spain†.*
Amoxicillin trihydrate (p.155·3).
*Bacterial infections.*

**Damoxicil Mucolitico** *Byk Elmu, Spain†.*
Amoxicillin trihydrate (p.155·3); bromhexine hydrochloride (p.1115·3).
*Respiratory-tract infections.*

**Damoxy** *Dabur, India.*
Amoxicillin trihydrate (p.155·3).
*Bacterial infections.*

**Dampo**
*Roche Consumer, Neth.*
*Ointment for inhalation:* Camphor (p.1665·3); menthol (p.1711·3); eucalyptus oil (p.1686·2).
*Cold symptoms.*
*Roche Nicholas, Neth.†.*
*Nasal spray:* Oxymetazoline hydrochloride (p.1126·1).
*Nasal congestion.*

**Dampo bij droge hoest** *Roche Consumer, Neth.*
Dextromethorphan hydrobromide (p.1117·3).
*Coughs.*

**Dampo Mucopect** *Roche Consumer, Neth.†.*
Acetylcysteine (p.1112·3).
*Respiratory-tract congestion.*

**Dampo Solvopect** *Roche Consumer, Neth.*
Carbocisteine (p.1116·2).
*Respiratory-tract congestion.*

**Danalem** *Lemery, Mex.*
Danazol (p.1545·2).

**Danantizol** *Gador, Arg.*
Thiamazole (p.1603·3).
*Hyperthyroidism.*

**Danatrol**
*Sanofi Synthelabo, Belg.; Sanofi Synthelabo, Fr.; Sanofi Synthelabo, Gr.; Sanofi Synthelabo, Ital.; Sanofi Synthelabo, Neth.; Sanofi Synthelabo, Port.; Sanofi Synthelabo, Spain; Sanofi Synthelabo, Switz.*
Danazol (p.1545·2).
*Benign breast disorders; endometriosis; hereditary angioedema; menorrhagia; precocious puberty.*

**Danazant**
*Antigen, Hong Kong†; Antigen, Irl.*
Danazol (p.1545·2).
*Benign breast disorders; dysfunctional uterine bleeding; endometriosis; gynaecomastia; precocious puberty.*

**Dancimin-C** *Dankos, Singapore.*
Vitamin C (p.1460·2).
*Vitamin C deficiency.*

**Dancor**
*Merck, Austria; Merck, Port.; Merck, Spain; Merck, Switz.*
Nicorandil (p.965·3).
*Angina pectoris.*

**Dandrazol** *Transdermal, UK.*
Ketoconazole (p.403·3).
*Dandruff; pityriasis versicolor; seborrhoeic dermatitis.*

**Dandrid** *Sandoz, UK.*
Ketoconazole (p.403·3).
*Dandruff; seborrhoeic dermatitis.*

**Dandruff Control Pert 2 in 1** *Procter & Gamble, Austral.†.*
Pyrithione zinc (p.1156·2).
*Dandruff.*

**Dandruff Shampoo plus Conditioner** *Sutton, Canad.*
Pyrithione zinc (p.1156·2).
*Dandruff.*

**Dandruff Treatment Shampoo** *Sutton, Canad.*
Pyrithione zinc (p.1156·2).

**Daneral** *Hoechst Marion Roussel, Irl.†.*
Pheniramine maleate (p.438·3).
*Hypersensitivity reactions.*

**Danferane** *Rivero, Arg.*
Co-trimoxazole (p.199·3).
*Bacterial infections; Pneumocystis carinii pneumonia.*

**Dan-Gard**
*Faulding, Austral.; Stiefel, Canad.*
Pyrithione zinc (p.1156·2).
*Dandruff; seborrhoeic dermatitis.*

**Danilax**
*Danipharm, Denm.; Danipharm, Hong Kong.*
Lactulose (p.1269·1).
*Constipation; hepatic encephalopathy.*

**Danilon**
*Note. This name is used for preparations of different composition.*
*Allergan-Frumtost, Braz.†.*
Ibuprofen (p.45·3).
*Fever; inflammation; pain.*
*Esteve, Spain.*
Suxibuzone (p.93·1).
*Musculoskeletal, joint, peri-articular, and soft-tissue disorders.*

**Danitin** *Carnot, Mex.†.*
Ranitidine (p.1285·2).

**Danka** *Angelini, Ital.*
Levodropropizine (p.1119·3).
*Coughs.*

**Danlax** *Sovereign, UK.*
Dantron (p.1261·1); poloxamer 188 (p.1414·2).
*Constipation.*

**Danlox** *Casasco, Arg.*
Omeprazole (p.1278·2).
*Gastro-oesophageal reflux; peptic ulcer; Zollinger-Ellison syndrome.*

**Danocrine**
*Sanofi Synthelabo, Austral.; Sanofi Winthrop, Denm.; Sanofi Synthelabo, Fin.; Sanofi Synthelabo, Hong Kong; Sanofi Winthrop, Israel; Sanofi Synthelabo, Norw.; Sanofi Synthelabo, NZ; Sanofi Synthelabo, Swed.; Sanofi Winthrop, USA.*
Danazol (p.1545·2).
*Benign breast disorders; endometriosis; female infertility; hereditary angioedema; menorrhagia; precocious puberty.*

**Danogar** *Sanofi Synthelabo, Chile.*
Danazol (p.1545·2).
*Benign breast disorders; dyfunctional uterine bleeding; endometrial thinning; endometriosis; hereditary angioedema.*

**Danogen**
*Cipla, India; Cipla-Medpro, S.Afr.*
Danazol (p.1545·2).
*Benign breast disorders; endometriosis; female infertility; hereditary angioedema; menorrhagia.*

**Danokrin** *Sanofi Synthelabo, Austria.*
Danazol (p.1545·2).
*Endometriosis; gynaecomastia; hereditary angioedema; precocious puberty.*

**Danol**
*Sanofi Synthelabo, Irl.; Sanofi Synthelabo, UK.*
Danazol (p.1545·2).
*Benign breast disorders; dysfunctional uterine bleeding; endometriosis; gynaecomastia.*

**Danovag** *Novag, Mex.*
Omeprazole (p.1278·2).
*Peptic ulcer.*

**Danovir** *Dankos, Singapore.*
Aciclovir (p.626·1).
*Herpes simplex infections.*

**Danruf** *Torrent, India.*
Ketoconazole (p.403·3).
*Dandruff; pityriasis versicolor; seborrhoeic dermatitis.*

**Danssan** *Duopharma, Hong Kong.*
Enalapril maleate (p.909·2).
*Heart failure; hypertension.*

**Dantalin** *Cazi, Braz.*
Phenytoin (p.370·2).
*Epilepsy.*

**Dantamacrin**
*Procter & Gamble, Austria; Procter & Gamble, Ger.; Vifor, Switz.*
Dantrolene sodium (p.1393·3).
*Skeletal muscle spasm; spasticity.*

**Dan-Tar Plus** *Stiefel, Canad.*
Polytar (a blend of wood and mineral tars) (p.1159·2); pyrithione disulfide (p.1156·2).
*Seborrhoeic dermatitis.*

**Dantenk** *Biotenk, Arg.*
Ondansetron hydrochloride (p.1281·1).
*Nausea and vomiting.*

**D-Antihist** *Raza, Malaysia; Pharmaniaga, Malaysia.*
Dexchlorpheniramine maleate (p.427·3).
*Hypersensitivity reactions.*

**Dantrium**
*Pharmacia, Austral.; Procter & Gamble, Belg.; Procter & Gamble, Canad.; Procter & Gamble, Denm.; Lipha Sante, Fr.; Procter & Gamble, Hong Kong; Procter & Gamble, Irl.; Procter & Gamble, Israel; Formenti, Ital.; Procter & Gamble, Neth.; Pharmacia, NZ; Normal, Port.; Pharmaco, S.Afr.; Procter & Gamble, UK; Procter & Gamble, USA.*
Dantrolene sodium (p.1393·3).
*Malignant hyperthermia; skeletal muscle spasm; spasticity.*

**Dantrolen**
*Cristalia, Braz.; IFET (ΙΦΕΤ), Gr.*
Dantrolene sodium (p.1393·3).
*Malignant hyperthermia; skeletal muscle spasm.*

**Danubial** *Atlantis, Mex.*
Ornidazole (p.612·2).
*Amoebiasis.*

**Dany** *The Forty-Two, Thai.*
Domperidone (p.1263·2).
*Digestive disorders; dyspepsia; nausea and vomiting.*

**Danzen**
*Casasco, Arg.; Allergan-Frumtost, Braz.†; Takeda, Hong Kong; Takeda, Ital.; Takeda, Malaysia; Hormona, Mex.; Takeda, Singapore; Takeda, Thai.*
Serrapeptase (p.1743·2).
*Inflammation; respiratory-tract congestion.*

**Danzyme** *Progress, Thai.*
Serrapeptase (p.1743·2).
*Inflammation; respiratory-tract congestion.*

**Daohair-S** *Pharmex (Φαρμεξ), Gr.*
Pyrithione zinc (p.1156·2).
*Pityriasis; seborrhoeic dermatitis.*

**Daonil**
*Aventis, Arg.; Aventis, Austral.; Aventis, Austria; Aventis, Belg.; Aventis, Braz.; Aventis, Chile; Aventis, Denm.; Aventis, Fin.; Aventis, Fr.; Hoechst Marion Roussel, Gr.; Aventis, Hong Kong; Aventis, India; Aventis, Irl.; Aventis, Israel; Aventis, Ital.; Aventis, Malaysia; Aventis, Mex.; Aventis, Neth.; Aventis, Norw.; Aventis, NZ†; Aventis, Port.; Aventis, S.Afr.; Aventis, Singapore; Aventis, Spain; Aventis, Swed.; Aventis, Switz.; Aventis, Thai.; Aventis, UK.*
Glibenclamide (p.331·2).
*Diabetes mellitus.*

**Daono** *Milano, Thai.*
Glibenclamide (p.331·2).
*Diabetes mellitus.*

**Dapa** *Alphapharm, Malaysia; Merck, Malaysia.*
Indapamide (p.938·2).
*Hypertension.*

**Dapacin Cold** *Ferndale, USA†.*
Phenylpropanolamine hydrochloride (p.1127·3); chlorphenamine maleate (p.427·3); paracetamol (p.76·2).
*Upper respiratory-tract symptoms.*

**Dapamax** *Parke-Med, S.Afr.*
Indapamide (p.938·2).
*Hypertension; oedema.*

**Dapa-Tabs**
*Alphapharm, Austral.; Alphapharm, Hong Kong; Alphapharm, Singapore; Merck, Singapore.*
Indapamide (p.938·2).
*Hypertension.*

**Dapaz** *Alter, Spain†.*
Meprobamate (p.706·2).
*Anxiety; insomnia; skeletal muscle spasm.*

**Dapotum**
*Sanofi Synthelabo, Austria; Bristol-Myers Squibb, Ger.; Sanofi Synthelabo, Ger.; Bristol-Myers Squibb, Switz.*
Fluphenazine decanoate (p.699·3) or fluphenazine hydrochloride (p.699·3).
*Psychoses.*

**Daprox** *Nycomed, Denm.†.*
Naproxen (p.65·1).
*Inflammation; musculoskeletal and joint disorders; pain.*

**Daps** *Pharmacia, Arg.*
Dapsone (p.202·2).
*Leprosy.*

**Dapsoderm-X** *Remexa, Mex.*
Dapsone (p.202·2).
*Bacterial mycetoma; dermatitis herpetiformis; leprosy.*

**Daptacel** *Aventis Pasteur, USA.*
A diphtheria, tetanus, and pertussis vaccine (p.1613·3).
*Active immunisation.*

**Daptaral** *Wyeth-Ayerst, Thai.*
Multivitamin and mineral preparation (p.1417·1).

**Daptril** *Qestmed, S.Afr.*
Indapamide (p.938·2).
*Hypertension.*

**Daralix** *Quatromed, S.Afr.*
Promethazine hydrochloride (p.439·1).
*Hypersensitivity reactions; nausea; vomiting.*

**Daram** *Bittner, Austria.*
Homoeopathic preparation.

**Daramal** *GlaxoSmithKline, S.Afr.*
Chloroquine sulfate (p.448·2).
*Discoid lupus erythematosus; malaria; rheumatoid arthritis.*

**Daramal-Paludrine** *Zeneca, S.Afr.*
Chloroquine sulfate (p.448·2); proguanil hydrochloride (p.457·1).
*Malaria.*

**Daranide**
*Sigma, Austral.†; Merck Sharp & Dohme, Irl.†; Merck, USA.*
Diclofenamide (p.894·1).
*Glaucoma.*

**Daraprim**
*GlaxoSmithKline, Arg.; GlaxoSmithKline, Austral.; GlaxoSmithKline, Austria; GlaxoSmithKline, Belg.; Glaxo Wellcome, Braz.†; GlaxoSmithKline, Canad.; GlaxoSmithKline, Chile; GlaxoSmithKline, Ger.; Wellcome, Irl.; Wellcome, Israel; Glaxo Wellcome, Mex.; GlaxoSmithKline, Neth.; GlaxoSmithKline, S.Afr.; GlaxoSmithKline, Spain; GlaxoSmithKline, Switz.; GlaxoSmithKline, Thai.; GlaxoSmithKline, UK; Glaxo Wellcome, USA.*
Pyrimethamine (p.458·1).
*Malaria; toxoplasmosis.*

**Daraprin** *Zest, Braz.*
Pyrimethamine (p.458·1).
*Malaria.*

**Darax** *Pond's, Thai.*
Hydroxyzine hydrochloride (p.434·3).
*Anxiety; hypersensitivity reactions.*

**Darbalan** *Merck, Austria.*
Bisoprolol fumarate (p.875·1).
*Angina pectoris; hypertension.*

**Darbalan Plus** *Merck, Austria.*
Bisoprolol fumarate (p.875·1); hydrochlorothiazide (p.933·2).
*Hypertension.*

**Darcipireno** *Fabra, Arg.*
Biperiden (p.479·3).
*Parkinsonism.*

**Dardex** *Pliva, Spain.*
Captopril (p.879·2).
*Diabetic nephropathy; heart failure; hypertension; myocardial infarction.*

**Dardum**
*Lisapharma, Ital.; Lisapharma, Singapore.*
Cefoperazone sodium (p.174·3).
Lidocaine hydrochloride (p.1377·3) may be included in the intramuscular injection to alleviate the pain of injection.
*Bacterial infections.*

**Darebon**
*Novartis, Austria; Novartis, Ger.*
Chlortalidone (p.882·3); reserpine (p.995·1).
*Hypertension.*

**Daren**
*Note. This name is used for preparations of different composition.*
*Organon, Jpn.*
Emedastine fumarate (p.433·2).
*Allergic rhinitis; allergic skin disorders.*

Delta, Singapore.
Enalapril maleate (p.909·2).
*Heart failure; hypertension.*

**Dari** Vita Elan, Spain†.
Nifedipine (p.966·2).
*Angina pectoris; hypertension; Raynaud's syndrome.*

**Daricon**
Pfizer, Hong Kong; Pfizer, Thai.
Oxyphencyclimine hydrochloride (p.487·2).
*Irritable bowel syndrome; peptic ulcer.*

**Dariseb** Darier, Mex.
Coal tar (p.1159·2); menthol (p.1711·3).
*Scalp disorders.*

**Darkene** Bayer, Ital.
Flunitrazepam (p.698·2).
*Insomnia.*

**Darleton** Anpharm (Ανφαρμ), Gr.
Sulpiride (p.722·2).
*Psychoses.*

**Darlin** Sandipro, Belg.
Senna fruit (p.1288·2).
*Constipation.*

**Darmen Salt** Ern, Spain.
Magnesium sulfate (p.1228·2); sodium bicarbonate (p.1223·2); dibasic sodium phosphate (p.1231·1); sodium sulfate (p.1290·1).
*Constipation; dyspepsia; gastric hyperacidity.*

**Darmol**
Note. This name is used for preparations of different composition.
Schmidgall, Austria; Iromedica, Switz.
Senna (p.1288·2).
*Bowel evacuation; constipation.*

Omegin, Ger.
Sodium picosulfate (p.1289·3).
Formerly contained phenolphthalein.
*Constipation.*

**Darmol Bisacodyl** Omegin, Ger.†.
Bisacodyl (p.1251·3).
*Constipation.*

**Darmol Lactulose** Schmidgall, Austria.
Lactulose (p.1269·1).
*Constipation; stool softener.*

**Darmol Pico** Omegin, Ger.
Sodium picosulfate (p.1289·3).
*Constipation.*

**Daro** Heco, Neth.†.
Paracetamol (p.76·2).
*Fever; pain.*

**Daro Hoofdpijnpoeders** Heco, Neth.†.
Paracetamol (p.76·2); propyphenazone (p.85·3); caffeine (p.782·1).
*Headache.*

**Daro Thijm** Heco, Neth.†.
Thyme (p.1755·2).
*Coughs.*

**Darob**
Abbott, Arg.; Ebewe, Austria; Abbott, Ger.; Abbott, Port.; Meda, Swed.†.
Sotalol hydrochloride (p.1001·3).
*Arrhythmias.*

**Darocet** Heco, Neth.†.
Paracetamol (p.76·2).
*Fever; pain.*

**Darocillin** Hoechst Marion Roussel, S.Afr.†.
Phenoxymethylpenicillin potassium (p.242·1).
*Bacterial infections.*

**Darolan Hoestprikkeldempende** Heco, Neth.†.
Dextromethorphan hydrobromide (p.1117·3).
*Coughs.*

**Darolan Slijmplossende** Heco, Neth.†.
Bromhexine hydrochloride (p.1115·3).
*Respiratory-tract disorders with viscous mucus.*

**Daromide** Quatromed, S.Afr.
Merbromin (p.1185·3); sulfanilamide (p.263·2); acriflavinium chloride (p.1165·3); cod-liver oil (p.1425·2); zinc oxide (p.1163·2).
*Skin infections; wounds.*

**Daronda** Abbott, Gr.
Leuprorelin acetate (p.1331·1).
*Endometriosis; female infertility; prostatic cancer; uterine fibroids.*

**Darosed** Hoechst Marion Roussel, S.Afr.†.
Promethazine hydrochloride (p.439·1); codeine phosphate (p.27·1); ephedrine hydrochloride (p.1120·1).
*Coughs.*

**Darrow-Liq** Brunel, S.Afr.
Sodium chloride; potassium chloride; sodium citrate dihydrate; glucose (p.1222·2).
*Oral rehydration therapy.*

**Darrowped** Aspen Consumer, S.Afr.†.
Potassium chloride; sodium chloride; sodium citrate; glucose (p.1222·2).
*Diarrhoea; oral rehydration therapy.*

**Dart** Bergamo, Braz.†.
Metoclopramide (p.1274·3).
*Nausea and vomiting.*

**Dartrox** Pisa, Mex.†.
Naproxen (p.65·1).

**Daruma** Wyeth Lederle, Ital.
Idebenone (p.1700·3).
*Mental and movement disturbances associated with cerebrovascular disorders.*

**Darvocet** aai, USA.
Dextropropoxyphene napsilate (p.28·3); paracetamol (p.76·2).
*Pain.*

**Darvocet-N** Lilly, USA.
Dextropropoxyphene napsilate (p.28·3); paracetamol (p.76·2).
*Fever; pain.*

**Darvon**
Lilly, Spain.
Dextropropoxyphene napsilate (p.28·3).
*Pain.*

Lilly, USA.
Dextropropoxyphene hydrochloride (p.28·3).
*Pain.*

**Darvon Compound** aai, USA.
Dextropropoxyphene hydrochloride (p.28·3); aspirin (p.15·1); caffeine (p.782·1).
*Fever; pain.*

**Darvon Simple** Lilly, Mex.
Dextropropoxyphene hydrochloride (p.28·3).
*Pain.*

**Darvon-N**
Lilly, Canad.; Lilly, Mex.†; Lilly, USA.
Dextropropoxyphene napsilate (p.28·3).
*Pain.*

**Darvon-N Compuesto** Lilly, Mex.
Dextropropoxyphene napsilate (p.28·3); aspirin (p.15·1); caffeine (p.782·1).
*Pain.*

**Darzitil** Fabra, Arg.
Amoxicillin (p.155·3).
*Bacterial infections.*

**Darzitil Plus** Fabra, Arg.
Amoxicillin trihydrate (p.155·3); potassium clavulanate (p.193·3).
*Bacterial infections.*

**Darzitil SB** Fabra, Arg.
Amoxicillin (p.155·3); sulbactam (p.257·2).
*Bacterial infections.*

**Dasc** EMS, Braz.
Pancrelipase (p.1725·3); bile salts (p.1660·3); cellulase (p.1669·1).
*Digestive disorders.*

**Dasen** Takeda, Jpn.
Serrapeptase (p.1743·2).
*Inflammation; respiratory-tract congestion.*

**Daskil**
Novartis, Austria; LPB, Ital.
Terbinafine hydrochloride (p.408·2).
*Fungal skin and nail infections.*

**Daskyl** Azevedos, Port.
Terbinafine hydrochloride (p.408·2).
*Fungal skin and nail infections.*

**Daslin** RPG, India.
Diphenhydramine (p.431·3); ammonium chloride (p.1115·2); alcohol (p.1166·1); sodium citrate (p.1223·2); menthol (p.1711·3).
*Coughs.*

**Dasmetrol** Tocogino, Mex.†.
Metronidazole (p.607·2).

**Dasolin** Yauquimia, Mex.†.
Metronidazole (p.607·2).

**Dasten** Asta Medica, Braz.†.
Mazindol (p.1589·1).
*Obesity.*

**Dastonil** Montpellier, Arg.
Cyanocobalamin (p.1458·2) or hydroxocobalamin (p.1458·2); prasterone sodium sulfate (p.1566·1) procaine hydrochloride (p.1383·2).
*Tonic.*

**Dastosin** Yamanouchi, Spain.
Dimemorfan phosphate (p.1118·3).
*Coughs.*

**Dastusin** Shiwa, Thai.
Diphenhydramine hydrochloride (p.431·3); ammonium chloride (p.1115·2); sodium citrate (p.1223·2).
*Cold symptoms; coughs.*

**Dasuglor** Fada, Arg.
Cefalotin (p.168·3).
*Bacterial infections.*

**Datisan** Duncan, Arg.
Mitomycin (p.573·3).
*Malignant neoplasms.*

**Datolan** Faes, Spain.
Zopiclone (p.729·3).
*Insomnia.*

**Datril** Bristol-Myers Squibb, Mex.
Paracetamol (p.76·2).
*Fever; pain.*

**DaTSCAN**
Nycomed, Ital.; Nycomed Amersham, UK.
Iodine-123 (p.1524·1) as ioflupane.
*Diagnosis of parkinsonism.*

**Daunoblastin**
Pharmacia, Austria; Pharmacia, Ger.; Pharmacia, S.Afr.
Daunorubicin hydrochloride (p.545·3).
*Leukaemias.*

**Daunoblastina**
Pharmacia, Arg.; Pharmacia, Braz.; Pharmacia, Hong Kong; Pharmacia Upjohn, Ital.; Pharmacia, Port.; Pharmacia, Singapore; Kenfarma, Spain.
Daunorubicin hydrochloride (p.545·3).
*Malignant neoplasms.*

**Daunocin** BPL-Meizler, Braz.
Daunorubicin hydrochloride (p.545·3).
*Malignant neoplasms.*

**DaunoXome**
Gilead, Austral.; Gilead, Fr.; Gilead, Irl.
Liposomal daunorubicin hydrochloride (p.545·3) (p.545·3).
*AIDS-related Kaposi's sarcoma.*

Calea, Austria; Nexstar, Belg.†; United Medical, Braz.†; Gilead, Denm.; Orphan, Fin.; Gilead, Ger.; Gilead, Gr.; Gilead, Ital.; Gilead, Neth.; Gilead, Spain; Swedish Orphan, Swed.; Fresenius, Switz.; Gilead, UK; Nexstar, USA.
Liposomal daunorubicin citrate (p.546·1) (p.545·3).
*HIV-related Kaposi's sarcoma.*

**Daurocina** Laboratorios Chile, Chile.
Daunorubicin (p.546·1).
*Malignant neoplasms.*

**Dauxona** Northia, Arg.
Glyceryl trinitrate (p.923·2).

**Davedax** Bracco, Ital.
Reboxetine mesilate (p.316·3).
*Depression.*

**D'Aveia** Dermoteca, Port.
A range of skin, scalp, and vaginal preparations containing avena (p.1658·2).

**Daverium** Monsanto, Ital.
α-Dihydroergocryptine mesilate (p.1680·1).
*Age-related mental and movement disorders; headache; hyperprolactinaemia; lactation inhibition; migraine; parkinsonism.*

**Davicaina** Davi, Port.†.
Metamfetamine (p.1589·3); tetracaine (p.1385·1).

**David Morton's Quintessential** Lifeplan, UK†.
A range of multivitamin and mineral supplements (p.1417·1).

**Davilla** Rekah, Israel.
Opium (p.74·2); rhubarb (p.1287·3); cinnamon (p.1672·2); peppermint oil (p.1283·2).
*Gastrointestinal disorders.*

**Davilose** Davi, Port.
Methylcellulose (p.1580·2).
*Dry eyes.*

**Davimicina** Davi, Port.
Bacitracin (p.161·3); hydrocortisone (p.1103·3); neomycin (p.235·1).
*Infected eye disorders.*

**Davinefrina** Davi, Port.
Phenylephrine (p.1126·3).

**Davistar** Dansk-Flama, Braz.†.
Magnesium clofibrate (p.885·1); pyricarbate (p.1737·1).
*Hyperlipidaemias.*

**Davitamon AD** Chefaro, Neth.†.
Vitamin A palmitate (p.1453·1); colecalciferol (p.1461·3).

**Davitamon AD Fluor** Chefaro, Neth.†.
Vitamin A palmitate (p.1453·1); colecalciferol (p.1461·3); sodium fluoride (p.1444·3).
*Dental caries prophylaxis; rickets.*

**Davitamon E** Chefaro, Neth.†.
*dl*-Alpha tocoferil acetate (p.1465·1).

**Davitamon Fem** Chefaro, UK.
A range of vitamin, mineral, and nutritional supplements (p.1417·1).

**Davitamon fluor** Chefaro, Neth.†.
Sodium fluoride (p.1444·3).
*Dental caries prophylaxis.*

**Davixolol** Davi, Port.
Betaxolol hydrochloride (p.873·1).
*Glaucoma; ocular hypertension.*

**Daxon** Columbia, Mex.
Nitazoxanide (p.612·1).
*Amoebiasis; giardiasis; nematode infections.*

**Daxotel**
Note. This name is used for preparations of different composition.
Laboratorios Chile, Chile.
Doxorubicin hydrochloride (p.547·3).
*Malignant neoplasms.*

Dabur, India; Dabur, Thai.
Docetaxel (p.547·1).
*Breast cancer; non-small cell lung cancer.*

**Day Cold Comfort** Boots, UK†.
Paracetamol (p.76·2); pseudoephedrine hydrochloride (p.1129·2); pholcodine (p.1128·3).
*Cold symptoms.*

**Day & Night** Warner-Lambert, Irl.
15 Tablets, paracetamol (p.76·2); phenylpropanolamine hydrochloride (p.1127·3); 5 tablets, paracetamol; diphenhydramine hydrochloride (p.431·3).
*Cold and influenza symptoms.*

**Day & Night Cold & Flu**
Pfizer Consumer, Austral.; Pfizer, NZ.
Day capsules, paracetamol (p.76·2); pseudoephedrine hydrochloride (p.1129·2); dextromethorphan hydrobromide (p.1117·3); night capsules, paracetamol; chlorphenamine maleate (p.427·3); dextromethorphan hydrobromide.
*Cold and influenza symptoms.*

**Day & Night Nurse** GlaxoSmithKline Consumer, UK.
Day capsules, paracetamol (p.76·2); pseudoephedrine hydrochloride (p.1129·2); pholcodine (p.1128·3); night capsules, paracetamol; promethazine hydrochloride (p.439·1); dextromethorphan hydrobromide (p.1117·3).
*Cold and influenza symptoms.*

**Day Nurse**
Note. This name is used for preparations of different composition.
SmithKline Beecham Consumer, Irl.
Paracetamol (p.76·2); phenylpropanolamine hydrochloride (p.1127·3); dextromethorphan hydrobromide (p.1117·3).
*Cold and influenza symptoms.*

GlaxoSmithKline Consumer, UK.
Paracetamol (p.76·2); pholcodine (p.1128·3); pseudoephedrine hydrochloride (p.1129·2).
Formerly contained paracetamol, dextromethorphan hydrobromide, and phenylpropanolamine hydrochloride.
*Cold and influenza symptoms.*

**Day Time Liquigels** Scherer, Braz.†.
Guaifenesin (p.1122·1); paracetamol (p.76·2); pseudoephedrine (p.1129·2).
*Cold and influenza symptoms.*

**Dayalets**
Abbott, Hong Kong; Abbott, USA.
Multivitamin preparation (p.1417·1).

**Dayalets + Iron** Abbott, USA.
Multivitamin preparation with iron and folic acid (p.1417·1).

**Dayalets plus Iron** Abbott, Hong Kong.
Multivitamin preparation with iron (p.1417·1).

**Dayamin** Atlantic, Thai.†.
Astemizole (p.424·2).
*Hypersensitivity reactions.*

**Dayamineral**
Abbott, Arg.; Abbott, Chile; Abbott, Spain.
Multivitamin and mineral preparation (p.1417·1).

**Daycef** Elbea, Ital.
Cefonicid sodium (p.174·2).
Lidocaine hydrochloride (p.1377·3) is included in this preparation to alleviate the pain of injection.
*Gram-negative bacterial infections.*

**Dayhist** The Forty-Two, Thai.
Mebhydrolin napadisilate (p.436·3).
*Hypersensitivity reactions.*

**Dayhist-1** Major, USA.
Clemastine fumarate (p.429·1).
*Allergic rhinitis; urticaria.*

**Daypro**
Pharmacia, Canad.; Pharmacia, USA.
Oxaprozin (p.75·1).
*Osteoarthritis; rheumatoid arthritis.*

**Dayquil** Procter & Gamble, Canad.
Pseudoephedrine hydrochloride (p.1129·2); dextromethorphan hydrobromide (p.1117·3); paracetamol (p.76·2).
*Cold and influenza symptoms.*

**Dayquil Sinus and Pain Relief** Procter & Gamble, Canad.
Pseudoephedrine hydrochloride (p.1129·2); ibuprofen (p.45·3).

**Days** Merck, Mex.
Ibuprofen (p.45·3).
*Fever; inflammation; pain.*

**Daytime Cold & Flu** Stanley, Canad.
Pseudoephedrine hydrochloride (p.1129·2); dextromethorphan hydrobromide (p.1117·3); paracetamol (p.76·2).
Formerly contained pseudoephedrine hydrochloride, dextromethorphan hydrobromide, guaifenesin, and paracetamol.

**Dayto Himbin** Dayton, USA†.
Yohimbine hydrochloride (p.1766·2).

**Dayto Sulf** Dayton, USA†.
Sulfathiazole (p.264·1); sulfacetamide (p.257·3); sulfabenzamide (p.257·3); urea (p.1162·2).
*Vaginitis due to Gardnerella vaginalis.*

**Dayvit** Ache, Braz.
Vitamin and mineral preparation (p.1417·1).

**Daywear** Estee Lauder, Canad.
*SPF 15:* Octinoxate (p.1154·3); titanium dioxide (p.1160·3).
*Sunscreen.*

**Dazamide** Major, USA.
Acetazolamide (p.849·1).
*Epilepsy; glaucoma; oedema; symptoms associated with acute mountain sickness.*

**Dazen** Takeda, Fr.
Serrapeptase (p.1743·2).
*Oedema; respiratory-tract congestion.*

**Dazid** Macrophar, Thai.
Triamterene (p.1016·2); hydrochlorothiazide (p.933·2).
*Hypertension; oedema.*

**Dazine** PP Lab, Thai.
Thioridazine hydrochloride (p.724·2).
*Anxiety; mania; schizophrenia.*

**Dazocan** Protein, Mex.†.
Albendazole (p.101·2).

**Dazol** Darrow, Braz.†.
Albendazole (p.101·2).
*Worm infections.*

**Dazolin**
Note. This name is used for preparations of different composition.
Roux-Ocefa, Arg.
Naphazoline hydrochloride (p.1124·3).
*Nasal congestion.*

Drugtech, Chile.
Donepezil (p.1490·1).
*Alzheimer's disease.*

Offenbach, Mex.
Albendazole (p.101·2).
*Worm infections.*

**DBI** USV, India.
Phenformin hydrochloride (p.344·1).
*Diabetes mellitus.*

**DBI AP** Montpellier, Arg.
Metformin hydrochloride (p.342·3).
*Diabetes mellitus.*

**DC Softgels** Goldline, USA.
Docusate calcium (p.1262·1).
*Constipation.*

**DC Vin** Medicamed, Port.†.
Vinpocetine (p.1764·2).
*Vascular disorders.*

**D-Calsor** Orion, Fin.
Calcium hydrogen phosphate (p.1225·2); colecalciferol (p.1461·3).
*Calcium supplement; vitamin D deficiency.*

**DCCK** Shire, Ger.
Co-dergocrine mesilate (p.1674·1).
*Cerebral and peripheral vascular disorders; cervical disc syndrome; hypertension; migraine; shock.*

**D-Coate** Hua, Thai.
Dextromethorphan hydrobromide (p.1117·3); guaifenesin (p.1122·1); terpin hydrate (p.1131·1).
*Coughs.*

**D-Cure** SMB, Belg.†.
Colecalciferol (p.1461·3).
*Dietary supplement; hypoparathyroidism; pseudohypoparathyroidism; vitamin D deficiency.*

**DDAVP**
Ferring, Braz.†; Ferring, Canad.; Ferring, Chile; Ferring, Ger.†; IFET (ΙΦΕΤ), Gr.; Ferring, Irl.; Remexa, Mex.; Ferring, Port.; Ferring, S.Afr.; Ferring, UK; Aventis, USA.
Desmopressin (p.1322·3) or desmopressin acetate (p.1322·3).
*Diabetes insipidus; haemophilia; headache resulting from lumbar puncture; multiple sclerosis associated nocturia; polydipsia; polyuria; test of fibrinolytic response; test of renal concentrating capacity; von Willebrand's disease.*

**DDD**
Note. This name is used for preparations of different composition.
Austroplant, Austria.
Salicylic acid (p.1157·1); methyl salicylate (p.59·3); thymol (p.1194·2); camphor (p.1665·3).
*Skin disorders.*

delta pronatura, Ger.†.
Thymol (p.1194·2); salicylic acid (p.1157·1); methyl salicylate (p.59·3).
*Skin disorders.*

DDD, UK.
*Cream:* Thymol (p.1194·2); menthol (p.1711·3); methyl salicylate (p.59·3); chlorobutanol (p.1176·3); titanium dioxide (p.1160·3).
*Cuts; grazes; rashes; spots.*
*Lotion:* Thymol (p.1194·2); menthol (p.1711·3); salicylic acid (p.1157·1); chlorobutanol (p.1176·3); methyl salicylate (p.59·3).
*Rashes; spots.*

**De A a Zinc Grossesse** Arkopharma, Fr.
Multivitamin and mineral preparation (p.1417·1).

**De Icin** Viatris, Belg.
Dexamethasone sodium metasulfobenzoate (p.1097·2); neomycin sulfate (p.235·1); polymyxin B sulfate (p.245·1).
*Infected eye disorders.*

**De Icol**
Viatris, Belg.; Alcon Cusi, Malaysia.
Dexamethasone sodium phosphate (p.1097·2); chloramphenicol (p.185·1).
*Infected eye disorders.*

**de STAT** Sherman, USA.
Range of solutions for contact lenses (p.1164·2).

**De Witt's Analgesic** De Witt, UK.
Paracetamol (p.76·2); caffeine (p.782·1).
*Fever; pain.*

**De Witt's Antacid**
Note. This name is used for preparations of different composition.
Fleet, Austral.†.
*Oral powder:* Magnesium trisilicate (p.1272·3); magnesium carbonate (p.1272·1); calcium carbonate (p.1254·2); sodium bicarbonate (p.1223·2); kaolin (p.1268·3); aluminium hydroxide (p.1249·2).
*Gastrointestinal hyperacidity.*
*Tablets:* Magnesium trisilicate (p.1272·3); magnesium carbonate (p.1272·1); calcium carbonate (p.1254·2); sodium bicarbonate (p.1223·2); aluminium hydroxide (p.1249·2).
*Hyperacidity.*

De Witt, UK.
*Oral powder:* Magnesium trisilicate (p.1272·3); light magnesium carbonate (p.1272·1); calcium carbonate (p.1254·2); sodium bicarbonate (p.1223·2); light kaolin (p.1268·3); peppermint oil (p.1283·2).
*Tablets:* Calcium carbonate (p.1254·2); magnesium carbonate (p.1272·1); magnesium trisilicate (p.1272·3); peppermint oil (p.1283·2).
*Dyspepsia; gastric hyperacidity; heartburn.*

**De Witt's K & B Pills** De Witt, UK.
Bearberry (p.1659·2); buchu (p.1663·1).
*Fluid retention.*

**De Witt's Lozenges** De Witt, UK†.
Benzocaine (p.1370·3); cetylpyridinium chloride (p.1173·1).
Formerly contained tyrothricin, benzocaine, and cetylpyridinium chloride.
*Sore throat.*

**De Witts New Pills** Fleet, Austral.†.
Bearberry (p.1659·2); buchu (p.1663·1).
*Fluid retention.*

**De Witts Pills** De Witt, NZ.
Bearberry (p.1659·2); buchu (p.1663·1); caffeine (p.782·1); methylthioninium chloride (p.1042·2).
*Fluid retention.*

**Deacos** Indian Drugs, India.
Chlorphenamine maleate (p.427·3); ammonium chloride (p.1115·2); sodium citrate (p.1223·2); menthol (p.1711·3).
*Cold symptoms; coughs.*

**Deacura** Dermapharm, Ger.
Biotin (p.1423·2).
*Biotin deficiency.*

**Deafort** Collins, Mex.
Multivitamin preparation (p.1417·1).

**Deaftol avec lidocaine** Wild, Switz.
Aluminium lactate (p.1653·1); lidocaine hydrochloride (p.1377·3).
*Mouth and throat disorders.*

**Dealan** Silanes, Mex.
Coal tar (p.1159·2); clioquinol (p.196·3); allantoin (p.1141·3).
*Seborrhoeic dermatitis.*

**Dealgic** Monsanto, Ital.
Diclofenac sodium (p.32·1).
*Inflammation; musculoskeletal and joint disorders; pain.*

**Dealyd** Rosch & Handel, Austria.
Polyphloroglucinol phosphate (p.1156·1).
*Burns; skin disorders; wounds.*

**Deanacaps** Collins, Mex.
Multivitamin preparation (p.1417·1).

**Deanxit**
Lundbeck, Austria; Lundbeck, Belg.; Lundbeck, Hong Kong; Lundbeck, Ital.; Lundbeck, Singapore; Lundbeck, Spain; Lundbeck, Switz.; Lundbeck, Thai.
Flupentixol hydrochloride (p.699·1); melitracen hydrochloride (p.306·3).
*Anxiety; asthenia; depression.*

**Deavynfar** Remir, Mex.†.
Chlorpropamide (p.330·3).
*Diabetes mellitus.*

**Deb** Monsanto, Ital.
Tetridamine maleate (p.93·2).
*Cervicitis; vulvovaginitis.*

**Debacterol** Northern Research, USA.
Sulfuric acid (p.1750·3); sulfonated phenols (p.1188·1).
*Mouth and gum disorders.*

**Debax** Gebro, Austria.
Captopril (p.879·2).
*Diabetic nephropathy; heart failure; hypertension; myocardial infarction.*

**Debefenium** UCI, Braz.†.
Bephenium hydroxynaphthoate (p.103·2).
*Ancylostomiasis; ascariasis.*

**Debei** Eurofarma, Braz.†.
Phenformin hydrochloride (p.344·1).
*Diabetes mellitus.*

**Debeina** CPH, Port.
Phenformin hydrochloride (p.344·1).
*Diabetes mellitus.*

**Debekacyl** Rhone-Poulenc Rorer, Fr.†.
Dibekacin sulfate (p.205·2).
*Bacterial infections.*

**Debela** Brasifa, Braz.†.
Dipyrone (p.35·3).
*Fever; pain.*

**Debelex** Pharmacia, Arg.
Azapropazone (p.20·1).
*Gout; inflammation.*

**Debeone** Armstrong, Mex.
Phenformin hydrochloride (p.344·1).
*Diabetes mellitus.*

**Debequin** Degorts, Mex.
Dextromethorphan (p.1117·3).
*Coughs.*

**Debequin-C** Degorts, Mex.
Dextromethorphan (p.1117·3); guaifenesin (p.1122·1).
*Coughs.*

**Debisor** Novag, Mex.
Isosorbide (p.941·1).

**Deblaston**
Madaus, Austria; Hoyer, Ger.; Byk Madaus, S.Afr.; Biomed, Switz.†.
Pipemidic acid (p.243·1).
*Bacterial infections of the urinary tract.*

**Debonal** Cryopharma, Mex.
Sodium bicarbonate (p.1223·2).
*Metabolic acidosis.*

**Debridat**
Armstrong, Arg.; Croma, Austria; Enila, Braz.; Saval, Chile; Pfizer, Fr.; Sigma-Tau, Ital.; SmithKline Beecham, Mex.; Pfizer, Port.; Parke, Davis, Singapore; Uhlmann-Eyraud, Switz.
Trimebutine (p.1758·1) or trimebutine maleate (p.1758·1).
*Gastrointestinal disorders.*

**Debridat B** Armstrong, Arg.
Trimebutine maleate (p.1758·1); bromazepam (p.671·3).
*Gastrointestinal disorders.*

**Debril** Monserrat, Arg.
Naproxen (p.65·1).
*Fever; inflammation; pain.*

**Debrisan**
Pharmacia, Belg.; Pharmacia Upjohn, Canad.†; Pharmacia Upjohn, Fr.†; Pharmacia, Hong Kong; Pharmacia, Irl.; Kabi Pharmacia, Israel†; Pharmacia Upjohn, Ital.; Pharmacia Upjohn, Mex.; Pharmacia Upjohn, Neth.†; Pharmacia Upjohn, S.Afr.†; Pharmacia Upjohn, Swed.†; Pharmacia Upjohn, Switz.†; Pharmacia, UK; Johnson & Johnson, USA.
Dextranomer (p.1145·2).
*Burns; skin ulcers; wounds.*

**Debrisorb**
Pharmacia, Austria; Pharmacia, Ger.
Dextranomer (p.1145·2).
*Wounds.*

**Debrox**
Farmila, Ital.; Marion Merrell Dow, USA.
Urea hydrogen peroxide (p.1195·3).
*Ear wax removal.*

**Debrum** Sigma-Tau, Ital.
Trimebutine maleate (p.1758·1); medazepam (p.706·1).
*Gastrointestinal spasm with a component of anxiety.*

**Debrumyl**
Pierre Fabre Sante, Fr.; Pierre Fabre, Port.
Deanol pidolate (p.1585·3); heptaminol hydrochloride (p.1697·1).
*Mental function disorders.*

**Debtan**
YSP, Malaysia; Yung Shin, Thai.
Glibenclamide (p.331·2).
*Diabetes mellitus.*

**DEC**
Note. A similar name is used for preparations of different composition (see below).
Synco, Hong Kong.
Codeine phosphate (p.27·1); ephedrine hydrochloride (p.1120·1); dexchlorpheniramine maleate (p.427·3); ammonium chloride (p.1115·2).
*Coughs.*

**Dec**
Note. A similar name is used for preparations of different composition (see above).
PP Lab, Thai.
Dextromethorphan hydrobromide (p.1117·3).
*Coughs.*

**Deca**
Atlantic, Malaysia; Atlantic, Thai.
Fluphenazine decanoate (p.699·3).
*Schizophrenia.*

**Decacef** Boniscontro & Gazzone, Ital.†.
Cefmetazole sodium (p.173·3).
Lidocaine hydrochloride (p.1377·3) is included in this preparation to alleviate the pain of injection.
*Bacterial infections.*

**Decadran** Merck Sharp & Dohme, Spain†.
Dexamethasone (p.1097·1), dexamethasone phosphate (p.1097·2), or dexamethasone sodium phosphate (p.1097·2).
*Corticosteroid.*

**Decadran Neomicina** Merck Sharp & Dohme, Spain.
Dexamethasone phosphate (p.1097·2); neomycin sulfate (p.235·1).
*Eye or ear disorders.*

**Decadron**
Sidus, Arg.; Merck Sharp & Dohme, Austral.†; Merck Sharp & Dohme, Belg.; Prodome, Braz.; Merck Frosst, Canad.; Merck Sharp & Dohme, Denm.; Merck Sharp & Dohme, Fin.; Merck Sharp & Dohme-Chibret, Fr.†; IFET (ΙΦΕΤ), Gr.; Merck Sharp & Dohme, Hong Kong†; Merck Sharp & Dohme, Irl.; Merck Sharp & Dohme, Ital.; Merck Sharp & Dohme, Malaysia; Merck Sharp & Dohme, Mex.; Merck Sharp & Dohme, Neth.; Merck Sharp & Dohme, Norw.; Merck Sharp & Dohme, NZ†; Merck Sharp & Dohme, Port.; Merck Sharp & Dohme, S.Afr.; Merck Sharp & Dohme, Swed.; Merck Sharp & Dohme, Switz.; Merck Sharp & Dohme, Thai.; Merck Sharp & Dohme, UK; Merck, USA.
Dexamethasone (p.1097·1), dexamethasone acetate (p.1097·1), or dexamethasone sodium phosphate (p.1097·2).
*Corticosteroid.*

**Decadron avec Neomycine** Merck Sharp & Dohme, Belg.†.
Dexamethasone sodium phosphate (p.1097·2); neomycin sulfate (p.235·1).
*Infected eye and external ear disorders.*

**Decadron com Neomicina** Merck Sharp & Dohme, Port.
Dexamethasone sodium phosphate (p.1097·2); neomycin sulfate (p.235·1).
*Infected eye and ear disorders.*

**Decadron con Neomicina**
Note. This name is used for preparations of different composition.
Sidus, Arg.
Dexamethasone sodium phosphate (p.1097·2); neomycin sulfate (p.235·1).
*Infected eye and ear disorders.*

Merck Sharp & Dohme, Mex.
*Eye and ear drops:* Dexamethasone sodium phosphate (p.1097·2); neomycin sulfate (p.235·1).
*Infected eye and ear disorders.*
*Nasal drops*†*:* Dexamethasone sodium phosphate (p.1097·2); neomycin sulfate (p.235·1); phenylephrine hydrochloride (p.1126·3).
*Rhinitis.*

**Decadron con Nistatina** Merck Sharp & Dohme, Mex.
Dexamethasone tebutate (p.1097·3); diiodohydroxyquinoline (p.603·3); nystatin (p.406·3).
*Vaginitis.*

**Decadron cum neomycin** Merck Sharp & Dohme, Swed.
Dexamethasone sodium phosphate (p.1097·2); neomycin sulfate (p.235·1).
*Infected eye and ear disorders.*

**Decadron med Neomycin** Merck Sharp & Dohme, Denm.
Dexamethasone sodium phosphate (p.1097·2); neomycin sulfate (p.235·1).
*Infected eye and ear disorders.*

**Decadron met neomycine** Merck Sharp & Dohme, Neth.
Dexamethasone sodium phosphate (p.1097·2); neomycin sulfate (p.235·1).
*Infected eye and ear disorders.*

**Decadron Nasal** Prodome, Braz.
Dexamethasone (p.1097·1); neomycin sulfate (p.235·1); phenylephrine hydrochloride (p.1126·3).
*Infected nasal disorders.*

**Decadron with Neomycin**
Merck Sharp & Dohme, Hong Kong†; Merck Sharp & Dohme, Thai.
Dexamethasone sodium phosphate (p.1097·2); neomycin sulfate (p.235·1).
*Infected eye and ear disorders.*

**Decadron Oftalmico** Prodome, Braz.
Dexamethasone sodium phosphate (p.1097·2); neomycin sulfate (p.235·1).
Formerly contained dexamethasone, neomycin sulfate, and phenylephrine.
*Infected eye disorders.*

**Decadron Phosphat** Merck Sharp & Dohme, Ger.†.
Dexamethasone phosphate (p.1097·2).
*Corticosteroid.*

**Decadronal**
Prodome, Braz.; Merck Sharp & Dohme, Mex.
Dexamethasone acetate (p.1097·1).
*Corticosteroid.*

**Deca-Durabol** Organon, Swed.
Nandrolone decanoate (p.1561·2).
*Anaemia; osteoporosis.*

**Deca-Durabolin**
Organon, Arg.; Organon, Austral.; Organon, Austria; Organon, Belg.; Organon, Braz.; Organon, Canad.; Organon, Chile; Organon, Fin.; Organon (Οργανον), Gr.; Organon, Ger.; Organon, Hong Kong; Infar, India; Organon, Irl.†; Organon, Israel†; Organon, Ital.; Organon, Malaysia; Organon, Mex.; Organon, Neth.; Organon, Norw.; Organon, NZ; Organon, Port.; Donmed, S.Afr.; Organon, Singapore; Organon, Spain; Organon, Switz.; Organon, Thai.; Organon, UK; Organon, USA.
Nandrolone decanoate (p.1561·2).
*Anabolic; anaemias; breast cancer; osteoporosis.*

**Decafar** Lafare, Ital.
Ubidecarenone (p.1760·2).
*Cardiac disorders.*

**Decagen** Goldline, USA.
Multivitamin and mineral preparation with iron and folic acid (p.1417·1).

**Decahist-DM** Cypress, USA.
Carbinoxamine maleate (p.426·3); dextromethorphan hydrobromide (p.1117·3); pseudoephedrine hydrochloride (p.1129·2).
*Coughs; upper respiratory-tract congestion.*

**Decaject** Mayrand, USA†.
Dexamethasone acetate (p.1097·1) or dexamethasone sodium phosphate (p.1097·2).
*Corticosteroid.*

**Decal** Rice Steele, Irl.
Calcium lactate (p.1225·3); calcium gluconate (p.1225·2); calcium phosphate (p.1225·3); ergocalciferol (p.1462·1).
*Calcium deficiencies; calcium supplement.*

**Decalcit**
Neves, Port.
Colecalciferol (p.1461·3); calcium hydrogen phosphate (p.1225·2).
*Calcium and vitamin D deficiency; osteomalacia; osteoporosis; rickets.*

Geistlich, Switz.
Ergocalciferol (p.1462·1); calcium hydrogen phosphate (p.1225·2).
*Calcium and vitamin D deficiencies.*

**Decalogiflox** Pharmacia, Fr.
Lomefloxacin hydrochloride (p.227·2).
*Urinary-tract infections.*

**Decaltrex** Ern, Spain†.
Amino-acid, vitamin, and mineral preparation (p.1417·1).

**Decan**
Note. This name is used for preparations of different composition.
Aguettant, Fr.; Baxter, Spain; Baxter, UK.
Electrolyte (p.1217·1) and trace element preparation (p.1417·1).
*Parenteral nutrition.*

YSP, Malaysia.
Dexamethasone (p.1097·1).
*Corticosteroid.*

**Decaneurabol** Cadila, India.
Nandrolone decanoate (p.1561·2).
*Anabolic; osteoporosis.*

**Deca-Noralone** Taro, Israel†.
Nandrolone decanoate (p.1561·2).
*Anabolic; breast cancer; osteoporosis; renal failure.*

**Decapeptyl**
Sidus, Arg.; Ferring, Austria; Ipsen, Belg.; Tecnofarma, Chile; Ferring, Denm.; Ferring, Fin.; Ipsen Biotech, Fr.; Ferring, Ger.; Ferring, Hong Kong; Ferring, India; Ipsen, Irl.; Ferring, Israel; Ipsen, Ital.; Ferring, Malaysia; Ferring, Neth.; Aventis, NZ†; Ipsen, Port.; Pharmaplan, S.Afr.;

*Ferring, Singapore; Ipsen, Spain; Ferring, Swed.; Ferring, Switz.; Ferring, Thai.; Ipsen, UK.*
Triptorelin (p.1341·2), triptorelin acetate (p.1341·2), or triptorelin embonate (p.1341·2).
*Breast cancer; endometriosis; female infertility; ovarian cancer; precocious puberty; prostatic cancer; uterine fibroids.*

**Decaprednil** *Orion, Ger.†.*
Prednisolone (p.1108·1) or prednisolone acetate (p.1108·1).
*Corticosteroid.*

**Decaquinon** *Eisai, Thai.*
Ubidecarenone (p.1760·2).
*Heart failure.*

**Decaris**
*Janssen, Hong Kong.*
Levamisole (p.107·1).
*Hookworm and roundworm infections.*

*Janssen, Mex.*
Levamisole hydrochloride (p.107·2).
*Nematode infections.*

**Deca-Scab** *Lafedar, Arg.*
Deltamethrin (p.1503·1); piperonyl butoxide (p.1509·2); butylated hydroxytoluene (p.1171·3); lavender oil (p.1705·2).
*Pediculosis; scabies.*

**Decasept N** *Streuli, Switz.*
Dequalinium chloride (p.1178·1); calcium pantothenate (p.1442·3); lauromacrogol 400 (p.1412·3).
Decasept formerly contained dequalinium chloride, calcium pantothenate, lauromacrogol 400, and ammonium gualenate.
*Mouth and throat disorders.*

**Decasona** *Alter, Spain.*
Beclometasone dipropionate (p.1091·1).
*Asthma.*

**Decasone** *Aspen, S.Afr.*
Dexamethasone phosphate (p.1097·2).
*Corticosteroid.*

**Decaspray** *Merck, USA.*
Dexamethasone (p.1097·1).
*Skin disorders.*

**Decatylen**
*Note. This name is used for preparations of different composition.*
*Mepha, Hong Kong; Mepha, Malaysia; Mepha, Singapore.*
Dequalinium chloride (p.1178·1); cinchocaine hydrochloride (p.1373·2).
*Mouth and throat disorders.*

*Protein, Mex.†.*
Dequalinium chloride (p.1178·1).

**Decatylene** *Mepha, Switz.*
Dequalinium chloride (p.1178·1).
*Mouth and throat disorders.*

**Decatylene Neo** *Mepha, Switz.*
Dequalinium chloride (p.1178·1); cinchocaine hydrochloride (p.1373·2).
*Mouth and throat disorders.*

**Decaugh** *Fortune, Hong Kong.*
Dextromethorphan hydrobromide (p.1117·3); guaifenesin (p.1122·1).
*Coughs.*

**Decaven** *Baxter, Ital.*
Mineral and trace-element preparation (p.1417·1).
*Parenteral nutrition.*

**Deca-Vi-Sol** *Bristol-Myers Squibb, Mex.*
Vitamin preparation (p.1417·1).

**Decavit** *Rowa, Irl.*
Multivitamin preparation (p.1417·1).

**Decdan** *Merind, India.*
Dexamethasone (p.1097·1) or dexamethasone sodium phosphate (p.1097·2).
*Corticosteroid.*

**Decdan-N** *Merind, India.*
Dexamethasone sodium phosphate (p.1097·2); neomycin sulfate (p.235·1).
*Eye disorders.*

**Decentan**
*Merck, Austria; Merck, Ger.; Merck, Spain.*
Perphenazine (p.714·2) or perphenazine enantate (p.714·2).
*Anxiety; depression; pain; psychoses; vomiting.*

**De-Chlor DM** *Cypress, USA.*
Dextromethorphan hydrobromide (p.1117·3); phenylephrine hydrochloride (p.1126·3); chlorphenamine maleate (p.427·3).
*Coughs; respiratory-tract congestion.*

**De-Chlor DR** *Cypress, USA.*
Dextromethorphan hydrobromide (p.1117·3); phenylephrine hydrochloride (p.1126·3); chlorphenamine maleate (p.427·3).
*Coughs; respiratory-tract congestion.*

**De-Chlor G** *Cypress, USA.*
Hydrocodone tartrate (p.45·1); phenylephrine hydrochloride (p.1126·3); guaifenesin (p.1122·1).
*Coughs; respiratory-tract congestion.*

**De-Chlor HC** *Cypress, USA.*
Hydrocodone tartrate (p.45·1); phenylephrine hydrochloride (p.1126·3); chlorphenamine maleate (p.427·3).
*Allergic rhinitis; cold symptoms.*

**De-Chlor HD** *Cypress, USA.*
Hydrocodone tartrate (p.45·1); phenylephrine hydrochloride (p.1126·3); chlorphenamine maleate (p.427·3).
*Allergic rhinitis; cold symptoms.*

**De-Chlor MR** *Cypress, USA.*
Hydrocodone tartrate (p.45·1); mepyramine maleate (p.437·1); phenylephrine hydrochloride (p.1126·3).
*Coughs; nasal congestion.*

**De-Chlor NX** *Cypress, USA.*
Hydrocodone tartrate (p.45·1); sulfogaiacol (p.1131·1).
*Coughs.*

**Decho** *Milano, Thai.*
Dequalinium chloride (p.1178·1).
*Mouth and throat infections.*

**Decholin**
*Riedel-Zabinka, Braz.†; Miles, USA.*
Dehydrocholic acid (p.1679·2).
*Biliary disorders; constipation.*

**Decidex** *Roemmers, Arg.*
Chlorphenamine maleate (p.427·3); pseudoephedrine sulfate (p.1129·2).
*Respiratory-tract congestion.*

**Decidex Compuesto** *Roemmers, Arg.*
Chlorphenamine maleate (p.427·3); pseudoephedrine sulfate (p.1129·2); paracetamol (p.76·2).
*Influenza symptoms.*

**Decidex Plus** *Roemmers, Arg.*
Loratadine (p.436·1); pseudoephedrine sulfate (p.1129·2).
*Allergic rhinitis.*

**Decilina** *Klonal, Arg.*
Ampicillin (p.157·1).
*Bacterial infections.*

**Decipar** *Italfarmaco, Spain.*
Enoxaparin sodium (p.910·3).
*Thromboembolic disorders.*

**Decitriol** *Richmond, Arg.*
Lysine aspirin (p.54·3).
*Inflammation; pain.*

**Decliten** *Ariston, Arg.*
Prazosin hydrochloride (p.985·1).
*Hypertension.*

**Decloban** *Farmacusi, Spain.*
Clobetasol propionate (p.1095·2).
*Skin disorders.*

**Declomycin**
*Wyeth-Ayerst, Canad.; ESP, USA.*
Demeclocycline hydrochloride (p.204·3).
*Bacterial infections; intestinal amoebiasis.*

**Declovir** *Hoe, Malaysia.*
Aciclovir (p.626·1).
*Herpes simplex infections.*

**Decme** *Italmex, Mex.†.*
Dihydroergocristine mesilate (p.1680·1).

**Decocort**
*Hoe, Malaysia; Hoe, Singapore.*
Miconazole nitrate (p.405·3); hydrocortisone (p.1103·3).
*Fungal and Gram-positive bacterial skin infections with inflammation.*

**Decoderm**
*Hermal, Austria; Boots Healthcare, Belg.; Hermal, Ger.; Boots Healthcare, Neth.†; Boots Healthcare, Spain†; Boots Healthcare, Switz.*
Fluprednidene acetate (p.1102·2).
*Skin disorders.*

**Decoderm Base** *Boots Healthcare, Switz.†.*
Emollient.
*Skin disorders.*

**Decoderm Basiscreme** *Hermal, Ger.*
Emollient.
*Skin disorders.*

**Decoderm bivalent** *Boots Healthcare, Switz.*
Fluprednidene acetate (p.1102·2); miconazole nitrate (p.405·3).
*Infected skin disorders.*

**Decoderm Comp**
*Boots Healthcare, Belg.; Hermal, Ger.*
Fluprednidene acetate (p.1102·2); gentamicin sulfate (p.217·1).
*Infected skin disorders.*

**Decoderm compositum** *Hermal, Austria.*
Fluprednidene acetate (p.1102·2); gentamicin sulfate (p.217·1).
*Infected skin disorders.*

**Decoderm tri** *Hermal, Ger.*
Fluprednidene acetate (p.1102·2); miconazole nitrate (p.405·3).
*Infected skin disorders.*

**Decoderm trivalent** *Hermal, Austria.*
Fluprednidene acetate (p.1102·2); gentamicin sulfate (p.217·1); cloxiquine (p.220·3).
*Infected skin disorders.*

**Decoderm Trivalente** *Boots Healthcare, Spain†.*
Fluprednidene acetate (p.1102·2); neomycin sulfate (p.235·1); cloxiquine (p.220·3).
*Infected skin disorders.*

**Decofam Cough** *DHA, Singapore.*
Ammonium chloride (p.1115·2); ephedrine hydrochloride (p.1120·1); guaifenesin (p.1122·1); menthol (p.1711·3).
*Coughs.*

**Decofed** *Barre-National, USA; Major, USA.*
Pseudoephedrine hydrochloride (p.1129·2).
*Nasal congestion.*

**Decohistine DH** *Morton Grove, USA.*
Pseudoephedrine hydrochloride (p.1129·2); chlorphenamine maleate (p.427·3); codeine phosphate (p.27·1).
*Coughs and cold symptoms.*

**Decolgen**
*Note. This name is used for preparations of different composition.*
*Westmont, Hong Kong†.*
Paracetamol (p.76·2); phenylpropanolamine hydrochloride (p.1127·3); chlorphenamine maleate (p.427·3).
*Cold symptoms; upper respiratory-tract disorders.*

*Westmont, Singapore.*
*Oral liquid†:* Chlorphenamine maleate (p.427·3); paracetamol (p.76·2); phenylpropanolamine hydrochloride (p.1127·3).
*Tablets:* Chlorphenamine maleate (p.427·3); paracetamol (p.76·2); phenylephrine hydrochloride (p.1126·3). Formerly contained ascorbic acid, chlorphenamine maleate, paracetamol, and phenylpropanolamine hydrochloride.
*Cold symptoms; upper respiratory-tract disorders.*

*Great Eastern, Thai.; Westmont, Thai.*
Paracetamol (p.76·2); chlorphenamine maleate (p.427·3).
Formerly contained phenylpropanolamine hydrochloride, paracetamol, and chlorphenamine maleate.
*Cold symptoms; hay fever; respiratory-tract disorders; sinusitis.*

**Decomit** *Beximco, Singapore.*
Beclometasone dipropionate (p.1091·1).
*Allergic rhinitis; nasal polyps.*

**Decon** *Cadila Pharma, India.*
Xylometazoline hydrochloride (p.1132·2).
*Nasal congestion.*

**Deconamine**
*Kenwood, Hong Kong; Kenwood, USA.*
Chlorphenamine maleate (p.427·3); pseudoephedrine hydrochloride (p.1129·2).
*Allergic rhinitis; nasal congestion; sinusitis.*

**Deconamine CX** *Bradley, USA.*
Guaifenesin (p.1122·1); hydrocodone tartrate (p.45·1); pseudoephedrine hydrochloride (p.1129·2).
*Coughs.*

**Deconex 50FF** *Borer, Thai.*
Glyoxal (p.1181·1); glutaral (p.1180·3); didecyldimethylammonium chloride (p.1178·3).
*Surface and instrument disinfection.*

**Deconex 53IN** *Borer, Thai.*
Alkylamine; didecyldimethylammonium chloride (p.1178·3).
*Instrument disinfection.*

**Decongest**
*Technilab, Canad.; Technilab, Hong Kong†.*
Xylometazoline hydrochloride (p.1132·2).
*Nasal congestion.*

**Decongestabs** *Parmed, USA†.*
Phenylpropanolamine hydrochloride (p.1127·3); phenylephrine hydrochloride (p.1126·3); chlorphenamine maleate (p.427·3); phenyltoloxamine citrate (p.439·1).
*Upper respiratory-tract symptoms.*

**Decongestant**
*Moore, USA†.*
Phenylpropanolamine hydrochloride (p.1127·3); phenylephrine hydrochloride (p.1126·3); chlorphenamine maleate (p.427·3); phenyltoloxamine citrate (p.439·1).
*Upper respiratory-tract symptoms.*

*Rugby, USA.*
Phenylephrine hydrochloride (p.1126·3); paracetamol (p.76·2); chlorphenamine maleate (p.427·3).
*Upper respiratory-tract symptoms.*

**Decongestant Antihistaminic Syrup** *Pharmascience, Canad.†.*
Brompheniramine maleate (p.426·1); phenylephrine hydrochloride (p.1126·3); phenylpropanolamine hydrochloride (p.1127·3).
*Antihistamine; decongestant.*

**Decongestant Expectorant** *Schein, USA†.*
Pseudoephedrine hydrochloride (p.1129·2); guaifenesin (p.1122·1); codeine phosphate (p.27·1).
*Coughs.*

**Decongestant Nasal Mist** *Prodemdis, Canad.*
Oxymetazoline hydrochloride (p.1126·1).

**Decongestant Nasal Spray** *Prodemdis, Canad.; Technilab, Canad.; Stanley, Canad.*
Xylometazoline hydrochloride (p.1132·2).

**Decongestant Nose Drops** *Prodemdis, Canad.*
Xylometazoline hydrochloride (p.1132·2).

**Decongestant SR** *Geneva, USA†.*
Phenylpropanolamine hydrochloride (p.1127·3); phenylephrine hydrochloride (p.1126·3); chlorphenamine maleate (p.427·3); phenyltoloxamine citrate (p.439·1).
*Upper respiratory-tract symptoms.*

**Decongestant Tablets**
*Stanley, Canad.; Unichem, UK†.*
Pseudoephedrine hydrochloride (p.1129·2).

**Decongex Plus** *Ache, Braz.*
Brompheniramine maleate (p.426·1); phenylephrine hydrochloride (p.1126·3).
*Nasal congestion.*

**Decongex Plus Expectorante** *Ache, Braz.*
Brompheniramine maleate (p.426·1); phenylephrine hydrochloride (p.1126·3); guaifenesin (p.1122·1).
*Nasal congestion.*

**Deconhist LA** *Goldline, USA†.*
Phenylephrine hydrochloride (p.1126·3); phenylpropanolamine hydrochloride (p.1127·3); chlorphenamine maleate (p.427·3); hyoscyamine sulfate (p.485·1); atropine sulfate (p.477·1); hyoscine hydrobromide (p.483·3).
*Upper respiratory-tract symptoms.*

**Decono** *Milano, Thai.*
Paracetamol (p.76·2); chlorphenamine maleate (p.427·3).
*Upper respiratory-tract disorders.*

**Deconomed** *Iopharm, USA.*
Pseudoephedrine hydrochloride (p.1129·2); chlorphenamine maleate (p.427·3).
*Upper respiratory-tract disorders.*

**Deconsal II** *Carolina, USA.*
Phenylephrine hydrochloride (p.1126·3); guaifenesin (p.1122·1).
Formerly contained pseudoephedrine hydrochloride and guaifenesin.
*Coughs; nasal congestion.*

**Deconsal Pediatric** *Adams, USA†.*
Codeine phosphate (p.27·1); pseudoephedrine hydrochloride (p.1129·2); guaifenesin (p.1122·1).

**Deconsal Sprinkle** *Adams, USA†.*
Phenylephrine hydrochloride (p.1126·3); guaifenesin (p.1122·1).
*Coughs; nasal congestion.*

**Decontractyl**
*Note. This name is used for preparations of different composition.*
*Synthelabo, Belg.†; Sanofi Synthelabo, Fr.*
*Ointment:* Mephenesin (p.1394·3); methyl nicotinate (p.59·2).
*Painful muscular disorders.*

*Sanofi Synthelabo, Fr.*
*Tablets:* Mephenesin (p.1394·3).
*Painful muscular disorders.*

**Decontractyl New** *Sanofi Synthelabo, Belg.†.*
Ibuprofen (p.45·3).
*Peri-articular and soft-tissue disorders.*

**Decontril** *Pulitzer, Ital.*
Thiocolchicoside (p.1395·2).
*Neuromuscular pain; parkinsonism; spasticity.*

**Decorenone** *Italfarmaco, Ital.*
Ubidecarenone (p.1760·2).
*Cardiac disorders; co-enzyme Q deficiency.*

**Decorex** *Pisa, Mex.*
Dexamethasone (p.1097·1).
*Corticosteroid.*

**Decorpa** *Pierre Fabre, Ger.*
Sterculia (p.1290·2).
*Obesity.*

**Decortilen** *Merck, Ger.*
Prednylidene (p.1109·3).
*Corticosteroid.*

**Decortin** *Merck, Ger.*
Prednisone (p.1109·3).
*Oral corticosteroid.*

**Decortin H** *Merck, Ger.*
Prednisolone (p.1108·1).
*Oral corticosteroid.*

**Decos** *Sriprasit, Thai.*
Promethazine hydrochloride (p.439·1); codeine phosphate (p.27·1).
*Coughs.*

**Decosil** *Collins, Mex.*
Naproxen sodium (p.65·1); paracetamol (p.76·2).
*Inflammation; pain.*

**Decostriol** *Jenapharm, Ger.*
Calcitriol (p.1461·2).
*Hypoparathyroidism; pseudohypoparathyroidism; renal osteodystrophy; rickets.*

**Decozol**
*Hoe, Malaysia; Hoe, Singapore.*
Miconazole nitrate (p.405·3).
*Fungal skin and nail infections.*

**Decrelip** *Ferrer, Spain.*
Gemfibrozil (p.923·1).
*Hyperlipidaemias.*

**Decresco** *Pharmacia, Spain.*
Captopril (p.879·2); hydrochlorothiazide (p.933·2).
*Hypertension.*

**Decrin** *Roche Consumer, Austral.†.*
Aspirin (p.15·1); codeine phosphate (p.27·1).
*Fever; pain.*

**Dectancyl** *Aventis, Fr.*
Dexamethasone acetate (p.1097·1).
*Corticosteroid.*

**Decubal**
*Alpharma, Fin.; Alpharma, Port.; Dumex, UK.*
Emollient.
*Dry skin disorders.*

**Decurin** *Gray, Arg.*
Tubocurarine chloride (p.1409·2).
*Competitive neuromuscular blocker.*

**Decylenes** *Rugby, USA.*
Undecenoic acid (p.410·3); zinc undecenoate (p.411·1).
*Bromhidrosis; fungal skin infections; hyperhidrosis; minor skin irritation; nappy rash.*

**Dedile** *Elvetium, Arg.*
Flutamide (p.556·2).

**Dediol** *Aventis, Ital.*
Alfacalcidol (p.1461·2).
*Hypoparathyroidism; osteomalacia; osteoporosis; renal osteodystrophy; rickets.*

**Dedolor** *Klinge, Austria.*
Diclofenac (p.32·1).
*Inflammation; musculoskeletal and joint disorders; pain.*

**Dedostryl** *Antor, Gr.*
Budesonide (p.1094·2).
*Topical corticosteroid.*

**Dedralen** *Italfarmaco, Ital.*
Doxazosin mesilate (p.908·3).
*Hypertension.*

**Dedrei** *Opfermann, Ger.*
Colecalciferol (p.1461·3).
*Osteoporosis; vitamin D deficiency.*

**Dedrogyl**
*Aventis, Belg.; Aventis, Fr.; Aventis, Ger.; IFET (ΙΦΕΤ), Gr.; Aventis, Port.*
Calcifediol (p.1461·2).
*Hypocalcaemia; hypoparathyroidism; osteomalacia; renal osteodystrophy; rickets; vitamin D deficiency.*

**Deep Cold** *Mentholatum, Canad.*
Menthol (p.1711·3).

**Deep Freeze** *Mentholatum, UK.*
Menthol (p.1711·3); pentane.
*Musculoskeletal, joint, and soft-tissue disorders.*

**Deep Freeze Cold Gel** *Mentholatum, UK.*
Menthol (p.1711·3).
*Musculoskeletal, joint, and peri-articular disorders.*

**Deep Heat** *Mentholatum, Austral.*
*Cream:* Methyl salicylate (p.59·3); menthol (p.1711·3).
*Topical spray:* Methyl salicylate (p.59·3); ethyl salicylate (p.37·3); glycol salicylate (p.44·3); methyl nicotinate (p.59·2).
*Muscular aches and pains.*

**Deep Heat Massage** *Mentholatum, UK†.*
Menthol (p.1711·3); methyl salicylate (p.59·3).
*Musculoskeletal, joint, and soft-tissue disorders.*

**Deep Heat Maximum Strength** *Mentholatum, UK.*
Menthol (p.1711·3); methyl salicylate (p.59·3).
*Musculoskeletal, joint, and soft-tissue disorders.*

**Deep Heat Rub**
*Mentholatum, Israel; Mentholatum, UK.*
Menthol (p.1711·3); eucalyptus oil (p.1686·2); methyl salicylate (p.59·3); turpentine oil (p.1760·1).
*Musculoskeletal, joint, and soft-tissue disorders.*

**Deep Heat Spray**
*Mentholatum, Israel; Mentholatum, UK.*
Methyl nicotinate (p.59·2); glycol salicylate (p.44·3); methyl salicylate (p.59·3); ethyl salicylate (p.37·3).
*Musculoskeletal, joint, peri-articular, and soft-tissue disorders.*

**Deep Heating** *Mentholatum, Canad.*
Methyl salicylate (p.59·3); menthol (p.1711·3).

**Deep Heating Rub** *Mentholatum, Singapore.*
Methyl salicylate (p.59·3); menthol (p.1711·3).
*Musculoskeletal, joint, and soft-tissue pain.*

**Deep Heating Spray** *Mentholatum, Singapore.*
Methyl salicylate (p.59·3); ethyl salicylate (p.37·3); glycol salicylate (p.44·3); methyl nicotinate (p.59·2).
*Musculoskeletal, joint, and soft-tissue pain.*

**Deep Relief**
*Gezzi, Arg.; Mentholatum, UK.*
Ibuprofen (p.45·3); menthol (p.1711·3).
*Musculoskeletal, joint, and soft-tissue disorders.*

**Deep-Down Rub** *SmithKline Beecham, USA.*
Methyl salicylate (p.59·3); menthol (p.1711·3); camphor (p.1665·3).
*Muscle, joint, and soft-tissue pain; neuralgia.*

**Deetipat** *Ferrosan, Fin.*
Colecalciferol (p.1461·3).
*Vitamin D deficiency.*

**Defanac** *Ranbaxy, UK.*
Diclofenac sodium (p.32·1).
*Gout; musculoskeletal, joint, peri-articular, and soft-tissue disorders; pain.*

**Defanyl** *Biodim, Fr.*
Amoxapine (p.286·3).
*Depression.*

**Defarol** *Adipharm (Αδηφαρμ), Gr.*
Tamoxifen citrate (p.584·1).
*Breast cancer.*

**Defatig** *Allergan-Frumtost, Braz.†.*
Vitamin B substances; potassium aspartate; magnesium aspartate (p.1417·1).
*Nutritional supplement.*

**Defaxina** *Smaller, Spain.*
Cefalexin (p.168·1).
*Bacterial infections.*

**DeFed** *Ferndale, USA.*
Pseudoephedrine hydrochloride (p.1129·2).
*Nasal congestion.*

**Defencid** *Duopharm, Ger.†.*
Devil's claw root (p.28·2).
*Musculoskeletal and joint disorders.*

**Defen-LA** *Horizon, USA.*
Pseudoephedrine hydrochloride (p.1129·2); guaifenesin (p.1122·1).

**Defibrase** *Gerot, Austria.*
Batroxobin (p.743·3).
*Thromboembolic disorders.*

**Deficical B12** *Gross, Braz.*
Calcium phosphate; sodium fluoride; colecalciferol; cyanocobalamin (p.1417·1).
*Nutritional supplement.*

**Defiltran** *Alpharma, Fr.*
Acetazolamide (p.849·1).
*Soft-tissue injury.*

**Definity** *Bristol-Myers Squibb, USA.*
Perflutren (p.1067·2) in lipid-coated microspheres.
*Contrast medium for echocardiography.*

**Defirin** *Chemipharma, Gr.*
Desmopressin acetate (p.1322·3).
*Diabetes insipidus; haemophilia; von Willebrand's disease.*

**Defix** *SNBTS, UK.*
Factor VIII inhibitor bypassing fraction (p.752·2).
*Haemorrhagic disorders.*

**Deflam** *Akromed, S.Afr.*
Oxaprozin (p.75·1).
*Musculoskeletal and joint disorders.*

**Deflamat**
*Klinge, Austria; Andromaco, Chile; Sankyo, Ital.; Klinge, Switz.*
Diclofenac (p.32·1) or diclofenac sodium (p.32·1).
*Fever; gout; inflammation; musculoskeletal, joint, peri-articular, and soft-tissue disorders; oedema; pain.*

**Deflamm** *Klinge, Austria.*
Diclofenac sodium (p.32·1).
*Musculoskeletal pain and inflammation.*

**Deflamol** *Fumouze, Fr.*
Titanium dioxide (p.1160·3); zinc oxide (p.1163·2).
*Nappy rash; skin irritation.*

**Deflamon** *SPA, Ital.*
Metronidazole (p.607·2).
*Anaerobic bacterial infections.*

**Deflamox** *Sanfer, Mex.*
Naproxen sodium (p.65·1).
*Inflammation; pain.*

**Deflan** *Guidotti, Ital.*
Deflazacort (p.1096·2).
*Oral corticosteroid.*

**Deflanil** *Libbs, Braz.*
Deflazacort (p.1096·2).
*Corticosteroid.*

**Deflaren** *Sanval, Braz.*
Dexamethasone (p.1097·1) or dexamethasone acetate (p.1097·1).
*Corticosteroid.*

**Deflogen** *Biolab Sanus, Braz.*
Nimesulide (p.67·1).
*Fever; inflammation; pain.*

**Deflogix** *Vedim, Port.*
Ketoprofen lysine (p.51·3).
*Inflammation; musculoskeletal, joint, and peri-articular disorders.*

**Deflox**
*Note. This name is used for preparations of different composition.*
*Merck, Mex.*
Diclofenac potassium (p.32·1) or diclofenac resinate (p.33·1).
*Inflammation; pain.*

*Abbott, Spain.*
Terazosin hydrochloride (p.1010·3).
*Benign prostatic hyperplasia; hypertension.*

**Defluin** *Merck, Arg.*
Enalapril maleate (p.909·2).
*Heart failure; hypertension.*

**Defluin Plus** *Merck, Arg.*
Enalapril maleate (p.909·2); hydrochlorothiazide (p.933·2).
*Hypertension.*

**Defluina**
*Note. This name is used for preparations of different composition.*
*Ebewe, Austria.*
Raubasine (p.994·3) or raubasine hydrochloride (p.994·3); dihydroergocristine mesilate (p.1680·1); dihydroergotamine mesilate (p.465·3).
*Cerebral and peripheral vascular disease.*

*Aventis, Ger.*
Buflomedil hydrochloride (p.877·2).
*Peripheral vascular disorders.*

*Teofarma, Ital.*
Dihydroergocristine mesilate (p.1680·1).
*Cerebral and peripheral vascular disorders; headache; hypertension.*

**Defluina N** *Aventis, Ger.*
Co-dergocrine mesilate (p.1674·1).
*Mental function disorders.*

**Defomil** *Nakornpatana, Thai.*
Aluminium hydroxide-magnesium carbonate co-dried gel (p.1250·1); magnesium hydroxide (p.1272·2); simeticone (p.1289·2).
*Flatulence; gastric hyperacidity; heartburn; peptic ulcer.*

**Deftan** *Merck, Spain.*
Lofepramine hydrochloride (p.305·3).
*Depression.*

**Defungo** *Siam Bheasach, Thai.*
Clotrimazole (p.396·2).
*Fungal skin and vaginal infections; trichomoniasis.*

**Degabina** *Rivero, Arg.*
Dexamethasone (p.1097·1).
*Corticosteroid.*

**DeGalin** *Degab, Ger.*
Calcium folinate (p.1431·1).
*Folic acid deficiency; prevention of methotrexate toxicity.*

**De-Gas** *Whitehall, NZ.*
Simeticone (p.1289·2).
*Flatulence.*

**Degas**
*Whitehall, Austral.; Invamed, USA.*
Simeticone (p.1289·2).
*Flatulence.*

**Degas Extra** *Whitehall, Austral.*
Simeticone (p.1289·2); calcium carbonate (p.1254·2); light magnesium carbonate (p.1272·1); sodium bicarbonate (p.1223·2).
*Dyspepsia; flatulence.*

**Degas Infant Drops** *Whitehall, Austral.*
Simeticone (p.1289·2).
*Infant colic.*

**Degest** *Akorn, USA.*
Naphazoline hydrochloride (p.1124·3).
*Minor eye irritation.*

**Degest 2** *Barnes Hind, NZ.*
Naphazoline hydrochloride (p.1124·3); phenazone (p.82·3).
*Eye irritation.*

**Degona** *Prodotti, Braz.†.*
Ampicillin (p.157·1).
Probenecid (p.416·3) is included in this preparation to reduce renal tubular excretion of the antibiotic.
*Bacterial infections.*

**Degoran** *Novartis Consumer, S.Afr.*
*Effervescent tablets:* Phenylephrine hydrochloride (p.1126·3); paracetamol (p.76·2); pheniramine maleate (p.438·3).
Formerly contained phenylpropanolamine hydrochloride, paracetamol, and pheniramine maleate.
*Tablets†; oral liquid†:* Chlorphenamine maleate (p.427·3); phenylpropanolamine hydrochloride (p.1127·3); dextromethorphan hydrobromide (p.1117·3); paracetamol (p.76·2).
*Cold and influenza symptoms.*

**Degoran C** *Novartis Consumer, S.Afr.*
Paracetamol (p.76·2); vitamin C (p.1460·2); phenylephrine hydrochloride (p.1126·3); chlorphenamine maleate (p.427·3); caffeine (p.782·1).
*Cold and influenza symptoms.*

**Degoran Cold & Flu** *Novartis Consumer, S.Afr.*
Paracetamol (p.76·2); chlorphenamine maleate (p.427·3); pseudoephedrine hydrochloride (p.1129·2).
*Cold and influenza symptoms.*

**Degoran Cough** *Novartis Consumer, S.Afr.*
Dextromethorphan hydrobromide (p.1117·3); phenylephrine hydrochloride (p.1126·3); ammonium chloride (p.1115·2); sodium citrate (p.1223·2).
*Coughs.*

**Degoran Plus** *Novartis Consumer, S.Afr.*
Paracetamol (p.76·2); phenylephrine hydrochloride (p.1126·3); caffeine (p.782·1); chlorphenamine maleate (p.427·3).
*Cold and influenza symptoms.*

**Degorflan** *Degorts, Mex.*
Nimesulide (p.67·1).
*Fever; inflammation; pain.*

**Degran** *Ranbaxy, Thai.*
Ergotamine tartrate (p.467·2); caffeine (p.782·1).
*Migraine and other vascular headaches.*

**Degranol** *Aspen, S.Afr.*
Carbamazepine (p.353·3).
*Epilepsy; trigeminal neuralgia.*

**Dehidrobenzperidol** *Kern, Spain.*
Droperidol (p.697·2).
*General anaesthesia; neuroleptanalgesia; premedication.*

**Dehistine** *Cypress, USA.*
Chlorphenamine maleate (p.427·3); phenylephrine hydrochloride (p.1126·3); hyoscine methonitrate (p.483·3).
*Upper respiratory-tract disorders.*

**Dehydral** *Trans Canaderm, Canad.*
Methenamine (p.230·1).
*Bacterial infections; hyperhidrosis.*

**dehydro sanol tri** *Sanol, Ger.*
Bemetizide (p.867·1); triamterene (p.1016·2).
*Leg pain associated with venous insufficiency.*

**dehydro tri mite** *Sanol, Ger.*
Bemetizide (p.867·1); triamterene (p.1016·2).
*Leg pain associated with venous insufficiency.*

**Dehydrobenzperidol**
*Janssen-Cilag, Austria†; Janssen-Cilag, Denm.†; Orion, Fin.; Janssen-Cilag, Ger.†; IFET (ΙΦΕΤ), Gr.; Janssen, Hong Kong†; Janssen, Mex.†; Janssen-Cilag, Neth.†; Janssen-Cilag, Switz.†; Janssen-Cilag, Thai.†.*
Droperidol (p.697·2).
*Nausea and vomiting; neuroleptanalgesia; premedication.*

*Janssen-Cilag, Belg.†.*
Droperidol tartrate (p.697·2).
*Agitation; nausea and vomiting; neuroleptanalgesia; shock.*

**Deiten** *ABC, Ital.*
Nitrendipine (p.973·3).
*Hypertension.*

**Dekamega** *Omega, Spain†.*
Piroxicam choline (p.85·1).
*Gout; musculoskeletal, joint, and peri-articular disorders; pain.*

**Dekamin** *Monico, Ital.*
Amino-acid infusion (p.1417·1).
*Parenteral nutrition.*

**Dekar 2** *Pentamedical, Ital.*
Benzyl benzoate (p.1500·2); quassia (p.1737·2).

**Dekatin** *Ativus, Braz.*
Crataegus (p.1677·1).
*Heart failure.*

**Dekinet** *Rafa, Israel.*
Biperiden hydrochloride (p.479·3).
*Drug-induced extrapyramidal disorders; parkinsonism.*

**Dekka** *Pond's, Thai.*
Chlorhexidine gluconate (p.1173·2); cetrimide (p.1172·1).
*Disinfection of skin, wounds, and instruments.*

**Dekristol** *Jenapharm, Ger.*
Colecalciferol (p.1461·3).
*Hypoparathyroidism; osteomalacia; osteoporosis; pseudohypoparathyroidism; rickets; vitamin D deficiency.*

**Del Aqua** *Del-Ray, USA.*
Benzoyl peroxide (p.1143·2).
*Acne.*

**Delabarre** *Fumouze, Fr.*
Tamarind (p.1293·2).
*Teething pain.*

**De-Lact**
*Nutricia, Austral.; Sharpe, NZ†.*
Infant feed (p.1417·1).
*Lactose intolerance.*

**Delagil** *Dermapharm, Ger.*
Phenol-formaldehyde-urea polycondensate sodium sulfate.
*Skin disorders.*

**Delak** *Raffo, Arg.*
Oxybutynin (p.487·1).
*Urinary-tract disorders.*

**Delaket** *Chiesi, Ital.*
Delapril (p.892·2).
*Heart failure; hypertension.*

**Delakete** *Formalab, Braz.*
Delapril hydrochloride (p.892·2).
*Hypertension.*

**Delakmin** *Albert-Roussel, Ger.†; Hoechst, Ger.†.*
(5*E*,7*E*)-9,10-Secocholesta-5,7,10(19)-triene-3β,25-diol.
*Renal osteopathy.*

**Delapride** *Chiesi, Ital.*
Delapril (p.892·2); indapamide (p.938·2).
*Hypertension.*

**Delatestryl**
*Theramed, Canad.; BTG, USA.*
Testosterone enantate (p.1570·1).
*Breast cancer; delayed puberty (males); male hypogonadism.*

**Delbiase** *Chiesi, Fr.*
Magnesium chloride (p.1228·1); magnesium bromide (p.1229·1).
*Magnesium deficiency.*

**Delbulasa** *Alpharma, Mex.*
Phenylbutazone (p.83·2).
*Inflammation; musculoskeletal and joint disorders.*

**Delcoprep** *DeltaSelect, Ger.*
Macrogol 4000 (p.1709·1); electrolytes (p.1217·1).
*Bowel evacuation.*

**Delecit** *MDM, Ital.*
Choline alfoscerate (p.1488·3).
*Mental function impairment.*

**Delegol** *Bayer, Ital.*
Partially chlorinated benzylphenol.
*Surface disinfection.*

**Delepsine** *Orion, Denm.*
Sodium valproate (p.380·1).
*Epilepsy.*

**Deleptin** *Stada, Austria.*
Carbamazepine (p.353·3).
*Alcohol withdrawal syndrome; diabetes insipidus; diabetic neuropathy; epilepsy; mania; neuralgias.*

**Delestrogen**
*Theramed, Canad.; Monarch, USA.*
Estradiol valerate (p.1550·2).
*Breast cancer; menopausal disorders; menstrual disorders; prostatic cancer.*

**Deletus** *Nicholas Piramal, India.*
Dextromethorphan hydrobromide (p.1117·3); triprolidine hydrochloride (p.442·3); pseudoephedrine hydrochloride (p.1129·2).
*Coughs.*

**Deletus A** *Nicholas Piramal, India.*
Salbutamol sulfate (p.791·3); guaifenesin (p.1122·1).
*Asthmatic cough.*

**Deletus D** *Nicholas Piramal, India.*
Dextromethorphan hydrobromide (p.1117·3); triprolidine hydrochloride (p.442·3); pseudoephedrine hydrochloride (p.1129·2); menthol (p.1711·3).
*Coughs.*

**Deletus P** *Nicholas Piramal, India.*
Bromhexine hydrochloride (p.1115·3); pseudoephedrine hydrochloride (p.1129·2); guaifenesin (p.1122·1).
*Coughs.*

**Delfen**
*Janssen-Cilag, Arg.; Janssen-Cilag, Austral.†; Janssen-Cilag, Austria; Johnson & Johnson, Canad.; Ethnor, India; Janssen-Cilag, Irl.; Janssen-Cilag, Israel; Janssen-Cilag, Port.; Janssen-Cilag, S.Afr.; Janssen-Cilag, Switz.; Janssen-Cilag, UK; Advanced Care, USA.*
Nonoxinol 9 (p.1413·3).
*Contraceptive.*

**Delfos** *AGIPS, Ital.*
Nimesulide (p.67·1).
*Fever; inflammation; pain.*

**Delgacin Fibras** *Higate, Arg.*
Lecithin; glucomannan; bladderwrack (p.1417·1).
*Dietary supplement.*

**Delgafen** *Geva, Mex.†.*
Fenproporex (p.1588·3).

**Delgamer** *Marion Merrell, Spain†.*
Diethylpropion hydrochloride (p.1587·1).
*Obesity.*

**Delical** *DHN, Fr.*
Food for special diets (p.1417·1).
*Diarrhoea; lactose intolerance; nutritional supplement.*

**Delicate Skin Pasta** *RCA, Ital.*
Zinc oxide (p.1163·2).
*Skin irritation.*

**Delidose** *Orion, Fr.*
Estradiol (p.1550·1).
*Menopausal disorders.*

**delimmun** *Sanofi Synthelabo, Ger.*
Inosine pranobex (p.640·2).
*Viral infections.*

**Delimon** *Pharmaten (Φαρματεν), Gr.*
Diclofenac sodium (p.32·1).
*Prevention of miosis in ophthalmic surgery.*

**Delin**
*Atlantic, Hong Kong; Atlantic, Malaysia.*
Dequalinium chloride (p.1178·1).
*Gingivitis; sore throat.*

**Delinar** *Teva Tuteur, Arg.*
Mesna (p.1041·2).

**Delipoderm** *Reig Jofre, Spain.*
Promestriene (p.1568·2).
*Acne; seborrhoea.*

**Deliproct** *Schering, Fr.*
Prednisolone caproate (p.1108·1); cinchocaine hydrochloride (p.1373·2).
*Anorectal disorders.*

**Delirex** *Sanova, Austria.*
Caroverine hydrochloride (p.1668·1).
*Alcohol and drug withdrawal syndromes.*

**Delitan** *Gynopharm, Chile.*
Esterified oestrogens (p.1549·3); methyltestosterone (p.1559·3).
*Menopausal disorders.*

**Delitex N** *Infectopharm, Ger.*
Lindane (p.1506·3).
*Pediculosis.*

**Delitroxin** *Pharmaten (Φαρματεν), Gr.*
Roxithromycin (p.254·2).
*Bacterial infections.*

**Deliver**
*Mead Johnson, Austral.; Mead Johnson, Hong Kong†; Mead Johnson, NZ.*
Preparation for enteral nutrition (p.1417·1).
*Fluid or volume restriction; hypermetabolic states.*

**Delix**
*Note. This name is used for preparations of different composition.*
*Aventis, Ger.*
Ramipril (p.994·1).
*Heart failure; hypertension.*
*Xepa-Soul Pattinson, Singapore†.*
Phenylpropanolamine hydrochloride (p.1127·3); pholcodine (p.1128·3); promethazine hydrochloride (p.439·1).
*Coughs.*

**Delix plus** *Aventis, Ger.*
Ramipril (p.994·1); hydrochlorothiazide (p.933·2).
*Hypertension.*

**Delixi** *Infectopharm, Ger.†.*
Permethrin (p.1508·3).
*Pediculosis.*

**Delixir** *Hamilton, Austral.†.*
Diphenhydramine hydrochloride (p.431·3); ammonium chloride (p.1115·2); sodium citrate (p.1223·2).
*Coughs and cold symptoms.*

**Del-Lend** *Eversil, Braz.*
Deltamethrin (p.1503·1).

**Dellova** *Clement Thionville, Fr.*
Bladderwrack (p.1742·3); java tea (p.1702·3).
*Obesity.*

**Delmuno** *Aventis, Ger.*
Felodipine (p.914·3); ramipril (p.994·1).
*Hypertension.*

**Del-Mycin** *Del-Ray, USA.*
Erythromycin (p.208·1).

**Delonal**
*Essex, Ger.; Essex, Switz.*
Alclometasone dipropionate (p.1090·3).
*Skin disorders.*

**Delos** *Dallas, Arg.*
Roxithromycin (p.254·2).
*Bacterial infections.*

**Delph Sun Lotion** *Fenton, UK.*
*SPF 15:* Octinoxate (p.1154·3); oxybenzone (p.1154·3); titanium dioxide (p.1160·3).
*Sunscreen.*

**Delphi**
*Wyeth Lederle, Belg.; Lederle, Neth.†.*
Triamcinolone acetonide (p.1110·2).
*Skin disorders.*

**Delphicol** *Wyeth Lederle, India.*
Tricholine citrate (p.1424·3); acetyl dimethionine; inositol (p.1701·2); vitamin $B_{12}$ (p.1458·2).
*Liver disorders.*

**Delphicort**
*Wyeth Lederle, Austria; Lederle, Ger.*
Triamcinolone (p.1110·2), triamcinolone acetonide (p.1110·2), or triamcinolone diacetate (p.1110·2).
*Corticosteroid.*

**Delphimix** *Lederle, Ger.*
Triamcinolone diacetate (p.1110·2).
*Musculoskeletal and joint disorders.*

**Delphinac** *Lederle, Ger.*
Diclofenac sodium (p.32·1).
*Gout; inflammation; musculoskeletal, joint, and soft-tissue disorders; pain.*

**Delpral** *Sanofi Synthelabo, Austria.*
Tiapride hydrochloride (p.725·1).
*Alcohol withdrawal syndrome; movement disorders.*

**Delrosa** *ICN, Hong Kong.*
Vitamin C (p.1460·2).
*Vitamin C supplement.*

**Delsacid** *Selvi, Ital.*
Cefonicid sodium (p.174·2).
Lidocaine hydrochloride (p.1377·3) is included in this preparation to alleviate the pain of injection.
*Gram-negative bacterial infections.*

**Delsym**
*Novartis Consumer, Canad.*
Dextromethorphan hydrobromide (p.1117·3).
*Coughs.*
*Roche Consumer, Irl.*
Dextromethorphan resinate (p.1117·3).
*Coughs.*
*Rhone-Poulenc Rorer, Mex.†.*
Dextromethorphan (p.1117·3).
*Celltech, USA.*
Dextromethorphan polistirex (p.1118·1).
*Coughs.*

**Delta 80** *IDI, Ital.*
Benzoyl peroxide (p.1143·2); cetylpyridinium chloride (p.1173·1).
*Acne; skin disinfection.*

**Delta Charcoal** *Sriprasit, Thai.*
Charcoal (p.1030·2); magnesium hydroxide (p.1272·2); belladonna (p.479·1); peppermint oil (p.1283·2).
*Flatulence; gastrointestinal disorders.*

**Delta 80 Plus** *IDI, Ital.*
Benzoyl peroxide (p.1143·2); cetylpyridinium chloride (p.1173·1).
*Acne; skin disinfection.*

**Delta Tomanil B12** *Byk, Arg.*
Diclofenac sodium (p.32·1); prednisolone (p.1108·1); cyanocobalamin (p.1458·2) or hydroxocobalamin (p.1458·2).
*Musculoskeletal and joint disorders; pain.*

**Deltacef** *Pulitzer, Ital.*
Cefuroxime sodium (p.184·1).
*Gram-negative bacterial infections.*

**Deltacid** *Sintofarma, Braz.*
Deltamethrin (p.1503·1).
*Scabies.*

**Deltacid Plus** *Sintofarma, Braz.*
Deltamethrin (p.1503·1); piperonyl butoxide (p.1509·2).
*Pediculosis; scabies.*

**Deltacina** *Upsamedica, Spain†.*
Neomycin sulfate (p.235·1); thiomersal (p.1194·1).
*Skin infections.*

**Delta-Cortef** *Upjohn, USA.*
Prednisolone (p.1108·1).
*Corticosteroid.*

**Deltacortene** *Bruno, Ital.*
Prednisone (p.1109·3).
*Oral corticosteroid.*

**Deltacortril**
*Pfizer, Belg.; Pfizer, Gr.; Pfizer, Irl.; Pfizer, UK.*
Prednisolone (p.1108·1).
*Corticosteroid.*

**Delta-D** *Freeda, USA.*
Colecalciferol (p.1461·3).
*Dietary supplement; vitamin D deficiency.*

**Delta-Diona** *Reuffer, Mex.†.*
Prednisolone (p.1108·1).
*Corticosteroid.*

**Deltaflan** *Delta, Braz.*
Nimesulide (p.67·1).

**Deltaflogin** *Delta, Braz.*
Diclofenac diethylamine (p.32·1), diclofenac resinate (p.33·1), or diclofenac sodium (p.32·1).
*Gout; inflammation; musculoskeletal, joint, and periarticular disorders; pain.*

**Delta-Hadensa** *Kolassa, Austria.*
Prednisolone sodium metasulfobenzoate (p.1108·1); chlorcarvacrol; ichthammol (p.1148·2); menthol (p.1711·3); with or without chamomile oil (p.1669·3).
*Anorectal disorders.*

**Deltalaf** *Lafage, Arg.*
Betamethasone (p.1093·1).
*Corticosteroid.*

**Deltalipid** *DeltaSelect, Ger.*
Soya oil (p.1447·2).
Contains egg phospholipids.
*Lipid infusion for parenteral nutrition.*

**Deltamid** *Sophia, Mex.*
Prednisolone acetate (p.1108·1); sulfacetamide sodium (p.257·3).
*Eye disorders.*

**Deltamidrina** *Tubilux, Ital.*
Prednisolone acetate (p.1108·1); atropine sulfate (p.477·1); phenylephrine hydrochloride (p.1126·3).
*Inflammatory eye disorders.*

**Deltamitren** *Teuto, Braz.*
Deltamethrin (p.1503·1).

**Deltapio** *Luper, Braz.*
Deltamethrin (p.1503·1).
*Pediculosis; scabies.*

**Deltaran** *Strathmann, Ger.*
Dexibuprofen (p.46·1).
*Musculoskeletal and joint disorders; pain.*

**Deltaren** *Delta, Braz.*
Diclofenac diethylamine (p.32·1), diclofenac potassium (p.32·1), or diclofenac resinate (p.33·1).
*Gout; inflammation; musculoskeletal, joint, and periarticular disorders; pain.*

**Deltarhinol-Mono** *Aventis, Belg.*
Naphazoline nitrate (p.1124·3).
*Nasal congestion.*

**Deltarinolo** *Aventis, Ital.*
Ephedrine hydrochloride (p.1120·1); naphazoline nitrate (p.1124·3).
*Nasal congestion.*

**Deltasone**
*Pharmacia Upjohn, Canad.†; Pharmacia Upjohn, Hong Kong†; Pharmacia Upjohn, NZ†; Upjohn, USA.*
Prednisone (p.1109·3).
*Corticosteroid.*

**Deltasoralen** *Delta, Irl.*
Methoxsalen (p.1152·1).
*Leucoderma; psoriasis; vitiligo.*

**Deltastab** *Sovereign, UK.*
Prednisolone acetate (p.1108·1).
*Corticosteroid.*

**Delta-Tritex** *Dermol, USA.*
Triamcinolone acetonide (p.1110·2).
*Skin disorders.*

**Deltavac** *Trimen, USA.*
Sulfanilamide (p.263·2); aminoacridine hydrochloride (p.1165·3); allantoin (p.1141·3).
*Vaginal infections.*

**Deltavagin** *Finderm, Ital.*
Betamethasone (p.1093·1); tyrothricin (p.275·1); norvaline.
*Vaginitis.*

**Deltavit** *Delta, Braz.*
Amino-acid, vitamin, and mineral preparation (p.1417·1).

**Deltazen** *Irex, Fr.*
Diltiazem hydrochloride (p.900·1).
*Hypertension.*

**Deltisan** *Valma, Chile.*
Zinc (p.1469·2); cod-liver oil (p.1425·2).
*Skin disorders.*

**Deltison** *Recip, Swed.*
Prednisone (p.1109·3).
Magnesium trisilicate (p.1272·3) and calcium hydrogen phosphate (p.1225·2) are included in this preparation in an attempt to limit adverse effects on the gastrointestinal mucosa.
*Corticosteroid.*

**Deltisona B** *Aventis, Arg.*
Meprednisone (p.1106·1) or meprednisone hemisuccinate.
*Corticosteroid.*

**Delto-cyl Ho-Len-Complex** *Liebermann, Ger.*
Homoeopathic preparation.

**Deltrox** *Dupomar, Arg.*
Cefuroxime (p.184·1) or cefuroxime axetil (p.184·1).
*Bacterial infections.*

**Delufen** *Bittner, Austria.*
Homoeopathic preparation.

**Delursan** *Aventis, Fr.*
Ursodeoxycholic acid (p.1760·3).
*Gallstones; liver and biliary disorders.*

**Delvas** *Berk, UK†.*
Amiloride hydrochloride (p.858·2); hydrochlorothiazide (p.933·2).
These ingredients can be described by the British Approved Name Co-amilozide.
*Cirrhosis with ascites; heart failure; hypertension.*

**Del-Vi-A** *Del-Ray, USA†.*
Vitamin A (p.1451·2).
*Vitamin A deficiency.*

**Demac** *Osotspa, Thai.*
Diclofenac diethylamine (p.32·1) or diclofenac sodium (p.32·1).
*Fever; inflammation; musculoskeletal, joint, peri-articular, and soft-tissue disorders; pain.*

**Demadex**
*Boehringer Mannheim, Canad.†; Jouveinal, Canad.†; Roche, USA.*
Torasemide (p.1015·3).
*Hypertension; oedema.*

**Demazin**
*Note. This name is used for preparations of different composition.*
*Schering-Plough, Austral.; Schering-Plough, NZ; Schering-Plough, S.Afr.†.*
*Delayed-release tablets; sustained-release capsules:* Dexchlorpheniramine maleate (p.427·3); pseudoephedrine sulfate (p.1129·2).
*Upper respiratory-tract congestion.*
*Schering-Plough, Austral.; Schering-Plough, NZ; Schering-Plough, S.Afr.; Schering-Plough, USA†.*
*Syrup:* Chlorphenamine maleate (p.427·3); phenylpropanolamine hydrochloride (p.1127·3).
*Upper respiratory-tract congestion.*
*Schering-Plough, Austral.*
*Tablets:* Chlorphenamine maleate (p.427·3); pseudoephedrine sulfate (p.1129·2).
*Upper respiratory tract congestion.*

**Demazin Anti-Allergy** *Schering-Plough, S.Afr.*
Loratadine (p.436·1).
*Allergic rhinitis; urticaria.*

**Demazin Anti-Tussive** *Schering-Plough, S.Afr.*
Chlorphenamine maleate (p.427·3); dextromethorphan hydrobromide (p.1117·3); phenylpropanolamine hydrochloride (p.1127·3).
*Coughs.*

**Demazin Clear** *Schering-Plough, Austral.*
Chlorphenamine maleate (p.427·3); phenylephrine hydrochloride (p.1126·3).
*Upper respiratory tract congestion.*

**Demazin Cold & Flu** *Schering-Plough, Austral.*
Chlorphenamine maleate (p.427·3); pseudoephedrine sulfate (p.1129·2); paracetamol (p.76·2).
*Cold and influenza symptoms; sinusitis.*

**Demazin Day/Night Relief**
*Schering-Plough, Austral.; Schering-Plough, NZ.*
Day tablets, pseudoephedrine sulfate (p.1129·2); night tablets, pseudoephedrine sulfate; dexchlorpheniramine maleate (p.427·3).
*Upper respiratory-tract congestion.*

**Demazin Decongestant** *Schering-Plough, S.Afr.*
Pseudoephedrine sulfate (p.1129·2).
*Upper respiratory-tract congestion.*

**Demazin Expectorant** *Schering-Plough, S.Afr.*
Dexchlorpheniramine maleate (p.427·3) pseudoephedrine sulfate (p.1129·2) guaifenesin (p.1122·1).
*Coughs.*

**Demazin Non-Drowsy** *Schering-Plough, NZ.*
Pseudoephedrine sulfate (p.1129·2); loratadine (p.436·1).
*Upper respiratory-tract congestion.*

**Demazin NS** *Schering-Plough, S.Afr.*
Loratadine (p.436·1); pseudoephedrine sulfate (p.1129·2).
*Rhinitis.*

**Demazin Sinus** *Schering-Plough, Austral.*
Pseudoephedrine sulfate (p.1129·2).
*Upper respiratory-tract congestion.*

**Demdec** *Rougier, Canad.†.*
Pseudoephedrine hydrochloride (p.1129·2); dextromethorphan hydrobromide (p.1117·3).
*Coughs; respiratory-tract congestion.*

**De-menthasin** *Scheurich, Ger.†.*
Dequalinium salicylate (p.1178·1); hexetidine (p.1182·1).
*Mouth and throat inflammation.*

**Demergin** *Demo, Gr.*
Methylergometrine maleate (p.1714·2).
*Postpartum haemorrhage.*

**Demerol**
*Sanofi Winthrop, Braz.†; Abbott, Canad.; Sanofi Synthelabo, Canad.; Abbott, Chile; Sanofi Winthrop, USA.*
Pethidine hydrochloride (p.80·2).
*Pain.*

**Demetil** *Farmila, Ital.*
Tetryzoline hydrochloride (p.1131·2).
*Eye congestion.*

**Demetrin**
*Pfizer, Austria; Parke, Davis, Ger.; Pfizer, Port.; Pfizer, S.Afr.; Pfizer, Switz.*
Prazepam (p.716·2).
*Anxiety; sleep disorders.*

**Demex** *Berlin-Chemie, Ger.*
Propyphenazone (p.85·3).
*Fever; pain.*

**Demiax** *Merck, Spain.*
Xipamide (p.1029·2).
*Hypertension; oedema.*

**Demi-Regroton** *Rhone-Poulenc Rorer, USA.*
Chlortalidone (p.882·3); reserpine (p.995·1).
*Hypertension.*

**Demix** *Ashbourne, UK.*
Doxycycline hyclate (p.206·2).

**Demo baume** *Demopharm, Switz.†.*
Chlorobutanol (p.1176·3); ephedrine hydrochloride (p.1120·1); lidocaine hydrochloride (p.1377·3); camphor (p.1665·3); menthol (p.1711·3); lavender oil (p.1705·2); niaouli oil (p.1719·3).
*Rhinitis.*

**Demo elixir pectoral N** *Democal, Switz.*
Ephedrine hydrochloride (p.1120·1); guaifenesin (p.1122·1); belladonna (p.479·1); drosera (p.1683·1); hedera helix; ipecacuanha (p.1122·3).
Demo elixir pectoral formerly contained ephedrine hydrochloride, guaifenesin, belladonna, drosera, hedera helix, ipecacuanha, and codeine phosphate.
*Coughs.*

**Demo gouttes bronchiques** *Demopharm, Switz.†.*
Thyme (p.1755·2); ground ivy (p.1696·1); liquorice (p.1270·2).
*Coughs with viscous mucus.*

**Demo gouttes contre la toux** *Demopharm, Switz.†.*
Codeine phosphate (p.27·1); ephedrine hydrochloride (p.1120·1); guaifenesin (p.1122·1); drosera (p.1683·1);

hedera helix; ipecacuanha (p.1122·3); thyme oil (p.1755·3).
*Coughs; respiratory-tract disorders with increased or viscous mucus.*

**Demo pates pectorales** *Demopharm, Switz.†.*
Codeine phosphate (p.27·1); benzoic acid (p.1169·3); ipecacuanha (p.1122·3); tolu balsam (p.1131·3); drosera (p.1683·1); hedera helix; plantaginis (p.1738·2); menthol (p.1711·3); anise oil (p.1655·2); bitter orange oil (p.1723·3); eucalyptus oil (p.1686·2); peppermint oil (p.1283·2).
*Bronchitis; coughs.*

**Demo pommade contre les refroidissements** *Democal, Switz.*
Eucalyptus oil (p.1686·2); pine needle oil; peru balsam (p.1730·2); camphor (p.1665·3); thyme oil (p.1755·3).
*Cold symptoms.*

**Demo pommade contre les refroidissements pour bebes** *Democal, Switz.†.*
Eucalyptus oil (p.1686·2); pine needle oil; sage oil (p.1741·2); thyme oil (p.1755·3); juniper oil (p.1703·1); peru balsam (p.1730 2).
*Respiratory-tract disorders.*

**Demo sirop bronchique N** *Demopharm, Switz.†.*
Thyme (p.1755·2); cowslip rhizome (p.1735·1); hedera helix.
*Coughs.*

**Demo sirop contre la toux** *Demopharm, Switz.†.*
Ephedrine hydrochloride (p.1120·1); guaifenesin (p.1122·1); tolu balsam (p.1131·3); drosera (p.1683·1); ipecacuanha (p.1122·3); thyme (p.1755·2); belladonna (p.479·1); liquorice (p.1270·2).
*Bronchitis; catarrh; coughs.*

**Demo-Cineol** *Sabex, Canad.*
Cineole (p.1672·1); guaiacol (p.1122·1); camphor (p.1665·3).
*Coughs.*

**Democyl** *Democal, Switz.*
Paracetamol (p.76·2).
*Fever; pain.*

**Demodek** *Drag, Chile.*
Nitrofurazone (p.238·2).
*Bacterial skin infections.*

**Demodenal** *Demopharm, Switz.†.*
Dimenhydrinate (p.431·1).
*Motion sickness.*

**Demodenal compositum** *Democal, Switz.†.*
Dimenhydrinate (p.431·1); pyridoxine hydrochloride (p.1456·3); caffeine (p.782·1).
*Motion sickness.*

**Demoderhin** *Demopharm, Switz.†.*
Diphenhydramine hydrochloride (p.431·3); mepyramine maleate (p.437·1); caffeine (p.782·1).
*Nasal congestion; rhinitis.*

**Demodon Neo** *Democal, Switz.*
Senna (p.1288·2).
*Constipation.*

**Demogripal** *Democal, Switz.*
Paracetamol (p.76·2).
*Fever; pain.*

**Demogripal C** *Democal, Switz.*
Paracetamol (p.76·2); ascorbic acid (p.1460·2).
*Cold symptoms.*

**Demolaxin** *Democal, Switz.*
Bisacodyl (p.1251·3).
*Constipation.*

**Demolibral** *Democal, Switz.*
Acetylcysteine (p.1112·3).
*Coughs.*

**Demolox**
*Wyeth Lederle, Denm.; Wyeth Lederle, India; Wyeth, Spain†.*
Amoxapine (p.286·3).
*Depression.*

**Demonatur Capsules contre les refroidissements** *Democal, Switz.*
Brown capsules, thyme oil (p.1755·3); origanum oil; savory oil; green capsules, echinacea purpurea (p.1683·2).
*Influenza symptoms.*

**Demonatur Dragees pour les reins et la vessie** *Democal, Switz.*
Bearberry (p.1659·2); solidago virgaurea (p.1748·3); ononis (p.1723·3); echinacea (p.1683·2); Java tea (p.1702·3).
*Urinary-tract disorders.*

**Demonatur Ginkgo** *Democal, Switz.*
Ginkgo biloba (p.1692·3).
*Cerebrovascular disorders.*

**Demonatur Gouttes pour le foie et la bile** *Democal, Switz.*
Vial no 1: gentian (p.1692·2); taraxacum (p.1751·3); cynara (p.1678·3); vial no 2: silybum marianum (p.1043·3); celandine (p.1695·3); berberis.
*Gastrointestinal disorders.*

**Demopart** *Ferring, Ital.†.*
Demoxytocin (p.1322·3).
*Induction of labour; lactation induction.*

**DemoPectol** *Democal, Switz.*
*Oral drops:* Thyme (p.1755·2); hedera helix; liquorice (p.1270·2).
*Syrup:* Thyme (p.1755·2); primula root (p.1735·1); hedera helix.
*Coughs.*

**Demoplas** *Godecke, Ger.†.*
Phenylbutazone (p.83·2).
Lidocaine hydrochloride (p.1377·3) is included in this preparation to alleviate the pain of injection.
*Acute ankylosing spondylitis; rheumatism.*

**Demoprin nouvelle formule** *Democal, Switz.†.*
Aspirin (p.15·1).
*Fever; pain.*

**Demostan** *Demopharm, Switz.†.*
*Ointment:* Diphenhydramine hydrochloride (p.431·3); lidocaine hydrochloride (p.1377·3); menthol (p.1711·3).
*Topical gel:* Diphenhydramine hydrochloride (p.431·3); lidocaine hydrochloride (p.1377·3).
*Burns; insect bites; skin irritation.*

**Demostan N** *Democal, Switz.*
*Cream:* Mepyramine maleate (p.437·1); lidocaine hydrochloride (p.1377·3); calcium levulinate (p.1225·3); menthol (p.1711·3).
*Topical gel:* Mepyramine maleate (p.437·1); lidocaine hydrochloride (p.1377·3); dexpanthenol (p.1727·2).
*Allergic, pruritic and inflamed skin conditions.*

**Demosvelte N** *Demopharm, Switz.†.*
Agar (p.1576·3); guar gum (p.333·2); sodium alginate (p.1577·1); pectin (p.1580·3); soya (p.1447·2).
*Obesity.*

**Demotest** *Pierre Fabre, Spain.*
Budesonide (p.1094·2).
*Skin disorders.*

**Demotherm Pommade contre le rhumatisme** *Democal, Switz.*
Benzyl nicotinate (p.21·2); glycol salicylate (p.44·3).
*Musculoskeletal and joint pain.*

**Demotussil** *Democal, Switz.*
Noscapine (p.1125·3); drosera (p.1683·1); liquorice (p.1270·2); eucalyptus oil (p.1686·2); peppermint oil (p.1283·2).
Formerly contained codeine phosphate, ephedrine hydrochloride, ipecacuanha, guaifenesin, and cineole.
*Bronchitis; coughs; laryngitis; sinusitis.*

**Demotussol** *Democal, Switz.*
Butamirate citrate (p.1116·2).
*Coughs.*

**Demovarin** *Democal, Switz.*
Heparin sodium (p.928·1).
*Superficial vascular disorders.*

**Demoven N** *Democal, Switz.*
Troxerutin (p.1688·3); aesculus (p.1648·2).
*Venous insufficiency.*

**Demovit** *Democal, Switz.*
A range of multivitamin and mineral preparations (p.1417·1).
*Dietary supplementation.*

**Demovit C** *Democal, Switz.*
Ascorbic acid (p.1460·2).
*Vitamin C deficiency.*

**Dempol** *Esoform, Ital.*
Chlorhexidine gluconate (p.1173·2).
*Hand disinfection.*

**Demser**
*Merck Sharp & Dohme, UK†; Merck, USA.*
Metirosine (p.956·1).
Available on a named patient basis in the *UK.*
*Phaeochromocytoma.*

**Demulcin** *Ferraton, Denm.*
Codeine phosphate (p.27·1); ammonium chloride (p.1115·2).
*Coughs.*

**Demulen**
*Pharmacia, Canad.; Searle, USA.*
Etynodiol diacetate (p.1554·2); ethinylestradiol (p.1553·2).
28-Day packs also contain 7 inert tablets.
*Combined oral contraceptive.*

**Demusin** *Reig Jofre, Spain.*
Albumin tannate (p.1248·1); amylase (p.1654·2); ethylmorphine hydrochloride (p.37·3).
*Diarrhoea.*

**Denacen** *Marjan, Braz.*
Deflazacort (p.1096·2).
*Corticosteroid.*

**Denaclof** *Novartis, Gr.*
Diclofenac sodium (p.32·1).
*Prevention of miosis in ophthalmic surgery.*

**Denan** *Boehringer Ingelheim, Ger.*
Simvastatin (p.997·1).
*Hypercholesterolaemia.*

**Denapril** *Medinfar, Port.*
Enalapril maleate (p.909·2).
*Heart failure; hypertension.*

**Denavir**
*SmithKline Beecham, Fr.†; SmithKline Beecham Consumer, USA.*
Penciclovir (p.651·2).
*Herpes labialis.*

**Denaxpren** *Smaller, Spain.*
Naproxen (p.65·1).
*Fever; gout; musculoskeletal and joint disorders; pain.*

**Denazox** *Remedica, Thai.*
Diltiazem hydrochloride (p.900·1).
*Angina pectoris.*

**Dencorub** *Carter-Wallace, Austral.†.*
Camphor (p.1665·3); menthol (p.1711·3); eucalyptus oil (p.1686·2); methyl salicylate (p.59·3).
*Musculoskeletal pain.*

**Dencorub Anti-Inflammatory** *Carter-Wallace, Austral.*
Diclofenac sodium (p.32·1).
*Peri-articular and soft-tissue disorders.*

**Dencorub Arthritis** *Carter-Wallace, Austral.*
Trolamine salicylate (p.95·3).
*Arthritis; muscle pain.*

**Dencorub Arthritis Ice** *Carter-Wallace, Austral.*
Menthol (p.1711·3).
*Musculoskeletal pain.*

**Dencorub Extra Strength** *Carter-Wallace, Austral.†.*
Methyl salicylate (p.59·3); menthol (p.1711·3).
*Muscle pain.*

**Dencorub Pain Relieving Cream** *Carter-Wallace, Austral.*
Camphor (p.1665·3); menthol (p.1711·3); eucalyptus oil (p.1686·2); methyl salicylate (p.59·3).

**Denerel**
*Medochemie, Malaysia; Medochemie, Singapore†; Medochemie, Thai.*
Ketotifen fumarate (p.788·1).
*Allergic bronchitis; allergic rhinitis; allergic skin disorders; asthma.*

**Denex**
*Medochemie, Hong Kong; Medochemie, Malaysia; Medochemie, Singapore†; Medochemie, Thai.*
Metoprolol tartrate (p.957·1).
*Angina pectoris; hypertension; myocardial infarction.*

**Deniban** *Sanofi Synthelabo, Ital.*
Amisulpride (p.669·3).
*Dysthymia.*

**Denim** *Hua, Thai.*
Dimenhydrinate (p.431·1).
*Motion sickness; nausea and vomiting.*

**Deniren** *Searle, Mex.†.*
Amoxicillin (p.155·3).
*Bacterial infections.*

**Denisoline** *Aerocid, Fr.†.*
Precipitated sulfur (p.1158·2); alum (p.1652·1).
*Acne.*

**Denium** *Strand, Malaysia.*
Dequalinium chloride (p.1178·1).
*Mouth and throat infections.*

**Denkacort** *Denk, Hong Kong.*
Triamcinolone acetonide (p.1110·2).
*Corticosteroid.*

**De-Nol**
*Parke, Davis, Austral.†; Yamanouchi, Belg.†; Gerolimatos (Γερολυματος), Gr.; Gerolymatos, Hong Kong; Yamanouchi, Irl.†; Agis, Israel†; Yamanouchi, Ital.; Yamanouchi, Neth.; Yamanouchi, Norw.†; CSL, NZ; Yamanouchi, NZ; Yamanouchi, Port.; Pharmaplan, S.Afr.; Yamanouchi, Switz.†; Gerolymatos, Thai.†.*
Tripotassium dicitratobismuthate (p.1252·2).
*Dyspepsia; gastritis; peptic ulcer.*

**De-Noltab**
*Yamanouchi, Irl.; Yamanouchi, UK.*
Tripotassium dicitratobismuthate (p.1252·2).
*Dyspepsia; gastritis; peptic ulcer.*

**Denoral**
*Note. This name is used for preparations of different composition.*
*Aventis, Belg.†; Theraplix, Fr.†; Rhone-Poulenc Rorer, Hong Kong†; Aventis, Ital.*
Buzepide metiodide (p.480·2); clocinizine hydrochloride (p.429·2); phenylpropanolamine hydrochloride (p.1127·3).
*Allergic rhinitis; nasal congestion; sinusitis.*

*Theraplix, Fr.*
*Syrup:* Clocinizine hydrochloride (p.429·2); pholcodine (p.1128·3).
Formerly contained buzepide metiodide, clocinizine hydrochloride, and pholcodine.
*Coughs.*

*Rhone-Poulenc Rorer, Hong Kong†.*
*Syrup:* Buzepide metiodide (p.480·2); pholcodine (p.1128·3); clocinizine hydrochloride (p.429·2).
*Coughs.*

**Denorex**
*Note. This name is used for preparations of different composition.*
*Whitehall-Robins, Canad.; Wyeth, Irl.; Wyeth Consumer, Neth.; Wyeth Consumer, Singapore; Whitehall, UK†; Whitehall, USA†.*
Coal tar (p.1159·2); menthol (p.1711·3).
*Dandruff; psoriasis; seborrhoeic dermatitis.*

*Whitehall, Israel.*
Coal tar (p.1159·2).
*Dandruff; psoriasis; seborrhoeic dermatitis.*

**Denorex Daily** *Whitehall, Braz.*
Salicylic acid (p.1157·1).
*Scalp disorders.*

**Denorex Herbal** *Wyeth Consumer, Chile.*
Coal tar (p.1159·2); menthol (p.1711·3).
*Scalp disorders.*

**Denorex Plus** *Whitehall, Braz.*
Salicylic acid (p.1157·1).
*Scalp disorders.*

**Denosol** *Doerenkamp, Ger.†.*
Cineole (p.1672·1); menthol (p.1711·3); camphor (p.1665·3); thymol (p.1194·2).
*Colds; influenza.*

**Denpru** *Foda, Arg.*
Protamine (p.1050·3).
*Heparin overdose.*

**Denquel** *Procter & Gamble, USA.*
Potassium nitrate (p.1190·1).
*Sensitive teeth.*

**Densical**
*Zambon, Fr.; Rubio, Spain.*
Calcium carbonate (p.1254·2).
*Calcium deficiency; osteoporosis.*

**Densical D** *Vitoria, Port.*
Calcium carbonate (p.1254·2); colecalciferol (p.1461·3).
*Calcium and vitamin D deficiencies; osteoporosis.*

**Densical vitamine $D_3$** *Laphal, Fr.*
Calcium carbonate (p.1254·2); colecalciferol (p.1461·3).
*Calcium and vitamin D deficiencies; osteoporosis.*

**Denson** *Siam Bheasach, Thai.*
Prednisolone (p.1108·1); nitrofurazone (p.238·2).
*Infected skin disorders.*

**Densopax** *Justesa Imagen, Arg.*
Meglumine amidotrizoate (p.1060·2).
*Radiographic contrast medium.*

**Denta Plus** *Rising Pharmaceuticals, USA.*
Sodium fluoride (p.1444·3).
*Dental caries prophylaxis.*

**DentaGel** *Rising Pharmaceuticals, USA.*
Sodium fluoride (p.1444·3).
*Dental caries prophylaxis.*

**Dentagesic** *Maver, Chile.*
Clonixin lysine (p.26·3).
*Pain.*

**Dentalgar** *Marc-O, Canad.†.*
Benzocaine (p.1370·3); camphor (p.1665·3); guaiacol (p.1122·1); menthol (p.1711·3); clove oil (p.1673·3).

**Dentaliv** *Mintlab, Chile.*
Lidocaine hydrochloride (p.1377·3).
*Local anaesthesia.*

**Dentalivio** *IMA, Braz.*
Benzocaine (p.1370·3); cetylpyridinium chloride (p.1173·1).
*Mouth disorders.*

**Dental-Phenjoca** *Worndli, Switz.†.*
Iodine (p.1598·1); camphor (p.1665·3); thymol (p.1194·2); anethole (p.1654·3); safrole (p.1742·1); eugenol (p.1686·2); chlorobutanol (p.1176·3); phenol (p.1188·1).
*Dental extraction pain.*

**Dentan** *Ipex, Swed.*
Sodium fluoride (p.1444·3).
*Dental caries prophylaxis.*

**Dentapaine** *Reese, USA.*
Benzocaine (p.1370·3); clove oil (p.1673·3).
*Toothache.*

**Dentaton Antisettico** *Ghimas, Ital.†.*
Chlorhexidine gluconate (p.1173·2); benzalkonium chloride (p.1168·3).
*Oral disinfection.*

**Dentecalcio** *Melpoejo, Braz.†.*
Vitamin and mineral preparation (p.1417·1).

**Dentex** *Colgate-Palmolive, Fr.*
Hydrogen peroxide (35%) (p.1182·2).
*Mouth irritation; oral hygiene.*

**Denticare** *Trima, Israel.*
Sodium fluoride (p.1444·3).
*Dental caries prophylaxis.*

**Dentigoa** *Scheurich, Ger.†.*
Ibuprofen (p.45·3).
*Fever; pain.*

**Dentikrisos** *Quimifar, Spain.*
Creosote (p.1117·2); benzocaine (p.1370·3); tetracaine hydrochloride (p.1385·1); menthol (p.1711·3).
*Toothache.*

**Dentin** *Rekah, Israel.*
Eugenol (p.1686·2); benzocaine (p.1370·3); chlorobutanol (p.1176·3).
*Toothache.*

**Dentinale** *Montefarmaco, Ital.*
Amylocaine hydrochloride (p.1370·2); sodium benzoate (p.1169·3).
*Teething pain.*

**Dentinox**
*Note. This name is used for preparations of different composition.*
*Byk, Austria.*
*Dental gel:* Chamomile (p.1669·3); lidocaine hydrochloride (p.1377·3); lauromacrogol 400 (p.1412·3).
*Oral drops:* Chamomile tincture (p.1669·3); myrrh tincture (p.1718·3); cetylpyridinium chloride (p.1173·1); lauromacrogol 400 (p.1412·3).
*Teething pain.*

*DDD, Israel; DDD, Singapore.*
Simeticone (p.1289·2); dill oil (p.1680·2).
*Infant colic.*

*Vemedia, Neth.*
Lidocaine hydrochloride (p.1377·3).
*Teething pain.*

*Dentinox, Switz.†.*
Chamomile (p.1669·3); lidocaine hydrochloride (p.1377·3); lauromacrogol 400 (p.1412·3).
*Dental pain.*

**Dentinox Colic Drops**
*DDD, Hong Kong; DDD, Malaysia; DDD, UK.*
Simeticone (p.1289·2).
*Infant colic.*

**Dentinox Cradle Cap**
*DDD, Malaysia; DDD, Singapore; DDD, UK.*
Sodium lauril ether sulfosuccinate; sodium lauril ether sulfate (p.1574·3).
*Cradle cap.*

**Dentinox N** *Dentinox, Ger.*
Chamomile (p.1669·3); lidocaine hydrochloride (p.1377·3); lauromacrogol 400 (p.1412·3).
*Teething pain.*

**Dentinox Teething Gel**
*DDD, Hong Kong; DDD, Malaysia; DDD, Singapore; DDD, UK.*
Lidocaine hydrochloride (p.1377·3); cetylpyridinium chloride (p.1173·1).
*Denture irritation; sore gums; teething pain.*

**Dentipatch** *Noven, USA.*
Lidocaine (p.1377·3).
*Local anaesthesia.*

**Dentispray**
*Master, Chile; Ferraz, Lynce, Port.; Vinas, Spain.*
Benzocaine (p.1370·3).
*Mouth pain; toothache.*

**Dentogen** *Anglian, UK.*
Clove oil (p.1673·3).
*Toothache.*

**Dentohexine** *Streuli, Switz.*
Chlorhexidine gluconate (p.1173·2).
*Mouth and throat disorders.*

**Dentol Topico** *Perez Gimenez, Spain.*
Camphor (p.1665·3); saffron (p.1058·2); clove oil (p.1673·3); cloral hydrate (p.684·1); procaine hydrochloride (p.1383·2); menthol (p.1711·3).
*Toothache.*

**Dentolamina** *Inibsa, Port.†.*
Sodium perborate (p.1192·2); sodium tartrate (p.1290·1).
*Mouth disorders; oral hygiene.*

**Dentolina Plus** *Fucus, Arg.*
Dipyrone (p.35·3); caffeine (p.782·1).
*Fever; pain.*

**Dentomicin** *Seid, Spain.*
Saffron (p.1058·2); tamarind (p.1293·2).
*Toothache.*

**Dentomycin**
*Note. This name is used for preparations of different composition.*
*Kreussler, Ger.*
Clindamycin hydrochloride (p.194·2).
*Bacterial infections.*

*Wyeth, Irl.†; Blackwell, UK.*
Minocycline hydrochloride (p.231·3).
*Bacterial mouth infections.*

**Dentophar** *Qualiphar, Belg.*
Amylocaine hydrochloride (p.1370·2); cloral hydrate (p.684·1); chloroform (p.1296·3); menthol (p.1711·3); thymol (p.1194·2); eugenol (p.1686·2) =CSP.02.
*Dental pain.*

**Dentosan Azione Intensiva** *Pfizer Consumer, Ital.*
Chlorhexidine gluconate (p.1173·2); peppermint oil (p.1283·2); geranium oil (p.1692·2); melissa oil (p.1711·2); clove oil (p.1673·3); spearmint oil (p.1749·1).
*Oral hygiene.*

**Dentosan Carie & Alito** *Pfizer Consumer, Ital.*
Sanguinaria (p.1741·3); sodium monofluorophosphate (p.1446·2).
*Dental caries prophylaxis.*

**Dentosan Clorexidina** *Pfizer Consumer, Ital.*
Chlorhexidine (p.1173·2).
*Gum disorders.*

**Dentosan Extra Fluor** *Pfizer Consumer, Ital.*
Sodium fluoride (p.1444·3).
*Dental caries prophylaxis.*

**Dentosan Junior** *Pfizer Consumer, Ital.*
Sodium monofluorophosphate (p.1446·2); sodium fluoride (p.1444·3).
*Dental caries prophylaxis.*

**Dentosan Mese** *Pfizer Consumer, Ital.*
Peppermint oil (p.1283·2); geranium oil (p.1692·2); melissa oil (p.1711·2); clove oil (p.1673·3); spearmint oil (p.1749·1); chlorhexidine gluconate (p.1173·2).
*Oral hygiene.*

**Dentosan Parodontale** *Pfizer Consumer, Ital.*
Chlorhexidine gluconate (p.1173·2).
*Oral hygiene.*

**Dentosan Placca & Carie** *Pfizer Consumer, Ital.*
Chlorhexidine gluconate (p.1173·2); sodium fluoride (p.1444·3); peppermint oil (p.1283·2).
*Oral hygiene.*

**Dentosan Sensibile** *Pfizer Consumer, Ital.*
Potassium nitrate (p.1190·1) sodium fluoride (p.1444·3).
*Gingivitis; hypersensitive teeth.*

**Dentosedina** *Teofarma, Ital.*
Procaine hydrochloride (p.1383·2); benzocaine (p.1370·3).
Formerly contained procaine, procaine hydrochloride, benzocaine hydrochloride, and ephedrine hydrochloride.
*Dental pain.*

**Dentovax** *Bouty, Ital.†.*
Inactivated cells of: *Escherichia coli*; *Streptococcus ovalis*; *Staphylococcus pyog. aur.*; *Proteus vulgaris*; chlorophyll (p.1057·1).
*Gingivitis.*

**Dentoxil** *Master, Chile.*
Strontium chloride (p.1749·3).
*Hypersensitive teeth.*

**Dent's Extra Strength Toothache Gum** *Dent, USA.*
Benzocaine (p.1370·3).

**Dent's Maximum Strength Toothache Drops** *Dent, USA.*
Benzocaine (p.1370·3).

**Dentsiblen** *Glaxo Wellcome, Mex.*
*Mouthwash:* Potassium nitrate (p.1190·1); sodium monofluorophosphate (p.1446·2); xylitol (p.1469·1).
*Toothpaste:* Potassium nitrate (p.1190·1); sodium monofluorophosphate (p.1446·2); aldioxa (p.1141·2).
*Dental hypersensitivity; oral hygiene.*

**Dentyl pH** *Grafton, UK.*
Triclosan (p.1195·2); fluoride (p.1444·3).
*Oral hygiene.*

**Denubil** *Pierre Fabre, Spain.*
Heptaminol hydrochloride (p.1697·1); deanol pidolate (p.1585·3).
*Mental function disorders.*

**Denulcer** *Ciclum, Spain.*
Ranitidine hydrochloride (p.1285·2).
*Acid aspiration; gastro-oesophageal reflux; gastrointestinal hyperacidity; peptic ulcer; Zollinger-Ellison syndrome.*

**Denvar**
*Merck, Mex.; Merck, Spain.*
Cefixime (p.172·3).
*Bacterial infections.*

**Denvercrem** *Denver, Arg.*
Gentamicin sulfate (p.217·1); miconazole nitrate (p.405·3); betamethasone valerate (p.1093·2).
*Infected skin disorders.*

**Denyl** *Cristalia, Braz.*
Citalopram (p.289·1).
*Depression; obsessive-compulsive disorder; panic attacks.*

**Denzo** *TO-Chemicals, Thai.*
Serrapeptase (p.1743·2).
*Inflammation; oedema.*

**Deo** *Milano, Thai.*
Dequalinium chloride (p.1178·1).
*Mouth and throat infections.*

**Deolin** *Unison, Thai.*
Drotaverine hydrochloride (p.1683·1).
*Smooth muscle spasm.*

**Deopens** *Brunel, S.Afr.*
Magnesium hydroxide (p.1272·2).
*Gastro-oesophageal reflux.*

**Deopid** *Masa, Thai.*
Gemfibrozil (p.923·1).
*Hyperlipidaemias.*

**Deotrin** *Bunker, Braz.*
Deltamethrin (p.1503·1).

**Depacon** *Abbott, USA.*
Sodium valproate (p.380·1).
*Epilepsy.*

**Depade** *Mallinckrodt, USA.*
Naltrexone hydrochloride (p.1046·1).
*Alcohol withdrawal syndrome; opioid withdrawal.*

**Depain Plus** *Vesta, S.Afr.†.*
Paracetamol (p.76·2); codeine phosphate (p.27·1); phenobarbital (p.367·3).
*Pain and associated tension.*

**Depakene**
*Abbott, Arg.; Abbott, Braz.; Abbott, Canad.; Abbott, Chile; Kyowa, Jpn; Abbott, Mex.; Abbott, USA.*
Valproic acid (p.380·1) or sodium valproate (p.380·1).
*Bipolar disorder; epilepsy; mania.*

**Depakin** *Sanofi Synthelabo, Ital.*
Sodium valproate (p.380·1).
*Epilepsy.*

**Depakin Chrono** *Sanofi Synthelabo, Ital.*
Sodium valproate (p.380·1); valproic acid (p.380·1).
*Epilepsy.*

**Depakine**
*Sanofi Synthelabo, Austria; Sanofi Synthelabo, Belg.; Sanofi Synthelabo, Fr.; Sanofi Synthelabo, Gr.; Sanofi Synthelabo, Neth.; Sanofi Synthelabo, Port.; Sanofi Synthelabo, Spain; Sanofi Synthelabo, Switz.; Sanofi Synthelabo, Thai.*
Sodium valproate (p.380·1).
*Epilepsy.*

**Depakine Chrono**
*Sanofi Synthelabo, Austria; Sanofi Synthelabo, Fr.; Sanofi Synthelabo, Gr.; Sanofi Synthelabo, Neth.; Sanofi Synthelabo, Port.; Sanofi Synthelabo, Switz.*
Sodium valproate (p.380·1); valproic acid (p.380·1).
*Epilepsy.*

**Depakine Crono** *Sanofi Synthelabo, Spain.*
Sodium valproate (p.380·1); valproic acid (p.380·1).
*Epilepsy.*

**Depakote**
*Abbott, Braz.; Sanofi Synthelabo, Fr.; Sanofi Synthelabo, UK; Abbott, USA.*
Valproate semisodium (p.380·1).
*Bipolar disorder; epilepsy; migraine.*

**Depalept** *CTI, Israel.*
Sodium valproate (p.380·1).
*Epilepsy; porphyria.*

**Depalept Chrono** *CTI, Israel.*
Sodium valproate (p.380·1); valproic acid (p.380·1).
*Epilepsy.*

**Depamag** *Sigma-Tau, Ital.*
Magnesium valproate (p.382·2).
*Epilepsy.*

**Depamide**
*Sanofi Synthelabo, Fr.; Sanofi Synthelabo, Ital.; Sanofi Synthelabo, Spain.*
Valpromide (p.380·1).
*Bipolar disorder; epilepsy; mania.*

**depAndro** *Forest Pharmaceuticals, USA†.*
Testosterone cipionate (p.1569·3).
*Breast cancer; delayed puberty (males); male hypogonadism.*

**depAndrogyn** *Forest Pharmaceuticals, USA†.*
Estradiol cipionate (p.1550·1); testosterone cipionate (p.1569·3).
*Menopausal vasomotor symptoms; prevention of postpartum breast engorgement.*

**Deparon** *Great Eastern, Thai.; Westmont, Thai.*
Dipyrone (p.35·3).
*Pain.*

**Depas**
*Fournier, Ital.; Mitsubishi, Jpn.*
Etizolam (p.698·1).
*Anxiety states; psychosomatic disorders; sleep disorders.*

**Depen**
*Carter Horner, Canad.; Wallace, USA.*
Penicillamine (p.1046·3).
*Cystinuria; rheumatoid arthritis; Wilson's disease.*

**depGynogen** *Forest Pharmaceuticals, USA.*
Estradiol cipionate (p.1550·1).
*Female hypogonadism; menopausal vasomotor symptoms.*

**Depicor** *Merck, India.*
Nifedipine (p.966·2).
*Angina pectoris; hypertension.*

**Depiderm** *Uriage, Fr.*
Liquorice (p.1270·2).
*Skin hyperpigmentation.*

**Depin** *Cadila, India.*
Nifedipine (p.966·2).
*Angina pectoris; hypertension.*

**Depixol**
*Lundbeck, Irl.; Lundbeck, NZ†; Lundbeck, UK.*
Flupentixol decanoate (p.699·1) or flupentixol hydrochloride (p.699·1).
*Psychoses.*

**Depizide** *Pond's, Thai.*
Glipizide (p.332·2).
*Diabetes mellitus.*

**Deplecat** *Baxter, Mex.*
Potassium phosphate (p.1230·3).

**depMedalone** *Forest Pharmaceuticals, USA.*
Methylprednisolone acetate (p.1106·1).
*Corticosteroid.*

**Depnil** *Cipla-Medpro, S.Afr.*
Moclobemide (p.308·2).
*Depression; social phobia.*

**Depnon** *Infar, India.*
Mianserin hydrochloride (p.306·3).
*Depression.*

**Depo Moderin** *Pharmacia, Spain.*
Methylprednisolone acetate (p.1106·1).
*Corticosteroid.*

**Depo-Clinovir** *Pharmacia, Ger.*
Medroxyprogesterone acetate (p.1557·2).
*Progestogen-only injectable contraceptive.*

**Depocon** *Pharmacia, Austria.*
Medroxyprogesterone acetate (p.1557·2).
*Progestogen-only injectable contraceptive.*

**DepoCyt**
*Paladin, Canad.; Enzon, USA.*
Liposomal cytarabine (p.543·1) (p.543·1).
*Lymphomatous meningitis.*

**DepoCyte** *Napp, UK.*
Liposomal cytarabine (p.543·1) (p.543·1).
*Lymphomatous meningitis.*

**Depofin** *Allen, Mex.*
Diiodohydroxyquinoline (p.603·3).
*Amoebiasis.*

**Depogen** *Hyrex, USA.*
Estradiol cipionate (p.1550·1).
*Female hypogonadism; menopausal vasomotor symptoms.*

**Depo-Gestin** *ANB, Thai.*
Medroxyprogesterone acetate (p.1557·2).
*Dysfunctional uterine bleeding; endometriosis; progestogen-only injectable contraceptive.*

**Depoject** *Mayrand, USA†.*
Methylprednisolone acetate (p.1106·1).
*Corticosteroid.*

**Depolan**
*Lannacher, Denm.; Nordic Drugs, Fin.; Nordic, Swed.*
Morphine hydrochloride (p.60·1).
*Pain.*

**Depolut** *Taro, Israel.*
Hydroxyprogesterone caproate (p.1556·3).
*Amenorrhoea; endometriosis; functional uterine bleeding; uterine cancer.*

**Depo-Medrate** *Pharmacia, Ger.*
Methylprednisolone acetate (p.1106·1).
*Parenteral corticosteroid.*

**Depo-Medrol**
*Pharmacia, Austral.; Pharmacia, Austria; Pharmacia, Belg.; Pharmacia, Braz.; Pharmacia, Canad.; Pharmacia, Chile; Pharmacia, Denm.; Pharmacia, Fin.; Pharmacia, Fr.; Pharmacia-Upjohn, Gr.; IFET (ΙΦΕΤ), Gr.; Pharmacia, Hong Kong; Pharmacia Upjohn, Israel; Pharmacia Upjohn, Ital.; Pharmacia, Malaysia; Pharmacia Upjohn, Mex.; Pharmacia, Neth.; Pharmacia, Norw.; Pharmacia, NZ; Pharmacia, Port.; Pharmacia, S.Afr.; Pharmacia, Swed.; Pharmacia, Switz.; Pharmacia, Thai.; Pharmacia Upjohn, USA.*
Methylprednisolone acetate (p.1106·1).
Lidocane hydrochloride (p.1377·3) is included in some injections to alleviate the pain of injection.
*Corticosteroid.*

**Depo-Medrol com Lidocaina** *Pharmacia, Port.*
Methylprednisolone acetate (p.1106·1); lidocaine hydrochloride (p.1377·3).
*Musculoskeletal, joint, and peri-articular disorders.*

**Depo-Medrol cum Lidocain**
*Pharmacia, Fin.; Pharmacia, Norw.*
Methylprednisolone acetate (p.1106·1); lidocaine hydrochloride (p.1377·3).
*Musculoskeletal, joint, and peri-articular disorders.*

**Depo-Medrol cum Lidokain** *Pharmacia, Swed.*
Methylprednisolone acetate (p.1106·1); lidocaine hydrochloride (p.1377·3).
*Peri-articular disorders.*

**Depo-Medrol + Lidocaina** *Pharmacia Upjohn, Ital.*
Methylprednisolone acetate (p.1106·1); lidocaine hydrochloride (p.1377·3).
*Musculoskeletal, joint, and peri-articular disorders.*

**Depo-Medrol Lidocaine** *Pharmacia, Switz.*
Methylprednisolone acetate (p.1106·1); lidocaine hydrochloride (p.1377·3).
*Musculoskeletal, joint, and peri-articular disorders.*

**Depo-Medrol + Lidocaine**
*Pharmacia, Belg.; Pharmacia, Neth.*
Methylprednisolone acetate (p.1106·1); lidocaine hydrochloride (p.1377·3).
*Musculoskeletal, joint, and peri-articular disorders.*

**Depo-Medrol mit Lidocain** *Pharmacia, Austria.*
Methylprednisolone acetate (p.1106·1); lidocaine hydrochloride (p.1377·3).
*Musculoskeletal and joint disorders.*

**Depo-Medrol with Lidocaine**
*Pharmacia, Canad.; Pharmacia, Hong Kong; Pharmacia Upjohn, Israel; Pharmacia, NZ; Pharmacia, S.Afr.; Pharmacia, Thai.*
Methylprednisolone acetate (p.1106·1); lidocaine hydrochloride (p.1377·3).
*Musculoskeletal, joint, and peri-articular disorders.*

**Depo-Medrone**
*Pharmacia, Irl.; Pharmacia, UK.*
Methylprednisolone acetate (p.1106·1).
*Corticosteroid.*

**Depo-Medrone with Lidocaine**
*Pharmacia, Irl.; Pharmacia, UK.*
Methylprednisolone acetate (p.1106·1); lidocaine hydrochloride (p.1377·3).
*Musculoskeletal, joint, and peri-articular disorders.*

**Depon** *Bristol-Myers Squibb, Gr.*
Paracetamol (p.76·2).
*Fever; pain.*

**Depon Maximum** *Bristol-Myers Squibb, Gr.*
Paracetamol (p.76·2).
*Fever; pain.*

**Depo-Nisolone** *Pharmacia, Austral.*
Methylprednisolone acetate (p.1106·1).
*Corticosteroid.*

**Deponit**
*Gebro, Austria; Byk, Belg.; Schering, Braz.†; Pharmacal, Fin.; Schwarz, Ger.; Schwarz, Hong Kong; Schwarz, Irl.; Medis, Israel; Schwarz, Ital.; Schwarz, Malaysia; Byk, Neth.; Ranbaxy, Singapore; Schwarz, Singapore; Schwarz, Switz.; Schwarz, Thai.†; Schwarz, UK; Schwarz, USA†.*
Glyceryl trinitrate (p.923·2).
*Angina pectoris; heart failure; prophylaxis of phlebitis and extravasation.*

**Depopred** *Hyrex, USA.*
Methylprednisolone acetate (p.1106·1).
*Corticosteroid.*

**Depo-Prodasone**
*Pharmacia, Chile; Pharmacia, Fr.*
Medroxyprogesterone acetate (p.1557·2).
*Endometriosis; malignant neoplasms.*

**Depo-Progesno** *Milano, Thai.*
Medroxyprogesterone acetate (p.1557·2).
*Progestogen-only injectable contraceptive.*

**Depo-Progesta** *General Drugs, Thai.*
Medroxyprogesterone acetate (p.1557·2).
*Endometriosis; progestogen-only injectable contraceptive.*

**Depo-Progevera** *Pharmacia, Spain.*
Medroxyprogesterone acetate (p.1557·2).
*Endometrial cancer; progestogen-only injectable contraceptive.*

**Depo-Provera**
*Pharmacia, Arg.; Pharmacia, Austral.; Pharmacia, Austria; Pharmacia, Belg.; Pharmacia, Braz.; Pharmacia, Canad.; Pharmacia, Denm.; Pharmacia, Fin.; Pharmacia, Fr.; Pharmacia-Upjohn, Gr.; Pharmacia, Hong Kong; Pharmacia Upjohn, India; Pharmacia, Irl.; Pharmacia Upjohn, Israel; Pharmacia Upjohn, Ital.; Pharmacia, Malaysia; Pharmacia Upjohn, Mex.; Pharmacia, Neth.; Pharmacia, Norw.; Pharmacia, NZ; Pharmacia, Port.; Pharmacia, S.Afr.; Pharmacia, Singapore; Pharmacia, Swed.; Pharmacia, Switz.; Pharmacia, Thai.; Pharmacia, UK; Pharmacia Upjohn, USA.*
Medroxyprogesterone acetate (p.1557·2).
*Breast cancer; endometrial cancer; endometriosis; menopausal disorders; progestogen-only injectable contraceptive; renal cancer.*

**Depo-Ralovera** *Pharmacia, Austral.*
Medroxyprogesterone acetate (p.1557·2).
*Endometriosis; malignant neoplasms; progestogen-only injectable contraceptive.*

**Depostat**
*Schering, Ger.; Schering, Ital.; Schering, Spain; Schering, Switz.*
Gestonorone caproate (p.1556·2).
*Breast cancer; endometrial cancer; prostatic adenoma.*

**Deposteron** *Sigma, Braz.*
Testosterone cipionate (p.1569·3).
*Androgen deficiency; breast cancer; delayed puberty (males); male hypogonadism.*

**Depotest** *Hyrex, USA†.*
Testosterone cipionate (p.1569·3).
*Breast cancer; delayed puberty (males); male hypogonadism.*

**Depo-Testadiol** Upjohn, USA.
Estradiol cipionate (p.1550·1); testosterone cipionate (p.1569·3).
*Menopausal vasomotor symptoms; prevention of postpartum breast engorgement.*

**Depotestogen** Hyrex, USA.
Estradiol cipionate (p.1550·1); testosterone cipionate (p.1569·3).
*Menopausal vasomotor symptoms; prevention of postpartum breast engorgement.*

**Depot-Hal**
Hal, Ger.
Allergen extracts of pollen, fungi, house dust mites (p.1650·2) and skin (p.1650·2) (p.1650·1).
*Allergen immunotherapy.*

Hal, Neth.
Allergen extracts (p.1650·1).
*Allergen immunotherapy.*

**Depot-H-Insulin** Hoechst, Ger.†.
Neutral insulin suspension (human, highly-purified)(75% crystalline) (p.333·3).
*Diabetes mellitus.*

**Depot-H15-Insulin** Hoechst, Ger.†.
Neutral insulin suspension (human, highly-purified)(85% crystalline) (p.333·3).
*Diabetes mellitus.*

**Depot-Insulin**
Aventis, Austria; Aventis, Ger.
Insulin injection (bovine) (p.333·3).
*Diabetes mellitus.*

**Depot-Insulin S** Aventis, Ger.
Insulin injection (porcine) (p.333·3).
*Diabetes mellitus.*

**Depotrone** Propan, S.Afr.
Testosterone cipionate (p.1569·3).
*Gynaecomastia; lactation suppression; male hypogonadism; mastitis; menstrual disorders.*

**Depot-Thrombophob-N** Knoll, Ger.†.
Heparin sodium (p.928·1).
Formerly contained heparin sodium and ephedrine hydrochloride.
*Thromboembolic disorders.*

**Deprakine**
Sanofi Winthrop, Denm.; Sanofi Synthelabo, Fin.; Sanofi Synthelabo, Norw.
Sodium valproate (p.380·1).
*Bipolar disorder; epilepsy.*

**Deprakine Depot** Sanofi Synthelabo, Fin.
Sodium valproate (p.380·1); valproic acid (p.380·1).
*Bipolar disorder; epilepsy.*

**Depramina** Teuto, Braz.
Imipramine hydrochloride (p.300·1).
*Depression.*

**Deprancol** Parke, Davis, Spain.
Dextropropoxyphene hydrochloride (p.28·3).
*Pain.*

**Depraser** Farma Lepori, Spain†.
Etoperidone (p.292·1) or etoperidone hydrochloride (p.292·1).
*Depression.*

**Deprax**
Note. This name is used for preparations of different composition.
Ache, Braz.
Fluoxetine hydrochloride (p.292·1).
*Depression; obsessive-compulsive disorder.*

Saval, Chile.
Sertraline (p.317·3).
*Depression; obsessive-compulsive disorder; panic attacks.*

Farma Lepori, Spain.
Trazodone hydrochloride (p.319·1).
*Depression; dyskinesias; mood disorders; premedication; tremor.*

**Deprece** Tecnobio, Spain.
Almagate (p.1248·2).
*Dyspepsia; gastritis; gastro-oesophageal reflux; peptic ulcer.*

**Deprefax** Pharmacia, Arg.
Nefazodone (p.310·1).
*Depression.*

**Deprelio** Estedi, Spain.
Amitriptyline hydrochloride (p.280·3).
Formerly contained amitriptyline hydrochloride and perphenazine.
*Bulimia nervosa; depression; neuropathic pain; nocturnal enuresis; postherpetic neuralgia.*

**Deprenyl**
Orion, Fr.; Sanofi Winthrop, Ger.†.
Selegiline hydrochloride (p.1214·1).
*Parkinsonism.*

**Depress** Uniao Quimica, Braz.
Fluoxetine hydrochloride (p.292·1).
*Depression.*

**Depressan** OPW, Ger.
Dihydralazine sulfate (p.899·3).
*Hypertension.*

**Deprexan** Unipharm, Israel.
Desipramine hydrochloride (p.290·2).
*Depression.*

**Deprexen** Lisapharma, Ital.
Fluoxetine hydrochloride (p.292·1).
*Depression.*

**Deprexin**
Gedeon Richter, Hong Kong; Gedeon Richter, Singapore.
Fluoxetine hydrochloride (p.292·1).
*Depression; obsessive-compulsive disorder.*

**Deprilan** Biosintetica, Braz.
Selegiline hydrochloride (p.1214·1).
*Parkinsonism.*

**Deprilept** Lundbeck, Ger.
Maprotiline hydrochloride (p.306·1).
*Depression.*

**Deprimil** Merck, Port.
Lofepramine hydrochloride (p.305·3).
*Depression.*

**Deprocid** Aventis Pasteur, Chile.
Metronidazole (p.607·2).
*Anaerobic bacterial infections; protozoal infections.*

**Deproic** Technilab, Canad.†.
Valproic acid (p.380·1) or sodium valproate (p.380·1).
*Epilepsy.*

**Deproist Expectorant with Codeine** Geneva, USA.
Pseudoephedrine hydrochloride (p.1129·2); guaifenesin (p.1122·1); codeine phosphate (p.27·1).
*Coughs.*

**Depronal**
Pfizer, Belg.; Parke, Davis, Neth.; Warner-Lambert, Switz.†.
Dextropropoxyphene hydrochloride (p.28·3).
*Pain.*

**Deproxin** Siam Bheasach, Thai.
Fluoxetine hydrochloride (p.292·1).
*Depression; obsessive-compulsive disorder.*

**Deprozol** Ache, Braz.
Secnidazole (p.615·3).
*Bacterial infections; protozoal infections.*

**Depsonil** Sarabhai Piramal, India.
Imipramine hydrochloride (p.300·1) or imipramine embonate (p.300·1).
*Depression; nocturnal enuresis.*

**Depsonil-DZ** Sarabhai Piramal, India.
Imipramine hydrochloride (p.300·1); diazepam (p.690·1).
*Mixed anxiety depressive states.*

**Depten** Cadila, India.
Atenolol (p.865·2); nifedipine (p.966·2).
*Hypertension.*

**Deptran**
Note. This name is used for preparations of different composition.
Alphapharm, Austral.
Doxepin hydrochloride (p.291·2).
*Depression.*

Enila, Braz.
Bromazepam (p.671·3).
*Anxiety; insomnia.*

**Depuran**
Woelm, Ger.; Aspen, S.Afr.; Aventis, Spain†.
Senna (p.1288·2).
*Constipation.*

**Depuratif des Alpes** Sodia, Fr.
Frangula bark (p.1266·3).
Formerly contained senna, frangula bark, liquorice, and magnesium chloride.
*Constipation.*

**Depuratif Parnel** Phytoprevent, Fr.
Lappa (p.1704·3); viola tricolor; saponaria; fumitory (p.1690·1).
*Gastrointestinal disorders.*

**Depuratif Richelet** Richelet, Fr.
Walnut leaves; cresson leaves; cochlearia armoracia root; cochlearia officinalis leaves; menyanthes leaves; cinnamon bark; bitter orange; gentian; tannic acid; magnesium chloride; magnesium bromide; nicotinamide (p.1417·1).
*Tonic.*

**Depurativo** IDI, Ital.†.
Sarsaparilla (p.1742·1); fumitory (p.1690·1); borrana; saponaria; viola; walnut leaves; clover; rhubarb (p.1287·3); senna (p.1288·2); cascara (p.1255·1); lappa (p.1704·3); chicory; dulcamara (p.1683·1); couchgrass (p.1676·2); bitter-orange (p.1723·3); gentian (p.1692·2); salix (p.87·3).
*Constipation.*

**Depurativo Richelet** Vitafarma, Spain.
Gentian (p.1692·2); potassium iodide (p.1598·1); salicylic acid (p.1157·1); tannic acid (p.1751·2); iodine (p.1598·1); cinnamon oil (p.1672·2); magnesium chloride (p.1228·1); magnesium bromide (p.1229·1); nicotinamide (p.1441·2).
*Detoxification.*

**Depuratum** Lehning, Fr.
Birch leaf (p.1660·3); rosemary leaf (p.1740·2); juniper (p.1703·1); rhapontic root (p.1288·1); fumitory (p.1690·1); thyme (p.1755·2); ononis (p.1723·3).
*Gastrointestinal disorders.*

**Depurfat** Herbaline, Ital.†.
Rosemary (p.1740·2); silver birch (p.1660·3); taraxacum (p.1751·3); cupressus sempervirens; juniper (p.1703·1).
*Adjuvant in obesity; biliary disorders; liver disorders; venous disorders; water retention.*

**Depurol** Royal, Chile.
Venlafaxine hydrochloride (p.321·3).
*Depression.*

**Depygon** Sriprasit, Thai.
Paracetamol (p.76·2); chlorphenamine maleate (p.427·3).
*Cold symptoms.*

**Depyrel** Abic, Israel.
Trazodone hydrochloride (p.319·1).
*Depression.*

**Deq**
Atlantic, Hong Kong; Atlantic, Malaysia; Atlantic, Singapore; Atlantic, Thai.
Dequalinium chloride (p.1178·1); tyrothricin (p.275·1).
*Mouth and throat disorders.*

**Dequacaine**
Boots Healthcare, Irl.; Crookes Healthcare, UK.
Benzocaine (p.1370·3); dequalinium chloride (p.1178·1).
*Sore throat.*

**Dequa-Coff** Quatromed, S.Afr.
Promethazine hydrochloride (p.439·1); codeine phosphate (p.27·1); ephedrine hydrochloride (p.1120·1).
*Coughs.*

**Dequa/Delin** Atlantic, Thai.†.
Dequalinium chloride (p.1178·1).
*Mouth and throat disorders.*

**Dequadin**
Glaxo Wellcome, Austria†; Wellspring, Canad.; GlaxoSmithKline, Hong Kong; Boots Healthcare, Irl.; Eurospital, Ital.; Boots Healthcare, NZ†; Aspen, S.Afr.; GlaxoSmithKline, Singapore; Inibsa, Spain; GlaxoSmithKline, Thai.; Crookes Healthcare, UK.
Dequalinium chloride (p.1178·1).
*Mouth and throat infections.*

**Dequadin C** Zest, Braz.
Dequalinium chloride (p.1178·1); benzocaine (p.1370·3).
*Mouth and throat disorders.*

**Dequadin Complex** Inibsa, Spain†.
Lidocaine hydrochloride (p.1377·3); cetylpyridinium chloride (p.1173·1); dequalinium chloride (p.1178·1).
*Mouth and throat infections.*

**Dequadin Mouth Paint** Aspen, S.Afr.
Dequalinium chloride (p.1178·1); lidocaine (p.1377·3).
*Mouth and throat disorders.*

**Dequa-Flu** Quatromed, S.Afr.
Paracetamol (p.76·2); phenylephrine hydrochloride (p.1126·3); phenyltoloxamine citrate (p.439·1); caffeine (p.782·1); chlorphenamine maleate (p.427·3).
*Cold and influenza symptoms; rhinitis; sinusitis.*

**Dequafungan** Provita, Austria.
Dequalinium chloride (p.1178·1); undecenoic acid (p.410·3).
*Skin infections.*

**Dequalid** Wolfs, Belg.
Dequalinium chloride (p.1178·1); lidocaine hydrochloride (p.1377·3).
*Mouth and throat disorders.*

**Dequalinetten** Provita, Austria.
Dequalinium chloride (p.1178·1); benzocaine (p.1370·3).
*Mouth and throat disorders.*

**Dequalinium** Wolfs, Belg.†.
Dequalinium chloride (p.1178·1); amylocaine (p.1370·3).
*Mouth and throat disorders.*

**Dequamed** Rhone-Poulenc Rorer, S.Afr.†.
Dequalinium chloride (p.1178·1); lidocaine hydrochloride (p.1377·3).
*Sore throat.*

**Dequasept** Vitamed, Israel.
Dequalinium chloride (p.1178·1); vitamin C (p.1460·2).
*Mouth and throat infections.*

**Dequasine** Miller, USA.
Vitamin C with minerals and amino-acids (p.1417·1).

**Dequaspray** Crookes Healthcare, UK.
Lidocaine hydrochloride (p.1377·3).
Formerly known as Strepsils Pain Relief Spray.
*Sore throat.*

**Dequavagyn** Provita, Austria.
Dequalinium chloride (p.1178·1).

**Dequin** Degorts, Mex.
Dextromethorphan (p.1117·3); guaifenesin (p.1122·1); phenylpropanolamine (p.1127·3).
*Coughs; respiratory-tract congestion.*

**Dequonal**
Nycomed, Austria; Kreussler, Ger.; Kreussler, Switz.
Dequalinium chloride (p.1178·1); benzalkonium chloride (p.1168·3).
*Mouth and throat infections.*

**Dequosangola** Eurospital, Ital.
Dequalinium chloride (p.1178·1).
*Mouth disinfection.*

**Deralbine** Andromaco, Arg.
Miconazole nitrate (p.405·3).
*Fungal infections.*

**Deralin**
Alphapharm, Austral.; Abic, Israel.
Propranolol hydrochloride (p.989·3).
*Angina pectoris; arrhythmias; hypertension; hyperthyroidism; hypertrophic obstructive cardiomyopathy; migraine; myocardial infarction; phaeochromocytoma; tremor.*

**Deratin** Normon, Spain.
Chlorhexidine gluconate (p.1173·2).
*Mouth and throat infections; skin and wound disinfection.*

**Derbac-C** Seton, Irl.†.
Carbaryl (p.1501·2).
*Pediculosis.*

**Derbac-M**
SSL, Irl.; SSL, NZ; SSL, UK.
Malathion (p.1507·1).
*Pediculosis; scabies.*

**Dercolina** Casasco, Arg.
Choline salicylate (p.26·2).
*Mouth disorders.*

**Dercome** Wolff, Ger.
Benzoyl peroxide (p.1143·2).
*Acne.*

**Dercusan** Viatris, Belg.†.
Tosylchloramide sodium (p.1194·3).
*Burns; ulcers.*

**Dercut** Pekana, Ger.
Homoeopathic preparation.

**Dereme** Menarini, Spain.
Beclometasone salicylate (p.1092·1).
*Skin disorders.*

**Derifil** Rystan, USA.
Chlorophyllin copper complex (p.1057·1).
*Ostomy deodorant; reduction of faecal or urinary odour in incontinence.*

**Deril** Ibirn, Ital.
Alfacalcidol (p.1461·2).
*Hypoparathyroidism; osteomalacia; osteoporosis; renal osteodystrophy; rickets.*

**Derilate** Hosbon, Spain†.
Tiaprofenic acid (p.93·3).
*Inflammation; musculoskeletal, joint, and peri-articular disorders; pain.*

**Derinase Plus** Bioindustria, Ital.†.
Deoxyribonuclease (p.1119·1); bromelains (p.1662·2).
*Inflammatory disorders.*

**Derinox**
Note. This name is used for preparations of different composition.
Therabel, Fr.
Prednisolone (p.1108·1); naphazoline nitrate (p.1124·3).
Formerly contained prednisolone, phenylephrine hydrochloride, and naphazoline nitrate.
*Rhinopharyngitis.*

Sodip, Switz.†.
Prednisolone (p.1108·1); phenylephrine hydrochloride (p.1126·3); naphazoline nitrate (p.1124·3).
*Inflammatory and allergic disorders of upper respiratory tract.*

**Deriphyllin** German Remedies, India.
Etofylline (p.785·1); theophylline (p.798·3).
*Cardiac disorders; oedema; respiratory disorders.*

**Deripil** Galderma, Spain.
Erythromycin (p.208·1).
*Acne.*

**Derivatio H** Pfluger, Ger.
Homoeopathic preparation.

**Derivoco** Defuen, Arg.
Hydrocortisone acetate (p.1103·3); vitamin A (p.1451·2); neomycin sulfate (p.235·1).
*Infected skin disorders.*

**Derivon** Gerot, Austria.
*Cream:* Benzyl nicotinate (p.21·2); diethylamine salicylate (p.34·1); heparin (p.927·3).
*Musculoskeletal and joint disorders; neuralgia; soft-tissue disorders.*

*Liniment:* Benzyl nicotinate (p.21·2); camphor (p.1665·3); methyl salicylate (p.59·3).
*Soft-tissue, peri-articular, musculoskeletal, and joint disorders.*

**Derm Hydralin** Roche Nicholas, Fr.
Glycine (p.1433·3).
*Pruritus.*

**Derma Care** Fischer, Israel.
Salicylic acid (p.1157·1); hamamelis (p.1696·3); chamomile (p.1669·3); provitamin $B_5$.
*Seborrhoea; skin cleansing.*

**Derma Keri** Darier, Mex.
Urea (p.1162·2).
*Hyperkeratotic skin disorders.*

**Derma Viva** Rugby, USA.
Emollient and moisturiser.

**Dermabase** Paddock, USA.
Vehicle for topical preparations.

**Dermabaz** Sanofi Synthelabo, Hong Kong.
Tretinoin (p.1161·1); erythromycin (p.208·1).
*Acne.*

**Dermabel** Laboratorios Chile, Chile.
Clindamycin phosphate (p.194·2).
*Acne.*

**Dermabiotico** Saval, Chile.
Polymyxin B sulfate (p.245·1); bacitracin zinc (p.161·3).
*Burns; infected skin disorders; wounds.*

**Dermablend**
Sephytal, Fr.†; Brodie & Stone, UK.
A covering cream.
*Concealment of birth marks, scars, and disfiguring skin disease.*

**Dermabond** Ethicon, UK.
Ocrilate (p.1678·1).
*Tissue adhesive for wound closure.*

**Dermac** Stiefel, Mex.
*Cream:* Sulfur (p.1158·2); resorcinol (p.1156·3).
*Acne.*

*Soap:* Sulfated castor oil (p.1575·3).
*Seborrhoea.*

**Dermac Crema** Stiefel, Chile.
Sulfur (p.1158·2); resorcinol (p.1156·3); chloroxylenol (p.1177·2).
*Acne.*

**Dermac Jabon** *Stiefel, Chile.*
Soap substitute.
*Acne.*

**Dermacalm-d** *Roche, Switz.*
Hydrocortisone acetate (p.1103·3); dexpanthenol (p.1727·2).
*Skin disorders.*

**Dermacare**
*Note. A similar name is used for preparations of different composition (see below).*
*Darrow, Braz.*
Clobetasol propionate (p.1095·2).
*Skin disorders.*

**Derma-Care**
*Note. A similar name is used for preparations of different composition (see above).*
*Hermal, Israel.*
Lauromacrogol 400 (p.1412·3); urea (p.1162·2).
*Skin disorders.*

**Dermacerium** *Silvestre, Braz.†.*
Sulfadiazine silver (p.259·1); cerous nitrate (p.1144·3).
*Bacterial skin infections.*

**Dermacetin-Ped** *Stiefel, Braz.*
Neomycin sulfate (p.235·1); bacitracin zinc (p.161·3).
*Bacterial skin infections.*

**Dermachrome** *Sanofi Synthelabo OTC, Fr.*
Thiomersal (p.1194·1); lidocaine hydrochloride (p.1377·3).
Formerly contained thiomersal, lidocaine hydrochloride, and phenylephrine hydrochloride.
*Burns; wounds.*

**Dermacide** *CS, Fr.*
*Soap:* Tartaric acid (p.1752·1); salicylic acid (p.1157·1); benzoic acid (p.1169·3).
*Cleansing of skin.*
*Topical solution:* Hydroxyquinoline sulfate (p.1700·1); sodium propionate (p.408·1); salicylic acid (p.1157·1); tartaric acid (p.1752·1).
*Bacterial skin infections; cleansing of skin.*

**Dermacne** *Bio-Sante, Canad.†.*
Benzoyl peroxide (p.1143·2).
*Acne.*

**Dermacoat** *Century, USA.*
Benzocaine (p.1370·3); chloroxylenol (p.1177·2); menthol (p.1711·3).
*Skin disorders.*

**Dermacol** *Vitamed, Israel.*
Emollient.
*Dry skin.*

**Dermacolor** *Fox, UK.*
A covering cream.
*Concealment of birth marks, scars, and disfiguring skin disease.*

**Dermacombin**
*Taro, Israel.*
Triamcinolone acetonide (p.1110·2); nystatin (p.406·3); neomycin sulfate (p.235·1); gramicidin (p.220·2).
*Skin disorders.*
*Taro, Thai.*
Nystatin (p.406·3); neomycin (p.235·1); gramicidin (p.220·2); triamcinolone acetonide (p.1110·2).
*Infected skin disorders.*

**Dermacort**
*Note. This name is used for preparations of different composition.*
*Medinovum, Fin.†; Sankyo, UK.*
Hydrocortisone (p.1103·3).
*Skin disorders.*
*DHA, Hong Kong; DHA, Malaysia; DHA, Singapore.*
Triamcinolone acetonide (p.1110·2).
*Skin disorders.*

**Dermacreme** *Potter's, UK.*
Menthol (p.1711·3); methyl salicylate (p.59·3); liquefied phenol (p.1188·1).
*Antiseptic for minor skin injuries.*

**Dermacure** *Taxandria, Neth.*
Miconazole nitrate (p.405·3).
*Fungal skin and nail infections.*

**Dermacyd** *Sanofi Synthelabo, Braz.†.*
Lactoserum; lactic acid (p.1704·1).
*Skin disorders.*

**Dermadex**
*Note. This name is used for preparations of different composition.*
*GlaxoSmithKline, Arg.*
Clobetasol propionate (p.1095·2).
*Skin disorders.*
*Teofarma, Ital.*
Dexamethasone valerate (p.1097·3).
*Skin disorders.*

**Dermadex NN** *GlaxoSmithKline, Arg.*
Clobetasol propionate (p.1095·2); neomycin sulfate (p.235·1); nystatin (p.406·3).
*Infected skin disorders.*

**Dermadine** *Medpro, S.Afr.*
Povidone-iodine (p.1190·3).
*Mouth and throat disorders; skin disinfection.*

**Dermadrate**
*Dermatech, Austral.; Balmar, NZ; Dermatech, Singapore.*
Lactic acid (p.1704·1); urea (p.1162·2); sodium pidolate (p.1158·1).
*Dry skin.*

**Dermaflex** *Neolab, Canad.*
Urea (p.1162·2).
*Emollient; moisturiser.*

**Dermaflogil** *NCSN, Ital.*
Diflucortolone valerate (p.1099·3); kanamycin sulfate (p.225·1).
*Skin disorders.*

**Dermaflor**
*Note. This name is used for preparations of different composition.*
*ICN, Arg.*
Ciclopirox olamine (p.396·1).
*Fungal skin and nail infections.*
*NCSN, Ital.*
Diflorasone diacetate (p.1099·3).
*Skin disorders.*

**Dermaglos**
*Note. This name is used for preparations of different composition.*
*Andromaco, Arg.*
A range of moisturisers with or without sunscreens.
*Dry skin.*
*Andromaco, Chile.*
Vitamin A palmitate (p.1453·1); ergocalciferol (p.1462·1); benzethonium chloride (p.1169·2); allantoin (p.1141·3).
*Burns; skin disorders; wounds.*

**Dermaglos Plus** *Andromaco, Chile.*
Vitamin A palmitate (p.1453·1); ergocalciferol (p.1462·1); benzethonium chloride (p.1169·2); allantoin (p.1141·3); vitamin E acetate (p.1465·1); centella (p.1144·3).
*Burns; skin disorders; wounds.*

**Dermagor**
*Note. This name is used for preparations of different composition.*
*Coryne de Bruynes, Mon.*
Aluminium chlorohydrate (p.1142·1).
*Hyperhidrosis.*
*Dermoteca, Port.*
Emollient.

**Dermagor Ecran Solar** *Dermoteca, Port.†.*
Titanium dioxide (p.1160·3).
*Sunscreen.*

**Dermagor-Antitranspirante** *Dermoteca, Port.*
Aluminium chlorohydrate (p.1142·1).
*Hyperhidrosis.*

**Dermagraft**
*Smith & Nephew, UK; Smith & Nephew, USA.*
Human dermal tissue (p.1158·1).
*Diabetic foot ulcers.*

**Derm-Aid**
*Ego, Austral.; Ego, Malaysia; Ego, NZ; Ego, Singapore.*
Hydrocortisone (p.1103·3).
*Skin disorders.*

**Dermal C** *Raza, Malaysia; Pharmaniaga, Malaysia.*
Betamethasone dipropionate (p.1093·1); clotrimazole (p.396·2).
*Fungal skin infections.*

**Dermal Care** *Bayer Diagnostici, Ital.*
Urea (p.1162·2).
*Dry skin and nail disorders.*

**Dermal G** *Raza, Malaysia; Pharmaniaga, Malaysia.*
Betamethasone (p.1093·1); gentamicin sulfate (p.217·1).
*Infected skin disorders.*

**Dermal SA** *Raza, Malaysia; Pharmaniaga, Malaysia.*
Betamethasone dipropionate (p.1093·1); salicylic acid (p.1157·1).
*Skin disorders.*

**Dermalar** *Teva, Israel.*
Fluocinolone acetonide (p.1101·2).
*Skin disorders.*

**Dermalibour**
*Pierre Fabre Dermo-Cosmetique, Arg.; Ducray, Fr.*
Avena (p.1658·2); zinc oxide (p.1163·2); copper sulfate (p.1426·1); zinc sulfate (p.1469·3).
*Skin disorders.*

**Dermalife**
*Pharmacia Upjohn, Austral.†.*
Vitamin A palmitate (p.1453·1).
*Burns; minor skin lesions; nappy rash.*
*Orion, NZ.*
Vitamin A (p.1451·2).
*Skin disorders.*

**Dermalife Plus**
*Orion, Austral.*
Calamine (p.1144·1); vitamin A palmitate (p.1453·1); dimethicone (p.1482·1).
*Burns; cradle cap; minor skin lesions; nappy rash; skin disorders.*
*Pharmacia Upjohn, NZ†.*
Calamine (p.1144·1); vitamin A (p.1451·2); dimethicone (p.1482·1).
*Skin disorders.*

**Dermalisan** *Prodotti, Braz.*
Vitamin A (p.1451·2); vitamin D (p.1461·2); zinc oxide (p.1163·2).
*Skin disorders.*

**Dermallerg** *Ratiopharm, Ger.*
Hydrocortisone (p.1103·3).
*Skin disorders.*

**Dermalo** *Dermal Laboratories, UK.*
Liquid paraffin (p.1479·1); acetylated wool alcohols (p.1483·1).
Formerly known as Emmolate.
*Dry skin.*

**Dermalog** *Bristol-Myers Squibb, Mex.*
Halcinonide (p.1103·2).
*Skin disorders.*

**Dermalog-C** *Bristol-Myers Squibb, Mex.*
Halcinonide (p.1103·2); nystatin (p.406·3); neomycin sulfate (p.235·1).
*Infected skin disorders.*

**derma-loges N** *Loges, Ger.†.*
Peru balsam (p.1730·2); arnica (p.1656·3); hamamelis (p.1696·3); chamomile (p.1669·3); sunflower oil (p.1451·1).
*Burns; haemorrhoids; skin disorders; wounds.*

**Dermamina** *EMS, Braz.*
Calamine (p.1144·1); zinc oxide (p.1163·2); diphenhydramine hydrochloride (p.431·3); camphor (p.1665·3); glycerol (p.1694·3).
*Skin disorders.*

**Dermamist**
*Yamanouchi, Ital.*
Emollient.
*Dry skin disorders.*
*Yamanouchi, UK.*
White soft paraffin (p.1479·3); liquid paraffin (p.1479·1).
*Dry skin disorders.*

**Dermamycin** *Pfeiffer, USA.*
Diphenhydramine hydrochloride (p.431·3).

**Derma-Mykotral** *Rosen, Ger.*
Miconazole nitrate (p.405·3).
*Fungal infections of the skin and mucous membranes.*

**Dermana** *Milte, Port.†.*
A range of emollient and barrier preparations.

**Dermana Pasta** *Humana, Ital.*
Gamolenic acid (p.1690·2); omega-3 triglyceride (p.976·1); vitamin E (p.1464·3); vitamin A (p.1451·2); zinc oxide (p.1163·2).
*Dry skin disorders; skin irritation.*

**DermaNail** *Summers, USA.*
Alpha acetoxy acid.
*Nail disorders.*

**Dermanatur** *Sofex, Port.†.*
Emollient.
*Barrier preparation; dry skin.*

**Derman-Oil** *Humana, Ital.*
Gamolenic acid (p.1690·2); omega-3 triglycerides (p.976·1); vitamins A (p.1451·2); vitamin E (p.1464·3).
*Bath additive.*

**Dermaor** *Sam-On, Israel†.*
Chlorhexidine gluconate (p.1173·2); cetrimide (p.1172·1).
*Skin, hand, and instrument disinfection.*

**Derma-Pax** *Recsei, USA.*
Mepyramine maleate (p.437·1); chlorphenamine (p.428·1).
*Pruritus.*

**Dermapro** *Raza, Malaysia; Pharmaniaga, Malaysia.*
Clobetasol propionate (p.1095·2).
*Skin disorders.*

**Dermarell** *Sanorell, Ger.*
Homoeopathic preparation.

**Dermaren** *Areu, Spain.*
Dichlorisone acetate (p.1099·3).
*Skin disorders.*

**Dermarest** *Del, USA.*
Diphenhydramine hydrochloride (p.431·3); resorcinol (p.1156·3).
*Pruritus.*

**Dermarest Dri-Cort** *Del, USA.*
Hydrocortisone acetate (p.1103·3).
*Skin disorders.*

**Dermarest Dricort Anti-Itch** *Del, Canad.*
Hydrocortisone (p.1103·3).
*Skin disorders.*

**Dermarest Plus**
*Del, Canad.; Del, USA.*
Diphenhydramine hydrochloride (p.431·3); menthol (p.1711·3).
*Pruritus.*

**Dermase** *Sanval, Braz.*
Neomycin sulfate (p.235·1); bacitracin zinc (p.161·3).
*Skin infections.*

**Dermaseb** *Cassara, Arg.*
Sulfacetamide (p.257·3).
*Acne.*

**Dermasept Antifungal** *Pharmakon, USA.*
Tannic acid (p.1751·2); zinc chloride (p.1469·2); benzocaine (p.1370·3); methylbenzethonium chloride (p.1186·1); tolnaftate (p.410·1); undecenoic acid (p.410·3).
*Fungal skin infections.*

**Dermasil** *Silom, Thai.*
Clobetasol propionate (p.1095·2).
*Skin disorders.*

**Derma-Smoothe/FS** *Hill, USA.*
Fluocinolone acetonide (p.1101·2).
*Skin disorders.*

**Dermasol** *Olan-Kemed, Thai.*
Chloramphenicol (p.185·1); hydrocortisone acetate (p.1103·3).
*Infected skin disorders.*

**Dermasole** *Raza, Malaysia; Pharmaniaga, Malaysia.*
Betamethasone valerate (p.1093·2).
*Skin disorders.*

**Dermasole DP** *Raza, Malaysia; Pharmaniaga, Malaysia.*
Betamethasone dipropionate (p.1093·1).
*Skin disorders.*

**Dermasole N** *Raza, Malaysia; Pharmaniaga, Malaysia.*
Betamethasone valerate (p.1093·2); neomycin sulfate (p.235·1).
*Infected skin disorders.*

**Dermasone**
*Technilab, Canad.; Technilab, Hong Kong.*
Clobetasol propionate (p.1095·2).
*Skin and scalp disorders.*

**Dermaspraid Antiseptique** *Roche Nicholas, Fr.*
Chlorhexidine gluconate (p.1173·2); benzalkonium chloride (p.1168·3); benzyl alcohol (p.1170·2).
Formerly known as Dermaspray.
*Wound and burn disinfection.*

**Dermaspraid Demangeaison** *Roche Nicholas, Fr.*
Hydrocortisone acetate (p.1103·3).
*Nettle and insect stings; sunburn.*

**Dermaspray**
*Roche, Austria; Roche, Belg.*
Chlorhexidine gluconate (p.1173·2); benzalkonium chloride (p.1168·3); benzyl alcohol (p.1170·2).
*Wound disinfection.*

**Dermaspray demangeaison** *Roche Nicholas, Fr.†.*
Hydrocortisone (p.1103·3).
*Skin disorders.*

**Dermasten** *Offenbach, Mex.*
Clotrimazole (p.396·2).
*Fungal skin infections.*

**Dermatar** *IDI, Ital.*
Betamethasone valero-acetate (p.1093·2); salicylic acid (p.1157·1); ichthammol (p.1148·2).
*Skin disorders.*

**Dermatech Liquid** *Dermatech, Austral.*
Alcohol (p.1166·1); propylene glycol (p.1735·2).
*Vehicle for topical drugs.*

**Dermatech Wart Treatment**
*Dermatech, Austral.; Dermatech, Singapore.*
Lactic acid (p.1704·1); salicylic acid (p.1157·1).
*Warts.*

**Dermatitis Relief** *Brauer, Austral.†.*
Homoeopathic preparation.

**Dermatix** *ICN, UK.*
Silicone liquid gel (p.1482·1).
*Hypertrophic and keloid scars.*

**Dermatodoron**
*Note. This name is used for preparations of different composition.*
*Weleda, Austria; Weleda, Ger.*
Dulcamara (p.1683·1); lysimachia nummularia.
*Eczema.*
*Weleda, UK.*
Homoeopathic preparation.

**Dermatofides** *Fides, Ger.†.*
Homoeopathic preparation.

**Dermatol** *Chinosolfabrik, Ger.*
Bismuth subgallate (p.1252·2).
*Burns; excoriations.*

**Dermatop**
*Aventis, Braz.; Aventis, Chile; Aventis, Ger.; Aventis, Ital.; Aventis, Thai.; Dermik, USA.*
Prednicarbate (p.1107·3).
*Skin disorders.*

**Dermatovate** *Glaxo Wellcome, Mex.*
Clobetasol propionate (p.1095·2).
*Skin disorders.*

**Dermatrans**
*Note. This name is used for preparations of different composition.*
*Rottapharm, Chile.*
Estradiol (p.1550·1).
*Menopausal disorders.*
*Bayer, Ital.; Recordati, Spain.*
Glyceryl trinitrate (p.923·2).
*Angina pectoris.*

**Derm'attive** *Sidone, Braz.*
Theophylline glycolate; centella (p.1144·3); guarana (p.1765·3).

**Derm'attive Solaire** *Sidone, Braz.*
Octinoxate (p.1154·3); oxybenzone (p.1154·3); titanium dioxide (p.1160·3); zinc oxide (p.1163·2); ginkgo biloba (p.1692·3); aloe vera (p.1141·3).

**Dermaval** *FIRMA, Ital.*
Diflucortolone valerate (p.1099·3).
*Skin disorders.*

**Dermaveen** *Balmar, NZ.*
Colloidal oatmeal (p.1658·2).
*Dry skin; pruritus; soap-free cleanser.*

**DermaVeen Acne** *Dermatech, Singapore.*
Colloidal oatmeal (p.1658·2); salicylic acid (p.1157·1).
*Soap-free cleanser.*

**DermaVeen Bath**
*Dermatech, Austral.†; Dermatech, Singapore.*
Colloidal oatmeal (p.1658·2).
*Bath additive; skin irritation.*

**DermaVeen Dry Skin**
*Dermatech, Austral.†; Dermatech, Singapore.*
Colloidal oatmeal (p.1658·2).
*Skin irritation; soap-free cleanser.*

**DermaVeen Moisturising**
*Note. This name is used for preparations of different composition.*
*Dermatech, Austral.†.*
Colloidal oatmeal (p.1658·2); sodium pidolate (p.1158·1); white soft paraffin (p.1479·3).
*Dry skin; pruritus.*
*Dermatech, Singapore.*
Colloidal oatmeal (p.1658·2).
*Dry skin; skin irritation.*

**DermaVeen Oatmeal Shampoo** *Dermatech, Singapore.*
Colloidal oatmeal (p.1658·2).
*Scalp disorders.*

**DermaVeen Shower & Bath** *Dermatech, Austral.†; Dermatech, Singapore.*
Colloidal oatmeal (p.1658·2); sodium pidolate (p.1158·1); liquid paraffin (p.1479·1).
*Bath additive; dry skin; soap-free skin cleanser.*

**DermaVeen Soap Free** *Dermatech, Singapore.*
Colloidal oatmeal (p.1658·2).
*Soap-free skin cleanser.*

**DermaVite** *Stiefel, USA.*
Multivitamin and mineral preparation (p.1417·1).

**Dermax**
*Note. This name is used for preparations of different composition.*
*Galderma, Braz.*
Sulfur (p.1158·2); salicylic acid (p.1157·1).
*Acne.*
*Fischer, Israel.*
Triclosan (p.1195·2).
*Skin disinfectant.*

**Dermazellon** *Kohler, Ger.*
Silver salt of 2-aminoethyl dihydrogen phosphate.
*Burns; skin infections; wounds.*

**Dermazin**
*Pharmascience, Canad.; Lek, Hong Kong; Lek, Thai.*
Sulfadiazine silver (p.259·1).
*Bacterial skin infections; burns; infected wounds.*

**Dermazinc** *Sivaderm, Arg.*
Pyrithione zinc (p.1156·2).
*Pityriasis.*

**Dermazine** *Silvestre, Braz.†.*
Sulfadiazine silver (p.259·1).
*Bacterial skin infections; infected burns; skin ulceration.*

**Dermazol**
*Sanval, Braz.; Bailleul, Fr.*
Econazole nitrate (p.397·2).
*Fungal skin infections.*

**Dermazole**
*Ego, Austral.; Ego, Hong Kong; Ego, NZ; Ego, Singapore.*
Econazole nitrate (p.397·2).
*Fungal skin infections.*

**Dermazon** *Dinafarma, Braz.†.*
Dexamethasone (p.1097·1); neomycin sulfate (p.235·1).
*Skin disorders.*

**Dermdryl** *Teuto, Braz.*
Calamine (p.1144·1); diphenhydramine hydrochloride (p.431·3); camphor (p.1665·3).
*Skin disorders.*

**Der-med** *Permamed, Switz.*
Soap substitute.
*Skin disorders.*

**Dermedal** *Farmec, Ital.*
Tosylchloramide sodium (p.1194·3).
*Disinfection of burns, wounds, and surfaces; genital hygiene.*

**Dermenet** *Essex, Chile.*
Mometasone furoate (p.1107·2).
*Skin disorders.*

**Dermeol** *Cooperation Pharmaceutique, Fr.†.*
Dodeclonium bromide (p.1178·3); enoxolone (p.36·2).
*Skin disorders.*

**Dermestril**
*Mayne, Austral.; CSC, Austria; Besins, Belg.; Rottapharm, Fin.; Rottapharm, Fr.; Opfermann, Ger.; Faran, Gr.; Rotta, Hong Kong; Rottapharm, Irl.; LTS, Israel; Rotta, Israel; Rottapharm, Ital.; Sigma-Tau, Neth.; Delta, Port.; Rottapharm, Spain; Sigma-Tau, Switz.; Strakan, UK†.*
Estradiol (p.1550·1).
*Menopausal disorders; osteoporosis.*

**Dermex** *Hamilton, Austral.*
Range of barrier creams.

**Dermeze** *Royal Childrens Hospital, Austral.†.*
Liquid paraffin (p.1479·1); white soft paraffin (p.1479·3).
*Dry skin.*

**Derm-Freeze** *Eagle, Austral.†.*
Trichlorofluoromethane (p.1236·1); dichlorodifluoromethane (p.1236·1).
*Local anaesthesia; pain.*

**Dermic** *Kinder, Braz.*
Salicylic acid (p.1157·1); sulfur (p.1158·2).
*Acne.*

**Dermichthol** *Ichthyol, Ger.*
Ictasol (p.1148·3).
*Skin disorders.*

**Dermicin** *Heralds, Braz.†.*
Polymyxin B sulfate (p.245·1); prednisolone (p.1108·1).
*Skin disorders.*

**Dermicon** *Bunker, Braz.*
Benzoic acid (p.1169·3); salicylic acid (p.1157·1); iodine (p.1598·1); licor de Hoffman (alcohol, solvent ether).
*Fungal skin infections.*

**Dermi-cyl** *Liebermann, Ger.*
Calcium hydroxide solution (p.1664·3).
*Burns; skin disorders.*

**Dermi-cyl Allerg** *Liebermann, Austria.*
Calcium hydroxide solution (p.1664·3).
*Skin disorders.*

**Dermi-cyl Ho-Lens-Complex** *Liebermann, Ger.*
Homoeopathic preparation.

**Dermi-cyl Schrunden** *Liebermann, Austria.*
Salicylic acid (p.1157·1).
*Skin disorders.*

**Dermidex** *Thornton & Ross, UK.*
Lidocaine (p.1377·3); alcloxa (p.1141·2); chlorobutanol (p.1176·3); cetrimide (p.1172·1).
*Skin irritation.*

**Dermifun** *Fustery, Mex.*
Miconazole nitrate (p.405·3).
*Fungal skin and nail infections.*

**Dermil** *Nettopharma, Denm.†.*
Hydrocortisone (p.1103·3).
*Skin disorders.*

**Dermilan** *Hearst, Braz.†.*
Nitrofurazone (p.238·2); hydrocortisone acetate (p.1103·3).
*Skin disorders.*

**Dermilia Flebozin** *Depofarma, Ital.*
Zinc oxide (p.1163·2); myrtillus (p.1718·3); echinacea (p.1683·2); hamamelis (p.1696·3); melilotus; centella (p.1144·3).
*Tired legs.*

**Dermilon**
*Caesaro, Austria; Cesra, Ger.*
Zinc oxide (p.1163·2); cod-liver oil (p.1425·2).
*Skin disorders.*

**Dermimade Bacitracina** *Esfar, Port.*
Bacitracin (p.161·3); neomycin (p.235·1).
*Skin infections.*

**Dermimade Cloranfenicol** *Esfar, Port.*
Chloramphenicol (p.185·1).
*Skin infections.*

**Dermimade Hidrocortisona** *Esfar, Port.*
Hydrocortisone (p.1103·3).
*Skin disorders.*

**Derminiol** *Schwabe, Spain.*
Hamamelis (p.1696·3).
*Skin irritation.*

**Derminovag** *Novag, Spain†.*
Hydrocortisone acetate (p.1103·3).
*Skin disorders.*

**Dermirex** *Irex, Fr.†.*
Minocycline (p.231·3).
*Acne.*

**Dermirit** *Medisint, Ital.*
Hydrocortisone acetate (p.1103·3).
*Skin disorders.*

**Dermisdin** *Isdin, Spain.*
Fenticlor (p.397·3); miconazole nitrate (p.405·3); salicylic acid (p.1157·1).
Formerly contained sulfur, fenticlor, miconazole nitrate, and salicylic acid.
*Acne; scalp disorders; seborrhoea.*

**Dermisone Beclo** *Zyma, Spain†.*
Beclometasone dipropionate (p.1091·1).
*Skin disorders.*

**Dermisone Epitelizante** *Novartis Consumer, Spain.*
Amino acids (p.1417·1); chloramphenicol (p.185·1); vitamin A palmitate; vitamin F.
*Wound healing.*

**Dermisone Tri Antibiotic** *Novartis Consumer, Spain.*
Bacitracin (p.161·3); neomycin sulfate (p.235·1); polymyxin B sulfate (p.245·1).
*Skin infections.*

**Dermitina** *Donini, Ital.*
Hamamelis (p.1696·3); sodium glutamate; fatty acids (p.1417·1).
*Soap substitute.*

**Dermizan** *Bunker, Braz.*
Azelaic acid (p.1142·3).
*Acne.*

**Dermizol** *Roux-Ocefa, Arg.*
Betamethasone benzoate (p.1093·1).
*Skin disorders.*

**Dermizol G** *Roux-Ocefa, Arg.*
Betamethasone benzoate (p.1093·1); gentamicin sulfate (p.217·1).
*Infected skin disorders.*

**Dermizol Trio** *Roux-Ocefa, Arg.*
Betamethasone valerate (p.1093·2); gentamicin sulfate (p.217·1); miconazole (p.405·2).
*Infected skin disorders.*

**Dermo 6** *Pharmadeveloppement, Fr.*
Pyridoxine hydrochloride (p.1456·3).
*Seborrhoea.*

**Dermo Base Grassa** *Restiva, Ital.†.*
Product basis.

**Dermo Base Magra** *Restiva, Ital.†.*
Product basis.

**Dermo Halibut Infantil** *Novartis Consumer, Spain.*
Dimethicone (p.1482·1); benzalkonium chloride (p.1168·3); vitamin A (p.1451·2); zinc oxide (p.1163·2).
Formerly known as Dermo H Infantil.
*Burns; skin disorders; wounds.*

**Dermo Hubber** *Teofarma, Spain.*
Bacitracin zinc (p.161·3); hydrocortisone acetate (p.1103·3); neomycin sulfate (p.235·1).
*Infected skin disorders.*

**Dermo Lassar** *Remexa, Mex.†.*
Zinc oxide (p.1163·2).

**Dermo Posterisan** *Kade, Ger.*
Hydrocortisone (p.1103·3).
*Skin disorders.*

**Dermo Silanols** *Sedifa, Mon.*
A range of preparations containing silicones (p.1482·1).
*Skin disorders.*

**Dermo WAS** *Montavit, Austria.*
Lecithin (p.1706·1).
*Skin disorders.*

**Dermoangiopan** *Abiogen, Ital.*
Troxerutin (p.1688·3); sulodexide (p.1009·2).
*Soft-tissue disorders; vascular disorders.*

**Dermobacter** *Innotech, Fr.*
Benzalkonium chloride (p.1168·3); chlorhexidine gluconate (p.1173·2).
*Bacterial skin infections.*

**Dermobarrina** *Reccius, Chile.*
*Cream:* Resorcinol (p.1156·3).
*Lotion:* Benzalkonium chloride (p.1168·3); menthol (p.1711·3).

**Dermobase** *Key, Arg.*
Emollient.
*Skin disorders.*

**Dermobel**
*Note. A similar name is used for preparations of different composition (see below).*
*Sedabel, Braz.*
Fluocinolone acetonide (p.1101·2); neomycin (p.235·1).
*Infected skin disorders.*

**Dermo-Bell**
*Note. A similar name is used for preparations of different composition (see above).*
*Remexa, Mex.*
Araquida oil.

**Dermobene** *Legrand, Braz.*
Clotrimazole (p.396·2).
*Fungal skin infections.*

**Dermobet** *Infabra, Braz.†.*
Betamethasone valerate (p.1093·2).
*Skin disorders.*

**Dermobeta** *Krugher, Ital.*
Fluocinolone acetonide (p.1101·2).
*Skin disorders.*

**Dermobion**
*Note. This name is used for preparations of different composition.*
*Bergamo, Braz.†.*
Zinc oxide (p.1163·2); boric acid (p.1662·1); dogfish-liver oil.
*Barrier preparation; skin disorders.*
*Serral, Mex.*
Filiferine; papain (p.1727·3).
*Burns; wounds.*

**Dermobios** *Biotekfarma, Ital.†.*
Diflucortolone valerate (p.1099·3); tetracycline (p.266·2); polymyxin B sulfate (p.245·1).
*Infected skin disorders.*

**Dermobiotico** *Davi, Port.*
Neomycin sulfate (p.235·1); bacitracin (p.161·3).
*Skin infections.*

**Dermobras** *Remexa, Mex.*
Aluminium oxide (p.1140·1); triclosan (p.1195·2).
*Skin cleansing.*

**Dermocaine**
*Note. This name is used for preparations of different composition.*
*Ego, Austral.†.*
Lidocaine hydrochloride (p.1377·3); menthol (p.1711·3); phenoxypropanol (p.1189·1); cetrimide (p.1172·1).
*Bites and stings.*
*Ego, NZ†.*
Lidocaine (p.1377·3); cetrimide (p.1172·1); phenoxypropanol (p.1189·1).
*Insect bites and stings; pruritus; skin irritation.*

**Dermocal** *Panalab, Arg.*
Calcipotriol (p.1144·1).
*Psoriasis.*

**Dermocalm** *Pharmadeveloppement, Fr.†.*
Vitamin A (p.1451·2); lidocaine (p.1377·3); framycetin sulfate (p.215·1); hydrocortisone acetate (p.1103·3).
*Burns.*

**Dermocica** *Phytomedica, Fr.*
Arnica (p.1656·3); melaleuca oil (p.1710·2); mimosa; vervain oil.
*Burns; scars; wounds.*

**Dermocinetic** *Geymonat, Ital.*
Levothyroxine sodium (p.1600·1); aescin (p.1648·2).
*Cellulite; local build up of adipose tissue.*

**Dermocortal** *Pfizer Consumer, Ital.*
Hydrocortisone (p.1103·3).
*Burns; eczema; erythema; insect stings; pruritus.*

**Dermocrem** *Ache, Braz.†.*
Wheat germ.
*Wounds.*

**Dermocreme** *Chauvin, Fr.†.*
Zinc oxide (p.1163·2); copper sulfate (p.1426·1).
*Skin irritation.*

**Dermocridin** *Neo Dermos, Arg.*
Lactic acid (p.1704·1); menthol (p.1711·3); panthenol (p.1727·2); vegetable extracts.
*Seborrhoeic dermatitis.*

**Dermocuivre** *Chauvin, Fr.*
Copper sulfate (p.1426·1); zinc oxide (p.1163·2).
*Skin disorders.*

**Dermodan** *ITF, Chile.*
Tretinoin (p.1161·1).
*Acne; light-induced skin damage.*

**Dermodex** *Bristol-Myers Squibb, Braz.*
Zinc oxide (p.1163·2); nystatin (p.406·3).
*Infected skin disorders.*

**Dermodis** *Farmades, Ital.†.*
Rifaximin (p.254·1).
*Bacterial skin infections.*

**Dermodrin** *Montavit, Austria.*
Diphenhydramine hydrochloride (p.431·3).
*Skin disorders.*

**Dermofenac** *Whitehall, Fr.*
Hydrocortisone (p.1103·3).
*Skin disorders.*

**Dermofibrin C** *Biochimico, Braz.*
Fibrinolysin (p.916·2); dornase alfa (p.1119·1); chloramphenicol (p.185·1).
*Wounds.*

**Dermofilm** *Innovatec, Singapore†.*
Topical barrier preparation.

**Dermofix**
*Azevedos, Port.; Ferrer, Spain.*
Sertaconazole nitrate (p.408·1).
*Fungal skin and nail infections; vulvovaginal candidiasis.*

**Dermofug** *Wolff, Ger.†.*
Dodecylbenzolsulphonic acid trolamine; ammonium laurilsulfate (p.1574·3).
*Acne; fungal infections; seborrhoeic dermatitis.*

**Dermofytol** *Sedar, Braz.†.*
Salicylic acid (p.1157·1); benzoic acid (p.1169·3); iodine (p.1598·1).
*Skin infections.*

**Dermogaze** *Ache, Braz.†.*
Wheat germ.
*Wounds.*

**Dermogen** *Dermopen, Braz.†.*
Dexamethasone sodium phosphate (p.1097·2); neomycin sulfate (p.235·1).
*Skin disorders.*

**Dermoglos** *Galderma, Braz.†.*
Zinc oxide (p.1163·2); cod-liver oil (p.1425·2).
*Barrier preparation; skin disorders.*

**Dermoil** *Dermofarma, Ital.*
Emollient.
*Bath additive; dry skin disorders.*

**Dermojela** *Jean-Marie, Hong Kong.*
Choline salicylate (p.26·2); benzalkonium chloride (p.1168·3); menthol (p.1711·3).
*Mouth disorders.*

**Dermojuventus** *Juventus, Spain.*
Tretinoin (p.1161·1).
*Acne; sunlight-induced skin damage.*

**Dermokin** *Kinder, Braz.*
Zinc oxide (p.1163·2); nystatin (p.406·3).
*Skin disorders.*

**Dermol**
*Note. This name is used for preparations of different composition.*
*Simoes, Braz.*
Benzalkonium chloride (p.1168·3); salicylic acid (p.1157·1); camphor (p.1665·3); iodo iodetata (p.1598·1); siam benzoin (p.1744·1); arnica (p.1656·3).
*Pruritic skin disorders.*
*Pacific, NZ.*
Clobetasol propionate (p.1095·2).
*Skin and scalp disorders.*
*Dermal Laboratories, UK.*
Benzalkonium chloride (p.1168·3); chlorhexidine hydrochloride (p.1173·3); liquid paraffin (p.1479·1); isopropyl myristate (p.1481·2).
*Dry and pruritic skin disorders.*

**Dermol HC** *Dermol, USA.*
Hydrocortisone (p.1103·3).

**Dermolate** *Schering-Plough, USA.*
Hydrocortisone (p.1103·3).
*Skin disorders.*

**Dermolin**
*Note. This name is used for preparations of different composition.*
*Lafare, Ital.*
Fluocinolone acetonide (p.1101·2).
*Skin disorders.*
*Roberts, USA.*
Methyl salicylate (p.59·3); camphor (p.1665·3); menthol (p.1711·3); mustard oil (p.1718·2).
*Muscle, joint, and soft-tissue pain; neuralgia.*

**Dermomycin** *Sigma-Tau, Ital.*
Sodium fusidate (p.215·2).
*Bacterial skin infections.*

**Dermomycose Liquido** *Reig Jofre, Spain.*
Boric acid (p.1662·1); phenol (p.1188·1); rosaniline; resorcinol (p.1156·3).
*Fungal infections.*

**Dermomycose Talco** *Reig Jofre, Spain.*
Neomycin undecylenate (p.235·2); menthol (p.1711·3).
*Skin infections.*

**Dermon** *Unison, Hong Kong.*
Miconazole nitrate (p.405·3).
*Fungal skin and nail infections.*

**Dermopan** *Pierre Fabre Dermo-Cosmetique, Arg.*
Avena (p.1658·2).
*Skin cleansing.*

**Dermoper** *Defuen, Arg.*
Permethrin (p.1508·3).
*Scabies.*

**Dermoperative** *Giscard, Arg.*
Hydrocortisone (p.1103·3); gentamicin (p.219·1).
*Infected skin disorders.*

**Dermophil Indien** *Dermophil Indien, Fr.*
Peru balsam (p.1730·2); levomenol (p.1707·1); salol (p.88·1).
*Lipstick:* Enzacamene (p.1147·1); isopropyldibenzoylmethane (p.1148·3).
*Sunscreen.*
*Lipstick SPF 7:* Enzacamene (p.1147·1).
*Sunscreen.*
*Maxi-stick:* Enzacamene (p.1147·1); avobenzone (p.1142·3); titanium dioxide (p.1160·3).
*Sunscreen.*

**Dermophil Indien Nouvelle formule** *Dermophil Indien, Switz.; Girard, Switz.*
Peru balsam (p.1730·2); levomenol (p.1707·1); salol (p.88·1).
*Emollient.*

**Dermoplast**
*Note. This name is used for preparations of different composition.*
*Wyeth-Ayerst, Canad.†.*
Benzocaine (p.1370·3); benzethonium chloride (p.1169·2); menthol (p.1711·3); hydroxyquinoline benzoate (p.1700·1).
*Local anaesthesia.*
*Remexa, Mex.*
Urea (p.1162·2).
*Dry skin disorders.*
*Whitehall, USA.*
Benzocaine (p.1370·3).
*Painful conditions of the skin and perineum.*

**Dermoplex Antifungal** *Upha, Malaysia.*
Tolnaftate (p.410·1).
*Fungal skin infections.*

**Dermoplex Antiseptic** *Upha, Malaysia.*
Cetrimide (p.1172·1).
*Insect bites and stings; minor wounds and burns; nappy rash.*

**Dermoplex Calamine** *Upha, Malaysia.*
Calamine (p.1144·1); zinc oxide (p.1163·2).
*Insect bites; nappy rash; skin irritation.*

**Dermoprolyn** *Infosint, Ital.*
Aescin (p.1648·2); hamamelis (p.1696·3); ruscus aculeatus; hedera helix.
*Skin disorders.*

**Dermoquinol** *East India Pharma, India.*
Clioquinol (p.196·3).
*Fungal skin infections.*

**Dermorelle** *IPRAD, Fr.*
*dl*-Alpha tocoferil acetate (p.1465·1).
*Vitamin E deficiency.*

**Dermoretin** *Sintofarma, Braz.†.*
Tretinoin (p.1161·1).
*Acne.*

**Dermosa Aureomicina** *Farmacusi, Spain.*
Chlortetracycline hydrochloride (p.187·3).
*Skin infections.*

**Dermosa Hidrocortisona** *Farmacusi, Spain.*
Hydrocortisone acetate (p.1103·3).
*Skin disorders.*

**Dermosalic** *Bunker, Braz.*
Betamethasone dipropionate (p.1093·1); salicylic acid (p.1157·1).
*Skin disorders.*

**Dermosed** *Makros, Braz.†.*
Tyrothricin (p.275·1); salicylic acid (p.1157·1); boric acid (p.1662·1).
*Skin infections.*

**Dermoseptic** *GlaxoSmithKline, Spain.*
Sertaconazole nitrate (p.408·1).
*Fungal skin and nail infections.*

**Dermoskin** *Remexa, Mex.*
Almond oil (p.1651·1).
*Moisturiser.*

**Dermoskin C** *Remexa, Mex.*
Sodium ascorbate (p.1460·2); ascorbic acid (p.1460·2).
*UV-induced skin damage.*

**Dermosol**
*YSP, Malaysia; Yung Shin, Singapore.*
Clobetasol propionate (p.1095·2).
*Skin disorders.*

**Dermosolon** *Dermapharm, Ger.*
Prednisolone (p.1108·1).
*Corticosteroid.*

**Dermosona**
*Note. This name is used for preparations of different composition.*
*Fecofar, Arg.*
Miconazole (p.405·2); betamethasone (p.1093·1); gentamicin (p.219·1).
*Infected skin disorders.*
*Saval, Chile.*
Mometasone furoate (p.1107·2).
*Skin disorders.*

**Dermo-Steril** *Ghimas, Ital.†.*
Triclosan (p.1195·2).
*Acne.*

**Dermo-Sulfuryl** *Richelet, Fr.*
Precipitated sulfur (p.1158·2); copper sulfate (p.1426·1); zinc sulfate (p.1469·3).
*Acne.*

**Dermovagisil** *Combe, Spain.*
Lidocaine (p.1377·3).
*Vaginal disorders.*

**Dermoval**
*Note. This name is used for preparations of different composition.*
*Luper, Braz.*
Betamethasone valerate (p.1093·2).
*Skin disorders.*
*GlaxoSmithKline, Fr.*
Clobetasol propionate (p.1095·2).
*Skin disorders.*
*Tocogino, Mex.†.*
Betamethasone (p.1093·1).
*Skin disorders.*

**Dermovan** *Healthpoint, USA.*
Vehicle for topical preparations.

**Dermovat**
*GlaxoSmithKline, Denm.; GlaxoSmithKline, Fin.; GlaxoSmithKline, Norw.; GlaxoSmithKline, Swed.*
Clobetasol propionate (p.1095·2).
*Skin and scalp disorders.*

**Dermovate**
*Note. This name is used for preparations of different composition.*
*GlaxoSmithKline, Austria; GlaxoSmithKline, Belg.; GlaxoSmithKline, Canad.; GlaxoSmithKline, Chile; GlaxoSmithKline, Hong Kong; GlaxoSmithKline, Irl.; GlaxoSmithKline, Israel; GlaxoSmithKline, Malaysia; GlaxoSmithKline, Neth.; Glaxo Wellcome, NZ†; Glaxo Wellcome, Port.; Glaxo Wellcome, S.Afr.; GlaxoSmithKline, Singapore; GlaxoSmithKline, Switz.; GlaxoSmithKline, Thai.; GlaxoSmithKline, UK.*
Clobetasol propionate (p.1095·2).
*Skin and scalp disorders.*
*Baldassari, Braz.†.*
Betamethasone (p.1093·1).
*Skin disorders.*

**Dermovate-NN**
*Glaxo Wellcome, Port.; GlaxoSmithKline, Switz.; GlaxoSmithKline, UK.*
Clobetasol propionate (p.1095·2); neomycin sulfate (p.235·1); nystatin (p.406·3).
*Skin disorders with bacterial or fungal infection.*

**Dermovit**
*Note. This name is used for preparations of different composition.*
*White, Arg.*
Betamethasone dipropionate (p.1093·1); clotrimazole (p.396·2); gentamicin sulfate (p.217·1).
*Infected skin disorders.*
*Kemiprogress, Ital.†.*
Vitamin, selenium, yeast, and coenzyme Q10 (p.1417·1).
*Nutritional supplement.*

**Dermovitamina** *Pasquali, Ital.*
Cod-liver oil (p.1425·2).
*Skin disorders.*

**Dermowas**
*Wolff, Ger.†.*
Soap substitute.
*Wolff, Ger.*
Dodecylbenzolsulfonic acid trolamine; ammonium laurilsulfate (p.1574·3).
*Skin disorders.*

**Dermowund** *Adler, Austria.*
Acriflavinium chloride (p.1165·3); diacetylaminoazotoluene (p.1178·2); cod-liver oil (p.1425·2); linseed oil (p.1707·2); sodium propionate (p.408·1); zinc oxide (p.1163·2).
*Wounds.*

**Dermox** *Remexa, Mex.*
Methoxsalen (p.1152·1).
*Psoriasis; vitiligo.*

**Dermoxin**
*Note. This name is used for preparations of different composition.*
*Bunker, Braz.*
Fluocinolone acetonide (p.1101·2); neomycin sulfate (p.235·1).
*Skin disorders.*
*GlaxoSmithKline, Ger.*
Clobetasol propionate (p.1095·2).
*Skin disorders.*

**Dermoxinale** *GlaxoSmithKline, Ger.*
Clobetasol propionate (p.1095·2).
*Skin disorders.*

**Dermoxyl**
*Note. This name is used for preparations of different composition.*
*ICN, Canad.*
Benzoyl peroxide (p.1143·2).
*Acne.*
*Laboratorios Chile, Chile.*
Terbinafine hydrochloride (p.408·2).
*Fungal skin and nail infections.*
*Euroderm-RDC, Ital.*
Urea hydrogen peroxide (p.1195·3).
*Skin disinfection and cleansing.*

**Derms** *Uniao Quimica, Braz.*
Tiabendazole (p.114·2); neomycin sulfate (p.235·1).
*Skin infections.*

**Dermtex HC with Aloe** *Pfeiffer, USA.*
Hydrocortisone (p.1103·3); aloe vera (p.1141·3).
*Skin disorders.*

**Dermum** *Dermophil Indien, Fr.*
Hypericum (p.299·1).
*Skin irritation.*

**Dermuspray** *Warner Chilcott, USA.*
Trypsin (p.1758·3); peru balsam (p.1730·2); castor oil (p.1668·2).
*Wounds.*

**Dermycose** *Prima, Braz.*
Iodine (p.1598·1); sodium iodide (p.1598·1); salicylic acid (p.1157·1); benzoic acid (p.1169·3).
*Fungal skin infections.*

**Derobin Skin** *USV, India.*
Dithranol (p.1146·1); salicylic acid (p.1157·1); coal tar (p.1159·2).
*Corns; psoriasis; ringworm.*

**Deroctyl** *Gap, Gr.*
Glibenclamide (p.331·2).
*Diabetes mellitus.*

**Derofen Miel** *Sanofi Synthelabo, Mex.*
Dextromethorphan (p.1117·3); guaifenesin (p.1122·1).
*Coughs.*

**Deronga Heilpaste** *Galderma, Ger.*
Natamycin (p.406·2).
*Fungal skin infections.*

**Deroxat**
*GlaxoSmithKline, Fr.; SmithKline Beecham, Switz.*
Paroxetine hydrochloride (p.311·2).
*Depression; obsessive-compulsive disorder; panic attacks; social phobia.*

**Derozin** *Gap, Gr.*
Cinnarizine (p.428·3).
*Vertigo.*

**Derrumal** *Finadiet, Arg.*
Avocado; soya (p.1447·2).
*Arthritis.*

**Derso TCC** *Pfizer, Braz.*
Triclocarban (p.1195·1).
*Skin infections.*

**Dertrase** *UCB, Spain.*
Carbamoylglutamic acid; inositol (p.1701·2); methionine (p.1042·1); chymotrypsin (p.1671·2); ribonucleic acid (p.1738·2); trypsin (p.1758·3); nitrofurazone (p.238·2).
*Burns; skin disorders; ulcers; wounds.*

**Dertrin** *Iqfasa, Mex.*
Co-trimoxazole (p.199·3).

**Dervin** *Boniscontro & Gazzone, Ital.*
Diflucortolone valerate (p.1099·3).
*Skin disorders.*

**Derzid**
*Unison, Hong Kong; Unison, Singapore; Unison, Thai.*
Betamethasone valerate (p.1093·2).
*Skin disorders.*

**Derzid-C** *Unison, Thai.*
Betamethasone valerate (p.1093·2); clotrimazole (p.396·2).
*Skin disorders with fungal infection.*

**Desacil** *Zambon, Braz.†.*
Deslanoside (p.893·1).
*Arrhythmias; heart failure.*

**Desalark** *Farmacologico Milanese, Ital.†.*
Dexamethasone sodium phosphate (p.1097·2).
*Eye/ear disorders.*

**Desalex** *Schering-Plough, Braz.*
Desloratadine (p.431·1).
*Allergic rhinitis.*

**Desalfa** *INTES, Ital.*
*Cream; ointment:* Dexamethasone isonicotinate (p.1097·2); lidocaine hydrochloride (p.1377·3).
*Haemorrhoids; skin disorders.*
*Eye drops; eye ointment:* Dexamethasone isonicotinate (p.1097·2); phenylephrine hydrochloride (p.1126·3); neomycin (p.235·1).
*Eye disorders.*
*Lotion:* Dexamethasone isonicotinate (p.1097·2); neomycin (p.235·1).
Formerly contained dexamethasone isonicotinate, neomycin, and nystatin.
*Skin disorders.*
*Nasal/ear drops:* Dexamethasone isonicotinate (p.1097·2); neomycin (p.235·1).
Formerly contained dexamethasone isonicotinate, neomycin, lidocaine hydrochloride, phenylephrine hydrochloride, and nystatin.
*Nasal and ear infections.*

**Desamin Same** *Savoma, Ital.*
Naphazoline hydrochloride (p.1124·3).
*Nasal congestion.*

**Desamix Effe** *Savoma, Ital.*
Dexamethasone (p.1097·1); clotrimazole (p.396·2).
*Infected skin disorders.*

**Desamix-Neomicina** *Savoma, Ital.*
Dexamethasone (p.1097·1); neomycin sulfate (p.235·1).
*Skin disorders.*

**Desamon** *Streuli, Switz.*
Didecyldiammonium chloride; isopropyl alcohol (p.1184·3).
*Disinfection of instruments, clothing, hands, skin, and mucous membranes.*

**Desanden** *Nycomed, Switz.†.*
Benzoyl peroxide (p.1143·2).
*Acne.*

**Desarell** *Sanorell, Ger.*
Homoeopathic preparation.

**Desarrol** *Iquinosa, Spain.*
Cyproheptadine hydrochloride (p.430·1); amino acids (p.1417·1).
*Tonic.*

**Desatura** *Sanofi Winthrop, Fr.†.*
Allopurinol (p.412·2); benzbromarone (p.414·3).
*Hyperuricaemia.*

**Desbly** *Medeva, Fr.†.*
Guaifenesin (p.1122·1); senega (p.1130·2).
Formerly contained drosera, grindelia, sodium bromide, sodium benzoate, magnesium sulfate, and wild thyme.
*Respiratory-tract disorders.*

**Desclidium** *Nattermann, Ger.†.*
Viquidil hydrochloride (p.1764·3).
*Circulatory and metabolic disorders of the brain, eyes, and inner ear.*

**Descon** *Hoechst Marion Roussel, Braz.†.*
Chlorphenamine maleate (p.427·3); phenylpropanolamine hydrochloride (p.1127·3); paracetamol (p.76·2).
*Nasal congestion.*

**Descon AP** *Hoechst Marion Roussel, Braz.†.*
Chlorphenamine maleate (p.427·3); phenylpropanolamine hydrochloride (p.1127·3); isopropamide iodide (p.485·2).
*Nasal congestion.*

**Descon Expectorante** *Hoechst Marion Roussel, Braz.†.*
Chlorphenamine maleate (p.427·3); phenylpropanolamine hydrochloride (p.1127·3); guaifenesin (p.1122·1).
*Respiratory-tract congestion.*

**Desconasal** *Warner-Lambert, Spain†.*
Xylometazoline hydrochloride (p.1132·2).
*Nasal congestion.*

**Desconex** *Reig Jofre, Spain.*
Loxapine hydrochloride (p.705·2) or loxapine succinate (p.705·2).
*Psychoses.*

**Descongestan** *Merck, Spain†.*
Oxymetazoline hydrochloride (p.1126·1).
*Nasal congestion.*

**Descongestivo Cuve Nasal** *Perez Gimenez, Spain.*
Phenylephrine hydrochloride (p.1126·3); menthol (p.1711·3).
*Nasal congestion.*

**Desconphar** *ICN, Arg.*
Salicylic acid (p.1157·1).
*Eye irritation.*

**Descutan** *Fresenius Kabi, Swed.*
Chlorhexidine gluconate (p.1173·2).
*Skin disinfection.*

**Desderman N** *Schulke & Mayr, Ger.*
Orthophenylphenol (p.1187·2); alcohol (p.1166·1).
*Hand disinfection.*

**Desdol** *Medipharm, Chile.*
Paracetamol (p.76·2); chlorzoxazone (p.1392·3).
*Musculoskeletal spasm.*

**Desec** *TO-Chemicals, Thai.*
Omeprazole (p.1278·2).
*Gastro-oesophageal reflux, Zollinger-Ellison syndrome; peptic ulcer.*

**Deselex** *Schering-Plough, S.Afr.*
Desloratadine (p.431·1).
*Allergic rhinitis.*

**Desenex**
*Novartis Consumer, Canad.; Roche Consumer, Irl.*
Zinc undecenoate (p.411·1); undecenoic acid (p.410·3).
*Fungal skin infections.*
*Ciba, USA.*
Undecenoic acid (p.410·3) and/or zinc undecenoate (p.411·1).
*Fungal skin infections; minor skin disorders.*

**DesenexMax** *Novartis, USA.*
Terbinafine hydrochloride (p.408·2).
*Fungal skin infections.*

**Desenfriol**
*Key, Arg.; Schering-Plough, Spain.*
Aspirin (p.15·1); caffeine (p.782·1); chlorphenamine maleate (p.427·3).
*Cold and influenza symptoms.*

**Desenfriol C** *Schering-Plough, Spain.*
Aspirin (p.15·1); ascorbic acid (p.1460·2); caffeine (p.782·1); chlorphenamine maleate (p.427·3).
*Fever; nasal congestion; pain.*

**Desenfriol Caramelos** *Key, Arg.*
Cetylpyridinium chloride (p.1173·1); propyl aminobenzoate; gramicidin (p.220·2).
*Sore throat.*

**Desenfriol Con Paracetamol** *Schering-Plough, Chile.*
Chlorphenamine maleate (p.427·3); paracetamol (p.76·2).
*Upper respiratory-tract disorders.*

**Desenfriol D**
*Note. This name is used for preparations of different composition.*
*Schering-Plough, Mex.*
Aspirin (p.15·1); chlorphenamine maleate (p.427·3); pseudoephedrine sulfate (p.1129·2).
Formerly contained aspirin, chlorphenamine maleate, and phenylpropanolamine hydrochloride.
*Allergic rhinitis.*
*Schering-Plough, Spain.*
Aspirin (p.15·1); caffeine (p.782·1); chlorphenamine maleate (p.427·3); phenylephrine hydrochloride (p.1126·3).
*Fever; nasal congestion; pain.*

**Desenfriol Decongestivo** *Key, Arg.*
Paracetamol (p.76·2); phenylephrine hydrochloride (p.1126·3).
*Cold and influenza symptoms.*

**Desenfriol Hiper T** *Key, Arg.*
Paracetamol (p.76·2); chlorphenamine maleate (p.427·3).
*Allergic respiratory-tract disorders; cold symptoms.*

**Desenfriol Infantil** *Schering-Plough, Spain†.*
Aspirin (p.15·1); chlorphenamine maleate (p.427·3); phenylephrine hydrochloride (p.1126·3).
*Fever; nasal congestion; pain.*

**Desenfriolito** *Key, Arg.*
Aspirin (p.15·1).
*Cold and influenza symptoms.*

**Desenfriolito con Paracetamol** Schering-Plough, Chile.
Chlorphenamine maleate (p.427·3); paracetamol (p.76·2).
*Cold symptoms.*

**Desenfriol-Ito Plus** Schering-Plough, Mex.
Paracetamol (p.76·2); chlorphenamine maleate (p.427·3); pseudoephedrine sulfate (p.1129·2).
Formerly contained paracetamol, chlorphenamine maleate, and phenylpropanolamine hydrochloride.
*Allergic rhinitis.*

**Desenfriol-Ito TF** Schering-Plough, Mex.
Dextromethorphan hydrobromide (p.1117·3); guaifenesin (p.1122·1).
*Coughs.*

**Desensib** Wiedemann, Ger.
Homoeopathic preparation.

**Desensibilizante Chauvin** Primo, Braz.
Sodium thiosulfate (p.1053·3); magnesium thiosulfate (p.1054·1).
*Hypersensitivity reactions.*

**Desentol** Ipex, Swed.
Diphenhydramine hydrochloride (p.431·3).
*Hypersensitivity reactions.*

**Deseril**
Novartis, Austral.; Novartis, Belg.; Novartis, Ger.; Novartis, Irl.†; Novartis, Neth.; Novartis, S.Afr.; Novartis, Switz.; Alliance, UK.
Methysergide maleate (p.469·3).
*Cluster headache; diarrhoea associated with carcinoid disease; migraine.*

**Deserila** Novartis, Braz.
Methysergide maleate (p.469·3).
*Migraine.*

**Desernil** Novartis, Fr.
Methysergide maleate (p.469·3).
*Migraine; vascular facial pain.*

**Deserril** Sandoz, Ital.†.
Methysergide maleate (p.469·3).
*Migraine.*

**Desert Pure Calcium** Cal-White, USA.
Calcium carbonate (p.1254·2); vitamin D (p.1461·2).

**Desfatigan** IMA, Braz.†.
Arginine aspartate (p.1421·1).
*Nutritional supplement.*

**Desfatin** Heralds, Braz.†.
Multivitamin and mineral preparation (p.1417·1).

**Desferal**
Novartis, Arg.; Novartis, Austral.; Novartis, Austria; Novartis, Belg.; Novartis, Braz.; Novartis, Canad.; Novartis, Chile; Novartis, Denm.; Novartis, Fin.; Novartis, Fr.; Novartis, Ger.; Novartis, Gr.; Novartis, Hong Kong; Novartis, India; Novartis, Irl.; Novartis, Israel; Novartis, Ital.; Novartis, Malaysia; Novartis, Neth.; Novartis, Norw.; Novartis, NZ; Novartis, Port.; Novartis, S.Afr.; Novartis, Singapore†; Novartis, Swed.; Novartis, Switz.; Novartis, Thai.; Novartis, UK; Novartis, USA.
Desferrioxamine mesilate (p.1033·1).
*Aluminium overload; iron overload.*

**Desferin** Padro, Spain.
Desferrioxamine mesilate (p.1033·1).
*Aluminium overload; iron overload.*

**Desflam** Merck, Mex.
Bumadizone calcium (p.21·3).
*Inflammation; peri-articular and soft-tissue disorders.*

**Desfrin** Uniao Quimica, Braz.
Oxymetazoline hydrochloride (p.1126·1).
*Nasal congestion.*

**Desicort** Taro, Israel.
Desoximetasone (p.1096·3).
*Skin disorders.*

**Desidoxepin** Declimed, Ger.†.
Doxepin hydrochloride (p.291·2).
*Anxiety; depression.*

**Desifluvoxamin** Declimed, Ger.
Fluvoxamine maleate (p.298·2).
*Depression.*

**Desiken** Kendrick, Mex.
Ribavirin (p.652·1).
*Viral infections.*

**Desinflam** Pharmacia, Arg.
Diclofenac sodium (p.32·1).
*Musculoskeletal, joint, and peri-articular disorders.*

**Desinflam Biotic** Pharmacia, Arg.
Amoxicillin trihydrate (p.155·3); diclofenac sodium (p.32·1).
*Bacterial infections.*

**Desinflex** Diffucap, Braz.
Diclofenac diethylamine (p.32·1).
*Inflammation.*

**Desintan P** Stafford-Miller, Port.†.
Permethrin (p.1508·3).
*Pediculosis.*

**Desintex** Richard, Fr.
Sodium thiosulfate (p.1053·3); magnesium thiosulfate (p.1054·1).
*Dyspepsia; rhinitis; rhinopharyngitis.*

**Desintex Infantile** Richard, Fr.
Sodium thiosulfate (p.1053·3); magnesium thiosulfate (p.1054·1); calcium gluconate (p.1225·2); calcium carbonate (p.1254·2).
*Dyspepsia; rhinitis; rhinopharyngitis.*

**Desintex-Choline** Richard, Fr.
Sodium thiosulfate (p.1053·3); magnesium thiosulfate (p.1054·1); choline chloride (p.1424·3).
*Dyspepsia.*

**Desinvag** Casen Fleet, Spain.
Benzalkonium chloride (p.1168·3); furazolidone (p.605·2).
*Vaginal antiseptic; vulvovaginal trichomoniasis.*

**Desiperiden** Desitin, Ger.†.
Biperiden hydrochloride (p.479·3) or biperiden lactate (p.479·3).
*Drug-induced extrapyramidal disorders; nicotine poisoning; parkinsonism.*

**Desirel** Codal Synto, Thai.
Trazodone hydrochloride (p.319·1).
*Anxiety; depression.*

**Desisulpid** Desitin, Ger.†.
Sulpiride (p.722·2).
*Depression; schizophrenia; vestibular disorders.*

**Desiticlopidin** Desitin, Ger.
Ticlopidine hydrochloride (p.1011·2).
*Thromboembolic disorders.*

**Desitin**
Note. This name is used for preparations of different composition.
Sigmapharm, Austria; Pfizer Consumer, Canad.; Desitin, Ger.; Pfizer, Hong Kong; Pfizer, Israel; Pfizer, Mex.; Pfizer Consumer, Singapore; Leeming, USA.
Cod-liver oil (p.1425·2); zinc oxide (p.1163·2).
*Burns; cuts; nappy rash; skin disorders.*

Desitin, Ger.
*Topical powder:* Zinc oxide (p.1163·2).
*Burns; skin disorders.*

**Desitin Creamy**
Note. This name is used for preparations of different composition.
Pfizer Consumer, Singapore.
Zinc oxide (p.1163·2); aloe vera (p.1141·3); vitamin E (p.1464·3).
*Nappy rash.*

Pfizer, USA.
Zinc oxide (p.1163·2); liquid paraffin (p.1479·1); white soft paraffin (p.1479·3).
Formerly known as Daily Care.
*Nappy rash.*

**Desitin Daily Care** Pfizer, Hong Kong.
Zinc oxide (p.1163·2).
*Nappy rash.*

**Desitin Nappy Rash Ointment** Pfizer Consumer, Austral.
Cod-liver oil (p.1425·2); zinc oxide (p.1163·2).
*Nappy rash.*

**Desitin with Zinc Oxide** Pfizer, USA.
Corn starch (p.1449·1); zinc oxide (p.1163·2).

**Desitur** Turimed, Switz.
Alcohol (p.1166·1); cetrimonium bromide (p.1173·1).
*Hand disinfection.*

**Desketo** Malesci, Ital.
Dexketoprofen trometamol (p.51·2).
*Pain.*

**Deslor** Sun, India.
Desloratadine (p.431·1).
*Allergic rhinitis; urticaria.*

**Desmanol** Schulke & Mayr, Ger.
Chlorhexidine gluconate (p.1173·2); propyl alcohol (p.1191·2); isopropyl alcohol (p.1184·3).
*Hand disinfection.*

**Desmanol G** Merck, Thai.; Schulke & Mayr, Thai.
Chlorhexidine gluconate (p.1173·2).
*Hand disinfection.*

**Desmin** Grunenthal, Ger.
Ethinylestradiol (p.1553·2); desogestrel (p.1547·2).
*Combined oral contraceptive.*

**Desmogalen** Galen, Ger.
Desmopressin acetate (p.1322·3).
*Diabetes insipidus; nocturnal enuresis; polydipsia; polyuria; test of renal concentrating capacity.*

**Desmoline** Schering-Plough, Port.†.
Dithranol (p.1146·1).
*Psoriasis.*

**Desmospray**
Ferring, Irl.; Ferring, Port.; Ferring, UK.
Desmopressin acetate (p.1322·3).
*Diabetes insipidus; nocturia associated with multiple sclerosis; nocturnal enuresis; test of renal concentrating capacity.*

**Desmotabs**
Ferring, Irl.; Ferring, UK.
Desmopressin acetate (p.1322·3).
*Diabetes insipidus; nocturnal enuresis; post-hypophysectomy polyuria or polydipsia.*

**Desobesi-M** Asta Medica, Braz.
Fenproporex hydrochloride (p.1588·3).
*Obesity.*

**Desocol** Lampugnani, Ital.
Ursodeoxycholic acid (p.1760·3).
*Biliary dyspepsia; cholesterol gallstones.*

**Desocort**
Note. This name is used for preparations of different composition.
Galderma, Canad.
Desonide (p.1096·3).
*Skin disorders.*

Chauvin, Fr.
*Ear drops:* Dexamethasone sodium phosphate (p.1097·2).
*Otitis externa.*
*Eye drops†:* Prednisolone metasulfobenzoate sodium (p.1108·1); chlorhexidine gluconate (p.1173·2).
*Eye disorders.*

**Desoform** Lysoform, Ger.
Glyoxal (p.1181·1); formaldehyde (p.1179·3); glutaral (p.1180·3); didecyldimethylammonium chloride (p.1178·3).
*Instrument disinfection.*

**Desogen**
Note. This name is used for preparations of different composition.
Hoechst Marion Roussel, Ital.†.
Toloconium metilsulfate (p.1194·3).
*Skin, burn, and wound disinfection.*

Organon, USA.
21 Tablets, desogestrel (p.1547·2); ethinylestradiol (p.1553·2); 7 tablets, inert.
*Combined oral contraceptive.*

**Desol** Geno, India.
Docusate sodium (p.1262·2).
*Ear wax removal.*

**Desolett** Organon, Swed.
Desogestrel (p.1547·2); ethinylestradiol (p.1553·2).
28-Day packs also contain 7 inert tablets.
*Combined oral contraceptive.*

**Desomedine**
Sidus, Arg.; Chauvin, Fr.; Chauvin, Hong Kong†; Chauvin, Singapore; Bausch & Lomb, Switz.
Hexamidine isetionate (p.1181·3).
*Infections of the eye or nose.*

**Deson** Unison, Thai.
Metformin hydrochloride (p.342·3).
*Diabetes mellitus.*

**Desonax** LPB, Ital.
Budesonide (p.1094·2).
*Asthma.*

**Desonol** Medley, Braz.
Desonide (p.1096·3).
*Skin disorders.*

**Desoplus** Lagos, Arg.
Desonide (p.1096·3).
*Skin disorders.*

**Desorelle** Durascan, Denm.
Desogestrel (p.1547·2); ethinylestradiol (p.1553·2).
*Combined oral contraceptive.*

**Desoren**
Note. This name is used for preparations of different composition.
Grunenthal, Chile.
Desogestrel (p.1547·2); ethinylestradiol (p.1553·2).
*Combined oral contraceptive.*

Vitamed, Israel.
Dexamethasone sodium phosphate (p.1097·2); neomycin sulfate (p.235·1); polymyxin B sulfate (p.245·1).
*Ear infections.*

**DesOwen**
Galderma, Arg.; Galderma, Austral.; Galderma, Braz.; Galderma, Chile; Galderma, Hong Kong; Galderma, India; Galderma, Mex.; Galderma, NZ†; Galderma, Singapore; Galderma, USA.
Desonide (p.1096·3).
*Skin disorders.*

**Desoxi** Optimapharma, Canad.
Desoximetasone (p.1096·3).
*Skin disorders.*

**Desoxil** Boniscontro & Gazzone, Ital.
Ursodeoxycholic acid (p.1760·3).
*Biliary disorders.*

**Desoxyn** Abbott, USA.
Metamfetamine hydrochloride (p.1589·2).
*Attention deficit hyperactivity disorder; obesity.*

**Despacilina** Bristol-Myers Squibb, Braz.
Procaine benzylpenicillin (p.246·1); benzylpenicillin potassium (p.163·2).
*Bacterial infections.*

**Despamen** AF, Mex.
Estradiol valerate (p.1550·2); testosterone enantate (p.1570·1).
*Menopausal disorders; osteoporosis.*

**Desparasil** Rimsa, Mex.
Piperazine hydrate (p.111·2).
*Nematode infections.*

**Despex** Alcon, Arg.
Budesonide (p.1094·2).
*Nasal polyps; rhinitis.*

**Despigmentante** Dermoteca, Port.
Lactic acid (p.1704·1); kojic acid (p.1151·2); enoxolone (p.36·2); arbutin.
*Skin hyperpigmentation.*

**Desquam** Westwood-Squibb, USA.
Benzoyl peroxide (p.1143·2).
*Acne.*

**Desquaman**
Hermal, Austria; Hermal, Israel; Hermal, Port.†.
Pyrithione zinc (p.1156·2).
*Scalp infections; seborrhoeic dermatitis.*

**De-squaman N** Hermal, Ger.
Pyrithione zinc (p.1156·2).
*Scalp disorders.*

**Desquam-X** Westwood-Squibb, Canad.
Benzoyl peroxide (p.1143·2).
*Acne.*

**Dessolets** SMB, Chile.
Naphazoline hydrochloride (p.1124·3); pheniramine maleate (p.438·3).
*Eye congestion.*

**Destamin** Medifarma, Mex.
Histamine hydrochloride (p.1697·1).

**Destap** Laboratorios Chile, Chile.
Beclometasone dipropionate (p.1091·1).
*Allergic rhinitis; asthma; nasal polyps.*

**deSTAT 3**
Sherman, Israel†.
Cleaning and storage solution for gas permeable contact lenses (p.1164·2).

Sherman, USA.
Cleaning, disinfectant, and storage solution for gas permeable contact lenses (p.1164·2).

**Destilbenol** Apsen, Braz.
Diethylstilbestrol (p.1548·1).
*Prostatic cancer.*

**Destolit**
Aventis, Fr.†; Aventis, Port.; Norgine, UK.
Ursodeoxycholic acid (p.1760·3).
*Biliary tract disorders; cholesterol gallstones.*

**Destoxican** Pentafarma, Port.
Naltrexone hydrochloride (p.1046·1).
*Opioid dependence.*

**Destrobac**
Rusch, Ital.; Gebro, Switz.
Povidone-iodine (p.1190·3).
*Skin disinfection; wounds.*

**Desuric**
Sanofi Synthelabo, Belg.; Sanofi Synthelabo, Fr.†; Sanfer, Mex.; Sanofi Synthelabo, Neth.; Sanofi Synthelabo, Switz.
Benzbromarone (p.414·3).
*Gout; hyperuricaemia.*

**Desyrel**
Bristol, Canad.; Apothecon, USA.
Trazodone hydrochloride (p.319·1).
*Depression.*

**DET MS** Shire, Ger.
Dihydroergotamine mesilate (p.465·3).
*Hypotension; migraine and other vascular headaches.*

**DET MS spezial** Shire, Ger.
Dihydroergotamine mesilate (p.465·3).
*Chronic venous insufficiency; hypotension; migraine and other vascular headaches.*

**Detamol** PD, Thai.
Paracetamol (p.76·2).
Lidocaine hydrochloride (p.1377·3) is included in this preparation to alleviate the pain of injection.
*Fever; pain; post-immunisation reactions.*

**Detane** Del, USA.
Benzocaine (p.1370·3).
*Genital desensitising lubricant.*

**Detantol**
Eisai, Jpn; Eisai, Thai.
Bunazosin hydrochloride (p.878·1).
*Hypertension.*

**Detebencil** Roux-Ocefa, Arg.
*Cream:* Permethrin (p.1508·3); benzyl benzoate (p.1500·2); benzocaine (p.1370·3).
*Lotion:* Permethrin (p.1508·3); benzyl benzoate (p.1500·2).
*Pediculosis.*

**Deteclo**
Wyeth, Irl.†; Goldshield, UK.
Tetracycline hydrochloride (p.266·2); chlortetracycline hydrochloride (p.187·3); demeclocycline hydrochloride (p.204·3).
*Bacterial infections.*

**Detect Baby** Blausiegel, Braz.
Pregnancy test (p.1734·3).

**Detemes** Sanova, Austria.
Dihydroergotamine mesilate (p.465·3).
*Hypotension; migraine and related vascular headaches; venous insufficiency.*

**Detensiel** Lipha Sante, Fr.
Bisoprolol fumarate (p.875·1).
*Angina pectoris; hypertension.*

**Detensor** Novartis Consumer, Switz.
Diphenhydramine hydrochloride (p.431·3); 8-chlorotheophylline.
*Sleep disorders.*

**Detergil** Manetti Roberts, Ital.
Benzalkonium chloride (p.1168·3).
*Instrument disinfection; wound disinfection.*

**Dethamycin** Vitamed, Israel.
Dexamethasone sodium phosphate (p.1097·2); neomycin sulfate (p.235·1).
*Infected eye, ear, and nose disorders.*

**Dethaphrine** Vitamed, Israel.
Dexamethasone sodium phosphate (p.1097·2); neomycin sulfate (p.235·1); phenylephrine hydrochloride (p.1126·3).
*Infected eye, ear, and nose disorders.*

**Deticene**
Aventis, Arg.; Aventis, Fr.; Aventis, Gr.; Rhone-Poulenc Rorer, Hong Kong†; Aventis, Israel; Aventis, Ital.; Aventis, Mex.; Aventis, Neth.; Aventis, Port.
Dacarbazine (p.544·2).
*Malignant neoplasms.*

**Detilem** Lemery, Mex.
Dacarbazine (p.544·2).
*Malignant neoplasms.*

**Detimedac** Medac, Ger.
Dacarbazine (p.544·2).
*Malignant neoplasms.*

**Detoch** PD, Thai.
Dequalinium chloride (p.1178·1); ascorbic acid (p.1460·2).
*Mouth and throat infections.*

**Detox** Reese, USA.
Red clover; liquorice; peach bark; orange grape root; stillingla; cascara; sarsaparilla; lappa root; buckthorn (p.1417·1).
*Dietary supplement.*

**Detox Thuja** Homeocan, Canad.
Homoeopathic preparation.

**Detoxalgine** Organon, Fr.
Glucuronamide; aspirin (p.15·1); ascorbic acid (p.1460·2).
*Fever; musculoskeletal and joint disorders; pain.*

**Detoxergon** Baldacci, Port.
Pirglutargine (p.1732·3); taurine (p.1752·1); pyridoxine hydrochloride (p.1456·3); electrolytes.
*Liver disorders.*

**Detoxicon** SIT, Ital.
Glycine (p.1433·3); acetylmethionine.
*Tonic.*

**Detraine** Seid, Spain.
Hydrocortisone (p.1103·3); propanocaine hydrochloride (p.1383·3).
*Insect bites and stings; pruritus; skin disorders.*

**Detrixin** Astra, Swed.†.
Colecalciferol (p.1461·3).
*Osteoporosis; vitamin D deficiency.*

**Detrol**
Pharmacia, Canad.; Pharmacia Upjohn, USA.
Tolterodine tartrate (p.489·3).
*Bladder instability.*

**Detrunorm** Schering-Plough, UK.
Propiverine hydrochloride (p.489·1).
*Bladder instability; neurogenic bladder.*

**Detrusan** Stada, Austria.
Oxybutynin hydrochloride (p.486·3).
*Bladder instability.*

**Detrusitol**
Pharmacia, Arg.; Pharmacia, Austria; Pharmacia, Belg.; Pharmacia, Braz.; Pharmacia, Chile; Pharmacia, Denm.; Pharmacia, Fin.; Pharmacia, Fr.; Pharmacia, Ger.; Pharmacia-Upjohn, Gr.; Pharmacia, Hong Kong; Pharmacia, Irl.; Pharmacia Upjohn, Israel; Pharmacia, Ital.; Pharmacia, Malaysia; Pharmacia Upjohn, Mex.; Pharmacia, Neth.; Pharmacia, Norw.; Pharmacia, NZ; Pharmacia, Port.; Pharmacia, S.Afr.; Pharmacia, Singapore; Pharmacia, Spain; Pharmacia, Swed.; Pharmacia, Switz.; Pharmacia, Thai.; Pharmacia, UK.
Tolterodine tartrate (p.489·3).
*Bladder instability.*

**Detsel** Pharmacia, Neth.
Tolterodine tartrate (p.489·3).
*Bladder instability.*

**Dettol**
Note. This name is used for preparations of different composition.
Reckitt & Colman, Belg.†; Reckitt Benckiser, Hong Kong; Reckitt Benckiser, Irl.; Reckitt Benckiser, Malaysia; Reckitt Benckiser, NZ; Reckitt & Colman, S.Afr.†; Reckitt & Colman, Singapore†; Reckitt Benckiser, Thai.; Reckitt Benckiser, UK.
*Topical solution:* Chloroxylenol (p.1177·2).
*Disinfection of skin and wounds.*

Reckitt Benckiser, Hong Kong; Reckitt Benckiser, Irl.; Reckitt Benckiser, Malaysia; Reckitt Benckiser, NZ; Reckitt & Colman, S.Afr.†; Reckitt & Colman, Singapore†; Reckitt Benckiser, Thai.; Reckitt Benckiser, UK.
*Cream:* Chloroxylenol (p.1177·2); triclosan (p.1195·2).
*Disinfection of skin and wounds.*

Reckitt Benckiser, NZ.
*Topical spray:* Benzalkonium chloride (p.1168·3).
*Skin disinfection.*

Reckitt & Colman, Singapore†.
*Medicated dressing:* Ethacridine lactate (p.1165·3).
*Wounds.*

Reckitt & Colman, Singapore†; Reckitt Benckiser, UK.
*Topical spray:* Benzalkonium chloride (p.1168·3); lidocaine hydrochloride (p.1377·3).
*Bites and stings; minor burns; minor wounds.*

**Dettol Antiseptic Spray** Reckitt Benckiser, Austral.
Benzalkonium chloride (p.1168·3).
Formerly known as Dettol Fresh.
*Bites and stings; burns; minor abrasions; skin disorders; skin infections.*

**Dettol Antiseptic Wash** Reckitt Benckiser, UK.
Benzalkonium chloride (p.1168·3).
*Wound disinfection.*

**Dettol Classic** Reckitt Benckiser, Austral.
Chloroxylenol (p.1177·2).
*Bath additive; bites and stings; burns; minor abrasions; skin disorders; skin infections.*

**Dettol Cream** Reckitt Benckiser, Austral.
Chloroxylenol (p.1177·2); triclosan (p.1195·2).
*Bites and stings; burns; minor abrasions; skin disorders; skin infections.*

**Dettol Fresh**
Reckitt Benckiser, Irl.; Reckitt Benckiser, NZ; Reckitt Benckiser, UK.
Benzalkonium chloride (p.1168·3).
*Skin disinfection.*

**Dettol Liquid Wash**
Reckitt Benckiser, Austral.; Reckitt & Colman, Belg.†.
Triclosan (p.1195·2).
*Skin disinfection.*

**Dettol Obstetric** Reckitt Piramal, India.
Chloroxylenol (p.1177·2); terpineol (p.1752·2).
*Skin disinfection; vaginal lubricant.*

**Dettolin** Reckitt Piramal, India.
Chloroxylenol (p.1177·2); menthol (p.1711·3); alcohol (p.1166·1).
*Gingivitis; oral hygiene; periodontitis.*

**Dettonjab** Defuen, Arg.
Undecenoic acid diethanolamide; triclosan (p.1195·2).
*Acne.*

**Detulin** Woelm, Ger.
*dl*-Alpha tocoferil acetate (p.1465·1).
*Vitamin E deficiency.*

**Deturgylone** Sanofi Synthelabo, Fr.
Prednisolone sodium phosphate (p.1108·1); oxymetazoline hydrochloride (p.1126·1).
Formerly contained prednazoline.
*Rhinitis.*

**Detuss** Siam Bheasach, Thai.†.
*Syrup:* Dextromethorphan hydrobromide (p.1117·3); ammonium chloride (p.1115·2); dexpanthenol (p.1727·2).
*Tablets:* Dextromethorphan (p.1117·3).
*Coughs.*

**Deucoaler** Medipharm, Chile.
Dexchlorpheniramine maleate (p.427·3); betamethasone (p.1093·1).
*Hypersensitivity reactions.*

**Deucodol** Medipharm, Chile.
Ibuprofen (p.45·3).
*Fever; inflammation.*

**Deucotos** Medipharm, Chile.
Codeine (p.27·1); pseudoephedrine (p.1129·2); chlorphenamine (p.428·1).
*Bronchitis; cold symptoms; coughs.*

**Deucoval** Medipharm, Chile.
Naproxen sodium (p.65·1).
*Inflammation; pain.*

**Deursil**
Sanofi Synthelabo, Ital.; Synthelabo, Switz.
Ursodeoxycholic acid (p.1760·3).
*Biliary-tract disorders.*

**Devaron** Solvay, Neth.
Colecalciferol (p.1461·3).
*Vitamin D deficiency.*

**Develanid** Klonal, Arg.
Lanatoside C (p.945·1).

**Develin** Godecke, Ger.†.
Dextropropoxyphene hydrochloride (p.28·3).
*Pain.*

**Deverol** Sanochemia, Austria†.
Spironolactone (p.1003·1).
*Hyperaldosteronism; hypertension; liver cirrhosis with ascites; nephrotic syndrome; oedema.*

**Deverol mit Thiazid** Sanochemia, Austria.
Spironolactone (p.1003·1); hydrochlorothiazide (p.933·2).
*Ascites; heart failure; nephrotic syndrome; oedema.*

**Devils Claw Plus** Eagle, Austral.†.
Devil's claw root (p.28·2); murraya; celery (p.1669·1); hesperidin (p.1688·2).
*Arthritis; rheumatism.*

**Devincal** Almirall, Spain.
Piracetam (p.1732·1); vincamine (p.1764·2).
*Cerebrovascular disorders.*

**Devitol** Orion, Fin.
Ergocalciferol (p.1462·1).
*Vitamin D deficiency.*

**Devitre** Nycomed, Swed.
Colecalciferol (p.1461·3).
*Osteoporosis; vitamin D deficiency.*

**Devix** Phoinix Pharm (Φοινιξ Φαρμ), Gr.
Butamirate citrate (p.1116·2).
*Cough.*

**Devorfungi** Combe, Spain†.
Tolnaftate (p.410·1).
*Fungal skin infections.*

**Devrom** Parthenon, USA.
Bismuth subgallate (p.1252·2).
*Ostomy deodorant.*

**Dewax** Ranbaxy, Thai.
Docusate sodium (p.1262·2).
*Ear wax removal.*

**Dex** PP Lab, Thai.
Dextromethorphan hydrobromide (p.1117·3).
*Coughs and cold symptoms.*

**Dex4 Glucose** Can-Am Care, USA.
Glucose (p.1432·2).
*Hypoglycaemia.*

**Dexa**
CT, Ger.; Jenapharm, Ger.; Shiwa, Thai.
Dexamethasone sodium phosphate (p.1097·2).
*Corticosteroid.*

**Dexa Aminofilin** Phoenix, Arg.
Theophylline (p.798·3); dexamethasone (p.1097·1) or dexamethasone sodium phosphate (p.1097·2).
*Asthma.*

**Dexa ANB** ANB, Thai.
Dexamethasone sodium phosphate (p.1097·2).
*Corticosteroid.*

**Dexa Biciron** Alcon, Ger.
Dexamethasone isonicotinate (p.1097·2); tramazoline hydrochloride (p.1131·3).
*Allergic and inflammatory disorders of the eye.*

**Dexa in der Ophtiole** Mann, Ger.†.
Dexamethasone sodium phosphate (p.1097·2).
*Eye disorders.*

**Dexa Fenic** Ciba Vision, Spain†.
Chloramphenicol (p.185·1); dexamethasone (p.1097·1).
*Infected eye disorders.*

**Dexa Loscon mono** Galderma, Ger.
Dexamethasone isonicotinate (p.1097·2).
*Scalp disorders.*

**Dexa Polyspectran** Alcon, Ger.
Polymyxin B sulfate (p.245·1); neomycin sulfate (p.235·1); dexamethasone sodium phosphate (p.1097·2).
*Infected eye and ear disorders.*

**Dexa Tavegil** Novartis Consumer, Spain.
Clemastine (p.429·2); dexamethasone (p.1097·1).
*Hypersensitivity reactions; inflammatory eye disorders; insect bites and stings; sunburn.*

**Dexa Teosona** Phoenix, Arg.
Theophylline (p.798·3); dexamethasone (p.1097·1).
*Obstructive airways disease.*

**Dexa Vasoc** Ciba Vision, Spain†.
Dexamethasone (p.1097·1); naphazoline hydrochloride (p.1124·3); zinc sulfate (p.1469·3).
*Eye congestion; inflammatory eye disorders.*

**Dexa-Allvoran** TAD, Ger.
Dexamethasone sodium phosphate (p.1097·2).
*Corticosteroid.*

**Dexabene**
Ratiopharm, Austria; Merckle, Ger.
Dexamethasone sodium phosphate (p.1097·2).
*Corticosteroid.*

**Dexabion**
Note. This name is used for preparations of different composition.
Merck, Arg.; Merck, Mex.
Ampoule 1: thiamine hydrochloride (p.1455·1); pyridoxine hydrochloride (p.1456·3); cyanocobalamin (p.1458·2); ampoule 2: dexamethasone sodium phosphate (p.1097·2).
Lidocaine hydrochloride (p.1377·3) may be included in ampoule 2 to alleviate the pain of injection.
*Inflammation; neuralgias; neuritis; peri-articular disorders; rheumatoid arthritis.*

Merck, Arg.
*Tablets:* Vitamin $B_1$ (p.1455·2); vitamin $B_6$ (p.1457·2); vitamin $B_{12}$ (p.1458·2); dexamethasone (p.1097·1).
*Inflammation; joint and peri-articular disorders; neuralgia; neuritis.*

**Dexa-Brachialin N** Steigerwald, Ger.†.
Dexamethasone sodium phosphate (p.1097·2).
*Acute inflammatory rheumatic disorders.*

**Dexacap** Dexa, Hong Kong.
Captopril (p.879·2).
*Heart failure; hypertension.*

**Dexacidin** Novartis Ophthalmics, USA.
Dexamethasone (p.1097·1); neomycin sulfate (p.235·1); polymyxin B sulfate (p.245·1).
*Eye inflammation with bacterial infection.*

**Dexacin** ANB, Thai.
Dexamethasone sodium phosphate (p.1097·2); neomycin sulfate (p.235·1).
*Infected eye or ear disorders.*

**Dexacine** Novartis Ophthalmics, USA.
Dexamethasone (p.1097·1); neomycin sulfate (p.235·1); polymyxin B sulfate (p.245·1).
*Infected eye disorders.*

**Dexa-Citoneurin** Merck, Braz.
Thiamine hydrochloride (p.1455·1) or thiamine nitrate (p.1455·1); pyridoxine hydrochloride (p.1456·3); cyanocobalamin (p.1458·2); dexamethasone (p.1097·1) or dexamethasone acetate (p.1097·1).
*Neuritis.*

**dexa-clinit** Hormosan, Ger.
Dexamethasone sodium phosphate (p.1097·2).
*Parenteral corticosteroid.*

**Dexaclor** Hebron, Braz.
Dexamethasone (p.1097·1); chloramphenicol (p.185·1).
*Infected skin disorders.*

**Dexacloran** Dansk-Flama, Braz.†.
Dexamethasone (p.1097·1); diiodohydroxyquinoline (p.603·3); chloramphenicol (p.185·1).
*Vulvovaginal disorders.*

**Dexacobal** Uniao Quimica, Braz.
Thiamine hydrochloride (p.1455·1); pyridoxine hydrochloride (p.1456·3); cyanocobalamin (p.1458·2); dexamethasone acetate (p.1097·1).
*Neuritis.*

**Dexacollyre** Cooper (Κοπερ), Gr.
Dexamethasone sodium phosphate (p.1097·2).
*Inflammatory eye disorders.*

**Dexacort**
Note. This name is used for preparations of different composition.
Gemballa, Braz.
Dexamethasone (p.1097·1); neomycin (p.235·1).
*Skin disorders.*

Biogal, Israel; Medeva, USA†.
Dexamethasone sodium phosphate (p.1097·2).
Formerly known as Decadron in the *USA*.
*Allergic rhinitis; corticosteroid; nasal polyps.*

**Dexacortal** Organon, Swed.
Dexamethasone (p.1097·1).
*Corticosteroid.*

**Dexacortin** Streuli, Switz.
Dexamethasone (p.1097·1) or dexamethasone sodium phosphate (p.1097·2).
*Corticosteroid.*

**Dexacortin-K** Streuli, Switz.
Dexamethasone (p.1097·1); lidocaine hydrochloride (p.1377·3).
*Joint and peri-articular disorders.*

**Dexacortisone** ANB, Thai.†.
Dexamethasone sodium phosphate (p.1097·2).
*Corticosteroid.*

**Dexacrinin** Pharmagalen, Ger.†.
Dexamethasone (p.1097·1); salicylic acid (p.1157·1); coal tar (p.1159·2).
*Scalp disorders.*

**Dexa-Cronobe** Biolab Sanus, Braz.
Ampoule A, cyanocobalamin (p.1458·2); pyridoxine hydrochloride (p.1456·3); thiamine hydrochloride (p.1455·1); ampoule B, dexamethasone acetate (p.1097·1).
*Neuritis.*

**Dexadermil** Legrand, Braz.
Dexamethasone (p.1097·1) or dexamethasone acetate (p.1097·1).
*Skin disorders.*

**Dexador** Ativus, Braz.
Cyanocobalamin (p.1458·2); thiamine hydrochloride (p.1455·1) or thiamine nitrate (p.1455·1); pyridoxine hydrochloride (p.1456·3); dexamethasone phosphate (p.1097·2).
Procaine hydrochloride (p.1383·2) is included in the injection to alleviate the pain of injection.
*Neuritis.*

**Dexadoze** Teuto, Braz.
Dexamethasone acetate (p.1097·1); thiamine hydrochloride (p.1455·1); pyridoxine (p.1457·2); cyanocobalamin (p.1458·2).
*Neuritis.*

**DexaEDO** Mann, Ger.
Dexamethasone sodium phosphate (p.1097·2).
*Inflammatory eye disorders.*

**Dexa-Effekton** Teofarma, Ger.
Dexamethasone sodium phosphate (p.1097·2).
*Rheumatic disorders.*

**Dexafarm** ICN, Arg.
Dexamethasone sodium phosphate (p.1097·2).
*Inflammatory eye disorders.*

**Dexafed Cough** Mallard, USA.
Phenylephrine hydrochloride (p.1126·3); dextromethorphan hydrobromide (p.1117·3); guaifenesin (p.1122·1).
*Coughs.*

**Dexafenicol**
Allergan, Braz.; Ciba Vision, Spain†.
Chloramphenicol (p.185·1); dexamethasone (p.1097·1).
*Infected eye disorders.*

**Dexaflam** Lichtenstein, Ger.†.
Dexamethasone (p.1097·1).
*Corticosteroid.*

**Dexaflam N** Lichtenstein, Ger.
Dexamethasone sodium phosphate (p.1097·2).
*Musculoskeletal, joint, and peri-articular disorders.*

**Dexaflan** Hebron, Braz.
Dexamethasone (p.1097·1).
*Corticosteroid.*

**Dexafrin** Sophia, Mex.
Dexamethasone sodium phosphate (p.1097·2); phenylephrine hydrochloride (p.1126·3).
*Eye disorders.*

**Dexafurazon** Allergan, Arg.
Dexamethasone phosphate (p.1097·2); neomycin sulfate (p.235·1); naphazoline hydrochloride (p.1124·3).
*Infected eye disorders.*

**Dexagalen** Galen, Ger.†.
Dexamethasone (p.1097·1).
*Scalp disorders.*

**Dexagel** Mann, Ger.
Dexamethasone sodium phosphate (p.1097·2).
*Eye disorders.*

**Dexagenta** Croma, Austria.
Dexamethasone (p.1097·1) or dexamethasone sodium phosphate (p.1097·2); gentamicin sulfate (p.217·1).
*Infected eye disorders.*

**Dexa-Gentamicin**
Ursapharm, Ger.; Ursapharm, Malaysia.
Dexamethasone (p.1097·1) or dexamethasone sodium phosphate (p.1097·2); gentamicin sulfate (p.217·1).
*Infected eye disorders.*

**Dexagenta-POS** Ursapharm, Neth.†.
Dexamethasone (p.1097·1) or dexamethasone sodium phosphate (p.1097·2); gentamicin sulfate (p.217·1).
*Infected eye disorders.*

**Dexagil** Marjan, Braz.
Dexamethasone phosphate (p.1097·2); cyanocobalamin (p.1458·2); thiamine hydrochloride (p.1455·1); pyridoxine hydrochloride (p.1456·3).
Procaine hydrochloride (p.1383·2) is included in the injection to alleviate the pain of injection.
*Neuritis.*

**Dexagrane** Ioltech, Fr.
Dexamethasone sodium phosphate (p.1097·2); neomycin sulfate (p.235·1).
*Infected eye disorders.*

**Dexagrin** Grin, Mex.
Dexamethasone (p.1097·1) or dexamethasone phosphate (p.1097·2).
*Corticosteroid.*

**Dexa-Helvacort** Helvepharm, Switz.†.
Dexamethasone sodium phosphate (p.1097·2).
Now known as Dexamethasone Helvepharm.
*Corticosteroid.*

**Dexahexal** Hexal, Ger.
Dexamethasone sodium phosphate (p.1097·2).
*Corticosteroid.*

**Dexalergin** Armstrong, Arg.
*Cream:* Dexamethasone (p.1097·1); neomycin sulfate (p.235·1); chlorphenamine maleate (p.427·3).
*Skin disorders.*

*Injection:* Dexamethasone sodium phosphate (p.1097·2).
*Corticosteroid.*

*Nasal spray; nose drops:* Dexamethasone (p.1097·1) or dexamethasone sodium phosphate (p.1097·2); neomycin sulfate (p.235·1); chlorphenamine maleate (p.427·3); naphazoline hydrochloride (p.1124·3).
*Nasal disorders.*

*Syrup; tablets:* Dexamethasone (p.1097·1) or dexamethasone sodium phosphate (p.1097·2); chlorphenamine maleate (p.427·3).
*Hypersensitivity reactions.*

**Dexalgen** *Eurofarma, Braz.*
Hydroxocobalamin (p.1458·2); dipyrone (p.35·3); dexamethasone sodium phosphate (p.1097·2).
*Neuritis.*

**Dexalin** *General Drugs, Thai.*
Methyl salicylate (p.59·3); menthol (p.1711·3); cajuput oil (p.1664·1); cineole (p.1672·1).
*Lumbago; rheumatic conditions; sciatica.*

**Dexalocal**
*Medinova, Hong Kong†; Medinova, Switz.*
Dexamethasone (p.1097·1).
*Skin and scalp disorders.*

**Dexalocal-F** *Medinova, Switz.*
Dexamethasone (p.1097·1); framycetin sulfate (p.215·1).
*Infected skin disorders.*

**Dexalone**
*Note. A similar name is used for preparations of different composition (see below).*
*Upha, Malaysia.*
Dexamethasone (p.1097·1) or dexamethasone sodium phosphate (p.1097·2).
*Corticosteroid.*

**DexAlone**
*Note. A similar name is used for preparations of different composition (see above).*
*DexGen, USA.*
Dextromethorphan hydrobromide (p.1117·3).
*Coughs.*

**Dexaltin**
*Kayaku, Malaysia; Kayaku, Singapore; ANB, Thai.*
Dexamethasone (p.1097·1).
*Mouth ulcers.*

**Dexam Constric** *Alcon Cusi, Spain.*
Chloramphenicol succinate (p.186·3); dexamethasone sodium phosphate (p.1097·2); tetryzoline hydrochloride (p.1131·2).
*Eye disorders.*

**Dexambutol** *SERP, Mon.*
Ethambutol hydrochloride (p.211·3).
*Opportunistic mycobacterial infections; tuberculosis.*

**Dexambutol-INH** *SERP, Mon.*
Ethambutol hydrochloride (p.211·3); isoniazid (p.222·2).
*Opportunistic mycobacterial infections; tuberculosis.*

**Dexamed**
*Medochemie, Hong Kong; Medochemie, Singapore†.*
Dexamethasone (p.1097·1).
*Corticosteroid.*

**Dexameral** *Kampel Martian, Arg.*
Dexamethasone (p.1097·1).
*Corticosteroid.*

**Dexameson** *Cristalia, Braz.*
Dexamethasone acetate (p.1097·1).
*Corticosteroid.*

**Dexametax** *Galenogal, Braz.†.*
Dexamethasone (p.1097·1).
*Skin disorders.*

**Dexameth** *Major, USA.*
Dexamethasone (p.1097·1).
*Corticosteroid.*

**Dexametonal** *Hexal, Braz.*
Dexamethasone (p.1097·1).
*Corticosteroid.*

**Dexamicin** *Grin, Mex.*
Dexamethasone sodium phosphate (p.1097·2); neomycin sulfate (p.235·1).
*Infected eye disorders.*

**Dexamin** *Streuli, Switz.*
Dexamfetamine sulfate (p.1585·3).
*Obesity.*

**Dexaminor** *Allergan, Braz.*
Dexamethasone (p.1097·1).
*Eye disorders.*

**Dexamol** *Dexxon, Israel.*
Paracetamol (p.76·2).
*Fever; pain.*

**Dexamol Cold Day** *Dexxon, Israel.*
Paracetamol (p.76·2); guaifenesin (p.1122·1); dextromethorphan hydrobromide (p.1117·3); pseudoephedrine hydrochloride (p.1129·2).
*Coughs and cold symptoms.*

**Dexamol Cold Night** *Dexxon, Israel.*
Paracetamol (p.76·2); dextromethorphan hydrobromide (p.1117·3); pseudoephedrine hydrochloride (p.1129·2); chlorphenamine maleate (p.427·3).
*Coughs and cold symptoms.*

**Dexamol Kid** *Dexxon, Israel.*
Paracetamol (p.76·2).
*Fever; pain.*

**Dexamol Plus** *Dexxon, Israel.*
Paracetamol (p.76·2); caffeine (p.782·1).
*Fever; pain.*

**Dexamol PM** *Dexxon, Israel.*
Paracetamol (p.76·2); diphenhydramine hydrochloride (p.431·3).
*Insomnia; pain.*

**Dexamol Sinus Day** *Dexxon, Israel.*
Paracetamol (p.76·2); pseudoephedrine hydrochloride (p.1129·2).
*Cold symptoms.*

**Dexamol Sinus Night** *Dexxon, Israel.*
Paracetamol (p.76·2); pseudoephedrine hydrochloride (p.1129·2); chlorphenamine maleate (p.427·3).
*Cold symptoms.*

**Dexamonozon** *Medice, Ger.*
Dexamethasone (p.1097·1).
*Oral corticosteroid.*

**Dexamonozon N** *Medice, Ger.*
Dexamethasone (p.1097·1).
Lidocaine hydrochloride (p.1377·3) is included in the intramuscular injection to alleviate the pain of injection.
*Musculoskeletal and joint disorders.*

**Dexamycin** *Teva, Israel.*
Dexamethasone sodium phosphate (p.1097·2); neomycin sulfate (p.235·1).
*Infected eye disorders.*

**Dexamytrex**
*Bausch & Lomb, Braz.; Mann, Ger.; Tramedico, Neth.; Lepori, Port.; Mann, Singapore; Bausch & Lomb, Thai.; Mann, Thai.*
Gentamicin sulfate (p.217·1); dexamethasone (p.1097·1) or dexamethasone sodium phosphate (p.1097·2).
*Infected eye disorders.*

**Dexamytrex Ophtiole** *Mann, Malaysia.*
Gentamicin sulfate (p.217·1); dexamethasone sodium phosphate (p.1097·2).
*Infected eye disorders.*

**Dexa-Neuriberi** *Haller, Braz.*
Dexamethasone (p.1097·1); cyanocobalamin (p.1458·2); thiamine hydrochloride (p.1455·1); pyridoxine hydrochloride (p.1456·3).
Procaine hydrochloride (p.1383·2) is included in this preparation to alleviate the pain of injection.
*Neuritis.*

**Dexaneurin** *Uniao Quimica, Braz.*
Dexamethasone acetate (p.1097·1); cyanocobalamin (p.1458·2); thiamine hydrochloride (p.1455·1); pyridoxine hydrochloride (p.1456·3).
Procaine hydrochloride (p.1383·2) is included in this preparation to alleviate the pain of injection.
*Neuritis.*

**Dexanevral** *Hebron, Braz.*
Dexamethasone (p.1097·1); thiamine nitrate (p.1455·1); pyridoxine hydrochloride (p.1456·3); cyanocobalamin (p.1458·2).
*Neuritis.*

**Dexanil** *Ducto, Braz.*
*Cream:* Dexamethasone acetate (p.1097·1); neomycin sulfate (p.235·1).
*Tablets; injection:* Dexamethasone acetate (p.1097·1) or dexamethasone sodium phosphate (p.1097·2).
*Corticosteroid.*

**Dexano** *Milano, Thai.*
Dexamethasone (p.1097·1).
*Corticosteroid.*

**Dex-Antihist** *Raza, Malaysia.*
Dexchlorpheniramine maleate (p.427·3).
*Hypersensitivity reactions.*

**Dexa-P** *PP Lab, Thai.*
Dexamethasone (p.1097·1) or dexamethasone sodium phosphate (p.1097·2).
*Corticosteroid.*

**Dexaphen-SA** *Major, USA.*
Pseudoephedrine sulfate (p.1129·2); dexbrompheniramine maleate (p.426·1).
*Upper respiratory-tract symptoms.*

**Dexa-Phlogont L** *Azupharma, Ger.*
Prednisolone (p.1108·1); dexamethasone (p.1097·1); lidocaine hydrochloride (p.1377·3).
*Musculoskeletal and joint disorders.*

**Dexa-Polyspectran** *Thilo, Hong Kong†.*
Polymyxin B sulfate (p.245·1); neomycin sulfate (p.235·1); gramicidin (p.220·2); dexamethasone sodium phosphate (p.1097·2).
*Infected eye disorders.*

**Dexapos** *Ursapharm, Ger.*
Dexamethasone sodium metasulfobenzoate (p.1097·2).
*Allergic and inflammatory disorders of the eye.*

**Dexa-POS** *Ursapharm, Neth.†.*
Dexamethasone phosphate (p.1097·2).
*Inflammatory eye disorders.*

**Dexaprof D** *Elvetium, Arg.*
Astemizole (p.424·2); dexamethasone (p.1097·1).
*Hypersensitivity reactions.*

**Dexa-ratiopharm** *Ratiopharm, Ger.*
Dexamethasone sodium phosphate (p.1097·2).
*Corticosteroid.*

**Dexa-Rhinaspray** *Boehringer Ingelheim, Irl.†.*
Tramazoline hydrochloride (p.1131·3); dexamethasone isonicotinate (p.1097·2); neomycin sulfate (p.235·1).
*Allergic rhinitis.*

**Dexa-Rhinaspray Duo**
*Boehringer Ingelheim, Irl.; Boehringer Ingelheim, UK.*
Tramazoline hydrochloride (p.1131·3); dexamethasone isonicotinate (p.1097·2).
*Allergic rhinitis.*

**Dexa-Rhinospray** *Boehringer Ingelheim, Belg.*
Tramazoline hydrochloride (p.1131·3); dexamethasone isonicotinate (p.1097·2).
Formerly contained tramazoline hydrochloride, dexamethasone isonicotinate, and neomycin sulfate.
*Rhinitis.*

**Dexa-Rhinospray M** *Mann, Ger.*
Dexamethasone isonicotinate (p.1097·2).
*Allergic rhinitis.*

**Dexa-Rhinospray N**
*Boehringer Ingelheim, Arg.; Boehringer Ingelheim, Ger.†.*
Tramazoline hydrochloride (p.1131·3); dexamethasone isonicotinate (p.1097·2).
*Rhinitis.*

**Dexasalyl**
*Mayrhofer, Austria; Nourypharma, Ger.†; Medinova, Hong Kong†; Medinova, Switz.*
Dexamethasone (p.1097·1) or dexamethasone acetate (p.1097·1); salicylic acid (p.1157·1).
*Skin and scalp disorders.*

**Dexasil** *Silom, Thai.*
Dexamethasone sodium phosphate (p.1097·2); neomycin sulfate (p.235·1).
*Infected eye disorders.*

**Dexa-sine** *Alcon, Ger.*
Dexamethasone sodium phosphate (p.1097·2).
*Eye disorders.*

**Dexa-Siozwo** *Febena, Ger.*
Dexamethasone acetate (p.1097·1); peppermint oil (p.1283·2).
Formerly contained dexamethasone acetate, naphazoline hydrochloride, and peppermint oil.
*Catarrh; rhinitis; sinusitis.*

**Dexason** *Teuto, Braz.*
Dexamethasone (p.1097·1), dexamethasone acetate (p.1097·1), or dexamethasone sodium phosphate (p.1097·2).
*Corticosteroid.*

**Dexasone**
*ICN, Canad.; Atlantic, Hong Kong; Atlantic, Malaysia; Atlantic, Singapore; Atlantic, Thai.; Hauck, USA.*
Dexamethasone (p.1097·1), dexamethasone acetate (p.1097·1), or dexamethasone sodium phosphate (p.1097·2).
*Corticosteroid.*

**Dexasporin** *Moore, USA; Rugby, USA; URL, USA.*
Dexamethasone (p.1097·1); neomycin sulfate (p.235·1); polymyxin B sulfate (p.245·1).
*Eye inflammation with bacterial infection.*

**Dexatam** *Euromex, Mex.†.*
Dexamethasone (p.1097·1).
*Corticosteroid.*

**Dexatopic**
*Organon, Arg.; Organon, Fin.†; Organon, Neth.†.*
Dexamethasone (p.1097·1); nandrolone decanoate (p.1561·2); chlorhexidine hydrochloride (p.1173·3).
*Skin disorders.*

**Dexatrim**
*Note. This name is used for preparations of different composition.*
*Chattem, Canad.*
Benzocaine (p.1370·3).
*Obesity.*

*Stella, Canad.†.*
Benzocaine (p.1370·3); ferrous fumarate (p.1427·3); carmellose sodium (p.1577·3).
*Obesity.*

*Roche, Switz.†; Thompson, USA†; Chattem, USA†.*
Phenylpropanolamine hydrochloride (p.1127·3).
*Obesity.*

**Dexatrim Plus Vitamin C** *Chattem, USA†.*
Phenylpropanolamine hydrochloride (p.1127·3); ascorbic acid (p.1460·2).
*Obesity.*

**Dexatrim Plus Vitamins** *Thompson, USA.*
*Caplets:* Multivitamin and mineral preparation (p.1417·1).
*Controlled release caplets†:* Phenylpropanolamine (p.1127·3); vitamin C (p.1460·2).
*Obesity.*

**Dexaval** *Tecnifar, Port.*
Dexamethasone valerate (p.1097·3).
*Skin disorders.*

**Dexaval V** *Tecnifar, Port.*
Dexamethasone valerate (p.1097·3); clioquinol (p.196·3).
*Infected skin disorders.*

**Dexaval A** *Tecnifar, Port.*
Dexamethasone valerate (p.1097·3); chlorphenamine maleate (p.427·3).
*Skin disorders with pruritus.*

**Dexaval N** *Tecnifar, Port.*
Dexamethasone valerate (p.1097·3); neomycin sulfate (p.235·1).
*Infected skin disorders.*

**Dexaval O** *Tecnifar, Port.*
Dexamethasone sodium phosphate (p.1097·2); neomycin sulfate (p.235·1).
*Infected eye and ear disorders.*

**Dexa-Vastrictol** *Allergan-Frumtost, Braz.†.*
Dexamethasone (p.1097·1); naphazoline nitrate (p.1124·3); zinc sulfate (p.1469·3).
*Infected eye disorders.*

**Dexavison** *Teuto, Braz.*
Dexamethasone phosphate (p.1097·2); neomycin sulfate (p.235·1).
*Infected eye disorders.*

**Dexazen** *Luper, Braz.*
Dexamethasone acetate (p.1097·1), dexamethasone phosphate (p.1097·2), or dexamethasone sodium phosphate (p.1097·2).
*Corticosteroid.*

**Dexazona** *Bunker, Braz.*
*Cream:* Dexamethasone phosphate (p.1097·2); neomycin sulfate (p.235·1).
*Injection:* Dexamethasone phosphate (p.1097·2).
*Corticosteroid.*

**Dexchloramine** *Upha, Malaysia.*
Dexchlorpheniramine maleate (p.427·3).
*Hypersensitivity reactions.*

**Dexclor** *Cristalia, Braz.*
Dexchlorpheniramine maleate (p.427·3).
*Hypersensitivity reactions.*

**Dexcophan** *Hovid, Malaysia.*
Dextromethorphan hydrobromide (p.1117·3).
*Coughs.*

**Dexcophan Cough** *Hovid, Malaysia.*
Ammonium chloride (p.1115·2); dextromethorphan hydrobromide (p.1117·3); ephedrine hydrochloride (p.1120·1).
*Coughs; nasal congestion.*

**Dexedrine**
*GlaxoSmithKline, Canad.; Celltech, UK; GlaxoSmithKline, USA.*
Dexamfetamine sulfate (p.1585·3).
*Attention deficit hyperactivity disorder; narcoleptic syndrome.*

**Dexef** *Dexo, Fr.*
Cefradine (p.179·3).
*Bacterial infections.*

**Dexefrin** *Fischer, Israel.*
Dexamethasone sodium phosphate (p.1097·2); phenylephrine (p.1126·3); neomycin sulfate (p.235·1).
*Infected eye disorders.*

**Dexelle** *ITF, Chile.*
Dexibuprofen (p.46·1).
*Fever; pain.*

**Dexemel** *ML Laboratories, UK.*
Icodextrin (p.1427·1).
*Vehicle for peritoneal drug administration.*

**Dexeryl**
*Note. This name is used for preparations of different composition.*
*Pierre Fabre Sante, Fr.*
Glycerol (p.1694·3); white soft paraffin (p.1479·3); liquid paraffin (p.1479·1).
*Dry skin disorders; minor burns.*

*Pascual, Hong Kong.*
Dextromethorphan hydrobromide (p.1117·3); guaifenesin (p.1122·1); phenylephrine hydrochloride (p.1126·3); chlorphenamine maleate (p.427·3).
*Respiratory-tract disorders.*

**DexFerrum** *American Regent, USA.*
Iron dextran (p.1436·3).
*Iron deficiency.*

**Dexicam** *OFF, Ital.*
Piroxicam (p.84·2).
*Gout; musculoskeletal, joint, and peri-articular disorders.*

**Dexicar** *Provit, Mex.*
Dexamethasone (p.1097·1).
*Corticosteroid.*

**Dexide**
*Sanofi Synthelabo, Ital.†; Rottapharm, Spain.*
Colextran hydrochloride (p.890·3).
*Hyperlipidaemias.*

**Deximune** *Dexcel, Israel.*
Ciclosporin (p.1351·2).
*Atopic eczema; psoriasis; transplant rejection; uveitis.*

**Dexipan** *Julphar, UAE.*
Dexpanthenol (p.1727·2).
*Skin irritation; wounds.*

**Dexir**
*Bristol-Myers Squibb, Belg.; Oberlin, Fr.*
Dextromethorphan hydrobromide (p.1117·3).
*Coughs.*

**Dexiron** *Genpharm, Canad.*
Iron dextran (p.1436·3).
*Iron deficiency.*

**Dexit** *Leiras, Fin.*
Dexibuprofen (p.46·1).
*Fever; pain.*

**Dexi-Tuss** *3M, Austral.*
Dextromethorphan hydrobromide (p.1117·3).
*Coughs.*

**Dexium** *Sanofi Synthelabo, Ger.*
Calcium dobesilate (p.1664·2).
*Vascular disorders.*

**Dexiven** *Rivero, Arg.*
Calcitriol (p.1461·2).
*Hypocalcaemia in dialysis patients.*

**Dexlerg** *Cazi, Braz.*
Dexchlorpheniramine maleate (p.427·3).
*Hypersensitivity reactions.*

**Dexmethsone**
*Aspen, Austral.; Aspen, Hong Kong.*
Dexamethasone (p.1097·1).
*Corticosteroid.*

**Dexmin**
*Note. This name is used for preparations of different composition.*
*Neckerman, Braz.†.*
Dexchlorpheniramine maleate (p.427·3).
*Hypersensitivity reactions.*

Daewon, Hong Kong.
Betamethasone (p.1093·1); dexchlorpheniramine maleate (p.427·3).
*Allergic rhinitis; asthma; skin disorders.*

**Dexne** Offenbach, Mex.
*Ear drops:* Dexamethasone (p.1097·1); neomycin (p.235·1); lidocaine (p.1377·3).
*Inflammatory ear disorders.*
*Eye drops:* Dexamethasone (p.1097·1); neomycin (p.235·1).
*Inflammatory eye disorders.*
Offenbach, Mex.
*Nose drops:* Dexamethasone (p.1097·1); neomycin (p.235·1); phenylephrine (p.1126·3).
*Inflammatory nose disorders.*

**Dexnon** Kern, Spain.
Levothyroxine sodium (p.1600·1).
*Hypothyroidism.*

**Dexo** Dominguez, Arg.
Ursodeoxycholic acid (p.1760·3).
*Biliary-tract disorders; cholesterol gallstones.*

**Dexodin** IQFA, Mex.
Astemizole (p.424·2).
*Hypersensitivity.*

**Dexodon** Tika, Swed.†.
Dextropropoxyphene hydrochloride (p.28·3); paracetamol (p.76·2).
*Pain.*

**Dexofan** Nycomed, Denm.
Dextromethorphan hydrobromide (p.1117·3).
*Coughs.*

**Dexofen** Astra, Swed.
Dextropropoxyphene napsilate (p.28·3).
*Pain.*

**Dexol**
Note. This name is used for preparations of different composition.
SMB, Chile.
Borage (p.1661·3).
*Barrier preparation; dry skin.*
Andromaco, Mex.
Ambroxol (p.1114·3); dextromethorphan (p.1117·3).
*Respiratory-tract congestion.*

**Dexolan** Streuli, Switz.
Dexamethasone (p.1097·1); zinc oxide (p.1163·2).
*Skin disorders.*

**Dexoline** Ciba Vision, Ital.
Chloramphenicol (p.185·1); dexamethasone sodium phosphate (p.1097·2); tetryzoline hydrochloride (p.1131·2).
*Eye disorders.*

**Dexomon** Hillcross, UK.
Diclofenac sodium (p.32·1).
*Gout; inflammation; musculoskeletal, joint, peri-articular, and soft-tissue disorders; pain.*

**Dexon** General Drugs, Thai.
Dexamethasone sodium phosphate (p.1097·2).
*Corticosteroid.*

**Dexona**
Cadila, India; Jofrain, Mex.†.
Dexamethasone (p.1097·1) or dexamethasone sodium phosphate (p.1097·2).
*Corticosteroid.*

**Dexona Eye/Ear** Cadila, India.
Dexamethasone sodium phosphate (p.1097·2); neomycin sulfate (p.235·1).
*Bacterial eye infections; inflammatory ear disorders.*

**Dexoph**
Seng, Hong Kong.
Dexamethasone phosphate (p.1097·2); neomycin sulfate (p.235·1).
*Infected ear disorders; infected eye disorders.*
Seng, Thai.
Dexamethasone sodium phosphate (p.1097·2); neomycin sulfate (p.235·1).
*Infected eye and ear disorders.*

**DexOptifen** Spirig, Switz.
Dexibuprofen (p.46·1).
*Fever; inflammation; musculoskeletal, joint, and periarticular disorders; pain.*

**Dexorange** Franco-Indian, India.
Ferric ammonium citrate (p.1427·2); vitamin $B_{12}$ (p.1458·2); folic acid (p.1429·1).
*Anaemias.*

**Dexosyn-C** Bell, India.
Chloramphenicol (p.185·1); dexamethasone (p.1097·1).
*Corneal lesions; infected inflammatory eye disorders.*

**Dexosyn-N** Bell, India.
Neomycin sulfate (p.235·1); dexamethasone (p.1097·1).
*Corneal lesions; infected inflammatory eye disorders.*

**Dex-Otic**
Teva, Israel; Teva, Thai.†.
Dexamethasone sodium phosphate (p.1097·2); neomycin sulfate (p.235·1); polymyxin B sulfate (p.245·1).
*Infected ear disorders.*

**DexPak** ECR, USA.
Dexamethasone (p.1097·1).
*Poison ivy dermatitis.*

**Dex-Panol** Stada, Austria.
Dexpanthenol (p.1727·2).
*Wounds.*

**Dexpanol** Stada, Ger.†.
Dexpanthenol (p.1727·2).
*Wounds.*

**Dexpin** Greater Pharma, Thai.
Dextromethorphan hydrobromide (p.1117·3); terpin hydrate (p.1131·1); chlorphenamine maleate (p.427·3).
*Coughs.*

**Dexsal**
Reckitt Benckiser, Austral.
*Oral granules:* Sodium citrotartrate (p.1224·1); tartaric acid (p.1752·1); glucose (p.1432·2); sodium bicarbonate (p.1223·2).
*Dyspepsia.*
Reckitt & Colman, Austral.†.
*Oral liquid:* Calcium carbonate (p.1254·2); simeticone (p.1289·2).
*Dyspepsia; flatulence.*

**Dexsol** Rosemont, UK.
Dexamethasone sodium phosphate (p.1097·2).
*Corticosteroid.*

**Dexsul** Parggon, Mex.
Dexamethasone sodium phosphate (p.1097·2); neomycin sulfate (p.235·1); polymyxin B sulfate (p.245·1).
*Infected eye disorders.*

**Dextasona** Blausiegel, Braz.
Dexamethasone sodium phosphate (p.1097·2).
*Corticosteroid.*

**Dexthasol** Olan-Kemed, Thai.
Dexamethasone sodium phosphate (p.1097·2).
*Corticosteroid.*

**Dextolyte-E** Tablets, India.
Electrolyte infusion (p.1217·1).
*Fluid and electrolyte imbalance.*

**Dextoma** Ferrier, Fr.†.
Aluminium hydroxide (p.1249·2); aluminium carbonate (p.1249·1); magnesium hydroxide (p.1272·2); magnesium carbonate (p.1272·1).
*Gastrointestinal disorders.*

**Dexton** TP, Thai.
Dexamethasone sodium phosphate (p.1097·2).
*Corticosteroid.*

**Dextracin**
Xepa-Soul Pattinson, Hong Kong; Xepa-Soul Pattinson, Malaysia; Xepa-Soul Pattinson, Singapore.
Dexamethasone sodium phosphate (p.1097·2); neomycin sulfate (p.235·1).
*Infected eye and ear disorders.*

**Dextralpha** Alpha, Mex.†.
Glucose (p.1432·2).
*Hypoglycaemia.*

**Dextrarine Phenylbutazone** Sanofi Synthelabo, Fr.
Dextran sulfate (p.1679·2); phenylbutazone (p.83·2).
*Tendinitis.*

**Dextrevit** ICN, Mex.
Vitamin B substances; vitamin C; glucose (p.1417·1).
*Neuritis; vitamin deficiencies.*

**Dextricea** Durban, Spain.
Rice; gelatin tannate (p.1751·3); pectin (p.1580·3); wheat germ.
*Diarrhoea.*

**Dextro** Osoth, Thai.
Dextromethorphan (p.1117·3); guaifenesin (p.1122·1); chlorphenamine maleate (p.427·3).
*Coughs.*

**Dextro BS** Osoth, Thai.
Dextromethorphan (p.1117·3); terpin hydrate (p.1131·1); chlorphenamine maleate (p.427·3).
*Coughs.*

**Dextro + Dipirona** Richmond, Arg.
Dextropropoxyphene (p.28·3); dipyrone (p.35·3).
*Fever.*

**Dextro GG** Jean-Marie, Hong Kong.
Dextromethorphan hydrobromide (p.1117·3); guaifenesin (p.1122·1).
*Coughs.*

**Dextro OG-T** Roche, Ger.
Mono- and oligosaccharide mixture.
*Glucose tolerance test.*

**Dextro Plus** Jean-Marie, Hong Kong.
Dextromethorphan hydrobromide (p.1117·3); guaifenesin (p.1122·1); pseudoephedrine hydrochloride (p.1129·2).
*Coughs; nasal congestion.*

**Dextrocalmine** Democal, Switz.†.
Dextromethorphan hydrobromide (p.1117·3).
*Coughs.*

**Dextrodip** Drawer, Arg.
Dextropropoxyphene (p.28·3); dipyrone (p.35·3).
*Pain.*

**Dextrodyl** Upha, Malaysia.
Dextromethorphan hydrobromide (p.1117·3); promethazine hydrochloride (p.439·1).
*Coughs.*

**Dextrolyte** Tablets, India.
Calcium lactate; potassium chloride; magnesium sulfate; sodium chloride; monobasic sodium phosphate; sodium citrate; glucose (p.1222·2).
*Oral rehydration therapy.*

**Dextrolyte-G** Tablets, India.
Electrolyte infusion (p.1217·1).
*Forced diuresis; loss of gastric juice; mild alkalosis.*

**Dextrolyte-M** Tablets, India.
Electrolyte infusion (p.1217·1).
*Fluid and electrolyte imbalance; metabolic acidosis.*

**Dextrolyte-P** Tablets, India.
Electrolyte infusion (p.1217·1).
*Fluid and electrolyte imbalance; mild acidosis.*

**Dextromine** General Drugs, Thai.
Dextromethorphan hydrobromide (p.1117·3); chlorphenamine maleate (p.427·3).
*Coughs.*

**Dextropirac** Montpellier, Arg.
Dexibuprofen (p.46·1).
*Fever; gout; inflammation; musculoskeletal and joint disorders; pain.*

**Dextroral** General Drugs, Thai.
Dextromethorphan hydrobromide (p.1117·3).
*Coughs.*

**Dextrostat** Shire Richwood, USA.
Dexamfetamine sulfate (p.1585·3).
*Attention deficit hyperactivity disorder; narcoleptic syndrome.*

**Dextrostix**
Bayer, Arg.; Bayer Diagnostics, Fr.†; Ames, Irl.†; Bayer, Ital.†; Bayer Diagnostics, Mex.; Bayer, USA†.
Test for glucose in blood (p.1694·2).

**Dextrotos** Lafedar, Arg.
Dextromethorphan hydrobromide (p.1117·3).
*Coughs.*

**Dextrovitase** Ache, Braz.
Vitamin B substances; ascorbic acid; glucose (p.1417·1).
*Nutritional supplement.*

**Dexylin** General Drugs, Thai.
Dexamethasone sodium phosphate (p.1097·2); neomycin sulfate (p.235·1).
*Infected eye and ear disorders.*

**Dezacor** Aventis, Spain.
Deflazacort (p.1096·2).
*Corticosteroid.*

**Dezartal** Andromaco, Chile.
Deflazacort (p.1096·2).
*Corticosteroid.*

**Dezepan** Klonal, Arg.
Diazepam (p.690·1).
*Anxiety.*

**Dezol** Farmion, Braz.†.
Tioconazole (p.409·3).
*Fungal skin infections.*

**Dezor** Hoe, Malaysia.
Ketoconazole (p.403·3).
*Fungal skin and scalp infections.*

**Dezoral** Hoe, Singapore.
Ketoconazole (p.403·3).
*Fungal skin infections; seborrhoeic dermatitis.*

**DF 118**
GlaxoSmithKline, Hong Kong; Galen, Irl.; GlaxoSmithKline, Malaysia; GlaxoSmithKline, S.Afr.; Martindale Pharmaceuticals, UK.
Dihydrocodeine tartrate (p.34·3).
NOTE. There is no connection between Martindale, The Complete Drug Reference and Martindale Pharmaceuticals.
*Pain.*

**DF Multi-Symptom** Merck, Hong Kong.
Paracetamol (p.76·2); brompheniramine maleate (p.426·1); phenylephrine hydrochloride (p.1126·3); bromhexine hydrochloride (p.1115·3); salicylamide (p.87·3); caffeine (p.782·1).
*Upper respiratory-tract disorders.*

**D-Feda II** WE, USA.
Pseudoephedrine hydrochloride (p.1129·2); guaifenesin (p.1122·1).

**D-Fluoretten** Aventis, Ger.
Colecalciferol (p.1461·3); sodium fluoride (p.1444·3).
*Dental caries prophylaxis; rickets prophylaxis.*

**DFN** Bajer, Arg.
Diclofenac diethylamine (p.32·1) or diclofenac sodium (p.32·1).
*Inflammation; musculoskeletal and joint disorders; pain.*

**DG-6** Craveri, Arg.
Lapyrium chloride.
*Burns; skin infections; skin, surface, and equipment disinfection.*

**DG-6 Iodopovidona** Craveri, Arg.
Povidone-iodine (p.1190·3).
*Instrument disinfection; skin infections; wounds.*

**D-Gam** BPL, UK.
An anti-D immunoglobulin (p.1608·1).
*Prevention of rhesus sensitisation.*

**Dhabesol** DHA, Singapore.
Clobetasol propionate (p.1095·2).
*Skin disorders.*

**Dhacillin**
DHA, Hong Kong; DHA, Singapore.
Ampicillin trihydrate (p.157·2).
*Bacterial infections.*

**Dhacodine** DHA, Malaysia.
Pholcodine (p.1128·3).
*Coughs.*

**Dhacold** DHA, Singapore.
Caffeine (p.782·1); chlorphenamine maleate (p.427·3); paracetamol (p.76·2); pseudoephedrine hydrochloride (p.1129·2).
*Cold symptoms.*

**Dhacopan**
DHA, Hong Kong; DHA, Malaysia; DHA, Singapore.
Hyoscine butylbromide (p.483·3).
*Smooth muscle spasm.*

**Dhacort**
DHA, Malaysia; DHA, Singapore.
Hydrocortisone acetate (p.1103·3).
*Skin disorders.*

**Dhactulose** DHA, Singapore.
Lactulose (p.1269·1).
*Constipation; hepatic encephalopathy.*

**Dhaflu** DHA, Singapore†.
Caffeine (p.782·1); chlorphenamine maleate (p.427·3); paracetamol (p.76·2); phenylpropanolamine hydrochloride (p.1127·3).
*Cold symptoms.*

**Dhalgesic**
DHA, Hong Kong; DHA, Singapore.
Methyl salicylate (p.59·3); menthol (p.1711·3); camphor (p.1665·3).
*Musculoskeletal, joint, and soft-tissue disorders.*

**Dhalumag**
DHA, Malaysia; DHA, Singapore.
Aluminium hydroxide (p.1249·2); magnesium trisilicate (p.1272·3).
*Gastric hyperacidity; peptic ulcer.*

**Dhamol**
DHA, Hong Kong; DHA, Malaysia; DHA, Singapore.
Paracetamol (p.76·2).
*Fever; pain.*

**Dhamotil**
DHA, Hong Kong; DHA, Malaysia; DHA, Singapore.
Diphenoxylate hydrochloride (p.1261·3).
Atropine sulfate (p.477·1) is included in this preparation to discourage abuse.
*Diarrhoea.*

**Dhaperazine**
DHA, Hong Kong; DHA, Malaysia; DHA, Singapore.
Prochlorperazine maleate (p.716·3).
*Emotional and mental disturbances; Ménière's disease; migraine; nausea and vomiting.*

**Dhasedyl**
DHA, Hong Kong; DHA, Singapore.
Codeine phosphate (p.27·1); ephedrine hydrochloride (p.1120·1); promethazine hydrochloride (p.439·1).
*Coughs.*

**Dhasedyl DM** DHA, Singapore.
Dextromethorphan hydrobromide (p.1117·3); ephedrine hydrochloride (p.1120·1); promethazine hydrochloride (p.439·1).
*Coughs.*

**Dhasolone**
DHA, Hong Kong; DHA, Malaysia; DHA, Singapore.
Prednisolone (p.1108·1).
*Corticosteroid.*

**Dhatalin** DHA, Hong Kong.
Terbutaline sulfate (p.797·2).
*Asthma; bronchitis.*

**Dhatifen**
DHA, Malaysia; DHA, Singapore.
Ketotifen (p.788·2).
*Asthma; hypersensitivity reactions.*

**Dhatracin** DHA, Malaysia.
Tetracycline hydrochloride (p.266·2).
*Bacterial infections.*

**Dhatrin**
DHA, Hong Kong; DHA, Singapore.
Co-trimoxazole (p.199·3).
*Bacterial infections.*

**DHC** Mundipharma, Ger.
Dihydrocodeine tartrate (p.34·3).
*Pain.*

**DHC Continus**
Napp, Irl.; Rafa, Israel†; Douglas, NZ; Napp, UK.
Dihydrocodeine tartrate (p.34·3).
*Pain.*

**DHC Plus** Purdue Frederick, USA.
Dihydrocodeine tartrate (p.34·3); paracetamol (p.76·2); caffeine (p.782·1).

**DHE**
Alpharma-Isis, Ger.; Ratiopharm, Ger.; Xcel, USA.
Dihydroergotamine mesilate (p.465·3).
*Cluster headache; hypotension; migraine.*

**DHS Sal** Dispolab, Chile.
Salicylic acid (p.1157·1).
*Dandruff.*

**DHS Tar** Person & Covey, USA.
Coal tar (p.1159·2).
*Scalp disorders; seborrhoea.*

**DHS Tar Gel** Dispolab, Chile.
Coal tar (p.1159·2).
*Psoriasis.*

**DHS Zinc**
Dispolab, Chile; Person & Covey, USA.
Pyrithione zinc (p.1156·2).
*Scalp disorders.*

**DHT** Roxane, USA.
Dihydrotachysterol (p.1461·3).
*Hypoparathyroidism; postoperative and idiopathic tetany.*

**Di Anatoxal** Berna, NZ.
A diphtheria vaccine (p.1612·3).
*Active immunisation.*

**Di Dolko** Therabel, Fr.
Paracetamol (p.76·2); dextropropoxyphene hydrochloride (p.28·3).
*Pain.*

**Di Retard** Llorens, Spain.
Diclofenac sodium (p.32·1).
*Dysmenorrhoea; gout; musculoskeletal, joint, and peri-articular disorders; pain; renal colic.*

**Di Te Anatoxal**
Berna, Singapore†; Berna, Thai.
An adsorbed diphtheria and tetanus vaccine (p.1613·1).
*Active immunisation.*

**Di Te Per Anatoxal**
*Berna, Hong Kong†; Berna, Singapore†; Berna, Thai.†.*
A diphtheria, tetanus, and pertussis vaccine (p.1613·3).
*Active immunisation of infants and young children.*

**Dia-Aktivanad-N** *Rentschler, Ger.*
Bovine liver extract; yeast extract; caffeine (p.1417·1).
*Tonic.*

**DiaB Gel** *Carrington, USA.*
Acemannan (p.1645·2).
*Diabetic ulcers.*

**Diabact UBT**
*Diabact, Swed.; Medical Diagnostics, UK.*
Carbon-13 (p.1667·3) labelled urea.
*Test for Helicobacter pylori infection.*

**Diabamyl** *Expanpharm, Fr.*
Metformin hydrochloride (p.342·3).
*Diabetes mellitus.*

**Dia-BASF** *BASF, Ger.†.*
Glibenclamide (p.331·2).
*Diabetes mellitus.*

**Diabecontrol** *Sanval, Braz.*
Chlorpropamide (p.330·3).
*Diabetes mellitus.*

**Diabeedol** *Sriprasit, Thai.*
Chlorpropamide (p.330·3).
*Diabetes mellitus.*

**Diabemet** *YSP, Malaysia.*
Metformin hydrochloride (p.342·3).
*Diabetes mellitus.*

**Diabemide** *Guidotti, Ital.*
Chlorpropamide (p.330·3).
*Diabetes mellitus.*

**Diabemin** *Lacefa, Arg.*
Glibenclamide (p.331·2).
*Diabetes mellitus.*

**Diaben** *Kinder, Braz.*
Glibenclamide (p.331·2).
*Diabetes mellitus.*

**Diabene** *Lehning, Fr.*
Homoeopathic preparation.

**Diabenol** *Greater Pharma, Thai.*
Glibenclamide (p.331·2).
*Diabetes mellitus.*

**Diabenor** *IFI, Ital.*
Glisolamide (p.333·1).
*Diabetes mellitus.*

**Diabenyl T** *Chauvin ankerpharm, Ger.*
Tetryzoline hydrochloride (p.1131·2).
*Eye irritation.*

**Diabenyl-Rhinex** *Wernigerode, Ger.*
Diphenhydramine hydrochloride (p.431·3); naphazoline hydrochloride (p.1124·3).
*Allergic rhinitis.*

**Diabeside** *Chew, Thai.*
Gliclazide (p.332·1).
*Diabetes mellitus.*

**Diabesin** *TAD, Ger.*
Metformin hydrochloride (p.342·3).
*Diabetes mellitus.*

**Diabesor** *Soria Natural, Spain.*
Centaurea aspera; eucalyptus (p.1686·1); phaseolus vulgaris; sage (p.1741·2); lappa (p.1704·3).
*Diabetes mellitus.*

**Diabestat** *Andromaco, Chile.*
Pioglitazone hydrochloride (p.344·1).
*Diabetes mellitus.*

**DiaBeta**
*Aventis, Canad.; Hoechst Marion Roussel, USA.*
Glibenclamide (p.331·2).
*Diabetes mellitus.*

**Diabetamide** *Ashbourne, UK.*
Glibenclamide (p.331·2).
*Diabetes mellitus.*

**Diabetan S** *Schuck, Ger.*
Homoeopathic preparation.

**Diabetase** *Azupharma, Ger.*
Metformin hydrochloride (p.342·3).
*Diabetes mellitus.*

**Diabetex** *Germania, Austria.*
Metformin hydrochloride (p.342·3).
*Diabetes mellitus.*

**Diabetic Tussin** *Roberts, USA.*
Dextromethorphan hydrobromide (p.1117·3); guaifenesin (p.1122·1); phenylephrine (p.1126·3).
*Coughs.*

**Diabetic Tussin DM** *Roberts, USA.*
Dextromethorphan hydrobromide (p.1117·3); guaifenesin (p.1122·1).
*Coughs.*

**Diabetic Tussin EX** *Health Care Products, USA†.*
Guaifenesin (p.1122·1).
*Coughs.*

**Diabetiks** *Green Turtle Bay Vitamin Co., USA.*
Vitamins; minerals; bioflavonoids; myrtillus; ginkgo biloba; green tea; pine bark; acetylcysteine; taurine; ubidecarenone; lipoic acid (p.1417·1).
*Tonic.*

**Diabetisource com Nutrishield** *Novartis, Braz.*
Preparation for enteral nutrition (p.1417·1).

**Diabetmin**
*Hovid, Hong Kong; Hovid, Malaysia; Hovid, Singapore.*
Metformin hydrochloride (p.342·3).
*Diabetes mellitus.*

**Diabe-Tuss DM** *Paddock, USA.*
Dextromethorphan hydrobromide (p.1117·3).
*Coughs.*

**Diabex** *Alphapharm, Austral.*
Metformin hydrochloride (p.342·3).
*Diabetes mellitus.*

**Diabexan** *Crosara, Ital.†.*
Chlorpropamide (p.330·3).
*Diabetes mellitus.*

**Diabexil** *Dansk-Flama, Braz.*
Glibenclamide (p.331·2).
*Diabetes mellitus.*

**Diabiclor** *Mavi, Mex.*
Chlorpropamide (p.330·3).
*Diabetes mellitus.*

**Diabiformine** *Pfizer, Switz.*
Chlorpropamide (p.330·3); metformin hydrochloride (p.342·3).
*Diabetes mellitus.*

**Diabines** *Pfizer, Swed.†.*
Chlorpropamide (p.330·3).
*Diabetes mellitus.*

**Diabinese**
*Pfizer, Arg.; Pfizer, Austral.†; Pfizer, Belg.; Pfizer, Braz.; Pfizer, Canad.†; Pfizer, Chile; Pfizer, Gr.; Pfizer, Hong Kong; Pfizer, Irl.†; Pfizer, Israel; Pfizer, Malaysia; Pfizer, Mex.; Pfizer, Norw.†; Pfizer, S.Afr.†; Pfizer, Singapore; Farmasierra, Spain; Pfizer, Switz.†; Pfizer, Thai.; Pfizer, USA.*
Chlorpropamide (p.330·3).
*Diabetes insipidus; diabetes mellitus.*

**Diabitex**
*Rekah, Israel; Salters, S.Afr.†.*
Chlorpropamide (p.330·3).
*Diabetes mellitus.*

**Diaborale** *Pharmacia Upjohn, Ital.*
Glycyclamide (p.333·1).
*Diabetes mellitus.*

**Diabrezide**
*Helsinn Birex, Irl.; Molteni, Ital.*
Gliclazide (p.332·1).
*Diabetes mellitus.*

**Diabur-5000** *Roche Diagnostics, NZ.*
Test for glucose in urine (p.1694·2).

**Diabur-Test 5000**
*Roche Diagnostics, Austral.; Roche Diagnostics, Irl.; Roche Diagnostics, Ital.; Roche, Mex.; Roche Diagnostics, UK.*
Test for glucose in urine (p.1694·2).

**Diacard** *Madaus, Ger.*
Homoeopathic preparation.

**Diacare** *Be-Tabs, S.Afr.*
Glibenclamide (p.331·2).
*Diabetes mellitus.*

**Diaceplex** *Salvat, Spain†.*
Diazepam (p.690·1).
*Alcohol withdrawal syndrome; anxiety; febrile convulsions; insomnia; skeletal muscle spasm.*

**Diaceplex Simple** *Salvat, Spain†.*
Diazepam (p.690·1).
*Alcohol withdrawal syndrome; anxiety; epilepsy; febrile convulsions; general anaesthesia; insomnia; skeletal muscle spasm.*

**Dia-Chek** *Pharmacia, Austral.†.*
Codeine phosphate (p.27·1); aluminium hydroxide (p.1249·2).
*Diarrhoea.*

**Diaclaron** *Siam Bheasach, Thai.*
Gliclazide (p.332·1).
*Diabetes mellitus.*

**Diaclide** *Gerard, Irl.*
Gliclazide (p.332·1).
*Diabetes mellitus.*

**Diacol** *Bial, Port.*
Dextromethorphan hydrobromide (p.1117·3).
Formerly contained ethylmorphine hydrochloride, sodium benzoate, belladonna, and ephedrine hydrochloride.
*Coughs.*

**Dia-Colon** *Piam, Ital.*
Lactulose (p.1269·1).
*Gastrointestinal disorders; liver disorders.*

**Diacor**
*Note. This name is used for preparations of different composition.*
*Pasteur, Chile.*
Mebendazole (p.108·2).
*Worm infections.*

*Dexo, Fr.*
Diltiazem hydrochloride (p.900·1).
*Angina pectoris.*

**Diacron** *Tempo Scan Pacific, Malaysia.*
Gliclazide (p.332·1).
*Diabetes mellitus.*

**Diactal** *Neuropharma, Arg.*
Diazepam (p.690·1).

**Di-Actane** *Menarini, Fr.*
Naftidrofuryl oxalate (p.964·1).
*Cerebral and peripheral vascular disorders; mental function impairment in the elderly.*

**Diacure**
*Note. This name is used for preparations of different composition.*
*Lehning, Fr.*
Taraxacum (p.1751·3); berberis; juglans; millefolium; myrtillus (p.1718·3); centaury (p.1669·2); natrum phosphoricum.
*Metabolic disorders.*

*Taxandria, Neth.*
Loperamide hydrochloride (p.1271·1).
*Diarrhoea.*

**Diacure Plus** *Taxandria, Neth.*
Loperamide hydrochloride (p.1271·1); simeticone (p.1289·2).
*Diarrhoea.*

**Diadermina** *Dermopen, Braz.†.*
Emollient.
*Barrier preparation; dry skin.*

**Diadicon** *Labomed, Chile Compuesto.*
Bromhexine hydrochloride (p.1115·3); clofedanol hydrochloride (p.1117·1).
*Coughs; respiratory-tract congestion.*

**Diadin M** *Diadin, Ger.†.*
Mofebutazone (p.60·1).
*Musculoskeletal, joint, and soft-tissue disorders.*

**Di-Adreson-F**
*Organon, Fin.; Nourypharma, Neth.*
Prednisolone sodium succinate (p.1108·2).
*Corticosteroid.*

*Organon, Hong Kong; Organon, Thai.*
Prednisolone (p.1108·1).
*Corticosteroid.*

**Diadupsan** *UPSA, Fr.†.*
Dextropropoxyphene hydrochloride (p.28·3); paracetamol (p.76·2).
*Pain.*

**Dia-Eptal** *Montavit, Austria.*
Glibenclamide (p.331·2).
*Diabetes mellitus.*

**Diaformin**
*Alphapharm, Austral.; Alphapharm, Hong Kong.*
Metformin hydrochloride (p.342·3).
*Diabetes mellitus.*

**Diafuran** *Cazi, Braz.*
Loperamide hydrochloride (p.1271·1).
*Diarrhoea.*

**Diafusor**
*Schering-Plough, Belg.; Pierre Fabre, Fr.; Pierre Fabre, Spain.*
Glyceryl trinitrate (p.923·2).
*Angina pectoris.*

**Diagesil** *Berk, UK†.*
Diamorphine hydrochloride (p.30·2).
*Pain.*

**Diaglucide** *Tema, S.Afr.*
Gliclazide (p.332·1).
*Diabetes mellitus.*

**Diaglyk** *Ashbourne, UK.*
Gliclazide (p.332·1).
*Diabetes mellitus.*

**Diagnosis** *Rottapharm, Ital.*
Pregnancy test (p.1734·3).

**Diagnostic Skin Testing Kit** *Bayer, S.Afr.†.*
Allergen extracts (p.1650·1).
*Diagnostic agent.*

**Diagran** *Teofarma, Ital.*
Multivitamin preparation (p.1417·1).

**Diagran Minerale** *Bristol-Myers Squibb, Ital.*
Multivitamin and mineral preparation (p.1417·1).

**Diagrin** *Makros, Braz.†.*
Metoclopramide hydrochloride (p.1274·3); vitamin $B_6$ (p.1456·3).
*Nausea and vomiting.*

**Diahalt** *Wampole, Canad.*
Loperamide hydrochloride (p.1271·1).
*Diarrhoea.*

**Diah-Limit** *Wallis, UK.*
Loperamide hydrochloride (p.1271·1).
*Diarrhoea.*

**Dialacid** *Collins, Mex.*
Loperamide (p.1271·2).
*Diarrhoea.*

**Dialamine**
*Scientific Hospital Supplies, Austral.; SHS, Fr.; Scientific Hospital Supplies, Irl.†; Nutricia, NZ; Scientific Hospital Supplies, NZ; Scientific Hospital Supplies, UK.*
Amino acid, carbohydrate, ascorbic acid, and mineral preparation (p.1417·1).
*Enteral nutrition.*

**Dialar** *Sandoz, UK.*
Diazepam (p.690·1).

**Dialens**
*Note. This name is used for preparations of different composition.*
*Specia, Fr.†; Bausch & Lomb, Switz.*
Dextran 60-85 (p.746·1).
*Dry eyes; wetting agent for contact lenses.*

*Chauvin, Port.*
Chlorhexidine gluconate (p.1173·2).
*Contact lens care; tear deficiency.*

**Dialgin** *Collins, Mex.*
Diiodohydroxyquinoline (p.603·3); furazolidone (p.605·2); homatropine (p.483·2).
*Amoebiasis; diarrhoea.*

**Dialgine forte** *Intermedica, Switz.*
Paracetamol (p.76·2); propyphenazone (p.85·3); caffeine (p.782·1).
*Fever; pain.*

**Dialgirex** *Irex, Fr.*
Dextropropoxyphene hydrochloride (p.28·3); paracetamol (p.76·2).
*Pain.*

**Dialibra** *Dieterba, Ital.†.*
Dietary fibre supplement (p.1253·2).
*Disorders of glucose and lipid metabolism.*

**Dialine** *Teva, Israel.*
Glucose; sodium chloride; sodium lactate; calcium chloride; magnesium chloride (p.1221·1).
*Peritoneal dialysis.*

**Dialisis Perit** *Bieffe, Spain.*
Electrolytes; glucose monohydrate (p.1221·1).
*Peritoneal dialysis.*

**Dialisol** *Antibioticos, Spain†.*
Calcium chloride; anhydrous glucose; magnesium chloride; sodium chloride; sodium lactate (p.1221·1).
*Peritoneal dialysis.*

**Dialoc** *Masa, Thai.†.*
Gliclazide (p.332·1).
*Diabetes mellitus.*

**Dialon** *Julphar, UAE.*
Metformin hydrochloride (p.342·3).
*Diabetes mellitus.*

**Dialster** *Esoform, Ital.*
Sodium dichloroisocyanurate (p.1191·3).
*Disinfection of surfaces, water, food, and feeding bottles.*

**Dialudon** *Sigma, Braz.*
Phenytoin (p.370·2); diazepam (p.690·1).
*Epilepsy.*

**Dialume**
*Aventis, Spain†; Rhone-Poulenc Rorer, USA.*
Aluminium hydroxide (p.1249·2).
*Hyperacidity; hyperphosphataemia.*

**Dialvit** *Bichsel, Switz.*
Multivitamin preparation (p.1417·1).
*Dietary supplement in renal failure.*

**Dialycare** *Abbott, Ital.*
Preparation for enteral nutrition (p.1417·1).
*Renal dialysis.*

**Dialysol Acide** *Soludia, Fr.†.*
Sodium chloride; potassium chloride; calcium chloride; magnesium chloride; acetic acid (p.1221·1).
*Haemodialysis solution.*

**Dialysol Bicarbonate** *Soludia, Fr.†.*
Sodium bicarbonate; sodium chloride (p.1221·1).
*Haemodialysis solution.*

**Dialytan H** *Aguettant, Fr.*
Haemodialysis solution (p.1221·1).

**Dialyte**
*GHP, Thai.; Gambro, USA.*
Glucose; electrolytes (p.1221·1).
*Peritoneal dialysis solution.*

**Diamaze** *Macrophar, Thai.*
Gliclazide (p.332·1).
*Diabetes mellitus.*

**Diameb** *Precimex, Mex.†.*
Diiodohydroxyquinoline (p.603·3).

**Diamet** *Weifa, Thai.*
Metformin hydrochloride (p.342·3).
*Diabetes mellitus.*

**Diamexon** *TO-Chemicals, Thai.*
Gliclazide (p.332·1).
*Diabetes mellitus.*

**Diamicron**
*Servier, Arg.; Servier, Austral.; Servier, Austria; Servier, Belg.; Servier, Braz.; Servier, Canad.; Servier, Denm.; Servier, Fr.; Servier, Ger.; Servier, Gr.; Servier, Hong Kong; Serdia, India; Servier, Irl.; Servier, Ital.; Servier, Malaysia; Byk Gulden, Mex.; Servier, Neth.; Servier, NZ; Servier, Port.; Servier, S.Afr.; Servier, Singapore; Servier, Spain; Servier, Switz.; Servier, Thai.; Servier, UK.*
Gliclazide (p.332·1).
*Diabetes mellitus.*

**Diamin** *Malaysia Chemist, Singapore.*
Metformin hydrochloride (p.342·3).
*Diabetes mellitus.*

**Diaminocillina** *Fournier, Ital.*
Benzathine benzylpenicillin (p.162·3).
*Bacterial infections.*

**Diamitex** *Duopharma, Hong Kong.*
Gliclazide (p.332·1).
*Diabetes mellitus.*

**Diamorf** *Medeva, UK†.*
Diamorphine hydrochloride (p.30·2).
*Pain.*

**Diamoril** *Chiesi, Fr.*
Benzquercin (p.1688·2).
*Peripheral vascular disorders.*

**Diamox**
*Wyeth, Arg.; Wyeth, Austral.; Wyeth Lederle, Austria; Wyeth Lederle, Belg.; Wyeth, Braz.; Wyeth-Ayerst, Canad.; Wyeth Lederle, Denm.; Wyeth Lederle, Fin.; Theraplix, Fr.; Lederle, Ger.; IFET (ΙΦΕΤ), Gr.; Lederle, Hong Kong; Wyeth Lederle, India; Goldshield, Irl.; Lederle, Israel; Wyeth Lederle, Ital.; Wyeth, Mex.; Goldshield, Neth.; Wyeth Lederle, Norw.; Wyeth, NZ; Wyeth, S.Afr.†; Wyeth, Spain†; Goldshield, Swed.; Vifor, Switz.; Wyeth-Ayerst, Thai.; Goldshield, UK; Barr, USA.*
Acetazolamide (p.849·1) or acetazolamide sodium (p.849·1).
*Acute mountain sickness; eclampsia; epilepsy; glaucoma; Ménière's disease; oedema; pancreatic disorders; premenstrual syndrome; respiratory insufficiency.*

**Diamplicil** *Pharmacia Upjohn, Ital.*
Ampicillin (p.157·1); dicloxacillin (p.205·2).
*Bacterial infections.*

**Dianben** *Roche, Spain.*
Metformin hydrochloride (p.342·3).
*Diabetes mellitus.*

**Diane**
*Schering, Arg.; Schering, Austral.; Schering, Austria; Schering, Belg.; Schering, Braz.; Berlex, Canad.; Schering, Chile; Schering, Denm.; Schering, Fin.; Schering, Fr.; Schering, Ger.; Schering, Hong Kong;*

Schering, Israel; Schering, Ital.; Schering, Malaysia; Schering, Mex.; Schering, Neth.; Schering, Norw.; Schering, NZ; Schering, Port.; Schering, S.Afr.; Schering, Singapore; Schering, Spain; Schering, Swed.; Schering, Switz.; Schering, Thai.
Cyproterone acetate (p.1544·1); ethinylestradiol (p.1553·2).
28-Day packs also contain 7 inert tablets.
*Androgen-dependent acne, alopecia, hirsutism, and seborrhoea in women; oral contraceptive in women with androgenic symptoms; polycystic ovary syndrome.*

**Dianeal**
Baxter, Austral.; Baxter, Austria; Baxter, Denm.; Baxter, Fin.; Baxter, Israel; Baxter, Port.†; Baxter, Spain; Baxter, Swed.; Baxter, Switz.; Baxter, UK†.
Glucose; sodium chloride; sodium lactate; calcium chloride; magnesium chloride (p.1221·1).
*Peritoneal dialysis.*

**Dianette**
Schering, Irl.; Schering, UK.
Cyproterone acetate (p.1544·1); ethinylestradiol (p.1553·2).
These ingredients can be described by the British Approved Name Co-cyprindiol.
*Acne and hirsutism in females.*

**Dianicotyl** IFET (ΙΦΕΤ), Gr.
Isoniazid (p.222·2).
*Tuberculosis.*

**Dianid**
Biolab, Malaysia; Biolab, Thai.
Gliclazide (p.332·1).
*Diabetes mellitus.*

**Diano** Milano, Thai.
Diazepam (p.690·1).
*Anxiety; insomnia; skeletal muscle spasm.*

**Dianoct** Silesia, Chile.
Day tablets, paracetamol (p.76·2); pseudoephedrine hydrochloride (p.1129·2); night tablets, paracetamol; pseudoephedrine hydrochloride; chlorphenamine maleate.
*Cold and influenza symptoms.*

**Dianormax** Servier, Chile.
Gliclazide (p.332·1).
*Diabetes mellitus.*

**Di-Antalvic** Aventis, Fr.
Dextropropoxyphene hydrochloride (p.28·3); paracetamol (p.76·2).
*Pain.*

**Diapam**
Note. This name is used for preparations of different composition.
Pasteur, Chile.
Chlormezanone (p.675·1); diazepam (p.690·1).
*Anxiety; musculoskeletal spasm; sleep disorders.*
Orion, Fin.; Greater Pharma, Thai.
Diazepam (p.690·1).
*Alcohol withdrawal syndromes; anxiety disorders; insomnia; muscle spasms; pain; premedication; status epilepticus.*

**Diapanil** Randall, Mex.
Diazepam (p.690·1).

**Diaparene Corn Starch** Personal Care, USA.
Corn starch (p.1449·1); aloes (p.1248·2).
*Nappy rash.*

**Diaparene Diaper Rash** Personal Care, USA.
Zinc oxide (p.1163·2).
*Nappy rash.*

**Diapatol** Teofarma, Ital.
Amitriptyline hydrochloride (p.280·3); chlordiazepoxide hydrochloride (p.674·2).
*Anxiety disorders; depression; insomnia.*

**Diaper Guard**
Note. This name is used for preparations of different composition.
Del, Canad.†.
Dimethicone (p.1482·1); soft paraffin (p.1479·3); zinc oxide (p.1163·2).
Del, USA.
Dimethicone (p.1482·1); white soft paraffin (p.1479·3); vitamin A (p.1451·2); vitamin $D_3$ (p.1461·2); vitamin E (p.1464·3).
*Nappy rash.*

**Diaper Rash**
Note. This name is used for preparations of different composition.
DC Labs, Canad.
Zinc oxide (p.1163·2).
Goldline, USA; Rugby, USA.
Zinc oxide (p.1163·2); cod-liver oil (p.1425·2).
*Nappy rash.*

**Diaphal** Pierre Fabre, Ger.
Furosemide (p.919·3); amiloride hydrochloride (p.858·2).
*Ascites; hypertension; oedema.*

**Diapid**
Sandoz, Fr.†; Novartis, USA†.
Lypressin (p.1342·3).
*Diabetes insipidus.*

**Diapine**
Atlantic, Malaysia; Atlantic, Singapore; Atlantic, Thai.
Diazepam (p.690·1).
*Alcohol withdrawal syndrome; anxiety; epilepsy; skeletal muscle spasm.*

**Diapo** Upha, Malaysia.
Diazepam (p.690·1).
*Anxiety; skeletal muscle spasm; sleep disorders.*

**Diapool** Dovalle, Braz.†.
Attapulgite (p.1251·1); pectin (p.1580·3); aluminium hydroxide (p.1249·2); homatropine (p.483·2).
*Diarrhoea.*

**Diaquitte** Peach, UK.
Loperamide hydrochloride (p.1271·1).
*Diarrhoea.*

**Diarcalm** McGloin, Austral.†.
Light kaolin (p.1268·3); pectin (p.1580·3); catechu (p.1668·3); aluminium hydroxide (p.1249·2).
*Diarrhoea; stomach pain.*

**Diaren** Saval, Chile.
Nifuroxazide (p.237·2); activated attapulgite (p.1251·1).
*Diarrhoea.*

**Diarent** Chew, Thai.
Loperamide hydrochloride (p.1271·1).
*Diarrhoea.*

**Diaretyl** Cooperation Pharmaceutique, Fr.
Loperamide hydrochloride (p.1271·1).
*Diarrhoea.*

**Diarex** Pharmavite, Canad.†.
Kaolin (p.1268·3); pectin (p.1580·3).

**Diareze**
Note. This name is used for preparations of different composition.
Key, Austral.
*Oral suspension*†: Attapulgite (p.1251·1); pectin (p.1580·3); simeticone (p.1289·2).
*Tablets:* Attapulgite (p.1251·1); pectin (p.1580·3); aluminium hydroxide (p.1249·2).
*Diarrhoea.*
Boots, UK.
Loperamide hydrochloride (p.1271·1).
*Diarrhoea.*

**Diarfin** Laboratorios Chile, Chile.
Nifuroxazide (p.237·2); activated attapulgite (p.1251·1).
*Diarrhoea.*

**Diargal** Gallia, Fr.
Infant feed; food for special diets (p.1417·1).
*Diarrhoea; lactose intolerance; sucrose intolerance.*

**Diarigoz** Guigoz, Fr.
Infant feed (p.1417·1).
*Diarrhoea.*

**Diaril** MC, Ital.
Glutaral (p.1180·3); phenol (p.1188·1); orthophenylphenol (p.1187·2).
*Instrument disinfection.*

**Diarim** Rimsa, Mex.
Nifuroxazide (p.237·2).

**Diarlac** Urgo, Fr.
*Lactobacillus acidophilus* (p.1704·2).
*Diarrhoea.*

**Diarlop** Jagson, India.
*Capsules:* Loperamide hydrochloride (p.1271·1).
*Oral suspension:* Nalidixic acid (p.234·1).
*Diarrhoea.*

**Diarman** Berman, Mex.
Chloramphenicol palmitate (p.185·1).
*Bacterial infections.*

**Diaro** Madaus, Austria.
Tormentil (p.1757·2).
*Diarrhoea.*

**Diarodil** Greater Pharma, Thai.
Loperamide hydrochloride (p.1271·1).
*Diarrhoea.*

**Diarona** Cimed, Braz.†.
Dipyrone (p.35·3); papaverine hydrochloride (p.1728·1).
*Smooth muscle spasm.*

**Diaront mono** Chephasaar, Ger.
Colistin sulfate (p.198·3).
*Selective gastrointestinal tract decontamination.*

**Diarresec** Farmion, Braz.
Loperamide hydrochloride (p.1271·1).
*Diarrhoea.*

**Diarrest** Galen, UK†.
Codeine phosphate (p.27·1); dicycloverine hydrochloride (p.481·2); sodium chloride; potassium chloride; sodium citrate.
*Diarrhoea.*

**Diarrest RF** Galen, Irl.
Loperamide hydrochloride (p.1271·1); potassium chloride; sodium chloride; sodium citrate.
*Diarrhoea.*

**Diarret** Geymonat, Ital.
Nifuroxazide (p.237·2).
*Acute infective diarrhoea.*

**Diarrex** Hylands, Canad.
Homoeopathic preparation.

**Diarr-Eze** Pharmascience, Canad.
Loperamide hydrochloride (p.1271·1).
*Diarrhoea.*

**Diarrhea Relief** Stanley, Canad.
Loperamide hydrochloride (p.1271·1).

**Diarrheel S** Heel, Ger.†.
Homoeopathic preparation.

**Diarrhoea Complex** Brauer, Austral.†.
Homoeopathic preparation.

**Diarrhoea Relief Tablets** Brauer, Austral.†.
Homoeopathic preparation.

**Diarrhoesan**
Vitasan, Austria; Loges, Ger.
Apple pectin (p.1580·3); chamomile (p.1669·3).
*Diarrhoea.*

**Diarrhoesan SC** Loges, Ger.†.
Saccharomyces boulardii (p.1704·2).
*Acne; diarrhoea.*

**Diarril** Hebron, Braz.†.
*Saccharomyces cerevisiae* (p.1469·1).
*Diarrhoea; restoration of gastrointestinal flora.*

**Diarrocalmol** Benitol, Arg.
Phthalylsulfathiazole (p.242·3); activated charcoal (p.1030·2).
*Diarrhoea.*

**Diarsed** Sanofi Synthelabo, Fr.
Diphenoxylate hydrochloride (p.1261·3).
Atropine sulfate (p.477·1) is included in this preparation to discourage abuse.
*Diarrhoea.*

**Diarstop** Giuliani, Ital.
Loperamide hydrochloride (p.1271·1).
*Diarrhoea.*

**Diarzero** Uniform, Ital.
Loperamide hydrochloride (p.1271·1).
*Diarrhoea.*

**Diascan** Home Diagnostics, USA.
Test for glucose in blood (p.1694·2).

**Diascreen 3** Marco, Austral.
Test for glucose, protein, and pH in urine.

**Diascreen 5** Marco, Austral.
Test for glucose, protein, ketones, pH, and blood in urine.

**Diascreen 6** Marco, Austral.
Test for glucose, protein, ketones, pH, blood, and bilirubin in urine.

**Diascreen 7** Marco, Austral.
Test for glucose, protein, ketones, pH, blood, bilirubin, and urobilinogen in urine.

**Diascreen 8** Marco, Austral.
Test for glucose, protein, ketones, pH, blood, bilirubin, urobilinogen, and nitrite in urine.

**Diascreen 9** Marco, Austral.
Test for glucose, protein, ketones, pH, blood, bilirubin, urobilinogen, nitrite, and leucocytes in urine.

**Diascreen 10** Marco, Austral.
Test for glucose, protein, ketones, pH, blood, bilirubin, urobilinogen, nitrite, leucocytes, and specific gravity in urine.

**Diascreen 40BL** Marco, Austral.
Test for glucose, protein, blood, and leucocytes in urine.

**Diascreen 2GK** Marco, Austral.
Test for glucose and ketones in urine.

**Diascreen Glucose** Marco, Austral.
Test for glucose in urine (p.1694·2).
Formerly known as Diascreen 1G.

**Diascreen 2GP** Marco, Austral.
Test for glucose and protein in urine.

**Diascreen 1K** Marco, Austral.
Test for ketones in urine.

**Diascreen 4NL** Marco, Austral.
Test for glucose, protein, nitrite, and leucocytes in urine.

**Diascreen 4PH** Marco, Austral.
Test for glucose, protein, pH, and blood in urine.

**Diasec** Hexal, Braz.
Loperamide hydrochloride (p.1271·1).
*Diarrhoea.*

**Diasectral**
Aventis, Denm.; Aventis, Fin.
Acebutolol hydrochloride (p.848·1).
*Angina pectoris; arrhythmias; hypertension; myocardial infarction.*

**Diasef**
Unison, Hong Kong; Unison, Singapore; Unison, Thai.
Glipizide (p.332·2).
*Diabetes mellitus.*

**Diaseptyl** Ducray, Fr.
Chlorhexidine gluconate (p.1173·2).
*Skin disinfection.*

**Diasgest** Siam Bheasach, Thai.
Amylase (p.1654·2); sodium bicarbonate (p.1223·2); calcium carbonate (p.1254·2); aluminium magnesium silicate (p.1577·1); scopolia; vitamin $B_1$ (p.1455·2).
*Dyspepsia; gastric hyperacidity; gastritis; gastrointestinal motility disorders; heartburn.*

**Diasorb**
Note. This name is used for preparations of different composition.
Norton Healthcare, UK†.
Loperamide hydrochloride (p.1271·1).
*Diarrhoea.*
Columbia, USA.
Activated attapulgite (p.1251·1).
*Diarrhoea.*

**Diastabol**
Sanofi Synthelabo, Austria; Sanofi Synthelabo, Braz.†; Sanofi Winthrop, Fin.†; Sanofi Synthelabo, Fr.; Sanofi Synthelabo, Ger.; Sanofi Synthelabo, Mex.; Sanofi Synthelabo, Port.†; Sanofi Synthelabo, Spain; Sanofi Synthelabo, Swed.; Sanofi Synthelabo, Switz.
Miglitol (p.343·2).
*Diabetes mellitus.*

**Diastat**
Draxis, Canad.; Xcel, USA.
Diazepam (p.690·1).
*Convulsions; epilepsy.*

**Diastix**
Bayer, Arg.; Bayer, Austral.; Bayer, Canad.; Bayer, India; Bayer Diagnostics, Irl.; Bayer Diagnostici, Ital.; Bayer Diagnostics, Mex.; Bayer, NZ; Bayer Diagnostics, UK; Bayer, USA.
Test for glucose in urine (p.1694·2).

**Diastone** Microsules, Arg.
Diclofenac sodium (p.32·1).
*Fever; inflammation; pain.*

**Diastop** Pacific, NZ.
Diphenoxylate hydrochloride (p.1261·3).
Atropine sulfate (p.477·1) is included in this preparation to discourage abuse.
*Diarrhoea.*

**Diatabs** Biomedis, Hong Kong.
Attapulgite (p.1251·1).
*Diarrhoea.*

**Diatec** Neckerman, Braz.†.
Meloxicam (p.56·1).

**Diatelan** Reuffer, Mex.†.
Tolbutamide (p.348·1).
*Diabetes mellitus.*

**Diatex** Medix, Mex.
Diazepam (p.690·1).
*Anxiety.*

**Diathynil** Sigma-Tau, Ital.
Biotin (p.1423·2).
*Skin disorders.*

**Diatil** Mer-National, S.Afr.†.
Diltiazem hydrochloride (p.900·1).
*Angina pectoris; hypertension.*

**Diatin** Ferrer, Spain.
Elcatonin (p.768·3).
*Hypercalcaemia; osteoporosis; Paget's disease of bone.*

**Diatol**
Pacific, Hong Kong; Pacific, NZ.
Tolbutamide (p.348·1).
*Diabetes mellitus.*

**Diatolil** Fardi, Spain†.
Buphenine hydrochloride (p.1663·2).
*Dysmenorrhoea; peripheral and cerebral circulatory disorders.*

**Diatracin** Dista, Spain.
Vancomycin hydrochloride (p.275·2).
*Bacterial infections.*

**Diatrum** Romilo, Canad.†.
Multivitamin and mineral preparation (p.1417·1).

**Diatussin** Propan, S.Afr.
Diphenhydramine hydrochloride (p.431·3); sodium citrate (p.1223·2); menthol (p.1711·3); ammonium chloride (p.1115·2); theophylline (p.798·3).
*Coughs.*

**Diatx** Pan American, USA.
Vitamin B substances and vitamin C (p.1417·1).

**Diatx Fe** Pan American, USA.
Vitamin B substances; vitamin C; ferrous fumarate (p.1417·1).

**Diaval** Valdecasas, Mex.
Tolbutamide (p.348·1).
*Diabetes mellitus.*

**Dia-Vite** R&D, Canad.†.
Vitamin B substances with ascorbic acid (p.1417·1).

**Diawern** Wernigerode, Ger.†.
Crataegus (p.1677·1); valerian (p.1762·2).
*Heart failure.*

**Diaz** Taro, Israel.
Diazepam (p.690·1).
*Anxiety; insomnia; skeletal muscle spasm.*

**Diazelong** Cazi, Braz.†.
Diazepam (p.690·1).
*Alcohol withdrawal syndrome; anxiety; epilepsy; insomnia; sedative; skeletal muscle spasm.*

**Diazemuls**
Pharmacia, Austral.†; Pharmacia, Canad.; Pharmacia, Hong Kong; Dumex, Irl.; Teva, Ital.; CSL, NZ; Dumex, NZ; Alpharma, UK.
Diazepam (p.690·1).
*Alcohol withdrawal syndrome; anxiety; convulsions; premedication; sedative; status epilepticus; skeletal muscle spasm; tetanus.*

**Diazep** CT, Ger.; ABZ, Ger.
Diazepam (p.690·1).
*Anxiety; premedication; skeletal muscle spasm; status epilepticus.*

**Diazepan** Cazi, Braz.; Sigma, Braz.
Diazepam (p.690·1).
*Anxiety.*

**Diazol** EMS, Braz.
Co-trimoxazole (p.199·3); calcium carbonate (p.1254·2); attapulgite (p.1251·1).
*Diarrhoea.*

**Diazolen** Degorts, Mex.
Mebendazole (p.108·2).
*Worm infections.*

**Diazon**
Unison, Hong Kong; Unison, Singapore; Unison, Thai.
Ketoconazole (p.403·3).
*Fungal infections; seborrhoeic dermatitis.*

**Diba** Manetti Roberts, Ital.
Glutaral (p.1180·3).
*Instrument disinfection; surface disinfection.*

**Dibacilina** Diba, Mex.
Ampicillin trihydrate (p.157·2).
*Bacterial infections.*

**Dibagesic** Diba, Mex.†.
Dextropropoxyphene (p.28·3).
*Pain.*

**Diban** *Wyeth-Ayerst, Canad.†.*
Activated attapulgite (p.1251·1); pectin (p.1580·3); prepared opium (p.74·2); hyoscyamine sulfate (p.485·1); atropine sulfate (p.477·1); hyoscine hydrobromide (p.483·3).
*Diarrhoea.*

**Dibapec Compuesto** *Diba, Mex.*
Furazolidone (p.605·2); kaolin (p.1268·3); pectin (p.1580·3).
*Diarrhoea.*

**Dibaprim** *Diba, Mex.*
Co-trimoxazole (p.199·3).
*Bacterial infections.*

**Dibasona** *Diba, Mex.*
Dexamethasone sodium phosphate (p.1097·2).
*Corticosteroid.*

**Dibasul** *Diba, Mex.†.*
Sulfamethoxypyridazine (p.263·1).
*Bacterial infections.*

**Dibaterr** *Diba, Mex.*
Tetracycline hydrochloride (p.266·2).
*Bacterial infections.*

**Dibecon** *Pharmasant, Thai.*
Chlorpropamide (p.330·3).
*Diabetes mellitus.*

**Dibelet**
*Atlantic, Malaysia; Atlantic, Singapore; Atlantic, Thai.*
Glibenclamide (p.331·2).
*Diabetes mellitus.*

**Dibendril** *EMS, Braz.†.*
Ampicillin benzathine (p.158·1); ampicillin sodium (p.157·1).
*Bacterial infections.*

**Dibendyl** *Malaysia Chemist, Singapore.*
Diphenhydramine hydrochloride (p.431·3); ammonium chloride (p.1115·2).
*Coughs; respiratory-tract congestion; sneezing.*

**Dibendyl Forte CD** *Malaysia Chemist, Singapore.*
Diphenhydramine hydrochloride (p.431·3); codeine phosphate (p.27·1); ammonium chloride (p.1115·2); sodium citrate (p.1223·2).
*Coughs; respiratory-tract congestion; sneezing.*

**Dibent** *Hauck, USA.*
Dicycloverine hydrochloride (p.481·2).
*Functional bowel/irritable bowel syndrome.*

**Dibenyline**
*Link, Austral.; SmithKline Beecham, Belg.†; IFET (ΙΦΕΤ), Gr.; Goldshield, Hong Kong; Goldshield, Israel; SmithKline Beecham, Neth.; Link, NZ; Forley, UK.*
Phenoxybenzamine hydrochloride (p.981·2).
*Benign prostatic hyperplasia; neurogenic bladder; phaeochromocytoma; shock.*

**Dibenzyline** *Wellspring, USA.*
Phenoxybenzamine hydrochloride (p.981·2).
*Phaeochromocytoma.*

**Dibenzyran**
*Procter & Gamble, Austria; Esparma, Ger.*
Phenoxybenzamine hydrochloride (p.981·2).
*Neurogenic bladder; phaeochromocytoma.*

**Dibertil** *Sandipro, Belg.*
Metoclopramide hydrochloride (p.1274·3).
*Adjunct in gastrointestinal examination; gastrointestinal motility disorders; nausea and vomiting.*

**Dibetasol** *Shin Poong, Singapore.*
Betamethasone dipropionate (p.1093·1); betamethasone sodium phosphate (p.1093·1).
*Parenteral corticosteroid.*

**Dibetid** *Arlex, Mex.†.*
Glibenclamide (p.331·2).
*Diabetes mellitus.*

**Dibetop** *Davi, Port.*
Betamethasone dipropionate (p.1093·1).
*Skin disorders.*

**Dibetop Q** *Davi, Port.*
Betamethasone dipropionate (p.1093·1); salicylic acid (p.1157·1).
*Skin disorders.*

**Dibilan F** *Byk Gulden, Mex.†.*
Bumadizone (p.21·3).

**Dibional** *Rivero, Arg.*
Amoxicillin trihydrate (p.155·3); potassium clavulanate (p.193·3).
*Bacterial infections.*

**Dibistic** *Elvetium, Arg.*
Didanosine (p.630·3).
*HIV infection.*

**Diblocin** *AstraZeneca, Ger.*
Doxazosin mesilate (p.908·3).
*Benign prostatic hyperplasia; hypertension.*

**Dibondrin** *Montavit, Austria.*
Diphenhydramine hydrochloride (p.431·3).
*Hypersensitivity disorders; prophylaxis against anaphylactic shock; sedative.*

**Dibro-Be Mono** *Dibropharm, Ger.*
Potassium bromide (p.1663·1).
*Epilepsy.*

**Dibromol** *Trommsdorff, Ger.*
Sodium 3,5-dibromo-4-hydroxybenzenesulphonate; bromchlorophen (p.1171·1); isopropyl alcohol (p.1184·3).
*Skin disinfection; wounds.*

**Dibroxin** *Tecnofarma, Mex.*
Bromhexine (p.1115·3).
*Respiratory-tract congestion.*

**Dibtrigen** *Diba, Mex.*
Vitamin and mineral preparation (p.1417·1).

**Dibufen** *Diba, Mex.*
Ibuprofen (p.45·3).
*Inflammation; musculoskeletal, joint and peri-articular disorders; pain.*

**Dibunafon** *Alpes Chemie, Chile.*
Sodium dibunate (p.1130·2); chlorphenamine maleate (p.427·3); paracetamol (p.76·2); sodium benzoate (p.1169·3).
*Coughs.*

**Dical**
*Note. This name is used for preparations of different composition.*
*Abbott, Mex.*
Calcium carbonate (p.1254·2); colecalciferol (p.1461·3).
*Calcium and vitamin D deficiency; calcium and vitamin D supplement.*

*Abbott, USA.*
Calcium with vitamin D and phosphorus (p.1417·1).
*Calcium deficiency; dietary supplement.*

**Di-Calcii-Plex** *Khandelwal, India.*
Multivitamin and mineral preparation (p.1417·1).

**Dicalcium** *Abiogen, Ital.*
Vitamin A palmitate (p.1453·1); colecalciferol (p.1461·3); calcium carbonate (p.1254·2).
*Vitamin or mineral deficiency.*

**Dical-D**
*Note. This name is used for preparations of different composition.*
*Abbott, Chile.*
Calcium carbonate (p.1254·2); colecalciferol (p.1461·3).
*Calcium and vitamin D deficiency; hypocalcaemia; osteomalacia; osteoporosis; rickets.*

*Abbott, Hong Kong.*
Calcium with vitamin D and phosphorus (p.1417·1).
*Dietary supplement.*

**Dicalm** *Mavena, Switz.*
Valerian (p.1762·2); lupulus (p.1708·1); ballota; passion flower (p.1729·1).
*Anxiety; nervousness.*

**Dicalmir** *Dicofarm, Ital.*
Fennel (p.1687·2); chamomile (p.1669·3); aniseed (p.1655·2); liquorice (p.1270·2); cumin; coriander (p.1676·1).
*Colic; meteorism.*

**Dicalys 11** *Dicamed, Swed.*
Sodium chloride; potassium chloride; calcium chloride; magnesium chloride; sodium lactate; glucose (p.1221·1).
*Haemofiltration.*

**Dicalys 17** *Dicamed, Swed.*
Sodium chloride; potassium chloride; calcium chloride; magnesium chloride; sodium lactate (p.1221·1).
*Haemofiltration.*

**Dicap** *Pacific, NZ.*
Loperamide hydrochloride (p.1271·1).
*Diarrhoea.*

**Dicavin** *Quimica y Farmacia, Mex.†.*
Difenidol (p.1261·1).
*Nausea and vomiting.*

**Dicentril** *Degorts, Mex.*
Aluminium (p.1652·2); magnesium (p.1227·3).
*Gastrointestinal hyperacidity.*

**Dicepin B6** *Ipsen, Spain†.*
Diazepam (p.690·1).
Contains pyridoxine hydrochloride.
*Alcohol withdrawal syndrome; anxiety; febrile convulsions; insomnia; skeletal muscle spasm.*

**Dicetel**
*Raffo, Arg.; Solvay, Austria; Solvay, Belg.; Byk, Braz.; Solvay, Canad.; Solvay, Fr.; Solvay, Gr.; Solvay, Hong Kong†; Solvay, Ital.; Byk Gulden, Mex.; Solvay, Neth.†; Solvay, Port.; Solvay, Switz.; Solvay, Thai.*
Pinaverium bromide (p.1732·1).
*Biliary-tract disorders; irritable bowel syndrome; preparation for barium enema; smooth muscle spasm.*

**Dicfafena** *IQFA, Mex.*
Diclofenac (p.32·1).
*Inflammation; musculoskeletal and joint disorders; pain.*

**Dichlor-Stapenor** *Bayer, Ger.†.*
Dicloxacillin sodium (p.205·2).
*Benzylpenicillin-resistant staphylococcal infections.*

**Dichlotride**
*Merck Sharp & Dohme, Austral.; Merck Sharp & Dohme, Belg.†; Merck Sharp & Dohme, Denm.; Merck Sharp & Dohme, Malaysia; Merck Sharp & Dohme, Neth.†; Merck Sharp & Dohme, Norw.†; Merck Sharp & Dohme, Port.; Merck Sharp & Dohme, S.Afr.†; Merck Sharp & Dohme, Swed.†; Merck Sharp & Dohme, Thai.*
Hydrochlorothiazide (p.933·2).
*Hypertension; oedema; premenstrual syndrome.*

**Dicillin** *Durascan, Denm.*
Dicloxacillin sodium (p.205·2).
*Bacterial infections.*

**Dicinone**
*Sanofi Synthelabo, Braz.*
Etamsylate (p.749·3).
*Haemorrhage.*

*Pensa, Spain.*
Etamsylate (p.749·3).
*Haemorrhage.*

**Dicitrate** *Pharmascience, Singapore.*
Sodium citrate (p.1223·2); citric acid monohydrate (p.1673·1).
*Acid aspiration; acidosis; gout; renal calculi.*

**Diclac**
*Hexal, Arg.; Hexal, Austral.; Hexal, Austria; Hexal, Braz.; Hexal, Ger.; Rowex, Irl.*
Diclofenac (p.32·1) or diclofenac sodium (p.32·1).
*Gout; inflammation; musculoskeletal, joint, peri-articular, and soft-tissue disorders; pain.*

**Dicladox** *Elvetium, Arg.*
Doxorubicin (p.547·3).
*Malignant neoplasms.*

**Diclamina** *Esteve, Spain.*
Cinnarizine (p.428·3); heptaminol acefyllinate (p.786·3).
*Vascular headache; vertigo.*

**Diclanil** *Condrugs, Thai.*
Glibenclamide (p.331·2).
*Diabetes mellitus.*

**Diclax** *Douglas, NZ.*
Diclofenac sodium (p.32·1).
*Osteoarthritis; rheumatoid arthritis.*

**Diclaxol** *Hexal, Austria.*
Diclofenac sodium (p.32·1).
*Gout; inflammation; musculoskeletal, joint, and peri-articular disorders; pain.*

**Diclectin** *Duchesnay, Canad.*
Doxylamine succinate (p.432·3); pyridoxine hydrochloride (p.1456·3).
*Nausea and vomiting of pregnancy.*

**Diclen** *Frasca, Arg.*
Clonixin lysine (p.26·3).
*Fever; inflammation; pain.*

**Diclex** *Meiji, Thai.*
Dicloxacillin sodium (p.205·2).
*Bacterial infections.*

**Diclo**
*Note. This name is used for preparations of different composition.*
*Uniao Quimica, Braz.†.*
Quinine dihydrochloride (p.460·1).
*Arrhythmias.*

*Kade, Ger.; CT, Ger.; Betapharm, Ger.; ABZ, Ger.; Eu Rho, Ger.; Sudmedica, Ger.; 1A, Ger.; Wolff, Ger.; Ratiopharm, Ger.†; Pinewood, Irl.; Cophar, Switz.*
Diclofenac sodium (p.32·1).
*Gout; inflammation; musculoskeletal, joint, peri-articular, and soft-tissue disorders; pain.*

*FIRMA, Ital.†.*
Dicloxacillin sodium (p.205·2).
*Bacterial infections.*

**Diclo P** *Uniao Quimica, Braz.*
Diclofenac potassium (p.32·1).

**Diclo-B** *Lannacher, Austria.*
Diclofenac sodium (p.32·1); thiamine hydrochloride (p.1455·1); pyridoxine hydrochloride (p.1456·3); cyanocobalamin (p.1458·2).
*Gout; musculoskeletal, joint, and peri-articular disorders; neuralgia; neuritis; pain.*

**diclo-basan** *Schonenberger, Switz.*
Diclofenac sodium (p.32·1).
*Gout; inflammation; musculoskeletal and joint disorders; pain; soft-tissue injuries.*

**Diclobene** *Ratiopharm, Austria.*
Diclofenac potassium (p.32·1) or diclofenac sodium (p.32·1).
*Gout; inflammation; musculoskeletal, joint, peri-articular, and soft-tissue disorders; pain; renal and biliary colic.*

**Diclocil**
*Bristol-Myers Squibb, Austral.; Bristol-Myers Squibb, Denm.; Bristol-Myers Squibb, Fin.; Bristol-Myers Squibb, Gr.; Bristol-Myers Squibb, Hong Kong†; Bristol-Myers Squibb, Norw.; Bristol-Myers Squibb, NZ; Bristol-Myers Squibb, Port.; Bristol-Myers Squibb, Swed.; Bristol-Myers Squibb, Thai.*
Dicloxacillin sodium (p.205·2).
*Bacterial infections.*

**Diclocillin** *TO-Chemicals, Thai.*
Dicloxacillin sodium (p.205·2).
*Bacterial infections.*

**Diclocular** *Angelini, Ital.*
Diclofenac sodium (p.32·1).
*Pain and inflammation of the eye.*

**Diclodan** *Pharmacodane, Denm.*
Diclofenac (p.32·1).
*Gout; inflammation; musculoskeletal and joint disorders; pain.*

**Diclo-Denk**
*Denk, Hong Kong; Denk, Singapore.*
Diclofenac sodium (p.32·1).
*Gout; inflammation; musculoskeletal, joint, and soft-tissue disorders.*

**Dicloderm Forte** *Cruz, Spain.*
Dichlorisone acetate (p.1099·3).
*Skin disorders.*

**Diclo-Divido** *Alpharma-Isis, Ger.*
Diclofenac sodium (p.32·1).
*Gout; inflammation; musculoskeletal, joint, and soft-tissue disorders.*

**Diclodoc** *Docpharm, Ger.*
Diclofenac sodium (p.32·1).
*Gout; inflammation; musculoskeletal, joint, and soft-tissue disorders.*

**Diclodol** *IPFI, Ital.†.*
Diclofenac sodium (p.32·1).
*Inflammation; musculoskeletal and joint disorders; pain.*

**Diclofan** *Boniscontro & Gazzone, Ital.*
Diclofenac sodium (p.32·1).
*Inflammation; musculoskeletal and joint disorders; pain.*

**Diclofen**
*Pharmacia, Braz.*
Diclofenac potassium (p.32·1).
*Gout; inflammation; musculoskeletal, joint, and peri-articular disorders; pain.*

*Jean-Marie, Hong Kong; Berlin Pharm, Thai.*
Diclofenac sodium (p.32·1).
*Inflammation; musculoskeletal, joint, peri-articular, and soft-tissue disorders; pain.*

**Diclofenax** *Infabra, Braz.†.*
Diclofenac potassium (p.32·1).

**Diclofenbeta** *Betapharm, Ger.*
Diclofenac sodium (p.32·1).
*Gout; inflammation; musculoskeletal, joint, and soft-tissue disorders; pain.*

**Diclofetamol** *Ducto, Braz.*
Caffeine (p.782·1); carisoprodol (p.1392·1); diclofenac sodium (p.32·1); paracetamol (p.76·2).

**Dicloflam** *Garec, S.Afr.*
Diclofenac sodium (p.32·1).
*Inflammation; musculoskeletal and joint disorders; pain.*

**Dicloflex** *Dexcel, UK.*
Diclofenac sodium (p.32·1).
*Gout; inflammation; musculoskeletal, joint, peri-articular, and soft-tissue disorders; pain.*

**Dicloftal** *Lepori, Port.*
Diclofenac sodium (p.32·1).
*Inflammatory eye disorders.*

**Dicloftil** *Farmigea, Ital.*
Diclofenac sodium (p.32·1).
*Inflammatory eye disorders.*

**Diclogea** *Gea, Denm.*
Diclofenac sodium (p.32·1).
*Gout; inflammation; musculoskeletal and joint disorders; pain.*

**Diclogel** *Polipharm, Thai.*
Diclofenac diethylamine (p.32·1).
*Inflammation; pain.*

**Diclogenom** *Genom, Braz.*
Diclofenac sodium (p.32·1).
*Eye disorders.*

**Diclogenta** *Centaur, India.*
Diclofenac sodium (p.32·1); gentamicin sulfate (p.217·1).
*Infected inflammatory eye disorders.*

**Diclogesic**
*TRB, Arg.; Dar Al Dawa, Hong Kong.*
Diclofenac diethylamine (p.32·1) or diclofenac sodium (p.32·1).
*Biliary and renal colic; gout; inflammation; musculoskeletal, joint, peri-articular, and soft-tissue disorders; pain.*

**Diclogesic Relax** *TRB, Arg.*
Diclofenac sodium (p.32·1); pridinol mesilate (p.1395·2).
*Musculoskeletal and joint disorders.*

**Diclogrand** *Ahimsa, Arg.*
Diclofenac (p.32·1).
*Inflammation; pain.*

**Diclogrun** *Grunenthal, Ger.†.*
Diclofenac sodium (p.32·1).
*Inflammatory eye disorders.*

**Diclohexal**
*Hexal, Austral.; Hexal, S.Afr.*
Diclofenac sodium (p.32·1).
*Gout; inflammation; musculoskeletal and joint disorders; pain.*

**Diclokin** *Kinder, Braz.*
Chloroquine phosphate (p.448·2).
*Malaria.*

**Diclolan** *Olan-Kemed, Thai.*
Diclofenac sodium (p.32·1).
*Musculoskeletal, joint, and peri-articular disorders.*

**Diclomar** *Mar, Arg.*
Diclofenac (p.32·1).
*Inflammation; pain.*

**Diclomar Flex** *Mar, Arg.*
Diclofenac (p.32·1); pridinol (p.1395·2).
*Inflammation; muscle spasm; pain.*

**Diclomax** *Provalis, UK.*
Diclofenac sodium (p.32·1).
*Inflammation; musculoskeletal, joint, peri-articular and soft-tissue disorders; pain.*

**Diclomel** *Clonmel, Irl.*
Diclofenac sodium (p.32·1).
*Gout; musculoskeletal and joint disorders; pain.*

**Diclomelan** *Lannacher, Austria.*
Diclofenac sodium (p.32·1).
*Gout; inflammation; musculoskeletal, joint, and peri-articular disorders; pain; renal and biliary colic.*

**Diclomerck** *Merck, Ger.†.*
Diclofenac sodium (p.32·1).
*Gout; inflammation; musculoskeletal and joint disorders; pain.*

**Diclometin** *Pharmacia, Fin.*
Diclofenac sodium (p.32·1).
*Musculoskeletal and joint disorders; pain.*

**Diclomex** *Ratiopharm, Fin.*
Diclofenac potassium (p.32·1) or diclofenac sodium (p.32·1).
*Inflammation; musculoskeletal and joint disorders; pain.*

**Diclomin** *Atlantis, Mex.*
Dicycloverine hydrochloride (p.481·2).
*Gastrointestinal spasm and hypermotility.*

**Diclomol**
*Note. This name is used for preparations of different composition.*
*Win-Medicare, India.*
*Injection; slow-release tablets:* Diclofenac sodium (p.32·1).
*Tablets:* Diclofenac sodium (p.32·1); paracetamol (p.76·2).
*Gout; inflammation; musculoskeletal and joint disorders; pain.*
*Win-Medicare, Thai.*
Diclofenac diethylamine (p.32·1) or diclofenac sodium (p.32·1).
*Inflammation; musculoskeletal and joint disorders; pain.*

**Diclon** *Durascan, Denm.*
Diclofenac sodium (p.32·1).
*Gout; inflammation; musculoskeletal and joint disorders; pain.*

**Diclonac** *Lupin, India.*
Diclofenac sodium (p.32·1).
*Gout; musculoskeletal and joint disorders; pain.*

**Diclophlogont**
*Azupharma, Ger.; Novartis, Gr.*
Diclofenac sodium (p.32·1).
*Gout; inflammation; musculoskeletal, joint, peri-articular, and soft-tissue disorders; pain.*

**Dicloplast** *CTI, Israel.*
Diclofenac epolamine (p.33·1).
*Inflammation; musculoskeletal and joint disorders; pain.*

**Diclo-Puren** *Alpharma-Isis, Ger.*
Diclofenac sodium (p.32·1).
*Inflammation; musculoskeletal, joint, peri-articular, and soft-tissue disorders; pain.*

**Dicloral** *Formenti, Ital.*
Diclofenac (p.32·1) or diclofenac sodium (p.32·1).
*Mouth and throat disorders.*

**Dicloran**
*Unique, India; Randall, Mex.*
Diclofenac diethylamine (p.32·1) or diclofenac sodium (p.32·1).
*Gout; inflammation; musculoskeletal, joint, peri-articular, and soft-tissue disorders; pain.*

**Dicloran-A** *Unique, India.*
Diclofenac sodium (p.32·1); paracetamol (p.76·2).
*Gout; musculoskeletal and joint disorders.*

**Diclorektal** *Sanorania, Ger.†.*
Diclofenac sodium (p.32·1).
*Gout; inflammation; musculoskeletal and joint disorders.*

**Diclorengel** *Trima, Israel.*
Diclofenac sodium (p.32·1).
*Inflammation; musculoskeletal and joint disorders; pain.*

**Dicloreum** *Wassermann, Ital.*
Diclofenac epolamine (p.33·1) or diclofenac sodium (p.32·1).
*Inflammation; musculoskeletal, joint, and peri-articular disorders; pain.*

**Diclo-saar** *Chephasaar, Ger.*
Diclofenac sodium (p.32·1).
*Gout; inflammation; musculoskeletal, joint, and soft-tissue disorders; pain.*

**Diclosian** *Asian Pharm, Thai.*
Diclofenac sodium (p.32·1).
*Musculoskeletal, joint, and peri-articular disorders.*

**Diclosifar** *Siphar, Switz.*
Diclofenac sodium (p.32·1).
*Gout; inflammation; musculoskeletal and joint disorders; oedema; pain.*

**Dicloson** *Unison, Thai.*
Dicloxacillin sodium (p.205·2).
*Bacterial infections.*

**Diclo-Spondyril** *Orion, Ger.†.*
Diclofenac sodium (p.32·1).
*Acute gout; inflammation; neuralgia; neuritis; pain; rheumatic disorders; soft-tissue disorders.*

**Diclostad** *Stada, Austria.*
Diclofenac sodium (p.32·1).
*Gout; inflammation; musculoskeletal, joint, peri-articular, and soft-tissue disorders; pain; renal and biliary colic.*

**Diclosyl** *Medicopharm, Austria.*
Diclofenac sodium (p.32·1).
*Musculoskeletal, joint, peri-articular, and soft-tissue disorders.*

**Diclo-Tablinen** *Sanorania, Ger.†.*
Diclofenac sodium (p.32·1).
*Gout; inflammation; musculoskeletal and joint disorders.*

**Diclotard** *Galen, UK†.*
Diclofenac sodium (p.32·1).
*Inflammation; musculoskeletal, joint, peri-articular, and soft-tissue disorders; pain.*

**Diclotec**
*Technilab, Canad.*
Diclofenac sodium (p.32·1).
*Inflammation; pain.*
*Lepori, Port.*
Diclofenac sodium (p.32·1).
Misoprostol (p.1519·2) is included in this preparation in an attempt to limit adverse effects on the gastrointestinal mucosa.
*Osteoarthritis; rheumatoid arthritis.*

**Diclo-Tecno** *Tecnofarma, Mex.*
Dicloxacillin (p.205·2).
*Staphylococcal infections.*

**Diclotride** *Merck Sharp & Dohme, Mex.†.*
Hydrochlorothiazide (p.933·2).
*Hypertension; oedema.*

**Diclovit** *Lannacher, Austria.*
Diclofenac sodium (p.32·1); thiamine hydrochloride (p.1455·1); pyridoxine hydrochloride (p.1456·3); cyanocobalamin (p.1458·2).
*Gout; musculoskeletal, joint, and soft-tissue disorders; neuralgia; neuritis.*

**Diclovol** *Arun, UK.*
Diclofenac sodium (p.32·1).
*Gout; musculoskeletal, joint, peri-articular, and soft-tissue disorders; pain.*

**Diclowal**
*Ritter, Hong Kong; Ritter, Singapore.*
Diclofenac sodium (p.32·1).
*Gout; inflammation; musculoskeletal and joint disorders; pain.*

**Diclox** *PP Lab, Thai.*
Dicloxacillin sodium (p.205·2).
*Bacterial infections.*

**Dicloxia** *Asian Pharm, Thai.*
Dicloxacillin sodium (p.205·2).
*Bacterial infections.*

**Dicloxin** *Olan-Kemed, Thai.*
Dicloxacillin sodium (p.205·2).
*Bacterial infections.*

**Dicloxman** *T Man, Thai.*
Dicloxacillin sodium (p.205·2).
*Gram-positive bacterial infections.*

**Dicloxno** *Milano, Thai.*
Dicloxacillin sodium (p.205·2).
*Bacterial infections.*

**Dicloxsig** *Sigma, Austral.*
Dicloxacillin sodium (p.205·2).
*Gram-positive bacterial infections.*

**Diclozip** *Ashbourne, UK.*
Diclofenac sodium (p.32·1).
*Inflammation; pain.*

**Dicodid**
*Abbott, Ger.; Knoll, Switz.*
Hydrocodone hydrochloride (p.45·1) or hydrocodone tartrate (p.45·1).
*Coughs; pain.*

**Dicodin** *Viatris, Fr.*
Dihydrocodeine tartrate (p.34·3).
*Pain.*

**Dicodral** *Dicofarm, Ital.*
Sodium chloride; potassium chloride; sodium bicarbonate or sodium citrate; glucose (p.1222·2).
*Diarrhoea; oral rehydration therapy.*

**Dicofan** *Rivero, Arg.*
Sodium phosphate (p.1231·1).
*Bowel evacuation.*

**Dicofarm** *Continentales, Mex.†.*
Pipemidic acid (p.243·1).

**Dicoflor** *Dicofarm, Ital.*
Food containing lactic-acid-producing organisms (p.1704·2).
*Disturbances of the gastrointestinal flora.*

**Dicogel** *Mintlab, Chile.*
Diclofenac diethylamine (p.32·1).
*Inflammation.*

**Dicoman** *Dicofarm, Ital.*
Dietary fibre supplement (p.1417·1).

**Dicomin** *Berlin Pharm, Thai.*
Dicycloverine hydrochloride (p.481·2).
*Gastrointestinal spasm.*

**Diconal**
*Wellcome, Irl.; CeNeS, UK.*
Dipipanone hydrochloride (p.35·3); cyclizine hydrochloride (p.429·3).
*Pain.*

**Diconpin** *TAD, Ger.*
Isosorbide dinitrate (p.941·1).
*Angina pectoris; heart failure; pulmonary hypertension.*

**Dicopac** *Nycomed Amersham, UK.*
1 capsule, cyanocobalamin (cobalt-57) (p.1523·2); 1 capsule, cyanocobalamin (cobalt-58) (p.1523·2); 1 ampoule, cyanocobalamin (p.1458·2).
*Diagnosis of vitamin $B_{12}$ malabsorption.*

**Dicoplus** *Dicofarm, Ital.*
Glucomannan (p.1693·3).
*Constipation; diverticulitis; irritable bowel syndrome.*

**Dicorantil** *Aventis, Braz.*
Disopyramide phosphate (p.903·3).
*Arrhythmias.*

**Dicortal** *Avantgarde, Ital.*
Diflucortolone valerate (p.1099·3).
*Skin disorders.*

**Dicorten** *Trima, Israel.*
Betamethasone dipropionate (p.1093·1).
*Skin disorders.*

**Dicorvin** *ICN, Spain.*
Acetylspiramycin (p.256·1).
*Bacterial infections.*

**Dicorynan** *Aventis, Spain.*
Disopyramide (p.903·3).
*Arrhythmias.*

**Dicton** *Dolorgiet, Ger.†.*
Codeine polistirex (p.27·3).
*Coughs.*

**Dicynene**
*Sanofi Synthelabo, Irl.; Sanofi Synthelabo, UK.*
Etamsylate (p.749·3).
*Menorrhagia; periventricular haemorrhage.*

**Dicynone**
*Sanofi Synthelabo, Belg.; Sanofi Synthelabo, Fr.; Sanofi Synthelabo, Ital.; Knoll, Mex.; Sanofi Synthelabo, Singapore†; OM, Switz.*
Etamsylate (p.749·3).
*Haemorrhagic disorders; menorrhagia; metrorrhagia.*

**Didamega** *Larkhall Laboratories, UK.*
Multivitamin and mineral preparation (p.1417·1).

**Di-Delamine** *Del, USA; Commerce, USA.*
Diphenhydramine hydrochloride (p.431·3); tripelennamine hydrochloride (p.442·3).
*Pruritus.*

**Didor** *Viatris, Port.*
Dihydrocodeine tartrate (p.34·3).
*Pain.*

**Didralin**
*Medochemie, Singapore†; Medochemie, Thai.†.*
Hydrochlorothiazide (p.933·2).
*Heart failure; hypertension; oedema.*

**Didrex** *Upjohn, USA.*
Benzfetamine hydrochloride (p.1585·2).
*Obesity.*

**Didrica** *Pensa, Spain.*
Calcium chloride; potassium chloride; sodium chloride; sodium lactate; glucose (p.1222·2).
*Oral rehydration therapy.*

**Didrocal**
*Pharmacia, Austral.; Procter & Gamble, Canad.*
White tablets, disodium etidronate (p.771·2); blue tablets, calcium carbonate (p.1254·2).
*Osteoporosis.*

**Didrogyl** *Bruno, Ital.*
Calcifediol (p.1461·2).
*Hypocalcaemia; hypoparathyroidism; osteomalacia; osteoporosis; renal osteodystrophy; rickets.*

**Didro-Kit** *Procter & Gamble, Ital.†.*
White tablets, disodium etidronate (p.771·2); blue tablets, calcium carbonate (p.1254·2).
*Osteoporosis.*

**Didrokit** *Procter & Gamble, Neth.*
Tablets, disodium etidronate (Didronel) (p.771·2); tablets, calcium carbonate (Cacit) (p.1254·2).
*Osteoporosis.*

**Didronate**
*Procter & Gamble, Denm.; Roche, Fin.; Procter & Gamble, Norw.†; Roche, Swed.*
Disodium etidronate (p.771·2).
*Ectopic ossification; osteoporosis; Paget's disease of bone.*

**Didronate Calcium** *Procter & Gamble, Denm.*
14 Tablets, disodium etidronate (p.771·2); 76 tablets, calcium carbonate (p.1254·2).
*Osteoporosis.*

**Didronate + Calcium**
*Roche, Fin.; Roche, Swed.*
14 Tablets, disodium etidronate (p.771·2) (Didronate); 76 tablets, calcium carbonate (p.1254·2).
*Osteoporosis.*

**Didronate + Calsium** *Procter & Gamble, Norw.*
14 Didronate tablets, disodium etidronate (p.771·2); 76 calcium tablets, calcium carbonate (p.1254·2).
*Osteoporosis.*

**Didronel**
*Pharmacia, Austral.; Aventis, Austria; Procter & Gamble, Belg.; Procter & Gamble, Canad.; Knoll, Canad.; Procter & Gamble, Fr.; Procter & Gamble, Ger.; Procter & Gamble, Hong Kong; Procter & Gamble, Irl.; Procter & Gamble, Israel; Procter & Gamble, Ital.; Sumitomo, Jpn; Pharmacia Upjohn, NZ†; Normal, Port.; Boehringer Mannheim, S.Afr.†; Vifor, Switz.; Procter & Gamble, UK; Procter & Gamble, USA; MGI, USA.*
Disodium etidronate (p.771·2).
*Ectopic ossification; hypercalcaemia of malignancy; osteoporosis; Paget's disease of bone.*

**Didronel Kit** *Aventis, Ger.; Procter & Gamble, Ger.*
White tablets, disodium etidronate (p.771·2); blue tablets, calcium carbonate (p.1254·2).
*Osteoporosis.*

**Didronel PMO**
*Procter & Gamble, Irl.; Procter & Gamble, UK.*
Tablets, disodium etidronate (Didronel) (p.771·2); tablets, calcium carbonate (Cacit) (p.1254·2).
*Osteoporosis.*

**Diele** *Diele, Fr.†.*
Food for special diets (p.1417·1).
*A range of foods for patients with amino acid metabolic disorders.*

**Diemil** *Almirall, Spain.*
Dihydroergocristine mesilate (p.1680·1); piracetam (p.1732·1).
*Cerebrovascular disorders; head injury.*

**Diemon** *Pharmacia, Arg.*
Tamoxifen citrate (p.584·1).
*Breast cancer.*

**Dienpax** *Sanofi Synthelabo, Braz.*
Diazepam (p.690·1).
*Alcohol withdrawal syndrome; anxiety; epilepsy; insomnia; premedication; sedative; skeletal muscle spasm; tetanus.*

**Dientrin** *Sanofi Synthelabo, Braz.*
Co-trimoxazole (p.199·3).
Formerly contained co-trimoxazole, attapulgite, and calcium carbonate.
*Diarrhoea.*

**Diergo** *Novartis, Belg.*
Dihydroergotamine mesilate (p.465·3).
Formerly contained dihydroergotamine mesilate and caffeine.
*Migraine.*

**Diergospray** *Novartis, Fr.*
Dihydroergotamine mesilate (p.465·3); caffeine (p.782·1).
*Migraine.*

**Diertina**
*Mundipharma, Austria†; Monsanto, Ital.; Sankyo, Port.; Poli, Switz.†.*
Dihydroergocristine mesilate (p.1680·1).
*Cerebral and peripheral vascular disorders; dopamine deficiency; headache; hypertension; migraine; tinnitus; vertigo.*

**Diertine** *Yamanouchi, Spain.*
Dihydroergocristine mesilate (p.1680·1).
*Cerebrovascular disorders; tinnitus; vascular eye disorders; vertigo.*

**Di-Ertride** *Malaysia Chemist, Singapore.*
Hydrochlorothiazide (p.933·2).
*Diabetes insipidus; hypertension; oedema.*

**Diesan** *CT, Ital.*
Fluoxetine hydrochloride (p.292·1).
*Bulimia nervosa; depression; obsessive-compulsive disorders.*

**Diesel** *Neves, Port.†.*
Multivitamin and mineral preparation (p.1417·1).

**Diespor** *Biomedica, Ital.*
Cefonicid sodium (p.174·2).
Lidocaine hydrochloride (p.1377·3) is included in this preparation to alleviate the pain of injection.
*Gram-negative bacterial infections.*

**Diestet** *Searle, Mex.*
Mazindol (p.1589·1).
*Obesity.*

**Diet Ayds** *DEP, USA†.*
Benzocaine (p.1370·3).
*Obesity.*

**Diet Complet** *Natural Life, Arg.*
Multivitamin preparation (p.1417·1).

**Diet Sucaryl** *Abbott, Ital.*
Sodium cyclamate (p.1426·2); saccharin (p.1443·2).
*Sugar substitute.*

**Dietacil** *IMA, Braz.*
Aspartame (p.1422·1).
*Sugar substitute.*

**Dietamina** *Neckerman, Braz.†.*
Aspartame (p.1422·1).
*Sugar substitute.*

**Dietasal** *Libbs, Braz.*
Sodium chloride; potassium chloride (p.1222·2).
*Oral rehydration solution.*

**Dietene** *Restan, S.Afr.*
Cathine hydrochloride (p.1585·2).
*Obesity.*

**Diethizine** *Pond's, Thai.*
Diethylcarbamazine citrate (p.104·1).
*Filariasis; loiasis.*

**Dietil**
*Trenker, Belg.†; Trenker, Thai.*
Diethylpropion hydrochloride (p.1587·1).
*Obesity.*

**Dietmann** *Zydus, India.*
Glucomannan (p.1693·3).
*Constipation; diabetes mellitus; hyperlipidaemias; obesity.*

**Dietoman**
*Note. This name is used for preparations of different composition.*
*Schering-Plough, Braz.†.*
Bran (p.1253·2).
*Constipation; diverticular disease; irritable bowel syndrome.*
*Teofarma, Ital.; Armstrong, Mex.*
Glucomannan (p.1693·3).
*Diabetes mellitus; lipid disorders; obesity.*

**Dieutrim** *Legere, USA†.*
Phenylpropanolamine hydrochloride (p.1127·3); benzocaine (p.1370·3); carmellose sodium (p.1577·3).
*Obesity.*

**Dievril** *FIRMA, Ital.†.*
Vitamin B preparation (p.1417·1).
Lidocaine hydrochloride (p.1377·3) is included in the intramuscular injection to alleviate the pain of injection.
*Neuralgia; neuritis.*

**Diezime** *Recordati, Ital.*
Cefodizime sodium (p.174·1).
Lidocaine hydrochloride (p.1377·3) is included in the intramuscular injection to alleviate the pain of injection.
*Gram-negative bacterial infections.*

**Dif Vitamin A Masivo** *Roche, Spain.*
Vitamin A acetate (p.1453·1).
*Vitamin A deficiency.*

**Difarben** *Rayere, Mex.*
Pancreatin (p.1725·3); ox bile (p.1660·3); dimeticone (p.1289·2).
*Digestive disorders.*

**Difaterol** *Bial, Spain.*
Bezafibrate (p.873·2).
*Hyperlipidaemias.*

**Difedram** *Mavi, Mex.†.*
Diphenhydramine (p.431·3).

**Difelene** *Nakorn, Thai.*
Diclofenac diethylamine (p.32·1) or diclofenac sodium (p.32·1).
*Inflammation; musculoskeletal, joint, peri-articular, and soft-tissue disorders; pain.*

**Difemic** *Pharmasant, Thai.*
Dicycloverine hydrochloride (p.481·2); mefenamic acid (p.55·2).
*Gastrointestinal spasm.*

**Difen**
*Note. This name is used for preparations of different composition.*
*Allergan, Braz.*
Pranoprofen (p.85·2).
*Inflammatory eye disorders.*

*Nakorn, Thai.*
Diclofenac sodium (p.32·1).
*Gout; inflammation; musculoskeletal, joint, and peri-articular disorders; pain.*

**Difena** *Standard, Hong Kong†.*
Diclofenac sodium (p.32·1).
*Inflammation; musculoskeletal, joint, and soft-tissue disorders.*

**Difenac**
*DHA, Hong Kong; DHA, Singapore; TP, Thai.*
Diclofenac sodium (p.32·1).
*Inflammation; musculoskeletal and joint disorders; pain.*

**Difenan** *Royton, Braz.*
Diclofenac sodium (p.32·1).
*Inflammation; pain.*

**Difene**
*Klinge, Austria; Klinge, Irl.*
Diclofenac sodium (p.32·1).
*Gout; inflammation; musculoskeletal, joint, peri-articular, and soft-tissue disorders; pain; renal colic.*

**Difenet** *Nettopharma, Denm.*
Diclofenac sodium (p.32·1).
*Gout; inflammation; musculoskeletal and joint disorders; pain.*

**Difenhistat** *Precimex, Mex.†.*
Diphenhydramine (p.431·3).

**Difenidrin** *Cristalia, Braz.*
Diphenhydramine hydrochloride (p.431·3).

**Difeno** *Milano, Thai.*
Diclofenac sodium (p.32·1).
*Inflammation; musculoskeletal and joint disorders.*

**Difenol** *Merck, Hong Kong.*
Diclofenac sodium (p.32·1).
*Musculoskeletal and joint disorders.*

**Diferbest** *Best, Mex.*
Naproxen sodium (p.65·1).
*Gout; inflammation; musculoskeletal and joint disorders; pain.*

**Diferin** *Grossman, Mex.*
Ampicillin (p.157·1).
*Bacterial infections.*

**Difexon**
*Note. This name is used for preparations of different composition.*
*Bago, Chile Espumante.*
Povidone-iodine (p.1190·3).
*Burns; disinfection of mucous membranes and skin; skin infections; ulcers; vaginal infections; wounds.*

*Armstrong, Mex.*
Deltamethrin (p.1503·1).
*Pediculosis; scabies.*

**Differin**
*Galderma, Arg.; Galderma, Austral.; AB-Consult, Austria; Galderma, Belg.; Galderma, Braz.; Galderma, Canad.; Galderma, Chile; Galderma, Fin.; Galderma, Ger.; Galderma, Hong Kong; Galderma, Irl.; Galderma, Ital.; Galderma, Malaysia; Galderma, Norw.; Galderma, NZ; Galderma, Port.; Galderma, S.Afr.; Galderma, Singapore; Galderma, Swed.; Galderma, Switz.; Galderma, Thai.; Galderma, UK; Galderma, USA.*
Adapalene (p.1141·1).
*Acne.*

**Differine**
*Galderma, Fr.; Galderma, Spain.*
Adapalene (p.1141·1).
*Acne.*

**Difflam**
*3M, Austral.; 3M, Hong Kong; 3M, Irl.; 3M, NZ; 3M, Singapore; 3M, Thai.; 3M, UK.*
Benzydamine hydrochloride (p.21·1).
*Inflammation; pain.*

**Difflam Anti-inflammatory Antibacterial Lozenges** *3M, NZ†.*
Benzydamine hydrochloride (p.21·1); cetylpyridinium chloride (p.1173·1).
*Mouth and throat disorders.*

**Difflam Anti-inflammatory Cough Lozenges**
*3M, Austral.*
Benzydamine hydrochloride (p.21·1); cetylpyridinium chloride (p.1173·1); pholcodine (p.1128·3).
*Coughs; sore throat.*

**Difflam Anti-inflammatory Lozenges** *3M, Malaysia.*
Benzydamine hydrochloride (p.21·1).
*Mouth and throat pain and inflammation.*

**Difflam Anti-inflammatory Lozenges (with Antibacterial)** *3M, Malaysia.*
Benzydamine hydrochloride (p.21·1); cetylpyridinium chloride (p.1173·1).
*Mouth and throat disorders.*

**Difflam Anti-inflammatory Throat Spray** *3M, Austral.*
Benzydamine hydrochloride (p.21·1).
*Mouth and throat pain.*

**Difflam Cough** *3M, NZ.*
Benzydamine hydrochloride (p.21·1); cetylpyridinium chloride (p.1173·1); pholcodine (p.1128·3).
formerly called Difflam Anti-inflammatory Cough Lozenges.
*Coughs; mouth and throat disorders.*

**Difflam Lozenges** *3M, Austral.*
Benzydamine hydrochloride (p.21·1); cetylpyridinium chloride (p.1173·1).
*Mouth and throat pain.*

**Difflam Mouth Gel**
*3M, Austral.; 3M, Malaysia; 3M, NZ; 3M, Singapore.*
Benzydamine hydrochloride (p.21·1); cetylpyridinium chloride (p.1173·1).
*Painful inflammatory mouth disorders.*

**Difflam Solution**
*3M, Austral.; 3M, Malaysia.*
Benzydamine hydrochloride (p.21·1).
Formerly known as Difflam Anti-Inflammatory Solution in *Austral.*
*Mouth and throat pain and inflammation.*

**Difflam-C**
*3M, Austral.; 3M, Hong Kong; 3M, Malaysia; 3M, NZ; 3M, Singapore.*
Benzydamine hydrochloride (p.21·1); chlorhexidine gluconate (p.1173·2).
*Mouth and throat pain.*

**Diffu-K** *UCB, Fr.*
Potassium chloride (p.1232·2).
*Hypokalaemia.*

**Diffumal** *Malesci, Ital.*
Theophylline (p.798·3).
*Asthma; bronchospasm.*

**Diffusyl** *Farmasan, Ger.*
Sodium cromoglicate (p.795·3).
*Asthma.*

**Difilina Asmorax** *Liade, Spain†.*
Diprophylline (p.784·3); ephedrine hydrochloride (p.1120·1); hydroxyzine hydrochloride (p.434·3).
*Obstructive airways disease.*

**Difiram** *Pharmasant, Thai.*
Disulfiram (p.1681·3).
*Chronic alcoholism.*

**Difix** *Promedica, Ital.*
Calcitriol (p.1461·2).
*Hypoparathyroidism; osteoporosis; pseudohypoparathyroidism; renal osteodystrophy; rickets.*

**Diflamil** *Belmac, Spain†.*
Oxyphenbutazone piperazine (p.76·1).
*Gout; musculoskeletal and joint disorders.*

**Diflerix**
*Medochemie, Hong Kong; Medochemie, Malaysia.*
Indapamide (p.938·2).
*Hypertension.*

**Diflonid**
*Dumex-Alpharma, Denm.†; Dumex, Norw.†.*
Diflunisal (p.34·1).
*Musculoskeletal and joint disorders; pain.*

**Diflucan**
*Pfizer, Austral.; Pfizer, Austria; Pfizer, Belg.; Pfizer, Canad.; Pfizer, Chile; Pfizer, Denm.; Pfizer, Fin.; Pfizer, Ger.; Pfizer, Hong Kong; Pfizer, Irl.; Pfizer, Israel; Pfizer, Ital.; Pfizer, Jpn; Pfizer, Malaysia; Pfizer, Mex.; Pfizer, Neth.; Pfizer, Norw.; Pfizer, NZ; Pfizer, Port.; Pfizer, S.Afr.; Pfizer, Singapore; Pfizer, Spain; Pfizer, Swed.; Pfizer, Switz.; Pfizer, Thai.; Pfizer, UK; Pfizer, USA.*
Fluconazole (p.398·1).
*Fungal infections.*

**Difludol** *Edmond Pharma, Ital.†.*
Diflunisal (p.34·1).
*Musculoskeletal disorders; pain.*

**Difluid** *Bioprogress, Ital.*
Dihydroergocristine mesilate (p.1680·1).
*Cerebral and peripheral disorders; headache; hypertension; migraine.*

**Diflusal** *Merck Sharp & Dohme, Belg.*
Diflunisal (p.34·1).
*Pain.*

**Diflux** *Merck, Arg.*
Furosemide (p.919·3); amiloride hydrochloride (p.858·2).
*Hypertension.*

**Difmecor** *Solvay, Ital.†.*
Fendiline hydrochloride (p.915·1).
*Cardiac disorders.*

**Difmedol** *Faran, Gr.*
Loratadine (p.436·1).
*Allergic rhinitis; pruritus.*

**Difmetre** *Solvay, Ital.*
Indometacin (p.47·3); caffeine (p.782·1); prochlorperazine maleate (p.716·3).
*Headache; migraine.*

**Difmetus Compositum** *Solvay, Ital.†.*
Noscapine embonate (p.1125·3); noscapine (p.1125·3); promethazine embonate (p.440·1).
*Coughs.*

**Difnal**
*Ranbaxy, Malaysia; Ranbaxy, Singapore.*
Diclofenac sodium (p.32·1).
*Inflammation; musculoskeletal, joint, peri-articular, and soft-tissue disorders; pain.*

**Difnan** *Hikma, Port.*
Diclofenac (p.32·1).

**Diformil** *Faes, Spain.*
Formaldehyde (p.1179·3).
*Mouth infections.*

**Diformiltricina** *Faes, Spain.*
Cetrimonium bromide (p.1173·1); benzocaine (p.1370·3); formaldehyde (p.1179·3); tyrothricin (p.275·1).
*Mouth and throat disorders.*

**Diformin** *Leiras, Fin.*
Metformin hydrochloride (p.342·3).
*Diabetes mellitus.*

**Difosfen**
*Omedir, Arg.; Rubio, Singapore; Rubio, Spain.*
Disodium etidronate (p.771·2).
*Ectopic ossification; osteoporosis; Paget's disease of bone.*

**Difosfocin** *Magis, Ital.*
Citicoline (p.1672·3).
*Cerebrovascular disorders; parkinsonism.*

**Difosfonal** *SPA, Ital.*
Disodium clodronate (p.770·2).
*Hyperparathyroidism; multiple myeloma; osteolytic tumours; osteoporosis.*

**Difosquin** *Vitamed, Braz.†.*
Chloroquine phosphate (p.448·2).
*Malaria; rheumatoid arthritis.*

**Difoxacil** *Quimica y Farmacia, Mex.*
Norfloxacin (p.238·3).
*Bacterial infections.*

**Dif-Per-Tet-All**
*Chiron Vaccines, Ital.†; Chiron, Thai.†.*
An adsorbed diphtheria, tetanus, and pertussis vaccine (p.1613·3).
*Active immunisation.*

**Difrarel**
*Note. This name is used for preparations of different composition.*
*Leurquin, Fr.*
Myrtillus (p.1718·3); betacarotene (p.1422·3).
*Peripheral vascular disorders.*

*Sigma-Tau, Ger.; Tecnifar, Port.; Sigma-Tau, Spain†.*
Myrtillus (p.1718·3).
*Eye disorders; vascular disorders.*

**Difrarel E**
*Note. This name is used for preparations of different composition.*
*Leurquin, Fr.; Sigma-Tau, Spain†.*
Myrtillus (p.1718·3); vitamin E (p.1464·3).
*Myopias; vascular disorders.*

*Leurquin, Hong Kong.*
Vitamin E (p.1464·3); anthrocyanosides.
*Myopias.*

**Difrin** *Vitamed, Israel.*
Dipivefrine hydrochloride (p.1681·2).
*Glaucoma.*

**Diftavax**
*Aventis Pasteur, Arg.; Pasteur Merieux, Fr.†; Aventis Pasteur, Irl.; Aventis Pasteur, Ital.; Aventis Pasteur, Spain; Aventis Pasteur, UK.*
An adsorbed diphtheria and tetanus vaccine (p.1613·1).
*Active immunisation.*

**Dif-Tet-All**
*Chiron Vaccines, Ital.; Chiron, Thai.*
An adsorbed diphtheria and tetanus vaccine (p.1613·1).
*Active immunisation.*

**Difur** *Cantabria, Spain.*
Polypodium leucotomos.
*Skin disorders.*

**Difuran** *The Forty-Two, Thai.*
Furazolidone (p.605·2); kaolin (p.1268·3); pectin (p.1580·3).
*Gastrointestinal infections.*

**Difusil** *Elvetium, Arg.*
Co-dergocrine mesilate (p.1674·1); cinnarizine (p.428·3).
*Mental function impairment.*

**Digacin** *Lilly, Ger.*
Digoxin (p.895·2).
*Arrhythmias; heart failure.*

**Digaol** *Ioltech, Fr.*
Timolol maleate (p.1012·2).
*Glaucoma; ocular hypertension.*

**Digaril** *Solvay, Spain.*
Fluvastatin sodium (p.918·2).
*Atherosclerosis; hyperlipidaemias.*

**Digassim** *Vitoria, Port.*
Fluoxetine hydrochloride (p.292·1).
*Bulimia nervosa; depression; mixed anxiety depressive states; obsessive-compulsive disorder.*

**Digastril** *Brasmedica, Braz.†.*
Aluminium hydroxide (p.1249·2); magnesium hydroxide (p.1272·2); kaolin (p.1268·3).
*Gastrointestinal hyperacidity.*

**Digecap** *Sigma, Braz.†.*
Bromopride (p.1254·1).
*Nausea and vomiting.*

**Digecap-Zimatico** *Sigma, Braz.*
Bromopride (p.1254·1); dimeticone (p.1289·2); pancreatin (p.1725·3).
*Digestive disorders; nausea and vomiting.*

**Digedryl** *Merck Medication Familiale, Fr.*
Anhydrous sodium sulfate (p.1290·1); monobasic sodium phosphate (p.1230·3).
*Dyspepsia.*

**Digeflash** *Boehringer Ingelheim, Fr.†.*
Pancreas.
*Dyspepsia.*

**Di-Gel**
*Note. This name is used for preparations of different composition.*
*Plough, Port.*
Aluminium hydroxide-magnesium carbonate co-dried gel (p.1250·1); magnesium hydroxide (p.1272·2); simeticone (p.1289·2).
*Dyspepsia; gastric hyperacidity.*

*Schering-Plough, USA.*
Aluminium hydroxide (p.1249·2); magnesium hydroxide (p.1272·2); simeticone (p.1289·2).
*Hyperacidity.*

**Di-Gel Forte** *Plough, Port.*
Aluminium hydroxide-magnesium carbonate co-dried gel (p.1250·1); magnesium hydroxide (p.1272·2); calcium carbonate (p.1254·2); simeticone (p.1289·2).
*Dyspepsia; flatulence; gastric hyperacidity.*

**Digelax** *Monsanto, Ital.*
Boldo (p.1661·2); rhubarb (p.1287·3); cascara (p.1255·1); cynara (p.1678·3); croton eleuteria; inositol (p.1701·2).
*Constipation.*

**Digene** *Knoll, India.*
Simeticone (p.1289·2); magnesium hydroxide (p.1272·2); aluminium hydroxide (p.1249·2); carmellose sodium (p.1577·3).
*Gastro-oesophageal reflux; gastrointestinal hyperacidity; heartburn; peptic ulcer.*

**Digenil** *Saval, Chile.*
Pancreatin (p.1725·3); simeticone (p.1289·2).
*Digestive disorders; flatulence.*

**Digenor Plus** *Rudefsa, Mex.*
Metoclopramide hydrochloride (p.1274·3); dimeticone (p.1289·2); papain (p.1727·3).
*Adjunct in gastrointestinal procedures; gastrointestinal disorders.*

**Digenorflat** *Baliarda, Arg.*
Pancreatin (p.1725·3); simeticone (p.1289·2); dehydrocholic acid (p.1679·2).
*Digestive disorders.*

**Digenormotil** *Baliarda, Arg.*
Cisapride (p.1259·2).
*Gastrointestinal motility disorders.*

**Digenormotil Plus** *Baliarda, Arg.*
Cisapride (p.1259·2); simeticone (p.1289·2).
*Gastrointestinal disorders.*

**Digepepsin** *Kenwood, USA.*
Pepsin (p.1729·3); pancreatin (p.1725·3); bile salts (p.1660·3).

**Digeplex** *Amadeus, India.*
*Oral drops:* Amylase (p.1654·2); pepsin (p.1729·3); cardamom oil (p.1668·1); cinnamon oil (p.1672·2).
*Oral liquid:* Amylase (p.1654·2); pepsin (p.1729·3).
*Digestive disorders.*

**Digeplex-T** *Amadeus, India.*
Pancreatin (p.1725·3); ox-bile (p.1660·3); pepsin (p.1729·3); amylase (p.1654·2); dimethicone (p.1289·2).
*Digestive disorders.*

**Digeplus** *Ache, Braz.*
Metoclopramide hydrochloride (p.1274·3); dimethicone (p.1289·2); dehydrocholic acid (p.1679·2); cellulase (p.1669·1); pepsin (p.1729·3); pancreatin (p.1725·3).
*Digestive disorders.*

**Digerall** *Falqui, Ital.*
Alginic acid (p.1576·3); aluminium hydroxide (p.1249·2); magnesium trisilicate (p.1272·3); sodium bicarbonate (p.1223·2).
*Gastro-oesophageal reflux; gastrointestinal hyperacidity; peptic ulcer.*

**Digerent** *Poliframa, Ital.*
Trimebutine maleate (p.1758·1).
*Gastrointestinal spasm; irritable colon; oesophageal motility disorders.*

**Digerex** *De Mayo, Braz.*
Bromopride (p.1254·1).
*Nausea and vomiting.*

**Digerfit** *Body Spring, Ital.*
Papaya; pineapple; fennel; amino acids; pyridoxine (p.1417·1).
*Digestive disorders; nutritional supplement.*

**Digervin** *Alacan, Spain.*
Famotidine (p.1265·2).
*Gastro-oesophageal reflux; peptic ulcer; Zollinger-Ellison syndrome.*

**Digesan** *Sanofi Synthelabo, Braz.*
Bromopride (p.1254·1).
*Nausea and vomiting.*

**Di-Gesic**
*Dista, Austral.*
Dextropropoxyphene hydrochloride (p.28·3); paracetamol (p.76·2).
*Pain.*

*Lilly, NZ†.*
Dextropropoxyphene napsilate (p.28·3); paracetamol (p.76·2).
*Pain.*

**Digesnorma** *INQ, Braz.†.*
Amylase (p.1654·2); aluminium hydroxide (p.1249·2); magnesium hydroxide (p.1272·2); dimethicone (p.1289·2).
*Flatulence; gastrointestinal disorders.*

**Digespar** *Sanofi Synthelabo, Chile.*
Metoclopramide hydrochloride (p.1274·3); simeticone (p.1289·2).
*Gastrointestinal disorders.*

**Digesplen** *Craveri, Arg.*
Pancreatin (p.1725·3); metoclopramide (p.1274·3); simeticone (p.1289·2); deoxycholic acid (p.1660·3).
*Gastrointestinal disorders.*

**Digesprid** *Neo Quimica, Braz.*
Bromopride (p.1254·1).
*Nausea and vomiting.*

**Digess** *Axcan, Canad.†.*
Pancrelipase (p.1725·3).
*Pancreatic insufficiency.*

**Digest**
*Note. This name is used for preparations of different composition.*
*Heralds, Braz.†.*
Metoclopramide (p.1274·3); dimethicone (p.1289·2).
*Nausea and vomiting.*
*Modern Health Products, UK†.*
Parsley (p.1728·3); centaury (p.1669·2); althaea root (p.1651·3).
*Dyspepsia; flatulence.*

**Digest Plus** *Nutravite, Canad.*
Bromelain; catnip; fennel seed; ginger root; glutamic acid; pancreatin; papain; papaya fruit complex and leaf; peppermint root; pepsin; saw palmetto berries.

**Digestaid** *Eagle, Austral.†.*
Betaine hydrochloride (p.1660·2); pepsin (p.1729·3); pancreatin (p.1725·3); ox bile salt (p.1660·3); bromelain (p.1662·2); papain (p.1727·3); maltase (p.1646·2); potassium chloride (p.1232·2); gentian (p.1692·2); fennel; peppermint oil (p.1283·2); chromium chelate (p.1425·1).
*Gastrointestinal disorders.*

**Digestal** *Odontofarma, Braz.†.*
Pancreatin (p.1725·3); ox bile (p.1660·3).
*Digestive disorders.*

**Digestar** *Brasmedica, Braz.†.*
Chamomile (p.1669·3); gentian (p.1692·2).
*Gastrointestinal disorders.*

**Digestbem** *Eurofarma, Braz.*
Sodium bicarbonate (p.1223·2); sodium carbonate (p.1747·1); citric acid (p.1673·1).
*Gastrointestinal hyperacidity.*

**Digestelact** *Nutricia, Austral.*
Food for special diets (p.1417·1).
*Lactose intolerance.*

**Digestif Marga** *Cooperation Pharmaceutique, Fr.*
Magnesium hydroxide (p.1272·2); dried aluminium hydroxide (p.1249·2); calcium carbonate (p.1254·2).
*Gastrointestinal disorders.*

**Digestif Rennie**
*Note. This name is used for preparations of different composition.*
*Roche, Austria.*
Papain (p.1727·3); pancreatin (p.1725·3); calcium carbonate (p.1254·2); magnesium carbonate (p.1272·1).
*Dyspepsia.*
*Roche Consumer, Irl.†; Roche Consumer, S.Afr.*
Calcium carbonate (p.1254·2); magnesium carbonate (p.1272·1).
*Dyspepsia; gastric hyperacidity; heartburn.*

**Digestif-Ara** *Rafa, Israel.*
Magnesium carbonate (p.1272·1); magnesium peroxide (p.1185·2); magnesium oxide (p.1272·3); calcium carbonate (p.1254·2); kaolin (p.1268·3); peppermint oil (p.1283·2).
*Calcium supplement; dyspepsia; flatulence; gastrointestinal hyperacidity.*

**Digestil** *Teuto, Braz.†.*
Bromopride (p.1254·1).
*Gastrointestinal disorders.*

**Digestin** *Chew, Thai.*
Mamylase; amylase (p.1654·2); thiamine nitrate (p.1455·1); scopolia; sodium bicarbonate (p.1223·2); calcium carbonate (p.1254·2); dried aluminium hydroxide gel (p.1249·2).
*Gastrointestinal disorders.*

**Digestina** *Uniao Quimica, Braz.*
Bromopride (p.1254·1).
*Nausea and vomiting.*

**Digestinas Super** *Geminis, Spain†.*
Aluminium glycinate (p.1249·1); aluminium hydroxide (p.1249·2).
*Gastrointestinal hyperacidity.*

**Digestion L114** *Homeocan, Canad.*
Homoeopathic preparation.

**Digestive** *Dorwest, UK.*
Ginger (p.1267·1); hydrastis (p.1698·3); rhubarb (p.1287·3); valerian (p.1762·2).
*Dyspepsia; gastric hyperacidity; heartburn; nausea.*

**Digestive Aid** *Blackmores, Austral.†.*
Slippery elm (p.1747·1); fennel (p.1687·2); ginger (p.1267·1); gentian (p.1692·2); papain (p.1727·3); bromelains (p.1662·2); peppermint leaf (p.1283·2); anise oil (p.1655·2).
*Digestive disorders.*

**Digestive Rennie** *Roche Consumer, Austral.†.*
Calcium carbonate (p.1254·2); heavy magnesium carbonate (p.1272·1).
*Dyspepsia; flatulence.*

**Digestivo Antonetto** *Antonetto, Ital.*
Anionic resin; glycine (p.1433·3); calcium carbonate (p.1254·2).
*Gastric hyperacidity.*

**Digestivo Giuliani** *Giuliani, Ital.*
Domperidone (p.1263·2).
*Dyspepsia.*

**Digestivo Rennie** *Roche Nicholas, Spain†.*
Calcium carbonate (p.1254·2); magnesium carbonate (p.1272·1); peppermint oil (p.1283·2).
*Gastrointestinal hyperacidity; heartburn; meteorism.*

**Digestivum-Hetterich S** *Galenika, Ger.*
Gentian (p.1692·2).
*Bloating; flatulence; loss of appetite.*

**Digest-Merz** *Merz, Ger.*
Turmeric (p.1058·3); dimethicone (p.1289·2).
Formerly contained porcine pancreatin, Javanese turmeric, and dimethicone.
*Digestive system disorders.*

**Digestodoron**
*Note. This name is used for preparations of different composition.*
*Weleda, Austria.*
Male fern (p.108·2); polypodium leaf; scolopendrium vulgare; salix leaf (p.87·3).
*Gastrointestinal disorders.*
*Weleda, Fr.; Weleda, UK.*
Homoeopathic preparation.

**Digestol** *Richter, Austria.*
Gentian (p.1692·2); bitter-orange peel (p.1723·3); taraxacum (p.1751·3).
*Gastrointestinal disorders.*

**Digestol Sanatorium** *Santiveri, Spain†.*
Aniseed (p.1655·2); centaurium erythraea (p.1669·2); gentian (p.1692·2); chamomile (p.1669·3); melissa (p.1711·1); peppermint (p.1283·2).
*Digestive disorders; gastric hyperacidity.*

**Digestomen** *Menarini, Belg.*
Betaine hydrochloride (p.1660·2); pepsin (p.1729·3); papain (p.1727·3); amylase (p.1654·2); pancreatin (p.1725·3); pancrelipase (p.1725·3); cellulase (p.1669·1).
*Digestive disorders due to pancreatic insufficiency.*

**Digestomen Complex** *Menarini, Spain.*
White tablets, pepsin (p.1729·3); red tablets, papain (p.1727·3); amylase (p.1654·2); green tablets, pancreatin (p.1725·3).
*Digestive disorders.*

**Digeston** *Hexal, Braz.*
Bromopride (p.1254·1).
*Nausea and vomiting.*

**Digestopan** *Menarini, Ital.*
Pepsin (p.1729·3); papain (p.1727·3); amylase (p.1654·2); pancreatin (p.1725·3); pancreatic lipase; cellulase (p.1669·1).
*Digestive disorders.*

**Digestosan** *Fresenius Kabi, Austria†.*
Ranitidine hydrochloride (p.1285·2).
*Acid aspiration; gastro-oesophageal reflux; gastrointestinal haemorrhage; peptic ulcer; Zollinger-Ellison syndrome.*

**Digestovital** *Puerto Galiano, Spain.*
Belladonna (p.479·1); opium (p.74·2); sodium bicarbonate (p.1223·2); sodium citrate (p.1223·2); sodium sulfate (p.1290·1); star anise; aniseed (p.1655·2) cardamom (p.1667·3).
*Gastritis; gastrointestinal hyperacidity; peptic ulcer.*

**Digestron** *Loprofar, Braz.*
Dehydrocholic acid (p.1679·2); aesculus (p.1648·2); drimys winterii; erythroxylon catuaba; cynara (p.1678·3); cnicus benedictus (p.1673·3); sodium phosphate (p.1231·1); liver extract.
*Liver disorders.*

**Digest-X Yucca L110** *Homeocan, Canad.*
Homoeopathic preparation.

**Digezanol** *Hormona, Mex.*
Albendazole (p.101·2).
*Giardiasis; worm infections.*

**Digezin** *Recalcine, Chile.*
Fenipentol (p.1687·2); benoctonium bromide.
*Gastrointestinal disorders.*

**Digezyme** *Contassium Co., UK†.*
Betaine hydrochloride (p.1660·2); ox bile (p.1660·3); pepsin (p.1729·3); pancrelipase (p.1725·3); bromelain (p.1662·2).

**Digherbal** *Knop, Chile.*
Homoeopathic preparation.

**Digi-Aldopur** *Kwizda, Austria.*
Spironolactone (p.1003·1); β-acetyldigoxin (p.851·1).
*Arrhythmias; heart failure.*

**Digibind**
*GlaxoSmithKline, Austral.; GlaxoSmithKline, Canad.; IFET (IΦET), Gr.; GlaxoSmithKline, UK; Glaxo Wellcome, USA.*
Digoxin-specific antibody fragments (p.1036·3).
*Digoxin or digitoxin toxicity.*

**Digidot** *Roche, Fr.*
Digoxin-specific antibody fragments (p.1036·3).
*Digoxin or digitoxin toxicity.*

**DigiFab** *Protherics, USA.*
Digoxin-specific antibody fragments (p.1036·3).
*Digoxin toxicity.*

**Digifar** *Farmila, Ital.*
Digitalin (p.1680·1); vitamin P (p.1688·2).
*Eye disorders.*

**Digimed** *corax, Ger.*
Digitoxin (p.894·3).
*Heart failure.*

**Digimerck**
*Merck, Austria; Merck, Ger.*
Digitoxin (p.894·3).
*Arrhythmias; heart failure.*

**Digitaline**
*Procter & Gamble, Belg.; Barrenne, Braz.; Welcker-Lyster, Canad.†; Procter & Gamble, Fr.†; Rougier, Hong Kong†.*
Digitoxin (p.894·3).
*Arrhythmias; heart failure.*

**Digitalis Antidot**
*Roche, Austria; Roche, Belg.; Roche, Ger.; Roche, Swed.*
Digoxin-specific antibody fragments (p.1036·3).
*Digitalis poisoning.*

**Digitalis Antidote**
*Roche, Hong Kong; Roche, Singapore†.*
Digoxin-specific antibody fragments (p.1036·3).
*Digitalis poisoning.*

**Digitalysat Scilla-Digitaloid** *Ysatfabrik, Ger.*
Squill (p.1130·3).
*Cardiac disorders.*

**Digitrin**
*Astra, Norw.†; Tika, Swed.*
Digitoxin (p.894·3).
*Arrhythmias; heart failure.*

**Diglexol** *IQFA, Mex.*
Glibenclamide (p.331·2).
*Diabetes mellitus.*

**Dignobeta** *Luitpold, Ger.†.*
Atenolol (p.865·2).
*Arrhythmias; hypertension; ischaemic heart disease.*

**Dignobroxol** *Luitpold, Ger.†.*
Ambroxol hydrochloride (p.1114·3).
*Respiratory-tract disorders associated with increased or viscous mucus.*

**Dignodolin** *Sankyo, Ger.*
Flufenamic acid (p.43·2).
*Musculoskeletal and joint disorders.*

**Dignofenac** *Deutsche Pharma, Chile.*
Diclofenac sodium (p.32·1).
*Inflammation; musculoskeletal and joint disorders; pain.*

**Dignoflex** *Luitpold, Ger.†.*
Ibuprofen (p.45·3).
*Gout; inflammation; musculoskeletal and joint disorders; pain.*

**Dignokonstant** *Sankyo, Ger.*
Nifedipine (p.966·2).
*Angina pectoris; hypertension.*

**Dignometoprol** *Luitpold, Ger.†.*
Metoprolol tartrate (p.957·1).
*Angina pectoris; arrhythmias; hypertension; migraine; myocardial infarction.*

**Dignonitrat** *Luitpold, Ger.†.*
Isosorbide dinitrate (p.941·1).
*Angina pectoris; heart failure; pulmonary hypertension.*

**Dignoretik** *Sankyo, Ger.†.*
Amiloride hydrochloride (p.858·2); hydrochlorothiazide (p.933·2).
*Hypertension; oedema.*

**Dignotrimazol** *Luitpold, Ger.†.*
Clotrimazole (p.396·2).
*Fungal skin infections.*

**Dignover** *Luitpold, Ger.†.*
Verapamil hydrochloride (p.1019·1).
*Angina pectoris; arrhythmias; hypertension.*

**Dignowell** *Luitpold, Ger.†.*
Phenylephrine hydrochloride (p.1126·3); a heparinoid (p.931·1).
*Venous insufficiency.*

**Digocard-G** *Klonal, Arg.*
Digoxin (p.895·2).

**Digomal** *Malesci, Ital.†.*
Digoxin (p.895·2).
*Cardiac disorders.*

**Digophton** *Chauvin ankerpharm, Ger.*
Digitalis (p.894·2).
*Eye strain.*

**Digosin** *Chugai, Jpn.*
Digoxin (p.895·2).
*Arrhythmias; heart failure.*

**Digostada** *Stada, Ger.*
β-Acetyldigoxin (p.851·1).
*Arrhythmias; heart failure.*

**Digotab** *AWD, Ger.*
β-Acetyldigoxin (p.851·1).
*Arrhythmias; heart failure.*

**Digox** *CT, Ger.*
β-Acetyldigoxin (p.851·1).
*Arrhythmias; heart failure.*

**Digoxil** *Legrand, Braz.*
Digoxin (p.895·2).

**Digoxin "Didier"** *Hormosan, Ger.*
β-Acetyldigoxin (p.851·1).
*Heart failure.*

**Digton** *Areu, Spain.*
Sulpiride (p.722·2).
*Anxiety disorders; psychoses; vertigo.*

**Di-Hydan**
*Synthelabo, Belg.†; Genopharm, Fr.†.*
Phenytoin (p.370·2).
*Arrhythmias; epilepsy; facial neuralgias.*

**Dihydergot**
*Note. This name is used for preparations of different composition.*
*Novartis, Austral.; Novartis, Austria; Novartis, Belg.; Novartis, Braz.; Novartis, Ger.; Novartis, Gr.; Novartis, India; Novartis, Mex.; Novartis, Neth.; Novartis, Port.; Novartis, S.Afr.†; Novartis, Spain; Novartis, Switz.*
Dihydroergotamine mesilate (p.465·3).
*Chronic fatigue; hypotension; migraine and related vascular headache; urinary retention; venous insufficiency; vertigo.*
*Novartis, Austria; Novartis, Switz.*
*Nasal spray:* Dihydroergotamine mesilate (p.465·3); caffeine (p.782·1).
*Migraine.*

**Dihydergot plus**
*Novartis, Ger.; Novartis, Switz.*
Dihydroergotamine mesilate (p.465·3); etilefrine hydrochloride (p.914·1).
*Hypotension.*

**Dihydral**
*Solvay, Belg.†; Solvay, Neth.*
Dihydrotachysterol (p.1461·3).
*Hypoparathyroidism; renal osteodystrophy; rickets.*

**DiHydro-CP** *Cypress, USA.*
Dihydrocodeine tartrate (p.34·3); chlorphenamine maleate (p.427·3); pseudoephedrine hydrochloride (p.1129·2).
*Coughs; nasal congestion.*

**DiHydro-GP** *Cypress, USA.*
Dihydrocodeine tartrate (p.34·3); guaifenesin (p.1122·1); pseudoephedrine hydrochloride (p.1129·2).
*Coughs; nasal congestion.*

**Dihytamin** *Wernigerode, Ger.; Temmler, Ger.*
Dihydroergotamine mesilate (p.465·3).
*Hypotension; migraine and other vascular headaches.*

**Dihyzin** *Henning, Ger.†.*
Dihydralazine sulfate (p.899·3).
*Hypertension.*

**Diidergot** *Novartis, Ital.*
Dihydroergotamine mesilate (p.465·3).
*Headache; vascular disorders.*

**Dijex** *SSL, UK†.*
*Oral liquid:* Aluminium hydroxide (p.1249·2); magnesium hydroxide (p.1272·2).
These ingredients can be described by the British Approved Name Co-magaldrox.
*Tablets:* Aluminium hydroxide-magnesium carbonate co-dried gel (p.1250·1).
*Dyspepsia.*

**Dikacine** *Continental Pharma, Belg.*
Dibekacin sulfate (p.205·2).
*Gram-negative bacterial infections; staphylococcal infections.*

**Dilabar** *Vita, Spain.*
Captopril (p.879·2).
*Diabetic nephropathy; heart failure; hypertension; myocardial infarction.*

**Dilabar Diu** *Vita, Spain.*
Hydrochlorothiazide (p.933·2); captopril (p.879·2).
*Hypertension.*

**Dilacard** *Royton, Braz.*
Verapamil hydrochloride (p.1019·1).
*Arrhythmias; hypertension.*

**Dilaclan** *CEPA, Spain.*
Diltiazem hydrochloride (p.900·1).
*Angina pectoris; hypertension.*

**Dilacor**
*Note. This name is used for preparations of different composition.*
*Temis, Arg.*
Barnidipine hydrochloride (p.866·3).
*Hypertension.*
*Teuto, Braz.*
Verapamil hydrochloride (p.1019·1).
*Arrhythmias; hypertension.*
*Watson, USA.*
Diltiazem hydrochloride (p.900·1).
*Angina pectoris; hypertension.*

**Dilacoran** *Knoll, Mex.*
Verapamil hydrochloride (p.1019·1).
*Angina pectoris; arrhythmias; heart failure; hypertension; myocardial infarction.*

**Dilacoron** *Abbott, Braz.*
Verapamil hydrochloride (p.1019·1).
*Angina pectoris; arrhythmias; hypertension; hypertrophic cardiomyopathy; migraine and other vascular headaches.*

**Diladel** *Sanofi Synthelabo, Ital.*
Diltiazem hydrochloride (p.900·1).
*Angina pectoris; hypertension.*

**Dilaescol** *Kolassa, Austria.*
Buphenine hydrochloride (p.1663·2); thiamine hydrochloride (p.1455·1); aesculus (p.1648·2).
*Migraine; peripheral vascular disease; premenstrual syndrome; reflex sympathetic dystrophy.*

**Dilaflux** *Medley, Braz.*
Nifedipine (p.966·2).
*Angina pectoris; hypertension.*

**Dilafurane** *Sanofi Synthelabo, Spain.*
Benziodarone (p.415·1).
*Gout; hyperuricaemia.*

**Dilamax** *Bialfar, Port.*
Salmeterol xinafoate (p.795·1).
*Asthma.*

**Dilamet** *Gramon, Arg.*
Lormetazepam (p.705·2).
*Anxiety.*

**Dilamol** *Sanval, Braz.*
Salbutamol sulfate (p.791·3).
*Obstructive airways disease.*

**Dilanacin** *AWD, Ger.*
Digoxin (p.895·2).
*Arrhythmias; heart failure.*

**Dilanorm** *Aventis, Neth.*
Celiprolol hydrochloride (p.881·3).
*Angina pectoris; hypertension.*

**Dilantin**
*Pfizer, Austral.; Pfizer, Canad.; Pfizer, Fr.; Pfizer, Hong Kong; Parke, Davis, India; Parke, Davis, Israel; Pfizer, Malaysia; Pfizer, NZ; Pfizer, Singapore; Pfizer, Thai.; Parke, Davis, USA.*
Phenytoin (p.370·2) or phenytoin sodium (p.370·2).
*Arrhythmias; epilepsy; migraine; seizures during neurosurgery; trigeminal neuralgia.*

**Dilantin with Phenobarbital** *Parke, Davis, Canad.†; Parke, Davis, India.*
Phenytoin sodium (p.370·2); phenobarbital (p.367·3).
*Epilepsy.*

**Dilaplus** *Roche, Austria.*
Carvedilol (p.881·1); hydrochlorothiazide (p.933·2).
*Hypertension.*

**Dilapres** *Quimifar, Spain†.*
Bencyclane fumarate (p.867·3); clonidine hydrochloride (p.885·2); hydrochlorothiazide (p.933·2).
*Hypertension.*

**Dilar**
*Cassenne, Fr.†; Syntex, Mex.*
Paramethasone acetate (p.1107·3).
*Corticosteroid.*

**Dilarmine** *Syntex, Mex.*
Paramethasone acetate (p.1107·3); chlorphenamine maleate (p.427·3).
*Hypersensitivity; inflammation.*

**Dilartan** *Duncan, Arg.*
Bamethan (p.866·3).
*Varices.*

**Dilarterial** *Llorente, Spain†.*
Vincamine (p.1764·2).
*Cerebral trauma; cerebrovascular disorders.*

**Dilatam**
*Abic, Israel; Aspen, S.Afr.; Novopharm, Singapore; Pharmachemie, Singapore; Teva, Singapore; Abic, Thai.†.*
Diltiazem hydrochloride (p.900·1).
*Angina pectoris; hypertension.*

**Dilatol**
*Note. This name is used for preparations of different composition.*
*Kolassa, Austria.*
Buphenine hydrochloride (p.1663·2).
*Inhibition of labour; peripheral vascular disease; uterine relaxant; vascular headache.*

*Jaba, Port.*
Isradipine (p.942·2).
*Hypertension.*

**Dilatol-Chinin** *Kolassa, Austria.*
Buphenine hydrochloride (p.1663·2); quinine sulfate (p.460·2).
*Cramp.*

**Dilatrane** *SERP, Mon.*
Theophylline (p.798·3) or theophylline sodium acetate (p.804·3).
*Obstructive airways disease.*

**Dilatrat** *Cazi, Braz.*
Isosorbide dinitrate (p.941·1).
*Angina pectoris.*

**Dilatrate** *Schwarz, USA.*
Isosorbide dinitrate (p.941·1).
*Angina pectoris.*

**Dilatrend**
*Roche, Arg.; Roche, Austral.; Roche, Austria; Asta Medica, Braz.; Roche, Chile; Roche, Ger.; Roche, Gr.; Roche, Hong Kong; Roche, Ital.; Roche, Mex.; Boehringer Mannheim, Norw.†; Roche, NZ; Roche, S.Afr.; Roche, Singapore; Roche, Switz.; Roche, Thai.*
Carvedilol (p.881·1).
*Angina pectoris; heart failure; hypertension.*

**Dilaudid**
*Abbott, Austral.; Ebewe, Austria; Abbott, Canad.; Abbott, Ger.; Abbott, USA.*
Hydromorphone hydrochloride (p.45·2).
*Pain.*

**Dilaudid Cough** *Knoll, USA.*
Hydromorphone hydrochloride (p.45·2); guaifenesin (p.1122·1).
*Coughs.*

**Dilaudid-Atropin**
*Knoll, Ger.†; Abbott, Swed.; Knoll, Switz.*
Hydromorphone hydrochloride (p.45·2); atropine sulfate (p.477·1).
*Pain; smooth muscle spasm.*

**Dilbloc** *Roche, Port.*
Carvedilol (p.881·1).
*Heart failure; hypertension; ischaemic heart disease.*

**Dilcard**
*Alphapharm, Malaysia; Merck, Malaysia; Pacific, NZ.*
Diltiazem hydrochloride (p.900·1).
*Angina pectoris.*

**Dilcardia**
*Unique, India; Generics, UK.*
Diltiazem hydrochloride (p.900·1).
*Angina pectoris.*

**Dilclor** *Diba, Mex.*
Chloramphenicol (p.185·1).
*Bacterial infections.*

**Dilcontin** *Modi-Mundipharma, India.*
Diltiazem hydrochloride (p.900·1).
*Angina pectoris; hypertension.*

**Dilcor**
*Note. This name is used for preparations of different composition.*
*Norpharma, Denm.*
Diltiazem hydrochloride (p.900·1).
*Angina pectoris; hypertension.*

*BOI, Spain.*
Nifedipine (p.966·2).
*Angina pectoris; hypertension; Raynaud's syndrome.*

**Dilcoran** *Alpharma-Isis, Ger.*
Pentaerithrityl tetranitrate (p.979·1).
*Angina pectoris.*

**Dilem**
*Douglas, Hong Kong†; Ist. Chim. Inter., Ital.; Douglas, Malaysia; Douglas, Thai.; TTN, Thai.*
Diltiazem hydrochloride (p.900·1).
*Angina pectoris; hypertension.*

**Dilena**
*Organon, Arg.; Organon, Hong Kong; Organon, Port.*
11 Tablets, estradiol valerate (p.1550·2); 10 tablets, estradiol valerate; medroxyprogesterone acetate (p.1557·2).
*Menopausal disorders; osteoporosis.*

*Organon, Braz.; Organon, Mex.*
White tablets, estradiol valerate (p.1550·2); blue tablets, estradiol valerate; medroxyprogesterone acetate (p.1557·2).
*Menopausal disorders; osteoporosis.*

**Diletan** *Vitoria, Port.*
Sumatriptan succinate (p.471·2).
*Cluster headache; migraine.*

**Dilfar** *Fournier, Port.*
Diltiazem hydrochloride (p.900·1).
*Angina pectoris; hypertension.*

**Diligan**
*Note. This name is used for preparations of different composition.*
*UCB, Austria.*
Hydroxyzine hydrochloride (p.434·3); meclozine hydrochloride (p.436·3); nicotinic acid (p.1441·1).
*Vestibular disorders.*

*UCB, Ger.*
Hydroxyzine hydrochloride (p.434·3); meclozine hydrochloride (p.436·3).
*Ménière's disease; vertigo.*

*UCB, India.*
Meclozine hydrochloride (p.436·3); nicotinic acid (p.1441·1).
*Labyrinthitis; vertigo.*

*UCB, Port.*
Hydroxyzine (p.435·1); meclozine (p.436·3); nicotinic acid (p.1441·1).

**Dilinct** *Restan, S.Afr.*
Etofylline (p.785·1); diphenhydramine hydrochloride (p.431·3); ammonium chloride (p.1115·2); polysorbate 20 (p.1415·1).
*Bronchodilator; coughs.*

**Diliter** *Pulitzer, Ital.*
Diltiazem hydrochloride (p.900·1).
*Angina pectoris; heart failure; hypertension.*

**Dilizem**
*Berlin Pharm, Singapore†; Berlin Pharm, Thai.*
Diltiazem hydrochloride (p.900·1).
*Angina pectoris; hypertension.*

**Dilmin** *Ratiopharm, Fin.*
Diltiazem hydrochloride (p.900·1).
*Angina pectoris; hypertension.*

**Diloc** *Tramedico, Neth.*
Diltiazem hydrochloride (p.900·1).
*Angina pectoris; hypertension.*

**Dilocaine** *Hauck, USA.*
Lidocaine hydrochloride (p.1377·3).
*Local anaesthesia.*

**Dilomil** *Siam Bheasach, Thai.*
Diphenoxylate hydrochloride (p.1261·3).
Atropine sulfate (p.477·1) is included in this preparation to discourage abuse.
*Diarrhoea.*

**Dilongo** *IPI, Port.*
Diltiazem hydrochloride (p.900·1).
*Angina pectoris; hypertension.*

**Dilor** *Savage, USA.*
Diprophylline (p.784·3).
*Obstructive airways disease.*

**Dilor-G** *Savage, USA†.*
Diprophylline (p.784·3); guaifenesin (p.1122·1).
*Bronchospasm.*

**Dilospir** *Boehringer Ingelheim, Austria.*
Sodium cromoglicate (p.795·3).
*Asthma.*

**Dilostop** *Collins, Mex.*
Loperamide (p.1271·2).
*Diarrhoea.*

**Dilosyn**
*Sigma, Austral.; GlaxoSmithKline, India.*
Methdilazine hydrochloride (p.437·2).
*Hypersensitivity reactions; neurodermatitis; pruritus.*

**Dilosyn Expectorant** *GlaxoSmithKline, India.*
Methdilazine hydrochloride (p.437·2); ammonium chloride (p.1115·2); sodium citrate (p.1223·2); menthol (p.1711·3).
*Coughs.*

**Dilotab**
*Note. This name is used for preparations of different composition.*
*Zee, Canad.†.*
Phenylpropanolamine hydrochloride (p.1127·3); paracetamol (p.76·2).

*Zee, USA.*
Paracetamol (p.76·2); pseudoephedrine hydrochloride (p.1129·2).
*Upper respiratory-tract disorders.*

**Dilox** *Recalcine, Chile.*
Ketorolac trometamol (p.52·1).
*Pain.*

**Diloxin** *Pond's, Thai.*
Dicloxacillin sodium (p.205·2).
*Gram-positive bacterial infections.*

**Dilpral** *Orion, Fin.*
Diltiazem hydrochloride (p.900·1).
*Angina pectoris; hypertension.*

**Dilrene** *Irex, Fr.*
Diltiazem hydrochloride (p.900·1).
*Angina pectoris; hypertension.*

**Dilsal** *TAD, Ger.*
Diltiazem hydrochloride (p.900·1).
*Angina pectoris; hypertension.*

**Dilsana**
*Milupa, Hong Kong†.*
Nutritional supplement with vitamins and minerals (p.1417·1).
*Pregnancy and lactation.*

*Milupa, Switz.†.*
Preparation for enteral nutrition (p.1417·1).

**Dil-Sanorania** *Lichtenstein, Ger.*
Diltiazem hydrochloride (p.900·1).
*Angina pectoris; hypertension.*

**Dilta** *ABZ, Ger.; 1A, Ger.*
Diltiazem hydrochloride (p.900·1).
*Angina pectoris; hypertension.*

**Diltabeta** *Betapharm, Ger.*
Diltiazem hydrochloride (p.900·1).
*Angina pectoris; hypertension.*

**Diltahexal**
*Hexal, Austral.; Hexal, Austria; Hexal, Ger.*
Diltiazem hydrochloride (p.900·1).
*Angina pectoris; hypertension.*

**Diltam** *Rowex, Irl.*
Diltiazem hydrochloride (p.900·1).
*Angina pectoris; hypertension.*

**Diltan**
*Mepha, Hong Kong; Mepha, Thai.†.*
Diltiazem hydrochloride (p.900·1).
*Angina pectoris; hypertension.*

**Diltapham** *Phamos, Ger.*
Diltiazem hydrochloride (p.900·1).
*Angina pectoris; hypertension.*

**Diltaretard** *Betapharm, Ger.*
Diltiazem hydrochloride (p.900·1).
*Angina pectoris; hypertension.*

**Diltec** *Utopian, Thai.*
Diltiazem hydrochloride (p.900·1).
*Angina pectoris; hypertension.*

**Diltelan** *Faran, Gr.*
Diltiazem (p.901·3).
*Angina; hypertension.*

**Diltenk** *Biotenk, Arg.*
Diltiazem (p.901·3).
*Angina pectoris; hypertension.*

**Dilti** *CT, Ger.*
Diltiazem hydrochloride (p.900·1).
*Angina pectoris; hypertension.*

**Diltia** *Andrx, USA.*
Diltiazem hydrochloride (p.900·1).
*Angina pectoris; hypertension.*

**Diltiacor**
*Hexal, Arg.; Biolab Sanus, Braz.*
Diltiazem hydrochloride (p.900·1).
*Arrhythmias; hypertension.*

**Diltiagamma** *Worwag, Ger.*
Diltiazem hydrochloride (p.900·1).
*Angina pectoris; hypertension.*

**Diltiamax** *PMC, Austral.†.*
Diltiazem hydrochloride (p.900·1).
*Angina pectoris.*

**Diltiamerck** *Merck, Ger.†.*
Diltiazem hydrochloride (p.900·1).
*Angina pectoris; hypertension.*

**Diltiangina** *Tecnimede, Port.*
Diltiazem hydrochloride (p.900·1).

**Diltiastad** *Stada, Austria.*
Diltiazem hydrochloride (p.900·1).
*Angina pectoris; hypertension.*

**Diltiem** *Sanofi Synthelabo, Port.*
Diltiazem hydrochloride (p.900·1).
*Angina pectoris; hypertension.*

**Diltikard** *Nycomed, Norw.†.*
Diltiazem hydrochloride (p.900·1).
*Angina pectoris; hypertension.*

**Diltin** *Cimed, Braz.*
Sodium picosulfate (p.1289·3).
*Bowel evacuation; constipation.*

**Diltipress** *Sigma, Braz.*
Diltiazem hydrochloride (p.900·1).
*Angina pectoris; hypertension.*

**Diltiuc** *Merck dura, Ger.*
Diltiazem hydrochloride (p.900·1).
*Angina pectoris; hypertension.*

**Diltiwas** *Chiesi, Spain.*
Diltiazem hydrochloride (p.900·1).
*Angina pectoris; hypertension.*

**Diltix** *Pliva, Spain.*
Ibuprofen (p.45·3).
*Fever; musculoskeletal, joint, peri-articular, and soft-tissue disorders; pain.*

**Diltizem** *Searle, Braz.†.*
Diltiazem hydrochloride (p.900·1).
*Angina pectoris; hypertension; supraventricular arrhythmias.*

**Diltotal** *Mintlab, Chile.*
Ginseng; lecithin; procaine hydrochloride (p.1383·2); vitamins; rutin; minerals (p.1417·1).

**Dilubrin** *UCI, Braz.†.*
Dipyrone (p.35·3); metixene hydrochloride (p.485·3).
*Fever; pain.*

**Dilucid** *Collins, Mex.*
Lovastatin (p.949·1).
*Hypercholesterolaemia.*

**Dilucort** *Triomed, S.Afr.*
Hydrocortisone acetate (p.1103·3).
*Skin disorders.*

**Dilum** *Tecnifar, Port.*
Isoxsuprine hydrochloride (p.1702·2).
*Cerebral and peripheral vascular disorders; relaxation of the uterus.*

**Diluplex** *Steierl, Ger.*
Homoeopathic preparation.

**Dilusol** *Dermtek, Canad.*
Alcohol (p.1166·1); isopropyl alcohol; propylene glycol; laureth-4.
*Topical vehicle.*

**Dilusol AHA** *Dermtek, Canad.*
Alcohol (p.1166·1); glycolic acid (p.1147·3); polyquaternium 10; polysorbate 20; propylene glycol.
*Topical vehicle.*

**Dilutol** *Roche, Spain.*
Torasemide (p.1015·3) or torasemide sodium (p.1015·3).
*Hypertension; oedema.*

**Dilydrin** *Willvonseder, Austria†.*
Buphenine hydrochloride (p.1663·2).
*Dysmenorrhoea; premature labour.*

**Dilydrine Retard** *Medichemie, Switz.†.*
Buphenine hydrochloride (p.1663·2).
*Peripheral vascular disorders.*

**Dilzanol** *Remedina, Gr.*
Diltiazem (p.901·3).
*Angina; hypertension.*

**Dilzatyrol** *Tyrol, Austria.*
Diltiazem hydrochloride (p.900·1).
*Angina pectoris; hypertension.*

**Dilzem**
*Douglas, Austral.; Parke, Davis, Austria; Orion, Fin.; Godecke, Ger.; Douglas, Hong Kong†; Torrent, India; Elan, Irl.; Douglas, NZ; Pfizer, Switz.; Pharmasant, Thai.; Elan, UK.*
Diltiazem hydrochloride (p.900·1).
*Angina pectoris; arrhythmias; hypertension.*

**Dilzene** *Sigma-Tau, Ital.*
Diltiazem hydrochloride (p.900·1).
*Arrhythmias; hypertension; ischaemic heart disease.*

**Dilzen-G** *Klonal, Arg.*
Diltiazem (p.901·3).
*Angina pectoris.*

**Dilzereal** *Realpharma, Ger.†.*
Diltiazem hydrochloride (p.900·1).
*Angina pectoris; hypertension.*

**Dilzicardin** *Azupharma, Ger.*
Diltiazem hydrochloride (p.900·1).
*Angina pectoris; hypertension.*

**Dima** *Medochemie, Singapore†.*
Nitrazepam (p.710·1).
*Insomnia.*

**Dimac** *Lilly, Austria†.*
Dirithromycin (p.206·1).
*Bacterial infections.*

**Dimacol**
*Wyeth, Mex.; Robins, USA.*
Guaifenesin (p.1122·1); pseudoephedrine hydrochloride (p.1129·2); dextromethorphan hydrobromide (p.1117·3).
*Coughs; nasal congestion.*

**Dimafit** *Body Spring, Ital.*
Garcinia, chromium tripicolinate; taraxacum; birch leaf; camelia sinensis (p.1417·1).
*Nutritional supplement; obesity.*

**Dimagrasi** *Giuliani, Ital.*
Avena; soya lecithin; oligopeptides; vitamin E; betacarotene; chromium-rich yeast (p.1417·1).
*Nutritional supplement; obesity.*

**Dimagrasicell** *Giuliani, Ital.*
Bladderwrack; java tea; bioflavonoids; tilia; ginkgo biloba; chronium-rich yeast; centella; vitamin E (p.1417·1).
*Cellulite; nutritional supplement.*

**Dimagress** *Heralds, Braz.†.*
Tiratricol (p.1604·3).
*Lipolytic.*

**Dimagrir Triac** *Gador, Arg.*
Mazindol (p.1589·1); tiratricol (p.1604·3).
*Obesity.*

**Dimalosio** *Tipomark, Ital.†.*
Lactulose (p.1269·1); glucomannan (p.1693·3).
*Gastrointestinal disorders.*

**Dimanin R** *Bayer, Ital.*
Benzalkonium chloride (p.1168·3).
*Surface disinfection.*

**Dim-Antos** *Pharmonta, Austria.*
Propyphenazone (p.85·3).
*Fever; pain.*

**Dimaphen** *Major, USA†.*
Phenylpropanolamine hydrochloride (p.1127·3); brompheniramine maleate (p.426·1).
*Upper respiratory-tract symptoms.*

**Dimate** *Merck, Hong Kong.*
Dimenhydrinate (p.431·1).
*Motion sickness.*

**Dimaval**
*Note. This name is used for preparations of different composition.*
*Lazar, Arg.*
Homatropine methylbromide (p.483·2); benactyzine hydrochloride (p.287·1); pentobarbital (p.713·2).
*Smooth muscle spasm.*

*Heyl, Ger.*
Unithiol (p.1055·3).
*Heavy-metal poisoning.*

**Dimaxin** *Medipharma, Hong Kong.*
Brompheniramine maleate (p.426·1); phenylephrine hydrochloride (p.1126·3); phenylpropanolamine hydrochloride (p.1127·3).
*Cold and influenza symptoms.*

**Dimayon** *Sabater, Spain†.*
Camphor (p.1665·3); cineole (p.1672·1); niaouli oil (p.1719·3); oxolamine citrate (p.1126·1); paracetamol (p.76·2); choline theophyllinate (p.784·2); vitamin A (p.1451·2).
*Influenza and cold symptoms.*

**Dimecaina** *Grunenthal, Chile.*
Lidocaine hydrochloride (p.1377·3).
*Arrhythmias; local anaesthesia.*

**Dimefor**
*Farmoquimica, Braz.; Lilly, Mex.*
Metformin hydrochloride (p.342·3).
*Diabetes mellitus.*

**Dimegan**
*Dexo, Fr.; Kreussler, Ger.†.*
Brompheniramine maleate (p.426·1).
*Allergic disorders.*

**Dimelor**
*Lilly, Canad.†; Lilly, Hong Kong†; Quatromed, S.Afr.†.*
Acetohexamide (p.329·2).
*Diabetes mellitus.*

**Dimen** *Heumann, Ger.*
Dimenhydrinate (p.431·1).
*Dizziness; motion sickness; nausea; vomiting.*

**Dimenate**
*DHA, Hong Kong; DHA, Singapore.*
Dimenhydrinate (p.431·1).
*Ménière's syndrome; motion sickness; nausea and vomiting.*

**Dimenformon** *Organon, Belg.*
Estradiol benzoate (p.1550·1); estradiol phenylpropionate (p.1550·2).
*Menstrual disorders; oestrogen replacement therapy.*

**Dimeno** *Milano, Thai.*
Dimenhydrinate (p.431·1).
*Motion sickness; nausea and vomiting; vertigo.*

**Dimertest** *Agen, Austral.†.*
Test for fibrin derivatives in plasma.

**Dimesul** *Lafare, Ital.*
Nimesulide (p.67·1).
*Fever; inflammation; pain.*

**Dimetabs** *Jones, USA.*
Dimenhydrinate (p.431·1).
*Motion sickness.*

**Dimetane**
*Note. This name is used for preparations of different composition.*
*Whitehall-Robins, Canad.†; Whitehall, Thai.; Robins, USA.*
Brompheniramine maleate (p.426·1).
*Hypersensitivity reactions.*

*Whitehall, Fr.*
Brompheniramine maleate (p.426·1); pholcodine (p.1128·3).
Formerly contained brompheniramine maleate, pholcodine, phenylephrine hydrochloride, guaifenesin, and sodium benzoate.
*Coughs.*

*Wyeth, Switz.†.*
Codeine phosphate (p.27·1); phenylephrine hydrochloride (p.1126·3); phenylpropanolamine hydrochloride (p.1127·3); guaifenesin (p.1122·1).
*Coughs and associated respiratory-tract disorders.*

**Dimetane DC** *Robins, USA†.*
Brompheniramine maleate (p.426·1); phenylpropanolamine hydrochloride (p.1127·3); codeine phosphate (p.27·1).
*Coughs.*

**Dimetane Decongestant** *Robins, USA.*
Brompheniramine maleate (p.426·1); phenylephrine hydrochloride (p.1126·3).
*Upper respiratory-tract symptoms.*

**Dimetane DX** *Robins, USA†.*
Brompheniramine maleate (p.426·1); pseudoephedrine hydrochloride (p.1129·2); dextromethorphan hydrobromide (p.1117·3).
*Coughs.*

**Dimetane Expect** *Wyeth Lederle, Fin.†.*
Brompheniramine maleate (p.426·1); guaifenesin (p.1122·1); phenylpropanolamine hydrochloride (p.1127·3); phenylephrine hydrochloride (p.1126·3).
*Respiratory-tract disorders.*

**Dimetane Expect DC** *Wyeth Lederle, Fin.†.*
Codeine phosphate (p.27·1); brompheniramine maleate (p.426·1); guaifenesin (p.1122·1); phenylpropanolamine hydrochloride (p.1127·3); phenylephrine hydrochloride (p.1126·3).
*Respiratory-tract disorders.*

**Dimetane Expectorant**
*Whitehall-Robins, Canad.†; Whitehall, Thai.†.*
Brompheniramine maleate (p.426·1); phenylephrine hydrochloride (p.1126·3); phenylpropanolamine hydrochloride (p.1127·3); guaifenesin (p.1122·1).
*Coughs; hypersensitivity reactions.*

**Dimetane Expectorant C** *Whitehall-Robins, Canad.*
Brompheniramine maleate (p.426·1); phenylephrine hydrochloride (p.1126·3); guaifenesin (p.1122·1); codeine phosphate (p.27·1).
Formerly contained brompheniramine maleate, phenylephrine hydrochloride, guaifenesin, codeine phosphate, and phenylpropanolamine hydrochloride.
*Upper respiratory-tract disorders.*

**Dimetane Expectorant DC**
*Note. This name is used for preparations of different composition.*
*Whitehall-Robins, Canad.*
Brompheniramine maleate (p.426·1); hydrocodone tartrate (p.45·1); guaifenesin (p.1122·1); phenylephrine hydrochloride (p.1126·3); phenylpropanolamine hydrochloride (p.1127·3).
Formerly contained brompheniramine maleate, hydrocodone tartrate, guaifenesin, phenylephrine hydrochloride, and phenylpropanolamine hydrochloride.
*Upper respiratory-tract disorders.*

*Whitehall, Thai.†.*
Brompheniramine maleate (p.426·1); phenylephrine hydrochloride (p.1126·3); phenylpropanolamine hydrochloride (p.1127·3); guaifenesin (p.1122·1); codeine phosphate (p.27·1).
*Coughs; hypersensitivity reactions.*

**Dimetane Expectorant Enfant** *Whitehall, Fr.*
Brompheniramine maleate (p.426·1); guaifenesin (p.1122·1); sodium benzoate (p.1169·3).
*Upper respiratory-tract congestion.*

**Dimetapp**
*Note. This name is used for preparations of different composition.*
*Whitehall Consumer, Austral.; Robins, Hong Kong; Whitehall, NZ; Wyeth Consumer, Singapore; Whitehall, Thai.*
*Elixir; oral drops:* Brompheniramine maleate (p.426·1); phenylephrine hydrochloride (p.1126·3).
Formerly contained brompheniramine maleate, phenylephrine hydrochloride, and phenylpropanolamine hydrochloride in *Hong Kong* and *Thai.*
*Respiratory-tract disorders.*

*Whitehall, Braz.; Whitehall-Robins, Canad.†; Whitehall, S.Afr.; Wyeth, Switz.†.*
Brompheniramine maleate (p.426·1); phenylephrine hydrochloride (p.1126·3); phenylpropanolamine hydrochloride (p.1127·3).
*Cold and influenza symptoms.*

*Robins, Hong Kong†; Wyeth, Mex.; Whitehall, Thai.†.*
*Extentabs:* Brompheniramine maleate (p.426·1); phenylpropanolamine hydrochloride (p.1127·3).
*Upper respiratory-tract symptoms.*

*Whitehall-Robins, USA.*
Brompheniramine maleate (p.426·1); pseudoephedrine hydrochloride (p.1129·2).
Formerly contained brompheniramine maleate and phenylpropanolamine hydrochloride.
*Allergic rhinitis; nasal congestion.*

**Dimetapp Chewables** *Whitehall-Robins, Canad.†.*
Brompheniramine maleate (p.426·1); phenylpropanolamine hydrochloride (p.1127·3).
*Upper respiratory-tract disorders.*

**Dimetapp Children's Cough & Cold** *Whitehall-Robins, Canad.*
Dextromethorphan hydrobromide (p.1117·3); pseudoephedrine hydrochloride (p.1129·2).
*Coughs.*

**Dimetapp Clear** *Whitehall-Robins, Canad.†.*
Brompheniramine maleate (p.426·1); phenylpropanolamine hydrochloride (p.1127·3).
*Upper respiratory-tract disorders.*

**Dimetapp Cold** *Whitehall-Robins, Canad.*
Brompheniramine maleate (p.426·1); phenylephrine hydrochloride (p.1126·3).
*Allergic rhinitis; cold symptoms.*

**Dimetapp Cold & Allergy Chewable** *Robins, USA†.*
Brompheniramine maleate (p.426·1); phenylpropanolamine hydrochloride (p.1127·3).
*Upper respiratory-tract symptoms.*

**Dimetapp Cold, Cough & Flu** *Whitehall Consumer, Austral.*
*Day & Night Liquid Capsules:* Day capsules, dextromethorphan hydrobromide (p.1117·3); pseudoephedrine hydrochloride (p.1129·2); paracetamol (p.76·2); night capsules, dextromethorphan hydrobromide; pseudoephedrine hydrochloride; doxylamine succinate (p.432·3); paracetamol.
*Cold and influenza symptoms.*
*Liquid Capsules:* Dextromethorphan hydrobromide (p.1117·3); pseudoephedrine hydrochloride (p.1129·2); guaifenesin (p.1122·1); paracetamol (p.76·2).
*Cold and influenza symptoms; coughs.*

**Dimetapp Cold, Cough & Flu Day & Night** *Whitehall, NZ.*
Day capsules, dextromethorphan hydrobromide (p.1117·3); pseudoephedrine hydrochloride (p.1129·2); paracetamol (p.76·2); night capsules, dextromethorphan hydrobromide; pseudoephedrine hydrochloride; doxylamine succinate (p.432·3); paracetamol.
*Cold and influenza symptoms; cough.*

**Dimetapp Cold, Cough & Sinus** *Whitehall Consumer, Austral.*
Dextromethorphan hydrobromide (p.1117·3); pseudoephedrine hydrochloride (p.1129·2); guaifenesin (p.1122·1).
*Coughs; nasal congestion.*

**Dimetapp Cold & Fever** *Whitehall-Robins, USA.*
Pseudoephedrine hydrochloride (p.1129·2); brompheniramine maleate (p.426·1); paracetamol (p.76·2).
*Cold symptoms.*

**Dimetapp Cold & Flu**
*Note. This name is used for preparations of different composition.*
*Whitehall Consumer, Austral.; Whitehall, NZ.*
Dextromethorphan hydrobromide (p.1117·3); pseudoephedrine hydrochloride (p.1129·2); paracetamol (p.76·2).
*Cold and influenza symptoms; cough.*

*Robins, USA†.*
Brompheniramine maleate (p.426·1); phenylpropanolamine hydrochloride (p.1127·3); paracetamol (p.76·2).
*Upper respiratory-tract symptoms.*

**Dimetapp Cough & Cold Liqui-Gels** *Whitehall-Robins, Canad.†.*
Brompheniramine maleate (p.426·1); phenylpropanolamine hydrochloride (p.1127·3); dextromethorphan hydrobromide (p.1117·3).
*Coughs and cold symptoms.*

**Dimetapp Cough & Congestion** *Whitehall-Robins, Canad.*
Guaifenesin (p.1122·1); dextromethorphan hydrobromide (p.1117·3); pseudoephedrine hydrochloride (p.1129·2).
*Coughs.*

**Dimetapp Daytime Cold** *Whitehall-Robins, Canad.*
Paracetamol (p.76·2); pseudoephedrine hydrochloride (p.1129·2).
*Cold symptoms.*

**Dimetapp Decongestant** *Whitehall-Robins, USA.*
Pseudoephedrine hydrochloride (p.1129·2).
*Nasal congestion.*

**Dimetapp Decongestant Plus Cough** *Whitehall-Robins, USA.*
Pseudoephedrine hydrochloride (p.1129·2); dextromethorphan hydrobromide (p.1117·3).
*Coughs; nasal congestion.*

**Dimetapp DM**
*Note. This name is used for preparations of different composition.*
*Whitehall Consumer, Austral.; Whitehall-Robins, Canad.*
Brompheniramine maleate (p.426·1); phenylephrine hydrochloride (p.1126·3); dextromethorphan hydrobromide (p.1117·3).
*Cold symptoms; upper respiratory-tract disorders.*

*Whitehall-Robins, USA.*
Brompheniramine maleate (p.426·1); pseudoephedrine hydrochloride (p.1129·2); dextromethorphan hydrobromide (p.1117·3).
Formerly contained brompheniramine maleate, phenylpropanolamine hydrochloride, and dextromethorphan hydrobromide.
*Coughs and cold symptoms.*

**Dimetapp DM Cold & Cough** *Whitehall, NZ.*
Brompheniramine maleate (p.426·1); phenylephrine hydrochloride (p.1126·3); dextromethorphan hydrobromide (p.1117·3).
*Cold symptoms; cough; hay fever; nasal congestion.*

**Dimetapp Expectorante** *Whitehall, Braz.†.*
Brompheniramine maleate (p.426·1); phenylephrine hydrochloride (p.1126·3); phenylpropanolamine hydrochloride (p.1127·3); guaifenesin (p.1122·1).
*Nasal congestion.*

**Dimetapp 12 Hour Nasal** *Whitehall Consumer, Austral.*
Oxymetazoline hydrochloride (p.1126·1).
*Nasal congestion.*

**Dimetapp Liqui-Gels** *Whitehall-Robins, Canad.†.*
Brompheniramine maleate (p.426·1); phenylpropanolamine hydrochloride (p.1127·3).
*Upper respiratory-tract disorders.*

**Dimetapp Long Actine Cough Plus Cold** *Wyeth, USA.*
Dextromethorphan hydrobromide (p.1117·3); pseudoephedrine hydrochloride (p.1129·2).
*Upper respiratory-tract disorders.*

**Dimetapp New** *Wyeth, Gr.*
Brompheniramine maleate (p.426·1); phenylpropanolamine hydrochloride (p.1127·3).
*Hypersensitivity reactions.*

**Dimetapp Nighttime Cold** *Whitehall-Robins, Canad.*
Phenylephrine hydrochloride (p.1126·3); chlorphenamine maleate (p.427·3); paracetamol (p.76·2).
*Cold symptoms.*

**Dimetapp Nighttime Flu** *Whitehall-Robins, USA.*
Pseudoephedrine hydrochloride (p.1129·2); dextromethorphan hydrobromide (p.1117·3); paracetamol (p.76·2); brompheniramine maleate (p.426·1).
*Coughs and cold symptoms.*

**Dimetapp Non-Drowsy Flu** *Whitehall-Robins, USA.*
Pseudoephedrine hydrochloride (p.1129·2); dextromethorphan hydrobromide (p.1117·3); paracetamol (p.76·2).
*Coughs and cold symptoms.*

**Dimetapp Oral Infant Drops** *Whitehall-Robins, Canad.*
Brompheniramine maleate (p.426·1); phenylephrine hydrochloride (p.1126·3).
Formerly contained brompheniramine maleate, phenylephrine hydrochloride, and phenylpropanolamine hydrochloride.
*Cold symptoms; hypersensitivity reactions.*

**Dimetapp Quick Dissolve** *Whitehall-Robins, Canad.†.*
Brompheniramine maleate (p.426·1); phenylpropanolamine hydrochloride (p.1127·3).
*Respiratory-tract disorders.*

**Dimetapp Sinus**
*Note. This name is used for preparations of different composition.*
*Whitehall Consumer, Austral.; Whitehall, NZ.*
Pseudoephedrine hydrochloride (p.1129·2).
*Nasal and sinus congestion.*

*Robins, USA.*
Pseudoephedrine hydrochloride (p.1129·2); ibuprofen (p.45·3).
*Nasal congestion.*

**Dimetapp-A Sinus** *Whitehall-Robins, Canad.†.*
Phenylephrine hydrochloride (p.1126·3); phenylpropanolamine hydrochloride (p.1127·3); paracetamol (p.76·2).
*Cold symptoms.*

**Dimetapp-C** *Whitehall-Robins, Canad.*
Brompheniramine maleate (p.426·1); phenylephrine hydrochloride (p.1126·3); codeine phosphate (p.27·1).
Formerly contained brompheniramine maleate, phenylephrine hydrochloride, codeine phosphate, and phenylpropanolamine hydrochloride.
*Cold symptoms; upper respiratory-tract disorders.*

**Dimethicream** *Hamilton, Austral.*
Dimethicone (p.1482·1); cetrimide (p.1172·1).
*Emollient barrier cream.*

**Dimetigal** *Galen, Mex.†.*
Cimetidine (p.1255·3).

**Dime-Time** *Time-Cap, Hong Kong†.*
Brompheniramine maleate (p.426·1); phenylephrine hydrochloride (p.1126·3); phenylpropanolamine hydrochloride (p.1127·3).
*Upper respiratory-tract symptoms.*

**Dimetin-F** *Farcoral, Mex.*
Dimenhydrinate (p.431·1).
*Nausea and vomiting.*

**Dimetirol** *Offenbach, Mex.*
Metamizole magnesium (p.36·1).
*Fever; muscle spasm; pain.*

**Dimetriose**
*Aventis, Austral.; Aventis, Malaysia; Aventis, NZ; Aventis, Port.; Aventis, Singapore; Aventis, Thai.; Distriphar, UK.*
Gestrinone (p.1556·2).
*Endometriosis.*

**Dimetrose**
*Piette, Belg.†; Aventis, Braz.; Monsanto, Ital.*
Gestrinone (p.1556·2).
*Endometriosis.*

**Dimex** *Cazi, Braz.*
Dipyrone (p.35·3); diphenhydramine hydrochloride (p.431·3).
*Fever; pain.*

**Dimezin** *Teuto, Braz.*
Dimeticone (p.1289·2).
*Flatulence.*

**Dimicaps** *Pharmacaps, Mex.†.*
Dimenhydrinate (p.431·1).

**Dimicin** *Bergamo, Braz.†.*
Phthalylsulfacetamide; neomycin (p.235·1); aluminium hydroxide (p.1249·2).
*Diarrhoea.*

**Dimicina** *Codilab, Port.*
Bacitracin (p.161·3); neomycin sulfate (p.235·1).
*Diarrhoea.*

**DiMill** *SIT, Ital.*
Benzalkonium chloride (p.1168·3).
*Eye disinfection; eye irritation.*

**Diminex** *Rhone-Poulenc Rorer, Mex.†.*
Phentermine (p.1592·2).

**Diminex Antitusigeno** *Vinas, Spain.*
Cineole (p.1672·1); chlorcyclizine hydrochloride (p.427·2); codeine phosphate (p.27·1); guaifenesin (p.1122·1).
*Coughs.*

**Diminex Balsamico** *Vinas, Spain†.*
Cineole (p.1672·1); chlorcyclizine hydrochloride (p.427·2); chlorpromazine hydrochloride (p.675·2); dextromethorphan hydrobromide (p.1117·3); niaouli oil (p.1719·3); guaifenesin (p.1122·1).
*Respiratory-tract disorders.*

**Diminon** *Master, Chile.*
Clonixin lysine (p.26·3).
*Inflammation; pain.*

**Diminual** *Labocean, Fr.*
Avena; citrus documana murra; camelia sinensis; ananas tige; pectin; yeast; laminaria digitata; sweet marjoram (p.1417·1).
*Nutritional supplement.*

**Diminut** *Libbs, Braz.*
Ethinylestradiol (p.1553·2); gestodene (p.1556·1).
*Combined oral contraceptive.*

**Dimirel** *Aventis, Austral.*
Glimepiride (p.332·2).
*Diabetes mellitus.*

**Dimiril** *Chowgule, India.*
Diphenhydramine hydrochloride (p.431·3).
*Hypersensitivity reactions.*

**Dimitone**
*Roche, Belg.; Roche, Denm.; Abic, Israel.*
Carvedilol (p.881·1).
*Angina pectoris; heart failure; hypertension.*

**Dimodan** *Aventis, Mex.*
Disopyramide (p.903·3).
*Arrhythmias.*

**Dimol** *Wallace, India.*
Simeticone (p.1289·2).
*Adjunct in gastroscopy and abdominal x-ray; flatulence; infant colic.*

**Dimophen** *Nakornpatana, Thai.*†.
Dextromethorphan hydrobromide (p.1117·3); phenylpropanolamine hydrochloride (p.1127·3); chlorphenamine maleate (p.427·3); terpin hydrate (p.1131·1).
*Coughs.*

**Dimophen DC** *Nakornpatana, Thai.*
Diphenhydramine hydrochloride (p.431·3); ammonium chloride (p.1115·2); sodium citrate (p.1223·2).
*Coughs.*

**Dimor** *Nordic, Swed.*
Loperamide hydrochloride (p.1271·1).
*Diarrhoea.*

**Dimorf** *Cristalia, Braz.*
Morphine sulfate (p.60·2).
*Pain.*

**Dimotane**
*Wyeth, Irl.*†; *Goldshield, UK.*
Brompheniramine maleate (p.426·1).
*Allergic rhinitis; urticaria.*

**Dimotane Co**
*Wyeth, Irl.; Wyeth Consumer, UK.*
Brompheniramine maleate (p.426·1); codeine phosphate (p.27·1); pseudoephedrine hydrochloride (p.1129·2).
*Coughs.*

**Dimotane Expectorant**
*Whitehall, Irl.*†; *Wyeth Consumer, UK.*
Brompheniramine maleate (p.426·1); guaifenesin (p.1122·1); pseudoephedrine hydrochloride (p.1129·2).
Formerly contained phenylephrine hydrochloride, phenylpropanolamine hydrochloride, brompheniramine maleate, and guaifenesin in *Irl.*
*Coughs; respiratory-tract congestion.*

**Dimotane Plus** *Goldshield, UK.*
Brompheniramine maleate (p.426·1); pseudoephedrine hydrochloride (p.1129·2).
*Allergic rhinitis.*

**Dimotapp**
*Whitehall, Irl.*†; *Whitehall, UK*†.
Brompheniramine maleate (p.426·1); phenylephrine hydrochloride (p.1126·3); phenylpropanolamine hydrochloride (p.1127·3).
*Rhinitis; sinusitis.*

**Dimotapp Expectorant** *Whitehall, Fr.*
Carbocisteine (p.1116·2).
*Respiratory-tract disorders.*

**Dina** *San Carlo, Ital.*
Cimetidine (p.1255·3).
*Gastrointestinal disorders associated with hyperacidity.*

**Dinabac** *Lilly, Ital.*†.
Dirithromycin (p.206·1).
*Bacterial infections.*

**Dinac**
*Douglas, Austral.; Sriprasit, Thai.*
Diclofenac sodium (p.32·1).
*Gout; inflammation; musculoskeletal, joint, and soft-tissue disorders; pain.*

**Dinacode** *Picot, Fr.*
*Cream:* Turpentine oil (p.1760·1); pine oil; rosemary oil (p.1740·2); wild thyme oil; white thyme oil; niaouli oil (p.1719·3); cineole (p.1672·1); quinine sulfate (p.460·2).
*Respiratory congestion.*
*Paediatric suppositories:* Potassium borotartrate (p.1734·1); sodium benzoate (p.1169·3); sodium bromide (p.1663·1); phenobarbital (p.367·3).
*Coughs.*
*Paediatric syrup:* Sodium benzoate (p.1169·3); grindelia (p.1696·1); wild thyme; tolu balsam (p.1131·3).
*Coughs.*

**Dinacode avec codeine** *Picot, Fr.*
*Suppositories:* Codeine (p.27·1); cineole (p.1672·1).
*Syrup; paediatric syrup:* Sodium benzoate (p.1169·3); wild thyme; tolu balsam (p.1131·3); codeine (p.27·1).
*Coughs.*

**Dinacode N** *Picot, Switz.*
*Syrup:* Codeine (p.27·1); sodium benzoate (p.1169·3); thyme (p.1755·2); tolu balsam (p.1131·3).
*Tablets:* Codeine (p.27·1); sodium benzoate (p.1169·3).
*Coughs.*

**Dinaflex**
*Zodiac, Braz.; Tecnofarma, Chile.*
Glucosamine sulfate (p.1694·1).
*Degenerative joint disorders.*

**Dinaflex Duo** *Tecnofarma, Chile.*
Glucosamine sulfate (p.1694·1); chondroitin sulfate.
*Degenerative joint disorders.*

**Dinagen** *Hormona, Mex.*
Piracetam (p.1732·1).
*Cerebrovascular disease.*

**Dinalexin** *Pharmaten (Φαρματεν), Gr.*
Fluoxetine hydrochloride (p.292·1).
*Depression; obsessive-compulsive disorder; panic disorder.*

**Dinamotonic** *Pharma Investi, Chile.*
Vitamin E; vitamin C; zinc; selenium (p.1417·1).
*Tonic.*

**Dinapres** *Master Pharma, Ital.*
Delapril (p.892·2); indapamide (p.938·2).
*Hypertension.*

**Dinasepte** *Cosmofarma, Port.*
Povidone-iodine (p.1190·3).
*Skin and vulvovaginal infections; skin, burn, and vaginal disinfection.*

**Dinate**
*Jaapharm, Canad.; Seatrace, USA.*
Dimenhydrinate (p.431·1).
*Motion sickness.*

**Dinaton** *Asta Medica, Braz.*
Ginkgo biloba (p.1692·3).
*Vascular disorders.*

**Dinavir** *Cristalia, Braz.*†.
Indinavir sulfate (p.638·2).
*HIV infection.*

**Dinavital Ginseng** *Raffo, Arg.*
Ginseng; pyritinol; B vitamins (p.1417·1).
*Tonic.*

**Dinavital Q10** *Raffo, Arg.*
Betacarotene; ascorbic acid; *dl*-alpha tocoferol acetate; ubidecarenone (p.1417·1).
*Antoxidant.*

**Dinavital Vascular** *Raffo, Arg.*
Co-dergocrine; pyritinol; B vitamins; ginseng (p.1417·1).
*Cerebrovascular disorders; tonic.*

**Dinaxil** *Tecnifar, Port.*
Triprolidine hydrochloride (p.442·3); pseudoephedrine hydrochloride (p.1129·2).
*Allergic rhinitis; asthma; hypersensitivity; urticaria.*

**Dinaxil Capilar** *Serra Pamies, Spain.*
Minoxidil (p.960·1).
*Alopecia androgenetica.*

**Dinaxin** *Rayere, Mex.*
Ranitidine (p.1285·2).
*Peptic ulcer.*

**Dinazide** *TO-Chemicals, Thai.*
Triamterene (p.1016·2); hydrochlorothiazide (p.933·2).
*Hypertension; oedema.*

**Dindevan**
*Boots Healthcare, Austral.; Biological E, India; Goldshield, UK*†.
Phenindione (p.981·1).
*Thromboembolic disorders.*

**Dinefec** *British Dispensary, Thai.*
Diclofenac diethylamine (p.32·1).
*Inflammation; musculoskeletal, joint, peri-articular, and soft-tissue disorders; pain.*

**Di-Neumobron** *Roemmers, Arg.*
*Oral solution:* Paracetamol (p.76·2); chlorphenamine maleate (p.427·3).
*Soluble tablets:* Paracetamol (p.76·2); chlorphenamine maleate (p.427·3); tipepidine hibenzate (p.1131·3).
*Suppositories:* Paracetamol (p.76·2); guaifenesin (p.1122·1); niaouli oil (p.1719·3); cineole (p.1672·1); camphor (p.1665·3); terpineol (p.1752·2).
*Respiratory-tract disorders.*

**Dineurin** *Drugtech, Chile.*
Gabapentin (p.362·2).
*Epilepsy.*

**Diniket** *Schwarz, Ital.*
Isosorbide dinitrate (p.941·1).
*Angina pectoris; heart failure.*

**Dinill** *Allergan, Braz.*
Benzalkonium chloride (p.1168·3); boric acid (p.1662·1); borax (p.1661·3); hamamelis (p.1696·3); chamomile (p.1669·3).
*Eye disorders.*

**Dinintel**
*Diamant, Port.*†; *Diamant, Singapore*†.
Clobenzorex hydrochloride (p.1585·3).
*Obesity.*

**Dinisor** *Pfizer, Spain.*
Diltiazem hydrochloride (p.900·1).
*Angina pectoris; hypertension.*

**Dinistenile** *Lepori, Port.*
Prasterone sodium sulfate (p.1566·1).
*Anabolic; tonic.*

**Dinit** *Leiras, Fin.*
Isosorbide dinitrate (p.941·1).
*Angina pectoris; heart failure.*

**Dinnefords Teejel** *SSL, UK.*
Choline salicylate (p.26·2).
*Denture irritation; herpes labialis; mouth ulcers; teething pain.*

**Dinobroxol** *Sankyo, Spain.*
Ambroxol hydrochloride (p.1114·3).
*Respiratory-tract disorders.*

**Dinostral** *Helvepharm, Switz.*
Pentoxifylline (p.979·3).
*Vascular disorders.*

**Dinoven** *Sankyo, Spain.*
A heparinoid (p.931·1).
*Soft-tissue disorders; varices.*

**Dintoina** *Recordati, Ital.*
Phenytoin sodium (p.370·2).
*Arrhythmias; epilepsy; trigeminal neuralgia.*

**Dintoinale** *Recordati, Ital.*
Phenytoin sodium (p.370·2); methylphenobarbital (p.366·3).
*Epilepsy.*

**Dinul** *Tecnifar, Port.*
Famotidine (p.1265·2).
*Gastro-oesophageal reflux; peptic ulcer; Zollinger-Ellison syndrome.*

**Dio** *Sciencex, Fr.*
Diosmin (p.1688·2).
*Capillary fragility; haemorrhoids; venous insufficiency.*

**Dioalgo** *Bouchara-Recordati, Fr.*
Dextropropoxyphene hydrochloride (p.28·3); paracetamol (p.76·2).
*Pain.*

**Diocaine** *Dioptic, Canad.*
Proxymetacaine hydrochloride (p.1384·1).
*Local anaesthesia.*

**Diocalm Dual Action** *SSL, UK.*
Morphine hydrochloride (p.60·1); attapulgite (p.1251·1).
*Diarrhoea.*

**Diocalm Replenish** *Seton, UK*†.
Anhydrous glucose; sodium chloride; sodium citrate; potassium chloride (p.1222·2).
Formerly known as Diocalm Junior.
*Diarrhoea; oral rehydration therapy.*

**Diocalm Ultra** *SSL, UK.*
Loperamide hydrochloride (p.1271·1).
*Diarrhoea.*

**Diocam** *Elisium, Arg.*
Clonazepam (p.359·1).
*Anxiety; epilepsy; panic attacks; social phobia.*

**Diocaps** *Berk, UK.*
Loperamide hydrochloride (p.1271·1).
*Diarrhoea.*

**Diocarpine** *Dioptic, Canad.*
Pilocarpine hydrochloride (p.1495·1).
*Cholinergic; production of miosis.*

**Diochloram** *Dioptic, Canad.*
Chloramphenicol (p.185·1).
*Bacterial eye infections.*

**Diocimex** *Cimex, Switz.*
Doxycycline hyclate (p.206·2).
*Bacterial infections.*

**Diocla** *Oriental, Arg.*
Co-trimoxazole (p.199·3).
*Bacterial infections.*

**Dioctosal** *Libbs, Braz.*†.
Docusate sodium (p.1262·2); phenolphthalein (p.1284·1); dehydrocholic acid (p.1679·2); cascara (p.1255·1); magnesium sulfate (p.1228·2).
*Constipation.*

**Dioctyl**
*Everest, Canad.*†; *Schwarz, UK.*
Docusate sodium (p.1262·2).
*Constipation.*

**Diodarone** *Prodotti, Braz.*
Amiodarone hydrochloride (p.859·2).
*Arrhythmias.*

**Dioderm**
*Dermal Laboratories, Irl.; Dermal Laboratories, UK.*
Hydrocortisone (p.1103·3).
*Skin disorders.*

**Diodex** *Dioptic, Canad.*
Dexamethasone sodium phosphate (p.1097·2).
*Corticosteroid.*

**Diodine** *Marc-O, Canad.*†.
Iodine (p.1598·1); isopropyl alcohol (p.1184·3); potassium iodide (p.1598·1).

**Diodolina** *Mayo, Mex.*†.
Diiodohydroxyquinoline (p.603·3).

**Diodoquin**
*Glenwood, Canad.; Searle, Mex.*
Diiodohydroxyquinoline (p.603·3).
*Amoebiasis.*

**Dioeze** *Century, USA*†.
Docusate sodium (p.1262·2).
*Constipation.*

**Diofen** *Liptis, USA.*
Glibenclamide (p.331·2); metformin hydrochloride (p.342·3).
*Diabetes.*

**Diofluor** *Dioptic, Canad.*
Fluorescein sodium (p.1689·1).
*Aid to ophthalmic examination.*

**Diogent** *Dioptic, Canad.*
Gentamicin sulfate (p.217·1).
*Bacterial eye infections.*

**Diolaxil** *Sanofi Synthelabo, Spain.*
Sennosides A and B (p.1288·2).
*Constipation.*

**Diolin** *Chinta, Thai.*†.
*Syrup:* Streptomycin sulfate (p.256·2); furazolidone (p.605·2); kaolin (p.1268·3); pectin (p.1580·3); belladonna tincture (p.479·1); ipecacuanha tincture (p.1122·3).
*Tablets:* Diiodohydroxyquinoline (p.603·3); furazolidone (p.605·2); kaolin (p.1268·3); pectin (p.1580·3); atropine sulfate (p.477·1).
*Gastrointestinal infections.*

**Diomicete** *Edol, Port.*
Clotrimazole (p.396·2).
*Fungal eye infections.*

**Diomycin** *Dioptic, Canad.*
Erythromycin (p.208·1).
*Bacterial eye infections.*

**Diondel**
*Note. This name is used for preparations of different composition.*
*Roemmers, Arg.*
Flecainide (p.917·3).
*Arrhythmias.*
*Sanofi Synthelabo, Spain*†.
Metolazone (p.956·2).
*Hypertension; oedema.*

**Dionephrine** *Dioptic, Canad.*
Phenylephrine hydrochloride (p.1126·3).

**Dionina** *Merck, Arg.*
Ethylmorphine hydrochloride (p.37·3).
*Coughs.*

**Dionosil** *GlaxoSmithKline, Israel.*
Propyliodone (p.1067·3).
*Radiographic contrast medium for bronchography.*

**Dioparine**
*Thea, Fr.*†; *Ciba Vision, Switz.*†.
Sodium iodoheparinate (p.1748·1).
*Burns to the eye; corneal damage.*

**Diopentolate** *Dioptic, Canad.*
Cyclopentolate hydrochloride (p.480·3).
*Production of mydriasis and cycloplegia.*

**Diophenyl-T** *Dioptic, Canad.*
Phenylephrine hydrochloride (p.1126·3); tropicamide (p.491·1).
*Production of mydriasis and cycloplegia.*

**Diopine**
*Alvia (Αλβια), Gr.; Allergan, Mex.; Allergan, Spain; Allergan, Switz.*
Dipivefrine hydrochloride (p.1681·2).
*Glaucoma; ocular hypertension.*

**Diopred** *Dioptic, Canad.*
Prednisolone acetate (p.1108·1).
*Eye inflammation.*

**Dioptears** *Dioptic, Canad.*
Polysorbate 80 (p.1415·2).
*Dry eyes.*

**Dioptec** *Dergam, Fr.*
Evening primrose oil (p.1686·3); salmon oil (p.976·1); calendula (p.1665·2); vitamins; minerals (p.1417·1).
*Dry eyes.*

**Diopticon** *Dioptic, Canad.*
Naphazoline hydrochloride (p.1124·3).

**Diopticon A** *Dioptic, Canad.*
Naphazoline hydrochloride (p.1124·3); pheniramine maleate (p.438·3).

**Dioptimyd** *Dioptic, Canad.*
Sulfacetamide sodium (p.257·3); prednisolone acetate (p.1108·1).
*Eye disorders.*

**Dioptrol** *Dioptic, Canad.*
Neomycin sulfate (p.235·1); polymyxin B sulfate (p.245·1); dexamethasone (p.1097·1).
*Eye disorders.*

**Dioralyte**
*Aventis, Irl.; Rhone-Poulenc Rorer, Neth.; Korangi, Port.; Aventis, UK.*
Sodium chloride; potassium chloride; sodium acid citrate; glucose (p.1222·2).
*Diarrhoea; oral rehydration therapy.*

**Dioralyte Effervescent** *Aventis, UK.*
Sodium chloride; sodium bicarbonate; potassium chloride; citric acid; glucose (p.1222·2).
*Diarrhoea; oral rehydration therapy.*

**Dioralyte Relief** *Aventis, UK.*
Rice powder; sodium citrate; sodium chloride; potassium chloride (p.1222·2).
*Diarrhoea; oral rehydration therapy.*

**Dioralyte Rice** *Aventis, Neth.*
Rice powder; sodium chloride; potassium chloride; sodium citrate (p.1222·2).
*Diarrhoea; oral rehydration therapy.*

**Dioran** *Andromaco, Chile.*
Ibuprofen (p.45·3); dipyrone (p.35·3); chlormezanone (p.675·1).
*Musculoskeletal spasm; pain.*

**Diosmectal** *Malesci, Ital.*
Diosmectite.
*Gastrointestinal disorders.*

**Diosmil** *Cooperation Pharmaceutique, Fr.*
Diosmin (p.1688·2).
*Capillary fragility; haemorrhoids; venous insufficiency.*

**Diosminil** *Teofarma, Spain*†.
Diosmin (p.1688·2).
*Chronic venous insufficiency; haemorrhoids.*

**Diospor HC** *Dioptic, Canad.*†.
Neomycin sulfate (p.235·1); polymyxin B sulfate (p.245·1); hydrocortisone (p.1103·3).
*Eye disorders.*

**Diosporin** *Dioptic, Canad.*†.
Neomycin sulfate (p.235·1); polymyxin B sulfate (p.245·1); gramicidin (p.220·2).
*Bacterial eye infections.*

**Diostate** *Roberts, USA.*
Calcium with vitamin D and phosphorus (p.1417·1).
*Calcium deficiency; dietary supplement.*

**Diosulf** *Dioptic, Canad.*
Sulfacetamide sodium (p.257·3).
*Bacterial eye infections.*

**Diosven** *CT, Ital.*
Diosmin (p.1688·2).
*Peripheral vascular disorders.*

**Diotrope** *Dioptic, Canad.*
Tropicamide (p.491·1).
*Production of mydriasis and cycloplegia.*

**Diotroxin** *GlaxoSmithKline, S.Afr.*
Levothyroxine sodium (p.1600·1); liothyronine sodium (p.1602·2).
*Hypothyroidism.*

**Diotul** *Faes, Spain.*
Dosmalfate (p.1264·1).
*NSAID-induced peptic ulcer.*

**Diovan**
*Novartis, Arg.; Novartis, Austria; Novartis, Braz.; Novartis, Canad.; Novartis, Denm.; Novartis, Fin.; Novartis, Ger.; Novartis, Gr.; Novartis, Hong Kong; Novartis, Irl.; Novartis, Israel; Novartis, Malaysia; Novartis, Mex.; Novartis, Neth.; Novartis, Norw.; Novartis, NZ†; Novartis, Port.; Novartis, S.Afr.; Novartis, Singapore; Novartis, Spain; Novartis, Swed.; Novartis, Switz.; Novartis, Thai.; Novartis, UK; Novartis, USA.*
Valsartan (p.1018·3).
*Hypertension.*

**Diovan Comp**
*Novartis, Denm.; Novartis, Fin.; Novartis, Norw.; Novartis, Swed.*
Valsartan (p.1018·3); hydrochlorothiazide (p.933·2).
*Hypertension.*

**Diovan D** *Novartis, Arg.*
Valsartan (p.1018·3); hydrochlorothiazide (p.933·2).
*Hypertension.*

**Diovan HCT**
*Novartis, Braz.; Novartis, Canad.; Novartis, Mex.†; Novartis, USA.*
Valsartan (p.1018·3); hydrochlorothiazide (p.933·2).
*Hypertension.*

**Diovane** *Novartis, Belg.*
Valsartan (p.1018·3).
*Hypertension.*

**Diovenor** *Innothera, Fr.*
Diosmin (p.1688·2).
*Capillary fragility; haemorrhoids; venous insufficiency.*

**Diovol**
*Note. This name is used for preparations of different composition.*
*Carter Horner, Canad.*
*Oral suspension; caplets:* Aluminium hydroxide (p.1249·2); magnesium hydroxide (p.1272·2).
*Tablets:* Aluminium hydroxide-magnesium carbonate co-dried gel (p.1250·1); magnesium hydroxide (p.1272·2).
*Dyspepsia; heartburn.*
*Wallace, India.*
Aluminium hydroxide (p.1249·2); magnesium hydroxide (p.1272·2); magnesium carbonate (p.1272·1); simeticone (p.1289·2).
*Gastritis; gastrointestinal hyperacidity; hiatus hernia; peptic ulcer.*
*Carter Horner, Thai.*
*Oral suspension:* Aluminium hydroxide (p.1249·2); magnesium hydroxide (p.1272·2); simeticone (p.1289·2).
*Tablets:* Aluminium hydroxide-magnesium carbonate co-dried gel (p.1250·1); magnesium hydroxide (p.1272·2); simeticone (p.1289·2).
*Flatulence; gastric hyperacidity; gastritis; gastro-oesophageal reflux; heartburn; peptic ulcer.*
*Pharmax, UK†.*
Aluminium hydroxide (p.1249·2); magnesium hydroxide (p.1272·2); simeticone (p.1289·2).
*Flatulence; gastrointestinal hyperacidity.*

**Diovol EX** *Carter Horner, Canad.*
Aluminium hydroxide (p.1249·2); magnesium hydroxide (p.1272·2).
*Dyspepsia; gastro-oesophageal reflux; heartburn.*

**Diovol Forte** *Wallace, India.*
Aluminium hydroxide (p.1249·2); magnesium hydroxide (p.1272·2); simeticone (p.1289·2).
*Gastritis; gastrointestinal hyperacidity; hiatus hernia; peptic ulcer.*

**Diovol Forte DGL** *Wallace, India.*
Aluminium hydroxide (p.1249·2); magnesium hydroxide (p.1272·2); simeticone (p.1289·2); liquorice (p.1270·2).
*Gastritis; gastrointestinal hyperacidity; hiatus hernia; peptic ulcer.*

**Diovol Plus**
*Carter Horner, Canad.; Carter Horner, Hong Kong.*
*Oral suspension:* Aluminium hydroxide (p.1249·2); magnesium hydroxide (p.1272·2); simeticone (p.1289·2).
*Tablets:* Aluminium hydroxide-magnesium carbonate co-dried gel (p.1250·1); magnesium hydroxide (p.1272·2); simeticone (p.1289·2).
*Dyspepsia; flatulence; gastrointestinal hyperacidity; peptic ulcer.*

**Diovol Plus AF** *Carter Horner, Canad.*
Calcium carbonate (p.1254·2); magnesium hydroxide (p.1272·2); simeticone (p.1289·2).
*Dyspepsia; flatulence; heartburn.*

**Dioxadol** *Bago, Arg.*
*Injection; syrup; tablets:* Dipyrone (p.35·3).
*Oral drops:* Dipyrone (p.35·3); paracetamol (p.76·2).
*Pain.*

**Dioxaflex**
*Bago, Arg.*
Diclofenac (p.32·1).
*Inflammation; pain.*
*Armstrong, Mex.*
Diclofenac epolamine (p.33·1).
*Musculoskeletal, joint, and soft-tissue disorders.*

**Dioxaflex B12** *Bago, Arg.*
Diclofenac sodium (p.32·1); betamethasone (p.1093·1); cyanocobalamin (p.1458·2) or hydroxocobalamin (p.1458·2).
*Joint pain.*

**Dioxaflex Forte** *Bago, Arg.*
Diclofenac sodium (p.32·1); codeine phosphate (p.27·1).
*Pain.*

**Dioxaflex Gesic** *Bago, Arg.*
Diclofenac potassium (p.32·1); paracetamol (p.76·2).
*Dysmenorrhoea; soft-tissue disorders.*

**Dioxaflex Plus** *Bago, Arg.*
Diclofenac sodium (p.32·1); pridinol mesilate (p.1395·2).
*Musculoskeletal, joint, and peri-articular disorders.*

**Dioxicolagol** *Fabra, Arg.*
Cynara (p.1678·3); boldo (p.1661·2); belladonna (p.479·1); valerian (p.1762·2); espina colorada.
*Digestive disorders.*

**Dipasic** *Atlantis, Mex.†.*
Isoniazid aminosalicylate (p.224·2).

**Dipatropin** *Pasteur, Chile.*
Atropine sulfate (p.477·1); papaverine hydrochloride (p.1728·1).
*Muscle spasm.*

**Dipaverina** *Geyer, Braz.*
Papaverine hydrochloride (p.1728·1).

**Dipazide** *Siam Bheasach, Thai.*
Glipizide (p.332·2).
*Diabetes mellitus.*

**Dipedyne** *Wayne, Mex.†.*
Zidovudine (p.658·2).
*HIV infection.*

**Dipen** *Elpen (Ελπεν), Gr.*
Diltiazem (p.901·3).
*Angina; hypertension.*

**Dipentum**
*Pharmacia, Arg.; Pharmacia, Austral.; Pharmacia, Austria; Pharmacia, Canad.; Pharmacia, Chile; Pharmacia, Denm.; Pharmacia, Fin.; Pharmacia, Fr.; Pharmacia, Ger.; Pharmacia-Upjohn, Gr.; Pharmacia, Hong Kong; Celltech, Irl.; Sequus, Israel; Pharmacia Upjohn, Ital.; Pharmacia, Neth.; Pharmacia, Norw.; Pharmacia, NZ; Pharmacia, S.Afr.; Pharmacia, Swed.; Pharmacia, Switz.; Celltech, UK; Celltech, USA.*
Olsalazine sodium (p.1278·1).
*Ulcerative colitis.*

**Dipep** *Serum Institute, India.*
Papain (p.1727·3); amylase (p.1654·2); pepsin (p.1729·3); lipase; cellulase (p.1669·1).
*Dyspepsia.*

**Dipeptamin** *Fresenius Kabi, Ger.*
L-Alanyl-L-glutamine (p.1433·2).
*Parenteral nutrition.*

**Dipeptiven**
*Roux-Ocefa, Arg.; Fresenius Kabi, Austria; Fresenius, Braz.†; Fresenius Kabi, Denm.; Fresenius Kabi, Fin.; Fresenius Kabi, Fr.; Fresenius Kabi, Gr.; Fresenius Kabi, Ital.; Fresenius Kabi, Mex.; Fresenius Kabi, Norw.; Fresenius Kabi, Port.; Fresenius Kabi, Spain; Fresenius Kabi, Swed.; Fresenius Kabi, Switz.; Fresenius Kabi, Thai.; Fresenius Kabi, UK.*
L-Alanyl-L-glutamine (p.1433·2).
*Parenteral nutrition.*

**Diperflox** *Francia, Ital.*
Norfloxacin pivoxil (p.239·1).
*Urinary-tract infections.*

**Dipergon** *Shepa, Gr.*
Lisuride (p.1211·1).
*Acromegaly; hyperprolactinaemia; lactation inhibition; prolactinoma.*

**Diperil** *Nutrifar, Ital.*
Piperacillin sodium (p.243·1).
Lidocaine hydrochloride (p.1377·3) is included in this preparation to alleviate the pain of injection.
*Bacterial infections.*

**Diperpen** *Francia, Ital.*
Pipemidic acid (p.243·1).
*Bacterial infections of the urinary tract.*

**Dipervina** *Farma Lepori, Spain†.*
Dihydroergocristine mesilate (p.1680·1); vincamine (p.1764·2) or vincamine hydrochloride (p.1764·2).
*Cerebrovascular disorders; head injury.*

**Dipezona** *Omega, Arg.*
Diazepam (p.690·1).
*Anxiety; epilepsy; muscle spasm; sedation.*

**Diphamine** *Medgenix, Belg.*
Diphenhydramine hydrochloride (p.431·3).
*Hypersensitivity reactions; insect stings; pruritus; sunburn; urticaria.*

**Diphantoine** *Wolfs, Belg.*
Phenytoin sodium (p.370·2).
*Arrhythmias; epilepsy.*

**Diphemin** *Alcon, Switz.†.*
Dipivefrine hydrochloride (p.1681·2).
*Glaucoma.*

**Diphen AF** *Morton Grove, USA.*
Diphenhydramine hydrochloride (p.431·3).

**Diphen Cough** *Morton Grove, USA†.*
Diphenhydramine hydrochloride (p.431·3).
*Coughs.*

**Diphenamill** *Brunel, S.Afr.*
Aminophylline (p.780·2); diphenhydramine hydrochloride (p.431·3); ammonium chloride (p.1115·2); sodium citrate (p.1223·2).
*Coughs.*

**Diphenazol** *Vitamed, Israel.*
Diphenhydramine hydrochloride (p.431·3); naphazoline (p.1124·3).
*Allergic conjunctivitis.*

**Diphenhist** *Rugby, USA.*
Diphenhydramine hydrochloride (p.431·3).

**Diphenhydramine Compound Linctus** *Medipharma, Hong Kong.*
Diphenhydramine hydrochloride (p.431·3); ammonium chloride (p.1115·2).

**Diphenhydramine Constrictor** *Viatris, Belg.*
Diphenhydramine hydrochloride (p.431·3); naphazoline hydrochloride (p.1124·3).
*Hypersensitivity reactions.*

**Diphereline**
*Ipsen, Hong Kong; Beaufour-Ipsen, Hong Kong; Beaufour-Ipsen, Thai.*
Triptorelin (p.1341·2).
*Endometriosis; female infertility; precocious puberty; prostatic cancer; uterine fibroids.*
*Pharma Biotech, Israel.*
Triptorelin embonate (p.1341·2).
*Endometriosis; female infertility; precocious puberty, uterine fibroids; prostate cancer.*

**Diphlogen** *Novartis Consumer, Austria.*
Aluminium sodium silicate (p.1250·2); eucalyptus oil (p.1686·2); menthol (p.1711·3); methyl salicylate (p.59·3).
Formerly contained ethyl salicylate, eucalyptus oil, and menthol.
*Musculoskeletal, joint, peri-articular, and soft-tissue disorders.*

**Diphos** *Procter & Gamble, Ger.*
Disodium etidronate (p.771·2).
*Ectopic ossification; Paget's disease of bone.*

**Dipidolor**
*Janssen-Cilag, Austria; Janssen-Cilag, Belg.; Janssen-Cilag, Ger.; Janssen-Cilag, Neth.*
Piritramide (p.84·1).
*Pain.*

**Dipigrand** *Ahimsa, Arg.*
Dipyrone (p.35·3).
*Fever; inflammation; pain.*

**Dipimax** *Cimed, Braz.*
Dipyrone (p.35·3).
*Fever; pain.*

**Dipine** *Sanfer, Mex.†.*
Dipivefrine (p.1681·2).

**Dipiperon**
*Janssen-Cilag, Belg.; Janssen-Cilag, Denm.; Janssen-Cilag, Fr.; Janssen-Cilag, Ger.; Janssen-Cilag, Neth.; Janssen-Cilag, Switz.*
Pipamperone hydrochloride (p.716·1).
*Psychoses.*

**Dipiperon R-3345** *Janssen-Cilag, Gr.*
Pipamperone hydrochloride (p.716·1).
*Psychoses.*

**Dipiraxil** *Wayne, Mex.†.*
Dipyrone (p.35·3).

**Dipirex** *Geyer, Braz.*
Dipyrone (p.35·3).
*Fever; pain.*

**Dipirol** *Royton, Braz.*
Dipyrone (p.35·3); adiphenine hydrochloride (p.1648·1); homatropine methylbromide (p.483·2); papaverine hydrochloride (p.1728·1).
*Muscle spasm; pain.*

**Dipiron** *IMA, Braz.*
Dipyrone (p.35·3).
*Fever; pain.*

**Dipironax** *Royton, Braz.*
Dipyrone (p.35·3).
*Fever; pain.*

**Diplexil** *Tecnifar, Port.*
Sodium valproate (p.380·1).
*Epilepsy.*

**Diplexil-R** *Tecnifar, Port.*
Valproate semisodium (p.380·1).
*Bipolar disorder; epilepsy; migraine and other headaches.*

**Diplovax** *Biovac, S.Afr.*
A measles vaccine (Edmonston-Zagreb strain) (p.1623·1).
*Active immunisation.*

**Dipni** *Omega, Arg.*
Nystatin (p.406·3).
*Candidiasis.*

**Dipofen** *Arlex, Mex.†.*
Ibuprofen (p.45·3).

**Dipoquin**
*Ioquin, Austral.; Alcon, NZ†.*
Dipivefrine hydrochloride (p.1681·2).
*Glaucoma.*

**Diposef** *Unison, Thai.*
Dipotassium clorazepate (p.685·1).
*Anxiety.*

**Dipot** *Asian Pharm, Thai.*
Dipotassium clorazepate (p.685·1).
*Anxiety; insomnia.*

**Dipres** *Precimex, Mex.†.*
Dipyridamole (p.903·1).

**Diprin**
*Alcon, Denm.†; Alcon, Swed.†.*
Dipivefrine hydrochloride (p.1681·2).
*Glaucoma.*

**Diprivan**
*AstraZeneca, Arg.; AstraZeneca, Austral.; AstraZeneca, Austria; AstraZeneca, Belg.; AstraZeneca, Braz.; AstraZeneca, Canad.; AstraZeneca, Chile; AstraZeneca, Denm.; AstraZeneca, Fin.; AstraZeneca, Fr.; Cana, Gr.; AstraZeneca, Hong Kong; AstraZeneca, Irl.; Zeneca, Israel; AstraZeneca, Ital.; AstraZeneca, Malaysia; AstraZeneca, Mex.; AstraZeneca, Neth.; AstraZeneca, Norw.; AstraZeneca, NZ; AstraZeneca, Port.; AstraZeneca, S.Afr.; AstraZeneca, Singapore; AstraZeneca, Spain; Astra, Swed.; AstraZeneca, Thai.; AstraZeneca, UK; AstraZeneca, USA.*
Propofol (p.1305·3).
*General anaesthesia; sedative.*

**Dipro AS** *Delta, Braz.*
Betamethasone dipropionate (p.1093·1); salicylic acid (p.1157·1).
*Psoriasis.*

**Diprobase**
*Essex, Chile; Schering-Plough, Fr.; Schering-Plough, Irl.; Schering-Plough, Port.; Schering-Plough, UK.*
Emollient.
*Dry skin conditions; topical vehicle.*
*Schering-Plough, UK.*
*Ointment:* White soft paraffin (p.1479·3); liquid paraffin (p.1479·1).
*Emollient.*

**Diprobath**
*Schering-Plough, Irl.†; Schering-Plough, UK.*
Light liquid paraffin (p.1479·1); isopropyl myristate (p.1481·2); laureth 4.
*Bath additive; dry skin; hyperkeratosis.*

**Diprobet** *Polipharm, Thai.*
Betamethasone dipropionate (p.1093·1).
*Skin disorders.*

**Diprobeta** *Bunker, Braz.*
Betamethasone dipropionate (p.1093·1); betamethasone sodium phosphate (p.1093·1).
*Corticosteroid.*

**Diprocel**
*Key, Arg.; Schering-Plough, Hong Kong; Schering-Plough, Malaysia; Schering-Plough, Singapore.*
Betamethasone dipropionate (p.1093·1).
*Skin disorders.*

**Diproderm**
*Aesca, Austria; Schering-Plough, Denm.; Schering-Plough, Fin.; Schering-Plough, Norw.; Schering-Plough, Spain; Schering-Plough, Swed.*
Betamethasone dipropionate (p.1093·1).
*Otitis externa; skin disorders.*

**Diprodol** *Sons, Mex.*
Ibuprofen (p.45·3).
*Gout; inflammation; musculoskeletal and joint disorders; pain.*

**Diprofol** *Taro, Israel.*
Propofol (p.1305·3).
*General anaesthesia; sedative.*

**Diproform**
*Schering-Plough, Denm.†; Schering-Plough, Ital.*
Betamethasone dipropionate (p.1093·1); clioquinol (p.196·3).
*Infected skin disorders.*

**Diproforte** *Aesca, Austria.*
Betamethasone dipropionate (p.1093·1).
*Skin disorders.*

**Diprofos** *Schering-Plough, Port.*
Betamethasone dipropionate (p.1093·1); betamethasone sodium phosphate (p.1093·1).
*Corticosteroid.*

**Diprogen** *Schering, Canad.*
Betamethasone dipropionate (p.1093·1); gentamicin sulfate (p.217·1).
*Infected skin disorders.*

**Diprogenta**
*White, Arg.; Aesca, Austria; Schering-Plough, Braz.; Essex, Ger.; Schering-Plough, Hong Kong; Schering-Plough, Israel; Essex, Ital.†; Schering-Plough, Malaysia; Schering-Plough, Port.; Schering-Plough, S.Afr.; Schering-Plough, Singapore; Schering-Plough, Spain; Essex, Switz.; Schering-Plough, Thai.*
Betamethasone dipropionate (p.1093·1); gentamicin sulfate (p.217·1).
*Infected skin disorders.*

**Diprolen**
*Schering-Plough, Denm.; Schering-Plough, Fin.; Schering-Plough, Swed.*
Betamethasone dipropionate (p.1093·1).
*Skin disorders.*

**Diprolene**
*Schering-Plough, Belg.; Essex, Chile; Schering-Plough, Fr.; Schering-Plough, Israel; Schering-Plough, Neth.; Schering-Plough, NZ; Schering-Plough, S.Afr.; Essex, Switz.; Schering, USA.*
Betamethasone dipropionate (p.1093·1).
*Skin disorders.*

**Diprolene Glycol** *Schering, Canad.*
Betamethasone dipropionate (p.1093·1).
*Skin disorders.*

**Di-Promal** *Mundipharma, Austria.*
Ipratropium bromide (p.787·1); salbutamol (p.791·3).
*Obstructive airways disease.*

**Diprophos**
*Aesca, Austria; Schering-Plough, Belg.; Essex, Switz.*
Betamethasone dipropionate (p.1093·1); betamethasone sodium phosphate (p.1093·1).
*Corticosteroid.*

**Diproquin** *Essex, Chile.*
Betamethasone dipropionate (p.1093·1); hydroxyquinoline iodochloride (p.1700·1).
*Infected skin disorders.*

**Diprosalic**
*Key, Arg.; Aesca, Austria; Schering-Plough, Belg.; Schering-Plough, Braz.; Schering, Canad.; Essex, Chile; Schering-Plough, Denm.; Schering-Plough, Fin.; Schering-Plough, Fr.; Essex, Ger.; Schering-Plough, Hong Kong; Schering-Plough, Irl.; Schering-Plough, Israel; Schering-Plough, Ital.; Schering-Plough, Mex.; Schering-Plough, Neth.; Schering-Plough, Norw.; Schering-Plough, NZ; Schering-Plough, Port.; Schering-Plough, S.Afr.; Schering-Plough, Singapore; Schering-Plough, Spain; Schering-Plough, Swed.; Essex, Switz.; Schering-Plough, Thai.; Schering-Plough, UK.*
Betamethasone dipropionate (p.1093·1); salicylic acid (p.1157·1).
*Skin and scalp disorders.*

**Diprosept** *Schering-Plough, Fr.*
Betamethasone dipropionate (p.1093·1); clioquinol (p.196·3).
*Infected skin disorders.*

**Diprosis** *Essex, Ger.*
Betamethasone dipropionate (p.1093·1).
*Skin disorders.*

**Diprosone**
*Key, Arg.; Schering-Plough, Austral.; Schering-Plough, Belg.; Schering-Plough, Braz.; Schering, Canad.; Schering-Plough, Fr.; Essex, Ger.; Schering-Plough, Hong Kong; Schering-Plough, Irl.; Schering-Plough, Israel; Schering-Plough, Ital.; Schering-Plough, Malaysia; Schering-Plough, Mex.; Schering-Plough, Neth.; Schering-Plough, NZ; Schering-Plough, Port.; Schering-Plough, S.Afr.; Schering-Plough, Singapore; Essex, Switz.; Schering-Plough, Thai.; Schering-Plough, UK; Schering, USA.*
Betamethasone dipropionate (p.1093·1).
*Skin disorders.*

**Diprosone Depot** *Essex, Ger.*
Betamethasone dipropionate (p.1093·1); betamethasone sodium phosphate (p.1093·1).
*Parenteral corticosteroid.*

**Diprosone G** *Schering-Plough, Mex.*
Betamethasone dipropionate (p.1093·1); gentamicin sulfate (p.217·1).
*Infected skin disorders.*

**Diprosone Neomycine** *Schering-Plough, Fr.*
Betamethasone dipropionate (p.1093·1); neomycin sulfate (p.235·1).
*Infected skin disorders.*

**Diprosone Y** *Schering-Plough, Mex.*
Betamethasone dipropionate (p.1093·1); clioquinol (p.196·3).
*Infected skin disorders.*

**Diprospan**
*Note. This name is used for preparations of different composition.*
*Schering-Plough, Braz.; Essex, Chile; Schering-Plough, Denm.; Schering-Plough, Hong Kong; Schering-Plough, Israel; Schering-Plough, Malaysia; Schering-Plough, Mex.; Schering-Plough, Singapore; Schering-Plough, Thai.*
Betamethasone dipropionate (p.1093·1); betamethasone sodium phosphate (p.1093·1).
*Corticosteroid.*

*Essex, Chile.*
*Cream; lotion; ointment:* Betamethasone dipropionate (p.1093·1).
*Skin disorders.*

**Diprospan G** *Essex, Chile Crema.*
Betamethasone dipropionate (p.1093·1); gentamicin sulfate (p.217·1).
*Infected skin disorders.*

**Diprostene** *Schering-Plough, Fr.*
Betamethasone dipropionate (p.1093·1); betamethasone sodium phosphate (p.1093·1).
*Corticosteroid.*

**Diprotop** *Schering-Plough, Thai.*
Betamethasone dipropionate (p.1093·1).
*Skin disorders.*

**Diprox** *Sintofarma, Braz.†.*
Lansoprazole (p.1269·3).
*Peptic ulcer.*

**Dipsin** *CPH, Port.*
Famotidine (p.1265·2).
*Peptic ulcer; Zollinger-Ellison syndrome.*

**Dipulmin** *Allen, Spain†.*
Salbutamol sulfate (p.791·3).
*Obstructive airways disease.*

**Dipxapen** *Liferpal, Mex.*
Dicloxacillin (p.205·2).
*Bacterial infections.*

**Dipydol** *Valdecasas, Mex.*
Dipyrone (p.35·3).
*Pain.*

**Dipyridan** *Aventis, Belg.*
Dipyridamole (p.903·1).
*Angina pectoris; thromboembolism prophylaxis.*

**Dipyrin** *Ratiopharm, Fin.*
Dipyridamole (p.903·1).
*Thromboembolic disorders.*

**Dirahist** *Teofarma, Ital.*
Triamcinolone (p.1110·2); chlorphenamine maleate (p.427·3).
*Hypersensitivity reactions.*

**Directim** *Azevedos, Port.*
Amineptine hydrochloride (p.280·3).
*Depression.*

**Direktan** *Gerot, Austria.*
Sodium nicotinate (p.1442·1).
*Decubitus ulcer; peripheral vascular disease; sports massage.*

**Dirfaben** *Rayere, Mex.*
Pancreatin (p.1725·3); ox bile (p.1660·3); dimeticone (p.1289·2).
*Digestive disorders.*

**Dirine**
*Atlantic, Malaysia; Atlantic, Singapore; Atlantic, Thai.*
Furosemide (p.919·3).
*Hypertension; oedema.*

**Dirinol** *Cryopharma, Mex.†.*
Dipyridamole (p.903·1).
*Thromboembolic disorders.*

**Diroquine** *Atlantic, Thai.*
Chloroquine phosphate (p.448·2).
*Amoebiasis; malaria; rheumatoid arthritis.*

**Dirosea** *Pierre Fabre Dermo-Cosmetique, Arg.*
Retinal; HMC; dextran sulfate (p.1679·2).
*Skin disorders.*

**Diroseal** *Avene, Fr.*
Retinal; HMC; dextran sulfate (p.1679·2).
*Skin redness.*

**Dirox** *Gramon, Arg.*
Paracetamol (p.76·2).
*Fever; pain.*

**Dirret** *Best, Mex.*
Diclofenac sodium (p.32·1).
*Musculoskeletal, joint, and peri-articular disorders; pain.*

**Dirtop** *Medipharm, Chile.*
Sildenafil (p.1744·2).
*Erectile dysfunction.*

**Dirythmin** *AstraZeneca, UK†.*
Disopyramide phosphate (p.903·3).
*Arrhythmias.*

**Dirytmin**
*Astra, Belg.†; AstraZeneca, Neth.; Hassle, Swed.*
Disopyramide phosphate (p.903·3).
*Arrhythmias.*

**Disalcid**
*3M, Canad.†; 3M, USA.*
Salsalate (p.88·1).
*Musculoskeletal and joint disorders.*

**Disalgil** *Also, Ital.*
Glycol salicylate (p.44·3); camphor (p.1665·3); capsaicin (p.24·2).
*Musculoskeletal, joint, and soft-tissue disorders.*

**Disalgyl** *Monin, Fr.*
Methyl salicylate (p.59·3); capsicum oleoresin (p.1667·1); camphor (p.1665·3).
*Musculoskeletal and joint pain.*

**Disalpin** *AWD, Ger.*
Hydrochlorothiazide (p.933·2); reserpine (p.995·1).
*Hypertension.*

**Disalunil** *Berlin-Chemie, Ger.*
Hydrochlorothiazide (p.933·2).
*Diabetes insipidus; heart failure; hypertension; oedema.*

**Disanal** *Humana, Ital.*
Food for special diets (p.1417·1).
*Gastrointestinal disorders.*

**Disbuspan** *Prodotti, Braz.*
Dipyrone (p.35·3); hyoscine butylbromide (p.483·3).
*Pain; smooth muscle spasm.*

**Discase** *Knoll, Belg.†.*
Chymopapain (p.1671·1).
*Herniated lumbar intervertebral disc.*

**Dis-Cinil Complex** *Menarini, Ital.*
Dihydroxydibutylether (p.1680·2); cascara (p.1255·1); rhubarb (p.1287·3); boldo (p.1661·2).
*Constipation.*

**Dis-Cinil Ilfi** *Menarini, Ital.†.*
Dihydroxydibutylether (p.1680·2).
*Constipation with digestive disorders.*

**Disclar** *Casen Fleet, Spain†.*
Tocoferil nicotinate (p.1015·1).
*Hyperlipidaemias.*

**Disclo-Gel** *Colgate Oral Care, Austral.†.*
Erythrosine (p.1057·2).
*Disclosing agent for dental plaque.*

**Disclo-Plaque** *Colgate Oral Care, Austral.†.*
Fluorescein (p.1689·1).
*Disclosing agent for dental plaque.*

**Disclo-Tabs** *Colgate Oral Care, Austral.†.*
Erythrosine (p.1057·2).
*Disclosing agent for dental plaque.*

**Discmigon** *Zilly, Ger.†.*
Hypericum oil (p.299·2); wheat-germ oil; avocado oil; birch tar oil (p.1159·2); beef hoof oil; thiamine hydrochloride (p.1455·1); formic acid (p.1689·3); garlic juice (p.1691·1); birch leaf (p.1660·3); juniper berry (p.1703·1); gentian root (p.1692·2); lupulus (p.1708·1); clove (p.1673·2); male fern leaf (p.108·2).
*Joint disorders; keloid scars; rheumatism.*

**Disco-cyl Ho-Len-Complex** *Liebermann, Ger.*
Homoeopathic preparation.

**Discorid** *Bros, Gr.*
Nimesulide (p.67·1).
*Inflammation; musculoskeletal disorders; pain.*

**Discotrine**
*3M, Denm.; 3M, Fr.*
Glyceryl trinitrate (p.923·2).
*Angina pectoris; prevention of phlebitis and extravasation during intravenous infusion.*

**Discover** *Carter-Wallace, UK.*
Pregnancy test (p.1734·3).

**Discover One Step** *Wilson, NZ.*
Pregnancy test (p.1734·3).

**Discover Onestep** *Carter-Wallace, Austral.†.*
Pregnancy test (p.1734·3).

**Discover Onestep Ovulation Prediction** *Carter-Wallace, Austral.*
Fertility test (p.1734·3).

**Discretal** *Beta, Arg.*
Tibolone (p.1572·3).
*Menopausal disorders; osteoporosis.*

**Discromil** *Pergam, Ital.†.*
Hydroquinone (p.1148·1).
*Skin hyperpigmentation.*

**Discus compositum** *Heel, Ger.†.*
Homoeopathic preparation.

**Disdolen** *Uriach, Spain.*
Fosfosal (p.44·2).
*Fever; musculoskeletal, joint, peri-articular, and soft-tissue disorders; pain.*

**Disdolen Codeina** *Uriach, Spain.*
Codeine phosphate (p.27·1); fosfosal (p.44·2).
*Pain.*

**Disebrin** *Tubilux, Ital.*
Heparin sodium (p.928·1).
*Eye disorders.*

**Disel** *Andromaco, Arg.*
Naphazoline hydrochloride (p.1124·3).
*Nasal congestion.*

**Disel Hidrocortisona** *Andromaco, Arg.*
Naphazoline hydrochloride (p.1124·3); hydrocortisone (p.1103·3).

**Disento** *Nakornpatana, Thai.*
Diiodohydroxyquinoline (p.603·3); furazolidone (p.605·2); neomycin sulfate (p.235·1); phthalylsulfathiazole (p.242·3); light kaolin (p.1268·3).
*Diarrhoea; gastrointestinal infections.*

**Disento PF** *Nakornpatana, Thai.*
Furazolidone (p.605·2); pectin (p.1580·3); light kaolin (p.1268·3).
*Bacterial diarrhoea; enteritis.*

**Diseon** *Teva, Ital.*
Alfacalcidol (p.1461·2).
*Hypoparathyroidism; osteomalacia; osteoporosis; renal osteodystrophy; rickets.*

**Diseptil** *Gedis, Ital.*
Benzalkonium chloride (p.1168·3).
*Skin disinfection.*

**Diseptyl** *Rekah, Israel.*
Co-trimoxazole (p.199·3).
*Bacterial infections.*

**Diserim** *Apsen, Braz.*
Bendroflumethiazide (p.867·3); fluphenazine hydrochloride (p.699·3).
*Obesity; oedema; premenstrual syndrome.*

**Diserinal** *Pulitzer, Ital.*
Alfacalcidol (p.1461·2).
*Hypoparathyroidism; osteomalacia; osteoporosis; renal osteodystrophy; rickets.*

**Disfil** *Llorente, Spain†.*
Ectylurea; phenytoin (p.370·2); phenobarbital (p.367·3); aminohydroxybutyric acid (p.353·2).
*Epilepsy.*

**Disflatyl**
*Note. This name is used for preparations of different composition.*
*Solco, Austria; Solco, Fin.; Solco, Hong Kong; Solco, Malaysia; Inibsa, Spain†; Solco, Switz.; Merck, Thai.; Solco, Thai.*
Simeticone (p.1289·2).
*Flatulence; preparation for gastrointestinal investigations.*

*Solco, Hong Kong; Solco, Singapore.*
Dimeticone (p.1289·2); silicon dioxide (p.1581·3).
*Flatulence; preparation for gastrointestinal investigations.*

**Disfruta** *Maver, Chile.*
Citric acid (p.1673·1); sodium bicarbonate (p.1223·2).
*Antacid.*

**Disgren**
*Note. This name is used for preparations of different composition.*
*Biosintetica, Braz.; Poli, Ital.†; Hormona, Mex.; Uriach, Spain.*
Triflusal (p.1017·3).
*Thromboembolic disorders.*

*Pasteur, Chile.*
Aspirin (p.15·1).
*Thromboembolism prophylaxis.*

**Disifelit** *Fada, Arg.*
Droperidol (p.697·2); fentanyl (p.40·1).
*Neuroleptanalgesia.*

**Disinal** *Silanes, Mex.*
Clonixin lysine (p.26·3).
*Pain.*

**Disinclor** *Tipomark, Ital.†.*
Tosylchloramide sodium (p.1194·3).
*Disinfection of wounds and external genitals.*

**Disintyl** *Zeta, Ital.*
Benzalkonium chloride (p.1168·3).
*Disinfection of wounds, burns, and external genitals.*

**Disipal**
*Yamanouchi, Belg.; 3M, Canad.; Yamanouchi, Denm.; Gerolimatos (Γερολυματος), Gr.; Yamanouchi, Irl.†; Yamanouchi, Ital.; Yamanouchi, Norw.; CSL, NZ; Yamanouchi, NZ; 3M, S.Afr.; Yamanouchi, Swed.; Sovereign, UK.*
Orphenadrine hydrochloride (p.486·1).
*Drug-induced extrapyramidal disorders; parkinsonism; senile or presenile depression; vertigo.*

**Disipan** *Microsules Bernabo, Arg.*
Diclofenac sodium (p.32·1).
*Inflammation; musculoskeletal, joint, peri-articular, and soft-tissue disorders.*

**Diskin** *Federfarma, Ital.*
Dihydroxydibutylether (p.1680·2).
*Constipation with digestive disorders.*

**Diskinebyl** *Laphal, Hong Kong†.*
Dihydroxydibutylether (p.1680·2).
*Biliary-tract disorders; liver disorders.*

**Dislax** *Makros, Braz.†.*
Bisacodyl (p.1251·3).
*Constipation.*

**Dislembral** *Sanofi Synthelabo, Arg.*
Hyoscine butylbromide (p.483·3); diazepam (p.690·1).
*Muscle spasm with anxiety.*

**Dislep** *Silesia, Chile.*
Levosulpiride (p.722·2).
*Gastrointestinal motility disorders; nausea and vomiting; vertigo.*

**Dislipina** *Merck, Port.*
Simvastatin (p.997·1).
*Hyperlipidaemias.*

**Dislipor** *Andromaco, Chile.*
Atorvastatin calcium (p.866·1).
*Hypercholesterolaemia.*

**Disman Sobres** *Merck, Chile.*
Lactulose (p.1269·1).
*Constipation; hepatic encephalopathy.*

**Dismaren** *Sanofi Synthelabo, Arg.*
Cinnarizine (p.428·3).
*Cerebral and peripheral vascular disorders; vestibular disorders.*

**Dismenol N**
*Simons, Ger.; Adroka, Switz.*
Ibuprofen (p.45·3).
*Fever; inflammation; pain.*

**Dismenol Neu** *Medra, Austria.*
Ibuprofen (p.45·3).
*Pain.*

**Dismifen** *Best, Mex.*
Paracetamol (p.76·2).
*Fever; pain.*

**Dismolan** *Rivero, Arg.*
Ondansetron hydrochloride (p.1281·1).
*Nausea and vomiting.*

**Dismozon pur** *Bode, Ger.*
Magnesium monoperoxyphthalate.
*Surface disinfection.*

**Disnal** *Ferrer, Spain.*
Calcium carbonate (p.1254·2); colecalciferol (p.1461·3).
*Calcium deficiency; osteoporosis.*

**Disne Asmol** *Berenguer Infale, Spain†.*
Ipratropium bromide (p.787·1).
*Obstructive airways disease.*

**Disneumon Pernasal** *Solvay, Spain.*
Phenylephrine hydrochloride (p.1126·3).
*Nasal and sinus congestion.*

**D-Iso** *Ratiopharm, Ger.†.*
Sodium chloride; sodium citrate; potassium chloride; glucose (p.1222·2).
*Diarrhoea; oral rehydration therapy.*

**Disobrom**
*Cord, Hong Kong†; Geneva, USA.*
Pseudoephedrine sulfate (p.1129·2); dexbrompheniramine maleate (p.426·1).
*Upper respiratory-tract symptoms.*

**Disocor** *Janssen-Cilag, Port.*
Carnitine (p.1423·3).

**Disoderme** *Plough, Port.†.*
Benzocaine (p.1370·3); triclosan (p.1195·2); aloe vera (p.1141·3); *dl*-alpha tocopherol (p.1464·3); menthol (p.1711·3); camphor (p.1665·3).
*Burns; insect bites; sunburn.*

**Diso-Duriles** *AstraZeneca, Ger.*
Disopyramide phosphate (p.903·3).
*Arrhythmias.*

**Disofarin** *Wayne, Mex.†.*
Disopyramide (p.903·3).

**Disofrin** *Essex, Chile.*
Dexbrompheniramine maleate (p.426·1); pseudoephedrine sulfate (p.1129·2).
*Upper respiratory-tract disorders.*

**Disofrol**
*Schering-Plough, Braz.†; Schering-Plough, Fin.; Schering-Plough, Spain; Schering-Plough, Swed.; Essex, Switz.*
Pseudoephedrine sulfate (p.1129·2); dexbrompheniramine maleate (p.426·1).
*Upper respiratory-tract congestion.*

**Disogel** *Concept, India.*
Aluminium hydroxide (p.1249·2); magnesium hydroxide (p.1272·2); liquorice (p.1270·2); simeticone (p.1289·2).
*Gastro-oesophageal reflux; peptic ulcer.*

**Disogram** *Ranbaxy, UK.*
Diltiazem hydrochloride (p.900·1).
*Angina pectoris; hypertension.*

**Disol** *Siam Bheasach, Thai.*
Bromhexine hydrochloride (p.1115·3).
*Respiratory-tract disorders associated with increased or viscous mucus.*

**Di-Solvente** *Miller, Braz.†.*
Glibenclamide (p.331·2).
*Diabetes mellitus.*

**Disomet** *Orion, Fin.*
Disopyramide phosphate (p.903·3).
*Arrhythmias.*

**Disonorm** *Solvay, Ger.†.*
Disopyramide (p.903·3) or disopyramide phosphate (p.903·3).
*Arrhythmias.*

**Disopam** *Dexxon, Israel†.*
Diazepam (p.690·1).
*Alcohol withdrawal syndrome; anxiety; epilepsy; insomnia; lumbago; psychosomatic disorders; slipped disc; tremor.*

**Disophrol**
*Aesca, Austria†; Schering-Plough, USA.*
Pseudoephedrine sulfate (p.1129·2); dexbrompheniramine maleate (p.426·1).
*Upper respiratory-tract symptoms.*

**Disopranil** Prater, Chile.
Betamethasone (p.1093·1).
*Skin disorders.*

**Disoprivan**
AstraZeneca, Ger.; AstraZeneca, Switz.
Propofol (p.1305·3).
*General anaesthesia; sedative.*

**Disotat** Alpharma-Isis, Ger.
Di-isopropylammonium dichloroacetate (p.900·1) or di-isopropylammonium hydrochloride (p.900·1).
*Hypertension.*

**Disotate** Forest Pharmaceuticals, USA†.
Disodium edetate (p.1037·3).
*Digitalis-induced cardiac arrhythmias; hypercalcaemia.*

**Disothiazide** Dexxon, Israel.
Hydrochlorothiazide (p.933·2).
*Hypertension; oedema.*

**Disotron** Ariston, Braz.
Heparin sodium (p.928·1).

**Dispaclonidin** Novartis Ophthalmics, Ger.
Clonidine hydrochloride (p.885·2).
*Glaucoma; ocular hypertension.*

**Dispacromil** Novartis Ophthalmics, Ger.
Sodium cromoglicate (p.795·3).
*Allergic conjunctivitis.*

**Dispadex comp** Novartis Ophthalmics, Ger.
Dexamethasone sodium phosphate (p.1097·2); neomycin sulfate (p.235·1).
*Bacterial infections and inflammation of the eye.*

**Dispagent** Ciba Vision, Ger.†.
Gentamicin sulfate (p.217·1).
*Bacterial eye infections.*

**Dispasan** Ciba Vision, Ger.
Sodium hyaluronate (p.1697·3).
*Adjunct in ocular surgery.*

**Dispasmol** Andromaco, Chile.
Phenobarbital (p.367·3); atropine (p.476·3).
*Muscle spasm.*

**Dispatenol** Novartis Ophthalmics, Ger.
Dexpanthenol (p.1727·2); polyvinyl alcohol (p.1581·1).
*Dry eyes.*

**Dispatim**
Novartis, Austria; Novartis Ophthalmics, Ger.
Timolol maleate (p.1012·2).
*Glaucoma; ocular hypertension.*

**Dispello** Ayrton, UK.
Salicylic acid (p.1157·1); zinc chloride (p.1469·2); hypophosphorous acid (p.1700·2); pyroxylin (p.1156·2); colophony resin (p.1675·1).
*Corns; warts.*

**Dispeptal** Nicholas Piramal, India.
Pancreatin (p.1725·3); vegetable enzymes; bile salts (p.1660·3).
*Dyspepsia; eructation; flatulence; heartburn.*

**Dispeptrin** Ciformo, Braz.†.
Co-trimoxazole (p.199·3); calcium carbonate (p.1254·2); attapulgite (p.1251·1).
*Bacterial infections.*

**Disperbarium** Rovi, Spain.
Barium sulfate (p.1061·1).
*Contrast medium for gastrointestinal radiography.*

**Dispercarpine** Novartis, Gr.
Pilocarpine hydrochloride (p.1495·1).
*Glaucoma; production of mydriasis.*

**Disperin** Orion, Fin.
Aspirin (p.15·1).
*Fever; musculoskeletal and joint disorders; pain; thromboembolism prophylaxis.*

**DisperMox** Ranbaxy, USA.
Amoxicillin (p.155·3).
*Bacterial infections.*

**Displata** Serono, Mex.†.
Carboplatin (p.533·3).

**Display** Solea, Ital.
Benzalkonium chloride (p.1168·3).
*Eye disinfection; eye irritation.*

**Dispneitrat** IMA, Braz.
Aminophylline (p.780·2); guaifenesin (p.1122·1).
*Obstructive airways disease.*

**Dispon** Monsanto, Ital.
Liothyronine (p.1602·2).
*Cellulite; local accumulation of adipose tissue.*

**Dispril**
Reckitt & Colman, Belg.†; Reckitt Benckiser, Norw.; Meda, Swed.†.
Aspirin (p.15·1).
*Fever; inflammation; pain.*

**Disprin**
Reckitt Benckiser, Austral.; Reckitt Benckiser, Hong Kong; Reckitt Benckiser, Irl.; Reckitt Benckiser, Malaysia; Reckitt Benckiser, NZ; Reckitt Benckiser, S.Afr.; Reckitt Benckiser, Singapore; Reckitt Benckiser, UK.
Aspirin (p.15·1).
*Fever; inflammation; pain; thromboembolic disorders.*

**Disprin CV** Reckitt & Colman, UK†.
Aspirin (p.15·1).
*Thromboembolism prophylaxis.*

**Disprin Direct**
Reckitt Benckiser, Austral.
Aspirin (p.15·1).
Glycine (p.1433·3) is included in this preparation in an attempt to limit adverse effects on the gastrointestinal mucosa.
*Fever; inflammation; pain.*

Reckitt Benckiser, UK.
Aspirin (p.15·1).
*Fever; pain.*

**Disprin Extra**
Reckitts, Irl.†; Reckitt Benckiser, UK.
Aspirin (p.15·1); paracetamol (p.76·2).
*Fever; pain.*

**Disprin Forte** Reckitt Benckiser, Austral.
Aspirin (p.15·1); codeine phosphate (p.27·1).
*Fever; inflammation; pain.*

**Disprina** Sanofi Synthelabo, Mex.
Aspirin (p.15·1).
*Fever; pain.*

**Disprol**
Reckitt Benckiser, Irl.; Reckitt Benckiser, NZ; Reckitt Benckiser, UK.
Paracetamol (p.76·2).
*Fever; pain.*

**Dispromil** Diviser Aquilea, Spain.
Famotidine (p.1265·2).
*Gastro-oesophageal reflux; peptic ulcer; Zollinger-Ellison syndrome.*

**Disques Coricides** SSL, Fr.
Salicylic acid (p.1157·1).
*Calluses; corns.*

**Dissenten** SPA, Ital.
Loperamide hydrochloride (p.1271·1).
*Diarrhoea.*

**Dissolursil** Uno, Ital.
Ursodeoxycholic acid (p.1760·3).
*Biliary dyspepsia; cholesterol gallstones.*

**Dissolvurol** Dissolvurol, Mon.
Colloidal silicon dioxide (p.1581·3).
*Musculoskeletal and joint disorders.*

**Distaclor**
Lilly, Irl.; Lilly, Malaysia; Lilly, Singapore; Lilly, Thai.; Dista, UK.
Cefaclor (p.167·1).
*Bacterial infections.*

**Distalene** Elvetium, Arg.
Anastrozole (p.528·1).

**Distalgesic**
Lilly, Hong Kong; Napp, Irl.; Lilly, Swed.; Dista, Switz.; Meda, UK.
Dextropropoxyphene hydrochloride (p.28·3); paracetamol (p.76·2).
These ingredients can be described by the British Approved Name Co-proxamol.
*Pain.*

Aspen, S.Afr.
Dextropropoxyphene napsilate (p.28·3); paracetamol (p.76·2).
*Fever; pain.*

**Distalgic** Lilly, Belg.
Dextropropoxyphene hydrochloride (p.28·3); paracetamol (p.76·2).
*Fever; pain.*

**Distamine**
Alliance, Irl.; Lilly, Neth.†; Lilly, NZ; Alliance, UK.
Penicillamine (p.1046·3).
*Cystinuria; heavy metal poisoning; hepatitis; rheumatoid arthritis; Wilson's disease.*

**Distaph** Alphapharm, Austral.
Dicloxacillin sodium (p.205·2).
*Gram-positive bacterial infections.*

**Distaquaine V-K** Lilly, UK†.
Phenoxymethylpenicillin potassium (p.242·1).
*Bacterial infections.*

**Distasil** Milana, Ital.
Benzalkonium chloride (p.1168·3).
*Skin disinfection.*

**Distaxid** Norgine, Spain.
Nizatidine (p.1277·2).
*Gastro-oesophageal reflux; peptic ulcer.*

**Distenil** Sun, India.
Simeticone (p.1289·2); activated charcoal (p.1030·2).
*Aerophagia; dyspepsia; food intolerance; gastrointestinal spasm; malabsorption syndrome; meteorism.*

**Distensan** Esteve, Spain.
Clotiazepam (p.685·2).
*Anxiety; neuroleptanalgesia; premedication.*

**Disteril** Lachifarma, Ital.
Benzalkonium chloride (p.1168·3).
*Genital hygiene; skin, wound, and burn disinfection.*

**Distex** Pharmafina, Chile.
Flurbiprofen (p.43·3).

**Distilbene** Gerda, Fr.
Diethylstilbestrol (p.1548·1).
*Prostatic cancer.*

**Distinon** Samarth, India.
Pyridostigmine bromide (p.1496·1).
*Myasthenia gravis.*

**Distobram** Lilly, Port.
Tobramycin (p.271·2).
*Bacterial infections.*

**Distonal** Royal, Chile.
Desipramine hydrochloride (p.290·2).
*Attention-deficit hyperactivity disorder; bulimia; cocaine withdrawal syndrome; depression; narcoleptic syndrome; pain; panic attacks.*

**Distovagal** Tedec Meiji, Spain†.
Belladonna alkaloids (p.479·1); ergotamine tartrate (p.467·2); phenobarbital (p.367·3).
*Cardiovascular disorders; gastrointestinal disorders; genito-urinary disorders; menopausal disorders; premenstrual syndrome; vascular headaches.*

**Distraneurin**
Astra, Austria†; AstraZeneca, Ger.; AstraZeneca, Switz.
Clomethiazole (p.683·1) or clomethiazole edisilate (p.683·1).
*Alcohol withdrawal syndrome; insomnia; mania; pre-eclampsia and eclampsia; sedative; status epilepticus.*

**Distraneurine**
AstraZeneca, Belg.; IFET (ΙΦΕΤ), Gr.; AstraZeneca, Spain.
Clomethiazole (p.683·1).
*Alcohol withdrawal syndrome; insomnia; sedative.*

AstraZeneca, Neth.†.
Clomethiazole edisilate (p.683·1).
*Alcohol withdrawal syndrome; sedative; status epilepticus.*

**Di-Su-Frone** Hua, Thai.
Furazolidone (p.605·2); pectin (p.1580·3); kaolin (p.1268·3).
*Gastrointestinal infections.*

**Disulone** Aventis, Fr.
Dapsone (p.202·2); ferrous oxalate (p.1428·2).
*Dermatitis herpetiformis; leprosy; Pneumocystis carinii pneumonia; polychondritis.*

**Disupril** Faria, Braz.
Amino acids; vitamin B substances (p.1417·1).
*Nutritional supplement.*

**Diswart** Dermatech, Austral.
Glutaral (p.1180·3).
*Common warts.*

**DIT I-2** Dunhall, USA.
Sulfanilamide (p.263·2); aminoacridine hydrochloride (p.1165·3); allantoin (p.1141·3).
*Vaginal infections.*

**Ditanrix**
SmithKline Beecham, Austria†; GlaxoSmithKline, Ital.; GlaxoSmithKline, Spain; SmithKline Beecham, Switz.
An adsorbed diphtheria and tetanus vaccine (p.1613·1).
Separate preparations are available for infants and young children and for children and adults.
*Active immunisation.*

**Ditaven**
Merck, Austria; Merck, Ger.†.
Digitoxin (p.894·3).
*Haematomas; leg oedema; peripheral vascular disease; varicose ulcers; venous insufficiency.*

**Ditaven comp** Merck, Austria†.
Digitoxin (p.894·3); heparin sodium (p.928·1).
*Leg oedema; soft-tissue injuries; varicose ulcers; venous insufficiency.*

**Ditavene** Pharmadeveloppement, Fr.
Melilotus officinalis; red vine.
*Capillary disorders.*

**Ditayod** Solfran, Mex.†.
Phthalylsulfathiazole (p.242·3); clioquinol (p.196·3).
*Amoebiasis.*

**DiTe Anatoxal**
Berna, Hong Kong; Berna, NZ.
An adsorbed diphtheria and tetanus vaccine (p.1613·1).
*Active immunisation.*

**DiTe Booster**
Statens Serum Institut, Denm.; Statens Serum Institut, Fin.; SSI, Swed.
A diphtheria and tetanus vaccine (p.1613·1).
*Active immunisation.*

**Ditec**
Boehringer Ingelheim, Austria; Boehringer Ingelheim, Ger.
Fenoterol hydrobromide (p.785·2); sodium cromoglicate (p.795·3).
*Obstructive airways disease.*

**Di-Te-Kik**
Statens Serum Institut, Fin.; SSI, Swed.
A diphtheria, tetanus, and pertussis vaccine (p.1613·3).
*Active immunisation.*

**Di-Te-Ki-Pol**
Statens Serum Institut, Denm.; Statens Serum Institut, Fin.; SSI, Swed.
A diphtheria, tetanus, pertussis, and poliomyelitis vaccine (p.1615·1).
*Active immunisation.*

**Ditemer** Aventis Pasteur, Belg.
An adsorbed diphtheria and tetanus vaccine (p.1613·1).
*Active immunisation.*

**Ditenate N** Herbert, Ger.†.
Theophylline (p.798·3).
*Obstructive airways disease.*

**Ditenside** Almirall, Spain.
Enalapril maleate (p.909·2); hydrochlorothiazide (p.933·2).
*Hypertension.*

**Ditensor** Almirall, Spain.
Enalapril maleate (p.909·2).
*Heart failure; hypertension.*

**Di-Te-Per Anatoxal** Faran, Gr.
An adsorbed diphtheria, tetanus, and pertussis vaccine (p.1613·3).
*Active immunisation.*

**DiTePer Anatoxal** Pharmabroker, NZ†.
A diphtheria, tetanus, and pertussis vaccine (p.1613·3).
*Active immunisation.*

**DiTePerPol Vaccin** Berna, Switz.†.
A diphtheria, tetanus, pertussis, and poliomyelitis vaccine (p.1615·1).
*Active immunisation.*

**Di-Te-Pol** Statens Serum Institut, Denm.†.
A diphtheria, tetanus, and poliomyelitis vaccine (p.1615·2).
*Active immunisation.*

**Diteutrin** Teuto, Braz.†.
Co-trimoxazole (p.199·3); aluminium silicate (p.1250·2); magnesium hydroxide (p.1272·2).
*Diarrhoea.*

**Dithiazid** Merck, Austria†.
Hydrochlorothiazide (p.933·2).
*Hypertension; oedema.*

**Dithiazide** Pharmalab, Austral.
Hydrochlorothiazide (p.933·2).
*Hypertension; oedema.*

**Dithiol** Galephar, Fr.
Ethylmorphine hydrochloride (p.37·3).
*Coughs.*

**Dithrasal**
Dermatech, Austral.; Dermatech, Singapore.
Dithranol (p.1146·1); salicylic acid (p.1157·1).
*Psoriasis.*

**Dithrocream**
Hamilton, Austral.; Dermal Laboratories, Irl.; Dermal, Israel; Dermal Laboratories, UK.
Dithranol (p.1146·1).
*Psoriasis.*

**Ditizem** Siam Bheasach, Thai.
Diltiazem hydrochloride (p.900·1).
*Angina pectoris; hypertension.*

**Ditoin**
Atlantic, Hong Kong; Atlantic, Malaysia; Atlantic, Thai.
Phenytoin sodium (p.370·2).
*Epilepsy; migraine; trigeminal neuralgia.*

**Ditomed** Medifive, Thai.
Phenytoin sodium (p.370·2).
*Epilepsy.*

**Ditonal** Athenstaedt & Redeker, Hong Kong†.
Trichlor-dimethylethyl-salicylate; paracetamol (p.76·2).
*Fever; pain.*

**Ditonal N** Athenstaedt, Ger.
Paracetamol (p.76·2); caffeine (p.782·1).
*Pain.*

**Ditopax**
Note. This name is used for preparations of different composition.
Key, Arg.
*Chewable tablets:* Simeticone (p.1289·2); calcium carbonate (p.1254·2); magnesium hydroxide (p.1272·2).
*Flatulence; gastric hyperacidity.*

Key, Arg.; Essex, Chile; Schering-Plough, Mex.
*Oral suspension:* Simeticone (p.1289·2); aluminium hydroxide (p.1249·2); magnesium hydroxide (p.1272·2).
*Flatulence; gastric hyperacidity.*

Essex, Chile; Schering-Plough, Mex.
*Chewable tablets:* Simeticone (p.1289·2); aluminium hydroxide-magnesium carbonate co-dried gel (p.1250·1); magnesium hydroxide (p.1272·2).
*Flatulence; gastric hyperacidity.*

**Ditopax-F** Schering-Plough, Mex.
Aluminium hydroxide-magnesium carbonate co-dried gel (p.1250·1); magnesium hydroxide (p.1272·2); calcium carbonate (p.1254·2); dimeticone (p.1289·2).
*Flatulence; gastrointestinal hyperacidity.*

**Ditral**
Note. This name is used for preparations of different composition.
LA, Arg.; Sanitas, Arg.
Dipyrone (p.35·3).
*Fever; pain.*

Berman, Mex.
Tetrametamizole guaiacol; vitamins (p.1417·1).
*Bacterial infections.*

**Ditran** Breves, Braz.†.
Tenitramine (p.1010·3).
*Angina pectoris.*

**Ditrei** Italmex, Mex.
Di-isopropylammonium dichloroacetate (p.900·1).
*Angina pectoris; myocardial infarction; vascular disorders.*

**Ditrenil** Siam Bheasach, Thai.
Nitrendipine (p.973·3).
*Hypertension.*

**Ditrim** Orion, Fin.
Trimethoprim (p.272·2); sulfadiazine (p.258·2).
*Bacterial infections; Pneumocystis carinii pneumonia.*

**Ditripentat-Heyl** Heyl, Ger.
Calcium trisodium pentetate (p.1050·1).
*Poisoning with heavy or radioactive metals.*

**Ditropan**
Phoenix, Arg.; Aventis, Austral.; Sanofi Synthelabo, Austria; Sanofi Synthelabo, Belg.; Alza, Canad.; Sanofi Synthelabo, Fin.; Sanofi Synthelabo, Fr.; Sanofi Synthelabo, Gr.; Aventis, Hong Kong; Sanofi Synthelabo, Irl.; Sanofi Synthelabo, Ital.; Sanofi Synthelabo, Malaysia; Aventis, NZ†; Sanofi Synthelabo, Port.; Sanofi Synthelabo, S.Afr.; Sanofi Synthelabo, Singapore; Sanofi Synthelabo, Spain; Sanofi Synthelabo, Swed.; Synthelabo, Switz.; Janssen-Cilag, UK; Alza, USA.
Oxybutynin hydrochloride (p.486·3).
*Neurogenic bladder; urinary incontinence.*

**Ditropine** Asian Pharm, Thai.†.
Diphenoxylate hydrochloride (p.1261·3).
Atropine sulfate (p.477·1) is included in this preparation to discourage abuse.
*Diarrhoea.*

**Ditterolina** Fustery, Mex.
Dicloxacillin (p.205·2) or dicloxacillin sodium (p.205·2).
*Bacterial infections.*

**Ditum** Nakorn, Thai.
Dicloxacillin (p.205·2).
*Bacterial infections.*

**Diu Rauwiplus** *Lacer, Spain†.*
Ajmaline (p.856·1); hydrochlorothiazide (p.933·2); methylrauhimbine; sarpagine (p.994·3); rescinnamine (p.994·3); reserpine hydrochloride (p.995·2).
*Hypertension.*

**Diu Venostasin** *Fujisawa, Ger.*
Tablets, triamterene (p.1016·2); hydrochlorothiazide (p.933·2); controlled-release capsules, aesculus (p.1648·2).
*Venous insufficiency.*

**Diu-Atenolol** *Verla, Ger.*
Atenolol (p.865·2); chlortalidone (p.882·3).
*Hypertension.*

**Diube** *SIT, Ital.*
Atenolol (p.865·2); chlortalidone (p.882·3).
*Hypertension.*

**Diubeloc** *AstraZeneca, Arg.*
Metoprolol tartrate (p.957·1); hydrochlorothiazide (p.933·2).
*Hypertension.*

**Diucardin** *Wyeth-Ayerst, USA†.*
Hydroflumethiazide (p.937·2).
*Hypertension; oedema.*

**Diucomb**
*Gebro, Austria†; Byk, Belg.; Sanofi Synthelabo, Ger.; Schwarz, Switz.†.*
Bemetizide (p.867·1); triamterene (p.1016·2).
*Hypertension; oedema.*

**Diucontin-K** *Modi-Mundipharma, India.*
Furosemide (p.919·3); potassium chloride (p.1232·2).
*Oedema.*

**Diulo** *Pharmacia, Port.*
Metolazone (p.956·2).
*Ascites associated with liver cirrhosis; hypertension; oedema.*

**diu-melusin** *Schwarz, Ger.*
Hydrochlorothiazide (p.933·2).
*Hypertension; oedema.*

**Diumide-K Continus**
*Napp, Irl.; Asta Medica, UK†.*
Furosemide (p.919·3); potassium chloride (p.1232·2).
*Oedema.*

**Diupres**
*Note. A similar name is used for preparations of different composition (see below).*
*Merck, USA.*
Reserpine (p.995·1); chlorothiazide (p.882·1).
*Hypertension.*

**Diupress**
*Note. A similar name is used for preparations of different composition (see above).*
*Eurofarma, Braz.*
Chlortalidone (p.882·3); amiloride hydrochloride (p.858·2).
*Hypertension; oedema.*

**Diuprol** *Protein, Mex.†.*
Chlortalidone (p.882·3).

**Diuprotect** *Silesia, Chile.*
Copper-wound plastic (p.1425·3).
*Intra-uterine contraceptive device.*

**Diurace** *Bristol-Myers Squibb, Neth.*
Fosinopril sodium (p.919·1); hydrochlorothiazide (p.933·2).
*Hypertension.*

**Diural**
*Note. This name is used for preparations of different composition.*
*LA, Arg.*
Hydrochlorothiazide (p.933·2).
*Hypertension.*

*Alpharma, Denm.; Alpharma, Norw.*
Furosemide (p.919·3).
*Forced diuresis; hypertension; oedema; renal failure.*

*Silanes, Mex.*
Piretanide (p.983·3).

**Diuramid** *Medphano, Ger.*
Acetazolamide (p.849·1).
*Glaucoma.*

**Diuramin** *Ratiopharm, Fin.*
Amiloride hydrochloride (p.858·2); hydrochlorothiazide (p.933·2).
*Ascites; hypertension; oedema.*

**Diurana** *Sanofi Synthelabo, Braz.*
Furosemide (p.919·3); triamterene (p.1016·2).
*Hypertension; oedema.*

**Diurapid** *Jenapharm, Ger.*
Furosemide (p.919·3) or furosemide sodium (p.921·2).
*Oedema; oliguria.*

**Diurek** *Pulitzer, Ital.*
Potassium canrenoate (p.984·2).
*Hyperaldosteronism; hypertension.*

**Diuremid** *Guidotti, Ital.*
Torasemide (p.1015·3) or torasemide sodium (p.1015·3).
*Ascites; heart failure; oedema; renal failure.*

**Diurene** *Irex, Port.*
Amiloride hydrochloride (p.858·2); hydrochlorothiazide (p.933·2).
*Ascites associated with liver cirrhosis; heart failure; hypertension.*

**Diurepina** *Prodotti, Braz.*
Hydrochlorothiazide (p.933·2).
*Hypertension.*

**Diuresal** *Lagap, Switz.†.*
Furosemide (p.919·3).
*Hypertension; oedema; renal failure.*

**Diurese** *American Urologicals, USA.*
Trichlormethiazide (p.1017·2).
*Hypertension; oedema.*

**Diuresix** *Menarini, Ital.*
Torasemide (p.1015·3) or torasemide sodium (p.1015·3).
*Ascites; heart failure; kidney disorders; oedema.*

**Diuret** *Ibfarma, Braz.†.*
Furosemide (p.919·3).
*Hypertension.*

**Diuretabs** *Potter's, UK.*
Buchu leaf (p.1663·1); juniper berry oil (p.1703·1); parsley piert (p.1729·1); bearberry (p.1659·2).
*Fluid retention.*

**Diuretic** *Royton, Braz.*
Hydrochlorothiazide (p.933·2).

**Diuretikum Verla** *Verla, Ger.*
Triamterene (p.1016·2); hydrochlorothiazide (p.933·2).
*Hypertension; oedema.*

**Diuretil** *Ducto, Braz.*
Hydrochlorothiazide (p.933·2).
*Hypertension.*

**Diuret-P** *PP Lab, Thai.*
Hydrochlorothiazide (p.933·2).
*Diuretic.*

**Diurevit Mono** *Bional, Ger.*
Java tea (p.1702·3).
*Urinary-tract disorders.*

**Diurex**
*Note. This name is used for preparations of different composition.*
*Bago, Arg.*
Hydrochlorothiazide (p.933·2).
*Ascites; heart failure; hypertension; nephrotic syndrome; pre-eclampsia.*

*Cimed, Braz.†.*
Furosemide (p.919·3).
*Hypercalcaemia; hypertension; oedema.*

*Orion, Fin.*
Amiloride hydrochloride (p.858·2); hydrochlorothiazide (p.933·2).
*Cirrhosis with ascites; heart failure; hypertension.*

*Lacer, Spain.*
Xipamide (p.1029·2).
*Hypertension; oedema.*

**Diurexan**
*Asta Medica, Belg.†; Asta Medica, Hong Kong†; Asta Medica, Irl.†; Viatris, Port.; Mer-National, S.Afr.; Viatris, UK.*
Xipamide (p.1029·2).
*Hypertension; oedema.*

**Diurezin** *Cazi, Braz.*
Hydrochlorothiazide (p.933·2).
*Diabetes insipidus; hypertension; oedema; renal calculi.*

**Diurid** *Laevosan, Austria†.*
Triamterene (p.1016·2); hydrochlorothiazide (p.933·2).
*Heart failure; hypertension; oedema.*

**Diurigen** *Goldline, USA.*
Chlorothiazide (p.882·1).
*Hypertension; oedema.*

**Diuril** *Merck, USA.*
Chlorothiazide (p.882·1) or chlorothiazide sodium (p.882·2).
*Hypertension; oedema.*

**Diurin** *Pacific, NZ.*
Furosemide (p.919·3).
*Hypertension; oedema; severe renal impairment.*

**Diurinat** *Soria Natural, Spain.*
Betula alba (p.1660·3); equisetum (p.1684·1); corn silk (p.1676·1); couch-grass (p.1676·2).
*Gout; rheumatism; urinary-tract disorders.*

**Diurisa** *Eurofarma, Braz.*
Furosemide (p.919·3); amiloride hydrochloride (p.858·2).
*Hypertension; oedema.*

**Diurit** *Neckerman, Braz.†.*
Furosemide (p.919·3).
*Hypertension.*

**Diurix**
*Teuto, Braz.; Helvepharm, Switz.†.*
Furosemide (p.919·3).
Now known as Furosemide Helvepharm in *Switz.*
*Forced diuresis; hypertension; oedema.*

**Diurolan** *Rayere, Mex.†.*
Furosemide (p.919·3).

**Diursan** *TAD, Ger.*
Hydrochlorothiazide (p.933·2); amiloride hydrochloride (p.858·2).
*Hypertension; oedema.*

**Diutec** *Garec, S.Afr.†.*
Amiloride hydrochloride (p.858·2); hydrochlorothiazide (p.933·2).
*Hypertension; oedema.*

**Diutensat** *Azupharma, Ger.*
Triamterene (p.1016·2); hydrochlorothiazide (p.933·2).
*Hypertension; oedema.*

**Diutensat comp** *Azupharma, Ger.*
Triamterene (p.1016·2); hydrochlorothiazide (p.933·2); propranolol hydrochloride (p.989·3).
*Hypertension.*

**Diutensen-R** *Wallace, USA.*
Methyclothiazide (p.953·2); reserpine (p.995·1).
*Hypertension.*

**Diutropan** *Prima, Thai.*
Oxybutynin hydrochloride (p.486·3).
*Neurogenic bladder disorders.*

**Diuzine** *I Farmacologia, Spain.*
Amiloride hydrochloride (p.858·2); hydrochlorothiazide (p.933·2).
*Hypertension; liver cirrhosis with ascites; oedema.*

**Divacuna DT** *Leti, Spain†.*
A diphtheria and tetanus vaccine (p.1613·1).
Formerly known as Divacuna TD.
*Active immunisation of infants and young children.*

**Divalol W** *Wernigerode, Ger.*
Javanese turmeric (p.1759·3); peppermint oil (p.1283·2).
*Biliary disorders.*

**Divanon** *Tecnofarma, Chile.*
Clindamycin phosphate (p.194·2).
*Bacterial vaginitis.*

**Divaril** *Tecnofarma, Chile.*
Mirtazapine (p.307·3).
*Depression.*

**Divarius** *Chiesi, Fr.*
Paroxetine hydrochloride (p.311·2).

**Divascan** *Berlin-Chemie, Ger.*
Iprazochrome (p.469·2).
*Diabetic retinopathy; headache; migraine.*

**Divegal** *Sanochemia, Austria.*
Dihydroergotamine tartrate (p.466·1).
*Migraine and related vascular headaches.*

**Divelol** *Baldacci, Braz.*
Carvedilol (p.881·1).
*Angina pectoris; hypertension.*

**Divermil** *Gross, Braz.*
Mebendazole (p.108·2).
*Worm infections.*

**Divial** *Merck, Spain†.*
Lorazepam pivalate (p.705·1).
*Alcohol withdrawal syndrome; anxiety; chemotherapy-induced nausea and vomiting; epilepsy; insomnia.*

**Divical** *Rottapharm, Ital.*
Calcium folinate (p.1431·1).
*Folate deficiency.*

**Divicil** *BA Farma, Port.*
Aciclovir (p.626·1).
*Herpesvirus infections.*

**Dividol**
*Zambon, Braz.*
Viminol para-aminobenzoate.
*Pain.*

*Zambon, Ital.*
Viminol hydroxybenzoate (p.96·3).
*Pain.*

**Divigel**
*Orion, Denm.; Orion, Fin.; Orion, Irl.; Orion, Malaysia; Orion, Singapore; Orion, Swed.; Orion, Switz.; Orion, Thai.*
Estradiol (p.1550·1).
*Menopausal disorders; osteoporosis.*

**Divina**
*Organon, Austral.†; Orion, Denm.; Orion, Fin.; Innotech, Fr.; Organon (Οργανον), Gr.; Organon, Neth.; Aspen, S.Afr.; Orion, Swed.*
11 Tablets, estradiol valerate (p.1550·2); 10 tablets, estradiol valerate; medroxyprogesterone acetate (p.1557·2).
*Menopausal disorders; menstrual disorders; osteoporosis.*

**Divina Plus**
*Orion, Denm.; Orion, Swed.*
16 Tablets, estradiol valerate (p.1550·2); 12 tablets, estradiol valerate; medroxyprogesterone acetate (p.1557·2).
*Menopausal disorders; osteoporosis.*

**Diviplus** *Pharmacia, Belg.*
16 Tablets, estradiol valerate (p.1550·2); 12 tablets, estradiol valerate; medroxyprogesterone acetate (p.1557·2).
*Menopausal disorders; osteoporosis.*

**Diviseq**
*Orion, Fr.; Orion, Irl.; Orion, Norw.; Orion, Switz.*
16 Tablets, estradiol valerate (p.1550·2); 12 tablets, estradiol valerate; medroxyprogesterone acetate (p.1557·2).
*Menopausal disorders.*

**Divitren** *Orion, Fin.*
70 Tablets, estradiol valerate (p.1550·2); 14 tablets, estradiol valerate; medroxyprogesterone acetate (p.1557·2); 7 tablets, inert.
*Menopausal disorders; osteoporosis.*

**Diviva** *Pharmacia, Belg.*
11 Tablets, estradiol valerate (p.1550·2); 10 tablets, estradiol valerate; medroxyprogesterone acetate (p.1557·2).
*Menopausal disorders; oestrogen replacement therapy.*

**Dixarit**
*Boehringer Ingelheim, Belg.; Boehringer Ingelheim, Canad.; Boehringer Ingelheim, Ger.; Boehringer Ingelheim, Hong Kong; Boehringer Ingelheim, Irl.; Boehringer Ingelheim, Malaysia; Boehringer Ingelheim, Neth.; Boehringer Ingelheim, NZ; Boehringer Ingelheim, S.Afr.; Boehringer Ingelheim, Singapore; Boehringer Ingelheim, UK.*
Clonidine hydrochloride (p.885·2).
*Menopausal flushing; migraine and other vascular headache.*

**Dixen** *Maver, Mex.*
Dicloxacillin (p.205·2).
*Bacterial infections.*

**Dixeran**
*Lundbeck, Austria; Lundbeck, Belg.*
Melitracen hydrochloride (p.306·3).
*Depression.*

**Dixi-35** *Gynopharm, Chile.*
Cyproterone acetate (p.1544·1); ethinylestradiol (p.1553·2).

**Dixidrol** *Rivero, Arg.*
Glucose; sodium chloride; potassium chloride; sodium citrate (p.1222·2).
*Oral rehydration therapy.*

**Dixiflen** *Farcoral, Mex.*
Ox bile (p.1660·3); pancreatin (p.1725·3); cellulase (p.1669·1); dimeticone (p.1289·2).
*Digestive disorders; flatulence.*

**Dixocillin** *Siam Bheasach, Thai.*
Dicloxacillin sodium (p.205·2).
*Gram-positive bacterial infections.*

**Dixonal** *Medix, Mex.*
Piroxicam (p.84·2).
*Gout; musculoskeletal, joint, peri-articular, and soft-tissue disorders.*

**Diyomex** *Ofimex, Mex.†.*
Diiodohydroxyquinoline (p.603·3).

**Diyosul** *Jofrain, Mex.†.*
Diiodohydroxyquinoline (p.603·3).

**Diyowil** *Willmar, Mex.†.*
Diiodohydroxyquinoline (p.603·3).

**Dizan** *Pharmaland, Thai.*
Diazepam (p.690·1).
*Anxiety; skeletal muscle spasm.*

**Dizem** *IQFA, Mex.*
Di-iodohomatropine.
*Amoebiasis.*

**Dizepam** *Masa, Thai.*
Diazepam (p.690·1).
*Anxiety.*

**Dizinil** *Julphar, UAE.*
Dimenhydrinate (p.431·1).
*Nausea and vomiting; vestibular disorders.*

**Dizmiss** *JMI, USA.*
Meclozine hydrochloride (p.436·3).
*Motion sickness; vertigo.*

**Dizolam**
*Atlantic, Singapore; Atlantic, Thai.*
Alprazolam (p.668·3).
*Anxiety; mixed anxiety depressive states.*

**Dizolvin** *Rayere, Mex.*
Bromhexine hydrochloride (p.1115·3).
*Respiratory-tract disorders congestion.*

**D-Lisin** *Collins, Mex.*
Vitamin preparation (p.1417·1).

**DLPA** *Cantassium Co., UK†.*
DL-Phenylalanine.

**DM Cough Syrup**
*Note. This name is used for preparations of different composition.*
*Prodemdis, Canad.†.*
Diphenhydramine hydrochloride (p.431·3); dextromethorphan hydrobromide (p.1117·3); ammonium chloride (p.1115·2).
*Coughs.*

*Technilab, Canad.; DC Labs, Canad.*
Dextromethorphan hydrobromide (p.1117·3).
*Coughs.*

**DM Cough Syrup Decongestant** *Prometic, Canad.†.*
Pseudoephedrine hydrochloride (p.1129·2); dextromethorphan hydrobromide (p.1117·3).
*Coughs.*

**DM Cough Syrup Expectorant** *Prometic, Canad.†.*
Dextromethorphan hydrobromide (p.1117·3); guaifenesin (p.1122·1).
*Coughs.*

**DM Creme** *Byk, Port.*
Glycol salicylate (p.44·3); menthol (p.1711·3).
*Musculoskeletal, joint, peri-articular, and soft-tissue disorders; neuralgia; neuritis.*

**DM E Suppressant Expectorant** *Drug Trading, Canad.†.*
Dextromethorphan hydrobromide (p.1117·3); guaifenesin (p.1122·1).

**DM Expectorant Cough** *DC Labs, Canad.*
Dextromethorphan hydrobromide (p.1117·3); guaifenesin (p.1122·1).
*Coughs.*

**DM Gel** *Byk, Port.*
Glycol salicylate (p.44·3); menthol (p.1711·3); heparin sodium (p.928·1).
*Muscular pain; neuralgia; soft-tissue injury.*

**DM Plus** *Technilab, Canad.*
Dextromethorphan hydrobromide (p.1117·3); diphenhydramine hydrochloride (p.431·3); ammonium chloride (p.1115·2).
Formerly known as DM Syrup.
*Coughs.*

**DM Plus Decongestant** *Technilab, Canad.*
Dextromethorphan hydrobromide (p.1117·3); pseudoephedrine hydrochloride (p.1129·2).
*Coughs.*

**DM Plus Decongestant Expectorant** *Technilab, Canad.*
Dextromethorphan hydrobromide (p.1117·3); pseudoephedrine hydrochloride (p.1129·2); guaifenesin (p.1122·1).
*Coughs.*

**DM Plus Expectorant** *Technilab, Canad.*
Dextromethorphan hydrobromide (p.1117·3); guaifenesin (p.1122·1).
*Coughs.*

**DM Sans Sucre** *Trianon, Canad.*
Dextromethorphan hydrobromide (p.1117·3).
*Coughs.*

**DM Termo** *Byk, Port.†.*
Glycol salicylate (p.44·3); benzyl nicotinate (p.21·2).
*Musculoskeletal and joint disorders; neuritis; peripheral vascular disorders.*

**4-DMAP**
*Kohler, Ger.; Tramedico, Neth.*
Dimethylaminophenol hydrochloride (p.1037·3).
*Cyanide, hydrocyanic acid, nitrile, hydrogen sulfide, or prussic acid poisoning.*

**DMax** *Great Southern, USA.*
Dextromethorphan hydrobromide (p.1117·3); phenylephrine hydrochloride (p.1126·3); carbinoxamine maleate (p.426·3).
*Upper respiratory-tract disorders.*

**DM-D Expectorant Cough & Cold** *DC Labs, Canad.*
Pseudoephedrine hydrochloride (p.1129·2); dextromethorphan hydrobromide (p.1117·3); guaifenesin (p.1122·1).
*Cold symptoms; coughs.*

**DMG-B15** *Cantassium Co., UK†.*
Calcium gluconate (p.1225·2); NN-dimethylglycine hydrochloride.

**DML** *Person & Covey, USA.*
A range of moisturisers.

**DML Facial** *Dispolab, Chile.*
*SPF 25:* Octinoxate (p.1154·3); homosalate (p.1148·1); avobenzone (p.1142·3); octocrilene (p.1154·3).
*Sunscreen.*

**DML Forte Con Pantenol** *Dispolab, Chile.*
Emollient.
*Dry skin.*

**D-Mulsin** *Mucos, Ger.†.*
Colecalciferol (p.1461·3).
*Osteoporosis; vitamin D deficiency.*

**D/N PR** *Magis, Ital.†.*
Naproxen aminobutanol (p.65·3).
*Gynaecological disorders.*

**Dnaren** *Ariston, Braz.*
Diclofenac sodium (p.32·1).
*Inflammation; pain.*

**DNCG** *Mundipharma, Ger.; Stada, Ger.; Trommsdorff, Ger.; Penta, Ger.; Padia, Ger.*
Sodium cromoglicate (p.795·3).
*Asthma; conjunctivitis; hypersensitivity reactions; rhinitis.*

**Doak-Oil** *Trans Canaderm, Canad.*
Liquid paraffin; isopropyl palmitate; coal tar (p.1159·2).
*Skin disorders.*

**Doans**
*Note. This name is used for preparations of different composition.*
*Medipharma, Hong Kong.*
Zinc oxide (p.1163·2); phenol (p.1188·1).
*Skin disorders.*

*Ciba Consumer, USA.*
Magnesium salicylate (p.55·1).
*Fever; inflammation; pain.*

**Doans Backache Pills**
*Note. This name is used for preparations of different composition.*
*Novartis Consumer, Canad.†.*
Magnesium salicylate (p.55·1).
*Muscular back pain.*

*Eastern Pharmaceuticals, UK.*
Paracetamol (p.76·2); sodium salicylate (p.90·1).
*Pain.*

**Dobacen** *Brandt, Switz.*
Diphenhydramine hydrochloride (p.431·3).
*Insomnia.*

**Dobendan**
*Hoechst Marion Roussel, Austria; Boots Healthcare, Ger.*
Cetylpyridinium chloride (p.1173·1).
*Mouth and throat disorders.*

**Dobesifar** *Alcon, Hong Kong.*
Calcium dobesilate (p.1664·2).
*Haemorrhagic eye disorders.*

**Dobesin** *Abigo, Denm.†.*
Diethylpropion hydrochloride (p.1587·1).
*Obesity.*

**Dobesix** *Brasmedica, Braz.†.*
Mazindol (p.1589·1); diazepam (p.690·1).
*Obesity.*

**Dobetin** *Angelini, Ital.*
Cyanocobalamin (p.1458·2).
*Tonic; vitamin $B_{12}$ deficiency.*

**Dobetin con Vitamina B1** *Angelini, Ital.*
Cyanocobalamin (p.1458·2); thiamine hydrochloride (p.1455·1).
*Neuralgia; neuritis.*

**Dobetin Totale** *Angelini, Ital.*
Hydroxocobalamin (p.1458·2); thiamine (p.1455·2); pyridoxine (p.1457·2).
*Neuralgia.*

**Dobica** *OPW, Ger.*
Calcium dobesilate (p.1664·2).
*Capillary fragility and leakage; venous insufficiency.*

**Dobil** *Pharmaland, Thai.*
Paracetamol (p.76·2); chlorphenamine maleate (p.427·3).
Formerly contained paracetamol, chlorphenamine maleate, and phenylpropanolamine hydrochloride.
*Cold symptoms; hay fever; nasal congestion; rhinitis.*

**Dobiron** *Legrand, Braz.*
Ferrous sulfate (p.1428·2); vitamin B substances; liver extract; gastric mucosa extract (p.1417·1).
Ascorbic acid (p.1460·2) is included in this preparation to increase the absorption and availability of iron.
*Anaemias.*

**Doblexan** *Quimifar, Spain.*
Piroxicam (p.84·2).
*Gout; musculoskeletal, joint, and peri-articular disorders; pain.*

**Dobren** *Teofarma, Ital.*
Sulpiride (p.722·2).
*Dysthymia; psychoses.*

**Dobriciclin** *Quimifar, Spain.*
Amoxicillin trihydrate (p.155·3).
*Bacterial infections.*

**Dobtan** *Uniao Quimica, Braz.†.*
Dobutamine hydrochloride (p.905·3).
*Heart failure; shock.*

**Dobucard**
*Scott-Cassara, Arg.; Solvay, Malaysia; Solvay, Thai.†.*
Dobutamine hydrochloride (p.905·3).
*Heart failure.*

**Dobucor** *Juste, Spain.*
Dobutamine hydrochloride (p.905·3).
*Heart failure; shock.*

**Dobuject**
*Gautier, Arg.; Leiras, Denm.†; Leiras, Fin.; Leiras, Israel; Pisa, Mex.; Probios, Port.†; Leiras, Singapore; Leiras, Swed.†; Leiras, Thai.*
Dobutamine hydrochloride (p.905·3).
*Heart failure; shock.*

**Dobupal** *Almirall, Spain.*
Venlafaxine hydrochloride (p.321·3).
*Anxiety; depression.*

**Dobutabbott** *Abbott, Braz.*
Dobutamine hydrochloride (p.905·3).
*Heart failure.*

**Dobutal** *Biochimico, Braz.*
Dobutamine (p.906·1).
*Heart failure.*

**Dobutam** *Rafa, Israel.*
Dobutamine hydrochloride (p.905·3).
*Heart failure.*

**Dobutil** *BPL-Meizler, Braz.*
Dobutamine hydrochloride (p.905·3).
*Heart failure; shock.*

**Dobutina** *Faulding, Port.*
Dobutamine hydrochloride (p.905·3).

**Dobuton** *Ariston, Braz.*
Dobutamine (p.906·1).

**Dobutrex**
*Lilly, Arg.; Lilly, Austral.; Lilly, Austria†; Lilly, Belg.; Lilly, Braz.; Lilly, Canad.; Lilly, Chile; Lilly, Denm.; Lilly, Fin.; Lilly, Fr.; Lilly, Ger.†; Lilly, Hong Kong; Lilly, India; Lilly, Irl.; Lilly, Israel†; Bayer, Ital.; Lilly, Malaysia; Lilly, Mex.; Lilly, Neth.†; Lilly, Norw.; Lilly, NZ; Rolab, S.Afr.; Irisfarma, Spain; Lilly, Swed.; Lilly, Switz.; Lilly, Thai.; Lilly, UK†; Lilly, USA.*
Dobutamine hydrochloride (p.905·3).
*Cardiac stress testing; heart failure.*

**Doc** *Lacoer, Ger.*
Arnica (p.1656·3).
*Musculoskeletal, joint, and soft-tissue disorders.*

**Docaine** *M & H, Thai.*
Lidocaine hydrochloride (p.1377·3).
*Local anaesthesia.*

**Docard** *Dexxon, Israel.*
Dopamine hydrochloride (p.907·1).
*Shock.*

**Docatone** *Wyeth, Spain.*
Doxapram (p.1587·3).
*CNS depression; respiratory depression.*

**Docdol** *Adcock Ingram, S.Afr.*
Paracetamol (p.76·2); codeine phosphate (p.27·1); caffeine (p.782·1).
*Pain.*

**Doce Vida** *Marjan, Braz.*
Aspartame (p.1422·1).
*Sugar substitute.*

**Docetril** *Loren, Mex.*
Liver extract; vitamin B substances (p.1417·1).

**Docgel** *Docmed, S.Afr.†.*
Dried aluminium hydroxide gel (p.1249·2); magnesium oxide (p.1272·3); simeticone (p.1289·2).
*Dyspepsia; gastritis; gastro-oesophageal reflux; peptic ulcer.*

**Docidrazin** *AstraZeneca, Ger.*
Propranolol hydrochloride (p.989·3); hydralazine hydrochloride (p.931·2); bendroflumethiazide (p.867·3).
*Hypertension.*

**Dociretic** *AstraZeneca, Ger.*
Propranolol hydrochloride (p.989·3); bendroflumethiazide (p.867·3).
*Hypertension.*

**Dociteren** *AstraZeneca, Ger.*
Propranolol hydrochloride (p.989·3); triamterene (p.1016·2); hydrochlorothiazide (p.933·2).
*Hypertension.*

**Dociton** *AstraZeneca, Ger.*
Propranolol hydrochloride (p.989·3).
*Angina pectoris; anxiety; arrhythmias; essential tremor; hypertension; hyperthyroidism; migraine; myocardial infarction.*

**Docline** *Atlantic, Thai.*
Doxycycline (p.206·2).
*Bacterial infections.*

**Doclis** *Bial, Spain.*
Diltiazem hydrochloride (p.900·1).
*Angina pectoris; hypertension.*

**Docostyl** *Pentafarm, Spain.*
Doxycycline hyclate (p.206·2).
*Bacterial infections; malaria.*

**Docrub** *Aspen Consumer, S.Afr.*
Camphor (p.1665·3); menthol (p.1711·3); methyl salicylate (p.59·3); eucalyptus oil (p.1686·2); buchu oil (p.1663·1).
*Cold symptoms; coughs; soft-tissue disorders.*

**Docsed** *Aspen, S.Afr.*
Mepyramine maleate (p.437·1); codeine phosphate (p.27·1); pholcodine (p.1128·3); ephedrine hydrochloride (p.1120·1).
*Coughs.*

**Doctar** *Savage, USA†.*
Coal tar (p.1159·2).
*Scalp disorders.*

**Docticam** *Doctum, Gr.*
Tenoxicam (p.93·1).
*Dysmenorrhoea; gout; inflammation; osteoarthritis; pain; rheumatoid arthritis; spondyloarthropathies.*

**Doctodermis** *Medea, Spain.*
Biotin (p.1423·2); triclosan (p.1195·2).
Formerly contained biotin, methyl hydroxybenzoate, and trolamine laurilsulfate.
*Skin cleansing.*

**Doctofril Antiinflamat** *Medea, Spain.*
Phenylbutazone (p.83·2); lidocaine (p.1377·3); methyl nicotinate (p.59·2); vitamin F.
*Chilblains; rheumatic and muscle pain.*

**Doctogaster** *Medea, Spain†.*
Aluminium silicate (p.1250·2); frangula bark (p.1266·3); magnesium carbonate (p.1272·1); magnesium polygalacturonate; liquorice (p.1270·2); sodium bicarbonate (p.1223·2).
*Gastritis; hyperacidity; peptic ulcer.*

**Doctomitil** *Medea, Spain.*
Cineole (p.1672·1); diethylamine salicylate (p.34·1); methyl nicotinate (p.59·2).
*Soft-tissue disorders.*

**Doctril**
*Martin, Fr.†; Abello, Spain.*
Ibuprofen lysine (p.46·3).
*Fever; pain.*

**Doctrim** *Docmed, S.Afr.†.*
Co-trimoxazole (p.199·3).
*Bacterial infections.*

**Docusoft**
*Taro, Israel†; Reese, USA.*
Docusate sodium (p.1262·2).
*Constipation.*

**Docusoft Plus** *Reese, USA.*
Docusate sodium (p.1262·2); casanthranol (p.1255·1).
*Constipation.*

**Docusol** *Typharm, UK.*
Docusate sodium (p.1262·2).
*Bowel evacuation; constipation.*

**Dodds** *Stella, Canad.*
Sodium salicylate (p.90·1).
*Musculoskeletal pain.*

**Dodds Back Ease** *Stella, Canad.*
Paracetamol (p.76·2); methocarbamol (p.1395·1).

**Dodecatol N** *Heyl, Ger.†.*
Procaine hydrochloride (p.1383·2); cyanocobalamin (p.1458·2).
*Inflammation; pain.*

**Dodecavit** *SERB, Fr.*
Hydroxocobalamin acetate (p.1458·2).
*Vitamin $B_12$ deficiency.*

**Dodemox** *Fadim, Ital.*
Amoxicillin trihydrate (p.155·3).
*Bacterial infections.*

**Dodepar** *ABC, Port.*
Vitamin B substances (p.1417·1).
*Anaemias; tonic.*

**Doderlein Med** *Novartis Consumer, Ger.*
*Lactobacillus gasseri.*
*Vaginal disorders.*

**Dodesept** *Merck, Austria.*
Orthophenylphenol (p.1187·2); alcohol (p.1166·1); isopropyl alcohol (p.1184·3); propyl alcohol (p.1191·2).
*Skin disinfection.*

**Dodesept Gefarbt** *Merck, Austria.*
Orthophenylphenol (p.1187·2); alcohol (p.1166·1); isopropyl alcohol (p.1184·3).
*Skin disinfection.*

**Dodesept N** *Merck, Austria.*
Alcohol (p.1166·1); isopropyl alcohol (p.1184·3).
*Skin disinfection.*

**Do-Do ChestEze** *Novartis Consumer, UK.*
Theophylline (p.798·3); ephedrine hydrochloride (p.1120·1); caffeine (p.782·1).
*Bronchial coughs; respiratory-tract congestion; wheezing.*

**Do-Do Expectorant Linctus** *Novartis Consumer, UK†.*
Guaifenesin (p.1122·1).
*Coughs.*

**Doederlein** *Novartis Consumer, Austria.*
*Lactobacillus acidophilus* (p.1704·2).
*Vaginal candidiasis.*

**Dofedrin** *Knoll, Mex.*
Pseudoephedrine (p.1129·2).
*Upper respiratory-tract congestion.*

**Dofen**
*Note. This name is used for preparations of different composition.*
*Knoll, Mex.†.*
Pseudoephedrine (p.1129·2).

*Parggon, Mex.*
Diclofenac sodium (p.32·1).
*Inflammation; musculoskeletal and joint disorders.*

**Doferol** *Tocogino, Mex.†.*
Ergocalciferol (p.1462·1).

**Dofisan** *Berman, Mex.*
Dipyrone (p.35·3).
*Fever; pain.*

**Doflex** *Jagson, India.*
Diclofenac sodium (p.32·1).
*Gout; musculoskeletal and joint disorders.*

**Dogistin** *Temis, Arg.*
Ambroxol acefyllinate (p.1114·3).
*Obstructive airways disease.*

**Dogmatil**
*Sanofi Synthelabo, Austria; Sanofi Synthelabo, Belg.; Sanofi Synthelabo, Braz.; Sanofi Winthrop, Denm.; Sanofi Synthelabo, Fr.; Sanofi Synthelabo, Ger.; Sanofi Synthelabo, Hong Kong; Carnot, Mex.†; Sanofi Synthelabo, Neth.; Sanofi Synthelabo, Port.; Sanofi Synthelabo, Singapore†; Sanofi Synthelabo, Spain; Synthelabo, Switz.*
Sulpiride (p.722·2).
*Anxiety disorders; depression; obsessive-compulsive disorder; peptic ulcer; psychoses; vertigo.*

**Dogmatyl**
*Sanofi Synthelabo, Gr.; Fujisawa, Jpn.*
Sulpiride (p.722·2).
*Depression; peptic ulcer; psychoses.*

**Dogoxine** *Rudefsa, Mex.†.*
Digoxin (p.895·2).

**Dohyfral Vitamine AD3** *Solvay, Neth.†.*
Vitamin A (p.1451·2); colecalciferol (p.1461·3).
*Vitamin A and vitamin D deficiency.*

**DOK** *Major, USA.*
Docusate sodium (p.1262·2).
*Constipation.*

**Doketrol** *Rivero, Arg.*
Sodium nitroprusside (p.1000·2).
*Hypertension.*

**Doktacillin**
*AstraZeneca, Denm.; AstraZeneca, Norw.†; AstraZeneca, Swed.*
Ampicillin sodium (p.157·1).
*Bacterial infections.*

**Dolac** *Syntex, Mex.*
Ketorolac trometamol (p.52·1).
*Pain.*

**Dolacet** *Roberts, USA.*
Hydrocodone tartrate (p.45·1); paracetamol (p.76·2).
*Pain.*

**Dolak** *Bama, Spain.*
Isosorbide mononitrate (p.942·1).
*Angina pectoris.*

**Dolal**
*Note. This name is used for preparations of different composition.*
*Biocodex, Fr.*
Ethylmethoxy salicylate; phenylpropyl salicylate.
*Musculoskeletal and joint pain.*

*Remek, Gr.*
Paracetamol (p.76·2).
*Fever; pain.*

**Dolalgial**
*Grunenthal, Chile; Sanofi Synthelabo, Spain.*
Clonixin lysine (p.26·3).
*Pain; peri-articular disorders.*

**Dolamin** *Sintofarma, Braz.*
Clonixin lysine (p.26·3).
*Pain.*

**Dolan** *Leiras, Fin.*
Orphenadrine citrate (p.486·1); paracetamol (p.76·2).
*Skeletal muscle spasm and pain.*

**Dolanaest**
*Gebro, Austria; Strathmann, Ger.*
Bupivacaine hydrochloride (p.1371·1).
*Local anaesthesia; pain syndromes.*

**Dolanet** *Sanofi Synthelabo, Arg.*
Paracetamol (p.76·2); caffeine (p.782·1).
*Fever; pain.*

**Dolantin** *Aventis, Ger.*
Pethidine hydrochloride (p.80·2).
*Pain.*

**Dolantina**
*Aventis, Braz.; Bayer, Spain.*
Pethidine hydrochloride (p.80·2).
*Pain; premedication; smooth muscle spasm.*

**Dolantine** *Aventis, Belg.*
Pethidine hydrochloride (p.80·2).
*Pain.*

**Dolaren** AF, Mex.
*Cream:* Diclofenac diethylamine (p.32·1).
*Inflammation; musculoskeletal, joint, peri-articular and soft-tissue disorders; pain.*
*Tablets:* Diclofenac sodium (p.32·1); carisoprodol (p.1392·1).
*Gout; inflammation; musculoskeletal, joint, peri-articular and soft-tissue disorders; pain.*

**Dolased Analgesic Calmative** Herron, Austral.
Paracetamol (p.76·2); codeine phosphate (p.27·1); doxylamine succinate (p.432·3).
*Pain.*

**Dolased Day/Night Pain Relief** Herron, Austral.
Day tablets, paracetamol (p.76·2); codeine phosphate (p.27·1); night tablets, paracetamol; codeine phosphate; doxylamine succinate (p.432·3).
Formerly known as Chemists Own Dolased.
*Pain.*

**Dolaut** GiEnne, Ital.
Diclofenac sodium (p.32·1).
*Musculoskeletal, joint, and peri-articular disorders.*

**Dolcevita** Codilab, Port.
Aspartame (p.1422·1).
*Sugar substitute.*

**Dolcidium** SMB, Belg.
Indometacin (p.47·3).
*Gout; musculoskeletal, joint and peri-articular disorders; pain.*

**Dolcin** EciFarma, Chile.
Mefenamic acid (p.55·2).
*Pain.*

**Dolcol** Dainippon, Jpn.
Pipemidic acid (p.243·1).
*Bacterial infections.*

**Dolcontin**
Mundipharma, Fin.; Pharmacia, Norw.; Pharmacia, Swed.
Morphine sulfate (p.60·2).
*Pain.*

**Dolcopin**
Note. This name is used for preparations of different composition.
Pasteur, Chile.
Dipyrone (p.35·3); hyoscine butylbromide (p.483·3).
*Smooth muscle spasm.*
Rottapharm, Spain.
Magnesium trisilicate (p.1272·3); sodium bicarbonate (p.1223·2); almasilate (p.1248·2); alginic acid (p.1576·3).
*Dyspepsia; gastro-oesophageal reflux.*

**Dolcor** Gazzoni, Ital.†.
Aspartame (p.1422·1).
*Sugar substitute.*

**Dolcoxx** Merck Sharp & Dohme, Ital.
Rofecoxib (p.86·3).
*Pain.*

**Dolean** Recalcine, Chile.
Paracetamol (p.76·2); codeine phosphate (p.27·1).
*Pain.*

**Dolectran** Kampel Martian, Arg.
Docetaxel (p.547·1).
*Malignant neoplasms.*

**Dolefin Paracetamol** Pharmacia, Spain†.
Paracetamol (p.76·2).
*Fever; pain.*

**Dolemicin** Dreiman, Spain†.
Metamizole magnesium (p.36·1).
*Fever; pain.*

**Dolenon** Strathmann, Ger.
Cayenne pepper (p.1667·1).
*Muscle pain; nerve pain.*

**Dolenso** Kwizda, Austria.
Paracetamol (p.76·2); aspirin (p.15·1).
*Fever; pain.*

**Doleron** Astra, Swed.
Aspirin (p.15·1); dextropropoxyphene napsilate (p.28·3); phenazone (p.82·3).
*Pain.*

**Doleside** FD, Ital.
Nimesulide (p.67·1).
*Fever; inflammation; pain.*

**Dolestan** Krewel, Ger.
Diphenhydramine hydrochloride (p.431·3).
*Sleep disorders.*

**Dolestan forte comp** Whitehall-Much, Ger.
Diphenhydramine hydrochloride (p.431·3); guaifenesin (p.1122·1).
*Sleep disorders.*

**Dolestine** Biogal, Israel.
Pethidine hydrochloride (p.80·2).
*Pain.*

**Dolex**
Note. This name is used for preparations of different composition.
Armstrong, Arg.
Clonixin lysine (p.26·3).
*Pain.*
Terramin, Austria†.
Glycol salicylate (p.44·3); salicylic acid (p.1157·1); camphor (p.1665·3); turpentine oil (p.1760·1).
*Rheumatic and muscle pain.*
IFI, Ital.
Furprofen (p.44·3).
*Pain.*

**Dolexaderm H** Strathmann, Ger.†.
Dulcamara (p.1683·1).
*Eczema.*

**Dolexamed N** Strathmann, Ger.†.
Eucalyptus oil (p.1686·2); peppermint oil (p.1283·2); rosemary oil (p.1740·2).
*Myalgia; neuralgia; rheumatism.*

**Dolflam** Rayere, Mex.
Diclofenac sodium (p.32·1).
*Gout; musculoskeletal, joint, peri-articular, and soft-tissue disorders; pain.*

**Dolflash** Sanofi Winthrop, Fr.†.
Paracetamol (p.76·2).
*Fever; pain.*

**Dolgan** Bioresearch, Mex.
Dipyrone (p.35·3).
*Fever; pain.*

**Dolgenal** Tecnofarma, Chile.
Ketorolac trometamol (p.52·1).
*Pain.*

**Dolgesic** Novag, Spain.
Paracetamol (p.76·2).
*Fever; pain.*

**Dolgesic Codeina** Novag, Spain.
Codeine phosphate (p.27·1); paracetamol (p.76·2).
*Pain.*

**Dolgic** Athlon, USA.
Paracetamol (p.76·2); butalbital (p.673·3).
*Pain.*

**Dolgic LQ** Athlon, USA.
Paracetamol (p.76·2); butalbital (p.673·3); caffeine (p.782·1).
*Pain.*

**Dolgit**
Sanova, Austria; Lipha Sante, Fr.; Dolorgiet, Ger.; Dolorgiet, Switz.†.
Ibuprofen (p.45·3).
*Fever; inflammation; musculoskeletal, joint, and peri-articular disorders; pain; soft-tissue injury.*

**Dolgit-Diclo** Dolorgiet, Ger.
Diclofenac sodium (p.32·1).
*Gout; inflammation; musculoskeletal, joint, and soft-tissue disorders; pain.*

**Dolgosin** Pulitzer, Ital.
Ketoprofen (p.51·2).
*Musculoskeletal and joint disorders.*

**Doli Rhume** Theraplix, Fr.
Paracetamol (p.76·2); pseudoephedrine hydrochloride (p.1129·2).
*Cold symptoms.*

**Dolib** Panacea, India.
Rofecoxib (p.86·3).
*Dysmenorrhoea; musculoskeletal and joint disorders; pain.*

**Dolibu** Klinge, Austria.
Ibuprofen (p.45·3).
*Fever; musculoskeletal and joint disorders; pain.*

**Dolical** Rekah, Israel.
Morpholine salicylate (p.63·3).
*Skeletal muscle spasm.*

**Dolicoccil** Dolisos, Canad.
Homoeopathic preparation.

**Dolidermil** Dolisos, Fr.
Homoeopathic preparation.

**Dolidon** Medifa, Fr.†.
Paracetamol (p.76·2); caffeine (p.782·1).
*Pain.*

**Dolifebril** Dolisos, Fr.
Homoeopathic preparation.

**Dolilux** Uno, Ital.
Ranitidine hydrochloride (p.1285·2).
*Gastro-oesophageal reflux; peptic ulcer; Zollinger-Ellison syndrome.*

**Dolinac**
Note. This name is used for preparations of different composition.
Whitehall, Denm.†; Teofarma, Ital.; Whitehall, S.Afr.†.
Felbinac (p.39·1).
*Inflammation; pain; soft-tissue disorders.*
Durachemie, Ger.†.
Diisopropanolamine felbinac (p.39·1).
*Muscle, joint, and soft-tissue pain and inflammation.*

**Doline**
Note. This name is used for preparations of different composition.
Alphapharm, Malaysia; Merck, Malaysia.
Doxycycline hyclate (p.206·2).
*Bacterial infections.*
Ferrer, Spain†.
Benorilate (p.20·3).
*Fever; musculoskeletal and joint disorders; pain.*

**Doliprane**
Theraplix, Fr.; Nicholas Piramal, India.
Paracetamol (p.76·2).
*Fever; pain.*

**Dolirelax** Dolisos, Fr.
Homoeopathic preparation.

**Dolisedal** Dolisos, Fr.
Homoeopathic preparation.

**Dolistamine** Dolisos, Fr.
Homoeopathic preparation.

**Dolitabs** Theraplix, Fr.
Paracetamol (p.76·2).
*Fever; pain.*

**Dolitravel** Dolisos, Fr.
Homoeopathic preparation.

**Dolium** Utopian, Thai.
Domperidone (p.1263·2).
*Flatulence; nausea and vomiting.*

**Dolkin** Caber, Ital.
Disodium clodronate (p.770·2).
*Hyperparathyroidism; multiple myeloma; osteolysis of malignancy; osteoporosis.*

**Dolko** Therabel, Fr.
Paracetamol (p.76·2).
*Fever; pain.*

**Dolmatil**
Sanofi Synthelabo, Irl.; Sanofi Synthelabo, UK.
Sulpiride (p.722·2).
*Schizophrenia.*

**Dolmed** Leiras, Fin.
Methadone hydrochloride (p.57·2).
*Opioid dependence; pain.*

**Dolmen**
Note. This name is used for preparations of different composition.
Sigma-Tau, Ital.
Tenoxicam (p.93·1).
*Musculoskeletal disorders.*
Uriach, Spain.
Aspirin (p.15·1); ascorbic acid (p.1460·2); codeine phosphate (p.27·1).
*Fever; pain.*

**Dolmex** Ofimex, Mex.†.
Aspirin (p.15·1).

**Dolmigral** Abbott, Spain.
Sumatriptan succinate (p.471·2).
*Migraine.*

**Dol-Mite** Swiss Herbal, Canad.
Calcium carbonate; magnesium carbonate (p.1417·1).

**Dolmitin** Medea, Spain.
Cineole (p.1672·1); diethylamine salicylate (p.34·1).
*Soft-tissue disorders.*

**Dolmix** Apomedica, Austria.
Ethenzamide (p.37·2); paracetamol (p.76·2); caffeine (p.782·1).
*Fever; pain.*

**Dolnaxen** Arlex, Mex.†.
Naproxen (p.65·1).

**Dolnefort** Farcoral, Mex.
Dipyrone (p.35·3); vitamin B substances (p.1417·1).
*Neuritis; pain.*

**Dolnix** Recalcine, Chile.
Ibuprofen (p.45·3); dipyrone (p.35·3); chlormezanone (p.675·1).
*Musculoskeletal, joint, peri-articular, and soft-tissue disorders; pain.*

**Dolnot** ICN, Arg.
Clonixin lysine (p.26·3).
*Fever; inflammation; pain.*

**Dolo Demotherm** Democal, Switz.
Dimethyl sulfoxide (p.1473·2); benzyl nicotinate (p.21·2); glycol salicylate (p.44·3).
*Musculoskeletal and joint pain.*

**Dolo Mobilat** Sankyo, Ger.
Phenylephrine hydrochloride (p.1126·3); a heparinoid (p.931·1); glycol salicylate (p.44·3).
*Musculoskeletal, joint, peri-articular, and soft-tissue disorders.*

**Dolo neos** Optimed, Ger.†.
Ibuprofen (p.45·3).
*Fever; inflammation; musculoskeletal and joint disorders; pain.*

**Dolo Nervobion**
Note. This name is used for preparations of different composition.
Merck, Arg.
Diclofenac sodium (p.32·1); thiamine (p.1455·2); pyridoxine hydrochloride (p.1456·3); mecobalamin (p.1459·1).
*Inflammation; pain.*
Merck, Spain.
Diclofenac sodium (p.32·1).
*Gout; musculoskeletal, joint, and peri-articular disorders; pain; renal colic.*

**Dolo Nervobion 10000** Merck, Arg.
Ampoule 1, thiamine hydrochloride (p.1455·1); pyridoxine hydrochloride (p.1456·3); cyanocobalamin (p.1458·2); ampoule 2, dipyrone (p.35·3).
*Musculoskeletal, joint, and peri-articular disorders; neuralgia; neuritis.*

**Dolo Sanol** Sanol, Ger.; Schwarz, Ger.
Ibuprofen (p.45·3).
*Fever; pain.*

**Dolo Target** Whitehall-Robins, Switz.
Felbinac (p.39·1).
*Musculoskeletal, joint, peri-articular, and soft-tissue injuries and disorders.*

**Dolo Tomanil** Byk, Arg.
Diclofenac (p.32·1).
*Gout; inflammation; musculoskeletal, joint, peri-articular, and soft-tissue disorders; pain.*

**Doloana** Quimifar, Spain†.
Aspirin (p.15·1); salicylamide (p.87·3).
*Fever; pain.*

**Dolo-Arthrodynat** Ziethen, Ger.
Devil's claw root (p.28·2).
*Musculoskeletal and joint disorders.*

**Dolo-Arthrosenex** Whitehall-Robins, Switz.
Glycol salicylate (p.44·3); heparin sodium (p.928·1); camphor (p.1665·3).
*Musculoskeletal, joint, peri-articular, and soft-tissue disorders.*

**Dolo-Arthrosenex N** Riemser, Ger.
Glycol salicylate (p.44·3).
*Muscle, joint, peri-articular, and soft-tissue disorders.*

**Dolo-Arthrosenex sine Heparino** Whitehall-Robins, Switz.
Glycol salicylate (p.44·3); camphor (p.1665·3); isopropyl alcohol (p.1184·3); lavender oil (p.1705·2); thyme oil (p.1755·3); Siberian fir oil.
*Musculoskeletal, joint, peri-articular, and soft-tissue injuries and disorders.*

**Dolo-Arthrosetten H** Riemser, Ger.
Devil's claw root (p.28·2).
*Musculoskeletal and joint disorders.*

**Doloatrixen** Zerboni, Mex.†.
Naproxen (p.65·1).

**Dolobene**
Ratiopharm, Austria; Mepha, Braz.; Merckle, Ger.; Mepha, Hong Kong; Mepha, Switz.
Dimethyl sulfoxide (p.1473·2); heparin sodium (p.928·1); dexpanthenol (p.1727·2).
*Musculoskeletal, joint, peri-articular, and soft-tissue disorders; neuralgia.*

**Dolobid**
Merck Sharp & Dohme, Austral.; Merck Frosst, Canad.†; Merck Sharp & Dohme, Hong Kong†; Merck Sharp & Dohme, Irl.; Merck Sharp & Dohme, Israel; Merck Sharp & Dohme, Ital.; Merck Sharp & Dohme, Mex.; Merck Sharp & Dohme, Port.; Merck Sharp & Dohme, S.Afr.†; Frosst, Spain; Merck Sharp & Dohme, Thai.; Merck Sharp & Dohme, UK; Merck, USA.
Diflunisal (p.34·1).
*Inflammation; musculoskeletal, joint, and peri-articular disorders; pain.*

**Dolobis** Merck Sharp & Dohme-Chibret, Fr.
Diflunisal (p.34·1).
*Pain.*

**Doloc** Instituto Sanitas, Chile.
Nimesulide (p.67·1).
*Fever; inflammation; pain.*

**Dolocalma** Neves, Port.
Metamizole magnesium (p.36·1).
*Colic; fever; pain.*

**Dolocibal** Novartis, Mex.†.
Ibuprofen (p.45·3); caffeine (p.782·1).
*Fever; inflammation; pain.*

**Dolocid** Merck Sharp & Dohme, Neth.
Diflunisal (p.34·1).
*Musculoskeletal and joint disorders; pain.*

**DoloCitran C** Novartis Consumer, Switz.
Paracetamol (p.76·2); ascorbic acid (p.1460·2).
*Fever; pain.*

**Dolocod** Klinge, Austria.
Aspirin (p.15·1); paracetamol (p.76·2); codeine phosphate (p.27·1).
*Fever; pain.*

**Doloctaprin** Elvetium, Arg.
Nimesulide (p.67·1).
*Musculoskeletal, joint, and peri-articular disorders.*

**Doloctaprin Plus** Elvetium, Arg.
Nimesulide (p.67·1); orphenadrine (p.486·2).
*Musculoskeletal pain and spasm.*

**Dolo-cyl**
Note. A similar name is used for preparations of different composition (see below).
Liebermann, Ger.
Arnica oil (p.1656·3); eucalyptus oil (p.1686·2); hypericum oil (p.299·2); juniper oil (p.1703·1); lavender oil (p.1705·2); pumilio pine oil (p.1737·1); rosemary oil (p.1740·2).
*Musculoskeletal and joint disorders; sports injuries.*

**Dolocyl**
Note. A similar name is used for preparations of different composition (see above).
Novartis Consumer, Ital.; Novartis Consumer, Port.; Novartis Consumer, Switz.
Ibuprofen (p.45·3).
*Fever; pain.*

**Dolodens** Reig Jofre, Spain.
Codeine phosphate (p.27·1); hydroxyzine hydrochloride (p.434·3); propyphenazone (p.85·3).
*Pain.*

**Dolodent**
Note. This name is used for preparations of different composition.
OBA, Denm.
Benzocaine (p.1370·3); myrrh (p.1718·3).
*Mouth pain.*
Gilbert, Fr.
Amylocaine hydrochloride (p.1370·2).
Formerly contained amylocaine hydrochloride and cloral hydrate.
*Teething pain.*

**Doloderm**
Theraplix, Fr.†; Aventis, Ital.
Methyl butetisalicylate (p.59·2).
*Musculoskeletal and joint pain.*

**Dolo-Dismenol** Adroka, Switz.
Ibuprofen (p.45·3).
*Pain.*

**Dolo-Dobendan** Boots Healthcare, Ger.
Cetylpyridinium chloride (p.1173·1); benzocaine (p.1370·3).
*Mouth and throat disorders.*

**Dolodoc** Docpharm, Ger.
Ibuprofen (p.45·3).
*Fever; pain.*

**Dolofar** Medipharm, Chile.
Ketoprofen (p.51·2).
*Gout; musculoskeletal and joint disorders; pain.*

**Dolofarma** *Maxfarma, Spain.*
Aspirin (p.15·1); caffeine (p.782·1); paracetamol (p.76·2).
*Fever; pain.*

**Dolofast** *Bracco, Ital.*
Ibuprofen lysine (p.46·3).
*Musculoskeletal pain; soft-tissue disorders.*

**Dolofenac** *Arlex, Mex.†.*
Diclofenac (p.32·1).

**Doloflex** *Byk Gulden, Ital.*
Paracetamol (p.76·2); aspirin (p.15·1).
*Pain.*

**Dolofort** *Klinge, Austria.*
Ibuprofen (p.45·3).
*Pain.*

**Dolofrix** *Richmond, Arg.*
Paracetamol (p.76·2); codeine (p.27·1).
*Pain.*

**Dolofur** *Fustery, Mex.*
Dipyrone (p.35·3).
*Fever; pain.*

**Dologel**
*Note. This name is used for preparations of different composition.*
*Medicamed, Port.†.*
Capsicum (p.1667·1); eucalyptus oil (p.1686·2); methyl salicylate (p.59·3); menthol (p.1711·3).
*Muscular pain.*

*Wander OTC, Switz.†.*
Ibuprofen (p.45·3).
*Musculoskeletal, joint, and soft-tissue disorders.*

**Dologen** *Kenyaku, Thai.*
Ibuprofen (p.45·3); paracetamol (p.76·2).
*Musculoskeletal, joint, peri-articular, and soft-tissue disorders.*

**Dologesic** *Lilly, Hong Kong†.*
Paracetamol (p.76·2); dextropropoxyphene napsilate (p.28·3).
*Pain.*

**Dologex** *Cinfa, Spain.*
Turpentine oil (p.1760·1); menthol (p.1711·3); camphor (p.1665·3); methyl salicylate (p.59·3).
*Musculoskeletal, joint, and soft-tissue disorders.*

**Dologyne** *Arkopharma, Fr.†.*
Artemisia vulgaris; chamomile (p.1669·3).
*Pain.*

**Doloject** *Syxyl, Ger.*
Homoeopathic preparation.

**Dolokapton** *Strallhofer, Austria.*
Paracetamol (p.76·2); codeine phosphate (p.27·1).
*Coughs; fever; pain.*

**Dolo-Ketazon** *Recalcine, Chile.*
Ketoprofen (p.51·2).
*Gout; musculoskeletal, joint, peri-articular, and soft-tissue disorders; pain.*

**Dolokey** *Inkeysa, Spain.*
Camphor (p.1665·3); lavender oil (p.1705·2); methyl salicylate (p.59·3); expressed mustard oil (p.1718·2); rosemary oil (p.1740·2); eucalyptus oil (p.1686·2); belladonna (p.479·1); capsicum (p.1667·1); menthol (p.1711·3).
*Musculoskeletal and joint disorders.*

**Dolol**
*Nycomed, Austria; Nycomed, Denm.*
Tramadol hydrochloride (p.94·3).
*Pain.*

**Dolomedil** *Almirall, Spain.*
Codeine phosphate (p.27·1); paracetamol (p.76·2).
*Pain.*

**Dolo-Menthoneurin**
*Byk, Austria; Roland, Ger.; Byk Gulden, Ger.*
Diethylamine salicylate (p.34·1); heparin sodium (p.928·1); menthol (p.1711·3).
*Musculoskeletal, joint, and soft-tissue disorders; neuralgia.*

**Dolo-Menthoneurin CreSa** *Tosse, Ger.†.*
Glycol salicylate (p.44·3); benzyl nicotinate (p.21·2); camphor (p.1665·3).
*Muscle, joint, and peri-articular disorders.*

**Dolomin** *Bago, Arg.*
Dexibuprofen (p.46·1).
*Fever; inflammation; musculoskeletal, joint, and peri-articular disorders; pain.*

**Dolomine** *Frega, Canad.†.*
Aspirin (p.15·1); caffeine (p.782·1).

**Dolomite** *Nature's Bounty, USA.*
Calcium salts (p.1225·1); magnesium salts (p.1227·3).
*Dietary supplement.*

**Dolomo** *Klinge, Austria.*
Aspirin (p.15·1); paracetamol (p.76·2); caffeine (p.782·1).
*Fever; pain.*

**Dolomo TN** *Fujisawa, Ger.*
White tablets, aspirin (p.15·1); paracetamol (p.76·2); caffeine (p.782·1); blue tablets, aspirin; paracetamol; codeine phosphate (p.27·1).
*Pain.*

**Dolonase** *Medipharm, Chile.*
Ibuprofen (p.45·3); dipyrone (p.35·3); chlormezanone (p.675·1).
*Dysmenorrhoea; musculoskeletal and joint disorders.*

**Dolonerv** *Gerot, Austria.*
Paracetamol (p.76·2); vitamin B substances (p.1417·1).
*Pain.*

**Doloneuro** *Merck, Ger.*
Diethylamine salicylate (p.34·1); glycol salicylate (p.44·3); methyl nicotinate (p.59·2).
*Musculoskeletal, joint, and soft-tissue injury; neuralgia.*

**Dolo-Neurobion**
*Note. This name is used for preparations of different composition.*
*Merck, Austria.*
Diclofenac sodium (p.32·1); thiamine nitrate (p.1455·1); pyridoxine hydrochloride (p.1456·3).
*Musculoskeletal and joint disorders; neuralgia; neuritis; pain.*

*Merck, Mex.*
Diclofenac sodium (p.32·1); thiamine nitrate (p.1455·1); pyridoxine hydrochloride (p.1456·3); cyanocobalamin (p.1458·2).
*Neuralgia; neuritis; neuropathy.*

**Dolo-Neurobion forte** *Merck, Ger.*
Paracetamol (p.76·2); thiamine nitrate (p.1455·1); pyridoxine hydrochloride (p.1456·3); cyanocobalamin (p.1458·2).
*Arthritis; back pain; neuralgia.*

**Dolo-Neurobion N**
*Merck, Ger.*
Paracetamol (p.76·2); thiamine nitrate (p.1455·1); pyridoxine hydrochloride (p.1456·3).
*Joint disorders; lumbago; neuralgia; neuritis; sciatica.*

*Merck, Hong Kong†.*
Vitamin B substances (p.1417·1); paracetamol (p.76·2).
*Neuralgia; neuritis.*

**Dolo-Neurobionta** *Merck, Chile.*
Dipyrone (p.35·3); vitamin B substances.
Procaine (p.1383·2) is included in the injection to alleviate the pain of injection.
*Musculoskeletal, joint, and peri-articular disorders; neuralgia; neuritis.*

**Dolonex** *Pfizer, India.*
Piroxicam (p.84·2).
*Dysmenorrhoea; gout; musculoskeletal, joint, and peri-articular disorders; pain.*

**Dolono** *RID, USA.*
Paracetamol (p.76·2).
*Fever; pain.*

**Dolonovag** *Gobbi, Arg.*
Hydromorphone hydrochloride (p.45·2).
*Pain.*

**Dolo-Octirona** *Laboratorios Chile, Chile.*
Ibuprofen (p.45·3); paracetamol (p.76·2).
*Inflammation; musculoskeletal and joint disorders; pain.*

**Dolo-Pangavit** *Carter-Wallace, Mex.*
Diclofenac sodium (p.32·1); cyanocobalamin (p.1458·2); thiamine nitrate (p.1455·1); pyridoxine hydrochloride (p.1456·3).
*Musculoskeletal, joint, and peri-articular disorders; neuritis; neuropathy; pain.*

**Dolopharm** *Interpharm, Austria.*
Paracetamol (p.76·2); aspirin (p.15·1).
*Fever; pain.*

**Dolophine** *Roxane, USA.*
Methadone hydrochloride (p.57·2).
*Detoxification and treatment of opioid addiction; pain.*

**DoloPosterine N** *Kade, Ger.*
Cinchocaine hydrochloride (p.1373·2).
*Anorectal disorders.*

**Doloproct**
*Schering, Denm.; Schering, Ger.; Asche, Ger.*
Fluocortolone pivalate (p.1102·1); lidocaine hydrochloride (p.1377·3).
*Anorectal disorders.*

**Doloproct Comp** *Schering, Denm.*
Fluocortolone pivalate (p.1102·1); lidocaine hydrochloride (p.1377·3); benzyl alcohol (p.1170·2).
*Anorectal disorders.*

**Dolo-Prolixan** *Siegfried, Switz.†.*
Yellow tablets, azapropazone (p.20·1); dextropropoxyphene hydrochloride (p.28·3); blue tablets, azapropazone; phenprobamate (p.715·1).
*Musculoskeletal, joint, and peri-articular pain.*

**Dolo-Puren** *Alpharma-Isis, Ger.*
Ibuprofen (p.45·3).
*Fever; gout; inflammation; musculoskeletal, joint, and soft-tissue disorders; pain.*

**Dolopyrine** *Streuli, Switz.*
Propyphenazone (p.85·3); atropine methobromide (p.476·3); papaverine hydrochloride (p.1728·1); diphenhydramine hydrochloride (p.431·3); codeine phosphate (p.27·1).
*Pain.*

**Dolorac**
*Note. This name is used for preparations of different composition.*
*Lesvi, Spain.*
Ibuprofen lysine (p.46·3).
*Inflammation; pain.*

*GenDerm, USA.*
Capsaicin (p.24·2).
*Pain.*

**Doloreduct** *Azupharma, Ger.*
Paracetamol (p.76·2).
*Fever; pain.*

**Dolorelax** *Silesia, Chile.*
Paracetamol (p.76·2); chlormezanone (p.675·1).
*Musculoskeletal spasm; pain.*

**Dolorex**
*Note. This name is used for preparations of different composition.*
*S Med, Austria.*
Diethylamine salicylate (p.34·1); menthol (p.1711·3); camphor (p.1665·3).
*Musculoskeletal, joint, peri-articular, and soft-tissue disorders.*

*Whitehall-Robins, Switz.†.*
Glycol salicylate (p.44·3); camphor (p.1665·3); lavender oil (p.1705·2); thyme oil (p.1755·3); siberian fir oil; isopropyl alcohol (p.1184·3).
*Musculoskeletal, joint, peri-articular, and soft-tissue disorders.*

**Dolorex Neo** *Whitehall-Robins, Switz.†.*
Glycol salicylate (p.44·3); allantoin (p.1141·3).
*Musculoskeletal and joint disorders; superficial circulatory disorders.*

**Dolorgiet** *Dolorgiet, Ger.†.*
Glycol salicylate (p.44·3); benzyl nicotinate (p.21·2).
*Musculoskeletal and joint disorders.*

**Dolor-loges** *Loges, Ger.*
Homoeopathic preparation.

**Dolormin** *Woelm, Ger.*
Ibuprofen (p.45·3) or ibuprofen lysine (p.46·3).
*Fever; pain.*

**Dolorol** *Aspen, S.Afr.*
Paracetamol (p.76·2).
*Fever; pain.*

**Dolorol Forte** *Aspen, S.Afr.*
Paracetamol (p.76·2); codeine phosphate (p.27·1).
*Fever; pain.*

**Dolorsan-Balsam** *Opfermann, Ger.†.*
Methyl salicylate (p.59·3); menthol (p.1711·3); camphor (p.1665·3).
*Catarrh; musculoskeletal, joint, and soft-tissue disorders; neuralgia.*

**Dolorsin** *Recalcine, Chile.*
Paracetamol (p.76·2); caffeine (p.782·1).
*Pain.*

**Dolorsyn** *Omega, Arg.*
Ibuprofen (p.45·3).
*Fever; inflammation; pain.*

**Dolorub** *Maver, Chile.*
*Cream:* Ibuprofen (p.45·3).
*Inflammation; pain.*
*Transdermal patch:* Capsicum (p.1667·1).
*Pain.*

**Dolo-Rubriment H** *Riemser, Ger.*
Glycol salicylate (p.44·3).
Dolo-Rubriment formerly contained glycol salicylate, benzyl nicotinate, and heparin sodium.
*Musculoskeletal, joint, and soft-tissue disorders; neuritis.*

**Dolosal**
*Cristalia, Braz.; Aventis, Fr.†.*
Pethidine hydrochloride (p.80·2).
*Pain; premedication.*

**Dolosarto** *Biosarto, Spain.*
Aspirin (p.15·1); benzydamine hydrochloride (p.21·1).
*Fever; inflammation; musculoskeletal and joint disorders; pain.*

**Dolospam** *Laboratorios Chile, Chile.*
Atropine sulfate (p.477·1); papaverine hydrochloride (p.1728·1).
*Smooth muscle spasm.*

**Dolo-Spedifen** *Inpharzam, Switz.*
Ibuprofen arginine (p.46·3).
*Fever; pain.*

**Dolostop**
*Note. This name is used for preparations of different composition.*
*Bayer, Spain.*
Paracetamol (p.76·2).
*Fever; pain.*

*Zeller, Switz.*
Propyphenazone (p.85·3); paracetamol (p.76·2); caffeine (p.782·1).
*Fever; pain.*

**Dolosul** *Soria Natural, Spain.*
Devil's claw root (p.28·2); salix (p.87·3); meadowsweet (p.1710·1).
*Rheumatic disorders.*

**Dolotandax** *Novartis, Mex.*
Naproxen sodium (p.65·1); paracetamol (p.76·2).
*Fever; pain.*

**Dolotard** *Nycomed, Swed.†.*
Dextropropoxyphene chloride (p.28·3).
*Pain.*

**Dolotec** *Innotech, Fr.*
Paracetamol (p.76·2).
*Fever; pain.*

**Doloteffin**
*Chemists Own, Austral.†; Ardeypharm, Ger.*
Devil's claw root (p.28·2).
*Musculoskeletal and joint disorders.*

**Dolotemp** *Glaxo Wellcome, Mex.*
Paracetamol (p.76·2).
*Fever; pain.*

**Dolo-Tiaminal** *Silanes, Mex.*
Dipyrone (p.35·3); cyanocobalamin (p.1458·2); thiamine nitrate (p.1455·1); pyridoxine hydrochloride (p.1456·3).
*Neuralgia; neuritis.*

**Dolotol 12** *Saval, Chile.*
Lysine aspirin (p.54·3); glycine (p.1433·3); hydroxocobalamin (p.1458·2); thiamine hydrochloride (p.1455·1); pyridoxine hydrochloride (p.1456·3).
Lidocaine hydrochloride (p.1377·3) is included in this preparation to alleviate the pain of injection.
*Musculoskeletal, joint, and peri-articular disorders; neuralgia; neuritis.*

**Dolotor** *Roche, Mex.*
Ketorolac trometamol (p.52·1).
*Pain.*

**Dolotren** *Faes, Spain.*
Diclofenac (p.32·1); diclofenac diethylamine (p.32·1) or diclofenac sodium (p.32·1).
*Gout; musculoskeletal, joint, peri-articular, and soft-tissue disorders; pain; renal colic.*

**Dolo-Veniten** *Whitehall-Robins, Switz.*
Glycol salicylate (p.44·3); a heparinoid (p.931·1); aescin (p.1648·2).
*Vascular disorders.*

**Doloverina** *Saval, Chile.*
Mebeverine hydrochloride (p.1273·1).
*Gastrointestinal pain and spasm.*

**Dolovin** *Atral, Port.*
Indometacin (p.47·3).
*Gout; musculoskeletal and joint disorders.*

**DoloVisano M** *Kade, Ger.*
Mephenesin (p.1394·3).
*Cervical syndrome; lumbago; skeletal muscle spasm.*

**DoloVisano Salbe** *Kade, Ger.*
Glycol salicylate (p.44·3); benzyl nicotinate (p.21·2).
*Circulatory disorders of the skin; muscle, joint, and soft-tissue disorders.*

**Dolo-Voltaren** *Novartis, Spain.*
Diclofenac sodium (p.32·1).
*Gout; musculoskeletal, joint, and peri-articular disorders; pain; renal colic.*

**Doloxene**
*Lilly, Austral.; Lilly, Denm.; Lilly, Hong Kong†; Lilly, Irl.; Lilly, NZ; Lilly, Swed.; Lilly, UK†.*
Dextropropoxyphene napsilate (p.28·3).
*Pain.*

*Aspen, S.Afr.*
Dextropropoxyphene hydrochloride (p.28·3).
*Pain.*

**Doloxene Co** *Quatromed, S.Afr.*
Dextropropoxyphene hydrochloride (p.28·3); aspirin (p.15·1); caffeine (p.782·1).

**Doloxene Compound**
*Lilly, Hong Kong†; Lilly, Irl.†.*
Dextropropoxyphene napsilate (p.28·3); aspirin (p.15·1); caffeine (p.782·1).
*Pain.*

**Doloxene-A** *Lilly, Braz.*
Dextropropoxyphene napsilate (p.28·3); aspirin (p.15·1).
*Pain.*

**Doloxtren** *Sintactica, Ital.*
Nimesulide (p.67·1).
*Fever; inflammation; pain.*

**Dolpasse** *Fresenius Kabi, Austria.*
Diclofenac sodium (p.32·1).
*Gout; inflammation; musculoskeletal, joint, and peri-articular disorders; pain.*

**Dolpic Forte** *Pasteur, Chile.*
Trimebutine maleate (p.1758·1).
*Irritable bowel syndrome.*

**Dolpocetmol** *Synco, Hong Kong.*
Dextropropoxyphene hydrochloride (p.28·3); paracetamol (p.76·2).
*Pain.*

**Dolprin** *Collins, Mex.*
Ibuprofen (p.45·3).
*Inflammation.*

**Dolprofen** *Collins, Mex.*
Ibuprofen (p.45·3).
*Inflammation.*

**Dolprone**
*Aventis, Belg.; Aventis, Switz.*
Paracetamol (p.76·2).
*Fever; pain.*

**Dolpyc**
*Note. This name is used for preparations of different composition.*
*Bournonville, Belg.†.*
Capsicum oleoresin (p.1667·1); chloroform (p.1296·3).
*Muscle and joint pain.*

*Warner-Lambert, Fr.†.*
Capsicum (p.1667·1); chloroform (p.1296·3).
*Pain and bruising.*

*Teofarma, Ital.*
Capsicum oleoresin (p.1667·1).
*Musculoskeletal, joint, and soft-tissue pain.*

**Dolquine** *Rubio, Spain.*
Hydroxychloroquine sulfate (p.452·3).
*Lupus erythematosus; malaria; rheumatoid arthritis.*

**Dolsed** *American Urologicals, USA.*
Methenamine (p.230·1); salol (p.88·1); atropine sulfate (p.477·1); hyoscyamine sulfate (p.485·1); benzoic acid (p.1169·3); methylthioninium chloride (p.1042·2).
*Urinary-tract infections.*

**Dolsinal** *Ferrer, Spain†.*
Nabumetone (p.63·3).
*Osteoarthritis; rheumatoid arthritis.*

**Doltard** *Nycomed, Denm.*
Morphine sulfate (p.60·2).
*Pain.*

**Dolten** *Pharmacia, Arg.*
Ketorolac trometamol (p.52·1).
*Pain.*

The symbol † denotes a preparation no longer actively marketed

**Dol-u-ron** *Neo-Farmaceutica, Port.*
Paracetamol (p.76·2); codeine phosphate (p.27·1).
*Pain.*

**Doluvital** *Valdecasas, Mex.*
Paracetamol (p.76·2).
*Fever; pain.*

**Dolval** *Randall, Mex.*
Ibuprofen (p.45·3).
*Fever; pain.*

**Dolvan** *Norma, UK.*
Diphenhydramine hydrochloride (p.431·3); ephedrine hydrochloride (p.1120·1); paracetamol (p.76·2); caffeine (p.782·1).
*Cold and influenza symptoms; nasal congestion.*

**Dolver** *Maver, Mex.*
Ibuprofen (p.45·3).
*Inflammation; pain.*

**Dolviran**
*Note. This name is used for preparations of different composition.*
*Bayer, Belg.; Bayer, Port.; Bayer, Spain.*
Aspirin (p.15·1); codeine phosphate (p.27·1); caffeine (p.782·1).
*Fever; pain.*

*Bayer, Mex.*
Paracetamol (p.76·2).
*Fever; pain.*

**Dolviran N**
*Note. This name is used for preparations of different composition.*
*Hexal, Ger.; Tropon, Ger.*
Aspirin (p.15·1); codeine phosphate (p.27·1).
*Pain.*

*Bayer, Neth.*
Aspirin (p.15·1); codeine phosphate (p.27·1); caffeine (p.782·1).
*Fever; pain.*

**Dolxen** *Maver, Mex.*
Naproxen (p.65·1).
*Inflammation; musculoskeletal and joint disorders; pain.*

**Dolzam** *Zambon, Belg.*
Tramadol hydrochloride (p.94·3).
*Pain.*

**Dolzycam** *Sons, Mex.*
Piroxicam (p.84·2).
*Gout; musculoskeletal, joint, peri-articular, and soft-tissue disorders; pain.*

**Doma Grip** *Dallas, Arg.*
Guaifenesin (p.1122·1); chlorphenamine maleate (p.427·3); phenylephrine hydrochloride (p.1126·3); paracetamol (p.76·2).

**Doma Grip NF** *Dallas, Arg.*
Astemizole (p.424·2); paracetamol (p.76·2); phenylephrine hydrochloride (p.1126·3); guaifenesin (p.1122·1).

**Domar**
*Eurodrug, Hong Kong; Teofarma, Ital.; Eurodrug, Singapore; Eurodrug, Thai.*
Pinazepam (p.715·3).
*Anxiety; chronic alcoholism; depression; epilepsy.*

**Domeboro**
*Serral, Mex.; Miles, USA.*
Aluminium sulfate (p.1653·1); calcium acetate (p.1225·1).
*Inflammatory skin conditions.*

**Domenal** *Collins, Mex.*
Dipyrone (p.35·3).
*Fever; pain.*

**Domenan** *Kissei, Jpn.*
Ozagrel hydrochloride (p.1725·2).
*Asthma.*

**Domeni** *Tafir, Spain.*
Vincamine (p.1764·2).
*Cerebral trauma; cerebrovascular disorders; circulatory disorders of the eye, ear, nose, and throat; vestibular disorders.*

**Dome-Paste** *Miles, USA.*
Zinc oxide (p.1163·2); calamine (p.1144·1); gelatin (p.754·3).
*Conditions of the extremities requiring protection and support.*

**Domer** *Best, Mex.*
Omeprazole (p.1278·2).
*Gastro-oesophageal reflux; gastrointestinal hyperacidity; peptic ulcer; Zollinger-Ellison syndrome.*

**Domerdon** *Asian Pharm, Thai.*
Domperidone (p.1263·2).
*Delayed gastric emptying; dyspepsia; flatulence; gastro-oesophageal reflux; heartburn; nausea and vomiting.*

**Domes** *SoSe, Ital.*
Nimesulide (p.67·1).
*Fever; inflammation; pain.*

**Domex** *Sante Naturelle, Canad.†.*
Calcium and magnesium (p.1417·1).

**Domical** *Rhone-Poulenc Rorer, Hong Kong†.*
Amitriptyline hydrochloride (p.280·3).
*Depression.*

**Domicap** *Raza, Malaysia; Pharmaniaga, Malaysia.*
Indometacin (p.47·3).
*Gout; musculoskeletal, joint, and peri-articular disorders.*

**Domicetina** *Wiener, Mex.†.*
Chloramphenicol (p.185·1).
*Bacterial infections.*

**Domidone** *Milano, Thai.*
Domperidone (p.1263·2).
*Digestive disorders; dyspepsia; flatulence; gastro-oesophageal reflux; heartburn; nausea and vomiting.*

**Domiken** *Kendrick, Mex.*
Doxycycline hyclate (p.206·2).
*Bacterial infections.*

**Domilium** *LSP, Thai.†.*
Domperidone (p.1263·2) or domperidone maleate (p.1263·2).
*Delayed gastric emptying; digestive disorders; dyspepsia; nausea and vomiting.*

**Domin** *Boehringer Ingelheim, Jpn.*
Talipexole hydrochloride (p.1215·3).
*Parkinsonism.*

**Dominal**
*Asta Medica, Austria; Viatris, Belg.; AWD, Ger.*
Prothipendyl hydrochloride (p.718·1).
*Atopic dermatitis; eclampsia; gastrointestinal spasm; postoperative vomiting; premedication; pruritus; psychiatric disorders; sedative.*

**Dominans** *Lundbeck, Ital.*
Nortriptyline hydrochloride (p.310·2); fluphenazine hydrochloride (p.699·3).
*Mixed anxiety depressive states.*

**Dominium** *Tecnofarma, Chile.*
Fluoxetine (p.296·3).
*Bulimia; depression; obsessive-compulsive disorder.*

**Domnamid** *Lundbeck, Denm.*
Estazolam (p.697·3).
*Premedication; sleep disorders.*

**Domol** *Miles, USA.*
Bath additive.
*Lubrication of the skin; pruritus.*

**Dompel** *Samnam, Singapore.*
Domperidone (p.1263·2).
*Dyspepsia.*

**Dompenyl** *Korea United, Singapore.*
Domperidone (p.1263·2).
*Nausea and vomiting.*

**Dompeon** *Merck, Hong Kong.*
Domperidone (p.1263·2).
*Digestive disorders; dyspepsia; flatulence; gastro-oesophageal reflux; heartburn; nausea and vomiting.*

**Domper**
*YSP, Malaysia; Yung Shin, Singapore.*
Domperidone (p.1263·2).
*Meteorism; nausea and vomiting.*

**Domperamol** *Servier, UK.*
Paracetamol (p.76·2); domperidone maleate (p.1263·2).
*Migraine.*

**Domperdone** *Polipharm, Thai.*
Domperidone (p.1263·2).
*Digestive disorders; dyspepsia; nausea and vomiting.*

**Domper-M** *Bangkok Lab & Cosmetic, Thai.*
Domperidone maleate (p.1263·2).
*Digestive disorders; nausea and vomiting.*

**Domperol** *Farmion, Braz.†.*
Domperidone (p.1263·2).
*Nausea and vomiting.*

**Dompil** *Spyfarma, Spain†.*
Metampicillin sodium (p.229·3).
*Bacterial infections.*

**Dom-Polienzim** *Sanitas, Arg.*
Domperidone (p.1263·2); lipase; amylase (p.1654·2); protease; cellulase (p.1669·1); simeticone (p.1289·2).
*Gastrointestinal disorders; pancreatic insufficiency.*

**Domstal** *Torrent, India.*
Domperidone (p.1263·2).
*Dyspepsia; nausea and vomiting.*

**Domutussina** *Proge, Ital.*
Dropropizine (p.1119·3).
*Coughs.*

**Domuvar** *Bioprogress, Ital.*
Spores of *Bacillus subtilis*.
*Gastrointestinal disorders.*

**Dona**
*Helsinn Birex, Irl.; Rottapharm, Ital.*
Glucosamine sulfate (p.1694·1).
*Osteoarthritis.*

**Dona 200-S** *Opfermann, Ger.*
Glucosamine sulfate (p.1694·1).
*Degenerative joint disorders.*

**Donalg** *Dynacren, Ital.*
Tetracaine hydrochloride (p.1385·1); sulfogaiacol (p.1131·1); salicylic acid (p.1157·1); menthol (p.1711·3); sage (p.1741·2); chamomile (p.1669·3); salix (p.87·3); ginger (p.1267·1).
*Dental pain.*

**Donamet** *Abbott, Ital.*
Ademetionine butanedisulfonate (p.1647·2).
*Hepatic cholestasis.*

**Donaprox** *Reuffer, Mex.†.*
Naproxen (p.65·1).

**Donaren** *Apsen, Braz.*
Trazodone hydrochloride (p.319·1).
*Depression; neurogenic pain.*

**Donataxel** *Gautier, Arg.*
Docetaxel (p.547·1).
*Breast cancer; non-small cell lung cancer.*

**Donatiol** *AGIPS, Ital.*
Mecysteine hydrochloride (p.1124·1); guaifenesin (p.1122·1); camphor (p.1665·3).
*Respiratory-tract disorders.*

**Donatussin** *Laser, USA.*
*Oral drops:* Chlorphenamine maleate (p.427·3); phenylephrine hydrochloride (p.1126·3); guaifenesin (p.1122·1).
*Syrup:* Chlorphenamine maleate (p.427·3); phenylephrine hydrochloride (p.1126·3); dextromethorphan hydrobromide (p.1117·3); guaifenesin (p.1122·1).
*Coughs.*

**Donatussin DC** *Laser, USA.*
Hydrocodone tartrate (p.45·1); phenylephrine hydrochloride (p.1126·3); guaifenesin (p.1122·1).
*Coughs.*

**Doncef** *Pharma 2000, Fr.†.*
Cefradine (p.179·3).
*Bacterial infections.*

**Donegal** *Medipharm, Chile.*
Domperidone (p.1263·2).
*Gastro-oesophageal reflux; hiccups; nausea; vomiting.*

**Doneka** *Vita, Spain.*
Lisinopril (p.946·3).
*Diabetic nephropathy; heart failure; hypertension; myocardial infarction.*

**Doneka Plus** *Vita, Spain.*
Lisinopril (p.946·3); hydrochlorothiazide (p.933·2).
*Hypertension.*

**Doneurin** *Hexal, Ger.*
Doxepin hydrochloride (p.291·2).
*Anxiety; depression; withdrawal syndromes.*

**Dong Quai Complex** *Blackmores, Austral.†.*
Angelica sinensis (p.1655·1); avena (p.1658·2); cimicifuga (p.1671·3); vitex agnus castus (p.1649·1); vitamins and minerals (p.1417·1).
*Menopausal disorders; premenstrual syndrome; uterine cramping.*

**Donicer** *Novag, Spain†.*
Amiloride hydrochloride (p.858·2); hydrochlorothiazide (p.933·2).
*Hypertension; oedema.*

**Donix** *Llorens, Spain.*
Lorazepam (p.704·1).
*Alcohol withdrawal syndrome; anxiety disorders; chemotherapy induced nausea and vomiting; insomnia; premedication.*

**Donna** *Eurofarma, Braz.*
Tibolone (p.1572·3).
*Menopausal disorders.*

**Donnagel**
*Note. This name is used for preparations of different composition.*
*Whitehall, Austral.*
Hyoscyamine sulfate (p.485·1); atropine sulfate (p.477·1); hyoscine hydrobromide (p.483·3); kaolin (p.1268·3); pectin (p.1580·3).
*Gastrointestinal disorders.*

*IQB, Braz.*
Metronidazole (p.607·2); nystatin (p.406·3); benzalkonium chloride (p.1168·3); urea (p.1162·2).
*Vulvovaginal infections.*

*Wyeth-Ayerst, USA†.*
Attapulgite (p.1251·1).
*Diarrhoea.*

**Donnagel-PG** *Wyeth-Ayerst, Canad.†.*
*Capsules:* Activated attapulgite (p.1251·1); pectin (p.1580·3); prepared opium (p.74·2).
*Oral suspension:* Kaolin (p.1268·3); pectin (p.1580·3); prepared opium (p.74·2).
*Diarrhoea.*

**Donnalix** *Whitehall, Austral.*
Hyoscyamine sulfate (p.485·1); atropine sulfate (p.477·1); hyoscine hydrobromide (p.483·3).
*Gastrointestinal disorders.*

**Donnamar** *Marnel, USA.*
Hyoscyamine sulfate (p.485·1).

**Donnatab** *Whitehall, Austral.*
Hyoscyamine sulfate (p.485·1); atropine sulfate (p.477·1); hyoscine hydrobromide (p.483·3).
*Gastrointestinal disorders.*

**Donnatal**
*Wyeth-Ayerst, Canad.†; Aspen, S.Afr.; Whitehall, Thai.; Robins, USA†.*
Hyoscyamine sulfate (p.485·1); atropine sulfate (p.477·1); hyoscine hydrobromide (p.483·3); phenobarbital (p.367·3).
*Motion sickness; smooth muscle spasm.*

**Donnazyme** *Robins, USA†.*
Pancreatin (p.1725·3).
*Pancreatic insufficiency.*

**Donobid**
*Merck Sharp & Dohme, Denm.; Merck Sharp & Dohme, Fin.; Merck Sharp & Dohme, Norw.; Merck Sharp & Dohme, Swed.*
Diflunisal (p.34·1).
*Inflammation; musculoskeletal and joint disorders; pain.*

**Donodol** *Armstrong, Mex.*
Clonixin lysine (p.26·3).
*Pain.*

**Donodol Compuesto** *Armstrong, Mex.*
Clonixin lysine (p.26·3); hyoscine butylbromide (p.483·3).
*Smooth muscle pain and spasm.*

**Donomix** *Laboratorios Chile, Chile.*
Clotrimazole (p.396·2); betamethasone (p.1093·1).
*Fungal skin infections with inflammation.*

**Donorest**
*Wyeth Lederle, Port.; Wyeth, Spain†.*
Fentiazac (p.43·1).
*Musculoskeletal, joint, and peri-articular disorders; pain.*

**Donormyl**
*Oberlin, Fr.; Upsamedica, Spain†.*
Doxylamine succinate (p.432·3).
*Insomnia.*

**Dontisolon D** *Aventis, Ger.*
Prednisolone (p.1108·1) or prednisolone acetate (p.1108·1).
*Inflammatory disorders of the mouth.*

**Dontopivalone** *Parke, Davis, Fr.†.*
Tixocortol pivalate (p.1110·1); chlorhexidine acetate (p.1173·2).
*Mouth disorders.*

**Dontuxin** *Continentales, Mex.†.*
Dextromethorphan (p.1117·3).

**Donulide** *Wyeth Lederle, Port.*
Nimesulide (p.67·1).
*Fever; pain.*

**Donum** *M & H, Thai.*
Domperidone (p.1263·2).
*Dyspepsia; gastro-oesophageal reflux; heartburn; nausea and vomiting.*

**Dopabane** *Ariston, Braz.*
Dopamine hydrochloride (p.907·1).

**Dopacard**
*Ipsen, Denm.; Ipsen, Fin.; Elan, Fr.; Elan, Ger.; Elan, Irl.; NZ Medical & Scientific, NZ†; Ipsen, Swed.; Vifor, Switz.; Elan, UK.*
Dopexamine hydrochloride (p.908·2).
*Heart failure.*

**Dopacris** *Cristalia, Braz.*
Dopamine hydrochloride (p.907·1).

**Dopadura C** *Merck dura, Ger.*
Levodopa (p.1205·2); carbidopa (p.1204·3).
*Parkinsonism.*

**Dopaflex** *Medphano, Ger.*
Levodopa (p.1205·2).
*Parkinsonism.*

**Dopagon** *Schering, Arg.*
Lisuride maleate (p.1210·3).
*Acromegaly; female infertility; hyperprolactinaemia; lactation inhibition; menstrual disorders.*

**Dopagrand** *Ahimsa, Arg.*
Methyldopa (p.953·2).
*Hypertension.*

**Dopagyt** *Themis Chemicals, India.*
Methyldopa (p.953·2).
*Hypertension.*

**Dopamed**
*Note. This name is used for preparations of different composition.*
*Kolassa, Austria.*
Levodopa (p.1205·2); benserazide hydrochloride (p.1200·2).
*Parkinsonism.*

*General Drugs, Thai.*
Methyldopa (p.953·2).
*Hypertension.*

**Dopamet**
*Dumex-Alpharma, Denm.†; Medochemie, Hong Kong; Raza, Malaysia; Pharmaniaga, Malaysia; Dumex, Norw.†; Dumex, Switz.†.*
Methyldopa (p.953·2).
*Hypertension.*

**Dopametil** *Bunker, Braz.*
Methyldopa (p.953·2).
*Hypertension.*

**Dopamex** *Biolab, Thai.*
Dopamine hydrochloride (p.907·1).
*Acute poisoning; hypotension; shock.*

**Dopaminex**
*Solvay, Hong Kong†; Solvay, Thai.*
Dopamine hydrochloride (p.907·1).
*Hypotension; shock.*

**Dopar** *Procter & Gamble, USA.*
Levodopa (p.1205·2).
*Parkinsonism.*

**Doparid** *Rafa, Israel.*
Tiapride hydrochloride (p.725·1).
*Choreas; dyskinesias; tics; tremor.*

**Dopasian** *Asian Pharm, Thai.*
Methyldopa (p.953·2).
*Hypertension.*

**Dopatral** *LA, Arg.*
Methyldopa (p.953·2).
*Hypertension.*

**Dopatropin** *Scott-Cassara, Arg.*
Dopamine (p.907·3).

**Dopegyt**
*Thiemann, Ger.; Egis, Hong Kong; Egis, Malaysia; Egis, Singapore; Egis, Thai.*
Methyldopa (p.953·2).
*Hypertension.*

**Dopergin**
*Schering, Austria; Schering, Braz.†; Schering, Ger.; Schering, Israel; Schering, Ital.; Schering, Mex.; Schering, Neth.; Schering, NZ; Schering, Spain; Schering, Switz.; Schering, Thai.*
Lisuride maleate (p.1210·3).
*Acromegaly; hyperprolactinaemia; infertility; lactation inhibition; male hypogonadism; mastitis; menstrual disorders; parkinsonism; premenstrual syndrome; prolactinoma.*

**Dopergine** *Schering, Fr.*
Lisuride maleate (p.1210·3).
*Erectile dysfunction; galactorrhoea; gynaecomastia in males; infertility; menstrual disorders; parkinsonism.*

**Dopicar** *Merck Sharp & Dohme, Israel.*
Carbidopa (p.1204·3); levodopa (p.1205·2).
*Parkinsonism.*

**Dopin** *Pharmaland, Thai.*
Dosulepin hydrochloride (p.291·1).
*Depression; mixed anxiety depressive states.*

**Dopinga** *Inga, India.*
Dopamine hydrochloride (p.907·1).
*Shock.*

**Dopmin**
*Orion, Denm.; Orion, Fin.; Orion, Malaysia; Orion, Singapore; Orion, Thai.*
Dopamine hydrochloride (p.907·1).
*Heart failure; open heart surgery; shock.*

**Dopo Pik** *Tipomark, Ital.*
Triclosan (Irgasan 300) (p.1195·2); trolamine (p.1758·2); propylene glycol (p.1735·2).
*Skin disinfection.*

**Doppelherz Energie-Tonikum N** *Queisser, Ger.*
Vitamin B substances; crataegus; valerian; lupulus (p.1417·1).
*Tonic.*

**Doppelherz Ginseng Aktiv** *Queisser, Ger.*
Ginseng; pyridoxine hydrochloride; nicotinamide; caffeine (p.1417·1).
*Tonic.*

**Doppelherz Magenstarkung** *Queisser, Ger.†.*
Peppermint leaf (p.1283·2); absinthium (p.1645·1); silybum marianum (p.1043·3).
*Gastrointestinal disorders.*

**Doppelherz Melissengeist** *Queisser, Ger.*
Melissa (p.1711·1); angelica (p.1655·1); cinnamon (p.1672·2); nutmeg (p.1722·2); bitter-orange peel (p.1723·3); clove (p.1673·2); lemon peel (p.1706·2).
*Digestive disorders; skin circulatory disorders.*

**Doppelherz Tonikum** *Queisser, Austria†.*
Crataegus (p.1677·1); melissa (p.1711·1); lupulus (p.1708·1).
*Tonic.*

**Doppel-Spalt Compact** *Whitehall-Much, Ger.*
Aspirin (p.15·1); caffeine (p.782·1).
*Fever; inflammation; pain.*

**Dopram**
*Wyeth, Austral.; Wyeth Lederle, Austria; Wyeth Lederle, Belg.; Wyeth-Ayerst, Canad.†; Meda, Denm.; Wyeth Lederle, Fin.; Riemser, Ger.; IFET (ΙΦΕΤ), Gr.; Robins, Hong Kong; Antigen, Irl.; Bournonville, Neth.; Wyeth Lederle, Norw.; Wyeth, NZ; Bodene, S.Afr.; Wyeth, Switz.; Anpharm, UK; Robins, USA.*
Doxapram hydrochloride (p.1587·2).
*Respiratory depression.*

**Dopress** *Pacific, NZ.*
Dosulepin hydrochloride (p.291·1).
*Depression.*

**Doprit** *Farcoral, Mex.†.*
Hydroxocobalamin (p.1458·2).

**Doproct** *Continental Pharma, Thai.*
Hydrocortisone acetate (p.1103·3); zinc oxide (p.1163·2); benzocaine (p.1370·3).
*Anorectal disorders.*

**Dops**
*Note. This name is used for preparations of different composition.*
*Fuca, Fr.*
Sodium bicarbonate (p.1223·2); calcium carbonate (p.1254·2); calcium phosphate (p.1225·3); magnesium hydroxide (p.1272·2); titanium dioxide (p.1160·3); magnesium carbonate (p.1272·1).
*Gastrointestinal hyperacidity.*
*Sumitomo, Jpn.*
Droxidopa (p.1204·3).
*Familial amyloid polyneuropathy; parkinsonism.*

**Dopsan** *Pond's, Thai.*
Dapsone (p.202·2).
*Dermatitis herpetiformis; leprosy.*

**Doqua** *Sriprasit, Thai.*
Triamphenicol.
*Bacterial infections.*

**Doraine** *Labortecne, Braz.†.*
Aspirin (p.15·1).
*Fever; pain.*

**Doral**
*Mitsubishi, Jpn; Wallace, USA.*
Quazepam (p.718·2).
*Insomnia; premedication.*

**Doralem** *Farmedica, Braz.†.*
Aspirin (p.15·1); paracetamol (p.76·2); caffeine (p.782·1).
Aluminium hydroxide (p.1249·2) is included in this preparation in an attempt to limit adverse effects on the gastrointestinal mucosa.
*Fever; pain.*

**Doralese**
*GlaxoSmithKline, Irl.*
Indoramin (p.939·3).
*Benign prostatic hyperplasia.*
*GlaxoSmithKline, UK.*
Indoramin hydrochloride (p.939·2).
*Benign prostatic hyperplasia.*

**Doralgina** *Neo Quimica, Braz.*
Isometheptene mucate (p.1702·1); dipyrone (p.35·3); caffeine (p.782·1).
*Muscle spasm; pain.*

**Doralin** *Menarini, Gr.*
Otilonium bromide (p.1725·1).
*Aid in gastrointestinal endoscopy; gastrointestinal smooth muscle spasm.*

**Doralon** *Heralds, Braz.†.*
Dipyrone (p.35·3); diphenhydramine (p.431·3).
*Fever; pain.*

**Doran** *QIF, Braz.†.*
Dipyrone (p.35·3).
*Fever; pain.*

**Doraplax** *Luper, Braz.*
Ibuprofen (p.45·3).
*Fever; musculoskeletal and joint disorders; pain.*

**Dorbantil** *Drugtech, Chile.*
Doxazosin mesilate (p.908·3).
*Benign prostatic hyperplasia; hypertension.*

**Dorbid** *Prodome, Braz.†.*
Diflunisal (p.34·1).
*Gout; inflammation; musculoskeletal, joint, and periarticular disorders; pain.*

**Dorcalor** *BA Farma, Port.*
Diclofenac sodium (p.32·1).
*Inflammation; musculoskeletal, joint, and peri-articular disorders; pain.*

**Dorcol Children's Cold Formula** *Novartis, USA.*
Pseudoephedrine hydrochloride (p.1129·2); chlorphenamine maleate (p.427·3).
*Cold symptoms.*

**Dorcol Children's Cough Syrup** *Novartis, USA.*
Pseudoephedrine hydrochloride (p.1129·2); guaifenesin (p.1122·1); dextromethorphan hydrobromide (p.1117·3).
*Coughs.*

**Dorcol Children's Decongestant** *Novartis, USA.*
Pseudoephedrine hydrochloride (p.1129·2).
*Nasal congestion.*

**Dordendril** *Heralds, Braz.†.*
Paracetamol (p.76·2).
*Fever; pain.*

**Dordente** *Hearst, Braz.†.*
Phenol (p.1188·1); menthol (p.1711·3); procaine (p.1383·2).
*Local anaesthesia.*

**Dore Immun** *Rentschler, Ger.†.*
Echinacea (p.1683·2).
*Immunostimulant.*

**Doregrippin** *Rentschler, Ger.*
Paracetamol (p.76·2); phenylephrine hydrochloride (p.1126·3).
*Cold and influenza symptoms.*

**Dorehydrin** *Sanova, Austria.*
Co-dergocrine mesilate (p.1674·1).
*Cervical syndrome; hypertension; mental function impairment; migraine and related vascular headache; peripheral vascular disorders.*

**Dorenasin** *Rentschler, Ger.†.*
Xylometazoline hydrochloride (p.1132·2).
*Nasal congestion.*

**Dorend** *Teuto, Braz.*
Paracetamol (p.76·2); phenylbutazone (p.83·2).

**Doreperol N** *Rentschler, Ger.*
Hexetidine (p.1182·1).
*Mouth and throat disorders; oral hygiene.*

**Doretrim** *Novartis, Braz.*
Ibuprofen (p.45·3).
*Fever; inflammation; pain.*

**Dorex** *Catarinense, Braz.†.*
Paracetamol (p.76·2); caffeine (p.782·1).
*Fever; pain.*

**Dorf** *Ibirn, Ital.*
Cefaclor (p.167·1).
*Bacterial infections.*

**Dorfen** *Cazi, Braz.*
Paracetamol (p.76·2).
*Fever; pain.*

**Dorflan** *Cazi, Braz.*
Diclofenac (p.32·1), diclofenac potassium (p.32·1), or diclofenac resinate (p.33·1).
*Inflammation; pain.*

**Dorflex** *Aventis, Braz.*
Dipyrone (p.35·3); orphenadrine citrate (p.486·1); caffeine (p.782·1).
*Skeletal muscle spasm.*

**Dorgen** *Cazi, Braz.*
Diclofenac sodium (p.32·1).
*Gout; inflammation; musculoskeletal, joint, and periarticular disorders; pain.*

**Dori** *Rentschler, Ger.†.*
Benzocaine (p.1370·3); cetylpyridinium chloride (p.1173·1); tyrothricin (p.275·1).
*Mouth and throat inflammation.*

**Dorib** *Ibfarma, Braz.†.*
Paracetamol (p.76·2).
*Fever; pain.*

**Doribel** *Luper, Braz.*
Aspirin (p.15·1); caffeine (p.782·1).
*Fever; pain.*

**Dorical** *Legrand, Braz.*
Vitamins; rutin; minerals (p.1417·1).
*Nutritional supplement.*

**Doricin** *EMS, Braz.*
Orphenadrine citrate (p.486·1); dipyrone (p.35·3); caffeine citrate (p.782·1).
*Skeletal muscle spasm.*

**Dorico** *Sanofi Synthelabo, Braz.*
Paracetamol (p.76·2).
*Fever; pain.*

**Doricoflu** *Farmila, Ital.*
Flunisolide (p.1101·1).
*Asthma; bronchitis; rhinitis.*

**Doricum** *Farmila, Ital.*
Fluocinolone acetonide (p.1101·2); neomycin sulfate (p.235·1).
*Eye, ear, and nose disorders.*

**Doridamina** *Angelini, Ital.*
Lonidamine (p.565·3).
*Malignant neoplasms.*

**Doridina** *Bunker, Braz.*
Isometheptene hydrochloride (p.1702·1) or isometheptene mucate (p.1702·1); dipyrone (p.35·3); caffeine (p.782·1).
*Pain.*

**Doridone** *DHA, Singapore.*
Domperidone (p.1263·2).
*Nausea and vomiting.*

**Doriflan** *Luper, Braz.*
Diclofenac diethylamine (p.32·1), diclofenac potassium (p.32·1), or diclofenac resinate (p.33·1).
*Gout; inflammation; musculoskeletal, joint, and periarticular disorders; pain.*

**Doril** *DM, Braz.†.*
Aspirin (p.15·1); caffeine (p.782·1).
*Fever; pain.*

**Dorilan** *Luper, Braz.*
Dipyrone (p.35·3).
*Fever; pain.*

**Dorilax** *Ache, Braz.*
Paracetamol (p.76·2); carisoprodol (p.1392·1); caffeine (p.782·1).
*Skeletal muscle spasm.*

**Doriman** *Vir, Spain.*
Ciprofloxacin hydrochloride (p.188·2).
*Bacterial infections.*

**Dorithricin**
*Note. This name is used for preparations of different composition.*
*Provita, Austria.*
*Eye ointment:* Tyrothricin (p.275·1); neomycin sulfate (p.235·1).
*Rentschler, Austria.*
*Lozenges:* Tyrothricin (p.275·1); benzalkonium chloride (p.1168·3); benzocaine (p.1370·3).
*Mouth and throat disorders.*
*Rentschler, Singapore.*
Tyrothricin (p.275·1); benzalkonium chloride (p.1168·3); benzocaine (p.1370·3).
*Sore throat.*

**Dorithricin Limone** *Rentschler, Ger.*
Tyrothricin (p.275·1); lidocaine hydrochloride (p.1377·3).
*Mouth and throat disorders.*

**Dorithricin Original** *Rentschler, Ger.*
Tyrothricin (p.275·1); benzalkonium chloride (p.1168·3); benzocaine (p.1370·3).
*Mouth and throat disorders.*

**Dorival** *Bayer, Spain.*
Ibuprofen (p.45·3).
*Fever; pain.*

**Dorixina**
*Roemmers, Arg.; Rhein, Mex.*
Clonixin lysine (p.26·3).
*Musculoskeletal, joint, peri-articular, and soft-tissue disorders; pain.*

**Dorixina B1 B6 B12** *Roemmers, Arg.*
Clonixin lysine (p.26·3); thiamine hydrochloride (p.1455·1) or thiamine nitrate (p.1455·1); pyridoxine hydrochloride (p.1456·3); cyanocobalamin (p.1458·2) or hydroxocobalamin acetate (p.1458·2).
*Inflammation; pain.*

**Dorixina Relax** *Roemmers, Arg.*
Clonixin lysine (p.26·3); cyclobenzaprine hydrochloride (p.1393·1).
*Musculoskeletal pain.*

**Dorken** *Vedim, Spain.*
Dipotassium clorazepate (p.685·1); aminohydroxybutyric acid (p.353·2); pyridoxine hydrochloride (p.1456·3).
*Anxiety disorders; insomnia.*

**Dorless** *Uniao Quimica, Braz.†.*
Tramadol (p.95·2).
*Pain.*

**Dorm** *Norma (Νορμα), Gr.*
Lorazepam (p.704·1).
*Anxiety disorders; insomnia; status epilepticus.*

**Dormalon** *Wernigerode, Ger.*
Nitrazepam (p.710·1).
*Sleep disorders.*

**Dormarist** *Steiner, Ger.*
Valerian (p.1762·2); melissa (p.1711·1).
*Sleep disorders.*

**Dorme** *Hoechst Marion Roussel, S.Afr.†.*
Quazepam (p.718·2).
*Insomnia.*

**Dormeasan**
*Bioforce, Ger.; Bioforce, Switz.*
Lupulus (p.1708·1); valerian (p.1762·2).
*Agitation; insomnia; irritability.*

**Dormelox** *Delta, Braz.*
Meloxicam (p.56·1).

**Dormen** *Labima, Belg.†.*
Pyrithyldione (p.718·1); diphenhydramine hydrochloride (p.431·3).
*Insomnia.*

**Dormer 211** *Dormer, Canad.*
Emollient.
*Dry skin.*

**Dormex**
*Note. This name is used for preparations of different composition.*
*Nobel, Canad.*
Diphenhydramine hydrochloride (p.431·3).
*Insomnia.*
*Lafi, Chile.*
Brotizolam (p.672·1).
*Insomnia.*

**Dormicum**
*Roche, Arg.; Roche, Austria; Roche, Belg.; Roche, Denm.; Roche, Fin.; Roche, Ger.; Roche, Gr.; Roche, Hong Kong; Roche, Israel; Roche, Mex.; Roche, Neth.; Roche, Norw.; Roche, Port.; Roche, S.Afr.; Roche, Singapore; Roche, Spain; Roche, Swed.; Roche, Switz.; Roche, Thai.*
Midazolam (p.707·1), midazolam hydrochloride (p.707·2), or midazolam maleate (p.707·2).
*General anaesthesia; insomnia; premedication; sedative; status epilepticus.*

**Dormid** *Scott-Cassara, Arg.*
Midazolam (p.707·1).
*Premedication; sedative.*

**Dormidina** *Pensa, Spain.*
Doxylamine succinate (p.432·3).
*Insomnia.*

**Dormi-Gastreu S R14** *Reckeweg, Ger.*
Homoeopathic preparation.

**Dormigoa N** *Scheurich, Ger.†.*
Diphenhydramine hydrochloride (p.431·3).
Dormigoa formerly contained diphenhydramine hydrochloride and guaifenesin.
*Sleep disorders.*

**Dormilam** *Laboratorios Chile, Chile.*
Zolpidem tartrate (p.728·3).
*Insomnia.*

**Dormin** *Randob, USA.*
Diphenhydramine hydrochloride (p.431·3).
*Insomnia.*

**Dorminoctil** *Recalcine, Chile.*
Doxylamine succinate (p.432·3).
*Sleep disorders.*

**Dormiphen** *Lalco, Canad.*
Diphenhydramine hydrochloride (p.431·3).
*Insomnia.*

**Dormiplant** *Schwabe, Switz.*
Valerian (p.1762·2); melissa (p.1711·1).
*Nervous disorders; sleep disorders.*

**Dormire** *Cristalia, Braz.*
Midazolam maleate (p.707·2).
*Insomnia; premedication.*

**Dormium** *Uniao Quimica, Braz.*
Midazolam (p.707·1).
*Insomnia.*

**Dormodor** *ICN, Spain.*
Flurazepam hydrochloride (p.700·3).
*Insomnia.*

**Dormonid**
*Roche, Braz.; Roche, Chile.*
Midazolam (p.707·1) or midazolam hydrochloride (p.707·2).
*General anaesthesia; insomnia; premedication; sedative.*

**Dormonoct**
*Aventis, Arg.; Aventis, Belg.; Aventis, Neth.; Aventis, Port.; Aventis, S.Afr.*
Loprazolam mesilate (p.704·1).
*Insomnia; premedication.*

**Dormo-Puren** *Alpharma-Isis, Ger.*
Nitrazepam (p.710·1).
*Sleep disorders.*

**Dormo-Sern** *Riemser, Ger.*
Valerian (p.1762·2); passion flower (p.1729·1).
*Nervous disorders; sleep disorders.*

**Dormosol** *Raffo, Chile.*
Zolpidem tartrate (p.728·3).
*Insomnia.*

**Dormosyx** *Syxyl, Ger.*
Homoeopathic preparation.

**Dormoverlan** *Verla, Ger.*
Valerian (p.1762·2); lupulus (p.1708·1); passion flower (p.1729·1).
*Agitation; insomnia.*

**Dormplus** *Pensa, Spain†.*
Diphenhydramine hydrochloride (p.431·3).
*Insomnia.*

**Dormutil N** *Alpharma-Isis, Ger.*
Diphenhydramine hydrochloride (p.431·3).
*Sleep disorders.*

**Dornal** *Klinger, Braz.*
Dipyrone (p.35·3).
*Fever; pain.*

**Dorner**
*Toray, Jpn; Yamanouchi, Thai.*
Beraprost sodium (p.1514·1).
*Thromboembolic disorders.*

**Dorocoff-ASS plus** *Hevert, Ger.†.*
Aspirin (p.15·1); caffeine (p.782·1).
*Pain.*

**Dorocoff-Paracetamol** *Hevert, Ger.*
Paracetamol (p.76·2).
*Fever; pain.*

**Dorofen** *Liptis, USA.*
Glucosamine sulfate (p.1694·1); ginkgo biloba (p.1692·3).
*Intermittent claudication; osteoarthritis.*

**Dorona** *Ducto, Braz.*
Dipyrone (p.35·3).
*Fever; pain.*

**Dorox** *M & H, Thai.*
Dicloxacillin sodium (p.205·2).
*Bacterial infections.*

**Dorpane** *Macrophar, Thai.*
Orphenadrine citrate (p.486·1); paracetamol (p.76·2).
*Peri-articular disorders; skeletal muscle pain; tension headache.*

**Dorpiel** *Fortbenton, Arg.*
Tretinoin (p.1161·1).
*Acne.*

**Dorpinol** *Heralds, Braz.†.*
Paracetamol (p.76·2); diclofenac sodium (p.32·1); caffeine (p.782·1); carisoprodol (p.1392·1).
*Skeletal muscle spasm.*

**Dorpiren** *Heralds, Braz.†.*
Diclofenac potassium (p.32·1).
*Gout; inflammation; musculoskeletal, joint, and peri-articular disorders; pain.*

**Dorscopena** *Ariston, Braz.*
Dipyrone (p.35·3); chlorophenothiazinylscopine.
*Skeletal muscle spasm.*

**Dorsedin** *EMS, Braz.*
Isometheptene mucate (p.1702·1); dipyrone (p.35·3); caffeine (p.782·1).
*Pain.*

**Dorserol** *Heralds, Braz.†.*
Carisoprodol (p.1392·1); paracetamol (p.76·2); caffeine (p.782·1).
*Skeletal muscle spasm.*

**Dorsiflex** *Will-Pharma, Neth.*
Mephenoxalone (p.1395·1).
*Muscle pain.*

**Dorsof T** *Laboratorios Chile, Chile.*
Dorzolamide hydrochloride (p.908·3); timolol maleate (p.1012·2).
*Glaucoma; ocular hypertension.*

**Dorspan** *EMS, Braz.*
Butylhyoscine (p.484·2); dipyrone (p.35·3).
*Skeletal muscle spasm.*

**Dorvan** *Simoes, Braz.*
Paracetamol (p.76·2).
*Fever; pain.*

**Dorveran** *Hexal, Braz.*
Belladonna (p.479·1); hyoscyamus (p.485·2); star anise; boldo (p.1661·2).
*Smooth muscle spasm.*

**Doryl**
*Merck, Fin.; Merck, Ger.; Merck, Switz.*
Carbachol (p.1488·1).
*Gastrointestinal motility disorders; urinary retention.*

**Doryx**
*Faulding, Austral.; Parke, Davis, Canad.†; Gerard, Norw.; Parke, Davis, NZ†; Parke-Med, S.Afr.†; Faulding, Singapore; Scand Pharm, Swed.; Warner Chilcott, USA.*
Doxycycline hyclate (p.206·2).
*Bacterial infections.*

**Dorzoflax** *Sidus, Arg.*
Dorzolamide hydrochloride (p.908·3); timolol maleate (p.1012·2).
*Glaucoma; ocular hypertension.*

**Dorzone** *Delta, Braz.*
Orphenadrine citrate (p.486·1); dipyrone (p.35·3); caffeine (p.782·1).
Formerly contained dipyrone and caffeine.
*Pain.*

**Dos Dias N** *Elea, Arg.*
*Injection:* Estradiol benzoate (p.1550·1); hydroxyprogesterone caproate (p.1556·3).
*Tablets:* Levonorgestrel (p.1563·2); ethinylestradiol (p.1553·2).
*Amenorrhoea.*

**DOS Softgel** *Goldline, USA.*
Docusate sodium (p.1262·2).
*Constipation.*

**Dosaflex** *Richwood, USA.*
Senna (p.1288·2).
*Constipation.*

**Dosalax** *Richwood, USA†.*
Senna (p.1288·2).
*Constipation.*

**Dosamont** *Medinova (Μεντινοβα), Gr.*
Gemfibrozil (p.923·1).
*Hyperlipidaemias.*

**Dosan** *Pacific, NZ.*
Doxazosin mesilate (p.908·3).
*Benign prostatic hyperplasia; hypertension.*

**Dosanac** *Siam Bheasach, Thai.*
Diclofenac diethylamine (p.32·1) or diclofenac sodium (p.32·1).
*Inflammation; musculoskeletal, joint, peri-articular, and soft-tissue disorders; pain.*

**Dosate** *Pharmasant, Thai.*
Omeprazole (p.1278·2).
*Gastro-oesophageal reflux, Zollinger-Ellison syndrome; peptic ulcer.*

**Dosberotec** *Boehringer Ingelheim, Ital.*
Fenoterol hydrobromide (p.785·2).
*Respiratory-tract disorders.*

**Doscafis** *Llorens, Spain.*
Aspirin (p.15·1); caffeine (p.782·1); paracetamol (p.76·2).
*Fever; inflammation; musculoskeletal and joint disorders; pain.*

**Doses-O-Son** *Realdyme, Fr.*
Bran (p.1253·2).
*Dietary fibre supplement.*

**Dosier**
*Note. This name is used for preparations of different composition.*
*Casasco, Arg.*
Ticlopidine hydrochloride (p.1011·2).
*Thromboembolic disorders.*

*Tecnofarma, Chile.*
Bupropion hydrochloride (p.287·2).
*Aid to smoking withdrawal; depression.*

**Dosil** *Llorens, Spain.*
Doxycycline hyclate (p.206·2).
*Bacterial infections; malaria.*

**Dosil Enzimatico** *Llorens, Spain.*
Doxycycline hyclate (p.206·2); chymotrypsin (p.1671·2); trypsin (p.1758·3).
*Bacterial infections.*

**Dosin** *Andromaco, Chile.*
Domperidone (p.1263·2).
*Diabetic gastroparesis; gastro-oesophageal reflux; nausea; vomiting.*

**Dosiseptine** *Gifrer Barbezat, Fr.*
Chlorhexidine gluconate (p.1173·2).
*Wounds disinfection.*

**Dosodos** *Beta, Arg.*
Butamirate citrate (p.1116·2).
*Coughs.*

**Dosoxygenee** *Gifrer Barbezat, Fr.*
Hydrogen peroxide (p.1182·2).
*Wound disinfection.*

**Dospan Pento** *Elvetium, Arg.*
Pentoxifylline (p.979·3).
*Cerebral and peripheral vascular disorders; circulatory disorders of the eye and ear.*

**Dospir** *Boehringer Ingelheim, Switz.*
Ipratropium bromide (p.787·1); salbutamol sulfate (p.791·3).
*Obstructive airways disease.*

**Doss**
*Note. This name is used for preparations of different composition.*
*SmithKline Beecham, Canad.†.*
Dantron (p.1261·1); docusate sodium (p.1262·2).
*Constipation.*

*Byk Tosse, Ger.; Byk Gulden, Ger.*
Alfacalcidol (p.1461·2).
*Bone disorders; hypoparathyroidism.*

**Dostein** *Glaxo Wellcome, Mex.*
Erdosteine (p.1121·1).
*Respiratory-tract congestion.*

**Dostil** *Triomed, S.Afr.*
Paracetamol (p.76·2); codeine phosphate (p.27·1).
*Pain.*

**Dostinex**
*Pharmacia, Arg.; Pharmacia, Austral.; Pharmacia, Austria; Pharmacia, Belg.; Pharmacia, Braz.; Pharmacia, Chile; Pharmacia, Denm.; Pharmacia, Fin.; Pharmacia, Fr.; Pharmacia, Ger.; Pharmacia-Upjohn, Gr.; Pharmacia, Hong Kong; Pharmacia, Irl.; Agis, Israel; Pharmacia Upjohn, Ital.; Pharmacia, Malaysia; Pharmacia Upjohn, Mex.; Pharmacia, Neth.; Pharmacia, Norw.; Pharmacia, NZ; Pharmacia, Port.; Pharmacia, S.Afr.; Pharmacia, Singapore; Kenfarma, Spain; Pharmacia, Swed.; Pharmacia, Switz.; Pharmacia, UK; Pharmacia Upjohn, USA.*
Cabergoline (p.1203·3).
*Hyperprolactinaemia; lactation inhibition; prolactinomas.*

**Dosulfin Bronquial** *Labinca, Arg.*
Co-trimoxazole (p.199·3); bromhexine (p.1115·3); etamivan (p.1588·1); guaifenesin (p.1122·1).
*Respiratory-tract infections.*

**Dosulfin Fuerte** *Labinca, Arg.*
Co-trimoxazole (p.199·3); aluminium hydroxide (p.1249·2); magnesium trisilicate (p.1272·3).
*Bacterial infections.*

**Dosyklin** *Leiras, Fin.*
Doxycycline (p.206·2).
*Bacterial infections.*

**Dotalsec** *Hexa-Medinova, Arg.*
Loperamide hydrochloride (p.1271·1).
*Diarrhoea.*

**Dotarem**
*Temis, Arg.; Aspen, Austral.; Guerbet, Austria; Codali, Belg.; Guerbet, Braz.; Rider, Chile; Guerbet, Denm.; Guerbet, Fin.; Guerbet, Fr.; R+N, Gr.; Guerbet, Israel; Guerbet, Ital.; Guerbet, Neth.†; Guerbet, Norw.; Guerbet, Port.; Guerbet, Spain; Gothia, Swed.; Guerbet, Switz.*
Meglumine gadoterate (p.1062·3).
*Contrast medium for magnetic resonance imaging.*

**Dotest** *Mentholatum, Austral.*
Pregnancy test (p.1734·3).

**Dothapax** *Ashbourne, UK.*
Dosulepin hydrochloride (p.291·1).

**Dothep**
*Alphapharm, Austral.; Gerard, Irl.; Alphapharm, Malaysia; Merck, Malaysia.*
Dosulepin hydrochloride (p.291·1).
*Depression.*

**Dotur** *Biochemie, Austria.*
Doxycycline hyclate (p.206·2).
*Bacterial infections; protozoal infections.*

**Double Check** *Family Planning Sales, UK†.*
Nonoxinol 9 (p.1413·3).
*Contraceptive.*

**Double-Action Toothache Kit** *Dent, USA.*
Liquid, benzocaine (p.1370·3); tablets, paracetamol (p.76·2) (Maranox).

**Doublebase** *Dermal Laboratories, UK.*
Isopropyl myristate (p.1481·2); liquid paraffin (p.1479·1).
*Dry skin; pruritus.*

**Doublecap** *Breckenridge, USA.*
Capsaicin (p.24·2).
*Musculoskeletal and joint pain.*

**Double-Tussin DM** *Reese, USA.*
Guaifenesin (p.1122·1); dextromethorphan hydrobromide (p.1117·3).
*Coughs.*

**Douglas Protein Plus** *Douglas, NZ†; Nutricia, NZ†.*
Protein preparation with electrolytes (p.1417·1).
*Nutritional supplement.*

**Doulax**
*Note. This name is used for preparations of different composition.*
*Bio-Sante, Canad.†.*
Cascara (p.1255·1); phenolphthalein (p.1284·1).

*Bio-Sante, Canad.*
Cascara (p.1255·1); senna (p.1288·2).

**Douleurs & Fievre** *Pharmacard, Switz.*
Paracetamol (p.76·2).
*Fever; pain.*

**Douzabox** *Sriprasit, Thai.*
Vitamin $B_1$ (p.1455·2); vitamin $B_6$ (p.1457·2); vitamin $B_{12}$ (p.1458·2).
*Vitamin B deficiency.*

**Doval** *Pharmaceutical Enterprises, S.Afr.*
Diazepam (p.690·1).
*Alcohol withdrawal syndrome; anxiety; depression; premedication.*

**Dovate** *Aspen, S.Afr.*
Clobetasol propionate (p.1095·2).
*Skin disorders.*

**Dovavixin** *Help, Gr.*
Zipeprol hydrochloride (p.1132·3).
*Cough.*

**Doven** *Eurofarmaco, Ital.*
Diosmin (p.1688·2).
*Haemorrhoids; phlebitis; venous insufficiency.*

**Doveri** *Rekah, Israel.*
Opium (p.74·2); ipecacuanha (p.1122·3).
*Coughs; dyspnoea.*

**Dovobet**
*Leo, Irl.; Leo, UK.*
Calcipotriol (p.1144·1); betamethasone dipropionate (p.1093·1).
*Psoriasis.*

**Dovonex**
*Leo, Canad.; Leo (Λεο), Gr.; Leo, Irl.; Teikoku Seiyaku, Jpn; Adcock Ingram, S.Afr.; Leo, UK; Westwood-Squibb, USA.*
Calcipotriol (p.1144·1).
*Psoriasis.*

**Doxacard** *Cipla, India.*
Doxazosin (p.909·1).
*Benign prostatic hyperplasia; hypertension.*

**Doxacor** *Hexal, Ger.*
Doxazosin mesilate (p.908·3).
*Hypertension.*

**Doxacyne** *Raza, Malaysia; Pharmaniaga, Malaysia.*
Doxycycline hyclate (p.206·2).
*Bacterial infections.*

**Doxadura** *Schein, UK.*
Doxazosin mesilate (p.908·3).
*Hypertension.*

**Doxagamma** *Worwag, Ger.*
Doxazosin mesilate (p.908·3).
*Hypertension.*

**Doxakne** *Bioglan, Ger.*
Doxycycline (p.206·2).
*Acne.*

**Doxal**
*Note. This name is used for preparations of different composition.*
*Agepha, Austria.*
Doxycycline hyclate (p.206·2).
*Bacterial infections.*

*Sigma, Braz.*
Pyridoxine hydrochloride (p.1456·3); thiamine hydrochloride (p.1455·1).
*Vitamin supplement.*

*Orion, Fin.*
Doxepin hydrochloride (p.291·2).
*Anxiety; depression; insomnia.*

**Doxaloc** *Unipharm, Israel.*
Doxazosin mesilate (p.908·3).
*Benign prostatic hyperplasia; hypertension.*

**Doxam** *TAD, Ger.*
Doxycycline hyclate (p.206·2); ambroxol hydrochloride (p.1114·3).
*Respiratory-tract infections.*

**Doxamil** *Quimica y Farmacia, Mex.*
Amoxicillin trihydrate (p.155·3).
*Bacterial infections.*

**Doxapril** *Bago, Arg.*
Lisinopril (p.946·3).
*Hypertension.*

**Doxa-Puren** *Alpharma-Isis, Ger.*
Doxazosin mesilate (p.908·3).
*Hypertension.*

**Doxasin** *Fortbenton, Arg.*
Doxazosin (p.909·1).
*Benign prostatic hyperplasia; hypertension.*

**Doxasyn** *Genthon, Hong Kong.*
Doxazosin mesilate (p.908·3).
*Benign prostatic hyperplasia; hypertension.*

**Doxate-C** *Richmond, Canad.†.*
Docusate calcium (p.1262·1).
*Constipation.*

**Doxatensa** *Ciclum, Spain.*
Doxazosin mesilate (p.908·3).
*Benign prostatic hyperplasia; hypertension.*

**Doxate-S** *Richmond, Canad.†.*
Docusate sodium (p.1262·2).
*Constipation.*

**Doxazobene** *Ratiopharm, Austria.*
Doxazosin mesilate (p.908·3).
*Hypertension.*

**Doxazomerck** *Merck dura, Ger.*
Doxazosin mesilate (p.908·3).
*Hypertension.*

**Doxederm** *Lazar, Arg.*
Doxepin (p.291·2).
*Pruritus.*

**Doxemina** *Collins, Mex.*
Vitamin preparation (p.1417·1).
*Neuritis.*

**Doxepia** *Temmler, Ger.*
Doxepin hydrochloride (p.291·2).
*Anxiety; depression; sleep disorders.*

**Doxergan** *Aventis, Belg.†.*
Oxomemazine (p.438·2).
*Coughs; gastritis; hypersensitivity reactions; insomnia.*

**Doxetal** *Richmond, Arg.*
Docetaxel (p.547·1).
*Malignant neoplasms.*

**Doxi Crisol** *Quimifar, Spain.*
Doxycycline hyclate (p.206·2).
*Bacterial infections; malaria.*

**Doxi Sergo** *Inexfa, Spain†.*
Doxycycline hyclate (p.206·2).
*Bacterial infections; malaria.*

**Doxibiot** *Hexal, Arg.*
Doxycycline (p.206·2).
*Bacterial infections.*

**Doxibiotic** *CTI, Israel.*
Doxycycline hyclate (p.206·2).
*Bacterial infections; malaria.*

**Doxican** *Azevedos, Port.*
Tenoxicam (p.93·1).
*Inflammation; musculoskeletal and joint disorders.*

**Doxiclat** *Pierre Fabre, Spain.*
Doxycycline hyclate (p.206·2).
*Bacterial infections; malaria.*

**Doxidan**
*Note. This name is used for preparations of different composition.*
*Hoechst Marion Roussel, Canad.†.*
Docusate calcium (p.1262·1); yellow phenolphthalein (p.1284·1).
*Constipation.*

*Pharmacia, USA.*
*Capsules†:* Docusate calcium (p.1262·1); phenolphthalein (p.1284·1).
*Delayed-release tablets:* Bisacodyl (p.1251·3).
*Constipation.*

**Doxifen** *Bago, Chile.*
Miconazole nitrate (p.405·3); tinidazole (p.617·1).
*Balanitis; vaginal infections.*

**Doxil** *Sequus, USA.*
Liposomal doxorubicin hydrochloride (p.547·3) (p.547·3).
*AIDS-related Kaposi's sarcoma.*

**Doxilin** *Malayan, Singapore.*
Doxycycline hyclate (p.206·2).
*Bacterial infections.*

**Doximal** *Cipla-Medpro, S.Afr.*
Doxycycline hyclate (p.206·2).
*Bacterial infections; malaria.*

**Doximed** *Ratiopharm, Fin.*
Doxycycline (p.206·2).
*Bacterial infections.*

**Doximucol** *Lichtenstein, Ger.*
Doxycycline hyclate (p.206·2); ambroxol hydrochloride (p.1114·3).
*Bacterial infections of the respiratory tract associated with increased or viscous mucus.*

**Doximycin** *Orion, Fin.*
Doxycycline hyclate (p.206·2).
*Bacterial infections.*

**Doxin** *Asian Pharm, Thai.*
Doxycycline hyclate (p.206·2).
*Bacterial infections.*

**Doxina**
*Eurofarma, Braz.†.*
Doxycycline (p.206·2).
*Bacterial infections.*

*IPFI, Ital.†.*
Doxycycline hyclate (p.206·2).
*Bacterial infections.*

**Doxinate**
*Note. This name is used for preparations of different composition.*
*Sigma, India.*
Doxylamine succinate (p.432·3).
*Nausea and vomiting in pregnancy.*

*Torlan, Spain.*
Doxycycline hyclate (p.206·2).
*Bacterial infections; malaria.*

**Doxine**
*Pacific, NZ; Merck, Singapore; Pacific, Singapore.*
Doxycycline hyclate (p.206·2).
*Bacterial infections.*

**Doxi-Om** *OM, Port.*
Calcium dobesilate (p.1664·2).
*Vascular disorders.*

**Doxiproct**
*Note. This name is used for preparations of different composition.*
*Ebewe, Austria; OM, Port.; OM, Switz.*
Calcium dobesilate (p.1664·2); lidocaine hydrochloride (p.1377·3).
*Anorectal disorders.*

*Abiogen, Ital.*
Calcium dobesilate (p.1664·2); lidocaine hydrochloride (p.1377·3); dexamethasone acetate (p.1097·1).
Formerly known as Doxiproct Plus.
*Anorectal disorders.*

**Doxiproct mit Dexamethason** *Ebewe, Austria.*
Calcium dobesilate (p.1664·2); lidocaine hydrochloride (p.1377·3); dexamethasone acetate (p.1097·1).
*Anorectal disorders.*

**Doxiproct Plus** *OM, Switz.*
Calcium dobesilate (p.1664·2); lidocaine hydrochloride (p.1377·3); dexamethasone acetate (p.1097·1).
*Anorectal disorders.*

**Doxitab** *Medpro, S.Afr.*
Doxycycline hyclate (p.206·2).
*Bacterial infections; malaria.*

**Doxiten** *Zyma, Spain†.*
Doxycycline hyclate (p.206·2).
*Bacterial infections.*

**Doxiten Bio** *Teofarma, Spain.*
Doxycycline hyclate (p.206·2).
*Bacterial infections; malaria.*

**Doxiten Enzimatico** *Teofarma, Spain.*
Doxycycline hyclate (p.206·2); chymotrypsin (p.1671·2); trypsin (p.1758·3).
*Bacterial infections.*

**Doxithal** *Grunenthal, Chile.*
Doxycycline (p.206·2).
*Bacterial infections.*

**Doxitin** *Vitabalans, Fin.*
Doxycycline hyclate (p.206·2).
*Bacterial infections.*

**Doxium**
*Byk, Arg.; Ebewe, Austria; Sanofi Synthelabo, Belg.†; Allergan-Frumtost, Braz.†; Labomed, Chile; Ebewe, Hong Kong; Abiogen, Ital.; OM, Malaysia; Knoll, Mex.; Europhta, Mon.; Esteve, Spain; OM, Switz.*
Calcium dobesilate (p.1664·2).
*chronic venous insufficiency; diabetic retinopathy; microcirculatory disorders.*

**Doxivenil**
*OM, Port.; OM, Switz.*
Calcium dobesilate (p.1664·2); dextran sulfate potassium (p.1679·2).
*Peripheral vascular disorders.*

**Doxmil** *Biotenk, Arg.*
Docetaxel (p.547·1).
*Breast cancer; non-small cell lung cancer.*

**DOXO-cell** *Cell Pharm, Ger.*
Doxorubicin hydrochloride (p.547·3).
*Malignant neoplasms.*

**Doxocris** *Kampel Martian, Arg.*
Doxorubicin (p.547·3).
*Malignant neoplasms.*

**Doxolbran** *Phoenix, Arg.*
Doxazosin mesilate (p.908·3).
*Benign prostatic hyperplasia; hypertension.*

**Doxolem**
*CSC, Austria; Zodiac, Braz.; Lemery, Mex.; Lemery, Thai.*
Doxorubicin hydrochloride (p.547·3).
*Malignant neoplasms.*

**Doxorbin** *Bristol-Myers Squibb, Arg.*
Doxorubicin hydrochloride (p.547·3).
*Malignant neoplasms.*

**Doxorubin**
*Asta Medica, Austral.†; Nycomed, Austria; Nettopharma, Denm.†; Pharmachemie, Malaysia; Asta Medica, NZ; NZ Medical & Scientific, NZ; Pharmachemie, Singapore; Pharmachemie, Thai.; Teva, Thai.*
Doxorubicin hydrochloride (p.547·3).
*Malignant neoplasms.*

**Doxotec** *Columbia, Mex.†.*
Doxorubicin hydrochloride (p.547·3).
*Malignant neoplasms.*

**Doxsig** *Sigma, Austral.*
Doxycycline hyclate (p.206·2).
*Adjunct in amoebiasis; bacterial infections; malaria.*

**Doxtie** *Gautier, Arg.*
Doxorubicin hydrochloride (p.547·3).
*Malignant neoplasms.*

**Doxtran** *Phoenix-Elea, Arg.*
Rofecoxib (p.86·3).
*Osteoarthritis; pain.*

**Doxy**
*Douglas, Austral.; Elerte, Fr.; 1A, Ger.; CT, Ger.; ABZ, Ger.; Acis, Ger.; Herbert, Ger.; S & K, Ger.; Douglas, Hong Kong; Vitamed, Israel; Strand, Malaysia; Douglas, NZ; Masa, Thai.; Edwards, USA†.*
Doxycycline (p.206·2) or doxycycline hyclate (p.206·2).
*Bacterial infections.*

**Doxy-1** *Sterling, India.*
Doxycycline (p.206·2).
*Bacterial infections.*

**Doxy-100** *Douglas, Thai.†; TTN, Thai.†.*
Doxycycline (p.206·2).
*Bacterial infections.*

**Doxy Comp** *CT, Ger.*
Doxycycline hyclate (p.206·2); ambroxol hydrochloride (p.1114·3).
*Respiratory-tract infections.*

**Doxy Komb** *Herbert, Ger.*
Doxycycline hyclate (p.206·2).
*Bacterial infections.*

**Doxy Lindoxyl** *Lindopharm, Ger.*
Doxycycline hyclate (p.206·2); ambroxol hydrochloride (p.1114·3).
*Bacterial infections of the respiratory-tract associated with increased or viscous mucus.*

**Doxy M** *CT, Ger.; Ratiopharm, Ger.*
Doxycycline (p.206·2).
*Bacterial infections.*

**Doxy Plus** *Stada, Ger.*
Doxycycline hyclate (p.206·2); ambroxol hydrochloride (p.1114·3).
*Respiratory-tract infections.*

**Doxy-basan** *Schonenberger, Switz.*
Doxycycline hyclate (p.206·2).
*Bacterial infections.*

**Doxybene** *Ratiopharm, Austria.*
Doxycycline (p.206·2) or doxycycline hyclate (p.206·2).
*Bacterial infections.*

**Doxybiocin** *Orion, Ger.†.*
Doxycycline hyclate (p.206·2).
*Bacterial infections.*

**Doxycap** *Hovid, Singapore.*
Doxycycline hyclate (p.206·2).
*Bacterial infections.*

**Doxychel** *Rachelle, USA†.*
Doxycycline hyclate (p.206·2).
*Bacterial infections.*

**Doxycillin** *Upha, Malaysia.*
Doxycycline hyclate (p.206·2).
*Bacterial infections.*

**Doxycin** *Riva, Canad.*
Doxycycline hyclate (p.206·2).
*Bacterial infections.*

**Doxycline**
*Spirig, Switz.*
Doxycycline hyclate (p.206·2).
*Bacterial infections.*

*General Drugs, Thai.*
Doxycycline (p.206·2).
*Bacterial infections.*

**Doxycyl** *Aspen, S.Afr.*
Doxycycline hyclate (p.206·2).
*Bacterial infections.*

**Doxy-Dagra** *Viatris, Neth.*
Doxycycline fosfatex (p.206·2).
*Bacterial infections.*

**Doxyderm** *Klinge, Austria.*
Doxycycline hyclate (p.206·2).
*Acne.*

**Doxyderma** *Dermapharm, Ger.*
Doxycycline (p.206·2).
*Bacterial infections.*

**Doxy-Diolan** *Brahms, Ger.*
Doxycycline hyclate (p.206·2).
*Bacterial infections.*

**Doxydoc** *Docpharm, Ger.*
Doxycycline (p.206·2).
*Bacterial infections.*

**Doxy-duramucal** *Merck dura, Ger.†.*
Doxycycline hyclate (p.206·2); ambroxol hydrochloride (p.1114·3).
*Bacterial infections of the respiratory-tract associated with increased or viscous mucus.*

**Doxydyn** *Klinge, Austria.*
Doxycycline hyclate (p.206·2).
*Bacterial infections.*

**Doxyfene** *Covan, S.Afr.*
Dextropropoxyphene hydrochloride (p.28·3); paracetamol (p.76·2).
*Fever; pain.*

**Doxyferm** *Nordic, Swed.*
Doxycycline (p.206·2) or doxycycline hyclate (p.206·2).
*Bacterial infections.*

**Doxyfim** *Wolfs, Belg.†.*
Doxycycline hyclate (p.206·2).
*Bacterial infections.*

**Doxygram** *Pharma 2000, Fr.†.*
Doxycycline hyclate (p.206·2).
*Bacterial infections.*

**Doxyhexal**
*Hexal, Austral.; Hexal, Austria; Hexal, Ger.; Hexal, S.Afr.*
Doxycycline (p.206·2) or doxycycline hyclate (p.206·2).
*Adjunct in amoebiasis; bacterial infections; malaria.*

**Doxy-HP** *Hefa, Ger.*
Doxycycline (p.206·2).
*Bacterial infections.*

**Doxylag** *Lagap, Switz.*
Doxycycline hyclate (p.206·2).
*Bacterial infections.*

**Doxylan** *Lannacher, Austria.*
Doxycycline (p.206·2) or doxycycline hyclate (p.206·2).
*Bacterial infections.*

**Doxylar** *Sandoz, UK.*
Doxycycline hyclate (p.206·2).
*Bacterial infections.*

**Doxylets**
*SMB, Belg.; Galephar, Fr.†.*
Doxycycline hyclate (p.206·2).
*Bacterial infections.*

**Doxylin**
*Alphapharm, Austral.; Dexxon, Israel; Alpharma, Norw.; TP, Thai.*
Doxycycline (p.206·2) or doxycycline hyclate (p.206·2).
*Amoebiasis; bacterial infections; malaria.*

**Doxyline** *Yung Shin, Singapore.*
Doxycycline hyclate (p.206·2).
*Bacterial infections.*

**Doxymerck** *Merck dura, Ger.*
Doxycycline (p.206·2).
*Bacterial infections.*

**Doxymono** *Betapharm, Ger.*
Doxycycline (p.206·2).
*Bacterial infections.*

**Doxymycin**
*YSP, Malaysia; Beacons, Singapore; Yung Shin, Thai.†.*
Doxycycline hyclate (p.206·2).
*Bacterial infections.*

**Doxy-N-Tablinen** *Lichtenstein, Ger.*
Doxycycline (p.206·2).
*Bacterial infections.*

**Doxy-P**
*Ratiopharm, Ger.†; PP Lab, Thai.*
Doxycycline hyclate (p.206·2).
*Bacterial infections.*

**Doxypal-DR** *Jagson, India.*
Doxycycline hyclate (p.206·2).
*Bacterial infections.*

**Doxypalu** *Biorga, Fr.*
Doxycycline (p.206·2).
*Malaria.*

**Doxypol** *Beige, S.Afr.†.*
Dextropropoxyphene hydrochloride (p.28·3); paracetamol (p.76·2); caffeine (p.782·1).
*Pain.*

**Doxy-Puren** *Alpharma-Isis, Ger.*
Doxycycline hyclate (p.206·2).
*Bacterial infections.*

**Doxysol**
*Ecosol, Norw.; Ecosol, Switz.*
Doxycycline (p.206·2).
*Bacterial infections.*

**Doxysolvat** *Betapharm, Ger.*
Doxycycline hyclate (p.206·2); ambroxol hydrochloride (p.1114·3).
*Respiratory-tract infections.*

**Doxystad** *Stada, Austria.*
Doxycycline (p.206·2) or doxycycline hyclate (p.206·2).
*Bacterial infections.*

**Doxy-Tablinen** *Sanorania, Ger.†.*
Doxycycline hyclate (p.206·2).
*Bacterial infections.*

**Doxytec** *Technilab, Canad.*
Doxycycline hyclate (p.206·2).
*Bacterial infections.*

**Doxytem** *Temmler, Ger.†.*
Doxycycline hyclate (p.206·2).
*Bacterial infections.*

**Doxytrex** *Helfarma, Port.*
Doxycycline hyclate (p.206·2).
*Bacterial infections.*

**Doxytrim** *Trima, Israel.*
Doxycycline hyclate (p.206·2).
*Amoebiasis; bacterial infections; malaria.*

**Doxy-Wolff** *Wolff, Ger.*
Doxycycline (p.206·2) or doxycycline hyclate (p.206·2).
*Bacterial infections.*

**Doxy-Wolff Mucolyt** *Wolff, Ger.*
Doxycycline hyclate (p.206·2); ambroxol hydrochloride (p.1114·3).
*Respiratory-tract infections associated with increased or viscous mucus.*

**Doyle** *Asofarma, Arg.*
Azithromycin (p.159·1).
*Bacterial infections.*

**Dozbe** *Profarb, Braz.†.*
Vitamin $B_1$; vitamin $B_6$; vitamin $B_{12}$ (p.1417·1).
*Vitamin B deficiency.*

**Dozebion** *Baldacci, Braz.†.*
Vitamin B substances; iron molybdate; copper chloride; liver extract (p.1417·1).
*Vitamin and mineral supplement.*

**Dozelin Junior** *Sigma, Braz.†.*
Multivitamin and amino-acid preparation (p.1417·1).

**Dozelin Lisina** *Sigma, Braz.†.*
Vitamin B substances; lysine hydrochloride (p.1417·1).

**Dozeneurin** *Sigma, Braz.*
Cyanocobalamin (p.1458·2); thiamine hydrochloride (p.1455·1).
*Vitamin $B_1$ and $B_{12}$ deficiency.*

**Dozic** *Rosemont, UK.*
Haloperidol (p.701·2).
*Anxiety; intractable hiccup; motor tics; nausea and vomiting; psychoses.*

**Dozile**
*Pharmacia, Austral.; Pharmacia, NZ.*
Doxylamine succinate (p.432·3).
*Insomnia.*

**Dozol**
*Rice Steele, Irl.; Typharm, UK.*
Paracetamol (p.76·2); diphenhydramine hydrochloride (p.431·3).
*Cold and influenza symptoms; fever; pain.*

**D-P**
*Note. A similar name is used for preparations of different composition (see below).*
*Klonal, Arg.*
Dextropropoxyphene (p.28·3); dipyrone (p.35·3).
*Pain.*

**DP**
*Note. A similar name is used for preparations of different composition (see above and below).*
*Douglas, NZ.*
Liquid paraffin (p.1479·1); wool fat (p.1483·1).
*Dry skin; pruritus.*

*Douglas, Singapore†.*
Dimeticone (p.1482·1).
*Topical barrier preparation.*

**dp**
*Note. A similar name is used for preparations of different composition (see above).*
*Scientific Hospital Supplies, UK†.*
Low-protein food for special diets (p.1417·1).

**DP Barrier Cream** *Douglas, NZ.*
Dimethicone (p.1482·1).

**DP Hand Rub** *Douglas, NZ.*
Chlorhexidine (p.1173·2).
*Skin disinfection.*

**DP Hydrocortisone** *Douglas, NZ.*
Hydrocortisone (p.1103·3).
*Skin disorders.*

**DP Lotion - HC** *Douglas, NZ.*
Hydrocortisone (p.1103·3); liquid paraffin (p.1479·1); wool fat (p.1483·1).
*Skin disorders.*

**DP Lubricating Gel** *Douglas, NZ.*
Lubricating gel.

**DP Warm Up** *Douglas, NZ†.*
Methyl salicylate (p.59·3); eucalyptus oil (p.1686·2); camphor (p.1665·3).
*Muscular rub.*

**D-Pam** *Douglas, NZ†.*
Diazepam (p.690·1).
*Alcohol withdrawal syndrome; anxiety; epilepsy; sedative; skeletal muscle spasm.*

**DPCA** *Fresenius Medical, Switz.*
Electrolytes; anhydrous glucose (p.1221·1).
*Peritoneal dialysis.*

**DPCA 2** *Fresenius, Fr.†.*
Sodium chloride; sodium lactate; calcium chloride; magnesium chloride; glucose monohydrate (p.1221·1).
*Peritoneal dialysis.*

**DPE** *Alcon, Canad.†.*
Dipivefrine hydrochloride (p.1681·2).
*Glaucoma.*

**D-Penamine**
*Alphapharm, Austral.; Dista, NZ†.*
Penicillamine (p.1046·3).
*Cystinuria; heavy metal poisoning; rheumatoid arthritis; Wilson's disease.*

**DPH** *Propan, S.Afr.*
Diphenhydramine hydrochloride (p.431·3); ammonium chloride (p.1115·2); sodium citrate (p.1223·2).
*Coughs.*

**DPN** *Alclin, S.Afr.*
Nadide (p.1719·1).
*Alcoholism; drug addiction.*

**DPT Merieux** *Pasteur Merieux, Ger.†.*
An adsorbed diphtheria, tetanus, and pertussis vaccine (p.1613·3).
*Active immunisation of infants and young children.*

**DPT-Impfstoff** *Chiron Behring, Ger.†.*
An adsorbed diphtheria, tetanus, and pertussis vaccine (p.1613·3).
*Active immunisation of infants and young children.*

**DPT-Vaccinol** *Procter & Gamble, Ger.†.*
An adsorbed diphtheria, tetanus, and pertussis vaccine (p.1613·3).
*Active immunisation of infants and young children.*

**DQM** *Raza, Malaysia; Pharmaniaga, Malaysia.*
Dequalinium chloride (p.1178·1).
*Mouth and throat infections.*

**Dr Calm** *Wunderpharm, Arg.*
Thiamine (p.1455·2); melissa (p.1711·1); tilia (p.1756·2).
*Sedative.*

**Dr Dermi-Heal** *Quality Formulations, USA.*
Allantoin (p.1141·3); zinc oxide (p.1163·2); peru balsam (p.1730·2); castor oil (p.1668·2).
*Skin disorders.*

**Dr Ernst Richter's Abfuhrtee** *Sanova, Austria†.*
Senna (p.1288·2); frangula bark (p.1266·3).
*Constipation.*

**Dr. Ernst Richter's Abfuhrtee-Filterbeutel** *Hermes, Austria†.*
Senna (p.1288·2); frangula (p.1266·3); calcatrippae; calendula (p.1665·2); centaurea cyanus; helianthus; rubus fruticosus; coriander (p.1676·1).
*Bowel evacuation; constipation.*

**Dr Ernst Richter's Abfuhrtee-tassenfertig** *Sanova, Austria†.*
Senna (p.1288·2); frangula bark (p.1266·3); peppermint oil (p.1283·2); liquorice (p.1270·2).
*Constipation.*

**Dr Grandel Brennessel Vital Tonikum** *Grandel-Synpharma, Ger.†.*
Urtica (p.1762·1).
*Tonic.*

**Dr Grandel Granobil** *Grandel, Ger.*
Usnea barbata (p.1762·1).
*Bacterial infections of the mouth and throat.*

**Dr. Hotz Vollbad** *Hotz, Ger.†.*
Whey; sorbitol (p.1446·3); lactic acid (p.1704·1); alum (p.1652·1); gentian (p.1692·2); achillea (p.1646·2); crataegus (p.1677·1); olive oil (p.1723·2); arachis oil (p.1656·1); sage oil (p.1741·2); rosemary oil (p.1740·2); chamomile oil (p.1669·3); alpha tocoferil acetate (p.1465·1).
*Bath additive; skin disorders.*

**Dr Janssens Teebohnen** *Dr Janssen, Ger.*
Aloes (p.1248·2).
*Constipation.*

**Dr Schmidgall Halsweh** *Schmidgall, Austria.*
*dl*-Alpha tocoferil acetate (p.1465·1); benzalkonium chloride (p.1168·3).
*Mouth and throat inflammation.*

**Dr Scholl's Athlete's Foot** *Schering-Plough, USA.*
Tolnaftate (p.410·1).
*Tinea pedis.*

**Dr Scholl's Callus Removers** *Schering-Plough, USA.*
Salicylic acid (p.1157·1).

**Dr Scholl's Clear Away** *Schering-Plough, USA.*
Salicylic acid (p.1157·1).
*Hyperkeratosis.*

**Dr Scholl's Corn Removers** *Schering-Plough, USA.*
Salicylic acid (p.1157·1).

**Dr Scholl's Corn/Callus Remover** *Schering-Plough, USA.*
Salicylic acid (p.1157·1).
*Hyperkeratosis.*

**Dr Scholl's Cracked Heel Relief** *Schering-Plough, USA.*
Lidocaine (p.1377·3).

**Dr Scholl's Wart Remover** *Schering-Plough, USA.*
Salicylic acid (p.1157·1).

**Dr Selby** *Sidus, Arg.*
Zinc oxide (p.1163·2); vitamin D (p.1461·2); wool fat (p.1483·1); talc (p.1159·1).
*Skin disorders.*

**Dr Smiths** *Beta, USA.*
Zinc oxide (p.1163·2).
*Skin disorders.*

**Dr Wiemanns Rheumatonikum** *Beethoven, Ger.*
Birch leaf (p.1660·3); salix (p.87·3); devil's claw root (p.28·2); heisteriae.
*Musculoskeletal and joint disorders.*

**Dracanyl** *Astra-Zeneca, Gr.*
Terbutaline sulfate (p.797·2).
*Asthma.*

**Dracodermalin** *Richter, Austria.*
Camphor (p.1665·3); rosemary oil (p.1740·2); turpentine oil (p.1760·1).
*Frostbite; musculoskeletal and joint disorders; respiratory-tract disorders.*

**Drafilyn-Z** *Zafiro, Mex.*
Aminophylline (p.780·2).
*Obstructive airways disease.*

**Draganon** *Roche, Ital.*
Aniracetam (p.1655·1).
*Mental function disorders.*

**Dragee Vauban** *Monot, Fr.†.*
Lidocaine hydrochloride (p.1377·3); borax (p.1661·3).

**Dragees antirhumatismales** *Zeller, Switz.*
Salix (p.87·3); passion flower (p.1729·1).
*Musculoskeletal and joint disorders.*

**Dragees aux figues avec du sene** *Zeller, Switz.*
Fig (p.1266·3); senna (p.1288·2); petasites officinalis (p.1663·3).
*Constipation.*

**Dragees contre la toux no 536** *Renapharm, Switz.†.*
Butetamate citrate (p.1116·2); codeine phosphate (p.27·1); thyme (p.1755·2).
*Coughs.*

**Dragees contre les maux de tete** *Zeller, Switz.†.*
Salix (p.87·3); kola (p.1765·3).
*Headache.*

**Dragees contre les maux de voyage no 537** *Iromedica, Switz.*
Dimenhydrinate (p.431·1); caffeine (p.782·1).
*Motion sickness.*

**Dragees Fuca** *Fuca, Fr.*
Frangula bark (p.1266·3); cascara (p.1255·1); bladderwrack (p.1742·3).
*Constipation.*

**Dragees laxatives no 510** *Renapharm, Switz.†.*
Aloes (p.1248·2); belladonna (p.479·1); rhubarb (p.1287·3).
*Constipation.*

**Dragees Neunzehn** *Wyeth Lederle, Austria.*
Aloes (p.1248·2); frangula (p.1266·3); cascara (p.1255·1); fel suis (p.1660·3).
*Constipation.*

**Dragees Neunzehn Senna** *Wyeth Lederle, Austria.*
Senna (p.1288·2).
*Constipation.*

**Dragees pour la detente nerveuse** *Zeller, Switz.*
Petasites officinalis (p.1663·3); valerian (p.1762·2); passion flower (p.1729·1); melissa (p.1711·1).
*Nervous disorders.*

**Dragees pour le coeur et les nerfs** *Zeller, Switz.*
Crataegus (p.1677·1); passion flower (p.1729·1); lupulus (p.1708·1); valerian (p.1762·2).
*Nervous disorders.*

**Dragees pour le sommeil nouvelle formule** *Zeller, Switz.*
Valerian (p.1762·2); lupulus (p.1708·1).
*Sleep disorders.*

**Dragees pour reins et vessie S** *Synpharma, Switz.†.*
Java tea (p.1702·3); solidago virgaurea (p.1748·3); ononis (p.1723·3); bearberry (p.1659·2); boldo (p.1661·2).
*Urinary-tract disorders.*

**Dragees Vegetales Rex** *Lehning, Fr.*
Frangula bark (p.1266·3); cascara (p.1255·1).
*Constipation.*

**Dragon Balm** *Peter Black, UK.*
Camphor (p.1665·3); menthol (p.1711·3); turpentine oil (p.1760·1); nutmeg oil (p.1722·3); eucalyptus oil (p.1686·2); cassia oil (p.1668·2); pine oil; thymol (p.1194·2); guaiacol (p.1122·1); peru balsam (p.1730·2).
*Muscular aches.*

**Dragosil** *Daker Farmasimes, Spain†.*
Creatinolfosfate (p.1677·3) or creatinolfosfate sodium (p.1677·3).
*Cardiac disorders.*

**Drainactil** *Aerocid, Fr.*
Boldo (p.1661·2); birch leaf (p.1660·3); black currant leaf (p.1661·1).
*Gastrointestinal disorders; kidney disorders.*

**Draituss-Ped** *Stiefel, Braz.†.*
Dimenhydrinate (p.431·1).
*Nausea and vomiting.*

**Dralen** *Specifar (Σπεσιφαρ), Gr.*
Disodium etidronate (p.771·2).
*Osteoporosis; Paget's disease of bone.*

**Dralinsa** *Duopharm, Ger.†.*
Linseed (p.1707·2); senna leaf (p.1288·2).
*Constipation.*

**Dramamine**
*Temis, Arg.; Pharmacia, Austral.; Searle, Belg.†; Pharmacia, Fr.; Pharmacia Upjohn, Hong Kong†; Pharmacia, Irl.; Searle, Israel; Pharmacia, Malaysia; Pharmacia Upjohn, Mex.; Pharmacia, Neth.; Pharmacia, NZ; Pharmacia, Port.; Pharmacia, Singapore; Pharmacia, Switz.; Pharmacia, Thai.; Pharmacia Upjohn, UK†; Upjohn, USA.*
Dimenhydrinate (p.431·1).
*Motion sickness; nausea and vomiting; vestibular disorders.*

**Dramamine II** *Upjohn, USA.*
Meclozine hydrochloride (p.436·3).
*Motion sickness.*

**Dramamine-compositum** *Pharmacia, Switz.*
Dimenhydrinate (p.431·1); caffeine (p.782·1).
*Motion sickness.*

**Dramanate** *Pasadena, USA.*
Dimenhydrinate (p.431·1).
*Motion sickness.*

**Dramavit** *Luper, Braz.*
Dimenhydrinate (p.431·1).
*Nausea and vomiting.*

**Dramavit B6** *Luper, Braz.*
Vitamin $B_6$ (p.1456·3); dimenhydrinate (p.431·1).
*Nausea and vomiting.*

**Dramigel** *Drug Research, Ital.*
Amikacin sulfate (p.154·1).
*Gram-negative bacterial infections.*

**Dramin** *Altana, Braz.*
Dimenhydrinate (p.431·1).
*Hypersensitivity reactions; motion sickness; nausea and vomiting; vertigo.*

**Dramin B-6** *Altana, Braz.*
Dimenhydrinate (p.431·1); pyridoxine hydrochloride (p.1456·3).
*Motion sickness; nausea and vomiting; vestibular disorders.*

**Dramin B-6 DL** *Altana, Braz.*
Dimenhydrinate (p.431·1); pyridoxine hydrochloride (p.1456·3); glucose (p.1432·2); fructose (p.1431·3).
*Nausea and vomiting; vertigo.*

**Dramine** *Uriach, Spain.*
Meclozine hydrochloride (p.436·3).
*Motion sickness.*

**Dramnate** *RPG, India.*
Dimenhydrinate (p.431·1).
*Ménière's syndrome; nausea and vomiting; vertigo.*

**Dranat** *Remedina, Gr.*
Tenoxicam (p.93·1).
*Dysmenorrhoea; gout; inflammation; osteoarthritis; pain; rheumatoid arthritis; spondyloarthropathies.*

**Drapix** *Doctum, Gr.*
Povidone-iodine (p.1190·3).
*Disinfection of vagina, vulva, and mouth.*

**Drapolene**
*Note. This name is used for preparations of different composition.*
*Zest, Braz.*
Benzalkonium chloride (p.1168·3); cetrimonium bromide (p.1173·1).
*Barrier preparation; skin disorders.*

*GlaxoSmithKline, Hong Kong; Wellcome, Irl.; GlaxoSmithKline, Malaysia; GlaxoSmithKline, Singapore; GlaxoSmithKline, Thai.; Pfizer Consumer, UK.*
Benzalkonium chloride (p.1168·3); cetrimide (p.1172·1).
*Minor burns and wounds; napkin rash; skin irritation caused by urine.*

**Dravyr**
*Drug Research, Ital.; Drug Research, Singapore.*
Aciclovir (p.626·1).
*Herpesvirus infections.*

**Draxon** *Inibsa, Port.†.*
Flutamide (p.556·2).
*Prostatic cancer.*

**Drazine** *Pharmasant, Thai.*
Hydroxyzine hydrochloride (p.434·3).
*Anxiety; hypersensitivity reactions; motion sickness.*

**Dreemon** *Peach, UK.*
Diphenhydramine hydrochloride (p.431·3).
*Insomnia.*

**Dreierlei** *Hofmann & Sommer, Ger.*
Valerian (p.1762·2); mint oil (p.1715·2).
*Digestive disorders.*

**Dreisacarb**
*Brady, Austria; Gry, Ger.*
Calcium carbonate (p.1254·2).
*Calcium supplement; hyperphosphataemia.*

**Dreisafer** *Gry, Ger.*
Ferrous sulfate (p.1428·3).
*Iron deficiency.*

**DreisaFol** *Gry, Ger.*
Folic acid (p.1429·1).
*Folic acid deficiency; megaloblastic anaemia.*

**Dreisavit** *Brady, Austria.*
Multivitamin preparation (p.1417·1).

**Dreisavit N**
*Gry, Ger.; Bichsel, Switz.*
Vitamin B substances with ascorbic acid (p.1417·1).
*Dietary supplement.*

**Drenalin** *Ariston, Braz.*
Adrenaline (p.852·2).

**Drenian** *Ern, Spain†.*
Diazepam (p.690·1).
*Alcohol withdrawal syndrome; anxiety; epilepsy; premedication; skeletal muscle spasticity; sleep disorders.*

**Drenidra** *Cazi, Braz.*
Chlortalidone (p.882·3).
*Hypertension.*

**Dreniformio** *Biolab Sanus, Braz.*
Fludroxycortide (p.1100·3); clioquinol (p.196·3).
*Skin disorders.*

**Drenison**
*Biolab Sanus, Braz.; Lilly, Canad.†; Derly, Spain†.*
Fludroxycortide (p.1100·3).
*Skin disorders.*

**Drenison N**
*Biolab Sanus, Braz.; Lilly, Hong Kong†.*
Fludroxycortide (p.1100·3); neomycin sulfate (p.235·1).
*Infected skin disorders.*

**Drenison Neomicina** *Derly, Spain†.*
Fludroxycortide (p.1100·3); neomycin sulfate (p.235·1).
*Infected skin disorders.*

**Dren'it** *Wassen, Ital.*
Pineapple; urtica; java tea; ruscus (p.1417·1).
*Nutritional supplement.*

**Drenocol** *Lafage, Arg.*
Magnesium sulfate (p.1228·2); boldo (p.1661·2) peptone.
*Biliary-tract disorders.*

**Drenoflux** *Zeller, Port.†.*
Diphenhydramine hydrochloride (p.431·3); ammonium chloride (p.1115·2); sodium citrate (p.1223·2); menthol (p.1711·3); sodium benzoate (p.1169·3).
*Coughs; respiratory-tract congestion.*

**Drenol** *Searle, Braz.†.*
Hydrochlorothiazide (p.933·2).
*Diabetes insipidus; hypertension; oedema; renal calculi.*

**Drenomade** *Esfar, Port.†.*
Dehydrocholic acid (p.1679·2); methionine (p.1042·1).

**Drenotosse** *Odontofarma, Braz.†.*
Diphenhydramine hydrochloride (p.431·3); ammonium chloride (p.1115·2).
*Coughs.*

**Drenovac** *Nikkho, Braz.*
Procaine benzylpenicillin (p.246·1); benzylpenicillin potassium (p.163·2).
*Bacterial infections.*

**Drenoxol** *Vitoria, Port.*
Ambroxol hydrochloride (p.1114·3).
*Respiratory-tract congestion.*

**Drenur** *Merck, Port.†.*
Fenproporex hydrochloride (p.1588·3).
*Obesity.*

**Drenural** *Grossman, Mex.*
Bumetanide (p.877·2).
*Hypertension; oedema; premenstrual syndrome.*

**Drepatil** *Fada, Arg.*
Diphenhydramine (p.431·3).
*Hypersensitivity reactions.*

**Dresan** *Phoenix, Arg.*
Dipyrone (p.35·3); benzydamine hydrochloride (p.21·1).
*Fever; inflammation; pain.*

**Dresan Biotic** *Phoenix, Arg.*
Dipyrone (p.35·3); benzydamine hydrochloride (p.21·1); tetracycline (p.266·2).
*Bacterial infections.*

**Dresplan** *Seid, Spain.*
Oxybutynin hydrochloride (p.486·3).
*Neurogenic bladder.*

**Driclor**
*Stiefel, Austral.; Stiefel, Fr.; Stiefel, Hong Kong; Stiefel, Irl.; Stiefel, Malaysia; Stiefel, Singapore; Stiefel, UK.*
Aluminium chloride (p.1142·1).
*Hyperhidrosis.*

**Dridase**
*Sanofi Synthelabo, Ger.; Byk, Neth.*
Oxybutynin hydrochloride (p.486·3).
*Bladder disorders.*

**Dridol**
*Janssen-Cilag, Norw.†; Janssen-Cilag, Swed.†.*
Droperidol (p.697·2).
*Nausea; neuroleptanalgesia; premedication; vomiting.*

**Dri/Ear** *Pfeiffer, USA.*
Boric acid (p.1662·1); isopropyl alcohol (p.1184·3).
*Ear disorders.*

**Drifen** *Richmond, Arg.*
Paclitaxel (p.577·3).
*Malignant neoplasms.*

**DriHist** *Prasco, USA.*
Phenylephrine hydrochloride (p.1126·3); chlorphenamine maleate (p.427·3); hyoscine methonitrate (p.483·3).
*Upper respiratory-tract disorders.*

**Driken** *Kendrick, Mex.*
Iron dextran (p.1436·3).
*Iron-deficiency anaemia.*

**Drilix** *Be-Tabs, S.Afr.*
Pseudoephedrine hydrochloride (p.1129·2).
*Upper respiratory-tract congestion.*

**Drill**
*Note. This name is used for preparations of different composition.*
*Sidus, Arg.; Pierre Fabre Sante, Fr.; Pierre Fabre, Port.*
Chlorhexidine gluconate (p.1173·2); tetracaine hydrochloride (p.1385·1).
*Mouth and throat infections.*

*Pierre Fabre, Spain.*
Chlorhexidine gluconate (p.1173·2); benzocaine (p.1370·3).
*Mouth and throat infections.*

**Drill Expectorant** *Pierre Fabre Sante, Fr.*
Carbocisteine (p.1116·2).
*Respiratory-tract congestion.*

**Drill Mucolitico** *Pierre Fabre, Port.*
Carbocisteine (p.1116·2).
*Respiratory-tract disorders associated with increased or viscous mucus.*

**Drill rhinites** *Pierre Fabre Sante, Fr.†.*
Pseudoephedrine hydrochloride (p.1129·2).
*Nasal congestion.*

**Drill Tosse Seca** *Pierre Fabre, Port.*
Dextromethorphan hydrobromide (p.1117·3).
*Coughs.*

**Drill toux seche** *Pierre Fabre Sante, Fr.*
Dextromethorphan hydrobromide (p.1117·3).
*Coughs.*

**Drilyna** *Bago, Arg.*
Theophylline (p.798·3) or theophylline sodium glycinate (p.804·3).
*Obstructive airways disease.*

**Drimen** *Coup, Gr.*
Dimenhydrinate (p.431·1).
*Motion sickness; nausea and vomiting; vertigo.*

**Drimnorth** *Northia, Arg.*
Midazolam (p.707·1).

**Drimpam** *Alliance, S.Afr.*
Alprazolam (p.668·3).
*Anxiety; mixed anxiety depressive states; panic attacks.*

**Drin** *Wassermann, Ital.*
Aspirin (p.15·1); paracetamol (p.76·2); caffeine (p.782·1).
*Fever; pain.*

**Drina** *Silesia, Chile.*
Cyproterone acetate (p.1544·1); ethinylestradiol (p.1553·2).
*Androgen-dependent acne, alopecia, and hirsutism in women.*

**Drioquilen** *Columbia, Mex.†.*
Diiodohydroxyquinoline (p.603·3).

**Driptane**
*Fournier, Belg.; Fournier, Fr.*
Oxybutynin hydrochloride (p.486·3).
*Enuresis; neurogenic bladder.*

**Drisdol**
*Sanofi Synthelabo, Canad.; Sanofi Winthrop, USA.*
Ergocalciferol (p.1462·1).
*Familial hypophosphataemia; hypoparathyroidism; rickets.*

**Drisi-Ven** *Truw, Ger.*
Troxerutin (p.1688·3).
*Vascular disorders.*

**Drisofal** *Help, Gr.*
Gemfibrozil (p.923·1).
*Hyperlipidaemias.*

**Dristal Cold** *Whitehall, Hong Kong.*
Chlorphenamine maleate (p.427·3); phenylephrine hydrochloride (p.1126·3); paracetamol (p.76·2).
*Cold symptoms; upper respiratory-tract symptoms.*

**Dristan**
Note. This name is used for preparations of different composition.
*Whitehall-Robins, Canad.*
*Caplets; tablets:* Paracetamol (p.76·2); phenylephrine hydrochloride (p.1126·3); chlorphenamine maleate (p.427·3).
*Cold symptoms.*
*Capsules*†: Phenylpropanolamine hydrochloride (p.1127·3); chlorphenamine maleate (p.427·3); aspirin (p.15·1); caffeine (p.782·1).
*Cold symptoms; fever; headache; pain; upper respiratory-tract disorders.*
*Nasal spray:* Phenylephrine hydrochloride (p.1126·3); pheniramine maleate (p.438·3).
*Nasal congestion.*
*Whitehall-Robins, Canad.; Whitehall, Fin.*†*; Wyeth, Irl.; Whitehall, UK*†.
*Long-acting nasal spray; nasal spray:* Oxymetazoline hydrochloride (p.1126·1).
*Nasal congestion.*
*Wyeth Consumer, Chile.*
Chlorphenamine maleate (p.427·3); phenylephrine hydrochloride (p.1126·3).
*Respiratory-tract congestion.*
*Whitehall, Irl.*†*; Whitehall, UK*†.
*Tablets:* Aspirin (p.15·1); caffeine (p.782·1); chlorphenamine maleate (p.427·3); phenylephrine hydrochloride (p.1126·3).
*Cold symptoms; nasal congestion.*

**Dristan Allergy** *Whitehall, USA.*
Pseudoephedrine hydrochloride (p.1129·2); brompheniramine maleate (p.426·1).
*Hypersensitivity reactions.*

**Dristan Analgesico** *Wyeth-Whitehall, Arg.*
Aspirin (p.15·1); caffeine (p.782·1); ascorbic acid (p.1460·2).
Aluminium hydroxide (p.1249·2) and magnesium carbonate (p.1272·1) are included in this preparation in an attempt to limit adverse effects on the gastrointestinal mucosa.
*Fever; pain.*

**Dristan Cold** *Whitehall, USA.*
Chlorphenamine maleate (p.427·3); phenylephrine hydrochloride (p.1126·3); paracetamol (p.76·2).
Formerly known as Advanced Formula Dristan.
*Cold symptoms.*

**Dristan Cold Caplets** *Whitehall, USA.*
Pseudoephedrine hydrochloride (p.1129·2); paracetamol (p.76·2).
*Upper respiratory-tract symptoms.*

**Dristan Cold & Flu** *Whitehall, USA.*
Chlorphenamine maleate (p.427·3); dextromethorphan hydrobromide (p.1117·3); paracetamol (p.76·2); pseudoephedrine hydrochloride (p.1129·2).
*Coughs and cold symptoms.*

**Dristan Cold Maximum Strength** *Whitehall, Hong Kong.*
Paracetamol (p.76·2); pseudoephedrine hydrochloride (p.1129·2).
*Cold symptoms.*

**Dristan Cold Maximum Strength Multi-symptom Formula** *Whitehall, USA.*
Paracetamol (p.76·2); pseudoephedrine hydrochloride (p.1129·2); brompheniramine maleate (p.426·1).
*Cold symptoms; hypersensitivity reactions.*

**Dristan Cold Maximum Strength No Drowsiness Formula** *Whitehall, USA.*
Paracetamol (p.76·2); pseudoephedrine hydrochloride (p.1129·2).
*Cold symptoms.*

**Dristan Cold Multi-Symptom Formula** *Whitehall, USA.*
Phenylephrine hydrochloride (p.1126·3); paracetamol (p.76·2); chlorphenamine maleate (p.427·3).
*Upper respiratory-tract symptoms.*

**Dristan Compuesto** *Wyeth-Whitehall, Arg.*
Aspirin (p.15·1); caffeine (p.782·1); chlorphenamine maleate (p.427·3); ascorbic acid (p.1460·2).
Aluminium hydroxide (p.1249·2) and magnesium carbonate (p.1272·1) are included in this preparation in an attempt to limit adverse effects on the gastrointestinal mucosa.
*Influenza symptoms.*

**Dristan Descongestivo** *Wyeth-Whitehall, Arg.*
Paracetamol (p.76·2); phenylephrine hydrochloride (p.1126·3).

**Dristan Expectorant** *Wyeth, India.*
*Oral liquid:* Codeine phosphate (p.27·1); guaifenesin (p.1122·1); sodium citrate (p.1223·2); citric acid (p.1673·1); phenylephrine hydrochloride (p.1126·3); chlorphenamine maleate (p.427·3).
*Tablets:* Phenylephrine hydrochloride (p.1126·3); caffeine (p.782·1); chlorphenamine maleate (p.427·3); aspirin (p.15·1).
*Coughs.*

**Dristan 12-hr Nasal Decongestant Spray** *Whitehall, USA.*
Oxymetazoline hydrochloride (p.1126·1).
Formerly known as Dristan Long Lasting.
*Nasal congestion.*

**Dristan Juice Mix-in** *Whitehall, USA.*
Paracetamol (p.76·2); pseudoephedrine hydrochloride (p.1129·2); dextromethorphan hydrobromide (p.1117·3).
*Coughs and cold symptoms.*

**Dristan Long Lasting** *Whitehall, USA.*
Oxymetazoline hydrochloride (p.1126·1).
*Nasal congestion.*

**Dristan N D** *Whitehall-Robins, Canad.*
Pseudoephedrine hydrochloride (p.1129·2); paracetamol (p.76·2).
Formerly known as Dristan Non Drowsy.
*Cold symptoms; fever; headache; pain; upper respiratory-tract disorders.*

**Dristan Nasal** *Wyeth-Whitehall, Arg.*
Oxymetazoline hydrochloride (p.1126·1).
*Nasal congestion.*

**Dristan Nasal Drops** *Wyeth, India.*
Phenylephrine hydrochloride (p.1126·3); pheniramine maleate (p.438·3); menthol (p.1711·3); cineole (p.1672·1).
*Nasal congestion.*

**Dristan Nasal Spray** *Whitehall, USA.*
Phenylephrine hydrochloride (p.1126·3); pheniramine maleate (p.438·3).
*Nasal congestion.*

**Dristan Saline Spray** *Whitehall, USA.*
Sodium chloride (p.1233·3).
*Inflammation and dryness of nasal membranes.*

**Dristan Sinus**
*Whitehall-Robins, Canad.; Whitehall, USA.*
Pseudoephedrine hydrochloride (p.1129·2); ibuprofen (p.45·3).
*Cold and influenza symptoms; sinusitis.*

**Dristancito** *Wyeth-Whitehall, Arg.*
Paracetamol (p.76·2).
*Fever; pain.*

**Drithocreme** *Dermik, USA.*
Dithranol (p.1146·1).
*Psoriasis.*

**Dritho-Scalp** *Dermik, USA.*
Dithranol (p.1146·1).
*Psoriasis.*

**Drivermide** *Nakornpatana, Thai.*
Mebendazole (p.108·2).
*Worm infections.*

**Drix** *Pharmacal, Switz.*†.
Bisacodyl (p.1251·3); frangula bark (p.1266·3); senna (p.1288·2); sodium sulfate (p.1290·1).
*Constipation.*

**Drix Abfuhr-Dragees** *Hermes, Ger.*†.
Senna leaf (p.1288·2).
*Constipation.*

**Drix Bisacodyl** *Hermes, Ger.*
Bisacodyl (p.1251·3).
*Constipation.*

**Drixin** *Schering-Plough, Denm.*
Oxymetazoline hydrochloride (p.1126·1).
*Nasal congestion.*

**Drixine**
*Schering-Plough, NZ; Schering-Plough, S.Afr.*
Oxymetazoline hydrochloride (p.1126·1).
*Nasal congestion.*

**Drixine Nasal** *Schering-Plough, Austral.*
Oxymetazoline hydrochloride (p.1126·1).
*Nasal congestion.*

**Drixomed** *Iopharm, USA.*
Dexbrompheniramine maleate (p.426·1); pseudoephedrine sulfate (p.1129·2).
*Respiratory-tract disorders.*

**Drixora** *Schering-Plough, S.Afr.*†.
Pseudoephedrine sulfate (p.1129·2).
*Upper respiratory-tract congestion.*

**Drixoral**
Note. This name is used for preparations of different composition.
*Schering, Canad.*†.
*Capsules:* Dextromethorphan hydrobromide (p.1117·3).
*Coughs.*
*Schering-Plough, Canad.*
*Nasal spray:* Oxymetazoline hydrochloride (p.1126·1).
*Sustained release tablets:* Dexbrompheniramine maleate (p.426·1); pseudoephedrine sulfate (p.1129·2).
*Upper respiratory-tract congestion.*
*Schering-Plough, Hong Kong; Schering-Plough, Malaysia; Schering-Plough, Singapore.*
Dexbrompheniramine maleate (p.426·1); pseudoephedrine sulfate (p.1129·2).
*Upper respiratory-tract congestion.*
*Schering-Plough, USA.*
Pseudoephedrine sulfate (p.1129·2); brompheniramine maleate (p.426·1).
*Upper respiratory-tract symptoms.*

**Drixoral Cold & Allergy** *Schering-Plough, USA.*
Pseudoephedrine sulfate (p.1129·2); dexbrompheniramine maleate (p.426·1).
*Upper respiratory-tract symptoms.*

**Drixoral Cold & Flu** *Schering-Plough, USA.*
Pseudoephedrine sulfate (p.1129·2); paracetamol (p.76·2); dexbrompheniramine maleate (p.426·1).
*Upper respiratory-tract symptoms.*

**Drixoral Cough** *Schering, Canad.*†.
Dextromethorphan hydrobromide (p.1117·3).
*Coughs.*

**Drixoral Cough & Congestion** *Schering-Plough, USA.*
Pseudoephedrine hydrochloride (p.1129·2); dextromethorphan hydrobromide (p.1117·3).

**Drixoral Cough & Sore Throat** *Schering-Plough, USA.*
Dextromethorphan hydrobromide (p.1117·3); paracetamol (p.76·2).

**Drixoral Day/Night** *Schering-Plough, Canad.*
Yellow tablets, pseudoephedrine sulfate (p.1129·2); white tablets, dexbrompheniramine maleate (p.426·1); pseudoephedrine sulfate.
*Ear disorders; upper respiratory-tract congestion.*

**Drixoral ND** *Schering-Plough, Canad.*
Pseudoephedrine sulfate (p.1129·2).
*Ear disorders; upper respiratory-tract congestion.*

**Drixoral Non-Drowsy Formula** *Schering, USA.*
Pseudoephedrine sulfate (p.1129·2).
*Nasal congestion.*

**Drixoral Plus** *Schering-Plough, USA.*
Pseudoephedrine sulfate (p.1129·2); paracetamol (p.76·2); dexbrompheniramine maleate (p.426·1).
Formerly known as Drixoral Allergy Sinus.
*Upper respiratory-tract symptoms.*

**Drixtab** *Schering, Canad.*†.
Dexbrompheniramine maleate (p.426·1); pseudoephedrine sulfate (p.1129·2).
*Upper respiratory-tract congestion.*

**Drize** *Jones, USA*†.
Chlorphenamine maleate (p.427·3); phenylpropanolamine hydrochloride (p.1127·3).
*Cold symptoms.*

**Droal** *Vita, Spain.*
Ketorolac trometamol (p.52·1).
*Pain.*

**Drocef** *Eurofarma, Braz.*†.
Cefadroxil (p.167·2).
*Bacterial infections.*

**Droclina** *Vitae, Mex.*†.
Tetracycline (p.266·2).
*Bacterial infections.*

**Drocon-CS** *Cypress, USA.*
Hydrocodone tartrate (p.45·1); brompheniramine maleate (p.426·1); pseudoephedrine hydrochloride (p.1129·2).
*Coughs; upper respiratory-tract congestion.*

**Drofaron** *Democal, Switz.*
Aluminium hydroxide (p.1249·2); magnesium trisilicate (p.1272·3); dimethicone (p.1289·2).
*Flatulence; gastric hyperacidity; gastritis.*

**Drofaxil** *Royton, Braz.*
Cefadroxil (p.167·2).
*Bacterial infections.*

**Drogenil**
*Essex, Chile; Schering-Plough, Irl.; Essex, Ital.; Schering-Plough, Neth.; Schering-Plough, UK.*
Flutamide (p.556·2).
*Prostatic cancer.*

**Drogimed** *Synpharma, Austria.*
Birch leaf (p.1660·3); equisetum (p.1684·1).
*Urinary-tract disorders.*

**Drolasona** *Alter, Spain.*
Fluticasone propionate (p.1102·3).
*Skin disorders.*

**Droleptan**
*Janssen-Cilag, Austral.*†*; Pharmalab, Austral.; OTL, Fr.; Janssen-Cilag, Irl.*†*; HSL, NZ; Janssen-Cilag, NZ*†*; Janssen-Cilag, UK*†.
Droperidol (p.697·2).
*Adjunct in neuroleptanalgesia; nausea and vomiting; premedication; psychoses.*

**Dromadol** *Ivax, UK.*
Tramadol hydrochloride (p.94·3).
*Pain.*

**Dromos** *Sigma-Tau, Ital.*
Propionyl-L-carnitine hydrochloride.
*Cardiac disorders.*

**Dronal** *Sigma-Tau, Ital.*
Alendronate sodium (p.765·3).
*Osteoporosis.*

**Dronate-OS** *BDH, India.*
Disodium etidronate (p.771·2).
*Hypercalcaemia of malignancy; Paget's disease of bone.*

**Dropcina** *Plough, Port.*
Gramicidin (p.220·2); cetylpyridinium chloride (p.1173·1); dichlorobenzyl alcohol (p.1178·3); benzocaine (p.1370·3).
*Mouth and throat disorders.*

**Droperdal** *Cristalia, Braz.*
Droperidol (p.697·2).
*Psychoses.*

**Droperol** *Troikaa, India.*
Droperidol (p.697·2).
*Agitation; neuroleptanalgesia; premedication.*

**Dropgel** *Farmila, Ital.*
Carbomer 980 (p.1577·2).
*Dry eyes.*

**Dropicine** *Beta, Arg.*
Risperidone (p.719·2).
*Psychoses.*

**Dropid** *Progress, Thai.*
Gemfibrozil (p.923·1).
*Hyperlipidaemias.*

**Dropilton** *Bruschettini, Ital.*
Pilocarpine hydrochloride (p.1495·1).
*Glaucoma.*

**Dropovit** *Wyeth, India.*
Multivitamin preparation (p.1417·1).

**Dropstar**
*Poen, Arg.; Farmigea, Ital.*
Sodium hyaluronate (p.1697·3).
*Dry eyes.*

**Droptimol** *Farmigea, Ital.*
Timolol maleate (p.1012·2).
*Glaucoma; ocular hypertension.*

**Dropyal** *Bruschettini, Ital.*
Sodium hyaluronate (p.1697·3); carbomer 941 (p.1577·2); glycerol (p.1694·3).
*Dry eyes.*

**Drosana Hyperflorin** *Democal, Switz.*†.
Hypericum (p.299·1); passion flower (p.1729·1).
*Depression.*

**Drosana Resiston** *Democal, Switz.*
Echinacea purpurea (p.1683·2).
*Cold symptoms.*

**Drosera Komplex** *Richter, Austria.*
Homoeopathic preparation.

**Droserapect** *Weber & Weber, Ger.*
Homoeopathic preparation.

**Drosera-Weliplex** *Weber & Weber, Ger.*
Homoeopathic preparation.

**Drosetux**
*Dolisos, Canad.; Dolisos, Fr.*
Homoeopathic preparation.

**Drosinula** *Bioforce, Switz.*
Norway spruce buds; drosera (p.1683·1); hedera helix; pear.
*Respiratory-tract disorders.*

**Drosithym-N** *Ysatfabrik, Ger.*
Cowslip rhizome (p.1735·1); thyme (p.1755·2); drosera (p.1683·1).
*Catarrh; coughs.*

**Drossadin** *Drossapharm, Switz.*
Hexetidine (p.1182·1).
*Mouth and throat disorders.*

**Drossanose** *Drossapharm, Israel.*
Sea salt (p.1233·3).
*Nasal disorders.*

**Drossa-Nose** *Drossapharm, Switz.*
Sea salt (p.1233·3).
*Nasal dryness.*

**Drosten** *Vocate, Gr.*
Butamirate citrate (p.1116·2).
*Cough.*

**Drosyn** *FDC, India.*
Phenylephrine hydrochloride (p.1126·3).
*Production of cycloplegia and mydriasis; synechiae.*

**Drotin** *Bushnell, India.*
Drotaverine hydrochloride (p.1683·1).
*Smooth muscle spasm.*

**Drovitol** *Synpharma, Austria.*
Myrrh (p.1718·3); clove (p.1673·2); tormentil (p.1757·2).
*Mouth and throat disorders.*

**Droxaine** *Daudt, Braz.*
Aluminium hydroxide (p.1249·2); magnesium hydroxide (p.1272·2); oxetacaine (p.1382·1).
*Gastrointestinal hyperacidity.*

**Droxaryl**
Note. This name is used for preparations of different composition.
*Sanova, Austria.*
*Cream:* Bufexamac (p.21·3).
*Ointment:* Bufexamac (p.21·3); alfa tocoferil acetate (p.1465·1).
*Skin disorders.*
*Continental Pharma, Belg.; Continental Pharma, Thai.*†.
Bufexamac (p.21·3).
*Skin disorders.*

**Droxel** *Recalcine, Chile.*
Propyphenazone (p.85·3); calcium ascorbate (p.1460·2); chlorphenamine maleate (p.427·3); pseudoephedrine hydrochloride (p.1129·2); vitamin a (p.1451·2).
*Cold and influenza symptoms.*

**Droxia** *Bristol-Myers Squibb Oncology, USA.*
Hydroxycarbamide (p.559·1).
*Sickle-cell anaemia.*

**Droxil** *Klonal, Arg.*
Cefadroxil (p.167·2).
*Bacterial infections.*

**Droximag** *PP Lab, Thai.*
Aluminium hydroxide (p.1249·2); magnesium trisilicate (p.1272·3); kaolin (p.1268·3); atropine sulfate (p.477·1).
*Alkaloid poisoning; gastrointestinal infection; peptic ulcer.*

**Droxitop** *Synpharma, Austria.*
Java tea (p.1702·3); solidago virgaurea (p.1748·3); equisetum (p.1684·1).
*Kidney and urinary-tract disorders.*

**Droxiurea** *Pharmacia, Arg.*
Hydroxycarbamide (p.559·1).
*Malignant neoplasms.*

**Droxivit** *Pizzard, Mex.*
Hydroxocobalamin (p.1458·2).

**Droxol** *Microsules Bernabo, Arg.*
Pirenzepine hydrochloride (p.488·1).
*Peptic ulcer.*

**Droxyl** *Pharmaland, Thai.*
Aluminium hydroxide (p.1249·2); magnesium hydroxide (p.1272·2); simeticone (p.1289·2).
*Gastric hyperacidity; peptic ulcer.*

**Drufusan N** *Syxyl, Ger.*
Homoeopathic preparation.

**Druisel** *Northia, Arg.*
Ibuprofen (p.45·3).
*Fever; inflammation; pain.*

**Dry Cough Syrup** *AAH, UK.*
Dextromethorphan hydrobromide (p.1117·3).
*Coughs.*

**Dry Eyes** *Bausch & Lomb, USA.*
*Eye drops:* Polyvinyl alcohol (p.1581·1).
*Eye ointment:* White soft paraffin (p.1479·3); liquid paraffin (p.1479·1); wool fat (p.1483·1).
*Dry eyes.*

**Drylin** *Merckle, Ger.*
Co-trimoxazole (p.199·3).
*Bacterial infections; Pneumocystis carinii pneumonia.*

**Drynalken** *Kendrick, Mex.*
Dopamine hydrochloride (p.907·1).
*Extracorporeal circulation; hypotension; shock.*

**Drynalquin** *Kendrick, Mex.†.*
Dopamine hydrochloride (p.907·1).

**Drynisan** *Fecofar, Arg.*
Naphazoline (p.1124·3); mepyramine (p.437·1).

**Dryptal** *Rhone-Poulenc Rorer, Hong Kong†.*
Furosemide (p.919·3).
*Hypertension; oedema.*

**Drysol**
*Note. This name is used for preparations of different composition.*
*Dispolab, Chile; Person & Covey, USA.*
Aluminium chloride (p.1142·1).
*Hyperhidrosis.*

*Darier, Mex.*
Aluminium chlorohydrate (p.1142·1).
*Hyperhidrosis.*

**Drytergent** *C & M, USA.*
Skin cleanser.

**Drytex** *C & M, USA.*
Salicylic acid (p.1157·1); methylbenzethonium chloride (p.1186·1).
*Acne.*

**Dryvax** *Wyeth-Ayerst, USA.*
A smallpox vaccine (p.1639·1).
*Active immunisation.*

**DS Emulsion**
*Biorga, Fr.; Saninter, Port.†.*
Copper pidolate; zinc pidolate.
*Seborrhoeic dermatitis; skin irritation.*

**D-Seb**
*Rydelle, Fr.†; Johnson & Johnson, Ital.†.*
Chlorhexidine gluconate (p.1173·2).
*Acne; seborrhoea.*

**D-S-S** *Warner Chilcott, USA.*
Docusate sodium (p.1262·2).
*Constipation.*

**D-Stop** *Ratiopharm, Ger.†.*
Loperamide hydrochloride (p.1271·1).
*Diarrhoea.*

**D-Stress** *Fontovit, Braz.*
Ginseng; vitamin B substances; ascorbic acid; rutoside (p.1417·1).

**DT Bis** *Merieux, Fr.†.*
A diphtheria and tetanus vaccine (p.1613·1).
*Active immunisation of older children and adults.*

**DT Coq** *Pasteur Merieux, Fr.†.*
An adsorbed diphtheria, tetanus, and pertussis vaccine (p.1613·3).
*Active immunisation.*

**DT Polio** *Aventis Pasteur, Fr.*
A diphtheria, tetanus, and poliomyelitis vaccine (p.1615·2).
*Active immunisation.*

**DT Vax**
*Aventis Pasteur, Arg.; Aventis Pasteur, Braz.; Aventis, S.Afr.; Aventis Pasteur, Thai.*
An adsorbed diphtheria and tetanus vaccine (p.1613·1).
*Active immunisation.*

**D-Tabs** *Riva, Canad.†.*
Colecalciferol (p.1461·3).
*Vitamin D supplement.*

**DTap-IPV** *SSI, Swed.†.*
A diphtheria, tetanus, pertussis, and poliomyelitis vaccine (p.1615·1).
*Active immunisation.*

**D-Tato** *Protein, Mex.†.*
Benzonatate (p.1115·3).

**DTCoq/DTP**
*Aventis Pasteur, Braz.; Pasteur Merieux, Israel; Aventis Pasteur, Thai.*
An adsorbed diphtheria, tetanus, and pertussis vaccine (p.1613·3).
*Active immunisation.*

**DTI** *Korean United, Malaysia.*
Dacarbazine (p.544·2).
*Malignant melanoma; sarcoma.*

**DTIC**
*Bayer, Austral.; Bayer, Canad.; VHB, India; Bayer, Swed.; Dome, Switz.*
Dacarbazine (p.544·2).
*Malignant neoplasms.*

*Rhone-Poulenc Rorer, Ger.†.*
Dacarbazine citrate (p.544·3).
*Hodgkin's disease; melanomas; sarcomas.*

**DTIC-Dome**
*Bayer, Austria; Bayer, Belg.†; Bayer, Irl.†; Bayer, NZ; Bayer, S.Afr.; Bayer, Spain†; Bayer, UK; Bayer, USA.*
Dacarbazine (p.544·2).
*Malignant neoplasms.*

**DT-Impfstoff** *Aventis Pasteur, Ger.; Chiron Behring, Ger.*
An adsorbed diphtheria and tetanus vaccine (p.1613·1).
*Active immunisation of infants and young children.*

**DTM** *Biochem, India.*
Diltiazem (p.901·3).
*Angina pectoris.*

**DTP** *Aventis Pasteur, Braz.†.*
A diphtheria, tetanus, and pertussis vaccine (p.1613·3).
*Active immunisation.*

**DTP-Merieux**
*Aventis, S.Afr.; Aventis Pasteur, Spain.*
An adsorbed diphtheria, tetanus, and pertussis vaccine (p.1613·3).
*Active immunisation.*

**DTP-Rix** *SmithKline Beecham, Ger.†.*
An adsorbed diphtheria, tetanus, and pertussis vaccine (p.1613·3).
*Active immunisation.*

**D-Tracetten** *Hoechst Marion Roussel, Ger.†.*
Colecalciferol (p.1461·3).
*Vitamin D deficiency.*

**DT-reduct** *Aventis Pasteur, Austria.*
An adsorbed diphtheria and tetanus vaccine (p.1613·1).
*Active immunisation.*

**DT-Rix** *SmithKline Beecham, Ger.†.*
An adsorbed diphtheria and tetanus vaccine (p.1613·1).
*Active immunisation of infants and young children.*

**D-Tussin** *Pharmco, S.Afr.†.*
Etofylline (p.785·1); diphenhydramine hydrochloride (p.431·3); ammonium chloride (p.1115·2); sodium citrate (p.1223·2).
*Coughs; obstructive airways disease.*

**DT-Vaccinol** *Procter & Gamble, Ger.†.*
An adsorbed diphtheria and tetanus vaccine (p.1613·1).
*Active immunisation of infants and young children.*

**D.T.Vax Adsorbe** *Vianex (Βιανέξ), Gr.*
An adsorbed diphtheria and tetanus vaccine (p.1613·1).
*Active immunisation.*

**Duac** *Stiefel, USA.*
Benzoyl peroxide (p.1143·2); clindamycin (p.194·2).
*Acne.*

**Duac Once Daily** *Stiefel, UK.*
Benzoyl peroxide (p.1143·2); clindamycin phosphate (p.194·2).
*Acne.*

**Duact**
*GlaxoSmithKline, Austria; GlaxoSmithKline, Denm.; GlaxoSmithKline, Fin.*
Acrivastine (p.423·3); pseudoephedrine hydrochloride (p.1129·2).
*Allergic rhinitis.*

**Duadacin** *Kenwood, USA†.*
Paracetamol (p.76·2); chlorphenamine maleate (p.427·3); phenylpropanolamine hydrochloride (p.1127·3).
*Upper respiratory-tract symptoms.*

**Duadacin Extra Strength Cold & Flu** *Bradley, USA.*
Pseudoephedrine hydrochloride (p.1129·2); chlorphenamine maleate (p.427·3); paracetamol (p.76·2).
*Upper respiratory-tract disorders.*

**Duafen** *Pharmed, Austria.*
Ibuprofen (p.45·3).
*Fever; pain.*

**Dual Antigen** *Serum Institute, India.*
A diphtheria and tetanus vaccine (p.1613·1).
*Active immunisation.*

**Dualgan** *ITF, Port.*
Etodolac (p.37·3).
*Musculoskeletal, joint, and peri-articular disorders; pain.*

**Dualid** *Duncan, Arg.*
Ranitidine (p.1285·2).
*Peptic ulcer.*

**Dualid S** *Asta Medica, Braz.*
Diethylpropion hydrochloride (p.1587·1).
*Obesity.*

**Dualizol** *Degorts, Mex.*
Metronidazole (p.607·2).
*Amoebiasis; giardiasis; trichomoniasis.*

**Dual-Lax Extra Strong** *Lane, UK.*
Senna (p.1288·2); aloin (p.1248·3); cascara (p.1255·1).
*Constipation.*

**Dual-Lax Normal Strength** *Lane, UK.*
Senna (p.1288·2); cape aloes (p.1248·2); cascara (p.1255·1).
*Constipation.*

**Dualten** *Saval, Chile.*
Carvedilol (p.881·1).
*Heart failure; hypertension; ischaemic heart disease.*

**Duan** *Pharmed, Austria.*
Aspirin (p.15·1); paracetamol (p.76·2); caffeine (p.782·1).
*Fever; pain.*

**Duaneo** *Pharmed, Austria.*
Paracetamol (p.76·2).
*Fever; pain.*

**Duaneo mit Codein** *Pharmed, Austria.*
Aspirin (p.15·1); paracetamol (p.76·2); codeine hydrochloride (p.27·1).
*Pain.*

**Dubam** *Norma, UK.*
*Cream:* Methyl salicylate (p.59·3); menthol (p.1711·3); cineole (p.1672·1).
*Topical spray:* Methyl salicylate (p.59·3); ethyl salicylate (p.37·3); glycol salicylate (p.44·3); methyl nicotinate (p.59·2).
*Musculoskeletal pain.*

**Dube** *Korean Drug, Singapore.*
Lidocaine (p.1377·3).
*Local anaesthesia.*

**Dublon** *Fada, Arg.*
Esmolol (p.913·2).

**Ducene** *Sauter, Austral.*
Diazepam (p.690·1).
*Alcohol withdrawal syndrome; anxiety disorders; skeletal muscle spasm; spasticity.*

**Duciclon** *Degorts, Mex.*
Diclofenac sodium (p.32·1); thiamine hydrochloride (p.1455·1); pyridoxine hydrochloride (p.1456·3); cyanocobalamin (p.1458·2).
*Neuralgia; neuritis; neuropathy.*

**Ductelmin** *Ducto, Braz.*
Mebendazole (p.108·2).
*Worm infections.*

**Ductogel** *Ducto, Braz.*
Aluminium hydroxide (p.1249·2).
*Antacid.*

**Ductomet** *Ducto, Braz.*
Methyldopa (p.953·2).
*Hypertension.*

**Ductopan** *Neo Quimica, Braz.*
Hyoscine butylbromide (p.483·3); dipyrone (p.35·3).
*Smooth muscle spasm.*

**Ductopril** *Ducto, Braz.*
Captopril (p.879·2).
*Hypertension.*

**Ductoveran** *Ducto, Braz.*
Papaverine hydrochloride (p.1728·1); belladonna (p.479·1); hyoscyamus (p.485·2); boldo (p.1661·2); star anise.

**Duebien** *PQS, Spain†.*
Doxylamine succinate (p.432·3).
*Insomnia.*

**Duet** *Integrity, USA.*
Multivitamin and mineral preparation (p.1417·1).

**Dueva** *Menarini, Ital.*
Desogestrel (p.1547·2); ethinylestradiol (p.1553·2).
*Biphasic oral contraceptive.*

**Dufaston** *Solvay, Ital.*
Dydrogesterone (p.1549·2).
*Endometriosis; female infertility; menopausal disorders; menstrual disorders; threatened or recurrent miscarriage.*

**Dufine** *Inibsa, Port.*
Clomifene citrate (p.1542·2).
*Anovulatory infertility; oligospermia.*

**Duflemina** *Janssen-Cilag, Arg.*
Calcium dobesilate (p.1664·2).
*Haemorrhoids; venous insufficiency.*

**Duinum**
*Medochemie, Hong Kong; Medochemie, Malaysia; Medochemie, Singapore†; Medochemie, Thai.*
Clomifene citrate (p.1542·2).
*Amenorrhoea; anovulatory infertility; oligospermia; polycystic ovary syndrome.*

**Dukoral**
*Statens Serum Institut, Denm.; SBL, Norw.; CSL, NZ; SBL, Swed.; Chiron Vaccines, UK.*
An oral cholera vaccine (p.1611·2).
*Active immunisation.*

**Dularell Classic** *Sanorell, Ger.*
Homoeopathic preparation.

**Dularell N** *Sanorell, Ger.*
Homoeopathic preparation.

**Dulax** *Antigen, Irl.*
Lactulose (p.1269·1).
*Constipation; hepatic encephalopathy.*

**Dulcamara-Homaccord** *Peithner, Austria.*
Homoeopathic preparation.

**Dulceril** *Codilab, Port.*
Sodium cyclamate (p.1426·2); saccharin (p.1443·2).
*Sugar substitute.*

**Dulcilarmes** *Allergan, Fr.*
Povidone (p.1581·2).
*Dry eyes; eye examinations.*

**Dulciphak** *Allergan, Fr.*
Sodium monomethyltrisilanol orthohydroxybenzoate; parahydroxycinnamic acid.
*Lens opacities.*

**Dulcivit** *Abigo, Swed.*
Multivitamin preparation (p.1417·1).

**Dulco Laxo** *Fher, Spain.*
Bisacodyl (p.1251·3).
*Constipation.*

**Dulcodruppels** *Boehringer Ingelheim, Neth.*
Sodium picosulfate (p.1289·3).
*Constipation.*

**Dulcolan** *Boehringer Ingelheim, Mex.*
Bisacodyl (p.1251·3).
*Bowel evacuation; constipation.*

**Dulcolax**
*Note. This name is used for preparations of different composition.*
*Boehringer Ingelheim, Arg.; Boehringer Ingelheim, UK.*
*Capsules; oral drops:* Sodium picosulfate (p.1289·3).
*Bowel evacuation; constipation.*

*Boehringer Ingelheim, Arg.; Boehringer Ingelheim, Austria; Boehringer Ingelheim, Belg.; Boehringer de Angeli, Braz.; Boehringer Ingelheim, Canad.; Boehringer Ingelheim, Denm.; Boehringer Ingelheim, Fr.; Boehringer Ingelheim, Ger.; Boehringer Ingelheim, Gr.; Boehringer Ingelheim, Hong Kong; German Remedies, India; Boehringer Ingelheim, Irl.; Boehringer Ingelheim, Ital.; Boehringer Ingelheim, Malaysia; Boehringer Ingelheim, Neth.; Boehringer Ingelheim, Norw.; Boehringer Ingelheim, NZ; Boehringer Ingelheim, Port.; Boehringer Ingelheim, S.Afr.; Boehringer Ingelheim, Singapore; Boehringer Ingelheim, Swed.; Boehringer Ingelheim, Switz.; Boehringer Ingelheim, Thai.; Boehringer Ingelheim, UK; Novartis Consumer, USA.*
Bisacodyl (p.1251·3).
*Bowel evacuation; constipation.*

**Dulcolax Liquid** *Boehringer de Angeli, Braz.†.*
Sodium picosulfate (p.1289·3).
*Bowel evacuation; constipation.*

**Dulcolax NP** *Boehringer Ingelheim, Ger.*
Sodium picosulfate (p.1289·3).
*Constipation.*

**Dulcolax Picosulphate** *Boehringer Ingelheim, Belg.*
Sodium picosulfate (p.1289·3).
*Constipation.*

**Dulconatur** *Boehringer Ingelheim, Switz.†.*
Psyllium seed (p.1268·1).
*Constipation; gastrointestinal disorders.*

**Dulcosol** *Medifood, Ital.*
A nutritional supplement for infants (p.1417·1).

**Dulinas** *Alpes Chemie, Chile.*
Cod-liver oil (p.1425·2); zinc oxide (p.1163·2).
*Skin disorders.*

**Dull-C** *Freeda, USA.*
Ascorbic acid (p.1460·2).
*Scurvy; vitamin C deficiency.*

**Dul-X** *Biokosma, Braz.†.*
Methyl salicylate (p.59·3).
*Pain.*

**Dumesil** *Dumex-Alpharma, Denm.†.*
Ammonium chloride (p.1115·2); diphenhydramine hydrochloride (p.431·3); menthol (p.1711·3).
*Coughs; hypersensitivity reactions.*

**Dumex Lactose-Free**
*Dumex, Malaysia; Dumex, Singapore.*
Lactose-free infant feed (p.1417·1).
*Diarrhoea; lactose intolerance.*

**Dumex Plus** *Dumex, Singapore.*
A range of nutritional supplements (p.1417·1).

**Dumicoat**
*Dumex-Alpharma, Denm.†; Dumex-Alpharma, Fin.†; Dumex, Ger.†; Alpharma, Norw.†; Dumex-Alpharma, Swed.†; Alpharma, Switz.; Dumex, UK†.*
Miconazole (p.405·2).
*Candidal stomatitis.*

**Dumin** *Alpharma, Malaysia.*
Paracetamol (p.76·2).
*Fever; pain.*

**Dumirox**
*Solvay, Belg.; Solvay, Ital.; Solvay, Spain.*
Fluvoxamine maleate (p.298·2).
*Depression; obsessive-compulsive disorder.*

**Dumocalcin**
*Alpharma, Malaysia.*
Calcium hydrogen phosphate (p.1225·2); ergocalciferol (p.1462·1).
*Dental caries; rickets.*

*Alpharma, Singapore.*
Calcium hydrogen phosphate (p.1225·2); colecalciferol (p.1461·3).
*Nutritional supplement.*

**Dumocyclin** *Dumex-Alpharma, Denm.†.*
Tetracycline hydrochloride (p.266·2).
*Bacterial infections.*

**Dumolid** *Dumex-Alpharma, Denm.†.*
Nitrazepam (p.710·1).
*Epilepsy; sleep disorders.*

**Dumovit C**
*Alpharma, Malaysia; Alpharma, Singapore.*
Ascorbic acid (p.1460·2); sodium ascorbate (p.1460·2).
*Vitamin C supplement.*

**Dumovital** *Dumex, Port.†.*
Multivitamin and mineral preparation (p.1417·1).

**Dumoxin**
*Dumex-Alpharma, Denm.†; Aspen, S.Afr.*
Doxycycline hyclate (p.206·2).
*Bacterial infections.*

*Alpharma, Norw.; Dumex-Alpharma, Thai.*
Doxycycline (p.206·2).
*Bacterial infections.*

**Dumozol** *Alpharma, Port.*
Metronidazole (p.607·2).
*Anaerobic bacterial infections; rosacea.*

**Dumyrox**
*Solvay, Gr.; Solvay, Port.*
Fluvoxamine maleate (p.298·2).
*Depression; obsessive-compulsive disorder.*

**Duna** *Tedec Meiji, Spain.*
Pinazepam (p.715·3).
*Anxiety.*

**Dunason**
*Note. This name is used for preparations of different composition.*
*Alcon, Arg.*
Chondroitin sulfate; aprotinin (p.742·3).
*Dry eyes.*
*Alcon, Braz.*
Chondroitin sulfate (p.1670·2).
*Dry eyes.*

**Duncan** *Pharmaland, Thai.*
Chlorpromazine hydrochloride (p.675·2).
*Mania; schizophrenia; sedative.*

**Duncankil** *Duncan, Arg.*
Permethrin (p.1508·3).
*Pediculosis.*

**Dunox** *Duncan, Arg.*
Amoxicillin (p.155·3).
*Bacterial infections.*

**Duo Celloids CPIP** *Blackmores, Austral.†.*
Calcium phosphate (p.1225·3); iron phosphate.

**Duo Celloids CPMP** *Blackmores, Austral.†.*
Calcium phosphate (p.1225·3); magnesium phosphate (p.1228·1).

**Duo Celloids PCCP** *Blackmores, Austral.†.*
Potassium chloride (p.1232·2); calcium phosphate (p.1225·3).

**Duo Celloids PCIP** *Blackmores, Austral.†.*
Potassium chloride (p.1232·2); iron phosphate.

**Duo Celloids PCMP** *Blackmores, Austral.†.*
Potassium chloride (p.1232·2); magnesium phosphate (p.1228·1).

**Duo Celloids PPIP** *Blackmores, Austral.†.*
Potassium phosphate (p.1230·3); iron phosphate.

**Duo Celloids PPMP** *Blackmores, Austral.†.*
Potassium phosphate (p.1230·3); magnesium phosphate (p.1228·1).

**Duo Celloids PSMP** *Blackmores, Austral.†.*
Potassium sulfate (p.1232·2); magnesium phosphate (p.1228·1).

**Duo Celloids PSPC** *Blackmores, Austral.†.*
Potassium sulfate (p.1232·2); potassium chloride (p.1232·2).

**Duo Celloids SCF** *Blackmores, Austral.†.*
Silicon dioxide (p.1581·3); calcium fluoride.

**Duo Celloids SPCF** *Blackmores, Austral.†.*
Dibasic sodium phosphate (p.1231·1); calcium fluoride.

**Duo Celloids SPCP** *Blackmores, Austral.†.*
Dibasic sodium phosphate (p.1231·1); calcium phosphate (p.1225·3).

**Duo Celloids SPIP** *Blackmores, Austral.†.*
Dibasic sodium phosphate (p.1231·1); iron phosphate.

**Duo Celloids SPMP** *Blackmores, Austral.†.*
Dibasic sodium phosphate (p.1231·1); magnesium phosphate (p.1228·1).

**Duo Celloids SPPC** *Blackmores, Austral.†.*
Dibasic sodium phosphate (p.1231·1); potassium chloride (p.1232·2).

**Duo Celloids SPPP** *Blackmores, Austral.†.*
Dibasic sodium phosphate (p.1231·1); potassium phosphate (p.1230·3).

**Duo Celloids SPPS** *Blackmores, Austral.†.*
Dibasic sodium phosphate (p.1231·1); potassium sulfate (p.1232·2).

**Duo Celloids SPS** *Blackmores, Austral.†.*
Dibasic sodium phosphate (p.1231·1); silicon dioxide (p.1581·3).

**Duo Celloids SPSS** *Blackmores, Austral.†.*
Dibasic sodium phosphate (p.1231·1); sodium sulfate (p.1290·1).

**Duo Celloids SSMP** *Blackmores, Austral.†.*
Sodium sulfate (p.1290·1); magnesium phosphate (p.1228·1).

**Duo Celloids SSPC** *Blackmores, Austral.†.*
Sodium sulfate (p.1290·1); potassium chloride (p.1232·2).

**Duo Celloids SSS** *Blackmores, Austral.†.*
Sodium sulfate (p.1290·1); silicon dioxide (p.1581·3).

**Duo Decadron** *Sidus, Arg.*
Dexamethasone acetate (p.1097·1); dexamethasone sodium phosphate (p.1097·2).
*Corticosteroid.*

**Duo Gobens** *Normon, Spain†.*
Doxycycline hyclate (p.206·2).
Formerly contained doxycycline hyclate, chymotrypsin, and trypsin.
*Bacterial infections.*

**Duo Minoxi** *Finadiet, Arg.*
Ketoconazole (p.403·3); trolamine salicylate (p.95·3).
*Dandruff.*

**Duo Vizerul** *Montpellier, Arg.*
Ranitidine hydrochloride (p.1285·2); pirenzepine hydrochloride (p.488·1).
*Gastritis; gastro-oesophageal reflux; peptic ulcer.*

**Duobact** *Orion, Irl.*
Co-trimoxazole (p.199·3).
*Bacterial infections.*

**Duobar**
*Scientific Hospital Supplies, Austral.; Scientific Hospital Supplies, Irl.†; Nutricia, Ital.; Nutricia, NZ†; Scientific Hospital Supplies, NZ†; Scientific Hospital Supplies, UK.*
Food for special diets (p.1417·1).
*Protein restriction.*

**Duo-C** *Geymonat, Ital.*
Ascorbic acid (p.1460·2).
*Vitamin C deficiency; vitamin C supplement.*

**Duocal**
*Note. This name is used for preparations of different composition.*
*Scientific Hospital Supplies, Austral.; Nutricia, Fin.; SHS, Fr.; Scientific Hospital Supplies, Irl.; Piam, Ital.†; Nutricia, NZ; Scientific Hospital Supplies, NZ; SHS, Singapore; Scientific Hospital Supplies, UK.*
Food for special diets (p.1417·1).
*Serag-Wiessner, Ger.†.*
Glucose monohydrate (p.1432·2); xylitol (p.1469·1).
*Parenteral nutrition.*

**Duocet** *Mason, USA.*
Hydrocodone tartrate (p.45·1); paracetamol (p.76·2).
*Pain.*

**Duocort** *Orion, Fin.*
Hydrocortisone butyrate (p.1104·1); chlorhexidine gluconate (p.1173·2).
*Skin disorders.*

**Duoctrin** *Haller, Braz.*
Co-trimoxazole (p.199·3).
*Bacterial infections; Pneumocystis carinii pneumonia; protozoal infections.*

**Duoctrin Balsamico** *Haller, Braz.†.*
Co-trimoxazole (p.199·3); guaifenesin (p.1122·1); ammonium chloride (p.1115·2).
*Bacterial infections.*

**Duoctrin Enterico** *Haller, Braz.†.*
Co-trimoxazole (p.199·3); attapulgite (p.1251·1).
*Diarrhoea.*

**Duo-CVP**
*Aventis, Canad.; Aventis, Chile.*
Bioflavonoids (p.1688·2); ascorbic acid (p.1460·2).
*Capillary fragility; haemorrhage.*

**Duo-Cyp** *Keene, USA†.*
Estradiol cipionate (p.1550·1); testosterone cipionate (p.1569·3).
*Menopausal vasomotor symptoms; prevention of postpartum breast engorgement.*

**Duo-Decadron** *Prodome, Braz.*
Dexamethasone sodium phosphate (p.1097·2); dexamethasone acetate (p.1097·1).
*Parenteral corticosteroid.*

**Duoderm**
*Note. This name is used for preparations of different composition.*
*Bristol-Myers Squibb, Arg.; Convatec, Austral.; Bristol-Myers Squibb, Belg.†; Convatec, Fr.; Convatec, UK.*
Hydrocolloid dressing.
*Burns; ulcers; wounds.*
*Schering-Plough, S.Afr.*
Tolnaftate (p.410·1); nystatin (p.406·3).
*Fungal skin infections.*

**Duodexa N** *Kade, Ger.*
Dexamethasone (p.1097·1); dexamethasone sodium metasulfobenzoate (p.1097·2).
*Skin disorders.*

**Duodil** *Solvay, India.*
Chlorzoxazone (p.1392·3); paracetamol (p.76·2).
*Skeletal muscle spasm.*

**Duo-Extolen** *Specifar (Σπεσιφαρ), Gr.*
Zipeprol hydrochloride (p.1132·3).
*Cough.*

**Duofem** *Hexal, Ger.*
Levonorgestrel (p.1563·2).
*Progestogen-only oral contraceptive.*

**Duofer** *Andreabal, Switz.*
Ferrous fumarate (p.1427·3); ferrous gluconate (p.1428·1).
Ascorbic acid (p.1460·2) is included in this preparation to increase the absorption and availability of iron.
*Iron deficiency.*

**Duofer Fol** *Andreabal, Switz.*
Ferrous fumarate (p.1427·3); ferrous gluconate (p.1428·1); folic acid (p.1429·1).
Ascorbic acid (p.1460·2) is included in this preparation to increase the absorption and availability of iron.
*Iron and folic acid deficiency.*

**Duofilm**
*Note. This name is used for preparations of different composition.*
*Stiefel, Arg.; Stiefel, Austral.; Stiefel, Canad.; Stiefel, NZ; Schering-Plough, USA.*
*Topical gel:* Salicylic acid (p.1157·1).
*Corns; warts.*
*Stiefel, Arg.; Stiefel, Austral.; Stiefel, Chile.*
*Topical solution:* Salicylic acid (p.1157·1); lactic acid (p.1704·1); flexible collodion.
*Warts.*
*Sanova, Austria; Stiefel, Braz.; Stiefel, Canad.; Stiefel, Fr.; Stiefel, Ger.; Stiefel, Hong Kong; Stiefel, Irl.; Stiefel, Ital.; Stiefel, Malaysia; Stiefel, Mex.; Stiefel, NZ; Stiefel, Port.; Stiefel, S.Afr.; Stiefel, Singapore; Stiefel, Switz.; Stiefel, Thai.; Stiefel, UK.*
*Topical solution:* Salicylic acid (p.1157·1); lactic acid (p.1704·1).
*Calluses; corns; warts.*

**Duoflam**
*Note. This name is used for preparations of different composition.*
*Cristalia, Braz.*
Betamethasone dipropionate (p.1093·1); betamethasone sodium phosphate (p.1093·1).
*Corticosteroid.*
*Sigma, India.*
Ibuprofen (p.45·3); paracetamol (p.76·2).
*Fever; inflammation; pain.*

**Duoflam Gel** *Sigma, India.*
Diclofenac diethylamine (p.32·1); linseed oil (p.1707·2); methyl salicylate (p.59·3); menthol (p.1711·3).
*Musculoskeletal and soft-tissue disorders.*

**Duoflam Plus** *Sigma, India.*
Ibuprofen (p.45·3); paracetamol (p.76·2); caffeine (p.782·1).
*Fever; inflammation; pain.*

**Duoflex** *Rayere, Mex.*
Diclofenac sodium (p.32·1); carisoprodol (p.1392·1).
*Inflammation; musculoskeletal pain with muscle spasm; pain.*

**Duoform Novo** *Mauermann, Ger.*
Ruscus aculeatus.
*Haemorrhoids.*

**Duoforte**
*Stiefel, Arg.; Stiefel, Braz.; Stiefel, Canad.*
Salicylic acid (p.1157·1).
*Warts.*

**Duogas**
*Note. This name is used for preparations of different composition.*
*Bracco, Ital.*
Sodium bicarbonate (p.1223·2); anhydrous citric acid (p.1673·1); dimeticone (p.1289·2).
*Double-contrast radiography of the oesophagus and stomach.*
*Bracco, Port.†.*
Barium sulfate (p.1061·1).
*Macrophar, Thai.*
Omeprazole (p.1278·2).
*Gastro-oesophageal reflux; peptic ulcer; Zollinger-Ellison syndrome.*

**Duogastral** *ISM, Ital.†.*
Pirenzepine hydrochloride (p.488·1).
*Gastroduodenitis; peptic ulcer.*

**Duogink** *Duopharm, Ger.*
Ginkgo biloba (p.1692·3).
*Cerebrovascular disorders.*

**Duokapton** *Strallhofer, Austria.*
Aspirin (p.15·1); paracetamol (p.76·2).
*Fever; pain.*

**Duolax** *Almirall, Spain†.*
Lactulose (p.1269·1).
*Constipation; hepatic encephalopathy.*

**Duolaxan** *Carlo Erba OTC, Ital.*
Ispaghula (p.1268·1); liquid paraffin (p.1479·1).
*Constipation.*

**Duolin**
*Cipla, India; Rex, NZ.*
Ipratropium bromide (p.787·1); salbutamol (p.791·3).
*Obstructive airways disease.*

**Duolip**
*Ratiopharm, Austria; Merckle, Ger.; Mepha, Hong Kong; Mepha, Malaysia; Mepha, Switz.*
Etofylline clofibrate (p.914·2).
*Hyperlipidaemias.*

**Duolube** *Bausch & Lomb, Canad.*
White soft paraffin (p.1479·3); liquid paraffin (p.1479·1).
*Corneal dryness.*

**Duoluton** *Schering, Hong Kong†.*
Norgestrel (p.1563·2); ethinylestradiol (p.1553·2).
*Endometriosis; menstrual disorders.*

**Duoluton-L** *German Remedies, India.*
Levonorgestrel (p.1563·2); ethinylestradiol (p.1553·2).
*Endometriosis; menstrual disorders.*

**Duolys A** *Dicamed, Swed.†.*
A range of haemodialysis solutions (p.1221·1).

**Duolys B** *Dicamed, Swed.†.*
Sodium bicarbonate; disodium edetate (p.1221·1).
*Haemodialysis solution.*

**Duomet**
*Uniao Quimica, Braz.; Pacific, NZ†; Propan, S.Afr.†.*
Cimetidine (p.1255·3).
*Acid aspiration; gastric hyperacidity; gastrointestinal haemorrhage; gastro-oesophageal reflux; peptic ulcer; Zollinger-Ellison syndrome.*

**Duonalc** *ICN, Canad.*
Isopropyl alcohol (p.1184·3).
*Skin cleanser.*

**Duonalc-E** *ICN, Canad.*
Alcohol (p.1166·1); isopropyl alcohol (p.1184·3).
*Skin cleanser.*

**Duonasa** *Normon, Spain.*
Amoxicillin trihydrate (p.155·3); potassium clavulanate (p.193·3).
*Bacterial infections.*

**Duonate** *URL, USA.*
Phenylephrine tannate (p.1127·2); mepyramine tannate (p.437·1).
*Upper respiratory-tract disorders.*

**DuoNeb** *Dey, USA.*
Ipratropium bromide (p.787·1); salbutamol sulfate (p.791·3).
*Obstructive airways disease.*

**Duo-Ormogyn** *Amsa, Ital.†.*
Estradiol benzoate (p.1550·1); progesterone (p.1566·2).
*Menstrual disorders.*

**Duopack** *Danes, Arg.*
Salbutamol (p.791·3).
*Obstructive airways disease.*

**Duoplant**
*Note. This name is used for preparations of different composition.*
*Stiefel, Canad.*
Salicylic acid (p.1157·1); lactic acid (p.1704·1); formaldehyde (p.1179·3).
*Plantar warts.*
*Stiefel, Mex.; Schering-Plough, USA.*
Salicylic acid (p.1157·1).
*Moluscum contagiosum; warts.*

**Duoplant Gel** *Stiefel, Chile.*
Salicylic acid (p.1157·1).
*Warts.*

**Duoran** *Lisapharma, Ital.*
Ranitidine hydrochloride (p.1285·2).
*Acid aspiration; gastro-oesophageal reflux; gastrointestinal haemorrhage; peptic ulcer; Zollinger-Ellison syndrome.*

**Duorol** *Pharmacia, Spain.*
Paracetamol (p.76·2).
*Fever; pain.*

**Duo-Scabil** *Agis, Israel.*
Crotamiton (p.1145·1); sulfur (p.1158·2).
*Scabies.*

**Duotec** *Boehringer Ingelheim, Arg.*
Fenoterol hydrobromide (p.785·2) sodium cromoglicate (p.795·3).
*Obstructive airways disease.*

**Duoton** *TP, Thai.*
Progesterone (p.1566·2); estradiol benzoate (p.1550·1).
*Menstrual disorders.*

**Duo-Trach Kit** *Astra, USA.*
Lidocaine hydrochloride (p.1377·3).
*Local anaesthesia.*

**Duotric** *Asian Pharm, Thai.*
Cimetidine (p.1255·3).
*Gastric hyperacidity; peptic ulcer.*

**Duova** *Orion, Fr.*
Estradiol valerate (p.1550·2); medroxyprogesterone acetate (p.1557·2).
*Menopausal disorders.*

**Duoval** *Saval, Chile.*
Chlorphenamine maleate (p.427·3); pseudoephedrine hydrochloride (p.1129·2).
*Respiratory-tract congestion.*

**Duovax** *Merck Sharp & Dohme, Belg.†.*
A live measles and mumps vaccine (Enders' attenuated Edmonston strain and Jeryl Lynn B strain, respectively) (p.1624·3).
*Active immunisation.*

**Duovent**
*Boehringer Ingelheim, Belg.; Boehringer de Angeli, Braz.; Boehringer Ingelheim, Canad.; Boehringer Ingelheim, Irl.; Boehringer Ingelheim, Ital.; Boehringer Ingelheim, Malaysia; Boehringer Ingelheim, NZ†; Boehringer Ingelheim, S.Afr.; Boehringer Ingelheim, Singapore; Boehringer Ingelheim, UK.*
Fenoterol hydrobromide (p.785·2); ipratropium bromide (p.787·1).
*Obstructive airways disease.*

**Duoventrin** *Schwörer, Ger.*
Bismuth subnitrate (p.1252·2); linseed (p.1707·2); lactose.
*Gastrointestinal disorders.*

**Duoventrinetten N** *Schwörer, Ger.*
Aluminium hydroxide-magnesium carbonate co-dried gel (p.1250·1); magnesium trisilicate (p.1272·3); magnesium hydroxide (p.1272·2).
*Gastrointestinal hyperacidity.*

**Duovir**
*Cristalia, Braz.; Cipla, India.*
Lamivudine (p.648·2); zidovudine (p.658·2).
*HIV infection.*

**Duovisc**
*Alcon, Austral.; Alcon, Ger.; Alcon, Hong Kong; Alcon, S.Afr.; Alcon, Singapore; Alcon, Thai.*
1 Syringe, sodium hyaluronate (p.1697·3) (Provisc); 1 syringe, sodium hyaluronate; chondroitin sulfate sodium (p.1670·2) (Viscoat).
*Adjunct in eye surgery.*

**Duovitan** *Asta Medica, Austria.*
Allopurinol (p.412·2); benzbromarone (p.414·3).
*Gout; hyperuricaemia.*

**Duozol** *Blausiegel, Braz.*
Tinidazole (p.617·1); tioconazole (p.409·3).
*Vaginal infections.*

**Duphalac**
*Solvay, Austral.; Solvay, Austria; Solvay, Belg.; Solvay, Canad.†; Grunenthal, Chile; Solvay, Fin.; Solvay, Fr.; Solvay, Gr.; Solvay, Hong Kong; Solvay, Irl.; Solvay, Ital.; Solvay, Malaysia; Vemedia, Neth.; Solvay, Norw.; Solvay, NZ†; Solvay, Port.; Solvay, S.Afr.; Solvay, Singapore; Solvay, Spain; Solvay, Swed.; Solvay, Switz.; Solvay, Thai.; Solvay, UK; Solvay, USA.*
Lactulose (p.1269·1).
*Constipation; hepatic encephalopathy; salmonella enteritis.*

**Duphaston**
*Solvay, Austral.; Solvay, Austria; Solvay, Belg.; Grunenthal, Chile; Solvay, Fr.; Solvay, Ger.; Solvay, Gr.; Solvay, Hong Kong; Solvay, India; Solvay, Irl.; Solvay, Malaysia; Solvay, Neth.; Duphar, NZ; Solvay, Port.; Solvay, S.Afr.; Solvay, Singapore; Solvay, Spain†; Solvay, Swed.; Solvay, Switz.; Solvay, Thai.; Solvay, UK.*
Dydrogesterone (p.1549·2).
*Dysfunctional uterine bleeding; endometriosis; female infertility; menopausal disorders; menstrual disorders; progestogen deficiency; threatened or recurrent miscarriage.*

**Duplamin** *Bruschettini, Ital.†.*
Promethazine hydrochloride (p.439·1).
*Skin irritation.*

**Duplex**
*Note. This name is used for preparations of different composition.*
*SBL, Swed.†.*
A diphtheria and tetanus vaccine (p.1613·1).
*Active immunisation.*

*C & M, USA.*
Skin cleanser.

**Duplex T** *C & M, USA†.*
Coal tar (p.1159·2).
*Scalp disorders.*

**Duplexcillina** *Metapharma, Ital.†.*
Ampicillin (p.157·1); dicloxacillin (p.205·2).
*Bacterial infections.*

**Duplexil** *Euroformaco, Ital.†.*
Ampicillin trihydrate (p.157·2); dicloxacillin sodium (p.205·2).
*Bacterial infections.*

**Duplicalcio** *Medical, Spain†.*
Calcium levulinate (p.1225·3); vitamin B substances (p.1417·1); ergocalciferol (p.1462·1); liver extract; isoniazid (p.222·2).
*Anaemias; bone and dental disorders; calcium deficiency; osteomalacia; rickets; tonic.*

**Duplicalcio 150** *Medical, Spain†.*
Isoniazid (p.222·2); pyridoxine (p.1457·2); calcium gluconate (p.1225·2).
*Tuberculosis.*

**Duplicalcio B12** *Medical, Spain.*
Calcium gluconate (p.1225·2); cyanocobalamin (p.1458·2); isoniazid (p.222·2).
*Anaemias; tonic; tuberculosis.*

**Duplicalcio Hidraz** *Medical, Spain†.*
Calcium gluconate (p.1225·2); calcium levulinate (p.1225·3); isoniazid (p.222·2).
*Tonic; tuberculosis.*

**Duplide** *Euro-Labor, Port.†; Grunenthal, Port.†.*
Diltiazem hydrochloride (p.900·1).

**Duplobar** *Enila, Braz.†.*
Barium sulfate (p.1061·1).
*Contrast medium for gastrointestinal radiography.*

**Duplocitrin** *QIF, Braz.†.*
Neomycin (p.235·1); bacitracin (p.161·3).
*Skin infections.*

**Duplo-Penicillin** *Teva, Israel.*
Procaine benzylpenicillin (p.246·1); benzylpenicillin (p.163·2).
*Bacterial infections.*

**Duplotrast** *Gerot, Austria.*
Sodium bicarbonate (p.1223·2); simeticone (p.1289·2).
*Adjunct in double contrast radiography.*

**Duplotrast Z** *Gerot, Austria.*
Citric acid (p.1673·1); sodium bicarbonate (p.1223·2); simeticone (p.1289·2).
*Adjunct in double contrast radiography.*

**Duponil** *Inkeysa, Spain†.*
Ammonium chloride (p.1115·2); codeine phosphate (p.27·1); diphenhydramine hydrochloride (p.431·3); ephedrine hydrochloride (p.1120·1).
*Respiratory-tract disorders.*

**dura AL** *Merck dura, Ger.*
Allopurinol (p.412·2).
*Gout; hyperuricaemia; renal calculi.*

**dura AX** *Durachemie, Ger.†.*
Amoxicillin trihydrate (p.155·3).
*Bacterial infections.*

**duraampicillin** *Durachemie, Ger.†.*
Ampicillin trihydrate (p.157·2).
*Bacterial infections.*

**Durabezur** *Durachemie, Ger.†.*
Bezafibrate (p.873·2).
*Hyperlipidaemias.*

**Durabiotic** *Teva, Israel.*
Benzathine benzylpenicillin (p.162·3).
*Bacterial infections.*

**Durabolin**
*Infar, India; Organon, Israel†; Organon, USA.*
Nandrolone phenylpropionate (p.1561·3).
*Anabolic; breast cancer; osteoporosis.*

**Durabronchal** *Merck dura, Ger.*
Acetylcysteine (p.1112·3).
*Respiratory-tract disorders associated with increased or viscous mucus.*

**Duracain** *Sintetica, Switz.*
Bupivacaine hydrochloride (p.1371·1).
*Local anaesthesia.*

**Duracaine**
*AstraZeneca, Arg.; AstraZeneca, Chile.*
Bupivacaine hydrochloride (p.1371·1).
Adrenaline (p.852·2) is included in some injections as a vasoconstrictor to diminish absorption and localise the effect of the local anaesthetic.
*Local anaesthesia.*

**Duracare**
*Allergan, Austral.†.*
Disinfecting and storage solution for hard and gas permeable contact lenses (p.1164·2).

*Allergan, Austria†.*
Disinfecting and storage solution for hard contact lenses (p.1164·2).

*Allergan, Braz.*
Polyvinyl alcohol (p.1581·1) (p.1164·2).
*Cleansing solution for contact lenses.*

*Allergan, Canad.†.*
Polyvinyl alcohol (p.1581·1) (p.1164·2).
*A wetting and soaking solution for gas permeable contact lenses.*

*Allergan, Ger.†.*
Polyvinyl alcohol (p.1581·1); disodium edetate (p.1037·3)(p.1164·2).
*Disinfection and storage solution for gas-permeable hard contact lenses.*

*Blairex, USA.*
Cleansing solution for soft contact lenses (p.1164·2).

**duracebrol** *Merck dura, Ger.†.*
Nicergoline (p.1719·3).
*Mental function disorders.*

**Duracef**
*Bristol-Myers Squibb, Austria; Bristol-Myers Squibb, Belg.; Bristol-Myers Squibb, Fin.; Bristol-Myers Squibb, Hong Kong; Bristol-Myers Squibb, Israel; Bristol-Myers Squibb, Mex.; Bristol-Myers Squibb, S.Afr.†; Juste, Spain; Bristol-Myers Squibb, Switz.†.*
Cefadroxil (p.167·2).
*Bacterial infections.*

**duracetamol** *Merck dura, Ger.†.*
Paracetamol (p.76·2).
*Fever; pain.*

**Duraclean**
*Allergan, Austral.†; Allergan, Canad.†.*
Cleansing solution for hard and gas permeable contact lenses (p.1164·2).

**Duraclon** *aai, USA.*
Clonidine hydrochloride (p.885·2).
*Pain.*

**Duracoll** *Schering-Plough, Belg.*
Gentamicin sulfate (p.217·1); collagen (bovine) (p.1674·3).
*Bone infections.*

**duracoron** *Merck dura, Ger.*
Molsidomine (p.961·3).
*Angina pectoris.*

**Duracreme** *LRC Products, UK†.*
Nonoxinol 9 (p.1413·3).
*Contraceptive.*

**duracroman** *Merck dura, Ger.*
Sodium cromoglicate (p.795·3).
*Allergic conjunctivitis; allergic rhinitis.*

**duradermal** *Merck dura, Ger.*
Bufexamac (p.21·3).
*Skin disorders.*

**duradiuret** *Merck dura, Ger.*
Triamterene (p.1016·2); hydrochlorothiazide (p.933·2).
*Hypertension; oedema.*

**Duradoce** *Atlantis, Mex.*
Hydroxocobalamin (p.1458·2).
*Neuritis; pernicious anaemia.*

**Duradox** *Julphar, UAE.*
Doxycycline hyclate (p.206·2).
*Bacterial infections.*

**duradoxal** *Durachemie, Ger.†.*
Doxycycline (p.206·2) or doxycycline hyclate (p.206·2).
*Bacterial infections.*

**Duradrin** *Duramed, USA.*
Isometheptene mucate (p.1702·1); dichloralphenazone (p.697·1); paracetamol (p.76·2).
*Migraine; tension headache.*

**duraerythromycin** *Merck dura, Ger.†.*
Erythromycin stearate (p.208·2).
*Bacterial infections.*

**durafenat** *Merck dura, Ger.*
Fenofibrate (p.915·2).
*Hyperlipidaemias.*

**Duraflor** *Pharmascience, Canad.†.*
Sodium fluoride (p.1444·3).

**Duraflu** *Proethic, USA.*
Dextromethorphan hydrobromide (p.1117·3); guaifenesin (p.1122·1); pseudoephedrine hydrochloride (p.1129·2); paracetamol (p.76·2).
*Upper respiratory-tract disorders.*

**durafungol** *Merck dura, Ger.*
Clotrimazole (p.396·2).
*Fungal skin infections; vaginal infections.*

**durafurid** *Merck dura, Ger.*
Furosemide (p.919·3) (p.921·2).
*Hypertension; oedema.*

**Duragel** *SSL, UK.*
Nonoxinol 9 (p.1413·3).
*Contraceptive.*

**duragentamicin** *Merck dura, Ger.†.*
Gentamicin sulfate (p.217·1).
*Bacterial infections.*

**Duragesic**
*Janssen-Ortho, Canad.; Janssen, USA.*
Fentanyl (p.40·1).
*Pain.*

**Dura-Gest** *DJ, USA†.*
Phenylephrine hydrochloride (p.1126·3); phenylpropanolamine hydrochloride (p.1127·3); guaifenesin (p.1122·1).
*Coughs and cold symptoms; nasal congestion.*

**duraglucon N** *Merck dura, Ger.*
Glibenclamide (p.331·2).
*Diabetes mellitus.*

**duraH2** *Merck dura, Ger.*
Cimetidine (p.1255·3).
*Gastro-oesophageal reflux; peptic ulcer; Zollinger-Ellison syndrome.*

**Durahist** *Proethic, USA.*
Pseudoephedrine hydrochloride (p.1129·2); chlorphenamine maleate (p.427·3); hyoscine methonitrate (p.483·3).
*Upper respiratory-tract disorders.*

**dura-Ibu** *Durachemie, Ger.†.*
Ibuprofen (p.45·3).
*Inflammation; musculoskeletal, joint, and soft-tissue disorders; pain.*

**duralbuprofen** *Merck dura, Ger.†.*
Ibuprofen (p.45·3).
*Gout; inflammation; musculoskeletal, joint, and soft-tissue disorders.*

**durakne** *Merck dura, Ger.†.*
Minocycline hydrochloride (p.231·3).
*Acne.*

**Duralex** *American Urologicals, USA.*
Pseudoephedrine hydrochloride (p.1129·2); chlorphenamine maleate (p.427·3).
*Upper respiratory-tract symptoms.*

**Duralgin** *Ethypharm, Denm.†.*
Morphine sulfate (p.60·2).
*Pain.*

**duralipon** *Merck dura, Ger.*
Thioctic acid (p.1754·3).
*Diabetic polyneuropathy.*

**Duralith** *Janssen-Ortho, Canad.*
Lithium carbonate (p.301·1).
*Bipolar disorder.*

**Duralmor** *Sanfer, Mex.*
Morphine sulfate (p.60·2).
*Pain.*

**Duralone** *Hauck, USA†.*
Methylprednisolone acetate (p.1106·1).
*Corticosteroid.*

**duralopid** *Merck dura, Ger.*
Loperamide hydrochloride (p.1271·1).
*Diarrhoea.*

**duralozam** *Merck dura, Ger.*
Lorazepam (p.704·1).
*Anxiety; sleep disorders.*

**duraMCP** *Merck dura, Ger.†.*
Metoclopramide hydrochloride (p.1274·3).
*Gastrointestinal disorders.*

**duramipress** *Merck dura, Ger.*
Prazosin hydrochloride (p.985·1).
*Heart failure; hypertension; Raynaud's syndrome.*

**Duramist Plus** *Pfeiffer, USA.*
Oxymetazoline hydrochloride (p.1126·1).
*Nasal congestion.*

**duramonitat** *Merck dura, Ger.*
Isosorbide mononitrate (p.942·1).
*Angina pectoris; heart failure.*

**Duramorph**
*Gray, Arg.; Elkins-Sinn, USA; Baxter, USA.*
Morphine sulfate (p.60·2).
*Pain.*

**duramucal** *Merck dura, Ger.*
Ambroxol hydrochloride (p.1114·3).
*Respiratory-tract disorders associated with increased or viscous mucus.*

**Duran** *Nakorn, Thai.*
Ibuprofen (p.45·3).
*Fever; inflammation; musculoskeletal and joint disorders; pain.*

**Duranest**
*AstraZeneca, Fr.†; Astra, Ger.†; Astra, USA†.*
Etidocaine hydrochloride (p.1376·3).
Adrenaline acid tartrate (p.852·2) is included in some injections as a vasoconstrictor to diminish absorption and localise the effect of the local anaesthetic.
*Local anaesthesia.*

**duranifin** *Merck dura, Ger.*
Nifedipine (p.966·2).
*Angina pectoris; hypertension; Raynaud's syndrome.*

**duranifin Sali** *Merck dura, Ger.*
Nifedipine (p.966·2); mefruside (p.951·3).
*Hypertension.*

**Duranil** *Interbelle, Arg.*
Hexetidine (p.1182·1).
*Mouth and throat disorders.*

**duranitrat** *Merck dura, Ger.*
Isosorbide dinitrate (p.941·1).
*Angina pectoris; heart failure; pulmonary hypertension.*

**durapaediat** *Merck dura, Ger.†.*
Erythromycin ethyl succinate (p.208·1).
*Bacterial infections.*

**Durapen** *De Mayo, Braz.*
Ampicillin benzathine (p.158·1); ampicillin sodium (p.157·1).
*Bacterial infections.*

**Durapen Balsamico** *De Mayo, Braz.†.*
Ampicillin (p.157·1); guaiacol (p.1122·1); cineole (p.1672·1); niaouli oil (p.1719·3).
*Bacterial infections.*

**durapenicillin** *Merck dura, Ger.*
Phenoxymethylpenicillin potassium (p.242·1).
*Bacterial infections.*

**durapental** *Merck dura, Ger.*
Pentoxifylline (p.979·3).
*Peripheral vascular disorders.*

**Duraphat**
*Austrodent, Austria; Colgate-Palmolive, Denm.; Inpharma, Fin.; Colgate-Palmolive, Ger.; Woelm, Israel; Colgate-Palmolive, Norw.; Colgate-Palmolive, Swed.; Colgate-Palmolive, UK.*
Sodium fluoride (p.1444·3).
*Dental caries prophylaxis; sensitive teeth.*

**duraphyllin** *Merck dura, Ger.*
Theophylline (p.798·3).
*Obstructive airways disease.*

**durapindol** *Merck dura, Ger.*
Pindolol (p.983·2).
*Cardiac hyperkinesis; hypertension; ischaemic heart disease.*

**durapirenz** *Durachemie, Ger.†.*
Pirenzepine hydrochloride (p.488·1).
*Gastrointestinal disorders.*

**durapirox** *Merck dura, Ger.*
Piroxicam (p.84·2).
*Gout; musculoskeletal, joint, and soft-tissue disorders.*

**durapitrop** *Merck dura, Ger.†.*
Piracetam (p.1732·1).
*Mental function disorders.*

**duraprednisolon** *Merck dura, Ger.*
Prednisolone (p.1108·1).
*Corticosteroid.*

**Duraprox** *Aventis Pasteur, Chile.*
Oxaprozin (p.75·1).
*Gout; musculoskeletal, joint, and peri-articular disorders.*

**durarese** *Merck dura, Ger.*
Amiloride hydrochloride (p.858·2); hydrochlorothiazide (p.933·2).
*Hypertension; oedema.*

**Durasal** *Prasco, USA.*
Pseudoephedrine hydrochloride (p.1129·2); guaifenesin (p.1122·1).
*Upper respiratory-tract disorders.*

**Durascreen**
*Note. This name is used for preparations of different composition.*
*Pharmascience, Canad.*
*SPF 15:* Octinoxate (p.1154·3); octisalate (p.1154·3); oxybenzone (p.1154·3); titanium dioxide (p.1160·3).
*SPF 30:* Octinoxate (p.1154·3); octisalate (p.1154·3); oxybenzone (p.1154·3); titanium dioxide (p.1160·3); ensulizole (p.1147·1).
*Sunscreen.*

*Pierre Fabre, USA.*
*SPF 15:* Octinoxate (p.1154·3); octisalate (p.1154·3); oxybenzone (p.1154·3).
*SPF 30:* Octinoxate (p.1154·3); octisalate (p.1154·3); oxybenzone (p.1154·3); ensulizole (p.1147·1); titanium dioxide (p.1160·3).
*Sunscreen.*

**durasilymarin** *Merck dura, Ger.*
Silybum marianum (p.1043·3).
*Liver disorders.*

**Durasina** *SmithKline Beecham, Spain†.*
Chlorphenamine maleate (p.427·3); phenylpropanolamine hydrochloride (p.1127·3).
*Nasal congestion; sinus congestion.*

**Durasolets** *SMB, Chile.*
White soft paraffin (p.1479·3); liquid paraffin (p.1479·1).
*Dry eyes.*

**durasoptin** *Merck dura, Ger.*
Verapamil hydrochloride (p.1019·1).
*Angina pectoris; arrhythmias; hypertension.*

**duraspiron** *Merck dura, Ger.*
Spironolactone (p.1003·1).
*Hyperaldosteronism; liver cirrhosis with ascites; oedema.*

**duraspiron-comp** *Merck dura, Ger.*
Spironolactone (p.1003·1); furosemide (p.919·3).
*Ascites; hyperaldosteronism; hypertension; oedema.*

**duratamoxifen** *Durachemie, Ger.†.*
Tamoxifen citrate (p.584·1).
*Breast cancer.*

**Dura-Tap/PD** *Dura, USA.*
Chlorphenamine maleate (p.427·3); pseudoephedrine hydrochloride (p.1129·2).
*Allergic rhinitis; nasal congestion.*

**Duratears**
*Note. This name is used for preparations of different composition.*
*Alcon, Austral.; Alcon, Switz.†.*
Liquid paraffin (p.1479·1); wool fat (p.1483·1).
*Dry eyes.*

*Alcon, Belg.; Alcon, Canad.; Alcon, Chile; Alkon (Αλκον), Gr.; Alcon, Hong Kong; Alcon, Israel; Alcon, Singapore; Alcon, Thai.*
White soft paraffin (p.1479·3); wool fat (p.1483·1); liquid paraffin (p.1479·1).
*Dry eyes.*

*Alcon, NZ†.*
Liquid paraffin (p.1479·1); white soft paraffin (p.1479·3).
*Dry eyes.*

*Alcon, S.Afr.*
Anhydrous liquid lanolin (p.1483·1).
*Dry eyes.*

**Duratears Naturale**
*Alcon, Malaysia; Alcon, USA.*
Liquid paraffin (p.1479·1); wool fat (p.1483·1); white soft paraffin (p.1479·3).
*Dry eyes.*

**duratenol** *Merck dura, Ger.*
Atenolol (p.865·2).
*Angina pectoris; arrhythmias; hypertension.*

**duratenol comp** Merck dura, Ger.
Atenolol (p.865·2); chlortalidone (p.882·3).
*Hypertension.*

**Durater** Senosiain, Mex.
Famotidine (p.1265·2).
*Gastro-oesophageal reflux; gastrointestinal hyperacidity; peptic ulcer; Zollinger-Ellison syndrome.*

**Duratest** Roberts, USA†; Hauck, USA†.
Testosterone cipionate (p.1569·3).
*Breast cancer; delayed puberty (males); male hypogonadism.*

**Durateston** Organon, Braz.
Testosterone propionate (p.1570·1); testosterone phenylpropionate (p.1570·1); testosterone isocaproate (p.1570·1); testosterone caproate (p.1571·2).
*Anaemia; androgenic; breast cancer; delayed puberty; male hypogonadism.*

**Duratestrin** Hauck, USA†.
Estradiol cipionate (p.1550·1); testosterone cipionate (p.1569·3).
*Menopausal vasomotor symptoms; prevention of postpartum breast engorgement.*

**Durathate** Roberts, USA†; Hauck, USA†.
Testosterone enantate (p.1570·1).
*Breast cancer; delayed puberty (males); male hypogonadism.*

**duratimol** Durachemie, Ger.†.
Timolol maleate (p.1012·2).
*Glaucoma; ocular hypertension.*

**Duration**
Schering-Plough, Hong Kong; Schering-Plough, USA.
Oxymetazoline hydrochloride (p.1126·1).
*Nasal congestion.*

**Duratirs** Alcon, Ital.
Liquid paraffin (p.1479·1).
*Dry eyes.*

**Duratocin**
Ferring, Arg.; Ferring, Canad.
Carbetocin (p.1320·2).
*Postpartum haemorrhage; uterine atony.*

**Duratuss** UCB, USA†.
Pseudoephedrine hydrochloride (p.1129·2); guaifenesin (p.1122·1).
*Nasal congestion.*

**Duratuss DM** UCB, USA†.
Dextromethorphan hydrobromide (p.1117·3); guaifenesin (p.1122·1).
*Coughs.*

**Duratuss G** UCB, USA†.
Guaifenesin (p.1122·1).
*Respiratory-tract congestion.*

**Duratuss GP** UCB, USA†.
Guaifenesin (p.1122·1); pseudoephedrine hydrochloride (p.1129·2).
*Coughs.*

**Duratuss HD** UCB, USA†.
Pseudoephedrine hydrochloride (p.1129·2); guaifenesin (p.1122·1); hydrocodone tartrate (p.45·1).
*Coughs; nasal congestion.*

**duraultra** Ciba Vision, Ger.
Vitamin A (p.1451·2); actinoquinol sodium (p.1647·2); naphazoline nitrate (p.1124·3).
*Eye disorders.*

**Dura-Vent** DJ, USA†.
Phenylpropanolamine hydrochloride (p.1127·3); guaifenesin (p.1122·1).
*Respiratory-tract congestion.*

**Dura-Vent/A** Dura, USA†.
Phenylpropanolamine hydrochloride (p.1127·3); chlorphenamine maleate (p.427·3).
*Upper respiratory-tract symptoms.*

**Dura-Vent/DA** Dura, USA.
Chlorphenamine maleate (p.427·3); phenylephrine hydrochloride (p.1126·3); hyoscine methonitrate (p.483·3).
*Upper respiratory-tract symptoms.*

**duravolten** Merck dura, Ger.
Diclofenac sodium (p.32·1).
*Gout; inflammation; musculoskeletal, joint, and soft-tissue disorders; pain.*

**durazanil** Merck dura, Ger.
Bromazepam (p.671·3).
*Anxiety disorders; insomnia.*

**durazepam** Merck dura, Ger.
Oxazepam (p.712·2).
*Anxiety disorders; sleep disorders.*

**durazidum** Merck dura, Ger.
Magnesium hydroxide gel (p.1272·2); aluminium hydroxide gel (p.1249·2).
*Gastrointestinal disorders.*

**Durazina** Maggioni, Ital.†.
Chlorphenamine maleate (p.427·3); phenylpropanolamine hydrochloride (p.1127·3).
*Nasal congestion.*

**Dura-Zok** Durascan, Denm.
Metoprolol succinate (p.957·1).
*Angina pectoris; arrhythmias; hypertension; hyperthyroidism; migraine; myocardial infarction.*

**Durbis**
Aventis, Denm.; Hoechst Marion Roussel, Fin.†; Aventis, Norw.; Aventis, Swed.
Disopyramide (p.903·3) or disopyramide phosphate (p.903·3).
*Arrhythmias.*

**Durekal** Leo, Fin.
Potassium chloride (p.1232·2).
*Hypokalaemia.*

**Dur-Elix**
3M, Austral.†; 3M, S.Afr.†.
Bromhexine hydrochloride (p.1115·3).
*Respiratory-tract disorders associated with viscous mucus.*

**Dur-Elix Plus** 3M, Austral.†.
Bromhexine hydrochloride (p.1115·3); pseudoephedrine hydrochloride (p.1129·2).
*Nasal congestion; respiratory-tract disorders associated with excess mucus.*

**Duremesan** Streuli, Switz.
*Suppositories:* Meclozine hydrochloride (p.436·3).
*Tablets:* Meclozine hydrochloride (p.436·3); caffeine (p.782·1).
*Nausea and vomiting.*

**Duremid** Chobet, Arg.
Indapamide (p.938·2).
*Hypertension.*

**Durex Sensilube** SSL, UK.
Vaginal lubricant.
Formerly known as Senselle.

**Duricef**
Bristol, Canad.; Bristol-Myers Squibb, Singapore; Bristol-Myers Squibb, Thai.†; Bristol-Myers Squibb, USA.
Cefadroxil (p.167·2).
*Bacterial infections.*

**Duride**
Alphapharm, Austral.; Pacific, NZ.
Isosorbide mononitrate (p.942·1).
*Angina pectoris.*

**Durin** Farmasa, Mex.†.
Bumetanide (p.877·2).

**Durobac** Pharmaceutical Enterprises, S.Afr.
Co-trimoxazole (p.199·3).
*Bacterial infections.*

**Duroferon**
AstraZeneca, Fin.; AstraZeneca, Norw.; Hassle, Swed.
Ferrous sulfate (p.1428·2).
Ascorbic acid (p.1460·2) may be included in this preparation to increase the absorption and availability of iron.
*Iron deficiency; iron-deficiency anaemia.*

**Duroferon Vitamin**
Astra, Denm.†; Hassle, Swed.
Multivitamin preparation with iron (p.1417·1).
*Iron-deficiency anaemia in pregnancy.*

**Durogesic**
Janssen-Cilag, Arg.; Janssen-Cilag, Austral.; Janssen-Cilag, Austria; Janssen-Cilag, Belg.; Janssen-Cilag, Braz.; Janssen-Cilag, Chile; Janssen-Cilag, Denm.; Janssen-Cilag, Fin.; Janssen-Cilag, Fr.; Janssen-Cilag, Ger.; Janssen-Cilag, Gr.; Janssen, Hong Kong; Janssen-Cilag, India; Janssen-Cilag, Irl.; Janssen-Cilag, Israel; Janssen-Cilag, Ital.; Janssen-Cilag, Malaysia; Janssen, Mex.; Janssen-Cilag, Neth.; Janssen-Cilag, Norw.; Janssen-Cilag, NZ; Janssen-Cilag, Port.; Janssen-Cilag, S.Afr.; Janssen-Cilag, Singapore; Janssen-Cilag, Spain; Janssen-Cilag, Swed.; Janssen-Cilag, Switz.; Janssen-Cilag, Thai.; Janssen-Cilag, UK.
Fentanyl (p.40·1).
*Pain.*

**Duro-K** Biochemie, Austral.
Potassium chloride (p.1232·2).
*Hypokalaemia.*

**Durolax** Boehringer Ingelheim, Austral.
Bisacodyl (p.1251·3).
*Bowel evacuation; constipation.*

**Durolax X-Pack** Boehringer Ingelheim, Austral.
*Combination pack:* 3 Tablets, bisacodyl (p.1251·3); 1 suppository, bisacodyl; 1 sachet, citric acid (p.1673·1); heavy magnesium carbonate (p.1272·1).
*Bowel evacuation.*

**Durolax SP** Boehringer Ingelheim, Austral.
Sodium picosulfate (p.1289·3).
*Constipation.*

**Duromine**
3M, Austral.; 3M, Hong Kong; 3M, Malaysia; 3M, NZ; 3M, S.Afr.; 3M, Singapore; 3M, Thai.; 3M, UK†.
Phentermine (as an ion-exchange resin complex) (p.1592·2).
*Obesity.*

**Duronitrin** AstraZeneca, Ital.
Isosorbide mononitrate (p.942·1).
*Angina pectoris; cardiac stenosis; heart failure; myocardial infarction.*

**Durotan** Lilly, Ger.
Xipamide (p.1029·2); reserpine (p.995·1).
*Hypertension.*

**Duro-Tuss**
3M, Austral.; 3M, Hong Kong; 3M, Malaysia; 3M, NZ; 3M, Singapore.
Pholcodine (p.1128·3).
*Coughs.*

**Duro-Tuss Cold & Allergy** 3M, Austral.
Phenylephrine hydrochloride (p.1126·3); chlorphenamine maleate (p.427·3).
*Upper respiratory-tract congestion.*

**Duro-Tuss Cough Lozenges** 3M, Austral.
Pholcodine (p.1128·3); cetylpyridinium chloride (p.1173·1).
*Coughs; sore throat.*

**Duro-Tuss Decongestant**
3M, Austral.; 3M, Hong Kong; 3M, NZ; 3M, Singapore.
Pholcodine (p.1128·3); pseudoephedrine hydrochloride (p.1129·2).
*Coughs; nasal congestion.*

**Duro-Tuss Expectorant**
3M, Austral.; 3M, Hong Kong; 3M, NZ; 3M, Singapore.
Pholcodine (p.1128·3); bromhexine hydrochloride (p.1115·3).
*Coughs.*

**Duro-Tuss Lozenges** 3M, NZ.
Pholcodine (p.1128·3); cetylpyridinium chloride (p.1173·1).
*Coughs; sore throat.*

**Duro-Tuss Mucolytic** 3M, NZ.
Bromhexine hydrochloride (p.1115·3).
Formerly known as Dur-Elix.
*Respiratory-tract congestion.*

**Duro-Tuss Mucolytic Cough Liquid** 3M, Austral.
Bromhexine hydrochloride (p.1115·3).
*Respiratory-tract congestion.*

**Duro-Tuss Sinus** 3M, Austral.
Bromhexine hydrochloride (p.1115·3); pseudoephedrine hydrochloride (p.1129·2).
*Upper respiratory-tract congestion.*

**Durvitan** Seid, Spain.
Caffeine (p.782·1).
*Asthenia.*

**Dusil**
Alpharma, Malaysia; Alpharma, Singapore.
Aspirin (p.15·1).
*Fever; pain.*

**Dusodril**
Merck, Austria; Merck, Ger.
Naftidrofuryl oxalate (p.964·1).
*Peripheral vascular disorders; vascular disorders of the brain, ears, and eyes.*

**Duspatal**
Grunenthal, Chile; Solvay, Ger.; Solvay, Ital.; Solvay, Neth.; Solvay, Port.
Mebeverine embonate (p.1273·1) or mebeverine hydrochloride (p.1273·1).
*Gastrointestinal spasm; irritable bowel syndrome.*

**Duspatalin**
Byk, Arg.; Solvay, Belg.; Sintofarma, Braz.; Solvay, Denm.; Solvay, Fr.; Solvay, Gr.; Solvay, Hong Kong; Solvay, Malaysia; Solvay, Singapore; Solvay, Spain; Solvay, Switz.
Mebeverine embonate (p.1273·1) or mebeverine hydrochloride (p.1273·1).
*Gastrointestinal spasm; irritable bowel syndrome.*

**Duspatin** Berlin Pharm, Thai.
Mebeverine hydrochloride (p.1273·1).
*Gastrointestinal pain and spasm.*

**Dutacor** Durascan, Denm.
Sotalol hydrochloride (p.1001·3).
*Arrhythmias.*

**Dutimelan** Hoechst Marion Roussel, Ital.†.
10 Tablets, prednisolone acetate (p.1108·1); prednisolone (p.1108·1); 10 tablets, prednisolone; cortisone acetate (p.1096·1).
*Oral corticosteroid.*

**Dutonin**
Bristol-Myers Squibb, Austria†; Bristol-Myers Squibb, Irl.†; Bristol-Myers Squibb, Neth.†; Bristol-Myers, Spain†; Bristol-Myers Squibb, UK†.
Nefazodone hydrochloride (p.309·2).
*Depression.*

**Dutross** Nakorn, Thai.
Bromhexine hydrochloride (p.1115·3).
*Respiratory-tract disorders associated with increased or viscous mucus.*

**Duvadilan**
Byk, Arg.; Solvay, Belg.†; Solvay, Gr.; Solvay, Hong Kong†; Solvay, India; Solvay, Irl.†; Solvay, Ital.†; Solvay, Neth.†; Duphar, Spain†; Duphar-Interfran, Thai.
Isoxsuprine hydrochloride (p.1702·2) or isoxsuprine resinate (p.1702·3).
*Cerebral and peripheral vascular disorders; premature labour.*

**Duvaxan** Labinca, Arg.
Ifosfamide (p.561·1).
*Malignant neoplasms.*

**Duvig** Fada, Arg.
Dobutamine (p.906·1).

**Duvium**
Zambon, Belg.; Inpharzam, Switz.
Benorilate (p.20·3).
*Fever; musculoskeletal and joint disorders; pain.*

**Duvoid**
Shire, Canad.; Roberts, USA†.
Bethanechol chloride (p.1487·3).
*Urinary retention.*

**Duxaril**
Servier, Hong Kong; Servier, Singapore; Servier, Thai.
Almitrine (p.1584·2) or almitrine dimesilate (p.1584·2); raubasine (p.994·3).
*Cochleovestibular ischaemia; mental function impairment; retinal ischaemia; stroke.*

**Duxil**
Ardix, Fr.; Servier, Port.
Almitrine (p.1584·2) or almitrine dimesilate (p.1584·2); raubasine (p.994·3).
*Cerebral ischaemia; mental function impairment; retinal ischaemia; vestibular ischaemia.*

**Duxima** Ecobi, Ital.
Cefuroxime sodium (p.184·1).
*Gram-negative bacterial infections.*

**Duxor** Servier, Spain.
Raubasine (p.994·3); almitrine (p.1584·2) or almitrine dimesilate (p.1584·2).
*Cerebrovascular disorders; vestibular disorders.*

**D-Vi-Sol** Mead Johnson Nutritionals, Canad.
Colecalciferol (p.1461·3).
*Vitamin supplement.*

**D-Vital** Will-Pharma, Belg.
Calcium carbonate (p.1254·2); colecalciferol (p.1461·3).
*Calcium and vitamin D deficiency; osteoporosis.*

**D-Void** Tamilnadu Dadha, India.
Desmopressin acetate (p.1322·3).
*Diabetes insipidus; nocturia; nocturnal enuresis; test of renal concentrating capacity.*

**D-Worm** Triomed, S.Afr.
Mebendazole (p.108·2).
*Worm infections.*

**Dyazide**
SmithKline Beecham, Austral.†; SmithKline Beecham, Canad.†; Goldshield, Hong Kong; Goldshield, Irl.; SmithKline Beecham, Mex.; SmithKline Beecham, NZ†; Decomed, Port.; Pharmafrica, S.Afr.; SmithKline Beecham, Singapore†; Doetsch, Grether, Switz.; SmithKline Beecham, Thai.†; Goldshield, UK; SmithKline Beecham, USA.
Hydrochlorothiazide (p.933·2); triamterene (p.1016·2).
These ingredients can be described by the British Approved Name Co-triamterzide.
*Hypertension; oedema.*

**Dycholium** Novartis Consumer, Canad.†.
Dehydrocholic acid (p.1679·2).
*Biliary-tract disorders.*

**Dycill** SmithKline Beecham, USA†.
Dicloxacillin sodium (p.205·2).
*Bacterial infections.*

**Dyclone** Astra, USA†.
Dyclonine hydrochloride (p.1376·2).
*Local anaesthesia.*

**Dyflex-G** Econo Med, USA.
Diprophylline (p.784·3); guaifenesin (p.1122·1).
*Bronchospasm.*

**Dy-G** Cypress, USA.
Diprophylline (p.784·3); guaifenesin (p.1122·1).
*Asthma.*

**Dygratyl**
Solvay, Denm.; Solvay, Fin.; Solvay, Swed.
Dihydrotachysterol (p.1461·3).
*Hypocalcaemia; hypoparathyroidism; osteomalacia; pseudohypoparathyroidism; renal osteodystrophy; rickets; secondary hyperparathyroidism; vitamin D deficiency.*

**Dyka-D** Covan, S.Afr.†.
Chlorphenamine maleate (p.427·3); phenylephrine hydrochloride (p.1126·3); hyoscine methonitrate (p.483·3).
*Hypersensitivity reactions; nasal congestion.*

**Dykatuss Co** Covan, S.Afr.†.
Mepyramine maleate (p.437·1); ephedrine hydrochloride (p.1120·1); codeine phosphate (p.27·1).
*Cold symptoms; coughs.*

**Dyline GG** Seatrace, USA.
Diprophylline (p.784·3); guaifenesin (p.1122·1).
*Bronchospasm.*

**Dylix** Lunsco, USA.
Diprophylline (p.784·3).

**Dymadon** Pfizer Consumer, Austral.
Paracetamol (p.76·2).
*Fever; pain.*

**Dymadon Co** Pfizer Consumer, Austral.
Paracetamol (p.76·2); codeine phosphate (p.27·1).
*Pain.*

**Dymadon Forte** GlaxoSmithKline, Austral.
Paracetamol (p.76·2); codeine phosphate (p.27·1).
*Pain.*

**Dymelor** Lilly, USA.
Acetohexamide (p.329·2).
*Diabetes mellitus.*

**Dymenate** Keene, USA.
Dimenhydrinate (p.431·1).
*Motion sickness.*

**Dymion** Pulitzer, Ital.†.
Ubidecarenone (p.1760·2).
*Cardiac disorders; co-enzyme Q deficiency.*

**Dymotil** Goldshield, UK.
Diphenoxylate hydrochloride (p.1261·3).
Atropine sulfate (p.477·1) is included in this preparation to discourage abuse.
These ingredients can be described by the British Approved Name Co-phenotrope.
*Diarrhoea.*

**Dyna Jets** Roche, S.Afr.
Multivitamin preparation (p.1417·1).

**Dyna-Ampcil** Salters, S.Afr.†.
Ampicillin trihydrate (p.157·2).
*Bacterial infections.*

**Dynabac**
Lilly, Braz.†; Lilly, Chile; Pharmafarm, Fr.; Pharmaserve Lilly (Φαρμασερβ Λιλλυ), Gr.; Lilly, Hong Kong†; Lilly, Malaysia; Muro, USA.
Dirithromycin (p.206·1).
*Bacterial infections.*

**Dynabolon** Fournier, Ital.
Nandrolone undecylate (p.1561·3).
*Osteoporosis.*

**Dynacide** Rivadis, Fr.
Peracetic acid (p.1187·3).
*Instrument disinfection.*

**Dynacil** Schwarz, Ger.; Sanol, Ger.
Fosinopril sodium (p.919·1).
*Heart failure; hypertension.*

**Dynacil comp** *Schwarz, Ger.; Sanol, Ger.*
Fosinopril sodium (p.919·1); hydrochlorothiazide (p.933·2).
*Hypertension.*

**Dynacin** *Medicis, USA.*
Minocycline hydrochloride (p.231·3).
*Bacterial infections.*

**Dynacirc**
*Novartis, Arg.; Novartis, Chile; Novartis, Hong Kong; Novartis, Malaysia; Novartis, Mex.; Novartis, NZ†; Novartis, S.Afr.; Novartis, Singapore; Novartis, Thai.; Novartis, USA.*
Isradipine (p.942·2).
*Hypertension.*

**Dynacold** *Thuasne, Fr.†.*
Dichlorodifluoromethane (p.1236·1); trichlorofluoromethane (p.1236·1).
*Joint and muscle pain.*

**Dynadol** *Salters, S.Afr.†.*
Paracetamol (p.76·2).
*Fever; pain.*

**Dynafed Asthma Relief** *BDI, USA.*
Ephedrine hydrochloride (p.1120·1); guaifenesin (p.1122·1).
*Coughs.*

**Dynafed EX** *BDI, USA.*
Paracetamol (p.76·2).
*Fever; pain.*

**Dynafed Plus** *BDI, USA.*
Paracetamol (p.76·2); pseudoephedrine hydrochloride (p.1129·2).
Formerly known as Maximum Strength Dynafed.
*Upper respiratory-tract symptoms.*

**Dynafed Pseudo** *BDI, USA†.*
Pseudoephedrine hydrochloride (p.1129·2).
*Nasal congestion.*

**Dynafemme** *Diepharmex, Fr.*
Vitamin, mineral, bladderwrack, and evening primrose oil preparation (p.1417·1).
*Nutritional supplement.*

**Dynagastrin** *Salters, S.Afr.†.*
Dicycloverine hydrochloride (p.481·2); dried aluminium hydroxide gel (p.1249·2); light magnesium oxide (p.1272·3).
*Gastric hyperacidity.*

**Dyna-Hex** *Western Medical, USA.*
Chlorhexidine gluconate (p.1173·2).
*Skin disinfection.*

**Dynalert** *Restan, S.Afr.†.*
Pemoline (p.1591·2).
*Fatigue.*

**Dynametron** *Salters, S.Afr.†.*
Metronidazole (p.607·2).
*Anaerobic bacterial infections; protozoal infections.*

**Dynamin**
*Note. This name is used for preparations of different composition.*
*Ern, Spain.*
Vitamin B substances; caffeine; glutamine (p.1417·1).
*Tonic.*
*Berk, UK.*
Isosorbide mononitrate (p.942·1).
*Angina pectoris; heart failure.*

**Dynamisan**
*Wander, Belg.†; Novartis Consumer, Switz.*
Arginine aspartate (p.1421·1).
*Tonic.*
*Novartis Sante, Fr.; Mipharm, Ital.; Novartis Consumer, Port.†.*
Arginine glutamate (p.1421·1).
*Tonic.*

**Dynamo** *Key, Austral.†.*
Caffeine (p.782·1); glucose; thiamine hydrochloride; nicotinic acid (p.1417·1).
*Drowsiness; mental fatigue.*

**Dynamogen** *Faes, Spain.*
Arginine aspartate (p.1421·1); glutodina.
*Anorexia; tonic; weight loss.*

**Dynamucil** *Siphar, Switz.*
Acetylcysteine (p.1112·3).
*Respiratory-tract disorders with viscous mucus.*

**Dynapayne** *Salters, S.Afr.†.*
*Syrup:* Paracetamol (p.76·2); codeine phosphate (p.27·1); promethazine hydrochloride (p.439·1).
*Fever; pain.*
*Tablets:* Paracetamol (p.76·2); codeine phosphate (p.27·1); caffeine (p.782·1); meprobamate (p.706·2).
*Pain and associated tension.*

**Dynapen**
*Note. This name is used for preparations of different composition.*
*Leo, Austria†.*
Sultamicillin (p.264·2) or sultamicillin tosilate (p.264·2).
*Bacterial infections.*
*Dynamed, S.Afr.†.*
Phenoxymethylpenicillin potassium (p.242·1).
*Bacterial infections.*
*Apothecon, USA†.*
Dicloxacillin sodium (p.205·2).
*Bacterial infections.*

**Dynaphos-C** *Sofar, Ital.*
Ascorbic acid (p.1460·2).
*Gingivitis; stomatitis; vitamin C deficiency.*

**Dynaspor** *Salters, S.Afr.†.*
Clotrimazole (p.396·2).
*Fungal infections.*

**Dynasprin** *USV, India.*
Aspirin (p.15·1); dipyridamole (p.903·1).
*Thromboembolic disorders.*

**Dynastat**
*Pharmacia, Austral.; Pharmacia, Irl.; Pharmacia, Norw.; Pharmacia, Port.; Pharmacia, UK.*
Parecoxib sodium (p.79·2).
*Postoperative pain.*

**Dynatra**
*Almirall, Belg.; Zambon, Neth.*
Dopamine hydrochloride (p.907·1).
*Hypotension; shock.*

**Dynavital** *Monal, Fr.†.*
A range of trace element preparations (p.1417·1).

**Dynazole** *Salters, S.Afr.†.*
Co-trimoxazole (p.199·3).
*Bacterial infections.*

**Dynef** *Sigma-Tau, Ger.*
Anthocyanins from myrtillus; alpha tocoferil acetate (p.1465·1).
*Eye disorders.*

**Dynergum** *Sanobia, Port.*
Citrulline malate (p.1425·2).
*Tonic.*

**Dyneric** *Henning, Ger.†.*
Clomifene citrate (p.1542·2).
*Anovulatory infertility.*

**Dynese** *Galen, UK†.*
Magaldrate (p.1271·3).
*Dyspepsia.*

**Dynexan**
*Note. This name is used for preparations of different composition.*
*Nycomed, Austria.*
Tetracaine hydrochloride (p.1385·1); chamomile (p.1669·3); sage (p.1741·2); arnica (p.1656·3); aluminium formate.
*Mouth and throat disorders.*
*Kreussler, Fr.; Kreussler, Ger.*
Lidocaine hydrochloride (p.1377·3).
*Local anaesthesia; painful mouth lesions.*
*Restan, S.Afr.; Kreussler, Switz.†.*
Tetracaine hydrochloride (p.1385·1); chamomile (p.1669·3); arnica (p.1656·3); sage (p.1741·2); aluminium formate.
*Local anaesthesia; mouth and throat disorders.*

**Dynexan Herpescreme** *Kreussler, Ger.*
Aciclovir (p.626·1).
*Herpes infections of the skin.*

**Dynexan Mundgel** *Kreussler, Ger.*
Lidocaine hydrochloride (p.1377·3); benzalkonium chloride (p.1168·3).
*Painful inflammatory disorders of the mouth.*

**Dynexan Zahnfleischtropfen** *Kreussler, Ger.*
Aluminium formate.
Formerly known as Cional S.
*Mouth and throat inflammation.*

**Dynofen** *Salters, S.Afr.†.*
Ibuprofen (p.45·3).
*Musculoskeletal and joint disorders.*

**Dynorm** *Roche, Ger.*
Cilazapril (p.883·3).
*Hypertension.*

**Dynorm Plus** *Roche, Ger.*
Cilazapril (p.883·3); hydrochlorothiazide (p.933·2).
*Hypertension.*

**Dynos** *Intramed, S.Afr.†.*
Dopamine hydrochloride (p.907·1).
*Heart failure; shock.*

**Dynothel** *Henning, Ger.†.*
Dextrothyroxine sodium (p.893·2).
*Hyperlipidaemias.*

**Dynoxytet** *Salters, S.Afr.†.*
Oxytetracycline hydrochloride (p.241·1).
*Bacterial infections.*

**Dyphylline-GG** *Cypress, USA.*
Diprophylline (p.784·3); guaifenesin (p.1122·1).
*Asthma with associated cough.*

**Dyprotex**
*Note. This name is used for preparations of different composition.*
*Blistex, Hong Kong.*
Dimethicone (p.1482·1); zinc oxide (p.1163·2); soft paraffin (p.1479·3).
*Nappy rash.*
*Blistex, Israel.*
Zinc oxide (p.1163·2).
*Nappy rash.*
*Blistex, USA.*
Dimethicone (p.1482·1); zinc oxide (p.1163·2); cod-liver oil (p.1425·2).
*Nappy rash.*

**Dyrade-M** *Cipla, India.*
Diloxanide furoate (p.604·1); metronidazole (p.607·2) or metronidazole benzoate (p.607·2).
*Amoebiasis; giardiasis.*

**Dyrenium**
*GlaxoSmithKline, Canad.; Doetsch, Grether, Switz.†; SmithKline Beecham, USA.*
Triamterene (p.1016·2).
*Heart failure; oedema.*

**Dyrenium compositum** *Doetsch, Grether, Switz.*
Triamterene (p.1016·2); benzthiazide (p.868·2).
*Hypertension; oedema.*

**Dyrexan-OD** *Trimen, USA†.*
Phendimetrazine tartrate (p.1592·1).
*Obesity.*

**Dyrosol** *Propan, S.Afr.†.*
Bismuth salicylate (p.1252·1); codeine phosphate (p.27·1); atropine sulfate (p.477·1).
*Diarrhoea.*

**Dysalfa** *Fournier, Fr.*
Terazosin hydrochloride (p.1010·3).
*Benign prostatic hyperplasia.*

**Dyscornut** *Weber & Weber, Ger.*
Homoeopathic preparation.

**Dysetrin** *Hua, Thai.†.*
Diiodohydroxyquinoline (p.603·3).
*Amoebiasis.*

**Dysfur-M** *Biological E, India.*
Furazolidone (p.605·2); metronidazole (p.607·2); homatropine methylbromide (p.483·2).
*Intestinal infections.*

**Dyskinebyl** *Zyma, Fr.†.*
Dihydroxydibutylether (p.1680·2).
*Dyspepsia.*

**Dyskinon** *Nicholas Piramal, India.*
Biperiden hydrochloride (p.479·3).
*Cranial trauma; drug-induced extrapyramidal disorders; nicotine poisoning; parkinsonism; trigeminal neuralgia.*

**Dysman** *Ashbourne, UK.*
Mefenamic acid (p.55·2).
*Dysfunctional menorrhagia; fever; pain.*

**Dysmen** *Sigma, India.*
*Injection:* Dicycloverine hydrochloride (p.481·2).
*Tablets:* Mefenamic acid (p.55·2); dicycloverine hydrochloride (p.481·2).
*Smooth muscle spasm.*

**Dysmen-500** *Sigma, India.*
Mefenamic acid (p.55·2).
*Dysmenorrhoea; pain.*

**Dysmen Forte** *Sigma, India.*
Mefenamic acid (p.55·2); paracetamol (p.76·2).
*Pain.*

**Dysmenalgit** *Krewel, Ger.*
Naproxen (p.65·1).
*Dysmenorrhoea.*

**Dysmenorrhoe-Gastreu S R75** *Reckeweg, Ger.*
Homoeopathic preparation.

**Dyspagon** *Pierre Fabre Sante, Fr.*
Loperamide hydrochloride (p.1271·1).
*Diarrhoea.*

**Dyspamet**
*Goldshield, Irl.; Goldshield, UK.*
Cimetidine (p.1255·3).
*Gastric hyperacidity; gastro-oesophageal reflux; peptic ulcer; Zollinger-Ellison syndrome.*

**Dyspen**
*Biolab, Hong Kong; Biolab, Thai.*
Mefenamic acid (p.55·2).
*Fever; inflammation; pain.*

**Dyspne-Inhal** *Augot, Fr.†.*
Adrenaline (p.852·2).
*Glottal oedema.*

**Dysport**
*Ipsen, Austral.; Croma, Austria; Ipsen, Belg.; Biosintetica, Braz.; Ipsen, Denm.; Ipsen, Fin.; Ipsen Biotech, Fr.; Ipsen, Ger.; Ipsen, Gr.; Beaufour-Ipsen, Hong Kong; Ipsen, Irl.; Ipsen, Israel; Ipsen, Ital.; Beaufour-Ipsen, Malaysia; Emerging Pharma, Malaysia; NZ Medical & Scientific, NZ; Ipsen, NZ; Beaufour-Ipsen, Singapore; Ipsen, Spain; Ipsen, Swed.; Ipsen, Switz.; Ipsen, UK.*
Botulinum A toxin (p.1388·3).
*Arm spasticity following stroke; blepharospasm; foot spasticity associated with paediatric cerebral palsy; hemifacial spasm; spasmodic torticollis.*

**dysto-L 90 N** *Loges, Ger.*
Homoeopathic preparation.

**Dystolise** *Motima, Fr.*
Melissa (p.1711·1); angelica (p.1655·1); sweet marjoram.
*Tonic.*

**dysto-loges** *Loges, Ger.*
Homoeopathic preparation.

**dysto-lux** *Loges, Ger.*
Hypericum (p.299·1).
*Anxiety; depression.*

**Dystonal** *Pharmethic, Belg.†.*
Dihydroergotamine mesilate (p.465·3).
Formerly contained belladonna, ergotamine tartrate, and phenobarbital.
*Migraine and other vascular headaches; orthostatic hypotension.*

**Dystophan** *Kattwiga, Ger.*
Homoeopathic preparation.

**Dystrol** *Wyeth Lederle, Denm.†.*
Levonorgestrel (p.1563·2); ethinylestradiol (p.1553·2).
*Endometriosis; menstrual disorders.*

**Dysurgal** *Disperga, Austria†.*
Atropine sulfate (p.477·1); ephedrine hydrochloride (p.1120·1); strychnine nitrate (p.1750·1).
*Urinary-tract disorders.*

**Dysurgal N** *Galenika, Ger.*
Atropine sulfate (p.477·1).
Dysurgal formerly contained atropine sulfate, ephedrine hydrochloride, and strychnine nitrate.
*Dysmenorrhoea; urinary-tract disorders.*

**Dytac**
*GlaxoSmithKline, Neth.; Goldshield, UK.*
Triamterene (p.1016·2).
*Hypertension; oedema.*

**Dytan** *Hawthorn, USA.*
Diphenhydramine tannate (p.432·2).
*Hypersensitivity reactions.*

**Dytan-D** *Hawthorn, USA.*
Diphenhydramine tannate (p.432·2); phenylephrine tannate (p.1127·2).
*Cold symptoms; nasal congestion.*

**Dyta-Urese**
*SMB, Belg.†; SmithKline Beecham, Neth.*
Triamterene (p.1016·2); epitizide (p.911·3).
*Hypertension; oedema.*

**Dytenzide**
*Yamanouchi, Belg.; SmithKline Beecham, Neth.*
Triamterene (p.1016·2); hydrochlorothiazide (p.933·2).
*Hypertension; oedema.*

**Dyterene** *Pharmasant, Thai.*
Hydrochlorothiazide (p.933·2); triamterene (p.1016·2).
*Hypertension; oedema.*

**Dytide** *Goldshield, UK.*
Triamterene (p.1016·2); benzthiazide (p.868·2).
*Oedema.*

**Dytide H**
*Procter & Gamble, Austria; Procter & Gamble, Ger.*
Triamterene (p.1016·2); hydrochlorothiazide (p.933·2).
*Heart failure; hypertension; oedema.*

**Dytuss** *Lunsco, USA.*
Diphenhydramine hydrochloride (p.431·3).

**Dyzole** *Douglas, NZ.*
Tinidazole (p.617·1).
*Bacterial infections; protozoal infections.*

**D-Zol** *Pacific, NZ.*
Danazol (p.1545·2).
*Benign breast disease; endometriosis; hereditary angioedema; menorrhagia.*

**E45**
*Note. This name is used for preparations of different composition.*
*Boots, Austral.†.*
White soft paraffin (p.1479·3); light liquid paraffin (p.1479·1); wool fat (p.1483·1).
*Dry skin.*
*Boots Healthcare, Irl.; Boots Healthcare, S.Afr.; Crookes Healthcare, UK.*
Emollient.
*Dry skin disorders.*
*Boots Healthcare, NZ†.*
*Bath oil:* Liquid paraffin (p.1479·1); dimethicone (p.1482·1).
*Bath additive; dry skin; pruritus.*
*Wash:* Liquid paraffin (p.1479·1); zinc oxide (p.1163·2).
*Cleansing agent for dry skin.*

**E45 Itch Relief** *Crookes Healthcare, UK.*
Macrogol lauril ethers (p.1412·3); urea (p.1162·2).
*Pruritus; scaling skin conditions.*

**E Mal** *Themis Chemicals, India.*
Artemotil (p.447·2).
*Malaria.*

**E Plus** *Delta, Braz.*
dl-Alpha tocoferil acetate (p.1465·1).

**E Radicaps** *Legrand, Braz.*
Vitamin E (p.1464·3).
*Vitamin E supplement.*

**E45 Sun** *Crookes Healthcare, UK.*
*SPF 15:* Octinoxate (p.1154·3); avobenzone (p.1142·3); titanium dioxide (p.1160·3).
Formerly contained titanium dioxide and zinc oxide.
*SPF 30:* Octinoxate (p.1154·3); avobenzone (p.1142·3); enzacamene (p.1147·1); titanium dioxide (p.1160·3).
*Sunscreen.*

**E45 Sun Block** *Crookes Healthcare, UK.*
*SPF 25; SPF 50:* Titanium dioxide (p.1160·3); zinc oxide (p.1163·2).
*Sunscreen.*

**Eaca Balsamico** *Nikkho, Braz.*
Aminocaproic acid (p.741·3); sodium benzoate (p.1169·3); guaifenesin (p.1122·1); ammonium chloride (p.1115·2).
*Respiratory-tract congestion.*

**Eanox** *Desitin, Denm.*
Zolpidem tartrate (p.728·3).
*Insomnia.*

**EAP-61** *Hanosan, Ger.*
Homoeopathic preparation.

**Ear Clear** *Key, Austral.†.*
Urea hydrogen peroxide (p.1195·3).
*Ear wax removal.*

**Ear Clear for Swimmer's Ear** *Key, Austral.†.*
Acetic acid (p.1645·2); isopropyl alcohol (p.1184·3).
*Otitis externa.*

**Earache** *Hylands, Canad.*
Homoeopathic preparation.

**Earache Pain** *Homeocan, Canad.*
Homoeopathic preparation.

**EarCalm** *GlaxoSmithKline Consumer, UK.*
Glacial acetic acid (p.1645·2).
*Superficial ear infections.*

**Earclear** *Wilson, NZ.*
Urea hydrogen peroxide (p.1195·3).
*Ear wax removal.*

**Ear-Dry** *Scherer, USA.*
Boric acid (p.1662·1); isopropyl alcohol (p.1184·3).
*Ear disorders.*

**Earex** SSL, UK.
Arachis oil (p.1656·1); almond oil (p.1651·1); rectified camphor oil.
*Ear wax removal.*

**Earex Plus** SSL, UK.
Choline salicylate (p.26·2); glycerol (p.1694·3).
*Ear wax removal; earache.*

**Ear-Eze** Hyrex, USA.
Hydrocortisone (p.1103·3); neomycin sulfate (p.235·1); polymyxin B (p.245·2).
*Bacterial ear infections.*

**Early Bird**
Note. This name is used for preparations of different composition.
Mentholatum, Austral.
Pyrantel embonate (p.113·2).
*Enterobiasis.*

Kent, UK.
Pregnancy test (p.1734·3).

**EarSol** Parnell, USA†.
Alcohol (p.1166·1).
*Ear disorders.*

**EarSol-HC** Parnell, USA.
Hydrocortisone (p.1103·3).
*Ear inflammation.*

**EAS** Fresenius Kabi, Switz.†.
Amino-acid preparation (p.1417·1).
*Nutritional supplement in renal failure.*

**Ease Pain Away** RMC, Canad.†.
Menthol (p.1711·3); trolamine salicylate (p.95·3).

**Easiko** Medipharma, Hong Kong.
Mepyramine maleate (p.437·1); menthol (p.1711·3); camphor (p.1665·3).

**Easistix BG** Eastern Pharmaceuticals, UK†.
Test for glucose in blood (p.1694·2).

**Easistix UG** Eastern Pharmaceuticals, UK†.
Test for glucose in urine (p.1694·2).

**Easprin** Lotus, USA.
Aspirin (p.15·1).
*Fever; inflammation; pain.*

**Easy gel** Abic, Israel.
Benzydamine hydrochloride (p.21·1).
*Musculoskeletal and joint disorders.*

**Easylax** Sam-On, Israel.
Phenolphthalein (p.1284·1).
*Constipation.*

**Eatan N** Desitin, Ger.
Nitrazepam (p.710·1).
*Sleep disorders.*

**Eau Precieuse** Pfizer Sante, Fr.
Boric acid (p.1662·1); resorcinol (p.1156·3); salicylic acid (p.1157·1); tannic acid (p.1751·2); lysol (p.1177·3); phenol (p.1188·1); menthol (p.1711·3).
*Seborrhoea.*

**Eau-de-vie de France avec huile de pin nain du Tirol** Doetsch, Grether, Switz.
Menthol (p.1711·3); pumilio pine oil (p.1737·1).
*Muscular pain and fatigue.*

**Eavit** Terapeutico, Ital.
Gelatin; wheat-germ oil; carrot oil; soya lecithin; royal jelly; beeswax (p.1417·1).
*Nutritional supplement.*

**Eavit Plus** Terapeutico, Ital.
Gelatin; wheat-germ oil; carrot oil; lecithin; royal jelly; soya oil (p.1417·1).
*Nutritional supplement.*

**Ebamin** Jin Yang, Hong Kong.
Ginkgo biloba (p.1692·3).
*Cerebral disorders; peripheral vascular disorders.*

**E-Base** Barr, USA.
Erythromycin (p.208·1).
*Bacterial infections.*

**Ebastel**
Byk, Arg.; Eurofarma, Braz.; Grunenthal, Chile; Dainippon, Jpn; Almirall, Spain.
Ebastine (p.433·1).
*Hypersensitivity reactions.*

**Ebastel D**
Byk, Arg.; Eurofarma, Braz.
Ebastine (p.433·1); pseudoephedrine hydrochloride (p.1129·2).
*Allergic rhinitis.*

**Ebefen** Ebewe, Austria.
Tamoxifen citrate (p.584·1).
*Breast cancer; endometrial cancer.*

**Ebenol** Strathmann, Ger.
Hydrocortisone acetate (p.1103·3).
*Skin disorders.*

**Ebersept** Bros, Gr.
Ketoconazole (p.403·3).
*Fungal infections.*

**Ebertuss** Bros, Gr.
Ambroxol hydrochloride (p.1114·3).
*Respiratory disorders associated with viscous mucus.*

**Ebexid** Sigma, India.
Thyroid (p.1604·2); vitamin B substances; vitamin E (p.1417·1).
*Hypothyroidism.*

**Ebixa**
Lundbeck, Austral.; Lundbeck, Fr.; Lundbeck, Irl.; Lundbeck, Norw.; Lundbeck, UK.
Memantine hydrochloride (p.1711·2).
*Alzheimer's disease.*

**Ebrantil**
Byk, Austria; Byk, Belg.; Byk, Braz.†; Byk Gulden, Ger.; Byk Gulden, Ital.; Byk, Neth.; Byk, Port.; Altana, Switz.
Urapidil (p.1018·1), urapidil fumarate (p.1018·2), or urapidil hydrochloride (p.1018·1).
*Hypertension; production of controlled hypotension.*

**Ebromin** Degorts, Mex.
Ambroxol hydrochloride (p.1114·3).
*Respiratory-tract disorders with viscous mucus.*

**Ebromin-P** Degorts, Mex.
Ambroxol hydrochloride (p.1114·3); clenbuterol hydrochloride (p.784·2).
*Respiratory-tract congestion.*

**Ebufac** DDSA Pharmaceuticals, UK.
Ibuprofen (p.45·3).

**Eburdent** Acro, Ital.
Sodium fluoride (p.1444·3).
*Gum disorders.*

**Eburdent F** Acro, Ital.
Miristalkonium saccharinate (p.1186·3); sodium fluoride (p.1444·3).
*Dental caries prophylaxis; oral hygiene.*

**Eburnal** Chiesi, Ital.
Vinburnine (p.1764·2).
*Cerebrovascular disorders.*

**Eburnate** Vannier, Arg.
Fluoxetine hydrochloride (p.292·1).
*Depression.*

**Eburnoxin** Astra, Spain†.
Vinburnine (p.1764·2).
*Cerebrovascular disorders; retinopathies.*

**Eburos** Acro, Ital.
Chlorhexidine gluconate (p.1173·2).
*Oral hygiene.*

**EC + Complex** Seroyal, Canad.†.
Vitamin preparation with zinc (p.1417·1).

**Ecabil** Biologici Italia, Ital.
Heparin calcium (p.927·3).
*Thromboembolic disorders.*

**Ecadiu** Elan, Spain.
Hydrochlorothiazide (p.933·2); captopril (p.879·2).
*Hypertension.*

**Ecafast** Crinos, Ital.
Heparin calcium (p.927·3).
*Thromboembolic disorders.*

**Ecamannan** CaDiGroup, Ital.
Glucomannan (p.1693·3); vitamin E (p.1464·3); vitamin C (p.1460·2); betacarotene (p.1422·3).
*Gastrointestinal disorders; hypercholesterolaemia; obesity.*

**Ecanol** Sarabhai Piramal, India.
Econazole nitrate (p.397·2).
*Fungal and Gram-positive bacterial skin infections; vulvovaginal candidiasis.*

**Ecapresan** Bristol-Myers Squibb, Mex.
Captopril (p.879·2).
*Hypertension.*

**Ecapril**
Note. This name is used for preparations of different composition.
Promeco, Mex.†.
Captopril (p.879·2).

Atral, Port.
Lisinopril (p.946·3).
*Heart failure; hypertension.*

**Ecaprilat** Lazar, Arg.
Enalapril (p.909·2).
*Heart failure; hypertension.*

**Ecasil** Biolab Sanus, Braz.
Aspirin (p.15·1).
*Fever; inflammation; pain; thromboembolism prophylaxis.*

**Ecasolv** Benedetti, Ital.
Heparin calcium (p.927·3).
*Thromboembolic disorders.*

**Ecaten** Fustery, Mex.
Captopril (p.879·2).
*Heart failure; hypertension; myocardial infarction.*

**Ecax** Bago, Chile.
Meloxicam (p.56·1).
*Inflammation; pain.*

**Ecazide**
Bristol-Myers Squibb, Fr.; Squibb, Spain.
Captopril (p.879·2); hydrochlorothiazide (p.933·2).
*Hypertension.*

**Eccarvit Plus** CaDiGroup, Ital.
Vitamin C; vitamin E; betacarotene; ginkgo biloba; chromium tripicolinate (p.1417·1).
*Nutritional supplement.*

**Eccelium** Manetti Roberts, Ital.
Econazole sulfosalicylate (p.397·2).
*Fungal infections; Gram-positive bacterial superinfections.*

**Eccoxolac** Viatris, UK.
Etodolac (p.37·3).
*Osteoarthritis; rheumatoid arthritis.*

**Ecee2** German Remedies, India.
Levonorgestrel (p.1563·2).
*Postcoital contraceptive.*

**Ecee Plus** Edwards, USA.
Vitamins C and E with minerals (p.1417·1).

**Echan** Biocur, Ger.
Echinacea purpura (p.1683·2).
*Respiratory- and urinary-tract infections.*

**Echifit** Krewel, Ger.
Echinacea purpurea (p.1683·2).
*Respiratory- and urinary-tract infections.*

**Echiherb** Duopharm, Ger.
Echinacea purpurea (p.1683·2).
*Respiratory- and urinary- tract infections.*

**Echina Pro** Planta, Canad.†.
Echinacea (p.1683·2).
*Cold and influenza symptoms.*

**Echinacea** Potter's, UK.
*Elixir:* Echinacea (p.1683·2); baptisia tinctoria; fumitory (p.1690·1).
*Catarrh; immunostimulant; minor skin disorders.*
*Tablets:* Echinacea (p.1683·2).
*Immunostimulant; skin disorders.*

**Echinacea 4000** Procare, Austral.†.
Echinacea (p.1683·2); calcium ascorbate (p.1460·2); zinc amino acid chelate (p.1469·3).
*Upper respiratory-tract symptoms.*

**Echinacea ACE Plus Zinc** Blackmores, Austral.†.
Echinacea angustifolia (p.1683·2); vitamins (p.1417·1); zinc amino acid chelate (p.1469·3); garlic oil (p.1691·2).
*Tonic.*

**Echinacea ACE + Zinc** Blackmores, Austral.†.
Echinacea pallida (p.1683·2); vitamins (p.1417·1); zinc (p.1469·2).
*Cold and influenza symptoms.*

**Echinacea akut** Hevert, Ger.†.
Homoeopathic preparation.

**Echinacea & Antioxidants** Vitaplex, Austral.†.
Ascorbic acid (p.1460·2); *d*-alpha tocoferil acid succinate (p.1465·1); zinc gluconate (p.1469·2); echinacea (p.1683·2); garlic (p.1691·1).
*Upper respiratory-tract disorders.*

**Echinacea comp**
Hevert, Ger.; Steigerwald, Ger.
Homoeopathic preparation.

**Echinacea Complex** Cenovis, Austral.†.
Echinacea (p.1683·2); vitamins (p.1417·1); zinc amino acid chelate (p.1469·3).
*Skin disorders; upper respiratory-tract infections; wounds.*

**Echinacea Herbal Plus Formula** Vitelle, Austral.†.
Multivitamins with echinacea and zinc amino acid chelate (p.1417·1) (p.1683·2) (p.1469·3).
*Minor upper respiratory-tract disorders; skin disorders.*

**Echinacea L40** Homeocan, Canad.
Homoeopathic preparation.

**Echinacea Lozenge** Blackmores, Austral.†.
Echinacea purpurea (p.1683·2); sodium ascorbate (p.1460·2); eucalyptus oil (p.1686·2).
*Cold and influenza symptoms.*

**Echinacea Med Complex** Dynamit, Austria.
Homoeopathic preparation.

**Echinacea Oligoplex** Madaus, Ger.
Homoeopathic preparation.

**Echinacea Plus** Eagle, Austral.†.
Echinacea (p.1683·2); astragalus membranaceus; schizandra chinensis; tabebuia avellanedae.
*Minor infections; tonic.*

**Echinacea Ro-Plex (Rowo-415)** Pharmakon, Ger.
Homoeopathic preparation.

**Echinacea Urtinktur** Hevert, Ger.
Homoeopathic preparation.

**Echinacea-Complex** Weber & Weber, Ger.
Homoeopathic preparation.

**Echinacea-Cosmoplex** Peithner, Austria.
Homoeopathic preparation.

**Echinacin**
Polcopharma, Austral.†; Madaus, Austria; Madaus, Belg.; Madaus, Ger.; Madaus, Spain; Biomed, Switz.
Echinacea purpurea (p.1683·2).
*Respiratory- and urinary-tract infections; wounds.*

**Echinaforce**
Bio-Garten, Austria†; Bioforce, Ger.; Bioforce, Switz.; Bioforce, UK.
Echinacea purpura (p.1683·2).
*Respiratory- and urinary-tract infections.*

**EchinaMed** Bioforce, Switz.
Echinacea (p.1683·2).
*Immunostimulant.*

**Echinapur** Scheffler, Ger.
Echinacea purpura (p.1683·2).
*Respiratory- and urinary-tract infections.*

**Echinarell** Sanorell, Ger.
Homoeopathic preparation.

**Echinart** Ceom, Ital.
Homoeopathic preparation.

**Echinasyx** Syxyl, Ger.
Homoeopathic preparation.

**Echinatur** Ritsert, Ger.
Echinacea purpurea (p.1683·2).
*Respiratory- and urinary-tract infections.*

**Echine** Eagle, Austral.†.
Herbal and homoeopathic antiseptic.

**Echnatol** Gerot, Austria.
Cyclizine hydrochloride (p.429·3).
*Motion sickness; nausea and vomiting.*

**Echnatol B$_6$** Gerot, Austria.
Cyclizine hydrochloride (p.429·3); pyridoxine hydrochloride (p.1456·3).
*Motion sickness; nausea and vomiting; vestibular disorders.*

**Echovist**
Schering, Austria; Berlex, Canad.; Schering, Denm.†; Schering, Fin.; Schering, Fr.; Schering, Ger.; Schering, Israel; Schering, Neth.; Schering, Norw.†; Schering, NZ†; Schering, S.Afr.†; Schering, Swed.; Schering, Switz.†; Schering, UK.
Galactose (p.1063·1).
*Ultrasound contrast medium.*

**Echte Sodener Mineral-Pastillen** Twardy, Ger.
Minerals from spring or stream (p.1217·1).
*Respiratory-tract congestion.*

**Echtroferment-N** Weber & Weber, Ger.†.
Aniseed (p.1655·2); caraway (p.1667·2); fennel (p.1687·2); potentilla anserina.
*Gastrointestinal disorders.*

**Echtronerval-N** Weber & Weber, Ger.
Homoeopathic preparation.

**Echtrosept-N** Weber & Weber, Ger.
Homoeopathic preparation.

**Echtrovit** Weber & Weber, Ger.
Vitamins; rutoside (p.1417·1).
*Tonic.*

**Echtrovit-K** Weber & Weber, Ger.†.
Procaine hydrochloride (p.1383·2); vitamins (p.1417·1); rutoside (p.1688·2).
*Tonic.*

**Eciclean** EciFarma, Chile.
Chamomile flowers (p.1669·3); sage leaf (p.1741·2).
*Dry mouth; mouth disorders.*

**Eclaran**
Pierre Fabre, Arg.; Pierre Fabre, Fr.; Pierre Fabre, Port.
Benzoyl peroxide (p.1143·2).
*Acne.*

**Eclipse Lip and Face** Triangle, USA.
*SPF 15:* Padimate O (p.1155·1); oxybenzone (p.1154·3).
*Sunscreen.*

**Eclipsol** Darier, Mex.
*SPF 40:* Octocrilene (p.1154·3); octinoxate (p.1154·3); titanium dioxide (p.1160·3); avobenzone (p.1142·3).
*SPF 50:* Octocrilene (p.1154·3); octinoxate (p.1154·3); avobenzone (p.1142·3).
*SPF 15; gel SPF 30:* Octinoxate (p.1154·3); oxybenzone (p.1154·3).
*SPF 20; SPF 27; cream SPF 30:* Octinoxate (p.1154·3); avobenzone (p.1142·3).
*Sunscreen.*

**Eclorion** Norma (Νορμα), Gr.
Sulpiride (p.722·2).
*Psychoses.*

**Ecnagel** LDA, Arg.
Salicylic acid (p.1157·1); resorcinol (p.1156·3); hamamelis (p.1696·3).
*Skin disorders.*

**Ecnagel E** LDA, Arg.
Salicylic acid (p.1157·1); resorcinol (p.1156·3); erythromycin (p.208·1).
*Infected skin disorders.*

**Ecnagel PB** LDA, Arg.
Benzoyl peroxide (p.1143·2).
*Acne.*

**Eco Mi** Geymonat, Ital.
Econazole nitrate (p.397·2).
*Fungal skin or vulvovaginal infections.*

**Ecobec** CSP, Fr.
Beclometasone dipropionate (p.1091·1).
*Asthma.*

**Ecocain**
Katsoupas, Gr.; Molteni, Ital.; Julphar, UAE.
Lidocaine hydrochloride (p.1377·3).
Adrenaline acid tartrate (p.852·2) is included in some injections to reduce absorption and localise the effect of the local anaesthetic.
*Local anaesthesia.*

**Ecocillin** Proge, Ital.
*Lactobacillus plantarum.*
*Vaginitis.*

**Ecocort**
Hoe, Malaysia; Hoe, Singapore.
Econazole nitrate (p.397·2); triamcinolone acetonide (p.1110·2).
*Fungal skin infections.*

**Ecodax** Unique, India.
Beclometasone dipropionate (p.1091·1); econazole nitrate (p.397·2); gentamicin sulfate (p.217·1).
*Infected skin disorders.*

**Ecodergin** Farmigea, Ital.
Econazole nitrate (p.397·2).
*Vulvovaginal or dermatological fungal and Gram-positive bacterial infections.*

**Ecoderm**
Note. This name is used for preparations of different composition.
Hoe, Malaysia; Hoe, Singapore†.
Econazole nitrate (p.397·2).
*Fungal skin infections.*

Chew, Thai.
Econazole nitrate (p.397·2); triamcinolone acetonide (p.1110·2).
*Fungal skin infections.*

**Ecodipine** Ecosol, Switz.
Nifedipine (p.966·2).
*Hypertension; ischaemic heart disease; Raynaud's syndrome.*

**Ecodolor** Ecosol, Switz.
Tramadol hydrochloride (p.94·3).
*Pain.*

**Ecodurex** *Ecosol, Switz.*
Hydrochlorothiazide (p.933·2); amiloride hydrochloride (p.858·2).
*Hypertension; oedema.*

**Ecoendocilli Testimonia** *Istoria, Ital.†.*
Lactic-acid-producing organisms (p.1704·2); vitamins (p.1417·1).
*Disturbances of the gastrointestinal flora; nutritional supplement.*

**Ecofenac** *Ecosol, Switz.*
Diclofenac sodium (p.32·1).
*Gout; inflammation; musculoskeletal, joint, and peri-articular disorders; pain.*

**Ecofermenti** *Echo, Ital.*
Lactic-acid-producing organisms (p.1704·2); vitamins (p.1417·1).
*Disturbances of the gastrointestinal flora.*

**Ecofibra** *Echo, Ital.*
Dietary fibre supplement (p.1417·1) (p.1253·2).
*Delayed gastrointestinal transit; obesity.*

**Ecoflorina** *Ecobi, Ital.*
Lactic-acid-producing organisms (p.1704·2).
*Nutritional supplement.*

**Ecofol** *Ecobi, Ital.*
Calcium folinate (p.1431·1).
*Anaemias; antidote to overdosage with folic acid antagonists; folic acid deficiency.*

**Ecolicin** *Chauvin ankerpharm, Ger.*
Erythromycin lactobionate (p.208·2); colistimethate sodium (p.199·1).
*Bacterial eye infections.*

**Ecomucyl** *Ecosol, Switz.*
Acetylcysteine (p.1112·3).
*Paracetamol overdosage; respiratory-tract disorders.*

**Econ**
*Note. This name is used for preparations of different composition.*
*Orion, Denm.*
Ethinylestradiol (p.1553·2); norethisterone acetate (p.1562·2).
*Combined oral contraceptive.*
*General Drugs, Thai.*
Econazole nitrate (p.397·2).
*Fungal skin infections.*

**Econac** *Goldshield, UK.*
Diclofenac sodium (p.32·1).
*Gout; musculoskeletal, joint, and peri-articular disorders; pain.*

**Econacort** *Bristol-Myers Squibb, UK.*
Econazole nitrate (p.397·2); hydrocortisone (p.1103·3).
*Infected skin disorders.*

**Econazine**
*YSP, Malaysia; Yung Shin, Singapore.*
Econazole nitrate (p.397·2); triamcinolone acetonide (p.1110·2).
*Infected skin disorders.*

**Economycin** *DDSA Pharmaceuticals, UK†.*
Tetracycline hydrochloride (p.266·2).

**Econopred** *Alcon, USA.*
Prednisolone acetate (p.1108·1).
*Eye disorders.*

**Ecopace** *Goldshield, UK.*
Captopril (p.879·2).
*Heart failure; hypertension; myocardial infarction.*

**Ecophane**
*Biorga, Fr.*
Nutritional supplement (p.1417·1).
*Nail and hair tonic.*
*Saninter, Port.†.*
Amino acids; magnesium oxoproline; vitamin B substances; zinc gluconate (p.1417·1).
*Hair and nail disorders.*

**Ecoprin** *Sam-On, Israel.*
Aspirin (p.15·1).
*Thrombosis prophylaxis.*

**Ecoprofen** *Ecosol, Switz.*
Ibuprofen (p.45·3).
*Inflammation; musculoskeletal, joint, and peri-articular disorders; pain.*

**Ecorex** *Zambon, Ital.*
Econazole nitrate (p.397·2).
*Fungal or bacterial skin or vulvovaginal infections.*

**Ecos** *Uniao Quimica, Braz.*
Dropropizine (p.1119·3).
*Coughs.*

**Ecosette** *Ecobi, Ital.*
Piperacillin sodium (p.243·1).
Lidocaine hydrochloride (p.1377·3) is included in this preparation to alleviate the pain of injection.
*Bacterial infections.*

**Ecoshampoo** *ICN, Arg.*
Acetic acid (p.1645·2).
*Pediculosis.*

**Ecosporina** *Ecobi, Ital.*
Cefradine (p.179·3).
*Bacterial infections.*

**Ecosprin** *Sidmak, India.*
Aspirin (p.15·1).
*Thromboembolism prophylaxis.*

**Ecostatin**
*Bristol-Myers Squibb, Austral.†; Westwood-Squibb, Canad.; Bristol-Myers Squibb, Irl.; Bristol-Myers Squibb, NZ†; Bristol-Myers Squibb, UK.*
Econazole nitrate (p.397·2).
*Fungal infections.*

**Ecosteril** *Amsa, Ital.*
Econazole nitrate (p.397·2).
*Fungal and Gram-positive skin and nail infections; vulvovaginitis.*

**Ecotam** *Alacan, Spain.*
Econazole nitrate (p.397·2).
*Fungal infections.*

**Ecotrin**
*Link, Austral.; GlaxoSmithKline, Chile; Goldshield, Hong Kong; SmithKline Beecham, Mex.; Link, NZ; Pharmafrica, S.Afr.; SmithKline Beecham Consumer, USA.*
Aspirin (p.15·1).
*Fever; inflammation; pain; thrombosis prophylaxis.*

**Ecoval** *GlaxoSmithKline, Ital.*
Betamethasone valerate (p.1093·2).
*Skin and scalp disorders.*

**Ecoval con Neomicina** *GlaxoSmithKline, Ital.*
Betamethasone valerate (p.1093·2); neomycin sulfate (p.235·1).
*Infected skin disorders.*

**Ecovent** *Ecosol, Switz.*
Salbutamol (p.791·3).
*Obstructive airways disease.*

**Ecovist** *Schering, Braz.†.*
Galactose (p.1063·1).
*Ultrasound contrast medium.*

**Eco-Vita-Min** *Ecobi, Ital.*
Multivitamin and mineral preparation (p.1417·1).

**Ecran Anti-Solaire** *Clarins, Canad.†.*
*SPF 25:* Octinoxate (p.1154·3); oxybenzone (p.1154·3); ensulizole (p.1147·1); titanium dioxide (p.1160·3).
*Sunscreen.*

**Ecran Extreme** *Lutsia, Fr.†.*
*SPF 30+:* Octinoxate (p.1154·3); enzacamene (p.1147·1); ensulizole (p.1147·1); avobenzone (p.1142·3); titanium mica (p.1160·3).
*Sunscreen.*

**Ecran Lutsia** *Lutsia, Fr.†.*
*SPF 8; SPF 10; SPF 15; SPF 25:* Octinoxate (p.1154·3); enzacamene (p.1147·1); ensulizole (p.1147·1); avobenzone (p.1142·3); with or without titanium mica (p.1160·3).
*Sunscreen.*

**Ecran Teinte** *Lutsia, Fr.†.*
*SPF 30+:* Octinoxate (p.1154·3); enzacamene (p.1147·1); ensulizole (p.1147·1); avobenzone (p.1142·3); titanium mica (p.1160·3).
*Sunscreen.*

**Ecran Total** *Vichy, Canad.*
*SPF 45:* Avobenzone (p.1142·3); enzacamene (p.1147·1); ecamsule (p.1146·3); titanium dioxide (p.1160·3).
*Sunscreen.*

**Ecrans Anti-Solaires** *Juvex, Fr.†.*
Octinoxate (p.1154·3); ensulizole (p.1147·1); avobenzone (p.1142·3).
*Sunscreen.*

**Ecreme** *Pacific, NZ.*
Econazole nitrate (p.397·2).
*Fungal skin infections.*

**Ectaprim** *Liomont, Mex.*
Co-trimoxazole (p.199·3).
*Bacterial infections.*

**Ectinex** *20th Century, Mex.†.*
Suxamethonium chloride (p.1406·2).
*Depolarising neuromuscular blocker.*

**Ectiva**
*Bracco, Ital.; Byk Gulden, Mex.*
Sibutramine hydrochloride (p.1593·1).
*Obesity.*

**Ectodyne** *Wigglesworth, UK†.*
Piperazine citrate (p.111·2).
*Ascariasis; enterobiasis.*

**Ectofus** *Coup, Gr.*
Carbocisteine (p.1116·2).
*Respiratory disorders associated with viscous mucus.*

**Ectopal** *Codal Synto, Thai.*
Danazol (p.1545·2).
*Benign breast disorders; endometriosis; female infertility; gynaecomastia; hereditary angioedema; menorrhagia; precocious puberty.*

**Ectosone**
*Technilab, Canad.; Technilab, Hong Kong.*
Betamethasone valerate (p.1093·2).
*Scalp disorders.*

**Ectren** *Menarini, Spain.*
Quinapril hydrochloride (p.991·1).
*Heart failure; hypertension.*

**Ectrin** *EMS, Braz.*
Co-trimoxazole (p.199·3).
*Bacterial infections; Pneumocystis carinii pneumonia; protozoal infections.*

**Ectrin Balsamico** *EMS, Braz.*
Co-trimoxazole (p.199·3); guaifenesin (p.1122·1); ammonium chloride (p.1115·2).
*Bacterial infections.*

**Ecuamon** *Lazar, Arg.*
Domperidone (p.1263·2).
*Dyspepsia; nausea and vomiting.*

**Ecur Test** *Roche Diagnostics, Austral.*
Test for glucose, protein, and blood in urine.

**Ecur Test and Leucocytes** *Roche Diagnostics, Austral.*
Test for protein, glucose, blood, and leucocytes in urine.

**Ecural** *Essex, Ger.*
Mometasone furoate (p.1107·2).
*Scalp disorders; skin disorders.*

**Eczema** *Homeocan, Canad.*
Homoeopathic preparation.

**Eczema Cream** *Hamilton, Austral.*
Coal tar (p.1159·2); dimethicone (p.1482·1); zinc oxide (p.1163·2).
*Dermatitis; eczema.*

**Eczema L87** *Homeocan, Canad.*
Homoeopathic preparation.

**Eczema Ointment**
*Note. This name is used for preparations of different composition.*
*Stanley, Canad.†.*
Bismuth subcarbonate (p.1252·1); salicylic acid (p.1157·1); zinc oxide (p.1163·2).
*Potter's, UK.*
Zinc oxide (p.1163·2); salicylic acid (p.1157·1); benzoic acid (p.1169·3); stellaria media.
*Eczema.*

**Eczo-Wokadine** *Wockhardt, India.*
Fluocinolone acetonide (p.1101·2); povidone-iodine (p.1190·3).
*Infected skin disorders.*

**Ed A-Hist** *Edwards, USA.*
Phenylephrine hydrochloride (p.1126·3); chlorphenamine maleate (p.427·3).
*Allergic rhinitis; nasal congestion.*

**ED Tuss HC** *Edwards, USA.*
Phenylephrine hydrochloride (p.1126·3); chlorphenamine maleate (p.427·3); hydrocodone tartrate (p.45·1).
*Coughs and cold symptoms.*

**Edamox** *Remedica, Hong Kong.*
Amoxicillin trihydrate (p.155·3).
*Bacterial infections.*

**Edason** *Medicus, Gr.*
Clindamycin phosphate (p.194·2).
*Acne.*

**Eddia** *Pierre Fabre Sante, Fr.†.*
Metformin hydrochloride (p.342·3).
*Diabetes mellitus.*

**Ede** *Teofarma, Ital.†.*
Metoclopramide (p.1274·3); simeticone (p.1289·2).
*Gastrointestinal disorders.*

**Ede 6** *Teofarma, Ital.*
Dimeticone (p.1289·2); pancreatin (p.1725·3).
*Digestive disorders.*

**Edecril**
*Merck Sharp & Dohme, Austral.; Merck Sharp & Dohme, NZ†.*
Etacrynic acid (p.913·2).
*Heart failure; hepatic cirrhosis with ascites; nephrotic syndrome; oedema.*

**Edecrin**
*Merck Sharp & Dohme, Austria; Merck Frosst, Canad.; Merck Sharp & Dohme, Irl.†; Merck Sharp & Dohme, Ital.†; Merck Sharp & Dohme, Neth.†; Merck, USA.*
Etacrynic acid (p.913·2) or sodium etacrynate (p.913·3).
*Oedema.*

**Edecrina** *Merck Sharp & Dohme, Swed.*
Sodium etacrynate (p.913·3).
*Oedema.*

**Edefen** *Diba, Mex.*
Oxyphenbutazone (p.76·1).
*Rheumatoid disorders.*

**Edemax** *SIFI, Ital.*
Nimesulide (p.67·1).
*Fever; inflammation; pain.*

**Edemox** *Chiesi, Spain.*
Acetazolamide (p.849·1).
*Epilepsy; glaucoma; high-altitude disorders; oedema.*

**Edenil** *Zambon, Ital.*
Ibuprofen isobutanolammoniun (p.46·3).
*Gynaecological disorders.*

**Edenol** *Randall, Mex.*
Furosemide (p.919·3).
*Hypertension; liver cirrhosis with ascites; nephrotic syndrome; oedema.*

**Ederal** *Esteve, Spain†.*
Cinnarizine (p.428·3); calcium dobesilate (p.1664·2).
*Cerebrovascular disorders; vestibular disorders.*

**Ederphyt** *Mavena, Switz.*
*Cream:* Phenol undecenoate; thymol (p.1194·2); salicylic acid (p.1157·1).
*Topical spray:* Phenol undecenoate; menthol (p.1711·3); thymol (p.1194·2); salicylic acid (p.1157·1); phenoxyethanol (p.1189·1); isopropyl alcohol (p.1184·3).
*Fungal foot infections.*

**Edeven** *Ibi, Ital.*
*Tablets; injection:* Sodium aescinate (p.1648·2).
*Oedema.*
*Topical gel:* Aescin (p.1648·2); heparin sodium (p.928·1); diethylamine salicylate (p.34·1).
*Soft-tissue injury; superficial vascular disorders.*

**Edex**
*Schwarz, Fr.; Schwarz, USA.*
Alprostadil (p.1512·3).
*Erectile dysfunction.*

**Edhanol** *Sintofarma, Braz.*
Phenobarbital (p.367·3).
*Epilepsy.*

**Edicin** *Lek, Thai.*
Vancomycin hydrochloride (p.275·2).
*Staphylococcal infections.*

**Edifaringen** *Edigen, Spain.*
Bacitracin zinc (p.161·3); benzocaine (p.1370·3); hydrocortisone acetate (p.1103·3); neomycin sulfate (p.235·1); potassium chlorate (p.1734·2).
*Mouth and throat disorders.*

**Edigastrol** *Edigen, Spain.*
Aluminium hydroxide (p.1249·2); magnesium oxide (p.1272·3).
*Dyspepsia; gastrointestinal hyperacidity.*

**Ediluna** *Vinas, Spain†.*
Ibuprofen (p.45·3).
*Fever; musculoskeletal and joint disorders; pain; peri-articular disorders.*

**Edinol** *Bayer, India.*
Multivitamin and mineral preparation (p.1417·1).

**Ed-in-Sol** *Edwards, USA.*
Ferrous sulfate (p.1428·2).
*Iron deficiency.*

**Edirel** *Laphal, Fr.*
Erdosteine (p.1121·1).
*Respiratory-tract congestion.*

**Ediston** *Pierre Fabre Sante, Fr.*
Nifuroxazide (p.237·2).
*Diarrhoea.*

**Edmilla** *Hanseler, Switz.†.*
Chamomile (p.1669·3).
*Inflammatory disorders of the skin and mouth.*

**Ednyt**
*Pinewood, Irl.; Dominion, UK†.*
Enalapril maleate (p.909·2).
*Heart failure; hypertension.*

**Edolfene** *Edol, Port.*
Flurbiprofen sodium (p.44·1).
*Ocular inflammation; prevention of intra- and postoperative miosis.*

**Edolglau** *Edol, Port.*
Clonidine hydrochloride (p.885·2).
*Glaucoma.*

**Edoltar** *Edol, Port.*
Undecenoic acid monoethanolamide (p.411·1); coal tar (p.1159·2); salicylic acid (p.1157·1); resorcinol (p.1156·3); thymol (p.1194·2).
*Skin and scalp disorders.*

**Edolzine** *Oftalder, Port.†.*
Tetryzoline hydrochloride (p.1131·2).
*Eye disorders.*

**Edoxil** *Inibsa, Spain.*
Amoxicillin trihydrate (p.155·3).
*Bacterial infections.*

**Edoxil Mucolitico** *Inibsa, Spain.*
Amoxicillin trihydrate (p.155·3); bromhexine hydrochloride (p.1115·3).
*Respiratory-tract infections.*

**EDP-Evans Dermal Powder** *Boots, Austral.†.*
Povidone-iodine (p.1190·3).
*Burns; chafing; tinea pedis; ulcers; wounds.*

**Edrigyl** *Allen, Gr.*
Nimesulide (p.67·1).
*Inflammation; musculoskeletal disorders; pain.*

**Edronax**
*Pharmacia, Austral.; Pharmacia, Austria; Pharmacia, Belg.; Pharmacia, Denm.; Pharmacia, Fin.; Pharmacia, Ger.; Pharmacia, Irl.; Pharmacia Upjohn, Israel; Pharmacia Upjohn, Ital.; Pharmacia Upjohn, Mex.; Pharmacia, Norw.; Pharmacia, NZ; Pharmacia, Port.; Pharmacia, S.Afr.; Pharmacia, Swed.; Pharmacia, Switz.; Pharmacia, UK.*
Reboxetine mesilate (p.316·3).
*Depression.*

**E-Drops** *Ranbaxy, Thai.*
*dl*-Alpha tocoferil acetate (p.1465·1).
*Vitamin E deficiency.*

**ED-SPAZ** *Edwards, USA.*
Hyoscyamine sulfate (p.485·1).

**ED-TLC** *Edwards, USA.*
Phenylephrine hydrochloride (p.1126·3); chlorphenamine maleate (p.427·3); hydrocodone tartrate (p.45·1).
*Coughs and cold symptoms.*

**Edual** *Pharmafina, Chile.*
Hypericum (p.299·1).
*Depression.*

**Eductyl** *Techni-Pharma, Mon.*
Potassium acid tartrate (p.1284·3); sodium bicarbonate (p.1223·2).
*Bowel evacuation; constipation.*

**Edul K-200** *Knop, Chile.*
Chromium tripicolinate (p.1425·1).
*Chromium deficiency.*

**Eduprim** *F5 Profas, Spain.*
Co-trimoxazole (p.199·3).
*Bacterial infections; Pneumocystis carinii pneumonia.*

**Eduprim Mucolitico** *F5 Profas, Spain.*
Carbocisteine (p.1116·2); guaifenesin (p.1122·1); co-trimoxazole (p.199·3).
*Respiratory-tract infections.*

**Edurid** *Iromedica, Switz.*
Edoxudine (p.632·1).
*Herpes simplex infections.*

**Edusan Fte Rectal** *Casen Fleet, Spain†.*
Camphor (p.1665·3); cineole (p.1672·1); niaouli oil (p.1719·3); guaiacol (p.1122·1).
*Respiratory-tract disorders.*

**Edym Sedante** *Vita, Spain†.*
Diazepam (p.690·1); dimethicone (p.1289·2); metoclopramide hydrochloride (p.1274·3); pancreatin (p.1725·3).
*Gastrointestinal disorders.*

**EES**
*Abbott, Austral.; Abbott, Canad.; Abbott, Hong Kong; Abbott, Malaysia; Abbott, NZ†; Abbott, Singapore; Abbott, USA.*
Erythromycin ethyl succinate (p.208·1).
*Bacterial infections; intestinal amoebiasis.*

**Eetless** *Adcock Ingram, S.Afr.*
Cathine hydrochloride (p.1585·2).
*Obesity.*

**EFA Steri** *Pharmavite, Canad.†.*
Sodium chloride (p.1233·3).

**Efabetic** *Express Care, NZ.*
Essential fatty acids; gamolenic acid; vitamin E (p.1417·1).
*Dietary supplement in diabetic neuropathy.*

**Efacal**
*Efamol, Austral.†; Nutricia, NZ; Efamol, UK†.*
Evening primrose oil (p.1686·3); fish oil (p.976·2); calcium (p.1225·1).
*Calcium supplement; osteoporosis.*

**Efadermin** *Widmer, Ger.*
Lithium succinate (p.1151·2); zinc sulfate (p.1469·3).
*Seborrhoeic dermatitis.*

**Efagel** *Mavi, Ital.*
Gamolenic acid (p.1690·2); vitamin E (p.1464·3).
*Nutritional supplement.*

**Efalex**
*Efamol, Austral.; Nutricia, Canad.; Nutricia, NZ; Nutricia Dietary, UK.*
Marine fatty acids (p.976·2); evening primrose oil (p.1686·3); thyme oil (p.1755·3).
*Dietary supplement.*

**Efalex Focus** *Efamol, Canad.†.*
Evening primrose oil (p.1686·3).

**Efalith**
*Widmer, Austria; Scotia, Irl.; Scotia, NZ†; Widmer, Switz.; United Drug, UK†.*
Lithium succinate (p.1151·2); zinc sulfate (p.1469·3).
*Seborrhoeic dermatitis.*

**Efamarine**
*Efamol, Austral.; Nutricia, NZ; Efamol, UK.*
Evening primrose oil (p.1686·3); marine fish oil (p.976·2).
Formerly known as Efamol Marine in *NZ*.
*Dietary supplement.*

**Efamast**
*Scotia, Hong Kong†.*
Gamolenic acid (p.1690·2).
*Dysmenorrhoea; mastalgia.*

*Express Care, NZ.*
Essential fatty acids; gamolenic acid (p.1690·2).
*Mastalgia.*

*Pharmacia, UK†.*
Evening primrose oil (p.1686·3).
*Mastalgia.*

**Efamax** *Nutricia, NZ.*
Evening primrose oil (p.1686·3); fish oil (p.976·2); vitamins and minerals (p.1417·1); herbs.
*Dietary supplement.*

**Efamol**
*Primula, Arg.; Efamol, Canad.; Nutricia, NZ; Sidroga, Switz.; Efamol, UK.*
Evening primrose oil (p.1686·3).
*Dietary supplement.*

**Efamol Fortify** *Efamol, Canad.†.*
Evening primrose oil (p.1686·3); calcium carbonate (p.1254·2).

**Efamol G** *Covan, S.Afr.*
Gamolenic acid (p.1690·2); linoleic acid (p.1690·2).
*Nutritional supplement.*

**Efamol Plus Coenzyme Q10** *Efamol, UK†.*
Evening primrose oil (p.1686·3); ubidecarenone (p.1760·2).
*Tonic.*

**Efamol PMP** *Nutricia Dietary, UK.*
Evening primrose oil (p.1686·3); vitamins; minerals (p.1417·1).
*Premenstrual syndrome.*

**Efamol Safflower & Linseed** *Efamol, UK†.*
Evening primrose oil (p.1686·3); linseed oil (p.1707·2); safflower oil (p.1443·3).

**Efanatal**
*Efamol, Austral.†; Nutricia Dietary, UK.*
Evening primrose oil; fish oil (p.1417·1).
*Nutritional supplement in pregnancy and lactation.*

*Nutricia, NZ.*
Polyunsaturated fatty acids; docosahexaenoic acid; arachidonic acid; gamolenic acid (p.1417·1).
*Dietary supplement during pregnancy and breast feeding.*

**Efaprost** *Efamol, NZ†.*
Fatty acids; evening primrose oil; gamolenic acid; saw palmetto; sitosterol (p.1417·1).
*Dietary supplement; prostatic disorders.*

**Efargen** *Teofarma, Ital.†.*
Cyanocobalamin (p.1458·2); folic acid (p.1429·1); nicotinamide (p.1441·2); pyridoxine hydrochloride (p.1456·3).
*Vitamin deficiency.*

**Efasit N** *Togal, Ger.†.*
*Plaster:* Salicylic acid (p.1157·1).
*Tincture:* Salicylic acid (p.1157·1); lactic acid (p.1704·1).
*Calluses; corns; hard skin.*

**Efatime** *Efamol, UK†.*
Fatty acids (p.976·2); vitamin E (p.1464·3); red thyme oil.

**Efavir** *Cipla, India.*
Efavirenz (p.632·2).
*HIV infection.*

**Efavite** *Efamol, UK†.*
Multivitamin and mineral preparation (p.1417·1).

**Efcorlin** *GlaxoSmithKline, India.*
Hydrocortisone (p.1103·3); naphazoline nitrate (p.1124·3).
*Nasal congestion.*

**Efcortelan** *GlaxoSmithKline, UK.*
Hydrocortisone (p.1103·3).
*Skin disorders.*

**Efcortesol** *Sovereign, UK.*
Hydrocortisone sodium phosphate (p.1104·1).
*Corticosteroid.*

**Efectin** *Wyeth Lederle, Austria.*
Venlafaxine hydrochloride (p.321·3).
*Depression.*

**Efederm** *Hertz, Braz.†.*
Boric acid (p.1662·1); triclosan (p.1195·2); zinc (p.1469·2).
*Antiseptic.*

**Efedronal** *Baldassari, Braz.†.*
Diphenhydramine hydrochloride (p.431·3); sodium benzoate (p.1169·3); belladonna (p.479·1); lobelia (p.1589·1); guaifenesin (p.1122·1); ephedrine hydrochloride (p.1120·1).
*Respiratory-tract congestion.*

**Efedrosan** *Pasteur, Chile.*
Ephedrine hydrochloride (p.1120·1).
*Asthma; bronchitis.*

**Efektolol** *Alpharma-Isis, Ger.*
Propranolol hydrochloride (p.989·3).
*Angina pectoris; arrhythmias; essential tremor; hypertension; hyperthyroidism; migraine.*

**Efemida** *Llorens, Spain†.*
Cefalexin (p.168·1).
*Bacterial infections.*

**Efemolin** *Novartis Ophthalmics, Ger.*
Fluorometholone (p.1102·2); tetryzoline hydrochloride (p.1131·2).
*Allergic and inflammatory disorders of the eye.*

**Efemolina** *Novartis Ophthalmics, Arg.*
Fluorometholone (p.1102·2); tetryzoline hydrochloride (p.1131·2).
*Eye disorders.*

**Efemoline**
*Novartis Ophthalmics, Hong Kong; Ciba Vision, Ital.; Novartis Ophthalmics, Malaysia; Restan, S.Afr.; Novartis Ophthalmics, Singapore; Novartis Ophthalmics, Switz.; Ciba Vision, Thai.*
Fluorometholone (p.1102·2); tetryzoline hydrochloride (p.1131·2).
*Allergic and inflammatory disorders of the eye.*

**Efensol** *Ipsen, Spain.*
Filicol.
*Hypercholesterolaemia; pruritus associated with partial biliary obstruction.*

**Eferox** *Hexal, Ger.*
Levothyroxine sodium (p.1600·1).
*Hypothyroidism.*

**Efexor**
*Wyeth, Arg.; Wyeth, Austral.; Wyeth Lederle, Austria†; Wyeth Lederle, Belg.; Wyeth, Braz.; Wyeth, Chile; Wyeth Lederle, Denm.; Wyeth Lederle, Fin.; Wyeth, Gr.; Wyeth, Hong Kong; Wyeth, Irl.; Dexcel, Israel; Wyeth Lederle, Ital.; Wyeth, Malaysia; Wyeth, Mex.; Wyeth, Neth.; Wyeth Lederle, Norw.; Wyeth, NZ; Wyeth Lederle, Port.; Wyeth, S.Afr.; Wyeth, Singapore; Wyeth Lederle, Swed.; Cross, Swed.; Netpharma, Swed.; Wyeth, Switz.; Wyeth-Ayerst, Thai.; Wyeth, UK.*
Venlafaxine hydrochloride (p.321·3).
*Anxiety; depression; mixed anxiety depressive states.*

**Effaclar**
*Note. This name is used for preparations of different composition.*
*Roche-Posay, Arg.*
Zinc pidolate.
*Acne.*

*Roche-Posay, Braz.*
Zinc pidolate; iodopropynyl butyl carbamate (Glycacil); chlorhexidine gluconate (p.1173·2).

*Roche-Posay, Irl.*
Iodopropynyl butyl carbamate (Glycacil); zinc pidolate.
*Acne.*

**Effacne**
*Roche-Posay, Fr.; Roche-Posay, Switz.*
Benzoyl peroxide (p.1143·2).
*Acne.*

**Effagel** *Roche-Posay, Fr.†.*
Pharmaceutical gel base.

**Effalpha** *Roche-Posay, Arg.*
Glycolic acid (p.1147·3); zinc pidolate.
*Acne.*

**Effcal** *Ranbaxy, Thai.*
Calcium carbonate (p.1254·2); colecalciferol (p.1461·3).
*Calcium supplement; osteoporosis.*

**Effective Strength Cough Formula** *Barre-National, USA.*
Chlorphenamine maleate (p.427·3); dextromethorphan hydrobromide (p.1117·3).
*Coughs and cold symptoms.*

**Effective Strength Cough Formula Liquid With Decongestant** *Barre-National, USA.*
Dextromethorphan hydrobromide (p.1117·3); pseudoephedrine hydrochloride (p.1129·2).
*Coughs and cold symptoms.*

**Effectsal** *Shin Poong, Singapore.*
Norfloxacin (p.238·3).
*Bacterial infections.*

**Effederm** *CS, Fr.*
Tretinoin (p.1161·1).
*Acne; keratinisation disorders; warts.*

**Effekton** *Teofarma, Ger.*
Diclofenac sodium (p.32·1).
*Gout; inflammation; musculoskeletal, joint, and soft-tissue disorders; pain.*

**Efferalgan**
*Upsamedica, Belg.†; UPSA, Fr.; Bristol-Myers Squibb, Israel; Upsa, Ital.; Bristol-Myers Squibb, Port.; Upsamedica, Spain.*
Paracetamol (p.76·2).
*Fever; pain.*

**Efferalgan C**
*Bristol-Myers Squibb, Belg.; Upsamedica, Ital.; Upsamedica, Switz.†.*
Paracetamol (p.76·2); ascorbic acid (p.1460·2).
*Fever; pain.*

**Efferalgan Codeine**
*UPSA, Fr.; Bristol-Myers Squibb, Israel.*
Paracetamol (p.76·2); codeine phosphate (p.27·1).
*Pain.*

**Efferalgan Vit C** *Upsamedica, Spain.*
Paracetamol (p.76·2); ascorbic acid (p.1460·2).
*Fever; pain.*

**Efferalgan Vitamine C** *UPSA, Fr.*
Paracetamol (p.76·2); ascorbic acid (p.1460·2).
*Fever; pain.*

**Efferalganodis** *UPSA Conseil, Fr.*
Paracetamol (p.76·2).
*Fever; pain.*

**Efferbalgine** *Pharmethic, Belg.†.*
Aspirin (p.15·1); codeine phosphate (p.27·1); ascorbic acid (p.1460·2).
*Fever; pain.*

**Effercal**
*Note. This name is used for preparations of different composition.*
*Piam, Ital.†.*
Calcium carbonate (p.1254·2).
*Calcium deficiency; calcium supplement.*

*Akromed, S.Afr.†.*
Vitamin $B_6$ and mineral preparation (p.1417·1).

**Effercal D3** *Piam, Ital.*
Calcium carbonate (p.1254·2); colecalciferol (p.1461·3).
*Calcium and vitamin D deficiency.*

**Effercet** *Doctum, Gr.*
Ambroxol hydrochloride (p.1114·3).
*Respiratory disorders associated with viscous mucus.*

**Effercitrate** *Typharm, UK.*
Potassium citrate (p.1223·1); citric acid (p.1673·1).
*Cystitis.*

**Effer-K** *Nomax, USA.*
Potassium bicarbonate (p.1223·1); potassium citrate (p.1223·1).
*Hypokalaemia; potassium depletion.*

**Effersol** *Aspen, S.Afr.*
Sodium bicarbonate (p.1223·2); citric acid (p.1673·1).
*Acidosis; urinary alkalinisation.*

**Effersyllium** *Johnson & Johnson, Austria†.*
Ispaghula (p.1268·1).
*Constipation.*

**Efferzyme** *Bausch & Lomb, Canad.*
Subtilisin (p.1164·2).
*Protein remover for soft contact lenses.*

**Effetre** *Farmatre, Ital.†.*
Chlorhexidine gluconate (p.1173·2).
*Disinfection of skin, wounds, burns, hands, and surgical materials; skin irritation.*

**Effexor**
*Wyeth-Ayerst, Canad.; Wyeth Lederle, Fr.; Wyeth-Ayerst, USA.*
Venlafaxine hydrochloride (p.321·3).
*Anxiety; depression.*

**Efficlean** *Bausch & Lomb, Fr.†.*
Subtilisin-A(p.1164·2).
*Protein remover for contact lenses.*

**Effico**
*Pharmax, Irl.*
Nicotinamide; thiamine hydrochloride; caffeine (p.1417·1).
*Tonic.*

*Forest Laboratories, UK.*
Nicotinamide; thiamine hydrochloride; caffeine; compound gentian infusion (p.1417·1).
*Tonic.*

**Efficort**
*Galderma, Arg.; Galderma, Chile; Galderma, Fr.; Galderma, Hong Kong; Galderma, Israel; Galderma, Ital.; Galderma, Malaysia; Galderma, Mex.; Galderma, Singapore.*
Hydrocortisone aceponate (p.1104·2).
*Skin disorders.*

**Effidigest**
*Yves Ponroy, Fr.; Ceuta, UK†.*
Nutritional supplement (p.1417·1).
*Gastrointestinal disorders.*

**Effidrate**
*Roche-Posay, Arg.*
Glycerol; octoxin; aluminium (p.1652·2).
*Acne.*

*Roche-Posay, Braz.*
Glycerol; octoxyglycerin; aluminium amido-octenylsuccinate.

**Effiplen** *Effik, Spain.*
Buspirone hydrochloride (p.672·2).
*Anxiety; mixed anxiety depressive states.*

**Effiprev** *Effik, Fr.*
Norgestimate (p.1563·2); ethinylestradiol (p.1553·2).
*Combined oral contraceptive.*

**Efflumidex** *Allergan, Ger.*
Fluorometholone (p.1102·2).
*Allergic and inflammatory disorders of the eye.*

**Efflumycin** *Allergan, Ger.*
Fluorometholone (p.1102·2); neomycin sulfate (p.235·1).
*Infected eye disorders.*

**Effortil**
*Boehringer Ingelheim, Arg.; Boehringer Ingelheim, Austria; Boehringer Ingelheim, Belg.; Boehringer Ingelheim, Chile; Boehringer Ingelheim, Fin.; Boehringer Ingelheim, Fr.†; Boehringer Ingelheim, Ger.; Boehringer Ingelheim, Gr.; IFET (ΙΦΕΤ), Gr.; Boehringer Ingelheim, Ital.; Boehringer Ingelheim, Mex.; Boehringer Ingelheim, Norw.; Boehringer Ingelheim, Port.; Boehringer Ingelheim, S.Afr.; Boehringer Ingelheim, Swed.; Boehringer Ingelheim, Switz.; Boehringer Ingelheim, Thai.*
Etilefrine hydrochloride (p.914·1).
*Hypotension.*

**Effortil comp** *Boehringer Ingelheim, Austria.*
Etilefrine hydrochloride (p.914·1); dihydroergotamine mesilate (p.465·3).
*Hypotension.*

**Effortil plus**
*Boehringer Ingelheim, Ger.; Boehringer Ingelheim, Switz.*
Etilefrine hydrochloride (p.914·1); dihydroergotamine mesilate (p.465·3).
*Hypotension.*

**Efherol** *Vitemat, Braz.*
Vitamin E (p.1464·3).

**Efical** *Irex, Fr.†.*
Calcium pidolate (p.1226·1); calcium carbonate (p.1254·2).
*Calcium deficiency; osteoporosis.*

**Efidac 24 Chlorpheniramine** *Hogil, USA.*
Chlorphenamine maleate (p.427·3).
*Hypersensitivity reactions.*

**Efidac 24 Pseudoepehdrine** *Hogil, USA.*
Pseudoephedrine hydrochloride (p.1129·2).

**Efiken** *Kendrick, Mex.*
Ketoprofen (p.51·2).
*Fever; osteoarthritis; pain; rheumatoid arthritis.*

**Efimag** *Fornet, Fr.*
Magnesium pidolate (p.1228·2).
*Magnesium deficiency.*

**Efisol S** *Roland, Ger.†.*
Dequalinium chloride (p.1178·1).
*Mouth and throat inflammation.*

**Efixano** *Dosa, Arg.*
Irinotecan (p.564·3).
*Malignant neoplasms.*

**Eflevar** *Byk, Arg.*
Calcium dobesilate (p.1664·2).
*Haemorrhoids; venous insufficiency.*

**Eflone** *Ciba Vision, USA.*
Fluorometholone acetate (p.1102·2).
*Eye disorders.*

**Efluvium Anti-caspa** *Dermoteca, Port.*
Salicylic acid (p.1157·1); ichthammol (p.1148·2); saw palmetto (p.1569·1); climbazole (p.396·2); acetamide monoethanolamide.
*Scalp disorders.*

**Efluvium Anti-seborreico** *Dermoteca, Port.*
*Lotion:* Salicylic acid (p.1157·1); panthenol (p.1727·2); azeoglycine; acetamide monoethanolamide.
*Shampoo:* Salicylic acid (p.1157·1); ichthammol (p.1148·2); saw palmetto (p.1569·1); acetamide monoethanolamide.
*Scalp disorders.*

**Efodil** *Lafage, Arg.*
Ephedrine (p.1120·1); silver (p.1746·1).
*Nasal congestion.*

**Efodine** *Fougera, USA.*
Povidone-iodine (p.1190·3).
*Skin disinfection.*

**Efortil**
*Boehringer de Angeli, Braz.; Boehringer Ingelheim, Spain.*
Etilefrine hydrochloride (p.914·1).
*Hypotension.*

**Efrane**
*Abbott, Denm.; Abbott, Fin.; Abbott, Norw.†Abbott, Swed.*
Enflurane (p.1298·1).
*General anaesthesia.*

**Efridol** *Aesculapius, Ital.*
Nimesulide (p.67·1).
*Fever; inflammation; pain.*

**Efrin** *Fischer, Israel.*
Phenylephrine hydrochloride (p.1126·3).
*Eye congestion; production of mydriasis.*

**Efriviral** *Aesculapius, Ital.*
Aciclovir (p.626·1).
*Herpesvirus infections.*

**Eftab** *Thornton & Ross, UK†.*
Peppermint oil (p.1283·2); clove oil (p.1673·3); spearmint oil (p.1749·1); menthol (p.1711·3); thymol (p.1194·2); methyl salicylate (p.59·3).
*Oral hygiene.*

**Eftapan**
*Ratiopharm, Austria; Merckle, Ger.*
Eprazinone hydrochloride (p.1121·1).
*Coughs.*

**Eftapan Tetra** *Ratiopharm, Austria.*
Eprazinone hydrochloride (p.1121·1); tetracycline hydrochloride (p.266·2).
*Bacterial respiratory-tract infections.*

**Eftazid** *Mundogen, Spain†.*
Paracetamol (p.76·2).
*Fever; pain.*

**Eftiar Decalin** *DORC, Neth.*
Perflunafene (p.1730·1).
*Ophthalmic tamponade.*

**Eftiar Octane** *DORC, Neth.*
Perfluoroctane (p.1730·2).
*Ophthalmic tamponade.*

**Efudex**
*ICN, Canad.; Roche, USA.*
Fluorouracil (p.554·2).
*Skin cancer; solar keratoses.*

**Efudix**
*ICN, Arg.; ICN, Austral.; Sanico, Belg.†; CSP, Fr.; ICN, Ger.; ICN, Hong Kong; ICN, Irl.; ICN, Israe; ICN, Ital.; ICN, Mex.; ICN, Neth.; ICN, NZ; Pacific, NZ; Pharmaco, S.Afr.; ICN, Singapore; ICN, Spain; ICN, Switz.; ICN, Thai.†; ICN, UK.*
Fluorouracil (p.554·2).
*Anogenital warts; premalignant skin lesions; skin cancer; solar and senile keratoses.*

**Efurix** *ICN, Braz.*
Fluorouracil (p.554·2).
*Skin cancer; solar and senile keratoses.*

**Efxine** *Pharmasant, Thai.*
Etilefrine hydrochloride (p.914·1).
*Hypotension.*

**Egacene** *AstraZeneca, Neth.†.*
Hyoscyamine sulfate (p.485·1).
*Bradycardia; gastrointestinal spasm; hyperhidrosis.*

**Egarone** *Farmalider, Spain.*
Allantoin (p.1141·3); benzalkonium chloride (p.1168·3); muramidase hydrochloride (p.1717·2); oxymetazoline (p.1126·2).
*Cold symptoms; rhinitis; sinusitis.*

**Egarone Oximetazolina** *Alcala, Spain†.*
Oxymetazoline hydrochloride (p.1126·1).
*Nasal congestion; sinus congestion.*

**Egazil**
*AstraZeneca, Denm.; AstraZeneca, Fin.; AstraZeneca, Norw.; Hassle, Swed.*
Hyoscyamine sulfate (p.485·1).
*Biliary colic; bladder tenesmus; hypersecretion; irritable bowel syndrome.*

**E-Gems** *Carlson, USA.*
*d*-Alpha tocoferil acetate (p.1465·1).
*Vitamin E supplement.*

**E-Gen-C** *Schering, S.Afr.*
Levonorgestrel (p.1563·2); ethinylestradiol (p.1553·2).
*Postcoital oral contraceptive.*

**Egery** *Biorga, Fr.*
Erythromycin (p.208·1).
*Bacterial infections.*

**Egibren** *Chiesi, Ital.*
Selegiline hydrochloride (p.1214·1).
*Psychiatric disorders.*

**Egicalm** *Sanofi Synthelabo, Gr.*
Lysine aspirin (p.54·3).
*Fever; inflammation; pain.*

**Eglandin** *Welfide, Singapore.*
Alprostadil (p.1512·3).
*Maintenance of patent ductus arteriosus.*

**Eglidon** *Merck, Arg.*
Terazosin hydrochloride (p.1010·3).
*Benign prostatic hyperplasia.*

**Eglonyl** *Sanofi Synthelabo, S.Afr.*
Sulpiride (p.722·2).
*Depression; disturbed behaviour; peptic ulcer; psychoses; vertigo.*

**Egmovit** *Schmidgall, Austria.*
Plantago lanceolata (p.1738·2); thyme (p.1755·2); cowslip (p.1735·1).
*Coughs.*

**Ego Skin Cream**
*Ego, Austral.†; Ego, Malaysia.*
Emollient.
*Dry skin.*

*Ego, Hong Kong; Ego, NZ.*
Cetyl alcohol (p.1480·3); glycerol (p.1694·3); liquid paraffin (p.1479·1).
*Barrier cream; emollient.*

**Egocort**
*Ego, Austral.; Ego, Hong Kong; Ego, Malaysia; Ego, NZ; Ego, Singapore.*
Hydrocortisone (p.1103·3).
*Skin disorders.*

**Egoderm**
*Note. This name is used for preparations of different composition.*
*Ego, Austral.*
*Cream:* Ichthammol (p.1148·2).
*Skin disorders.*

*Ego, Austral.; Ego, Hong Kong; Ego, Malaysia; Ego, NZ; Ego, Singapore.*
*Ointment:* Ichthammol (p.1148·2); zinc oxide (p.1163·2).
*Skin disorders.*

*Ego, Hong Kong; Ego, Malaysia; Ego, NZ; Ego, Singapore.*
*Cream:* Ichthammol (p.1148·2); allantoin (p.1141·3).
*Skin disorders.*

**Egogyn**
*Note. A similar name is used for preparations of different composition (see below).*
*Osteolab, Chile.*
Vitamin E (p.1464·3).
*Dietary supplement.*

**Egogyn 30**
*Note. A similar name is used for preparations of different composition (see above).*
*Schering, Ital.*
Levonorgestrel (p.1563·2); ethinylestradiol (p.1553·2).
*Combined oral contraceptive.*

**Egomycol**
*Ego, Austral.†; Ego, NZ.*
Undecylenic alkanolamide (p.411·1); chlorhexidine gluconate (p.1173·2); salicylic acid (p.1157·1); benzoic acid (p.1169·3); resorcinol (p.1156·3).
*Fungal and bacterial skin and nail infections.*

**Egopsoryl TA**
*Note. This name is used for preparations of different composition.*
*Ego, Austral.*
Sulfur (p.1158·2); phenol (p.1188·1); menthol (p.1711·3); glycerol (p.1694·3); coal tar (p.1159·2).
*Psoriasis.*

*Ego, Hong Kong.*
Sulfur (p.1158·2); phenol (p.1188·1); coal tar (p.1159·2); menthol (p.1711·3).
*Eczema; psoriasis.*

*Ego, Malaysia; Ego, Singapore.*
Sulfur (p.1158·2); phenol (p.1188·1); coal tar (p.1159·2).
*Eczema; psoriasis.*

*Ego, NZ.*
Allantoin (p.1141·3); sulfur (p.1158·2); menthol (p.1711·3); coal tar (p.1159·2); phenol (p.1188·1).
*Psoriasis.*

**Egosona** *Danes, Arg.*
Beclometasone dipropionate (p.1091·1).
*Asthma; rhinitis.*

**Egotussano** *Sedabel, Braz.*
Sodium sulfonate; sodium benzoate (p.1169·3); guaiacol (p.1122·1).
*Coughs.*

**Egozinc**
*Pharmascience, Canad; Pharmascience, Hong Kong.*
Zinc oxide (p.1163·2) or zinc sulfate (p.1469·3).
*Burns; haemorrhoids; ulcers; wounds.*

**Egozite Baby** *Ego, NZ.*
Zinc oxide (p.1163·2); dimethicone (p.1482·1); light liquid paraffin (p.1479·1).
*Barrier cream; nappy rash.*

**Egozite Baby Cream**
*Note. This name is used for preparations of different composition.*
*Ego, Austral.*
Zinc oxide (p.1163·2); dimethicone (p.1482·1); light liquid paraffin (p.1479·1).
*Skin disorders.*

*Ego, Hong Kong.*
Zinc oxide (p.1163·2); dimethicone (p.1482·1); light liquid paraffin (p.1479·1); dexpanthenol (p.1727·2).
*Skin disorders.*

*Ego, Malaysia; Ego, Singapore.*
Zinc oxide (p.1163·2); dimeticone (p.1482·1); light liquid paraffin (p.1479·1); glycerol (p.1694·3); dexpanthenol (p.1727·2).
*Skin disorders.*

**Egozite Cradle Cap**
*Ego, Austral.; Ego, Hong Kong; Ego, Malaysia; Ego, NZ.*
Salicylic acid (p.1157·1) in an oil basis.
*Cradle cap.*

**Egozite Protective Baby Lotion**
*Ego, Austral.; Ego, Hong Kong; Ego, Malaysia; Ego, NZ; Ego, Singapore.*
Dimeticone (p.1482·1).
*Barrier preparation; nappy rash.*

**EH Retard** *Eco, S.Afr.*
Allergen extracts (p.1650·1).
*Hyposensitisation.*

**Ehlifena** *Ehlinger, Mex.†.*
Diclofenac (p.32·1).

**Ehlifung** *Ehlinger, Mex.†.*
Ketoconazole (p.403·3).

**Ehlindopa** *Ehlinger, Mex.†.*
Methyldopa (p.953·2).

**Ehliten** *Ehlinger, Mex.†.*
Praziquantel (p.112·2).

**Ehlixacin** *Ehlinger, Mex.†.*
Ciprofloxacin (p.188·2).
*Bacterial infections.*

**Ehrenhofer-Salbe** *Ehrenhofer, Austria.*
Colophony (p.1675·1); lovage root (p.1708·1).
*Bronchitis; skin disorders; soft-tissue, peri-articular, musculoskeletal, and joint disorders.*

**Ehrmann's Entschlackungstee** *Ehrmann, Austria.*
Prunus spinosa; equisetum (p.1684·1); birch leaf (p.1660·3); urtica (p.1762·1); taraxacum (p.1751·3); peppermint leaf (p.1283·2); chamomile (p.1669·3).
*Urinary disorders.*

**Eicosan** *Redino, Ger.*
Marine fish oil (p.976·2).
*Hyperlipidaemias.*

**Eicosapen**
*Nefro, Austria; Redino, Ger.; Altana, Switz.*
Marine fish oil (p.976·2).
*Hyperlipidaemias.*

**Eicovis** *C & RF, Ital.*
Omega-3 triglycerides, vitamins, and minerals (p.1417·1).
*Eye disorders; nutritional supplement.*

**Eifel** *Rafarm, Gr.*
Betaxolol hydrochloride (p.873·1).
*Glaucoma; raised intra-ocular pressure.*

**Eifelfango-Neuenahr** *Eifelfango, Ger.*
Medicinal mud.
*Gastrointestinal disorders; gout; musculoskeletal and joint disorders; neuralgia.*

**EinsAlpha** *Leo, Ger.*
Alfacalcidol (p.1461·2).
*Osteodystrophy; osteomalacia; osteoporosis; rickets; vitamin D deficiency.*

**Einschlafkapseln** *Twardy, Austria.*
Valerian (p.1762·2); lupulus (p.1708·1).
*Nervous disorders; sleep disorders.*

**Einschlaf-Kapseln biologisch** *Twardy, Ger.†.*
Valerian (p.1762·2); lupulus (p.1708·1).
*Nervous disorders; sleep disorders.*

**Eiquinon** *Eisai, Hong Kong.*
Ubidecarenone (p.1760·2).
*Heart failure.*

**Eisen-Diasporal** *Protina, Ger.†.*
Ferrous sulfate (p.1428·2).
*Iron deficiency; iron-deficiency anaemia.*

**Eisendragees-ratiopharm** *Ratiopharm, Ger.*
Ferrous sulfate (p.1428·2).
*Iron deficiency; iron-deficiency anaemia.*

**Eisenkapseln** *Forster, Ger.*
Ferrous sulfate (p.1428·2); yeast; nicotinamide; folic acid; cyanocobalamin; copper sulfate; manganese sulfate (p.1417·1).
*Iron deficiency.*

**Eisen-Sandoz** *Novartis Consumer, Ger.*
Ferrous gluconate (p.1428·1).
*Iron deficiency.*

**EK Burger** *Ysatfabrik, Ger.*
Homoeopathic preparation.

**Ekanin** *Romer, Mex.†.*
Vitamin E (p.1464·3).

**Ekilid** *Aventis, Mex.*
Sulpiride (p.722·2).
*Depression; schizophrenia; vertigo.*

**Eksalb** *Kade, Ger.†.*
Cell components and metabolic products of *Staphylococcus aureus*; *Enterococcus faecalis* (p.1704·2); *Pseudomonas aeruginosa*; *Escherichia coli*; hydrocortisone (p.1103·3).
*Skin disorders.*

**Eksalb Simplex** *Kade, Ger.†.*
Cell components and metabolic products of *Staphylococcus aureus*; *Enterococcus faecalis* (p.1704·2); *Pseudomonas aeruginosa*; *Escherichia coli*.
*Skin disorders.*

**ektebin** *Hefa, Ger.*
Protionamide (p.246·3).
*Tuberculosis.*

**Ektogan**
*Hoechst, Fr.†; Teofarma, Ital.*
Zinc peroxide (p.1195·3); zinc oxide (p.1163·2); magnesium peroxide (p.1185·2).
*Skin disorders; wound disinfection.*

**Ektoselene** *Robapharm, Switz.*
Selenium disulfide (p.1157·3); sulfur (p.1158·2).
*Scalp disorders.*

**Ektrofil** *Ecobi, Ital.*
Zinc oxide (p.1163·2); aloe vera (p.1141·3).
*Emollient.*

**Ekuba** *Teofarma, Ital.*
Chlorhexidine gluconate (p.1173·2).
*Personal hygiene.*

**Ekvacillin**
*AstraZeneca, Denm.†; AstraZeneca, Fin.; AstraZeneca, Norw.; AstraZeneca, Swed.*
Cloxacillin sodium (p.198·2).
*Bacterial infections.*

**Ekxine** *Strand, Malaysia.*
Bromhexine hydrochloride (p.1115·3).
*Respiratory-tract disorders associated with viscous mucus.*

**Ekzemase** *Azupharma, Ger.†.*
Bufexamac (p.21·3).
*Eczema; neurodermatitis.*

**Ekzemsalbe F** *Agepha, Austria.*
Hydrocortisone acetate (p.1103·3).
*Eczema.*

**Ekzevowen** *Weber & Weber, Ger.*
Homoeopathic preparation.

**EL Diet** *Support, Braz.*
Preparation for enteral nutrition (p.1417·1).

**Elacto** *Novartis Consumer, Spain†.*
Infant feed (p.1417·1).
*Eczema in infants; food-related respiratory-tract disorders.*

**Elacur** *Riemser, Ger.*
Propyl nicotinate (p.85·3).
*Musculoskeletal and joint disorders; neuralgia.*

**Elacutan** *Riemser, Ger.*
Urea (p.1162·2).
*Skin disorders.*

**Elafax** *Gador, Arg.*
Venlafaxine (p.322·3).
*Anxiety; depression.*

**Elagen** *Eladon, UK.*
Eleutherococcus senticosis (p.1744·1).
*Tonic.*

**Elageno OS** *Mavi, Ital.*
Folic acid; magnesium; omega 6 and omega 3 triglycerides; fatty acids (p.1417·1).
Formerly known as Pufolic.
*Nutritional supplement.*

**Elamax** *Biolab Sanus, Braz.*
11 Tablets, estradiol valerate (p.1550·2); 10 tablets, cyproterone acetate (p.1544·1); estradiol valerate.
*Menopausal disorders.*

**Elan** *Schwarz, Ital.*
Isosorbide mononitrate (p.942·1).
*Angina pectoris; cardiac stenosis; heart failure; myocardial infarction.*

**Elana** *OTW, Ger.*
Homoeopathic preparation.

**Elana mono** *OTW, Ger.*
Homoeopathic preparation.

**Elandur** *Sidus, Arg.*
Alendronate sodium (p.765·3).
*Osteoporosis; Paget's disease of bone.*

**Elan-Forte** *YSP, Malaysia.*
Chlorhexidine hydrochloride (p.1173·3); tolnaftate (p.410·1).
*Fungal skin infections.*

**Elantan**
*Note. This name is used for preparations of different composition.*
*Gebro, Austria; Sanofi Synthelabo, Ger.; Schwarz, Hong Kong; Schwarz, Irl.; Schwarz, Malaysia; Knoll, Mex.; Omnimed, S.Afr.; Schwarz, Singapore; Schwarz, Switz.†; Schwarz, Thai.; Schwarz, UK.*
Isosorbide mononitrate (p.942·1).
*Angina pectoris; heart failure; myocardial infarction; pulmonary hypertension.*

*Schering, Braz.†.*
Isosorbide dinitrate (p.941·1).
*Angina pectoris.*

**Elanver** *Remedina, Gr.*
Verapamil hydrochloride (p.1019·1).
*Angina; arrythmias; hypertension.*

**Elase**
*Parke, Davis, Canad.†; Parke, Davis, Chile; Pfizer, Fr.; Parke, Davis, Ital.; Pfizer, Malaysia; Parke, Davis, Neth.*
Fibrinolysin (p.916·2); deoxyribonuclease (p.1119·1).
*Cervicitis; debridement of wounds; vaginitis.*

**Elase-Chloromycetin** *Parke, Davis, Canad.†.*
Fibrinolysin (bovine) (p.916·2); deoxyribonuclease (bovine) (p.1119·1); chloramphenicol (p.185·1).
*Debridement of infected lesions.*

**Elaspol** *Ono, Jpn.*
Sivelestat sodium (p.1746·3).
*Acute lung injury associated with septicaemia.*

**Elastab** *TO-Chemicals, Thai.*
Pentoxifylline (p.979·3).
*Cerebral and peripheral vascular disorders.*

**Elatrol** *Teva, Israel.*
Amitriptyline hydrochloride (p.280·3).
*Depression; nocturnal enuresis.*

**Elatrolet** *Teva, Israel.*
Amitriptyline hydrochloride (p.280·3).
*Depression; nocturnal enuresis.*

**Elavil**
*Merck Frosst, Canad.; Merck Sharp & Dohme-Chibret, Fr.; DDSA Pharmaceuticals, UK; Zeneca, USA†.*
Amitriptyline hydrochloride (p.280·3).
*Depression; nocturnal enuresis.*

**Elavil Plus** *Merck Frosst, Canad.†.*
Amitriptyline hydrochloride (p.280·3); perphenazine (p.714·2).
*Depression.*

**Elawox** *Riemser, Ger.*
Urea hydrogen peroxide (p.1195·3).
*Infected wounds.*

**Elazor** *Sigma-Tau, Ital.*
Fluconazole (p.398·1).
*Fungal infections.*

**Elbat** *Genepharm, Gr.*
Flutamide (p.556·2).
*Prostatic cancer.*

**Elbrol** *Pfleger, Ger.*
Propranolol hydrochloride (p.989·3).
*Essential tremor; hypertension; hyperthyroidism; ischaemic heart disease; migraine.*

**Elcal** *Andromaco, Chile.*
Calcium carbonate (p.1254·2).
*Calcium deficiency; osteoporosis.*

**Elcal I** *Andromaco, Chile.*
Calcium gluconate (p.1225·2); calcium lactobionate (p.1225·3).
*Calcium deficiency.*

**Elcal-D** *Andromaco, Chile.*
Calcium carbonate (p.1254·2) or calcium phosphate (p.1225·3); colecalciferol (p.1461·3).
*Calcium and vitamin D deficiency; osteomalacia; osteoporosis; rickets.*

**Elcarn** *Co-Pharma, UK†.*
Carnitine (p.1423·3).
*Carnitine deficiency.*

**Elcimen** *Nycomed, Austria.*
Elcatonin (p.768·3).
*Hypercalcaemia; osteoporosis; Paget's disease of bone; reflex sympathetic dystrophy.*

**Elcion** *Ranbaxy, India.*
Diazepam (p.690·1).
*Alcohol withdrawal; anxiety; muscle spasm.*

**Elcoman** *Labinca, Arg.*
Loperamide hydrochloride (p.1271·1).
*Diarrhoea.*

**Elcrit** *Parke, Davis, Ger.; Pfizer, Ger.*
Clozapine (p.685·3).
*Schizophrenia.*

**Eldepryl**
*Douglas, Austral.; Viatris, Belg.; Draxis, Canad.; Orion, Denm.; Orion, Fin.; Orion, Irl.; Viatris, Neth.; Orion, Norw.; Douglas, NZ; Reckitt Benckiser, S.Afr.; Orion, Swed.; Orion, UK; Somerset, USA.*
Selegiline hydrochloride (p.1214·1).
*Parkinsonism.*

**Eldercaps** *Merz, USA†.*
Multivitamin and mineral preparation (p.1417·1).

**Elderin** *Lek, Hong Kong†.*
Etodolac (p.37·3).
*Musculoskeletal, joint, and peri-articular disorders.*

**Eldertonic** *Merz, USA.*
Vitamin B substances with minerals (p.1417·1).

**Eldicet**
*Recalcine, Chile; Infar, India; Solvay, Spain.*
Pinaverium bromide (p.1732·1).
*Biliary-tract dyskinesia; gastrointestinal spasm; irritable bowel syndrome.*

**Eldisin** *Lilly, Austria.*
Vindesine sulfate (p.593·3).
*Malignant neoplasms.*

**Eldisine**
*Lilly, Arg.; Lilly, Austral.; Lilly, Belg.; Lilly, Canad.†; Lilly, Fin.; Lilly, Fr.; Lilly, Ger.; Lilly, Hong Kong†; Lilly, Irl.; Lilly, Ital.; Centrapharm, Neth.; Lilly, S.Afr.; Lilly, Swed.; Lilly, Switz.; Clonmel, UK.*
Vindesine sulfate (p.593·3).
*Malignant neoplasms.*

**Eldopaque**
*ICN, Canad.; ICN, Hong Kong; ICN, Malaysia; ICN, Mex.; ICN, Singapore; Crawford, UK; ICN, USA.*
Hydroquinone (p.1148·1) in a sunblocking basis.
*Hyperpigmented skin conditions.*

**Eldoquin**
*ICN, Canad.; ICN, Hong Kong; ICN, Malaysia; ICN, Mex.; ICN, NZ; ICN, Singapore; Crawford, UK; ICN, USA.*
Hydroquinone (p.1148·1).
*Hyperpigmented skin conditions.*

**Eldox** *Aspen Consumer, S.Afr.†.*
Diphenoxylate hydrochloride (p.1261·3).
Atropine sulfate (p.477·1) is included in this preparation to discourage abuse.
*Diarrhoea.*

**Elebloc**
*Alcon, Arg.; Alcon, Braz.†; Alcon Cusi, Spain.*
Carteolol hydrochloride (p.880·3).
*Glaucoma; ocular hypertension.*

**EleCare** *Ross, USA.*
Elemental amino-acid based food for special diets (p.1417·1).
*Food allergies; malabsorption; maldigestion; whole protein intolerance.*

**Electopen** *Alter, Spain†.*
Ampicillin sodium (p.157·1) or ampicillin trihydrate (p.157·2).
*Bacterial infections.*

**Electopen Balsam Retard** *Alter, Spain†.*
Ampicillin sodium (p.157·1); ampicillin benzathine (p.158·1); niaouli oil (p.1719·3); guaifenesin (p.1122·1).
*Respiratory-tract infections.*

**Electopen Retard** *Alter, Spain†.*
Ampicillin sodium (p.157·1); ampicillin benzathine (p.158·1).
*Bacterial infections.*

**Electral** *FDC, India.*
Potassium chloride; sodium chloride; sodium citrate; anhydrous glucose (p.1222·2).
*Oral rehydration therapy.*

**Electric Blue Headlice** *Apotex, NZ.*
*Conditioner:* Brilliant blue (p.1056·2); clove oil (p.1673·3); lavender oil (p.1705·2); lemon oil (p.1706·2); rosemary oil (p.1740·2); melaleuca oil (p.1710·2).
*Detection of pediculosis.*
*Cream:* Clove oil (p.1673·3); rosemary oil (p.1740·2); melaleuca oil (p.1710·2).
*Pediculosis.*

**Electrobion** *Merck, India.*
Sodium chloride; potassium chloride; sodium citrate; anhydrous glucose (p.1222·2).
*Oral rehydration therapy.*

**Electrolade**
*Eastern Pharmaceuticals, Irl.; Thornton & Ross, UK.*
Sodium chloride; potassium chloride; sodium bicarbonate; glucose (p.1222·2).
*Diarrhoea; oral rehydration therapy.*

**Electrolit** *Pisa, Mex.*
Sodium chloride; potassium chloride; calcium chloride; magnesium chloride; sodium lactate; glucose (p.1222·2).
*Oral rehydration therapy.*

**Electrolit Pediatrico** *Pisa, Mex.*
Glucose; sodium chloride; sodium citrate; potassium chloride (p.1222·2).
*Diarrhoea; oral rehydration therapy.*

**Electrona** *Aspen Consumer, S.Afr.†.*
Potassium chloride; sodium chloride; sodium bicarbonate; calcium lactate; sodium acid phosphate; magnesium sulfate; heavy magnesium carbonate; glucose (p.1222·2).
*Diarrhoea; oral rehydration therapy.*

**Electropak** *Mirren, S.Afr.*
Potassium chloride; sodium chloride; sodium bicarbonate; glucose (p.1222·2).
*Diarrhoea; oral rehydration therapy.*

**Electrorice** *Naveh, Israel.*
Electrolytes in rice flour base (p.1222·2).
*Diarrhoea; oral rehydration therapy.*

**Elegelin**
*Sun, Singapore†; Sun, Thai.*
Selegiline hydrochloride (p.1214·1).
*Parkinsonism.*

**Elem** *Andromaco, Chile.*
Methylphenidate hydrochloride (p.1590·2).
*Attention-deficit hyperactivity disorder; narcoleptic syndrome.*

**Elemental 028**
*Scientific Hospital Supplies, Austral.; Nutricia, Fin.; Scientific Hospital Supplies, Irl.; Nutricia, Ital.; Nutricia, NZ; Scientific Hospital Supplies, NZ; Scientific Hospital Supplies, UK.*
Preparation for enteral nutrition (p.1417·1).

**Elemental Zinc** *DBL, NZ; Baxter, NZ.*
Zinc chloride (p.1469·2).
*Zinc deficiency.*

**Elenol** *Gerda, Fr.*
Lindane (p.1506·3); amylocaine hydrochloride (p.1370·2).
*Scabies.*

**Elental** *Ajinomoto, Thai.†.*
Preparation for enteral nutrition (p.1417·1).

**Elentol** *Gerda, Fr.†.*
Lindane (p.1506·3).
*Disinfection of clothing and bedding; pediculosis.*

**Eleparon** *Sankyo, Braz.*
Silymarin (p.1043·3).
*Liver disorders.*

**Elepril** *Farmasa, Braz.*
Selegiline (p.1214·3).
*Parkinsonism.*

**Elepsin** *Andromaco, Arg.*
Imipramine hydrochloride (p.300·1).
*Depression.*

**Elequine** *Cilag, Mex.*
Levofloxacin (p.225·3).
*Bacterial infections.*

**Elestat** *Allergan, USA.*
Epinastine hydrochloride (p.433·3).
*Allergic conjunctivitis.*

**Eleu** *Harras-Curarina, Ger.*
Eleutherococcus senticosis (p.1744·1).
*Tonic.*

**Eleu-Kokk**
*Pharmaton, Ger.; Pharmaton, Switz.†.*
Eleutherococcus senticosis (p.1744·1).
*Tonic.*

**Eleuphrat** *Essex, Austral.*
Betamethasone dipropionate (p.1093·1).
*Skin disorders.*

**Eleutheroforce** *Bioforce, Ger.*
Eleutherococcus senticosis root (p.1744·1).
*Tonic.*

**Eleutherokokk** *Arko, Ger.*
Eleutherococcus senticosis root (p.1744·1).
*Tonic.*

**Eleutherokokk-Aktiv-Kapseln SenticoMega**
*Twardy, Ger.†.*
Eleutherococcus senticosis root (p.1744·1).
*Tonic.*

**Eleu-Twardypharm** *Twardy, Ger.*
Eleutherococcus senticosis (p.1744·1).
*Tonic.*

**Eleval** *Recalcine, Chile.*
Sertraline (p.317·3).
*Depression.*

**Elevat** *Lagamed, S.Afr.†.*
Dronabinol (p.1264·2).
*Anorexia with weight loss in AIDS; nausea and vomiting.*

**Elevit**
*Roche, Austria; Roche, NZ; Roche, Switz.*
Range of multivitamin or multivitamin and mineral preparations (p.1417·1).

**Elevit Geriatrico** *Roche, Braz.*
Multivitamin and mineral preparation (p.1417·1).

**Elevit Pronatal** *Roche, Austria.*
Multivitamin and mineral preparation (p.1417·1).

**Elevit Vitamine B$_9$** *Roche Nicholas, Fr.*
Multivitamin and mineral preparation (p.1417·1).

**Elex** *Verla, Ger.†.*
*dl*-Alpha tocoferil acetate (p.1465·1); magnesium oxide (p.1272·3).
*Vitamin E and magnesium deficiency.*

**Elex E** *Verla, Ger.*
*d*-Alpha tocopherol (p.1464·3).
*Vitamin E deficiency.*

**Elfanex** *Novartis, Austria†.*
Reserpine (p.995·1); dihydralazine sulfate (p.899·3); hydrochlorothiazide (p.933·2); potassium chloride (p.1232·2).
*Hypertension.*

**Elfer** *Zerboni, Mex.†.*
Ferrous sulfate (p.1428·2).

**Elferri** *Sigma, India.*
Vitamin B substances (p.1454·3); ferrous gluconate (p.1428·1); yeast (p.1469·1).
*Tonic.*

**Elferri-Z** *Sigma, India.*
Ferrous fumarate (p.1427·3); folic acid (p.1429·1); vitamin $B_{12}$ (p.1458·2); zinc sulfate (p.1469·3).
*Iron and folic acid deficiency during pregnancy.*

**Elgadil** *Altana, Spain.*
Urapidil hydrochloride (p.1018·1).
*Hypertension.*

**Elgam** *Sankyo, Spain.*
Omeprazole (p.1278·2).
*Gastro-oesophageal reflux; peptic ulcer; Zollinger-Ellison syndrome.*

**Elgydium**
*Sidus, Arg.; Pierre Fabre Sante, Fr.; Ceuta, UK.*
Chlorhexidine gluconate (p.1173·2).
*Dental caries prophylaxis; mouth disorders.*

**Elgydium Bicarbonate** *Pierre Fabre Sante, Fr.*
Sodium bicarbonate (p.1223·2).
*Dental hygiene.*

**Elgyfluor**
*Note. This name is used for preparations of different composition.*
*Sidus, Arg.*
Nicomethanol hydrofluoride; chlorhexidine gluconate (p.1173·2).
*Dental caries prophylaxis.*

*Pierre Fabre Sante, Fr.*
*Dental gel:* Nicomethanol hydrofluoride; chlorhexidine gluconate (p.1173·2).
*Oral hygiene; sensitive gums.*
*Toothpaste:* Nicomethanol hydrofluoride.
*Oral hygiene.*

**Elgyfluor Junior** *Pierre Fabre Sante, Fr.*
Nicomethanol hydrofluoride.
*Dental caries prophylaxis.*

**Elian** *Infirmarius-Rovit, Ger.*
Homoeopathic preparation.

**Elibet** *Willmar, Mex.†.*
Vitamin E (p.1464·3).

**Elica**
*Undra, Mex.; Schering-Plough, S.Afr.; Schering-Plough, Spain.*
Mometasone furoate (p.1107·2).
*Skin and scalp disorders.*

**Elicodil** *Menarini, Ital.*
Ranitidine bismuth citrate (p.1287·2).
*Peptic ulcer.*

**Elicor** *Pharmanik (Φαρμανικ), Gr.*
Acetylcysteine (p.1112·3).
*Respiratory disorders associated with viscous mucus.*

**Elidel**
*Novartis, NZ; Novartis, UK; Novartis, USA.*
Pimecrolimus (p.1155·1).
*Atopic eczema.*

**Elidiur** *Upsa, Ital.*
Fosinopril sodium (p.919·1); hydrochlorothiazide (p.933·2).
*Hypertension.*

**Eligard**
*Mayne, Austral.; Atrix, USA; Sanofi Synthelabo, USA.*
Leuprorelin acetate (p.1331·1).
Formerly known as Leuprogel One-Month Depot in the USA.
*Prostatic cancer.*

**Elimin** *Cantabria, Spain†.*
Sodium picosulfate (p.1289·3).
*Constipation.*

**Elimite** *Allergan, USA.*
Permethrin (p.1508·3).
*Scabies.*

**Elimitona** *Brauer, Austral.†.*
Homoeopathic preparation.

**Elina** *Reddy's, India.*
Mizolastine (p.437·3).
*Allergic rhinoconjunctivitis; hay fever; urticaria.*

**Elinap** *Kleva, Gr.*
Nimesulide (p.67·1).
*Inflammation; musculoskeletal disorders; pain.*

**Elingrip** *Wasserman, Spain†.*
Aspirin (p.15·1); ascorbic acid (p.1460·2); chlorphenamine maleate (p.427·3); kola (p.1765·3).
*Cold and influenza symptoms.*

**Elios** *Rydelle, Fr.†.*
Amino-acid, fatty-acid, and vitamin preparation (p.1417·1).
*UV-induced skin damage.*

**Elisir Depurativo Ambrosiano** *Alckamed, Ital.†.*
Aesculus hippocastanum (p.1648·2); hypericum perforatum (p.299·1); arnica montana (p.1656·3); knotgrass; hamamelis virginiana (p.1696·3); gentiana lutea (p.1692·2).
*Circulatory disorders.*

**Elisir Terpina** *Teofarma, Ital.*
Terpin hydrate (p.1131·1); dropropizine (p.1119·3).
*Coughs.*

**Elisor** *Bristol-Myers Squibb, Fr.*
Pravastatin sodium (p.984·3).
*Hypercholesterolaemia.*

**Elissan** *Dermofarm, Spain.*
Loperamide hydrochloride (p.1271·1).
*Diarrhoea.*

**Elitan** *Medochemie, Thai.†.*
Metoclopramide hydrochloride (p.1274·3).
*Gastrointestinal motility disorders; nausea and vomiting.*

**Elitar** *Daquimed, Port.*
Nabumetone (p.63·3).
*Musculoskeletal, joint, and peri-articular disorders.*

**Elite** *Bayer, Port.*
Test for glucose in blood (p.1694·2).
*For use with Glucometer Elite.*

**Elitek** *Sanofi Synthelabo, USA.*
Rasburicase (p.418·3).
*Hyperuricaemia.*

**Eliten** *Bristol-Myers Squibb, Ital.*
Fosinopril sodium (p.919·1).
*Heart failure; hypertension.*

**Elitiran** *Mintlab, Chile.*
Diclofenac (p.32·1) or diclofenac sodium (p.32·1).
*Inflammation; pain.*

**Elitos** *Andromaco, Arg.*
Oxeladin citrate (p.1126·1).
*Coughs.*

**Elitos Et** *Andromaco, Chile.*
Codeine phosphate (p.27·1); pseudoephedrine hydrochloride (p.1129·2); chlorphenamine maleate (p.427·3); tolu (p.1131·3).
*Coughs.*

**Elityran** *Vianex (Βιανεξ), Gr.*
Leuprorelin acetate (p.1331·1).
*Endometriosis; female infertility; prostatic cancer; uterine fibroids.*

**Eliur** *Northia, Arg.*
Furosemide (p.919·3).

**Elixifilin** *Yamanouchi, Spain.*
Theophylline (p.798·3).
Formerly contained potassium iodide and theophylline.
*Obstructive airways disease.*

**Elixine** *Saval, Chile.*
Theophylline (p.798·3).
*Obstructive airways disease.*

**Elixir 914** *Simoes, Braz.*
Potassium iodide (p.1598·1); star anise.

**Elixir Americano** *Labortecne, Braz.†.*
Potassium iodide (p.1598·1).
*Coughs.*

**Elixir Bonjean** *Dexo, Fr.*
Melissa (p.1711·1); bitter-orange peel (p.1723·3); aniseed (p.1655·2); cumin seed; catechu (p.1668·3); peppermint oil (p.1283·2).
*Digestive disorders.*

**Elixir Contre La Toux Weleda** *Weleda, Fr.†.*
Aniseed (p.1655·2); dulcamara (p.1683·1); drosera; althaea (p.1651·3); ipecacuanha (p.1122·3); malt (p.1439·2); white marrubium (p.1124·1); pulsatilla; thyme (p.1755·2).
*Coughs.*

**Elixir Damiana and Saw Palmetto** *Potter's, UK.*
Corn silk (p.1676·1); damiana (p.1679·1); saw palmetto (p.1569·1).
*Tonic.*

**Elixir de Inhame** *Goulart, Braz.†.*
Colocassia antiquarum; sarsaparilla (p.1742·1); honey (p.1434·2).

**Elixir de Maracuja Composto** *Kanda, Braz.†.*
Casimiroa; passion flower (p.1729·1); erythrina mulungu (p.1717·2).
*Sedative.*

**Elixir de Marinheiro** *Phos-Kola, Braz.†.*
Potassium iodide (p.1598·1); cocillana (p.1117·2); sarsaparilla (p.1742·1); camphorated opium (p.74·2); anacardium occidentale.
*Respiratory-tract congestion.*

**Elixir de Passiflora** *Sinterapico, Braz.†.*
Passion flower (p.1729·1); erythrina mulungu (p.1717·2); melissa (p.1711·1).

**Elixir fortifiant** *Phytomed, Switz.*
Ginkgo biloba; ginseng; calcium lactophosphate (p.1417·1).
*Tonic.*

**Elixir Grez** *Monin, Fr.*
Bitter-orange (p.1723·3); gentian (p.1692·2); cinnamon (p.1672·2); citric acid monohydrate (p.1673·1).
*Digestive disorders.*

**Elixir Paregorico** *Granado, Braz.; Catarinense, Braz.*
Camphorated opium (p.74·2).
*Diarrhoea; opioid withdrawal syndrome.*

**Elixir Rebleuten** *Pharmacal, Switz.†.*
Aloes (p.1248·2).
*Constipation.*

**Elixir Spark** *Phytoprevent, Fr.*
Boldo (p.1661·2); cynara (p.1678·3).
*Constipation; dyspepsia.*

**Elixofilina** *Schering, Mex.†.*
Theophylline (p.798·3).

**Elixomin** *Cenci, USA.*
Theophylline (p.798·3).
*Obstructive airways disease.*

**Elixophyllin**
*Note. This name is used for preparations of different composition.*
*Sam-On, Israel†.*
Aminophylline (p.780·2).
*Heart failure; obstructive airways disease.*

*Forest Pharmaceuticals, USA.*
Theophylline (p.798·3).
*Obstructive airways disease.*

**Elixophyllin-GG** *Forest Pharmaceuticals, USA.*
Theophylline (p.798·3); guaifenesin (p.1122·1).
*Obstructive airways disease.*

**Elixophyllin-KI** *Forest Pharmaceuticals, USA.*
Theophylline (p.798·3); potassium iodide (p.1598·1).
*Tenacious mucus in asthma and bronchitis.*

**Elizabeth Arden Suncare** *Arden, NZ†.*
*SPF 15:* Octinoxate (p.1154·3); titanium dioxide (p.1160·3); avobenzone (p.1142·3).
*Sunscreen.*

**Elkamol** *Kendon, UK†.*
Paracetamol (p.76·2).

**Elkapin**
*Godecke, Ger.†; Parke, Davis, Ital.; Parke, Davis, Spain†.*
Etozolin (p.914·2).
*Hypertension; oedema.*

**Elkin** *Byk, Neth.†.*
Furosemide (p.919·3); amiloride hydrochloride (p.858·2).
*Hypertension; oedema.*

**ELKO** *Baxter, Ger.*
Electrolyte infusion (p.1217·1).
*Parenteral nutrition.*

**Elkostop** *Minerva (Μινερβα), Gr.*
Omeprazole (p.1278·2).
*Acid aspiration; eradication of Helicobacter pylori in combination with antimicrobials; peptic ulcer; reflux oesophagitis; Zollinger-Ellison syndrome.*

**Elkotheran** *Bros, Gr.*
Omeprazole (p.1278·2).
*Acid aspiration; eradication of Helicobacter pylori in combination with antimicrobials; peptic ulcer; reflux oesophagitis; Zollinger-Ellison syndrome.*

**Ellanco** *Duopharma, Hong Kong.*
Lovastatin (p.949·1).
*Atherosclerosis; hypercholesterolaemia.*

**Ellatun** *Alcon, Ger.*
Tramazoline hydrochloride (p.1131·3).
*Nasal congestion.*

**Ell-Cranell** *Galderma, Ger.†.*
Estradiol (p.1550·1); dexamethasone (p.1097·1); salicylic acid (p.1157·1).
*Hair loss; scalp disorders.*

**Ell-Cranell alpha** *Galderma, Ger.*
Alfatradiol.
*Alopecia androgenetica.*

**Ell-Cranell dexa** *Galderma, Ger.*
Alfatradiol; dexamethasone (p.1097·1).
*Hair loss.*

**Elle-care** *Geistlich, Switz.†.*
Lactic acid (p.1704·1); sodium lactate (p.1223·2); docusate sodium (p.1262·2).
*Vaginal disorders.*

**Elleci** *Lampugnani, Ital.*
Levocarnitine (p.1423·3).
*Carnitine deficiency.*

**Ellence** *Pharmacia Upjohn, USA.*
Epirubicin hydrochloride (p.550·2).
*Breast cancer.*

**Elleste Duet Conti** *Shire, UK.*
Estradiol (p.1550·1); norethisterone acetate (p.1562·2).
*Menopausal disorders; osteoporosis.*

**Elleste-Duet** *Shire, UK.*
16 Tablets, estradiol (p.1550·1); 12 tablets, estradiol; norethisterone acetate (p.1562·2).
*Menopausal disorders; osteoporosis.*

**Elleste-Solo** *Shire, UK.*
Estradiol (p.1550·1).
*Menopausal disorders; osteoporosis.*

**Elle-Test** *Gilbert, Fr.*
Pregnancy test (p.1734·3).

**Ellimans** *Thornton & Ross, UK.*
Turpentine oil (p.1760·1); acetic acid (p.1645·2).
*Musculoskeletal pain.*

**Elliots B** *Orphan Medical, Israel.*
Electrolyte solution with glucose (p.1217·1).
*Diluent for intrathecal administration of methotrexate sodium and cytarabine.*

**Ellsurex** *Galderma, Ger.*
Selenium sulfide (p.1157·3); colloidal sulfur (p.1158·2); allantoin (p.1141·3).
*Scalp disorders.*

**Elmego** *Chinta, Thai.*
Indometacin (p.47·3).
*Musculoskeletal, joint, and peri-articular disorders.*

**Elmetacin**
*Sankyo, Ger.; Wilson, NZ; Sankyo, Port.; Pharmafrica, S.Afr.; Sankyo, Switz.; Sankyo, Thai.*
Indometacin (p.47·3).
*Inflammation; musculoskeletal, joint, peri-articular, and soft-tissue disorders; pain.*

**Elmetin**
*Medochemie, Hong Kong; Medochemie, Thai.†.*
Mebendazole (p.108·2).
*Worm infections.*

**Elmetrin** *Merck, Braz.†.*
Elcometrine (p.1549·3).

**Elmex**
*Note. This name is used for preparations of different composition.*
*Gebro, Austria; GABA, Belg.; Orion, Fin.; GABA, Ger.; Teva, Israel; Vebas, Ital.; GABA, Neth.; Dental Warehouse, S.Afr.†; Inibsa, Spain†; GABA, Switz.*
*Topical gel:* Olaflur (p.1442·3); dectaflur (p.1427·1); sodium fluoride (p.1444·3).
*Dental caries prophylaxis; sensitive teeth.*

*Gebro, Austria; Orion, Fin.; GABA, Ger.; GABA, Switz.*
*Topical solution:* Olaflur (p.1442·3); dectaflur (p.1427·1).
*Dental caries prophylaxis; sensitive teeth.*

*GABA, Fr.; Teva, Israel.*
*Mouthwash:* Olaflur (p.1442·3); sodium fluoride (p.1444·3).
*Dental caries prophylaxis.*

*GABA, Fr.; Teva, Israel.*
*Toothpaste:* Olaflur (p.1442·3); hetaflur (p.1434·2).
*Dental caries prophylaxis.*

*Teva, Israel.*
*Toothpaste for sensitive teeth:* Olaflur (p.1442·3).
*Dental caries prophylaxis.*

*Inibsa, Port.†.*
Amine fluoride.
*Dental caries prophylaxis.*

**Elmex Sensitive** *GABA, Fr.*
*Mouthwash:* Olaflur (p.1442·3); potassium fluoride (p.1445·3).
*Toothpaste:* Olaflur (p.1442·3).
*Dental caries prophylaxis; dental hypersensitivity.*

**Elmiron**
*Elvetium, Arg.; Arthropharm, Austral.; Alza, Canad.; Ivax, Hong Kong; Alza, USA.*
Pentosan polysulfate sodium (p.979·2).
*Interstitial cystitis.*

**Elmogan** *Lek, Hong Kong†.*
Gemfibrozil (p.923·1).
*Hyperlipidaemias.*

**Elmuten** *Byk Elmu, Spain†.*
Aceglutamide; acetylaspartic acid; cyanocobalamin; citrulline; inositol; thiamine nitrate; magnesium potassium aspartate; pyridoxal phosphate; serine phosphate (p.1417·1).
Lidocaine hydrochloride (p.1377·3) is included in this preparation to alleviate the pain of injection.
*Tonic.*

**Elo-admix** *Fresenius Kabi, Austria.*
Electrolyte infusion (p.1217·1).
*Fluid and electrolyte disorders.*

**Eloamin** *Fresenius Kabi, Austria.*
Amino-acid and electrolyte infusion (p.1417·1).
*Parenteral nutrition.*

**Elobact** *Cascan, Ger.; GlaxoSmithKline, Ger.*
Cefuroxime axetil (p.184·1).
*Bacterial infections.*

**Elocin** *Shiwa, Thai.*
Erythromycin stearate (p.208·2).
*Bacterial infections.*

**Elocom**
*Schering-Plough, Belg.; Schering-Plough, Braz.; Schering, Canad.; Schering-Plough, Chile; Schering-Plough, Israel; Schering-Plough, Port.; Schering-Plough, Spain; Essex, Switz.*
Mometasone furoate (p.1107·2).
*Skin disorders.*

**Elocon**
*White, Arg.; Schering-Plough, Austral.; Aesca, Austria; Schering-Plough, Denm.; Schering-Plough, Fin.; Schering-Plough, Gr.; Fulford, India; Schering-Plough, Irl.; Schering-Plough, Ital.; Schering-Plough, Neth.; Schering-Plough, Norw.; Schering-Plough, NZ; Schering-Plough, S.Afr.; Schering-Plough, Swed.; Schering-Plough, UK; Schering, USA.*
Mometasone furoate (p.1107·2).
*Skin disorders.*

**Elocor** *Ehlinger, Mex.†.*
Nifedipine (p.966·2).

**Elocort** *Elofar, Braz.†.*
Hydrocortisone (p.1103·3); nitrofurazone (p.238·2).
*Skin disorders.*

**Elofuran** *Elofar, Braz.*
Pipemidic acid (p.243·1).
*Urinary-tract infections.*

**Eloglucose** *Fresenius Kabi, Austria†.*
Electrolyte infusion with glucose (p.1217·1).
*Carbohydrate source; fluid and electrolyte disorders.*

**Elohaes**
*Fresenius, Belg.†; Fresenius Kabi, UK.*
Hexastarch (p.750·1) in sodium chloride.
*Extracorporeal circulation; hypovolaemic shock; leucopheresis.*

**Elohast**
*Fresenius Kabi, Austria.*
An etherified starch (p.750·1) in sodium chloride.
*Hypovolaemia; plasma volume expansion.*

*Fresenius Kabi, Switz.†.*
An etherified starch (p.750·1) in electrolytes.
*Hypovolaemia; shock.*

**Elohes**
*Fresenius Kabi, Fr.†; Fresenius Kabi, Spain.*
An etherified starch (p.750·1) in sodium chloride.
*Haemodilution; hypovolaemia; plasma exchange.*

**Eloisin** *Alcon Cusi, Spain.*
Eledoisin trifluoroacetate (p.1683·3).
*Dry eyes.*

**Elolipid**
*Fresenius Kabi, Austria; Fresenius Kabi, Ital.*
Soya oil (p.1447·2).
Contains egg lecithin.
*Lipid infusion for parenteral nutrition.*

**ELO-MEL** *Fresenius Kabi, Austria.*
A range of electrolyte infusions with or without glucose (p.1217·1).
*Carbohydrate source; fluid and electrolyte disorders.*

**Elomet**
*Schering-Plough, Hong Kong; Schering-Plough, Malaysia; Schering-Plough, Mex.; Schering-Plough, Singapore; Schering-Plough, Thai.*
Mometasone furoate (p.1107·2).
*Skin disorders.*

**Elongal** *Royal, Chile.*
Diazepam (p.690·1).
*Epilepsy.*

**ELO-oral** *Fresenius Kabi, Austria†.*
Electrolytes (p.1217·1).
*Fluid and electrolyte disorders.*

**Elopram** *Recordati, Ital.*
Citalopram hydrobromide (p.289·1) or citalopram hydrochloride (p.289·1).
*Anxiety disorders; depression.*

**Elorgan** *Aventis, Spain.*
Pentoxifylline (p.979·3).
*Vascular disorders.*

**Elorheo** *Fresenius Kabi, Austria.*
Dextran 40 (p.745·3) in electrolytes.
*Fluid and electrolyte disorders.*

**Elosalic**
*White, Arg.; Schering-Plough, Braz.†; Schering-Plough, Hong Kong; Schering-Plough, S.Afr.; Schering-Plough, Swed.; Schering-Plough, Thai.*
Mometasone furoate (p.1107·2); salicylic acid (p.1157·1).
*Psoriasis.*

**Elotin** *Elofar, Braz.*
Fluocinolone acetonide (p.1101·2); polymyxin B sulfate (p.245·1); neomycin sulfate (p.235·1); lidocaine hydrochloride (p.1377·3).
Formerly contained fluocinolone and neomycin.
*Ear disorders.*

**Elotrace** *Fresenius Kabi, Austria.*
Electrolyte infusion with trace elements (p.1217·1).
*Parenteral nutrition; trace element deficiency.*

**Elotrans**
*Niddapharm, Ger.; Helvepharm, Switz.*
Anhydrous glucose; sodium chloride; sodium citrate; potassium chloride (p.1222·2).
*Diarrhoea; oral rehydration therapy.*

**Eloverlan** *Mayrhofer, Austria.*
Anhydrous glucose; sodium chloride; potassium chloride; sodium bicarbonate (p.1222·2).
*Diarrhoea; oral rehydration therapy.*

**Elovol** *Fresenius Kabi, Austria†.*
Electrolyte infusion (p.1217·1).
*Fluid and electrolyte disorders.*

**Eloxatin**
*Sanofi Synthelabo, Austral.; Sanofi Synthelabo, Belg.; Sanofi Synthelabo, Braz.; Sanofi Synthelabo, Ger.; Sanofi Synthelabo, Hong Kong; Sanofi Synthelabo, Ital.; Sanofi Synthelabo, Malaysia; Sanofi Synthelabo, Mex.; Sanofi Synthelabo, Neth.; Sanofi Synthelabo, Singapore; Sanofi Synthelabo, Spain; Sanofi Synthelabo, Swed.; Sanofi Synthelabo, Thai.; Sanofi Synthelabo, UK; Sanofi Synthelabo, USA.*
Oxaliplatin (p.577·1).
*Colorectal cancer.*

**Eloxatine**
*Sanofi Synthelabo, Fr.; Sanofi Synthelabo, Switz.*
Oxaliplatin (p.577·1).
*Colorectal cancer.*

**Elozell** *Fresenius Kabi, Austria.*
Magnesium aspartate (p.1227·3); potassium aspartate (p.1233·1).
*Cardiac disorders; digitalis toxicity; potassium and magnesium deficiency.*

**Elozell spezial** *Fresenius Kabi, Austria.*
Potassium chloride (p.1232·2); potassium aspartate (p.1233·1); magnesium aspartate (p.1227·3).
*Cardiac disorders; digitalis toxicity; potassium and magnesium deficiency.*

**Elozima** *Elofar, Braz.*
Pancreatin (p.1725·3); dimethicone (p.1289·2).
*Digestive disorders.*

**Elpi** *Elea, Arg.*
Clofibrate (p.884·3).
*Hyperlipidaemias; thrombosis prophylaxis.*

**Elpi Lip** *Elea, Arg.*
Bezafibrate (p.873·2).
*Hyperlipidaemias.*

**Elroquil N** *Rodleben, Ger.*
Hydroxyzine hydrochloride (p.434·3).
*Anxiety disorders; premedication; pruritus; sleep disorders.*

**Elspar**
*Prodome, Braz.; Merck Sharp & Dohme, Hong Kong; Merck, USA.*
Asparaginase (p.528·3).
*Acute lymphocytic leukaemia.*

**Elstatin** *Glenmark, Singapore.*
Lovastatin (p.949·1).
*Hypercholesterolaemia.*

**Eltair**
*Douglas, Hong Kong†; Scharper, Ital.; Douglas, Malaysia; Douglas, NZ; Douglas, Singapore; Douglas, Thai.; TTN, Thai.*
Budesonide (p.1094·2).
*Nasal polyps; rhinitis.*

**Elteans** *Jaldes, Fr.*
Salmon oil (p.976·1); borage oil (p.1661·3); carrot and soya oils.
*Nutritional fatty acid supplement.*

**Elthyrone** *Knoll, Belg.*
Levothyroxine sodium (p.1600·1).
*Hypothyroidism.*

**Eltocin** *Ipca, India.*
Erythromycin estolate (p.208·1).
*Bacterial infections.*

**Eltor** *Aventis, Canad.*
Pseudoephedrine hydrochloride (p.1129·2).
*Nasal and sinus congestion.*

**Eltroxin**
*GlaxoSmithKline, Canad.; GlaxoSmithKline, Denm.; Sigma, Hong Kong; GlaxoSmithKline, India; Goldshield, Irl.; GlaxoSmithKline, Israel; GlaxoSmithKline, Neth.; GlaxoSmithKline, NZ; GlaxoSmithKline, S.Afr.; GlaxoSmithKline, Singapore; GlaxoSmithKline, Thai.; Goldshield, UK; Roberts, USA†.*
Levothyroxine sodium (p.1600·1).
*Hypothyroidism.*

**Eltroxine** *Sigma-Tau, Switz.*
Levothyroxine sodium (p.1600·1).
*Hypothyroidism.*

**Elucent Skin Refining Day Cream** *Ego, Austral.†.*
*SPF 20:* Titanium dioxide (p.1160·3); octinoxate (p.1154·3); avobenzone (p.1142·3); emollients.
*Dry skin; sunscreen.*

**Eludril**
*Note. This name is used for preparations of different composition.*
*Sidus, Arg.; Inava, Fr.; Pierre Fabre, Port.; Pierre Fabre, Singapore; Pierre Fabre, Spain; Pierre Fabre, Switz.; Ceuta, UK.*
*Mouthwash:* Chlorhexidine gluconate (p.1173·2); chlorobutanol (p.1176·3).
Formerly contained chlorhexidine gluconate, chlorobutanol, and chloroform in *Fr.*
*Mouth and throat disorders.*

*Inava, Fr.; Pierre Fabre, Switz.; Ceuta, UK.*
*Throat spray:* Chlorhexidine gluconate (p.1173·2); tetracaine hydrochloride (p.1385·1).
*Mouth and throat disorders.*

**Elugan** *Menadier, Ger.*
Simeticone (p.1289·2).
*Gastrointestinal disorders with excess gas.*

**Elugel**
*Pierre Fabre Sante, Fr.; Pierre Fabre, Singapore.*
Chlorhexidine gluconate (p.1173·2).
*Gum disorders; oral hygiene.*

**Elum** *Farmasa, Braz.*
Cloxazolam (p.685·3).
*Anxiety.*

**Elusanes** *Dolisos, Fr.*
A range of herbal preparations.

**Elusanes Espino Albar** *Pierre Fabre, Spain†.*
Crataegus (p.1677·1).
*Nervous disorders; sleep disorders.*

**Elutit-Calcium** *Felgentrager, Ger.*
Calcium polystyrene sulfonate (p.1032·3).
*Hyperkalaemia.*

**Elutit-Natrium** *Felgentrager, Ger.*
Sodium polystyrene sulfonate (p.1053·1).
*Hyperkalaemia.*

**Elvecis** *Elvetium, Arg.*
Cisplatin (p.538·1).
*Malignant neoplasms.*

**Elvefocal** *Elvetium, Arg.*
Calcium folinate (p.1431·1).

**Elvenavir** *Elvetium, Arg.*
Indinavir sulfate (p.638·2).
*HIV infection.*

**Elvesil** *Biomedica-Chemica, Gr.*
Diltiazem (p.901·3).
*Angina; hypertension.*

**Elvorine**
*Wyeth Lederle, Belg.; Wyeth Lederle, Fr.*
Calcium levofolinate (p.1431·1).
*Adjuvant to fluorouracil therapy; drug-induced megaloblastic anaemia; folic acid deficiency; prevention of methotrexate-induced toxicity.*

**E-Lyte**
*Fleet, Austral.; Regional Health, NZ.*
Glucose; citric acid; sodium bicarbonate; potassium chloride; sodium chloride (p.1222·2).
*Diarrhoea; oral rehydration therapy.*

**Elyzol**
*Chemomedica, Austria; Colgate-Palmolive, Denm.; Alpharma, Fin.; Pharmadent, Fr.; Colgate-Palmolive, Ger.; Alpharma, Hong Kong; Dumex, Irl.†; CTI, Israel; Cabon, Ital.; Alpharma, Mex.; Colgate-Palmolive, Norw.; Dumex-Alpharma, Singapore†; Alpharma, Swed.; Colgate-Palmolive, Swed.; Colgate-Palmolive, Switz.; Dumex-Alpharma, Thai.; Dumex, UK†.*
Metronidazole (p.607·2) or metronidazole benzoate (p.607·2).
*Anaerobic bacterial infections; bacterial mouth infections; Crohn's disease; protozoal infections; rosacea; vaginal trichomoniasis.*

**Elzogram** *Lilly, Ger.*
Cefazolin sodium (p.170·3).
*Bacterial infections.*

**Elzym**
*Sankyo, Switz.†; Sankyo, Thai.*
Enzyme concentrate from *Aspergillus oryzae*; simeticone (p.1289·2); ethaverine hydrochloride (p.1685·2).
*Gastrointestinal disorders with excess gas; preparation of gastrointestinal tract for radiological examination.*

**EM Eukal** *Sohan, Canad.†.*
Eucalyptus oil (p.1686·2); menthol (p.1711·3).

**Emadine**
*Alcon, Austria; Alcon, Belg.; Alcon, Braz.; Alcon, Canad.; Alcon, Denm.; Alcon, Fin.; Alcon, Fr.; Alcon, Ger.; Alkon (Αλκον), Gr.; Alcon,*

Hong Kong; Alcon, Irl.; Alcon, Israel; Alcon, Ital.; Alcon, Norw.; Alcon, Port.; Alcon, S.Afr.; Alcon Cusi, Spain; Alcon, Swed.; Alcon, Switz.; Alcon, Thai.; Alcon, UK; Alcon, USA.
Emedastine fumarate (p.433·2).
*Allergic conjunctivitis.*

**Emaftol** Ogna, Ital.
Policresulen (p.1190·1).
*Mouth disinfection.*

**Emagel** Aventis, Ital.
Polygeline (p.759·1).
*Plasma volume expansion.*

**Emagrevit** Viternat, Braz.
Bladderwrack (p.1742·3); cynara (p.1678·3); cascara (p.1255·1); centella (p.1144·3); bearberry (p.1659·2); dried yeast (p.1469·1); boldo (p.1661·2); passion flower (p.1729·1).
*Obesity.*

**Emagrex** Dinafarma, Braz.†.
Bladderwrack (p.1742·3); thyroid (p.1604·2); bile salts (p.1660·3); phenolphthalein (p.1284·1).
*Constipation; obesity.*

**Emanthal** MM, India.
Albendazole (p.101·2).
*Worm infections.*

**Emantid** MM, India.
Furazolidone (p.605·2); berberine hydrochloride (p.1659·3); belladonna (p.479·1).
*Gastrointestinal infections.*

**Emasex A** Eurim, Ger.
Bamethan sulfate (p.866·3).
*Erectile dysfunction.*

**Emasex-N** Eurim, Ger.
Bamethan sulfate (p.866·3); benzyl nicotinate (p.21·2).
*Erectile dysfunction; tonic.*

**Emazian B12** Pfizer, Ital.
Thiamine hydrochloride (p.1455·1); riboflavin (p.1456·1); panthenol (p.1727·2); nicotinamide (p.1441·2); calcium folinate (p.1431·1); cyanocobalamin (p.1458·2).
*Deficiency states; macrocytic anaemia.*

**EMB** Fatol, Ger.; Hefa, Ger.
Ethambutol hydrochloride (p.211·3).
*Tuberculosis.*

**Embeline** Healthpoint, USA.
Clobetasol propionate (p.1095·2).
*Skin disorders.*

**Embial** Merck, Ger.
*dl*-Alpha tocoferil acetate (p.1465·1).
*Vitamin E deficiency.*

**EMB-INH** Fatol, Ger.
Ethambutol hydrochloride (p.211·3); isoniazid (p.222·2).
*Tuberculosis.*

**Emblon** Berk, UK†.
Tamoxifen citrate (p.584·1).
*Anovulatory infertility; breast cancer.*

**Embol** Yung Shin, Thai.
Piracetam (p.1732·1).
*Alcohol withdrawal syndrome; cerebrovascular disorders; mental function impairment.*

**Embolex** Novartis, Austria.
Certoparin sodium (p.882·1) dihydroergotamine mesilate (p.465·3).
Lidocaine hydrochloride (p.1377·3) is included in this preparation to alleviate the pain of injection.
*Thromboembolic disorders.*

**Embolex NM** Novartis, Ger.
Certoparin sodium (p.882·1); dihydroergotamine mesilate (p.465·3).
Lidocaine hydrochloride (p.1377·3) is included in this preparation to alleviate the pain of injection.
*Thromboembolism prophylaxis.*

**Embrex** Andrx, USA.
Multivitamin and mineral preparation with iron and folic acid (p.1417·1).

**Embrocacion Gras** Quimifar, Spain.
Alcohol (p.1166·1); methyl salicylate (p.59·3); turpentine oil (p.1760·1).
Formerly contained alcohol, capsicum oleoresin, methyl salicylate, and turpentine oil.
*Muscle and joint pain.*

**Embropax** Taphlan, Switz.†.
Methyl salicylate (p.59·3); isopropyl nicotinate; capsicum (p.1667·1); camphor (p.1665·3); turpentine oil (p.1760·1); eucalyptus oil (p.1686·2); lavender oil (p.1705·2).
*Peri-articular and soft-tissue disorders.*

**Emconcor**
Merck, Belg.; Merck, Denm.; Merck, Fin.; Merck, Spain; Merck, Swed.
Bisoprolol fumarate (p.875·1).
*Angina pectoris; arrhythmias; heart failure; hypertension.*

**Emconcor Comp** Merck, Fin.
Bisoprolol fumarate (p.875·1); hydrochlorothiazide (p.933·2).
*Hypertension.*

**Emcor**
Merck, Irl.; Merck, Neth.; Merck, UK.
Bisoprolol fumarate (p.875·1).
*Angina pectoris; heart failure; hypertension.*

**Emcoretic**
Merck, Belg.; Merck, Neth.; Merck, Spain.
Bisoprolol fumarate (p.875·1); hydrochlorothiazide (p.933·2).
*Hypertension.*

**Emcredil** Unichem, India.
Ethacridine lactate (p.1165·3).
*Termination of pregnancy.*

**Emcyt**
Pharmacia, Canad.; Pharmacia Upjohn, Mex.; Pharmacia Upjohn, USA.
Estramustine sodium phosphate (p.551·1).
*Prostatic cancer.*

**Emdalen** Merck, S.Afr.
Lofepramine hydrochloride (p.305·3).
*Depression.*

**Emdar** Merck, Mex.
Astemizole (p.424·2).
*Hypersensitivity.*

**Emecort** Merck, Braz.
Fluprednidene acetate (p.1102·2); gentamicin sulfate (p.217·1).
Formerly contained methylprednisolone acetate and gentamicin sulfate.
*Infected skin disorders.*

**Emedal** Norma (Νορμα), Gr.
Metronidazole (p.607·2).
*Acne rosacea.*

**Emediba** Diba, Mex.
Meclozine hydrochloride (p.436·3); pyridoxine hydrochloride (p.1456·3).
*Infant colic; nausea; vertigo; vomiting.*

**Emedrin N** Streuli, Switz.
Dextromethorphan hydrobromide (p.1117·3).
*Coughs.*

**Emedyl** Montavit, Austria.
Dimenhydrinate (p.431·1).
*Nausea and vomiting; vestibular disorders.*

**Emelis**
Clintec, Fr.†.
High protein food supplement with vitamins and minerals (p.1417·1).

Clintec, Irl.†.
High-protein semi-solid dietary supplement (p.1417·1).
*Chewing or swallowing disorders.*

**Emend**
Merck Sharp & Dohme, UK; Merck, USA.
Aprepitant (p.1250·3).
*Nausea and vomiting.*

**Eme-Ped** Stiefel, Braz.†.
Bromopride (p.1254·1).
*Nausea and vomiting.*

**Emeproton** Cantabria, Spain.
Omeprazole (p.1278·2).
*Gastro-oesophageal reflux; peptic ulcer; Zollinger-Ellison syndrome.*

**Emercol** Pharmavite, Canad.†.
Benzocaine (p.1370·3); cetalkonium chloride (p.1172·1); cetylpyridinium chloride (p.1173·1).

**Emercreme No 4** Pharmavite, Canad.†.
Cetylpyridinium chloride (p.1173·1); bacitracin (p.161·3); tyrothricin (p.275·1); diphenylpyraline hydrochloride (p.432·3); benzocaine (p.1370·3).

**Emereze Plus** Pharmavite, Canad.†.
Cetylpyridinium chloride (p.1173·1).

**Emergen** Laboratorios Chile, Chile.
Sertraline (p.317·3).
*Depression.*

**Emergent-Ez** Healthfirst, USA.
*Combination pack:* 2 Ampoules, adrenaline (p.852·2); 1 ampoule, aminophylline (p.780·2); 3 inhalants, ammonia (p.1653·3); 2 inhalants, amyl nitrite (p.1032·1); 2 ampoules, atropine (p.476·3); 2 ampoules, diphenhydramine hydrochloride (Benadryl) (p.431·3); tablets, glyceryl trinitrate (p.923·2); 1 vial, hydrocortisone sodium succinate (Solu-Cortef) (p.1104·1); 1 ampoule, pentazocine lactate (Talwin) (p.79·3); 1 ampoule, trimethobenzamide hydrochloride (Tigan) (p.442·2); 2 ampoules, diazepam (Valium) (p.690·1); 2 ampoules, mephentermine sulfate (Wyamine) (p.952·1).
*Emergency treatment.*

**Emersal** Medco, USA†.
Ammoniated mercury (p.1152·1); salicylic acid (p.1157·1).
*Psoriasis.*

**Emesafene** Ace, Neth.
Meclozine hydrochloride (p.436·3); pyridoxine hydrochloride (p.1456·3).
*Nausea; vomiting.*

**Emesan** Betapharm, Ger.
Diphenhydramine hydrochloride (p.431·3).
*Nausea; vertigo; vomiting.*

**Emeset**
Cipla, India; Cipla, Thai.
Ondansetron hydrochloride (p.1281·1).
*Nausea and vomiting induced by radiotherapy or chemotherapy; postoperative nausea and vomiting.*

**Emeside** Laboratories for Applied Biology, UK.
Ethosuximide (p.360·1).
*Absence seizures; myoclonic seizures.*

**Emetal** Asian Pharm, Thai.
Metoclopramide hydrochloride (p.1274·3).
*Nausea and vomiting.*

**Emetic** Elofar, Braz.†.
Metoclopramide (p.1274·3).
*Gastrointestinal motility disorders; nausea and vomiting.*

**Emetostop** Specifar (Σπεσιφαρ), Gr.
Meclozine hydrochloride (p.436·3).
*Vertigo.*

**Emetrol**
Note. This name is used for preparations of different composition.
Aventis, Austral.; Sanofi Winthrop, USA.
Fructose (p.1431·3); glucose (p.1432·2); phosphoric acid (p.1731·2).
*Nausea; vomiting.*

Gemballa, Braz.
Metoclopramide (p.1274·3); pyridoxine (p.1457·2).
*Nausea and vomiting.*

Aspen, S.Afr.
Sucrose (p.1450·1); phosphoric acid (p.1731·2).
*Nausea; vomiting.*

**Em-eukal** Soldan, Ger.
*Balsam:* Eucalyptus oil (p.1686·2); menthol (p.1711·3); pumilio pine oil (p.1737·1); thyme oil (p.1755·3); turpentine oil (p.1760·1); camphor (p.1665·3).
*Coughs and cold symptoms.*
*Oral drops:* Eucalyptus leaf (p.1686·1); aniseed (p.1655·2); fennel (p.1687·2); thyme (p.1755·2).
*Coughs.*
*Oral liquid:* Dextromethorphan hydrobromide (p.1117·3); menthol (p.1711·3); cetylpyridinium chloride (p.1173·1); anise oil (p.1655·2); gypsophila saponin; thymol (p.1194·2).
*Catarrh; coughs.*

**Em-eukal forte N** Soldan, Ger.
Dextromethorphan hydrobromide (p.1117·3).
Em-eukal forte formerly contained dextromethorphan hydrobromide, menthol, cetylpyridinium chloride, eucalyptus oil, gypsophila saponin, and benzocaine.
*Catarrh; coughs.*

**Em-eukal Husten- und Brusttee** Soldan, Ger.
Althaea (p.1651·3); fennel (p.1687·2); aniseed (p.1655·2); liquorice (p.1270·2); fennel oil (p.1687·3); anise oil (p.1655·2).
*Coughs.*

**Em-eukal Mono** Soldan, Ger.
Oxymetazoline hydrochloride (p.1126·1).
*Rhinitis.*

**Emex** Mirren, S.Afr.
Invert sugar (p.1434·3); phosphoric acid (p.1731·2).
*Nausea.*

**Emflam** Merck, India.
Ibuprofen (p.45·3).
*Inflammation; pain.*

**Emflam Plus** Merck, India.
Ibuprofen (p.45·3); paracetamol (p.76·2).
*Inflammation; pain.*

**Emflex** Merck, UK.
Acemetacin (p.11·3).
*Inflammation; pain; rheumatoid arthritis.*

**Emforal** Remedica, Thai.
Propranolol hydrochloride (p.989·3).
*Angina pectoris; anxiety; arrhythmias; hypertension; hyperthyroidism; migraine; obstructive cardiomyopathy; tremor.*

**Emgecard** Mayrhofer, Austria.
Magnesium aspartate hydrochloride (p.1229·1).
*Magnesium deficiency.*

**Emgel** Glaxo Wellcome, USA.
Erythromycin (p.208·1).
*Acne.*

**Emgesan**
Recip, Fin.; Recip, Swed.
Magnesium hydroxide (p.1272·2).
*Magnesium deficiency; renal calculi.*

**Emican** Alter, Spain.
Salbutamol sulfate (p.791·3).
*Obstructive airways disease.*

**Emicilin** EMS, Braz.
Ampicillin (p.157·1) or ampicillin sodium (p.157·1).
Probenecid (p.416·3) is included in some of preparations to reduce renal tubular excretion of the antibiotic.
*Bacterial infections.*

**Emidoxin** Magis, Ital.
Cefonicid sodium (p.174·2).
Lidocaine hydrochloride (p.1377·3) is included in this preparation to alleviate the pain of injection.
*Gram-negative bacterial infections.*

**Emidoxyn** Amadeus, India.
Prochlorperazine maleate (p.716·3).
*Nausea and vomiting.*

**Emidrat** EMS, Braz.
Sodium chloride; potassium chloride; sodium citrate; sodium phosphate; calcium lactate; magnesium citrate; citric acid; saccharin sodium; glucose (p.1222·2).
*Diarrhoea; oral rehydration solution.*

**Emifol** Solfran, Mex.†.
Vitamin B substances (p.1417·1).

**Emiken** Kener, Mex.†.
Domperidone (p.1263·2).

**E-Mil** Fontovit, Braz.
dl-Alpha tocoferil acetate (p.1465·1).

**Emilace** Yamanouchi, Jpn.
Nemonapride (p.710·1).
*Schizophrenia.*

**Eminase**
Torrex, Austria†; Tramedico, Belg.; Roberts, Canad.†; Carinopharm, Ger.; Roberts, Israel; Tramedico, Neth.; Monmouth, UK†; Roberts, USA†.
Anistreplase (p.863·3).
*Myocardial infarction.*

**Emistin** EMS, Braz.
Clemastine fumarate (p.429·1); dexamethasone acetate (p.1097·1).
*Hypersensitivity reactions.*

**Emitex** Garec, S.Afr.
Cyclizine hydrochloride (p.429·3).
*Motion sickness; nausea; vestibular disorders; vomiting.*

**Emivox** Phoenix, Arg.
Ondansetron (p.1281·1).
*Vomiting.*

**Emizol** Lemery, Mex.†.
Astemizole (p.424·2).

**Emko** Schering, USA†.
Nonoxinol 9 (p.1413·3).
*Contraceptive.*

**Emla**
AstraZeneca, Arg.; AstraZeneca, Austral.; AstraZeneca, Austria; AstraZeneca, Belg.; AstraZeneca, Braz.; AstraZeneca, Canad.; AstraZeneca, Denm.; AstraZeneca, Fin.; AstraZeneca, Fr.; AstraZeneca, Ger.; Cana, Gr.; AstraZeneca, Hong Kong; AstraZeneca, Irl.; Astra, Israel; AstraZeneca, Ital.; AstraZeneca, Malaysia; AstraZeneca, Neth.; AstraZeneca, Norw.; AstraZeneca, NZ; AstraZeneca, Port.; Astra, S.Afr.; AstraZeneca, Singapore; AstraZeneca, Spain; Astra, Swed.; AstraZeneca, Switz.; AstraZeneca, Thai.; AstraZeneca, UK; AstraZeneca, USA.
Lidocaine (p.1377·3); prilocaine (p.1382·3).
*Local anaesthesia.*

**Emlapatch** AstraZeneca, Fr.
Lidocaine (p.1377·3); prilocaine (p.1382·3).
*Local anaesthesia.*

**Emlyte** MM, India.
Sodium chloride; sodium citrate; potassium chloride (p.1222·2).
*Oral rehydration therapy.*

**Emlyte-S** MM, India.
Sodium chloride; sodium citrate; potassium chloride; glucose; lactobacillus (p.1222·2).
*Oral rehydration therapy.*

**Emmenoiasi** Palmares, Ital.
Centella asiatica (p.1144·3); couch-grass (p.1676·2); lupulus (p.1708·1); melissa (p.1711·1); zinc (p.1469·2); copper (p.1425·3).
*Nutritional supplement.*

**Emmenovis** Vitoria, Port.
Estradiol benzoate (p.1550·1); progesterone (p.1566·2).
*Menstrual disorders; recurrent miscarriage.*

**Emmetipi** Sicor, Ital.†.
Methylprednisolone sodium succinate (p.1106·2).
*Parenteral corticosteroid.*

**Emoantitossina** Piam, Ital.
Calcium folinate (p.1431·1); cyanocobalamin (p.1458·2); monophosphothiamine chloride (p.1455·2); riboflavin sodium phosphate (p.1456·1); pyridoxine hydrochloride (p.1456·3); nicotinamide (p.1441·2); panthenol (p.1727·2).
*Anaemias; deficiency states.*

**Emoclot**
Scott-Cassara, Arg.; BBC, Braz.†; Cristalia, Braz.†; Kedrion, Ital.; Serono, Mex.
A factor VIII preparation (p.751·1).
*Haemorrhagic disorders.*

**Emo-Cort** Trans Canaderm, Canad.
Hydrocortisone (p.1103·3).
*Skin disorders.*

**Emocrat forte** Hevert, Ger.
Crataegus; rutoside sodium sulfate (p.1688·3).
*Arrhythmias; ischaemic heart disease.*

**Emodella** GABA, Switz.†.
Frangula bark (p.1266·3).
*Constipation.*

**Emoderm** Igefarma, Braz.†.
Urea (p.1162·2); vitis vinifera oil; borage oil (p.1661·3).

**Emoferrina** Piam, Ital.†.
Sodium ferric gluconate complex (p.1444·3).
*Iron deficiency; iron-deficiency anaemias.*

**Emoflux** Metapharma, Ital.†.
Buflomedil hydrochloride (p.877·2).
*Vascular disorders.*

**Emoform**
Note. This name is used for preparations of different composition.
Altana, Braz.
Electrolytes (p.1217·1).
Formerly contained formaldehyde.
*Dental caries prophylaxis; hypersensitive teeth.*

Pfizer Sante, Fr.
Stannous fluoride (p.1448·3).
*Dental caries prophylaxis; sensitive gums.*

Warner-Lambert, Fr.†.
Formaldehyde (p.1179·3).
*Bleeding gums; hypersensitive teeth.*

**Emoform Gencives** Pfizer Sante, Fr.
Potassium nitrate (p.1190·1); sodium bicarbonate (p.1223·2); sodium chloride (p.1233·3).
*Gingivitis; sensitive gums.*

**Emoform nouvelle formule** Wild, Switz.
Electrolytes (p.1217·1).
*Oral hygiene; sensitive teeth.*

**Emoform Sensibles** Pfizer Sante, Fr.
Potassium nitrate (p.1190·1); sodium monofluorophosphate (p.1446·2).
*Dental caries prophylaxis; sensitive gums.*

**Emoform-F au fluor** Wild, Switz.
Electrolytes (p.1217·1); sodium monofluorophosphate (p.1446·2).
*Dental caries prophylaxis; oral hygiene; sensitive teeth.*

**Emoform-Tat** *Byk Gulden, Ital.*
Sodium monofluorophosphate (p.1446·2); sodium fluoride (p.1444·3).
*Dental tartar.*

**Emoklar** *Savio, Ital.*
Heparin calcium (p.927·3).
*Thromboembolic disorders.*

**Emol** *Fischer, Israel†.*
Bath additive.
*Dry skin; skin irritation.*

**Emolan** *Mediderm, Chile.*
Soap substitute.
*Dermatitis.*

**Emolan Bloqueador Solar** *Mediderm, Chile.*
*SPF 60:* Enzacamene (p.1147·1); titanium dioxide (p.1160·3); ensulizole (p.1147·1); avobenzone (p.1142·3).
*Sunscreen.*

**Emolan H** *Mediderm, Chile.*
Padimate O (p.1155·1).
*Sunscreen.*

**Emolan Protector Solar** *Mediderm, Chile.*
*SPF 20:* Octinoxate (p.1154·3); octisalate (p.1154·3); benzophenone.
*Sunscreen.*

**Emollia** *Gordon, USA.*
Emollient and moisturiser.

**Emolytar** *Stiefel, Spain.*
Tar (p.1159·3); juniper oil (p.1703·1); coal tar (p.1159·2); arachis oil (p.1656·1).
*Skin disorders.*

**Emonorm** *Aesculapius, Ital.*
Ferrous gluconate (p.1428·1).
Ascorbic acid (p.1460·2) is included in this preparation to increase the absorption and availability of iron.
*Iron-deficiency anaemia.*

**Emopads** *Farmalight, Port.†.*
Aloes (p.1248·2); propylene glycol (p.1735·2); aesculus (p.1648·2); ruscus aculeatus; sage (p.1741·2); melaleuca alternifolia (p.1710·2).
*Anal discomfort.*

**Emopon** *Terapeutico, Ital.*
Calcium folinate (p.1431·1); cyanocobalamin (p.1458·2); ferric ammonium citrate (p.1427·2); thiamine hydrochloride (p.1455·1); nicotinamide (p.1441·2).
*Macrocytic anaemia; tonic.*

**Emopremarin** *Wyeth Lederle, Ital.*
Conjugated oestrogens (p.1543·2).
*Haemorrhage.*

**Emoren** *IFI, Ital.*
Oxetacaine hydrochloride (p.1382·1).
*Haemorrhoids.*

**Emorril** *Monsanto, Ital.*
Hydrocortisone acetate (p.1103·3); lidocaine hydrochloride (p.1377·3).
Formerly contained troxerutin, hydrocortisone acetate, nifuratel, and lidocaine or lidocaine hydrochloride.
*Adjunct in anorectal surgery; haemorrhoids.*

**Emortrofine** *Alphrema, Ital.*
Vitamin E (p.1464·3); bioflavonoids (p.1688·2).
*Capillary disorders; haemorrhoids.*

**Emorzim** *Pharmacia-Upjohn, Gr.*
Carboplatin (p.533·3).
*Ovarian cancer; small-cell lung cancer.*

**Emosint**
*Scott-Cassara, Arg.; Kedrion, Ital.*
Desmopressin acetate (p.1322·3).
*Haemorrhagic disorders.*

**Emotion** *Picot, Fr.*
Pregnancy test (p.1734·3).

**Emotival**
*Note. This name is used for preparations of different composition.*
*Armstrong, Arg.*
Lorazepam (p.704·1).
*Anxiety; insomnia.*
*Klinger, Braz.*
Hypericum (p.299·1).
*Depression.*

**Emoton** *Tentan, Switz.†.*
Agnus castus (p.1649·1).
*Premenstrual disorders.*

**Emotonico** *EMS, Braz.†.*
Ferric ammonium citrate (p.1427·2); vitamin B substances (p.1417·1).
*Anaemias.*

**Emotpin** *Meda, Swed.*
Aspirin (p.15·1).
*Fever; pain.*

**Emovat**
*GlaxoSmithKline, Denm.; GlaxoSmithKline, Fin.; GlaxoSmithKline, Swed.*
Clobetasone butyrate (p.1095·3).
*Skin disorders.*

**Emovate**
*GlaxoSmithKline, Austria; GlaxoSmithKline, Ger.; GlaxoSmithKline, Neth.; Glaxo Wellcome, Port.; Celltech, Spain; GlaxoSmithKline, Switz.*
Clobetasone butyrate (p.1095·3).
*Skin disorders.*

**Emovis** *Boniscontro & Gazzone, Ital.*
Calcium folinate (p.1431·1).
*Anaemias; antidote to overdosage with folic acid antagonists; folate deficiency; reduction of aminopterin and methotrexate toxicity.*

**Emoxiron** *Caber, Ital.*
Ferrous gluconate (p.1428·1).

**Empacod** *Byk Madaus, S.Afr.*
Paracetamol (p.76·2); codeine phosphate (p.27·1).
*Fever; pain.*

**Empaped** *Byk Madaus, S.Afr.*
Paracetamol (p.76·2).
*Fever; pain.*

**Empapol** *Vilardell, Spain†.*
Terpineol (p.1752·2); cresol (p.1177·3); pinus sylvestris resin (p.1675·1).
*Mouth and throat disorders; wounds.*

**Empecid** *Bayer, Arg.*
Clotrimazole (p.396·2).
*Fungal skin infections; vaginal candidiasis.*

**Empecid Cort** *Bayer, Arg.*
Clotrimazole (p.396·2); dexamethasone acetate (p.1097·1).
*Infected skin disorders.*

**Emperal** *Orion, Denm.*
Metoclopramide hydrochloride (p.1274·3).
*Gastro-oesophageal reflux; irritable bowel syndrome; nausea and vomiting.*

**Empirin** *Wellcome, USA.*
Aspirin (p.15·1).
*Fever; inflammation; myocardial infarction; pain; transient ischaemic attacks.*

**Empirin with Codeine** *Wellcome, USA.*
Aspirin (p.15·1); codeine phosphate (p.27·1).
*Pain.*

**Emplasto Monopolis** *Grisi, Mex.*
Copper acetate; lead monoxide (p.1706·1).
*Medicated dressing.*

**Emplastro Salonpas** *Hisamitsu, Braz.†.*
Camphor (p.1665·3); thymol (p.1194·2); methyl salicylate (p.59·3); glycol salicylate (p.44·3); menthol (p.1711·3).
*Pain.*

**Emplatre Croix D** *Democal, Switz.†.*
Cayenne pepper (p.1667·1); methyl salicylate (p.59·3); venice turpentine.
*Musculoskeletal and joint pain.*

**Emportal** *Novartis Consumer, Spain.*
Lactitol (p.1269·1).
*Constipation; hepatic encephalopathy.*

**Empracet** *GlaxoSmithKline, Canad.*
Paracetamol (p.76·2); codeine phosphate (p.27·1).
*Pain.*

**Emprazil-A** *Glaxo Wellcome, S.Afr.†.*
Triprolidine hydrochloride (p.442·3); pseudoephedrine hydrochloride (p.1129·2); caffeine (p.782·1); paracetamol (p.76·2).
*Cold and influenza symptoms.*

**Empynase** *Kaken, Jpn.*
Pronase.
*Inflammation; respiratory-tract congestion.*

**Emquin** *Merck, India.*
Chloroquine phosphate (p.448·2).
*Hepatic amoebiasis; lupus erythematosus; malaria; rheumatoid arthritis.*

**EMS Expectorante** *EMS, Braz.*
Guaifenesin (p.1122·1); etafedrine hydrochloride (p.1121·2); bufylline (p.781·3); doxylamine succinate (p.432·3).
*Respiratory-tract disorders.*

**Emscab** *MM, India.*
Lindane (p.1506·3); aminoacridine hydrochloride (p.1165·3).
*Pediculosis; scabies.*

**Emser Erkaltungsgel** *Siemens, Ger.†.*
Pumilio pine oil (p.1737·1); eucalyptus oil (p.1686·2); camphor (p.1665·3).
*Cold symptoms.*

**Emser Inhalationslosung** *Siemens, Ger.*
Natural emser salt (see Emser Salz) in isotonic solution.
*Respiratory-tract disorders.*

**Emser Nasensalbe** *Hexal, Austria.*
Natural emser salt; azulene (p.1658·3); nutmeg oil (p.1722·3); oleum pini sylvestris; pumilio pine oil (p.1737·1); eucalyptus oil (p.1686·2); cedar wood oil; turpentine oil (p.1760·1); camphor (p.1665·3).
*Colds; hay fever.*

**Emser Nasensalbe N** *Siemens, Ger.*
Natural emser salz; azulene (p.1658·3); nutmeg oil (p.1722·3); pine needle oil; pumilio pine oil (p.1737·1); eucalyptus oil (p.1686·2); cedar wood oil; camphor (p.1665·3); turpentine oil (p.1760·1).
*Colds; hay fever.*

**Emser Nasenspray** *Siemens, Ger.*
Natural emser salt (see Emser Salz) in isotonic solution.
*Cold symptoms; rhinosinusitis.*

**Emser Pastillen**
*Hexal, Austria; Siemens, Ger.*
Natural emser salt (see Emser Salz).
*Respiratory-tract disorders.*

**Emser Pastillen mit Menthol** *Hexal, Austria.*
Natural emser salt; menthol (p.1711·3); peppermint oil (p.1283·2).
*Respiratory-tract disorders.*

**Emser Salz** *Siemens, Ger.*
Natural emser salt (containing lithium, sodium, potassium, magnesium, calcium, manganese, ferrous, ferric, fluoride, chloride, bromide, iodide, nitrite, sulfate, bicarbonate, and carbonate ions).
*Dyspepsia; respiratory-tract disorders.*

**Emsilat** *Siemens, Ger.†.*
Eucalyptus oil (p.1686·2); pine needle oil.
*Cold symptoms.*

**Emsogen**
*Scientific Hospital Supplies, Austral.; Scientific Hospital Supplies, Irl.; Nutricia, NZ; Scientific Hospital Supplies, NZ.*
Preparation for enteral nutrition (p.1417·1).

**Emsyn** *Aspen, S.Afr.*
Erythromycin estolate (p.208·1).
*Bacterial infections.*

**Emtec-30** *Technilab, Canad.*
Paracetamol (p.76·2); codeine phosphate (p.27·1).
*Cold symptoms; pain; upper respiratory-tract disorders.*

**Emthexat**
*Nycomed, Fin.; Nycomed, Norw.; Nycomed, Swed.*
Methotrexate (p.568·2).
*Malignant neoplasms; psoriasis; rheumatoid arthritis.*

**Emthexate**
*Nycomed, Austria; Asta Oncologia, Braz.; Nettopharma, Denm.; Chemipharma, Gr.; Pharmachemie, Israel†; Pharmachemie, Malaysia; Asta Medica, NZ†; Pharmachemie, S.Afr.; Pharmachemie, Singapore†; Pras, Spain; Pharmachemie, Thai.; Teva, Thai.*
Methotrexate (p.568·2) or methotrexate sodium (p.568·3).
*Graft-versus-host disease; malignant neoplasms; psoriasis; rheumatoid arthritis.*

**Emtriva**
*Gilead, UK; Gilead, USA.*
Emtricitabine (p.632·3).
*HIV infection.*

**Emuclens** *Ovelle, Irl.†.*
Cleanser in an emollient base.
*Water-free cleansing.*

**Emucream** *Ovelle, Irl.†.*
Emollient.
*Dry skin.*

**Emulave**
*Rydelle, Fr.†; Ovelle, Irl.; Johnson & Johnson, Ital.; Dermoteca, Port.†.*
Avena (p.1658·2).
*Dry skin disorders; soap substitute.*
*Ovelle, Irl.*
Soap substitute.

**Emulax**
*Note. This name is used for preparations of different composition.*
*Hassle, Swed.*
Cascara (p.1255·1); docusate sodium (p.1262·2).
*Constipation.*
*British Dispensary, Thai.*
*Oral liquid:* Liquid paraffin (p.1479·1); phenolphthalein (p.1284·1); carmellose sodium (p.1577·3).
*Tablets:* Bisacodyl (p.1251·3).
*Constipation.*

**Emuliquen Laxante** *Lainco, Spain.*
Sodium picosulfate (p.1289·3); paraffin (p.1479·1).
Formerly contained phenolphthalein and paraffin.
*Constipation.*

**Emuliquen Simple** *Lainco, Spain.*
Paraffin (p.1479·1).
*Constipation.*

**Emulsan** *Pisa, Mex.*
Lipid infusion (p.1417·1).

**Emulsao de Lipidos** *Grifols, Port.*
Soya oil (p.1447·2).
Contains egg phospholipids.
*Lipid emulsion for parenteral nutrition.*

**Emulsao Scott** *GlaxoSmithKline, Braz.*
Cod-liver oil; soya oil; vitamin A; vitamin D; electrolytes (p.1417·1).
*Nutritional supplement.*

**Emulsao Universal** *Merck, Braz.*
Emollient.

**Emulsiderm**
*Dermal Laboratories, Irl.; Dermal, Israel; Dermal Laboratories, UK.*
Isopropyl myristate (p.1481·2); liquid paraffin (p.1479·1); benzalkonium chloride (p.1168·3).
*Dry skin conditions.*

**E-Mulsin** *Mucos, Ger.*
Alpha tocoferil acetate (p.1465·1).
*Vitamin E deficiency.*

**Emulsoil** *Paddock, USA.*
Castor oil (p.1668·2).
*Constipation.*

**Emu-V**
*Pharmacia, Austral.†; Pharmacia Upjohn, S.Afr.†.*
Erythromycin (p.208·1).
*Bacterial infections.*

**E-Mycin**
*Alphapharm, Austral.; Pacific, NZ.*
Erythromycin ethyl succinate (p.208·1).
*Bacterial infections.*
*Pharmacia Upjohn, Canad.†; Pharmacia, Hong Kong; Pharmacia Upjohn, Israel†; Pharmacia Upjohn, Singapore†; Knoll, USA.*
Erythromycin (p.208·1).
*Bacterial infections.*
*Themis, India; Docmed, S.Afr.†.*
Erythromycin estolate (p.208·1).
*Bacterial infections.*

**En** *Ravizza, Ital.†.*
Delorazepam (p.689·3).
*Anxiety disorders; premedication; sleep disorders.*

**Ena** *ABZ, Ger.; Hennig, Ger.*
Enalapril maleate (p.909·2).
*Heart failure; hypertension.*

**Enabeta** *Betapharm, Ger.*
Enalapril maleate (p.909·2).
*Heart failure; hypertension.*

**Enac** *Hexal, Austria.*
Enalapril maleate (p.909·2).
*Heart failure; hypertension.*

**Enacard** *Approved Prescription Services, UK†.*
Enalapril maleate (p.909·2).
*Heart failure; hypertension.*

**EnAce** *Nicholas Piramal, India.*
Enalapril maleate (p.909·2).
*Heart failure; hypertension; myocardial infarction.*

**EnAce-D** *Nicholas Piramal, India.*
Enalapril maleate (p.909·2); hydrochlorothiazide (p.933·2).
*Hypertension.*

**Enada** *Health & Diet Food Co., UK†.*
Nadide (p.1719·1).
*Chronic fatigue syndrome.*

**Enadil** *United Nordic, Denm.*
Enalapril maleate (p.909·2).
*Heart failure; hypertension.*

**Enadiol** *Laboratorios Chile, Chile.*
Estradiol valerate (p.1550·2).
*Menopausal disorders.*

**Enadiol CC** *Laboratorios Chile, Chile.*
Estradiol valerate (p.1550·2); medroxyprogesterone acetate (p.1557·2).
*Menopausal disorders; osteoporosis.*

**Enadiol MP** *Laboratorios Chile, Chile.*
12 tablets, estradiol valerato (p.1550·2); medroxyprogesterone acetate (p.1557·2); 18 tablets, estradiol valerate.
*Menopausal disorders.*

**enadura** *Merck dura, Ger.*
Enalapril maleate (p.909·2).
*Heart failure; hypertension.*

**Enahexal**
*Hexal, Austral.; Hexal, Ger.; Hexal, NZ.*
Enalapril maleate (p.909·2).
*Heart failure; hypertension.*

**Enal** *1A, Ger.*
Enalapril maleate (p.909·2).
*Heart failure; hypertension.*

**Enalabal** *Baldacci, Braz.*
Enalapril maleate (p.909·2).

**Enalabene** *Ratiopharm, Austria.*
Enalapril maleate (p.909·2).
*Heart failure; hypertension.*

**Enaladex** *Dexcel, Israel.*
Enalapril maleate (p.909·2).
*Heart failure; hypertension.*

**Enaladil** *Rhein, Mex.*
Enalapril maleate (p.909·2).
*Heart failure; hypertension.*

**Enalafel** *Asofarma, Arg.*
Enalapril maleate (p.909·2).
*Heart failure; hypertension.*

**Enalagamma** *Worwag, Ger.*
Enalapril maleate (p.909·2).
*Heart failure; hypertension.*

**Enalamed** *Cimed, Braz.*
Enalapril (p.909·2).
*Hypertension.*

**Enalapril Comp** *Ratiopharm, Swed.*
Enalapril maleate (p.909·2); hydrochlorothiazide (p.933·2).
*Hypertension.*

**Enalapril/HCT** *Kwizda, Austria.*
Enalapril maleate (p.909·2); hydrochlorothiazide (p.933·2).
*Hypertension.*

**Enaldun** *Duncan, Arg.*
Enalapril (p.909·2).
*Hypertension.*

**Enalind** *Lindopharm, Ger.*
Enalapril maleate (p.909·2).
*Heart failure; hypertension.*

**Enaloc** *Leiras, Fin.*
Enalapril maleate (p.909·2).
*Heart failure; hypertension.*

**Enaloc Comp** *Leiras, Fin.*
Enalapril maleate (p.909·2); hydrochlorothiazide (p.933·2).
*Hypertension.*

**Enalprin** *Royton, Braz.*
Enalapril maleate (p.909·2).
*Hypertension.*

**Enalten** *Saval, Chile.*
Enalapril maleate (p.909·2).
*Heart failure; hypertension.*

**Enalten D** *Saval, Chile.*
Enalapril maleate (p.909·2); hydrochlorothiazide (p.933·2).
*Hypertension.*

**Enalten DN** *Saval, Chile.*
Enalapril maleate (p.909·2); hydrochlorothiazide (p.933·2).
*Hypertension.*

**Enam** *Neopharm, Thai.*
Enalapril maleate (p.909·2).
*Heart failure; hypertension.*

**Enaminoleban** *Otsuka, Jpn.*
Amino acid preparation for enteral nutrition (p.1417·1).
*Hepatic encephalopathy; liver failure.*

**Enangel** *Menarini, Spain.*
Dexketoprofen trometamol (p.51·2).
*Inflammation; pain.*

**Enanton**
*Orion, Denm.; Orion, Fin.; Orion, Norw.; Orion, Swed.*
Leuprorelin acetate (p.1331·1).
*Endometriosis; prostatic cancer; uterine leiomyomas.*

**Enantone**
*Takeda, Austria; Takeda, Fr.; Takeda, Ger.; Takeda, Hong Kong; Takeda, Ital.; Takeda, Thai.*
Leuprorelin acetate (p.1331·1).
*Breast cancer; endometriosis; precocious puberty; prostatic cancer; stimulation of ovulation; uterine fibroids.*

**Enantone-Gyn** *Takeda, Ger.*
Leuprorelin acetate (p.1331·1).
*Breast cancer; endometriosis.*

**Enantyum**
*Menarini, Arg.; Menarini, Ital.; Menarini, Spain.*
Dexketoprofen trometamol (p.51·2).
*Pain.*

**Enap**
*Rowex, Irl.; Pharma Dynamics, S.Afr.; KRKA, Singapore.*
Enalapril maleate (p.909·2).
*Heart failure; hypertension.*

**Enap HL** *KRKA, Singapore.*
Enalapril maleate (p.909·2); hydrochlorothiazide (p.933·2).
*Hypertension.*

**Enap-Co** *Pharma Dynamics, S.Afr.*
Enalapril maleate (p.909·2); hydrochlorothiazide (p.933·2).
*Hypertension.*

**Enapren** *Merck Sharp & Dohme, Ital.*
Enalapril maleate (p.909·2).
*Heart failure; hypertension; ischaemic heart disease.*

**Enapress** *Berner, Fin.*
Enalapril maleate (p.909·2).
*Heart failure; hypertension.*

**Enapril**
*Sintofarma, Braz.†; Intas, Thai.*
Enalapril maleate (p.909·2).
*Heart failure; hypertension.*

**Enaprotec** *Hexal, Braz.*
Enalapril maleate (p.909·2).
*Hypertension.*

**Ena-Puren** *Alpharma-Isis, Ger.*
Enalapril maleate (p.909·2).
*Heart failure; hypertension.*

**Enaran** *Kwizda, Austria.*
Enalapril maleate (p.909·2).
*Heart failure; hypertension.*

**Enaril**
*Biolab, Singapore; Biolab, Thai.*
Enalapril maleate (p.909·2).
*Heart failure; hypertension.*

**Enasifar** *Siphar, Switz.*
Enalapril maleate (p.909·2).
*Heart failure; hypertension.*

**Enatec**
*Hebron, Braz.; Mepha, Switz.*
Enalapril maleate (p.909·2).
*Heart failure; hypertension.*

**Enatec F** *Hebron, Braz.*
Enalapril maleate (p.909·2); hydrochlorothiazide (p.933·2).
*Hypertension.*

**Enatia** *Pentafarma, Port.*
Enalapril maleate (p.909·2); hydrochlorothiazide (p.933·2).
*Hypertension.*

**Enatral** *LA, Arg.*
Enalapril (p.909·2).
*Hypertension.*

**Enatrial** *Hexal, Arg.*
Enalapril maleate (p.909·2).
*Heart failure; hypertension.*

**Enatus** *Medisint, Ital.*
Iceland moss; plantago; althaea; aesculus; thyme; melissa; drosera; papaver.
*Coughs.*

**Enatyrol** *Tyrol, Austria.*
Enalapril maleate (p.909·2).
*Heart failure; hypertension.*

**Enbrel**
*Wyeth, Arg.; Wyeth, Austral.; Wyeth Lederle, Belg.; Wyeth-Ayerst, Canad.; Wyeth, Chile; Wyeth Lederle, Fin.; Wyeth Lederle, Fr.; Wyeth, Ger.; Wyeth, Israel; Wyeth Lederle, Ital.; Wyeth, Mex.; Wyeth Lederle, Norw.; Wyeth, NZ; Wyeth Lederle, Port.; Wyeth, Spain; Wyeth Lederle, Swed.; Wyeth, Switz.; Wyeth, UK; Amgen, USA.*
Etanercept (p.36·3).
*Ankylosing spondylitis; psoriatic arthritis; rheumatoid arthritis.*

**Encare**
*Stella, Canad.†; Thompson, USA.*
Nonoxinol 9 (p.1413·3).
*Contraceptive.*

**Encaskin Cream** *APR, Switz.*
Salnacedin (p.1157·2).
*Acne.*

**Encaskin Creme** *Farmalight, Port.*
Salnacedin (p.1157·2).
*Acne.*

**Encaskin Detergente** *Farmalight, Port.*
Salnacedin (p.1157·2).
*Skin wash.*

**Encaskin Liquid Detergent** *APR, Switz.*
Salnacedin (p.1157·2).
*Skin wash.*

**Encebrin** *Lilly, Hong Kong†.*
Multivitamin and mineral preparation (p.1417·1).

**Encefabol**
*Merck, Braz.†; Merck, Chile; Bracco, Ital.†.*
Pyritinol (p.1737·2) or pyritinol hydrochloride (p.1737·2).
*Cerebrovascular disorders; mental function impairment.*

**Encegam** *Centeon, Ger.†; Chiron Behring, Ger.†.*
A tick-borne encephalitis immunoglobulin (p.1642·1).
*Passive immunisation.*

**Encelin** *Crosara, Ital.†.*
Citicoline sodium (p.1672·3).
*Cerebrovascular disorders; parkinsonism.*

**Encephabol**
*Merck, Austria; Lipha Sante, Fr.†; Merck, Ger.; Merck, Hong Kong; Merck, India; Merck, Malaysia; Merck, Mex.; Merck, S.Afr.; Merck, Singapore; Merck, Thai.*
Pyritinol (p.1737·2) or pyritinol hydrochloride (p.1737·2).
*Cerebrovascular disorders; mental function impairment.*

**Encepur**
*Grunenthal, Austria; Chiron Behring, Fin.; Chiron Behring, Ger.; Meda, Swed.; Berna, Switz.*
An inactivated tick-borne encephalitis vaccine (p.1642·1).
*Active immunisation.*

**Encetrop** *Dumex, Ger.†.*
Piracetam (p.1732·1).
*Mental function disorders.*

**Encialina** *Bucca, Spain.*
Aconite (p.1646·3); arnica (p.1656·3); ipecacuanha (p.1122·3); chamomile (p.1669·3); rhatany (p.1738·1); iodine (p.1598·1).
*Mouth inflammation; pyorrhoea.*

**Encorate** *Sun, Singapore†.*
Sodium valproate (p.380·1).
*Epilepsy.*

**Encypalmed** *Trima, Israel.*
Pancreatin (p.1725·3); ox bile (p.1660·3); rhubarb (p.1287·3); frangula bark (p.1266·3); sodium bicarbonate (p.1223·2).
*Dyspepsia; gastro-enteritis; meteorism.*

**End Lice** *Thompson, USA†.*
Pyrethrins (p.1509·3); piperonyl butoxide (p.1509·2).
*Pediculosis.*

**Endace** *Samarth, India.*
Megestrol (p.1558·3).
*Breast cancer; endometrial cancer.*

**Endacil** *Sydenham, Mex.†.*
Indometacin (p.47·3).

**Endafed** *UAD, USA.*
Pseudoephedrine hydrochloride (p.1129·2); brompheniramine maleate (p.426·1).
*Allergic rhinitis; nasal congestion.*

**Endagen-HD** *Abana, USA.*
Phenylephrine hydrochloride (p.1126·3); chlorphenamine maleate (p.427·3); hydrocodone tartrate (p.45·1).
*Coughs and cold symptoms.*

**Endak**
*Madaus, Austria; Madaus, Ger.*
Carteolol hydrochloride (p.880·3).
*Angina pectoris; arrhythmias; hypertension; myocardial infarction.*

**Endal** *Pediamed, USA.*
Phenylephrine hydrochloride (p.1126·3); guaifenesin (p.1122·1).
*Coughs.*

**Endal Expectorant** *Pediamed, USA.*
Phenylephrine hydrochloride (p.1126·3); guaifenesin (p.1122·1); codeine phosphate (p.27·1).
Formerly contained phenylpropanolamine hydrochloride, guaifenesin, and codeine phosphate.
*Coughs.*

**Endal HD** *Pediamed, USA.*
Diphenhydramine hydrochloride (p.431·3); phenylephrine hydrochloride (p.1126·3); hydrocodone tartrate (p.45·1).
*Upper respiratory-tract disorders.*

**Endalbumin** *Alfa Biotech, Ital.†.*
Albumin (p.740·3).
*Hypoalbuminaemia.*

**Endal-HD** *Pediamed, USA†.*
Chlorphenamine maleate (p.427·3); phenylephrine hydrochloride (p.1126·3); hydrocodone tartrate (p.45·1).
*Coughs and cold symptoms.*

**Endal-HD Plus** *Pediamed, USA.*
Chlorphenamine maleate (p.427·3); phenylephrine hydrochloride (p.1126·3); hydrocodone tartrate (p.45·1).
*Coughs and cold symptoms.*

**Endantadine** *Endo, Canad.*
Amantadine hydrochloride (p.1197·2).
*Influenza A; parkinsonism.*

**Endcol Cold & Flu** *Aspen, S.Afr.*
Paracetamol (p.76·2); vitamin C (p.1460·2); phenylephrine hydrochloride (p.1126·3); chlorphenamine maleate (p.427·3); caffeine (p.782·1).
*Cold and influenza symptoms.*

**Endcol Cough Linctus** *Aspen, S.Afr.*
Triprolidine hydrochloride (p.442·3); pseudoephedrine hydrochloride (p.1129·2); codeine phosphate (p.27·1).
*Coughs.*

**Endcol DM** *Aspen, S.Afr.*
Triprolidine hydrochloride (p.442·3); pseudoephedrine hydrochloride (p.1129·2); dextromethorphan hydrobromide (p.1117·3).
*Coughs.*

**Endcol Expectorant** *Aspen, S.Afr.*
Triprolidine hydrochloride (p.442·3); pseudoephedrine hydrochloride (p.1129·2); guaifenesin (p.1122·1).
Formerly contained triprolidine hydrochloride, pseudoephedrine hydrochloride, guaifenesin, and codeine phosphate.
*Coughs.*

**Endcol Lozenges** *Aspen, S.Afr.*
Cetylpyridinium chloride (p.1173·1); benzocaine (p.1370·3).
*Sore throat.*

**En-De-Kay** *Manx, UK.*
Sodium fluoride (p.1444·3).
*Dental caries prophylaxis.*

**Endep**
*Alphapharm, Austral.; Alphapharm, Malaysia; Merck, Malaysia.*
Amitriptyline hydrochloride (p.280·3).
*Depression; nocturnal enuresis.*

**Endermyl** *Galderma, Canad.†.*
Emollient.
*Dry skin.*

**Endial** *Roemmers, Arg.*
Glimepiride (p.332·2).
*Diabetes mellitus.*

**Endiaron** *Medphano, Ger.*
Loperamide hydrochloride (p.1271·1).
*Diarrhoea.*

**Endium** *Dexo, Fr.*
Diosmin (p.1688·2).
*Haemorrhoids; peripheral vascular disorders.*

**Endobil** *Merck, Irl.†.*
Meglumine iodoxamate (p.1064·1).
*Contrast medium for cholecystography and cholangiography.*

**Endobon** *Biomet Merck, Ger.*
Calcium hydroxide phosphate (p.1225·3).
*Bone defects.*

**Endobulin**
*Baxter Immuno, Arg.; Immuno, Austria; Baxter, Denm.; Baxter, Fin.; Baxter, Ger.; Immuno, Israel; Baxter, Ital.; Adcock Ingram Critical Care, S.Afr.; Baxter, Spain; Baxter, Swed.; Baxter, Switz.†.*
A normal immunoglobulin (p.1627·2).
*Guillain-Barré syndrome; hypogammaglobulinaemia; idiopathic thrombocytopenic purpura; immunodeficiency disorders; Kawasaki disease; passive immunisation.*

**Endobuline** *Baxter, Fr.*
A normal immunoglobulin (p.1627·2).
*Hypogammaglobulinaemia; passive immunisation.*

**Endocaina** *Lafage, Arg.*
Procaine (p.1383·2).
*Local anaesthesia.*

**Endocal** *Pisa, Mex.*
Calcitonin (salmon) (p.768·2).

**Endocet**
*Endo, Canad.; Endo, USA.*
Oxycodone hydrochloride (p.75·2); paracetamol (p.76·2).
*Pain.*

**Endocodone** *Endo, USA.*
Oxycodone hydrochloride (p.75·2).
*Pain.*

**Endocorion** *Elea, Arg.*
Chorionic gonadotrophin (p.1320·3).
*Benign breast disorders; cryptorchidism; delayed puberty; habitual and threatened miscarriage; male and female infertility; menstrual disorders.*

**Endocris** *Cristalia, Braz.†.*
Sodium laurilsulfate (p.1574·2).
*Dental disorders.*

**Endodan** *Endo, Canad.*
Oxycodone hydrochloride (p.75·2); aspirin (p.15·1).
*Fever; inflammation; pain.*

**Endofalk** *Falk, Ger.*
Macrogol 3350 (p.1709·1); electrolytes (p.1217·1).
*Bowel cleansing for endoscopy.*

**Endofolin** *Marjan, Braz.*
Folic acid (p.1429·1).
*Anaemias; folic acid deficiency.*

**Endogel Esteril** *Rider, Chile.*
Lidocaine hydrochloride (p.1377·3); chlorhexidine gluconate (p.1173·2).
*Endoscopy; urethral disinfection and anaesthesia.*

**Endogest** *Siam Bheasach, Thai.*
Amylase (p.1654·2); vitamin $B_1$ (p.1455·2); scopolia; sodium bicarbonate (p.1223·2); calcium carbonate (p.1254·2).
*Dyspepsia; gastric hyperacidity; gastritis; gastrointestinal motility disorders; heartburn.*

**Endol** *Cruz, Spain†.*
Tiadenol (p.1011·2).
*Hyperlipidaemias.*

**Endolac** *Proge, Ital.*
*Lactobacillus acidophilus* (p.1704·2); *Lactobacillus delbrueckii*; *Streptococcus thermophilus* (p.1704·2).
*Gastrointestinal disorders.*

**Endolipid** *Darrow, Braz.*
Fractionated soya oil (p.1447·2).
Contains egg lecithin.
*Lipid infusion for parenteral nutrition.*

**Endolipide** *Braun, Fr.*
Soya oil (p.1447·2).
Contains egg lecithin.
*Lipid infusion for parenteral nutrition.*

**Endolor** *Keene, USA.*
Paracetamol (p.76·2); caffeine (p.782·1); butalbital (p.673·3).
*Pain.*

**Endomethasone** *Septodont, Switz.†.*
Powder, hydrocortisone acetate (p.1103·3); thymol iodide (p.1194·3); barium sulfate (p.1061·1); liquid, eugenol (p.1686·2); peppermint oil (p.1283·2); anise oil (p.1655·2).
*Root canal sealant.*

**Endomethazone** *Austrodent, Austria†.*
Dexamethasone (p.1097·1); hydrocortisone acetate (p.1103·3).
*Root canal filling.*

**Endometrin** *Lapidot, Israel.*
Progesterone (p.1566·2).

**Endomicina** *Key, Arg.*
Neomycin (p.235·1); furazolidone (p.605·2); pectin (p.1580·3); kaolin (p.1268·3).
*Diarrhoea.*

**Endomina** *Farma Lepori, Spain.*
Estradiol (p.1550·1).
*Menopausal disorders; osteoporosis.*

**Endone** *Boots Healthcare, Austral.*
Oxycodone hydrochloride (p.75·2).
*Pain.*

**Endoneutralio** *SoSe, Ital.*
Sodium citrate (p.1223·2); potassium citrate (p.1223·1).
*Gastric hyperacidity.*

**Endopancrine 40** *Organon, Fr.†.*
Insulin injection (crystalline) (porcine, highly purified) (p.333·3).
*Diabetes mellitus.*

**Endopancrine 100** *Organon, Fr.†.*
Insulin zinc suspension (porcine, highly purified) (p.333·3).
*Diabetes mellitus.*

**Endopancrine Protamine** *Organon, Fr.†.*
Isophane insulin injection (crystalline) (porcine, highly purified) (p.333·3).
*Diabetes mellitus.*

**Endopancrine Zinc Protamine** *Organon, Fr.†.*
A protamine zinc insulin suspension (porcine, highly purified) (p.333·3).
*Diabetes mellitus.*

**Endo-Paractol** *Temmler, Ger.*
Simeticone (p.1289·2).
*Adjuvant for endoscopy and double contrast radiography.*

**Endophleban** *Rentschler, Ger.†.*
Dihydroergotamine mesilate (p.465·3).
*Chronic venous insufficiency; hypotension; migraine and related vascular headache.*

**Endoprost** *Italfarmaco, Ital.*
Iloprost trometamol (p.1518·2).
*Arterial ischaemia; Raynaud's syndrome; thromboangiitis obliterans.*

**Endorem**
*Guerbet, Austria; Codali, Belg.; Guerbet, Denm.; Guerbet, Fin.; Guerbet, Fr.; Guerbet, Ger.; R+N, Gr.; Guerbet, Ital.; Guerbet, Neth.†; Guerbet, Norw.; Guerbet, Port.; Guerbert, Spain; Gothia, Swed.; Guerbet, Switz.*
Ferumoxides (p.1061·3).
*Contrast medium for magnetic resonance imaging.*

**Endosalil** *Elofar, Braz.†.*
Aspirin (p.15·1).
*Fever; inflammation; pain; thromboembolism prophylaxis.*

**Endosgel**
*Solco, Austria; Farco, Ger.; Almed, Switz.†.*
Chlorhexidine gluconate (p.1173·2); sodium lactate (p.1223·2).
*Aid to endoscopy and catheterisation.*

**Endosporine** *Peters, Fr.†.*
Glutaral (p.1180·3).
*Instrument disinfection.*

**Endospray** *Axcan, Canad.*
Benzocaine (p.1370·3); tetracaine hydrochloride (p.1385·1).
*Local anaesthesia.*

**Endotelon**
*Sanofi Synthelabo, Chile; Sanofi Synthelabo, Fr.*
Grape seeds.
*Lymphoedema; peripheral vascular disorders; venous insufficiency.*

**Endotropina** *Fada, Arg.*
Atropine (p.476·3).

**Endotussin** *Prodotti, Braz.*
Potassium iodide (p.1598·1); theophylline calcium salicylate (p.804·3).
*Respiratory-tract congestion.*

**Endoxan**
*Labinca, Arg.; Baxter, Austral.; Asta Medica, Austria; Baxter, Belg.; Asta Médica, Chile; Baxter, Chile; Baxter Oncology, Fr.; Baxter, Ger.;*

Asta, Gr.; Baxter, Hong Kong; German Remedies, India; Asta Medica, Israel; Asta Medica, Ital.; Baxter Oncology, Malaysia; Viatris, Neth.; Asta Medica, NZ; Baxter, NZ; Asta Medica, Port.; Aventis, S.Afr.; Baxter Oncology, Singapore; Asta Medica, Switz.; Baxter, Thai.
Cyclophosphamide (p.540·2).
*Auto-immune disorders; malignant neoplasms; transplant rejection.*

**Endoxana** Asta Medica, Irl.; Asta Medica, Thai.†; Baxter, UK.
Cyclophosphamide (p.540·2).
*Malignant neoplasms.*

**Endrate** Abbott, USA.
Disodium edetate (p.1037·3).
*Digitalis-induced cardiac arrhythmias; hypercalcaemia.*

**Endrine**
Wyeth Lederle, Austria†; Christiaens, Belg.; Wyeth, India.
Ephedrine (p.1120·1); camphor (p.1665·3); menthol (p.1711·3); cineole (p.1672·1).
*Catarrh; nasal congestion; rhinitis.*

**Endrine Doux** Christiaens, Belg.
Ephedrine (p.1120·1); camphor (p.1665·3); cineole (p.1672·1).
*Cold symptoms.*

**Endrine Mild**
Wyeth Lederle, Austria†; Wyeth, India.
Ephedrine (p.1120·1); camphor (p.1665·3); cineole (p.1672·1).
*Catarrh; nasal congestion; rhinitis.*

**Endronax** Sintofarma, Braz.
Alendronate sodium (p.765·3).
*Bone metastases; hypercalcaemia; osteoporosis; Paget's disease of bone.*

**Enduron**
Abbott, Austral.†; Abbott, Hong Kong; Abbott, USA.
Methyclothiazide (p.953·2).
*Hypertension; oedema.*

**Enduronil** Abbott, Ital.†.
Methyclothiazide (p.953·2); deserpidine (p.892·3).
*Hypertension.*

**Enduronyl**
Abbott, Hong Kong; Abbott, USA†.
Methyclothiazide (p.953·2); deserpidine (p.892·3).
*Hypertension.*

**Enduxan** Abbott, Braz.†.
Cyclophosphamide (p.540·2).
*Malignant neoplasms.*

**Eneas** Vita, Spain.
Enalapril maleate (p.909·2); nitrendipine (p.973·3).
*Hypertension.*

**Enecat** Lafayette, USA†.
Barium sulfate (p.1061·1).
*Contrast medium for gastrointestinal radiography.*

**Enelbin-Paste N** Cassella-med, Ger.
Zinc oxide (p.1163·2); salicylic acid (p.1157·1); aluminium silicate (p.1250·2).
*Inflammation; musculoskeletal and joint disorders.*

**Enelbin-Salbe N** Cassella-med, Ger.
Heparin sodium (p.928·1); salicylic acid (p.1157·1).
*Musculoskeletal, joint, peri-articular and soft-tissue disorders; superficial vascular disorders.*

**Enelfa**
Sanova, Austria; Dolorgiet, Ger.
Paracetamol (p.76·2).
*Fever; pain.*

**Enema Casen** Casen Fleet, Spain.
Dibasic sodium phosphate (p.1231·1); monobasic sodium phosphate (p.1230·3).
*Bowel evacuation.*

**Enema Cooper** Cooper (Κοπερ), Gr.
Dibasic sodium phosphate (p.1231·1); monobasic sodium phosphate (p.1230·3).
*Bowel evacuation; constipation.*

**Enemac** Eurospital, Ital.
Monobasic sodium phosphate (p.1230·3); dibasic sodium phosphate (p.1231·1).
*Bowel evacuation; constipation.*

**Enemol**
Gador, Arg.; Dominion, Canad.
Dibasic sodium phosphate (p.1231·1); monobasic sodium phosphate (p.1230·3).
*Bowel evacuation.*

**Ener-B** Nature's Bounty, USA†.
Vitamin $B_{12}$ (p.1458·2).
*Dietary supplement.*

**Enerbody** Body Spring, Ital.
Maltodextrin; fructose; vitamins; minerals (p.1417·1).
*Nutritional supplement; obesity.*

**Enercal Plus**
Wyeth, Hong Kong; Wyeth, Malaysia; Wyeth, Singapore.
Lactose-free preparation for enteral nutrition (p.1417·1).

**Enercomplex** Provita, Ital.†.
Mineral preparation with vitamin C, carnitine, creatine, and ginseng (p.1417·1).
*Tonic.*

**Enerday** Pharmafina, Chile.
Ginseng; vitamins; erythroxylon catuaba; marapuama (p.1417·1).
*Tonic.*

**Ener-E** Wassen, Ital.
Vitamin E (p.1464·3); ubidecarenone (p.1760·2).
*Nutritional supplement.*

**Ener-G** General Dietary, UK.
Gluten-free bread, rice bran, and pasta (p.1417·1).
*Gluten-sensitive enteropathies.*

**Energeia** Sanitalia, Ital.
Ginseng; ginkgo biloba; eleutherococcus; minerals (p.1417·1).
*Nutritional supplement.*

**Energen** Volchem, Ital.
Glucose (p.1432·2) or maltodextrin (p.1439·3).
*Energy loss; hypoglycaemia.*

**Energex Fort** Frega, Canad.†.
Multivitamin and mineral preparation (p.1417·1).

**Energiclin** Hebron, Braz.
Piracetam (p.1732·1); vitamins (p.1417·1).
*Tonic.*

**Energil C** Novamed, Braz.
Ascorbic acid (p.1460·2).
*Vitamin C supplement.*

**Energisan** Ache, Braz.†.
Vitamin B substances; fructose; succinic dinitrile (p.1417·1).
*Tonic.*

**Energitum** Zambon, Fr.
Arginine glutamate (p.1421·1).
*Asthenia.*

**Energivit**
Note. This name is used for preparations of different composition.
Scientific Hospital Supplies, Austral.; Nutricia, NZ; Scientific Hospital Supplies, NZ; Scientific Hospital Supplies, UK.
Nutritional supplement for infants and children (p.1417·1).

Ache, Braz.
Piracetam (p.1732·1); fructose; vitamin B substances; ascorbic acid; tocopherol acetate (p.1417·1).
*Alcoholism; behaviour disorders in children; cerebrovascular disorders; senile dementia; vertigo.*

**Energizante** AM, Arg.
Vitamins; minerals; arginine; choline; royal jelly; guarana; pollen (p.1417·1).
*Tonic.*

**Energona** Maurer, Ger.†.
Norfenefrine hydrochloride (p.975·3).
*Hypotension.*

**Energoplex** Libbs, Braz.
Vitamins; fructose; arginine (p.1417·1).
*Nutritional supplement.*

**Energy Alfa** Dolisos, Canad.
Homoeopathic preparation.

**Energy Plus** Nutravite, Canad.
Ginseng (p.1693·1); kola (p.1765·3).

**Energyn-T** DHA, Singapore.
Multivitamin and mineral preparation (p.1417·1).

**Energysor** Soria Natural, Spain.
Ginseng (p.1693·1); eleutherococcus senticosis (p.1744·1); damiana (p.1679·1).
*Fatigue; tonic.*

**Enerjets** Chilton, USA.
Caffeine (p.782·1).
*Fatigue.*

**Ener-Mix** Also, Ital.
Multivitamin and mineral preparation (p.1417·1).

**Enertonic** Bifarma, Ital.†.
Eleutherococcus senticosis (p.1744·1); ginkgo biloba (p.1692·3); guarana (p.1765·3); echinacea (p.1683·2).
*Dietary supplement.*

**Enervit**
EMS, Braz.
Succinic dinitrile; vitamin B substances (p.1417·1).
*Nutritional supplement.*

Also, Ital.
A range of nutritional supplements (p.1417·1).

**Enervon-C**
United American, Hong Kong; United American, Malaysia; United American, Singapore; Great Eastern, Thai.; United American, Thai.
Vitamin B substances and vitamin C (p.1417·1).

United American, Singapore.
*Syrup:* Multivitamin preparation (p.1417·1).

**Enervon-C Plus**
United American, Hong Kong; United American, Malaysia.
Multivitamin preparation (p.1417·1).

**Enetege** Fada, Arg.
Glyceryl trinitrate (p.923·2).

**Enfalac AR**
Mead Johnson, Austral.†; Mead Johnson Nutritionals, Canad.; Mead Johnson, Malaysia; Mead Johnson, NZ†; Mead Johnson, Singapore; Mead Johnson Nutritionals, Thai.
Infant feed (p.1417·1).
*Gastro-oesophageal reflux.*

**Enfalac Enfalyte** Mead Johnson Nutritionals, Canad.
Rice syrup; sodium chloride; potassium citrate; sodium citrate; citric acid (p.1222·2).
*Diarrhoea; oral rehydration therapy.*

**Enfalac HA** Mead Johnson, Port.
Infant feed (p.1417·1).
*Milk intolerance.*

**Enfalac Lactofree** Mead Johnson Nutritionals, Canad.
Lactose-free infant feed (p.1417·1).
Formerly known as Enfalac Lactose Free.
*Lactose intolerance.*

**Enfalac Lytren** Mead Johnson Nutritionals, Canad.†.
Glucose; potassium citrate; sodium chloride; sodium citrate; citric acid (p.1222·2).
*Diarrhoea.*

**Enfalac Nutramigen** Mead Johnson Nutritionals, Canad.
Gluten-free, lactose-free casein hydrolysate preparation for special diets (p.1417·1).
*Galactosaemia; protein sensitivity.*

**Enfalac Pregestimil** Mead Johnson Nutritionals, Canad.
Infant feed (p.1417·1).
*Malabsorption syndromes.*

**Enfalac Prosobee Soy** Mead Johnson Nutritionals, Canad.
Soy based infant feed (p.1417·1).
*Hypersensitivity to cow's milk.*

**Enfamil AR**
Bristol-Myers Squibb, Arg.; Mead Johnson, Braz.; Mead Johnson, Chile; Mead Johnson, Fr.; Bristol-Myers Squibb, Hong Kong; Mead Johnson, Irl.; Mead Johnson, Israel; Bristol-Myers Squibb, Mex.; Mead Johnson, Port.; Mead Johnson Nutritionals, UK†.
Infant feed (p.1417·1).
*Gastro-oesophageal reflux.*

**Enfamil Lactofree** Mead Johnson, Irl.
Infant feed (p.1417·1).
*Lactose intolerance.*

**Enfamil Natalins Rx** Mead Johnson Nutritionals, USA.
Multivitamin and mineral preparation (p.1417·1).
Formerly known as Natalins Rx.

**Enfamil Nutramigen** Bristol-Myers Squibb, Arg.
Infant feed (p.1417·1).
*Diarrhoea; frustosaemia; galactosaemia; protein sensitivity.*

**Enfamil Pregestimil** Bristol-Myers Squibb, Arg.
Infant feed (p.1417·1).
*Diarrhoea; galactosaemia; lactose intolerance; pancreatic insufficiency; protein sensitivity; sucrose intolerance.*

**Enfamil sin Lactosa**
Bristol-Myers Squibb, Arg.; Mead Johnson, Chile; Bristol-Myers Squibb, Mex.
Infant feed (p.1417·1).
*Lactose intolerance.*

**Enfamil Soya**
Bristol-Myers Squibb, Arg.; Mead Johnson, Chile; Bristol-Myers Squibb, Mex.
Infant feed (p.1417·1).
*Diarrhoea; lactose intolerance.*

**Enfluthane** Baxter, Braz.
Enflurane (p.1298·1).
*General anaesthesia.*

**Enforan** Richmond, Arg.
Enflurane (p.1298·1).
*General anaesthesia.*

**Enfran** Pisa, Mex.
Enflurane (p.1298·1).
*General anaesthesia.*

**En-Ga-Lax** Omega, Arg.
Casanthranol (p.1255·1); bisacodyl (p.1251·3).
*Bowel evacuation; constipation.*

**Engerix** SmithKline Beecham, Gr.
A hepatitis B vaccine (p.1618·1).
*Active immunisation.*

**Engerix-B**
GlaxoSmithKline, Arg.; GlaxoSmithKline, Austral.; GlaxoSmithKline, Austria; GlaxoSmithKline, Belg.; GlaxoSmithKline, Braz.; GlaxoSmithKline, Canad.; GlaxoSmithKline, Chile; GlaxoSmithKline, Denm.; GlaxoSmithKline, Fin.; GlaxoSmithKline, Fr.; GlaxoSmithKline, Ger.; GlaxoSmithKline, Hong Kong; GlaxoSmithKline, India; GlaxoSmithKline, Irl.; SmithKline Beecham, Israel; GlaxoSmithKline, Ital.; GlaxoSmithKline, Malaysia; SmithKline Beecham, Mex.; GlaxoSmithKline, Neth.; GlaxoSmithKline, Norw.; GlaxoSmithKline, NZ; Smith Kline & French, Port.; GlaxoSmithKline, S.Afr.; GlaxoSmithKline, Singapore; GlaxoSmithKline, Spain; GlaxoSmithKline, Swed.; SmithKline Beecham, Switz.; GlaxoSmithKline, Thai.; GlaxoSmithKline, UK; SmithKline Beecham, USA.
A hepatitis B vaccine (recombinant DNA) (p.1618·1).
*Active immunisation.*

**Engov** DM, Braz.†.
Aspirin (p.15·1); caffeine (p.782·1); mepyramine (p.437·1).
Aluminium hydroxide (p.1249·2) is included in this preparation in an attempt to limit adverse effects on the gastrointestinal mucosa.
*Fever; pain.*

**Engystol**
Peithner, Austria; Heel, Ger.
Homoeopathic preparation.

**Engystol N** Heel, S.Afr.
Homoeopathic preparation.

**Enhancin**
Ranbaxy, Malaysia; Ranbaxy, Singapore.
Amoxicillin (p.155·3) or amoxicillin trihydrate (p.155·3); clavulanic acid (p.193·3) or potassium clavulanate (p.193·3).
*Bacterial infections.*

**Eni** Grossman, Mex.
Ciprofloxacin hydrochloride (p.188·2).
*Bacterial infections.*

**Enicul** Apomedica, Austria.
Magnesium trisilicate (p.1272·3); algeldrate (p.1249·2); ammonium glycyrrhizinate (p.1115·2).
*Gastrointestinal disorders.*

**Enidazol** East India Pharma, India.
Tinidazole (p.617·1).
*Amoebiasis; giardiasis.*

**Enidin** Allergan, Austral.
Brimonidine tartrate (p.876·3).
*Glaucoma; ocular hypertension.*

**Eniflex** Bogo, Chile.
Glucosamine hydrochloride; ascorbic acid (p.1460·2); lucerne; minerals.
*Joint disorders.*

**Enirant** Gepepharm, Ger.†.
Co-dergocrine mesilate (p.1674·1).
*Cerebral circulatory disorders; hypertension.*

**Enison** Ciclum, Spain.
Vindesine sulfate (p.593·3).
*Malignant neoplasms.*

**Enit** Lesvi, Spain.
Enalapril maleate (p.909·2); nitrendipine (p.973·3).
*Hypertension.*

**Enjomin** Codilab, Port.
Dimenhydrinate (p.431·1).
*Motion sickness; nausea; vertigo; vomiting.*

**Enjoy** Heralds, Braz.†.
Aspirin (p.15·1); mepyramine (p.437·1).
Aluminium hydroxide (p.1249·2) is included in this preparation in an attempt to limit adverse effects on the gastrointestinal mucosa.
*Fever; pain.*

**Enlinea** Elhoim, Arg.
Centella (p.1144·3); caffeine (p.782·1); levocarnitine (p.1423·3); seaweed extract.

**Enlirane** Zeneca, Mex.†.
Enflurane (p.1298·1).
*General anaesthesia.*

**Enlive**
Abbott, Austral.; Abbott, Fin.; Abbott, Fr.; Abbott, Irl.; Abbott, Ital.†; Abbott, Mex.; Abbott Nutrition, UK.
A range of products for enteral nutrition (p.1417·1).

**Enlon**
AstraZeneca, Canad.; Baxter, USA.
Edrophonium chloride (p.1490·3).
*Differential diagnosis of myasthenia gravis; reversal of competitive neuromuscular blockade.*

**Enlon-Plus** Baxter, USA.
Edrophonium chloride (p.1490·3).
Atropine sulfate (p.477·1) is included in this preparation to protect against the muscarinic actions.
*Curare antagonist; reversal of competitive neuromuscular blockade.*

**Eno**
Note. This name is used for preparations of different composition.
GlaxoSmithKline Consumer, Austral.; GlaxoSmithKline, Hong Kong; SmithKline Beecham, Ital.†; GlaxoSmithKline Consumer, UK.
Citric acid (p.1673·1); sodium bicarbonate (p.1223·2); sodium carbonate (p.1747·1).
*Dyspepsia; flatulence; nausea.*

GlaxoSmithKline Consumer, Canad.
Sodium citrate (p.1223·2).
*Dyspepsia.*

SmithKline Beecham, Israel.
Sodium bicarbonate (p.1223·2); tartaric acid (p.1752·1); citric acid (p.1673·1).
*Dyspepsia; flatulence.*

GlaxoSmithKline Consumer, Port.
Citric acid (p.1673·1); sodium carbonate (p.1747·1).

**Enofosforina Vigor** Serra Pamies, Spain.
Calcium lactophosphate; magnesium glycerophosphate; kola; pyridoxine; sodium glycerophosphate; potassium glycerophosphate; nicotinamide; glycerol; manganese glycerophosphate (p.1417·1).
*Tonic.*

**Enomdan** Pharmacia, Swed.
Multivitamin preparation (p.1417·1).

**Enomine** Major, USA†.
Phenylpropanolamine hydrochloride (p.1127·3); guaifenesin (p.1122·1); phenylephrine hydrochloride (p.1126·3).
*Coughs.*

**Enorden** Finadiet, Arg.
Amisulpride (p.669·3).
*Depression.*

**Enoton** Pensa, Spain.
Cyproheptadine aspartate (p.430·2); mecobalamin (p.1459·1).
*Anorexia; tonic; weight loss.*

**Enoval** Novag, Mex.
Enalapril (p.909·2).
*Hypertension.*

**Enoxen** EG, Ital.
Enoxacin (p.207·2).
*Bacterial infections.*

**Enoxin** Faulding, Austral.†.
Enoxacin (p.207·2).
*Bacterial infections.*

**Enoxor**
Germania, Austria; Sinbio, Fr.; Pierre Fabre, Ger.
Enoxacin (p.207·2).
*Bacterial infections.*

**Enper** Elea, Arg.
Zidovudine (p.658·2).
*HIV infection.*

**Enpott** Ranbaxy, Thai.
Potassium chloride (p.1232·2).
*Hypokalaemia.*

**Enpovax HDC** CSL, Austral.
An inactivated poliomyelitis vaccine (p.1633·3).
*Active immunisation.*

**Enpresse** Barr, USA.
Levonorgestrel (p.1563·2); ethinylestradiol (p.1553·2). 28-Day packs also contain 7 inert tablets.
*Triphasic oral contraceptive.*

**Enprin** Galpharm, UK.
Aspirin (p.15·1).
*Thrombosis prophylaxis.*

**Enrich**
Abbott, Fin.; Abbott, Fr.†; Abbott, Irl.; Abbott, Ital.; Abbott, Switz.†; Abbott Nutrition, UK.
Preparation for enteral nutrition (p.1417·1).

**Enromic** *Microsules, Arg.*
Losartan potassium (p.947·2).
*Hypertension.*

**Ensinger Schiller-Quelle Heilwasser** *Ensinger, Ger.*
Electrolytes (p.1217·1); silicic acid; boric acid (p.1662·1); carbon dioxide (p.1235·2).
*Gastrointestinal disorders; urinary-tract infections.*

**Ensini** *Nutricia, Fin.*
Preparation for enteral nutrition (p.1417·1).

**Ensure**
*Abbott, Arg.; Abbott, Austral.; Abbott, Braz.; Abbott, Chile; Abbott, Fin.; Abbott, Fr.; Abbott, Hong Kong; Abbott, Irl.; Abbott, Israel; Abbott, Ital.; Abbott, Malaysia; Abbott, Mex.; Abbott, NZ; Abbott, Singapore; Abbott, Switz.†; Abbott, Thai.; Abbott Nutrition, UK; Ross, USA.*
A range of preparations for enteral nutrition (p.1417·1).

**Ensure Plus**
*Abbott, Hong Kong; Abbott, Irl.; Abbott, Ital.; Abbott, Singapore; Abbott, Switz.†; Abbott Nutrition, UK.*
High calorie preparation for enteral nutrition (p.1417·1).

**ENT**
*Note. This name is used for preparations of different composition.*
*Iomed, Hong Kong.*
Phenylpropanolamine hydrochloride (p.1127·3); brompheniramine maleate (p.426·1).
*Nasal congestion; sinusitis.*
*Covan, S.Afr.*
Phenylephrine hydrochloride (p.1126·3); naphazoline nitrate (p.1124·3).
*Nasal congestion.*

**Entacyl** *Shire, Canad.*
Piperazine adipate (p.111·2).
*Ascariasis; enterobiasis.*

**Entalgic** *Salters, S.Afr.†.*
Paracetamol (p.76·2).
*Fever; pain.*

**Entamizole** *Knoll, India.*
Diloxanide furoate (p.604·1); metronidazole (p.607·2).
*Amoebiasis; giardiasis.*

**Entecet** *Sorin-Maxim, Fr.*
Hordeum sativum germ; enzymes derived from aspergillus including amylase and protease; lipase derived from rhizopus.
*Dyspepsia.*

**Entera**
*Rowa, Irl.†; Fresenius Kabi, Mex.*
Preparation for enteral nutrition (p.1417·1).
Formerly known as Fresenius High Energy in *Irl.*

**Enteral 400** *Scientific Hospital Supplies, UK†.*
Preparation for enteral nutrition (p.1417·1).

**Enterasin** *Crinos, Ital.*
Mesalazine (p.1273·2).
*Crohn's disease; ulcerative colitis.*

**Entercal** *Luper, Braz.†.*
Co-trimoxazole (p.199·3); attapulgite (p.1251·1).
*Diarrhoea.*

**Enterex** *Pisa, Mex.*
Preparation for enteral nutrition (p.1417·1).

**Entermid** *Nakornpatana, Thai.*
Loperamide hydrochloride (p.1271·1).
*Diarrhoea.*

**Entero Heractrin** *Heralds, Braz.†.*
Co-trimoxazole (p.199·3); calcium carbonate (p.1254·2).
*Diarrhoea.*

**Entero Micinovo** *Bago, Chile.*
Co-trimoxazole (p.199·3); attapulgite (p.1251·1).
*Diarrhoea.*

**Entero VU** *Temis, Arg.*
Barium sulfate (p.1061·1).
*Contrast medium for gastrointestinal radiography.*

**Enterobacilli** *Proge, Ital.*
*Lactobacillus paracasei*; *Lactobacillus salivarius*; vitamins (p.1417·1).
*Disturbances of the intestinal flora.*

**Enterobacticel**
*Note. This name is used for preparations of different composition.*
*Bago, Arg.*
Co-trimoxazole (p.199·3); attapulgite (p.1251·1).
*Diarrhoea.*
*Armstrong, Mex.†.*
Co-trimoxazole (p.199·3).

**Enterobene** *Ratiopharm, Austria.*
Loperamide hydrochloride (p.1271·1).
*Diarrhoea.*

**Enterobion** *Makros, Braz.†.*
Furazolidone (p.605·2); homatropine (p.483·2); pectin (p.1580·3).
*Diarrhoea.*

**Enterocare** *Phytocare, Austral.†.*
Ispaghula (p.1268·1); plum; black currant (p.1661·1); slippery elm (p.1747·1); *Lactobacillus acidophilus* (p.1704·2); pectin (p.1580·3); sterculia (p.1290·2).
*Constipation.*

**Enterocid** *Teuto, Braz.*
Pyrvinium embonate (p.113·3).
*Worm infections.*

**Enterocir** *AstraZeneca, Ital.*
Budesonide (p.1094·2).
*Crohn's disease.*

**Enterocler** *Heralds, Braz.†.*
Neomycin (p.235·1); attapulgite (p.1251·1); pectin (p.1580·3); electroytes (p.1217·1).
*Diarrhoea.*

**Enterodina** *Luper, Braz.†.*
Neomycin (p.235·1); sulfadiazine (p.258·2); phthalylsulfathiazole (p.242·3); pectin (p.1580·3).
*Diarrhoea.*

**Entero-Diyod** *Serral, Mex.*
Diiodohydroxyquinoline (p.603·3).
*Amoebiasis; giardiasis; shigellosis; trichomoniasis.*

**Enterodrip** *Diepal, Fr.†.*
Preparation for enteral nutrition (p.1417·1).

**Enterodyne** *Adcock Ingram, S.Afr.*
Bismuth carbonate (p.1252·1); calcium carbonate (p.1254·2); chloroform and morphine tincture (p.60·1); aromatic ammonia liquid (p.1653·3); nutmeg oil (p.1722·3); clove oil (p.1673·3); cardamom tincture (p.1667·3); catechu tincture (p.1668·3); conc. cinnamon water; cinnamon oil (p.1672·2).
*Gastrointestinal disorders.*

**Enterofigon** *Hertz, Braz.†.*
Adenosine (p.851·2); betaine (p.1660·1); choline (p.1424·3); methionine (p.1042·1); pyridoxine (p.1457·2).
*Liver disorders.*

**Enteroftal** *Windson, Braz.†.*
Neomycin (p.235·1); sulfaguanidine (p.260·3); phthalylsulfathiazole (p.242·3); ceratonia (p.1579·1).
*Diarrhoea.*

**Enterogermina** *Sanofi Synthelabo OTC, Ital.*
Spores of *Bacillus subtilis*.
*Gastrointestinal disorders.*

**Enterogil** *Diepal, Fr.†.*
Preparation for enteral nutrition (p.1417·1).

**Enterol**
*Note. This name is used for preparations of different composition.*
*Instituto Sanitas, Chile.*
Phthalylsulfacetamide; activated attapulgite (p.1251·1); pectin (p.1580·3).
*Diarrhoea.*
*Merck, Port.*
*Saccharomyces boulardii* (p.1704·2).
*Gastrointestinal disorders.*

**Enterol Con Nifuroxacida** *Instituto Sanitas, Chile.*
Phthalylsulfacetamide; nifuroxazide (p.237·2).
*Gastrointestinal infections; gastrointestinal sterilisation.*

**Enterolidon** *Ortoquimica, Braz.†.*
Furazolidone (p.605·2).

**Enterolyte** *Propan, S.Afr.*
Kaolin (p.1268·3); pectin (p.1580·3); sodium lactate; potassium chloride; sodium chloride (p.1222·2).
*Diarrhoea.*

**Enteromicina**
*Note. This name is used for preparations of different composition.*
*Gross, Braz.†.*
Streptomycin sulfate (p.256·2); phthalylsulfathiazole (p.242·3); menadione (p.1466·3).
*Diarrhoea.*
*Confar, Port.*
Neomycin sulfate (p.235·1).
*Gastro-enteritis.*

**Enteromix** *Bioprogress, Ital.*
Piromidic acid (p.244·1).
*Bacterial infections of the gastrointestinal tract.*

**Enteromucilage** *Bayer, Fr.†.*
Sterculia (p.1290·2).
*Constipation.*

**Enterone** *Heralds, Braz.†.*
Co-trimoxazole (p.199·3).
*Bacterial infections; Pneumocystis carinii pneumonia; protozoal infections.*

**Enteronorm** *Apsen, Braz.†.*
Loperamide hydrochloride (p.1271·1).
*Diarrhoea.*

**Enteropathyl** *Merck Medication Familiale, Fr.*
Sulfaguanidine (p.260·3).

**Enteropen** *Cazi, Braz.†.*
Attapulgite (p.1251·1); pectin (p.1580·3); homatropine (p.483·2).
*Diarrhoea.*

**Enteroplant** *Spitzner, Ger.*
Peppermint oil (p.1283·2); caraway oil (p.1667·3).
*Dyspepsia.*

**Enteropride**
*Janssen-Cilag, Braz.†; Cilag, Mex.*
Cisapride (p.1259·2).
*Gastro-oesophageal reflux; gastrointestinal motility disorders.*

**Entero-Quinol** *East India Pharma, India.*
Clioquinol (p.196·3).
*Amoebic dysentery.*

**Enterosan** *Monmouth, UK†.*
Light kaolin (p.1268·3); morphine hydrochloride (p.60·1); belladonna (p.479·1).
*Diarrhoea.*

**Enteroseven** *Pharma Italia, Ital.*
Lactic-acid-producing organisms (p.1704·2); vitamins; minerals; inulin (p.1417·1).
*Disturbances of the intestinal flora; nutritional supplement.*

**Enterosilicona** *Estedi, Spain.*
Dimethicone (p.1289·2).
*Flatulence; infant colic; meteorism.*

**Enterostop** *Teofarma, Ital.*
Bacitracin (p.161·3); neomycin sulfate (p.235·1).
*Gastrointestinal infections.*

**Entero-Teknosal** *Taco, Ger.*
Colloidal silicon dioxide (p.1581·3).
*Diarrhoea.*

**Enterotonus** *Breves, Braz.†.*
Physostigmine (p.1494·1); atropine (p.476·3); cascara (p.1255·1).
*Constipation.*

**Enterovaccino ISI (Antitifico)** *ISI, Ital.†.*
A killed oral typhoid vaccine (p.1642·2).
*Active immunisation.*

**Enterovaccino Nuovo ISM** *ISM, Ital.†.*
A killed oral typhoid vaccine (p.1642·2).
*Active immunisation.*

**Enterovit** *Sedabel, Braz.†.*
Attapulgite (p.1251·1); broxyquinoline (p.165·3); neomycin (p.235·1); homatropine (p.483·2); sulfadiazine (p.258·2); phthalylsulfathiazole (p.242·3).
*Diarrhoea.*

**Enterozol** *Dinafarma, Braz.†.*
Neomycin sulfate (p.235·1); sulfadiazine (p.258·2).
*Diarrhoea.*

**Entertainer's Secret** *KLI, USA.*
Aloe vera (p.1141·3); carmellose sodium (p.1577·3); glycerol (p.1694·3).
Formerly known as Moi-Stir 10.
*Throat discomfort.*

**Enterum** *Angelini, Ital.*
Spores of *Bacillus subtilis*.
*Gastrointestinal disorders.*

**Entex**
*Note. This name is used for preparations of different composition.*
*Purdue Frederick, Canad.†.*
Phenylpropanolamine hydrochloride (p.1127·3); guaifenesin (p.1122·1).
*Upper respiratory-tract congestion.*
*Andrx, USA.*
Phenylephrine hydrochloride (p.1126·3); guaifenesin (p.1122·1).
Formerly contained phenylephrine hydrochloride, phenylpropanolamine hydrochloride, and guaifenesin.
*Coughs and cold symptoms; nasal congestion.*

**Entex HC** *Andrx, USA.*
Hydrocodone tartrate (p.45·1); phenylephrine hydrochloride (p.1126·3); guaifenesin (p.1122·1).
*Coughs.*

**Entex LA** *Andrx, USA.*
Phenylephrine hydrochloride (p.1126·3); guaifenesin (p.1122·1).
Formerly contained phenylpropanolamine hydrochloride and guaifenesin.
*Respiratory-tract congestion.*

**Entex PSE** *Andrx, USA.*
Pseudoephedrine hydrochloride (p.1129·2); guaifenesin (p.1122·1).
*Coughs; nasal congestion.*

**Entianthe** *Rafarm, Gr.*
Gemfibrozil (p.923·1).
*Hyperlipidaemias.*

**Entir**
*Unison, Hong Kong; Unison, Singapore; Unison, Thai.*
Aciclovir (p.626·1).
*Herpesvirus infections.*

**Entocir** *AstraZeneca, Ital.*
Budesonide (p.1094·2).
*Crohn's disease.*

**Entocord**
*Astra, S.Afr.; AstraZeneca, Spain.*
Budesonide (p.1094·2).
*Crohn's disease; ulcerative colitis.*

**Entocort**
*AstraZeneca, Arg.; AstraZeneca, Austral.; AstraZeneca, Austria; AstraZeneca, Belg.; AstraZeneca, Braz.; AstraZeneca, Canad.; AstraZeneca, Chile; AstraZeneca, Denm.; AstraZeneca, Fin.; AstraZeneca, Fr.; AstraZeneca, Ger.; AstraZeneca, Hong Kong; AstraZeneca, Irl.; AstraZeneca, Israel; AstraZeneca, Mex.; AstraZeneca, Neth.; AstraZeneca, Norw.; AstraZeneca, NZ; AstraZeneca, Port.; AstraZeneca, Singapore; Hassle, Swed.; AstraZeneca, Switz.; AstraZeneca, UK; AstraZeneca, USA.*
Budesonide (p.1094·2).
*Inflammatory bowel disease.*

**Entodiba** *Diba, Mex.*
Diiodohydroxyquinoline (p.603·3).
*Amoebiasis.*

**Entom** *Dynacren, Ital.†.*
Diethyltoluamide (p.1503·3); piperonyl butoxide (p.1509·2); pyrethrum (p.1509·3).
*Insect repellent.*

**Entom Nature** *Dynacren, Ital.*
Geranium oil (p.1692·2).
*Insect repellent.*

**Entonox**
*Afrox, S.Afr.; BOC, UK.*
Nitrous oxide (p.1304·3); oxygen (p.1236·3).
*Obstructive airways disease; pain.*

**Entoplus** *Diba, Mex.*
Albendazole (p.101·2).
*Worm infections.*

**Entosorbine-N** *Roche Consumer, Neth.*
Albumin tannate (p.1248·1).
*Diarrhoea.*

**Entox-P**
*Wyeth Consumer, Malaysia; Wyeth-Ayerst, Thai.*
Activated attapulgite (p.1251·1).
*Diarrhoea.*

**Entrarin** *Asian Pharm, Thai.*
Aspirin (p.15·1).
*Fever; inflammation; pain.*

**Entrition** *Clintec, USA.*
A range of lactose-free preparations for enteral nutrition (p.1417·1).

**Entrobar** *Lafayette, USA.*
Barium sulfate (p.1061·1).
*Contrast medium for gastrointestinal radiography.*

**Entrocalm** *Galpharm, UK.*
*Capsules:* Loperamide hydrochloride (p.1271·1).
*Tablets:* Kaolin (p.1268·3).
*Diarrhoea.*

**Entrocalm Replace** *Galpharm, UK.*
Glucose monohydrate; sodium chloride; potassium chloride; sodium citrate; citric acid (p.1222·2).
*Oral rehydration therapy.*

**Entrodyn** *Ravensberg, Ger.*
Phenylephrine (p.1126·3); caffeine (p.782·1).
*Hypotension.*

**Entrolate** *Stadmed, India.*
Tinidazole (p.617·1); diloxanide furoate (p.604·1).
*Amoebiasis.*

**Entrolax** *Galpharm, UK.*
Bisacodyl (p.1251·3).
*Constipation.*

**Entrophen** *Johnson & Johnson, Canad.*
Aspirin (p.15·1).
*Fever; musculoskeletal and joint disorders; myocardial infarction; pain; transient ischaemic attacks.*

**Entrotabs** *Monmouth, UK†.*
Aluminium hydroxide (p.1249·2); attapulgite (p.1251·1); pectin (p.1580·3).
*Diarrhoea; dyspepsia.*

**Entrozyme Plain** *Stadmed, India.*
Clioquinol (p.196·3).
*Amoebic dysentery.*

**Entrydil** *Orion, Irl.*
Diltiazem hydrochloride (p.900·1).
*Angina pectoris; hypertension.*

**Entschlackender Abfuhrtee EF-EM-ES** *Smetana, Austria.*
Senna (p.1288·2); equisetum (p.1684·1); sambucus (p.1741·3); calcatrippae flowers.
*Constipation.*

**ENTsol** *Bradley, Singapore.*
Sodium chloride (p.1233·3); monobasic potassium phosphate (p.1230·3); dibasic sodium phosphate (p.1231·1).
*Nasal congestion; throat disorders.*

**Entumin** *Novartis, Ital.*
Clotiapine (p.685·2).
*Anxiety disorders; psychoses.*

**Entumine** *Novartis, Switz.*
Clotiapine (p.685·2).
*Alcohol withdrawal syndrome; anxiety disorders; hyperactivity; psychoses; sleep disorders.*

**Enturen** *Ciba Vision, Ital.*
Sulfinpyrazone (p.417·3).
*Thromboembolic disorders.*

**Entuss Expectorant** *Roberts, USA; Hauck, USA.*
*Oral liquid:* Hydrocodone tartrate (p.45·1); sulfogaiacol (p.1131·1).
*Tablets:* Hydrocodone tartrate (p.45·1); guaifenesin (p.1122·1).
*Coughs.*

**Entuss-D** *Roberts, USA.*
*Liquid:* Hydrocodone tartrate (p.45·1); pseudoephedrine hydrochloride (p.1129·2).
*Tablets:* Hydrocodone tartrate (p.45·1); pseudoephedrine hydrochloride (p.1129·2); guaifenesin (p.1122·1).
*Coughs.*

**Entuss-D Jr** *Roberts, USA.*
Hydrocodone tartrate (p.45·1); pseudoephedrine hydrochloride (p.1129·2); guaifenesin (p.1122·1).
*Coughs.*

**Entwasserungs-Tabletten** *Hexal, Austria.*
Birch leaf (p.1660·3).
*Diuretic.*

**Entzundungstropfen** *Cosmochema, Ger.*
Homoeopathic preparation.

**Enuclen** *Alcon, Ger.*
Tyloxapol (p.1416·3).
*Cleansing and lubrication of eye prostheses.*

**Enuclene**
*Alcon, Canad.; Alcon, NZ; Alcon, USA.*
Tyloxapol (p.1416·3).
*Lubrication, cleaning, and wetting of artificial eyes.*

**Enulid** *Rottapharm, Ital.*
Moexipril hydrochloride (p.961·2).
*Hypertension.*

**Enulose** *Barre-National, USA.*
Lactulose (p.1269·1).
*Hepatic encephalopathy.*

**EnurAid** *Hylands, Canad.*
Homoeopathic preparation.

**Enuretine** *Le Marchand, Fr.†.*
Isopropamide iodide (p.485·2); vitamin E (p.1464·3); thiamine (p.1455·2); ephedrine hydrochloride (p.1120·1); phenobarbital (p.367·3).
*Urinary incontinence.*

**Europlant** *DHU, Ger.*
Homoeopathic preparation.

**Envas** *Cadila Pharma, India.*
Enalapril maleate (p.909·2).
*Heart failure; hypertension; myocardial infarction.*

**Enveloppements ECR** *ECR, Switz.†.*
Hay flowers; chamomile (p.1669·3); achillea (p.1646·2); linseed (p.1707·2); equisetum (p.1684·1).
*Cold symptoms.*

**Enviro-Stress** *Vitaline, USA.*
Vitamin B substances with vitamin C and minerals (p.1417·1).

**Enxak** *Luitpold, Braz.†.*
Ergotamine tartrate (p.467·2).
*Migraine and other vascular headaches.*

**Enzace** *Sigma, Austral.*
Captopril (p.879·2).
*Diabetic nephropathy; heart failure; hypertension; myocardial infarction.*

**Enzaprost** *Faran, Gr.*
Dinoprost (p.1514·3).
*Therapeutic abortion in second trimester of pregnancy.*

**Enziagil Magenplus** *Riemser, Ger.*
Gentian (p.1692·2).
*Digestive system disorders.*

**Enzicoba** *Farmasa, Braz.*
Cobamamide (p.1459·1).
*Reduced appetite; tonic.*

**Enzipan** *Abbott, Ital.*
Pancrelipase (p.1725·3).
*Pancreatic disorders.*

**Enziprid** *Brasmedica, Braz.†.*
Bromopride (p.1254·1); lipase; amylase (p.1654·2).
*Digestive-system disorders; nausea and vomiting.*

**Enzivital** *Farmasa, Braz.†.*
Cobamamide; carnitine; lysine; vitamin B substances (p.1417·1).
*Tonic.*

**Enzogenol** *MD, Singapore.*
Pinus radiata; vitamin C; vitamin E; linseed oil (p.1417·1).
*Antioxidant preparation.*

**Enzone** *UAD, USA.*
Hydrocortisone acetate (p.1103·3); pramocaine (p.1382·2).

**Enzyflat** *Solvay, Austria.*
Pancreatin (p.1725·3); dimethicone (p.1289·2).
*Flatulence; meteorism; preparation for gastrointestinal radiography and ultrasound.*

**Enzymatic Cleaner** *Alcon, USA.*
Pancreatin (p.1725·3) (p.1164·2).
*Cleansing solution for soft contact lenses.*

**Enzyme**
*Note. This name is used for preparations of different composition.*
*GNLD, Austral.†.*
Pancreatin (p.1725·3); pepsin (p.1729·3); ox bile (p.1660·3); papain (p.1727·3); amylase (p.1654·2).
*Digestive disorders.*
*Nature's Bounty, USA.*
Amylase (p.1654·2); cellulase (p.1669·1); lipase; protease.
*Gastrointestinal disorders.*

**Enzyme Digest** *Quest, UK.*
Betaine hydrochloride (p.1660·2); papain (p.1727·3); bromelain (p.1662·2); amylase (p.1654·2).

**Enzyme Plus** *Lifeplan, UK.*
Betaine hydrochloride (p.1660·2); amylase (p.1654·2); pepsin (p.1729·3); lipase.
*Dietary supplement.*

**Enzymet** *Ranbaxy, Thai.*
Pancreatin (p.1725·3); simeticone (p.1289·2).
*Digestive system disorders; flatulence.*

**Enzym-Harongan** *Schwabe, Ger.*
Haronga; Javanese turmeric (p.1759·3); pancreas.
*Digestive system disorders.*

**Enzym-Lefax** *Bayer, Ger.*
Pancreatin (p.1725·3); simeticone (p.1289·2).
*Digestive system disorders.*

**Enzym-Wied** *Wiedemann, Ger.*
Pancreatin (p.1725·3); bromelains (p.1662·2); papain (p.1727·3); triacylglycerollipase; amylase (p.1654·2); trypsin (p.1758·3); chymotrypsin (p.1671·2); rutoside (p.1688·2).
*Atherosclerosis; soft-tissue injury; thrombosis; venous inflammation.*

**Enzynorm**
*Pharmaselect, Austria; Knoll, Ger.†; Hoechst Marion Roussel, S.Afr.†.*
Stomach extract.
*Anaemia; digestive disorders.*

**Enzynorm forte** *Abbott, Ger.*
Gastric mucous membrane extract; amino acids (p.1417·1).
*Gastrointestinal disorders.*

**Enzyplex**
*Westmont, Hong Kong; Westmont, Malaysia; Westmont, Singapore; Great Eastern, Thai.; Westmont, Thai.*
Lipase; amylase (p.1654·2); protease; deoxycholic acid (p.1660·3); simeticone (p.1289·2); vitamin B substances (p.1417·1).
*Digestive system disorders with excess gas.*

**Eogran** *Synpharma, Austria.*
Chamomile (p.1669·3); peppermint leaf (p.1283·2); tormentil (p.1757·2).
*Diarrhoea.*

**Eoline** *Pfizer, Belg.*
Hydrocortisone (p.1103·3); nystatin (p.406·3); oxytetracycline calcium (p.241·1).
*Infected skin disorders.*

**Eolus** *Sigma-Tau, Ital.*
Formoterol fumarate (p.786·1).
*Obstructive airways disease.*

**E.P.** *Pharmax, UK†.*
Paracetamol (p.76·2); caffeine (p.782·1); codeine phosphate (p.27·1).
*Pain.*

**Epabetina** *OFF, Ital.*
Betaine glucuronate (p.1660·2); trigonelline.
*Liver disorders.*

**Epa-Bon** *Sifarma, Ital.†.*
Cyclobutyrol sodium (p.1678·2).
*Biliary disorders.*

**Epacalcica** *Ibirn, Ital.*
Heparin calcium (p.927·3).
*Thromboembolic disorders.*

**Epacaps** *Altana, Switz.*
Marine fish oil (p.976·2).
*Hyperlipidaemias; nutritional supplement.*

**Epacrosil** *Uniao Quimica, Braz.†.*
Adenosine (p.851·2); methionine (p.1042·1); choline citrate (p.1424·3); vitamin $B_6$ (p.1456·3).
*Liver disorders.*

**Epadel** *Mochida, Jpn.*
Ethyl icosapentate.
*Arteriosclerosis obliterans; hyperlipidaemias.*

**Epaderm** *SSL, UK.*
Yellow soft paraffin (p.1479·3); emulsifying wax (p.1481·1); liquid paraffin (p.1479·1).
*Dry skin.*

**Epadoren** *Demo, Gr.*
Ranitidine hydrochloride (p.1285·2).
*Conditions where gastric acid reduction is beneficial; gastric hypersecretion including Zollinger-Ellison syndrome; peptic ulcer.*

**Epagest** *Lampugnani, Ital.*
Fennel (p.1687·2); silybum marianum (p.1043·3); cynara (p.1678·3); vitamin B substances (p.1417·1).
*Dietary supplement; liver disorders.*

**Epagogo** *Kopkins, Braz.†.*
Boldo (p.1661·2); rhubarb (p.1287·3); cynara (p.1678·3); cascara (p.1255·1).
*Liver disorders.*

**Epailis** *DHN, Fr.*
Nutritional supplement (p.1417·1).
*Regurgitation.*

**Epalat EPS** *OFF, Ital.*
Lactulose (p.1269·1).
*Liver disorders.*

**Epalfen** *Zambon, Ital.*
Lactulose (p.1269·1).
*Bacterial gastrointestinal infections; constipation; digestive disorders; liver disorders.*

**Epamin**
*Parke, Davis, Arg.; Parke, Davis, Chile; Parke, Davis, Mex.*
Phenytoin (p.370·2) or phenytoin sodium (p.370·2).
*Arrhythmias; epilepsy; seizures associated with neurosurgery.*

**Epanutin**
*Pfizer, Austria; Parke, Davis, Belg.; Parke, Davis, Ger.; Pfizer, Gr.; Parke, Davis, Irl.; Parke, Davis, Israel; Parke, Davis, Neth.; Pfizer, S.Afr.; Davis, Spain; Pfizer, Swed.; Pfizer, Switz.; Pfizer, UK.*
Phenytoin (p.370·2) or phenytoin sodium (p.370·2).
*Arrhythmias; epilepsy; seizures associated with neurosurgery or head injury; trigeminal neuralgia.*

**Epaplex 40** *Uno, Ital.*
Sodium ferric gluconate complex (p.1444·3).
*Sideropenic anaemia.*

**Epaq**
*Note. This name is used for preparations of different composition.*
*3M, Arg.; 3M, Mex.*
Metronidazole (p.607·2).
*Vaginitis.*
*Arrow, Austral.; Kolassa, Austria†; 3M, Ger.*
Salbutamol sulfate (p.791·3).
*Obstructive airways disease.*

**Eparema**
*Altana, Braz.; SIT, Ital.*
Cascara (p.1255·1); boldo (p.1661·2); rhubarb (p.1287·3).
*Constipation; liver disorders.*

**Eparema-Levul** *SIT, Ital.*
Cascara (p.1255·1); boldo (p.1661·2); rhubarb (p.1287·3); fructose (p.1431·3).
*Constipation.*

**Eparex** *DM, Braz.†.*
Adenosine (p.851·2); methionine (p.1042·1); betaine hydrochloride (p.1660·2).
*Liver disorders.*

**Epargriseovit**
*Pharmacia Upjohn, Hong Kong†; Pharmacia Upjohn, Ital.*
Cyanocobalamin (p.1458·2); folic acid (p.1429·1); nicotinamide (p.1441·2); ascorbic acid (p.1460·2).
*Anaemias; liver disorders; peripheral neuropathies; tonic.*

**Eparical** *Aventis, Ital.*
Heparin calcium (p.927·3).
*Thromboembolic disorders.*

**Eparinlider** *Scharper, Ital.*
Heparin calcium (p.927·3).
*Thromboembolic disorders.*

**Eparinovis** *INTES, Ital.*
Heparin sodium (p.928·1).
*Eye disorders.*

**Eparmefolin** *Bracco, Ital.*
Cyanocobalamin (p.1458·2); calcium folinate (p.1431·1).
*Folate and vitamin $B_{12}$ deficiency.*

**Eparsil** *Pulitzer, Ital.†.*
Silymarin (p.1043·3).
*Liver disorders.*

**Eparven** *Pantafarm, Ital.*
Heparin calcium (p.927·3).
*Thromboembolic disorders.*

**Epasan 30% Omega 3** *Maver, Chile.*
Marine fish oils (p.976·1).
*Dietary supplement; hyperlipidaemias.*

**Epasol** *Mendelejeff, Ital.*
Ursodeoxycholic acid (p.1760·3).
*Biliary dyspepsia; cholesterol gallstones.*

**Epativan B6** *Cimed, Braz.*
Adenosine (p.851·2); methionine (p.1042·1); choline (p.1424·3); vitamin $B_6$ (p.1456·3).
*Liver disorders.*

**Epatovis** *DM, Braz.†.*
Cynara (p.1678·3); cascara (p.1255·1); persea americana; rhubarb (p.1287·3); boldo (p.1661·2).
*Liver disorders.*

**Epatoxil** *C & RF, Ital.*
Cogalactoisomerase sodium (p.1674·3).
*Liver disorders.*

**Epa-Treis** *Ecobi, Ital.†.*
Calcium oxoglurate; choline orotate (p.1724·3).
*Liver disorders.*

**Epaxal**
*Berna, Belg.†; Berna, Canad.; Berna, Denm.; Berna, Fin.; Niddapharm, Ger.; Berna, Hong Kong; Berna, Ital.; Berna, Norw.; Berna, NZ; Pharmabroker, NZ; Cortec, Swed.; Berna, Switz.; Masta, UK.*
An inactivated hepatitis A vaccine (RG-SB strain) (p.1617·1).
*Active immunisation.*

**EP&C Essence** *Potter's, UK.*
Bayberry bark (p.1659·2); hemlock spruce; sambucus (p.1741·3); peppermint oil (p.1283·2).
*Colds; sore throat.*

**Epelin** *Pfizer, Braz.; Ache, Braz.*
Phenytoin (p.370·2) or phenytoin sodium (p.370·2).
*Epilepsy; trigeminal neuralgia.*

**Ephed 20th** *20th Century, Mex.†.*
Ephedrine (p.1120·1).

**Ephedroides** *Richelet, Fr.*
Pseudoephedrine hydrochloride (p.1129·2).
*Nasal congestion.*

**Ephedronguent** *Pharmacobel, Belg.*
Ephedrine (p.1120·1).
*Nasal congestion.*

**Ephedyl** *Synco, Hong Kong.*
Promethazine hydrochloride (p.439·1); codeine phosphate (p.27·1); ephedrine hydrochloride (p.1120·1).
*Coughs and cold symptoms; rhinitis.*

**Ephelia**
*Niddapharm, Ger.; Ipsen, Ital.*
Estradiol (p.1550·1).
*Menopausal disorders.*

**Ephepect** *Bolder, Ger.†.*
Ephedrine hydrochloride (p.1120·1); ammonium chloride (p.1115·2); thyme (p.1755·2); cowslip rhizome (p.1735·1); anise oil (p.1655·2); fennel oil (p.1687·3); peppermint oil (p.1283·2); eucalyptus oil (p.1686·2).
*Bronchitis; catarrh.*

**Ephepect-Blocker-Pastillen N** *Bolder, Ger.*
Sodium dibunate (p.1130·2); dequalinium chloride (p.1178·1).
*Coughs.*

**Ephepect-Pastillen N** *Bolder, Ger.*
Thyme (p.1755·2); anise oil (p.1655·2); eucalyptus oil (p.1686·2); fennel oil (p.1687·3); peppermint oil (p.1283·2); ammonium chloride (p.1115·2).
*Respiratory-tract disorders.*

**Ephydion** *Theratech, Fr.*
*Syrup:* Ethylmorphine hydrochloride (p.37·3); sulfogaiacol (p.1131·1); grindelia (p.1696·1).
*Tablets; oral drops:* Ethylmorphine hydrochloride (p.37·3); sodium benzoate (p.1169·3); grindelia (p.1696·1).
*Coughs.*

**Ephydrol** *CS, Fr.*
*Cream:* Fioravanti; lavender oil (p.1705·2); bergamot oil (p.1659·3); lemon oil (p.1706·2); camphor (p.1665·3); menthol (p.1711·3); salicyl alcohol; formaldehyde solution (p.1179·3).
*Topical solution (with brush or aeosol spray):* Fioravanti; camphor (p.1665·3); menthol (p.1711·3); salicyl alcohol; bergamot oil (p.1659·3); lemon oil (p.1706·2); lavender oil (p.1705·2); formaldehyde solution (p.1179·3); plantain (p.1733·1).
*Topical spray:* Sanicula; fioravanti; camphor (p.1665·3); lavender oil (p.1705·2); bergamot oil (p.1659·3); lemon oil (p.1706·2); menthol (p.1711·3); salicyl alcohol; formaldehyde solution (p.1179·3).
*Hyperhidrosis.*

**Ephynal**
*Roche, Arg.; Roche, Austria; Roche, Belg.; Roche, Braz.; Roche Nicholas, Fr.; Roche Nicholas, Ger.; Roche Consumer, Irl.; Roche, Israel†; Roche, Ital.; Roche, Mex.†; Roche, Port.; Roche Consumer, S.Afr.; Roche, Spain; Roche, Switz.; Roche Consumer, UK.*
Vitamin E (p.1465·1).
*Nutritional supplement; vitamin E deficiency.*

**Epi EZ** *Allerex, Canad.†.*
Adrenaline (p.852·2).
*Anaphylactic shock.*

**Epi-Aberel** *Janssen-Cilag, Ger.†.*
Tretinoin (p.1161·1).
*Acne.*

**Epianal** *Will-Pharma, Neth.*
Sodium oleate (p.1574·3); oxypolyethoxydodecanum; chlorocarvacrol.
*Haemorrhoids.*

**Epi-C** *Lafayette, USA.*
Barium sulfate (p.1061·1).
*Contrast medium for gastrointestinal radiography.*

**Epicef** *FD, Ital.*
Cefonicid sodium (p.174·2).
Lidocaine hydrochloride (p.1377·3) is included in the intramuscular preparation to alleviate the pain of injection.
*Gram-negative bacterial infections.*

**Epi-Cell** *Cell Pharm, Ger.*
Epirubicin hydrochloride (p.550·2).
*Malignant neoplasms.*

**Epiclodina** *Piso, Mex.*
Clonidine (p.885·2).
*Pain.*

**Epicol** *Loren, Mex.*
Dextromethorphan (p.1117·3); guaifenesin (p.1122·1); tolu balsam (p.1131·3).
*Coughs.*

**Epicol NF** *Loren, Mex.*
Dextromethorphan (p.1117·3); ambroxol (p.1114·3).
*Coughs.*

**Epicol Pediatrico** *Loren, Mex.*
Guaifenesin (p.1122·1); dextromethorphan hydrobromide (p.1117·3).
*Coughs.*

**Epicordin**
*Note. This name is used for preparations of different composition.*
*Solvay, Austria.*
Isosorbide mononitrate (p.942·1).
*Angina pectoris; heart failure; pulmonary hypertension.*
*Solvay, Ger.*
Captopril (p.879·2).
*Heart failure; hypertension.*

**Epicrin** *Gebro, Switz.†.*
Vitamin A; biotin; dexpanthenol; zinc amino acid chelate; millet extract; cystine; wheat-germ oil (p.1417·1).
*Hair and nail disorders.*

**Epident** *Grands Espaces, Fr.*
Tooth extract.
*Mucous membrane disorders of the nose and throat.*

**Epidermil** *Kinder, Braz.†.*
Betamethasone (p.1093·1).
*Skin disorders.*

**Epidex** *Kinder, Braz.†.*
Desonide (p.1096·3).
*Skin disorders.*

**Epidona** *Wyeth, Braz.*
Primidone (p.376·3).
*Epilepsy.*

**Epidosin**
*Solvay, Ger.†; TTK, India.*
Valethamate bromide (p.491·3).
*Smooth muscle spasm.*

**Epidoxo** *Kampel Martian, Arg.*
Epirubicin (p.550·3).
*Malignant neoplasms.*

**Epidropal** *Teofarma, Ger.*
Allopurinol (p.412·2).
*Gout; hyperuricaemia; renal calculi.*

**Epiestrol**
*Rottapharm, Chile; Helsinn Birex, Irl.; Pfizer, Ital.; Rottapharm, Switz.*
Estradiol (p.1550·1).
*Menopausal disorders; osteoporosis.*

**Epiferol** *Juventus, Spain†.*
Reproterol hydrochloride (p.791·2).
*Obstructive airways disease.*

**Epifil** *Filaxis, Arg.*
Epirubicin (p.550·3).
*Malignant neoplasms.*

**Epifoam**
*Medis, Israel; Schwarz, USA.*
Hydrocortisone acetate (p.1103·3); pramocaine hydrochloride (p.1382·2).
*Skin disorders.*

**Epifrin**
*Allergan, Canad.†; Allergan, USA.*
Adrenaline hydrochloride (p.852·3).
*Open-angle glaucoma.*

**Epigen**
*Catalysis, Arg.; Medix, Mex.*
Glycyrrhizinic acid.
*Herpes simplex infections.*

**Epiglu**
*Meyer-Haake, Ger.; ICN, UK.*
Ethyl 2-cyanoacrylate (p.1678·1); polymethylmethacrylate (p.1714·3).
*Skin wounds.*

**Epiject** *Abbott, Canad.*
Sodium valproate (p.380·1).
*Epilepsy.*

**Epikebir** *Aspen, Arg.*
Epirubicin (p.550·3).
*Malignant neoplasms.*

**Epikur** *Agepha, Austria.*
Meprobamate (p.706·2).
*Anxiety; sleep disturbances.*

**Epilan**
*Note. This name is used for preparations of different composition.*
*Gerot, Austria.*
Mephenytoin (p.366·2).
*Epilepsy.*

*Anglo-French Drugs, India.*
Phenytoin sodium (p.370·2); phenobarbital (p.367·3).
*Epilepsy.*

**Epilan-D** *Gerot, Austria.*
Phenytoin (p.370·2).
*Epilepsy.*

**Epilantin** *Otsuka, Spain.*
Phenytoin (p.370·2); phenobarbital (p.367·3).
*Epilepsy.*

**Epilantine** *Streuli, Switz.*
Phenytoin sodium (p.370·2).
*Epilepsy.*

**Epilem**
*Lemery, Mex.; Lemery, Thai.*
Epirubicin hydrochloride (p.550·2).
*Malignant neoplasms.*

**Epilenil** *Biolab Sanus, Braz.*
Valproic acid (p.380·1).
*Epilepsy.*

**Epilex** *Knoll, India.*
Sodium valproate (p.380·1).
*Epilepsy.*

**Epilim**
*Sanofi Synthelabo, Austral.; Sanofi Synthelabo, Hong Kong; Sanofi Synthelabo, Irl.; Sanofi Synthelabo, Malaysia; Sanofi Synthelabo, NZ; Sanofi Synthelabo, S.Afr.; Sanofi Synthelabo, Singapore; Sanofi Synthelabo, UK.*
Sodium valproate (p.380·1).
*Epilepsy; mania.*

**Epilim Chrono**
*Sanofi Synthelabo, Irl.; Sanofi Synthelabo, UK.*
Sodium valproate (p.380·1); valproic acid (p.380·1).
*Epilepsy.*

**E-Pilo**
*Ciba Vision, Canad.†; Ciba Vision, USA.*
Adrenaline acid tartrate (p.852·2); pilocarpine hydrochloride (p.1495·1).
*Glaucoma; raised intra-ocular pressure.*

**Epi-Lyt**
*Stiefel, Canad.; Stiefel, USA.*
Glycerol (p.1694·3); lactic acid (p.1704·1).
*Dry skin.*

**Epimaz** *Ivax, UK.*
Carbamazepine (p.353·3).

**Epi-Monistat** *Janssen-Cilag, Ger.†.*
Miconazole nitrate (p.405·3).
*Fungal infections.*

**Epinal** *Alcon, USA.*
Adrenaline borate complex (p.854·1).
*Open-angle glaucoma.*

**Epinat** *Nycomed, Norw.*
Phenytoin (p.370·2).
*Epilepsy.*

**Epinitril**
*Bouchara-Recordati, Fr.; Rottapharm, Irl.; Rottapharm, Ital.; Rottapharm, Spain.*
Glyceryl trinitrate (p.923·2).
*Angina pectoris.*

**Epione** *Schering-Plough, Port.*
Betamethasone valerate (p.1093·2); gentamicin sulfate (p.217·1).
*Infected skin disorders.*

**Epipak** *3M Espe, Ger.*
Aluminium chlorohydrate (p.1142·1); polyethyleneimine hydrochloride.
*Mouth disorders.*

**Epipen**
*CSL, Austral.; ALK, Austria; ALK, Belg.†; Allerex, Canad.; ALK, Denm.; ALK, Fin.; Center, Israel; ALK, Norw.; CSL, NZ; Merck, Port.; Merck, S.Afr.; ALK, Swed.; Trimedal, Switz.; ALK, UK; Dey, USA.*
Adrenaline (p.852·2).
*Anaphylaxis.*

**Epi-Pevaryl** *Janssen-Cilag, Ger.*
Econazole nitrate (p.397·2).
*Fungal skin and nail infections.*

**Epi-Pevaryl Heilpaste** *Janssen-Cilag, Ger.*
Econazole nitrate (p.397·2); zinc oxide (p.1163·2).
*Fungal skin infections.*

**Epi-Pevaryl Pv** *Janssen-Cilag, Ger.*
Econazole (p.397·1).
*Pityriasis versicolor.*

**Epipevisone** *Janssen-Cilag, Ger.*
Econazole nitrate (p.397·2); triamcinolone acetonide (p.1110·2).
*Fungal and Gram-positive bacterial skin infections.*

**Epiphane**
*Note. This name is used for preparations of different composition.*
*Biorga, Fr.†.*
Gelatin (p.754·3).
*Fragile nails and hair.*

*Uriage, Fr.*
*Shampoo:* Piroctone olamine (p.1155·2); cade oil (p.1159·2); levomenol (p.1707·1).
*Scalp disorders.*

**Epiphane 7** *Saninter, Port.†.*
Gelatin (p.754·3).
*Fragile hair and nails.*

**Epiphysan** *Dispergo, Austria†.*
Bovine pineal gland extract (p.1709·3).
*Hypersexuality; psychoses.*

**Epiplaie Epitege** *Euromedex, Fr.*
Barrier cream.

**Epiprocto** *Epicaris, Arg.*
Lidocaine (p.1377·3); hydrocortisone acetate (p.1103·3); aluminium acetate (p.1652·3); zinc oxide (p.1163·2).
*Anorectal disorders.*

**Epipropane** *Medgenix, Belg.*
Phenobarbital magnesium (p.369·2); amfetamine sulfate (p.1584·3).
*Agitation; epilepsy; hypertension.*

**EpiQuin** *SkinMedica, USA.*
Hydroquinone (p.1148·1).
*Skin pigmentation disorders.*

**Episcorit** *Sanum-Kehlbeck, Ger.*
Echinacea purpura (p.1683·2).
*Respiratory- and urinary-tract infections.*

**Episec** *Odan, Canad.*
Liquid paraffin (p.1479·1); propylene glycol (p.1735·2); trolamine stearate.

**Episoft** *LED, Fr.*
Moisturiser.
*Dry skin disorders.*

**Episol** *Schering-Plough, Port.†.*
*SPF 15:* Padimate O (p.1155·1); oxybenzone (p.1154·3).
*Sunscreen.*

**Epistaxol** *Medical, Spain.*
Adrenaline (p.852·2); phenazone (p.82·3); naphazoline hydrochloride (p.1124·3); rutoside (p.1688·2).
*Epistaxis; mucous membrane haemorrhage.*

**Epitaloe** *Mediwhite, Ital.*
Aloe vera (p.1141·3).
*Corneal trauma.*

**Epiteliol-C** *Spedrog, Arg.*
Vitamin C (p.1460·2); hesperidin (p.1688·2); vitamins A and E (p.1417·1).
*Skin and capillary disorders.*

**Epitelizante** *Novartis, Spain.*
Methionine (p.1042·1); gentamicin sulfate (p.217·1); vitamin A palmitate (p.1453·1).
Formerly contained amino acids, chloramphenicol, and vitamin A palmitate.
*Corneal damage.*

**Epitezan** *Allergan, Braz.*
Vitamin A (p.1451·2); chloramphenicol (p.185·1); amino acids.
*Eye infections.*

**Epithea** *Thea, Fr.*
Cyanocobalamin (p.1458·2).
*Corneal scarring.*

**Epithelial** *Pierre Fabre Dermo-Cosmetique, Arg.*
Avena (p.1658·2); vitamins A and E (p.1417·1).
*Skin disorders.*

**Epitheliale** *Ducray, Fr.*
Avena (p.1658·2); vitamins A and E (p.1417·1).
*Skin disorders.*

**Epitol** *Lemmon, USA.*
Carbamazepine (p.353·3).
*Epilepsy; trigeminal neuralgia.*

**Epitomax** *Janssen-Cilag, Fr.*
Topiramate (p.378·3).
*Epilepsy.*

**Epitopic** *Gerda, Fr.*
Difluprednate (p.1100·1).
*Skin disorders.*

**Epitril** *Novartis, India.*
Clonazepam (p.359·1).
*Epilepsy.*

**Epival**
*Abbott, Canad.; Abbott, Mex.*
Valproate semisodium (p.380·1).
*Epilepsy; mania; migraine.*

**Epivir**
*GlaxoSmithKline, Austria; GlaxoSmithKline, Belg.; GlaxoSmithKline, Braz.; Glaxo Wellcome, Denm.; GlaxoSmithKline, Fin.; GlaxoSmithKline, Fr.; GlaxoSmithKline, Ger.; Glaxo Wellcome, Gr.; GlaxoSmithKline, Irl.; GlaxoSmithKline, Israel; GlaxoSmithKline, Ital.; Glaxo, Jpn; GlaxoSmithKline, Neth.; GlaxoSmithKline, Norw.; Glaxo Wellcome, Port.; GlaxoSmithKline, Singapore; GlaxoSmithKline, Spain; GlaxoSmithKline, Swed.; GlaxoSmithKline, Thai.; GlaxoSmithKline, UK; GlaxoSmithKline, USA.*
Lamivudine (p.648·2).
*Hepatitis B; HIV infection.*

**Epixian** *UCB, Spain†.*
Cocarboxylase (p.1455·2); magnesium phosphate (p.1228·1); magnesium succinate; pyridoxal phosphate (p.1456·3); chymotrypsin (p.1671·2); trypsin (p.1758·3).
*Renal calculi.*

**Epizon** *Mepha, Hong Kong.*
*Rectocaps for children:* Paracetamol (p.76·2); propyphenazone (p.85·3); guaifenesin (p.1122·1).
*Rectocaps for infants:* Paracetamol (p.76·2); propyphenazone (p.85·3); guaifenesin (p.1122·1); valerian (p.1762·2); passion flower (p.1729·1).
*Fever; pain.*

**Eplonat** *Infirmarius-Rovit, Ger.*
*d*-Alpha tocopherol (p.1464·3).
*Vitamin E deficiency.*

**E.P.O. & E** *Quest, UK†.*
Evening primrose oil (p.1686·3); vitamin E.

**Epo + Maxepa + Vitamin E Herbal Plus Formula 8** *Vitelle, Austral.†.*
*d*-Alpha tocopherol (p.1464·3); evening primrose oil (p.1686·3); marine fish oil (p.976·2).
*Nutritional supplement.*

**Epocan** *Merck, Arg.*
Pyritinol hydrochloride (p.1737·2).
*Cerebrovascular disorders.*

**Epocelin**
*Orion, Fin.†; Fujisawa, Jpn; CEPA, Spain†; Fujisawa, Thai.†.*
Ceftizoxime sodium (p.182·2).
Lidocaine (p.1377·3) or lidocaine hydrochloride (p.1377·3) may be included in the intramuscular injection to alleviate the pain of injection.
*Bacterial infections.*

**Epocler**
*Note. This name is used for preparations of different composition.*
*Whitehall, Braz.*
Adenosine (p.851·2); methionine (p.1042·1); choline (p.1424·3); betaine hydrochloride (p.1660·2); vitamin $B_6$ (p.1456·3).
*Liver disorders.*

*Whitehall, Ital.†.*
Hydroquinone (p.1148·1).
*Skin hyperpigmentation.*

**Epogam**
*Searle, Austral.†; Strathmann, Ger.; Pharmacia, Irl.; Whitehall, Ital.†; Sidroga, Switz.; Pharmacia, UK†.*
Evening primrose oil (p.1686·3).
*Eczema.*

*Scotia, Denm.†; Scotia, NZ†; Covan, S.Afr.†; Leti, Spain†.*
Gamolenic acid (p.1690·2).
*Atopic eczema.*

**Epogen** *Amgen, USA.*
Epoetin alfa (p.747·2).
*Anaemia in cancer patients on chemotherapy; anaemia in zidovudine-treated HIV-infected patients; anaemia of chronic renal failure.*

**Epogin** *Chugai, Jpn.*
Epoetin beta (p.747·2).
*Anaemias; autologous blood transfusion.*

**Epokelan** *Medochemie, Malaysia.*
Minoxidil (p.960·1).
*Alopecia androgenetica.*

**Epomax** *Cryopharma, Mex.*
Epoetin (p.747·1).
*Anaemias.*

**Epopa** *Vitalia, UK†.*
Safflower oil (p.1443·3); salmon oil (p.976·1); evening primrose oil (p.1686·3); borage oil (p.1661·3); nicotinic acid (p.1441·1).

**Epopen** *Pensa, Spain.*
Epoetin alfa (p.747·2).
*Anaemias; autologous blood transfusions.*

**Eposal** *Sanofi Synthelabo, Chile.*
Carbamazepine (p.353·3).
*Epilepsy; trigeminal neuralgia.*

**Eposerin** *Pharmacia Upjohn, Ital.*
Ceftizoxime sodium (p.182·2).
Lidocaine hydrochloride (p.1377·3) is included in the intramuscular injection to alleviate the pain of injection.
*Gram-negative bacterial infections.*

**Eposid** *Nettopharma, Denm.†.*
Etoposide (p.551·3).
*Malignant neoplasms.*

**Eposido** *Blausiegel, Braz.*
Etoposide (p.551·3).
*Malignant neoplasms.*

**Eposin**
*Nycomed, Fin.; Pharmachemie, Malaysia; Nycomed, Norw.; Pharmachemie, S.Afr.; Tedec Meiji, Spain; Nycomed, Swed.; Pharmachemie, Thai.; Teva, Thai.; Medac, UK.*
Etoposide (p.551·3).
*Malignant neoplasms.*

**Epotin** *Julphar, UAE.*
Epoetin (p.747·1).
*Anaemias; autologous blood transfusions.*

**Epoxide** *PP Lab, Thai.*
Chlordiazepoxide hydrochloride (p.674·2).
*Anxiety.*

**Epoxitin** *JC Healthcare, Ital.*
Epoetin alfa (p.747·2).
*Anaemias; autologous blood transfusions.*

**Eppy**
*Allergan, Fr.†; Chauvin, Irl.; Visufarma, Ital.†; Smith & Nephew, S.Afr.†; Abigo, Swed.; Chauvin, UK†.*
Adrenaline (p.852·2).
*Glaucoma.*

**EPR** *Elvetium, Arg.*
Epirubicin (p.550·3).
*Malignant neoplasms.*

**Epresat** *Salus, Fr.†.*
Multivitamin preparation with plant extracts and yeast (p.1417·1).
*Tonic.*

**Eprex**
*Janssen-Cilag, Arg.; Janssen-Cilag, Austral.; Janssen-Cilag, Belg.; Janssen-Cilag, Braz.; Janssen-Ortho, Canad.; Pentafarma, Chile; Janssen-Cilag, Denm.; Janssen-Cilag, Fin.; Janssen-Cilag, Fr.; Janssen-Cilag, Ger.; Janssen-Cilag, Gr.; Cilag, Hong Kong; Janssen-Cilag, Irl.; Janssen-Cilag, Israel; Janssen-Cilag, Ital.; Janssen-Cilag, Malaysia; Cilag, Mex.; Janssen-Cilag, Neth.; Janssen-Cilag, Norw.; Janssen-Cilag, NZ; Janssen-Cilag, S.Afr.; Janssen-Cilag, Singapore; Janssen-Cilag, Spain; Janssen-Cilag, Swed.; Janssen-Cilag, Switz.; Janssen-Cilag, Thai.; Janssen-Cilag, UK.*
Epoetin alfa (p.747·2).
*Anaemias; autologous blood transfusions.*

**Epril** *Ecosol, Switz.*
Enalapril maleate (p.909·2).
*Heart failure; hypertension; left ventricular dysfunction.*

**E-Prime** *Usana, Hong Kong.*
Vitamin E substances (p.1464·3).
*Vitamin E supplement.*

**Eprodine** *Pond's, Thai.*
Povidone-iodine (p.1190·3).
*Skin disinfection.*

**Eprofil**
*Note. This name is used for preparations of different composition.*
*Andromaco, Chile.*
Ketoconazole (p.403·3).
*Dandruff; seborrhoeic dermatitis.*

*Columbia, Mex.†.*
Tiabendazole (p.114·2).

**Epsicaprom** *Bial, Port.*
Aminocaproic acid (p.741·3).
*Fibrinolysis.*

**Epsidox** *Laboratorios Chile, Chile.*
Etoposide (p.551·3).
*Malignant neoplasms.*

**Epsilat** *Coup, Gr.*
Buspirone hydrochloride (p.672·2).
*Generalised anxiety.*

**Epsin** *Glaxo Wellcome, Mex.*
Aciclovir (p.626·1).
*Herpesvirus infections.*

**Epsitron**
*Remedica, Hong Kong; Remedica, Thai.*
Captopril (p.879·2).
*Heart failure; hypertension.*

**Epsoclar** *Biologici Italia, Ital.*
Heparin sodium (p.928·1).
*Thromboembolic disorders.*

**Epsodil** *Biologici Italia, Ital.*
Heparin sodium (p.928·1).
*Maintenance of patency of catheters and cannulas.*

**Epsolin** *Cadila, India.*
Phenytoin sodium (p.370·2).
*Epilepsy; trigeminal neuralgia; ventricular arrhythmias.*

**ept Stick Test** *Warner-Lambert, USA.*
Pregnancy test (p.1734·3).

**Eptadone** *Zambon, Ital.*
Methadone hydrochloride (p.57·2).
*Opioid withdrawal; pain.*

**Eptico** *Watsons, Canad.†.*
Camphor (p.1665·3); zinc oxide (p.1163·2).

**Eptoin** *Knoll, India.*
Phenytoin sodium (p.370·2).
*Epilepsy; trigeminal neuralgia.*

**Epulor** *Vistapharm, USA.*
Preparation for enteral nutrition (p.1417·1).

**Epuram** *Pharmafarm, Fr.*
Citrulline (p.1425·2); arginine hydrochloride (p.1421·1); ornithine hydrochloride (p.1442·3).
*Liver disorders.*

**Equagesic**
*Note. This name is used for preparations of different composition.*
*Wyeth-Ayerst, Canad.†; Akromed, S.Afr.†; Wyeth, UK†.*
Aspirin (p.15·1); meprobamate (p.706·2); ethoheptazine citrate (p.37·2).
*Pain; skeletal muscle spasm.*

*Wyeth, India.*
Aspirin (p.15·1); ethoheptazine citrate (p.37·2).
*Dysmenorrhoea; pain.*

*Wyeth-Ayerst, USA†.*
Aspirin (p.15·1); meprobamate (p.706·2).
*Musculoskeletal pain.*

**Equal**
*Nutrasweet, NZ; Merisant, Thai.*
Aspartame (p.1422·1).
*Sugar substitute.*

**Equalactin** *Numark, USA.*
Polycarbophil calcium (p.1284·2).
*Constipation; diarrhoea.*

**Equanil**
*Wyeth, Austral.†; Wyeth-Ayerst, Canad.†; Sanofi Synthelabo, Fr.; Akromed, S.Afr.; Wyeth-Ayerst, USA†.*
Meprobamate (p.706·2).
*Alcohol withdrawal sydrome; anxiety; premedication; sedative; skeletal muscle spasm.*

**Equanox** *Linde, UK.*
Nitrous oxide (p.1304·3); oxygen (p.1236·3).

**Equasym** *Celltech, UK.*
Methylphenidate hydrochloride (p.1590·2).
*Attention-deficit hyperactivity disorder.*

**Equiday** *Algol, Fin.*
*d*-Alpha tocopherol (p.1464·3).
*Vitamin E deficiency.*

**Equiday E** *Solvay, Ger.†.*
*d*-Alpha tocopherol (p.1464·3).
*Vitamin E deficiency.*

**Equiderm** *Galderma, Mex.*
Emollient; moisturiser.

**Equidral** *Scherer, Ital.†.*
Maltodextrin; electrolytes (p.1217·1).
*Electrolyte depletion in hyperhidrosis.*

**Equilet** *Mission Pharmacal, USA.*
Calcium carbonate (p.1254·2).
*Hyperacidity.*

**Equilibra** *Darrow, Braz.*
Hypericum (p.299·1).
*Depression.*

**Equilibrane** *Temis, Arg.*
Fluoxetine (p.296·3).
*Depression.*

**Equilibrin** *Aventis, Ger.*
Amitriptylinoxide (p.285·2).
*Depression.*

**Equilibrium**
*Note. This name is used for preparations of different composition.*
*Jagson, India.*
Chlordiazepoxide (p.674·2).
*Alcohol withdrawal syndrome; anxiety.*
*SFD, Port.*†.
A range of emollients, moisturisers, and shampoos.

**Equilibrium Creme Anti-transpirante** *SFD, Port.*†.
Aluminium chlorohydrate (p.1142·1); centella (p.1144·3); aloe vera (p.1141·3).
*Hyperhidrosis.*

**Equilid**
*Aventis, Braz.; Bruno, Ital.*
Sulpiride (p.722·2).
*Adjuvant in gastric ulcer; depression; nausea and vomiting; nervous disorders; psychoses.*

**Equilium** *Fumouze, Fr.*
Tiapride (p.725·1).
*Aggressive states; agitation; choreiform movements; pain.*

**Equilon** *Chefaro, UK.*
Mebeverine hydrochloride (p.1273·1).
*Irritable bowel syndrome.*

**Equilon Herbal** *Chefaro, UK.*
Peppermint oil (p.1283·2).
*Irritable bowel syndrome.*

**Equin**
*Aldo-Union, Hong Kong; Aldo, Spain.*
Conjugated oestrogens (p.1543·2).
*Dysfunctional uterine haemorrhage; female hypogonadism; lactation inhibition; menopausal disorders; osteoporosis.*

**Equinacea** *Herbarium, Braz.*
Echinacea (p.1683·2).

**Equinorm** *Aspen, S.Afr.*
Clomipramine hydrochloride (p.289·3).
*Depression; narcoleptic syndrome.*

**Equipax** *Parke, Davis, Spain*†.
Gabapentin (p.362·2).
*Epilepsy.*

**Equipur** *Medipharma, Ger.*†.
Vincamine (p.1764·2).
*Ménière's disease; mental function disorders; metabolic and circulatory disorders of the brain, retina, and inner ear.*

**Equirex** *Jagson, India.*
Chlordiazepoxide (p.674·2); clidinium bromide (p.480·2).
*Dyspepsia; gastritis; inflammatory bowel disorders; peptic ulcer.*

**Equisedin** *Lazar, Arg.*
Bromazepam (p.671·3).
*Anxiety.*

**Equisil N** *Klein, Ger.*
Equisetum (p.1684·1); plantago lanceolata (p.1738·2); castanea vulgaris; cowslip rhizome (p.1735·1); verbascum flowers (p.1764·1); thyme (p.1755·2); colloidal silicon dioxide (p.1581·3).
Equisil formerly contained equisetum, plantago lanceolata, castanea vulgaris, cowslip rhizome, verbascum flowers, thyme, colloidal silicon dioxide, and ephedrine hydrochloride.
*Coughs and associated respiratory-tract disorders.*

**Equi-Sleep** *Equity, S.Afr.*
Doxylamine succinate (p.432·3).
*Insomnia.*

**Equitam**
*Note. This name is used for preparations of different composition.*
*Eurofarma, Braz.*
Ginkgo biloba (p.1692·3).
*Cerebrovascular disorders.*
*Biotherapie, Fr.*
Lorazepam (p.704·1).
*Alcohol withdrawal syndrome; anxiety.*

**Equiton** *Bruschettini, Ital.*
Timolol maleate (p.1012·2); pilocarpine hydrochloride (p.1495·1).
*Glaucoma; ocular hypertension.*

**ER Cream** *Curacel, Austral.*
Allantoin (p.1141·3); alpha tocoferil acetate (p.1465·1); eicosapentaenoic acid (p.976·2); coal tar (p.1159·2); vitamin A palmitate (p.1453·1); zinc oxide (p.1163·2).
*Skin disorders.*

**Era** *Abbott, NZ.*
Erythromycin lactobionate (p.208·2) or erythromycin stearate (p.208·2).
*Bacterial infections.*

**Eracillin** *Chew, Thai.*
Ampicillin trihydrate (p.157·2).
*Bacterial infections.*

**Eracine** *Sanofi Synthelabo, Fr.*†.
Rosoxacin (p.254·1).
*Bacterial infections.*

**Eradacil**
*Sanofi Synthelabo, Braz.; Sanofi Synthelabo, Mex.; Sanofi Synthelabo, Port.*
Rosoxacin (p.254·1).
*Gonorrhoea.*

**Eradix** *Kwizda, Austria.*
Famotidine (p.1265·2).
*Peptic ulcer.*

**Eralga** *Chew, Thai.*
Hyoscine butylbromide (p.483·3).
*Smooth muscle spasm.*

**Eramox** *Nycomed, Austria.*
Amoxicillin trihydrate (p.155·3).
*Bacterial infections.*

**Eramycin** *Wesley, USA.*
Erythromycin stearate (p.208·2).
*Bacterial infections.*

**Erantin** *Boehringer Mannheim, Spain*†.
Epoetin beta (p.747·2).
*Anaemia of chronic renal failure; cisplatin-induced anaemia.*

**Eranz**
*Wyeth, Arg.; Wyeth, Braz.; Wyeth, Braz.; Wyeth, Chile; Wyeth, Mex.*
Donepezil hydrochloride (p.1489·2).
*Alzheimer's disease.*

**Erasis** *Orion, Fin.*†.
Erythromycin acistrate (p.208·1).
*Bacterial infections.*

**Erasol** *McGloin, Austral.*†.
Phenazone (p.82·3).
*Ear ache.*

**Erathrom** *Asian Pharm, Thai.*
Erythromycin estolate (p.208·1) or erythromycin stearate (p.208·2).
*Bacterial infections.*

**Eraverm** *Gemballa, Braz.*
Mebendazole (p.108·2).
*Worm infections.*

**Eraxil** *Gepepharm, Ger.*
Crotamiton (p.1145·1).
*Scabies.*

**Erbazid** *Pharmacia Upjohn, Mex.*†.
Isoniazid (p.222·2).

**Erbazide** *Mac, India.*
Methaniazide calcium (p.230·1).
*Tuberculosis.*

**Erbesil** *Bittner, Austria.*
Melissa (p.1711·1); sage (p.1741·2); thyme (p.1755·2).
*Mouth disorders.*

**Erbitux** *Bristol-Myers Squibb, USA.*
Cetuximab (p.536·1).
*Colorectal cancer.*

**Erbonda Noche** *Boehringer Ingelheim, Arg.*
Valerian (p.1762·2); melissa (p.1711·1).
*Insomnia.*

**Ercaf** *Geneva, USA.*
Ergotamine tartrate (p.467·2); caffeine (p.782·1).
*Migraine and related vascular headache.*

**Ercal** *Syntex, Mex.*†.
Fluocinolone acetonide (p.1101·2); bismuth subgallate (p.1252·2); lidocaine hydrochloride (p.1377·3).
*Anorectal disorders.*

**Ercar** *Almirall, Spain.*
Carboplatin (p.533·3).
*Bladder cancer; head and neck cancer; ovarian cancer; small-cell lung cancer.*

**Ercefuryl**
*Sanofi Synthelabo, Belg.; Sanofi Synthelabo, Fr.; Sanofi Synthelabo, Hong Kong; Luitpold, Ital.*†*; Sanofi Synthelabo, Singapore*†*; Sanofi Synthelabo, Thai.*
Nifuroxazide (p.237·2).
*Gastrointestinal infections.*

**Erceryl** *Sanofi Synthelabo OTC, Fr.*
Nifuroxazide (p.237·2).
*Diarrhoea.*

**Ercestop** *Sanofi Synthelabo, Fr.*
Loperamide hydrochloride (p.1271·1).
Formerly known as Delalande Diarrhee.
*Diarrhoea.*

**Ercestopyl** *Sanofi Synthelabo, Belg.*†.
Loperamide hydrochloride (p.1271·1).
*Diarrhoea.*

**Ercevit** *Synthelabo, Fr.*†.
Rutoside (p.1688·2); rutoside propylsulfonate sodium.
*Peripheral vascular disorders.*

**Erco-Fer** *Orion, Swed.*
Ferrous fumarate (p.1427·3).
*Iron deficiency; iron-deficiency anaemia.*

**Erco-Fer vitamin** *Orion, Swed.*†.
Multivitamin preparation with ferrous fumarate (p.1427·3)(p.1417·1).
*Iron deficiency; iron-deficiency anaemia.*

**Ercolax** *Ercopharm, Switz.*†.
Bisacodyl (p.1251·3).
*Bowel evacuation; constipation.*

**Ercoquin**
*Medic, Denm.; Nycomed, Norw.*†.
Hydroxychloroquine sulfate (p.452·3).
*Lupus erythematosus; malaria; photosensitivity; rheumatoid arthritis; Sjögren's syndrome.*

**Ercorax Roll-on** *Ercopharm, Switz.*†.
Propantheline bromide (p.489·1).
*Hyperhidrosis.*

**Ercoril** *Medic, Denm.*
Propantheline bromide (p.489·1).
*Gastrointestinal spasm.*

**Ercotina** *Orion, Swed.*†.
Propantheline bromide (p.489·1).
*Gastrointestinal disorders.*

**Erdopect** *Pharmacal, Fin.*
Erdosteine (p.1121·1).
*Respiratory-tract disorders.*

**Erdotin**
*Asta Medica, Braz.; Edmond Pharma, Ital.*
Erdosteine (p.1121·1).
*Respiratory-tract congestion.*

**Eremfat**
*Fatol, Austria; Fatol, Ger.*
Rifampicin (p.250·2) or rifampicin sodium (p.252·3).
*Brucellosis; leprosy; meningococcal meningitis prophylaxis; staphylococcal infections; tuberculosis.*

**Eres N** *Muller Goppingen, Ger.*
Verbascum flowers (p.1764·1).
*Bronchial catarrh.*

**Erevan** *Fournier, Ital.*
A heparinoid (p.931·1).
*Superficial vascular disorders; thrombosis prophylaxis.*

**Erfolgan** *Roche, Spain*†.
Ibopamine hydrochloride (p.937·3).
*Heart failure.*

**Erg XXI** *Farmorcore, Port.*
Nicergoline (p.1719·3).
*Cerberal and peripheral vascular disorders; hypertension.*

**Ergamisol**
*Janssen-Cilag, Austral.; Janssen-Cilag, Belg.; Janssen-Ortho, Canad.; Janssen-Cilag, Ger.; Janssen-Cilag, Israel; Janssen-Cilag, Ital.*†*; Janssen-Cilag, Neth.; Janssen-Cilag, S.Afr.; Janssen, USA.*
Levamisole hydrochloride (p.107·2).
*Adjunct to fluorouracil in colon cancer.*

**Ergenyl**
*Sanofi Synthelabo, Ger.; Sanofi Synthelabo, Swed.*
Sodium valproate (p.380·1).
*Epilepsy; mania.*

**Ergenyl Chrono** *Sanofi Synthelabo, Ger.*
Sodium valproate (p.380·1); valproic acid (p.380·1).
*Epilepsy.*

**Ergix** *Merck Medication Familiale, Fr.*
*Capsules:* Dextromethorphan hydrobromide (p.1117·3).
*Coughs.*
*Lozenges:* Tyrothricin (p.275·1); lidocaine hydrochloride (p.1377·3).
*Sore throat.*
*Syrup:* Carbocisteine (p.1116·2).
*Respiratory-tract congestion.*
*Tablets:* Ibuprofen (p.45·3).
*Fever; pain.*

**ergo sanol spezial N** *Sanol, Ger.*
Ergotamine tartrate (p.467·2).
*Migraine and other vascular headache.*

**ergobel** *Hormosan, Ger.*
Nicergoline (p.1719·3).
*Mental function disorders.*

**Ergobelan** *Labomed, Chile.*
Belladonna (p.479·1); ergotamine tartrate (p.467·2); phenobarbital (p.367·3).
*Vascular headache.*

**Ergocaf** *Galen, Mex.*
Ergotamine tartrate (p.467·2); caffeine (p.782·1).
*Migraine.*

**Ergocalm**
*Note. This name is used for preparations of different composition.*
*Mayrhofer, Austria*†.
Lorazepam (p.704·1).
*Anxiety disorders; premedication; sleep disorders.*
*Teofarma, Ger.*
Lormetazepam (p.705·2).
*Premedication; sleep disorders.*

**Ergoclavin** *Bros, Gr.*
Diltiazem (p.901·3).
*Angina; hypertension.*

**Ergocris** *Magis, Ital.*†.
Dihydroergocristine mesilate (p.1680·1).
*Cerebral and peripheral vascular disorders; dopaminergic deficiency; headache; hypertension; migraine.*

**Ergodavur** *Davur, Spain.*
Dihydroergocristine mesilate (p.1680·1).
*Cerebrovascular disorders; vascular ear, nose, throat and eye disorders; vestibular disorders.*

**Ergodesit** *Desitin, Ger.*
Co-dergocrine mesilate (p.1674·1).
*Hypertension; mental function disorders.*

**Ergodilat** *Diviser Aquilea, Spain.*
Co-dergocrine mesilate (p.1674·1).
*Cerebrovascular disorders; circulatory disorders.*

**Ergodose** *Shire, Fr.*
Co-dergocrine mesilate (p.1674·1).
*Mental function impairment in the elderly.*

**Ergodryl**
*Pfizer, Austral.; Pfizer, Canad.; Pfizer, NZ*†.
Ergotamine tartrate (p.467·2); caffeine citrate (p.782·1); diphenhydramine hydrochloride (p.431·3).
*Migraine and other vascular headaches.*

**Ergodryl Mono** *Pfizer, Austral.*
Ergotamine tartrate (p.467·2).
*Migraine and other vascular headaches.*

**Ergofar** *Continentales, Mex.*†.
Ergometrine (p.1684·2).

**Ergoffin** *Temmler, Ger.*
Ergotamine tartrate (p.467·2); caffeine (p.782·1).
*Headache; migraine.*

**Ergofit** *Bonomelli, Ital.*†.
Vitamin C (p.1460·2).
*Nutritional supplement.*

**Ergo-Fort** *Odontofarma, Braz.*†.
Amino acids; vitamin B substances (p.1417·1).

**Ergohepat B12** *IMA, Braz.*†.
Acetylmethionine; choline (p.1424·3); vitamin $B_{12}$ (p.1458·2).
*Liver disorders.*

**Ergohydrine** *Streuli, Switz.*
Co-dergocrine mesilate (p.1674·1).
*Cerebrovascular disorders.*

**Ergokapton** *Strallhofer, Austria.*
Ergotamine tartrate (p.467·2).
*Migraine and related vascular headaches.*

**Ergokoffin** *OBA, Denm.*
Ergotamine tartrate (p.467·2); caffeine (p.782·1).
*Migraine.*

**Ergo-Kranit** *Krewel, Ger.*
Ergotamine tartrate (p.467·2); propyphenazone (p.85·3); paracetamol (p.76·2).
*Headache; migraine.*

**Ergo-Kranit mono** *Krewel, Ger.*
Ergotamine tartrate (p.467·2).
*Migraine and other vascular headaches.*

**Ergolefrin** *Gepepharm, Ger.*
Dihydroergotamine mesilate (p.465·3); etilefrine hydrochloride (p.914·1).
*Hypotension.*

**Ergolin** *Boniscontro & Gazzone, Ital.*†.
Nicergoline (p.1719·3).
*Cerebrovascular disorders.*

**Ergo-Lonarid PD** *Boehringer Ingelheim, Ger.*
Dihydroergotamine tartrate (p.466·1); paracetamol (p.76·2).
*Headache; migraine.*

**Ergomar**
*Rhone-Poulenc Rorer, Canad.*†*; Lotus, USA.*
Ergotamine tartrate (p.467·2).
*Migraine and related vascular headache.*

**Ergomed** *Kwizda, Austria.*
Co-dergocrine mesilate (p.1674·1).
*Cerebral insufficiency; hypertension; migraine and related vascular headache.*

**Ergomemor** *Hexal, Braz.*
Glutamic acid; calcium glycerophosphate; tribasic calcium phosphate; vitamin B substances (p.1417·1).
*Dietary supplement.*

**Ergomicon** *Offenbach, Mex.*
Ketoconazole (p.403·3).
*Fungal infections.*

**Ergomimet** *Fujisawa, Ger.*
Dihydroergotamine mesilate (p.465·3).
*Hypotension; migraine and other vascular headaches; vascular disorders.*

**Ergomimet plus** *Fujisawa, Ger.*
Dihydroergotamine mesilate (p.465·3); etilefrine hydrochloride (p.914·1).
*Hypotension.*

**Ergonef** *ITF, Chile.*
Clonixin lysine (p.26·3); ergotamine tartrate (p.467·2).
*Headache; migraine.*

**Ergont**
*Sigmapharm, Austria; Desitin, Ger.*
Dihydroergotamine mesilate (p.465·3).
*Hypotension; migraine and related vascular headache; vascular disorders.*

**ergoplus** *Hormosan, Ger.*†.
Co-dergocrine mesilate (p.1674·1).
*Cervical disc syndrome; hypertension; mental function disorders.*

**Ergoram** *Bonomelli, Ital.*†.
Amino-acid preparation (p.1417·1).
*Nutritional supplement.*

**Ergosanol a la cafeine** *Schwarz, Switz.*†.
*Suppositories:* Ergotamine tartrate (p.467·2); ethenzamide (p.37·2); caffeine (p.782·1); caffeine citrate (p.782·1).
*Tablets:* Ergotamine tartrate (p.467·2); ethenzamide (p.37·2); caffeine (p.782·1).
*Cluster headache; migraine and related vascular headache.*

**Ergosanol special** *Schwarz, Switz.*†.
Ergotamine tartrate (p.467·2); phenyltoloxamine citrate (p.439·1); ethenzamide (p.37·2); caffeine (p.782·1).
*Cluster headache; migraine and related vascular headache.*

**Ergosanol special a la cafeine** *Schwarz, Switz.*†.
Ergotamine tartrate (p.467·2); ethenzamide (p.37·2); caffeine (p.782·1); caffeine citrate (p.782·1); phenyltoloxamine citrate (p.439·1).
*Cluster headache; migraine and other vascular headaches.*

**Ergosia** *Asian Pharm, Thai.*
Ergotamine tartrate (p.467·2).
*Migraine.*

**Ergotab** *Jagson, India.*
Ergot (p.1685·1).
*Menopausal haemorrhage; menorrhagia; postpartum haemorrhage; uterine atony.*

**ergotam** *CT, Ger.*
Dihydroergotamine mesilate (p.465·3).
*Hypotension; migraine and other vascular headaches; vascular disorders.*

**Ergotan** *Salf, Ital.*
Ergotamine tartrate (p.467·2).
*Migraine and related vascular headache.*

**Ergotonine** *Streuli, Switz.*
Dihydroergotamine mesilate (p.465·3).
*Fatigue; hypotension; migraine.*

**Ergotop** *Kwizda, Austria.*
Nicergoline (p.1719·3).
*Peripheral and cerebral vascular disorders.*

**ergotox** *CT, Ger.*
Co-dergocrine mesilate (p.1674·1).
*Mental function disorders.*

**Ergotrate**
*Biolab Sanus, Braz.; Lilly, Canad.†; Lilly, Mex.; Bedford, USA.*
Ergometrine maleate (p.1684·1).
*Postpartum or postabortal haemorrhage.*

**Ergotyl** *Lek, Thai.*
Methylergometrine maleate (p.1714·2).
*Management of third stage of labour; postpartum haemorrhage; postpartum uterine atony.*

**Ergovasan** *Klinge, Austria.*
Dihydroergotamine mesilate (p.465·3).
*Circulatory disorders; hypotension; migraine and related vascular headaches.*

**Ergovis** *Bonomelli, Ital.†.*
A range of nutritional supplements (p.1417·1).

**Ergoxina** *Klonal, Arg.*
Co-dergocrine (p.1674·1).

**Ergybiol** *Nutergia, Fr.*
Mineral preparation (p.1417·1).

**Ergymag** *Nutergia, Fr.*
Vitamin B and mineral preparation (p.1417·1).

**Ergyphilus** *Nutergia, Fr.*
*Lactobacillus* species, fibre, and mineral preparation (p.1417·1).
*Maintenance of normal gastrointestinal flora.*

**Eribec** *Collins, Mex.*
Erythromycin (p.208·1).
*Bacterial infections.*

**Eriber** *Berman, Mex.*
Erythromycin (p.208·1).
*Bacterial infections.*

**Eribiotic** *Teuto, Braz.*
Erythromycin estolate (p.208·1).
*Bacterial infections.*

**Eribus** *Welfer, Mex.†.*
Erythromycin (p.208·1).
*Bacterial infections.*

**Ericin** *Chew, Thai.*
Erythromycin stearate (p.208·2).
*Bacterial infections.*

**Ericosol** *Ecosol, Switz.†.*
Erythromycin stearate (p.208·2).
*Bacterial infections.*

**Eridamin** *Brasmedica, Braz.†.*
Benzydamine hydrochloride (p.21·1).
*Fever; inflammation; pain.*

**Eridan** *SIT, Ital.†.*
Diazepam (p.690·1).
*Adjuvant in epilepsy; anxiety disorders.*

**Eridosis** *Orravan, Spain.*
Erythromycin (p.208·1).
*Acne.*

**Eriflogin** *Asta Medica, Braz.*
Erythromycin estolate (p.208·1).
*Bacterial infections.*

**Erifoscin** *I Farmacologia, Spain†.*
Erythromycin estolate (p.208·1); fosfomycin calcium (p.214·2).
*Bacterial infections.*

**Erifostine** *Teva Tuteur, Arg.*
Amifostine (p.1031·3).
*Reduction of haematotoxicity and nephrotoxicity associated with chemotherapy.*

**Eriglobin** *Max Farma, Ital.*
Ferrous gluconate (p.1428·1).
Ascorbic acid (p.1460·2) is included in this preparation to increase the absorption and availability of the iron.
*Iron-deficiency anaemia.*

**Erigrand** *Ahimsa, Arg.*
Erythromycin (p.208·1).
*Bacterial infections.*

**Eriken** *Kendrick, Mex.*
Cisapride (p.1259·2).
*Gastro-oesophageal reflux; gastrointestinal motility disorders.*

**Eril**
*Note. This name is used for preparations of different composition.*
*Savio, Ital.*
Piperacillin sodium (p.243·1).
Lidocaine hydrochloride (p.1377·3) is included in this preparation to alleviate the pain of injection.
*Bacterial infections.*

*Asahi, Jpn.*
Fasudil hydrochloride (p.914·3).
*Cerebral vasospasm following subarachnoid haemorrhage.*

**Erimicin** *Cassara, Arg.*
Benzoyl peroxide (p.1143·2); erythromycin (p.208·1).
*Acne.*

**Erimicina** *Medifarma, Mex.†.*
Erythromycin (p.208·1).
*Bacterial infections.*

**Erimit** *TP, Thai.*
Erythromycin estolate (p.208·1) or erythromycin stearate (p.208·2).
*Bacterial infections.*

**Erimycin** *Siam Bheasach, Thai.*
Erythromycin ethyl succinate (p.208·1) or erythromycin stearate (p.208·2).
*Bacterial infections.*

**Erios** *Mepha, Switz.*
Erythromycin ethyl succinate (p.208·1) or erythromycin stearate (p.208·2).
*Bacterial infections.*

**Erisol** *Cassara, Arg.*
Erythromycin (p.208·1).
*Acne.*

**Erisuspen** *Medifarma, Mex.†.*
Erythromycin (p.208·1).
*Bacterial infections.*

**Eritina**
*Note. This name is used for preparations of different composition.*
*Cristalia, Braz.*
Epoetin (p.747·1).
*Anaemias.*

*Sanitas, Port.*
Erythromycin propionate (p.208·2).
*Bacterial infections.*

**Eritolat** *Marcel, Mex.†.*
Erythromycin (p.208·1).
*Bacterial infections.*

**Eritos** *Biolab Sanus, Braz.*
Dropropizine (p.1119·3).
*Coughs.*

**Eritrax** *Luper, Braz.*
Erythromycin estolate (p.208·1).
*Bacterial infections.*

**Eritrerba** *Pharmacia Upjohn, Mex.†.*
Erythromycin (p.208·1).
*Bacterial infections.*

**Eritrex** *Ache, Braz.*
Erythromycin estolate (p.208·1).
*Bacterial infections.*

**Eritrex A** *Ache, Braz.*
Erythromycin (p.208·1); azulene (p.1658·3).
Formerly contained erythromycin estolate and oxolamine.
*Bacterial skin infections.*

**Eritril** *Ortoquimica, Braz.†.*
Erythromycin (p.208·1).
*Bacterial infections.*

**Eritrin** *Hebron, Braz.*
Erythromycin estolate (p.208·1).
*Bacterial infections.*

**Eritrobron** *Casasco, Arg.*
Erythromycin estolate (p.208·1); bromhexine hydrochloride (p.1115·3).
*Respiratory-tract disorders.*

**Eritrocin** *Sobral, Braz.†.*
Erythromycin estolate (p.208·1).
*Bacterial infections.*

**Eritrocina**
*Abbott, Ital.; Abbott, Port.*
Erythromycin ethyl succinate (p.208·1) or erythromcyin lactobionate (p.208·2).
*Bacterial infections.*

**Eritrocist** *Edmond Pharma, Ital.†.*
Erythromycin stinoprate (p.210·3).
*Bacterial infections.*

**Eritroderm** *ICN, Arg.*
Erythromycin (p.208·1).
*Acne.*

**Eritrofar** *Elofar, Braz.†.*
Erythromycin estolate (p.208·1).
*Bacterial infections.*

**Eritrofarm** *ICN, Arg.*
Erythromycin lactobionate (p.208·2).
*Bacterial conjunctivitis.*

**Eritrofarmin** *Rayere, Mex.*
Erythromycin (p.208·1).
*Bacterial infections.*

**Eritrogen** *Boehringer Mannheim, Ital.†.*
Epoetin beta (p.747·2).
*Anaemia associated with renal impairment; autologous blood transfusion.*

**Eritrogobens** *Normon, Spain.*
Erythromycin ethyl succinate (p.208·1).
*Bacterial infections.*

**Eritrolat** *Liferpal, Mex.*
Erythromycin (p.208·1).
*Bacterial infections.*

**Eritromax** *Blausiegel, Braz.*
Epoetin (p.747·1).
*Anaemias.*

**Eritromed** *Biocumed, Arg.*
Erythromycin (p.208·1) or erythromycin lactobionate (p.208·2).
*Bacterial eye infections.*

**Eritromicina** *Sanofi Synthelabo, Port.†.*
Erythromycin lactobionate (p.208·2).
*Bacterial infections.*

**Eritropiu** *Uno, Ital.*
Ferrous gluconate (p.1428·1).
Ascorbic acid (p.1460·2) is included in this preparation to increase the absorption and availability of the iron.
*Iron-deficiency anaemia.*

**Eritroquim** *Quimica y Farmacia, Mex.*
Erythromycin (p.208·1).
*Bacterial infections.*

**Eritrosima** *Quimioterapica, Braz.†.*
Erythromycin estolate (p.208·1); muramidase hydrochloride (p.1717·2).
*Bacterial infections.*

**Eritrosol** *Solfran, Mex.*
Erythromycin (p.208·1).
*Bacterial infections.*

**Eritroveinte** *Madariaga, Spain.*
Erythromycin estolate (p.208·1).
*Bacterial infections.*

**Eritrovier** *Tecnofarma, Mex.*
Erythromycin ethyl succinate (p.208·1) or erythromycin stearate (p.208·2).
*Bacterial infections.*

**Eritrovit B12** *Lisapharma, Ital.*
Cyanocobalamin (p.1458·2).
*Anaemia; neuritis.*

**Eritrowel** *Welfer, Mex.†.*
Erythromycin (p.208·1).
*Bacterial infections.*

**Erjean** *Erjean, Fr.*
Sodium chloride (p.1233·3).
*Fluid and electrolyte disorders.*

**Erkaltungsbad** *Agepha, Austria.*
Eucalyptus oil (p.1686·2); pumilio pine oil (p.1737·1); menthol (p.1711·3).
*Catarrh.*

**Erkaltungsbalsam**
*Note. This name is used for preparations of different composition.*
*Agepha, Austria.*
Peppermint oil (p.1283·2); camphor (p.1665·3); menthol (p.1711·3).
*Catarrh.*

*Genericon, Austria.*
Menthol (p.1711·3); camphor (p.1665·3); methyl salicylate (p.59·3).
*Cold symptoms; musculoskeletal and joint disorders.*

*Sanofi Synthelabo, Austria.*
Eucalyptus oil (p.1686·2); pumilio pine oil (p.1737·1); oleum pini sylvestris; camphor (p.1665·3); menthol (p.1711·3).
*Cold symptoms.*

**Erkaltungsbalsam forte Salbe** *Twardy, Ger.†.*
Camphor (p.1665·3); menthol (p.1711·3); clove oil (p.1673·3).
*Bronchitis; cold symptoms; coughs.*

**Erkaltungsbalsam-ratiopharm E Salbe** *Ratiopharm, Ger.*
Eucalyptus oil (p.1686·2); camphor (p.1665·3); turpentine oil (p.1760·1).
*Cold symptoms.*

**Erkaltungstee** *Sanova, Austria.*
Thyme leaf (p.1755·2); althaea (p.1651·3); verbascum flowers (p.1764·1); drosera (p.1683·1); plantago lanceolata leaf (p.1738·2).
*Mouth and throat disorders; respiratory-tract disorders.*

**Erladexone** *Malaysia Chemist, Singapore.*
Dexamethasone (p.1097·1).
*Corticosteroid.*

**Erlecit** *Doctum, Gr.*
Nimesulide (p.67·1).
*Inflammation; musculoskeletal disorders; pain.*

**Erliten** *Malaysia Chemist, Singapore.*
Ketotifen fumarate (p.788·1).
*Allergic bronchitis; allergic conjunctivitis; allergic rhinitis; allergic skin disorders; asthma; hay fever.*

**Erlivin** *Malaysia Chemist, Singapore†.*
Griseofulvin (p.400·3).
*Fungal skin, hair, and nail infections.*

**Erlmetin** *Malaysia Chemist, Singapore.*
Cimetidine (p.1255·3).
*Acid aspiration; adjunct in pancreatic insufficiency; gastro-oesophageal reflux; peptic ulcer; Zollinger-Ellison syndrome.*

**Erloric** *Malaysia Chemist, Singapore.*
Allopurinol (p.412·2).
*Gout; hyperuricaemia; renal calculi.*

**Erlotyl** *Malaysia Chemist, Singapore†.*
Diphenoxylate hydrochloride (p.1261·3).
Atropine sulfate (p.477·1) is included in this preparation to discourage abuse.
*Diarrhoea.*

**Erlvirax** *Malaysia Chemist, Singapore.*
Aciclovir (p.626·1).
*Herpesvirus infections.*

**Ermofan** *Chrispa (Χρισπα), Gr.*
Ofloxacin (p.239·3).
*Bacterial infections.*

**Ermsech** *Pharmacia, Ger.*
Calcium lactate (p.1225·3); echinacea (p.1683·2).
*Hypersensitivity disorders; increase of immune capacity.*

**Ermycin** *Remedica, Singapore.*
Erythromycin stearate (p.208·2).
*Bacterial infections.*

**Ermysin** *Orion, Fin.*
Erythromycin (p.208·1) or erythromycin ethyl succinate (p.208·1).
*Bacterial infections.*

**Ernex** *Casasco, Arg.*
Benzydamine hydrochloride (p.21·1).
*Mouth and throat disorders; vulvovaginal disorders.*

**Ernodasa** *Ern, Spain.*
Streptodornase (p.1749·3); streptokinase (p.1005·2).
*Inflammation; soft-tissue damage; ulcers.*

**ERO** *Scherer, USA.*
Urea hydrogen peroxide (p.1195·3).
*Ear wax removal.*

**Ero Test** *Heralds, Braz.†.*
Conjugated oestrogens (p.1543·2); methyltestosterone (p.1559·3); vitamin C (p.1460·2).
*Erectile dysfunction.*

**Erocap** *Lilly, Austral.*
Fluoxetine hydrochloride (p.292·1).
*Depression; obsessive-compulsive disorder; premenstrual dysphoric disorder.*

**Erogran** *Hovid, Malaysia.*
Erythromycin ethyl succinate (p.208·1).
*Bacterial infections; protozoal infections.*

**Erole Forte** *Orion, Fin.*
*d*-Alpha tocopherol; selenium yeast (p.1417·1).
*Dietary supplement.*

**Erole-C** *Orion, Fin.*
Capsules, *d*-alpha tocopherol; selenium yeast; tablets, ascorbic acid (p.1417·1).
*Dietary supplement.*

**Eromel** *Aspen, S.Afr.*
Erythromycin stearate (p.208·2).
*Bacterial infections.*

**Eromel-S** *Lagamed, S.Afr.†.*
Erythromycin ethyl succinate (p.208·1).
*Bacterial infections.*

**Eromycin**
*Dista, NZ†.*
Erythromycin estolate (p.208·1).
*Bacterial infections.*

*Julphar, UAE.*
Erythromycin (p.208·1), erythromycin ethyl succinate (p.208·1), or erythromycin stearate (p.208·2).
*Bacterial infections.*

**Erosfil** *Andromaco, Chile.*
Sildenafil (p.1744·2).
*Erectile dysfunction.*

**Erotab**
*Hovid, Malaysia; Hovid, Singapore.*
Erythromycin stearate (p.208·2).
*Bacterial infections.*

**Eroxade** *Osoth, Thai.*
Roxithromycin (p.254·2).
*Bacterial infections.*

**Erpalfa** *INTES, Ital.*
Cytarabine (p.543·1).
*Viral keratitis.*

**Erpecalm** *Prisfar, Port.*
Thyme oil (p.1755·3); oregao oil; sweet marjoram oil; lavender (p.1705·1); lemon (p.1706·2); chamomile (p.1669·3); thuja (p.1755·1); lappa (p.1704·3); plantain (p.1733·1).
*Herpes labialis.*

**Erradic** *Libbs, Braz.*
4 Capsules, amoxicillin (p.155·3); 2 tablets, clarithromycin (p.192·2); 2 capsules, omeprazole (p.1278·2).
Formerly contained amoxicillin, azithromycin, and omeprazole.
*Peptic ulcer.*

**Erreclor** *Errekappa, Ital.*
Cefaclor (p.167·1).
*Bacterial infections.*

**Erremox** *Errekappa, Ital.*
Amoxicillin trihydrate (p.155·3).
*Bacterial infections.*

**Errevit Combi** *Erredici, Ital.†.*
Vitamin E; betacarotene; selenium (p.1417·1).
*Nutritional supplement.*

**Errevit Forte Gamma** *Erredici, Ital.†.*
Betacarotene; vitamin E; selenium; gamolenic acid (p.1690·2).
*Nutritional supplement.*

**Errolon** *Labinca, Arg.*
Furosemide (p.919·3).
*Hypertension.*

**Errolon A** *Labinca, Arg.*
Furosemide (p.919·3); amiloride hydrochloride (p.858·2).

**Ertaczo** *Neutrogena Dermatologicals, USA.*
Sertaconazole nitrate (p.408·1).
*Tinea pedis.*

**Erthiol** *American de Mexico, Mex.†.*
Merbromin (p.1185·3).

**Ervemin** *Elvetium, Arg.*
Methotrexate (p.568·2).
*Malignant neoplasms; psoriasis; rheumatoid arthritis.*

**Ervevax**
*GlaxoSmithKline, Austral.; GlaxoSmithKline, Austria; SmithKline Beecham, Belg.†; SmithKline Beecham, Ger.†; Dresden, Ger.†; GlaxoSmithKline, Irl.; GlaxoSmithKline, Ital.; GlaxoSmithKline, Malaysia; SmithKline Beecham, Mex.; SmithKline Beecham, NZ†; SmithKline Beecham, Switz.; SmithKline Beecham, Thai.†; GlaxoSmithKline, UK†.*
A rubella vaccine (Wistar RA 27/3 strain) (p.1637·3).
*Active immunisation.*

**Ervin** *Nakorn, Thai.†.*
Thiamphenicol (p.269·2).
*Bacterial infections.*

**Erwinase**
*Ipsen, Denm.; Ipsen, Fin.; Ipsen, Ger.; Ipsen, Gr.; Ipsen, Irl.; Beaufour-Ipsen, Malaysia; Emerging Pharma, Malaysia; NZ Medical & Scientific, NZ; Beaufour-Ipsen, Singapore; Ipsen, Swed.; Beaufour-Ipsen, Thai.; Ipsen, UK.*
Crisantaspase (asparaginase) (p.528·3).
*Acute lymphocytic leukaemia.*

**Erxetilan** *Leovan, Gr.*
Enalapril maleate (p.909·2).
*Heart failure; hypertension.*

**Ery**
*Bouchara-Recordati, Fr.*
Erythromycin ethyl succinate (p.208·1) or erythromycin propionate (p.208·2).
*Bacterial infections.*

*1A, Ger.; Astrapin, Ger.; Curasan, Ger.; Hameln, Ger.*
Erythromycin lactobionate (p.208·2) or erythromycin stearate (p.208·2).
*Bacterial infections.*

*Bouchara, Switz.†.*
Erythromycin ethyl succinate (p.208·1).
*Bacterial infections.*

**Eryacne**
*Galderma, Arg.; Galderma, Austral.; Galderma, Fr.; Galderma, Hong Kong; Galderma, Ital.; Galderma, Neth.; Galderma, NZ; Galderma, Singapore; Galderma, Thai.; Galderma, UK†.*
Erythromycin (p.208·1).
*Acne.*

**Eryacnen**
*Galderma, Braz.; Galderma, Chile; Galderma, Mex.*
Erythromycin (p.208·1).
*Acne.*

**Eryaknen**
*AB-Consult, Austria; Galderma, Ger.; Galderma, Switz.*
Erythromycin (p.208·1).
*Acne.*

**Eryase** *Ducray, Fr.*
Avena (p.1658·2); zinc oxide (p.1163·2); copper sulfate (p.1426·1).
*Nappy rash.*

**Erybesan** *Biochemie, Austria.*
Erythromycin ethyl succinate (p.208·1) or erythromycin stearate (p.208·2).
*Bacterial infections.*

**Erybeta** *Betapharm, Ger.*
Erythromycin ethyl succinate (p.208·1) or erythromycin stearate (p.208·2).
*Bacterial infections.*

**Erybid** *Abbott, Canad.*
Erythromycin (p.208·1).
*Bacterial infections.*

**Erybros** *Bros, Gr.*
Roxithromycin (p.254·2).
*Bacterial infections.*

**Eryc**
*Faulding, Austral.; Pfizer, Canad.; Faulding, Hong Kong†; Taro, Israel; Parke, Davis, Neth.; Parke, Davis, NZ†; Warner Chilcott, USA.*
Erythromycin (p.208·1).
*Bacterial infections.*

*Faulding, Port.*
Erythromycin lactobionate (p.208·2).
*Bacterial infections.*

**Erycette**
*Janssen-Cilag, S.Afr.; Ortho Dermatological, USA.*
Erythromycin (p.208·1).
*Acne.*

**Erycin**
*Nycomed, Denm.*
Erythromycin (p.208·1) or erythromycin ethyl succinate (p.208·1).
*Bacterial infections.*

*Atlantic, Thai.*
Erythromycin stearate (p.208·2).
*Bacterial infections.*

**Erycinum** *CytoChemia, Ger.*
Erythromycin lactobionate (p.208·2).
*Bacterial infections.*

**Erycocci** *Pharmafarm, Fr.†.*
Erythromycin ethyl succinate (p.208·1).
*Bacterial infections.*

**Erycytol** *Lannacher, Austria.*
Hydroxocobalamin (p.1458·2).
*Herpes zoster infections; liver disorders; macrocytic anaemias; neuralgia; neuritis; tobacco amblyopia; vitamin $B_{12}$ deficiency.*

**Eryderm**
*Abbott, Belg.; Abbott, Israel; Abbott, Malaysia; Abbott, Mex.; Abbott, Neth.; Abbott, S.Afr.; Abbott, Singapore; Abbott, Switz.; Abbott, USA.*
Erythromycin (p.208·1).
*Acne.*

**Erydermec** *Bioglan, Ger.*
Erythromycin (p.208·1).
*Acne.*

**Ery-Diolan** *Brahms, Ger.*
Erythromycin ethyl succinate (p.208·1) or erythromycin stearate (p.208·2).
*Bacterial infections.*

**Eryfer** *Cassella-med, Ger.*
Ferrous sulfate (p.1428·2).
*Iron deficiency; iron-deficiency anaemias.*

**Eryfer comp** *Cassella-med, Ger.*
Ferrous sulfate (p.1428·2); cyanocobalamin (p.1458·2); folic acid (p.1429·1).
*Iron and vitamin deficiency.*

**Eryfluid**
*Pierre Fabre, Arg.; Pierre Fabre, Fr.; Pierre Fabre, Port.*
Erythromycin (p.208·1).
*Acne.*

**Erygel** *Merz, USA.*
Erythromycin (p.208·1).
*Acne; skin infections.*

**Eryhexal**
*Hexal, Austral.; Hexal, Austria; Hexal, Ger.*
Erythromycin ethyl succinate (p.208·1) or erythromycin stearate (p.208·2).
*Bacterial infections.*

**Erylar** *Arlex, Mex.†.*
Erythromycin (p.208·1).
*Bacterial infections.*

**Erylik**
*Biorga, Fr.; Biorga, Hong Kong.*
Erythromycin (p.208·1); tretinoin (p.1161·1).
*Acne.*

**Erymax**
*Elan, Irl.; Parke-Med, S.Afr.†; Elan, UK; Allergan, USA.*
Erythromycin (p.208·1).
*Bacterial infections.*

**Ery-Max**
*AstraZeneca, Norw.; I Farmacologia, Spain†; Astra, Swed.*
Erythromycin (p.208·1), or erythromycin ethyl succinate (p.208·1), or erythromycin lactobionate (p.208·2).
*Bacterial infections.*

**Erymin** *Milano, Thai.*
Erythromycin estolate (p.208·1).
*Bacterial infections.*

**Erymycin** *Triomed, S.Afr.*
Erythromycin estolate (p.208·1) or erythromycin stearate (p.208·2).
*Bacterial infections.*

**Eryped**
*Abbott, Hong Kong†; Abbott, Malaysia; Abbott, Singapore.*
Erythromycin ethyl succinate (p.208·1).
*Bacterial infections.*

**Ery-Ped** *Abbott, USA.*
Erythromycin ethyl succinate (p.208·1).
*Bacterial infections.*

**Eryplast** *Boots Healthcare, Fr.*
Barrier cream.
*Nappy rash.*

**Erypo**
*Janssen-Cilag, Austria; Janssen-Cilag, Ger.*
Epoetin alfa (p.747·2).
*Anaemias; autologous blood transfusion.*

**Ery-Reu** *Reusch, Ger.†.*
Erythromycin lactobionate (p.208·2).
*Bacterial infections.*

**Erysafe** *USV, India.*
Erythromycin (p.208·1).
*Bacterial infections.*

**Erysec** *Lindopharm, Ger.*
Erythromycin stinoprate (p.210·3).
*Bacterial infections.*

**Ery-Set** *Ebewe, Austria.*
Sodium chloride (p.1233·3).
*Diluent for concentrated erythrocyte suspensions.*

**Erysidoron**
*Weleda, Austria; Weleda, Ger.; Weleda, UK.*
A range of homoeopathic preparations.

**Erysil** *Silom, Thai.*
Erythromycin estolate (p.208·1).
*Bacterial infections.*

**Erysol**
*Stiefel, Canad.*
Erythromycin (p.208·1).
*Acne.*

*Xepa-Soul Pattinson, Hong Kong†; Xepa-Soul Pattinson, Singapore.*
Erythromycin ethyl succinate (p.208·1).
*Bacterial infections.*

**Erysolvan** *Fresenius Kabi, Austria†.*
Erythromycin stinoprate (p.210·3).
*Bacterial infections.*

**Eryson**
*Upha, Malaysia.*
Erythromycin ethyl succinate (p.208·1) or erythromycin stearate (p.208·2).
*Bacterial infections.*

*Beacons, Singapore.*
Erythromycin (p.208·1) or erythromycin ethyl succinate (p.208·1).
*Bacterial infections.*

**Erystad** *Stada, Austria.*
Erythromycin stearate (p.208·2).
*Bacterial infections.*

**Erystamine-K** *Biostam (Βιοσταμ), Gr.*
Sodium cromoglicate (p.795·3).
*Allergic conjunctivitis; allergic rhinitis.*

**Erystat** *Medpro, S.Afr.†.*
Erythromycin estolate (p.208·1).
*Bacterial infections.*

**Erystrat** *Orion, Denm.†.*
Erythromycin acistrate (p.208·1).
*Bacterial infections.*

**Erytab** *Abbott, Israel†.*
Erythromycin (p.208·1).
*Bacterial infections.*

**Ery-Tab**
*Abbott, Thai.; Abbott, USA.*
Erythromycin (p.208·1).
*Bacterial infections.*

**Erytab-S** *Xepa-Soul Pattinson, Singapore†.*
Erythromycin stearate (p.208·2).
*Bacterial infections.*

**Eryteal** *Pierre Fabre, Fr.†.*
Cod-liver oil (p.1425·2); halibut-liver oil (p.1434·1); zinc oxide (p.1163·2); cetrimonium bromide (p.1173·1).
*Burns; nappy rash.*

**Eryth-mycin** *Pond's, Thai.*
Erythromycin estolate (p.208·1) or erythromycin stearate (p.208·2).
*Bacterial infections.*

**Erythra-Derm** *Paddock, USA†.*
Erythromycin (p.208·1).
Formerly known as ETS-2%.
*Acne.*

**Erythro**
*CT, Ger.; DHA, Hong Kong.*
Erythromycin ethyl succinate (p.208·1) or erythromycin stearate (p.208·2).
*Bacterial infections.*

**Erythrocin**
*Abbott, Austral.; Abbott, Austria; Abbott, Canad.; Abbott, Ger.; Abbott, Gr.; Abbott, Hong Kong; Abbott, India; Abbott, Irl.; Abbott, Israel; Abbott, Malaysia; Abbott, S.Afr.; Abbott, Singapore; Abbott, Thai.; Abbott, UK; Abbott, USA.*
Erythromycin (p.208·1), erythromycin ethyl succinate (p.208·1), erythromycin lactobionate (p.208·2), or erythromycin stearate (p.208·2).
*Bacterial infections.*

**Erythrocin Neo** *Abbott, Ger.*
Erythromycin ethyl succinate (p.208·1).
*Bacterial infections.*

**Erythrocine**
*Abbott, Belg.; Abbott, Fr.; Abbott, Neth.; Abbott, Switz.*
Erythromycin ethyl succinate (p.208·1), erythromycin lactobionate (p.208·2), or erythromycin stearate (p.208·2).
*Bacterial infections.*

**Erythroderm** *Agis, Israel†.*
Erythromycin (p.208·1).
*Acne.*

**Erythroforte** *Abbott, Belg.*
Erythromycin ethyl succinate (p.208·1).
*Bacterial infections.*

**Erythrogel** *Biorga, Fr.*
Erythromycin (p.208·1).
*Acne.*

**Erythrogenat** *Azupharma, Ger.*
Erythromycin ethyl succinate (p.208·1) or erythromycin stearate (p.208·2).
*Bacterial infections.*

**Erythrogram** *Pharma 2000, Fr.*
Erythromycin ethyl succinate (p.208·1).
*Bacterial infections.*

**Erythro-Hefa** *Hefa, Ger.*
Erythromycin stearate (p.208·2).
*Bacterial infections.*

**Erythrol** *Vitamed, Israel.*
Erythromycin ethyl succinate (p.208·1).
*Bacterial infections.*

**Erythromid**
*Abbott, Canad.†; Abbott, Irl.†; Abbott, S.Afr.†; Abbott, UK†.*
Erythromycin (p.208·1).
*Bacterial infections.*

**Erythroped**
*Abbott, Irl.; Abbott, Israel; Abbott, S.Afr.; Abbott, UK.*
Erythromycin ethyl succinate (p.208·1).
*Bacterial infections.*

**Erythro-Teva** *Teva, Israel.*
Erythromycin (p.208·1), erythromycin ethyl succinate (p.208·1), or erythromycin stearate (p.208·2).
*Bacterial infections.*

**Erytop** *Stada, Ger.†.*
Erythromycin (p.208·1).
*Acne.*

**Erytran** *Spirig, Switz.†.*
Erythromycin stearate (p.208·2).
*Bacterial infections.*

**Erytrociclin** *Lisapharma, Ital.*
Erythromycin stearate (p.208·2).
*Bacterial infections.*

**Eryval** *Smetana, Austria.*
Absinthium (p.1645·1); centaury (p.1669·2); hypericum (p.299·1); peppermint leaf (p.1283·2); valerian (p.1762·2).
*Gastrointestinal disorders.*

**Eryzole** *Alra, USA.*
Erythromycin ethyl succinate (p.208·1); acetyl sulfafurazole (p.260·1).
*Otitis media.*

**ES Bronchial Mixture** *Torbet Laboratories, UK†.*
Squill (p.1130·3); ipecacuanha tincture (p.1122·3); senega (p.1130·2); ammonium bicarbonate (p.1115·1).
*Coughs.*

**Esacinone** *Lisapharma, Ital.*
Fluocinolone acetonide (p.1101·2).
*Skin disorders.*

**Esafosfina**
*Biomedica, Hong Kong; Biomedica, Ital.; Biomedica, Thai.*
Sodium fructose-1,6-diphosphate.
*Hypophosphataemia; ischaemia of lower limbs; myocardial infarction; regional ischaemia; shock.*

**Esafosfina Glutammica** *Biomedica, Hong Kong.*
Calcium fructose-1,6-diphosphate; vitamin B substances (p.1417·1); glutamine (p.1433·2).
*Metabolic disorders.*

**Esaglut** *Biomedica, Ital.*
Glutamine (p.1433·2); dicalcium fructose-1,6-diphosphate; thiamine nitrate (p.1455·1); pyridoxine hydrochloride (p.1456·3); calcium pantothenate (p.1442·3).
*Asthenia; mental function impairment; tonic.*

**Esalfon** *Recalcine, Chile.*
Enalapril maleate (p.909·2).
*Heart failure; hypertension.*

**Esalfon-D** *Recalcine, Chile.*
Enalapril maleate (p.909·2); hydrochlorothiazide (p.933·2).
*Hypertension.*

**Esametone** *Lisapharma, Ital.*
Methylprednisolone (p.1106·1).
*Oral corticosteroid.*

**Esanic** *Merck, Arg.*
Idebenone (p.1700·3).
*Dementia.*

**Esapent** *Pharmacia, Ital.*
Omega-3 triglycerides (p.976·1).
*Hypertriglyceridaemia.*

**Esarondil** *Terapeutico, Ital.*
Methacycline hydrochloride (p.230·1).
*Bacterial infections.*

**Esavir** *Boniscontro & Gazzone, Ital.*
Aciclovir (p.626·1).
*Herpesvirus infections.*

**Esbelcaps** *Medix, Mex.*
Fenproporex hydrochloride (p.1588·3); diazepam (p.690·1).
*Obesity.*

**Esbelt** *Virtus, Braz.†.*
Thyroid (p.1604·2); bladderwrack (p.1742·3); bile salts (p.1660·3); phenolphthalein (p.1284·1).

**Esbeltex** *Medix, Mex.*
Glucomannan (p.1693·3).
*Hyperglycaemia; hyperlipidaemias; obesity.*

**Esbeltrat** *Luper, Braz.†.*
Thyroid (p.1604·2); bladderwrack (p.1742·3); phenolphthalein (p.1284·1).

**Esbericard**
*Europharm, Austria; Asta Medica, Switz.†.*
Crataegus (p.1677·1).
*Cardiac disorders.*

**Esbericard novo** *Schaper & Brummer, Ger.*
Crataegus (p.1677·1).
*Heart failure.*

**Esbericum**
*Europharm, Austria; Schaper & Brummer, Ger.*
Hypericum (p.299·1).
*Anxiety; depression.*

**Esberitop** *Zeller, Switz.*
*Oral drops:* Thuja (p.1755·1); echinacea (p.1683·2); baptisia tinctoria.
*Tablets:* Thuja (p.1755·1); echinacea (p.1683·2); baptisia tinctoria; vitamin C (p.1460·2).
*Cold symptoms.*

**Esberitox mono** *Schaper & Brummer, Ger.*
Echinacea purpurea (p.1683·2).
*Respiratory-tract infections.*

**Esberitox N**
*Schaper & Brummer, Ger.; Asta Medica, Switz.†.*
Thuja (p.1755·1); baptisia tinctoria; echinacea purpurea et pallida (p.1683·2).
*Respiratory-tract infections; tonic.*

**Esberiven**
*Note. This name is used for preparations of different composition.*
*Craveri, Arg.*
*Tablets:* Coumarin (p.1676·2); troxerutin (p.1688·3).
*Venous insufficiency.*
*Topical application:* Coumarin (p.1676·2).
*Soft-tissue disorders.*

*Knoll, Fr.*
Melilot; heparin sodium (p.928·1).
*Peripheral vascular disorders.*

*Iquinosa, Spain.*
Melilot; troxerutin (p.1688·3).
*Peripheral vascular disorders.*

**Esberiven Fort** *Knoll, Fr.*
Melilot; rutoside (p.1688·2).
*Haemorrhoids; venous insufficiency.*

**Escabin** *Virtus, Braz.†.*
Lindane (p.1506·3).
*Pediculosis; scabies.*

**Escabron** *Hebron, Braz.*
Lindane (p.1506·3).
*Pediculosis; scabies.*

**Escacin** *Reuffer, Mex.†.*
Benzyl benzoate (p.1500·2).

**Escalgin sans codeine** *Streuli, Switz.*
Salicylamide (p.87·3); propyphenazone (p.85·3); caffeine (p.782·1).
*Fever; pain.*

**Escancil** *Grunenthal, Chile.*
Metamfetamine hydrochloride (p.1589·2).
*Attention-deficit hyperactivity disorder; obesity.*

**Escandine**
*Strallhofer, Austria; Zambon, Braz.; Pharmazam, Spain.*
Ibopamine hydrochloride (p.937·3).
*Heart failure.*

**Escapin-N** *Streger, Mex.*
Hyoscine butylbromide (p.483·3); paracetamol (p.76·2).
*Smooth muscle pain and spasm.*

**Escar T** *Prater, Chile.*
Centella (p.1144·3).

**Escar T-Neomicina** *Prater, Chile.*
Neomycin (p.235·1); centella (p.1144·3).

**Escarbicida** *Stafford, Mex.*†.
Lindane (p.1506·3).

**Escarine** *Rivadis, Fr.*
Barrier preparation.

**Escarol** *Muller Goppingen, Ger.*
Asarabacca (p.1658·1).
*Respiratory-tract disorders.*

**Escatitona** *Madaus, Austria.*
Homoeopathic preparation.

**Escina Forte** *Omega, Arg.*
Aescin (p.1648·2); hesperidin (p.1688·2).
*Haemorrhoids; venous insufficiency.*

**Escina Omega** *Omega, Arg.*
Aescin (p.1648·2); hesperidin (p.1688·2).
*Haemorrhoids; venous insufficiency.*

**Escinogel** *Bouchara-Recordati, Fr.*
Bamethan sulfate (p.866·3); aescin (p.1648·2).
*Peripheral vascular disorders.*

**Esclama** *Pharmacia, Ger.*
Nimorazole (p.611·3).
*Protozoal infections.*

**Esclebin** *Smaller, Spain.*
Norfloxacin (p.238·3).
*Bacterial infections.*

**Esclerobion** *Merck, Port.*
Vitamin A acetate (p.1453·1); pyridoxine hydrochloride (p.1456·3); *dl*-alpha tocoferil acetate (p.1465·1).
*Atherosclerosis; vascular disorders.*

**Esclerovitan** *Merck, Braz.*
Vitamins A, $B_6$, and E (p.1417·1).

**Esclerovitan A O** *Merck, Mex.*
Multivitamin and mineral preparation (p.1417·1).

**Esclerovitan Antioxidante** *Merck, Arg.*
Multivitamin and mineral preparation (p.1417·1).

**Esclerovitan E** *Merck, Arg.*
Vitamin A palmitate; pyridoxine hydrochloride; alpha tocoferil acetate (p.1417·1).

**Esclim** *Women First, USA.*
Estradiol (p.1550·1).
*Menopausal disorders; osteoporosis.*

**Esclima** *Takeda, Ital.*
Estradiol (p.1550·1).
*Menopausal disorders.*

**Escodarone** *Streuli, Switz.*
Amiodarone hydrochloride (p.859·2).
*Arrhythmias.*

**Escogripp sans codeine** *Streuli, Switz.*
Propyphenazone (p.85·3); salicylamide (p.87·3); caffeine (p.782·1); ascorbic acid (p.1460·2); mepyramine maleate (p.437·1).
*Cold and influenza symptoms.*

**Esconitro** *Streuli, Switz.*
Isosorbide dinitrate (p.941·1).
*Ischaemic heart disease.*

**Escophylline** *Streuli, Switz.*
Aminophylline (p.780·2).
*Obstructive airways disease.*

**Escoprim** *Streuli, Switz.*
Co-trimoxazole (p.199·3).
*Bacterial infections.*

**Escor**
*E. Merck, Denm.†; Pharmacal, Fin.; Trommsdorff, Ger.; Merck, Hong Kong†.*
Nilvadipine (p.972·2).
*Hypertension.*

**Escoretic** *Streuli, Switz.*
Amiloride hydrochloride (p.858·2); hydrochlorothiazide (p.933·2).
*Hypertension; oedema.*

**Escotussin** *Streuli, Switz.*
Dihydrocodeine thiocyanate (p.35·2); belladonna (p.479·1); drosera (p.1683·1); guaifenesin (p.1122·1).
*Coughs.*

**Escozem** *Streuli, Switz.*
Diltiazem hydrochloride (p.900·1).
*Hypertension; ischaemic heart disease.*

**Escudo** *Lampugnani, Ital.*
Sucralfate (p.1290·2).
*Gastritis; gastro-oesophageal reflux; peptic ulcer.*

**Esculeol P** *Medical, Arg.*
Benzocaine (p.1370·3); hamamelis (p.1696·3); camphor (p.1665·3); rhatany (p.1738·1).
*Haemorrhoids.*

**Escumycin** *Orion, Denm.*
Erythromycin (p.208·1) or erythromycin ethyl succinate (p.208·1).
*Bacterial infections.*

**ESE** *Abbott, Port.*
Erythromycin ethyl succinate (p.208·1).
*Bacterial infections.*

**Esedril** *Lipha, Ital.*†.
Naftidrofuryl oxalate (p.964·1).
*Cerebral and peripheral vascular disorders.*

**Eselan** *Anpharm (Ανφαρμ), Gr.*
Omeprazole (p.1278·2).
*Acid aspiration; eradication of Helicobacter pylori in combination with antimicrobials; peptic ulcer; reflux oesophagitis; Zollinger-Ellison syndrome.*

**Eselin** *Abbott, Ital.*
Etamsylate (p.749·3).
*Haemorrhage; vascular disorders.*

**Esforza** *Normon, Spain.*
Ginseng (p.1693·1); eleutherococcus senticosis (p.1744·1).
*Tonic.*

**Esgic** *Forest Pharmaceuticals, USA.*
Butalbital (p.673·3); paracetamol (p.76·2); caffeine (p.782·1).
*Tension headache.*

**Esgic-Plus** *Forest Pharmaceuticals, USA.*
Butalbital (p.673·3); paracetamol (p.76·2); caffeine (p.782·1).
*Tension headache.*

**Esgipyrin** *Sarabhai Piramal, India.*
Diclofenac sodium (p.32·1); paracetamol (p.76·2).
*Musculoskeletal and joint disorders; pain.*

**Esgipyrin DS** *Sarabhai Piramal, India.*
Diclofenac sodium (p.32·1).
*Pain.*

**Esidrex**
*Novartis, Austria; Ciba-Geigy, Belg.†; Novartis, Fr.; Novartis, India; Novartis, Ital.; Novartis, Neth.; Novartis, Norw.; Geminis, Spain; Novartis, Swed.; Novartis, Switz.*
Hydrochlorothiazide (p.933·2).
*Diabetes insipidus; heart failure; hypercalciuria; hypertension; oedema.*

**Esidrix**
*Novartis, Ger.; Ciba, USA.*
Hydrochlorothiazide (p.933·2).
*Hypertension; oedema.*

**Esilgan** *Takeda, Ital.*
Estazolam (p.697·3).
*Insomnia.*

**Esimil**
*Novartis, Ger.; Ciba, USA.*
Guanethidine monosulfate (p.926·3); hydrochlorothiazide (p.933·2).
*Hypertension.*

**Esiteren** *Novartis, Ger.*†.
Hydrochlorothiazide (p.933·2); triamterene (p.1016·2).
*Hypertension; oedema.*

**Eskaflam** *SmithKline Beecham, Mex.*
Nimesulide (p.67·1).
*Fever; inflammation; pain; peri-articular and soft-tissue disorders.*

**Eskalith** *SmithKline Beecham, USA.*
Lithium carbonate (p.301·1).
*Bipolar disorder.*

**Eskamel**
*Dermatech, Austral.; Goldshield, UK.*
Resorcinol (p.1156·3); precipitated sulfur (p.1158·2).
*Acne.*

**Eskapar** *SmithKline Beecham, Mex.*†.
Nifuroxazide (p.237·2).
*Diarrhoea.*

**Eskazine** *SmithKline Beecham, Spain.*
Trifluoperazine hydrochloride (p.726·3).
*Anxiety; psychoses.*

**Eskazole**
*GlaxoSmithKline, Austral.; GlaxoSmithKline, Austria; SmithKline Beecham, Fr.†; GlaxoSmithKline, Ger.; SmithKline Beecham, Israel; Armstrong, Mex.; GlaxoSmithKline, Neth.; Morrith, Spain; SmithKline Beecham, UK†.*
Albendazole (p.101·2).
*Cestode infections; giardiasis; intestinal nematode infections.*

**Eskim** *Sigma-Tau, Ital.*
Omega-3 triglycerides (p.976·1).
*Hypertriglyceridaemia.*

**Eskold** *GlaxoSmithKline, India.*
Phenylpropanolamine hydrochloride (p.1127·3); diphenylpyraline hydrochloride (p.432·3).
*Cold symptoms; hypersensitivity reactions; nasal congestion; rhinitis.*

**Eskold Expectorant** *GlaxoSmithKline, India.*
Phenylpropanolamine hydrochloride (p.1127·3); diphenylpyraline hydrochloride (p.432·3); guaifenesin (p.1122·1).
*Cold symptoms; hypersensitivity reactions; nasal congestion; rhinitis.*

**Eskornade**
*Pharmaco, S.Afr.†; Goldshield, UK†.*
Phenylpropanolamine hydrochloride (p.1127·3); diphenylpyraline hydrochloride (p.432·3).
*Nasal and sinus congestion.*

**Esmacen** *Smaller, Spain.*
Astemizole (p.424·2).
*Hypersensitivity reactions.*

**Esmalorid** *Merck, Ger.*
Trichlormethiazide (p.1017·2); amiloride hydrochloride (p.858·2).
*Hypertension; oedema.*

**Esme Topico** *Esme, Arg.*
Strontium chloride (p.1749·3); lidocaine hydrochloride (p.1377·3).
*Hypersensitive teeth.*

**Esmedent con Fluor** *Esme, Arg.*
Triclosan (p.1195·2); sodium fluoride (p.1444·3); benzocaine (p.1370·3); allantoin (p.1141·3).
*Dental hygiene; sensitive teeth.*

**Esmeron**
*Organon, Austral.; Organon Teknika, Austria; Organon, Belg.; Organon, Braz.; Organon, Chile; Organon, Denm.; Organon, Fin.; Organon, Fr.; Organon, Ger.; Organon (Οργκανον), Gr.; Organon, Hong Kong; Organon Teknika, Irl.; Organon Teknika, Israel; Organon, Ital.; Organon, Malaysia; Organon Teknika, Neth.; Organon Teknika, Norw.; Organon, NZ; Organon, Port.; Sanofi Synthelabo, S.Afr.; Organon, Singapore; Organon, Spain; Organon, Swed.; Organon, Switz.; Organon, Thai.; Organon, UK.*
Rocuronium bromide (p.1405·2).
*Competitive neuromuscular blocker.*

**Eso 70** *Esoform, Ital.*
Paraformaldehyde (p.1187·3); hydrogen peroxide 40/45 (p.1182·2).
*Room disinfection.*

**Eso Cem** *Esoform, Ital.*
Glutaral (p.1180·3).
*Instrument disinfection.*

**Eso Deterferri** *Esoform, Ital.*
Benzalkonium chloride (p.1168·3).
*Instrument disinfection.*

**Eso Din** *Esoform, Ital.*
Glutaral (p.1180·3); phenol (p.1188·1).
*Instrument disinfection.*

**Eso Ferri** *Esoform, Ital.*
Benzalkonium chloride (p.1168·3).
*Instrument disinfection.*

**Eso Ferri Alcolico** *Esoform, Ital.*
Benzalkonium chloride (p.1168·3); alcohol (p.1166·1).
*Instrument disinfection.*

**Eso Ferri Alcolico Plus** *Esoform, Ital.*
Benzalkonium chloride (p.1168·3); isopropyl alcohol (p.1184·3).
*Instrument disinfection.*

**Eso Ferri Plus** *Esoform, Ital.*
Chlorhexidine gluconate (p.1173·2); isopropyl alcohol (p.1184·3).
*Instrument disinfection and storage.*

**Eso H1, HP, and HP1** *Esoform, Ital.*
Glutaral (p.1180·3).
*Instrument disinfection.*

**Eso S 80** *Esoform, Ital.*
Benzalkonium chloride (p.1168·3); chlorhexidine gluconate (p.1173·2).
*Instrument disinfection.*

**Eso Zim** *Esoform, Ital.*
Proteolytic enzymes; sodium laurilsulfate (p.1574·2); cocoamidopropylbetaine.
*Instrument disinfection.*

**Esoalcolico Incolore** *Esoform, Ital.*
Benzalkonium chloride (p.1168·3); alcohol (p.1166·1).
*Skin, hand, burn, and wound disinfection.*

**Esocetic** *Esoform, Ital.*
Peracetic acid (p.1187·3); isopropyl alcohol (p.1184·3).
*Instrument disinfection.*

**Esodar** *Biocumed, Arg.; Cassara, Arg.*
Prednisolone (p.1108·1); chloramphenicol (p.185·1).
*Infected eye and ear disorders.*

**Esodrox** *Esoform, Ital.*
Peracetic acid (p.1187·3).
*Instrument disinfection.*

**Esofenol 60** *Esoform, Ital.*
Sodium *o*-phenylphenol (p.1187·2).
*Waste disinfection.*

**Esofenol Ferri** *Esoform, Ital.*
Orthobenzyl parachlorophenol (p.1187·3); orthophenylphenol (p.1187·2).
*Instrument disinfection.*

**Esofex** *Leiras, Fin.*
Ranitidine hydrochloride (p.1285·2).
*Dyspepsia; heartburn; peptic ulcer.*

**Esoform 92** *Esoform, Ital.*
Benzalkonium chloride (p.1168·3); glutaral (p.1180·3); alkylphenoxypolyglycol ether.
*Surface disinfection.*

**Esoform Alcolico** *Esoform, Ital.*
Benzalkonium chloride (p.1168·3); methyl salicylate; camphor; thyme oil; alcohol (p.1166·1); acetone; chloroform.
*Skin disinfection.*

**Esoform Deterferri** *Esoform, Ital.*†.
Benzalkonium chloride (p.1168·3).
*Instrument disinfection.*

**Esoform Ferri** *Esoform, Ital.*†.
Benzalkonium chloride (p.1168·3); sodium nitrite (p.1052·3); methylthioninium chloride.
*Instrument disinfection.*

**Esoform Ferri Alcolico** *Esoform, Ital.*†.
Benzalkonium chloride (p.1168·3); alcohol (p.1166·1); sodium nitrite (p.1052·3); acetone; chloroform.
*Instrument disinfection.*

**Esoform Jod 25** *Esoform, Ital.*
Alkylphenoxypolyglycol-iodine-ether complex.
*Room and surface disinfection.*

**Esoform Jod 35 and 75** *Esoform, Ital.*
Povidone-iodine (p.1190·3).
*Skin, wound, and hand disinfection.*

**Esoform Jod 20 and 50** *Esoform, Ital.*
Iodine (p.1598·1); potassium iodide (p.1598·1); alcohol; chloroform; isopropyl alcohol.
*Skin and hand disinfection.*

**Esoform Mani** *Esoform, Ital.*
Chlorhexidine gluconate (p.1173·2); isopropyl alcohol; chloroform; alcohol.
*Skin and hand disinfection.*

**Esoform Maniferri** *Esoform, Ital.*†.
Chlorhexidine gluconate (p.1173·2); isopropyl alcohol (p.1184·3).
*Skin, hand, and instrument disinfection.*

**Esoform 7 mc** *Esoform, Ital.*
Paraformaldehyde (p.1187·3); hydrogen peroxide (40-45 volume) (p.1182·2).
*Surface and room disinfection.*

**Esoform 70 mc** *Esoform, Ital.*
Paraformaldehyde (p.1187·3); hydrogen peroxide (40-45 volume) (p.1182·2).
*Room disinfection.*

**Eso-Jod** *Esoform, Ital.*
Povidone-iodine (p.1190·3).
*Wound disinfection.*

**Esol** *Leiras, Fin.*
*d*-Alpha tocopherol (p.1464·3).
*Vitamin E deficiency.*

**Esolut** *Angelini, Ital.*
Progesterone (p.1566·2).
*Luteal insufficiency.*

**E-Solve** *Syosset, USA.*
Vehicle for topical preparations.

**Esonide** *Kleva, Gr.*
Budesonide (p.1094·2).
*Allergic rhinitis; topical corticosteroid.*

**Esopral** *Bracco, Ital.*
Esomeprazole magnesium (p.1265·1).
*Gastro-oesophageal reflux; peptic ulcer.*

**Esorid** *Sun, Thai.*
Cisapride (p.1259·2).
*Dyspepsia; gastro-oesophageal reflux; gastrointestinal motility disorders.*

**Esosan** *Esoform, Ital.*
Benzalkonium chloride (p.1168·3).
*Skin and surface disinfection.*

**Esosan Casa** *Esoform, Ital.*
Benzalkonium chloride (p.1168·3).
*Surface disinfection.*

**Esosan Pronto** *Esoform, Ital.*
Chlorhexidine gluconate (p.1173·2); benzalkonium chloride (p.1168·3).
*Disinfection.*

**Esoterica**
*Medicis, Canad.*
Hydroquinone (p.1148·1); oxybenzone (p.1154·3); padimate O (p.1155·1).
*Skin pigmentation disorders.*

*Lentheric, UK†.*
Hydroquinone (p.1148·1).

**Esoterica Facial and Sunscreen** *Medicis, USA.*
Hydroquinone (p.1148·1); padimate O (p.1155·1); oxybenzone (p.1154·3).
*Hyperpigmentation.*

**Esoterica Regular**
*Medicis, Canad.; Medicis, USA.*
Hydroquinone (p.1148·1).
*Skin pigmentation disorders.*

**Esoterica Unscented** *Medicis, Canad.*
Hydroquinone (p.1148·1).
*Skin pigmentation disorders.*

**Esotran** *Almirall, Spain*†.
Estradiol (p.1550·1).
*Menopausal disorders; osteoporosis.*

**Esoxid** *Esoform, Ital.*
Glutaral (p.1180·3).
*Instrument disinfection.*

**Espabion** *Degorts, Mex.*
Trimebutine (p.1758·1).
*Gastrointestinal motility disorders.*

**espa-butyl** *Esparma, Ger.*†.
Hyoscine butylbromide (p.483·3).
*Smooth muscle spasm.*

**Espacil** *ICN, Mex.*
Hyoscine butylbromide (p.483·3).
*Smooth muscle spasm.*

**Espacil Compuesto** *ICN, Mex.*
Hyoscine butylbromide (p.483·3); clonixin lysine (p.26·3).
*Smooth muscle pain and spasm.*

**Espadol** *Reckitt & Colman, Arg.*
Chloroxylenol (p.1177·2).
*Disinfection.*

**espa-dorm** *Esparma, Ger.*
Zopiclone (p.729·3).
*Sleep disorders.*

**espa-formin** *Esparma, Ger.*
Metformin hydrochloride (p.342·3).
*Diabetes mellitus.*

**espa-lepsin** *Esparma, Ger.*
Carbamazepine (p.353·3).
*Alcohol withdrawal syndrome; bipolar disorder; diabetic neuropathy; epilepsy; multiple sclerosis; neuralgias.*

**espa-lipon** *Esparma, Ger.*
Thioctic acid (p.1754·3) or ethylenediamine thioctate (p.1754·3).
*Diabetic polyneuropathy.*

**espa-moxin** *Esparma, Ger.*
Amoxicillin trihydrate (p.155·3).
*Bacterial infections.*

**Espar** *Greater Pharma, Thai.*
Aspartame (p.1422·1).
*Sugar substitute.*

**Esparil** *Esparma, Ger.*†.
Captopril (p.879·2).
*Heart failure; hypertension.*

**Esparon** *Orion, Ger.†.*
Alprazolam (p.668·3).
*Anxiety.*

**Espasal** *Offenbach, Mex.*
Dimeticone (p.1289·2); pipenzolate (p.487·3).
*Smooth muscle spasm.*

**Espasantral** *Carnot, Mex.†.*
Hyoscine methobromide (p.483·3).

**Espasevit** *Richmond, Arg.*
Ondansetron (p.1281·1).
*Nausea and vomiting.*

**Espasmacid** *Gemballa, Braz.*
Aluminium hydroxide (p.1249·2); magnesium hydroxide (p.1272·2); dimethicone (p.1289·2).
*Flatulence; gastrointestinal hyperacidity.*

**Espasmalgon** *Dovalle, Braz.*
Papaverine hydrochloride (p.1728·1); phenobarbital (p.367·3); homatropine methylbromide (p.483·2); phenazone (p.82·3); hyoscyamus (p.485·2).
*Smooth muscle spasm.*

**Espasmo Biotenk** *Biotenk, Arg.*
Hyoscine butylbromide (p.483·3); dipyrone (p.35·3).
*Painful smooth muscle spasm.*

**Espasmo Canulase** *Novartis Consumer, Port.*
Cellulase (p.1669·1); dimeticone (p.1289·2); glutamic acid hydrochloride (p.1433·2); metixene hydrochloride (p.485·3); pancreatin (p.1725·3); pepsin (p.1729·3); sodium dehydrocholate (p.1679·2).

**Espasmo Cibalena** *Novartis, Arg.*
Propyphenazone (p.85·3); drofenine hydrochloride (p.482·1).

**Espasmo Cibalena Fuerte** *Novartis, Arg.*
Propyphenazone (p.85·3); drofenine hydrochloride (p.482·1); codeine phosphate (p.27·1).

**Espasmo Cibalgina**
*Novartis, Chile; Novartis, Mex.*
Drofenine hydrochloride (p.482·1); propyphenazone (p.85·3).
*Smooth muscle pain and spasm.*

**Espasmo Cibalgina Compuesta** *Novartis, Chile.*
Propyphenazone (p.85·3); drofenine hydrochloride (p.482·1); codeine phosphate (p.27·1).
*Smooth muscle spasm and pain.*

**Espasmo Colic** *Makros, Braz.†.*
Homatropine methylbromide (p.483·2); dimethicone (p.1289·2).
*Smooth muscle spasm.*

**Espasmo Digestomen** *Menarini, Spain†.*
Amylase (p.1654·2); methionine phenylbutyrate; nicotinic acid (p.1441·1); papain (p.1727·3); pepsin (p.1729·3); flopropione (p.1689·1); betaine hydrochloride (p.1660·2); pancreatin (p.1725·3); lipase; bile extract (p.1660·3); cellulase (p.1669·1); hemicellulase (p.1669·1).
*Biliary-tract disorders; digestive system insufficiency; dyspepsia; meteorism.*

**Espasmo Dioxadol** *Bago, Arg.*
Octatropine methylbromide (p.486·1); dipyrone (p.35·3).
*Painful smooth muscle spasm.*

**Espasmo Dolex** *Armstrong, Arg.*
Clonixin lysine (p.26·3); pargeverine (p.487·3).
*Smooth muscle spasm.*

**Espasmo Ibupirac** *Pharmacia, Arg.*
Ibuprofen (p.45·3); homatropine methylbromide (p.483·2).
*Painful smooth muscle spasm.*

**Espasmo Luftal** *Bristol-Myers Squibb, Braz.*
Homatropine methylbromide (p.483·2); dimethicone (p.1289·2).
*Smooth muscle spasm.*

**Espasmo Motrax** *Labinca, Arg.*
Ciclonium bromide (p.480·2); ibuprofen (p.45·3).
*Painful smooth muscle spasm.*

**Espasmo Novozyme** *Novartis, Braz.†.*
Metixene hydrochloride (p.485·3); dimethicone (p.1289·2); cellulase (p.1669·1); pepsin (p.1729·3); glutamic acid hydrochloride (p.1433·2); pancreatin (p.1725·3); sodium dehydrocholate (p.1679·2).
*Digestive-system disorders.*

**Espasmo Silidron** *GlaxoSmithKline, Braz.*
Dimeticone (p.1289·2); camylofin (p.1666·1).
*Smooth muscle spasm.*

**Espasmobel** *Opofarm, Braz.†.*
Dipyrone (p.35·3); adiphenine hydrochloride (p.1648·1); papaverine (p.1728·1); homatropine (p.483·2).
*Smooth muscle spasm.*

**Espasmocron** *Delta, Braz.*
Atropine sulfate (p.477·1); papaverine hydrochloride (p.1728·1); thiamine hydrochloride (p.1455·1); dipyrone (p.35·3).
*Smooth muscle spasm.*

**Espasmodid Composto** *Uniao Quimica, Braz.*
Hyoscine butylbromide (p.483·3); dipyrone (p.35·3).
*Smooth muscle spasm.*

**Espasmofin**
*Note. This name is used for preparations of different composition.*
*Oriental, Arg.*
Homatropine (p.483·2); ibuprofen (p.45·3).
*Painful smooth muscle spasm.*

*Elofar, Braz.†.*
Homatropine methylbromide (p.483·2).
*Smooth muscle spasm.*

**Espasmolex** *Bergamo, Braz.†.*
Papaverine hydrochloride (p.1728·1); belladonna (p.479·1); star anise; hyoscyamus (p.485·2); boldo (p.1661·2).
*Smooth muscle spasm.*

**Espasmo-Ped** *Stiefel, Braz.†.*
Pargeverine hydrochloride (p.487·3).
*Nausea and vomiting.*

**Espasmosan** *Leofarma, Braz.†.*
Belladonna (p.479·1); papaverine hydrochloride (p.1728·1).
*Smooth muscle spasm.*

**Espasmosan Composto** *Leofarma, Braz.†.*
Belladonna (p.479·1); papaverine hydrochloride (p.1728·1); dipyrone (p.35·3).
*Smooth muscle spasm.*

**Espasmotropin** *Sintesina, Arg.*
Homatropine (p.483·2).
*Smooth muscle spasm.*

**Espa-Valept** *Esparma, Ger.*
Sodium valproate (p.380·1).
*Epilepsy.*

**Espaven** *ICN, Mex.*
Dimeticone (p.1289·2); calcium pantothenate (p.1442·3).
*Gastrointestinal disorders.*

**Espaven Alcalino** *ICN, Mex.*
Aluminium hydroxide (p.1249·2); magnesium hydroxide (p.1272·2); dimeticone (p.1289·2).
*Gastrointestinal disorders.*

**Espaven Enzimatico** *ICN, Mex.*
Pancreatin (p.1725·3); dimeticone (p.1289·2); ox bile (p.1660·3); *Aspergillus niger* cellulase (p.1669·1).
*Gastrointestinal disorders.*

**Espaven MD** *ICN, Mex.*
Metoclopramide hydrochloride (p.1274·3); dimeticone (p.1289·2).
*Gastrointestinal disorders.*

**Espaven Pediatrico** *ICN, Mex.*
Dimeticone (p.1289·2).
*Dyspepsia; flatulence; meteorism.*

**Especies Calmantes** *Bergamo, Braz.†.*
Passion flower (p.1729·1); erythrina mulungu (p.1717·2); melissa (p.1711·1).
*Sedative.*

**Espectocural** *Raymos, Arg.*
Bromhexine (p.1115·3); benzydamine (p.21·1).
*Coughs.*

**Espectral** *Centrum, Spain.*
Ampicillin trihydrate (p.157·2); muramidase hydrochloride (p.1717·2).
*Bacterial infections.*

**Espectral Balsamico** *Centrum, Spain†.*
Ampicillin trihydrate (p.157·2); guaifenesin (p.1122·1); muramidase hydrochloride (p.1717·2).
*Respiratory-tract infections.*

**Espectrin** *GlaxoSmithKline, Braz.*
Co-trimoxazole (p.199·3).
*Bacterial infections; Pneumocystis carinii pneumonia; protozoal infections.*

**Espectrosira** *Clariana, Spain.*
Ampicillin sodium (p.157·1); ampicillin benzathine (p.158·1); bromhexine hydrochloride (p.1115·3); guaifenesin (p.1122·1).
Lidocaine hydrochloride (p.1377·3) is included in this preparation to alleviate the pain of injection.
*Respiratory-tract infections.*

**Espeden** *Vita, Spain.*
Norfloxacin (p.238·3).
*Bacterial infections.*

**Esperal**
*Sanofi Synthelabo, Fr.; Torrent, India.*
Disulfiram (p.1681·3).
*Chronic alcoholism.*

**Espercil** *Grunenthal, Chile.*
Tranexamic acid (p.760·3).
*Haemorrhage; hyperfibrinolysis.*

**Espermicida Preserv** *Blausiegel, Braz.*
Nonoxinol 9 (p.1413·3).
*Contraceptive.*

**Esperson**
*Aventis, Braz.; Hoechst Marion Roussel, Hong Kong†; Aventis, Thai.*
Desoximetasone (p.1096·3).
*Skin disorders.*

**Esperson N** *Aventis, Braz.*
Desoximetasone (p.1096·3); neomycin sulfate (p.235·1).
*Infected skin disorders.*

**Espesil** *Orion, Fin.*
Acebutolol hydrochloride (p.848·1).
*Angina pectoris; arrhythmias; hypertension; myocardial infarction.*

**Espidifen** *Zambon, Spain.*
Ibuprofen arginine (p.46·3).
*Fever; musculoskeletal, joint, and peri-articular disorders; pain.*

**Espin** *Taejoon, Singapore.*
Dosulepin hydrochloride (p.291·1).
*Depression.*

**Espiran** *ICT, Ital.†.*
Fenspiride hydrochloride (p.786·1).
*Respiratory-tract disorders.*

**Espiride** *Aspen, S.Afr.*
Sulpiride (p.722·2).
*Behaviour disorders; depression; peptic ulcer; psychoses; vertigo.*

**Espirolona** *Cazi, Braz.*
Spironolactone (p.1003·1).
*Hypertension.*

**Espledol** *Fher, Spain.*
Acemetacin (p.11·3).
*Musculoskeletal and joint disorders; peri-articular disorders.*

**Espo** *Kirin, Jpn.*
Epoetin alfa (p.747·2).
*Anaemia; autologous blood transfusion.*

**Espongostan** *Byk Leo, Spain†.*
Gelatin (p.754·3).
*Mucous membrane haemorrhage.*

**Espotabs** *Combe, Canad.†.*
Yellow phenolphthalein (p.1284·1).

**Esprenit** *Hennig, Ger.*
Ibuprofen (p.45·3) or ibuprofen sodium (p.46·3).
*Fever; inflammation; musculoskeletal, joint, and soft-tissue disorders; pain.*

**Esprit** *Bayer, Austral.*
Test for glucose in blood (p.1694·2).

**Esprit Sensor** *Bayer Diagnostics, Irl.*
Test for glucose in blood.
For use with Esprit Glucometer.

**Espritin** *Petrasch, Austria.*
Lactic acid (p.1704·1).
*Psoriasis.*

**Espumisan** *Berlin-Chemie, Ger.*
Simeticone (p.1289·2).
*Defoaming agent in radiography and endoscopy of the gastrointestinal tract.*

**Esracain** *Rafa, Israel.*
Lidocaine hydrochloride (p.1377·3).
*Arrhythmias; local anaesthesia.*

**Esradin** *Sigma-Tau, Ital.*
Isradipine (p.942·2).
*Hypertension.*

**Essamin** *Torre, Ital.†.*
Amino-acid preparation (p.1417·1).
*Renal failure.*

**Essaven**
*Note. This name is used for preparations of different composition.*
*Nattermann, Ger.; Aventis, S.Afr.*
*Topical gel:* Aescin (p.1648·2); heparin sodium (p.928·1); essential phospholipids.
*Soft-tissue trauma; vascular disorders.*

*Rhone-Poulenc Rorer, Hong Kong†; Aventis, S.Afr.; Aventis, Thai.*
*Capsules:* Aescin (p.1648·2); rutoside (p.1688·2); essential phospholipids.
*Vascular disorders.*

*Aventis, Ital.*
*Capsules:* Aescin (p.1648·2); phosphatidyl choline (p.1731·1).
*Topical gel:* Aescin (p.1648·2); heparin sodium (p.928·1); phosphatidyl choline (p.1731·1).
*Venous insufficiency.*

**Essaven 60 000** *Nattermann, Ger.*
Heparin sodium (p.928·1).
*Soft-tissue disorders; superficial vascular disorders.*

**Essaven Mono** *Nattermann, Ger.†.*
Aesculus (p.1648·2).
*Chronic venous insufficiency.*

**Essaven N** *Nattermann, Ger.*
Aesculus (p.1648·2); trimethylhesperidin chalcone (p.1688·3).
*Soft-tissue disorders; vascular disorders.*

**Essaven Sport** *Nattermann, Ger.*
Glycol salicylate (p.44·3); arnica tincture (p.1656·3).
*Sports injuries.*

**Essaven Tri-Complex** *Nattermann, Ger.*
Heparin sodium (p.928·1); allantoin (p.1141·3); dexpanthenol (p.1727·2).
*Soft-tissue disorders; superficial vascular disorders.*

**Essaven ultra** *Nattermann, Ger.*
Aesculus (p.1648·2); trimethylhesperidin chalcone (p.1688·3); essential phospholipids.
*Soft-tissue injury; vascular disorders.*

**Essavenon** *Aventis, Spain.*
Aescin (p.1648·2); phospholipids; heparin sodium (p.928·1).
*Peripheral vascular disorders; soft-tissue disorders.*

**Esseldon** *Anpharm (Ανφαρμ), Gr.*
Famotidine (p.1265·2).
*Conditions where gastric acid reduction is beneficial; gastric hypersecretion including Zollinger-Ellison syndrome; peptic ulcer.*

**Essen** *Farmasa, Braz.*
Metoclopramide hydrochloride (p.1274·3); dimethicone (p.1289·2); dehydrocholic acid (p.1679·2); cellulase (p.1669·1); pepsin (p.1729·3); lipase; amylase (p.1654·2); pancreatin (p.1725·3).
*Digestive-system disorders.*

**Essen Enzimatico** *EG, Ital.*
Pepsin (p.1729·3); amylase (p.1654·2); lipase; trypsin (p.1758·3); chymotrypsin (p.1671·2); cellulase (p.1669·1).
*Dyspepsia.*

**Essence Algerienne** *Toulade, Fr.*
Cineole (p.1672·1); menthol (p.1711·3); guaiacol (p.1122·1).
*Upper respiratory-tract congestion.*

**Essential 50+** *Pharmavite, Canad.*
Multivitamin and mineral preparation (p.1417·1).

**Essential B** *General Nutrition, Canad.*
Vitamin B substances (p.1417·1).

**Essential Balance** *Pharmavite, Canad.*
Multivitamin and mineral preparation (p.1417·1).

**Essential ProPlus** *Nutrisoy, USA.*
Preparation for enteral nutrition (p.1417·1).

**Essentiale**
*Note. This name is used for preparations of different composition.*
*Gerot, Austria; Aventis, Hong Kong; Aventis, Malaysia; Aventis, S.Afr.; Aventis, Thai.*
Essential phospholipids; vitamins (p.1417·1).
*Liver disorders.*

*Aventis, Ital.*
Phosphatidyl choline (p.1731·1).
*Liver disorders.*

**Essentiale N** *Nattermann, Ger.*
Essential phospholipids.
*Gallstones; liver disorders; psoriasis; radiation trauma.*

**Essentiale-L** *Nicholas Piramal, India.*
Lecithin (p.1706·1).
*Liver disorders.*

**Essentielle Aminosauren** *Fresenius Kabi, Ger.*
Amino-acid preparation (p.1417·1).
*Dietary supplement in renal failure.*

**Essex**
*Schering-Plough, Denm.; Essex, Ger.; Essex, Switz.*
Emollient.
*Skin disorders.*

*Schering-Plough, Fin.*
A range of vehicles for topical preparations.

**Essigsaure Tonerde-Salbe** *Michallik, Ger.*
Aluminium acetotartrate (p.1652·3).
*Soft-tissue disorders.*

**Essitol** *Athenstaedt, Ger.*
Aluminium acetotartrate (p.1652·3).
*Hyperhidrosis; soft-tissue injury.*

**EST** *Rosch & Handel, Austria.*
Alum (p.1652·1); calcium acetate (p.1225·1); calcium carbonate (p.1254·2).
*Bruises; insect bites; sprains; swelling.*

**Establix** *BA Farma, Port.*
Buspirone hydrochloride (p.672·2).
*Anxiety; insomnia.*

**Estac** *Gross, Braz.*
Metoclopramide hydrochloride (p.1274·3); pyridoxine hydrochloride (p.1456·3).
*Nausea and vomiting.*

**Estafan** *Heralds, Braz.†.*
Arginine; vitamin C (p.1417·1).
*Nutritional supplement.*

**Estafiloide** *IQB, Braz.*
A staphylococcal vaccine (toxoid) (p.1640·2).
*Active immunisation.*

**Estalis**
*Novartis, Austria; Novartis, Braz.; Novartis, Canad.; Novartis, Fin.; Novartis, Irl.; Novartis, Norw.; Novartis, Port.; Novartis, Spain; Novartis, Swed.; Novartis, Switz.*
Estradiol (p.1550·1); norethisterone acetate (p.1562·2).
*Menopausal disorders; osteoporosis.*

**Estalis Continuous** *Novartis, Austral.*
Estradiol (p.1550·1); norethisterone acetate (p.1562·2).
*Menopausal disorders; osteoporosis.*

**Estalis Sekvens**
*Novartis, Fin.*
4 Patches, estradiol (p.1550·1); 4 patches, estradiol; norethisterone acetate (p.1562·2).
*Menopausal disorders; osteoporosis.*

*Novartis, Norw.; Novartis, Swed.*
Patch I, estradiol (p.1550·1); Patch II, estradiol; norethisterone acetate (p.1562·2).
*Menopausal disorders; osteoporosis.*

**Estalis Sequens** *Novartis, Austria.*
4 Patches, estradiol (p.1550·1); 4 patches, estradiol; norethisterone acetate (p.1562·2).
*Menopausal disorders; osteoporosis.*

**Estalis Sequi**
*Novartis, Austral.; Novartis, Irl.; Novartis, Port.; Novartis, Spain; Novartis, Switz.*
4 Patches, estradiol (p.1550·1); 4 patches, estradiol; norethisterone acetate (p.1562·2).
*Menopausal disorders; osteoporosis.*

*Novartis, Canad.*
Patches, estradiol (Vivelle) (p.1550·1); patches, estradiol; norethisterone acetate (Estalis) (p.1562·2).
*Menopausal disorders.*

*Novartis, Ger.; Novartis, Ital.*
Patch I, estradiol (p.1550·1); patch II, estradiol; norethisterone acetate (p.1562·2).
*Menopausal disorders; osteoporosis.*

**Estandron P** *Organon, Braz.*
Estradiol benzoate (p.1550·1); estradiol phenylpropionate (p.1550·2); testosterone propionate (p.1570·1); testosterone phenylpropionate (p.1570·1); testosterone isocaproate (p.1570·1).
*Menopausal disorders.*

**Estandron Prolongado** *Organon, Chile Solución oleosa inyectable para uso IM.*
Estradiol benzoate (p.1550·1); estradiol phenylpropionate (p.1550·2); testosterone propionate (p.1570·1); testosterone phenylpropionate (p.1570·1); testosterone isocaproate (p.1570·1).
*Menopausal disorders.*

**Estaprol**
*Sanofi Synthelabo, Arg.; Sanofi Synthelabo, Chile.*
Ciprofibrate (p.884·2).
*Hyperlipidaemias.*

**Estar**
Westwood-Squibb, Canad.; Westwood-Squibb, USA.
Coal tar (p.1159·2).
*Psoriasis.*

**Estecina**
APS, Port.
Ciprofloxacin (p.188·2) or ciprofloxacin hydrochloride (p.188·2).
*Bacterial infections.*
Normon, Spain.
Ciprofloxacin hydrochloride (p.188·2) or ciprofloxacin lactate (p.188·3).
*Bacterial infections.*

**Esteclin** Syntex, Mex.
Erdosteine (p.1121·1).
*Respiratory-tract disorders with viscous mucus.*

**Esteclin Bac** Syntex, Mex.
Amoxicillin trihydrate (p.155·3); erdosteine (p.1121·1).
*Respiratory-tract infections.*

**Estelle** Douglas, NZ.
21 Tablets, cyproterone acetate (p.1544·1); ethinylestradiol (p.1553·2); 7 tablets, inert.
*Androgen-dependent acne, alopecia, and hirsutism in females; oral contraceptive in women with androgenic symptoms; polycystic ovary syndrome.*

**Esteprim** Solfran, Mex.
Co-trimoxazole (p.199·3).
*Bacterial infections.*

**Ester Aces** Sisu, Canad.
Betacarotene, selenium, vitamin C, and vitamin E (p.1417·1).

**Ester C EVC** Sisu, Canad.
Vitamins A, B, and C with zinc (p.1417·1).

**Esterasine** Baxter, Fr.
Complement C1 esterase inhibitor (p.1675·2).
*Hereditary angioedema.*

**Esterbiol** Inexfa, Spain†.
Pyricarbate (p.1737·1).
*Hypercholesterolaemia.*

**Ester-C**
Quest, Canad.; Sisu, Canad.; Stanley, Canad.
Calcium ascorbate (p.1460·2).
Solgar, UK†.
Vitamin C with bioflavonoids (p.1417·1).

**Ester-C Plus** Solgar, USA.
Vitamin C (p.1460·2); citrus bioflavonoids complex (p.1688·2); acerola; rose hips (p.1740·1); rutoside (p.1688·2); calcium (p.1225·1).
*Capillary bleeding.*

**Ester-C Plus Multi-Mineral** Solgar, USA.
Vitamin C (p.1460·2); citrus bioflavonoids complex (p.1688·2); acerola; rose hips (p.1740·1); rutoside (p.1688·2); calcium; magnesium; potassium; zinc (p.1217·1).
*Capillary bleeding.*

**Estericlean** Braun, Spain†.
Sodium chloride (p.1233·3).
*Fluid and electrolyte replacement; hypovolaemia.*

**Esterofundina** Braun, Port.
Electrolyte infusion with or without glucose (p.1217·1).
*Fluid and electrolyte disorders.*

**Esterol** Laborest, Ital.
Rice oil; vitamin E; oleic acid; linoleic acid; linolenic acid; gamma-orizanol (p.1417·1).
*Nutritional supplement.*

**Esterol Plus** Laborest, Ital.†.
Rice oil; tocotrienol; vitamin E; gamma-orizanol (p.1417·1).
*Nutritional supplement.*

**Esteromicin** Universales, Mex.†.
Erythromycin (p.208·1).
*Bacterial infections.*

**Esteronide** Galderma, Arg.
Desonide (p.1096·3).
*Skin disorders.*

**Estigyn** Glaxo Wellcome, Austral.†.
Ethinylestradiol (p.1553·2).
*Amenorrhoea; menopausal disorders.*

**Estilomicin** Beta, Arg.
Metronidazole (p.607·2); spiramycin (p.255·3).
*Mouth infections.*

**Estilsona** Ern, Spain.
Prednisolone steaglate (p.1108·2).
*Corticosteroid.*

**Estima** Effik, Fr.
Progesterone (p.1566·2).
*Female infertility; menopausal disorders; menstrual disorders; threatened or recurrent miscarriage.*

**Estimulocel** Synthelabo, Spain†.
Procodazole ethyl ester (p.1735·2).
*Immunotherapy.*

**Estinyl**
Schering, Canad.†; Schering-Plough, S.Afr.; Schering, USA.
Ethinylestradiol (p.1553·2).
*Breast cancer; female hypogonadism; menopausal disorders; prostatic cancer.*

**Estival** Specifar (Σπεσιφαρ), Gr.
Carbocisteine (p.1116·2).
*Respiratory disorders associated with viscous mucus.*

**Estivan** Almirall, Belg.
Ebastine (p.433·1).
*Allergic conjunctivitis; allergic rhinitis; urticaria.*

**Esto** Angelini, Ital.
Alfoscerate olamine.
*Anxiety disorders.*

**Estomafitino** Jofadel, Braz.†.
Chamomile (p.1669·3); condurango (p.1675·3); gentian (p.1692·2); glycerol (p.1694·3); nux vomica (p.1722·3); senna (p.1288·2).
*Constipation.*

**Estomagel** Neo Quimica, Braz.
*Oral suspension:* Aluminium hydroxide (p.1249·2); magnesium hydroxide (p.1272·2).
*Antacid.*
*Tablets:* Aluminium hydroxide (p.1249·2); magnesium hydroxide (p.1272·2); dimeticone (p.1289·2).
*Flatulence; gastrointestinal hyperacidity.*

**Estomaplus** QIF, Braz.†.
Metoclopramide (p.1274·3).
*Gastrointestinal motility disorders; nausea and vomiting.*

**Estomazil** DM, Braz.†.
Sodium carbonate (p.1747·1); sodium bicarbonate (p.1223·2); citric acid (p.1673·1).
*Gastrointestinal hyperacidity.*

**Estomepe** Bunker, Braz.
Omeprazole (p.1278·2).
*Peptic ulcer.*

**Estomil** Merck, Spain.
Lansoprazole (p.1269·3).
*Gastro-oesophageal reflux; peptic ulcer.*

**Estomina** Fabra, Arg.
Bromazepam (p.671·3).
*Anxiety.*

**Estomycin** Columbia, S.Afr.†.
Erythromycin estolate (p.208·1).
*Bacterial infections.*

**Estopause** Faran, Gr.
Estradiol (p.1550·1); medroxyprogesterone (p.1557·3).
*Hormone replacement therapy.*

**Estopein** Diba, Mex.
Ketorolac trometamol (p.52·1).
*Pain.*

**Estovyn-T** Grossman, Mex.
Tinidazole (p.617·1).

**Estrabeta** Betapharm, Ger.
Estradiol (p.1550·1).
*Menopausal disorders; osteoporosis.*

**Estrace**
Shire, Canad.; Bristol-Myers Squibb, USA.
Estradiol (p.1550·1).
*Breast cancer; female castration; female hypogonadism; menopausal vasomotor symptoms; osteoporosis; primary ovarian failure; prostatic cancer; vulval and vaginal atrophy.*

**Estracomb**
Novartis, Arg.; Novartis, Austria; Novartis, Canad.; Novartis, Hong Kong; Byk Gulden, Mex.; Novartis, Neth.; Novartis, Singapore; Novartis, Switz.
4 Patches, estradiol (p.1550·1) (Estraderm); 4 patches, estradiol; norethisterone acetate (p.1562·2) (Estragest).
*Menopausal disorders; osteoporosis.*
Novartis, Braz.; Novartis, Fin.; Novartis, Ger.; Novartis, Port.
4 Patches, estradiol (p.1550·1); 4 patches, estradiol; norethisterone acetate (p.1562·2).
*Menopausal disorders; osteoporosis.*
Novartis, Chile.
4 Patches, estradiol (p.1550·1) (Femiderm TTS); 4 patches, estradiol; norethisterone acetate (p.1562·2) (Estragest TTS).
*Menopausal disorders; osteoporosis.*
Novartis, Denm.; Novartis, Ital.; Novartis, Norw.†; Novartis, Spain; Novartis, Swed.
Patch I, estradiol (p.1550·1); patch II, estradiol; norethisterone acetate (p.1562·2).
*Menopausal disorders; osteoporosis.*

**Estracomb TTS** Novartis, Gr.
Estradiol (p.1550·1); norethisterone (p.1562·2).
*Hormone replacement therapy.*

**Estracombi**
Novartis, Austral.; Novartis, Belg.; Novartis, Irl.; Novartis, S.Afr.; Novartis, UK.
4 Patches, estradiol (p.1550·1) (Estraderm TTS); 4 patches, estradiol; norethisterone acetate (p.1562·2) (Estragest TTS).
*Menopausal disorders; osteoporosis.*

**Estracutan** Hexal, Austria.
Estradiol (p.1550·1).
*Menopausal disorders.*

**Estracyt**
Pharmacia, Arg.; Pharmacia Upjohn, Austral.†; Pharmacia, Austria; Pharmacia, Belg.; Pharmacia, Braz.†; Pharmacia, Chile; Pharmacia, Denm.; Pharmacia, Fin.; Pharmacia, Fr.; Pharmacia, Ger.; Pharmacia-Upjohn, Gr.; Pharmacia, Hong Kong; Pharmacia, Irl.; Pharmacia Upjohn, Israel; Pharmacia Upjohn, Ital.; Shinyaku, Jpn; Pharmacia, Malaysia; Pharmacia, Neth.; Pharmacia, Norw.; Pharmacia, Port.; Pharmacia, S.Afr.; Pharmacia, Singapore; Pharmacia, Spain; Pharmacia, Swed.; Pharmacia, Switz.; Pharmacia, UK.
Estramustine meglumine phosphate (p.551·2), estramustine phosphate (p.551·2), or estramustine sodium phosphate (p.551·1).
*Prostatic cancer.*

**Estradelle** Sigma, Braz.
Estradiol (p.1550·1).
*Menopausal disorders.*

**Estraderm**
Novartis, Arg.; Novartis, Austral.; Novartis, Austria; Novartis, Belg.; Novartis, Braz.; Novartis, Canad.; Novartis, Denm.; Novartis, Fin.; Novartis, Fr.; Novartis, Ger.; Novartis, Hong Kong; Novartis, India; Novartis, Irl.; Novartis, Israel; Novartis, Ital.; Byk Gulden, Mex.; Novartis, Neth.; Novartis, Norw.; Novartis, NZ; Novartis, Port.; Novartis, S.Afr.; Novartis, Singapore; Novartis, Spain; Novartis, Swed.; Novartis, Switz.; Novartis, UK; Novartis, USA.
Estradiol (p.1550·1).
*Menopausal disorders; osteoporosis.*

**Estraderm TTS** Novartis, Gr.
Estradiol (p.1550·1).
*Menopausal disorders; oestrogen deficiency.*

**Estradot**
Novartis, Canad.; Novartis, Irl.; Novartis, Norw.; Novartis, Port.
Estradiol (p.1550·1).
*Menopausal disorders; osteoporosis.*

**Estradurin**
Pharmacia, Austria; Pharmacia, Denm.; Pharmacia, Fin.; Pharmacia, Ger.; Pharmacia, Neth.; Pharmacia, Norw.; Pharmacia Upjohn, Spain†; Pharmacia, Swed.; Pharmacia, Switz.
Polyestradiol phosphate (p.1565·3).
Mepivacaine hydrochloride (p.1381·2) may be included in this preparation to alleviate the pain of injection.
*Amenorrhoea; breast cancer; menopausal disorders; prostatic cancer.*

**Estradurine** Pharmacia, Belg.
Polyestradiol phosphate (p.1565·3).
Mepivacaine hydrochloride (p.1381·2) is included in this preparation to alleviate the pain of injection.
*Prostatic cancer.*

**Estrafemol** Henning, Ger.
12 Capsules, estradiol valerate (p.1550·2); 14 capsules, estradiol valerate; medroxyprogesterone acetate (p.1557·2).
*Menopausal disorders.*

**Estragest**
Novartis, Arg.; Ciba-Geigy, Austria†; Novartis, Braz.; Novartis, Chile; Novartis, Ger.; Novartis, Switz.
Estradiol (p.1550·1); norethisterone acetate (p.1562·2).
*Menopausal disorders; osteoporosis.*

**Estramon**
Hexal, Austria; Hexal, Ger.; Rowex, Irl.†; Ecosol, Switz.
Estradiol (p.1550·1).
*Menopausal disorders; osteoporosis.*

**Estranova CC** Silesia, Chile.
Estradiol valerate (p.1550·2); medroxyprogesterone acetate (p.1557·2).
*Menopausal disorders.*

**Estranova E** Silesia, Chile.
Estradiol valerate (p.1550·2).
*Menopausal disorders.*

**Estranova 30 Simple** Silesia, Chile.
13 Tablets, estradiol valerate (p.1550·2); medroxyprogesterone acetate (p.1557·2); 17 tablets, estradiol valerate.
*Menopausal disorders.*

**Estrapak**
Note. This name is used for preparations of different composition.
Novartis, Austral.†; Novartis, Irl.; Novartis, Mex.†; Novartis, NZ; Novartis, UK†.
Transdermal patches, estradiol (p.1550·1); tablets, norethisterone acetate (p.1562·2).
*Menopausal disorders; osteoporosis.*

**Estrapatch** Pierre Fabre, Fr.
Estradiol (p.1550·1).
*Menopausal disorders.*

**Estrarona** Silesia, Chile.
Conjugated oestrogens (p.1543·2).
*Menopausal disorders; osteoporosis; prostatic cancer.*

**Estrasorb** Novavax, USA.
Estradiol (p.1550·1).
*Menopausal vasomotor disorders.*

**Estratab** Solvay, USA.
Esterified oestrogens (p.1549·3).
*Breast cancer; menopausal vasomotor symptoms; oestrogen deficiency; osteoporosis; prostatic cancer; vulval and vaginal atrophy.*

**Estratest** Solvay, USA.
Esterified oestrogens (p.1549·3); methyltestosterone (p.1559·3).
*Menopausal disorders.*

**Estrefen** Solfran, Mex.
Dihydrostreptomycin (p.206·1); sulfadiazine (p.258·2).
*Diarrhoea.*

**Estregur** Tegur, Mex.†.
Chlorotrianisene (p.1542·1).

**Estrena** Merck, Fin.
Estradiol (p.1550·1).
*Menopausal disorders.*

**Estreptocarbocaftiazol** Bago, Arg.
*Oral suspension:* Phthalylsulfathiazole (p.242·3); streptomycin sulfate (p.256·2); charcoal (p.1030·2); menadione (p.1466·3).
*Tablets:* Phthalylsulfathiazole (p.242·3); streptomycin sulfate (p.256·2); charcoal (p.1030·2); simeticone (p.1289·2); menadione (p.1466·3).
*Diarrhoea; flatulence.*

**Estreptoenterol** Juste, Spain.
Dihydrostreptomycin sulfate (p.205·3); phthalylsulfathiazole (p.242·3); pectin (p.1580·3).
*Gastrointestinal infections.*

**Estreva**
Merck, Arg.; Merck, Belg.; Merck, Braz.; Merck, Chile; Merck, Ger.; Merck-Theramex, Hong Kong; Theramex, Mon.
Estradiol (p.1550·1).
*Menopausal disorders; osteoporosis.*

**Estrex** Lake, USA.
Homoeopathic preparation.

**Estriagel** Medicamed, Port.†.
Collagen (p.1674·3); cerais oil; placenta filatol.
*Firming cream.*

**Estrifam** Novo Nordisk, Ger.
Estradiol (p.1550·1).
*Menopausal disorders; oestrogen deficiency; osteoporosis.*

**Estring**
Pharmacia, Arg.; Pharmacia, Austral.†; Pharmacia, Austria; Pharmacia, Canad.; Pharmacia, Denm.; Pharmacia, Fin.; Pharmacia, Ger.; Pharmacia, Neth.; Pharmacia, Norw.; Pharmacia Upjohn, NZ†; Pharmacia, S.Afr.; Pharmacia, Switz.; Pharmacia, UK; Pharmacia Upjohn, USA.
Estradiol (p.1550·1).
*Postmenopausal atrophy of the vagina or lower urinary-tract.*

**Estrocare** Pharmanex, USA.
Cordyceps sinensis; cimicifuga (p.1671·3).
*Menopausal disorders.*

**Estroclim** Sigma-Tau, Ital.
Estradiol (p.1550·1).
*Menopausal disorders; osteoporosis.*

**Estrodose** Wyeth Lederle, Ital.
Estradiol (p.1550·1).
*Menopausal disorders.*

**Estrofem**
Elea, Arg.; Novo Nordisk, Austral.; Novo Nordisk, Austria; Novo Nordisk, Belg.; Medley, Braz.; Novo Nordisk, Denm.; Novo Nordisk, Fin.; Novo Nordisk, Fr.; Novo Nordisk, Hong Kong; Novo Nordisk, Irl.; Novo Nordisk, Israel; Novo Nordisk, Ital.; Novo Nordisk, Malaysia; Novo Nordisk, Neth.; Novo Nordisk, NZ; Isdin, Port.; Novo Nordisk, S.Afr.; Novo Nordisk, Singapore; Novo Nordisk, Thai.
Estradiol (p.1550·1).
Formerly contained estradiol and estriol in *Fr.* and *S.Afr.*
*Menopausal disorders; osteoporosis.*

**Estrofem N** Novo Nordisk, Switz.
Estradiol (p.1550·1).
Estrofem formerly contained estradiol and estriol.
*Oestrogen deficiency.*

**Estrogel**
Asta Medica, Austria; Schering, Canad.; Leiras, Denm.; Leiras, Fin.
Estradiol (p.1550·1).
*Menopausal disorders; osteoporosis.*

**EstroGel** Solvay, USA.
Estradiol (p.1550·1).
*Menopausal disorders.*

**Estrogenon** Sanval, Braz.
Conjugated oestrogens (p.1543·2).
*Menopausal disorders.*

**Estro-Logic** Quest, Canad.
Astragalus; black cohosh; chastetree berry; motherwort; sage; soy bean; vervain; wild yam (p.1417·1).

**Estronar** Menarini, Port.
Estradiol (p.1550·1).
*Menopausal disorders; prostatic cancer.*

**Estronorm** Jenapharm, Ger.
Estradiol (p.1550·1).
*Menopausal disorders; osteoporosis.*

**Estro-Pause** Adcock Ingram, S.Afr.
Estradiol valerate (p.1550·2).
*Menopausal disorders.*

**Estroplus** Sintofarma, Braz.
Conjugated oestrogens (p.1543·2).
*Menopausal disorders.*

**Estroquin** Richmond, Arg.
Calcium folinate (p.1431·1).

**Estrostep** Warner Chilcott, USA.
Norethisterone acetate (p.1562·2); ethinylestradiol (p.1553·2).
*Triphasic oral contraceptive.*

**Estrostep Fe** Warner Chilcott, USA.
21 Tablets, norethisterone acetate (p.1562·2); ethinylestradiol (p.1553·2); 7 tablets, ferrous fumarate (p.1427·3).
*Triphasic oral contraceptive.*

**Estroxyn** Pharmacia, Austral.†.
Tamoxifen citrate (p.584·1).
*Breast cancer.*

**Estulic**
Novartis, Belg.; Novartis, Fr.; Novartis, Ger.†; Viatris, Neth.
Guanfacine hydrochloride (p.927·2).
*Hypertension.*

**Esucos**
UCB, Austria;.UCB, Belg.†; UCB, Denm.†; UCB, Fin.; SIT, Ital.; UCB, Norw.; UCB, Swed.
Dixyrazine (p.697·2).
*Alcohol withdrawal syndrome; anxiety; postoperative vomiting; premedication; senile agitation; sleep disorders.*

**Esvit C** Laboratorios Chile, Chile.
Ascorbic acid (p.1460·2).
*Vitamin C deficiency; vitamin C supplement.*

**Eta Biocortilen** SIFI, Ital.
Dexamethasone sodium phosphate (p.1097·2); neomycin sulfate (p.235·1).
*Infected eye disorders.*

**Eta Biocortilen VC** SIFI, Ital.
Dexamethasone sodium phosphate (p.1097·2); neomycin sulfate (p.235·1); gramicidin (p.220·2); tetryzoline hydrochloride (p.1131·2).
*Infected eye disorders.*

**Eta Cortilen** SIFI, Ital.†.
Dexamethasone sodium phosphate (p.1097·2).
*Eye disorders.*

**Etabus** Columbia, Mex.†.
Disulfiram (p.1681·3).

**Etaconil** Tecnofarma, Chile.
Flutamide (p.556·2).
*Benign prostatic hyperplasia; prostatic cancer.*

**Etacril** Beta, Arg.
Cisapride (p.1259·2).
*Gastro-oesophageal reflux.*

**Etalpha**
Leo, Austria; Pentafarma, Chile; Leo, Denm.; Leo, Fin.; Leo, Neth.; Leo, Norw.; Leo, Port.; Farmacusi, Spain; Leo, Swed.
Alfacalcidol (p.1461·2).
*Calcium metabolic disorders; hyperparathyroidism; hypoparathyroidism; osteomalacia; renal osteodystrophy; rickets; vitamin D deficiency.*

**Etamucin** Etapharm, Austria.
Sodium hyaluronate (p.1697·3).
*Adjunct in ophthalmic surgery.*

**Etanicozid B6** Piam, Ital.
Ethambutol hydrochloride (p.211·3); isoniazid (p.222·2).
Pyridoxine hydrochloride (p.1456·3) is included in this preparation for the prophylaxis of peripheral neuropathy.
*Tuberculosis.*

**Etapiam** Piam, Ital.
Ethambutol hydrochloride (p.211·3).
*Tuberculosis.*

**Etaretin** Etapharm, Austria.
Retinal phosphatides; sodium bicarbonate (p.1223·2).
*Eye disorders.*

**Etasisen** Rafarm, Gr.
Aciclovir (p.626·1).
*Labial and genital herpes simplex infections.*

**Etaverol** Dinafarma, Braz.†.
Homatropine (p.483·2); belladonna (p.479·1).
*Smooth muscle spam.*

**Etaxene**
Wassermann, Ital.
Somatostatin (p.1339·3).
*Gastrointestinal haemorrhage.*
Alfa Wassermann, Thai.
Somatostatin acetate (p.1339·3).
*Gastrointestinal haemorrhage; prevention of complications following pancreatic surgery.*

**ETDR** SIFI, Ital.
Vitamin C; vitamin E; rutoside; sambucus (p.1417·1).
*Nutritional supplement.*

**Etec** Raffo, Arg.
Vitamin E (p.1464·3).
*Vitamin E supplement.*

**Etec 1000** Tecnofarma, Chile.
Vitamin E (p.1464·3).
*Vitamin E supplement.*

**Eterciclina** Uniao Quimica, Braz.†.
Guaifenesin (p.1122·1); potassium iodide (p.1598·1).
*Respiratory-tract congestion.*

**Etermol** Quimpe, Spain†.
Aconite (p.1646·3); calcium lactophosphate; ephedrine hydrochloride (p.1120·1); beech; lemon; sulfogaiacol (p.1131·1).
*Upper-respiratory-tract disorders.*

**Etermol Antitusivo** Quimpe, Spain.
Benzydamine hydrochloride (p.21·1); dextromethorphan hydrobromide (p.1117·3); guaifenesin (p.1122·1); sodium benzoate (p.1169·3).
*Coughs.*

**Eternex** Dabur, India.
Melatonin (p.1710·2); vitamin $B_6$ (p.1457·2).
*Circadian rhythm disorders; jet lag; sleep disorders.*

**Etfariol** Vilco, Gr.
Ticlopidine (p.1012·1).
*Thromboembolic disorders.*

**Ethacid** Stadmed, India.
Etamsylate (p.749·3).
*Menorrhagia.*

**Etham** Pond's, Thai.
Ethambutol hydrochloride (p.211·3).
*Tuberculosis.*

**Ethamolin**
Zest, Braz.; Reed & Carnrick, Canad.†; Questcor, USA.
Monoethanolamine oleate (p.1716·1).
*Haemorrhoids; oesophageal varices; varicose veins.*

**Ethasyl** FDC, India.
Etamsylate (p.749·3).
*Haemorrhage.*

**Ethatyl** Aventis, S.Afr.
Ethionamide (p.212·3).
*Tuberculosis.*

**Ethbutol** Pharmasant, Thai.
Ethambutol hydrochloride (p.211·3).
*Tuberculosis.*

**EtheDent** Ethex, USA.
Sodium fluoride (p.1444·3).
*Dental caries prophylaxis.*

**Etheophyl** Lindopharm, Ger.†.
Theophylline (p.798·3).
*Obstructive airways disease.*

**Ethezyme** Ethex, USA.
Papain (p.1727·3); urea (p.1162·2).
*Debridement of wounds and ulcers.*

**Ethibloc**
Ethicon, Ger.; Johnson & Johnson, Switz.†.
Sodium amidotrizoate (p.1060·2).
*Packing of pancreatic duct following partial pancreatic resection; pre-operative vascular embolisation for renal tumours.*

**Ethical Nutrients 45+** Health World, Austral.†.
Multivitamin and mineral supplement (p.1417·1).

**Ethical Nutrients Antioxidant Fish Oil Garlic Plus** Health World, Austral.†.
Fish oil (p.976·2); garlic oil (p.1691·2); betacarotene; folic acid; vitamin $B_{12}$; vitamin $B_6$; vitamin E (p.1417·1).
*Peripheral vascular disorders.*

**Ethical Nutrients Bioflavonoids Plus** Health World, Austral.†.
Ascorbic acid (p.1460·2); bioflavonoids (p.1688·2).
*Cold and influenza symptoms; peripheral vascular disorders.*

**Ethical Nutrients HRT Support** Health World, Austral.†.
Multivitamin and mineral preparation (p.1417·1).

**Ethical Nutrients Inner Health Powder** Health World, Austral.†.
*Lactobacillus acidophilus* (p.1704·2).
*Maintenance of normal gastrointestinal flora.*

**Ethical Nutrients Iron Plus** Health World, Austral.†.
Iron amino-acid chelate; vitamin B substances; calcium ascorbate; calcium succinate (p.1417·1).
*Iron supplement.*

**Ethical Nutrients Maxepa** Health World, Austral.†.
Omega-3 marine triglycerides (p.976·2).
*Premenstrual disorder; psoriasis.*

**Ethical Nutrients Maxi Bifidus** Health World, Austral.†.
*Bifidobacterium bifidum* (p.1704·2).
*Maintenance of normal gastrointestinal flora.*

**Ethical Nutrients Maxi Dophilus** Health World, Austral.†.
*Lactobacillus acidophilus* (p.1704·2).
*Maintenance of normal gastrointestinal flora.*

**Ethical Nutrients Super Multi** Health World, Austral.†.
Vitamins; minerals; bladderwrack; vanadium; molybdenum (p.1417·1).

**Ethical Nutrients Womens Multi** Health World, Austral.†.
Vitamins; minerals; taraxacum (p.1417·1).

**Ethicholine**
Baxter, NZ; DBL, NZ; Bull, Singapore.
Suxamethonium chloride (p.1406·2).
*Depolarising neuromuscular blocker.*

**Ethicoline** Faulding, Malaysia.
Suxamethonium chloride (p.1406·2).
*Depolarising neuromuscular blocker.*

**Ethimil** Dexcel, UK†.
Verapamil hydrochloride (p.1019·1).
*Angina pectoris; hypertension.*

**Ethiodol** Savage, USA.
Iodised oil (p.1063·2).
*Contrast medium for hysterosalpingography and lymphography.*

**Ethipramine** Aspen, S.Afr.
Imipramine hydrochloride (p.300·1).
*Alcohol withdrawal syndrome; behaviour disorders; depression; parkinsonism.*

**Ethmozine**
Monmouth, Irl.†; Monmouth, UK†; Roberts, USA.
Moracizine hydrochloride (p.962·1).
*Ventricular arrhythmias.*

**Ethrane**
Abbott, Austral.; Abbott, Austria; Abbott, Belg.†; AstraZeneca, Canad.†; Abbott, Ger.; Abbott, Hong Kong†; Abbott, Irl.; Abbott, Israel; Abbott, Mex.; Abbott, Neth.; Abbott, S.Afr.; Abbott, Switz.; Baxter, USA.
Enflurane (p.1298·1).
*Anaesthesia and analgesia in obstetrics; general anaesthesia.*

**Ethyol**
Essex, Arg.; Schering-Plough, Austral.; Schering-Plough, Belg.; Schering-Plough, Braz.; Lilly, Canad.†; Schering-Plough, Chile; Medimmune, Denm.; Schering-Plough, Fin.; Schering-Plough, Fr.; Essex, Ger.; Medimmune, Gr.; Schering-Plough, Hong Kong; Medimmune, Israel; Schering-Plough, Ital.; Schering-Plough, Malaysia; Schering-Plough, Mex.; Schering-Plough, Neth.; Schering-Plough, NZ; Schering-Plough, Port.†; Schering-Plough, S.Afr.; Schering-Plough, Singapore; Schering-Plough, Spain; Schering-Plough, Swed.; Essex, Switz.; Schering-Plough, Thai.; Schering-Plough, UK†; Alza, USA; US Bioscience, USA.
Amifostine (p.1031·3).
*Radiation-associated xerostomia; reduction of nephrotoxicity due to cisplatin; reduction of neutropenia due to cyclophosphamide and cisplatin therapy for ovarian cancer.*

**Etiaxil** Interdelta, Switz.
Aluminium chloride (p.1142·1).
*Hyperhidrosis.*

**Etibi**
Gerot, Austria; ICN, Canad.; Zoja, Hong Kong†.
Ethambutol hydrochloride (p.211·3).
*Tuberculosis.*

**Etidrate** Pacific, NZ.
Disodium etidronate (p.771·2).
*Ectopic ossification; osteoporosis; Paget's disease of the bone.*

**Etidron** Abiogen, Ital.
Disodium etidronate (p.771·2).
*Paget's disease of bone.*

**Etifollin** Nycomed, Norw.†.
Ethinylestradiol (p.1553·2).
*Menopausal disorders; prostatic cancer.*

**etil** CT, Ger.
Etilefrine hydrochloride (p.914·1).
*Hypotension.*

**Etil Adrianol** Klonal, Arg.
Etilefrine (p.914·1).
*Hypotension.*

**Etildopanan** Neo Quimica, Braz.
Methyldopa (p.953·2).
*Hypertension.*

**Etiles** Microsules Bernabo, Arg.
Tiapride hydrochloride (p.725·1).

**Etiltox** AFOM, Ital.
Disulfiram (p.1681·3).
*Alcoholism.*

**Etimonis** Ecosol, Switz.†.
Isosorbide mononitrate (p.942·1).
*Heart failure; ischaemic heart disease.*

**Etindrax** Valdecasas, Mex.
Allopurinol (p.412·2).
*Calcium oxalate calculi; hyperuricaemia.*

**Etioven** Aventis, Fr.
Naftazone (p.757·1).
*Peripheral vascular disorders.*

**Etiplus** Zekides, Gr.
Disodium etidronate (p.771·2).
*Osteoporosis; Paget's disease of bone.*

**Eti-Puren** Alpharma-Isis, Ger.
Etilefrine hydrochloride (p.914·1).
*Hypotension.*

**Etizem** Neo-Farmaceutica, Port.
Diltiazem hydrochloride (p.900·1).
*Angina pectoris; hypertension.*

**Etmoren** Evers, Ger.†.
Silver birch (p.1660·3); java tea (p.1702·3); solidago virgaurea (p.1748·3).
*Diuretic.*

**Etnoderm** Koni-Cofarm, Chile.
Hydroquinone (p.1148·1).

**ETO CS** Pharmacia, Ger.
Etoposide (p.551·3).
*Malignant neoplasms.*

**Etocin** Malaysia Chemist, Singapore†.
Erythromycin ethyl succinate (p.208·1) or erythromycin stearate (p.208·2).
*Bacterial infections.*

**Etocoderm** Richter, Austria.
Alpha tocopherol (p.1464·3).
*Skin disorders.*

**Etocovit** Richter, Austria.
*d*-Alpha-tocopherol (p.1464·3).
*Vitamin E deficiency.*

**Etocris** Kampel Martian, Arg.
Etoposide (p.551·3).
*Malignant neoplasms.*

**Etofen** Ecosol, Switz.
Etofenamate (p.38·1).
*Musculoskeletal, joint, and soft-tissue disorders.*

**Eto-Gry** Gry, Ger.
Etoposide (p.551·3).
*Malignant neoplasms.*

**Etoina** Klonal, Arg.
Phenytoin (p.370·2).
*Arrhythmias; epilepsy.*

**Etomedac** Medac, Ger.
Etoposide (p.551·3).
*Malignant neoplasms.*

**Etomine** Novartis, S.Afr.
Clotiapine (p.685·2).
*Agitation; anxiety; depression; psychoses.*

**E-Tonil** APS, Ger.
*d*-Alpha tocopherol (p.1464·3).
*Vitamin E deficiency.*

**Etono** Chefaro, Fin.
Tripelennamine hydrochloride (p.442·3).
*Insect stings and bites.*

**Etonox** Charoen, Thai.
Etodolac (p.37·3).
*Musculoskeletal and joint disorders; pain.*

**Etopan** Taro, Israel.
Etodolac (p.37·3).
*Osteoarthritis; pain; rheumatoid arthritis.*

**Etophylate** Martin & Harris, India.
Acefylline piperazine (p.780·1).
*Bronchitis; bronchospasm.*

**Etopofos**
Bristol-Myers Squibb, Arg.; Bristol-Myers Squibb, Austria; Bristol-Myers Squibb, Denm.; Bristol-Myers Squibb, Fin.; Bristol-Myers Squibb, Norw.; Bristol-Myers Squibb, Swed.
Etoposide phosphate (p.551·3).
*Malignant neoplasms.*

**Etopophos**
Bristol-Myers Squibb, Austral.; Bristol-Myers Squibb, Belg.; Bristol-Myers Squibb, Fr.; Bristol-Myers Squibb, Ger.; Bristol-Myers Squibb, Irl.; Bristol-Myers Squibb, Israel; Bristol-Myers Squibb, Neth.†; Bristol-Myers Squibb, NZ; Bristol-Myers Squibb, S.Afr.; Bristol-Myers Squibb, Switz.; Bristol-Myers Squibb, UK; Bristol-Myers Squibb Oncology, USA.
Etoposide phosphate (p.551·3).
*Malignant neoplasms.*

**Etopos**
Eurofarma, Braz.; Lemery, Mex.
Etoposide (p.551·3).
*Malignant neoplasms.*

**Etopul** BPL-Meizler, Braz.
Etoposide (p.551·3).
*Malignant neoplasms.*

**Etosid** Cipla, India.
Etoposide (p.551·3).
*Leukaemias; lymphomas.*

**Etosin** Asta Oncologia, Braz.
Etoposide (p.551·3).
*Malignant neoplasms.*

**Etoxisclerol** Bama, Spain.
Lauromacrogol 400 (p.1412·3).
*Varices.*

**Etrafon**
Schering, Canad.†; Schering-Plough, S.Afr.; Schering, USA.
Perphenazine (p.714·2); amitriptyline hydrochloride (p.280·3).
*Mixed anxiety depressive states.*

**Etramon** Janssen-Cilag, Spain†.
Econazole nitrate (p.397·2).
*Fungal infections.*

**Etrane** Abbott, Braz.
Enflurane (p.1298·1).
*General anaesthesia.*

**Etrat**
Note. This name is used for preparations of different composition.
Klinge, Austria; Novartis Consumer, Port.†.
Heparin sodium (p.928·1); menthol (p.1711·3); glycol salicylate (p.44·3).
*Musculoskeletal, joint, peri-articular, and soft-tissue disorders.*
Gemballa, Braz.
A heparinoid (p.931·1); glycol salicylate (p.44·3); benzyl nicotinate (p.21·2).
*Soft-tissue injury.*

**Etrat Sportgel** Fujisawa, Ger.
Heparin sodium (p.928·1); menthol (p.1711·3); glycol salicylate (p.44·3).
*Sports injuries.*

**Etrat Sportsalbe MPS** Fujisawa, Ger.
A heparinoid (p.931·1).
*Soft-tissue injury; superficial vascular disorders.*

**Etro** Inexfa, Spain†.
Ampicillin sodium (p.157·1); ampicillin benzathine (p.158·1).
Lidocaine hydrochloride (p.1377·3) is included in this preparation to alleviate the pain of injection.
*Bacterial infections.*

**Etro Balsamico** Inexfa, Spain†.
Ampicillin sodium (p.157·1); ampicillin benzathine (p.158·1); cineole (p.1672·1); niaouli oil (p.1719·3); guaifenesin (p.1122·1).
Lidocaine hydrochloride (p.1377·3) is included in this preparation to alleviate the pain of injection.
*Respiratory-tract infections.*

**E-Trocima-P** Columbia, Mex.
Erythromycin (p.208·1).
*Bacterial infections.*

**Etrogran** Raza, Malaysia; Pharmaniaga, Malaysia.
Erythromycin ethyl succinate (p.208·1).
*Bacterial infections.*

**Etrolate** Pharmasant, Thai.
Erythromycin (p.208·1).
*Bacterial infections.*

**Etronil** Klonal, Arg.
Metronidazole (p.607·2).

**Etrosteron** Elea, Arg.
Estradiol undecylate (p.1551·1).
*Menopausal disorders.*

**Etrotab** Raza, Malaysia; Pharmaniaga, Malaysia.
Erythromycin stearate (p.208·2).
*Bacterial infections.*

**Etumina**
Novartis, Arg.; Novartis, Spain.
Clotiapine (p.685·2).
*Alcohol withdrawal syndrome; anxiety; insomnia; psychoses.*

**Etumine** Novartis, Belg.
Clotiapine (p.685·2).
*Agitation; alcohol withdrawal syndrome; anxiety; psychoses.*

**Etumin/Entumin** Novartis, Israel.
Clotiapine (p.685·2).
*Alcohol withdrawal syndrome; anxiety; bipolar disorder; schizophrenia.*

**Etyofil** FDC, India.
Theophylline (p.798·3); etofylline (p.785·1).
*Cardiac disorders; cerebrovascular disorders.*

**Etyzem** Caber, Ital.
Diltiazem hydrochloride (p.900·1).
*Angina pectoris; heart failure; hypertension.*

**Eubetal** SIFI, Ital.†.
Betamethasone sodium phosphate (p.1093·1); antazoline phosphate (p.424·2).
*Eye disorders.*

**Eubetal Antibiotico** SIFI, Ital.
*Eye drops:* Betamethasone sodium phosphate (p.1093·1); rolitetracycline (p.254·1); chloramphenicol (p.185·1); colistimethate sodium (p.199·1).
*Eye ointment:* Betamethasone sodium phosphate (p.1093·1); tetracycline (p.266·2); chloramphenicol (p.185·1); colistimethate sodium (p.199·1).
*Eye disorders.*

**Eubetal Biotic** *Craveri, Arg.*
Betamethasone sodium phosphate (p.1093·1); rolitetracycline (p.254·1) or tetracycline (p.266·2); chloramphenicol (p.185·1); colistimethate sodium (p.199·1).
*Eye disorders.*

**Eubine** *Chiesi, Fr.*
Oxycodone hydrochloride (p.75·2).
*Pain.*

**Eubiol** *Chephasaar, Ger.*
Arginine aspartate (p.1421·1).
*Liver disorders.*

**Eubiolac** *Verla, Ger.*
Calcium lactate (p.1225·3).
*Vaginal disorders.*

**Euboral** *Reig Jofre, Spain.*
Naphazoline hydrochloride (p.1124·3); borax (p.1661·3).
*Eye irritation.*

**Eubos**
*Hobein, Hong Kong; Hobein, Malaysia.*
Range of emollients, moisturisers and soap substitutes.
*Dry skin.*

**Eubucal** *Sanopharm, Switz.*
Chlorhexidine gluconate (p.1173·2); myrrh (p.1718·3); chamomile (p.1669·3); arnica (p.1656·3); rhatany (p.1738·1); menthol (p.1711·3).
*Mouth disorders.*

**Eucabal** *Esparma, Ger.*
Plantago lanceolata (p.1738·2); thyme (p.1755·2).
*Catarrh.*

**Eucabal-Balsam S** *Esparma, Ger.*
Eucalyptus oil (p.1686·2); oleum pini sylvestris.
*Respiratory-tract disorders.*

**Eucafluid N** *Steigerwald, Ger.†.*
Eucalyptus oil (p.1686·2); oleum pini sylvestris; peppermint oil (p.1283·2); rosemary oil (p.1740·2).
*Musculoskeletal and joint disorders; neuralgia.*

**Eucalcic** *Byk, Fr.*
Calcium carbonate (p.1254·2).
*Renal osteodystrophy.*

**Eucalin** *Farcoral, Mex.*
Guaiacol (p.1122·1); cineole (p.1672·1).
*Respiratory-tract disorders.*

**Eucaliptan** *Bunker, Braz.*
Ampoule A, cineole (p.1672·1); guaifenesin (p.1122·1); dipyrone (p.35·3); terpineol (p.1752·2); chlorophyll (p.1057·1); ampoule B, chlorphenamine maleate (p.427·3); vitamin C (p.1460·2).
*Influenza symptoms.*

**Eucalipto Composto** *Dynacren, Ital.*
Eucalyptus oil (p.1686·2); camphor (p.1665·3); levomenthol (p.1711·3); thymol (p.1194·2).
*Nasal congestion.*

**Eucaliptol**
*Note. This name is used for preparations of different composition.*
*Bunker, Braz.†.*
Dipyrone (p.35·3); guaifenesin (p.1122·1); cineole (p.1672·1).
*Cold and influenza symptoms.*

*Neo Quimica, Braz.†.*
Dipyrone (p.35·3); guaifenesin (p.1122·1); cineole (p.1672·1); sodium camsilate; ascorbic acid (p.1460·2).
Lidocaine hydrochloride (p.1377·3) is included in this preparation to alleviate the pain of injection.
*Cold and influenza symptoms.*

**Eucaliptol Composto**
*Note. This name is used for preparations of different composition.*
*Bunker, Braz.†.*
Dipyrone (p.35·3); cineole (p.1672·1); guaifenesin (p.1122·1).
*Cold and influenza symptoms.*

*INQ, Braz.†.*
Dipyrone (p.35·3); guaifenesin (p.1122·1); cineole (p.1672·1); terpineol (p.1752·2); ascorbic acid (p.1460·2); chlorphenamine maleate (p.427·3).
*Cold and influenza symptoms.*

**Eucalyptamint** *Ciba, USA.*
Menthol (p.1711·3); eucalyptus oil (p.1686·2).

**Eucalyptine**
*Note. This name is used for preparations of different composition.*
*Millet Roux, Braz.†.*
Camphor (p.1665·3); cineole (p.1672·1); phenol (p.1188·1); guaiacol (p.1122·1).
*Respiratory-tract congestion.*

*Martin, Fr.*
*Adult suppositories:* Cineole (p.1672·1); guaifenesin (p.1122·1); camphor (p.1665·3).
Formerly contained cineole, guaiacol, phenol, camphor, and codeine phosphate.
*Infant suppositories:* Cineole (p.1672·1); guaifenesin (p.1122·1).
*Coughs.*

**Eucalyptine Le Brun**
*Note. This name is used for preparations of different composition.*
*Medgenix, Belg.*
*Capsules:* Cineole (p.1672·1); codeine (p.27·1).
Formerly contained cineole, guaiacol, phenol, codeine, camphor, and bromoform.
*Coughs.*
*Suppositories for adults and children:* Codeine phosphate (p.27·1); cineole (p.1672·1).
Formerly contained camphor, phenol, cineole, and guaiacol.
*Coughs.*
*Suppositories for infants:* Codeine phosphate (p.27·1); cineole (p.1672·1).
*Respiratory disorders.*
*Syrup:* Codeine (p.27·1); cineole (p.1672·1).
Formerly contained sulfogaiacol, sodium phenolsulfonate, sodium camsilate, codeine, belladonna, aconite, bromoform, and cineole.
*Coughs.*

*Martin, Fr.*
*Infant suppositories:* Cineole (p.1672·1); sulfogaiacol (p.1131·1).
Formerly contained cineole, sulfogaiacol, and sodium camsilate.
*Respiratory-tract disorders.*
*Syrup:* Cineole (p.1672·1); codeine (p.27·1).
Formerly contained eucalyptus oil, sodium phenolsulfonate, sodium camsilate, sulfogaiacol, bromoform, codeine, belladonna, and aconite.
*Coughs.*

**Eucalyptine Pholcodine** *Martin, Fr.†.*
Cineole (p.1672·1); pholcodine (p.1128·3).
Formerly contained cineole, guaiacol, phenol, camphor, and pholcodine.
*Coughs.*

**Eucalyptine Pholcodine Le Brun** *Medgenix, Belg.*
*Suppositories for adults and children:* Cineole (p.1672·1); camphor (p.1665·3); phenol (p.1188·1); guaiacol (p.1122·1); pholcodine (p.1128·3).
*Suppositories for infants:* Cineole (p.1672·1); camphor (p.1665·3); guaiacol (p.1122·1); pholcodine (p.1128·3).
*Syrup:* Sulfogaiacol (p.1131·1); sodium camsilate; sodium phenolsulfonate; pholcodine (p.1128·3); belladonna (p.479·1); aconite (p.1646·3); cineole (p.1672·1).
Formerly contained sulfogaiacol, sodium camsilate, sodium phenolsulfonate, pholcodine, belladonna, aconite, bromoform, and cineole.
*Respiratory disorders.*

**Eucalyptospirine** *Pfizer Lambert, Spain.*
Aspirin (p.15·1); cineole (p.1672·1); guaiacol (p.1122·1).
Formerly contained aspirin, amylocaine hydrochloride, cineole, ethylmorphine, guaiacol, and sodium camsilate.
*Influenza and cold symptoms.*

**Eucalyptospirine Lact** *Rovi, Spain†.*
Aspirin (p.15·1); amylocaine hydrochloride (p.1370·2); cineole (p.1672·1); guaiacol (p.1122·1); sodium camsilate.
*Influenza and cold symptoms.*

**Eucalyptrol L** *Medopharm, Ger.†.*
Eucalyptus oil (p.1686·2).
*Cold symptoms.*

**Eucalytux** *Tilman, Belg.*
Codeine (p.27·1); sulfogaiacol (p.1131·1); eucalyptus oil (p.1686·2); pumilio pine oil (p.1737·1).
*Coughs.*

**Eucament** *Catarinense, Braz.†.*
Benzocaine (p.1370·3); camphor (p.1665·3); cetylpyridinium chloride (p.1173·1); tyrothricin (p.275·1).
*Mouth and throat disorders.*

**Eucamenth** *Planta, Canad.†.*
Camphor oil; eucalyptus oil (p.1686·2); menthol (p.1711·3).
*Coughs; nasal and sinus congestion.*

**Eucanol** *Pharma Nord, UK.*
*Cream:* Eucalyptus oil (p.1686·2); lavender oil (p.1705·2); calendula oil (p.1665·2).
*Insect bites; skin irritation.*
*Topical rub; topical spray:* Eucalyptus oil (p.1686·2); lavender oil (p.1705·2); sweet birch oil (p.60·1).
*Musculoskeletal and joint pain.*

**Eucar** *Salus, Ital.*
Levocarnitine hydrochloride (p.1424·1).
*Carnitine deficiency.*

**Eucarbon**
*Note. This name is used for preparations of different composition.*
*Trenka, Austria; Trenker, Belg.†.*
Senna (p.1288·2); rhubarb (p.1287·3); vegetable charcoal (p.1030·3); sulfur (p.1158·2); peppermint oil (p.1283·2); fennel oil (p.1687·3).
*Constipation; dyspepsia; flatulence.*

*Trenka, Israel; Giuliani, Ital.; Trenka, Malaysia; Bio-Pharmaceuticals, Malaysia.*
Senna (p.1288·2); rhubarb (p.1287·3); charcoal (p.1030·3); sulfur (p.1158·2).
*Bowel evacuation; constipation; flatulence.*

*Trenka, Switz.†.*
Senna (p.1288·2); rhubarb (p.1287·3); vegetable charcoal (p.1030·3); peppermint oil (p.1283·2); fennel oil (p.1687·3).
*Constipation; flatulence.*

**Eucardic**
*Roche, Irl.; Roche, Neth.; Boehringer Mannheim, Swed.†; Roche, UK.*
Carvedilol (p.881·1).
*Angina pectoris; heart failure; hypertension.*

**Eucardina** *Italmex, Mex.*
Tripsepar.
*Thromboembolic disorders.*

**Eucardion** *Dompe Biotec, Ital.†.*
Dexrazoxane hydrochloride (p.1036·2).
*Prevention of doxorubicin cardiotoxicity.*

**Eucarnil** *Pulitzer, Ital.*
Levocarnitine (p.1423·3).
*Carnitine deficiency; myocardial ischaemia.*

**Eucerin**
*Note. This name is used for preparations of different composition.*
*Beiersdorf, Austral.; Smith & Nephew, Canad.†; Beiersdorf, Irl.; Beiersdorf, Thai.; Beiersdorf, UK; Beiersdorf, USA.*
A range of skin cleansing and emollient preparations.

*Beiersdorf, Chile.*
*Cream:* Zinc oxide (p.1163·2); panthenol (p.1727·2); levomenol (p.1707·1); diazolidinyl urea; phenoxyethanol (p.1189·1).
*Acne.*
*Cream-gel:* Lactic acid (p.1704·1); sodium lactate (p.1223·2).
*Acne.*
*SPF 15:* Enzacamene (p.1147·1); octil triazone (p.1154·3); avobenzone (p.1142·3); titanium dioxide (p.1160·3).
*Sunscreen.*
*SPF 25 cream:* Enzacamene (p.1147·1); titanium dioxide (p.1160·3); octil triazone (p.1154·3); avobenzone (p.1142·3).
*Sunscreen.*
*SPF 25 pigmented cream:* Zinc oxide (p.1163·2); titanium dioxide (p.1160·3).
*Sunscreen.*
*Topical gel:* Salicylic acid (p.1157·1).
*Acne.*

*Beiersdorf, USA.*
*SPF 25:* Octinoxate (p.1154·3); octisalate (p.1154·3); titanium dioxide (p.1160·3); zinc oxide (p.1163·2).
*Dry skin; sunscreen.*

**Eucerin Baby & Mom** *Beiersdorf, Chile.*
A range of skin cleansing and emollient preparations.

**Eucerin Dry Skin Care Daily Facial** *Beiersdorf, USA.*
*SPF 20:* Octinoxate (p.1154·3); titanium dioxide (p.1160·3); ensulizole (p.1147·1); octisalate (p.1154·3).
*Sunscreen.*

**Eucerin Itch-Relief** *Beiersdorf, USA.*
Menthol (p.1711·3); evening primrose oil (p.1686·3).
*Pruritus.*

**Eucerin Omega Fettsauren Olbad** *Beiersdorf, Ger.*
Soya oil (p.1447·2).
*Bath additive; dry skin.*

**Eucerin peau seche** *Beiersdorf, Switz.*
Urea (p.1162·2).
*Dry skin disorders.*

**Eucerin Pele com tendencia para o acne** *Beiersdorf, Port.*
A range of cleansing and moisturising preparations.
*Acne.*

**Eucerin Pele com tendencia para o acne creme anti-borbulhas** *Beiersdorf, Port.†.*
Zinc oxide (p.1163·2); panthenol (p.1727·2).
*Acne.*

**Eucerin Pele Seca** *Beiersdorf, Port.*
Urea (p.1162·2).
*Dry skin.*

**Eucerin Pele Sensivel** *Beiersdorf, Port.*
A range of soap substitutes and moisturisers.

**Eucerin pH5** *Beiersdorf, Arg.*
A range of skin cleansing and emollient preparations.

**Eucerin Piel con Tendencia Acneica** *BDF, Mex.*
Lactic acid (p.1704·1).
*Acne.*

**Eucerin Piel Seca/Reseca** *BDF, Mex.*
Urea (p.1162·2); sodium lactate (p.1223·2).
*Dry skin disorders.*

**Eucerin Piel Sensible al Sol** *BDF, Mex.*
*SPF 20; SPF 25; SPF 35:* Titanium dioxide (p.1160·3); octil triazone (p.1154·3); zinc oxide (p.1163·2); avobenzone (p.1142·3).
*Sunscreen.*

**Eucerin Plus** *Beiersdorf, USA.*
*SPF 15:* Octinoxate (p.1154·3); oxybenzone (p.1154·3); octisalate (p.1154·3).
*Dry skin; sunscreen.*

**Eucerin Salbe** *Beiersdorf, Ger.*
Urea (p.1162·2).
*Dry skin.*

**Eucerin Solar** *Beiersdorf, Chile.*
*Cream SPF 15:* Titanium dioxide (p.1160·3).
*Cream SPF 20:* Zinc oxide (p.1163·2); titanium dioxide (p.1160·3).
*Gel SPF 25:* Enzacamene (p.1147·1); titanium dioxide (p.1160·3); octil triazone (p.1154·3); avobenzone (p.1142·3).
*SPF 35:* Enzacamene (p.1147·1); titanium dioxide (p.1160·3); octil triazone (p.1154·3); avobenzone (p.1142·3).
*Spray SPF 20:* Enzacamene (p.1147·1); octil triazone (p.1154·3); avobenzone (p.1142·3); dicaprylyl ether; dietheylhexyl butamido triazone; ensulizole (p.1147·1).
*Stick SPF 25:* Enzacamene (p.1147·1); octylmethoxyferyl acetate; avobenzone (p.1142·3); titanium dioxide (p.1160·3).
*Sunscreen.*

**Eucerinum** *Beiersdorf, Chile.*
Dry skin; pharmaceutical base.

**Euceta**
*Sandoz, Ital.†; Novartis Consumer, Switz.*
Aluminium acetotartrate (p.1652·3).
*Skin disorders.*

**Euceta avec camomille et arnica** *Novartis Consumer, Switz.*
Aluminium acetotartrate (p.1652·3); chamomile (p.1669·3); arnica (p.1656·3).
*Skin disorders.*

**Euceta mit Kamille** *Novartis Consumer, Austria.*
Aluminium acetotartrate (p.1652·3); chamomile (p.1669·3).
*Skin disorders.*

**Euceta Pic** *Novartis Consumer, Switz.*
Aluminium acetotartrate (p.1652·3); mepyramine maleate (p.437·1); lidocaine hydrochloride (p.1377·3).
*Insect bites.*

**Euchessina** *Antonetto, Switz.†.*
Phenolphthalein (p.1284·1).
*Constipation.*

**Euchessina CM** *Antonetto, Ital.*
Sodium picosulfate (p.1289·3).
*Constipation.*

**Euci** *Falqui, Ital.†.*
Paracetamol (p.76·2); ascorbic acid (p.1460·2); pseudoephedrine hydrochloride (p.1129·2); dextromethorphan hydrobromide (p.1117·3).
*Cold symptoms.*

**Eucid** *Greater Pharma, Thai.*
Omeprazole (p.1278·2).
*Gastro-oesophageal reflux, Zollinger-Ellison syndrome; peptic ulcer.*

**Eucil** *Farmasa, Braz.*
Metoclopramide hydrochloride (p.1274·3).
*Gastrointestinal motility disorders; nausea and vomiting.*

**Eucillin** *Petrasch, Austria.*
Bacitracin (p.161·3); dequalinium chloride (p.1178·1); diphenylpyraline hydrochloride (p.432·3).
*Infected skin disorders.*

**Euciton** *Roux-Ocefa, Arg.*
Domperidone (p.1263·2).
*Gastrointestinal disorders.*

**Euciton Complex** *Roux-Ocefa, Arg.*
Domperidone (p.1263·2); dipotassium clorazepate (p.685·1).
*Gastrointestinal disorders.*

**Euclorina** *Bracco, Ital.*
Tosylchloramide sodium (p.1194·3).
*Skin, wound, and genital disinfection.*

**Eucol** *Augot, Fr.†.*
Arginine oxoglurate (p.1421·2).
*Hepatic encephalopathy; tonic.*

**Eucoprost** *Frosst, Spain.*
Finasteride (p.1554·2).
*Benign prostatic hyperplasia.*

**Eucor** *Greater Pharma, Thai.*
Simvastatin (p.997·1).
*Hypercholesterolaemia.*

**Eucorten** *Trima, Israel.*
Clobetasone butyrate (p.1095·3).
*Skin disorders.*

**Eucycline** *Demo, Gr.*
Ketotifen fumarate (p.788·1).
*Allergic rhinitis; asthma.*

**Eudal-SR** *UAD, USA.*
Pseudoephedrine hydrochloride (p.1129·2); guaifenesin (p.1122·1).
*Coughs.*

**Eudemine**
*Celltech, UK.*
*Tablets:* Diazoxide (p.893·2).
*Hypoglycaemia.*

*Goldshield, UK.*
*Injection:* Diazoxide (p.893·2).
*Hypertensive crises.*

**Eudent con Glysan** *Kemiprogress, Ital.*
Glysan (enoxolone (p.36·2); sanguinaria (p.1741·3)); sodium monofluorophosphate (p.1446·2) or sodium fluoride (p.1444·3).
*Gum disorders; oral hygiene.*

**Euderm**
*Xepa-Soul Pattinson, Hong Kong; Xepa-Soul Pattinson, Malaysia; Xepa-Soul Pattinson, Singapore.*
Urea (p.1162·2).
*Dry skin disorders.*

**Eudermal Pasta** *Pentaderm, Ital.†.*
Barrier cream.

**Eudermal Sapone Allo Zolfo pH 5** *Pentaderm, Ital.†.*
Sulfur (p.1158·2).
*Skin cleansing.*

**Eudermico** *Novogaleno, Ital.*
Urea (p.1162·2); lactic acid (p.1704·1).
*Dry skin disorders.*

**Eudextran** *Clarmed, Ital.*
Dextran 40 (p.745·3) in sodium chloride or glucose.
*Plasma volume expansion; thromboembolic disorders.*

**Eudigestio** *Ogna, Ital.*
Pancreatin (p.1725·3); pepsin (p.1729·3).
*Dyspepsia.*

**Eudigox** *Teofarma, Ital.*
Digoxin (p.895·2).
*Arrhythmias; heart failure.*

**Eudipar** *CT, Ital.*
Heparin calcium (p.927·3).
*Thromboembolic disorders.*

**Eudolene** *Savio, Ital.*
Nimesulide (p.67·1).
*Fever; inflammation; pain.*

**Eudon**
*Note. This name is used for preparations of different composition.*
*Baliarda, Arg.*
Bromazepam (p.671·3); clebopride (p.1260·3); simeticone (p.1289·2).
*Gastrointestinal disorders.*

*Eurofarmaco, Ital.*
Glutathione (p.1040·3).
*Drug and alcohol intoxication; reduction of radiation-induced damage.*

**Eudorlin** *Berlin-Chemie, Ger.*
Propyphenazone (p.85·3); paracetamol (p.76·2); caffeine (p.782·1).
*Pain.*

**Eudorlin Extra** *Berlin-Chemie, Ger.*
Ibuprofen (p.45·3).
*Fever; pain.*

**Eudur** *Astra, Ger.†.*
Terbutaline sulfate (p.797·2); theophylline (p.798·3).
*Obstructive airways disease.*

**Eudyna**
*Ebewe, Austria; BASF, Ger.†; Knoll, Hong Kong†; German Remedies, India; Knoll, Mex.†; Knoll, Singapore†.*
Tretinoin (p.1161·1).
*Acne.*

**Eufans** *Sigma-Tau, Ital.*
Amtolmetin guacil (p.14·3).
*Musculoskeletal and joint disorders; pain.*

**Eufenil** *Pharmacaps, Mex.†.*
Ibuprofen (p.45·3).

**Eufermen** *Sankyo, Braz.*
Enzymes from *Aspergillus oryzae*; ethaverine hydrochloride (p.1685·2); dimethicone (p.1289·2).
*Digestive-system disorders.*

**Eufibron** *Berlin-Chemie, Ger.*
Propyphenazone (p.85·3).
*Fever; pain.*

**Eufilin** *Byk, Braz.†.*
Aminophylline (p.780·2).
*Neonatal apnoea; obstructive airways disease.*

**Eufilina**
*Byk, Port.; Byk Elmu, Spain.*
Theophylline (p.798·3).
Formerly contained aminophylline in *Spain*.
*Cor pulmonale; obstructive airways disease.*

**Eufimenth N mild** *Lichtenstein, Ger.†.*
Eucalyptus oil (p.1686·2); Norway spruce oil.
*Respiratory-tract disorders.*

**Eufimenth-Balsam N** *Lichtenstein, Ger.*
Cineole (p.1672·1); Norway spruce oil; menthol (p.1711·3).
*Respiratory-tract disorders.*

**Euflat I** *Stegopharm, Ger.*
Dimethicone (p.1289·2); caraway oil (p.1667·3); fennel oil (p.1687·3).
*Digestive system disorders.*

**Euflat-E** *Sudmedica, Ger.*
Pancreatin (p.1725·3).
*Digestive system disorders.*

**Euflex** *Schering, Canad.*
Flutamide (p.556·2).
*Prostatic cancer.*

**Euflux-N** *Sudmedica, Ger.*
Pumilio pine oil (p.1737·1); camphor (p.1665·3).
*Catarrh; rheumatic disorders.*

**Eufor** *Farmasa, Braz.*
Fluoxetine (p.296·3).
*Depression; obsessive-compulsive disorder.*

**Eufusin** *Clarmed, Ital.*
Succinylated gelatin (p.754·3).
*Hypovolaemia.*

**Eugalac** *Topfer, Ger.*
Lactulose (p.1269·1).
*Constipation; hepatic encephalopathy.*

**Eugalan Topfer forte** *Topfer, Ger.*
Bifidum bacteria; lactulose (p.1269·1).
*Cirrhosis; gastrointestinal disorders.*

**Eugenol-Guaiacolo Composto** *Ogna, Ital.*
Eugenol (p.1686·2); guaiacol (p.1122·1); lidocaine hydrochloride (p.1377·3); thymol (p.1194·2).
*Dental extraction pain.*

**Eugerial**
*Bago, Arg.; Merck, Braz.*
Nimodipine (p.972·3).
*Cerebrovascular disorders; hypertension; mental function impairment.*

**Eugerminal** *Medix, Mex.*
Vitamin E (p.1464·3).
*Vitamin E supplement.*

**Eugiron** *Denolin, Belg.†.*
Clove flower (p.1673·2); althaea root and leaf (p.1651·3); raspberry leaf (p.1737·3); tilia flower (p.1756·2); eucalyptus leaf (p.1686·1); aniseed fruit (p.1655·2); fennel fruit (p.1687·2).
*Mouth and throat disorders.*

**Euglamin** *Ratiopharm, Fin.*
Glibenclamide (p.331·2).
*Diabetes mellitus.*

**Euglim** *Zydus, India.*
Glimepiride (p.332·2).
*Diabetes mellitus.*

**Euglucan** *Roche, Fr.*
Glibenclamide (p.331·2).
*Diabetes mellitus.*

**Euglucon**
*Roche, Arg.; Roche, Austria; Roche, Belg.; Roche, Braz.; Pharmascience, Canad.; Roche, Denm.†; Roche, Fin.; Roche, Hong Kong; Nicholas Piramal, India; Roche, Ital.; Roche, Mex.; Boehringer Mannheim, Neth.†; Roche, Norw.†; Roche, Port.; Roche, S.Afr.; Roche, Singapore†; Roche, Spain; Roche, Swed.; Roche, Switz.; Roche, Thai.; Aventis, UK.*
Glibenclamide (p.331·2).
*Diabetes mellitus.*

**Euglucon N** *Aventis, Ger.*
Glibenclamide (p.331·2).
*Diabetes mellitus.*

**Euglusid** *Roche, Chile.*
Glibenclamide (p.331·2).
*Diabetes mellitus.*

**Eugrippine** *Synthelabo, Belg.†.*
Diphenhydramine hydrochloride (p.431·3); caffeine (p.782·1); quinine sulfate (p.460·2); ascorbic acid (p.1460·2).
*Fever associated with influenza.*

**Eugune** *Palmares, Ital.*
Magnesium; bioflavonoids; proline oxide; lupulus; hydroxyapatite (p.1417·1).
*Menopausal disorders.*

**Eugusal** *Nutricia-Bago, Arg.*
Potassium chloride; potassium tartrate; ammonium chloride; citric acid; calcium phosphate (p.1217·1).
*Salt substitute.*

**Eugynol** *Hearst, Braz.†.*
Plumeria; gossypium; hypericum (p.299·1).

**Eugynon**
*Schering, Hong Kong; Schering, Ital.; Schering, Norw.†.*
Norgestrel (p.1563·2); ethinylestradiol (p.1553·2).
*Combined oral contraceptive; endometriosis; menstrual disorders.*

**Eugynon 30** *Schering, UK.*
Levonorgestrel (p.1563·2); ethinylestradiol (p.1553·2).
*Combined oral contraceptive.*

**Eugynon 250** *Schering, Thai.*
Levonorgestrel (p.1563·2); ethinylestradiol (p.1553·2).
28-Day packs also contain 7 inert tablets.
*Combined oral contraceptive.*

**Euhypnos**
*Sigma, Austral.; Pharmacia, Belg.; Pharmacia, Irl.; Sigma, NZ; Pharmacia, Thai.; Farmitalia Carlo Erba, UK†.*
Temazepam (p.723·2).
*Insomnia; premedication.*

**Euipnos** *Teva, Ital.*
Temazepam (p.723·2).
*Insomnia.*

**Euka** *Pharmonta, Austria.*
Fennel (p.1687·2); aniseed (p.1655·2); rosemary (p.1740·2); eucalyptus (p.1686·1); lavender flowers (p.1705·1); laurel leaves; camphor (p.1665·3); peppermint oil (p.1283·2); spearmint oil (p.1749·1).
*Gastrointestinal disorders.*

**Eukalisan forte** *Steigerwald, Ger.†.*
Cyanocobalamin (p.1458·2); nicotinamide (p.1441·2); rutoside sodium sulfate (p.1688·3).
Lidocaine hydrochloride (p.1377·3) is included in this preparation to alleviate the pain of injection.
*Liver disorders.*

**Eukalisan N** *Steigerwald, Ger.*
Cyanocobalamin (p.1458·2); nicotinamide (p.1441·2); rutoside sodium sulfate (p.1688·3).
Procaine hydrochloride (p.1383·2) is included in this preparation to alleviate the pain of injection.
*Liver disorders; neuralgia; peripheral vascular disorders; tonic.*

**Eukamillat** *Biocur, Ger.*
Chamomile (p.1669·3).
*Gastrointestinal, anogenital, mouth, respiratory-tract, and skin disorders.*

**Eukavan** *Duopharm, Ger.†.*
Kava (p.1703·2).
*Anxiety disorders.*

**Euketos** *CT, Ital.*
Ketoprofen (p.51·2).
*Inflammation; musculoskeletal, joint, peri-articular, and soft-tissue disorders; pain; phlebitis; thrombophlebitis.*

**Euky Bear Cough Syrup** *Felton, Austral.†.*
Chlorphenamine (p.428·1); dextromethorphan (p.1117·3); sodium citrate (p.1223·2).
*Coughs and cold symptoms.*

**Euky Bear Eu-Clear Inhalant** *Felton, Austral.†.*
Eucalyptus oil (p.1686·2); menthol (p.1711·3).
*Cold symptoms; respiratory-tract congestion.*

**Euky Bear Nasex** *Felton, Austral.†.*
Oxymetazoline hydrochloride (p.1126·1); cineole (p.1672·1); menthol (p.1711·3).
*Nasal congestion.*

**Euky Bearub** *Felton, Austral.†.*
Eucalyptus oil (p.1686·2); cineole (p.1672·1); menthol (p.1711·3); camphor (p.1665·3); rosemary oil (p.1740·2).
*Cold and influenza symptoms; insect bites; muscular aches and pains; nasal congestion.*

**Eulactol** *Eulactol, S.Afr.†.*
Urea (p.1162·2).
*Dry skin.*

**Eulactol Antifungal** *Eulactol, Austral.*
Miconazole (p.405·2).
Formerly known as Leuko Fungex Antifungal.
*Fungal skin infections.*

**Eulatin N** *Riemser, Ger.*
Lidocaine (p.1377·3); bismuth subgallate (p.1252·2).
*Anorectal disorders.*

**Eulatin NN** *Riemser, Ger.*
Hamamelis (p.1696·3); bismuth subgallate (p.1252·2); benzocaine (p.1370·3).
*Anorectal disorders.*

**Eulexin**
*Essex, Arg.; Schering-Plough, Austral.; Schering-Plough, Belg.; Schering-Plough, Braz.; Schering-Plough, Denm.; Schering-Plough, Fin.; Schering-Plough, Israel; Schering-Plough, Ital.; Schering-Plough, Mex.; Schering-Plough, Neth.; Schering-Plough, Norw.; Schering-Plough, NZ†; Schering-Plough, Port.; Schering-Plough, S.Afr.; Schering-Plough, Spain; Schering-Plough, Swed.; Schering, USA.*
Flutamide (p.556·2).
*Prostatic cancer.*

**Eulexine** *Schering-Plough, Fr.*
Flutamide (p.556·2).
*Prostatic cancer.*

**Eulip** *SIT, Ital.†.*
Tiadenol (p.1011·2).
*Hyperlipidaemias.*

**Eulitop**
*Roche, Belg.; Roche, Spain.*
Bezafibrate (p.873·2).
*Hyperlipidaemias.*

**Eulux** *Mediwhite, Ital.*
Chamomile (p.1669·3); euphrasia (p.1686·3); centaurea cyanus; hamamelis (p.1696·3).
*Eye irritation.*

**Eulyptan** *Labima, Belg.*
Codeine (p.27·1).
*Coughs.*

**Eu-Med**
*Note. This name is used for preparations of different composition.*
*Novartis Consumer, Austria.*
Paracetamol (p.76·2); caffeine (p.782·1); propyphenazone (p.85·3).
Formerly contained salacetamide, caffeine, propyphenazone, and phenazone.
*Fever; pain.*

*Zyma, Ger.†.*
Phenazone (p.82·3).
*Fever; pain.*

**Eumetic** *Pharmacia, Arg.*
Granisetron hydrochloride (p.1267·1).
*Nausea and vomiting.*

**Eumetinex** *Lakeside, Mex.†.*
Amoxicillin trihydrate (p.155·3); clavulanic acid (p.193·3).
*Bacterial infections.*

**Euminz** *Lichtwer, Ger.*
Peppermint oil (p.1283·2).
*Tension-type headache.*

**Eumol** *Arlex, Mex.†.*
Oxolamine (p.1126·1).

**Eumosone** *GlaxoSmithKline, India.*
Clobetasone butyrate (p.1095·3).
*Skin disorders.*

**Eumotol** *Byk, Braz.†.*
Bumadizone calcium (p.21·3).
*Gout; musculoskeletal and joint disorders.*

**Eumovate**
*GlaxoSmithKline, Arg.; GlaxoSmithKline, Belg.; Zest, Braz.; GlaxoSmithKline, Canad.; GlaxoSmithKline, Chile; GlaxoSmithKline, Hong Kong; GlaxoSmithKline, Irl.; GlaxoSmithKline, Israel; GlaxoSmithKline, Ital.; GlaxoSmithKline, Malaysia; GlaxoSmithKline, NZ; Glaxo Wellcome, S.Afr.; GlaxoSmithKline, Singapore; GlaxoSmithKline, Thai.; GlaxoSmithKline Consumer, UK.*
Clobetasone butyrate (p.1095·3).
*Skin disorders.*

**EuMunil** *Madaus, Ital.*
Echinacea (p.1683·2).
*Immunostimulant; respiratory-tract infections.*

**Eunades** *Pharmacia, Braz.*
Etoposide (p.551·3).
*Malignant neoplasms.*

**Eunasin** *Bracco, Ital.†.*
Metizoline hydrochloride (p.1124·3).
*Upper respiratory-tract disorders.*

**Eunerpan** *Abbott, Ger.*
Melperone hydrochloride (p.706·1).
*Psychiatric disorders; sleep disorders.*

**Eunova** *GlaxoSmithKline Consumer, Ger.*
Multivitamin and mineral preparation (p.1417·1).

**Eupantol** *Altana, Fr.*
Pantoprazole sodium (p.1283·1).
*Gastro-oesophageal reflux; peptic ulcer; Zollinger-Ellison syndrome.*

**Eupatal** *Madaus, Ger.*
Thyme (p.1755·2); star anise oil.
*Cold symptoms.*

**Eupatol** *Donini, Ital.*
Cascara (p.1255·1); boldo (p.1661·2); rhubarb (p.1287·3).
*Constipation.*

**Eupatorium Oligoplex** *Madaus, Ger.*
Homoeopathic preparation.

**Eupeclanic** *Uriach, Spain.*
Amoxicillin trihydrate (p.155·3); potassium clavulanate (p.193·3).
*Bacterial infections.*

**Eupen** *Uriach, Spain.*
Amoxicillin trihydrate (p.155·3).
*Bacterial infections.*

**Eupen Bronquial** *Uriach, Spain.*
Amoxicillin trihydrate (p.155·3); brovanexine hydrochloride (p.1116·1).
*Respiratory-tract infections.*

**Eupept** *Cifarma, Braz.†.*
Omeprazole (p.1278·2).
*Peptic ulcer.*

**Eupeptina** *Almirall, Spain.*
Dibasic sodium phosphate (p.1231·1); magnesium carbonate (p.1272·1); magnesium phosphate (p.1228·1); magnesium oxide (p.1272·3); pepsin carbonate.
*Constipation; dyspepsia.*

**Euphidra G2 Radical** *Zeta, Ital.†.*
Multivitamin and mineral preparation (p.1417·1).
*Nutritional supplement.*

**Euphon**
*Note. This name is used for preparations of different composition.*
*ACP, Belg.*
Codeine (p.27·1); aconite (p.1646·3); sodium formate (p.1689·3); erysimin; elecampane (p.1119·3).
*Throat disorders.*

*Mayoly-Spindler, Fr.†.*
*Oral solution:* Codeine (p.27·1); aconite (p.1646·3); sodium formate (p.1689·3); erysimin.
*Coughs.*

*Mayoly-Spindler, Fr.; Jaba, Port.; Mayoly-Spindler, Singapore.*
*Pastilles:* Erysimin.
*Catarrh; cough; throat disorders.*

*Mayoly-Spindler, Fr.*
*Syrup; capsules:* Erysimin; codeine (p.27·1).
*Coughs.*

*Mayoly-Spindler, Malaysia.*
Erysimin; menthol (p.1711·3).
*Sore throat.*

*Jaba, Port.*
*Syrup:* Codeine (p.27·1); erysimin.
*Coughs.*

**Euphon N** *Mayoly-Spindler, Switz.; Uhlmann-Eyraud, Switz.*
Codeine (p.27·1); tolu balsam (p.1131·3).
*Coughs and associated respiratory-tract disorders.*

**Euphorbia Complex** *Blackmores, Austral.†.*
Passion flower (p.1729·1); thyme (p.1755·2); grindelia (p.1696·1); euphorbia (p.1686·3); vitamins (p.1417·1).
*Asthma; bronchitis; catarrh.*

**Euphorbium Compositum** *Peithner, Austria.*
Homoeopathic preparation.

**Euphorbium Compositum S** *Heel, S.Afr.*
Homoeopathic preparation.

**Euphorbium compositum-Nasentropfen SN** *Heel, Ger.*
Homoeopathic preparation.

**Euphyllin**
*Byk, Austria; Byk, Belg.; Meda, Fin.; Byk Gulden, Ger.†; Byk, Neth.; Byk Gulden, Norw.†; Byk Madaus, S.Afr.; Altana, Switz.*
Aminophylline (p.780·2) or theophylline (p.798·3).
*Obstructive airways disease.*

**Euphyllina** *Byk Gulden, Ital.*
Aminophylline (p.780·2) or theophylline (p.798·3).
*Obstructive airways disease.*

**Euphylline** *Byk, Fr.*
Theophylline (p.798·3).
*Obstructive airways disease.*

**Euphylong**
*Byk Gulden, Ger.; Altana, Hong Kong; Byk, Neth.†; Swedish Orphan, Swed.*
Theophylline (p.798·3).
*Obstructive airways disease.*

**Euphytose** *Roche Nicholas, Fr.*
Crataegus (p.1677·1); passion flower (p.1729·1); valerian (p.1762·2); ballota.
Formerly contained crataegus, passion flower, guarana, kola, valerian, and ballota.
*Nervous disorders.*

**Euplix** *Desitin, Ger.*
Paroxetine mesilate (p.311·2).
*Bipolar disorder; depression; panic attacks.*

**Eupneron** *Lyocentre, Fr.*
Eprozinol hydrochloride (p.1121·1).
*Obstructive airways disease.*

**Eupnol** *Rottapharm, Spain.*
Benzethonium chloride (p.1169·2); cineole (p.1672·1); cherry-laurel; procaine hydrochloride (p.1383·2); terpineol (p.1752·2); menthol (p.1711·3).
*Mouth and throat inflammation.*

**Eupragin** *Alcon, Ger.†.*
Erythromycin estolate (p.208·1).
*Bacterial eye infections.*

**Eupres** *Monsanto, Ital.*
Atenolol (p.865·2); chlortalidone (p.882·3).
*Hypertension.*

**Eupressin** *Biosintetica, Braz.*
Enalapril maleate (p.909·2).
*Heart failure; hypertension.*

**Eupressin H** *Biosintetica, Braz.*
Enalapril maleate (p.909·2); hydrochlorothiazide (p.933·2).
*Hypertension.*

**Eupressyl** *Byk, Fr.*
Urapidil (p.1018·1) or urapidil hydrochloride (p.1018·1).
*Hypertension.*

**Euproct** *Andromaco, Chile.*
Tribenoside (p.1757·3); lidocaine (p.1377·3).
*Anorectal disorders.*

**Euproctol** *Sanopharm, Switz.*
Resorcinol (p.1156·3); ephedrine hydrochloride (p.1120·1); lidocaine hydrochloride (p.1377·3); menthol (p.1711·3).
*Anorectal disorders.*

**Euproctol N** *Sanopharm, Switz.*
Bismuth oxychloride (p.1253·1); ethacridine lactate (p.1165·3); zinc oxide (p.1163·2); menthol (p.1711·3); lidocaine hydrochloride (p.1377·3); ephedrine hydrochloride (p.1120·1); hamamelis (p.1696·3); peru balsam (p.1730·2).
*Anorectal disorders.*

**Euprotin** *Prasfarma, Spain.*
Lenograstim (p.755·3).
*Mobilisation of autologous peripheral blood progenitor cells; reduction of neutropenia associated with cancer chemotherapy.*

**Euradal** *Lacer, Spain.*
Bisoprolol fumarate (p.875·1).
*Angina pectoris; hypertension.*

**Euralben** *Reuffer, Mex.†.*
Albendazole (p.101·2).

**Eurax**
*Novartis Consumer, Austral.; Novartis Consumer, Austria; Novartis Consumer, Belg.; Novartis Consumer, Canad.; Novartis, Chile; Novartis Sante, Fr.; Novartis, Hong Kong; Novartis Consumer, Irl.; Novartis, Israel; Novartis Consumer, Ital.; Novartis, Malaysia; Novartis, Mex.; Novartis, Norw.; Novartis, NZ; Novartis Consumer, Port.; Novartis Consumer, S.Afr.; Novartis Nutrition, Singapore; Novartis Consumer, Switz.; Novartis Consumer, UK; Westwood-Squibb, USA.*
Crotamiton (p.1145·1).
*Pediculosis; pruritus; scabies.*

**Eurax-Hydrocortisone**
*Novartis Consumer, Irl.; Novartis Consumer, UK.*
Crotamiton (p.1145·1); hydrocortisone (p.1103·3).
*Pruritic skin disorders.*

**Euraxil**
*Gepepharm, Ger.†; Novartis Consumer, Spain.*
Crotamiton (p.1145·1).
*Pediculosis; pruritus; scabies.*

**Euraxil Hidrocort** *Padro, Spain†.*
Crotamiton (p.1145·1); hydrocortisone (p.1103·3).
*Skin disorders.*

**Eureceptor** *Zambon, Ital.†.*
Cimetidine (p.1255·3).
*Gastrointestinal disorders.*

**Eurelix** *Aventis, Fr.*
Piretanide (p.983·3).
*Hypertension.*

**Euretico** *Casasco, Arg.*
Chlortalidone (p.882·3).
*Diuretic.*

**Eurex** *Sanofi Synthelabo, Ger.†.*
Prazosin hydrochloride (p.985·1).
*Heart failure; hypertension.*

**Eurhyton** *Adima, Switz.†.*
Crataegus (p.1677·1).
*Cardiac disorders.*

**Eurifam** *Euromex, Mex.†.*
Rifampicin (p.250·2).

**Euritmin** *Rhein, Mex.†.*
Verapamil (p.1021·1).

**Euritsin** *Sanofi Synthelabo, Arg.*
Adenosine (p.851·2).
*Supraventricular tachycardia.*

**Eurixor**
*Richter, Austria; Biosyn, Ger.*
Mistletoe (p.1715·3).
*Joint disorders; malignant neoplasms.*

**Eurobiol**
*Pfizer, Fr.; Interdelta, Switz.†.*
Pancreas extract.
*Digestive disorders; pancreatic insufficiency.*

**Eurocal D3** *Promedica, Ital.*
Calcium carbonate (p.1254·2); colecalciferol (p.1461·3).
*Calcium and vitamin D deficiency; osteoporosis.*

**Eurocefix** *Uno, Ital.*
Cefaclor (p.167·1).
*Bacterial infections.*

**Eurocoal** *Euroderm, Arg.*
Salicylic acid (p.1157·1); benzalkonium chloride (p.1168·3); coal tar (p.1159·2).
*Dandruff; seborrhoea.*

**Eurocolor** *Euroderm, Arg.*
*SPF 4:* Benzophenone (p.1143·1).
*SPF 15:* Titanium dioxide (p.1160·3).
*SPF 34:* Titanium dioxide (p.1160·3); zinc oxide (p.1163·2).
*Sunscreen.*

**Eurocolor Post Solar** *Euroderm, Arg.*
Aloe vera (p.1141·3); calendula (p.1665·2).
*Emollient.*

**Eurocolor Sin Sol** *Euroderm, Arg.*
Dihydroxyacetone (p.1145·2).
*Tanning agent.*

**Euroderm-A** *Euroderm, Arg.*
Vitamin A; vitamin E; vitamin D; allantoin.
*Moisturiser.*

**Eurodin** *Takeda, Jpn.*
Estazolam (p.697·3).
*Insomnia; premedication.*

**Eurofer** *Euroderm, Arg.*
Ferrous sulfate (p.1428·2).
*Iron supplement.*

**Euroflash** *Lifescan, Port.*
Test for glucose in blood (p.1694·2).

**Euroflu** *Euro-Pharma, Ital.*
Flunisolide (p.1101·1).
*Allergic rhinitis; asthma; bronchitis.*

**Eurogel** *Cielle, Ital.*
Royal jelly (p.1740·3); dried yeast (p.1469·1); vitamin E (p.1464·3).
*Nutritional supplement.*

**Eurogesic Gel** *Saval, Chile.*
Naproxen (p.65·1) or naproxen sodium (p.65·1).
*Musculoskeletal, joint, peri-articular, and soft-tissue disorders; pain.*

**Eurolase** *Europharm, Hong Kong.*
Papain (p.1727·3).
*Inflammation; oedema.*

**Eurolat** *Euromex, Mex.†.*
Ketoconazole (p.403·3).

**Eurolol** *Euromex, Mex.†.*
Metoprolol (p.956·3).

**Euromicina** *Saval, Chile.*
Clarithromycin (p.192·2).
*Bacterial infections; Helicobacter pylori eradication.*

**Euromucil** *Saval, Chile.*
Psyllium (p.1268·1).
*Constipation.*

**Euronac** *Europhta, Mon.*
Acetylcysteine (p.1112·3).
*Eye ulceration.*

**Europiel** *Euroderm, Arg.*
Silicone oil (p.1482·1).
*Barrier preparation.*

**Europranolol** *Euromex, Mex.†.*
Propranolol (p.990·1).

**Europrazosin** *Euromex, Mex.†.*
Prazosin (p.986·1).

**Europrotec P** *Euroderm, Arg.*
*SPF 15:* Titanium dioxide (p.1160·3).
*Sunscreen.*

**Europrotec Post Solar** *Euroderm, Arg.*
Aloe vera (p.1141·3); calendula (p.1665·2).
*Emollient.*

**Europrotec Ultra** *Euroderm, Arg.*
*SPF 34:* Titanium dioxide (p.1160·3); zinc oxide (p.1163·2).
*Sunscreen.*

**Eurosan** *Mepha, Switz.*
Clotrimazole (p.396·2).
*Fungal skin and nail infections.*

**Euroton** *Cielle, Ital.*
Withania somnifera; maca; muira puama; ginseng; damiana; rhodiola.

**Eurotretin** *Euroderm, Arg.*
Tretinoin (p.1161·1).
*Photodamaged skin.*

**Eurovan** *Europharm, Hong Kong.*
Zopiclone (p.729·3).
*Insomnia.*

**Eurovir** *Saval, Chile.*
Aciclovir (p.626·1).
*Herpesvirus infections.*

**Euroxi** *Copernico, Ital.*
Piroxicam (p.84·2).
*Musculoskeletal, joint, and peri-articular disorders.*

**Eurozyme** *Europharm, Hong Kong.*
Muramidase hydrochloride (p.1717·2).
*Haemorrhage; inflammation; upper respiratory-tract disorders.*

**Eurythmic** *Troikaa, India.*
Amiodarone hydrochloride (p.859·2).
*Arrhythmias.*

**Eusaprim**
*GlaxoSmithKline, Austria; GlaxoSmithKline, Belg.; GlaxoSmithKline, Fr.; GlaxoSmithKline, Ger.; GlaxoSmithKline, Ital.; GlaxoSmithKline, Neth.; GlaxoSmithKline, Swed.; Wellcome, Switz.†.*
Co-trimoxazole (p.199·3).
*Bacterial infections; Pneumocystis carinii pneumonia; toxoplasmosis.*

**Eusedon mono** *Krewel, Ger.*
Promethazine hydrochloride (p.439·1).
*Hypersensitivity reactions; nausea; nervous disorders; sleep disorders; vomiting.*

**Euserpina Cellulite** *Biogena, Ital.*
Aristolochia (p.1656·3).
*Cellulite.*

**Euskin** *Sankyo, Spain.*
Erythromycin (p.208·1).
*Acne.*

**Eusovit** *Strathmann, Ger.*
*dl*-Alpha tocoferil acetate (p.1465·1).
*Vitamin E deficiency.*

**Euspirax** *Asche, Ger.*
Choline theophyllinate (p.784·2).
*Obstructive airways disease.*

**Eustidil** *Vitoria, Port.*
Fluticasone propionate (p.1102·3).
*Allergic rhinitis.*

**Eutalgic** *Pierre Fabre Sante, Fr.†.*
Menthol (p.1711·3); methyl salicylate (p.59·3); camphor (p.1665·3).
*Soft-tissue injury.*

**Eutecaina** *Silesia, Chile.*
Lidocaine hydrochloride (p.1377·3); prilocaine (p.1382·3).
*Local anaesthesia.*

**Euthyral** *Lipha Sante, Fr.*
Liothyronine sodium (p.1602·2); levothyroxine sodium (p.1600·1).
*Hypothyroidism.*

**Euthyrox**
*Euroderm, Arg.; Merck, Austria†; Merck, Belg.; Merck, Braz.; Merck, Ger.; Merck, Neth.; Merck, Singapore; Merck, Switz.*
Levothyroxine sodium (p.1600·1).
*Goitre; hypothyroidism; thyroid cancer.*

**Eutirox**
*Merck, Chile.*
Levothyroxine (p.1601·3).
*Hypothyroidism.*

*Bracco, Ital.; Merck, Mex.*
Levothyroxine sodium (p.1600·1).
*Hypothyroidism.*

**Eutiz** *Merck, Arg.*
Finasteride (p.1554·2).
*Benign prostatic hyperplasia.*

**Eutocol** *Gador, Arg.*
Estradiol hemisuccinate (p.1551·1).
*Labour induction.*

**Eutrodin** *GD, Ital.*
Zinc oxide (p.1163·2); titanium dioxide (p.1160·3).
*Barrier cream.*

**Eutrofic** *Dermoteca, Port.*
A range of moisturisers.

**Eutrofic Forte Gel Despigmentante** *Dermoteca, Port.†.*
Glycolic acid (p.1147·3); hydroquinone (p.1148·1).
*Hyperpigmentation; keratoses.*

**Eutroid** *Parke, Davis, Arg.*
Levothyroxine sodium (p.1600·1); liothyronine sodium (p.1602·2).
*Hypothyroidism.*

**Eutroxsig** *Fawns & McAllan, Austral.*
Levothyroxine sodium (p.1600·1).
*Hypothyroidism.*

**Eutys-Kili** *Farmila, Ital.†.*
Vitamin $B_6$; chromium; citrin; kelp; kola (p.1417·1).
*Nutritional supplement.*

**Euvaderm**
*Note. This name is used for preparations of different composition.*
*Parke, Davis, Ger.†.*
*Cream:* Betamethasone benzoate (p.1093·1).
*Ointment:* Betamethasone benzoate (p.1093·1); salicylic acid (p.1157·1).
*Skin disorders.*

*Raza, Malaysia; Pharmaniaga, Malaysia.*
Clobetasone butyrate (p.1095·3).
*Skin disorders.*

**Euvaderm N** *Parke, Davis, Ger.†.*
Betamethasone benzoate (p.1093·1); salicylic acid (p.1157·1).
*Skin disorders.*

**Euvalon** *Hotz, Ger.†.*
Crataegus (p.1677·1); valerian (p.1762·2).
*Cardiac disorders.*

**Euvanol** *Monot, Fr.†.*
Geranium oil (p.1692·2); niaouli oil (p.1719·3); camphor (p.1665·3); benzalkonium bromide (p.1169·1).
*Rhinopharyngeal infections.*

**Euvax-B**
*Aventis Pasteur, Malaysia; LG Chem, Thai.*
A hepatitis B vaccine (recombinant DNA) (p.1618·1).
*Active immunisation.*

**Euvaxon** *Teva Tuteur, Arg.*
Etoposide (p.551·3).
*Malignant neoplasms.*

**Euvegal Balance** *Schwabe, Ger.*
Valerian (p.1762·2).
*Insomnia; nervous disorders.*

**Euvegal Entspannungs- und Einschlafdragees** *Schwabe, Ger.*
Valerian (p.1762·2); melissa (p.1711·1).
*Nervous disorders; sleep disorders.*

**Euvegal Entspannungs- und Einschlaftropfen**
*Schwabe, Ger.*
Valerian (p.1762·2); melissa (p.1711·1).
*Nervous disorders; sleep disorders.*

**Euvegal forte** *Spitzner, Ger.†.*
Valerian (p.1762·2); melissa (p.1711·1).
*Insomnia; nervous disorders.*

**Euvegal N** *Spitzner, Ger.†.*
Valerian (p.1762·2); melissa (p.1711·1); passion flower (p.1729·1).
*Neurosedative.*

**Euvifor** *Vedim, Port.*
Piracetam (p.1732·1); co-dergocrine mesilate (p.1674·1).
*Cerebrovascular disorders; mental function disorders; vestibular disorders.*

**Euvitan** *Baer, Ger.†.*
Caffeine and sodium benzoate (p.783·1); rutoside sodium sulfate (p.1688·3); tinct. amara; angelica (p.1655·1); calluna vulgaris; juglans regia; valerian (p.1762·2).
*Dystonias; reduced appetite.*

**Euvitol** *Bracco, Ital.*
Vitamin A palmitate (p.1453·1).
*Skin disorders.*

**Euxat** *PH&T, Ital.*
Nifedipine (p.966·2).
*Angina pectoris; hypertension.*

**Euzymina Lisina I** *Menarini, Spain.*
Lysine hydrochloride (p.1439·2); nicotinic acid (p.1441·1); pepsin (p.1729·3); bitter orange (p.1723·3); lactic acid (p.1704·1).
*Digestive enzyme deficiency.*

**Euzymina Lisina II** *Menarini, Spain.*
Lysine hydrochloride (p.1439·2); nicotinic acid (p.1441·1); pepsin (p.1729·3); bitter orange (p.1723·3).
*Digestive disorders.*

**Evacode** *Norton, UK†.*
Codeine phosphate (p.27·1).

**Evac-Q-Kwik**
*Note. This name is used for preparations of different composition.*
*Pharmacia Upjohn, Canad.†.*
*Combination preparation:* Solution, magnesium citrate (p.1272·1); tablets, phenolphthalein (p.1284·1); suppository, bisacodyl (p.1251·3).
*Colonic evacuation.*

*Savage, USA†.*
*Combination pack:* Evac-Q-Mag; Evac-Q-Tabs, 2 tablets; Evac-Q-Kwik Suppositories, 1 suppository.
*Bowel evacuation.*

**Evac-Q-Kwik Suppository** *Savage, USA†.*
Bisacodyl (p.1251·3).

**Evac-Q-Mag** *Savage, USA.*
Magnesium citrate (p.1272·1).

**Evac-Q-Tabs** *Savage, USA.*
Bisacodyl (p.1251·3).
Formerly contained phenolphthalein.

**Evacream** *Gambar, Ital.*
Sodium carboxymethyl betaglucan.
*Stretch marks.*

**Evacrine** *Motima, Fr.*
Wild cherry (p.1058·1); ginger (p.1267·1); viola tricolor.
*Gastrointestinal disorders.*

**Evacuante** *Bohm, Spain; Lainco, Spain.*
Macrogol (p.1708·2); electrolytes (p.1217·1).
*Bowel evacuation.*

**Evacuol** *Almirall, Spain.*
Sodium picosulfate (p.1289·3).
*Constipation.*

**Evadene** *Wyeth Lederle, Ital.†.*
Butriptyline hydrochloride (p.289·1).
*Depression.*

**Evadermin** *Gambar, Ital.†.*
Povidone-iodine (p.1190·3).
*Genital hygiene.*

**Evadol**
*Note. This name is used for preparations of different composition.*
*Andromaco, Chile.*
Mebeverine hydrochloride (p.1273·1).
*Gastrointestinal spasm.*

*Degorts, Mex.*
Diclofenac sodium (p.32·1).
*Gout; inflammation; musculoskeletal and joint disorders; pain.*

**Evafer** *Gambar, Ital.*
Iron (p.1434·3); folic acid (p.1429·1).
*Anaemia during pregnancy.*

**Evafilm** *Laphal, Fr.*
Estradiol (p.1550·1).
*Menopausal disorders.*

**Evagelin** *Help, Gr.*
Bromazepam (p.671·3).
*Anxiety disorders.*

**Evagrip**
*Temis, Arg.; Celltech, Spain.*
An influenza vaccine (p.1620·2).
*Active immunisation.*

**Evalgan** *Perstorp, Austria.*
Dimeticone (p.1482·1); zinc oxide (p.1163·2).
*Skin disorders.*

**Evalin** *Queisser, Ger.*
Cimicifuga (p.1671·3).
*Menopausal disorders.*

**Evalon** *Infar, India.*
Estriol (p.1552·3).
*Adjunct in vaginal operations; menopausal disorders.*

**Evalose** *Copley, USA†.*
Lactulose (p.1269·1).

**Evamilk** *Gambar, Ital.*
Fennel (p.1687·2); myrtillus (p.1718·3); wild carrot (p.1765·1).
*Lactation stimulation.*

**Evana** *Pharmaton, Switz.†.*
Agnus castus (p.1649·1).
*Premenstrual syndrome.*

**Evanor** *Wyeth, Braz.*
Levonorgestrel (p.1563·2); ethinylestradiol (p.1553·2).
*Combined oral contraceptive.*

**Evanor-D** *Wyeth Lederle, Ital.*
Levonorgestrel (p.1563·2); ethinylestradiol (p.1553·2).
*Combined oral contraceptive.*

**Evapause** *Laphal, Fr.*
Progesterone (p.1566·2).
*Female infertility; menopausal disorders; menstrual disorders; threatened or habitual miscarriage.*

**Evaphol** *Norton, UK†.*
Pholcodine (p.1128·3).

**Evaplan**
*Roche, Arg.; Roche Diagnostics, Austral.†.*
Fertility test (p.1734·3).

**Evarose** *Bailly, Fr.*
Arnica (p.1656·3); hamamelis (p.1696·3); melilot; aesculus (p.1648·2); ruscus.
*Skin redness.*

**Evasen Crema** *Gambar, Ital.*
Vitamin E (p.1464·3).
*Cracked nipples.*

**Evasen Dischetti** *Gambar, Ital.*
Potassium sorbate (p.1192·3); glycerol (p.1694·3).
*Cracked nipples.*

**Evasen Liquido** *Gambar, Ital.*
Potassium sorbate (p.1192·3); glycerol (p.1694·3).
*Nipple care during lactation.*

**Evasidol** *Wyeth Lederle, Austria†.*
Butriptyline hydrochloride (p.289·1).
*Anxiety; depression.*

**Evasprin** *Euro-Labor, Port.†; Grunenthal, Port.†.*
Lysine aspirin (p.54·3).
*Fever; pain.*

**Evastel** *Aventis, Mex.*
Ebastine (p.433·1).
*Hypersensitivity.*

**Evatest** *Roche, Arg.*
Pregnancy test (p.1734·3).

**Evatest One Step** *Roche Diagnostics, Austral.†.*
Pregnancy test (p.1734·3).

**Evavit** *Gambar, Ital.*
Multivitamin preparation containing folic acid (p.1417·1).
*Nutritional supplement during pregnancy.*

**Evazol**
*Petrasch, Austria; Ravensberg, Ger.*
Dequalinium chloride (p.1178·1).
*Infected wounds; skin infections.*

**EVC** *Sisu, Canad.*
Vitamin and mineral preparation (p.1417·1).

**Eve** *Grunenthal, Ger.*
Ethinylestradiol (p.1553·2); norethisterone (p.1562·2).
*Combined oral contraceptive.*

**Evelea** *Elea, Arg.*
Levonorgestrel (p.1563·2); ethinylestradiol (p.1553·2).
*Combined oral contraceptive; menstrual disorders.*

**Evening Gold** *Larkhall Laboratories, UK.*
Evening primrose oil (p.1686·3).

**Evercid** *Boniscontro & Gazzone, Ital.*
Flucloxacillin sodium (p.213·3).
*Bacterial infections.*

**Ever-fit Cardio** *Prisfar, Port.*
Multivitamin and mineral preparation (p.1417·1).

**Ever-Fit Plus** *Prisfar, Port.*
Vitamin and mineral preparation (p.1417·1).

**Evergin** *Eversil, Braz.†.*
Metamizole magnesium (p.36·1).
*Fever; pain.*

**Everon** *Weleda, Austria†.*
Pepsin (p.1729·3); lemon juice (p.1706·2); menthol (p.1711·3).
*Colds.*

**Everone** *Hyrex, USA†.*
Testosterone enantate (p.1570·1).
*Breast cancer; delayed puberty (males); male hypogonadism.*

**Eversun** *Pfizer, NZ†.*
*SPF 30+:* Avobenzone (p.1142·3); octinoxate (p.1154·3); oxybenzone (p.1154·3).
*Sunscreen.*

**Evestrel**
*Theramex, Ital.*
Phytoestrogens (genistein, daidzein) (p.1692·1).
*Menopausal disorders.*

*Theramex, Mon.*
Soya bean (p.1447·2).
*Nutritional supplement during menopause.*

**Eviantrina** *Korhispana, Spain.*
Famotidine (p.1265·2).
*Gastro-oesophageal reflux; peptic ulcer; Zollinger-Ellison syndrome.*

**Evicer** *Sanofi Synthelabo, Port.*
Cimetidine (p.1255·3).
*Gastro-oesophageal reflux; gastrointestinal haemorrhage; peptic ulcer; Zollinger-Ellison syndrome.*

**E-Vicotrat** *Heyl, Ger.*
Alpha tocoferil acetate (p.1465·1).
*Vitamin E deficiency.*

**E-Vicotrat + Magnesium** *Heyl, Ger.†.*
*dl*-Alpha tocoferil acetate (p.1465·1); magnesium oxide (p.1272·3).
*Vitamin E and magnesium deficiency.*

**Evicyl** *Sanofi Synthelabo, Arg.*
Inositol nicotinate (p.939·3).
*Hyperlipidaemias; peripheral vascular disorders.*

**E-vidon** *Abigo, Swed.*
*d*-Alpha tocoferil acetate (p.1465·1).
*Vitamin E deficiency.*

**Eviepar** *Eversil, Braz.†.*
Adenosine (p.851·2); methionine (p.1042·1); betaine (p.1660·1); choline citrate (p.1424·3); pyridoxine hydrochloride (p.1456·3).
*Liver disorders.*

**Eviletten N** *Evers, Ger.†.*
Modified keratin.
*Haemorrhoids; varicose veins.*

**Evilin** *Merck, Chile.*
Cyproterone acetate (p.1544·1); ethinylestradiol (p.1553·2).
*Androgen-associated acne, alopecia, and hirsutism in women.*

**Evimal** *Andromaco, Chile.*
Donepezil hydrochloride (p.1489·2).
*Alzheimer's disease.*

**E-vimin** *Astra, Swed.*
*dl*-Alpha-tocoferil acetate (p.1465·1).
*Vitamin E deficiency.*

**Evina**
*Note. This name is used for preparations of different composition.*
*Klonal, Arg.*
Ergometrine (p.1684·2).

*Rodisma, Ger.*
*d*-Alpha tocopherol with ascorbic acid (p.1417·1).
*Vitamin E and C deficiency.*

**Evinopon** *Bros, Gr.*
Diclofenac sodium (p.32·1).
*Dysmenorrhoea; inflammation; musculoskeletal and joint disorders; pain; prevention of miosis in ophthalmic surgery.*

**Eviol** *Gap, Gr.*
*dl*-Alfa tocoferyl acetate.
*Vitamin E deficiency.*

**Eviol-A** *Gap, Gr.*
*dl*-Alpha tocoferil acetate (p.1465·1); vitamin A acetate (p.1453·1).
*Vitamin A and E deficiency.*

**Evion**
*Merck, Arg.; Merck, Ger.; Merck, India; Bracco, Ital.*
Vitamin E (p.1464·3).
*Vitamin E deficiency.*

**Eviprostat**
*Note. This name is used for preparations of different composition.*
*Eversil, Braz.†.*
Manganese amino acid chelate (p.1440·2); populus tremula (p.1733·3); pulsatilla (p.1737·1); salicylic acid (p.1157·1); kaolin (p.1268·3).
*Urinary-tract disorders.*

*Evers, Hong Kong†.*
Wheat-germ oil; manganese chloride (p.1440·1); chimaphila umbellata; populus tremulula (p.1733·3); pulsatilla (p.1737·1); equisetum (p.1684·1); sodium taurocholate.
*Benign prostatic hyperplasia.*

*Shinyaku, Jpn; Interdelta, Switz.†.*
Wheat-germ oil; chimaphila umbellata; populus tremula (p.1733·3); pulsatilla (p.1737·1); equisetum (p.1684·1).
*Benign prostatic hyperplasia.*

*Shinyaku, Singapore.*
Wheat-germ oil; chimaphila umbellata; populus tremula (p.1733·3); pulsatilla (p.1737·1); equisetum (p.1684·1); choleinic sodium; manganese chloride (p.1440·1).
*Benign prostatic hyperplasia.*

**Eviprostat N** *Evers, Ger.*
Chimaphila umbellata; populus tremula (p.1733·3); pulsatilla (p.1737·1); equisetum (p.1684·1).
*Prostatic hyperplasia.*

**Eviprostat-S** *Evers, Ger.*
Saw palmetto (p.1569·1).
*Micturition disorders associated with benign prostatic hyperplasia.*

**Evisco Mistel Urtinktur** *Evisco, Ger.*
Homoeopathic preparation.

**Evisco Misteltropfen N** *Evisco, Ger.*
Homoeopathic preparation.

**Evista**
*Lilly, Arg.; Lilly, Austral.; Lilly, Austria; Lilly, Belg.; Lilly, Braz.; Lilly, Canad.; Lilly, Chile; Lilly, Denm.; Lilly, Fin.; Lilly, Fr.; Lilly, Ger.; Pharmaserve Lilly (Φαρμασερβ Λιλλυ), Gr.; Lilly, Hong Kong; Lilly, Irl.; Lilly, Israel; Lilly, Ital.; Lilly, Malaysia; Lilly, Mex.; Lilly, Neth.; Lilly, Norw.; Lilly, NZ; Lilly, Port.; Lilly, S.Afr.; Lilly, Singapore; Lilly, Spain; Lilly, Swed.; Lilly, Switz.; Lilly, UK; Lilly, USA.*
Raloxifene hydrochloride (p.1568·3).
*Osteoporosis.*

**Evit**
*Europharm, Austria; Chefaro, Ger.†; Mavena, Switz.*
*Vitamin E* (p.1464·3).
*Vitamin E deficiency.*

**Evitas** *Heralds, Braz.†.*
Algestone acetophenide (p.1541·3); estradiol enantate (p.1550·1).
*Injectable contraceptive.*

**Evitex**
*Note. This name is used for preparations of different composition.*
*Stanley, Israel.*
*d*-Alpha tocoferil acetate (p.1465·1).
*Vitamin E supplement.*

*Alcon, Ital.*
Vitamin A (p.1451·2); tocoferil nicotinate (p.1015·1).
*Vitamin A and E deficiency.*

**Evitex A E Fuerte** *Alcon Cusi, Spain.*
Vitamin A palmitate (p.1453·1); tocoferil nicotinate (p.1015·1).
*Deficiency of vitamins A and E; eye disorders; infertility; recurrent miscarriage; skin disorders.*

**Evitina** *CT, Ital.†.*
*dl*-Alpha tocoferil acetate (p.1465·1).

**Evitocor** *Apogepha, Ger.*
Atenolol (p.865·2).
*Angina pectoris; arrhythmias; cardiovascular disorders; hypertension.*

**Evitocor plus** *Apogepha, Ger.†.*
Atenolol (p.865·2); chlortalidone (p.882·3).
*Hypertension.*

**Evitol**
*Lannacher, Austria; Teva, Israel.*
Alpha tocoferil acetate (p.1465·1).
*Vitamin E deficiency; vitamin E supplement.*

**E-Vitum** *Merck, Ital.*
*d*-Alpha tocoferil acetate (p.1465·1).
*Haemolytic anaemia; intermittent claudication; vitamin E deficiency.*

**Evo-Conti** *Janssen-Cilag, Denm.*
Estradiol (p.1550·1); norethisterone acetate (p.1562·2).
*Menopausal disorders.*

**Evolis** *Solvay, Fr.*
Betahistine hydrochloride (p.1660·1).
*Vestibular disorders.*

**Evopad** *Janssen-Cilag, Spain.*
Estradiol (p.1550·1).
*Menopausal disorders; osteoporosis.*

**Evoprim** *Bioceuticals, UK.*
Evening primrose oil (p.1686·3).

**Evoquin** *Elvetium, Arg.*
Hydroxychloroquine sulfate (p.452·3).
*Lupus erythematosus; rheumatoid arthritis.*

**Evorel**
*Janssen-Cilag, Arg.; Janssen-Cilag, Denm.; Janssen-Cilag, Fin.; Janssen-Cilag, Ger.; Janssen-Cilag, Irl.; Janssen-Cilag, Israel; Janssen, Mex.; Janssen-Cilag, Norw.; Janssen-Cilag, S.Afr.; Janssen-Cilag, Swed.; Janssen-Cilag, UK.*
Estradiol (p.1550·1).
*Menopausal disorders; osteoporosis.*

**Evorel Conti**
*Janssen-Cilag, Arg.; Janssen-Cilag, Fin.; Janssen-Cilag, Irl.; Janssen-Cilag, Israel; Janssen-Cilag, S.Afr.; Janssen-Cilag, UK.*
Estradiol (p.1550·1); norethisterone acetate (p.1562·2).
*Menopausal disorders; osteoporosis.*

**Evorel Micronor** *Janssen-Cilag, Swed.*
Patches, estradiol (p.1550·1); tablets, norethisterone (p.1562·2).
*Oestrogen deficiency; osteoporosis.*

**Evorel Pak** *Janssen-Cilag, UK.*
Transdermal patches, estradiol (p.1550·1); tablets, norethisterone (p.1562·2).
*Menopausal disorders; osteoporosis.*

**Evorel Sequi**
*Janssen-Cilag, Arg.; Janssen-Cilag, Fin.; Janssen-Cilag, Israel; Janssen-Cilag, S.Afr.; Janssen-Cilag, UK.*
4 Patches, estradiol (Evorel) (p.1550·1); 4 patches, estradiol; norethisterone acetate (Evorel Conti) (p.1562·2).
*Menopausal disorders; osteoporosis.*

**Evorelconti** *Janssen, Mex.*
Estradiol (p.1550·1); norethisterone acetate (p.1562·2).
*Menopausal disorders.*

**Evo-Sequi** *Janssen-Cilag, Denm.*
Patch I, estradiol (p.1550·1); patch II, estradiol; norethisterone acetate (p.1562·2).
*Menopausal disorders.*

**Evoxac** *Daiichi, USA.*
Cevimeline hydrochloride (p.1488·3).
*Dry mouth associated with Sjögren's syndrome.*

**Evra**
*Janssen-Cilag, Fr.; Janssen-Cilag, UK.*
Norelgestromin (p.1562·1); ethinylestradiol (p.1553·2).
*Combined transdermal contraceptive.*

**Evril** *Boehringer de Angeli, Braz.†.*
Flurbiprofen (p.43·3).
*Dysmenorrhoea; musculoskeletal, joint, and peri-articular disorders.*

**Ewadyl** *Masa, Thai.*
Diphenhydramine hydrochloride (p.431·3); ammonium chloride (p.1115·2); sodium citrate (p.1223·2).
*Cold symptoms; coughs; nasal congestion.*

**Exabrol** *Pharmacos, Mex.*
Ambroxol hydrochloride (p.1114·3).
*Respiratory-tract congestion.*

**Exacol** *Pharmacos, Mex.*
Chloramphenicol (p.185·1).
*Bacterial eye infections.*

**Exacor** *Pharmacia, Fr.*
Cibenzoline succinate (p.883·2).
*Arrhythmias.*

**Exact** *Premier, USA†.*
Benzoyl peroxide (p.1143·2).
*Acne.*

**ExacTech**
*Medisense, Austral.; Medisense, UK.*
Test for glucose in blood (p.1694·2).

**Exacyl**
*Bournonville, Belg.; Sanofi Synthelabo, Fr.*
Tranexamic acid (p.760·3).
*Haemorrhagic disorders.*

**Exafenil** *Grin, Mex.*
Dexamethasone (p.1097·1); phenylephrine (p.1126·3).
*Eye disorders.*

**Exafil** *Degorts, Mex.*
Salbutamol sulfate (p.791·3).
*Asthma; bronchitis; emphysema.*

**Ex'ail**
*Solvay, Belg.†; Warner-Lambert, Fr.†.*
Garlic (p.1691·1); rutoside (p.1688·2); copper chlorophyll (p.1057·1).
*Circulatory disorders.*

**Exalamin** *Pharmacos, Mex.†.*
Oxolamine (p.1126·1).
*Coughs.*

**Exaler** *Pharmacos, Mex.*
Sodium cromoglicate (p.795·3).
*Inflammatory eye disorders.*

**Exalgin** *Sons, Mex.*
Dipyrone (p.35·3).
*Fever; pain.*

**Exaliver** *Pharmacos, Mex.*
Aciclovir (p.626·1).
*Herpesvirus infections of the eye.*

**Exalver** *Maver, Mex.*
Paracetamol (p.76·2); pseudoephedrine hydrochloride (p.1129·2); dextromethorphan hydrobromide (p.1117·3).
*Coughs; nasal congestion.*

**Examicyn** *Pharmacos, Mex.†.*
Erythromycin (p.208·1).
*Bacterial infections.*

**Examida** *Pharmacos, Mex.*
Sulfacetamide sodium (p.257·3).
*Bacterial eye infections.*

**Examolin** *Pharmacos, Mex.*
Amoxicillin trihydrate (p.155·3).
*Bacterial infections.*

**Exangina N** *Muller Goppingen, Ger.*
Homoeopathic preparation.

**Exarex** *Rolab, S.Afr.*
Coal tar (p.1159·2).
*Eczema.*

**Exastrin** *Pharmacos, Mex.*
Zinc sulfate (p.1469·3); phenylephrine hydrochloride (p.1126·3).
*Eye disorders.*

**Exasul** *Pharmacos, Mex.†.*
Sulfamethoxypyridazine (p.263·1).
*Bacterial infections.*

**Exatech** *Medica, NZ†.*
Test for glucose in blood (p.1694·2).

**Exaverm** *Pharmacos, Mex.†.*
Mebendazole (p.108·2).
*Worm infections.*

**Exavir** *UCI, Braz.*
Aciclovir (p.626·1).
*Herpesvirus infections.*

**Exavit** *Pharmacos, Mex.*
Vitamin and mineral preparation (p.1417·1).

**Exazen** *Vocate, Gr.*
Azelaic acid (p.1142·3).
*Acne.*

**Exbenzol** *Sons, Mex.*
Mebendazole (p.108·2).
*Worm infections.*

**Excedrin**
*Note. This name is used for preparations of different composition.*
*Bristol-Myers Squibb, Braz.; Bristol-Myers Squibb, Canad.*
Paracetamol (p.76·2); caffeine (p.782·1).
*Fever; pain.*

*Bristol-Myers Squibb, USA.*
Aspirin (p.15·1); paracetamol (p.76·2); caffeine (p.782·1).
*Pain.*

**Excedrin Migraine** *Bristol-Myers Squibb, USA.*
Paracetamol (p.76·2); aspirin (p.15·1); caffeine (p.782·1).
*Migraine.*

**Excedrin PM** *Bristol-Myers Squibb, USA.*
Paracetamol (p.76·2); diphenhydramine citrate (p.431·3) or diphenhydramine hydrochloride (p.431·3).
*Pain associated with sleeplessness.*

**Excedrin QuickTabs** *Bristol-Myers Squibb, USA.*
Paracetamol (p.76·2); caffeine (p.782·1).
*Pain.*

**Excedrin Tension Headache** *Bristol-Myers Squibb, USA.*
Paracetamol (p.76·2); caffeine (p.782·1).
*Headache.*

**Excegran** *Dainippon, Jpn.*
Zonisamide (p.384·3).
*Epilepsy.*

**Excel ET** *Inverness Medical, Austral.†.*
Test for glucose in blood (p.1694·2).

**Excelcur MF1** *Maeil, Hong Kong.*
Preparation for enteral nutrition (p.1417·1).
*Gastro-enteritis.*

**Excelsior** *Grisi, Mex.*
*Ointment:* Salicylic acid (p.1157·1).
*Warts.*
*Topical solution:* Tolnaftate (p.410·1).
*Fungal skin infections.*

**Excillin** *Propan, S.Afr.†.*
Ampicillin trihydrate (p.157·2).
*Bacterial infections.*

**Excipial** *Spirig, Switz.*
Emollient.
*Skin disorders.*

**Excipial U** *Spirig, Switz.*
Urea (p.1162·2).
*Skin disorders.*

**Excivit** *Gallia, Braz.†.*
Multivitamin and mineral preparation (p.1417·1).

**Excough** *Fortune, Hong Kong.*
Guaifenesin (p.1122·1).
*Coughs.*

**Exdol** Lioh, Canad.
Paracetamol (p.76·2); caffeine citrate (p.782·1); codeine phosphate (p.27·1).
*Fever; pain.*

**Exe-Cort** Pinewood, UK.
Hydrocortisone (p.1103·3).
*Skin disorders.*

**Executive B** Cenovis, Austral.†; Vitelle, Austral.†.
Vitamins and minerals (p.1417·1); valerian (p.1762·2); passion flower (p.1729·1).
*Stress; vitamin and mineral deficiencies.*

**Exel** Senosiain, Mex.
Meloxicam (p.56·1).
*Gout; inflammation; musculoskeletal and joint disorders; pain.*

**Exelderm**
Bioglan, Irl.; Schwarz, Ital.†; Syntex, Mex.†; Centrapharm, UK; Westwood-Squibb, USA.
Sulconazole nitrate (p.408·2).
*Fungal skin infections.*

**Exelmin** UCI, Braz.
Cambendazole (p.103·3); mebendazole (p.108·2).
*Worm infections.*

**Exelon**
Novartis, Arg.; Novartis, Austral.; Novartis, Austria; Novartis, Belg.; Novartis, Braz.; Novartis, Canad.; Novartis, Chile; Novartis, Denm.; Novartis, Fin.; Novartis, Fr.; Novartis, Ger.; Novartis, Gr.; Novartis, Hong Kong; Novartis, India; Novartis, Irl.; Novartis, Israel; Novartis, Ital.; Novartis, Malaysia; Novartis, Mex.; Novartis, Neth.; Novartis, Norw.; Novartis, NZ; Novartis, Port.; Novartis, S.Afr.; Novartis, Singapore; Novartis, Spain; Novartis, Swed.; Novartis, Switz.; Novartis, Thai.; Novartis, UK; Novartis, USA.
Rivastigmine tartrate (p.1497·1).
*Alzheimer's disease.*

**Exempla** Fada, Arg.
Ceftriaxone (p.183·3).
*Bacterial infections.*

**Exertial** Baliarda, Arg.
Ciprofloxacin (p.188·2).
*Bacterial infections.*

**Exetin-A** Pisa, Mex.
Epoetin (p.747·1).
*Anaemias.*

**Exeu**
Hexal, Austria; Biocur, Ger.
Eucalyptus oil (p.1686·2).
*Catarrh; cold symptoms; coughs.*

**Exflam** Merck, Chile.
Diclofenac potassium (p.32·1).
*Inflammation; pain.*

**Exflem** Prima, Thai.
Carbocisteine (p.1116·2).
*Respiratory-tract disorders associated with increased or viscous mucus.*

**Exfoliac** Liphaderm, Fr.
A range of skin-care preparations.
*Acne; seborrhoea.*

**Exfolium** Wyeth, Arg.
Triamcinolone acetonide (p.1110·2); salicylic acid (p.1157·1).
*Skin disorders.*

**Exgest LA** Carnrick, USA†.
Phenylpropanolamine hydrochloride (p.1127·3); guaifenesin (p.1122·1).
*Respiratory-tract congestion.*

**Exhirud**
Sanofi Synthelabo, Austria; Sanofi Synthelabo, Ger.
Leech extract (p.931·2).
*Soft-tissue disorders; superficial vascular disorders.*

**Ex-Histine** WE, USA.
Phenylephrine (p.1126·3); chlorphenamine (p.428·1); hyoscine (p.483·3).
*Upper respiratory-tract disorders.*

**Exibral** Bago, Arg.
Valproic acid (p.380·1) or magnesium valproate (p.382·2).
*Bipolar disorder; epilepsy; migraine.*

**Exidine** Baxter, USA.
Chlorhexidine gluconate (p.1173·2).
*Skin disinfection.*

**Exido** Prater, Chile.
Lidocaine hydrochloride (p.1377·3).
*Erectile dysfunction.*

**Exidol** Galephar, Fr.
Paracetamol (p.76·2); caffeine (p.782·1).
*Fever; pain.*

**Exil** Esoform, Ital.
Cetylpyridinium chloride (p.1173·1).
*Genital hygiene.*

**Exipan** Agis, Israel.
Piroxicam (p.84·2).
*Inflammation; pain.*

**Exiplon** Khandelwal, India.
Codeine phosphate (p.27·1); chlorphenamine maleate (p.427·3).
*Coughs.*

**Exirel** Byk, Austria.
Pirbuterol acetate (p.790·3).
*Obstructive airways disease.*

**Exit**
Note. This name is used for preparations of different composition.
Farmasa, Braz.
Cinnarizine (p.428·3); piracetam (p.1732·1).
*Cerebral and peripheral vascular disorders; impaired mental function.*

Stadmed, India.
Monobasic sodium phosphate (p.1230·3); dibasic sodium phosphate (p.1231·1).
*Bowel evacuation; constipation.*

**Exitop**
Asta Medica, Austria†; Asta Medica, Fin.; Baxter, Ger.; Asta Medica, Swed.
Etoposide (p.551·3).
*Malignant neoplasms.*

**Ex-Lax**
Novartis Consumer, Canad.
Sennosides (p.1288·2).
Formerly contained yellow phenolphthalein.

Novartis Consumer, UK; Novartis Consumer, USA.
Senna (p.1288·2).
Formerly contained phenolphthalein in the *USA*.
*Constipation.*

**Ex-Lax Extra Gentle Pills** Novartis, USA†.
Docusate sodium (p.1262·2); phenolphthalein (p.1284·1).
*Constipation.*

**Ex-Lax Gentle Nature** Novartis, USA†.
Calcium sennoside A (p.1288·3); calcium sennoside B (p.1288·3).
*Constipation.*

**Ex-Lax Gentle Strength**
Novartis Consumer, Canad.
Senna (p.1288·2); docusate sodium (p.1262·2).
*Constipation.*

Novartis, USA.
Sennosides (p.1288·2); docusate sodium (p.1262·2).
*Constipation.*

**Ex-Lax Light** Sandoz, Canad.†.
Yellow phenolphthalein (p.1284·1); docusate sodium (p.1262·2).

**Ex-Lax Stool Softener**
Novartis Consumer, Canad.; Novartis Consumer, USA.
Docusate sodium (p.1262·2).
*Constipation.*

**Exlutena** Organon, Swed.
Lynestrenol (p.1557·1).
*Progestogen-only oral contraceptive.*

**Exluton**
Organon, Arg.; Organon, Belg.†; Organon, Braz.; Organon, Chile; Organon, Fin.; Organon, Fr.†; Organon, Mex.; Organon, Neth.†; Organon, Port.; Organon, Thai.
Lynestrenol (p.1557·1).
*Progestogen-only oral contraceptive.*

**Exlutona**
Organon, Denm.†; Organon, Ger.†; Organon, Norw.; Organon, Switz.†.
Lynestrenol (p.1557·1).
*Progestogen-only oral contraceptive.*

**Exmykehl** Sanum-Kehlbeck, Ger.
Homoeopathic preparation.

**Exna** Robins, USA†.
Benzthiazide (p.868·2).
*Hypertension; oedema.*

**Exneural** BASF, Ger.†.
Ibuprofen (p.45·3).
*Fever; inflammation; musculoskeletal, joint, and soft-tissue disorders; pain.*

**Exocaine** Del, USA; Commerce, USA.
Methyl salicylate (p.59·3).
*Muscle and joint pain.*

**Exocin**
Allergan, Denm.; Allergan, Fin.; Alvia (Αλβια), Gr.; Allergan, Irl.; Allergan, Ital.; Allergan, Port.; Allergan, S.Afr.; Allergan, Spain; Allergan, UK.
Ofloxacin (p.239·3).
*Bacterial eye infections.*

**Exocine** Allergan, Fr.
Ofloxacin (p.239·3).
*Bacterial eye infections.*

**Exodalina** Sons, Mex.
Dipyrone (p.35·3).
*Pain.*

**Exoderil**
Biochemie, Austria; Rentschler, Ger.; Biochemie, Hong Kong; Merck, Israel; Biochemie, Malaysia; Biochemie, Singapore.
Naftifine hydrochloride (p.406·2).
*Fungal skin and nail infections.*

**Exofat** Sunspot, Austral.†.
Poliglusam; oligofructose; ascorbic acid (p.1460·2).
*Obesity.*

**Exo'Fat** Sidus, Arg.
Poliglusam; oligofructose; calcium carbonate (p.1417·1).
*Obesity.*

**Exofur** Sons, Mex.
Furazolidone (p.605·2).
*Diarrhoea.*

**Exolise**
Arkopharma, Fr.†; Arkochim, Spain†.
Camellia sinensis (p.1765·3).
*Obesity.*

**Exolit**
Medochemie, Hong Kong; Medochemie, Singapore†; Medochemie, Thai.
Bromhexine hydrochloride (p.1115·3).
*Respiratory-tract disorders associated with increased or viscous mucus.*

**Exolyt** Abigo, Swed.
Chlorcyclizine hydrochloride (p.427·2); guaifenesin (p.1122·1); ammonium chloride (p.1115·2).
*Coughs.*

**Exomega**
Pierre Fabre Dermo-Cosmetique, Arg.; Ducray, Fr.
Avena (p.1658·2); omega-6 fatty acids (p.1690·2).
*Skin disorders.*

**Exomuc** Bouchara-Recordati, Fr.
Acetylcysteine (p.1112·3).
*Respiratory-tract congestion.*

**Exorex**
Trans Dermal, Austral.; Cybermed, Austria; Forest, Irl.; Forest Laboratories, UK.
Coal tar (p.1159·2).
*Psoriasis.*

**Exormin** Health Care, Hong Kong†.
Ginkgo biloba (p.1692·3).
*Cerebral disorders; peripheral vascular disorders; tinnitis; vertigo.*

**Exorvit** Sons, Mex.
Cyanocobalamin (p.1458·2).
*Anaemias; neuritis.*

**Exorvit VM** Sons, Mex.
Vitamin and mineral preparation (p.1417·1).

**Exoseptoplix** Diepharmex, Fr.
Chlorhexidine gluconate (p.1173·2).
*Bacterial skin infections.*

**Exostrept** Biomedica-Chemica, Gr.
Fluoxetine hydrochloride (p.292·1).
*Depression; obsessive-compulsive disorder; panic disorder.*

**Exosurf**
GlaxoSmithKline, Arg.; GlaxoSmithKline, Austral.; GlaxoSmithKline, Austria; GlaxoSmithKline, Belg.†; GlaxoSmithKline, Braz.; GlaxoSmithKline, Canad.; GlaxoSmithKline, Chile; Glaxo Wellcome, Denm.†; Glaxo Wellcome, Fin.†; GlaxoSmithKline, Ger.†; GlaxoSmithKline, Hong Kong; Wellcome, Irl.; Wellcome, Israel; GlaxoSmithKline, Ital.; Glaxo Wellcome, Mex.; GlaxoSmithKline, Neth.; Glaxo Wellcome, S.Afr.†; Glaxo Wellcome, Singapore†; Glaxo Wellcome, Spain†; GlaxoSmithKline, Swed.†; Wellcome, Switz.†; Glaxo Wellcome, Thai.†; Wellcome, UK†; Glaxo Wellcome, USA.
Colfosceril palmitate (p.1736·2).
*Neonatal respiratory distress syndrome.*

**Exova** Montebello, Fr.
Sorbitol (p.1446·3); xylitol (p.1469·1).
*Halitosis.*

**Exovir** Pharmacia, Arg.
Zidovudine (p.658·2).
*HIV infection.*

**44 Exp** Procter & Gamble, Mex.
Guaifenesin (p.1122·1).
*Coughs.*

**Expafusin**
Fresenius Kabi, Austria; Baxter, Ger.; Fresenius Kabi, Spain†.
An etherified starch (p.750·1) with electrolytes.
*Plasma volume expansion; vascular disorders.*

**Expahes**
Fresenius Kabi, Austria; Fresenius Kabi, Switz.
Hetastarch (p.750·1) in sodium chloride.
*Blood-volume expansion.*

**Expal** Sons, Mex.
Pipenzolate (p.487·3).
*Gastrointestinal disorders.*

**Expanden** Master, Chile.
Menthol (p.1711·3); camphor (p.1665·3); methyl salicylate (p.59·3); bornyl acetate (p.1662·2); eucalyptus oil (p.1686·2).
*Nasal congestion.*

**Expandox** Expanpharm, Fr.
Paracetamol (p.76·2).
Formerly known as Expandol.
*Fever; pain.*

**Expanfen** Expanpharm, Fr.
Ibuprofen (p.45·3).
*Fever; pain.*

**Expec** Legrand, Braz.
Oxomemazine hydrochloride (p.438·2); potassium iodide (p.1598·1); sodium benzoate (p.1169·3); guaifenesin (p.1122·1); ipecacuanha (p.1122·3).
*Respiratory-tract congestion.*

**Expectal N** Biocur, Ger.
Thyme (p.1755·2).
*Catarrh; coughs.*

**Expectal-Balsam** Kolassa, Austria.
Pumilio pine oil (p.1737·1); camphor (p.1665·3); eucalyptus oil (p.1686·2); nutmeg oil (p.1722·3); thyme oil (p.1755·3); benzyl nicotinate (p.21·2).
*Respiratory-tract disorders.*

**Expectalin** Parke-Med, S.Afr.
Diphenhydramine hydrochloride (p.431·3); ammonium chloride (p.1115·2).
*Coughs.*

**Expectalin with Codeine** Parke-Med, S.Afr.
Diphenhydramine hydrochloride (p.431·3); ammonium chloride (p.1115·2); codeine phosphate (p.27·1).
*Coughs.*

**Expectal-Tropfen** Kolassa, Austria.
Codeine (p.27·1); thyme extract (p.1755·2); orange extract (p.1723·3); anise oil (p.1655·2).
*Respiratory-tract disorders.*

**Expectamin** Legrand, Braz.
Dexchlorpheniramine maleate (p.427·3); pseudoephedrine sulfate (p.1129·2); guaifenesin (p.1122·1).
*Respiratory-tract disorders.*

**Expectil** Bunker, Braz.
Diphenhydramine hydrochloride (p.431·3); ammonium chloride (p.1115·2); sulfogaiacol (p.1131·1); sodium citrate (p.1223·2).
*Respiratory-tract congestion.*

**Expectobron** Hebron, Braz.
Guaifenesin (p.1122·1); sodium benzoate (p.1169·3); potassium iodide (p.1598·1); lobelia (p.1589·1).
*Coughs.*

**Expectocilin** EMS, Braz.
Ampicillin benzathine (p.158·1); ampicillin sodium (p.157·1).
*Bacterial infections.*

**Expectocilin Balsamico** EMS, Braz.†.
Ampicillin sodium (p.157·1); ampicillin benzathine (p.158·1); guaifenesin (p.1122·1); cineole (p.1672·1).
*Bacterial infections.*

**Expectofar** Esfar, Port.†.
Codeine (p.27·1); ephedrine (p.1120·1); mepiraxamine; vitamin C (p.1460·2).

**Expectol** Teuto, Braz.
Lobelia (p.1589·1); erysimum; stramonium (p.489·2).
*Coughs.*

**Expectolu** Bergamo, Braz.†.
Potassium iodide (p.1598·1); lobelia (p.1589·1); hyoscyamus (p.485·2).
*Respiratory-tract congestion.*

**Expectomel** Cazi, Braz.
Rorippa nasturtium aquaticum; aconite (p.1646·3); ipecacuanha (p.1122·3); senega (p.1130·2); tolu balsam (p.1131·3); honey (p.1434·2); guaco.
*Respiratory-tract congestion.*

**Expectoral** Hebron, Braz.
Bromelains (p.1662·2); invertase; glucose oxidase (p.1694·2); ribonuclease (p.1738·1).
*Coughs.*

**Expectoran Codein** Grossmann, Switz.
Codeine phosphate (p.27·1); thyme (p.1755·2); senega (p.1130·2); quillaia (p.1416·1).
*Adjuvant in bronchitis; coughs.*

**Expectorant Cough Formula** Tanta, Canad.
Guaifenesin (p.1122·1).

**Expectorant Cough Syrup**
Technilab, Canad.; DC Labs, Canad.; AAH, UK.
Guaifenesin (p.1122·1).
*Coughs.*

**Expectorant and Decongestant Cough Syrup** AAH, UK.
Guaifenesin (p.1122·1); pseudoephedrine hydrochloride (p.1129·2).
*Coughs.*

**Expectorant Syrup** Marc-O, Canad.†.
Guaifenesin (p.1122·1).

**Expectosan Hierbas y Miel** Excelentia, Arg.
Grindelia (p.1696·1); pimpinella major; cowslip (p.1735·1); rosa gallica (p.1058·1); thyme (p.1755·2).
*Coughs.*

**Expectotussin C** Adcock Ingram, S.Afr.
Mepyramine maleate (p.437·1); ammonium chloride (p.1115·2); sodium citrate (p.1223·2); phenylephrine hydrochloride (p.1126·3); ascorbic acid (p.1460·2).
*Coughs.*

**Expectovac** Nikkho, Braz.
Procaine benzylpenicillin (p.246·1); benzylpenicillin potassium (p.163·2); aminocaproic acid (p.741·3); bacterial antigens.
*Bacterial infections.*

**Expectuss** EMS, Braz.
Ambroxol hydrochloride (p.1114·3).
*Respiratory-tract congestion.*

**Expectussin** Dinafarma, Braz.†.
Noscapine (p.1125·3); mepyramine maleate (p.437·1).
*Coughs.*

**Expectysat N** Ysatfabrik, Ger.
Primula root (p.1735·1); thyme (p.1755·2).
*Cold symptoms.*

**Expeflen** Diba, Mex.
Ambroxol hydrochloride (p.1114·3).
*Respiratory-tract disorders with viscous mucus.*

**Expelinct** Propan, S.Afr.
Guaifenesin (p.1122·1).
*Coughs.*

**Expergesic** Win-Medicare, India.
Paracetamol (p.76·2); pentazocine hydrochloride (p.79·3).
*Pain.*

**Expicin** Sons, Mex.
Ampicillin (p.157·1).
*Bacterial infections.*

**Expigen**
Note. This name is used for preparations of different composition.
Sanova, Austria.
Polysorbate 20 (p.1415·1); ammonium chloride (p.1115·2); sodium benzoate (p.1169·3); anise oil (p.1655·2); niaouli oil (p.1719·3); thyme oil (p.1755·3); menglytate (p.1124·2).
*Coughs; respiratory congestion.*

Pharmacia, Fin.; Pharmacia Upjohn, Norw.†; Adcock Ingram, S.Afr.
Polysorbate 20 (p.1415·1); ammonium chloride (p.1115·2).
*Coughs.*

**Expiran** British Dispensary, Thai.†.
Chlorphenamine maleate (p.427·3); ammonium chloride (p.1115·2); sulfogaiacol (p.1131·1).
*Coughs.*

**Expit** Ritsert, Ger.
Ambroxol hydrochloride (p.1114·3).
*Respiratory-tract disorders associated with increased or viscous mucus.*

**Exposis** *Osler, Fr.*
*SPF 20; SPF 30:* Octinoxate (p.1154·3); titanium dioxide (p.1160·3); avobenzone (p.1142·3).
*Sunscreen.*

**Exprep** *Mundipharma, Fin.*
Senna (p.1288·2).
*Bowel evacuation.*

**Expron** *Pharmaserve Lilly (Φαρμασερβ Λιλλυ), Gr.*
Fenoprofen calcium (p.39·2).
*Inflammation; musculoskeletal and joint disorders; pain.*

**Expros** *Orion, Fin.*
Tamsulosin hydrochloride (p.1009·2).
*Benign prostatic hyperplasia.*

**Expulin**
*Shire, Irl.; Shire, UK†.*
Pholcodine (p.1128·3); pseudoephedrine hydrochloride (p.1129·2); chlorphenamine maleate (p.427·3).
*Coughs; respiratory-tract congestion.*

**Expulin Chesty Cough** *Shire, UK†.*
Guaifenesin (p.1122·1).
*Coughs.*

**Expulin Childrens Cough**
*Shire, Irl.; Monmouth, UK†.*
Pholcodine (p.1128·3); chlorphenamine maleate (p.427·3).
*Coughs.*

**Expulin Decongestant** *Monmouth, UK†.*
Ephedrine hydrochloride (p.1120·1); chlorphenamine maleate (p.427·3).
*Nasal congestion.*

**Expulin Dry Cough**
*Shire, Irl.; Monmouth, UK†.*
Pholcodine (p.1128·3).
*Coughs.*

**Expuryl** *Codifra, Fr.*
Cynara; ash; black currant; meadowsweet; green tea (p.1417·1).
*Tonic.*

**Exputex** *Shire, Irl.*
Carbocisteine (p.1116·2).
*Respiratory-tract disorders with excessive or viscous mucus.*

**exrheudon OPT** *Optimed, Ger.*
*Ointment†:* Glycol salicylate (p.44·3); benzyl nicotinate (p.21·2).
*Frostbite; inflammatory disorders; soft-tissue, nerve, and joint disorders; sports injuries.*
*Tablets:* Phenylbutazone (p.83·2).
*Acute ankylosing spondylitis; gout; rheumatism.*

**Exrhinin** *Wernigerode, Ger.†.*
Tetryzoline hydrochloride (p.1131·2).
*Nasal congestion.*

**Exsel** *Allergan, USA.*
Selenium sulfide (p.1157·3).
*Dandruff; pityriasis versicolor; seborrhoeic dermatitis.*

**Extencilline** *Aventis, Fr.*
Benzathine benzylpenicillin (p.162·3).
*Bacterial infections.*

**Extendryl** *Fleming, USA.*
Phenylephrine hydrochloride (p.1126·3); hyoscine methonitrate (p.483·3); chlorphenamine maleate (p.427·3).
*Allergic rhinitis; respiratory congestion; urticaria and angioedema.*

**Exteny** *IQFA, Mex.*
Mebendazole (p.108·2).
*Worm infections.*

**Exterol**
*Dermal Laboratories, Irl.; Dermal, Israel; Dermal Laboratories, UK.*
Urea hydrogen peroxide (p.1195·3).
*Ear wax removal.*

**Extin N** *Opfermann, Ger.*
Ammonium chloride (p.1115·2).
Extin formerly contained adipic acid and ammonium chloride.
*Urinary-tract infections.*

**Extiser Q** *Serral, Mex.*
Praziquantel (p.112·2).
*Cysticercosis.*

**Extosen** *Instituto Sanitas, Chile.*
Codeine phosphate (p.27·1); pseudoephedrine hydrochloride (p.1129·2); chlorphenamine maleate (p.427·3).
*Coughs.*

**Extovyl** *Dexo, Fr.*
Betahistine mesilate (p.1660·1).
*Vertigo.*

**Extra Action Cough** *Rugby, USA.*
Dextromethorphan hydrobromide (p.1117·3); guaifenesin (p.1122·1).
*Coughs.*

**Extra Once A Day** *Quest, Canad.*
Multivitamin, mineral, and trace element preparation (p.1417·1).

**Extra Power Pain Reliever** *AAH, UK.*
Paracetamol (p.76·2); aspirin (p.15·1); caffeine (p.782·1).
*Pain.*

**Extra Strength Acetaminophen with Codeine** *WestCan, Canad.†.*
Paracetamol (p.76·2); caffeine (p.782·1); codeine phosphate (p.27·1).
*Fever; pain.*

**Extra Strength Alenic Alka** *Rugby, USA.*
Aluminium hydroxide (p.1249·2); magnesium carbonate (p.1272·1).
*Hyperacidity.*

**Extra Strength Alka-Seltzer Effervescent Tablets** *Bayer, USA.*
Sodium bicarbonate (p.1223·2); citric acid (p.1673·1); aspirin (p.15·1).
*Hyperacidity.*

**Extra Strength Allergy Sinus** *Stanley, Canad.; WestCan, Canad.*
Pseudoephedrine hydrochloride (p.1129·2); chlorphenamine maleate (p.427·3); paracetamol (p.76·2).

**Extra Strength Analgesic** *Prodemdis, Canad.*
Methyl salicylate (p.59·3); camphor (p.1665·3); menthol (p.1711·3); eucalyptus oil (p.1686·2).

**Extra Strength Bayer Plus** *Sterling Health, USA.*
Aspirin (p.15·1).
Calcium carbonate (p.1254·2), magnesium carbonate (p.1272·1), and magnesium oxide (p.1272·3) are included in this preparation in an attempt to limit adverse effects on the gastrointestinal mucosa.

**Extra Strength Cold Medication Daytime Relief** *Stanley, Canad.; WestCan, Canad.*
Pseudoephedrine hydrochloride (p.1129·2); dextromethorphan hydrobromide (p.1117·3); paracetamol (p.76·2).

**Extra Strength Cold Medication Nightime**
*Stanley, Canad.*
Pseudoephedrine hydrochloride (p.1129·2); chlorphenamine maleate (p.427·3); dextromethorphan hydrobromide (p.1117·3); paracetamol (p.76·2).

**Extra Strength Cold Medication Nighttime Relief** *WestCan, Canad.*
Pseudoephedrine hydrochloride (p.1129·2); chlorphenamine maleate (p.427·3); dextromethorphan hydrobromide (p.1117·3); paracetamol (p.76·2).

**Extra Strength Cough Syrup Expectorant**
*Stanley, Canad.*
Guaifenesin (p.1122·1).
*Coughs.*

**Extra Strength Doans PM** *Ciba, USA.*
Magnesium salicylate (p.55·1); diphenhydramine hydrochloride (p.431·3).

**Extra Strength Genaton** *Goldline, USA.*
Aluminium hydroxide (p.1249·2); magnesium carbonate (p.1272·1).
*Hyperacidity.*

**Extra Strength Maalox Antacid/Anti-Gas** *Novartis Consumer, USA.*
Aluminium hydroxide (p.1249·2); magnesium hydroxide (p.1272·2); simeticone (p.1289·2).
*Hyperacidity.*

**Extra Strength Mintox Plus** *Major, USA.*
Simeticone (p.1289·2).

**Extra Strength Multi-Symptom PMS Relief**
*Stanley, Canad.*
Paracetamol (p.76·2); pamabrom (p.978·2); mepyramine maleate (p.437·1).

**Extra Strength Pyrroxate** *Roberts, USA†.*
Phenylpropanolamine hydrochloride (p.1127·3); chlorphenamine maleate (p.427·3); paracetamol (p.76·2).
*Upper respiratory-tract symptoms.*

**Extra Strength Sinus and Congestion Relief**
*WestCan, Canad.*
Pseudoephedrine hydrochloride (p.1129·2); paracetamol (p.76·2).

**Extra Strength Sinus Medication** *Stanley, Canad.*
Pseudoephedrine hydrochloride (p.1129·2); paracetamol (p.76·2).

**Extra Strength Tylenol Headache Plus** *McNeil Consumer, USA†.*
Paracetamol (p.76·2); calcium carbonate (p.1254·2).
*Gastrointestinal pain associated with hyperacidity.*

**Extra Strength Tylenol PM** *McNeil Consumer, USA.*
Diphenhydramine hydrochloride (p.431·3); paracetamol (p.76·2).
*Insomnia.*

**Extra Strength Vicks Cough Drops** *Procter & Gamble, USA.*
Menthol (p.1711·3).

**Extra Strong Formula 12** *Hilarys, Canad.*
Aloes (p.1248·2); bisacodyl (p.1251·3); cascara (p.1255·1); frangula (p.1266·3); rhubarb (p.1287·3); senna (p.1288·2).
*Constipation.*

**Extraboline** *Genepharm, Gr.*
Nandrolone decanoate (p.1561·2).
*Anabolic.*

**Extracort** *Galderma, Ger.†.*
Triamcinolone acetonide (p.1110·2).
*Skin disorders.*

**Extracort Rhin sine** *Alcon, Ger.†.*
Triamcinolone acetonide (p.1110·2); phenylephrine hydrochloride (p.1126·3).
*Allergic nasal disorders.*

**Extracort Tinktur** *Galderma, Ger.*
Triamcinolone acetonide (p.1110·2); salicylic acid (p.1157·1).
*Skin disorders.*

**Extrafer** *SoSe, Ital.*
Sodium ferric gluconate complex (p.1444·3).
*Anaemias.*

**Extralife Arthri-Care** *Felton, Austral.†.*
Turmeric (p.1058·3); ginger (p.1267·1); feverfew (p.469·1); devil's claw root (p.28·2); lecithin (p.1706·1).
*Musculoskeletal and joint disorders.*

**Extralife Extra-Brite** *Felton, Austral.†.*
Ginkgo biloba (p.1692·3); ginseng (p.1693·1); lecithin (p.1706·1).
*Alzheimer's disease; mental function disorders.*

**Extralife Eye-Care** *Felton, Austral.†.*
Myrtillus (p.1718·3); ginkgo biloba (p.1692·3); big marigold; riboflavin (p.1456·1); zinc gluconate (p.1469·2).
*Eye disorders.*

**Extralife Flow-Care** *Felton, Austral.†.*
Saw palmetto (p.1569·1); urtica (p.1762·1); pyridoxine hydrochloride (p.1456·3); zinc gluconate (p.1469·2).
*Benign prostatic hyperplasia; micturition disorders in men.*

**Extralife Fluid-Care** *Felton, Austral.†.*
Taraxacum (p.1751·3); equisetum (p.1684·1); parsley (p.1728·3); bearberry (p.1659·2); solidago virgaurea (p.1748·3); pyridoxine hydrochloride (p.1456·3).
*Fluid retention.*

**Extralife Leg-Care** *Felton, Austral.†.*
Aesculus (p.1648·2); ruscus aculeatus; centella (p.1144·3); ginkgo biloba (p.1692·3); myrtillus (p.1718·3); hesperidin (p.1688·2); rutoside (p.1688·2); ascorbic acid (p.1460·2).
*Varicose veins.*

**Extralife Liva-Care** *Felton, Austral.†.*
Silybum marianum (p.1043·3); greater celandine (p.1695·3); cynara (p.1678·3); turmeric (p.1058·3); astragalus; taraxacum (p.1751·3); lecithin (p.1706·1).
*Acne; gastrointestinal disorders; halitosis; hyperlipidaemias; hypersensitivity disorders; hypoglycaemia; menopausal disorders; migraine; obesity; premenstrual syndrome.*

**Extralife Meno-Care** *Felton, Austral.†.*
Soya bean (p.1447·2); cimicifuga (p.1671·3); chaste tree; angelica sinensis (p.1655·1); calcium phosphate (p.1225·3).
*Menopausal disorders; osteoporosis.*

**Extralife Migrai-Care** *Felton, Austral.†.*
Feverfew (p.469·1); salix (p.87·3); magnesium phosphate (p.1228·1).
*Migraine and other headaches.*

**Extra-life Nasex** *Felton, Austral.*
Cineole (p.1672·1); oxymetazoline hydrochloride (p.1126·1); menthol (p.1711·3).
*Nasal congestion.*

**Extralife PMS-Care** *Felton, Austral.†.*
Salix (p.87·3); chaste tree; cimicifuga (p.1671·3); viburnum opulus; bearberry (p.1659·2); pyridoxine hydrochloride (p.1456·3); ferrous fumarate (p.1427·3).
*Premenstrual syndrome.*

**Extralife Sleep-Care** *Felton, Austral.†.*
Valerian (p.1762·2); passion flower (p.1729·1); gentian (p.1692·2); lupulus (p.1708·1); magnesium phosphate (p.1228·1); calcium phosphate (p.1225·3).
*Nervous disorders; sleep disorders.*

**Extralife Uri-Care** *Felton, Austral.†.*
Cranberry (p.1676·3); bearberry (p.1659·2); buchu (p.1663·1); pyridoxine hydrochloride (p.1456·3); ascorbic acid (p.1460·2); potassium sulfate (p.1232·2).
*Cystitis.*

**Extranase** *Rottapharm, Fr.*
Bromelains (p.1662·2).
*Post-traumatic and postoperative oedema.*

**Extraneal**
*Baxter, Austral.; Baxter, Austria; Baxter, Braz.†; Baxter, Denm.; Baxter, Fin.; Baxter, Ger.; Baxter, Ital.; Baxter, Spain; Baxter, Swed.; Baxter, Switz.; Baxter, USA.*
Icodextrin; sodium chloride; sodium lactate; calcium chloride; magnesium chloride (p.1221·1).
*Peritoneal dialysis.*

**Extrapan** *Qualiphar, Belg.*
Ibuprofen (p.45·3).
*Peri-articular and soft-tissue disorders.*

**Extraplus** *Pierre Fabre, Spain.*
Ketoprofen (p.51·2).
*Musculoskeletal, joint disorders, peri-articular, and soft-tissue disorders.*

**Extrato Hepatico Composto**
*Note. This name is used for preparations of different composition.*
*Delta, Braz.*
Methionine (p.1042·1); choline (p.1424·3); liver extract.
*Liver disorders.*
*Heralds, Braz.†.*
Methionine (p.1042·1); choline (p.1424·3); pyridoxine hydrochloride (p.1456·3).
*Liver disorders.*

**Extrato Hepatico Vitaminado** *Granado, Braz.*
Methionine (p.1042·1); liver extract; choline (p.1424·3).
*Liver disorders.*

**Extravite** *Vitalia, UK†.*
Multivitamin and mineral preparation (p.1417·1).

**Extravits** *Lifeplan, UK†.*
Multivitamin and mineral preparation (p.1417·1).

**Extur** *Normon, Spain.*
Indapamide (p.938·2).
*Hypertension; oedema.*

**Exuracid** *Rosch & Handel, Austria.*
Tisopurine (p.418·2).
*Gout; hyperuricaemia; urinary calculi.*

**Exviral** *Kwizda, Austria.*
Aciclovir (p.626·1).
*Herpes labialis.*

**Exzem Oil** *Pharmadass, UK†.*
Vitamin E oil (p.1464·3); evening primrose oil (p.1686·3); castor oil (p.1668·2); olive oil (p.1723·2); safflower oil (p.1443·3); grapeseed oil; chamomile oil (p.1669·3).

**Eye Dew** *Crookes Healthcare, UK.*
Hamamelis (p.1696·3); naphazoline hydrochloride (p.1124·3).
Formerly known as Optrex Eye Dew.
*Eye irritation.*

**Eye Drops**
*Zee, Canad.; Reese, USA.*
Tetryzoline hydrochloride (p.1131·2).
*Eye irritation.*

**Eye Drops Extra** *Ocusoft, USA†.*
Phenylephrine hydrochloride (p.1126·3).

**Eye Eze** *Pharmavite, Canad.†.*
Boric acid (p.1662·1); borax (p.1661·3).

**Eye Formula Euphr** *Homeocan, Canad.*
Homoeopathic preparation.

**Eye Health Herbal Plus Formula 4** *Vitelle, Austral.†.*
Euphrasia (p.1686·3); ginkgo biloba (p.1692·3); betacarotene (p.1422·3); *d*-alpha tocoferil acid succinate (p.1465·1); ascorbic acid (p.1460·2); rutoside (p.1688·2); hesperidin (p.1688·2).
*Eye strain.*

**Eye Mo**
*SmithKline Beecham, Hong Kong†; GlaxoSmithKline, Singapore; GlaxoSmithKline, Thai.*
Boric acid (p.1662·1); borax (p.1661·3).
*Eye irritation.*

**Eye Mo 36** *SmithKline Beecham, Hong Kong†.*
Boric acid (p.1662·1); tetryzoline hydrochloride (p.1131·2).
*Eye irritation.*

**Eye Mo Moist** *GlaxoSmithKline, Singapore.*
Hypromellose (p.1579·3).
*Dry eyes.*

**Eye Scrub** *Novartis Ophthalmics, USA.*
Eyelid cleanser.

**Eye Vites** *Natural Life, Arg.*
Vitamin and mineral preparation (p.1417·1).

**Eye Wash**
*Note. This name is used for preparations of different composition.*
*Rivex, Canad.†.*
Boric acid (p.1662·1).
*Zee, Canad.*
Electrolytes (p.1217·1).
*Eye irrigation.*

**Eyebrex** *Alvia (Αλβια), Gr.*
Tobramycin (p.271·2).
*Eye infections.*

**Eyecon** *Ciba Vision, Israel.*
Sodium hyaluronate (p.1697·3).
*Dry eyes.*

**Eyedex** *Siam Bheasach, Thai.*
Dexamethasone sodium phosphate (p.1097·2); neomycin sulfate (p.235·1).
*Infected eye and ear disorders.*

**Eye-Gene** *JDH Borneo, Thai.*
Phenylephrine hydrochloride (p.1126·3); boric acid (p.1662·1); borax (p.1661·3); sodium chloride (p.1233·3).
*Eye irritation.*

**Eye-Gene Soft** *JDH Borneo, Thai.*
Boric acid (p.1662·1); borax (p.1661·3); sodium chloride (p.1233·3).
*Eye irritation.*

**Eyelube** *Sabex, Canad.*
Hypromellose (p.1579·3).
*Dry eyes.*

**Eye-Lube-A** *Optopics, USA.*
Glycerol (p.1694·3).
*Dry eyes.*

**Eye-Sed** *Scherer, USA†.*
Zinc sulfate (p.1469·3).
*Minor eye irritation.*

**Eyesine** *Akorn, USA†.*
Tetryzoline hydrochloride (p.1131·2).
*Minor eye irritation.*

**Eyestil** *Ophtapharma, Canad.*
Sodium hyaluronate (p.1697·3).
*Dry eyes.*

**Eye-Stream**
*Alcon, Austral.; Alcon, Canad.; Alcon, Hong Kong; Alcon, Malaysia; Alcon, NZ.; Alcon, Singapore; Alcon Cusi, Spain; Alcon, USA.*
Electrolyte preparation (p.1217·1).
*Eye irrigation.*

**Eyetobrin** *Cooper (Κοπερ), Gr.*
Tobramycin (p.271·2).
*Eye infections.*

**EyeVit** *Pharmadass, UK.*
Multivitamin, mineral, and amino-acid preparation (p.1417·1).

**Eyevite**
*Allergan, Austral.; Allergan, NZ.*
Vitamin and mineral preparation (p.1417·1).
*Eye disorders.*

**Eyewash** *Sabex, Canad.; Zee, Canad.*
Electrolyte solution (p.1217·1).
*Eye irrigation.*

**Eye-Zine** Ocumed, USA.
Tetryzoline hydrochloride (p.1131·2).
*Eye irritation.*

**Eykosacol** Knop, Chile.
Fish oil.
*Hyperlipidaemias; hypertension.*

**EZ Detect**
Step, Arg.; Marco, Austral.; Biomerica, USA.
Test for occult blood in faeces or urine.

**EZ HP** Marco, Austral.
Test for *Helicobacter pylori* antibodies in blood, serum or plasma.

**E-Z-Cat**
Temis, Arg.; Therapex, Canad.†; E-Z-EM, Port.; E-Z-EM, UK.
Barium sulfate (p.1061·1).
*Contrast medium for computerised axial tomography of the gastrointestinal tract.*

**Ezede** Xepa-Soul Pattinson, Malaysia.
Loratadine (p.436·1).
*Allergic conjunctivitis; allergic rhinitis; allergic skin disorders.*

**Ezetrol**
Merck Sharp & Dohme, Ger.; Merck Sharp & Dohme, UK.
Ezetimibe (p.914·2).
*Hypercholesterolaemia.*

**E-Z-Gas II**
Therapex, Canad.
Sodium bicarbonate (p.1223·2); tartaric acid (p.1752·1); simeticone (p.1289·2).
*Production of $CO_2$ in double contrast radiography of the gastrointestinal tract.*

Bracco, Switz.
Sodium bicarbonate (p.1223·2); citric acid (p.1673·1); simeticone (p.1289·2).
*Production of $CO_2$ in double contrast radiography of the gastrointestinal tract.*

**Ez-HBT** Metabolic Solutions, USA.
Carbon-13 (p.1667·3) labelled urea (Helicosol); test meal (Ensure).
*Diagnosis of Helicobacter pylori infection.*

**E-Z-HD**
E-Z-EM, Israel; E-Z-EM, Port.; E-Z-EM, UK.
Barium sulfate (p.1061·1).
*Contrast medium for gastrointestinal radiography.*

**Ezipol** Kleva, Gr.
Omeprazole (p.1278·2).
*Acid aspiration; eradication of Helicobacter pylori in combination with antimicrobials; peptic ulcer; reflux oesophagitis; Zollinger-Ellison syndrome.*

**Ezon-T** Unison, Thai.
*Ointment:* Tolnaftate (p.410·1).
*Topical solution:* Tolnaftate (p.410·1); triacetin (p.410·2).
*Fungal skin infections.*

**Ezopen** Teuto, Braz.
Aciclovir (p.626·1).
*Herpesvirus infections.*

**Ezopta** Biomedica-Chemica, Gr.
Ranitidine hydrochloride (p.1285·2).
*Conditions where gastric acid reduction is beneficial; gastric hypersecretion including Zollinger-Ellison syndrome; peptic ulcer.*

**Ezosina** Fournier, Ital.
Terazosin hydrochloride (p.1010·3).
*Hypertension.*

**E-Z-Paque**
E-Z-EM, Belg.; E-Z-EM, UK.
Barium sulfate (p.1061·1).
*Contrast medium for gastrointestinal radiography.*

**I + I-F** Dunhall, USA.
Hydrocortisone (p.1103·3); clioquinol (p.196·3); pramocaine (p.1382·2).
*Skin disorders.*

**F9** Loren, Mex.
Loperamide (p.1271·2).
*Diarrhoea.*

**F080** Baxter, Ital.†.
Amino-acid infusion for parenteral nutrition (p.1417·1).
*Liver disorders.*

**F 99 Sulgan N** Divapharma, Ger.†.
Hamamelis (p.1696·3).
*Anorectal disorders.*

**FAB** Medical Research, Austral.†.
Iron and vitamin B substances (p.1417·1).

**FAB Co** Medical Research, Austral.†.
Iron, vitamin B substances, and vitamin C (p.1417·1).

**FAB Tri-Cal** Medical Research, Austral.†.
Calcium hydrogen phosphate (p.1225·2); calcium carbonate (p.1254·2); calcium gluconate (p.1225·2); zinc oxide (p.1163·2); magnesium oxide (p.1272·3); colecalciferol (p.1461·3).
*Nutritional supplement.*

**Fabopxicam** Fabop, Arg.
Piroxicam (p.84·2).
*Fever; inflammation; pain.*

**Fabracin** Fabra, Arg.
Cinnarizine (p.428·3).
*Cerebrovascular disorders.*

**Fabralgina** Fabra, Arg.
Naproxen (p.65·1).
*Inflammation; pain.*

**Fabramicina** Fabra, Arg.
Azithromycin (p.159·1).
*Bacterial infections.*

**Fabrapride** Fabra, Arg.
Cisapride (p.1259·2).
*Gastrointestinal motility disorders.*

**Fabrazol** Fabra, Arg.
Omeprazole (p.1278·2).

**Fabrazyme**
Genzyme, Denm.; Genzyme, Fr.; Genzyme, Ger.; Genzyme, Israel; Genzyme, Ital.; Genzyme, Spain; Genzyme, UK; Genzyme, USA.
Agalsidase beta (p.1651·1).
*Fabry disease.*

**Fabroven**
Note. This name is used for preparations of different composition.
Schering-Plough, Mex.
Ascorbic acid (p.1460·2); hesperidin methyl chalcone (p.1688·3); ruscus aculeatus.
*Haemorrhoids; metrorrhagia; peripheral vascular disorders.*

Pierre Fabre, Spain.
*Capsules:* Ascorbic acid (p.1460·2); hesperidin methyl chalcone (p.1688·3); ruscus aculeatus.
*Cream:* Melilotus; ruscus aculeatus.
Formerly contained dextran sulfate, melilotus, and ruscus aculeatus.
*Peripheral vascular disorders.*

**Fabubac** Brunel, S.Afr.
Co-trimoxazole (p.199·3).
*Bacterial infections.*

**Fabudol** Volta, Chile.
Piroxicam (p.84·2).

**Fabulaxol** Master, Chile.
Monobasic sodium phosphate (p.1230·3); dibasic sodium phosphate (p.1231·1).
*Constipation.*

**Fabutin** Pharmacos Abug, Mex.
Famotidine (p.1265·2).
*Peptic ulcer.*

**Face Foundation** Avon, Canad.†.
*SPF 15:* Octinoxate (p.1154·3); titanium dioxide (p.1160·3).
*Sunscreen.*

**Face Zone** Clinique, Canad.
*SPF 30:* Homosalate (p.1148·1); octinoxate (p.1154·3); octisalate (p.1154·3); titanium dioxide (p.1160·3); zinc oxide (p.1163·2).
Formerly contained homosalate, octinoxate, octisalate, and oxybenzone.
*Sunscreen.*

**Facelit** Collins, Mex.
Cefalexin (p.168·1).
*Bacterial infections.*

**Faces Only** Schering-Plough, USA.
*SPF 6; SPF 15:* Octinoxate (p.1154·3); oxybenzone (p.1154·3).
*Sunscreen.*

**Facetin-D** Ifusa, Mex.
Diiodohydroxyquinoline (p.603·3); phthalylsulfacetamide; homatropine (p.483·2); kaolin (p.1268·3); pectin (p.1580·3).
*Amoebiasis.*

**Facicam** Senosiain, Mex.
Piroxicam (p.84·2).
*Gout; musculoskeletal, joint, peri-articular and soft-tissue disorders.*

**Facilgest** Raffo, Arg.
Metoclopramide (p.1274·3); pancreatin (p.1725·3); simeticone (p.1289·2).
*Digestive disorders; flatulence; gastrointestinal motility disorders.*

**Facilit** Fides Ecopharma, Spain.
Allopurinol (p.412·2); benzbromarone (p.414·3).
*Gout; hyperuricaemia.*

**Facitor** Mintlab, Chile.
Aspirin (p.15·1); chlorphenamine (p.428·1); caffeine (p.782·1).
*Cold and influenza symptoms.*

**Faclor** Novartis, Braz.
Cefaclor (p.167·1).
*Bacterial infections.*

**Facogen** NBF-Lanes, Ital.†.
Lipid, protein, carbohydrate, multivitamin, and trace-element preparation (p.1417·1).
*Nutritional supplement.*

**Facort** Biolab, Thai.
Triamcinolone acetonide (p.1110·2).
*Skin disorders.*

**Facovit** Teofarma, Ital.
Testosterone propionate (p.1570·1); rubidium iodide (p.1741·1); potassium iodide (p.1598·1); riboflavin (p.1456·1).
*Cataract; vitreous turbidity.*

**Fact Plus**
Medisense, Canad.; Advanced Care, USA.
Pregnancy test (p.1734·3).

**Factane** Lab Francais du Fractionnement, Fr.
A factor VIII preparation (p.751·1).
*Haemorrhagic disorders.*

**Faction** Maigal, Arg.
Ketoconazole (p.403·3).
*Fungal infections.*

**Factioneye** Maigal, Arg.
Naphazoline (p.1124·3); neomycin (p.235·1); dexamethasone (p.1097·1).
*Eye disorders.*

**Factive** Genesoft, USA.
Gemifloxacin mesilate (p.216·3).
*Bacterial infections of the respiratory tract.*

**Factodin** Faran, Gr.
Clotrimazole (p.396·2).
*Fungal skin infections.*

**Factofer** Raymos, Arg.
Ferrous sulfate (p.1428·2).
*Anaemias.*

**Factofer B12** Raymos, Arg.
Vitamin $B_{12}$ (p.1458·2); folic acid (p.1429·1); ferrous sulfate (p.1428·2).
*Anaemias.*

**Factor AF2** Biosyn, Ger.
Liver and spleen extract.
*Supportive tumour therapy.*

**Factor AG** Casasco, Arg.
Simeticone (p.1289·2).
*Meteorism.*

**Factor AG Antiacido** Casasco, Arg.
Aluminium hydroxide (p.1249·2); magnesium hydroxide (p.1272·2); simeticone (p.1289·2).
*Flatulence; gastric hyperacidity.*

**Factor AG Antiespasmodico** Casasco, Arg.
Simeticone (p.1289·2); homatropine methylbromide (p.483·2).
*Gastrointestinal spasm.*

**Factor Antigripal** Inmunolab, Arg.
Astemizole (p.424·2); paracetamol (p.76·2); phenylephrine (p.1126·3).
*Influenza symptoms.*

**Factor Dermico** Casasco, Arg.
Gentamicin sulfate (p.217·1); betamethasone valerate (p.1093·2); miconazole nitrate (p.405·3).
*Infected skin disorders.*

**Factorine** Casasco, Arg.
Metoclopramide (p.1274·3); simeticone (p.1289·2).
*Dyspepsia; flatulence; nausea and vomiting.*

**Factoss** Laboratorios Chile, Chile.
Noscapine hydrochloride (p.1125·3).
*Coughs.*

**Factrel**
Wyeth-Ayerst, Canad.†; Wyeth-Ayerst, USA.
Gonadorelin hydrochloride (p.1325·2).
*Diagnostic evaluation of anterior pituitary function.*

**Factus** Roux-Ocefa, Arg.
*Oral drops:* Phenylpropanolamine hydrochloride (p.1127·3); chlorphenamine maleate (p.427·3).
*Allergic rhinitis; cold and influenza symptoms.*
*Tablets:* Phenylpropanolamine (p.1127·3); paracetamol (p.76·2); moroxydine; dexbrompheniramine (p.426·2) vitamin C (p.1460·2); muramidase (p.1717·2).
*Influenza symptoms.*

**Fa-Cyl** Medley, Braz.
Tinidazole (p.617·1).
*Anaerobic bacterial infections; protozoal infections.*

**Facyl M** Medley, Braz.
Tinidazole (p.617·1); miconazole nitrate (p.405·3).
*Vulvovaginal infections.*

**FAD Ophthalmic Soln** Santen, Hong Kong.
Flavine adenine dinucleotide disodium.
*Blepharitis; keratitis.*

**Fadacaina** Fada, Arg.
Procaine (p.1383·2).
*Local anaesthesia.*

**Fadaespasmol** Fada, Arg.
Isoxsuprine (p.1702·3).

**Fadafilina** Fada, Arg.
Aminophylline (p.780·2).
*Obstructive airways disease.*

**Fadaflumaz** Fada, Arg.
Flumazenil (p.1038·3).

**Fadalefrina** Fada, Arg.
Phenylephrine (p.1126·3).

**Fadalivio** Fada, Arg.
Naproxen (p.65·1).
*Fever; pain.*

**Fadametasona** Fada, Arg.
Dexamethasone (p.1097·1).
*Corticosteroid.*

**Fadamine** Fada, Arg.
Metaraminol (p.952·3).

**Fadanasal** Fada, Arg.
Naphazoline (p.1124·3); nitrofurazone (p.238·2); mepyramine (p.437·1).
*Nasal congestion.*

**Fadastigmina** Fada, Arg.
Neostigmine (p.1492·2).

**Fade Cream** Cosmofarma, Port.
Kojic acid (p.1151·2); achillea (p.1646·2); octinoxate (p.1154·3); titanium dioxide (p.1160·3).
*Skin pigmentation disorders.*

**Fadiamone** CS, Fr.
Phytoestrogens; centella (p.1144·3).
*Skin ageing.*

**Fadig** Dansk-Flama, Braz.
Amino acids and vitamin B substances (p.1417·1).

**Fadina** Cantabria, Spain.
Loratadine (p.436·1).
*Allergic rhinitis; urticaria.*

**Fadine**
Biolab, Hong Kong; Biolab, Malaysia; Biolab, Thai.
Famotidine (p.1265·2).
*Gastric hyperacidity; gastro-oesophageal reflux; peptic ulcer; Zollinger-Ellison syndrome.*

**Fadol** Lemery, Mex.
Hydrocortisone (p.1103·3).
*Corticosteroid.*

**Fadul** Hexal, Ger.
Famotidine (p.1265·2).
*Peptic ulcer; Zollinger-Ellison syndrome.*

**Faelac** Inmunolab, Arg.
Lactobacillus acidophilus (p.1704·2); Lactobacillus casei; Enterococcus faecium (p.1704·2); simeticone (p.1289·2).
*Restoration of normal gastrointestinal flora.*

**Faexojodan** Kanoldt, Ger.†.
*Saccharomyces cerevisiae* (non-fermentable) (p.1469·1).
*Skin disorders.*

**Fagastril** Quimifar, Spain.
Famotidine (p.1265·2).
*Gastro-oesophageal reflux; peptic ulcer; Zollinger-Ellison syndrome.*

**Fagatrim** Collins, Mex.
Famotidine (p.1265·2).
*Peptic ulcer.*

**Fagizol** Continentales, Mex.†.
Metronidazole (p.607·2).

**Fagolipo** Libbs, Braz.
Mazindol (p.1589·1).
*Obesity.*

**Fagorutin Buchweizen** GlaxoSmithKline Consumer, Ger.
*Tablets:* Fagopyrum esculentum; troxerutin (p.1688·3).
*Tea:* Fagopyrum esculentum.
*Venous insufficiency.*

**Fagorutin Rosskastanien-Balsam N** GlaxoSmithKline Consumer, Ger.
Aesculus (p.1648·2); rutoside sodium sulfate (p.1688·3); menthol (p.1711·3).
Formerly contained aesculus, rutoside sodium sulfate, menthol, arnica, and rosemary oil.
*Venous insufficiency.*

**Fagorutin Ruscus** GlaxoSmithKline Consumer, Ger.
Ruscus aculeatus.
*Chronic venous insufficiency; haemorrhoids.*

**Fagus** Abbott, Spain.
Ranitidine hydrochloride (p.1285·2).
*Acid aspiration; gastro-oesophageal reflux; gastrointestinal hyperacidity; peptic ulcer; short-bowel syndrome; Zollinger-Ellison syndrome.*

**Fagusan** Spreewald, Ger.†.
Guaifenesin (p.1122·1).
*Coughs and related respiratory-tract disorders.*

**Faifloc** TS, Ital.
Flucloxacillin sodium (p.213·3).
*Bacterial infections.*

**Fairgenol** FDC, India.
Dichloroxylenol (p.1178·3); terpineol (p.1752·2).
*Skin disinfection.*

**Fairy ADE** YSP, Malaysia.
Vitamin A (p.1451·2); vitamin D (p.1461·2); vitamin E (p.1464·3).
*Dry skin.*

**Faktu**
Meda, Fin.; Byk Gulden, Ger.; Roland, Ger.; Altana, Hong Kong; Byk, Port.; Byk Gulden, Singapore; Altana, Switz.; Byk Gulden, Thai.†.
Policresulen (p.1190·1); cinchocaine hydrochloride (p.1373·2).
*Anorectal disorders.*

**Faktu akut** Byk Gulden, Ger.; Roland, Ger.
Bufexamac (p.21·3); bismuth subgallate (p.1252·2); titanium dioxide (p.1160·3); lidocaine hydrochloride (p.1377·3).
*Anorectal disorders.*

**Falacid** Collins, Mex.
Quinfamide (p.615·2).
*Amoebiasis.*

**Falcigo** Cadila, India.
Artesunate (p.447·2).
*Malaria.*

**Falcol** Farma Lepori, Spain.
Aceclofenac (p.11·2).
*Gout; musculoskeletal, joint, and peri-articular disorders; pain.*

**Falexol** Protein, Mex.†.
Cefalexin (p.168·1).
*Bacterial infections.*

**Falgos** Gramon, Arg.
Aspirin (p.15·1); paracetamol (p.76·2); caffeine (p.782·1); aluminium hydroxide (p.1249·2); magnesium hydroxide (p.1272·2).
*Dyspepsia; hangover; pain.*

**Falicard** AWD, Ger.
Verapamil hydrochloride (p.1019·1).
*Arrhythmias; hypertension; ischaemic heart disease.*

**Falimint** Berlin-Chemie, Ger.
Acetylaminopropoxybenzene.
*Mouth and throat disorders.*

**Falithrom** Hexal, Ger.
Phenprocoumon (p.981·3).
*Thromboembolism prophylaxis.*

**Falitonsin** AWD, Ger.
Atenolol (p.865·2).
*Arrhythmias; hypertension; ischaemic heart disease.*

**Falkamin**
Note. This name is used for preparations of different composition.
Falk, Ger.; Abbott, Ital.
Leucine (p.1439·1); valine (p.1451·2); isoleucine (p.1438·2).
*Liver disorders.*

*Falk, Hong Kong.*
Amino-acid, vitamin and trace element preparation preparation (p.1417·1).
*Hepatic failure.*

*Falk, Malaysia; Falk, Singapore.*
Amino-acid preparation (p.1417·1).
*Nutritional supplement in liver disorders.*

**Falmonox** *Sanofi Synthelabo, Braz.*
Teclozan (p.616·3).
*Intestinal amoebiasis.*

**Falot** *Pisa, Mex.*
Cefalotin sodium (p.168·3).
*Bacterial infections.*

**Falquigut** *Falqui, Ital.*
Sodium picosulfate (p.1289·3).
*Constipation.*

**Falquilax** *Falqui, Ital.*
Senna (p.1288·2).
*Constipation.*

**Faltium** *Almirall, Spain†.*
Veralipride (p.727·2).
*Menopausal disorders.*

**Falvin** *Theramex, Ital.*
Fenticonazole nitrate (p.397·3).
*Dermatological and gynaecological fungal infections.*

**Famcod** *Salters, S.Afr.†.*
Paracetamol (p.76·2); codeine phosphate (p.27·1).
*Pain.*

**Famel**
*Note. This name is used for preparations of different composition.*
*Boots Healthcare, Ital.*
Lactocreosote (p.1117·2); calcium lactophosphate; ephedrine hydrochloride (p.1120·1).
*Bronchial catarrh.*

*Boots Healthcare, Neth.†.*
Creosote (p.1117·2); ephedrine hydrochloride (p.1120·1).
*Coughs.*

*Boots Healthcare, Switz.*
Lactocreosote (p.1117·2); calcium lactophosphate; codeine (p.27·1); drosera (p.1683·1); grindelia (p.1696·1).
*Bronchitis; coughs; sore throat.*

**Famel Broomhexine** *Boots Healthcare, Neth.*
Bromhexine hydrochloride (p.1115·3).
*Coughs.*

**Famel cum Codein** *Brady, Austria.*
Lactocreosote (p.1117·2); calcium lactophosphate; codeine hydrochloride (p.27·1).
*Asthma; bronchitis; catarrh; cold symptoms.*

**Famel cum Ephedrin** *Brady, Austria.*
Lactocreosote (p.1117·2); calcium lactophosphate; ephedrine hydrochloride (p.1120·1).
*Asthma; bronchitis; catarrh; cold symptoms.*

**Famel Expectorant** *SSL, UK†.*
Guaifenesin (p.1122·1).
*Coughs.*

**Famel Original** *SSL, UK.*
Creosote (p.1117·2); codeine phosphate (p.27·1).
*Coughs.*

**Famidal** *Andromaco, Chile.*
Miconazole (p.405·2); tinidazole (p.617·1).
*Balanitis; vulvovaginal infections.*

**Famidal Ad** *Andromaco, Chile.*
Tinidazole (p.617·1); miconazole nitrate (p.405·3).
*Balanitis; vulvovaginal infections.*

**Family Medic First Aid Treatment** *Tender, Canad.*
Benzalkonium chloride (p.1168·3); lidocaine hydrochloride (p.1377·3).

**Family Medicated Sunburn Relief** *Tender, Canad.†.*
Lidocaine (p.1377·3).

**Famine** *Merck, Hong Kong.*
Famotidine (p.1265·2).
*Peptic ulcer; Zollinger-Ellison syndrome.*

**Fam-Lax** *Torbet Laboratories, UK.*
Yellow phenolphthalein (p.1284·1); rhubarb (p.1287·3).
*Constipation.*

**Fam-Lax Senna** *Torbet Laboratories, UK.*
Turkey rhubarb (p.1287·3); senna leaf (p.1288·2); carrageenan (p.1578·2).
*Constipation.*

**Famo**
*IA, Ger.; ABZ, Ger.; CTI, Israel.*
Famotidine (p.1265·2).
*Gastro-oesophageal reflux; peptic ulcer; Zollinger-Ellison syndrome.*

**Famobeta** *Betapharm, Ger.*
Famotidine (p.1265·2).
*Peptic ulcer; Zollinger-Ellison syndrome.*

**Famoc**
*Berlin Pharm, Singapore; Berlin Pharm, Thai.*
Famotidine (p.1265·2).
*Gastro-oesophageal reflux; peptic ulcer; Zollinger-Ellison syndrome.*

**Famocid**
*Sun, Singapore†; Sun, Thai.*
Famotidine (p.1265·2).
*Peptic ulcer; Zollinger-Ellison syndrome.*

**Famodil** *Sigma-Tau, Ital.*
Famotidine (p.1265·2).
*Gastro-oesophageal reflux; peptic ulcer; Zollinger-Ellison syndrome.*

**Famodine**
*Farmasa, Braz.; Duopharma, Hong Kong.*
Famotidine (p.1265·2).
*Acid aspiration; gastro-oesophageal reflux; peptic ulcer; Zollinger-Ellison syndrome.*

**Famokey** *Inkeysa, Spain.*
Famotidine (p.1265·2).
*Gastric hyperacidity; gastro-oesophageal reflux; peptic ulcer; Zollinger-Ellison syndrome.*

**Famolta** *Jean-Marie, Hong Kong.*
Famotidine (p.1265·2).
*Gastro-oesophageal reflux; peptic ulcer; Zollinger-Ellison syndrome.*

**Famonerton** *Dolorgiet, Ger.*
Famotidine (p.1265·2).
*Peptic ulcer; Zollinger-Ellison syndrome.*

**Famonox** *Charoen, Thai.*
Famotidine (p.1265·2).
*Peptic ulcer; Zollinger-Ellison syndrome.*

**Famopril** *BPRL, Singapore.*
Famotidine (p.1265·2).
*Peptic ulcer; Zollinger-Ellison syndrome.*

**Famopsin**
*Remedica, Hong Kong; Remedica, Malaysia; Remedica, Singapore; Remedica, Thai.*
Famotidine (p.1265·2).
*Dyspepsia; gastrointestinal hyperacidity; heartburn; peptic ulcer; Zollinger-Ellison syndrome.*

**Famoset** *Sintofarma, Braz.*
Famotidine (p.1265·2).
*Acid aspiration; gastro-oesophageal reflux; peptic ulcer; Zollinger-Ellison syndrome.*

**Famotab** *Bangkok Lab & Cosmetic, Thai.*
Famotidine (p.1265·2).
*Peptic ulcer; Zollinger-Ellison syndrome.*

**Famotal** *Alpharma, Norw.*
Famotidine (p.1265·2).
*Gastro-oesophageal reflux; peptic ulcer; Zollinger-Ellison syndrome.*

**Famotec** *Julphar, UAE.*
Famotidine (p.1265·2).
*Gastro-oesophageal reflux; peptic ulcer; Zollinger-Ellison syndrome.*

**Famotid** *Neo Quimica, Braz.*
Famotidine (p.1265·2).
*Peptic ulcer.*

**Famotil** *Farmion, Braz.*
Famotidine (p.1265·2).
*Peptic ulcer.*

**Famotin**
*DHA, Singapore; LSP, Thai.*
Famotidine (p.1265·2).
*Gastro-oesophageal reflux; peptic ulcer; Zollinger-Ellison syndrome.*

**Famowal** *Wallace, India.*
Famotidine (p.1265·2).
*Gastro-oesophageal reflux; peptic ulcer; Zollinger-Ellison syndrome.*

**Famox**
*Ache, Braz.; Pacific, Hong Kong; Pacific, NZ; Merck, Singapore; Pacific, Singapore.*
Famotidine (p.1265·2).
*Acid aspiration; gastro-oesophageal reflux; peptic ulcer; Zollinger-Ellison syndrome.*

**Famoxal** *Silanes, Mex.*
Famotidine (p.1265·2).
*Acid aspiration; gastro-oesophageal reflux; peptic ulcer; Zollinger-Ellison syndrome.*

**Famoxil** *Hebron, Braz.*
Famotidine (p.1265·2).
*Peptic ulcer.*

**Fampin** *Wayne, Mex.†.*
Rifampicin (p.250·2).

**Famstim** *Genpharm, S.Afr.†.*
Ammonium bicarbonate (p.1115·1); aromatic ammonium spirit (p.1653·3); spirit of ether (p.1474·2).
*Coughs.*

**Famtac** *Nicholas Piramal, India.*
Famotidine (p.1265·2).
*Gastro-oesophageal reflux; peptic ulcer; Zollinger-Ellison syndrome.*

**Famtuss** *Genpharm, S.Afr.*
Diphenhydramine hydrochloride (p.431·3); ammonium chloride (p.1115·2); sodium citrate (p.1223·2); menthol (p.1711·3).
*Coughs.*

**Famucaps** *Brunel, S.Afr.*
Phenylephrine hydrochloride (p.1126·3); chlorphenamine maleate (p.427·3); ascorbic acid (p.1460·2); caffeine (p.782·1); paracetamol (p.76·2); atropine sulfate (p.477·1).
*Upper respiratory-tract disorders.*

**Famulan** *Bittner, Austria.*
Homoeopathic preparation.

**Famulcer** *Inkeysa, Spain.*
Famotidine (p.1265·2).
*Gastro-oesophageal reflux; peptic ulcer; Zollinger-Ellison syndrome.*

**Famvir**
*Note. This name is used for preparations of different composition.*
*Novartis, Austral.; Novartis, Belg.; Novartis, Canad.; Novartis, Denm.; Novartis, Fin.; Novartis, Ger.; Novartis, Gr.; Novartis, Hong Kong; Novartis, Irl.; Novartis, Israel; Novartis, Ital.; SmithKline Beecham, NZ†; Novartis, S.Afr.; Novartis, Singapore; Novartis, Spain; Novartis, Swed.; Novartis, Thai.; Novartis, UK; SmithKline Beecham, USA.*
Famciclovir (p.633·2).
*Herpesvirus infections.*

*Novartis, Austria; Novartis, Braz.; SmithKline Beecham, Neth.; Novartis, Switz.*
Famciclovir (p.633·2), penciclovir (p.651·2), or penciclovir sodium (p.651·3).
*Herpesvirus infections.*

**Fanaletas** *Lazar, Arg.*
Benzocaine (p.1370·3); tyrothricin (p.275·1); chlorophyllin (p.1057·1); hexylresorcinol (p.1182·1).
*Mouth and throat infections.*

**Fanalgic** *Mitchell, UK†.*
Paracetamol (p.76·2).
*Fever; pain.*

**Fanalgin** *Weifa, Norw.*
Phenazone (p.82·3); caffeine (p.782·1).
*Pain.*

**Fanasil** *Roche, Ital.†.*
Sulfadoxine (p.259·3).
*Bacterial infections.*

**Fanaxal** *Esteve, Spain.*
Alfentanil hydrochloride (p.12·2).
*General anaesthesia.*

**Fanciadazol** *Novag, Mex.*
Mebendazole (p.108·2).
*Worm infections.*

**Fanclomax** *Blausiegel, Braz.*
Famciclovir (p.633·2).

**Fandall** *Maver, Mex.*
Dipyrone (p.35·3).
*Fever; pain.*

**Fangan** *Lazar, Arg.*
Ketoconazole (p.403·3).
*Vulvovaginal candidiasis.*

**Fangopress** *Geistlich, Switz.†.*
Compress.
*Musculoskeletal and joint disorders.*

**Fango-Rubriment** *Riemser, Ger.*
Medicinal mud; sulfur (p.1158·2).
*Musculoskeletal and joint disorders.*

**Fangotherm**
*Eifelfango, Ger.; Eifelfango, Switz.†.*
Medicinal mud.
*Gastrointestinal, liver, and kidney disorders; gout; musculoskeletal and joint disorders; neuralgia.*

**Fanhdi**
*Grifols, Arg.; Grifols, Chile; Grifols, Ger.; Grifols, Ital.; Grifols, Port.; Grifols, Singapore; Grifols, Spain; Grifols, UK.*
A factor VIII preparation (p.751·1).
*Haemophilia A.*

**Fanolyte** *Bioprojet, Fr.*
Glucose; sodium chloride; potassium citrate; citric acid (p.1222·2).
*Diarrhoea; oral rehydration therapy.*

**Fanosin** *Abello, Spain.*
Famotidine (p.1265·2).
*Gastro-oesophageal reflux; peptic ulcer; Zollinger-Ellison syndrome.*

**Fanox** *Lesvi, Spain.*
Famotidine (p.1265·2).
*Gastro-oesophageal reflux; peptic ulcer; Zollinger-Ellison syndrome.*

**Fansamac** *Farmigea, Ital.*
Bufexamac (p.21·3).
*Pruritus; skin disorders; sunburn.*

**Fansia** *Eurodrug, Thai.†.*
Phenylpropanolamine hydrochloride (p.1127·3).
*Obesity.*

**Fansidar**
*Roche, Austral.; Roche, Belg.†; Roche, Braz.; Roche, Canad.; Roche, Denm.; Roche, Fr.; Roche, Irl.; Roche, Israel; Roche, S.Afr.; Roche, Swed.†; Roche, Switz.; Roche, UK; Roche, USA.*
Sulfadoxine (p.259·3); pyrimethamine (p.458·1).
*Malaria; Pneumocystis carinii pneumonia; toxoplasmosis.*

**Fansidol** *NCSN, Ital.*
Nimesulide (p.67·1).
*Fever; inflammation; pain.*

**Fansimef** *Roche, Switz.*
Mefloquine hydrochloride (p.453·3); sulfadoxine (p.259·3); pyrimethamine (p.458·1).
*Malaria.*

**Fantomalt**
*Nutricia, Fin.; Nutricia, Ital.; Nutricia, Port.*
Maltodextrin (p.1439·3).
*Preparation for enteral nutrition.*

**Fantrodol** *Farmaco, Mex.*
Ambroxol (p.1114·3).
*Respiratory-tract disorders.*

**Faradil** *Sidus, Arg.*
Metoclopramide (p.1274·3); diazepam (p.690·1); simeticone (p.1289·2).
*Gastrointestinal disorders.*

**Faradil Enzimatico** *Sidus, Arg.*
Metoclopramide (p.1274·3); pancreatin (p.1725·3); simeticone (p.1289·2).
*Gastrointestinal disorders.*

**Faradil Novo** *Sidus, Arg.*
Bromazepam (p.671·3); domperidone (p.1263·2); simeticone (p.1289·2).
*Gastrointestinal disorders.*

**Farakil** *Chew, Thai.*
Prednisolone (p.1108·1); neomycin (p.235·1).
*Infected skin disorders.*

**Faraxen** *Randall, Mex.†.*
Naproxen (p.65·1).

**Farbee with Vitamin C** *Major, USA.*
Vitamin B substances with vitamin C (p.1417·1).

**Farbovil** *Pharmaten (Φαρματεν), Gr.*
Ketoprofen (p.51·2).
*Inflammation; musculoskeletal and joint disorders; pain.*

**Farcef** *Faran, Gr.*
Ceftriaxone sodium (p.182·3).
*Bacterial infections.*

**Farcolan** *Farcoral, Mex.*
Dicycloverine hydrochloride (p.481·2); aluminium hydroxide (p.1249·2); magnesium hydroxide (p.1272·2); dimeticone (p.1289·2).
*Dyspepsia; flatulence; gastritis; meteorism; peptic ulcer.*

**Farco-Oxicyanid-Tupfer** *Farco, Ger.†.*
Mercuric oxycyanide (p.1713·3).
*Disinfection of skin and mucous membranes.*

**Farco-Tril** *Farco, Ger.*
Oxytetracycline calcium (p.241·1); polymyxin B sulfate (p.245·1); hydrocortisone (p.1103·3).
*Genito-urinary-tract disorders.*

**Farco-Uromycin** *Farco, Ger.*
Neomycin sulfate (p.235·1); lidocaine hydrochloride (p.1377·3).
*Urinary-tract infections.*

**Farcyclin** *Faran, Gr.*
Amikacin sulfate (p.154·1).
*Bacterial infections.*

**Fardixon** *Farcoral, Mex.*
Nalidixic acid (p.234·1).
*Urinary-tract infections.*

**Fardolpin** *Farcoral, Mex.*
Dipyrone (p.35·3).
*Fever; pain.*

**Farecef** *Lafare, Ital.*
Cefoperazone sodium (p.174·3).
Lidocaine hydrochloride (p.1377·3) is included in this preparation to alleviate the pain of injection.
*Gram-negative bacterial infections.*

**Farecillin** *Lafare, Ital.*
Piperacillin sodium (p.243·1).
Lidocaine hydrochloride (p.1377·3) is included in some injections to alleviate the pain of injection.
*Bacterial infections.*

**Fareclox** *Lafare, Ital.*
Flucloxacillin sodium (p.213·3).
*Bacterial infections.*

**Faremicin** *Lafare, Ital.*
Fosfomycin calcium (p.214·2).
*Bacterial infections.*

**Faremid** *Lafare, Ital.*
Pipemidic acid (p.243·1).
*Bacterial infections.*

**Fareston**
*Essex, Arg.; Schering-Plough, Austral.; Orion, Austria; Baxter, Belg.; Schering-Plough, Braz.†; Ercopharm, Denm.†; Orion, Fin.; Orion, Fr.; Baxter, Ger.; Orion, Gr.; Orion, Irl.; Schering-Plough, Ital.; Schering-Plough, Mex.; Asta Medica, Neth.†; Schering-Plough, NZ; Schering-Plough, Port.; Schering-Plough, S.Afr.†; Schering-Plough, Spain; Orion, Swed.; Orion, Switz.; Schering-Plough, Thai.; Orion, UK; Schering-Plough, USA.*
Toremifene citrate (p.589·2).
*Breast cancer.*

**Faretrizin** *Lafare, Ital.*
Propylene glycol cefatrizine (p.170·3).
*Bacterial infections.*

**Fargan** *Carlo Erba OTC, Ital.*
Promethazine (p.439·1).
*Skin irritation.*

**Farganesse** *Pharmacia Upjohn, Ital.*
Promethazine hydrochloride (p.439·1).
*Hypersensitivity reactions; premedication.*

**Fargestium** *Cazi, Braz.†.*
Rhubarb (p.1287·3); aniseed (p.1655·2); melissa (p.1711·1); clove (p.1673·2); quassia (p.1737·2); pichurim; gentian (p.1692·2); nux vomica (p.1722·3).
*Digestive-system disorders.*

**Farial** *Riemser, Ger.*
Indanazoline hydrochloride (p.1122·3).
*Colds.*

**Farin Gola** *Montefarmaco, Ital.*
Cetylpyridinium chloride (p.1173·1).
*Mouth and throat disinfection.*

**Faringesic** *Diafarm, Spain.*
Chlorhexidine hydrochloride (p.1173·3); benzocaine (p.1370·3).
*Mouth and throat disorders.*

**Faringina** *SIT, Ital.*
Dequalinium chloride (p.1178·1).
*Mouth disinfection.*

**Faringotricina** *SIT, Ital.*
Tyrothricin (p.275·1).
*Stomatitis.*

**Farizym** *Infar, India.*
Lipase; protease; amylase (p.1654·2); cellulase (p.1669·1); bile extract (p.1660·3).
*Fermentative dyspepsia; pancreatic deficiency; phytobezoar.*

**Farlac** *Farmasa, Braz.*
Lactulose (p.1269·1).
*Constipation; hepatic encephalopathy.*

**Farlin** *Continentales, Mex.†.*
Dipyrone (p.35·3).

**Farludiol** Pharmacia, Arg.
Estradiol valerate (p.1550·2); medroxyprogesterone acetate (p.1557·2).
*Menopausal disorders; osteoporosis.*

**Farludiol Ciclo** Pharmacia, Arg.
16 Tablets, estradiol valerate (p.1550·2); 12 tablets, estradiol valerate; medroxyprogesterone acetate (p.1557·2).
*Menopausal disorders; osteoporosis.*

**Farlupost** Pharmacia, Chile.
Estradiol valerate (p.1550·2); medroxyprogesterone acetate (p.1557·2).

**Farlutal**
Pharmacia, Austria; Pharmacia, Belg.; Pharmacia, Braz.; Pharmacia, Chile; Pharmacia, Fin.; Pharmacia, Fr.; Pharmacia, Ger.; Pharmacia-Upjohn, Gr.; IFET (ΙΦΕΤ), Gr.; Pharmacia, Hong Kong; Carlo Erba OTC, Ital.; Pharmacia, Malaysia; Pharmacia Upjohn, Mex.; Pharmacia, Neth.; Pharmacia, Norw.; Pharmacia, NZ; Pharmacia Upjohn, S.Afr.†; Pharmacia, Singapore; Kenfarma, Spain; Pharmacia, Swed.; Pharmacia, Switz.; Pharmacia, Thai.; Pharmacia, UK.
Medroxyprogesterone acetate (p.1557·2).
*Cachexia; endometriosis; malignant neoplasms; metrorrhagia; progestogen-only injectable contraceptive; secondary amenorrhoea.*

**Farlutal Estrogeno** Pharmacia, Chile.
11 Tablets, ethinylestradiol (p.1553·2); 10 tablets, ethinylestradiol; medroxyprogesterone acetate (p.1557·2).

**Farlutale** Pharmacia, Arg.
Medroxyprogesterone acetate (p.1557·2).
*Adenosis; malignant neoplasms; mastodynia; menopausal disorders; metrorrhagia; secondary amenorrhoea.*

**Farlutes** Pharmacia, Chile.
18 Tablets, estradiol valerate (p.1550·2); 13 tablets, estradiol valerate; medroxyprogesterone acetate (p.1557·2).

**Farmabroxol** Farmasan, Ger.†.
Ambroxol hydrochloride (p.1114·3).
*Respiratory disorders associated with viscid or excessive mucus.*

**Farmacetamol** Docmed, S.Afr.†.
Paracetamol (p.76·2).
*Fever; pain.*

**Farmacola** Roche Nicholas, Spain†.
Ginseng (p.1693·1); multivitamins and minerals (p.1417·1); caffeine (p.782·1).
*Tonic.*

**Farmacrom** Alcon Cusi, Spain.
Sodium cromoglicate (p.795·3).
*Allergic rhinitis; hay fever.*

**Farmadiuril** Farmacusi, Spain†.
Bumetanide (p.877·2).
*Oedema, hypertension.*

**Farmaflebon** Farmasa, Mex.
Hydroxypolyethoxydodecanol (p.1412·3).
*Oesophageal varices; telangiectasis.*

**Farmagola** Ribex, Ital.
Cetylpyridinium chloride (p.1173·1); dichlorobenzyl alcohol (p.1178·3).
*Mouth and throat irritation; mouth disinfection.*

**Farmagripine** Cinfa, Spain†.
Chlorphenamine maleate (p.427·3); phenylephrine hydrochloride (p.1126·3); paracetamol (p.76·2).
Formerly contained chlorphenamine maleate, phenylpropanolamine hydrochloride, and paracetamol.
*Fever; influenza and cold symptoms; pain.*

**Farmalcohol** Cinfa, Spain.
Alcohol (p.1166·1); cetylpyridinium chloride (p.1173·1).
*Disinfection.*

**Farmalex** Farmaline, Thai.
Cefalexin (p.168·1).
*Bacterial infections.*

**Farmaproina** Reig Jofre, Spain.
Procaine benzylpenicillin (p.246·1).
*Bacterial infections.*

**Farmeban** Farmasa, Mex.
Diiodohydroxyquinoline (p.603·3); dimeticone (p.1289·2).
*Amoebiasis.*

**Farmiblastina** Kenfarma, Spain.
Doxorubicin hydrochloride (p.547·3).
*Malignant neoplasms.*

**Farmicam** Continentales, Mex.†.
Piroxicam (p.84·2).

**Farmicetina**
Rontag, Arg.; Darrow, Braz.
Chloramphenicol (p.185·1).
*Bacterial infections.*

**Farmidal S** Continentales, Mex.†.
Astemizole (p.424·2).

**Farmifeno** Pharmacia, Arg.
Tamoxifen citrate (p.584·1).
*Breast cancer.*

**Farmigras** Bajer, Arg.
Sulfur (p.1158·2); resorcinol (p.1156·3).
*Skin cleanser.*

**Farmin** Farcoral, Mex.†.
Diazepam (p.690·1).

**Farmistin** Pharmacia, Ger.
Vincristine sulfate (p.592·2).
*Malignant neoplasms.*

**Farmitrexat** Pharmacia, Ger.
Methotrexate sodium (p.568·3).
*Malignant neoplasms; psoriasis.*

**Farmiz** Neo-Farmaceutica, Port.
Azithromycin (p.159·1).
*Bacterial infections.*

**Farmorrubicina** Pharmacia, Chile.
Epirubicin hydrochloride (p.550·2).
*Malignant neoplasms.*

**Farmorubicin**
Pharmacia, Arg.; Pharmacia, Austria; Pharmacia, Denm.; Pharmacia, Fin.; Pharmacia, Ger.; Pharmacia-Upjohn, Gr.; Pharmacia, Israel; Pharmacia Upjohn, Mex.; Pharmacia, Norw.; Pharmacia, S.Afr.; Pharmacia, Swed.; Pharmacia, Switz.; Pharmacia, Thai.
Epirubicin hydrochloride (p.550·2).
*Malignant neoplasms.*

**Farmorubicina**
Pharmacia, Braz.; Pharmacia, Ital.; Pharmacia, Port.; Kenfarma, Spain.
Epirubicin hydrochloride (p.550·2).
*Malignant neoplasms.*

**Farmorubicine**
Pharmacia, Belg.; Pharmacia, Fr.; Pharmacia, Neth.
Epirubicin hydrochloride (p.550·2).
*Malignant neoplasms.*

**Farmospasmina** Giuliani, Ital.†.
Papaverine hydrochloride (p.1728·1); belladonna (p.479·1).
*Gastrointestinal spasm.*

**Farmotal** Pharmacia Upjohn, Ital.
Thiopental sodium (p.1309·1).
*General anaesthesia.*

**Farmotex** Liomont, Mex.†.
Famotidine (p.1265·2).
*Peptic ulcers.*

**Farmoxil** Elofar, Braz.
Amoxicillin trihydrate (p.155·3).
*Bacterial infections.*

**Farm-X** Bajer, Arg.
Zinc undecenoate (p.411·1); zinc oxide (p.1163·2); salicylic acid (p.1157·1); sodium propionate (p.408·1); coal tar (Alcoderm) (p.1159·2).
*Burns; fungal skin infections; skin disorders; wounds.*

**Farm-X Duo** Bajer, Arg.
Metronidazole (p.607·2); nystatin (p.406·3).
*Vaginal infections.*

**Farm-X Ginecologico** Bajer, Arg.
Metronidazole (p.607·2); neomycin sulfate (p.235·1).
*Vaginal infections.*

**Farnerate** Kuraray, Jpn.
Prednisolone farnesil (p.1109·1).
*Skin disorders.*

**Farnezone** Taiho, Jpn.
Prednisolone farnesil (p.1109·1).
*Skin disorders.*

**Farnitin** Lafare, Ital.
Levocarnitine (p.1423·3).
*Carnitine deficiency; myocardial ischaemia.*

**Farnitran** Fariberica, Port.
Nitrendipine (p.973·3).
*Hypertension.*

**Farocid** Faromed, Austria.
Aciclovir (p.626·1).
*Herpesvirus infections.*

**Farom** Suntory, Jpn.
Faropenem sodium (p.213·1).
*Bacterial infections.*

**Faros**
Lichtwer, Ger.; Medichemie Bioline, Switz.
Crataegus (p.1677·1).
*Cardiac disorders.*

**Farpectol** Farcoral, Mex.
Kaolin (p.1268·3); pectin (p.1580·3).
*Gastrointestinal disorders.*

**Farpik** Farcoral, Mex.
Paracetamol (p.76·2).
*Fever; pain.*

**Farpresse** Fariberica, Port.
Lisinopril (p.946·3).
*Heart failure; hypertension.*

**Fartoxol** Farcoral, Mex.
Oxolamine citrate (p.1126·1).
*Coughs.*

**Fartricon** Farcoral, Mex.
Metronidazole benzoate (p.607·2).
*Amoebiasis; giardiasis; trichomoniasis.*

**Fartussin** Farmaline, Thai.
Dextromethorphan hydrobromide (p.1117·3); guaifenesin (p.1122·1); terpin hydrate (p.1131·1).
*Coughs.*

**Farvicett** Farmec, Ital.
Chlorhexidine gluconate (p.1173·2); cetrimide (p.1172·1).
*Skin, wound, burn, and mucous membrane disinfection.*

**Farviran** Farmigea, Ital.
Inosine pranobex (p.640·2).
*Viral gynaecological infections.*

**Farxen** Farcoral, Mex.
Naproxen (p.65·1); paracetamol (p.76·2).
*Fever; pain.*

**Fasarax** Prater, Chile.
Hydroxyzine (p.435·1).

**Fasax** BASF, Ger.†.
Piroxicam (p.84·2).
*Gout; musculoskeletal, joint, and soft-tissue disorders.*

**Fase** Schwarz, Ital.†.
Aprotinin (p.742·3).
*Oedema; pancreatic disorders; prevention of post-surgical adhesions; pulmonary embolism; shock.*

**Faselut** ICN, Arg.
Progesterone (p.1566·2).

**Fasidine** Siam Medicare, Thai.
Famotidine (p.1265·2).
*Peptic ulcer; Zollinger-Ellison syndrome.*

**Fasigin** Pfizer, Ital.
Tinidazole (p.617·1).
*Trichomoniasis.*

**Fasigin N** Pfizer, Ital.
Tinidazole (p.617·1); nystatin (p.406·3).
*Vulvovaginal trichomoniasis and candidiasis.*

**Fasigyn**
Pfizer, Arg.; Pfizer, Austral.; Pfizer, Belg.; Pfizer, Braz.; Pfizer, Chile; Pfizer, Gr.; Pfizer, Hong Kong; Pfizer, India; Pfizer, Israel; Pfizer, Malaysia; Pfizer, Mex.; Pfizer, Neth.; Pfizer, Port.; Pfizer, S.Afr.; Pfizer, Singapore; Pfizer, Swed.; Pfizer, Thai.; Pfizer, UK.
Tinidazole (p.617·1).
*Anaerobic bacterial infections; protozoal infections.*

**Fasigyn Nistatina** Pfizer, Arg.
Tinidazole (p.617·1); nystatin (p.406·3).
*Vaginal trichomoniasis and candidiasis.*

**Fasigyn VT** Pfizer, Mex.
Tinidazole (p.617·1); tioconazole (p.409·3).
*Vaginal fungal and bacterial infections.*

**Fasigyne**
Teofarma, Fr.; Pfizer, Switz.
Tinidazole (p.617·1).
*Anaerobic bacterial infections; protozoal infections.*

**Faslodex**
AstraZeneca, UK; AstraZeneca, USA.
Fulvestrant (p.557·3).
*Breast cancer.*

**Fasolan** Cilag, Mex.
Flunarizine hydrochloride (p.434·1).
*Cerebral and peripheral vascular disorders; migraine; vertigo.*

**Faspic**
Zambon, Ital.; Robapharm, Spain†; Inpharzam, Switz.†; Zambon, Thai.; Sermmitr, Thai.
Ibuprofen (p.45·3).
*Fever; gout; musculoskeletal, joint, and peri-articular disorders; pain.*

**Fast Powder** Medochemie, Singapore†.
Bacitracin zinc (p.161·3); neomycin sulfate (p.235·1).
*Bacterial skin infections.*

**Fast-Acting Mylanta** J&J-Merck, USA.
*Oral liquid:* Aluminium hydroxide (p.1249·2); magnesium hydroxide (p.1272·2); simeticone (p.1289·2).
*Flatulence; hyperacidity.*
*Tablets:* Calcium carbonate (p.1254·2); magnesium hydroxide (p.1272·2).
*Hyperacidity.*

**Fastenyl** Sarget, Fr.
Arginine aspartate (p.1421·1); vitamin C (p.1460·2).
*Tonic.*

**Fastfen** Cristalia, Braz.
Sufentanil citrate (p.90·2).
*Pain.*

**Fastin**
SmithKline Beecham, Canad.†; SmithKline Beecham, USA†.
Phentermine hydrochloride (p.1592·2).
*Obesity.*

**Fastium** Biolab Sanus, Braz.†.
Diethylpropion hydrochloride (p.1587·1); diazepam (p.690·1).
*Obesity.*

**Fastjekt**
Allergopharma, Ger.
Adrenaline hydrochloride (p.852·3).
*Anaphylaxis.*
Merck, Ital.
Adrenaline (p.852·2).
*Anaphylactic shock.*

**Fastum**
Menarini, Belg.; Raffo, Chile; Menarini, Hong Kong; Menarini, Irl.; Menarini, Ital.; Menarini, Malaysia; Menarini, Port.; Restan, S.Afr.; Menarini, Singapore; Guidotti, Spain; Menarini, Switz.; Menarini, Thai.
Ketoprofen (p.51·2).
*Gout; inflammation; musculoskeletal, joint, peri-articular, and soft-tissue disorders; pain.*

**Fasturtec**
Sanofi Synthelabo, Austral.; Sanofi Synthelabo, Belg.; Sanofi Synthelabo, Chile; Sanofi Synthelabo, Denm.; Sanofi Synthelabo, Fin.; Sanofi Synthelabo, Fr.; Sanofi Synthelabo, Ger.; Sanofi Synthelabo, Gr.; Sanofi Synthelabo, Hong Kong; Sanofi Synthelabo, Ital.; Sanofi Synthelabo, Norw.; Sanofi Synthelabo, NZ; Sanofi Synthelabo, Port.; Sanofi Synthelabo, Spain; Sanofi Synthelabo, Swed.; Sanofi Synthelabo, Switz.; Sanofi Synthelabo, UK.
Rasburicase (p.418·3).
*Hyperuricaemia.*

**Fasulide** Bunker, Braz.
Nimesulide (p.67·1).

**Fasupond** Eu Rho, Ger.†.
Phenylpropanolamine hydrochloride (p.1127·3).
*Obesity.*

**Fate Low Protein** Fate, UK.
A range of low-protein foods for special diets (p.1417·1).

**Fatec** Fascino, Thai.
Cetirizine hydrochloride (p.427·1).
*Hypersensitivity reactions.*

**Father John's Medicine Plus** Oakhurst, USA.
Phenylephrine hydrochloride (p.1126·3); dextromethorphan hydrobromide (p.1117·3); chlorphenamine maleate (p.427·3); ammonium chloride (p.1115·2); guaifenesin (p.1122·1).
*Coughs.*

**Fatidin** Cipan, Port.
Famotidine (p.1265·2).
*Peptic ulcer; Zollinger-Ellison syndrome.*

**Fatigan Bronquial** Phoenix, Arg.
Salbutamol sulfate (p.791·3); theophylline (p.798·3); ketotifen fumarate (p.788·1).
*Obstructive airways disease.*

**Fatigue** Homeocan, Canad.
Homoeopathic preparation.

**Fatigue L5** Homeocan, Canad.
Homoeopathic preparation.

**Fatol** Lisfarma, Braz.†.
Terizidone (p.266·2).
*Tuberculosis.*

**Fatori 8Y** BPL-Meizler, Braz.
A factor VIII preparation (p.751·1).
*Haemorrhagic disorders.*

**Fatoril** Farmaco, Mex.
Famotidine (p.1265·2).
*Gastro-oesophageal reflux; gastrointestinal hyperacidity; peptic ulcer; Zollinger-Ellison syndrome.*

**Fat-Solv** Cantassium Co., UK†.
Inositol (p.1701·2); choline bitartrate (p.1424·3); methionine (p.1042·1); betaine hydrochloride (p.1660·2); alfalfa (p.1649·1); kelp (p.1742·3); glutamic acid hydrochloride (p.1433·2); vitamin $B_6$ (p.1456·3).

**Faulcris** Faulding, Port.
Vincristine sulfate (p.592·2).

**Faulcurium** Faulding, Port.
Atracurium besilate (p.1399·1).
*Competitive neuromuscular blocker.*

**Fauldetic** Faulding, Port.
Dacarbazine (p.544·2).

**Fauldexato** Faulding, Port.
Methotrexate (p.568·2).

**Fauldoxo** Faulding, Port.
Doxorubicin hydrochloride (p.547·3).

**Faulplatin** Faulding, Port.
Cisplatin (p.538·1).

**Faulviral** Faulding, Port.
Aciclovir (p.626·1).

**Faustan** Temmler, Ger.
Diazepam (p.690·1).
*Anxiety disorders; premedication; skeletal muscle spasm; sleep disorders; status epilepticus.*

**Fave di Fuca** Roche, Ital.
Bladderwrack (p.1742·3); cascara (p.1255·1); frangula (p.1266·3).
*Constipation.*

**Faverin**
Arrow, Austral.; Solvay, Hong Kong; Solvay, Irl.; Solvay, Singapore; Solvay, Thai.; Solvay, UK.
Fluvoxamine maleate (p.298·2).
*Depression; obsessive-compulsive disorder.*

**Favistan**
Biochemie, Austria; Temmler, Ger.
Thiamazole (p.1603·3).
*Hyperthyroidism.*

**Favorex** TAD, Ger.
Sotalol hydrochloride (p.1001·3).
*Arrhythmias.*

**Favoxil** Agis, Israel.
Fluvoxamine maleate (p.298·2).
*Depression; obsessive-compulsive disorder.*

**Fawodin** Wayne, Mex.†.
Famotidine (p.1265·2).

**Faxet** Volta, Chile.
Lidocaine hydrochloride (p.1377·3); methylrosanilinium chloride (p.1186·1).
*Antiseptic.*

**Fazol** Aventis, Fr.
Isoconazole nitrate (p.401·3).
*Fungal skin infections.*

**Fazol G** Aventis, Fr.
Isoconazole nitrate (p.401·3).
*Vaginal candidiasis.*

**Fazolin** Siam Bheasach, Thai.
Cefazolin (p.170·3).
*Bacterial infections.*

**Fazoplex** Inkeysa, Spain.
Cefazolin sodium (p.170·3).
*Bacterial infections.*

**FBC** Ranbaxy, Thai.
Ferrous fumarate (p.1427·3); vitamins; calcium phosphate (p.1417·1).
*Anaemias.*

**FBC Plus** Ranbaxy, Thai.
Ferrous fumarate (p.1427·3); vitamins; calcium phosphate; sodium fluoride (p.1417·1).
*Iron-deficiency anaemia.*

**FBIC** Pond's, Thai.
Ferrous fumarate (p.1427·3); vitamins; calcium phosphate (p.1417·1).
*Anaemia.*

**18F-FDG** BSM, Austria.
Fluorine-18 labelled fludeoxyglucose (p.1523·3).
*Assessment of regional glucose metabolism.*

**FDP** Fisiopharma, Ital.
Trisodium fructose-1,6-diphosphate.
*Hypophosphataemia; ischaemic heart disease.*

**Fe$^{50}$** UCB, USA.
Dried ferrous sulfate (p.1428·3).
*Iron-deficiency anaemia.*

**Fealin** Bros, Gr.
Atenolol (p.865·2).
*Angina; arrythmias; hypertension.*

**Febichol** Medphano, Ger.
Fenipentol (p.1687·2).
*Biliary disorders.*

**Febmil** Milte, Ital.
Dietary fibre supplement with vitamins (p.1417·1).
*Fever; nutritional supplement.*

**Febracyl** Vifor, Switz.†.
Propyphenazone (p.85·3); paracetamol (p.76·2).
*Fever; pain.*

**Febralgin** Boehringer de Angeli, Braz.†.
Paracetamol (p.76·2).
Formerly contained dipyrone.
*Fever; pain.*

**Febran** Columbia, Mex.
Paracetamol (p.76·2).
*Fever; pain.*

**Febranine** Roche Nicholas, Spain†.
Paracetamol (p.76·2).
*Fever; pain.*

**Febratic**
Roemmers, Arg.; Rhein, Mex.
Ibuprofen (p.45·3).
*Fever; inflammation; pain.*

**Febrax** Syntex, Mex.
Naproxen sodium (p.65·1); paracetamol (p.76·2).
*Fever; pain.*

**Febrectal**
Note. This name is used for preparations of different composition.
Almirall, Spain.
Paracetamol (p.76·2).
Formerly known as Febrectal Simple.
*Fever; pain.*
Funk, Spain†.
Mucopolysaccharidases; paracetamol (p.76·2); oleum pini sylvestris.
*Fever; pain.*

**Febrectol** Irex, Fr.
*Suppositories:* Paracetamol (p.76·2); pine needle oil. Paediatric and infant suppositories formerly contained paracetamol, pine needle oil, and phenobarbital.
*Tablets:* Paracetamol (p.76·2).
*Fever; pain.*

**Febricol**
Note. This name is used for preparations of different composition.
Xepo-Soul Pattinson, Hong Kong.
Paracetamol (p.76·2); phenylpropanolamine hydrochloride (p.1127·3); chlorphenamine maleate (p.427·3).
*Catarrh; cold and influenza symptoms.*
Xepa-Soul Pattinson, Singapore.
Paracetamol (p.76·2); pseudoephedrine hydrochloride (p.1129·2); chlorphenamine maleate (p.427·3).
Formerly contained chlorphenamine maleate, paracetamol, and phenylpropanolamine hydrochloride (.
*Cold symptoms.*

**Febridol** Genpharm, Austral.
Paracetamol (p.76·2).
*Fever; pain.*

**Febrigrip** Monserrat, Arg.
Paracetamol (p.76·2); butetamate citrate (p.1116·2); pseudoephedrine (p.1129·2); chlorphenamine maleate (p.427·3).
*Allergic rhinitis; cold and influenza symptoms.*

**Febrim** Rimsa, Mex.†.
Paracetamol (p.76·2).
*Fever; pain.*

**Febrimicina** Lazar, Arg.
Tetracycline (p.266·2); dipyrone (p.35·3).
*Bacterial infections.*

**Febrinal** Singer, Switz.†.
Paracetamol (p.76·2); dextromethorphan hydrobromide (p.1117·3); phenylephrine hydrochloride (p.1126·3).
*Cold and influenza symptoms.*

**Febro-cyl Ho-Len-Complex** Liebermann, Ger.
Homoeopathic preparation.

**Febronyl** Rhone-Poulenc Rorer, Mex.†.
Paracetamol (p.76·2).
*Fever; pain.*

**Febs** Boots, Singapore.
Paracetamol (p.76·2); ascorbic acid (p.1460·2); caffeine (p.782·1); phenylephrine hydrochloride (p.1126·3).
*Cold and influenza symptoms; fever; pain; sinus congestion.*

**Febupen** EMS, Braz.
Oxyphenbutazone (p.76·1); paracetamol (p.76·2).
*Fever; inflammation; pain.*

**Fecinole** Dosa, Arg.
Letrozole (p.565·1).

**Fecol** Nakornpatana, Thai.
*Syrup:* Paracetamol (p.76·2); salicylamide (p.87·3); chlorphenamine maleate (p.427·3); phenylephrine hydrochloride (p.1126·3).
*Tablets:* Paracetamol (p.76·2); chlorphenamine maleate (p.427·3); phenylephrine hydrochloride (p.1126·3).
*Cold symptoms; nasal congestion.*

**Fecontin-F** Modi-Mundipharma, India.
Ferrous glycine sulfate (p.1428·2); folic acid (p.1429·1).
*Iron and folic acid deficiency in pregnancy.*

**Fecontin-Z** Modi-Mundipharma, India.
Ferrous glycine sulfate (p.1428·2); zinc sulfate (p.1469·3); folic acid (p.1429·1).
*Iron, zinc, and folic acid deficiency in pregnancy.*

**Fectri** Parggon, Mex.
Co-trimoxazole (p.199·3).
*Bacterial infections.*

**Fectrim** DDSA Pharmaceuticals, UK.
Co-trimoxazole (p.199·3).
*Bacterial infections; Pneumocystis carinii pneumonia.*

**Fedac**
DHA, Hong Kong; DHA, Malaysia; DHA, Singapore.
Pseudoephedrine hydrochloride (p.1129·2); triprolidine hydrochloride (p.442·3).
*Allergic rhinitis; cold symptoms; sinusitis; upper respiratory-tract congestion.*

**Fedac Compound**
DHA, Hong Kong; DHA, Singapore.
Codeine phosphate (p.27·1); pseudoephedrine hydrochloride (p.1129·2); triprolidine hydrochloride (p.442·3).
*Coughs; nasal congestion.*

**Fedip** Gebro, Austria.
Nifedipine (p.966·2).
*Angina pectoris; hypertension; Raynaud's syndrome.*

**Fedolen** Viofar, Gr.
Calcium folinate (p.1431·1).
*Antidote to folic acid antagonists; megaloblastic anaemia.*

**Fedra** Schering, Ital.
Gestodene (p.1556·1); ethinylestradiol (p.1553·2).
*Combined oral contraceptive.*

**Feel Naturale** L'Oreal, Canad.
*SPF 15:* Octinoxate (p.1154·3).
*Sunscreen.*

**Feel Perfecte** L'Oreal, Canad.†.
*SPF 15:* Octinoxate (p.1154·3).
*Sunscreen.*

**Feen-A-Mint**
Note. This name is used for preparations of different composition.
Interbelle, Arg.
Sodium picosulfate (p.1289·3).
*Constipation.*
Schering-Plough, Canad.; Schering-Plough, USA.
Bisacodyl (p.1251·3).
Formerly contained phenolphthalein.
*Constipation.*

**Fefol**
Key, Arg.; Pfizer Consumer, Austral.; GlaxoSmithKline, India; Medeva, Irl.; SmithKline Beecham, S.Afr.; ICN, Singapore†; Intropharm, UK.
Ferrous sulfate (p.1428·3); folic acid (p.1429·1).
*Iron and folic acid deficiency in pregnancy.*

**Fefol-Z** GlaxoSmithKline, India.
Dried ferrous sulfate (p.1428·3); zinc sulfate (p.1469·3); folic acid (p.1429·1).
*Iron and folic acid deficiency in pregnancy and lactation.*

**FegaCoren** Vitorgan, Ger.
Protein extracts from hepar, pancreas, thymus, lien, cor, ren, aorta, gland. suprarenal., mucosa intest., amnion, testes, gland. thyreoidea, diencephalon.
*Cardiovascular and liver disorders.*

**FegaCoren N** Vitorgan, Ger.
Protein extracts from hepar, pancreas, thymus, lien, cor, ren, aorta, gland. suprarenal., mucosa intest., amnion, testes, gland. thyreoidea, diencephalon; metenolone acetate; prednisolone acetate; liothyronine hydrochloride; deslanoside; alpha-tocoferil acetate; cyanocobalamin; pyridoxine hydrochloride.
*Cardiovascular and liver disorders.*

**Fegatex** Vifor, Switz.†.
Vegetable extracts.
*Digestive disorders.*

**Fegenor** Leurquin, Fr.
Fenofibrate (p.915·2).
*Hyperlipidaemias.*

**Fegran** Dovalle, Braz.
Omeprazole (p.1278·2).
*Peptic ulcer.*

**Feiba**
Baxter, Belg.†; Immuno, Braz.†; Baxter, Canad.; Baxter, Denm.; Baxter, Fin.; Baxter, Fr.; Immuno, Israel; Baxter, Ital.; Baxter, Swed.; Baxter, Switz.; Baxter BioScience, UK; Immuno, USA.
A factor VIII inhibitor bypassing fraction (p.752·2).
*Haemorrhagic disorders.*

**Feiba S-TIM 4**
Immuno, Austria; Baxter, Ger.
A factor VIII inhibitor bypassing fraction (p.752·2).
*Haemorrhagic disorders.*

**Feiba TIM 4**
Baxter Immuno, Arg.; Immuno, Hong Kong; Adcock Ingram Critical Care, S.Afr.; Baxter, Spain.
A factor VIII inhibitor bypassing fraction (p.752·2).
*Haemorrhagic disorders.*

**Felaxen** Labomed, Chile.
Aloin (p.1248·3); belladonna (p.479·1); phenolphthalein (p.1284·1).
*Constipation.*

**Felbamyl** Key, Arg.
Felbamate (p.361·1).
*Epilepsy.*

**Felbatol** Wallace, USA.
Felbamate (p.361·1).
*Epilepsy.*

**Felcam** Asian Pharm, Thai.
Piroxicam (p.84·2).
*Gout; musculoskeletal and joint disorders.*

**Feldegel** Pfizer Lambert, Spain.
Piroxicam (p.84·2).
*Musculoskeletal, joint, peri-articular, and soft-tissue disorders.*

**Felden**
Pfizer, Austria; Pfizer, Denm.; Pfizer, Fin.; Mack, Illert., Ger.; Pfizer, Ger.; Pfizer, Norw.; Pfizer, Swed.; Pfizer, Switz.
Piroxicam (p.84·2).
*Gout; inflammation; musculoskeletal, joint, peri-articular, and soft-tissue disorders; pain.*

**Feldene**
Pfizer, Arg.; Pfizer, Austral.; Roerig, Austral.; Pfizer, Belg.; Pfizer, Braz.; Pfizer, Canad.; Pfizer, Chile; Pfizer, Fr.; Pfizer, Gr.; Pfizer, Hong Kong; Pfizer, Irl.; Pfizer, Israel; Pfizer, Ital.; Pfizer, Malaysia; Pfizer, Mex.; Pfizer, Neth.; Pfizer, NZ†; Pfizer, Port.; Pfizer, S.Afr.; Pfizer, Singapore; Nefox, Spain; Pfizer, Thai.; Pfizer, UK; Pfizer, USA.
Piroxicam (p.84·2).
*Gout; inflammation; musculoskeletal, joint, peri-articular, and soft-tissue disorders; pain.*

**Feldexican** INQ, Braz.†.
Piroxicam (p.84·2).
*Gout; musculoskeletal, joint, peri-articular, and soft-tissue disorders; pain.*

**Feldox** Farmion, Braz.
Piroxicam (p.84·2).
*Gout; musculoskeletal, joint, peri-articular, and soft-tissue disorders; pain.*

**Felexin**
Remedica, Hong Kong; Remedica, Malaysia; Remedica, Singapore; Remedica, Thai.
Cefalexin (p.168·1).
*Bacterial infections.*

**Felfar** Faran, Gr.
Magaldrate (p.1271·3).
*Antacid.*

**Feliberal** Silanes, Mex.
Enalapril maleate (p.909·2).
*Angina pectoris; heart failure; hypertension; myocardial infarction.*

**Felicium**
Stada, Austria; Opus, UK†.
Fluoxetine hydrochloride (p.292·1).
*Bulimia nervosa; depression; obsessive-compulsive disorder.*

**Felidon neu** Sanova, Austria.
Absinthium (p.1645·1); achillea (p.1646·2); taraxacum (p.1751·3).
*Hepatobiliary disorders.*

**Felis**
Hexal, Arg.; Hexal, Austria; Biocur, Ger.; Ecosol, Switz.†.
Hypericum (p.299·1).
*Anxiety; depression; insomnia.*

**Felison** Bayer, Ital.
Flurazepam monohydrochloride (p.700·3).
*Insomnia.*

**Felix** Apotheke Heiligen Josef, Austria.
Hamamelis (p.1696·3); panthenol (p.1727·2); zinc oxide (p.1163·2).
*Haemorrhoids; pruritus ani.*

**Felixene** Quimifar, Spain.
Ciprofloxacin hydrochloride (p.188·2).
*Bacterial infections.*

**Felixsan** Stada, Austria.
Fluvoxamine maleate (p.298·2).
*Depression; obsessive-compulsive disorder.*

**Feller** Makros, Braz.†.
Mebendazole (p.108·2).
*Worm infections.*

**Fellesan**
Recip, Fin.†; Recip, Swed.†.
Cholic acid (p.1660·3); dehydrocholic acid (p.1679·2).
*Biliary-tract disorders.*

**Felnan** EMS, Braz.†.
Piroxicam (p.84·2).
*Gout; musculoskeletal, joint, peri-articular, and soft-tissue disorders; pain.*

**Felo** Pacific, NZ.
Felodipine (p.914·3).
*Angina pectoris; hypertension.*

**Felobits** Duncan, Arg.
Atenolol (p.865·2).
*Hypertension.*

**Felocor** Hexal, Ger.
Felodipine (p.914·3).
*Hypertension.*

**Feloday** Novartis, Ital.
Felodipine (p.914·3).
*Angina pectoris; hypertension.*

**Felodur** Alphapharm, Austral.
Felodipine (p.914·3).
*Hypertension.*

**Felogard** Cipla, India.
Felodipine (p.914·3).
*Hypertension.*

**Felo-Puren** Alpharma-Isis, Ger.
Felodipine (p.914·3).
*Hypertension.*

**Felotens** Genus, UK.
Felodipine (p.914·3).
*Angina pectoris; hypertension.*

**Felrox** Seng, Thai.
Piroxicam (p.84·2).
*Gout; musculoskeletal, joint, peri-articular, and soft-tissue disorders.*

**Felsol** Pasteur, Chile.
Fluconazole (p.398·1).
*Fungal infections.*

**Felsol Neo** Roland, Ger.†.
Phenazone (p.82·3); nikethamide calcium thiocyanate (p.1591·2); ephedrine hydrochloride (p.1120·1).
*Asthma; bronchitis; dyspnoea; emphysema; silicosis.*

**Felxicam** Hovid, Hong Kong.
Piroxicam (p.84·2).
*Gout; musculoskeletal and joint disorders.*

**Fem-1** BDI, USA.
Paracetamol (p.76·2); pamabrom (p.978·2).
*Pain.*

**Fem 7**
Merck, Arg.; Merck, Braz.; Merck, Chile; Merck, Ger.; Merck, Hong Kong; Merck, Mex.; Merck, Neth.; Merck, Singapore.
Estradiol (p.1550·1).
*Menopausal disorders; osteoporosis.*

**Fem 7 Combi**
Merck, Chile; Merck, Ger.; Golaz, Switz.
Phase I patch, estradiol (p.1550·1); phase II patch, estradiol; levonorgestrel (p.1563·2).
*Menopausal disorders; osteoporosis.*

**Fem pH** Pharmics, USA.
Glacial acetic acid (p.1645·2); hydroxyquinoline sulfate (p.1700·1).
*Vaginal disorders.*

**Fem 7 Sequi** Merck, Neth.
Patch I, estradiol (p.1550·1); patch II, estradiol; levonorgestrel (p.1563·2).
*Menopausal disorders.*

**Femalon** Silesia, Chile.
Estradiol (p.1550·1).
*Menopausal disorders; osteoporosis.*

**Femanest**
Durascan, Denm.; AstraZeneca, Swed.
Estradiol (p.1550·1).
*Menopausal disorders; osteoporosis.*

**Femanor**
Durascan, Denm.; AstraZeneca, Swed.
Estradiol (p.1550·1); norethisterone acetate (p.1562·2).
*Menopausal disorders; osteoporosis.*

**Femapak** Solvay, UK.
*Combination pack:* Patches, estradiol (p.1550·1) (Fematrix); tablets, dydrogesterone (p.1549·2) (Duphaston).
*Menopausal disorders; osteoporosis.*

**Femapirin** Chefaro, Neth.†.
Ibuprofen (p.45·3).
*Dysmenorrhoea.*

**Femaplus spezial Dr Hagedorn** Naturarzneimittel, Ger.
Homoeopathic preparation.

**Femaprin** Chefaro, Spain†.
Ibuprofen (p.45·3).
*Fever; musculoskeletal, joint, and peri-articular disorders; pain.*

**Femar**
Novartis, Denm.; Novartis, Fin.; Novartis, Norw.; Novartis, Swed.
Letrozole (p.565·1).
*Breast cancer.*

**Femara**
Novartis, Arg.; Novartis, Austral.; Novartis, Austria; Novartis, Belg.; Novartis, Braz.; Novartis, Canad.; Novartis, Chile; Novartis, Fr.; Novartis, Ger.; Novartis, Gr.; Novartis, Hong Kong; Novartis, Irl.; Novartis, Israel; Novartis, Ital.; Novartis, Malaysia; Novartis, Mex.; Novartis, Neth.; Novartis, NZ; Novartis, Port.; Novartis, S.Afr.; Novartis, Singapore†; Novartis, Spain; Novartis, Switz.; Novartis, Thai.; Novartis, UK; Novartis, USA.
Letrozole (p.565·1).
*Breast cancer.*

**Femasekvens**
Durascan, Denm.; AstraZeneca, Swed.
16 Tablets, estradiol (p.1550·1); 12 tablets, estradiol; norethisterone acetate (p.1562·2).
*Menopausal disorders; osteoporosis.*

**Femaston** Solvay, Gr.
Estradiol (p.1550·1); dydrogesterone (p.1549·2).
*Hormone replacement therapy.*

**Fematab** Solvay, Irl.
Estradiol (p.1550·1).
*Menopausal disorders.*

**Fematrix**
Solvay, Irl.†; Solvay, UK.
Estradiol (p.1550·1).
*Menopausal disorders; osteoporosis.*

**Femavit** Pharmacia, Ger.
21 Tablets, conjugated oestrogens (p.1543·2); 7 tablets, inert.
*Menopausal disorders; osteoporosis.*

**FemCal** Freeda, USA†.
Calcium carbonate (p.1254·2); colecalciferol (p.1461·3); vitamin B; minerals (p.1417·1).

**Femcet** Russ, USA†.
Paracetamol (p.76·2); caffeine (p.782·1); butalbital (p.673·3).
*Pain.*

**Femease** Robinson, UK.
Self-heating adhesive pad.
*Dysmenorrhoea.*

**Femen** Osotspa, Thai.
Mefenamic acid (p.55·2).
*Pain.*

**Femepen** Nycomed, Norw.†.
Phenoxymethylpenicillin potassium (p.242·1).
*Bacterial infections.*

**Femerital** Asta Medica, Neth.†.
Ambucetamide (p.1653·1); paracetamol (p.76·2); caffeine hydrate (p.782·1).
*Dysmenorrhoea.*

**Femeron** Johnson & Johnson MSD Consumer, UK†.
Miconazole nitrate (p.405·3).
*Vaginal candidiasis.*

**Femex** Roche, Neth.
Naproxen sodium (p.65·1).
*Fever; inflammation; musculoskeletal and joint disorders; pain.*

**Femexin** Elea, Arg.
Levonorgestrel (p.1563·2); ethinylestradiol (p.1553·2).
*Combined oral contraceptive.*

**FemHRT**
Pfizer, Austria; Pfizer, Canad.; Warner Chilcott, USA.
Ethinylestradiol (p.1553·2); norethisterone acetate (p.1562·2).
*Menopausal disorders; osteoporosis.*

**Femiane**
Schering, Arg.; Schering, Braz.
Ethinylestradiol (p.1553·2); gestodene (p.1556·1).
*Combined oral contraceptive.*

**Femibel** Silesia, Chile.
Esterified oestrogens (p.1549·3).
*Menopausal disorders; osteoporosis.*

**Femibion** Merck, Chile.
Vitamin and mineral preparation (p.1417·1).

**Femicin** Democal, Switz.
Cimicifuga (p.1671·3).
Formerly known as Drosana Femicin.
*Menopausal disorders.*

**Femicur N** Schaper & Brummer, Ger.
Agnus castus (p.1649·1).
*Mastalgia; menstrual disorders.*

**Femi-cyl Ho-Len-Complex** Liebermann, Ger.
Homoeopathic preparation.

**Femiderm** Novartis, Chile.
Estradiol (p.1550·1).
*Menopausal disorders; osteoporosis.*

**Femidol** Merck, Spain†.
Ibuprofen (p.45·3).
*Fever; pain.*

**Femigel** Scientific, S.Afr.
Estradiol (p.1550·1).
*Menopausal disorders.*

**Femigoa** Wyeth, Ger.; Lederle, Ger.
Levonorgestrel (p.1563·2); ethinylestradiol (p.1553·2).
*Combined oral contraceptive.*

**Femikliman uno** Biocur, Ger.
Cimicifuga (p.1671·3).
*Menopausal disorders.*

**Femilar** Schering, Fin.
Cyproterone acetate (p.1544·1); estradiol valerate (p.1550·2).
*Biphasic oral contraceptive.*

**Femilla N** Steigerwald, Ger.
Cimicifuga (p.1671·3).
*Dysmenorrhoea.*

**Femina** Ache, Braz.
Desogestrel (p.1547·2); ethinylestradiol (p.1553·2).
*Combined oral contraceptive.*

**Feminalin** Farma Lepori, Spain.
Ibuprofen (p.45·3).
*Fever; pain.*

**Feminax**
Roche Consumer, Irl.; Roche Consumer, UK.
Paracetamol (p.76·2); codeine phosphate (p.27·1); caffeine (p.782·1); hyoscine hydrobromide (p.483·3).
*Dysmenorrhoea.*

**Femin-Do** Grasler, Ger.
Homoeopathic preparation.

**Feminease** Parnell, USA.
Vaginal moisturising and lubricating cream with eriodictyon (p.1121·2).

**Femineo** Ducto, Braz.
Algestone acetophenide (p.1541·3); estradiol enantate (p.1550·1).
*Injectable contraceptive.*

**Feminesse** Anglian, UK.
Sorbic acid; glycerol; liquid paraffin; polycarbophil.
*Vaginal odour.*

**Feminex** Sante Naturelle, Canad.
Multivitamin and mineral preparation (p.1417·1).

**Feminine Herbal Complex** GNLD, Austral.†.
Wild yam root; red sage (p.1741·2); hypericum (p.299·1); vitex agnus castus (p.1649·1); alchemilla vulgaris; angelica sinensis (p.1655·1); skullcap (p.1746·3); ginger (p.1267·1); taraxacum (p.1751·3); liquorice (p.1270·2).
*Menstrual disorders.*

**Feminique** QHP, USA.
Sodium benzoate (p.1169·3); sorbic acid (p.1192·3); lactic acid (p.1704·1); octoxinol 9 (p.1414·1).
*Vaginal disorders.*

The symbol † denotes a preparation no longer actively marketed

Vinegar (p.1645·2).
*Vaginal disorders.*

**Feminique with Iron and Calcium** Stanley, Canad.†.
Multivitamin preparation with calcium and iron (p.1417·1).

**Feminoflex** Medicus, Gr.
Disodium etidronate (p.771·2).
*Osteoporosis; Paget's disease of bone.*

**Feminol** Laboratorios Chile, Chile.
Gestodene (p.1556·1); ethinylestradiol (p.1553·2).
*Combined oral contraceptive; menstrual disorders.*

**Feminon A** Cesra, Ger.
Agnus castus (p.1649·1).
*Mastalgia; menstrual disorders.*

**Feminon C** Cesra, Ger.
Cimicifuga (p.1671·3).
*Menopausal disorders.*

**Feminon N** Cesra, Ger.
Homoeopathic preparation.

**Feminosan** Pasteur, Chile.
Propyphenazone (p.85·3); caffeine (p.782·1).
*Dysmenorrhoea.*

**Feminova** Merck, Belg.
Estradiol (p.1550·1).
*Menopausal disorders; osteoporosis.*

**Feminova Plus** Merck, Belg.
Phase I patch, estradiol (p.1550·1); phase II patch, estradiol; levonorgestrel (p.1563·2).
*Menopausal disorders.*

**Feminova-T** Silesia, Chile.
Esterified oestrogens (p.1549·3); methyltestosterone (p.1559·3).
*Menopausal disorders; osteoporosis.*

**Feminvit** Ativus, Braz.
Multivitamin and mineral preparation (p.1417·1).

**Femipak** Sanova, Austria.
16 Tablets, estradiol (p.1550·1); 12 tablets, estradiol; medroxyprogesterone acetate (p.1557·2).
*Menopausal disorders; osteoporosis.*

**Femiplexe** Lehning, Fr.†.
Copper gluconate (p.1425·3); zinc gluconate (p.1469·2).
*Menopausal disorders; menstrual disorders.*

**Femiplus** Quesada, Arg.
Vitamin E; vitamin $B_6$; vitamin A (p.1417·1).

**Femipres** Schwarz, Ital.
Moexipril hydrochloride (p.961·2).
*Hypertension.*

**Femipres Plus** Schwarz, Ital.
Moexipril hydrochloride (p.961·2); hydrochlorothiazide (p.933·2).
*Hypertension.*

**Femiron** Menley & James, USA.
Ferrous fumarate (p.1427·3).
*Iron-deficiency anaemias.*

**Femiron Multi-Vitamins and Iron** Menley & James, USA.
Multivitamin preparation with iron and folic acid (p.1417·1).

**Femisan** Grossman, Mex.
Ketoconazole (p.403·3); clindamycin phosphate (p.194·2).
*Vaginitis.*

**Femisana** Riemser, Ger.
Agnus castus (p.1649·1); greater celandine (p.1695·3); cimicifuga (p.1671·3); phosphorus.
*Gynaecological disorders.*

**Femisana H** Riemser, Ger.
Homoeopathic preparation.

**Femit** Mitim, Ital.†.
Ferritin (p.1427·2).
*Iron deficiency; iron-deficiency anaemias.*

**Femixol** Omega, Arg.
Fluconazole (p.398·1).
*Fungal infections.*

**Femizol-M** Lake, USA.
Miconazole nitrate (p.405·3).
*Fungal vaginal infections.*

**Femme** Ache, Braz.
Multivitamin and mineral preparation (p.1417·1).

**Fem-Mono**
Generics, Denm.; Scand Pharm, Swed.
Isosorbide mononitrate (p.942·1).
*Angina pectoris.*

**Femnet** Inibsa, Port.
Genistein (p.1692·1); daizein; glicetein.
*Menopausal disorders.*

**Femodeen** Schering, Neth.
Ethinylestradiol (p.1553·2); gestodene (p.1556·1).
*Combined oral contraceptive.*

**Femoden** Schering, Fin.
Ethinylestradiol (p.1553·2); gestodene (p.1556·1).
*Combined oral contraceptive.*

**Femoden ED** Schering, Austral.
21 Tablets, ethinylestradiol (p.1553·2); gestodene (p.1556·1); 7 tablets, inert.
*Combined oral contraceptive.*

**Femodene**
Schering, Belg.; Schering, Irl.; Schering, NZ; Schering, UK.
Ethinylestradiol (p.1553·2); gestodene (p.1556·1).
28-Day packs also contain 7 inert tablets.
*Combined oral contraceptive.*

**Femodene ED** Schering, S.Afr.
21 Tablets, ethinylestradiol (p.1553·2); gestodene (p.1556·1); 7 tablets, inert.
*Combined oral contraceptive.*

**Femodette** Schering, UK.
Ethinylestradiol (p.1553·2); gestodene (p.1556·1).
*Combined oral contraceptive.*

**Femogex** Germiphene, Canad.†.
Estradiol valerate (p.1550·2).
*Oestrogenic.*

**Femoston**
Solvay, Austral.; Solvay, Austria; Solvay, Belg.; Solvay, Fin.; Solvay, Ger.; Solvay, Hong Kong; Solvay, Irl.; Solvay, Ital.; Solvay, Malaysia; Solvay, Neth.; Solvay, Port.; Solvay, Singapore; Solvay, Switz.; Solvay, UK.
14 Tablets, estradiol (p.1550·1); 14 tablets, estradiol; dydrogesterone (p.1549·2).
*Menopausal disorders; osteoporosis.*

**Femoston 1/5** Solvay, Port.
Estradiol (p.1550·1); dydrogesterone (p.1549·2).
*Menopausal disorders; osteoporosis.*

**Femoston Conti**
Solvay, Austria; Solvay, Belg.; Solvay, Fin.; Solvay, Irl.; Solvay, Ital.; Solvay, Switz.; Solvay, UK.
Estradiol (p.1550·1); dydrogesterone (p.1549·2).
*Menopausal disorders; osteoporosis.*

**Femoston mono** Solvay, Ger.
Estradiol (p.1550·1).
*Menopausal disorders; osteoporosis.*

**Femovan** Schering, Ger.
Ethinylestradiol (p.1553·2); gestodene (p.1556·1).
*Combined oral contraceptive.*

**FemPatch** Parke, Davis, USA.
Estradiol (p.1550·1).
*Menopausal disorders; oestrogen deficiency.*

**Femphascyl** Solvay, Austria.
14 Tablets, estradiol (p.1550·1); 14 tablets, estradiol; dydrogesterone (p.1549·2).
*Menopausal disorders; osteoporosis.*

**Femphascyl conti** Solvay, Austria.
Estradiol (p.1550·1); dydrogesterone (p.1549·2).
*Menopausal disorders; osteoporosis.*

**Femplan-MA** Antigen, Irl.†.
Estradiol (p.1550·1); medroxyprogesterone acetate (p.1557·2).
*Menopausal disorders; osteoporosis.*

**Fempress**
Alpharma-Isis, Ger.; Schwarz, Switz.†.
Moexipril hydrochloride (p.961·2).
*Hypertension.*

**Fempress Plus** Alpharma-Isis, Ger.
Moexipril hydrochloride (p.961·2); hydrochlorothiazide (p.933·2).
*Hypertension.*

**Femranette mikro** Wyeth, Ger.
Ethinylestradiol (p.1553·2); levonorgestrel (p.1563·2).
*Combined oral contraceptive.*

**Femring** Galen, USA.
Estradiol acetate (p.1551·1).
*Menopausal disorders.*

**Femsept** Lipha Sante, Fr.
Estradiol (p.1550·1).
*Menopausal disorders.*

**FemseptCombi** Theramex, Mon.
Patch 1, estradiol (p.1550·1); patch 2, estradiol; levonorgestrel (p.1563·2).
*Menopausal disorders.*

**FemSeven**
Merck, Austria; Merck, Denm.†; Merck, Fin.; Bracco, Ital.; Merck, Swed.; Golaz, Switz.; Merck, UK.
Estradiol (p.1550·1).
*Menopausal disorders; osteoporosis.*

**FemSeven Combi** Merck, Austria.
Phase 1 patch, estradiol (p.1550·1); phase 2 patch, estradiol; levonorgestrel (p.1563·2).
*Menopausal disorders.*

**FemSeven Conti** Merck, UK.
Estradiol (p.1550·1); levonorgestrel (p.1563·2).
*Menopausal disorders.*

**FemSeven Sequi** Merck, UK.
Phase 1, estradiol (p.1550·1); phase 2, estradiol; levonorgestrel (p.1563·2).
*Menopausal disorders.*

**FemSieben** Merck, Austria.
Estradiol (p.1550·1).
*Menopausal disorders; osteoporosis.*

**Femstal** Syntex, Mex.†.
Butoconazole nitrate (p.395·2).
*Vulvovaginal candidiasis.*

**Femstat** Bayer Consumer, USA†.
Butoconazole nitrate (p.395·2).
*Vulvovaginal candidiasis.*

**FemTab** Merck, UK.
Estradiol valerate (p.1550·2).
*Menopausal disorders; osteoporosis.*

**FemTab Continuous** Merck, UK.
Estradiol (p.1550·1); norethisterone acetate (p.1562·2).
*Menopausal disorders; osteoporosis.*

**FemTab Sequi** Merck, UK.
16 Tablets, estradiol valerate (p.1550·2); 12 tablets, estradiol valerate; levonorgestrel (p.1563·2).
*Menopausal disorders; osteoporosis.*

**Femtran**
3M, Austral.; 3M, NZ.
Estradiol (p.1550·1).
*Menopausal disorders; osteoporosis.*

**Femulen**
Searle, Israel; Pharmacia, NZ; Pharmacia, UK.
Etynodiol diacetate (p.1554·2).
*Progestogen-only oral contraceptive.*

**Fenac**
Alphapharm, Austral.; LBS, Thai.
Diclofenac diethylamine (p.32·1) or diclofenac sodium (p.32·1).
*Inflammation; musculoskeletal, joint, peri-articular, and soft-tissue disorders.*

**Fenactol** Discovery, UK.
Diclofenac sodium (p.32·1).
*Gout; musculoskeletal, joint, peri-articular, and soft-tissue disorders; pain.*

**Fenadium** Sunward, Malaysia.
Diclofenac sodium (p.32·1).
*Gout; inflammation; musculoskeletal and joint disorders; pain.*

**Fenadol** Proge, Ital.
Diclofenac sodium (p.32·1).
*Inflammation; musculoskeletal and joint disorders; pain.*

**Fenaflan** Teuto, Braz.
Diclofenac potassium (p.32·1) or diclofenac resinate (p.33·1).
*Gout; inflammation; musculoskeletal, joint, and peri-articular disorders; pain.*

**Fenagel** SM, Thai.
Diclofenac diethylamine (p.32·1).
*Musculoskeletal, joint, and peri-articular disorders.*

**Fenalgin** Geminis, Spain†.
Caffeine (p.782·1); paracetamol (p.76·2); propyphenazone (p.85·3).
*Pain.*

**Fenam** Solvay, Ital.†.
Isoxsuprine resinate (polistirex) (p.1702·3).
*Cerebrovascular disorders.*

**Fenamic**
Note. This name is used for preparations of different composition.
Enila, Braz.
Tolfenamic acid (p.94·2).
*Inflammation.*

Siam Bheasach, Thai.
Mefenamic acid (p.55·2).
*Pain.*

**Fenamide** Farmigea, Ital.
Diclofenamide (p.894·1).
*Glaucoma.*

**Fenamin** Aspen, S.Afr.
Mefenamic acid (p.55·2).
*Dysmenorrhoea; musculoskeletal, joint, and soft-tissue disorders.*

**Fenamine** Fawns & McAllan, Austral.
Pheniramine maleate (p.438·3).
*Hypersensitivity reactions; motion sickness; vestibular disorders.*

**Fenamon**
Medochemie, Hong Kong; Medochemie, Malaysia; Medochemie, Singapore†; Medochemie, Thai.
Nifedipine (p.966·2).
*Angina pectoris; heart failure; hypertension; myocardial infarction.*

**Fenantoin** Recip, Swed.
Phenytoin (p.370·2).
*Epilepsy.*

**Fenaplus** Modi-Mundipharma, India.
Diclofenac sodium (p.32·1); paracetamol (p.76·2).
*Inflammation; musculoskeletal and joint disorders; pain.*

**Fenaplus-MR** Modi-Mundipharma, India.
Diclofenac sodium (p.32·1); paracetamol (p.76·2); chlorzoxazone (p.1392·3).
*Painful muscle spasm; premenstrual syndrome.*

**Fenaren**
Mundipharma, Austria; Uniao Quimica, Braz.
Diclofenac diethylamine (p.32·1), diclofenac sodium (p.32·1), or diclofenac resinate (p.33·1).
*Gout; inflammation; musculoskeletal, joint, and peri-articular disorders; pain; renal and biliary colic.*

**Fenarol-S** Sanofi Synthelabo, Chile.
Chlorzoxazone (p.1392·3).
*Musculoskeletal spasm.*

**Fenasil** Sintofarma, Braz.†.
Terfenadine (p.441·1).
*Hypersensitivity reactions.*

**Fenason**
Unison, Hong Kong; Unison, Thai.†.
Terfenadine (p.441·1).
*Hypersensitivity reactions.*

**Fenasten** Sintofarma, Braz.†.
Cinasteride.
*Malignant neoplasms.*

**Fenatrop** Quesada, Arg.
Trimebutine (p.1758·1).

**Fenatrop-A** Quesada, Arg.
Trimebutine (p.1758·1); bromazepam (p.671·3).

**Fenax** Andromaco, Chile.
Fexofenadine hydrochloride (p.433·3).
*Allergic rhinitis.*

**Fenazil** Sella, Ital.
Promethazine hydrochloride (p.439·1).
*Allergic skin reactions.*

**Fenbid** Goldshield, UK.
Ibuprofen (p.45·3).
*Inflammation; pain.*

**Fenburil** De Mayo, Braz.
Diclofenac sodium (p.32·1).
*Gout; inflammation; musculoskeletal, joint, and peri-articular disorders; pain.*

**Fenchelsaft N** Chauvin ankerpharm, Ger.†.
Fennel oil (p.1687·3).
*Catarrh.*

**Fendazol** Lepori, Port.
Ditazole (p.905·3).
*Thromboembolic disorders.*

**Fender** Krugher, Ital.
Diclofenac sodium (p.32·1).
*Inflammation; musculoskeletal and joint disorders; pain.*

**Fendibina** Northia, Arg.
Ranitidine (p.1285·2).
*Peptic ulcer.*

**Fendin** Ranbaxy, S.Afr.†.
Terfenadine (p.441·1).
*Hypersensitivity reactions.*

**Fendiprazol** Northia, Arg.
Omeprazole (p.1278·2).
*Peptic ulcer.*

**Fendyl** Jean-Marie, Hong Kong.
Promethazine hydrochloride (p.439·1); codeine phosphate (p.27·1); ephedrine hydrochloride (p.1120·1).
*Cold symptoms; coughs.*

**Fenemal**
Nycomed, Denm.; Nycomed, Norw.; Recip, Swed.
Phenobarbital (p.367·3).
*Epilepsy; pre-eclampsia; withdrawal syndromes.*

**Fenergan**
Aventis, Arg.; Aventis, Braz.; Vitoria, Port.
Promethazine (p.439·1) or promethazine hydrochloride (p.439·1).
*Adjunct to analgesia and anaesthesia; hypersensitivity reactions; insomnia; nausea and vomiting; sedative.*

**Fenergan Expectorante**
Aventis, Braz.; Aventis, Spain.
Promethazine hydrochloride (p.439·1); sulfogaiacol (p.1131·1); ipecacuanha (p.1122·3).
*Upper-respiratory-tract disorders.*

**Fenergan Topico** Aventis, Spain.
Promethazine (p.439·1).
*Cutaneous hypersensitivity reactions.*

**Fenesin** DJ, USA.
Guaifenesin (p.1122·1).
*Coughs.*

**Fenesin DM** Biovail, USA.
Dextromethorphan hydrobromide (p.1117·3); guaifenesin (p.1122·1).
*Coughs.*

**Fenfedrin**
Xepa-Soul Pattinson, Hong Kong; Xepa-Soul Pattinson, Singapore.
Chlorphenamine maleate (p.427·3); pseudoephedrine hydrochloride (p.1129·2).
*Allergic rhinitis; cold symptoms.*

**Fengam** Pharmasant, Thai.
Tiaprofenic acid (p.93·3).
*Gout; inflammation; musculoskeletal, joint, and soft-tissue disorders; pain.*

**Feniben** Zerboni, Mex.†.
Phenylbutazone (p.83·2).

**Feniclor** Luper, Braz.
Chloramphenicol (p.185·1).
*Bacterial eye infections.*

**Fenicol**
Offenbach, Mex.; Pharmasant, Thai.
Chloramphenicol (p.185·1).
*Bacterial infections.*

**Fenidantal** Teuto, Braz.†.
Phenytoin (p.370·2).
*Epilepsy.*

**Fenidantoin S** Byk Gulden, Mex.
Phenytoin sodium (p.370·2).
*Epilepsy.*

**Fenidex** Allergan, Braz.
Dexamethasone (p.1097·1); chloramphenicol (p.185·1); tetryzoline hydrochloride (p.1131·2).
Formerly contained dexamethasone and chloramphenicol.
*Infected eye disorders.*

**Fenidina** Boniscontro & Gazzone, Ital.
Nifedipine (p.966·2).
*Angina pectoris; hypertension.*

**Fenigramon** Gramon, Arg.
Phenytoin sodium (p.370·2).
*Epilepsy.*

**Feniken** Kener, Mex.†.
Nifedipine (p.966·2).

**Fenil-Livre** Mead Johnson, Port.
Preparation for enteral nutrition (p.1417·1).
*Phenylketonuria.*

**Fenil-V** Vitoria, Port.
Diclofenac sodium (p.32·1).
*Musculoskeletal, joint, and soft-tissue disorders; neuralgia; neuritis.*

**Fenint** Pharmacia, Ger.
Thioctic acid (p.1754·3).
*Diabetic polyneuropathy.*

**Fenipencil** Marcel, Mex.†.
Ampicillin (p.157·1).
*Bacterial infections.*

**Fenisal** Sofar, Ital.†.
Nimesulide (p.67·1).
*Inflammation; musculoskeletal and joint disorders; pain.*

**Fenisec** Hoechst Marion Roussel, Mex.†.
Fenproporex (p.1588·3).

**Fenisol** Reuffer, Mex.†.
Chloramphenicol (p.185·1).
*Bacterial infections.*

**Fenistil**
Note. This name is used for preparations of different composition.
Novartis Consumer, Austria; Novartis Consumer, Belg.; Novartis Consumer, Ger.; Novartis, Gr.; Novartis, Israel; Novartis Consumer, Ital.; Novartis Consumer, Neth.; Novartis, Norw.; Novartis Consumer, Port.; Novartis Consumer, Spain; Novartis Consumer, Switz.; Novartis, Thai.
Dimetindene maleate (p.431·2).
*Hypersensitivity reactions; pruritic skin disorders.*

Novartis Consumer, Ger.
*Cream:* Tripelennamine hydrochloride (p.442·3).
*Pruritic skin disorders.*
*Eye drops:* Sodium cromoglicate (p.795·3).
*Allergic conjunctivitis.*
*Ointment:* Hydrocortisone acetate (p.1103·3).
*Skin disorders.*

**Fenital** Pharmacon, Braz.
Phenytoin (p.370·2) or phenytoin sodium (p.370·2).
*Epilepsy.*

**Fenitenk** Biotenk, Arg.
Phenytoin (p.370·2).
*Epilepsy.*

**Feniton** Teuto, Braz.
Phenytoin (p.370·2).
*Epilepsy.*

**Fenitron** Psicofarma, Mex.
Phenytoin sodium (p.370·2).
*Epilepsy.*

**Fenizolan**
Grunenthal, Austria†; Nourypharma, Ger.
Fenticonazole nitrate (p.397·3).
*Genital candidiasis; vulvovaginal Gram-positive bacterial infections.*

**Fenizzard** Pizzard, Mex.
Chloramphenicol (p.185·1).
*Bacterial eye infections.*

**Fenn** Sriprasit, Thai.
Paracetamol (p.76·2).
*Fever; pain.*

**Fennings Childrens Cooling Powders** Anglian, UK.
Paracetamol (p.76·2).
*Fever; pain.*

**Feno** YSP, Malaysia.
Fenoterol hydrobromide (p.785·2).
*Obstructive airways disease.*

**Fenobeta** Betapharm, Ger.
Fenofibrate (p.915·2).
*Hyperlipidaemias.*

**Fenobrate** Sanofi Synthelabo, Arg.
Fenofibrate (p.915·2).
*Atherosclerosis; hyperlipidaemias.*

**Fenoclof** Pharmanel, Gr.
Diclofenac sodium (p.32·1).
*Dysmenorrhoea; inflammation; musculoskeletal and joint disorders; pain.*

**Fenocris** Cristalia, Braz.
Phenobarbital (p.367·3).
*Anxiety; epilepsy; hyperbilirubinaemia; insomnia; premedication; sedation.*

**Fenocriz** Fustery, Mex.†.
Phenobarbital (p.367·3).

**Fenodid** Pisa, Mex.
Fentanyl citrate (p.40·1).
*General anaesthesia; neuroleptanalgesia.*

**Fenogal**
SMB, Belg.; Genus, UK.
Fenofibrate (p.915·2).
*Hyperlipidaemias.*

**Fenogar** Ibefar, Braz.†.
Agar (p.1576·3); dantron (p.1261·1); phenolphthalein (p.1284·1); liquid paraffin (p.1479·1).
*Constipation.*

**Fenogel** Basi, Port.
Etofenamate (p.38·1).

**Fenoket** Opus, UK†.
Ketoprofen (p.51·2).
*Gout; musculoskeletal, joint, and peri-articular disorders; pain.*

**Fenokomp 39** Knop, Chile.
Phenolphthalein (p.1284·1); citric acid (p.1673·1); nux vomica (p.1722·3); belladonna (p.479·1).
*Constipation.*

**Fenolftaleina Compuesta** Hochstetter, Chile.
Phenolphthalein (p.1284·1); belladonna (p.479·1); nux vomica (p.1722·3).
*Constipation.*

**Fenolip**
Note. This name is used for preparations of different composition.
Hexal, Arg.; Lannacher, Austria.
Fenofibrate (p.915·2).
*Hyperlipidaemias.*

Lepori, Port.
Sodium cromoglicate (p.795·3).
*Allergic rhinitis; conjunctivitis.*

**Fenomel** Clonmel, Irl.†.
Flurbiprofen (p.43·3).
*Musculoskeletal and joint disorders.*

**Fenopron**
Lilly, Hong Kong†; Dista, Irl.†; Aspen, S.Afr.; Typharm, UK.
Fenoprofen calcium (p.39·2).
*Fever; gout; musculoskeletal and joint disorders; pain.*

**Fenoptic** Allergan, Port.
Chloramphenicol (p.185·1).
*Bacterial eye infections.*

**Fenorit** Scharper, Ital.
Propafenone hydrochloride (p.988·3).
*Arrhythmias.*

**Fenospen** Pharmacia, Ital.†.
Phenoxymethylpenicillin (p.242·1).
*Bacterial infections.*

**Fenostad** Stada, Austria.
Fenoterol hydrobromide (p.785·2).
*Obstructive airways disease.*

**Fenotricin** Dinafarma, Braz.†.
Cetylpyridinium chloride (p.1173·1); benzocaine (p.1370·3).
*Mouth and throat disorders.*

**Fenox**
Note. This name is used for preparations of different composition.
Knoll, India; Boots Healthcare, Ital.†; Boots Healthcare, S.Afr.†.
Phenylephrine hydrochloride (p.1126·3); naphazoline nitrate (p.1124·3).
*Nasal congestion; sinusitis.*

Thornton & Ross, UK.
Phenylephrine hydrochloride (p.1126·3).
*Nasal congestion.*

**Fenoxcillin** Novo Nordisk, Denm.†.
Phenoxymethylpenicillin potassium (p.242·1).
*Bacterial infections.*

**Fenoxene** Samarth, India.
Phenoxybenzamine hydrochloride (p.981·2).
*Neuropathic bladder; phaeochromocytoma.*

**Fenoxypen** Novo Nordisk, Switz.†.
Phenoxymethylpenicillin potassium (p.242·1).
*Bacterial infections.*

**Fenozan** Zambon, Braz.
Fenoterol hydrobromide (p.785·2).
*Obstructive airways disease.*

**Fenpaed** Pinewood, UK.
Ibuprofen (p.45·3).
*Fever; pain.*

**Fenpic** Andromaco, Chile.
Ibuprofen (p.45·3).
*Musculoskeletal, joint, and peri-articular disorders; pain.*

**Fensaide** Nicholas Piramal, India.
Diclofenac sodium (p.32·1).
*Gout; inflammation; musculoskeletal and joint disorders; pain.*

**Fensaide-P** Nicholas Piramal, India.
Diclofenac sodium (p.32·1); paracetamol (p.76·2).
*Musculoskeletal and joint disorders; pain.*

**Fensedyl** Microsules Bernabo, Arg.
Oxatomide (p.438·1).
*Hypersensitivity reactions.*

**Fensel** Pharmacia, Spain.
Felodipine (p.914·3).
*Angina pectoris; hypertension.*

**Fenspin** Basi, Port.
Fenspiride hydrochloride (p.786·1).

**Fenspir** Ibirn, Ital.†.
Fenspiride hydrochloride (p.786·1).
*Respiratory-tract disorders.*

**Fensum** Merckle, Ger.
Paracetamol (p.76·2).
*Fever; pain.*

**Fentabbott** Abbott, Braz.
Fentanyl citrate (p.40·1).
*Anaesthesia.*

**Fenta-Hameln** Astrapin, Ger.; Curasan, Ger.; Hameln, Ger.
Fentanyl citrate (p.40·1).
*Analgesia during anaesthesia; general anaesthesia; neuroleptanalgesia; premedication.*

**Fentalim** Angelini, Ital.
Alfentanil hydrochloride (p.12·2).
*General anaesthesia; neuroleptanalgesia.*

**Fentanest**
Note. This name is used for preparations of different composition.
Cristalia, Braz.; Pharmacia Upjohn, Ital.; Janssen, Mex.
Fentanyl citrate (p.40·1).
*Analgesia during anaesthesia; general anaesthesia; neuroleptanalgesia.*

Kern, Spain.
Fentanyl (p.40·1).
*Analgesia during anaesthesia; premedication.*

**Fentatienil** Angelini, Ital.
Sufentanil citrate (p.90·2).
*General anaesthesia; neuroleptanalgesia.*

**Fentax** Richmond, Arg.
Fentanyl citrate (p.40·1).
*Pain.*

**Fentazin**
Goldshield, Irl.†; Forley, UK.
Perphenazine (p.714·2).
*Anxiety; nausea; psychoses; vomiting.*

**Fentiderm** Pharmarecord, Ital.
Fenticonazole nitrate (p.397·3).
*Fungal skin and anogenital infections.*

**Fentigyn** Novartis, Ital.
Fenticonazole nitrate (p.397·3).
*Fungal vulvovaginal infections.*

**Fentizol** Asta Medica, Braz.
Fenticonazole nitrate (p.397·3).
*Fungal infections.*

**Fentos** Sanofi Synthelabo, Chile.
Codeine phosphate (p.27·1); caffeine (p.782·1); chlorphenamine (p.428·1).
*Coughs.*

**Fentrinol** Fresenius Kabi, Austria.
Amidefrine mesilate (p.1115·1).
*Rhinitis.*

**Fentul** Elvetium, Arg.
Ifosfamide (p.561·1).
*Malignant neoplasms.*

**Fenugrene** Richelet, Fr.
Fenugreek (p.1688·1).
*Appetite stimulant.*

**Fenulin** Gerard House, UK†.
Fenugreek (p.1688·1); slippery elm (p.1747·1); hydrastis (p.1698·3).
*Gastrointestinal disorders.*

**Fenuril**
Pharmacia, Fin.; Pharmacia, Swed.
Urea (p.1162·2).
*Dry skin.*

**Fenuril-Hydrokortison** Pharmacia, Swed.
Urea (p.1162·2); hydrocortisone (p.1103·3).
*Eczema.*

**Fenwal ACD** Baxter, Denm.†.
Citric acid monohydrate (p.1673·1); anhydrous glucose (p.1432·2); sodium citrate (p.1223·2).
*Anticoagulant for blood transfusions.*

**Feocyte** Dunhall, USA.
Iron (p.1434·3); liver extracts; folic acid (p.1429·1); vitamin B substances (p.1417·1); copper.
Vitamin C (p.1460·2) is included in this preparation to increase the absorption and availability of iron.
*Iron-deficiency anaemias.*

**Feofol** Vianex (Βιανεξ), Gr.
Ferrous sulfate (p.1428·2); folic acid (p.1417·1).
*Iron and folic acid deficiency in pregnancy.*

**FeoGen** Rising Pharmaceuticals, USA.
Iron (p.1434·3); vitamin $B_{12}$ (p.1458·2); stomach extract.
Vitamin C (p.1460·2) is included in this preparation to increase the absorption and availability of iron.
*Anaemias.*

**FeoGen FA** Rising Pharmaceuticals, USA.
Iron; vitamin $B_{12}$; vitamin C; folic acid (p.1417·1).

**Feosol** SmithKline Beecham Consumer, USA.
Ferrous sulfate (as dried or hydrate) (p.1428·2).
*Iron deficiency; iron-deficiency anaemia.*

**Feospan**
ICN, Hong Kong; Intrapharm, Irl.; ICN, Malaysia; ICN, Singapore; Intropharm, UK.
Dried ferrous sulfate (p.1428·3).
*Iron deficiency; iron-deficiency anaemia.*

**Feostat** Forest Pharmaceuticals, USA.
Ferrous fumarate (p.1427·3).
*Iron-deficiency anaemias.*

**Fepalitan** Madaus, Spain†.
Aescin (p.1648·2).
*Oedema; venous insufficiency.*

**Feparil**
Note. This name is used for preparations of different composition.
Phoenix, Arg.
Aescin (p.1648·2); diethylamine salicylate (p.34·1).
*Soft-tissue injury; venous disorders.*

Madaus, Spain.
*Tablets*†: Aescin (p.1648·2).
*Oedema; peripheral vascular disorders.*
*Topical gel:* Diethylamine salicylate (p.34·1); aescin (p.1648·2); sodium aescin polysulfate (p.1648·2).
*Peripheral vascular disorders.*

**Feprapax** Ashbourne, UK.
Lofepramine hydrochloride (p.305·3).
*Depression.*

**Fepron** Lilly, Ital.†.
Fenoprofen calcium (p.39·2).
*Inflammation; musculoskeletal, joint, and peri-articular disorders.*

**Fer UCB** UCB, Fr.
Ferrous chloride (p.1427·3).
*Iron deficiency; iron-deficiency anaemia.*

**Feraken** Kendrick, Mex.
Moclobemide (p.308·2).
*Depression.*

**Feratab** Upsher-Smith, USA.
Ferrous sulfate (p.1428·2).
*Iron-deficiency anaemias.*

**Fercayl** Pharmacobel, Belg.†.
Iron dextran (p.1436·3).
*Iron-deficiency anaemia.*

**Fercovit** Andromaco, Chile.
Ferrous fumarate; calcium carbonate; magnesium oxide; vitamins (p.1417·1).
*Dietary supplement.*

**Ferdek** Ranbaxy, Thai.
Ferrous fumarate (p.1427·3).
*Iron-deficiency anaemia.*

**Ferdromaco** Andromaco, Arg.
Ferrous succinate (p.1428·2).

Succinic acid is included in this preparation to increase the absorption and availability of iron.
*Anaemias.*

**Ferfolic SV** *Durbin, UK.*
Ferrous gluconate (p.1428·1); folic acid (p.1429·1).
*Iron and folic acid deficiency; neural tube defect prophylaxis.*

**Fer-gen-sol** *Goldline, USA.*
Ferrous sulfate (p.1428·2).
*Iron deficiency anaemia.*

**Fergon**
*Sanofi Synthelabo, Austral.; Sanofi Winthrop, Irl.†; ICN, NZ; Winthrop Consumer, USA.*
Ferrous gluconate (p.1428·1).
*Iron deficiency; iron-deficiency anaemia.*

**Feridex**
*Temis, Arg.; Advanced Magnetics, Israel; Eiken, Jpn; Berlex, USA.*
Ferumoxides (p.1061·3).
*Contrast medium for magnetic resonance imaging of the liver.*

**Ferifer** *Streger, Mex.*
Ferrous sulfate (p.1428·2).
*Iron-deficiency anaemia.*

**Ferig** *CT, Ital.*
Ferrous gluconate (p.1428·1).
Ascorbic acid (p.1460·2) is included in this preparation to increase the absorption and availability of iron.
*Iron-deficiency anaemia.*

**Ferin** *Collins, Mex.*
Vitamin preparation with iron (p.1417·1).

**Fer-In-Sol**
*Bristol-Myers Squibb, Arg.; Mead Johnson, Braz.; Mead Johnson Nutritionals, Canad.; Mead Johnson, Chile; Bristol-Myers Squibb, Gr.; Mead Johnson, Hong Kong†; Bristol-Myers Squibb, Irl.; Mead Johnson, Ital.; Bristol-Myers Squibb, Mex.; Mead Johnson Nutritionals, Thai.; Mead Johnson Nutritionals, USA.*
Ferrous sulfate (p.1428·2).
*Iron deficiency; iron-deficinecy anaemia.*

**Fer-Iron** *Rugby, USA.*
Ferrous sulfate (p.1428·2).
*Iron-deficiency anaemias.*

**Ferlactis** *AGIPS, Ital.*
*Streptococcus lactis.*
*Gastrointestinal disorders.*

**Ferlasin** *Martin, Spain†.*
Multivitamin, mineral, and amino-acid preparation (p.1417·1).
*Tonic.*

**Ferlatum** *Lifepharma, Ital.*
Iron succinyl-protein complex (p.1438·1).
*Anaemias; iron deficiency.*

**Ferlea** *Elea, Arg.*
Ferrous sulfate (p.1428·2).
*Iron-deficiency anaemia.*

**Ferli-6** *Continental Pharma, Thai.*
Ferrous fumarate (p.1427·3); folic acid (p.1429·1); pyridoxine hydrochloride (p.1456·3).
*Anaemia; vitamin and iron supplement.*

**Ferlis B12** *Iodo Suma, Braz.†.*
Ferrous citrate (p.1436·1); copper; vitamin B substances (p.1417·1).
*Iron deficiency; iron-deficiency anaemia.*

**Ferlixir** *Aspen, S.Afr.*
Multivitamin and mineral preparation (p.1417·1).

**Ferlixit** *Aventis, Ital.*
Sodium ferric gluconate complex (p.1444·3).
*Anaemias; iron deficiency.*

**Ferlor AF** *Loren, Mex.*
Ferrous fumarate (p.1427·3); folic acid (p.1429·1).
*Folic-acid deficiency; iron deficiency.*

**Fermalac** *Rougier, Canad.†.*
*Lactobacillus acidophilus* (p.1704·2); *Lactobacillus bulgaricus* (p.1704·2); *Streptococcus lactis.*
*Diarrhoea.*

**Fermalac Vaginal** *Rougier, Canad.*
*Lactobacillus acidophilus* (p.1704·2); *Lactobacillus bulgaricus* (p.1704·2); *Streptococcus lactis.*
*Adjunct in treatment of vaginal infections.*

**Fermasian** *Asian Pharm, Thai.*
Ferrous fumarate (p.1427·3).
*Iron-deficiency anaemia.*

**Fermate** *Kenyaku, Thai.*
Ferrous fumarate (p.1427·3).
*Iron-deficiency anaemia.*

**Fermathron**
*Biomet, Austral.; Biomet Merck, UK.*
Sodium hyaluronate (p.1697·3).
*Osteoarthritis of the knee.*

**Fermavisc** *Novartis Ophthalmics, Switz.*
Sodium hyaluronate (p.1697·3) (p.1164·2).
*Contact lens lubricant.*

**Fermentmycin** *Intramed, S.Afr.†.*
Gentamicin sulfate (p.217·1).
*Bacterial infections.*

**Fermento duodenal**
*Note. This name is used for preparations of different composition.*
*Hommel, Ger.*
Pancreatin (p.1725·3).
Formerly contained pancreatin and dimethicone.
*Digestive enzyme deficiency disorders.*

*Schwarz, Switz.*
Pancreatin (p.1725·3); dimethicone (p.1289·2).
*Digestive disorders.*

**Fermentol** *Carter Horner, Canad.*
Pepsin (p.1729·3).
*Dyspepsia without hyperacidity; oral vehicle.*

**Fermenturto-Lio** *Teknofarma, Ital.*
*Lactobacillus bulgaricus* (p.1704·2); *Lactobacillus casei.*
*Gastrointestinal disorders.*

**Fermetone Composto** *Lepori, Port.*
Bile extract (p.1660·3); dimethicone (p.1289·2); hemicellulose (p.1578·3); pancreatin (p.1725·3).
*Digestive disorders.*

**Fernadin** *Liferpal, Mex.*
Ferrous fumarate (p.1427·3).
*Anaemias.*

**Fernore** *Knoll, Belg.†.*
Ferrous gluconate (p.1428·1).
*Iron-deficiency anaemia.*

**Ferodan** *Odan, Canad.*
Ferrous sulfate (p.1428·2).
*Anaemias.*

**Fero-Folic**
*Abbott, S.Afr.; Abbott, Switz.; Abbott, USA.*
Ferrous sulfate (p.1428·2); folic acid (p.1429·1).
Ascorbic acid (p.1460·2) or sodium ascorbate (p.1460·2) is included in this preparation to increase the absorption and availability of iron.
*Folic acid deficiency; iron deficiency.*

**Fero-folic-500** *Abbott, Gr.*
Ferrous sulfate (p.1428·2); folic acid (p.1417·1).
*Iron and folic acid deficiency in pregnancy.*

**Feroglobin**
*Vitabiotics, Hong Kong.*
Iron, vitamin B, and mineral preparation (p.1417·1).
*Anaemias.*

*Vitabiotics, UK.*
*Capsules:* Vitamin B substances; folic acid; iron; copper; zinc (p.1417·1).
*Oral liquid:* Vitamin B substances; vitamin C; minerals; honey; malt; lysine (p.1417·1).

**Fero-Grad**
*Abbott, Belg.; Abbott, Canad.; Abbott, S.Afr.; Abbott, USA.*
Ferrous sulfate (p.1428·2).
Ascorbic acid (p.1460·2) or sodium ascorbate (p.1460·2) is included in this preparation to increase the absorption and availability of iron.
*Iron deficiency; iron-deficiency anaemia.*

**Fero-Grad vitamine C** *Abbott, Fr.*
Ferrous sulfate (p.1428·2).
Ascorbic acid (p.1460·2) is included in this preparation to increase the absorption and availability of iron.
*Iron deficiency; iron-deficiency anaemia.*

**Fero-Gradumet**
*Abbott, Belg.; Abbott, Neth.; Abbott, Spain.*
Ferrous sulfate (p.1428·2).
*Iron deficiency; iron-deficiency anaemia.*

**Feromiel** *Herbaxt, Fr.*
Honey (p.1434·2); iron pidolate.
*Nutritional supplement.*

**Feron** *Toray, Jpn.*
Interferon beta (p.645·3).
*Hepatitis; malignant neoplasms.*

**Ferona** *Sidus, Arg.*
Fluoxymesterone (p.1555·3); yohimbine hydrochloride (p.1766·2); caffeine (p.782·1); lysine hydrochloride; vitamins; minerals.
*Male impotence.*

**Ferosof** *Banner, Hong Kong†.*
Ferrous fumarate (p.1427·3).
Docusate sodium (p.1262·2) is included in this preparation to reduce the constipating effects of iron.
*Iron-deficiency anaemia.*

**Ferotrinsic** *Rugby, USA.*
Ferrous fumarate (p.1427·3); folic acid (p.1429·1); intrinsic factor; vitamin $B_{12}$ substances (p.1458·2).
Vitamin C (p.1460·2) is included in this preparation to increase the absorption and availability of iron.
*Anaemias.*

**Ferplex**
*Bago, Arg.; Italfarmaco, Ital.; Italfarmaco, Spain.*
Iron succinyl-protein complex (p.1438·1).
*Iron-deficiency anaemia.*

**Ferplus-B** *Chew, Thai.*
Ferrous fumarate (p.1427·3); vitamins; minerals (p.1417·1).
*Iron-deficiency anaemia; vitamin deficiency.*

**Ferquifa $B_{12}$** *Merck, Port.*
Ferrous citrate; copper sulfate; liver extract; folic acid; cyanocobalamin (p.1417·1).
*Anaemias.*

**Ferradol** *Parke, Davis, India.*
Ferric ammonium citrate (p.1427·2); vitamins (p.1417·1).
*Tonic.*

**Ferralet Plus** *Mission Pharmacal, USA.*
Ferrous gluconate (p.1428·1); folic acid (p.1429·1); vitamin $B_{12}$ substances (p.1458·2).
Vitamin C (p.1460·2) is included in this preparation to increase the absorption and availability of iron.
*Iron-deficiency anaemias.*

**Ferranem** *Chemopharma, Chile.*
Ferrous sulfate (p.1428·2); cyanocobalamin (p.1458·2); folic acid (p.1429·1).
Ascorbic acid (p.1460·2) is included in this preparation to increase the absorption and availability or iron.
*Iron-deficiency anaemia.*

**Ferranim** *Instituto Sanitas, Chile.*
Ferrous fumarate (p.1427·3); vitamin $B_{12}$ (p.1458·2); folic acid (p.1429·1).
Ascorbic acid (p.1460·2) is included in this preparation to increase the absorption and availability or iron.
*Iron deficiency; iron-deficiency anaemia.*

**Ferranin** *Byk, Arg.*
Iron polymaltose (p.1437·3).
*Iron-deficiency anaemia.*

**Ferranin Complex** *Byk, Arg.*
Iron polymaltose (p.1437·3); cyanocobalamin (p.1458·2) or hydroxocobalamin (p.1458·2); folic acid (p.1429·1).
*Anaemias.*

**Ferranina** *Byk Gulden, Mex.*
Iron polymaltose (p.1437·3).
*Iron deficiency; iron-deficiency anaemia.*

**Ferranina Fol** *Byk Gulden, Mex.*
Iron polymaltose (p.1437·3); folic acid (p.1429·1).
*Iron-deficiency anaemias.*

**Ferrascorbin** *Streuli, Switz.*
*Oral drops:* Ferrous chloride (p.1427·3).
Ascorbic acid (p.1460·2) is included in this preparation to increase the absorption and availability of iron.
*Tablets:* Ferrous chloride (p.1427·3); ferrous gluconate (p.1428·1).
Ascorbic acid (p.1460·2) is included in this preparation to increase the absorption and availability of iron.
*Iron deficiency; iron-deficiency anaemia.*

**Ferrematos** *Boniscontro & Gazzone, Ital.†.*
Ferrous gluconate (p.1428·1).
*Iron deficiency; iron-deficiency anaemias.*

**Ferremon** *San Carlo, Ital.*
Iron succinyl-protein complex (p.1438·1).
*Anaemias; iron deficiency.*

**Ferretab**
*Lannacher, Austria; Ridupharm, Switz.†.*
Ferrous fumarate (p.1427·3).
Ascorbic acid (p.1460·2) is included in this preparation to increase the absorption and availability of iron.
*Iron-deficiency anaemia.*

**Ferretab comp** *Lannacher, Austria.*
Ferrous fumarate (p.1427·3); sodium folate (p.1429·3).
*Iron and folic acid deficiency.*

**Ferretab Compuesto** *Biol, Arg.*
Ferrous fumarate (p.1427·3); sodium folate (p.1429·3).
*Iron and folic acid deficiency.*

**Ferretts** *Pharmics, USA.*
Ferrous fumarate (p.1427·3).

**Ferrex** *Breckenridge, USA.*
Polysaccharide-iron complex (p.1443·2).
*Iron-deficiency anaemia.*

**Ferrex Forte** *Breckenridge, USA.*
Polysaccharide-iron complex (p.1443·2); folic acid (p.1429·1); cyanocobalamin (p.1458·2).
*Iron-deficiency anaemia.*

**Ferrex Forte Plus** *Breckenridge, USA.*
Iron (p.1443·2); vitamin $B_{12}$ (p.1458·2); folic acid (p.1429·1).
Vitamin C (p.1460·2) is included in this preparation to increase the absorption and availability of iron.
*Anaemias.*

**Ferrex PC** *Breckenridge, USA.*
Multivitamin and mineral preparation with polysaccharide-iron complex (p.1443·2) (p.1417·1).
*Nutritional supplement.*

**Ferrex Plus** *Breckenridge, USA.*
Iron (p.1443·2).
Vitamin C (p.1460·2) is included in this preparation to increase the absorption and availability of iron.
*Iron deficiency.*

**Ferricure** *Trenker, Belg.*
Polysaccharide-iron complex (p.1443·2).
*Iron-deficiency anaemia.*

**Ferri-Emina** *Lafare, Ital.*
Sodium ferric gluconate complex (p.1444·3).
*Anaemias; iron deficiency.*

**Ferrifol** *Sanico, Belg.†.*
Ferrous succinate (p.1428·2); folic acid (p.1429·1).
*Iron and folic acid deficiencies; megaloblastic anaemia.*

**Ferrifol-3** *CTI, Israel.*
Iron polymaltose (p.1437·3); folic acid (p.1429·1).
*Anaemias.*

**Ferrifol B12** *Sanico, Belg.†.*
Ferric ammonium citrate (p.1427·2); folic acid (p.1429·1); vitamin $B_{12}$ (p.1458·2).
*Anaemias; growth disorders.*

**Ferrigot** *Pasteur, Chile.*
Ferrous sulfate (p.1428·2).
*Iron deficiency; iron-deficiency anaemia.*

**Ferrimed** *Byk Madaus, S.Afr.*
*Capsules:* Iron polymaltose (p.1437·3); folic acid (p.1429·1).
*Injection; syrup:* Iron polymaltose (p.1437·3).
*Iron-deficiency anaemia.*

**Ferrimed DS** *Byk Madaus, S.Afr.*
Iron polymaltose (p.1437·3).
*Iron-deficiency anaemias.*

**Ferrin** *Ativus, Braz.†.*
Ferrous fumarate (p.1427·3) or ferrous gluconate (p.1428·1).
*Iron deficiency; iron-deficiency anaemia.*

**Ferripel-3** *CTI, Israel.*
Iron polymaltose (p.1437·3).
*Iron-deficiency anaemia.*

**Ferriprox**
*Orphan, Austral.; Apotex, Denm.; Chiesi, Fr.; Orphan, Ger.; Apotex, Gr.; Swedish Orphan, Irl.; Chiesi, Ital.; Chiesi, Spain; Swedish Orphan, Swed.; PFC, Switz.; Orphan, UK.*
Deferiprone (p.1033·1).
*Iron overload.*

**Ferriseltz**
*Bracco, Ital.†; Rovi, Spain.*
Ferric ammonium citrate (p.1427·2).
*Contrast medium for magnetic resonance imaging.*

**Ferriseptil** *Gedis, Ital.*
Glutaral (p.1180·3).
*Disinfection.*

**Ferrister** *Gedis, Ital.*
Peracetic acid (p.1187·3).
*Instrument disinfection.*

**Ferritamin** *Abigo, Swed.*
Multivitamin preparation with iron and caffeine (p.1417·1).

**Ferritin Complex** *ABC, Ital.*
Sodium ferric gluconate complex (p.1444·3); calcium folinate (p.1431·1).
*Anaemias.*

**Ferritin Oti** *ABC, Ital.*
Sodium ferric gluconate complex (p.1444·3).
*Anaemias; iron deficiency.*

**Ferrlecit**
*Aventis, Ger.; Aventis, Israel; Schein, USA.*
Sodium ferric gluconate complex (p.1444·3).
*Iron deficiency; iron-deficiency anaemias.*

**Ferrlecit 2** *Aventis, Ger.*
Ferrous succinate (p.1428·2).
*Iron deficiency; iron-deficiency anaemias.*

**Ferro**
*Note. This name is used for preparations of different composition.*
*AstraZeneca, Denm.*
Ferrous sulfate (p.1428·2).
*Iron deficiency.*

*Sam-On, Israel.*
Ferrous gluconate (p.1428·1).
*Iron-deficiency anaemia.*

**Ferro-12** *Wassen, Ital.†.*
Ferrous fumarate (p.1427·3).
Vitamin C (p.1460·2) is included in this preparation to increase the absorption and availability of iron.
*Iron supplement.*

**Ferro 66** *Byk Gulden, Ger.†.*
Ferrous chloride (p.1427·3).
*Iron deficiency; iron-deficiency anaemias.*

**Ferro Complex** *Pharmafar, Ital.*
Ferrous gluconate (p.1428·1).
Ascorbic acid (p.1460·2) is included in some dosage forms to increase the absorption and availability of iron.
Formerly contained sodium feredetate.
*Iron-deficiency anaemia.*

**Ferro Drops L** *Aspen, S.Afr.*
Ferrous lactate (p.1428·2).
*Iron-deficiency anaemias.*

**Ferro F-500 Gradumet** *Abbott, Chile.*
Ferrous sulfate (p.1428·2); folic acid (p.1429·1).
Ascorbic acid (p.1460·2) is included in this preparation to increase the absorption and availability or iron.
*Iron and folate deficiency.*

**Ferro Folic** *Abbott, Arg.*
Ferrous sulfate (p.1428·2); folic acid (p.1429·1).
Ascorbic acid (p.1460·2) is included in this preparation to increase the absorption and availability of iron.
*Iron and folic acid deficiency.*

**Ferro Folico** *Abbott, Mex.*
Ferrous sulfate (p.1428·2); folic acid (p.1429·1).
Ascorbic acid (p.1460·2) is included in this preparation to increase the absorption and availability of iron.
*Iron and folic acid deficiency.*

**Ferro sanol** *Sanol, Ger.*
Ferrous glycine sulfate (p.1428·2).
*Iron deficiency; iron-deficiency anaemias.*

**Ferro sanol comp** *Sanol, Ger.*
Ferrous glycine sulfate (p.1428·2); folic acid (p.1429·1); cyanocobalamin (p.1458·2).
*Iron and vitamin B deficiency; iron-deficiency anaemias.*

**Ferro sanol duodenal** *Sanol, Ger.; Schwarz, Ger.*
Ferrous glycine sulfate (p.1428·2).
*Iron deficiency; iron-deficiency anaemias.*

**Ferro sanol gyn** *Sanol, Ger.; Schwarz, Ger.*
Ferrous glycine sulfate (p.1428·2); folic acid (p.1429·1).
*Iron and folic acid deficiency.*

**Ferro Semar** *Midy, Spain†.*
Ferrous ascorbate (p.1427·3).
*Iron-deficiency anaemia.*

**Ferro Vitaminico** *Laboratorios Chile, Chile.*
Ferrous fumarate (p.1427·3); folic acid (p.1429·1); pyridoxine hydrochloride (p.1456·3).
Ascorbic acid (p.1460·2) is included in this preparation to increase the absorption and availability or iron.
*Iron-deficiency anaemia.*

**Ferro-Agepha** *Agepha, Austria.*
Ferrous gluconate (p.1428·1).
*Iron deficiency anaemia.*

**Ferroben** *Teuto, Braz.*
*Oral solution:* Ferric ammonium citrate (p.1427·2); vitamin B substances; copper sulfate (p.1417·1).
*Tablets†:* Ferrous sulfate (p.1428·2); vitamin B substances (p.1417·1).
*Iron deficiency; iron-deficiency anaemia.*

**Ferro-Be-Sian** *Asian Pharm, Thai.*
Ferrous gluconate (p.1428·1); vitamins (p.1417·1).
*Iron-deficiency anaemia.*

**Ferrobet** *Montavit, Austria.*
Ferrous fumarate (p.1427·3).
*Iron deficiency anaemias.*

**Ferrocal** *Rekah, Israel.*
Calcium ferrous citrate (p.1436·1).
*Iron-deficiency anaemia.*

**Ferrocap F** *Consolidated Chemicals, Irl.*
Ferrous fumarate (p.1427·3); folic acid (p.1429·1).
*Anaemia during pregnancy.*

**Ferro-C-Calcium** *Riemser, Ger.*
Ferrous gluconate (p.1428·1); calcium gluconate (p.1225·2); ascorbic acid (p.1460·2).
*Iron and calcium deficiency.*

**Ferrocebrina** *Bajer, Arg.*
*Capsules:* Ferrous fumarate (p.1427·3); folic acid (p.1429·1); vitamin $B_{12}$ (p.1458·2).
Ascorbic acid (p.1460·2) is included in this preparation to increase the absorption and availability of iron.
*Anaemias.*
*Oral solution; syrup:* Ferrous sulfate (p.1428·2).
*Iron deficiency; iron-deficiency anaemia.*

**Ferrocel** *Medifarma, Mex.†.*
Iron dextran (p.1436·3).

**Ferrochelate** *David, India.*
Ferric ammonium citrate (p.1427·2); vitamin $B_{12}$ (p.1458·2); folic acid (p.1429·1); lysine hydrochloride (p.1439·2).
*Anaemias.*

**Ferrochelate-Z** *David, India.*
Dried ferrous sulfate (p.1428·3); folic acid (p.1429·1); zinc (p.1469·2).
*Anaemias.*

**Ferrocitol** *Delta, Braz.†.*
Iron (p.1434·3); copper; vitamin B substances (p.1417·1).
*Iron deficiency; iron-deficiency anaemia.*

**Ferrocomplex** *Farmalab, Braz.*
Ferrous sulfate (p.1428·2); vitamin B substances; panthenol; liver extract (p.1417·1).
Ascorbic acid (p.1460·2) is included in this preparation to increase the absorption and availability of iron.
Formerly contained ferrous sulfate, aluminium hydroxide, magnesium hydroxide, and thiamine.
*Iron deficiency; iron-deficiency anaemia.*

**Ferrocur** *CIC, Spain.*
Iron succinyl-protein complex (p.1438·1).
*Iron-deficiency anaemia.*

**Ferrocutid** *Labocor, Port.*
Ferrous glycine sulfate (p.1428·2).
*Iron deficiency; iron-deficiency anaemia.*

**Ferrocyte**
*Eisai, Malaysia; Eisai, Singapore; Eisai, Thai.*
Ferrous sodium citrate (p.1436·1).
*Iron-deficiency anaemia.*

**Ferrodix** *Duopharm, Ger.*
Ferrous fumarate (p.1427·3); ferric sodium citrate (p.1436·1); ferrous gluconate (p.1428·1).
*Iron-deficiency anaemia.*

**Ferro-Dok** *Major, USA.*
Ferrous fumarate (p.1427·3).
Docusate sodium (p.1262·2) is included in this preparation to reduce the constipating effects of iron.
*Iron-deficiency anaemias.*

**Ferro-Folgamma** *Worwag, Ger.*
Ferrous sulfate (p.1428·3); folic acid (p.1429·1); cyanocobalamin (p.1458·2).
*Iron and vitamin deficiency.*

**Ferrofolin** *Farmades, Ital.*
Iron succinyl-protein complex (p.1438·1); calcium folinate (p.1431·1).
*Anaemias; folic acid deficiency; iron deficiency.*

**Ferrofolin Simplex** *Farmades, Ital.†.*
Iron succinyl-protein complex (p.1438·1).
*Anaemias; iron deficiency.*

**Ferro-Folsan**
*Desma, Ger.; Solvay, Port.*
Ferrous sulfate (p.1428·2); folic acid (p.1429·1).
*Iron and folic acid deficiency.*

**Ferrofran** *Faria, Braz.†.*
Ferrous sulfate (p.1428·2); aluminium hydroxide (p.1249·2); magnesium hydroxide (p.1272·2); thiamine.
Ascorbic acid (p.1460·2) is included in this preparation to increase the absorption and availability of iron.
*Iron deficiency; iron-deficiency anaemia.*

**Ferrogamma** *Worwag, Ger.*
Ferrous sulfate (p.1428·2).
*Iron deficiency.*

**Ferrogels Forte** *Cypress, USA.*
Ferrous fumarate (p.1427·3); folic acid (p.1429·1); cyanocobalamin (p.1458·2).
Ascorbic acid (p.1460·2) is included in this preparation to increase the absorption and availability of iron.
*Iron and folat deficiency.*

**Ferrograd**
*Abbott, Irl.; Abbott, Ital.; Abbott, UK.*
Ferrous sulfate (p.1428·3).
*Iron deficiency; iron-deficiency anaemia.*

**Ferrograd C**
*Abbott, Austral.; Abbott, Austria; Abbott, Irl.; Abbott, Ital.; Abbott, NZ; Abbott, UK.*
Ferrous sulfate (p.1428·3).
Ascorbic acid (p.1460·2) or sodium ascorbate (p.1460·2) is included in this preparation to increase the absorption and availability of iron.
*Iron-deficiency anaemia.*

**Ferrograd Fol** *Abbott, Austria.*
Ferrous sulfate (p.1428·2); folic acid (p.1429·1).
*Iron and folic acid deficiency.*

**Ferrograd Folic**
*Abbott, Irl.; Abbott, Israel; Abbott, Ital.; Abbott, NZ; Abbott, UK.*
Ferrous sulfate (p.1428·3); folic acid (p.1429·1).
Ascorbic acid (p.1460·2) may be included in this preparation to increase the absorption and availability of iron.
*Iron and folic acid deficiency in pregnancy.*

**Ferrograd Folico** *Abbott, Port.*
Ferrous sulfate (p.1428·2); folic acid (p.1429·1).
*Iron and folic acid deficiency in pregnancy.*

**Ferro-Gradumet**
*Abbott, Austral.; Abbott, Austria; Abbott, Israel; Abbott, NZ; Abbott, Port.; Abbott, Switz.*
Ferrous sulfate (p.1428·2).
*Iron deficiency; iron-deficiency anaemia.*

**Ferrogyn** *SoSe, Ital.*
Ferrous gluconate (p.1428·1).
Ascorbic acid (p.1460·2) is included in this preparation to increase the absorption and availability of iron.
*Iron-deficiency anaemia.*

**Ferroin** *Pisa, Mex.*
Iron dextran (p.1436·3).
*Anaemias.*

**FERROinfant N** *Rubiepharm, Ger.*
Ferrous sulfate (p.1428·2).
*Iron deficiency; iron-deficiency anaemias.*

**FERROinfant Neu** *Rubiepharm, Ger.*
Iron sucrose (p.1438·2).
*Iron deficiency; iron-deficiency anaemias.*

**Ferrokapsul** *Strathmann, Ger.*
Ferrous fumarate (p.1427·3).
*Iron deficiency; iron-deficiency anaemias.*

**Ferrokatabios** *SIT, Ital.*
Multivitamin preparation with iron (p.1417·1).

**Ferroklinge** *Ariston, Braz.*
Ferrous sulfate (p.1428·2).
Succinic acid is included in this preparation to increase the absorption and availability of iron.
*Iron deficiency; iron-deficiency anaemia.*

**Ferrol-Cal** *YSP, Malaysia.*
Ascorbic acid; calcium carbonate; ferrous fumarate; magnesium carbonate; vitamin E (p.1417·1).
*Vitamin and mineral supplement.*

**Ferromalt** *Knop, Chile.*
Ferrous sulfate (p.1428·2).
*Iron deficiency; iron-deficiency anaemia.*

**Ferromas** *Mertens, Arg.*
Ferrous sulfate (p.1428·2).
*Iron deficiency; iron-deficiency anaemia.*

**Ferromax** *Weifa, Norw.*
Ferrous sulfate (p.1428·2).
*Iron deficiency; iron-deficiency anaemia.*

**Ferrometion** *Northia, Arg.*
Ferrous sulfate (p.1428·2).
*Iron deficiency.*

**Ferromex** *Dumex-Alpharma, Singapore†.*
Ferrous sulfate (p.1428·2); copper sulfate (p.1426·1); manganese sulfate (p.1440·1).
*Iron-deficiency anaemia.*

**Ferromia** *Eisai, Jpn.*
Ferrous sodium citrate (p.1436·1).
*Iron-deficiency anaemia.*

**Ferromina** *Provita, Ital.*
Ferrous gluconate; vitamin C; magnesium stearate; folic acid; vitamin $B_{12}$ (p.1417·1).
*Nutritional supplement.*

**Ferromyn** *Astra, Denm.†.*
Ferrous succinate (p.1428·2).
Succinic acid is included in this preparation to increase the absorption and availability of iron.
*Iron deficiency.*

**Ferromyn S** *Hassle, Swed.*
Ferrous succinate (p.1428·2).
*Iron deficiency; iron-deficiency anaemia.*

**Ferronil** *Teuto, Braz.*
Ferrous sulfate (p.1428·2).
*Iron-deficiency anaemia.*

**Ferroplex** *Cimed, Braz.*
Ferrous sulfate (p.1428·2); cyanocobalamin (p.1458·2); folic acid (p.1429·1).
Ascorbic acid (p.1460·2) is included in this preparation to increase the absorption and availability of iron.
*Iron deficiency; iron-deficiency anaemia.*

**Ferroplex-frangula** *ERA, Denm.*
Iron salts (p.1434·3); frangula bark (p.1266·3).
*Iron deficiency.*

**Ferropro** *Progress, Thai.*
Ferrous fumarate (p.1427·3); vitamins; calcium phosphate (p.1417·1).
*Iron-deficiency anaemia.*

**Ferroprotina**
*AF, Mex.†; Faes, Spain.*
Ferritin (p.1427·2).
*Iron-deficiency anaemia.*

**Ferro-Retard** *Nycomed, Norw.†.*
Ferrous sulfate (p.1428·2).
*Iron deficiency; iron-deficiency anaemia.*

**Ferrosanol duodenal** *Schwarz, Switz.*
Ferrous glycine sulfate (p.1428·2).
*Iron deficiency; iron-deficiency anaemia.*

**Ferrosig** *Sigma, Austral.*
Iron polymaltose (p.1437·3).
*Iron-deficiency anaemias.*

**Ferrosprint** *Monsanto, Ital.*
Sodium ferric gluconate complex (p.1444·3).
*Anaemias.*

**Ferrostrane** *Pfizer, Fr.*
Sodium feredetate (p.1444·3).
*Iron deficiency; iron-deficiency anaemia.*

**Ferrotab** *Antigen, Irl.*
Dried ferrous sulfate (p.1428·3); copper sulfate (p.1426·1); manganese sulfate (p.1440·1).
*Iron-deficiency anaemia.*

**Ferrotabs** *Thaipharmed, Thai.*
Ferrous sulfate (p.1428·2).
*Iron-deficiency anaemia.*

**Ferrotemp** *Medix, Mex.*
Ferrous fumarate (p.1427·3); thiamine hydrochloride (p.1455·1).
*Iron-deficiency anaemia.*

**Ferro-Terapina** *Degorts, Mex.*
Ferrous fumarate (p.1427·3).
*Iron-deficiency anaemia.*

**Ferrotonico** *Neo Quimica, Braz.*
Ferrous sulfate (p.1428·2); phosphoric acid; aloes; myrrh; cinnamon; nutmeg.
*Tonic.*

**Ferrotonico B12** *Neo Quimica, Braz.*
*Oral solution:* Ferrous sulfate (p.1428·2); vitamin B substances (p.1417·1).
Sodium ascorbate (p.1460·2) is included in this preparation to increase the absorption and availability of iron.
*Tablets:* Ferrous sulfate (p.1428·2); folic acid (p.1429·1); vitamin B substances (p.1417·1).
Ascorbic acid (p.1460·2) is included in this preparation to increase the absorption and availability of iron.
*Anaemias.*

**Ferrototal** *Sanval, Braz.*
Ferrous sulfate (p.1428·2).

**Ferrotrat** *Medley, Braz.*
Ferrous sulfate (p.1428·2); folic acid (p.1429·1); vitamin $B_{12}$ (p.1458·2).
*Iron deficiency; iron-deficiency anaemia.*

**Ferrotrat B12** *Medley, Braz.*
Ferric ammonium citrate (p.1427·2); vitamin $B_{12}$; liver extract; stomach extract; carnitine hydrochloride; lysine; sodium glycerophosphate; manganese sulfate; copper sulfate (p.1417·1).
*Anaemias.*

**Ferro-Tre** *Mediolanum, Ital.*
Iron acetyltransferrin.
Formerly contained ferritin and folic acid.
*Iron-deficiency anaemias.*

**Ferrotron**
*Note. This name is used for preparations of different composition.*
*Ariston, Braz.*
Ferrous sulfate (p.1428·2).
*Iron-deficiency anaemia.*

*VAAS, Ital.*
Amino-acid preparation with vitamins and minerals (p.1417·1).
*Nutritional supplement.*

**Ferroven** *Geymonat, Ital.†.*
Iron sucrose (p.1438·2).
*Iron-deficiency anaemias.*

**Ferrovin-Chinaeisenwein** *Pharmonta, Austria.*
Ferric ammonium citrate (p.1427·2); manganese hypophosphite; cinchona bark (p.1671·3); bitter orange (p.1723·3).
*Anaemias; iron deficiency; tonic.*

**Ferrovin-Eisenelixier** *Pharmonta, Austria.*
Iron sucrose (p.1438·2); aromatic tincture; bitter orange tincture (p.1723·3).
*Iron deficiency; tonic.*

**Ferrum** *Hausmann, Irl.*
Iron polymaltose (p.1437·3).
*Iron-deficiency anaemia.*

**Ferrum Fol** *Ferraz, Lynce, Port.*
Iron polymaltose (p.1437·3); folic acid (p.1429·1).
*Iron and folic acid deficiency.*

**Ferrum Fol Hausmann** *Nycomed, Gr.*
Iron polymaltose (p.1437·3); folic acid (p.1417·1).
*Iron and folic acid deficiency in pregnancy.*

**Ferrum H**
*Baxter, Austral.; Sigma, NZ.*
Iron polymaltose (p.1437·3).
*Iron-deficiency anaemias.*

**Ferrum Hausmann**
*Richter, Austria; Nycomed, Gr.; Vifor, Hong Kong; Ferraz, Lynce, Port.; Vifor, Singapore.*
Iron polymaltose (p.1437·3).
*Iron deficiency; iron-deficiency anaemia.*

*Bio-Therabel, Belg.†.*
Ferrous fumarate (p.1427·3).
*Iron deficiency.*

*Yamanouchi, Ger.*
Ferrous fumarate (p.1427·3) or iron polymaltose (p.1437·3).
*Iron deficiency; iron-deficiency anaemias.*

*Geymonat, Ital.*
Iron sucrose (p.1438·2).
*Iron-deficiency anaemias.*

*Vifor International, Switz.*
Ferrous fumarate (p.1427·3), iron dextran (p.1436·3), or iron polymaltose (p.1437·3).
*Iron deficiency; iron-deficiency anaemia.*

**Ferrum phosphoricum comp** *Weleda, Ger.*
Homoeopathic preparation.

**Ferrum Verla** *Verla, Ger.*
Ferrous gluconate (p.1428·1).
*Iron deficiency.*

**Ferrum-Quarz** *Weleda, Austria.*
Ferrous sulfate (p.1428·2); quartz.
*Migraine and related vascular headaches; tonic.*

**Ferrumvit** *Viternat, Braz.*
Iron chelate (p.1434·3); folic acid (p.1429·1).
*Anaemias.*

**Fersaday** *Goldshield, UK.*
Ferrous fumarate (p.1427·3).
*Iron deficiency.*

**Fersamal** *Goldshield, UK.*
Ferrous fumarate (p.1427·3).
*Iron deficiency.*

**Fertibion** *Tegur, Mex.†.*
Arginine (p.1421·1).

**Fertilan** *Codal Synto, Hong Kong.*
Clomifene citrate (p.1542·2).
*Anovulatory infertility.*

**Fertility Day** *Blausiegel, Braz.*
Pregnancy test (p.1734·3).

**Fertility Score** *FertiPro, Irl.†.*
Test for male fertility (p.1734·3).

**Fertinex** *Serono, USA.*
Urofollitropin (p.1342·1).
*Female infertility.*

**Fertinic** *Desbergers, Canad.†.*
Ferrous gluconate (p.1428·1).
*Iron-deficiency anaemias.*

**Fertinorm**
*Serono, Canad.; Serono, Ger.†.*
Urofollitropin (p.1342·1).
*Male and female infertility.*

**Fertodur**
*Schering, Braz.†; Schering, Mex.*
Cyclofenil (p.1544·1).
*Anovulatory infertility.*

**Fertomcidina-U** *Theriaca, Ital.*
Magnesium glycerophosphate (p.1228·1); salicylic acid (p.1157·1); sodium iodide (p.1598·1); ammonium bromide (p.1663·1).
*Wound disinfection.*

**Fertomid**
*Cipla, India; Cipla-Medpro, S.Afr.*
Clomifene citrate (p.1542·2).
*Anovulatory infertility.*

**Ferumat** *Continental Pharma, Belg.†.*
Ferrous fumarate (p.1427·3).
*Iron deficiency; iron-deficiency anaemias.*

**Ferval** *Valdecasas, Mex.*
Ferrous fumarate (p.1427·3).
*Iron-deficiency anaemia.*

**Fervex**
*Note. This name is used for preparations of different composition.*
*Hertz, Braz.†.*
Paracetamol (p.76·2).
*Fever; pain.*

*Oberlin, Fr.*
Pheniramine maleate (p.438·3); paracetamol (p.76·2); ascorbic acid (p.1460·2).
*Upper respiratory-tract disorders.*

**Fervex Rhume** *Oberlin, Fr.†.*
Paracetamol (p.76·2); phenylpropanolamine hydrochloride (p.1127·3).
*Cold symptoms.*

**Fervical** *Garant, Ital.*
Calcium carbonate (p.1254·2).
*Calcium deficiency; calcium supplement.*

**Fervit**
*Note. This name is used for preparations of different composition.*
*Bushnell, India.*
Ferrous fumarate (p.1427·3); vitamin $B_{12}$ (p.1458·2); folic acid (p.1429·1); vitamin C (p.1460·2).
*Anaemias.*

*Vitoria, Port.*
Iron succinyl-protein complex (p.1438·1).
*Iron deficiency; iron-deficiency anaemias.*

**Ferxal** *Silanes, Mex.*
Iron succinyl-protein complex (p.1438·1).
*Iron-deficiency anaemia.*

**Ferybar** *Pinewood, Irl.*
Liver extract; vitamin B substances; minerals (p.1417·1).
*Vitamin and mineral supplement.*

**Fesema** *Etex, Chile.*
Salbutamol (p.791·3) or salbutamol sulfate (p.791·3).
*Obstructive airways disease.*

**Fesovit**
*Note. This name is used for preparations of different composition.*
*GlaxoSmithKline, India.*
*Capsules:* Folic acid (p.1429·1); vitamin B substances (p.1417·1); dried ferrous sulfate (p.1428·3).
*Iron-deficiency anaemia; tonic.*
*Elixir:* Vitamin B substances (p.1417·1); dried ferrous sulfate (p.1428·3).
*Nutritional supplement.*

*Evans Medical, Irl.†.*
Dried ferrous sulfate (p.1428·3); vitamin B and C substances (p.1417·1).
*Iron deficiency.*

**Fess** *Paedpharm, Austral.*
Sodium chloride (p.1233·3).
*Nasal congestion; sinusitis.*

**Festal N**
Aventis, India; Hoechst Marion Roussel, Ital.†.
Pancreatin (p.1725·3).
*Digestive system disorders.*

**Fe-Tinic** Ethex, USA.
Polysaccharide-iron complex (p.1443·2).
*Iron-deficiency anaemia.*

**Fe-Tinic Forte** Ethex, USA.
Polysaccharide-iron complex (p.1443·2); folic acid (p.1429·1); vitamin $B_{12}$ (p.1458·2).
*Iron-deficiency anaemia.*

**Feto-Longoral** Artesan, Ger.; Cassella-med, Ger.
Multivitamin and mineral preparation (p.1417·1).

**Fetrin** Lunsco, USA.
Ferrous fumarate (p.1427·3); cyanocobalamin (p.1458·2); intrinsic factor.
Ascorbic acid (p.1460·2) is included in this preparation to increase the absorption and availability of iron.

**Fetrival** Probios, Port.
Iron succinyl-protein complex (p.1438·1).
*Iron deficiency; iron-deficiency anaemia.*

**Feudoftal** Biocumed, Arg.
Ascorbic acid; alpha tocoferil acetate; vitamin A palmitate (p.1417·1).
*Antoxidant preparation.*

**Feuille de Saule** Gilbert, Fr.
Salicylic acid (p.1157·1).
*Callus; corns; verrucas.*

**Fevamol** Garec, S.Afr.
Paracetamol (p.76·2).
*Fever; pain.*

**Fevarin**
Solvay, Denm.; Solvay, Fin.; Solvay, Ger.; Solvay, Ital.; Solvay, Neth.; Solvay, Norw.; Solvay, Swed.
Fluvoxamine maleate (p.298·2).
*Anxiety disorders; depression; obsessive-compulsive disorder.*

**Fever & Inflammation Relief** Brauer, Austral.†.
Homoeopathic preparation.

**Feverall** Alpharma, USA.
Paracetamol (p.76·2).
*Fever; pain.*

**Feverfen** Wise, UK.
Ibuprofen (p.45·3).
*Fever; pain.*

**Fevital Simplex** Prospa, Ital.
Sodium ferric gluconate complex (p.1444·3).
*Iron deficiency; iron-deficiency anaemias.*

**Fexicam** Technilab, Canad.
Piroxicam (p.84·2).
*Fever; inflammation; pain.*

**Fexin** Aspen, S.Afr.
Cefalexin (p.168·1).
*Bacterial infections.*

**Fexiron** Rivero, Arg.
Iron dextran (p.1436·3).
*Iron-deficiency anaemia.*

**Fexofen** Elvetium, Arg.
Fexofenadine hydrochloride (p.433·3).
*Allergic rhinitis.*

**Fezona** Diba, Mex.
Phenylbutazone (p.83·2).
*Musculoskeletal and joint disorders; pain.*

**FGF Tabs** Abbott, Austral.
Dried ferrous sulfate (p.1428·3); folic acid (p.1429·1).
*Iron and folate deficiency; iron-deficiency anaemia; megaloblastic anaemia.*

**Fhbc** Baxter, Ital.
Amino-acid infusion (p.1417·1).
*Parenteral nutrition.*

**Fiacin** Biosarto, Spain.
Indometacin (p.47·3); prednisone (p.1109·3).
*Musculoskeletal, joint, and peri-articular disorders.*

**Fialetta Odontalgica Dr Knapp** Montefarmaco, Ital.
Benzocaine (p.1370·3); chlorobutanol (p.1176·3); clove oil (p.1673·3); colophony (p.1675·1).
*Toothache.*

**Fiamelis** Teclapharm, Ger.
Hamamelis (p.1696·3).
*Skin disorders.*

**Fibalip** Pacific, NZ.
Bezafibrate (p.873·2).
*Hyperlipidaemias.*

**Fiberall** Ciba Consumer, USA.
*Chewable tablets*†: Polycarbophil calcium (p.1284·2).
*Constipation; diarrhoea; stool softener in haemorrhoids.*
*Oral powder; wafers:* Psyllium hydrophilic mucilloid (p.1268·1).
*Constipation; stool softener in haemorrhoids.*

**Fibercon**
Wyeth-Whitehall, Arg.; Wyeth Lederle, Austria; Lederle, Israel; Wyeth, Mex.; Whitehall, Thai.; Lederle, USA.
Polycarbophil calcium (p.1284·2).
*Bowel disorders; constipation.*

**Fiberform**
Solvay, Neth.; Recip, Swed.
Wheat germ.
*Constipation.*

**Fiberform Mix** Recip, Swed.
Wheat germ.
*Constipation.*

**Fibergy** Usana, Hong Kong.
Preparation for enteral nutrition (p.1417·1).

**Fiberlan** Galagen, USA.
Lactose-free, gluten-free preparation for enteral nutrition (p.1417·1).

**Fiber-Lax** Rugby, USA.
Polycarbophil calcium (p.1284·2).
*Constipation; diarrhoea.*

**FiberNorm** G & W, USA.
Polycarbophil calcium (p.1284·2).
*Constipation.*

**Fibersource**
Novartis, Arg.; Novartis Consumer, Austral.; Novartis, Braz.; Novartis Nutrition, Singapore.
Preparation for enteral nutrition with fibre (p.1417·1).

**Fibion** Asta Medica, Switz.
Soya bran (p.1253·2).
*Constipation.*

**Fiblaferon** Biosyn, Ger.
Interferon beta (human) (p.645·3).
*Viral infections.*

**Fibonel** Pharma Investi, Chile.
Famotidine (p.1265·2).
*Gastro-oesophageal reflux; peptic ulcer; Zollinger-Ellison syndrome.*

**Fiboran**
Christiaens, Belg.; Nycomed, Fr.; Amersham, Spain†.
Aprindine hydrochloride (p.864·2).
*Arrhythmias.*

**Fibra Light** Farmalight, Port.
Fibre; arabinogalactan.
Formerly contained fibre and guar gum.
*Dietary fibre supplement.*

**Fibra Line** Investigacion, Mex.
A range of dietary fibre supplements (p.1417·1).
*Gastrointestinal disorders; obesity.*

**Fibrabene** Legrand, Braz.
Dornase alfa (p.1119·1); fibrinolysin (bovine) (p.916·2).
*Wounds.*

**Fibracap** Hebron, Braz.
Dietary fibre preparation (p.1417·1).
*Constipation; fibre supplement.*

**Fibracol** Johnson & Johnson Medical, UK†.
Collagen alginate (p.1674·3).
*Wounds.*

**Fibraflex** Orion, Ger.†.
*Ointment:* Heparin sodium (p.928·1); glycol salicylate (p.44·3); benzyl nicotinate (p.21·2).
*Musculoskeletal, joint, and nerve disorders; sports injuries.*
*Tablets:* Ibuprofen (p.45·3).
*Fever; musculoskeletal, joint, and soft-tissue disorders; pain.*
*Topical gel:* Heparin sodium (p.928·1); glycol salicylate (p.44·3); menthol (p.1711·3).
*Musculoskeletal and joint disorders; sports injuries.*

**Fibraguar** Fardi, Spain.
Guar gum (p.333·2).
*Diabetes mellitus.*

**Fibral** Aliud, Austria.
Aciclovir (p.626·1).
*Herpes labialis.*

**Fibralime** Bio2, Fr.
Dietary fibre supplement (p.1417·1).
*Obesity.*

**Fibramucil** Procter & Gamble, Spain†.
Ispaghula (p.1268·1).
*Constipation.*

**Fibrasan** Errekappa, Ital.
Cellulose (p.1578·3).
*Gastrointestinal disorders.*

**Fibrase**
Note. This name is used for preparations of different composition.
Ache, Braz.; Parke, Davis, Mex.
Fibrinolysin (p.916·2); dornase alfa (p.1119·1); chloramphenicol (p.185·1).
Formerly known as Fibrase com Cloranfenicol in *Braz.*
*Infected burns, ulcers, and wounds; skin infections.*
Teofarma, Ital.
Pentosan polysulfate sodium (p.979·2).
*Peripheral vascular disorders; soft-tissue disorders; thrombosis prophylaxis.*

**Fibrase SA** Parke, Davis, Mex.
Fibrinolysin (bovine) (p.916·2); dornase alfa (p.1119·1).
*Burns; ulcers; wounds.*

**Fibrasol** Maver, Chile.
Psyllium hydrophillic mucilloid (p.1268·1).
*Constipation.*

**Fibrax** Whitehall-Robins, Canad.†.
Grain and citrus fibre.
*Constipation.*

**Fibre Dophilus** Pharmadass, UK.
*Lactobacillus acidophilus* (p.1704·2); Acidophilus bifidus; ispaghula (p.1268·1).
*Fibre supplement; maintenance of gastrointestinal flora.*

**Fibre Plus** Pharmadass, UK.
Ispaghula (p.1268·1); senna (p.1288·2).
*Constipation; fibre supplement.*

**Fibreline** DHN, Fr.
Dietary fibre supplement (p.1417·1).
*Gastrointestinal disorders.*

**Fibrepur** Hoechst Marion Roussel, Canad.†.
Ispaghula (p.1268·1).
*Constipation.*

**Fibresource** Novartis Nutrition, Hong Kong.
Preparation for enteral nutrition (p.1417·1).

**Fibre-Vit** Vitalia, UK†.
Multivitamin, mineral, and fibre preparation (p.1417·1).

**Fibrex Hot Drink** Berlin-Chemie, Ger.
Aspirin (p.15·1); ascorbic acid (p.1460·2).
*Fever; inflammation; pain.*

**Fibrex Tabletten** Berlin-Chemie, Ger.
Aspirin (p.15·1); paracetamol (p.76·2).
*Fever; pain.*

**Fibrexin** Menarini, Singapore.
Paracetamol (p.76·2).
*Fever; pain.*

**Fibrezym** Bene, Ger.
Pentosan polysulfate sodium (p.979·2).
*Thrombosis prophylaxis.*

**Fibrimol** Andromaco, Chile.
Paracetamol (p.76·2).
*Fever; pain.*

**Fibrin Glue** National Blood Centre, Thai.
Thrombin (p.760·1); fibrinogen (p.753·2).
*Haemostatic.*

**Fibrinol** Baldacci, Braz.†.
Fibrin (bovine) (p.753·1).
*Haemorrhage.*

**Fibrinomer** ISI, Ital.†.
Fibrinogen (p.753·2).
*Haemorrhagic disorders; hypofibrinogenaemia.*

**Fibrit** Neo-Farmaceutica, Port.†.
Anistreplase (p.863·3).
*Myocardial infarction.*

**Fibrocid** Lacer, Spain†.
Pentosan polysulfate sodium (p.979·2).
*Hyperlipidaemias; thromboembolic disorders.*

**Fibrocide** Neo-Farmaceutica, Port.
Pentosan polysulfate sodium (p.979·2).
*Hyperlipidaemias; thromboembolic disorders.*

**Fibrocit** CT, Ital.
Gemfibrozil (p.923·1).
*Hyperlipidaemias.*

**Fibrocol** Zambon, Braz.†.
Bran (p.1253·2).
*Constipation; diverticulitis; irritable bowel syndrome; nutritional supplement.*

**Fibroderm** Torlan, Spain†.
Acedoben potassium (p.1645·2).
*Skin disorders.*

**Fibrogammin**
Aventis Behring, Austria; Aventis Behring, Braz.; Aventis Behring, Ger.
A factor XIII preparation (p.753·1).
*Factor XIII deficiency; haemorrhagic disorders.*

**Fibrogammin P**
Aventis Behring, Hong Kong; Aventis, Israel; Aventis Behring, UK.
A factor XIII preparation (p.753·1).
*Factor XIII deficiency; haemorrhagic disorders.*

**Fibrol** Raza, Malaysia; Pharmaniaga, Malaysia.
Gemfibrozil (p.923·1).
*Hyperlipidaemias.*

**Fibrolan**
Pfizer, Austria; Parke, Davis, Ger.; Pfizer, Ger.; Pfizer, Switz.
Fibrinolysin (bovine) (p.916·2); deoxyribonuclease (p.1119·1).
*Wounds.*

**Fibrolax** Giuliani, Ital.
Ispaghula (p.1268·1).
*Constipation.*

**Fibrolax Complex** Giuliani, Ital.
Ispaghula (p.1268·1); senna (p.1288·2).
*Constipation.*

**Fibrolip** Anpharm (Ανφαρμ), Gr.
Gemfibrozil (p.923·1).
*Hyperlipidaemias.*

**Fibromucil** Collins, Mex.
Ispaghula (p.1268·1).
*Constipation; hypercholesterolaemia.*

**Fibronevrina** Ceccarelli, Ital.
Thiamine hydrochloride (p.1455·1); cyanocobalamin (p.1458·2).
*Peripheral neuralgia and neuritis.*

**Fibroquel** Aspid, Mex.
Collagen (p.1674·3).
*Burns; haemorrhage; ulcers; wounds.*

**Fibroral** Novartis Nutrition, Fr.†.
Preparation for enteral nutrition (p.1417·1).

**Fibrorelax** Silesia, Chile.
Chlormezanone (p.675·1); paracetamol (p.76·2); glucametacin (p.44·3).
*Musculoskeletal, joint, and soft-tissue disorders.*

**Fibros** Boniscontro & Gazzone, Ital.†.
Gemfibrozil (p.923·1).
*Hyperlipidaemias.*

**Fibrosine**
Note. This name is used for preparations of different composition.
Whitehall, Irl.†; Whitehall, Port.†.
Maltodextrin (p.1439·3).
*Constipation.*
Wyeth Consumer, Singapore.
Dietary fibre preparation (p.1417·1).
Whitehall, Thai.†.
Soluble fibre (p.1417·1).
*Fibre supplement.*

**Fibrospes** Specifar (Σπεσιφαρ), Gr.
Gemfibrozil (p.923·1).
*Hyperlipidaemias.*

**Fibro-Vein**
Craveri, Arg.; Australasian Medical, Austral.; STD, Irl.; Mac, Ital.; NZ Medical & Scientific, NZ; STD Pharmaceutical Products, UK.
Sodium tetradecyl sulfate (p.1575·1).
Formerly known as STD Injection in the *UK*.
*Varicose veins.*

**Fibrovein** Intramed, S.Afr.†.
Sodium tetradecyl sulfate (p.1575·1).
*Varicose veins.*

**Fibrovit** Provita, Ital.†.
Glucomannan (p.1693·3); pectin; inulin; guar; garcinia cambogia (p.1253·2).
*Dietary fibre supplement.*

**Fibroxyn** Garec, S.Afr.
Naproxen (p.65·1).
*Gout; musculoskeletal and joint disorders; pain.*

**Fibsol** Arrow, Austral.
Lisinopril (p.946·3).
*Heart failure; hypertension; myocardial infarction.*

**Fibyrax**
Rhone-Poulenc Rorer, Austral.†; Whitehall-Robins, Canad.†.
Grain and citrus fibres (p.1253·2).
*Constipation; dietary fibre supplement.*

**Fichtensirup N** Jukunda, Ger.
Spruce needles; thyme (p.1755·2); sage (p.1741·2); liquorice (p.1270·2); thyme oil (p.1755·3); sage oil (p.1741·2).
*Respiratory-tract disorders; tonic.*

**Ficortril**
Mann, Ger.; Pfizer, Swed.
Hydrocortisone (p.1103·3) or hydrocortisone acetate (p.1103·3).
*Anogenital pruritus; eczema; inflammatory eye disorders.*

**Fideine** Bergamo, Braz.†.
Phenolphthalein (p.1284·1); rhubarb (p.1287·3); cascara (p.1255·1); gentian (p.1692·2); papain (p.1727·3).
*Constipation.*

**Fidium** Fides Ecopharma, Spain.
Betahistine hydrochloride (p.1660·1).
*Vertigo.*

**Fiebrolito** Fabop, Arg.
Paracetamol (p.76·2).
*Fever; pain.*

**Fienamina** Recordati, Ital.
Chlorphenamine maleate (p.427·3); ephedrine hydrochloride (p.1120·1).
*Hypersensitivity reactions.*

**Fiery Jack** Pickles, UK.
*Cream:* Glycol salicylate (p.44·3); diethylamine salicylate (p.34·1); capsicum oleoresin (p.1667·1); methyl nicotinate (p.59·2).
*Ointment:* Capsicum oleoresin (p.1667·1).
*Musculoskeletal and joint disorders.*

**Figadobil** DM, Braz.†.
Adenosine (p.851·2); methionine (p.1042·1); betaine hydrochloride (p.1660·2); choline citrate (p.1424·3); pyridoxine hydrochloride (p.1456·3).
*Liver disorders.*

**Figadosan** La-Sante, Braz.†.
Cynara (p.1678·3); cascara (p.1255·1); boldo (p.1661·2); rhubarb (p.1287·3); persea americana.
*Liver disorders.*

**Figalol** Biomedica-Chemica, Gr.
Fluconazole (p.398·1).
*Fungal infections.*

**Figatil** Catarinense, Braz.†.
Cynara (p.1678·3); boldo (p.1661·2); ox bile (p.1660·3).
*Liver disorders.*

**Figen** ERA, Denm.
Senna (p.1288·2); fig (p.1266·3).
*Constipation.*

**Figozant** Chrispa (Χρισπα), Gr.
Nimodipine (p.972·3).
*Neurological deficit following subarachnoid haemorrhage.*

**FIII Hc** Baxter, Ital.
Amino-acid infusion (p.1417·1).
*Parenteral nutrition.*

**Fijacid** Bajer, Arg.
Coal tar (Alcoderm) (p.1159·2).
*Scalp disorders.*

**Fil Olor** Andromaco, Arg.
Camphor (p.1665·3); menthol (p.1711·3); methyl salicylate (p.59·3).

**Filair**
3M, Chile; 3M, UK.
Beclometasone dipropionate (p.1091·1).
*Obstructive airways disease.*

**Filartros** Armstrong, Arg.
Leflunomide (p.53·2).
*Rheumatoid arthritis.*

**Filcrin**
Note. This name is used for preparations of different composition.
Filaxis, Arg.
Vinorelbine (p.594·2).
*Malignant neoplasms.*
Serono, Mex.†.
Vincristine (p.593·2).

**File** Bouzen, Arg.
Sildenafil citrate (p.1744·2).
*Erectile dysfunction.*

**Fileen** *Sriprasit, Thai.*
Aminophylline (p.780·2).
*Asthma.*

**Filena**
*Organon, Austria.*
11 White tablets, estradiol valerate (p.1550·2); 10 blue tablets, estradiol valerate; medroxyprogesterone acetate (p.1557·2).
*Menopausal disorders; osteoporosis.*

*Organon, Ital.*
White tablets, estradiol valerate (p.1550·2); blue tablets, estradiol valerate; medroxyprogesterone acetate (p.1557·2).
*Menopausal disorders.*

**Filesna** *Serono, Mex.†.*
Mesna (p.1041·2).

**Filgen** *Gautier, Arg.*
Filgrastim (p.753·3).
*Mobilisation of peripheral blood progenitor cells; neutropenia.*

**Filginase** *Filaxis, Arg.*
Efavirenz (p.632·2).
*HIV infection.*

**Filibon**
*Wyeth Lederle, India; Wyeth, Mex.†; Wyeth, S.Afr.†.*
Multivitamin and mineral preparation (p.1417·1).

**Filicine** *Adelco, Gr.*
Folic acid (p.1429·1).
*Megaloblastic anaemia; neural tube defects.*

**Filide** *Filaxis, Arg.*
Nevirapine (p.650·2).
*HIV infection.*

**Filigel** *Codifra, Fr.*
Ispaghula (p.1268·1); glucomannan (p.1693·3); fructose (p.1431·3); guarana (p.1765·3).
*Obesity.*

**Filinasma** *Uniao Quimica, Braz.†.*
Theophylline (p.798·3); ephedrine hydrochloride (p.1120·1); phenobarbital (p.367·3); homatropine (p.483·2).
*Respiratory-tract disorders.*

**Filivir** *Serono, Mex.†.*
Aciclovir (p.626·1).

**Filmagene** *Confar, Port.†.*
Barrier cream.

**Filmcel** *Allergan, Braz.*
Hypromellose (p.1579·3).
*Dry eyes.*

**Filmexil** *Pharmacos, Mex.*
Hypromellose (p.1579·3).
*Dry eyes.*

**Filmogen Same** *Savoma, Ital.*
Barrier cream.

**Filnarine** *Approved Prescription Services, UK; Berk, UK.*
Morphine sulfate (p.60·2).
*Pain.*

**Filocot** *Sanofi Synthelabo, Gr.*
Hydrocortisone acetate (p.1103·3).
*Topical corticosteroid.*

**Filoderma** *Armstrong, Arg.*
Diflorasone diacetate (p.1099·3); gentamicin sulfate (p.217·1).
*Infected skin disorders.*

**Filoderma Plus** *Armstrong, Arg.*
Diflorasone diacetate (p.1099·3); gentamicin sulfate (p.217·1); econazole nitrate (p.397·2).
*Infected skin disorders.*

**Filogargan** *Heralds, Braz.†.*
Tyrothricin (p.275·1); benzocaine (p.1370·3); cetylpyridinium chloride (p.1173·1).
*Mouth and throat disorders.*

**Filogaster** *Climax, Braz.*
Amylase (p.1654·2); papain (p.1727·3); pepsin (p.1729·3); homocysteine thiolactone; pancreatin (p.1725·3); sodium dehydrocholate (p.1679·2); vitamin B substances (p.1417·1); magnesium chloride.
*Digestive-system disorders.*

**Filoklin** *Generfarma, Spain.*
Cefazolin sodium (p.170·3).
Lidocaine hydrochloride (p.1377·3) is included in this preparation to alleviate the pain of injection.
*Bacterial infections.*

**Filosfil** *Filaxis, Arg.*
Nelfinavir (p.650·1).
*HIV infection.*

**Filotempo** *Viatris, Port.*
Aminophylline (p.780·2).
*Asthma.*

**Filotricin A** *Dupomar, Arg.*
Tyrothricin (p.275·1); benzocaine (p.1370·3).
*Mouth and throat disorders.*

**Filter Oil Free** *Dermoteca, Port.*
*SPF 16:* Amiloxate (p.1142·2); zinc oxide (p.1163·2).
*SPF 30:* Amiloxate (p.1142·2); zinc oxide (p.1163·2); titanium dioxide (p.1160·3); ferric oxide (p.1057·3).
*Sunscreen.*

**Filter OTC** *Dermoteca, Port.*
*SPF 40:* Amiloxate (p.1142·2); padimate (p.1155·1); enzacamene (p.1147·1); zinc oxide (p.1163·2).
*Topical emulsion SPF 15; SPF 20:* Amiloxate (p.1142·2); zinc oxide (p.1163·2); titanium dioxide (p.1160·3).
*Topical spray SPF 15:* Amiloxate (p.1142·2); zinc oxide (p.1163·2).
*Sunscreen.*

**Filtrax** *Ipso, Ital.*
Pipemidic acid (p.243·1).
*Bacterial urinary-tract infections.*

**Fimdor** *Climax, Braz.†.*
Dipyrone (p.35·3).
*Fever; pain.*

**Fin-A** *Ehlinger, Mex.†.*
Ketotifen (p.788·2).

**Finaber** *Microsules, Arg.*
Ondansetron (p.1281·1).
*Nausea and vomiting.*

**Finac** *C & M, USA.*
Sulfur (p.1158·2); methylbenzethonium chloride (p.1186·1).
*Acne.*

**Finacea** *Berlex, USA.*
Azelaic acid (p.1142·3).
*Rosacea.*

**Finacilen** *Microsules, Arg.*
Nimodipine (p.972·3).
*Cerebrovascular disorders.*

**Finagrip** *Finadiet, Arg.*
Paracetamol (p.76·2); salicylamide (p.87·3); phenylephrine hydrochloride (p.1126·3); ascorbic acid (p.1460·2).
*Influenza symptoms.*

**Finalgon**
*Boehringer Ingelheim, Austral.; Boehringer Ingelheim, Austria; Boehringer Ingelheim, Canad.; Boehringer Ingelheim, Ger.; Boehringer Ingelheim, NZ; Boehringer Ingelheim, Port.; Boehringer Ingelheim, Spain.*
Nonivamide (p.67·2); nicoboxil (p.66·3).
*Musculoskeletal, joint, peri-articular, and soft-tissue disorders; peripheral vascular disorders.*

**Finalgon N Schmerzpflaster** *Thomae, Ger.†.*
Cayenne pepper (p.1667·1); methyl salicylate (p.59·3).
*Musculoskeletal and joint disorders; sprains.*

**Finalop** *Libbs, Braz.*
Finasteride (p.1554·2).
*Benign prostatic hyperplasia.*

**Finamicina** *Fustery, Mex.*
Rifampicin (p.250·2).
*Tuberculosis.*

**Finan** *Solfran, Mex.*
Multivitamin and mineral preparation (p.1417·1).

**Finap** *Raffo, Chile.*
Citalopram (p.289·1).
*Depression.*

**Finaplac** *Epicaris, Arg.*
Chlorhexidine gluconate (p.1173·2).
*Dental hygiene.*

**Finasept** *Microsules, Arg.*
Clarithromycin (p.192·2).
*Bacterial infections.*

**Finasterin** *Finadiet, Arg.*
Finasteride (p.1554·2).

**Finastid** *Neopharmed, Ital.*
Finasteride (p.1554·2).
*Benign prostatic hyperplasia.*

**Finastil** *Sigma, Braz.*
Finasteride (p.1554·2).

**Finaten** *Microsules, Arg.*
Bromazepam (p.671·3).
*Anxiety; muscle relaxant; sedative.*

**Finater** *Fustery, Mex.*
Rifampicin (p.250·2); isoniazid (p.222·2).
*Tuberculosis.*

**Finatux** *Jaba, Port.*
Carbocisteine (p.1116·2).
*Respiratory-tract congestion.*

**Fincar** *Cipla, India.*
Finasteride (p.1554·2).
*Benign prostatic hyperplasia.*

**Fincoid** *Orion, Switz.†.*
Copper-wound polyethylene (p.1425·3).
*Intra-uterine contraceptive device.*

**Findaler** *Medipharm, Chile.*
Cetirizine hydrochloride (p.427·1).
*Hypersensitivity reactions.*

**Findaler-D** *Medipharm, Chile.*
Cetirizine (p.427·2); pseudoephedrine (p.1129·2).

**Findeclin** *Microsules, Arg.*
Alendronate sodium (p.765·3).
*Osteoporosis.*

**Findedol** *Pharmafina, Chile.*
Ketorolac trometamol (p.52·1).
*Pain.*

**Findol** *Senosiain, Mex.*
Ketorolac trometamol (p.52·1).
*Pain.*

**Findol N** *Mundipharma, Ger.*
Tilidine hydrochloride (p.94·1).
Naloxone hydrochloride (p.1044·3) is included in this preparation to discourage abuse.
*Pain.*

**Findor** *Climax, Braz.*
Dipyrone (p.35·3).
*Fever; pain.*

**Finedal** *Llorente, Spain†.*
Clobenzorex hydrochloride (p.1585·3).
*Obesity.*

**Finelium** *PP Lab, Thai.*
Flunarizine hydrochloride (p.434·1).
*Cerebral and peripheral vascular disorders; vestibular disorders.*

**Fineural N** *Molimin, Ger.†.*
Aspirin (p.15·1); paracetamol (p.76·2); caffeine (p.782·1).
*Cold symptoms; fever; neuralgia; pain.*

**Finevin** *Berlex, USA.*
Azelaic acid (p.1142·3).
*Acne.*

**Finex**
*Sintofarma, Braz.*
Terbinafine hydrochloride (p.408·2).
*Fungal infections.*

*Saval, Chile.*
Terbinafine (p.408·2).
*Fungal skin and nail infections.*

**Finfo** *Osotspa, Thai.†.*
Piroxicam (p.84·2).
*Fever; inflammation; musculoskeletal and joint disorders; pain.*

**Fingras** *Dexter, Arg.*
Carnitine; chromium tripicolinate (p.1417·1).
*Dietary supplement.*

**Finidol** *Novartis, Fr.*
Aspirin (p.15·1); caffeine (p.782·1).
Colloidal aluminium hydroxide (p.1249·2) is included in this preparation in an attempt to limit adverse effects on the gastrointestinal mucosa.
*Fever; pain.*

**Finigas** *Apsen, Braz.*
Dimeticone (p.1289·2).
*Flatulence.*

**Finil** *Coradol, Ger.*
Homoeopathic preparation.

**Finimal**
*Roche, Belg.†; Roche Consumer, Neth.*
Paracetamol (p.76·2); caffeine (p.782·1).
*Fever; pain.*

**Finipect** *Roche Nicholas, Neth.†.*
Noscapine (p.1125·3).
*Coughs.*

**Finiweh** *Dentinox, Ger.†.*
Paracetamol (p.76·2).
*Fever; pain.*

**Finlepsin** *AWD, Ger.*
Carbamazepine (p.353·3).
*Alcohol withdrawal syndrome; bipolar disorder; diabetic neuropathy; epilepsy; multiple sclerosis; neuralgias.*

**Finn** *Boehringer de Angeli, Braz.*
Aspartame (p.1422·1).
*Sugar substitute.*

**Finn Cristal** *Boehringer Ingelheim, Braz.*
Saccharin sodium (p.1443·3); sodium cyclamate (p.1426·2).
*Sugar substitute.*

**Finnferon-Alpha** *Veripalvelu, Fin.*
Interferon alfa (p.640·3).
*Malignant neoplasms.*

**Finoxi** *Finadiet, Arg.*
Ondansetron (p.1281·1).
*Nausea and vomiting.*

**Finprob** *Farcoral, Mex.*
Pipenzolate (p.487·3); dimeticone (p.1289·2).
*Gastrointestinal disorders.*

**Finprostat** *Kampel Martian, Arg.*
Finasteride (p.1554·2).

**Finrexin** *Leiras, Fin.*
Aspirin (p.15·1); caffeine (p.782·1); ascorbic acid (p.1460·2).
*Fever; pain.*

**Fintal** *Nicholas Piramal, India.*
Sodium cromoglicate (p.795·3).
*Allergic conjunctivitis; allergic rhinitis; asthma; vernal keratoconjunctivitis.*

**Fintaxim** *Finn Vita, Chile.*
Metformin hydrochloride (p.342·3).
*Diabetes mellitus.*

**Finuret** *Microsules Bernabo, Arg.*
Pipemidic acid (p.243·1).
*Bacterial infections of the urinary tract.*

**Fioricet** *Watson, USA.*
Butalbital (p.673·3); paracetamol (p.76·2); caffeine (p.782·1).
*Tension headache.*

**Fioricet with Codeine** *Novartis, USA.*
Codeine phosphate (p.27·1); butalbital (p.673·3); paracetamol (p.76·2); caffeine (p.782·1).
*Tension headache.*

**Fiorinal**
*Note. This name is used for preparations of different composition.*
*Novartis Consumer, Austral.*
Codeine phosphate (p.27·1); doxylamine succinate (p.432·3); paracetamol (p.76·2).
*Pain.*

*Paladin, Canad.; Novartis, USA.*
Aspirin (p.15·1); butalbital (p.673·3); caffeine (p.782·1).
*Pain; vascular or tension headaches.*

*Novartis, Spain†.*
Aspirin (p.15·1); caffeine (p.782·1); paracetamol (p.76·2).
*Pain.*

**Fiorinal C** *Paladin, Canad.*
Butalbital (p.673·3); caffeine (p.782·1); aspirin (p.15·1); codeine phosphate (p.27·1).
*Anxiety; pain; tension.*

**Fiorinal Codeina** *Novartis, Spain.*
Aspirin (p.15·1); caffeine (p.782·1); codeine phosphate (p.27·1); paracetamol (p.76·2).
*Pain.*

**Fiorinal with Codeine** *Novartis, USA.*
Aspirin (p.15·1); butalbital (p.673·3); caffeine (p.782·1); codeine phosphate (p.27·1).
*Tension headache.*

**Fioritina** *Fada, Arg.*
Noradrenaline (p.974·3).

**Fiormil** *Inpharzam, Switz.*
*Enterococcus faecium* (p.1704·2).
*Restoration of normal gastrointestinal flora.*

**Fiorpap** *Geneva, USA†.*
Butalbital (p.673·3); paracetamol (p.76·2); caffeine (p.782·1).
*Pain.*

**Fiortal** *Geneva, USA†.*
Aspirin (p.15·1); caffeine (p.782·1); butalbital (p.673·3).
*Pain.*

**Fiortal with Codeine** *Geneva, USA†.*
Aspirin (p.15·1); caffeine (p.782·1); butalbital (p.673·3); codeine (p.27·1).

**Fiosen Plus** *Frasca, Arg.*
Alpha tocoferol; vitamin A; pyridoxine (p.1417·1).
*Vitamin supplement.*

**Fiosen-A** *Medica, Arg.*
Vitamin A (p.1451·2).
*Skin disorders.*

**Fiotan** *Altana, Braz.*
Hypericum (p.299·1).
*Depression.*

**Fioton** *Phoenix, Arg.*
Ginkgo biloba; vitamin E (p.1417·1).
*Tonic.*

**FiProFLAX** *Arkopharma, UK.*
Flax oil; fibre; protein; carbohydrate; lignans (p.1417·1).
*Dietary supplement.*

**Firac** *Grossman, Mex.*
Clonixin lysine (p.26·3).
*Pain.*

**Firac Plus** *Grossman, Mex.*
Clonixin lysine (p.26·3); pargeverine hydrochloride (p.487·3).
*Smooth muscle pain and spasm.*

**Firin** *Hoyer, Ger.*
Norfloxacin (p.238·3).
*Bacterial infections.*

**Firmacef** *FIRMA, Ital.†.*
Cefazolin sodium (p.170·3).
Lidocaine hydrochloride (p.1377·3) is included in the intramuscular injection to alleviate the pain of injection.
*Bacterial infections.*

**Firmacort** *FIRMA, Ital.†.*
Methylprednisolone (p.1106·1) or methylprednisolone sodium succinate (p.1106·2).
*Corticosteroid.*

**Firmavit** *FIRMA, Ital.†.*
Cobamamide (p.1459·1); pyridoxal phosphate (p.1456·3); thiamine diphosphate (p.1455·2).
*Neuritis.*

**Firmel** *Craveri, Arg.*
Sildenafil (p.1744·2).
*Erectile dysfunction.*

**Firon** *Raza, Malaysia; Pharmaniaga, Malaysia.*
Ferrous fumarate (p.1427·3).
*Iron-deficiency anaemia.*

**Fironetta** *Schering, Denm.*
21 Tablets, ethinylestradiol (p.1553·2); levonorgestrel (p.1563·2); 7 tablets, inert.
*Triphasic oral contraceptive.*

**First Choice** *Polymer Technology, USA.*
Test for glucose in blood (p.1694·2).

**First Response**
*Carter-Wallace, Austral.†; Carter Horner, Canad.; Carter-Wallace, UK; Carter-Wallace, USA.*
Fertility test or pregnancy test (p.1734·3).

**Fisamox** *Aspen, Austral.*
Amoxicillin sodium (p.155·3).
*Bacterial infections.*

**Fish Factor** *Farmila, Ital.*
Omega-3 marine triglycerides (p.976·2).
*Hyperlipidaemias.*

**Fishaphos** *Felton, Austral.†.*
Omega-3 marine triglycerides (p.976·2).
*Dietary supplement.*

**Fisherman's Friend** *Lofthouse of Fleetwood, Canad.*
Menthol (p.1711·3).
*Coughs; sore throat.*

**Fisherman's Friend Original** *Lofthouse of Fleetwood, Canad.*
Menthol (p.1711·3); eucalyptus oil (p.1686·2).
*Cold symptoms.*

**Fisherman's Friend Zinc** *Lofthouse of Fleetwood, Canad.*
Zinc gluconate (p.1469·2).
*Cold symptoms; zinc supplement.*

**Fisher's Phospherine** *Felton, Austral.†.*
Vitamins and minerals; alstonia constricta; quassia; valerian (p.1417·1).
*Tonic.*

**Fishogar** *Self-Care Products, UK.*
Fish oil; garlic (p.1691·1).

**Fisifax** *Reig Jofre, Spain.*
Nicergoline (p.1719·3).
*Cerebral and peripheral vascular disorders; vascular headache.*

**Fisifer Folico** *Eurofarma, Braz.†.*
Iron succinyl-protein complex (p.1438·1); calcium folinate (p.1431·1).
*Anaemias.*

**Fisiobil** *Salvat, Spain.*
Dimecrotic acid, magnesium salt (p.1680·3).
*Hepatobiliary disorders.*

**Fisiodar** *Abiogen, Ital.*
Diacerein (p.30·1).
*Osteoarthritis.*

**Fisiofer**
*Note. This name is used for preparations of different composition.*
*Eurofarma, Braz.; Labomed, Chile.*
Iron succinyl-protein complex (p.1438·1).
*Iron deficiency; iron-deficiency anaemia.*

*Molteni, Ital.†.*
Sodium ferric gluconate complex (p.1444·3).
*Iron deficiency; iron-deficiency anaemias.*

**Fisiogastrol** *Salvat, Spain.*
Cisapride (p.1259·2).
*Gastro-oesophageal reflux; gastroparesis.*

**Fisiolimp** *Pasteur, Chile.*
Sodium chloride (p.1233·3).
*Nasal congestion; nasal hygiene.*

**Fisiologica** *Fardi, Spain.*
Sodium chloride (p.1233·3).
*Nasal congestion.*

**Fisiologico**
*Labormedica, Braz.†.*
Sodium chloride (p.1233·3).
*Fluid and electrolyte depletion.*

*Betamadrileño, Spain; Neusc, Spain; Perez Gimenez, Spain.*
Sodium chloride (p.1233·3).
*Nasal congestion.*

**Fisiologico Bieffe M** *Baxter, Spain.*
Sodium chloride (p.1233·3).
*Fluid and electrolyte depletion; hypovolaemia.*

**Fisiologico Braun** *Braun, Spain†.*
Sodium chloride (p.1233·3).
*Fluid and electrolyte depletion; hypovolaemia.*

**Fisiologico Farmacelsia** *Farmacelsia, Spain.*
Sodium chloride (p.1233·3).
*Fluid and electrolyte disorders.*

**Fisiologico Isoton** *Braun, Spain.*
Sodium chloride (p.1233·3).
*Fluid and electrolyte disorders.*

**Fisiologico Mein** *Fresenius Kabi, Spain.*
Sodium chloride (p.1233·3).
*Fluid and electrolyte depletion; hypovolaemia.*

**Fisiologico Vitulia** *Ern, Spain.*
Sodium chloride (p.1233·3).
*Fluid and electrolyte depletion; hypovolaemia.*

**Fisioren** *Ducto, Braz.*
Diclofenac resinate (p.33·1).

**Fisiotens** *Solvay, Gr.*
Moxonidine (p.962·3).
*Hypertension.*

**Fisohex** *GlaxoSmithKline, Braz.*
Triclosan (p.1195·2).
*Skin disinfection.*

**Fisopred** *Aventis, Mex.*
Prednisolone sodium phosphate (p.1108·1).
*Corticosteroid.*

**Fissan** *Uhlmann-Eyraud, Switz.*
Casein hydrolysate; bismuth subnitrate (p.1252·2); kaolin (p.1268·3); silica clay (p.1581·3); titanium dioxide (p.1160·3); zinc oxide (p.1163·2).
*Skin irritation.*

**Fissan-Silberpuder** *Salitine, Ger.*
Methenamine silver nitrate compound.
*Umbilical cord care; wounds.*

**Fissan-Zinkschuttelmixtur** *Salitine, Ger.*
Zinc oxide (p.1163·2).
*Skin disorders.*

**Fitacnol** *Arkopharma, Fr.*
Lappa (p.1704·3); viola tricolor; urtica (p.1762·1).
*Seborrhoea.*

**Fitaxal** *Phygiene, Fr.†.*
Lactulose (p.1269·1).
*Constipation.*

**Fito Stomygen** *Stomygen, Ital.*
Mallow; hamamelis; chamomile; sage; calendula.
*Herbal toothpaste.*

**Fitocalmin** *Hochstetter, Chile.*
Homoeopathic preparation.

**Fitocrem** *Andromaco, Spain†.*
Paraffin; wheat germ; phenoxyethanol.
*Burns; ulcers; wounds.*

**Fitocreme** *Fariberica, Port.*
Wheat germ; phenoxyethanol.
*Burns; ulcers; wounds.*

**Fitoderme** *Hebron, Braz.*
Erigeron bonariensis.
*Fungal infections.*

**Fitodorf Alghe Marine** *Fitodorfarma, Ital.†.*
Quercia marine extract; frangula (p.1266·3); rhubarb (p.1287·3).
*Constipation; dietary supplement.*

**Fitodorf Rabarbaro** *Fitodorfarma, Ital.†.*
Boldo (p.1661·2); rhubarb (p.1287·3).
*Digestive disorders; reduced intestinal motility.*

**Fitoestimulina** *Grossman, Mex.*
Wheat germ; phenoxyethanol (p.1189·1).
*Burns; ulcers; vaginal lesions; wounds.*

**Fitogen** *Scherer, Ital.*
Soya oil (p.1447·2); calcium carbonate (p.1254·2); colecalciferol (p.1461·3).
*Menopausal disorders; nutritional supplement.*

**Fitokey Ginkgo** *Inkeysa, Spain.*
Ginkgo biloba (p.1692·3).
*Cerebral and peripheral circulatory disorders.*

**Fitokey Harpagophytum** *Inkeysa, Spain.*
Devil's claw root (p.28·2).
*Musculoskeletal and joint disorders.*

**Fitolax** *IMA, Braz.*
Senna (p.1288·2); cassia pulp (p.1255·2); tamarind (p.1293·2); coriander (p.1676·1).
*Constipation.*

**Fitolinea** *Pharbenia, Ital.†.*
Bladderwrack (p.1742·3); senna (p.1288·2).
*Constipation; obesity.*

**Fitonal** *Andromaco, Arg.*
Ketoconazole (p.403·3).
*Fungal infections.*

**Fitosonno** *Pharbenia, Ital.*
Eschscholtzia californica; passion flower (p.1729·1); valerian (p.1762·2).
*Insomnia.*

**Fitostimoline** *Damor, Ital.*
*Cream; medicated dressing; pessaries; vaginal wash:* Wheat germ; phenoxyethanol (p.1189·1).
*Burns; skin disorders; vaginal disorders; vascular disorders; wounds.*
*Injection:* Wheat germ.
*Burns; skin disorders; vascular disorders; wounds.*

**Fitostress** *Pharbenia, Ital.†.*
Ginseng (p.1693·1); kola (p.1765·3).
*Tonic.*

**Fitosvelt** *Arkochim, Spain.*
Black currant (p.1661·1); tea (p.1765·3).
*Diuretic.*

**Fitotos** *Koni-Cofarm, Chile.*
Tolu balsam (p.1131·3); drosera (p.1683·1); quillaia (p.1416·1).
*Coughs.*

**Fittig** *Andromaco, Chile.*
Undecenoic acid (p.410·3); zinc undecenoate (p.411·1); hexylresorcinol (p.1182·1); calcium propionate (p.408·1) or sodium propionate (p.408·1).
*Fungal skin infections.*

**Fitton** *Teva, Israel†.*
Fenetylline (p.1588·2).
*CNS stimulant.*

**Fittydent** *Hoeveler, Austria.*
Eucalyptus oil (p.1686·2); sage oil (p.1741·2); clove oil (p.1673·3).
*Mouth and throat inflammation; toothache.*

**Fitzecalm** *Julphar, UAE.*
Carbamazepine (p.353·3).
*Bipolar disorder; epilepsy.*

**Fivasa** *Norgine, Fr.*
Mesalazine (p.1273·2).
*Inflammatory bowel disease.*

**Fivefluro** *GlaxoSmithKline, India.*
Fluorouracil (p.554·2).
*Malignant neoplasms.*

**Fiverocil** *Serono, Mex.†.*
Fluorouracil (p.554·2).

**Fivoflu** *Dabur, Thai.*
Fluorouracil (p.554·2).
*Malignant neoplasms.*

**Fixateur phospho-calcique** *Bichsel, Switz.*
Calcium carbonate (p.1254·2).
*Hyperphosphataemia.*

**Fixca** *Lesvi, Spain†.*
Ondansetron hydrochloride (p.1281·1).
*Nausea and vomiting.*

**Fixical** *Pharmascience, Fr.*
Calcium carbonate (p.1254·2).
*Calcium deficiency; osteoporosis.*

**Fixical Vitamine $D_3$** *Pharmascience, Fr.*
Calcium carbonate (p.1254·2); colecalciferol (p.1461·3).
*Calcium and vitamin D deficiency; osteoporosis.*

**Fixim** *Yamanouchi, Neth.*
Cefixime (p.172·3).
*Bacterial infections.*

**Fixime** *Merck, S.Afr.*
Cefixime (p.172·3).
*Bacterial infections.*

**Fixoten** *Cryopharma, Mex.*
Pentoxifylline (p.979·3).
*Vascular disorders.*

**Fixx** *Unichem, India.*
Cefixime (p.172·3).
*Bacterial infections.*

**Fizz** *Stanley, Canad.†.*
Multivitamin preparation (p.1417·1).

**Fizziclean** *Bausch & Lomb, Braz.*
Subtilisin A(p.1164·2).
*Cleansing of contact lenses.*

**Flacar** *Schwabe, Ger.*
Betaine dihydrogen citrate (p.1660·2); sorbitol (p.1446·3).
*Liver disorders.*

**Fladex** *Dexa, Singapore.*
Metronidazole (p.607·2).
*Amoebiasis; giardiasis; trichomoniasis.*

**Flagass** *Ache, Braz.*
Simeticone (p.1289·2).
*Flatulence.*

**Flagass Baby** *Ache, Braz.*
Simeticone (p.1289·2); homatropine methylbromide (p.483·2).
*Flatulence.*

**Flagenase** *Liomont, Mex.*
Metronidazole (p.607·2) or metronidazole benzoate (p.607·2).
*Anaerobic bacterial infections; protozoal infections.*

**Flagenase 400** *Liomont, Mex.*
Metronidazole (p.607·2) or metronidazole benzoate (p.607·2); diiodohydroxyquinoline (p.603·3).
*Amoebiasis.*

**Flagenol** *Allen, Mex.*
Metronidazole (p.607·2) or metronidazole benzoate (p.607·2).
*Amoebiasis; giardiasis; trichomoniasis.*

**Flagentyl**
*Aventis, Arg.; Aventis, Fr.†; Vitoria, Port.*
Secnidazole (p.615·3).
*Protozoal infections.*

**Flaginazol** *Vitae, Mex.†.*
Metronidazole (p.607·2).
*Amoebiasis; giardiasis; trichomoniasis.*

**Flagosil** *Collins, Mex.*
Diiodohydroxyquinoline (p.603·3); metronidazole (p.607·2).
*Protozoal infections.*

**Flagyl**
*Aventis, Arg.; Aventis, Austral.; Rhone-Poulenc Rorer, Austria†; Aventis, Belg.; Aventis, Braz.; Aventis, Canad.; Aventis, Chile; Aventis, Denm.; Aventis, Fin.; Aventis, Fr.; Aventis, Ger.; Aventis, Gr.; Aventis, Hong Kong; Nicholas Piramal, India; Aventis, Irl.; Aventis, Israel; Zambon, Ital.; Aventis, Malaysia; Aventis, Mex.; Aventis, Neth.; Aventis, Norw.; Aventis, NZ; Vitoria, Port.; Aventis, S.Afr.; Aventis, Singapore; Aventis, Spain; Aventis, Swed.; Aventis, Switz.; Aventis, Thai.; Hawgreen, UK; Aventis, UK; SCS, USA; Searle, USA.*
Metronidazole (p.607·2), metronidazole benzoate (p.607·2), or metronidazole hydrochloride (p.607·2).
*Anaerobic bacterial infections; Crohn's disease; protozoal infections; rosacea.*

**Flagyl Comp** *Aventis, Fin.*
Metronidazole (p.607·2); nystatin (p.406·3).
*Bacterial vaginosis; vaginal trichomoniasis.*

**Flagyl Compak**
*Rhone-Poulenc Rorer, Irl.†; Hawgreen, UK†.*
*Combination preparation:* Tablets, metronidazole (p.607·2); pessaries, nystatin (p.406·3).
*Vaginitis.*

**Flagyl Nistatina** *Aventis, Braz.*
Metronidazole (p.607·2); nystatin (p.406·3).
*Vulvovaginal candidiasis and trichomoniasis.*

**Flagyl-F** *Nicholas Piramal, India.*
Metronidazole (p.607·2) or metronidazole benzoate (p.607·2); furazolidone (p.605·2).
*Amoebiasis.*

**Flagystatin**
*Aventis, Arg.; Aventis, Canad.; Aventis, Singapore.*
Metronidazole (p.607·2); nystatin (p.406·3).
*Vulvovaginal infections.*

**Flagystatin V** *Aventis, Mex.*
Metronidazole (p.607·2); nystatin (p.406·3).
*Vaginal trichomoniasis and candidiasis.*

**Flamadene** *Heralds, Braz.†.*
Piroxicam (p.84·2).
*Dysmenorrhoea; gout; musculoskeletal, joint, and peri-articular disorders.*

**Flamanan** *Legrand, Braz.*
Paracetamol (p.76·2); oxyphenbutazone (p.76·1).
*Fever; inflammation; pain.*

**Flamar** *Indoco, India.*
Methyl nicotinate (p.59·2); methyl salicylate (p.59·3); mephenesin (p.1394·3); menthol (p.1711·3).
*Musculoskeletal and joint disorders.*

**Flamarene** *Biolab Sanus, Braz.†.*
Piroxicam (p.84·2).
*Dysmenorrhoea; gout; musculoskeletal, joint, and peri-articular disorders.*

**Flamaret** *Xixia, S.Afr.*
Indometacin (p.47·3).
*Dysmenorrhoea; gout; musculoskeletal and joint disorders.*

**Flamar-MX** *Indoco, India.*
Diclofenac sodium (p.32·1); paracetamol (p.76·2); chlorzoxazone (p.1392·3).
*Painful skeletal muscle spasm.*

**Flamatak** *Alpharma, UK.*
Diclofenac sodium (p.32·1).
*Gout; inflammation; musculoskeletal, joint, peri-articular, and soft-tissue disorders; pain.*

**Flamatec** *Uniao Quimica, Braz.†.*
Meloxicam (p.56·1).

**Flamatrol**
*Teva, Hong Kong; Berk, UK†.*
Piroxicam (p.84·2).
*Inflammation; musculoskeletal and joint disorders; pain.*

**Flamazine**
*Smith & Nephew, Canad.; Smith & Nephew, Denm.; Smith & Nephew, Fin.; IFET (ΙΦΕΤ), Gr.; Smith & Nephew, Hong Kong; Smith & Nephew, Irl.; Smith & Nephew, Norw.; Solvay, Port.; Smith & Nephew, S.Afr.; Smith & Nephew, Singapore; Smith & Nephew, Thai.; Smith & Nephew Healthcare, UK.*
Sulfadiazine silver (p.259·1).
*Infected wounds and burns.*

**Flamazine C** *Smith & Nephew, Canad.*
Sulfadiazine silver (p.259·1); chlorhexidine gluconate (p.1173·2).
*Burns; ulcers; wounds.*

**Flamecid** *Propan, S.Afr.*
Indometacin (p.47·3).
*Gout; musculoskeletal and joint disorders.*

**Flameril**
*Novartis, NZ; Biochemie, NZ; Normal, Port.*
Diclofenac (p.32·1), diclofenac diethylamine (p.32·1), or diclofenac sodium (p.32·1).
*Gout; inflammation; musculoskeletal and joint disorders; pain.*

**Flamic** *Siam Bheasach, Thai.*
Piroxicam (p.84·2).
*Gout; musculoskeletal, joint, peri-articular, and soft-tissue disorders.*

**Flamicina** *Fustery, Mex.*
Ampicillin (p.157·1), ampicillin sodium (p.157·1), or ampicillin trihydrate (p.157·2).
*Bacterial infections.*

**Flamide** *Rayere, Mex.*
Nimesulide (p.67·1).
*Fever; inflammation; pain.*

**Flamin** *Loren, Mex.*
Metronidazole (p.607·2).
*Amoebiasis.*

**Flamin 400** *Loren, Mex.†.*
Metronidazole (p.607·2); clioquinol (p.196·3).
*Amoebiasis.*

**Flaminase** *Formenti, Ital.*
Promelase (p.1735·2).
*Respiratory-tract disorders.*

**Flamirex**
*Note. This name is used for preparations of different composition.*
*Sanofi Synthelabo, Arg.*
Deflazacort (p.1096·2).
*Corticosteroid.*

*Irex, Fr.†.*
Tiaprofenic acid (p.93·3).
*Musculoskeletal and joint disorders.*

**Flammacerium**
*Solvay, Belg.; Solvay, Fr.; Solvay, Israel†; Solvay, Neth.; Solvay, UK.*
Sulfadiazine silver (p.259·1); cerous nitrate (p.1144·3).
Available on a named patient basis in the UK.
*Infected burns.*

**Flammazine**
*Solvay, Austria; Solvay, Belg.; Solvay, Fr.; Solvay, Ger.; Solvay, Neth.; Solvay, Spain; Solvay, Switz.*
Sulfadiazine silver (p.259·1).
*Burns; infected wounds.*

**Flamon** *Mepha, Switz.*
Verapamil hydrochloride (p.1019·1).
*Arrhythmias; hypertension; ischaemic heart disease.*

**Flamostat** *Cimed, Braz.*
Piroxicam (p.84·2).
*Dysmenorrhoea; gout; musculoskeletal, joint, and peri-articular disorders.*

**Flamrase** *Berk, UK.*
Diclofenac sodium (p.32·1).
*Musculoskeletal, joint, peri-articular, and soft-tissue disorders; pain.*

**Flanakin** *Kinder, Braz.*
Diclofenac potassium (p.32·1).

**Flanamox** *Wolff, Ger.*
Amoxicillin trihydrate (p.155·3); flucloxacillin sodium (p.213·3).
*Bacterial infections.*

**Flanaren** *Teuto, Braz.*
Diclofenac sodium (p.32·1).
*Gout; inflammation; musculoskeletal, joint, and peri-articular disorders; pain.*

**Flanax**
*Aventis, Braz.†; Syntex, Mex.*
Naproxen sodium (p.65·1).
*Fever; gout; inflammation; pain.*

**Flancox** *Apsen, Braz.†.*
Etodolac (p.37·3).

**Flanders Buttocks** *Flanders, USA.*
Zinc oxide (p.1163·2); peru balsam (p.1730·2).
*Nappy rash.*

**Flanid** *Pierre Fabre Sante, Fr.*
Tiaprofenic acid (p.93·3).
*Musculoskeletal and joint disorders; pain.*

**Flanil**
*Biolab, Malaysia; Biolab, Singapore; Biolab, Thai.*
Methyl salicylate (p.59·3); menthol (p.1711·3); eugenol (p.1686·2).
*Insect bites; muscle pain; pruritus.*

**Flanizol** *Delta, Braz.*
Metronidazole (p.607·2) or metronidazole benzoate (p.607·2).
*Vaginal infections.*

**Flankol** *Pharmacos, Mex.*
Diclofenac sodium (p.32·1).
*Inflammatory eye disorders.*

**Flanoquin** *Liomont, Mex.†.*
Diiodohydroxyquinoline (p.603·3).

**Flantadin** *Lepetit, Ital.*
Deflazacort (p.1096·2).
*Oral corticosteroid.*

**Flanzen** *Sigma, India.*
Serrapeptase (p.1743·2).
*Hyphaema; inflammation or oedema associated with infection or trauma; respiratory-tract congestion; subconjunctival bleeding.*

**Flapex** *Silesia, Chile.*
Simeticone (p.1289·2).
*Adjunct in gastrointestinal radiography; gastrointestinal disorders with excess gas.*

**Flapex E** *Silesia, Chile.*
Simeticone (p.1289·2); pancreatin (p.1725·3); pepsin (p.1729·3); amylase (p.1654·2); bile (p.1660·3).
*Digestive disorders; flatulence.*

**Flar** *ISM, Ital.†.*
*Streptococcus lactis; Lactobacillus acidophilus* (p.1704·2); nicotinamide (p.1441·2).
*Gastrointestinal disorders.*

**Flarex**
*Alcon, Arg.; Alcon, Austral.; Alcon, Austria; Alcon, Canad.; Alcon, Israel; Alcon, Ital.; Alcon, Mex.†; Pacific, NZ†; Alcon, Switz.†; Alcon, Thai.; Alcon, USA.*
Fluorometholone acetate (p.1102·2).
*Inflammatory eye disorders.*

**Flaspas** *Daito, Jpn.*
Aranidipine (p.864·2).
*Hypertension.*

**Flatex** *Farmasa, Braz.*
Dimeticone (p.1289·2).
*Flatulence.*

**Flatol** *Legrand, Braz.*
Dimeticone (p.1289·2).
*Flatulence.*

**Flatoril** *Almirall, Spain.*
Clebopride malate (p.1260·3); simeticone (p.1289·2).
*Dyspepsia; gastro-oesophageal reflux; hiatus hernia.*

**Flatulence Gastulence** *Greater Pharma, Thai.*
Cascara (p.1255·1); capsicum (p.1667·1); amylase (p.1654·2); ginger (p.1267·1); nux vomica (p.1722·3); asafetida (p.1658·1).
*Constipation; flatulence.*

**Flatulex**
*Note. This name is used for preparations of different composition.*
*Globopharm, Switz.*
*Chewable tablets:* Simeticone (p.1289·2); caraway oil (p.1667·3); fennel oil (p.1687·3); peppermint oil (p.1283·2).
*Adjunct prior to gastrointestinal examination; flatulence.*
*Globopharm, Switz.; Dayton, USA.*
*Oral drops:* Simeticone (p.1289·2).
*Adjunct prior to gastrointestinal examination; detergent poisoning; flatulence.*
*Dayton, USA.*
*Tablets:* Simeticone (p.1289·2); activated charcoal (p.1030·2).
*Flatulence.*

**Flaval** *Cetus, Arg.*
Bamethan (p.866·3); diclofenac (p.32·1); esculoside (p.1648·2).

**Flavamed Halstabletten** *Berlin-Chemie, Ger.*
Benzocaine (p.1370·3).
*Sore throat.*

**Flavan** *Pharmafarm, Fr.*
Leucocianidol (p.1688·2).
*Capillary fragility; haemorrhoids; venous insufficiency.*

**Flavangin** *Streuli, Switz.†.*
Ethacridine lactate (p.1165·3); cetylpyridinium chloride (p.1173·1); lidocaine hydrochloride (p.1377·3); menthol (p.1711·3).
*Mouth and throat disorders.*

**Flavedon** *Serdia, India.*
Trimetazidine hydrochloride (p.1018·1).
*Ischaemic heart disease.*

**Flaveric** *Pfizer, Jpn.*
Benproperine phosphate (p.1115·2).
*Coughs.*

**Flavettes**
*CCM, Hong Kong; Upha, Singapore.*
Vitamin C (p.1460·2).
*Vitamin C deficiency.*

**Flavettes Neuroforte** *Upha, Malaysia.*
Vitamin $B_1$ (p.1455·2); vitamin $B_6$ (p.1457·2); vitamin $B_{12}$ (p.1458·2).
*Neuralgias; neuritis; neuropathy; vitamin B supplement.*

**Flaviastase** *Iphym, Fr.†.*
Enzymes derived from Aspergillus.
*Digestive disorders.*

**Flavicina** *Pharmacia, Arg.*
Doxorubicin hydrochloride (p.547·3).
*Malignant neoplasms.*

**Flavinol** *Chew, Thai.*
Acriflavinium monochloride (p.1165·3); thymol (p.1194·2).
*Burns; wounds.*

**Flavion** *Terapeutico, Ital.*
*Tablets:* Aesculus; centella; lemon; red vine (p.1417·1).
*Nutritional supplement.*
*Topical gel:* Aesculus (p.1648·2); catechu (p.1668·3); solidago virgaurea (p.1748·3).
*Peripheral vascular disorders.*

**Flavis** *Pulitzer, Ital.†.*
Piracetam (p.1732·1).
*Mental function impairment.*

**Flavit** *Hormona, Mex.*
Bioflavonoids (p.1688·2); ascorbic acid (p.1460·2).
*Capillary fragility.*

**Flavit-AV** *Hormona, Mex.*
Paracetamol (p.76·2); phenylephrine hydrochloride (p.1126·3); chlorphenamine maleate (p.427·3).
*Hypersensitivity; nasal congestion; pain.*

**Flavix** *Wockhardt, India.*
Venlafaxine hydrochloride (p.321·3).
*Anxiety; depression.*

**Flavodrei** *Dreiman, Spain.*
Soya bean (p.1447·2).
*Menopausal disorders.*

**Flavogin** *Baif, Ital.*
Ginkgo biloba; bioflavonoids; dog rose; myrtillus; vitamin C (p.1417·1).
*Tonic.*

**Flavon** *General Drugs, Thai.*
Flavonoids (p.1688·2).
*Haemorrhoids; vascular insufficiency.*

**Flavone 500** *Ecobi, Ital.†.*
Ascorbic acid (p.1460·2); hesperidin (p.1688·2).

**Flavonex** *Ross, USA†.*
Preparation for enteral nutrition (p.1417·1).

**Flavonoid Complex** *Neo-Life, Austral.†.*
Cranberry; kale; green tea; red beetroot; mixed berry; oregon grape; grape; orange extract; lemon extract; grapefruit (p.1688·2).
*Flavonoid supplement.*

**Flavons**
*Note. This name is used for preparations of different composition.*
*Eagle, Austral.†.*
Ascorbic acid (p.1460·2); sodium ascorbate (p.1460·2); calcium ascorbate (p.1460·2); hesperidin (p.1688·2); bioflavonoids (p.1688·2); rutoside (p.1688·2); rose fruit (p.1740·1); boneset (p.1661·3); echinacea (p.1683·2); achillea (p.1646·2).
*Minor wounds; tonic.*
*Freeda, USA.*
Citrus bioflavonoids complex (p.1688·2); hesperidin (p.1688·2).
*Capillary bleeding.*

**Flavoquine** *Aventis, Fr.*
Amodiaquine hydrochloride (p.446·3).
*Malaria.*

**Flavorin** *TO-Chemicals, Thai.*
Flavoxate hydrochloride (p.482·2).
*Urinary-tract disorders.*

**Flavorola C** *Lifeplan, UK†.*
Vitamin C (p.1460·2); bioflavonoids (p.1688·2).
*Nutritional supplement.*

**Flavo-Spa** *Utopian, Thai.*
Flavoxate hydrochloride (p.482·2).
*Urinary-tract disorders.*

**Flavostat** *Lafedar, Arg.*
Vitamin A (p.1451·2).
*Vitamin supplement.*

**Flavoton** *GD, Ital.*
Bioflavonoids; calcium; magnesium; colecalciferol (p.1417·1).
*Nutritional supplement.*

**Flavovenyl** *Plan, Switz.*
*Capsules; oral drops:* Bioflavonoids (p.1688·2); hesperidin methyl chalcone (p.1688·3); esculoside (p.1648·2).
*Ointment:* Bioflavonoids (p.1688·2); hesperidin methyl chalcone (p.1688·3); esculoside (p.1648·2); menthol (p.1711·3).
*Peripheral vascular disorders.*

**Flavo-Zinc** *Solgar, UK.*
Zinc gluconate (p.1469·2); zinc citrate.
*Dietary supplement.*

**Flaxedil**
*Rhone-Poulenc Rorer, Austral.†; Aventis, Braz.†; Rhone-Poulenc Rorer, Canad.†; Rhone-Poulenc Rorer, Neth.†; Concord, UK.*
Gallamine triethiodide (p.1403·2).
*Competitive neuromuscular blocker.*

**Flaxin** *Merck, Braz.*
Finasteride (p.1554·2).
*Benign prostatic hyperplasia.*

**Flebeside** *Jorba, Spain.*
Carbazochrome (p.745·1); troxerutin (p.1688·3).
*Vascular disorders.*

**Flebil** *Molteni, Ital.†.*
Troxerutin (p.1688·3).
*Haemorrhoids; peripheral vascular disorders.*

**Flebior** *Therasophia, Fr.*
Myrtillus (p.1718·3); buckwheat; red vine; vitamin E; vitamin C (p.1417·1).
*Capillary disorders; nutritional supplement.*

**Flebitol** *Phoenix, Arg.*
Ginkgo biloba (p.1692·3); heptaminol hydrochloride (p.1697·1); troxerutin (p.1688·3).
*Phlebitis; premenstrual disorders; venous insufficiency.*

**Flebo Stop** *Inexfa, Spain†.*
Bromelains (p.1662·2); esculoside (p.1648·2); etofylline (p.785·1); hydrochlorothiazide (p.933·2).
*Oedema; vascular disorders.*

**Flebobag Fisio** *Grifols, Spain.*
Sodium chloride infusion (p.1233·3).
*Fluid and electrolyte depletion; hypovolaemia.*

**Flebobag Glucosa** *Grifols, Spain.*
Glucose infusion (p.1432·2).
*Parenteral nutrition.*

**Flebobag Glucosal** *Grifols, Spain.*
Sodium chloride infusion (p.1233·3) with glucose (p.1432·2).
*Fluid and electrolyte depletion; hypovolaemia.*

**Flebobag Ring Lact** *Grifols, Spain.*
Electrolyte infusion (p.1217·1).
*Fluid and electrolyte disorders.*

**Flebocortid**
*Aventis, Braz.†; Lepetit, Ital.; Cilag, Mex.*
Hydrocortisone sodium succinate (p.1104·1).
*Corticosteroid.*

**Fleboderma** *Labinca, Arg.*
A heparinoid (p.931·1).

**Flebogamma**
*Grifols, Arg.; Grifols, Chile; Grifols, Ger.; Demo, Gr.; Grifols, Ital.; Grifols, Port.; Grifols, Singapore; Grifols, Spain; Grifols, UK; Grifols, USA.*
A normal immunoglobulin (p.1627·2).
*Hypogammglobulinaemia; idiopathic thrombocytopenic purpura; Kawasaki disease; passive immunisation.*

**Flebon** *Elvetium, Arg.*
Diosmin (p.1688·2).
*Haemorrhoids; venous insufficiency.*

**Flebopex** *Bago, Chile.*
Rutoside (p.1688·2).
*Haemorrhoids; metrorrhagia; retinal haemorrhage; venous insufficiency.*

**Fleboplast Fisio** *Grifols, Spain.*
Sodium chloride infusion (p.1233·3).
*Fluid and electrolyte depletion; hypovolaemia.*

**Fleboplast Glucosa** *Grifols, Spain.*
Glucose infusion (p.1432·2).
*Parenteral nutrition.*

**Fleboplast Glucosal** *Grifols, Spain.*
Sodium chloride infusion (p.1233·3) with glucose (p.1432·2).
*Fluid and electrolyte depletion; hypovolaemia.*

**Fleboplast Levulosa** *Grifols, Spain†.*
Fructose infusion (p.1431·3).
*Parenteral nutrition.*

**Fleboplast Plurisal** *Grifols, Spain.*
Electrolyte infusion (p.1217·1) with sodium lactate (p.1223·2).
*Fluid and electrolyte depletion; hypovolaemia.*

**Flebopom** *Typen, Arg.*
Ruscogenin (p.1741·1).
*Inflammation; phlebitis.*

**Fleboside** *Pharmafar, Ital.*
Troxerutin (p.1688·3); carbazochrome (p.745·1).
*Capillary fragility; haemorrhoids; varicose ulcers.*

**Flebosmil** *Socopharm, Fr.*
Diosmin (p.1688·2).
*Haemorrhoids; peripheral vascular disorders; venous insufficiency.*

**Flebostasin**
*Sankyo, Ital.*
Aesculus (p.1648·2).
*Chronic venous insufficiency.*
*Sankyo, Spain.*
Aescin (p.1648·2).
*Oedema; peripheral vascular disorders.*

**Fleboton** *Sanofi Winthrop, Port.†.*
Hidrosmin (p.1688·3).
*Oedema; vascular disorders.*

**Flebotrat** *Neckerman, Braz.†.*
Coumarin (p.1676·2); troxerutin (p.1688·3).
*Varices.*

**Flebotropin** *Bago, Arg.*
*Cream:* Flavonoids (p.1688·2); benzocaine (p.1370·3).
*Tablets:* Flavonoids (p.1688·2).
*Haemorrhoids; venous insufficiency.*

**Flebovis** *Amnol, Ital.*
Hedera; birch; aesculus; equisetum; myrtillus; centella; vitamin E.
*Circulatory disorders of the skin; emollient.*
Soya oil; centella; melilotus; cumin; *dl*-alfa tocoferil acetate; rutoside; triglycerides (p.1417·1).
*Circulatory disorders; haemorrhoids; nutritional supplement; oedema.*

**Flebozin** *Depofarma, Ital.*
Melilot; aesculus; centella (p.1417·1).
*Nutritional supplement.*

**Flebs** *Pierre Fabre, Ital.*
Heparin sodium (p.928·1); a heparinoid (p.931·1).
*Haemorrhoids; phlebitis; soft-tissue injury; thrombophlebitis.*

**Flecaine** *3M, Fr.*
Flecainide acetate (p.916·2).
*Arrhythmias.*

**Flecatab** *Alphapharm, Austral.*
Flecainide acetate (p.916·2).
*Arrhythmias.*

**Flecor-N** *Zekides, Gr.*
Nifedipine (p.966·2).
*Angina; hypertension.*

**Flectadol**
*Note. This name is used for preparations of different composition.*
*Recalcine, Chile.*
Chlorzoxazone (p.1392·3); paracetamol (p.76·2).
*Musculoskeletal, joint, and peri-articular disorders; tension headache.*
*Sanofi Synthelabo, Ital.*
Lysine aspirin (p.54·3).
*Musculoskeletal and joint disorders; pain.*

**Flector**
*Sanova, Austria; Therabel, Belg.; Genevrier, Fr.; IBSA, Hong Kong; IBSA, Ital.; IBSA, Switz.*
Diclofenac epolamine (p.33·1) or diclofenac sodium (p.32·1).
*Inflammation; musculoskeletal, joint, peri-articular, and soft-tissue disorders; oedema; pain.*

**Fleet**
*De Witt, Denm.; De Witt, Irl.; Pisa, Mex.*
Monobasic sodium phosphate (p.1230·3); dibasic sodium phosphate (p.1231·1).
*Bowel evacuation; constipation.*

**Fleet Babylax**
*Rider, Chile; Fleet, Malaysia; Dewitt, Malaysia; Fleet, Singapore; Fleet, USA.*
Glycerol (p.1694·3).
*Constipation in children.*

**Fleet Bagenema** *Fleet, USA.*
Liquid castile soap (p.1575·2).

**Fleet Bisacodyl** *Fleet, USA.*
Bisacodyl (p.1251·3).
*Bowel evacuation; constipation.*

**Fleet Enema**
*Note. This name is used for preparations of different composition.*
*Raymos, Arg.; Wolfs, Belg.; Whitehall, Braz.; Johnson & Johnson, Canad.; Pharmakochimiki (Φαρμακοχημική), Gr.; Fleet-Dewitt, Hong Kong; Dexxon, Israel; Fleet, Malaysia; Dewitt, Malaysia; Fleet, Singapore; Fleet, USA.*
Dibasic sodium phosphate (p.1231·1); monobasic sodium phosphate (p.1230·3).
*Bowel evacuation; constipation.*
*Rider, Chile.*
Monobasic sodium phosphate (p.1230·3); tribasic sodium phosphate (p.1231·1).
*Bowel evacuation; constipation.*

**Fleet Enema Mineral Oil** *Johnson & Johnson, Canad.*
Liquid paraffin (p.1479·1).
*Bowel evacuation; constipation.*

**Fleet Fosfosoda** *Rider, Chile.*
Monobasic sodium phosphate (p.1230·3); tribasic sodium phosphate (p.1231·1).
*Bowel evacuation; constipation.*

**Fleet Laxative**
*Fleet, Austral.; Baxter, NZ; Fleet, NZ; Fleet, USA.*
Bisacodyl (p.1251·3).
*Bowel evacuation; constipation.*

**Fleet Medicated Pads** *Fleet, USA.*
Hamamelis water (p.1696·3); alcohol; glycerol.
*Anorectal disorders.*

**Fleet Micro** *Ferring, Swed.*
Sodium citrate (p.1223·2); sodium lauril sulfoacetate (p.1574·3).
*Constipation.*

**Fleet Micro-Enema**
*Note. This name is used for preparations of different composition.*
*Fleet, Austral.*
Sodium citrate (p.1223·2); sodium lauril sulfoacetate (p.1574·3); sorbitol (p.1446·3).
*Bowel evacuation; constipation.*
*Fleet-Dewitt, Hong Kong; Baxter, NZ; Fleet, NZ.*
Sodium citrate (p.1223·2); sodium lauril sulfoacetate (p.1574·3).
*Bowel evacuation; constipation.*

**Fleet Mineral Enema** *Baxter, NZ; Fleet, NZ.*
Liquid paraffin (p.1479·1).
*Bowel evacuation; constipation.*

**Fleet Pain Relief** *Fleet, USA.*
Pramocaine hydrochloride (p.1382·2).
*Anorectal disorders.*

**Fleet Phosphate Enema** *Baxter, NZ; Fleet, NZ.*
Monobasic sodium phosphate (p.1230·3); dibasic sodium phosphate (p.1231·1).
*Bowel evacuation; constipation.*

**Fleet Phospho-Soda**
*Fleet, Austral.; De Witt, Austria; Wolfs, Belg.; Johnson & Johnson, Canad.; Ferring, Fr.; Ferring, Ger.; Fleet-Dewitt, Hong Kong; Fleet, Malaysia; Dewitt, Malaysia; Baxter, NZ; Fleet, NZ; Fleet, Singapore; De Witt, UK; Fleet, USA.*
Monobasic sodium phosphate (p.1230·3); dibasic sodium phosphate (p.1231·1).
*Bowel evacuation; constipation.*

**Fleet Prep Kit No. 1** *Fleet, USA.*
*Combination pack:* Fleet Phospho-Soda; Fleet Bisacodyl Tablets (p.1251·3), 4 tablets; Fleet Bisacodyl Suppositories, 1 suppository.
*Bowel evacuation.*

**Fleet Prep Kit No. 2** *Fleet, USA.*
*Combination pack:* Fleet Phospho-Soda; Fleet Bisacodyl Tablets (p.1251·3), 4 tablets; Fleet Bagenema, 1 enema.
*Bowel evacuation.*

**Fleet Prep Kit No. 3** *Fleet, USA.*
*Combination pack:* Fleet Phospho-Soda; Fleet Bisacodyl Tablets (p.1251·3), 4 tablets; Fleet Bisacodyl Enema.
*Bowel evacuation.*

**Fleet Ready-to-Use**
*Fleet, Austral.; De Witt, UK.*
Monobasic sodium phosphate (p.1230·3); dibasic sodium phosphate (p.1231·1).
*Bowel evacuation; constipation.*

**Flemex**
*Note. This name is used for preparations of different composition.*
*Precimex, Mex.†.*
Hydrocortisone (p.1103·3).
*Corticosteroid.*

*Pfizer Consumer, S.Afr.; Gemardi, Thai.*
Carbocisteine (p.1116·2).
*Respiratory-tract disorders associated with increased or viscous mucus.*

**Flemex Jat** *Recalcine, Chile.*
Codeine phosphate (p.27·1); pseudoephedrine hydrochloride (p.1129·2); chlorphenamine maleate (p.427·3); tolu (p.1131·3); herbs.
*Coughs.*

**Flemex-AC** *Gemardi, Thai.*
Acetylcysteine (p.1112·3).
*Respiratory-tract disorders associated with increased or viscous mucus.*

**Flemeze** *Pfizer Consumer, S.Afr.*
Orciprenaline sulfate (p.790·2); bromhexine hydrochloride (p.1115·3).
*Coughs.*

**Flemgo** *Alliance, S.Afr.*
Carbocisteine (p.1116·2).
*Respiratory-tract disorders with increased or viscous mucus.*

**Flemina** *Precimex, Mex.†.*
Dopamine (p.907·3).

**Fleminosan** *Pharmathen, Hong Kong.*
Clindamycin phosphate (p.194·2).
*Acne.*

**Flemizyme** *Pascual, Hong Kong.*
Muramidase hydrochloride (p.1717·2).
*Haemorrhage; sinusitis.*

**Flemlite** *Garec, S.Afr.*
Carbocisteine (p.1116·2).
*Respiratory-tract disorders with increased or viscous mucus.*

**Flemoxin**
*Yamanouchi, Belg.; Yamanouchi, Denm.; Yamanouchi, Fin.; Gerolimatos (Γερολυματος), Gr.; East India Pharma, India; Yamanouchi, Neth.; Yamanouchi, Port.; Yamanouchi, Swed.†; Yamanouchi, Switz.*
Amoxicillin (p.155·3), amoxicillin sodium (p.155·3), or amoxicillin trihydrate (p.155·3).
*Bacterial infections.*

**Flemoxine** *Yamanouchi, Fr.*
Amoxicillin trihydrate (p.155·3).
*Bacterial infections.*

**Flemoxon**
*Temis, Arg.; Merck, Braz.; Merck, Mex.*
Amoxicillin trihydrate (p.155·3).
*Bacterial infections.*

**Flemun** *Intermuti, Ger.*
Sitosterol (p.982·3).
*Rheumatic disorders.*

**Flenalgin** *Kanda, Braz.†.*
Metixene hydrochloride (p.485·3); dipyrone (p.35·3).
*Smooth muscle spasm.*

**Flenid** *Merckle, Ger.*
Sodium cromoglicate (p.795·3).
*Hypersensitivity reactions.*

**Flenin** *Schuck, Ger.*
Homoeopathic preparation.

**Flenverme** *Hipolabor, Braz.†.*
Mebendazole (p.108·2); tiabendazole (p.114·2).
*Worm infections.*

**Flepin X-3** *Farcoral, Mex.*
Paracetamol (p.76·2); phenylephrine (p.1126·3); chlorphenamine (p.428·1); moroxydine hydrochloride (p.649·3).
*Cold symptoms.*

**Flerox**
*Note. This name is used for preparations of different composition.*
*Pharmacia, Arg.*
Leucocianidol (p.1688·2).
*Capillary disorders; haemorrhoids; venous insufficiency.*

*Instituto Sanitas, Chile.*
Flunarizine (p.434·2).
*Mental function impairment; migraine; motion sickness; peripheral vascular disorders; vestibular disorders.*

**Flerudin** *Janssen-Cilag, Spain.*
Flunarizine hydrochloride (p.434·1).
*Migraine; vertigo.*

**Fletanol** *Sante Naturelle, Canad.*
Vitamin A and vitamin D (p.1417·1).

**Fletchers Arachis Oil Retention Enema** *Forest Laboratories, UK.*
Arachis oil (p.1656·1).
*Constipation.*

**Fletchers Castoria** *Mentholatum, USA.*
Senna (p.1288·2).
*Constipation.*

**Fletchers Enemette**
*Pharmax, Irl.†; Forest Laboratories, UK.*
Docusate sodium (p.1262·2).
*Bowel evacuation; constipation.*

**Fletchers Phosphate Enema**
*Pharmax, Irl.; Forest Laboratories, UK.*
Monobasic sodium phosphate (p.1230·3); dibasic sodium phosphate (p.1231·1).
*Bowel evacuation; constipation.*

**Fletchers Sore Mouth Medicine** *Nasmark, Canad.*
Alum (p.1652·1); potassium chlorate (p.1734·2).
*Canker sores; denture irritation; herpes labialis.*

**Flevic** *Microsules Bernabo, Arg.*
*Enterococcus faecium* (p.1704·2).
*Maintenance of normal gastrointestinal flora.*

**Flexafen** *Diba, Mex.*
Ibuprofen (p.45·3).
*Inflammation; musculoskeletal, joint, and peri-articular disorders; pain.*

**Flexagen** *Aspen, S.Afr.†.*
Diclofenac sodium (p.32·1).
*Inflammation; musculoskeletal and joint disorders; pain.*

**Flexagil** *Kern, Spain.*
Carisoprodol (p.1392·1); propyphenazone (p.85·3).
*Musculoskeletal spasms.*

**Flexal Brennessel** *Biocur, Ger.*
Urtica (p.1762·1).
*Rheumatic pain.*

**Flexal Vitamin E** *Biocur, Ger.*
*d*-Alpha tocopherol (p.1464·3).
*Vitamin E deficiency.*

**Flex-All**
*Note. This name is used for preparations of different composition.*
*Martin, Arg.*
Menthol (p.1711·3).

*Chattem, Canad.*
*Topical gel:* Menthol (p.1711·3).
*Muscle and joint pain.*
*Topical stick:* Menthol (p.1711·3); methyl salicylate (p.59·3).
*Musculoskeletal, joint, peri-articular, and soft-tissue disorders.*

**Flex-all 454** *Chattem, USA.*
Menthol (p.1711·3); methyl salicylate (p.59·3).
*Musculoskeletal pain and stiffness.*

**Flexamina** *Climax, Braz.*
Diclofenac sodium (p.32·1).

**Flexaphen** *Trimen, USA.*
Chlorzoxazone (p.1392·3); paracetamol (p.76·2).
*Musculoskeletal pain.*

**Flexar** *Menarini, Port.*
Piroxicam (p.84·2).
*Gout; musculoskeletal, joint, and peri-articular disorders; pain.*

**Flexase** *TAD, Ger.*
Piroxicam (p.84·2).
*Gout; musculoskeletal, joint, and soft-tissue disorders.*

**Flex-Care**
*Alcon, Braz.†.*
Chlorhexidine (p.1173·2); thiomersal (p.1194·1); disodium edetate (p.1037·3) (p.1164·2).
*Cleansing solution for contact lenses.*

*Alcon, Mex.*
Solution for complete care of soft contact lenses (p.1164·2).

*Alcon, USA.*
Range of solutions for contact lenses (p.1164·2).

**Flexdor** *Bunker, Braz.*
Orphenadrine citrate (p.486·1); dipyrone (p.35·3); caffeine (p.782·1).
*Skeletal muscle spasm.*

**Flexelite** *Bros, Gr.*
Amikacin sulfate (p.154·1).
*Bacterial infections.*

**Flexen**
*Note. This name is used for preparations of different composition.*
*Italfarmaco, Ital.*
Ketoprofen (p.51·2).
*Gout; musculoskeletal, joint, peri-articular, and soft-tissue disorders.*

*Rayere, Mex.*
Naproxen (p.65·1).
*Inflammation; musculoskeletal and joint disorders.*

**Flexeril**
*Alza, Canad.; McNeil, USA.*
Cyclobenzaprine hydrochloride (p.1393·1).
*Skeletal muscle spasm.*

**Flexeze** *Goldshield, Singapore.*
Glucosamine sulfate (p.1694·1); chondroitin sulfate (p.1670·2); vitamin C (p.1460·2); calcium (p.1225·1).
*Maintenance of joint and connective tissue function.*

**Flexfree** *Whitehall, Belg.†.*
Felbinac (p.39·1).
*Soft-tissue, peri-articular, and joint pain and inflammation.*

**Flexiban**
*SIT, Ital.; Frosst, Port.*
Cyclobenzaprine hydrochloride (p.1393·1).
*Skeletal muscle spasm.*

**Flexicamin** *Sidus, Arg.*
Piroxicam (p.84·2); carisoprodol (p.1392·1).
*Musculoskeletal, joint, and peri-articular disorders.*

**Flexicamin A** *Sidus, Arg.*
Piroxicam (p.84·2); carisoprodol (p.1392·1); dipyrone (p.35·3).
*Musculoskeletal, joint, and peri-articular disorders; pain.*

**Flexicamin B12** *Sidus, Arg.*
Piroxicam (p.84·2); carisoprodol (p.1392·1); dexamethasone (p.1097·1); pyridoxine (p.1457·2); hydroxocobalamin (p.1458·2).
*Musculoskeletal, joint, peri-articular, and soft-tissue disorders; neuritis.*

**Flexicamin Crema** *Sidus, Arg.*
Piroxicam (p.84·2); myrtecaine (p.1381·3).
*Musculoskeletal, joint, peri-articular, and soft-tissue disorders.*

**Flexican** *Libbs, Braz.†.*
Meloxicam (p.56·1).

**Flexidin** *Mundipharma, Austria.*
Indometacin (p.47·3).
*Gout; inflammation; musculoskeletal, joint, and peri-articular disorders; oedema; pain.*

**Flexidol**
*Note. This name is used for preparations of different composition.*
*Raffo, Arg.*
Meloxicam (p.56·1).
*Inflammation; pain.*

*Almirall, Spain.*
Fepradinol hydrochloride (p.43·1).
*Peri-articular disorders; soft-tissue disorders.*

**Flexidon** *Cosmopharm, Gr.*
Nizatidine (p.1277·2).
*Gastro-oesophageal reflux disease; peptic ulcer.*

**Flexidone** *Poli, Ital.†.*
Carisoprodol (p.1392·1); propyphenazone (p.85·3).
*Musculoskeletal and joint disorders.*

**Flexifer** *Pulitzer, Ital.*
Ferrous gluconate (p.1428·1).
Ascorbic acid (p.1460·2) is included in this preparation to increase the absorption and availability of iron.
*Iron-deficiency anaemia.*

**flexi-loges** *Loges, Ger.*
Devil's claw root (p.28·2).
*Musculoskeletal and joint disorders.*

**Flexin**
*Note. This name is used for preparations of different composition.*
*Taro, Israel.*
Orphenadrine citrate (p.486·1).
*Skeletal muscle spasm.*

*Douglas, Thai.†; TTN, Thai.†.*
Naproxen (p.65·1).
*Dysmenorrhoea; gout; musculoskeletal, joint, and peri-articular disorders.*

**Flexin Continus**
*Napp, Irl.; Napp, UK.*
Indometacin (p.47·3).
*Gout; inflammation; musculoskeletal, joint, and peri-articular disorders; pain.*

**Flexirox** *Viatris, Fr.†.*
Piroxicam (p.84·2).
*Musculoskeletal, joint, and peri-articular disorders.*

**Flexital**
*Sun, Singapore†; Sun, Thai.*
Pentoxifylline (p.979·3).
*Cerebral, ocular, and peripheral vascular disorders.*

**Flexitec** *Technilab, Canad.*
Cyclobenzaprine hydrochloride (p.1393·1).

**Flexium** *Aventis, Belg.*
Etofenamate (p.38·1).
*Lumbar spondylosis; peri-articular disorders; soft-tissue injury.*

**Flexocutan N** *Orion, Ger.†.*
Flufenamic acid (p.43·2); glycol salicylate (p.44·3); benzyl nicotinate (p.21·2).
*Bruising; muscle and joint disorders; neuralgia.*

**Flexogyne** *Biogyne, Fr.†.*
Benzalkonium chloride (p.1168·3).
*Contraceptive.*

**Flexoject** *Mayrand, USA†.*
Orphenadrine citrate (p.486·1).
*Musculoskeletal pain.*

**Flexon** *Keene, USA.*
Orphenadrine citrate (p.486·1).
*Musculoskeletal pain.*

**Flexono** *Instituto Sanitas, Chile.*
Indometacin (p.47·3).
Aluminium glycinate (p.1249·1) is included in this preparation in an attempt to limit adverse effects on the gastrointestinal mucosa.
*Inflammation; pain.*

**Flexotard** *Pharmacia, UK†.*
Diclofenac sodium (p.32·1).
*Gout; inflammation; musculoskeletal, joint, peri-articular, and soft-tissue disorders; pain.*

**Flex-Power Performance Sports** *Flex-Power, USA.*
Trolamine salicylate (p.95·3).
*Musculoskeletal and joint disorders.*

**Flextoss** *Teuto, Braz.*
Dropropizine (p.1119·3).
*Coughs.*

**Flextra** *Poly, USA.*
Paracetamol (p.76·2); phenyltoloxamine citrate (p.439·1).
*Pain.*

**Flexurat**
*Note. This name is used for preparations of different composition.*
*Nycomed, Austria†.*
Suprarenal cortex (p.1110·1); pentosan polysulfate sodium (p.979·2).
*Peri-articular, and soft-tissue disorders.*

*Truw, Ger.†.*
Bovine suprarenal cortex (p.1110·1); diethylamine salamidacetate (p.87·3); pentosan polysulfate sodium (p.979·2).
*Joint and soft-tissue disorders.*

**Flezol** *Ferrer, Spain.*
Zolmitriptan (p.473·3).
*Migraine.*

**Flicum** *Distriquimica, Spain.*
Flubendazole (p.105·2).
*Ascariasis; enterobiasis; hookworm infections; trichuriasis.*

**Flindix** *Vitoria, Port.*
Isosorbide dinitrate (p.941·1).
*Angina pectoris; heart failure; myocardial infarction.*

**flint** *Togal, Ger.*
Poly(butylmethacrylate, methylmethacrylate) (p.1714·3).
*Wounds.*

**Flintstones**
*Bayer Consumer, Canad.; Bayer, Singapore; Miles Consumer Healthcare, USA.*
Multivitamins or multivitamins and minerals (p.1417·1).

**Flipal** *Alpes Chemie, Chile.*
Mefenamic acid (p.55·2).
*Pain.*

**Flivas** *Asahi, Jpn.*
Naftopidil (p.964·1).

**Flixoderm** *GlaxoSmithKline, Ital.*
Fluticasone propionate (p.1102·3).
*Skin disorders.*

**Flixonase**
*GlaxoSmithKline, Arg.; GlaxoSmithKline, Austria; GlaxoSmithKline, Belg.; GlaxoSmithKline, Braz.; GlaxoSmithKline, Chile; GlaxoSmithKline, Denm.; GlaxoSmithKline, Fin.; GlaxoSmithKline, Fr.; GlaxoSmithKline, Hong Kong; Allen & Hanburys, Irl.; GlaxoSmithKline, Israel; GlaxoSmithKline, Ital.; GlaxoSmithKline, Malaysia; Glaxo Wellcome, Mex.; GlaxoSmithKline, Neth.; GlaxoSmithKline, NZ; GlaxoSmithKline, S.Afr.; GlaxoSmithKline, Singapore; GlaxoSmithKline, Spain; GlaxoSmithKline, Thai.; GlaxoSmithKline Consumer, UK.*
Fluticasone propionate (p.1102·3).
*Allergic rhinitis; nasal polyps.*

**Flixotaide** *Glaxo Wellcome, Port.*
Fluticasone propionate (p.1102·3).
*Asthma.*

**Flixotide**
*GlaxoSmithKline, Arg.; Allen & Hanburys, Austral.; GlaxoSmithKline, Austria; GlaxoSmithKline, Belg.; GlaxoSmithKline, Braz.; GlaxoSmithKline, Chile; GlaxoSmithKline, Denm.; GlaxoSmithKline, Fin.; GlaxoSmithKline, Fr.; Glaxo Wellcome, Gr.; GlaxoSmithKline, Hong Kong; Allen & Hanburys, Irl.; GlaxoSmithKline, Israel; GlaxoSmithKline, Ital.; GlaxoSmithKline, Malaysia; Glaxo Wellcome, Mex.; GlaxoSmithKline, Neth.; GlaxoSmithKline, NZ; GlaxoSmithKline, S.Afr.; GlaxoSmithKline, Singapore; GlaxoSmithKline, Spain; GlaxoSmithKline, Thai.; Allen & Hanburys, UK.*
Fluticasone propionate (p.1102·3).
*Allergic rhinitis; asthma; skin disorders.*

**Flixovate** *GlaxoSmithKline, Fr.*
Fluticasone propionate (p.1102·3).
*Skin disorders.*

**Flobac** *Pharmus, Braz.†.*
Ciprofloxacin (p.188·2).
*Bacterial infections.*

**Flobacin** *Sigma-Tau, Ital.*
Ofloxacin (p.239·3).
*Bacterial infections.*

**Flocet** *Collins, Mex.*
Fluoxetine (p.296·3).
*Depression.*

**Flociprin**
*Phoinix Pharm (Φοινιξ Φαρμ), Gr.; Ibi, Ital.*
Ciprofloxacin hydrochloride (p.188·2) or ciprofloxacin lactate (p.188·3).
*Bacterial infections.*

**Flo-Coat** *Lafayette, USA.*
Barium sulfate (p.1061·1).
*Contrast medium for gastrointestinal radiography.*

**Flocofil** *Serono, Mex.†.*
Mercaptopurine (p.567·2).

**Flocur**
*Beta, Arg.; Pharmacia Upjohn, Mex.†.*
Tolfenamic acid (p.94·2).
*Pain.*

**Flodeneu** *Remedina, Gr.*
Piroxicam (p.84·2).
*Dysmenorrhoea; gout; inflammation; musculoskeletal and joint disorders; pain.*

**Flodermol** *Juventus, Spain.*
Fluocinolone acetonide (p.1101·2); gramicidin (p.220·2); neomycin sulfate (p.235·1).
*Infected skin disorders.*

**Flodil** *AstraZeneca, Fr.*
Felodipine (p.914·3).
*Angina pectoris; hypertension.*

**Flodol** *Uno, Ital.*
Piroxicam (p.84·2).
*Musculoskeletal, joint, and peri-articular disorders.*

**Flogan** *Merck, Braz.*
Diclofenac (p.32·1), diclofenac potassium (p.32·1), or diclofenac resinate (p.33·1).
*Gout; inflammation; musculoskeletal, joint, and peri-articular disorders; pain.*

**Flogecyl** *Wild, Switz.*
Aescin beta (p.1648·2); carrageenan (p.1578·2).
*Mouth disorders.*

**Flogen** *Fustery, Mex.*
Naproxen sodium (p.65·1).
*Inflammation; pain.*

**Flogencyl** *Expanpharm, Fr.*
Aescin (p.1648·2).
*Mouth ulcers.*

**Flogene**
*Note. This name is used for preparations of different composition.*
*Ache, Braz.*
Piroxicam betadex (p.84·2).
*Dysmenorrhoea; gout; musculoskeletal, joint, and peri-articular disorders.*

*Polifarma, Ital.†.*
Fentiazac (p.43·1) or fentiazac calcium (p.43·1).
*Fever; inflammation; pain.*

**Flogesic** *Klinger, Braz.*
Diclofenac sodium (p.32·1).

**Flogiatrin** *Sanofi Synthelabo, Arg.*
Carisoprodol (p.1392·1); piroxicam (p.84·2).
*Musculoskeletal and joint disorders.*

**Flogiatrin B12** *Sanofi Synthelabo, Arg.*
Carisoprodol (p.1392·1); piroxicam (p.84·2); dexamethasone (p.1097·1); pyridoxine (p.1457·2); hydroxocobalamin (p.1458·2).
*Musculoskeletal, joint, and soft-tissue disorders; neuritis.*

**Flogiftalmina** *Davi, Port.*
Phenylephrine hydrochloride (p.1126·3); prednisolone metasulfobenzoate sodium (p.1108·1).
*Eye disorders.*

**Flogilid** *Luper, Braz.*
Nimesulide (p.67·1).

**Floginax** *Teofarma, Ital.*
Naproxen (p.65·1).
*Musculoskeletal and joint disorders; pain.*

**Flogin-Ped** *Stiefel, Braz.*
Benzydamine hydrochloride (p.21·1).
*Fever; inflammation; pain.*

**Flogiren** *Sanval, Braz.*
Diclofenac (p.32·1).
*Gout; inflammation; musculoskeletal, joint, and peri-articular disorders; pain.*

**Flogo Rosa** *Asta Medica, Braz.*
Benzydamine hydrochloride (p.21·1).
*Vaginal irritation.*

**Flogobene** *Upsamedica, Ital.†.*
Piroxicam (p.84·2).
*Musculoskeletal and joint disorders.*

**Flogocan** *Quimedical, Port.*
Piroxicam (p.84·2).
*Gout; musculoskeletal, joint, and peri-articular disorders; pain.*

**Flogocefal** *Lacefa, Arg.*
Naproxen (p.65·1).
*Fever; inflammation; pain.*

**Flogocid**
*Note. This name is used for preparations of different composition.*
*Continental Pharma, Belg.†.*
Bufexamac (p.21·3); neomycin sulfate (p.235·1); nystatin (p.406·3).
*Infected skin disorders.*

*Continental Pharma, Switz.†.*
Bufexamac (p.21·3).
*Skin disorders.*

**Flogocid NN** *Continental Pharma, Switz.†.*
Bufexamac (p.21·3); nystatin (p.406·3); neomycin sulfate (p.235·1).
*Infected skin disorders.*

**Flogocort** *Bago, Chile.*
Mometasone furoate (p.1107·2).
*Skin disorders.*

**Flogodisten** *Bago, Arg.*
Niflumic acid (p.67·1); orphenadrine citrate (p.486·1); aluminium hydroxide (p.1249·2).

**Flogofenac** *Ecobi, Ital.*
Diclofenac diethylamine (p.32·1) or diclofenac sodium (p.32·1).
*Musculoskeletal, joint, and soft-tissue disorders.*

**Flogofin** *Laboratorios Chile, Chile.*
Ketoprofen (p.51·2).
*Gout; musculoskeletal, joint, and peri-articular disorders; pain.*

**Flogogin**
*Note. This name is used for preparations of different composition.*
*Angelini, Ital.*
*Injection; suppositories:* Naproxen sodium (p.65·1). Lidocaine hydrochloride (p.1377·3) and lidocaine (p.1377·3) are included in the intramuscular injection to alleviate the pain of injection.
*Musculoskeletal and joint disorders; pain.*

*Tosi, Ital.†.*
*Topical gel:* Naproxen sodium (p.65·1); a heparinoid (p.931·1).
*Inflammation; musculoskeletal and joint disorders; pain.*

**Flogojet** *Andromaco, Chile.*
Etofenamate (p.38·1).
*Musculsoskeletal, joint, peri-articular, and soft-tissue disorders.*

**Flogoken** *Kener, Mex.*
Diclofenac (p.32·1).
*Inflammation.*

**Flogol-gel** *Lazar, Arg.*
Etofenamate (p.38·1).
*Musculoskeletal, joint, and soft-tissue disorders.*

**Flogonac** *Haller, Braz.*
Diclofenac potassium (p.32·1) or diclofenac resinate (p.33·1).
*Fever; inflammation; pain.*

**Flogoprofen** *Chiesi, Spain.*
Etofenamate (p.38·1).
*Pain; peri-articular disorders.*

**Flogoral**
*Asta Medica, Braz.; Lepori, Port.*
Benzydamine hydrochloride (p.21·1).
*Mouth and throat disorders.*

**Flogosan** *Liomont, Mex.†.*
Piroxicam (p.84·2).
*Inflammation; musculoskeletal and joint disorders; pain.*

**Flogosine** *Ahimsa, Arg.*
Piroxicam (p.84·2).
*Inflammation; pain.*

**Flogostop** *Zekides, Gr.*
Nimesulide (p.67·1).
*Inflammation; musculoskeletal disorders; pain.*

**Flogoter** *Estedi, Spain.*
Indometacin (p.47·3).
*Gout; inflammation; musculoskeletal and joint disorders; pain; peri-articular disorders.*

**Flogotisol**
*Zambon, Braz.†; Zambon, Ital.†.*
Thiamphenicol sodium glycinate isophthalolate (p.269·3).
Lidocaine (p.1377·3) may be included in the injection to alleviate the pain of injection.
*Bacterial infections.*

**Flogovis** *Amnol, Ital.*
Aesculus; bromelains; pineapple; zinc sulfate; copper sulfate (p.1417·1).
*Inflammation; nutritional supplement; oedema.*

**Flogovis IdroGel** *Amnol, Ital.*
Aescin (p.1648·2); bromelains (p.1662·2).
*Inflammation; oedema.*

**Flogovital** *Bago, Arg.*
Niflumic acid (p.67·1).
*Inflammation.*

**Flogovital NF** *Bago, Arg.*
Nimesulide (p.67·1).
*Inflammation.*

**Flogoxen** *Medley, Braz.*
Piroxicam (p.84·2).
*Dysmenorrhoea; gout; musculoskeletal, joint, and peri-articular disorders.*

**Flogozen** *Valeas, Ital.†.*
Imidazole salicylate (p.47·2).
*Fever; otorhinolaryngeal inflammation.*

**Flogozyme** *Norma (Νορμα), Gr.*
Betamethasone valerate (p.1093·2).
*Topical corticosteroid.*

**Flohale** *Cipla, India.*
Fluticasone propionate (p.1102·3).
*Asthma.*

**Flolan**
*GlaxoSmithKline, Austral.; GlaxoSmithKline, Austria; GlaxoSmithKline, Belg.; GlaxoSmithKline, Canad.; GlaxoSmithKline, Denm.; GlaxoSmithKline, Fr.; Wellcome, Irl.; GlaxoSmithKline, Israel; GlaxoSmithKline, Ital.; GlaxoSmithKline, Neth.; GlaxoSmithKline, Norw.; GlaxoSmithKline, Singapore; GlaxoSmithKline, Spain; GlaxoSmithKline, Switz.; GlaxoSmithKline, UK; Glaxo Wellcome, USA.*
Epoprostenol sodium (p.1516·3).
*Pulmonary hypertension; thrombosis prophylaxis during renal dialysis.*

**Flolid** *CT, Ital.*
Nimesulide (p.67·1).
*Fever; inflammation; pain.*

**Flomax**
*Note. This name is used for preparations of different composition.*
*CSL, Austral.; Boehringer Ingelheim, Canad.; Pharmaco, NZ; Yamanouchi, NZ; Pharmaplan, S.Afr.; Yamanouchi, UK; Boehringer Ingelheim, USA.*
Tamsulosin hydrochloride (p.1009·2).
Formerly known as Omnic in *NZ.*
*Benign prostatic hyperplasia.*

*Chiesi, Ital.*
Morniflumate (p.60·1).
*Fever; inflammation; pain.*

**Flomed** *Pulitzer, Ital.*
Buflomedil hydrochloride (p.877·2).
*Cerebral and peripheral vascular disorders.*

**Flomox** *Shionogi, Jpn.*
Cefcapene pivoxil hydrochloride (p.171·3).
*Bacterial infections.*

**Flonase**
*GlaxoSmithKline, Canad.; Glaxo Wellcome, USA.*
Fluticasone propionate (p.1102·3).
*Allergic rhinitis.*

**Flonital** *Anpharm (Ανφαρμ), Gr.*
Fluoxetine hydrochloride (p.292·1).
*Depression; obsessive-compulsive disorder; panic disorder.*

**Flonorm** *Schering-Plough, Mex.*
Rifaximin (p.254·1).
*Bacterial infections of the gastro-intestinal tract; diarrhoea; diverticular disease; hyperammonaemia secondary to hepatic encephalopathy.*

**Flopen** *CSL, Austral.*
Flucloxacillin magnesium (p.213·3) or flucloxacillin sodium (p.213·3).
*Gram-positive coccal infections.*

**florabio Mann-Feigen-Sirup mit Senna** *Florabio, Ger.*
Fig (p.1266·3); cassia; manna (p.1273·1).
*Constipation.*

**florabio naturreiner Heilpflanzensaft** *Florabio, Ger.*
A range of plant extracts.

**Floradix** *Salus, Fr.†.*
Nutritional supplement with iron (p.1417·1).

**Floradix Krauterblut** *Salushaus, Ger.*
*Oral liquid:* Ferrous gluconate (p.1428·1); thiamine hydrochloride; riboflavine sodium phosphate; pyridoxine hydrochloride; cyanocobalamin (p.1417·1).
*Iron deficiency; tonic.*
*Tablets:* Ferrous gluconate; folic acid; thiamine hydrochloride; riboflavin; nicotinamide (p.1417·1).
*Tonic.*

**Floradix Maskam** *Duopharm, Ger.†.*
Frangula bark (p.1266·3); rhubarb (p.1287·3); senna (p.1288·2); fennel (p.1687·2).
*Constipation.*

**Floradix Multipretten N** *Salushaus, Ger.*
Caraway (p.1667·2); caraway oil (p.1667·3); fennel (p.1687·2); fennel oil (p.1687·3); aniseed (p.1655·2) anise oil (p.1655·2); coriander (p.1676·1); coriander oil (p.1676·1); peppermint leaf (p.1283·2); peppermint oil (p.1283·2); absinthium (p.1645·1); achillea (p.1646·2).
*Gastrointestinal disorders.*

**Floralac** *Fresenius Kabi, Austria.*
Lactulose (p.1269·1).
*Constipation.*

**Floralax** *Flora, Canad.†.*
Ispaghula (p.1268·1).

**Floralaxative** *Lalco, Canad.†.*
Buckthorn (p.1254·1); senna (p.1288·2).

**Floraquin**
*Searle, Austral.†; Searle, Thai.†.*
Diiodohydroxyquinoline (p.603·3); boric acid (p.1662·1); phosphoric acid (p.1731·2).
*Vaginal infections.*

**Florate** *Alcon, Braz.*
Fluorometholone acetate (p.1102·2).
*Eye disorders.*

**Floratil**
*Merck, Arg.; Merck, Braz.; Merck, Mex.*
Lysate of *Saccharomyces boulardii* (p.1704·2).
*Diarrhoea; restoration of gastrointestinal flora.*

**Florax** *Hebron, Braz.*
*Saccharomyces cerevisiae* (p.1469·1).
*Diarrhoea; restoration of gastrointestinal flora.*

**Floraxina** *Amhof, Arg.*
Ciprofloxacin hydrochloride (p.188·2).
*Bacterial eye infections.*

**Florbiox** *Crinos, Ital.*
Multivitamin and mineral preparation with *Lactobacillus acidophilus* (p.1417·1)(p.1704·2).
*Maintenance of gastrointestinal flora.*

**Floregin** *Abbott, Braz.†.*
Muramidase hydrochloride (p.1717·2); nimorazole (p.611·3).
*Vulvovaginal infections.*

**Floregin Composto** *Abbott, Braz.†.*
Nimorazole (p.611·3); clotrimazole (p.396·2); muramidase (p.1717·2).
*Vulvovaginal infections.*

**Florelax** *Sanofi Synthelabo, Ital.*
Dried yeast (p.1469·1); lactic-acid-producing organisms (p.1704·2); chamomile (p.1669·3); angelica (p.1655·1); valerian (p.1762·2); peppermint leaf (p.1283·2); caraway (p.1667·2); vitamin B substances (p.1417·1).
*Gastrointestinal disorders.*

**Florelax Stomaco** *Sanofi Synthelabo, Ital.*
Pineapple stem; rice starch; dog rose; green tea (p.1417·1).
*Gastrointestinal disorders.*

**Florerbe Lassativa** *Bonomelli, Ital.†.*
Senna (p.1288·2); boldo (p.1661·2); cynara (p.1678·3); aniseed (p.1655·2); liquorice (p.1270·2).
*Constipation.*

**Floresse** *Roche Consumer, UK.*
Borage oil (p.1661·3) with or without vitamins.

**Florexal** *Silanes, Mex.*
Fluoxetine hydrochloride (p.292·1).
*Bulimia; depression; obsessive-compulsive disorder.*

**Florgynal** *Lyocentre, Fr.*
Estriol (p.1552·3); progesterone (p.1566·2); *Lactobacillus casei* var. *Rhamnosus* (p.1704·2).
*Adjunct in gynaecological surgery during menopause; vulvovaginitis.*

**Florical** *Mericon, USA.*
Calcium carbonate (p.1254·2); sodium fluoride (p.1444·3).
*Dietary supplement.*

**Floridine** *DHN, Fr.†.*
Preparation for enteral nutrition (p.1417·1).

**Floridral** *Dicofarm, Ital.*
Glucose; sodium citrate; potassium chloride; sodium chloride; aspartame; *Lactobacillus* (p.1222·2)(p.1704·2).
*Diarrhoea; disturbances of the gastrointestinal microbial flora; oral rehydration therapy.*

**Florigien** *Schering, Ital.†.*
Nonoxinol 9 (p.1413·3); phenoxyethanol (p.1189·1); sodium laurilsulfate (p.1574·2); thymol (p.1194·2).
*Vaginal infections.*

**Florilax**
*Note. This name is used for preparations of different composition.*
*Floris, Israel.*
Senna (p.1288·2).
*Constipation.*

*Confar, Port.*
Glucomannan (p.1693·3).
*Constipation; hyperlipidaemias; obesity.*

**Florinef**
*Bristol-Myers Squibb, Austral.; Shire, Canad.; Bristol-Myers Squibb, Chile; Bristol-Myers Squibb, Denm.; Bristol-Myers Squibb, Fin.; IFET (ΙΦΕΤ), Gr.; Bristol-Myers Squibb, Hong Kong; Bristol-Myers Squibb, Irl.; Bristol-Myers Squibb, Israel; Bristol-Myers Squibb, Malaysia; Bristol-Myers Squibb, Neth.; Bristol-Myers Squibb, Norw.; Bristol-Myers Squibb, NZ; Bristol-Myers Squibb, S.Afr.; Bristol-Myers Squibb, Singapore; Bristol-Myers Squibb, Swed.; Bristol-Myers Squibb, Switz.; Bristol-Myers Squibb, Thai.; Bristol-Myers Squibb, UK; Monarch, USA.*
Fludrocortisone acetate (p.1100·1).
*Adrenocortical insufficiency; congenital adrenal hyperplasia.*

**Florinefe** *Bristol-Myers Squibb, Braz.*
Fludrocortisone acetate (p.1100·1).
*Adrenocortical insufficiency; congenital adrenal hyperplasia; orthostatic hypotension.*

**Florisan** *Boehringer Ingelheim, Gr.*
Docusate sodium (p.1262·2); bisacodyl (p.1251·3).
*Constipation.*

**Florisan N** *Boehringer Ingelheim, Ger.*
Bisacodyl (p.1251·3).
*Constipation.*

**Florisene** *Lamberts Healthcare, UK.*
Ferrous glycine sulfate; vitamin C; vitamin $B_{12}$; lysine (p.1417·1).
*Hair loss in women.*

**Florissamol** *Andrae, Austria.*
Urtica (p.1762·1); camphor (p.1665·3).
*Chilblains; muscle and joint pain; scalp disorders; soft-tissue disorders.*

**Florlax** *Cazi, Braz.*
Senna (p.1288·2); tamarind (p.1293·2); coriander (p.1676·1); cassia pulp (p.1255·2).
*Constipation.*

**Florocycline** *SmithKline Beecham, Fr.†.*
Tetracycline hydrochloride (p.266·2).
*Bacterial infections.*

**Florone**
*Pharmacia Upjohn, Canad.†; Galderma, Ger.; Dermik, USA.*
Diflorasone diacetate (p.1099·3).
*Skin disorders.*

**Florvite** *Everett, USA.*
A range of vitamin and fluoride (p.1444·3) preparations with or without minerals (p.1417·1).
*Dental caries prophylaxis; dietary supplement.*

**Flosa** *Merckle, Ger.*
Ispaghula (p.1268·1).
*Constipation; stool softener.*

**Flosef** *Milmet, India.*
Fluorometholone (p.1102·2).
*Inflammatory eye disorders.*

**Flosine** *Bittermedizin, Ger.*
Ispaghula (p.1268·1).
*Constipation; stool softener.*

**Flossac** *Caber, Ital.*
Norfloxacin (p.238·3).
*Bacterial urinary-tract infections.*

**Flotac**
*Novartis, Arg.; Novartis, Braz.; Novartis, Chile; Novartis, Mex.*
Diclofenac colestyramine (p.33·1).
*Gout; inflammation; musculoskeletal and joint disorders; pain.*

**Flotina** *Lampugnani, Ital.*
Fluoxetine hydrochloride (p.292·1).
*Bulimia nervosa; depression; obsessive-compulsive disorder.*

**Flotiran** *Schering-Plough, Port.*
Betamethasone dipropionate (p.1093·1); clotrimazole (p.396·2).
*Infected skin disorders.*

**Flotrin** *Abbott, Ger.*
Terazosin hydrochloride (p.1010·3).
*Benign prostatic hyperplasia.*

**Flovent**
*GlaxoSmithKline, Canad.; Glaxo Wellcome, USA.*
Fluticasone propionate (p.1102·3).
*Asthma.*

**Flowmega** *Lifeplan, UK†.*
Omega-3 marine triglycerides (p.976·2).

**Flox** *Hexal, Braz.*
Norfloxacin (p.238·3).
*Bacterial infections.*

**Floxacin**
*Riel, Austria; Merck Sharp & Dohme, Braz.; Medix, Mex.*
Norfloxacin (p.238·3).
*Bacterial infections.*

**Floxacipron** *BA Farma, Port.*
Ciprofloxacin (p.188·2).
*Bacterial infections.*

**Floxager** *Streger, Mex.*
Ciprofloxacin hydrochloride (p.188·2).
*Bacterial infections.*

**Floxakin** *Kener, Mex.†.*
Ciprofloxacin (p.188·2).
*Bacterial infections.*

**Floxal** *Riel, Austria; Mann, Ger.; Bausch & Lomb, Switz.*
Ofloxacin (p.239·3).
*Bacterial eye infections.*

**Floxalin** *Salus, Ital.*
Naproxen sodium (p.65·1).
*Musculoskeletal and joint disorders; pain.*

**Floxamicin** *Biotenk, Arg.*
Norfloxacin (p.238·3).
*Bacterial infections.*

**Floxan** *Prodotti, Braz.*
Ciprofloxacin (p.188·2).
*Bacterial infections.*

**Floxanor** *Delta, Braz.*
Norfloxacin (p.238·3).
*Bacterial infections.*

**Floxantina** *Degorts, Mex.*
Ciprofloxacin hydrochloride (p.188·2).
*Bacterial infections.*

**Floxapen**
*GlaxoSmithKline, Austral.; GlaxoSmithKline, Austria; GlaxoSmithKline, Belg.; GlaxoSmithKline, Irl.; SmithKline Beecham, Mex.; GlaxoSmithKline, Neth.; GlaxoSmithKline, NZ; Beecham, Port.; GlaxoSmithKline, S.Afr.; SmithKline Beecham, Switz.; GlaxoSmithKline, UK.*
Flucloxacillin magnesium (p.213·3) or flucloxacillin sodium (p.213·3).
*Bacterial infections.*

**Floxaquil** *Decomed, Port.*
Lomefloxacin hydrochloride (p.227·2).
*Bacterial infections.*

**Floxatral** *LA, Arg.*
Norfloxacin (p.238·3).
*Bacterial infections.*

**Floxatrat** *Luper, Braz.*
Norfloxacin (p.238·3).
*Bacterial infections.*

**Floxedol** *Edol, Port.*
Ofloxacin (p.239·3).
*Bacterial eye infections.*

**Floxelena** *Pharmacos Abug, Mex.*
Ciprofloxacin (p.188·2).
*Bacterial infections.*

**Floxen** *Raza, Malaysia; Pharmaniaga, Malaysia.*
Norfloxacin (p.238·3).
*Bacterial infections.*

**Floxenor** *Pose, Thai.†.*
Norfloxacin (p.238·3).
*Bacterial infections.*

**Flox-ex** *Ecosol, Switz.*
Fluvoxamine maleate (p.298·2).
*Depression; obsessive-compulsive disorder.*

**Floxicam** *Neo Quimica, Braz.*
Piroxicam (p.84·2).

**Floxid** *Sintofarma, Braz.*
Roxithromycin (p.254·2).
*Bacterial infections.*

**Floxil**
*Note. This name is used for preparations of different composition.*
*Janssen-Cilag, Arg.; Janssen, Mex.*
Ofloxacin (p.239·3).
*Bacterial infections.*

*Dumex-Alpharma, Hong Kong†.*
Menthol (p.1711·3); tartaric acid (p.1752·1).
*Sore throat.*

*Tecnimede, Port.*
Flucloxacillin sodium (p.213·3).
*Bacterial infections.*

*Dumex-Alpharma, Singapore†.*
Dichlorobenzyl alcohol (p.1178·3); amylmetacresol (p.1168·2); menthol (p.1711·3).
*Sore throat.*

**Floxin**
*Note. This name is used for preparations of different composition.*
*Janssen-Ortho, Canad.; Ortho McNeil, USA; Daiichi, USA.*
Ofloxacin (p.239·3).
*Bacterial infections.*

*Sriprasit, Thai.*
Flunarizine hydrochloride (p.434·1).
*Cerebral and peripheral vascular disorders.*

**Floxinol** *Millet Roux, Braz.*
Norfloxacin (p.238·3).
*Bacterial infections.*

**Floxinon** *Ariston, Braz.*
Pefloxacin (p.241·3).
*Bacterial infections.*

**Floxlevo** *Biotenk, Arg.*
Levofloxacin (p.225·3).
*Bacterial infections.*

**Floxsig** *Sigma, Austral.*
Flucloxacillin sodium (p.213·3).
*Gram-positive coccal infections.*

**Floxstat**
*Janssen-Cilag, Braz.; Cilag, Mex.*
Ofloxacin (p.239·3).
*Bacterial infections.*

**Floxur** *Merind, India.*
Ofloxacin (p.239·3).
*Bacterial infections.*

**Floxyfral**
*Solvay, Austria; Solvay, Belg.; Solvay, Fr.; Solvay, Switz.*
Fluvoxamine maleate (p.298·2).
*Depression; obsessive-compulsive disorder.*

**Flu-21** *Uno, Ital.*
Fluocinonide (p.1101·3).
*Skin disorders.*

**Flu, Cold & Cough Medicine** *Major, USA.*
Chlorphenamine maleate (p.427·3); dextromethorphan hydrobromide (p.1117·3); paracetamol (p.76·2); pseudoephedrine hydrochloride (p.1129·2).
*Coughs and cold symptoms.*

**Flu & Fever Relief** *Brauer, Austral.†.*
Homoeopathic preparation.

**Flu Oph** *Seng, Thai.*
Fluorometholone (p.1102·2).
*Inflammatory eye disorders.*

**Fluad**
*Grunenthal, Austria; Chiron Vaccines, Ital.; Chiron, Singapore; Pacific Biosciences, Singapore; Meda, Swed.*
An inactivated influenza vaccine (p.1620·2).
*Active immunisation.*

**Fluagel** *EMS, Braz.*
Aluminium hydroxide (p.1249·2).
*Gastrointestinal hyperacidity.*

**Flu-Amp** *Generics, UK†.*
Ampicillin trihydrate (p.157·2); flucloxacillin sodium (p.213·3).
These ingredients can be described by the British Approved Name Co-fluampicil.
*Bacterial infections.*

**Fluanxol**
*Lundbeck, Austral.; Lundbeck, Austria; Lundbeck, Belg.; Lundbeck, Canad.; Silesia, Chile; Lundbeck, Denm.; Lundbeck, Fin.; Lundbeck, Fr.; Bayer, Ger.; Lundbeck, Hong Kong; Lundbeck, India; Lundbeck, Irl.; Lundbeck, Israel; Lundbeck, Malaysia; Organon, Mex.; Lundbeck, Neth.; Lundbeck, Norw.; Lundbeck, NZ; Zuellig, NZ; Lundbeck, Port.; Lundbeck, S.Afr.; Lundbeck, Singapore; Lundbeck, Swed.; Lundbeck, Switz.; Lundbeck, Thai.; Lundbeck, UK.*
Flupentixol (p.699·2), flupentixol decanoate (p.699·1), or flupentixol hydrochloride (p.699·1).
*Alcohol or opioid withdrawal syndromes; anxiety; depression; psychoses.*

**Fluarix**
*GlaxoSmithKline, Arg.; GlaxoSmithKline, Austral.; GlaxoSmithKline, Austria; GlaxoSmithKline, Braz.; GlaxoSmithKline, Chile; SmithKline Beecham, Denm.; GlaxoSmithKline, Fin.; GlaxoSmithKline, Fr.; SmithKline Beecham, Gr.; GlaxoSmithKline, Hong Kong; GlaxoSmithKline, Irl.; GlaxoSmithKline, Ital.; SmithKline Beecham, Mex.; SmithKline Beecham, Neth.; GlaxoSmithKline, Norw.; GlaxoSmithKline, NZ; Smith Kline & French, Port.; GlaxoSmithKline, S.Afr.; GlaxoSmithKline, Singapore; GlaxoSmithKline, Spain; GlaxoSmithKline, Swed.; SmithKline Beecham, Switz.; GlaxoSmithKline, Thai.; GlaxoSmithKline, UK.*
An inactivated influenza vaccine (split virion) (p.1620·2).
*Active immunisation.*

**Fluaton** *Tubilux, Ital.*
Fluorometholone (p.1102·2).
*Inflammatory eye disorders.*

**Flubason**
*Aventis, Ital.; Aventis, Spain.*
Desoximetasone (p.1096·3).
*Skin disorders.*

**Flubilar** *Byk, Fr.*
Sodium methylcamphorate.
*Constipation; dyspepsia.*

**Flubiotic NF** *Pharmazam, Spain.*
Amoxicillin trihydrate (p.155·3).
Flubiotic formerly contained acetylcysteine and amoxicillin trihydrate.
*Bacterial infections.*

**Flucacid** *Euro-Pharma, Ital.*
Flucloxacillin sodium (p.213·3).
*Bacterial infections.*

**Flucalin** *Ariston, Arg.*
Calcium gluceptate (p.1225·2); calcium gluconate (p.1225·2); vitamin C (p.1460·2).
*Nutritional supplement.*

**Flucam** *Pfizer, Jpn.*
Ampiroxicam (p.14·2).
*Inflammation; musculoskeletal, joint, and peri-articular disorders; pain.*

**Flucanol**
*Zeus, Braz.; Rafa, Israel.*
Fluconazole (p.398·1).
*Fungal infections.*

**Flucazol** *Cristalia, Braz.*
Fluconazole (p.398·1).
*Fungal infections.*

**Flucef** *Max Farma, Ital.*
Flucloxacillin sodium (p.213·3).
*Bacterial infections.*

**Fluciderm** *Shiwa, Thai.*
Fluocinolone acetonide (p.1101·2).
*Skin disorders.*

**Fluciderm-N** *Shiwa, Thai.*
Fluocinolone acetonide (p.1101·2); neomycin sulfate (p.235·1).
*Infected skin disorders.*

**Flucil**
*Note. This name is used for preparations of different composition.*
*Aspen, Austral.*
Flucloxacillin sodium (p.213·3).
*Gram-positive coccal infections.*

*Masa, Thai.*
Acetylcysteine (p.1112·3).
*Respiratory-tract disorders associated with increased or viscous mucus.*

**Flucillin** *Pinewood, Irl.*
Flucloxacillin sodium (p.213·3).
*Gram-positive bacterial infections.*

**Flucin** *Wayne, Mex.†.*
Fluocinolone (p.1101·2).
*Skin disorders.*

**Flucinal** *Selvi, Ital.*
Flucloxacillin sodium (p.213·3).
*Bacterial infections.*

**Flucinar** *Medphano, Ger.*
Fluocinolone acetonide (p.1101·2).
*Skin disorders.*

**Flucinom** *Schering-Plough, Gr.*
Flutamide (p.556·2).
*Prostatic cancer.*

**Flucinome** *Essex, Switz.*
Flutamide (p.556·2).
*Prostatic cancer.*

**Flucistein** *Uniao Quimica, Braz.*
Acetylcysteine (p.1112·3).
*Respiratory-tract congestion.*

**Fluclomix** *Ashbourne, UK.*
Flucloxacillin sodium (p.213·3).
*Bacterial infections.*

**Fluclon** *Clonmel, Irl.†.*
Flucloxacillin sodium (p.213·3).
*Gram-positive bacterial infections.*

**Fluclox** *Uno, Ital.*
Flucloxacillin sodium (p.213·3).
*Bacterial infections.*

**Flucloxa** *Astrapin, Ger.; Hameln, Ger.*
Flucloxacillin sodium (p.213·3).
*Bacterial infections.*

**Flucloxil** *Duopharma, Hong Kong.*
Flucloxacillin (p.213·3).
*Bacterial infections.*

**Flucloxin**
*Douglas, NZ; Rivopharm, Switz.†.*
Flucloxacillin sodium (p.213·3).
*Gram-positive bacterial infections.*

**Fluclox-Reu** *Reusch, Ger.†.*
Flucloxacillin sodium (p.213·3).
*Bacterial infections.*

**Flucol** *Apotex, S.Afr.†; Garec, S.Afr.†.*
Paracetamol (p.76·2); codeine phosphate (p.27·1); caffeine (p.782·1); mepyramine maleate (p.437·1); phenylephrine hydrochloride (p.1126·3).
*Cold and influenza symptoms; sinusitis.*

**Flucoltrix** *Gallia, Braz.†.*
Fluconazole (p.398·1).
*Fungal infections.*

**Flucon**
*Alcon, Austral.; Alcon, Belg.; Alcon, Fr.; Alkon (Αλκον), Gr.; Alcon, Hong Kong; Alcon, NZ; Alcon, S.Afr.; Alcon, Thai.*
Fluorometholone (p.1102·2).
*Inflammatory eye disorders.*

**Fluconal** *Libbs, Braz.*
Fluconazole (p.398·1).
*Fungal infections.*

**Fluconax** *Ariston, Braz.*
Fluconazole (p.398·1).
*Fungal infections.*

**Fluconeo** *Neo Quimica, Braz.*
Fluconazole (p.398·1).
*Fungal infections.*

**Flucort** *Glenmark, India.*
Fluocinolone acetonide (p.1101·2).
*Skin disorders.*

**Flu-Cortanest** *Piam, Ital.*
Diflucortolone valerate (p.1099·3).
*Burns; insect stings; skin disorders.*

**Flucort-C** *Glenmark, India.*
Fluocinolone acetonide (p.1101·2); ciclopirox olamine (p.396·1).
*Skin disorders.*

**Flucort-H** *Glenmark, India.*
Fluocinolone acetonide (p.1101·2).
*Skin disorders.*

**Flucort-MZ** *Glenmark, India.*
Miconazole nitrate (p.405·3); fluocinolone acetonide (p.1101·2).
*Infected skin disorders.*

**Flucort-N** *Glenmark, India.*
Fluocinolone acetonide (p.1101·2); neomycin sulfate (p.235·1).
*Infected skin disorders.*

**Flucoxan** *Instituto Sanitas, Chile.*
Fluconazole (p.398·1).
*Candidiasis.*

**Flucozal** *Aegis, Hong Kong.*
Fluconazole (p.398·1).
*Candidiasis.*

**Flucozen** *Cazi, Braz.*
Fluconazole (p.398·1).
*Fungal infections.*

**Flucozole** *Siam Bheasach, Thai.*
Fluconazole (p.398·1).
*Fungal infections.*

**Flucreme NM** *Concept, India.*
Fluocinolone acetonide (p.1101·2); neomycin sulfate (p.235·1); miconazole nitrate (p.405·3).
*Infected skin disorders.*

**Fluctin**
*Note. This name is used for preparations of different composition.*
*Osteolab, Chile.*
Fluconazole (p.398·1).
*Fungal infections.*

*Lilly, Ger.*
Fluoxetine hydrochloride (p.292·1).
*Bulimia nervosa; depression; obsessive-compulsive disorder.*

**Fluctine**
*Lilly, Austria; Lilly, Switz.*
Fluoxetine hydrochloride (p.292·1).
*Bulimia nervosa; depression; obsessive-compulsive disorder.*

**Flucur** *Shigaken, Singapore.*
Chlorphenamine maleate (p.427·3); naphazoline hydrochloride (p.1124·3).
*Cold symptoms; rhinitis; sinusitis.*

**Fludac** *Cadila Pharma, India.*
Fluoxetine hydrochloride (p.292·1).
*Depression.*

**Fludactil** *Garec, S.Afr.*
Triprolidine hydrochloride (p.442·3); pseudoephedrine hydrochloride (p.1129·2).
*Cold and influenza symptoms.*

**Fludactil Co** *Garec, S.Afr.*
Triprolidine hydrochloride (p.442·3); pseudoephedrine hydrochloride (p.1129·2); codeine phosphate (p.27·1).
*Coughs.*

**Fludactil Expectorant** *Garec, S.Afr.*
Triprolidine hydrochloride (p.442·3); pseudoephedrine hydrochloride (p.1129·2); guaifenesin (p.1122·1).
*Coughs.*

**Fludan**
*Biolab, Hong Kong; Biopharm, Hong Kong.*
Flunarizine hydrochloride (p.434·1).
*Migraine; vestibular disorders.*

*Biolab, Malaysia; Biolab, Thai.*
Flunarizine (p.434·2).
*Cerebrovascular disorders; migraine.*

**Fludan Codeina** *Ipsen, Spain.*
Codeine phosphate (p.27·1).
*Coughs; diarrhoea; pain.*

**Fludapamide** *Spirig, Switz.*
Indapamide (p.938·2).
*Hypertension.*

**Fludara**
*Schering, Arg.; Schering, Austral.; Schering, Austria; Schering, Belg.; Schering, Braz.; Schering, Chile; Schering, Denm.; Schering, Fin.; Schering, Fr.; MSO, Ger.; Schering, Ger.; Shepa, Gr.; Schering, Hong Kong; Schering, Irl.; Schering, Israel; Schering, Ital.; Schering, Malaysia; Schering, Mex.; Schering, Neth.; Schering, Norw.; Berlex, NZ; Schering, NZ; Schering, Port.; Schering, S.Afr.; Schering, Singapore; Schering, Swed.; Schering, Switz.; Schering, Thai.; Schering, UK; Berlex, USA.*
Fludarabine phosphate (p.553·2).
*Chronic lymphocytic leukaemia.*

*Berlex, Canad.*
Fludarabine phosphate sodium (p.554·1).
*Chronic lymphocytic leukaemia.*

**Fludarene** *Thea, Ital.*
Chromocarb diethylamine (p.1670·3).
*Capillary fragility.*

**Fludecate**
*Unipharm, Israel; Intramed, S.Afr.†.*
Fluphenazine decanoate (p.699·3).
*Psychoses.*

**Fluden** *Rekah, Israel.*
Sodium fluoride (p.1444·3).
*Dental caries prophylaxis.*

**Fludent**
*Alpharma, Fin.; Alpharma, Swed.*
Sodium fluoride (p.1444·3).
*Dental caries prophylaxis.*

**Fludestrin** *Bristol-Myers Squibb, Ger.*
Testolactone (p.587·3).
*Breast cancer.*

**Fludeten**
*Alter, Port.; Alter, Spain.*
Paracetamol (p.76·2); codeine phosphate (p.27·1).
*Fever; pain.*

**Fludex**
*Servier, Austria; Servier, Belg.; Servier, Denm.; Eutherapie, Fr.; Servier, Gr.; Servier, Neth.; Servier, Port.; Servier, Switz.*
Indapamide (p.938·2).
*Hypertension.*

**Fludilat**
*Organon, Braz.; Thiemann, Ger.; Organon, Hong Kong†; Organon, Port.; Organon, Thai.*
Bencyclane fumarate (p.867·3).
*Vascular disorders.*

**Fluditec** *Innotech, Fr.*
Carbocisteine (p.1116·2).
*Respiratory-tract congestion.*

**Fludizol** *M & H, Thai.*
Fluconazole (p.398·1).
*Fungal infections.*

**Fludocel** *CPH, Port.*
Fluconazole (p.398·1).
*Fungal infections.*

**Fludren** *Diafarm, Spain.*
Dextromethorphan hydrobromide (p.1117·3); ephedrine hydrochloride (p.1120·1); chlorphenamine maleate (p.427·3).
*Coughs.*

**Fludronef** *Iquinosa, Spain.*
Fludrocortisone acetate (p.1100·1); gramicidin (p.220·2); neomycin sulfate (p.235·1).
*Eye disorders; infected skin disorders.*

**Fludrop** *Andromaco, Chile.*
Sodium chloride (p.1233·3).
*Nasal congestion; nasal hygiene.*

**Fluend** *Herbaline, Ital.†.*
Silver birch (p.1660·3); salix (p.87·3); thyme (p.1755·2); tilia (p.1756·2); cynara (p.1678·3); rose fruit (p.1740·1); bitter orange (p.1723·3).
*Cold and influenza symptoms.*

**Fluental** *Aventis, Ital.*
Sobrerol (p.1130·2); paracetamol (p.76·2).
*Respiratory-tract disorders.*

**Fluenzen** *Ecupharma, Ital.†.*
Imidazole salicylate (p.47·2).
*Fever; otorhinolaryngeal inflammation.*

**Flufenal** *Roux-Ocefa, Arg.*
Flunarizine (p.434·2).
*Cerebral and peripheral vascular disorders.*

**Flufenan** *Cristalia, Braz.*
Fluphenazine enantate (p.699·3) or fluphenazine hydrochloride (p.699·3).
*Psychoses.*

**Fluforte**
*Allergan, Chile; Allergan, Mex.*
Fluorometholone (p.1102·2).
*Inflammatory eye disorders.*

**Fluforte N**
*Allergan, Chile; Allergan, Mex.*
Fluorometholone (p.1102·2); neomycin sulfate (p.235·1).
*Infected eye disorders.*

**Flufran** *Unique, India.*
Fluoxetine hydrochloride (p.292·1).
*Depression.*

**Flugen** *Novartis, Spain.*
Fluorometholone (p.1102·2); gentamicin sulfate (p.217·1).
*Ocular inflammation following cataract surgery.*

**Flugeral** *Italfarmaco, Ital.*
Flunarizine hydrochloride (p.434·1).
*Migraine; vertigo.*

**Flui-Amoxicillin** *Zambon, Ger.*
Amoxicillin trihydrate (p.155·3).
*Bacterial infections.*

**Fluibil** *Zambon, Braz.†.*
Chenodeoxycholic acid (p.1670·1).
*Cholesterol gallstones.*

**Fluibron**
*Farmalab, Braz.; Andromaco, Chile; Chiesi, Ital.; Chiesi, Singapore†; Chiesi, Switz.*
Ambroxol hydrochloride (p.1114·3).
*Respiratory-tract disorders associated with increased or viscous mucus.*

**Fluibrox** *Medichrom, Gr.*
Ambroxol hydrochloride (p.1114·3).
*Respiratory disorders associated with viscous mucus.*

**Fluid Loss**
*Note. This name is used for preparations of different composition.*
*Vitaglow, Austral.†.*
Celery (p.1669·1); juniper (p.1703·1); bearberry (p.1659·2); parsley (p.1728·3); potassium chloride (p.1232·2).
*Fluid retention.*

*Vitaplex, Austral.†.*
Celery (p.1669·1); buchu (p.1663·1); taraxacum (p.1751·3); bearberry (p.1659·2).
*Fluid retention.*

**Fluidabak** *Thea, Fr.*
Povidone (p.1581·2).
*Dry eyes.*

**Fluidasa**
*Note. This name is used for preparations of different composition.*
*Montpellier, Arg.*
Erdosteine (p.1121·1).
*Respiratory-tract congestion.*

*Knoll, Mex.; Abbott, Spain.*
Mepyramine acefyllinate (p.437·1).
*Obstructive airways disease.*

**Fluide Hydratant Matifiant** *Vichy, Canad.†.*
*SPF 13:* Octinoxate (p.1154·3); ensulizole (p.1147·1).
*Sunscreen.*

**Fluide Hydratant Quotidien** *L'Oreal, Canad.*
*SPF 15:* Octinoxate (p.1154·3); ensulizole (p.1147·1).
*Sunscreen.*

**Fluide Multi-Confort** *Clarins, Canad.*
*SPF 15:* Octinoxate (p.1154·3); oxybenzone (p.1154·3); titanium dioxide (p.1160·3).
*Sunscreen.*

**Fluide Multi-Regenerant Lift Jour** *Clarins, Canad.*
*SPF 15:* Octinoxate (p.1154·3); oxybenzone (p.1154·3); titanium dioxide (p.1160·3).
Formerly contained octinoxate and oxybenzone.
*Sunscreen.*

**Fluide Protecteur Jeunesse des Mains** *Clarins, Canad.*
*SPF 15:* Avobenzone (p.1142·3); octinoxate (p.1154·3); octisalate (p.1154·3); oxybenzone (p.1154·3).
*Sunscreen.*

**Fluidema** *Baldacci, Port.*
Indapamide (p.938·2).
*Hypertension.*

**Fluiden** *Legon, Ital.†.*
Fenspiride hydrochloride (p.786·1).
*Respiratory-tract disorders.*

**Fluidin**
*Note. This name is used for preparations of different composition.*
*Ativus, Braz.*
Ambroxol (p.1114·3).
*Respiratory-tract congestion.*

*Lasa, Spain†.*
Guaifenesin (p.1122·1).
*Coughs.*

**Fluidin Adulto** *Merck, Port.†.*
Codeine (p.27·1); guaifenesin (p.1122·1); sodium benzoate (p.1169·3); ammonium acetate (p.1115·1); ephedrine hydrochloride (p.1120·1); caffeine (p.782·1); sodium iodide (p.1598·1); ipecacuanha (p.1122·3).
*Coughs and other respiratory-tract disorders.*

**Fluidin Antiasmatico** *Merck, Port.†.*
Aminophylline (p.780·2); potassium iodide (p.1598·1); ephedrine hydrochloride (p.1120·1); phenobarbital (p.367·3); sodium benzoate (p.1169·3); senega (p.1130·2); ipecacuanha (p.1122·3); belladonna (p.479·1); thyme (p.1755·2).
*Asthma.*

**Fluidin Infantil** *Merck, Port.†.*
Guaifenesin (p.1122·1); sodium benzoate (p.1169·3); ammonium acetate (p.1115·1); cowslip (p.1735·1); senega (p.1130·2); pine oil; drosera (p.1683·1); belladonna (p.479·1).
*Coughs and other respiratory-tract disorders.*

**Fluidin Mucolitico NF** *Ipsen, Spain.*
Carbocisteine (p.1116·2).
Fluidin Mucolitico formerly contained butetamate citrate, carbocisteine, diprophylline, and guaifenesin.
*Respiratory-tract disorders.*

**Fluidin Nocturno** *Merck, Port.†.*
Codeine (p.27·1); ethylmorphine hydrochloride (p.37·3); terpin hydrate (p.1131·1); homatropine methylbromide (p.483·2); phenobarbital (p.367·3); cineole (p.1672·1).
*Coughs.*

**Flui-DNCG** *Zambon, Ger.*
Sodium cromoglicate (p.795·3).
*Asthma.*

**Fluidox** *Baldacci, Port.*
Ambroxol hydrochloride (p.1114·3).
*Respiratory-tract disorders.*

**Fluidrenol** *Sofex, Port.*
Ambroxol hydrochloride (p.1114·3).
*Respiratory-tract disorders associated with increased or viscous mucus.*

**Fluifort** *Dompe, Ital.*
Carbocisteine lysine (p.1116·3).
*Respiratory disorders associated with excessive or viscous mucus.*

**Fluilast** *Boniscontro & Gazzone, Ital.*
Ticlopidine hydrochloride (p.1011·2).
*Thrombosis prophylaxis.*

**Fluimare** *Inpharzam, Switz.*
Sea water (p.1233·3).
*Nasal irrigation.*

**Fluimucil**
*Kirby, Arg.; Strallhofer, Austria; Zambon, Braz.; Zambon, Fr.; Zambon, Ger.; Zambon, Hong Kong; Zambon, Ital.; Zambon, Neth.; Zambon, Port.; Zambon, Singapore; Boots Healthcare, Spain; Inpharzam, Switz.; Sermmitr, Thai.; Zambon, Thai.*
Acetylcysteine (p.1112·3).
*Adjunct to cyclophosphamide treatment; haemorrhagic cystitis; poisoning with paracetamol, acrylonitrile, methacrynitrile, or methyl bromide; respiratory-tract disorders associated with increased or viscous mucus.*

**Fluimucil Antibiotic**
*Zambon, Belg.*
Thiamphenicol glycine acetylcysteinate (p.269·3).
*Bacterial infections of the respiratory tract associated with increased or viscous mucus.*

*Zambon, Fr.†.*
Thiamphenicol acetylcysteinate (p.269·3).
*Respiratory-tract infections.*

*Sermmitr, Thai.; Zambon, Thai.*
Thiamphenicol (p.269·2); acetylcysteine (p.1112·3).
*Respiratory-tract infections associated with increased or viscous mucus.*

**Fluimucil Antibiotico**
*Zambon, Ital.; Zambon, Spain.*
Thiamphenicol glycine acetylcysteinate (p.269·3).
*Respiratory-tract infections.*

**Fluimucil Biotic**
*Note. This name is used for preparations of different composition.*
*Kirby, Arg.*
Amoxicillin trihydrate (p.155·3); acetylcysteine (p.1112·3).
*Respiratory-tract infections.*

*Zambon, Braz.†.*
Acetylcysteine (p.1112·3); thiamphenicol (p.269·2).
*Respiratory-tract infections.*

**Fluimucil Solucao Nasal** *Zambon, Braz.†.*
Acetylcysteine (p.1112·3); benzalkonium chloride (p.1168·3); sodium chloride (p.1233·3).
*Nasal congestion.*

**Fluinol** *Almirall, Spain.*
Fluticasone propionate (p.1102·3).
*Nasal polyps; rhinitis.*

**Fluir** *Schering-Plough, Braz.*
Formoterol fumarate (p.786·1).
*Obstructive airways disease.*

**Fluirespir** *Zambon, Ital.*
Camphor (p.1665·3); cineole (p.1672·1).
*Nasal congestion.*

**Fluisedal** *Elerte, Fr.*
Meglumine benzoate; polysorbate 20 (p.1415·1); promethazine hydrochloride (p.439·1).
*Coughs.*

**Fluisedal sans promethazine** *Elerte, Fr.*
Meglumine benzoate; polysorbate 20 (p.1415·1).
*Respiratory-tract congestion.*

**Fluitoss** *Teuto, Braz.*
Carbocisteine (p.1116·2).
*Respiratory-tract congestion.*

**Fluiven** *Herbaline, Ital.†.*
Achillea (p.1646·2); centella (p.1144·3); hamamelis (p.1696·3); myrtillus (p.1718·3).
*Peripheral vascular disorders.*

**Fluixol** *Sintofarm, Ital.*
Ambroxol hydrochloride (p.1114·3).
*Respiratory-tract disorders.*

**Fluizan** *Klinger, Braz.*
Carbocisteine (p.1116·2).
*Respiratory-tract congestion.*

**Flukazol** *Kener, Mex.*
Fluconazole (p.398·1).
*Fungal infections.*

**Fluken** *Kendrick, Mex.*
Flutamide (p.556·2).
*Prostatic cancer.*

**Flukenol** *Kendrick, Mex.†.*
Fluconazole (p.398·1).
*Fungal infections.*

**Flukit** *Julphar, UAE.*
*Syrup:* Paracetamol (p.76·2); pseudoephedrine hydrochloride (p.1129·2); chlorphenamine maleate (p.427·3).
*Cold and influenza symptoms.*
*Tablets:* Paracetamol (p.76·2); salicylamide (p.87·3); promethazine hydrochloride (p.439·1); phenylephrine hydrochloride (p.1126·3).
*Cold and influenza symptoms; rhinitis.*

**Flulem**
*Laboratorios Chile, Chile; Lemery, Mex.*
Flutamide (p.556·2).
*Prostatic cancer.*

**Flulium**
*Note. This name is used for preparations of different composition.*
*Pharmasant, Thai.*
Dipotassium clorazepate (p.685·1).
*Anxiety; depression; dystonias.*

*Utopian, Thai.*
Flunarizine (p.434·2).
*Cerebrovascular disorders.*

**Flulone** *Panalab, Arg.*
Fluocinolone acetonide (p.1101·2).
*Skin disorders.*

**Flumach** *Mayoly-Spindler, Fr.*
Spironolactone (p.1003·1).
*Hyperaldosteronism; hypertension; myasthenia gravis; oedema.*

**Flumadine**
*Forest, Israel; Forest Pharmaceuticals, USA.*
Rimantadine hydrochloride (p.653·1).
*Influenza A.*

**Flumage** *Gemepe, Arg.*
Flumazenil (p.1038·3).

**Flumanovag** *Gobbi, Arg.*
Flumazenil (p.1038·3).

**Flumarc** *Raffo, Arg.*
Terazosin hydrochloride (p.1010·3).
*Benign prostatic hyperplasia; hypertension.*

**Flumarin** *Shionogi, Jpn.*
Flomoxef sodium (p.213·2).
*Bacterial infections.*

**Flumark** *Dainippon, Jpn.*
Enoxacin (p.207·2).
*Bacterial infections.*

**Flumasalen** *TO-Chemicals, Thai.*
Flumetasone pivalate (p.1101·1); salicylic acid (p.1157·1).
*Skin disorders.*

**Flumates** *Mintlab, Chile.*
Beclometasone dipropionate (p.1091·1).

**Flumazen** *Scott-Cassara, Arg.*
Flumazenil (p.1038·3).

**Flumed**
*Note. This name is used for preparations of different composition.*
*Andromaco, Chile.*
Bromhexine (p.1115·3).
*Respiratory-tract congestion.*

*Medifive, Thai.*
Fluoxetine (p.296·3).
*Depression; obsessive-compulsive disorder.*

**Flumetholon** *Santen, Hong Kong.*
Fluorometholone (p.1102·2).
*Inflammatory eye disorders.*

**Flumetol**
*Note. This name is used for preparations of different composition.*
*Faran, Gr.*
Timolol maleate (p.1012·2).
*Glaucoma.*

*Farmila, Ital.*
Fluorometholone (p.1102·2); tetryzoline hydrochloride (p.1131·2).
*Inflammatory eye disorders.*

**Flumetol Antibiotico** *Farmila, Ital.*
Fluorometholone (p.1102·2); tetracycline (p.266·2).
*Infected eye disorders.*

**Flumetol NF** *Sophia, Mex.*
Fluorometholone acetate (p.1102·2).
*Inflammatory eye disorders.*

**Flumetol Semplice** *Farmila, Ital.*
Fluorometholone (p.1102·2).
*Inflammatory eye disorders.*

**Flumex** *Allergan, Braz.*
Fluorometholone (p.1102·2).
*Eye disorders.*

**Flumex N** *Allergan, Braz.*
Neomycin sulfate (p.235·1); fluorometholone (p.1102·2).
*Infected eye disorders.*

**Flumid** *Hexal, Ger.*
Flutamide (p.556·2).
*Prostatic cancer.*

**Flumil**
*Note. This name is used for preparations of different composition.*
*Senosiain, Mex.*
Aminophenazone (p.14·2); buphenine hydrochloride (p.1663·2); diphenylpyraline hydrochloride (p.432·3).
*Rhinitis; sinusitis.*

*Pharmazam, Spain.*
Acetylcysteine (p.1112·3).
*Respiratory-tract disorders associated with excessive or viscous mucus.*

**Flumil Antibiotico** *Zambon, Spain.*
Acetylcysteine (p.1112·3); thiamphenicol (p.269·2).
*Respiratory-tract infections.*

**Flumil Antidoto** *Zambon, Spain.*
Acetylcysteine (p.1112·3).
*Paracetamol poisoning.*

**Fluminex** *Fournier, Ital.*
Flunisolide (p.1101·1).
*Asthma; bronchitis; rhinitis.*

**FluMist** *Medimmune, USA; Wyeth-Ayerst, USA.*
A live influenza vaccine (p.1620·2).
*Active immunisation.*

**Flumoxal** *Janssen-Cilag, Arg.*
Flubendazole (p.105·2).
*Worm infections.*

**Flumural** *SPA, Ital.†.*
Flumequine (p.214·2).
*Urinary-tract infections.*

**Flunagen** *Gentili, Ital.*
Flunarizine hydrochloride (p.434·1).
*Migraine; vertigo.*

**Flunal** *Rayere, Mex.*
Fluocinolone acetonide (p.1101·2); clioquinol (p.196·3).
*Infected skin disorders.*

**Flunal-Neo** *Rayere, Mex.*
Fluocinolone acetonide (p.1101·2); neomycin (p.235·1).
*Infected skin disorders.*

**Flunarin** *Asta Medica, Braz.*
Flunarizine hydrochloride (p.434·1).
*Hemiplegia; migraine and other vascular headaches; subarachnoid haemorrhage.*

**Flunarium**
*Jacoby, Austria; Greater Pharma, Thai.*
Flunarizine hydrochloride (p.434·1).
*Cerebrovascular disorders; migraine; motion sickness; vertigo.*

**Flunase** *Teva, Israel.*
Flunisolide (p.1101·1).
*Rhinitis.*

**Flunavert** *Hennig, Ger.*
Flunarizine hydrochloride (p.434·1).
*Migraine; vertigo.*

**Flunaza** *Pharmaland, Thai.*
Flunarizine (p.434·2).
*Cerebrovascular disorders.*

**Flunazine** *Shiwa, Thai.*
Flunarizine (p.434·2).
*Cerebral and peripheral vascular disorders; vestibular disorders.*

**Flunazol** *Sintofarma, Braz.*
Fluconazole (p.398·1).
*Fungal infections.*

**Flunco** *TO-Chemicals, Thai.*
Fluconazole (p.398·1).
*Fungal infections.*

**Fluneurin** *Hexal, Ger.*
Fluoxetine hydrochloride (p.292·1).
*Bulimia; depression; obsessive-compulsive disorder.*

**Fluni** *1A, Ger.*
Flunitrazepam (p.698·2).
*Sleep disorders.*

**Flunibeta** *Betapharm, Ger.*
Flunitrazepam (p.698·2).
*Sleep disorders.*

**Flunidor** *Chibret, Port.*
Diflunisal (p.34·1).
*Inflammation; pain.*

**Flunigar** *Farminvest, Ital.*
Flunisolide (p.1101·1).
*Asthma; bronchitis allergic rhinitis.*

**Fluniget**
*Merck Sharp & Dohme, Austria; Merck Sharp & Dohme, Ger.†.*
Diflunisal (p.34·1).
*Musculoskeletal and joint disorders; pain.*

**Flunimerck** *Merck dura, Ger.*
Flunitrazepam (p.698·2).
*Insomnia.*

**Fluninoc** Hexal, Ger.
Flunitrazepam (p.698·2).
*Insomnia.*

**Flunipam**
Alpharma, Denm.; Alpharma, Norw.
Flunitrazepam (p.698·2).
*Insomnia; premedication.*

**Flunir** Oberlin, Fr.
Niflumic acid (p.67·1).
*Sprains.*

**Flunitec**
Boehringer Ingelheim, Arg.; Boehringer de Angeli, Braz.†; Boehringer Ingelheim, Denm.†; Boehringer Ingelheim, Norw.†.
Flunisolide (p.1101·1).
*Asthma; nasal congestion.*

**Flunitop** Pierre Fabre, Ital.
Flunisolide (p.1101·1).
*Asthma, bronchitis; rhinitis.*

**Flunolone**
Atlantic, Hong Kong; Atlantic, Singapore; Vana, Thai.
Fluocinolone acetonide (p.1101·2); neomycin sulfate (p.235·1).
*Infected skin disorders.*

**Flunolone-V**
Atlantic, Hong Kong; Atlantic, Singapore; Vana, Thai.
Fluocinolone acetonide (p.1101·2).
*Skin disorders.*

**Flunox**
Note. This name is used for preparations of different composition.
Eurofarma, Braz.†.
Enoxaparin (p.910·3).

Roche, Ital.
Flurazepam monohydrochloride (p.700·3).
*Insomnia.*

**Fluo Fenic** Novartis, Spain.
Chloramphenicol (p.185·1); fluocinolone acetonide (p.1101·2).
*Infected eye disorders.*

**Fluo Grin** Grin, Mex.
Fluocinolone acetonide (p.1101·2); neomycin sulfate (p.235·1).
*Infected eye disorders.*

**Fluo Vasoc** Ciba Vision, Spain†.
Fluocinolone acetonide (p.1101·2); naphazoline hydrochloride (p.1124·3); neomycin sulfate (p.235·1); zinc sulfate (p.1469·3).
*Infected eye disorders.*

**Fluocal com Pectina** Breves, Braz.†.
Neomycin sulfate (p.235·1); dihydrostreptomycin sulfate (p.205·3); pectin (p.1580·3); apple juice; attapulgite (p.1251·1); calcium lactate (p.1225·3).
*Diarrhoea.*

**Fluo-calc** Pharmacia, Switz.
Sodium monofluorophosphate (p.1446·2); calcium carbonate (p.1254·2).
*Osteoporosis.*

**Fluocalcic**
Raffo, Arg.; Asta Medica, Austria; Yamanouchi, Belg.; Yamanouchi, Fr.†.
Sodium monofluorophosphate (p.1446·2); calcium carbonate (p.1254·2).
*Osteoporosis.*

**Fluocaril**
Note. This name is used for preparations of different composition.
Asta Medica, Braz.†; Kramer, Switz.
Sodium fluoride (p.1444·3).
*Dental caries prophylaxis.*

Sanofi Synthelabo OTC, Ital.
Potassium fluoride (p.1445·3); potassium nitrate (p.1190·1); enoxolone (p.36·2).
*Gum hypersensitivity and pain.*

**Fluocaril Bi-Fluore**
Rider, Chile; Sanofi Synthelabo OTC, Fr.; Sanofi Synthelabo OTC, Ital.
Sodium monofluorophosphate (p.1446·2); sodium fluoride (p.1444·3).
*Dental caries prophylaxis.*

**Fluocaril blancheur** Sanofi Synthelabo OTC, Fr.
Calcium carbonate (p.1254·2); sodium benzoate (p.1169·3); sodium monofluorophosphate (p.1446·2).
*Dental discoloration.*

**Fluocaril dents sensibles** Sanofi Synthelabo OTC, Fr.
Potassium fluoride (p.1445·3); potassium nitrate (p.1190·1); enoxolone (p.36·2).
*Sensitive teeth.*

**Fluocaril Junior and Fluocaril Kids** Sanofi Synthelabo, Fr.
Sodium monofluorophosphate (p.1446·2); sodium fluoride (p.1444·3).
*Dental caries prophylaxis.*

**Fluocid Forte** Inkeysa, Spain.
Fluocinolone acetonide (p.1101·2).
*Skin disorders.*

**Fluocim** Medika, Switz.
Fluoxetine hydrochloride (p.292·1).
*Bulimia; depression.*

**Fluoclox** Ranbaxy, Singapore†.
Flucloxacillin sodium (p.213·3).
*Bacterial infections.*

**Fluocortan** Centrum, Spain†.
Fluocinolone acetonide (p.1101·2).
*Skin disorders.*

**Fluodel** QIF, Braz.†.
Sodium fluoride (p.1444·3).
*Dental caries prophylaxis.*

**Fluodent** Scherer, Ital.†.
Sodium fluoride (p.1444·3).
*Dietary-fluoride deficiency.*

**Fluoderm** Taro, Canad.
Fluocinolone acetonide (p.1101·2).
*Skin disorders.*

**Fluodermo Fuerte** Reig Jofre, Spain.
Fluocinolone acetonide (p.1101·2).
*Skin disorders.*

**Fluodonil** Biologici Italia, Ital.†.
Diflunisal (p.34·1).
*Musculoskeletal and joint disorders; pain.*

**Fluodont** Gebro, Austria.
Sodium fluoride (p.1444·3).
*Dental caries prophylaxis.*

**Fluodontyl**
Sanofi Synthelabo OTC, Fr.; Sanofi Synthelabo, Spain.
Sodium fluoride (p.1444·3).
Formerly contained sodium fluoride and formaldehyde in *Fr.*
*Dental caries prophylaxis.*

**Fluodrazin F** Breves, Braz.†.
Isoniazid (p.222·2); ascorbic acid (p.1460·2).
*Tuberculosis.*

**Fluo-Fenicol** Allergan-Frumtost, Braz.†.
Fluocinolone acetonide (p.1101·2); chloramphenicol (p.185·1).
*Infected eye disorders.*

**Flu-Off** Europharm, Hong Kong.
Paracetamol (p.76·2); chlorphenamine maleate (p.427·3); phenylephrine hydrochloride (p.1126·3); caffeine (p.782·1).
*Cold and influenza symptoms.*

**Fluoftal** Agepha, Austria.
Fluorescein sodium (p.1689·1).
*Diagnosis of corneal disorders.*

**Fluogel** Sanofi Synthelabo OTC, Fr.
Sodium fluoride (p.1444·3); ammonium difluoride (p.1445·3).
*Dental caries prophylaxis following radiotherapy.*

**Fluogen** Parkedale, USA†.
An influenza vaccine (p.1620·2).
*Active immunisation.*

**Fluogum** Sanofi Synthelabo OTC, Fr.
Sodium fluoride (p.1444·3).
*Dental caries prophylaxis.*

**Fluohexal** Hexal, Austral.
Fluoxetine hydrochloride (p.292·1).
*Depression; obsessive-compulsive disorder.*

**Fluomint** Daudt, Braz.
Sodium monofluorophosphate (p.1446·2); cineole (p.1672·1); thymol (p.1194·2); methyl salicylate (p.59·3); menthol (p.1711·3).
*Dental caries prophylaxis; oral hygeine.*

**Fluomit** Laboratorios Chile, Chile.
Ambroxol hydrochloride (p.1114·3).
*Respiratory-tract congestion.*

**Fluomix Same** Savoma, Ital.
Fluocinolone acetonide (p.1101·2).
*Skin disorders.*

**Fluomycin N** Nourypharma, Ger.
Dequalinium chloride (p.1178·1).
*Vaginal infections.*

**Fluon** Aerocid, Fr.
Metesculetol sodium (p.1714·1); hamamelis (p.1696·3); aesculus (p.1648·2); viburnum.
*Haemorrhoids; peripheral vascular disorders; venous insufficiency.*

**Fluonid** Allergan, USA.
Fluocinolone acetonide (p.1101·2).
*Skin disorders.*

**Fluonid-N**
Biolab, Hong Kong; Biopharm, Hong Kong; Biolab, Malaysia; Biolab, Thai.
Fluocinolone acetonide (p.1101·2); neomycin sulfate (p.235·1).
*Infected skin disorders.*

**Fluopate** Laphal, Fr.†.
Sodium fluoride (p.1444·3); calcium fluoride (p.1423·3).
*Dental caries prophylaxis.*

**Fluopiram** Ariston, Arg.
Fluoxetine hydrochloride (p.292·1).
*Depression.*

**Fluoplexe** Lehning, Fr.
Sodium fluoride (p.1444·3).
*Peri-articular disorders.*

**Fluor**
Or-Dov, Austral.†; Crinex, Fr.†; Lacer, Spain; Kin, Spain.
Sodium fluoride (p.1444·3).
*Dental caries prophylaxis.*

**Fluor Microsol** Herbaxt, Fr.
Sodium fluoride (p.1444·3).
*Peri-articular disorders.*

**Fluor Verde** Angelini, Ital.
Sodium fluoride (p.1444·3).
*Dental caries prophylaxis.*

**Fluoracaine**
Dioptic, Canad.; Akorn, Canad.; Akorn, USA.
Fluorescein sodium (p.1689·1); proxymetacaine hydrochloride (p.1384·1).
*Aid to eye examination; local anaesthesia.*

**Fluor-A-Day**
Pharmascience, Canad.; Dental Health Products, UK.
Sodium fluoride (p.1444·3).
*Dental caries prophylaxis.*

**Fluoralfa** INTES, Ital.
Fluorescein sodium (p.1689·1).
*Diagnosis of eye disorders.*

**Fluordent**
Microsules Bernabo, Arg.; Warner-Lambert, Ital.†.
Sodium fluoride (p.1444·3).
*Dental caries prophylaxis.*

**Fluore Stain Strips** Bell, India.
Fluorescein sodium (p.1689·1).
*Aid to eye examination.*

**Fluorescite**
Alcon, Arg.; Alcon, Austral.; Alcon, Canad.; Alcon, Hong Kong; Alcon, Malaysia; Alcon, NZ; Alcon, S.Afr.; Alcon, Singapore; Alcon, Thai.; Alcon, USA.
Fluorescein sodium (p.1689·1).
*Aid to eye examination.*

**Fluorets**
Smith & Nephew, Austral.; Novartis Ophthalmics, Canad.; Dioptic, Canad.; Chauvin, Hong Kong; Chauvin, Irl.; Smith & Nephew, NZ; SofLens, S.Afr.; Chauvin, Singapore; Bausch & Lomb, UK; Akorn, USA.
Fluorescein sodium (p.1689·1).
*Aid to eye examination.*

**Fluorette**
Fertin, Denm.; Fertin, Norw.; Meda, Swed.
Sodium fluoride (p.1444·3).
*Dental caries prophylaxis.*

**Fluoretten** Aventis, Ger.
Sodium fluoride (p.1444·3).
*Dental caries prophylaxis.*

**Fluorex** Crinex, Fr.
Sodium fluoride (p.1444·3).
*Dental caries prophylaxis.*

**Fluorex Plus** Gerot, Austria.
Tetracycline hydrochloride (p.266·2); dequalinium chloride (p.1178·1); prednisone (p.1109·3).
*Colpitis.*

**Fluorexidina** Careiatrics, Arg.
Sodium fluoride (p.1444·3); chlorhexidine (p.1173·2).
*Dental caries prophylaxis.*

**Fluorhinose** Monot, Fr.†.
Benzododecinium bromide (p.1170·2); sodium chloride (p.1233·3).

**Fluoridrops** WestCan, Canad.
Sodium fluoride (p.1444·3).
*Fluoride supplement.*

**Fluorigard**
Colgate-Palmolive, Ital.†; Colgate-Palmolive, UK; Colgate-Palmolive, USA.
Sodium fluoride (p.1444·3).
*Dental caries prophylaxis.*

**Fluorigard Gel-Kam** Colgate-Palmolive, UK.
Stannous fluoride (p.1448·3).
*Dental caries prophylaxis.*

**Fluorigard Ortho** Asta Medica, Port.†.
Sodium fluoride (p.1444·3).
*Dental caries prophylaxis.*

**Fluoril** Novartis, Ger.
Sodium monofluorophosphate (p.1446·2); calcium lactate gluconate (p.1225·3); calcium carbonate (p.1254·2).
*Osteoporosis.*

**Fluorilette** Leiras, Fin.
Sodium fluoride (p.1444·3).
*Dental caries prophylaxis.*

**Fluori-Methane** Gebauer, USA.
Dichlorodifluoromethane (p.1236·1); trichlorofluoromethane (p.1236·1).
*Local anaesthesia.*

**Fluor-In**
Sanofi Synthelabo, Ital.; Sanofi Synthelabo, Port.†.
Sodium fluoride (p.1444·3).
*Dental caries prophylaxis.*

**Fluorinse**
Oral-B, Canad.; Oral-B, USA.
Sodium fluoride (p.1444·3).
*Dental caries prophylaxis.*

**Fluor-I-Strip** Bausch & Lomb, USA.
Fluorescein sodium (p.1689·1).
*Aid to eye examination.*

**Fluor-I-Strip AT** Bausch & Lomb, Canad.†.
Fluorescein sodium (p.1689·1).
*Aid to eye examination.*

**Fluoritab** Fluoritab, USA.
Sodium fluoride (p.1444·3).
*Dental caries prophylaxis.*

**Fluoritabs** WestCan, Canad.
Sodium fluoride (p.1444·3).

**Fluornatrium** Odontomed, Braz.
Sodium fluoride (p.1444·3).
*Dental caries prophylaxis.*

**Fluorobioptal** Farmila, Ital.†.
Dexamethasone (p.1097·1); chloramphenicol (p.185·1).
*Inflammatory eye disorders.*

**Fluorocaine** Medical Ophthalmics, USA.
Fluorescein sodium (p.1689·1); proxymetacaine hydrochloride (p.1384·1).

**Fluorocalciforte** Serozym, Fr.†.
Calcium chloride (p.1225·1); calcium gluceptate (p.1225·2); calcium gluconate (p.1225·2); calcium lactate (p.1225·3); calcium carbonate (p.1254·2); sodium monofluorophosphate (p.1446·2); yeast (p.1469·1).
*Osteoporosis.*

**Fluorocare** Colgate Oral Care, Austral.†.
Sodium monofluorophosphate (p.1446·2).
*Dental caries prophylaxis; sensitive teeth.*

**Fluorogel** Naf, Arg.
Sodium fluoride (p.1444·3).
*Dental caries prophylaxis.*

**Fluoro-Ophtal** Winzer, Ger.
Fluorometholone (p.1102·2).
*Inflammatory eye disorders.*

**Fluor-Op** Novartis Ophthalmics, USA.
Fluorometholone (p.1102·2).
*Inflammatory eye disorders.*

**Fluoroplat** Naf, Arg.
Diamino silver fluoride.
*Dental caries prophylaxis.*

**Fluoroplex**
Allergan, Austral.†; Allergan, Canad.†; Allergan, USA.
Fluorouracil (p.554·2).
*Actinic keratoses.*

**Fluoropoen** Poen, Arg.
Dexamethasone (p.1097·1); chloramphenicol (p.185·1); phenylephrine (p.1126·3).
*Conjunctivitis.*

**Fluoropos** Ursapharm, Ger.
Fluorometholone (p.1102·2).
*Inflammatory eye disorders.*

**Fluororinil** Farmila, Ital.
Betamethasone (p.1093·1); chlorphenamine maleate (p.427·3).
*Rhinitis.*

**Fluoros** Jenapharm, Ger.
Sodium fluoride (p.1444·3).
*Osteoporosis.*

**Fluorosol** WestCan, Canad.
Sodium fluoride (p.1444·3).

**Fluorox** Medical Ophthalmics, USA.
Fluorescein sodium (p.1689·1); oxybuprocaine (p.1382·2).

**Fluorthyrin** Agepha, Austria.
Fluorotyrosine (p.1598·1).
*Hyperthyroidism.*

**Fluortop** GABA, Switz.†.
Sodium fluoride (p.1444·3).
*Dental caries prophylaxis.*

**Fluorvas** Llorens, Spain.
Fluorometholone (p.1102·2); tetryzoline hydrochloride (p.1131·2).
*Eye disorders.*

**Fluor-Vigantoletten** Merck, Ger.
Colecalciferol (p.1461·3); sodium fluoride (p.1444·3).
*Dental caries prophylaxis; rickets; vitamin D deficiency.*

**Fluorvitin** IPFI, Ital.†.
Sodium fluoride (p.1444·3).
*Dental caries prophylaxis.*

**Fluoselgine** Teofarma, Fr.
Domiphen bromide (p.1179·1); sodium fluoride (p.1444·3).
*Dental hygiene; gingivitis.*

**Fluosept** Inava, Fr.†.
Ammonium difluoride (p.1445·3); benzyl salicylate.
*Dental caries prophylaxis.*

**Fluotec** Bergamo, Braz.†.
Fluconazole (p.398·1).
*Fungal infections.*

**Fluotest**
Alcon, Port.; Alcon Cusi, Spain.
Fluorescein sodium (p.1689·1); oxybuprocaine hydrochloride (p.1382·1).
*Aid to eye examination.*

**Fluothane**
AstraZeneca, Austral.; AstraZeneca, Austria; Zeneca, Belg.†; AstraZeneca, Braz.; AstraZeneca, Chile; AstraZeneca, Fr.; AstraZeneca, Ger.; Astra-Zeneca, Gr.; Zeneca, Hong Kong†; ICI, India; Zeneca, Irl.†; Zeneca, Israel; Zeneca, Ital.†; AstraZeneca, Malaysia; Zeneca, Mex.†; AstraZeneca, Neth.†; Zeneca, Norw.†; AstraZeneca, NZ; Zeneca, Port.†; AstraZeneca, S.Afr.; AstraZeneca, Spain; Astra, Swed.; Zeneca, Switz.†; AstraZeneca, Thai.†; AstraZeneca, UK†; Wyeth-Ayerst, USA.
Halothane (p.1299·3).
*General anaesthesia.*

**Fluotic** Aventis, Canad.
Sodium fluoride (p.1444·3).
*Otospongiosis.*

**Fluotrat** Biolab Sanus, Braz.
Sodium fluoride (p.1444·3).
*Dental caries prophylaxis.*

**Fluo-Vaso** Allergan, Braz.
Fluocinolone acetonide (p.1101·2); naphazoline hydrochloride (p.1124·3); neomycin sulfate (p.235·1); zinc sulfate (p.1469·3).
*Infected eye disorders.*

**Fluovitef** Teofarma, Ital.
Fluocinolone acetonide (p.1101·2).
*Skin disorders.*

**Fluox**
ABZ, Ger.; Pacific, NZ.
Fluoxetine hydrochloride (p.292·1).
*Bulimia nervosa; depression; obsessive-compulsive disorder; premenstrual dysphoric disorder.*

**Fluoxa** 1A, Ger.
Fluoxetine hydrochloride (p.292·1).
*Depression.*

**Fluoxac** Psicofarma, Mex.
Fluoxetine hydrochloride (p.292·1).
*Depression.*

**flux-basan** Schonenberger, Switz.
Fluoxetine hydrochloride (p.292·1).
*Bulimia; depression.*

**Fluoxemerck** *Merck dura, Ger.*
Fluoxetine hydrochloride (p.292·1).
*Depression.*

**Fluoxeren** *Menarini, Ital.*
Fluoxetine hydrochloride (p.292·1).
*Bulimia nervosa; depression; obsessive-compulsive disorder.*

**Fluoxgamma** *Worwag, Ger.*
Fluoxetine hydrochloride (p.292·1).
*Depression.*

**Fluoxibene** *Ratiopharm, Austria.*
Fluoxetine hydrochloride (p.292·1).
*Bulimia nervosa; depression; obsessive-compulsive disorder.*

**Fluoxifar** *Siphar, Switz.*
Fluoxetine hydrochloride (p.292·1).
*Bulimia; depression.*

**Fluoxin** *Ibirn, Ital.*
Fluoxetine hydrochloride (p.292·1).
*Bulimia nervosa; depression; obsessive-compulsive disorder.*

**Flu-Oxinate** *Pasadena, USA.*
Fluorescein sodium (p.1689·1); oxybuprocaine hydrochloride (p.1382·1).

**Fluoxine** *TO-Chemicals, Thai.*
Fluoxetine (p.296·3).
*Depression.*

**Fluoxistad** *Stada, Austria.*
Fluoxetine hydrochloride (p.292·1).
*Bulimia nervosa; depression; obsessive compulsive disorder.*

**Fluoxityrol** *Tyrol, Austria.*
Fluoxetine hydrochloride (p.292·1).
*Depression.*

**Fluox-Puren** *Alpharma-Isis, Ger.*
Fluoxetine hydrochloride (p.292·1).
*Depression.*

**Fluoxytil** *Glaxo Wellcome, Mex.*
*Dental gel:* Sodium monofluorophosphate (p.1446·2); calcium glycerophosphate (p.1225·2).
*Oral drops:* Sodium fluoride (p.1444·3); xylitol (p.1469·1).
*Dental caries prophylaxis.*

**Flupar** *Orion, Fin.*
An inactivated influenza vaccine (p.1620·2).
*Active immunisation.*

**Flupazine** *Psicofarma, Mex.*
Trifluoperazine hydrochloride (p.726·3).
*Nausea and vomiting; psychoses.*

**Flupid** *Damor, Ital.*
Ticlopidine hydrochloride (p.1011·2).
*Thrombosis prophylaxis.*

**Flupidol** *Janssen-Cilag, Gr.*
Penfluridol (p.713·2).
*Psychoses.*

**Flupress** *Drug Research, Ital.†.*
Buflomedil pyridoxal phosphate compound (p.877·2).
*Cerebral and peripheral vascular disorders.*

**Fluprim Tosse** *Roche, Ital.†.*
Dextromethorphan hydrobromide (p.1117·3).
*Coughs.*

**Fluprosin** *Pharmacodane, Denm.*
Flutamide (p.556·2).
*Prostatic cancer.*

**Fluprost** *Lisapharma, Ital.*
Flutamide (p.556·2).
*Prostatic cancer.*

**Flura** *Kirkman, USA.*
Sodium fluoride (p.1444·3).
*Dental caries prophylaxis.*

**Flurablastin**
*Pharmacia, Denm.; Pharmacia, Fin.; Pharmacia, Norw.*
Fluorouracil (p.554·2).
*Malignant neoplasms.*

*Pharmacia, Swed.*
Fluorouracil sodium (p.555·2).
*Malignant neoplasms.*

**Fluracedyl**
*Pharmachemie, Israel†; Nycomed, Norw.†; Pharmachemie, Thai.; Teva, Thai.*
Fluorouracil (p.554·2).
*Malignant neoplasms.*

*Nycomed, Swed.*
Fluorouracil sodium (p.555·2).
*Malignant neoplasms.*

**Fluracil** *Biochem, India.*
Fluorouracil (p.554·2).
*Malignant neoplasms.*

**Flurate** *Bausch & Lomb, USA.*
Fluorescein sodium (p.1689·1); oxybuprocaine hydrochloride (p.1382·1).
*Local anaesthesia.*

**Fluraz** *Brown & Burk, India.*
Flurazepam dihydrochloride (p.700·3).
*Anxiety; insomnia.*

**Flurbid** *Klonal, Arg.*
Flurbiprofen (p.43·3).
*Inflammation; pain.*

**Flurekain** *Croma, Austria.*
Oxybuprocaine hydrochloride (p.1382·1); fluorescein sodium (p.1689·1).
*Local anaesthesia.*

**Fluress**
*AMO, Austral.; Allergan, Canad.†; Barnes Hind, NZ; Abigo, Swed.; Akorn, USA.*
Fluorescein sodium (p.1689·1); oxybuprocaine hydrochloride (p.1382·1).
*Aid to eye examination; local anaesthesia.*

**Flurets** *Oral-B, Austral.†.*
Sodium fluoride (p.1444·3).
*Prevention of tooth decay.*

**Fluricin** *Seng, Thai.*
Flunarizine hydrochloride (p.434·1).
*Cerebral and peripheral vascular disorders; vestibular disorders.*

**Flurinol**
*Boehringer Ingelheim, Arg.; Boehringer Ingelheim, Chile; Promeco, Mex.*
Epinastine (p.433·3) or epinastine hydrochloride (p.433·3).
*Allergic rhinitis; asthma; pruritus.*

**Flurizic** *Pantafarm, Ital.*
Flurithromycin ethyl succinate (p.214·2).
*Bacterial infections.*

**Fluroblastin**
*Pharmacia Upjohn, Ger.†; Pharmacia, S.Afr.*
Fluorouracil (p.554·2).
*Malignant neoplasms.*

**Fluroblastine** *Pharmacia, Belg.*
Fluorouracil sodium (p.555·2).
*Malignant neoplasms.*

**Fluro-Ethyl** *Gebauer, USA.*
Ethyl chloride (p.1376·2); cryofluorane (p.1235·3).
*Topical anaesthesia.*

**Flurofen**
*Abbott, Denm.; Vianex (Βιανεξ), Gr.*
Flurbiprofen (p.43·3).
*Inflammation; musculoskeletal and joint disorders; pain.*

**Flurolon** *Allergan, Denm.*
Fluorometholone (p.1102·2).
*Inflammatory eye disorders.*

**Flurop** *Davi, Port.*
Fluorometholone (p.1102·2).
*Eye disorders.*

**Fluroptic** *Cooper (Κοπερ), Gr.*
Flurbiprofen sodium (p.44·1).
*Prevention of miosis in ophthalmic surgery.*

**Flurosyn** *Rugby, USA.*
Fluocinolone acetonide (p.1101·2).
*Skin disorders.*

**Flurox**
*Note. This name is used for preparations of different composition.*
*Lemery, Mex.*
Fluorouracil (p.554·2).
*Malignant neoplasms.*

*Ocusoft, USA.*
Fluorescein sodium (p.1689·1); oxybuprocaine hydrochloride (p.1382·1).

**Flurozin** *Remedica, Thai.*
Flurbiprofen (p.43·3).
*Musculoskeletal and joint disorders.*

**Flurpax** *Aventis, Spain.*
Flunarizine hydrochloride (p.434·1).
*Migraine; vertigo.*

**Flusac** *Sriprasit, Thai.*
Fluoxetine hydrochloride (p.292·1).
*Mixed anxiety depressive states.*

**Flusan**
*Note. This name is used for preparations of different composition.*
*Eurofarma, Braz.†.*
Fluconazole (p.398·1).
*Fungal infections.*

*Novag, Mex.*
Tolbutamide (p.348·1).
*Diabetes mellitus.*

**Fluscand** *Enapharm, Swed.*
Flunitrazepam (p.698·2).
*Premedication; sleep disorders.*

**Flusemide** *Vedim, Spain.*
Nicardipine hydrochloride (p.965·1).
*Angina pectoris; cerebral vasospasm; hypertension.*

**Fluseminal** *Anpharm (Ανφαρμ), Gr.*
Norfloxacin (p.238·3).
*Urinary tract infections.*

**Flusenil** *Anpharm (Ανφαρμ), Gr.*
Fluconazole (p.398·1).
*Fungal infections.*

**Fluserin** *Sigma, Braz.†.*
Flunitrazepam (p.698·2).
*Adjunct in general anaesthesia; insomnia; premedication.*

**Flushield**
*Wyeth, Mex.†; Wyeth-Ayerst, USA†.*
An inactivated influenza vaccine (split virion) (p.1620·2).
*Active immunisation.*

**Flusin** *Aspen, S.Afr.*
Chlorphenamine maleate (p.427·3); ephedrine hydrochloride (p.1120·1); paracetamol (p.76·2); caffeine (p.782·1).
*Cold and influenza symptoms.*

**Flusin C** *Aspen, S.Afr.*
Chlorphenamine maleate (p.427·3); pseudoephedrine hydrochloride (p.1129·2); vitamin C (p.1460·2).
*Cold and influenza symptoms.*

**Flusin DM** *Aspen, S.Afr.*
Chlorphenamine maleate (p.427·3); pseudoephedrine hydrochloride (p.1129·2); dextromethorphan hydrobromide (p.1117·3); ascorbic acid (p.1460·2).
*Coughs; upper respiratory-tract congestion.*

**Flusin S** *Aspen, S.Afr.*
Chlorphenamine maleate (p.427·3); paracetamol (p.76·2); pseudoephedrine hydrochloride (p.1129·2); vitamin C (p.1460·2).
*Cold and influenza symptoms.*

**Flusol** *Ecosol, Switz.*
Fluoxetine hydrochloride (p.292·1).
*Bulimia; depression.*

**Flusolgen** *Geni, Spain.*
Fluocinolone acetonide (p.1101·2).
*Skin disorders.*

**Flusolv** *Ecobi, Ital.*
Heparin calcium (p.927·3).
*Thromboembolic disorders.*

**Flusona** *Recalcine, Chile.*
Fluticasone (p.1103·1).
*Asthma.*

**Flusonal** *Almirall, Spain.*
Fluticasone propionate (p.1102·3).
*Asthma.*

**Fluspi** *Hexal, Ger.*
Fluspirilene (p.701·1).
*Schizophrenia.*

**Fluspiral** *Menarini, Ital.*
Fluticasone propionate (p.1102·3).
*Obstructive airways disease.*

**Flusporan**
*Menarini, Arg.; Menarini, Spain.*
Flutrimazole (p.400·3).
*Fungal skin infections.*

**Fluss 40** *Scharper, Ital.*
Furosemide (p.919·3); triamterene (p.1016·2).
*Ascites; hyperaldosteronism; hypertension; oedema.*

**Flussorex** *Lampugnani, Ital.*
Citicoline sodium (p.1672·3).
*Cerebrovascular disorders; mental function disorders; parkinsonism.*

**Flu-Stat** *Be-Tabs, S.Afr.*
*Capsules:* Paracetamol (p.76·2); ascorbic acid (p.1460·2); phenylephrine hydrochloride (p.1126·3); chlorphenamine maleate (p.427·3); caffeine (p.782·1).
*Syrup:* Paracetamol (p.76·2); phenylpropanolamine hydrochloride (p.1127·3); dextromethorphan hydrobromide (p.1117·3).
*Cold and influenza symptoms.*

**Flusten** *Eurofarma, Braz.*
Erdosteine (p.1121·1).
*Respiratory-tract congestion.*

**Fluta** *1A, Ger.; Cell Pharm, Ger.; Gry, Ger.*
Flutamide (p.556·2).
*Prostatic cancer.*

**Flutabene** *Ratiopharm, Austria.*
Flutamide (p.556·2).
*Prostatic cancer.*

**Flutacan**
*Leiras, Denm.; Ferring, Swed.*
Flutamide (p.556·2).
*Prostatic cancer.*

**Flutaide** *Glaxo Wellcome, Port.*
Fluticasone propionate (p.1102·3).
*Rhinitis.*

**Flutamex** *Sanofi Synthelabo, Ger.†.*
Flutamide (p.556·2).
*Prostatic cancer.*

**Flutamin**
*Alphapharm, Austral.; Pacific, NZ.*
Flutamide (p.556·2).
*Prostatic cancer.*

**Flutan**
*Medochemie, Hong Kong; Medochemie, Malaysia; Medochemie, Thai.*
Flutamide (p.556·2).
*Prostatic cancer.*

**Flutandrona** *Ciclum, Spain.*
Flutamide (p.556·2).
*Prostatic cancer.*

**Flutaplex**
*Teva Tuteur, Arg.; Abbott, Belg.†; Nettopharma, Denm.†; Pharmachemie, Malaysia; Pharmachemie, S.Afr.; Tedec Meiji, Spain.*
Flutamide (p.556·2).
*Prostatic cancer.*

**Flutastad** *Stada, Austria.*
Flutamide (p.556·2).
*Prostatic cancer.*

**Flutax** *Hexal, Arg.*
Flutamide (p.556·2).
*Prostatic cancer.*

**Flutec** *Hexal, Braz.*
Fluconazole (p.398·1).
*Fungal infections.*

**Flutenal** *Recordati, Spain.*
Flupamesone (p.1110·3).
*Skin disorders.*

**Flutenal Gentamicina** *Recordati, Spain.*
Flupamesone (p.1110·3); gentamicin sulfate (p.217·1).
*Infected skin disorders.*

**Flutenal Sali** *Recordati, Spain.*
Flupamesone (p.1110·3); salicylic acid (p.1157·1).
*Skin disorders.*

**Flutepan** *Labinca, Arg.*
Flutamide (p.556·2).
*Prostatic cancer.*

**Flutex**
*Note. This name is used for preparations of different composition.*
*Aspen, S.Afr.*
*Capsules:* Ascorbic acid (p.1460·2); salicylamide (p.87·3); paracetamol (p.76·2); caffeine (p.782·1); phenylephrine hydrochloride (p.1126·3); chlorphenamine maleate (p.427·3).
*Cold and influenza symptoms.*

*Aspen Consumer, S.Afr.†.*
*Syrup:* Paracetamol (p.76·2); phenylephrine hydrochloride (p.1126·3).
*Cold and influenza symptoms.*

*Syosset, USA.*
Triamcinolone acetonide (p.1110·2).
*Skin disorders.*

**Flutex Cough Linctus** *Aspen, S.Afr.*
Diphenhydramine hydrochloride (p.431·3); codeine phosphate (p.27·1); ammonium chloride (p.1115·2).
*Coughs.*

**Flutex Decon-S** *Apotex, S.Afr.*
Pseudoephedrine hydrochloride (p.1129·2).
*Upper respiratory-tract congestion.*

**Flutiamik** *Microsules, Arg.*
Finasteride (p.1554·2).
*Benign prostatic hyperplasia.*

**Flutide**
*GlaxoSmithKline, Ger.; Cascan, Ger.; GlaxoSmithKline, Norw.; GlaxoSmithKline, Swed.*
Fluticasone propionate (p.1102·3).
*Allergic rhinitis; asthma; nasal polyps.*

**Flutin**
*Orion, Denm.; Julphar, UAE.*
Fluoxetine hydrochloride (p.292·1).
*Bulimia; depression; obsessive-compulsive disorder.*

**Flutinase** *GlaxoSmithKline, Switz.*
Fluticasone propionate (p.1102·3).
*Nasal polyps; rhinitis.*

**Flutine**
*Teva, Israel; Pharmasant, Thai.*
Fluoxetine hydrochloride (p.292·1).
*Depression; obsessive-compulsive disorder.*

**Flutivate**
*GlaxoSmithKline, Braz.; GlaxoSmithKline, Chile; GlaxoSmithKline, Ger.; GlaxoSmithKline, Norw.; GlaxoSmithKline, Swed.*
Fluticasone propionate (p.1102·3).
*Skin disorders.*

**Flutol** *Douglas, NZ.*
Flutamide (p.556·2).

**Flutox** *Pharmazam, Spain.*
Cloperastine fendizoate (p.1117·2) or cloperastine hydrochloride (p.1117·2).
*Coughs.*

**Flutrax** *Gautier, Arg.*
Flutamide (p.556·2).
*Prostatic cancer.*

**Flutraz** *Tika, Norw.†.*
Flunitrazepam (p.698·2).
*Insomnia.*

**Fluvaleas** *Valeas, Ital.†.*
Isopropamide iodide (p.485·2); paracetamol (p.76·2); diphenhydramine hydrochloride (p.431·3); caffeine (p.782·1).
*Fever; inflammation; pain.*

**Fluvax**
*CSL, Austral.; Commonwealth Serum, Hong Kong; CSL, NZ.*
An inactivated influenza vaccine (split virion) (p.1620·2).
*Active immunisation.*

**Fluvean** *Formenti, Ital.*
Fluocinolone acetonide (p.1101·2).
*Skin disorders.*

**Fluvermal**
*Janssen-Cilag, Fr.; Janssen-Cilag, Port.*
Flubendazole (p.105·2).
Veterinary names include Flubenol.
*Worm infections.*

**Fluvert** *Medley, Braz.*
Flunarizine hydrochloride (p.434·1).
*Cerebral and peripheral vascular disorders; vestibular disorders.*

**Fluvet** *Vianex (Βιανεξ), Gr.*
Sodium cromoglicate (p.795·3).
*Allergic conjunctivitis.*

**Fluvic** *Pierre Fabre Sante, Fr.*
Carbocisteine (p.1116·2).
*Respiratory-tract congestion.*

**Fluviral**
*Note. This name is used for preparations of different composition.*
*Virtus, Braz.†.*
Paracetamol (p.76·2); pentoxyverine citrate (p.1126·2); phenylephrine hydrochloride (p.1126·3); carbinoxamine maleate (p.426·3).
Formerly contained mepyramine maleate, caffeine, phenylpropanolamine hydrochloride, and dipyrone.
*Cold and influenza symptoms.*

*Shire Biologics, Canad.*
An inactivated influenza vaccine (split virion) (p.1620·2).
*Active immunisation.*

**Fluvirin**
*Thomson, Austral.†; Celltech, Belg.; Evans, Fin.; Evans, Irl.; Medeva,*

*Israel; Farmarekord, Ital.†; Evans, Norw.; Helsinn, Port.; Medpro, S.Afr.; SBL, Swed.; Chiron Vaccines, UK; Powderject, USA.*
An inactivated influenza vaccine (surface antigen) (p.1620·2).
*Active immunisation.*

**Fluvirine** *Celltech, Fr.*
An influenza vaccine (p.1620·2).
*Active immunisation.*

**Fluvium** *Rekah, Israel.*
Sodium fluoride (p.1444·3).
*Osteoporosis.*

**Fluvohexal** *Hexal, Ger.*
Fluvoxamine maleate (p.298·2).
*Depression.*

**Fluvosol** *Berner, Fin.*
Fluvoxamine maleate (p.298·2).
*Depression; obsessive-compulsive disorder.*

**Fluvoxadura** *Merck dura, Ger.*
Fluvoxamine maleate (p.298·2).
*Depression; obsessive-compulsive disorder.*

**Fluvoxin** *Sun, India.*
Fluvoxamine maleate (p.298·2).
*Depression; obsessive-compulsive disorder.*

**Flux**
*Note. This name is used for preparations of different composition.*
*Hexal, Austria.*
Fluoxetine hydrochloride (p.292·1).
*Bulimia nervosa; depression; obsessive-compulsive disorder.*
*Alpharma, Norw.*
Sodium fluoride (p.1444·3).
*Dental caries prophylaxis.*

**Fluxacil** *Uno, Ital.*
Flucloxacillin sodium (p.213·3).
*Bacterial infections.*

**Fluxacina** *Laboratorios Chile, Chile.*
Flucloxacillin (p.213·3).
*Staphylococcal infections.*

**Fluxadir** *Antor, Gr.*
Fluoxetine hydrochloride (p.292·1).
*Depression; obsessive-compulsive disorder; panic disorder.*

**Fluxal** *Pfizer Lambert, Spain.*
Lysine aspirin (p.54·3); calcium ascorbate (p.1460·2); chlorphenamine maleate (p.427·3); phenylephrine hydrochloride (p.1126·3).
*Influenza and cold symptoms.*

**Fluxantin**
*Gea, Denm.; Gea, Fin.; Gea, Swed.*
Fluoxetine hydrochloride (p.292·1).
*Bulimia; depression.*

**Fluxapril**
*Wyeth Lederle, Austria†; Lederle, Ger.†.*
Flucloxacillin sodium (p.213·3); piperacillin sodium (p.243·1).
*Bacterial infections.*

**Fluxarten** *GlaxoSmithKline, Ital.*
Flunarizine hydrochloride (p.434·1).
*Migraine; vertigo.*

**Fluxedan** *AF, Mex.*
Bromhexine hydrochloride (p.1115·3); oxeladin citrate (p.1126·1).
*Respiratory-tract disorders with viscous mucus.*

**Fluxema** *Zimaia, Port.†.*
Bencyclane fumarate (p.867·3).

**Fluxene** *Eurofarma, Braz.*
Fluoxetine hydrochloride (p.292·1).
*Depression; obsessive-compulsive disorder.*

**Fluxet** *Krewel, Ger.*
Fluoxetine hydrochloride (p.292·1).
*Depression.*

**Fluxetil**
*Unison, Singapore; Unison, Thai.*
Fluoxetine hydrochloride (p.292·1).
*Depression; obsessive-compulsive disorder.*

**Fluxetin**
*Atlantic, Singapore; Atlantic, Thai.*
Fluoxetine hydrochloride (p.292·1).
*Depression.*

**Fluxifarm** *Richmond, Arg.*
Flumazenil (p.1038·3).

**Fluxil**
*Note. This name is used for preparations of different composition.*
*UCB, Austria; Aegis, Hong Kong.*
Fluoxetine hydrochloride (p.292·1).
*Bulimia nervosa; depression; obsessive-compulsive disorder.*
*Teuto, Braz.*
Furosemide (p.919·3).

**Fluxinam** *Vilco, Gr.*
Fluorometholone (p.1102·2).
*Inflammatory eye disorders.*

**Fluxine** *Rudefsa, Mex.†.*
Aesculus (p.1648·2).

**Fluxocor** *Cibran, Braz.†.*
Dipyridamole (p.903·1).
*Adjunct in myocardial imaging; ischaemic heart disease; thromboembolism prophylaxis.*

**Fluxol** *UCI, Braz.*
Ambroxol hydrochloride (p.1114·3).
*Respiratory-tract congestion.*

**FluxoMed** *S Med, Austria.*
Fluoxetine hydrochloride (p.292·1).
*Bulimia nervosa; depression; obsessive-compulsive disorder.*

**Fluxoten** *Herbaline, Ital.†.*
Melissa (p.1711·1); centaury (p.1669·2); calendula (p.1665·2); artemisia vulgaris; saffron (p.1058·2).
*Menstrual disorders.*

**Fluxpiren** *Ariston, Arg.*
Diclofenac sodium (p.32·1).
*Musculoskeletal and joint disorders.*

**Fluxum**
*Wassermann, Ital.; Armstrong, Mex.*
Parnaparin sodium (p.978·3).
*Thromboembolic disorders.*

**Fluxus** *Tecnofarma, Chile.*
Flunarizine (p.434·2).
*Mental function impairment; peripheral vascular disorders; vestibular disorders.*

**Fluzac** *LBS, Thai.*
Fluoxetine hydrochloride (p.292·1).
*Depression; obsessive-compulsive disorder.*

**Fluzal** *Julphar, UAE†.*
Carbinoxamine maleate (p.426·3); phenylpropanolamine hydrochloride (p.1127·3).
*Upper respiratory-tract disorders.*

**Fluzerit** *De Salute, Ital.*
Flucloxacillin sodium (p.213·3).
*Bacterial infections.*

**Fluzine** *PP Lab, Thai.*
Fluphenazine hydrochloride (p.699·3).
*Anxiety; schizophrenia.*

**Fluzix** *Cazi, Braz.*
Flunarizine hydrochloride (p.434·1).

**Fluzol** *Kampel Martian, Arg.*
Fluconazole (p.398·1).
*Fungal infections.*

**Fluzone**
*Aventis, Arg.; Aventis Pasteur, Braz.†; Aventis Pasteur, Canad.; Pasteur Merieux, Irl.†; Connaught, Norw.†; Pasteur Merieux, UK†; Pasteur Merieux, USA.*
An inactivated influenza vaccine (split virion) (p.1620·2).
*Active immunisation.*

**Fluzor** *Collins, Mex.*
Fluconazole (p.398·1).
*Fungal infections.*

**Flynoken A** *Kendrick, Mex.*
Calcium folinate (p.1431·1).
*Antidote to folic acid antagonists; megaloblastic anaemia; reduction of methotrexate toxicity.*

**FM7 E** *Rubiepharm, Ger.*
Vitamins; minerals; caffeine; cinchona; rutoside sodium sulfate; spigelia; fructose; glucose; honey (p.1417·1).
*Tonic.*

**FML**
*Allergan, Arg.; Allergan, Austral.; Allergan, Belg.; Allergan, Canad.; Allergan, Fin.; Alvia (Αλβια), Gr.; Allergan, Hong Kong; Allergan, Irl.; Allergan, Israel; Allergan, Malaysia; Allergan, Mex.†; Allergan, NZ; Allergan, Port.; Allergan, S.Afr.; Allergan, Singapore; Allergan, Spain; Allergan, Switz.; Allergan, Thai.; Allergan, UK; Allergan, USA.*
Fluorometholone (p.1102·2).
*Inflammatory eye disorders.*

**FML Neo**
*Allergan, Arg.; Allergan, Israel†; Allergan, Port.; Allergan, S.Afr.; Allergan, Spain†; Allergan, Switz.; Allergan, Thai.*
Fluorometholone (p.1102·2); neomycin sulfate (p.235·1).
*Inflammatory eye infections.*

**FML Neo Liquifilm** *Allergan, UK†.*
Fluorometholone (p.1102·2); neomycin sulfate (p.235·1).
*Inflammatory eye infections.*

**FML-S** *Allergan, USA.*
Fluorometholone (p.1102·2); sulfacetamide sodium (p.257·3).
*Inflammatory eye infections.*

**FMP** *Nakorn, Thai.*
21 Tablets, norgestrel (p.1563·2); ethinylestradiol (p.1553·2); 7 tablets, inert.
*Combined oral contraceptive.*

**FNZ** *Pose, Thai.†.*
Flunarizine hydrochloride (p.434·1).
*Cerebrovascular disorders.*

**Foamicon** *Invamed, USA.*
Aluminium hydroxide (p.1249·2); magnesium trisilicate (p.1272·3); sodium bicarbonate (p.1223·2); alginic acid (p.1576·3).
*Hyperacidity.*

**Foban**
*Hoe, Malaysia; Hoe, Singapore.*
Fusidic acid (p.215·2).
*Staphylococcal skin infections; streptococcal skin infections.*

**Fobancort**
*Hoe, Malaysia; Hoe, Singapore.*
Fusidic acid (p.215·2) or sodium fusidate (p.215·2); betamethasone dipropionate (p.1093·1).
*Skin disorders infected with staphylococci or streptococci.*

**Fobidon** *IBN, Ital.*
Domperidone (p.1263·2).
*Gastric discomfort; nausea; vomiting.*

**Focalin** *Novartis, USA.*
*d*-Methylphenidate hydrochloride (p.1587·1).
*Attention deficit hyperactivity disorder.*

**Focam** *YSP, Malaysia.*
Piroxicam (p.84·2).
*Gout; musculoskeletal and joint disorders.*

**Focus** *Swiss Herbal, Canad.*
Linoleic acid; gamolenic acid; vitamin E (p.1417·1).

**Focus Care All-in-One**
*Ciba Vision, Austral.†; Ciba Vision, NZ.*
Cleansing, rinsing, disinfecting, and storage solution for soft contact lenses (p.1164·2).

**Focus Care One Step**
*Ciba Vision, Austral.†; Ciba Vision, NZ.*
Hydrogen peroxide (p.1182·2) (p.1164·2).
*Disinfection, neutralisation, and storage of contact lenses.*

**Fohn- und Wettertropfen N** *Biomedica, Ger.†.*
Homoeopathic preparation.

**Fohnetten N** *Ziethen, Ger.*
Benzyl mandelate; caffeine (p.782·1); paracetamol (p.76·2).
*Migraine; pain.*

**Foille**
*Note. This name is used for preparations of different composition.*
*Blistex, Canad.†.*
Benzocaine (p.1370·3); benzyl alcohol (p.1170·2).
*Burns; insect bites; wounds.*
*Rider, Chile.*
Benzocaine (p.1370·3).
*Skin irritation.*
*Blistex, USA.*
Benzocaine (p.1370·3); chloroxylenol (p.1177·2).
*Local anaesthesia.*

**Foille Insetti** *Sanofi Synthelabo OTC, Ital.*
Hydrocortisone (p.1103·3).
*Insect stings; skin irritation.*

**Foille Scottature** *Sanofi Synthelabo OTC, Ital.*
Benzocaine (p.1370·3); benzyl alcohol (p.1170·2); chloroxylenol (p.1177·2).
Formerly contained benzocaine, benzyl alcohol, hydroxyquinoline, and colloidal sulfur.
*Burns; skin irritation; wounds.*

**Foille Sole** *Sanofi Synthelabo OTC, Ital.*
Benzocaine (p.1370·3); benzyl alcohol (p.1170·2); chloroxylenol (p.1177·2).
*Burns; skin irritation; wounds.*

**Foipan** *Ono, Jpn.*
Camostat mesilate (p.1665·2).
*Gastro-oesophageal reflux; pancreatitis.*

**Fokalepsin** *Lundbeck, Ger.*
Carbamazepine (p.353·3).
*Alcohol withdrawal syndrome; diabetic neuropathy; epilepsy; multiple sclerosis; neuralgias.*

**Fokeston** *Rafarm, Gr.*
Fluoxetine hydrochloride (p.292·1).
*Depression; obsessive-compulsive disorder; panic disorder.*

**Fol Sang** *IQB, Braz.*
Cyanocobalamin (p.1458·2); hydroxocobalamin (p.1458·2); thiamine hydrochloride (p.1455·1); folic acid (p.1429·1) liver extract.
*Megaloblastic anaemia.*

**Folacid** *ITF, Chile.*
Folic acid (p.1429·1).
*Prevention of neural tube defects in pregnancy; raised plasma homocysteine.*

**Folacin**
*Note. This name is used for preparations of different composition.*
*Ativus, Braz.*
*Oral drops; oral solution:* Folic acid (p.1429·1); ascorbic acid (p.1460·2).
*Tablets:* Folic acid (p.1429·1).
*Folic acid deficiency; megaloblastic anaemia.*
*Pharmacia, Swed.*
Folic acid (p.1429·1).
*Folate deficiency; megaloblastic anaemia.*

**Folacin 12** *Quest, Canad.†.*
Vitamin $B_{12}$ (p.1458·2); folic acid (p.1429·1).

**Folarell** *Sanorell, Ger.*
Folic acid (p.1429·1).
*Antidote to treatment with folic acid antagonists; folate deficiency; megaloblastic anaemia.*

**Folaren** *Ist. Chim. Inter., Ital.*
Calcium folinate (p.1431·1).
*Antidote to folic acid antagonists; folate deficiency; reduction of aminopterin and methotrexate toxicity.*

**Fol-Asmedic** *Dyckerhoff, Ger.*
Folic acid (p.1429·1).
*Folic acid deficiency; megaloblastic anaemia.*

**Folatine** *Lifeplan, UK†.*
Folic acid (p.1429·1).
*Nutritional supplement.*

**Folavit** *Wolfs, Belg.*
Folic acid (p.1429·1).
*Anaemias; prevention of neural tube defects in pregnancy.*

**Folaxin** *Zambon, Spain.*
Calcium folinate (p.1431·1).
*Adjunct to fluorouracil therapy; antidote to folic acid antagonists; reduction of methotrexate toxicity.*

**Folcane** *Rhone-Poulenc Rorer, Mex.†.*
Folinic acid (p.1431·1).

**Folcodal** *Armstrong, Arg.*
Cinnarizine (p.428·3).
*Cerebral and peripheral vascular disorders.*

**Folcodex** *Sanico, Belg.†.*
Pholcodine (p.1128·3); ephedrine hydrochloride (p.1120·1); belladonna (p.479·1); aconite (p.1646·3); sulfogaiacol (p.1131·1); ipecacuanha (p.1122·3); tolu balsam (p.1131·3).
*Bronchopulmonary disorders.*

**Folcofen** *Alliance, S.Afr.*
Diphenhydramine hydrochloride (p.431·3); pholcodine (p.1128·3); guaifenesin (p.1122·1).
*Coughs.*

**Folcress** *Grisi, Mex.*
Minoxidil (p.960·1).
*Alopecia.*

**Folcur** *1A, Ger.*
Folic acid (p.1429·1).
*Folic acid deficiency.*

**Foldan**
*Andromaco, Arg.; Uniao Quimica, Braz.*
Tiabendazole (p.114·2).
*Nematode infections.*

**Folderm** *Kinder, Braz.†.*
Tiabendazole (p.114·2).
*Nematode infections.*

**Folderm Pomada** *Kinder, Braz.*
Tiabendazole (p.114·2); neomycin sulfate (p.235·1).
*Scabies.*

**Foldox**
*Note. A similar name is used for preparations of different composition (see below).*
*Roerig, Chile.*
Piroxicam (p.84·2).
*Inflammation; pain.*

**Foldoxx**
*Note. A similar name is used for preparations of different composition (see above).*
*Sidus, Arg.*
Rofecoxib (p.86·3).
*Osteoarthritis; pain.*

**Folepar B12** *Lisapharma, Ital.*
Folic acid (p.1429·1); nicotinamide (p.1441·2); thiamine hydrochloride (p.1455·1); cyanocobalamin (p.1458·2).
*Deficiency states; macrocytic anaemia.*

**Folergot-DF** *Marnel, USA.*
Phenobarbital (p.367·3); ergotamine tartrate (p.467·2); belladonna (p.479·1).
*Gastrointestinal disorders.*

**Folex**
*Note. This name is used for preparations of different composition.*
*Qualiphar, Belg.*
Pholcodine (p.1128·3); ephedrine hydrochloride (p.1120·1); sodium citrate (p.1223·2).
*Bronchitis; coughs; laryngitis.*
*Rybar, Irl.†; Pharmateam, Israel; Pharmateam, UK†.*
Ferrous fumarate (p.1427·3); folic acid (p.1429·1).
*Iron and folic acid deficiency in pregnancy.*

**Folgamma** *Worwag, Ger.*
Cyanocobalamin (p.1458·2); folic acid (p.1429·1).
*Vitamin $B_{12}$ and folic acid deficiency.*

**Folgamma Mono** *Worwag, Ger.†.*
Folic acid (p.1429·1).
*Folic acid deficiency.*

**Folgard** *Upsher-Smith, USA.*
Folic acid; cyanocobalamin; pyridoxine hydrochloride; riboflavin (p.1417·1).
*Dietary supplement.*

**Foli Doce** *Italfarmaco, Spain.*
Folic acid (p.1429·1); cyanocobalamin (p.1458·2).
*Prevention of neural-tube defects.*

**Foliamin**
*Takeda, Hong Kong†; Takeda, Thai.*
Folic acid (p.1429·1).
*Anaemias.*

**Foliben** *Shire, Ital.*
Calcium folinate (p.1431·1).
*Antidote to folic acid antagonists; folate deficiency; reduction of aminopterin and methotrexate toxicity.*

**Folic Acid Plus** *Cenovis, Austral.†; Vitelle, Austral.†.*
Vitamin and mineral preparation with iron and folic acid (p.1417·1).

**Folic Plus** *Peter Black, UK†.*
Folic acid (p.1429·1); calcium (p.1225·1); vitamin D (p.1461·2).

**Folicalgyn** *Amsa, Ital.*
Calcium folinate (p.1431·1).
*Folate deficiency; reduction of aminopterin and methotrexate toxicity.*

**Folicare** *Rosemont, UK.*
Folic acid (p.1429·1).

**FOLI-cell** *Cell Pharm, Ger.*
Calcium folinate (p.1431·1).
*Antidote to treatment with folic acid antagonists; folate deficiency.*

**Folicil** *Bial, Port.*
Folic acid (p.1429·1).
*Folic acid deficiency.*

**Folicombin** *Jenapharm, Ger.*
Ammonium iron sulfate (p.1436·1); folic acid (p.1429·1).
*Iron and folate deficiency.*

**Folicorin** *Uniao Quimica, Braz.*
Calcium folinate (p.1431·1).

**Folicron** *Julphar, UAE.*
Ferrous sulfate (p.1428·2); folic acid (p.1429·1).
*Iron and folic acid deficiency in pregnancy.*

**Folicum** *Julphar, UAE.*
Folic acid (p.1429·1).
*Folate deficiency.*

**Folidan** *Prasfarma, Spain.*
Calcium folinate (p.1431·1).
*Adjunct to fluorouracil therapy; megaloblastic anaemia; methotrexate poisoning.*

**Folidar** *Italfarmaco, Ital.*
Calcium folinate (p.1431·1).
*Folate deficiency; reduction of aminopterin and methotrexate toxicity.*

**Folifer**
*Note. This name is used for preparations of different composition.*
*Ativus, Braz.*
Iron-amino acid chelate (p.1434·3); folic acid (p.1429·1).
*Anaemias.*

*Rider, Chile.*
Ferrous fumarate (p.1427·3); folic acid (p.1429·1); cyanocobalamin (p.1458·2).
Ascorbic acid (p.1460·2) is included in this preparation to increase the absorption and availability of iron.
*Anaemias; iron deficiency.*

*Bial, Port.*
Ferrous sulfate (p.1428·2); folic acid (p.1429·1).
*Iron and folic acid deficiency.*

**Foliferron** *Wyeth, Spain.*
Folic acid (p.1429·1); ferrous fumarate (p.1427·3).
*Iron and folic acid deficiency.*

**Foligan**
*Desma, Ger.; Synthelabo, Switz.†.*
Allopurinol (p.412·2).
*Gout; hyperuricaemia; renal calculi.*

**Foliglobin** *Pharmaceutical Enterprises, S.Afr.*
Ferrous sulfate (p.1428·2); folic acid (p.1429·1); vitamin $B_{12}$ (p.1458·2).
Ascorbic acid (p.1460·2) is included in this preparation to increase the absorption and availability of iron.
*Anaemias; iron deficiency.*

**Foliment** *Chrispa (Χρισπα), Gr.*
Calcium folinate (p.1431·1).
*Antidote to folic acid antagonists; megaloblastic anaemia.*

**Folimet** *Nycomed, Denm.*
Folic acid (p.1429·1).
*Folate deficiency.*

**Folin** *Geyer, Braz.*
Folic acid (p.1429·1).

**Folina** *Schwarz, Ital.*
Folic acid (p.1429·1) or sodium folate (p.1429·3).
*Folate deficiency.*

**Folinac** *Bioprogress, Ital.*
Calcium folinate (p.1431·1).
*Antidote to overdosage with folic acid antagonists; folate deficiency; reduction of aminopterin and methotrexate toxicity.*

**Folinato** *Faran, Gr.*
Calcium folinate (p.1431·1).
*Antidote to folic acid antagonists; megaloblastic anaemia.*

**Folinemic Ferro** *FIRMA, Ital.*
Iron succinyl-protein complex (p.1438·1).
*Iron deficiency; iron-deficiency anaemias.*

**Folinfabra** *Fabra, Arg.*
Calcium folinate (p.1431·1).
*Antidote to folic acid antagonists.*

**Folingrav** *Amnol, Ital.*
Folic acid (p.1429·1).
*Folic acid supplement.*

**Folinoral** *Therabel, Fr.*
Calcium folinate (p.1431·1).
*Drug-induced megaloblastic anaemia; methotrexate toxicity.*

**Folinovo** *Faulding, Port.*
Calcium folinate (p.1431·1).

**Folinvit** *Garant, Ital.*
Calcium folinate (p.1431·1).
*Anaemias; folate deficiency; reduction of aminopterin and methotrexate toxicity.*

**Foliper** *Ativus, Braz.†.*
Iron-amino acid chelate (p.1434·3); folic acid (p.1429·1).
*Anaemias.*

**Foliplus** *Sanofi Synthelabo, Ital.*
Calcium folinate (p.1431·1).
*Anaemias; folate deficiency; reduction of aminopterin and methotrexate toxicity.*

**Foli-Rivo** *Rivopharm, Switz.*
Folic acid (p.1429·1).
*Megaloblastic anaemias.*

**Folisanin** *Instituto Sanitas, Chile.*
Folic acid (p.1429·1).
*Folic acid deficiency.*

**Folitab** *Rhone-Poulenc Rorer, Mex.†.*
Folic acid (p.1429·1).

**Folitabs** *Abello, Spain†.*
Finasteride (p.1554·2).
*Alopecia androgenetica.*

**Folium** *Defuen, Arg.*
Vaginal lubricant.

**Folivit** *Siam Bheasach, Thai.*
Folic acid (p.1429·1).
*Anaemias.*

**Folix** *Caber, Ital.†.*
Calcium folinate (p.1431·1).
*Antidote to overdosage with folic acid antagonists; folate deficiency; reduction of aminopterin and methotrexate toxicity.*

**Folix-Mater** *IQB, Braz.*
Ascorbic acid; folic acid; cyanocobalamin; ferrous fumarate (p.1417·1).

**Folizol** *Pharmacodane, Denm.*
Fluoxetine (p.296·3).
*Bulimia nervosa; depression.*

**Follegon** *Organon, Neth.*
Urofollitropin (p.1342·1).
*Male and female infertility.*

**Follimin**
*Wyeth Lederle, Norw.; Wyeth Lederle, Swed.*
Levonorgestrel (p.1563·2); ethinylestradiol (p.1553·2).
28-Day packs also contain 7 inert tablets.
*Combined oral contraceptive.*

**Follimon** *LG Pharm, Hong Kong.*
Urofollitropin (p.1342·1).
*Female infertility.*

**Follinett** *Wyeth Lederle, Swed.*
Levonorgestrel (p.1563·2); ethinylestradiol (p.1553·2).
*Combined oral contraceptive.*

**Follistim** *Organon, USA.*
Follitropin beta (p.1324·2).
*Male and female infertility.*

**Follistrel** *Wyeth Lederle, Swed.*
Levonorgestrel (p.1563·2).
*Progestogen-only oral contraceptive.*

**Follitrin**
*Ferring, Arg.; Fustery, Mex.†.*
Urofollitropin (p.1342·1).
*Male and female infertility.*

**Folmigor** *Medinova (Μεντνοβα), Gr.*
Calcium folinate (p.1431·1).
*Antidote to folic acid antagonists; megaloblastic anaemia.*

**Folsan**
*Solvay, Austria; Solvay, Ger.*
Folic acid (p.1429·1).
*Folic acid deficiency.*

**Folsana** *Hotz, Ger.†.*
Ferrous gluconate (p.1428·1); folic acid (p.1429·1).
Formerly known as Ferro-Folsan.
*Iron-deficiency anaemia.*

**Foltene** *Crinos, Hong Kong†.*
Tricosaccaride.
*Alopecia.*

**Foltene Research Anticaspa** *Silesia, Chile.*
Tricosaccharides; piroctone olamine (p.1155·2); pantothenic acid (p.1442·3); salicylic acid (p.1157·1).
*Dandruff.*

**Foltran** *Armstrong, Arg.*
Zopiclone (p.729·3).
*Insomnia.*

**FOLTX** *Pan American, USA.*
Folic acid (p.1429·1); cyanocobalamin (p.1458·2); pyridoxine hydrochloride (p.1456·3).
*Homocysteinaemia; homocystinuria; nutritional supplement.*

**Folverlan** *Verla, Ger.*
Folic acid (p.1429·1).
*Antidote to treatment with folic acid antagonists; folic acid deficiency; increased need for folic acid; megaloblastic anaemia.*

**Folvite**
*Wyeth-Ayerst, Canad.†; Wyeth Lederle, Fin.; ICN, Switz.; Lederle, USA.*
Folic acid (p.1429·1) or sodium folate (p.1429·3).
*Folate deficiency; megaloblastic anaemia.*

**Fomagrippin N** *Michallik, Ger.*
Propyphenazone (p.85·3); ephedrine hydrochloride (p.1120·1); ascorbic acid (p.1460·2).
*Cold symptoms.*

**Fomene** *Almirall, Spain.*
Tetridamine maleate (p.93·2).
*Vaginitis.*

**Fomentil** *SIT, Ital.*
Eucalyptus oil (p.1686·2); menthol (p.1711·3); thyme oil (p.1755·3); peru balsam (p.1730·2); benzoin (p.1751·1).
*Laryngitis; respiratory congestion; rhinitis; sore throat.*

**Fomos** *Luitpold, Ger.†.*
Terfenadine (p.441·1).
*Hypersensitivity reactions.*

**Fon Wan Eleuthero** *Giuliani, Ital.*
Honey (p.1434·2); eleutherococcus senticosis (p.1744·1).
*Nervous tension.*

**Fon Wan Energy** *Giuliani, Ital.*
Multivitamin and mineral preparation with ginseng (p.1417·1).
*Nutritional supplement.*

**Fon Wan Ginsenergy** *Giuliani, Ital.*
Honey (p.1434·2); royal jelly (p.1740·3); ginseng (p.1693·1).
*Nutritional supplement.*

**Fon Wan Memory** *Giuliani, Ital.*
Multivitamin preparation with eleutherococcus and ginkgo biloba (p.1417·1).
*Mental function disorders; nutritional supplement.*

**Fon Wan Pocket Energy** *Giuliani, Ital.†.*
Ginseng (p.1693·1); honey (p.1434·2).
*Nutritional supplement.*

**Fon Wan Pollen** *Giuliani, Ital.†.*
Pollen; honey (p.1434·2); royal jelly (p.1740·3); ginseng (p.1693·1).
*Nutritional supplement.*

**Foncitril** *Lafon, Fr.*
Citric acid monohydrate (p.1673·1); monobasic potassium citrate (p.1224·1); monosodium citrate (p.1224·1).
Formerly contained trimethylphloroglucinol, citric acid monohydrate, monobasic potassium citrate, and monosodium citrate.
*Metabolic acidosis; urinary alkalinisation.*

**Fonderyl** *Raymos, Arg.*
Metoclopramide (p.1274·3).
*Nausea and vomiting.*

**Fondril** *Procter & Gamble, Ger.*
Bisoprolol fumarate (p.875·1).
*Angina pectoris; hypertension.*

**Fondril HCT** *Procter & Gamble, Ger.*
Bisoprolol fumarate (p.875·1); hydrochlorothiazide (p.933·2).
*Hypertension.*

**Fondur** *Durascan, Denm.*
Fluoxetine hydrochloride (p.292·1).
*Bulimia nervosa; depression.*

**Fonergin** *Aventis, Braz.*
Prednisolone (p.1108·1); framycetin sulfate (p.215·1); gramicidin (p.220·2); amylocaine hydrochloride (p.1370·2); procaine hydrochloride (p.1383·2).
*Mouth disorders.*

**Fonergine** *Benitol, Arg.*
Benzocaine (p.1370·3); tyrothricin (p.275·1); bithionol (p.103·3).
*Mouth and throat disorders.*

**Fonergoral** *Ducto, Braz.*
Benzydamine hydrochloride (p.21·1).

**Fonexel** *Francia, Ital.*
Cefonicid sodium (p.174·2).
Lidocaine hydrochloride (p.1377·3) is included in this preparation to alleviate the pain of injection.
*Gram-negative bacterial infections.*

**Fongamil**
*Biorga, Fr.; Remek, Gr.; Juste, Spain†.*
Omoconazole nitrate (p.407·2).
*Fungal infections.*

**Fongarex**
*Piette, Belg.†; Besins, Fr.*
Omoconazole nitrate (p.407·2).
*Fungal skin and vulvovaginal infections.*

**Fongeryl** *SERB, Fr.*
Econazole nitrate (p.397·2).
*Fungal skin infections.*

**Fongitar**
*Note. This name is used for preparations of different composition.*
*Stiefel, Austral.; Stiefel, Hong Kong; Stiefel, NZ; Stiefel, Singapore; Stiefel, Thai.*
Pyrithione zinc (p.1156·2); tar (p.1159·3); cade oil (p.1159·2); coal tar (p.1159·2).
*Scalp disorders.*

*Stiefel, Ital.†.*
Pyrithione zinc (p.1156·2); tar (p.1159·3).
*Seborrhoeic dermatitis.*

*Stiefel, Port.*
Pyrithione zinc (p.1156·2); Polytar (p.1159·2).
*Scalp disorders.*

**Fonicef** *Errekappa, Ital.*
Cefonicid sodium (p.174·2).
Lidocaine hydrochloride (p.1377·3) is included in this preparation to alleviate the pain of injection.
*Gram-negative bacterial infections.*

**Fonicid** *Lafare, Ital.*
Cefonicid sodium (p.174·2).
Lidocaine hydrochloride (p.1377·3) is included in the intramuscular injection to alleviate the pain of injection.
*Gram-negative bacterial infections.*

**Fonigen** *Opco, Denm.*
Fluoxetine (p.296·3).
*Bulimia nervosa; depression.*

**Fonisal** *Salus, Ital.*
Cefonicid sodium (p.174·2).
Lidocaine hydrochloride (p.1377·3) is included in this preparation to alleviate the pain of injection.
*Gram-negative bacterial infections.*

**Fonlipol** *Lafon, Fr.*
Tiadenol (p.1011·2).
*Hypercholesterolaemia.*

**Fonofos** *Pulitzer, Ital.†.*
Fosfomycin calcium (p.214·2).
*Bacterial infections.*

**Fontego** *Polifarma, Ital.†.*
Bumetanide (p.877·2).
*Oedema.*

**Fontex**
*Lilly, Belg.; Lilly, Denm.; Lilly, Fin.; Lilly, Norw.; Lilly, Swed.*
Fluoxetine hydrochloride (p.292·1).
*Anxiety disorders; bulimia; depression; obsessive-compulsive disorder.*

**Fontol** *Altana, Braz.*
Aspirin (p.15·1); caffeine (p.782·1).
*Fever; pain.*

**Fontolax** *Fontovit, Braz.*
Cassia (p.1255·2); coriander (p.1676·1); senna (p.1288·2); liquorice (p.1270·2); tamarind (p.1293·2).
*Constipation.*

**Fonto-Vit B6** *Fontovit, Braz.*
Pyridoxine hydrochloride (p.1456·3).

**Fonto-Vit C** *Fontovit, Braz.*
Ascorbic acid (p.1460·2).

**Fonto-Vit E** *Fontovit, Braz.*
Vitamin E (p.1464·3).

**Fonx** *Yamanouchi, Fr.*
Oxiconazole nitrate (p.407·3).
*Fungal skin infections.*

**Fonzac** *Gemelli, Denm.*
Fluoxetine hydrochloride (p.292·1).
*Bulimia nervosa; depression.*

**Fonzylane**
*Lafon, Fr.; Lafon, Hong Kong.*
Buflomedil hydrochloride (p.877·2).
*Cerebral and peripheral vascular disorders.*

**Foot Zeta** *Zeta, Ital.*
Undecenoic acid (p.410·3); usnic acid (p.1762·1).
*Burns; fungal skin infections; wounds.*

**Footworks** *Avon, Canad.*
Tolnaftate (p.410·1).
*Fungal skin infections.*

**For Gas** *Uniao Quimica, Braz.*
Dimeticone (p.1289·2).
*Flatulence.*

**For Kids Only** *Stanley, Canad.*
Multivitamin preparation (p.1417·1).

**For Liver** *Tosi, Ital.†.*
*Injection:* Uridine (p.1760·3); inosine (p.1701·2); guanosine; cytidine; cyanocobalamin (p.1458·2); riboflavin sodium phosphate (p.1456·1); pyridoxine hydrochloride (p.1456·3); nicotinamide (p.1441·2); calcium folinate (p.1431·1).
*Oral liquid:* Uridine (p.1760·3); inosine (p.1701·2); guanosine; cytidine; cyanocobalamin (p.1458·2); thiamine hydrochloride (p.1455·1); riboflavin sodium phosphate (p.1456·1); pyridoxine hydrochloride (p.1456·3); nicotinamide (p.1441·2); calcium folinate (p.1431·1).
*Anaemias; liver disorders.*

**For Men** *Jamieson, Canad.†.*
Multivitamin and mineral preparation (p.1417·1).

**For Peripheral Circulation Herbal Plus Formula 5** *Vitelle, Austral.†.*
Ginkgo biloba (p.1692·3); crataegus (p.1677·1); zanthoxylum (p.1766·3); capsicum (p.1667·1); rutoside (p.1688·2); hesperidin (p.1688·2).
*Peripheral vascular disorders.*

**For the Post-Menopausal Years** *Jamieson, Canad.†.*
Multivitamin and mineral preparation (p.1417·1).

**For Women Active Woman Formula** *Blackmores, Austral.†.*
Eleutherococcus senticosis; damiana; avena; centella; minerals; vitamin C (p.1417·1).
*Dietary supplement.*

**For Women Multi Plus EPO** *Blackmores, Austral.†.*
Evening primrose oil (p.1686·3); vitamins; minerals; choline bitartrate; bioflavonoids; rutoside (p.1417·1).
*Dietary supplement.*

**Foracet** *Solus, India.*
Pentazocine hydrochloride (p.79·3); paracetamol (p.76·2).
*Pain.*

**Foracort** *Cipla, India.*
Formoterol (p.786·2); budesonide (p.1094·2).
*Asthma.*

**Foradil**
*Novartis, Austria; Novartis, Belg.; Novartis, Braz.; Novartis, Canad.; Novartis, Denm.; Novartis, Fin.; Novartis, Fr.; Novartis, Ger.; Novartis, Gr.; Novartis, Hong Kong; Novartis, Irl.; Novartis, Israel; Novartis, Ital.; Novartis, Malaysia; Novartis, Mex.; Novartis, Neth.; Novartis, Norw.; Novartis, NZ; Novartis, Port.; Novartis, S.Afr.; Novartis, Singapore; Novartis, Spain; Novartis, Swed.; Novartis, Switz.; Novartis, UK; Schering, USA.*
Formoterol fumarate (p.786·1).
*Obstructive airways disease.*

**Foradile** *Novartis, Austral.*
Formoterol fumarate (p.786·1).
*Obstructive airways disease.*

**Foral** *Grossmann, Switz.*
Codeine phosphate (p.27·1); ephedrine hydrochloride (p.1120·1); sodium benzoate (p.1169·3); hedera helix; senega (p.1130·2); liquorice (p.1270·2); star anise oil.
*Coughs.*

**Forane**
*Abbott, Arg.; Abbott, Austria; Abbott, Braz.; AstraZeneca, Canad.; Abbott, Hong Kong; Abbott, Irl.; Abbott, Israel; Abbott, Ital.; Abbott, Malaysia; Abbott, Mex.; Abbott, NZ; Abbott, S.Afr.; Abbott, Singapore; Abbott, Spain; Abbott, Thai.; Baxter, USA.*
Isoflurane (p.1301·1).
*General anaesthesia.*

**Forapin**
*Mack, Belg.†; Mack, Switz.*
Bee venom (p.1655·3); benzyl nicotinate (p.21·2); bornyl salicylate (p.21·2); nonivamide (p.67·2).
*Musculoskeletal, joint, and peri-articular pain.*

**Forapin E** *Mack, Illert., Ger.*
*Liniment:* Bee venom (p.1655·3); bornyl salicylate (p.21·2); methyl nicotinate (p.59·2).
*Ointment:* Bee venom (p.1655·3); benzyl nicotinate (p.21·2); bornyl salicylate (p.21·2).
*Cold damage; musculoskeletal and joint disorders; sports injuries.*

**Foraseq** *Novartis, Braz.*
Treatment 1, formoterol fumarate (p.786·1); treatment 2, budesonide (p.1094·2).
*Asthma.*

**Forbrand** *Uragme, Ital.*
Zinc chloride (p.1469·2); alcohol (p.1166·1).
*Mouth hygiene.*

**Forcaltonin** *Strakan, UK†.*
Calcitonin (salmon) (p.768·2).
*Hypercalcaemia of malignancy; Paget's disease of bone.*

**Forcan** *Cipla, India.*
Fluconazole (p.398·1).
*Fungal infections.*

**Forcapil** *Arkopharma, Fr.*
Calcium pantothenate (p.1442·3); biotin (p.1423·2); pyridoxine (p.1457·2); vitamin $B_{12}$ (p.1458·2); zinc pidolate; cystine (p.1426·3); methionine (p.1042·1).
*Hair and nail tonic.*

**Forcemil** *Normon, Spain.*
Multivitamin and mineral preparation with ginseng (p.1417·1).

**Forceval**
*Unigreg, Irl.; Unigreg, UK.*
Multivitamin and mineral preparation (p.1417·1).

**Forceval Protein**
*Unigreg, Irl.†; Unigreg, UK.*
Lactose- and gluten-free nutritional preparation (p.1417·1).
*Hypoproteinaemia; malabsorption states; nutritional supplement.*

**Forcicline** *Tocogino, Mex.†.*
Tetracycline (p.266·2).
*Bacterial infections.*

**Forcil** *Continentales, Mex.†.*
Ferrous sulfate (p.1428·2).

**Forcilen** *Specifar (Σπεσιφαρ), Gr.*
Azelaic acid (p.1142·3).
*Acne.*

**Forclina** *Kampel Martian, Arg.*
Fludarabine (p.554·1).
*Malignant neoplasms.*

**Forcremol** *Ifusa, Mex.*
Borax (p.1661·3); phenol (p.1188·1); alum (p.1652·1); potassium (p.1232·1).

**Ford Fibre** *Vitelle, Austral.†.*
Ispaghula (p.1268·1).
*Constipation; digestive disorders.*

**Ford Pills** *Faulding, Austral.†.*
Aloin (p.1248·3); phenolphthalein (p.1284·1).
*Constipation.*

**Fordilen** *Novartis, Arg.*
Formoterol fumarate (p.786·1).
*Obstructive airways disease.*

**Fordiuran** *Farmacusi, Spain.*
Bumetanide (p.877·2).
*Hypertension; oedema.*

**Fordrim** *Montpellier, Arg.*
Flurazepam hydrochloride (p.700·3).
*Hypnotic.*

**Fordtran** *Hanseler, Switz.; Streuli, Switz.*
Macrogol 4000 (p.1709·1) with electrolytes.
*Bowel evacuation.*

**Forehead-C** *Lina, UK†.*
Aloe vera (p.1141·3).
*Fever.*

**Forene**
*Abbott, Belg.; Abbott, Denm.; Abbott, Fin.; Abbott, Ger.; Abbott, Neth.; Abbott, Norw.; Abbott, Swed.; Abbott, Switz.*
Isoflurane (p.1301·1).
*General anaesthesia.*

**Forenium** *Abbott, Gr.*
Isoflurane (p.1301·1).
*General anaesthesia.*

**Foresight** *Cantassium Co., UK.*
Multivitamin preparation (p.1417·1).

**Foresight Iron Formula** *Cantassium Co., UK.*
Ferrous gluconate (p.1428·1); copper gluconate (p.1425·3).

**Forexin** *Pharmaland, Thai.*
Ciprofloxacin (p.188·2).
*Bacterial infections.*

**Forgenac** *Formenti, Ital.*
Diclofenac sodium (p.32·1).
*Inflammation; musculoskeletal and joint disorders; oedema.*

**Forgrip** *Ortoquimica, Braz.†.*
Paracetamol (p.76·2); ascorbic acid (p.1460·2); phenylephrine (p.1126·3); cinnarizine (p.428·3).
*Cold and influenza symptoms.*

**Foric** *Sam-On, Israel.*
Ferrous fumarate (p.1427·3); folic acid (p.1429·1).
*Anaemias; folic acid supplement.*

**Forilin** *Novo Nordisk, Denm.*
Roxithromycin (p.254·2).
*Bacterial infections.*

**Forimycin** *Durascan, Denm.*
Roxithromycin (p.254·2).
*Bacterial infections.*

**Foristal** *Novartis, India.*
Dimetindene maleate (p.431·2).
*Allergic eye disorders; allergic skin disorders; pruritus.*

**Forken** *Kendrick, Mex.*
Amiodarone hydrochloride (p.859·2).
*Arrhythmias.*

**Forknow**
*YSP, Malaysia; Yung Shin, Singapore.*
Flunarizine hydrochloride (p.434·1).
*Migraine; peripheral vascular disease.*

**Forlax**
*Note. This name is used for preparations of different composition.*
*Ipsen, Belg.; Beaufour, Fr.; Intersan, Ger.; Beaufour-Ipsen, Hong Kong; Beaufour-Ipsen, Malaysia; Emerging Pharma, Malaysia; Beaufour-Ipsen, Thai.*
Macrogol 4000 (p.1709·1).
*Constipation.*

*IMA, Braz.*
Sodium picosulfate (p.1289·3); cassia (p.1255·2).
*Constipation.*

**Forli** *Filaxis, Arg.*
Indinavir (p.640·1).
*HIV infection.*

**Formadon** *Gordon, USA.*
Formaldehyde (p.1179·3).
*Hyperhidrosis.*

**Formalyde** *Pedinol, USA.*
Formaldehyde (p.1179·3).
*Drying agent in surgical removal of warts; hyperhidrosis and offensive odour of the feet.*

**Formance**
*Abbott, Hong Kong; Abbott, Irl.; Abbott, Mex.; Abbott, Thai.†; Abbott Nutrition, UK.*
Preparation for enteral nutrition (p.1417·1).

**Formasan** *Sanum-Kehlbeck, Ger.*
Homoeopathic preparation.

**Format** *Northia, Arg.*
Metronidazole (p.607·2).

**Formedico** *Uragme, Ital.*
Zinc chloride (p.1469·2); alcohol (p.1166·1); sodium monofluorophosphate (p.1446·2).
*Mouth disorders.*

**Formicain** *DHU, Ger.*
Homoeopathic preparation.

**Formidium** *DHU, Ger.*
Homoeopathic preparation.

**Formin**
*Stadmed, India; Pharmaland, Thai.*
Metformin hydrochloride (p.342·3).
*Diabetes mellitus.*

**Formisoton** *Staufen, Ger.*
Homoeopathic preparation.

**Formistin** *Lusofarmaco, Ital.*
Cetirizine hydrochloride (p.427·1).
*Hypersensitivity reactions.*

**Formitonicum** *Simoes, Braz.†.*
Chinaria officinalis; sterculia (p.1290·2); gentian (p.1692·2); iodine (p.1598·1); cinnamon (p.1672·2).

**Formitrol** *Mipharm, Ital.*
Dextromethorphan hydrobromide (p.1117·3).
*Coughs.*

**Formocarbine** *GlaxoSmithKline Sante, Fr.*
Activated charcoal (p.1030·2).
*Gastrointestinal disorders.*

**Formo-Cresol Mitis** *Colgate Oral Care, Austral.†.*
Formaldehyde (p.1179·3); cresol (p.1177·3).
*Endodontics.*

**Formoftil** *Farmigea, Ital.*
Formocortal (p.1103·2).
*Inflammatory eye disorders.*

**Formomicin** *Farmigea, Ital.*
Formocortal (p.1103·2); gentamicin sulfate (p.217·1).
*Infected inflammatory eye disorders.*

**Formula 2** *Nutrifarma, Mex.†.*
Preparation for enteral nutrition (p.1417·1).

**Formula IV** *GNLD, Austral.†.*
Nutritional supplement with vitamins and minerals (p.1417·1).

**Formula 28** *QIF, Braz.†.*
Vitamin, mineral, and enzyme preparation (p.1417·1).

**Formula 44** *Procter & Gamble, Canad.*
Dextromethorphan hydrobromide (p.1117·3).
*Coughs.*

**Formula 405** *Doak, USA.*
Skin cleanser.

**Formula A-C-E & Selenium** *Sante Naturelle, Canad.*
Vitamin C; calcium; betacarotene; selenium (p.1417·1).

**Formula B Plus** *Major, USA.*
Ferrous fumarate (p.1427·3); folic acid (p.1429·1); multivitamins and minerals (p.1417·1).
*Iron-deficiency anaemias.*

**Formula CDC** *Seroyal, Canad.†.*
Vitamin C, manganese, and zinc (p.1417·1).

**Formula CI** *Seroyal, Canad.†.*
Chromium proteinate (p.1425·1); inositol nicotinate (p.939·3).

**Formula 44D** *Procter & Gamble, Canad.*
Dextromethorphan hydrobromide (p.1117·3); pseudoephedrine hydrochloride (p.1129·2).
*Coughs and cold symptoms.*

**Formula E** *Procter & Gamble, Mex.†.*
Guaifenesin (p.1122·1).

**Formula 44E** *Procter & Gamble, Canad.*
Dextromethorphan hydrobromide (p.1117·3); guaifenesin (p.1122·1).
*Coughs.*

**Formula EM** *Major, USA.*
Glucose (p.1432·2); fructose (p.1431·3); phosphoric acid (p.1731·2).
*Nausea and vomiting.*

**Formula II Especial** *Knop, Chile.*
Homoeopathic preparation.

**Formula Forte Senior** *Hall, Canad.*
Multivitamin and mineral preparation (p.1417·1).

**Formula Gly** *Seroyal, Canad.†.*
Multivitamin and mineral preparation (p.1417·1).

**Formula Gyn** *Seroyal, Canad.†.*
Vitamin $B_6$ (p.1457·2); magnesium proteinate (p.1227·3).

**Formula 44M** *Procter & Gamble, Canad.†.*
Dextromethorphan hydrobromide (p.1117·3); pseudoephedrine hydrochloride (p.1129·2); chlorphenamine maleate (p.427·3); paracetamol (p.76·2).
*Coughs and cold symptoms.*

**Formula 44M Pediatric** *Procter & Gamble, Canad.†.*
Dextromethorphan hydrobromide (p.1117·3); pseudoephedrine hydrochloride (p.1129·2); chlorphenamine maleate (p.427·3).
*Cold symptoms.*

**Formula O** *General Nutrition, Canad.*
Multivitamin preparation with zinc (p.1417·1).

**Formula OSG** *Seroyal, Canad.†.*
Vitamins A, C, and D, and minerals (p.1417·1).

**Formula OSX** *Seroyal, Canad.†.*
Mineral preparation (p.1417·1).

**Formula S** *Procter & Gamble, Mex.†.*
Dextromethorphan (p.1117·3).

**Formula 33 SE** *Nutrition Care, Austral.†.*
Vitamins; minerals; selenium; bladderwrack; echinacea purpurea; hydrastis (p.1417·1).
*Dietary supplement.*

**Formula Stress** *Sante Naturelle, Canad.*
Multivitamin and mineral preparation (p.1417·1).

**Formula VM** *Solgar, USA.*
A range of vitamin preparations (p.1417·1).

**Formula VM-75** *Solgar, UK.*
Multivitamin and mineral preparation (p.1417·1).

**Formulaexpec** *Procter & Gamble, Spain.*
Guaifenesin (p.1122·1).
*Coughs.*

**Formula-S** *Nutricia, Singapore†.*
Lactose-free, soya-based infant feed (p.1417·1).

**Formulat Biosoya** *Dicofarm, Ital.*
Infant feed (p.1417·1).
*Cow's milk intolerance; lactose intolerance.*

**Formulat Pregel** *Dicofarm, Ital.*
Infant feed (p.1417·1).
*Gastro-oesophageal reflux.*

**Formulation R** *G & W, USA.*
Glycerol (p.1694·3); soft paraffin (p.1479·3); phenylephrine hydrochloride (p.1126·3).
*Anorectal disorders.*

**Formulatus** *Procter & Gamble, Spain.*
Dextromethorphan hydrobromide (p.1117·3).
*Coughs.*

**Formule de l'Abbe Chaupitre** *Arkopharma, Fr.*
A range of homoeopathic preparations.

**Formule 115 DM** *Frega, Canad.†.*
Pseudoephedrine hydrochloride (p.1129·2); chlorphenamine maleate (p.427·3); dextromethorphan hydrobromide (p.1117·3).

**Formule No 203 Profil** *Pharmalab, Canad.†.*
Multivitamin and mineral preparation (p.1417·1).

**Formule No 204 Profil** *Pharmalab, Canad.†.*
Vitamin C, iron, and potassium (p.1417·1).

**Formule W** *Wyeth Consumer, Neth.*
Salicylic acid (p.1157·1).
*Corns; warts.*

**Formulex** *ICN, Canad.*
Dicycloverine hydrochloride (p.481·2).
*Antispasmodic.*

**Formulix** *Ortho, UK†.*
Paracetamol (p.76·2); codeine phosphate (p.27·1).
These ingredients can be described by the British Approved Name Co-codamol.
*Pain.*

**Formuly-Piel** *Assistance, Arg.*
Vitamins; minerals; cystine (p.1417·1).
*Nutritional supplement.*

**Formyxan** *Pisa, Mex.*
Mitoxantrone hydrochloride (p.575·2).
*Breast cancer; non-Hodgkin's lymphoma; non-lymphoblastic leukaemia.*

**Forpyn** *Rolab, S.Afr.*
Paracetamol (p.76·2); codeine phosphate (p.27·1); caffeine (p.782·1); doxylamine succinate (p.432·3).
*Pain and associated tension.*

**Forsalil** *UCI, Braz.†.*
Cetylpyridinium chloride (p.1173·1); borax (p.1661·3); benzocaine (p.1370·3); phenosalyl; menthol (p.1711·3); eucalyptus oil (p.1686·2); mallow (p.1709·3).
*Mouth and throat disorders.*

**Forsteo** *Lilly, UK.*
Teriparatide (p.775·2).
*Osteoporosis.*

**Forta** *Ross, USA.*
A range of nutritional supplement preparations (p.1417·1).

**Forta B** *Pharmacia, Belg.*
Hydroxocobalamin acetate (p.1458·2).
*Megaloblastic anaemia; neuralgia; vitamin $B_{12}$ deficiency.*

**Fortacet** *Interdelta, Switz.*
Aluminium acetotartrate (p.1652·3); chamomile (p.1669·3); arnica (p.1656·3).
*Insect bites; skin irritation; soft-tissue injuries.*

**Fortacil** *Manuell, Mex.*
Amino-acid and mineral preparation (p.1417·1).
*Anaemia; tonic.*

**Fortagesic** *Sanofi Synthelabo, Irl.*
Pentazocine hydrochloride (p.79·3); paracetamol (p.76·2).
*Musculoskeletal pain.*

**Fortakehl** *Sanum-Kehlbeck, Ger.*
Homoeopathic preparation.

**Fortal**
*Note. This name is used for preparations of different composition.*
*Sanofi Synthelabo, Belg.; Sanofi Synthelabo, Fr.; Sanofi Synthelabo, Gr.; IFET (ΙΦΕΤ), Gr.*
Pentazocine (p.79·3), pentazocine hydrochloride (p.79·3), or pentazocine lactate (p.79·3).
*Pain.*

*Prisfar, Port.†.*
Calcium and magnesium preparation (p.1417·1).
*Nutritional supplement.*

**Fortal Vision** *Prisfar, Port.*
Multivitamin and mineral supplement (p.1417·1).
*Eye disorders.*

**Fortalgesic**
*Sanofi Winthrop, Swed.†; Sanofi Synthelabo, Switz.*
Pentazocine (p.79·3), pentazocine hydrochloride (p.79·3), or pentazocine lactate (p.79·3).
*Neuroleptanalgesia; pain; premedication.*

**Fortalgex GH** *Laborsil, Braz.†.*
Multivitamin and mineral preparation (p.1417·1).

**Fortalidon P** *Novartis Consumer, Switz.†.*
Paracetamol (p.76·2).
*Fever; pain.*

**Fortalis** *Interdelta, Switz.*
Methyl salicylate (p.59·3); salicylic acid (p.1157·1); formic acid (p.1689·3); camphor (p.1665·3); spike lavender oil (p.1749·2).
*Musculoskeletal and joint pain.*

**Fortam**
*GlaxoSmithKline, Spain; GlaxoSmithKline, Switz.*
Ceftazidime (p.180·2).
*Bacterial infections.*

**Fortamines 10** *Rougier, Canad.*
Multivitamin preparation (p.1417·1).

**Fortamol** *Nordic Drugs, Denm.*
Codeine phosphate (p.27·1); paracetamol (p.76·2).
*Pain.*

**Fortaneurin** *Continental Pharma, Belg.*
Vitamin B substances (p.1417·1).
*Megaloblastic anaemia; neuralgia; polyneuritis; vitamin $B_1$ and/or $B_{12}$ deficiency.*

**Fortapal** *GlaxoSmithKline, Chile.*
Ibuprofen (p.45·3).
*Fever; pain.*

**Fortasec** *Esteve, Spain.*
Loperamide hydrochloride (p.1271·1).
*Diarrhoea.*

**Fortathrin** *Gap, Gr.*
Indometacin (p.47·3).
*Gout; inflammation; musculoskeletal and joint disorders; pain.*

**Fortavil** *Instituto Sanitas, Chile.*
Vitamins; minerals; ginseng; rutin; deanol tartrate (p.1417·1).
*Tonic.*

**Fortax** *Dankos, Thai.*
Cefotaxime sodium (p.175·3).
*Bacterial infections.*

**Fortaz**
*GlaxoSmithKline, Braz.; GlaxoSmithKline, Canad.; Glaxo Wellcome, USA.*
Ceftazidime (p.180·2).
*Bacterial infections.*

**Fortcinolona** *Fortbenton, Arg.*
Triamcinolone (p.1110·2).
*Corticosteroid.*

**Fortecortin**
*Merck, Austria; Merck, Ger.; Merck, Spain; Merck, Switz.*
Dexamethasone (p.1097·1) or dexamethasone sodium phosphate (p.1097·2).
*Corticosteroid.*

**Fortefog** *Agropharm, UK.*
Pyrethrins (p.1509·3); piperonyl butoxide (p.1509·2).
Formerly contained cypermethrin (Fortemethrin), piperonyl butoxide, bioallethrin, and *N*-octylbicycloheptene dicarboximide.
*Insecticide.*

**Fortel**
*Marco, Austral.; Biomerica, USA.*
Fertility test or pregnancy test (p.1734·3).

**Forten** *Farmalab, Braz.*
Amino-acid preparation with hydroxocobalamin (p.1417·1).
*Nutritional supplement.*

**Fortenac** *Interdelta, Switz.*
Diclofenac sodium (p.32·1).
*Musculoskeletal, joint, and peri-articular disorders.*

**Forteo** *Lilly, USA.*
Teriparatide (p.775·2).
*Osteoporosis.*

**Fortepen** *Biochemie, Austria.*
Procaine benzylpenicillin (p.246·1); benzylpenicillin sodium (p.163·2).
*Bacterial infections.*

**Forterra** *Help, Gr.*
Ciprofloxacin hydrochloride (p.188·2).
*Bacterial infections.*

**Fortevital** *Tentan, Switz.*
Multivitamin and mineral preparation with caffeine, ginseng, and ginkgo biloba (p.1417·1).
*Tonic.*

**Fortfen** *Aspen, S.Afr.*
Diclofenac sodium (p.32·1).
*Gout; inflammation; musculoskeletal and joint disorders; pain.*

**Forthane** *Abbott, Austral.*
Isoflurane (p.1301·1).
*General anaesthesia.*

**Fortical** *Rubio, Spain.*
Calcium carbonate (p.1254·2).
*Hypocalcaemia; osteoporosis.*

**Forticine** *Wolfs, Belg.*
Nutritional supplement (p.1417·1).

**Forticol** *Medinfar, Port.*
Deanol acetoglutamate (p.1585·3); heptaminol hydrochloride (p.1697·1).
*Mental function disorders.*

**Forticreme**
*Nutricia, Austral.; Nutricia, Fin.; Nutricia, Fr.; Nutricia, Irl.; Nutricia, Ital.; Nutricia, Port.; Nutricia Clinical, UK.*
Preparation for enteral nutrition (p.1417·1).

**Forticrin** *Panzera, Ital.*
Vitamin B substances (p.1417·1); vitamin E (p.1464·3); achillea (p.1646·2); ginkgo biloba (p.1692·3); ginseng (p.1693·1).
*Hair loss.*

**Fortidrink** *Support, Braz.*
Preparation for enteral nutrition (p.1417·1).

**Fortifer** *United American, Hong Kong.*
Ferrous fumarate (p.1427·3); vitamin B substances; liver (p.1417·1).
*Anaemias.*

**Fortifresh**
*Nutricia, Fin.†; Nutricia, Fr.; Nutricia, Irl.; Nutricia, Ital.; Nutricia, Port.†.*
Preparation for enteral nutrition (p.1417·1).

**Fortijuice**
*Nutricia, Austral.; Nutricia, Irl.; Baxter, NZ; Nutricia, NZ; Nutricia, Singapore†; Nutricia Clinical, UK.*
Preparation for enteral nutrition (p.1417·1).

**Fortilut** *Gap, Gr.*
Norethisterone (p.1562·2).
*Breast or endometrial cancer; endometriosis; hormone replacement therapy; secondary amenorrhoea.*

**Fortimel**
*Nutricia, Fin.; Nutricia, Fr.; Nutricia, Irl.; Nutricia, Ital.; Baxter, NZ; Nutricia, NZ; Nutricia, Port.; Nutricia Clinical, UK.*
High protein nutritional supplement (p.1417·1).

**Fortimicin** *Kyowa, Jpn.*
Astromicin sulfate (p.158·3).
*Bacterial infections.*

**Fortini**
*Nutricia, Irl.; Baxter, NZ; Nutricia, NZ; Nutricia, Port.; Nutricia Clinical, UK.*
Preparation for enteral nutrition (p.1417·1).

**Fortini Multi Fibre** *Nutricia, Austral.*
Preparation for enteral nutrition (p.1417·1).

**Fortinol** *Pharmanel, Gr.*
Carteolol hydrochloride (p.880·3).
*Glaucoma; raised intra-ocular pressure.*

**Fortipine** *Goldshield, UK.*
Nifedipine (p.966·2).
*Angina pectoris; hypertension; Raynaud's syndrome.*

**Fortiplex**
*Note. This name is used for preparations of different composition.*
*Cazi, Braz.†.*
Multivitamin and mineral preparation (p.1417·1).
*Sante Naturelle, Canad.*
Vitamin $B_{12}$ (p.1458·2); ferrous fumarate (p.1427·3).

**Fortipudding**
*Nutricia, Fr.†; Nutricia, Irl.†; Nutricia, Ital.†; Nutricia, Port.†; Nutricia Clinical, UK†.*
High-protein nutritional supplement (p.1417·1).

**Fortisip**
*Nutricia-Bago, Arg.; Nutricia, Austral; Nutricia, Fr.; Nutricia, Irl.; Nutricia, Ital.†; Baxter, NZ; Nutricia, NZ; Nutricia, Singapore†; Nutricia Clinical, UK.*
A range of preparations for enteral nutrition (p.1417·1).

**Fortistress** *Sante Naturelle, Canad.*
Vitamin B substances and vitamin C (p.1417·1).

**Fortolin** *Fortune, Hong Kong.*
Paracetamol (p.76·2).
*Fever; pain.*

**Fortonal** *Medic, Braz.†.*
Ferrous sulfate (p.1428·2); calcium glycerophosphate; sodium glycerophosphate.
*Iron deficiency; iron-deficiency anaemia.*

**Fortovase**
*Roche, Arg.; Roche, Austral.; Roche, Austria; Roche, Belg.; Roche, Braz.; Roche, Canad.; Roche, Chile; Roche, Denm.; Roche, Fin.; Roche, Fr.; Roche, Ger.; Roche, Hong Kong; Roche, Irl.; Roche, Israel; Roche, Ital.; Roche, Mex.; Roche, Neth.; Roche, Norw.; Roche, NZ; Roche, Port.; Roche, S.Afr.; Roche, Spain; Roche, Swed.; Roche, Switz.; Roche, Thai.; Roche, UK; Roche, USA.*
Saquinavir (p.653·3).
*HIV infection.*
*Roche, Gr.*
Saquinavir mesilate (p.653·3).
*HIV infection.*

**Fortplex** *Cazi, Braz.†.*
Multivitamin and mineral preparation (p.1417·1).

**Fortradol** *Bayer, Ital.*
Tramadol hydrochloride (p.94·3).
*Pain.*

**Fortral**
*Sanofi Synthelabo, Austral.; Sanofi Synthelabo, Austria; Sanofi Winthrop, Denm.; Sanofi Synthelabo, Ger.; Sanofi Winthrop, Irl.†; Sanofi Synthelabo, Neth.; Sanofi Synthelabo, NZ; Sanofi Synthelabo, UK.*
Pentazocine (p.79·3), pentazocine hydrochloride (p.79·3), or pentazocine lactate (p.79·3).
*Pain.*

**Fortralin** *Sanofi Synthelabo, Norw.*
Pentazocine (p.79·3), pentazocine hydrochloride (p.79·3), or pentazocine lactate (p.79·3).
*Pain.*

**Fortrans**
*Beaufour, Fr.; Beaufour-Ipsen, Hong Kong†; Beaufour-Ipsen, Malaysia; Emerging Pharma, Malaysia; Beaufour-Ipsen, Singapore; Emerging Pharma, Singapore.*
Macrogol 4000 (p.1709·1); anhydrous sodium sulfate; sodium bicarbonate; sodium chloride; potassium chloride (p.1217·1).
*Bowel evacuation.*

**Fortravel** *Asta Medica, Austria.*
Cyclizine hydrochloride (p.429·3).
*Motion sickness.*

**Fortum**
*GlaxoSmithKline, Arg.; GlaxoSmithKline, Austral.; GlaxoSmithKline, Austria; GlaxoSmithKline, Chile; GlaxoSmithKline, Denm.; GlaxoSmithKline, Fr.; Cascan, Ger.; GlaxoSmithKline, Ger.; GlaxoSmithKline, Hong Kong; GlaxoSmithKline, India; GlaxoSmithKline, Irl.; GlaxoSmithKline, Israel; GlaxoSmithKline, Malaysia; Glaxo Wellcome, Mex.; GlaxoSmithKline, Neth.; GlaxoSmithKline, Norw.; GlaxoSmithKline, NZ; Glaxo Wellcome, S.Afr.†; GlaxoSmithKline, Singapore; GlaxoSmithKline, Swed.; GlaxoSmithKline, Thai.; GlaxoSmithKline, UK.*
Ceftazidime (p.180·2).
*Bacterial infections.*

**Fortumset** *GlaxoSmithKline, Fr.*
Ceftazidime (p.180·2).
*Bacterial infections.*

**Fortwin**
*Ranbaxy, India; Ranbaxy, Thai.*
Pentazocine lactate (p.79·3).
*Pain; premedication.*

**Fortyplan** *Lifeplan, UK†.*
Vitamin, mineral, and nutritional preparation (p.1417·1).

**Fortzaar**
*Merck Sharp & Dohme, Denm.; Merck Sharp & Dohme-Chibret, Fr.; Merck Sharp & Dohme, Malaysia; Merck Sharp & Dohme, Port.; Merck Sharp & Dohme, S.Afr.; Merck Sharp & Dohme, Spain; Merck Sharp & Dohme, Thai.*
Losartan potassium (p.947·2); hydrochlorothiazide (p.933·2).
*Hypertension.*

**Forverm** *Elofar, Braz.*
Mebendazole (p.108·2); tiabendazole (p.114·2).
*Worm infections.*

**Forvital** *Whitehall, Fr.†.*
Multivitamin and iron preparation (p.1417·1).

**Forzaar** *Merck Sharp & Dohme, Ital.*
Losartan potassium (p.947·2); hydrochlorothiazide (p.933·2).
*Hypertension.*

**Forzid** *Atlantic, Thai.*
Ceftazidime (p.180·2).
*Bacterial infections.*

**Fosalan** *Merck Sharp & Dohme, Israel.*
Alendronate sodium (p.765·3).
*Osteoporosis.*

**Fosamax**
*Merck Sharp & Dohme, Arg.; Merck Sharp & Dohme, Austral.; Merck Sharp & Dohme, Austria; Merck Sharp & Dohme, Belg.; Merck Sharp & Dohme, Braz.; Merck Frosst, Canad.; Merck Sharp & Dohme, Chile; Merck Sharp & Dohme, Denm.; Merck Sharp & Dohme, Fin.; Merck Sharp & Dohme-Chibret, Fr.; Merck Sharp & Dohme, Ger.; Vianex (Βιανέξ), Gr.; Merck Sharp & Dohme, Hong Kong; Merck Sharp & Dohme, Irl.; Merck Sharp & Dohme, Ital.; Merck Sharp & Dohme, Malaysia; Merck Sharp & Dohme, Mex.; Merck Sharp & Dohme, Neth.; Merck Sharp & Dohme, Norw.; Merck Sharp & Dohme, NZ; Merck Sharp & Dohme, Port.; Merck Sharp & Dohme, S.Afr.; Merck Sharp & Dohme, Singapore; Merck Sharp & Dohme, Spain; Merck Sharp & Dohme, Swed.; Merck Sharp & Dohme, Switz.; Merck Sharp & Dohme, Thai.; Merck Sharp & Dohme, UK; Merck, USA.*
Alendronate sodium (p.765·3).
*Osteoporosis; Paget's disease of bone.*

**Foscald3** *FIRMA, Ital.*
Calcium phosphate (p.1225·3); colecalciferol (p.1461·3).
*Calcium and vitamin D deficiency; osteoporosis.*

**Foscan** *Biolitec, UK.*
Temoporfin (p.586·3).
*Photodynamic therapy of head and neck cancers.*

**Foscavir**
*AstraZeneca, Austral.; AstraZeneca, Austria; AstraZeneca, Belg.; AstraZeneca, Braz.; AstraZeneca, Fin.†; AstraZeneca, Fr.; AstraZeneca, Ger.; IFET (ΙΦΕΤ), Gr.; Astra, Hong Kong†; Astra, Israel; AstraZeneca, Ital.; Astra, Jpn; AstraZeneca, Neth.; AstraZeneca, Norw.; AstraZeneca, Port.; AstraZeneca, Spain; Astra, Swed.; AstraZeneca, Switz.; AstraZeneca, Thai.†; AstraZeneca, UK; Astra, USA.*
Foscarnet sodium (p.634·2).
*Cytomegalovirus retinitis; herpes simplex infections.*

**Foscovir** *AstraZeneca, Denm.†.*
Foscarnet sodium (p.634·2).
*Cytomegalovirus infections; herpes simplex infections.*

**Fosfalugel** *Yamanouchi, Ital.*
Aluminium phosphate (p.1250·1).
*Gastric hyperacidity.*

**Fosfalumina** *Schering-Plough, Spain†.*
Aluminium phosphate (p.1250·1).
*Gastrointestinal hyperacidity; phosphate deficiency.*

**Fosfarsile Forte** *Fitobucaneve, Ital.*
*Oral liquid:* Royal jelly (p.1740·3); propolis (p.1735·2); selenium (p.1444·1); ginseng (p.1693·1).
*Tablets:* Glucose (p.1432·2); royal jelly (p.1740·3); ginseng (p.1693·1).
*Nutritional supplement.*

**Fosfarsile Junior** *Fitobucaneve, Ital.*
Royal jelly (p.1740·3); vitamins (p.1417·1); phosphorus proteinate; cod-liver oil (p.1425·2).
*Nutritional supplement.*

**Fosfaserin** *Amnol, Ital.*
Phosphatidlyserine; glutamine; vitamin B substances; lecithin; caffeine; ginseng; ginkgo biloba (p.1417·1).
*Mental function disorders; nutritional supplement.*

**Fosfaseron** *Serono, Mex.†.*
Cyclophosphamide (p.540·2).

**Fosfatan** *Farmavy, Braz.*
Thiamine hydrochloride; magnesium glycerophosphate; calcium glycerophosphate; sodium glycerophosphate; guarana; kola; cinchona bark; nux vomica (p.1417·1).
*Tonic.*

**Fosfitone** *Fada, Arg.*
Suxamethonium (p.1408·3).
*Depolarising neuromuscular blocker.*

**Fosfo Plus** *FAMA, Ital.*
Glutamine (p.1433·2); DL-phosphoserine; cyanocobalamin (p.1458·2).
*Tonic.*

**Fosfo-Acutil** *Montpellier, Arg.*
L-Asparagine; glutamine or N-acetyl-L-glutamine; pyridoxine hydrochloride; D-phosphorylserine (p.1417·1).
*Tonic.*

**Fosfoadital** *Gobbi, Arg.*
Monobasic sodium phosphate (p.1230·3); dibasic sodium phosphate (p.1231·1).
*Bowel evacuation; constipation.*

**Fosfo-Astenil** *Sanofi Synthelabo, Port.†.*
Sodium hydroxybenzylphosphinate; phosphoric acid; manganese chloride; calcium glycerophosphate; magnesium glycerophosphate; potassium glycerophosphate; sodium glycerophosphate; totamine; thiamine hydrochloride (p.1417·1).
*Tonic.*

**Fosfocaps** *Sigma, Braz.*
Amino-acid, vitamin, and mineral preparation (p.1417·1).

**Fosfocil** *Senosiain, Mex.*
Fosfomycin calcium (p.214·2) or fosfomycin disodium (p.214·3).
Lidocaine hydrochloride (p.1377·3) is included in the intramuscular injection to alleviate the pain of injection.
*Bacterial infections.*

**Fosfocin**
*Infectopharm, Ger.†; Crinos, Ital.; Boehringer Mannheim, Switz.†.*
Fosfomycin calcium (p.214·2) or fosfomycin disodium (p.214·3).
*Bacterial infections.*

**Fosfocina** *Ern, Spain.*
Fosfomycin calcium (p.214·2) or fosfomycin disodium (p.214·3).
Lidocaine hydrochloride (p.1377·3) is included in the intramuscular injection to alleviate the pain of injection.
*Bacterial infections.*

**Fosfocine** *Sanofi Synthelabo, Fr.*
Fosfomycin sodium (p.214·3).
*Bacterial infections.*

**Fosfocrisolo** *Zambon, Ital.*
Sodium aurotiosulfate (p.90·1).
*Rheumatoid arthritis.*

**Fosfo-Dom** *Dominguez, Arg.*
Monobasic sodium phosphate (p.1230·3); dibasic sodium phosphate (p.1231·1).
*Bowel evacuation; constipation.*

**Fosfoevac** *Bohm, Spain.*
Monobasic sodium phosphate (p.1230·3); dibasic sodium phosphate (p.1231·1).
*Bowel evacuation.*

**Fosfoglutina B6** *Baldacci, Port.*
Calcium pyrrolidonecarboxylate; glutamine; tetraethylamonium phosphate; pyridoxine hydrochloride (p.1417·1).
*Mental function impairment.*

**Fosfoguaiacol** *Ogna, Ital.*
Guaiacol (p.1122·1); eucalyptus (p.1686·1).
*Respiratory congestion.*

**Fosfomik** *Finadiet, Arg.*
Terazosin (p.1011·1).

**Fosfor**
*Consolidated Chemicals, Irl.; Ayrton, UK.*
Phosphorylcolamine.
*Tonic.*

**Fosforal** *Fournier, Ital.†.*
Fosfomycin calcium (p.214·2).
*Bacterial infections.*

**Fosforil Calcium** *SPA, Ital.†.*
Calcium glucose-1-phosphate; pyridoxine hydrochloride (p.1456·3); ergocalciferol (p.1462·1).
*Calcium and vitamin deficiency.*

**Fosforilasi** *Polifarma, Ital.*
Cocarboxylase (p.1455·2); riboflavin sodium phosphate (p.1456·1); pyridoxal phosphate (p.1456·3); nicotinamide (p.1441·2).
Lidocaine hydrochloride (p.1377·3) is included in this preparation to alleviate the pain of injection.
*Neuritis; toxicosis.*

**Fosforina** *Francia, Ital.†.*
Vitamin B substances; vitamin E (p.1417·1).
*Nutritional supplement.*

**Fosfosoda** *Casen Fleet, Spain.*
Monobasic sodium phosphate (p.1230·3); dibasic sodium phosphate (p.1231·1).
*Bowel evacuation.*

**Fosfo-Soda Fleet** *Bergamon, Ital.*
Monobasic sodium phosphate (p.1230·3); dibasic sodium phosphate (p.1231·1).
*Constipation.*

**Fosfosol** *Virtus, Braz.†.*
Kola; guarana; nux vomica; sodium glycerophosphate; glutamic acid; phosphoric acid (p.1417·1).

**Fosfosol Stress** *Virtus, Braz.†.*
Glutamic acid; phosphoric acid; sodium glycerophosphate; vitamin B substances (p.1417·1).
*Tonic.*

**Fosfostilben** *Labinca, Arg.*
Fosfestrol (p.1555·3).

**Fosfotonico** *Hexal, Braz.†.*
Ferrous sulfate (p.1428·2); phosphoric acid; aloes; myrrh; nutmeg; cinnamon.
*Anaemias.*

**Fosfoutipi Vitaminico** *Terapeutico, Ital.*
Uridine triphosphate (p.1760·3); cyanocobalamin (p.1458·2); thiamine hydrochloride (p.1455·1).
*Peripheral neuropathies.*

**Fosfovita** *Wierhom, Arg.*
Lecithin; phenylalanine; vitamin B substances (p.1417·1).
*Nutritional supplement.*

**Fosfree** *Mission Pharmacal, USA.*
Multivitamin preparation with iron and calcium (p.1417·1).
*Calcium supplement; nocturnal leg cramping.*

**Fosgluten Reforzado** *Alter, Spain.*
Calcium magnesium fytate; vitamin B substances; glutamine (p.1417·1).
*Tonic.*

**Fosgluten Super Reforcado** *Alter, Port.†.*
Glutamine; calcium glycerophosphate; vitamin B substances (p.1417·1).

**Fosicomb** *Bristol-Myers Squibb, Austria.*
Fosinopril sodium (p.919·1); hydrochlorothiazide (p.933·2).
*Hypertension.*

**Fosicombi** *Menarini, Ital.*
Fosinopril sodium (p.919·1); hydrochlorothiazide (p.933·2).
*Hypertension.*

**Fosicomp** *Bristol-Myers Squibb, Switz.*
Fosinopril sodium (p.919·1); hydrochlorothiazide (p.933·2).
*Hypertension.*

**Foside** *Solvay, Belg.*
Fosinopril sodium (p.919·1); hydrochlorothiazide (p.933·2).
*Hypertension.*

**Fosinil**
*Solvay, Belg.; Squibb, Spain.*
Fosinopril sodium (p.919·1).
*Heart failure; hypertension.*

**Fosinorm** *Bristol-Myers Squibb, Ger.*
Fosinopril sodium (p.919·1).
*Heart failure; hypertension.*

**Fosinorm comp** *Bristol-Myers Squibb, Ger.*
Fosinopril sodium (p.919·1); hydrochlorothiazide (p.933·2).
*Heart failure; hypertension.*

**Fosipres** *Menarini, Ital.*
Fosinopril sodium (p.919·1).
*Heart failure; hypertension.*

**Fositen**
*Bristol-Myers Squibb, Port.; Bristol-Myers Squibb, Switz.*
Fosinopril sodium (p.919·1).
*Heart failure; hypertension.*

**Fositens**
*Bristol-Myers Squibb, Austria; Squibb, Spain.*
Fosinopril sodium (p.919·1).
*Heart failure; hypertension.*

**Fositens Plus** *Squibb, Spain.*
Fosinopril sodium (p.919·1); hydrochlorothiazide (p.933·2).
*Hypertension.*

**Foslainco** *Lainco, Spain.*
Monobasic sodium phosphate (p.1230·3); dibasic sodium phosphate (p.1231·1).
*Bowel evacuation.*

**Fosmicin** *Meiji, Thai.*
Fosfomycin sodium (p.214·3).
*Bacterial infections.*

**Fosmicin-S** *Meiji, Jpn.*
Fosfomycin sodium (p.214·3).
*Bacterial infections.*

**Fospartan Ginseng** *Craveri, Arg.*
Ginseng; magnesium aspartate; potassium aspartate; adenosine triphosphate; vitamin B substances (p.1417·1).
*Tonic.*

**Fossyol** *Merckle, Ger.*
Metronidazole (p.607·2).
*Trichomoniasis.*

**Fostex** *Westwood, USA.*
Benzoyl peroxide (p.1143·2).
*Acne.*

**Fostex Acne Medication Cleansing** *Bristol-Myers Products, USA.*
Salicylic acid (p.1157·1).
*Acne; hyperkeratosis.*

**Fostex Medicated** *Westwood-Squibb, USA.*
Salicylic acid (p.1157·1); sulfur (p.1158·2).
*Acne.*

**Fostex Medicated Cleansing** *Bristol-Myers Squibb, Canad.†.*
Salicylic acid (p.1157·1).
*Acne; oily skin.*

**Fostimon**
*Genevrier, Fr.; IBSA, Hong Kong; IBSA, Ital.; IBSA, Switz.*
Urofollitropin (p.1342·1).
*Female infertility.*

**Fostril** *Westwood, USA.*
Sulfur (p.1158·2); zinc oxide (p.1163·2).
*Acne.*

**Fosval** *Saval, Chile.*
Alendronate sodium (p.765·3).
*Osteoporosis.*

**Fosvital** *IMA, Braz.*
Vitamin B substances; amino acids; minerals (p.1417·1).
*Tonic.*

**Fotax** *M & H, Thai.*
Cefotaxime sodium (p.175·3).
*Bacterial infections.*

**Fotexina** *Pisa, Mex.*
Cefotaxime sodium (p.175·3).
Lidocaine (p.1377·3) is included in the intramuscular injection to alleviate the pain of injection.
*Bacterial infections.*

**Fotil**
*Croma, Austria; Santen, Denm.; Santen, Fin.; Novartis Ophthalmics, Ger.; Santen, Norw.; Santen, Swed.; Novartis Ophthalmics, Switz.; Santen, Thai.*
Pilocarpine hydrochloride (p.1495·1); timolol maleate (p.1012·2).
*Glaucoma; ocular hypertension.*

**Fotocollyre** *Rafarm, Gr.*
Neomycin sulfate (p.235·1); polymyxin B sulfate (p.245·1).
*Eye infections.*

**Fotocrem 8** *ICN, Arg.*
*SPF 15:* Octinoxate (p.1154·3); avobenzone (p.1142·3).
*Sunscreen.*

**Fotocrem P** *ICN, Arg.*
*SPF 24:* Octinoxate (p.1154·3); oxybenzone (p.1154·3).
*SPF 34:* Octinoxate (p.1154·3); oxybenzone (p.1154·3); titanium dioxide (p.1160·3).
*Sunscreen.*

**Fotocrem Ultra** *ICN, Arg.*
*SPF 42:* Octinoxate (p.1154·3); meradimate (p.1151·3); avobenzone (p.1142·3); biomelanin.
*Sunscreen.*

**Fotocrem-P** *ITF, Chile.*
Titanium dioxide (p.1160·3).
*Sunscreen.*

**Fotofil** *INTES, Ital.*
Sodium aminobenzoate (p.1747·1); actinoquinol (p.1647·2); naphazoline nitrate (p.1124·3); borax (p.1661·3).
*Blepharitis; conjunctivitis; corneal damage.*

**Fotoprotector 15** *Ingens, Arg.*
Octinoxate (p.1154·3); Eusolex 6300 (p.1147·1); avobenzone (p.1142·3).
*Sunscreen.*

**Fotoprotector Extrem** *Ingens, Arg.*
*Cream:* Octinoxate (p.1154·3); Eusolex 6300 (p.1147·1); avobenzone (p.1142·3); methylene bis-benzotriazolyl tetramethylbutylphenol; titanium dioxide (p.1160·3).
*Lotion:* Octinoxate (p.1154·3); Eusolex 6300 (p.1147·1); methylene bis-benzotriazolyl tetramethylbutylphenol; titanium dioxide (p.1160·3).
*Topical gel:* Octinoxate (p.1154·3); Eusolex 6300 (p.1147·1); avobenzone (p.1142·3); methylene bis-benzotriazolyl tetramethylbutylphenol.
*Sunscreen.*

**Fotoprotector Isdin-25** *Andromaco, Chile.*
*SPF 25:* Octinoxate (p.1154·3); titanium dioxide (p.1160·3); avobenzone (p.1142·3).
*Sunscreen.*

**Fotoprotector Isdin-50** *Andromaco, Chile.*
*SPF 50:* Octinoxate (p.1154·3); titanium dioxide (p.1160·3); enzacamene (p.1147·1); zinc oxide (p.1163·2).
*Sunscreen.*

**Fotoprotector Isdin Dry Oil** *Andromaco, Chile.*
Octinoxate (p.1154·3); octisalate (p.1154·3); enzacamene (p.1147·1); dioctylbutamidotriazone; avobenzone (p.1142·3).
*Sunscreen.*

**Fotoprotector Isdin Extrem** *Andromaco, Chile.*
*Gel-cream:* Octinoxate (p.1154·3); enzacamene (p.1147·1); isopropyl palmitate (p.1481·2); avobenzone (p.1142·3).
*Lotion:* Octinoxate (p.1154·3); enzacamene (p.1147·1); titanium dioxide (p.1160·3); avobenzone (p.1142·3).
*Sunscreen.*

**Fotoprotector Isdin F-15** *Andromaco, Chile.*
Octinoxate (p.1154·3); enzacamene (p.1147·1); avobenzone (p.1142·3).
*Sunscreen.*

**Fotoprotectores**
*Note. This name is used for preparations of different composition.*
*Silesia, Chile.*
*Cream SPF 20:* Mpi; cinnamate.
*Sunscreen.*
*Cream SPF 50:* Mpi.
*Sunscreen.*
*Milk:* Dihydroxyacetone (p.1145·2).
*Tanning aid.*
*Stick SPF 20:* Titanium dioxide (p.1160·3); cinnamate.
*Sunscreen.*

*Isdin, Port.*
*SPF 15; SPF 20; SPF 25; SPF 50:* A range of sunscreen preparations.

**Fotoral** *ICN, Arg.*
Vitamin E; vitamin C; betacarotene; zinc; selenium (p.1417·1).
*Antoxidant.*

**Fotorretin** *Poen, Arg.*
Phenylephrine (p.1126·3); tropicamide (p.491·1).
*Production of mydriasis.*

**Fotot ar** *ICN, USA.*
Coal tar (p.1159·2).
*Psoriasis; seborrhoeic dermatitis.*

**Fotrec DHA** *Visufarma, Ital.*
Docosahexaenoic acid (p.976·1); omega-3 triglycerides (p.976·1).
*Nutritional supplement.*

**Fournox** *Charoen Bhaesaj, Thai.*
Ceftazidime (p.180·2).
*Bacterial infections.*

**Four-Ton** *Body Spring, Ital.*
Guarana (p.1765·3); damiana (p.1679·1); ginseng (p.1693·1); royal jelly (p.1740·3).
*Nutritional supplement.*

**Fovas** *Cadila Pharma, India.*
Fosinopril sodium (p.919·1).
*Heart failure; hypertension.*

**Fovysat** *Ysatfabrik, Ger.*
Crataegus (p.1677·1); ginger (p.1267·1).
*Dystonias; neuroses.*

**Fowlers** *Novartis Consumer, Canad.*
Attapulgite (p.1251·1).

**Foxetin** *Gador, Arg.*
Fluoxetine hydrochloride (p.292·1).
*Bulimia; depression; obsessive-compulsive disorder; premenstrual syndrome.*

**Foxil** *Ibirn, Ital.*
Cefadroxil (p.167·2).
*Bacterial infections.*

**Foximin** *Euro-Pharma, Ital.†.*
Fosfomycin calcium (p.214·2).
*Bacterial infections.*

**Foxin** *Pharmaland, Thai.*
Norfloxacin (p.238·3).
*Bacterial infections.*

**Foxinon** *M & H, Thai.*
Norfloxacin (p.238·3).
*Bacterial infections.*

**Foxolin** *Gap, Gr.*
Calcium folinate (p.1431·1).
*Antidote to folic acid antagonists; megaloblastic anaemia.*

**Foxtil** *Uniao Quimica, Braz.*
Cefoxitin sodium (p.177·2).
*Bacterial infections.*

**Foy**
*Lepetit, Ital.; Ono, Jpn.*
Gabexate mesilate (p.1690·1).
*Disseminated intravascular coagulation; pancreatitis.*

**Foziretic** *Lipha Sante, Fr.*
Fosinopril sodium (p.919·1); hydrochlorothiazide (p.933·2).
*Hypertension.*

**Fozitec** *Lipha Sante, Fr.*
Fosinopril sodium (p.919·1).
*Heart failure; hypertension.*

**FP 20** *Pisa, Mex.*
Electrolyte infusion (p.1217·1).

**Fracidin** *Rayere, Mex.*
Oxymetazoline (p.1126·2).
*Nasal congestion.*

**Fractal** *Sinbio, Fr.*
Fluvastatin sodium (p.918·2).
*Hypercholesterolaemia.*

**Frademicina**
*Janssen-Cilag, Arg.; Pharmacia, Braz.*
Lincomycin (p.226·2).
*Bacterial infections.*

**Fradilen** *Chibret, Port.*
Chromocarb diethylamine (p.1670·3).
*Capillary fragility.*

**Frador**
*Note. This name is used for preparations of different composition.*
*Wilson, NZ.*
Menthol (p.1711·3); chlorobutanol (p.1176·3); storax (p.1749·3).
*Mouth ulcers.*

*Trinity, UK.*
Menthol (p.1711·3); chlorobutanol (p.1176·3); storax (p.1749·3); benzoin (p.1751·1).
*Mouth ulcers.*

**Fragador** *Weleda, UK.*
Homoeopathic preparation.

**Fragmin**
*Pharmacia, Austral.; Pharmacia, Austria; Pharmacia, Belg.; Pharmacia, Braz.; Pharmacia, Canad.; Pharmacia, Chile; Pharmacia, Denm.; Pharmacia, Fin.; Pharmacia, Ger.; Pharmacia-Upjohn, Gr.; Pharmacia, Hong Kong; Kabi Pharmacia, Israel; Pharmacia Upjohn, Ital.; Pharmacia, Neth.; Pharmacia, Norw.; Pharmacia, NZ; Pharmacia, Port.; Pharmacia, S.Afr.; Pharmacia, Singapore; Pharmacia, Spain; Pharmacia, Swed.; Pharmacia, Switz.; Pharmacia, UK; Pharmacia, USA.*
Dalteparin sodium (p.891·1).
*Prevention of clotting during haemodialysis or haemofiltration; thromboembolic disorders; unstable angina.*

**Fragmine** *Pharmacia, Fr.*
Dalteparin sodium (p.891·1).
*Prevention of clotting during haemodialysis; thromboembolic disorders.*

**Fragonal** *Phygiene, Fr.†.*
Ruscus aculeatus; esculoside (p.1648·2).
*Circulatory disorders; haemorrhoids.*

**Frakidex**
*Chauvin, Fr.; Chauvin, Hong Kong; Chauvin, Singapore; Bausch & Lomb, Switz.*
Dexamethasone sodium phosphate (p.1097·2); framycetin sulfate (p.215·1).
*Infected eye disorders.*

*Chauvin, Port.*
Dexamethasone phosphate (p.1097·2); framycetin sulfate (p.215·1).
*Infected eye disorders.*

**Frakitacine** *Bausch & Lomb, Switz.*
Framycetin sulfate (p.215·1).
*Bacterial eye infections.*

**Framecef** *Levofarma, Ital.*
Cefonicid sodium (p.174·2).
Lidocaine hydrochloride (p.1377·3) is included in this preparation to alleviate the pain of injection.
*Gram-negative bacterial infections.*

**Framil** *Francia, Ital.†.*
Bicarnitine chloride (p.1424·1).
*Anorexia; dyspepsia.*

**Framin** *SIFRA, Ital.†.*
Amino-acid infusion (p.1417·1).
*Parenteral nutrition.*

**Framybiotal** *Martin, Fr.†.*
Framycetin sulfate (p.215·1).
*Rhinopharyngeal infections.*

**Framyxone** *Theratech, Fr.*
Dexamethasone sodium phosphate (p.1097·2); framycetin sulfate (p.215·1); polymyxin B sulfate (p.245·1).
Formerly known as Dexapolyfra.
*Ear and nose infections.*

**Francital** *Francia, Ital.*
Fosfomycin calcium (p.214·2).
*Bacterial infections.*

**Frangulina** *Ottolenghi, Ital.*
Frangula (p.1266·3); boldo (p.1661·2).
*Constipation.*

**Franol**
*Note. This name is used for preparations of different composition.*
*Sanofi Synthelabo, Braz.*
Ephedrine sulfate (p.1120·1); theophylline (p.798·3).
*Bronchospasm.*

*Sanofi Winthrop, Irl.†; Sanofi Synthelabo, UK.*
Ephedrine hydrochloride (p.1120·1); theophylline (p.798·3).
Formerly contained phenobarbital, ephedrine hydrochloride, and theophylline in the *UK.*
*Obstructive airways disease.*

*Sanofi Synthelabo, Thai.*
Theophylline (p.798·3).
*Obstructive airways disease.*

**Franol Expectorant** *Sanofi Synthelabo, Irl.*
Theophylline hydrate (p.798·3); guaifenesin (p.1122·1).
*Obstructive airways disease.*

**Franol Plus** *Sanofi Synthelabo, UK.*
Ephedrine sulfate (p.1120·1); theophylline (p.798·3).
*Obstructive airways disease.*

**Franolyn Expectorant** *Johnson & Johnson MSD Consumer, UK†.*
Ephedrine (p.1120·1); guaifenesin (p.1122·1); theophylline (p.798·3).
*Coughs.*

**Franolyn Sedative** *Johnson & Johnson MSD Consumer, UK†.*
Dextromethorphan hydrobromide (p.1117·3).
*Coughs.*

**Franzbranns** *Hilarys, Canad.*
Menthol (p.1711·3); alcohol (p.1166·1); eucalyptus oil (p.1686·2); salol (p.88·1).

**Franzbranntwein** *Klosterfrau, Ger.*
Camphor (p.1665·3); pumilio pine oil (p.1737·1).
*Musculoskeletal and joint pain; soft-tissue disorders.*

**Franzbranntwein mit Fichtennadelol** *Hetterich, Ger.*
Camphor (p.1665·3); alcohol (p.1166·1); Norway spruce oil.
*Musculoskeletal and joint pain; soft-tissue disorders.*

**Fraurs** *Francia, Ital.*
Ursodeoxycholic acid (p.1760·3).
*Biliary disorders; gallstones.*

**Fravitan** *Degorts, Mex.*
Vitamin and mineral preparation (p.1417·1).

**Fraxidol** *Edmond Pharma, Ital.*
Tramadol hydrochloride (p.94·3).
*Pain.*

**Fraxiforte** *Sanofi Synthelabo, Switz.*
Nadroparin calcium (p.963·3).
*Deep-vein thrombosis.*

**Fraxiparin**
*Sanofi Synthelabo, Austria; Kwizda, Austria; Sanofi Synthelabo, Ger.*
Nadroparin calcium (p.963·3).
*Thromboembolic disorders.*

**Fraxiparina**
*Sanofi Synthelabo, Braz.; Sanofi Synthelabo, Ital.; Sanofi Synthelabo, Port.; Sanofi Synthelabo, Spain.*
Nadroparin calcium (p.963·3).
*Prevention of clotting during haemodialysis; thromboembolic disorders; unstable angina.*

**Fraxiparine**
*Sanofi Synthelabo, Arg.; Sanofi Synthelabo, Austral.†; Sanofi Synthelabo, Belg.; Sanofi Synthelabo, Canad.; Sanofi Synthelabo, Chile; Sanofi Winthrop, Denm.†; Sanofi Winthrop, Fin.†; Sanofi Synthelabo, Fr.; Sanofi Synthelabo, Gr.; Sanofi Synthelabo, Hong Kong; Sanofi Synthelabo, Israel; Sanofi Synthelabo, Malaysia; Sanofi Synthelabo, Mex.; Sanofi Synthelabo, Neth.; Sanofi Synthelabo, Norw.; Sanofi Synthelabo, NZ; Sanofi Synthelabo, S.Afr.; Sanofi Synthelabo, Singapore; Sanofi Synthelabo, Swed.; Sanofi Synthelabo, Switz.; Sanofi Synthelabo, Thai.*
Nadroparin calcium (p.963·3).
*Prevention of clotting during haemodialysis; thromboembolic disorders; unstable angina.*

**Fraxodi**
*Sanofi Synthelabo, Fr.; Sanofi Synthelabo, Ger.; Sanofi Synthelabo, Mex.; Sanofi Synthelabo, Neth.*
Nadroparin calcium (p.963·3).
*Thromboembolic disorders.*

**Frazim** *Francia, Ital.*
Pirenzepine hydrochloride (p.488·1).
*Peptic ulcer.*

**Frazoline** *Bouchara-Recordati, Fr.†.*
Framycetin sulfate (p.215·1); naphazoline nitrate (p.1124·3); amylocaine hydrochloride (p.1370·2).
*Nasal infection and congestion.*

**FreAmine**
*McGaw, NZ†.*
Amino-acid infusion (p.1417·1).
*Parenteral nutrition.*

*Fresenius Kabi, UK†.*
Amino-acid and electrolyte infusions (p.1417·1).
*Parenteral nutrition.*

**FreAmine III**
*Braun McGaw, Hong Kong†; Braun, USA.*
A range of amino-acid infusions (p.1417·1).
*Parenteral nutrition.*

*Baxter, Ital.*
Amino-acid and electrolyte infusions (p.1417·1).
*Parenteral nutrition.*

**FreAmine 3% Electrolitos** *Pharmacia Upjohn, Spain†.*
Amino-acid and electrolyte infusion (p.1417·1).
*Parenteral nutrition.*

**FreAmine HBC** *McGaw, USA.*
Amino-acid infusion (p.1417·1).
*Parenteral nutrition in hepatic encephalopathy.*

**FreAmine Hepatico** *Pharmacia Upjohn, Spain†.*
Amino-acid infusion (p.1417·1).
*Parenteral nutrition in hepatic encephalopathy.*

**Frebac** *Macrophar, Thai.*
Chlorhexidine gluconate (p.1173·2); cetrimide (p.1172·1).
*Disinfection od skin, wounds, and instruments.*

**Frebini**
*Fresenius Kabi, Irl.; Fresenius Kabi, UK.*
A range of preparations for enteral nutrition in children (p.1417·1).

**Fre-bre** *Self-Care Products, UK.*
Parsley seed (p.1728·3); peppermint oil (p.1283·2); spearmint oil (p.1749·1).

**Frecuental** *Lacefa, Arg.*
Furosemide (p.919·3).

**Fredcina** *Bunker, Braz.†.*
Lincomycin (p.226·2).
*Bacterial infections.*

**Fredol** *Medipharm, Chile.*
Ergotamine tartrate (p.467·2); dipyrone (p.35·3); caffeine (p.782·1); chlorphenamine (p.428·1).
*Vascular headache.*

**Fredyr** *Rafarm, Gr.*
Cefuroxime sodium (p.184·1).
*Bacterial infections.*

**Free & Clear** *Pharmaceutical Specialties, USA.*
Skin cleanser.

**Freecad** *Wockhardt, India.*
Betacarotene; vitamin E; vitamin C; zinc; copper; manganese; selenium (p.1417·1).
*Ischaemic heart disease; prevention of cataract and macular degeneration; skin disorders.*

**Freedavite** *Freeda, USA.*
Multivitamin and mineral preparation with iron (p.1417·1).

**Freedox**
*Pharmacia Upjohn, Austral.†; Pharmacia, Austria; Pharmacia, Belg.; Pharmacia Upjohn, Denm.†; Pharmacia Upjohn, Fin.†; Pharmacia Upjohn, Norw.†; Pharmacia, S.Afr.; Pharmacia Upjohn, Swed.†; Pharmacia, Switz.*
Tirilazad mesilate (p.1013·2).
*Subarachnoid haemorrhage in males.*

**Freeflex Cloruro Sodico** *Fresenius Kabi, Spain.*
Sodium chloride (p.1233·3).
*Fluid and electrolyte disorders.*

**Freeflex Ringer Lactato** *Fresenius Kabi, Spain.*
Electrolyte infusion (p.1217·1).
*Fluid and electrolyte disorders.*

**Freenal** *Ache, Braz.*
Oxymetazoline hydrochloride (p.1126·1).
*Nasal congestion.*

**Freesept** *Rider, Chile.*
Cetylpyridinium chloride (p.1173·1).
*Mouth and throat hygiene.*

**Freezone**
*Medtech, Canad.; Whitehall, Irl.†; Whitehall, USA.*
Salicylic acid (p.1157·1).
*Hyperkeratosis.*

**Freimax** *Caldeira & Marques, Port.*
Methyl salicylate (p.59·3); turpentine oil (p.1760·1); camphor (p.1665·3); thymol (p.1194·2); pine oil.
*Inflammation; musculoskeletal and joint disorders.*

**Freka-cid**
*Niddapharm, Ger.; Stada, Hong Kong; Stada, Malaysia.*
Povidone-iodine (p.1190·3).
*Burns; skin disinfection; wounds.*

**Freka-Clyss** *Fresenius Kabi, Switz.*
Dibasic sodium phosphate (p.1231·1); monobasic sodium phosphate (p.1230·3).
*Bowel evacuation; constipation.*

**Frekaderm**
*Fresenius, Fr.†; Fresenius Kabi, Switz.*
Alcohol (p.1166·1); benzalkonium chloride (p.1168·3); orthophenylphenol (p.1187·2); clorophene (p.1177·3).
*Skin disinfection.*

**Freka-Derm** *Fresenius Kabi, Ger.*
Alcohol (p.1166·1); benzalkonium chloride (p.1168·3); orthophenylphenol (p.1187·2); clorophene (p.1177·3).
*Skin disinfection.*

**Freka-Drainjet** *Fresenius Kabi, Ger.*
Sodium chloride (p.1233·3).
*Irrigation fluid.*

**Freka-Drainjet Purisole** *Fresenius Kabi, Ger.*
Sorbitol (p.1446·3); mannitol (p.950·2).
*Bladder irrigation.*

**Freka-Nol** *Fresenius Kabi, Ger.*
Alcohol (p.1166·1); glyoxal (p.1181·1); didecyldimethylammonium chloride (p.1178·3).
*Surface and instrument disinfection.*

**Freka-Sept 80** *Fresenius Kabi, Ger.*
Alcohol (p.1166·1); orthophenylphenol (p.1187·2); clorophene (p.1177·3); benzalkonium chloride (p.1168·3).
*Hand disinfection.*

**Freka-Steril** *Fresenius Kabi, Ger.*
Propyl alcohol (p.1191·2); isopropyl alcohol (p.1184·3).
*Hand disinfection; skin disinfection.*

**FrekaVit** *Fresenius Kabi, Ger.*
Multivitamin infusion (p.1417·1).
*Parenteral nutrition.*

**Fremet** *Recordati, Spain.*
Cimetidine (p.1255·3).
*Acid aspiration; gastro-oesophageal reflux; gastrointestinal haemorrhage; gastrointestinal hyperacidity; peptic ulcer; short-bowel syndrome; Zollinger-Ellison syndrome.*

**Frenacol** *Sanofi Synthelabo, Chile Solución oral.*
Paracetamol (p.76·2); pseudoephedrine hydrochloride (p.1129·2); chlorphenamine maleate (p.427·3).
*Cold symptoms; nasal congestion; sinusitis.*

**Frenactil**
*Janssen-Cilag, Belg.; Janssen-Cilag, Neth.*
Benperidol (p.671·2).
*Agitation; delirium; hallucinations; nausea and vomiting; psychoses; sexually deviant behaviour.*

**Frenadol** *Abello, Spain.*
Paracetamol (p.76·2); chlorphenamine maleate (p.427·3); dextromethorphan hydrobromide (p.1117·3).
*Coughs; fever; influenza and cold symptoms; pain.*

**Frenadol Complex** *Abello, Spain.*
Ascorbic acid (p.1460·2); caffeine citrate (p.782·1); chlorphenamine maleate (p.427·3); dextromethorphan hydrobromide (p.1117·3); paracetamol (p.76·2).
*Cold and influenza symptoms; coughs; fever; pain.*

**Frenadol PS** *Abello, Spain.*
Paracetamol (p.76·2); pseudoephedrine hydrochloride (p.1129·2); dextromethorphan hydrobromide (p.1117·3); chlorphenamine maleate (p.427·3).
*Cold and influenza symptoms; coughs; fever; pain.*

**Frenal**
*Monsanto, Ital.; Sigma-Tau, Spain.*
Sodium cromoglicate (p.795·3).
*Asthma; bronchospasm.*

**Frenal Compositum** *Sigma-Tau, Spain.*
Sodium cromoglicate (p.795·3); isoprenaline sulfate (p.940·2).
*Allergic bronchitis; asthma.*

**Frenal Rinologico** *Searle, Ital.†.*
Sodium cromoglicate (p.795·3).
*Allergic rhinitis.*

**Frenaler** *Laboratorios Chile, Chile.*
Loratadine (p.436·1).
*Hypersensitivity reactions.*

**Frenaler-D** *Laboratorios Chile, Chile.*
Loratadine (p.436·1); pseudoephedrine hydrochloride (p.1129·2) or pseudoephedrine sulfate (p.1129·2).
*Nasal congestion; rhinitis; sinusitis.*

**Frenaseltz** *Abello, Spain.*
Paracetamol (p.76·2); chlorphenamine maleate (p.427·3).
Formerly contained paracetamol, chlorphenamine maleate, and phenylpropanolamine hydrochloride.
*Cold and influenza symptoms.*

**Frenasma** *Faran, Gr.*
Ketotifen fumarate (p.788·1).
*Allergic rhinitis; asthma.*

**Frenatus** *Abello, Spain.*
Dextromethorphan hydrobromide (p.1117·3).
*Coughs.*

**Frendox** *Errekappa, Ital.†.*
Bioflavonoids; vitamin E (p.1417·1).
*Nutritional supplement.*

**frenopect** *Hefa, Ger.*
Ambroxol hydrochloride (p.1114·3).
*Respiratory-tract disorders associated with increased or viscous mucus.*

**Frenotos**
*Note. This name is used for preparations of different composition.*
*Disprovent, Arg.*
Oxeladin citrate (p.1126·1).
*Coughs.*

*Lafi, Chile.*
Zipeprol hydrochloride (p.1132·3).
*Coughs.*

**Frenotos Muc** *Disprovent, Arg.*
Oxeladin citrate (p.1126·1); bromhexine hydrochloride (p.1115·3).
*Coughs; respiratory-tract congestion.*

**Frenotosse** *Cimed, Braz.*
Bromoform (p.1663·1); tolu balsam (p.1131·3); sodium benzoate (p.1169·3).
*Coughs.*

**Frenotossil** *Infabra, Braz.†.*
Potassium iodide (p.1598·1); sulfogaiacol (p.1131·1); tolu balsam (p.1131·3).
*Respiratory-tract congestion.*

**Frenovex** *Hearst, Braz.†.*
Rutoside (p.1688·2); menadione (p.1466·3); ascorbic acid (p.1460·2).
*Haemorrhagic disorders.*

**Frenurin** *UCI, Braz.*
Oxybutynin hydrochloride (p.486·3).
*Urinary-tract disorders.*

**Frerichs Maldifassi** *Pharbenia, Ital.*
Aloes (p.1248·2); rhubarb (p.1287·3); calamus (p.1664·1); gentian (p.1692·2).
*Constipation.*

**Frescansol** *Volta, Chile.*
Borax (p.1661·3); sodium bicarbonate (p.1223·2); boric acid (p.1662·1).
*Hyperhidrosis.*

**Fresco** *Rekah, Israel.*
Calcium carbonate (p.1254·2); magnesium carbonate (p.1272·1); magnesium trisilicate (p.1272·3).
*Gastrointestinal hyperacidity; peptic ulcer.*

**Fresenius OPD** *Rowa, Irl.†.*
Preparation for enteral nutrition (p.1417·1).
*Inflammatory bowel disease.*

**Fresenizol** *Fresenius Kabi, Mex.*
Metronidazole (p.607·2).
*Anaerobic bacterial infections.*

**Fresh Tears** *Allergan, Braz.*
Carmellose sodium (p.1577·3).
*Dry eyes.*

**FreshBurst Listerine** *Warner-Lambert, USA.*
Thymol (p.1194·2); cineole (p.1672·1); methyl salicylate (p.59·3); menthol (p.1711·3).
*Mouth disorders.*

**Freshmel** *Laboratorios Chile, Chile.*
Chlorhexidine hydrochloride (p.1173·3).
*Mouth and throat infections.*

**Freshmel Tos** *Laboratorios Chile, Chile.*
Chlorhexidine hydrochloride (p.1173·3); noscapine (p.1125·3).
*Coughs; mouth and throat infections.*

**Fresofol** *Fresenius Kabi, Mex.*
Propofol (p.1305·3).
*General anaesthesia; sedative.*

**Fresubin**
*Fresenius Kabi, Fin.; Fresenius Kabi, Irl.; Fresenius Kabi, Ital.; Fresenius Kabi, Mex.; Fresenius Kabi, Port.; Fresenius Kabi, Switz.; Fresenius Kabi, Thai.; Fresenius Kabi, UK.*
A range of preparations for enteral nutrition (p.1417·1).

**Freudal** *Ifusa, Mex.*
Diazepam (p.690·1).

**Frialgina** *Prodes, Spain†.*
Aspirin (p.15·1); ascorbic acid (p.1460·2); caffeine (p.782·1).
*Fever; pain.*

**Friax** *Zeller, Port.†.*
Cetrimide (p.1172·1); benzyl alcohol (p.1170·2); eucalyptus oil (p.1686·2).
*Chilblains.*

**Friccex** *Bergamo, Braz.†.*
Methacholine; thymol (p.1194·2); menthol (p.1711·3); methyl salicylate (p.59·3); camphor (p.1665·3).
*Musculoskeletal and joint disorders.*

**Friction Rub** *Mathieu, Canad.†.*
Isopropyl alcohol (p.1184·3).

**Fridalit** *Fada, Arg.*
Hydrocortisone (p.1103·3).
*Corticosteroid.*

**Frigol** *Brady, Austria.*
Xantinol nicotinate (p.1029·1).
*Cerebral and peripheral vascular disorders.*

**Frigoplasma** *Kropf, Switz.*
Aluminium acetotartrate (p.1652·3); chamomile (p.1669·3); hamamelis (p.1696·3); camphor (p.1665·3); cajuput oil (p.1664·1); rosemary oil (p.1740·2); thyme oil (p.1755·3).
*Phlebitis; soft-tissue and peri-articular disorders.*

**Frilen** *Offenbach, Mex.*
Paracetamol (p.76·2).
*Fever; pain.*

**Friliver** *Bracco, Ital.*
Amino-acid preparations (p.1417·1).
*Hepatic failure; tonic.*

**Frinova** *Aventis, Spain.*
Promethazine (p.439·1).
*Hypersensitivity reactions; motion sickness; nausea and vomiting.*

**Friobax** *Degorts, Mex.*
Paracetamol (p.76·2); phenylpropanolamine (p.1127·3); chlorphenamine (p.428·1).

**Frionex** *Wierhom, Arg.*
Pentane; butane (p.1235·1).
*Pain.*

**Frionex Plus** *Wierhom, Arg.*
Menthol (p.1711·3); camphor (p.1665·3).
*Inflammation; pain.*

**Friosmin N** *Michallik, Ger.*
Bismuth subgallate (p.1252·2); emplastrum lithargyri.
*Burns; wounds.*

**Fripi** *Monserrat, Arg.*
Permethrin (p.1508·3).
*Pediculosis.*

**Friral** *Farcoral, Mex.*
Moroxydine hydrochloride (p.649·3); phenylephrine (p.1126·3); chlorphenamine (p.428·1).
*Cold symptoms.*

**Frisin** *Aventis, Chile.*
Clobazam (p.358·2).
*Anxiety; epilepsy.*

**Frisium**
*Aventis, Austral.; Aventis, Austria; Aventis, Belg.; Aventis, Braz.; Aventis, Canad.; Aventis, Denm.; Aventis, Fin.; Aventis, Ger.; Hoechst Marion Roussel, Gr.; Aventis, Hong Kong; Aventis, India; Aventis, Irl.; Hoechst Marion Roussel, Israel†; Aventis, Ital.; Aventis, Malaysia; Aventis, Mex.; Aventis, Neth.; Aventis, NZ; Hoechst Marion Roussel, Singapore†; Aventis, Thai.; Aventis, UK.*
Clobazam (p.358·2).
*Anxiety; epilepsy; insomnia.*

**Frisogrow** *Friesland, Singapore†.*
Nutritional supplement (p.1417·1).

**Frisol** *BA Farma, Port.*
Ketoconazole (p.403·3).

**Frisolac** *BA Farma, Port.*
Ketoconazole (p.403·3).
*Fungal infections.*

**Frisolona** *Allergan, Port.*
Prednisolone acetate (p.1108·1).
*Eye disorders.*

**Frisomum**
*Friesland, Hong Kong; Friesland, Singapore.*
Preparation for enteral nutrition (p.1417·1).
*Pregnancy and lactation.*

**Frisosoy**
*Friesland, Hong Kong; Friesland, Singapore.*
Infant feed (p.1417·1).
*Cow's milk protein allergy; lactose intolerance.*

**Frisovom**
*Friesland, Hong Kong; Friesland, Malaysia; Friesland, Singapore.*
Infant feed (p.1417·1).
*Colic; constipation; vomiting.*

**Fristamin** *FIRMA, Ital.*
Loratadine (p.436·1).
*Allergic rhinitis; hypersensitivity reactions.*

**Frivent** *Dompe, Ital.*
Theophylline (p.798·3).
*Asthma; bronchospasm.*

**Frixio** *Laboratorios Chile, Chile.*
Methyl salicylate (p.59·3); methyl nicotinate (p.59·2).
*Musculoskeletal and joint disorders.*

**Frixodon** *Brasmedica, Braz.†.*
Methacholine hydrochloride (p.1492·1); thymol (p.1194·2); menthol (p.1711·3); methyl salicylate (p.59·3).
*Musculoskeletal and joint disorders.*

**Frixopel** *EMS, Braz.*
Turpentine oil (p.1760·1); methyl salicylate (p.59·3); camphor (p.1665·3); menthol (p.1711·3).
*Musculoskeletal and joint disorders.*

**Froben**
*Ebewe, Austria; Knoll, Belg.; Abbott, Canad.; Kanoldt, Ger.†; Boots, Hong Kong†; Knoll, India; Abbott, Irl.; Abbott, Ital.; Promeco, Mex.†; Knoll, Neth.; Abbott, NZ†; Abbott, Port.; Knoll, S.Afr.; Knoll, Singapore†; Cantabria, Spain; Knoll, Switz.; Abbott, UK.*
Flurbiprofen (p.43·3).
*Inflammation; musculoskeletal, joint, peri-articular, and soft-tissue disorders; pain.*

**Froidir** *Orion, Fin.*
Clozapine (p.685·3).
*Schizophrenia.*

**Fromentyl** *Medinova (Μενινοβα), Gr.*
Amikacin sulfate (p.154·1).
*Bacterial infections.*

**Frone**
*Serono, Braz.†; Serono, Ital.†; Serono, Spain†.*
Interferon beta (p.645·3).
*Anogenital warts; hepatitis B or C; malignant neoplasms; viral infections.*

**Frontal**
*Pharmacia, Braz.; Solvay, Ital.*
Alprazolam (p.668·3).
*Anxiety disorders; insomnia; panic disorders; tremor.*

**Froop** *Ashbourne, UK.*
Furosemide (p.919·3).
*Oedema; oliguria.*

**Froop Co** *Ashbourne, UK.*
Furosemide (p.919·3); amiloride hydrochloride (p.858·2).
These ingredients can be described by the British Approved Name Co-amilofruse.
*Ascites with cirrhosis; oedema.*

**Frosinor** *Novartis, Spain.*
Paroxetine hydrochloride (p.311·2).
*Anxiety disorders; depression; obsessive-compulsive disorder; social phobia.*

**Frost Cream** *Weleda, UK.*
Homoeopathic preparation.

**Frostsalbe** *Weleda, Austria.*
Homoeopathic preparation.

**Frotin** *YSP, Malaysia.*
Metronidazole (p.607·2).
*Vaginal trichomoniasis.*

**Frova** *Elan, USA.*
Frovatriptan (p.469·2).
*Migraine.*

**Frovex** *Menarini, Irl.*
Frovatriptan succinate (p.469·2).
*Migraine.*

**Froxal** *Galen, Mex.*
Cefuroxime sodium (p.184·1).
*Bacterial infections.*

**Frubiase** *Boehringer de Angeli, Braz.†.*
Citric acid (p.1673·1); sodium bicarbonate (p.1223·2); calcium carbonate (p.1254·2).
*Gastrointestinal hyperacidity.*

**Frubiase Calcium** *Boehringer Ingelheim, Ger.†.*
Calcium carbonate (p.1254·2).
*Calcium deficiency; osteoporosis.*

**Frubiase Calcium forte 500** *Boehringer Ingelheim, Ger.*
Calcium gluconate (p.1225·2); calcium lactate (p.1225·3); ergocalciferol (p.1462·1).
*Osteomalacia; osteoporosis.*

**Frubiase Calcium T** *Boehringer Ingelheim, Ger.*
Calcium gluconate (p.1225·2); calcium lactate (p.1225·3).
*Calcium deficiency.*

**Frubienzym** *Boehringer Ingelheim, Ger.*
Muramidase (p.1717·2); cetylpyridinium chloride (p.1173·1).
*Mouth and throat disorders.*

**Frubilurgyl** *Boehringer Ingelheim, Ger.*
Chlorhexidine gluconate (p.1173·2).
*Mouth and throat disorders.*

**Frubiose Calcium** *Wild, Switz.†.*
Calcium gluconate (p.1225·2); calcium lactate (p.1225·3); ergocalciferol (p.1462·1); phosphoric acid (p.1731·2).
*Calcium deficiency.*

**Frubiose Vitamine D** *Boehringer Ingelheim, Fr.*
Ergocalciferol (p.1462·1); calcium gluconate (p.1225·2); calcium lactate (p.1225·3).
*Vitamin D and calcium deficiency.*

**Frubizin** *Boehringer Ingelheim, Ger.†.*
Cetylpyridinium chloride (p.1173·1).
*Mouth and throat disorders.*

**Frubizin Forte** *Boehringer Ingelheim, Ger.*
Cetylpyridinium chloride (p.1173·1); benzocaine (p.1370·3).
*Mouth and throat disorders.*

**Frucalde** *Euro-Labor, Port.†.*
Ergocalciferol (p.1462·1); calcium gluconate (p.1225·2); calcium lactate (p.1225·3).
*Hypocalcaemia; osteomalacia; osteoporosis.*

**Fru-Co**
*Ivax, Irl.; Ivax, UK.*
Furosemide (p.919·3); amiloride hydrochloride (p.858·2).
These ingredients can be described by the British Approved Name Co-amilofruse.
*Ascites; heart failure; nephrotic syndrome; oedema.*

**Fructal** *Bieffe, Ital.*
Fructose (p.1431·3).
*Diabetes; liver disorders; post-operative care.*

**Fructan** *Monsanto, Ital.*
Fructose (p.1431·3).
*Sugar substitute.*

**Fructines**
*Note. This name is used for preparations of different composition.*
*Fucus, Arg.*
Phenolphthalein (p.1284·1).
*Constipation.*
*Pharmethic, Belg.†; DB, Fr.; DB, Switz.*
Sodium picosulfate (p.1289·3).
*Constipation.*

**Fructofin** *Also, Ital.*
Fructose (p.1431·3).
*Sugar substitute.*

**Fructogenase** *Luper, Braz.*
Fructose; vitamins (p.1417·1).
*Vitamin supplement.*

**Fructopiran** *Monico, Ital.*
Fructose (p.1431·3).
*Cardiac disorders; kidney disorders; liver disorders.*

**Fructosil** *Volchem, Ital.*
Fructose (p.1431·3).
*Supplementation of glycogen reserves.*

**Frudemisan** *Bioquimico, Mex.†.*
Furosemide (p.919·3).

**Frugelletten** *Bregenzer, Austria.*
Fig (p.1266·3); senna (p.1288·2); tamarind (p.1293·2).
*Constipation.*

**Fruhjahrs-Elixier ohne Alkohol** *Ehrmann, Austria.*
Urtica (p.1762·1); birch leaf (p.1660·3); taraxacum (p.1751·3).
*Diuretic.*

**Fruit of the Earth Block-Up Baby Sunblock**
*Fruit of the Earth, Canad.*
*SPF 30:* Octinoxate (p.1154·3); octisalate (p.1154·3); oxybenzone (p.1154·3).
*Sunscreen.*

**Fruit of the Earth Block-Up Kids** *Fruit of the Earth, Canad.*
*SPF 30:* Octinoxate (p.1154·3); octisalate (p.1154·3); oxybenzone (p.1154·3).
*SPF 45:* Homosalate (p.1148·1); octinoxate (p.1154·3); octisalate (p.1154·3); oxybenzone (p.1154·3).
*Sunscreen.*

**Fruit of the Earth Block-Up Regular** *Fruit of the Earth, Canad.*
*SPF 45:* Homosalate (p.1148·1); octinoxate (p.1154·3); octisalate (p.1154·3); oxybenzone (p.1154·3).
*Sunscreen.*

**Fruit of the Earth Block-Up Regular Sunblock** *Fruit of the Earth, Canad.*
*SPF 15:* Octinoxate (p.1154·3); oxybenzone (p.1154·3).
*Sunscreen.*

**Fruit of the Earth Block-Up Sport** *Fruit of the Earth, Canad.*
*SPF 15:* Octinoxate (p.1154·3); oxybenzone (p.1154·3).
*SPF 30:* Octinoxate (p.1154·3); octisalate (p.1154·3); oxybenzone (p.1154·3).
*Sunscreen.*

**Fruit of the Earth Block-Up Sunblock** *Fruit of the Earth, Canad.*
*SPF 30:* Octinoxate (p.1154·3); octisalate (p.1154·3); oxybenzone (p.1154·3).
*Sunscreen.*

**Fruit of the Earth Moisturizing Aloe** *Fruit of the Earth, Canad.†.*
*SPF 8; SPF 15:* Octinoxate (p.1154·3); oxybenzone (p.1154·3).
*SPF 30; SPF 45:* Octinoxate (p.1154·3); octocrilene (p.1154·3); octisalate (p.1154·3); oxybenzone (p.1154·3); titanium dioxide (p.1160·3).
*Sunscreen.*

**Fruit of the Earth Moisturizing Aloe Baby**
*Fruit of the Earth, Canad.†.*
*SPF 45:* Octinoxate (p.1154·3); octocrilene (p.1154·3); octisalate (p.1154·3); oxybenzone (p.1154·3); titanium dioxide (p.1160·3).
*Sunscreen.*

**Fruit of the Earth Moisturizing Aloe Kids** *Fruit of the Earth, Canad.†.*
*Topical liquid SPF 30:* Octinoxate (p.1154·3); octocrilene (p.1154·3); octisalate (p.1154·3); oxybenzone (p.1154·3); titanium dioxide (p.1160·3).
*Topical spray SPF 30:* Octinoxate (p.1154·3); octocrilene (p.1154·3); octisalate (p.1154·3); oxybenzone (p.1154·3); DEA-methoxycinnamate.
*Sunscreen.*

**Fruit of the Earth Moisturizing Aloe Sport**
*Fruit of the Earth, Canad.†.*
*SPF 30:* Octinoxate (p.1154·3); octisalate (p.1154·3); oxybenzone (p.1154·3).
*SPF 8; SPF 15:* Octinoxate (p.1154·3); oxybenzone (p.1154·3).
*Sunscreen.*

**Fruitatives** *Rogers, Canad.*
Bisacodyl (p.1251·3); docusate sodium (p.1262·2); prune (p.1285·1).

**Fruity Chews** *Goldline, USA.*
A range of vitamin preparations (p.1417·1).

**Frumax** *Ashbourne, UK†.*
Furosemide (p.919·3).
*Oedema.*

**Frumeron**
*Remedica, Hong Kong; Remedica, Thai.*
Indapamide (p.938·2).
*Hypertension.*

**Frumil**
*Aventis, Gr.; Rhone-Poulenc Rorer, Hong Kong†; Geno, India; Aventis, Irl.; Aventis, NZ; Aventis, Switz.; Helios, UK.*
Furosemide (p.919·3); amiloride hydrochloride (p.858·2).
These ingredients can be described by the British Approved Name Co-amilofruse.
*Ascites; heart failure; hypertension; oedema.*

**Frunalia** *Pasteur, Chile.*
Tartaric acid (p.1752·1); sodium bicarbonate (p.1223·2).
*Antacid; constipation.*

**Frusamil**
*Aventis, Belg.; Aventis, Denm.*
Furosemide (p.919·3); amiloride hydrochloride (p.858·2).
*Hypertension; oedema.*

**Frusehexal** *Hexal, Austral.*
Furosemide (p.919·3).
*Hypertension; oedema.*

**Frusemek** *Berk, UK†.*
Furosemide (p.919·3); amiloride hydrochloride (p.858·2).
These ingredients can be described by the British Approved Name Co-amilofruse.
*Ascites; fluid retention; heart failure.*

**Frusene** *Orion, UK.*
Furosemide (p.919·3); triamterene (p.1016·2).
*Ascites; heart failure; oedema.*

**Frusenex** *Geno, India.*
Furosemide (p.919·3).
*Hypertension; oedema.*

**Frusid**
*Douglas, Austral.; Douglas, Hong Kong†; Douglas, NZ; Douglas, Singapore†; Douglas, Thai.; TTN, Thai.; DDSA Pharmaceuticals, UK.*
Furosemide (p.919·3).
*Ascites; hypertension; oedema.*

**Frusol** *Rosemont, UK.*
Furosemide (p.919·3).
*Hypertension; oedema.*

**Frut** *Infosint, Ital.*
Trisodium fructose diphosphate.
*Hypophosphataemia; ischaemic heart disease.*

**Frutalax** *Hexal, Braz.*
Senna (p.1288·2); cassia pulp (p.1255·2); tamarind (p.1293·2); coriander (p.1676·1); liquorice (p.1270·2).
*Constipation.*

**Frutarine** *Farmalab, Braz.†.*
Senna (p.1288·2); cassia pulp (p.1255·2); tamarind (p.1293·2); liquorice (p.1270·2).
*Constipation.*

**Frutasal Knop** *Knop, Chile.*
Tartaric acid (p.1752·1); sodium bicarbonate (p.1223·2).
*Antacid.*

**Frutin** *Prisfar, Port.†.*
Natural dolomite.
*Gastric hyperacidity.*

**Frutoplex** *Marjan, Braz.*
Fructose; ascorbic acid; riboflavin; pyridoxine hydrochloride; nicotinamide (p.1417·1).
*Vitamin supplement.*

**Frutovena** *Farmalab, Braz.*
Fructose; riboflavin sodium phosphate; pyridoxine hydrochloride; ascorbic acid; nicotinamide (p.1417·1).
*Vitamin supplement.*

**Frutovitam** *Cristalia, Braz.*
Multivitamin preparation (p.1417·1).

**Fruttasan** *Graf Fruttasan, Switz.*
Senna (p.1288·2); fig (p.1266·3).
*Constipation.*

**Fruttocal** *Sigma-Tau, Ital.†.*
Ergocalciferol (p.1462·1); calcium ascorbate (p.1460·2); calcium gluconate (p.1225·2); inosine (p.1701·2).
*Dental caries prophylaxis; osteoporosis; rickets.*

**Fruver** *EG, Ital.*
Multivitamin preparation (p.1417·1).

**Fruxucre** *Etajesa, Fr.†.*
Fructose (p.1431·3).
*Sugar substitute.*

**FSME-Bulin**
*Baxter, Austria; Baxter, Ger.; Baxter, Switz.†.*
A tick-borne encephalitis immunoglobulin (p.1642·1).
*Passive immunisation.*

**FSME-Immun**
*Baxter, Austria; Immuno, Belg.†; Baxter, Switz.; Baxter BioScience, UK.*
A tick-borne encephalitis vaccine (p.1642·1).
*Active immunisation.*

**F-Tab** *Ranbaxy, Thai.*
Ferrous fumarate (p.1427·3).
*Iron-deficiency anaemia.*

**Ftazidime** *Pharmaserve Lilly (Φαρμασερβ Λιλλυ), Gr.*
Ceftazidime (p.180·2).
*Bacterial infections.*

**FTDA** *Cassara, Arg.*
Flutamide (p.556·2).

**Ftoral**
*Abic, Hong Kong†; Abic, Israel.*
Tegafur (p.586·2).
*Malignant neoplasms.*

**Ftoralon** *Sanova, Austria.*
Tegafur (p.586·2).
*Malignant neoplasms.*

**Ftorocort** *Gedeon Richter, Thai.*
Triamcinolone acetonide (p.1110·2).
*Skin disorders.*

**Fuca** *Cassella-med, Switz.†.*
Frangula bark (p.1266·3); cascara (p.1255·1).
*Constipation.*

**Fuca N** *Melisana, Switz.*
Senna (p.1288·2).
*Constipation.*

**Fucafibres** *Fuca, Fr.†.*
Fruit and cereal fibres (p.1417·1); lactitol (p.1269·1).
*Gastrointestinal disorders.*

**Fucerox** *Pisa, Mex.*
Cefuroxime sodium (p.184·1).
*Bacterial infections.*

**Fucibet**
*Leo, Irl.; Farmacusi, Spain; Leo, UK.*
Betamethasone valerate (p.1093·2); fusidic acid (p.215·2).
*Infected skin disorders.*

**Fucicort**
*Andromaco, Arg.; Leo, Belg.; Andromaco, Chile; Leo, Denm.; Leo, Fin.; Leo, Ger.; Leo (Λεο), Gr.; Leo, Hong Kong; Leo, Israel; Formenti, Ital.; Leo, Malaysia; Senosiain, Mex.; CSL, NZ; Leo, NZ; Leo, Port.; Leo, Singapore; Leo, Switz.; Leo, Thai.*
Fusidic acid (p.215·2); betamethasone valerate (p.1093·2).
*Infected skin disorders.*

**Fucidin**
*Andromaco, Arg.; CSL, Austral.; Leo, Austria; Leo, Belg.; Leo, Canad.; Andromaco, Chile; Leo, Denm.; Leo, Fin.; Leo (Λεο), Gr.; Leo, Hong Kong; Leo, Irl.; Leo, Israel; Formenti, Ital.; Leo, Malaysia; Senosiain, Mex.; Leo, Neth.; Leo, Norw.; CSL, NZ; Leo, NZ; Adcock Ingram, S.Afr.; Leo, Singapore; Leo, Swed.; Leo, Thai.; Leo, UK.*
Fusidic acid (p.215·2) or sodium fusidate (p.215·2).
*Gram-positive bacterial infections.*

**Fucidin H**
*Leo, Canad.; Leo (Λεο), Gr.; Leo, Hong Kong; Leo, Irl.; Discotrade, Israel; Formenti, Ital.; Leo, Malaysia; Adcock Ingram, S.Afr.; Leo, Singapore; Leo, Switz.; Leo, Thai.; Leo, UK.*
Fusidic acid (p.215·2) or sodium fusidate (p.215·2); hydrocortisone acetate (p.1103·3).
*Infected skin disorders.*

**Fucidin Hydrocortisone** *Leo, Belg.†.*
Fusidic acid (p.215·2); hydrocortisone acetate (p.1103·3).
*Infected skin disorders.*

**Fucidine**
*Leo, Fr.; Leo, Ger.; Leo, Port.; Farmacusi, Spain; Leo, Switz.*
Fusidic acid (p.215·2) or sodium fusidate (p.215·2).
*Bacterial infections.*

**Fucidine H**
*Andromaco, Chile; Leo, Port.; Farmacusi, Spain†.*
Fusidic acid (p.215·2); hydrocortisone acetate (p.1103·3).
*Infected skin disorders.*

**Fucidine plus** *Boehringer Ingelheim, Ger.*
Sodium fusidate (p.215·2); hydrocortisone butyrate (p.1104·1).
*Infected skin disorders.*

**Fucidin-Hydrocortison**
*Leo, Denm.; Leo, Swed.*
Fusidic acid (p.215·2); hydrocortisone (p.1103·3).
*Infected skin disorders.*
*Leo, Fin.; Leo, Norw.*
Fusidic acid (p.215·2); hydrocortisone acetate (p.1103·3).
*Infected skin disorders.*

**Fucithalmic**
*Andromaco, Arg.; Leo, Austria; Leo, Belg.; Leo, Canad.; Andromaco, Chile; Leo, Denm.; Leo, Fin.; Leo, Fr.; Alcon, Ger.; Leo, Hong Kong; Leo, Irl.; Leo, Israel; Formenti, Ital.; Leo, Malaysia; Leo, Neth.; Leo, Norw.; CSL, NZ; Leo, NZ; Leo, Port.; Adcock Ingram, S.Afr.; Leo, Singapore; Alcon Cusi, Spain; Leo, Swed.; Leo, Switz.; Leo, Thai.; Leo, UK.*
Fusidic acid (p.215·2).
*Bacterial eye infections.*

**Fuclode** *Bioprogress, Ital.*
Cefaclor (p.167·1).
*Bacterial infections.*

**Fucon**
*YSP, Malaysia; Yung Shin, Singapore.*
Hyoscine butylbromide (p.483·3).
*Smooth muscle spasm.*

**Fucsina Fenica** *AFOM, Ital.; Farmacologico Milanese, Ital.; Farmatre, Ital.; Farmed, Ital.; Marco Viti, Ital.; NewFaDem, Ital.; Nova Argentia, Ital.; Ogna, Ital.; Ottolenghi, Ital.; Ramini, Ital.; Sella, Ital.; Zeta, Ital.*
Boric acid (p.1662·1); phenol (p.1188·1); magenta (p.1185·1); resorcinol (p.1156·3).
*Fungal skin infections.*

**Fucus** *Homeocan, Canad.*
Homoeopathic preparation.

**Fucus Composto** *Simoes, Braz.†.*
Pokeroot (p.1733·1); bladderwrack (p.1742·3); calotropis gigantea.

**Fucus Compuesto** *Hochstetter, Chile.*
Bladderwrack (p.1742·3); marrubium (p.1124·1); alfalfa (p.1649·1); avena (p.1658·2); carica papaya.
*Obesity.*

**Fucus Especial** *Knop, Chile.*
Homoeopathic preparation.

**Fucusor** *Soria Natural, Spain.*
Bladderwrack (p.1742·3); laminaria (p.1704·3).
*Dietary supplement; slimming aid.*

**Fudermex** *Prater, Chile.*
Lansoprazole (p.1269·3).

**Fudimun** *Kanoldt, Ger.†.*
Echinacea purpura (p.1683·2).
*Respiratory- and urinary-tract infections.*

**Fudirine** *PP Lab, Thai.*
Furosemide (p.919·3).
*Hypertension; oedema.*

**Fudone** *Wockhardt, India.*
Famotidine (p.1265·2).
*Gastro-oesophageal reflux; peptic ulcer; Zollinger-Ellison syndrome.*

**FUDR**
*Roche, Singapore†; Roche, USA.*
Floxuridine (p.553·1).
*Gastrointestinal adenocarcinoma metastatic to the liver.*

**Fugacar** *Janssen-Cilag, Thai.*
Mebendazole (p.108·2).
*Worm infections.*

**Fugaten** *Lysoform, Ger.*
Alcohol (p.1166·1).
*Surface disinfection.*

**Fugentin**
*Elpen (Ελπεν), Gr.; Elpen, Singapore.*
Amoxicillin trihydrate (p.155·3); potassium clavulanate (p.193·3).
*Bacterial infections.*

**Fugerel**
*Essex, Austral.; Aesca, Austria; Essex, Ger.; Schering-Plough, Hong Kong; Schering-Plough, Malaysia; Schering-Plough, Singapore†; Schering-Plough, Thai.*
Flutamide (p.556·2).
*Prostatic cancer.*

**Fugisept** *Lysoform, Ger.*
Didecyldimethylammonium chloride (p.1178·3); glyoxal (p.1181·1).
*Fungal and bacterial skin infections.*

**Fulcin**
*Zeneca, Austral.†; AstraZeneca, Braz.; AstraZeneca, Denm.†; Astra-Zeneca, Fin.†; Zeneca, Hong Kong†; AstraZeneca, Irl.; SIT, Ital.; Zeneca, Mex.; AstraZeneca, Norw.†; Zeneca, Port.; Zeneca, S.Afr.†; AstraZeneca, Singapore†; Teofarma, Spain; Zeneca, Swed.†; Zeneca, Switz.†; AstraZeneca, Thai.†; AstraZeneca, UK†.*
Griseofulvin (p.400·3).
*Fungal skin, hair, and nail infections.*

**Fulcin S** *AstraZeneca, Ger.*
Griseofulvin (microfine) (p.400·3).
*Fungal skin, hair, and nail infections.*

**Fulcine** *AstraZeneca, Fr.†.*
Griseofulvin (p.400·3).
*Fungal infections.*

**Fulcro** *Fournier, Ital.*
Fenofibrate (p.915·2).
*Hyperlipidaemias.*

**Fulgium** *Teofarma, Spain.*
Benzydamine salicylate (p.21·1).
*Peri-articular and soft-tissue disorders.*

**Ful-Glo**
*Allergan, Austral.†; Barnes Hind, NZ†; Akorn, USA.*
Fluorescein sodium (p.1689·1).
*Aid to eye examination.*

**Fulgram** *ABC, Ital.*
Norfloxacin (p.238·3).
*Urinary-tract infections.*

**Fulgram 400** *Labomed, Chile.*
Norfloxacin (p.238·3).
*Bacterial infections.*

**Full Marks**
*SSL, NZ; SSL, UK.*
Phenothrin (p.1509·1).
*Pediculosis.*

**Full Service Sunblock** *Clinique, Canad.*
*SPF 15:* Octinoxate (p.1154·3); octisalate (p.1154·3); oxybenzone (p.1154·3).
*Sunscreen.*

**Fullcilina** *Elea, Arg.*
Amoxicillin trihydrate (p.155·3).
*Bacterial infections.*

**Fullcilina Duo** *Elea, Arg.*
Amoxicillin trihydrate (p.155·3).
*Bacterial infections.*

**Fullcilina Plus** *Elea, Arg.*
Amoxicillin trihydrate (p.155·3); potassium clavulanate (p.193·3).
*Bacterial infections.*

**Full-Fort** *Kopkins, Braz.†.*
Ptychopetalum uncinatum; erythroxylon catuaba.
*Tonic.*

**Fullgrip T** *Elea, Arg.*
Levophenylephrine (p.1127·2); paracetamol (p.76·2); vitamin C (p.1460·2).
*Influenza symptoms.*

**Fullvita Multivitaminas e Minerais** *Farmalight, Port.†.*
Multivitamin and mineral preparation (p.1417·1).

**Fulsed**
*Ranbaxy, India.*
Midazolam hydrochloride (p.707·2).
*Sedative.*

Ranbaxy, Malaysia; Ranbaxy, Singapore.
Midazolam (p.707·1).
*Induction of anaesthesia; premedication; sedative.*

**Fulsivin** Collins, Mex.
Griseofulvin (p.400·3).
*Fungal infections.*

**Fulvicin**
Schering, Canad.; Schering, USA†.
Griseofulvin (p.400·3).
*Fungal infections of the skin, hair, and nails.*

**Fulvina** Schering-Plough, Mex.
Griseofulvin (p.400·3).
*Fungal infections.*

**Fulvistatin P/G** Essex, Chile.
Griseofulvin (p.400·3).
*Fungal skin and nail infections.*

**Fulzoltec** Tecnofarma, Mex.
Itraconazole (p.401·3).
*Fungal infections.*

**Fumaderm** Fumedica, Ger.; Hermal, Ger.
Dimethyl fumarate (p.1147·3); calcium monoethyl fumarate (p.1147·3); magnesium monoethyl fumarate (p.1147·3); zinc monoethyl fumarate (p.1147·3).
*Psoriasis.*

**Fumafer** Sanofi Synthelabo, Fr.
Ferrous fumarate (p.1427·3).
*Iron deficiency; iron-deficiency anaemia.*

**Fumarol** Offenbach, Mex.
Ferrous fumarate (p.1427·3); vitamin B substances (p.1417·1).
Vitamin C (p.1460·2) is included in this preparation to increase the absorption and availability of iron.
*Anaemias.*

**Fumasil** Sidepal, Braz.
Homoeopathic preparation.

**Fumatinic** Laser, USA.
Ferrous fumarate (p.1427·3); cyanocobalamin (p.1458·2).
Ascorbic acid (p.1460·2) is included in this preparation to increase the absorption and availability of iron.
*Iron-deficiency anaemias.*

**Fumavit** IQFA, Mex.
Ferrous fumarate (p.1427·3).
*Iron-deficiency anaemia.*

**Funa** LBS, Thai.
Fluconazole (p.398·1).
*Fungal infections.*

**Funazole** Khandelwal, India.
Ketoconazole (p.403·3).
*Fungal infections.*

**Funcenal** Farma Lepori, Spain.
Flutrimazole (p.400·3).
*Fungal skin infections.*

**Funchicorea** Melpoejo, Braz.†.
Cichorium intybus; rhubarb (p.1287·3); aniseed (p.1655·2).
*Gastrointestinal spasm.*

**Funcort** Nakorn, Thai.
Miconazole nitrate (p.405·3).
*Fungal skin and nail infections.*

**Fundamin**
Biomedis, Hong Kong; Biomedis, Malaysia; Biomedis, Singapore.
Vitamin B substances (p.1417·1).
*Nausea and vomiting; neuritis; tonic.*

**Fundamin-E**
Biomedis, Hong Kong; Biomedis, Malaysia; Biomedis, Singapore; Biomedis, Thai.; Great Eastern, Thai.
Vitamin B substances; vitamin E (p.1417·1).
*Nausea and vomiting; neuritis; tonic.*

**Fundan** Ipex, Swed.
Ketoconazole (p.403·3).
*Seborrhoeic dermatitis.*

**Funduscein**
Ciba Vision, Canad.†; Iolab, USA.
Fluorescein sodium (p.1689·1).
*Aid to eye examination.*

**Funga** Vida, Hong Kong.
Miconazole nitrate (p.405·3).
*Fungal skin infections.*

**Fungamizol** Ofimex, Mex.†.
Ketoconazole (p.403·3).
*Fungal infections.*

**Funganiline** Squibb, Spain.
Amphotericin B (p.391·2).
*Oropharyngeal candidiasis.*

**Fungarest**
Janssen-Cilag, Chile; Janssen-Cilag, Spain.
Ketoconazole (p.403·3).
*Fungal infections.*

**Fungata**
Pfizer, Austria; Mack, Illert., Ger.
Fluconazole (p.398·1).
*Vaginal candidiasis.*

**Fungazol**
Biolab, Hong Kong; Biolab, Malaysia; Ofimex, Mex.†; Biolab, Thai.
Ketoconazole (p.403·3).
*Fungal infections.*

**Fungederm** Nucare, UK.
Clotrimazole (p.396·2).
*Fungal skin infections.*

**Fungex** Streuli, Switz.
*Ointment:* Undecenoic acid (p.410·3); zinc undecenoate (p.411·1).
*Topical powder:* Undecenoic acid (p.410·3); zinc undecenoate (p.411·1); aluminium acetotartrate (p.1652·3); calcium lactate (p.1225·3).
*Fungal skin infections.*

**Fungi B** Eurofarma, Braz.
Amphotericin B (p.391·2).
*Fungal infections.*

**Fungibacid** Asche, Ger.†.
Tioconazole (p.409·3).
*Fungal infections.*

**Fungicida** Lauria, Arg.
Zinc undecenoate (p.411·1); calcium propionate (p.408·1); sodium propionate (p.408·1); hexylresorcinol (p.1182·1); salicylic acid (p.1157·1); benzoic acid (p.1169·3); thymol (p.1194·2).
*Fungal infections.*

**Fungicide**
Torrent, India; Torrent, Thai.†.
Ketoconazole (p.403·3).
*Fungal infections.*

**Fungicil** Labinca, Arg.
Ketoconazole (p.403·3).
*Fungal infections.*

**Fungicon** Continental Pharma, Thai.
Clotrimazole (p.396·2).
*Trichomoniasis; vaginal candidiasis.*

**Fungicrem** Andromaco, Mex.
Miconazole (p.405·2).
*Fungal skin infections.*

**Fungiderm**
Note. This name is used for preparations of different composition.
Nycomed, Austria; Zekides, Gr.
Bifonazole (p.395·1).
*Fungal skin and nail infections.*

Terra-Bio, Ger.; Greater Pharma, Thai.
Clotrimazole (p.396·2).
*Fungal skin and vaginal infections; trichomoniasis.*

Janssen-Cilag, Ital.†.
Miconazole nitrate (p.405·3).
*Fungal infections.*

**Fungiderm comp** Nycomed, Austria.
Bifonazole (p.395·1); urea (p.1162·2).
*Fungal nail infections.*

**Fungiderm-B** Greater Pharma, Thai.
Clotrimazole (p.396·2); betamethasone (p.1093·1).
*Fungal skin infections.*

**Fungiderm-K** Greater Pharma, Thai.
Ketoconazole (p.403·3).
*Fungal skin infections.*

**Fungidermo** Cinfa, Spain.
Clotrimazole (p.396·2).
*Fungal skin infections.*

**Fungidexan** Hermal, Ger.
Clotrimazole (p.396·2); urea (p.1162·2).
*Fungal and bacterial skin infections.*

**Fungifax** Medipharma, Hong Kong.
*Cream:* Zinc undecenoate (p.411·1); undecenoic acid (p.410·3); benzoic acid (p.1169·3); camphor (p.1665·3); methyl salicylate (p.59·3); chlorobutanol (p.1176·3).
*IMP Cream:* Zinc undecenoate (p.411·1); undecenoic acid (p.410·3).
*Fungal skin infections.*

**Fungifos** Combustin, Ger.
Tolciclate (p.410·1).
*Fungal skin infections.*

**Fungilin**
Bristol-Myers Squibb, Austral.; Bristol-Myers Squibb, Denm.; Bristol-Myers Squibb, Hong Kong†; Bristol-Myers Squibb, Israel; Bristol-Myers Squibb, Ital.; Bristol-Myers Squibb, NZ; Bristol-Myers Squibb, UK.
Amphotericin B (p.391·2).
*Candidiasis.*

**Fungi-M** Nakornpatana, Thai.
Miconazole nitrate (p.405·3).
*Fungal skin, nail, and hair infections.*

**Fungimax** Neo Quimica, Braz.
Metronidazole (p.607·2); nystatin (p.406·3).
*Vulvovaginal infections.*

**Fungimon** Trima, Israel.
Zinc undecenoate (p.411·1); undecenoic acid (p.410·3); aluminium chlorohydrate (p.1142·1).
*Fungal skin infections.*

**Fungi-Nail** Kramer, USA.
Resorcinol (p.1156·3); salicylic acid (p.1157·1); chloroxylenol (p.1177·2); benzocaine (p.1370·3); isopropyl alcohol (p.1184·3).
*Fungal and bacterial skin infections; fungal nail infections.*

**Funginox**
Charoen Bhaesaj, Malaysia; Charoen, Thai.
Ketoconazole (p.403·3).
*Fungal infections.*

**Fungiquim** Quimica y Farmacia, Mex.
Miconazole (p.405·2).
*Fungal infections.*

**Fungireduct** Azupharma, Ger.
Nystatin (p.406·3).
*Candidiasis.*

**Fungirox** UCI, Braz.
Ciclopirox (p.396·1).
*Fungal vaginal infections.*

**Fungisan** Galderma, Ger.†.
Omoconazole nitrate (p.407·2).
*Fungal skin infections.*

**Fungisdin** Isdin, Spain.
Miconazole (p.405·2) or miconazole nitrate (p.405·3).
*Candidiasis; fungal skin infections.*

**Fungisil** Silom, Thai.
Miconazole nitrate (p.405·3).
*Fungal infections of the skin, nails, and mucous membranes.*

**Fungisil-T** Silom, Thai.
Miconazole nitrate (p.405·3); triamcinolone acetonide (p.1110·2).
*Fungal infections of the skin, nails, and mucous membranes.*

**Fungistat** Cilag, Mex.
Terconazole (p.409·3).
*Vulvovaginal candidiasis.*

**Fungisten** Weifa, Norw.†.
Clotrimazole (p.396·2).
*Fungal infections.*

**Fungium** Saval, Chile.
Ketoconazole (p.403·3).
*Fungal infections.*

**Fungizid**
Ratiopharm, Ger.; Ratiopharm, Hong Kong; Douglas, NZ†.
Clotrimazole (p.396·2).
*Fungal and bacterial vaginal infections; fungal skin infections.*

**Fungizon**
Bristol-Myers Squibb, Braz.; Bristol-Myers Squibb, Chile.
Amphotericin B (p.391·2).
*Fungal infections.*

**Fungizona** Squibb, Spain.
Amphotericin B (p.391·2).
*Fungal infections.*

**Fungizone**
Bristol-Myers Squibb, Austral.; Bristol-Myers Squibb, Belg.; Squibb, Canad.; Bristol-Myers Squibb, Fin.; Bristol-Myers Squibb, Fr.; IFET (ΙΦΕΤ), Gr.; Bristol-Myers Squibb, Hong Kong; Sarabhai Piramal, India; Bristol-Myers Squibb, Irl.; Bristol-Myers Squibb, Israel; Bristol-Myers Squibb, Ital.; Bristol-Myers Squibb, Malaysia; Bristol-Myers Squibb, Neth.; Bristol-Myers Squibb, Norw.; Bristol-Myers Squibb, NZ; Bristol-Myers Squibb, S.Afr.; Bristol-Myers Squibb, Singapore; Bristol-Myers Squibb, Swed.; Bristol-Myers Squibb, Switz.; Bristol-Myers Squibb, Thai.; Bristol-Myers Squibb, UK; Bristol-Myers Squibb Oncology, USA.
Amphotericin B (p.391·2).
*Fungal infections; leishmaniasis.*

**Fungo**
Ego, Hong Kong; Ego, Malaysia; Ego, NZ; Ego, Singapore.
Miconazole nitrate (p.405·3).
*Fungal and bacterial infections.*

**Fungo Hubber** Farmasierra, Spain.
Ketoconazole (p.403·3).
*Fungal infections.*

**Fungocina** Lazar, Arg.
Fluconazole (p.398·1).
*Fungal infections.*

**Fungocop** Fecofar, Arg.
Boric acid (p.1662·1); undecenoic acid (p.410·3); zinc undecenoate (p.411·1).
*Fungal infections.*

**Fungocort** Douglas, NZ.
Miconazole nitrate (p.405·3); hydrocortisone (p.1103·3).
*Infected skin disorders.*

**Fungodermol** Sedabel, Braz.†.
Benzoic acid (p.1169·3); iodine (p.1598·1).
*Fungal skin infections.*

**Fungoid** Pedinol, USA.
*Topical solution*†: Clotrimazole (p.396·2).
*Fungal infections.*
*Topical tincture:* Miconazole nitrate (p.405·3).
*Fungal nail infections.*

**Fungoid AF** Pedinol, USA†.
Undecenoic acid (p.410·3).
*Fungal skin infections.*

**Fungoid HC** Pedinol, USA.
Miconazole nitrate (p.405·3); hydrocortisone (p.1103·3).
*Bacterial and fungal skin infections.*

**Fungol** Aventis, Braz.†.
Iodine (p.1598·1); potassium iodide (p.1598·1); salicylic acid (p.1157·1); boric acid (p.1662·1); magenta (p.1185·1).
*Fungal skin infections.*

**Fungopirox** Laboratorios Chile, Chile.
Ciclopirox olamine (p.396·1).
*Fungal skin infections.*

**Fungoral**
Janssen-Cilag, Austria; Farmion, Braz.; Janssen-Cilag, Gr.; Cilag, Mex.; Janssen-Cilag, Norw.; Janssen-Cilag, Swed.
Ketoconazole (p.403·3).
*Fungal infections; seborrhoeic dermatitis.*

**Fungos** Pasteur, Chile.
Miconazole nitrate (p.405·3).
*Fungal balanitis; fungal vulvovaginal infections.*

**Fungotox** Mepha, Switz.
Clotrimazole (p.396·2).
*Fungal skin and vaginal infections.*

**Fungowas** Chiesi, Spain.
Ciclopirox olamine (p.396·1).
*Cutaneous, mucosal and nail fungal infections.*

**Funguard** Fujisawa, Jpn.
Micafungin sodium.
*Fungal infections.*

**Fungur M** Hexal, Ger.
Miconazole nitrate (p.405·3).
*Fungal skin and vaginal infections.*

**Fungusol** Roche, Spain.
Boric acid (p.1662·1); zinc oxide (p.1163·2).
*Fungal skin infections; intertrigo.*

**Fungustatin** Pfizer, Gr.
Fluconazole (p.398·1).
*Fungal infections.*

**Fungusteril** Zekides, Gr.
Fluconazole (p.398·1).
*Fungal infections.*

**Funida** Nakornpatana, Thai.
Tinidazole (p.617·1).
*Amoebiasis; anaerobic bacterial infections; giardiasis; trichomoniasis.*

**Funzal** Gynopharm, Chile.
Clotrimazole (p.396·2).
*Fungal vaginal infections.*

**Furabid** Procter & Gamble, Neth.
Nitrofurantoin (p.237·2).
*Urinary-tract infections.*

**Furacin**
Key, Arg.; Schering-Plough, Braz.; Boehringer Ingelheim, Chile; GlaxoSmithKline, India; Rhein, Mex.; GlaxoSmithKline, S.Afr.; Seid, Spain; Procter & Gamble, USA; Roberts, USA.
Nitrofurazone (p.238·2).
*Burns; skin disinfection; ulcers; wounds.*

**Furacine**
Norgine, Belg.; Norgine, Neth.
Nitrofurazone (p.238·2).
*Infected wounds and burns; infection prophylaxis for skin grafts.*

**Furacin-S** GlaxoSmithKline, India.
Nitrofurazone (p.238·2); hydrocortisone acetate (p.1103·3).
*Infected skin disorders.*

**Furacin-Sol** Bioglan, Ger.
Nitrofurazone (p.238·2).
*Skin infections; wounds.*

**Furadantin**
Pharmacia, Austral.; Procter & Gamble, Austria; Goldshield, Ger.; GlaxoSmithKline, India; Goldshield, Irl.; Formenti, Ital.; Recip, Norw.; Pharmacia, NZ; GlaxoSmithKline, S.Afr.; Recip, Swed.; Goldshield, UK; Dura, USA.
Nitrofurantoin (p.237·2).
*Urinary-tract infections.*

**Furadantina**
Key, Arg.; Boehringer Ingelheim, Mex.; Normal, Port.
Nitrofurantoin (p.237·2).
*Urinary-tract infections.*

**Furadantine**
Procter & Gamble, Belg.†; Lipha Sante, Fr.; Vifor, Switz.
Nitrofurantoin (p.237·2).
*Urinary-tract infections.*

**Furadantine MC** Procter & Gamble, Neth.
Nitrofurantoin (macrocrystalline) (p.237·2).
*Urinary-tract infections.*

**Furadoine** Lipha Sante, Fr.
Nitrofurantoin (p.237·2).
*Cystitis.*

**Furagrand** Ahimsa, Arg.
Furosemide (p.919·3).

**Fural** Aliud, Austria.
Furosemide (p.919·3).
*Hypertension; oedema.*

**Furamid** Knoll, Switz.†.
Diloxanide furoate (p.604·1).
*Amoebiasis.*

**Furamide**
Knoll, Irl.†; Sovereign, UK†.
Diloxanide furoate (p.604·1).
*Amoebiasis.*

**Furanthril** Medphano, Ger.
Furosemide (p.919·3) or furosemide sodium (p.921·2).
*Forced diuresis; hypertension; oedema; oliguria.*

**Furantoina** Uriach, Spain.
Nitrofurantoin (p.237·2).
*Urinary-tract infections.*

**Furanton** Randall, Mex.†.
Nitrofurantoin (p.237·2); methenamine mandelate (p.230·2).
*Urinary-tract infections.*

**Furanvit** SIFI, Ital.†.
Nitrofurazone (p.238·2); pyridoxine hydrochloride (p.1456·3).
*Bacterial eye infections.*

**Furasept** Beige, S.Afr.†.
Nitrofurazone (p.238·2).
*Burns; skin infections; ulcers; wounds.*

**Furasian** Asian Pharm, Thai.
*Syrup:* Furazolidone (p.605·2); kaolin (p.1268·3); pectin (p.1580·3).
*Tablets:* Furazolidone (p.605·2).
*Diarrhoea; enteritis.*

**Furazolidona** Laboratorios Chile, Chile.
Furazolidone (p.605·2); kaolin (p.1268·3); pectin (p.1580·3).
*Bacterial gastrointestinal infections; giardiasis.*

**Furazolin** De Mayo, Braz.†.
Furazolidone (p.605·2); phthalylsulfathiazole (p.242·3); pectin (p.1580·3).
*Diarrhoea.*

**Furazolon** Heralds, Braz.†.
Hydrocortisone (p.1103·3); nitrofurazone (p.238·2).
*Infected skin disorders.*

**Furdiuren**
Bristol-Myers Squibb, Arg.; Chemopharma, Chile.
Furosemide (p.919·3); amiloride (p.858·3).
*Heart failure; hepatic cirrhosis with ascites; hypertension; odema.*

**Furedan** Scharper, Ital.
Nitrofurantoin (p.237·2).
*Urinary-tract infections.*

**Furese** Durascan, Denm.
Furosemide (p.919·3).
*Hypertension; oedema.*

**Furesin** Prodotti, Braz.†.
Furosemide (p.919·3).
*Hypertension.*

**Furesis** Orion, Fin.
Furosemide (p.919·3).
*Hypertension; oedema; renal failure.*

**Furesis comp**
Orion, Fin.; Orion, Ger.†.
Furosemide (p.919·3); triamterene (p.1016·2).
*Hypertension; oedema.*

**Furetic** Siam Bheasach, Thai.
Furosemide (p.919·3).
*Ascites; barbiturate poisoning; eclampsia; oedema.*

**Furex** Aspen, S.Afr.
Nitrofurazone (p.238·2).
*Burns; skin infections; ulcers; wounds.*

**Furide** Polipharm, Thai.
Furosemide (p.919·3).
*Ascites; hypertension; oedema.*

**Furil** OFF, Ital.
Nitrofurantoin (p.237·2).
*Urinary-tract infections.*

**Furine** Progress, Thai.
Furosemide (p.919·3).
*Hypertension; oedema.*

**Furion** Chew, Thai.
Furazolidone (p.605·2).
*Diarrhoea; enteritis.*

**Furital** Rivero, Arg.
Furosemide (p.919·3).

**Furix**
Hexal, Arg.; Nycomed, Denm.; Nycomed, Norw.; Nycomed, Swed.
Furosemide (p.919·3).
*Forced diuresis; hypertension; nephrotic syndrome; oedema; renal insufficiency.*

**Furmidal** Sydenham, Mex.†.
Furosemide (p.919·3).

**Furmide** Upha, Malaysia.
Furosemide (p.919·3).
*Hypertension; oedema.*

**Furo** 1A, Ger.; ABZ, Ger.; CT, Ger.
Furosemide (p.919·3) or furosemide sodium (p.921·2).
*Ascites; hypertension; oedema; oliguria.*

**Furo-Aldopur**
Kwizda, Austria; Hormosan, Ger.
Furosemide (p.919·3); spironolactone (p.1003·1).
*Ascites; oedema.*

**Furobactina** Dexter, Spain.
Nitrofurantoin (p.237·2).
*Urinary-tract infections.*

**furo-basan** Schonenberger, Switz.
Furosemide (p.919·3).
*Hypertension; oedema.*

**Furo-BASF** BASF, Ger.†.
Furosemide (p.919·3).
*Ascites; hypertension; oedema; oliguria.*

**Furobeta** Betapharm, Ger.
Furosemide (p.919·3).
*Ascites; hypertension; oedema; oliguria.*

**Furocloran** AF, Mex.†.
Chloramphenicol (p.185·1).
*Bacterial infections.*

**Furocombin** Streuli, Switz.
Spironolactone (p.1003·1); furosemide (p.919·3).
*Ascites; oedema.*

**Furodermal** Streuli, Switz.
Camphor (p.1665·3); ichthammol (p.1148·2); bismuth oxyiodogallate (p.1253·1); thymol (p.1194·2).
*Skin infections.*

**Furodermil** Vifor, Switz.†.
Ichthammol (p.1148·2); salicylic acid (p.1157·1); bismuth hydroxyquinoline (p.1253·1); peru balsam (p.1730·2).
*Skin disorders.*

**Furodrix** Streuli, Switz.
Furosemide (p.919·3) or furosemide sodium (p.921·2).
*Forced diuresis; heart failure; hypertension; oedema; oliguria in pregnancy; renal failure.*

**Furogamma** Worwag, Ger.
Furosemide (p.919·3).
*Ascites; hypertension; oedema; oliguria.*

**Furohexal** Hexal, Austria.
Furosemide (p.919·3).
*Hypertension; oedema.*

**Furoic** Monsanto, Ital.
Calcium mefolinate (p.1431·2).
*Antidote in overdosage with folic acid antagonists; folate deficiency; reduction of aminopterin and methotrexate toxicity.*

**Furolacton** Lannacher, Austria.
Spironolactone (p.1003·1); furosemide (p.919·3).
*Oedema.*

**Furolin** Pharmanik (Φαρμανικ), Gr.
Nitrofurantoin (p.237·2).
*Urinary tract infections.*

**Furomed** Wolff, Ger.
Furosemide (p.919·3).
*Hypertension; oedema.*

**Furomil** Euromex, Mex.†.
Furosemide (p.919·3).

**Furomin** Ratiopharm, Fin.
Furosemide (p.919·3).
*Hypertension; oedema.*

**Furon** Ratiopharm, Austria.
Furosemide (p.919·3) or furosemide sodium (p.921·2).
*Forced diuresis; hypercalcaemic crises; hypertension; oedema; renal failure.*

**Furonet** Nettopharma, Denm.†.
Furosemide (p.919·3).
*Hypertension; oedema.*

**Furonex** Zerboni, Mex.†.
Furosemide (p.919·3).

**Furopectin** PP Lab, Thai.
Furazolidone (p.605·2); kaolin (p.1268·3); pectin (p.1580·3).
*Bacterial diarrhoea; enteritis.*

**Furo-Puren** Alpharma-Isis, Ger.
Furosemide (p.919·3).
*Ascites; hypertension; oedema; oliguria.*

**Furorese** Hexal, Ger.
Furosemide (p.919·3) or furosemide sodium (p.921·2).
*Ascites; forced diuresis; hypertension; oedema; oliguria.*

**Furorese Comp** Hexal, Ger.
Furosemide (p.919·3); spironolactone (p.1003·1).
*Ascites; oedema.*

**Furosal** TAD, Ger.
Furosemide (p.919·3).
*Ascites; hypertension; oedema; oliguria.*

**Furosan**
Sanval, Braz.; Fustery, Mex.
Furosemide (p.919·3).

**Furoscand** Enapharm, Swed.†.
Furosemide (p.919·3).
*Hypertension; oedema.*

**Furosem** Medley, Braz.
Furosemide (p.919·3).
*Hypertension; oedema.*

**Furosemid comp** Upsamedica, Switz.†.
Furosemide (p.919·3); spironolactone (p.1003·1).
*Ascites; oedema.*

**Furosemida Composta** Heralds, Braz.†.
Furosemide (p.919·3); potassium chloride (p.1232·2).
*Hypertension; oedema.*

**Furosetron** Ariston, Braz.
Furosemide (p.919·3).

**Furosifar** Siphar, Switz.
Furosemide (p.919·3).
*Hypertension; oedema; renal failure.*

**Furosix** Delta, Braz.
Furosemide (p.919·3).

**Furospir** Mepha, Switz.
Furosemide (p.919·3); spironolactone (p.1003·1).
*Oedema.*

**Furo-Spirobene** Ratiopharm, Austria.
Furosemide (p.919·3); spironolactone (p.1003·1).
*Aldosteronism; oedema.*

**Furostad** Stada, Austria.
Furosemide (p.919·3).
*Hypertension; oedema.*

**Furoter** Protein, Mex.†.
Furosemide (p.919·3).

**Furotricina** Finderm, Ital.
Tyrothricin (p.275·1); nitrofurazone (p.238·2).
*Gynaecological infections.*

**Furotyrol** Tyrol, Austria.
Furosemide (p.919·3).
*Hypertension; oedema.*

**Furovite** Vitamed, Israel†.
Furosemide (p.919·3).
*Hypertension; oedema.*

**Furoxim** Lannacher, Austria.
Cefuroxime axetil (p.184·1) or cefuroxime sodium (p.184·1).
*Bacterial infections.*

**Furoxime** Siam Bheasach, Thai.
Cefuroxime axetil (p.184·1) or cefuroxime sodium (p.184·1).
*Bacterial infections.*

**Furoxona**
Boehringer Ingelheim, Chile; Boehringer Ingelheim, Mex.
Furazolidone (p.605·2).
*Gastrointestinal infections.*

**Furoxone**
GlaxoSmithKline, India; Formenti, Ital.†; Roberts, USA.
Furazolidone (p.605·2).
*Gastrointestinal infections.*

**Furozix** Bunker, Braz.
Furosemide (p.919·3).

**Fursemida**
Biocrom, Arg.; Fabra, Arg.; Sintesina, Arg.; Veinfar, Arg.; Legrand, Braz.
Furosemide (p.919·3).
*Hypercalcaemia; hypertension; oedema.*

**Fursol** Ecosol, Switz.
Furosemide (p.919·3).
*Hypertension; oedema.*

**Furtenk** Biotenk, Arg.
Furosemide (p.919·3).
*Hypertension; oedema.*

**Furtulon** Roche, Jpn.
Doxifluridine (p.547·3).
*Malignant neoplasms.*

**Furunkulosin** Merckle, Ger.
Yeast (p.1469·1).
*Furunculosis.*

**Fusalar** Fustery, Mex.
Fluocinolone (p.1101·2).
*Skin disorders.*

**Fusaloyos** Danval, Spain.
Fusafungine (p.215·2).
*Upper respiratory-tract infections and inflammation.*

**Fusanidazol** Universales, Mex.†.
Metronidazole (p.607·2).

**Fusepina** Fustery, Mex.
Nifedipine (p.966·2).
*Hypertension.*

**Fusid**
Note. This name is used for preparations of different composition.
Gry, Ger.; Teva, Israel.
Furosemide (p.919·3) or furosemide sodium (p.921·2).
*Ascites; hypertension; oedema; oliguria.*

Chew, Thai.
Fusidic acid (p.215·2).
*Bacterial skin infections.*

**Fusimed** Cassara, Arg.
Fusidic acid (p.215·2).
*Burns; skin infections; ulcers; wounds.*

**Fusimed B** Cassara, Arg.
Fusidic acid (p.215·2); betamethasone (p.1093·1).
*Infected skin, ear, and nose disorders.*

**Fusitop** Ingens, Arg.
Fusidic acid (p.215·2).
*Skin infections; ulcers; wounds.*

**Fusiwal** Wallace, India.
Sodium fusidate (p.215·2).
*Bacterial skin infections.*

**Fustaren** Fustery, Mex.
Diclofenac sodium (p.32·1).
*Inflammation; musculoskeletal and joint disorders; pain.*

**Fustermicina** Fustery, Mex.
Gentamicin (p.219·1).
*Bacterial infections.*

**Fustermid** Fustery, Mex.†.
Pipemidic acid (p.243·1).

**Fustermizol** Fustery, Mex.
Astemizole (p.424·2).
*Hypersensitivity.*

**Fuston** YSP, Malaysia.
Guaifenesin (p.1122·1).
*Coughs.*

**Futasole** Julphar, UAE.
Fusidic acid (p.215·2).
*Bacterial skin infections.*

**Futasone** Julphar, UAE.
Fusidic acid (p.215·2); betamethasone valerate (p.1093·2).
*Infected skin disorders.*

**Futraful** Otsuka, Hong Kong†.
Tegafur (p.586·2).
*Malignant neoplasms.*

**Futroken** Kener, Mex.†.
Nitrofurantoin (p.237·2).

**Futura** Marano, Ital.
Aspartame (p.1422·1).
*Sugar substitute.*

**Futuran**
Note. This name is used for preparations of different composition.
Madaus, Ger.†.
Hypericum (p.299·1).
*Depression.*

Madaus, Spain.
Eprosartan mesilate (p.912·1).
*Hypertension.*

**Future E** L'Oreal, Canad.
*SPF 15:* Ensulizole (p.1147·1); octocrilene (p.1154·3). Formerly contained avobenzone and octocrilene.
*Sunscreen.*

**Fuviron** Proge, Ital.
Aciclovir (p.626·1).
*Herpesvirus infections.*

**Fuxen** Fustery, Mex.
Naproxen (p.65·1).
*Gout; inflammation; musculoskeletal, joint, and periarticular disorders; pain.*

**Fuxol** Columbia, Mex.†.
Furazolidone (p.605·2).
*Gastrointestinal infections.*

**Fuzeon**
Roche, Fr.; Roche, UK; Roche, USA.
Enfuvirtide (p.633·1).
*HIV infection.*

**Fuzoltec** Tecnofarma, Mex.
Itraconazole (p.401·3).
*Fungal infections.*

**Fuzotyl** Rayere, Mex.
Furazolidone (p.605·2); homatropine (p.483·2); kaolin (p.1268·3); pectin (p.1580·3).
*Gastrointestinal disorders.*

**FX Passage**
Hestag, Austria; Worwag, Ger.
Magnesium sulfate (p.1228·2).
*Constipation; stool softener.*

**Fybogel**
Reckitt Benckiser, Austral.; Reckitt & Colman, Belg.; Reckitt Benckiser, Hong Kong; Reckitt Benckiser, Irl.; Reckitt Benckiser, Malaysia; Schering-Plough, Mex.; Reckitt Benckiser, S.Afr.; Reckitt Benckiser, Singapore; Reckitt Benckiser, Spain†; Reckitt Benckiser, Thai.; Reckitt Benckiser, UK.
Ispaghula (p.1268·1).
*Constipation; diarrhoea; diverticular disease; irritable bowel syndrome.*

**Fybogel Mebeverine**
Reckitt Benckiser, Hong Kong; Reckitt Benckiser, Irl.; Reckitt & Colman, Singapore†; Reckitt Benckiser, UK.
Ispaghula (p.1268·1); mebeverine hydrochloride (p.1273·1).
*Inflammatory bowel disease; irritable bowel syndrome.*

**Fybozest** Reckitt Benckiser, UK†.
Ispaghula (p.1268·1).
*Hypercholesterolaemia.*

**Fymnal** Farmasa, Braz.
Ibuprofen (p.45·3); fenoterol hydrobromide (p.785·2).
*Dysmenorrhoea.*

**Fynnon Salt** SSL, UK†.
Sodium sulfate (p.1290·1).
*Constipation.*

**Fysiofer** ITF, Gr.
Iron succinyl-protein complex (p.1438·1).
*Iron-deficiency anaemia.*

**Fysionorm** Pharmaselect, Ger.
Fluoxetine hydrochloride (p.292·1).
*Depression.*

**Fysioquens**
Aaciphar, Belg.†; Nourypharma, Neth.
7 Tablets, ethinylestradiol (p.1553·2); 15 tablets, ethinylestradiol; lynestrenol (p.1557·1).
*Sequential-type oral contraceptive.*

**Fytosid** Dabur, Thai.
Etoposide (p.551·3).
*Malignant neoplasms.*

**G-204** Teva, Israel.
Electrolyte solution (p.1221·1).
*Haemodialysis.*

**G-248** Teva, Israel.
Electrolyte solution (p.1221·1).
*Haemodialysis.*

**G Tril** Vinas, Spain†.
Febarbamate (p.698·2).
*Alcohol withdrawal syndrome; insomnia; tremor.*

**Gab** Gufic, India.
Lindane (p.1506·3).
*Pediculosis; scabies.*

**Gaba** Nikkho, Braz.
Gamma-aminobutyric acid (p.1690·2); papaverine hydrochloride (p.1728·1); nicotinic acid (p.1441·1); calcium pantothenate (p.1442·3).
*Impaired mental function.*

**Gabacet** Sanofi Synthelabo, Fr.
Piracetam (p.1732·1).
*Cerebrovascular disorders; vertigo.*

**Gaballon** Nikkho, Braz.
Gamma-aminobutyric acid; lysine hydrochloride; thiamine hydrochloride; pyridoxine hydrochloride; calcium pantothenate (p.1417·1).
*Nutritional supplement.*

**Gabatril** Abbott, Mex.
Tiagabine hydrochloride (p.378·1).
*Epilepsy.*

**Gabax** Nikkho, Braz.
Gamma-aminobutyric acid (p.1690·2); pyridoxine hydrochloride (p.1456·3).
*Impaired mental function.*

**Gabbromicina** Pharmacia Upjohn, Hong Kong†.
Paromomycin sulfate (p.612·3).
*Amoebiasis; bacterial infections.*

**Gabbroral**
Pharmacia, Belg.; Pharmacia Upjohn, Ital.
Paromomycin sulfate (p.612·3).
*Amoebiasis; bacterial intestinal infections; giardiasis.*

**Gabecon M** Dovalle, Braz.
Methyltestosterone (p.1559·3); vitamin E.

**Gabil** Tecnifar, Port.†.
Barbetonium iodide; idanpramine; chlordiazepoxide (p.674·2).
*Gastrointestinal motility disorders.*

**Gabimex** Sanofi Synthelabo, Arg.
4-Amino-3-hydroxybutyric acid (p.353·2).
*Behaviour disorders; mental function impairment.*

**Gabimex Plus** Sanofi Synthelabo, Arg.
4-Amino-3-hydroxybutyric acid (p.353·2); pyritinol (p.1737·2).
*Mental function impairment.*

**Gabisedil** Seber, Port.
Amino-hydroxybutyric acid (p.353·2); valerian (p.1762·2); passion flower (p.1729·1); chamomile (p.1669·3); crataegus (p.1677·1).
*Anxiety; excitability; infantile convulsions; insomnia.*

**Gabitran** Solfran, Mex.
Multivitamin preparation (p.1417·1).

**Gabitril** Sanofi Synthelabo, Austral.; Sanofi Synthelabo, Austria; Sanofi Synthelabo, Belg.; Abbott, Braz.†; Sanofi Winthrop, Denm.; Sanofi Synthelabo, Fin.; Sanofi Synthelabo, Fr.; Sanofi Synthelabo, Ger.; Sanofi Synthelabo, Gr.; Cephalon, Irl.; Sanofi Synthelabo, Ital.; Sanofi Synthelabo, Port.; Sanofi Synthelabo, Spain; Sanofi Synthelabo, Switz.; Cephalon, UK; Cephalon, USA.
Tiagabine hydrochloride (p.378·1).
*Epilepsy.*

**Gabomade** Esfar, Port.
4-Amino-3-hydroxybutyric acid (p.353·2).
*Convulsions; headache; mental function disorders; nocturnal enuresis.*

**Gabormon** Nikkho, Braz.†.
Gamma-aminobutyric acid (p.1690·2); methyltestosterone (p.1559·3).
*Androgen deficiency; breast cancer (females); delayed growth; delayed puberty (males).*

**Gabrene** Synthelabo, Fr.†.
Progabide (p.377·2).
*Epilepsy.*

**Gabrilen** Kreussler, Ger.
Ketoprofen (p.51·2).
*Inflammation; musculoskeletal, joint, peri-articular, and soft-tissue disorders; pain.*

**Gabunat** Strathmann, Ger.
Biotin (p.1423·2).
*Biotin deficiency.*

**Gacida** Aventis, Thai.
Magnesium trisilicate (p.1272·3); dried aluminium hydroxide gel (p.1249·2).
*Gastric hyperacidity; gastritis; heartburn; peptic ulcer.*

**Gadograf** Juste, Spain.
Gadobutrol (p.1062·1).
*Contrast medium for magnetic resonance imaging.*

**Gadopril** Gador, Arg.
Enalapril (p.909·2).
*Heart failure; hypertension.*

**Gadovist**
Schering, Austral.; Schering, Austria; Schering, Denm.; Schering, Fin.; Schering, Ger.; Schering, Ital.; Schering, Norw.; Schering, Port.; Schering, S.Afr.; Schering, Spain; Schering, Swed.; Schering, Switz.; Schering, UK.
Gadobutrol (p.1062·1).
*Contrast medium for magnetic resonance imaging.*

**Gadral** GiEnne, Ital.
Magaldrate (p.1271·3).
*Gastro-oesophageal reflux; peptic ulcer.*

**Gaduol** Climax, Braz.
Vitamin A palmitate (p.1453·1); ergocalciferol (p.1462·1).
*Vitamin supplement.*

**Gaiarsol** Monin, Fr.†.
Methylarsinic acid; guaiacol (p.1122·1); aconite root (p.1646·3); codeine (p.27·1); tolu balsam (p.1131·3).
*Coughs.*

**Galacordin** Biomo, Ger.
Potassium aspartate (p.1233·1); magnesium aspartate (p.1227·3).
*Potassium and magnesium deficiency.*

**Galactogil** IPRAD, Fr.
Galega; calcium phosphate (p.1225·3); malt extract (p.1439·2).
*Lactation insufficiency.*

**Galactomin**
Scientific Hospital Supplies, Irl.; Piam, Ital.; Scientific Hospital Supplies, UK.
Food for special diets (p.1417·1).
*Lactose, glucose, or galactose intolerance.*

**Galake** Galen, UK†.
Dihydrocodeine tartrate (p.34·3); paracetamol (p.76·2).
These ingredients can be described by the British Approved Name Co-dydramol.
*Pain.*

**Galama Entschlackungselixier** Pharmonta, Austria.
Birch leaf (p.1660·3).
*Kidney disorders.*

**Galamila** Mavena, Switz.
Dexpanthenol (p.1727·2); chlorhexidine gluconate (p.1173·2) or chlorhexidine hydrochloride (p.1173·3).
*Nipple care during breastfeeding.*

**Galanol GLX** Lifeplan, UK†.
Evening primrose oil (p.1686·3).
*Nutritional supplement.*

**Galanol Gold** Lifeplan, UK†.
Evening primrose oil (p.1686·3); borage oil (p.1661·3).
*Nutritional supplement.*

**Galantase**
Mitsubishi, Jpn; Hoechst Marion Roussel, S.Afr.†.
Tilactase (p.1756·2).
*Lactose intolerance.*

**Galaren** Fada, Arg.
Vecuronium (p.1409·3).
*Competitive neuromuscular blocker.*

**Galcdexan** Grin, Mex.†.
Aluminium hydroxide (p.1249·2).

**Galciclina** Sant Gall, Arg.
Ampicillin (p.157·1).
*Bacterial infections.*

**Galcodine** Thornton & Ross, UK.
Codeine phosphate (p.27·1).
*Dry coughs.*

**Galebiron** Biomedica-Chemica, Gr.
Ranitidine hydrochloride (p.1285·2).
*Conditions where gastric acid reduction is beneficial; gastric hypersecretion including Zollinger-Ellison syndrome; peptic ulcer.*

**Galecin** Galen, Mex.
Clindamycin phosphate (p.194·2).
*Bacterial infections.*

**Galedol** Galen, Mex.
Diclofenac sodium (p.32·1).
*Gout; musculoskeletal, joint, peri-articular and soft-tissue disorders; pain.*

**Galemin** Biomedica-Chemica, Gr.
Cefuroxime sodium (p.184·1).
*Bacterial infections.*

**Galenamet**
Galen, Irl.; Galen, UK.
Cimetidine (p.1255·3).
*Gastric hyperacidity; peptic ulcer; Zollinger-Ellison syndrome.*

**Galenamox**
Galen, Irl.; Galen, UK.
Amoxicillin trihydrate (p.155·3).
*Bacterial infections.*

**Galenat Kamill N** Hetterich, Ger.
Chamomile (p.1669·3).
*Gastrointestinal disorders; inflammatory disorders of skin and mucous membranes.*

**Galenavowen** Weber & Weber, Ger.
Homoeopathic preparation.

**Galenpamil** Galen, Mex.†.
Verapamil (p.1021·1).
*Angina pectoris.*

**Galenphol** Thornton & Ross, UK.
Pholcodine (p.1128·3).
Formerly known as Galphol.
*Coughs.*

**Galentromicina** Galen, Mex.†.
Erythromycin (p.208·1).
*Bacterial infections.*

**Galfer**
Galen, Irl.; Thornton & Ross, UK.
Ferrous fumarate (p.1427·3).
*Iron-deficiency anaemia.*

**Galfer FA**
Galen, Irl.; Thornton & Ross, UK.
Ferrous fumarate (p.1427·3); folic acid (p.1429·1).
*Iron and folic acid deficiency in pregnancy.*

**Galfloxin** Galen, UK†.
Flucloxacillin sodium (p.213·3).
*Bacterial infections.*

**Galidrin** Galen, Mex.
Ranitidine hydrochloride (p.1285·2).
*Gastro-oesophageal reflux; peptic ulcer; Zollinger-Ellison syndrome.*

**Galinocort** Vilco, Gr.
Betamethasone valerate (p.1093·2).
*Topical corticosteroid.*

**Galirene** Alpharma, Fr.
Calcium bromide (p.1663·1); calcium lactate (p.1225·3).
*Insomnia; nervous disorders.*

**Galium Complex** Blackmores, Austral.†.
Clivers (p.1673·2); echinacea angustifolia (p.1683·2); calendula (p.1665·2); baptisia tinctoria; vitamins (p.1417·1); zinc amino acid chelate (p.1469·3).
*Tonic.*

**Galivert** Luhr-Lehrs, Ger.†.
Homoeopathic preparation.

**Galleb S** Hoyer, Ger.†.
Taraxacum (p.1751·3).
*Biliary-tract disorders; dyspepsia.*

**Galle-Donau** Sanova, Austria.
*p*,α-Dimethylbenzyl alcohol nicotinate (p.1680·3); α-naphthylacetic acid (p.1719·1).
*Biliary-tract disorders.*

**Gallemolan forte** Cesra, Ger.
Greater celandine (p.1695·3); absinthium (p.1645·1); taraxacum (p.1751·3).
*Biliary-tract disorders; dyspepsia.*

**Gallemolan G** Cesra, Ger.
Absinthium (p.1645·1); boldo leaves (p.1661·2); chamomile flowers (p.1669·3); greater celandine (p.1695·3); taraxacum (p.1751·3).
*Biliary-tract disorders; dyspepsia.*

**Gallen- und Lebertee EF-EM-ES** Smetana, Austria.
Agrimony herb (p.1649·1); marrubium vulgare (p.1124·1); peppermint leaf (p.1283·2); achillea (p.1646·2); taraxacum (p.1751·3).
*Biliary-tract disorders.*

**Gallenja** OTW, Ger.
Homoeopathic preparation.

**Gallenperlen** Agepha, Austria.
Phenylpropanol (p.1731·1).
*Biliary-tract disorders.*

**Gallesyn** Wenig, Austria.
*Oral drops:* Frangula (p.1266·3); herba teucrii; peppermint oil (p.1283·2).
*Tablets:* Frangula (p.1266·3); herba teucrii; menthol (p.1711·3).
*Biliary-tract disorders.*

**Gallesyn neu** Wenig, Austria.
*Oral drops:* Cynara (p.1678·3); taraxacum (p.1751·3); peppermint leaf (p.1283·2).
*Tablets:* Cynara (p.1678·3); taraxacum (p.1751·3); menthol (p.1711·3).
*Biliary-tract disorders.*

**Gallexier**
Note. This name is used for preparations of different composition.
Salus, Fr.
Cynara (p.1678·3).
*Gastrointestinal and liver disorders.*

Salushaus, Ger.
*Oral liquid:* Cynara (p.1678·3); Javanese turmeric (p.1759·3); gentian (p.1692·2); ginger (p.1267·1); cnicus benedictus (p.1673·3); menyanthes (p.1712·1); absinthium (p.1645·1); fennel (p.1687·2); cardamom (p.1667·3); bitter-orange peel (p.1723·3); chamomile (p.1669·3); achillea (p.1646·2); taraxacum (p.1751·3).
*Gastrointestinal disorders.*
*Tablets:* Javanese turmeric (p.1759·3); cynara (p.1678·3); silybum marianum (p.1043·3); taraxacum (p.1751·3); chamomile (p.1669·3); peppermint leaf (p.1283·2).
*Biliary disorders.*

**Gallia HA** Gallia, Fr.
Infant feed (p.1417·1).
*Milk-protein intolerance.*

**Gallia Lactofidus** Gallia, Fr.
Infant feed (p.1417·1).
*Gastrointestinal disorders.*

**Gallia Soja** Gallia, Fr.
Infant feed (p.1417·1).
*Diarrhoea; gluten intolerance; milk-intolerance.*

**Galliagene** Gallia, Fr.
Infant feed (p.1417·1).
*Diarrhoea; malabsorption syndromes; milk-protein intolerance.*

**Gallifugo** Mediplants, Gr.
Salicylic acid (p.1157·1).
*Hyperkeratosis.*

**Gallith** Evers, Ger.
Hedera helix.
*Cholesterol gallstones.*

**Gallo Merz** Kolassa, Austria†.
Dehydrocholic acid (p.1679·2); pancreatin (p.1725·3); cellulase (p.1669·1); dimethicone (p.1289·2); turmeric (p.1058·3).
*Biliary-tract and pancreatic disorders.*

**Gallo Merz N** Merz, Ger.
Dimethicone (p.1289·2); turmeric (p.1058·3).
*Biliary-tract disorders.*

**Gallo Merz Spasmo** Merz, Ger.
Hymecromone (p.1700·1).
*Biliary-tract spasm.*

**Gallobeta** Betapharm, Ger.
Gallopamil hydrochloride (p.922·3).
*Angina pectoris; arrhythmias; hypertension.*

**Gallogen** Torii, Hong Kong†.
Tocamphyl.
*Biliary-tract disorders; liver disorders.*

**Gallogran** Synpharma, Austria.
Taraxacum (p.1751·3); achillea (p.1646·2); absinthium (p.1645·1).
*Biliary- and gastrointestinal tract disorders.*

**Gallopas** Pascoe, Ger.
Greater celandine (p.1695·3).
*Gastrointestinal and biliary-tract spasm.*

**Galloselect** Dreluso, Ger.
Homoeopathic preparation.

**Galloselect M** Dreluso, Ger.
Greater celandine (p.1695·3); taraxacum (p.1751·3); silybum marianum (p.1043·3); cynara (p.1678·3); chamomile (p.1669·3); peppermint oil (p.1283·2); caraway oil (p.1667·3).
*Biliary-tract disorders.*

**Galloway's Cough Syrup** Pfizer Consumer, UK.
Ipecacuanha liquid extract (p.1122·3); squill vinegar (p.1130·3).
*Coughs.*

**Galmarin** Lifeplan, UK†.
Evening primrose oil (p.1686·3); borage oil (p.1661·3); omega-3 marine triglycerides (p.976·2).
*Nutritional supplement.*

**Galmax** Max Farma, Ital.
Sodium succinate ursodeoxycholate (p.1761·1).
*Biliary disorders; gallstones.*

**Galopran** Microsules Bernabo, Arg.
Mosapride citrate (p.1276·3).
*Gastro-oesophageal reflux; gastrointestinal motility disorders; nausea and vomiting.*

**Galpamol** Galpharm, UK.
Paracetamol (p.76·2).
*Pain.*

**Galpharm Flu Relief** Galpharm, UK.
Paracetamol (p.76·2); phenylephrine hydrochloride (p.1126·3).
*Cold and influenza symptoms.*

**Galprofen** Galpharm, UK.
Ibuprofen (p.45·3).
*Fever; pain.*

**Galpseud** Galen, Irl.†.
Pseudoephedrine hydrochloride (p.1129·2).
*Respiratory-tract congestion.*

**Galpseud Plus** Thornton & Ross, UK.
Pseudoephedrine hydrochloride (p.1129·2); chlorphenamine maleate (p.427·3).
*Allergic rhinitis.*

**Galsud** Thornton & Ross, UK.
Pseudoephedrine hydrochloride (p.1129·2).
Formerly known as Galpseud.
*Respiratory-tract congestion.*

**Galtamicina** Northia, Arg.
Benzathine benzylpenicillin (p.162·3).
*Bacterial infections.*

**Galusan** Almirall, Spain.
Pipemidic acid (p.243·1).
*Urinary-tract infections.*

**Galutec** Master, Chile.
Salol (p.88·1); menthol (p.1711·3); thymol (p.1194·2).
*Mouth and throat disorders.*

**Gama Venina** Aventis Behring, Braz.
A normal immunoglobulin (p.1627·2).
*Agammaglobulinaemia; chronic demyelinated polyneuropathy; hypogammaglobulinaemia; idiopathic thrombocytopenic purpura; Kawasaki disease; lymphocytic leukaemia; passive immunisation.*

**Gamactrin** Delta, Braz.
Co-trimoxazole (p.199·3).
*Bacterial infections; Pneumocystis carinii pneumonia; protozoal infections.*

**Gamafine** Haffkine, India.
A normal immunoglobulin (p.1627·2).
*Hypogammaglobulinaemia; passive immunisation.*

**Gamalat** Novaquimica, Braz.†.
Dimethicone (p.1289·2); aluminium hydroxide (p.1249·2); magnesium hydroxide (p.1272·2).
*Flatulence; gastrointestinal hyperacidity.*

**Gamalate B6**
Andromaco, Chile.
Gamma-aminobutyric acid (p.1690·2); gamma-amino beta hydroxybutyric acid; magnesium glutamate hydrobromide (p.1709·2); pyridoxine hydrochloride (p.1456·3).
*Mental function impairment.*

Novag, Spain.
Gamma-aminobutyric acid (p.1690·2); aminohydroxybutyric acid (p.353·2); magnesium glutamate hydrobromide (p.1709·2); pyridoxine (p.1457·2).
*Mental function impairment; senility.*

**Gamaline-V** Herbarium, Braz.
Gamolenic acid (p.1690·2); oleic acid (p.1481·3); linoleic acid (p.1690·2); polyunsaturated acids.
*Essential fatty acid deficiency.*

**Gamanil**
Merck, Irl.; Merck, UK.
Lofepramine hydrochloride (p.305·3).
*Depression.*

**Gamatol** LED, Fr.
Borage oil (p.1661·3).
*Dry skin disorders.*

**Gamavate** Julphar, UAE.
Clobetasol propionate (p.1095·2).
*Skin disorders.*

**Gamax** Hebron, Braz.
Linoleic acid; linolenic acid; fatty acids (p.1417·1).
*Nutritional supplement.*

**Gambex** Aspen, S.Afr.
Lindane (p.1506·3).
*Pediculosis.*

**Gambrolys** Gambro, Swed.†.
Sodium chloride; sodium hydroxide; potassium chloride; magnesium chloride; calcium chloride; acetic acid (p.1221·1).
*Haemodialysis solution.*

**Gambrosol**
Gambro, Denm.; Gambro, Fin.; Gambro, Spain; Gambro, Swed.; Bichsel, Switz.†.
Glucose; sodium chloride; sodium lactate; calcium chloride; magnesium chloride (p.1221·1).
*Peritoneal dialysis solution.*

**Gamespir** Cosmopharm, Gr.
Acemetacin (p.11·3).
*Dysmenorrhoea; gout; inflammation; musculoskeletal disorders; pain; spondyloarthritis.*

**Gamibetal**
Dansk-Flama, Braz.; SIT, Ital.; Italmex, Mex.
Gamma-aminohydroxybutyric acid (p.353·2).
*Epilepsy; neurosis; premenstrual syndrome.*

Seber, Port.
4-Amino-3-hydroxybutyric acid (p.353·2).
*Behaviour disorders; infantile convulsions.*

**Gamibetal Complex**
Dansk-Flama, Braz.
Aminohydroxybutyric acid (p.353·2); phenobarbital (p.367·3); phenytoin (p.370·2).
*Epilepsy.*

SIT, Ital.
Aminohydroxybutyric acid (p.353·2); phenobarbital (p.367·3); phenytoin sodium (p.370·2).
*Epilepsy.*

**Gamibetal Compositum** Seber, Port.
4-Amino-3-hydroxybutyric acid (p.353·2); diazepam (p.690·1).
*Epilepsy; excitability.*

**Gamibetal Plus** SIT, Ital.
Aminohydroxybutyric acid (p.353·2); diazepam (p.690·1).
*Childhood behaviour disorders; epilepsy.*

**Gamikal** Galen, Mex.
Amikacin sulfate (p.154·1).
*Bacterial infections.*

**Gamimune**
Gador, Arg.; Sintofarma, Braz.
A normal immunoglobulin (p.1627·2).
*Idiopathic thrombocytopenic purpura; immunodeficiency; passive immunisation.*

**Gamimune N**
Bayer, Canad.; Bayer, Chile; Bayer Biological, Hong Kong†; Bayer, Israel; Bayer, USA.
A normal immunoglobulin (p.1627·2).
*Idiopathic thrombocytopenic purpura; immunodeficiency; passive immunisation.*

**Gamma Anti D** Grifols, Spain.
An anti-D immunoglobulin (p.1608·1).
*Prevention of rhesus sensitisation.*

**Gamma Antihep B** Grifols, Spain.
A hepatitis B immunoglobulin (p.1617·2).
*Passive immunisation.*

**Gamma Antitenos** Grifols, Spain†.
A tetanus immunoglobulin (p.1640·3).
*Passive immunisation.*

**Gamma Antitetanos** Grifols, Spain.
A tetanus immunoglobulin (p.1640·3).
*Passive immunisation.*

**Gamma EPA** Quest, UK†.
Concentrated fish oil (p.976·2).

**Gamma Glob Antihepa B** Alonga, Spain†.
A hepatitis B immunoglobulin (p.1617·2).
*Passive immunisation.*

**Gamma Marine** Quest, UK†.
Evening primrose oil (p.1686·3); borage oil (p.1661·3); fish oil (p.976·1).

**Gamma Oil**
Quest, Canad.†; Quest, UK†.
Evening primrose oil (p.1686·3).
*Nutritional supplement.*

**Gamma Oil Marine** Quest, Canad.†.
Gamolenic acid (p.1690·2); linoleic acid (p.1690·2); vitamins (p.1417·1).

**Gammabulin**
Immuno, Ger.†; Immuno, Hong Kong†; Immuno, Irl.†; Immuno, Ital.†; Baxter BioScience, UK†.
A normal immunoglobulin (p.1627·2).
*Agammaglobulinaemia; hypogammaglobulinaemia; passive immunisation.*

**Gammabulin A** Immuno, Ger.†.
A hepatitis A immunoglobulin (p.1617·1).
*Passive immunisation.*

**Gammacur** Biocur, Ger.
Evening primrose oil (p.1686·3).
*Eczema.*

**Gammaderm** Linderma, UK.
Evening primrose oil (p.1686·3).
*Dry skin disorders.*

**Gammadin** OFF, Ital.
Povidone-iodine (p.1190·3).
*Skin, wound, and mucous membrane disinfection.*

**Gammagard**
Baxter, Austria; Baxter, Belg.†; Baxter, Canad.; Baxter, Denm.; Baxter, Fin.; Baxter, Fr.; Baxter, Ger.; Baxter-Hyland, Hong Kong; Baxter, Israel; Baxter, Ital.; Baxter, Malaysia; Baxter, Singapore†; Baxter, Spain; Baxter, Swed.; Baxter, Switz.; Baxter BioScience, UK; Baxter, USA.
A normal immunoglobulin (p.1627·2).
*Guillain-Barré syndrome; hypogammaglobulinaemia; idiopathic thrombocytopenic purpura; immunodeficiency; Kawasaki syndrome; passive immunisation.*

**Gammagard SD** Baxter, Gr.
A normal immunoglobulin (p.1627·2).
*Hypogammglobulinaemia; idiopathic thrombocytopenic purpura; Kawasaki disease; passive immunisation.*

**Gammaglob** Grifols, Spain.
A normal immunoglobulin (p.1627·2).
*Passive immunisation.*

**Gammaglob Anti D** Grifols, Spain†.
An anti-D immunoglobulin (p.1608·1).
*Prevention of rhesus sensitisation.*

**Gammaglob Antihep B P BE** Aventis Behring, Spain.
A hepatitis B immunoglobulin (p.1617·2).
*Passive immunisation.*

**Gammaglob Antite** ICN, Spain†; Centeon, Spain†.
A tetanus immunoglobulin (p.1640·3).
*Passive immunisation.*

**Gammaglobulin**
Pharmacia Upjohn, Denm.†; Biovitrum, Norw.
A normal immunoglobulin (p.1627·2).
*Hypogammaglobulinaemia; passive immunisation.*

**Gammaglobulin SPR** Veripalvelu, Fin.
A normal immunoglobulin (p.1627·2).
*Hypogammaglobulinaemia; passive immunisation.*

**Gammaglobulina** Hemoderivados, Arg.
A normal immunoglobulin (p.1627·2).
*Passive immunisation.*

**Gammakine** Dompe Biotec, Ital.
Interferon gamma-1b (p.647·2).
*Chronic granulomatous disease.*

**Gammalon**
Daiichi, Hong Kong; Daiichi, Thai.
Gamma-aminobutyric acid (p.1690·2).
*Cerebrovascular disorders; head injury; hypertension; mental function impairment.*

**Gamma-Men** Nuovo ISM, Ital.†.
An anti-D immunoglobulin (p.1608·1).
*Prevention of rhesus sensitisation.*

**Gammamida Complex** Laproquifar, Spain†.
Cyanocobalamin (p.1458·2); glutamic acid (p.1433·2); pyridoxine (p.1457·2); thiamine (p.1455·2).
*Alcoholism; muscular dystrophies; nausea and vomiting in pregnancy; vitamin B deficiency.*

**Gammanorm**
Biovitrum, Denm.; Biovitrum, Norw.; Biovitrum, Swed.
A normal immunoglobulin (p.1627·2).
*Hypogammaglobulinaemia.*

**Gammanova** Elvetium, Arg.
Immunoglobulin A-11-S; muramidase hydrochloride (p.1717·2).

**Gamma-OH** SERB, Fr.
Sodium oxybate (p.1308·3).
*General anaesthesia; sedative.*

**GammaOil Premium** Quest, UK†.
Evening primrose oil (p.1686·3).

**Gammaplus** Fidia, Ital.
Omega-3 triglycerides (p.976·1); omega-6 triglycerides.
*Nutritional supplement.*

**Gammar** Nikkho, Braz.
Gamma-aminobutyric acid (p.1690·2).
*Impaired mental function.*

**Gammariza** Toyo, Hong Kong†.
Oryzanol (p.1725·1).
*Autonomic nervous-system disorders; menopausal disorders.*

**Gammar-P** Centeon, USA.
A normal immunoglobulin (p.1627·2).
*Immunoglobulin deficiency; passive immunisation.*

**Gamma-Scab** Lafedar, Arg.
*Lotion:* Lindane (p.1506·3); lidocaine hydrochloride (p.1377·3).
*Pediculosis; scabies.*
*Shampoo:* Lindane (p.1506·3).
*Pediculosis.*

**Gammatet** Gador, Arg.
A tetanus immunoglobulin (p.1640·3).
*Passive immunisation.*

**Gamma-Tet P** Aventis Behring, Ital.
A tetanus immunoglobulin (p.1640·3).
*Passive immunisation.*

**Gammatetanos** Lab Francais du Fractionnement, Fr.
A tetanus immunoglobulin (p.1640·3).
*Passive immunisation.*

**Gamma-Venin**
Aventis Behring, Austria; Aventis Behring, Ger.; Behringwerke, Israel†; Centeon, Spain†.
A normal immunoglobulin (p.1627·2).
*Hypogammaglobulinaemia; passive immunisation.*

**Gamma-Venin P**
Gerolimatos (Γερολυματος), Gr.; Aventis Behring, Ital.
A normal immunoglobulin (p.1627·2).
*Hypogammaglobulinaemia; idiopathic thrombocytopenic purpura; Kawasaki disease; passive immunisation.*

**Gammavit** Sessa, Ital.†.
Borage oil (p.1661·3).
*Nutritional supplement.*

**Gammonativ**
Biovitrum, Denm.; Pharmacia, Ger.; Pharmacia Upjohn, Norw.†; Biovitrum, Swed.
A normal immunoglobulin (p.1627·2).
*Hypogammaglobulinaemia; idiopathic thrombocytopenic purpura.*

**Gamonil**
Merck, Ger.; Merck, Switz.
Lofepramine hydrochloride (p.305·3).
*Depression.*

**Gamophen**
Johnson & Johnson, Austral.†; Johnson & Johnson Medical, UK.
Triclosan (p.1195·2).
*Skin cleanser.*

**Gamulin Rh** Armour, USA†.
An anti-D immunoglobulin (p.1608·1).
*Prevention of rhesus sensitisation.*

**Gamunex** Bayer, USA.
A normal immunoglobulin (p.1627·2).
*Idiopathic thrombocytopenic purpura; immunodeficiency.*

**Ganaprofene** Ganassini, Ital.
Ibuprofen sodium (p.46·3).
*Fever; influenza symptoms; pain.*

**Ganaton** Hokuriku, Jpn.
Itopride hydrochloride (p.1268·2).
*Gastrointestinal symptoms of chronic gastritis.*

**Ganavit** Pharmaton, Switz.†.
Guarana (p.1765·3); caffeine (p.782·1); vitamins; minerals (p.1417·1).
*Tonic.*

**Ganazolo** Ganassini, Ital.
Econazole (p.397·1) or econazole nitrate (p.397·2).
*Fungal and Gram-positive bacterial infections.*

**Gancivir** Eurofarma, Braz.†.
Ganciclovir sodium (p.635·3).
*Viral infections.*

**Ganda**
Chauvin, Irl.; Chauvin, UK†.
Guanethidine monosulfate (p.926·3); adrenaline (p.852·2).
*Glaucoma.*

**Gandhour** Dermoteca, Port.†.
A range of soap substitutes and moisturisers.

**Gandin** Polipharm, Thai.
Mefenamic acid (p.55·2).
*Pain.*

**Ganidin NR** Cypress, USA.
Guaifenesin (p.1122·1).

**Ganite** Genta, USA.
Gallium nitrate (p.772·2).
*Hypercalcaemia of malignancy.*

**Gani-Tuss NR** Cypress, USA.
Guaifenesin (p.1122·1); codeine phosphate (p.27·1).
*Coughs.*

**Gani-Tuss-DM NR** Cypress, USA.
Guaifenesin (p.1122·1); dextromethorphan hydrobromide (p.1117·3).
*Coughs.*

**Ganor** Boehringer Ingelheim, Ger.†.
Famotidine (p.1265·2).
*Peptic ulcer; Zollinger-Ellison syndrome.*

**Gantanol** Roche, USA†.
Sulfamethoxazole (p.261·1).
*Adjunct in falciparum malaria; bacterial infections.*

**Gantil** Elpen (Ελπεν), Gr.
Tolfenamic acid (p.94·2).
*Dysmenorrhoea; inflammation; musculoskeletal and joint disorders; pain.*

**Gantin** Arrow, Austral.
Gabapentin (p.362·2).
*Epilepsy; neuropathic pain.*

**Gantrim** Geymonat, Ital.
Co-trimoxazole (p.199·3).
*Bacterial infections; Pneumocystis carinii pneumonia.*

**Gantrimex** Geymonat, Ital.
Oxolamine citrate (p.1126·1) or oxolamine phosphate (p.1126·1).
*Respiratory-tract disorders.*

**Gantrisin** Roche, USA.
Acetyl sulfafurazole (p.260·1) or sulfafurazole diolamine (p.260·1).
*Bacterial eye infections; urinary-tract infections.*

**Ganvirax** Blausiegel, Braz.
Ganciclovir sodium (p.635·3).

**Ganvirel** Elvetium, Arg.
Lamivudine (p.648·2).
*HIV infection.*

**Ganvirel Duo** Elvetium, Arg.
Lamivudine (p.648·2); zidovudine (p.658·2).
*HIV infection.*

**Gaopathyl** Monot, Fr.†.
Aluminium hydroxide (p.1249·2); magnesium hydroxide (p.1272·2).
*Antacid.*

**Gaoptol** Europhta, Mon.
Timolol maleate (p.1012·2).
*Glaucoma; ocular hypertension.*

**Gaosedal Codeine** Monot, Fr.†.
Paracetamol (p.76·2); codeine phosphate (p.27·1).

**Gaproxen** Gap, Gr.
Ranitidine hydrochloride (p.1285·2).
*Conditions where gastric acid reduction is beneficial; gastric hypersecretion including Zollinger-Ellison syndrome; peptic ulcer.*

**Garacin** Delta, Braz.
Gentamicin sulfate (p.217·1).
*Bacterial infections.*

**Garacol** Schering-Plough, Neth.
Gentamicin sulfate (p.217·1).
*Bacterial infections.*

**Garacoll**
Schering-Plough, Mex.; Schering-Plough, S.Afr.
Gentamicin sulfate (p.217·1).
*Bone infections.*

**Garalen** Galen, Mex.
Gentamicin sulfate (p.217·1).
*Bacterial infections.*

**Garalone** Schering-Plough, Port.
Gentamicin sulfate (p.217·1).
*Bacterial infections.*

**Garamicina**
Schering-Plough, Braz.; Schering-Plough, Mex.
Gentamicin (p.219·1) or gentamicin sulfate (p.217·1).
*Bacterial infections.*

**Garamicina-V** Schering-Plough, Mex.
Gentamicin sulfate (p.217·1); betamethasone valerate (p.1093·2).
*Infected skin disorders.*

**Garamycin**
Aesca, Austria; Schering, Canad.; Schering-Plough, Denm.; Schering-Plough, Gr.; Schering-Plough, Hong Kong; Fulford, India; Schering-Plough, Israel†; Schering-Plough, Malaysia; Schering-Plough, Neth.; Schering-Plough, Norw.; Schering-Plough, S.Afr.; Schering-Plough, Singapore; Schering-Plough, Swed.; Essex, Switz.; Schering-Plough, Thai.; Schering-Plough, UK†; Schering, USA.
Gentamicin (p.219·1) or gentamicin sulfate (p.217·1).
*Bacterial infections.*

**Garanil** Zambon, Spain.
Captopril (p.879·2).
*Diabetic nephropathy; heart failure; hypertension; myocardial infarction.*

**Garapepsin** Medichrom, Gr.
Trimebutine (p.1758·1).
*Gastrointestinal and gallbladder pain.*

**Garasone**
Schering-Plough, Belg.; Schering-Plough, Braz.; Schering, Canad.; Schering-Plough, Hong Kong; Schering-Plough, Malaysia; Schering-Plough, Mex.; Schering-Plough, S.Afr.; Schering-Plough, Singapore.
Gentamicin sulfate (p.217·1); betamethasone sodium phosphate (p.1093·1).
*External ear disorders; inflammatory eye infections.*

**Garatec** Technilab, Canad.
Gentamicin sulfate (p.217·1).
*Bacterial infections.*

**Garceptol** Grunenthal, Chile.
Dimeticone (p.1289·2); metoclopramide (p.1274·3); chlordiazepoxide (p.674·2).
*Gastrointestinal disorders.*

**Garcinol Max** Garden House, Arg.
*Tablets:* Centella (p.1144·3); carnitine (p.1423·3); garcinia cambogia.
*Cellulitis; dietary supplement; slimming aid.*
*Topical gel:* Centella (p.1144·3); ginkgo biloba (p.1692·3); hedera helix.
*Cellulitis.*

**Garde Gomas** Grisi, Mex.
Benzocaine (p.1370·3).
*Mouth and throat pain.*

**Garde Jarabe** Grisi, Mex.
Dextromethorphan (p.1117·3).
*Coughs.*

**Gardenal**
Aventis, Arg.; Aventis, Belg.; Aventis, Braz.; Aventis, Fr.; Aventis, Gr.; Rhone-Poulenc Rorer, Hong Kong†; Nicholas Piramal, India; Aventis, NZ; Aventis, S.Afr.; Aventis, Spain; Aventis, Thai.; Concord, UK.
Phenobarbital (p.367·3) or phenobarbital sodium (p.367·3).
*Epilepsy; febrile convulsions; insomnia; sedative.*

**Gardenale** Aventis, Ital.
Phenobarbital (p.367·3) or phenobarbital sodium (p.367·3).
*Epilepsy; insomnia; sedative.*

**Gardoton**
Note. This name is used for preparations of different composition.
Raffo, Arg.
Glibenclamide (p.331·2).
*Diabetes mellitus.*

Raffo, Chile.
Ondansetron (p.1281·1).
*Nausea and vomiting.*

**GA-301-Redskin 301** Madaus, Ger.†.
Histamine hydrochloride (p.1697·1); clove oil (p.1673·3); juniper oil (p.1703·1).
*Migraine; musculoskeletal and joint disorders; neuritis; respiratory-tract disorders.*

**Garfield**
Whitehall-Robins, Canad.; Menley & James, USA.
A range of multivitamin preparations with or without minerals (p.1417·1).

**Gargaletas** Monserrat, Arg.
Gramicidin (p.220·2); neomycin sulfate (p.235·1); benzocaine (p.1370·3).
*Mouth and throat disorders.*

**Gargaril** Puerto Galiano, Spain.
Chlorhexidine (p.1173·2); benzocaine (p.1370·3).
Formerly contained formaldehyde and menthol.
*Mouth and throat disorders.*

**Gargarisma zum Gurgeln** Krewel, Ger.
Aluminium chloride (p.1142·1).
*Mouth inflammation.*

**Gargarol** Boiron, Canad.
Homoeopathic preparation.

**Gargaron** Sam-On, Israel†.
Cetylpyridinium chloride (p.1173·1).
*Mouth and throat infections.*

**Gargilon** Vemedia, Neth.
Dequalinium chloride (p.1178·1).
*Sore throat.*

**Gargocetil** Bunker, Braz.
Cetylpyridinium chloride (p.1173·1).
*Mouth and throat disorders.*

**Gargol** Rekah, Israel.
Boric acid (p.1662·1); thymol (p.1194·2); menthol (p.1711·3); terpineol (p.1752·2); cineole (p.1672·1); methyl salicylate (p.59·3); chloroxylenol (p.1177·2).
*Mouth and throat disorders.*

**Gargosedans** INQ, Braz.†.
Tyrothricin (p.275·1); neomycin sulfate (p.235·1); sulfadiazine (p.258·2); benzocaine (p.1370·3); chlorophyll (p.1057·1).
*Mouth and throat disorders.*

**Gargotan** Ibefar, Braz.†.
Tyrothricin (p.275·1); sulfanilamide (p.263·2); thymol (p.1194·2); cineole (p.1672·1); menthol (p.1711·3); benzocaine (p.1370·3).

**Gargotrat** Bergamo, Braz.†.
Cetylpyridinium chloride (p.1173·1); allantoin (p.1141·3); benzocaine (p.1370·3); chlorophyll (p.1057·1); peppermint leaf (p.1283·2); cineole (p.1672·1).
*Mouth and throat disorders.*

**Garia** Sankyo, Spain.
Cefpodoxime proxetil (p.178·3).
*Bacterial infections.*

**Garlic Allium Complex** GNLD, Austral.†.
Garlic (p.1691·1); onion (p.1723·2); chive; leek; rosemary (p.1740·2).
*Upper respiratory-tract congestion.*

**Garlic, Horseradish, A & C Capsules** Vitaplex, Austral.†.
Garlic oil (p.1691·2); horseradish (p.1697·3); ascorbic acid (p.1460·2); vitamin A palmitate (p.1453·1).
*Excess body fluids; excess mucus formation.*

**Garlic and Horseradish + C Complex** Cenovis, Austral.†; Vitelle, Austral.†.
Horseradish (p.1697·3); garlic (p.1691·1); sodium ascorbate (p.1460·2); ascorbic acid (p.1460·2); fenugreek (p.1688·1); althaea (p.1651·3).
*Upper respiratory-tract symptoms.*

**Garlimega** Cantassium Co., UK.
Garlic (p.1691·1).

**Garlix** *Blackmores, Austral.†.*
Garlic (p.1691·1).
*Cold and influenza symptoms.*

**Garlodex** *Modern Health Products, UK†.*
Althaea root (p.1651·3); parsley (p.1728·3); garlic oil (p.1691·2).
*Catarrh; colds.*

**Garmastan**
*Austroplant, Austria; Protina, Ger.†.*
Guaiazulene (p.1696·2).
*Mastitis prophylaxis.*

**Garoin**
*Nicholas Piramal, India; Rhone-Poulenc Rorer, S.Afr.†.*
Phenytoin sodium (p.370·2); phenobarbital sodium (p.367·3).
*Epilepsy.*

**Garonsept**
*Note. This name is used for preparations of different composition.*
*Master, Chile.*
Chlorhexidine gluconate (p.1173·2).
*Mouth and throat infections.*
*Sam-On, Israel.*
Benzalkonium chloride (p.1168·3); menthol (p.1711·3); thymol (p.1194·2); lemon oil (p.1706·2).
*Mouth and throat infections.*

**Gartech** *Eagle, Austral.†.*
Astragalus; echinacea pallida (p.1683·2); garlic (p.1691·1); berberis vulgaris; paraformaldehyde (p.1187·3); garlic oil (p.1691·2); anise oil (p.1655·2); thymol (p.1194·2); savory oil.
*Cold and influenza symptoms.*

**Gartricin** *Cantabria, Spain.*
Benzocaine (p.1370·3).
*Mouth and throat disorders.*

**Garydol** *Cinfa, Spain†.*
Chlorhexidine gluconate (p.1173·2); benzocaine (p.1370·3).
*Sore throat.*

**Garze Disinfettanti alla Pomata Betadine**
*Asta Medica, Ital.†.*
Povidone-iodine (p.1190·3).
*Medicated dressing.*

**Gas Ban** *Roberts, USA.*
Calcium carbonate (p.1254·2); simeticone (p.1289·2).
*Flatulence.*

**Gas Ban DS** *Roberts, USA.*
Aluminium hydroxide (p.1249·2); magnesium hydroxide (p.1272·2); simeticone (p.1289·2).
*Flatulence.*

**Gas Relief** *Rugby, USA.*
Simeticone (p.1289·2).
*Flatulence.*

**Gasam** *Sriprasit, Thai.†.*
Tiaprofenic acid (p.93·3).
*Gout; musculoskeletal, joint, and soft-tissue disorders.*

**Gasbrand-Antitoxin** *Chiron Behring, Ger.†.*
A gas-gangrene antitoxin (p.1615·3).
*Gas gangrene.*

**Gascoal**
*YSP, Malaysia; Yung Shin, Singapore.*
Simeticone (p.1289·2).
*Flatulence; preparation for gastrointestinal examination.*

**Gascop** *Valdecasas, Mex.*
Albendazole (p.101·2).
*Worm infections.*

**Gasec**
*Mepha, Braz.; Mepha, Malaysia; Mepha, Port.*
Omeprazole (p.1278·2).
*Gastro-oesophageal reflux; peptic ulcer; Zollinger-Ellison syndrome.*

**Gaseofin** *Andromaco, Chile.*
Metoclopramide hydrochloride (p.1274·3); chlordiazepoxide hydrochloride (p.674·2); simeticone (p.1289·2).
*Gastrointestinal disorders.*

**Gaslon N** *Shinyaku, Jpn.*
Irsogladine maleate (p.1267·3).
*Gastritis; peptic ulcer.*

**Gasmilen** *Elvetium, Arg.*
Ganciclovir (p.635·3).
*Viral infections.*

**Gas-MM** *Milano, Thai.*
Simeticone (p.1289·2).
*Flatulence; preparation for gastrointestinal examination.*

**Gasmol** *Hilarys, Canad.†.*
Magnesium carbonate (p.1272·1); magnesium hydroxide (p.1272·2); magnesium trisilicate (p.1272·3); calcium carbonate (p.1254·2); rhubarb (p.1287·3).

**Gasmotin** *Dainippon, Jpn.*
Mosapride citrate (p.1276·3).
*Gastritis.*

**Gas-Nep** *Sriprasit, Thai.*
Catnep; sodium bicarbonate (p.1223·2); caraway oil (p.1667·3); fennel oil (p.1687·3); cardamom oil (p.1668·1); anise oil (p.1655·2).
*Flatulence; gastrointestinal disorders.*

**Gasorbol** *Andromaco, Chile.*
*Oral drops:* Simeticone (p.1289·2); pipenzolate bromide (p.487·3).
*Aerophagia; infant colic.*
*Tablets:* Simeticone (p.1289·2).
*Abdominal distension; aerophagia; meteorism.*

**Gasorbol Plus** *Andromaco, Chile.*
Simeticone (p.1289·2); aluminium hydroxide (p.1249·2); magnesium trisilicate (p.1272·3).
*Gastrointestinal disorders.*

**Gaspiren** *Biolab Sanus, Braz.*
Omeprazole (p.1278·2).
*Gastro-oesophageal reflux; gastrointestinal hyperacidity; peptic ulcer.*

**Gassi** *Progress, Thai.*
Simeticone (p.1289·2).
*Flatulence.*

**Gastab**
*Note. This name is used for preparations of different composition.*
*Merck, Hong Kong.*
Cimetidine (p.1255·3).
*Dyspepsia; peptic ulcer.*
*Greater Pharma, Thai.*
Sodium bicarbonate (p.1223·2); cataria.
*Flatulence.*

**Gastec** *Microsules Bernabo, Arg.*
Omeprazole (p.1278·2).
*Acid aspiration; gastro-oesophageal reflux; peptic ulcer; Zollinger-Ellison syndrome.*

**Gasteel**
*Note. This name is used for preparations of different composition.*
*Fuso, Hong Kong.*
Dimethicone (p.1289·2).
*Flatulence.*
*Shinfuso, Thai.†.*
Simeticone (p.1289·2); dried aluminium hydroxide gel (p.1249·2).
*Flatulence; preparation for gastrointestinal examinations.*

**Gaster**
*Note. This name is used for preparations of different composition.*
*SoSe, Ital.†.*
Sodium cromoglicate (p.795·3).
*Food hypersensitivity; proctitis; ulcerative colitis.*
*Yamanouchi, Jpn.*
Famotidine (p.1265·2).
*Gastro-oesophageal reflux; gastrointestinal haemorrhage; peptic ulcer; premedication; Zollinger-Ellison syndrome.*

**Gasterogen** *Faran, Gr.*
Famotidine (p.1265·2).
*Conditions where gastric acid reduction is beneficial; gastric hypersecretion including Zollinger-Ellison syndrome; peptic ulcer.*

**Gastidin** *Neckerman, Braz.†.*
Cimetidine (p.1255·3).
*Peptic ulcer.*

**Gastidine** *Vida, Hong Kong.*
Cimetidine (p.1255·3).
*Peptic ulcer.*

**Gastop** *Bajer, Arg.*
Simeticone (p.1289·2); bismuth carbonate (p.1252·1).
*Gastrointestinal disorders.*

**Gastopride** *Solvay, Port.*
Famotidine (p.1265·2).
*Peptic ulcer; Zollinger-Ellison syndrome.*

**Gastracol** *Streuli, Switz.*
Aluminium hydroxide (p.1249·2).
*Gastric hyperacidity.*

**Gastral** *Novag, Spain†.*
Sucralfate (p.1290·2).
*Gastrointestinal haemorrhage; peptic ulcer.*

**Gastralgin** *De Angeli, Ital.*
Roxatidine acetate hydrochloride (p.1288·1).
*Gastro-oesophageal reflux; peptic ulcer.*

**Gastralgine** *UPSA, Fr.†.*
Aluminium hydroxide (p.1249·2); aluminium glycinate (p.1249·1); magnesium trisilicate (p.1272·3); simeticone (p.1289·2).
*Gastrointestinal disorders.*

**Gastralon N** *Cesra, Ger.*
Chamomile (p.1669·3); gentian (p.1692·2); absinthium (p.1645·1).
*Gastrointestinal disorders.*

**Gastralsan**
*Note. This name is used for preparations of different composition.*
*Dolisos, Canad.†.*
Homoeopathic preparation.
*Dolisos, Fr.†.*
Cynara (p.1678·3); boldo (p.1661·2); fumitory (p.1690·1).
*Biliary-tract disorders.*

**Gastran**
*Note. This name is used for preparations of different composition.*
*Johnson & Johnson, Braz.*
Simeticone (p.1289·2); aluminium hydroxide (p.1249·2); magnesium hydroxide (p.1272·2).
*Flatulence; gastrointestinal hyperacidity.*
*Delta, Singapore.*
Ranitidine (p.1285·2).
*Gastro-oesophageal reflux; peptic ulcer.*

**Gastranil** *Lafage, Arg.*
Bismuth hydroxide; papaverine (p.1728·1); kaolin (p.1268·3); magnesium trisilicate (p.1272·3); titanium dioxide (p.1160·3).
*Gastrointestinal disorders.*

**Gastrarctin N** *Serum-Werk Bernburg, Ger.*
Colloidal silver (p.1746·2); chamomile flowers (p.1669·3); peppermint leaf (p.1283·2).
*Gastrointestinal disorders.*

**Gastrat** *Ibfarma, Braz.†.*
Ranitidine (p.1285·2).
*Peptic ulcer.*

**Gastrax** *Asche, Ger.*
Nizatidine (p.1277·2).
*Peptic ulcer.*

**Gastrec** *Tecnofarma, Mex.*
Ranitidine (p.1285·2).

**Gastregan** *Synpharma, Austria.*
Chamomile flower (p.1669·3); melissa leaf (p.1711·1); peppermint leaf (p.1283·2).
*Gastrointestinal pain and inflammation.*

**Gastrex**
*Note. This name is used for preparations of different composition.*
*Simoes, Braz.*
Aluminium hydroxide (p.1249·2); magnesium hydroxide (p.1272·2); calcium carbonate (p.1254·2).
*Gastrointestinal hyperacidity.*
*Boehringer Ingelheim, Fr.†.*
Aluminium histidinate; magnesium hydroxide (p.1272·2).
*Gastrointestinal disorders.*
*OM, Port.*
Lansoprazole (p.1269·3).
*Gastro-oesophageal reflux; peptic ulcer; Zollinger-Ellison syndrome.*

**Gastrial** *Sanofi Synthelabo, Arg.*
Ranitidine (p.1285·2).
*Gastritis; gastro-oesophageal reflux; peptic ulcer; Zollinger-Ellison syndrome.*

**Gastrib** *Ibfarma, Braz.†.*
Omeprazole (p.1278·2).
*Peptic ulcer.*

**Gastribien** *Cinfa, Spain.*
Aluminium hydroxide (p.1249·2); magnesium trisilicate (p.1272·3).
*Dyspepsia; peptic ulcer.*

**Gastricalm** *Novum, Belg.*
Magaldrate (p.1271·3).
*Gastrointestinal disorders associated with hyperacidity.*

**Gastricard** *Ysatfabrik, Ger.*
*Oral drops:* Ginger oil (p.1667·1); fennel oil (p.1687·3); peppermint oil (p.1283·2); caraway oil (p.1667·3); coriander oil (p.1676·1).
Gastricard N formerly contained ginger oil, fennel oil, peppermint oil, caraway oil, coriander oil, gentian, and crataegus.
*Tablets:* Peppermint oil (p.1283·2); caraway oil (p.1667·3); fennel oil (p.1687·3); coriander oil (p.1676·1).
Gastricard N formerly contained peppermint oil, caraway oil, fennel oil, coriander oil, dimethicone, and crataegus.
*Gastrointestinal disorders.*

**Gastricholan-L** *Sudmedica, Ger.*
Chamomile flowers (p.1669·3); peppermint leaf (p.1283·2); fennel (p.1687·2).
*Gastrointestinal disorders.*

**Gastricin** *Odontofarma, Braz.†.*
Dicycloverine hydrochloride (p.481·2); aluminium hydroxide (p.1249·2); magnesium hydroxide (p.1272·2); simeticone (p.1289·2).
*Flatulence; gastrointestinal hyperacidity.*

**Gastricumeel** *Peithner, Austria.*
Homoeopathic preparation.

**Gastricur** *Heumann, Ger.*
Pirenzepine hydrochloride (p.488·1).
*Dyspepsia; gastritis; peptic ulcer.*

**Gastricure** *Bio-Familia, Switz.†.*
Ceratonia (p.1579·1); marine algae; magnesium trisilicate (p.1272·3).
*Bloating; gastric hyperacidity; gastric irritation.*

**Gastride** *Laboratorios Chile, Chile.*
Lansoprazole (p.1269·3).
*Gastro-oesophageal reflux; peptic ulcer; Zollinger-Ellison syndrome.*

**Gastridin**
*Note. This name is used for preparations of different composition.*
*Microsules Bernabo, Arg.*
Clebopride (p.1260·3).
*Merck Sharp & Dohme, Ital.*
Famotidine (p.1265·2).
*Gastro-oesophageal reflux; peptic ulcer; Zollinger-Ellison syndrome.*

**Gastridina** *Medibial, Port.*
Ranitidine hydrochloride (p.1285·2).
*Acid aspiration; dyspepsia; gastro-oesophageal reflux; peptic ulcer; Zollinger-Ellison syndrome.*

**Gastridin-E** *Microsules Bernabo, Arg.*
Gastric capsules, clebopride malate (p.1260·3); pepsin (p.1729·3); simeticone (p.1289·2); enteric capsules, pancreatin (p.1725·3); amylase (p.1654·2); lipase; cellulase (p.1669·1).
*Gastrointestinal disorders.*

**Gastrifam** *Helsinn, Port.*
Famotidine (p.1265·2).
*Dyspepsia; gastro-oesophageal reflux; peptic ulcer; Zollinger-Ellison syndrome.*

**Gastrifom** *Tanta, Canad.*
Aluminium hydroxide (p.1249·2); alginic acid (p.1576·3).

**Gastril** *Duopharma, Hong Kong.*
Ranitidine hydrochloride (p.1285·2).
*Acid aspiration; dyspepsia; gastrointestinal haemorrhage; peptic ulcer.*

**gastri-L 90 N** *Loges, Ger.*
Homoeopathic preparation.

**Gastrimagal** *Azupharma, Ger.†.*
Magaldrate (p.1271·3).
*Gastrointestinal disorders associated with hyperacidity.*

**Gastrimet** *Raffo, Arg.*
Cisapride (p.1259·2); dimeticone (p.1289·2).
*Gastrointestinal disorders.*

**Gastrimet Enzimatico** *Raffo, Arg.*
Cisapride (p.1259·2); simeticone (p.1289·2); pancreatin (p.1725·3).
*Gastrointestinal disorders.*

**Gastrimut** *Normon, Spain.*
Omeprazole (p.1278·2).
*Gastro-oesophageal reflux; peptic ulcer; Zollinger-Ellison syndrome.*

**Gastrimuto** *Medibial, Port.†.*
Ranitidine bismuth citrate (p.1287·2).
*Peptic ulcer.*

**Gastrin-Do** *Grasler, Ger.*
Homoeopathic preparation.

**Gastrinol** *Frega, Canad.†.*
Magnesium hydroxide (p.1272·2); aluminium hydroxide-magnesium carbonate co-dried gel (p.1250·1); simeticone (p.1289·2).

**Gastrion** *Vita, Spain.*
Famotidine (p.1265·2).
*Gastro-oesophageal reflux; peptic ulcer; Zollinger-Ellison syndrome.*

**Gastri-P** *Sanorania, Ger.†.*
Pirenzepine hydrochloride (p.488·1).
*Gastrointestinal disorders.*

**Gastripan**
*Note. This name is used for preparations of different composition.*
*Ratiopharm, Austria.*
Aluminium glycinate (p.1249·1); almasilate (p.1248·2); liquorice (p.1270·2); ethaverine hydrochloride (p.1685·2).
*Gastrointestinal disorders.*
*Merckle, Ger.*
Magaldrate (p.1271·3).
*Gastric hyperacidity; heartburn; peptic ulcer.*

**Gastriselect** *Dreluso, Ger.*
Homoeopathic preparation.

**Gastritol** *Klein, Ger.*
Potentilla anserina; absinthium (p.1645·1); cnicus benedictus (p.1673·3); liquorice (p.1270·2); angelica (p.1655·1); chamomile (p.1669·3); hypericum (p.299·1).
*Gastrointestinal disorders.*

**Gastrium**
*Note. This name is used for preparations of different composition.*
*Ache, Braz.*
Omeprazole (p.1278·2).
*Gastro-oesophageal reflux; gastrointestinal hyperacidity; peptic ulcer.*
*Saval, Chile.*
Famotidine (p.1265·2).
*Acid aspiration; gastritis; gastro-oesophageal reflux; gastrointestinal haemorrhage; peptic ulcer; Zollinger-Ellison syndrome.*

**Gastriveran** *Finadiet, Arg.*
Alizapride (p.1248·1).
*Nausea and vomiting.*

**Gastri-Vyr** *Cazi, Braz.*
Magnesium hydroxide (p.1272·2); aluminium hydroxide (p.1249·2).
Formerly contained calcium carbonate and aluminium hydroxide.
*Gastrointestinal hyperacidity.*

**Gastro** *Unipharm, Israel.*
Famotidine (p.1265·2).
*Gastrointestinal hyperacidity; heartburn; peptic ulcer; Zollinger-Ellison syndrome.*

**Gastro Gobens** *Normon, Spain†.*
Aluminium hydroxide (p.1249·2); dimethicone (p.1289·2); glutamine (p.1433·2); metoclopramide hydrochloride (p.1274·3).
*Dyspepsia; gastritis; meteorism; nausea; oesophagitis; peptic ulcer.*

**Gastro H2** *Lesvi, Spain†.*
Cimetidine (p.1255·3).
*Acid aspiration; gastro-oesophageal reflux; gastrointestinal haemorrhage; gastrointestinal hyperacidity; peptic ulcer; short-bowel syndrome; Zollinger-Ellison syndrome.*

**Gastroalgine** *Novag, Spain.*
Aluminium hydroxide (p.1249·2); dimethicone (p.1289·2); enoxolone aluminium (p.1264·3); magnesium hydroxide (p.1272·2).
*Dyspepsia; flatulence; gastritis; gastrointestinal hyperacidity.*

**Gastrobario** *Bial, Port.*
Barium sulfate (p.1061·1).
*Radiographic contrast medium.*

**Gastrobene** *Legrand, Braz.*
*Oral powder:* Calcium carbonate (p.1254·2); belladonna (p.479·1); magnesium trisilicate (p.1272·3); aluminium hydroxide (p.1249·2); dimeticone (p.1289·2); kaolin (p.1268·3).
*Tablets:* Calcium carbonate (p.1254·2); belladonna (p.479·1); magnesium trisilicate (p.1272·3); aluminium hydroxide (p.1249·2); dimeticone (p.1289·2).
Formerly contained calcium carbonate, belladonna, and magnesium trisilicate.
*Gastrointestinal hyperacidity.*

**Gastrobid Continus**
Napp, Irl.; Napp, UK.
Metoclopramide hydrochloride (p.1274·3).
*Gastrointestinal disorders; nausea and vomiting.*

**Gastrobion** Galenogal, Braz.†.
Simeticone (p.1289·2); aluminium hydroxide (p.1249·2); magnesium hydroxide (p.1272·2).
*Flatulence; gastroinestinal hyperacidity.*

**Gastrobitan** Geo, Norw.†.
Cimetidine (p.1255·3).
*Aspiration syndrome; gastro-oesophageal reflux; peptic ulcer; Zollinger-Ellison syndrome.*

**Gastrobon** Byk Madaus, S.Afr.†.
Magaldrate (p.1271·3).
*Dyspepsia; gastritis; gastro-oesophageal reflux disease; peptic ulcer.*

**Gastrobul**
Codali, Belg.†; Guerbet, Fr.
Betaine hydrochloride (p.1660·2); sodium bicarbonate (p.1223·2); dimeticone (p.1289·2).
*Gas production for double-contrast radiography.*

**Gastrocaine** Europharm, Hong Kong.
Oxetacaine (p.1382·1); aluminium hydroxide (p.1249·2); magnesium hydroxide (p.1272·2).
*Gastritis; gastro-oesophageal reflux; peptic ulcer.*

**Gastrocalm** Bio-Sante, Canad.
Aluminium hydroxide-magnesium carbonate co-dried gel (p.1250·1); simeticone (p.1289·2).
*Chewable tablets:* Calcium carbonate (p.1254·2); simeticone (p.1289·2).

**Gastrocaps A** Riemser, Ger.†.
Aluminium hydroxide (p.1249·2).
*Gastrointestinal disorders associated with hyperacidity; hyperphosphaturia.*

**Gastroccult** SmithKline Diagnostics, USA.
Test for occult blood in gastric contents.

**Gastrocol** Grunenthal, Chile.
Sucralfate (p.1290·2).
*Peptic ulcer.*

**Gastrocote**
Stanley, Canad.†; Thornton & Ross, UK.
Alginic acid (p.1576·3) or sodium alginate (p.1577·1); aluminium hydroxide (p.1249·2); magnesium trisilicate (p.1272·3); sodium bicarbonate (p.1223·2).
*Gastro-oesophageal reflux; heartburn; hiatus hernia.*

**Gastrocrom** Celltech, USA.
Sodium cromoglicate (p.795·3).
*Mastocytosis.*

**Gastrocure** Taxandria, Neth.
Domperidone maleate (p.1263·2).
*Gastrointestinal disorders.*

**Gastrocynesine**
Boiron, Fr.; Boiron, Port.
Homoeopathic preparation.

**Gastrodenol** Yamanouchi, Spain.
Tripotassium dicitratobismuthate (p.1252·2).
*Gastritis; peptic ulcer.*

**Gastrodin** Shiwa, Thai.
Cimetidine (p.1255·3).
*Gastric hyperacidity; peptic ulcer; Zollinger-Ellison syndrome.*

**Gastrodina** Degorts, Mex.
Cimetidine (p.1255·3).
*Peptic ulcer.*

**Gastrodine**
Note. This name is used for preparations of different composition.
Apsen, Braz.†.
Cimetidine (p.1255·3).
*Acid aspiration; gastro-oesophageal reflux; gastrointestinal haemorrhage; peptic ulcer; Zollinger-Ellison syndrome.*

Medipharm, Chile.
Rabeprazole sodium (p.1285·1).
*Gastro-oesophageal reflux; peptic ulcer; Zollinger-Ellison syndrome.*

**Gastrodomina**
Almirall, Hong Kong; Almirall, Spain.
Famotidine (p.1265·2).
*Gastro-oesophageal reflux; peptic ulcer; Zollinger-Ellison syndrome.*

**Gastrodue** MDM, Ital.
Oxetacaine (p.1382·1); aluminium oxide (p.1140·1); magnesium carbonate (p.1272·1) or magnesium oxide (p.1272·3).
*Gastric hyperacidity.*

**Gastrodyn** Leiras, Fin.†.
Glycopyrronium bromide (p.482·3).
*Premedication; protection against muscarinic effects of anticholinesterases used to reverse neuromuscular blockade.*

**Gastrodyn comp** Leiras, Fin.
Glycopyrronium bromide (p.482·3); diazepam (p.690·1).
*Gastrointestinal disorders.*

**Gastroenterol** Dermofarma, Ital.
Lactic-acid-producing organisms (p.1704·2); vitamins; minerals; plant extracts (p.1417·1).
*Nutritional supplement.*

**Gastrofilm** Will-Pharma, Belg.
Algeldrate (p.1249·2); magnesium carbonate (p.1272·1); calcium carbonate (p.1254·2); magnesium trisilicate (p.1272·3); bismuth subnitrate (p.1252·2); belladonna (p.479·1).
*Dyspepsia; gastric hyperacidity.*

**Gastroflat** Bunker, Braz.
Dimethicone (p.1289·2).
*Flatulence.*

**Gastrofloral** Silesia, Chile.
*Enterococcus faecium* (p.1704·2).
*Diarrhoea.*

**Gastroflux** Ashbourne, UK.
Metoclopramide hydrochloride (p.1274·3).
*Gastrointestinal disorders.*

**Gastrofrenal**
Monsanto, Ital.; Sigma-Tau, Spain.
Sodium cromoglicate (p.795·3).
*Food hypersensitivity; inflammatory bowel disease.*

**Gastrofusine** Braun, Switz.†.
Electrolyte infusion with glucose (p.1217·1).
*Fluid and electrolyte disorders.*

**Gastrogard-R** Nutricia, Austral.†.
Antirotavirus hyperimmune bovine colostrum (p.1611·1).
*Diarrhoea due to rotavirus.*

**Gastroge** Klonal, Arg.
Aluminium hydroxide (p.1249·2); magnesium hydroxide (p.1272·2); simeticone (p.1289·2).
*Gastric hyperacidity.*

**Gastrogel**
Note. This name is used for preparations of different composition.
Fawns & McAllan, Austral.; Sigma, Hong Kong.
*Oral liquid:* Aluminium hydroxide (p.1249·2); magnesium trisilicate (p.1272·3); magnesium hydroxide (p.1272·2).
*Dyspepsia.*

Fawns & McAllan, Austral.; Sigma, Hong Kong.
*Tablets:* Aluminium hydroxide (p.1249·2); magnesium trisilicate (p.1272·3); magnesium hydroxide (p.1272·2); simeticone (p.1289·2).
*Dyspepsia.*

Medquimica, Braz.†.
Aluminium hydroxide (p.1249·2); magnesium hydroxide (p.1272·2); dimethicone (p.1289·2).
*Flatulence; gastrointestinal hyperacidity.*

Giuliani, Ital.; Synthelabo, Switz.†.
Sucralfate (p.1290·2).
*Gastritis; gastro-oesophageal reflux; peptic ulcer.*

Sigma, NZ†.
Aluminium hydroxide (p.1249·2); magnesium trisilicate (p.1272·3); magnesium hydroxide (p.1272·2); simeticone (p.1289·2).
*Antacid; flatulence.*

**Gastrogenol** Profarb, Braz.†.
Guarana (p.1765·3); kola (p.1765·3); cinchona bark (p.1671·3).

**Gastroglutal** Tedec Meiji, Spain.
Magnesium oxide (p.1272·3); glutamine (p.1433·2); aluminium glycinate (p.1249·1).
*Gastrointestinal hyperacidity.*

**Gastrografin**
Schering, Austral.; Schering, Austria; Squibb Diagnostics, Canad.†; Schering, Fin.; Schering, Ger.; Shepa, Gr.; Schering, Ital.; Schering, Neth.; Schering, Norw.; Schering, NZ; Schering, S.Afr.; Schering, Spain; Schering, Swed.; Schering, Switz.; Schering, UK; Squibb Diagnostics, USA.
Meglumine amidotrizoate (p.1060·2); sodium amidotrizoate (p.1060·2).
*Contrast medium for gastrointestinal radiography; meconium ileus.*

**Gastrografina** Schering, Port.
Meglumine amidotrizoate (p.1060·2); sodium amidotrizoate (p.1060·2).
*Contrast medium for gastrointestinal radiography.*

**Gastrografine** Schering, Fr.
Meglumine amidotrizoate (p.1060·2); sodium amidotrizoate (p.1060·2).
*Contrast medium for gastrointestinal radiography.*

**Gastrokin** Instituto Sanitas, Chile.
Cisapride (p.1259·2).
*Constipation; dyspepsia; gastro-oesophageal reflux; gastroparesis; irritable colon; postoperaticve ileus.*

**Gastrol**
Note. This name is used for preparations of different composition.
Luper, Braz.
Aluminium hydroxide (p.1249·2); magnesium hydroxide (p.1272·2); calcium carbonate (p.1254·2).
*Gastrointestinal hyperacidity.*

Salus, Ital.†.
Pirenzepine hydrochloride (p.488·1).
*Gastroduodenitis; peptic ulcer.*

**Gastrol S** Fides, Ger.
Gentian (p.1692·2); chamomile (p.1669·3); melissa (p.1711·1); caraway (p.1667·2); fennel (p.1687·2); coriander (p.1676·1); sweet basil; absinthium (p.1645·1); hypericum (p.299·1); cinchona bark (p.1671·3); juniper (p.1703·1); calamus (p.1664·1); turmeric (p.1058·3).
*Gastrointestinal disorders.*

**Gastrol TC** Luper, Braz.
Aluminium hydroxide (p.1249·2); magnesium hydroxide (p.1272·2); simeticone (p.1289·2).
*Gastrointestinal hyperacidity.*

**Gastrolav** Vitoria, Port.
Ranitidine hydrochloride (p.1285·2).
*Acid aspiration; dyspepsia; gastro-oesophageal reflux; gastrointestinal haemorrhage; peptic ulcer; Zollinger-Ellison syndrome.*

**Gastrolem** Lemery, Mex.†.
Cimetidine (p.1255·3).

**Gastrolen** Chemopharma, Chile.
Clidinium bromide (p.480·2); chlordiazepoxide (p.674·2).
*Gastrointestinal pain; genitourinary disorders; irritable colon.*

**Gastrolene** Faran, Gr.
Cimetidine (p.1255·3).
*Conditions where gastric acid reduction is beneficial; gastric hypersecretion including Zollinger-Ellison syndrome; peptic ulcer.*

**Gastrolets** Hexa-Medinova, Arg.
Ranitidine hydrochloride (p.1285·2).
*Peptic ulcer.*

**Gastroliber** Tecnimede, Port.
Lansoprazole (p.1269·3).

**Gastroloc** Stern, Ger.†.
Omeprazole (p.1278·2).
*Gastro-oesophageal reflux; peptic ulcer; Zollinger-Ellison syndrome.*

**Gastroluft**
Fuji, Swed.†; Nycomed, Switz.†.
Sodium bicarbonate (p.1223·2); tartaric acid (p.1752·1); dimethicone (p.1289·2).
*Adjunct in gastrointestinal double-contrast radiography.*

**Gastrolux** Goldham, Ger.
Sodium amidotrizoate (p.1060·2); meglumine amidotrizoate (p.1060·2) or lysine amidotrizoate (p.1061·1).
*Contrast medium for gastrointestinal radiography.*

**Gastrolyte**
Aventis, Austral.
*Effervescent tablet:* Sodium chloride; potassium chloride; anhydrous citric acid; glucose; sodium bicarbonate (p.1222·2).
*Oral solution; powder for oral solution:* Sodium chloride; potassium chloride; sodium acid citrate; glucose (p.1222·2).
*Diarrhoea; oral rehydration therapy.*

Aventis, Canad.; Aventis, NZ.
Sodium chloride; potassium chloride; sodium acid citrate; glucose (p.1222·2).
*Diarrhoea; oral rehydration therapy.*

**Gastrolyte-R**
Aventis, Austral.; Rhone-Poulenc Rorer, Hong Kong†.
Rice powder; sodium chloride; sodium citrate; potassium chloride (p.1222·2).
*Diarrhoea; oral rehydration therapy.*

**Gastrom** Tanabe, Jpn.
Ecabet sodium (p.1264·3).
*Gastritis; peptic ulcer.*

**Gastromag** Windson, Braz.†.
Dicycloverine hydrochloride (p.481·2); aluminium hydroxide (p.1249·2); magnesium hydroxide (p.1272·2); simeticone (p.1289·2).
*Flatulence; gastrointestinal hyperacidity.*

**Gastromax**
Note. This name is used for preparations of different composition.
Quesada, Arg.
Pantoprazole (p.1283·1).

Pfizer, UK†.
Metoclopramide hydrochloride (p.1274·3).
*Gastrointestinal disorders; nausea and vomiting.*

**Gastromet**
Note. This name is used for preparations of different composition.
Recalcine, Chile.
Cisapride (p.1259·2).
*Constipation; dyspepsia; gastro-oesophageal reflux; gastroparesis; irritable colon; postoperaticve ileus.*

Bayer, Ital.†; Malayan, Singapore.
Cimetidine (p.1255·3) or cimetidine hydrochloride (p.1255·3).
*Peptic ulcer; Zollinger-Ellison syndrome.*

**Gastromiro**
Gerot, Austria; Merck, Irl.; Bracco, Israel; Bracco, Ital.; Bracco, Port.; Bracco, UK.
Iopamidol (p.1064·3).
*Contrast medium for gastrointestinal radiography.*

**Gastromol** Cantabria, Spain.
Magaldrate (p.1271·3).
*Dyspepsia; gastric hyperacidity; gastro-oesophageal reflux; peptic ulcer.*

**Gastron** Aspen, S.Afr.
Loperamide hydrochloride (p.1271·1).
*Colostomies; diarrhoea; ileostomies.*

**Gastron Fuerte** Sanofi Synthelabo, Arg.
Pancreatin (p.1725·3); hemicellulase (p.1669·1); ox bile (p.1660·3); simeticone (p.1289·2).
*Dyspepsia.*

**Gastronerton**
Sanova, Austria; Dolorgiet, Ger.
Metoclopramide (p.1274·3) or metoclopramide hydrochloride (p.1274·3).
*Gastrointestinal motility disorders; nausea and vomiting.*

**Gastronol** Bioforce, Switz.
Homoeopathic preparation.

**Gastronorm** Janssen-Cilag, Ital.
Domperidone (p.1263·2).
*Dyspepsia; nausea.*

**Gastropaque** Temis, Arg.
Barium sulfate (p.1061·1).
*Contrast medium for gastrointestinal radiography.*

**Gastro-Pasc** Pascoe, Ger.
Homoeopathic preparation.

**Gastropax** Lehning, Fr.
Kaolin (p.1268·3); calcium carbonate (p.1254·2); magnesium trisilicate (p.1272·3); magnesium carbonate (p.1272·1); calcium phosphate (p.1225·3); sodium bicarbonate (p.1223·2); magnesium hydroxide (p.1272·2).
Formerly contained belladonna, star anise, kaolin, calcium carbonate, magnesium trisilicate, magnesium carbonate, vegetable charcoal, thyme, calcium phosphate, liquorice, sodium bicarbonate, sodium sulfate, and magnesium hydroxide.
*Gastrointestinal disorders.*

**Gastropeache Susp** Italfarmaco, Spain.
Aluminium hydroxide (p.1249·2); magnesium hydroxide (p.1272·2).
*Dyspepsia; gastrointestinal hyperacidity; peptic ulcer.*

**Gastropect** Aspen, S.Afr.
Kaolin (p.1268·3); pectin (p.1580·3).
*Diarrhoea.*

**Gastropen** I Farmacologia, Spain.
Famotidine (p.1265·2).
*Gastro-oesophageal reflux; peptic ulcer; Zollinger-Ellison syndrome.*

**Gastro-Pepsin** Ceccarelli, Ital.
Pepsin (p.1729·3); gastric mucosa; hydrochloric acid (p.1699·1); lactic acid (p.1704·1); bitter orange (p.1723·3).
*Dyspepsia; hypoacidity.*

**Gastropin** Boehringer Ingelheim, Mex.†.
Pirenzepine hydrochloride (p.488·1).

**Gastropiren** AGIPS, Ital.
Pirenzepine hydrochloride (p.488·1).
*Gastrointestinal disorders.*

**Gastroplant** DHU, Ger.
Homoeopathic preparation.

**Gastroplex** Codilab, Port.†.
Bismuth carbonate (p.1252·1); calcium carbonate (p.1254·2); magnesium carbonate (p.1272·1); sodium bicarbonate (p.1223·2); aluminium silicate (p.1250·2).
*Gastrointestinal disorders.*

**Gastroplus** Hexal, Braz.
Magnesium hydroxide (p.1272·2); aluminium hydroxide (p.1249·2); dimethicone (p.1289·2).
*Flatulence; gastrointestinal hyperacidity.*

**Gastroprotect** Riemser, Ger.
Cimetidine (p.1255·3).
*Acid aspiration; gastro-oesophageal reflux; peptic ulcer; Zollinger-Ellison syndrome.*

**Gastropulgit** Spitzner, Ger.†.
Attapulgite (p.1251·1); aluminium hydroxide-magnesium carbonate co-dried gel (p.1250·1).
*Gastrointestinal disorders.*

**Gastropulgite**
Ipsen, Belg.†; Beaufour, Fr.; Beaufour-Ipsen, Switz.
Attapulgite (p.1251·1); aluminium hydroxide-magnesium carbonate co-dried gel (p.1250·1).
*Gastrointestinal disorders.*

**Gastrosan**
Note. This name is used for preparations of different composition.
Inkeysa, Spain†.
Aluminium hydroxide (p.1249·2); magnesium hydroxide (p.1272·2).
*Dyspepsia; gastrointestinal hyperacidity.*

Bioforce, Switz.
Achillea (p.1646·2); taraxacum (p.1751·3); melissa (p.1711·1); gentian (p.1692·2); cnicus benedictus (p.1673·3); angelica (p.1655·1); centaury (p.1669·2).
*Digestive disorders.*

**Gastrosecur** Duopharm, Ger.
Chirata; gentian (p.1692·2); ginger (p.1267·1); cinnamon (p.1672·2); dried bitter-orange peel (p.1723·3); caraway (p.1667·2).
*Gastrointestinal disorders.*

**Gastrosed**
Note. This name is used for preparations of different composition.
Amsa, Ital.†.
Pirenzepine hydrochloride (p.488·1).
*Gastritis; peptic ulcer.*

Roberts, USA.
Hyoscyamine sulfate (p.485·1).

**Gastrosedol** Bristol-Myers Squibb, Arg.
Ranitidine hydrochloride (p.1285·2).
*Gastro-oesophageal reflux; pathological gastric hypersecretion; peptic ulcer.*

**Gastrosedyl** Monin, Fr.†.
Belladonna (p.479·1); hyoscyamus (p.485·2).
*Gastrointestinal and biliary-tract disorders.*

**Gastrosil**
Sanova, Austria; Heumann, Ger.; Heumann, Switz.
Metoclopramide (p.1274·3) or metoclopramide hydrochloride (p.1274·3).
*Adjunct in gastrointestinal examination; gastrointestinal disorders.*

**Gastrosine** Boiron, Canad.
Homoeopathic preparation.

**Gastrostad** Stada, Ger.†.
Magaldrate (p.1271·3).
*Gastrointestinal disorders associated with hyperacidity.*

**Gastro-Stop**
Note. A similar name is used for preparations of different composition (see below).
Aspen, Austral.
Loperamide hydrochloride (p.1271·1).
*Diarrhoea.*

**Gastrostop**
Note. A similar name is used for preparations of different composition (see above).
Biomedica, Ital.†.
Aluminium glycinate (p.1249·1); magnesium hydroxide (p.1272·2).
*Hyperchlorhydria.*

**Gastrotem** Temis, Arg.
Omeprazole (p.1278·2).

The symbol † denotes a preparation no longer actively marketed

**Gastrotest** *Sanochemia, Austria†.*
2 White tablets, caffeine and sodium benzoate (p.783·1); 3 yellow tablets, phenazopyridine (p.83·2).
*Test for gastric acid production.*

**Gastro-Timelets**
*Sanova, Austria; Temmler, Denm.; Temmler, Ger.†; Asta Medica, Switz.†.*
Metoclopramide hydrochloride (p.1274·3).
*Gastrointestinal disorders.*

**Gastrotranquil** *Azupharma, Ger.*
Metoclopramide hydrochloride (p.1274·3).
*Gastrointestinal disorders.*

**Gastrovegetalin** *Verla, Ger.*
Melissa (p.1711·1).
*Gastrointestinal disorders; sleep disorders.*

**Gastrovison**
*Note. This name is used for preparations of different composition.*
*Shepa, Gr.*
Citric acid (p.1673·1); sodium bicarbonate (p.1223·2); colloidal silicon dioxide (p.1581·3); hypromellose; dimeticone (p.1289·2).
*Gas production for double-contrast radiography.*

*Schering, Ital.†.*
Sodium bicarbonate (p.1223·2); citric acid (p.1673·1); simeticone (p.1289·2); silicon dioxide (p.1581·3).
*Gas production for double-contrast radiography.*

**Gastrozac** *Klonal, Arg.*
Ranitidine (p.1285·2).
*Peptic ulcer.*

**Gastrozepin**
*Boehringer Ingelheim, Austria; Boehringer Ingelheim, Ger.; Boehringer Ingelheim, Gr.; Boehringer Ingelheim, Ital.†.*
Pirenzepine hydrochloride (p.488·1).
*Duodenitis; gastritis; gastrointestinal haemorrhage; peptic ulcer; Zollinger-Ellison syndrome.*

**Gastrozepina** *Boehringer Ingelheim, Port.*
Pirenzepine hydrochloride (p.488·1).

**Gastrozepine** *Boehringer Ingelheim, Switz.†.*
Pirenzepine hydrochloride (p.488·1).
*Gastroduodenitis; peptic ulcer.*

**Gastrozol** *Delta, Braz.*
Omeprazole (p.1278·2).
*Peptic ulcer.*

**Gastrulcer** *Fariberica, Port.*
Ranitidine hydrochloride (p.1285·2).
*Gastro-oesophageal reflux; gastrointestinal haemorrhage; peptic ulcer; Zollinger-Ellison syndrome.*

**Gastyl**
*ANB, Malaysia; ANB, Thai.*
Simeticone (p.1289·2).
*Excess gastrointestinal gas.*

**Gasulsol** *Herbes Universelles, Canad.*
Aluminium hydroxide (p.1249·2); magnesium trisilicate (p.1272·3).

**Gasva** *Gerbex, Canad.†.*
Aluminium hydroxide (p.1249·2); magnesium trisilicate (p.1272·3).

**Gas-X**
*Novartis Consumer, Canad.; General Drugs, Thai.; Novartis, USA.*
Simeticone (p.1289·2).
*Excess gastrointestinal gas.*

**Gasyran** *Loren, Mex.*
Ranitidine (p.1285·2).
*Peptic ulcer.*

**Gaszym** *Ranbaxy, Thai.*
Simeticone (p.1289·2); pancreatin (p.1725·3).
*Digestive system disorders; flatulence.*

**Gat Globulina Antitimocitaria** *Butantan, Braz.†.*
An antilymphocyte immunoglobulin (p.1348·3).

**Gatiflo** *Kyorin, Jpn.*
Gatifloxacin (p.216·2).
*Bacterial infections.*

**Gatinar**
*Novartis, Spain†; Melisana, Switz.*
Lactulose (p.1269·1).
*Constipation; hepatic encephalopathy; salmonella enteritis.*

**Gavicid** *Grisi, Mex.*
Aluminium (p.1652·2); magnesium (p.1227·3).
*Gastrointestinal hyperacidity.*

**Gavilast** *Reckitt Benckiser, UK.*
Ranitidine hydrochloride (p.1285·2).
*Dyspepsia; heartburn.*

**Gaviscon**
*Note. This name is used for preparations of different composition.*
*Key, Arg.; Reckitt Benckiser, Austral.; Novartis Consumer, Belg.; Essex, Chile; GlaxoSmithKline, Fr.; Reckitt Benckiser, Irl.; Novartis Consumer, Ital.; Reckitt Benckiser, Malaysia; Novartis Consumer, Neth.; Reckitt Benckiser, S.Afr.; Reckitt Benckiser, Singapore; Reckitt Benckiser, UK.*
*Oral suspension:* Sodium alginate (p.1577·1); calcium carbonate (p.1254·2); sodium bicarbonate (p.1223·2).
*Gastro-oesophageal reflux; heartburn.*

*Reckitt Benckiser, Austral.; Novartis Consumer, Belg.; Reckitt Benckiser, Hong Kong; Reckitt Benckiser, India; Reckitt Benckiser, Irl.; Novartis Consumer, Ital.; Reckitt Benckiser, Malaysia; Reckitt Benckiser, NZ; Helsinn, Port.†; Reckitt Benckiser, S.Afr.; Reckitt Benckiser, Singapore; Reckitt Benckiser, UK; SmithKline Beecham Consumer, USA.*
*Tablets:* Alginic acid (p.1576·3); aluminium hydroxide (p.1249·2); magnesium trisilicate (p.1272·3); sodium bicarbonate (p.1223·2).
*Gastro-oesophageal reflux; heartburn.*

*Novartis Consumer, Belg.*
*Oral powder:* Alginic acid (p.1576·3); algeldrate (p.1249·2); sodium bicarbonate (p.1223·2); magnesium trisilicate (p.1272·3).
*Gastro-oesophageal reflux.*

*Essex, Chile.*
*Tablets:* Alginic acid (p.1576·3); sodium bicarbonate (p.1223·2); aluminium hydroxide (p.1249·2); magnesium trisilicate (p.1272·3); calcium carbonate (p.1254·2).
*Gastro-oesophageal reflux.*

*Ferring, Denm.; Ferring, Fin.; Ferring, Israel†; Ferring, Norw.; Ferring, Swed.*
*Oral liquid:* Sodium alginate (p.1577·1); sodium bicarbonate (p.1223·2); aluminium hydroxide (p.1249·2); calcium carbonate (p.1254·2).
*Gastro-oesophageal reflux; heartburn.*

*Ferring, Denm.; Ferring, Fin.; Ferring, Israel†; Ferring, Norw.; Ferring, Swed.; Novartis Consumer, Switz.*
*Chewable tablets:* Alginic acid (p.1576·3); aluminium hydroxide (p.1249·2); sodium bicarbonate (p.1223·2).
*Gastro-oesophageal reflux; heartburn.*

*GlaxoSmithKline, Fr.*
*Tablets:* Alginic acid (p.1576·3); sodium alginate (p.1577·1); dried colloidal aluminium hydroxide (p.1249·2); sodium bicarbonate (p.1223·2); magnesium trisilicate (p.1272·3).
*Gastro-oesophageal reflux.*

*Pohl, Ger.*
*Tablets:* Alginic acid (p.1576·3).
*Gastro-oesophageal reflux.*

*Reckitt Benckiser, Hong Kong.*
*Oral liquid:* Sodium alginate (p.1577·1); sodium bicarbonate (p.1223·2).
*Flatulence; gastro-oesophageal reflux; heartburn.*

*Novartis Consumer, Neth.*
*Tablets:* Alginic acid (p.1576·3); algeldrate (p.1249·2); sodium bicarbonate (p.1223·2); calcium carbonate (p.1254·2); magnesium trisilicate (p.1272·3).
*Gastro-oesophageal reflux.*

*Reckitt Benckiser, NZ.*
*Infant oral powder:* Magnesium alginate (p.1577·1); sodium alginate (p.1577·1).
*Gastro-oesophageal reflux.*

*Reckitt Benckiser, NZ.*
*Oral liquid:* Sodium alginate (p.1577·1); calcium carbonate (p.1254·2); potassium bicarbonate (p.1223·1) or sodium bicarbonate (p.1223·2).
*Gastro-oesophageal reflux.*

*Reckitt Benckiser, S.Afr.*
*Oral liquid (peppermint):* Sodium alginate (p.1577·1).
*Gastrointestinal disorders.*

*Novartis Consumer, Spain†.*
Alginic acid (p.1576·3); sodium bicarbonate (p.1223·2).
*Gastro-oesophageal reflux.*

*Novartis Consumer, Switz.*
*Oral suspension:* Sodium alginate (p.1577·1); potassium bicarbonate (p.1223·1); calcium carbonate (p.1254·2).
Formerly contained sodium alginate, aluminium hydroxide, sodium bicarbonate, and calcium carbonate.
*Gastric hyperacidity; gastro-oesophageal reflux; heartburn.*

*SmithKline Beecham Consumer, USA.*
*Oral liquid:* Aluminium hydroxide (p.1249·2); magnesium carbonate (p.1272·1); sodium alginate (p.1577·1).
*Dyspepsia.*

**Gaviscon Acid** *SmithKline Beecham Consumer, Canad.†.*
Magnesium hydroxide (p.1272·2); calcium carbonate (p.1254·2).

**Gaviscon Advance**
*Note. This name is used for preparations of different composition.*
*Novartis Consumer, Belg.; Reckitt Benckiser, Irl.; Novartis Consumer, Ital.; Reckitt Benckiser, UK.*
Sodium alginate (p.1577·1); potassium bicarbonate (p.1223·1).
*Gastro-oesophageal reflux; heartburn; hiatus hernia.*

*Pohl, Ger.*
Sodium alginate (p.1577·1).
Formerly contained sodium alginate, sodium bicarbonate, aluminium hydroxide, and calcium carbonate.
*Gastro-oesophageal reflux.*

**Gaviscon Double Strength** *Reckitt Benckiser, Austral.*
Sodium alginate (p.1577·1); potassium bicarbonate (p.1223·1); calcium carbonate (p.1254·2).
*Gastro-oesophageal reflux.*

**Gaviscon Extra Strength** *SmithKline Beecham Consumer, USA.*
Aluminium hydroxide (p.1249·2); magnesium carbonate (p.1272·1).
*Dyspepsia.*

**Gaviscon Extra Strength Relief Formula**
*SmithKline Beecham Consumer, USA.*
Aluminium hydroxide (p.1249·2); magnesium carbonate (p.1272·1); simeticone (p.1289·2).
*Hyperacidity.*

**Gaviscon Heartburn Relief** *GlaxoSmithKline Consumer, Canad.*
*Oral liquid:* Sodium alginate (p.1577·1); aluminium hydroxide (p.1249·2).
*Oral suspension:* Sodium alginate (p.1577·1); aluminium hydroxide (p.1249·2).
*Tablets:* Alginic acid (p.1576·3); magnesium carbonate (p.1272·1).
Formerly known as Gaviscon Heartburn Relief Aluminium-Free.
*Gastro-oesophageal reflux; heartburn.*

**Gaviscon Infant**
*Note. This name is used for preparations of different composition.*
*Reckitt Benckiser, Irl.*
Alginic acid (p.1576·3); magnesium alginate (p.1577·1); aluminium hydroxide (p.1249·2).
*Gastro-oesophageal reflux.*

*Reckitt Benckiser, UK.*
Magnesium alginate (p.1577·1); sodium alginate (p.1577·1).
Formerly known as Infant Gaviscon and contained aluminium hydroxide, magnesium alginate, and sodium alginate.
NOTE. In view of its high sodium content this preparation should not be used in premature infants or in situations where excess water-loss is likely, such as fever or high room-temperature; some sources have recommended that it should be avoided altogether in children less than 6 months of age.
*Gastro-oesophageal reflux.*

**Gaviscon Prevent** *GlaxoSmithKline Consumer, Canad.*
Cimetidine (p.1255·3).

**Gaviz** *Uniao Quimica, Braz.*
*Oral liquid:* Aluminium hydroxide (p.1249·2); magnesium carbonate (p.1272·1).
*Tablets:* Aluminium hydroxide (p.1249·2); magnesium trisilicate (p.1272·3).
*Gastrointestinal hyperacidity.*

**Gaz Away** *Swiss Herbal, Canad.*
Alpha galactosidase A (p.1651·1).

**Gazyme** *Cifarma, Braz.†.*
Dimeticone (p.1289·2).
*Flatulence.*

**GB Tablets** *Potter's, UK.*
Leptandra virginica; euonymus (p.1265·2); lappa root (p.1704·3).
Formerly contained leptandra virginica, euonymus, lappa root, and kava root.
*Abdominal discomfort; gall bladder disorders.*

**GBN**
*Malpharm, Hong Kong†; Malaysia Chemist, Singapore.*
Glibenclamide (p.331·2).
*Diabetes mellitus.*

**G-Dil** *Gap, Gr.*
Isosorbide mononitrate (p.942·1).
*Angina; heart failure.*

**GDP-Ex** *Cypress, USA.*
Dextromethorphan hydrobromide (p.1117·3); phenylephrine hydrochloride (p.1126·3); guaifenesin (p.1122·1).
*Coughs; respiratory-tract congestion.*

**GE** *Thai Otsuka, Thai.*
Carbohydrate, electrolyte, and trace element infusion (p.1417·1).
*Parenteral nutrition.*

**Geangin**
*Gea, Denm.; Gea, Norw.†.*
Verapamil hydrochloride (p.1019·1).
*Angina pectoris; arrhythmias; hypertension; myocardial infarction.*

**Geasalol** *Gea, Denm.*
Methenamine hippurate (p.230·2).
*Urinary-tract infections.*

**Geavir**
*Gea, Denm.; Gea, Fin.; Gea, Norw.†; Gea, Swed.*
Aciclovir (p.626·1) or aciclovir sodium (p.626·1).
*Herpesvirus infections.*

**Gebrozil** *Cooper (Κοπερ), Gr.*
Gemfibrozil (p.923·1).
*Hyperlipidaemias.*

**Gedol** *Lafi, Chile.*
Ibuprofen (p.45·3); paracetamol (p.76·2).
*Pain.*

**Gedun** *Duncan, Arg.*
Gemfibrozil (p.923·1).
*Hyperlipidaemias.*

**Gee-Gee** *Jones, USA†.*
Guaifenesin (p.1122·1).
*Coughs.*

**Geepenil** *Orion, Fin.*
Benzylpenicillin sodium (p.163·2).
*Bacterial infections.*

**Geffer** *Roche, Ital.*
Metoclopramide hydrochloride (p.1274·3); dimeticone (p.1289·2); potassium citrate (p.1223·1); citric acid (p.1673·1); tartaric acid (p.1752·1); sodium bicarbonate (p.1223·2).
*Gastrointestinal disorders associated with hyperacidity.*

**Gefina** *Gea, Fin.*
Finasteride (p.1554·2).
*Benign prostatic hyperplasia.*

**Gegorvit** *Fher, Ital.*
Multivitamin and mineral preparation with ginseng (p.1417·1).
*Nutritional supplement.*

**Gegrip** *Gemballa, Braz.*
Paracetamol (p.76·2); pentoxyverine (p.1126·2); phenylephrine (p.1126·3); carbinoxamine (p.426·3).
*Cold and influenza symptoms.*

**Gehwol Fungizid** *Gerlach, Ger.*
*Cream:* Undecenoic acid monoethanolamide (p.411·1); chloroxylenol (p.1177·2); 3,4,5,6-tetrabromo-*o*-cresol (p.1193·3).
*Topical liquid:* Undecenoic acid monoethanolamide (p.411·1); chloroxylenol (p.1177·2); 3,4,5,6-tetrabromo-*o*-cresol (p.1193·3); copper-trolamine complex.
*Topical powder:* Bromosalicylic acid (p.1157·2); undecenoic acid monoethanolamide (p.411·1); chloroxylenol (p.1177·2); 3,4,5,6-tetrabromo-*o*-cresol (p.1193·3).
*Fungal foot infections.*

**Gehwol Huhneraugen Pflaster** *Gerlach, Ger.*
Salicylic acid (p.1157·1); lactic acid (p.1704·1).
*Callouses; corns.*

**Gehwol Huhneraugen Tinktur** *Gerlach, Ger.*
Salicylic acid (p.1157·1); glacial acetic acid (p.1645·2).
*Callouses; corns.*

**Gehwol Nagelpilz** *Gerlach, Ger.*
Zinc chloride (p.1469·2); bromosalicylic acid (p.1157·2); salicylic acid (p.1157·1); undecenoic acid monoethanolamide (p.411·1).
*Fungal nail infections.*

**Gehwol Schalpaste** *Gerlach, Ger.*
Salicylic acid (p.1157·1).
*Callouses; corns.*

**Gel 4000** *Bruschettini, Ital.*
Hypromellose (p.1579·3).
*Aid in ophthalmic procedures.*

**Gel a la consoude** *Phytomed, Switz.*
Comfrey (p.1675·2); calendula (p.1665·2); hypericum (p.299·1); echinacea (p.1683·2); mint (p.1749·1).
*Soft-tissue injuries.*

**Gel a l'Acetotartrate d'Alumine Defresne**
*Sanofi Synthelabo OTC, Fr.*
Hesperidin methyl chalcone (p.1688·3); aluminium acetotartrate (p.1652·3).
*Soft-tissue injury; venous insufficiency.*

**Gel Antiinflamatorio** *Sertex, Arg.*
Diclofenac diethylamine (p.32·1).
*Musculoskeletal, joint, and soft-tissue disorders; neuralgia; neuritis.*

**Gel Carpina** *Alcon, Arg.*
Pilocarpine hydrochloride (p.1495·1).
*Production of miosis.*

**Gel Creme Protector** *Vichy, Canad.*
*SPF 15:* Avobenzone (p.1142·3); octocrilene (p.1154·3) ecamsule (p.1146·3); titanium dioxide (p.1160·3).
Formerly contained avobenzone, enzacamene, ecamsule, and titanium dioxide.
*Sunscreen.*

**Gel de Calamine** *Bailleul, Fr.*
Calamine (p.1144·1); zinc oxide (p.1163·2).
*Skin irritation.*

**Gel Kam**
*Asta Medica, Port.†; Scherer, USA.*
Stannous fluoride (p.1448·3).
*Dental caries prophylaxis.*

**Gel Rubefiant** *Ducray, Fr.*
Methyl nicotinate (p.59·2); essential oils.
*Scalp disorders.*

**Gel Solaire Bronzage** *Clarins, Canad.†.*
*SPF 3:* Ensulizole (p.1147·1).
*Sunscreen.*

**Gel Solaire Bronzage Securite** *Clarins, Canad.†.*
*SPF 15:* Octocrilene (p.1154·3); octinoxate (p.1154·3); octisalate (p.1154·3) oxybenzone (p.1154·3).
*Sunscreen.*

**Gel Solaire Bronzage Securite Special Sport**
*Clarins, Canad.†.*
*SPF 15:* Avobenzone (p.1142·3); octinoxate (p.1154·3); octisalate (p.1154·3); oxybenzone (p.1154·3).
*Sunscreen.*

**Gelacet**
*Hermal, Austria; Boots Healthcare, Switz.*
Vitamin A acetate (p.1453·1); L-cystine (p.1426·3); gelatin (p.754·3).
*Hair and nail disorders.*

**Gelacet N** *Hermal, Ger.*
Vitamin A acetate (p.1453·1); cystine (p.1426·3); gelatin (p.754·3).
*Hair and nail disorders.*

**Gelacid** *Xeragen, S.Afr.*
Alginic acid (p.1576·3); magnesium trisilicate (p.1272·3); aluminium hydroxide (p.1249·2); sodium bicarbonate (p.1223·2).
*Dyspepsia; gastro-oesophageal reflux; heartburn.*

**Gelafundin**
*Braun, Arg.; Braun, Ger.; Braun, Hong Kong†; Braun, Thai.*
Gelatin polysuccinate (p.754·3) with electrolytes.
*Extracorporeal circulation; haemodilution; hypotension; hypovolaemia.*

**Gelafundina** *Braun, Port.†.*
Modified gelatin (p.754·3) with electrolytes.
*Extracorporeal circulation; hypovolaemia.*

**Gelafusal-N in Ringeracetat** *Serum-Werk Bernburg, Ger.*
Gelatin polysuccinate (p.754·3) in electrolytes.
*Hypovolaemia; pre-operative haemodilution.*

**Gelamel** *Morado, Ital.*
Royal jelly (p.1740·3).
*Nutritional supplement.*

**Gelan Plus** *Chinoin, Mex.*
Aluminium hydroxide (p.1249·2); magnesium hydroxide (p.1272·2); dimeticone (p.1289·2).
*Flatulence; gastrointestinal hyperacidity.*

**Gelasim** *Berman, Mex.*
Aluminium hydroxide-magnesium carbonate co-dried gel (p.1250·1).
*Gastrointestinal hyperacidity.*

**Gelaspon** *Chauvin ankerpharm, Ger.*
Gelatin (p.754·3).
*Haemorrhage; haemostatic.*

**Gelastypt** *Aventis, Ger.*
Gelatin (p.754·3).
*Dental dressing.*

**Gelbiotic** *Kampel Martian, Arg.*
Fusidic acid (p.215·2).
*Bacterial skin infections.*

**Gelbiotic Plus** *Kampel Martian, Arg.*
Fusidic acid (p.215·2); betamethasone (p.1093·1).
*Bacterial skin infections.*

**Gelcain** *Valma, Chile.*
Lidocaine (p.1377·3).
*Local anaesthesia.*

**Gelcen** *Centrum, Spain.*
Capsaicin (p.24·2).
*Muscle and joint pain.*

**Gelclair** *Sinclair, UK.*
Povidone (p.1581·2); sodium hyaluronate (p.1697·3); enoxolone (p.36·2).
*Painful mouth lesions.*

**Gelcosal** *Quinoderm, UK†.*
Coal tar (p.1159·2); tar (p.1159·3); salicylic acid (p.1157·1).
*Dermatitis; psoriasis.*

**Gelcotar**
*Note. This name is used for preparations of different composition.*
*Quinoderm, Hong Kong†; Quinoderm, Irl.; Quinoderm, UK†.*
*Shampoo:* Coal tar (p.1159·2); cade oil (p.1159·2).
*Dandruff; psoriasis of the scalp; seborrhoeic dermatitis.*

*Quinoderm, Irl.; Quinoderm, UK†.*
*Topical gel:* Coal tar (p.1159·2); tar (p.1159·3).
*Dermatitis; psoriasis.*

**Geldene** *Pfizer, Fr.*
Piroxicam (p.84·2).
*Soft-tissue disorders; tendinitis.*

**Geldrox Plus** *Pharmacos, Mex.*
Aluminium hydroxide (p.1249·2); magnesium hydroxide (p.1272·2); dimeticone (p.1289·2).
*Gastrointestinal hyperacidity.*

**Gelee Solaire Haute Protection** *Clarins, Canad.*
*SPF 15:* Octinoxate (p.1154·3); octisalate (p.1154·3); oxybenzone (p.1154·3); ensulizole (p.1147·1).
*Sunscreen.*

**Gelenkja** *OTW, Ger.*
Homoeopathic preparation.

**Gelerit** *Koni-Cofarm, Chile.*
Erythromycin (p.208·1).
*Acne.*

**Gelestra** *Abiogen, Ital.*
Estradiol (p.1550·1).
*Menopausal disorders.*

**Gelfilm**
*Pharmacia, Austral.; Pharmacia, Canad.; Pharmacia Upjohn, Hong Kong†; Pharmacia, Neth.; Pharmacia, NZ; Upjohn, USA.*
Gelatin (p.754·3).
*Haemostatic.*

**Gelflex** *Bunker, Braz.*
Turpentine oil (p.1760·1); methyl salicylate (p.59·3); camphor (p.1665·3); mustard oil (p.1718·2); rosemary oil (p.1740·2); lavender oil (p.1705·2); menthol (p.1711·3).
*Musculoskeletal and joint disorders.*

**Gelfoam**
*Pharmacia, Austral.; Pharmacia, Belg.; Pharmacia, Braz.; Pharmacia, Canad.; Pharmacia, Chile; Pharmacia, Hong Kong; Pharmacia Upjohn, Israel; Pharmacia, Malaysia; Pharmacia, Neth.; Pharmacia, NZ; Pharmacia, Singapore; Pharmacia Upjohn, Switz.†; Upjohn, USA.*
Gelatin (p.754·3).
*Haemostatic.*

**Gelhist** *Econolab, USA.*
Phenylephrine tannate (p.1127·2); chlorphenamine tannate (p.428·1); mepyramine tannate (p.437·1).
*Nasal congestion; rhinitis.*

**Gelicain** *Curasan, Ger.*
Lidocaine hydrochloride (p.1377·3).
*Local anaesthesia.*

**Gelictar** *Nigy, Fr.*
Ichthammol (p.1148·2).
*Seborrhoeic dermatitis.*

**Gelictar Fort** *Nigy, Fr.*
Ichthammol (p.1148·2); salicylic acid (p.1157·1); resorcinol (p.1156·3).
*Keratinisation disorders; seborrhoeic dermatitis.*

**Gelidina** *Yamanouchi, Spain.*
Fluocinolone acetonide (p.1101·2).
*Skin disorders.*

**Gelifundol**
*Biogam, Arg.; Biotest, Austria; Biotest, Ger.; Biotest, Hong Kong; Mednostica, S.Afr.; Biotest, Thai.*
Oxypolygelatin (p.757·2).
*Hypovolaemia; resuspension of concentrated erythrocytes; thrombosis prophylaxis.*

**Gelimag** *British Dispensary, Thai.†.*
Magnesium trisilicate (p.1272·3); aluminium hydroxide (p.1249·2).
*Gastric hyperacidity; peptic ulcer.*

**Geliofil**
*Effik, Fr.; Effik, Ital.*
Lactic acid (p.1704·1); glycogen.
*Vaginal hygiene.*

**Geliperm**
*Yamanouchi, Ger.†; Geistlich, Switz.†; Geistlich, UK.*
Hydrogel dressing.
*Burns; ulcers; wounds.*

**Gelisyn** *Syntex, Mex.†.*
Fluocinonide (p.1101·3).
*Skin disorders.*

**Gel-Kam**
*Colgate-Palmolive, Ital.; Colgate-Palmolive, USA.*
Stannous fluoride (p.1448·3).
*Dental caries prophylaxis; sensitive gums..*

**Gel-Larmes** *Thea, Fr.*
Carbomer 934 P (p.1577·2).
*Dry eyes.*

**Gellodex** *Miller, Braz.†.*
Methyl salicylate (p.59·3).
*Musculoskeletal and joint disorders.*

**Gelmax** *Novamed, Braz.*
Aluminium hydroxide (p.1249·2); calcium carbonate (p.1254·2); magnesium hydroxide (p.1272·2).
*Gastrointestinal hyperacidity.*

**Gelmicin** *Collins, Mex.*
Clotrimazole (p.396·2); betamethasone (p.1093·1).
*Infected skin disorders.*

**Geloalumin** *Gelos, Spain.*
Aluminium hydroxide (p.1249·2); dimethicone (p.1289·2); magnesium hydroxide (p.1272·2).
*Gastrointestinal hyperacidity and flatulence.*

**Geloboll** *Sinteropico, Braz.†.*
Turpentine; methyl salicylate (p.59·3); camphor (p.1665·3); menthol (p.1711·3).
*Musculoskeletal and joint disorders.*

**Gelobronchial** *Pohl, Ger.*
Thyme (p.1755·2).
*Bronchitis; catarrh.*

**Gelocast** *Beiersdorf, Ital.*
Zinc oxide (p.1163·2).
*Medicated dressing.*

**Gelocatil** *Gelos, Spain.*
Paracetamol (p.76·2).
*Fever; pain.*

**Gelocatil Codeina** *Gelos, Spain.*
Paracetamol (p.76·2); codeine phosphate (p.27·1).
*Pain.*

**Geloderm** *SMB, Chile.*
Metronidazole (p.607·2).
*Anaerobic bacterial infections; malodorous wounds; rosacea.*

**Gelodiet** *DHN, Fr.*
Gelatin (p.754·3); sucrose (p.1450·1).
*Dehydration.*

**Gelodrin** *Pohl, Ger.†.*
Sodium cromoglicate (p.795·3).
*Allergic conjunctivitis; allergic rhinitis.*

**Gelodrox** *Gelos, Spain.*
Dried aluminium hydroxide (p.1249·2); calcium carbonate (p.1254·2); magnesium carbonate (p.1272·1); magnesium trisilicate (p.1272·3).
*Gastrointestinal hyperacidity.*

**Gelodual** *Gelos, Spain.*
Dried aluminium hydroxide (p.1249·2); magnesium hydroxide (p.1272·2); magnesium trisilicate (p.1272·3).
*Gastrointestinal hyperacidity.*

**Gelodurat** *Pohl, Ger.*
Eucalyptus oil (p.1686·2).
*Bronchitis; cold symptoms.*

**Gelofalk** *Falk, Ger.†.*
Smectite; aluminium hydroxide gel (p.1249·2); magnesium hydroxide (p.1272·2).
*Gastrointestinal disorders.*

**Gelofeno** *Gelos, Spain.*
Ibuprofen (p.45·3).
*Fever; musculoskeletal and joint disorders; pain.*

**Geloflex** *Braun, UK†.*
Succinylated gelatin (p.754·3) in sodium chloride.
*Hypovolaemia.*

**Gelofrix** *Delta, Braz.*
Turpentine oil (p.1760·1); methyl salicylate (p.59·3); camphor (p.1665·3); menthol (p.1711·3).
Formerly contained turpentine oil, mustard oil, rosemary oil, lavender oil, methyl salicylate, camphor, and menthol.
*Musculoskeletal and joint disorders.*

**Gelofusin** *Braun, Austria.*
Gelatin (p.754·3) with electrolytes.
*Haemodilution; hypovolaemia.*

**Gelofusine**
*Braun, Austral.; Braun, Belg.; Braun, Chile; Braun, Fin.; Braun, Fr.; Bioser (Βιοσερ), Gr.; Braun, Hong Kong; Biomed, NZ; Braun, Port.; Braun, S.Afr.; Braun, Singapore; Braun, Thai.; Braun, UK.*
Succinylated gelatin (p.754·3) in sodium chloride.
*Extracorporeal circulation; hypovolaemia; plasma volume expansion.*

**Gelogastrine** *Monot, Fr.†.*
Agar (p.1576·3); gelatin (p.754·3); kaolin (p.1268·3).
*Gastrointestinal disorders.*

**Gelogel** *Stevia, Braz.†.*
Methyl salicylate (p.59·3); camphor (p.1665·3); menthol (p.1711·3); turpentine oil (p.1760·1).
*Musculoskeletal and joint disorders.*

**Gelol** *DM, Braz.†.*
Methyl salicylate (p.59·3); camphor (p.1665·3); menthol (p.1711·3); turpentine oil (p.1760·1); mustard oil (p.1718·2); rosemary oil (p.1740·2); lavender oil (p.1705·2).
*Musculoskeletal and joint disorders.*

**Gelolagar** *Fada, Arg.*
Atracurium (p.1402·2).
*Competitive neuromuscular blocker.*

**Gelomyrtol**
*Sanova, Austria; Pohl, Ger.; Pohl, Hong Kong.*
Myrtol.
*Bronchitis; sinusitis.*

**Gelonasal** *Pohl, Ger.*
Xylometazoline hydrochloride (p.1132·2).
*Nasal congestion.*

**Gelonevral** *Teuto, Braz.*
Turpentine oil (p.1760·1); methyl salicylate (p.59·3); camphor (p.1665·3); mustard oil (p.1718·2); menthol (p.1711·3); rosemary oil (p.1740·2); lavender oil (p.1705·2).
*Musculoskeletal and joint disorders.*

**Gelonic** *Dermoteca, Port.†.*
Amino-acid and mineral preparation (p.1417·1).
*Hair and nail disorders.*

**Gelonic Forte** *Dermoteca, Port.†.*
Amino-acid, vitamin and mineral preparation (p.1417·1).
*Hair and nail disorders.*

**Gelonida**
*Note. This name is used for preparations of different composition.*
*Lundbeck, Denm.†.*
Aspirin (p.15·1); codeine phosphate (p.27·1).
*Pain.*

*Godecke, Ger.*
Paracetamol (p.76·2); codeine phosphate (p.27·1).
*Pain.*

**Gelonida NA** *Godecke, Ger.*
*Oral liquid:* Sodium salicylate (p.90·1); paracetamol (p.76·2); codeine phosphate (p.27·1).
*Cold symptoms; fever; neuralgia; neuritis; pain.*
*Suppositories:* Aspirin (p.15·1); paracetamol (p.76·2); codeine phosphate (p.27·1).
*Fever; pain.*

**Gelopectose** *IPRAD, Fr.*
Pectin (p.1580·3); microcrystalline cellulose (p.1578·3); hydrated colloidal silicon dioxide (p.1581·3).
*Regurgitation in infants.*

**Geloplasma**
*Pasteur Merieux, Belg.†; Rhone-Poulenc Rorer, Spain†.*
Gelatin (p.754·3) with electrolytes.
*Blood-volume expansion.*

**Gelora** *Reckitt Piramal, India.*
Choline salicylate (p.26·2).
*Cold sores; mouth ulcers; teething pain.*

**Geloril** *Farmion, Braz.†.*
Aescin (p.1648·2); diethylamine salicylate (p.34·1).
*Varices.*

**Gelostretch** *Beiersdorf, Ital.*
Zinc oxide (p.1163·2).
*Medicated dressing.*

**Gelotricar** *Gelos, Spain.*
Calcium carbonate (p.1254·2); magnesium carbonate (p.1272·1); sodium bicarbonate (p.1223·2).
*Gastrointestinal hyperacidity.*

**Gelotrisin** *Gelos, Spain.*
Aluminium hydroxide (p.1249·2); magnesium trisilicate (p.1272·3).
*Dyspepsia; gastrointestinal hyperacidity; peptic ulcer.*

**Gelovit** *Almirall, Spain†.*
Androstanolone (p.1541·3).
*Atrophic vaginitis; gynaecomastia; male hypogonadism and androgen deficiency.*

**Gelovital** *Pohl, Ger.*
Cod-liver oil (p.1425·2).
*Tonic.*

**Gelox** *Beaufour, Fr.*
Montmorillonite; aluminium hydroxide (p.1249·2); magnesium hydroxide (p.1272·2).
*Gastrointestinal disorders.*

**Gelpan** *Neckerman, Braz.†.*
Aluminium hydroxide (p.1249·2).
*Gastrointestinal hyperacidity.*

**Gelparine** *Streuli, Switz.*
Heparin sodium (p.928·1).
*Soft-tissue injury; superficial inflammation and thrombosis.*

**Gel-Phan** *Pierre Fabre, Fr.*
Gelatin (p.754·3).
*Fragile hair or nails.*

**Gelpirin** *Alra, USA†.*
Paracetamol (p.76·2); aspirin (p.15·1); caffeine (p.782·1).

**Gelpirin-CCF** *Alra, USA†.*
Paracetamol (p.76·2); guaifenesin (p.1122·1); phenylpropanolamine hydrochloride (p.1127·3); chlorphenamine maleate (p.427·3).
*Coughs and cold symptoms.*

**Gelplex** *Fresenius Kabi, Ital.*
Polygeline (p.759·1) with electrolytes.
*Plasma volume expansion.*

**Gelsemium Comp** *Hevert, Ger.*
Homoeopathic preparation.

**Gelsemium Oligoplex** *Madaus, Ger.*
Homoeopathic preparation.

**Gelsica** *Resinag, Switz.*
Aluminium chlorohydrate (p.1142·1).
*Wounds.*

**Gelsolets** *SMB, Chile.*
Carbomer (p.1577·2); mannitol (p.950·2).
*Dry eyes.*

**GelTears**
*Smith & Nephew, Austral.†; Chauvin, Irl.; Bausch & Lomb, UK.*
Carbomer (p.1577·2).
*Dry eyes.*

**Gel-Tin** *Young, USA.*
Stannous fluoride (p.1448·3).
*Dental caries prophylaxis.*

**Gelucystine** *Pfizer, Fr.*
Cystine (p.1426·3).
*Fragile nails and hair.*

**Gelufene** *Cooperation Pharmaceutique, Fr.*
Ibuprofen (p.45·3).
*Fever; pain.*

**Gelum** *Dreluso, Ger.*
*Oral drops; topical gel:* Potassium-iron (III)-citrate-phosphate complex.
*Liver disorders; musculoskeletal, joint, peri-articular, and soft-tissue disorders.*
*Suppositories:* Potassium-iron (III)-citrate-phosphate complex; benzocaine (p.1370·3).
*Anorectal disorders.*

**Gelumag** *Synco, Hong Kong.*
Magnesium trisilicate (p.1272·3); aluminium hydroxide (p.1249·2).
*Gastrointestinal hyperacidity; peptic ulcer.*

**Gelumaline** *Solvay, Fr.*
Belladonna (p.479·1); codeine (p.27·1); caffeine (p.782·1); paracetamol (p.76·2).
*Fever; pain.*

**Gelumen** *Medpro, S.Afr.*
Dicycloverine hydrochloride (p.481·2); dried aluminium hydroxide gel (p.1249·2); light magnesium oxide (p.1272·3).
*Gastric hyperacidity.*

**Gelumina** *Sanitas, Port.*
*Oral liquid:* Aluminium hydroxide (p.1249·2).
*Tablets:* Aluminium hydroxide (p.1249·2); calcium carbonate (p.1254·2).
*Gastrointestinal disorders.*

**Geluprane** *Theraplix, Fr.*
Paracetamol (p.76·2).
*Fever; pain.*

**Gelusil**
*Note. This name is used for preparations of different composition.*
*Pfizer Consumer, Austral.; Parke, Davis, USA.*
Aluminium hydroxide (p.1249·2); magnesium hydroxide (p.1272·2); simeticone (p.1289·2).
*Dyspepsia; gastro-oesophageal reflux.*

*Pfizer, Austria; Pfizer Consumer, Ger.; Warner-Lambert Consumer, Switz.†.*
Almasilate (p.1248·2).
*Gastrointestinal disorders.*

*Pfizer Consumer, Belg.†; Pfizer Consumer, Canad.*
Aluminium hydroxide (p.1249·2); magnesium hydroxide (p.1272·2).
*Gastrointestinal hyperacidity.*

*Pfizer Sante, Fr.; Pfizer, Hong Kong; Pfizer, Malaysia; Pfizer Consumer, S.Afr.; Pfizer Consumer, Singapore; Pfizer, Thai.*
Aluminium hydroxide (p.1249·2); magnesium trisilicate (p.1272·3).
*Gastric hyperacidity.*

*Warner-Lambert Consumer, Port.†.*
Aluminium hydroxide (p.1249·2); calcium phosphate (p.1225·3); magnesium trisilicate (p.1272·3).
Formerly contained aluminium hydroxide, magnesium hydroxide, and magnesium trisilicate.
*Gastrointestinal disorders.*

**Gelusil Forte** *Pfizer, Malaysia.*
Magnesium hydroxide (p.1272·2); aluminium hydroxide (p.1249·2); simeticone (p.1289·2).
*Dyspepsia; flatulence; gastric hyperacidity; heartburn.*

**Gelusil M** *Pfizer, Braz.*
Aluminium hydroxide (p.1249·2); magnesium hydroxide (p.1272·2); dimethicone (p.1289·2).
*Flatulence; gastrointestinal hyperacidity.*

**Gelusil MPS**
*Parke, Davis, India; Pfizer, Thai.*
Aluminium hydroxide (p.1249·2); magnesium hydroxide (p.1272·2); simeticone (p.1289·2).
*Flatulence; gastric hyperacidity; peptic ulcer.*

**Gelusil Plus**
*Pfizer, Hong Kong; Pfizer, Malaysia; Pfizer Consumer, Singapore.*
Aluminium hydroxide (p.1249·2); magnesium hydroxide (p.1272·2); simeticone (p.1289·2).
*Dyspepsia; flatulence; gastric hyperacidity; gastritis; peptic ulcer.*

**Gelusil S** *Pfizer Consumer, S.Afr.*
Aluminium hydroxide (p.1249·2); magnesium hydroxide (p.1272·2); simeticone (p.1289·2).
*Bloating; gastric hyperacidity; peptic ulcer.*

**Gelusil Simethicone** *Pfizer Consumer, Belg.*
Aluminium hydroxide (p.1249·2); magnesium hydroxide (p.1272·2); simeticone (p.1289·2).
*Flatulence; gastrointestinal disorders associated with hyperacidity.*

**Gelusil-Lac**
*Pfizer Consumer, Ger.; Pfizer, Switz.*
Almasilate (p.1248·2); milk powder.
*Gastrointestinal disorders.*

**Gely** *Ipsen, Spain.*
Glycerol (p.1694·3).
*Barrier preparation; lubricant.*

**Gem** *Nycomed, Norw.*
Sodium chloride; potassium chloride; sodium citrate; glucose (p.1222·2).
*Diarrhoea; oral rehydration therapy.*

**Gemalt** *Pharmavite, Canad.†.*
Multivitamin preparation with iron (p.1417·1).

**Gemcite** *Lilly, India.*
Gemcitabine hydrochloride (p.558·1).
*Bladder cancer; non-small-cell lung cancer; pancreatic cancer.*

**Gemd** *Yung Shin, Singapore.*
Gemfibrozil (p.923·1).
*Hyperlipidaemias.*

**Gemfi** *IA, Ger.*
Gemfibrozil (p.923·1).
*Hyperlipidaemias.*

**Gemfibril** *Siam Bheasach, Thai.*
Gemfibrozil (p.923·1).
*Hyperlipidaemias.*

**Gemfibromax** *PMC, Austral.†.*
Gemfibrozil (p.923·1).
*Hyperlipidaemias.*

**Gemfolid** *Genepharm, Gr.*
Gemfibrozil (p.923·1).
*Hyperlipidaemias.*

**Gemhexal** *Hexal, Austral.*
Gemfibrozil (p.923·1).
*Hyperlipidaemias.*

**Gemicina** *Gastroenterologicos, Mex.†.*
Neomycin (p.235·1).

**Gemini** *Restan, S.Afr.*
Antazoline hydrochloride (p.424·2); tetryzoline hydrochloride (p.1131·2).
*Eye irritation; inflammatory eye disorders.*

**Gemipasmol** *Geminis, Arg.*
Dihydrostreptomycin (p.206·1); phthalylsulphathiazole (p.242·3).
*Gastrointestinal infections.*

**Gemitin** *SMB, Chile.*
Chloramphenicol (p.185·1).
*Bacterial eye and skin infections.*

**Gemitin con Prednisolona** *SMB, Chile.*
Chloramphenicol (p.185·1); prednisolone acetate (p.1108·1).
*Bacterial skin infections; otitis externa.*

**Gemizol** *Pacific, NZ.*
Gemfibrozil (p.923·1).
*Hyperlipidaemias.*

**Gemlipid**
*Medichrom, Gr.; FIRMA, Ital.*
Gemfibrozil (p.923·1).
*Hyperlipidaemias.*

**Gemnpid** *CCPC, Hong Kong†.*
Gemfibrozil (p.923·1).
*Hyperlipidaemias.*

**Gemtro** *Lilly, Arg.*
Gemcitabine hydrochloride (p.558·1).
*Bladder cancer; non-small cell lung cancer; pancreatic cancer.*

**Gemvites** *Pharmavite, Canad.†.*
Multivitamin preparation (p.1417·1).

**Gemzar**
*Lilly, Austral.; Lilly, Austria; Lilly, Belg.; Lilly, Braz.; Lilly, Canad.; Lilly, Chile; Lilly, Denm.; Lilly, Fin.; Lilly, Fr.; Lilly, Ger.; Pharmaserve Lilly (Φαρμασερβ Λιλλυ), Gr.; Lilly, Hong Kong; Lilly, Irl.; Lilly, Israel; Lilly, Ital.; Lilly, Malaysia; Lilly, Mex.; Lilly, Neth.; Lilly, Norw.; Lilly, NZ; Lilly, Port.; Lilly, S.Afr.; Lilly, Singapore; Spaly, Spain; Lilly, Swed.; Lilly, Switz.; Lilly, Thai.; Lilly, UK; Lilly, USA.*
Gemcitabine hydrochloride (p.558·1).
*Bladder cancer; non-small cell lung cancer; pancreatic cancer.*

**Gemzil**
*Note. This name is used for preparations of different composition.*
*Merck, Hong Kong.*
Gemfibrozil (p.923·1).
*Hyperlipidaemias.*

*Pharmasant, Thai.*
Captopril (p.879·2).
*Heart failure; hypertension.*

**Gen H-B-Vax**
*Aventis Pasteur, Austria; Chiron Behring, Ger.; Aventis Pasteur, Ger.; Pro Vaccine, Switz.*
A hepatitis B vaccine (recombinant DNA) (p.1618·1).
Separate preparations are available for children, adults, and adult dialysis patients.
*Active immunisation.*

**Genac**
*Note. This name is used for preparations of different composition.*
*Genevrier, Fr.*
Acetylcysteine (p.1112·3).
*Corneal ulceration.*

*Goldline, USA.*
Pseudoephedrine hydrochloride (p.1129·2); triprolidine hydrochloride (p.442·3).
*Upper respiratory-tract symptoms.*

**Genacol** *Goldline, USA.*
Chlorphenamine maleate (p.427·3); dextromethorphan hydrobromide (p.1117·3); paracetamol (p.76·2); pseudoephedrine hydrochloride (p.1129·2).
*Coughs and cold symptoms.*

**Genahist** *Goldline, USA.*
Diphenhydramine hydrochloride (p.431·3).
*Insomnia; motion sickness; parkinsonism.*

**Genalen** *Gentili, Ital.*
Alendronate sodium (p.765·3).
*Osteoporosis.*

**Genalfa** *INTES, Ital.*
Gentamicin sulfate (p.217·1); naphazoline nitrate (p.1124·3).
*Eye infections.*

**Genalgen** *Farmaco, Mex.*
Naproxen (p.65·1).
*Inflammation; musculoskeletal and joint disorders; pain.*

**Genalin** *Great Eastern, Thai.; Therapharma, Thai.*
Multivitamin and mineral preparation (p.1417·1).

**Genamin** *Goldline, USA†.*
Phenylpropanolamine hydrochloride (p.1127·3); chlorphenamine maleate (p.427·3).
*Upper respiratory-tract symptoms.*

**Genapap** *Goldline, USA.*
Paracetamol (p.76·2).
*Fever; pain.*

**Genaphed** *Goldline, USA.*
Pseudoephedrine hydrochloride (p.1129·2).
*Nasal congestion.*

**Genaprost** *Gentili, Ital.*
Finasteride (p.1554·2).
*Benign prostatic hyperplasia.*

**Genasal** *Goldline, USA.*
Oxymetazoline hydrochloride (p.1126·1).
*Nasal congestion.*

**Genasoft Plus Softgels** *Goldline, USA†.*
Docusate sodium (p.1262·2); casanthranol (p.1255·1).
*Constipation.*

**Genaspor** *Goldline, USA.*
Tolnaftate (p.410·1).
*Fungal skin infections.*

**Genaton** *Goldline, USA.*
*Oral liquid:* Aluminium hydroxide (p.1249·2); magnesium carbonate (p.1272·1).
*Tablets:* Aluminium hydroxide (p.1249·2); magnesium trisilicate (p.1272·3); sodium bicarbonate (p.1223·2); alginic acid (p.1576·3).
*Hyperacidity.*

**Genatrop** *INTES, Ital.*
Gentamicin sulfate (p.217·1); atropine sulfate (p.477·1).
*Bacterial eye infections.*

**Genatropine** *Amido, Fr.†.*
Atropine oxide hydrochloride (p.478·1).
*Biliary tract disorders; gastrointestinal disorders.*

**Genatuss** *Goldline, USA†.*
Guaifenesin (p.1122·1).
*Coughs.*

**Genatuss DM** *Goldline, USA.*
Dextromethorphan hydrobromide (p.1117·3); guaifenesin (p.1122·1).
*Coughs.*

**Genavit** *General Drugs, Thai.*
Vitamin $B_1$ (p.1455·2); vitamin $B_6$ (p.1457·2); vitamin $B_{12}$ (p.1458·2).
*Anaemia; beri-beri; nausea and vomiting; vitamin B deficiency.*

**Gen-Beclo** *Genpharm, Canad.*
Beclometasone dipropionate (p.1091·1).
*Corticosteroid.*

**Gen-bee with C** *Goldline, USA.*
Vitamin B substances with vitamin C (p.1417·1).

**Gencalc** *Goldline, USA†.*
Calcium carbonate (p.1254·2).
*Calcium deficiency; dietary supplement.*

**Gencardia** *Genus, UK†.*
Aspirin (p.15·1).

**Gencefal** *Llorente, Spain.*
Cefazolin sodium (p.170·3).
*Bacterial infections.*

**Gencifrice Baume 1re Dents** *Synthelabo, Fr.†.*
Casein hydrolysate.
*Teething pain.*

**Gencin** *Curasan, Ger.*
Gentamicin sulfate (p.217·1).
*Bacterial infections.*

**Gencolax** *General Drugs, Thai.*
Bisacodyl (p.1251·3).
*Bowel evacuation; constipation.*

**Gencold** *Goldline, USA†.*
Phenylpropanolamine hydrochloride (p.1127·3); chlorphenamine maleate (p.427·3).
*Upper respiratory-tract symptoms.*

**Gen-Cromolyn** *Genpharm, Canad.*
Sodium cromoglicate (p.795·3).

**Gencydo**
*Note. This name is used for preparations of different composition.*
*Weleda, Austria; Weleda, Ger.*
Lemon (p.1706·2); cydonia.
*Hypersensitivity reactions.*

*Weleda, UK.*
Homoeopathic preparation.

**Gendazel** *General Drugs, Thai.*
Albendazole (p.101·2).
*Worm infections.*

**Gendecon**
*Note. This name is used for preparations of different composition.*
*General Drugs, Thai.†.*
Phenylpropanolamine hydrochloride (p.1127·3); paracetamol (p.76·2); chlorphenamine maleate (p.427·3).
*Fever; muscle pain; nasal congestion; rhinitis.*

*Goldline, USA.*
Phenylephrine hydrochloride (p.1126·3); paracetamol (p.76·2); chlorphenamine maleate (p.427·3).
*Upper respiratory-tract symptoms.*

**Genebs** *Goldline, USA.*
Paracetamol (p.76·2).
*Fever; pain.*

**Genecalcin** *Genepharm, Gr.*
Calcitonin (p.768·2).
*Osteoporosis.*

**Genefadrone** *Genepharm, Gr.*
Mitoxantrone hydrochloride (p.575·2).
*Malignant neoplasms.*

**Genemicin** *Diba, Mex.*
Gentamicin (p.219·1).
*Bacterial infections.*

**Generaid**
*Scientific Hospital Supplies, Austral.; Scientific Hospital Supplies, Irl.†; Nutricia, NZ; Scientific Hospital Supplies, NZ; Scientific Hospital Supplies, UK.*
Amino-acid and protein preparation (p.1417·1).
*Hepatic encephalopathy; liver disorders.*

**Genercin** *General Drugs, Thai.*
Chloramphenicol (p.185·1).
*Bacterial infections.*

**Generet** *Goldline, USA.*
Ferrous sulfate (p.1428·2); vitamin B substances with vitamin C (p.1417·1).
*Iron-deficiency anaemias.*

**Energin** *General Drugs, Thai.*
Dipyrone (p.35·3).
*Fever; pain.*

**Generix-T** *Goldline, USA.*
Multivitamin and mineral preparation with iron (p.1417·1).

**Generlog** *General Drugs, Thai.*
Triamcinolone acetonide (p.1110·2).
*Oral lesions.*

**Generman** *Byk Gulden, Ital.*
Multivitamin preparation with calcium glycerophosphate and sodium fluoride (p.1417·1).
*Bone and dental weakness.*

**Genes Vit** *Wassen, Ital.*
A range of vitamin and mineral preparations (p.1417·1).

**Genesa**
*Gensia, Swed.†; Gensia, USA.*
Arbutamine hydrochloride (p.864·2).
*Pharmacological cardiac stress test.*

**Geneserine** *Biodim, Fr.*
Eseridine salicylate (p.1491·2).
*Dyspepsia.*

**Genesis** *Wassen, UK†.*
Multivitamin and mineral preparation (p.1417·1).

**Genevis** *Andromaco, Chile.*
Ergocalciferol (p.1462·1).
*Osteomalacia; rickets; vitamin D deficiency.*

**Genevis D2**
*Andromaco, Chile; Rudefsa, Mex.†.*
Vitamin D (p.1462·1).
*Osteomalacia; rickets; vitamin D deficiency.*

**Genexal** *Medifarma, Mex.†.*
Gentamicin (p.219·1).
*Bacterial infections.*

**Geneye Extra** *Goldline, USA.*
Tetryzoline hydrochloride (p.1131·2).
*Eye irritation.*

**Gen-Formula** *Thai Otsuka, Thai.*
Preparation for enteral nutrition (p.1417·1).

**Gengigel**
*Esme, Arg.; Oraldent, UK.*
Hyaluronic acid (p.1697·3).
*Mouth disorders.*

*Abbott, Port.*
Sodium hyaluronate (p.1697·3).
*Mouth lesions.*

**Gengisyl** *Master, Chile.*
Sodium monofluorophosphate (p.1446·2); sodium fluoride (p.1444·3).
*Dental caries prophylaxis.*

**Gengivario** *Farmatre, Ital.; Iema, Ital.; AFOM, Ital.*
Myrrh (p.1718·3); rhatany root (p.1738·1).
*Astringent.*

**Gengivarium** *Kemyos, Ital.†.*
Benzocaine (p.1370·3).
*Mouth disorders.*

**Gen-Glybe** *Genpharm, Canad.*
Glibenclamide (p.331·2).
*Diabetes mellitus.*

**Gengraf**
*Abbott, Arg.; Abbott, Braz.; Abbott, Hong Kong; Abbott, USA.*
Ciclosporin (p.1351·2).
*Psoriasis; rheumatoid arthritis; transplant rejection.*

**GenHevac B** *Pasteur Vaccins, Fr.*
A hepatitis B vaccine (recombinant DNA) (p.1618·1).
*Active immunisation.*

**Geniad** *Infosint, Ital.*
Alfacalcidol (p.1461·2).
*Osteomalacia; osteoporosis; renal osteodystrophy; rickets.*

**Geniceral** *Casasco, Arg.*
Idebenone (p.1700·3).
*Cerebrovascular disorders.*

**Genimox** *Ecobi, Ital.*
Amoxicillin trihydrate (p.155·3).
*Bacterial infections.*

**Genin** *General Drugs, Thai.*
Quinine sulfate (p.460·2).
*Malaria.*

**Geniol** *GlaxoSmithKline, Arg.*
Aspirin (p.15·1); caffeine (p.782·1).
*Fever; pain.*

**Geniol AP** *GlaxoSmithKline, Arg.*
Aspirin (p.15·1).
*Pain.*

**Geniol Flex** *GlaxoSmithKline, Arg.*
Trolamine salicylate (p.95·3).
*Musculoskeletal, joint, and peri-articular disorders.*

**Geniol SC sin Cafeina** *GlaxoSmithKline, Arg.*
Aspirin (p.15·1).
*Fever; pain.*

**Geniolito** *GlaxoSmithKline, Arg.*
Aspirin (p.15·1).
*Fever; pain.*

**Geniol-P** *Mintlab, Chile.*
Paracetamol (p.76·2).
*Fever; pain.*

**Genisol**
*Note. This name is used for preparations of different composition.*
*Fisons, Irl.†.*
Coal tar (p.1159·2); sodium sulfosuccinated undecenoic acid monoethanolamide (p.411·1).
*Dandruff; scalp psoriasis.*

*Teofarma, Ital.*
Piroctone olamine (p.1155·2); sodium sulfosuccinated undecenoic acid monoethanolamide (p.411·1).
Formerly contained coal tar and sodium sulfosuccinated undecenoic acid monoethanolamide.
*Seborrhoeic dermatitis.*

**Genite** *Goldline, USA.*
Pseudoephedrine hydrochloride (p.1129·2); dextromethorphan hydrobromide (p.1117·3); doxylamine succinate (p.432·3); paracetamol (p.76·2).
*Coughs and cold symptoms.*

**Genitoflox** *IQB, Braz.*
Norfloxacin (p.238·3).
*Bacterial infections.*

**Genitopen** *IQB, Braz.†.*
Ampicillin benzathine (p.158·1); ampicillin sodium (p.157·1); antigens from *Neisseria, Escherichia, Streptococcus, Staphylococcus, Proteus,* and *Pseudomonas.*
*Bacterial infections.*

**Gen-K** *Goldline, USA.*
Potassium chloride (p.1232·2).
*Hypokalaemia; potassium depletion.*

**Genkova** *Sons, Mex.*
Gentamicin sulfate (p.217·1).
*Bacterial infections.*

**Genlac** *Arrow, Austral.*
Lactulose (p.1269·1).
*Constipation; hepatic encephalopathy.*

**Gen-Lac** *Genpharm, Canad.*
Lactulose (p.1269·1).
*Constipation.*

**Genlip** *Teofarma, Ital.*
Gemfibrozil (p.923·1).
*Hyperlipidaemias.*

**Gen-Medroxy** *Genpharm, Canad.*
Medroxyprogesterone acetate (p.1557·2).

**Genocin** *General Drugs, Thai.*
Chloroquine phosphate (p.448·2).
*Amoebiasis; malaria.*

**Genocolan** *Craveri, Arg.*
Lactulose (p.1269·1).
*Constipation; gastrointestinal infections; hepatic encephalopathy.*

**Genogris** *Vita, Spain†.*
Piracetam (p.1732·1).
*Cerebrovascular disorders; cortical myoclonia; mental function impairment.*

**Genola** *CCD, Fr.†.*
Hexylresorcinol (p.1182·1); benzododecinium bromide (p.1170·2); allantoin (p.1141·3); boric acid (p.1662·1).
*Spermicide.*

**Genolaxante** *Craveri, Arg.*
Phenolphthalein (p.1284·1); aloes (p.1248·2); simeticone (p.1289·2).
*Constipation.*

**Genoptic**
*Allergan, Austral.; Allergan, Hong Kong; Allergan, NZ; Allergan, S.Afr.; Allergan, Singapore; Allergan, USA.*
Gentamicin sulfate (p.217·1).
*Bacterial eye infections.*

**Genora 0.5/35 and 1/35** *Rugby, USA†.*
Ethinylestradiol (p.1553·2); norethisterone (p.1562·2).
28-Day packs also contain 7 inert tablets.
*Combined oral contraceptive.*

**Genora 1/50** *Rugby, USA†.*
Mestranol (p.1559·2); norethisterone (p.1562·2).
28-Day packs also contain 7 inert tablets.
*Combined oral contraceptive.*

**Genoral** *Pharmacia, Austral.*
Estropipate (p.1553·1).
*Menopausal disorders; oestrogen deficiency.*

**Genoscopolamine** *Amido, Fr.†.*
Hyoscine oxide hydrobromide (p.484·2).
*Parkinsonism.*

**Genotonorm**
*Pharmacia, Belg.; Pharmacia, Chile; Pharmacia, Fr.; Pharmacia, Spain.*
Somatropin (p.1327·2).
*Growth disorders in renal failure; growth hormone deficiency; Prader-Willi syndrome; Turner's syndrome.*

**Genotropin**
*Pharmacia, Arg.; Pharmacia, Austral.; Pharmacia, Austria; Pharmacia, Braz.; Pharmacia, Denm.; Pharmacia, Fin.; Pharmacia, Ger.; Pharmacia-Upjohn, Gr.; Pharmacia, Hong Kong; Pharmacia, Irl.;*

*Pharmacia Upjohn, Israel; Pharmacia Upjohn, Ital.; Pharmacia, Malaysia; Pharmacia Upjohn, Mex.; Pharmacia, Neth.; Pharmacia, Norw.; Pharmacia, NZ; Pharmacia, Port.; Pharmacia, S.Afr.; Pharmacia, Singapore; Pharmacia, Swed.; Pharmacia, Switz.; Pharmacia, UK; Pharmacia, USA.*
Somatropin (p.1327·2).
*Growth disorders in renal failure; growth hormone deficiency; Prader-Willi syndrome; Turner's syndrome.*

**Genovox** *Kleva, Gr.*
Nimodipine (p.972·3).
*Neurological deficit following subarachnoid haemorrhage.*

**Genox**
*Alphapharm, Austral.; Alphapharm, Malaysia; Merck, Malaysia; Pacific, NZ.*
Tamoxifen citrate (p.584·1).
*Breast cancer; endometrial cancer.*

**Genoxal**
*Kampel Martian, Arg.; Sanfer, Mex.; Prasfarma, Spain.*
Cyclophosphamide (p.540·2).
*Auto-immune disorders; malignant neoplasms; transplant rejection.*

**Genoxal Trofosfamida** *Prasfarma, Spain.*
Trofosfamide (p.590·2).
*Malignant neoplasms.*

**Genoxen** *Antigen, Hong Kong†.*
Naproxen (p.65·1).
*Gout; musculoskeletal, joint, peri-articular, and soft-tissue disorders.*

**Genozil** *Pulitzer, Ital.*
Gemfibrozil (p.923·1).
*Hyperlipidaemias.*

**Genozym** *Bristol-Myers Squibb, Arg.*
Clomifene citrate (p.1542·2).
*Female infertility.*

**Genpril** *Goldline, USA.*
Ibuprofen (p.45·3).
*Fever; osteoarthritis; pain; rheumatoid arthritis.*

**Genprin** *Goldline, USA.*
Aspirin (p.15·1).
*Fever; inflammation; myocardial infarction; pain; transient ischaemic attacks.*

**Genprol** *Geminis, Spain.*
Citalopram hydrobromide (p.289·1).
*Anxiety; depression; obsessive-compulsive disorder.*

**Genquin** *Seng, Thai.*
Gentamicin sulfate (p.217·1); bacitracin (p.161·3); clioquinol (p.196·3); glycine; threonine; cystine.
*Infected skin disorders.*

**Genrex** *Rayere, Mex.*
Gentamicin sulfate (p.217·1).
*Bacterial infections.*

**Genrex-B** *Rayere, Mex.†.*
Gentamicin sulfate (p.217·1); betamethasone (p.1093·1).
*Infected skin disorders.*

**Gensan** *Goldline, USA†.*
Aspirin (p.15·1); caffeine (p.782·1).

**Genser Sweet** *Genser, Arg.*
Aspartame (p.1422·1); acesulfame potassium (p.1420·3).
*Sugar substitute.*

**Gensil** *General Drugs, Thai.*
Metoclopramide (p.1274·3).
*Nausea and vomiting.*

**Gensumycin**
*Aventis, Denm.†; Aventis, Fin.; Aventis, Norw.; Aventis, Swed.*
Gentamicin sulfate (p.217·1).
*Bacterial infections.*

**Genta**
*CT, Ger.; Grin, Mex.; M & H, Thai.; Shiwa, Thai.*
Gentamicin sulfate (p.217·1).
*Bacterial infections.*

**Genta Gobens**
*APS, Port.; Normon, Spain.*
Gentamicin sulfate (p.217·1).
*Bacterial infections.*

**Gentabac** *Infan, Mex.†.*
Gentamicin (p.219·1).
*Bacterial infections.*

**Gentabilles** *Schering-Plough, Fr.†.*
Gentamicin sulfate (p.217·1).
*Bacterial infections.*

**Gentac**
*Sanval, Braz.; Samakeephaesaj, Thai.*
Gentamicin sulfate (p.217·1).
*Bacterial infections.*

**Gentacarnot** *Carnot, Mex.†.*
Gentamicin (p.219·1).
*Bacterial infections.*

**Gentacidin**
*Ciba Vision, Canad.†; Novartis Ophthalmics, USA.*
Gentamicin sulfate (p.217·1).
*Bacterial eye infections.*

**Gentacin**
*Carter-Wallace, Mex.†; Olan-Kemed, Thai.*
Gentamicin sulfate (p.217·1).
*Bacterial infections.*

**Gentacoll**
*Schering-Plough, Denm.; Schering-Plough, Fin.*
Gentamicin sulfate (p.217·1).
*Bone infection.*

**Gentacort**
*Note. This name is used for preparations of different composition.*
*Allergan, Braz.*
Gentamicin sulfate (p.217·1); betamethasone sodium phosphate (p.1093·1).
*Infected eye disorders.*

*Ciba Vision, Ital.*
Gentamicin sulfate (p.217·1); fluorometholone (p.1102·2).
*Infected eye disorders.*

**Gentadexa**
*Alcon Cusi, Malaysia; Alcon, Port.; Alcon Cusi, Spain.*
Dexamethasone sodium phosphate (p.1097·2); gentamicin sulfate (p.217·1); tetryzoline hydrochloride (p.1131·2).
*External ear infections; eye infections with inflammation.*

**Gentagran** *Legrand, Braz.*
Gentamicin sulfate (p.217·1).
*Bacterial eye infections.*

**Gentak** *Akorn, USA.*
Gentamicin sulfate (p.217·1).
*Bacterial infections.*

**Gental**
*General Drugs, Thai.; Julphar, UAE.*
Gentamicin sulfate (p.217·1).
*Bacterial infections.*

**Gental-F** *General Drugs, Thai.*
Gentamicin sulfate (p.217·1); fluocinolone acetonide (p.1101·2).
*Infected skin disorders.*

**Gentalline** *Schering-Plough, Fr.*
Gentamicin sulfate (p.217·1).
*Bacterial infections.*

**Gentalodina** *Rhone-Poulenc Rorer, Spain†.*
Gentamicin sulfate (p.217·1).
*Bacterial infections.*

**Gentalyn**
*Schering-Plough, Chile; Schering-Plough, Ital.*
Gentamicin sulfate (p.217·1).
*Bacterial infections.*

**Gentalyn Beta** *Schering-Plough, Ital.*
Gentamicin sulfate (p.217·1); betamethasone valerate (p.1093·2).
*Infected skin disorders.*

**Gentamed** *Medochemie, Malaysia.*
Gentamicin (p.219·1).
*Bacterial infections.*

**Gentamedical** *Medical, Spain.*
Gentamicin sulfate (p.217·1).
*Bacterial infections.*

**Gentamen** *Fournier, Ital.*
Gentamicin sulfate (p.217·1).
*Bacterial infections.*

**Gentamil** *Ducto, Braz.*
Gentamicin sulfate (p.217·1).
*Bacterial infections.*

**Gentamina** *Key, Arg.*
Gentamicin sulfate (p.217·1).
*Bacterial infections.*

**Gentamival** *Rovi, Spain.*
Gentamicin sulfate (p.217·1).
*Bacterial infections.*

**Gentamytrex**
*Tramedico, Belg.†; Mann, Ger.; Mann, Malaysia; Tramedico, Neth.; Mann, Singapore.*
Gentamicin sulfate (p.217·1).
*Bacterial eye infections.*

**Gentanacin** *Loren, Mex.*
Gentamicin (p.219·1).
*Bacterial infections.*

**Genta-Oph** *Seng, Thai.*
Gentamicin sulfate (p.217·1).
*Bacterial eye infections.*

**Gentapat** *Parggon, Mex.*
Gentamicin (p.219·1).
*Bacterial infections.*

**Gentapharma** *Fada, Arg.*
Gentamicin (p.219·1).
*Bacterial infections.*

**Gentaplex** *Liptis, USA.*
Lyophilised fish roe; ginkgo biloba (p.1692·3).
*Decreased libido in men.*

**Gentaplus** *Abbott, Braz.†.*
Gentamicin sulfate (p.217·1).
*Bacterial infections.*

**Gentarim** *Rimsa, Mex.*
Gentamicin sulfate (p.217·1).
*Bacterial infections.*

**Gentaron** *Ariston, Braz.*
Gentamicin (p.219·1).
*Bacterial infections.*

**Gentasol**
*Note. This name is used for preparations of different composition.*
*Monserrat, Arg.*
Gentamicin sulfate (p.217·1); betamethasone valerate (p.1093·2); miconazole nitrate (p.405·3).
*Infected skin disorders.*

*Ocusoft, USA.*
Gentamicin sulfate (p.217·1).
*Bacterial eye infections.*

**Gentasone**
*Schering-Plough, Chile; Schering-Plough, Fr.†.*
Gentamicin sulfate (p.217·1); betamethasone sodium phosphate (p.1093·1).
*Bacterial eye infections with inflammation; infected external ear disorders.*

**Gentasporin** *Pharmaceutical Co, India.*
Gentamicin sulfate (p.217·1).
*Bacterial infections.*

**Gentatenk** *Biotenk, Arg.*
Gentamicin sulfate (p.217·1).
*Bacterial infections.*

**Gentatrim** *Trima, Israel.*
Gentamicin sulfate (p.217·1).
*Bacterial skin infections.*

**Gentavasor** *Alcon Cusi, Spain†.*
Gentamicin sulfate (p.217·1); tetryzoline hydrochloride (p.1131·2).
*Eye disorders.*

**Gentavivant** *Vivant, Mex.†.*
Gentamicin (p.219·1).
*Bacterial infections.*

**Gentax**
*Agepha, Austria; Luper, Braz.*
Gentamicin sulfate (p.217·1).
*Bacterial infections.*

**Gentaxil** *Haller, Braz.†.*
Gentamicin (p.219·1).
*Bacterial infections.*

**Gentazaf Z** *Zafiro, Mex.*
Gentamicin sulfate (p.217·1).
*Bacterial infections.*

**Genteal**
*Novartis Ophthalmics, Arg.; Novartis Ophthalmics, Braz.; Novartis Ophthalmics, Canad.; Novartis, Chile; Novartis Ophthalmics, Ger.; Novartis Ophthalmics, Hong Kong; Novartis, Israel; Novartis, Ital.; Novartis, NZ; Novartis Ophthalmics, USA.*
Hypromellose (p.1579·3).
*Dry eyes; wetting solution for contact lenses.*

**Genteal Lubricant** *Novartis, Austral.*
Hypromellose (p.1579·3).
*Dry eyes; eye irritation.*

**Genteal Moisturising** *Novartis, Austral.*
Hypromellose (p.1579·3); carbomer (p.1577·2).
*Dry eyes; eye irritation.*

**Gentiabron** *Bristol-Myers Squibb, Arg.*
Clofedanol hydrochloride (p.1117·1); ambroxol hydrochloride (p.1114·3); pseudoephedrine sulfate (p.1129·2); astemizole (p.424·2).
*Respiratory-tract disorders with increased or viscous mucus.*

**Gentialoquin** *Collins, Mex.*
Gentamicin (p.219·1).
*Bacterial infections.*

**Gentibioptal** *Farmila, Ital.*
Gentamicin sulfate (p.217·1).
*Bacterial eye infections.*

**Genticin**
*Roche, Irl.; Roche, UK.*
Gentamicin sulfate (p.217·1).
*Bacterial infections.*

**Genticina** *Pharmacia, Spain.*
Gentamicin sulfate (p.217·1).
*Bacterial infections.*

**Genticol**
*Craveri, Arg.; SIFI, Ital.*
Gentamicin sulfate (p.217·1).
*Bacterial eye infections.*

**Genticyn** *Nicholas Piramal, India.*
Gentamicin sulfate (p.217·1).
*Bacterial infections.*

**Genticyn B Eye/Ear** *Nicholas Piramal, India.*
Gentamicin sulfate (p.217·1); betamethasone sodium phosphate (p.1093·1).
*Allergic and inflammatory eye and ear disorders.*

**Genticyn Eye/Ear** *Nicholas Piramal, India.*
Gentamicin sulfate (p.217·1).
*Bacterial eye infections; ear infections; earache.*

**Genticyn HC** *Nicholas Piramal, India.*
Gentamicin sulfate (p.217·1); hydrocortisone acetate (p.1103·3).
*Allergic and inflammatory eye and ear disorders.*

**Gentipress** *Gentili, Ital.*
Enalapril maleate (p.909·2); hydrochlorothiazide (p.933·2).
*Hypertension.*

**Gentiran** *Vocate, Gr.*
Cetirizine hydrochloride (p.427·1).
*Allergic conjunctivitis; allergic rhinitis; pruritus.*

**Gentisone HC**
*Roche, Irl.; Roche, UK.*
Gentamicin sulfate (p.217·1); hydrocortisone acetate (p.1103·3).
*Bacterial ear infections.*

**Gentlax** *Purdue Frederick, USA.*
Bisacodyl (p.1251·3).
*Constipation.*

**Gentle C with Bioflavonoids** *Cenovis, Austral.†.*
Calcium ascorbate (p.1460·2); lemon bioflavonoids (p.1688·2); rutoside (p.1688·2); hesperidin (p.1688·2).
*Capillary disorders; cold and influenza symptoms; wounds.*

**Gentlees** *Delamac, Austral.†.*
Hamamelis water (p.1696·3); glycerol; cetylpyridinium chloride (p.1173·1).
*Anogenital wounds; anorectal disorders; nappy rash; nipple care.*

**Gent-L-Tip** *Chester, Canad.*
Monobasic sodium phosphate (p.1230·3); dibasic sodium phosphate (p.1231·1).
*Bowel evacuation.*

**Gentocelina** *Roux-Ocefa, Arg.*
Metampicillin (p.229·3); gentamicin (p.219·1).
*Bacterial infections.*

**Gentocil** *Edol, Port.*
Gentamicin sulfate (p.217·1).
*Bacterial infections.*

**Gentoler** *Lersan, Arg.*
Gentamicin sulfate (p.217·1).
*Bacterial eye infections.*

**Gentomil** *Biologici Italia, Ital.*
Gentamicin sulfate (p.217·1).
*Bacterial infections.*

**Gent-Ophtal** *Winzer, Ger.*
Gentamicin sulfate (p.217·1).
*Bacterial eye infections.*

**Gentos**
*Note. This name is used for preparations of different composition.*
*Bittner, Austria.*
Homoeopathic preparation.

*Llorente, Spain.*
Clofedanol hydrochloride (p.1117·1).
*Coughs.*

**Gentralay** *Plevifarma, Spain†.*
Gentamicin sulfate (p.217·1).
*Bacterial infections.*

**Gentran 40**
*Baxter, Canad.; Baxter, UK; Baxter, USA.*
Dextran 40 (p.745·3) in glucose or sodium chloride.
*Extracorporeal circulation; plasma volume expansion; thromboembolism prophylaxis.*

**Gentran 70**
*Baxter, Canad.; Baxter, UK; Baxter, USA.*
Dextran 70 (p.746·2) in glucose or sodium chloride.
*Plasma volume expansion.*

**Gentrisone** *Shin Poong, Singapore.*
Betamethasone dipropionate (p.1093·1); clotrimazole (p.396·2); gentamicin sulfate (p.217·1).
*Infected skin disorders.*

**Gentus** *Gentili, Ital.†.*
Dimemorfan phosphate (p.1118·3).
*Coughs.*

**Gentussiin** *General Drugs, Thai.*
Guaifenesin (p.1122·1); dextromethorphan hydrobromide (p.1117·3).
*Coughs.*

**Genu-cyl Ho-Len-Complex** *Liebermann, Ger.*
Homoeopathic preparation.

**Genuine Australian Eucalyptus Drops** *Felton, Austral.†.*
Eucalyptus oil (p.1686·2); menthol (p.1711·3); lemon oil (p.1706·2).
*Cough; nasal congestion; sore throat.*

**Genurat** *Soria Natural, Spain.*
Bearberry (p.1659·2); betula alba (p.1660·3); oleum pini sylvestris; calluna vulgaris.
*Urinary-tract infections.*

**Genurin**
*Recordati, Hong Kong; Recordati, Ital.; Recordati, Singapore.*
Flavoxate hydrochloride (p.482·2).
*Genito-urinary tract disorders.*

**Genurin-S** *Aventis, Braz.*
Flavoxate hydrochloride (p.482·2).
*Urinary-tract spasm.*

**Genuxal** *Asta Oncologia, Braz.*
Cyclophosphamide (p.540·2).
*Malignant neoplasms.*

**Gen-Xene** *Alra, USA†.*
Dipotassium clorazepate (p.685·1).
*Alcohol withdrawal syndrome; anxiety; epilepsy.*

**Genziana (Specie Composta)** *Dynacren, Ital.*
Gentian (p.1692·2); bitter orange (p.1723·3); absinthium (p.1645·1); centaury (p.1669·2).
*Appetite loss.*

**Geo Vit H3** *Sedabel, Braz.*
Vitamin preparation (p.1417·1).

**Geocillin** *Pfizer, USA.*
Carindacillin sodium (p.166·3).
*Bacterial infections.*

**Geodon**
*Pfizer, Irl.; Mack, Israel; Pfizer, USA.*
Ziprasidone hydrochloride (p.728·1).
*Schizophrenia.*

**Geo-magnit** *Biomo, Ger.*
Magnesium glutamate (p.1229·1); dibasic magnesium phosphate (p.1229·1).
*Magnesium deficiency.*

**Geomicina** *Atral, Port.*
Oxytetracycline hydrochloride (p.241·1).
*Bacterial infections.*

**Geomycine** *Schering-Plough, Belg.*
Gentamicin sulfate (p.217·1).
*Bacterial infections.*

**Geopen**
*Note. This name is used for preparations of different composition.*
Pfizer, Hong Kong†.
Carindacillin sodium (p.166·3).
*Bacterial infections of the urinary tract.*

Pfizer, Ital.†; Pfizer, Spain†.
Carbenicillin sodium (p.166·2).
*Bacterial infections.*

**Geophagol** Sanval, Braz.
Mebendazole (p.108·2).
*Worm infections.*

**Georkacina** Ehlinger, Mex.†.
Amikacin (p.154·1).
*Bacterial infections.*

**Gepan** Pharmapol, Ger.
Glyceryl trinitrate (p.923·2).
*Angina pectoris; coronary spasm; heart failure; myocardial infarction.*

**Gepeprostin** Labinca, Arg.
Bicalutamide (p.530·1).

**Gepromi** Fustery, Mex.
Progesterone (p.1566·2).
*Female infertility; menopausal disorders; threatened miscarriage.*

**Geracin** Reuffer, Mex.†.
Gentamicin (p.219·1).
*Bacterial infections.*

**Geralen** Gerot, Austria.
5-Methoxypsoralen (p.1154·1).
*Psoriasis.*

**Geram** Vedim, Fr.
Piracetam (p.1732·1).
*Cerebrovascular disorders; dyslexia in childhood; mental function disorders in the elderly; myoclonus; vertigo.*

**Geramet** Gerard, Irl.
Cimetidine (p.1255·3).
*Gastric hyperacidity; gastro-oesophageal reflux; peptic ulcer; Zollinger-Ellison syndrome.*

**Geramox** Gerard, Irl.
Amoxicillin (p.155·3) or amoxicillin trihydrate (p.155·3).
*Bacterial infections.*

**Geranil** Neuropharma, Arg.
Pergolide (p.1211·3).
*Parkinsonism.*

**Gerard 99** Gerard House, UK†.
Lupulus (p.1708·1); passion flower (p.1729·1); valerian (p.1762·2).
*Irritability; tenseness.*

**Gerard House Buchu Compound** Peter Black, UK†.
Taraxacum (p.1751·3); buchu (p.1663·1); bearberry (p.1659·2); clivers (p.1673·2).
*Fluid retention.*

**Gerard House Cranesbill** Peter Black, UK†.
Geranium maculatum.
*Diarrhoea.*

**Gerard House Curzon** Peter Black, UK†.
Damiana (p.1679·1).
*Tonic.*

**Gerard House Gladlax** Peter Black, UK†.
Aloes (p.1248·2); fennel (p.1687·2); valerian (p.1762·2); cnicus benedictus (p.1673·3).
*Constipation.*

**Gerard House Golden Seal Compound** Peter Black, UK†.
Althaea root (p.1651·3); hydrastis (p.1698·3); geranium maculatum; taraxacum (p.1751·3).
*Gastrointestinal disorders.*

**Gerard House Helonias Compound** Peter Black, UK†.
Helonias (p.1696·3); parsley (p.1728·3); cimicifuga (p.1671·3); raspberry leaf (p.1737·3).
*Fluid retention.*

**Gerard House Ligvites** Peter Black, UK†.
Guaiacum (p.1696·2); cimicifuga (p.1671·3); white willow bark (p.87·3); sarsaparilla (p.1742·1); poplar bark (p.1733·3).
*Musculoskeletal and joint disorders.*

**Gerard House Motherwort Compound** Peter Black, UK†.
Passion flower (p.1729·1); motherwort (p.1717·1); tilia flower (p.1756·2).
*Stresses and strains.*

**Gerard House Reumalex** Chefaro, UK.
Guaiacum resin (p.1696·2); cimicifuga (p.1671·3); salix (p.87·3); sarsaparilla (p.1742·1); poplar bark (p.1733·3).
*Musculoskeletal and joint disorders.*

**Gerard House Serenity** Chefaro, UK.
Lupulus (p.1708·1); passion flower (p.1729·1); valerian (p.1762·2).
*Irritability; stress.*

**Gerard House Skin** Chefaro, UK.
Lappa (p.1704·3); wild pansy.
*Eczema; skin blemishes.*

**Gerard House Somnus** Chefaro, UK.
Valerian (p.1762·2); lupulus (p.1708·1); wild lettuce (p.1765·2).
*Insomnia.*

**Gerard House Valerian Compound** Peter Black, UK†.
Lupulus (p.1708·1); passion flower (p.1729·1); valerian (p.1762·2); wild lettuce (p.1765·2); Jamaica dogwood (p.1702·3); skullcap (p.1746·3).
*Insomnia; restlessness.*

**Gerard House Water Relief Tablets** Chefaro, UK.
Bladderwrack (p.1742·3); clivers (p.1673·2); ground ivy (p.1696·1); lappa (p.1704·3).
*Premenstrual water retention.*

**Gerard House Waterlex** Peter Black, UK†.
Taraxacum (p.1751·3); equisetum (p.1684·1); bearberry (p.1659·2).
*Water retention.*

**Geratam** UCB, Belg.
Piracetam (p.1732·1).
*Mental function impairment.*

**Geratar** UCB, S.Afr.†.
Inositol nicotinate (p.939·3); multivitamins (p.1417·1); meclozine (p.436·3); hydroxyzine hydrochloride (p.434·3).
*Vascular disorders; vertigo.*

**Geravim** Major, USA.
Vitamin B substances with minerals (p.1417·1).

**Geravitine** Dinafarma, Braz.†.
Erythroxylon catuaba; liriosma ovata; vitamin E; vitamin B substances (p.1417·1); yohimbine hydrochloride (p.1766·2).

**Gerax** Gerard, Irl.
Alprazolam (p.668·3).
*Alcohol withdrawal syndrome; anxiety disorders; depression; mixed anxiety-depressive states; panic attacks; phobias.*

**Gerbin** ICN, Spain.
Aceclofenac (p.11·2).
*Gout; inflammation; musculoskeletal, joint, peri-articular, and soft-tissue disorders; pain.*

**Gercid forte** Henkel, Ger.
Didecyldimethylammonium chloride (p.1178·3); isopropyl alcohol (p.1184·3).
*Fungal foot infections; surface disinfection.*

**Geref**
Serono, Austria; Serono, Canad.†; Serono, Fin.; Serono, Hong Kong; Serono, Irl.; Serono, Israel†; Serono, Ital.; Serono, Mex.†; Serono, Norw.; Serono, Port.; Serono, S.Afr.†; Serono, Spain; Serono, Swed.; Serono, Switz.; Serono, Thai.†; Serono, UK; Serono, USA.
Sermorelin (p.1339·2) or sermorelin acetate (p.1339·2).
*Test for growth hormone secretion.*

**Gerelax**
Gerard, Irl.; Gerard, Israel.
Lactulose (p.1269·1).
*Constipation; hepatic encephalopathy.*

**Geri** Gisand, Switz.
Vitamin, mineral, and amino-acid preparation (p.1417·1) with ginseng (p.1693·1).
*Tonic.*

**Geriac** Klinger, Braz.†.
Ginseng; erythroxylon catuaba; vitamin E; vitamin B substances (p.1417·1).
*Nutritional supplement.*

**Geriaforce**
*Note. This name is used for preparations of different composition.*
Bioforce, Ger.
Homoeopathic preparation.

Bioforce, Switz.
Ginkgo biloba (p.1692·3).
*Atherosclerosis.*

**Gerial B12** Allen, Mex.
Amino-acids and vitamin B substances with iron (p.1417·1).

**Gerialong** Heralds, Braz.†.
Multivitamin, amino-acid, and mineral preparation (p.1417·1).

**Geriaplasma** Ardeypharm, Ger.
Bovine heart extract; bovine liver extract; bovine spleen extract.
*Tonic.*

**Geriaton** Ache, Braz.
Multivitamin and mineral preparation with ginseng (p.1417·1).

**Geriatric** Stanley, Canad.; Herbes Universelles, Canad.
Multivitamin and mineral preparation (p.1417·1).

**Geriatric Pharmaton**
Boehringer Ingelheim, Austria.
Ginseng; vitamins; minerals; lecithin (p.1417·1).
Formerly known as Geriatric Pharmaton-neu.
*Tonic.*

Pharmaton, Israel.
Multivitamin and mineral preparation with ginseng (p.1417·1).
*Tonic; vitamin and mineral deficiency.*

Pharmaton, Thai.
Deanol tartrate; vitamins; minerals; rutoside; linoleic acid; linolenic acid (p.1417·1).
*Tonic.*

**Geriatrie-Mulsin** Mucos, Ger.
Multivitamin preparation (p.1417·1).

**Geriavit** Pharmaton, Switz.
Ginseng; deanol bitartrate; multivitamins; minerals; rutoside; lecithin (p.1417·1).
*Tonic.*

**Geriavite** Sintofarma, Braz.
Multivitamins with ginseng, inositol, and rutoside (p.1417·1).

**Gericaps** Pharmadass, UK.
Multivitamin and mineral preparation (p.1417·1).

**Gericarb** Gerard, Irl.
Carbamazepine (p.353·3).
*Alcohol withdrawal syndrome; epilepsy; pain.*

**Gericin** Seid, Spain.
Nitrendipine (p.973·3).
*Angina pectoris; hypertension; Raynaud's syndrome.*

**Gericomplex**
Boehringer Ingelheim, Austria.
Ginseng; vitamins; minerals; trace elements (p.1417·1).
*Tonic.*

Boehringer Ingelheim, S.Afr.
Multivitamins; minerals; dimethylaminoethanol bitartrate; ginseng (p.1417·1).
*Tonic.*

**Geriflox** Gerard, Irl.
Flucloxacillin sodium (p.213·3).
*Gram-positive bacterial infections.*

**Gerigoa** Sanova, Austria†.
Procaine resinate; procaine hydrochloride; buphenine resinate; haematoporphyrin; orotic acid; vitamins (p.1417·1).
*Tonic.*

**Geri-Kan H3** Kanda, Braz.†.
Etofylline (p.785·1); procaine hydrochloride (p.1383·2); potassium aspartate; magnesium aspartate; adenosine; linoleic acid; linolenic acid; choline bitartrate; methionine; biotin; vitamin E acetate; vitamin A; vitamin C; vitamin B substances; folic acid; inositol (p.1417·1).
*Tonic.*

**Gerilide** CPH, Port.
Nimesulide (p.67·1).
*Fever; pain.*

**Gerimal** Rugby, USA.
Co-dergocrine mesilate (p.1674·1).
*Senile dementia.*

**Gerimax** Vitalia, UK†.
Multivitamin and mineral preparation with ginseng (p.1417·1).

**Gerimax adultes** Richelet, Fr.
Multivitamin and mineral preparation with ginseng (p.1417·1).

**Gerimax enfants** Richelet, Fr.
Multivitamin and mineral preparation (p.1417·1).

**Gerimax Junior** Dansk, Israel.
Multivitamin and mineral preparation (p.1417·1).

**Gerimax NF** Dansk, Israel.
Multivitamin and mineral preparation with ginseng (p.1417·1).

**Gerimax Tonique** Richelet, Fr.
Ginseng (p.1693·1).
*Tonic.*

**Gerimed** Fielding, USA.
Multivitamin and mineral preparation (p.1417·1).
*Osteoporosis.*

**Gerin** Legrand, Braz.
Amino acids; minerals; vitamins (p.1417·1); ginseng (p.1693·1).
*Tonic.*

**Gerinap** Gerard, Irl.
Naproxen (p.65·1).
*Gout; musculoskeletal and joint disorders.*

**Geriot** Goldline, USA.
Ferrous fumarate (p.1427·3); folic acid (p.1429·1); multivitamins and minerals (p.1417·1).
*Iron-deficiency anaemias.*

**Geripan** Heralds, Braz.†.
Guarana (p.1765·3); erythroxylon catuaba; liriosma ovata; ginger (p.1267·1).
*Nutritional supplement.*

**Geri-Plus** Herbes Universelles, Canad.
Betacarotene, selenium, vitamin C, and vitamin E (p.1417·1).

**Geriso** Sidefarma, Port.
Linoleic acid (p.1690·2); vitamin A; vitamin E; pyridoxine; lecithin (p.1417·1).
*Atherosclerosis; hypercholesterolaemia; vascular disorders.*

**Geritol**
GlaxoSmithKline Consumer, Canad.
Ferric ammonium citrate (p.1427·2); vitamin B substances (p.1417·1).

SmithKline Beecham Consumer, USA.
Ferric ammonium citrate (p.1427·2); vitamin B substances with methionine (p.1417·1).
*Iron-deficiency anaemias.*

**Geritol Complete** SmithKline Beecham Consumer, USA.
Iron (p.1434·3); folic acid (p.1429·1); multivitamins and minerals (p.1417·1).
*Iron-deficiency anaemias.*

**Geritol Extend** SmithKline Beecham Consumer, USA.
Multivitamin and mineral preparation with iron and folic acid (p.1417·1).

**Geriton** Gerbex, Canad.
Vitamin B substances, calcium, and iron (p.1417·1).

**Geritonic** Geriatric Pharm. Corp., USA.
Ferric ammonium citrate (p.1427·2); liver fraction; vitamin B substances and minerals (p.1417·1).
*Iron-deficiency anaemias.*

**Gerivent** Gerard, Irl.
Salbutamol (p.791·3).
*Obstructive airways disease.*

**Gerivit**
*Note. This name is used for preparations of different composition.*
Sanoreform, Ger.†.
Ginseng (p.1693·1).
*Tonic.*

Westmont, Hong Kong†.
Methyltestosterone (p.1559·3); ethinylestradiol (p.1553·2); vitamins; minerals; amino acids (p.1417·1).
*Geriatric nutritional supplement.*

**Gerivite** Goldline, USA.
Multivitamin and mineral preparation (p.1417·1).

**Gerivites** Rugby, USA.
Ferrous sulfate (p.1428·2); vitamin B substances with vitamin C (p.1417·1).
*Iron-deficiency anaemias.*

**Gerivix** Neo Quimica, Braz.†.
Multivitamin and mineral preparation (p.1417·1).

**Germacid** Raza, Malaysia; Pharmaniaga, Malaysia.
Sodium fusidate (p.215·2).
*Bacterial skin infections.*

**Germacort** Raza, Malaysia; Pharmaniaga, Malaysia.
Fusidic acid (p.215·2); betamethasone valerate (p.1093·2).
*Infected skin disorders.*

**Germanin** Bayer, Ger.
Suramin sodium (p.615·3).
*Onchocerciasis; trypanosomiasis.*

**Germentin** Gerard, Irl.
Amoxicillin trihydrate (p.155·3); potassium clavulanate (p.193·3).
*Bacterial infections.*

**Germic** Finadiet, Arg.
Rimantadine (p.653·2) or rimantadine hydrochloride (p.653·1).
*Influenza A.*

**Germicidin** IMS, Ital.
Benzalkonium chloride (p.1168·3).
*Surface and instrument disinfection.*

**Germisdin Antiseptico** Isdin, Port.
Antiseptic cleanser for skin and hair.

**Germisdin Higiene Intima** Isdin, Port.
Preparation for vaginal hygiene.

**Germolene**
*Note. This name is used for preparations of different composition.*
SmithKline Beecham Consumer, Irl.†.
Zinc oxide (p.1163·2); methyl salicylate (p.59·3); octafonium chloride (p.1187·1); phenol (p.1188·1).
*Skin disinfection.*

Bayer Consumer, UK.
*Cream:* Chlorhexidine gluconate (p.1173·2); phenol (p.1188·1).
*Burns; skin irritation; wounds.*
*Ointment:* Zinc oxide (p.1163·2); methyl salicylate (p.59·3); octafonium chloride (p.1187·1); phenol (p.1188·1).
*Burns; skin irritation; wounds.*
*Topical spray:* Triclosan (p.1195·2); dichlorophen (p.104·1).
*Skin disinfection.*
*Topical wipes:* Benzalkonium chloride (p.1168·3); chlorhexidine gluconate (p.1173·2).
*Skin disinfection.*

**Germolene First Aid** SmithKline Beecham Consumer, Irl.†.
Chlorhexidine gluconate (p.1173·2); phenol (p.1188·1).
*Skin disinfections.*

**Germoloids** Bayer Consumer, UK.
*Cream; ointment; suppositories:* Lidocaine hydrochloride (p.1377·3); zinc oxide (p.1163·2).
*Topical wipes:* Chlorhexidine gluconate (p.1173·2); benzalkonium chloride (p.1168·3); menthol (p.1711·3).
*Haemorrhoids.*

**Germoloids HC** Bayer Consumer, UK.
Hydrocortisone (p.1103·3); lidocaine hydrochloride (p.1377·3).
*Anorectal disorders.*

**Germose** Besins, Fr.
Sodium benzoate (p.1169·3); sulfogaiacol (p.1131·1); grindelia (p.1696·1); crataegus (p.1677·1); peppermint (p.1283·2); thyme (p.1755·2).
*Respiratory-tract congestion.*

**Germosept** Medipharm, Chile.
Benzalkonium chloride (p.1168·3).
*Disinfection of instruments and skin.*

**Germozero** Carlo Erba OTC, Ital.
Tosylchloramide sodium (p.1194·3).
*Skin disinfection.*

**Germozero Dermo** Carlo Erba OTC, Ital.
Benzalkonium chloride (p.1168·3); orthophenylphenol (p.1187·2); alkyl isoquinoline bromide.
*Wound disinfection.*

**Germozero Hospital** Carlo Erba OTC, Ital.†.
Chlorhexidine gluconate (p.1173·2); cetrimide (p.1172·1).
*Disinfection of wounds, external genitalia, surfaces, and instruments.*

**Germozero Plus** Carlo Erba OTC, Ital.
Benzalkonium chloride (p.1168·3); orthophenylphenol (p.1187·2).
*Wounds disinfection.*

**Gernebcin** Lilly, Ger.
Tobramycin sulfate (p.271·3).
*Bacterial infections.*

**Gernel** Gerbex, Canad.
Cresol (p.1177·3); zinc oxide (p.1163·2).

**Gero H3** Sedabel, Braz.
Multivitamins, amino acids, and minerals with erythroxylon catuaba and adenosine (p.1417·1).

**Gero H3 Aslan**
Phoenix, Arg.; Chefaro, Ger.
Procaine hydrochloride (p.1383·2); benzoic acid; potassium disulfite; sodium phosphate (p.1417·1).
*Tonic.*

**Geroaslan H3** Sanova, Austria.
Procaine hydrochloride (p.1383·2).
*Tonic.*

**Geroderm** Avantgarde, Ital.
Triclosan (p.1195·2).
*Skin cleansing.*

**Geroderm Zolfo** Avantgarde, Ital.
Sulfur (p.1158·2); lactic acid (p.1704·1); triclosan (p.1195·2).
*Skin cleansing in acne.*

**Gerodorm** Gerot, Austria.
Cinolazepam (p.683·1).
*Sleep disorders.*

**Geroforte** IMA, Braz.
Multivitamins with guarana and erythroxylon catuaba (p.1417·1).

**Gerogelat** Metochem, Austria.
Vitamin A palmitate (p.1453·1); tocoferil acetate (p.1465·1).
*Hearing loss; mucous membrane disorders; tinnitus; vitamin A and E deficiency.*

**Gerolin** CT, Ital.
Citicoline sodium (p.1672·3).
*Cerebrovascular disorders; parkinsonism.*

**Gerontamin** Heilit, Ger.†.
Gelatin (p.754·3); cystine (p.1426·3).
*Joint disorders.*

**Gerontex** Marjan, Braz.
Multivitamin, amino-acid, and mineral preparation (p.1417·1).

**Gerontin** Pharmonta, Austria.
Procaine hydrochloride (p.1383·2); caffeine (p.782·1).
*Tonic.*

**Geroplus** Pharmafina, Chile.
Co-dergocrine mesilate (p.1674·1).
*Mental function impairment.*

**Gerosenil** Delta, Braz.†.
Methyltestosterone (p.1559·3); alpha tocoferil acetate (p.1465·1); yohimbine (p.1766·2); caffeine (p.782·1); ephedrine (p.1120·1).
*Erectile dysfunction.*

**Geroten** Gerard, Irl.
Captopril (p.879·2).
*Heart failure; hypertension.*

**Gerotrex H3** Bunker, Braz.
Multivitamin, amino-acid, and mineral preparation (p.1417·1).

**Gerovital** EMS, Braz.
Ginseng; rutoside; vitamins; minerals (p.1417·1).
*Nutritional supplement.*

**Gerovital H3**
Sanova, Austria; Sicomed, Hong Kong.
Procaine hydrochloride (p.1383·2).
*Tonic.*

**Geroxalen**
Galderma, Denm.; Sanofi Synthelabo, Neth.; Galderma, Norw.
Methoxsalen (p.1152·1).
*Mycosis fungoides; psoriasis.*

**Geroxicam** Gerard, Irl.†.
Piroxicam (p.84·2).
*Dysmenorrhoea; gout; musculoskeletal and joint disorders.*

**Gerozac** Gerard, Irl.
Fluoxetine hydrochloride (p.292·1).
*Depression.*

**Gerskin**
YSP, Malaysia; Yung Shin, Singapore.
Magnesium oxide (p.1272·3); aluminium hydroxide (p.1249·2); simeticone (p.1289·2).
*Flatulence; gastric hyperacidity; gastritis; peptic ulcer.*

**Gertac** Gerard, Irl.
Ranitidine hydrochloride (p.1285·2).
*Gastro-oesophageal reflux; peptic ulcer; Zollinger-Ellison syndrome.*

**Gertalgin** Faran, Gr.
Omeprazole (p.1278·2).
*Acid aspiration; eradication of Helicobacter pylori in combination with antimicrobials; peptic ulcer; reflux oesophagitis; Zollinger-Ellison syndrome.*

**Gertemycin** Faran, Gr.
Cefatrizine (p.170·3) or cefatrizine propylene glycol (p.170·3).
*Bacterial infections.*

**Gertocalm** Faran, Gr.
Ranitidine hydrochloride (p.1285·2).
*Conditions where gastric acid reduction is beneficial; gastric hypersecretion including Zollinger-Ellison syndrome; peptic ulcer.*

**Gervaken** Kendrick, Mex.
Clarithromycin (p.192·2).
*Bacterial infections.*

**GES 45**
Milupa, Fr.; Milupa, Hong Kong†; Milupa, Singapore†; Milupa, Switz.
Oral rehydration solution (p.1222·2).
*Diarrhoea.*

**Gesamtnahrlosung** Fresenius Kabi, Austria.
A range of amino-acid, glucose, and lipid (from soya oil (p.1447·2)) infusions (p.1417·1).
Contains egg lecithin.
*Parenteral nutrition.*

**Gesicain** Sarabhai Piramal, India.
Lidocaine (p.1377·3) or lidocaine hydrochloride (p.1377·3).
Adrenaline (p.852·2) is included in some injections as a vasoconstrictor to diminish absorption and localise the effect of the local anaesthetic.
*Local anaesthesia.*

**Gesidine**
Pharmaserve Lilly (Φαρμασερβ Λιλλυ), Gr.; Lilly, Port.
Vindesine sulfate (p.593·3).
*Malignant neoplasms.*

**Gesiprox** Kalbe, Singapore.
Naproxen sodium (p.65·1).
*Gout; musculoskeletal and joint disorders; pain.*

**Geslutin** Asofarma, Mex.
Progesterone (p.1566·2).
*Benign breast disorders; dysfunctional uterine haemorrhage; female infertility; habitual or threatened miscarriage; menopausal disorders.*

**Gestadinona** Schering, Braz.
Hydroxyprogesterone caproate (p.1556·3); estradiol valerate (p.1550·2).
*Endometriosis; menopausal disorders; menstrual disorders.*

**Gestaferron** Arlex, Mex.†.
Ferrous fumarate (p.1427·3).

**Gestafortin** Merck, Ger.
Chlormadinone acetate (p.1542·1).
*Endometriosis; menstrual disorders.*

**Gestageno** Elea, Arg.
Hydroxyprogesterone acetate (p.1556·3).
*Female infertility; hypertrichosis; menstrual disorders; premature labour; threatened or recurrent miscarriage.*

**Gestakadin** Kade, Ger.
Norethisterone acetate (p.1562·2).
*Menopausal disorders; menstrual disorders.*

**Gestamater** Wyeth, Spain.
Multivitamin and mineral preparation (p.1417·1).

**Gestamestrol N** Hermal, Ger.
Chlormadinone acetate (p.1542·1); mestranol (p.1559·2).
*Androgen-dependent acne, alopecia, hirsutism, and seborrhoea in women.*

**Gestamine** Nadeau, Canad.†.
Multivitamin preparation with calcium and iron (p.1417·1).

**Gestanon** Organon, Mex.†.
Allylestrenol (p.1541·3).

**GestaPolar** Orion, Ger.†.
Medroxyprogesterone acetate (p.1557·2).

**Gestapuran**
Leo, Fin.; Leo, Swed.
Medroxyprogesterone acetate (p.1557·2).
*Endometriosis; menopausal disorders; menstrual disorders.*

**Gestarelle** IPRAD-Sante, Fr.
Multivitamin and mineral preparation (p.1417·1).

**Gestatest** Polychaco, Arg.
Pregnancy test (p.1734·3).

**Gestavit** Recalcine, Chile.
Multivitamin and mineral preparation (p.1417·1).

**Gester** Merck, Arg.
Progesterone (p.1566·2).
*Benign breast disorders; female infertility; menopausal disorders; menstrual disorders; threatened or recurrent miscarriage.*

**Gesterol** Germiphene, Canad.†.
Progesterone (p.1566·2).
*Progestogenic.*

**Gestid** Ranbaxy, Singapore.
*Oral suspension:* Aluminium hydroxide (p.1249·2); magnesium hydroxide (p.1272·2); simeticone (p.1289·2).
*Tablets:* Aluminium hydroxide (p.1249·2); magnesium trisilicate (p.1272·3); magnesium hydroxide (p.1272·2); simeticone (p.1289·2).
*Flatulence; gastric hyperacidity; gastritis; gastro-oesophageal reflux; peptic ulcer.*

**Gestiferrol** Wolfs, Belg.
Ferrous fumarate (p.1427·3); folic acid (p.1429·1).
*Anaemias; dietary supplement during pregnancy.*

**Gestinol** Libbs, Braz.
Gestodene (p.1556·1); ethinylestradiol (p.1553·2).
*Combined oral contraceptive.*

**Gestone**
Ferring, Israel; Paines & Byrne, NZ; Paines & Byrne, Thai.; Nordic, UK.
Progesterone (p.1566·2).
*Adjunct in infertility disorders; dysfunctional uterine bleeding; premenstrual syndrome; threatened or recurrent miscarriage.*

**Gestoral**
Novartis, Fr.; IFET (ΙΦΕΤ), Gr.
Medroxyprogesterone acetate (p.1557·2).
*Cancer of breast, kidney, and endometrium; contraception; endometriosis; menopausal disorders.*

**Gestrelan** Biolab Sanus, Braz.
Levonorgestrel (p.1563·2); ethinylestradiol (p.1553·2).
*Combined oral contraceptive.*

**Gets-It**
Note. This name is used for preparations of different composition.
Schering-Plough, Braz.
Salicylic acid (p.1157·1); balsamo FIR Oregon; betacarotene; acetone.
*Keratinisation disorders.*

Oakhurst, USA.
Salicylic acid (p.1157·1); zinc chloride (p.1469·2).
*Hyperkeratosis.*

**Getup** Rafarm, Gr.
Bezafibrate (p.873·2).
*Hyperlipidaemias.*

**Gevatran** Lipha Sante, Fr.
Naftidrofuryl oxalate (p.964·1).
*Peripheral and cerebral vascular disorders.*

**Gevilon**
Pfizer, Austria; Orion, Fin.; Parke, Davis, Ger.; Pfizer, Switz.
Gemfibrozil (p.923·1).
*Hyperlipidaemias.*

**Gevirol** Gerbex, Canad.
Multivitamin and mineral preparation (p.1417·1).

**Gevrabon** Lederle, USA.
Vitamin B substances with minerals (p.1417·1).

**Gevral**
Whitehall, Braz.; Cyanamid, Ital.†; Whitehall, S.Afr.†; Lederle, USA.
Multivitamin and mineral preparation (p.1417·1).

**Gevral Instant Protein**
Whitehall, Irl.; Whitehall-Robins, Switz.
Multivitamin, mineral, and protein preparation (p.1417·1).
*Tonic.*

**Gevral Protein** Lederle, USA.
Dietary protein supplement (p.1417·1).

**Gevral Proteina**
Wyeth, Mex.; Wyeth, Spain†.
Protein, vitamin, and mineral preparation (p.1417·1).
*Nutritional supplement.*

**Gevral T** Lederle, USA.
Ferrous fumarate (p.1427·3); folic acid (p.1429·1); multivitamins and minerals (p.1417·1).
*Iron-deficiency anaemias.*

**Gevral Tablets** Whitehall, Irl.†.
Multivitamin and mineral preparation (p.1417·1).

**Gevramycin** Schering-Plough, Spain.
Gentamicin sulfate (p.217·1).
*Bacterial infections.*

**Gevramycin Topica** Schering-Plough, Spain.
Gentamicin sulfate (p.217·1).
*Bacterial skin infections; ulcers.*

**Gewacalm** Nycomed, Austria.
Diazepam (p.690·1).
*Anxiety disorders; eclampsia; neuroses; panic attacks; phobias; premedication; skeletal muscle spasm; sleep disorders; status epilepticus.*

**Gewacyclin** Nycomed, Austria.
Doxycycline hyclate (p.206·2).
*Bacterial infections.*

**Gewadal** Nycomed, Austria.
Paracetamol (p.76·2); propyphenazone (p.85·3); caffeine (p.782·1).
*Fever; pain.*

**Gewaglucon** Nycomed, Austria.
Glibenclamide (p.331·2).
*Diabetes mellitus.*

**Gewamol** Nycomed, Austria.
Paracetamol (p.76·2).
*Fever; pain.*

**Gewapurol** Pharmaselect, Austria.
Allopurinol (p.412·2).
*Gout; hyperuricaemia; renal calculi.*

**Gewazem** Nycomed, Austria.
Diltiazem hydrochloride (p.900·1).
*Angina pectoris.*

**Gewodin** Gewo, Ger.†.
Famprofazone (p.38·3); paracetamol (p.76·2); propyphenazone (p.85·3); caffeine (p.782·1).
*Pain.*

**Gewodine** Geistlich, Switz.
Paracetamol (p.76·2); caffeine (p.782·1); propyphenazone (p.85·3).
*Fever; pain.*

**Gewusst wie Darmtee** Kottas-Heldenberg, Austria.
Mallow leaf (p.1709·3); fennel (p.1687·2); achillea (p.1646·2); peppermint leaf (p.1283·2); taraxacum (p.1751·3); calendula (p.1665·2).
*Gastrointestinal disorders.*

**Gewusst wie Entschlackungstee** Kottas-Heldenberg, Austria.
Viola tricolor; java tea (p.1702·3); taraxacum (p.1751·3); peppermint leaf (p.1283·2); ononis (p.1723·3).
*Diuretic.*

**Gewusst wie Gruner Fastentee** Kottas-Heldenberg, Austria.
Rose fruit (p.1740·1); taraxacum (p.1751·3); urtica (p.1762·1); maté (p.1765·3); fennel (p.1687·2); bellis perennis.
*Gastrointestinal and renal disorders.*

**Gewusst wie Husten-Bronchialtee** Kottas-Heldenberg, Austria.
Plantago lanceolata (p.1738·2); thyme (p.1755·2); althaea (p.1651·3); tilia (p.1756·2); aniseed (p.1655·2); eucalyptus (p.1686·1).
*Catarrh; coughs; sore throat.*

**Gewusst wie Leber-Gallentee** Kottas-Heldenberg, Austria.
Fennel (p.1687·2); peppermint leaf (p.1283·2); taraxacum (p.1751·3); centaury (p.1669·2); calendula (p.1665·2).
*Liver and biliary-tract disorders.*

**Gewusst wie Magentee mild** Kottas-Heldenberg, Austria.
Mallow leaf (p.1709·3); chamomile (p.1669·3); peppermint leaf (p.1283·2); calendula (p.1665·2).
*Gastrointestinal disorders.*

**Gewusst wie Nerven-Schlaftee** Kottas-Heldenberg, Austria.
Valerian (p.1762·2); melissa (p.1711·1); mallow leaf (p.1709·3); chamomile (p.1669·3); orange flower (p.1723·3).
*Nervous disorders; sleep disorders.*

**Geyderm** Geymonat, Ital.†.
Benzalkonium chloride (p.1168·3).
*Disinfection of mucous membranes, wounds, burns, surfaces, and instruments.*

**Geyderm Sepsi** Geymonat, Ital.†.
Cetylpyridinium chloride (p.1173·1).
*Disinfection of wounds and burns.*

**Geyfritz** Geymonat, Ital.
Aspirin (p.15·1); caffeine (p.782·1).
Glycine (p.1433·3) is included in this preparation in an attempt to limit adverse effects on the gastrointestinal mucosa.
*Cold symptoms; pain.*

**Gezon** Laborsil, Braz.†.
Diclofenac potassium (p.32·1).
*Gout; inflammation; musculoskeletal, joint, and periarticular disorders; pain.*

**G-Farlutal** Pharmacia, Ger.
Medroxyprogesterone acetate (p.1557·2).
*Menstrual disorders; test of ovarian function.*

**G-Fen** General Drugs, Thai.
Ibuprofen (p.45·3).
*Fever; inflammation; pain.*

**GFN Phenylephrine** Cypress, USA.
Guaifenesin (p.1122·1); phenylephrine hydrochloride (p.1126·3).
*Coughs; rhinitis; sinusitis.*

**GFN PSE DM** Cypress, USA.
Guaifenesin (p.1122·1); pseudoephedrine hydrochloride (p.1129·2); dextromethorphan hydrobromide (p.1117·3).
*Coughs; nasal congestion.*

**GFN/DM** Cypress, USA.
Guaifenesin (p.1122·1); dextromethorphan hydrobromide (p.1117·3).
*Coughs.*

**GFN/DM/PE** Cypress, USA.
Guaifenesin (p.1122·1); dextromethorphan hydrobromide (p.1117·3); phenylephrine hydrochloride (p.1126·3).
*Coughs; nasal congestion.*

**GFN/PSE** Cypress, USA.
Guaifenesin (p.1122·1); pseudoephedrine hydrochloride (p.1129·2).
*Coughs; nasal congestion.*

**GHRH**
Ferring, Belg.; Ferring, Ger.; Ferring, Ital.; Ferring, Neth.; Ferring, UK.
Somatorelin acetate (p.1339·2).
*Diagnosis of growth hormone deficiency.*

**GI**
Note. This name is used for preparations of different composition.
Sankyo, Hong Kong†.
Taka-diastase (p.1654·2); lipase; aluminium magnesium silicate (p.1577·1); hydrotalcite (p.1267·3); sodium bicarbonate (p.1223·2); calcium carbonate (p.1254·2); scopolia; cinnamon (p.1672·2); fennel (p.1687·2); ginger (p.1267·1); menthol (p.1711·3); liquorice (p.1270·2); clove (p.1673·2); phellodendron.
*Gastrointestinal disorders.*

Provit, Mex.
Gentamicin sulfate (p.217·1).
*Bacterial infections.*

**Giamebil** Hebron, Braz.
Spearmint (p.1749·1).
*Smooth muscle spasm.*

**Gianda** Grunenthal, Ger.
12 Capsules, estradiol valerate (p.1550·2); 14 capsules, estradiol valerate; medroxyprogesterone acetate (p.1557·2).
*Menopausal disorders.*

**Giarcid** Teuto, Braz.
Furazolidone (p.605·2).

**Giardil** Phoenix, Arg.
Furazolidone (p.605·2).
*Giardiasis.*

**Giarlam** UCI, Braz.
Furazolidone (p.605·2).
*Cholera; diarrhoea; giardiasis.*

**Gibicef** Metapharma, Ital.†.
Cefuroxime sodium (p.184·1).
*Bacterial infections.*

**Gibifer** Metapharma, Ital.†.
Sodium ferric gluconate complex (p.1444·3).
*Iron-deficiency anaemias.*

**Gibiflu** Metapharma, Ital.
Flunisolide (p.1101·1).
*Rhinitis.*

**Gibilon** Delta, Braz.
Ginkgo biloba (p.1692·3).

**Gibinap** Metapharma, Ital.†.
Naproxen sodium (p.65·1).
Lidocaine hydrochloride (p.1377·3) is included in the intramuscular injection to alleviate the pain of injection.
*Musculoskeletal and joint disorders; pain.*

**Gibixen** *Metapharma, Ital.*
Naproxen (p.65·1).
*Musculoskeletal and joint disorders; pain.*

**Gichtex** *Gerot, Austria.*
Allopurinol (p.412·2).
*Gout; hyperuricaemia; renal calculi.*

**Gichtex plus** *Gerot, Austria.*
Allopurinol (p.412·2); benzbromarone (p.414·3).
*Gout; hyperuricaemia.*

**Giflorex** *Errekappa, Ital.*
*Lactobacillus casei* var *rhamnosus* (p.1704·2); maltodextrin (p.1439·3); fructose (p.1431·3).
*Maintenance of gastrointestinal flora.*

**Gigasept** *Schulke & Mayr, Ger.†.*
Succinic dialdehyde (p.1180·2); dimethoxytetrahydrofuran; formaldehyde (p.1179·3).
*Instrument disinfection.*

**Gigasept AF** *Schulke & Mayr, Ger.†.*
Didecyldimethylammonium chloride (p.1178·3); phenoxypropanol (p.1189·1); aminoalkylglycine.
*Instrument disinfection.*

**Gigasept FF** *Schulke & Mayr, Ger.†.*
Succinic dialdehyde (p.1180·2); dimethoxytetrahydrofuran.
*Instrument disinfection.*

**Gigasept Med** *Schulke & Mayr, Ger.*
Didecyldimethylammonium chloride (p.1178·3); phenoxypropanol (p.1189·1); aminoalkylglycine.
*Instrument disinfection.*

**Gigatrom** *Baldacci, Port.*
Azithromycin (p.159·1).
*Bacterial infections.*

**Gilemal** *Enzypharm, Austria.*
Glibenclamide (p.331·2).
*Diabetes mellitus.*

**Gilex** *Rekah, Israel.*
Doxepin hydrochloride (p.291·2).
*Depression; mixed anxiety depressive states.*

**Gillazyme** *Sandoz OTC, Switz.†.*
Pancreatin (p.1725·3); dehydrocholic acid (p.1679·2); dimethicone (p.1289·2).
*Digestive-system disorders.*

**Gillazyme plus** *Sandoz OTC, Switz.†.*
Pancreatin (p.1725·3); dehydrocholic acid (p.1679·2); dimethicone (p.1289·2); metixene hydrochloride (p.485·3).
*Digestive-system disorders.*

**Gilt** *Lacoer, Ger.*
Clotrimazole (p.396·2).
*Fungal skin infections.*

**Gilucor** *Solvay, Ger.*
Sotalol hydrochloride (p.1001·3).
*Arrhythmias.*

**Giludop**
*Solvay, Denm.; Solvay, Gr.; Solvay, Swed.*
Dopamine hydrochloride (p.907·1).
*Shock.*

**Gilurytmal**
*Solvay, Austria; Solvay, Ger.; Lacer, Spain†.*
Ajmaline (p.856·1).
*Arrhythmias.*

**Gilustenon** *Solvay, Ger.†.*
Glyceryl trinitrate (p.923·2).
*Angina pectoris; heart failure.*

**Gimabrol** *Collins, Mex.*
Amoxicillin (p.155·3); ambroxol (p.1114·3).
*Respiratory-tract infections.*

**Gimalxina** *Collins, Mex.*
Amoxicillin trihydrate (p.155·3).
*Bacterial infections.*

**Gin Pain** *Stella, Canad.*
Paracetamol (p.76·2); chlorzoxazone (p.1392·3).

**Ginal Cent** *Beta, Arg.*
Metronidazole (p.607·2); miconazole nitrate (p.405·3); neomycin sulfate (p.235·1); centella (p.1144·3); polymyxin B sulfate (p.245·1).
*Vulvovaginal infections.*

**Ginal Gel** *Beta, Arg.*
Vaginal moisturiser.
*Vaginal dryness.*

**Ginarsan** *Elvetium, Arg.*
Tamoxifen citrate (p.584·1).

**Ginatex** *Baliarda, Arg.*
Estradiol (p.1550·1).
*Menopausal disorders.*

**Ginatren** *LPB, Ital.†.*
A trichomonal vaccine containing *Lactobacillus acidophilus* (p.1642·1).
*Vaginitis.*

**Ginbiloba** *Bunker, Braz.*
Ginkgo biloba (p.1692·3).
*Vascular disorders.*

**Gincaps** *Medix, Mex.*
Ginseng (p.1693·1).
*Tonic.*

**Gincare**
*YSP, Malaysia; Yung Shin, Singapore.*
Ginkgo biloba (p.1692·3).
*Peripheral vascular disorders.*

**Gincoben** *Ipsen, Port.*
Ginkgo biloba (p.1692·3).
*Cerebral and peripheral vascular disorders; vestibular disorders.*

**Gincola** *Biocontrolfarm, Ital.†.*
Ginseng (p.1693·1); kola (p.1765·3).

**Gincolin** *Teuto, Braz.*
Ginkgo biloba (p.1692·3).

**Ginconazol** *Hebron, Braz.*
Terconazole (p.409·3).
*Fungal vaginal infections.*

**Gincosan**
*Boehringer Ingelheim, Chile; Pharmaton, Switz.*
Ginkgo biloba (p.1692·3); ginseng (p.1693·1).
*Mental function impairment.*

**Gine Canesten** *Bayer, Spain.*
Clotrimazole (p.396·2).
*Balanitis; vulvovaginal candidiasis.*

**Gine Heyden** *Squibb, Spain.*
Amphotericin B (p.391·2); tetracycline hydrochloride (p.266·2).
*Vulvovaginal infections.*

**Gine Zalain** *Robert, Spain†.*
Sertaconazole nitrate (p.408·1).
*Vulvovaginal candidiasis.*

**Gineburno** *Dovalle, Braz.*
Estrone (p.1553·1); aminophenazone (p.14·2); viburnum prunifolium.
*Dysmenorrhoea.*

**Ginec** *Klinger, Braz.*
Neomycin sulfate (p.235·1); polymyxin B sulfate (p.245·1); nystatin (p.406·3); tinidazole (p.617·1).

**Ginecofuran** *Crosara, Ital.†.*
Nifuroxime (p.406·3); furazolidone (p.605·2).
*Vaginitis.*

**Ginecopast** *Pasteur, Chile.*
Miconazole nitrate (p.405·3); tinidazole (p.617·1).
*Fungal balanitis; vulvovaginal infections.*

**Ginecoside** *Darrow, Braz.*
*Injection:* Progesterone (p.1566·2); estradiol (p.1550·1).
*Tablets:* Normethandrone; methyloestradiol (p.1551·1).
*Menopausal disorders.*

**Ginecrin** *Abbott, Spain.*
Leuprorelin acetate (p.1331·1).
*Endometriosis; female infertility; precocious puberty; prostatic cancer; uterine fibroma.*

**Ginedak** *Organon, Braz.*
Miconazole nitrate (p.405·3).
*Vulvovaginal candidiasis.*

**Ginedazol Dual** *Laboratorios Chile, Chile.*
Tinidazole (p.617·1); miconazole nitrate (p.405·3).
*Vulvovaginal infections.*

**Ginedermofix** *Ferrer, Spain.*
Sertaconazole nitrate (p.408·1).
*Vulvovaginal candidiasis.*

**Ginedisc**
*Schering, Braz.; Schering, Mex.*
Estradiol (p.1550·1).
*Menopausal disorders; osteoporosis.*

**Ginedisc 50 Plus** *Schering, Braz.*
Patch 1, estradiol (p.1550·1); patch 2, estradiol; norethisterone acetate (p.1562·2).
*Menopausal disorders.*

**Gineflor** *Medestea, Ital.*
Ibuprofen isobutanolammonium (p.46·3).
*Gynaecological disorders.*

**Ginejuvent** *Juventus, Spain.*
Benzalkonium chloride (p.1168·3); calcium lactate (p.1225·3); lactic acid (p.1704·1); chamomile (p.1669·3).
*Vulvovaginal candidiasis; vulvovaginal trichomoniasis.*

**Ginelea** *Elea, Arg.*
Gestodene (p.1556·1); ethinylestradiol (p.1553·2).
*Combined oral contraceptive.*

**Ginelea T** *Elea, Arg.*
Gestodene (p.1556·1); ethinylestradiol (p.1553·2).
*Triphasic oral contraceptive.*

**Ginemaxim** *Knop, Chile.*
Cimicifuga (p.1671·3).
*Menopausal disorders; menstrual disorders; osteoporosis.*

**Ginenorm** *Aesculapius, Ital.*
Ibuprofen isobutanolammonium (p.46·3).
*Gynaecological inflammatory disorders.*

**Ginesal** *Farmigea, Ital.*
Benzydamine hydrochloride (p.21·1).
*Gynaecological disorders; vaginal hygiene.*

**Gineseptina** *Lafage, Arg.*
Zinc phenolsulfonate (p.1163·3); tyrothricin (p.275·1); borax (p.1661·3); aluminium sulfate (p.1653·1).

**Ginesse** *Farmoquimica, Braz.*
Gestodene (p.1556·1); ethinylestradiol (p.1553·2).
*Combined oral contraceptive.*

**Ginestatin** *Organon, Braz.*
Metronidazole (p.607·2); nystatin (p.406·3); benzalkonium chloride (p.1168·3).
Formerly contained metronidazole and benzalkonium chloride.
*Vulvovaginal infections.*

**Ginetris** *Pharmacia, Hong Kong.*
Chloramphenicol (p.185·1); myralact (p.1186·3); clopoxone (p.1177·3).
*Vaginal disorders.*

**Ginevit** *Gambar, Ital.*
Vitamin and mineral preparations (p.1417·1).
*Menopausal disorders; menstrual disorders.*

**Ginex** *Raza, Malaysia; Pharmaniaga, Malaysia.*
Selegiline hydrochloride (p.1214·1).
*Parkinsonism.*

**Ginexin-F** *SK, Singapore.*
Ginkgo biloba (p.1692·3).
*Organic brain disorders; peripheral vascular disorders; tinnitus; vertigo.*

**Gingeron** *Baliarda, Arg.*
Ginseng; magnesium glycerophosphate; procaine hydrochloride (p.1383·2); zinc; copper; cobalt; manganese (p.1417·1).
*Tonic.*

**Gingicain D** *Aventis, Ger.*
Tetracaine (p.1385·1); benzalkonium chloride (p.1168·3).
*Local anaesthesia; skin disinfection.*

**Gingilacer** *Andromaco, Chile.*
*Mouthwash:* Triclosan (p.1195·2); zinc chloride (p.1469·2).
*Dental caries prophylaxis; dental hygiene.*
*Toothpaste:* Triclosan (p.1195·2); zinc citrate; enoxolone (p.36·2); sodium monofluorophosphate (p.1446·2).
*Dental caries prophylaxis.*

**Gingiloba** *1A, Ger.*
Ginkgo biloba (p.1692·3).
*Dizziness; mental function disorders; peripheral vascular disorders; tinnitus.*

**Gingilone**
Note. This name is used for preparations of different composition.
*Farmasa, Braz.*
Hydrocortisone acetate (p.1103·3); neomycin sulfate (p.235·1); troxerutin (p.1688·3); ascorbic acid (p.1460·2); benzocaine (p.1370·3).
*Mouth disorders.*
*Teofarma, Spain.*
Ascorbic acid (p.1460·2); cortisone acetate (p.1096·1); neomycin sulfate (p.235·1); rutoside (p.1688·2).
*Bleeding gums; mouth ulcers; stomatitis.*

**Gingi-Pak** *Gingi-Pak, Switz.†.*
A range of threads and tampons impregnated with adrenaline hydrochloride (p.852·3).
*Dental haemorrhage.*

**Gingisan** *Teva, Israel.*
*Mouthwash:* Chamomile (p.1669·3); eucalyptus (p.1686·1); liquorice (p.1270·2).
*Ointment:* Chamomile (p.1669·3); eucalyptus (p.1686·1); liquorice (p.1270·2); benzocaine (p.1370·3).
*Mouth disorders.*

**Gingium** *Biocur, Ger.*
Ginkgo biloba (p.1692·3).
*Dizziness; mental function disorders; peripheral vascular disorders; tinnitus.*

**Gingivan** *Provita, Austria.*
Tyrothricin (p.275·1); thymol (p.1194·2); pancreatin (p.1725·3) lauromacrogol 400 (p.1412·3).
*Mouth disorders.*

**Gingivitol N** *Hennig, Ger.*
Hydrastis (p.1698·3).
*Inflammatory disorders of the mouth.*

**Gingo A** *Eagle, Austral.†.*
Ginkgo biloba (p.1692·3); crataegus (p.1677·1); eleutherococcus senticosis (p.1744·1); liquorice (p.1270·2); choline bitartrate (p.1424·3); cayenne (p.1667·1); nicotinic acid (p.1441·1); potassium phosphate (p.1230·3).

**Gingobeta** *Betapharm, Ger.*
Ginkgo biloba (p.1692·3).
*Dizziness; headache; mental function disorders; peripheral vascular disorders; tinnitus.*

**Gingohexal** *Hexal, Austria.*
Ginkgo biloba (p.1692·3).
*Cerebral and peripheral vascular disorders; cervical syndrome.*

**Gingol** *Hexal, Austria.*
Ginkgo biloba (p.1692·3).
*Cerebral and peripheral vascular disorders; cervical syndrome.*

**Gingopret** *Bionorica, Ger.*
Ginkgo biloba (p.1692·3).
*Headache; mental function disorders; peripheral vascular disorders; tinnitus; vertigo.*

**Gingosol** *Ecosol, Switz.*
Ginkgo biloba (p.1692·3).
*Mental function impairment.*

**Gingo-Ther** *Laboratorios Chile, Chile.*
Ginkgo biloba (p.1692·3); eleutherococcus senticosis (p.1744·1); myrtillus (p.1718·3).
*Cerebral and peripheral vascular disorders.*

**Gingviton** *Sam Chun Dang, Singapore.*
Multivitamin and mineral preparation with ginseng and lecithin (p.1417·1).

**Ginil** *Wassen, Ital.*
*Topical liquid:* Soya (p.1447·2); mimosa tenuiflora.
*Vaginal tablets: Lactobacillus acidophilus* (p.1704·2); lactic acid (p.1704·1).

**Ginkan** *Baliarda, Arg.*
*Pessaries:* Metronidazole (p.607·2); miconazole nitrate (p.405·3); neomycin sulfate (p.235·1); polymyxin B sulfate (p.245·1); centella (p.1144·3).
*Vaginal infections.*
*Tablets:* Metronidazole (p.607·2).
*Anaerobic bacterial infections; protozoal infections.*

**Ginkapran** *Yungjin, Singapore.*
Ginkgo biloba (p.1692·3).
*Cerebral disorders; peripheral vascular disorders.*

**Ginkgo biloba comp** *Hevert, Ger.*
Homoeopathic preparation.

**Ginkgo Biloba Plus** *Eagle, Austral.†.*
Ginkgo biloba (p.1692·3); crataegus (p.1677·1); eleutherococcus senticosis (p.1744·1); ginseng (p.1693·1).
*Peripheral circulatory disorders; tinnitus.*

**Ginkgo Complex** *Blackmores, Austral.†.*
Ginkgo biloba (p.1692·3); crataegus (p.1677·1); ginseng (p.1693·1); *d*-alpha tocoferil acid succinate (p.1465·1).
*Cerebral and peripheral vascular disorders.*

**Ginkgo Plus** *Biohorma, Ital.†.*
Hamamelis (p.1696·3); aesculus (p.1648·2); ginkgo biloba (p.1692·3); cupressus sempervirens.
*Peripheral vascular disorders.*

**Ginkgo Plus Herbal Plus Formula 10** *Vitelle, Austral.†.*
Ginkgo biloba (p.1692·3); ginger (p.1267·1); potassium phosphate (p.1230·3); magnesium oxide (p.1272·3).
*Peripheral vascular disorders.*

**Ginkgo Plus Vivo-Livo** *Panpharma, Hong Kong.*
Ginkgo biloba (p.1692·3); crataegus (p.1677·1); garlic (p.1691·1).
*Peripheral and cerebral circulatory disorders.*

**Ginkgobakehl** *Sanum-Kehlbeck, Ger.*
Homoeopathic preparation.

**Ginkgoforce** *Weber & Weber, Ger.*
Homoeopathic preparation.

**Ginkgo-PS** *Usana, Hong Kong.*
Ginkgo biloba (p.1692·3); lecithin (p.1706·1).
*Mental function disorders.*

**Ginkgorell** *Sanorell, Ger.*
Homoeopathic preparation.

**Ginkoba**
*Nikkho, Braz.; Fher, Ital.; Pharmaton, Switz.†.*
Ginkgo biloba (p.1692·3).
*Mental function disorders; vascular disorders.*

**Ginkoba M/E** *Quest, Canad.*
Ginseng (p.1693·1); ginkgo biloba (p.1692·3).

**Ginkobil**
*Infabra, Braz.†; Ratiopharm, Ger.*
Ginkgo biloba (p.1692·3).
*Headache; mental function disorders; peripheral vascular disorders; tinnitus; vertigo.*

**Ginkocer** *Ranbaxy, Malaysia.*
Ginkgo biloba (p.1692·3).
*Peripheral circulation disorders.*

**Ginkodilat** *Azupharma, Ger.*
Ginkgo biloba (p.1692·3).
*Headache; intermittent claudication; mental function disorders; tinnitus; vertigo.*

**Ginkoftal** *Tubilux, Ital.*
Bioflavonoids (p.1688·2); ginkgo biloba (p.1692·3).
*Eye disorders; nutritional supplement.*

**Ginkogink** *URPAC, Fr.*
Ginkgo biloba (p.1692·3).
*Mental function impairment in the elderly; peripheral and cerebral vascular disorders; vertigo.*

**Ginkoplus** *Fontovit, Braz.*
Ginkgo biloba (p.1692·3).
*Vascular disorders.*

**Ginkopur** *Spitzner, Ger.*
Ginkgo biloba (p.1692·3).
*Dizziness; headache; intermittent claudication; mental function disorders; tinnitus.*

**Ginkor** *Beaufour, Fr.*
Ginkgo biloba (p.1692·3); troxerutin (p.1688·3).
*Peripheral vascular disorders.*

**Ginkor Fort**
*Beaufour, Fr.; Beaufour-Ipsen, Hong Kong; Beaufour-Ipsen, Malaysia; Emerging Pharma, Malaysia.*
Ginkgo biloba (p.1692·3); heptaminol hydrochloride (p.1697·1); troxerutin (p.1688·3).
*Haemorrhoids; venous insufficiency.*
*Beaufour-Ipsen, Thai.*
Ginkgo biloba (p.1692·3); heptaminol (p.1697·1); troxerutin (p.1688·3).
*Haemorrhoids; venous insufficiency.*

**Ginkoret** *Tubilux, Ital.*
Ginkgo biloba (p.1692·3); vitamins; lutein (p.1417·1).
*Circulatory disorders.*

**Ginkosen** *Tai Guk, Singapore.*
Ginkgo biloba (p.1692·3).
*Circulatory disorders.*

**Ginkovital** *Pharmadass, UK.*
Ginkgo biloba (p.1692·3).

**Gino Clotrimix** *Eversil, Braz.*
Clotrimazole (p.396·2).
*Vulvovaginal candidiasis.*

**Gino Conazol** *Kinder, Braz.*
Tioconazole (p.409·3).

**Gino Loprox** *Aventis, Braz.*
Ciclopirox olamine (p.396·1).
*Vulvovaginal candidiasis.*

**Gino Monipax** *Haller, Braz.*
Isoconazole nitrate (p.401·3).
*Vaginal infections.*

**Gino Pletil** *Searle, Braz.*
Tinidazole (p.617·1); miconazole nitrate (p.405·3).
*Vulvovaginal infections.*

**Gino Tralen** *Pfizer, Braz.*
Tioconazole (p.409·3).
*Vulvovaginal candidiasis.*

**Gino-Canesten** *Bayer, Braz.; Bayer, Port.*
Clotrimazole (p.396·2).
*Vaginal infections.*

**Ginocap** *Biocontrolfarm, Ital.†.*
Bearberry (p.1659·2).

**Gino-Cauterex** *Ache, Braz.*
Fibrinolysin (p.916·2); dornase alfa (p.1119·1); gentamicin sulfate (p.217·1).
Formerly contained fibrinolysin (human), dornase alfa, and chloramphenicol.
*Vulvovaginal infections.*

**Ginoday** *Biocontrolfarm, Ital.†.*
Birch (p.1660·3); alga clorella.

**Ginoden** *Schering, Ital.*
Gestodene (p.1556·1); ethinylestradiol (p.1553·2).
*Combined oral contraceptive.*

**Ginoderm** *Osteolab, Chile.*
Estradiol (p.1550·1).

**Gino-Fibrase** *Ache, Braz.*
Fibrinolysin (p.916·2); dornase alfa (p.1119·1); chloramphenicol (p.185·1).
*Vulvovaginal infections.*

**Ginoflorax** *Hebron, Braz.*
*Saccharomyces cerevisiae* (p.1469·1).
*Diarrhoea; restoration of gastrointestinal flora.*

**Ginolax** *Biocontrolfarm, Ital.†.*
Psyllium seed (p.1268·1); frangula (p.1266·3).

**Gino-Lotremine** *Schering-Plough, Port.*
Clotrimazole (p.396·2).

**Ginomains** *Gandhour, Fr.†.*
Emollient.
*Dry skin disorders.*

**Ginometrim** *Nikkho, Braz.†.*
Tinidazole (p.617·1); nystatin (p.406·3); gentamicin (p.219·1); benzalkonium chloride (p.1168·3).
*Vulvovaginal infections.*

**Ginometrim Oral** *Nikkho, Braz.*
Tinidazole (p.617·1); mepyramine maleate (p.437·1).
*Protozoal infections.*

**Ginomineral** *Biocontrolfarm, Ital.†.*
Mineral preparation (p.1417·1).
*Nutritional supplement.*

**Ginomizol** *Tocogino, Mex.†.*
Astemizole (p.424·2).

**Gino-Panflogin** *Farmion, Braz.†.*
Benzydamine hydrochloride (p.21·1).

**Ginopil** *Biocontrolfarm, Ital.†.*
Pilosella.

**Ginoplan** *Carnot, Mex.*
Algestone (p.1541·3); estradiol (p.1550·1).
*Injectable contraceptive.*

**Ginorectol** *Kleva, Gr.*
Ciprofloxacin hydrochloride (p.188·2).
*Bacterial infections.*

**Ginosutin** *Organon, Braz.*
Tinidazole (p.617·1).
*Vulvovaginal infections.*

**Ginosutin M** *Organon, Braz.*
Tinidazole (p.617·1); miconazole nitrate (p.405·3).
*Vulvovaginal infections.*

**Ginotarin** *Bunker, Braz.*
Miconazole nitrate (p.405·3).
*Fungal skin infections.*

**Gino-Teracin** *Neo Quimica, Braz.*
Tetracycline hydrochloride (p.266·2); amphotericin B (p.391·2).
*Vaginal infections.*

**Gino-Travogen** *Schering, Port.*
Isoconazole nitrate (p.401·3).
*Vulvovaginal infections.*

**Ginotrax** *Ativus, Braz.*
Isoconazole nitrate (p.401·3).
*Fungal infections.*

**Gino-Trosyd** *Pfizer, Port.*
Tioconazole (p.409·3).
*Fungal vaginal infections.*

**Ginovagin** *Neo Quimica, Braz.†.*
Metronidazole (p.607·2).
*Vaginal infections.*

**Ginoven** *Biocontrolfarm, Ital.†.*
Aesculus (p.1648·2).

**Ginoxil** *RDC, Ital.*
Urea hydrogen peroxide (p.1195·3).
*Vaginal disorders; vaginal hygiene.*

**Ginoxil Ecoschiuma** *Euroderm-RDC, Ital.*
Hamamelis (p.1696·3); aloe vera (p.1141·3); allantoin (p.1141·3).
*Personal hygiene.*

**Ginroy** *Medisculab, Ger.†.*
Ginseng (p.1693·1).
*Tonic.*

**Ginsactiv** *Azevedos, Port.*
Nutritional supplement (p.1417·1).

**Ginsana**
*Boehringer Ingelheim, Arg.; Boehringer Ingelheim, Austria; Boehringer Ingelheim, Belg.; Boehringer de Angeli, Braz.; Boehringer Ingelheim Consumer, Canad.; Boehringer Ingelheim, Fr.; Pharmaton, Ger.; Fher, Ital.; Pharmaton, Malaysia; Boehringer Ingelheim, Port.; Boehringer Ingelheim, S.Afr.†; Pharmaton, Singapore; Fher, Spain; GPL, Switz.; Boehringer Ingelheim, Thai.*
Ginseng (p.1693·1).
*Tonic.*

**Ginsana Ton** *Fher, Ital.*
Ginseng (p.1693·1); zinc (p.1469·2).
*Tonic.*

**Ginsatonic** *Arkopharma, Fr.†.*
Ginseng (p.1693·1).
*Tonic.*

**Ginsavit** *Julphar, UAE.*
Multivitamin and mineral preparation with ginseng (p.1417·1).

**Ginseng Med Complex** *Dynamit, Austria.*
Homoeopathic preparation.

**Ginseng-Complex "Schuh"** *Coradol, Ger.*
Panax ginseng (p.1693·1); chlorophyllin (p.1057·1); crataegus (p.1677·1).
*Tonic.*

**GinsengSure** *Abbott, Hong Kong.*
Preparation for enteral nutrition with ginseng (p.1693·1) (p.1417·1).

**Ginsex** *Delta, Braz.*
Ginseng (p.1693·1).
*Tonic.*

**Ginsroy** *Schumit, Thai.*
Ginseng (p.1693·1).
*Tonic.*

**Gintonal** *Biocom, Fr.*
Ginseng (p.1693·1); royal jelly (p.1740·3).
*Tonic.*

**Ginurovac** *Nikkho, Braz.*
Ampoule 1, procaine benzylpenicillin (p.246·1); benzylpenicillin potassium (p.163·2); ampoule 2, aminocaproic acid (p.741·3); antigens from *Neisseria gonorrhoea, Escherichia coli, Staphylococcus aureus, Streptococcus pyogenes, Proteus vulgaris,* and *Pseudomonas aeruginosa.*
*Bacterial infections.*

**Ginvapast**
*Note. This name is used for preparations of different composition.*
*Ogna, Ital.*
Calcium gluconate (p.1225·2); procaine hydrochloride (p.1383·2); cetylpyridinium chloride (p.1173·1).
*Gum disorders; skin ulcers.*

*Wild, Switz.*
Calcium gluconate (p.1225·2); procaine hydrochloride (p.1383·2); vitamins A and D (p.1417·1).
*Gum disorders.*

**Ginzing** *Vitaglow, Austral.†.*
Ginseng (p.1693·1).
*Tonic.*

**Ginzing E** *Vitaglow, Austral.†.*
Ginseng (p.1693·1); *d*-alpha tocopherol (p.1464·3).
*Tonic.*

**Ginzing G** *Vitaglow, Austral.†.*
Ginseng (p.1693·1); ginkgo biloba (p.1692·3).
*Tonic.*

**Gipzide** *Sriprasit, Thai.*
Glipizide (p.332·2).
*Diabetes mellitus.*

**Girha "Schuh"** *Coradol, Ger.*
Homoeopathic preparation.

**Girheulit HM** *Pfluger, Ger.*
Homoeopathic preparation.

**Giroflox** *Tecnimede, Port.*
Ciprofloxacin (p.188·2).
*Bacterial infections.*

**Gi-Sen** *Giuliani, Ital.*
Ginseng (p.1693·1).

**Gittalun** *Boehringer Ingelheim, Ger.*
Doxylamine succinate (p.432·3).
*Sleep disorders.*

**Gityl** *Krewel, Ger.*
Bromazepam (p.671·3).
*Anxiety; sleep disorders.*

**Givalex**
*Norgine, Belg.; Norgine, Fr.; Norgine, Ger.*
Hexetidine (p.1182·1); choline salicylate (p.26·2); chlorobutanol (p.1176·3).
*Mouth and throat disorders.*

**Givitol**
*Galen, Irl.; Galen, UK†.*
Ferrous fumarate (p.1427·3); folic acid (p.1429·1); vitamin B and C substances (p.1417·1).
*Iron and folic acid deficiency in pregnancy.*

**GLA-130** *Shaklee, Canad.†.*
Borage oil (p.1661·3); safflower oil (p.1443·3).

**Glaan** *Neo-Farmaceutica, Port.†.*
Emollient.
*Skin disorders.*

**Gladase** *Glades, USA.*
Papain (p.1727·3); urea (p.1162·2).
*Debridement of necrotic tissue.*

**Gladem**
*Boehringer Ingelheim, Austria; Boehringer Ingelheim, Ger.; Boehringer Ingelheim, Switz.*
Sertraline hydrochloride (p.317·2).
*Depression; obsessive-compulsive disorder; panic attacks; post-traumatic stress disorder.*

**Gladiaton** *Sedar, Braz.†.*
Ferric ammonium citrate (p.1427·2); phosphoric acid; dibasic sodium phosphate; melissa; vitamin B substances; vitamin C (p.1417·1).
*Iron deficiency; iron-deficiency anaemia.*

**Gladius** *Biomedica-Chemica, Gr.*
Ceftriaxone sodium (p.182·3).
*Bacterial infections.*

**Gladixol** *Kolassa, Austria.*
β-Acetyldigoxin (p.851·1); potassium aspartate (p.1233·1); magnesium aspartate (p.1227·3).
*Arrhythmias; heart failure.*

**Gladixol N** *corax, Ger.†.*
β-Acetyldigoxin (p.851·1).
*Heart failure.*

**Glafemak** *Alvia (Αλβια), Gr.*
Timolol maleate (p.1012·2).
*Glaucoma.*

**Glafornil** *Merck, Chile.*
Metformin hydrochloride (p.342·3).
*Diabetes mellitus.*

**Glakay**
*Eisai, Jpn; Eisai, Thai.*
Menatetrenone (p.1467·1).
*Osteoporosis.*

**Glamidolo**
*Angelini, Israel; Angelini, Ital.*
Dapiprazole hydrochloride (p.1679·1).
*Glaucoma; reversal of mydriasis.*

**Glamin**
*Fresenius Medical, Austral.; Baxter, Ger.; Fresenius Kabi, Hong Kong; Pharmacia Upjohn, Irl.†; Fresenius Kabi, Ital.; Fresenius Kabi, Malaysia; Fresenius Kabi, Neth.; Baxter, NZ; Fresenius Kabi, NZ; Fresenius Kabi, Port.; Fresenius Kabi, Singapore; Fresenius Kabi, Spain; Fresenius Kabi, Switz.; Fresenius Kabi, UK.*
Amino-acid infusion (p.1417·1).
*Parenteral nutrition.*

**Glandicin** *Degorts, Mex.*
Piroxicam (p.84·2).
*Inflammation; pain.*

**Glandol** *Boots Healthcare, Switz.†.*
Borage oil (p.1661·3).
*Dietary supplement.*

**Glandosane**
*Calea, Austria; Cell Pharm, Ger.; Fresenius, Israel; Fresenius Kabi, Port.; Helvepharm, Switz.; Fresenius Kabi, Thai.; Fresenius Kabi, UK; Kenwood, USA†.*
Carmellose sodium (p.1577·3); sorbitol (p.1446·3); electrolytes (p.1217·1).
*Dry mouth.*

**Glandulae-F-Gastreu R20** *Reckeweg, Ger.†.*
Homoeopathic preparation.

**Glandulae-M-Gastreu R19** *Reckeweg, Ger.†.*
Homoeopathic preparation.

**GLA-Plus Vitamin E** *Shaklee, Canad.*
Essential fatty acids with vitamin E (p.1417·1).
*Nutritional supplement.*

**Glatim** *Amhof, Arg.*
Timolol maleate (p.1012·2).
*Glaucoma; ocular hypertension.*

**Glaucadrine**
*Merck Sharp & Dohme-Chibret, Fr.†; Merck Sharp & Dohme, Switz.†.*
Aceclidine hydrochloride (p.1487·1); adrenaline (p.852·2).
*Glaucoma.*

**Glaucocare**
*Bournonville, Belg.†.*
Aceclidine (p.1487·1).
*Glaucoma.*

*Bournonville, Neth.†.*
Aceclidine hydrochloride (p.1487·1).
*Glaucoma; raised intra-ocular pressure.*

**Glaucocarpine** *Taro, Israel.*
Pilocarpine hydrochloride (p.1495·1).
*Glaucoma.*

**Glaucocin** *Klonal, Arg.*
Pilocarpine (p.1494·3); timolol (p.1012·3).
*Glaucoma.*

**Glaucofrin**
*Bournonville, Belg.†.*
Aceclidine (p.1487·1); adrenaline (p.852·2).
*Glaucoma.*

*Bournonville, Neth.†.*
Aceclidine hydrochloride (p.1487·1); adrenaline (p.852·2).
*Glaucoma; raised intra-ocular pressure.*

**Glaucol**
*Note. This name is used for preparations of different composition.*
*Croma, Austria†.*
Diclofenamide (p.894·1).
*Glaucoma.*

*Norton, UK†.*
Timolol maleate (p.1012·2).
*Ocular hypertension.*

**Glaucon** *Alcon, USA.*
Adrenaline hydrochloride (p.852·3).
*Open-angle glaucoma.*

**Glauconex**
*Alcon, Austria; Bournonville, Belg.†; Alcon, Ger.†.*
Befunolol hydrochloride (p.867·1).
*Glaucoma.*

**Glauconide** *Llorens, Spain.*
Diclofenamide (p.894·1).
*Glaucoma.*

**Glauco-Oph**
*Seng, Hong Kong; Seng, Thai.*
Timolol maleate (p.1012·2).
*Glaucoma; ocular hypertension.*

**Glaucosan** *Hexal, S.Afr.*
Timolol maleate (p.1012·2).
*Glaucoma; ocular hypertension.*

**Glaucostat**
*Merck Sharp & Dohme-Chibret, Fr.†; IFET (ΙΦΕΤ), Gr.; Chibret, Port.; Merck Sharp & Dohme, Spain†; Merck Sharp & Dohme, Switz.†.*
Aceclidine hydrochloride (p.1487·1).
*Glaucoma; ocular hypertension.*

**Glauco-Stulln** *Stulln, Ger.*
Pindolol (p.983·2).
*Glaucoma.*

**Glaucotat** *Chibret, Ger.†.*
Aceclidine hydrochloride (p.1487·1).
*Glaucoma.*

**Glaucotensil**
*Note. This name is used for preparations of different composition.*
*Poen, Arg.*
Pilocarpine hydrochloride (p.1495·1); timolol maleate (p.1012·2).
*Glaucoma.*

*Poen, Chile.*
Dorzolamide hydrochloride (p.908·3).
*Glaucoma; ocular hypertension.*

**Glaucotensil T** *Poen, Chile.*
Dorzolamide hydrochloride (p.908·3); timolol maleate (p.1012·2).
*Glaucoma; ocular hypertension.*

**Glaucotensil TD** *Poen, Arg.*
Dorzolamide (p.908·3); timolol maleate (p.1012·2).
*Glaucoma; ocular hypertension.*

**Glaucothil**
*Alcon, Austria; Alcon, Ger.*
Dipivefrine hydrochloride (p.1681·2).
*Glaucoma.*

**GlaucTabs** *Akorn, USA†.*
Methazolamide (p.953·1).
*Glaucoma.*

**Glaudrops** *Alcon Cusi, Spain.*
Dipivefrine hydrochloride (p.1681·2).
*Glaucoma; ocular hypertension.*

**Glaufrin** *Allergan, Swed.†.*
Adrenaline hydrochloride (p.852·3).
*Open-angle glaucoma.*

**Glauko Biciron** *S & K, Ger.*
Pilocarpine hydrochloride (p.1495·1); phenylephrine hydrochloride (p.1126·3).
*Glaucoma.*

**Glaumetax** *Novartis Ophthalmics, Arg.*
Methazolamide (p.953·1).

**Glaumid** *SIFI, Ital.*
Diclofenamide (p.894·1).
*Glaucoma.*

**Glaunorm** *Farmigea, Ital.*
Aceclidine hydrochloride (p.1487·1).
*Glaucoma.*

**Glau-opt** *Trinity, UK.*
Timolol maleate (p.1012·2).
*Glaucoma; ocular hypertension.*

**Glaupax**
*Orion, Denm.†; Novartis Ophthalmics, Ger.; Orion, Irl.†; Novartis, Neth.; Orion, Norw.†; Novartis Ophthalmics, Switz.; Ercopharm, Thai.†.*
Acetazolamide (p.849·1).
*Epilepsy; glaucoma.*

**Glausine** *Agepha, Austria.*
Clonidine hydrochloride (p.885·2).
*Glaucoma.*

**Glausolets** *SMB, Chile.*
Timolol maleate (p.1012·2).
*Glaucoma; ocular hypertension.*

**Glautarakt** *Pekana, Ger.*
Homoeopathic preparation.

**Glauteolol** *ICN, Arg.*
Carteolol hydrochloride (p.880·3).
*Ocular hypertension.*

**Glautimol**
*Note. This name is used for preparations of different composition.*
*Alcon, Braz.*
Timolol maleate (p.1012·2).
*Glaucoma; ocular hypertension.*

*Farmigea, Ital.*
Aceclidine hydrochloride (p.1487·1); timolol maleate (p.1012·2).
*Glaucoma; ocular hypertension.*

**Glavamin**
*Fresenius Kabi, Austria; Fresenius Kabi, Denm.; Fresenius Kabi, Fin.; Fresenius Kabi, Norw.; Fresenius Kabi, Swed.*
Amino-acid infusion (p.1417·1).
*Parenteral nutrition.*

**Glaveral** *Help, Gr.*
Omeprazole (p.1278·2).
*Acid aspiration; eradication of Helicobacter pylori in combination with antimicrobials; peptic ulcer; reflux oesophagitis; Zollinger-Ellison syndrome.*

**Glavit** *Fontovit, Braz.*
Gamolenic acid (p.1690·2); linolenic acid; oleic acid (p.1481·3).
*Premenstrual syndrome.*

**Glaxal Base** *Wellspring, Canad.*
Moisturiser.
*Dermatological base.*

**Glazidim**
*GlaxoSmithKline, Belg.; GlaxoSmithKline, Fin.; GlaxoSmithKline, Ital.*
Ceftazidime (p.180·2).
*Bacterial infections.*

**Gleevec** *Novartis, S.Afr.; Novartis, USA.*
Imatinib mesilate (p.562·1).
*Chronic myeloid leukaemia; gastrointestinal stromal tumours.*

**Glefos** *Grunenthal, Spain.*
Misoprostol (p.1519·2).
*Peptic ulcer.*

**Gleitgelen** *Wolff, Ger.*
Liquid paraffin (p.1479·1); medium-chain triglycerides (p.1440·3).
*Vaginal dryness.*

**Gleitmittel** *Bichsel, Switz.*
Chlorhexidine gluconate (p.1173·2); macrogol (p.1709·1).
*Lubrication before catheterisation or endoscopy.*

**Glemaz** *Montpellier, Arg.*
Glimepiride (p.332·2).
*Diabetes mellitus.*

**Glemicid** *Collins, Mex.*
Glibenclamide (p.331·2).
*Diabetes mellitus.*

**Glencamide** *Pond's, Thai.*
Glibenclamide (p.331·2).
*Diabetes mellitus.*

**Glenol** *Alpes Chemie, Chile.*
Paracetamol (p.76·2); pseudoephedrine hydrochloride (p.1129·2).
*Cold and influenza symptoms.*

**Glevomicina** *Bago, Arg.*
Gentamicin sulfate (p.217·1).
*Bacterial infections.*

**Gliadel**
*Orphan, Austral.; Aventis, Braz.†; Rhone-Poulenc Rorer, Canad.†; Aventis, Chile; Rhone-Poulenc Rorer, Fr.†; Guilford, Israel; Aventis, NZ†; Aventis, Port.†; Rhone-Poulenc Rorer, Singapore†; Link, UK; Guildford, USA.*
Carmustine (p.535·1).
*Glioblastoma multiforme; malignant glioma.*

**Glianimon**
*Bayer, Ger.; Menarini, Gr.*
Benperidol (p.671·2).
*Psychoses.*

**Gliatilin**
*Montpellier, Arg.; Italfarmaco, Ital.*
Choline alfoscerate (p.1488·3).
*Mental function impairment.*

**Glib** *ABZ, Ger.*
Glibenclamide (p.331·2).
*Diabetes mellitus.*

**gli-basan** *Schonenberger, Switz.*
Glibenclamide (p.331·2).
*Diabetes mellitus.*

**Glibediab** *Hexal, Arg.*
Glibenclamide (p.331·2).
*Diabetes mellitus.*

**Glibemid** *Malayan, Singapore.*
Glibenclamide (p.331·2).
*Diabetes mellitus.*

**Gliben**
*Cristalia, Braz.; CT, Ger.; Lichtenstein, Ger.; Biolab, Hong Kong; Biopharm, Hong Kong; Abiogen, Ital.; Biolab, Malaysia; Pacific, NZ; Biolab, Thai.*
Glibenclamide (p.331·2).
*Diabetes mellitus.*

**Gliben F** *Abiogen, Ital.*
Glibenclamide (p.331·2); phenformin hydrochloride (p.344·1).
*Diabetes mellitus.*

**Gliben-Azu** *Azupharma, Ger.*
Glibenclamide (p.331·2).
*Diabetes mellitus.*

**Glibenbeta** *Betapharm, Ger.*
Glibenclamide (p.331·2).
*Diabetes mellitus.*

**Glibenclamon** *Sanval, Braz.*
Glibenclamide (p.331·2).
*Diabetes mellitus.*

**Glibendoc** *Docpharm, Ger.*
Glibenclamide (p.331·2).
*Diabetes mellitus.*

**Glibenese**
*Pfizer, Austria; Pfizer, Belg.; Pfizer, Denm.; Pfizer, Fin.; Pfizer, Fr.; Pfizer, Ger.†; Pfizer, Gr.; Pfizer, Irl.; Pfizer, Neth.; Pfizer, Spain; Mack, Switz.; Pfizer, UK.*
Glipizide (p.332·2).
*Diabetes mellitus.*

**Glibenhexal** *Hexal, Ger.*
Glibenclamide (p.331·2).
*Diabetes mellitus.*

**Glibenil** *Cryopharma, Mex.*
Glibenclamide (p.331·2).
*Diabetes mellitus.*

**Gliben-Puren N** *Alpharma-Isis, Ger.*
Glibenclamide (p.331·2).
*Diabetes mellitus.*

**Glibenval** *Valdecasas, Mex.*
Glibenclamide (p.331·2).
*Diabetes mellitus.*

**Glibesifar** *Siphar, Switz.*
Glibenclamide (p.331·2).
*Diabetes mellitus.*

**Glibesyn**
*Medochemie, Malaysia; Medochemie, Singapore†; Medochemie, Thai.†.*
Glibenclamide (p.331·2).
*Diabetes mellitus.*

**Glibetic**
*Teva, Israel; The Forty-Two, Thai.*
Glibenclamide (p.331·2).
*Diabetes mellitus.*

**Glibexil** *Royton, Braz.*
Glibenclamide (p.331·2).
*Diabetes mellitus.*

**Glibic** *Progress, Thai.*
Glibenclamide (p.331·2).
*Diabetes mellitus.*

**Glibomet** *Guidotti, Ital.*
Glibenclamide (p.331·2); metformin hydrochloride (p.342·3).
*Diabetes mellitus.*

**Gliboral**
*Menarini, Hong Kong; Guidotti, Ital.*
Glibenclamide (p.331·2).
*Diabetes mellitus.*

**Glib-ratiopharm** *Ratiopharm, Ger.*
Glibenclamide (p.331·2).
*Diabetes mellitus.*

**Glicacil** *Bioprogress, Ital.†.*
Sodium cromoglicate (p.795·3).
*Asthma; chronic intestinal inflammatory disease; food hypersensitivity.*

**Glicalox** *Dominguez, Arg.*
Alginic acid (p.1576·3); sodium alginate (p.1577·1); magnesium trisilicate (p.1272·3); aluminium hydroxide (p.1249·2).
*Gastric hyperacidity; gastro-oesophageal reflux.*

**Glicamin** *Lafare, Ital.*
A heparinoid (p.931·1).
*Thrombosis prophylaxis.*

**Glicel** *Brasterapica, Braz.†.*
Glycerol (p.1694·3).
*Constipation.*

**Glicemin** *Apsen, Braz.†.*
Diazoxide (p.893·2).
*Hypertension.*

**Glicermina** *Bescansa, Spain†.*
Stearic acid; glycerol.
*Skin disorders.*

**Glicerolax** *Dynacren, Ital.*
Glycerol (p.1694·3); mallow (p.1709·3) (p.1709·3).
*Constipation.*

**Glicerolo microclismi** *Mediplants, Gr.*
Glycerol (p.1694·3).
*Bowel evacuation.*

**Glicerotens** *Llorens, Spain.*
Glycerol (p.1694·3).
*Glaucoma; ocular hypertension; ocular surgery.*

**Glicero-Valerovit** *Teofarma, Ital.*
Sodium glycerophosphate (p.1695·2); valerian (p.1762·2).
Lidocaine hydrochloride (p.1377·3) is included in the intramuscular injection to alleviate the pain of injection.
*Hyperexcitability; tonic.*

**Glicima** *Atlantis, Mex.*
Ketorolac trometamol (p.52·1).
*Pain.*

**Glicinal** *Ogera, Switz.*
Sodium cromoglicate (p.795·3).
*Asthma.*

**Glico Test** *Callegari, Ital.†.*
Test for glucose in blood (p.1694·2).

**Glico Urine B** *Callegari, Ital.†.*
Test for glucose in urine (p.1694·2).

**Glicobase** *Formenti, Ital.*
Acarbose (p.328·3).
*Diabetes mellitus.*

**Glicoben** *Cazi, Braz.*
Chlorpropamide (p.330·3).
*Diabetes mellitus.*

**Glicoderm** *Remexa, Mex.*
Glycolic acid (p.1147·3).
*Dry skin disorders.*

**Glicodin** *Novaquimica, Braz.†.*
Potassium iodide (p.1598·1); ammonium chloride (p.1115·2); hyoscyamus (p.485·2).
*Respiratory-tract congestion.*

**Glicofisiologica** *Aster, Braz.*
Sodium chloride (p.1233·3); glucose (p.1432·2).
*Fluid and electrolyte disorders.*

**Glico-Fita** *Lilly, Braz.*
Test for glucose in urine (p.1694·2).

**Gliconorm** *Abiogen, Ital.*
Glibenclamide (p.331·2); metformin hydrochloride (p.342·3).
*Diabetes mellitus.*

**Glicorest** *Fournier, Ital.*
Glibenclamide (p.331·2); metformin hydrochloride (p.342·3).
*Diabetes mellitus.*

**Glicorp** *Neo Quimica, Braz.*
Chlorpropamide (p.330·3).
*Diabetes mellitus.*

**Glicosado** *Labormedica, Braz.†.*
Glucose infusion (p.1432·2).
*Parenteral nutrition.*

**Glicoxem** *Precimex, Mex.†.*
Glibenclamide (p.331·2).
*Diabetes mellitus.*

**Glicron** *Siam Medicare, Thai.*
Gliclazide (p.332·1).
*Diabetes mellitus.*

**Glidanil** *Montpellier, Arg.*
Glibenclamide (p.331·2).
*Diabetes mellitus.*

**Glide** *Franco-Indian, India.*
Glipizide (p.332·2).
*Diabetes mellitus.*

**Glidiab** *CCPC, Hong Kong†.*
Glipizide (p.332·2).
*Diabetes mellitus.*

**Glifage** *Merck, Braz.*
Metformin (p.342·3).
*Diabetes mellitus.*

**Glifarcal** *Farcoral, Mex.*
Glibenclamide (p.331·2).
*Diabetes mellitus.*

**Gliformin** *Guidotti, Ital.*
Glibenclamide (p.331·2); phenformin hydrochloride (p.344·1).
*Diabetes mellitus.*

**Glifortex** *Andromaco, Chile.*
Metformin hydrochloride (p.342·3).
*Diabetes mellitus.*

**Glikeyer** *Keyerson, Mex.*
Glibenclamide (p.331·2).
*Diabetes mellitus.*

**Glimbal** *CSC, Austria.*
Clocortolone pivalate (p.1096·1).
*Skin disorders.*

**Glimel**
*Alphapharm, Austral.; Alphapharm, Hong Kong.*
Glibenclamide (p.331·2).
*Diabetes mellitus.*

**Glimepil** *Farmoquimica, Braz.*
Glimepiride (p.332·2).
*Diabetes mellitus.*

**Glimesec** *Marjan, Braz.*
Glimepiride (p.332·2).
*Diabetes mellitus.*

**Glimial** *Neves, Port.*
Glimepiride (p.332·2).
*Diabetes mellitus.*

**Glimicron**
*Hovid, Hong Kong; Hovid, Malaysia; Hovid, Singapore.*
Gliclazide (p.332·1).
*Diabetes mellitus.*

**Glimide**
*Note. This name is used for preparations of different composition.*
*Beta, Arg.*
Rosiglitazone maleate (p.345·2).
*Diabetes melitus.*
*Upha, Malaysia; Beacons, Singapore.*
Glibenclamide (p.331·2).
*Diabetes mellitus.*

**Glimidstada** *Stada, Ger.*
Glibenclamide (p.331·2).
*Diabetes mellitus.*

**Glimiton** *Mead Johnson, Braz.*
Mineral preparation with vitamin B substances (p.1417·1).

**Glinate** *Glenmark, India.*
Nateglinide (p.343·3).
*Diabetes mellitus.*

**Glineon** *Dovalle, Braz.*
Potassium aspartate; magnesium aspartate; fructose; ascorbic acid (p.1417·1).

**Glinor** *Ratiopharm, Fin.*
Sodium cromoglicate (p.795·3).
*Allergic conjunctivitis; allergic rhinitis.*

**Glinorboral** *Silanes, Mex.*
Glibenclamide (p.331·2); phenformin (p.329·2).
*Diabetes mellitus.*

**Glionil** *Neo Quimica, Braz.*
Glibenclamide (p.331·2).
*Diabetes mellitus.*

**Glios** *Pharmacia Upjohn, Ital.†.*
Serine alfoscerate.
*Cerebrovascular disorders; mental function impairment.*

**Gliosartan** *Bago, Arg.*
Telmisartan (p.1010·1).
*Hypertension.*

**Glioten**
*Bago, Arg.; Merck Bago, Braz.; Bago, Chile; Armstrong, Mex.*
Enalapril maleate (p.909·2) or enalaprilat (p.909·3).
*Heart failure; hypertension.*

**Gliotenzide**
*Bago, Arg.; Merck Bago, Braz.*
Enalapril maleate (p.909·2); hydrochlorothiazide (p.933·2).
*Hypertension.*

**Glipep** *Faulding, Port.*
Vancomycin (p.275·2).

**Glipgen** *Teuto, Braz.*
Glipizide (p.332·2).
*Diabetes mellitus.*

**Glipicontin** *Modi-Mundipharma, India.*
Glipizide (p.332·2).
*Diabetes mellitus.*

**Glipid** *Pacific, NZ.*
Glipizide (p.332·2).
*Diabetes mellitus.*

**Glipiscand** *Scand Pharm, Swed.*
Glipizide (p.332·2).
*Diabetes mellitus.*

**Gliplex** *Farmasa, Braz.*
Vitamin B substances; vitamin C (p.1417·1).

**Glipressina** *Ferring, Ital.*
Terlipressin acetate (p.1340·1).
*Haemorrhage from oesophageal varices.*

**Gliptide** *Crinos, Ital.*
Sulglicotide (p.1293·2).
*Gastrointestinal disorders; peptic ulcer.*

**Glisuret** *Pisa, Mex.*
Glycine (p.1433·3).
*Transurethral irrigation.*

**Glitisol**
*Zambon, Braz.*
Thiamphenicol (p.269·2).
*Bacterial infections.*
*Zambon, Ital.*
Thiamphenicol glycinate hydrochloride (p.269·2).
*Bacterial infections.*

**Glitral** *LA, Arg.*
Glibenclamide (p.331·2).
*Diabetes mellitus.*

**Glivec**
*Novartis, Austral.; Novartis, Braz.; Novartis, Chile; Novartis, Denm.; Novartis, Fin.; Novartis, Fr.; Novartis, Irl.; Novartis, Israel; Novartis, Ital.; Novartis, Malaysia; Novartis, Norw.; Novartis, NZ; Novartis, Port.; Novartis, Spain; Novartis, Switz.; Novartis, Thai.; Novartis, UK.*
Imatinib mesilate (p.562·1).
*Chronic myeloid leukaemia; gastrointestinal stromal tumours.*

**Glix** *YSP, Malaysia.*
Glipizide (p.332·2).
*Diabetes mellitus.*

**Gliza** *Stadmed, India.*
Gliclazide (p.332·1).
*Diabetes mellitus.*

**Glizide** *Fascino, Thai.*
Glipizide (p.332·2).
*Diabetes mellitus.*

**Glizone** *Zydus, India.*
Pioglitazone (p.344·2).
*Diabetes mellitus.*

**Globac-Z** *Zydus, India.*
Glycerinated haemoglobin (p.755·2); ferric ammonium citrate (p.1427·2) or ferrous fumarate (p.1427·3); copper sulfate; zinc sulfate; manganese sulfate (p.1417·1); vitamin $B_{12}$ (p.1458·2); folic acid (p.1429·1).
*Iron-deficiency anaemia.*

**Globenicol** *Yamanouchi, Neth.*
Chloramphenicol (p.185·1).
*Bacterial eye infections.*

**Globentyl** *Nycomed, Norw.†.*
Aspirin (p.15·1).
*Fever; pain; rheumatic disorders.*

**Globocef**
*Roche, Braz.; Roche, Ger.; Roche, Hong Kong; Roche, Ital.; Roche, Mex.†; Roche, Port.; Roche, Switz.*
Cefetamet pivoxil hydrochloride (p.172·3).
*Bacterial infections.*

**Globoid** *Nycomed, Norw.*
Aspirin (p.15·1).
*Fever; pain; rheumatic disorders.*

**Globovit** *Andromaco, Chile.*
Multivitamin and mineral preparation (p.1417·1).

**Globuce** *Sigma-Tau, Spain.*
Ciprofloxacin hydrochloride (p.188·2).
*Bacterial infections.*

**Globuli gegen Gelenkschmerzen** *Jacoby, Austria.*
Homoeopathic preparation.

**Globuli gegen Grippe** *Jacoby, Austria.*
Homoeopathic preparation.

**Globuli gegen Halsweh** *Jacoby, Austria.*
A range of homoeopathic preparations.

**Globuli gegen Hautausschlage** *Jacoby, Austria.*
Homoeopathic preparation.

**Globuli gegen Heiserkeit** *Jacoby, Austria.*
Homoeopathic preparation.

**Globuli gegen Husten** *Jacoby, Austria.*
A range of homoeopathic preparations.

**Globuli gegen Schnupfen** *Jacoby, Austria.*
A range of homoeopathic preparations.

**Globuli gegen Sonnenallergie** *Jacoby, Austria.*
Homoeopathic preparation.

**Globulina Lloren Anti RH** *Llorente, Spain†.*
An anti-D immunoglobulin (p.1608·1).
*Prevention of rhesus sensitivity.*

**Globuman**
*Berna, Belg.†; Berna, Hong Kong; Berna, Ital.; Berna, Malaysia; Swiss Serum, Malaysia; Berna, Port.; Byk Madaus, S.Afr.†; Berna, Spain; Berna, Switz.; Berna, Thai.†.*
A normal immunoglobulin (p.1627·2).
*Idiopathic thrombocytopenic purpura; immune deficiency; passive immunisation.*

**Globuman Hepatite A**
*Berna, Belg.†; Berna, Port.; Berna, Switz.†.*
A hepatitis A immunoglobulin (p.1617·1).
*Passive immunisation.*

**Globuman Hepatitis A** Berna, Hong Kong†; Byk Madaus, S.Afr.†; Berna, Thai.†.
A hepatitis A immunoglobulin (p.1617·1).
*Passive immunisation.*

**Globuman iv CMV** Berna, Switz.†.
A cytomegalovirus immunoglobulin (p.1612·1).
*Passive immunisation.*

**Globuren** Dompe Biotec, Ital.
Epoetin alfa (p.747·2).
*Anaemias; autologous blood transfusions.*

**Gloceda** Medgenix, Belg.
Codeine (p.27·1).
Formerly contained erysimin, aconite, belladonna, euphorbia, drosera, cherry-laurel, and codeine phosphate.
*Coughs.*

**Glofil** Cypros, USA.
Iodine-125 (p.1524·2) as sodium iotalamate.
*Evaluation of glomerular filtration rate.*

**Glogama Antihepatitis B** Evans, Spain†.
A hepatitis B immunoglobulin (p.1617·2).
*Passive immunisation.*

**Glonoin** Coradol, Ger.
Herbal and homoeopathic preparation.

**Glonoinum** Hevert, Ger.†.
Homoeopathic preparation.

**Glopir** Gap, Gr.
Nifedipine (p.966·2).
*Angina; hypertension.*

**Glorixone** Help, Gr.
Ceftriaxone sodium (p.182·3).
*Bacterial infections.*

**Glossderm** Columbia, Mex.
Cod-liver oil (p.1425·2); benzalkonium chloride (p.1168·3); zinc oxide (p.1163·2); allantoin (p.1141·3).
*Napkin rash.*

**Glossithiase** Jolly-Jatel, Fr.
Thenoate monoethanolamine (p.269·2); muramidase hydrochloride (p.1717·2).
*Infections of the mouth and throat.*

**Glossware & Brush** Clinique, Canad.†.
*SPF 8:* Octinoxate (p.1154·3).
*Sunscreen.*

**Glossyfin** Doctum, Gr.
Ciprofloxacin hydrochloride (p.188·2).
*Bacterial infections.*

**Glotil** Brasifa, Braz.†.
Sodium dibunate (p.1130·2); phenethylamine citrate; homatropine methylbromide (p.483·2).
*Coughs.*

**Glotone** Vita, Spain.
Cyproheptadine hydrochloride (p.430·1); arginine hydrochloride; carnitine; cyanocobalamin (p.1417·1).
Formerly contained cyproheptadine hydrochloride, embryo extract, gastric mucosa extract, and muscle extract.
*Tonic.*

**Glottyl**
Note. This name is used for preparations of different composition.
Viatris, Belg.
Codeine phosphate (p.27·1).
Formerly contained aconite, codeine phosphate, cherry-laurel, belladonna, drosera, erysimin, and euphorbia.
*Coughs.*

Marion Merrell, Fr.†.
Amylocaine hydrochloride (p.1370·2); erysimum; grindelia (p.1696·1).
*Sore throat.*

**Glovan** Teva, Israel.
Nonoxinol 9 (p.1413·3); ricinoleic acid (p.1738·3).
*Contraceptive.*

**Gluben** Dexcel, Israel.
Glibenclamide (p.331·2).
*Diabetes mellitus.*

**Gluborid**
Sanochemia, Austria†; Grunenthal, Ger.; Grunenthal, Switz.
Glibornuride (p.331·3).
*Diabetes mellitus.*

**GlucaGen**
Novo Nordisk, Arg.; Novo Nordisk, Austral.; Novo Nordisk, Austria; Novo Nordisk, Belg.; Novo Nordisk, Denm.; Novo Nordisk, Fin.; Novo Nordisk, Fr.; Novo Nordisk, Ger.; Novo Nordisk, Gr.; Novo Nordisk, Hong Kong; Knoll, India; Novo Nordisk, Irl.; Novo Nordisk, Israel; Novo Nordisk, Ital.; Novo Nordisk, Malaysia; Novo Nordisk, NZ; Novo Nordisk, Port.; Novo Nordisk, S.Afr.; Novo Nordisk, Singapore; Novo Nordisk, Switz.; Novo Nordisk, Thai.†; Novo Nordisk, UK; Bedford, USA.
Glucagon hydrochloride (p.1040·1).
*Aid in gastrointestinal examination; beta-blocker poisoning; hypoglycaemia.*

**Glucal** Galen, Mex.
Glibenclamide (p.331·2).
*Diabetes mellitus.*

**Glucal B12** Dansk-Flama, Braz.
Cyanocobalamin; colecalciferol; minerals; lysine hydrochloride (p.1417·1).
*Nutritional supplement.*

**Glucalbott Rth** Abbott, Chile.
Preparation for enteral nutrition in diabetes mellitus (p.1417·1).

**Glucalcium** Renaudin, Fr.†.
Calcium gluconate (p.1225·2); calcium gluceptate (p.1225·2).
*Hypocalcaemia.*

**Glucamet** Opus, UK†.
Metformin hydrochloride (p.342·3).
*Diabetes mellitus.*

**Glucaminol** Roche, Arg.
Metformin hydrochloride (p.342·3).
*Diabetes mellitus.*

**Glucanet**
Note. This name is used for preparations of different composition.
Noos, Ital.
Glucan.
*Nasal cleansing.*

Formalight, Port.
Sodium chloride (p.1233·3); carboxymethyl-beta-glucan.
*Nasal congestion; rhinitis.*

**Glucantim** Aventis, Ital.
Meglumine antimonate (p.600·3).
*Leishmaniasis.*

**Glucantime**
Aventis, Braz.; Aventis, Fr.; Aventis, Spain.
Meglumine antimonate (p.600·3).
*Leishmaniasis.*

**Gluceride** Klonal, Arg.
Glimepiride (p.332·2).
*Diabetes mellitus.*

**Glucerna**
Abbott, Arg.; Abbott, Austral.; Abbott, Braz.; Abbott, Canad.; Abbott, Fin.; Abbott, Hong Kong; Abbott, Irl.; Ross, Israel; Abbott, Ital.; Abbott, Mex.; Abbott, NZ; Abbott, Singapore; Abbott, Thai.; Ross, USA.
A range of preparations for enteral nutrition (p.1417·1).
*Glucose intolerance.*

**Glucidoral** Servier, Fr.
Carbutamide (p.330·3).
*Diabetes mellitus.*

**Glucinan** Lipha Sante, Fr.†.
Metformin chlorophenoxyacetate (p.342·3).
*Diabetes mellitus.*

**Glucobay**
Bayer, Arg.; Bayer, Austral.; Bayer, Austria; Bayer, Belg.; Bayer, Braz.; Bayer, Chile; Bayer, Denm.; Bayer, Fin.†; Bayer, Ger.; Asche, Ger.; Bayer, Gr.; Bayer, Hong Kong; Bayer, India; Bayer, Irl.; Bayer, Ital.; Bayer, Malaysia; Bayer, Mex.; Bayer, Neth.; Bayer, Norw.; Bayer, NZ; Bayer, Port.; Bayer, S.Afr.; Bayer, Singapore; Bayer, Spain; Bayer, Swed.; Bayer, Switz.; Bayer, Thai.; Bayer, UK.
Acarbose (p.328·3).
*Diabetes mellitus.*

**Glucobene** Ratiopharm, Austria.
Glibenclamide (p.331·2).
*Diabetes mellitus.*

**Glucobon** Biomo, Ger.
Metformin hydrochloride (p.342·3).
*Diabetes mellitus.*

**Gluco-Calcium**
Note. A similar name is used for preparations of different composition (see below).
Lilly, Hong Kong.
Calcium (p.1225·1).
*Alkalosis; hypocalcaemia; parathyroid deficiency; vitamin D deficiency.*

Lilly, Thai.
Calcium (p.1225·1); glucose (p.1432·2).
*Hypocalcaemia.*

**Glucocalcium**
Note. A similar name is used for preparations of different composition (see above).
Streuli, Switz.
Calcium gluconate (p.1225·2); calcium sucrate.
*Hypocalcaemia; poisoning.*

**Glucocard**
NZ Medical & Scientific, NZ; Menarini Diagnostics, Port.
Test for glucose in blood (p.1694·2).

**Glucochaux** Darci, Belg.†.
Calcium gluconate (p.1225·2); calcium hydrogen phosphate (p.1225·2).
*Calcium deficiency; calcium supplement.*

**Gluco-Cinta** Lilly, Mex.
Test for glucose in urine (p.1694·2).

**Glucocron** Farmaline, Thai.
Gliclazide (p.332·1).
*Diabetes mellitus.*

**Glucodex** Rougier, Canad.
Glucose (p.1432·2).
*Oral glucose tolerance test.*

**Glucodiab** Bangkok Lab & Cosmetic, Thai.
Glipizide (p.332·2).
*Diabetes mellitus.*

**Glucodin** Boots Healthcare, Irl.†.
Glucose (p.1432·2); vitamin C (p.1460·2).

**Glucoferro** Guidotti, Ital.
Ferrous gluconate (p.1428·1).
*Iron deficiency; iron-deficiency anaemias.*

**Glucoferro K** Knop, Chile.
Ferrous gluconate (p.1428·1).
*Iron deficiency; iron deficiency anaemia.*

**Glucofilm**
Bayer, Austral.†; Miles, Canad.†; Bayer Diagnostics, Fr.†; Bayer Diagnostici, Ital.; Bayer, NZ†; Bayer, USA.
Test for glucose in blood (p.1694·2).

**Glucoflex-R** Technostic, Austral.
Test for glucose in blood (p.1694·2).

**Glucoformin** Biobras, Braz.
Metformin hydrochloride (p.342·3).
*Diabetes mellitus.*

**Glucohex** Eurofarma, Braz.
Chlorhexidine gluconate (p.1173·2).
*Antiseptic.*

**Glucohexal** Hexal, Austral.
Metformin hydrochloride (p.342·3).
*Diabetes mellitus.*

**Glucoles-500** T Man, Thai.
Metformin hydrochloride (p.342·3).
*Diabetes mellitus.*

**Glucolin** GlaxoSmithKline, Arg.
Preparation for enteral nutrition (p.1417·1).

**Glucolip** Wallace, India.
Glipizide (p.332·2).
*Diabetes mellitus.*

**Glucolon** Generfarma, Spain.
Glibenclamide (p.331·2).
*Diabetes mellitus.*

**Glucolyte** Thai Otsuka, Thai.
Electrolyte infusion with glucose (p.1217·1).
*Carbohydrate source; fluid and electrolyte disorders.*

**Glucoman** Volchem, Ital.
Dietary fibre supplement containing glucomannan (p.1693·3), galactomannan, and minerals (p.1417·1).
*Disorders of carbohydrate and lipid metabolism; gastrointestinal disorders; obesity.*

**Glucomed** Parke-Med, S.Afr.
Gliclazide (p.332·1).
*Diabetes mellitus.*

**Glucomen** Menarini, Irl.
Test for glucose in blood (p.1694·2).

**Glucomet**
Douglas, Austral.; Douglas, NZ; Hua, Thai.
Metformin hydrochloride (p.342·3).
*Diabetes mellitus.*

**Glucometer**
Bayer, Austral.; Bayer Diagnostici, Ital.
Test for glucose in blood (p.1694·2).
*For use with Glucometer Elite blood glucose meter.*

**Glucometer Elite**
Bayer, Arg.; Bayer Diagnostics, Irl.; Bayer, NZ.
Test for glucose in blood (p.1694·2).
For use with Glucometer Elite blood glucose meter.

**Glucometer Esprit** Bayer, NZ.
Test for glucose in blood (p.1694·2).
For use with Glucometer Esprit blood glucose meter.

**Glucomide** Merck, Ital.
Metformin hydrochloride (p.342·3); glibenclamide (p.331·2).
*Diabetes mellitus.*

**Glucomin**
Stada, Austria; Dexcel, Israel.
Metformin hydrochloride (p.342·3).
*Diabetes mellitus.*

**Glucomol** Allergan, India.
Timolol maleate (p.1012·2).
*Glaucoma; ocular hypertension.*

**Glucomore** Hayes, Israel.
Glucose polymers (p.1417·1).
*High-calorie supplement.*

**Gluconil** Utopian, Thai.
Glibenclamide (p.331·2).
*Diabetes mellitus.*

**Gluconorm**
Note. This name is used for preparations of different composition.
Roche, Braz.; Novo Nordisk, Canad.
Repaglinide (p.344·3).
*Diabetes mellitus.*

Wolff, Ger.†.
Glibenclamide (p.331·2).
*Diabetes mellitus.*

**Glucophage**
Merck, Arg.; Arrow, Austral.; Merck, Austria; Merck, Belg.; Aventis, Canad.; Roche, Chile; Lipha, Denm.; Merck, Fin.; Lipha Sante, Fr.; Merck, Ger.; Petsiavas (Πετσιαβας), Gr.; Merck-Lipha, Hong Kong; Lipha, Irl.; Abic, Israel; Merck, Ital.; Merck Sante, Malaysia; Roche, Mex.; Merck, Neth.; Lipha, Norw.; Pacific, NZ; Merck, Port.; Merck, S.Afr.; Merck, Singapore; Boehringer Mannheim, Spain†; Merck, Swed.; Lipha, Switz.; Merck, Thai.; Merck, UK; Bristol-Myers Squibb, USA.
Metformin hydrochloride (p.342·3).
*Diabetes mellitus.*

**Glucopirida** Biotenk, Arg.
Glimepiride (p.332·2).
*Diabetes mellitus.*

**Glucoplasmal**
Braun, Austria; Braun, Ger.; Braun, Spain.
Amino-acid, glucose, and electrolyte infusion (p.1417·1).
*Parenteral nutrition.*

**Glucoplex** Geistlich, UK†.
Carbohydrate, electrolyte, and trace element infusion (p.1417·1).
*Parenteral nutrition.*

**Glucoplurisalina** Fresenius Kabi, Spain.
Electrolyte infusion with glucose (p.1217·1).
*Fluid and electrolyte depletion.*

**Glucopolielectrol** Baxter, Spain.
Electrolyte infusion with glucose (p.1417·1).
*Fluid and electrolyte depletion.*

**Glucopotasica** Braun, Spain†; Mein, Spain†.
Potassium chloride infusion (p.1232·2) with glucose (p.1432·2).
*Fluid and electrolyte depletion.*

**Glucopotasico** Bieffe, Spain.
Potassium chloride infusion (p.1232·2) with glucose (p.1432·2).
*Fluid and electrolyte depletion.*

**Glucor** Bayer, Fr.
Acarbose (p.328·3).
*Diabetes mellitus.*

**Glucoremed** Lichtenstein, Ger.
Glibenclamide (p.331·2).
*Diabetes mellitus.*

**Gluco-Rite** Agis, Israel.
Glipizide (p.332·2).
*Diabetes mellitus.*

**Glucosada** Grifols, Port.†.
Glucose (p.1432·2).
*Carbohydrate source; fluid depletion.*

**Glucosado** Braun, Port.
Glucose (p.1432·2).
*Carbohydrate source; fluid depletion.*

**Glucosalin** Bioren, Switz.
Anhydrous glucose (p.1432·2); sodium chloride (p.1233·3).
*Carbohydrate source; fluid and electrolyte disorders.*

**Glucosalina** Braun, Spain; Grifols, Spain; Instituto Farmacologico, Spain; Fresenius Kabi, Spain.
Sodium chloride infusion (p.1233·3) with glucose (p.1432·2).
*Fluid and electrolyte depletion.*

**Glucosalina Modific** Mein, Spain†.
Sodium chloride (p.1233·3) and sodium lactate (p.1223·2) infusion with glucose (p.1432·2).
*Fluid and electrolyte depletion.*

**Glucosaline** Baxter, Switz.; Braun, Switz.; Infosint, Switz.
Anhydrous glucose (p.1432·2); sodium chloride (p.1233·3).
*Carbohydrate source; fluid and electrolyte disorders.*

**Glucosalino**
Braun, Port.; Bieffe, Spain; Ern, Spain; Braun, Spain; Baxter, Spain.
Sodium chloride (p.1233·3) infusion with glucose (p.1432·2).
*Fluid and electrolyte depletion.*

**Glucosan** Ortho, Ital.
Test for glucose in blood (p.1694·2).

**GlucoSelene** Wassen, UK.
Glucosamine sulfate; selenium; vitamins (p.1417·1).

**Glucoseral** Streuli, Switz.
Electrolyte infusion with glucose (p.1217·1).
*Fluid and electrolyte disorders; parenteral nutrition.*

**Glucosmon** Altana, Spain.
Glucose (p.1432·2).
*Carbohydrate source; hypoglycaemia.*

**Glucostad** Stada, Austria.
Glibenclamide (p.331·2).
*Diabetes mellitus.*

**Glucosteril**
Baxter, Fin.; Fresenius Kabi, Ger.; Fresenius Kabi, Port.
Glucose (p.1432·2) with or without sodium chloride.
*Carbohydrate source; fluid depletion.*

**Glucostix**
Bayer, Arg.; Bayer, Austral.; Bayer, Canad.†; Bayer Diagnostics, Fr.†; Bayer Diagnostics, Irl.; Bayer Diagnostici, Ital.; Bayer Diagnostics, Mex.; Bayer, NZ; Bayer, Port.†; Bayer Diagnostics, UK; Bayer, USA.
Test for glucose in blood (p.1694·2).

**Glucostrip** Biodiagnostics, Austral.†.
Test for glucose in blood (p.1694·2).

**Glucosulfa** Lipha, Ital.†.
Metformin (p.342·3); tolbutamide (p.348·1).
*Diabetes mellitus.*

**Gluco-Tablinen** Sanorania, Ger.†.
Glibenclamide (p.331·2).
*Diabetes mellitus.*

**Glucotard** Boehringer Mannheim, Ger.†.
Guar gum (p.333·2).
*Diabetes mellitus.*

**Glucotem** Temis, Arg.
Glucose monohydrate (p.1432·2).
*Hypoglycaemia.*

**Glucotide**
Bayer, Arg.; Bayer Diagnostics, Fr.; Bayer Diagnostics, Irl.; Bayer Diagnostics, Mex.; Bayer Diagnostics, UK.
Test for glucose in blood (p.1694·2).

**Glucotouch** Lifescan, Port.
Test for glucose in blood (p.1694·2).

**Glucotrend**
Roche, Arg.; Roche Diagnostics, Austral.†; Roche Diagnostics, Irl.†; Roche Diagnostics, Ital.
Test for glucose in blood (p.1694·2).

**Glucotrol**
Pfizer, Hong Kong; Pfizer, USA.
Glipizide (p.332·2).
*Diabetes mellitus.*

**Glucovance**
Merck, Chile; Merck, Port.; Bristol-Myers Squibb, USA.
Glibenclamide (p.331·2); metformin hydrochloride (p.342·3).
*Diabetes mellitus.*

**Glucoven** Chinoin, Mex.
Glibenclamide (p.331·2).
*Diabetes mellitus.*

**Glucoven infant** Fresenius Kabi, Ger.
Carbohydrate and electrolyte infusion (p.1417·1).
Formerly known as Glucovenos pad.
*Parenteral nutrition.*

**Glucovitan Ginseng** *Elvetium, Arg.*
Ginseng; thiamine hydrochloride; pyridoxine hydrochloride; cyanocobalamin; magnesium glycerophosphate (p.1417·1).
*Tonic.*

**Glucozide**
*Unison, Malaysia; Unison, Singapore; Unison, Thai.†.*
Gliclazide (p.332·1).
*Diabetes mellitus.*

**Glufcaps** *Belfar, Braz.†.*
Vitamins; minerals; lecithin; yeast (p.1417·1).

**Glufer-C** *Nakornpatana, Thai.*
Ferrous gluconate (p.1428·1); manganese sulfate; copper sulfate (p.1417·1).
Ascorbic acid (p.1460·2) is included in this preparation to increase the absorption and availability of iron.
*Iron-deficiency anaemia.*

**Glufor** *CTI, Israel.*
Metformin hydrochloride (p.342·3).
*Diabetes mellitus.*

**Gluformin** *Condrugs, Thai.*
Metformin hydrochloride (p.342·3).
*Diabetes mellitus.*

**Glukacel** *Braun, Norw.*
Electrolyte infusion with glucose (p.1217·1).
*Carbohydrate source; fluid and electrolyte disorders.*

**Gluketur** *Nicholas Piramal, India.*
Test for glucose and ketones in urine.

**Gluketurtest** *Roche Diagnostics, Ital.*
Test for glucose and ketone bodies in urine.

**Gluko** *Savio, Ital.†.*
Glutathione sodium (p.1040·3).
*Alcohol and drug poisoning; radiation trauma.*

**Glukolyt** *Kohler, Ger.*
Carbohydrate and electrolyte infusion (p.1417·1).
*Carbohydrate source; fluid depletion.*

**Glukoreduct** *Sanofi Synthelabo, Ger.*
Glibenclamide (p.331·2).
*Diabetes mellitus.*

**Glukos-El** *Braun, Swed.*
Carbohydrate and electrolyte infusion (p.1417·1).
*Parenteral nutrition.*

**Glukotest**
*Roche, Arg.; Roche, Chile.*
Test for glucose in urine (p.1694·2).

**Glukovital** *Wolff, Ger.*
Glibenclamide (p.331·2).
*Diabetes mellitus.*

**Glukurtest** *Roche Diagnostics, Ital.*
Test for glucose in urine (p.1694·2).

**Glumal**
*Kyowa, Jpn; Knoll, Spain†.*
Aceglutamide aluminium (p.1248·1).
*Gastrointestinal hyperacidity; peptic ulcer.*

**Glumet**
*Raza, Hong Kong; Raza, Malaysia; Pharmaniaga, Malaysia.*
Metformin hydrochloride (p.342·3).
*Diabetes mellitus.*

**Glumida** *Pensa, Spain.*
Acarbose (p.328·3).
*Diabetes mellitus.*

**Gluparin** *Locatelli, Ital.†.*
A heparinoid (p.931·1).
*Hyperlipidaemias; peripheral vascular disorders; thrombosis prophylaxis.*

**Glu-Phos** *SPA, Ital.*
Disodium glucose-1-phosphate.
*Glucose deficiency.*

**Glupitel** *Lilly, Mex.*
Glipizide (p.332·2).
*Diabetes mellitus.*

**Glupozide** *Merck, Hong Kong.*
Gliclazide (p.332·1).
*Diabetes mellitus.*

**Glurenor**
*Guidotti, Ital.; Boehringer Ingelheim, Port.; Yamanouchi, Spain; Menarini, Thai.*
Gliquidone (p.332·3).
*Diabetes mellitus.*

**Glurenorm**
*Boehringer Ingelheim, Austria; Menarini, Belg.; Yamanouchi, Ger.; Sanofi Synthelabo, UK.*
Gliquidone (p.332·3).
*Diabetes mellitus.*

**Glustress** *Pond's, Thai.*
Metformin hydrochloride (p.342·3).
*Diabetes mellitus.*

**Gluta Complex** *UCB, Ital.*
Cobamamide (p.1459·1); amino acids (p.1417·1).
*Tonic.*

**Glutabeina A** *Allergan-Frumtost, Braz.†.*
Glutamic acid; vitamin A acetate; thiamine; pyridoxine (p.1417·1).
*Nutritional supplement.*

**Glutabeina E** *Allergan-Frumtost, Braz.†.*
Glutamic acid; tocoferil acetate; thiamine; pyridoxine (p.1417·1).
*Nutritional supplement.*

**Glutacerebro** *AFOM, Ital.*
Glutamine (p.1433·2).
*Mental function impairment.*

**Glutacid** *Nycomed, Norw.†.*
Glutamic acid (p.1433·2).
*Achlorhydria; hypochlorhydria.*

**Glutacyl Vitaminado** *Instituto Sanitas, Chile.*
Monosodium glutamate (p.1441·1); pyridoxine hydrochloride (p.1456·3); glutamic acid (p.1433·2).
*Mental function impairment.*

**Glutaferro** *Medix, Spain.*
Ferrous glutamate (p.1436·1) or ferrous glycine sulfate (p.1428·2).
Ascorbic acid (p.1460·2) is included in the capsules to increase absorption and availability of iron and docusate sodium (p.1262·2) is included to reduce the constipating effects of iron.
*Anaemias.*

**Glutafin**
*Nutricia, Irl.; Nutricia, Ital.; Nutricia, NZ†; Nutricia Dietary, UK.*
A range of gluten-free foods (p.1417·1).
*Gluten sensitivity.*

**Glutamag Vitamine** *Euform, Fr.†.*
Magnesium glutamate (p.1229·1); riboflavin sodium phosphate (p.1456·1); nicotinamide (p.1441·2).
*Tonic.*

**Glutamed** *Boehringer Mannheim, Ital.†.*
Glutathione sodium (p.1040·3).
*Alcohol and drug poisoning; protection against toxicity induced by cytotoxic chemotherapy; radiation trauma.*

**Glutamin** *Verla, Ger.*
Glutamic acid (p.1433·2).
*Tonic.*

**Glutamin Fosforo** *SIT, Ital.*
Glutamine (p.1433·2); DL-phosphoserine; cyanocobalamin (p.1458·2).
*Mental function impairment.*

**Glutanil** *Bioprogress, Ital.*
Reduced glutathione sodium (p.1040·3).
*Alcohol and drug poisoning; radiation trauma.*

**Glutarex** *Ross, USA.*
A range of lysine- and tryptophan-free preparations for enteral nutrition including an infant feed (p.1417·1).
*Glutaric aciduria type I.*

**Glutargin** *Terapeutico, Ital.*
Arginine glutamate (p.1421·1); arginine aspartate (p.1421·1).
*Liver disorders.*

**Glutarin** *Pharmaland, Thai.†.*
Glutaral (p.1180·3).
*Instrument disinfection.*

**Glutarol**
*Dermal Laboratories, Irl.; Vifor, Switz.†; Dermal Laboratories, UK.*
Glutaral (p.1180·3).
*Warts.*

**Glutarsin E** *Berlin-Chemie, Ger.*
Glutamic acid (p.1433·2); arginine hydrochloride (p.1421·1); potassium hydroxide (p.1734·2); sodium hydroxide (p.1747·3).
*Hyperammonaemia.*

**Glutasan** *San Carlo, Ital.†.*
Glutathione sodium (p.1040·3).
*Alcohol and drug poisoning; radiation trauma.*

**Glutasedan** *Northia, Arg.*
Diazepam (p.690·1).
*Anxiety; muscle spasm.*

**Glutasey** *Alacan, Spain.*
Simvastatin (p.997·1).
*Hyperlipidaemias; secondary prophylaxis of ischaemic heart disease.*

**Glutasorb** *Hormel, Hong Kong.*
A glutamine-rich preparation for enteral nutrition (p.1417·1).

**Glutaven** *Teofarma, Ital.*
Glutamine (p.1433·2).
*Mental function impairment.*

**Glutavigon** *Delta, Braz.*
Calcium phosphate; calcium glycerophosphate; glutamic acid; vitamin B substances (p.1417·1).

**Gluthion** *CT, Ital.*
Reduced glutathione sodium (p.1040·3).
*Alcohol and drug poisoning; radiation trauma.*

**Gluti-Agil mono** *Riemser, Ger.*
Glutamic acid (p.1433·2).
*Mental function disorders.*

**Glutilage** *Beacons, Singapore.*
Glucosamine sulfate (p.1694·1).
*Joint and cartilage disorders.*

**Glutisal** *Ravensberg, Ger.*
Salicylamide (p.87·3); ethenzamide (p.37·2).
*Fever; gout; pain.*

**Glutofac**
*Kenwood, Hong Kong; Kenwood, USA.*
A range of vitamin and mineral preparations (p.1417·1).

**Glutose** *Paddock, USA.*
Glucose (p.1432·2).
*Hypoglycaemia.*

**Glutoxil** *Rottapharm, Ital.†.*
Glutathione sodium (p.1040·3).
*Alcohol and drug poisoning; radiation trauma.*

**Glutril**
*ICN, Austria; CSP, Fr.; ICN, Ger.; ICN, Switz.*
Glibornuride (p.331·3).
*Diabetes mellitus.*

**Gluzo** *Pharmasant, Thai.*
Glibenclamide (p.331·2).
*Diabetes mellitus.*

**Gluzolyte** *Pharmasant, Thai.*
Metformin hydrochloride (p.342·3).
*Diabetes mellitus.*

**Gly Derm Super Sunblock** *ICN, Canad.*
Meradimate (p.1151·3); octinoxate (p.1154·3); octisalate (p.1154·3); titanium dioxide (p.1160·3).
*Sunscreen.*

**Glyade**
*Alphapharm, Austral.; Alphapharm, Malaysia; Merck, Malaysia.*
Gliclazide (p.332·1).
*Diabetes mellitus.*

**Glyate** *Geneva, USA†.*
Guaifenesin (p.1122·1).
*Coughs.*

**Glycemin** *Siam Bheasach, Thai.*
Chlorpropamide (p.330·3).
*Diabetes mellitus.*

**Glycemirex** *Irex, Fr.†.*
Gliclazide (p.332·1).
*Diabetes mellitus.*

**Glyceol**
*Chugai, Hong Kong; Chugai, Thai.*
Glycerol (p.1694·3) with fructose and sodium chloride.
*Cerebral oedema; raised intracranial pressure.*

*Chugai, Jpn.*
Glycerol (concentrated) (p.1694·3).
*Cerebral oedema; ocular hypertension; raised intracranial pressure.*

**Glycerosteril**
*Fresenius Kabi, Ger.*
Glycerol (p.1694·3).
*Cerebral oedema.*

*Fresenius Kabi, Thai.*
Glycerol (p.1694·3) with glucose and sodium chloride.
*Cerebral oedema.*

**Glycerotone** *Novartis, Fr.†.*
Glycerol (p.1694·3).
*Ocular hypertension; raised intracranial pressure.*

**Glyceryl-T** *Rugby, USA.*
Theophylline (p.798·3); guaifenesin (p.1122·1).
*Bronchospasm.*

**Glycifer** *Nycomed, Denm.*
Ferrous glycine sulfate (p.1428·2).
*Iron deficiency.*

**Glycilax** *Engelhard, Ger.*
Glycerol (p.1694·3).
*Constipation.*

**Glyciphage** *Franco-Indian, India.*
Metformin hydrochloride (p.342·3).
*Diabetes mellitus.*

**Glycirenan** *Dispergo, Austria†.*
Adrenaline hydrochloride (p.852·3).
*Bronchospasm.*

**Glycobal** *Nadeau, Canad.†.*
Multivitamin and mineral preparation (p.1417·1).

**Glycocortison** *Novartis Ophthalmics, Ger.*
Hydrocortisone acetate (p.1103·3).
*Eye disorders.*

**Glycocortisone H** *Ciba Vision, Switz.*
Hydrocortisone acetate (p.1103·3) in glucose.
*Corneal disorders.*

**Glycofed** *Pal-Pak, USA.*
Pseudoephedrine hydrochloride (p.1129·2); guaifenesin (p.1122·1).
*Coughs.*

**glycolande N** *Sanofi Synthelabo, Ger.*
Glibenclamide (p.331·2).
*Diabetes mellitus.*

**Glycomin** *Aspen, S.Afr.*
Glibenclamide (p.331·2).
*Diabetes mellitus.*

**Glycon**
*Note. This name is used for preparations of different composition.*
*Farmalab, Braz.*
Potassium iodide (p.1598·1); ammonium benzoate; tolu balsam (p.1131·3).
*Respiratory-tract congestion.*

*ICN, Canad.*
Metformin hydrochloride (p.342·3).
*Diabetes mellitus.*

*Siam Bheasach, Thai.*
Gliclazide (p.332·1).
*Diabetes mellitus.*

**Glyconon** *DDSA Pharmaceuticals, UK†.*
Tolbutamide (p.348·1).
*Diabetes mellitus.*

**Glycophos**
*Fresenius Kabi, Austria; Fresenius Kabi, Fin.†; Fresenius Kabi, Gr.; Fresenius Kabi, Port.; Fresenius Kabi, Swed.; Fresenius Kabi, Switz.; Fresenius Kabi, UK.*
Sodium glycerophosphate (p.1695·2).
*Phosphate supplement for parenteral nutrition.*

**Glycoplex** *Vitaplex, Austral.†.*
Vitamins, minerals, and amino acids (p.1417·1); liquorice (p.1270·2); taraxacum (p.1751·3).
*Dietary supplement.*

**Glycoprep**
*Pharmatel, Austral.; Bamford, NZ.*
Macrogol 3350 (p.1709·1); electrolytes (p.1217·1).
*Bowel evacuation.*

**Glycoprep-C** *Pharmatel, Austral.*
Macrogol 3350 (p.1709·1); electrolytes (p.1217·1); ascorbic acid (p.1460·2).
*Bowel evacuation.*

**Gly-Coramin** *Novartis Consumer, Switz.*
Nikethamide (p.1591·2); glucose and other reduced sugars (p.1432·2).
*Tonic.*

**Glycoran** *Shinyaku, Singapore.*
Metformin hydrochloride (p.342·3).
*Diabetes mellitus.*

**Glycostigmin** *Leiras, Fin.*
Neostigmine metilsulfate (p.1492·2).
Glycopyrronium bromide (p.482·3) is included in this preparation to protect against muscarinic actions.
*Reversal of competitive neuromuscular blockade.*

**Glyco-Thymoline** *SERP, Mon.*
Sodium benzoate (p.1169·3); sodium bicarbonate (p.1223·2); borax (p.1661·3); sodium salicylate (p.90·1); thymol (p.1194·2); cineole (p.1672·1); oleum pini sylvestris; menthol (p.1711·3); glycerol (p.1694·3).
*Mouth disorders.*

**Glycotuss** *Pal-Pak, USA.*
Guaifenesin (p.1122·1).
*Coughs.*

**Glycotuss-dM** *Pal-Pak, USA.*
Dextromethorphan hydrobromide (p.1117·3); guaifenesin (p.1122·1).
*Coughs.*

**Glycovit** *Alifarma, Ital.*
Amino-acid, multivitamin, and mineral preparation (p.1417·1).
*Nutritional supplement.*

**Glycron** *Aspen, S.Afr.*
Gliclazide (p.332·1).
*Diabetes mellitus.*

**Glycylpressin**
*Ferring, Arg.; Ferring, Austria; Ferring, Ger.*
Terlipressin acetate (p.1340·1).
*Haemorrhagic gastritis; variceal haemorrhage.*

**Glycyrrhiza Complex** *Blackmores, Austral.†.*
Liquorice (p.1270·2); avena (p.1658·2); rose fruit (p.1740·1); vitamins (p.1417·1); ginseng (p.1693·1).
*Tonic.*

**Glyderm**
*ICN, Hong Kong; ICN, Malaysia; ICN, Singapore.*
Esterified glycolic acid (p.1147·3).
*Dry skin disorders.*

**Glyfucan** *Legrand, Braz.*
Fluconazole (p.398·1).
*Fungal infections.*

**Glygen** *General Drugs, Thai.*
Glipizide (p.332·2).
*Diabetes mellitus.*

**Glykola** *Durbin, UK.*
Calcium glycerophosphate (p.1225·2); caffeine (p.782·1); kola liquid extract (p.1765·3); ferric chloride (p.1688·1).
*Tonic.*

**Glymax** *LPN, Fr.†.*
Metformin hydrochloride (p.342·3).
*Diabetes mellitus.*

**Glymese** *DDSA Pharmaceuticals, UK†.*
Chlorpropamide (p.330·3).
*Diabetes mellitus.*

**Glynase**
*Note. This name is used for preparations of different composition.*
*USV, India.*
Glipizide (p.332·2).
*Diabetes mellitus.*

*Julphar, UAE; Pharmacia Upjohn, USA.*
Glibenclamide (p.331·2).
*Diabetes mellitus.*

**Glyoktyl** *Medic, Denm.*
Docusate sodium (p.1262·2); glycerol (p.1694·3).
*Bowel evacuation; constipation.*

**Gly-Oxide** *SmithKline Beecham Consumer, USA.*
Urea hydrogen peroxide (p.1195·3).
*Oral hygiene; oral inflammation.*

**Glyphyllin** *Rekah, Israel.*
Theophylline sodium glycinate (p.804·3).
*Obstructive airways disease.*

**Glypressin**
*Ferring, Belg.; Ferring, Braz.†; Ferring, Denm.; Ferring, Fin.; Ferring, Irl.; Ferring, Neth.; Ferring, Spain; Ferring, UK.*
Terlipressin acetate (p.1340·1).
*Variceal haemorrhage.*

*Ferring, Hong Kong; Ferring, Malaysia; Ferring, Singapore; Ferring, Thai.†.*
Terlipressin (p.1340·1).
*Variceal haemorrhage.*

**Glypressine**
*Ferring, Fr.; Ferring, Switz.*
Terlipressin acetate (p.1340·1).
*Variceal haemorrhage.*

**Glyprin** *CCM, Malaysia.*
Aspirin (p.15·1).
Glycine (p.1433·3) is included in this preparation in an attempt to limit adverse effects on the gastrointestinal mucosa.
*Thromboembolism prophylaxis.*

**Glyquin**
*Note. This name is used for preparations of different composition.*
*ICN, Hong Kong.*
Hydroquinone (p.1148·1); padimate O (p.1155·1); oxybenzone (p.1154·3); octinoxate (p.1154·3); glycolic acid (p.1147·3).
*Hyperpigmented skin disorders.*

*ICN, Singapore.*
Hydroquinone (p.1148·1); glycolic acid (p.1147·3).
*Hyperpigmentation of the skin.*

**Glyquin-XM** *ICN, USA.*
Hydroquinone (p.1148·1); octocrilene (p.1154·3); oxybenzone (p.1154·3); avobenzone (p.1142·3); glycolic acid (p.1147·3).
*Hyperpigmented skin disorders.*

**Gly-Rectal** *Valmo, Canad.†.*
Glycerol (p.1694·3).

**Glysan** *Riemser, Ger.*
Magaldrate (p.1271·3).
*Gastric hyperacidity; heartburn; peptic ulcer.*

**Glysennid** *Novartis Consumer, Canad.*
Sennosides (p.1288·2).
*Constipation.*

**Glyset** *Bayer, USA.*
Miglitol (p.343·2).
*Diabetes mellitus.*

**Glyteol Balsamico** *Hertz, Braz.†.*
Guaifenesin (p.1122·1); potassium iodide (p.1598·1); menthol (p.1711·3).
*Coughs.*

**Glytop** *Pharmatrix, Arg.*
Triamcinolone acetonide (p.1110·2).
*Skin disorders.*

**Glytoss** *Sibras, Braz.†.*
Ammonium chloride (p.1115·2); cetylpyridinium chloride (p.1173·1).
*Coughs.*

**Glytrin**
*Bioglan, Denm.; Bioglan, Hong Kong†; Sanofi Synthelabo, Irl.; Bioglan, Malaysia; Tramedico, Neth.; AFT, NZ; Bioglan, Singapore†; Bioglan, Swed.; Bioglan, Thai.; Sanofi Synthelabo, UK.*
Glyceryl trinitrate (p.923·2).
*Angina pectoris.*

**Glytuss** *Mayrand, USA†.*
Guaifenesin (p.1122·1).
*Coughs.*

**Glyvenol**
*Novartis, Austria†; Novartis, Belg.; Novartis, Braz.; Novartis, Hong Kong†; Novartis, Mex.; Novartis, Switz.†; Novartis, Thai.†.*
Tribenoside (p.1757·3).
*Haemorrhoids; venous insufficiency.*

**Glyzide** *Julphar, UAE.*
Gliclazide (p.332·1).
*Diabetes mellitus.*

**Glyzip** *Stadmed, India.*
Glipizide (p.332·2).
*Diabetes mellitus.*

**G-Myticin** *Pedinol, USA†.*
Gentamicin sulfate (p.217·1).
*Bacterial infections.*

**GNC** *General Nutrition, Canad.*
Range of vitamin and mineral preparations (p.1417·1).

**GNC Herbal Laxative** *General Nutrition, Canad.*
Senna (p.1288·2).
*Constipation.*

**GNO** *Arion, Arg.*
Morphine (p.60·1).
*Pain.*

**GNO CP** *Arion, Arg.*
Paracetamol (p.76·2); codeine (p.27·1).
*Fever; pain.*

**Gnostocardin** *Bros, Gr.*
Enalapril maleate (p.909·2).
*Heart failure; hypertension.*

**Gnostol** *Bros, Gr.*
Metronidazole (p.607·2).
*Anaerobic bacterial infections.*

**Gnostoval** *Bros, Gr.*
Lisinopril (p.946·3).
*Heart failure; hypertension; myocardial infarction.*

**Go Kit** *Pharmatel, Austral.*
3 Tablets, bisacodyl (p.1251·3); 1 sachet, magnesium citrate (p.1272·1).
*Bowel evacuation.*

**Go Kit Plus** *Pharmatel, Austral.*
3 Tablets, bisacodyl (p.1251·3); 1 suppository, bisacodyl (p.1251·3); 1 sachet, magnesium citrate (p.1272·1).
*Bowel evacuation.*

**Goanna Analgesic Ice** *Herron, Austral.*
Glycol salicylate (p.44·3); menthol (p.1711·3).
*Musculoskeletal and joint pain.*

**Goanna Arthritis Cream** *Herron, Austral.*
Trolamine salicylate (p.95·3).
*Musculoskeletal and joint pain.*

**Goanna Bite-Eze** *Herron, Austral.†.*
Eucalyptus (p.1686·1); citronella oil (p.1673·2); peppermint flower (p.1283·2).
*Bites; cold and influenza symptoms; skin disorders.*

**Goanna Heat Cream** *Herron, Austral.†.*
Methyl salicylate (p.59·3); menthol (p.1711·3); camphor (p.1665·3); eucalyptus oil (p.1686·2); pumilio pine oil (p.1737·1); turpentine oil (p.1760·1); peppermint oil (p.1283·2); cajuput oil (p.1664·1); capsicum oleoresin (p.1667·1).
*Musculoskeletal, joint, and soft-tissue pain.*

**Goanna Liniment** *Herron, Austral.†.*
Methyl salicylate (p.59·3); turpentine oil (p.1760·1); eucalyptus oil (p.1686·2); camphor (p.1665·3); peppermint oil (p.1283·2); pumilio pine oil (p.1737·1); menthol (p.1711·3).
*Musculoskeletal and joint pain.*

**Goanna Salve** *Herron, Austral.†.*
Eucalyptus oil (p.1686·2); pumilio pine oil (p.1737·1); peppermint oil (p.1283·2); camphor (p.1665·3); methyl salicylate (p.59·3); menthol (p.1711·3); turpentine oil (p.1760·1).
*Musculoskeletal and joint pain.*

**Gobanal** *Normon, Spain.*
Diazepam (p.690·1).
Contains pyridoxine hydrochloride.
*Alcohol withdrawal syndrome; anxiety; febrile convulsions; insomnia; skeletal muscle spasm.*

**Gobbicaina** *Gobbi, Arg.*
Lidocaine (p.1377·3) or lidocaine hydrochloride (p.1377·3).
Adrenaline (p.852·2) is included in some injections as a vasoconstrictor to diminish absorption and localise the effect of the local anaesthetic.
*Local anaesthesia.*

**Gobbidona** *Gobbi, Arg.*
Methadone hydrochloride (p.57·2).
*Opioid withdrawal syndrome; pain.*

**Gobbizolam** *Gobbi, Arg.*
Midazolam (p.707·1).
*General anaesthesia; sedative.*

**Gobemicina** *Normon, Spain.*
Ampicillin trihydrate (p.157·2) or ampicillin sodium (p.157·1).
*Bacterial infections.*

**Gobemicina Retard** *Normon, Spain.*
Ampicillin sodium (p.157·1); ampicillin benzathine (p.158·1).
Lidocaine hydrochloride (p.1377·3) is included in this preparation to alleviate the pain of injection.
*Bacterial infections.*

**Gobens Trim** *Normon, Spain.*
Co-trimoxazole (p.199·3).
*Bacterial infections; Pneumocystis carinii pneumonia.*

**Gobrosan** *Protein, Mex.†.*
Ibuprofen (p.45·3).

**Gocce Antonetto** *Antonetto, Ital.†.*
Sodium picosulfate (p.1289·3).
*Constipation.*

**Gocce Lassative Aicardi** *SIT, Ital.*
Sodium picosulfate (p.1289·3).
*Constipation.*

**Goccemed** *Iodosan, Ital.*
Iodine (p.1598·1).
*Oral hygiene.*

**Gocox-3** *Ipca, India.*
Rifampicin (p.250·2); isoniazid (p.222·2); pyrazinamide (p.246·3).
*Tuberculosis.*

**Gocox Compound** *Ipca, India.*
Rifampicin (p.250·2); isoniazid (p.222·2); vitamin $B_6$ (p.1457·2).
*Tuberculosis.*

**Godabion B6** *Merck, Spain.*
Pyridoxine hydrochloride (p.1456·3).
*Vitamin B6 deficiency.*

**Godal** *Merck, Spain†.*
Bisoprolol fumarate (p.875·1).
*Angina pectoris; hypertension.*

**Godamed**
*Pfleger, Ger.*
Aspirin (p.15·1).
Glycine (p.1433·3) is included in this preparation in an attempt to limit adverse effects on the gastrointestinal mucosa.
*Fever; pain; thromboembolic disorders.*

*Pfleger, Israel.*
Aspirin (p.15·1).
*Thromboembolic disorders.*

**Goddards Embrocation** *Thornton & Ross, UK.*
Turpentine oil (p.1760·1); dilute acetic acid (p.1645·2); dilute ammonia solution (p.1653·3).
*Musculoskeletal and soft-tissue disorders.*

**Go-Evac** *Copley, USA†.*
Macrogol 3350 (p.1709·1); electrolytes (p.1217·1).
*Bowel evacuation.*

**Gofreely** *Promedical, Ital.†.*
Macrogol 3350 (p.1709·1); electrolytes (p.1217·1).
*Bowel evacuation.*

**Gola Action** *Iodosan, Ital.*
Benzydamine hydrochloride (p.21·1); cetylpyridinium chloride (p.1173·1).
*Mouth and throat disorders.*

**Golac** *Elofar, Braz.†.*
Potassium citrate; sodium chloride; sodium citrate; calcium lactate; magnesium citrate; glucose (p.1222·2).
*Diarrhoea; oral rehydration therapy.*

**Golacetin** *Vaillant, Ital.*
Cetylpyridinium chloride (p.1173·1).
*Oral disinfection.*

**Goladin** *Sofar, Ital.†.*
Dequalinium chloride (p.1178·1).
*Oral disinfection.*

**Golamed** *Iodosan, Ital.*
Cicliomenol (p.1177·3).
*Mouth and throat disinfection.*

**Golamed Due** *Iodosan, Ital.*
Cicliomenol (p.1177·3); hexylresorcinol (p.1182·1).
*Mouth and throat disinfection; sore throat.*

**Golamed Oral** *Iodosan, Ital.†.*
Iodinated glycerol (p.1122·3); domiphen bromide (p.1179·1).
*Oropharyngeal disinfection.*

**Golamixin** *Teofarma, Ital.*
Tyrothricin (p.275·1); cetrimonium bromide (p.1173·1); benzocaine (p.1370·3).
*Bacterial stomatitis.*

**Golan** *Mavi, Mex.†.*
Furosemide (p.919·3).

**Golapiol** *Antipiol, Ital.*
Propolis (p.1735·2).

**Golapiol C** *Antipiol, Ital.*
Propolis (p.1735·2); rose fruit (p.1740·1).

**Golasan** *Dynacren, Ital.*
Chlorhexidine gluconate (p.1173·2) or chlorhexidine hydrochloride (p.1173·3).
*Mouth and throat disinfection; oral hygiene.*

**Golasept** *Zeta, Ital.*
Povidone-iodine (p.1190·3).
*Oral disinfection.*

**Golaseptine** *SMB, Belg.*
Chlorhexidine hydrochloride (p.1173·3).
*Mouth and throat disorders.*

**Golasol** *Gambar, Ital.†.*
Chlorhexidine gluconate (p.1173·2).
*Mouth and throat disinfection; oral hygiene.*

**Golatux** *Antipiol, Ital.*
Hedera helix; echinacea (p.1683·2).

**Golaval** *Carlo Erba OTC, Ital.*
Cetrimonium tosilate (p.1173·1).
*Mouth and throat disinfection.*

**Gold-50** *Schering-Plough, Austral.†.*
Aurothioglucose (p.19·3).
*Rheumatoid arthritis.*

**Gold Alka-Seltzer** *Bayer, USA.*
Sodium bicarbonate (p.1223·2); citric acid (p.1673·1); potassium bicarbonate (p.1223·1).
*Hyperacidity.*

**Gold Cross Antihistamine Elixir** *Biotech, Austral.*
Promethazine hydrochloride (p.439·1).
*Hypersensitivity reactions; insomnia; motion sickness.*

**Gold Cross BOZ Ointment** *Biotech, Austral.*
Boric acid (p.1662·1); olive oil (p.1723·2); zinc oxide (p.1163·2).
Formerly known as Boz.
*Eczema; psoriasis.*

**Gold Cross Cough Medicine** *Biotech, Austral.*
Ammonium chloride (p.1115·2); diphenhydramine hydrochloride (p.431·3); menthol (p.1711·3); sodium citrate (p.1223·2).
*Coughs.*

**Gold Cross Gluco-lyte** *Biotech, Austral.*
Glucose; sucrose; sodium chloride; potassium chloride; sodium citrate; citric acid (p.1222·2).
*Diarrhoea; oral rehydration.*

**Gold Cross Skin Basics Zinc Cream** *Biotech, Austral.*
*SPF 15+:* Arachis oil (p.1656·1); white soft paraffin (p.1479·3); zinc oxide (p.1163·2).
*Skin disorders.*

**Gold Cross Vaporiser Fluid** *Biotech, Austral.*
Camphor (p.1665·3); eucalyptus oil (p.1686·2); menthol (p.1711·3); methyl salicylate (p.59·3).
*Nasal congestion.*

**Goldar** *Zydus, India.*
Auranofin (p.19·1).
*Rheumatoid arthritis.*

**Goldcare** *Vitabiotics, UK.*
Multivitamin and mineral preparation with ginkgo biloba and bioflavonoids (p.1417·1).

**Golden Eye Drops** *Typharm, UK.*
Propamidine isetionate (p.1191·2).
*Eye infections.*

**Golden Eye Ointment**
*Note. This name is used for preparations of different composition.*
*Sigma, Austral.*
Yellow mercuric oxide (p.1712·3).
*Bacterial eye infections.*

*Typharm, UK.*
Dibrompropamidine isetionate (p.1178·2).
*Eye infections.*

**Golden Star** *Duopharm, Ger.†.*
Vitamin A palmitate (p.1453·1); riboflavin sodium phosphate (p.1456·1).
*Eye disorders.*

**Goldgeist** *Gerlach, Ger.*
Pyrethrum (p.1509·3); piperonyl butoxide (p.1509·2).
*Pediculosis.*

**Goldgesic** *Ranbaxy, S.Afr.*
Paracetamol (p.76·2); codeine phosphate (p.27·1); promethazine hydrochloride (p.439·1).
*Fever; pain.*

**Gold-Komplex** *Steigerwald, Ger.*
Homoeopathic preparation.

**Goldtropfen N** *DHU, Ger.†.*
Homoeopathic preparation.

**Goldtropfen S** *DHU, Ger.*
Homoeopathic preparation.

**Goldtropfen-Hetterich** *Galenika, Ger.†.*
Crataegus (p.1677·1); valerian (p.1762·2); convallaria (p.1675·3); scoparium (p.1742·2); camphor (p.1665·3); gold chloride.
*Cardiac disorders.*

**GoLytely**
*Stafford-Miller, Austral.†; Braintree, Canad.; Stafford-Miller, NZ†; Kloster, S.Afr.; Braintree, USA.*
Macrogol 3350 (p.1709·1); electrolytes (p.1217·1).
*Bowel evacuation.*

**Gomec** *General Drugs, Thai.*
Omeprazole (p.1278·2).
*Gastro-oesophageal reflux, Zollinger-Ellison syndrome; peptic ulcer.*

**Gomenol** *Gomenol, Fr.*
Niaouli oil (p.1719·3).
*Respiratory-tract disorders.*

**Gomenoleo** *Gomenol, Fr.*
Niaouli oil (p.1719·3).
*Burns; infections; instrument lubrication; ulcers; wounds.*

**Gomenol-Syner-Penicilline** *Gomenol, Fr.†.*
Benzylpenicillin sodium (p.163·2); niaouli oil (p.1719·3).
*Bacterial infections.*

**Gon** *Sanitas, Arg.*
Glibenclamide (p.331·2).
*Diabetes mellitus.*

**Gonablok** *Win-Medicare, India.*
Danazol (p.1545·2).
*Endometriosis; female infertility; fibrocystic breast disease; gynaecomastia; menorrhagia; precocious puberty.*

**Gonacor** *Ferring, Arg.*
Chorionic gonadotrophin (p.1320·3).
*Crytporchidism; delayed puberty; female infertility; hypogonadism.*

**Gonadotraphon LH** *Paines & Byrne, Irl.†.*
Chorionic gonadotrophin (p.1320·3).
*Anovulatory infertility; delayed male puberty; oligospermia; undescended testes.*

**Gonadotropyl C** *Aventis, Mex.*
Chorionic gonadotrophin (p.1320·3).
*Cryptorchidism; delayed puberty; hypogonadism; male and female infertility.*

**Gonak** *Akorn, USA.*
Hypromellose (p.1579·3).
*Gonioscopic examination.*

**Gonakor** *Sanfer, Mex.*
Chorionic gonadotrophin (p.1320·3); hydroxocobalamin (p.1458·2).
*Erectile dysfunction; hypogonadism; oligospermia.*

**Gonal-F**
*Serono, Arg.; Serono, Austral.; Serono, Austria; Serono, Braz.; Serono, Canad.; Serono, Denm.; Serono, Fin.; Serono, Fr.; Serono, Ger.; Serono, Gr.; Serono, Hong Kong; Serum Institute, India; Serono, Irl.; Serono, Israel; Serono, Ital.; Serono, Malaysia; Serono, Mex.; Serono, Neth.; Serono, Norw.; Douglas, NZ; Serono, Port.; Serono, S.Afr.; Serono, Singapore; Serono, Spain; Serono, Swed.; Serono, Switz.; Serono, Thai.; Serono, UK; Serono, USA.*
Follitropin alfa (p.1324·2).
*Male and female infertility.*

**Gonapeptyl**
*Ferring, Arg.; Ferring, UK.*
Triptorelin (p.1341·2).
*Endometriosis; precocious puberty; prostatic cancer; uterine fibroids.*

**Gonaplex** *Carter-Wallace, Mex.†.*
Chorionic gonadotrophin (p.1320·3).

**Gonasi HP** *Amsa, Ital.*
Chorionic gonadotrophin (p.1320·3).
Formerly known as Gonadotrafon LH.
*Amenorrhoea; cryptorchidism; hypogonadism; infertility; threatened or recurrent miscarriage.*

**Gonasone** *Fustery, Mex.†.*
Chorionic gonadotrophin (p.1320·3).
*Cryptorchidism; female infertility; hypogonadism and delayed puberty in the male; recurrent miscarriage.*

**Gonaxine** *Motima, Fr.*
Parsley piert (p.1729·1); sage (p.1741·2); achillea (p.1646·2); alfalfa (p.1649·1); avena (p.1658·2).
*Tonic for females.*

**Gondonar** *Teva Tuteur, Arg.*
Anastrozole (p.528·1).
*Malignant neoplasms.*

**Gonic** *Hauck, USA.*
Chorionic gonadotrophin (p.1320·3).
*Male and female infertility; male hypogonadism; prepubertal cryptorchidism.*

**Gonif** *Kleva, Gr.*
Cefuroxime sodium (p.184·1).
*Bacterial infections.*

**Gonioscopic** *Alcon, USA.*
Hyetellose (p.1579·2).
*Gonioscopic examination.*

**Goniosoft** *Ocusoft, USA.*
Hypromellose (p.1579·3).

**Goniosol** *Novartis Ophthalmics, USA.*
Hypromellose (p.1579·3).
*Gonioscopic examination.*

**Gonne Balm** *Lane, UK.*
Camphor (p.1665·3); menthol (p.1711·3); eucalyptus oil (p.1686·2); methyl salicylate (p.59·3); turpentine oil (p.1760·1).
*Joint and muscular pain.*

**Gonocilin** *Uniao Quimica, Braz.†.*
Ampicillin (p.157·1).
Probenecid (p.416·3) is included in this preparation to reduce renal tubular excretion of the antibiotic.
*Bacterial infections.*

**Gonoform** *Ratiopharm, Austria.*
Amoxicillin trihydrate (p.155·3).
*Bacterial infections.*

**Gonol** *Neo Quimica, Braz.*
Ampicillin (p.157·1).

Probenecid (p.416·3) is included in this preparation to reduce renal tubular excretion of the antibiotic.
*Bacterial infections.*

**Gonorcin** *General Drugs, Thai.*
Norfloxacin (p.238·3).
*Bacterial infections.*

**Gonorrels** *Gilton, Braz.†.*
Ampicillin (p.157·1).
Probenecid (p.416·3) is included in this preparation to reduce renal tubular excretion of the antibiotic.
*Bacterial infections.*

**Gonotrop F** *Win-Medicare, India.*
Urofollitropin (p.1342·1).
*Stimulation of ovulation.*

**Goodnight** *Aventis, NZ†.*
Promethazine hydrochloride (p.439·1).
*Insomnia.*

**Goodnight Formula** *Vitaplex, Austral.†.*
Valerian (p.1762·2); chamomile (p.1669·3); passion flower (p.1729·1); skullcap (p.1746·3); vitamin B substances (p.1417·1); zinc sulfate (p.1469·3).
*Insomnia.*

**Goodnight StopSnore** *Swisshealth, UK.*
Sunflower oil (p.1451·1); peppermint oil (p.1283·2); sesame oil (p.1743·3); vitamins $B_6$, C, and E (p.1417·1).
*Snoring.*

**Goodypops** *Health Imports, UK.*
Echinacea (p.1683·2); vitamin C (p.1460·2); pectin (p.1580·3).
*Sore throat.*

**Goody's Headache Powders** *Goodys, USA.*
Aspirin (p.15·1); paracetamol (p.76·2); caffeine (p.782·1).

**Go-On**
*Opfermann, Ger.; Rottapharm, Ital.*
Sodium hyaluronate (p.1697·3).
*Joint disorders; knee and shoulder synovial fluid replacement.*

**Go-Pain** *PD Pharm, S.Afr.*
*Syrup:* Paracetamol (p.76·2); codeine phosphate (p.27·1); promethazine hydrochloride (p.439·1).
*Fever; pain.*
*Tablets:* Paracetamol (p.76·2); codeine phosphate (p.27·1); caffeine (p.782·1); meprobamate (p.706·2).
*Pain with tension.*

**Go-Pain P** *PD Pharm, S.Afr.*
Paracetamol (p.76·2).
*Fever; pain.*

**Gopten**
*Abbott, Austral.; Ebewe, Austria; Abbott, Braz.; Abbott, Denm.; Abbott, Fin.; Knoll, Fr.; Abbott, Ger.; Abbott, Irl.; Abbott, Ital.; Knoll, Mex.; Knoll, Neth.; Abbott, Norw.; Abbott, NZ; Abbott, Port.; Knoll, S.Afr.; Abbott, Spain; Abbott, Swed.; Knoll, Switz.; Abbott, UK.*
Trandolapril (p.1016·1).
*Hypertension; left ventricular dysfunction following myocardial infarction.*

**Gordobalm** *Gordon, USA.*
Methyl salicylate (p.59·3); menthol (p.1711·3); camphor (p.1665·3).
*Muscle, joint, and soft-tissue pain; neuralgia.*

**Gordochom** *Gordon, USA.*
Undecenoic acid (p.410·3); chloroxylenol (p.1177·2).
*Fungal skin infections.*

**Gordofilm** *Gordon, USA.*
Salicylic acid (p.1157·1).
*Verrucas.*

**Gordogesic** *Gordon, USA.*
Methyl salicylate (p.59·3).
*Muscle, joint, and soft-tissue pain; neuralgia.*

**Gorgonium** *Drossopharm, Switz.*
Heparin (p.927·3); allantoin (p.1141·3); dexpanthenol (p.1727·2); collagen (p.1674·3).
*Scars.*

**Gormel** *Gordon, USA.*
Urea (p.1162·2).
*Dry skin; hyperkeratosis.*

**Gota Cebrina** *Irisfarma, Spain.*
Multivitamin preparation (p.1417·1).

**Gotabiotic** *Poen, Arg.*
Tobramycin (p.271·2).
*Bacterial eye infections.*

**Gotabiotic D** *Poen, Arg.*
Tobramycin (p.271·2); naphazoline hydrochloride (p.1124·3); dexamethasone phosphate (p.1097·2).
*Conjunctivitis.*

**Gotabiotic F** *Poen, Arg.*
Tobramycin (p.271·2); dexamethasone (p.1097·1).
*Infected eye disorders.*

**Gotadex** *Collins, Mex.*
Dexamethasone (p.1097·1); neomycin (p.235·1).
*Infected eye disorders.*

**Gotalax** *Mertens, Arg.*
Sodium picosulfate (p.1289·3).
*Constipation.*

**Gotalgic** *Laboratorios Chile, Chile.*
Polymyxin b (p.245·2); neomycin (p.235·1); betamethasone phosphate (p.1093·2); lidocaine hydrochloride (p.1377·3).
*Otitis externa; otitis media.*

**Gotas Binelli** *Daudt, Braz.*
Fedrilate (p.1121·2).
*Coughs.*

**Gotas Digestivas** *Bunker, Braz.*
Chamomile (p.1669·3); gentian (p.1692·2); nux vomica (p.1722·3); boldo (p.1661·2).
*Liver disorders.*

**Gotas Hepaticas** *Ariston, Braz.†.*
Cascara (p.1255·1); rhubarb (p.1287·3); boldo (p.1661·2); cynara (p.1678·3); belladonna (p.479·1).
*Liver disorders.*

**Gotas Nican**
*Note. This name is used for preparations of different composition.*
*Prima, Braz.*
Belladonna (p.479·1); grindelia (p.1696·1); aconite (p.1646·3); bromoform (p.1663·1); sodium dibunate (p.1130·2); passion flower (p.1729·1); sodium benzoate (p.1169·3).
*Coughs.*

*Andromaco, Chile.*
Codeine (p.27·1); bromoform (p.1663·1); aconite (p.1646·3); belladonna (p.479·1); grindelia (p.1696·1); drosera (p.1683·1); sodium benzoate (p.1169·3); cherry laurel water.
*Coughs.*

**Gotas Otologicas**
*Drag, Chile.*
Lidocaine (p.1377·3); sulfathiazole (p.264·1).
*Bacterial ear infections.*

*Volta, Chile.*
Lidocaine (p.1377·3); sulfathiazole sodium (p.264·1).
*Bacterial ear infections.*

**Gotas Ototilan** *Prodotti, Braz.†.*
Fluocinolone (p.1101·2); neomycin (p.235·1); lidocaine (p.1377·3).
*Infected ear disorders.*

**Gotas Preciosas** *Hertz, Braz.†.*
Cynara (p.1678·3); belladonna (p.479·1); boldo (p.1661·2); carqueja; gentian (p.1692·2); rhubarb (p.1287·3).
*Liver disorders.*

**Gotas Zimaia** *Zimaia, Port.†.*
Ephedrine (p.1120·1); ethylmorphine (p.37·3).
*Coughs.*

**Gotavit** *Berman, Mex.*
Multivitamin preparation (p.1417·1).

**Gothaplast Capsicum-Warmepflaster** *Gothaplast, Ger.*
Nonivamide (p.67·2).
*Musculoskeletal and joint disorders.*

**Gothaplast Rheumamed AC** *Gothaplast, Ger.*
Capsicum (p.1667·1); arnica (p.1656·3).
*Musculoskeletal and joint disorders.*

**Gotil-AD** *Laborsil, Braz.†.*
Vitamin A (p.1451·2); vitamin D (p.1461·2).
*Vitamin supplement.*

**Gotinal** *Boehringer Ingelheim, Arg.*
Naphazoline hydrochloride (p.1124·3).
*Nasal congestion.*

**Gotir** *Hexal, Arg.*
Allopurinol (p.412·2).
*Gout; hyperuricaemia; renal calculi.*

**Gotu Kola** *Natural Life, Arg.*
Centella (p.1144·3).
*Dietary supplement.*

**Goutichine** *Farmaline, Thai.*
Colchicine (p.415·1).
*Gout.*

**Goutnil**
*Inga, India; Inga, Malaysia.*
Colchicine (p.415·1).
*Gout.*

**Gouttes aux Essences** *Dolisos, Fr.*
Peppermint oil (p.1283·2); clove oil (p.1673·3); thyme oil (p.1755·3); cinnamon oil (p.1672·2); lavender oil (p.1705·2).
*Respiratory-tract disorders.*

**Gouttes contre la toux "S"** *Synpharma, Switz.*
Codeine phosphate (p.27·1); aromatic tincture; hyoscyamus (p.485·2); ipecacuanha (p.1122·3); drosera (p.1683·1); plantago lanceolata (p.1738·2).
*Coughs.*

**Gouttes contre le rhume des foins** *Phytomed, Switz.*
Homoeopathic preparation.

**Gouttes Dentaires** *Valmo, Canad.†.*
Benzocaine (p.1370·3); camphor (p.1665·3); guaiacol (p.1122·1); menthol (p.1711·3); clove oil (p.1673·3).

**Gouttes homeopathiques contre le rhume des foins** *Herbamed, Switz.†.*
Homoeopathic preparation.

**Gouttes nasales** *Spirig, Switz.*
Phenylephrine (p.1126·3).
*Nasal congestion; rhinitis; sinusitis.*

**Gouttes nasales N** *Spirig, Switz.*
Naphazoline nitrate (p.1124·3); phenylephrine (p.1126·3).
*Nasal congestion; rhinitis; sinusitis.*

**Gouttes pour le coeur et les nerfs Concentrees** *Zeller, Switz.*
Crataegus (p.1677·1); passion flower (p.1729·1).
*Cardiac disorders; nervous disorders.*

**Gouttes pour Mal d'Orreilles** *Valmo, Canad.†.*
Benzocaine (p.1370·3); camphor (p.1665·3); chlorobutanol (p.1176·3).

**Goval** *Pharma Investi, Chile.*
Risperidone (p.719·2).
*Psychoses.*

**Goxil** *Pharmacia, Spain.*
Azithromycin (p.159·1).
*Bacterial infections.*

**Gozid** *General Drugs, Thai.*
Gemfibrozil (p.923·1).
*Hyperlipidaemias.*

**GP** *Cypress, USA.*
Pseudoephedrine hydrochloride (p.1129·2); guaifenesin (p.1122·1).
*Coughs; respiratory-tract congestion.*

**G-Press** *Gap, Gr.*
Nitrendipine (p.973·3).
*Hypertension.*

**Gracial**
*Organon, Austria; Organon, Belg.; Organon, Braz.; Organon, Chile; Organon, Denm.; Organon, Fin.; Organon (Οργανον), Gr.; Organon, Hong Kong; Organon, Ital.; Organon, Neth.; Organon, Port.; Organon, Spain; Organon, Switz.*
Desogestrel (p.1547·2); ethinylestradiol (p.1553·2).
*Biphasic oral contraceptive.*

**Gradient** *Polifarma, Ital.*
Flunarizine hydrochloride (p.434·1).
*Migraine; vertigo.*

**Gradin Del D Andreu** *Roche, Spain.*
Benzalkonium chloride (p.1168·3); benzocaine (p.1370·3); tyrothricin (p.275·1).
*Mouth and throat disorders.*

**Grafco batonnets de bois** *Salzmann, Switz.†.*
Silver nitrate (p.1746·1); potassium nitrate (p.1190·1).
*Granulation tissue; verrucas.*

**Grafin** *IQFA, Mex.*
Butylhyoscine (p.484·2).

**Grains de Vals**
*Note. This name is used for preparations of different composition.*
*Qualiphar, Belg.*
Aloes (p.1248·2); belladonna (p.479·1); cascara (p.1255·1); frangula bark (p.1266·3); intestinal mucosa extract; ox bile extract (p.1660·3); phenolphthalein (p.1284·1).
*Constipation.*

*Nogues, Fr.; Nogues, Switz.†.*
Boldo (p.1661·2); cascara (p.1255·1); senna (p.1288·2).
*Constipation.*

**Grains de Vals Nouvelle formule** *Nogues, Switz.*
Senna (p.1288·2).
*Constipation.*

**Gral** *Boniscontro & Gazzone, Ital.†.*
Dihydroergocristine mesilate (p.1680·1).
*Cerebrovascular disorders; dopaminergic deficiency; headache; hypertension; migraine; peripheral vascular disorders.*

**Gramal** *Probiomed, Mex.*
Molgramostim (p.756·1).
*Reduction of neutropenia associated with cytotoxic therapy or bone marrow transplants.*

**Gramalil** *Fujisawa, Jpn.*
Tiapride hydrochloride (p.725·1).
*Behaviour disorders associated with stroke; dyskinesias.*

**Gramaxin**
*Roche, Austria†; Boehringer Mannheim, Ger.†.*
Cefazolin sodium (p.170·3).
Lidocaine hydrochloride (p.1377·3) may be included in the intramuscular preparation to alleviate the pain of injection.
*Bacterial infections.*

**Gramcal** *Sandoz, Canad.†.*
Calcium lactate gluconate (p.1225·3); calcium carbonate (p.1254·2).
*Calcium supplement; osteoporosis.*

**Gramcilina** *Medley, Braz.*
Ampicillin (p.157·1) or ampicillin sodium (p.157·1).
*Bacterial infections.*

**Gramibiotic** *Cordoba, Arg.*
Neomycin (p.235·1); gramicidin (p.220·2).
*Mouth and throat infections.*

**Gramicortil** *Allergan, Arg.*
Neomycin sulfate (p.235·1); hydrocortisone (p.1103·3); naphazoline hydrochloride (p.1124·3).
*Eye infections.*

**Gramidil** *Dexo, Fr.*
Amoxicillin trihydrate (p.155·3).
*Bacterial infections.*

**Gramigna (Specie Composta)** *Dynacren, Ital.*
Couch-grass (p.1676·2); birch leaf (p.1660·3); solidago (p.1748·3); ononis (p.1723·3); liquorice (p.1270·2).
*Urinary-tract disorders.*

**Graminflor** *Adroka, Switz.*
*Bath additive:* Hay flower.
*Musculoskeletal and joint disorders.*

**Gramipan** *Mayoly-Spindler, Switz.*
Dequalinium chloride (p.1178·1); ascorbic acid (p.1460·2).
*Mouth and throat infections.*

**Gramixina** *Merck, Port.†.*
Polymyxin B sulfate (p.245·1); gramicidin (p.220·2); chlorphenamine maleate (p.427·3); naphazoline hydrochloride (p.1124·3); procaine hydrochloride (p.1383·2).

**Grammicin** *Siam Bheasach, Thai.*
Gentamicin sulfate (p.217·1).
*Bacterial infections.*

**Grammixin** *Siam Bheasach, Thai.*
Gentamicin sulfate (p.217·1).
*Bacterial skin infections.*

**Gramoce A** *Vir, Spain.*
Ascorbic acid (p.1460·2); vitamin A (p.1451·2).
*Deficiency of vitamins A and C.*

**Gramoneg** *Ranbaxy, India.*
Nalidixic acid (p.234·1).
*Diarrhoea; urinary-tract infections.*

**Gramostim** *Cristalia, Braz.*
Molgramostim (p.756·1).

**Grampenil** *Bristol-Myers Squibb, Arg.*
Ampicillin sodium (p.157·1) or ampicillin trihydrate (p.157·2).
*Bacterial infections.*

**Grampenil Bronquial** *Bristol-Myers Squibb, Arg.*
Ampicillin sodium (p.157·1); ampicillin benzathine (p.158·1); guaifenesin (p.1122·1); chlorphenamine maleate (p.427·3).
*Respiratory-tract infections.*

**Gramplus** *Chiesi, Ital.*
Clofoctol (p.198·1).
*Bacterial infections of the respiratory tract.*

**Gram-Val** *Polifarma, Ital.†.*
Doxycycline hyclate (p.206·2).
*Bacterial infections.*

**Gran** *Kirin, Jpn.*
Filgrastim (p.753·3).
*Mobilisation of autologous peripheral progenitor cells; neutropenia.*

**Granamon** *Norgine, Ger.*
Sterculia (p.1290·2).
*Constipation.*

**Grandaxin**
*EGIS, Hung.; Egis, Thai.*
Tofisopam (p.725·3).
*Alcohol withdrawal syndrome; anxiety; menopausal disorders.*

**Graneodin**
*Note. This name is used for preparations of different composition.*
*Bristol-Myers Squibb, Arg.*
Gramicidin (p.220·2); neomycin sulfate (p.235·1); benzocaine (p.1370·3).
*Mouth and throat disorders.*

*Bristol-Myers Squibb, Chile.*
Chlorhexidine hydrochloride (p.1173·3).
*Mouth and throat infections.*

*Bristol-Myers Squibb, Irl.; Bristol-Myers Squibb, UK.*
Neomycin sulfate (p.235·1); gramicidin (p.220·2).
*Bacterial infections of the skin and ear.*

**Graneodin Expectorante** *Bristol-Myers Squibb, Arg.*
Ambroxol hydrochloride (p.1114·3).
*Respiratory-tract congestion.*

**Graneodin N**
*Note. This name is used for preparations of different composition.*
*Bristol-Myers Squibb, Arg.*
Gramicidin (p.220·2); neomycin sulfate (p.235·1); benzocaine (p.1370·3); noscapine (p.1125·3).
*Coughs; mouth and throat disorders.*

*Bristol-Myers Squibb, Chile.*
Chlorhexidine hydrochloride (p.1173·3); noscapine (p.1125·3).
*Coughs; mouth and throat infections.*

**Graneodin-Tos** *Bristol-Myers Squibb, Chile.*
Noscapine (p.1125·3); chlorhexidine hydrochloride (p.1173·3).
*Coughs; mouth and throat infections.*

**Grani di Vals** *Geymonat, Ital.*
Cascara (p.1255·1); aloes (p.1248·2); aloin (p.1248·3).
*Constipation.*

**Granicip** *Cipla, India.*
Granisetron (p.1267·2).
*Nausea and vomiting induced by cytotoxics; postoperative nausea and vomiting.*

**Granions** *Granions, Mon.*
A range of mineral supplements (p.1417·1).

**Granitron** *Richmond, Arg.*
Granisetron (p.1267·2).
*Nausea and vomiting.*

**Granobil** *Synpharma, Austria.*
Fennel (p.1687·2); primula root (p.1735·1); thyme leaf (p.1755·2).
*Catarrh; coughs.*

**Granocol**
*Schering, Austral.; Schering, NZ.*
Sterculia (p.1290·2); frangula bark (p.1266·3).
*Constipation.*

**Granocyte**
*Aventis, Arg.; Amrad, Austral.; Aventis, Austria; Aventis, Belg.; Aventis, Braz.; Chugai, Denm.; Aventis, Fin.; Aventis, Fr.; Chugai, Ger.; Rhone-Poulenc Rorer, Gr.; Aventis, Irl.; Aventis, Israel; Aventis, Ital.; Aventis, Malaysia; Aventis, Neth.; Chugai, Norw.; Amrad, NZ; Aventis, Port.; Aventis, S.Afr.; Aventis, Singapore; Aventis, Spain; Aventis, Swed.; Aventis, Switz.; Chugai, Thai.; Aventis, UK.*
Lenograstim (p.755·3).
*Mobilisation of autologous peripheral blood progenitor cells; reduction of neutropenia associated with cytotoxic therapy or bone marrow transplantation.*

**Granoleina** *SIFI, Ital.*
*dl*-Alpha tocoferil acetate (p.1465·1); linoleic acid (p.1690·2); vitamin A palmitate (p.1453·1); ergocalciferol (p.1462·1).
*Vitamin deficiencies.*

**Granon** *Nycomed, Denm.*
Acetylcysteine (p.1112·3).
*Respiratory-tract congestion.*

**Granoton** *Grandel-Synpharma, Ger.†.*
Tocopherol; tritici sativi e embryo; ethanol.
*Tonic.*

**Grans Remedy** *Grans Remedy, NZ.*
Zinc oxide (p.1163·2); zinc undecenoate (p.411·1); alum (p.1652·1); talc (p.1159·1).
*Foot odour.*

**Granu Fink Kurbiskern** *GlaxoSmithKline Consumer, Ger.*
Cucurbita (p.1677·3).
*Urinary-tract disorders.*

**Granu Fink Kurbiskern N** *GlaxoSmithKline Consumer, Ger.*
Cucurbita (p.1677·3); cucurbita oil (p.1677·3).
*Urinary-tract disorders.*

**Granu Fink Prosta**
*GlaxoSmithKline Consumer, Ger.; SmithKline Beecham Consumer, Switz.*
Cucurbita (p.1677·3); cucurbita oil (p.1677·3); saw palmetto (p.1569·1).
*Benign prostatic hyperplasia; urinary-tract disorders.*

**Granudoxy** *Pierre Fabre, Fr.*
Doxycycline (p.206·2).
*Bacterial infections; rosacea.*

**Granuflex**
*Note. This name is used for preparations of different composition.*
*Convatec, Israel; Convatec, UK.*
Hydrocolloid dressing.
*Burns; skin ulcers; wounds.*

*Bristol-Myers Squibb, S.Afr.*
Gelatin (p.754·3); pectin (p.1580·3); carmellose sodium (p.1577·3).
*Burns; wounds.*

**Granugel**
*Note. This name is used for preparations of different composition.*
*Convatec, Israel.*
Hydrocolloid gel.
*Skin ulcers; wounds.*

*Bristol-Myers Squibb, S.Afr.*
Pectin (p.1580·3); carmellose sodium (p.1577·3).
*Wounds.*

**Granugen** *Knoll, Austral.*
Paraffin oil (p.1479·1); zinc oxide (p.1163·2); titanium dioxide (p.1160·3); paraffin viscous; ethyl vanillin; soft paraffin.
*Minor wounds and ulcers.*

**Granulax** *Lacefa, Arg.*
Sodium picosulfate (p.1289·3).
*Constipation.*

**Granulderm** *Copley, USA.*
Trypsin (p.1758·3); peru balsam (p.1730·2); castor oil (p.1668·2).
*Wounds.*

**Granulen** *Eurofarma, Braz.*
Filgrastim (p.753·3).
*Neutropenia.*

**Granules Boripharm** *Dolisos, Fr.*
A range of homoeopathic preparations.

**Granulex** *Bertek, USA.*
Trypsin (p.1758·3); peru balsam (p.1730·2); castor oil (p.1668·2).
*Wound dressing.*

**Granulokine**
*Roche, Braz.; Roche, Gr.; Amgen, Ital.; Pensa, Spain†.*
Filgrastim (p.753·3).
*Mobilisation of autologous peripheral blood progenitor cells; neutropenia.*

**GranuMed** *Rugby, USA.*
Trypsin (p.1758·3); peru balsam (p.1730·2); castor oil (p.1668·2).
*Wounds.*

**Gran-Verm** *Brasmedica, Braz.†.*
Mebendazole (p.108·2).
*Worm infections.*

**Granvit** *Plants, Ital.*
Royal jelly (p.1740·3) with wheat-germ oil, carrot oil, and soya lecithin (p.1417·1).
*Nutritional supplement.*

**Grasmin** *Almirall, Spain†.*
Fenproporex resinate (p.1588·3).
*Obesity.*

**Grassolind Neutral** *Hartmann, Fr.*
White soft paraffin (p.1479·3); wool fat (p.1483·1); hard paraffin (p.1479·1).
*Burns; wounds.*

**Graten** *Pisa, Mex.*
Morphine sulfate (p.60·2).
*Pain.*

**Gratusminal**
*Note. This name is used for preparations of different composition.*
*Zambon, Braz.†.*
Phenobarbital diethylamine (p.369·2); deslanoside (p.893·1).
*Cardiac disorders.*

*Almirall, Spain.*
Phenobarbital diethylamine (p.369·2).
*Agitation; convulsive disorders; depression; insomnia; smooth muscle spasm.*

**Gravergol**
*Carter Horner, Canad.; Carter Horner, Hong Kong.*
Ergotamine tartrate (p.467·2); caffeine (p.782·1); dimenhydrinate (p.431·1).
*Migraine and other vascular headaches.*

**Gravibinan** *Schering, Ital.*
Hydroxyprogesterone caproate (p.1556·3); estradiol valerate (p.1550·2).
*Threatened or recurrent miscarriage.*

**Gravibinon**
*Schering, Austria†; Schering, Ger.*
Hydroxyprogesterone caproate (p.1556·3); estradiol valerate (p.1550·2).
*Threatened or recurrent miscarriage.*

**Gravidex**
*Note. This name is used for preparations of different composition.*
*Provita, Ital.†.*
Multivitamin and mineral preparation (p.1417·1).

*Almirall, Spain†.*
Dinoprostone (p.1515·1).
*Hydatidiform mole; labour induction; termination of pregnancy.*

**Gravidinona**
*Schering, Chile; Schering, Mex.*
Hydroxyprogesterone caproate (p.1556·3); estradiol valerate (p.1550·2).
*Threatened and recurrent miscarriage.*

**Gravi-Fol** *Asconex, Ger.*
Folic acid (p.1429·1).
*Folic acid deficiency.*

**Gravigard** *SPA, Ital.*
Copper-wound plastic (p.1425·3).
*Intra-uterine contraceptive device.*

**Gravigen Plus** *Byk Gulden, Ital.*
Multivitamin and mineral preparation (p.1417·1).

**Gravindex** *Ortho, Israel.*
Pregnancy test (p.1734·3).

**Gravistat** *Jenapharm, Ger.*
Ethinylestradiol (p.1553·2); levonorgestrel (p.1563·2).
*Combined oral contraceptive; menstrual disorders.*

**Gravitamon** *Chefaro, Neth.†.*
Multivitamin and mineral preparation (p.1417·1).

**Gravitest** *Scidia, Arg.*
Pregnancy test (p.1734·3).

**Gravitest Crual** *Cruciani, Ital.*
Pregnancy test (p.1734·3).

**Gravol**
*Carter Horner, Canad.; Carter Horner, Hong Kong; Wallace, India; Carter Horner, Thai.*
Dimenhydrinate (p.431·1).
*Ménière's disease; motion sickness; nausea and vomiting; vertigo.*

**Grayxona** *Gray, Arg.*
Naloxone (p.1045·1).

**GRD** *Cadila, India.*
Dietary supplement (p.1417·1).

**Greatbloc** *Creative Brands, Austral.†.*
*SPF 15; SPF 30+:* Padimate O (p.1155·1); oxybenzone (p.1154·3); avobenzone (p.1142·3).
*Sunscreen.*

**Greater-Gloxa** *Greater Pharma, Thai.*
Cloxacillin sodium (p.198·2).
*Bacterial infections.*

**Greatofen** *Greater Pharma, Thai.*
Ibuprofen (p.45·3).
*Musculoskeletal and joint disorders.*

**Green Antiseptic Mouthwash & Gargle** *Lee-Adams, Canad.*
Alcohol (p.1166·1); cetylpyridinium chloride (p.1173·1).

**Green Diet** *Garden House, Arg.*
Glucomanan; seaweed extract (p.1417·1).
*Dietary supplement.*

**Green-A KGCC** *Interlab, Braz.†.*
Albumin (p.740·3).
*Plasma volume expansion.*

**Greenosan** *Bang & Tegner, Denm.†.*
Multivitamin and mineral preparation (p.1417·1).

**Grefen** *Doetsch, Grether, Switz.*
Ibuprofen (p.45·3).
*Fever; inflammation; musculoskeletal and joint disorders; pain.*

**Gregoderm** *Unigreg, UK.*
Neomycin sulfate (p.235·1); polymyxin B sulfate (p.245·1); hydrocortisone (p.1103·3); nystatin (p.406·3).
*Infected skin disorders.*

**Greini** *Fada, Arg.*
Amikacin (p.154·1).
*Bacterial infections.*

**Grenfung** *Cevallos, Arg.*
Ketoconazole (p.403·3).
*Fungal skin infections.*

**Grenin** *YSP, Malaysia.*
Theophylline sodium glycinate (p.804·3); guaifenesin (p.1122·1).
*Asthma; bronchitis.*

**Grenis** *Genepharm, Gr.*
Norfloxacin (p.238·3).
*Urinary tract infections.*

**Grenis-cipro** *Genepharm, Gr.*
Ciprofloxacin hydrochloride (p.188·2).
*Bacterial infections.*

**Grenovix** *Genepharm, Gr.*
Ambroxol hydrochloride (p.1114·3).
*Respiratory disorders associated with viscous mucus.*

**Greosin** *GlaxoSmithKline, Spain.*
Griseofulvin (p.400·3).
*Fungal skin and nail infections.*

**Gretivit** *Belfar, Braz.†.*
Multivitamin and mineral preparation (p.1417·1).

**G-Revm** *Gap, Gr.*
Nimesulide (p.67·1).
*Inflammation; musculoskeletal disorders; pain.*

**Grexin** *Pharmasant, Thai.*
Digoxin (p.895·2).
*Arrhythmias; heart failure.*

**Gricin**
*Dresden, Ger.†; Riemser, Ger.*
Griseofulvin (p.400·3).
*Fungal skin, hair, and nail infections.*

**Grietalgen** *Diviser Aquilea, Spain.*
Peru balsam (p.1730·2); bismuth subnitrate (p.1252·2); ergocalciferol (p.1462·1); estrone (p.1553·1); benzocaine (p.1370·3); vitamin A (p.1451·2).
*Cracked nipples; mastitis.*

**Grietalgen Hidrocort** *Diviser Aquilea, Spain.*
Bismuth subnitrate (p.1252·2); colecalciferol (p.1461·3); estrone (p.1553·1); benzocaine (p.1370·3); vitamin A (p.1451·2); hydrocortisone glycyrrhetinate (p.1104·2); neomycin sulfate (p.235·1).
*Burns; cracked nipples; mastitis; skin disorders; wounds.*

**Grifed** *Syntex, Mex.*
Naproxen sodium (p.65·1); pseudoephedrine hydrochloride (p.1129·2).
*Cold and influenza symptoms.*

**Grifenol** *Sibras, Braz.†.*
Paracetamol (p.76·2); phenylephrine hydrochloride (p.1126·3); chlorphenamine maleate (p.427·3).
*Cold and influenza symptoms.*

**Grifoalpram** *Laboratorios Chile, Chile.*
Alprazolam (p.668·3).
*Anxiety; panic attacks.*

**Grifobutol** *Laboratorios Chile, Chile.*
Acebutolol (p.848·1).
*Angina pectoris; arrhythmias; hypertension.*

**Grifociprox** *Laboratorios Chile, Chile.*
Ciprofloxacin (p.188·2).
*Bacterial infections.*

**Grifoclobam** *Laboratorios Chile, Chile.*
Clobazam (p.358·2).
*Anxiety; epilepsy.*

**Grifocriptina** *Laboratorios Chile, Chile.*
Bromocriptine mesilate (p.1200·3).
*Acromegaly; hyperprolactinaemia; lactation supression; mastodynia; parkinsonism; prolactinoma.*

**Grifodilzem** *Laboratorios Chile, Chile.*
Diltiazem hydrochloride (p.900·1).
*Angina pectoris; hypertension.*

**Grifoftal** *Laboratorios Chile, Chile.*
*Eye drops:* Polymyxin b sulfate (p.245·1); neomycin sulfate (p.235·1); gramicidin (p.220·2).
*Eye ointment:* Polymyxin b (p.245·2); neomycin sulfate (p.235·1); bacitracin (p.161·3).
*Bacterial eye infections.*

**Grifoftal-D** *Laboratorios Chile, Chile.*
Dexamethasone (p.1097·1); neomycin (p.235·1); polymyxin b (p.245·2).
*Bacterial eye infections with inflammation.*

**Grifogemzilo** *Laboratorios Chile, Chile.*
Gemfibrozil (p.923·1).
*Hyperlipidaemias.*

**Grifonimod** *Laboratorios Chile, Chile.*
Nimodipine (p.972·3).
*Ischaemic neurological deficit following cerebral vasospasm.*

**Grifonitren** *Laboratorios Chile, Chile.*
Nitrendipine (p.973·3).
*Hypertension.*

**Grifoparkin** *Laboratorios Chile, Chile.*
Levodopa (p.1205·2); carbidopa (p.1204·3).
*Parkinsonism.*

**Grifopril** *Laboratorios Chile, Chile.*
Enalapril maleate (p.909·2).
*Heart failure; hypertension.*

**Grifopril-D** *Laboratorios Chile, Chile.*
Enalapril maleate (p.909·2); hydrochlorothiazide (p.933·2).
*Hypertension.*

**Grifotaxima** *Laboratorios Chile, Chile.*
Cefotaxime (p.176·3).
*Bacterial infections.*

**Grifotenol** *Laboratorios Chile, Chile.*
Atenolol (p.865·2).
*Angina pectoris; arrhythmias; hypertension.*

**Grifotriaxona** *Laboratorios Chile, Chile.*
Ceftriaxone sodium (p.182·3).
*Bacterial infections.*

**Grifulin** *Teva, Israel.*
Griseofulvin (p.400·3).
*Fungal skin infections.*

**Grifulvin** *General Drugs, Thai.*
Griseofulvin (p.400·3).
*Fungal skin, hair, and nail infections.*

**Grifulvin V** *Ortho Dermatological, USA†.*
Griseofulvin (microsize) (p.400·3).
*Fungal skin, hair and nail infections.*

**Grilinctus** *Franco-Indian, India.*
*Capsules:* Dextromethorphan hydrobromide (p.1117·3); chlorphenamine maleate (p.427·3); phenylpropanolamine hydrochloride (p.1127·3).
*Syrup:* Dextromethorphan hydrobromide (p.1117·3); chlorphenamine maleate (p.427·3); guaifenesin (p.1122·1); ammonium chloride (p.1115·2).
*Coughs.*

**Grilinctus-BM** *Franco-Indian, India.*
Terbutaline sulfate (p.797·2); bromhexine hydrochloride (p.1115·3).
*Asthma; bronchitis; respiratory-tract disorders associated with increased or viscous mucus.*

**Grindocin** *Grin, Mex.*
Indometacin (p.47·3).
*Anterior eye inflammation following laser treatment or surgery; cystoid macular oedema following cataract surgery; intra-operative miosis.*

**Grinevel** *Filaxis, Arg.*
Ganciclovir sodium (p.635·3).
*Viral infections.*

**Grinflux** *Selvi, Ital.*
Fluoxetine hydrochloride (p.292·1).
*Bulimia nervosa; depression; obsessive-compulsive disorder.*

**Grinsil** *Bristol-Myers Squibb, Arg.*
Amoxicillin trihydrate (p.155·3).
*Bacterial infections.*

**Grinsil Clavulanico** *Bristol-Myers Squibb, Arg.*
Amoxicillin trihydrate (p.155·3); potassium clavulanate (p.193·3).
*Bacterial infections.*

**Grinsil Duo** *Bristol-Myers Squibb, Arg.*
Amoxicillin trihydrate (p.155·3).
*Bacterial infections.*

**Grinsil Respiratorio** *Bristol-Myers Squibb, Arg.*
Amoxicillin sodium (p.155·3) or amoxicillin trihydrate (p.155·3); bromhexine hydrochloride (p.1115·3).
*Respiratory-tract infections.*

**Gripakin** *Almi, Spain.*
Chlorphenamine maleate (p.427·3); paracetamol (p.76·2).
*Cold symptoms; nasal congestion.*

**Gripalgine** *Pharmethic, Belg.†.*
Aspirin (p.15·1); codeine phosphate (p.27·1); ascorbic acid (p.1460·2).
*Fever; pain.*

**Gripanil** *Ducto, Braz.*
*Injection:* Ampoule A, dipyrone (p.35·3); sodium camsilate; guaifenesin (p.1122·1); cineole (p.1672·1); niaouli oil (p.1719·3); ampoule B, ascorbic acid (p.1460·2); mepyramine maleate (p.437·1).
Lidocaine hydrochloride (p.1377·3) is included in this preparation to alleviate the pain of injection.
*Tablets:* Green tablets, dipyrone (p.35·3); camphor (p.1665·3); guaifenesin (p.1122·1); cineole (p.1672·1); niaouli oil (p.1719·3); white tablets, ascorbic acid (p.1460·2); mepyramine maleate (p.437·1).
Lidocaine hydrochloride (p.1377·3) is included in this preparation to alleviate the pain of injection.

**Gripanil C** *Ahimsa, Arg.*
Paracetamol (p.76·2); caffeine (p.782·1); ascorbic acid (p.1460·2).
*Fever; pain.*

**Gripasan Compuesto** *Laboratorios Chile, Chile.*
Paracetamol (p.76·2); propyphenazone (p.85·3); phenylpropanolamine hydrochloride (p.1127·3); chlorphenamine maleate (p.427·3); caffeine (p.782·1).
*Cold and influenza symptoms.*

**Gripasan Nueva Formula** *Laboratorios Chile, Chile.*
Paracetamol (p.76·2); chlorphenamine maleate (p.427·3); caffeine (p.782·1).
*Cold and influenza symptoms.*

**Gripavac** *Aventis Pasteur, Spain.*
An influenza vaccine (p.1620·2).
*Active immunisation.*

**Gripcaps C** *Infabra, Braz.†.*
Phenylephrine (p.1126·3); paracetamol (p.76·2); ascorbic acid (p.1460·2).
*Cold and influenza symptoms.*

**Gripe Mixture** *British Dispensary, Thai.*
Sodium bicarbonate (p.1223·2); dill oil (p.1680·2); caraway oil (p.1667·3); peppermint oil (p.1283·2).
*Flatulence; infant colic.*

**Gripe Water** *Beacons, Singapore.*
Sodium bicarbonate (p.1223·2).
*Flatulence; gastric hyperacidity.*

**Gripefago C** *Baldassari, Braz.†.*
Dipyrone (p.35·3); sodium camsilate; guaifenesin (p.1122·1); cineole (p.1672·1); niaouli oil (p.1719·3); ascorbic acid (p.1460·2); mepyramine maleate (p.437·1).
Lidocaine hydrochloride (p.1377·3) is included in this preparation to alleviate the pain of injection.
*Cold and influenza symptoms.*

**Gripefin** *Faria, Braz.†.*
Carbasalate calcium (p.25·1); phenylpropanolamine hydrochloride (p.1127·3); pheniramine maleate (p.438·3); mepyramine maleate (p.437·1).
*Cold and influenza symptoms.*

**Gripen** *EMS, Braz.*
Dimetindene maleate (p.431·2); rutoside (p.1688·2); ascorbic acid (p.1460·2); phenylephrine hydrochloride (p.1126·3); paracetamol (p.76·2).
*Cold and influenza symptoms.*

**Gripenil** *Windson, Braz.†.*
Phenylephrine (p.1126·3); carbinoxamine (p.426·3).
*Nasal congestion.*

**Gripeonil** *Faria, Braz.*
Paracetamol (p.76·2).
*Fever; pain.*

**Gripetral** *Atral, Port.*
Aspirin (p.15·1); ascorbic acid (p.1460·2); caffeine (p.782·1).
*Cold and influenza symptoms.*

**Gripexin Limonada Caliente** *Labomed, Chile.*
Paracetamol (p.76·2); sodium ascorbate (p.1460·2); caffeine (p.782·1); noscapine hydrochloride (p.1125·3); chlorphenamine maleate (p.427·3).
*Cold and influenza symptoms.*

**Gripexin Nueva Formula Compuesto** *Labomed, Chile.*
Paracetamol (p.76·2); sodium ascorbate (p.1460·2); caffeine (p.782·1); noscapine hydrochloride (p.1125·3); chlorphenamine maleate (p.427·3).
*Cold and influenza symptoms.*

**Gripexin Nueva Formula C/Pseudoefedrina** *Labomed, Chile.*
Paracetamol (p.76·2); pseudoephedrine hydrochloride (p.1129·2); chlorphenamine maleate (p.427·3).
*Cold and influenza symptoms.*

**Gripidor** *Medical, Port.*
Aspirin (p.15·1); paracetamol (p.76·2).
*Fever; pain.*

**Gripin C** *Medquimica, Braz.†.*
Salicylamide (p.87·3); chlorphenamine (p.428·1); caffeine (p.782·1); vitamin C (p.1460·2).
*Cold and influenza symptoms.*

**Gripion** *Makros, Braz.†.*
Diphenhydramine hydrochloride (p.431·3); dipyrone (p.35·3); ascorbic acid (p.1460·2).
*Cold and influenza symptoms.*

**Gripionex** *Delta, Braz.†.*
Paracetamol (p.76·2); caffeine (p.782·1); phenylephrine hydrochloride (p.1126·3); tripelennamine maleate (p.442·3).
*Cold and influenza symptoms.*

**Gripol C** *INQ, Braz.†.*
Dipyrone (p.35·3); mepyramine maleate (p.437·1); caffeine (p.782·1); ascorbic acid (p.1460·2).
*Cold and influenza symptoms.*

**Gripol C Capuride** *INQ, Braz.†.*
Dipyrone (p.35·3); guaifenesin (p.1122·1); sodium camsilate; cineole (p.1672·1).
*Cold and influenza symptoms.*

**Gripol Composto** *INQ, Braz.†.*
Dipyrone (p.35·3); mepyramine maleate (p.437·1); caffeine (p.782·1); ascorbic acid (p.1460·2).
*Cold and influenza symptoms.*

**Gripol Composto Xarope** *INQ, Braz.†.*
Dipyrone (p.35·3); ascorbic acid (p.1460·2).
*Cold and influenza symptoms.*

**Gripomatine** *Hexal, Braz.*
*Syrup:* Dipyrone (p.35·3); sodium camsilate; guaifenesin (p.1122·1); cineole (p.1672·1); vitamin C (p.1460·2).
*Tablets:* Green tablets, dipyrone (p.35·3); guaifenesin (p.1122·1); orange tablets, ascorbic acid (p.1460·2).
*Cold and influenza symptoms.*

**Griponal** *Merck, Port.†.*
Paracetamol (p.76·2); phenylephrine hydrochloride (p.1126·3); chlorphenamine maleate (p.427·3).
*Cold and influenza symptoms.*

**Griponia** *Bunker, Braz.*
Green tablets or ampoule 1, dipyrone (p.35·3); sodium camsilate; guaifenesin (p.1122·1); cineole (p.1672·1); niaouli oil (p.1719·3); yellow tablets or ampoule 2, ascorbic acid (p.1460·2).
*Cold and influenza symptoms.*

**Gripotermon** *Prodotti, Braz.*
Paracetamol (p.76·2).
*Fever; pain.*

**Gripp Heel** *Peithner, Austria.*
Homoeopathic preparation.

**Grippal** *Bayer, Spain.*
Aspirin (p.15·1); chlorphenamine maleate (p.427·3); phenylephrine (p.1126·3).
Formerly contained aspirin, chlorphenamine maleate, and phenylpropanolamine.
*Influenza and cold symptoms; nasal congestion.*

**Grippalgine N** *DP-Medica, Switz.*
Paracetamol (p.76·2); salicylamide (p.87·3); caffeine (p.782·1).
*Cold and influenza symptoms.*

**Grippalin** *Multi-Pro, Canad.*
Ephedrine hydrochloride (p.1120·1); paracetamol (p.76·2).

**Grippalin & C** *Multi-Pro, Canad.*
Ephedrine hydrochloride (p.1120·1); paracetamol (p.76·2).
Formerly contained chlorphenamine maleate, paracetamol, and ascorbic acid.

**Grippefloran** *Bioflora, Austria.*
Salix purpurea (p.87·3); tilia flower (p.1756·2); vitamin C (p.1460·2).
*Cold symptoms.*

**Grippe-Gastreu S R6** *Reckeweg, Ger.*
Homoeopathic preparation.

**Grippetee Dr Zeidler** *Apotheke Erzengel Michael, Austria.*
Tilia flower (p.1756·2); sambucus flower (p.1741·3); rose fruit (p.1740·1); thyme leaf (p.1755·2); drosera (p.1683·1).
*Cold symptoms.*

**Grippetee EF-EM-ES** *Smetana, Austria.*
Sambucus flower (p.1741·3); tilia flower (p.1756·2); plantago lanceolata (p.1738·2).
*Cold symptoms.*

**Gripp-Heel**
*Heel, Ger.; Heel, S.Afr.*
Homoeopathic preparation.

**Grippin-Merz** *Merz, Ger.†.*
Amantadine sulfate (p.1197·2).
*Influenza A.*

**Grippinon** *Nycomed, Austria.*
Aspirin (p.15·1); ascorbic acid (p.1460·2).
*Cold symptoms.*

**Grippogran** *Sympharma, Austria.*
Sambucus flower (p.1741·3); tilia flower (p.1756·2); centaury (p.1669·2).
*Cold symptoms.*

**Grippon** *Adcock Ingram, S.Afr.*
*Capsules:* Paracetamol (p.76·2); caffeine (p.782·1); ascorbic acid (p.1460·2); phenylephrine hydrochloride (p.1126·3); chlorphenamine maleate (p.427·3).
*Syrup:* Paracetamol (p.76·2); chlorphenamine maleate (p.427·3); ephedrine (p.1120·1).
*Cold and influenza symptoms.*

**Grippostad C**
*Note. This name is used for preparations of different composition.*
*Stada, Ger.*
Paracetamol (p.76·2); ascorbic acid (p.1460·2); caffeine (p.782·1); chlorphenamine maleate (p.427·3).
*Cold and influenza symptoms.*

*Medika, Switz.*
Paracetamol (p.76·2); ascorbic acid (p.1460·2).
*Cold symptoms.*

**Grippostad Gute Nacht-Saft** *Stada, Ger.*
Dextromethorphan hydrobromide (p.1117·3); paracetamol (p.76·2).
*Cold and influenza symptoms.*

**Grippostad Heissgetrank** *Stada, Ger.*
Paracetamol (p.76·2).
*Cold symptoms; pain.*

**Gripps** *Pascoe, Ger.*
Homoeopathic preparation.

**Gripsay** *Delta, Braz.*
Ampoule A, dipyrone (p.35·3); sodium camsilate; guaifenesin (p.1122·1); cineole (p.1672·1); niaouli oil (p.1719·3); lidocaine hydrochloride (p.1377·3); ampoule B, mepyramine maleate (p.437·1); ascorbic acid (p.1460·2).
*Cold and influenza symptoms.*

**Griptol** *Brasmedica, Braz.†.*
Aspirin (p.15·1); caffeine (p.782·1); vitamin C (p.1460·2).
*Fever; pain.*

**Grisactin**
*CFL, India; Wyeth-Ayerst, USA†.*
Griseofulvin (p.400·3).
*Fungal infections of the skin, hair, and nails.*

**Grise** *Cesam, Port.†.*
Emollient.
*Skin disorders.*

**Grisefuline** *Sanofi Synthelabo, Fr.*
Griseofulvin (p.400·3).
*Fungal infections.*

**Griseo** *CT, Ger.*
Griseofulvin (p.400·3).
*Fungal skin infections.*

**Griseocrem** *Armstrong, Arg.*
Diflorasone diacetate (p.1099·3); econazole nitrate (p.397·2); gentamicin sulfate (p.217·1).
*Infected skin disorders.*

**Griseoful** *Ofimex, Mex.†.*
Griseofulvin (p.400·3).
*Fungal infections.*

**Griseomed** *Sanochemia, Austria.*
Griseofulvin (p.400·3).
*Superficial fungal infections.*

**Griseoplus** *Armstrong, Arg.*
Griseofulvin (p.400·3); econazole nitrate (p.397·2); hydrocortisone (p.1103·3); salicylic acid (p.1157·1); neomycin undecenoate (p.235·2); boric acid (p.1662·1).
*Infected skin disorders.*

**Griseostatin**
*Schering-Plough, Austral.; Schering-Plough, Hong Kong†.*
Griseofulvin (p.400·3).
*Fungal infections of the skin, hair, and nails.*

**Grisetin**
*Note. This name is used for preparations of different composition.*
*Merck, Port.†.*
Vitamin $B_{12}$; vitamin $B_1$ (p.1417·1).
*Tonic.*

*Ipsen, Spain.*
Flutamide (p.556·2).
*Prostatic cancer.*

**Grisetin Con Carnitina** *Andromaco, Chile.*
Cyproheptadine hydrochloride (p.430·1); carnitine hydrochloride (p.1424·1).
*Reduced appetite.*

**Grisflavin** *Asian Pharm, Thai.*
Griseofulvin (p.400·3).
*Fungal skin, hair, and nail infections.*

**Grisical** *Grisi, Mex.*
Calcium carbonate (p.1254·2).

**Grisol** *Gebro, Switz.*
Griseofulvin (p.400·3).
*Tinea pedis.*

**Grisomicon** *Sanitas, Port.*
Griseofulvin (p.400·3).
*Fungal infections.*

**Grisovin**
*GlaxoSmithKline, Arg.; Sigma, Austral.; GlaxoSmithKline, Austria; Glaxo Wellcome, Hong Kong†; Glaxo Wellcome, Mex.; Glaxo Wellcome, NZ†; Glaxo Wellcome, Port.; Glaxo Wellcome, Thai.†; GlaxoSmithKline, UK.*
Griseofulvin (p.400·3).
*Fungal infections of the skin, hair, and nails.*

**Grisovin FP** *Roberts, Canad.†.*
Griseofulvin (p.400·3).
*Fungal skin infections.*

**Grisovina FP** *Teofarma, Ital.*
Griseofulvin (p.400·3).
*Fungal skin and nail infections.*

**Gris-PEG** *Pedinol, USA.*
Griseofulvin (ultramicrosize) (p.400·3).
*Fungal skin, hair, and nail infections.*

**Grisuvin** *DHA, Malaysia.*
Griseofulvin (p.400·3).
*Fungal skin, hair, and nail infections.*

**Grivin**
*Atlantic, Malaysia; Atlantic, Singapore; Atlantic, Thai.*
Griseofulvin (p.400·3).
*Fungal skin and nail infections.*

**Grodurex** *Grossmann, Switz.*
Hydrochlorothiazide (p.933·2); amiloride hydrochloride (p.858·2).
*Hypertension; oedema.*

**Grofenac**
*Grossmann, Hong Kong; Grossmann, Switz.*
Diclofenac sodium (p.32·1).
*Gout; inflammation; musculoskeletal, joint, and periarticular disorders; pain.*

**Gromazol** *Grossmann, Switz.*
Clotrimazole (p.396·2).
*Fungal foot infections.*

**Groprim** *Grossmann, Switz.*
Co-trimoxazole (p.199·3).
*Bacterial infections; blastomycosis; Pneumocystis carinii pneumonia.*

**Grotanat** *Schulke & Mayr, Ger.†.*
Chlorocresol (p.1177·1); clorophene (p.1177·3); orthophenylphenol (p.1187·2).
*Instrument disinfection.*

**Grovixim** *Torlan, Spain†.*
Carnitine chloride; cobamamide; cocarboxylase (p.1417·1).
*Tonic.*

**Growgen-GM** *Gautier, Arg.*
Molgramostim (p.756·1).
*Neutropenia.*

**Growject** *Sumitomo, Jpn.*
Somatropin (p.1327·2).
*Growth hormone deficiency; Turner's syndrome.*

**Gruben** *Pasteur, Chile.*
Codeine phosphate (p.27·1); bromoform (p.1663·1); sodium camsilate; belladonna (p.479·1); sodium benzoate (p.1169·3).
*Coughs.*

**Grumivit** *Piemont, Ital.*
Ascorbic acid (p.1460·2).
*Vitamin C deficiency.*

**Gruncef** *Grunenthal, Ger.*
Cefadroxil (p.167·2).
*Bacterial infections.*

**Grune Salbe "Schmidt" N** *Wider, Ger.†.*
Urea (p.1162·2); silver (p.1746·1); magnesium chloride (p.1228·1).
*Ulcers; wounds.*

**Grunicina** *Grunenthal, Mex.*
Amoxicillin trihydrate (p.155·3).
*Bacterial infections.*

**Grunlicht Dreierlei Tropfen** *Lichtenheldt, Ger.†.*
Peppermint oil (p.1283·2); valerian (p.1762·2).
*Dizziness; nausea; nervous disorders.*

**Grunlicht Hingfong Essenz** *Lichtenheldt, Ger.†.*
Peppermint oil (p.1283·2); anise oil (p.1655·2); cassia oil (p.1668·2); fennel oil (p.1687·3); rosemary oil (p.1740·2); thyme oil (p.1755·3); menthol (p.1711·3); camphor (p.1665·3); peppermint leaf (p.1283·2); bay leaf; arnica (p.1656·3); tilia (p.1756·2); chamomile (p.1669·3); aniseed (p.1655·2); fennel (p.1687·2); calamus (p.1664·1); valerian (p.1762·2).
*Cold symptoms; nausea; nervous disorders; neuralgias; rheumatic disorders.*

**Grunlicht Magenbalsam Tropfen** *Lichtenheldt, Ger.†.*
Anise oil (p.1655·2); fennel oil (p.1687·3); caraway oil (p.1667·3).
*Dyspepsia; gastrointestinal spasm; meteorism.*

**Gruntin Tropfen** *Grunenthal, Ger.*
Tilidine hydrochloride (p.94·1).
Naloxone hydrochloride (p.1044·3) is included in this preparation to discourage abuse.
*Pain.*

**G-Tase** *Unichem, India.*
Pioglitazone (p.344·2).
*Diabetes mellitus.*

**G.Test** *Sabiluc, Fr.*
Pregnancy test (p.1734·3).

**Guafen** *Agepha, Austria.*
Guaifenesin (p.1122·1).
*Catarrh; coughs.*

**Guaiacalcium Complex** *SIT, Ital.*
Dropropizine (p.1119·3); sulfogaiacol (p.1131·1).
*Coughs.*

**Guaiaspir** *Lampugnani, Ital.†.*
Guacetisal (p.1121·3).
*Respiratory-tract disorders.*

**Guaifed** *Verum, USA.*
Phenylephrine hydrochloride (p.1126·3); guaifenesin (p.1122·1).
Formerly contained pseudoephedrine hydrochloride and guaifenesin.
*Coughs; nasal congestion.*

**Guaifed-PD** *Verum, USA.*
Phenylephrine hydrochloride (p.1126·3); guaifenesin (p.1122·1).
Formerly contained pseudoephedrine hydrochloride and guaifenesin.
*Coughs; nasal congestion.*

**Guaifenesin DAC** *Cypress, USA.*
Codeine phosphate (p.27·1); pseudoephedrine hydrochloride (p.1129·2); guaifenesin (p.1122·1).
*Coughs and associated respiratory-tract disorders.*

**Guaifenesin DM** *Prasco, USA.*
Guaifenesin (p.1122·1); dextromethorphan hydrobromide (p.1117·3).
*Coughs.*

**Guaifenesin PSE** *Cypress, USA.*
Guaifenesin (p.1122·1); pseudoephedrine hydrochloride (p.1129·2).
*Coughs; nasal congestion.*

**Guaifenex DM** *Ethex, USA.*
Guaifenesin (p.1122·1); dextromethorphan hydrobromide (p.1117·3).
*Coughs.*

**Guaifenex G** *Ethex, USA.*
Guaifenesin (p.1122·1).
*Coughs.*

**Guaifenex LA** *Ethex, USA.*
Guaifenesin (p.1122·1).
*Coughs.*

**Guaifenex PPA** *Ethex, USA†.*
Guaifenesin (p.1122·1); phenylpropanolamine hydrochloride (p.1127·3).
*Coughs.*

**Guaifenex PSE**
*Ethex, Hong Kong; Ethex, USA.*
Guaifenesin (p.1122·1); pseudoephedrine hydrochloride (p.1129·2).
*Coughs; nasal congestion.*

**Guaifenex Rx** *Ethex, USA.*
AM tablets, guaifenesin (p.1122·1); pseudoephedrine hydrochloride (p.1129·2); PM tablets, guaifenesin.
*Coughs.*

**Guaifenex Rx DM** *Ethex, USA.*
AM tablets, guaifenesin (p.1122·1); pseudoephedrine hydrochloride (p.1129·2); PM tablets, guaifenesin; dextromethorphan hydrobromide (p.1117·3).
*Coughs.*

**Guaimax-D** *Schwarz, USA.*
Guaifenesin (p.1122·1); pseudoephedrine hydrochloride (p.1129·2).
*Coughs.*

**Guaipax** *Eon, USA†.*
Guaifenesin (p.1122·1); phenylpropanolamine hydrochloride (p.1127·3).
*Coughs.*

**Guaitab** *Muro, USA.*
Guaifenesin (p.1122·1); pseudoephedrine hydrochloride (p.1129·2).
*Coughs; nasal congestion.*

**Guaivent** *Ethex, USA.*
Guaifenesin (p.1122·1); pseudoephedrine hydrochloride (p.1129·2).
*Coughs.*

**Guai-Vent/PSE** *Dura, USA.*
Guaifenesin (p.1122·1); pseudoephedrine hydrochloride (p.1129·2).
*Coughs.*

**Guajabronc** *Molteni, Ital.†.*
Guacetisal (p.1121·3).
*Respiratory disorders.*

**Guanor** *Rosemont, UK†.*
Diphenhydramine hydrochloride (p.431·3); ammonium chloride (p.1115·2); sodium citrate (p.1223·2); menthol (p.1711·3).
*Coughs.*

**Guar Verlan** *Verla, Ger.*
Guar gum (p.333·2).
*Diabetes mellitus; hyperlipidaemias.*

**Guarana** *Wunderpharm, Arg.*
Caffeine (p.782·1).
*Fatigue.*

**Guaranace** *Tecnonat, Arg.*
Ascorbic acid; magnesium; guarana (p.1417·1).
*Tonic.*

**Guarasex** *Heralds, Braz.†.*
Vitamin preparation with guarana and erythroxylon catuaba (p.1417·1).

**Guaratuaba** *Belfar, Braz.†.*
Vitamins; erythroxylon catuaba; guarana (p.1417·1).
*Nutritional supplement.*

**Guarcol** *Orion, NZ.*
Food thickener (p.1417·1).
*Dysphagia.*

**Guarem**
*Orion, Fin.; Shire, Hong Kong; Rybar, Irl.; Orion, Israel†; Shire, UK†.*
Guar gum (p.333·2).
*Diabetes mellitus; dumping syndrome; hypercholesterolaemia.*

**Guastil** *Uriach, Spain.*
Sulpiride (p.722·2).
*Anxiety; psychoses; vertigo.*

**Guaxan** *Alcala, Spain†.*
Nimesulide (p.67·1).
*Fever; inflammation; pain.*

**Guayalin-Plus** *Farcoral, Mex.*
Guaiacol (p.1122·1); gordolobo; cineole (p.1672·1); honey (p.1434·2); vitamin C (p.1460·2).
*Respiratory-tract disorders.*

**Gubamine** *Gubler, Switz.†.*
Paracetamol (p.76·2); caffeine (p.782·1); propyphenazone (p.85·3).
*Fever; pain.*

**Guemusin** *Fada, Arg.*
Paracetamol (p.76·2).
*Fever; pain.*

**Guep'Away** *Clement, Fr.*
(N-Butyl-N-acetyl)-3-ethylaminopropionate; Frepylate.
*Insect repellent.*

**Guethural** *Elerte, Fr.*
Guaietolin (p.1122·1).
*Respiratory-tract congestion.*

**Gugecin** *Lilly, Mex.*
Cinoxacin (p.188·1).
*Urinary-tract infections.*

**GuiaCough CF** *Schein, USA†.*
Phenylpropanolamine hydrochloride (p.1127·3); dextromethorphan hydrobromide (p.1117·3); guaifenesin (p.1122·1).
*Coughs.*

**GuiaCough PE** *Schein, USA†.*
Pseudoephedrine hydrochloride (p.1129·2); guaifenesin (p.1122·1).
*Coughs.*

**Guiatex** *Rugby, USA†.*
Phenylephrine hydrochloride (p.1126·3); phenylpropanolamine hydrochloride (p.1127·3); guaifenesin (p.1122·1).
*Coughs.*

**Guiatex LA** *Rugby, USA†.*
Phenylpropanolamine hydrochloride (p.1127·3); guaifenesin (p.1122·1).
*Coughs.*

**Guiatex PSE** *Rugby, USA.*
Pseudoephedrine hydrochloride (p.1129·2); guaifenesin (p.1122·1).
*Coughs.*

**Guiatuss** *Goldline, USA.*
Guaifenesin (p.1122·1).
*Coughs; respiratory-tract congestion.*

**Guiatuss CF** *Barre-National, USA†.*
Phenylpropanolamine hydrochloride (p.1127·3); dextromethorphan hydrobromide (p.1117·3); guaifenesin (p.1122·1).
*Coughs.*

**Guiatuss PE** *Barre-National, USA.*
Pseudoephedrine hydrochloride (p.1129·2); guaifenesin (p.1122·1).
*Coughs.*

**Guiatussin with Codeine Expectorant** *Rugby, USA.*
Codeine phosphate (p.27·1); guaifenesin (p.1122·1).
*Coughs.*

**Guiatussin DAC** *Rugby, USA.*
Pseudoephedrine hydrochloride (p.1129·2); guaifenesin (p.1122·1); codeine phosphate (p.27·1).
*Coughs.*

**Guiatussin with Dextromethorphan** *Rugby, USA.*
Dextromethorphan hydrobromide (p.1117·3); guaifenesin (p.1122·1).
*Coughs.*

**Guigoz Hypoallergenique** *Guigoz, Fr.*
Infant feed (p.1417·1).
*Milk-protein allergy.*

**Guigoz Soja** *Guigoz, Fr.*
Infant feed (p.1417·1).
*Lactose intolerance.*

**Guigoz Transit** *Guigoz, Fr.*
Infant feed (p.1417·1).
*Gastrointestinal disorders.*

**Gumbaral** *AWD, Ger.*
Ademetionine sulfate tosilate (p.1647·2).
*Degenerative joint disorders.*

**Gumbix**
*Solvay, Austria; Cheplapharm, Ger.*
Aminomethylbenzoic acid (p.742·1).
*Haemorrhage.*

**Gum-Ese** *McGloin, Austral.†.*
Lidocaine hydrochloride (p.1377·3); benzalkonium chloride (p.1168·3).
*Mouth ulcers.*

**Gumilk** *Gallia, Fr.*
Ceratonia (p.1579·1); maltodextrin (p.1439·3).
*Regurgitation in infants.*

**Gunevax**
*Chiron Vaccines, Ital.; Chiron Behring, Malaysia; Fustery, Mex.; Chiron, Thai.*
A rubella vaccine (Wistar RA 27/3 strain) (p.1637·3).
*Active immunisation.*

**Gupisone** *Julphar, UAE.*
Prednisolone (p.1108·1).
*Corticosteroid.*

**Gurfi Fibras** *Oshima, Arg.*
Bran (p.1253·2); wheat; glucose.
*Fibre supplement.*

**Gurfix** *Novartis Consumer, Austria.*
Hexetidine (p.1182·1).
*Mouth and throat inflammation.*

**Gurgellosung Chauvin** *Chauvin ankerpharm, Ger.*
Chlorhexidine gluconate (p.1173·2).
*Mouth and throat disorders.*

**Gurgellosung-ratiopharm** *Ratiopharm, Ger.*
Dequalinium chloride (p.1178·1).
*Mouth and throat infections.*

**Gurgol** *DM, Braz.†.*
Cetylpyridinium chloride (p.1173·1).
*Mouth disinfection.*

**Guronsan**
*Note. This name is used for preparations of different composition.*
*Exel, Belg.; Organon, Fr.; Jaba, Port.*
Glucuronamide; ascorbic acid (p.1460·2); caffeine (p.782·1).
*Tonic.*

*Chugai, Hong Kong.*
*Injection:* Glucuronic acid.
*Oral liquid:* Vitamin $B_2$; vitamin $B_1$; glucuronolactone; vitamin $B_6$ (p.1417·1).
*Tablets:* Glucuronolactone; glucuronamide; vitamin C; thiamine disulfide (p.1417·1).
*Tonic.*

*Inibsa, Spain.*
Glucuronamide; ascorbic acid (p.1460·2).
*Tonic.*

**Gustase** *Geriatric Pharm. Corp., USA†.*
Standardised amylolytic enzyme (Gerilase) (p.1654·2); standardised proteolytic enzyme (Geriprotase); standardised cellulolytic enzyme (Gericellulase) (p.1669·1).
*Gastrointestinal disorders.*

**Gustase Plus** *Geriatric Pharm. Corp., USA†.*
Phenobarbital (p.367·3); homatropine methylbromide (p.483·2); standardised amylolytic enzyme (Gerilase) (p.1654·2); standardised proteolytic enzyme (Geriprotase); standardised cellulolytic enzyme (Gericellulase) (p.1669·1).
*Gastrointestinal disorders.*

**Gutalax** *Fher, Spain.*
Sodium picosulfate (p.1289·3).
*Constipation.*

**Gutnacht** *Salushaus, Ger.*
*Oral liquid:* Valerian (p.1762·2); passion flower (p.1729·1); hypericum (p.299·1); melissa (p.1711·1); chamomile (p.1669·3); peppermint leaf (p.1283·2).
*Tablets:* Valerian (p.1762·2); passion flower (p.1729·1); lupulus (p.1708·1); melissa (p.1711·1).
Formerly contained valerian, passion flower, lupulus, melissa, hypericum, and rhiz. jatamansi.
*Nervousness; sleep disorders.*

**Gutron**
*Nycomed, Austria; Silesia, Chile; Nycomed, Fr.; Nycomed, Ger.; Nycomed, Hong Kong; Rafa, Israel; Lusofarmaco, Ital.; Sanofi Winthrop, Mex.†; Douglas, NZ; Lab, Port.; Nycomed, Singapore; Nycomed, Switz.; Nycomed, Thai.*
Midodrine hydrochloride (p.959·2).
*Ejaculation disorders; hypotension; urinary incontinence.*

**Guttacor** *Galenika, Ger.†.*
Convallaria (p.1675·3); crataegus (p.1677·1); valerian (p.1762·2).
*Cardiac disorders.*

**Guttacor-Balsam N** *Galenika, Ger.†.*
Rosemary oil (p.1740·2); camphor (p.1665·3).
*Cardiovascular disorders.*

**Guttae 20 Hustentropfen N** *Palmicol, Ger.†.*
Thyme (p.1755·2); wild thyme; primrose flower (p.1735·1).
*Catarrh; coughs.*

**Guttalax**
*Boehringer Ingelheim, Austria; Wolfs, Belg.; Boehringer de Angeli, Braz.; Silesia, Chile; Boehringer Ingelheim, Gr.; Boehringer Ingelheim, Ital.; Boehringer Ingelheim, Port.; Byk, Switz.†.*
Sodium picosulfate (p.1289·3).
*Bowel evacuation; constipation.*

**Guttanotte** *Sigmapharm, Austria.*
Flunitrazepam (p.698·2).
*Insomnia.*

**Guttaplast** *Beiersdorf, Ger.*
Salicylic acid (p.1157·1).
*Hyperkeratosis.*

**G-well** *Goldline, USA†.*
Lindane (p.1506·3).
*Pediculosis; scabies.*

**GX** *Baxter, Ger.; Braun, Ger.; Delta, Ger.*
Carbohydrate infusion (p.1417·1).
*Parenteral nutrition.*

**GX E** *Baxter, Ger.; Braun, Ger.*
Carbohydrate and electrolyte infusion (p.1417·1).
*Parenteral nutrition.*

**Gyalme** *Effik, Fr.*
Sodium laurilsulfate (p.1574·2).
*Genito-urinary cleansing.*

**Gydrelle** *IPRAD, Fr.*
Estriol (p.1552·3).
*Menopausal disorders.*

**Gydrelle Phyto** *IPRAD-Sante, Fr.*
Soya bean (p.1447·2).

**Gynae-CVP** *Sterling, India.*
Citrus bioflavonoids (p.1688·2); vitamin C (p.1460·2); ferrous gluconate (p.1428·1); calcium lactate (p.1225·3).
*Gynaecological haemorrhage.*

**Gynaemine** *Sriprasit, Thai.*
Ergotamine tartrate (p.467·2); ergometrine maleate (p.1684·1).
*Oxytocic.*

**Gynalpha** *CCD, Fr.*
Soya bean (p.1447·2).
*Menopausal disorders.*

**Gynamon** *Jenapharm, Ger.*
Orange tablets, estradiol (p.1550·1); grey tablets, estradiol; norethisterone acetate (p.1562·2).
*Menopausal disorders; osteoporosis.*

**Gynasan** *Bastian, Ger.*
Estriol (p.1552·3).
*Menopausal disorders.*

**Gynaseptol** *Bravir, Braz.†.*
Hydroxyquinoline sulfate (p.1700·1); boric acid (p.1662·1).
*Vulvovaginal infections.*

**Gynasol** *Wild, Switz.†.*
Tartaric acid (p.1752·1); aluminium lactate (p.1653·1); aluminium sulfate (p.1653·1); anhydrous glucose (p.1432·2); sodium bicarbonate (p.1223·2).
*Vaginal disorders.*

**Gynatren** *Strathmann, Ger.*
A trichomonal vaccine (p.1642·1).

**Gynatrol** *Wyeth Lederle, Denm.*
Ethinylestradiol (p.1553·2); levonorgestrel (p.1563·2).
*Combined oral contraceptive.*

**Gynax-N** *Ativus, Braz.*
Dexamethasone sodium phosphate (p.1097·2); nystatin (p.406·3); neomycin sulfate (p.235·1); tyrothricin (p.275·1); sodium propionate (p.408·1); boric acid (p.1662·1).
*Vulvovaginal disorders.*

**Gynazole** *Ther-Rx, USA.*
Butoconazole nitrate (p.395·2).
*Vulvovaginal candidiasis.*

**Gynebo** *Chew, Thai.*
Clotrimazole (p.396·2).
*Trichomoniasis; vaginal fungal infections.*

**Gynecon** *Continental Pharma, Thai.*
Nystatin (p.406·3); diiodohydroxyquinoline (p.603·3); benzalkonium chloride (p.1168·3).
*Fungal, trichomonal and bacterial vaginitis.*

**Gynecort** *Combe, USA.*
Hydrocortisone acetate (p.1103·3).
*Skin disorders.*

**Gynecure** *Pfizer Consumer, Canad.*
Tioconazole (p.409·3).
*Vulvovaginal candidiasis.*

**Gynefix**
*Besins-Iscovesco, Fr.†; Family Planning Sales, UK.*
Copper-wound polypropylene thread (p.1425·3).
*Intra-uterine contraceptive device.*

**Gynegella P** *Rottapharm, Ital.*
Salicaria; α-ketoglutaric acid.
*Vaginal douche.*

**Gynelle 375** *CCD, Fr.*
Copper-wound polyethylene (p.1425·3).
*Intra-uterine contraceptive device.*

**Gyne-Lotremin**
*Schering-Plough, Hong Kong; Schering-Plough, Malaysia; Schering-Plough, Singapore.*
Clotrimazole (p.396·2).
*Vaginitis; vulvovaginal candidiasis.*

**Gyne-Lotrimin**
*Schering-Plough, Austral.; Schering-Plough, USA.*
Clotrimazole (p.396·2).
*Vulvovaginal candidiasis.*

**Gyne-Moistrin** *Schering-Plough, Canad.*
Polyglyceryl methacrylate; propylene glycol (p.1735·2).
*Vaginal dryness.*

**Gynera**
*Berlimed, Braz.; Schering, Chile; Schering, Denm.; Shepa, Gr.; Schering, Hong Kong; Schering, Israel; Schering, Malaysia; Schering, Port.; Schering, Singapore; Schering, Switz.; Schering, Thai.*
Gestodene (p.1556·1); ethinylestradiol (p.1553·2).
28-Day packs also contain 7 inert tablets.
*Combined oral contraceptive.*

**Gynergen Comp** *Novartis, Denm.*
Belladonna (p.479·1); butalbital (p.673·3); caffeine (p.782·1); ergotamine tartrate (p.467·2).
*Migraine.*

**Gynergene** *Novartis, Braz.†.*
Ergotamine tartrate (p.467·2).
*Migraine and other vascular headaches.*

**Gynergene Cafeine** *Novartis, Fr.*
Ergotamine tartrate (p.467·2); caffeine (p.782·1).
*Migraine.*

**Gynerium** *Armstrong, Arg.*
Ketoconazole (p.403·3); secnidazole (p.615·3).
*Bacterial infections; candidiasis; trichomoniasis.*

**Gynescal** *CCD, Fr.†.*
Paraformaldehyde (p.1187·3); salicylic acid (p.1157·1); benzoic acid (p.1169·3); borax (p.1661·3); sodium bicarbonate (p.1223·2).
*Topical antiseptic.*

**Gynesten-B** *Bangkok Lab & Cosmetic, Thai.*
Clotrimazole (p.396·2); betamethasone (p.1093·1).
*Infected skin disorders.*

**Gynestin** *Kenyaku, Thai.*
Clotrimazole (p.396·2); urea (p.1162·2).
*Trichomoniasis.*

**Gynestrel** *Recordati, Ital.*
Naproxen sodium (p.65·1).
*Gynaecological disorders.*

**Gyne-Sulf** *G & W, USA†.*
Sulfathiazole (p.264·1); sulfacetamide (p.257·3); sulfabenzamide (p.257·3).
*Vaginitis due to Gardnerella vaginalis.*

**Gyne-T**
*Janssen-Ortho, Canad.; Janssen-Cilag, Denm.†; Janssen-Cilag, Fr.†; Janssen-Cilag, Ger.†; Ortho, Hong Kong†; Ortho, Israel†; Janssen-Cilag, UK†.*
Copper-wound plastic (p.1425·3).
*Intra-uterine contraceptive device.*

**Gynezol** *Parke-Med, S.Afr.†.*
Clotrimazole (p.396·2).
*Vaginal fungal infections.*

**Gyn-Hydralin** *Roche Nicholas, Fr.*
Glycine (p.1433·3).
*Pruritus.*

**Gynintim Film** *Piette, Belg.†.*
Nonoxinol 9 (p.1413·3).
*Contraceptive.*

**Gynipral**
*Nycomed, Austria; Silesia, Chile; Nycomed, Switz.*
Hexoprenaline sulfate (p.786·3).
*Premature labour.*

**Gyno Icaden** *Schering, Braz.*
Isoconazole nitrate (p.401·3).
*Vulvovaginal candidiasis.*

**Gyno Iruxol** *Abbott, Braz.*
Chloramphenicol (p.185·1); collagenase (p.1675·1).
*Vulvovaginal infections.*

**Gyno Oceral** *Asta Medica, Austria†.*
Oxiconazole nitrate (p.407·3).
*Fungal and Gram-positive vaginal infections.*

**Gyno Zalain** *Pharmacia, Braz.*
Sertaconazole nitrate (p.408·1).
*Fungal vaginal infections.*

**Gynocanesten** *Bayer, Chile.*
Clotrimazole (p.396·2).
*Vaginal infections.*

**Gyno-Canesten**
*Bayer, Ger.; Bayer, Ital.*
Clotrimazole (p.396·2).
*Balanitis; fungal vulvovaginal infections.*

**Gyno-Canestene**
*Bayer, Belg.; Bayer, Switz.*
Clotrimazole (p.396·2).
*Fungal vaginal infections.*

**Gynocastus** *Zilly, Ger.*
Vitex agnus castus (p.1649·1).
*Mastalgia; menstrual disorders.*

**Gynoco** *TO-Chemicals, Thai.*
Nystatin (p.406·3); diiodohydroxyquinoline (p.603·3); benzalkonium chloride (p.1168·3).
*Trichomoniasis; vaginal fungal infections.*

**Gyno-Daktar** *Janssen-Cilag, Ger.*
Miconazole nitrate (p.405·3).
*Balanitis; fungal vaginal infections.*

**Gyno-Daktarin**
*Janssen-Cilag, Austral.†; Janssen-Cilag, Austria; Janssen-Cilag, Belg.; Janssen-Cilag, Braz.; Orion, Fin.; Janssen-Cilag, Fr.; Janssen, Hong Kong; Ethnor, India; Janssen-Cilag, Irl.; Janssen-Cilag, Israel; Janssen, Mex.†; Janssen-Cilag, Neth.; Janssen-Cilag, NZ†; Janssen-Cilag, Port.; Janssen-Cilag, S.Afr.; Janssen-Cilag, UK.*
Miconazole nitrate (p.405·3).
*Vulvovaginal candidiasis with Gram-positive bacterial infection.*

**Gynodal** *Asta Oncologia, Braz.*
Megestrol acetate (p.1558·2).
*Malignant neoplasms.*

**Gynodian Depot**
*Schering, Arg.; Schering, Austria; Schering, Chile; Schering, Ger.; Schering, Ital.; Schering, Spain†; Schering, Switz.*
Estradiol valerate (p.1550·2); prasterone enantate (p.1565·3).
*Menopausal disorders; osteoporosis.*

**Gynodiol** *Fielding, USA.*
Estradiol (p.1550·1).
*Breast cancer; menopausal disorders; oestrogen deficiency; osteoporosis; prostatic cancer.*

**Gynofen 35** *Shepa, Gr.*
Ethinylestradiol (p.1553·2); cyproterone acetate (p.1544·1).
*Androgen-related disorders in women; male-pattern alopecia; mild hirsutism; severe acne.*

**Gynoflor**
*Pharmacia, Austria; Grunenthal, Belg.; Nourypharma, Ger.; Medinova, Switz.*
*Lactobacillus acidophilus* (p.1704·2); estriol (p.1552·3).
*Restoration of vaginal flora; vaginal disorders.*

**Gyno-Flor E** *Medinova, Hong Kong†.*
*Lactobacillus acidophilus* (p.1704·2); estriol (p.1552·3).
*Restoration of vaginal flora; vaginal disorders.*

**Gynofug** *Wolff, Ger.*
Ibuprofen (p.45·3).
*Inflammation; pain.*

**Gyno-Fungistat** *Janssen-Cilag, Braz.†.*
Terconazole (p.409·3).
*Vulvovaginal candidiasis.*

**Gyno-Fungix** *Janssen-Cilag, Braz.*
Terconazole (p.409·3).
*Vulvovaginal candidiasis.*

**Gynokadin** Kade, Ger.; Besins, Ger.
Estradiol (p.1550·1) or estradiol valerate (p.1550·2).
*Menopausal disorders; osteoporosis.*

**Gynol** Advanced Care, USA.
Nonoxinol 9 (p.1413·3).
*Contraceptive.*

**Gynol II**
Janssen-Cilag, Irl.; Janssen-Cilag, UK.
Nonoxinol 9 (p.1413·3).
*Contraceptive.*

**Gyno-Liderman** Jacoby, Austria.
Oxiconazole nitrate (p.407·3).
*Fungal and Gram-positive vaginal infections.*

**Gynomax** Farmoquimica, Braz.
Tioconazole (p.409·3); tinidazole (p.617·1).
*Fungal infections.*

**Gyno-Mikozal** Julphar, UAE.
Miconazole nitrate (p.405·3).
*Vulvovaginal candidiasis.*

**Gyno-Monistat** Janssen-Cilag, Ger.†.
Miconazole nitrate (p.405·3).
*Balanitis; fungal vaginal infections.*

**Gyno-Mycel** Biolab Sanus, Braz.
Isoconazole nitrate (p.401·3).
*Vaginal candidiasis.*

**Gyno-Myfungar**
Rhein, Mex.; Klinge, Switz.†.
Oxiconazole nitrate (p.407·3).
*Fungal and Gram-positive vulvovaginal infections.*

**Gynomyk**
Will-Pharma, Belg.; Aventis, Fr.; Will-Pharma, Neth.
Butoconazole nitrate (p.395·2).
*Fungal vulvovaginal infections.*

**Gyno-Mykotral** Rosen, Ger.
Miconazole nitrate (p.405·3).
*Fungal genital infections.*

**Gyno-Neuralgin** Pfleger, Ger.
Ibuprofen (p.45·3).
*Dysmenorrhoea.*

**Gyno-Pevaryl**
Janssen-Cilag, Austria; Janssen-Cilag, Belg.; Janssen-Cilag, Fr.; Janssen-Cilag, Ger.; Cilag, Hong Kong; Janssen-Cilag, Irl.; Janssen-Cilag, Israel; Janssen-Cilag, Malaysia; ICN, NZ; Janssen-Cilag, Port.; Janssen-Cilag, S.Afr.; Janssen-Cilag, Singapore; Pensa, Spain; Janssen-Cilag, Switz.; Janssen-Cilag, UK.
Econazole nitrate (p.397·2).
*Fungal balanitis; fungal vulvovaginal infections.*

**Gynoplix** Bouchara-Recordati, Hong Kong.
Metronidazole (p.607·2).
*Vaginal infections.*

**Gynoplix Theraplix** Vaillant, Ital.†.
Acetarsol (p.600·2).
*Vaginal dryness.*

**Gynoplus** Gallia, Braz.†.
Isoconazole nitrate (p.401·3).
*Fungal vaginal infections.*

**Gynormal** Andromaco, Arg.
*Cream; pessaries:* Tinidazole (p.617·1); miconazole nitrate (p.405·3).
*Tablets:* Tinidazole (p.617·1).
*Anaerobic bacterial infections of the vagina; protozoal vaginal infections.*

**Gynosoja** Codifra, Fr.
Soya bean (p.1447·2); alfalfa (p.1649·1); folic acid (p.1429·1).
*Menopausal disorders.*

**Gynospasmine** Synthelabo, Fr.†.
Paracetamol (p.76·2).
*Fever; pain.*

**Gynospor** Garec, S.Afr.
Miconazole nitrate (p.405·3).
*Vaginal fungal infections.*

**Gynostat** Laboratorios Chile, Chile.
Desogestrel (p.1547·2); ethinylestradiol (p.1553·2).
*Combined oral contraceptive; menstrual disorders.*

**Gynosyl** Homberger, Switz.†.
Homoeopathic preparation.

**Gyno-Tardyferon**
Pharmafabre (Φαρμαφαμπρ), Gr.; Robapharm, Switz.
Ferrous sulfate (p.1428·2); folic acid (p.1429·1).
*Iron and folic acid deficiency; iron-deficiency anaemia.*

**Gyno-Terazol**
Janssen-Cilag, Belg.†; Janssen-Cilag, Neth.; Janssen-Cilag, Switz.
Terconazole (p.409·3).
*Fungal genital infections.*

**Gyno-Travogen**
Schering, Austria; Schering, Belg.†; Schering, Hong Kong; Schering, Israel; Schering, NZ†; Schering, Singapore; Schering, Switz.
Isoconazole nitrate (p.401·3).
*Fungal and Gram-positive vaginal infections.*

**Gyno-Trimaze** Garec, S.Afr.
Clotrimazole (p.396·2).
*Fungal vaginal infections.*

**Gyno-Trosyd**
Pfizer, Fin.; Teofarma, Fr.; Pfizer, Hong Kong; Pfizer, Malaysia; Pfizer, NZ; Pfizer, S.Afr.†; Pfizer, Singapore; Pfizer, Switz.
Tioconazole (p.409·3).
*Fungal vaginal infections; vaginal trichomoniasis.*

**Gynova** Milano, Thai.
Nystatin (p.406·3); diiodohydroxyquinoline (p.603·3); benzalkonium chloride (p.1168·3).
*Fungal, trichomonal and bacterial vaginitis.*

**Gynovin**
Schering, Arg.; Schering, Austria; Schering, Mex.; Schering, Spain.
Ethinylestradiol (p.1553·2); gestodene (p.1556·1).
*Combined oral contraceptive.*

**Gynovite Plus** Optimox, USA.
Multivitamin and mineral preparation with iron and folic acid (p.1417·1).

**GynPolar** Orion, Ger.
Estradiol (p.1550·1).
*Menopausal disorders.*

**Gyrablock**
Medochemie, Singapore†; Medochemie, Thai.†.
Norfloxacin (p.238·3).
*Bacterial infections.*

**Gyracon** Pond's, Thai.
Nystatin (p.406·3); diiodohydroxyquinoline (p.603·3); benzalkonium chloride (p.1168·3).
*Fungal, trichomonal and bacterial vaginitis.*

**Gyrol** Brasmedica, Braz.†.
Tyrothricin (p.275·1); thymol (p.1194·2); boric acid (p.1662·1).
*Vulvovaginal infections.*

**Gyrosan** CMS, Switz.
Heavy kaolin (p.1268·3); silver (p.1746·1).
*Burns; wounds.*

**Gy-Sol** Provit, Mex.†.
Gentamicin sulfate (p.217·1).
*Bacterial infections.*

**H I** Esoform, Ital.†.
Glutaral (p.1180·3).
*Instrument disinfection.*

**H 2 Blocker** Ratiopharm, Ger.
Cimetidine (p.1255·3) or cimetidine hydrochloride (p.1255·3).
*Acid aspiration; gastro-oesophageal reflux; gastrointestinal haemorrhage; hypersensitivity reactions; peptic ulcer; Zollinger-Ellison syndrome.*

**H Tussan** Inibsa, Spain.
Anise oil (p.1655·2); hedera helix; thyme oil (p.1755·3).
*Coughs.*

**Habitrol**
Novartis Consumer, Canad.; Novartis Consumer, USA.
Nicotine (p.1720·1).
*Aid to smoking withdrawal.*

**Habstal-Cor N** Steierl, Ger.
Homoeopathic preparation.

**Habstal-Nerv N** Steierl, Ger.
Passion flower (p.1729·1); valerian root (p.1762·2).
*Insomnia; nervous disorders.*

**Habstal-Pulm N** Steierl, Ger.
Homoeopathic preparation.

**HAC** Zeneca, Belg.†.
Cetrimonium bromide (p.1173·1); chlorhexidine gluconate (p.1173·2).
*Burns; disinfection of skin, instruments, textiles, and surfaces; wounds.*

**Hacdil-S** Zeneca, Belg.†.
Cetrimonium bromide (p.1173·1); chlorhexidine gluconate (p.1173·2).
*Disinfection of wounds and instruments.*

**Hachemina Fuerte** Medea, Spain.
Aminobenzoic acid (p.1142·2).
*Alopecia; leucopenia; skin disorders.*

**Hacks** Ernest Jackson, UK.
Menthol (p.1711·3); eucalyptus oil (p.1686·2); vitamin C (p.1460·2).
*Cold symptoms; coughs.*

**Hacks Blackcurrant** Ernest Jackson, UK.
Menthol (p.1711·3); vitamin C (p.1460·2).
*Cold symptoms; coughs.*

**Hactos** Hubert, UK.
Capsicum (p.1667·1); peppermint oil (p.1283·2); anise oil (p.1655·2); clove oil (p.1673·3).
*Catarrh; cold symptoms; coughs.*

**Hadarax** Greater Pharma, Thai.
Hydroxyzine hydrochloride (p.434·3).
*Pruritus.*

**Hadensa**
Note. This name is used for preparations of different composition.
Kolassa, Austria; Leiras, Fin.; Ferrer, Spain.
*Ointment:* Chlorocarvacrol; ichthammol (p.1148·2); menthol (p.1711·3).
*Anorectal disorders.*
Kolassa, Austria; Leiras, Fin.
*Suppositories:* Chlorocarvacrol; ichthammol (p.1148·2); menthol (p.1711·3); chamomile oil (p.1669·3).
*Anorectal disorders.*

**Hadiel** Piam, Ital.
Bezafibrate (p.873·2).
*Hyperlipidaemias.*

**H-Adiftal** ISM, Ital.†.
An adsorbed diphtheria vaccine (p.1612·3).
*Active immunisation.*

**H-Adiftetal** ISM, Ital.†.
An adsorbed diphtheria and tetanus vaccine (p.1613·1).
*Active immunisation.*

**Hadlinol** Help, Gr.
Fluconazole (p.398·1).
*Fungal infections.*

**Haelan**
Dista, Irl.†; Typharm, UK.
Fludroxycortide (p.1100·3).
*Skin disorders.*

**Haem Up** Cadila Pharma, India.
Glycerinated haemoglobin (p.755·2); copper sulfate; manganese sulfate; zinc sulfate (p.1417·1); ferric ammonium citrate (p.1427·2).
*Anaemia of pregnancy.*

**Haemaccel**
Aventis, Arg.; Aventis, Austral.; Aventis, Austria; Aventis, Belg.; Aventis, Braz.†; Aventis, Chile; Aventis, Denm.†; Hoechst Marion Roussel, Fin.†; Hoechst, Fr.†; Aventis, Ger.; Hoechst Marion Roussel, Gr.; Aventis, Hong Kong; Nicholas Piramal, India; Aventis, Irl.; Aventis, Israel; Aventis, Malaysia; Aventis, Mex.; Behring, Neth.; Aventis, Norw.; Aventis, NZ; Aventis, Port.; Aventis, S.Afr.; Hoechst Marion Roussel, Singapore†; Hoechst Marion Roussel, Swed.†; Aventis, Switz.; Aventis, Thai.; Beacon, UK†.
Polygeline (p.759·1) with electrolytes.
*Extra-corporeal circulation; organ perfusion; plasma exchange; plasma volume expansion; shock.*

**Haemanal** Sigmapharm, Austria.
Hydrastinine hydrochloride; chlorocarvacrol; zinc oxide (p.1163·2); tannic acid (p.1751·2); menthol (p.1711·3).
*Anorectal disorders.*

**Haemate**
Aventis Behring, Denm.; Aventis Behring, Ger.; Aventis Behring, Ital.; Aventis, Neth.; Aventis Behring, Spain; Aventis Behring, Swed.
A factor VIII preparation (p.751·1).
*Haemorrhagic disorders.*

**Haemate HS** Aventis Behring, Switz.
A factor VIII preparation (p.751·1).
*Haemorrhagic disorders.*

**Haemate P**
Aventis, Austria; Aventis Behring, Braz.; Aventis Behring, Hong Kong; Aventis Behring, Irl.; Aventis Behring, Israel; Aventis Behring, UK.
A factor VIII preparation (p.751·1).
*Haemorrhagic disorders.*

**Haematicum Glausch** Terramin, Austria†.
Iron; manganese (p.1417·1).
*Tonic.*

**Haemiton** AWD, Ger.
Clonidine hydrochloride (p.885·2).
*Hypertension.*

**Haemiton compositum** AWD, Ger.
Clonidine hydrochloride (p.885·2); triamterene (p.1016·2); hydrochlorothiazide (p.933·2).
*Hypertension.*

**Haemo Duoform** Mauermann, Ger.
Hamamelis leaves (p.1696·3).
*Haemorrhoids.*

**Haemocompletan**
Aventis Behring, Austria; Aventis Behring, Ger.; Aventis Behring, Switz.; Centeon, UK†.
Fibrinogen (p.753·2).
*Haemorrhagic disorders; hypofibrinogenaemia.*

**Haemocompletan-P** IFET (ΙΦΕΤ), Gr.
Fibrinogen (p.753·2).
*Haemorrhagic disorders associated with hypofibrinogenaemia.*

**Haemocortin** Streuli, Switz.
*Ointment:* Hydrocortisone acetate (p.1103·3); bismuth oxychloride (p.1253·1); lidocaine hydrochloride (p.1377·3); zinc oxide (p.1163·2).
*Suppositories:* Hydrocortisone acetate (p.1103·3); bismuth oxychloride (p.1253·1); lidocaine hydrochloride (p.1377·3); zinc oxide (p.1163·2); ethacridine lactate (p.1165·3); menthol (p.1711·3); adrenaline hydrochloride (p.852·3); hamamelis (p.1696·3); peru balsam (p.1730·2).
*Anorectal disorders.*

**Haemoctin SDH**
Biogam, Arg.; Biotest, Ger.; Boehringer Ingelheim, Port.; Biotest, Singapore.
A factor VIII preparation (p.751·1).
*Haemorrhagic disorders.*

**Haemoctin SDM** Biotest, Israel.
A factor VIII preparation (p.751·1).
*Haemophilia A.*

**Haemodyn** Klinge, Austria.
Pentoxifylline (p.979·3).
*Peripheral vascular disorders.*

**Haemo-Exhirud** Sanofi Synthelabo, Ger.
Leech extract (p.931·2); allantoin (p.1141·3); lauromacrogol 400 (p.1412·3).
*Anorectal disorders; urogenital venous disorders.*

**Haemo-Exhirud Bufexamac** Sanofi Synthelabo, Ger.
Bufexamac (p.21·3); bismuth subgallate (p.1252·2); titanium dioxide (p.1160·3); lidocaine hydrochloride (p.1377·3).
*Haemorrhoids.*

**Haemofusin** Baxter, Ger.
Pentastarch (p.750·1) in sodium chloride.
*Plasma volume expansion.*

**Haemo-Glukotest 20-800**
Roche, Arg.; Roche, Mex.
Test for glucose in blood (p.1694·2).

**Haemoglukotest 20-800** Roche Diagnostics, Ital.
Test for glucose in blood (p.1694·2).

**Haemolan** Streuli, Switz.
*Ointment:* Lidocaine hydrochloride (p.1377·3); bismuth oxychloride (p.1253·1); zinc oxide (p.1163·2); menthol (p.1711·3); peru balsam (p.1730·2).
*Suppositories:* Lidocaine hydrochloride (p.1377·3); bismuth oxychloride (p.1253·1); zinc oxide (p.1163·2); menthol (p.1711·3); peru balsam (p.1730·2); ethacridine lactate (p.1165·3); ephedrine hydrochloride (p.1120·1); hamamelis (p.1696·3).
*Anorectal disorders.*

**Haemomac** CT, Ger.†.
Bufexamac (p.21·3); lidocaine hydrochloride (p.1377·3); bismuth subgallate (p.1252·2); titanium dioxide (p.1160·3).
*Haemorrhoids.*

**Haemopressin** Curatis, Ger.; Meduna, Ger.
Terlipressin acetate (p.1340·1).
*Variceal haemorrhage.*

**Haemoproct** Julphar, UAE.
Tribenoside (p.1757·3); lidocaine (p.1377·3) or lidocaine hydrochloride (p.1377·3).
*Haemorrhoids.*

**Haemoprotect** Betapharm, Ger.
Ferrous sulfate (p.1428·2).
*Iron deficiency; iron-deficiency anaemia.*

**Haemo-Red Formula** Eagle, Austral.†.
Multivitamin and mineral preparation with yellow dock and urtica (p.1417·1).

**Haemorrhoid Cream** Nelson, UK.
Homoeopathic preparation.

**Haemosol** Eisai, Hong Kong†.
Alpha tocoferil calcium succinate (p.1465·3); phytomenadione (p.1467·1); rutoside (p.1688·2); muramidase hydrochloride (p.1717·2); pluronic F-68.
*Anorectal disorders.*

**Haemosolvate** NBI, S.Afr.
Factor VIII (p.751·1).
*Factor VIII deficiency.*

**Haemosolvex** NBI, S.Afr.
Factor IX (p.752·2).
*Coagulation disorders.*

**Haemovex 4** Gambro, Swed.
Sodium chloride; potassium chloride; calcium chloride; magnesium chloride; sodium lactate; glucose (p.1221·1).
*Haemofiltration.*

**Haemovex 8** Gambro, Swed.
Sodium chloride; calcium chloride; magnesium chloride; sodium lactate; glucose (p.1221·1).
*Haemofiltration.*

**Haemovital** Pharmadass, UK.
Vitamin, mineral, and nutritional preparation (p.1417·1).
*Tonic.*

**Haenal** Strathmann, Ger.†.
Quinisocaine hydrochloride (p.1384·2).
*Anorectal disorders; insect stings.*

**HAES Esteril** Fresenius Kabi, Spain.
Pentastarch (p.750·1).
*Plasma volume expansion.*

**HAES-Rheopond** Serag-Wiessner, Ger.
Pentastarch (p.750·1) in sodium chloride.
*Hypovolaemia; shock.*

**HAES-steril**
Fresenius Kabi, Austria; Fresenius, Belg.†; Fresenius Kabi, Denm.; Fresenius Kabi, Fin.; Fresenius Kabi, Ger.; Fresenius Kabi, Gr.; Fresenius Kabi, Ital.; Fresenius Kabi, Malaysia; Fresenius Kabi, Mex.; Fresenius Kabi, Norw.; Fresenius Kabi, Port.; Fresenius Kabi, S.Afr.; Fresenius Kabi, Singapore; Fresenius Kabi, Swed.; Fresenius Kabi, Switz.; Fresenius Kabi, Thai.; Fresenius Kabi, UK.
Pentastarch (p.750·1) in sodium chloride.
*Haemodilution; plasma volume expansion; shock.*

**HAES-sterile** Fresenius, Israel.
Pentastarch (p.750·1).
*Plasma volume expansion; shock.*

**Hafif** Biogal, Israel.
Carbaryl (p.1501·2).
*Pediculosis.*

**Hagevir** Cosmepharm, Gr.
Aciclovir (p.626·1).
*Herpes simplex infections.*

**Haimabig** Nuovo ISM, Ital.
A hepatitis B immunoglobulin (p.1617·2).
*Passive immunisation.*

**Haimacig** ISI, Ital.†.
A cytomegalovirus immunoglobulin (p.1612·1).
*Passive immunisation.*

**Haima-D** Nuovo ISM, Ital.
An anti-D immunoglobulin (p.1608·1).
*Prevention of rhesus sensitisation.*

**Haimaferone** Schiapparelli, Ital.
Interferon alfa (p.640·3).
*Malignant neoplasms; viral infections.*

**Haimalbumin** Nuovo ISM, Ital.†.
Albumin (p.740·3).
*Hypoalbuminaemia.*

**Haima-Parot** ISI, Ital.†.
A mumps immunoglobulin (p.1626·3).
*Passive immunisation.*

**Haimapertus** ISI, Ital.†.
A pertussis immunoglobulin (p.1631·2).
*Passive immunisation.*

**Haimarab** ISI, Ital.†.
A rabies immunoglobulin (p.1635·3).
*Passive immunisation.*

**Haimaserum** ISI, Ital.†.
Plasma protein fraction (p.758·2).
*Hypoproteinaemia; hypovolaemia.*

**Haima-Tetanus** ISI, Ital.†.
A tetanus immunoglobulin (p.1640·3).
*Passive immunisation.*

**Haimaven** Nuovo ISM, Ital.
A normal immunoglobulin (p.1627·2).
*Idiopathic thrombocytopenic purpura; immunodeficiency; passive immunisation.*

**Haimazig** *Nuovo ISM, Ital.†.*
A varicella-zoster immunoglobulin (p.1643·1).
*Passive immunisation.*

**Haiprex** *3M, Denm.*
Methenamine hippurate (p.230·2).
*Urinary-tract infections.*

**4 Hair** *Marlyn, USA.*
Multivitamin, mineral, and amino-acid preparation (p.1417·1).

**Hair Booster** *Nature's Bounty, USA.*
Vitamin B substances with minerals, iron, and folic acid (p.1417·1).

**Hair Nutrition** *Cantassium Co., UK.*
Multivitamin and mineral preparation (p.1417·1).

**Hair & Scalp**
*ICN, Canad.; ICN, Hong Kong†.*
Pyrithione zinc (p.1156·2).
*Scalp irritation; seborrhoeic dermatitis.*

**Hair and Skin Formula** *Vitaplex, Austral.†.*
Calcium pantothenate (p.1442·3); inositol (p.1701·2); aminobenzoic acid (p.1142·2); ascorbic acid (p.1460·2); *dl*-alpha tocoferil acetate (p.1465·1).
*Multivitamin preparation.*

**Hairclin** *Galderma, Arg.*
Permethrin (p.1508·3).
*Pediculosis.*

**Hairgaine** *Agis, Israel.*
Minoxidil (p.960·1).
*Alopecia androgenetica.*

**Hairgrow** *Dar Al Dawa, Hong Kong.*
Minoxidil (p.960·1).
*Alopecia androgenetica.*

**Hairplus** *Euroderm, Arg.*
Salicylic acid (p.1157·1); pyrithione zinc (p.1156·2); calcium pantothenate; jojoba oil; tricopeptides.
*Dandruff; seborrhoeic dermatitis.*

**Hairscience** *Ego, Singapore.*
Miconazole nitrate (p.405·3).
Formerly contained miconazole nitrate and salicylic acid.
*Dandruff; seborrhoeic dermatitis.*

**Hairscience Antidandruff** *Ego, NZ.*
Miconazole nitrate (p.405·3).
*Dandruff; seborrhoeic dermatitis.*

**Hairscience Conditioner** *Ego, NZ.*
Cetrimide (p.1172·1); lipids; cationic polymer.
*Scalp disorders.*

**Hairscience Shampoo** *Ego, NZ.*
Sodium salicylate (p.90·1).
*Dandruff.*

**HairVit** *Pharmadass, UK.*
Multivitamin, mineral, and trace element preparation (p.1417·1).

**Halamid** *Viatris, Ger.*
Nedocromil sodium (p.789·3).
*Obstructive airways disease.*

**Halbmond** *Whitehall-Much, Ger.*
Diphenhydramine hydrochloride (p.431·3).
*Sleep disorders.*

**Halcicomb** *Bristol-Myers Squibb, Braz.†.*
Halcinonide (p.1103·2); neomycin (p.235·1); nystatin (p.406·3).
*Infected skin disorders.*

**Halciderm**
*Note. This name is used for preparations of different composition.*
*Bristol-Myers Squibb, Austral.†; Rottapharm, Ital.; Bristol-Myers Squibb, UK.*
Halcinonide (p.1103·2).
*Skin disorders.*

*Rottapharm, Ital.*
*Tincture:* Halcinonide (p.1103·2); salicylic acid (p.1157·1).
*Skin disorders.*

**Halciderm Combi** *Rottapharm, Ital.*
Halcinonide (p.1103·2); neomycin sulfate (p.235·1).
*Infected skin disorders.*

**Halcion**
*Pharmacia, Austral.; Pharmacia, Austria; Pharmacia, Belg.; Pharmacia, Braz.; Pharmacia, Canad.; Pharmacia, Denm.; Pharmacia, Fin.; Pharmacia, Fr.; Pharmacia, Ger.; Pharmacia-Upjohn, Gr.; Pharmacia, Hong Kong; Pharmacia, Irl.; Pharmacia Upjohn, Israel; Pharmacia Upjohn, Ital.; Pharmacia Upjohn, Mex.; Pharmacia, Neth.; Pharmacia, NZ; Pharmacia, Port.; Pharmacia, S.Afr.; Pharmacia, Spain; Pharmacia, Swed.; Pharmacia, Switz.; Pharmacia, Thai.; Pharmacia Upjohn, USA.*
Triazolam (p.725·3).
*Insomnia.*

**Haldid** *Janssen-Cilag, Denm.*
Fentanyl citrate (p.40·1).
*Analgesia in anaesthesia.*

**Haldol**
*Janssen-Cilag, Austral.; Janssen-Cilag, Austria; Janssen-Cilag, Belg.; Janssen-Cilag, Braz.; Janssen-Ortho, Canad.; Janssen-Cilag, Chile; Janssen-Cilag, Fr.; Janssen-Cilag, Ger.; Janssen, Hong Kong; Janssen-Cilag, Irl.; Janssen-Cilag, Israel; Janssen-Cilag, Ital.; Janssen, Mex.; Janssen-Cilag, Neth.; Janssen-Cilag, Norw.; Janssen-Cilag, NZ; Janssen-Cilag, Swed.; Janssen-Cilag, Switz.; Janssen-Cilag, Thai.; Janssen-Cilag, UK; Ortho McNeil, USA.*
Haloperidol (p.701·2), haloperidol decanoate (p.701·3), or haloperidol lactate (p.702·1).
*Alcohol withdrawal syndrome; behaviour disorders in children; bipolar disorder; intractable hiccup; movement disorders; nausea; pain; psychoses; stuttering; Tourette syndrome; vomiting.*

**Halenol** *Halsey, USA.*
Paracetamol (p.76·2).
*Fever; pain.*

**Haley's M-O** *Sterling Health, USA.*
Magnesium hydroxide (p.1272·2); liquid paraffin (p.1479·1).
*Constipation.*

**Half Betadur CR** *Monmouth, UK†.*
Propranolol hydrochloride (p.989·3).

**Half Beta-Prograne** *Tillomed, UK.*
Propranolol hydrochloride (p.989·3).
*Angina pectoris; anxiety; essential tremor; hyperthyroidism; migraine; prophylaxis of gastrointestinal bleeding.*

**Half Capozide** *Bristol-Myers Squibb, Irl.*
Captopril (p.879·2); hydrochlorothiazide (p.933·2).
*Hypertension.*

**Half Inderal**
*AstraZeneca, Irl.; AstraZeneca, UK.*
Propranolol hydrochloride (p.989·3).
*Angina pectoris; anxiety; essential tremor; hypertension; hyperthyroidism; migraine; variceal haemorrhage.*

**Half Securon** *Abbott, UK.*
Verapamil hydrochloride (p.1019·1).
*Angina pectoris; hypertension; myocardial infarction.*

**Half Sinemet**
*Du Pont, Irl.; Bristol-Myers Squibb, UK.*
Carbidopa (p.1204·3); levodopa (p.1205·2).
These ingredients can be described by the British Approved Name Co-careldopa.
*Parkinsonism.*

**Halfan**
*GlaxoSmithKline, Belg.; GlaxoSmithKline, Fr.; GlaxoSmithKline, Ger.; GlaxoSmithKline, Neth.; Smith Kline & French, Port.; GlaxoSmithKline, S.Afr.; SmithKline, Spain; SmithKline Beecham, Switz.; SmithKline Beecham, UK†; SmithKline Beecham, USA†.*
Halofantrine hydrochloride (p.452·2).
*Malaria.*

**Halfprin** *Kramer, USA.*
Aspirin (p.15·1).
*Myocardial infarction.*

**Haliborange**
*Eurospital, Ital.; Inibsa, Spain; Seven Seas, UK.*
Vitamins A, C, and D (p.1417·1).

*Boots Healthcare, NZ.*
Multivitamin preparation (p.1417·1).

**Haliborange Calcium Plus Vitamin D** *Seven Seas, UK.*
Calcium (p.1225·1); vitamin D (p.1461·2).

**Haliborange Halibonbons** *Seven Seas, UK.*
Vitamin C (p.1460·2).

**Haliborange High Strength Vitamin C** *Seven Seas, UK.*
Vitamin C with or without vitamin E and bioflavonoids (p.1417·1).

**Haliborange Multivitamins** *Seven Seas, UK.*
Multivitamins with or without calcium and iron (p.1417·1).

**Halibut**
*Note. This name is used for preparations of different composition.*
*Andromaco, Port.; Grunenthal, Port.*
Halibut oil (p.1434·1); zinc oxide (p.1163·2).
*Anorectal disorders; skin disorders; vulvovaginal disorders.*

*Novartis Consumer, Spain.*
Benzethonium chloride (p.1169·2); vitamin A (p.1451·2); zinc oxide (p.1163·2).
*Burns; cracked nipples; skin irritation; ulcers; wounds.*

*Adroka, Switz.*
Halibut-liver oil (p.1434·1).
*Tonic; vitamin A and D deficiency.*

**Halibut Hidrocortisona** *Novartis Consumer, Spain.*
Hydrocortisone acetate (p.1103·3); vitamin A (p.1451·2); zinc oxide (p.1163·2); benzethonium chloride (p.1169·2).
*Insect bites; skin disorders.*

**Halibut Multivit** *Adroka, Switz.*
Halibut-liver oil with multivitamins (p.1417·1).

**Halicar**
*Peithner, Austria; DHU, Ger.*
Homoeopathic preparation.

**Halita** *Dentaid, Chile Colutorio.*
Zinc lactate; chlorhexidine gluconate (p.1173·2); cetylpyridinium chloride (p.1173·1).
*Halitosis.*

**Halitol** *Caldeira & Marques, Port.*
Salicylic acid (p.1157·1); benzocaine (p.1370·3); cineole (p.1672·1).
*Mouth disorders.*

**Halitol Mucolitico** *Reig Jofre, Spain†.*
Amoxicillin trihydrate (p.155·3); guaifenesin (p.1122·1).
Formerly known as Amoxyvinco Mucolitico.
*Respiratory-tract infections.*

**Halitran** *Roche Consumer, Neth.*
Vitamin A (p.1451·2); colecalciferol (p.1461·3).
*Vitamin A and D deficiency.*

**Halivite** *Whitehall, Fr.*
Cod-liver oil (p.1425·2); zinc oxide (p.1163·2).
*Skin disorders.*

**Halloo-Wach N** *Altana, Ger.*
Caffeine (p.782·1); glucose monohydrate.
*Fatigue.*

**Halls** *Adams, Canad.*
Eucalyptus oil (p.1686·2); menthol (p.1711·3).
*Coughs; nasal congestion.*

**Halls Mentholyptus** *Adams Confectionery, UK.*
Eucalyptus oil (p.1686·2); menthol (p.1711·3).
*Cold symptoms; nasal congestion; sore throat.*

**Halls Sugar Free Mentho-Lyptus** *Warner-Lambert, USA.*
Eucalyptus oil (p.1686·2); menthol (p.1711·3).
*Sore throats.*

**Halls Zinc Defense** *Warner-Lambert, USA.*
Zinc acetate (p.1469·2).
*Zinc supplement.*

**Halls-Plus Maximum Strength** *Warner-Lambert, USA.*
Menthol (p.1711·3).

**Halo** *Cristalia, Braz.*
Haloperidol (p.701·2).
*Psychoses.*

**Halodin** *TO-Chemicals, Thai.*
Loratadine (p.436·1).
*Allergic rhinitis; allergic skin disorders.*

**Halofed** *Halsey, USA.*
Pseudoephedrine hydrochloride (p.1129·2).
*Nasal congestion.*

**Halog**
*Bristol-Myers Squibb, Austria; Bristol-Myers Squibb, Braz.; Westwood-Squibb, Canad.; Bristol-Myers Squibb, Fr.†; Bristol-Myers Squibb, Ger.; Bristol-Myers Squibb, Hong Kong; Bristol-Myers Squibb, Norw.†; Squibb, Spain; Westwood-Squibb, USA.*
Halcinonide (p.1103·2).
*Skin disorders.*

**Halog Neomycine** *Bristol-Myers Squibb, Fr.†.*
Halcinonide (p.1103·2); neomycin sulfate (p.235·1).
*Infected skin disorders.*

**Halog Tri** *Bristol-Myers Squibb, Ger.*
Halcinonide (p.1103·2); neomycin sulfate (p.235·1); nystatin (p.406·3).
*Infected skin disorders.*

**Halogedol** *Fardi, Spain.*
Camphor (p.1665·3); methyl salicylate (p.59·3).
*Muscle and joint pain.*

**Halomed** *Medifive, Thai.*
Haloperidol (p.701·2).
*Alcohol withdrawal syndrome; anxiety; psychomotor agitation.*

**Halomycetin** *Kwizda, Austria.*
Chloramphenicol (p.185·1).
*Bacterial eye infections.*

**Haloneural** *Hexal, Ger.*
Haloperidol (p.701·2).
*Psychoses.*

**Halonix** *Cadila Pharma, India.*
Sodium hyaluronate (p.1697·3).
*Osteoarthritis of the knee.*

**Halo-P** *PP Lab, Thai.*
Haloperidol (p.701·2).
*Anxiety; psychomotor agitation.*

**Haloper**
*Teuto, Braz.; CT, Ger.; CTI, Israel.*
Haloperidol (p.701·2).
*Extrapyramidal disorders; hiccups; pain; psychoses; vomiting.*

**Haloperil** *Psicofarma, Mex.*
Haloperidol (p.701·2).
*Psychoses.*

**Halopidol** *Janssen-Cilag, Arg.*
Haloperidol (p.701·2) or haloperidol decanoate (p.701·3).
*Behaviour disorders; psychoses.*

**Halopol** *General Drugs, Thai.*
Haloperidol (p.701·2).
*Alcohol withdrawal syndrome; anxiety; behaviour disorders in children; psychomotor agitation.*

**Hal-oral** *Hal, Ger.†.*
Allergen extracts of pollen, fungi, house dust mites (p.1650·2) and skin (p.1650·2) (p.1650·1).
*Allergen immunotherapy.*

**Haloral** *Hal, Neth.†.*
Allergen extracts (p.1650·1).
*Allergen immunotherapy.*

**Halotestin**
*Pharmacia, Austral.†; Pharmacia Upjohn, Canad.†; Pharmacia Upjohn, Fr.†; Pharmacia, Hong Kong; Pharmacia Upjohn, Israel†; Pharmacia Upjohn, Ital.†; Pharmacia Upjohn, Neth.†; Pharmacia Upjohn, Norw.†; Pharmacia Upjohn, S.Afr.†; Pharmacia Upjohn, Singapore†; Pharmacia, Thai.; Upjohn, USA†.*
Fluoxymesterone (p.1555·3).
*Breast cancer; delayed puberty; male hypogonadism; prevention of postpartum breast engorgement.*

**Halotex** *Westwood, USA†.*
Haloprogin (p.401·2).
*Fungal skin infections.*

**Halotussin** *Halsey, USA.*
Guaifenesin (p.1122·1).
*Coughs.*

**Halotussin-DM** *Halsey, USA.*
Dextromethorphan hydrobromide (p.1117·3); guaifenesin (p.1122·1).
*Coughs.*

**Halozen** *Bouzen, Arg.*
Haloperidol (p.701·2).

**Halset** *Novartis Consumer, Austria.*
Cetylpyridinium chloride (p.1173·1).
*Mouth and throat inflammation.*

**Halset plus Dexpanthenol** *Novartis Consumer, Austria.*
Benzalkonium chloride (p.1168·3); dexpanthenol (p.1727·2).
*Mouth and throat disorders.*

**Haltran** *Roberts, USA.*
Ibuprofen (p.45·3).
*Fever; osteoarthritis; pain; rheumatoid arthritis.*

**Halycitrol**
*Tamar, Israel; Laboratories for Applied Biology, UK.*
Vitamin A and D substances (p.1417·1).
*Vitamin A and D deficiency; vitamin A and D supplement.*

**Hamadin** *Schwabe, Ger.*
*Saccharomyces boulardii* (p.1704·2).
*Acne; diarrhoea.*

**Hamamelis Complex** *Blackmores, Austral.†.*
Hamamelis (p.1696·3); stone root (p.1749·3); plantain seed (p.1733·1); rhubarb (p.1287·3); ascorbic acid (p.1460·2); rutoside (p.1688·2); hesperidin (p.1688·2).
*Haemorrhoids.*

**Hamamelis Compose** *Boiron, Fr.*
Homoeopathic preparation.

**Hamamelis-Homaccord** *Peithner, Austria.*
Homoeopathic preparation.

**Hamamilla** *Pharmasette, Ital.*
Benzalkonium chloride (p.1168·3); hamamelis (p.1696·3); chamomile (p.1669·3); hypromellose (p.1579·3).
*Eye disinfection; eye irritation.*

**Hamasana** *Robugen, Ger.*
Hamamelis (p.1696·3).
*Burns; haemorrhoids; skin disorders; varicose veins; wounds.*

**Hamatopan** *Wolff, Ger.*
Ferrous sulfate (p.1428·2).
*Iron deficiency; iron-deficiency anaemia.*

**Hamatopan F** *Wolff, Ger.*
Dried ferrous sulfate (p.1428·3); folic acid (p.1429·1).
*Iron and folic acid deficiency.*

**Hametum**
*Peithner, Austria; Spitzner, Ger.; Schwabe, Ger.; Schwabe, Switz.†; TTN, Thai.†; Willmar, Thai.†.*
Hamamelis (p.1696·3).
*Gingivitis; haemorrhoids; skin disorders.*

**Hametum-N**
*Note. This name is used for preparations of different composition.*
*Spitzner, Ger.; Schwabe, Ger.*
Hamamelis (p.1696·3); aesculus (p.1648·2).
*Anorectal disorders; haemorrhoids.*

*Schwabe, Switz.†.*
Hamamelis (p.1696·3).
*Haemorrhoids.*

**HAMFL** *Fresenius Medical, Austria.*
A range of electrolyte infusions with or without glucose (p.1221·1).
*Haemofiltration.*

**Hamilton Body Lotion** *Hamilton, Austral.*
Chlorhexidine gluconate (p.1173·2); glycerol (p.1694·3); liquid paraffin (p.1479·1).
*Emollient.*

**Hamilton Cleansing Lotion** *Hamilton, Austral.*
Glycerol (p.1694·3); liquid paraffin (p.1479·1); chlorhexidine gluconate (p.1173·2).
*Skin cleansing; skin disorders.*

**Hamilton Dry Skin** *Hamilton, Austral.*
*Bath oil:* Light liquid paraffin (p.1479·1).
*Bath additive; dry skin; eczema; psoriasis.*

*Cream:* Urea (p.1162·2).
*Dry skin.*

*Foam Wash; wash:* Light liquid paraffin (p.1479·1).
*Dry skin.*

*Lotion:* Liquid paraffin (p.1479·1); glycerol (p.1694·3).
*Dry skin.*

**Hamilton Lip Balm** *Hamilton, Austral.†.*
Octinoxate (p.1154·3); avobenzone (p.1142·3).
*Dry chapped lips; sunscreen.*

**Hamilton Sensitive Broad Spectrum Milk**
*Hamilton, Austral.†.*
*SPF 15:* Octinoxate (p.1154·3); titanium dioxide (p.1160·3).

*SPF 30+:* Octinoxate (p.1154·3); titanium dioxide (p.1160·3); zinc oxide (p.1163·2).

*Sunscreen.*

**Hamilton Skin Repair**
*Hamilton, Austral.; Hamilton, Hong Kong.*
Dimethicone (p.1482·1); cetrimide (p.1172·1).
*Dermatitis; dry skin.*

**Hamilton Solastick Broad Spectrum** *Hamilton, Austral.†.*
*SPF 15:* Octinoxate (p.1154·3); avobenzone (p.1142·3).

*SPF 30+:* Octinoxate (p.1154·3); avobenzone (p.1142·3); oxybenzone (p.1154·3); titanium dioxide (p.1160·3).

*Sunscreen.*

**Hamilton Sportblock Broad Spectrum Milk**
*Hamilton, Austral.†.*
*SPF 30+:* Octinoxate (p.1154·3); enzacamene (p.1147·1); avobenzone (p.1142·3); titanium dioxide (p.1160·3).
*Sunscreen.*

**Hamilton Sunscreen** *Intercare, NZ.*
*Clear Lotion:* Octinoxate (p.1154·3); oxybenzone (p.1154·3); avobenzone (p.1142·3).

*Cream; Solastick; Sunstick:* Octinoxate (p.1154·3); octisalate (p.1154·3); avobenzone (p.1142·3).

*Kidscreen; Low Allergy Milk:* Octinoxate (p.1154·3); titanium dioxide (p.1160·3).

*Quadblock Cream SPF 40:* Octinoxate (p.1154·3); oxybenzone (p.1154·3); padimate O (p.1155·1); titanium dioxide (p.1160·3).

*Quadblock Milk; Water Resistant Milk:* Octinoxate (p.1154·3); enzacamene (p.1147·1); titanium dioxide (p.1160·3).

*Quadblock Stick; Sunsport Lotion:* Octinoxate (p.1154·3); enzacamene (p.1147·1); avobenzone (p.1142·3).

*Sunscreen.*

**Hamilton Sunscreen Clear Lotion Broad Spectrum** *Hamilton, Austral.†.*
*SPF 15; SPF 30+:* Octinoxate (p.1154·3); oxybenzone (p.1154·3); avobenzone (p.1142·3).
*Sunscreen.*

**Hamilton Sunscreen Cream Broad Spectrum** *Hamilton, Austral.†.*
*SPF 15:* Octinoxate (p.1154·3); octisalate (p.1154·3); avobenzone (p.1142·3).

*SPF 30+:* Octinoxate (p.1154·3); enzacamene (p.1147·1); avobenzone (p.1142·3); titanium dioxide (p.1160·3).

*Sunscreen.*

**Hamilton Sunscreen Milk Broad Spectrum** *Hamilton, Austral.†.*
*SPF 15:* Octinoxate (p.1154·3); avobenzone (p.1142·3); enzacamene (p.1147·1).

*SPF 30+:* Octinoxate (p.1154·3); enzacamene (p.1147·1); avobenzone (p.1142·3); titanium dioxide (p.1160·3).

*Sunscreen.*

**Hamilton Superblock Broad Spectrum Milk** *Hamilton, Austral.†.*
*SPF 30+:* Octinoxate (p.1154·3); enzacamene (p.1147·1); avobenzone (p.1142·3); titanium dioxide (p.1160·3).
*Sunscreen.*

**Hamilton Toddler Broad Spectrum Milk** *Hamilton, Austral.†.*
*SPF 30+:* Octinoxate (p.1154·3); enzacamene (p.1147·1); avobenzone (p.1142·3); titanium dioxide (p.1160·3).
*Sunscreen.*

**Hamilton Watersport Broad Spectrum Milk** *Hamilton, Austral.†.*
*SPF 30+:* Octinoxate (p.1154·3); enzacamene (p.1147·1); titanium dioxide (p.1160·3).
*Sunscreen.*

**Hamitan** *Safire, Hong Kong.*
Mefenamic acid (p.55·2).
*Dysmenorrhoea; menorrhagia.*

**Hamoagil plus** *Chefaro, Ger.*
Bufexamac (p.21·3); lidocaine hydrochloride (p.1377·3); bismuth dihydroxide-(3,4,5-trihydroxybenzoate) or bismuth subgallate (p.1252·2); titanium dioxide (p.1160·3).
*Haemorrhoids.*

**Hamo-Europuran N** *Scheurich, Ger.†.*
Lauromacrogol 400 (p.1412·3).
*Anorectal disorders.*

**Hamofiltrasol** *Alte Kreis, Austria†.*
Anhydrous glucose; electrolytes (p.1221·1).
*Haemofiltration solution.*

**Hamo-ratiopharm** *Ratiopharm, Ger.†.*
Butoxycaine hydrochloride (p.1373·1); zinc oxide (p.1163·2); chamomile (p.1669·3).
*Anal fissure; haemorrhoids.*

**Hamo-ratiopharm N** *Ratiopharm, Ger.*
Bufexamac (p.21·3); bismuth subgallate (p.1252·2); lidocaine hydrochloride (p.1377·3); titanium dioxide (p.1160·3).
Hamo-ratiopharm suppositories formerly contained bismuth subgallate, zinc oxide, and chamomile.
*Anal fissure; haemorrhoids.*

**Hamorrhoidal-Zapfchen** *Weleda, Austria.*
Antimony.
*Anorectal disorders.*

**Hamos N** *Dr Janssen, Ger.*
Menthol (p.1711·3); aesculus (p.1648·2).
*Haemorrhoids.*

**Hamos-Tropfen-S** *Dr Janssen, Ger.*
Aesculus (p.1648·2).
*Thrombophlebitis; venous insufficiency.*

**Hamovannad** *Bastian, Ger.*
Inositol nicotinate (p.939·3).
*Haemorrhoids; peripheral vascular disorders.*

**Hamo-Vibolex** *Chephasaar, Ger.*
Cyanocobalamin (p.1458·2).
*Hyperchromic anaemia.*

**Hamoxillin** *Safire, Hong Kong.*
Amoxicillin (p.155·3).
*Bacterial infections.*

**Hand Cream with Sunscreen** *Kay, Canad.†.*
*SPF 4:* Octinoxate (p.1154·3).
*Sunscreen.*

**Handexin** *Rusch, Ital.*
Chlorhexidine gluconate (p.1173·2); aminoxide.
*Hand disinfection.*

**Hanotoxin N** *Hanosan, Ger.*
Homoeopathic preparation.

**Hanp** *Suntory, Jpn.*
Carperitide (p.880·2).
*Heart failure.*

**Hansamed Spray** *Beiersdorf, Ger.*
Chlorhexidine gluconate (p.1173·2).
*Wound disinfection.*

**Hansaplast Antimicotico** *Beiersdorf, Chile.*
Triclosan (p.1195·2); dichlorobenzyl alcohol (p.1178·3).

**Hansaplast Descongestionante** *Beiersdorf, Chile.*
Menthol (p.1711·3); camphor (p.1665·3); thymol (p.1194·2); pine oil; turpentine oil (p.1760·1); eucalyptus oil (p.1686·2); anfocerina K.
*Respiratory-tract congestion.*

**Hansaplast Footcare** *Beiersdorf, Chile.*
*Powder spray:* Purified talc (p.1159·1); camphor (p.1665·3); menthol (p.1711·3); undecenoic acid (p.410·3).

*Topical powder:* Triclosan (p.1195·2); aluminium stearate; camphor (p.1665·3); menthol (p.1711·3); purified talc (p.1159·1).

*Topical spray:* Aluminium chlorohydrate (p.1142·1).

*Hyperhidrosis of feet.*

**Hansaplast Herbal Heat Plaster** *Beiersdorf, UK.*
Capsicum (p.1667·1); arnica (p.1656·3).
*Musculoskeletal and joint pain.*

**Hansaplast Hornhaut-Pflaster** *Beiersdorf, Ger.*
Salicylic acid (p.1157·1).
*Keratinisation disorders.*

**Hansaplast Huhneraugen-Pflaster** *Beiersdorf, Ger.*
Salicylic acid (p.1157·1).
*Corns.*

**Hansaplast Spruhpflaster** *Beiersdorf, Ger.†.*
Methacrylate copolymer (p.1714·3).
*Wounds.*

**Hansepran** *Sarabhai Piramal, India.*
Clofazimine (p.197·1).
*Lepra reactions; leprosy.*

**Hantina** *Apsen, Braz.*
Nitrofurantoin (p.237·2).
*Urinary-tract infections.*

**Hapilux** *Biochemie, Thai.; Novartis, Thai.*
Fluoxetine hydrochloride (p.292·1).
*Bulimia nervosa; depression.*

**Happinose** *Dendron, UK.*
Menthol (p.1711·3).
*Nasal congestion.*

**Haricon** *Condrugs, Thai.*
Haloperidol (p.701·2).
*Alcohol withdrawal syndrome; anxiety; psychomotor agitation.*

**Haridol** *Atlantic, Thai.*
Haloperidol (p.701·2) or haloperidol decanoate (p.701·3).
*Anxiety; behaviour disorders in children; nausea and vomiting; psychoses; psychosomatic disorders.*

**Harmogen** *Abbott, Irl.; Pharmacia, UK.*
Estropipate (p.1553·1).
*Menopausal disorders; osteoporosis.*

**Harmomed** *Kwizda, Austria.*
Dosulepin hydrochloride (p.291·1); diazepam (p.690·1).
*Depression.*

**Harmonet** *Wyeth, Arg.; Wyeth Lederle, Belg.; Wyeth, Braz.; Wyeth, Chile; Wyeth Lederle, Denm.; Wyeth Lederle, Fin.; Wyeth Lederle, Fr.; Wyeth, Hong Kong; Wyeth, Israel; Wyeth Lederle, Ital.; Wyeth, Neth.; Wyeth Lederle, Port.; Wyeth, Spain; Wyeth, Switz.*
Gestodene (p.1556·1); ethinylestradiol (p.1553·2).
*Combined oral contraceptive.*

**Harmonette** *Wyeth Lederle, Austria; Wyeth, Gr.*
Ethinylestradiol (p.1553·2); gestodene (p.1556·1).
*Combined oral contraceptive.*

**Harmonise** *Hamilton, Austral.*
Loperamide hydrochloride (p.1271·1).
*Diarrhoea.*

**Harmosin** *Temmler, Ger.*
Melperone hydrochloride (p.706·1).
*Disturbed behaviour; psychoses; sleep disorders.*

**Harnal** *Yamanouchi, Jpn; Yamanouchi, Thai.*
Tamsulosin hydrochloride (p.1009·2).
*Benign prostatic hyperplasia.*

**Harnsauretropfen F** *Syxyl, Ger.*
Homoeopathic preparation.

**Harnsauretropfen N** *Syxyl, Ger.†.*
Homoeopathic preparation.

**Harntee 400** *TAD, Ger.*
Birch leaf (p.1660·3); calendula (p.1665·2); equisetum (p.1684·1); fennel (p.1687·2); couch-grass (p.1676·2); juniper (p.1703·1); liquorice (p.1270·2); ononis (p.1723·3); java tea (p.1702·3); phaseolus vulgaris; solidago virgaurea (p.1748·3); bearberry (p.1659·2).
*Urinary-tract infections.*

**Harntee 450** *Bad Heilbrunner, Ger.†.*
Birch leaf (p.1660·3); java tea (p.1702·3); solidago virgaurea (p.1748·3).
*Urinary-tract disorders.*

**Harntee STADA** *Stada, Ger.*
Bearberry (p.1659·2); birch leaf (p.1660·3); fructus phaseoli; solidago virgaurea (p.1748·3); java tea (p.1702·3); equisetum (p.1684·1).
*Urinary-tract disorders.*

**Harntee-Steiner** *Steiner, Ger.*
Silver birch (p.1660·3); java tea (p.1702·3); solidago virgaurea (p.1748·3).
*Urinary-tract disorders.*

**Harongan** *Schwabe, Ger.*
Haronga.
*Dyspepsia.*

**Harpadol** *Arkopharma, Fr.*
Devil's claw root (p.28·2).
*Joint pain.*

**Harpagin** *Merz, Ger.; Merz, Malaysia.*
Benzbromarone (p.414·3); allopurinol (p.412·2).
*Hyperuricaemia.*

**Harpagocid** *Phytomedica, Fr.*
Devil's claw root (p.28·2).
*Musculoskeletal and joint disorders.*

**Harpagofito Orto** *Normon, Spain.*
Devil's claw root (p.28·2).
*Rheumatic and joint pain.*

**Harpagoforte Asmedic** *Dyckerhoff, Ger.*
Devil's claw root (p.28·2).
*Gastrointestinal disorders; musculoskeletal and joint disorders.*

**HarpagoMega** *Twardy, Ger.*
Devil's claw root (p.28·2).
*Degenerative joint disorders; dyspepsia.*

**Harpagophytum Complex** *Blackmores, Austral.†.*
Salix alba (p.87·3); cimicifuga racemosa (p.1671·3); devil's claw root (p.28·2); bryonia alba (p.1663·1); vitamins and minerals (p.1417·1); hesperidin (p.1688·2); rutoside (p.1688·2).
*Musculoskeletal and joint disorders.*

**Hart** *Armstrong, Arg.*
Diltiazem hydrochloride (p.900·1).
*Angina pectoris; heart failure; hypertension.*

**Hartiosen** *Inkeysa, Spain†.*
Devil's claw root (p.28·2).
*Rheumatic and joint pain.*

**Hartmannsche** *Enzypharm, Austria.*
Electrolyte infusion (p.1217·1).
*Fluid and electrolyte disorders.*

**Hartsorb** *Siam Bheasach, Thai.*
Isosorbide dinitrate (p.941·1).
*Angina pectoris.*

**Harzer Hustenelixier** *Wernigerode, Ger.†.*
Plantago lanceolata (p.1738·2).
*Catarrh; mouth and throat inflammation.*

**Harzer Hustenloser** *Wernigerode, Ger.*
Thyme (p.1755·2); primula root (p.1735·1).
*Cold symptoms.*

**Harzol** *Europharm, Austria; Hoyer, Ger.*
Sitosterol (p.982·3).
*Benign prostatic hyperplasia.*

**Hassapirin Puro** *Mintlab, Chile.*
Aspirin (p.15·1).
*Fever; inflammation; pain.*

**HA-Tabletten N** *Boehringer Ingelheim, Ger.*
Aspirin (p.15·1); paracetamol (p.76·2); caffeine (p.782·1).
*Pain.*

**H-Atetal** *ISM, Ital.†.*
An adsorbed tetanus vaccine (p.1640·3).
*Active immunisation.*

**Hautfunktionstropfen S** *Cosmochema, Ger.*
Homoeopathic preparation.

**Hautplus N Dr Hagedorn** *Naturarzneimittel, Ger.*
Homoeopathic preparation.

**Haut-Vital N** *Twardy, Ger.†.*
Vitamins (p.1417·1); calcium lactate (p.1225·3); Saccharomyces cerevisiae (p.1469·1); lecithin (p.1706·1).
*Hair, skin, and nail disorders.*

**Havlane** *Aventis, Fr.*
Loprazolam mesilate (p.704·1).
*Insomnia.*

**Havpur** *Chiron Behring, Ger.*
A hepatitis A vaccine (p.1617·1).
*Active immunisation.*

**Havrix** *GlaxoSmithKline, Arg.; GlaxoSmithKline, Austral.; GlaxoSmithKline, Austria; GlaxoSmithKline, Belg.; GlaxoSmithKline, Braz.; GlaxoSmithKline, Canad.; GlaxoSmithKline, Chile; GlaxoSmithKline, Denm.; GlaxoSmithKline, Fin.; GlaxoSmithKline, Fr.; GlaxoSmithKline, Ger.; SmithKline Beecham, Gr.; GlaxoSmithKline, Hong Kong; GlaxoSmithKline, India; GlaxoSmithKline, Irl.; SmithKline Beecham, Israel; GlaxoSmithKline, Ital.; GlaxoSmithKline, Malaysia; SmithKline Beecham, Mex.; GlaxoSmithKline, Neth.; GlaxoSmithKline, Norw.; GlaxoSmithKline, NZ; Smith Kline & French, Port.; GlaxoSmithKline, S.Afr.; GlaxoSmithKline, Singapore; GlaxoSmithKline, Spain; GlaxoSmithKline, Swed.; SmithKline Beecham, Switz.; GlaxoSmithKline, Thai.; GlaxoSmithKline, UK; SmithKline Beecham, USA.*
An adsorbed inactivated hepatitis A vaccine (HM 175 strain) (p.1617·1).
Separate preparations are available for children and adults.
*Active immunisation.*

**Hawaiian Tropic**
*Note. This name is used for preparations of different composition.*
*Tanning Research, Canad.†.*
*SPF 10:* Meradimate (p.1151·3); octinoxate (p.1154·3); oxybenzone (p.1154·3).

*SPF 30; SPF 45:* Octinoxate (p.1154·3); octisalate (p.1154·3); titanium dioxide (p.1160·3).

*Sunscreen.*

*Solpro, Mex.*
*SPF 2:* Octinoxate (p.1154·3).

*SPF 4:* Octinoxate (p.1154·3); octisalate (p.1154·3).

*SPF 15+:* Octinoxate (p.1154·3); octisalate (p.1154·3); titanium dioxide (p.1160·3).

*Sunscreen.*

*Tanning Research, USA.*
*SPF 8+; SPF 10+:* Octinoxate (p.1154·3); oxybenzone (p.1154·3); meradimate (p.1151·3).

*Gel SPF 15+:* Octinoxate (p.1154·3); octocrilene (p.1154·3); oxybenzone (p.1154·3); meradimate (p.1151·3).

*Lotion SPF 15+:* Octinoxate (p.1154·3); oxybenzone (p.1154·3); meradimate (p.1151·3).

*SPF 30+:* Octinoxate (p.1154·3); meradimate (p.1151·3); oxybenzone (p.1154·3); octisalate (p.1154·3); homosalate (p.1148·1).

*SPF 45+:* Octinoxate (p.1154·3); octocrilene (p.1154·3); oxybenzone (p.1154·3); octisalate (p.1154·3); titanium dioxide (p.1160·3).

*SPF 45+:* Octinoxate (p.1154·3); oxybenzone (p.1154·3); octisalate (p.1154·3); titanium dioxide (p.1160·3); meradimate (p.1151·3).

*Sunscreen.*

**Hawaiian Tropic Baby Faces**
*Note. This name is used for preparations of different composition.*
*Tanning Research, Canad.*
*SPF 35; SPF 50:* Octinoxate (p.1154·3); octisalate (p.1154·3); titanium dioxide (p.1160·3).
*Sunscreen.*

*Tanning Research, USA.*
*SPF 20:* Octinoxate (p.1154·3); octocrilene (p.1154·3); oxybenzone (p.1154·3); meradimate (p.1151·3).

*SPF 35; SPF 50:* Octinoxate (p.1154·3); octocrilene (p.1154·3); oxybenzone (p.1154·3); octisalate (p.1154·3); titanium dioxide (p.1160·3).

*Sunscreen.*

**Hawaiian Tropic Bioshield** *Tanning Research, Canad.†.*
*SPF 15:* Octinoxate (p.1154·3); octisalate (p.1154·3); oxybenzone (p.1154·3).

*SPF 30:* Octinoxate (p.1154·3); octocrilene (p.1154·3); octisalate (p.1154·3); titanium dioxide (p.1160·3).

*Sunscreen.*

**Hawaiian Tropic Cool Aloe with I.C.E.** *Tanning Research, USA.*
Lidocaine (p.1377·3); menthol (p.1711·3); aloe vera (p.1141·3).

**Hawaiian Tropic Dark Tanning**
*Note. This name is used for preparations of different composition.*
*Tanning Research, Canad.*
*Lotion SPF 4:* Octinoxate (p.1154·3); octisalate (p.1154·3).
Formerly contained octinoxate and meradimate.

*Oil SPF 4:* Octinoxate (p.1154·3); padimate O (p.1155·1).

*Sunscreen.*

*Tanning Research, USA.*
*Gel SPF 2; gel SPF 4:* Ensulizole (p.1147·1).

*Oil SPF 2; oil SPF 4:* Octinoxate (p.1154·3); padimate O (p.1155·1).

*Sunscreen.*

**Hawaiian Tropic Herbal** *Tanning Research, Canad.*
*SPF 4:* Octinoxate (p.1154·3); oxybenzone (p.1154·3).

*SPF 2; SPF 15:* Ensulizole (p.1147·1); sulisobenzone (p.1158·3).

*Sunscreen.*

**Hawaiian Tropic Just For Kids**
*Note. This name is used for preparations of different composition.*
*Tanning Research, Canad.†.*
*SPF 30:* Octinoxate (p.1154·3); octisalate (p.1154·3); titanium dioxide (p.1160·3).
*Sunscreen.*

*Tanning Research, USA.*
*SPF 30:* Octinoxate (p.1154·3); oxybenzone (p.1154·3); octisalate (p.1154·3); homosalate (p.1148·1).

*SPF 45:* Octinoxate (p.1154·3); oxybenzone (p.1154·3); octisalate (p.1154·3); octocrilene (p.1154·3); titanium dioxide (p.1160·3).

*Sunscreen.*

**Hawaiian Tropic Lipbalm** *Tanning Research, Canad.†.*
*SPF 45:* Octinoxate (p.1154·3); meradimate (p.1151·3); octisalate (p.1154·3); oxybenzone (p.1154·3); titanium dioxide (p.1160·3).
*Sunscreen.*

**Hawaiian Tropic Plus** *Tanning Research, Canad.*
*SPF 15:* Octinoxate (p.1154·3); octisalate (p.1154·3); titanium dioxide (p.1160·3).
*Sunscreen.*

**Hawaiian Tropic Protective** *Tanning Research, Canad.*
*SPF 8:* Octinoxate (p.1154·3); octisalate (p.1154·3).

*SPF 12:* Octinoxate (p.1154·3); octisalate (p.1154·3); oxybenzone (p.1154·3).

*Sunscreen.*

**Hawaiian Tropic Protective Tanning** *Tanning Research, USA.*
*SPF 6:* Titanium dioxide (p.1160·3).
*Sunscreen.*

**Hawaiian Tropic Protective Tanning Dry** *Tanning Research, USA.*
*Gel SPF 6:* Ensulizole (p.1147·1); sulisobenzone (p.1158·3).

*Oil SPF 6:* Octinoxate (p.1154·3); homosalate (p.1148·1); meradimate (p.1151·3).
*Sunscreen.*

**Hawaiian Tropic Self Tanning Sunblock** *Tanning Research, USA.*
Octinoxate (p.1154·3); oxybenzone (p.1154·3).
*Sunscreen.*

**Hawaiian Tropic Shimmering** *Tanning Research, Canad.*
*SPF 6:* Ensulizole (p.1147·1).
*Sunscreen.*

**Hawaiian Tropic Sport**
*Note. This name is used for preparations of different composition.*
*Tanning Research, Canad.*†.
*SPF 8:* Octinoxate (p.1154·3); octocrilene (p.1154·3); oxybenzone (p.1154·3).
*SPF 15; SPF 30:* Octinoxate (p.1154·3); octisalate (p.1154·3); titanium dioxide (p.1160·3).
*Sunscreen.*
*Tanning Research, USA.*
*SPF 15:* Octinoxate (p.1154·3); octocrilene (p.1154·3); oxybenzone (p.1154·3).
*SPF 30:* Octinoxate (p.1154·3); octocrilene (p.1154·3); oxybenzone (p.1154·3); octisalate (p.1154·3); titanium dioxide (p.1160·3).
*Sunscreen.*

**Hawaiian Tropic Sport Sunblock** *Tanning Research, Canad.*
*SPF 30:* Octinoxate (p.1154·3); homosalate (p.1148·1); octisalate (p.1154·3); oxybenzone.
Formerly contained octinoxate, octocrilene, octisalate, oxybenzone, and titanium dioxide.
*Sunscreen.*

**Hawaiian Tropic Total Sport** *Tanning Research, Canad.*†.
*SPF 20:* Octinoxate (p.1154·3); octisalate (p.1154·3); oxybenzone (p.1154·3).
*Sunscreen.*

**Hawkmide** *LBS, Thai.*
Furosemide (p.919·3).
*Hypertension; oedema.*

**Hawkperan** *LBS, Thai.*
Metoclopramide (p.1274·3).
*Gastrointestinal motility disorders; nausea and vomiting.*

**Hay Fever**
*Homeocan, Canad.; Hylands, Canad.*
Homoeopathic preparation.

**Hay Fever Relief** *Brauer, Austral.*†.
Homoeopathic preparation.

**Hay Fever & Sinus Relief** *Herbal Concepts, UK.*
Echinacea (p.1683·2); sambucus (p.1741·3); garlic (p.1691·1).
*Catarrh; hay fever; sinus congestion.*

**Hayclear** *Novartis, NZ*†.
Budesonide (p.1094·2).
*Allergic rhinitis.*

**Hay-Crom**
*Ivax, Irl.; Norton, S.Afr.*†*; Ivax, UK.*
Sodium cromoglicate (p.795·3).
Formerly known as Eye-Crom in the *UK*.
*Allergic conjunctivitis.*

**Hayfebrol** *Scot-Tussin, USA.*
Pseudoephedrine hydrochloride (p.1129·2); chlorphenamine maleate (p.427·3).
*Upper respiratory-tract symptoms.*

**Hayfever & Allergy Relief** *Galpharm, UK.*
Cetirizine hydrochloride (p.427·1).
*Hypersensitivity reactions.*

**Hayfever Eye Drops** *Pliva, UK.*
Sodium cromoglicate (p.795·3).
*Ocular symptoms of hay fever.*

**Hayfever Relief**
*Note. This name is used for preparations of different composition.*
*Peach, UK.*
Cetirizine hydrochloride (p.427·1).
*Allergic rhinitis.*
*Thornton & Ross, UK.*
Beclometasone dipropionate (p.1091·1).
*Allergic rhinitis.*

**Hayfever & Sinus Relief** *Herbal Concepts, UK.*
Echinacea (p.1683·2); sambucus (p.1741·3); garlic (p.1691·1).
*Catarrh; hay fever; sinus congestion.*

**Hayleve** *Chatfield Laboratories, UK.*
Chlorphenamine (p.428·1).
*Hypersensitivity reactions.*

**Haymine** *Forest Laboratories, UK.*
Chlorphenamine maleate (p.427·3); ephedrine hydrochloride (p.1120·1).
*Hypersensitivity reactions.*

**HB Vac** *Cadila, India.*
A hepatitis B vaccine (p.1618·1).
*Active immunisation.*

**H-BIG** *Abbott, USA*†.
A hepatitis B immunoglobulin (p.1617·2).
*Passive immunisation.*

**H-B-Vax** *Aventis Pasteur, Denm.*
A hepatitis B vaccine (recombinant DNA) (p.1618·1).
*Active immunisation.*

**H-B-Vax II**
*Merck Sharp & Dohme, Arg.; Merck Sharp & Dohme, Austral.; Pasteur Merieux, Belg.*†*; Merck Sharp & Dohme, Hong Kong; Aventis Pasteur, Irl.; Merck Sharp & Dohme, Malaysia; Merck Sharp & Dohme, Mex.; Merck Sharp & Dohme, NZ; Merck Sharp & Dohme, S.Afr.; Merck Sharp & Dohme, Singapore; Merck Sharp & Dohme, Thai.; Aventis, UK*†.
A hepatitis B vaccine (recombinant DNA) (p.1618·1).
*Active immunisation.*

**HB-Vax-DNA**
*Aventis Pasteur, Fr.; Pasteur Merieux, Neth.*
An adsorbed hepatitis B vaccine (recombinant DNA) (p.1618·1).
*Active immunisation.*

**HBVaxPro**
*Aventis Pasteur, Belg.; Aventis Pasteur, Fin.; Aventis Pasteur, Fr.; Aventis Pasteur, Ger.; Vianex (Βιανέξ), Gr.; Merck Sharp & Dohme, Hong Kong; Aventis Pasteur, Ital.; Aventis Pasteur, Swed.; Aventis Pasteur, UK.*
A hepatitis B vaccine (recombinant) (p.1618·1).
*Active immunisation.*

**H-C** *Raza, Malaysia; Pharmaniaga, Malaysia.*
Hydrocortisone (p.1103·3); crotamiton (p.1145·1).
*Skin disorders.*

**Hc45**
*Boots Healthcare, Irl.; Crookes Healthcare, UK.*
Hydrocortisone acetate (p.1103·3).
*Dermatitis; eczema; insect bites.*

**HC Bidex** *Collins, Mex.*
Vitamin preparation (p.1417·1).

**HC Derma-Pax** *Recsei, USA.*
Hydrocortisone acetate (p.1103·3); mepyramine maleate (p.437·1); chlorphenamine maleate (p.427·3).
*Skin disorders.*

**HCT** *1A, Ger.; CT, Ger.; Hexal, Ger.*
Hydrochlorothiazide (p.933·2).
*Heart failure; hypertension; oedema.*

**HCT-Beta** *Betapharm, Ger.*
Hydrochlorothiazide (p.933·2).
*Heart failure; hypertension; oedema.*

**HCT-ISIS** *Alpharma-Isis, Ger.*
Hydrochlorothiazide (p.933·2).
*Heart failure; hypertension; oedema.*

**HD** *Braun, Braz.*†.
Electrolytes with or without glucose (p.1221·1).
*Dialysis solution.*

**HD 85** *Lafayette, USA.*
Barium sulfate (p.1061·1).
*Contrast medium for gastrointestinal radiography.*

**HD 200 Plus** *Lafayette, USA.*
Barium sulfate (p.1061·1).
*Contrast medium for gastrointestinal radiography.*

**HDCV** *Aventis Pasteur, Braz.*†.
A rabies vaccine (p.1635·3).
*Active immunisation.*

**4Head** *Diomed, UK.*
Levomenthol (p.1711·3).
*Headache.*

**Head Cold Relief** *Brauer, Austral.*†.
Homoeopathic preparation.

**Head & Shoulders**
*Procter & Gamble, Canad.; Procter & Gamble, USA.*
Pyrithione zinc (p.1156·2).
*Dandruff.*

**Head & Shoulders Intensive Treatment** *Procter & Gamble, USA.*
Selenium sulfide (p.1157·3).
*Dandruff; seborrhoeic dermatitis.*

**Headache Complex** *Brauer, Austral.*†.
Homoeopathic preparation.

**Headache & Migraine** *Homeocan, Canad.*
Homoeopathic preparation.

**Headache Relief** *Brauer, Austral.*†.
Homoeopathic preparation.

**Headache Tablets** *Romilo, Canad.*†.
Aspirin (p.15·1).

**Headgen**
*YSP, Malaysia; Yung Shin, Singapore.*
Co-dergocrine mesilate (p.1674·1).
*Mental function disorders in the elderly.*

**Headmaster** *SSL, Irl.*
Phenothrin (p.1509·1).
*Pediculosis.*

**Headrin Extra Strength** *Reese, USA.*
Aspirin (p.15·1); paracetamol (p.76·2); caffeine (p.782·1).

**Heads Shampoo** *Hamilton, Hong Kong.*
Econazole nitrate (p.397·2).
*Scalp irritation; seborrhoeic dermatitis.*

**Headway**
*Pacific, Hong Kong; Pacific, NZ.*
Minoxidil (p.960·1).
*Alopecia androgenetica.*

**Heafusine** *Braun, Fr.*
Pentastarch (p.750·1).
*Haemodilution; shock.*

**Heal Aid Plus** *Reese, USA.*
Resorcinol (p.1156·3); phenol (p.1188·1).

**Healex** *Amadeus, India.*
Polyvinyl polymer; benzocaine (p.1370·3).
*Wound dressing.*

**Healing Cream** *Nelson, UK.*
Homoeopathic preparation.

**Healon**
*Pharmacia, Austral.; Pharmacia, Belg.; Pharmacia, Braz.; Pharmacia, Canad.; Pharmacia, Chile; Pharmacia, Fin.; Pharmacia Upjohn, Fr.*†*; Pharmacia, Ger.; Pharmacia, Hong Kong; Pharmacia Upjohn, Israel; Pharmacia Upjohn, Ital.*†*; Pharmacia, Malaysia; Pharmacia Upjohn, Norw.*†*; Pharmacia, NZ; Pharmacia, S.Afr.; Pharmacia Upjohn, Singapore; Pharmacia Upjohn, Swed.*†*; Pharmacia Upjohn, Switz.; Pharmacia, Thai.; Pharmacia Upjohn, USA.*
Sodium hyaluronate (p.1697·3).
*Adjunct in eye surgery.*

**Healon Yellow**
*Pharmacia Upjohn, Ital.*†*; Kabi Pharmacia, USA.*
Sodium hyaluronate (p.1697·3); fluorescein sodium (p.1689·1).
*Adjunct in eye surgery.*

**Healonid**
*Pharmacia, Austria; Pharmacia Upjohn, Irl.*†*; Pharmacia, UK.*
Sodium hyaluronate (p.1697·3).
*Adjunct in eye surgery.*

**HealthAid Boldo-Plus** *Pharmadass, UK.*
Boldo (p.1661·2); taraxacum (p.1751·3); bladderwrack (p.1742·3); clivers (p.1673·2); bearberry (p.1659·2); juniper oil (p.1703·1); vitamin $B_6$ (p.1456·3).
Formerly known as HealthAid AquaFall.
*Water retention.*

**HealthAid FemmeVit PMS Formula** *Pharmadass, UK.*
Multivitamin and mineral preparation (p.1417·1).

**Healtheries Musseltone** *Optima, UK.*
Green-lipped mussel (p.1696·1).
*Musculoskeletal and joint disorders.*

**Healtheries Musseltone & Glucosamine** *Optima, UK.*
Green-lipped mussel (p.1696·1); glucosamine (p.1694·1).
*Musculoskeletal and joint disorders.*

**Healthy Feet** *Pickles, UK.*
Undecenoic acid (p.410·3); dibrompropamidine isetionate (p.1178·2).
*Fungal skin infections.*

**Heartburn & Indigestion Liquid** *Unichem, UK*†.
Sodium alginate (p.1577·1).
*Dyspepsia; heartburn.*

**Heartburn Relief** *Stanley, Canad.*
Aluminium hydroxide (p.1249·2); alginic acid (p.1576·3).

**Heat Cream** *General Drugs, Thai.*
Methyl salicylate (p.59·3); menthol (p.1711·3); eugenol (p.1686·2).
*Muscle pain; sprains.*

**Heat Rub** *Stanley, Canad.*
Methyl salicylate (p.59·3); camphor (p.1665·3); menthol (p.1711·3); eucalyptus oil (p.1686·2).

**Heath & Heather Becalm** *Peter Black, UK*†.
Valerian (p.1762·2); lupulus (p.1708·1); passion flower (p.1729·1).
*Stress.*

**Heath & Heather Inner Fresh Tablets** *Peter Black, UK*†.
Frangula bark (p.1266·3).
*Constipation.*

**Heath & Heather Quiet Night** *Peter Black, UK*†.
Valerian (p.1762·2); lupulus (p.1708·1); passion flower (p.1729·1).
*Insomnia.*

**Heath & Heather Skin Tablets** *Peter Black, UK*†.
Lappa root (p.1704·3); wild pansy.
*Eczema; skin blemishes.*

**Heath & Heather Water Relief Tablets** *Peter Black, UK*†.
Bladderwrack (p.1742·3); clivers (p.1673·2); ground ivy (p.1696·1); lappa (p.1704·3).
*Water retention.*

**Hebagam IM** *NBI, S.Afr.*
Hepatitis B immunoglobulin (p.1617·2).
*Passive immunisation.*

**Heberbiovac HB**
*Enila, Braz.; Bago, Chile; Fustery, Mex.; Heber, Thai.*
A hepatitis B vaccine (recombinant DNA) (p.1618·1).
*Active immunisation.*

**Hebermin** *Bago, Chile.*
Urogastrone (p.1294·2); sulfadiazine silver (p.259·1).
*Burns; ulcers.*

**Hebert Caramelos** *Fecofar, Arg.*
Cineole (p.1672·1); guaifenesin (p.1122·1); senega (p.1130·2).
*Respiratory-tract congestion.*

**Hebrin** *Uniao Quimica, Braz.*
Iodine (p.1598·1); cade oil (p.1159·2); salicylic acid (p.1157·1).
*Fungal skin infections.*

**Hebsbulin-IH** *Mitsubishi, Jpn.*
A hepatitis B immunoglobulin (p.1617·2).
*Passive immunisation.*

**Hebucol** *Chiesi, Fr.*†.
Cyclobutyrol sodium (p.1678·2).
*Dyspepsia.*

**HEC**
*Note. This name is used for preparations of different composition.*
*Chauvin, Fr.*
Tannic acid (p.1751·2); hamamelis (p.1696·3); phenazone (p.82·3).
*Burns; haemorrhoids; nose bleeds.*
*Chauvin, Singapore*†.
Tannin (p.1751·2); hamamelis (p.1696·3); phenazone (p.82·3).
*Haemorrhoids; nose bleeds; wounds.*
*Bausch & Lomb, Switz.*
Tannin (p.1751·2); pectin (p.1580·3); peru balsam (p.1730·2); hamamelis (p.1696·3).
*Mucous membrane disorders of the nose.*

**Heclivir** *Neo Quimica, Braz.*
Aciclovir (p.626·1).

**Hecrosine B12** *Ortoquimica, Braz.*†.
Methionine (p.1042·1); choline (p.1424·3); inositol (p.1701·2); liver extract; cynara (p.1678·3); solanum paniculatum.
*Liver disorders.*

**Hectonona** *Milo, Spain.*
Dried aluminium hydroxide (p.1249·2); magnesium carbonate (p.1272·1); sodium bicarbonate (p.1223·2); tartaric acid (p.1752·1).
*Dyspepsia.*

**Hectorol**
*Draxis, Canad.; Bone Care, USA.*
Doxercalciferol (p.1462·1).
*Hyperparathyroidism.*

**Hedazol** *Alpha, Mex.*†.
Mebendazole (p.108·2).

**Hedelix** *Krewel, Ger.*
Hedera helix.
*Respiratory-tract disorders.*

**Hederix**
*Note. This name is used for preparations of different composition.*
*SIT, Ital.*
Codeine hydrobromide (p.27·3); hedera helix.
*Coughs.*
*Plan, Switz.*
Noscapine hydrochloride (p.1125·3); hedera; senega (p.1130·2); helenium (p.1119·3); orris; marrubium (p.1124·1).
*Coughs.*

**Hedex**
*SmithKline Beecham Consumer, Irl.; SmithKline Beecham Consumer, Neth.*†*; SmithKline Beecham, Spain*†*; GlaxoSmithKline Consumer, UK.*
Paracetamol (p.76·2).
*Fever; pain.*

**Hedex Extra** *GlaxoSmithKline Consumer, UK.*
Paracetamol (p.76·2); caffeine (p.782·1).
*Fever; pain.*

**Hedex Ibuprofen** *GlaxoSmithKline Consumer, UK.*
Ibuprofen (p.45·3).
*Cold and influenza symptoms; fever; pain.*

**Hedonin** *Gerot, Austria.*
Phenylpropanol (p.1731·1); moxaverine hydrochloride (p.1717·2).
*Biliary-tract disorders; gastrointestinal disorders.*

**Heduline** *Costec, Arg.*
Salicylic acid (p.1157·1); triclosan (Irgasan DP-300) (p.1195·2); dexpanthenol (p.1727·2).
*Seborrhoeic dermatitis.*

**Heemex** *Lane, UK.*
Hamamelis (p.1696·3); compound benzoin tincture; zinc oxide (p.1163·2).
*Haemorrhoids.*

**Heer-More** *Eagle, Austral.*†.
Homoeopathic preparation.

**Heet**
*Medtech, Canad.; Whitehall, USA.*
Methyl salicylate (p.59·3); camphor (p.1665·3); capsaicin (p.24·2).
*Muscle, joint, and soft-tissue pain; neuralgia.*

**Hefaclor** *Hefa, Ger.*
Cefaclor (p.167·1).
*Bacterial infections.*

**hefasolon** *Hefa, Ger.*
Prednisolone (p.1108·1) or prednisolone sodium phosphate (p.1108·1).
*Corticosteroid.*

**Hegon** *Beta, Arg.*
Zaleplon (p.727·3).
*Insomnia.*

**Hegor** *Procter & Gamble, Austria.*
Shampoo.
*Scalp and hair disorders.*

**Hegor Antipoux** *Incomex, Mon.*
*d*-Phenothrin (p.1509·1).
*Pediculosis.*

**Hegor Climbazole** *Incomex, Mon.*
Climbazole (p.396·2).
*Dandruff.*

**Hegrimarin** *Strathmann, Ger.*†.
Silybum marianum (p.1043·3).
*Liver disorders.*

**Heidi** *Siam Bheasach, Thai.*
Ibuprofen (p.45·3).
*Musculoskeletal and joint disorders.*

**Heilit** *Heilit, Ger.*†.
Camphor (p.1665·3); methyl salicylate (p.59·3); benzyl nicotinate (p.21·2).
*Musculoskeletal and joint disorders.*

**Heilit Rheuma-Olbad** *Heilit, Ger.*†.
Camphor (p.1665·3); menthol (p.1711·3); methyl salicylate (p.59·3).
*Bath additive; musculoskeletal and joint disorders.*

**Heitrin** *Abbott, Ger.*
Terazosin hydrochloride (p.1010·3).
*Hypertension.*

**Hekabetol** *Fortbenton, Arg.*
Triclosan (Irgasan) (p.1195·2); betanaphthol (p.103·2).
*Seborrhoeic dermatitis.*

**Hekbilin Kapseln** *Strathmann, Ger.*†.
Cynara (p.1678·3).
*Dyspepsia.*

**Heksavit** Leiras, Fin.
Pyridoxine hydrochloride (p.1456·3).
*Vitamin $B_6$ deficiency.*

**Helago-Pflege-Oel** Helago, Ger.
Chamomile (p.1669·3); sage (p.1741·2).
Formerly known as Helago-oel N.
*Mouth and throat inflammation.*

**Helarium** Bionorica, Ger.
Hypericum (p.299·1).
*Depression; nervous disorders.*

**Helastop** Hamilton, Austral.†.
Propolis (p.1735·2).
*Herpes labialis.*

**Helberina** Galen, Mex.†.
Heparin (p.927·3).

**Helcon** Polipharm, Thai.
Co-dergocrine mesilate (p.1674·1).
*Mental function disorders.*

**Helenil** Roux-Ocefa, Arg.
Ketoprofen (p.51·2).
*Inflammation; pain.*

**Helfergin** Lundbeck, Ger.
Meclofenoxate hydrochloride (p.1710·1).
*Cerebral insufficiency; cerebrovascular disorders.*

**Helianthus comp** Infirmarius-Rovit, Ger.
Homoeopathic preparation.

**Heliclar** Abbott, Belg.
Clarithromycin (p.192·2).
*Helicobacter pylori-associated peptic ulcer.*

**Heliclear** Wyeth, UK.
Capsules, lansoprazole (Zoton) (p.1269·3); tablets, clarithromycin (Klaricid) (p.192·2); capsules, amoxicillin (p.155·3).
*Helicobacter pylori-associated duodenal ulcer.*

**Helicocin** Biochemie, Austria.
Oval tablet, amoxicillin trihydrate (p.155·3); round tablet, metronidazole (p.607·2).
*Helicobacter pylori infection.*

**Helicodid** Sigma, Braz.†.
Clarithromycin (p.192·2).

**Helicokit** Italchimici, Ital.
Carbon-13 (p.1667·3) labelled urea.
*Diagnosis of Helicobacter pylori infection.*

**Helicopac** Sigma, Braz.
Capsules, lansoprazole (p.1269·3); tablets, clarithromycin (p.192·2); tablets, amoxicillin (p.155·3).
*Peptic ulcer.*

**Helicosec** AstraZeneca, NZ†.
Capsules, omeprazole (p.1278·2); capsules, amoxicillin trihydrate (p.155·3); tablets, metronidazole (p.607·2).
*Helicobacter pylori-associated peptic ulcer.*

**Helicostad** Stada, Austria.
Omeprazole (p.1278·2).
*Gastro-oesophageal reflux; peptic ulcer; Zollinger-Ellison syndrome.*

**Helidac**
Note. This name is used for preparations of different composition.
Pharmacia, Austral.†.
Chewable tablets, tripotassium dicitratobismuthate (p.1252·2); tablets, metronidazole (p.607·2); capsules, tetracycline hydrochloride (p.266·2).
*Peptic ulcer.*
Procter & Gamble, USA.
Pink tablets, bismuth salicylate (p.1252·1); white tablets, metronidazole (p.607·2); orange/white capsules, tetracycline hydrochloride (p.266·2).
*Duodenal ulcer.*

**Helifenicol** Ariston, Braz.
Dextromethorphan hydrobromide (p.1117·3); helicin.
*Coughs.*

**Heli-Kit** Mayoly-Spindler, Fr.
Carbon-13 labelled urea (p.1667·3).
*Detection of Helicobacter pylori infection.*

**Heliklar**
Abbott, Arg.
Tablets, clarithromycin (Klaricid) (p.192·2); capsules, amoxicillin (p.155·3); capsules, lansoprazole (Ogasto) (p.1269·3).
*Helicobacter pylori-associated peptic ulcer.*
Abbott, Braz.
Capsules, lansoprazole (p.1269·3); tablets, clarithromycin (p.192·2); capsules, amoxicillin (p.155·3).

**HeliMet** Wyeth, UK.
Capsules, lansoprazole (Zoton) (p.1269·3); tablets, clarithromycin (Klaricid) (p.192·2); tablets, metronidazole (p.607·2).
*Peptic ulcer.*

**Helimox** Essex, Ital.†.
Amoxicillin (p.155·3).
*Bacterial infections.*

**Helioban** Galderma, Mex.†.
*SPF 15:* Octinoxate (p.1154·3); titanium dioxide (p.1160·3).
*Sunscreen.*

**Heliobloc** Galderma, Fr.†.
*SPF 25:* Titanium dioxide (p.1160·3); avobenzone (p.1142·3); ecamsule (p.1146·3).
*Sunscreen.*

**Heliobloc Fort** Galderma, Fr.†.
*SPF 60:* Titanium dioxide (p.1160·3); avobenzone (p.1142·3); ecamsule (p.1146·3); enzacamene (p.1147·1).
*Sunscreen.*

**Helioblock**
Note. This name is used for preparations of different composition.
Roche-Posay, Braz.
*SPF 30:* Drometrizole trisiloxane; avobenzone (p.1142·3); octocrilene (p.1154·3); titanium dioxide (p.1160·3); octil triazone (p.1154·3).
*SPF 20; SPF 40; SPF 50; SPF 60:* Drometrizole trisiloxane; ecamsule (p.1146·3); avobenzone (p.1142·3); octocrilene (p.1154·3); titanium dioxide (p.1160·3).
*Sunscreen.*
Galderma, Mex.†.
*SPF 25UVB/15UVA; SPF 60UVB/15UVA:* Ecamsule (p.1146·3); avobenzone (p.1142·3); enzacamene (p.1147·1); titanium dioxide (p.1160·3).
*Sunscreen.*
Galderma, Singapore†; Galderma, Thai.†.
*SPF 25; SPF 60:* Ecamsule (p.1146·3); avobenzone (p.1142·3); enzacamene (p.1147·1); titanium dioxide (p.1160·3).
*Sunscreen.*

**Heliofilm** Szama, Arg.
Benzophenone; enzacamene (p.1147·1).
*Sunscreen.*

**Heliopar** Orion, Fin.
Chloroquine phosphate (p.448·2).
*Amoebiasis; light-sensitive skin disorders; lupus erythematosus; malaria; musculoskeletal and joint disorders.*

**Helipak A** Orion, Fin.
Enteric-coated capsules, lansoprazole (Lanzo) (p.1269·3); tablets, amoxicillin (Amorion) (p.155·3); tablets, metronidazole (Trikozol) (p.607·2).
*Peptic ulcer.*

**Helipak K** Orion, Fin.
Enteric-coated capsules, lansoprazole (Lanzo) (p.1269·3); tablets, clarithromycin (Zeclar) (p.192·2); tablets, amoxicillin (Amorion) (p.155·3).
*Peptic ulcer.*

**Helipak T** Orion, Fin.
Enteric-coated capsules, lansoprazole (Lanzo) (p.1269·3); tablets, tetracycline (Oricyclin) (p.266·2); tablets, metronidazole (Trikozol) (p.607·2).
*Peptic ulcer.*

**Heliphenicol** Ariston, Arg.
Butetamate citrate (p.1116·2).
*Coughs.*

**Heliplant** Kanoldt, Ger.†.
Silybum marianum (p.1043·3).
*Liver disorders.*

**Helipur**
Braun, Ger.; Braun, Ital.
Chlorocresol (p.1177·1); clorophene (p.1177·3); orthophenylphenol (p.1187·2).
*Surface and instrument disinfection.*

**Helipur H plus** Braun, Ger.†.
Glyoxal (p.1181·1); glutaral (p.1180·3).
*Instrument disinfection.*

**Helipur H plus N** Braun, Ger.
Glutaral (p.1180·3); isopropyl alcohol (p.1184·3); ethylhexanal.
*Instrument disinfection.*

**Helirad** Allen, Austria.
Ranitidine bismuth citrate (p.1287·2).
*Peptic ulcer.*

**Helis** Bifarma, Ital.
Benzalkonium chloride (p.1168·3).
*Eye disinfection.*

**Heli-Sal**
Note. A similar name is used for preparations of different composition (see below).
Strallhofer, Austria.
Crataegus (p.1677·1); mistletoe (p.1715·3); garlic (p.1691·1).
*Cardiovascular disorders.*

**Helisal**
Note. A similar name is used for preparations of different composition (see above).
Cortecs, Irl.; Cortecs, UK†.
Test for *Helicobacter pylori* infection.

**Heliton**
Note. This name is used for preparations of different composition.
Disprovent, Arg.; Neckerman, Braz.†.
Nitazoxanide (p.612·1).
*Protozoal infections; worm infections.*
Columbia, Mex.
Nitazoxanide (p.612·1); tripotassium dicitratobismuthate (p.1252·2).
*Peptic ulcer.*

**Helix I** Braun, Ital.
Sodium *o*-phenylphenol (p.1187·2).
*Instrument disinfection.*

**Helixate**
Bayer, Austria; Bayer, Denm.; Centeon, Fin.†; Aventis Behring, Fr.; Aventis Behring, Ger.; Aventis Behring, Ital.; Bayer, Neth.; Aventis Behring, Spain; Aventis Behring, Swed.; Aventis Behring, Switz.; Aventis Behring, UK; Centeon, USA.
Octocog alfa (p.751·2).
*Haemophilia A.*

**Helixor**
Germania, Austria; Helixor, Ger.
A range of mistletoe (p.1715·3) preparations containing mistletoe from fir trees (Helixor A), from pine trees (Helixor P), or from apple trees (Helixor M).
*Malignant neoplasms.*

**Helmazan** Noel, India.
Diethylcarbamazine citrate (p.104·1); piperazine citrate (p.111·2).
*Worm infections.*

**Helmex** Infectopharm, Ger.
Pyrantel embonate (p.113·2).
*Worm infections.*

**Helmib** Ibfarma, Braz.†.
Mebendazole (p.108·2); tiabendazole (p.114·2).
*Worm infections.*

**Helmiben** Eurofarma, Braz.
Mebendazole (p.108·2); tiabendazole (p.114·2).
*Worm infections.*

**Helmicin** Sanval, Braz.
Fluconazole (p.398·1).
*Fungal infections.*

**Helmidrax** Haller, Braz.
Mebendazole (p.108·2); tiabendazole (p.114·2).
*Worm infections.*

**Helmifar** Farcoral, Mex.
Piperazine citrate (p.111·2).
*Worm infections.*

**Helmine** Allen, Spain†.
Ondansetron hydrochloride (p.1281·1).
*Nausea and vomiting.*

**Helmintal** Biolab Sanus, Braz.†.
Albendazole (p.101·2).
*Giardiasis; worm infections.*

**Helmintox** Innotech, Fr.
Pyrantel embonate (p.113·2).
*Intestinal nematode infections.*

**Helminzole** Randall, Mex.†.
Mebendazole (p.108·2).

**Helmi-Ped** Stiefel, Braz.
Mebendazole (p.108·2); tiabendazole (p.114·2).
*Worm infections.*

**Helmisons** Sons, Mex.
Albendazole (p.101·2).
*Worm infections.*

**Helmizil** Heralds, Braz.†.
Mebendazole (p.108·2).
*Worm infections.*

**Helmizol** Teuto, Braz.
Metronidazole (p.607·2) or metronidazole benzoate (p.607·2).

**Helo-acid** Rosch & Handel, Austria.
Citric acid (p.1673·1); tartaric acid (p.1752·1); lactic acid (p.1704·1); pepsin (p.1729·3).
*Digestive disorders.*

**Helopanflat**
Rosch & Handel, Austria; Knoll, Port.†; Knoll, Switz.
Pancreatin (p.1725·3); simeticone (p.1289·2).
*Gastrointestinal disorders; preparation for gastrointestinal radiography.*

**Helopanflat N** BASF, Ger.†.
Porcine pancreatin (p.1725·3); simeticone (p.1289·2).
*Digestive system disorders.*

**Helopanzym** Rosch & Handel, Austria.
Pepsin (p.1729·3); pancreatin (p.1725·3); porcine bile (p.1660·3).
*Digestive system disorders.*

**Helopyrin** Rosch & Handel, Austria.
Ethenzamide (p.37·2); ascorbic acid (p.1460·2); flavonoids (p.1688·2); rutoside (p.1688·2); ephedrine hydrochloride (p.1120·1).
*Cold symptoms.*

**Helpin**
Note. This name is used for preparations of different composition.
Drugtech, Chile.
Sildenafil (p.1744·2).
Berlin-Chemie, Ger.†.
Brivudine (p.629·2).
*Herpes and varicella infections.*

**Helporigin** Help, Gr.
Loratadine (p.436·1).
*Allergic rhinitis; pruritus.*

**Helposol** Help, Gr.
Aciclovir (p.626·1).
*Herpes simplex infections.*

**Helpp** ISA, Arg.
Permethrin (p.1508·3).
*Pediculosis.*

**Helvamox** Helvepharm, Switz.†.
Amoxicillin trihydrate (p.155·3).
Now known as Amoxicillin Helvepharm.
*Bacterial infections.*

**Helvecin** Helvepharm, Switz.†.
Indometacin (p.47·3).
Now known as Indometacin Helvepharm.
*Gout; musculoskeletal, joint, and peri-articular disorders.*

**Helvedoclyn** Helvepharm, Switz.†.
Doxycycline hyclate (p.206·2).
Now known as Doxycycline Helvepharm.
*Bacterial infections.*

**Helvedstensstifter** Braun, Denm.
Silver nitrate (p.1746·1).
*Hyperkeratosis.*

**Helvegeron** Helvepharm, Switz.
Amino-acid, multivitamin and mineral preparation with ginseng and lecithin (p.1417·1).
*Tonic.*

**Helvemycin** Helvepharm, Switz.†.
Erythromycin ethyl succinate (p.208·1) or erythromycin stearate (p.208·2).
*Bacterial infections.*

**Helveprim** Helvepharm, Switz.†.
Co-trimoxazole (p.199·3).
Now known as Co-trimoxazole Helvepharm.
*Bacterial infections; blastomycosis; malaria; Pneumocystis carinii pneumonia.*

**Helver Sal** Bouxili, Spain.
Aspirin (p.15·1).
*Fever; musculoskeletal, joint, and peri-articular disorders; pain; thromboembolism prophylaxis.*

**Helvevir** Helvepharm, Switz.
Aciclovir (p.626·1).
*Herpes labialis.*

**Hem Anth** Llorens, Spain.
Chlorphenamine maleate (p.427·3); dexamethasone phosphate (p.1097·2).
*Eye disorders.*

**Hem Fe** Wakefield, USA.
Ferrous fumarate (p.1427·3); vitamin $B_{12}$ (p.1458·2); desiccated gastric substance.
Ascorbic acid (p.1460·2) is included in this preparation to increase the absorption and availability of iron.
Docusate sodium (p.1262·2) is included in this preparation to reduce the constipating effects of iron.
*Iron deficiency anaemias.*

**Hemabate**
Pharmacia Upjohn, Hong Kong†; Pharmacia, UK; Upjohn, USA.
Carboprost trometamol (p.1514·2).
*Postpartum haemorrhage; termination of pregnancy.*

**Hema-Chek**
Bayer Diagnostics, UK; Bayer, USA.
Test for occult blood in faeces.

**Hema-Combistix**
Bayer, Austral.; Bayer Diagnostics, Irl.; Bayer Diagnostics, UK.
Test for pH, protein, glucose, and blood in urine.

**Hemafer** Unipharma, Gr.
Iron polymaltose (p.1437·3).
*Iron-deficiency anaemia.*

**Hemafer fol** Unipharma, Gr.
Iron polymaltose (p.1437·3); folic acid (p.1417·1).
*Iron and folic acid deficiency in pregnancy.*

**Hemagene Tailleur** Elerte, Fr.
Ibuprofen (p.45·3).
Formerly contained aspirin, phenacetin, menthol, and methyl nonyl ketone.
*Fever; pain.*

**Hemamina** Byk Gulden, Mex.
Vitamin preparation (p.1417·1).

**Hemarate** Biomedis, Thai.; Great Eastern, Thai.
Ferrous fumarate (p.1427·3); vitamins.
*Iron-deficiency anaemia.*

**Hemarexin** Technilab, Canad.
Multivitamins; minerals; kola (p.1417·1).
*Tonic.*

**Hemaspan** Sanofi Winthrop, USA.
Ferrous fumarate (p.1427·3).
Vitamin C (p.1460·2) is included in this preparation to increase the absorption and availability of iron.
Docusate sodium (p.1262·2) is included in this preparation to reduce the constipating effects of iron.
*Iron-deficiency anaemias.*

**Hemastix**
Bayer, Austral.; Bayer Diagnostics, Fr.; Bayer Diagnostics, Irl.; Bayer Diagnostici, Ital.; Bayer, NZ†; Bayer Diagnostics, UK; Bayer, USA.
Test for blood in urine.

**Hematest**
Bayer, Austral.; Bayer, Canad.†; Bayer Diagnostics, Mex.; Bayer, USA.
Test for blood in faeces.

**Hematiase B12** Gross, Braz.
Liver extract; gastric mucosa extract; ferric ammonium citrate (p.1427·2); cyanocobalamin (p.1458·2).
*Anaemias; iron-deficiency.*

**Hematinic**
Note. This name is used for preparations of different composition.
Solgar, UK.
Liver (desiccated); vitamin $B_{12}$ (p.1458·2); iron (p.1434·3); calcium ascorbate (p.1460·2); folic acid (p.1429·1).
*Dietary supplement.*
Cypress, USA.
Ferrous fumarate (p.1427·3); folic acid (p.1429·1).
*Anaemias.*

**Hematinic Plus** Cypress, USA.
Ferrous fumarate (p.1427·3); folic acid (p.1429·1); vitamin B substances; minerals (p.1417·1).
Vitamin C (p.1460·2) is included in this preparation to increase the absorption and availability of iron.
*Anaemias.*

**Hematiron** Ibefar, Braz.†.
Lysine hydrochloride; vitamin B substances; ferric ammonium citrate; copper sulfate; liver extract; gastric mucosa extract (p.1417·1).
*Nutritional supplement.*

**Hematon**
Note. This name is used for preparations of different composition.
Defuen, Arg.
Ferrous fumarate (p.1427·3); copper; vitamin B substances; intrinsic factor; liver extract (p.1417·1).
*Anaemias.*
Dexo, Fr.†.
Arginine aspartate; cobalt gluconate; manganese gluconate (p.1417·1).
*Tonic.*

**Hematone** Thuna, Canad.†.
Vitamin B substances, vitamin C, and iron (p.1417·1).

**Hematrine** Novartis, India.
Ferrous succinate (p.1428·2); vitamins (p.1417·1).
*Anaemias; nutritional supplement; tonic.*

**Hemax**
*Sidus, Arg.; Bio Sidus, Thai.*
Epoetin alfa (p.747·2).
*Anaemias.*

**Hemax-Eritron** *Biosintetica, Braz.*
Epoetin (p.747·1).
*Anaemias.*

**Hemcort HC**
*Technilab, Canad.; Technilab, Hong Kong.*
Hydrocortisone acetate (p.1103·3); zinc sulfate (p.1469·3).
*Anorectal disorders.*

**Hemedonine** *Creme d'Orient, Fr.†.*
Haematoporphyrin (p.1696·2).
*Tonic.*

**Hemeran**
*Note. This name is used for preparations of different composition.*
*Novartis, Arg.; Novartis Consumer, Austria; Novartis Consumer, Belg.; Novartis Consumer, Port.; Novartis Consumer, Switz.*
A heparinoid (p.931·1).
*Haematomas; thrombophlebitis; venous insufficiency.*

*Novartis Consumer, Ger.†.*
Heparin sodium (p.928·1).
*Skin trauma; soft-tissue injury.*

**Hemerven** *Interdelta, Switz.*
Diosmin (p.1688·2).
*Peripheral vascular disorders.*

**HemeSelect** *SmithKline Diagnostics, USA.*
Test for occult blood in faeces.

**Hemestal** *Silanes, Mex.*
Metronidazole hydrogen succinate (p.609·3).
*Anaerobic bacterial infections; protozoal infections.*

**Hemetiken** *Kener, Mex.†.*
Difenidol (p.1261·1).

**Hemibe** *Rider, Chile.*
Metoclopramide hydrochloride (p.1274·3).
*Gastrointestinal disorders; gastrointestinal radiography.*

**Hemicraneal** *Liade, Spain.*
Caffeine (p.782·1); ergotamine tartrate (p.467·2); paracetamol (p.76·2).
*Headache; migraine.*

**Hemi-Daonil**
*Aventis, Fr.; Aventis, Neth.*
Glibenclamide (p.331·2).
*Diabetes mellitus.*

**Hemigoxine Nativelle** *Procter & Gamble, Fr.*
Digoxin (p.895·2).
*Arrhythmias; heart failure.*

**Hemineurin**
*AstraZeneca, Austral.†; AstraZeneca, NZ†.*
Clomethiazole (p.683·1) or clomethiazole edisilate (p.683·1).
*Alcohol withdrawal syndrome; disturbed behaviour and sleep disorders in the elderly; insomnia; pre-eclampsia and eclampsia; sedative; status epilepticus.*

**Heminevrin**
*AstraZeneca, Denm.; AstraZeneca, Fin.; IFET (ΙΦΕΤ), Gr.; AstraZeneca, Hong Kong; AstraZeneca, Irl.; AstraZeneca, Norw.; Astra, S.Afr.†; Astra, Swed.; AstraZeneca, UK.*
Clomethiazole (p.683·1) or clomethiazole edisilate (p.683·1).
*Alcohol withdrawal syndrome; disturbed behaviour and sleep disorders in the elderly; insomnia; pre-eclampsia and eclampsia; sedative; status epilepticus.*

**Hemiphos** *Wyeth, India.*
Vitamin B substances; minerals (p.1417·1).

**Hemipralon** *URPAC, Fr.*
Propranolol hydrochloride (p.989·3).
*Cardiovascular disorders; migraine.*

**Hemo**
*Note. A similar name is used for preparations of different composition (see below).*
*Rekah, Israel.*
*Ointment:* Bismuth subgallate (p.1252·2); benzocaine (p.1370·3); zinc oxide (p.1163·2); chloroxylenol (p.1177·2); zinc sulfate (p.1469·3).
*Suppositories:* Bismuth subgallate (p.1252·2); benzocaine (p.1370·3); zinc oxide (p.1163·2); peru balsam (p.1730·2).
*Anorectal disorders.*

**Hemo 141**
*Note. A similar name is used for preparations of different composition (see above).*
*Esteve, Spain.*
Etamsylate (p.749·3).
*Haemorrhage.*

**Hemo Derminiol** *Schwabe, Spain.*
Hamamelis (p.1696·3).
*Haemorrhoids.*

**Hemoaenus** *Simoes, Braz.†.*
Rutoside (p.1688·2); hamamelis (p.1696·3); aesculus (p.1648·2); polygonum acre.
*Haemorrhoids.*

**Hemoal** *Combe, Spain.*
Ephedrine (p.1120·1); benzocaine (p.1370·3).
*Anorectal disorders.*

**Hemobion** *Merck, Mex.*
Ferrous sulfate (p.1428·2).
*Iron-deficiency anaemia.*

**Hemocalcin** *Vinas, Spain†.*
Disodium clodronate (p.770·2).
*Hypercalcaemia of malignancy; osteolytic bone metastases.*

**Hemocane**
*Note. This name is used for preparations of different composition.*
*Key, Austral.*
Lidocaine (p.1377·3); allantoin (p.1141·3); hamamelis (p.1696·3); zinc oxide (p.1163·2); chlorhexidine acetate (p.1173·2).
*Anal pruritus; haemorrhoids.*

*Eastern Pharmaceuticals, UK.*
Lidocaine hydrochloride (p.1377·3); zinc oxide (p.1163·2); bismuth oxide (p.1252·1); benzoic acid (p.1169·3); cinnamic acid (p.1177·3).
*Haemorrhoids.*

**Hemoccult**
*Prevention et Biologie, Fr.; SmithKline Diagnostics, USA.*
A range of tests for occult blood in faeces.

**Hemoce** *Aventis, Spain†.*
Polygeline (p.759·1).
*Perfusion fluid for extracorporeal circulation; plasma volume expansion; shock.*

**Hemocheck** *Matara, Fr.*
Test for blood in faeces.

**Hemocid** *GlaxoSmithKline, India.*
Aminocaproic acid (p.741·3).
*Haemorrhage.*

**Hemoclar** *Sanofi Synthelabo OTC, Fr.*
Pentosan polysulfate (p.979·2).
*Soft-tissue disorders; superficial vascular disorders.*

**Hemocol** *MBP, Ger.*
Collagen (porcine) (p.1674·3).
*Haemorrhage.*

**Hemocromo** *Francia, Ital.*
Sodium ferric gluconate complex (p.1444·3).
*Iron-deficiency anaemia.*

**Hemocyte** *US Pharmaceutical, USA.*
*Injection†:* Ferrous gluconate (p.1428·1); vitamin B substances (p.1417·1).
Procaine hydrochloride (p.1383·2) is included in this preparation to alleviate the pain of injection.
*Tablets:* Ferrous fumarate (p.1427·3).
*Iron-deficiency anaemias.*

**Hemocyte Plus** *US Pharmaceutical, USA.*
Ferrous fumarate (p.1427·3); folic acid (p.1429·1); sodium ascorbate (p.1460·2); vitamin B substances and minerals (p.1417·1).
*Iron-deficiency anaemias.*

**Hemocyte-F** *US Pharmaceutical, USA.*
*Elixir:* Polysaccharide-iron complex (p.1443·2); folic acid (p.1429·1); vitamin $B_{12}$ (p.1458·2).
*Anaemias.*
*Tablets:* Ferrous fumarate (p.1427·3); folic acid (p.1429·1).
*Iron-deficiency anaemias.*

**Hemocyte-V** *US Pharmaceutical, USA†.*
Ferrous gluconate (p.1428·1); vitamin B substances (p.1417·1).
*Iron-deficiency anaemias.*

**Hemo-Cyto-Serum** *Hua, Thai.*
Monosodium glutamate (p.1441·1); strychnine sulfate (p.1750·1); iron (p.1434·3).
*Anaemias; tonic.*

**Hemodex** *Pharmacia Upjohn, Fr.†.*
Dextran 60 (p.746·1) with electrolytes.
*Blood volume expansion.*

**Hemodotti** *Prodotti, Braz.*
Rutoside (p.1688·2); naphazoline hydrochloride (p.1124·3); hydrocortisone acetate (p.1103·3); hamamelis (p.1696·3); amylocaine hydrochloride (p.1370·2).
*Haemorrhoids.*

**Hemodren Compuesto** *Llorens, Spain.*
Bismuth subgallate (p.1252·2); aesculus (p.1648·2); hamamelis (p.1696·3); hydrocortisone acetate (p.1103·3); ruscogenin (p.1741·1); tyrothricin (p.275·1); amylocaine hydrochloride (p.1370·2); benzocaine (p.1370·3).
*Anorectal disorders.*

**Hemodren Simple** *Llorens, Spain†.*
Ruscogenin (p.1741·1).
*Anorectal disorders.*

**Hemofactor HT** *Grifols, Spain†.*
Factor IX (p.752·2); factor X; prothrombin; factor VII (p.750·3).
*Clotting-factor deficiencies; haemorrhage.*

**Hemofer**
*Note. This name is used for preparations of different composition.*
*Profarb, Braz.†.*
Iron (p.1434·3); intrinsic factor; liver extract; vitamins (p.1417·1).
*Iron deficiency; iron-deficiency anaemias.*

*Willmar, Mex.†.*
Ferrous sulfate (p.1428·2).

**Hemoferrol** *Sintesina, Arg.*
Ferrous sulfate (p.1428·2); ferrous fumarate (p.1427·3).
*Anaemias; iron supplement.*

**Hemofibrine Spugna** *Ogna, Ital.†.*
Fibrin (p.753·1).
*Absorbable haemostatic for dental use.*

**Hemofil**
*Baxter, Ger.; Baxter, Malaysia.*
A factor VIII preparation (p.751·1).
*Haemophilia A.*

**Hemofil HT** *Baxter, UK†.*
A factor VIII preparation (p.751·1).
*Haemophilia A.*

**Hemofil M**
*Baxter Immuno, Arg.; Baxter, Fr.; Baxter, Gr.; Baxter-Hyland, Hong Kong; Baxter, Israel; Baxter, Ital.; Baxter, Port.†; Baxter, Singapore†; Baxter, Spain; Baxter, Swed.; Baxter BioScience, UK; Baxter, USA.*
A factor VIII preparation (p.751·1).
*Haemorrhagic disorders.*

**Hemofiltracion E2 and E3** *Baxter, Spain.*
Sodium chloride; potassium chloride; calcium chloride; magnesium chloride; sodium lactate; glucose (p.1221·1).
*Haemofiltration solution.*

**Hemofiltracion E4 and E5** *Baxter, Spain.*
Sodium chloride; potassium chloride; calcium chloride; magnesium chloride; sodium lactate (p.1221·1).
*Haemofiltration solution.*

**Hemofiltracion HF 01** *Fresenius Medical, Spain.*
Sodium chloride; calcium chloride; magnesium chloride; sodium lactate; glucose (p.1221·1).
*Haemofiltration solution.*

**Hemofiltracion HF 02** *Fresenius Medical, Spain.*
Sodium chloride; calcium chloride; magnesium chloride; sodium acetate (p.1221·1).
*Haemofiltration solution.*

**Hemofiltracion HF 11 and HF 23** *Fresenius Medical, Spain.*
Sodium chloride; potassium chloride; calcium chloride; magnesium chloride; sodium lactate; glucose (p.1221·1).
*Haemofiltration solution.*

**Hemofiltrasol** *Gambro, Swed.*
Anhydrous glucose; electrolytes (p.1221·1).
*Haemofiltration.*

**Hemofiltrationslosning 401** *Baxter, Swed.*
Anhydrous glucose; sodium chloride; sodium lactate; calcium chloride; magnesium chloride; potassium chloride (p.1221·1).
*Haemofiltration.*

**Hemofissural** *Baldacci, Port.*
Zinc oxide (p.1163·2); titanium dioxide (p.1160·3); hamamelis (p.1696·3); tetracaine hydrochloride (p.1385·1).
*Anorectal disorders.*

**Hemofluss** *Fonten, Ital.*
Heparin calcium (p.927·3).
*Thromboembolic disorders.*

**Hemogenin** *Aventis, Braz.*
Oxymetholone (p.1565·2).
*Anaemias; growth retardation; hereditary angioedema.*

**Hemohes**
*Braun, Arg.; Braun, Chile; Braun, Fin.; Braun, Ger.; Braun, Norw.; Braun, Port.; Braun, Singapore; Braun, Spain; Braun, Swed.; Braun, Switz.; Braun, UK.*
Pentastarch (p.750·1) in sodium chloride or with electrolytes.
*Extracorporeal perfusion; haemodilution; plasma volume expansion.*

**Hemo-Ice** *Key, Israel.*
Freezable solution in plastic applicator.
*Haemorrhoids.*

**Hemolax** *Hua, Thai.*
Ferrous fumarate (p.1427·3); vitamin $B_1$ (p.1455·2); vitamin $B_6$ (p.1457·2); vitamin $B_{12}$ (p.1458·2); cascara (p.1255·1).
*Beri-beri; constipation; iron-deficiency anaemia; vitamin $B_{12}$ deficiency.*

**Hemoleven** *Lab Francais du Fractionnement, Fr.*
A factor XI preparation.
*Factor XI deficiency.*

**Hemoluol** *Warner-Lambert, Fr.†.*
Aesculus (p.1648·2); shepherd's purse (p.1744·1); cupressus sempervirens.
*Peripheral vascular disorders.*

**Hemon** *Norma (Νορμα), Gr.*
Atenolol (p.865·2).
*Angina; arrythmias; hypertension.*

**Hemonet** *Diafarm, Spain.*
Tetracaine hydrochloride (p.1385·1).
*Haemorrhoids.*

**Hemo-Ped** *Stiefel, Braz.†.*
Ferrous sulfate (p.1428·2); vitamin B substances (p.1417·1).
Sodium ascorbate (p.1460·2) is included in this preparation to increase the absorption and availability or iron.
*Anaemias.*

**Hemoplex** *Recalcine, Chile.*
Citrobioflavonoides (p.1688·2); ascorbic acid (p.1460·2).
*Haemorrhage; haemorrhoids; venous insufficiency.*

**Hemoray** *Varifarma, Arg.*
Iopamidol (p.1064·3).
*Radiographic contrast medium.*

**Hemorhin** *Hua, Thai.*
Docusate sodium (p.1262·2); spermaceti.
*Haemorrhoids.*

**Hemorid** *Upha, Malaysia.*
Diosmin (p.1688·2); hesperidin (p.1688·2).
*Haemorrhoids; venous insufficiency.*

**Hemorid For Women** *Thompson, USA.*
*Cream:* White soft paraffin (p.1479·3); liquid paraffin (p.1479·1); pramocaine hydrochloride (p.1382·2); phenylephrine hydrochloride (p.1126·3); aloe vera (p.1141·3).
*Lotion:* Liquid paraffin (p.1479·1); yellow soft paraffin (p.1479·3); glycerol (p.1694·3).
*Suppositories:* Zinc oxide (p.1163·2); phenylephrine hydrochloride (p.1126·3).
*Anorectal disorders.*

**Hemorrane** *Byk Elmu, Spain.*
Hydrocortisone acetate (p.1103·3).
Formerly contained aesculus, benzocaine, hydrocortisone acetate, and prednisone.
*Haemorroids.*

**Hemorrhoid Ointment** *Stanley, Canad.*
Pramocaine hydrochloride (p.1382·2); zinc sulfate (p.1469·3).
*Haemorrhoids.*

**Hemorrogel** *Arkopharma, Fr.*
*Capsules†:* Aesculus (p.1648·2).
*Haemorrhoids; peripheral vascular disorders.*
*Rectal gel:* Pilewort (p.1732·1); aesculus (p.1648·2); calendula (p.1665·2).
*Haemorrhoids.*

**Hemorroidex** *Medic, Braz.*
Rutoside (p.1688·2); hamamelis (p.1696·3); aesculus (p.1648·2).
*Haemorrhoids.*

**Hemorrol**
*Note. This name is used for preparations of different composition.*
*QIF, Braz.†.*
Rutoside (p.1688·2); aesculus (p.1648·2); hamamelis (p.1696·3).
*Venous insufficiency.*

*Hochstetter, Chile.*
Aescin (p.1648·2); hamamelis (p.1696·3); rhatany (p.1738·1).
*Haemorrhoids.*

**Hemosan** *Sanval, Braz.†.*
Hamamelis (p.1696·3); polygonum acre; aesculus (p.1648·2).
*Venous insufficiency.*

**Hemosedan** *Centrapharm, Belg.*
Prednisolone acetate (p.1108·1); lidocaine hydrochloride (p.1377·3).
Formerly contained prednisolone, hexachlorophene, cinchocaine hydrochloride, and belladonna.
*Haemorrhoids.*

**Hemoset A** *Pharmalink, Swed.†.*
Sodium chloride; potassium chloride; magnesium chloride; calcium chloride (p.1221·1).
*Haemodialysis.*

**Hemoset A glucos** *Pharmalink, Swed.†.*
Sodium chloride; potassium chloride; magnesium chloride; calcium chloride; anhydrous glucose (p.1221·1).
*Haemodialysis.*

**Hemosin-K** *Hormonas, Mex.*
Carbazochrome sodium sulfonate (p.745·1); vitamin K (p.1466·3).
*Haemorrhage.*

**Hemosol B0** *Gambro, Swed.*
Sodium chloride; calcium chloride; magnesium chloride; lactic acid or sodium lactate; sodium bicarbonate (p.1221·1).
*Haemofiltration.*

**Hemosol Bicar** *Hospal, Denm.*
Calcium chloride; magnesium chloride; sodium chloride; sodium bicarbonate; sodium lactate (p.1221·1).
*Haemodialysis; haemofiltration.*

**Hemo-Somaton** *Desbergers, Canad.†.*
*Combination preparation:* Oral solution, bovine plasma; tablets, multivitamins and minerals (p.1417·1).
*Tonic.*

**Hemo-Somaton with Vitamin C** *Desbergers, Canad.†.*
*Combination preparation:* Oral solution, bovine plasma; tablets multivitamins and minerals (p.1417·1).
*Tonic.*

**Hemostatico Antisep Asen** *Asens, Spain†.*
Benzalkonium chloride (p.1168·3); phenazone (p.82·3); hamamelis water (p.1696·3).
*Epistaxis; wounds.*

**Hemotene** *Astra, USA.*
Absorbable collagen (p.1674·3).
*Haemostatic.*

**Hemototal** *Euro-Labor, Port.; Grunenthal, Port.*
Ferrous gluconate (p.1428·1).
*Iron deficiency; iron-deficiency anaemia.*

**Hemovas** *Robert, Spain.*
Pentoxifylline (p.979·3).
*Vascular disorders.*

**Hemovasal** *Manetti Roberts, Ital.*
Suleparoid (p.1009·1).
*Soft-tissue disorders; superficial vascular disorders; thrombosis prophylaxis.*

**Hemovirtu's** *Virtus, Braz.†.*
Aesculus (p.1648·2); hamamelis (p.1696·3); polygonum.
*Haemorrhoids.*

**Hemovirtu's Pomada** *Virtus, Braz.†.*
Davila rugosa; belladonna (p.479·1).
*Haemorrhoids.*

**Hemovit** *Dayton, USA.*
Vitamin B substances; vitamin C (p.1417·1).

**Hem-Prep** *G & W, USA.*
Shark-liver oil; phenylmercuric nitrate (p.1189·2); bismuth subgallate (p.1252·2); zinc oxide (p.1163·2); benzocaine (p.1370·3).
*Anorectal disorders.*

**Hemril** *Upsher-Smith, USA.*
Bismuth subgallate (p.1252·2); bismuth resorcinol compound (p.1253·1); benzyl benzoate (p.1500·2); peru balsam (p.1730·2); zinc oxide (p.1163·2).

**Hemril-HC** *Upsher-Smith, USA.*
Hydrocortisone acetate (p.1103·3).

**Hemsi** *Serum Institute, India.*
Ferrous fumarate (p.1427·3); lysine hydrochloride; vitamins; minerals (p.1417·1).
*Iron-deficiency anaemia.*

**Hemsyl** *Indoco, India.*
Etamsylate (p.749·3).
*Haemorrhagic disorders.*

**Henetix** *Guerbet, Braz.*
Iobitridol (p.1063·1).
*Contrast media for angiography.*

**Henexal** *Pisa, Mex.*
Furosemide (p.919·3).

**Henofin** *Ehlinger, Mex.†.*
Astemizole (p.424·2).

**Hep Lok** *IFET (ΙΦΕΤ), Gr.*
Heparin sodium (p.928·1).
*Thromboembolic disorders.*

**Hepa** *Kolassa, Austria.*
Ornithine aspartate (p.1442·3).
*Hyperammonaemia associated with liver disorders.*

**Hepa Factor** *Sigma-Tau, Spain.*
Folic acid (p.1429·1); cobamamide (p.1459·1).
*Folic acid deficiency; liver disorders.*

**Hepabene** *Ratiopharm, Austria.*
Fumitory (p.1690·1); silybum marianum (p.1043·3).
*Biliary-tract disorders.*

**Hepabig** *Green Cross, Malaysia.*
A hepatitis B immunoglobulin (p.1617·2).
*Passive immunisation.*

**Hepabil** *Instituto Sanitas, Chile.*
Bile extract (p.1660·3); choline dihydrogen citrate (p.1424·3); inositol (p.1701·2); boldo (p.1661·2); vitamin K (p.1466·3); pancreatin (p.1725·3).
*Digestive disorders.*

**Hepabionta** *Merck, S.Afr.†.*
Vitamin B substances (p.1417·1); orotic acid (p.1724·3); folic acid (p.1429·1).
*Liver disorders.*

**Hepabuzone** *Spirig, Switz.*
Heparin sodium (p.928·1); phenylbutazone (p.83·2).
*Musculoskeletal, joint, peri-articular, and soft-tissue disorders; peripheral vascular disorders; thrombophlebitis.*

**Hepacal** *Benedetti, Ital.†.*
Heparin calcium (p.927·3).
*Thromboembolic disorders.*

**Hepacalmina** *Prisfar, Port.*
Bioflavonoids (p.1688·2).
*Liver disorders.*

**Hepacap** *Medicap, Thai.*
Essential phospholipids and multivitamins (p.1417·1).
*Liver disorders.*

**Hepaccine-B** *Biovac, S.Afr.*
A hepatitis B vaccine (p.1618·1).
*Active immunisation.*

**Hepachofril** *Sedabel, Braz.†.*
Cynara (p.1678·3); choline (p.1424·3); liver extract; methionine (p.1042·1).
*Liver disorders.*

**Hepachofril Solution** *Sedabel, Braz.†.*
Cynara (p.1678·3); choline (p.1424·3); liver extract.
*Liver disorders.*

**Hepacholan** *Hepacholan, Braz.†.*
Cynara (p.1678·3); solanum paniculatum.
*Digestive disorders.*

**Hepacholine** *Synthelabo, Fr.*
Choline citrate (p.1424·3); sorbitol (p.1446·3).
*Constipation; dyspepsia.*

**Hepacitol** *Andromaco, Spain†.*
Arginine timonacicate (p.1421·2).
*Liver disorders.*

**Hepacitron** *Ibefar, Braz.†.*
Adenosine (p.851·2); betaine (p.1660·1); methionine (p.1042·1); choline citrate (p.1424·3); pyridoxine hydrochloride (p.1456·3).
*Liver disorders.*

**Hepaclem** *Clement Thionville, Fr.*
Cynara (p.1678·3); boldo (p.1661·2); kinkeliba (p.1703·3); Javanese turmeric (p.1759·3).
*Digestive-system disorders; renal disorders.*

**Hepacoban B12** *Bohm, Spain†.*
Vitamin B substances (p.1417·1); liver extract.
*Tonic; vitamin B deficiency.*

**Hepacomplet B12 Triple** *Reig Jofre, Spain.*
Vitamin B substances (p.1417·1); liver; amino acids.
*Anaemias; tonic.*

**Hepactiv** *Rosch & Handel, Austria.*
Cynara (p.1678·3).
*Disorders of fat metabolism.*

**Hepacur** *Medical, Arg.*
Boldo (p.1661·2); carqueja; cynara (p.1678·3); hyoscyamus (p.485·2); belladonna (p.479·1).
*Gastrointestinal disorders.*

**Hepadial** *Biocodex, Fr.*
Dimecrotic acid, magnesium salt (p.1680·3).
*Dyspepsia.*

**Hepadif** *Reig Jofre, Spain.*
*Oral solution:* Carnitine orotate (p.1724·3); carnitine (p.1423·3); vitamin B substances (p.1417·1); liver extract.
*Tablets:* Carnitine orotate (p.1724·3); vitamin B substances (p.1417·1); liver extract; adenine hydrochloride (p.1647·3).
*Acetonaemia; hepatitis.*

**Hepadigenor** *Baliarda, Arg.*
Silymarin (p.1043·3); dehydrocholic acid (p.1679·2); pancreatin (p.1725·3); simeticone (p.1289·2).
*Digestive disorders; liver disorders.*

**Hepadoddi** *Merck, Port.*
Magnesium dimecrotate (p.1680·3).
*Biliary-tract disorders.*

**Hepaduran V** *OTW, Ger.*
Silybum marianum (p.1043·3).
*Liver disorders.*

**Hepa-Factor** *Max Farma, Ital.*
Folinic acid (p.1431·1); hydroxocobalamin (p.1458·2).
*Hyperchromic anaemia; liver disorders.*

**Hepaflex** *Baxter, Fin.*
Heparin sodium (p.928·1).
*Thrombosis prophylaxis.*

**Hepafol-F** *Farcoral, Mex.*
Multivitamin and mineral preparation with garlic and royal jelly (p.1417·1).

**Hepagallin N** *Pfluger, Ger.*
Cynara (p.1678·3).
*Dyspepsia.*

**Hepa-Gastreu S R7** *Reckeweg, Ger.*
Homoeopathic preparation.

**Hepa-Gel** *Lichtenstein, Ger.*
Heparin sodium (p.928·1).
*Soft-tissue injury; superficial vascular disorders.*

**HepaGel** *Spirig, Switz.*
Heparin sodium (p.928·1).
*Peripheral vascular disorders; soft-tissue disorders.*

**Hepagrisevit Forte-N** *Pharmacia, Ger.*
*Injection:* Cyanocobalamin (p.1458·2); folic acid (p.1429·1); nicotinamide (p.1441·2).
Lidocaine hydrochloride (p.1377·3) is included in this preparation to alleviate the pain of injection.
*Tablets:* Cyanocobalamin (p.1458·2); folic acid (p.1429·1); pyridoxine hydrochloride (p.1456·3).
*Liver disorders.*

**Hepagrume** *EG, Fr.*
Arginine (p.1421·1); betaine (p.1660·1); choline dihydrogen citrate (p.1424·3); inositol (p.1701·2); sorbitol (p.1446·3).
*Constipation; dyspepsia.*

**Hepal** *Rigers, Mex.†.*
Liver extract.

**hepa-L 90 N** *Loges, Ger.*
Homoeopathic preparation.

**Hepalac** *Berlin Pharm, Thai.*
Lactulose (p.1269·1).
*Constipation; hepatic encephalopathy.*

**Hepalean** *Organon Teknika, Canad.*
Heparin sodium (p.928·1).
*Thromboembolic disorders; thrombosis prophylaxis.*

**Hepalean-Lok** *Organon Teknika, Canad.*
Heparin sodium (p.928·1).
*To maintain patency of intravenous injection devices.*

**Hepalin** *Bergamo, Braz.†.*
Adenosine (p.851·2); methionine (p.1042·1); betaine hydrochloride (p.1660·2); choline (p.1424·3); pyridoxine (p.1457·2); sorbitol (p.1446·3).
*Liver disorders.*

**Hepalipon N** *Rhenomed, Ger.†.*
Methionine (p.1042·1); choline hydrogen tartrate (p.1424·3); inositol (p.1701·2).
*Liver disorders.*

**Hepa-Loges**
*Vitasan, Austria; Loges, Ger.*
Silybum marianum (p.1043·3).
*Liver disorders.*

**Hepa-Merz**
*Note. This name is used for preparations of different composition.*
*Searle, Braz.†; Grunenthal, Chile; Merz, Ger.; Merz, Hong Kong; Win-Medicare, India.*
Ornithine aspartate (p.1442·3).
*Hyperammonaemia.*

*Win-Medicare, India.*
*Syrup:* Ornithine aspartate (p.1442·3); nicotinamide (p.1441·2); vitamin $B_2$ (p.1456·1).
*Tablets:* Ornithine aspartate (p.1442·3); pancreatin (p.1725·3).
*Liver disorders.*

**Hepa-Merz KT** *Merz, Ger.*
Ornithine aspartate (p.1442·3).
*Liver disorders.*

**Hepa-Merz Lact** *Merz, Ger.*
Lactulose (p.1269·1).
*Constipation; liver disorders; salmonella enteritis.*

**Hepa-Merz Sil** *Merz, Ger.*
Silybum marianum (p.1043·3).
*Liver disorders.*

**Hepamig** *Welcker-Lyster, Canad.†.*
Tilia (p.1756·2).
*Biliary-tract disorders.*

**Hepanephrol**
*Zambon, Fr.; Knoll, Port.*
Cynara (p.1678·3).
*Dyspepsia; fluid retention.*

**Hepanisan** *Heralds, Braz.†.*
Carnitine (p.1423·3); liver extract; vitamin $B_2$; vitamin $B_6$; vitamin $B_{12}$ (p.1417·1).
*Liver disorders.*

**Hepanutrin**
*Fresenius, Braz.; Geistlich, UK†.*
Amino-acid infusion (p.1417·1).
*Parenteral nutrition.*

**Hepaplus** *Hexal, Ger.*
Heparin sodium (p.928·1).
*Soft-tissue injury; superficial vascular disorders.*

**Hepar 10%** *Baxter, Ger.*
Amino-acid infusion (p.1417·1).
*Liver disorders.*

**Hepar HM** *Pfluger, Ger.*
Homoeopathic preparation.

**Hepar 202 N** *Staufen, Ger.*
Homoeopathic preparation.

**Hepar Pasc Mono** *Koch, Austria.*
Silybum marianum (p.1043·3).
*Liver disorders.*

**Hepar SL** *Serturner, Ger.*
Cynara (p.1678·3).
*Dyspepsia.*

**Heparano N** *Pfluger, Ger.†.*
Silybum marianum (p.1043·3).
*Liver disorders.*

**Heparegen** *Drossapharm, Switz.*
Timonacic (p.1756·2).
*Liver disorders.*

**Heparexine** *Shire, Fr.†.*
Fosforylcholine magnesium (p.1690·1).
*Constipation; dyspepsia.*

**Hepargitol** *Elerte, Fr.*
Arginine hydrochloride (p.1421·1); sorbitol (p.1446·3); anhydrous sodium sulfate (p.1290·1); sodium phosphate (p.1230·3); citric acid (p.1673·1).
*Constipation; dyspepsia.*

**Hepar-Hevert** *Hevert, Ger.*
Homoeopathic preparation.

**Heparin Comp** *CT, Ger.*
Heparin sodium (p.928·1); arnica (p.1656·3); aesculus (p.1648·2).
*Soft-tissue injury; superficial vascular disorders.*

**Heparin Kombi-Gel** *Ratiopharm, Ger.*
Heparin sodium (p.928·1); arnica (p.1656·3); aesculus (p.1648·2).
*Soft-tissue injury; superficial vascular disorders.*

**Heparin Plus** *Heumann, Ger.*
Heparin sodium (p.928·1); glycol salicylate (p.44·3).
*Soft-tissue injury.*

**Heparinol** *Streuli, Switz.*
Heparin sodium (p.928·1); thymol.
*Haematomas; thrombophlebitis; ulcers; varicose veins.*

**Heparmin** *Tentan, Switz.*
Homoeopathic preparation.

**Heparon** *Nutricia, Ital.*
Preparation for enteral nutrition in liver disorders (p.1417·1).

**Heparos** *Desbergers, Canad.†.*
Cyanocobalamin (p.1458·2); ferric ammonium citrate (p.1427·2).
*Iron-deficiency anaemias.*

**Hepar-Pasc** *Pascoe, Ger.*
Silybum marianum (p.1043·3).
*Liver disorders.*

**Hepar-Pasc duo** *Pascoe, Ger.†.*
Silybum marianum (p.1043·3); methionine (p.1042·1).
*Liver disorders.*

**Hepar-Pasc N** *Pascoe, Ger.†.*
Methionine (p.1042·1); greater celandine (p.1695·3); silybum marianum (p.1043·3).
*Liver disorders.*

**Hepar-POS** *Ursapharm, Ger.*
Cynara (p.1678·3).
*Dyspepsia.*

**Heparstad**
*Stada, Austria; Stada, Ger.*
Cynara (p.1678·3).
*Biliary-tract disorders.*

**Heparsyx N** *Syxyl, Ger.*
Silybum marianum (p.1043·3).
*Liver disorders.*

**Heparth** *20th Century, Mex.†.*
Heparin sodium (p.928·1).

**Hepa-S**
*Lichtwer, Austria†; Medichemie Bioline, Switz.*
Cynara (p.1678·3).
*Digestive disorders; dyspepsia.*

**Hepa-Salbe** *Lichtenstein, Ger.*
Heparin sodium (p.928·1).
*Soft-tissue injury; superficial vascular disorders.*

**Hepasedan** *Delta, Braz.†.*
Vitamin $B_{12}$ (p.1458·2); methionine (p.1042·1); betaine tartrate (p.1660·2); choline tartrate (p.1424·3); liver extract; gastric mucosa extract; cynara (p.1678·3).
*Liver disorders.*

**Hepasil Composto** *Edmond Pharma, Ital.†.*
Fencibutirol sodium (p.1687·1); rhubarb (p.1287·3); frangula (p.1266·3); cascara (p.1255·1); boldo (p.1661·2).
*Constipation.*

**Hepasol** *G.P. Laboratories, Austral.†.*
Vitamin and mineral preparation with liver extract (p.1417·1).
*Tonic.*

**Hepasules** *Biological E, India.*
Ferrous fumarate (p.1427·3); vitamin $B_{12}$ (p.1458·2); folic acid (p.1429·1); docusate sodium (p.1262·2); vitamin C (p.1460·2).
*Anaemia.*

**Hepasulfol** *Franco-Indian, India.*
Anethole trithione (p.1655·1).
*Liver and biliary disorders.*

**Hepasulfol-AA** *Franco-Indian, India.*
Anethole trithione (p.1655·1); chlorphenamine maleate (p.427·3).
*Hypersensitivity reactions.*

**Hepatalgina** *Byk, Arg.*
*Oral drops:* Cynara (p.1678·3); boldo (p.1661·2); wild carrot (p.1765·1); menthol (p.1711·3).
*Tablets:* Cynara (p.1678·3); boldine (p.1661·2); wild carrot (p.1765·1); menthol (p.1711·3); dehydrocholic acid (p.1679·2); deoxycholic acid (p.1660·3).
*Dyspepsia.*

**Hepatamine**
*Scientific Hospital Supplies, Austral.; Scientific Hospital Supplies, Israel†; SHS, Singapore.*
Amino-acid preparation (p.1417·1).
*Nutritional supplement in liver disorders.*

*Braun McGaw, Hong Kong†; McGaw, NZ†; McGaw, USA.*
Amino-acid infusion (p.1417·1).
*Parenteral nutrition in hepatic encephalopathy.*

**Hepatect**
*Biotest, Austria; Biotest, Ger.; Biotest, Hong Kong; Intra Pharma, Irl.; Biotest, Israel; Biotest, Ital.†; Boehringer Ingelheim, Port.; Biotest, Switz.*
A hepatitis B immunoglobulin (p.1617·2).
*Passive immunisation.*

**Hepathromb** *Riemser, Ger.*
Heparin sodium (p.928·1).
*Soft-tissue injury; superficial vascular disorders.*

**Hepathrombin** *Teofarma, Ger.*
Heparin sodium (p.928·1).
*Soft-tissue injury; superficial vascular disorders.*

**Hepathrombine** *Lyron, Switz.*
Heparin sodium (p.928·1); allantoin (p.1141·3); dexpanthenol (p.1727·2).
*Scars; soft-tissue injury; venous insufficiency.*

**Hepatic-Aid** *McGaw, NZ†.*
Food for special diets (p.1417·1).
*Liver disease.*

**Hepatic-Aid II** *McGaw, USA.*
Preparation for enteral nutrition (p.1417·1).
*Liver disease.*

**Hepaticum novo** *Pascoe, Ger.*
Javanese turmeric (p.1759·3); peppermint leaf (p.1283·2); absinthium (p.1645·1).
*Biliary disorders.*

**Hepaticum-Lac-Medice** *Medice, Ger.*
Lactulose (p.1269·1).
*Constipation; hepatic encephalopathy.*

**Hepaticum-Medice H** *Medice, Ger.*
Cinchona bark (p.1671·3); silybum marianum (p.1043·3); greater celandine (p.1695·3); gentian (p.1692·2); turmeric (p.1058·3).
*Adjunct in skin disorders; constipation; liver and biliary disorders.*

**Hepatilon** *Galenogal, Braz.†.*
Avocado; cynara (p.1678·3); boldo (p.1661·2); carqueja.
*Liver disorders.*

**Hepationina** *Bunker, Braz.†.*
Methionine (p.1042·1); choline chloride (p.1424·3); vitamin B substances (p.1417·1).
*Digestive disorders.*

**Hepativax** *Aventis Pasteur, Arg.*
A hepatitis B vaccine (recombinant DNA) (p.1618·1).
*Active immunisation.*

**Hepato Diet** *Support, Braz.*
Preparation for enteral nutrition (p.1417·1).
*Liver disorders.*

**Hepato Fardi** *Fardi, Spain.*
Choline orotate (p.1724·3); almond milk.
*Liver disorders.*

**Hepatobe** *Sinterapico, Braz.†.*
Adenosine (p.851·2); betaine (p.1660·1); choline citrate (p.1424·3); pyridoxine hydrochloride (p.1456·3); sorbitol (p.1446·3).
*Digestive disorders.*

**Hepatobyl** *Breves, Braz.†.*
Dehydrocholic acid (p.1679·2); ox bile (p.1660·3); boldo (p.1661·2); belladonna (p.479·1).
*Liver disorders.*

**Hepatocler** *Heralds, Braz.†.*
Methionine (p.1042·1); choline chloride (p.1424·3); betaine hydrochloride (p.1660·2); thiamine nitrate; pyridoxine hydrochloride; riboflavin (p.1417·1).
*Liver disorders.*

**Hepatodirectol** *Sanitas, Arg.*
Homatropine methylbromide (p.483·2); papaverine hydrochloride (p.1728·1); boldo (p.1661·2); carqueja; cynara (p.1678·3); crataegus (p.1677·1); bitter orange peel (p.1723·3); belladonna (p.479·1).
*Gastrointestinal spasm; liver and biliary-tract disorders.*

**Hepatodoron**
*Weleda, Austria; Weleda, Ger.†.*
Fragaria vesca; vitis vinifera.
*Constipation; eczema; liver disorders.*

**Hepato-Drainol** *Boiron, Port.†.*
Homoeopathic preparation.

**Hepatofalk**
*Note. This name is used for preparations of different composition.*
*Falk, Ger.†.*
Choline orotate (p.1724·3); adenosine (p.851·2); cyanocobalamin (p.1458·2); hydroxocobalamin acetate (p.1458·2).
Lidocaine hydrochloride (p.1377·3) is included in the intramuscular injection to alleviate the pain of injection.
*Liver disorders.*

*Falk, Hong Kong.*
*Injection†:* Choline orotate (p.1724·3); adenosine (p.851·2); vitamin $B_{12}$ (p.1458·2).
Lidocaine (p.1377·3) is included in this preparation to alleviate the pain of injection.
*Tablets:* Choline orotate (p.1724·3); cysteine hydrochloride (p.1426·3); vitamin B substances (p.1417·1); folic acid (p.1429·1); ox bile (p.1660·3); greater celandine (p.1695·3); Javanese turmeric (p.1759·3); cynara (p.1678·3); taraxacum (p.1751·3); frangula (p.1266·3); rhubarb (p.1287·3).
*Liver disorders.*

**Hepatofalk Neu** *Falk, Ger.†.*
Choline orotate (p.1724·3); cysteine hydrochloride (p.1426·3); vitamins (p.1417·1); ox bile (p.1660·3); ammi visnaga (p.1653·3); absinthium (p.1645·1); boldo (p.1661·2); greater celandine (p.1695·3); Javanese turmeric (p.1759·3); cynara (p.1678·3); taraxacum (p.1751·3).
*Liver and biliary-tract disorders.*

**Hepatofalk Planta**
*Falk, Hong Kong.*
Silymarin (p.1043·3); turmeric (p.1058·3); greater celandine (p.1695·3).
*Liver disorders.*

*Falk, Singapore.*
Silybum marianum (p.1043·3); Javanese turmeric (p.1759·3); greater celandine (p.1695·3).
*Colic; dyspepsia; liver disorders.*

**Hepatofalk Planta N** *Falk, Ger.†.*
Silybum marianum (p.1043·3); Javanese turmeric (p.1759·3).
*Liver disorders.*

**Hepato-Flux** *Prodotti, Braz.†.*
Belladonna (p.479·1); boldo (p.1661·2); cascara (p.1255·1); colato; nicotinamide (p.1441·2).
*Liver disorders.*

**Hepatogenol** *Profarb, Braz.†.*
Inositol (p.1701·2); acetylmethionine; vitamin $B_{12}$ (p.1417·1).
*Liver disorders.*

**Hepatoglobine** *Raptakos, India.*
*Capsules:* Vitamin $B_{12}$ (p.1458·2); peptone; ferrous fumarate (p.1427·3); copper sulfate (p.1426·1); folic acid (p.1429·1).
*Oral drops:* Vitamin $B_{12}$ (p.1458·2); peptone; ferric ammonium citrate (p.1427·2); folic acid (p.1429·1).
*Oral liquid:* Liver extract (proteolysed); peptone; ferric ammonium citrate (p.1427·2); folic acid (p.1429·1).
*Anaemias.*

**Hepatophil** *Teuto, Braz.†.*
Avocado; boldo (p.1661·2); rhubarb (p.1287·3); cascara (p.1255·1); cynara (p.1678·3).
*Liver disorders.*

**Hepatoregius** *Dovalle, Braz.*
Pepsin (p.1729·3); pancreatin (p.1725·3); boldo (p.1661·2); cynara (p.1678·3).
*Digestive-system disorders.*

**Hepatorell** *Sanorell, Ger.†.*
Silybum marianum (p.1043·3).
*Liver disorders.*

**Hepatorell H Leber-Spezifikum** *Sanorell, Ger.*
Homoeopathic preparation.

**Hepatos**
*Note. This name is used for preparations of different composition.*
*Hevert, Ger.*
Silybum marianum (p.1043·3).
*Liver disorders.*

*Teofarma, Ital.*
Cascara (p.1255·1); boldo (p.1661·2).
*Constipation.*

**Hepatos B12** *Teofarma, Ital.*
Cascara (p.1255·1); boldo (p.1661·2); inositol (p.1701·2); cyanocobalamin (p.1458·2).
*Constipation.*

**Hepatotal Family** *Excelentia, Arg.*
Boldo (p.1661·2); chamomile (p.1669·3).
*Digestive disorders.*

**Hepatotris** *Medic, Braz.*
Methionine (p.1042·1); vitamin $B_{12}$ (p.1458·2); choline (p.1424·3).
*Liver disorders.*

**Hepatoum** *Hepatoum, Fr.*
*Oral liquid:* Pulsatilla (p.1737·1); turmeric (p.1058·3); peppermint oil (p.1283·2); alverine citrate (p.1250·2).
Formerly contained pulsatilla, turmeric, and peppermint oil.
*Gastrointestinal disorders.*
*Tablets†:* Pepsin (p.1729·3); pancreatin (p.1725·3); amylase (p.1654·2).
*Dyspepsia.*

**Hepatoxane** *Esplanade, Fr.†.*
Tocamphyl.
*Dyspepsia.*

**Hepatron C** *Schering-Plough, Mex.*
Capsules, ribavirin (p.652·1); injection, interferon alfa-2b (p.640·3).
*Chronic hepatitis C.*

**Hepatyrix** *GlaxoSmithKline, UK.*
A hepatitis A and typhoid vaccine (p.1620·1).
*Active immunisation.*

**Hepavax-Gene**
*Green Cross, Malaysia; Green Cross, Thai.*
A hepatitis B vaccine (recombinant DNA) (p.1618·1).
*Active immunisation.*

**Hepa-Vibolex** *MIP, Ger.*
Ornithine aspartate (p.1442·3).
*Hepatic encephalopathy.*

**Hepavirmo** *Cazi, Braz.†.*
Solanum paniculatum; cynara (p.1678·3); boldo (p.1661·2); cascara (p.1255·1); belladonna (p.479·1); liver extract; vitamin $B_{12}$; magnesium sulfate; nicotinamide (p.1417·1).
*Liver disorders.*

**Hepavit**
*Note. This name is used for preparations of different composition.*
*Calea, Austria.*
Hydroxocobalamin acetate (p.1458·2).
*Anaemias; neurologic disorders.*

*General Drugs, Thai.*
Liver extract.
*Anaemias.*

**Hepavite** *Covan, S.Afr.*
Choline bitartrate (p.1424·3); inositol (p.1701·2); methionine (p.1042·1); vitamin B substances; bioflavonoids; magnesium sulfate; zinc sulfate; potassium chloride (p.1417·1).
*Hepatic disorders.*

**Hepavitose** *Climax, Braz.*
Ferric ammonium citrate (p.1427·2); vitamin B substances; manganese hypophosphite; copper chloride (p.1417·1); liver extract; gastric mucosa extract.
*Iron deficiency; iron-deficiency anaemias.*

**Hepax** *UPSA Conseil, Fr.*
Cynara (p.1678·3); kinkeliba (p.1703·3); boldo (p.1661·2); rosemary (p.1740·2).
*Digestive disorders.*

**Hep-Flush** *Leo, UK†.*
Heparin sodium (p.928·1).
Now known as Heparin Sodium ampoules.
*To maintain patency of in-dwelling intravenous lines.*

**Hepflush** *American Pharmaceutical, USA.*
Heparin sodium (p.928·1).
*To maintain patency of indwelling intravenous catheters.*

**Hep-Forte** *Marlyn, USA.*
Multivitamin, amino-acid, and mineral preparation (p.1417·1).

**Hepirax** *Upha, Malaysia; CCM, Malaysia.*
Aciclovir (p.626·1).
*Herpesvirus infections.*

**Heplant** *Spitzner, Ger.*
Silybum marianum (p.1043·3).
*Liver disorders.*

**Hep-Lock** *Elkins-Sinn, USA.*
Heparin sodium (p.928·1).
*To maintain patency of in-dwelling intravenous lines.*

**Heplok**
*Leo, Irl.; Leo, UK†.*
Heparin sodium (p.928·1).
Now known as Heparin Sodium ampoules in the *UK.*
*To maintain patency of in-dwelling intravenous lines.*

**Hepofilina** *INQ, Braz.†.*
Adenosine (p.851·2); betaine hydrochloride (p.1660·2); choline (p.1424·3).
*Liver disorders.*

**Heprecomb** *Berna, Switz.*
A hepatitis B vaccine (recombinant DNA) (p.1618·1).
*Active immunisation.*

**Hep-Rinse** *Leo, Irl.*
Heparin sodium (p.928·1).
*To maintain patency of intravenous lines.*

**Hepro** *Casen Fleet, Spain.*
Allantoin (p.1141·3); aminoacridine hydrochloride (p.1165·3); hydrocortisone hydrogen succinate (p.1104·1); lidocaine hydrochloride (p.1377·3).
*Anorectal disorders.*

**Hepsal**
*IFET (ΙΦΕΤ), Gr.; CP Pharmaceuticals, Irl.; CP Pharmaceuticals, UK.*
Heparin sodium (p.928·1).
*To maintain patency of in-dwelling intravenous lines.*

**Hepsera**
*Gilead, Fr.; Gilead, UK; Gilead, USA.*
Adefovir dipivoxil (p.628·1).
*Hepatitis B.*

**Heptadon** *Ebewe, Austria.*
Methadone hydrochloride (p.57·2).
*Pain.*

**Heptalac** *Copley, USA†.*
Lactulose (p.1269·1).

**Hept-A-Myl**
*Synthelabo, Belg.†.*
Heptaminol (p.1697·1).
*Cardiovascular stimulant.*

*Sanofi Synthelabo, Fr.*
Heptaminol hydrochloride (p.1697·1).
*Hypotension.*

**Heptan** *Aguettant, Fr.*
Minerals and trace element preparation (p.1417·1).
*Parenteral nutrition.*

**Heptar** *Eurofarma, Braz.*
Heparin sodium (p.928·1).

**Heptovir** *GlaxoSmithKline, Canad.*
Lamivudine (p.648·2).
*Hepatitis B.*

**Heptylon** *Delalande, Port.†.*
Heptaminol hydrochloride (p.1697·1).
*Alcohol withdrawal syndrome; hypotension; neuromuscular and nervous disorders.*

**Hepuman**
*Berna, Belg.†; Berna, Hong Kong; Berna, Spain; Berna, Switz.; Berna, Thai.†.*
A hepatitis B immunoglobulin (p.1617·2).
*Passive immunisation.*

**Hepuman B** *Berna, Ital.*
A hepatitis B immunoglobulin (p.1617·2).
*Passive immunisation.*

**Heracillin**
*AstraZeneca, Denm.; Astra, Swed.*
Flucloxacillin magnesium (p.213·3) or flucloxacillin sodium (p.213·3).
*Bacterial infections.*

**Heracline** *Technilab, Canad.*
Adrenal cortex extract (p.1110·1); testis extract (p.1569·3); liver extract.
*Tonic.*

**Heractrin** *Heralds, Braz.†.*
Co-trimoxazole (p.199·3); guaifenesin (p.1122·1); ammonium chloride (p.1115·2).
*Bacterial infections.*

**Heralvent** *Luhr-Lehrs, Ger.†.*
Homoeopathic preparation.

**Herb and Honey Cough Elixir** *Weleda, UK.*
Honey (p.1434·2); althaea (p.1651·3); Iceland moss; marrubium (p.1124·1); pimpinella anisum; sambucus (p.1741·3); thyme (p.1755·2).
*Coughs.*

**Herbaccion Antioxidante** *ISA, Arg.*
Vitamin C; bearberry; betacarotene; vitamin E; selenium; zinc (p.1417·1).

**Herbaccion Bioenergizante** *ISA, Arg.*
Ginseng (p.1693·1).
*Tonic.*

**Herbaccion Cerebral** *ISA, Arg.*
Ginkgo biloba (p.1692·3).

**Herbaccion Circumax** *ISA, Arg.*
Selenium; garlic (p.1417·1).
*Dietary supplement.*

**Herbaccion Desinflamante** *ISA, Arg.*
Arnica (p.1656·3).

**Herbaccion Diet** *ISA, Arg.*
Chromium (p.1425·1); carnitine (p.1423·3); bladderwrack (p.1742·3).
*Obesity.*

**Herbaccion Dig Fresh** *ISA, Arg.*
Boldo (p.1661·2); cynara (p.1678·3); carqueja.
*Liver and biliary-tract disorders.*

**Herbaccion Digestivo** *ISA, Arg.*
Cynara (p.1678·3); boldo (p.1661·2); carqueja.

**Herbaccion Flex** *ISA, Arg.*
Devil's claw root (p.28·2).
*Joint disorders.*

**Herbaccion Laxante** *ISA, Arg.*
Ispaghula (p.1268·1).
*Constipation.*

**Herbaccion Menopausia** *ISA, Arg.*
Cimicifuga (p.1671·3).
*Menopausal disorders.*

**Herbaccion Motivante** *ISA, Arg.*
Hypericum (p.299·1).
*Depression.*

**Herbaccion Nutriderm** *ISA, Arg.*
Vitamin A (p.1451·2); aloe vera (p.1141·3).
*Skin disorders.*

**Herbaccion Prostatico** *ISA, Arg.*
Saw palmetto (p.1569·1).
*Prostate disorders.*

**Herbaccion Sedante** *ISA, Arg.*
Tilia (p.1756·2); passion flower (p.1729·1); valerian (p.1762·2).
*Anxiety; sedative.*

**Herbaccion Supervitaminico** *ISA, Arg.*
Vitamins; magnesium; guarana (p.1417·1).

**Herbaccion Venotonico** *ISA, Arg.*
Aesculus (p.1648·2).
*Vascular disorders.*

**Herbadon** *Mavena, Ger.*
Devil's claw root (p.28·2).
*Musculoskeletal and joint disorders.*

**Herbagola** *Gricar, Ital.†.*
Cetylpyridinium chloride (p.1173·1).
*Oral disinfection.*

**Herbagyn** *Mavena, Ger.†.*
Cimicifuga (p.1671·3).
*Menopausal disorders.*

**Herbal** *Rider, Chile.*
*SPF 15:* Octinoxate (p.1154·3); oxybenzone (p.1154·3).
*Sunscreen.*

**Herbal Anxiety Formula** *Faulding, Austral.†.*
Passion flower (p.1729·1); chamomile (p.1669·3).
*Anxiety; nervous tension.*

**Herbal Arthritis Formula** *Faulding, Austral.†.*
Ginkgo biloba (p.1692·3); devil's claw root (p.28·2).
*Arthritis; rheumatism.*

**Herbal Booster** *Pharmadass, UK.*
Herbal preparation with vitamins (p.1417·1).
*Tonic.*

**Herbal Capillary Care** *Faulding, Austral.†.*
Ginkgo biloba (p.1692·3); aesculus (p.1648·2).
*Nocturnal leg cramps; tinnitus; tired legs and feet.*

**Herbal Cleanse** *Vitaplex, Austral.†.*
Aloes (p.1248·2); taraxacum (p.1751·3); ispaghula (p.1268·1); yellow dock (p.1766·1); sarsaparilla (p.1742·1); lappa (p.1704·3); clivers (p.1673·2); hydrastis (p.1698·3); slippery elm (p.1747·1); echinacea purpurea (p.1683·2); ginger (p.1267·1); silybum marianum (p.1043·3).
*Constipation; liver disorders.*

**Herbal Cold & Flu Relief** *Faulding, Austral.†.*
Echinacea angustifolia (p.1683·2); liquorice (p.1270·2); garlic (p.1691·1).
*Catarrh; cold and influenza symptoms.*

**Herbal Cold Relief** *Jamieson, Canad.*
Ephedra (p.1119·3); eucalyptus oil (p.1686·2); grindelia (p.1696·1).

**Herbal Cough Expectorant** *Jamieson, Canad.†.*
Elm bark (p.1747·1); eucalyptus oil (p.1686·2); honey (p.1434·2); anise oil (p.1655·2); camphor oil; white pine.

**Herbal Digestive Formula** *Faulding, Austral.†.*
Liquorice (p.1270·2); turmeric (p.1058·3); ginger (p.1267·1).
*Dyspepsia; flatulence.*

**Herbal Diuretic Formula** *Faulding, Austral.†.*
Taraxacum (p.1751·3); bearberry (p.1659·2).
*Fluid retention.*

**Herbal Essence Anti-Dandruff** *Bristol-Myers Squibb, Canad.*
Salicylic acid (p.1157·1).
*Dandruff.*

**Herbal Expectorant** *Jamieson, Canad.†.*
Aclenophora; apricot; asparagus officinalis; citrus reticulata; ginger; liquorice; mulberry; ophiopogon japonicus; schizandra; skullcap.

**Herbal Eye Care Formula** *Faulding, Austral.†.*
Myrtillus (p.1718·3).
*Eye disorders.*

**Herbal Headache Relief** *Faulding, Austral.†.*
Feverfew (p.469·1).
*Headache.*

**Herbal Indigestion Naturtabs** *Cantassium Co., UK.*
Skullcap (p.1746·3); valerian (p.1762·2); fennel (p.1687·2); myrrh (p.1718·3); papain (p.1727·3); capsicum oleoresin (p.1667·1).

**Herbal Laxative**
*Note. This name is used for preparations of different composition.*
*Quest, Canad.*
Cascara (p.1255·1); rhubarb (p.1287·3).

*Shaklee, Canad.*
Senna (p.1288·2).
Formerly contained senna, buckthorn, and leptandra virginica.
*Constipation.*

*Swiss Herbal, Canad.*
Senna leaves (p.1288·2); cascara (p.1255·1); rhubarb root (p.1287·3); gentian root (p.1692·2); liquorice root (p.1270·2); juniper berries (p.1703·1); buchu leaves (p.1663·1); peppermint oil (p.1283·2).
*Constipation.*

**Herbal Liver Formula** *Faulding, Austral.†.*
Silybum marianum (p.1043·3).
*Digestive disorders; liver disorders.*

**Herbal Nerve** *Swiss Herbal, Canad.*
Valerian root (p.1762·2); skullcap (p.1746·3); gentian root (p.1692·2); liquorice (p.1270·2).

**Herbal Pain Relief** *Cantassium Co., UK.*
Salix bark (p.87·3); passion flower (p.1729·1); valerian (p.1762·2).
*Pain.*

**Herbal PMS Formula** *Faulding, Austral.†.*
Myrtillus (p.1718·3); liquorice (p.1270·2); cimicifuga (p.1671·3).
*Menstrual disorders.*

**Herbal Premens** *Swisshealth, UK.*
Agnus castus (p.1649·1).
*Premenstrual syndrome.*

**Herbal Sleep Aid** *Wampole, Canad.*
Lupulus (p.1708·1); passion flower (p.1729·1); valerian (p.1762·2).
*Sleep disorders.*

**Herbal Sleep Formula** *Faulding, Austral.†.*
Valerian (p.1762·2).
*Insomnia.*

**Herbal Stress Relief** *Faulding, Austral.†.*
Ginseng (p.1693·1).
*Stress.*

**Herbal Support for Active Lifestyles** *Nutravite, Canad.*
Bee pollen; guarana; ginseng; royal jelly; ginseng (p.1417·1).

**Herbal Support for Men Over 45** *Nutravite, Canad.*
Cayenne; chamomile; taraxacum; kelp; pygeum; saw palmetto berries skullcap; tribulus terrestris; yellow dock (p.1417·1).

**Herbal Support for Stressful Lifestyles** *Nutravite, Canad.*
Ginger root; lupulus; kava; passion flower; hypericum; skullcap; valerian root; wood betony (p.1417·1).

**Herbal Support for Women Over 45** *Nutravite, Canad.*
Black cohosh; dong quai; passion flower; red clover; raspberry leaves; squaw fine; wild yam; agnus castus (p.1417·1).

**Herbal Throat** *Jamieson, Canad.*
Camphor (p.1665·3); elm bark (p.1747·1); marrubium (p.1124·1); menthol (p.1711·3); parsley (p.1728·3); thyme (p.1755·2).

**Herb-a-Lax**
*Note. A similar name is used for preparations of different composition (see below).*
*Blooms, Austral.†.*
Senna (p.1288·2); frangula bark (p.1266·3); ispaghula (p.1268·1); dill seed (p.1680·2); liquorice (p.1270·2).
*Constipation.*

**Herbalax**
*Note. A similar name is used for preparations of different composition (see above).*
*Sante Naturelle, Canad.*
Cascara (p.1255·1); frangula (p.1266·3); rhubarb (p.1287·3); senna (p.1288·2); bile salts (p.1660·3).

**Herbalax Forte** *Sante Naturelle, Canad.†.*
Cascara (p.1255·1); phenolphthalein (p.1284·1); bile salts (p.1660·3); capsicum oleoresin (p.1667·1); papain (p.1727·3).

**HerbAllerg** *Herbamed, Switz.*
Homoeopathic preparation.

**Herbaneurin** *Mavena, Ger.*
Hypericum (p.299·1).
*Depression.*

**Herbapharm Rical** *Mavena, Switz.*
Castor oil (p.1668·2).
*Constipation.*

**Herbatar** *Erredici, Ital.†.*
*Cream:* Pine oil; birch oil (p.1159·2); castor oil (p.1668·2); chamomile (p.1669·3); allantoin (p.1141·3).
*Skin disorders.*
*Scalp application:* Pine oil; birch oil (p.1159·2); cedar oil.
*Seborrhoeic dermatitis.*

**Herbatar Plus** *Erredici, Ital.†.*
Ammonium lactate (p.1142·3); tar (p.1159·3); allantoin (p.1141·3).
*Hyperkeratosis.*

**Herbatorment** *Herbapharm, Ger.†.*
Tormentil (p.1757·2).
*Diarrhoea.*

**Herbavit** *Erredici, Ital.†.*
Biotin (p.1423·2); a heparinoid (p.931·1); arnica (p.1656·3); urtica (p.1762·1); polyglycopolyamine; dexpanthenol (p.1727·2); menthol (p.1711·3).
*Prevention of hair loss.*

**Herbe** *Recordati, Ital.*
Benzalkonium chloride (p.1168·3); hamamelis (p.1696·3).
*Eye disinfection.*

**Herbelax** *Sanochemia, Austria.*
Calcium sennoside A (p.1288·3); calcium sennoside B (p.1288·3); bran (p.1253·2); fig (p.1266·3).
*Bowel evacuation; constipation; stool softener.*

**Herbelix** *Lane, UK.*
Lobelia (p.1589·1); tolu solution; sodium bicarbonate (p.1223·2).
*Nasal congestion.*

**Herbesan** *Pfizer Sante, Fr.*
Senna (p.1288·2); aniseed (p.1655·2); peppermint leaf (p.1283·2); couch-grass (p.1676·2).
*Constipation.*

**Herbesan Instantane** *Pfizer Sante, Fr.*
Sennosides B (p.1288·2).
*Constipation.*

**Herbesser**
*Tanabe, Hong Kong; Tanabe, Jpn; Tanabe, Malaysia; Delta, Port.; Tanabe, Singapore; Tanabe, Thai.*
Diltiazem hydrochloride (p.900·1).
*Angina pectoris; arrhythmias; hypertension.*

**Herb-Fibe** *Shaklee, Canad.*
Fibre.
*Constipation.*

**Herbheal Ointment** *Potter's, UK.*
Colophony (p.1675·1); starch (p.1449·1); sublimed sulfur (p.1158·2); zinc oxide (p.1163·2); althaea root (p.1651·3); stellaria media.
*Skin irritation.*

**Herbogesic** *Seroyal, Canad.†.*
Magnesium salicylate (p.55·1).

**Herbolax** *Seroyal, Canad.†.*
Cascara (p.1255·1); rhubarb (p.1287·3); senna (p.1288·2); liquorice (p.1270·2).

**Herbopyrine** *Herbes Universelles, Canad.*
Aspirin (p.15·1); caffeine citrate (p.782·1).

**Herborex** *Rolmex, Canad.*
Cascara (p.1255·1); yellow dock (p.1766·1).

**Herbulax** *Chefaro, UK.*
Frangula bark (p.1266·3); taraxacum (p.1751·3).
*Constipation.*

**Herceptin**
*Roche, Arg.; Roche, Austral.; Roche, Belg.; Roche, Braz.; Roche, Canad.; Roche, Chile; Roche, Denm.; Roche, Fin.; Roche, Fr.; Roche, Ger.; Roche, Gr.; Roche, Irl.; Roche, Israel; Roche, Ital.; Roche, Mex.; Roche, Norw.; Roche, NZ; Roche, Port.; Roche, S.Afr.; Roche, Singapore; Roche, Spain; Roche, Swed.; Roche, Switz.; Roche, Thai.; Roche, UK; Genentech, USA.*
Trastuzumab (p.589·3).
*Breast cancer.*

**Herden** *Remedica, Thai.*
Pentoxifylline (p.979·3).
*Peripheral vascular disorders.*

**Herisan** *Rougier, Canad.†.*
Zinc oxide (p.1163·2).
*Superficial skin irritations.*

**Herivyl** *Libbs, Braz.*
Phentolamine mesilate (p.982·1).
*Erectile dysfunction.*

**Herklin** *Armstrong, Mex.*
*Lotion:* Lindane (p.1506·3); lidocaine (p.1377·3).
*Shampoo:* Lindane (p.1506·3).
*Pediculosis; scabies.*

**Hermal** *Merck-Clevenot, Fr.†.*
Pyrithione zinc (p.1156·2).
*Seborrhoeic dermatitis.*

**Hermalind** *Hermal, Ger.*
Dexpanthenol (p.1727·2); chlorhexidine gluconate (p.1173·2).
*Burns; wounds.*

**Hermes ASS** *Hermes, Ger.†.*
Aspirin (p.15·1).
*Fever; pain.*

**Hermes ASS plus** *Hermes, Ger.†.*
Aspirin (p.15·1); caffeine (p.782·1).
*Pain.*

**Hermes Cevitt** *Hermes, Ger.*
Ascorbic acid (p.1460·2).
*Vitamin C deficiency.*

**Hermes Cevitt + Calcium** *Hermes, Ger.†.*
Ascorbic acid (p.1460·2); calcium carbonate (p.1254·2).
*Vitamin C and calcium deficiency.*

**Hermes Drix Abfuhr-Tee** *Hermes, Ger.†.*
Senna (p.1288·2).
*Constipation.*

**Hermin** *Alembic, India.*
Amino-acid infusion (p.1417·1).
*Parenteral nutrition.*

**Hermixsofex** *Sofex, Port.*
Aciclovir (p.626·1).
*Herpes simplex infections.*

**Hermocil** *Edol, Port.*
Aciclovir (p.626·1).

**Hermodotti** *Prodotti, Braz.†.*
Amylocaine (p.1370·3); hamamelis (p.1696·3); hydrocortisone (p.1103·3); naphazoline (p.1124·3); rutoside (p.1688·2).
*Haemorrhoids.*

**Hermolepsin** *Orion, Swed.*
Carbamazepine (p.353·3).
*Alcohol withdrawal syndrome; epilepsy; trigeminal neuralgia.*

**Hernia-Tee** *Steierl, Ger.†.*
Bearberry (p.1659·2); herniaria (p.1697·1); equisetum (p.1684·1).
*Urinary-tract disorders.*

**Hernidisc** *Eagle, Austral.†.*
Homoeopathic preparation.

**Herniol** *Steierl, Ger.†.*
Bearberry (p.1659·2); herniaria (p.1697·1).
*Urinary-tract disorders.*

**Heroid** *Chew, Thai.*
Diosmin (p.1688·2); hesperidin (p.1688·2).
*Haemorrhoids; phlebitis; varicose veins; venous insufficiency.*

**Herolan Aerosol** *Laboratorios Chile, Chile.*
Beclometasone (p.1092·1); salbutamol (p.791·3).
*Obstructive airways disease.*

**Herpecin-L** *Chattem, USA.*
Allantoin (p.1141·3); padimate O (p.1155·1).
*Oral lesions.*

**Herpenon** *Polipharm, Thai.*
Aciclovir (p.626·1).
*Herpesvirus infections of the skin and mucous membranes.*

**Herpes Soothing Cream** *Homeocan, Canad.*
Homoeopathic preparation.

**Herpesan**
*Rowa, Hong Kong; Rowa, Malaysia; Rowa, Singapore.*
Carbenoxolone sodium (p.1254·3).
*Mouth ulcers; orofacial lesions.*

**Herpes-Gastreu R68** *Reckeweg, Ger.*
Homoeopathic preparation.

**Herpes-Gel** *Master Pharma, Ital.†.*
Ibacitabine (p.637·3).
*Herpesvirus infections.*

**Herpesil** *Hexal, Braz.*
Aciclovir (p.626·1).
*Herpesvirus infections.*

**Herpesine** *Nikkho, Braz.*
Idoxuridine (p.637·3).
*Herpesvirus skin infections.*

**Herpesnil** *Sofar, Ital.†.*
Aciclovir (p.626·1).
*Herpesvirus infections.*

**Herpetad**
*TAD, Ger.; Boehringer Ingelheim, UK.*
Aciclovir (p.626·1).
*Herpes simplex infections.*

**Herpetrol** *Alva, USA.*
Multivitamin preparation with zinc and lysine (p.1417·1).

**Herpex**
*Note. This name is used for preparations of different composition.*
*Pharmacia, Braz.*
Tromantadine hydrochloride (p.656·1).
*Viral skin infections.*
*Torrent, India.*
Aciclovir (p.626·1).
*Herpesvirus infections.*

**Herphonal** *Temmler, Ger.*
Trimipramine maleate (p.320·2).
*Depression; pain.*

**Herpid** *Yamanouchi, UK.*
Idoxuridine (p.637·3) in dimethyl sulfoxide.
*Herpesvirus skin infections.*

**Herpidu**
*Ciba Vision, Hong Kong†; Ciba Vision, Thai.†.*
Idoxuridine (p.637·3).
*Herpes simplex infections of the eye.*

**Herpilem** *Lemery, Mex.*
Aciclovir (p.626·1).
*Herpesvirus infections.*

**Herplex**
*Allergan, Canad.; Allergan, Hong Kong†.*
Idoxuridine (p.637·3).
*Herpes simplex infections.*

**Herplex-D** *Allergan, Austral.†.*
Idoxuridine (p.637·3).
*Herpes simplex skin infections.*

**Herpofug** *Wolff, Ger.†.*
Aciclovir (p.626·1).
*Herpesvirus infections.*

**Herpolips** *Berner, Fin.*
Aciclovir (p.626·1).
*Herpes labialis.*

**Herpomed** *S Med, Austria.*
Aciclovir (p.626·1).
*Herpes labialis.*

**Herposicc** *Medicopharm, Austria.*
Benzocaine (p.1370·3); sulfur (p.1158·2); zinc oxide (p.1163·2); talc (p.1159·1); phenol (p.1188·1).
*Herpes labialis.*

**Herpotern** *Rentschler, Ger.†.*
Aciclovir sodium (p.626·1).
*Herpes and varicella virus infections.*

**Herpoviric** *Azupharma, Ger.†.*
Aciclovir (p.626·1).
*Herpesvirus infections.*

**Herron Baby Teething Gel** *Herron, Austral.*
Choline salicylate (p.26·2).
*Sore gums; teething pain.*

**Herten** *Vir, Spain.*
Enalapril maleate (p.909·2).
*Heart failure; hypertension.*

**Herviros**
*Hermal, Austria; Hermal, Ger.; Hermal, Hong Kong†.*
Tetracaine hydrochloride (p.1385·1); aminoquinuride hydrochloride (p.1168·2).
*Infected mouth disorders.*

**Herz ASS** *Lannacher, Austria.*
Aspirin (p.15·1).
*Ischaemic heart disease; myocardial infarction.*

**Herz- und Kreislauftonikum Bioflora** *Bioflora, Austria.*
Crataegus (p.1677·1); mistletoe (p.1715·3); melissa (p.1711·1); rosemary (p.1740·2); lavender flower (p.1705·1).
*Cardiovascular disorders.*

**HerzASS** *Ratiopharm, Ger.*
Aspirin (p.15·1).
*Thrombosis prophylaxis.*

**Herzkur** *Chrispa (Χρισπα), Gr.*
Aciclovir (p.626·1).
*Herpes simplex infections.*

**Herz-Punkt Starkungstonikum mit Ginseng N** *Herzpunkt, Ger.†.*
Ginseng (p.1693·1).
*Tonic.*

**Herz-Punkt Vitaltonikum N** *Herzpunkt, Ger.†.*
Crataegus; melissa; ferrous gluconate (p.1417·1).
*Tonic.*

**Herz-Starkung N** *Jukunda, Ger.*
Crataegus (p.1677·1); lycopus virg.; cactus; kalmia latifolia; camphora.
*Cardiac disorders.*

**Herztropfen CM** *Cosmochema, Ger.*
Homoeopathic preparation.

**Herz-Tropfen Eu Rho** *Eu Rho, Ger.†.*
Crataegus (p.1677·1).
*Cardiac disorders.*

**Herztropfen Truw Gold** *Truw, Ger.†.*
Homoeopathic preparation.

**Hespan**
*Geistlich, UK†; Du Pont, USA.*
Hetastarch (p.750·1) in sodium chloride.
*Extracorporeal circulation; leucopheresis; plasma volume expansion.*

**Hespander**
*Kyorin, Jpn; Kyorin, Thai.*
Hetastarch (p.750·1) in glucose with electrolytes.
*Haemodiluent; haemorrhage; plasma volume expansion.*

**Hespercorbin** *Fides Ecopharma, Spain.*
Glucosamine sulfate (p.1694·1).
*Osteoarthritis.*

**Hesteril**
*Fresenius Kabi, Fr.; Fresenius Kabi, Spain.*
Pentastarch (p.750·1).
*Haemodilution; plasma volume expansion.*

**Hetaclox** *Faran, Gr.*
Cefaclor (p.167·1).
*Bacterial infections.*

**Hetacloxacin** *Faran, Gr.*
Ofloxacin (p.239·3).
*Bacterial infections.*

**Heteroid** *Chew, Thai.*
Diosmin (p.1688·2).
*Haemorrhoids; phlebitis; varicose veins; venous insufficiency.*

**Hetrazan**
*Wyeth-Ayerst, Canad.†; IFET (ΙΦΕΤ), Gr.; Wyeth Lederle, India; Lederle, UK†.*
Diethylcarbamazine citrate (p.104·1).
*Worm infections.*

**Hetrogalen** *Galenika, Ger.†.*
Hedera helix.
*Catarrh.*

**Hettytropin** *Elvetium, Arg.*
Dopamine hydrochloride (p.907·1).
*Heart failure.*

**Heumann Abfuhrtee Solubilax N** *Sanofi Synthelabo, Ger.*
Senna (p.1288·2); frangula bark (p.1266·3).
*Constipation.*

**Heumann Beruhigungstee Tenerval N** *Sanofi Synthelabo, Ger.*
Valerian root (p.1762·2); melissa (p.1711·1); valerian oil.
*Nervous disorders.*

**Heumann Blasen- und Nierentee Solubitrat S** *Sanofi Synthelabo, Ger.*
Java tea (p.1702·3); solidago virgaurea (p.1748·3); birch leaf (p.1660·3).
*Urinary-tract disorders.*

**Heumann Bronchialtee Solubifix** *Sanofi Synthelabo, Ger.*
Althaea (p.1651·3); liquorice (p.1270·2); primula root (p.1735·1); anise oil (p.1655·2); thyme oil (p.1755·3).
*Respiratory-tract disorders.*

**Heumann Leber- und Gallentee Solu-Hepar S** *Sanofi Synthelabo, Ger.*
Boldo (p.1661·2); silybum marianum (p.1043·3); peppermint oil (p.1283·2).
*Digestive disorders.*

**Heumann Magentee Solu-Vetan** *Sanofi Synthelabo, Ger.*
Liquorice root (p.1270·2); peppermint leaf (p.1283·2); peppermint oil (p.1283·2).
*Gastrointestinal disorders.*

**Heumann's Bronchialtee** *Sanova, Austria.*
Althaea (p.1651·3); liquorice (p.1270·2); primula root (p.1735·1); anise oil (p.1655·2); thyme oil (p.1755·3).
*Bronchitis; catarrh; coughs.*

**Heuschnupfenmittel**
*DHU, Ger.; Dreluso, Ger.*
Homoeopathic preparation.

**Heuschnupfenmittel DHU** *Peithner, Austria.*
Homoeopathic preparation.

**Heusin** *Riemser, Ger.*
Aesculus (p.1648·2); mistletoe (p.1715·3); crataegus (p.1677·1); hamamelis (p.1696·3); arnica (p.1656·3); silybum marianum (p.1043·3).
*Peripheral vascular disorders.*

**Hevac B** *Pasteur Merieux, Braz.†.*
A hepatitis B vaccine (recombinant) (p.1618·1).
*Active immunisation.*

**Hevert Enzym Novo** *Hevert, Ger.†.*
Dimethicone (p.1289·2); pancreatin (p.1725·3); trypsin (p.1758·3).
Hevert Enzym formerly contained thiamine hydrochloride, cholesterol, dimethicone, fel tauri, folic acid, pancreatin, papain, riboflavin, and trypsin.
*Digestive system disorders.*

**Hevert-Aktivon Mono** *Hevert, Ger.*
Ginseng (p.1693·1).
*Tonic.*

**Hevert-Blasen-Nieren-Tee N** *Hevert, Ger.*
Java tea (p.1702·3); birch leaf (p.1660·3); equisetum (p.1684·1); ononis (p.1723·3); couch-grass (p.1676·2).
*Urinary-tract disorders.*

**Hevert-Card forte** *Hevert, Ger.†.*
Herbal and homoeopathic preparation.

**Hevert-Carmin symbio** *Hevert, Ger.†.*
Vegetable charcoal (p.1030·3); aniseed (p.1655·2); caraway (p.1667·2); anise oil (p.1655·2); caraway oil (p.1667·3); fennel oil (p.1687·3); peppermint oil (p.1283·2).
*Gastrointestinal disorders.*

**Hevert-Dorm** *Hevert, Ger.*
Diphenhydramine hydrochloride (p.431·3).
*Sleep disorders.*

**Hevert-Entwasserungs-Tee** *Hevert, Ger.†.*
Pterocarpus santalinus; rosemary (p.1740·2); juniper (p.1703·1); asparagus; lovage (p.1708·1); ononis (p.1723·3); taraxacum (p.1751·3); rose fruit (p.1740·1); calendula (p.1665·2); squill (p.1130·3); birch leaf (p.1660·3); buchu (p.1663·1); centaurea cyanus.
*Cystitis; oedema; renal calculi.*

**Hevert-Enzym Plus** *Hevert, Ger.*
Dimeticone (p.1289·2); pancreas extract.
*Digestive disorders.*

**Hevert-Erkaltungs-Tee** *Hevert, Ger.†.*
Sambucus (p.1741·3); thyme (p.1755·2); salix bark (p.87·3).
*Cold symptoms.*

**Hevert-Gall S** *Hevert, Ger.†.*
Greater celandine (p.1695·3); cnicus benedictus (p.1673·3); chamomile (p.1669·3); taraxacum (p.1751·3); caraway oil (p.1667·3); peppermint oil (p.1283·2); boldo (p.1661·2); calamus (p.1664·1); silybum marianum (p.1043·3); turmeric (p.1058·3).
*Biliary disorders; duodenal disorders; liver disorders.*

**Hevert-Gicht-Rheuma-Tee comp** *Hevert, Ger.†.*
Salix (p.87·3); sambucus (p.1741·3); birch leaf (p.1660·3); juniper (p.1703·1); achillea (p.1646·2); liquorice (p.1270·2); ononis (p.1723·3).
*Rheumatic disorders.*

**Hevertigon** *Hevert, Ger.*
Homoeopathic preparation.

**Hevert-Mag** *Hevert, Ger.*
Magaldrate (p.1271·3).
*Gastric hyperacidity; heartburn; peptic ulcer.*

**Hevert-Magen-Galle-Leber-Tee** *Hevert, Ger.†.*
Calendula (p.1665·2); fennel (p.1687·2); absinthium (p.1645·1); centaurea (p.1669·2); greater celandine (p.1695·3); chichory; achillea (p.1646·2); thyme (p.1755·2); calamus (p.1664·1).
*Digestive system disorders.*

**Hevert-Migrane** *Hevert, Ger.*
Homoeopathic preparation.

**Hevert-Nerv plus Eisen** *Hevert, Ger.†.*
Minerals; kola; ginseng; iron phosphate; lecithin (p.1417·1).
*Tonic.*

**Hevert-Nier II** *Hevert, Ger.†.*
Homoeopathic preparation.

**Hevertnier Complex** *Hevert, Ger.*
Homoeopathic preparation.

**Hevertnier spasmo** *Hevert, Ger.†.*
Homoeopathic preparation.

**Hevertogyn** *Hevert, Ger.*
Agnus castus (p.1649·1).
*Mastalgia; menstrual disorders.*

**Hevertolax duo** *Hevert, Ger.*
Frangula bark (p.1266·3); senna (p.1288·2).
*Constipation.*

**Hevertolax Phyto** *Hevert, Ger.†.*
Senna fruit (p.1288·2).
*Constipation.*

**Hevertopect N** *Hevert, Ger.*
Anise oil (p.1655·2); eucalyptus oil (p.1686·2); fennel oil (p.1687·3); peppermint oil (p.1283·2); pumilio pine oil (p.1737·1); turpentine oil (p.1760·1); eucalyptus (p.1686·1); thyme (p.1755·2); verbascum (p.1764·1).
Hevertopect formerly contained anise oil, eucalyptus oil, fennel oil, peppermint oil, pumilio pine oil, turpentine oil, eucalyptus, thyme, verbascum, ammi visnaga, and ephedrine hydrochloride.
*Respiratory-tract disorders.*

**Hevertotox** *Hevert, Ger.*
Homoeopathic preparation.

**Hevertoval mono** *Hevert, Ger.*
Homoeopathic preparation.

**Hevertozym** *Hevert, Ger.*
Pancreatin (p.1725·3).
*Pancreatic insufficiency.*

**Hevert-Vitan N** *Hevert, Ger.†.*
Multivitamin and mineral preparation (p.1417·1).
*Calcium and vitamin deficiency.*

**Hewallergia** *Hevert, Ger.*
Homoeopathic preparation.

**Heweberberol-Tee** *Hevert, Ger.*
Birch leaf (p.1660·3); solidago virgaurea (p.1748·3); ononis (p.1723·3); java tea (p.1702·3); pterocarpus santalinus; liquorice root (p.1270·2).
*Urinary-tract disorders.*

**Hewechol Artischockendragees** *Hevert, Ger.*
Cynara (p.1678·3).
*Dyspepsia.*

**Hewedolor forte** *Hevert, Ger.†.*
Sodium salamidacetate (p.87·3).
*Nerve pain.*

**Hewedolor N** *Hevert, Ger.*
Methyl salicylate (p.59·3).
Hewedolor formerly contained rhus toxicodendron, capsicum, and methyl salicylate.
*Neuromuscular disorders; peri-articular and soft-tissue disorders.*

**Hewedolor neuro** *Hevert, Ger.*
Thiamine hydrochloride (p.1455·1); pyridoxine hydrochloride (p.1456·3); lidocaine hydrochloride (p.1377·3).
*Nerve pain.*

**Hewedolor plus Coffein** *Hevert, Ger.*
Procaine hydrochloride (p.1383·2); caffeine (p.782·1).
*Nerve pain.*

**Hewedolor Procain** *Hevert, Ger.*
Procaine hydrochloride (p.1383·2).
*Pain.*

**Hewedolor propy** *Hevert, Ger.*
Propyphenazone (p.85·3).
*Fever; pain.*

**Hewedormir** *Hevert, Ger.†.*
Valerian (p.1762·2).
*Nervousness; sleep disorders.*

**Hewedormir doxyl intens** *Hevert, Ger.*
Doxylamine succinate (p.432·3).
Formerly known as Hewedormir forte.
*Anxiety; hypersensitivity reactions; sleep disorders.*

**Heweformica** *Hevert, Ger.†.*
Homoeopathic preparation.

**Heweginkgo** *Hevert, Ger.*
Homoeopathic preparation.

**Hewekliman** *Hevert, Ger.*
Homoeopathic preparation.

**Hewekzem novo N** *Hevert, Ger.*
Chamomile oil (p.1669·3); dexpanthenol (p.1727·2); vitamin A palmitate (p.1453·1); alpha tocoferil acetate (p.1465·1).
*Skin disorders.*

**Hewelymphon N** *Hevert, Ger.*
Homoeopathic preparation.

**Hewenephron duo** *Hevert, Ger.*
Solidago virgaurea (p.1748·3); echinacea (p.1683·2).
*Renal calculi.*

**Heweneural** *Hevert, Ger.*
Lidocaine hydrochloride (p.1377·3).
*Migraine; neuromuscular disorders.*

**Hewepsychon duo** *Hevert, Ger.*
Kava (p.1703·2); hypericum (p.299·1).
*Depression; dystonias; hypertension; menopausal disorders; migraine; nocturnal enuresis; tonic.*

**Hewepsychon Mono** *Hevert, Ger.*
Homoeopathic preparation.

**Hewepsychon uno** *Hevert, Ger.*
Hypericum (p.299·1).
*Anxiety; depression.*

**Hewerheum N** *Hevert, Ger.*
Homoeopathic preparation.

**Hewesabal comp** *Hevert, Ger.*
Homoeopathic preparation.

**Hewesabal mono** *Hevert, Ger.*
Homoeopathic preparation.

**Heweselen** *Hevert, Ger.*
Homoeopathic preparation.

**Hewethyreon** *Hevert, Ger.*
Homoeopathic preparation.

**Hewetraumen** *Hevert, Ger.*
Homoeopathic preparation.

**Heweurat** *Hevert, Ger.*
Homoeopathic preparation.

**Heweven P 3** *Hevert, Ger.†.*
Hamamelis (p.1696·3); aesculus (p.1648·2); aescin (p.1648·2).
*Vascular disorders.*

**Heweven P 7** *Hevert, Ger.†.*
Hamamelis (p.1696·3); aesculus (p.1648·2); aescin; aesculin; echinacea.
*Vascular disorders.*

**Heweven Phyto** *Hevert, Ger.*
Aesculus (p.1648·2).
*Haemorrhoids; venous insufficiency.*

**Hewletts** *Kestrel, UK.*
Zinc oxide (p.1163·2); hydrous wool fat (p.1483·2); arachis oil (p.1656·1); white soft paraffin (p.1479·3).
*Dry skin; nappy rash.*

**Hexa-Blok** *Hexal, S.Afr.*
Atenolol (p.865·2).
*Angina pectoris; hypertension.*

**Hexabotin** *Durascan, Denm.*
Erythromycin stearate (p.208·2).
*Bacterial infections.*

**Hexabrix**
*Temis, Arg.; Mallinckrodt, Austral.; Guerbet, Austria; Codali, Belg.; Guerbet, Braz.; Mallinckrodt, Canad.; Rider, Chile; Guerbet, Denm.; Guerbet, Fin.; Guerbet, Fr.; Guerbet, Ger.; R+N, Gr.; Guerbet, Israel; Guerbet, Ital.; Guerbet, Neth.†; Guerbet, Norw.; Biotek, NZ; Guerbet, Port.; Guerbet, Spain; Gothia, Swed.; Guerbet, Switz.; May & Baker, UK; Mallinckrodt, USA.*
Meglumine ioxaglate (p.1066·2); sodium ioxaglate (p.1066·2).
*Radiographic contrast medium.*

**Hexacortone** *Spirig, Switz.*
Prednisolone acetate (p.1108·1).
*Skin disorders.*

**Hexacroman** *Durascan, Denm.*
Sodium cromoglicate (p.795·3).
*Allergic conjunctivitis.*

**Hexa-Defital** *Labinca, Arg.*
*Lotion:* Lindane (p.1506·3); benzocaine (p.1370·3).
*Pediculosis; scabies.*
*Shampoo:* Lindane (p.1506·3).
*Pediculosis.*

**Hexa-Defital NF** *Labinca, Arg.*
Deltamethrin (p.1503·1); piperonyl butoxide (p.1509·2).
*Pediculosis.*

**Hexadilat** *Durascan, Denm.*
Nifedipine (p.966·2).
*Angina pectoris; hypertension; Raynaud's syndrome.*

**Hexadrol**
*Organon Teknika, Canad.; Organon, USA.*
Dexamethasone (p.1097·1) or dexamethasone sodium phosphate (p.1097·2).
*Corticosteroid.*

**Hexafen** *EMS, Braz.*
Deltamethrin (p.1503·1).
*Scabies.*

**Hexafene** *Vifor, Switz.†.*
Inositol nicotinate (p.939·3); buclizine hydrochloride (p.426·3); hydroxyzine hydrochloride (p.434·3).
*Vertigo.*

**Hexafluid** *Diepha, Fr.†.*
Carbocisteine (p.1116·2).
*Respiratory-tract congestion.*

**Hexagastron** *Durascan, Denm.*
Sucralfate (p.1290·2).
*Gastro-oesophageal reflux; peptic ulcer.*

**Hexaglucon** *Durascan, Denm.*
Glibenclamide (p.331·2).
*Diabetes mellitus.*

**Hexakapron** *Teva, Israel.*
Tranexamic acid (p.760·3).
*Haemorrhage.*

**Hexal Comfarol Plus** *Hexal, Austral.*
Paracetamol (p.76·2); codeine phosphate (p.27·1).
*Fever; pain.*

**Hexal Compufen** *Hexal, Austral.*
Ibuprofen (p.45·3).

**Hexal Konazol Shampoo** *Hexal, Austral.*
Ketoconazole (p.403·3).
*Dandruff; seborrhoeic dermatitis.*

**Hexalacton** *Durascan, Denm.*
Spironolactone (p.1003·1).
*Ascites; hyperaldosteronism; oedema.*

**Hexalectol** *Rider, Chile.*
Glutamic acid (p.1433·2); pyridoxine (p.1457·2).
*Mental function impairment.*

**Hexalen**
*Note. This name is used for preparations of different composition.*
*Mayne, Austral.; Lilly, Canad.†; US Bio, Israel†; Medimmune, Norw.; Baxter, NZ; Faulding, NZ; Swedish Orphan, Swed.; Ipsen, UK†; MGI, USA.*
Altretamine (p.526·2).
*Ovarian cancer.*

*Lavipharm, Gr.*
Hexetidine (p.1182·1).
*Mouth infections.*

**Hexalense** *Ioltech, Fr.*
Aminocaproic acid (p.741·3).
*Eye irritation.*

**Hexalid** *Durascan, Denm.*
Diazepam (p.690·1).
*Alcohol withdrawal syndrome; anxiety; spasticity.*

**Hexalyse**
*Bouchara-Recordati, Fr.; Bouchara-Recordati, Hong Kong.*
Biclotymol (p.1171·1); muramidase hydrochloride (p.1717·2); enoxolone (p.36·2).
*Mouth and throat disorders.*

**Hexamet** *Hexal, S.Afr.*
Cimetidine (p.1255·3).
*Gastro-oesophageal reflux; peptic ulcer; Zollinger-Ellison syndrome.*

**Hexamon** *Schoning-Berlin, Ger.*
Hexylresorcinol (p.1182·1); lauromacrogol 400 (p.1412·3).
*Anorectal disorders.*

**Hexamycin** *Durascan, Denm.*
Gentamicin sulfate (p.217·1).
*Bacterial infections.*

**Hexanicit**
*Promed, Ger.†; Astra, Swed.†.*
Inositol nicotinate (p.939·3).
*Hyperlipidaemias; peripheral and central circulatory disorders.*

**Hexanios G+R** *Anios, Fr.*
Polihexanide (p.1190·1); didecyldimethylammonium chloride (p.1178·3).
*Instrument disinfection.*

**Hexanitrat** *Hexal, Austria.*
Isosorbide dinitrate (p.941·1).
*Angina pectoris; heart failure; myocardial infarction; pulmonary hypertension.*

**Hexanium** *Fides Ecopharma, Spain†.*
Emepronium bromide (p.482·1).
*Urinary-tract disorders.*

**Hexanurat** *Durascan, Denm.*
Allopurinol (p.412·2).
*Gout.*

**Hexaphane**
*Biorga, Fr.†; Saninter, Port.†.*
Gelatin; cystine; zinc gluconate; vitamin B substances (p.1417·1).
*Fragile hair and nails.*

**Hexaphenyl** *Ingram & Bell, Canad.†.*
Hexachlorophene sodium (p.1181·3).
*Disinfection.*

**Hexapindol**
*Durascan, Denm.; Tika, Norw.†; Tika, Swed.†.*
Pindolol (p.983·2).
*Angina pectoris; arrhythmias; hypertension; myocardial infarction.*

**Hexapneumine**
*Note. This name is used for preparations of different composition.*
*Bouchara-Recordati, Fr.*
*Adult suppositories; paediatric suppositories:* Biclotymol (p.1171·1); cineole (p.1672·1); pholcodine (p.1128·3).
Formerly contained biclotymol, cineole, pholcodine, and paracetamol.
*Coughs.*
*Adult syrup; paediatric syrup:* Biclotymol (p.1171·1); chlorphenamine maleate (p.427·3); pholcodine (p.1128·3).
Formerly contained biclotymol, chlorphenamine maleate, guaifenesin, and pholcodine.
*Coughs.*
*Infant suppositories:* Biclotymol (p.1171·1); cineole (p.1672·1).
Formerly contained biclotymol, cineole, and paracetamol.
*Respiratory-tract disorders.*
*Infant syrup:* Biclotymol (p.1171·1); chlorphenamine maleate (p.427·3); tolu balsam (p.1131·3).
Formerly contained biclotymol, chlorphenamine maleate, guaifenesin, paracetamol, and tolu balsam.
*Coughs.*
*Tablets:* Biclotymol (p.1171·1); chlorphenamine maleate (p.427·3); phenylephrine hydrochloride (p.1126·3).
*Nasal congestion.*

*Bouchara-Recordati, Hong Kong.*
*Adult syrup; paediatric syrup:* Biclotymol (p.1171·1); chlorphenamine maleate (p.427·3); guaifenesin (p.1122·1); pholcodine (p.1128·3).
*Coughs.*
*Infant syrup:* Biclotymol (p.1171·1); chlorphenamine maleate (p.427·3); guaifenesin (p.1122·1); paracetamol (p.76·2); tolu balsam (p.1131·3).
*Coughs; fever.*

*Doms-Adrian, Hong Kong.*
*Tablets:* Biclotymol (p.1171·1); chlorphenamine maleate (p.427·3); phenylephrine hydrochloride (p.1126·3).
*Nasal congestion.*

**Hexapress** *Durascan, Denm.*
Prazosin hydrochloride (p.985·1).
*Heart failure; hypertension; Raynaud's syndrome.*

**Hexaquart L** *Braun, Ger.*
Didecyldimethylammonium chloride (p.1178·3); benzalkonium chloride (p.1168·3).
*Surface disinfection.*

**Hexaquart plus** *Braun, Ger.*
Didecyldimethylammonium chloride (p.1178·3); laurydipropylene triamine; biguanidinium acetate.
*Surface and instrument disinfection.*

**Hexaquart S** *Braun, Ger.*
Didecyldimethylammonium chloride (p.1178·3); benzalkonium chloride (p.1168·3).
*Fungal skin infection prophylaxis; surface disinfection.*

**Hexaquine** *Gomenol, Fr.*
Quinine benzoate (p.462·1); thiamine hydrochloride (p.1455·1); niaouli oil (p.1719·3).
*Muscle cramps.*

**Hexaretic** *Hexal, S.Afr.*
Amiloride (p.858·3); hydrochlorothiazide (p.933·2).
*Hypertension; oedema.*

**Hexarone** *Hexal, S.Afr.*
Amiodarone hydrochloride (p.859·2).
*Arrhythmias.*

**Hexaseptine** *Gifrer Barbezat, Fr.*
Hexamidine isetionate (p.1181·3).
*Bacterial skin infections; skin and mucous membrane disinfection.*

**Hexasoptin** *Durascan, Denm.*
Verapamil hydrochloride (p.1019·1).
*Angina pectoris; arrhythmias; hypertension; myocardial infarction.*

**Hexaspray**
*Bouchara-Recordati, Fr.; Bouchara-Recordati, Hong Kong.*
Biclotymol (p.1171·1).
*Mouth and throat disorders.*

**Hexastat**
*Bellon, Fr.†; Rhone-Poulenc Rorer, Hong Kong†; Rhone-Poulenc Rorer, Ital.†; Rhone-Poulenc Rorer, Norw.†.*
Altretamine (p.526·2).
*Malignant neoplasms.*

**Hexatin** *Agepha, Austria.*
Hexetidine (p.1182·1).
*Mouth and throat inflammation.*

**Hexatrione** *Wyeth Lederle, Fr.*
Triamcinolone hexacetonide (p.1110·2).
*Musculoskeletal and joint disorders.*

**Hexavac**
*Aventis Pasteur, Arg.; Aventis Pasteur, Fr.; Aventis Pasteur, Ger.; Vianex (Βιανεξ), Gr.; Aventis Pasteur, Ital.; Aventis Pasteur, Spain; Pro Vaccine, Switz.*
A diphtheria, tetanus, pertussis, poliomyelitis, hepatitis B, and haemophilus influenzae vaccine (p.1614·3).
*Active immunisation.*

**Hexavitamin** *Upsher-Smith, USA.*
Multivitamin preparation (p.1417·1).

**Hexavitamins** *Novopharm, Canad.*
Multivitamin preparation (p.1417·1).

**Hexazide** *Hexal, S.Afr.*
Hydrochlorothiazide (p.933·2).
*Hypertension; oedema.*

**Hexene** *Osoth, Thai.*
Chlorhexidine gluconate (p.1173·2).
*Skin disinfection.*

**Hexiben Plus** *Sidus, Arg.*
Urea hydrogen peroxide (p.1195·3); sodium monofluorophosphate (p.1446·2).
*Dental whitener.*

**Hexide** *Milano, Thai.*
Chlorhexidine gluconate (p.1173·2).
*Antiseptic lubricant for vaginal examination.*

**Hexident** *Ipex, Swed.*
Chlorhexidine gluconate (p.1173·2).
*Mouth disinfection; oral hygiene.*

**Hexidin**
Note. This name is used for preparations of different composition.
Barnes Hind, Arg.
Chlorhexidine gluconate (p.1173·2) (p.1164·2).
*Disinfecting solution for soft contact lenses.*

Genericon, Austria; Nycomed, Norw.†.
Chlorhexidine gluconate (p.1173·2).
*Mouth and throat infections; oral hygiene.*

Fischer, Israel†.
Chlorhexidine gluconate (p.1173·2); thiomersal (p.1194·1)(p.1164·2).
*Disinfecting solution for soft contact lenses.*

**Hexifluor** Warner-Lambert, Port.†.
Hexetidine (p.1182·1).

**Hexil** Inmunolab, Arg.
Chlorhexidine (p.1173·2).
*Disinfection.*

**Hexilium** Pharmasant, Thai.
Flunarizine (p.434·2).
*Cerebral and peripheral vascular disorders; vestibular disorders.*

**Hexinawas** Wasserman, Spain†.
Altretamine (p.526·2).
*Lung cancer; ovarian cancer.*

**Hexit** Odan, Canad.
Lindane (p.1506·3).
*Pediculosis; scabies.*

**Hexobion** Merck, Ger.
Pyridoxine hydrochloride (p.1456·3).
*Vitamin $B_6$ deficiency.*

**Hexogen** Antigen, Irl.
Inositol nicotinate (p.939·3).
*Peripheral and cerebral vascular disorders.*

**Hexo-Imotryl** Cassenne, Fr.†.
Benzydamine hydrochloride (p.21·1); hexamidine isetionate (p.1181·3).
*Mouth and throat disorders.*

**Hexokain** Nycomed, Denm.
Benzocaine (p.1370·3); chlorhexidine hydrochloride (p.1173·3).
*Mouth disorders; oral hygiene.*

**Hexol**
Sigma, Austral.; Sigma, Hong Kong; Pharmaland, Thai.
Chlorhexidine gluconate (p.1173·2).
*Skin disinfection.*

**Hexoll** Asta Medica, Neth.†.
Acetic acid (p.1645·2); citric acid (p.1673·1).
*Pediculosis.*

**Hexolvon** Raza, Malaysia; Pharmaniaga, Malaysia.
Bromhexine hydrochloride (p.1115·3).
*Coughs.*

**Hexomedin** Aventis, Spain.
Hexamidine isetionate (p.1181·3).
*Burns; skin infections; wounds.*

**Hexomedin N** Nattermann, Ger.
Hexamidine isetionate (p.1181·3).
*Acne; paronychia.*

**Hexomedine**
Note. This name is used for preparations of different composition.
Aventis, Belg.; Theraplix, Fr.; Rhone-Poulenc Rorer, Neth.†; Rhone-Poulenc Rorer, Switz.†.
Hexamidine isetionate (p.1181·3).
*Infected skin disorders.*

Aventis, Braz.; Theraplix, Fr.
*Throat spray:* Hexamidine isetionate (p.1181·3); tetracaine hydrochloride (p.1385·1).
*Mouth and throat disorders.*

**Hexopal**
Sanofi Synthelabo, Irl.; Sanofi Synthelabo, UK.
Inositol nicotinate (p.939·3).
*Intermittent claudication; Raynaud's syndrome.*

**Hexoral**
Pfizer, Austria; Pfizer Consumer, Ger.
Hexetidine (p.1182·1).
*Mouth and throat disorders.*

**Hexoraletten N** Pfizer Consumer, Ger.
Chlorhexidine hydrochloride (p.1173·3); benzocaine (p.1370·3).
*Mouth and throat disorders.*

**Hextril**
Pfizer Consumer, Belg.; Pfizer Sante, Fr.; Warner-Lambert, Neth.; Pfizer Consumer, Port.; Pfizer Lambert, Spain; Pfizer, Switz.
Hexetidine (p.1182·1).
*Mouth and throat disorders.*

**Hextriletten** Pfizer, Switz.
Cetylpyridinium chloride (p.1173·1); dichlorobenzyl alcohol (p.1178·3); lidocaine hydrochloride (p.1377·3).
*Sore throat.*

**HF**
Fresenius, Braz.†; Fresenius Medical, Switz.
A range of electrolyte infusions with or without glucose (p.1221·1).
*Haemofiltration.*

**HF-BIC35+HF-EL010** Dicamed, Swed.
Sodium chloride; sodium bicarbonate; calcium chloride; magnesium chloride; glucose (p.1221·1).
*Haemofiltration.*

**HF-BIC35+HF-EL210** Dicamed, Swed.
Sodium chloride; sodium bicarbonate; calcium chloride; magnesium chloride; potassium chloride; glucose (p.1221·1).
*Haemofiltration.*

**HHT** Sidus, Arg.
Somatropin (p.1327·2).
*Cachexia; growth disorders in renal failure; growth hormone deficiency; Turner's syndrome.*

**Hi Potency B Compound** Swiss Herbal, Canad.
Vitamin B substances (p.1417·1).

**Hi Potency Cal** Swiss Herbal, Canad.
Calcium carbonate (p.1254·2).

**Hi Potency $KIB_6$** Swiss Herbal, Canad.
Pyridoxine hydrochloride (p.1456·3).

**Hi Potency Multi-Mineral** Swiss Herbal, Canad.
Mineral and trace element preparation (p.1417·1).

**Hi Potency Stress B with C** Lee-Adams, Canad.
Vitamin B substances; vitamin C (p.1417·1).

**Hialid**
Santen, Hong Kong; Santen, Singapore.
Sodium hyaluronate (p.1697·3).
*Keratoconjunctival epithelial disorders.*

**HIB Merieux** Pasteur Merieux, Ger.†.
A haemophilus influenzae conjugate vaccine (diphtheria toxoid conjugate) (p.1616·1).
*Active immunisation.*

**HIB-DPT** Pasteur Merieux, Ger.†.
A diphtheria, tetanus, pertussis and haemophilus influenzae vaccine (p.1614·2).
*Active immunisation.*

**HIB-DT** Pasteur Merieux, Ger.†.
A diphtheria, tetanus, and haemophilus influenzae vaccine (p.1613·3).
*Active immunisation.*

**Hiberix**
GlaxoSmithKline, Austral.; GlaxoSmithKline, Austria; GlaxoSmithKline, Belg.; GlaxoSmithKline, Braz.; GlaxoSmithKline, Fin.; SmithKline Beecham, Gr.; GlaxoSmithKline, Hong Kong; GlaxoSmithKline, India; GlaxoSmithKline, Irl.; GlaxoSmithKline, Ital.; GlaxoSmithKline, Malaysia; GlaxoSmithKline, NZ; GlaxoSmithKline, S.Afr.; GlaxoSmithKline, Singapore; GlaxoSmithKline, Spain; SmithKline Beecham, Switz.; GlaxoSmithKline, Thai.; GlaxoSmithKline, UK.
A haemophilus influenzae conjugate vaccine (tetanus toxoid conjugate) (p.1616·1).
*Active immunisation.*

**Hibernal** Aventis, Swed.
Chlorpromazine embonate (p.675·1) or chlorpromazine hydrochloride (p.675·2).
*Adjunct to analgesia; psychoses.*

**HIBest** Pasteur Vaccins, Fr.†.
A haemophilus influenzae conjugate vaccine (tetanus protein conjugate) (p.1616·1).
*Active immunisation.*

**Hibicet**
AstraZeneca, Austral.†; SSL, Irl.; Zeneca, Ital.†; SSL, Malaysia; AstraZeneca, NZ†; Zeneca, S.Afr.; SSL, Thai.; SSL, UK.
Chlorhexidine gluconate (p.1173·2); cetrimide (p.1172·1).
Formerly known as Savlon Hospital Concentrate in the UK.
*Disinfection.*

**Hibicet concentraat** AstraZeneca, Neth.†.
Chlorhexidine gluconate (p.1173·2); cetrimide (p.1172·1).
Formerly known as Savlon.
*Disinfection.*

**Hibicet Hospital Concentrate**
SSL, Hong Kong; AstraZeneca, Singapore†.
Chlorhexidine gluconate (p.1173·2); cetrimide (p.1172·1).
*Disinfection.*

**Hibicet verdunning** AstraZeneca, Neth.†.
Chlorhexidine gluconate (p.1173·2); cetrimide (p.1172·1).
Formerly known as Savlodil.
*Disinfection.*

**Hibiclens**
Zeneca, Austral.†; AstraZeneca, NZ†; Zeneca, USA.
Chlorhexidine gluconate (p.1173·2).
*Skin disinfection.*

**Hibicol** Zeneca, Austral.†.
Chlorhexidine gluconate (p.1173·2); isopropyl alcohol (p.1184·3).
*Hand disinfection.*

**Hibicrick** Master, Chile.
Chlorhexidine hydrochloride (p.1173·3).
*Mouth and throat infections.*

**Hibident**
SmithKline Beecham, Austria; SmithKline Beecham Consumer, Belg.†.
Chlorhexidine gluconate (p.1173·2).
*Mouth infections; oral hygiene.*

**Hibidil**
Zeneca, Belg.†; AstraZeneca, Canad.; SSL, Fr.; Zeneca, S.Afr.; SSL, Switz.
Chlorhexidine gluconate (p.1173·2).
*Skin, mucous membrane, wound, and instrument disinfection.*

**Hibiguard** Zeneca, Belg.†.
Chlorhexidine gluconate (p.1173·2).
*Disinfection of hands and skin.*

**Hibimax** AstraZeneca, Spain.
Chlorhexidine gluconate (p.1173·2).
*Burns; instrument disinfection; skin disinfection; skin disorders; wounds.*

**Hibiscrub**
Zeneca, Belg.†; AstraZeneca, Chile; AstraZeneca, Fin.†; SSL, Fr.; SSL, Hong Kong; SSL, Irl.; Zeneca, Ital.†; SSL, Malaysia; Zeneca, Mex.; AstraZeneca, Neth.†; SSL, Norw.; Zeneca, Port.†; Zeneca, S.Afr.; AstraZeneca, Singapore†; AstraZeneca, Spain; SSL, Swed.; SSL, Switz.; SSL, Thai.; SSL, UK.
Chlorhexidine gluconate (p.1173·2).
*Skin disinfection.*

**Hibisol**
Note. This name is used for preparations of different composition.
SSL, Hong Kong; SSL, Irl.; AstraZeneca, Neth.†; AstraZeneca, Singapore†; SSL, UK.
Chlorhexidine gluconate (p.1173·2); isopropyl alcohol (p.1184·3).
*Skin disinfection.*

SSL, Malaysia.
Chlorhexidine gluconate (p.1173·2).
*Skin disinfection.*

**Hibisprint** SSL, Fr.
Chlorhexidine gluconate (p.1173·2).
*Skin disinfection.*

**Hibistat** Zeneca, USA.
Chlorhexidine gluconate (p.1173·2).
*Skin disinfection.*

**Hibital** SSL, Switz.
Chlorhexidine gluconate (p.1173·2); isopropyl alcohol (p.1184·3).
*Skin and hand disinfection.*

**Hibitane**
Note. This name is used for preparations of different composition.
Zeneca, Austral.†; Tramedico, Belg.; AstraZeneca, Braz.†; AstraZeneca, Canad.; Bioglan, Denm.; SSL, Fr.; SSL, Hong Kong; SSL, Irl.; SSL, Malaysia; Bioglan, Norw.; AstraZeneca, NZ; CS, Port.†; Genop, S.Afr.†; Zeneca, S.Afr.†; AstraZeneca, Singapore†; Bioglan, Singapore†; Bioglan, Swed.; SSL, Switz.; SSL, Thai.; Centrapharm, UK.
Chlorhexidine gluconate (p.1173·2).
*Gynaecological and obstetric lubricant and disinfectant; wound, skin, and instrument disinfection.*

Zeneca, Austral.†.
*Tincture:* Chlorhexidine gluconate (p.1173·2); isopropyl alcohol (p.1184·3).
*Skin disinfection.*

GlaxoSmithKline Consumer, Belg.
*Pastilles:* Chlorhexidine hydrochloride (p.1173·3); lidocaine hydrochloride (p.1377·3).
Formerly contained chlorhexidine hydrochloride and benzocaine.
*Mouth and throat disorders.*

SmithKline Beecham Consumer, Neth.
Chlorhexidine gluconate (p.1173·2) or chlorhexidine hydrochloride (p.1173·3).
*Mouth infections; skin and wound disinfection.*

GlaxoSmithKline Consumer, Port.; GlaxoSmithKline, Spain.
*Pastilles:* Chlorhexidine hydrochloride (p.1173·3); benzocaine (p.1370·3).
*Mouth and throat disorders.*

**Hibitane Menta** GlaxoSmithKline Consumer, Port.
Benzocaine (p.1370·3); chlorhexidine hydrochloride (p.1173·3); menthol (p.1711·3).
*Mouth and throat disorders.*

**Hibitane Teinture** SSL, Switz.
Chlorhexidine gluconate (p.1173·2); isopropyl alcohol (p.1184·3).
*Skin disinfection.*

**Hibizene** SSL, Ital.
Cetrimide (p.1172·1); chlorhexidine gluconate (p.1173·2).
*Disinfection of burns, wounds, and external genitalia.*

**Hibon** Mitsubishi-Tokyo, Hong Kong.
Riboflavin tetrabutyrate (p.1456·2).
*Vitamin $B_2$ deficiency.*

**Hiboquad** Eczane, Arg.
Chlorhexidine gluconate (p.1173·2).
*Disinfection.*

**Hibor** Rovi, Spain.
Bemiparin sodium (p.867·1).
*Thromboembolism prophylaxis.*

**HibTITER**
Wyeth, Austral.; Wyeth Lederle, Austria; Wyeth Lederle, Belg.; Wyeth, Braz.†; Wyeth-Ayerst, Canad.†; Wyeth Lederle, Denm.; Wyeth Lederle, Fin.; Wyeth, Ger.; Pharmaserve Lilly (Φαρμασερβ Λιλλυ), Gr.; Wyeth, Irl.; Lederle, Israel; Wyeth Lederle, Ital.; Wyeth, Mex.; Lederle, NZ; Wyeth Lederle, Port.; Wyeth, S.Afr.†; Wyeth, Singapore†; Wyeth, Spain; Wyeth Lederle, Swed.; Lederle, Switz.†; Wyeth, UK†; Lederle, USA.
A haemophilus influenzae conjugate vaccine (diphtheria $CRM_{197}$ protein conjugate) (p.1616·1).
*Active immunisation.*

**HIB-Vaccinol** Procter & Gamble, Ger.†.
A haemophilus influenzae conjugate vaccine (diphtheria toxoid conjugate) (p.1616·1).
*Active immunisation.*

**Hicarlex** Ferrer, Spain†.
Fosinopril sodium (p.919·1).
*Heart failure; hypertension.*

**Hicee** Takeda, Thai.
Ascorbic acid (p.1460·2).
*Vitamin C deficiency.*

**Hicin** Douglas, Austral.†.
Indometacin (p.47·3).
*Gout; inflammation; musculoskeletal, joint, peri-articular, and soft-tissue disorders; oedema; pain.*

**Hicomp** GHP, Thai.
Vitamin B substances with glucose (p.1417·1).
*Nutritional supplement.*

**Hiconcil**
Bristol-Myers Squibb, Belg.; Bristol-Myers Squibb, Braz.; UPSA, Fr.; Bristol-Myers Squibb, Israel.
Amoxicillin trihydrate (p.155·3).
*Bacterial infections.*

**Hiconcil-NS** Bristol-Myers Squibb, S.Afr.†.
Amoxicillin trihydrate (p.155·3); nystatin (p.406·3).
*Bacterial infections; candidiasis.*

**Hi-Cor** C & M, USA.
Hydrocortisone (p.1103·3).
*Skin disorders.*

**Hicoseen** Piraud, Switz.†.
Butamirate citrate (p.1116·2); dextromethorphan (p.1117·3); guaifenesin (p.1122·1).
*Bronchitis; coughs.*

**Hicoton** Medika, Ger.
Ferric saccharose complex (p.1438·2); calcium glycerophosphate (p.1225·2); rhus toxicodendron (p.1738·1); lupulus (p.1708·1); cinchona bark (p.1671·3); lecithin (p.1706·1); camphor monobromide.
*Urinary-tract disorders.*

**Hidalone** Schering-Plough, Port.
Hydrocortisone (p.1103·3).
*Skin disorders.*

**Hidantal** Aventis, Braz.
Phenytoin (p.370·2) or phenytoin sodium (p.370·2).
*Arrhythmias; epilepsy; neuralgia; skeletal muscle spasm.*

**Hidantil** Ofimex, Mex.†.
Phenytoin sodium (p.370·2).

**Hidantina** Vitoria, Port.
Phenytoin sodium (p.370·2).
*Epilepsy; neuralgia.*

**Hidantina Composta** Vitoria, Port.
Phenytoin sodium (p.370·2); phenobarbital (p.367·3).
*Epilepsy.*

**Hidantoina** Rudefsa, Mex.
Phenytoin (p.370·2) or phenytoin sodium (p.370·2).
*Epilepsy.*

**Hiderm** Baypharm, Austral.†.
Clotrimazole (p.396·2).
*Fungal skin and vulvovaginal infections.*

**Hidil**
Berlin Pharm, Singapore; Berlin Pharm, Thai.
Gemfibrozil (p.923·1).
*Hyperlipidaemias.*

**Hidine** PD, Thai.
Chlorhexidine gluconate (p.1173·2).
*Disinfection.*

**Hidomin** Yung Shin, Singapore.
Hydroxocobalamin (p.1458·2).
*Anaemias.*

**Hidonac**
Zambon, Hong Kong; Zambon, Ital.
Acetylcysteine (p.1112·3).
*Paracetamol poisoning.*

**Hidra** Rydelle, Fr.†.
Amino-acid, fatty-acid, vitamin, and mineral preparation (p.1417·1).
*Skin disorders.*

**Hidra Plus** Luper, Braz.
Oral rehydration solution (p.1222·2).

**Hidrabene** Legrand, Braz.
Sodium chloride; potassium chloride; sodium citrate; anhydrous glucose (p.1222·2).
*Oral rehydration therapy.*

**Hidrafil**
Note. This name is used for preparations of different composition.
Stiefel, Arg.
Eusolex 4360; octinoxate (p.1154·3).
*Barrier preparation with sunscreens.*

Stiefel, Braz.
*Lotion:* Eusolex; octinoxate (p.1154·3).
*Sunscreen.*

Stiefel, Chile.
*SPF 14:* Oxybenzone (p.1154·3); octinoxate (p.1154·3).
*SPF 20:* Benzophenone; ensulizole (p.1147·1).
*Sunscreen.*

Stiefel, Mex.
*SPF 14:* Oxybenzone (p.1154·3); octinoxate (p.1154·3).
*Sunscreen.*

**Hidrafix** Altana, Braz.
Sodium citrate; sodium chloride; potassium chloride; glucose (p.1222·2).
*Oral rehydration therapy.*

**Hidrafix 90** Altana, Braz.
Potassium citrate; sodium citrate; sodium chloride; glucose (p.1222·2).
*Oral rehydration therapy.*

**Hidral** Biocontrol, Arg.
Hydralazine (p.933·1).
*Hypertension.*

**Hidralma** Wasserman, Spain†.
Hydrotalcite (p.1267·3).
*Hyperacidity.*

**Hidramox** Carter-Wallace, Mex.
Amoxicillin trihydrate (p.155·3).
*Bacterial infections.*

**Hidramox-M** Carter-Wallace, Mex.
Amoxicillin trihydrate (p.155·3); bromhexine hydrochloride (p.1115·3).
*Respiratory-tract infections.*

**Hidra-Ped** Stiefel, Braz.†.
Sodium chloride; potassium chloride; calcium chloride; magnesium chloride (p.1222·2).
*Oral rehydration therapy.*

**Hidrapel** *Stiefel, Braz.*
Urea (p.1162·2).
*Skin disorders.*

**Hidraplus** *Baxter, Mex.*
Sodium chloride; potassium chloride; sodium citrate; glucose; anhydrous citric acid (p.1222·2).
*Oral rehydration therapy.*

**Hidrasal** *Mediforma, Mex.†.*
Furosemide (p.919·3).

**Hidrasec** *GlaxoSmithKline, Thai.*
Racecadotril (p.1285·2).
*Diarrhoea.*

**Hidrasix** *Serral, Mex.*
Isoniazid (p.222·2).

**Hidratagel** *Barnes Hind, Arg.*
Hyetellose (p.1579·2); non-ionic surfactants (p.1164·2).
*Cleansing and wetting solution for soft contact lenses.*

**Hidratant** *Maurino, Arg.*
Benzalkonium chloride (p.1168·3) (p.1164·2).
*Cleansing solution for soft contact lenses.*

**Hidratante Enriquecida** *Silesia, Chile.*
Emollient.
*Dry skin.*

**Hidratante Ligera** *Silesia, Chile.*
Emollient.
*Dry skin.*

**Hidratante VG** *Isdin, Port.*
Polyglycerylmethacrylate; glycerol (p.1694·3); carbomer (p.1577·2).
*Vaginal lubricant.*

**Hidratante VV** *Isdin, Port.*
Polyglycerylmethacrylate; lauromacrogol (p.1412·3); borage oil (p.1661·3); levomenol (p.1707·1).
*Vulval lubricant.*

**Hidratoderme** *Sofex, Port.*
Urea (p.1162·2); allantoin (p.1141·3).
*Skin disorders.*

**Hidratoil Free** *Dermoteca, Port.*
A range of moisturisers and skin cleansers.

**Hidrazida** *Zimaia, Port.*
Isoniazid (p.222·2).
*Tuberculosis.*

**Hidrenox A** *Elvetium, Arg.*
Hydrochlorothiazide (p.933·2); amiloride hydrochloride (p.858·2).
*Heart failure; hypertension.*

**Hidrion** *Gross, Braz.*
Furosemide (p.919·3); potassium chloride (p.1232·2).
*Hypertension; oedema.*

**Hidrium** *Saval, Chile.*
Furosemide (p.919·3); amiloride (p.858·3).
*Heart failure; hepatic cirrhosis; hypertension.*

**Hidroaltesona** *Alter, Spain.*
Hydrocortisone (p.1103·3).
*Corticosteroid.*

**Hidroazer** *Zerboni, Mex.†.*
Ketotifen (p.788·2).

**Hidroc Cloranf** *Ciba Vision, Spain†.*
Chloramphenicol (p.185·1); hydrocortisone acetate (p.1103·3).
*Eye disorders.*

**Hidroc Neomic** *Ciba Vision, Spain†.*
Hydrocortisone acetate (p.1103·3); neomycin sulfate (p.235·1).
*Eye disorders.*

**Hidrocil** *Edol, Port.*
Hypromellose (p.1579·3).
*Dry eyes.*

**Hidrocilina** *Grossman, Mex.*
Procaine benzylpenicillin (p.246·1); benzylpenicillin sodium (p.163·2).
*Bacterial infections.*

**Hidrocin** *Asta Medica, Braz.*
Dexamethasone sodium phosphate (p.1097·2); neomycin sulfate (p.235·1); naphazoline hydrochloride (p.1124·3).
*Infected nasal disorders.*

**Hidrocisdin** *Isdin, Spain.*
Hydrocortisone acetate (p.1103·3).
*Skin disorders.*

**Hidroclorozil** *IMA, Braz.*
Hydrochlorothiazide (p.933·2).

**Hidrocol** *Apsen, Braz.†.*
Hydrocortisone (p.1103·3).
*Skin disorders.*

**Hidrocorte** *Legrand, Braz.*
Clioquinol (p.196·3); hydrocortisone (p.1103·3).
*Skin disorders.*

**Hidrocortin** *Alcon, Arg.*
Hydrocortisone (p.1103·3); neomycin sulfate (p.235·1).
*Infected eye disorders.*

**Hidrofall** *Sanval, Braz.*
Hydrochlorothiazide (p.933·2).
*Diuretic.*

**Hidrofenil** *Grin, Mex.*
Hydrocortisone (p.1103·3); phenylephrine (p.1126·3).
*Eye disorders.*

**Hidroferol** *Faes, Spain.*
Calcifediol (p.1461·2).
*Hypoparathyroidism; hypophosphataemia; osteodystrophy; osteomalacia; rickets.*

**Hidrofugal** *Beiersdorf, Chile.*
*Cream; roll-on:* Aluminium chlorohydrate (p.1142·1); aluminium chloride (p.1142·1).
*Topical spray:* Aluminium chlorohydrate (p.1142·1).
*Hyperhidrosis.*

**Hidrofugal Forte** *Beiersdorf, Chile.*
Aluminium chlorohydrate (p.1142·1); aluminium chloride (p.1142·1).
*Hyperhidrosis.*

**Hidrogel** *Omega, Arg.*
Vaginal lubricant.
*Vaginal dryness.*

**Hidrolac** *Lagos, Arg.*
Lactic acid (p.1704·1); urea (p.1162·2).
*Skin disorders.*

**Hidro-Lact**
*Cesam, Port.†.*
A range of moisturisers and soap substitutes.
*Cesam, Port.†.*
Sodium pidolate (p.1158·1); lactic acid (p.1704·1).
*Dry skin.*

**Hidrolyte** *QIF, Braz.†.*
Sodium chloride; acetylmethionine (p.1222·2).
*Oral rehydration therapy.*

**Hidromagma** *Mediforma, Mex.*
Kaolin (p.1268·3); pectin (p.1580·3); neomycin (p.235·1).
*Gastrointestinal infections.*

**Hidromens** *Dumont, Arg.*
Bendroflumethiazide (p.867·3); chlortrimeton maleate; meprobamate (p.706·2); potassium dihydrocholate.
*Premenstrual syndrome.*

**Hidrona** *Fustery, Mex.*
Chlortalidone (p.882·3).
*Hypertension; oedema.*

**Hidroneo** *Luper, Braz.*
Hydrocortisone acetate (p.1103·3); neomycin sulfate (p.235·1).
*Infected skin disorders.*

**Hidronovag Complex** *Gobbi, Arg.*
Hydrocodone tartrate (p.45·1); paracetamol (p.76·2).
*Pain.*

**Hidropid** *Recalcine, Chile.*
Furosemide (p.919·3); amiloride hydrochloride (p.858·2).
*Heart failure; hypertension; oedema.*

**Hidroplus** *Lagos, Arg.*
Urea (p.1162·2).
*Dry skin disorders.*

**Hidroplus CL** *Lagos, Arg.*
Collagen (p.1674·3).
*Skin disorders.*

**Hidroplus Nieve** *Lagos, Arg.*
*SPF 15:* Octinoxate (p.1154·3); oxybenzone (p.1154·3); titanium dioxide (p.1160·3); collagen (p.1674·3).
*Sunscreen.*

**Hidropolicin** *Grin, Mex.*
Polymyxin B sulfate (p.245·1); neomycin sulfate (p.235·1); hydrocortisone acetate (p.1103·3).
*Infected eye disorders.*

**Hidropolivit** *Menarini, Spain.*
Multivitamin preparation (p.1417·1).

**Hidropolivit Mineral** *Menarini, Spain.*
Multivitamins and minerals (p.1417·1); orotic acid; hesperidin.
*Tonic.*

**Hidropril** *Neo Quimica, Braz.*
Captopril (p.879·2); hydrochlorothiazide (p.933·2).
*Hypertension.*

**Hidroquilaude** *Dermofarm, Spain.*
Hydroquinone (p.1148·1).
*Skin hyperpigmentation.*

**Hidroquin** *Remexa, Mex.*
Hydroquinone (p.1148·1).
*Skin hyperpigmentation.*

**Hidroral** *Abbott, Braz.*
Sodium chloride; potassium chloride; sodium lactate; glucose (p.1222·2).
*Oral rehydration therapy.*

**Hidroronol** *Labomed, Chile.*
Hydrochlorothiazide (p.933·2).
*Hypertension; oedema.*

**Hidroronol T** *Labomed, Chile.*
Hydrochlorothiazide (p.933·2); triamterene (p.1016·2).
*Heart failure; hepatic cirrhosis; hypertension; nephrotic syndrome; oedema.*

**Hidrosaluretil** *Alcala, Spain.*
Hydrochlorothiazide (p.933·2).
*Diabetes insipidus; hypertension; oedema; renal calculi.*

**Hidrosam T** *Szama, Arg.*
Tretinoin (p.1161·1); collagen (p.1674·3); elastin; reticulin.
*Acne; photoaging; skin pigmentation disorders.*

**Hidrosol** *Pacific, NZ.*
Aluminium chloride (p.1142·1).
*Hyperhidrosis.*

**Hidrotisona** *Aventis, Arg.*
Hydrocortisone (p.1103·3).
*Corticosteroid.*

**Hidrowil** *Willmar, Mex.†.*
Hydroxocobalamin (p.1458·2).

**Hidroxid** *Elofar, Braz.†.*
Aluminium hydroxide (p.1249·2); magnesium hydroxide (p.1272·2); dimeticone (p.1289·2).
*Flatulence; gastrointestinal hyperacidity.*

**Hidroxil B12 B6 B1** *Almirall, Spain.*
Hydroxocobalamin (p.1458·2); pyridoxine hydrochloride (p.1456·3); thiamine hydrochloride (p.1455·1).
*Vitamin B deficiency.*

**Hidroxina** *ICN, Arg.*
Hydroxyzine hydrochloride (p.434·3).
*Hypersensitivity reactions; sedative.*

**Hidroxogel** *Delta, Braz.*
Aluminium hydroxide (p.1249·2); magnesium hydroxide (p.1272·2); dimeticone (p.1289·2).
*Flatulence; gastrointestinal hyperacidity.*

**Hidyn H** *Ativus, Braz.*
Hydrocortisone acetate (p.1103·3).
*Skin disorders.*

**Hierco** *Ern, Spain.*
Ferritin (p.1427·2).
*Iron-deficiency anaemia.*

**Hierroquick** *Purissimus, Arg.*
Iron (p.1434·3); folic acid (p.1429·1).
*Anaemias.*

**Hifamonil** *Raymos, Arg.*
Sodium perborate (p.1192·2).

**Hifamonil Crema** *Raymos, Arg.*
Miconazole (p.405·2); betamethasone (p.1093·1); gentamicin (p.219·1).
*Skin infections.*

**Higan** *Unison, Thai.*
Hyoscine butylbromide (p.483·3).
*Smooth muscle spasm.*

**Higesan** *Esoform, Ital.*
Sodium *o*-phenylphenol (p.1187·2).
*Surface disinfection.*

**High Potency Cal-Mag Plus** *Quest, Canad.*
Calcium; magnesium; zinc; vitamin C; vitamin D (p.1417·1).

**High Potency Lightening Serum** *Ocean Health, Singapore†.*
Lactic acid (p.1704·1); hydroquinone (p.1148·1); kojic acid (p.1151·2); liquorice (p.1270·2).
*Skin hyperpigmentation.*

**High Potency N-Vites** *Nion, USA.*
Vitamin B substances with vitamin C (p.1417·1).

**Higienex** *Sanval, Braz.†.*
Tyrothricin (p.275·1); thymol (p.1194·2); hydroxyquinoline sulfate (p.1700·1); menthol (p.1711·3); chlorophyll (p.1057·1); sodium bicarbonate (p.1223·2); alum (p.1652·1); lactic acid (p.1704·1).
*Vulvovaginal infections.*

**Higigripe** *CPH, Port.†.*
Aspirin (p.15·1); caffeine (p.782·1); ascorbic acid (p.1460·2).

**Higroton**
*Novartis, Braz.; Novartis, Mex.*
Chlortalidone (p.882·3).
*Ascites; heart failure; hypertension; oedema; renal calculi.*

**Higroton Reserpina** *Novartis, Braz.*
Chlortalidone (p.882·3); reserpine (p.995·1).
*Hypertension.*

**Higrotona** *Novartis, Spain.*
Chlortalidone (p.882·3).
*Diabetes insipidus; hypertension; oedema.*

**Higrotona Reserpina** *Novartis, Spain.*
Chlortalidone (p.882·3); reserpine (p.995·1).
*Hypertension.*

**Higroton-Res** *Novartis, Mex.*
Chlortalidone (p.882·3); reserpine (p.995·1).
*Hypertension.*

**Hijuven**
*Eisai, Hong Kong; Eisai, Malaysia; Eisai, Thai.†.*
*dl*-Alpha tocoferil nicotinate (p.1015·1).
*Cerebral and peripheral vascular disorders; hyperlipidaemias.*

**Hill's Balsam Chesty Cough** *Eastern Pharmaceuticals, UK.*
Guaifenesin (p.1122·1).
*Coughs.*

**Hill's Balsam Chesty Cough for Children** *Eastern Pharmaceuticals, UK.*
Citric acid (p.1673·1); ipecacuanha (p.1122·3).
*Coughs.*

**Hill's Balsam Chesty Cough Pastilles** *Eastern Pharmaceuticals, UK.*
Compound benzoin tincture; peppermint oil (p.1283·2); ipecacuanha (p.1122·3); menthol (p.1711·3).
*Cough and cold symptoms.*

**Hill's Balsam Dry Cough** *Eastern Pharmaceuticals, UK.*
Pholcodine (p.1128·3).
*Coughs.*

**Hill's Balsam Extra Strong** *Eastern Pharmaceuticals, UK.*
Compound benzoin tincture; peppermint oil (p.1283·2); ipecacuanha (p.1122·3); menthol (p.1711·3).
*Coughs and cold symptoms.*

**Hill's Balsam Nasal Congestion Pastilles** *Eastern Pharmaceuticals, UK.*
Eucalyptus oil (p.1686·2); menthol (p.1711·3).
*Nasal congestion.*

**Hima-Pasta nouvelle formule** *Mundipharma, Switz.*
Zinc sulfate (p.1469·3); zinc oxide (p.1163·2).
*Herpes labialis.*

**Himega**
*Sigma, Austral.; Sigma, Hong Kong.*
Eicosapentaenoic acid (p.976·2); docosahexaenoic acid (p.976·1).
*Dietary supplement.*

**Himelan** *Soria Natural, Spain.*
Fennel (p.1687·2); pimpinella; angelica (p.1655·1); melissa (p.1711·1).
*Aerophagia; dyspepsia; meteorism.*

**Himus** *Grossman, Mex.†.*
Thymomodulin (p.1756·1).

**Hincomox** *Teuto, Braz.*
Amoxicillin (p.155·3).
*Bacterial infections.*

**Hingfong-Essenz Hofmanns** *Hofmann & Sommer, Ger.*
Valerian (p.1762·2); peppermint oil (p.1283·2); rosemary oil (p.1740·2); fennel oil (p.1687·3); anise oil (p.1655·2); camphor (p.1665·3).
*Headache; nausea; pain; psychosomatic disorders.*

**Hinox** *Hebron, Braz.*
Multivitamin and mineral preparation (p.1417·1).

**H-Insulin** *Hoechst, Ger.†.*
Insulin injection (human, highly purified) (p.333·3).
*Diabetes mellitus.*

**Hiosinotil** *Loren, Mex.*
Hyoscine butylbromide (p.483·3).

**Hiosinotil Compuesto** *Loren, Mex.*
Hyoscine butylbromide (p.483·3); dipyrone (p.35·3).

**Hiospan** *Teuto, Braz.*
Hyoscine butylbromide (p.483·3).
*Skeletal muscle spasm.*

**Hiospan Composto** *Teuto, Braz.*
Dipyrone (p.35·3); hyoscine butylbromide (p.483·3).
*Pain; skeletal muscle spasm.*

**Hioxyl**
*Croma, Austria†; Quinoderm, Irl.; Ferndale, UK.*
Hydrogen peroxide (stabilised) (p.1182·2).
*Skin infections; skin ulcers; wounds.*

**Hipalen** *Braun, Chile.*
Preparation for enteral nutrition (p.1417·1).

**Hipax** *Baliardo, Arg.*
Hypericum (p.299·1).
*Depression.*

**Hipecor** *Bristol-Myers Squibb, Chile.*
Sotalol hydrochloride (p.1001·3).
*Arrhythmias.*

**Hipeksal** *Leiras, Fin.*
Methenamine hippurate (p.230·2).
*Urinary-tract infections.*

**Hipen** *Cadila, India.*
Amoxicillin (p.155·3) or amoxicillin trihydrate (p.155·3).
*Bacterial infections.*

**Hipenox** *Cadila, India.*
Amoxicillin sodium (p.155·3) or amoxicillin trihydrate (p.155·3); cloxacillin sodium (p.198·2).
*Bacterial infections.*

**Hiper Diet** *Support, Braz.*
A range of preparations for enteral nutrition (p.1417·1).

**Hiperbiotico** *Atral, Port.*
Ampicillin sodium (p.157·1) or ampicillin trihydrate (p.157·2).
*Bacterial infections.*

**Hiperbiotico Retard** *Atral, Port.*
Ampicillin sodium (p.157·1); ampicillin benzathine (p.158·1).
*Bacterial infections.*

**Hipercol** *Helfarma, Port.*
Citicoline (p.1672·3).
*Cerebrovascular disorders.*

**Hiperdipina** *Pentafarma, Port.*
Nitrendipine (p.973·3).

**Hiperex** *Eurofarma, Braz.*
Hypericum (p.299·1).
*Depression.*

**Hiperflex** *Recalcine, Chile.*
Glucosamine sulfate (p.1694·1); chondroitin sulfate.
*Osteoarthritis.*

**Hipericin** *Herbarium, Braz.*
Hypericum (p.299·1).
*Depression.*

**Hiperico**
*Herbarium, Braz.; Diviser Aquilea, Spain; Natysal, Spain.*
Hypericum (p.299·1).
*Depression; sleep disorders; tonic.*

**Hiperikan** *Farmasa, Mex.*
Hypericum (p.299·1).
*Depression.*

**Hiperil** *Teuto, Braz.*
Hypericum (p.299·1).
*Depression.*

**Hiperlex** *Cantabria, Spain.*
Fosinopril sodium (p.919·1).
*Heart failure; hypertension.*

**Hiperlex Plus** *Cantabria, Spain.*
Fosinopril sodium (p.919·1); hydrochlorothiazide (p.933·2).
*Hypertension.*

**Hiperogyn** *Madaus, Ital.*
Magnesium (p.1227·3); cimicifuga (p.1671·3); hypericum (p.299·1).
*Insomnia; menopausal disorders; menstrual disorders.*

**Hipersac** *Bunker, Braz.*
Hypericum (p.299·1).
*Depression.*

**Hipersex** *Medical, Port.*
Testis; pituitary; fitine; zinc phosphate; strychnine sulfate; adonis vernalis; boldo (p.1417·1).
*Tonic.*

**Hiperson** *Medipharm, Chile.*
Enalapril maleate (p.909·2).
*Heart failure; hypertension.*

**Hiperson-D** *Medipharm, Chile.*
Enalapril maleate (p.909·2); hydrochlorothiazide (p.933·2).
*Hypertension.*

**Hipersteno** *Hertz, Braz.†.*
Glycerophosphates; nicotinamide (p.1417·1).

**Hipertenol** *Sanofi Synthelabo, Port.*
Nitrendipine (p.973·3).

**Hipertex** *Rayere, Mex.*
Captopril (p.879·2).
*Hypertension.*

**Hipertil** *Normal, Port.*
Captopril (p.879·2).

**Hipertin** *Luper, Braz.*
Enalapril maleate (p.909·2).
*Hypertension.*

**Hiperton** *Grin, Mex.*
Sodium chloride (p.1233·3).
*Corneal oedema.*

**Hipfix** *SNBTS, UK.*
A factor IX preparation (p.752·2).
*Haemorrhagic disorders.*

**Hipnodem** *Armstrong, Arg.*
Zaleplon (p.727·3).
*Insomnia.*

**Hipnopento** *Gray, Arg.*
Thiopental sodium (p.1309·1).
*General anaesthesia; hypnotic.*

**Hipnosedon** *Roche, Gr.*
Flunitrazepam (p.698·2).
*Insomnia.*

**Hipoartel**
*Andromaco, Chile; Ipsen, Spain.*
Enalapril maleate (p.909·2).
*Heart failure; hypertension.*

**Hipoartel H** *Andromaco, Chile.*
Enalapril maleate (p.909·2); hydrochlorothiazide (p.933·2).
*Heart failure; hypertension.*

**Hipoartel Plus** *Ipsen, Spain.*
Enalapril maleate (p.909·2); hydrochlorothiazide (p.933·2).
*Hypertension.*

**Hipocatril** *Cibran, Braz.†.*
Captopril (p.879·2).
*Heart failure; hypertension.*

**Hipocol** *Valdecasas, Mex.*
Nicotinic acid (p.1441·1).
*Hypercholesterolaemia; pellagra.*

**Hipoderme** *Teuto, Braz.*
Vitamin A palmitate (p.1453·1); colecalciferol (p.1461·3); zinc oxide (p.1163·2).
*Barrier preparation.*

**Hipodermon** *Neo Quimica, Braz.*
Vitamin A palmitate (p.1453·1); colecalciferol (p.1461·3); boric acid (p.1662·1); zinc oxide (p.1163·2).
*Barrier preparation; emollient.*

**Hipodex** *Bunker, Braz.*
Vitamin A (p.1451·2); Ergocalciferol (p.1462·1); neomycin sulfate (p.235·1); benzethonium chloride (p.1169·2).
*Barrier preparation; infected skin disorders.*

**Hipodor** *Lepori, Port.*
Hexyl nicotinate (p.45·1); methyl salicylate (p.59·3).
*Musculoskeletal and joint disorders; neuritis; soft-tissue disorders.*

**Hipofagin S** *Sigma, Braz.*
Diethylpropion hydrochloride (p.1587·1).
*Obesity.*

**Hipofisina** *Biol, Arg.*
Oxytocin (p.1336·1).
*Postpartum haemorrhage.*

**Hipoge** *SMB, Chile.*
Hydrocortisone acetate (p.1103·3).
*Skin disorders.*

**Hipoglos**
Note. This name is used for preparations of different composition.
*Andromaco, Arg.*
Vitamin A (p.1451·2); zinc oxide (p.1163·2).
*Nappy rash; nipple care.*

*Procter & Gamble, Braz.*
Vitamin A (p.1451·2); colecalciferol (p.1461·3); zinc oxide (p.1163·2).
Formerly contained vitamin A palmitate, ergocalciferol, boric acid, zinc oxide, hydrocortisone, and aluminium magnesium silicate.
*Skin disorders.*

*Andromaco, Chile.*
Halibut-liver oil (p.1434·1); boric acid (p.1662·1); zinc oxide (p.1163·2).
*Burns; skin disorders; ulcers; wounds.*

**Hipoglos Cicatrizante** *Andromaco, Arg.*
Zinc undecenoate (p.411·1); sodium propionate (p.408·1); diiodohydroxyquinoline (p.603·3); boric acid (p.1662·1); zinc oxide (p.1163·2).
*Wounds.*

**Hipoglos con Hidrocortisona** *Andromaco, Arg.*
Hydrocortisone (p.1103·3); vitamin A (p.1451·2); cod-liver oil (p.1425·2); boric acid (p.1662·1).
*Skin disorders.*

**Hipoglos Oftalmico** *Procter & Gamble, Braz.†.*
Vitamin A palmitate (p.1453·1); ergocalciferol (p.1462·1); chloramphenicol (p.185·1); hydrocortisone (p.1103·3).
*Infected eye disorders.*

**Hipoglos Plus** *Andromaco, Mex.*
Vitamin A (p.1451·2); zinc oxide (p.1163·2); allantoin (p.1141·3); boric acid (p.1662·1); talc (p.1159·1).
*Skin disorders.*

**Hipoglucin** *Laboratorios Chile, Chile.*
Metformin hydrochloride (p.342·3).
*Diabetes mellitus.*

**Hipokinon** *Psicofarma, Mex.*
Trihexyphenidyl hydrochloride (p.490·2).
*Extrapyramidal disorders; parkinsonism.*

**Hipolixan**
Note. This name is used for preparations of different composition.
*Bago, Arg.*
Gemfibrozil (p.923·1).
*Hyperlipidaemias.*

*Pasteur, Chile.*
Atorvastatin (p.866·2).
*Hypercholesterolaemia.*

**Hiposan** *Sanval, Braz.*
Zinc oxide (p.1163·2); cod-liver oil (p.1425·2).
*Barrier preparation; skin disorders.*

**Hiposcler** *Basi, Port.*
Clofibrate nicotinyl alcohol.

**Hiposterol** *Laboratorios Chile, Chile.*
Lovastatin (p.949·1).
*Hypercholesterolaemia.*

**Hiposul** *Remexa, Mex.†.*
Sodium thiosulfate (p.1053·3).

**Hipoten** *Sanval, Braz.*
Captopril (p.879·2).
*Hypertension.*

**Hipotensil** *Medinfar, Port.*
Captopril (p.879·2).
*Heart failure; hypertension.*

**Hipotermal** *Sanval, Braz.*
Aspirin (p.15·1).
*Fever; pain.*

**Hipotest** *Marlop, USA.*
Multivitamin and mineral preparation with iron (p.1417·1).

**Hipotosse** *Clintex, Port.*
Ambroxol hydrochloride (p.1114·3).
*Respiratory-tract congestion.*

**Hipovastin** *Gador, Arg.*
Lovastatin (p.949·1).
*Atherosclerosis; hypercholesterolaemia.*

**Hi-Po-Vites** *Hudson, USA.*
Multivitamin and mineral preparation with iron and folic acid (p.1417·1).

**Hippophan** *Weleda, Fr.†.*
Sea buckthorn (p.1742·2).
*Tonic.*

**Hippramine** *3M, S.Afr.*
Methenamine hippurate (p.230·2).
*Urinary-tract infections.*

**Hipress** *Ache, Braz.†.*
Losartan potassium (p.947·2); hydrochlorothiazide (p.933·2).
*Hypertension.*

**Hiprex**
*3M, Austral.; Sanova, Austria; 3M, Belg.; 3M, Canad.; 3M, Fin.; 3M, Irl.; 3M, Israel; 3M, Norw.; 3M, NZ; 3M, Swed.; 3M, UK; Hoechst Marion Roussel, USA.*
Methenamine hippurate (p.230·2).
*Urinary-tract infections.*

**Hipten**
Note. This name is used for preparations of different composition.
*Ofimex, Mex.†.*
Methyldopa (p.953·2).

*Farmorcore, Port.*
Enalapril maleate (p.909·2).

**Hiremon** *Demo, Gr.*
Buspirone hydrochloride (p.672·2).
*Generalised anxiety.*

**Hirtonin** *Takeda, Jpn.*
Protirelin tartrate (p.1338·2).
*Prolonged disturbance of consciousness; spinocerebellar degeneration.*

**Hirucreme** *Roche Nicholas, Fr.*
Hirudin (p.931·2).
*Peripheral vascular disorders.*

**Hirudex** *Pharmafar, Ital.*
Leech extract (p.931·2); esculoside (p.1648·2).
*Bruises; inflammation; oedema; phlebitis; varices.*

**Hirudoid**
*Elvetium, Arg.; Key, Austral.; Sankyo, Austria; Sankyo, Belg.; Sankyo, Braz.; Sanofi Synthelabo, Chile; Sankyo, Denm.; Sankyo, Fin.; Sankyo, Ger.; Sankyo, Hong Kong; CFL, India; Sankyo, Ital.; Sankyo, Neth.; Sankyo, Norw.; Wilson, NZ; Sankyo, Port.; Sankyo, Singapore; Sankyo, Spain; Selena, Swed.; Sankyo, Switz.; Sankyo, Thai.; Sankyo, UK.*
A heparinoid (p.931·1).
*Soft-tissue injury; thrombophlebitis; venous insufficiency; wounds.*

**Hiscifed** *Greater Pharma, Thai.*
Pseudoephedrine hydrochloride (p.1129·2); triprolidine hydrochloride (p.442·3).
*Cold symptoms; hypersensitivity reactions; nasal congestion; otitis media; rhinitis.*

**Hiscolgen** *Greater Pharma, Thai.*
Paracetamol (p.76·2); chlorphenamine maleate (p.427·3).
Formerly contained paracetamol, phenylpropanolamine hydrochloride, and chlorphenamine maleate.
*Cold symptoms.*

**Hisdane** *Duopharma, Hong Kong.*
Terfenadine (p.441·1).
*Allergic rhinitis.*

**Hisfedin** *Wolff, Ger.*
Terfenadine (p.441·1).
*Allergic conjunctivitis; allergic rhinitis; allergic skin disorders.*

**Hismacon** *Condrugs, Thai.†.*
Astemizole (p.424·2).
*Allergic conjunctivitis; allergic rhinitis; allergic skin disorders.*

**Hismadrin** *Janssen-Cilag, Austria†.*
Astemizole (p.424·2); pseudoephedrine hydrochloride (p.1129·2).
*Hypersensitivity reactions.*

**Hismanal** *Janssen, USA†.*
Astemizole (p.424·2).
*Allergic rhinitis; idiopathic urticaria.*

**Hismizol** *TO-Chemicals, Thai.†.*
Astemizole (p.424·2).
*Allergic rhinitis; allergic skin disorders.*

**Hisno** *Milano, Thai.†.*
Astemizole (p.424·2).
*Hypersensitivity reactions.*

**Hisnot** *Farmasa, Braz.†.*
Astemizole (p.424·2).
*Hypersensitivity reactions.*

**Hisocel** *Fresenius, Braz.†.*
Gelatin (p.754·3) in electrolytes.
*Plasma volume expansion.*

**Hisof** *Banner, Hong Kong†.*
Docusate sodium (p.1262·2).
*Constipation; stool softener.*

**Hisoplex com Glicose** *Fresenius, Braz.†.*
Electrolyte infusion with glucose (p.1217·1).
*Plasma volume expansion.*

**Hispamicina Retard** *Inkeysa, Spain†.*
Ampicillin sodium (p.157·1); ampicillin benzathine (p.158·1).
*Bacterial infections.*

**Hisprin** *Shiwa, Thai.†.*
Paracetamol (p.76·2); chlorphenamine maleate (p.427·3); phenylpropanolamine (p.1127·3).
*Cold symptoms.*

**Histabloc** *Medley, Braz.†.*
Astemizole (p.424·2).
*Hypersensitivity reactions.*

**Histac**
*Ranbaxy, India; Ranbaxy, Malaysia; Ranbaxy, Singapore; Ranbaxy, Thai.*
Ranitidine hydrochloride (p.1285·2).
*Dyspepsia; gastric hyperacidity; gastro-oesophageal reflux; heartburn; peptic ulcer; Zollinger-Ellison syndrome.*

**Histaclar** *Gerard, Irl.*
Loratadine (p.436·1).
*Allergic rhinitis; idiopathic chronic urticaria.*

**Histacon** *Quatromed, S.Afr.*
Paracetamol (p.76·2); phenylephrine hydrochloride (p.1126·3); chlorphenamine maleate (p.427·3); caffeine (p.782·1).
*Allergic rhinitis; cold symptoms.*

**Histacyl Compositum** *Streuli, Switz.*
Diphenhydramine hydrochloride (p.431·3); mepyramine maleate (p.437·1).
*Hypersensitivity reactions.*

**Histacylettes** *Streuli, Switz.*
Diphenhydramine hydrochloride (p.431·3); mepyramine hydrochloride (p.437·1); caffeine (p.782·1).
*Hypersensitivity reactions.*

**Histadane** *Cibran, Braz.†.*
Terfenadine (p.441·1).
*Hypersensitivity reactions.*

**Histade** *Breckenridge, USA†.*
Phenylpropanolamine hydrochloride (p.1127·3); chlorphenamine maleate (p.427·3).
*Cold symptoms; rhinitis.*

**Histadestal** *Bioimmun, Ger.*
A normal immunoglobulin (p.1627·2); histamine hydrochloride (p.1697·1).
*Hypersensitivity reactions.*

**Histadex** *Vitamed, Israel.*
Dexchlorpheniramine maleate (p.427·3); pseudoephedrine hydrochloride (p.1129·2).
*Respiratory-tract congestion.*

**Histadin** *Uniao Quimica, Braz.*
Loratadine (p.436·1).
*Hypersensitivity reactions.*

**Histafed** *Trima, Israel.*
Triprolidine hydrochloride (p.442·3); pseudoephedrine hydrochloride (p.1129·2).
*Respiratory-tract congestion.*

**Histafed Comp** *Trima, Israel.*
Triprolidine hydrochloride (p.442·3); pseudoephedrine hydrochloride (p.1129·2); codeine phosphate (p.27·1).
*Coughs; upper respiratory-tract infections.*

**Histafed Expectorant** *Trima, Israel.*
Triprolidine hydrochloride (p.442·3); pseudoephedrine hydrochloride (p.1129·2); guaifenesin (p.1122·1).
*Coughs.*

**Histafen**
Note. This name is used for preparations of different composition.
*Xepa-Soul Pattinson, Hong Kong; Berk, UK†.*
Terfenadine (p.441·1).
*Allergic rhinitis; dermatologic hypersensitivity reactions; hay fever.*

*Douglas, NZ.*
Chlorphenamine maleate (p.427·3).
*Hypersensitivity reactions.*

**Histafilin** *Estedi, Spain.*
Theophylline (p.798·3).
*Heart failure; obstructive airways disease; paroxysmal dyspnoea.*

**Histafren** *Unipharma, Gr.*
Cetirizine hydrochloride (p.427·1).
*Allergic conjunctivitis; allergic rhinitis; pruritus.*

**Histagesic Modified** *Jones, USA.*
Phenylephrine hydrochloride (p.1126·3); paracetamol (p.76·2); chlorphenamine maleate (p.427·3).
*Upper respiratory-tract symptoms.*

**Histaglobin**
*Sidus, Arg.; Germania, Austria; Mirren, S.Afr.; Promedica, Thai.†.*
A normal immunoglobulin (p.1627·2); histamine hydrochloride (p.1697·1).
*Hypersensitivity reactions.*

**Histaglobulin** *Serum Institute, India.*
A normal immunoglobulin (p.1627·2); histamine hydrochloride (p.1697·1).
*Allergic skin disorders; asthma; migraine.*

**Histajodol N** *Kattwiga, Ger.†.*
Nonivamide (p.67·2); salicylic acid (p.1157·1); rosemary oil (p.1740·2).
*Circulatory disorders; neuralgia; rheumatism; sciatica.*

**Histak** *Ranbaxy, S.Afr.*
Ranitidine hydrochloride (p.1285·2).
*Acid aspiration; gastro-oesophageal reflux; peptic ulcer; Zollinger-Ellison syndrome.*

**Histalen** *Andromaco, Chile.*
Cetirizine (p.427·2).
*Hypersensitivity reactions.*

**Histaler** *Duncan, Arg.*
Diphenhydramine (p.431·3).
*Hypersensitivity reactions; sedative; vomiting.*

**Histalerg** *Dermopen, Braz.†.*
Fluocinolone acetonide (p.1101·2); neomycin (p.235·1).
*Infected skin disorders.*

**Histalerg Profen** *Dermopen, Braz.†.*
Pheniramine maleate (p.438·3).
*Hypersensitivity reactions.*

**Histalet** *Numark, USA.*
Pseudoephedrine hydrochloride (p.1129·2); chlorphenamine maleate (p.427·3).
*Upper respiratory-tract symptoms.*

**Histalet X** *Numark, USA.*
Pseudoephedrine hydrochloride (p.1129·2); guaifenesin (p.1122·1).
*Coughs.*

**Histalet Forte** *Numark, USA†.*
Phenylpropanolamine hydrochloride (p.1127·3); phenylephrine hydrochloride (p.1126·3); chlorphenamine maleate (p.427·3); mepyramine maleate (p.437·1).
*Upper respiratory-tract symptoms.*

**Histalgane** *Spirig, Switz.*
Nonivamide (p.67·2); benzyl nicotinate (p.21·2); glycol salicylate (p.44·3); dimethyl sulfoxide (p.1473·2).
*Musculoskeletal, joint, and peri-articular pain.*

**Histalgane mite** *Spirig, Switz.*
Glycol salicylate (p.44·3); dimethyl sulfoxide (p.1473·2).
*Musculoskeletal, joint, and peri-articular pain.*

**Histalino** *Arlex, Mex.†.*
Astemizole (p.424·2).

**Histalix**
Note. This name is used for preparations of different composition.
*Roche Consumer, S.Afr.*
Diphenhydramine hydrochloride (p.431·3); codeine phosphate (p.27·1).
*Coughs; nasal congestion.*

*Wallace Mfg Chem., UK.*
Diphenhydramine hydrochloride (p.431·3); ammonium chloride (p.1115·2); sodium citrate (p.1223·2); menthol (p.1711·3).
*Coughs.*

**Histalix-C** *Roche, S.Afr.†.*
Dextromethorphan hydrobromide (p.1117·3); paracetamol (p.76·2); pseudoephedrine hydrochloride (p.1129·2); ascorbic acid (p.1460·2).
*Cold symptoms.*

**Histaloc** *Julphar, UAE.*
Promethazine hydrochloride (p.439·1).
*Hypersensitivity; motion sickness.*

**Histalon** *ICN, Canad.†.*
Chlorphenamine maleate (p.427·3).

**Histalor**
Biochimico, Braz.†; Reddy, Singapore.
Loratadine (p.436·1).
*Allergic rhinitis; urticaria.*

**Histamed** Propan, S.Afr.
*Elixir*†: Chlorphenamine maleate (p.427·3).
*Hypersensitivity reactions.*
*Lotion:* Diphenhydramine hydrochloride (p.431·3); calamine (p.1144·1); camphor (p.1665·3); benzocaine (p.1370·3).
*Skin irritation.*

**Histamed Compound** Propan, S.Afr.
Chlorphenamine maleate (p.427·3); ascorbic acid (p.1460·2); salicylamide (p.87·3); paracetamol (p.76·2); caffeine (p.782·1); phenylephrine hydrochloride (p.1126·3).
*Cold symptoms.*

**Histamen** Polifarma, Ital.†.
Astemizole (p.424·2).
*Allergic conjunctivitis; rhinitis; urticaria.*

**Histamin** Neo Quimica, Braz.
Dexchlorpheniramine maleate (p.427·3).
*Hypersensitivity reactions.*

**Histamino Corteroid L** Montpellier, Arg.
Loratadine (p.436·1); betamethasone (p.1093·1).
*Hypersensitivity reactions.*

**Histaminos** Lesvi, Spain†.
Astemizole (p.424·2).
*Hypersensitivity reactions.*

**Histamix** Hebron, Braz.
Loratadine (p.436·1).
*Hypersensitivity reactions.*

**Histan** Siam Bheasach, Thai.
Hydroxyzine hydrochloride (p.434·3).
*Anxiety; hypersensitivity reactions.*

**Histantil** Pharmascience, Canad.
Promethazine hydrochloride (p.439·1).
*Antihistamine.*

**Histaoph** Seng, Thai.
Antazoline hydrochloride (p.424·2); tetryzoline hydrochloride (p.1131·2).
*Allergic eye disorders; conjunctivitis.*

**Histaplus** Pasteur, Chile.
Loratadine (p.436·1).
*Allergic rhinitis; allergic skin disorders; urticaria.*

**Histaser** Serral, Mex.
Astemizole (p.424·2).
*Hypersensitivity.*

**Histatab Plus** Century, USA.
Phenylephrine hydrochloride (p.1126·3); chlorphenamine maleate (p.427·3).
*Upper respiratory-tract symptoms.*

**Histatapp** Pharmasant, Thai.
Chlorphenamine maleate (p.427·3).
*Hypersensitivity reactions.*

**Histaterfen** Azupharma, Ger.†.
Terfenadine (p.441·1).
*Hypersensitivity reactions.*

**Histatex** Medix, Mex.
Pheniramine (p.438·3).
*Hypersensitivity.*

**Hista-Vadrin** Scherer, USA†.
Phenylpropanolamine hydrochloride (p.1127·3); phenylephrine hydrochloride (p.1126·3); chlorphenamine maleate (p.427·3).
*Upper respiratory-tract symptoms.*

**Hista-Vent DA** Ethex, USA.
Chlorphenamine maleate (p.427·3); phenylephrine hydrochloride (p.1126·3); hyoscine methonitrate (p.483·3).

**Histaverin** Estedi, Spain.
Codeine phosphate (p.27·1).
*Cough; diarrhoea; pain.*

**Histax** Recalcine, Chile.
Cetirizine hydrochloride (p.427·1).
*Hypersensitivity reactions.*

**Histaxin** Asta Medica, Austria.
Diphenhydramine hydrochloride (p.431·3).
*Allergic skin disorders.*

**Histazine** Trima, Israel.
Cetirizine (p.427·2).
*Hypersensitivity reactions.*

**Histema** Unison, Thai.†.
Astemizole (p.424·2).
*Allergic conjunctivitis; allergic rhinitis; allergic skin disorders.*

**Histenol Cold** Zee, Canad.
Pseudoephedrine hydrochloride (p.1129·2); dextromethorphan hydrobromide (p.1117·3); paracetamol (p.76·2).

**Histenol-Forte** Zee, USA.
Paracetamol (p.76·2); pseudoephedrine hydrochloride (p.1129·2); dextromethorphan hydrobromide (p.1117·3).
*Upper respiratory-tract disorders.*

**Histergan** Norma, UK.
Diphenhydramine hydrochloride (p.431·3).
*Hypersensitivity reactions.*

**Histerone** Roberts, USA†; Hauck, USA†.
Testosterone (p.1569·3).
*Androgen replacement therapy; delayed puberty.*

**Histex** Teamm, USA.
Pseudoephedrine hydrochloride (p.1129·2); chlorphenamine maleate (p.427·3).
*Upper respiratory-tract symptoms.*

**Histex CT** Teamm, USA.
Carbinoxamine maleate (p.426·3).
*Hypersensitivity reactions.*

**Histex HC** Teamm, USA.
Pseudoephedrine hydrochloride (p.1129·2); hydrocodone tartrate (p.45·1); carbinoxamine hydrochloride (p.426·3) or carbinoxamine maleate (p.426·3).
*Coughs; respiratory-tract congestion; rhinitis.*

**Histex PD** Teamm, USA.
Carbinoxamine (p.426·3).
*Allergic rhinitis.*

**Histex SR** Teamm, USA.
Paracetamol (p.76·2); phenylephrine (p.1126·3); chlorphenamine (p.428·1).
*Allergic rhinitis; cold symptoms; sinusitis.*

**Histiacil NF** Columbia, Mex.
Dextromethorphan hydrobromide (p.1117·3); ambroxol hydrochloride (p.1114·3).
*Respiratory-tract disorders.*

**Histica** M & H, Thai.
Cetirizine hydrochloride (p.427·1).
*Allergic conjunctivitis; allergic rhinitis; urticaria.*

**Histidanol** Geminis, Arg.
Boric acid (p.1662·1); bismuth salicylate (p.1252·1); diphenhydramine (p.431·3); resorcinol (p.1156·3).
*Skin disorders.*

**Histilos** UCB, Swed.†.
Nicotinic acid (p.1441·1); meclozine hydrochloride (p.436·3); hydroxyzine hydrochloride (p.434·3).
*Ménière's disease.*

**Histimet** Janssen-Cilag, Arg.
Levocabastine (p.435·3).
*Allergic conjunctivitis; allergic rhinitis.*

**Histin** Kenyaku, Thai.
Carbinoxamine maleate (p.426·3).
*Allergic rhinitis; allergic skin disorders.*

**Histine DM** Ethex, USA†.
Phenylpropanolamine hydrochloride (p.1127·3); brompheniramine maleate (p.426·1); dextromethorphan hydrobromide (p.1117·3).
*Coughs.*

**Histiness** Biomedica, Ger.†.
Homoeopathic preparation.

**Histinex D** Ethex, USA.
Hydrocodone tartrate (p.45·1); pseudoephedrine hydrochloride (p.1129·2).
*Coughs and cold symptoms.*

**Histinex DM** Ethex, USA†.
Dextromethorphan hydrobromide (p.1117·3); phenylpropanolamine hydrochloride (p.1127·3); brompheniramine maleate (p.426·1).
*Coughs and cold symptoms.*

**Histinex HC** Ethex, USA.
Hydrocodone tartrate (p.45·1); phenylephrine hydrochloride (p.1126·3); chlorphenamine maleate (p.427·3).
*Coughs.*

**Histinex PV** Ethex, USA.
Hydrocodone tartrate (p.45·1); pseudoephedrine hydrochloride (p.1129·2); chlorphenamine maleate (p.427·3).
*Cough and cold symptoms.*

**Histoacryl** Braun, UK.
Enbucrilate (p.1678·1).
*Tissue adhesive for closure of minor wounds.*

**Histodil** Gedeon Richter, Thai.†.
Cimetidine hydrochloride (p.1255·3).
*Gastro-oesophageal reflux; gastrointestinal haemorrhage; peptic ulcer; Zollinger-Ellison syndrome.*

**Histodor** Aspen, S.Afr.
*Cream:* Mepyramine maleate (p.437·1); diphenhydramine hydrochloride (p.431·3).
*Insect bites; skin disorders.*
*Tablets:* Mepyramine maleate (p.437·1); promethazine hydrochloride (p.439·1); caffeine (p.782·1).
*Hypersensitivity reactions.*

**Histodor Expectorant** Aspen, S.Afr.
Diphenhydramine hydrochloride (p.431·3); ammonium chloride (p.1115·2); sodium citrate (p.1223·2).
*Coughs.*

**Histodryl**
Biolab, Malaysia; Biolab, Thai.
Diphenhydramine hydrochloride (p.431·3); ammonium chloride (p.1115·2); sodium citrate (p.1223·2); menthol (p.1711·3).
*Cold symptoms; coughs.*

**Histo-Fluine P** Richard, Fr.
Aesculus (p.1648·2); hamamelis (p.1696·3); shepherd's purse (p.1744·1); pulsatilla (p.1737·1); esculoside (p.1648·2).
*Peripheral vascular disorders.*

**Histofreezer**
Note. This name is used for preparations of different composition.
Hamilton, Austral.
Dimethyl ether (p.1236·1); propane (p.1238·2); isobutane (p.1236·2).
*Warts.*
Braun, Fr.
Dimethyl ether (p.1236·1); propane (p.1238·2).
*Warts.*

**Histol** Julphar, UAE.
Pheniramine maleate (p.438·3).
*Hypersensitivity.*

**Histolyn-CYL** ALK, USA.
Histoplasmin (p.1697·2).
*Diagnostic test.*

**Histop** Salvat, Spain.
Simvastatin (p.997·1).
*Hyperlipidaemias.*

**Histopen** Microsules Bernabo, Arg.
Ampicillin sodium (p.157·1) or ampicillin trihydrate (p.157·2).
*Bacterial infections.*

**Histophtal** Metochem, Austria†.
Naphazoline hydrochloride (p.1124·3); antazoline hydrochloride (p.424·2).
*Eye disorders.*

**Histor-D** Roberts, USA.
Phenylephrine hydrochloride (p.1126·3); chlorphenamine maleate (p.427·3).
*Upper respiratory-tract symptoms.*

**Histor-D Timecelles** Roberts, USA.
Chlorphenamine maleate (p.427·3); phenylephrine hydrochloride (p.1126·3); hyoscine methonitrate (p.483·3).
*Upper respiratory-tract symptoms.*

**Histosal** Ferndale, USA†.
Phenylpropanolamine hydrochloride (p.1127·3); paracetamol (p.76·2); caffeine (p.782·1); mepyramine maleate (p.437·1).
*Upper respiratory-tract symptoms.*

**Histussin D** Sanofi Winthrop, USA.
Hydrocodone tartrate (p.45·1); pseudoephedrine hydrochloride (p.1129·2).
*Coughs; respiratory-tract congestion.*

**Histussin HC** Sanofi Winthrop, USA.
Chlorphenamine maleate (p.427·3); phenylephrine hydrochloride (p.1126·3); hydrocodone tartrate (p.45·1).
*Coughs and cold symptoms.*

**Hitocobamin** Hishiyama, Thai.
Mecobalamin (p.1459·1).
*Peripheral neuropathy.*

**Hitrechol** Evers, Hong Kong†.
Hedera helix.
*Gallstones.*

**Hi-Vegi-Lip** Freeda, USA.
Pancreatin (p.1725·3); pancrelipase (p.1725·3).
*Deficiency of digestive enzymes.*

**Hivensteril** Orion, Fin.†.
Mineral preparation for infusion (p.1417·1).

**Hivernum** Arkopharma, Fr.
Homoeopathic preparation.
Formerly known as Formule de l'Abbe Chaupitre no 5.

**Hives** Hylands, Canad.
Homoeopathic preparation.

**Hivid**
Roche, Arg.; Roche, Austral.; Roche, Austria; Roche, Belg.; Roche, Braz.; Roche, Canad.; Roche, Chile; Roche, Denm.; Roche, Fin.; Roche, Fr.; Roche, Ger.; Roche, Gr.; Roche, Hong Kong; Roche, Irl.; Roche, Israel; Roche, Ital.; Roche, Jpn; Roche, Mex.; Roche, Neth.; Roche, Norw.†; Roche, NZ†; Roche, Port.; Roche, S.Afr.; Roche, Singapore; Roche, Spain; Roche, Swed.; Roche, Switz.; Roche, Thai.; Roche, UK; Roche, USA.
Zalcitabine (p.657·1).
*HIV infection.*

**Hivirux** Labinca, Arg.
Lamivudine (p.648·2).
*HIV infection.*

**Hivirux Complex** Labinca, Arg.
Lamivudine (p.648·2); zidovudine (p.658·2).
*HIV infection.*

**Hivita** Mega Vitamin, Austral.†.
A range of multivitamin and mineral preparations (p.1417·1).

**Hivita Childvita** Mega Vitamin, Austral.†.
Multivitamin and mineral preparation with enzymes (p.1417·1).

**Hivita Liquivita** Mega Vitamin, Austral.†.
Multivitamin and mineral preparation with plant extracts (p.1417·1).

**Hivotex** Kleva, Gr.
Ambroxol hydrochloride (p.1114·3).
*Respiratory disorders associated with viscous mucus.*

**Hixizine** Igefarma, Braz.†.
Hydroxyzine hydrochloride (p.434·3).
*Hypersensitivity reactions.*

**Hizaar** Merck Sharp & Dohme, Ital.
Losartan potassium (p.947·2); hydrochlorothiazide (p.933·2).
*Hypertension.*

**Hizin** Ranbaxy, Thai.
Hydroxyzine hydrochloride (p.434·3).
*Hypersensitivity reactions.*

**Hjertealbyl** Leo, Denm.†.
Aspirin (p.15·1).
*Ischaemic heart disease; myocardial infarction.*

**Hjertemagnyl** Nycomed, Denm.
Aspirin (p.15·1).
*Ischaemic heart disease; myocardial infarction.*

**HMG** Farma Lepori, Spain.
Menotrophin (p.1330·1).
*Female infertility; male infertility.*

**HMG Massone**
Ferring, Arg.; Fustery, Mex.†.
Menotrophin (p.1330·1).
*Male and female infertility.*

**H-Mide** LBS, Thai.
Furosemide (p.919·3).
*Hypertension; oedema.*

**HMS**
Allergan, Austral.†; Allergan, Switz.†; Allergan, USA.
Medrysone (p.1106·1).
*Inflammatory eye disorders.*

**HN 25**
Milupa, Fr.; Milupa, Hong Kong†; Milupa, Irl.; Milupa, Port.; Milupa, Singapore†; Milupa, Switz.
Preparation for enteral nutrition (p.1417·1).
*Gastrointestinal disorders.*

**HN RL** Milupa, Fr.
Lactose-free infant feed (p.1417·1).
*Diarrhoea.*

**Hobaticam** Phoinix Pharm (Φοινιξ Φαρμ), Gr.
Tenoxicam (p.93·1).
*Dysmenorrhoea; gout; inflammation; osteoarthritis; pain; rheumatoid arthritis; spondyloarthropathies.*

**Hobatolex** Phoinix Pharm (Φοινιξ Φαρμ), Gr.
Gemfibrozil (p.923·1).
*Hyperlipidaemias.*

**Hobatstress** Phoinix Pharm (Φοινιξ Φαρμ), Gr.
Buspirone hydrochloride (p.672·2).
*Generalised anxiety.*

**Hocimin** Durascan, Denm.
Cimetidine (p.1255·3).
*Acid aspiration; gastro-oesophageal reflux; peptic ulcer; Zollinger-Ellison syndrome.*

**Hocura-Spondylose novo** Pascoe, Ger.†.
Hypericum (p.299·1); camphor (p.1665·3).
*Nerve and muscle pain.*

**Hodernal** Rottapharm, Spain.
Liquid paraffin (p.1479·1).
*Constipation.*

**Hoecutin Olbad** Hoernecke, Ger.†.
Soya oil (p.1447·2).
*Bath additive; dry skin; pruritus.*

**Hoecutin Olbad F** Hoernecke, Ger.†.
Arachis oil (p.1656·1); light liquid paraffin (p.1479·1).
*Bath additive; dry skin; pruritus.*

**Hoemarin Derma** Hoernecke, Ger.†.
Ichthammol (p.1148·2); sage oil (p.1741·2).
*Bath additive; eczema.*

**Hoemarin Rheuma** Hoernecke, Ger.†.
Methyl salicylate (p.59·3); turpentine oil (p.1760·1); eucalyptus oil (p.1686·2).
*Bath additive; circulatory disorders; musculoskeletal and joint disorders; neuralgia.*

**Hoepixin Bad N** Hoernecke, Ger.
Coal tar (p.1159·2).
*Bath additive; pruritic skin disorders.*

**Hoepixin N** Hoernecke, Ger.†.
Coal tar (p.1159·2); thyme oil (p.1755·3).
*Bath additive; eczema; psoriasis.*

**Hoevenol** Hoernecke, Ger.
*Capsules:* Aesculus (p.1648·2).
*Soft-tissue injury; venous insufficiency.*
*Topical emulsion*†: Methyl salicylate (p.59·3); aesculus (p.1648·2).
*Haemorrhoids; peripheral vascular disorders; venous insufficiency.*

**Hoevenol A** Hoernecke, Ger.†.
*Topical application:* Arnica (p.1656·3).
*Venous insufficiency.*
*Topical gel:* Arnica (p.1656·3); aesculus (p.1648·2).
*Circulatory disorders; phlebitis; venous insufficiency.*

**Hofcomant** Kolassa, Austria.
Amantadine sulfate (p.1197·2).
*Drug-induced extrapyramidal disorders; herpes zoster; parkinsonism.*

**Hofels White Willow and Burdock** Seven Seas, UK†.
Salix (p.87·3); lappa (p.1704·3); southern prickly ash (p.1766·3); bearberry (p.1659·2); poplar bark (p.1733·3).
*Musculoskeletal and joint pain.*

**Hoffmannstropfen** Hofmann & Sommer, Ger.
Ether; alcohol.
*Tonic.*

**Hoggar N** Stada, Ger.
Doxylamine succinate (p.432·3).
*Sleep disorders.*

**Hokunalin** Hokuriku, Jpn.
Tulobuterol (p.806·3).
*Obstructive airways disease.*

**Holadren** Laboratorios Chile, Chile.
Alendronate sodium (p.765·3).
*Bone metastases; hypercalcaemia; osteoporosis; Paget's disease of bone.*

**Hold DM** Ascher, USA.
Dextromethorphan hydrobromide (p.1117·3).
*Coughs.*

**Holfungin** Hollborn, Ger.
Clotrimazole (p.396·2).
*Fungal and bacterial skin infections.*

**Holgyeme** Effik, Fr.
Cyproterone acetate (p.1544·1); ethinylestradiol (p.1553·2).
*Acne in women.*

**Holofusine** Braun, Switz.
Electrolyte infusion with or without glucose (p.1217·1).
*Fluid and electrolyte disorders.*

**Holomagnesio** Phoenix, Arg.
Magnesium citrate (p.1272·1) or magnesium lactate (p.1228·1).
*Asthenia; dystonias; magnesium deficiency.*

**Holomagnesio Antioxidante** *Phoenix, Arg.*
Magnesium lactate; vitamin E (p.1417·1).

**Holomagnesio B6** *Phoenix, Arg.*
Magnesium lactate (p.1228·1); pyridoxine hydrochloride (p.1456·3).
*Atherosclerosis; muscular disorders.*

**Holomagnesio Ginseng** *Phoenix, Arg.*
Magnesium lactate; ginseng (p.1417·1).
*Tonic.*

**Holopon** *Byk Gulden, Hong Kong†.*
Hyoscine methobromide (p.483·3).
*Gastritis; motion sickness; peptic ulcer; smooth muscle spasm.*

**Holoxan**
*Kampel Martian, Arg.; Baxter, Austral.; Asta Medica, Austria; Baxter, Belg.; Asta Médica, Chile; Baxter, Chile; Baxter, Denm.; Asta Medica, Fin.; Baxter Oncology, Fr.; Baxter Oncology, Ger.; Asta, Gr.; Baxter, Hong Kong; Asta Medica, Ital.; Baxter Oncology, Malaysia; Sanfer, Mex.†; Viatris, Neth.; Asta Medica, Norw.; Asta Medica, NZ; NZ Medical & Scientific, NZ; Asta Medica, Port.; Aventis, S.Afr.; Baxter Oncology, Singapore; Asta Medica, Swed.; Asta Medica, Switz.; Baxter, Thai.*
Ifosfamide (p.561·1).
*Malignant neoplasms.*

**Holoxan Uromitexan** *German Remedies, India.*
Ifosfamide (p.561·1); mesna (p.1041·2).
*Malignant neoplasms.*

**Holoxane** *Asta Oncologia, Braz.*
Ifosfamide (p.561·1).
*Malignant neoplasms.*

**Holsten aktiv** *Holsten, Ger.†.*
Ethyl chloride (p.1376·2).
*Local anaesthesia.*

**Homa** *Upha, Malaysia.*
Homatropine hydrobromide (p.483·2).
*Production of mydriasis.*

**Homasedin** *Medifarma, Mex.*
Homatropine methylbromide (p.483·2).

**Homatrocil** *Oftalder, Port.†.*
Homatropine hydrobromide (p.483·2).
*Production of mydriasis and cycloplegia.*

**Homatrop** *Llorens, Spain.*
Homatropine hydrobromide (p.483·2).
*Production of mydriasis and cycloplegia; uveitis.*

**Homatropil** *Rhone-Poulenc Rorer, Mex.†.*
Homatropine (p.483·2).

**Homeoaftyl** *Boiron, Fr.*
Homoeopathic preparation.

**Homeocoksinum** *Homeocan, Canad.*
Homoeopathic preparation.

**Homeodent**
*Boiron, Canad.; Boiron, Port.†.*
Homoeopathic preparation.

**Homeodose**
*Dolisos, Canad.; Dolisos, Fr.*
A range of homoeopathic preparations.

**Homeofortil** *Dolisos, Fr.*
Homoeopathic preparation.

**Homeofortin III** *Hochstetter, Chile.*
Phosphoric acid (p.1731·2); avena (p.1658·2); strychnos ignatii (p.1722·3).
*Depression.*

**Homeogene 9**
*Boiron, Fr.; Boiron, Port.*
Homoeopathic preparation.

**Homeogene 46**
*Boiron, Canad.; Boiron, Fr.*
Homoeopathic preparation.

**Homeomunil** *Dolisos, Fr.*
Homoeopathic preparation.

**Homeoplasmina** *Hochstetter, Chile.*
Boric acid (p.1662·1); pokeroot (p.1733·1); calendula (p.1665·2).

**Homeoplasmine**
*Note. This name is used for preparations of different composition.*
*Boiron, Fr.*
Calendula (p.1665·2); pokeroot (p.1733·1); bryonia (p.1663·1); Siam benzoin (p.1744·1); boric acid (p.1662·1).
*Skin irritation.*

*Boiron, Port.*
Homoeopathic preparation.

**Homeoptic** *Boiron, Fr.*
Homoeopathic preparation.

**Homeovox**
*Boiron, Canad.; Boiron, Port.*
Homoeopathic preparation.

**Hominex** *Ross, USA.*
A range of methionine-free preparations for enteral nutrition including an infant feed (p.1417·1).
*Vitamin $B_6$-nonresponsive homocystinuria or hypermethioninaemia.*

**Homo** *Grin, Mex.*
Homatropine hydrobromide (p.483·2).
*Production of mydriasis.*

**Homocalmefyba** *Northia, Arg.*
Piroxicam (p.84·2).
*Inflammation.*

**Homocisteon Compuesto** *Purissimus, Arg.*
Amylase (p.1654·2); papain (p.1727·3); pancrelipase (p.1725·3); cysteine; vitamin B substances.
*Gastrointestinal disorders; pancreatic insufficiency.*

**Homoclomin**
*Eisai, Hong Kong; Eisai, Jpn; Eisai, Thai.*
Homochlorcyclizine hydrochloride (p.434·3).
*Allergic rhinitis; pruritus; urticaria.*

**Homoderma** *Brauer, Austral.†.*
Homoeopathic preparation.

**Homopafen** *Bioresearch, Mex.*
Propafenone (p.989·2).
*Arrhythmias.*

**Homopan** *Collins, Mex.*
Multivitamin preparation (p.1417·1).

**Homosismin** *Pharmavite, Canad.*
Multivitamin preparation with selenium (p.1417·1).

**Honey Lemon Cough Lozenges** *Sutton, Canad.*
Menthol (p.1711·3).

**Honey & Molasses** *Lane, UK.*
Ipecacuanha liquid extract (p.1122·3); marrubium (p.1124·1); squill vinegar (p.1130·3); capsicum (p.1667·1); peppermint oil (p.1283·2); tolu solution; honey (p.1434·2); molasses; glycerol (p.1694·3); liquorice (p.1270·2); anise oil (p.1655·2).
*Coughs.*

**Honeycold** *Whitehall, Ital.*
Paracetamol (p.76·2); pseudoephedrine hydrochloride (p.1129·2).
*Cold symptoms.*

**Honeyflu** *Home, Ital.*
Paracetamol (p.76·2); dextromethorphan hydrobromide (p.1117·3).
*Cough; fever.*

**Honeygola** *Whitehall, Ital.*
Cetylpyridinium chloride (p.1173·1).
*Mouth infections.*

**Honeytuss** *Whitehall, Ital.*
Dextromethorphan hydrobromide (p.1117·3).
*Coughs.*

**Hongosan** *Medea, Spain.*
Acedoben (p.1645·2); aluminium chlorohydrate (p.1142·1); cetrimonium bromide (p.1173·1); dexamethasone (p.1097·1); salicylic acid (p.1157·1).
*Fungal skin infections.*

**Hongoseril** *Isdin, Spain.*
Itraconazole (p.401·3).
*Fungal infections.*

**Honguil** *Raymos, Arg.*
Tioconazole (p.409·3).
*Fungal vaginal infections.*

**Honguil Plus** *Raymos, Arg.*
Fluconazole (p.398·1).
*Fungal infections.*

**Honsa** *M & H, Thai.*
Hydroxyzine hydrochloride (p.434·3).
*Anxiety; pruritus.*

**Honvan**
*Kampel Martian, Arg.; Asta Medica, Austral.†; Asta Medica, Austria; Baxter, Belg.; Abbott, Braz.†; Baxter Oncology, Ger.; Asta, Gr.; Baxter, Hong Kong; German Remedies, India; Sanfer, Mex.; Viatris, Neth.; Asta Medica, Norw.†; Asta Medica, NZ†; NZ Medical & Scientific, NZ†; Asta Medica, Port.; Asta Medica, Singapore†; Prasfarma, Spain; Asta Medica, Switz.; Baxter, UK†.*
Fosfestrol (p.1555·3) or fosfestrol sodium (p.1555·3).
*Prostatic cancer.*

**Honvol** *Asta Medica, Canad.*
Fosfestrol sodium (p.1555·3).
*Prostatic cancer.*

**Honzil** *Arlex, Mex.†.*
Ketoconazole (p.403·3).

**Hopacem** *Hommel, Ger.*
Mianserin hydrochloride (p.306·3).
*Depression.*

**Hopram** *IQFA, Mex.*
Omeprazole (p.1278·2).
*Peptic ulcer.*

**Hopranolol** *Hovid, Hong Kong.*
Propranolol hydrochloride (p.989·3).
*Angina pectoris; arrhythmias; hypertension; hyperthyroidism; hypertrophic subaortic stenosis; migraine; phaeochromocytoma; tremor.*

**Hordenol** *Aerocid, Fr.†.*
Hordenine sulfate; caffeine (p.782·1).
*Diarrhoea.*

**Horehound and Aniseed Cough Mixture** *Potter's, UK.*
Pleurisy root (p.1733·1); elecampane (p.1119·3); horehound (p.1124·1); skunk cabbage (p.1746·3); lobelia (p.1589·1).
*Coughs.*

**Horestyl** *Kleva, Gr.*
Loratadine (p.436·1).
*Allergic rhinitis; pruritus.*

**Horex** *Pharmacos, Mex.*
Timolol maleate (p.1012·2).
*Glaucoma.*

**Horf** *YSP, Malaysia.*
Chlorhexidine hydrochloride (p.1173·3); benzocaine (p.1370·3).
*Mouth and throat disorders.*

**Horizem** *Horizon, UK†.*
Diltiazem hydrochloride (p.900·1).
*Angina pectoris; hypertension.*

**Hormo Hepatico** *Iodo Suma, Braz.*
Adenosine (p.851·2); methionine (p.1042·1); betaine hydrochloride (p.1660·2); choline citrate (p.1424·3); inositol (p.1701·2); pyridoxine hydrochloride (p.1456·3); liver extract; sorbitol (p.1446·3).
*Liver disorders.*

**Hormocervix** *Millet Roux, Braz.†.*
Hydroxyestrone diacetate (p.1556·3).
*Vulvovaginal disorders.*

**Hormodausse** *Sabex, Canad.*
Vitamin B substances; iron; liver extract; beef serum (p.1417·1).

**Hormodausse plus Calcium and Vitamin D** *Charton, Canad.†.*
Multivitamin and mineral preparation (p.1417·1).

**Hormodiol** *Omega, Arg.*
Estradiol (p.1550·1).
*Menopausal disorders.*

**Hormodose** *Farmasa, Braz.*
Estradiol (p.1550·1).
*Menopausal disorders.*

**Hormoginase** *Sanval, Braz.†.*
Estradiol benzoate (p.1550·1); progesterone (p.1566·2); ergocalciferol (p.1462·1).
*Menopausal disorders.*

**Hormolax** *Hormona, Mex.*
Ispaghula (p.1268·1).
*Constipation.*

**Hormone Multicap** *Scherer, Thai.*
Methyltestosterone (p.1559·3); ethinylestradiol (p.1553·2); vitamins; rutoside; inositol; methionine; choline bitartrate (p.1417·1).
*Nutritional supplement.*

**Hormonin**
*Shire, Hong Kong; Shire, UK.*
Estriol (p.1552·3); estradiol (p.1550·1); estrone (p.1553·1).
*Menopausal disorders; osteoporosis.*

**Horon** *Scherer, Thai.*
Methyltestosterone (p.1559·3); ethinylestradiol (p.1553·2); vitamins; minerals; inositol; methionine; choline bitartrate (p.1417·1).
*Nutritional supplement.*

**Horse Radish and Garlic Tablets** *Vitaglow, Austral.†.*
Horseradish (p.1697·3); garlic (p.1691·1); ascorbic acid (p.1460·2); zinc sulfate (p.1469·3).
*Catarrh; coughs; hay fever; sinusitis; upper respiratory-tract congestion.*

**Horvilan N** *Schoning-Berlin, Ger.*
Turmeric (p.1058·3); peppermint oil (p.1283·2); greater celandine (p.1695·3).
*Biliary-tract disorders.*

**Hosboral** *Quimifar, Spain.*
Amoxicillin trihydrate (p.155·3).
*Bacterial infections.*

**Hosboral Bronquial** *Aventis, Spain†.*
Amoxicillin trihydrate (p.155·3); bromhexine hydrochloride (p.1115·3).
*Respiratory-tract infections.*

**Hospidermin** *Lysoform, Ger.*
Alcohol (p.1166·1); potassium thiocyanate; 5-chloro-2-hydroxybenzoic acid.
*Skin disinfection.*

**Hospisept** *Lysoform, Ger.*
Propyl alcohol (p.1191·2); alcohol (p.1166·1).
*Hand disinfection; skin disinfection.*

**Hostacyclin**
*Hoechst Marion Roussel, Austria†; Hoechst, Ger.†; Hoechst Marion Roussel, Gr.*
Tetracycline hydrochloride (p.266·2).
*Amoebiasis; bacterial infections.*

**Hostacycline**
*Aventis, India.*
Tetracycline (p.266·2).
*Bacterial infections.*

*Quatromed, S.Afr.†.*
Tetracycline hydrochloride (p.266·2).
*Bacterial infections.*

**Hostan** *Hovid, Hong Kong.*
Mefenamic acid (p.55·2).
*Musculoskeletal and joint disorders; pain.*

**Hosterona** *Gador, Arg.*
Progesterone (p.1566·2); estradiol hemisuccinate (p.1551·1).
*Menstrual disorders.*

**Hostid** *Fournier, Ger.†.*
Urtica root (p.1762·1).
*Micturition disorders associated with prostatic cancer.*

**Hostop** *Nettopharma, Denm.†.*
Acetylcysteine (p.1112·3).
*Respiratory-tract congestion.*

**Hot Coldrex** *SmithKline Beecham Consumer, Neth.*
Paracetamol (p.76·2); ascorbic acid (p.1460·2).
*Cold and influenza symptoms.*

**Hot Lemon** *Prodemdis, Canad.*
Phenylephrine hydrochloride (p.1126·3); pheniramine maleate (p.438·3); paracetamol (p.76·2); ascorbic acid (p.1460·2).

**Hot Lemon Relief** *Apotex, Canad.*
Phenylephrine hydrochloride (p.1126·3); pheniramine maleate (p.438·3); paracetamol (p.76·2); ascorbic acid (p.1460·2).

**Hot Thermo** *Merck dura, Ger.*
Glycol salicylate (p.44·3); benzyl nicotinate (p.21·2).
*Musculoskeletal, joint, and soft-tissue disorders; superficial vascular disorders.*

**Hotemin** *Egis, Hong Kong.*
Piroxicam (p.84·2).
*Gout; musculoskeletal and joint disorders.*

**12 Hour Antihistamine Nasal Decongestant**
*URL, USA.*
Pseudoephedrine sulfate (p.1129·2); dexbrompheniramine maleate (p.426·1).
*Upper respiratory-tract symptoms.*

**12 Hour Cold**
*Note. This name is used for preparations of different composition.*
*Goldline, USA.*
Pseudoephedrine sulfate (p.1129·2); dexbrompheniramine maleate (p.426·1).
*Upper respiratory-tract symptoms.*

*Hudson, USA†.*
Phenylpropanolamine hydrochloride (p.1127·3); chlorphenamine maleate (p.427·3).
*Upper respiratory-tract symptoms.*

**Hova**
*Novartis Consumer, Austria; Gebro, Switz.*
Valerian (p.1762·2); lupulus (p.1708·1).
*Nervous disorders; sleep disorders.*

**Hova Expectorant** *Hovid, Hong Kong.*
Diphenhydramine hydrochloride (p.431·3); ammonium chloride (p.1115·2); sodium citrate (p.1223·2).
*Coughs; respiratory-tract congestion.*

**Hovaletten N** *Zyma, Ger.†.*
Lupulus (p.1708·1); valerian (p.1762·2).
*Nervous disorders; sleep disorders.*

**Hovalin** *Astra, Gr.*
Fluvastatin (p.918·3).
*Primary hypercholesterolaemia.*

**Hovasin** *Novartis Consumer, Austria.*
Valerian (p.1762·2).
*Nervous disorders; sleep disorders.*

**Hovid Q10 Plus** *Hovid, Malaysia.*
Vitamins; ubidecarenone (p.1417·1).

**Hovite** *Raptakos, India.*
Multivitamin preparation (p.1417·1).

**Hox Alpha** *Strathmann, Ger.*
Urtica (p.1762·1).
*Rheumatic disorders.*

**$H_2$Oxyl** *Stiefel, Canad.†.*
Benzoyl peroxide (p.1143·2).
*Acne.*

**HPB** *Panalab, Arg.*
Finasteride (p.1554·2).
*Benign prostatic hyperplasia.*

**H-Peran** *LBS, Thai.*
Metoclopramide (p.1274·3).
*Gastrointestinal motility disorders; nausea and vomiting.*

**HPMC-Ophtal** *Winzer, Ger.*
Hypromellose (p.1579·3).
*Adjunct in ophthalmic surgery.*

**Hp-Pac** *Abbott, Canad.*
Capsules, lansoprazole (Prevacid) (p.1269·3); tablets, clarithromycin (Biaxin) (p.192·2); capsules, amoxicillin trihydrate (p.155·3).
*Helicobacter pylori-associated peptic ulcer.*

**H-R Lubricating Jelly** *Wallace, USA.*
Vaginal lubricant.

**HRF**
*Wyeth-Ayerst, Austral.†; Wyeth Lederle, Belg.†; Wyeth, Braz.†; Shire, Irl.; Sigma-Tau, Neth.; Wyeth, NZ; Akromed, S.Afr.†; Intropharm, UK.*
Gonadorelin (p.1325·1) or gonadorelin hydrochloride (p.1325·2).
*Anovulatory infertility; cryptorchidism; sterility or delayed puberty due to hypogonadotrophic hypogonadism; test of hypothalamic function.*

**HRI Calm Life** *Jessup, UK.*
Jamaica dogwood (p.1702·3); lupulus (p.1708·1); skullcap (p.1746·3); chamomile (p.1669·3); valerian (p.1762·2).
*Irritability; restlessness.*

**HRI Clear Complexion** *Jessup, UK.*
Sarsaparilla (p.1742·1); iris versicolor (p.1702·1); lappa (p.1704·3).
*Skin disorders.*

**HRI Golden Seal Digestive** *Jessup, UK.*
Ginger (p.1267·1); myrrh (p.1718·3); hydrastis (p.1698·3); rhubarb (p.1287·3); valerian (p.1762·2).
*Dyspepsia; flatulence.*

**HRI Night** *Jessup, UK.*
Valerian (p.1762·2); passion flower (p.1729·1); wild lettuce (p.1765·2); vervain (p.1764·1); lupulus (p.1708·1).
*Insomnia.*

**HRI Water Balance** *Jessup, UK.*
Taraxacum (p.1751·3); buchu (p.1663·1); parsley piert (p.1729·1); bearberry (p.1659·2).
*Water retention.*

**H-Sal** *Zambon, Braz.†.*
Homatropine (p.483·2); sodium; potassium; calcium; vitamin $B_2$; nicotinamide; glucose (p.1222·2).
*Gastrointestinal spasm; oral rehydration therapy.*

**HT903** *Optimal, Hong Kong†.*
Melatonin (p.1710·2).
*Jet lag; melatonin deficiency.*

**H-Tab** *Pharmaland, Thai.*
Haloperidol (p.701·2).
*Hypomania; mania; psychoses.*

**H-Tronin** *Aventis, Ger.*
Insulin injection (human) (p.333·3).
*Diabetes mellitus.*

**H-Tuss-D** *Cypress, USA.*
Hydrocodone tartrate (p.45·1); pseudoephedrine hydrochloride (p.1129·2).
*Coughs.*

**Huberdilat** *ICN, Spain†.*
Cetiedil (p.882·1).
*Peripheral vascular disorders.*

**Huberdoxina** *ICN, Spain.*
Ciprofloxacin hydrochloride (p.188·2) or ciprofloxacin lactate (p.188·3).
*Bacterial infections.*

**Hubergrip** *ICN, Spain.*
*Suppositories:* Caffeine (p.782·1); calcium pantothenate (p.1442·3); citiolone (p.1672·3); chlorphenamine maleate (p.427·3); paracetamol (p.76·2); vitamin A (p.1451·2).
*Tablets:* Caffeine (p.782·1); chlorphenamine maleate (p.427·3); propyphenazone (p.85·3); salicylamide (p.87·3).
*Influenza and cold symptoms.*

**Hubermizol** *Eight, Spain.*
Astemizole (p.424·2).
*Hypersensitivity reactions.*

**Huberplex** *Teofarma, Spain.*
Chlordiazepoxide hydrochloride (p.674·2).
*Alcohol withdrawal syndrome; anxiety; insomnia; skeletal muscle spasm.*

**Huile analgesique "Temple of Heaven" contre les maux de tete** *Panax, Switz.*
Mint oil (p.1715·2); camphor (p.1665·3); menthol (p.1711·3); eucalyptus oil (p.1686·2); methyl salicylate (p.59·3); thymol (p.1194·2).
Formerly known as Huile analgesique Polar-Bar.
*Headache.*

**Huile de Bain Therapeutique** *Atlas, Canad.*
Wool fat (p.1483·1); liquid paraffin (p.1479·1).

**Huile de Haarlem** *Lefevre, Fr.†.*
Sulfur (p.1158·2); linseed oil (p.1707·2); turpentine oil (p.1760·1).
*Arthritic disorders; respiratory-tract disorders.*

**Huile de millepertuis A. Vogel (huile de St. Jean)** *Bioforce, Switz.*
Hypericum (p.299·1); sunflower oil (p.1451·1).
*Superficial wounds.*

**Huile Gomenolee** *Gomenol, Fr.*
Niaouli oil (p.1719·3).
*Nasal infections.*

**Huile Po-Ho A. Vogel** *Bioforce, Switz.*
Peppermint oil (p.1283·2); eucalyptus oil (p.1686·2); juniper oil (p.1703·1); caraway oil (p.1667·3); fennel oil (p.1687·3).
*Cold symptoms; headache; muscular tension.*

**Huile Solaire Bronzage** *Clarins, Canad.†.*
*SPF 3:* Octinoxate (p.1154·3); oxybenzone (p.1154·3).
*Sunscreen.*

**Humacart 3/7** *Lilly, Jpn.*
A mixture of insulin injection (human, prb) and isophane insulin injection (human, prb) (p.333·3).
*Diabetes mellitus.*

**Humaject I** *Lilly, UK†.*
Injection device containing Humulin I (p.333·3).
*Diabetes mellitus.*

**Humaject 10/90, 20/80, 30/70, 40/60, 50/50** *Lilly, Neth.†.*
Mixtures of insulin injection (human) and isophane insulin injection (human) respectively in the proportions indicated (p.333·3).
*Diabetes mellitus.*

**Humaject 20/80, 30/70, 40/60, 50/50** *Lilly, Belg.*
Mixtures of insulin injection (human) and isophane insulin injection (human) respectively in the proportions indicated (p.333·3).
*Diabetes mellitus.*

**Humaject M1, M2, M3, M4, M5** *Lilly, UK†.*
Injection device containing Humulin M1, M2, M3, M4, and M5 respectively (p.333·3).
*Diabetes mellitus.*

**Humaject NPH**
*Lilly, Belg.; Lilly, Neth.†.*
Isophane insulin injection (human) (p.333·3).
*Diabetes mellitus.*

**Humaject Regular**
*Lilly, Belg.; Lilly, Neth.†.*
Insulin injection (human) (p.333·3).
*Diabetes mellitus.*

**Humaject S** *Lilly, UK.*
Injection device containing Humulin S (p.333·3).
*Diabetes mellitus.*

**Humal** *Rosch & Handel, Austria.*
Humic acid; salicylic acid (p.1157·1).
*Rheumatism.*

**Humalog**
*Lilly, Arg.; Lilly, Austral.; Lilly, Austria; Lilly, Belg.; Lilly, Braz.; Lilly, Canad.; Lilly, Chile; Lilly, Denm.; Lilly, Fin.; Lilly, Fr.; Lilly, Ger.; Pharmaserve Lilly (Φαρμασερβ Λιλλυ), Gr.; Lilly, Hong Kong; Lilly, Irl.; Lilly, Israel; Lilly, Ital.; Lilly, Malaysia; Lilly, Mex.; Lilly, Neth.; Lilly, Norw.; Lilly, NZ; Lilly, Port.†; Lilly, S.Afr.; Lilly, Singapore; Lilly, Spain; Lilly, Swed.; Lilly, Switz.; Lilly, Thai.; Lilly, UK; Lilly, USA.*
Insulin lispro (p.333·3).
*Diabetes mellitus.*

**Humalog Mix 25**
*Lilly, Austral.; Lilly, Braz.; Lilly, Canad.; Lilly, Israel; Lilly, Ital.; Lilly, Mex.; Lilly, Neth.; Lilly, Norw.; Lilly, NZ; Lilly, S.Afr.; Lilly, Singapore; Lilly, Thai.*
Mixture of insulin lispro 25% and protamine insulin lispro 75 % (p.333·3).
*Diabetes mellitus.*

**Humalog Mix 25 and 50**
*Lilly, Austria; Lilly, Denm.; Lilly, Fin.; Lilly, Fr.; Lilly, Ger.; Lilly, Irl.; Lilly, Spain; Lilly, Swed.; Lilly, UK.*
A mixture of insulin lispro 25% or 50% and isophane insulin lispro 75% or 50%, respectively (p.333·3).
*Diabetes mellitus.*

**Humalog Mix 75/25 and 50/50** *Lilly, USA.*
Mixtures of isophane insulin lispro 75% and 50% and insulin lispro 25% and 50% respectively (p.333·3).
*Diabetes mellitus.*

**Humalog NPL** *Lilly, Spain.*
Protamine insulin lispro (p.333·3).
*Diabetes mellitus.*

**Human Actrapid** *Knoll, India.*
Neutral insulin injection (human) (p.333·3).
*Diabetes mellitus.*

**Human Insultard** *Knoll, India.*
Isophane insulin injection (human) (p.333·3).
*Diabetes mellitus.*

**Human Mixtard 30 and 50** *Knoll, India.*
Mixture of neutral insulin injection (human) 30 or 50% and isophane insulin injection (human) 70 or 50%, respectively (p.333·3).
*Diabetes mellitus.*

**Human Monotard** *Knoll, India.*
Insulin zinc suspension (human) (p.333·3).
*Diabetes mellitus.*

**Humana AR** *Humana, Ital.*
Infant feed (p.1417·1).
*Gastro-oesophageal reflux; regurgitation.*

**Humana Disanal** *Humana, Ital.*
Food for special diets (p.1417·1).
*Gastrointestinal disorders.*

**Humana HA** *Humana, Ital.*
Infant feed (p.1417·1).
*Food intolerance.*

**Humana Sinelac** *Humana, Ital.*
Infant feed (p.1417·1).
*Milk intolerance.*

**Humanalbin** *Aventis Behring, Ger.*
Albumin (p.740·3).
*Hypovolaemia.*

**Humanilusin** *Cryopharma, Mex.*
Human insulin (p.333·3).
*Diabetes mellitus.*

**Humaplus 20/80, 30/70** *Lilly, Spain.*
Mixtures of insulin injection (human) and isophane insulin injection (human) respectively in the proportions indicated (p.333·3).
*Diabetes mellitus.*

**Humaplus NPH** *Lilly, Spain.*
Isophane insulin injection (human) (p.333·3).
*Diabetes mellitus.*

**Humaplus Regular** *Lilly, Spain.*
Insulin injection (human) (p.333·3).
*Diabetes mellitus.*

**Humate-P** *Aventis, USA.*
A factor VIII preparation (p.751·1).
*Haemophilia A; von Willebrand's disease.*

**Humatin**
*Pfizer, Austria; Pfizer, Canad.; Parke, Davis, Ger.; Parke, Davis, Ital.; Pfizer, Spain; Pfizer, Switz.; Parke, Davis, USA.*
Paromomycin sulfate (p.612·3).
*Hepatic encephalopathy and coma; intestinal amoebiasis; preoperative intestinal sterilisation; taeniasis.*

**Humatrope**
*Lilly, Austral.; Lilly, Austria; Lilly, Belg.; Lilly, Braz.; Lilly, Canad.; Lilly, Chile; Lilly, Denm.; Lilly, Fin.; Lilly, Ger.; Pharmaserve Lilly (Φαρμασερβ Λιλλυ), Gr; Lilly, Hong Kong; Lilly, Ital.; Lilly, Mex.; Lilly, Neth.; Lilly, Norw.; Lilly, Port.; Lilly, S.Afr.; Lilly, Singapore; Irisfarma, Spain; Lilly, Swed.; Lilly, Switz.; Lilly, UK; Lilly, USA.*
Somatropin (p.1327·2).
*Growth disorders in renal failure; growth hormone deficiency; Turner's syndrome.*

**Humatro-Pen** *Aza, Austral.*
Somatropin (p.1327·2).
*Growth hormone deficiency.*

**Humavent** *WE, USA.*
Guaifenesin (p.1122·1).

**Humectante** *Alcon Cusi, Spain.*
Hypromellose (p.1579·3); sodium chloride (p.1233·3).
Formerly contained methylcellulose and sodium chloride.
*Dry eyes in contact lens wearers.*

**Humectante Bucal** *Pharmatrix, Arg.*
Carmellose sodium (p.1577·3); sorbitol (p.1446·3); electrolytes (p.1217·1).
*Artificial saliva.*

**Humectol** *Virtus, Braz.†.*
Bisacodyl (p.1251·3); docusate (p.1262·1).
*Constipation.*

**Humedia** *APS, Ger.*
Glibenclamide (p.331·2).
*Diabetes mellitus.*

**Humegon**
*Organon, Austral.; Organon, Austria†; Organon, Belg.†; Akzo, Braz.†; Organon, Canad.; Organon, Ger.; Organon, Hong Kong†; Organon, Irl.; Organon, Israel; Organon, Ital.; Organon, Mex.†; Organon, Neth.†; Organon, Port.; Donmed, S.Afr.; Organon, Singapore†; Organon, Switz.†; Organon, Thai.†; Organon, USA.*
Menotrophin (p.1330·1).
*Male and female infertility.*

**Humektan** *Orion, Fin.*
Moisturiser; vehicle for topical drugs.

**Humex**
*Note. This name is used for preparations of different composition.*
*Urgo, Belg.*
Dextromethorphan hydrobromide (p.1117·3).
*Coughs.*

*Urgo, Fr.*
*Adult syrup:* Pholcodine (p.1128·3).
Formerly contained ethylmorphine hydrochloride, squill, ipecacuanha, and belladonna.
*Coughs.*
*Capsules†:* Carbinoxamine maleate (p.426·3); phenylpropanolamine hydrochloride (p.1127·3); paracetamol (p.76·2).
*Upper respiratory-tract disorders.*
*Lozenges:* Ethylmorphine hydrochloride (p.37·3); ipecacuanha (p.1122·3); belladonna (p.479·1).
*Coughs.*
*Nasal solution:* Benzalkonium chloride (p.1168·3).
Formerly contained benzododecinium bromide.
*Nasal infections.*
*Paediatric syrup:* Pholcodine (p.1128·3).
Formerly contained pholcodine, sodium benzoate, drosera, belladonna, and tolu balsam.
*Coughs.*
*Pastilles:* Biclotymol (p.1171·1).
*Sore throat.*
*Throat spray:* Benzalkonium chloride (p.1168·3); lidocaine hydrochloride (p.1377·3).
*Mouth and throat disorders.*

**Humex Expectorant** *Urgo, Fr.*
*Lozenges:* Acetylcysteine (p.1112·3).
*Syrup:* Carbocisteine (p.1116·2).
*Respiratory-tract congestion.*

**Humex Mal de Gorge sans sucre** *Urgo, Fr.*
Dequalinium chloride (p.1178·1); ascorbic acid (p.1460·2).
Formerly known as Humex Kinaldine.
*Mouth and throat disorders.*

**Humex Rhume** *Urgo, Fr.*
Tablets (daytime), paracetamol (p.76·2); pseudoephedrine hydrochloride (p.1129·2); capsules (evening), paracetamol; chlorphenamine maleate (p.427·3).
*Cold symptoms.*

**Humibid** *Carolina, USA.*
Guaifenesin (p.1122·1); sulfogaiacol (p.1131·1).
Formerly contained guaifenesin.
*Coughs.*

**Humibid DM** *Carolina, USA.*
Dextromethorphan hydrobromide (p.1117·3); guaifenesin (p.1122·1); sulfogaiacol (p.1131·1).
Formerly contained dextromethorphan hydrobromide and guaifenesin.
*Coughs.*

**Huminsulin Basal**
*Lilly, Austria; Lilly, Ger.*
Isophane insulin injection (human, prb) (p.333·3).
*Diabetes mellitus.*

**Huminsulin Basal (NPH)** *Lilly, Switz.*
Isophane insulin injection (human, prb) (p.333·3).
*Diabetes mellitus.*

**Huminsulin Long**
*Lilly, Austria; Lilly, Ger.†; Lilly, Switz.*
Insulin zinc suspension (crystalline 70%, amorphous 30%) (human, prb) (p.333·3).
*Diabetes mellitus.*

**Huminsulin Normal**
*Lilly, Austria; Lilly, Ger.; Lilly, Switz.*
Insulin injection (human, prb) (p.333·3).
*Diabetes mellitus.*

**Huminsulin Profil I, II, III, and IV**
*Lilly, Austria; Lilly, Switz.*
Mixtures of insulin injection (human, prb) 10%, 20%, 30%, and 40% and isophane insulin injection (human, prb) 90%, 80%, 70%, and 60% respectively (p.333·3).
*Diabetes mellitus.*

**Huminsulin Profil II and III** *Lilly, Ger.*
Mixtures of neutral insulin injection (human, prb) 20% and 30% and isophane insulin injection (human, prb) 80% and 70%, respectively (p.333·3).
*Diabetes mellitus.*

**Huminsulin Ultralong**
*Lilly, Austria; Lilly, Ger.†; Lilly, Switz.*
Insulin zinc suspension (crystalline) (human, prb) (p.333·3).
*Diabetes mellitus.*

**Humira**
*Abbott, Austral.; Abbott, Fr.; Abbott, UK; Abbott, USA.*
Adalimumab (p.12·1).
*Rheumatoid arthritis.*

**HuMist Nasal Mist** *Scherer, USA.*
Sodium chloride (p.1233·3).
*Nasal irritation.*

**Humoferon** *Sigma-Tau, Ital.*
Interferon alfa-n1 (p.640·3).
*Chronic hepatitis; leukaemias.*

**Humopin N** *Schoning-Berlin, Ger.*
Salicylic acid (p.1157·1).
*Bath additive; musculoskeletal and joint disorders.*

**Humorap** *Bago, Arg.*
Citalopram hydrobromide (p.289·1).
*Depression.*

**Humorsol** *Merck, USA.*
Demecarium bromide (p.1488·3).
*Open-angle glaucoma; strabismus.*

**Humoryl** *Sanofi Synthelabo, Fr.†.*
Toloxatone (p.318·2).
*Depression.*

**Humoxal** *Fredo, Port.†.*
Phenylephrine hydrochloride (p.1126·3).
*Nasal congestion.*

**Humulin I**
*Lilly, Irl.; Lilly, Ital.; Lilly, UK.*
Isophane insulin injection (human, prb) (p.333·3).
*Diabetes mellitus.*

**Humulin 10/90, 20/80, 30/70, 40/60, and 50/50** *Lilly, Ital.*
Mixtures of insulin injection (human) and isophane insulin injection (human) respectively in the proportions indicated (p.333·3).
*Diabetes mellitus.*

**Humulin 20/80, 30/70** *Lilly, Canad.*
Mixtures of insulin injection (human, prb) and isophane insulin injection (human, prb) (p.333·3) respectively in the proportions indicated.
*Diabetes mellitus.*

**Humulin 20/80, 30/70 and 50/50** *Lilly, Austral.*
Mixtures of insulin injection (human, prb) and isophane insulin (human, prb) (p.333·3), respectively, in the proportions indicated.
*Diabetes mellitus.*

**Humulin 30/70**
*Lilly, Malaysia; Lilly, S.Afr.; Lilly, Singapore.*
Mixture of insulin injection (human) 30% and isophane insulin injection (human) 70% (p.333·3).
*Diabetes mellitus.*

**Humulin 70/30**
*Lilly, Arg.; Lilly, Braz.; Lilly, Chile; Lilly, Hong Kong; Lilly, Thai.*
A mixture of isophane insulin injection (human) 70% and insulin injection (human) 30% (p.333·3).
*Diabetes mellitus.*

**Humulin 70/30, 50/50** *Lilly, USA.*
Mixture of isophane insulin suspension (human, crb) and insulin injection (human, crb) in the proportions indicated (p.333·3).
*Diabetes mellitus.*

**Humulin 70/30, 80/20**
*Lilly, Israel; Lilly, Mex.; Lilly, NZ.*
Mixtures of isophane insulin injection (human) and insulin injection (human) respectively in the proportions indicated (p.333·3).
*Diabetes mellitus.*

**Humulin L**
*Lilly, Arg.; Lilly, Austral.; Lilly, Canad.; Lilly, Chile; Lilly, Hong Kong; Lilly, Ital.; Lilly, Malaysia; Lilly, Mex.; Lilly, NZ; Lilly, S.Afr.; Lilly, Singapore; Lilly, USA.*
Insulin zinc suspension (human) (p.333·3).
*Diabetes mellitus.*

**Humulin L (Lente)** *Pharmaserve Lilly (Φαρμασερβ Λιλλυ), Gr.*
Insulin zinc suspension (human) (p.333·3).
*Diabetes mellitus.*

**Humulin Lenta**
*Lilly, Braz.; Lilly, Port.*
Insulin zinc suspension (30% amorphous, crystalline 70%) (human) (p.333·3).
*Diabetes mellitus.*

**Humulin Lente**
*Lilly, Irl.; Lilly, UK†.*
Insulin zinc suspension (30% amorphous, 70% crystalline) (human, prb) (p.333·3).
*Diabetes mellitus.*

**Humulin M2, M3, M4** *Lilly, Irl.*
Mixtures of insulin injection (human, prb) 20%, 30%, and 40% and isophane insulin injection (human, prb) 80%, 70%, and 60%, respectively (p.333·3).
*Diabetes mellitus.*

**Humulin M3** *Lilly, UK.*
A mixture of insulin injection (human, prb) 30% and isophane insulin injection (human, prb) 70% respectively (p.333·3).
*Diabetes mellitus.*

**Humulin M1, M2, M3, M4, M5**
*Pharmaserve Lilly (Φαρμασερβ Λιλλυ), Gr.; Lilly, Port.*
Mixtures of insulin injection (human) 10%, 20%, 30%, 40%, and 50% and isophane insulin injection (human) 90%, 80%. 70%, 60%, and 50%, respectively (p.333·3).
*Diabetes mellitus.*

**Humulin Mix 30/70**
*Lilly, Denm.; Lilly, Fin.†; Lilly, Norw.†; Lilly, Swed.*
A mixture of insulin injection (human) 30% and isophane insulin injection (human) 70% (p.333·3).
*Diabetes mellitus.*

**Humulin N**
*Lilly, Arg.; Lilly, Canad.; Lilly, Chile; Lilly, Hong Kong; Lilly, Israel; Lilly, Malaysia; Lilly, Mex.; Lilly, NZ; Lilly, S.Afr.; Lilly, Singapore; Lilly, Thai.; Lilly, USA.*
Isophane insulin injection (human) (p.333·3).
*Diabetes mellitus.*

**Humulin NPH**
*Lilly, Austral.; Lilly, Braz.; Lilly, Denm.; Lilly, Fin.; Lilly, Norw.; Lilly, Port.; Lilly, Swed.*
Isophane insulin injection (human) (p.333·3).
*Diabetes mellitus.*

**Humulin (NPH)** *Pharmaserve Lilly (Φαρμασερβ Λιλλυ), Gr.*
Isophane insulin (human, recombinant) (p.333·3).
*Diabetes mellitus.*

**Humulin R**
*Lilly, Arg.; Lilly, Austral.; Lilly, Canad.; Lilly, Chile; Lilly, Hong Kong; Lilly, Israel; Lilly, Ital.; Lilly, Malaysia; Lilly, Mex.; Lilly, NZ; Lilly, S.Afr.; Lilly, Singapore; Lilly, Thai.; Lilly, USA.*
Insulin injection (human) (p.333·3).
*Diabetes mellitus.*

**Humulin Regular** Lilly, Braz.; Lilly, Denm.; Lilly, Fin.; Pharmaserve Lilly (Φαρμασερβ Λιλλυ), Gr.; Lilly, Norw.†; Lilly, Port.; Lilly, Swed.
Insulin injection (human) (p.333·3).
*Diabetes mellitus.*

**Humulin S** Lilly, Irl.; Lilly, UK.
Insulin injection (human, prb) (p.333·3).
*Diabetes mellitus.*

**Humulin U** Lilly, Arg.; Lilly, Canad.; Lilly, Israel; Lilly, Ital.; Lilly, NZ; Lilly, S.Afr.†.
Insulin zinc suspension (crystalline) (human) (p.333·3).
*Diabetes mellitus.*

**Humulin U Ultralente** Lilly, USA.
Insulin zinc suspension, extended (human, crb) (p.333·3).
*Diabetes mellitus.*

**Humulin UL** Lilly, Austral.
Insulin zinc suspension (crystalline) (human, prb) (p.333·3).
*Diabetes mellitus.*

**Humulin UL (Utralente)** Pharmaserve Lilly (Φαρμασερβ Λιλλυ), Gr.
Insulin zinc suspension (human) (p.333·3).
*Diabetes mellitus.*

**Humulin Ultralenta** Lilly, Port.
Insulin zinc suspension (crystalline) (human) (p.333·3).
*Diabetes mellitus.*

**Humulin Zn** Lilly, Irl.; Lilly, UK†.
Insulin zinc suspension (crystalline) (human, prb) (p.333·3).
*Diabetes mellitus.*

**Humulina 20:80, 30:70, 50:50** Lilly, Spain.
Mixture of insulin injection (human, prb) and isophane insulin injection (human, prb) (p.333·3) respectively in the proportions indicated.
*Diabetes mellitus.*

**Humulina Lenta** Lilly, Spain.
Insulin zinc suspension (human) (p.333·3).
*Diabetes mellitus.*

**Humulina NPH** Lilly, Spain.
Isophane insulin injection (human, prb) (p.333·3).
*Diabetes mellitus.*

**Humulina Regular** Lilly, Spain.
Insulin injection (human, prb) (p.333·3).
*Diabetes mellitus.*

**Humulina Ultralenta** Lilly, Spain.
Insulin zinc suspension (crystalline 70%, amorphous 30%) (human) (p.333·3).
*Diabetes mellitus.*

**Humuline** Lilly, Neth.
Neutral insulin injection (human) (p.333·3).
*Diabetes mellitus.*

**Humuline 20/80, 30/70** Lilly, Neth.
Mixtures of insulin injection (human) and isophane insulin injection (human) respectively in the proportions indicated (p.333·3).
*Diabetes mellitus.*

**Humuline 20/80, 30/70, 40/60, 50/50** Lilly, Belg.
Mixtures of neutral insulin injection (human, biosynthetic) and insulin suspension (human, biosynthetic) respectively in the proportions indicated (p.333·3).
*Diabetes mellitus.*

**Humuline Long** Lilly, Belg.
Insulin suspension (human, biosynthetic) (p.333·3).
*Diabetes mellitus.*

**Humuline NPH** Lilly, Belg.; Lilly, Neth.
Isophane insulin injection (human) (p.333·3).
*Diabetes mellitus.*

**Humuline Regular** Lilly, Belg.
Neutral insulin injection (human, biosynthetic) (p.333·3).
*Diabetes mellitus.*

**Humuline Ultralong** Lilly, Belg.
Insulin suspension (human, biosynthetic) (p.333·3).
*Diabetes mellitus.*

**Humutard** Lilly, Fin.; Lilly, Swed.†.
Insulin zinc suspension (human) (amorphous 30%, crystalline 70%) (p.333·3).
*Diabetes mellitus.*

**Humutard Ultra** Lilly, Denm.†; Lilly, Fin.†.
Insulin zinc suspension (crystalline) (human)(p.333·3).
*Diabetes mellitus.*

**Hurricaine** Clarben, Spain; Beutlich, USA.
Benzocaine (p.1370·3).
*Local anaesthesia; mouth pain.*

**Hustagil** Master, Chile.
*Ointment:* Thyme oil (p.1755·3); eterea; pine oil; eucalyptus oil (p.1686·2) clove oil (p.1673·3).
*Respiratory-tract congestion.*
*Syrup:* Thyme (p.1755·2).
*Respiratory-tract disorders.*

**Hustagil Erkaltungsbalsam** Dentinox, Ger.
Thyme oil (p.1755·3); oleum pini sylvestris; eucalyptus oil (p.1686·2); clove oil (p.1673·3).
*Coughs and associated respiratory-tract disorders.*

**Hustagil Inhalationsol** Dentinox, Ger.†.
Thyme oil (p.1755·3); eucalyptus oil (p.1686·2); pumilio pine oil (p.1737·1); pine needle oil; clove oil (p.1673·3).
*Coughs and associated respiratory-tract disorders.*

**Hustagil Thymian-Hustensaft** Dentinox, Ger.
Thyme (p.1755·2).
*Coughs and associated respiratory-tract disorders.*

**Hustagil Thymiantropfen** Dentinox, Ger.
Thyme (p.1755·2).
*Coughs and associated respiratory-tract disorders.*

**Hustazol** Mitsubishi, Jpn.
Cloperastine fendizoate (p.1117·2) or cloperastine hydrochloride (p.1117·2).
*Coughs.*

**Hustazol-C** Takeda, Thai.
Cloperastine hydrochloride (p.1117·2); sulfogaiacol (p.1131·1); *dl*-methylephedrine hydrochloride (p.1124·2).
*Coughs.*

**Husten ACC** Hexal, Austria.
Acetylcysteine (p.1112·3).
*Respiratory-tract disorders with viscous secretions.*

**Husten- und Fieber-Saft** Ratiopharm, Ger.†.
Paracetamol (p.76·2); dextromethorphan hydrobromide (p.1117·3).
*Coughs; fever.*

**Hustensaft Weleda** Weleda, Austria.
Herbal and homoeopathic preparation.

**Hustensaft-Dr Schmidgall** Schmidgall, Austria†.
Plantago lanceolata (p.1738·2); thyme (p.1755·2); cowslip (p.1735·1).
*Catarrh; coughs and cold symptoms.*

**Hustenstiller** Ratiopharm, Ger.
Dextromethorphan hydrobromide (p.1117·3).
*Coughs.*

**Hustenstiller N** Palmicol, Ger.†.
Menthol (p.1711·3); benzocaine (p.1370·3).
*Catarrh; coughs.*

**Hustentabs** Ratiopharm, Ger.
Bromhexine hydrochloride (p.1115·3).
*Respiratory-tract disorders associated with increased or viscous mucus.*

**Husties** Eu Rho, Ger.
Thyme (p.1755·2).
*Catarrh; coughs.*

**Hustosol** Pharmeso, Switz.
Bromhexine hydrochloride (p.1115·3).
*Respiratory-tract disorders associated with increased or viscous mucus.*

**Hutrope** Lilly, Arg.
Somatropin (p.1327·2).
*Growth disorders in renal failure; growth hormone deficiency; Turner's syndrome.*

**HVM** Scherer, Singapore.
Multivitamin and mineral preparation (p.1417·1).

**Hya-ject** Hexal, Ger.
Sodium hyaluronate (p.1697·3).
*Joint disorders.*

**Hyalart** TRB, Arg.; Bayer, Ger.; Tropon, Ger.; Faran, Gr.; SPA, Ital.; Grunenthal, Port.
Sodium hyaluronate (p.1697·3).
*Musculoskeletal and joint disorders.*

**Hyalase** Aventis, Austral.; CP, Israel; Artex, NZ; Xixia, S.Afr.; CP Pharmaceuticals, UK.
Hyaluronidase (p.1698·2).
*Enhance absorption of intramuscular and subcutaneous injections; haematoma; oedema; promote tissue fluid and blood resorption.*

**Hyalcrom** Biocumed, Arg.
Sodium cromoglicate (p.795·3); naphazoline hydrochloride (p.1124·3); hyaluronic acid (p.1697·3).
*Eye disorders.*

**Hyal-Drop** Chauvin, Fr.; Bausch & Lomb, Switz.
Sodium hyaluronate (p.1697·3) (p.1164·2).
*Contact lens lubrication; dry eyes.*

**Hyalein** Santen, Jpn.
Sodium hyaluronate (p.1697·3).
*Keratoconjunctival disorders.*

**Hyalgan** Kolassa, Austria; Silesia, Chile; Nycomed, Denm.; Nycomed, Fin.; Fournier, Fr.†; Fidia, Hong Kong; Shire, Irl.; Fidia, Ital.; Fidia, Malaysia; Chemedica, Malaysia; TRB, Singapore; Bioiberica, Spain; Nycomed, Swed.; Shire, UK; Sanofi Winthrop, USA.
Sodium hyaluronate (p.1697·3).
*Osteoarthritis of the knee.*

**Hyalistil** SIFI, Ital.
Sodium hyaluronate (p.1697·3).
*Dry eyes.*

**Hyalofill** Convatec, Fr.; Convatec, Port.; Convatec, UK.
Hyaff (p.1697·3).
*Ulcers; wounds.*

**Hyalogran** Convatec, Fr.
Sodium alginate (p.1577·1); Hyaff (p.1697·3).
*Ulcers; wounds.*

**Hyalozima** Apsen, Braz.
Hyaluronidase (p.1698·2).
*Enhancement of absorption of intramuscular and subcutaneous injections; reduction of extravasation.*

**Hyal-System** Merz, Ger.
Sodium hyaluronate (p.1697·3).
*Skin regeneration.*

**Hyaludermin** TRB, Braz.
Sodium hyaluronate (p.1697·3).
*Ulcers; wounds.*

**Hyalugel** Pharmascience, Fr.
Hyaluronic acid (p.1697·3).
*Gum inflammation or injury.*

**Hyanac** Biocumed, Arg.
Diclofenac sodium (p.32·1); sodium hyaluronate (p.1697·3).
*Eye disorders.*

**Hyanit N** Strathmann, Ger.†.
Urea (p.1162·2).
*Skin disorders.*

**Hya-Ophtal** Winzer, Ger.
Sodium hyaluronate (p.1697·3).
*Aid in eye surgery.*

**Hyasol** Biocumed, Arg.
Sodium hyaluronate (p.1697·3).
*Dry eyes.*

**Hyason** Organon, Neth.
Hyaluronidase (p.1698·2).
*Adjunct to local anaesthesia of the eye.*

**Hyate:C** Porton, Israel; Speywood, Switz.†; Ipsen, UK; Speywood, USA.
A porcine factor VIII:C preparation (p.751·1).
*Haemophilia in patients with antibodies to human factor VIII.*

**Hy-Bio** Solgar, UK†.
Vitamin C with bioflavonoids (p.1417·1).

**Hybloc** Pacific, NZ.
Labetalol hydrochloride (p.943·3).
*Hypertension.*

**Hybolin** Hyrex, USA.
Nandrolone phenylpropionate (p.1561·3) or nandrolone decanoate (p.1561·2).
*Anaemia in renal disease; breast cancer.*

**Hybridil** Roche, Austria.
Carvedilol (p.881·1).
*Heart failure.*

**Hybutyl** Pharmaland, Thai.
Hyoscine butylbromide (p.483·3).
*Smooth muscle spasm.*

**Hycal** SmithKline Beecham, Irl.†.
Glucose syrup solids (p.1432·2).
*Food for special diets.*

**Hycamtin** GlaxoSmithKline, Arg.; GlaxoSmithKline, Austral.; SmithKline Beecham, Austria; GlaxoSmithKline, Belg.; GlaxoSmithKline, Braz.; GlaxoSmithKline, Canad.; GlaxoSmithKline, Chile; SmithKline Beecham, Denm.; GlaxoSmithKline, Fin.; GlaxoSmithKline, Fr.; GlaxoSmithKline, Ger.; SmithKline Beecham, Gr.; GlaxoSmithKline, Hong Kong; GlaxoSmithKline, Irl.; SmithKline Beecham, Israel; GlaxoSmithKline, Ital.; GlaxoSmithKline, Neth.; GlaxoSmithKline, Norw.; Beecham, Port.; GlaxoSmithKline, S.Afr.; GlaxoSmithKline, Singapore; GlaxoSmithKline, Spain; GlaxoSmithKline, Swed.; SmithKline Beecham, Switz.; GlaxoSmithKline, Thai.; Merck, UK; SmithKline Beecham, USA.
Topotecan hydrochloride (p.589·1).
*Ovarian cancer; small-cell lung cancer.*

**Hyceral** Condrugs, Thai.
Co-dergocrine mesilate (p.1674·1).
*Mental function impairment; peripheral vascular disorders.*

**Hycibex** Pharmed, India.
Vitamin B substances (p.1454·3).
*Vitamin B deficiency.*

**Hycocin** Rekah, Israel.
Hydrocortisone acetate (p.1103·3); neomycin sulfate (p.235·1).
*Infected eye, ear, and nose disorders.*

**HycoClear Tuss** Ethex, USA.
Hydrocodone tartrate (p.45·1); guaifenesin (p.1122·1).
*Coughs.*

**Hycodan**
Note. This name is used for preparations of different composition.
Du Pont, Canad.
Hydrocodone tartrate (p.45·1).
*Coughs.*
Endo, USA.
Hydrocodone tartrate (p.45·1); homatropine methylbromide (p.483·2).
*Coughs.*

**Hycomine**
Note. This name is used for preparations of different composition.
Du Pont, Canad.
Hydrocodone tartrate (p.45·1); mepyramine maleate (p.437·1); phenylephrine hydrochloride (p.1126·3); ammonium chloride (p.1115·2).
*Coughs; upper respiratory-tract congestion.*
Endo, USA†.
Hydrocodone tartrate (p.45·1); phenylpropanolamine hydrochloride (p.1127·3).
*Coughs and cold symptoms.*

**Hycomine Compound** Endo, USA.
Hydrocodone tartrate (p.45·1); chlorphenamine maleate (p.427·3); phenylephrine hydrochloride (p.1126·3); paracetamol (p.76·2); caffeine (p.782·1).
*Coughs and cold symptoms.*

**Hycomycin** Teva, Israel.
Hydrocortisone acetate (p.1103·3); neomycin sulfate (p.235·1).
*Infected skin disorders.*

**Hycor** Sigma, Austral.
Hydrocortisone (p.1103·3) or hydrocortisone acetate (p.1103·3).
*Inflammatory eye disorders.*

**Hycort** ICN, Canad.; Everett, USA.
Hydrocortisone (p.1103·3).
*Inflammatory diseases of the gastrointestinal tract; skin disorders.*

**Hycortin** Medipharma, Hong Kong.
Hydrocortisone (p.1103·3).
*Skin disorders.*

**Hycotuss** Endo, USA.
Hydrocodone tartrate (p.45·1); guaifenesin (p.1122·1).
*Coughs.*

**Hydac** Aventis, Denm.; Aventis, Fin.; Hoechst Marion Roussel, Swed.†.
Felodipine (p.914·3).
*Hypertension.*

**Hydal** Mundipharma, Austria.
Hydromorphone hydrochloride (p.45·2).
*Pain.*

**Hydantin** Orion, Fin.
Phenytoin (p.370·2).
*Epilepsy.*

**Hydeltrasol** Merck Sharp & Dohme, USA.
Prednisolone sodium phosphate (p.1108·1).
*Corticosteroid.*

**Hyderax** Rontag, Arg.
Hydroxyzine hydrochloride (p.434·3).
*Anxiety; premedication; pruritus.*

**Hydergin** Novartis, Austria; Novartis, Fin.; Novartis, Ger.; Novartis, Swed.
Co-dergocrine mesilate (p.1674·1).
*Cerebral and peripheral vascular disorders; cervical syndrome; hypertension; mental function impairment; migraine and other vascular headache; shock.*

**Hydergina** Novartis, Arg.; Novartis, Chile; Novartis, Ital.; Novartis, Mex.; Novartis, Spain.
Co-dergocrine mesilate (p.1674·1).
*Cerebral and peripheral vascular disorders; hypertension; mental function disorders; migraine and other vascular headache.*

**Hydergine** Novartis, Belg.; Novartis, Braz.; Novartis, Canad.; Novartis, Fr.; Novartis, Hong Kong; Novartis, Irl.†; Novartis, Israel; Novartis, Malaysia; Novartis, Neth.; Novartis, Port.; Novartis, Singapore; Novartis, Switz.; Novartis, Thai.; Novartis, UK; Novartis, USA.
Co-dergocrine mesilate (p.1674·1).
*Cerebral and peripheral vascular disorders; hypertension; mental function impairment; migraine and other vascular headache.*

**Hyderm**
Note. This name is used for preparations of different composition.
Taro, Canad.
Hydrocortisone acetate (p.1103·3).
*Skin disorders.*
Labomed, Chile.
Urea (p.1162·2).
*Skin disorders.*

**Hydiphen** Dresden, Ger.
Clomipramine hydrochloride (p.289·3).
*Depression; nocturnal enuresis; pain; psychoses; sleep disorders.*

**Hydoftal** Agepha, Austria.
Hydrocortisone (p.1103·3); hydrocortisone acetate (p.1103·3); neomycin sulfate (p.235·1).
*Inflammatory eye disorders.*

**Hydol** Napp, Irl.†.
Dihydrocodeine tartrate (p.34·3).
*Pain.*

**Hydopa** Alphapharm, Austral.
Methyldopa (p.953·2).
*Hypertension.*

**Hydra** Otsuka, Jpn.
Isoniazid (p.222·2).
*Tuberculosis.*

**Hydra Form Day** New Vision, Canad.
*SPF 15:* Avobenzone (p.1142·3); octinoxate (p.1154·3); octisalate (p.1154·3); oxybenzone (p.1154·3).
*Sunscreen.*

**Hydra Perfecte** L'Oreal, Canad.†.
*SPF 10:* Octinoxate (p.1154·3).
*Sunscreen.*

**Hydrabak**
Transphyto, Fr.†.
Wetting solution for contact lenses (p.1164·2).
Farmila, Ital.
Sodium chloride (p.1233·3) (p.1164·2).
*Comfort drops for contact lenses.*

**Hydracillin** SmithKline Beecham, Ger.†.
Procaine benzylpenicillin (p.246·1); benzylpenicillin sodium (p.163·2).
Lidocaine hydrochloride (p.1377·3) is included in this preparation to alleviate the pain of injection.
*Bacterial infections.*

**Hydracort** Galderma, Fr.
Hydrocortisone (p.1103·3).
*Skin disorders.*

**Hydracuivre** SVR, Fr.
Zinc pidolate; copper pidolate; sodium pidolate (p.1158·1); allantoin (p.1141·3).
*Dry skin; skin irritation.*

**Hydraderm** Sigma, Austral.
Moisturiser.

**Hydrafuca** Fuca, Fr.
Pentaerythritol (p.1283·2).
Formerly known as Combeylax.
*Constipation.*

**Hydragel** Roche Nicholas, Fr.
Vaginal lubricant.

**Hydragenic** Forder, Arg.
Glycolic acid (p.1147·3); triclosan (Irgasan) (p.1195·2).
*Skin hygiene.*

**Hydralift Day** Avon, Canad.
*SPF 15:* Octinoxate (p.1154·3); oxybenzone (p.1154·3).
*Sunscreen.*

**Hydralin**
Note. This name is used for preparations of different composition.
Roche Nicholas, Fr.; Roche Nicholas, Hong Kong.
*Powder for topical solution:* Sodium perborate (p.1192·2); borax (p.1661·3); sodium bicarbonate (p.1223·2); anhydrous sodium carbonate (p.1747·1).
*Skin cleansing in gynaecological care.*

Roche Nicholas, Fr.
*Soap:* Borax (p.1661·3).
*Skin cleansing in gynaecological care.*

Roche Nicholas, Hong Kong.
*Topical liquid:* Glycine (p.1433·3).
*Genital pruritus; soap substitute.*

**Hydralyte**
River Foods, Austral.; River, Singapore.
Oral rehydration solution (p.1222·2).
*Diarrhoea; oral rehydration therapy; vomiting.*

**Hydramine Cream** Medipharma, Hong Kong.
Diphenhydramine hydrochloride (p.431·3).

**Hydramine Expectorant** Medipharma, Hong Kong.
Diphenhydramine hydrochloride (p.431·3); ammonium chloride (p.1115·2); sodium citrate (p.1223·2).
*Cold and influenza symptoms; coughs.*

**Hydramox** Caber, Ital.
Amoxicillin trihydrate (p.155·3).
*Bacterial infections.*

**Hydran**
Note. This name is used for preparations of different composition.
Orion, Fin.
Vehicle for topical preparations.

Teva, Israel.
Sodium chloride; anhydrous trisodium citrate; potassium chloride; glucose (p.1222·2).
*Diarrhoea; oral rehydration therapy.*

**Hydranorme**
Roche-Posay, Braz.; Roche-Posay, Irl.
Emollient.
*Dry skin; psoriasis.*

**Hydrap-ES** Parmed, USA.
Hydrochlorothiazide (p.933·2); reserpine (p.995·1); hydralazine hydrochloride (p.931·2).
*Hypertension.*

**Hydraphase XL** Roche-Posay, Braz.
Emollient.

**Hydraplus** SFD, Port.†.
Emollient.
*Dry skin.*

**Hydrapres**
Omedir, Arg.; Rubio, Spain.
Hydralazine hydrochloride (p.931·2).
*Heart failure; hypertension.*

**Hydrares** Pharmasant, Thai.
Reserpine (p.995·1); hydralazine hydrochloride (p.931·2); hydrochlorothiazide (p.933·2).
*Hypertension.*

**Hydrasense** Schering, Canad.
Isotonic desalinated sea water.
*Nasal congestion; nasal dryness.*

**Hydrasor** Novag, Mex.
Oral rehydration therapy (p.1222·2).

**Hydrasorb** Knoll, Canad.†.
Polyurethane foam dressing.
*Wounds.*

**Hydrastis Complex** Blackmores, Austral.†.
Liquorice (p.1270·2); althaea (p.1651·3); chamomile (p.1669·3); hydrastis (p.1698·3); vitamin A acetate (p.1453·1).
*Gastrointestinal disorders.*

**Hydrastis Salbe N** Steigerwald, Ger.
Homoeopathic preparation.

**Hydrate** Hyrex, USA.
Dimenhydrinate (p.431·1).
*Motion sickness.*

**Hydrating B5 Gel** Dispolab, Chile.
Sodium hyaluronate (p.1697·3); pantothenic acid (p.1442·3).
*Skin disorders.*

**Hydrax** Klinger, Braz.
Oral rehydration solution (p.1222·2).

**Hydrazide**
Note. A similar name is used for preparations of different composition (see below).
Otsuka, Jpn.
Isoniazid (p.222·2).
*Tuberculosis.*

**Hydra-zide**
Note. A similar name is used for preparations of different composition (see above).
Par, USA.
Hydralazine hydrochloride (p.931·2); hydrochlorothiazide (p.933·2).

**Hydrea**
Bristol-Myers Squibb, Arg.; Bristol-Myers Squibb, Austral.; Bristol-Myers Squibb, Belg.; Bristol-Myers Squibb, Braz.; Squibb, Canad.; Bristol-Myers Squibb, Chile; Bristol-Myers Squibb, Denm.; Bristol-Myers Squibb, Fin.; Bristol-Myers Squibb, Fr.; Bristol-Myers Squibb, Hong Kong; Bristol-Myers Squibb, Irl.; Bristol-Myers Squibb, Israel; Bristol-Myers Squibb, Malaysia; Bristol-Myers Squibb, Mex.; Bristol-Myers Squibb, Neth.; Bristol-Myers Squibb, NZ; Bristol-Myers Squibb, Port.; Bristol-Myers Squibb, S.Afr.; Bristol-Myers Squibb, Singapore; Bristol-Myers, Spain; Bristol-Myers Squibb, Swed.; Bristol-Myers Squibb, Thai.; Bristol-Myers Squibb, UK; Bristol-Myers Squibb Oncology, USA.
Hydroxycarbamide (p.559·1).
*Essential thrombocytosis; malignant neoplasms; sickle-cell anaemia.*

**Hydrene** Alphapharm, Austral.
Triamterene (p.1016·2); hydrochlorothiazide (p.933·2).
*Hypertension; oedema.*

**Hydrex**
Note. This name is used for preparations of different composition.
Orion, Fin.
Hydrochlorothiazide (p.933·2).
*Diabetes insipidus; hypertension; oedema.*

Adams, Hong Kong; Unitech, Irl.†; Adams, Thai.; Adams, UK.
Chlorhexidine gluconate (p.1173·2).
*Skin disinfection.*

**Hydrigoz** Guigoz, Fr.
Maltodextrin; sucrose; sodium chloride; citric acid; potassium citrate (p.1222·2).
*Diarrhoea; oral dehydration.*

**Hydrinate** Upha, Malaysia.
Dimenhydrinate (p.431·1).
*Motion sickness; nausea and vomiting; vertigo.*

**Hydrine**
Note. This name is used for preparations of different composition.
BPL-Meizler, Braz.
Hydroxycarbamide (p.559·1).
*Malignant neoplasms.*

TO-Chemicals, Thai.
Co-dergocrine mesilate (p.1674·1).
*Cerebrovascular disorders; mental function impairment.*

**Hydrisalic** Pedinol, USA.
Salicylic acid (p.1157·1).
*Hyperkeratotic skin.*

**Hydrisea** Pedinol, USA.
Emollient and moisturiser.

**Hydrisinol** Pedinol, USA.
Emollient and moisturiser.

**Hydro Cobex** Pasadena, USA.
Hydroxocobalamin (p.1458·2).
*Schilling test; vitamin $B_{12}$ deficiency.*

**Hydro Cordes** Ichthyol, Ger.
Allantoin (p.1141·3); dexpanthenol (p.1727·2); ethyl linoleate.
*Skin disorders.*

**Hydro DP** Cypress, USA.
Hydrocodone tartrate (p.45·1); diphenhydramine hydrochloride (p.431·3); phenylephrine hydrochloride (p.1126·3).
*Coughs; upper respiratory-tract congestion.*

**Hydro PC** Cypress, USA.
Hydrocodone tartrate (p.45·1); phenylephrine hydrochloride (p.1126·3); chlorphenamine maleate (p.427·3).
*Coughs; upper respiratory-tract congestion.*

**Hydro-Adreson**
Organon, Neth.†; Organon, Singapore†; Organon, Thai.†.
Hydrocortisone sodium succinate (p.1104·1).
*Corticosteroid.*

**Hydroagisten** Agis, Israel.
Hydrocortisone acetate (p.1103·3); clotrimazole (p.396·2).
*Infected skin disorders.*

**Hydrocal** Bioglan, Irl.†.
Hydrocortisone acetate (p.1103·3); calamine (p.1144·1).
*Inflammatory skin disorders.*

**Hydrocare**
Allergan, Braz.; Allergan, Ger.†; Allergan, USA.
Range of solutions for soft contact lenses (p.1164·2).

**Hydrocare Cleaning/Soaking** Allergan, Israel†.
Solution for cleaning, soaking, and disinfecting soft contact lenses (p.1164·2).

**Hydrocare Enzymatic Protein Remover** Allergan, Austral.†.
Papain (p.1727·3) (p.1164·2).
*Cleanser for soft and gas permeable contact lenses.*

**Hydrocare Fizzy** Allergan, Port.†.
Solution for contact lenses (p.1164·2).

**Hydrocare Fizzy Protein Remover** Allergan, NZ†.
Papain (p.1727·3) (p.1164·2).
*Protein removal from soft and gas-permeable contact lenses.*

**Hydrocare Preserved Saline** Allergan, NZ†.
Sodium chloride (p.1233·3) (p.1164·2).

**Hydrocare Protein Remover**
Allergan, Canad.†.
Papain (p.1727·3)(p.1164·2).
*Protein remover for soft contact lenses.*

Allergan, Israel†.
Enzymatic protein remover for soft contact lenses (p.1164·2).

**Hydro-Cebral** Ratiopharm, Ger.
Co-dergocrine mesilate (p.1674·1).
*Mental function disorders.*

**Hydrocerin** Geritrex, USA.
*Cream:* White soft paraffin (p.1479·3); liquid paraffin (p.1479·1); wool alcohols (p.1482·3).
*Lotion:* Liquid paraffin (p.1479·1); wool alcohols (p.1482·3).
*Product basis.*

**Hydrocet** Carnrick, USA.
Hydrocodone tartrate (p.45·1); paracetamol (p.76·2).
*Pain.*

**Hydrocil Instant** Numark, USA.
Psyllium hydrophilic mucilloid (p.1268·1).
*Constipation.*

**Hydroclean** Hartmann, Fr.
Sodium polyacrylate; cellulose (p.1578·3).
*Burns; ulcers; wounds.*

**Hydroclonazone** Chiesi, Fr.
Tosylchloramide sodium (p.1194·3).
*Water purification.*

**Hydrocobamine** Byk, Neth.
Hydroxocobalamin (p.1458·2).
*Megaloblastic anaemia; vitamin $B_{12}$ deficiency.*

**Hydrocodeinon** Streuli, Switz.
Dihydrocodeine hydrochloride (p.35·2).
*Coughs.*

**Hydrocodone CP** Morton Grove, USA.
Hydrocodone tartrate (p.45·1); phenylephrine hydrochloride (p.1126·3); chlorphenamine maleate (p.427·3).
*Upper respiratory-tract symptoms.*

**Hydrocodone GF** Morton Grove, USA.
Hydrocodone tartrate (p.45·1); guaifenesin (p.1122·1).
*Upper respiratory-tract symptoms.*

**Hydrocodone HD** Morton Grove, USA.
Hydrocodone tartrate (p.45·1); phenylephrine hydrochloride (p.1126·3); chlorphenamine maleate (p.427·3).
*Upper respiratory-tract symptoms.*

**Hydrocodone PA** Morton Grove, USA†.
Hydrocodone tartrate (p.45·1); phenylpropanolamine hydrochloride (p.1127·3).
*Upper respiratory-tract symptoms.*

**Hydrocoll** Hartmann, Fr.
Carmellose sodium (p.1577·3); pectin (p.1580·3); gelatin (p.754·3).
*Burns; ulcers; wounds.*

**Hydrocomp** Lichtenstein, Ger.†.
Amiloride hydrochloride (p.858·2); hydrochlorothiazide (p.933·2).
*Hypertension; oedema.*

**Hydrocort**
Note. This name is used for preparations of different composition.
CT, Ger.; YSP, Malaysia; Yung Shin, Singapore.
Hydrocortisone acetate (p.1103·3).
*Skin disorders.*

Abic, Israel†.
Hydrocortisone sodium succinate (p.1104·1).
*Corticosteroid.*

**Hydrocort Mild** CT, Ger.†.
Hydrocortisone (p.1103·3).
*Skin disorders.*

**Hydrocortancyl** Aventis, Fr.
Prednisolone (p.1108·1) or prednisolone acetate (p.1108·1).
*Corticosteroid.*

**Hydrocortimycin** Kolassa, Austria.
Hydrocortisone acetate (p.1103·3); neomycin sulfate (p.235·1).
*Inflammatory eye disorders.*

**Hydrocortisone comp** Streuli, Switz.
Hydrocortisone acetate (p.1103·3); zinc stearate (p.1575·3).
*Skin disorders.*

**Hydrocortistab** Sovereign, UK.
Hydrocortisone acetate (p.1103·3).
*Corticosteroid.*

**Hydrocortisyl** Aventis, Irl.
Hydrocortisone (p.1103·3).
*Skin disorders.*

**Hydrocortone**
Merck Sharp & Dohme, Austria; Merck Sharp & Dohme, Irl.; Merck Sharp & Dohme, Port.; Merck Sharp & Dohme, Switz.; Merck Sharp & Dohme, UK; Merck, USA.
Hydrocortisone (p.1103·3), hydrocortisone acetate (p.1103·3), or hydrocortisone sodium phosphate (p.1104·1).
*Corticosteroid.*

**Hydrocream** Paddock, USA.
Vehicle for topical preparations.

**Hydro-Crysti-12** Roberts, USA; Hauck, USA.
Hydroxocobalamin (p.1458·2).
*Schilling test; vitamin $B_{12}$ deficiency.*

**Hydrocutan** Dermapharm, Ger.
Hydrocortisone (p.1103·3) or hydrocortisone acetate (p.1103·3).
*Corticosteroid.*

**Hydrocutan mild** Dermapharm, Ger.
Hydrocortisone (p.1103·3).
*Skin disorders.*

**Hydroderm**
Note. This name is used for preparations of different composition.
Aesca, Austria.
Hydrocortisone (p.1103·3).
*Skin disorders.*

Pacific, NZ.
Dewaxed oil-soluble lanolin fraction (p.1483·1); liquid paraffin (p.1479·1).
*Dry skin disorders; pruritus.*

**Hydroderm HC** Karrer, Ger.
Hydrocortisone (p.1103·3).
*Skin disorders.*

**Hydrodermed** Karrer, Ger.
Erythromycin (p.208·1).
*Acne.*

**Hydrodexan**
Procter & Gamble, Austria†; Hermal, Ger.
Hydrocortisone (p.1103·3); urea (p.1162·2).
*Skin and scalp disorders.*

**HydroDiuril**
Merck Frosst, Canad.; Merck, USA.
Hydrochlorothiazide (p.933·2).
*Hypertension; oedema.*

**Hydrofluoric Acid Antidote** Malaysia Chemist, Singapore.
Calcium gluconate (p.1225·2).
*Hydrofluoric acid burns.*

**Hydroflux** Unipharma, Gr.
Furosemide (p.919·3).
*Heart failure; hypertension; oedema; oliguria due to renal failure.*

**Hydroform** Stiefel, Austral.
Hydrocortisone (p.1103·3); clioquinol (p.196·3).
*Skin disorders.*

**Hydro-Funga** Vida, Hong Kong.
Miconazole nitrate (p.405·3); hydrocortisone (p.1103·3).
*Infected skin disorders.*

**Hydrogalen** Galen, Ger.
Hydrocortisone (p.1103·3).
*Skin disorders.*

**Hydrogesic** Edwards, USA.
Hydrocodone tartrate (p.45·1); paracetamol (p.76·2).
*Pain.*

**Hydro-GP** Cypress, USA.
Hydrocodone tartrate (p.45·1); phenylephrine hydrochloride (p.1126·3); guaifenesin (p.1122·1).
*Allergic rhinitis; cold symptoms; coughs.*

**Hydroheal Algin** Faulding, Austral.†.
Calcium alginate (p.745·1).
*Burns; ulcers; wounds.*

**Hydroheal Colloid** Faulding, Austral.†.
Hydrocolloid dressing.
*Burns; ulcers; wounds.*

**Hydroheal Gel** Faulding, Austral.†.
Hydrogel dressing.
*Burns; ulcers; wounds.*

**Hydrol** Janssen-Cilag, S.Afr.
Potassium chloride; sodium chloride; sodium citrate; glucose (p.1222·2).
*Oral rehydration therapy.*

**Hydrolac** Milk Industries, Israel.
Protein hydrolysate (p.1417·1).
*Nutritional supplement.*

**Hydro-Less** Aspen, S.Afr.
Indapamide (p.938·2).
*Hypertension.*

**Hydrolid** Helvepharm, Switz.†.
Amiloride hydrochloride (p.858·2); hydrochlorothiazide (p.933·2).
Now known as Amiloride HCTZ Helvepharm.
*Hypertension; oedema.*

**Hydro-long** Lichtenstein, Ger.
Chlortalidone (p.882·3).
*Diabetes insipidus; hypertension; oedema.*

**Hydrolotion** Pacific Biosciences, Singapore; Spirig, Singapore.
Emollient and moisturiser.

**Hydromedin** Merck Sharp & Dohme, Ger.
Sodium etacrynate (p.913·3).
*Ascites; oedema.*

**Hydromet**
Note. This name is used for preparations of different composition.
Prodome, Braz.; Merck Sharp & Dohme, Irl.†; Merck Sharp & Dohme, Swed.†.
Hydrochlorothiazide (p.933·2); methyldopa (p.953·2).
*Hypertension.*

Barre-National, USA.
Hydrocodone tartrate (p.45·1); homatropine methylbromide (p.483·2).
*Coughs.*

**Hydromol**
Note. This name is used for preparations of different composition.
Quinoderm, Hong Kong; Quinoderm, Irl.; Ferndale, UK.
*Emollient:* Light liquid paraffin (p.1479·1); isopropyl myristate (p.1481·2).
*Dry skin conditions.*

Quinoderm, Irl.
*Cream:* Sodium pidolate (p.1158·1); arachis oil (p.1656·1); isopropyl myristate (p.1481·2); liquid paraffin (p.1479·1); sodium lactate (p.1223·2).
*Dry skin.*

Ferndale, UK.
*Cream:* Isopropyl myristate (p.1481·2); liquid paraffin (p.1479·1); sodium pidolate (p.1158·1); sodium lactate (p.1223·2).
*Dry skin conditions.*

Ferndale, UK.
*Ointment:* Yellow soft paraffin (p.1479·3); emulsifying wax (p.1481·1).
*Dry skin; soap substitute.*

**Hydromorph** Purdue, Canad.
Hydromorphone hydrochloride (p.45·2).
*Pain.*

**Hydromox** *Lederle, USA†.*
Quinethazone (p.991·2).
*Hypertension; oedema.*

**Hydromycin** *PP Lab, Thai.*
Tetracycline hydrochloride (p.266·2).
*Bacterial infections.*

**Hydron CP** *Cypress, USA.*
Hydrocodone tartrate (p.45·1); phenylephrine hydrochloride (p.1126·3); chlorphenamine maleate (p.427·3).
*Allergic rhinitis; cold symptoms; coughs.*

**Hydron EX** *Cypress, USA.*
Hydrocodone tartrate (p.45·1); sulfogaiacol (p.1131·1).
*Coughs.*

**Hydron KGS** *Cypress, USA.*
Hydrocodone tartrate (p.45·1); sulfogaiacol (p.1131·1).
*Coughs.*

**Hydron PSC** *Cypress, USA.*
Hydrocodone tartrate (p.45·1); pseudoephedrine hydrochloride (p.1129·2); chlorphenamine maleate (p.427·3).
*Coughs; hay fever; respiratory-tract congestion.*

**Hydronet** *Nettopharma, Denm.†.*
Amiloride hydrochloride (p.858·2); hydrochlorothiazide (p.933·2).
*Hypertension; oedema.*

**Hy-Drop** *Fidia, Ital.*
Sodium hyaluronate (p.1697·3).
*Dry eyes.*

**Hydropane** *Halsey, USA.*
Hydrocodone tartrate (p.45·1); homatropine methylbromide (p.483·2).
*Coughs.*

**Hydropel** *C & M, USA.*
Topical barrier preparation.

**Hydrophed** *Rugby, USA.*
Theophylline (p.798·3); ephedrine sulfate (p.1120·1); hydroxyzine hydrochloride (p.434·3).
*Bronchospasm.*

**Hydrophil** *Omega, Canad.*
Urea (p.1162·2); white soft paraffin (p.1479·3).
*Dry skin.*

**Hydrophilic** *Rugby, USA.*
Vehicle for topical preparations.

**Hydroplus** *Eurofarma, Braz.†.*
Oral rehydration solution (p.1222·2).

**Hydropres**
*Merck Sharp & Dohme, Canad.†; Merck, USA.*
Hydrochlorothiazide (p.933·2); reserpine (p.995·1).
*Hypertension.*

**Hydro-rapid** *Lichtenstein, Ger.†.*
Furosemide (p.919·3).
*Hypertension; oedema; oliguria.*

**Hydros G** *Chaix et du Marais, Fr.*
Glucose, sodium chloride, and potassium chloride infusion (p.1217·1).
*Carbohydrate source; fluid and electrolyte disorders.*

**HydroSaluric**
*Merck Sharp & Dohme, Irl.†; Merck Sharp & Dohme, UK†.*
Hydrochlorothiazide (p.933·2).
*Hypertension; oedema.*

**Hydro-Serp** *Rugby, USA.*
Hydrochlorothiazide (p.933·2); reserpine (p.995·1).
*Hypertension.*

**Hydroserpine** *Rugby, USA.*
Hydrochlorothiazide (p.933·2); reserpine (p.995·1).
*Hypertension.*

**Hydrosil**
*Xepa-Soul Pattinson, Hong Kong; Xepa-Soul Pattinson, Singapore.*
Aluminium hydroxide (p.1249·2); magnesium hydroxide (p.1272·2); simeticone (p.1289·2).
*Dyspepsia; flatulence; gastric hyperacidity; gastro-oesophageal reflux; peptic ulcer.*

**HydroSkin** *Rugby, USA.*
Hydrocortisone (p.1103·3).
*Skin disorders.*

**Hydrosol Polyvitamin BON** *Doms-Adrian, Hong Kong†.*
Multivitamin preparation (p.1417·1).

**Hydrosol Polyvitamine** *Roche Nicholas, Fr.*
Multivitamin preparation (p.1417·1).

**Hydrosol Polyvitamine BON** *Bouchara-Recordati, Fr.*
Multivitamin preparation (p.1417·1).

**Hydrosone** *Technilab, Canad.*
Hydrocortisone (p.1103·3).

**HydroTex** *Syosset, USA†.*
Hydrocortisone (p.1103·3).
*Skin disorders.*

**Hydrotricine**
*Aventis, Ital.; Vitoria, Port.*
Tyrothricin (p.275·1).
*Bacterial stomatitis.*

**Hydrotrix**
*Kolassa, Austria; Trommsdorff, Ger.; Medice, Ger.; Medice, Switz.†.*
Furosemide (p.919·3); triamterene (p.1016·2).
*Heart failure; hypertension; oedema.*

**Hydro-Tussin DM** *Ethex, USA.*
Guaifenesin (p.1122·1); dextromethorphan hydrobromide (p.1117·3).
*Coughs and cold symptoms.*

**Hydro-Tussin HD** *Ethex, USA.*
Guaifenesin (p.1122·1); hydrocodone tartrate (p.45·1); pseudoephedrine hydrochloride (p.1129·2).
*Coughs and cold symptoms.*

**HydroVal** *Optimapharma, Canad.*
Hydrocortisone valerate (p.1104·2).
*Skin disorders.*

**Hydro-Wolff** *Wolff, Ger.*
Hydrocortisone (p.1103·3).
*Skin disorders.*

**Hydroxin** *Shiwa, Thai.*
Hydroxyzine hydrochloride (p.434·3).
*Anxiety; hypersensitivity reactions.*

**Hydroxy-Cal** *Sisu, Canad.*
Vitamin C and minerals (p.1417·1).

**Hydrozide**
*Note. This name is used for preparations of different composition.*
*Douglas, Austral.†; Douglas, Hong Kong†; Douglas, NZ†.*
Hydrochlorothiazide (p.933·2); amiloride hydrochloride (p.858·2).
*Hepatic cirrhosis with ascites; hypertension; oedema.*
*Atlantic, Hong Kong; Atlantic, Malaysia; Atlantic, Singapore; Atlantic, Thai.*
Hydrochlorothiazide (p.933·2).
*Hypertension; oedema.*

**Hydrozide Plus** *Progress, Thai.*
Hydrochlorothiazide (p.933·2); amiloride hydrochloride (p.858·2).
*Hepatic cirrhosis with ascites; hypertension; oedema.*

**Hydrozole** *Stiefel, Austral.*
Hydrocortisone (p.1103·3); clotrimazole (p.396·2).
*Skin disorders.*

**Hyfac** *Saninter, Port.†.*
Pyrithione zinc (p.1156·2); piroctone olamine (p.1155·2); vitamin E.
*Acne.*

**Hyfac AHA** *Saninter, Port.†.*
Piroctone olamine (p.1155·2); glycolic acid (p.1147·3); malic acid (p.1709·2).
*Acne.*

**Hyfac Plus** *Biorga, Fr.*
Glycolic acid (p.1147·3); alpha hydroxy acid ester; piroctone olamine (p.1155·2).
*Skin disorders.*

**Hyflex**
*Note. This name is used for preparations of different composition.*
*Laboratorios Chile, Chile.*
Meloxicam (p.56·1).
*Musculoskeletal and joint disorders.*
*Breckenridge, USA.*
Paracetamol (p.76·2); phenyltoloxamine citrate (p.439·1).
*Pain.*

**Hy-GAG** *Curasan, Ger.*
Sodium hyaluronate (p.1697·3).
*Degenerative joint disorders.*

**Hygeol** *Wampole, Canad.*
Sodium hypochlorite (p.1192·1).
*Disinfection; wound cleansing.*

**Hygienist** *Bayer, Ital.*
Chlorocresol (preventol CMK) (p.1177·1); clorophene (preventol BP) (p.1177·3); orthophenylphenol (preventol extra) (p.1187·2).
*Surface disinfection.*

**Hygienist Pavimenti e Piastrelle** *Bayer, Ital.*
Benzalkonium chloride (p.1168·3).
*Surface disinfection.*

**Hygine In** *Geymonat, Ital.†.*
*Lactobacillus acidophilus* (p.1704·2).
*Disturbances of vaginal flora.*

**Hygiodermil** *Vifor, Switz.*
Bornyl salicylate (p.21·2); neroli oil (p.1719·2); lavender oil (p.1705·2); menthol (p.1711·3).
*Skin disorders.*

**Hygroton**
*Novartis, Arg.; Novartis, Austral.; Novartis, Austria; Novartis, Belg.; Novartis, Denm.†; Novartis, Fr.†; Novartis, Ger.; Novartis, Gr.; Novartis, Hong Kong; Novartis, Israel†; Novartis, Malaysia; Novartis, Neth.; Novartis, NZ; Novartis, Port.; Novartis, S.Afr.; Novartis, Switz.; Alliance, UK; Rhone-Poulenc Rorer, USA.*
Chlortalidone (p.882·3).
*Diabetes insipidus; heart failure; hypertension; oedema; renal calculi.*

**Hygroton-Reserpina** *Novartis, Arg.*
Chlortalidone (p.882·3); reserpine (p.995·1).
*Hypertension.*

**Hygroton-Reserpine**
*Novartis, S.Afr.; Novartis, Switz.*
Chlortalidone (p.882·3); reserpine (p.995·1).
*Hypertension.*

**Hy-KXP** *Cypress, USA.*
Hydrocodone tartrate (p.45·1); sulfogaiacol (p.1131·1).
*Coughs.*

**Hylaform**
*Collagen, Ger.; McGhan, Ger.; Inamed, Singapore.*
Sodium hyaluronate (Hylan B) (p.1697·3).
*Skin contour defects.*

**Hylak** *Ratiopharm, Austria.*
Metabolic products of lactic-acid producing organisms (p.1704·2); lactic acid (p.1704·1); amino acids.
*Gastrointestinal disorders; liver disorders; skin disorders.*

**Hylak forte** *Ratiopharm, Austria.*
Metabolic products of lactic-acid producing organisms (p.1704·2); metabolic products of Gram-positive and Gram-negative intestinal flora; lactic acid (p.1704·1); amino acids.
*Gastrointestinal disorders; liver disorders; skin disorders.*

**Hylak forte N** *Merckle, Ger.†.*
Metabolic products of: *Lactobacillus helveticus* (p.1704·2); *Escherichia coli*; *Lactobacillus acidophilus* (p.1704·2).
*Gastrointestinal disorders.*

**Hylak N** *Merckle, Ger.*
Metabolic products of *Lactobacillus helveticus* (p.1704·2).
*Gastrointestinal disorders.*

**Hylak Plus** *Merckle, Ger.*
Metabolic products of *Lactobacillus helveticus* (p.1704·2); *Lactobacillus acidophilus* (p.1704·2).
*Gastrointestinal disorders.*

**Hylakombun** *Ratiopharm, Austria†.*
Phthalylsulfathiazole (p.242·3); ethaverine hydrochloride (p.1685·2); ox bile (p.1660·3); metabolic products of *Escherichia coli*; *Enterococcus faecalis* (p.1704·2); *Lactobacillus acidophilus* (p.1704·2).
*Bacterial infections of the gastrointestinal tract.*

**Hylands Preparations** *Hylands, Canad.*
A range of homoeopathic preparations.

**Hylase** *Dessau, Ger.*
Hyaluronidase (p.1698·2).
*Adjunct in ocular surgery; adjuvant to increase absorption and dispersion of drugs; inflammation.*

**Hylashield** *I-Med, Canad.†.*
Hylan A (p.1697·3).
*Eye disorders.*

**Hylocomod** *Ioltech, Fr.*
Sodium hyaluronate (p.1697·3).
*Dry eyes.*

**Hylo-Comod**
*Ioltech, Fr.; Ursapharm, Israel.*
Sodium hyaluronate (p.1697·3).
*Dry eyes.*

**Hylo-COMOD** *Ursapharm, Ger.*
Sodium hyaluronate (p.1697·3).
*Dry eyes.*

**Hylorel** *Medeva, USA†.*
Guanadrel sulfate (p.926·3).
*Hypertension.*

**Hylutin** *Hyrex, USA.*
Hydroxyprogesterone caproate (p.1556·3).
*Abnormal uterine bleeding; amenorrhoea; metrorrhagia.*

**Hymed** *Medifive, Thai.*
Co-dergocrine mesilate (p.1674·1).
*Cerebrovascular disorders; mental function impairment.*

**Hyneurin** *Korhispana, Spain.*
Hypericum (p.299·1).
*Tonic.*

**Hynidase** *Amadeus, India.*
Hyaluronidase (p.1698·2).
*Enhancement of absorption of intramuscular and subcutaneous injections; reduction of extravasation.*

**Hyomide**
*Upha, Malaysia; Beacons, Singapore.*
Hyoscine butylbromide (p.483·3).
*Smooth muscle spasm.*

**Hyoscal** *Steierl, Ger.*
Scopolia carniolica root.
*Smooth muscle spasm.*

**Hyosmed** *Medifive, Thai.*
Hyoscine butylbromide (p.483·3).
*Gastrointestinal motility disorders; smooth muscle spasm.*

**Hyosophen** *Rugby, USA.*
Atropine sulfate (p.477·1); hyoscine hydrobromide (p.483·3); hyoscyamine hydrobromide (p.485·1) or hyoscyamine sulfate (p.485·1); phenobarbital (p.367·3).
*Gastrointestinal disorders.*

**Hyospan** *Polipharm, Thai.*
Hyoscine butylbromide (p.483·3).
*Gastroduodenitis; peptic ulcer; postoperative nausea and vomiting; smooth muscle spasm.*

**Hyospasmol** *Aspen, S.Afr.*
Hyoscine butylbromide (p.483·3).
*Gastrointestinal spasm.*

**Hyostan** *Pharmaland, Thai.*
Hyoscine butylbromide (p.483·3).
*Gastro-duodenitis; nausea and vomiting; peptic ulcer; smooth muscle spasm.*

**Hyozin** *Samakeephaesaj, Thai.*
Hyoscine butylbromide (p.483·3).
*Nausea and vomiting; peptic ulcer; smooth muscle spasm.*

**Hypace** *Alchemy, S.Afr.*
Enalapril maleate (p.909·2).
*Heart failure; hypertension.*

**Hypadil** *Kowa, Jpn.*
Nipradilol (p.973·2).
*Glaucoma; ocular hypertension.*

**Hypam** *Pacific, NZ†.*
Triazolam (p.725·3).
*Insomnia.*

**Hypan** *Sandipro, Belg.*
Nifedipine (p.966·2).
*Angina pectoris; hypertension.*

**Hypaque**
*Sanofi Synthelabo, Braz.; Nycomed Imaging, Canad.; Intrapharm, UK; Nycomed, USA.*
Meglumine amidotrizoate (p.1060·2) or sodium amidotrizoate (p.1060·2).
*Radiographic contrast medium.*

**Hypaque 60%**
*Nycomed, Arg.; Sanofi Synthelabo, Chile.*
Meglumine amidotrizoate (p.1060·2).
*Radiographic contrast medium.*

**Hypaque 76%**
*Nycomed, Arg.; Sanofi Synthelabo, Chile.*
Meglumine amidotrizoate (p.1060·2); sodium amidotrizoate (p.1060·2).
*Radiographic contrast medium.*

**Hypaque-M**
*Sanofi Synthelabo, Braz.; Nycomed Imaging, Canad.*
Meglumine amidotrizoate (p.1060·2) or meglumine amidotrizoate and sodium amidotrizoate (p.1060·2).
*Radiographic contrast medium.*

**Hypaque-M, Hypaque-76** *Nycomed, USA.*
Meglumine amidotrizoate (p.1060·2); sodium amidotrizoate (p.1060·2).
*Radiographic contrast medium.*

**Hypen** *Shinyaku, Jpn.*
Etodolac (p.37·3).
*Inflammation; musculoskeletal and joint disorders; pain.*

**Hyperab**
*Bayer, Canad.†; Cutter, Israel†.*
A rabies immunoglobulin (p.1635·3).
*Passive immunisation.*

**Hyperamine**
*Braun, Fr.; Braun, UK.*
Amino-acid infusion (p.1417·1).
*Parenteral nutrition.*

**Hypercal**
*Note. This name is used for preparations of different composition.*
*Novartis Nutrition, Fr.†.*
Nutritional supplement (p.1417·1).
*Nelson, UK.*
Homoeopathic preparation.

**Hypercalcio** *Luper, Braz.*
Calcium, vitamin D, vitamin $B_{12}$, and fluoride supplement (p.1417·1).

**Hypercard** *Hotz, Ger.†.*
Olive leaves; mistletoe (p.1715·3); ginseng (p.1693·1); convallaria (p.1675·3); rauwolfia; silicea; sumbul. moschat.; conium.
*Cardiovascular disorders.*

**Hypercidin** *Electramed, Irl.†.*
Sodium hypochlorite (p.1192·1).
*Surface disinfection.*

**Hypercrit**
*Biolatina, Chile; Serono, Mex.*
Epoetin (p.747·1).
*Anaemias; autologous blood transfusion.*

**Hyperdine** *Masa, Thai.*
Clopamide (p.888·2); dihydroergocristine mesilate (p.1680·1); reserpine (p.995·1).
*Hypertension.*

**Hyperdix** *Servier, Thai.*
Rilmenidine phosphate (p.996·1).
*Hypertension.*

**Hyperesa** *Dolorgiet, Ger.*
Valerian (p.1762·2); hypericum (p.299·1).
*Insomnia; nervous disorders.*

**Hyperforat** *Klein, Ger.*
Hypericum (p.299·1).
*Depression; nervous disorders.*

**Hyperforat-forte** *Klein, Ger.*
Hypericum (p.299·1); rauwolfia vomitoria (p.994·3).
*Anxiety disorders.*

**Hypergel**
*SSL, Austral.*
Hypertonic saline debriding agent (p.1233·3).
*Wounds.*
*Molnlycke, Fr.*
Sodium chloride (p.1233·3).
*Ulcers; wounds.*

**HyperHAES**
*Fresenius Kabi, Ger.; Fresenius Kabi, Port.; Fresenius Kabi, UK.*
Pentastarch (p.750·1) in sodium chloride.
*Plasma volume expansion; shock.*

**HyperHep** *Bayer, Canad.†.*
A hepatitis B immunoglobulin (p.1617·2).
*Passive immunisation.*

**Hyperhes** *Fresenius Kabi, Austria.*
An etherified starch (p.750·1) in sodium chloride.
*Plasma volume expansion; shock.*

**Hypericaps** *Duopharm, Ger.*
Hypericum (p.299·1).
*Anxiety.*

**Hypericettes** *Kneipp, Switz.*
Hypericum (p.299·1).
*Depression; sleep disorders.*

**Hyperico** *Vitemat, Braz.*
Hypericum (p.299·1).
*Depression.*

**Hyperiforce**
*Bio-Garten, Austria; Bioforce, Switz.*
Hypericum (p.299·1).
*Anxiety; nervous disorders; sleep disorders.*

**Hyperiforce comp** *Bioforce, Switz.*
Hypericum (p.299·1); melissa (p.1711·1); lupulus (p.1708·1).
*Exhaustion; irritability; sleep disorders.*

**Hyperiforte** *Blackmores, Austral.†.*
Hypericum (p.299·1).
*Anxiety; depression; nervous disorders.*

**Hyperilex** *Medice, Ger.†.*
Pemoline (p.1591·2).
*Behaviour disorders in children.*

**HyperiMed** *Bioforce, Switz.*
Hypericum (p.299·1).
*Sleep disorders; tension.*

**Hyperimerck** *Merck dura, Ger.*
Hypericum (p.299·1).
*Anxiety; depression.*

**Hyperiplant** *Schwabe, Switz.*
Hypericum (p.299·1).
*Depression; insomnia; tension.*

**Hyperium**
*Servier, Arg.; Servier, Braz.; Biopharma, Fr.; Servier, Port.*
Rilmenidine phosphate (p.996·1).
*Hypertension.*

**Hyperlipen**
*Sanofi Synthelabo, Belg.; Sanofi Synthelabo, Switz.*
Ciprofibrate (p.884·2).
*Hyperlipidaemias.*

**Hyperlite** *Braun, Spain.*
Electrolyte infusion (p.1217·1).
*Fluid and electrolyte depletion.*

**Hyperlyte** *McGaw, USA.*
A range of electrolyte preparations (p.1217·1).
*Fluid and electrolyte disorders.*

**Hypermol** *Pacific, NZ.*
Timolol maleate (p.1012·2).
*Angina pectoris; hypertension; migraine; myocardial infarction.*

**Hypernol**
*DHA, Hong Kong; DHA, Singapore.*
Atenolol (p.865·2).
*Angina pectoris; arrhythmias; hypertension.*

**Hyperphen** *Aspen, S.Afr.*
Hydralazine hydrochloride (p.931·2).
*Hypertension.*

**Hyperprotidine** *NPC, Fr.*
Preparation for enteral nutrition (p.1417·1).

**Hyperpur** *Alpharma-Isis, Ger.*
Hypericum (p.299·1).
*Depression.*

**Hyperretic** *Pharmasant, Thai.*
Amiloride hydrochloride (p.858·2); hydrochlorothiazide (p.933·2).
*Hepatic cirrhosis with ascites; hypertension; oedema.*

**Hypersol** *Cassara, Arg.*
Sodium chloride (p.1233·3).
*Nasal dryness.*

**Hypersol B** *Cassara, Arg.*
Budesonide (p.1094·2).

**Hyperstat**
*Schering-Plough, Belg.†; Schering, Canad.; Schering-Plough, Fr.†; IFET (ΙΦΕΤ), Gr.; Schering-Plough, Ital.; Schering-Plough, Mex.; Schering-Plough, Neth.; Schering-Plough, S.Afr.†; Schering-Plough, Spain†; Schering-Plough, Swed.; Essex, Switz.†; Schering, USA.*
Diazoxide (p.893·2).
*Hypertension; hypoglycaemia.*

**Hyper-Tet** *Bayer, Canad.†.*
A tetanus immunoglobulin (p.1640·3).
*Passive immunisation.*

**Hypertonalum** *Essex, Ger.*
Diazoxide (p.893·2).
*Hypertension.*

**Hypertorr** *Henning, Ger.†.*
Triamterene (p.1016·2); hydrochlorothiazide (p.933·2).
*Heart failure; hypertension; oedema.*

**Hyperval** *Novartis Consumer, Switz.*
Hypericum (p.299·1).
*Anxiety; insomnia; tension.*

**Hypery** *Pond's, Thai.*
Reserpine (p.995·1); hydralazine hydrochloride (p.931·2); hydrochlorothiazide (p.933·2).
*Hypertension.*

**Hyphed** *Cypress, USA.*
Hydrocodone tartrate (p.45·1); pseudoephedrine hydrochloride (p.1129·2); chlorphenamine maleate (p.427·3).
*Coughs.*

**Hy-Phen** *Ascher, USA.*
Hydrocodone tartrate (p.45·1); paracetamol (p.76·2).

**Hypnasmine** *Elerte, Fr.*
Butobarbital (p.673·3); theophylline (p.798·3).
Formerly contained caffeine, butobarbital, and theophylline.
*Respiratory-tract disorders.*

**Hypnodorm**
*Alphapharm, Austral.; Teva, Israel.*
Flunitrazepam (p.698·2).
*General anaesthesia; insomnia; premedication.*

**Hypnol** *Cristalia, Braz.†.*
Pentobarbital (p.713·2).
*Cerebrovascular disorders; epilepsy; premedication.*

**Hypnomidate**
*Janssen-Cilag, Austria; Janssen-Cilag, Belg.; Janssen-Cilag, Braz.; Janssen-Cilag, Chile; Janssen-Cilag, Fr.; Janssen-Cilag, Ger.; Janssen-Cilag, Gr.; Janssen, Mex.; Janssen-Cilag, Neth.; Janssen-Cilag, S.Afr.; Janssen-Cilag, Spain; Janssen-Cilag, UK.*
Etomidate (p.1299·1).
*General anaesthesia.*

**Hypnor** *Rolab, S.Afr.*
Flunitrazepam (p.698·2).
*Insomnia.*

**Hypnorex** *Sanofi Synthelabo, Ger.*
Lithium carbonate (p.301·1).
*Bipolar disorder; depression; mania.*

**Hypnotex** *Pharmaceutical Co, India.*
Nitrazepam (p.710·1).
*Insomnia.*

**Hypnovel**
*Roche, Austral.; Roche, Fr.; Roche, Irl.; Roche, NZ; Roche, UK.*
Midazolam hydrochloride (p.707·2) or midazolam maleate (p.707·2).
*Induction of anaesthesia; premedication; sedative.*

**Hypo Tears** *Novartis, Spain.*
Polyvinyl alcohol (p.1581·1).
*Dry eyes.*

**Hypoca**
*Yamanouchi, Jpn; Yamanouchi, Thai.*
Barnidipine hydrochloride (p.866·3).
*Hypertension.*

**Hypocaina** *Hypoforma, Braz.†.*
Lidocaine hydrochloride (p.1377·3).
*Local anaesthesia.*

**Hypochylin**
*Recip, Fin.; Recip, Swed.*
Glutamic acid hydrochloride (p.1433·2).
*Hypochylia.*

**Hypodyn** *Novartis, Austria.*
Dihydroergotamine mesilate (p.465·3); etilefrine hydrochloride (p.914·1).
*Hypotension.*

**Hypoguard** *Hypoguard, Irl.*
Test for glucose in blood (p.1694·2).

**Hypoguard Supreme Plus** *Hypoguard, UK.*
Test for glucose in blood (p.1694·2).

**Hypol** *Felton, Austral.†.*
*Capsules:* Cod-liver oil (p.1425·2).
*Arthritis; cardiovascular disorders; cold and influenza symptoms; dietary supplement; inflammatory disorders.*
*Oral emulsion:* Cod-liver oil (p.1425·2); soya oil (p.1447·2); calcium hypophosphite; sodium hypophosphite.
*Arthritis; cardiovascular disorders; cold and influenza symptoms; dietary supplement; inflammatory disorders.*
*Tablets:* Vitamin A; colecalciferol; vitamin C; calcium dihydrogen phosphate (p.1417·1).
*Vitamin and calcium supplement.*

**Hypolac** *ALK, Ital.*
Infant feed (p.1417·1).
*Food intolerance.*

**Hypolar Retard** *Sandoz, UK.*
Nifedipine (p.966·2).
*Angina pectoris; hypertension.*

**Hypomed** *Interpharm, Austria.*
Lisinopril (p.946·3).
*Heart failure; hypertension; myocardial infarction.*

**Hypomide** *Aspen, S.Afr.*
Chlorpropamide (p.330·3).
*Diabetes mellitus.*

**Hyposedon N** *Harras-Curarina, Ger.*
Kava (p.1703·2); passion flower (p.1729·1).
*Agitation; sleep disorders.*

**Hypostamin** *Novartis Consumer, Austria.*
Tritoqualine (p.443·3).
*Hypersensitivity reactions.*

**Hypostamine** *Chiesi, Fr.*
Tritoqualine (p.443·3).
*Hypersensitivity reactions.*

**Hypotears**
*Note. This name is used for preparations of different composition.*
*Novartis Ophthalmics, Braz.; Restan, S.Afr.*
Povidone (p.1581·2).
*Contact lens lubricant; dry eyes.*

*Novartis Ophthalmics, Canad.; Ciba Vision, Israel; Novartis Ophthalmics, Singapore.*
*Eye drops:* Polyvinyl alcohol (p.1581·1).
*Dry eyes.*

*Novartis Ophthalmics, Canad.; Ciba Vision, Israel†; Novartis Ophthalmics, USA.*
*Eye ointment:* White soft paraffin (p.1479·3); light liquid paraffin (p.1479·1).
*Dry eyes.*

*Novartis Ophthalmics, Hong Kong; Ciba Vision, Ital.; Novartis Ophthalmics, Malaysia; Novartis Ophthalmics, Switz.; Novartis, UK; Novartis Ophthalmics, USA.*
*Eye drops:* Polyvinyl alcohol (p.1581·1); macrogol 400 (p.1709·1).
*Dry eyes.*

*Novartis Ophthalmics, Hong Kong.*
*Eye gel:* Vitamin A palmitate (p.1453·1); carbomer (p.1577·2).
*Dry eyes.*

**Hypotears E** *Ciba Vision, Israel.*
Povidone (p.1581·2).
*Dry eyes.*

**Hypotears PF** *Ciba Vision, Israel†.*
Polyvinyl alcohol (p.1581·1); macrogol 400 (p.1709·1).
*Dry eyes.*

**Hypotears Plus**
*Novartis Ophthalmics, Arg.; Novartis Ophthalmics, Hong Kong; Novartis, Mex.; Novartis, Thai.*
Povidone (p.1581·2).
*Dry eyes.*

**Hypoten** *Covan, S.Afr.*
Sodium nitroprusside (p.1000·2).
*Hypertension.*

**Hypotens** *Dexxon, Israel.*
Prazosin hydrochloride (p.985·1).
*Benign prostatic hyperplasia; hypertension.*

**Hypotensor** *Faran, Gr.*
Captopril (p.879·2).
*Heart failure; hypertension; myocardial infarction.*

**Hy-Po-Tone** *Aspen, S.Afr.*
Methyldopa (p.953·2).
*Hypertension.*

**Hypotonie-Gastreu R44** *Reckeweg, Ger.*
Homoeopathic preparation.

**Hypovase**
*Invicta, Irl.; Pfizer, UK.*
Prazosin hydrochloride (p.985·1).
*Benign prostatic hyperplasia; heart failure; hypertension; Raynaud's syndrome.*

**Hypren** *AstraZeneca, Austria.*
Ramipril (p.994·1).
*Heart failure; hypertension; myocardial infarction; nephropathy.*

**Hypren plus** *AstraZeneca, Austria.*
Ramipril (p.994·1); hydrochlorothiazide (p.933·2).
*Hypertension.*

**Hyprenan**
*Astra, Denm.†; Astra, Norw.†; Hassle, Swed.†.*
Prenalterol hydrochloride (p.986·3).
*Hypotension; reversal of beta blockade; shock.*

**HypRho-D** *Bayer, Canad.†.*
An anti-D immunoglobulin (p.1608·1).
*Prevention of rhesus sensitisation.*

**Hyprosia** *Asian Pharm, Thai.*
Etilefrine (p.914·1).
*Hypotension.*

**Hyprosin** *Pacific, NZ.*
Prazosin hydrochloride (p.985·1).
*Benign prostatic hyperplasia; heart failure; hypertension; Raynaud's disease.*

**Hyprosol** *Dzwon, India.*
Hypromellose (p.1579·3).
*Dry eyes.*

**Hypurin 30/70** *CP Pharmaceuticals, UK.*
Mixture of neutral insulin injection (porcine, highly purified) 30% and isophane insulin injection (porcine, highly purified) 70% (p.333·3).
*Diabetes mellitus.*

**Hypurin Isophane**
*Aspen, Austral.; CP Pharma, Switz.; CP Pharmaceuticals, UK.*
Isophane insulin injection (bovine or porcine, highly purified) (p.333·3).
*Diabetes mellitus.*

**Hypurin Lente** *CP Pharmaceuticals, UK.*
Insulin zinc suspension (30% amorphous, 70% crystalline) (bovine, highly purified) (p.333·3).
*Diabetes mellitus.*

**Hypurin 30/70 Mix** *CP Pharma, Switz.*
A mixture of insulin injection (porcine) and isophane insulin injection (porcine) respectively in the proportion indicated (p.333·3).
*Diabetes mellitus.*

**Hypurin Neutral**
*Aspen, Austral.; CP Pharma, Switz.; CP Pharmaceuticals, UK.*
Neutral insulin injection (bovine or porcine, highly purified) (p.333·3).
*Diabetes mellitus.*

**Hypurin Protamine Zinc** *CP Pharmaceuticals, UK.*
Protamine zinc insulin injection (bovine, highly purified) (p.333·3).
*Diabetes mellitus.*

**Hyrexin** *Hyrex, USA†.*
Diphenhydramine hydrochloride (p.431·3).
*Motion sickness; parkinsonism.*

**Hyrin** *Merckle, Ger.*
Metoclopramide (p.1274·3).
*Gastrointestinal motility disorders; nausea; vomiting.*

**Hyruan** *LG Pharm, Hong Kong.*
Sodium hyaluronate (p.1697·3).
*Osteoarthritis of the knee; periarthritis of the shoulder.*

**Hyrvalan** *Monot, Fr.†.*
Paracetamol (p.76·2); ascorbic acid (p.1460·2); chlorphenamine maleate (p.427·3).
*Upper respiratory-tract disorders.*

**Hysan** *Ursapharm, Ger.*
Sodium hyaluronate (p.1697·3).
*Nasal dryness.*

**Hyseke** *Saninter, Port.†.*
Sodium pidolate (p.1158·1); zinc pidolate; enoxolone (p.36·2).
*Dry skin.*

**Hyskon**
*Dermatech, Austral.; Pharmacia Upjohn, Canad.†; Reusch, Ger.†; Pharmacia, USA.*
Dextran 70 (p.746·2) in glucose.
*Aid to hysteroscopy.*

**Hysone**
*Note. This name is used for preparations of different composition.*
*Alphapharm, Austral.*
Hydrocortisone (p.1103·3).
*Corticosteroid.*

*Roberts, USA.*
Clioquinol (p.196·3); hydrocortisone (p.1103·3).
*Inflammatory skin disorders.*

**Hysopan** *Denk, Hong Kong.*
Hyoscine butylbromide (p.483·3).
*Smooth muscle spasm.*

**Hy-Spa** *Progress, Thai.*
Hyoscine butylbromide (p.483·3).
*Gastroduodenitis; peptic ulcer; smooth muscle spasm.*

**Hysticlar** *Mintlab, Chile.*
Loratadine (p.436·1).
*Hypersensitivity reactions.*

**Hytacand**
*AstraZeneca, Fr.; AstraZeneca, Port.*
Candesartan cilexetil (p.878·3); hydrochlorothiazide (p.933·2).
*Hypertension.*

**Hytakerol**
*Sanofi Synthelabo, Canad.; Sanofi Winthrop, USA.*
Dihydrotachysterol (p.1461·3).
*Hypoparathyroidism; postoperative and idiopathic tetany.*

**Hyteneze** *Opus, UK†.*
Captopril (p.879·2).
*Heart failure; hypertension.*

**Hythalton** *Sarabhai Piramal, India.*
Chlortalidone (p.882·3).
*Hypertension; oedema; premenstrual syndrome.*

**Hytic** *Seng, Thai.*
Hyoscine butylbromide (p.483·3).
*Smooth muscle spasm.*

**Hytinic** *Hyrex, USA.*
*Capsules:* Polysaccharide-iron complex (p.1443·2).
*Iron-deficiency anaemias.*
*Injection:* Ferrous gluconate (p.1428·1); vitamin B substances (p.1417·1).
Procaine hydrochloride (p.1383·2) is included in this preparation to alleviate the pain of injection.
*Iron-deficiency anaemias.*

**Hytisone**
*Atlantic, Hong Kong.*
Hydrocortisone (p.1103·3).
*Skin disorders.*

*Atlantic, Thai.*
Hydrocortisone acetate (p.1103·3).
*Inflammatory skin disorders.*

**Hytone** *Dermik, USA.*
Hydrocortisone (p.1103·3).
*Skin disorders.*

**Hytos Plus** *Uniao Quimica, Braz.*
Clobutinol hydrochloride (p.1117·1); doxylamine succinate (p.432·3).
*Coughs.*

**Hytrast** *Guerbet, Braz.†.*
Iopydol (p.1065·3); iopydone (p.1065·3).
*Contrast medium for upper respiratory-tract radiography.*

**Hytrin**
*Abbott, Austral.; Abbott, Belg.; Abbott, Braz.; Abbott, Canad.; Abbott, Chile; Abbott, Gr.; Abbott, Hong Kong; Abbott, India; Abbott, Irl.; Abbott, Israel; Abbott, Malaysia; Abbott, Mex.; Abbott, Neth.; Abbott, NZ; Abbott, Port.; Abbott, S.Afr.; Abbott, Singapore; Abbott, Thai.; Abbott, UK; Abbott, USA; Wellcome, USA.*
Terazosin hydrochloride (p.1010·3).
*Benign prostatic hyperplasia; hypertension.*

**Hytrin BPH** *Abbott, Switz.*
Terazosin hydrochloride (p.1010·3).
*Benign prostatic hyperplasia.*

**Hytrine** *Abbott, Fr.*
Terazosin hydrochloride (p.1010·3).
*Benign prostatic hyperplasia.*

**Hytrinex** *Abbott, Swed.*
Terazosin hydrochloride (p.1010·3).
*Benign prostatic hyperplasia; hypertension.*

**Hytuss** *Hyrex, USA.*
Guaifenesin (p.1122·1).
*Coughs.*

**Hyzaar**
*Merck Sharp & Dohme, Braz.; Merck Frosst, Canad.; Merck Sharp & Dohme, Chile; Merck Sharp & Dohme-Chibret, Fr.; Merck Sharp & Dohme, Hong Kong; Merck Sharp & Dohme, Malaysia; Merck Sharp & Dohme, Mex.; Merck Sharp & Dohme, Neth.; Merck Sharp & Dohme, Singapore; Merck Sharp & Dohme, Thai.; Merck, USA.*
Losartan potassium (p.947·2); hydrochlorothiazide (p.933·2).
*Hypertension.*

**Hyzan**
*Xepa-Soul Pattinson, Hong Kong; Xepa-Soul Pattinson, Malaysia; Xepa-Soul Pattinson, Singapore.*
Ranitidine hydrochloride (p.1285·2).
*Acid aspiration; gastric hyperacidity; gastro-oesophageal reflux; peptic ulcer; Zollinger-Ellison syndrome.*

**Hyzum N** *Merckle, Ger.*
Arnica (p.1656·3).
*Inflammation; muscle and joint pain; soft-tissue injury.*

**Ial**
*Fidia, Hong Kong†; Fidia, Ital.; Trans Bussan, Switz.; Fidia, Thai.*
Sodium hyaluronate (p.1697·3).
*Adjunct in ocular surgery.*

**Ialect** *Fidia, Ital.*
Sodium hyaluronate (p.1697·3).
*Adjunct in eye surgery.*

**Ialugen** *IBSA, Switz.*
Sodium hyaluronate (p.1697·3).
*Burns; wounds.*

**Ialugen Plus** *IBSA, Switz.*
Sodium hyaluronate (p.1697·3); sulfadiazine silver (p.259·1).
*Infected wounds and burns.*

**Ialum** *Fidia, Ital.*
Sodium hyaluronate (p.1697·3).
*Adjunct in eye surgery.*

**Ialurex** *Fidia, Ital.*
Sodium hyaluronate (p.1697·3).
*Dry eyes.*

**Ialuset** *Genevrier, Fr.*
Sodium hyaluronate (p.1697·3).
*Skin ulceration.*

**Iamin** *Merck, Mex.*
Prezatide copper acetate (p.1156·1).
*Burns; ulcers; wounds.*

**Iamin Hydrating Gel** *Procyte, USA.*
Prezatide copper acetate (p.1156·1).
*Burns; ulcers; wounds.*

**Iba-Cide** *Ingram & Bell, Canad.†.*
Chloroxylenol (p.1177·2); terpineol (p.1752·2); isopropyl alcohol (p.1184·3).
*Antiseptic.*

**Ibamoxil** *Ibfarma, Braz.†.*
Amoxicillin (p.155·3).
*Bacterial infections.*

**Ibaril**
*Aventis, Denm.; Aventis, Fin.; Bipharma, Neth.; Aventis, Norw.; Aventis, Swed.*
Desoximetasone (p.1096·3).
*Skin disorders.*

**Ibaril med salicylsyra** *Aventis, Swed.*
Desoximetasone (p.1096·3); salicylic acid (p.1157·1).
*Skin disorders.*

**Ibaril med salicylsyre**
*Aventis, Denm.; Aventis, Norw.*
Desoximetasone (p.1096·3); salicylic acid (p.1157·1).
*Skin disorders.*

**Ibarin** *Laboratorios Chile, Chile.*
Fluconazole (p.398·1).
*Fungal infections.*

**Ibdazol** *Ibfarma, Braz.†.*
Mebendazole (p.108·2).
*Worm infections.*

**Ibenon** *Diviser Aquilea, Spain†.*
Ibuprofen (p.45·3).
*Fever; pain.*

**Ibercal** *BOI, Spain.*
Calcium pidolate (p.1226·1).
*Hypocalcaemia; osteoporosis.*

**Iberet**
*Abbott, Canad.; Abbott, Hong Kong; Abbott, Malaysia; Abbott, Mex.; Abbott, S.Afr.†; Abbott, Singapore; Abbott, Spain†; Abbott, Thai.; Abbott, USA.*
Ferrous sulfate (p.1428·2); vitamin B substances (p.1417·1).
Vitamin C (p.1460·2) is included in this preparation to increase the absorption and availability of iron.
*Iron deficiency; iron-deficiency anaemias.*

**Iberet-Folic**
*Abbott, Hong Kong; Abbott, Malaysia; Abbott, Singapore; Abbott, USA.*
Ferrous sulfate (p.1428·2); folic acid (p.1429·1); vitamin B substances (p.1417·1).
Vitamin C (p.1460·2) is included in this preparation to increase the absorption and availability of iron.
*Folic acid deficiency; iron deficiency; iron-deficiency anaemias.*

**Iberin Folico** *Abbott, Braz.*
Ferrous sulfate (p.1428·2); folic acid (p.1429·1).
Ascorbic acid (p.1460·2) is included in this preparation to increase the absorption and availability of iron.
*Iron deficiency; iron-deficiency anaemia.*

**Iberogast**
*Steigerwald, Ger.*
Iberis amara; chamomile (p.1669·3); peppermint leaf (p.1283·2); greater celandine (p.1695·3); silybum marianum (p.1043·3); melissa (p.1711·1); caraway (p.1667·2); liquorice (p.1270·2); angelica (p.1655·1).
*Gastrointestinal disorders.*

*Steigerwald, Switz.*
Iberis amara; angelica (p.1655·1); silybum marianum (p.1043·3); cuminum cyminum; chamomile (p.1669·3); greater celandine (p.1695·3); liquorice (p.1270·2); melissa (p.1711·1); peppermint leaf (p.1283·2).
*Gastrointestinal disorders.*

**Iberol**
*Note. This name is used for preparations of different composition.*
*Abbott, Arg.; Abbott, Braz.*
*Oral drops:* Ferrous sulfate (p.1428·2).
*Iron deficiency; iron-deficiency anaemia.*

*Abbott, Arg.; Abbott, Braz.; Abbott, Chile; Abbott, Mex.*
*Oral liquid; tablets:* Ferrous sulfate (p.1428·2); vitamin B substances (p.1417·1).
Ascorbic acid (p.1460·2) is included in this preparation to increase the absorption and availability of iron.
*Iron deficiency; iron-deficiency anaemia; vitamin B deficiency.*

*Abbott, India.*
*Oral liquid:* Ferrous sulfate (p.1428·2); vitamins (p.1417·1).
*Tablets:* Ferrous sulfate (p.1428·2); desiccated liver; vitamins (p.1417·1).
*Anaemias.*

**Iberol Folico** *Abbott, Chile.*
Ferrous sulfate (p.1428·2); folic acid (p.1429·1); vitamin B substances (p.1417·1).
Ascorbic acid (p.1460·2) is included in this preparation to increase the absorption and availability of iron.
*Iron and folate deficiency; iron-deficiency anaemia.*

**Iberol Simple** *Abbott, Chile.*
Ferrous sulfate (p.1428·2).
*Iron deficiency.*

**Ibexone** *Sandipro, Belg.*
Co-dergocrine mesilate (p.1674·1).
*Mental function impairment.*

**Ibiamox**
*Ibi, Ital.; Douglas, NZ.*
Amoxicillin sodium (p.155·3).
*Bacterial infections.*

*IBI, Thai.*
Amoxicillin (p.155·3).
*Bacterial infections.*

**Ibifen** *Ibi, Ital.*
Ketoprofen (p.51·2).
*Inflammation; musculoskeletal, joint, peri-articular, and soft-tissue disorders; pain.*

**Ibilex**
*Alphapharm, Austral.; IBI, Thai.*
Cefalexin (p.168·1) or cefalexin sodium (p.168·2).
*Bacterial infections.*

**Ibimicyn**
*Note. A similar name is used for preparations of different composition (see below).*
*Ibi, Ital.*
*Injection:* Ampicillin sodium (p.157·1).
*Bacterial infections.*

**Ibimycin**
*Note. A similar name is used for preparations of different composition (see above).*
*IBI, Thai.†.*
Doxycycline (p.206·2).
*Bacterial infections.*

**Ibis** *Pharmaland, Thai.*
Ketotifen fumarate (p.788·1).
*Asthma; hypersensitivity reactions.*

**Iboflam** *MDI, S.Afr.*
Ibuprofen (p.45·3).
*Musculoskeletal and joint disorders.*

**Ibopain** *Docmed, S.Afr.†.*
Ibuprofen (p.45·3).
*Musculoskeletal and joint disorders.*

**Ibrofen** *TO-Chemicals, Thai.*
Ibuprofen (p.45·3).
*Musculoskeletal and joint disorders.*

**Ibrufhalal** *Halal, UK.*
Ibuprofen (p.45·3).
*Inflammation; pain.*

**IBS Relief** *Thornton & Ross, UK.*
Mebeverine hydrochloride (p.1273·1).
*Irritable bowel syndrome.*

**IB-Stat** *Inkine, USA.*
Hyoscyamine sulfate (p.485·1).

**Ibtrim** *Ibfarma, Braz.†.*
Co-trimoxazole (p.199·3).
*Bacterial infections.*

**Ibu**
*Master, Chile; 1A, Ger.; ABZ, Ger.; Acis, Ger.; Eu Rho, Ger.; Kade, Ger.; Hemopharm, Ger.; Pose, Thai.; Boots, USA.*
Ibuprofen (p.45·3) or ibuprofen lysine (p.46·3).
*Fever; gout; inflammation; musculoskeletal, joint, and soft-tissue disorders; pain.*

**Ibu-4** *Master, Chile.*
Ibuprofen (p.45·3).

**Ibu-6** *Master, Chile.*
Ibuprofen (p.45·3).

**Ibu-4, -6, -8** *Truxton, USA.*
Ibuprofen (p.45·3).

**Ibu Evanol** *GlaxoSmithKline, Arg.*
Ibuprofen (p.45·3).
*Fever; pain.*

**Ibualgic** *EG, Fr.*
Ibuprofen (p.45·3).
*Pain.*

**ibu-Attritin** *Tussin, Ger.*
Ibuprofen (p.45·3).
*Gout; inflammation; musculoskeletal, joint, and soft-tissue disorders; pain.*

**Ibubest** *CT, Ger.†.*
Ibuprofen (p.45·3).
*Fever; pain.*

**Ibubeta** *Betapharm, Ger.*
Ibuprofen (p.45·3).
*Fever; gout; inflammation; musculoskeletal, joint, and soft-tissue disorders; pain.*

**Ibu-Buscapina** *Boehringer Ingelheim, Arg.*
Ibuprofen (p.45·3); hyoscine butylbromide (p.483·3).
*Pain with muscle spasm.*

**Ibucler** *Monserrat, Arg.*
Ibuprofen (p.45·3).
*Fever; musculoskeletal and joint disorders; pain.*

**Ibudol** *Sanova, Austria†.*
Ibuprofen (p.45·3).
*Fever; inflammation; musculoskeletal and joint disorders; pain.*

**Ibudolofrix** *Richmond, Arg.*
Ibuprofen (p.45·3); codeine (p.27·1).
*Pain.*

**Ibudolor** *Stada, Ger.*
Ibuprofen (p.45·3).
*Fever; pain.*

**Ibudristan** *Wyeth-Whitehall, Arg.*
Ibuprofen (p.45·3); pseudoephedrine (p.1129·2).
*Fever; nasal congestion.*

**Ibudros** *Manetti Roberts, Ital.*
Ibuproxam (p.47·2).
*Musculoskeletal, joint, peri-articular, and soft-tissue disorders; phlebitis; superficial thrombophlebitis.*

**Ibufabra** *Fabra, Arg.*
Ibuprofen (p.45·3) or ibuprofen lysine (p.46·3).
*Fever; inflammation; pain.*

**Ibufac**
*Unison, Hong Kong; Unison, Thai.; DDSA Pharmaceuticals, UK†.*
Ibuprofen (p.45·3).
*Fever; musculoskeletal, joint, and soft-tissue disorders; pain.*

**Ibufem**
*Sanova, Austria; Galpharm, UK.*
Ibuprofen (p.45·3).
*Pain.*

**Ibufen**
*Dexxon, Israel; Upha, Malaysia; Beacons, Singapore; Cinfa, Spain; Siam Bheasach, Thai.†.*
Ibuprofen (p.45·3).
*Gout; inflammation; musculoskeletal and joint disorders; pain.*

**Ibufen-L** *Amino, Switz.*
*Suppositories:* Ibuprofen lysine (p.46·3); lidocaine hydrochloride (p.1377·3).
*Tablets:* Ibuprofen lysine (p.46·3).
*Gout; musculoskeletal, joint, and peri-articular disorders.*

**Ibufix** *Hexal, Arg.*
Ibuprofen (p.45·3).
*Fever; gout; musculoskeletal, joint, and soft-tissue disorders; pain.*

**Ibuflam**
*Lichtenstein, Ger.; 3M, Mex.*
Ibuprofen (p.45·3).
*Fever; gout; inflammation; musculoskeletal, joint, and peri-articular disorders; pain.*

**Ibuflamar-P** *Indoco, India.*
Ibuprofen (p.45·3); paracetamol (p.76·2).
*Musculoskeletal and joint disorders; pain.*

**Ibuflex** *Rayere, Mex.*
Ibuprofen (p.45·3).
*Inflammation; pain.*

**Ibufran** *Neo Quimica, Braz.*
Ibuprofen (p.45·3).

**Ibufug** *Wolff, Ger.†.*
Ibuprofen (p.45·3).
*Gout; inflammation; musculoskeletal and joint disorders; pain.*

**Ibugan** *Aventis, Thai.*
Ibuprofen (p.45·3).
*Musculoskeletal, joint, and soft-tissue disorders; pain.*

**Ibugel**
*Ebewe, Austria; Dermal Laboratories, Irl.; Medinova, Switz.†; Dermal Laboratories, UK.*
Ibuprofen (p.45·3).
*Musculoskeletal, joint, peri-articular, and soft-tissue disorders; neuralgia.*

**Ibugesic** *Cipla, India.*
Ibuprofen (p.45·3).
*Musculoskeletal and joint disorders; pain.*

**Ibugesic Plus** *Cipla, India.*
Ibuprofen (p.45·3); paracetamol (p.76·2).
*Musculoskeletal and joint disorders; pain.*

**Ibugesic-M** *Cipla, India.*
Methocarbamol (p.1395·1); ibuprofen (p.45·3).
*Skeletal muscle spasm.*

**Ibuhexal** *Hexal, Ger.*
Ibuprofen (p.45·3) or ibuprofen sodium (p.46·3).
*Fever; gout; inflammation; musculoskeletal, joint, and soft-tissue disorders; pain.*

**Ibu-Lady** *Microsules Bernabo, Arg.*
Ibuprofen (p.45·3).

**Ibulan** *Olan-Kemed, Thai.*
Ibuprofen (p.45·3).
*Fever; inflammation; musculoskeletal and joint disorders; pain.*

**Ibular** *Lagap, UK†.*
Ibuprofen (p.45·3).
*Inflammation; pain.*

**Ibuleve**
*Dermal, Israel; Pharmacia, S.Afr.; Dendron, UK.*
Ibuprofen (p.45·3).
*Musculoskeletal, joint, and soft-tissue disorders.*

**Ibuloid** *Reddy, Singapore.*
Ibuprofen (p.45·3).
*Musculoskeletal and joint disorders; pain.*

**Ibumac** *Belmac, Spain.*
Ibuprofen (p.45·3).
*Fever; musculoskeletal and joint disorders; pain.*

**Ibumar** *Mar, Arg.*
Ibuprofen (p.45·3).
*Inflammation; pain.*

**Ibumar Migra** *Mar, Arg.*
Ibuprofen (p.45·3); caffeine (p.782·1); ergotamine (p.468·3).
*Migraine.*

**Ibumax** *Vitabalans, Fin.*
Ibuprofen (p.45·3).
*Fever; gout; musculoskeletal and joint disorders; pain.*

**Ibumed**
*Pharmethic, Belg.†; GlaxoSmithKline, S.Afr.; Helvepharm, Switz.†.*
Ibuprofen (p.45·3).
*Fever; pain.*

**Ibumerck** *Merck dura, Ger.*
Ibuprofen (p.45·3).
*Fever; gout; inflammation; musculoskeletal, joint, and soft-tissue disorders; pain.*

**Ibumetin**
*Nycomed, Austria; Nycomed, Denm.; United Nordic, Denm.; Nycomed, Fin.; Nycomed, Norw.; Nycomed, Swed.*
Ibuprofen (p.45·3).
*Fever; gout; inflammation; musculoskeletal and joint disorders; pain.*

**Ibumousse** *Dermal Laboratories, UK.*
Ibuprofen (p.45·3).
*Musculoskeletal, joint, and soft-tissue pain; neuralgia.*

**Ibunet** *Nettopharma, Denm.†.*
Ibuprofen (p.45·3).
*Gout; musculoskeletal and joint disorders; pain.*

**Ibu-Novalgina** *Aventis, Arg.*
Ibuprofen (p.45·3).
*Fever; inflammation; pain.*

**Ibupax** *Alter, Port.*
Ibuprofen (p.45·3).
*Fever; gout; musculoskeletal, joint, peri-articular, and soft-tissue disorders; pain.*

**Ibupen** *Merck, Hong Kong.*
Ibuprofen (p.45·3).
*Fever; pain.*

**Ibuphlogont** *Azupharma, Ger.*
Ibuprofen (p.45·3).
*Gout; inflammation; musculoskeletal, joint, and soft-tissue disorders; pain.*

**Ibupirac**
*Pharmacia, Arg.; Chemopharma, Chile.*
Ibuprofen (p.45·3) or ibuprofen lysine (p.46·3).
*Fever; gout; inflammation; musculoskeletal, joint, peri-articular, and soft-tissue disorders; pain.*

**Ibupirac Compuesto** *Chemopharma, Chile.*
Ibuprofen (p.45·3); paracetamol (p.76·2).
*Fever; pain.*

**Ibupirac Fem** *Pharmacia, Arg.*
Ibuprofen (p.45·3); homatropine methylbromide (p.483·2).
*Pain with muscle spasm.*

**Ibupirac Flex** *Pharmacia, Arg.*
Ibuprofen (p.45·3); chlorzoxazone (p.1392·3).
*Musculoskeletal and joint disorders; pain.*

**Ibupirac Migra** *Pharmacia, Arg.*
Ibuprofen (p.45·3); caffeine (p.782·1); ergotamine tartrate (p.467·2).
*Migraine.*

**Ibupiretas** *Pharmacia, Arg.*
Ibuprofen (p.45·3).
*Fever; pain.*

**Ibupril**
*Teuto, Braz.; Liomont, Mex.†.*
Ibuprofen (p.45·3).
*Inflammation; pain.*

**Ibuprin** *Thompson, USA†.*
Ibuprofen (p.45·3).
*Fever; osteoarthritis; pain; rheumatoid arthritis.*

**Ibuprof** *CT, Ger.*
Ibuprofen (p.45·3) or ibuprofen lysine (p.46·3).
*Gout; inflammation; musculoskeletal, joint, and soft-tissue disorders; pain.*

**Ibuprofan** *Bunker, Braz.*
Ibuprofen (p.45·3).

**Ibuprohm** *Ohm, USA†.*
Ibuprofen (p.45·3).
*Fever; osteoarthritis; pain; rheumatoid arthritis.*

**Ibupron** *Ratiopharm, Austria.*
Ibuprofen (p.45·3).
*Fever; inflammation; musculoskeletal and joint disorders; pain.*

**Ibuprox** *Ferrer, Spain.*
Ibuprofen (p.45·3).
*Fever; musculoskeletal and joint disorders; pain.*

**Ibu-Proxyvon** *Wockhardt, India.*
Ibuprofen (p.45·3); dextropropoxyphene (p.28·3).
*Musculoskeletal and joint disorders; pain.*

**Ibu-ratiopharm** *Ratiopharm, Ger.*
Ibuprofen (p.45·3) or ibuprofen lysine (p.46·3).
*Fever; gout; inflammation; musculoskeletal, joint, and soft-tissue disorders; pain.*

**Iburem** *Sanova, Austria.*
Ibuprofen (p.45·3).
*Pain.*

**Iburen** *Hua, Thai.*
Ibuprofen (p.45·3).
*Gout; musculoskeletal and joint disorders.*

**Ibureumin** *Durascan, Denm.*
Ibuprofen (p.45·3).
*Gout; inflammation; musculoskeletal and joint disorders; pain.*

**Ibusal** *Orion, Fin.*
Ibuprofen (p.45·3).
*Fever; gout; musculoskeletal and joint disorders; pain.*

**Ibuscent** *Vita Elan, Spain†.*
Ibuprofen (p.45·3).
*Fever; pain.*

**Ibusi** *Mertens, Arg.*
Ibuprofen (p.45·3).
*Fever; inflammation; pain.*

**Ibusifar** *Siphar, Switz.*
Ibuprofen (p.45·3).
*Fever; inflammation; pain.*

**Ibu-Slow** *Therabel, Belg.*
Ibuprofen (p.45·3).
*Musculoskeletal, joint, and peri-articular disorders; pain.*

**Ibuslow** *Eurodrug, Hong Kong†.*
Ibuprofen (p.45·3).
*Dysmenorrhoea; fever; musculoskeletal, joint, peri-articular, and soft-tissue disorders.*

**Ibuspray** *Dermal Laboratories, UK.*
Ibuprofen (p.45·3).
*Musculoskeletal, joint, and soft-tissue disorders; neuralgia.*

**Ibustrin**
*Pharmacia, Austria; Pharmacia Upjohn, Ital.; Pharmacia Upjohn, Mex.; Pharmacia, Port.; Pharmacia Upjohn, Thai.†.*
Indobufen (p.939·1) or indobufen sodium (p.939·1).
*Thromboembolic disorders; thrombosis prophylaxis.*

**Ibusumal** *Purissimus, Arg.*
Ibuprofen (p.45·3).
*Dysmenorrhoea.*

**Ibu-Tab** *Alra, USA.*
Ibuprofen (p.45·3).
*Fever; osteoarthritis; pain; rheumatoid arthritis.*

**Ibutab** *Zee, USA.*
Ibuprofen (p.45·3).
*Fever; pain.*

**Ibutad** *TAD, Ger.*
Ibuprofen (p.45·3) or ibuprofen sodium (p.46·3).
*Gout; inflammation; musculoskeletal, joint, and soft-tissue disorders; pain.*

**Ibutenk** *Biotenk, Arg.*
Ibuprofen (p.45·3).
*Fever; pain.*

**Ibu-Tetralgin** *Craveri, Arg.*
Ibuprofen (p.45·3); ergotamine tartrate (p.467·2); caffeine (p.782·1).
*Migraine.*

**Ibutin** *Galenica, Gr.*
Trimebutine (p.1758·1).
*Gastrointestinal and gallbladder pain.*

**Ibutop**
*Sanova, Austria; Chefaro, Belg.; Dolorgiet, Denm.; Chefaro Ardeval, Fr.; Chefaro, Ger.*
Ibuprofen (p.45·3).
*Fever; inflammation; musculoskeletal, joint, peri-articular, and soft-tissue disorders; pain.*

**Ibutop Cuprofen** *SSL, UK.*
Ibuprofen (p.45·3).
*Musculoskeletal, joint, and soft-tissue disorders.*

**Ibutop Ralgex** *SSL, UK.*
Ibuprofen (p.45·3).
*Inflammation; musculoskeletal pain.*

**Ibu-Vivimed** *Mann, Ger.†.*
Ibuprofen (p.45·3).
*Fever; pain.*

**Ibux** *Weifa, Norw.*
Ibuprofen (p.45·3).
*Fever; musculoskeletal and joint disorders; pain.*

**Ibuxin** *Ratiopharm, Fin.*
Ibuprofen (p.45·3).
*Fever; gout; musculoskeletal and joint disorders; pain.*

**Ibuzidine** *Hexa-Medinova, Arg.*
Ibuprofen (p.45·3).
*Fever; gout; inflammation; musculoskeletal and joint disorders; pain.*

**IC Green**
*Akorn, Israel; Akorn, USA.*
Indocyanine green (p.1701·1).
*Determination of cardiac output and liver blood flow; ophthalmic angiography.*

**Icaden**
*Schering, Braz.; Schering, Mex.*
Isoconazole (p.401·3) or isoconazole nitrate (p.401·3).
*Fungal and Gram-positive vulvovaginal infections; fungal skin infections.*

**Icaps**
*Alcon, Canad.; Alcon, Hong Kong; Ciba Vision, USA.*
Multivitamin and mineral preparation (p.1417·1).

**Icaps Plus** *Alcon, Arg.*
Vitamins; minerals; cysteine (p.1417·1).

**Icar** *Hawthorn, USA.*
Carbonyl iron (p.1434·3).
*Iron deficiency; iron supplement.*

**Icar Prenatal** *Hawthorn, USA.*
Tablets, vitamins; minerals; chewable tablets, calcium carbonate; soft gel capsules, omega-3 marine triglycerides (p.1417·1).
*Nutritional supplement during pregnancy and lactation.*

**Icar-C Plus** *Hawthorn, USA.*
Carbonyl iron (p.1434·3); folic acid (p.1429·1); cyanocobalamin (p.1458·2).
Ascorbic acid (p.1460·2) is included in this preparation to increase the absorption and availability of iron.
*Folate deficiency; iron-deficiency anaemia.*

**Icavex** *Viatris, Fr.*
Moxisylyte hydrochloride (p.962·2).
*Erectile dysfunction.*

**Icaz** *Novartis, Fr.*
Isradipine (p.942·2).
*Hypertension.*

**Ice Cool Stress & Tension Relief** *Amirose, UK.*
Menthol (p.1711·3).
*Headache; tension.*

**Ice Gel**
*Mentholatum, Austral.†; Hyde, Canad.*
Menthol (p.1711·3).
*Muscular aches and pains.*

**Ice Gel Therapy** *Sutton, Canad.*
Menthol (p.1711·3).

**Ice Lipbalm** *Mentholatum, Canad.*
*SPF 12:* Padimate O (p.1155·1).
*Sunscreen.*

**Icespray** *Aventis, Spain†.*
Menthol (p.1711·3).
*Insect bites; pruritus; sprains.*

**Icetazol** *IQFA, Mex.*
Paracetamol (p.76·2).
*Fever; pain.*

**Ic-Gel** *Germiphene, Canad.†.*
Chlorhexidine gluconate (p.1173·2); isopropyl alcohol (p.1184·3).

**ICG-Pulsion**
*Pulsion, Ger.; Pulsion, Israel.*
Indocyanine green (p.1701·1).
*Diagnostic agent.*

**Ichthalgan** *Ichthyol, Ger.*
Heparin sodium (p.928·1); ictasol (p.1148·3).
*Musculoskeletal, joint, and peri-articular disorders; neuritis.*

**Ichthalgan forte** *Ichthyol, Austria.*
Heparin sodium (p.928·1); ictasol (p.1148·3).
*Musculoskeletal, joint, and peri-articular disorders.*

**Ichtho-Bad**
*Ichthyol, Austria; Ichthyol, Ger.; Ichthyol, Switz.*
Ichthammol (p.1148·2).
*Bath additive; genito-urinary disorders; hyperhidrosis; musculoskeletal and joint disorders; neuralgia; skin disorders; superficial circulatory disorders; wounds.*

**Ichtho-Bellol**
*Ichthyol, Austria; Ichthyol, Ger.*
Ictasol (p.1148·3); atropine sulfate (p.477·1).
*Anogenital disorders; urogenital disorders.*

**Ichtho-Bellol compositum S** *Ichthyol, Ger.*
Ictasol (p.1148·3); atropine sulfate (p.477·1); propyphenazone (p.85·3).
*Pelvic disorders.*

**Ichtho-Cadmin** *Ichthyol, Austria†.*
Ictasol (p.1148·3); cadmium sulfide (p.1663·3).
*Scalp disorders.*

**Ichtho-Cortin** *Ichthyol, Austria.*
Hydrocortisone (p.1103·3) or hydrocortisone acetate (p.1103·3); ictasol (p.1148·3).
*Skin disorders.*

**Ichthocortin** *Ichthyol, Ger.*
Hydrocortisone (p.1103·3) or hydrocortisone acetate (p.1103·3); ictasol (p.1148·3).
*Skin disorders.*

**Ichthoderm** *Ichthyol, Ger.*
Ictasol (p.1148·3).
*Scalp disorders.*

**Ichth-Oestren** *Ichthyol, Austria.*
Estradiol benzoate (p.1550·1); light ammonium bituminosulphonate (p.1148·2); urea (p.1162·2); lactose (p.1438·3).
*Vaginal disorders.*

**Ichtholan**
*Ichthyol, Austria; Ichthyol, Ger.; Ichthyol, Switz.*
Ichthammol (p.1148·2).
*Inflammatory skin disorders; musculoskeletal and joint disorders; thrombophlebitis.*

**Ichtholan spezial** *Ichthyol, Ger.*
Ichthammol (p.1148·2).
*Musculoskeletal and joint disorders.*

**Ichtholan T** *Ichthyol, Ger.*
Ictasol (p.1148·3).
*Skin disorders.*

**Ichthopaste**
*Smith & Nephew, Ital.; Smith & Nephew, UK.*
Ichthammol (p.1148·2); zinc oxide (p.1163·2).
*Medicated bandage.*

**Ichthoseptal** *Ichthyol, Ger.*
Chloramphenicol (p.185·1); ictasol (p.1148·3).
*Infected skin disorders.*

**Ichthosin** *Ichthyol, Ger.*
Ictasol (p.1148·3).
*Skin disorders.*

**Ichthraletten**
*Ichthyol, Austria; Ichthyol, Ger.*
Sodium bituminosulphonate (p.1148·3).
*Skin disorders.*

**Ichthyol** *Ichthyol, Ger.*
Ichthammol (p.1148·2).
*Skin disorders.*

**Ichtopur** *Ichthyol, Austria.*
Ichthammol (p.1148·2).
*Urogenital disorders.*

**Icht-Oral** *Ichthyol, Ger.†.*
Minocycline hydrochloride (p.231·3).
*Bacterial infections.*

**Ichtyosoft**
*Note. This name is used for preparations of different composition.*
*Fouchard, Chile.*
Ictasol (p.1148·3); ammonium lactate (p.1142·3); salicylic acid (p.1157·1).
*Seborrhoea.*

*LED, Fr.*
*Cream:* Ictasol (p.1148·3); ammonium lactate (p.1142·3).
Formerly contained ictasol, ammonium lactate, and gamolenic acid.
*Skin disorders.*
*Shampoo:* Ictasol (p.1148·3); ammonium lactate (p.1142·3); salicylic acid (p.1157·1).
*Scalp disorders.*

**Icodial**
*Bieffe, Ital.; Baxter, Spain.*
Icodextrin; sodium chloride; sodium lactate; calcium chloride; magnesium chloride (p.1221·1).
*Peritoneal dialysis.*

**Icol** *Alcon Cusi, Spain.*
Chloramphenicol (p.185·1) or chloramphenicol succinate (p.186·3); dexamethasone sodium phosphate (p.1097·2).
*Infected eye disorders.*

**Icolamida** *Alcon Cusi, Spain†.*
Chloramphenicol (p.185·1); sulfacetamide sodium (p.257·3).
*Eye infections.*

**Icoplax** *Richmond, Arg.*
Vancomycin (p.275·2).
*Bacterial infections.*

**Icoran** *Biomedica-Chemica, Gr.*
Lisinopril (p.946·3).
*Heart failure; hypertension; myocardial infarction.*

**Ictage 6** *Nuovo ICT, Ital.*
Gamolenic acid (p.1690·2).
*Skin disorders.*

**Ictan** *Sanofi Synthelabo, Spain†.*
Clotrimazole (p.396·2).
*Fungal skin infections.*

**Icthaband**
*SSL, Austral.; SSL, UK.*
Ichthammol (p.1148·2); zinc oxide (p.1163·2).
*Eczema; leg ulcers; medicated bandage.*

**Ictholin** *Hilarys, Canad.†.*
Ichthammol (p.1148·2); phenol (p.1188·1).

**Ictiomen** *Casen Fleet, Spain.*
Ichthammol (p.1148·2); talc (p.1159·1); menthol (p.1711·3).
*Skin disorders.*

**Ictom 3** *ICT, Ital.*
Omega-3 triglycerides (p.976·1); vitamin E (p.1464·3).
*Dry skin.*

**Ictotest**
*Bayer, Austral.; Bayer Diagnostics, Irl.†; Ames, Israel; Bayer Diagnostici, Ital.; Bayer Diagnostics, Mex.; Bayer Diagnostics, UK; Bayer, USA.*
Test for bilirubin in urine.

**Ictyane** *Ducray, Fr.*
Glycerol (p.1694·3); white soft paraffin (p.1479·3).
*Dry skin disorders.*

**Ictyoderm** *Bioderma, Fr.*
Urea (p.1162·2); lactic acid (p.1704·1).
*Dry skin; keratinisation disorders.*

**Icy Hot**
*Chattem, Singapore; Chattem, USA.*
Methyl salicylate (p.59·3); menthol (p.1711·3).
*Muscle, joint, and soft-tissue pain; neuralgia.*

**Id Sedin** *Nikkho, Braz.*
Gamma-aminobutyric acid (p.1690·2); reserpine (p.995·1).
*Cerebral disorders.*

**Ida** *The Forty-Two, Thai.*
Bromhexine hydrochloride (p.1115·3).
*Respiratory-tract disorders associated with increased or viscous mucus.*

**Ida-D** *The Forty-Two, Thai.*
Bromhexine hydrochloride (p.1115·3); dextromethorphan hydrobromide (p.1117·3).
*Respiratory-tract disorders associated with increased or viscous mucus.*

**Idalon** *Hoechst Marion Roussel, Neth.†.*
Floctafenine (p.43·2).
*Pain.*

**Idalprem** *Novartis Consumer, Spain.*
Lorazepam (p.704·1).
*Alcohol withdrawal syndrome; anxiety; insomnia; nausea and vomiting.*

**Idamycin**
*Pharmacia, Canad.; Pharmacia Upjohn, Mex.; Pharmacia Upjohn, USA.*
Idarubicin hydrochloride (p.560·2).
*Acute myeloid leukaemia; breast cancer.*

**Idaptan** *Danval, Spain.*
Trimetazidine hydrochloride (p.1018·1).
*Angina pectoris; neurosensorial ischaemia; retinal ischaemia; vestibular disorders.*

**Idarac**
*Hoechst Marion Roussel, Braz.†; Sanofi Synthelabo, Canad.; Aventis, Fr.; Aventis, Irl.; Hoechst Marion Roussel, Ital.†; Aventis, Spain†; Aventis, Thai.*
Floctafenine (p.43·2).
*Gout; inflammation; pain.*

**Idaralem** *Lemery, Mex.*
Idarubicin hydrochloride (p.560·2).
*Acute leukaemias; breast cancer.*

**Idarrux** *Richmond, Arg.*
Idarubicin (p.560·3).
*Malignant neoplasms.*

**Idasal Nebulizador** *Pfizer Lambert, Spain.*
Oxymetazoline hydrochloride (p.1126·1).
*Nasal congestion.*

**Idazole** *Chew, Thai.*
Tinidazole (p.617·1).
*Amoebiasis; bacterial mouth infections; giardiasis; trichomoniasis.*

**Idc** *Pharmaland, Thai.*
Indometacin (p.47·3).
*Gout; musculoskeletal and joint disorders.*

**Idealid**
*Note. This name is used for preparations of different composition.*
*Alterna, Ital.*
Nimesulide (p.67·1).
*Fever; inflammation; pain.*

*AF, Mex.*
Lidamidine (p.1270·2).
*Diarrhoea; irritable bowel syndrome.*

**Idecortex** *Pentafarma, Port.*
Idebenone (p.1700·3).

**Ideogrip** *Bioquimico, Arg.*
Astemizole (p.424·2); paracetamol (p.76·2); phenylephrine (p.1126·3).

**Ideolaxyl** *GlaxoSmithKline Sante, Fr.*
Aloes (p.1248·2); senna (p.1288·2).
*Constipation.*

**Ideolider** *IPFI, Ital.†.*
Acetylaspartic acid; citrulline (p.1425·2).
*Memory impairment.*

**Ideos**
*Innothera, Denm.; Meda, Fin.; Innotech, Fr.; Henning, Ger.; Sanofi Synthelabo, Ger.; Helsinn Birex, Irl.; Segix, Ital.; Innothera, Norw.; Helsinn, Port.; Lesvi, Spain; Meda, Swed.*
Calcium carbonate (p.1254·2); colecalciferol (p.1461·3).
*Calcium and vitamin D deficiency; osteoporosis.*

**Iderpes** *Pierre Fabre, Switz.*
Idoxuridine (p.637·3).

**Idesole** *Phoenix, Arg.*
Idebenone (p.1700·3).
*Cerebrovascular disorders.*

**Idesole Plus** *Phoenix, Arg.*
Idebenone (p.1700·3); nimodipine (p.972·3).
*Cerebrovascular disorders.*

**Idicin** *Indian Drugs, India.*
Indometacin (p.47·3).
*Dysmenorrhoea; gout; musculoskeletal and joint disorders.*

**Idina** *Grin, Mex.*
Idoxuridine (p.637·3).
*Herpes simplex infections.*

**Idle** *Klonal, Arg.*
Chlorpropamide (p.330·3).
*Diabetes mellitus.*

**IDM Solution** *Rougier, Canad.†.*
Guaifenesin (p.1122·1); potassium iodide (p.1598·1); ephedrine hydrochloride (p.1120·1); mepyramine maleate (p.437·1).
*Cold symptoms.*

**Ido A 50** *Byk Leo, Spain†.*
Vitamin A palmitate (p.1453·1).
*Vitamin A deficiency.*

**Ido-C** *Abigo, Swed.*
Ascorbic acid (p.1460·2).
Some tablets also contain sodium ascorbate.
*Vitamin C deficiency.*

**I-Doc** *Mentholatum, UK†.*
Hamamelis (p.1696·3).
*Sore eyes.*

**Ido-E**
*Pharmacia, Fin.; Pharmacia, Norw.; Pharmacia, Swed.*
*d*-Tocoferil acetate (p.1465·1).
*Vitamin E deficiency.*

**Idom** *Pharmaselect, Ger.*
Dosulepin hydrochloride (p.291·1).
*Depression.*

**Idomed** *Rowex, Irl.†.*
Indometacin (p.47·3).
*Gout; musculoskeletal, joint, and peri-articular disorders; pain.*

**Idon** *Saval, Chile.*
Domperidone (p.1263·2).
*Gastrointestinal disorders; gastrointestinal investigations; parkinsonism.*

**Idopamil** *Therabel, Belg.†.*
Ibopamine hydrochloride (p.937·3).
*Heart failure.*

**Idotrim** *Abigo, Swed.*
Trimethoprim (p.272·2).
*Urinary-tract infections.*

**Idotyl** *Ferrosan, Denm.*
Aspirin (p.15·1).
*Fever; inflammation; musculoskeletal and joint disorders; pain.*

**Idovit** *Vitamed, Israel.*
Povidone-iodine (p.1190·3).
*Bacterial and fungal skin infections; burns; skin disinfection; wounds.*

**IDR** *Sidefarma, Port.*
Fentiazac (p.43·1).
*Inflammation; pain.*

**Idracemi** *Farmigea, Ital.*
*Eye drops:* Hydrocortisone sodium phosphate (p.1104·1).
*Eye ointment:* Hydrocortisone hydrogen succinate (p.1104·1); neomycin sulfate (p.235·1); chloramphenicol (p.185·1).
*Eye disorders.*

**Idracemi Eparina** *Farmigea, Ital.†.*
Hydrocortisone sodium phosphate (p.1104·1); heparin sodium (p.928·1).
*Eye disorders.*

**Idratante Samil** *Sandoz, Ital.†.*
Emollient.

**Idril N sine** *Winzer, Ger.*
Naphazoline hydrochloride (p.1124·3).
Idril sine formerly contained actinoquinol sodium and naphazoline nitrate.
*Eye disorders.*

**Idro P2** *Sanofi Synthelabo, Ital.*
Sulmarin sodium; ascorbic acid (p.1460·2).
*Capillary disorders; haemorrhage.*

**Idrocet** *Lusofarmaco, Ital.*
Hydrocortisone acetate (p.1103·3); neomycin sulfate (p.235·1).
*Inflammatory eye and ear disorders.*

**Idrocol** *Lafon, Fr.†.*
Poloxamer 188 (p.1414·2).
*Constipation.*

**Idrolac** *Aesculapius, Ital.†.*
Lactulose (p.1269·1).
*Hepatic encephalopathy and cirrhosis.*

**Idrolax** *Schwarz, UK.*
Macrogol 4000 (p.1709·1).
*Constipation.*

**Idrolone** *Sanofi Synthelabo, Ital.*
Fenquizone potassium (p.916·2).
*Hypertension; oedema.*

**Idroneomicil** *Monsanto, Ital.*
Neomycin sulfate (p.235·1); hydrocortisone acetate (p.1103·3); naphazoline nitrate (p.1124·3).
*Infection and inflammation of the eye, nose, and ear.*

**Idropan B** *Lisapharma, Ital.*
Vitamin B substances (p.1417·1); calcium folinate (p.1431·1).
*Deficiency states; megaloblastic anaemia.*

**Idroplurivit** *Menarini, Ital.*
Multivitamin preparation (p.1417·1).

**Idropulmina** *ISI, Ital.†.*
Guaifenesin (p.1122·1).
*Coughs; respiratory-tract disorders.*

**Idroquark** *Polifarma, Ital.*
Ramipril (p.994·1); hydrochlorothiazide (p.933·2).
*Hypertension.*

**Idroskin** *Mavi, Ital.*
Collagen (p.1674·3).
*Dry skin.*

**Idroskin C** *Mavi, Ital.*
Hyaluronic acid (p.1697·3); vitamin C (p.1460·2).
*Dry skin.*

**Idrostamin** *Gap, Gr.*
Pefloxacin mesilate (p.241·3).
*Bacterial infections.*

**Idrovel** *Savoma, Ital.*
Emollient.

**Idrum** *FIRMA, Ital.†.*
Electrolytes (p.1217·1); carmellose sodium (p.1577·3).
*Dry mouth.*

**Iducher** *Farmigea, Ital.*
Idoxuridine (p.637·3).
*Herpesvirus infections of the eye.*

**Iducol** *SIFI, Ital.†.*
Idoxuridine (p.637·3); colistimethate sodium (p.199·1); rolitetracycline (p.254·1) or tetracycline (p.266·2); xanthopterin.
*Herpesvirus infections of the eye.*

**Iducutit** *Pharmagalen, Ger.†.*
Idoxuridine (p.637·3) in dimethyl sulfoxide.
*Herpes simplex and zoster infections.*

**Idulamine** *Schering-Plough, Mex.*
Azatadine maleate (p.425·1).
*Allergic skin reactions; rhinitis.*

**Idulanex** *Schering-Plough, Spain.*
Azatadine maleate (p.425·1); pseudoephedrine sulfate (p.1129·2).
*Allergic rhinitis.*

**Idulea** *Elea, Arg.*
Idoxuridine (p.637·3).
*Herpesvirus infections of the eye, face, lips, and genitals.*

**Iduridin**
*Geymonat, Ital.†; Ferring, Norw.†.*
Idoxuridine (p.637·3) in dimethyl sulfoxide.
*Herpesvirus skin infections.*

**Idustatin**
*Sanofi Synthelabo, Ital.†.*
*Ointment (1.5%):* Idoxuridine (p.637·3); neomycin sulfate (p.235·1); cod-liver oil (p.1425·2).
*Herpes simplex infections of the skin and mucous membranes.*
*Sanofi Synthelabo OTC, Ital.*
*Ointment (3%); topical solution:* Idoxuridine (p.637·3).
*Herpes simplex infections of the skin and mucous membranes.*

**Iduviran** *Chauvin, Fr.†.*
Idoxuridine (p.637·3).
*Herpes simplex eye infections.*

**Iduvo** *Dosa, Arg.*
Zidovudine (p.658·2).
*HIV infection.*

**Iecatec** *Tedec Meiji, Spain.*
Enalapril maleate (p.909·2).
*Heart failure; hypertension.*

**Ietepar** *Rottapharm, Ital.*
Betaine glucuronate (p.1660·2); diolamine glucuronate; nicotinamide ascorbate.
*Liver disorders; poisoning.*

**Ifa Dex** *Investigacion, Mex.†.*
Fenproporex (p.1588·3).
*Obesity.*

**Ifa Diety** *Investigacion, Mex.*
Fenproporex hydrochloride (p.1588·3).
*Obesity.*

**Ifa Norex** *Investigacion, Mex.*
Diethylpropion hydrochloride (p.1587·1).
*Obesity.*

**Ifa Reduccing S** *Investigacion, Mex.*
Phentermine hydrochloride (p.1592·2).
*Obesity.*

**Ifabla** *Andromaco, Mex.*
Vinblastine (p.592·1).
*Malignant neoplasms.*

**Ifacap** *Andromaco, Mex.*
Carboplatin (p.533·3).
*Ovarian cancer.*

**Ifacil** *Andromaco, Mex.*
Fluorouracil (p.554·2).
*Malignant neoplasms.*

**Ifacur** *Andromaco, Mex.*
Atracurium besilate (p.1399·1).

**Ifadac** *Andromaco, Mex.*
Dacarbazine (p.544·2).
*Malignant neoplasms.*

**Ifadox** *Andromaco, Mex.*
Doxorubicin hydrochloride (p.547·3).
*Malignant neoplasms.*

**Ifamet** *Andromaco, Mex.*
Methotrexate (p.568·2).
*Malignant neoplasms; psoriasis.*

**Ifamit** *Andromaco, Mex.*
Mitomycin (p.573·3).
*Malignant neoplasms.*

**Ifarab** *Andromaco, Mex.*
Cytarabine (p.543·1).
*Malignant neoplasms.*

**Ifavac** *Andromaco, Mex.*
Vancomycin hydrochloride (p.275·2).
*Bacterial infections.*

**Ifavin** *Andromaco, Mex.*
Vincristine (p.593·2).
*Malignant neoplasms.*

**Ifavor** *Andromaco, Mex.*
Calcium folinate (p.1431·1).
*Adjunct to fluorouracil therapy in colorectal cancer; antidote to folic acid antagonists; megaloblastic anaemia; reduction of methotrexate toxicity.*

**Ifaxol** *Andromaco, Mex.*
Paclitaxel (p.577·3).
*Breast cancer; ovarian cancer.*

**Ifecin** *Hormona, Mex.†.*
Ampicillin (p.157·1).
*Bacterial infections.*

**Ifemed** *Medifive, Thai.*
Piroxicam (p.84·2).
*Gout; musculoskeletal and joint disorders.*

**Ifenec** *Italfarmaco, Ital.*
Econazole (p.397·1) or econazole nitrate (p.397·2).
*Fungal infections; Gram-positive bacterial infections.*

**Ifersol** *Investigacion, Mex.†.*
Ferrous sulfate (p.1428·2).

**Ifex**
*Asta Medica, Canad.; Bristol-Myers Squibb Oncology, USA.*
Ifosfamide (p.561·1).
*Malignant neoplasms.*

**Ificipro** *Unique, India.*
Ciprofloxacin lactate (p.188·3).
*Bacterial infections.*

**Ifipef** *Unique, India.*
Pefloxacin (p.241·3).
*Gram-positive bacterial infections.*

**Ifiral** *Unique, Thai.†.*
Sodium cromoglicate (p.795·3).
*Allergic rhinitis; hay fever.*

**IFO-cell** *Cell Pharm, Ger.*
Ifosfamide (p.561·1).
*Malignant neoplasms.*

**Ifocid** *Richmond, Arg.*
Fluorouracil (p.554·2).
*Malignant neoplasms.*

**Ifocris** *Kampel Martian, Arg.*
Ifosfamide (p.561·1).
*Malignant neoplasms.*

**Ifolem**
*Laboratorios Chile, Chile; Lemery, Mex.*
Ifosfamide (p.561·1).
*Malignant neoplasms.*

**Ifomida** *Asofarma, Mex.*
Ifosfamide (p.561·1).
*Malignant neoplasms.*

**Ifos**
*Note. This name is used for preparations of different composition.*
*Zodiac, Braz.†.*
Ifosfamide (p.561·1).
*Malignant neoplasms.*
*Tecnofarma, Chile.*
Ofloxacin (p.239·3).
*Bacterial infections.*

**Ifosmixan** *Richmond, Arg.*
Ifosfamide (p.561·1).
*Malignant neoplasms.*

**Ifoxan**
*Teva, Israel; Sanfer, Mex.*
Ifosfamide (p.561·1).
*Malignant neoplasms.*

**Ifuchol** *Ifusa, Mex.*
Cynara (p.1678·3); boldo (p.1661·2); turmeric (p.1058·3).
*Digestive disorders.*

**Ifumelus** *Ifusa, Mex.*
Tolbutamide (p.348·1).
*Diabetes mellitus.*

**Ifupasil** *Ifusa, Mex.*
Passion flower (p.1729·1); salix (p.87·3); crataegus (p.1677·1).
*Nervous disorders.*

**Ifupeptol Magnesiado** *Ifusa, Mex.*
Magnesium sulfate (p.1228·2).
*Hypersensitivity.*

**Ifutemp** *Ifusa, Mex.*
Paracetamol (p.76·2).
*Fever; pain.*

**IFX** *Pharmacia, Arg.*
Ifosfamide (p.561·1).
*Malignant neoplasms.*

**Ig Gamma**
*Sclavo, Israel†; Nuovo ISM, Ital.*
A normal immunoglobulin (p.1627·2).
*Hypogammaglobulinaemia; passive immunisation.*

**Ig Tetano**
*Sclavo, Israel†; Nuovo ISM, Ital.*
A tetanus immunoglobulin (p.1640·3).
*Passive immunisation.*

**Ig Vena N** *Kedrion, Ital.*
A normal immunoglobulin (p.1627·2).
*Idiopathic thrombocytopenic purpura; immune deficiency; passive immunisation.*

**Igamad**
*Grifols, Chile; Grifols, Ital.*
An anti-D immunoglobulin (p.1608·1).
*Prevention of rhesus sensitisation.*

**Igantet**
*Grifols, Chile; Grifols, Ital.*
A tetanus immunoglobulin (p.1640·3).
*Passive immunisation.*

**Igantibe** *Grifols, Chile.*
Hepatitis B immunoglobulins (p.1617·2).
*Passive immunisation.*

**Igantid** *Grifols, Port.*
An anti-D immunoglobulin (p.1608·1).
*Prevention of rhesus sensitisation.*

**IgeE** *Grands Espaces, Fr.*
Black currant (p.1661·1); raspberry (p.1057·3).
*Cold symptoms.*

**I-Gesic** *Centaur, India.*
Diclofenac sodium (p.32·1).
*Eye inflammation and pain; inhibition of miosis in cataract surgery.*

**IgG** *Purissimus, Arg.*
A normal immunoglobulin (p.1627·2).
*Passive immunisation.*

**Igitur-antirheumatische** *Apomedica, Austria.*
Diethylamine salicylate (p.34·1); salicylic acid (p.1157·1); benzyl nicotinate (p.21·2); camphor (p.1665·3).
*Musculoskeletal, joint, and peri-articular disorders.*

**Igitur-Rheumafluid** *Apomedica, Austria.*
Diethylamine salicylate (p.34·1); salicylic acid (p.1157·1); glycol salicylate (p.44·3); benzyl nicotinate (p.21·2); camphor (p.1665·3).
*Musculoskeletal and joint disorders; peripheral vascular disorders.*

**I-Glo** *Aspen, S.Afr.*
Phenylephrine hydrochloride (p.1126·3).
*Eye irritation.*

**Ignatia-Homaccord** *Peithner, Austria.*
Homoeopathic preparation.

**IgRho** *Sclavo, Israel†.*
An anti-D immunoglobulin (p.1608·1).
*Prevention of rhesus sensitisation.*

**Igril** *Wellcome, Spain†.*
Caffeine hydrate (p.782·1); cyclizine hydrochloride (p.429·3); ergotamine tartrate (p.467·2).
*Headache; migraine.*

**Igroseles** *Schwarz, Ital.*
Atenolol (p.865·2); chlortalidone (p.882·3).
*Hypertension.*

**Igroton** *Novartis, Ital.*
Chlortalidone (p.882·3).
*Hypertension; oedema.*

**Igroton-Lopresor** *Novartis, Ital.*
Chlortalidone (p.882·3); metoprolol tartrate (p.957·1).
*Hypertension.*

**Igroton-Reserpina** *Novartis, Ital.*
Chlortalidone (p.882·3); reserpine (p.995·1).
*Hypertension.*

**Iguassina** *Zambon, Braz.*
Triamterene (p.1016·2); hydrochlorothiazide (p.933·2).
*Hypertension; oedema.*

**IHD** *Stadmed, India.*
Isosorbide mononitrate (p.942·1).
*Angina pectoris.*

**Iiyalgon** *Bioiberica, Spain†.*
Hyaluronic acid (p.1697·3).
*Osteoarthritis.*

**Ikaclomin** *Teva, Israel.*
Clomifene citrate (p.1542·2).
*Anovulatory infertility; oligospermia.*

**Ikacor** *Teva, Israel.*
Verapamil hydrochloride (p.1019·1).
*Angina pectoris; arrhythmias; hypertension.*

**Ikaflux** *Cifarma, Braz.†.*
Potassium iodide (p.1598·1); pinus palustris oil; guaifenesin (p.1122·1).
*Coughs.*

**Ikapress** *Teva, Israel.*
Verapamil hydrochloride (p.1019·1).
*Angina pectoris; hypertension.*

**Ikaran**
*Exel, Belg.†; Pierre Fabre, Fr.; Formenti, Ital.; Robapharm, Switz.*
Dihydroergotamine mesilate (p.465·3).
*Hypotension; migraine and vascular headache; venous insufficiency.*

**Ikatin** *Pisa, Mex.*
Gentamicin sulfate (p.217·1).
*Bacterial infections.*

**Ikatral** *Baliarda, Arg.*
OPC.
*Varices; venous disorders.*

**Ikatral Periferico** *Baliarda, Arg.*
OPC; pentoxifylline (p.979·3).
*Vascular disorders.*

**Ikeriane**
*Pierre Fabre Dermo-Cosmetique, Arg.; Ducray, Fr.*
Guanidine glycolate.
*Dry skin disorders.*

**Ikestatina** *Crinos, Ital.*
Somatostatin acetate (p.1339·3).
*Diabetic ketoacidosis; gastrointestinal haemorrhage; gastrointestinal radiography; prevention of complications following pancreatic surgery.*

**Iketoncid** *Iketon, Ital.†.*
Glutaral (p.1180·3); cetrimide (p.1172·1).
*Instrument disinfection.*

**Ikobel** *Rafarm, Gr.*
Tobramycin (p.271·2).
*Eye infections.*

**Ikolan** *Hexal, Arg.*
Clotrimazole (p.396·2).
*Fungal skin and vulvovaginal infections.*

**Ikoplex** *Knop, Chile.*
A range of homoeopathic preparations.

**Ikorel**
*Aventis, Austral.; Aventis, Fr.; Aventis, Irl.; Aventis, Neth.; Aventis, NZ; Merck, UK.*
Nicorandil (p.965·3).
*Angina pectoris.*

**Iktorivil** *Roche, Swed.*
Clonazepam (p.359·1).
*Epilepsy.*

**Ilagane** *Daker Farmasimes, Spain†.*
Naproxen (p.65·1).
*Musculoskeletal, joint, and peri-articular disorders.*

**Ila-med m** *Paesel, Ger.*
Pipenzolate bromide (p.487·3).
*Gastrointestinal disorders.*

**Ildamen**
*Asta Medica, Austria; AWD, Ger.; Asta Medica, Hong Kong†; German Remedies, India; Sidefarma, Port.*
Oxyfedrine hydrochloride (p.978·2).
*Angina pectoris; arrhythmias; heart failure; myocardial infarction.*

**Ilduc** *Baliarda, Arg.*
Amlodipine besilate (p.862·1).
*Angina pectoris; hypertension.*

**Iletin Lente** *Lilly, Canad.†.*
Insulin zinc suspension (bovine and porcine) (p.333·3).
*Diabetes mellitus.*

**Iletin NPH** *Lilly, Canad.†.*
Isophane insulin injection (bovine and porcine) (p.333·3).
*Diabetes mellitus.*

**Iletin II Pork Lente** *Lilly, Canad.*
Insulin zinc suspension (porcine) (p.333·3).
*Diabetes mellitus.*

**Iletin II Pork NPH** *Lilly, Canad.*
Isophane insulin injection (porcine) (p.333·3).
*Diabetes mellitus.*

**Iletin II Pork Regular** *Lilly, Canad.*
Neutral insulin injection (porcine) (p.333·3).
*Diabetes mellitus.*

**Iletin Regular** *Lilly, Canad.†.*
Neutral insulin injection (bovine and porcine) (p.333·3).
*Diabetes mellitus.*

**Ilgem** *Rafarm, Gr.*
Ketoconazole (p.403·3).
*Fungal infections.*

**Ilgen** *Gautier, Arg.*
Interleukin-2 (p.562·2).
*Metastatic melanoma; renal cancer.*

**Iliaclor** *Depofarma, Ital.*
Aciclovir (p.626·1).
*Herpesvirus infections.*

**Iliadin**
*Merck, Chile; Merck, Denm.; Merck, Hong Kong; Merck, Malaysia; Merck, Mex.; Merck, Neth.; Merck, Norw.; Merck, S.Afr.; Merck, Singapore; Merck, Swed.; Merck, Thai.*
Oxymetazoline hydrochloride (p.1126·1).
*Ear disorders; nasal congestion; rhinitis; sinusitis.*

**Iliocin** *Offenbach, Mex.*
Erythromycin estolate (p.208·1).
*Bacterial infections.*

**Ilio-Funkton** *Robugen, Ger.*
Dimethicone (p.1289·2).
*Reduction of gastrointestinal gas.*

**Ilja Rogoff** *Roche Nicholas, Ger.*
Garlic (p.1691·1); mistletoe (p.1715·3); crataegus (p.1677·1); sophora japonica; lupulus (p.1708·1).
*Vascular disorders.*

**Ilja Rogoff Forte** *Roche Nicholas, Ger.*
Garlic (p.1691·1).
*Hyperlipidaemia; vascular disorders.*

**Illings Bozner Maycur-Tee** *Esplanade, Austria.*
Senna (p.1288·2); magnesium sulfate (p.1228·2); chamomile (p.1669·3); fennel (p.1687·2).

**Ilman** *Demo, Gr.*
Flunitrazepam (p.698·2).
*Insomnia.*

**Iloban** *Merck, Braz.*
Cyanocobalamin (p.1458·2); ferrous fumarate (p.1427·3); folic acid (p.1429·1).
Ascorbic acid (p.1460·2) is included in this preparation to increase the absorption and availability of iron.
*Anaemias; iron deficiency.*

**Ilocin** *Haller, Braz.*
Erythromycin estolate (p.208·1).
*Bacterial infections.*

**Ilocit** *Juste, Spain†.*
Iloprost trometamol (p.1518·2).
*Thromboangitis obliterans.*

**Ilomedin**
*Schering, Austria; Schering, Denm.; Schering, Fin.; Schering, Ger.; Shepa, Gr.; Schering, Hong Kong; Schering, Israel; Schering, Ital.†; Schering, Norw.; Schering, NZ; Schering, Port.; Schering, Spain; Schering, Swed.; Schering, Switz.*
Iloprost trometamol (p.1518·2).
*Peripheral vascular disorders; thromboangiitis obliterans.*

**Ilomedine**
*Schering, Arg.; Schering, Fr.; Schering, Neth.*
Iloprost trometamol (p.1518·2).
*Peripheral ischaemia; thromboangiitis obliterans.*

**Ilon Abszess**
*Caesaro, Austria.*
Venice turpentine; turpentine oil (p.1760·1).
*Abscess; furunculosis; paranitium.*

*Cesra, Ger.*
Turpentine; turpentine oil (p.1760·1).
*Infected skin disorders.*

**Ilopan** *Savage, USA.*
Dexpanthenol (p.1727·2).
*Intestinal atony; paralytic ileus.*

**Ilopan-Choline** *Savage, USA†.*
Dexpanthenol (p.1727·2); choline bitartrate (p.1424·3).
*Flatulence.*

**Ilosin** *Collins, Mex.*
Erythromycin (p.208·1).
*Bacterial infections.*

**Ilosone**
*Lilly, Arg.; Lilly, Austral.†; Lilly, Austria†; ICN, Braz.; Lilly, Canad.†; Lilly, Hong Kong†; Dista, Irl.†; Lilly, Ital.†; Lilly, Mex.; Aspen, S.Afr.; Lilly, Thai.; Lilly, UK†; Dista, USA.*
Erythromycin (p.208·1) or erythromycin estolate (p.208·1).
*Bacterial infections.*

**Iloticina** *Lilly, Arg.*
Erythromycin (p.208·1).
*Bacterial infections.*

**Ilotrex** *Uniao Quimica, Braz.†.*
Erythromycin stearate (p.208·2).
*Bacterial infections.*

**Ilotycin**
*Lilly, Canad.†; Lilly, Switz.†; Dista, USA.*
Erythromycin (p.208·1) or erythromycin gluceptate (p.208·2).
*Bacterial infections.*

**Ilotycin TS** *Aspen, S.Afr.*
Erythromycin (p.208·1).
*Acne.*

**Ilotycin-A** *Quatromed, S.Afr.*
Tretinoin (p.1161·1).
*Acne.*

**Ilozyme** *Adria, USA†.*
Pancrelipase (p.1725·3).
*Pancreatic enzyme deficiency.*

**Ilsatec**
*Boehringer Ingelheim, Arg.; Boehringer de Angeli, Braz.†; Boehringer Ingelheim, Mex.*
Lansoprazole (p.1269·3).
*Gastro-oesophageal reflux; gastrointestinal hyperacidity; peptic ulcer; Zollinger-Ellison syndrome.*

**I-Lube**
*Note. A similar name is used for preparations of different composition (see below).*
*FDC, India.*
Polyvinyl alcohol (p.1581·1); povidone (p.1581·2).
*Dry eyes.*

**Ilube**
*Note. A similar name is used for preparations of different composition (see above).*
*Alcon, Irl.; Alcon, UK.*
Acetylcysteine (p.1112·3); hypromellose (p.1579·3).
*Dry eye syndromes.*

**Iluminoderm** *Hautel, Arg.*
Padimate O (Escalol 507) (p.1155·1).
*Sunscreen.*

**Iluminoderm Lips** *Hautel, Arg.*
Homosalate (p.1148·1); titanium dioxide (p.1160·3).
*Sunscreen.*

**Iluminoderm Plus** *Hautel, Arg.*
Homosalate (p.1148·1); titanium dioxide (p.1160·3).
*Sunscreen.*

**Ilvico**
*Note. This name is used for preparations of different composition.*
*Merck, Irl.†.*
Brompheniramine maleate (p.426·1); calcium ascorbate (p.1460·2); paracetamol (p.76·2); caffeine hydrate (p.782·1).
*Cold and influenza symptoms.*

*Merck, S.Afr.*
*Syrup:* Brompheniramine maleate (p.426·1); sodium ascorbate (p.1460·2); methylephedrine hydrochloride (p.1124·2); phenazone (p.82·3); sodium salicylate (p.90·1); codeine phosphate (p.27·1).
*Tablets:* Brompheniramine maleate (p.426·1); calcium ascorbate (p.1460·2); propyphenazone (p.85·3); salicylamide (p.87·3); quinine hydrochloride (p.460·2); caffeine (p.782·1).
*Allergic rhinitis; cold and influenza symptoms; sinusitis.*

*Merck, Spain.*
Brompheniramine maleate (p.426·1); caffeine (p.782·1); paracetamol (p.76·2).
*Fever; nasal congestion; pain.*

**Ilvico grippal** *Merck, Ger.*
Ibuprofen (p.45·3).
*Fever; pain.*

**Ilvico mit Vitamin C** *Merck, Austria†.*
Paracetamol (p.76·2); ascorbic acid (p.1460·2).
*Fever; pain.*

**Ilvico N**
*Merck, Ger.†; Merck, Port.†.*
Brompheniramine maleate (p.426·1); calcium ascorbate (p.1460·2); caffeine (p.782·1); paracetamol (p.76·2).
*Cold symptoms; fever; pain.*

**Ilvinax** *Merck, Spain.*
Oxymetazoline hydrochloride (p.1126·1).
*Nasal congestion.*

**Ilvispect** *Merck, S.Afr.†.*
Carbocisteine (p.1116·2).
*Respiratory-tract disorders.*

**Ilvitus** *Merck, Spain.*
Dextromethorphan hydrobromide (p.1117·3).
*Coughs.*

**I-L-X** *Kenwood, USA.*
A range of preparations containing iron (p.1434·3), liver extracts, and vitamin B substances (p.1417·1).
Vitamin C (p.1460·2) is included in some preparations to increase the absorption and availability of iron.
*Iron-deficiency anaemias.*

**I-L-X $B_{12}$** *Kenwood, USA.*
Iron preparation with multivitamins (p.1417·1).

**IM 75** *Montpellier, Arg.*
Indometacin (p.47·3).
*Musculoskeletal, joint, peri-articular, and soft-tissue disorders; pain.*

**Imacillin**
*AstraZeneca, Denm.; AstraZeneca, Norw.; Astra, Swed.*
Amoxicillin (p.155·3) or amoxicillin trihydrate (p.155·3).
*Bacterial infections.*

**Imacol** *Marcel, Mex.†.*
Tetracycline (p.266·2).
*Bacterial infections.*

**Imacort** *Spirig, Switz.*
Clotrimazole (p.396·2); hexamidine isetionate (p.1181·3); prednisolone acetate (p.1108·1).
*Infected skin disorders.*

**Imadrax** *Durascan, Denm.*
Amoxicillin trihydrate (p.155·3).
*Bacterial infections.*

**Imagent** *Alliance, USA.*
Perflexane lipid microspheres (p.1067·2).
*Contrast medium for echocardiography.*

**Imagent GI** *Alliance, USA.*
Perflubron (p.1730·1).
*Adjunct to magnetic resonance imaging of the gastrointestinal tract.*

**Imagopaque**
*Nycomed, Austria; Nycomed, Fin.†; Amersham Buchler, Ger.; Nycomed, Gr.; Nycomed, Ital.; Nycomed Imaging, Norw.†; Amersham, Spain; Nycomed, Switz.*
Iopentol (p.1065·1).
*Radiographic contrast medium.*

**Imanance** *Lancome, Canad.*
*SPF 15:* Octinoxate (p.1154·3); titanium dioxide (p.1160·3).
*Sunscreen.*

**Imanol** *Brobel, Arg.*
Diclofenac (p.32·1) or diclofenac diethylamine (p.32·1).
*Inflammation; pain.*

**Imap**
*Janssen-Cilag, Arg.; Janssen-Cilag, Belg.; Janssen-Ortho, Canad.†; Janssen-Cilag, Ger.; Abic, Israel†; Janssen-Cilag, Neth.*
Fluspirilene (p.701·1).
*Anxiety; insomnia; psychoses.*

**Imaplus** *MVM, Fr.†.*
Vegetable oils (p.1417·1).
*Gastrointestinal disorders; hypercholesterolaemia.*

**Imavermil** *IMA, Braz.*
Albendazole (p.101·2).
*Worm infections.*

**Imazin** *Napp, UK.*
Aspirin (p.15·1); isosorbide mononitrate (p.942·1).
*Angina pectoris; myocardial infarction.*

**Imazol**
*Note. This name is used for preparations of different composition.*
*Karrer, Ger.; Spirig, Switz.*
*Cream:* Clotrimazole (p.396·2); hexamidine isetionate (p.1181·3).
*Fungal skin infections.*

*Karrer, Ger.*
*Paste:* Clotrimazole (p.396·2); phenethyl alcohol (p.1188·1).
*Fungal skin infections.*

*Spirig, Switz.*
*Paste:* Clotrimazole (p.396·2).
*Skin disorders.*

**Imazol comp** *Karrer, Ger.*
Clotrimazole (p.396·2); hexamidine isetionate (p.1181·3); prednisolone acetate (p.1108·1).
*Fungal skin infections.*

**Imbak** *Mucos, Ger.†.*
Acidophilus-milk powder (p.1704·2); yeast (p.1469·1); juniper (p.1703·1); ginger (p.1267·1).
*Gastrointestinal disorders.*

**Imbrilon** *Rhone-Poulenc Rorer, Hong Kong†.*
Indometacin (p.47·3).
*Musculoskeletal and joint disorders.*

**Imbun**
*Ratiopharm, Austria; Merckle, Ger.*
Ibuprofen (p.45·3) or ibuprofen lysine (p.46·3).
*Fever; gout; inflammation; musculoskeletal, joint, and soft-tissue disorders; pain.*

**IMD** *Malaysia Chemist, Singapore.*
Loperamide hydrochloride (p.1271·1).
*Diarrhoea.*

**Imda** *Dosa, Arg.*
Bicalutamide (p.530·1).

**Imdex**
*CCM, Malaysia; CCM, Singapore.*
Isosorbide mononitrate (p.942·1).
*Angina pectoris.*

**Imdur**
*AstraZeneca, Austral.; Astra, Austria†; AstraZeneca, Canad.; Astra-Zeneca, Denm.; AstraZeneca, Fin.; Astra-Zeneca, Gr.; AstraZeneca, Hong Kong; AstraZeneca, Irl.; AstraZeneca, Malaysia; AstraZeneca, Mex.; AstraZeneca, Norw.; AstraZeneca, NZ†; AstraZeneca, Port.; AstraZeneca, S.Afr.; AstraZeneca, Singapore; Hassle, Swed.; Astra, Switz.†; AstraZeneca, Thai.; AstraZeneca, UK; Key, USA.*
Isosorbide mononitrate (p.942·1).
*Angina pectoris.*

**Imecol** *Andromaco, Chile.*
Phthalylsulfathiazole (p.242·3); nifuroxazide (p.237·2).
*Diarrhoea.*

**Imedeen** *Gobbi, Arg.*
Marine proteins; ascorbic acid; zinc gluconate (p.1417·1).
*Dietary supplement.*

**Imediat N** *Gador, Arg.*
Levonorgestrel (p.1563·2).
*Postcoital oral contraceptive.*

**Imegul** *Arkopharma, Fr.*
Cascara (p.1255·1); ispaghula (p.1268·1).
*Constipation.*

**Imepas** *Marcel, Mex.†.*
Diazepam (p.690·1).

**Imeron** *Byk Gulden, Ger.*
Iomeprol (p.1064·3).
*Radiographic contrast medium.*

**Imeson** *Taurus, Ger.*
Nitrazepam (p.710·1).
*Sleep disorders.*

**Imet** *FIRMA, Ital.*
Indometacin (p.47·3).
*Musculoskeletal and joint disorders.*

**Imex** *Merz, Ger.*
Tetracycline hydrochloride (p.266·2).
*Acne.*

**Imexim** *Cimex, Switz.†.*
Co-trimoxazole (p.199·3).
*Bacterial infections.*

**Imferon**
*Amadeus, India; Rhone-Poulenc Rorer, Mex.†; Llorente, Spain.*
Iron dextran (p.1436·3).
*Iron-deficiency anaemia.*

**Imflac** *Douglas, Austral.*
Diclofenac sodium (p.32·1).

**Imidazyl** *Recordati, Ital.*
Naphazoline nitrate (p.1124·3).
*Conjunctivitis.*

**Imidazyl Antistaminico** *Recordati, Ital.*
Naphazoline nitrate (p.1124·3); thonzylamine hydrochloride (p.442·2).
*Conjunctivitis.*

**Imidil** *Lyka, India.*
Clotrimazole (p.396·2).
*Fungal skin and vulvovaginal infections; nappy rash.*

**Imidin K** *Wernigerode, Ger.*
Xylometazoline hydrochloride (p.1132·2).
*Nasal congestion; rhinitis.*

**Imidin N** *Wernigerode, Ger.*
Xylometazoline hydrochloride (p.1132·2).
*Nasal congestion; rhinitis.*

**Imigran**
*GlaxoSmithKline, Arg.; GlaxoSmithKline, Austral.; GlaxoSmithKline, Austria; GlaxoSmithKline, Braz.; GlaxoSmithKline, Chile; GlaxoSmithKline, Denm.; GlaxoSmithKline, Fin.; GlaxoSmithKline, Ger.; Glaxo Wellcome, Gr.; GlaxoSmithKline, Hong Kong; Glaxo Wellcome, Irl.; GlaxoSmithKline, Ital.; GlaxoSmithKline, Malaysia; Glaxo Wellcome, Mex.; GlaxoSmithKline, Neth.; GlaxoSmithKline, Norw.; GlaxoSmithKline, NZ; Glaxo Wellcome, Port.; GlaxoSmithKline, S.Afr.; GlaxoSmithKline, Singapore; GlaxoSmithKline, Spain; GlaxoSmithKline, Swed.; GlaxoSmithKline, Switz.; GlaxoSmithKline, Thai.; GlaxoSmithKline, UK.*
Sumatriptan (p.473·1), sumatriptan hemisulfate (p.473·1), or sumatriptan succinate (p.471·2).
*Cluster headache; migraine.*

**Imigrane** *GlaxoSmithKline, Fr.*
Sumatriptan (p.473·1) or sumatriptan succinate (p.471·2).
*Migraine; vascular facial pain.*

**Imiject** *GlaxoSmithKline, Fr.*
Sumatriptan succinate (p.471·2).
*Vascular facial pain.*

**Imilgamma** *Worwag, Ger.†.*
Benfotiamine (p.1454·3).
Formerly known as Benfogamma.
*Vitamin $B_1$ deficiency.*

**Imin** *Yung Shin, Singapore.*
Inosine pranobex (p.640·2).
*Herpes zoster; measles.*

**Iminase** *Madaus, Spain†.*
Anistreplase (p.863·3).
*Myocardial infarction.*

**Imipem** *Neopharmed, Ital.*
Imipenem (p.221·1); cilastatin sodium (p.188·1).
Lidocaine (p.1377·3) is included in the intramuscular injection to alleviate the pain of injection.
*Bacterial infections.*

**Imipra** *Cristalia, Braz.*
Imipramine hydrochloride (p.300·1).
*Depression.*

**Imitrex**
*GlaxoSmithKline, Arg.; GlaxoSmithKline, Belg.; GlaxoSmithKline, Canad.; GlaxoSmithKline, Israel; Glaxo Wellcome, USA.*
Sumatriptan (p.473·1), sumatriptan hemisulfate (p.473·1), or sumatriptan succinate (p.471·2).
*Cluster headache; migraine.*

**Imizol** *Farmigea, Ital.†.*
Naphazoline nitrate (p.1124·3).
*Eye irritation.*

**Immediat** *Volta, Chile.*
Propyphenazone (p.85·3); adiphenine hydrochloride (p.1648·1); phenobarbital (p.367·3).

**Immignost** *GN, Ger.†.*
Tetanus toxoid; diphtheria toxoid; Streptococcal group C antigen; tuberculin (p.1759·1); Candida albicans antigen; Trichophyton mentagrophytes antigen; proteus mirabilis antigen.
*Assessment of cell-mediated immunity.*

**Immubron** *Bruschettini, Ital.*
Lysates of: *Staphylococcus aureus*; *Streptococcus pyogenes*; *Streptococcus viridans*; *Klebsiella pneumoniae*; *Klebsiella ozaenae*; *Haemophilus influenzae*; *Moraxella catarrhalis*; strains of *Streptococcus pneumoniae*.
*Respiratory-tract infections.*

**ImmuCyst**
*Aventis Pasteur, Arg.; Aventis, Austral.; Aventis Pasteur, Austria; Logistics, Belg.; Aventis Pasteur, Braz.; Aventis Pasteur, Canad.; Aventis Pasteur, Chile; Aventis Pasteur, Fr.; CytoChemia, Ger.; Aventis Pasteur, Hong Kong; Connaught, Israel; Wassermann, Ital.; Aventis Pasteur, Malaysia; Aventis, NZ; Inibsa, Port.; Aventis Pasteur, Singapore; Inibsa, Spain; Sanofi Synthelabo, Switz.†; Aventis Pasteur, Thai.; Cambridge, UK.*
A BCG vaccine (p.1609·2).
*Bladder cancer.*

**Immucytal** *Pierre Fabre, Ital.*
Ribosomal fractions of *Klebsiella pneumoniae*; *Streptococcus pneumoniae*; *Streptococcus pyogenes*; *Haemophilus influenzae*; membrane fraction of *Klebsiella pneumoniae*.
*Bronchial infections; otorhinolaryngeal infections.*

**Immudynal** *Ardeypharm, Ger.*
Homoeopathic preparation.

**Immugrip** *Pierre Fabre, Fr.*
An inactivated influenza vaccine (p.1620·2).
*Active immunisation.*

**Immukin**
*Boehringer Ingelheim, Hong Kong; Boehringer Ingelheim, Irl.; Boehringer Ingelheim, UK.*
Interferon gamma-1b (rbe) (p.647·2).
*Infections in chronic granulomatous disease.*

**Immukine**
*Boehringer Ingelheim, Belg.; Boehringer Ingelheim, Neth.*
Interferon gamma-1b (p.647·2).
*Infections in chronic granulomatous disease.*

**Immulem** *Lemery, Mex.*
Ciclosporin (p.1351·2).
*Transplant rejection.*

**Immumil** *Milte, Ital.*
Propolis (p.1735·2); echinacea (p.1683·2); thyme (p.1755·2).
*Cold symptoms.*

**Immunace** *Vitabiotics, UK.*
Multivitamin, mineral, and bioflavonoid preparation (p.1417·1).

**Immun-Aid**
*Pisa, Mex.; McGaw, NZ†; McGaw, USA.*
Preparation for enteral nutrition (p.1417·1).
*Immunosuppression.*

**Immunate**
*Baxter Immuno, Arg.; Baxter, Austria; Immuno, Braz.†; Baxter, Ger.; Baxter, Ital.; Baxter, Swed.; Baxter, Switz.*
A factor VIII preparation (p.751·1).
*Haemorrhagic disorders.*

**Immune Formula** *Nutravite, Canad.*
Astragalus; black seed; echinacea; grape seed (p.1417·1).

**Immunex CRP** *Wampole, USA.*
Test for C-reactive protein in serum.

**Immunine**
*Baxter Immuno, Arg.; Baxter, Austria; Immuno, Braz.†; Baxter, Canad.; Baxter, Denm.; Baxter, Ger.; Baxter, Ital.; Baxter, Spain; Baxter, Swed.; Baxter, Switz.*
A factor IX preparation (p.752·2).
*Haemorrhagic disorders.*

**Immunja** *OTW, Ger.*
Homoeopathic preparation.

**Immunocal** *Immunotec, USA.*
Preparation for enteral nutrition (p.1417·1).

**Immunoendocig** *Nuovo ISM, Ital.*
A cytomegalovirus immunoglobulin (p.1612·1).
*Passive immunisation.*

**Immunoendozig** *ISI, Ital.†.*
A varicella-zoster immunoglobulin (p.1643·1).
*Passive immunisation.*

**ImmunoHBs** *Kedrion, Ital.*
A hepatitis B immunoglobulin (p.1617·2).
*Passive immunisation.*

**Immunokine** *Oxo, Thai.*
Tetrachlorodecaoxide (p.1752·3).
*Post-radiation-therapy syndromes.*

**Immunomega** *Larkhall Laboratories, UK.*
Multivitamin and mineral preparation (p.1417·1).

**Immunomorb** *ISI, Ital.†.*
A measles immunoglobulin (p.1623·1).
*Passive immunisation.*

**Immunoparot** *ISI, Ital.†.*
A mumps immunoglobulin (p.1626·3).
*Passive immunisation.*

**Immunopertox** *ISI, Ital.†.*
A pertussis immunoglobulin (p.1631·2).
*Passive immunisation.*

**Immunopret** *Bionorica, Ger.†.*
Echinacea purpurea (p.1683·2).
*Respiratory- and urinary-tract infections.*

**Immunoprin** *Ashbourne, UK.*
Azathioprine (p.1349·1).
*Inflammatory disorders; organ transplants.*

**Immunorho** *Kedrion, Ital.*
An anti-D immunoglobulin (p.1608·1).
*Prevention of rhesus sensitisation.*

**Immunoros** *ISI, Ital.†.*
A rubella immunoglobulin (p.1637·3).
*Passive immunisation.*

**Immunotetan** *Kedrion, Ital.*
A tetanus immunoglobulin (p.1640·3).
*Passive immunisation.*

**Immunotrofina** *DMG, Ital.*
Fructose; arginine; vitamin B substances; potassium iodide (p.1417·1).

**Immunovac** *Artu, Neth.*
Allergen extracts (p.1650·1).
*Allergen immunotherapy.*

**Immunovir** *PRC, Ital.*
Aciclovir (p.626·1).
*Herpesvirus infections.*

**Immunozig** *ISI, Ital.†.*
A varicella-zoster immunoglobulin (p.1643·1).
*Passive immunisation.*

**Immunozima** *Valens, Ital.*
Muramidase hydrochloride (p.1717·2).
*Viral infections.*

**Immutone** *Pharmadass, UK.*
Shark-liver oil.

**Immuwash** *DMG, Ital.*
Glucan.
*Nasal cleansing.*

**Imocap** *Raza, Malaysia; Pharmaniaga, Malaysia.*
Loperamide hydrochloride (p.1271·1).
*Diarrhoea; ileostomy management.*

**Imoclone** *Orion, Denm.*
Zopiclone (p.729·3).
*Insomnia.*

**Imocur**
*Note. This name is used for preparations of different composition.*
*Pharmacia, Fin.*
Loperamide hydrochloride (p.1271·1).
*Diarrhoea; ileostomy management.*

*Zambon, Fr.*
Bacterial fractions of *Haemophilus influenzae*; *Streptococcus pneumoniae*; *Klebsiella ozaenae*; *Klebsiella pneumoniae*; *Staphylococcus aureus*; *Streptococcus viridans*; *Streptococcus pyogenes*; *Moraxella catarrhalis*.
*Prevention of upper respiratory-tract infection.*

**Imodium**
*Janssen-Cilag, Austral.; Janssen-Cilag, Austria; Janssen-Cilag, Belg.; McNeil Consumer, Canad.; Janssen-Cilag, Denm.; Orion, Fin.; Janssen-Cilag, Fr.; Janssen-Cilag, Ger.; Woelm, Ger.; Janssen-Cilag, Gr.; Janssen, Hong Kong; Janssen-Cilag, Irl.; Janssen-Cilag, Israel; Janssen-Cilag, Ital.; Janssen-Cilag, Malaysia; Janssen, Mex.; Janssen-Cilag, Neth.; Janssen-Cilag, Norw.; Janssen-Cilag, NZ; Janssen-Cilag, Port.; Janssen-Cilag, S.Afr.; Janssen-Cilag, Singapore; Abello, Spain; Janssen-Cilag, Swed.; Janssen-Cilag, Switz.; Janssen-Cilag, Thai.; Janssen-Cilag, UK; Johnson & Johnson MSD Consumer, UK; McNeil Consumer, USA; Janssen, USA.*
Loperamide hydrochloride (p.1271·1).
*Diarrhoea; ileostomy management.*

**Imodium Advanced**
*Janssen-Cilag, Austral.; McNeil Consumer, Canad.; Janssen-Cilag, NZ; McNeil Consumer, USA.*
Loperamide hydrochloride (p.1271·1); simeticone (p.1289·2).
*Diarrhoea; excess gastrointestinal gas.*

**Imodium med Simethicon** *Janssen-Cilag, Denm.*
Loperamide hydrochloride (p.1271·1); simeticone (p.1289·2).
*Diarrhoea.*

**Imodium Plus**
*Janssen-Cilag, Austria; Janssen-Cilag, Braz.; Woelm, Ger.; Janssen, Mex.; Janssen-Cilag, S.Afr.; Abello, Spain; Janssen-Cilag, Switz.; Johnson & Johnson MSD Consumer, UK.*
Loperamide hydrochloride (p.1271·1); simeticone (p.1289·2).
*Diarrhoea; flatulence.*

**Imogam**
*CSL, Austral.; Aventis Pasteur, Canad.*
A rabies immunoglobulin (p.1635·3).
*Passive immunisation.*

**Imogam Rabia**
*Aventis Pasteur, Arg.; Aventis Pasteur, Spain.*
A rabies immunoglobulin (p.1635·3).
*Passive immunisation.*

**Imogam Rabies**
*Pasteur Merieux, Israel; Pasteur Merieux, USA.*
A rabies immunoglobulin (p.1635·3).
*Passive immunisation.*

**Imogam Rage** *Aventis Pasteur, Fr.*
A rabies immunoglobulin (p.1635·3).
*Passive immunisation.*

**Imogam Tetano** *Pasteur Merieux, Ital.†.*
A tetanus immunoglobulin (p.1640·3).
*Passive immunisation.*

**Imosec**
*Janssen-Cilag, Braz.; Abello, Spain.*
Loperamide hydrochloride (p.1271·1).
*Diarrhoea.*

**Imossel** *Martin, Fr.*
Loperamide hydrochloride (p.1271·1).
*Diarrhoea.*

**Imosselduo**
*Martin, Fr.; Martin-Johnson & Johnson, Fr.*
Loperamide hydrochloride (p.1271·1); simeticone (p.1289·2).
*Diarrhoea; flatulence.*

**Imotab** *Raza, Malaysia; Pharmaniaga, Malaysia.*
Loperamide hydrochloride (p.1271·1).
*Diarrhoea; ileostomy management.*

**Imotoran** *Rayere, Mex.*
Enalapril (p.909·2).

**Imovane**
*Aventis, Arg.; Aventis, Austral.; Rhone-Poulenc Rorer, Austria†; Aventis, Belg.; Aventis, Braz.; Aventis, Canad.; Aventis, Chile; Aventis, Denm.; Aventis, Fin.; Aventis, Fr.; Aventis, Gr.; Aventis, Hong Kong; Aventis, Israel; Aventis, Ital.; Aventis, Malaysia; Aventis, Mex.; Aventis, Neth.; Aventis, Norw.; Aventis, NZ; Aventis, S.Afr.; Aventis Pasteur, Singapore; Aventis, Swed.; Aventis, Switz.*
Zopiclone (p.729·3).
*Sleep disorders.*

**Imovax** *Merieux, Fr.†.*
A mumps vaccine (Urabe Am 9 strain) (p.1626·3).
*Active immunisation.*

**Imovax BCG** *Aventis Pasteur, Ital.*
A BCG vaccine (p.1609·2).
*Active immunisation.*

**Imovax DT** *Pasteur Merieux, Ital.†.*
A diphtheria and tetanus vaccine (p.1613·1).
*Active immunisation.*

**Imovax DTP** *Pasteur Merieux, Ital.†.*
A diphtheria, tetanus, and pertussis vaccine (p.1613·3).
*Active immunisation.*

**Imovax Gripe** *Aventis, Arg.*
An influenza vaccine (p.1620·2).
*Active immunisation.*

**Imovax Meningo A & C** *Aventis, S.Afr.*
A meningococcal vaccine (p.1626·1).
*Active immunisation.*

**Imovax Mumps**
*Aventis Pasteur, Braz.; Pasteur Merieux, Hong Kong†.*
A mumps vaccine (live attenuated Urabe Am 9 strain) (p.1626·3).
*Active immunisation.*

**Imovax Parotiditis** *Aventis Pasteur, Arg.*
A mumps vaccine (Urabe Am 9 strain) (p.1626·3).
*Active immunisation.*

**Imovax Pneumo** *Aventis, Arg.*
A pneumococcal vaccine (23-valent) (p.1633·1).
*Active immunisation.*

**Imovax Pneumo 23** *Aventis, S.Afr.*
A pneumococcal vaccine (p.1633·1).
*Active immunisation.*

**Imovax Polio**
*Aventis Pasteur, Arg.; Aventis Pasteur, Belg.; Aventis Pasteur, Braz.; Aventis Pasteur, Fin.; Aventis Pasteur, Fr.; IFET (ΙΦΕΤ), Gr.; Aventis Pasteur, Hong Kong; Pasteur Merieux, Israel; Aventis Pasteur, Ital.; Aventis Pasteur, Norw.; Pasteur Merieux, Singapore†; Aventis Pasteur, Swed.*
An inactivated poliomyelitis vaccine (p.1633·3).
*Active immunisation.*

**Imovax Rabbia** *Aventis Pasteur, Ital.*
A rabies vaccine (p.1635·3).
*Active immunisation.*

**Imovax Rabies**
*Aventis Pasteur, Canad.; Pasteur Merieux, USA.*
A rabies vaccine (human diploid cell) (p.1635·3).
*Active immunisation.*

**Imovax Rubeola** *Aventis Pasteur, Arg.*
A rubella vaccine (Wistar RA 27/3-M strain) (p.1637·3).
*Active immunisation.*

**Imovax Tetano** *Aventis Pasteur, Ital.*
A tetanus vaccine (p.1640·3).
*Active immunisation.*

**Imovexil** *Medinova (Μεντνοβα), Gr.*
Trimetazidine (p.1018·1).
*Angina.*

**Imox** *Ipca, India.*
Amoxicillin trihydrate (p.155·3).
*Bacterial infections.*

**Imox-Clo** *Ipca, India.*
Amoxicillin trihydrate (p.155·3); cloxacillin sodium (p.198·2).
*Bacterial infections.*

**Imozop** *Durascan, Denm.*
Zopiclone (p.729·3).
*Insomnia.*

**Impact**
*Novartis, Arg.; Novartis Consumer, Austral.; Novartis, Braz.; Novartis, Fin.; Novartis Nutrition, Hong Kong; Novartis Consumer, Ital.; Novartis Consumer, Port.; Novartis Nutrition, Singapore; Novartis, UK; Novartis Nutrition, USA.*
A range of preparations for enteral nutrition (p.1417·1).

**Impalamycin** *Bros, Gr.*
Doxycycline hyclate (p.206·2).
*Bacterial infections.*

**Impalud** *Biolab Sanus, Braz.†.*
Quinine sulfate (p.460·2).
*Babesiosis; leg cramps; malaria.*

**Impedil** *Phoenix, Arg.*
Etamsylate (p.749·3).
*Haemorrhage.*

**Impelium** *TO-Chemicals, Thai.*
Loperamide hydrochloride (p.1271·1).
*Diarrhoea.*

**Impetex** *Roche, Ital.*
Diflucortolone valerate (p.1099·3); chlorquinaldol (p.187·3).
*Infected skin disorders.*

**Impidol** *Silesia, Chile.*
Nonoxinol 9 (p.1413·3).
*Contraceptive.*

**Implanon**
*Organon, Arg.; Organon, Austral.; Organon, Austria; Organon, Belg.; Organon, Braz.; Organon, Chile; Organon, Denm.; Organon, Fin.; Organon, Fr.; Nourypharma, Ger.; Organon, Irl.; Organon, Ital.; Organon, Malaysia; Organon, Mex.; Organon, Neth.; Organon, Norw.; Organon, Port.; Organon, Spain; Organon, Swed.; Organon, Switz.; Organon, Thai.; Organon, UK.*
Etonogestrel (p.1554·1).
*Progestogen-only implantable contraceptive.*

**Implementor** *Pentafarma, Port.*
Pirlindole hydrochloride (p.316·2).

**Impletol** *Bayer, Ger.†.*
Procaine hydrochloride (p.1383·2); caffeine (p.782·1).
*Nervous system disorders.*

**Implicane** *Tecnofarma, Chile.*
Sertraline (p.317·3).
*Depression.*

**Impore** *Unison, Thai.†.*
Loperamide hydrochloride (p.1271·1).
*Diarrhoea.*

**Importal**
*Novartis Consumer, Austria; Novartis Consumer, Belg.; Novartis, Denm.; Novartis, Fin.†; Novartis Sante, Fr.; Novartis Consumer, Ger.; Novartis, Gr.; Novartis, Israel; Novartis Consumer, Neth.; Novartis, Norw.; Novartis, NZ; Novartis Consumer, Port.; Novartis Consumer, S.Afr.†; Novartis, Swed.; Novartis Consumer, Switz.; Novartis, Thai.*
Lactitol (p.1269·1).
*Constipation; hepatic encephalopathy.*

**Imposergon** *Rafarm, Gr.*
Famotidine (p.1265·2).
*Conditions where gastric acid reduction is beneficial; gastric hypersecretion including Zollinger-Ellison syndrome; peptic ulcer.*

**Imposit N** *Madaus, Ger.†.*
Cetylpyridinium chloride (p.1173·1); benzocaine (p.1370·3).
*Mouth and throat disorders.*

**Impregon** *Fleming, USA.*
Tetrachlorosalicylanilide.
*Napkin disinfection.*

**Impresso** *Alpharma-Isis, Ger.*
Oxprenolol hydrochloride (p.978·1); hydralazine hydrochloride (p.931·2); chlortalidone (p.882·3).
*Hypertension.*

**Impril** *ICN, Canad.†.*
Imipramine hydrochloride (p.300·1).
*Depression.*

**Impromen**
*Janssen-Cilag, Belg.; Janssen-Cilag, Ger.; Formenti, Ital.; Janssen-Cilag, Neth.; Janssen, Thai.*
Bromperidol (p.672·1), bromperidol decanoate (p.672·1), or bromperidol lactate (p.672·1).
*Psychoses.*

**Improntal** *Fides Ecopharma, Spain.*
Piroxicam (p.84·2).
*Gout; musculoskeletal, joint, peri-articular, and soft-tissue disorders; pain.*

**Improved Analgesic** *Rugby, USA.*
Methyl salicylate (p.59·3); menthol (p.1711·3).
*Muscle, joint, and soft-tissue pain; neuralgia.*

**Improved Once A Day** *Quest, UK.*
Multivitamin and mineral preparation (p.1417·1).

**Improved Versal** *Clay Park, Hong Kong†.*
Zinc oxide (p.1163·2); calamine (p.1144·1).
*Anorectal disorders.*

**Improvil** *Pharmacia, Austral.*
21 Tablets, norethisterone (p.1562·2); ethinylestradiol (p.1553·2); 7 tablets, inert.
*Triphasic oral contraceptive.*

**Impugan**
*Dumex-Alpharma, Denm.†; Alpharma, Swed.; Alpharma, Switz.; Dumex-Alpharma, Thai.*
Furosemide (p.919·3).
*Forced diuresis; hypertension; nephrotic syndrome; oedema; renal insufficiency.*

**Imtrate**
*Douglas, Austral.; Douglas, NZ.*
Isosorbide mononitrate (p.942·1).
*Angina pectoris.*

**Imuderm** *Goldshield, UK.*
*Cream:* White soft paraffin (p.1479·3); fractionated coconut oil (p.1440·3); glycerol (p.1694·3).
*Skin disorders.*
*Hand & face wash; shower gel:* Soap substitute.
*Dry skin disorders.*
*Oil:* Light liquid paraffin (p.1479·1); almond oil (p.1651·1).
*Dry skin disorders.*

**Imudon** *Solvay, Fr.*
Lysates of *Lactobacillus acidophilus* (p.1704·2); *Lactobacillus helveticus* (p.1704·2); *Lactobacillus lactis* (p.1704·2); *Lactobacillus fermentum* (p.1704·2); *Streptococcus pyogenes*; *Enterococcus faecium* (p.1704·2); *Enterococcus faecalis* (p.1704·2); *Streptococcus sanguis*; *Staphylococcus aureus*; *Klebsiella pneumoniae*; *Corynebacterium pseudodiphtheriticum*; *Fusiformis fusiformis*; *Candida albicans*.
*Mouth disorders.*

**Imufor**
*Boehringer Ingelheim, Arg.; Boehringer Ingelheim, Austria.*
Interferon gamma-1b (p.647·2).
*Infections in chronic granulomatous disease.*

**Imuger** *Gerard, Irl.*
Azathioprine (p.1349·1).
*Immunosuppressant.*

**Imugins** *Schumit, Thai.*
Ginseng (p.1693·1); multivitamins and minerals (p.1417·1).
*Tonic.*

**Imukin**
*Boehringer Ingelheim, Austral.; Boehringer Ingelheim, Austria; Boehringer Ingelheim, Denm.; Boehringer Ingelheim, Fin.; Boehringer Ingelheim, Fr.; Boehringer Ingelheim, Ger.; Boehringer Ingelheim, Gr.; Boehringer Ingelheim, Ital.; Boehringer Ingelheim, Norw.; Boehringer Ingelheim, NZ; Boehringer Ingelheim, Port.; Boehringer Ingelheim, Spain; Boehringer Ingelheim, Swed.; Boehringer Ingelheim, Switz.*
Interferon gamma-1b (rbe) (p.647·2).
*Infections in chronic granulomatous disease.*

**Imunen** *Cristalia, Braz.*
Azathioprine (p.1349·1).
*Immunosuppressant.*

**Imuneprim** *IQB, Braz.*
Co-trimoxazole (p.199·3).
*Bacterial infections; Pneumocystis carinii pneumonia; protozoal infections.*

**Imuno Max-gel** *Herbarium, Braz.*
Plant alkaloids.
*Genital herpes; herpes labialis.*

**Imunoferon** *Fariberica, Port.*
Glicofosfopeptical (p.1693·3).
*Immunodeficiency.*

**Imunonutril** *Support, Braz.*
Preparation for enteral nutrition (p.1417·1).

**Imunoparvum** *Lafepe, Braz.†.*
*Corynebacterium parvum* (p.540·2).
*Immunostimulant.*

**Imunovir**
*Rivex, Canad.; Newport, Irl.; NZ Medical & Scientific, NZ; Ardern, UK.*
Inosine pranobex (p.640·2).
*Viral infections.*

**Imunoxa** *Gador, Arg.*
Lamivudine (p.648·2).
*HIV infection.*

**Imunoxa Complex** *Gador, Arg.*
Lamivudine (p.648·2); zidovudine (p.658·2).
*HIV infection.*

**Imuprel** *Adcock Ingram, S.Afr.*
Isoprenaline hydrochloride (p.940·2).
*Bronchospasm; heart block; shock.*

**Imuprin** *Pharmacia, Fin.*
Azathioprine (p.1349·1).
*Auto-immune disorders; lupus erythematosus; rheumatoid arthritis; transplant rejection.*

**Imuran**
*GlaxoSmithKline, Arg.; GlaxoSmithKline, Austral.; GlaxoSmithKline, Belg.; GlaxoSmithKline, Braz.; GlaxoSmithKline, Canad.; GlaxoSmithKline, Chile; Glaxo Wellcome, Gr.; GlaxoSmithKline, Hong Kong; GlaxoSmithKline, India; Wellcome, Irl.; Wellcome, Israel; GlaxoSmithKline, Malaysia; Glaxo Wellcome, Mex.; GlaxoSmithKline, Neth.; GlaxoSmithKline, NZ; Wellcome, Port.; GlaxoSmithKline, S.Afr.; GlaxoSmithKline, Singapore; GlaxoSmithKline, Thai.; GlaxoSmithKline, UK; Prometheus, USA.*
Azathioprine (p.1349·1) or azathioprine sodium (p.1350·1).
*Auto-immune disorders; transplant rejection.*

**Imurek**
*GlaxoSmithKline, Austria; GlaxoSmithKline, Ger.; GlaxoSmithKline, Switz.*
Azathioprine (p.1349·1) or azathioprine sodium (p.1350·1).
*Auto-immune disorders; transplant rejection.*

**Imurel**
*Glaxo Wellcome, Denm.; GlaxoSmithKline, Fin.; GlaxoSmithKline, Fr.; GlaxoSmithKline, Norw.; Celltech, Spain; GlaxoSmithKline, Swed.*
Azathioprine (p.1349·1).
*Auto-immune disorders; transplant rejection.*

**Imusporin** *Cipla, India.*
Ciclosporin (p.1351·2).
*Atopic dermatitis; graft-versus-host disease; nephrotic syndrome; psoriasis; rheumatoid arthritis; transplant rejection.*

**Imuvac** *Solvay, Spain.*
An influenza vaccine (p.1620·2).
*Active immunisation.*

**Imuvit**
*Adroka, Switz.; Rueckert, Thai.†.*
Ginseng (p.1693·1); multivitamins and minerals (p.1417·1).
*Tonic.*

**In A Wink**
*Note. This name is used for preparations of different composition.*
*Ciba Vision, Austral.†.*
Naphazoline nitrate (p.1124·3); zinc sulfate (p.1469·3).
*Conjunctivitis; eye irritation.*

*Ciba Vision, Canad.*
A range of solutions for contact lenses (p.1164·2).

*Ciba Vision, NZ†.*
Povidone (p.1581·2).
*Dry eyes.*

**In A Wink Allergy** *Ciba Vision, Austral.†.*
Antazoline hydrochloride (p.424·2); tetryzoline hydrochloride (p.1131·2).
*Allergic conjunctivitis; hay fever.*

**In A Wink Moisturing** *Ciba Vision, Austral.†.*
Povidone (p.1581·2).
*Dry eyes.*

**Inabrin**
*Pharmacia Upjohn, Belg.†; Pharmacia Upjohn, Port.†.*
Ibuprofen (p.45·3).
*Fever; pain.*

**Inabutol Forte** *Themis Chemicals, India.*
Isoniazid (p.222·2); ethambutol hydrochloride (p.211·3).
*Tuberculosis.*

**Inac** *Recon, Singapore.*
Diclofenac sodium (p.32·1).
*Gout; musculoskeletal, joint, peri-articular, and soft-tissue disorders.*

**Inacid** *Abello, Spain; Merck Sharp & Dohme, Spain.*
Indometacin (p.47·3) or indometacin sodium (p.47·3).
*Gout; inflammation; musculoskeletal, joint, peri-articular, and soft-tissue disorders; pain; patent ductus arteriosus.*

**Inacol** *Medifarma, Mex.†.*
Tetracycline (p.266·2).
*Bacterial infections.*

**Inadine**
*Johnson & Johnson, Ger.; Johnson & Johnson, Irl.; Ethicon, Ital.; Johnson & Johnson Medical, UK.*
Povidone-iodine (p.1190·3).
*Burns; skin ulcers; wounds.*

**Inadol** *Pharmagenus, Spain.*
Ibuprofen (p.45·3).
*Musculoskeletal pain and inflammation.*

**Inalacor** *Faes, Spain.*
Fluticasone propionate (p.1102·3).
*Asthma.*

**Inalador Vick** *Procter & Gamble, Braz.†.*
Menthol (p.1711·3); camphor (p.1665·3); methyl salicylate (p.59·3); siberian fir oil.
*Respiratory-tract congestion.*

**Inaladuo** *Faes, Spain.*
Salmeterol xinafoate (p.795·1); fluticasone propionate (p.1102·3).
*Asthma.*

**Inalar** *Montefarmaco, Ital.*
Xylometazoline hydrochloride (p.1132·2); domiphen bromide (p.1179·1).
*Nasal congestion.*

**Inalcort** *IBN, Ital.*
Flunisolide (p.1101·1).
*Asthma; bronchitis; rhinitis.*

**Inalgon Neu** *Calea, Austria.*
Dipyrone (p.35·3).
*Fever; pain.*

**Inalintra** *Diviser Aquilea, Spain†.*
Oxymetazoline hydrochloride (p.1126·1).
*Nasal congestion.*

**Inalobel** *Sedabel, Braz.†.*
Ephedrine (p.1120·1); cineole (p.1672·1); menthol (p.1711·3); niaouli oil (p.1719·3); tolu balsam (p.1131·3); sumatra benzoin (p.1751·1).
*Respiratory-tract congestion.*

**Inalpin** *Qualiphar, Belg.*
Codeine phosphate (p.27·1); guaifenesin (p.1122·1).
Formerly contained codeine phosphate, bromoform, sulfogaiacol, sodium camsilate, guaiacol, and aconite.
*Coughs.*

**Inamide** *Gerard, Irl.*
Indapamide (p.938·2).
*Hypertension.*

**Inapas** *Neo-Pharma, India.*
Sodium aminosalicylate (p.155·1); isoniazid (p.222·2).
*Tuberculosis.*

**Inapsin** *Janssen-Cilag, S.Afr.†.*
Droperidol (p.697·2).
*Neuroleptanalgesia; premedication.*

**Inapsine**
*Janssen-Ortho, Canad.†; Akorn, USA.*
Droperidol (p.697·2).
*Nausea and vomiting in surgical and diagnostic procedures; neuroleptanalgesia; premedication.*

**Inarub** *Frega, Canad.†.*
Methyl salicylate (p.59·3); menthol (p.1711·3); cineole (p.1672·1).

**Inaspir** *Almirall, Spain.*
Salmeterol xinafoate (p.795·1).
*Obstructive airways disease.*

**Inastmol** *Phoenix, Arg.*
Theophylline (p.798·3); ketotifen (p.788·2).
*Asthma.*

**Inatrex Balsamico** *Eurofarma, Braz.†.*
Dipyrone (p.35·3); niaouli oil (p.1719·3); cineole (p.1672·1); guaifenesin (p.1122·1); sodium camsilate; diphenhydramine hydrochloride (p.431·3).
*Cold and influenza symptoms.*

**Inazid** *Rekah, Israel.*
Isoniazid (p.222·2).
*Tuberculosis.*

**Incad** *Bushnell, India.*
Calcium carbonate (p.1254·2); colecalciferol (p.1461·3).
*Calcium supplement.*

**Inca's Gold** *Larkhall Laboratories, UK.*
Jojoba oil.

**Incena** *Bittner, Austria.*
Homoeopathic preparation.

**Incidal**
*Bayer, Hong Kong†; Bayer, Thai.†.*
Mebhydrolin napadisilate (p.436·3).
*Hypersensitivity reactions.*

**Incidal-OD** *Bayer, Thai.*
Cetirizine hydrochloride (p.427·1).
*Allergic rhinitis; allergic skin disorders.*

**Incidin** *Henkel, Ger.*
Isopropyl alcohol (p.1184·3); propyl alcohol (p.1191·2).
*Equipment disinfection.*

**Incidin Extra** *Henkel, Ger.*
Benzalkonium chloride (p.1168·3); oligo(di(iminoimidocarbonyl)iminohexamethylene); orthophenylphenol (p.1187·2).
*Surface disinfection.*

**Incidin extra N** *Henkel, Ger.*
Glucoprotamine (p.1180·3); benzalkonium chloride (p.1168·3).
*Surface disinfection.*

**Incidin M Spray Extra** *Henkel, Ger.*
Tributyltin benzoate; isopropyl alcohol (p.1184·3).
*Skin disinfection.*

**Incidin perfekt** *Henkel, Ger.*
Formaldehyde (p.1179·3); glyoxal (p.1181·1); glutaral (p.1180·3); benzalkonium chloride (p.1168·3); oligo(di(iminoimidocarbonyl)iminohexamethylene).
*Surface disinfection.*

**Incidin Plus** *Henkel, Ger.*
Glucoprotamine (p.1180·3).
*Surface disinfection.*

**Incidin Spezial**
*Note. This name is used for preparations of different composition.*
*Henkel, Ger.*
Formaldehyde (p.1179·3); glyoxal (p.1181·1); glutaral (p.1180·3); alcohol (p.1166·1).
*Surface disinfection.*

*Henkel, Ital.*
Alcohol (p.1166·1); glyoxal (p.1181·1); glutaral (p.1180·3); benzalkonium chloride (p.1168·3).
*Surface disinfection.*

**Incidine** *Paragerm, Fr.*
Glutaral (p.1180·3); formaldehyde (p.1179·3); glyoxal (p.1181·1).
*Surface and instrument disinfection.*

**Incidur** *Henkel, Ger.*
Glutaral (p.1180·3); glyoxal (p.1181·1).
*Surface disinfection.*

**Incidur Spray**
*Note. This name is used for preparations of different composition.*
*Henkel, Ger.*
Glutaral (p.1180·3); benzalkonium chloride (p.1168·3); 5-bromo-5-nitro-1,3-dioxacyclohexane; alcohol (p.1166·1); propyl alcohol (p.1191·2).
*Surface disinfection.*

*Henkel, Ital.*
Alcohol (p.1166·1); benzalkonium chloride (p.1168·3); 5-bromo-5-nitro-1,3-dioxacyclohexane.
*Disinfection of surfaces and instruments.*

**Incontinol** *Millet Roux, Braz.*
Oxybutynin hydrochloride (p.486·3).
*Urinary-tract disorders.*

**Inconturina** *OTW, Ger.*
Solidago virgaurea (p.1748·3); clove (p.1673·2).
*Urinary-tract disorders.*

**Incoril**
*Bago, Arg.; Merck Bago, Braz.; Bago, Chile.*
Diltiazem hydrochloride (p.900·1).
*Angina pectoris; arrhythmias; heart failure; hypertension.*

**Incremin**
*Note. This name is used for preparations of different composition.*
*Wyeth Consumer, Chile.*
Lysine hydrochloride; vitamin B substances; ferric pyrophosphate (p.1427·2) (p.1417·1).
*Iron-deficiency anaemia; reduced appetite.*

*Cyanamid, Ital.†; Wyeth, Mex.*
Lysine hydrochloride; vitamin B substances (p.1417·1).
*Nutritional supplement.*

*Wyeth Lederle, Port.*
Lysine (p.1439·1).

**Incremin Con Hierro** *Wyeth, Mex.*
Ferric pyrophosphate (p.1427·2); vitamin B substances; lysine hydrochloride (p.1417·1).
*Iron-deficiency anaemia.*

**Incremin Iron** *Whitehall, Austral.†.*
Ferric pyrophosphate (p.1427·2); vitamin B substances (p.1417·1); lysine hydrochloride.
*Dietary supplement.*

**Incremin with Iron** *Whitehall, NZ.*
Iron; vitamin B substances; lysine hydrochloride (p.1417·1).
*Dietary supplement.*

**Incremin with Vitamin C** *Whitehall, Austral.†.*
Vitamin B substances; lysine hydrochloride; vitamin C (p.1417·1).
*Dietary supplement.*

**Incutin** *Andreabal, Switz.†.*
Benzyl nicotinate (p.21·2); glycol salicylate (p.44·3); methyl salicylate (p.59·3); camphor (p.1665·3); capsicum (p.1667·1); pine oil; rosemary oil (p.1740·2).
*Musculoskeletal, joint, peri-articular, and soft-tissue pain and inflammation.*

**Indacar** *Pharmacodane, Denm.*
Indapamide (p.938·2).
*Hypertension.*

**Indaco** *Ciba Vision, Ital.*
Naphazoline nitrate (p.1124·3); zinc sulfate (p.1469·3).
*Eye irritation.*

**Indaflex** *Lampugnani, Ital.*
Indapamide (p.938·2).
*Hypertension.*

**Indahexal** *Hexal, Austral.*
Indapamide (p.938·2).
*Hypertension.*

**Indalgin** *Orion, Fin.*
Indometacin (p.47·3); ethylmorphine hydrochloride (p.37·3).
*Pain.*

**Indalix**
*Duopharma, Hong Kong; Triomed, S.Afr.*
Indapamide (p.938·2).
*Hypertension.*

**Indamol** *Aventis, Ital.*
Indapamide (p.938·2).
*Hypertension.*

**Indanorm** *Julphar, UAE.*
Indapamide (p.938·2).
*Hypertension.*

**Indapress** *Labomed, Chile.*
Indapamide (p.938·2).
*Hypertension.*

**Inda-Puren** *Alpharma-Isis, Ger.*
Indapamide (p.938·2).
*Hypertension.*

**Indarzona-N** *Streger, Mex.*
Dexamethasone (p.1097·1).
*Corticosteroid.*

**Inderal**
*AstraZeneca, Arg.; AstraZeneca, Austral.; AstraZeneca, Austria; AstraZeneca, Belg.; AstraZeneca, Braz.; Wyeth-Ayerst, Canad.; AstraZeneca, Denm.; AstraZeneca, Fin.; Cana, Gr.; IFET (ΙΦΕΤ), Gr.; AstraZeneca, Hong Kong; Nicholas Piramal, India; AstraZeneca, Irl.; Zeneca, Israel; AstraZeneca, Ital.; AstraZeneca, Malaysia; Zeneca, Neth.; AstraZeneca, Norw.; AstraZeneca, Port.; AstraZeneca, S.Afr.; AstraZeneca, Singapore; Hassle, Swed.; AstraZeneca, Switz.; AstraZeneca, Thai.; AstraZeneca, UK; Wyeth-Ayerst, USA.*
Propranolol hydrochloride (p.989·3).
*Angina pectoris; anxiety; arrhythmias; essential tremor; hypertension; hyperthyroidism; hypertrophic obstructive cardiomyopathy; migraine; myocardial infarction; phaeochromocytoma; variceal haemorrhage.*

**Inderal comp** *Zeneca, Austria†.*
Propranolol hydrochloride (p.989·3); triamterene (p.1016·2); hydrochlorothiazide (p.933·2).
*Hypertension.*

**Inderalici** *Zeneca, Mex.*
Propranolol hydrochloride (p.989·3).
*Angina pectoris; anxiety; arrhythmias; essential tremor; glaucoma; hypertension; hyperthyroidism; migraine; myocardial infarction; obstructive cardiomyopathy; phaeochromocytoma; variceal haemorrhage.*

**Inderetic**
*AstraZeneca, Austria; AstraZeneca, Belg.; Zeneca, Irl.†; Zeneca, Neth.; AstraZeneca, S.Afr.; AstraZeneca, Switz.; AstraZeneca, UK†.*
Propranolol hydrochloride (p.989·3); bendroflumethiazide (p.867·3).
*Hypertension.*

**Inderex** *AstraZeneca, UK†.*
Propranolol hydrochloride (p.989·3); bendroflumethiazide (p.867·3).
*Hypertension.*

**Inderide**
*Wyeth-Ayerst, Canad.†; Wyeth-Ayerst, USA.*
Propranolol hydrochloride (p.989·3); hydrochlorothiazide (p.933·2).
*Hypertension.*

**Inderm**
*Sankyo, Belg.; Dermapharm, Ger.; Will-Pharma, Neth.; Sankyo, Switz.*
Erythromycin (p.208·1).
*Acne.*

**Indermil** *Tyco, UK.*
Enbucrilate (p.1678·1).
*Wound closure.*

**Indian Brandee**
*Note. This name is used for preparations of different composition.*
*Anglian, UK.*
Capsicum (p.1667·1); compound cardamom tincture (p.1667·3).
*Dyspepsia; flatulence.*

*Potter's, UK.*
Capsicum (p.1667·1); ginger (p.1267·1); compound rhubarb tincture (p.1287·3).
*Colic; dyspepsia.*

**Indianische Frauenwurzel** *NAM, Ger.*
Cimicifuga (p.1671·3).
*Menopausal disorders.*

**Indiaral** *Gifrer Barbezat, Fr.*
Loperamide hydrochloride (p.1271·1).
*Diarrhoea.*

**Indican** *Sidus, Arg.*
Lidocaine hydrochloride (p.1377·3).
*Local anaesthesia.*

**Indicatest** *Polidis, Fr.*
Pregnancy test (p.1734·3).

**Indigestion** *Hylands, Canad.*
Homoeopathic preparation.

**Indigestion Complex** *Brauer, Austral.†.*
Homoeopathic preparation.

**Indigestion and Flatulence** *Cantassium Co., UK.*
Capsicum oleoresin (p.1667·1); valerian (p.1762·2); fennel (p.1687·2); myrrh (p.1718·3); papain (p.1727·3).

**Indigestion and Flatulence Tablets** *Healthcrafts, UK†.*
Peppermint oil (p.1283·2); fennel oil (p.1687·3); capsicum oleoresin (p.1667·1).
*Dyspepsia; flatulence.*

**Indigestion Mixture** *Potter's, UK.*
Meadowsweet (p.1710·1); gentian (p.1692·2); euonymus (p.1265·2).
*Dyspepsia; flatulence; heartburn.*

**Indigestion Relief**
*Note. This name is used for preparations of different composition.*
*Galpharm, UK†.*
Ranitidine (p.1285·2).
*Dyspepsia; heartburn.*

*Herbal Concepts, UK.*
Leptandra virginica; capsicum (p.1667·1); fringetree bark; ginger (p.1267·1).
*Colic; dyspepsia; nausea.*

**Indigestion Relief Liquid** *Boots, UK†.*
Simeticone (p.1289·2); aluminium hydroxide (p.1249·2); magnesium hydroxide (p.1272·2).
Formerly known as Double Action Indigestion Mixture.
*Dyspepsia.*

**Indigestion Relief Tablets** *Boots, UK†.*
Simeticone (p.1289·2); dried aluminium hydroxide gel (p.1249·2); magnesium hydroxide (p.1272·2).
Formerly known as Double Action Indigestion Tablets.
*Dyspepsia.*

**Indigestion Tablets** *Brauer, Austral.†.*
Homoeopathic preparation.

**Indigon** *IQFA, Mex.*
Dipyrone (p.35·3).
*Fever; inflammation; muscle spasm; pain.*

**Indilea** *Elea, Arg.*
Indinavir (p.640·1).
*HIV infection.*

**Indinax** *Eurofarma, Braz.*
Indinavir (p.640·1).

**Indivina** *Orion, Denm.; Orion, Fin.; Grunenthal, Ger.; Orion, Ger.; Orion, Irl.; Orion, Norw.; Orion, Swed.; Orion, Switz.; Orion, Thai.; Orion, UK.*
Estradiol valerate (p.1550·2); medroxyprogesterone acetate (p.1557·2).
*Menopausal disorders; osteoporosis.*

**Indo** *Agepha, Austria; CT, Ger.; Upha, Malaysia.*
Indometacin (p.47·3).
*Gout; inflammation; musculoskeletal, joint, and soft-tissue disorders; oedema; pain.*

**Indo Framan** *Inexfa, Spain†.*
Indometacin (p.47·3).
*Gout; musculoskeletal, joint, and peri-articular disorders; pain.*

**Indo Top** *Ratiopharm, Ger.*
Indometacin (p.47·3).
*Inflammation; musculoskeletal, joint, and soft-tissue disorders; pain.*

**Indobene** *Ratiopharm, Austria.*
Indometacin (p.47·3).
Aluminium glycinate (p.1249·1) is included in this preparation in an attempt to limit adverse effects on the gastrointestinal mucosa.
Formerly known as Gaurit.
*Gout; inflammation; musculoskeletal, joint, peri-articular, and soft-tissue disorders; pain.*

**Indobiotic** *Chauvin, Fr.; Chauvin, Port.; Bausch & Lomb, Switz.*
Indometacin (p.47·3); gentamicin sulfate (p.217·1).
*Infected eye disorders.*

**Indobloc** *Asta Medica, Ger.†.*
Propranolol hydrochloride (p.989·3).
*Anxiety; arrhythmias; essential tremor; hypertension; hyperthyroidism; migraine; myocardial infarction.*

**Indo-bros** *Bros, Gr.*
Tenoxicam (p.93·1).
*Dysmenorrhoea; gout; inflammation; osteoarthritis; pain; rheumatoid arthritis; spondyloarthropathies.*

**Indocaf** *Reig Jofre, Spain.*
Indometacin (p.47·3).
*Peri-articular and soft-tissue pain and inflammation.*

**Indocalm** *Koni-Cofarm, Chile.*
Lidocaine (p.1377·3); sulfathiazole (p.264·1).
*Ear infections.*

**Indocap** *Jagson, India.*
Indometacin (p.47·3).
*Dysmenorrhoea; gout: musculoskeletal and joint disorders; inhibition of intra-operative miosis.*

**Indocarsil** *Solfran, Mex.*
Indometacin (p.47·3).
*Musculoskeletal and joint disorders.*

**Indochron** *Inwood, USA†.*
Indometacin (p.47·3).
*Acute gouty arthritis; ankylosing spondylitis; bursitis; osteoarthritis; rheumatoid arthritis; tendinitis.*

**Indocid** *Merck Sharp & Dohme, Austral.; Merck Sharp & Dohme, Austria; Merck Sharp & Dohme, Belg.; Prodome, Braz.; Merck Frosst, Canad.; Merck Sharp & Dohme, Denm.; Merck Sharp & Dohme, Fin.; Merck Sharp & Dohme-Chibret, Fr.; IFET (ΙΦΕΤ), Gr.; Merck Sharp & Dohme, Hong Kong; Merck Sharp & Dohme, Irl.; Centra, Ital.; Merck Sharp & Dohme, Malaysia; Merck Sharp & Dohme, Mex.; Merck Sharp & Dohme, Neth.; Merck Sharp & Dohme, Norw.; Merck Sharp & Dohme, NZ†; Merck Sharp & Dohme, Port.; Merck Sharp & Dohme, S.Afr.; Merck Sharp & Dohme, Switz.; Merck Sharp & Dohme, Thai.; Merck Sharp & Dohme, UK†.*
Indometacin (p.47·3) or indometacin sodium (p.47·3).
*Fever; gout; inflammation; musculoskeletal, joint, and peri-articular disorders; pain; prevention of oedema and miosis during cataract extraction.*

**Indocid Colirio** *Merck Sharp & Dohme, Braz.*
Indometacin (p.47·3).
*Prevention of miosis and inflammation during ocular surgery.*

**Indocid PDA** *Merck Sharp & Dohme, Austral.; Merck Frosst, Canad.; Merck Sharp & Dohme, Hong Kong; Merck Sharp & Dohme, Irl.; Merck Sharp & Dohme, Neth.; Merck Sharp & Dohme, NZ; Merck Sharp & Dohme, UK.*
Indometacin sodium (p.47·3).
*Closure of patent ductus arteriosus.*

**Indocin** *Merck Sharp & Dohme, USA.*
*Injection:* Indometacin sodium (p.47·3).
*Closure of patent ductus arteriosus.*

*Merck, USA; Forte, USA.*
*Capsules; oral suspension; suppositories; sustained-release capsules:* Indometacin (p.47·3).
*Acute gouty arthritis; ankylosing spondylitis; bursitis; osteoarthritis; rheumatoid arthritis; tendinitis.*

**Indocolir** *Chauvin ankerpharm, Ger.*
Indometacin (p.47·3).
*Inflammation following eye surgery; prevention of miosis during eye surgery.*

**Indocollirio** *SIFI, Ital.*
Indometacin (p.47·3).
*Prevention of miosis and inflammation during cataract surgery.*

**Indocollyre** *Germania, Austria; Ophtapharma, Canad.†; Chauvin, Fr.; Chauvin, Hong Kong†; Chauvin, Israel; Chauvin, Port.; Chauvin, Singapore; Chauvin, Thai.*
Indometacin (p.47·3).
*Ocular inflammation following eye surgery; postoperative eye pain; prevention of intra-operative miosis.*

**Indocontin** *Note. This name is used for preparations of different composition.*
*Mundipharma, Ger.*
Indometacin (p.47·3).
*Inflammation; musculoskeletal, joint, and soft-tissue disorders; pain.*

*Modi-Mundipharma, India.*
Indapamide (p.938·2).
*Hypertension.*

**Indofeno** *Fada, Arg.*
Diclofenac (p.32·1).
*Inflammation; pain.*

**Indoflam** *Recon, Singapore†.*
Indometacin (p.47·3).
*Gout; musculoskeletal and joint disorders; pain.*

**Indoftol** *Merck Sharp & Dohme, Spain†.*
Indometacin (p.47·3).
*Postoperatve ocular inflammation.*

**Indogesic** *Dar Al Dawa, Hong Kong.*
Indometacin (p.47·3).
*Fever; inflammation; musculoskeletal, joint, and peri-articular disorders; oedema; pain.*

**Indohexal** *Hexal, Austria.*
Indometacin (p.47·3).
*Gout; inflammation; musculoskeletal, joint, and peri-articular disorders; oedema; pain.*

**Indolar SR** *Sandoz, UK.*
Indometacin (p.47·3).
*Inflammation; musculoskeletal, joint, and peri-articular disorders; pain.*

**Indolgina** *Uriach, Spain.*
Indometacin (p.47·3).
*Gout; inflammation; musculoskeletal, joint, and peri-articular disorders; pain.*

**Indolin** *Infosint, Ital.*
Indapamide (p.938·2).
*Hypertension.*

**Indom** *INTES, Ital.*
Indometacin (p.47·3).
*Prevention of miosis and inflammation during cataract surgery.*

**Indoman** *Berman, Mex.*
Indometacin (p.47·3).
*Inflammation; musculoskeletal and joint disorders.*

**Indomax** *Ashbourne, UK.*
Indometacin (p.47·3).
*Gout; inflammation; musculoskeletal and joint disorders; pain.*

**Indomed** *Merck Sharp & Dohme, Israel; Greater Pharma, Thai.*
Indometacin (p.47·3).
*Gout; inflammation; musculoskeletal and joint disorders; rheumatic fever.*

**Indomee** *Merck Sharp & Dohme, Swed.*
Indometacin (p.47·3).
*Gout; musculoskeletal, joint and peri-articular disorders.*

**Indomelan** *Lannacher, Austria.*
Indometacin (p.47·3).
*Gout; inflammation; musculoskeletal, joint, and peri-articular disorders; oedema; pain.*

**Indomen** *YSP, Malaysia; Yung Shin, Singapore.*
Indometacin (p.47·3).
*Inflammation; musculoskeletal and joint disorders.*

**Indo-Mepha** *Mepha, Switz.*
Indometacin (p.47·3).
*Musculoskeletal, joint, peri-articular, and soft-tissue pain and inflammation.*

**Indomet** *Heumann, Ger.; Ratiopharm, Hong Kong.*
Indometacin (p.47·3).
*Gout; inflammation; musculoskeletal, joint, peri-articular, and soft-tissue disorders; pain.*

**Indometacinum-mp** *Medphano, Ger.†.*
Indometacin (p.47·3).
*Gout; inflammation; musculoskeletal, joint, and soft-tissue disorders; pain.*

**Indometin** *Orion, Fin.*
Indometacin (p.47·3).
*Fever; gout; inflammation; musculoskeletal and joint disorders; pain.*

**Indomet-ratiopharm** *Ratiopharm, Ger.*
Indometacin (p.47·3).
*Gout; inflammation; musculoskeletal, joint, peri-articular, and soft-tissue disorders; pain.*

**Indomet-ratiopharm m** *Ratiopharm, Ger.*
Indometacin (p.47·3).
Aluminium glycinate (p.1249·1) is included in this preparation in an attempt to limit adverse effects on the gastrointestinal mucosa.
*Gout; inflammation; musculoskeletal, joint, and soft-tissue disorders; pain.*

**Indomisal** *Riemser, Ger.*
Indometacin (p.47·3).
*Gout; inflammation; musculoskeletal, joint, and soft-tissue disorders; pain.*

**Indomod** *Pharmacia Upjohn, Irl.†; Pharmacia, UK.*
Indometacin (p.47·3).
*Gout; musculoskeletal, joint, and peri-articular disorders.*

**Indon** *YSP, Malaysia.*
Propranolol (p.990·1).
*Angina pectoris; arrhythmias; hypertension; hypertrophic obstructive cardiomyopathy; phaeochromocytoma.*

**Indonet** *Nettopharma, Denm.†.*
Indometacin (p.47·3).
*Dysmenorrhoea; gout; musculoskeletal and joint disorders.*

**Indonilo** *Sigma-Tau, Spain.*
Indometacin (p.47·3).
*Gout; inflammation; musculoskeletal, joint, and peri-articular disorders; pain.*

**Indono** *Milano, Thai.*
Indometacin (p.47·3).
*Gout; musculoskeletal and joint disorders.*

**Indo-paed** *1A, Ger.*
Indometacin (p.47·3).
*Gout; inflammation; musculoskeletal, joint, peri-articular, and soft-tissue disorders; pain.*

**Indo-Phlogont** *Azupharma, Ger.*
Indometacin (p.47·3).
*Gout; inflammation; musculoskeletal, joint, and soft-tissue disorders; pain.*

**Indophtal** *Bausch & Lomb, Switz.*
Indometacin (p.47·3).
*Postoperative eye inflammation.*

**Indoptic** *Merck Sharp & Dohme, Israel; Merck Sharp & Dohme, Switz.†.*
Indometacin (p.47·3).
*Prevention of cystoid macular oedema after cataract surgery.*

**Indoptol** *Sigma, Austral.†; Merck Sharp & Dohme, Austria; Merck Sharp & Dohme, Belg.†; Merck Sharp & Dohme, Neth.*
Indometacin (p.47·3).
*Inhibition of intra-operative miosis; prevention of cystoid macular oedema after cataract surgery.*

**Indorektal** *Sanorania, Ger.†.*
Indometacin (p.47·3).
*Gout; inflammation; musculoskeletal and joint disorders; pain.*

**Indosan** *Sanfer, Mex.†.*
Indometacin (p.47·3).

**Indospray** *Rhone-Poulenc Rorer, Austral.†.*
Indometacin (p.47·3).
*Musculoskeletal, joint, peri-articular, and soft-tissue disorders.*

**Indostad** *Stada, Austria.*
Indometacin (p.47·3).
*Inflammation; musculoskeletal, joint, and peri-articular disorders; oedema; pain.*

**Indo-Tablinen** *Sanorania, Ger.†.*
Indometacin (p.47·3).
*Gout; inflammation; musculoskeletal and joint disorders; pain.*

**Indotard** *CTI, Israel; Galen, UK†.*
Indometacin (p.47·3).
*Inflammation; musculoskeletal, joint, and peri-articular disorders; pain.*

**Indotec** *Technilab, Canad.*
Indometacin (p.47·3).
*Gout; musculoskeletal and joint disorders; ovarian hyperstimulation syndrome; pain; renal calculi; renal colic.*

**Indotex** *Rontag, Arg.*
Indometacin (p.47·3).

**Indotrin** *Liferpal, Mex.*
Indometacin (p.47·3).
*Musculoskeletal and joint disorders.*

**Indovis** *CTI, Israel.*
Indometacin (p.47·3).
*Gout; musculoskeletal and joint disorders.*

**Indoxen** *Sigma-Tau, Ital.*
Indometacin (p.47·3).
*Musculoskeletal disorders.*

**Inducmina** *Gray, Arg.*
Ketamine hydrochloride (p.1302·1).
*General anaesthesia.*

**Inductal** *20th Century, Mex.†.*
Thiopental sodium (p.1309·1).

**Inductol** *20th Century, Mex.†.*
Propanidid (p.1305·3).

**InductOs** *Wyeth, UK.*
Dibotermin alfa (p.768·1).
*Tibia fracture.*

**Induken** *Kendrick, Mex.*
Tinidazole (p.617·1).
*Anaerobic bacterial infections; protozoal infections.*

**Indulfan** *Henkel, Ital.*
Glyoxal (p.1181·1); benzalkonium chloride (p.1168·3).
*Surface disinfection.*

**Indulfan plus** *Henkel, Ger.†.*
Formaldehyde (p.1179·3); glyoxal (p.1181·1); glutaral (p.1180·3); benzalkonium chloride (p.1168·3).
*Surface disinfection.*

**Indurgan** *Shire, Spain.*
Omeprazole (p.1278·2).
*Gastro-oesophageal reflux; peptic ulcer; Zollinger-Ellison syndrome.*

**Indusil** *Recordati, Ital.*
Cobamamide (p.1459·1).
*Vitamin $B_{12}$ deficiency.*

**Indusil T** *Diamant, Fr.†.*
Cobamamide (p.1459·1).
*Tonic.*

**Ineltano** *Richmond, Arg.*
Halothane (p.1299·3).
*General anaesthesia.*

**Inesfay** *Mavi, Mex.†.*
Cimetidine (p.1255·3).

**Inespecin** *Biol, Arg.*
*Salmonella typhi* glycolipids.
*Infection prophylaxis.*

**Inexbron** *Inexfa, Spain†.*
Amoxicillin trihydrate (p.155·3).
*Bacterial infections.*

**Inexbron Mucolitico** *Inexfa, Spain†.*
Amoxicillin trihydrate (p.155·3); bromhexine hydrochloride (p.1115·3).
*Respiratory-tract infections.*

**Inexfal** *Inexfa, Spain†.*
Cytidine; muramidase hydrochloride (p.1717·2); uridine (p.1760·3).
*Liver disorders.*

**Inexium** *AstraZeneca, Fr.*
Esomeprazole magnesium (p.1265·1).
*Gastro-oesophageal reflux; peptic ulcer.*

**INF** *Gautier, Arg.*
Interferon alfa-2b (p.640·3).
*Anogenital warts; hepatitis B and C; malignant neoplasms.*

**Infacol** *Pfizer Consumer, Austral.; Rosken, Hong Kong; Pharmax, Irl.; Pfizer, NZ; Pfizer Consumer, Singapore; Forest Laboratories, UK.*
Simeticone (p.1289·2).
*Infant colic.*

**Infa-C-Vit** *Pisa, Mex.†.*
Vitamin C (p.1460·2).

**Infaderm** *Ceuta, UK.*
Light liquid paraffin (p.1479·1); almond oil (p.1651·1).
*Dry skin disorders.*

**Infadrops** *Ceuta, UK.*
Paracetamol (p.76·2).
*Fever; pain.*

**Infafren Simple** *Pisa, Mex.†.*
Homatropine (p.483·2).

**Infalgina** *Pisa, Mex.*
Paracetamol (p.76·2).
*Fever; pain.*

**Infalivina** *Sibras, Braz.†.*
Solanum paniculatum; guacia; cibaruba.

**Infalyte** *Mead Johnson Nutritionals, USA.*
Electrolytes and rice syrup solids (p.1222·2).
Formerly known as Ricelyte.
*Oral rehydration therapy.*

**Infanolyte** *GHP, Thai.*
Calcium chloride; glucose; magnesium chloride; potassium chloride; sodium chloride; sodium citrate (p.1222·2).
*Diarrhoea; oral rehydration therapy.*

**Infanrix** *GlaxoSmithKline, Austral.; GlaxoSmithKline, Austria; GlaxoSmithKline, Belg.; GlaxoSmithKline, Braz.; GlaxoSmithKline, Fin.; GlaxoSmithKline, Ger.; SmithKline Beecham, Gr.; GlaxoSmithKline, Hong Kong; GlaxoSmithKline, Irl.; SmithKline Beecham, Israel; GlaxoSmithKline, Ital.; GlaxoSmithKline, Malaysia; SmithKline Beecham, Mex.; SmithKline Beecham, Norw.†; GlaxoSmithKline, NZ†; Smith Kline & French, Port.; GlaxoSmithKline, Singapore; GlaxoSmithKline, Spain; GlaxoSmithKline, Swed.; GlaxoSmithKline, Thai.; GlaxoSmithKline, UK; SmithKline Beecham, USA.*
A diphtheria, tetanus, and acellular pertussis vaccine (p.1613·3).
*Active immunisation.*

**Infanrix DTPa** *SmithKline Beecham, Switz.*
A diphtheria, tetanus, and pertussis vaccine (p.1613·3).
*Active immunisation.*

**Infanrix DTPa HB** *GlaxoSmithKline, Braz.†.*
A diphtheria, tetanus, pertussis, and hepatitis B vaccine (p.1614·3).
*Active immunisation.*

**Infanrix DTPa-HepB** *SmithKline Beecham, Switz.†.*
A diphtheria, tetanus, pertussis, and hepatitis B vaccine (p.1614·3).
*Active immunisation.*

**Infanrix DTPa-Hib** *SmithKline Beecham, Switz.*
A diphtheria, tetanus, pertussis, and haemophilus influenzae vaccine (p.1614·2).
*Active immunisation.*

**Infanrix DTPa-IPV** *SmithKline Beecham, Switz.*
A diphtheria, tetanus, pertussis, and poliomyelitis vaccine (p.1615·1).
*Active immunisation.*

**Infanrix DTPa-IPV+Hib** *SmithKline Beecham, Switz.*
A diphtheria, tetanus, pertussis, poliomyelitis, and haemophilus influenzae vaccine (p.1615·1).
*Active immunisation.*

**Infanrix HB** *GlaxoSmithKline, S.Afr.*
A diphtheria, tetanus, acellular pertussis, and hepatitis B vaccine (p.1614·3).
*Active immunisation.*

**Infanrix HepB** *GlaxoSmithKline, Austral.; GlaxoSmithKline, Fin.; SmithKline Beecham, Gr.; GlaxoSmithKline, Ital.; GlaxoSmithKline, NZ; SmithKline Beecham, Spain; GlaxoSmithKline, Swed.*
A diphtheria, tetanus, pertussis, and hepatitis B vaccine (p.1614·3).
*Active immunisation.*

**Infanrix Hexa** *GlaxoSmithKline, Arg.; GlaxoSmithKline, Belg.; GlaxoSmithKline, Chile; GlaxoSmithKline, Fin.; GlaxoSmithKline, Fr.; GlaxoSmithKline, Ger.; SmithKline Beecham, Gr.; GlaxoSmithKline, Ital.; SmithKline*

Beecham, Spain; GlaxoSmithKline, Swed.; SmithKline Beecham, Switz.
A diphtheria, tetanus, pertussis, hepatitis B, poliomyelitis, and haemophilus influenzae vaccine (p.1614·3).
*Active immunisation.*

**Infanrix Hib** SmithKline Beecham, Austral.; SmithKline Beecham, Israel; GlaxoSmithKline, NZ; GlaxoSmithKline, Singapore; GlaxoSmithKline, Spain; GlaxoSmithKline, UK.
A diphtheria, tetanus, acellular pertussis, and haemophilus influenzae vaccine (p.1614·2).
*Active immunisation.*

**Infanrix + Hib** GlaxoSmithKline, Austria; GlaxoSmithKline, Belg.; GlaxoSmithKline, Ger.
A diphtheria, tetanus, acellular pertussis, and haemophilus influenzae vaccine (p.1614·2).
*Active immunisation.*

**Infanrix IPV** GlaxoSmithKline, Belg.; GlaxoSmithKline, NZ.
A diphtheria, tetanus, pertussis, and poliomyelitis vaccine (p.1615·1).
*Active immunisation.*

**Infanrix IPV + Hib** GlaxoSmithKline, Austria; GlaxoSmithKline, Belg.; GlaxoSmithKline, Braz.; GlaxoSmithKline, Ger.; SmithKline Beecham, Gr.; GlaxoSmithKline, Hong Kong; GlaxoSmithKline, Singapore; GlaxoSmithKline, Thai.
A diphtheria, tetanus, acellular pertussis, poliomyelitis, and haemophilus influenzae vaccine (p.1615·1).
*Active immunisation.*

**Infanrix Penta** Glaxo Wellcome, Gr.; GlaxoSmithKline, Ital.
A diphtheria, tetanus, pertussis, poliomyelitis, and hepatitis B vaccine (p.1615·2).
*Active immunisation.*

**Infanrix Polio + Hib** GlaxoSmithKline, Fin.; SmithKline Beecham, Israel; GlaxoSmithKline, Norw.; GlaxoSmithKline, Swed.
A diphtheria, tetanus, pertussis, poliomyelitis, and haemophilus influenzae vaccine (p.1615·1).
*Active immunisation.*

**Infanrixhexa** GlaxoSmithKline, Fr.
A diphtheria, tetanus, acellular pertussis, poliomyelitis, hepatitis B, and haemophilus influenzae vaccine (p.1614·3).
*Active immunisation.*

**Infanrixquinta** GlaxoSmithKline, Fr.
A diphtheria, tetanus, pertussis, poliomyelitis, and haemophilus influenzae vaccine (p.1615·1).
Formerly known as Infanrix Polio-Hib.
*Active immunisation.*

**Infanrixtetra** GlaxoSmithKline, Fr.
A diphtheria, tetanus, pertussis, and poliomyelitis vaccine (p.1615·1).
Formerly known as Infanrix Polio.
*Active immunisation.*

**Infant Calm** Brauer, Austral.†.
Passion flower (p.1729·1); aconitum nap; belladonna; chamomilla.
*Insomnia; irritability or restlessness in children.*

**Infant Gaviscon**
Note. This name is used for preparations of different composition.
Reckitt Benckiser, Austral.
Magnesium alginate (p.1577·1); sodium alginate (p.1577·1).
Formerly contained alginic acid, aluminium hydroxide, magnesium trisilicate and sodium bicarbonate.
*Gastro-oesophageal reflux.*

Reckitt Benckiser, S.Afr.
Alginic acid (p.1576·3); magnesium trisilicate (p.1272·3); dried aluminium hydroxide gel (p.1249·2); sodium bicarbonate (p.1223·2).
*Gastro-oesophageal reflux.*

**Infant Multiple Vitamin** Stanley, Canad.
Vitamins A, C, and D (p.1417·1).

**Infant Tonic** Brauer, Austral.†.
Angelica (p.1655·1); ascorbic acid (p.1460·2); kola (p.1765·3); hypericum (p.299·1); ginseng (p.1693·1); urtica (p.1762·1); aven. sat.; calc. phos.; ferrum met.; ferrum phos.; kali phos.; mag. phos.; phosphoricum acidum.
*Tonic.*

**Infantaire** Altaire, USA.
Paracetamol (p.76·2).
*Fever; pain.*

**Infantol** Carter Horner, Canad.
Multivitamin preparation (p.1417·1).
*Dietary supplement.*

**Infantoss** Herbarium, Braz.
Grindelia (p.1696·1); guaco; tolu balsam (p.1131·3); propolis (p.1735·2); echinacea (p.1683·2); horseradish (p.1697·3).

**Infant's Tylenol** Johnson & Johnson, Hong Kong.
Paracetamol (p.76·2).
*Fever; pain.*

**Infants Tylenol Cold Decongestant & Fever Reducer** McNeil Consumer, USA.
Paracetamol (p.76·2); pseudoephedrine hydrochloride (p.1129·2).
*Congestion; fever; pain.*

**Infantussin N** Palmicol, Ger.†.
Anise oil (p.1655·2); fennel oil (p.1687·3); thyme (p.1755·2); althaea (p.1651·3).
*Coughs and cold symptoms.*

**Infapain** Alliance, S.Afr.
Paracetamol (p.76·2); codeine phosphate (p.27·1).
*Fever; pain.*

**Infapain Forte** Alliance, S.Afr.
Paracetamol (p.76·2); codeine phosphate (p.27·1); promethazine hydrochloride (p.439·1).
*Fever; pain.*

**Infasoy** Wyeth Health, Austral.†; Cow & Gate, Irl.; Wyeth, NZ; Cow & Gate, UK.
Infant feed (p.1417·1).
Formerly known as Nutrilon Soya in the *UK*.
*Galactosaemia; gluten intolerance; milk and lactose intolerance.*

**Infasoy Progress** Wyeth, NZ.
Infant feed (p.1417·1).
*Galactosaemia; lactose intolerance.*

**Infasurf** Ony, Israel; Forest Pharmaceuticals, USA.
Calfactant (p.1736·2).
*Neonatal respiratory distress syndrome.*

**Infa-Tardyferon** Germania, Austria.
Ferrous sulfate (p.1428·2).
*Iron deficiency; iron-deficiency anaemia.*

**Infatrini** Nutricia, Austral.; Nutricia, Fin.; Nutricia Clinical, UK.
Preparation for enteral nutrition in infants (p.1417·1).

**Infazinc** Atlas, Canad.
Zinc oxide (p.1163·2).

**Infecteracin** INQ, Braz.†.
Co-trimoxazole (p.199·3).
*Bacterial infections; Pneumocystis carinii pneumonia; protozoal infections.*

**InfectoBicillin** Infectopharm, Ger.
Benzathine phenoxymethylpenicillin (p.163·2).
*Bacterial infections.*

**InfectoBicillin H** Infectopharm, Ger.
Azidocillin sodium (p.159·1).
*Bacterial infections.*

**InfectoCef** Infectopharm, Ger.
Cefaclor (p.167·1).
*Bacterial infections.*

**InfectoCillin** Infectopharm, Ger.
Phenoxymethylpenicillin potassium (p.242·1).
*Bacterial infections.*

**Infectoclont** Infectopharm, Ger.
Metronidazole (p.607·2).
*Anaerobic bacterial infections.*

**Infectocortikrupp** Infectopharm, Ger.
Prednisolone acetate (p.1108·1).
*Corticosteroid.*

**Infectodiarrstop GG** Infectopharm, Ger.
Lactic-acid-producing organisms (p.1704·2).
*Gastrointestinal disorders.*

**InfectoDyspept** Infectopharm, Ger.†.
Carrot; rice; sodium chloride; sodium citrate; potassium citrate; citric acid (p.1222·2).
*Diarrhoea; oral rehydration.*

**Infectoflam** Ciba Vision, Braz.†; Ciba Vision, Hong Kong†; Novartis Ophthalmics, Malaysia; Novartis Ophthalmics, Singapore; Novartis Ophthalmics, Switz.; Novartis, Thai.
Fluorometholone (p.1102·2); gentamicin sulfate (p.217·1).
*Bacterial eye infections; inflammatory eye disorders.*

**InfectoFlu** Infectopharm, Ger.
Amantadine hydrochloride (p.1197·2).
Formerly known as Infectogripp.
*Influenza A.*

**InfectoFos** Infectopharm, Ger.
Fosfomycin sodium (p.214·3).
*Bacterial infections.*

**InfectoKrupp** Infectopharm, Ger.
Adrenaline (p.852·2).
*Obstructive airways disease.*

**InfectoMox** Infectopharm, Ger.
Amoxicillin (p.155·3).
*Bacterial infections.*

**InfectoMycin** Infectopharm, Ger.
Erythromycin estolate (p.208·1) or erythromycin ethyl succinate (p.208·1).
*Bacterial infections.*

**InfectoPedicul** Infectopharm, Ger.
Permethrin (p.1508·3).
*Pediculosis.*

**Infectoroxit** Infectopharm, Ger.
Roxithromycin (p.254·2).
*Bacterial infections.*

**InfectoSoor** Infectopharm, Ger.
*Ointment:* Miconazole nitrate (p.405·3); zinc oxide (p.1163·2).
*Napkin rash.*
*Oral gel:* Miconazole (p.405·2).
*Mouth and throat candidiasis.*

**Infectoss** Heralds, Braz.†.
Erythromycin (p.208·1).
*Bacterial infections.*

**InfectoStaph** Infectopharm, Ger.
Dicloxacillin sodium (p.205·2) or oxacillin sodium (p.240·2).
*Staphylococcal infections.*

**InfectoTop** Infectopharm, Ger.†.
Lodoxamide trometamol (p.1707·3).
*Allergic conjunctivitis.*

**InfectoTrimet** Infectopharm, Ger.
Trimethoprim (p.272·2).
*Urinary-tract infections.*

**Infectracina** Apsen, Braz.†.
Neomycin (p.235·1); bacitracin (p.161·3).
*Bacterial skin infections.*

**Infectrin**
Note. This name is used for preparations of different composition.
Boehringer de Angeli, Braz.
Co-trimoxazole (p.199·3).
*Bacterial infections; Pneumocystis carinii pneumonia; protozoal infections.*

Searle, Ital.†.
Ampicillin (p.157·1); flucloxacillin (p.213·3).
*Bacterial infections.*

**Infectrin Balsamico** Boehringer de Angeli, Braz.†.
Co-trimoxazole (p.199·3); guaifenesin (p.1122·1); ammonium chloride (p.1115·2).
*Bacterial infections.*

**INFeD** Schein, USA.
Iron dextran (p.1436·3).
*Iron deficiency.*

**Infekt-Komplex Ho-Fu-Complex** Liebermann, Ger.
Homoeopathic preparation.

**Infepan** Igefarma, Braz.†.
Clostebol acetate (p.1543·2); neomycin sulfate (p.235·1).
*Cicatrisation; skin infections.*

**Inferax** Yamanouchi, Ger.
Interferon alfacon-1 (p.643·1).
*Hepatitis C.*

**Infergen** Yamanouchi, Belg.; Amgen, Canad.; Chiesi, Fr.; Yamanouchi, Gr.; Yamanouchi, Ital.; Yamanouchi, Neth.; Amgen, USA.
Interferon alfacon-1 (p.643·1).
*Hepatitis C.*

**Inferil** Recofarma, Ital.
Sodium ferric gluconate complex (p.1444·3).
*Iron-deficiency anaemias.*

**Infesol** Berlin-Chemie, Ger.
Amino-acid, electrolyte, and xylitol infusion (p.1417·1).
*Protein and fluid deficiency.*

**Infex**
Note. This name is used for preparations of different composition.
Elofar, Braz.†.
Tetracycline (p.266·2).
*Bacterial infections.*

Pharmafina, Chile.
Clarithromycin (p.192·2).
*Respiratory-tract infections.*

Merz, Ger.
Amantadine sulfate (p.1197·2).
*Influenza A.*

**Infibran** Expanpharm, Fr.†; Menarini, Port.
Wheat bran (p.1253·2).
*Constipation.*

**Infi-China** Infirmarius-Rovit, Ger.
Homoeopathic preparation.

**Infidyston** Infirmarius-Rovit, Ger.
Homoeopathic preparation.

**Infi-Echinacea** Infirmarius-Rovit, Ger.
Homoeopathic preparation.

**Infifer** Infirmarius-Rovit, Ger.
Homoeopathic preparation.

**Infihepan** Infirmarius-Rovit, Ger.
Homoeopathic preparation.

**Infiltran B12** Sintofarma, Braz.†.
Methionine (p.1042·1); choline citrate (p.1424·3); inositol (p.1701·2); cyanocobalamin (p.1458·2); liver extract.
*Liver disorders.*

**Infi-Lymphect** Infirmarius-Rovit, Ger.
Homoeopathic preparation.

**Infiossan** Infirmarius-Rovit, Ger.
Homoeopathic preparation.

**Infi-Symphytum** Infirmarius-Rovit, Ger.
Homoeopathic preparation.

**Infi-tract** Infirmarius-Rovit, Ger.
*Capsules:* Javanese turmeric (p.1759·3).
*Dyspepsia.*
*Oral drops:* Scopolia carniolica; Javanese turmeric (p.1759·3); greater celandine (p.1695·3); gentian (p.1692·2); angelica (p.1655·1); manna (p.1273·1); saffron (p.1058·2); zedoary; myrrh (p.1718·3).
*Biliary disorders; digestive disorders; gastrointestinal spasm.*

**Infla-Ban** Triomed, S.Afr.
Diclofenac sodium (p.32·1).
*Gout; inflammation; musculoskeletal and joint disorders.*

**Inflaced** Dexo, Fr.
Piroxicam (p.84·2).
*Musculoskeletal, joint, and peri-articular disorders.*

**Inflacor** Pharmachemie, S.Afr.; Rolab, S.Afr.
Budesonide (p.1094·2).
*Asthma.*

**Infladase** Centaur, India.
Serrapeptase (p.1743·2); traces of cobalt, manganese, and zinc.
*Alveolar abscess; breast engorgement; inflammation; pain; pericoronitis.*

**Infladerm** Cazi, Braz.†.
Nitrofurazone (p.238·2); hydrocortisone acetate (p.1103·3).
*Infected skin disorders.*

**Infladoren** Hexal, Braz.
Diclofenac diethylamine (p.32·1) or diclofenac sodium (p.32·1).
*Gout; inflammation; musculoskeletal, joint, and peri-articular disorders; pain.*

**Inflalid** Legrand, Braz.
Nimesulide (p.67·1).

**Inflam** Lichtenstein, Ger.
*Capsules; slow-release capsules; topical spray:* Indometacin (p.47·3).
*Gout; inflammation; musculoskeletal, joint, and soft-tissue disorders; pain.*
*Ointment:* Indometacin (p.47·3); lauromacrogol 400 (p.1412·3).
*Inflammation; musculoskeletal, joint, and soft-tissue disorders; pain.*

**Inflamac** Spirig, Switz.
Diclofenac sodium (p.32·1).
*Fever; gout; inflammation; musculoskeletal, joint, and peri-articular disorders; pain.*

**Inflamase** Novartis Ophthalmics, Canad.; Novartis Ophthalmics, USA.
Prednisolone sodium phosphate (p.1108·1).
*Inflammatory eye disorders.*

**Inflamase IdroGel** Amnol, Ital.
Aescin (p.1648·2); bromelains (p.1662·2).
*Inflammation; oedema.*

**Inflamate** TO-Chemicals, Thai.
Indometacin (p.47·3).
*Gout; musculoskeletal and joint disorders; rheumatic fever.*

**Inflamax** Elofar, Braz.
Diclofenac sodium (p.32·1).

**Inflamene** Farmalab, Braz.
Piroxicam (p.84·2).
*Dysmenorrhoea; gout; musculoskeletal, joint, and peri-articular disorders.*

**Inflammide** Boehringer Ingelheim, Chile; Boehringer Ingelheim, Malaysia; Boehringer Ingelheim, S.Afr.; Boehringer Ingelheim, Singapore; Boehringer Ingelheim, Thai.
Budesonide (p.1094·2).
*Asthma; rhinitis.*

**Inflanac** Biolab, Hong Kong; Biolab, Singapore; Biolab, Thai.
Diclofenac sodium (p.32·1).
*Inflammation; musculoskeletal, joint, and peri-articular disorders.*

**Inflanan** Marjan, Braz.
Piroxicam (p.84·2).
*Dysmenorrhoea; gout; musculoskeletal, joint, and peri-articular disorders.*

**Inflanaze** Boehringer Ingelheim, S.Afr.
Budesonide (p.1094·2).
*Allergic rhinitis.*

**Inflanefran** Allergan, Ger.
Prednisolone acetate (p.1108·1).
*Eye disorders.*

**Inflanegent** Allergan, Ger.
Prednisolone acetate (p.1108·1); gentamicin sulfate (p.217·1).
*Infected eye disorders.*

**Inflanox** Formoquimica, Braz.
Piroxicam (p.84·2).
*Dysmenorrhoea; gout; musculoskeletal, joint, and peri-articular disorders.*

**Inflaren** Cibran, Braz.†.
Diclofenac potassium (p.32·1) or diclofenac sodium (p.32·1).
*Gout; inflammation; musculoskeletal, joint, and peri-articular disorders; pain.*

**Inflax** Ativus, Braz.
Piroxicam (p.84·2).
*Dysmenorrhoea; gout; musculoskeletal, joint, and peri-articular disorders.*

**Inflazone** Aspen, S.Afr.
Phenylbutazone (p.83·2).
*Ankylosing spondylitis.*

**Inflexal** Kwizda, Austria; Berna, Hong Kong†; Berna, Ital.; Berna, Port.; Byk Madaus, S.Afr.†; Berna, Singapore†; Berna, Spain†; Berna, Switz.; Aventis Pasteur, UK.
An inactivated influenza vaccine (surface antigen) (p.1620·2).
*Active immunisation.*

**Inflexal S** Niddapharm, Ger.
An influenza vaccine (p.1620·2).
*Active immunisation.*

**Infloran** Kwizda, Austria; Berna, Hong Kong; Vieira, Port.; Berna, Switz.; Berna, Thai.; Swiss Serum, Thai.
*Bifidobacterium infantis; Lactobacillus acidophilus* (p.1704·2).
*Constipation; digestive disorders in infants on artificial diets; enterocolitis; restoration of intestinal flora.*

SIT, Ital.; Berna, Spain.
*Bifidobacterium bifidum* (p.1704·2); *Lactobacillus acidophilus* (p.1704·2).
*Diarrhoea; restoration of gastrointestinal flora.*

**Infloxa** Alpharma, Mex.
Ciprofloxacin (p.188·2).
*Bacterial infections.*

**Influ-A** Trima, Israel.
Amantadine hydrochloride (p.1197·2).
*Influenza A.*

**Influaforce** Bioforce, Switz.
Homoeopathic preparation.

**Influamin** Serum-Werk Bernburg, Ger.†.
Amino-acid, electrolyte, and xylitol infusion (p.1417·1).
*Parenteral nutrition.*

**Influbene** Ratiopharm, Austria.
Paracetamol (p.76·2); etilefrine hydrochloride (p.914·1); butetamate citrate (p.1116·2); chlorphenamine maleate (p.427·3).
*Cold and influenza symptoms.*

**Influbene C** Mepha, Switz.
Paracetamol (p.76·2); ascorbic acid (p.1460·2).
*Fever; pain.*

**Influbene N** Mepha, Switz.
Paracetamol (p.76·2).
*Fever; pain.*

**Infludo**
Weleda, Austria; Weleda, Fr.; Weleda, Ger.; Weleda, UK.
Homoeopathic preparation.

**Influenzine** Hochstetter, Chile.
Influenzinum.
*Cold and influenza prophylaxis.*

**Influex** Steigerwald, Ger.
Homoeopathic preparation.

**Influk** Knop, Chile.
Homoeopathic preparation.

**Influpiol C** Antipiol, Ital.
Vitamin C; propolis; salix; dog rose (p.1417·1).

**Influpozzi** IVP, Ital.
An influenza vaccine (p.1620·2).
*Active immunisation.*

**Influrem** Edmond Pharma, Ital.
Propyphenazone (p.85·3); caffeine (p.782·1); paracetamol (p.76·2).
*Cold symptoms; pain.*

**Influsplit** Valda, Ital.
An inactivated influenza vaccine (p.1620·2).
*Active immunisation.*

**Influsplit SSW** GlaxoSmithKline, Ger.
An influenza vaccine (p.1620·2).
*Active immunisation.*

**Influtruw** Truw, Ger.
Homoeopathic preparation.

**Influtux** Antipiol, Ital.
Hedera; propolis; dog rose; echinacea (p.1417·1).

**Influvac**
Raffo, Arg.; Solvay, Austral.; Solvay, Austria; Solvay, Denm.; Solvay, Fin.; Solvay, Fr.; Solvay, Ger.; Solvay, Irl.; Solvay, Israel; Solvay, Neth.; Solvay, Norw.; Solvay, Port.; Solvay, S.Afr.; Solvay, Swed.; Solvay, Switz.; Solvay, UK.
An inactivated influenza vaccine (surface antigen) (p.1620·2).
*Active immunisation.*

**Influvac S**
Solvay, Belg.; Solvay, Ital.
An influenza vaccine (surface antigen) (p.1620·2).
*Active immunisation.*

**Influvac Sub-Unit** Solvay, Gr.
An influenza vaccine (p.1620·2).
*Active immunisation.*

**Influvidon** Sanochemia, Austria.
Salicylamide (p.87·3); caffeine (p.782·1); propyphenazone (p.85·3); hesperidin phosphate (p.1688·3); calcium ascorbate (p.1460·2); piprin hydrate (p.439·1).
*Cold and influenza symptoms.*

**Influvirus** Nuovo ISM, Ital.
An influenza vaccine (p.1620·2).
*Active immunisation.*

**Influvit**
Note. This name is used for preparations of different composition.
DHU, Ger.
Homoeopathic preparation.

Recordati, Ital.
Paracetamol (p.76·2); ascorbic acid (p.1460·2); propyphenazone (p.85·3).
*Fever; pain.*

**Influ-Zinc** Wassen, Ital.
Zinc gluconate (p.1469·2); vitamin C (p.1460·2); selenium (p.1444·1); echinacea (p.1683·2); salix (p.87·3).

**Influ-Zinc Gola** Wassen, Ital.
Zinc acetate (p.1469·2); zinc citrate; liquorice (p.1270·2).

**Inf-Oph** Seng, Thai.
Prednisolone acetate (p.1108·1).
*Conjunctivitis.*

**Infosan** Nycomed Imaging, Norw.†.
Albumin (p.740·3).
*Contrast medium for echocardiography.*

**Infostat** Gautier, Arg.
Interferon alfa-2a (p.640·3).
*Hepatitis C; malignant neoplasms.*

**Infraline** Rolmex, Canad.†.
Methyl salicylate (p.59·3); menthol (p.1711·3); cineole (p.1672·1).

**Inframin** Fresenius Kabi, Ital.
Amino-acid infusion (p.1417·1).
*Parenteral nutrition in renal failure.*

**Infrarub**
Note. This name is used for preparations of different composition.
Wyeth-Whitehall, Arg.
Glycol salicylate (p.44·3); methyl nicotinate (p.59·2); histamine hydrochloride (p.1697·1); capsicum oleoresin (p.1667·1).
*Musculoskeletal and joint disorders.*

Whitehall, Braz.†.
Methyl nicotinate (p.59·2); capsaicin (p.24·2); histamine hydrochloride (p.1697·1); glycol salicylate (p.44·3).
*Musculoskeletal and joint disorders.*

Whitehall, USA†.
Methyl salicylate (p.59·3); menthol (p.1711·3).
*Muscle, joint, and soft-tissue pain; neuralgia.*

**Infree** Eisai, Jpn.
Indometacin farnesil (p.48·3).
*Musculoskeletal, joint, and peri-articular disorders.*

**Infrotto Ultra** Cassella-med, Ger.
Glycol salicylate (p.44·3); nonivamide (p.67·2).
*Musculoskeletal, joint, and soft-tissue disorders; neuralgia.*

**Infufer** Sabex, Canad.
Iron dextran (p.1436·3).
*Iron deficiency.*

**Infukoll** Gobbi, Arg.
Succinylated gelatin (p.754·3) with electrolytes.
*Plasma volume expansion.*

**Infukoll HES**
Gobbi, Arg.; Serum-Werk Bernburg, Ger.; Schwarz, Ger.
Pentastarch (p.750·1) in sodium chloride.
*Haemodilution; hypovolaemia.*

**Infukoll M 40** Serum-Werk Bernburg, Ger.
Dextran 40 (p.745·3) in sodium chloride.
*Hypovolaemia; thrombosis prophylaxis.*

**Infumal** Serum-Werk Bernburg, Ger.†.
Arginine (p.1421·1); malic acid (p.1709·2); sodium hydroxide (p.1747·3).
*Hyperammonaemia.*

**Infumix** Orion, Fin.†.
A range of amino-acid, carbohydrate, lipid, and electrolyte infusions (p.1417·1).
*Parenteral nutrition.*

**Infumorph** Elkins-Sinn, USA.
Morphine sulfate (p.60·2).
*Pain.*

**Infuvite** Baxter, USA.
Multivitamin preparation (p.1417·1).
*Parenteral nutrition.*

**Ingafol** Inga, India.
Folic acid (p.1429·1).
*Folic acid supplement; megaloblastic anaemia.*

**Ingagen-M** Inga, India.
Methylergometrine maleate (p.1714·2).
*Uterine atony; uterine haemorrhage.*

**Ingastri** Ipsen, Spain.
Famotidine (p.1265·2).
*Gastro-oesophageal reflux; peptic ulcer; Zollinger-Ellison syndrome.*

**Ingelan**
Note. This name is used for preparations of different composition.
Germania, Austria; Boehringer Ingelheim, Ger.
*Topical gel:* Isoprenaline sulfate (p.940·2).
*Skin disorders.*

Germania, Austria; Boehringer Ingelheim, Ger.
*Topical powder:* Isoprenaline sulfate (p.940·2); salicylic acid (p.1157·1).
*Skin disorders.*

**Ingro** Farmacologico Milanese, Ital.†.
Sulfogaiacol (p.1131·1); dextromethorphan hydrobromide (p.1117·3); eucalyptus (p.1686·1).
*Coughs.*

**Ingrown Toe Nail Salve** Cress, Canad.†.
Boric acid (p.1662·1); camphor (p.1665·3); salicylic acid (p.1157·1).

**Inhacort** Boehringer Ingelheim, Ger.
Flunisolide (p.1101·1).
*Asthma.*

**Inhadrina** Ibefar, Braz.†.
Diphenhydramine hydrochloride (p.431·3); naphazoline hydrochloride (p.1124·3); menthol (p.1711·3); cineole (p.1672·1); sumatra benzoin (p.1751·1).
*Respiratory-tract congestion.*

**Inhalador** Fournier SA, Spain†.
Camphor (p.1665·3); methyl salicylate (p.59·3); oleum pini sylvestris; sassafras oil (p.1742·1); menthol (p.1711·3).
*Nasal congestion.*

**Inhalador Medex** Sidus, Arg.
Methyl salicylate (p.59·3); menthol (p.1711·3); camphor (p.1665·3); eucalyptus oil (p.1686·2); pine oil; sassafras oil (p.1742·1).
*Respiratory-tract congestion.*

**Inhalante Yatropan** Aventis, Braz.
Ephedrine (p.1120·1); menthol (p.1711·3); cineole (p.1672·1); tolu (p.1131·3); lavender oil (p.1705·2); benzoin (p.1751·1); sodium guaiacol sulfanilamide.
*Respiratory-tract congestion.*

**Inhalene** Sanofi Synthelabo, Belg.
Menthol (p.1711·3); cineole (p.1672·1).
*Cold symptoms; laryngitis; sinusitis.*

**Inhalosam** Hearst, Braz.†.
Ephedrine hydrochloride (p.1120·1); menthol (p.1711·3); cineole (p.1672·1).

**Inhelthran** Abbott, Arg.
Enflurane (p.1298·1).
*General anaesthesia.*

**Inhepar** Pisa, Mex.
Heparin sodium (p.928·1).

**Inhibac** Pharmaland, Thai.
Chlorhexidine gluconate (p.1173·2); cetrimide (p.1172·1).
*Disinfection.*

**Inhibace**
Note. This name is used for preparations of different composition.
Bayer, Austral.†; Roche, Austria; Merck, Austria; Roche, Belg.; Roche, Canad.; Roche, Chile; Roche, Hong Kong; Chugai, Jpn; Syntex, Mex.; Roche, NZ; Roche, S.Afr.; Roche, Singapore; Roche, Spain; Roche, Swed.; Roche, Switz.; Roche, Thai.
Cilazapril (p.883·3).
*Heart failure; hypertension.*

Bristol-Myers Squibb, Israel.
Captopril (p.879·2).
*Diabetic nephropathy; heart failure; hypertension; myocardial infarction.*

**Inhibace comp** Roche, Swed.
Cilazapril (p.883·3); hydrochlorothiazide (p.933·2).
*Hypertension.*

**Inhibace Plus**
Roche, Austria; Merck, Austria; Roche, Canad.; Roche, Chile; Roche, NZ; Roche, S.Afr.; Roche, Spain; Roche, Switz.
Cilazapril (p.883·3); hydrochlorothiazide (p.933·2).
*Hypertension.*

**Inhibin** Viatris, Neth.
Hydroquinine hydrobromide (p.1699·3).
*Nocturnal muscle cramps.*

**Inhibisam** Richmond, Arg.
Indinavir (p.640·1).
*HIV infection.*

**Inhibitron** Liomont, Mex.
Omeprazole (p.1278·2).
*Acid aspiration; gastro-oesophageal reflux; peptic ulcer; Zollinger-Ellison syndrome.*

**Inhibostamin** Novartis Consumer, Ger.
Tritoqualine (p.443·3).
*Hypersensitivity reactions; pruritus.*

**Inhiston** Biomedica, Ital.
Pheniramine maleate (p.438·3).
*Hypersensitivity reactions.*

**Inibace**
Roche, Ital.; Roche, Port.
Cilazapril (p.883·3).
*Heart failure; hypertension.*

**Inibace Plus**
Roche, Ital.; Roche, Port.
Cilazapril (p.883·3); hydrochlorothiazide (p.933·2).
*Hypertension.*

**Inib-Dor** Ibfarma, Braz.†.
Hyoscine butylbromide (p.483·3); dipyrone (p.35·3).
*Pain; smooth muscle spasm.*

**Inibex S** Medley, Braz.
Diethylpropion hydrochloride (p.1587·1).
*Obesity.*

**Inibina** Apsen, Braz.
Isoxsuprine (p.1702·3) or isoxsuprine hydrochloride (p.1702·2).
*Premature labour.*

**Inicox** Farmoquimica, Braz.
Meloxicam (p.56·1).
*Dysmenorrhoea; musculoskeletal and joint disorders.*

**Inimur** Taurus, Ger.
Nifuratel (p.611·2).
*Fungal infections; trichomoniasis.*

**Inimur Myko** Taurus, Ger.
Ciclopirox olamine (p.396·1).
*Fungal vaginal infections.*

**Inipomp** Sanofi Synthelabo, Fr.
Pantoprazole sodium (p.1283·1).
*Gastro-oesophageal reflux; peptic ulcer; Zollinger-Ellison syndrome.*

**Iniprol** Bournonville, Belg.†.
Aprotinin (p.742·3).
*Fatty emboli; haemorrhage; shock.*

**Inistolin Antitusivo Ped** Pfizer Lambert, Spain.
Dextromethorphan hydrobromide (p.1117·3); pseudoephedrine hydrochloride (p.1129·2).
*Coughs; nasal congestion.*

**Inistolin Expectoran Ped** Pfizer Lambert, Spain.
Pseudoephedrine hydrochloride (p.1129·2); guaifenesin (p.1122·1).
*Respiratory-tract congestion.*

**Iniston** Pfizer Lambert, Spain.
Pseudoephedrine hydrochloride (p.1129·2); triprolidine hydrochloride (p.442·3).
*Cold symptoms; nasal congestion.*

**Iniston Antitusivo** Pfizer Lambert, Spain.
Dextromethorphan hydrobromide (p.1117·3); pseudoephedrine hydrochloride (p.1129·2); triprolidine hydrochloride (p.442·3).
*Coughs; nasal congestion.*

**Iniston Expectorante** Pfizer Lambert, Spain.
Guaifenesin (p.1122·1); pseudoephedrine hydrochloride (p.1129·2); triprolidine hydrochloride (p.442·3).
*Coughs; nasal congestion.*

**Initiss** Pharmacia Upjohn, Ital.
Cilazapril (p.883·3).
*Hypertension.*

**Initiss Plus** Pharmacia Upjohn, Ital.
Cilazapril (p.883·3); hydrochlorothiazide (p.933·2).
*Hypertension.*

**Injectio Lymphatica N EKF** Biomedica, Ger.†.
Homoeopathic preparation.

**Inkamil** Ipsen, Spain†.
Ciprofloxacin hydrochloride (p.188·2).
*Bacterial infections.*

**Inmunoartro** Beta, Arg.
Leflunomide (p.53·2).
*Rheumatoid arthritis.*

**Inmunobalt** Rudefsa, Mex.
*Oral solution*†: A lysate of *Streptococcus pneumoniae*; *Klebsiella pneumoniae*; *Klebsiella ozaenae*; *Streptococcus viridans*; *Streptococcus pyogenes*; *Staphylococcus aureus*; *Moraxella catarrhalis*; *Haemophilus influenzae*.
*Tablets:* A lysate of *Streptococcus pneumoniae*; *Klebsiella pneumoniae*(p.0·0); *Streptococcus haemolyticus*; *Staphylococcus aureus*; *Moraxella catarrhalis*; *Haemophilus influenzae*.
*Respiratory-tract infections.*

**Inmunoferon**
Andromaco, Mex.†; Cantabria, Spain.
Glicofosfopeptical (p.1693·3).
*Immunotherapy.*

**Inmunogrip** Gezzi, Arg.
Paracetamol (p.76·2); caffeine (p.782·1); phenylephrine hydrochloride (p.1126·3).

**Inmunol** Andromaco, Mex.
Glicofosfopeptical (p.1693·3).
*Immunostimulant.*

**Inmupen** Llorente, Spain†.
Amoxicillin trihydrate (p.155·3); potassium clavulanate (p.193·3).
*Bacterial infections.*

**Inmutag** Pharmacia, Arg.
Interferon alfa (p.640·3).
*Anogenital warts; hepatitis B and C; malignant neoplasms.*

**Innersource** Quest, Canad.
Multivitamin and mineral preparation (p.1417·1).

**Inno Rheuma**
Note. This name is used for preparations of different composition.
Naturland, Austria.
*Oil:* Lavender oil (p.1705·2); menthol (p.1711·3); rosemary oil (p.1740·2).
*Musculoskeletal and joint disorders; nerve pain.*

Strallhofer, Austria.
*Cream:* Camphor (p.1665·3); menthol (p.1711·3); rosemary oil (p.1740·2).
*Musculoskeletal and joint disorders; nerve pain.*

**Innobrand** Lab Francais du Fractionnement, Fr.
A complex of factor VIII and von Willebrand's factor (p.751·1).
*Von Willebrand's disease.*

**InnoGel Plus** Hogil, USA†.
Pyrethrins (p.1509·3); piperonyl butoxide (p.1509·2).

**Innohep**
Purissimus, Arg.; Leo, Belg.; Leo, Canad.; Leo, Denm.; Leo, Fin.; Leo, Fr.; Braun, Ger.; Leo, Ger.; Leo (Λεο), Gr.; Leo, Hong Kong; Leo, Irl.; Leo, Israel; Formenti, Ital.†; Leo, Malaysia; Leo, Neth.; Leo, Norw.; CSL, NZ; Leo, NZ; Leo, Port.; Leo, Singapore; Farmacusi, Spain; Leo, Swed.; Leo, Thai.; Leo, UK; Pharmion, USA.
Tinzaparin sodium (p.1013·1).
*Thromboembolic disorders.*

**InnoLet N** Novo Nordisk, Jpn.
Isophane insulin injection (human, recombinant) (p.333·3).
*Diabetes mellitus.*

**InnoLet R** Novo Nordisk, Jpn.
Insulin injection (human, recombinant) (p.333·3).
*Diabetes mellitus.*

**InnoLet 30R** Novo Nordisk, Jpn.
Mixture of insulin injection (human, recombinant) 30% and isophane insulin (human, recombinant) 70% (p.333·3).
*Diabetes mellitus.*

**Innomel** Clonmel, Irl.
Enalapril maleate (p.909·2).
*Heart failure; hypertension.*

**InnoPran** Reliant, USA.
Propranolol hydrochloride (p.989·3).
*Hypertension.*

**Innova Cd** Laboratorios Chile, Chile.
21 Tablets, levonorgestrel (p.1563·2); ethinylestradiol (p.1553·2); 7 tablets, inert.
*Combined oral contraceptive.*

**Innovace**
Merck Sharp & Dohme, Irl.; Merck Sharp & Dohme, UK.
Enalapril maleate (p.909·2).
*Heart failure; hypertension; ischaemic heart disease.*

**Innovar** Janssen, USA†.
Fentanyl citrate (p.40·1); droperidol (p.697·2).
*Anaesthesia; neuroleptanalgesia; premedication.*

**Innozide**
Merck Sharp & Dohme, Irl.; Merck Sharp & Dohme, UK.
Enalapril maleate (p.909·2); hydrochlorothiazide (p.933·2).
*Hypertension.*

**Inobesin** Windson, Braz.†.
Fenproporex hydrochloride (p.1588·3).
*Obesity.*

**Inocar** Solvay, Spain.
Cilazapril (p.883·3).
*Heart failure; hypertension.*

**Inocar Plus** Solvay, Spain.
Cilazapril (p.883·3); hydrochlorothiazide (p.933·2).
*Hypertension.*

**Inocor**
Sanofi Winthrop, Belg.†; Sanofi Synthelabo, Braz.†; Sanofi Winthrop, Canad.†; Sanofi Winthrop, Fr.†; Sanofi Winthrop, Israel; Sanofi Synthelabo, Ital.; Sanofi Synthelabo, Malaysia; Sanofi Synthelabo, Port.; Sanofi Winthrop, Swed.†; Sanofi Winthrop, USA.
Amrinone (p.862·3) or amrinone lactate (p.862·3).
*Heart failure.*

**Inofer** *AJC, Fr.†.*
Ferrous succinate (p.1428·2).
Succinic acid is included in this preparation to increase the absorption and availability of iron.
*Anaemia.*

**Inoflox**
*Biomedis, Malaysia; Biomedis, Singapore.*
Ofloxacin (p.239·3).
*Bacterial infections.*

**Inolaxine**
*Fournier, Fr.; Dales, Hong Kong†; Fournier, Switz.*
Sterculia (p.1290·2).
*Constipation; inflammatory bowel disease.*

**Inolaxol** *Selena, Swed.*
Sterculia (p.1290·2).
*Adjunct in treatment of diarrhoea; constipation.*

**Inolin** *Tanabe, Jpn.*
Tretoquinol hydrochloride (p.806·3).
*Obstructive airways disease.*

**INOmax**
*AGA, Denm.; INO Therapeutics, Spain; INO Therapeutics, USA.*
Nitric oxide (p.973·3).
*Neonatal respiratory distress syndrome.*

**Inongan** *Fumouze, Fr.*
Menthol (p.1711·3); methyl salicylate (p.59·3); camphor (p.1665·3); eucalyptus oil (p.1686·2).
*Muscle pain.*

**Inopamil**
*Astra, Ital.†; Zambon, Neth.*
Ibopamine hydrochloride (p.937·3).
*Heart failure.*

**Inopin** *Siam Bheasach, Thai.*
Dopamine hydrochloride (p.907·1).
*Shock.*

**Inosital** *Toyo, Hong Kong†.*
Inositol (p.1701·2).
*Peripheral vascular disorders.*

**Inotan** *Eurofarma, Braz.†.*
Dobutamine hydrochloride (p.905·3).
*Heart failure; shock.*

**Inotop** *Torrex, Austria.*
Dobutamine hydrochloride (p.905·3).
*Heart failure; shock.*

**Inotrex**
*Pharmaserve Lilly (Φαρμασερβ Λιλλυ), Gr.; Lilly, Port.*
Dobutamine hydrochloride (p.905·3).
*Cardiac surgery; cardiomyopathy; heart failure; myocardial infarction; shock.*

**Inotropin** *Bago, Arg.*
Dopamine hydrochloride (p.907·1).
*Heart failure; shock.*

**Inotropisa** *Pisa, Mex.*
Dopamine hydrochloride (p.907·1).
*Cardiac surgery; hypovolaemia; shock.*

**Inotyol**
*Note. This name is used for preparations of different composition.*
*Brady, Austria; Aventis, Ital.*
*Ointment:* Ichthammol (p.1148·2); hamamelis (p.1696·3); zinc oxide (p.1163·2); titanium dioxide (p.1160·3).
*Burns; skin disorders; wounds.*

*Brady, Austria.*
*Topical powder:* Ichthammol (p.1148·2); hamamelis (p.1696·3); zinc oxide (p.1163·2); calcium carbonate (p.1254·2).
*Skin disorders.*

*Urgo, Belg.; Debat, Denm.; Debat, Norw.; Selena, Swed.*
Ichthammol (p.1148·2); zinc oxide (p.1163·2); titanium dioxide (p.1160·3).
Formerly contained ichthammol, hamamelis, zinc oxide, titanium dioxide, borax in *Belg.*
*Skin disorders.*

*Fournier, Fr.; Urgo, Israel.*
Ichthammol (p.1148·2); hamamelis (p.1696·3); zinc oxide (p.1163·2); titanium dioxide (p.1160·3); siam benzoin (p.1744·1).
*Burns; skin disorders; wounds.*

*Hoechst Marion Roussel, Ital.†.*
*Topical powder:* Ichthammol (p.1148·2); zinc oxide (p.1163·2); hamamelis (p.1696·3).
*Skin irritation.*

**Inova** *Inova, Ger.*
Dialkyldimethylammonium chloride (p.1178·3); alkyldimethylbenzylammonium chloride (p.1168·3); alkyldimethylethylbenzylammonium chloride.
*Surface disinfection.*

**Inoval** *Janssen, Braz.†.*
Fentanyl citrate (p.40·1); droperidol (p.697·2).
*Neuroleptanalgesia.*

**Inovan** *Kyowa, Jpn.*
Dopamine hydrochloride (p.907·1).
*Anuria; oliguria; shock.*

**Inovapar** *Zerboni, Mex.†.*
Bromocriptine (p.1202·3).

**Inovec** *Libbs, Braz.†.*
Amlodipine (p.862·2).
*Hypertension.*

**Inoven** *Johnson & Johnson MSD Consumer, UK†.*
Ibuprofen (p.45·3).
*Fever; inflammation; pain.*

**Inpanol**
*DHA, Hong Kong; DHA, Singapore.*
Propranolol hydrochloride (p.989·3).
*Angina pectoris; arrhythmias; hypertension; hyperthyroidism; myocardial infarction.*

**Inpront** *Laboratorios Chile, Chile.*
Moclobemide (p.308·2).
*Depression.*

**Insacial** *Byk Gulden, Mex.†.*
Cathine resinate (p.1585·2).

**Insadol**
*Sanofi Winthrop, Braz.†; Expanpharm, Fr.; Expanpharm, Switz.*
Maize (p.1676·1).
*Dental disorders.*

**Insect Ecran** *Osler, Fr.*
*Paediatric spray:* Ethohexadiol (p.1505·1).
*Insect repellent.*
*Solution:* Permethrin (p.1508·3).
*Insect repellent for clothing and bedding.*
*Spray:* Diethyltoluamide (p.1503·3).
*Insect repellent.*

**Insensye** *Merck Sharp & Dohme, Austral.*
Norfloxacin (p.238·3).
*Bacterial infections.*

**Insertec** *Baliarda, Arg.*
Sertraline (p.317·3).
*Depression.*

**Inside** *Antula, Swed.*
Ranitidine hydrochloride (p.1285·2).
*Gastro-oesophageal reflux; peptic ulcer; Zollinger-Ellison syndrome.*

**Insidon**
*Novartis, Austria; Ciba-Geigy, Belg.†; Novartis, Ger.; Novartis, Irl.†; Ciba, Ital.†; Novartis, Neth.†; Novartis, Switz.*
Opipramol hydrochloride (p.311·1).
*Anxiety; depression; sleep disorders.*

**Insig** *Sigma, Austral.*
Indapamide (p.938·2).
*Hypertension.*

**Insogen** *Byk Gulden, Mex.*
Chlorpropamide (p.330·3).
*Diabetes mellitus.*

**Insogen Plus** *Byk Gulden, Mex.*
Metformin hydrochloride (p.342·3); chlorpropamide (p.330·3).
*Diabetes mellitus.*

**Insom** *Lennon, S.Afr.†.*
Flunitrazepam (p.698·2).
*Insomnia.*

**Insoma** *Pacific, NZ.*
Nitrazepam (p.710·1).
*Insomnia.*

**Insomin** *Orion, Fin.*
Nitrazepam (p.710·1).
*Epilepsy; insomnia.*

**Insomnal**
*Note. This name is used for preparations of different composition.*
*Northia, Arg.*
Passion flower (p.1729·1); valerian (p.1762·2); tilia (p.1756·2).
*Insomnia.*

*Rougier, Canad.*
Diphenhydramine hydrochloride (p.431·3).
*Insomnia.*

**Insomn-Eze** *Aventis, Austral.*
Promethazine hydrochloride (p.439·1).
*Insomnia.*

**Insomnia** *Homeocan, Canad.*
Homoeopathic preparation.

**Insomnia Passiflora** *Homeocan, Canad.*
Homoeopathic preparation.

**Insomnium** *Gador, Arg.*
Zopiclone (p.729·3).
*Insomnia.*

**Inspirol Halsschmerztabletten** *Riemser, Ger.*
Tyrothricin (p.275·1); benzocaine (p.1370·3); dequalinium chloride (p.1178·1).
*Mouth and throat infections.*

**Inspirol Heilpflanzenol** *Riemser, Ger.*
Peppermint oil (p.1283·2).
*Cold symptoms; gastrointestinal disorders.*

**Inspirol Mundwasser konzentrat** *Hotz, Ger.†.*
Menthol (p.1711·3); eucalyptus oil (p.1686·2); peppermint oil (p.1283·2); pumilio pine oil (p.1737·1).
*Mouth and throat disorders.*

**Inspirol P** *Riemser, Ger.*
Myrrh (p.1718·3).
*Mouth and throat inflammation.*

**Inspiryl**
*Astra, Mex.†; AstraZeneca, Norw.†; Draco, Swed.†.*
Salbutamol sulfate (p.791·3).
*Obstructive airways disease.*

**Inspra** *Pfizer, USA.*
Eplerenone (p.911·3).
*Heart failure following myocardial infarction; hypertension.*

**Instacare**
*Ciba Vision, Austral.†; Ciba Vision, NZ.*
Cleansing and disinfecting solutions for soft contact lenses (p.1164·2).

**Instacyl** *Streuli, Switz.*
Aspirin (p.15·1); ascorbic acid (p.1460·2).
*Cold symptoms.*

**Insta-Glucose** *ICN, Austral.*
Glucose (p.1432·2).
*Hypoglycaemia.*

**Instana** *Farmacusi, Spain.*
Cefpodoxime proxetil (p.178·3).
*Bacterial infections.*

**Instant Rub** *Lioh, Canad.†.*
Methyl salicylate (p.59·3); menthol (p.1711·3).

**Instantine** *Bayer Consumer, Canad.*
Aspirin (p.15·1); caffeine (p.782·1).
*Fever; headache; pain.*

**Instaret** *Unipharma, Gr.*
Acetic acid (p.1645·2).
*Mild bacterial or fungal infections of the outer ear.*

**Instat**
*Johnson & Johnson, Austria†; Ethicon, Ital.†; Johnson & Johnson, Switz.†; Johnson & Johnson Medical, UK†.*
Collagen (bovine) (p.1674·3).
*Haemorrhage.*

**Instenon**
*Nycomed, Austria; Nycomed, Hong Kong; Nycomed, Thai.*
Hexobendine hydrochloride (p.931·2); etofylline (p.785·1); etamivan (p.1588·1).
*Cerebrovascular disorders.*

**Instillagel**
*Raffo, Arg.; Solco, Austria; Melisana, Belg.; Farco, Denm.; Fuca, Fr.; Farco, Ger.; Farco, Hong Kong; Farco, Irl.; Farco, Israel; Asofarma, Mex.; Selena, Swed.; Almed, Switz.†; CliniMed, UK.*
Lidocaine hydrochloride (p.1377·3); chlorhexidine gluconate (p.1173·2).
*Catheterisation; cystoscopy; endoscopy; urethroscopy.*

**Instrunet** *Inibsa, Port.*
A range of solutions for skin and instrument disinfection.

**Instru-Safe** *Eagle, Austral.†.*
Silicone (p.1482·1).
*Instrument lubrication.*

**Instruzyme** *Peters, Fr.†.*
Mixed quaternary ammonium salts; polihexanide (p.1190·1).
*Instrument disinfection.*

**Insuflen** *Fada, Arg.*
Ranitidine (p.1285·2).

**Insulatard**
*Pentafarma, Chile.*
Isophane insulin (porcine) (p.333·3).
*Diabetes mellitus.*

*Novo Nordisk, Denm.; Novo Nordisk, Fr.; Novo Nordisk, Irl.; Novo Nordisk, Malaysia; Novo Nordisk, Neth.; Novo Nordisk, Norw.; Novo Nordisk, Port.; Novo Nordisk, Swed.; Novo Nordisk, Thai.; Novo Nordisk, UK.*
Isophane insulin injection (human, pyr, highly purified) (p.333·3).
Formerly known as Human Insulatard in the *UK.*
*Diabetes mellitus.*

**Insulatard HM**
*Novo Nordisk, Arg.; Novo Nordisk, Austria; Novo Nordisk, Belg.; Pentafarma, Chile; Novo Nordisk, Singapore; Novo Nordisk, Switz.*
Isophane insulin injection (human, monocomponent) (p.333·3).
Formerly known as Protaphane HM in *Switz.*
*Diabetes mellitus.*

**Insulatard Human** *Novo Nordisk, Ger.*
Isophane insulin injection (human, ge) (p.333·3).
*Diabetes mellitus.*

**Insulatard MC**
*Novo Nordisk, Arg.; Novo Nordisk, Ger.†; Novo Nordisk, Hong Kong; Novo Nordisk, Switz.*
Isophane insulin injection (porcine, highly purified) (p.333·3).
*Diabetes mellitus.*

**Insulatard NPH** *Novo Nordisk, Spain.*
Isophane insulin injection (human) (p.333·3).
*Diabetes mellitus.*

**Insulex** *Pisa, Mex.*
Insulin (p.333·3).
*Diabetes mellitus.*

**Insulin 2** *Novo Nordisk, Austral.†.*
Acid insulin injection (bovine) (p.333·3).
*Diabetes mellitus.*

**Insulin Basal** *Hoechst Marion Roussel, Norw.†.*
Isophane insulin injection (human, emp) (p.333·3).
*Diabetes mellitus.*

**Insulin Infusat** *Hoechst Marion Roussel, Norw.†.*
Insulin injection (human, emp) (p.333·3).
*Diabetes mellitus.*

**Insulin Komb 25/75** *Hoechst Marion Roussel, Norw.†.*
Mixture of insulin injection (human, emp) and isophane insulin injection (human, emp) (p.333·3).
*Diabetes mellitus.*

**Insulin Lente MC** *Novo Nordisk, Fin.†.*
Insulin zinc suspension (porcine/bovine) (amorphous 34%, crystalline 66%) (p.333·3).
*Diabetes mellitus.*

**Insulin Lyhyt** *Orion, Fin.*
Insulin injection (human) (p.333·3).
*Diabetes mellitus.*

**Insulin Pitka** *Orion, Fin.*
Isophane insulin injection (human) (p.333·3).
*Diabetes mellitus.*

**Insulin Rapid** *Hoechst Marion Roussel, Norw.†.*
Insulin injection (human, emp) (p.333·3).
*Diabetes mellitus.*

**Insulin Reaction** *Sherwood, USA.*
Glucose (p.1432·2).
*Hypoglycaemia.*

**Insulin S** *Berlin-Chemie, Ger.; Hoechst, Ger.*
Insulin injection (pork) (p.333·3).
*Diabetes mellitus.*

**Insulin SNC** *Berlin-Chemie, Ger.*
Insulin injection (porcine) (p.333·3).
*Diabetes mellitus.*

**Insuline Semi Tardum** *Organon, Fr.†.*
Insulin zinc suspension (amorphous) (porcine, highly purified) (p.333·3).
*Diabetes mellitus.*

**Insuline Tardum MX** *Organon, Fr.†.*
Mixture of insulin zinc suspension (amorphous) (porcine, highly purified) 30% and insulin zinc suspension (crystalline) (bovine, highly purified) 70% (p.333·3).
*Diabetes mellitus.*

**Insuline Ultra Tardum** *Organon, Fr.†.*
Insulin zinc suspension (crystalline) (bovine, highly purified) (p.333·3).
*Diabetes mellitus.*

**Insuman Basal**
*Aventis, Austria; Aventis, Denm.; Aventis, Fin.; Aventis, Fr.; Aventis, Ger.; Aventis, Irl.; Aventis, Neth.; Aventis, Norw.; Aventis, Swed.; Aventis, Switz.; Aventis, UK.*
Isophane insulin injection (human) (p.333·3).
*Diabetes mellitus.*

**Insuman Comb 15, 25, and 50**
*Aventis, Austria; Aventis, Fr.; Aventis, Ger.; Aventis, Irl.; Aventis, Neth.; Aventis, Switz.; Aventis, UK.*
Mixtures of soluble insulin injection (human) 15%, 25%, and 50% and isophane insulin injection (human) 85%, 75%, and 50% respectively (p.333·3).
*Diabetes mellitus.*

**Insuman Comb 25**
*Aventis, Denm.; Aventis, Fin.; Aventis, Norw.; Aventis, Swed.*
A mixture of insulin injection (human) 25% and isophane insulin injection (human) 75% (p.333·3).
*Diabetes mellitus.*

**Insuman Comb 85N/15R and 75N/25R** *Aventis, Braz.*
Mixtures of isophane insulin injection (human) 85% and 75% and soluble insulin injection (human) 15% and 25% respectively (p.333·3).
*Diabetes mellitus.*

**Insuman Infusat**
*Aventis, Austria; Aventis, Fin.; Aventis, Fr.; Aventis, Ger.; Aventis, Norw.; Aventis, Swed.; Aventis, Switz.*
Soluble insulin injection (human) (p.333·3).
*Diabetes mellitus.*

**Insuman Intermediaire 25/75** *Hoechst, Fr.†.*
Mixture of insulin injection (human, emp, highly purified) 25% and isophane insulin injection (human, emp, highly purified) 75% (p.333·3).
*Diabetes mellitus.*

**Insuman Intermediaire 100%** *Hoechst, Fr.†.*
Isophane insulin injection (human, emp, highly purified) (p.333·3).
*Diabetes mellitus.*

**Insuman komb Typ 15, Typ 25, and Typ 50**
*Hoechst Marion Roussel, Austria†.*
Mixtures of soluble insulin injection (human) 15%, 25%, and 50% and isophane insulin injection (human) 85%, 75%, and 50% respectively (p.333·3).
*Diabetes mellitus.*

**Insuman N**
*Aventis, Arg.; Aventis, Braz.; Aventis, Chile.*
Isophane insulin (human) (p.333·3).
*Diabetes mellitus.*

**Insuman R**
*Aventis, Arg.; Aventis, Braz.; Aventis, Chile.*
Insulin injection (human) (p.333·3).
*Diabetes mellitus.*

**Insuman Rapid**
*Aventis, Austria; Aventis, Denm.; Aventis, Fin.; Aventis, Fr.; Aventis, Ger.; Aventis, Irl.; Aventis, Neth.; Aventis, Norw.; Aventis, Swed.; Aventis, Switz.; Aventis, UK.*
Neutral insulin injection (human) (p.333·3).
*Diabetes mellitus.*

**Insup** *Smaller, Spain.*
Enalapril maleate (p.909·2).
*Heart failure; hypertension.*

**Insuvac** *Biolab Sanus, Braz.†.*
Extracts of bacterial antigens and allergens (p.1650·1).
*Allergen immunotherapy.*

**Insuven**
*Grunenthal, Chile; Almirall, Spain†.*
Diosmin (p.1688·2).
*Capillary fragility; haemorrhoids; venous insufficiency.*

**Intacglobin** *Grossman, Mex.†.*
Immunoglobulin G (p.1627·2).

**Intal**
*Phoenix, Arg.; Aventis, Austral.; Sanova, Austria; Aventis, Braz.; Aventis, Canad.; Aventis, Ger.; Aventis, Hong Kong; Fisons, Irl.; Fujisawa, Jpn; Aventis, Malaysia; Aventis, Mex.; Aventis, NZ; Aventis, Port.; Aventis, Singapore; Aventis, Spain; Aventis, Thai.; Aventis, UK; Aventis, USA.*
Sodium cromoglicate (p.795·3).
*Allergic conjunctivitis; allergic rhinitis; asthma; food allergy.*

**Intapan** *Duopharma, Hong Kong.*
Nalbuphine hydrochloride (p.64·2).
*Adjunct in general anaesthesia; pain.*

**Intard** *Julphar, UAE.*
Diphenoxylate hydrochloride (p.1261·3).
Atropine sulfate (p.477·1) is included in this preparation to discourage abuse.
*Diarrhoea.*

**Intaxel**
*Dabur, India; Dabur, Thai.*
Paclitaxel (p.577·3).
*Breast cancer; ovarian cancer.*

**Inteflora** *Mer-National, S.Afr.*
*Saccharomyces boulardii* (p.1704·2).
*Gastrointestinal disorders.*

**Integrilin**
Schering-Plough, Belg.; Schering-Plough, Braz.†; Key, Canad.; Essex, Chile; Schering-Plough, Denm.; Schering-Plough, Fin.; Schering-Plough, Fr.; Essex, Ger.; Schering-Plough, Gr.; Schering-Plough, Hong Kong; Schering-Plough, Irl.; Schering-Plough, Israel; Schering-Plough, Ital.; Schering-Plough, Malaysia; Schering-Plough, Neth.; Schering-Plough, Norw.; Schering-Plough, NZ; Schering-Plough, Port.†; Schering-Plough, S.Afr.; Schering-Plough, Singapore; Schering-Plough, Spain; Schering-Plough, Swed.; Essex, Switz.; Schering-Plough, Thai.; Schering-Plough, UK; Cor Therapeutics, USA; Key, USA.
Eptifibatide (p.912·2).
*Adjunct in coronary angioplasty or atherectomy; myocardial infarction; unstable angina.*

**Integrobe** Northia, Arg.
Dipyrone (p.35·3).
*Inflammation; pain.*

**Inteligen** Phoenix, Arg.
Arginine acetylasparaginate (p.1421·2).
*Fatigue.*

**Inteligen Ginseng** Phoenix, Arg.
Arginine acetylasparaginate (p.1421·2); ginseng (p.1693·1).
*Asthenia.*

**Intensain** Hoechst, Ger.†.
Carbocromen hydrochloride (p.880·2).
*Cardiac disorders.*

**Inter IF** Biolab Sanus, Braz.†.
Interferon alfa (p.640·3).
*Viral skin infections.*

**Interacton** Enzypharm, Neth.†.
Amine oxidase; glutaminase; allyl sulfide.
*Asthma; bronchitis; hypersensitivity reactions; pertussis; sinusitis; skin disorders.*

**Interbion** Biospray, Gr.
Cefuroxime axetil (p.184·1).
*Bacterial infections.*

**Interceed**
Johnson & Johnson Medical, Fr.†; Johnson & Johnson, Ger.†; Johnson & Johnson Medical, UK†.
Oxidised cellulose (p.757·1).
*Postoperative adhesions.*

**Intercron** Laphal, Fr.
Sodium cromoglicate (p.795·3).
*Food hypersensitivity.*

**Intercyton**
Celltech, Fr.; Sanofi Synthelabo, Spain†.
Flavodate sodium (p.1688·2).
*Circulatory eye disorders; haemorrhoids; menometrorrhagia associated with intra-uterine devices; venous insufficiency.*

**Interderm** Interpharma, Spain.
Gentamicin sulfate (p.217·1); nystatin (p.406·3); triamcinolone acetonide (p.1110·2).
*Infected skin disorders.*

**Intermax-Alpha** Raffo, Chile.
Interferon alfa (p.640·3).

**Intersept** Interdelta, Switz.
Povidone-iodine (p.1190·3).
*Burns; skin disinfection; wounds.*

**Intestamin**
Fresenius Kabi, Ger.; Fresenius Kabi, Port.
Preparation for enteral nutrition (p.1417·1).

**Intestinol** Rasch & Handel, Austria.
Pancreatin (p.1725·3); sodium cholate; duodenum extract; charcoal (p.1030·2).
*Gastrointestinal disorders.*

**Intesul** Beta, Arg.
Mosapride citrate (p.1276·3).
*Gastritis; gastro-oesophageal reflux; gastroparesis.*

**Intetrix** Beaufour, Fr.
Tiliquinol (p.617·1); tiliquinol laurilsulfate (p.617·1); tilbroquinol (p.617·1).
*Intestinal amoebiasis.*

**Intetrix P** Beaufour, Fr.†.
Tilbroquinol (p.617·1).
Formerly contained tilbroquinol and furoylbromomethyloxine.
*Infective diarrhoea.*

**Inthacine** The Forty-Two, Thai.
Indometacin (p.47·3).
*Gout; musculoskeletal and joint disorders.*

**Intim** ICIM, Ital.
Hamamelis (p.1696·3); levomenol (p.1707·1).
*Personal hygiene.*

**Intimide** Novag, Mex.
Pregnancy test (p.1734·3).

**Intocel** Sidus, Arg.
Cladribine (p.539·3).
*Hairy-cell leukaemia.*

**Intracef** Aspen, S.Afr.
Cefuroxime sodium (p.184·1).
*Bacterial infections.*

**Intradermi** Eberth, Ger.
Troxerutin (p.1688·3); aesculus (p.1648·2).
Intradermi N formerly contained troxerutin, aesculus, and scoparium.
*Brachialgia paraesthetica; circulatory disorders.*

**Intradermi Fluid N** Eberth, Ger.†.
Dihydroxymethylrutin; aesculus (p.1648·2); benzyl nicotinate (p.21·2).
*Bath additive; musculoskeletal, joint, and soft-tissue disorders; neuralgia; peripheral vascular disorders.*

**Intradermi N** Eberth, Ger.†.
Bovine ovarian extract (p.1565·1); bovine testicular extract (p.1569·3); bovine adrenal extract.
*Musculoskeletal, joint, and soft-tissue disorders; neuralgia; peripheral vascular disorders.*

**Intradermo Cort Ant Fung** Cederroth, Spain.
Fluocinolone acetonide (p.1101·2); gramicidin (p.220·2); neomycin sulfate (p.235·1); nystatin (p.406·3).
*Infected skin disorders.*

**Intrafat** Nihon, Jpn.
Soya oil (p.1447·2).
Contains egg lecithin.
*Lipid infusion for parenteral nutrition.*

**Intrafer** Geymonat, Ital.
Iron polymaltose (p.1437·3).
*Iron deficiency; iron-deficiency anaemia.*

**Intrafusin**
Fresenius Kabi, Austria; Baxter, Ger.; Fresenius Kabi, Switz.†; Fresenius Kabi, UK.
Amino-acid infusion with or without electrolytes (p.1417·1).

**Intrafusin E** Baxter, Ger.
Amino-acid and electrolyte infusion (p.1417·1).
*Parenteral nutrition.*

**Intragam**
CSL, Austral.; Serotherapeutisches, Austria†; CSL, NZ; NBI, S.Afr.
A normal immunoglobulin (p.1627·2).
*Bone marrow transplantation; idiopathic thrombocytopenic purpura; immunodeficiency; Kawasaki disease; passive immunisation.*

**Intraglobin**
MDA, Austral.; Biotest, Austria; Biotest, Ger.; Intra Pharma, Irl.; Biotest, Thai.
A normal immunoglobulin (p.1627·2).
*Agammaglobulinaemia; Guillain-Barré syndrome; hypogammaglobulinaemia; idiopathic thrombocytopenic purpura; Kawasaki syndrome; passive immunisation; Wiskott-Aldrich syndrome.*

**Intraglobin F**
Marcos Pedrilson, Braz.†; Ionios (Ιονιος), Gr.; Biotest, Hong Kong; Biotest, Israel; Biotest, Ital.; Biotest, Malaysia; Mednostica, S.Afr.; Biotest, Singapore; Biotest, Switz.
A normal immunoglobulin (p.1627·2).
*Hypogammaglobulinaemia; idiopathic thrombocytopenic purpura; immunodeficiency disorders; Kawasaki disease; passive immunisation.*

**Intrait de Marron D'Inde P** Aerocid, Fr.
Aesculus (p.1648·2); metesculetol sodium (p.1714·1).
*Haemorrhoids.*

**Intralgin** 3M, UK†.
Benzocaine (p.1370·3); salicylamide (p.87·3).
*Musculoskeletal pain.*

**Intralgis** Urgo, Fr.
Ibuprofen (p.45·3).
*Fever; pain; peri-articular and soft-tissue disorders.*

**Intralipid**
Baxter, Austral.; Fresenius Kabi, Austria; Pharmacia Upjohn, Belg.†; Baxter, Canad.; Fresenius Kabi, Denm.; Fresenius Kabi, Fin.; Baxter, Ger.; Fresenius Kabi, Hong Kong; Pharmacia, Irl.; Pharmacia Upjohn, Israel; Fresenius Kabi, Ital.; Fresenius Kabi, Malaysia; Fresenius Kabi, Neth.; Fresenius Kabi, Norw.; Baxter, NZ; Fresenius Kabi, NZ; Fresenius Kabi, Port.; Fresenius Kabi, S.Afr.†; Fresenius Kabi, Singapore; Fresenius Kabi, Swed.; Fresenius Kabi, Switz.; Fresenius Kabi, Thai.; Fresenius Kabi, UK; Clintec, USA.
Soya oil (p.1447·2).
Contains egg phospholipids or egg lecithin.
*Lipid infusion for parenteral nutrition.*

**Intralipide** Fresenius Kabi, Fr.
Soya oil (p.1447·2).
Contains egg lecithin.
*Lipid infusion for parenteral nutrition.*

**Intralipos** Green Cross Guangzhou, Singapore.
Purified soya oil (p.1447·2).
Contains egg lecithin.
*Lipid infusion for parenteral nutrition.*

**Intramin** Baxter, Ger.
Amino-acid, carbohydrate, and electrolyte infusion (p.1417·1).
*Parenteral nutrition.*

**Intramin G** Fresenius Kabi, Austria.
Amino-acid, electrolyte, and glucose infusion (p.1417·1).
*Parenteral nutrition.*

**Intrasil** BASF, Ger.†.
Sulpiride (p.722·2).
*Depression; dizziness; Ménière's disease; schizophrenia.*

**Intrasite**
Note. This name is used for preparations of different composition.
Smith & Nephew, Austral.; Smith & Nephew, S.Afr.
Crilanomer (p.1145·1).
*Wound dressing.*

Smith & Nephew, Fr.
Carmellose sodium (p.1577·3); propylene glycol (p.1735·2).
*Leg ulcers.*

Smith & Nephew, Irl.
Hydrogel starch copolymer.
*Wounds.*

Smith & Nephew Healthcare, UK.
Carmellose (p.1577·3).
Formerly known as Scherisorb. Formerly contained hydrogel starch copolymer.
*Wound dressing.*

**Intrasol** Worndli, Switz.†.
Thymol iodide (p.1194·3).
*Oral hygiene.*

**Intrastigmina** Lusofarmaco, Ital.
Neostigmine metilsulfate (p.1492·2).
*Abdominal distension; post-operative intestinal atony; urinary retention.*

**Intraval** Aventis, NZ.
Thiopental sodium (p.1309·1).
*General anaesthesia.*

**Intraval Sodium**
Rhone-Poulenc Rorer, Hong Kong†; Aventis, Irl.; Rhone-Poulenc Rorer, S.Afr.†; Rhone-Poulenc Rorer, Thai.†; Rhone-Poulenc Rorer, UK†.
Thiopental sodium (p.1309·1).
*Convulsive states; general anaesthesia; raised intracranial pressure in neurosurgery.*

**Intra-Vite B Group plus Ascorbic Acid** Roche, Austral.
Vitamin B substances with vitamin C (p.1417·1).
*Vitamin deficiencies; vitamin supplement.*

**Intrazig** ISI, Ital.†.
A varicella-zoster immunoglobulin (p.1643·1).
*Passive immunisation.*

**Intrazolina** Torlan, Spain.
Cefazolin sodium (p.170·3).
Lidocaine hydrochloride (p.1377·3) is included in this preparation to alleviate the pain of injection.
*Bacterial infections.*

**Intricon** Great Eastern, Thai.; United American, Thai.
Ferrous fumarate (p.1427·3); vitamin B substances; liver (p.1417·1).
*Anaemias.*

**Intrimun** Biotest, Ger.†.
A normal immunoglobulin (p.1627·2).
*Immune deficiency.*

**Introcin** Andromaco, Chile.
Co-trimoxazole (p.199·3).
*Bacterial infections.*

**Introlan** Galagen, USA.
Lactose-free, gluten-free preparation for enteral nutrition (p.1417·1).

**Introlite**
Abbott, Irl.†; Abbott Nutrition, UK; Ross, USA.
Preparation for enteral nutrition (p.1417·1).

**Intron A**
Essex, Arg.; Schering-Plough, Austral.; Schering-Plough, Braz.; Schering, Canad.; Schering-Plough, Chile; Schering-Plough, Gr.; Schering-Plough, Hong Kong; Schering-Plough, Israel; Schering-Plough, Malaysia; Schering-Plough, Mex.; Schering-Plough, Neth.; Schering-Plough, NZ; Schering-Plough, Port.; Schering-Plough, S.Afr.; Schering-Plough, Singapore; Schering-Plough, Spain; Essex, Switz.; Schering, USA.
Interferon alfa-2b (rbe) (p.640·3).
*Chronic hepatitis; malignant neoplasms.*

**Intron A Peg** Essex, Arg.
Peginterferon alfa-2b (rbe) (p.643·1).
*Chronic hepatitis C.*

**Intron A/Rebetol** Essex, Switz.
Capsules, ribavirin (Rebetol) (p.652·1); injection, interferon alfa-2b (p.640·3).
*Hepatitis C.*

**IntronA**
Aesca, Austria; Schering-Plough, Norw.
Interferon alfa-2b (p.640·3).
Formerly known as Intron A in *Austria*.
*Anogenital warts; hepatitis; malignant neoplasms.*

**Introna**
Schering-Plough, Belg.; Schering-Plough, Chile; Schering-Plough, Denm.; Schering-Plough, Fin.; Schering-Plough, Fr.; Essex, Ger.; Schering-Plough, Irl.; Schering-Plough, Ital.; Schering-Plough, Swed.; Schering-Plough, Thai.; Schering-Plough, UK.
Interferon alfa-2b (rbe) (p.640·3).
Formerly known as Intron A.
*Chronic active hepatitis B; chronic hepatitis C; malignant neoplasms.*

**Intropin**
Du Pont, Canad.; Du Pont, Hong Kong; Boots, Hong Kong; Du Pont, Irl.†; Sanofi Synthelabo, S.Afr.; Du Pont, Singapore†; Bristol-Myers Squibb, Swed.; Du Pont, USA.
Dopamine hydrochloride (p.907·1).
*Shock.*

**Inulac** Corypharma, Ital.
Lactic-acid-producing organisms (p.1704·2).
*Maintenance of normal gastrointestinal flora.*

**Inutest**
Fresenius Kabi, Austria; Kemiflor, Swed.†.
Polyfructosan (Sinistrin) (p.1702·1).
*Determination of glomerular filtration rate.*

**Invanz**
Merck Sharp & Dohme, Austral.; Merck Sharp & Dohme-Chibret, Fr.; Merck Sharp & Dohme, Ger.; Merck Sharp & Dohme, Irl.; Merck Sharp & Dohme, NZ; Merck Sharp & Dohme, Singapore; Merck Sharp & Dohme, UK; Merck, USA.
Ertapenem sodium (p.207·3).
*Bacterial infections.*

**Inveoxel** Drag, Chile.
Naproxen (p.65·1).

**Inversine** Layton, USA.
Mecamylamine hydrochloride (p.951·3).
*Hypertension.*

**Invertos** Pharmacia Upjohn, Norw.†.
Anhydrous glucose (p.1432·2); fructose (p.1431·3).
*Carbohydrate source.*

**Invex** Sintofarma, Braz.
Prednicarbate (p.1107·3).
*Corticosteroid.*

**Invigan**
Note. This name is used for preparations of different composition.
Bago, Chile.
Ornidazole (p.612·2).
*Anaerobic bacterial infections; dracunculiasis; protozoal infections.*

Pliva, Spain.
Famotidine (p.1265·2).
*Gastro-oesophageal reflux; peptic ulcer; Zollinger-Ellison syndrome.*

**Invirase**
Roche, Austral.; Roche, Austria; Roche, Belg.; Roche, Braz.; Roche, Canad.; Roche, Denm.; Roche, Fin.; Roche, Fr.; Roche, Ger.; Roche, Gr.; Roche, Hong Kong; Roche, Irl.; Roche, Israel; Roche, Ital.; Roche, Jpn; Roche, Mex.†; Roche, Neth.; Roche, Norw.†; Roche, NZ; Roche, Port.†; Roche, S.Afr.; Roche, Singapore†; Roche, Spain; Roche, Swed.; Roche, Switz.; Roche, Thai.†; Roche, UK; Roche, USA.
Saquinavir mesilate (p.653·3).
*HIV infection.*

**Invoigin** Chew, Thai.
Dipyrone (p.35·3).
*Fever; pain.*

**Invoril**
Ranbaxy, Malaysia; Ranbaxy, Singapore; Ranbaxy, Thai.
Enalapril maleate (p.909·2).
*Heart failure; hypertension.*

**Invozide** Ranbaxy, India.
Enalapril maleate (p.909·2); hydrochlorothiazide (p.933·2).
*Hypertension.*

**Inxibir** Pharmacia, Arg.
Zalcitabine (p.657·1).
*HIV infection.*

**Inyesprin** Grunenthal, Spain.
Lysine aspirin (p.54·3).
*Fever; musculoskeletal, joint, and peri-articular disorders; pain; thromboembolism prophylaxis.*

**Inza**
Note. This name is used for preparations of different composition.
Alphapharm, Austral.; Alphapharm, Hong Kong; Alphapharm, Malaysia; Merck, Malaysia; Alphapharm, Singapore; Merck, Singapore.
Naproxen (p.65·1).
*Inflammation; musculoskeletal and joint disorders; pain.*

Aspen, S.Afr.
Ibuprofen (p.45·3).
*Gout; musculoskeletal and joint disorders.*

**Inzelloval** Kohler-Pharma, Ger.
Mineral preparation (p.1417·1).

**Inzitan** Kern, Spain.
Cyanocobalamin (p.1458·2); dexamethasone (p.1097·1); thiamine hydrochloride (p.1455·1).
Lidocaine hydrochloride (p.1377·3) is included in this preparation to alleviate the pain of injection.
*Musculoskeletal and joint disorders.*

**Inzolen** Kohler, Ger.
A range of electrolyte (p.1217·1) and trace element (p.1417·1) infusions.
*Electrolyte disorders; metabolic disorders.*

**Iobid DM** Iomed, USA.
Guaifenesin (p.1122·1); dextromethorphan hydrobromide (p.1117·3).
*Coughs.*

**Iocare** Ciba Vision, Ital.
Electrolytes (p.1217·1).
*Eye irrigation.*

**Iocare Balanced Salt Solution**
Iocom, UK; Novartis Ophthalmics, USA.
Electrolytes (p.1217·1).
*Eye irrigation.*

**Iocare BSS** Ciba Vision, Ger.
Electrolytes (p.1217·1).
*Eye irrigation.*

**Iocon** Healthpoint, USA†.
Coal tar (p.1159·2).
*Scalp disorders.*

**Iodal** Iomed, USA.
Hydrocodone tartrate (p.45·1); phenylephrine hydrochloride (p.1126·3); chlorphenamine maleate (p.427·3).
*Upper respiratory-tract symptoms.*

**Iodarsolo B12** Medifarma, Mex.
Iodine (p.1598·1); potassium iodide (p.1598·1); sodium arsenate (p.1747·1); vitamin $B_{12}$ (p.1458·2).

**Iodax** Rekah, Israel.
Iodine (p.1598·1); potassium iodide (p.1598·1).
*Disinfection of minor cuts and bruises.*

**Iode** Valmo, Canad.; Atlas, Canad.
Iodine (p.1598·1); potassium iodide (p.1598·1).

**Iodepol** Ache, Braz.
Potassium iodide (p.1598·1); guaifenesin (p.1122·1).
*Respiratory-tract congestion.*

**Iodermol** Heralds, Braz.†.
Iodine (p.1598·1); salicylic acid (p.1157·1); benzoic acid (p.1169·3).
*Fungal skin infections.*

**Iodesin** EMS, Braz.
Oxomemazine hydrochloride (p.438·2); potassium iodide (p.1598·1); sodium benzoate (p.1169·3); guaifenesin (p.1122·1); ipecacuanha (p.1122·3).
*Respiratory-tract congestion.*

**Iodetal**
Note. This name is used for preparations of different composition.
Sanval, Braz.†.
Potassium iodide (p.1598·1).
*Coughs.*

*Sanval, Braz.*
Sulfogaiacol (p.1131·1); potassium iodide (p.1598·1); tolu balsam (p.1131·3).
*Respiratory-tract congestion.*

**Iodeto de Potassio**
*Note. This name is used for preparations of different composition.*
*Delta, Braz.*
Potassium iodide (p.1598·1); belladonna (p.479·1); lobelia (p.1589·1); diphenhydramine hydrochloride (p.431·3).
*Coughs.*

*Sedar, Braz.*
Potassium iodide (p.1598·1); lobelia (p.1589·1); sodium benzoate (p.1169·3); sulfogaiacol (p.1131·1).
*Coughs.*

**Iodeto de Potassio Composto** *Delta, Braz.*
Potassium iodide (p.1598·1); guaifenesin (p.1122·1); carbinoxamine (p.426·3).
*Respiratory-tract congestion.*

**Iodeto de Potassium Composto** *Farmedica, Braz.*
Potassium iodide (p.1598·1); oxomemazine (p.438·2).
*Respiratory-tract congestion.*

**Iodeton** *Cazi, Braz.*
Potassium iodide (p.1598·1).
*Coughs.*

**Iodetoss** *Ducto, Braz.*
Potassium iodide (p.1598·1).
*Coughs.*

**Iodex**
*Qualiphar, Belg.; Lee, USA.*
Povidone-iodine (p.1190·3).
*Disinfection of skin and instruments; infected skin disorders.*

*Novamed, Braz.*
Iodine (p.1598·1).
*Skin infections.*

**Iodex com Salicilato de Metila** *Novamed, Braz.*
Iodine (p.1598·1); methyl salicylate (p.59·3).
*Musculoskeletal and joint disorders.*

**Iodex with Methyl Salicylate** *Medtech, USA.*
Iodine (p.1598·1); methyl salicylate (p.59·3).
*Muscle, joint, and soft-tissue pain; neuralgia.*

**Iodiflor** *Floris, Israel.*
Povidone-iodine (p.1190·3).
*Skin disinfection.*

**Iodina** *Orravan, Spain.*
Povidone-iodine (p.1190·3).
*Skin, wound, and burn disinfection.*

**Iodisis** *Prisfar, Port.*
Iodine (p.1598·1).
*Mouth and throat infections and inflammation.*

**Iodoasept** *ICN, Arg.*
Povidone-iodine (p.1190·3).
*Eye disinfection.*

**Iodobec** *Farmedica, Braz.†.*
Potassium iodide (p.1598·1); guaifenesin (p.1122·1); sodium benzoate (p.1169·3); oxomemazine (p.438·2); ipecacuanha (p.1122·3).
*Respiratory-tract congestion.*

**Iodocaine** *Sedabel, Braz.†.*
Lidocaine hydrochloride (p.1377·3); povidone (p.1190·3).
*Skin infections.*

**Iodocid** *Bergamon, Ital.†.*
Povidone-iodine (p.1190·3).
*Skin disinfection.*

**Iodoflex**
*Smith & Nephew, Austral.†; Smith & Nephew, Irl.; Smith & Nephew, Singapore; Smith & Nephew Healthcare, UK.*
Cadexomer-iodine (p.1172·1).
*Leg ulcers; wounds.*

**Iodomax** *Lafedar, Arg.*
Povidone-iodine (p.1190·3).
*Skin disinfection.*

**Iodopen** *American Pharmaceutical, USA.*
Sodium iodide (p.1598·1).
*Additive for intravenous total parenteral nutrition solutions.*

**Iodophil Viscous** *FDC, India.*
Sodium acetrizoate.
*Hysterosalpingography.*

**Iodopulmin** *Neckerman, Braz.†.*
Potassium iodide (p.1598·1); pepilamine maleate; ipecacuanha (p.1122·3); sodium benzoate (p.1169·3); guaifenesin (p.1122·1).
*Coughs.*

**Iodosan Collutorio** *SmithKline Beecham, Ital.†.*
Iodine (p.1598·1).
*Oral hygiene.*

**Iodosorb**
*Smith & Nephew, Austral.; Lannacher, Austria; Smith & Nephew, Canad.; Smith & Nephew, Denm.; Smith & Nephew, Fin.; Smith & Nephew, Ger.; Smith & Nephew, Ital.; Smith & Nephew, Singapore; Smith & Nephew, Spain; Smith & Nephew, Swed.; Smith & Nephew, Switz.; Smith & Nephew Healthcare, UK.*
Cadexomer-iodine (p.1172·1).
*Skin ulcers; wounds.*

**Iodosteril** *IMS, Ital.*
Povidone-iodine (p.1190·3).
*Skin disinfection.*

**Iodoten** *Pierrel, Ital.*
Povidone-iodine (p.1190·3).
*Wound disinfection.*

**Iodotiazol** *Ferro, Arg.*
Aminobenzene sulfonamide thiazol sodium; sulfanilamide (p.263·2) benzocaine (p.1370·3); iodine (p.1598·1); potassium iodide (p.1598·1).
*Mouth and throat disorders.*

**Iodotope** *Squibb Diagnostics, USA.*
Iodine-131 (p.1524·2) as sodium iodide.
*Hyperthyroidism; thyroid cancer.*

**Iodo-Vit** *Vitamed, Israel.*
Povidone-iodine (p.1190·3).
*Skin and wound disinfection.*

**Iofed** *Iomed, USA.*
Brompheniramine maleate (p.426·1); pseudoephedrine hydrochloride (p.1129·2).
*Upper respiratory-tract symptoms.*

**Iofoscal** *Virtus, Braz.†.*
Guarana (p.1765·3); kola (p.1765·3); minerals (p.1417·1).
*Nutritional supplement.*

**Iohist D** *Iomed, USA†.*
Phenylpropanolamine hydrochloride (p.1127·3); phenyltoloxamine citrate (p.439·1); mepyramine maleate (p.437·1); pheniramine maleate (p.438·3).
*Respiratory-tract disorders.*

**Iohist DM** *Iomed, USA†.*
Dextromethorphan hydrobromide (p.1117·3); phenylpropanolamine hydrochloride (p.1127·3); brompheniramine maleate (p.426·1).
*Upper respiratory-tract symptoms.*

**Ioimbina Composta**
*Note. This name is used for preparations of different composition.*
*Delta, Braz.†.*
Yohimbine hydrochloride (p.1766·2); vitamin B substances; inositol (p.1417·1).
*Erectile dysfunction.*

*Neo Quimica, Braz.†.*
Methyltestosterone (p.1559·3); yohimbine hydrochloride (p.1766·2); vitamin E (p.1464·3); caffeine (p.782·1); ephedrine (p.1120·1).
*Erectile dysfunction.*

**Ioiro** *Regional Health, NZ.*
Ioidol.
*Radiographic contrast medium.*

**Iol** *Quimioterapica, Braz.*
Potassium iodide (p.1598·1); guaifenesin (p.1122·1); sodium benzoate (p.1169·3); lobelia (p.1589·1).
*Coughs.*

**Iolin** *Quimioterapica, Braz.*
Potassium iodide (p.1598·1); lobelia (p.1589·1).
*Coughs.*

**Iolin NPH** *Biobras, Braz.†.*
Isophane insulin injection (bovine and porcine, highly purified) (p.333·3).
*Diabetes mellitus.*

**Iolin Regular** *Biobras, Braz.†.*
Insulin injection (bovine and porcine, highly purified) (p.333·3).
*Diabetes mellitus.*

**Iomeron**
*Regional Health, Austral.; Gerot, Austria; Byk, Belg.; Bracco, Denm.; Astra Tech, Fin.; Byk, Fr.; Gerolimatos (Γερολυματος), Gr.; Merck, Irl.; Bracco, Israel; Bracco, Ital.; Eisai, Jpn; Byk, Neth.; Astra Tech, Norw.; Regional Health, NZ; Bracco, Port.; Rovi, Spain; Astra Tech, Swed.; Bracco, Switz.; Merck, UK.*
Iomeprol (p.1064·3).
*Radiographic contrast medium.*

**Ionamin**
*Celltech, Belg.†; Aventis, Canad.; Pharmacia, Malaysia; Rhone-Poulenc Rorer, Mex.†; Pharmacia, Singapore; Cambridge Healthcare, UK†; Celltech, USA.*
Phentermine (as an ion-exchange resin complex) (p.1592·2).
*Obesity.*

**Ionamine** *Medeva, Switz.*
Phentermine (as an ion-exchange resin complex) (p.1592·2).
*Obesity.*

**Ionarthrol** *Picot, Fr.*
Copper gluconate (p.1425·3).
Formerly contained manganese sulfate, magnesium sulfate, calcium chloride, nickel chloride, ferrous sulfate, and sodium sulfate.
*Joint disorders; viral infections.*

**Ionax Astringent** *Healthpoint, USA.*
Salicylic acid (p.1157·1); allantoin (p.1141·3).
*Acne.*

**Ionax Foam** *Healthpoint, USA.*
Skin cleanser.

**Ionax P**
*Galderma, Fr.; Galderma, Spain.*
Piroctone olamine (p.1155·2); salicylic acid (p.1157·1).
*Scalp disorders.*

**Ionax Scrub**
*Galderma, Arg.; Galderma, Austral.†; Galderma, Braz.; Galderma, Chile; Galderma, Fr.; Galderma, Hong Kong; Galderma, Irl.; Galderma, Mex.; Galderma, Singapore; Galderma, Thai.†; Galderma, UK†; Healthpoint, USA.*
Polyethylene granules (abrasive) (p.1140·1).
*Acne.*

**Ionax T**
*Galderma, Fr.†; Galderma, Port.†.*
Coal tar (p.1159·2); salicylic acid (p.1157·1).
*Seborrhoeic dermatitis.*

**Ionet** *Cetus, Arg.*
Loperamide (p.1271·2).
*Diarrhoea.*

**Ionil**
*Note. This name is used for preparations of different composition.*
*Galderma, Austral.; Galderma, Braz.†; Galderma, Canad.†; Galderma, Mex.; Healthpoint, USA.*
Salicylic acid (p.1157·1).
*Seborrhoeic dermatitis.*

*Lavipharm, Gr.*
Coal tar (p.1159·2).
*Chronic eczema; psoriasis; seborrhoeic dermatitis.*

*Galderma, Spain.*
Coal tar (p.1159·2); salicylic acid (p.1157·1).
*Scalp disorders.*

**Ionil Champu** *Galderma, Spain.*
Coal tar (p.1159·2); salicylic acid (p.1157·1).
*Scalp disorders.*

**Ionil P** *Galderma, Port.*
Piroctone olamine (p.1155·2); salicylic acid (p.1157·1).
*Scalp disorders.*

**Ionil Plus**
*Galderma, Braz.†; Galderma, Mex.; Healthpoint, USA.*
Salicylic acid (p.1157·1).
*Scalp psoriasis; seborrhoeic dermatitis.*

**Ionil Rinse**
*Galderma, Austral.; Galderma, NZ.*
Hydrolised collagen proteins (p.1674·3).
*Dry brittle hair.*

**Ionil-T**
*Note. This name is used for preparations of different composition.*
*Galderma, Arg.; Galderma, Austral.; Galderma, Braz.†; Galderma, Chile; Galderma, Hong Kong; Galderma, Irl.; Galderma, Ital.†; Galderma, Mex.; Galderma, NZ; Galderma, Singapore; Galderma, Thai.; Galderma, UK†; Healthpoint, USA.*
Coal tar (p.1159·2); salicylic acid (p.1157·1).
*Scalp disorders.*

*Galderma, Canad.†.*
Coal tar (p.1159·2).
*Scalp disorders.*

**Ionil-T Plus**
*Note. This name is used for preparations of different composition.*
*Galderma, Arg.; Galderma, Austral.; Galderma, Canad.†; Galderma, Mex.; Healthpoint, USA.*
Coal tar (Owentar II) (p.1159·2).
*Scalp disorders.*

*Galderma, Braz.†.*
Salicylic acid (p.1157·1).
*Scalp psoriasis; seborrhoeic dermatitis.*

**Ionimag** *Byk, Fr.*
Magnesium lactate (p.1228·1).
*Magnesium deficiency.*

**Ionitan** *Aguettant, Fr.*
Electrolyte infusion (p.1217·1).
*Parenteral nutrition.*

**Ionosteril** *Fresenius Kabi, Port.*
Electrolyte infusion with or without glucose (p.1217·1).
*Plasma substitute.*

**Ion-Sol** *Berman, Mex.*
Electrolytes (p.1217·1).
*Electrolyte imbalance.*

**Ionyl** *Pharmadeveloppement, Fr.*
Phosphoric acid (p.1731·2); sodium glycerophosphate (p.1695·2); magnesium glycerophosphate (p.1228·1); manganese glycerophosphate (p.1695·2).
*Tonic.*

**Iopamiro**
*Astra Tech, Denm.; Astra Tech, Fin.†; Bracco, Israel; Bracco, Ital.; Astra Tech, Norw.; Regional Health, NZ; Bracco, Port.; Rovi, Spain; Astra Tech, Swed.; Bracco, Switz.*
Iopamidol (p.1064·3).
*Radiographic contrast medium.*

**Iopamiro 200, 300, and 370** *Gerolimatos (Γερολυματος), Gr.*
Iopamidol (p.1064·3).
*Radiographic contrast medium.*

**Iopamiron**
*Schering, Arg.; Schering, Braz.†; Schering, Fr.*
Iopamidol (p.1064·3).
*Radiographic contrast medium.*

**Iopanchol** *Genepharm, Gr.*
Sodium cromoglicate (p.795·3).
*Allergic conjunctivitis.*

**Iophen** *Rugby, USA.*
Iodinated glycerol (p.1122·3).
*Coughs.*

**Iopidine**
*Alcon, Arg.; Alcon, Austral.; Alcon, Austria; Alcon, Belg.; Alcon, Braz.; Alcon, Canad.; Alcon, Chile; Alcon, Denm.; Alcon, Fin.; Alcon, Fr.; Alcon, Ger.; Alkon (Αλκον), Gr.; Alcon, Hong Kong; Alcon, Irl.; Alcon, Israel; Alcon, Ital.; Alcon, Jpn; Alcon, Malaysia; Alcon, Mex.†; Alcon, Norw.; Alcon, NZ; Alcon, Port.; Alcon, S.Afr.; Alcon, Singapore; Alcon, Swed.; Alcon, Switz.; Alcon, UK; Alcon, USA.*
Apraclonidine hydrochloride (p.864·1).
*Control of intra-ocular pressure following eye surgery; glaucoma; ocular hypertension.*

**Iopimax** *Alcon Cusi, Spain.*
Apraclonidine hydrochloride (p.864·1).
*Glaucoma; prevention of ocular hypertension in laser surgery.*

**Ior T3**
*Bago, Chile; Pisa, Mex.*
Muromonab-CD3 (p.1360·3).
*Renal transplant rejection.*

**Iosal II** *Iomed, USA.*
Pseudoephedrine (p.1129·2); guaifenesin (p.1122·1).
*Coughs.*

**Iosalide** *Yamanouchi, Ital.*
Josamycin (p.224·3) or josamycin propionate (p.224·3).
*Bacterial infections.*

**Iosopan** *Goldline, USA.*
Magaldrate (p.1271·3).
*Hyperacidity.*

**Iosopan Plus** *Goldline, USA.*
Magaldrate (p.1271·3); simeticone (p.1289·2).
*Hyperacidity.*

**Iotrovist** *Schering, Port.†.*
Iotrolan (p.1066·1).
*Radiographic contrast medium.*

**Iotussin HC** *Iomed, USA.*
Hydrocodone tartrate (p.45·1); phenylephrine hydrochloride (p.1126·3); chlorphenamine maleate (p.427·3).
*Upper respiratory-tract symptoms.*

**Ipacef** *IPA, Ital.*
Cefuroxime sodium (p.184·1).
*Gram-negative bacterial infections.*

**Ipacid** *IPA, Ital.*
Cefonicid sodium (p.174·2).
Lidocaine hydrochloride (p.1377·3) is included in this preparation to alleviate the pain of injection.
*Gram-negative bacterial infections.*

**Ipagastril** *IPA, Ital.*
Sucralfate (p.1290·2).
*Gastritis; gastro-oesophageal reflux; peptic ulcer.*

**Ipalat** *Pfleger, Ger.†.*
*Ointment:* Pumilio pine oil (p.1737·1); eucalyptus oil (p.1686·2).
*Pastilles:* Primula root (p.1735·1).
*Respiratory-tract disorders.*

**Ipamicina** *IPA, Ital.*
Fosfomycin calcium (p.214·2).
*Bacterial infections.*

**Ipamix** *Gentili, Ital.*
Indapamide (p.938·2).
*Hypertension.*

**Iparen** *NCSN, Ital.†.*
Suleparoid (p.1009·1).
*Thrombosis prophylaxis.*

**Ipatox** *IPA, Ital.*
Reduced glutathione sodium (p.1040·3).
*Alcohol and drug poisoning; radiation trauma.*

**Ipatrizina** *IPA, Ital.*
Propylene glycol cefatrizine (p.170·3).
*Bacterial infections.*

**Ipaviran** *NCSN, Ital.*
Aciclovir (p.626·1).
*Herpesvirus infections.*

**Ipavit** *IPA, Ital.*
Vitamin B substances with calcium folinate (p.1417·1)(p.1431·1).

**Ipazone** *IPA, Ital.*
Cefoperazone sodium (p.174·3).
Lidocaine hydrochloride (p.1377·3) is included in this preparation to alleviate the pain of injection.
*Gram-negative bacterial infections.*

**Ipcacin Kid** *Ipca, India.*
Rifampicin (p.250·2); isoniazid (p.222·2); vitamin $B_6$ (p.1457·2).
*Tuberculosis.*

**Ipcamox** *Nat Druggists, S.Afr.*
Amoxicillin trihydrate (p.155·3).
*Bacterial infections.*

**Ipcazide** *Ipca, India.*
Isoniazid (p.222·2); vitamin $B_6$ (p.1457·2).
*Tuberculosis.*

**Ipeca**
*Note. This name is used for preparations of different composition.*
*Orion, Fin.*
Ipecacuanha (p.1122·3).
*Poisoning.*

*Amino, Switz.*
Emetine hydrochloride (p.604·3); ethylmorphine hydrochloride (p.37·3); ephedrine hydrochloride (p.1120·1); codeine phosphate (p.27·1); cherry-laurel water; tolu balsam (p.1131·3).
*Respiratory-tract disorders.*

**Ipecavom** *Elpen (Ελπεν), Gr.*
Ipecacuanha (p.1122·3).
*Induction of vomiting in poisoning.*

**Ipecol** *Simoes, Braz.*
Noscapine (p.1125·3); sodium benzoate (p.1169·3); sulfogaiacol (p.1131·1); tolu balsam (p.1131·3); ipecacuanha (p.1122·3).
*Coughs.*

**Ipercortis** *AGIPS, Ital.*
Triamcinolone (p.1110·2).
*Corticosteroid.*

**Iperisan** *Marjan, Braz.*
Hypericum (p.299·1).
*Depression.*

**Iperiton** *Lampugnani, Ital.†.*
Multivitamin and mineral preparation with hypericum and dog rose (p.1417·1).
*Nutritional supplement.*

**Iperix** *Palmares, Ital.†.*
Inositol; vitamin $B_6$; hypericum (p.1417·1).
*Nutritional supplement.*

**Iperplasin** *CSC, Austria.*
Mepartricin (p.405·2).
*Benign prostatic hyperplasia.*

**Iperten** Chiesi, Ital.
Manidipine hydrochloride (p.950·2).
*Hypertension.*

**Ipertrofan** SPA, Ital.
Mepartricin (p.405·2).
*Benign prostatic hyperplasia.*

**Ipervital** IDI, Ital.†.
Nutritional supplement (p.1417·1).

**Ipesandrine** Novartis Consumer, Port.
Dextromethorphan hydrobromide (p.1117·3); ephedrine hydrochloride (p.1120·1).
*Coughs.*

**Ipesil** Antigen, Irl.†.
Ipecacuanha (p.1122·3); squill (p.1130·3).
*Coughs.*

**Ipetitrin** Agepha, Austria.
Ipecacuanha (p.1122·3).
*Bronchitis; coughs.*

**Ipnopen** Recalcine, Chile.
Flunitrazepam (p.698·2).
*Insomnia.*

**Ipnovel** Roche, Ital.
Midazolam (p.707·1).
*General anaesthesia; premedication; sedative.*

**Ipoazotal** SIT, Ital.
Arginine hydrochloride (p.1421·1); ornithine hydrochloride (p.1442·3); citrulline (p.1425·2).
*Hyperammonaemia.*

**Ipoazotal Complex** SIT, Ital.
Arginine hydrochloride (p.1421·1); ornithine hydrochloride (p.1442·3); citrulline (p.1425·2); acetyl aspartate; aceglumic acid; calcium oxoglurate.
*Hyperammonaemia.*

**Ipocalcin** Salus, Ital.
Calcitonin (salmon) (p.768·2).
*Hypercalcaemia; osteoporosis; Paget's disease of bone; reflex sympathetic dystrophy.*

**Ipocol**
Note. This name is used for preparations of different composition.
Lagap, Switz.
Divistyramine (p.905·3).
*Biliary-tract disorders; hypercholesterolaemia.*

Sandoz, UK.
Mesalazine (p.1273·2).
*Ulcerative colitis.*

**Ipocromo** Ripari-Gero, Ital.†.
Sodium ferric gluconate complex (p.1444·3).
*Iron-deficiency anaemias.*

**Ipogen** Gentili, Ital.†.
Dihydralazine tartrate (p.900·1); chlorothiazide (p.882·1).
*Hypertension.*

**Ipoglusan** Bioquimico, Mex.†.
Tolbutamide (p.348·1).
*Diabetes mellitus.*

**Ipogras** Laboratorios Chile, Chile.
Sibutramine (p.1593·2).
*Obesity.*

**Ipol**
Aventis Pasteur, Austral.; CSL, NZ; Pasteur Merieux, USA.
An inactivated poliomyelitis vaccine (p.1633·3).
*Active immunisation.*

**Ipolab** Finmedical, Ital.
Labetalol hydrochloride (p.943·3).
*Hypertension.*

**Ipolipid**
Medochemie, Hong Kong; Medochemie, Malaysia; Medochemie, Singapore; Medochemie, Thai.†.
Gemfibrozil (p.923·1).
*Hyperlipidaemias.*

**Ipomex** Armstrong, Arg.
Sibutramine hydrochloride (p.1593·1).
*Obesity.*

**Iposeb** Rydelle, Fr.†.
Amino-acid, vitamin, and mineral preparation (p.1417·1).
*Seborrhoea.*

**Ippi Verde** Henkel, Ital.
Triclosan (Irgasan DP 300) (p.1195·2).
*Skin and hand disinfection.*

**Ipra** Pacific, NZ.
Ipratropium bromide (p.787·1).
*Obstructive airways disease.*

**Iprabon** Zambon, Braz.
Ipratropium bromide (p.787·1).
*Obstructive airways disease.*

**Iprabron** Prieto, Arg.
Ipratropium bromide (p.787·1).
*Obstructive airways disease.*

**Ipradol**
Nycomed, Austria; Nycomed, Hong Kong; Aspen, S.Afr.; Lacer, Spain†; Nycomed, Thai.
Hexoprenaline (p.786·3), hexoprenaline hydrochloride (p.786·3), or hexoprenaline sulfate (p.786·3).
*Obstructive airways disease; prevention of uterine contractions.*

**Iprafen** Chiesi, Ital.
Fenoterol hydrobromide (p.785·2); ipratropium bromide (p.787·1).
*Obstructive airways disease.*

**Ipragocce** Proge, Ital.
Benzalkonium chloride (p.1168·3); hypromellose (p.1579·3).
*Eye disinfection; eye irritation.*

**Ipral** Bristol-Myers Squibb, Irl.
Trimethoprim (p.272·2).
*Bacterial urinary- and respiratory-tract infections.*

**Ipraneo** Neo Quimica, Braz.
Ipratropium bromide (p.787·1).
*Obstructive airways disease.*

**Ipratrin** Alphapharm, Austral.
Ipratropium bromide (p.787·1).
*Obstructive airways disease.*

**Ipravent**
Pharmacia, Austral.; Apotex, Hong Kong; Cipla, India.
Ipratropium bromide (p.787·1).
*Obstructive airways disease.*

**Ipren**
Nycomed, Denm.; Pharmacia, Swed.
Ibuprofen (p.45·3).
*Fever; inflammation; musculoskeletal and joint disorders; pain.*

**Ipri V** Vannier, Arg.
Vitamin E acetate; vitamin C; betacarotene (p.1417·1).
*Antioxidant preparation.*

**Ipriosten** Pharmacia, Arg.
Ipriflavone (p.773·2).
*Osteoporosis.*

**Iprivask** Aventis, USA.
Desirudin (p.892·3).
*Deep-vein thrombosis prophylaxis following hip replacement.*

**Iproben** Mepha, Switz.
Ibuprofen (p.45·3).
*Fever; pain.*

**Iprogel** Mepha, Switz.
Ibuprofen (p.45·3).
*Musculoskeletal, joint, peri-articular and soft-tissue pain and inflammation.*

**Iprosten** Takeda, Ital.
Ipriflavone (p.773·2).
*Osteoporosis.*

**Ipsatol**
Note. A similar name is used for preparations of different composition (see below).
Orion, Fin.
Biperiden hydrochloride (p.479·3) or biperiden lactate (p.479·3).
*Drug-induced extrapyramidal disorders; parkinsonism; trigeminal neuralgia.*

**Ipsatol Cough Formula Liquid for Children and Adults**
Note. A similar name is used for preparations of different composition (see above).
Kenwood, USA†.
Guaifenesin (p.1122·1); dextromethorphan hydrobromide (p.1117·3); phenylpropanolamine hydrochloride (p.1127·3).
*Coughs.*

**Ipser Europe** Pasteur Vaccins, Fr.†.
A snake venom antiserum (*Vipera ammodytes, V. aspis,* and *V. berus*) (p.1639·1).
*Viper bites.*

**Ipsilon**
Bristol-Myers Squibb, Arg.; Nikkho, Braz.
Aminocaproic acid (p.741·3).
*Fibrinolytic haemorrhage.*

**Ipson** Saval, Chile.
Ibuprofen (p.45·3).
*Fever; inflammation; pain.*

**Ipsovir** Ipso, Ital.
Aciclovir (p.626·1).
*Herpesvirus infections.*

**Ipstyl**
Ipsen, Denm.; Ipsen, Ital.; Ipsen, Norw.
Lanreotide (p.1331·1) or lanreotide acetate (p.1330·3).
*Acromegaly; carcinoid tumours.*

**IPV** Aventis Pasteur, Braz.†.
An inactivated poliomyelitis vaccine (p.1633·3).
*Active immunisation.*

**IPV Merieux** Aventis Pasteur, Ger.
An inactivated poliomyelitis vaccine (type 1, 2, and 3) (p.1633·3).
*Active immunisation.*

**Ipvent** Cipla-Medpro, S.Afr.
Ipratropium bromide (p.787·1).
*Obstructive airways disease.*

**IPV-Virelon** Chiron Behring, Ger.
An inactivated poliomyelitis vaccine (type I, II, and III) (p.1633·3).
*Active immunisation.*

**Iqfacilina** IQFA, Mex.
Ampicillin (p.157·1).
*Bacterial infections.*

**Iqfadina** IQFA, Mex.
Ranitidine hydrochloride (p.1285·2).
*Acid aspiration; gastrointestinal haemorrhage; peptic ulcer; Zollinger-Ellison syndrome.*

**Iqfamicina** IQFA, Mex.
Erythromycin (p.208·1).
*Bacterial infections.*

**Iqfasol** IQFA, Mex.
Naproxen (p.65·1).
*Musculoskeletal and joint disorders.*

**Irban** Bristol-Myers Squibb, Israel.
Irbesartan (p.940·1).
*Hypertension.*

**Irban Plus** Bristol-Myers Squibb, Israel.
Irbesartan (p.940·1); hydrochlorothiazide (p.933·2).
*Hypertension.*

**Ircon** Kenwood, USA.
Iron carbonyl (p.1436·1).
Formerly contained ferrous fumarate.
*Iron-deficiency anaemias.*

**Ircon-FA** Kenwood, USA.
Iron carbonyl (p.1436·1); folic acid (p.1429·1).
Formerly contained ferrous fumarate and folic acid.
*Iron-deficiency anaemias.*

**Iremofar** Unipharma, Gr.
Hydroxyzine hydrochloride (p.434·3).
*Hypersensitivity reactions.*

**Irenat**
Kolassa, Austria; Bayer, Ger.
Sodium perchlorate (p.1603·3).
*Adjunct in radionuclide brain scanning; hyperthyroidism.*

**Irenax** Labinca, Arg.
Irinotecan hydrochloride (p.564·1).
*Malignant neoplasms.*

**Irene** Pharmaland, Thai.†.
Astemizole (p.424·2).
*Allergic conjunctivitis; allergic rhinitis; urticaria.*

**Irenor** Juste, Spain.
Reboxetine mesilate (p.316·3).
*Depression.*

**Iressa**
AstraZeneca, UK; AstraZeneca, USA.
Gefitinib (p.557·3).
*Non-small cell lung cancer.*

**Irfen** Mepha, Switz.
Ibuprofen (p.45·3).
*Musculoskeletal and joint disorders; pain.*

**Irgaman** Rusch, Ital.
Triclosan (Irgasan DP 300) (p.1195·2).
*Skin disinfection.*

**Irgamid**
Novartis, Denm.; Novartis, Fin.; Ciba Vision, Neth.†; Novartis Ophthalmics, Switz.
Sulfadicramide (p.259·2).
*Bacterial eye infections.*

**Iricalcin** Vocate, Gr.
Calcitonin (p.768·2).
*Hypercalcaemia; osteoporosis; Paget's disease of bone.*

**Iricil** Cantabria, Spain.
Lisinopril (p.946·3).
*Diabetic nephropathy; heart failure; hypertension; myocardial infarction.*

**Iricil Plus** Cantabria, Spain.
Lisinopril (p.946·3); hydrochlorothiazide (p.933·2).
*Hypertension.*

**Iridina Due** Montefarmaco, Ital.
Naphazoline hydrochloride (p.1124·3).
*Eye irritation.*

**Iridina Light** Montefarmaco, Ital.
Benzalkonium chloride (p.1168·3).
*Eye disinfection; eye irritation.*

**Iridus**
Aventis, Arg.
Naftidrofuryl oxalate (p.964·1).
*Cerebral and peripheral vascular disorders.*

Aventis, Mex.
Naftidrofuryl (p.964·1).
*Peripheral vascular disorders.*

**Iridux** Aventis, Braz.†.
Naftidrofuryl (p.964·1).
*Vascular disorders.*

**Irigal** Gobbi, Arg.
Neomycin sulfate (p.235·1); hydrocortisone (p.1103·3); lidocaine (p.1377·3); boric acid (p.1662·1); zinc oxide (p.1163·2).
*Wounds.*

**Irilens** Montefarmaco, Ital.
Sodium hyaluronate (p.1697·3).
*Dry eyes.*

**Iriniozol** Rafarm, Gr.
Dexamethasone dipropionate (p.1097·3).
*Allergic rhinitis.*

**Irinogen** Gautier, Arg.
Irinotecan hydrochloride (p.564·1).
*Colorectal cancer.*

**Irinotel** Dabur, India.
Irinotecan (p.564·3).
*Colorectal cancer.*

**Iris Med Complex** Dynamit, Austria.
Homoeopathic preparation.

**Iri-Sol** Ocumed, USA.
Eye irrigation.

**Iristamina** Montefarmaco, Ital.
Thonzylamine hydrochloride (p.442·2); naphazoline nitrate (p.1124·3).
*Conjunctivitis; eye irritation.*

**Irix** Gramon, Arg.
Ephedrine (p.1120·1); phenazone (p.82·3).
*Eye disorders.*

**Irix Lagrimas** Gramon, Arg.
Macrogol 400 (p.1709·1); hypromellose (p.1579·3); glycerol (p.1694·3).
*Dry eyes.*

**Irocombivit** Schmidgall, Austria†.
Multivitamin preparation (p.1417·1).

**Irocopar c C** Schmidgall, Austria.
Carbasalate calcium (p.25·1); paracetamol (p.76·2); codeine phosphate (p.27·1).
*Pain.*

**Irocophan** Schmidgall, Austria.
Carbasalate calcium (p.25·1); paracetamol (p.76·2); caffeine (p.782·1).
*Fever; pain.*

**Iromin** Schmidgall, Austria.
Carbasalate calcium (p.25·1).
*Cold symptoms; fever; pain.*

**Iromin-Chinin-C** Schmidgall, Austria.
Carbasalate calcium (p.25·1); quinine hydrochloride (p.460·2); calcium ascorbate (p.1460·2).
*Cold symptoms; fever; pain.*

**Iromin-G** Mission Pharmacal, USA.
Ferrous gluconate (p.1428·1); folic acid (p.1429·1); multivitamins and minerals (p.1417·1).
*Iron-deficiency anaemias.*

**Iron Complex** Jamieson, Canad.†.
Multivitamin and mineral preparation (p.1417·1).

**Iron Compound** Blackmores, Austral.†.
Sodium sulfate (p.1290·1); ferrous phosphate; potassium chloride (p.1232·2).
*Iron deficiency.*

**Iron Plus**
Cenovis, Austral.†; Vitelle, Austral.†.
Multivitamin preparation with iron (p.1417·1).
*Tonic; vitamin and iron supplement.*

Swiss Herbal, Canad.
Multivitamin and mineral preparation (p.1417·1).

**Ironax** Caber, Ital.†.
Ferrous gluconate (p.1428·1).
*Iron deficiency; iron-deficiency anaemia.*

**Ironfer** Uniao Quimica, Braz.
Ferrous sulfate (p.1428·2).
*Iron-deficiency anaemia.*

**Ironorm** Wallace Mfg Chem., UK.
*Capsules:* Dried ferrous sulfate (p.1428·3); folic acid (p.1429·1); vitamin B substances; vitamin C (p.1417·1).
*Oral drops:* Ferrous sulfate (p.1428·2).
*Syrup:* Ferric ammonium citrate (p.1427·2); vitamin B substances; minerals (p.1417·1).
*Iron deficiency.*

**Irontona** Brauer, Austral.†.
Angelica (p.1655·1); ascorbic acid (p.1460·2); kola (p.1765·3); ferrous sulfate (p.1428·2); hypericum (p.299·1); ginseng (p.1693·1); urtica (p.1762·1); aurum muriaticum; calcarea phosphorica; ferrum metallicum; ferrum phosphoricum; kali phosphoricum; magnesia phosphorica; phosphoric acid.
*Tonic.*

**Iroplex** Bioquimico, Arg.
Cinnarizine (p.428·3).
*Vertigo.*

**Irospan** Fielding, USA.
Ferrous sulfate (p.1428·2).
Ascorbic acid (p.1460·2) is included in this preparation to increase the absorption and availability of iron.
*Iron-deficiency anaemias.*

**Irovel** Sun, India.
Irbesartan (p.940·1).
*Hypertension.*

**Iroviton-Irocombivit** Schmidgall, Austria.
Multivitamin preparation with hesperidin (p.1417·1).

**Iroviton-Irocovit-C** Schmidgall, Austria.
Ascorbic acid (p.1460·2) or sodium ascorbate (p.1460·2).
*Vitamin C supplement.*

**Irradial** Armstrong, Arg.
Sertraline hydrochloride (p.317·2).
*Depression; obsessive-compulsive disorder; phobias.*

**Irriclens**
Convatec, Fr.; Convatec, UK.
Sodium chloride (p.1233·3).
*Wound cleansing and irrigation.*

**Irrigacion CLNA** Bieffe, Spain.
Sodium chloride (p.1233·3).
*Bladder irrigation.*

**Irrigor** Andromaco, Chile.
Flunarizine (p.434·2).
*Cerebral and peripheral vascular disorders; vestibular disorders.*

**Irritos** Faes, Spain†.
Phenylpropanolamine hydrochloride (p.1127·3); dextromethorphan hydrobromide (p.1117·3).
*Coughs; nasal congestion.*

**Irritren**
Byk, Austria; Tosse, Ger.†; Byk Gulden, Hong Kong†.
Lonazolac calcium (p.54·2).
*Inflammation; musculoskeletal, joint, and soft-tissue disorders; pain.*

**Irrodan**
Biomedica, Hong Kong; Biomedica, Ital.; Biomedica, Thai.
Buflomedil hydrochloride (p.877·2).
*Cerebral and peripheral vascular disorders.*

**IRS 19**
Solvay, Fr.
Lysates of *Streptococcus pneumoniae; Streptococcus* group G; *Streptococcus pyogenes; Staphylococcus aureus; Acinetobacter calcoaceticus; Neisseria subflava; Klebsiella pneumoniae; Moraxella catarrhalis; Haemophilus influenzae; Streptococcus dysgalactiae; Enterococcus faecium; Enterococcus faecalis* (p.1704·2).
*Respiratory-tract disorders.*

Hefa, Ger.
Lysate of: *Streptococcus pneumoniae; Streptococcus pyogenes; Enterococcus faecalis* (p.1704·2); *Staphylococcus aureus; Moraxella catarrhalis; Neisseria flava;*

*Neisseria perflava; Haemophilus influenzae; Klebsiella pneumoniae; Gaffkya tetragena; Moraxella.*
*Respiratory-tract infections.*

**Irtan** Aventis, Ger.; Rhone-Poulenc Rorer, Mex.†.
Nedocromil sodium (p.789·3).
*Allergic conjunctivitis; allergic rhinitis; keratoconjunctivitis.*

**Irtonin** Takeda, Ital.
Protirelin tartrate (p.1338·2).
*Mental function disorders.*

**Irudil** Roche, Austria†.
Hirudin (p.931·2).
*Peripheral vascular disorders.*

**Iruxol** Abbott, Arg.; Knoll, Braz.; Smith & Nephew, Fin.; Smith & Nephew, Ital.
Collagenase (p.1675·1); chloramphenicol (p.185·1).
*Skin infections; skin ulcers and wounds.*

**Iruxol Mono** Smith & Nephew, Fin.; Smith & Nephew, Hong Kong; Smith & Nephew, Irl.; Smith & Nephew, S.Afr.; Smith & Nephew, Spain; Smith & Nephew, Switz.
Collagenase (p.1675·1); proteases.
*Ulcers; wounds.*

**Iruxol N** Knoll, Ger.
Collagenase (p.1675·1); proteases.
Iruxol formerly contained collagenase and chloramphenicol.
*Skin ulcers.*

**Iruxol Neo** Smith & Nephew, Spain.
Collagenase (p.1675·1); neomycin sulfate (p.235·1).
*Burns; ulcers; wounds.*

**Iruxolum mono** Ebewe, Austria.
Enzymes from *Clostridium histolyticum*.
*Necrotic ulcers; wounds.*

**IS 5 Mono** Ratiopharm, Ger.
Isosorbide mononitrate (p.942·1).
*Angina pectoris; heart failure; myocardial infarction; pulmonary hypertension.*

**Isacilin** Eurofarma, Braz.†.
Benzylpenicillin potassium (p.163·2).
Procaine (p.1383·2) is included in this preparation to alleviate the pain of injection.
*Bacterial infections.*

**Isadol** Pisa, Mex.†.
Zidovudine (p.658·2).
*HIV infection.*

**Isairon** Pfizer, Ital.
Chondroitin sulfate–iron complex (p.1425·1).
*Iron deficiency; iron-deficiency anaemias.*

**Isangina** Pharmacal, Fin.
Isosorbide mononitrate (p.942·1).
*Angina pectoris; heart failure.*

**Isavir** Pisa, Mex.
Aciclovir sodium (p.626·1).
*Cytomegalovirus infections; herpesvirus infections.*

**Isaxion** Ferring, Port.
Ticlopidine hydrochloride (p.1011·2).
*Thromboembolism prophylaxis.*

**Iscador** Weleda, Austria; Weleda, Ger.; Weleda, Switz.
Mistletoe (p.1715·3) from apple trees, pine trees or oak trees.
*Malignant neoplasms.*

**Ischelium** Polifarma, Ital.
Co-dergocrine mesilate (p.1674·1).
*Cerebral and peripheral vascular disorders; hypertension.*

**Ischelium Papaverina** Polifarma, Ital.†.
Co-dergocrine mesilate (p.1674·1); papaverine hydrochloride (p.1728·1).
*Cerebral and peripheral vascular disorders; hypertension.*

**Ischemol** Rhone-Poulenc Rorer, Mex.†.
Tetryzoline hydrochloride (p.1131·2).

**Ischemol A** Farmila, Ital.
Tetryzoline hydrochloride (p.1131·2); chlorphenamine maleate (p.427·3).
*Eye disorders.*

**Isclofen** Isis, UK†.
Diclofenac sodium (p.32·1).
*Musculoskeletal and joint disorders.*

**Iscover** Bristol-Myers Squibb, Arg.; Bristol-Myers Squibb, Austral.; Bristol-Myers Squibb, Braz.; Bristol-Myers Squibb, Ger.; Bristol-Myers Squibb, Gr.; Bristol-Myers Squibb, Ital.; Bristol-Myers Squibb, Mex.; Bristol-Myers Squibb, Port.; Bristol-Myers, Spain; Bristol-Myers Squibb, Switz.†; Bristol-Myers Squibb, UK.
Clopidogrel bisulfate (p.888·3).
*Atherosclerosis.*

**Isdibudol** Isdin, Spain.
Ibuprofen (p.45·3).
*Musculoskeletal pain and inflammation.*

**Isdin Extrem** Medley, Braz.
*Lotion SPF 25:* Octinoxate (p.1154·3); enzacamene (p.1147·1); methylenebisbenzotriazolyl tetramethylbutyl phenol; titanium dioxide (p.1160·3).
*Topical gel/cream SPF 25:* Octinoxate (p.1154·3); enzacamene (p.1147·1); methylene bisbenzotriazolyl tetramethylbutyl phenol; avobenzone (p.1142·3).
*Sunscreen.*

**Isdin Infantil** Medley, Braz.
*SPF 30; SPF 40:* Titanium dioxide (p.1160·3); octinoxate (p.1154·3); enzacamene (p.1147·1); ensulizole (p.1147·1); avobenzone (p.1142·3).
*Sunscreen.*

**Isdinex** Isdin, Spain.
Benzethonium chloride (p.1169·2); diphenhydramine hydrochloride (p.431·3).
*Pruritus.*

**Isdinium** Isdin, Spain.
Hydrocortisone butyrate (p.1104·1) or hydrocortisone propionate (p.1104·2).
*Skin disorders.*

**Isdol** Isdin, Spain.
Ibuprofen (p.45·3).
*Fever; pain.*

**I-Sense** Akorn, USA.
Multivitamin preparation (p.1417·1).

**Isepacin** Calea, Austria; Schering-Plough, Ital.; Schering-Plough, Mex.; Schering-Plough, Port.†.
Isepamicin sulfate (p.222·2).
*Bacterial infections.*

**Isepacine** Schering-Plough, Belg.
Isepamicin sulfate (p.222·2).
*Bacterial infections.*

**Isepalline** Schering-Plough, Fr.
Isepamicin sulfate (p.222·2).
*Bacterial infections.*

**Isephca S** Iso, Ger.
Thyme (p.1755·2).
*Coughs.*

**Iset** Casasco, Arg.
Clarithromycin (p.192·2).
*Bacterial infections.*

**ISF 09338** ISF, Ital.
Temocillin sodium (p.266·1).
*Gram-negative bacterial infections.*

**Isib** Ashbourne, UK.
Isosorbide mononitrate (p.942·1).
*Angina pectoris.*

**Isi-Calcin** ISI, Ital.†.
Elcatonin (p.768·3).
*Hypercalcaemia; osteoporosis; Paget's disease of bone; reflex sympathetic dystrophy.*

**Isicom** Desitin, Ger.
Carbidopa (p.1204·3); levodopa (p.1205·2).
*Parkinsonism.*

**Isiferone** Kedrion, Ital.
Interferon alfa (p.640·3).
*Malignant neoplasms; viral infections.*

**Isiflu V** Berna, Ital.
An influenza vaccine (p.1620·2).
*Active immunisation.*

**Isiflu Zonale** Scott-Cassara, Arg.
An influenza vaccine (p.1620·2).
*Active immunisation.*

**ISI-F/2/ST** ISI, Ital.†.
Amino acids (p.1417·1).
*Nutritional supplement in renal insufficiency.*

**Isigrip Zonale** Kedrion, Ital.
An influenza vaccine (p.1620·2).
*Active immunisation.*

**Isilung** Exel, Belg.
Eprazinone hydrochloride (p.1121·1).
*Respiratory-tract disorders.*

**Isimet** Abbott, Ital.
Ademetionine busilate (p.1647·2).
*Depression.*

**Isimoxin** Kedrion, Ital.
Amoxicillin (p.155·3).
*Bacterial infections.*

**Isisfen** Isis, UK†.
Ibuprofen (p.45·3).
*Inflammation; pain.*

**Isitab** Agepha, Austria.
Disinfection tablets for soft contact lenses (p.1164·2).

**Isiven** Scott-Cassara, Arg.; Cristalia, Braz.†; Kedrion, Ital.; Serono, Mex.
A normal immunoglobulin (p.1627·2).
*Hypogammaglobulinaemia; idiopathic thrombocytopenic purpura; immunodeficiency disorders; passive immunisation.*

**Iskaemyl** Astra, Denm.†.
Aspirin (p.15·1).
*Ischaemic heart disease; thrombosis prophylaxis.*

**Iskedyl** Pierre Fabre, Fr.; Pierre Fabre, Spain†.
Dihydroergocristine mesilate (p.1680·1); raubasine (p.994·3).
*Cerebral and peripheral vascular disorders; head injury; mental function disorders of the elderly; vascular eye disorders.*

**Iskemil** Ache, Braz.
Dihydroergocristine mesilate (p.1680·1).
*Impaired mental function.*

**Isketam** Ache, Braz.
Piracetam (p.1732·1); dihydroergocristine mesilate (p.1680·1).
*Impaired mental function.*

**Iskevert** Eversil, Braz.
Dihydroergocristine mesilate (p.1680·1).
*Impaired mental function.*

**Iski** Stadmed, India.
Diltiazem (p.901·3).
*Angina pectoris.*

**Isla-Mint** Sanova, Austria†; Engelhard, Ger.; Engelhard, Hong Kong.
Iceland moss.
*Catarrh; coughs; sore throat.*

**Islamint** Ceuta, UK†.
Iceland moss.
*Dry throat; respiratory-tract congestion.*

**Isla-Mint Herbal** Engelhard, Singapore.
Iceland moss.
*Catarrh; coughs; sore throat.*

**Isla-Moos** Engelhard, Ger.; Engelhard, Hong Kong.
Iceland moss.
*Catarrh; coughs; sore throat.*

**Islopir** Craveri, Arg.
Glimepiride (p.332·2).
*Diabetes mellitus.*

**Islotin** Craveri, Arg.
Metformin (p.342·3) or metformin hydrochloride (p.342·3).
*Diabetes mellitus.*

**Isly** Alcon, Arg.; Alcon, Chile.
Oxymetazoline hydrochloride (p.1126·1).
*Dry eyes; eye congestion.*

**Ismelin** Novartis, Austral.; Novartis, Austria†; Novartis, Mex.†; Novartis, NZ†; Novartis, S.Afr.†; Ciba Vision, Switz.†; Sovereign, UK; Ciba, USA.
Guanethidine monosulfate (p.926·3).
*Hypertension; regional nerve blocks.*

**Ismeline** Ciba Vision, Fr.†.
Guanethidine sulfate (p.926·3).
*Eye disorders.*

**Ismexin** Ratiopharm, Fin.
Isosorbide mononitrate (p.942·1).
*Angina pectoris; heart failure.*

**Ismigen** Zambon, Ital.
Lysates of: *Staphylococcus aureus; Streptococcus pyogenes; Streptococcus viridans; Klebsiella pneumoniae; Klebsiella ozaenae; Haemophilus influenzae; Moraxella catarrhalis; Streptococcus pneumoniae.*
*Respiratory-tract infections.*

**Ismipur** ISM, Ital.†.
Mercaptopurine (p.567·2).
*Acute leukaemia.*

**Ismo** Wyeth-Ayerst, Canad.†; Roche, Chile; Ercopharm, Denm.†; Roche, Ger.; Roche, Hong Kong; Nicholas Piramal, India; Boehringer Mannheim, Israel†; Roche, Ital.; Boehringer Mannheim, Neth.†; Roche, Norw.; Roche, NZ; Roche, Port.; Roche, S.Afr.; Roche, Singapore†; Roche, Swed.; Roche, Switz.; Roche, Thai.; Roche, UK; ESP, USA.
Isosorbide mononitrate (p.942·1).
*Angina pectoris; heart failure; myocardial infarction; pulmonary hypertension.*

**Ismotic** Alcon, USA.
Isosorbide (p.941·1).
*Raised intra-ocular pressure.*

**Ismox** Roche, Fin.
Isosorbide mononitrate (p.942·1).
*Angina pectoris; heart failure.*

**Iso** Lacer, Spain.
Isosorbide dinitrate (p.941·1).
*Angina pectoris; heart failure.*

**Iso Mack** Pfizer, Austria; Mack, Denm.; Mack, Illert., Ger.; Mack, Hong Kong; Mack, Singapore; Mack, Switz.; Mack, Thai.
Isosorbide dinitrate (p.941·1).
*Angina pectoris; heart failure; myocardial infarction; pulmonary hypertension; pulmonary oedema.*

**Iso Triaupin** Roche, Hong Kong†.
Butizide (p.878·2); reserpine (p.995·1); rescinnamine (p.994·3); raubasine (p.994·3); potassium chloride (p.1232·2).
*Hypertension.*

**Isoacne** Schering-Plough, Braz.
Isotretinoin (p.1148·3).
*Acne.*

**ISO-Augentropfen C** Iso, Ger.
Homoeopathic preparation.

**Iso-B** Tyson, USA.
Multivitamin preparation (p.1417·1).

**Isobac** Carnot, Mex.†.
Co-trimoxazole (p.199·3).
*Bacterial infections.*

**Isobar** Chiesi, Fr.
Methyclothiazide (p.953·2); triamterene (p.1016·2).
*Hypertension.*

**Iso-Betadine** Viatris, Belg.
Povidone-iodine (p.1190·3).
*Burns; disinfection of the skin and mucous membranes; mouth and throat infections; skin infections; ulcers; vulvovaginal infections; wounds.*

**Isobin** Korea United, Singapore.
Isosorbide dinitrate (p.941·1).
*Angina pectoris; heart failure.*

**Isobinate** General Drugs, Thai.
Isosorbide dinitrate (p.941·1).
*Angina pectoris; heart failure.*

**Isobranch** Bieffe, Ital.
L-Isoleucine (p.1438·2); L-leucine (p.1439·1); L-valine (p.1451·2).
*Hepatic encephalopathy; post-trauma disorders.*

**Isobutil** Collins, Mex.
Isoprenaline (p.940·2); bufylline (p.781·3); bromhexine (p.1115·3).
*Respiratory-tract congestion.*

**Isocaine** Novocol, USA.
Mepivacaine hydrochloride (p.1381·2).
Corbadrine (p.1675·3) is included in some injections as a vasoconstrictor to diminish absorption and localise the effect of the local anaesthetic.
*Local anaesthesia.*

**Isocal** Mead Johnson, Austral.; Mead Johnson Nutritionals, Canad.; Mead Johnson, Hong Kong; Mead Johnson, Israel; Mead Johnson, Malaysia; Mead Johnson, NZ†; Mead Johnson, Singapore; Mead Johnson Nutritionals, Thai.; Mead Johnson Nutritionals, USA.
A range of preparations for enteral nutrition (p.1417·1).

**Isocar** Offenbach, Mex.
Kaolin (p.1268·3); pectin (p.1580·3).
*Diarrhoea.*

**Isocard**
Note. A similar name is used for preparations of different composition (see below).
Schwarz, Fr.; Eastern Pharmaceuticals, UK†.
Isosorbide dinitrate (p.941·1).
*Angina pectoris.*

**Iso-Card**
Note. A similar name is used for preparations of different composition (see above).
Triomed, S.Afr.†.
Verapamil hydrochloride (p.1019·1).
*Angina pectoris; arrhythmias; hypertension.*

**Isocardide** Sam-On, Israel.
Isosorbide dinitrate (p.941·1).
*Angina pectoris; heart failure.*

**Isocef** Recordati, Ital.
Ceftibuten (p.182·1).
*Bacterial infections.*

**IsoCell** Antonetto, Ital.
Multivitamin and mineral preparation with plant extracts (p.1417·1).

**Isocet** Rugby, USA†.
Paracetamol (p.76·2); caffeine (p.782·1); butalbital (p.673·3).

**Isochinol** Schwarzhaupt, Ger.; Democal, Switz.
Quinisocaine hydrochloride (p.1384·2).
*Burns; haemorrhoids; skin disorders; wounds.*

**Isochron** Forest Pharmaceuticals, USA.
Isosorbide dinitrate (p.941·1).
*Angina pectoris.*

**Isocillin** Aventis, Ger.
Phenoxymethylpenicillin potassium (p.242·1).
*Bacterial infections.*

**Isoclar** Boniscontro & Gazzone, Ital.
Heparin sodium (p.928·1).
*Thromboembolic disorders.*

**Isoclor** Ciba, USA†.
Chlorphenamine maleate (p.427·3); pseudoephedrine hydrochloride (p.1129·2).
*Cold symptoms.*

**Isoclor Expectorant** Fisons, USA†.
Codeine phosphate (p.27·1); pseudoephedrine hydrochloride (p.1129·2); guaifenesin (p.1122·1).
*Coughs.*

**Isocolan** Giuliani, Ital.; Synthelabo, Switz.
Macrogol 4000 (p.1709·1); electrolytes (p.1217·1).
*Bowel evacuation; constipation.*

**Isocom** Nutripharm, USA†.
Isometheptene mucate (p.1702·1); dichloralphenazone (p.697·1); paracetamol (p.76·2).
*Tension and vascular headaches.*

**Isocord** Asta Medica, Braz.
Isosorbide dinitrate (p.941·1).
*Angina pectoris.*

**Isocort** Pharma Clal, Israel.
Isoconazole nitrate (p.401·3); diflucortolone valerate (p.1099·3).
*Fungal skin infections.*

**Isoday** Tillotts, Switz.†.
Isosorbide dinitrate (p.941·1).
*Heart failure; ischaemic heart disease; myocardial infarction.*

**Isoderm** Alkapharm, Singapore.
Skin cleanser.

**Isodex** Braun, Braz.†.
Dextran 40 (p.745·3) in electrolytes.
*Plasma volume expansion.*

**Isodilan** Klonal, Arg.
Isoxsuprine (p.1702·3).

**Isodine** Faulding, Austral.; Boehringer Ingelheim Promeco, Mex.; Sidefarma, Port.; Meiji, Thai.
Povidone-iodine (p.1190·3).
*Mouth and throat infections; skin, mucous membrane, and instrument disinfection; vaginitis.*

**Isodinit** Hexal, Ger.†.
Isosorbide dinitrate (p.941·1).
*Angina pectoris; heart failure; pulmonary hypertension.*

**Isodiur** Italfarmaco, Spain.
Torasemide (p.1015·3) or torasemide sodium (p.1015·3).
*Hypertension; oedema.*

**Isodol** Magis, Ital.
Nimesulide (p.67·1).
*Fever; inflammation; pain.*

**Isodril** Monot, Fr.†.
Chlorhexidine gluconate (p.1173·2); phenylephrine hydrochloride (p.1126·3).
*Eye disorders.*

**Isodrink** *Volchem, Ital.*
Isotonic rehydration solution (p.1417·1).

**Isodur**
*Durascan, Denm.; Tika, Swed.; Galen, UK.*
Isosorbide mononitrate (p.942·1).
*Angina pectoris.*

**Iso-Eremfat** *Fatol, Ger.*
Rifampicin (p.250·2); isoniazid (p.222·2).
*Tuberculosis.*

**Isoess** *Bieffe, Ital.*
Amino-acid infusion (p.1417·1).
*Parenteral nutrition in renal failure.*

**Isoetam** *Ferrer, Spain†.*
Ethambutol (p.212·2); isoniazid (p.222·2).
Pyridoxine hydrochloride (p.1456·3) is included in this preparation for the prophylaxis of peripheral neuropathy.
*Tuberculosis.*

**Isoflurane** *Abbott, UK.*
Isoflurane (p.1301·1).
Formerly available as Forane.
*General anaesthesia.*

**Isoforine** *Cristalia, Braz.*
Isoflurane (p.1301·1).
*General anaesthesia.*

**Isofort** *Bieffe, Ital.*
Amino-acid infusion (p.1417·1).
*Parenteral nutrition.*

**Isofra** *Bouchara-Recordati, Fr.†.*
Framycetin sulfate (p.215·1).
*Bacterial nose and throat infections.*

**Isoftal** *Agepha, Austria.*
Naphazoline hydrochloride (p.1124·3).
*Conjunctivitis.*

**Isogaine** *Clarben, Spain.*
Mepivacaine hydrochloride (p.1381·2).
*Local anaesthesia.*

**Isogel**
*GlaxoSmithKline, India; GlaxoSmithKline, NZ; Charwell, Singapore†; Pfizer Consumer, UK.*
Ispaghula (p.1268·1).
*Colostomy management; constipation; diarrhoea; irritable bowel syndrome.*

**Isogen** *Pharma Clal, Israel.*
Isoconazole nitrate (p.401·3).
*Fungal skin infections.*

**Isoginkgo** *Merck dura, Ger.*
Ginkgo biloba (p.1692·3).
*Intermittent claudication; mental function impairment; tinnitus; vertigo.*

**Isoglaucon**
*Agepha, Austria; Alcon, Ger.; Alcon, Ital.; Alcon Cusi, Spain.*
Clonidine hydrochloride (p.885·2).
*Glaucoma.*

**Isogrow** *Bieffe, Ital.*
Amino-acid infusion (p.1417·1).
*Parenteral nutrition in neonates.*

**Isogutt** *Winzer, Ger.*
Monobasic sodium phosphate (p.1230·3); dibasic sodium phosphate (p.1231·1).
*Ocular burns.*

**Isogutt akut** *Winzer, Ger.*
Sodium chloride (p.1233·3).
*Eye injuries and burns.*

**Isogyn** *Finderm, Ital.*
Isoconazole nitrate (p.401·3).
*Fungal vulvovaginal infections.*

**Isohes**
*Fresenius Kabi, Austria; Fresenius Kabi, Switz.*
Pentastarch (p.750·1).
*Haemodilution; plasma volume expansion.*

**Isohexal** *Hexal, Austral.*
Isotretinoin (p.1148·3).
*Acne.*

**Isoket**
*Sidus, Arg.; ;Gebro, Austria; Schwarz, Ger.; Sanol, Ger.; Schwarz, Hong Kong; Schwarz, Irl.; Medis, Israel; Schwarz, Malaysia; Knoll, Mex.; Neo-Farmaceutica, Port.; Omnimed, S.Afr.; Ranbaxy, Singapore; Schwarz, Singapore; Schwarz, Switz.; Schwarz, Thai.; Schwarz, UK.*
Isosorbide dinitrate (p.941·1).
*Angina pectoris; coronary spasm; heart failure; myocardial infarction; pulmonary hypertension.*

**Isokin** *Parke, Davis, India.*
Isoniazid (p.222·2).
*Tuberculosis.*

**Isokin-300** *Parke, Davis, India.*
Isoniazid (p.222·2); vitamin $B_6$ (p.1457·2).
*Tuberculosis.*

**Isokin-T Forte** *Parke, Davis, India.*
Isoniazid (p.222·2); thioacetazone (p.269·3).
*Tuberculosis.*

**Isolan**
*Note. This name is used for preparations of different composition.*
*Hexal, Arg.*
Isosorbide mononitrate (p.942·1).
*Angina pectoris; heart failure.*

*Galagen, USA.*
Lactose-free, gluten-free preparation for enteral nutrition (p.1417·1).

**Isolin** *Samarth, India.*
Isoprenaline hydrochloride (p.940·2).
*Bradycardia; shock; Stokes-Adams attacks.*

**Isoliv** *Bieffe, Ital.†.*
An amino-acid infusion (p.1417·1).
*Parenteral nutrition in liver disease.*

**Isolyt** *CT, Ger.†.*
Glucose monohydrate; sodium chloride; sodium citrate; potassium chloride (p.1222·2).
*Diarrhoea; oral rehydration therapy.*

**Isolyte**
*Note. This name is used for preparations of different composition.*
*Darrow, Braz.†.*
Sodium lactate; potassium chloride; sodium chloride; calcium chloride; magnesium chloride (p.1222·2).
*Oral rehydration therapy.*

*Braun McGaw, Hong Kong†; Baxter, Ital.; McGaw, NZ†; McGaw, USA.*
A range of electrolyte infusions with or without glucose (p.1217·1).
*Fluid and electrolyte disorders.*

**Isomel** *Clonmel, Irl.*
Isosorbide mononitrate (p.942·1).
*Angina pectoris; heart failure.*

**Isomerine** *Key, Arg.*
Chlorphenamine (p.428·1).

**Isomerine N** *Key, Arg.*
Dexchlorpheniramine maleate (p.427·3); pseudoephedrine sulfate (p.1129·2); guaifenesin (p.1122·1).
*Coughs.*

**Isomet** *M & H, Thai.*
Methyldopa (p.953·2).
*Hypertension.*

**Isomide** *Monmouth, UK†.*
Disopyramide (p.903·3) or disopyramide phosphate (p.903·3).
*Arrhythmias.*

**Isomil**
*Abbott, Arg.; Abbott, Austral.†; Abbott, Braz.; Abbott, Canad.; Abbott, Chile; Abbott, Fin.†; Abbott, Hong Kong; Abbott, Israel; Abbott, Ital.; Abbott, Malaysia; Abbott, Mex.; Abbott, NZ†; Abbott, Singapore; Abbott, Thai.; Abbott Nutrition, UK; Ross, USA.*
Lactose-free soy protein infant feed (p.1417·1).
*Galactosaemia; lactose intolerance; milk intolerance.*

**Isomil DF**
*Abbott, NZ; Ross, USA.*
Lactose-free soy protein infant feed with fibre (p.1417·1).
*Diarrhoea.*

**Isomil SF** *Ross, USA†.*
Lactose-free, sucrose-free soy protein infant feed (p.1417·1).
*Milk intolerance; sucrose intolerance.*

**Isomol** *Schwarz, Ger.; Sanol, Ger.*
Macrogol 3350 (p.1709·1); electrolytes (p.1217·1).
*Constipation.*

**Isomon** *Roche, Gr.*
Isosorbide mononitrate (p.942·1).
*Angina; heart failure.*

**Isomonat** *Roche, Austria.*
Isosorbide mononitrate (p.942·1).
*Heart failure; ischaemic heart disease; pulmonary hypertension.*

**Isomonit**
*Hexal, Austral.; United Nordic, Denm.†; Hexal, Ger.; Rowex, Irl.*
Isosorbide mononitrate (p.942·1).
*Angina pectoris; heart failure; pulmonary hypertension.*

**Isomonoreal** *Realpharma, Ger.†.*
Isosorbide mononitrate (p.942·1).
*Angina pectoris; heart failure; myocardial infarction; pulmonary hypertension.*

**Isomyrtine** *Schwarz, Fr.*
Pholcodine (p.1128·3); isomyrtol.
*Coughs.*

**Isonefrine** *Tubilux, Ital.*
Phenylephrine hydrochloride (p.1126·3).
*Production of mydriasis.*

**Isonex** *Pfizer, India.*
Isoniazid (p.222·2).
*Tuberculosis.*

**Isoniac** *Klonal, Arg.*
Isoniazid (p.222·2).
*Tuberculosis.*

**Isonitril** *Rubio, Spain.*
Isosorbide mononitrate (p.942·1).
*Angina pectoris.*

**Isontyn** *Abbott, Arg.*
Terazosin hydrochloride (p.1010·3).
*Benign prostatic hyperplasia; hypertension.*

**Isopamil** *General Drugs, Thai.*
Verapamil hydrochloride (p.1019·1).
*Angina pectoris; arrhythmias; hypertension; myocardial infarction.*

**Isopap** *Geneva, USA†; Marsam, USA†.*
Isometheptene mucate (p.1702·1); dichloralphenazone (p.697·1); paracetamol (p.76·2).
*Tension and vascular headaches.*

**Isopaque** *Nycomed Imaging, Denm.†.*
Calcium metrizoate (p.1067·2); magnesium metrizoate (p.1067·2); meglumine metrizoate (p.1067·2); sodium metrizoate (p.1067·2).
*Radiographic contrast medium for cystography.*

**Isopaque Cysto**
*Nycomed Imaging, Norw.†; Nycomed, Swed.†; Nycomed Amersham, UK.*
Calcium metrizoate (p.1067·2); magnesium metrizoate (p.1067·2); meglumine metrizoate (p.1067·2); sodium metrizoate (p.1067·2).
*Radiographic contrast medium.*

**Isopen** *Siam Bheasach, Thai.*
Isosorbide mononitrate (p.942·1).
*Angina pectoris; heart failure; myocardial infarction.*

**Isophyllen** *Laevosan, Austria†.*
Diprophylline (p.784·3).
*Cardiovascular disorders; Cheyne Stokes respiration; oedema.*

**Isoplasmal G** *Braun, Spain.*
Amino-acid, carbohydrate, and electrolyte infusion (p.1417·1).
*Parenteral nutrition.*

**Isoprinosina** *Synthelabo, Ital.†.*
Inosine pranobex (p.640·2).
*Viral infections.*

**Isoprinosine**
*Sanofi Synthelabo, Belg.; Andromaco, Chile; Sanofi Synthelabo, Fr.; Degab, Ger.; Unipharma, Gr.; Newport, Irl.; Aventis, Mex.*
Inosine pranobex (p.640·2).
*Viral infections.*

**Isoprochin P** *Merckle, Ger.*
Propyphenazone (p.85·3).
*Fever; pain.*

**Isoprodian**
*Croma, Austria; Fatol, Ger.*
Isoniazid (p.222·2); protionamide (p.246·3); dapsone (p.202·2).
*Mycobacterial infections including leprosy.*

**Isopront** *Ferraz, Lynce, Port.*
Isosorbide dinitrate (p.941·1).
*Angina pectoris; heart failure; myocardial infarction; pulmonary oedema.*

**Isoptin**
*Abbott, Austral.; Ebewe, Austria; Abbott, Canad.; Abbott, Denm.; Abbott, Fin.; Abbott, Ger.; Vianex (Βιανεξ), Gr.; Knoll, Hong Kong; Abbott, Irl.; Abbott, Ital.; Abbott, Malaysia; Knoll, Neth.; Abbott, Norw.; Abbott, NZ; Abbott, Port.; Knoll, S.Afr.; Abbott, Singapore; Abbott, Swed.; Knoll, Switz.; Knoll, Thai.; Abbott, USA.*
Verapamil hydrochloride (p.1019·1).
*Angina pectoris; arrhythmias; coronary spasm; heart failure; hypertension; hypertrophic cardiomyopathy; myocardial infarction.*

**Isoptin plus** *Abbott, Ger.*
Verapamil hydrochloride (p.1019·1); hydrochlorothiazide (p.933·2).
*Hypertension.*

**Isoptina** *Abbott, Chile.*
Verapamil (p.1021·1).
*Angina pectoris; arrhythmias; hypertension.*

**Isoptine**
*Knoll, Belg.; Knoll, Fr.*
Verapamil hydrochloride (p.1019·1).
*Angina pectoris; arrhythmias; hypertension; myocardial infarction.*

**Isoptino** *Abbott, Arg.*
Verapamil (p.1021·1) or verapamil hydrochloride (p.1019·1).
*Arrhythmias; heart failure; hypertension; myocardial infarction.*

**Isopto Alkaline**
*Alcon, Fin.; Alcon, Irl.; Alcon, UK.*
Hypromellose (p.1579·3).
*Dry eyes.*

**Isopto B 12** *Alcon Cusi, Spain.*
Cyanocobalamin (p.1458·2).
*Corneal damage.*

**Isopto Biotic** *Alcon, Swed.*
Polymyxin B sulfate (p.245·1); neomycin sulfate (p.235·1); phenylephrine hydrochloride (p.1126·3).
*Bacterial eye infections.*

**Isopto Carpina**
*Alcon, Arg.; Alcon Cusi, Spain.*
Pilocarpine hydrochloride (p.1495·1).
*Glaucoma; ocular hypertension; reversal of mydriasis.*

**Isopto Carpine**
*Alcon, Austral.; Alcon, Belg.; Alcon, Braz.; Alcon, Canad.; Alkon (Αλκον), Gr.; Alcon, Fin.; Alcon, Hong Kong; Alcon, Irl.; Alcon, Israel; Alcon, Malaysia; Alcon, Norw.; Alcon, NZ†; Alcon, S.Afr.; Alcon, Singapore; Alcon, Switz.†; Alcon, Thai.; Alcon, UK†; Alcon, USA.*
Pilocarpine hydrochloride (p.1495·1).
*Glaucoma; ocular hypertension; production of miosis.*

**Isopto Cetamide**
*Alcon, Belg.†; Alcon, USA.*
Sulfacetamide sodium (p.257·3).
*Eye infections.*

**Isopto Cetapred**
*Alcon, Belg.†; Alcon, Braz.; Alcon, USA†.*
Prednisolone acetate (p.1108·1); sulfacetamide sodium (p.257·3).
*Infected eye disorders.*

**Isopto Dex** *Alcon, Ger.*
Dexamethasone (p.1097·1).
*Eye disorders.*

**Isopto Fenicol**
*Alcon, Arg.; Alcon, Hong Kong†; Alcon, NZ; Alcon, Singapore; Alcon Cusi, Spain†; Alcon, Swed.†.*
Chloramphenicol (p.185·1).
*Bacterial eye infections.*

**Isopto Flucon**
*Alcon, Ger.; Alcon Cusi, Spain.*
Fluorometholone (p.1102·2).
*Eye disorders.*

**Isopto Fluid** *Alcon, Ger.†.*
Hypromellose (p.1579·3).
*Dry eyes.*

**Isopto Frin**
*Alcon, Austral.; Sanofi Synthelabo, Belg.†; Alcon, Irl.; Alcon, Malaysia; Alcon, NZ; Alcon, Singapore; Alcon, UK†.*
Phenylephrine hydrochloride (p.1126·3).
*Eye irritation.*

**Isopto Karbakolin** *Alcon, Swed.*
Carbachol (p.1488·1).
*Glaucoma.*

**Isopto Max** *Alcon, Ger.*
Dexamethasone (p.1097·1); neomycin sulfate (p.235·1); polymyxin B sulfate (p.245·1).
*Infected eye disorders.*

**Isopto Maxidex**
*Alcon, Arg.; Alcon, Norw.; Alcon, Swed.*
Dexamethasone (p.1097·1).
*Inflammatory eye disorders.*

**Isopto Naturale** *Alcon, Ger.†.*
Dextran 70 (p.746·2); hypromellose (p.1579·3).
*Dry eyes.*

**Isopto Pilomin** *Alcon, Ger.†.*
Pilocarpine hydrochloride (p.1495·1); physostigmine salicylate (p.1494·1).
*Glaucoma.*

**Isopto Plain**
*Alcon, Fin.; Alcon, Irl.; Alcon, Swed.; Alcon, UK; Alcon, USA.*
Hypromellose (p.1579·3).
*Dry eyes; eye irritation.*

**Isopto Tears**
*Alcon, Austral.; Alcon, Belg.†; Alcon, Canad.; Alcon, Hong Kong; Alcon, NZ†; Alcon, Singapore†; Alcon, Switz.; Alcon, Thai.; Alcon, USA.*
Hypromellose (p.1579·3).
*Dry eyes; eye irritation.*

**Isoptomax** *Alcon, Arg.*
Dexamethasone (p.1097·1); neomycin sulfate (p.235·1); polymyxin B sulfate (p.245·1).
*Infected eye disorders.*

**Isopuramin** *Bieffe, Ital.*
A range of amino-acid infusions (p.1417·1).
*Parenteral nutrition.*

**Iso-Puren** *Alpharma-Isis, Ger.*
Isosorbide dinitrate (p.941·1).
*Heart failure; ischaemic heart disease.*

**Isoradin** *YSP, Malaysia.*
Isoconazole nitrate (p.401·3); diflucortolone valerate (p.1099·3).
*Fungal skin infections with inflammation.*

**Isoram** *Bieffe, Ital.*
L-Arginine (p.1421·1); L-isoleucine (p.1438·2); L-leucine (p.1439·1); L-valine (p.1451·2).
*Hepatic encephalopathy; post-trauma disorders.*

**Isorbid**
*Teuto, Braz.; Armstrong, Mex.*
Isosorbide dinitrate (p.941·1).
*Angina pectoris; heart failure.*

**Isordil**
*Wyeth, Arg.; Sigma, Austral.; Wyeth Lederle, Belg.; Sigma, Braz.; Wyeth-Ayerst, Canad.†; Wyeth, Hong Kong; Wyeth, India; Shire, Irl.; Wyeth, Malaysia; Wyeth, Neth.; Akromed, S.Afr.; Wyeth, Singapore; Wyeth-Ayerst, Thai.; Shire, UK†; Biovail, USA.*
Isosorbide dinitrate (p.941·1).
*Angina pectoris; heart failure; myocardial infarction.*

**Isorel** *Novipharm, Austria.*
Mistletoe (p.1715·3) from fir trees, apple trees or pine trees.
*Malignant neoplasms.*

**Isorem**
*Remedica, Hong Kong; Remedica, Thai.*
Isosorbide dinitrate (p.941·1).
*Angina pectoris; heart failure.*

**Isoren** *Bieffe, Ital.*
Amino-acid infusion (p.1417·1).
*Parenteral nutrition in renal failure.*

**Isorifam** *Biochem, India.*
Rifampicin (p.250·2); isoniazid (p.222·2).
*Tuberculosis.*

**Isoritmon** *Basi, Port.*
Chloroprocainamide.
*Arrhythmias.*

**Isorythm** *Lipha Sante, Fr.*
Disopyramide (p.903·3) or disopyramide phosphate (p.903·3).
*Arrhythmias.*

**Isosal** *Sanochemia, Austria.*
*Cream:* Salicylamide (p.87·3).
*Topical fluid:* Salicylamide (p.87·3); camphor (p.1665·3).
*Musculoskeletal, joint, and peri-articular disorders; neuralgia; soft-tissue injury.*

**Isoselect** *Bieffe, Ital.*
Amino-acid infusion (p.1417·1).
*Hepatic encephalopathy; parenteral nutrition.*

**Isosifar** *Siphar, Switz.*
Isosorbide dinitrate (p.941·1).
*Angina pectoris; heart failure.*

**Isosource**
*Novartis, Arg.; Novartis Consumer, Austral.; Novartis, Braz.; Novartis Nutrition, Canad.†; Novartis Nutrition, Fr.; Novartis Nutrition, Hong Kong; Novartis Consumer, Ital.; Novartis Consumer, Port.; Novartis Nutrition, Singapore; Sandoz Nutrition, USA.*
A range of preparations for enteral nutrition (p.1417·1).

**Isosource (Nutrodrip)** *Novartis, Fin.*
A range of preparations for enteral nutrition (p.1417·1).

**Isostad** *Stada, Austria.*
Isosorbide dinitrate (p.941·1).
*Angina pectoris; heart failure; hypertension; myocardial infarction.*

**Isostenase** Azupharma, Ger.
Isosorbide dinitrate (p.941·1).
*Angina pectoris.*

**Isosteril** Fresenius Kabi, Switz.
Electrolyte infusion with glucose (p.1217·1).
*Fluid and electrolyte disorders.*

**Isotamine** ICN, Canad.
Isoniazid (p.222·2).
*Tuberculosis.*

**Isotard**
Note. This name is used for preparations of different composition.
CTI, Israel.
Isosorbide dinitrate (p.941·1).
*Angina pectoris.*

Strakan, UK.
Isosorbide mononitrate (p.942·1).
*Angina pectoris.*

**Isotard MC** Novo Nordisk, Austral.†.
Isophane insulin injection (bovine, monocomponent) (p.333·3).
*Diabetes mellitus.*

**Isotein HN** Sandoz Nutrition, USA.
Lactose-free, gluten-free preparation for enteral nutrition (p.1417·1).

**Isoten** Wyeth Lederle, Belg.
Bisoprolol fumarate (p.875·1).
*Angina pectoris; cardiac hyperkinetic syndrome; heart failure; hypertension.*

**Isotenk** Biotenk, Arg.
Isoxsuprine hydrochloride (p.1702·2).
*Dysmenorrhoea; peripheral vascular disorders; premature labour; threatened miscarriage.*

**Isothane** Baxter, Braz.
Isoflurane (p.1301·1).
*General anaesthesia.*

**Isotol** Diaco, Ital.
Mannitol (p.950·2).
*Raised intra-ocular pressure; raised intracranial pressure.*

**Isotone Kochsalz** Baxter, Ger.
Sodium chloride (p.1233·3).
*Fluid and electrolyte disorders.*

**Isotonic** Ratiopharm, Ger.
Sodium chloride; sodium citrate; potassium chloride; glucose (p.1222·2).
*Diarrhoea; oral rehydration solution.*

**Isotrate**
Note. This name is used for preparations of different composition.
Bioglan, Hong Kong†; Helsinn Birex, Irl.†; Bioglan, Irl.†; Bioglan, Singapore†; Bioglan, UK.
Isosorbide mononitrate (p.942·1).
*Angina pectoris.*

Berlin Pharm, Thai.
Isosorbide dinitrate (p.941·1).
*Angina pectoris.*

**Isotrex**
Stiefel, Arg.; Stiefel, Austral.; Sanova, Austria; Stiefel, Braz.; Stiefel, Canad.; Stiefel, Denm.; Stiefel, Fr.†; Stiefel, Ger.; Stiefel, Hong Kong; Stiefel, Irl.; Stiefel, Israel; Stiefel, Ital.; Stiefel, Malaysia; Stiefel, Mex.; Stiefel, NZ; Stiefel, Port.; Stiefel, S.Afr.; Stiefel, Singapore; Stiefel, Spain; Stiefel, Thai.; Stiefel, UK.
Isotretinoin (p.1148·3).
*Acne.*

**Isotrex Eritromicina** Stiefel, Spain.
Isotretinoin (p.1148·3); erythromycin (p.208·1).
*Acne.*

**Isotrex Gel** Stiefel, Chile.
Isotretinoin (p.1148·3).
*Acne.*

**Isotrexin**
Sanova, Austria; Stiefel, Braz.; Stiefel, Ger.; Stiefel, Irl.; Stiefel, Ital.; Stiefel, Port.; Stiefel, UK.
Isotretinoin (p.1148·3); erythromycin (p.208·1).
*Acne.*

**Isotrexol** Stiefel, Braz.
Isotretinoin (p.1148·3); ensulizole (p.1147·1); avobenzone (p.1142·3); octinoxate (p.1154·3).

**Isotrim** Ghimas, Ital.†.
Co-trimoxazole (p.199·3).
*Bacterial infections.*

**Iso-Triraupin** Roche, Thai.
Butizide (p.878·2); reserpine (p.995·1); rescinnamine (p.994·3); raubasine (p.994·3).
*Hypertension.*

**Isovir** Sanofi Synthelabo, Port.
Inosine pranobex (p.640·2).
*Viral infections.*

**Isovist**
Schering, Austral.; Schering, Austria; Schering, Denm.; Schering, Fin.; Schering, Ger.; Schering, Ital.†; Schering, Neth.; Schering, Norw.†; Schering, NZ; Schering, S.Afr.; Schering, Swed.†; Schering, Switz.; Schering, UK.
Iotrolan (p.1066·1).
*Radiographic contrast medium.*

**Isovorin**
Wyeth Lederle, Austria; Wyeth, Braz.; Wyeth Lederle, Denm.; Wyeth Lederle, Fin.; Wyeth, Gr.; Wyeth, Irl.; Lederle, Neth.†; Wyeth Lederle, Norw.; Wyeth Lederle, Port.; Wyeth, S.Afr.; Wyeth, Spain; Wyeth Lederle, Swed.; Lederle, Switz.†; Wyeth, UK.
Calcium levofolinate (p.1431·1).
*Adjunct to fluorouracil therapy; antidote to folic acid antagonists.*

**Isovue**
Regional Health, Austral.; Squibb Diagnostics, Canad.†; Squibb Diagnostics, USA.
Iopamidol (p.1064·3).
*Radiographic contrast medium.*

**Isox**
Note. This name is used for preparations of different composition.
Saval, Chile.
Meloxicam (p.56·1).
*Musculoskeletal, joint, peri-articular, and soft-tissue disorders.*

Senosiain, Mex.
Itraconazole (p.401·3).
*Fungal infections.*

**Isoxan** NHS, Fr.
Multivitamin and mineral preparation (p.1417·1).

**I-Soyalac** Nutricia-Luma Lindar, USA.
Corn- and lactose-free soy protein infant feed (p.1417·1).

**Isozid** Fatol, Ger.
Isoniazid (p.222·2).
*Tuberculosis.*

**Isozid comp N** Fatol, Ger.
Isoniazid (p.222·2).
Pyridoxine hydrochloride (p.1456·3) is included in this preparation for the prophylaxis of peripheral neuropathy.
Formerly known as Isozid-compositum.
*Tuberculosis.*

**Isozid-H** Gebro, Austria.
Hexetidine (p.1182·1).
*Skin disinfection.*

**Ispagel** Richmond Pharmaceuticals, UK.
Ispaghula (p.1268·1).
*Constipation; diarrhoea; irritable bowel syndrome.*

**Ispenoral** Rosen, Ger.
Phenoxymethylpenicillin potassium (p.242·1).
*Bacterial infections.*

**Isquebral** Iquinosa, Spain†.
Dihydroergocristine mesilate (p.1680·1); raubasine (p.994·3).
*Cerebral and peripheral vascular disorders; head injury.*

**Isquelium** Rider, Chile.
Acenocoumarol (p.848·3).
*Thromboembolic disorders.*

**Issium** Lifepharma, Ital.
Flunarizine hydrochloride (p.434·1).
*Migraine; vertigo.*

**Istamex** Adelco, Gr.
Chlorphenamine maleate (p.427·3).
*Hypersensitivity reactions.*

**Istamyl** Monot, Fr.†.
Isothipendyl hydrochloride (p.435·2).
*Hypersensitivity reactions.*

**Isteropac** Bracco, Switz.
Iodamide (p.1063·2).
*Contrast medium for hysterosalpingography.*

**Isteropac ER** Bracco, Ital.
Meglumine iodamide (p.1063·2).
*Contrast medium for hysterosalpingography.*

**Isticilline** Norma (Νορμα), Gr.
Ampicillin sodium (p.157·1).
*Bacterial infections.*

**Istin**
Pfizer, Irl.; Pfizer, UK.
Amlodipine besilate (p.862·1).
*Angina pectoris; hypertension.*

**Istivac**
Aventis Pasteur, Arg.; Aventis Pasteur, Port.
An inactivated influenza vaccine (p.1620·2).
*Active immunisation.*

**Istix** Sons, Mex.
Tetracycline (p.266·2).
*Bacterial infections.*

**Istopar** Disperga, Austria†.
Mineral preparation with liver extract and thiamine hydrochloride (p.1417·1).
*Iron-deficiency anaemia; tonic.*

**Istopril** Codal Synto, Thai.
Enalapril maleate (p.909·2).
*Heart failure; hypertension.*

**Istotosal** Zekides, Gr.
Tenoxicam (p.93·1).
*Dysmenorrhoea; gout; inflammation; osteoarthritis; pain; rheumatoid arthritis; spondyloarthropathies.*

**Isudrine** Boehringer Ingelheim, Fr.†.
Aluminium phosphate (p.1250·1); magnesium oxide (p.1272·3).
*Gastrointestinal disorders.*

**Isugran** Synpharma, Austria.
Mistletoe (p.1715·3).
*Circulatory disorders.*

**Isuhuman Basal**
Hoechst Marion Roussel, Neth.†; Aventis, Port.; Hoechst Marion Roussel, Swed.†.
Isophane insulin injection (human) (p.333·3).
*Diabetes mellitus.*

**Isuhuman Comb 25** Aventis, Port.
Mixture of insulin injection (human) 25% and isophane insulin injection (human) 75% (p.333·3).
*Diabetes mellitus.*

**Isuhuman Comb 25/75, 50/50** Hoechst Marion Roussel, Swed.†.
Mixtures of insulin injection (human, emp) and isophane insulin injection (human, emp) respectively in the proportions indicated (p.333·3).
*Diabetes mellitus.*

**Isuhuman Comb 15, Comb 25, Comb 50**
Hoechst Marion Roussel, Neth.†.
Mixtures of isophane insulin injection (human) 85%, 75% and 50% and neutral insulin injection (human) 15%, 25% and 50% respectively (p.333·3).
*Diabetes mellitus.*

**Isuhuman Infusat**
Hoechst Marion Roussel, Neth.; Hoechst Marion Roussel, Swed.†.
Insulin injection (human) (p.333·3).
*Diabetes mellitus.*

**Isuhuman Rapid**
Hoechst Marion Roussel, Neth.†; Aventis, Port.; Hoechst Marion Roussel, Swed.†.
Insulin injection (human) (p.333·3).
*Diabetes mellitus.*

**Isuprel**
Abbott, Austral.; Abbott, Belg.; Sanofi Synthelabo, Canad.†; Abbott, Fr.; Abbott, Gr.; Abbott, Israel; Abbott, NZ; Abbott, Singapore; Abbott, Thai.; Sanofi Winthrop, USA.
Isoprenaline hydrochloride (p.940·2).
*Bronchospasm during anaesthesia; cardiac arrest; heart block; heart failure; shock; Stokes-Adams attacks.*

**IT SD-T** Purissimus, Arg.
A tetanus immunoglobulin (p.1640·3).
*Passive immunisation.*

**Itagil** Dumex, Port.†.
Buspirone hydrochloride (p.672·2).
*Anxiety.*

**Itaiflex** Ortoquimica, Braz.†.
Orphenadrine (p.486·2); dipyrone (p.35·3); caffeine (p.782·1).
*Pain.*

**Italdermol** Italmex, Mex.
Wheat germ; phenoxyethanol (p.1189·1).
*Burns; cervicitis; skin irritation; ulcers; vulvovaginitis; wounds.*

**Italmicin** Italmex, Mex.†.
Chloramphenicol (p.185·1).
*Bacterial infections.*

**Italnik** Italmex, Mex.
Ciprofloxacin (p.188·2).
*Bacterial infections.*

**Italon** Offenbach, Mex.
Indometacin (p.47·3).
*Inflammation.*

**Italprid** Teofarma, Ital.
Tiapride hydrochloride (p.725·1).
*Alcohol withdrawal syndrome; behaviour disorders; gastrointestinal motility disorders; headache; movement disorders.*

**Ital-Ultra** Italmex, Mex.
Ambroxol hydrochloride (p.1114·3).
*Respiratory-tract congestion.*

**Italviron** Italmex, Mex.
Asparagine; acetylglutamine; pyridoxine; phosphorylserine (p.1417·1).
*Memory disorders.*

**Itan** Saval, Chile.
Metoclopramide (p.1274·3).
*Gastrointestinal disorders.*

**Itapredin** Rafarm, Gr.
Indometacin (p.47·3).
*Gout; inflammation; musculoskeletal and joint disorders; pain.*

**Itax Antipoux**
Pierre Fabre, Fr.†.
*Topical spray:* Phenothrin (p.1509·1); tetramethrin (p.1510·2); piperonyl butoxide (p.1509·2).
*Pediculosis.*

Pierre Fabre Sante, Fr.
*Shampoo:* Phenothrin (p.1509·1).
*Pediculosis.*

**Itax Preventif** Pierre Fabre, Fr.†.
Repellent 3535.
*Head lice repellent.*

**ITC**
Note. This name is used for preparations of different composition.
Giscard, Arg.
Itraconazole (p.401·3).
*Fungal infections.*

Asta Medica, Belg.†.
Sodium iodide (p.1598·1); potassium iodide (p.1598·1); calcium chloride (p.1225·1); sodium thiosulfate (p.1053·3).
*Cataracts.*

**Itch-X** Ascher, USA.
Pramocaine hydrochloride (p.1382·2); benzyl alcohol (p.1170·2).
*Local anaesthesia.*

**ITE B12 Forte** Purissimus, Arg.
Cyanocobalamin (p.1458·2); folic acid (p.1429·1); ferric ammonium citrate (p.1427·2); liver extract.
*Anaemias.*

**Item Alphacade** Gandhour, Fr.
Alpha hydroxy acids; salicylic acid (p.1157·1); cedar oil; cade oil (p.1159·2).
*Dandruff; scalp psoriasis.*

**Item Alphakeptol** Gandhour, Fr.
Glycolic acid (p.1147·3); salicylic acid (p.1157·1); pyrithione zinc (p.1156·2); piroctone olamine (p.1155·2).
*Dandruff.*

**Item Alphazole** Gandhour, Fr.
Climbazole (p.396·2); glycine (p.1433·3); salicylic acid (p.1157·1); alpha hydroxy acids; cedar oil.
*Seborrhoeic dermatitis.*

**Item Antipoux** Gandhour, Fr.
*Lotion; shampoo:* Phenothrin (p.1509·1).
*Pediculosis.*
*Topical spray:* Diethyltoluamide (p.1503·3).
*Head lice repellent.*

**Iteol-3** AstraZeneca, India.
Chlorhexidine gluconate (p.1173·2); cetrimide (p.1172·1).
*Skin disinfection.*

**Iteor** Pierre Fabre Sante, Fr.†.
A range of vitamin and mineral preparations (p.1417·1).

**Iterium** Servier, Austria.
Rilmenidine phosphate (p.996·1).
*Hypertension.*

**Itinerol $B_6$** Vifor, Switz.
Meclozine hydrochloride (p.436·3); pyridoxine hydrochloride (p.1456·3); caffeine (p.782·1).
*Nausea; vomiting.*

**Itodal** Laboratorios Chile, Chile.
Itraconazole (p.401·3).
*Fungal infections.*

**Itorex** Pharma Italia, Ital.
Cefuroxime sodium (p.184·1).
*Gram-negative bacterial infections.*

**Itoxaril** Kampel Martian, Arg.
Irinotecan (p.564·3).
*Malignant neoplasms.*

**Itra** Macrophar, Thai.
Itraconazole (p.401·3).
*Fungal infections.*

**Itracon** Unison, Thai.
Itraconazole (p.401·3).
*Fungal infections.*

**Itracotan** Royton, Braz.
Itraconazole (p.401·3).
*Fungal infections.*

**Itranax**
Janssen-Cilag, Braz.; Cilag, Mex.
Itraconazole (p.401·3).
*Fungal infections.*

**Itraspor** Sigma, Braz.
Itraconazole (p.401·3).
*Fungal infections.*

**Itravil** Investigacion, Mex.
Clobenzorex hydrochloride (p.1585·3).
*Obesity.*

**Itrazol** Biolab Sanus, Braz.
Itraconazole (p.401·3).
*Fungal infections.*

**Itrin** Abbott, Ital.
Terazosin hydrochloride (p.1010·3).
*Hypertension.*

**Itrop**
Boehringer Ingelheim, Austria; Boehringer Ingelheim, Ger.
Ipratropium bromide (p.787·1).
*Arrhythmias.*

**Iuvacor** Inverni della Beffa, Ital.
Ubidecarenone (p.1760·2).
*Cardiac disorders; co-enzyme $Q_{10}$ deficiency.*

**Ivacin**
Wyeth Lederle, Denm.; Wyeth Lederle, Swed.†.
Piperacillin sodium (p.243·1).
*Bacterial infections.*

**Ivadal**
Sanofi Synthelabo, Austria; Grunenthal, Fr.†; Vita, Ital.†.
Zolpidem tartrate (p.728·3).
*Insomnia.*

**I-Valex** Ross, USA.
A range of leucine-free preparations for enteral nutrition including an infant feed (p.1417·1).
*Leucine catabolism disorders.*

**Ivaliten** Lavipharm, Gr.
Phenothrin (p.1509·1).
*Head, body, and crab lice.*

**Ivamix** Fresenius Kabi, Norw.
Amino-acid and lipid (from soya oil (p.1447·2)) infusion (p.1417·1).
*Parenteral nutrition.*

**Ivarest**
Rider, Chile; Blistex, USA.
Calamine (p.1144·1); diphenhydramine hydrochloride (p.431·3).
Formerly contained calamine and benzocaine in the USA.
*Minor skin irritation.*

**Iveegam**
Baxter, Canad.; Immuno, USA.
A normal immunoglobulin (p.1627·2).
*Hypogammaglobulinaemia; immunodeficiency; Kawasaki syndrome; passive immunisation.*

**Ivel** Knoll, Mex.
Lupulus (p.1708·1); valerian (p.1762·2).
*Anxiety; insomnia.*

**Ivel Schlaf** Kanoldt, Ger.†.
Lupulus (p.1708·1); valerian (p.1762·2).
*Restlessness; sleep disorders.*

**Ivelip**
Baxter, Austral.; Baxter, Belg.†; Baxter, Fr.; Clintec, Israel; Baxter, Ital.; Baxter, Mex.; Baxter, Spain; Baxter, UK.
Soya oil (p.1447·2).
Contains egg lecithin or egg phosphatides.
*Lipid infusion for parenteral nutrition.*

**Ivemix** *Clintec, Fr.†.*
Amino-acid, lipid (from soya oil (p.1447·2)), and glucose infusion (p.1417·1).
Contains egg lecithin.
*Parenteral nutrition.*

**Ivepaque** *Amersham, Fr.*
Iopentol (p.1065·1).
*Radiographic contrast medium.*

**Ivhebex** *Lab Francais du Fractionnement, Fr.*
A hepatitis B immunoglobulin (p.1617·2).
*Passive immunisation.*

**Ividol** *Rafarm, Gr.*
Amiloride hydrochloride (p.858·2); hydrochlorothiazide (p.933·2).
*Heart failure; hypertension; oedema.*

**Ivofol** *Juste, Spain.*
Propofol (p.1305·3).
*General anaesthesia; sedative.*

**Ivoran Pilot** *Eczane, Arg.*
Nitrofurazone (p.238·2).
*Bacterial infections.*

**Ivracain** *Sintetica, Switz.*
Chloroprocaine hydrochloride (p.1373·1).
*Local anaesthesia.*

**Ivy Block** *Enviroderm, USA.*
Bentoquatam (p.1143·1).
*Prophylaxis against poison ivy-, oak-, or sumac-induced contact dermatitis.*

**Ivy Dry** *Ivy Corp, USA.*
Zinc acetate (p.1469·2).
*Minor skin irritation.*

**Ivy-Chex** *JMI, USA†.*
Polyvinylpyrrolidone vinylacetate copolymers; methyl salicylate (p.59·3).
*Minor skin irritation.*

**Ivy-Rid** *Roberts, USA†.*
Polyvinylpyrrolidone vinylacetate copolymers.
*Minor skin irritation.*

**Iwamet** *Masa, Thai.*
Cimetidine (p.1255·3).
*Gastro-oesophageal reflux; hypersensitivity reactions; peptic ulcer; Zollinger-Ellison syndrome.*

**Iwazin** *Masa, Thai.*
Tyrothricin (p.275·1); benzethonium chloride (p.1169·2); benzocaine (p.1370·3).
*Mouth and throat infections.*

**Ixana** *Medical, Arg.*
*Lozenges:* Hexylresorcinol (p.1182·1) sodium benzoate (p.1169·3); senega (p.1130·2); ambay.
*Mouth and throat disorders.*
*Syrup:* Guaifenesin (p.1122·1); sodium benzoate (p.1169·3); senega (p.1130·2); aescin (p.1648·2); ambay.
*Coughs.*

**Ixel**
*Pierre Fabre, Arg.; Pierre Fabre, Austria; Pierre Fabre, Fin.; Pierre Fabre, Fr.; Pierre Fabre, Israel; Pierre Fabre, Port.*
Milnacipran hydrochloride (p.307·3).
*Depression.*

**Ixense**
*Takeda, Austria; Takeda, Fr.; Takeda, Ger.; Takeda, Ital.*
Apomorphine hydrochloride (p.1199·1).
*Erectile dysfunction.*

**Ixor** *Phoinix Pharm (Φοινιξ Φαρμ), Gr.*
Budesonide (p.1094·2).
Also known as Ιχωρ (Ichor).
*Topical corticosteroid.*

**Ixoten**
*Asta Medica, Austria; Baxter, Ger.*
Trofosfamide (p.590·2).
*Malignant neoplasms.*

**Ixprim** *Aventis, Fr.*
Paracetamol (p.76·2); tramadol hydrochloride (p.94·3).
*Pain.*

**Iyafin** *Nakorn, Thai.*
*Junior syrup:* Dextromethorphan hydrobromide (p.1117·3); pseudoephedrine hydrochloride (p.1129·2); chlorphenamine maleate (p.427·3); guaifenesin (p.1122·1); sodium citrate (p.1223·2).
*Syrup:* Dextromethorphan hydrobromide (p.1117·3); pseudoephedrine hydrochloride (p.1129·2); chlorphenamine maleate (p.427·3); guaifenesin (p.1122·1); ammonium chloride (p.1115·2); sodium citrate (p.1223·2).
*Tablets:* Dextromethorphan hydrobromide (p.1117·3); phenylpropanolamine hydrochloride (p.1127·3); chlorphenamine maleate (p.427·3); guaifenesin (p.1122·1).
*Coughs.*

**Izac** *Nakorn, Thai.*
Neomycin sulfate (p.235·1); bacitracin (p.161·3); amylocaine hydrochloride (p.1370·2).
*Mouth infections.*

**Izacef** *Intramed, S.Afr.†.*
Cefazolin sodium (p.170·3).
*Bacterial infections.*

**Izadima** *Pisa, Mex.*
Ceftazidime (p.180·2).
*Bacterial infections.*

**Izatax** *Durascan, Denm.*
Nizatidine (p.1277·2).
*Gastro-oesophageal reflux; peptic ulcer.*

**Izerin** *Rafarm, Gr.*
Propylene glycol cefatrizine (p.170·3).
*Bacterial infections.*

**Izilox** *Bayer, Fr.*
Moxifloxacin hydrochloride (p.233·1).
*Bacterial infections of the respiratory tract.*

**Izo** *Pond's, Thai.*
Isosorbide dinitrate (p.941·1).
*Angina pectoris; heart failure.*

**Izofran** *GlaxoSmithKline, Chile Comprimidos.*
Ondansetron (p.1281·1) or ondansetron hydrochloride (p.1281·1).
*Nausea and vomiting.*

**Jaa Pyral** *Jaapharm, Canad.*
Pyrantel embonate (p.113·2).

**Jaaps Health Salt** *Askit, UK.*
Sodium bicarbonate (p.1223·2); tartaric acid (p.1752·1); potassium sodium tartrate (p.1284·3).
*Constipation; dyspepsia; heartburn.*

**Jaba $B_{12}$** *Jaba, Port.*
Cobamamide (p.1459·1).
*Anaemias; liver disorders; neuralgia; neuritis.*

**Jabastatina** *Bonafarma, Port.*
Simvastatin (p.997·1).
*Hyperlipidaemias.*

**Jabasulide** *Jaba, Port.*
Nimesulide (p.67·1).
*Inflammation; musculoskeletal, joint, and peri-articular disorders; pain.*

**Jabobip** *Billiet, Arg.*
Triclocarban (p.1195·1).
*Skin disinfection.*

**Jabon Antiseptico Asens** *Asens, Spain†.*
Hexachlorophene (p.1181·2).
*Skin disinfection.*

**Jabonacid** *Bajer, Arg.*
Chloroxylenol (p.1177·2); cetrimide (p.1172·1); bornyl acetate (p.1662·2).
*Skin cleanser.*

**Jabonoil** *Panalab, Arg.*
Trichlorosalicylanilide.
*Emollient.*

**Jack and Jill** *Buckley, Canad.*
Guaifenesin (p.1122·1); mepyramine maleate (p.437·1).
Formerly known as Jack and Jill Cough Syrup.
*Cold symptoms; coughs.*

**Jack & Jill Bedtime** *Buckley, Canad.*
Diphenhydramine hydrochloride (p.431·3).

**Jack & Jill DM** *Buckley, Canad.*
Dextromethorphan hydrobromide (p.1117·3); chlorphenamine maleate (p.427·3).
Formerly known as Jack and Jill Children's Formula.
*Cold symptoms; coughs.*

**Jack & Jill Rub** *Buckley, Canad.†.*
Camphor (p.1665·3); menthol (p.1711·3); cineole (p.1672·1).
*Cold symptoms.*

**Jackson's All Fours** *Anglian, UK.*
Guaifenesin (p.1122·1).
*Coughs.*

**Jackson's Bronchial Balsam** *Anglian, UK.*
Guaifenesin (p.1122·1).
*Coughs.*

**Jacksons Herbal Laxative** *Anglian, UK.*
Cascara (p.1255·1); rhubarb (p.1287·3); senna (p.1288·2).
*Constipation.*

**Jackson's Lemon Linctus** *Anglian, UK.*
Glycerol (p.1694·3); honey (p.1434·2).
*Coughs; sore throat.*

**Jacksons Little Healers** *Anglian, UK.*
Ipecacuanha (p.1122·3).
Formerly known as Fennings Little Healers.
*Coughs.*

**Jacksons Mentholated Balm** *Anglian, UK.*
Eucalyptus oil (p.1686·2); methyl salicylate (p.59·3); camphor (p.1665·3); terpineol (p.1752·2); menthol (p.1711·3).
*Musculoskeletal pain; respiratory-tract congestion.*

**Jackson's Pain & Fever** *Anglian, UK.*
Sodium salicylate (p.90·1).
Formerly known as Jacksons Febrifuge.
*Cold and influenza symptoms; musculoskeletal, joint, and soft-tissue disorders.*

**Jackson's Troublesome Coughs** *Anglian, UK.*
Ipecacuanha (p.1122·3); glycerol (p.1694·3); honey (p.1434·2).
*Coughs.*

**Jactuss** *Coup, Gr.*
Zipeprol hydrochloride (p.1132·3).
*Cough.*

**Jacutin**
*Hermal, Austria; Hermal, Ger.; Hermal, Malaysia; Hermal, Singapore; Boots Healthcare, Switz.; Boots, Thai.; Hermal, Thai.*
Lindane (p.1506·3).
*Pediculosis; scabies.*

**Jacutin N** *Hermal, Ger.*
Bioallethrin (p.1500·3); piperonyl butoxide (p.1509·2).
*Pediculosis.*

**Jadelle** *Leiras, Fin.*
Levonorgestrel (p.1563·2).
*Progestogen-only contraceptive implant.*

**Jadit** *Hoechst Marion Roussel, Braz.†.*
Buclosamide (p.395·2); salicylic acid (p.1157·1).
*Fungal skin infections.*

**Jaikal** *S & K, Ger.*
Sodium thiosulfate (p.1053·3); salicylic acid (p.1157·1); resorcinol (p.1156·3).
*Acne.*

**Jaikin N** *Galderma, Ger.*
Dimethicone (p.1482·1).
*Acne.*

**Jakava** *Queisser, Ger.†.*
Kava (p.1703·2).
*Agitation; anxiety.*

**Jalapa comp** *Pfluger, Ger.*
Homoeopathic preparation.

**Jalapa Composta** *Granado, Braz.*
Jalap (p.1268·3); escamonea.

**Jalovis** *Coli, Ital.†.*
Hyaluronidase (p.1698·2); chlorhexidine hydrochloride (p.1173·3).
*Bruising; chilblains; haemorrhoids; skin ulceration; wounds.*

**Jaluran** *Pfizer, Ital.*
Hyaluronidase (p.1698·2).
*Facilitates subcutaneous absorption of drugs.*

**Jamaican Sarsaparilla** *Potter's, UK.*
Sarsaparilla root (p.1742·1); capsicum (p.1667·1); liquorice (p.1270·2); peppermint oil (p.1283·2).
*Skin disorders.*

**Jamylene** *Expanpharm, Fr.*
Docusate sodium (p.1262·2).
*Constipation.*

**Janacin**
*Biolab, Hong Kong; Biolab, Malaysia; Biolab, Thai.*
Norfloxacin (p.238·3).
*Bacterial infections.*

**Jantoven** *Upsher-Smith, USA.*
Warfarin sodium (p.1022·2).
*Thromboembolic disorders.*

**Japan Freeze-Dried Tuberculin** *Vaccina, S.Afr.†.*
Tuberculin purified protein derivative (p.1759·1).
*Tuberculosis test.*

**Japanol** *Liebermann, Ger.*
Mint oil (p.1715·2).
*Cold symptoms; dyspepsia; myalgia.*

**Japomin** *Bano, Austria.*
Peppermint oil (p.1283·2).
*Catarrh; gastrointestinal disorders; headache.*

**Jaquedryl**
*Parke, Davis, Arg.; Parke, Davis, Chile.*
Ergotamine tartrate (p.467·2); caffeine citrate (p.782·1); diphenhydramine hydrochloride (p.431·3).
*Migraine and other vascular headache.*

**Jaquesor** *Soria Natural, Spain.*
Salix (p.87·3); bitter orange (p.1723·3); melissa (p.1711·1); achillea (p.1646·2); tilia (p.1756·2).
*Migraine.*

**Jarabe Bago** *Bago, Arg.*
Noscapine hydrochloride (p.1125·3); guaifenesin (p.1122·1).
*Coughs.*

**Jarabe Manceau** *Alcor, Spain.*
Senna (p.1288·2); coriander (p.1676·1); pyrus malus.
*Constipation.*

**Jarabe Manzanas Siken** *Diafarm, Spain†.*
Senna (p.1288·2); coriander (p.1676·1); prune (p.1285·1); frangula (p.1266·3); fennel (p.1687·2).
*Constipation.*

**Jarabe Palto Compuesto Con Miel** *Maver, Chile.*
Avocado leaf; eucalyptus oil (p.1686·2); tolu balsam (p.1131·3); honey (p.1434·2).
*Coughs.*

**Jarsin**
*Kwizda, Austria; Biosintetica, Braz.; Lichtwer, Ger.; Medichemie Bioline, Switz.*
Hypericum (p.299·1).
*Agitation; anxiety; depression; insomnia; tension.*

**Jasicholin N** *Bolder, Ger.†.*
Butinoline phosphate (p.1663·3); dimethicone (p.1289·2).
*Gastrointestinal disorders.*

**Jasimenth CN** *Bolder, Ger.*
Dequalinium chloride (p.1178·1); ascorbic acid (p.1460·2).
*Mouth and throat disorders.*

**Jasmine** *Schering, Fr.*
Ethinylestradiol (p.1553·2); drospirenone (p.1549·1).
*Combined oral contraceptive.*

**Jatamansin** *Bristol-Myers Squibb, Arg.*
Troxerutin (p.1688·3).
*Haemorrhoids; venous insufficiency.*

**Jatroneural**
*Procter & Gamble, Austria†; Procter & Gamble, Ger.†.*
Trifluoperazine hydrochloride (p.726·3).
*Psychiatric disorders.*

**Jatropur** *Procter & Gamble, Ger.†.*
Triamterene (p.1016·2).
*Oedema.*

**Jatrosom N** *Esparma, Ger.*
Tranylcypromine sulfate (p.318·3).
*Depression.*

**Jatrox** *Procter & Gamble, Ger.†.*
Bismuth salicylate (p.1252·1).
*Gastritis; peptic ulcer; traveller's diarrhoea.*

**Jecobiase** *Pionneau, Fr.†.*
Sodium sulfate (p.1290·1); sodium citrate (p.1223·2); sodium bicarbonate (p.1223·2); magnesium chloride (p.1228·1).
*Gastrointestinal disorders.*

**Jecohepat** *Farmedica, Braz.†.*
Methionine (p.1042·1); choline citrate (p.1424·3); pyridoxine (p.1457·2); betaine (p.1660·1); adenosine (p.851·2); sorbitol (p.1446·3).
*Liver disorders.*

**Jecopeptol** *Alpharma, Fr.*
Aluminium hydroxide (p.1249·2); calcium carbonate (p.1254·2); magnesium hydroxide (p.1272·2); sodium bicarbonate (p.1223·2); boldo (p.1661·2); kinkeliba (p.1703·3); euonymus (p.1265·2).
*Digestive disorders.*

**Jectocos** *CFL, India.*
Iron sorbitol (p.1438·1).
*Iron-deficiency anaemia.*

**Jectocos Plus** *CFL, India.*
Iron sorbitol (p.1438·1); folic acid (p.1429·1); vitamin $B_{12}$ (p.1458·2).
*Iron-deficiency anaemia.*

**Jectofer**
*AstraZeneca, Austria; AstraZeneca, Canad.; AstraZeneca, Denm.†; AstraZeneca, Ger.; AstraZeneca, Irl.; AstraZeneca, Neth.†; AstraZeneca, Norw.; Astra, Swed.†; AstraZeneca, UK†.*
Iron sorbitol (p.1438·1).
*Iron deficiency; iron-deficiency anaemia.*

**Jedipin**
*Jenapharm, Ger.; Jenapharm, Thai.†.*
Nifedipine (p.966·2).
*Angina pectoris; hypertension; myocardial infarction; Raynaud's syndrome.*

**Jekovit** *Orion, Fin.*
Ergocalciferol (p.1462·1).
*Vitamin D deficiency.*

**Jellin** *Grunenthal, Ger.*
Fluocinolone acetonide (p.1101·2).
*Skin disorders.*

**Jellin polyvalent** *Grunenthal, Ger.*
Fluocinolone acetonide (p.1101·2); neomycin sulfate (p.235·1); nystatin (p.406·3).
*Infected skin disorders.*

**Jellin-Neomycin** *Grunenthal, Ger.*
Fluocinolone acetonide (p.1101·2); neomycin sulfate (p.235·1).
*Infected skin disorders.*

**Jelliproct** *Grunenthal, Ger.*
Fluocinonide (p.1101·3); lidocaine (p.1377·3) or lidocaine hydrochloride (p.1377·3).
*Anorectal disorders.*

**Jellisoft** *Grunenthal, Ger.*
Fluocinolone acetonide (p.1101·2).
*Skin disorders.*

**Jellisoft-Neomycin** *Grunenthal, Ger.†.*
Fluocinolone acetonide (p.1101·2); neomycin sulfate (p.235·1).
*Infected skin disorders.*

**Jelonet**
*Smith & Nephew, Austral.; Smith & Nephew, Fr.; Smith & Nephew, Ital.; Smith & Nephew, S.Afr.; Smith & Nephew Healthcare, UK.*
Soft paraffin (p.1479·3).
*Wound dressing.*

**Jemalt 13+13** *Wander Health Care, Switz.*
Multivitamin and mineral preparation (p.1417·1).

**Jemizym** *Jean-Marie, Hong Kong.*
Muramidase hydrochloride (p.1717·2).
*Haemorrhage; respiratory-tract disorders.*

**Jenabroxol** *Jenapharm, Ger.†.*
Ambroxol hydrochloride (p.1114·3).
*Respiratory disorders associated with viscous or excessive mucus.*

**Jenabroxol comp** *Jenapharm, Ger.*
Doxycycline hyclate (p.206·2); ambroxol hydrochloride (p.1114·3).
*Respiratory-tract infections.*

**Jenacard** *Jenapharm, Ger.*
Isosorbide dinitrate (p.941·1).
*Angina pectoris.*

**Jenacillin V** *Jenapharm, Ger.*
Phenoxymethylpenicillin potassium (p.242·1).
*Bacterial infections.*

**Jenacillin A** *Jenapharm, Ger.*
Benzylpenicillin sodium (p.163·2); procaine benzylpenicillin (p.246·1).
*Bacterial infections.*

**Jenacillin O** *Jenapharm, Ger.*
Procaine benzylpenicillin (p.246·1).
*Bacterial infections.*

**Jenacyclin** *Jenapharm, Ger.*
Doxycycline (p.206·2).
*Bacterial infections.*

**Jenacysteine** *Jenapharm, Ger.†.*
Acetylcysteine (p.1112·3).
*Respiratory disorders associated with viscous or excessive mucus.*

**Jenafenac** *Jenapharm, Ger.*
Diclofenac sodium (p.32·1).
*Gout; inflammation; musculoskeletal, joint, and soft-tissue disorders.*

**Jenamazol** *Jenapharm, Ger.*
Clotrimazole (p.396·2).
*Corynebacterium infections; fungal infections.*

**Jenametidin** Jenapharm, Ger.†.
Cimetidine (p.1255·3).
*Aspiration syndrome; gastro-oesophageal reflux; peptic ulcer; Zollinger-Ellison syndrome.*

**Jenamoxazol** Jenapharm, Ger.†.
Co-trimoxazole (p.199·3).
*Bacterial infections.*

**Jenampin** Jenapharm, Ger.†.
Ampicillin trihydrate (p.157·2).
*Bacterial infections.*

**Jenapamil** Jenapharm, Ger.
Verapamil hydrochloride (p.1019·1).
*Angina pectoris; hypertension; tachycardia.*

**Jenapirox** Jenapharm, Ger.
Piroxicam (p.84·2).
*Musculoskeletal and joint disorders.*

**Jenaprofen** Jenapharm, Ger.
Ibuprofen (p.45·3).
*Fever; inflammation; musculoskeletal, joint, and soft-tissue disorders; pain.*

**Jenapurinol** Jenapharm, Ger.
Allopurinol (p.412·2).
*Gout; hyperuricaemia; renal calculi.*

**Jenaspiron** Jenapharm, Ger.
Spironolactone (p.1003·1).
*Ascites; hyperaldosteronism; oedema.*

**Jenasteron** Jenapharm, Malaysia.
Testosterone enantate (p.1570·1).
*Breast cancer; delayed puberty and hypogonadism in males.*

**Jenatacin** Jenapharm, Ger.†.
Indometacin (p.47·3).
*Gout; musculoskeletal, joint, and soft-tissue disorders; pain.*

**Jenatenol** Jenapharm, Ger.
Atenolol (p.865·2).
*Angina pectoris; arrhythmias; myocardial infarction.*

**Jenateren comp** Jenapharm, Ger.
Triamterene (p.1016·2); hydrochlorothiazide (p.933·2).
*Heart failure; hypertension; oedema.*

**Jenest** Organon, USA†.
21 Tablets, norethisterone (p.1562·2); ethinylestradiol (p.1553·2); 7 tablets, inert.
*Biphasic oral contraceptive.*

**Jenoquine** Julphar, UAE.
Levofloxacin (p.225·3).
*Bacterial infections.*

**Jenoxifen** Jenapharm, Ger.
Tamoxifen citrate (p.584·1).
*Breast cancer.*

**Jephagynon** Jenapharm, Ger.
Estradiol benzoate (p.1550·1); progesterone (p.1566·2).
*Amenorrhoea.*

**Jephoxin** Jenapharm, Ger.†.
Amoxicillin trihydrate (p.155·3).
*Bacterial infections.*

**Jeprolol** Jenapharm, Ger.
Metoprolol tartrate (p.957·1).
*Arrhythmias; hypertension; migraine; myocardial infarction.*

**Jestryl** Chauvin ankerpharm, Ger.
Carbachol (p.1488·1).
*Glaucoma; production of miosis.*

**Jet Lag** Homeocan, Canad.
Homoeopathic preparation.

**Jetepar**
Rotta, Hong Kong; Rotta, Malaysia; Rotta, Singapore.
Betaine glucuronate (p.1660·2); diolamine glucuronate; nicotinamide ascorbate.
*Biliary-tract disorders; liver disorders.*

**Jetomisol-P** Ethnor, India.
Tetramisole (p.114·1); phenolphthalein (p.1284·1).
*Worm infections.*

**Jets** Freeda, USA.
Multivitamin preparation with lysine (p.1417·1).

**JE-Vaccine** Kaketsuken, Thai.
An inactivated Japanese encephalitis vaccine, Beijing strain (p.1621·2).
*Active immunisation.*

**JE-Vax**
Aventis Pasteur, Austral.; Aventis Pasteur, Canad.; Pasteur Merieux, USA.
An inactivated Japanese encephalitis vaccine (p.1621·2).
*Active immunisation.*

**Jevity**
Abbott, Arg.; Abbott, Austral.; Abbott, Braz.; Abbott, Canad.; Abbott, Fin.; Abbott, Fr.; Abbott, Hong Kong; Abbott, Irl.; Ross, Israel; Abbott, Ital.; Abbott, Mex.; Abbott, NZ; Abbott, Singapore; Abbott, Thai.; Abbott Nutrition, UK; Ross, USA.
Preparation for enteral nutrition (p.1417·1).

**Jezil** Alphapharm, Austral.
Gemfibrozil (p.923·1).
*Hyperlipidaemias.*

**JHP Rodler** Woelm, Ger.
Mint oil (p.1715·2).
*Cold symptoms; gastrointestinal disorders; headache.*

**Jiffy Toothache Drops** Block, Canad.†.
Benzocaine (p.1370·3); eugenol (p.1686·2).
*Toothache.*

**Jinda** Riemser, Ger.
Cimicifuga (p.1671·3).
*Menopausal disorders.*

**Jodetten** Henning, Ger.
Potassium iodide (p.1598·1).
*Iodine-deficiency disorders.*

**Jodgamma** Worwag, Ger.
Potassium iodide (p.1598·1).
*Iodine-deficiency disorders.*

**Jodid**
Merck, Austria; Merck, Ger.; Ratiopharm, Ger.; Verla, Ger.
Potassium iodide (p.1598·1).
*Iodine-deficiency disorders.*

**Jodieci** Esoform, Ital.
Povidone-iodine (p.1190·3); alcohol (p.1166·1).
*Disinfection of skin and superficial wounds; infected skin disorders.*

**Jodix** Orion, Fin.
Potassium iodide (p.1598·1).
*Protection of the thyroid from radio-iodine.*

**Jodlauge, Tolzer** Jodquellen, Ger.
Anions: chloride, bromide, iodide, bicarbonate; cations: sodium, magnesium, potassium, calcium.
*Circulatory disorders.*

**jodminerase** GN, Ger.†.
Potassium iodide (p.1598·1).
*Iodine-deficiency disorders.*

**Jodo Calcio Vitaminico** Bruschettini, Ital.
Sodium iodide (p.1598·1); potassium iodide (p.1598·1); rubidium iodide (p.1741·1); calcium gluconate (p.1225·2); ascorbic acid (p.1460·2).
*Cataracts.*

**Jodobac**
Note. This name is used for preparations of different composition.
Bode, Ger.
Povidone-iodine (p.1190·3).
*Catheter care; disinfection of the skin, mucous membranes, and hands; wounds.*

Beiersdorf, Switz.†.
Propyl alcohol (p.1191·2); povidone-iodine (p.1190·3).
*Skin and wound disinfection.*

**Jodocur** Farmacologico Milanese, Ital.
Povidone-iodine (p.1190·3).
*Disinfection of skin, wounds, and burns; mouth and throat infections; vaginal hygiene.*

**Jodoform** Lohmann, Ger.
Iodoform (p.1184·2).
*Wounds.*

**Jodogard** Gedis, Ital.
Povidone-iodine (p.1190·3).
*Skin and hand disinfection.*

**Jodonorm** Biochemie, Austria.
Sodium iodide (p.1598·1).
*Iodine-deficiency goitre.*

**Jodoplex** Streuli, Switz.
Povidone-iodine (p.1190·3).
*Burns; infected skin disorders; skin, hand, and mucous-membrane disinfection; ulcers; wounds.*

**Jodosan** Brenntag, Norw.
Iodine (p.1598·1).
Formerly known as Idu-Phor.
*Disinfection of skin and wounds.*

**Jodthyrox**
Merck, Austria; Merck, Ger.
Levothyroxine sodium (p.1600·1); potassium iodide (p.1598·1).
*Iodine-deficiency disorders.*

**Joggers** Solgar, UK†.
Multivitamin and mineral preparation with bee pollen and ginseng (p.1417·1).

**Johanicum** Apomedica, Austria.
Hypericum (p.299·1).
*Depression.*

**John Plunketts Protective Day Cream** Sunspot, Austral.†.
*SPF 25:* Elastin; collagen (p.1674·3); vitamin A (p.1451·2); Dermasome SOD; Dermasome E; Megasol Complex; oxybenzone (p.1154·3); octinoxate (p.1154·3).
*Emollient; sunscreen.*

**John Plunketts Super Wrinkle Cream** Sunspot, Austral.†.
Active soluble elastin; active soluble collagen (p.1674·3).
*Dry skin; wrinkles.*

**John Plunketts Vita-Pore** Sunspot, Austral.†.
Soluble bio-sulfur CLR (p.1158·2); vitamin B; hamamelis (p.1696·3).
*Oily skin.*

**Johnson & Johnson Burn Cream** Johnson & Johnson, Canad.†.
Benzocaine (p.1370·3).

**Johnson & Johnson First Aid Ointment** Johnson & Johnson, Canad.
Bacitracin zinc (p.161·3); polymyxin B sulfate (p.245·1).

**Johnson's Antiseptic Powder** Pharmedica, S.Afr.†.
Benzethonium chloride (p.1169·2).
*Skin disorders.*

**Johnsons Baby** Johnson & Johnson, Canad.
*SPF 15:* Meradimate (p.1151·3); octinoxate (p.1154·3); titanium dioxide (p.1160·3).
*Sunscreen.*

**Johnson's Baby Clear** Johnson & Johnson, Thai.
Ethyl butylacetylaminopropionate.
*Insect repellent.*

**Johnson's Baby Nappy Rash Ointment** Pharmedica, S.Afr.†.
Zinc oxide (p.1163·2).
*Napkin rash.*

**Johnson's Baby Prickly Heat Powder** Johnson & Johnson, Thai.
Eucalyptus oil (p.1686·2); zinc oxide (p.1163·2); chloroxylenol (p.1177·2).
*Heat rash.*

**Johnson's Baby Sunblock** Johnson & Johnson, USA.
*SPF 15:* Zinc oxide (p.1163·2); titanium dioxide (p.1160·3).
*SPF 30:* Oxybenzone (p.1154·3); octinoxate (p.1154·3) octisalate (p.1154·3); titanium dioxide (p.1160·3).
*Sunscreen.*

**Johnsons Clean & Clear Daily Facial Moisturiser** Johnson & Johnson, Austral.†.
*SPF 15:* Salicylic acid (p.1157·1); octinoxate (p.1154·3); enzacamene (p.1147·1); avobenzone (p.1142·3).
*Moisturiser; sunscreen.*

**Johnsons Clean & Clear Dual Action Moisturizer** Johnson & Johnson, Canad.
Salicylic acid (p.1157·1).
*Acne.*

**Johnsons Clean & Clear Facial Cleansing Bar** Johnson & Johnson, Austral.†.
Triclosan (p.1195·2).
*Acne; soap substitute.*

**Johnsons Clean & Clear Foaming Facial Wash** Johnson & Johnson, Austral.†.
Triclosan (p.1195·2).
*Acne; soap substitute.*

**Johnsons Clean & Clear Invisible Blemish Treatment** Johnson & Johnson, Austral.†.
Salicylic acid (p.1157·1); alcohol (p.1166·1).
*Acne.*

**Johnsons Clean & Clear Oil Controlling Toner** Johnson & Johnson, Austral.†.
Salicylic acid (p.1157·1); alcohol (p.1166·1).
*Acne.*

**Johnsons Clean & Clear Persa Gel** Johnson & Johnson, Canad.
Benzoyl peroxide (p.1143·2).
*Acne.*

**Johnsons Clean & Clear Pore Prep** Johnson & Johnson, Canad.
Salicylic acid (p.1157·1).
*Acne.*

**Johnsons Clean & Clear Skin Balancing Moisturiser** Johnson & Johnson, Austral.†.
Salicylic acid (p.1157·1).
*Acne.*

**Johnson's Diaper Rash** Johnson & Johnson, Canad.
Zinc oxide (p.1163·2).
*Nappy rash.*

**Johnson's Medicated** Johnson & Johnson, Canad.
Zinc oxide (p.1163·2).
*Nappy rash.*

**Johnson's Penaten Crema Disinfettante** Johnson & Johnson, Ital.†.
Cetylpyridinium chloride (p.1173·1).
*Nappy rash.*

**Joint** Pharmacia, Arg.
Oxaceprol (p.1725·1).
*Musculoskeletal and joint disorders.*

**Joint Action** Lifeplan, UK.
Glucosamine sulfate (p.1694·1); chondroitin sulfate; vitamin C; manganese (p.1417·1).
*Musculoskeletal and joint disorders.*

**Joint & Muscle Complex** Brauer, Austral.†.
Homoeopathic preparation.

**Joint & Muscle Oral Spray and Tablets** Brauer, Austral.†.
Homoeopathic preparation.

**Joint & Muscle Relief Cream** Brauer, Austral.†.
Arnica (p.1656·3); bellis perennis; bryonia (p.1663·1); hypericum (p.299·1); kalmia latifolia; ledum palustre; rue (p.1741·1); ranunculus bulbosus; toxicodendron radicans; belladonna; camphora; symphytum.
*Musculoskeletal, joint, peri-articular, and soft-tissue disorders.*

**Joint Support** Eurosup, Ital.
Glucosamine sulfate (p.1694·1); acetyl glucosamine; chondroitin sulfate (p.1670·2).
*Cartilage disorders.*

**Jointace** Vitabiotics, UK.
*Capsules:* Glucosamine; omega-3 fish oil; cod-liver oil; vitamins; trace elements (p.1417·1).
*Nutritional supplement.*
*Effervescent tablets:* Glucosamine sulfate (p.1694·1); chondroitin sulfate (p.1670·2); vitamin C; magnesium (p.1417·1).
*Nutritional supplement.*
*Topical gel:* Glucosamine (p.1694·1); chondroitin.
*Musculoskeletal and joint disorders.*

**Joint-e-Licious** Naturopathica, UK.
Glucosamine hydrochloride.
*Joint pain.*

**Jolivette** Watson, USA.
Norethisterone (p.1562·2).
*Progestogen-only oral contraceptive.*

**Jomax** Bioglan, Ger.
Bufexamac (p.21·3).
*Skin disorders.*

**Jomethid** Cox, UK†.
Ketoprofen (p.51·2).
*Gout; musculoskeletal, joint, and peri-articular disorders; pain.*

**Jonac** German Remedies, India.
Diclofenac diethylamine (p.32·1) or diclofenac sodium (p.32·1).
*Gout; musculoskeletal, joint, and soft-tissue disorders.*

**Jonctum** Aventis, Fr.
Oxaceprol (p.1725·1).
*Burns; rheumatic disorders.*

**Jonil T** Galderma, Switz.†.
Coal tar (p.1159·2); salicylic acid (p.1157·1); benzalkonium chloride (p.1168·3).
*Scalp disorders.*

**Jonosteril** Fresenius Kabi, Ger.
A range of electrolyte infusions with or without carbohydrate (p.1217·1).
*Fluid and electrolyte disorders.*

**Jopamiro** Gerot, Austria.
Iopamidol (p.1064·3).
*Radiographic contrast medium.*

**Jopinol** Bernhauer, Austria.
Iodine (p.1598·1); pumilio pine oil (p.1737·1).
*Catarrh.*

**Jorkil** Bohm, Spain†.
Silicone (p.1289·2); metoclopramide hydrochloride (p.1274·3); glutamine (p.1433·2); aluminium glycinate (p.1249·1); mannitol (p.950·2).
*Dyspepsia; meteorism.*

**Josacine**
Bayer, Fr.; Yamanouchi, Switz.†.
Josamycin (p.224·3) or josamycin propionate (p.224·3).
*Bacterial infections.*

**Josalid** Biochemie, Austria.
Josamycin (p.224·3).
*Bacterial infections; toxoplasmosis.*

**Josamina** Novag, Spain.
Josamycin (p.224·3) or josamycin propionate (p.224·3).
*Bacterial infections.*

**Josamy** Yamanouchi, Jpn.
Josamycin (p.224·3) or josamycin propionate (p.224·3).
*Bacterial infections.*

**Josaxin**
UCB, Ital.; Yamanouchi, Spain†.
Josamycin (p.224·3) or josamycin propionate (p.224·3).
*Bacterial infections.*

**Josir** Boehringer Ingelheim, Fr.
Tamsulosin hydrochloride (p.1009·2).
*Benign prostatic hyperplasia.*

**Jossalind** Hexal, Ger.†.
Sodium hyaluronate (p.1697·3).
*Ulcers; wounds.*

**Jour Apres Jour** Lactel, Fr.†.
Nutritional supplement (p.1417·1).

**Jouvence** Carmaran, Canad.†.
Hydroquinone (p.1148·1).

**Jouvence de l'Abbe Soury** Chefaro Ardeval, Fr.
*Oral solution; tablets:* Hamamelis (p.1696·3); calamus (p.1664·1); piscidia (p.1702·3); viburnum.
*Peripheral vascular disorders.*
*Topical gel:* Hamamelis (p.1696·3); viburnum.
*Peripheral vascular disorders; venous insufficiency.*

**Joy-Rides** GlaxoSmithKline Consumer, UK.
Hyoscine hydrobromide (p.483·3).
*Motion sickness.*

**Joysun** YSP, Malaysia.
Gentamicin sulfate (p.217·1); betamethasone sodium phosphate (p.1093·1).
*Infected eye and ear disorders.*

**Joyzol** Wockhardt, India.
Olanzapine (p.710·3).
*Bipolar disorder; psychoses.*

**JP Tone** Jagson, India.
Ferrous gluconate (p.1428·1); vitamin B substances (p.1454·3).
*Anaemias; tonic.*

**Jsoskleran** Iso, Ger.
Homoeopathic preparation.

**Jsostoma S** Iso, Ger.
Homoeopathic preparation.

**Juaflor** Terapia, Mex.†.
Metronidazole benzoate (p.607·2).

**JuBronchan C** Jukunda, Ger.
Homoeopathic preparation.

**JuCholan S** Jukunda, Ger.†.
Silybum marianum (p.1043·3); hypericum (p.299·1); taraxacum (p.1751·3); peppermint leaf (p.1283·2); cheldionium (p.1695·3).
*Liver and biliary-tract disorders.*

**JuCor** Jukunda, Ger.
Homoeopathic preparation.

**Jucurba** Strathmann, Ger.
Devil's claw root (p.28·2).
*Musculoskeletal and joint disorders.*

**JuCystan S** Jukunda, Ger.
Homoeopathic preparation.

**JuDorm** Jukunda, Ger.
Lupulus (p.1708·1); melissa (p.1711·1); valerian (p.1762·2); hypericum (p.299·1).
*Insomnia; stress.*

**JuGrippan** *Jukunda, Ger.†.*
Echinacea (p.1683·2); centaury (p.1669·2); chamomile (p.1669·3); calendula (p.1665·2); hamamelis; achillea; ysop; arnica; bryonia; aconit; belladonna; ferrum phos.; kalium chloratum; silicea; ammonium carb.
*Cold symptoms.*

**JuGrippan S** *Jukunda, Ger.*
Homoeopathic preparation.

**JuHepan** *Jukunda, Ger.*
Homoeopathic preparation.

**Jukunda Melissen-Krautergeist** *Jukunda, Ger.*
Melissa; sloe; ginger; melissa oil; rosemary oil; lavender oil; pimentol; cinnamon oil; clove oil (p.1417·1).
*Tonic.*

**Jukunda Rotol** *Jukunda, Ger.†.*
Hypericum (p.299·1).
*Gastrointestinal disorders; nervous disorders; wounds.*

**Julab**
*Biolab, Hong Kong; Biolab, Thai.*
Selegiline hydrochloride (p.1214·1).
*Parkinsonism.*

**JuLax** *Amadeus, India.*
Bisacodyl (p.1251·3).
*Constipation.*

**JuLax S** *Jukunda, Ger.†.*
Senna (p.1288·2).
*Constipation.*

**JuLax-M** *Amadeus, India.*
Bisacodyl (p.1251·3).
*Constipation.*

**Juliet** *Schering, Austral.*
21 Tablets, cyproterone acetate (p.1544·1); ethinylestradiol (p.1553·2); 7 tablets, inert.

**Julmentin** *Julphar, UAE.*
Amoxicillin trihydrate (p.155·3); potassium clavulanate (p.193·3).
*Bacterial infections.*

**Julphacef** *Julphar, UAE.*
Cefradine (p.179·3).
Formerly known as Eskacef.
*Bacterial infections.*

**Julphamox** *Julphar, UAE.*
Amoxicillin trihydrate (p.155·3).
*Bacterial infections.*

**Julphapen** *Julphar, UAE.*
Ampicillin trihydrate (p.157·2).
*Bacterial infections.*

**JuMenstran** *Jukunda, Ger.*
Homoeopathic preparation.

**Jumex**
*Armstrong, Arg.; Sanofi Synthelabo, Austria; Sanofi Synthelabo, Hong Kong; Dexxon, Israel; Chiesi, Ital.; Sanofi Synthelabo, Malaysia; Novartis, Port.; Sanofi Synthelabo, Singapore; Sanofi Synthelabo, Thai.*
Selegiline hydrochloride (p.1214·1).
*Parkinsonism.*

**Jumexal** *Sanofi Synthelabo, Switz.*
Selegiline hydrochloride (p.1214·1).
*Parkinsonism.*

**Jumexil** *Farmalab, Braz.*
Selegiline hydrochloride (p.1214·1).
*Parkinsonism.*

**Junamac** *Cantassium Co., UK.*
Multivitamin and mineral preparation (p.1417·1).

**Junel Fe** *Barr, USA.*
21 Tablets, norethisterone acetate (p.1562·2); ethinylestradiol (p.1553·2); 7 tablets, ferrous fumarate (p.1427·3).
*Combined oral contraceptive.*

**JuNeuron S** *Jukunda, Ger.†.*
Scopolaminum hydrobromic.; avena sativa; valerian (p.1762·2); passion flower (p.1729·1); lupulus (p.1708·1); hypericum (p.299·1); melissa (p.1711·1).
*Insomnia; nervousness.*

**Jungborn** *Taro, Israel.*
*Oral granules:* Senna (p.1288·2).
*Teabags:* Senna (p.1288·2); tilia (p.1756·2); caraway (p.1667·2); aniseed (p.1655·2); fennel (p.1687·2); bearberry (p.1659·2); chamomile (p.1669·3); peppermint leaf (p.1283·2).
*Constipation.*

**Jungle Formula Insect Repellent** *Chefaro, UK.*
Diethyltoluamide (p.1503·3).

**Jungle Formula Insect Repellent Plus U.V. Sunscreens** *Chefaro, UK†.*
Padimate O (p.1155·1); oxybenzone (p.1154·3); diethyltoluamide (p.1503·3).

**Jungle Formula Sting Relief Cream** *Chefaro, UK†.*
Hydrocortisone (p.1103·3).
*Insect bites and stings.*

**Junifen**
*Boots Healthcare, Belg.; Boots Healthcare, Spain; Boots, Thai.*
Ibuprofen (p.45·3).
*Fever; inflammation; pain.*

**Junik** *Fujisawa, Ger.*
Beclometasone dipropionate (p.1091·1).
*Asthma.*

**Junior Citrex** *Raza, Malaysia; Pharmaniaga, Malaysia.*
A range of multivitamin preparations with omega-3 marine triglycerides or lysine (p.1417·1).

**Junior Citrex Cal-Mag-D3** *Raza, Malaysia; Pharmaniaga, Malaysia.*
Calcium (p.1225·1); magnesium (p.1227·3); colecalciferol (p.1461·3).

**Junior Disprin** *Reckitt Benckiser, S.Afr.*
Paracetamol (p.76·2).
*Fever; pain.*

**Junior Ideal Quota** *Cantassium Co., UK.*
Multivitamin and mineral preparation (p.1417·1).

**Junior Kao-C** *Torbet Laboratories, UK.*
Calcium carbonate (p.1254·2); light kaolin (p.1268·3).
*Diarrhoea.*

**Junior Strength Cold DM** *WestCan, Canad.*
Pseudoephedrine hydrochloride (p.1129·2); chlorphenamine maleate (p.427·3); dextromethorphan hydrobromide (p.1117·3); paracetamol (p.76·2).

**Junior Strength Tylenol** *McNeil, Hong Kong.*
Paracetamol (p.76·2).
*Fever; pain.*

**Junior Time C** *Vitaplex, Austral.†.*
Vitamin C substances (p.1417·1).

**Juniormen** *Retrain, Spain†.*
Nicametate; ginseng; pyritinol hydrochloride; rutoside; vitamins (p.1417·1); deanol acid tartrate.
*Tonic.*

**Juniorvit** *Pharmadass, UK.*
Multivitamin and mineral preparation (p.1417·1).

**Juniperus-Komplex-Injektopas** *Pascoe, Ger.†.*
Homoeopathic preparation.

**Junisana** *Riemser, Ger.*
Althaea (p.1651·3); thyme (p.1755·2); guaiacum; liquorice (p.1270·2); iron(III)-sucrose-complex (p.1438·2); juniper (p.1703·1); calcium lactate (p.1225·3).
*Bronchitis; catarrh; coughs.*

**Junivite** *Boots, Thai.*
Multivitamin preparation (p.1417·1).

**Juno Junipah** *Torbet Laboratories, UK†.*
*Oral powders:* Sodium sulfate (p.1290·1); sodium phosphate (p.1231·1); sodium bicarbonate (p.1223·2); juniper oil (p.1703·1).
*Tablets:* Sodium sulfate (p.1290·1); sodium phosphate (p.1231·1); phenolphthalein (p.1284·1); juniper oil (p.1703·1).
*Constipation.*

**JuPhlebon S** *Jukunda, Ger.†.*
Melilotus; scoparium (p.1742·2); aesculus (p.1648·2); hamamelis; cuprum aceticum.
*Venous insufficiency.*

**Jurubileno** *Ibefar, Braz.†.*
Solanum paniculatum; boldo (p.1661·2); cascara (p.1255·1); cynara (p.1678·3); choline citrate (p.1424·3); sodium glycolate (p.1660·3).
*Liver disorders.*

**Jusline 70/30** *Julphar, UAE†.*
Insulin injection (human) (p.333·3).
*Diabetes mellitus.*

**Jusline N** *Julphar, UAE†.*
Insulin injection (human) (p.333·3).
*Diabetes mellitus.*

**Jusline R** *Julphar, UAE†.*
Insulin injection (human) (p.333·3).
*Diabetes mellitus.*

**Jusprin** *Julphar, UAE.*
Aspirin (p.15·1).
*Fever; inflammation; pain; thromboembolism prophylaxis.*

**Just One Per Day** *Reese, USA†.*
Phenylpropanolamine hydrochloride (p.1127·3).

**Justar** *Intersan, Ger.*
Cicletanine hydrochloride (p.883·2).
*Hypertension.*

**Justebarin** *Juste, Spain†.*
Barium sulfate (p.1061·1).
*Contrast medium for gastrointestinal radiography.*

**Justegas**
*Schering, Chile; Juste, Spain.*
Citric acid (p.1673·1); sodium bicarbonate (p.1223·2).
*Gastrointestinal hyperacidity.*

**Justelax** *Juste, Spain†.*
Sennosides A and B (p.1288·2).
*Bowel evacuation.*

**Justogen mono** *Wernigerode, Ger.†.*
Taraxacum (p.1751·3).
*Biliary-tract disorders; dyspepsia; reduced appetite.*

**Justor** *Chiesi, Fr.*
Cilazapril (p.883·3).
*Heart failure; hypertension.*

**Justum** *Labinca, Arg.*
Dipotassium clorazepate (p.685·1).
*Anxiety.*

**Jutussin N R8** *Reckeweg, Ger.*
Homoeopathic preparation.

**Jutussin neo** *Pharma Force, Austria.*
Plantago lanceolata (p.1738·2); thyme (p.1755·2); verbascum (p.1764·1).
*Coughs.*

**Juvela**
*Note. This name is used for preparations of different composition.*
*Scientific Hospital Supplies, Irl.; Scientific Hospital Supplies, UK.*
Food for special diets (p.1417·1).
*Gluten-sensitive enteropathies.*

*Eisai, Jpn.*
Tocoferil nicotinate (p.1015·1).
*Arteriosclerosis; cerebrovascular disorders; hyperlipidaemia; hypertension; peripheral circulatory disorders.*

*Eisai, Malaysia; Eisai, Singapore†.*
*dl*-Alpha tocoferil acetate (p.1465·1).
*Circulatory disorders; vitamin E deficiency.*

**Juvenit** *Andromaco, Chile.*
Vitis vinifera.

**Juvental** *Hennig, Ger.*
Atenolol (p.865·2).
*Angina pectoris; arrhythmias; hypertension.*

**Juvepirine** *Asta Medica, Fr.†.*
Aspirin (p.15·1).
Glycine (p.1433·3) is included in this preparation in an attempt to limit adverse effects on the gastrointestinal mucosa.
*Fever; musculoskeletal and joint disorders; pain.*

**Juvitan** *Elea, Arg.*
Ginsenosides (p.1693·1).
*Tonic.*

**JuViton** *Jukunda, Ger.*
Crataegus (p.1677·1); rosemary (p.1740·2); hypericum (p.299·1); primrose flower (p.1735·1); ginger (p.1267·1); primula veris; kola; cactus; kalmia; lilium tigrinum; ambra; aurum colloidale; lycopus virg.
*Cardiovascular disorders.*

**Juwoment Sport** *Serum-Werk Bernburg, Ger.†.*
Heparin sodium (p.928·1).
*Soft-tissue injury.*

**K1** *Sivaderm, Arg.*
Phytomenadione (p.1467·1).

**K-10** *GlaxoSmithKline, Canad.*
Potassium chloride (p.1232·2).
*Potassium depletion.*

**K-50** *ICN, Mex.*
Menadione sodium bisulfite (p.1466·3).
*Haemorrhagic disorders.*

**K + 8** *Alra, USA.*
Potassium chloride (p.1232·2).
*Hypokalaemia; potassium depletion.*

**K + 10** *Alra, USA.*
Potassium chloride (p.1232·2).
*Hypokalaemia; potassium depletion.*

**K + Care** *Alra, USA.*
Potassium bicarbonate (p.1223·1).
*Hypokalaemia; potassium depletion.*

**K5 Hair Tincture** *German Remedies, India.*
Benzyl nicotinate (p.21·2); vitamin $K_5$ (p.1466·3); salicylic acid (p.1157·1).
*Scalp disorders.*

**K 1000 T** *Hanosan, Ger.*
Homoeopathic preparation.

**K Thrombin** *Fawns & McAllan, Austral.*
Menadione sodium bisulfite (p.1466·3).
*Prothrombin deficiency.*

**Kabala** *IMA, Braz.†.*
Coal tar (p.1159·2); jaborandi.
*Keratinisation disorders; seborrhoeic dermatitis.*

**Kaban** *Asche, Ger.*
Clocortolone pivalate (p.1096·1); clocortolone caproate (p.1096·1).
*Burns; skin disorders.*

**Kabanimat** *Asche, Ger.*
Clocortolone pivalate (p.1096·1); clocortolone caproate (p.1096·1).
*Burns; skin disorders.*

**Kabiglobulin** *Pharmacia, UK†.*
A normal immunoglobulin (p.1627·2).
*Agammaglobulinaemia; hypogammaglobulinaemia; passive immunisation.*

**Kabikinase**
*Pharmacia, Austral.†; Pharmacia, Austria; Pharmacia Upjohn, Belg.†; Pharmacia, Braz.; Pharmacia Upjohn, Canad.†; Pharmacia Upjohn, Denm.†; Pharmacia Upjohn, Fin.†; Pharmacia Upjohn, Fr.†; Pharmacia Upjohn, Ger.†; Pharmacia Upjohn, Hong Kong†; Pharmacia Upjohn, Irl.†; Pharmacia Upjohn, Israel; Pharmacia Upjohn, Mex.†; Pharmacia Upjohn, Neth.†; Pharmacia, Norw.; Pharmacia Upjohn, NZ†; Pharmacia Upjohn, Port.†; Pharmacia Upjohn, S.Afr.†; Pharmacia Upjohn, Singapore†; Pharmacia, Spain; Pharmacia Upjohn, Swed.†; Pharmacia Upjohn, Switz.†; Pharmacia Upjohn, Thai.†; Pharmacia, UK†; Kabi Pharmacia, USA†.*
Streptokinase (p.1005·2).
*Thromboembolic disorders.*

**KabiMix**
*Fresenius Kabi, Austria; Fresenius Kabi, Denm.†; Fresenius Kabi, Fr.; Pharmacia Upjohn, Ital.; Fresenius Kabi, Neth.; Fresenius Kabi, Norw.; Fresenius Kabi, Port.†; Fresenius Kabi, Spain; Fresenius Kabi, Swed.; Fresenius Kabi, UK†.*
Amino-acid, carbohydrate, and lipid (from soya oil (p.1447·2)) infusion with or without electrolytes (p.1417·1).
Contains egg lecithin or egg phospholipids.
*Parenteral nutrition.*

**KabiMix Basal** *Fresenius Kabi, Fin.†.*
Amino-acid, glucose, lipid (from soya oil (p.1447·2)), and electrolyte infusion (p.1417·1).
Contains egg phospholipids.
*Parenteral nutrition.*

**Kabiven**
*Fresenius Kabi, Austria; Fresenius Kabi, Denm.; Fresenius Kabi, Fin.; Fresenius Kabi, Fr.; Fresenius Kabi, Ital.; Fresenius Kabi, Norw.; Fresenius Kabi, Port.; Fresenius Kabi, Singapore; Fresenius Kabi, Spain; Fresenius Kabi, Swed.; Fresenius Kabi, Switz.; Fresenius Kabi, UK.*
Amino-acid, glucose, lipid (from soyal oil (p.1447·2)) and electrolyte infusion (p.1417·1).
Contains egg phospholipids.
*Parenteral nutrition.*

**Kacerutin** *Purissimus, Arg.*
Vitamin K (p.1466·3); rutoside (p.1688·2); vitamin C (p.1460·2).
*Capillary haemorrhage.*

**KA-Cilone** *SM, Thai.*
Triamcinolone acetonide (p.1110·2); kanamycin sulfate (p.225·1).
*Infected skin disorders.*

**Kacinth** *Intramed, S.Afr.†.*
Amikacin sulfate (p.154·1).
*Bacterial infections.*

**Kadalex** *Diaco, Ital.*
Potassium chloride (p.1232·2).
*Hypokalaemia.*

**KadeFungin** *Kade, Ger.*
Clotrimazole (p.396·2).
*Fungal and bacterial infections of the vagina.*

**Kadian**
*Abbott, Canad.; Faulding, USA.*
Morphine sulfate (p.60·2).
*Pain.*

**Kadiur** *GiEnne, Ital.*
Potassium canrenoate (p.984·2); butizide (p.878·2).
*Hyperaldosteronism.*

**Kadol** *Teofarma, Ital.*
Phenylbutazone (p.83·2).
*Musculoskeletal and soft-tissue disorders; skin irritation.*

**Kadolax** *Hua, Thai.*
Bisacodyl (p.1251·3).
*Constipation.*

**Kaergona Hidrosoluble** *Ern, Spain.*
Menadione (p.1466·3).
*Hypoprothrombinaemia.*

**Kafa** *Democal, Switz.*
Propyphenazone (p.85·3); paracetamol (p.76·2); caffeine (p.782·1).
*Pain.*

**Kainever** *Seber, Port.*
Estazolam (p.697·3).
*Insomnia.*

**Kaion Retard** *Silesia, Chile.*
Potassium chloride (p.1232·2).
*Hypokalaemia.*

**Kaizem** *Wockhardt, India.*
Diltiazem hydrochloride (p.900·1).
*Angina pectoris.*

**Kajel** *Alacan, Spain†.*
Hypericum (p.299·1).
*Sleep disorders; tonic.*

**Kajos**
*AstraZeneca, Norw.; Hassle, Swed.*
Potassium citrate (p.1223·1).
*Potassium supplement.*

**Kal Sept** *Elofar, Braz.†.*
Kaolin (p.1268·3); pectin (p.1580·3); aluminium hydroxide (p.1249·2).
*Diarrhoea.*

**Kala** *Freeda, USA.*
Lactobacillus acidophilus (p.1704·2).
*Dietary supplement.*

**Kalaf** *Sam-On, Israel†.*
Xylometazoline hydrochloride (p.1132·2).
*Nasal congestion.*

**Kalaz D3** *Caber, Ital.*
Calcium carbonate (p.1254·2); colecalciferol (p.1461·3).

**Kalbeten** *Sam-On, Israel.*
Bismuth salicylate (p.1252·1).
*Abdominal cramps; diarrhoea; dyspepsia; flatulence; nausea.*

**Kal-Cee** *Hua, Thai.*
Vitamins; calcium carbonate (p.1417·1).

**Kalci-300** *Be-Tabs, S.Afr.†.*
Calcium gluconate (p.1225·2).
*Calcium supplement.*

**Kalcidon**
*Verman, Fin.; Abigo, Swed.*
Calcium carbonate (p.1254·2).
*Calcium deficiency; hyperphosphataemia; osteoporosis.*

**Kalcikidz** *Diepharmex, Fr.*
Calcium phosphate (p.1225·3).
*Calcium supplement.*

**Kalcipos**
*Recip, Fin.; Recip, Swed.*
Calcium carbonate (p.1254·2).
*Calcium deficiency; hyperphosphataemia; osteoporosis.*

**Kalcipos-D**
*Recip, Fin.; Recip, Swed.*
Calcium carbonate (p.1254·2); colecalciferol (p.1461·3).
*Calcium and vitamin D deficiencies; osteoporosis.*

**Kalcitena** *ACO, Swed.*
Calcium carbonate (p.1254·2).
*Calcium deficiency; hyperphosphataemia; osteoporosis.*

**Kaldil Diet** *Higate, Arg.*
Sodium cyclamate (p.1426·2).
*Sugar substitute.*

**Kaldor** *Finn Vita, Chile.*
Opuntia streptacantha lemaire.
*Dietary fibre supplement.*

**Kaleorid**
Leo, Denm.; Leo, Fr.; Leo, Norw.; Leo, Swed.
Potassium chloride (p.1232·2).
*Hypokalaemia; potassium supplement.*

**Kaletra**
Abbott, Arg.; Abbott, Austral.; Abbott, Belg.; Abbott, Braz.; Abbott, Canad.; Abbott, Chile; Abbott, Denm.; Abbott, Fin.; Abbott, Fr.; Abbott, Ger.; Abbott, Gr.; Abbott, Hong Kong; Abbott, Israel; Abbott, Ital.; Abbott, Norw.; Abbott, NZ; Abbott, Port.; Abbott, Spain; Abbott, Swed.; Abbott, Switz.; Abbott, Thai.; Abbott, UK; Abbott, USA.
Lopinavir (p.649·3); ritonavir (p.653·2).
*HIV infection.*

**Kalgaron** Rafa, Israel.
Tyrothricin (p.275·1); benzocaine (p.1370·3).
*Mouth and throat disorders.*

**Kalgut** Tanabe, Jpn.
Denopamine (p.892·2).
*Heart failure.*

**Kali Mag** Vitaplex, Austral.†.
Potassium amino acid chelate (p.1233·1); magnesium amino acid chelate (p.1229·1).
*Potassium and magnesium supplement.*

**Kalicet** Rhone-Poulenc Aventis, Ital.
Fexofenadine hydrochloride (p.433·3).
*Allergic rhinitis; urticaria.*

**Kalicitrine** Promedica, Fr.†.
Choline citrate (p.1424·3); potassium citrate (p.1223·1).
*Dyspepsia.*

**Kaliglutol** Streuli, Switz.
Potassium chloride (p.1232·2).
*Hypokalaemia.*

**Kaliject** Pharmadica, Thai.
Potassium chloride (p.1232·2).
*Hypokalaemia.*

**Kaliklora Jod med** Queisser, Ger.†.
Potassium iodide (p.1598·1).
*Iodine deficiency.*

**Kalimate** Nikken, Jpn.
Calcium polystyrene sulfonate (p.1032·3).
*Hyperkalaemia.*

**Kalinor** Abbott, Ger.
Potassium citrate (p.1223·1); potassium bicarbonate (p.1223·1).
*Potassium deficiency, particularly in association with metabolic acidosis.*

**Kalinorm**
Nycomed, Denm.†; Nycomed, Fin.; Nycomed, Norw.†.
Potassium chloride (p.1232·2).
*Hypokalaemia; potassium supplement.*

**Kalinor-retard P** Abbott, Ger.
Potassium chloride (p.1232·2).
*Potassium deficiency.*

**Kaliolite** Merck, Mex.
Potassium chloride (p.1232·2).
*Hypokalaemia.*

**Kalioral** Fresenius Kabi, Austria.
Anhydrous potassium citrate (p.1223·1); potassium bicarbonate (p.1223·1); citric acid (p.1673·1).
*Oedema; potassium deficiency.*

**Kalisol** Orion, Fin.
Potassium chloride (p.1232·2).
*Hypokalaemia.*

**Kalisteril** Orion, Fin.
Potassium chloride (p.1232·2).
*Potassium deficiency.*

**Kali-Sterop** Sterop, Belg.
Potassium chloride (p.1232·2).
*Hypokalaemia.*

**Kalitabs** Leo, Swed.
Potassium chloride (p.1232·2).
*Potassium deficiency; potassium supplement.*

**Kalitrans** Niddapharm, Ger.
Potassium bicarbonate (p.1223·1).
*Potassium deficiency.*

**Kalitrans retard** Fresenius, Ger.†.
Potassium chloride (p.1232·2).
*Potassium deficiency.*

**Kalium**
Apogepha, Ger.
Potassium adipate (p.1233·1).
*Potassium deficiency.*

Verla, Ger.
Potassium citrate (p.1223·1).
*Hypokalaemia.*

Vifor, Hong Kong.
Potassium chloride (p.1232·2).
*Potassium deficiency.*

**Kalium Duretter**
AstraZeneca, Fin.†; Hassle, Swed.
Potassium chloride (p.1232·2).
*Potassium deficiency; potassium supplement.*

**Kalium Durettes**
AstraZeneca, Belg.; AstraZeneca, Neth.
Potassium chloride (p.1232·2).
*Hypokalaemia; potassium supplement.*

**Kalium Durules**
Astra, Canad.†; AstraZeneca, Singapore†.
Potassium chloride (p.1232·2).
*Hypokalaemia.*

**Kalium Retard** Nycomed, Swed.
Potassium chloride (p.1232·2).
*Hypokalaemia; potassium supplement.*

**Kalium-Can** Ratiopharm, Ger.
Potassium canrenoate (p.984·2).
*Ascites; hyperaldosteronism; oedema.*

**Kalium-Duriles** AstraZeneca, Ger.
Potassium chloride (p.1232·2).
*Potassium deficiency.*

**Kalium-Magnesium** Apogepha, Ger.
Potassium adipate (p.1233·1); magnesium adipate (p.1229·1).
*Potassium and magnesium deficiency.*

**Kalium-Magnesium-Asparaginat** Berlin-Chemie, Ger.
Potassium hydroxide (p.1734·2); magnesium oxide (p.1272·3); DL-aspartic acid; xylitol (p.1469·1).
*Cardiac disorders.*

**Kalius** Fermenti, Ital.†.
Trimebutine maleate (p.1758·1).
*Gastrointestinal disorders.*

**Kalkurenal Goldrute** Muller Goppingen, Ger.
Solidago virgaurea (p.1748·3).
*Renal calculi.*

**Kalloplast** DM, Braz.†.
Salicylic acid (p.1157·1); zinc chloride (p.1469·2).
*Keratinisation disorders.*

**Kalma**
Note. This name is used for preparations of different composition.
Alphapharm, Austral.
Alprazolam (p.668·3).
*Anxiety; panic disorders.*

Stada, Austria; Niddapharm, Ger.
Tryptophan (p.320·3).
*Depression; sleep disorders.*

Schering-Plough, Spain†.
Ibuprofen (p.45·3).
*Fever; pain.*

**Kalmafta** Master, Chile.
Benzocaine (p.1370·3).
*Local anaesthesia.*

**Kalmalin** Montpellier, Arg.
Lorazepam (p.704·1).
*Alcohol withdrawal syndrome; anxiety.*

**Kalm-B** Cantassium Co., UK.
Multivitamin and mineral preparation (p.1417·1).

**Kalmiren** Aegis, Hong Kong.
Buspirone hydrochloride (p.672·2).
*Anxiety.*

**Kalmocaps** Medix, Mex.
Chlordiazepoxide (p.674·2).
*Skeletal muscle spasm.*

**Kalms** Lane, UK.
Lupulus (p.1708·1); valerian (p.1762·2); gentian (p.1692·2).
*Menopausal disorders; sleep disorders; stresses and strains.*

**Kaloplasmal** Braun, Ger.†.
Glucose monohydrate (p.1432·2); xylitol (p.1469·1).
*Parenteral nutrition.*

**Kaloplasmal E** Braun, Ger.†.
Electrolyte infusion with glucose and xylitol (p.1217·1).
*Parenteral nutrition.*

**Kalopsis** Roux-Ocefa, Arg.
Ephedrine (p.1120·1); phenazone (p.82·3).
*Eye disorders.*

**Kalostop** Hexal, Braz.
Salicylic acid (p.1157·1); lactic acid (p.1704·1); acetic acid (p.1645·2).
*Keratinisation disorders.*

**Kalovowen** Weber & Weber, Ger.
Homoeopathic preparation.

**Kalpastic** BDH, India.
Rutoside (p.1688·2); vitamin C (p.1460·2); acetomenaphthone (p.1466·3); calcium gluconate (p.1225·2).
*Capillary fragility.*

**Kalpress** Lacer, Spain.
Valsartan (p.1018·3).
*Hypertension.*

**Kalpress Plus** Lacer, Spain.
Valsartan (p.1018·3); hydrochlorothiazide (p.933·2).
*Hypertension.*

**Kalsimin** Altana, Spain†.
Calcitonin (salmon) (p.768·2).
*Hypercalcaemia; metastatic bone pain; osteoporosis; Paget's disease of bone.*

**Kalspare** Pliva, UK.
Chlortalidone (p.882·3); triamterene (p.1016·2).
*Ascites; hypertension; oedema.*

**Kalten**
AstraZeneca, Belg.; Teofarma, Spain; AstraZeneca, Switz.; AstraZeneca, UK.
Atenolol (p.865·2); amiloride hydrochloride (p.858·2); hydrochlorothiazide (p.933·2).
*Hypertension.*

**Kalter** Phoenix, Arg.
Ginkgo biloba (p.1692·3).
*Cerebral and peripheral vascular disorders.*

**Kaltiazem** Fabra, Arg.
Diltiazem (p.901·3).
*Angina pectoris.*

**Kaltin MF** Abbott, India.
Metronidazole (p.607·2); furazolidone (p.605·2).
*Gastrointestinal infections.*

**Kaltocarb** Convatec, Israel.
Calcium alginate (p.745·1); sodium alginate (p.1577·1); activated charcoal (p.1030·2).
*Malodorous wounds.*

**Kaltostat**
Bristol-Myers Squibb, Arg.; Convatec, UK.
Calcium alginate (p.745·1).
*Absorbable haemostatic.*

Convatec, Austral.; Convatec, Irl.; Convatec, Israel; Convatec, Ital.; Bristol-Myers Squibb, S.Afr.
Calcium alginate (p.745·1); sodium alginate (p.1577·1).
*Haemostatic wound dressing.*

Convatec, Port.
Calcium sodium alginate (p.1577·1) (p.745·1).
*Haemostatic wound dressing.*

**Kaltrim** Offenbach, Mex.
Co-trimoxazole (p.199·3).
*Bacterial infections.*

**Kaluril**
Note. This name is used for preparations of different composition.
Alphapharm, Austral.
Amiloride hydrochloride (p.858·2).
*Hypertension; oedema.*

Merck Sharp & Dohme, Israel.
Amiloride hydrochloride (p.858·2); hydrochlorothiazide (p.933·2).
*Hypertension; oedema.*

**Kalyamon B12** Janssen-Cilag, Braz.
Minerals; vitamin $B_{12}$; vitamin $D_3$ (p.1417·1).

**Kalymin** Temmler, Ger.
Pyridostigmine bromide (p.1496·1).
*Antimuscarinic toxicity; myasthenia gravis; reversal of competitive neuromuscular blockade; smooth muscle atony.*

**Kalzana** German Remedies, India.
Calcium phosphate (p.1225·3); colecalciferol (p.1461·3).
*Calcium supplement.*

**Kalzonorm** Merck, Austria†.
Calcium carbonate (p.1254·2).
*Hypocalcaemia; increased calcium requirements; osteoporosis.*

**Kam Rho-D** Teva Tuteur, Arg.
An anti-D immunoglobulin (p.1608·1).
*Prevention of rhesus sensitisation.*

**Kamacaine** Kamada, Israel.
Bupivacaine hydrochloride (p.1371·1).
Adrenaline (p.852·2) is included in some injections as a vasoconstrictor to diminish absorption and localise the effect of the local anaesthetic.
*Local anaesthesia.*

**Kaman** Savio, Ital.
Paromomycin sulfate (p.612·3).
*Gastro-enteritis; gastrointestinal sterilisation; hepatic coma; intestinal amoebiasis.*

**Kamfeine** Wolfs, Belg.
Sodium camsilate; ephedrine hydrochloride (p.1120·1); lobelia (p.1589·1); sodium benzoate (p.1169·3).
*Convalescence after influenza; dyspnoea.*

**Kamidex** Dexcel, Israel†.
Loperamide hydrochloride (p.1271·1).
*Diarrhoea.*

**Kamil Blue** Fischer, Israel.
*Liquid soap:* Azulene (p.1658·3); chamomile (p.1669·3).
*Skin cleansing; skin disorders.*
*Lotion:* Azulene (p.1658·3); glycerol (p.1694·3); silicone (p.1482·1); panthenol (p.1727·2).
*Barrier preparation; skin disorders.*
*Ointment:* Chamomile (p.1669·3); panthenol (p.1727·2); wool fat (p.1483·1); white soft paraffin (p.1479·3); silicone (p.1482·1); zinc oxide (p.1163·2).
*Barrier preparation; skin disorders.*
*Topical oil:* Azulene (p.1658·3).
*Barrier preparation; skin disorders.*

**Kamillan plus** Wernigerode, Ger.
Chamomile (p.1669·3); achillea (p.1646·2).
*Burns; gastrointestinal disorders; inflammation of mucous membranes; wounds.*

**Kamillan supra** Wernigerode, Ger.
Chamomile (p.1669·3).
*Gastrointestinal disorders; inflammation and infections of the skin and mucous membranes; respiratory-tract disorders.*

**Kamillat** Hexal, Austria.
Chamomile (p.1669·3).
*Mouth, throat, and anorectal disorders; respiratory-tract disorders; skin disorders.*

**Kamille N** Spitzner, Ger.
Chamomile (p.1669·3).
*Gastrointestinal disorders; inflammation of skin and mucous membranes; upper respiratory-tract inflammation.*

**Kamillen**
Agepha, Austria.
Chamomile oil (p.1669·3).
*Gastrointestinal disorders; mouth and throat disorders; skin disorders.*

Wernigerode, Austria.
Chamomile flowers (p.1669·3).
*Mouth, throat, gastrointestinal and anorectal disorders; skin disorders.*

Robugen, Ger.
Chamomile (p.1669·3).
*Skin disorders.*

**Kamillen-Bad** Iromedica, Switz.
Chamomile flowers (p.1669·3).
*Skin disorders.*

**Kamillenbad Intradermi** Eberth, Ger.
Chamomile oil (p.1669·3).
*Anogenital disorders; bath additive; skin and mucous membrane disorders.*

**Kamillen-Bad N Ritsert** Ritsert, Ger.
Chamomile oil (p.1669·3).
*Anorectal disorders; bath additive; inflammation of skin and mucous membranes.*

**Kamillen-Bad-Robugen** Robugen, Ger.
Chamomile (p.1669·3).
*Anogenital disorders; bath additive; skin and mucous membrane disorders; wounds.*

**Kamillencreme N** Ratiopharm, Ger.
Chamomile (p.1669·3).
*Skin disorders; wounds.*

**Kamillenextract** Steierl, Ger.
Chamomile (p.1669·3).
*Anogenital disorders; gastrointestinal disorders; respiratory-tract disorders; skin and mucous membrane disorders.*

**Kamillen-Heel** Peithner, Austria.
Homoeopathic preparation.

**Kamillin** Robugen, Ger.
Chamomile (p.1669·3).
*Gastrointestinal disorders; skin and mucous membrane disorders.*

**Kamillin Medipharm** Iromedica, Switz.
Chamomile (p.1669·3).
*Inflammation of skin and mucous membranes.*

**Kamillobad** Asta Medica, Ger.†.
Chamomile (p.1669·3); chamomile oil (p.1669·3).
*Bath additive; inflammation of skin and mucous membranes.*

**Kamilloderm** Serum-Werk Bernburg, Ger.
Chamomile (p.1669·3).
*Burns; skin irritation; wounds.*

**Kamillofluid** Amino, Switz.
Chamomile (p.1669·3).
*Mouth and throat disorders; skin disorders.*

**Kamillomed** Kottas-Heldenberg, Austria.
Chamomile (p.1669·3).
*Gastrointestinal disorders; skin and mucous membrane inflammation.*

**Kamillosan**
Note. This name is used for preparations of different composition.
Asta Medica, Austria.
*Drops; ointment:* Chamomile oil (p.1669·3).
*Anal disorders; gastrointestinal disorders; mouth and throat disorders; respiratory-tract disorders; skin disorders; vulvovaginal disorders.*

Asta Medica, Austria; Asta Medica, Switz.
*Mouth spray:* Chamomile oil (p.1669·3); peppermint oil (p.1283·2); anise oil (p.1655·2).
*Mouth and throat disorders.*

Viatris, Belg.; Asta Medica, Braz.; Grunenthal, Chile; Viatris, Ger.; German Remedies, India; Goldshield, Irl.; Sanfer, Mex.; CSL, NZ; Pharmafrica, S.Afr.; Asta Medica, Spain†; Asta Medica, Switz.; Goldshield, UK.
Chamomile (p.1669·3).
*Burns; gastrointestinal disorders; inflammation of mucous membranes; skin disorders; wounds.*

Asta Medica, Hong Kong; Asta Medica, Thai.
Chamazulene (p.1669·3); levomenol (p.1707·1).
*Burns; minor cuts and abrasions; mucous membrane disorders; nappy rash; skin irritation.*

Asta Medica, Switz.†.
*Topical gel:* Vitamin A (p.1451·2); chlorhexidine gluconate (p.1173·2); chamomile (p.1669·3).
*Skin disorders.*

**Kamillosan Mundspray** Viatris, Ger.
Chamomile (p.1669·3); peppermint oil (p.1283·2); anise oil (p.1655·2).
*Mouth and throat disorders.*

**Kamillosan-M** Asta Medica, Thai.
Chamomile (p.1669·3); chamazulene (p.1669·3); essential oil.
*Mouth and throat disorders.*

**Kamillosan-N** German Remedies, India.
Chamomile (p.1669·3); peppermint oil (p.1283·2); anise oil (p.1655·2).
*Mouth and throat disorders.*

**Kamiloderm** Remexa, Mex.
Chamomile (p.1669·3); vitamin A (p.1451·2).
*Skin disorders.*

**Kamilon** Offenbach, Mex.
Nalidixic acid (p.234·1).
*Urinary-tract disorders.*

**Kamilotract** Tamar, Israel.
Chamomile (p.1669·3); sage (p.1741·2).
*Mucous membrane inflammation.*

**Kamiltract Baby** Vitamed, Israel†.
Chamomile (p.1669·3); sage (p.1741·2); calamine (p.1144·1); zinc oxide (p.1163·2).
*Burns; insect bites; skin disorders; sore nipples; wounds.*

**Kamina** Hikma, Port.
Amikacin sulfate (p.154·1).
*Bacterial infections.*

**Kamistad**
Stada, Hong Kong; Stada, Singapore; Stada, Thai.
Lidocaine hydrochloride (p.1377·3); thymol (p.1194·2); chamomile (p.1669·3).
*Inflammatory disorders of the mouth.*

**Kamistad N** *Stada, Ger.*
Lidocaine hydrochloride (p.1377·3); chamomile (p.1669·3).
Kamistad formerly contained lidocaine hydrochloride, chamomile, and thymol.
*Mouth disorders.*

**Kamol** *Whitehall, Fr.*
Capsicum oleoresin (p.1667·1); menthol (p.1711·3); eucalyptus oil (p.1686·2); camphor (p.1665·3); methyl salicylate (p.59·3).
*Muscle and joint pain.*

**Kamoxin** *Chew, Thai.*
Amoxicillin trihydrate (p.155·3).
*Bacterial infections.*

**KamRho-D** *Kamada, Israel.*
An anti-D immunoglobulin (p.1608·1).
*Prevention of rhesus sensitisation.*

**Kamu Jay** *Jamieson, Canad.*
Ascorbic acid (p.1460·2).
*Vitamin supplement.*

**Kamu Jay Multi Complex** *Jamieson, Canad.†.*
Vitamin and mineral preparation (p.1417·1).

**Kamycine** *Bristol-Myers Squibb, Fr.†.*
Kanamycin sulfate (p.225·1).
*Bacterial infections.*

**Kanacil** *Collins, Mex.*
Kanamycin (p.225·2).
*Bacterial infections.*

**Kanacitrin** *Rider, Chile.*
Potassium citrate (p.1223·1); citric acid monohydrate (p.1673·1).
*Metabolic acidosis; urinary alkalinisation.*

**Kanacolirio** *Medical, Spain†.*
Kanamycin sulfate (p.225·1).
*Bacterial eye infections.*

**Kanacyl** *Edol, Port.*
Bekanamycin sulfate (p.162·2).
*Bacterial eye infections.*

**Kanadrex** *Collins, Mex.*
Kanamycin (p.225·2).
*Bacterial infections.*

**Kanafosal** *Medical, Spain.*
Ephedrine hydrochloride (p.1120·1); kanamycin sulfate (p.225·1); naphazoline hydrochloride (p.1124·3); procaine hydrochloride (p.1383·2); sulfanilamide sodium mesilate (p.263·3).
*Nasal congestion and infection.*

**Kanafosal Predni** *Medical, Spain.*
Ephedrine hydrochloride (p.1120·1); kanamycin sulfate (p.225·1); naphazoline hydrochloride (p.1124·3); prednisone (p.1109·3); procaine hydrochloride (p.1383·2); sulfanilamide sodium mesilate (p.263·3).
*Nasal congestion and infection.*

**Kanakion**
*Roche, Braz.; Roche, Port.*
Phytomenadione (p.1467·1).
*Haemorrhagic disorders; vitamin K deficiency.*

**Kanamytrex** *Alcon, Ger.*
Kanamycin sulfate (p.225·1).
*Bacterial eye infections.*

**Kanapat** *Parggon, Mex.*
Kanamycin (p.225·2).
*Bacterial infections.*

**Kanapomada** *Medical, Spain†.*
Kanamycin sulfate (p.225·1); prednisolone (p.1108·1); trypsin (p.1758·3); urea (p.1162·2); lidocaine (p.1377·3).
*Infected skin disorders.*

**Kana-Stulln** *Stulln, Ger.*
Kanamycin sulfate (p.225·1).
*Bacterial eye infections.*

**Kanavit** *Medphano, Ger.*
Phytomenadione (p.1467·1).
*Vitamin K deficiency.*

**Kanazima** *Kinder, Braz.*
Erythromycin estolate (p.208·1).
*Bacterial infections.*

**Kanazone** *SIT, Ital.†.*
Dexamethasone phosphate (p.1097·2); kanamycin sulfate (p.225·1); phenylephrine hydrochloride (p.1126·3).
*Eye, nose, and ear disorders.*

**Kanbine** *Rovi, Spain.*
Amikacin sulfate (p.154·1).
*Bacterial infections.*

**Kancin**
*Alembic, India.*
Kanamycin (p.225·2).
*Bacterial infections.*

*Atlantic, Malaysia; Atlantic, Singapore; Atlantic, Thai.*
Kanamycin sulfate (p.225·1).
*Bacterial infections.*

**Kancin-Gap** *Gap, Gr.*
Amikacin sulfate (p.154·1).
*Bacterial infections.*

**Kancin-L** *Atlantic, Singapore.*
Kanamycin sulfate (p.225·1).
*Bacterial infections.*

**Kandicin** *Microsules Bernabo, Arg.*
Cefadroxil (p.167·2).
*Bacterial infections.*

**Kandistat** *Kinder, Braz.*
Nystatin (p.406·3).
*Fungal infections.*

**Kandril** *Kinder, Braz.*
Sodium citrate (p.1223·2); ammonium chloride (p.1115·2); diphenhydramine hydrochloride (p.431·3).

**Kanebo Hochu-ekki-to** *Kanebo, Jpn.*
Ginseng; atractylodes rhizome; astragalus root; angelica acutiloba root; jujube; bupleurum root; liquorice; ginger; cimicifuga rhizome; citrus unshiu peel.
*Fatigue; malaise.*

**Kanebo Ninjin-yoei-to** *Kanebo, Jpn.*
Ginseng; angelica acutiloba root; peony root; rehmannia root; atractylodes rhizome; poria sclerotium; astragalus root; citrus unshiu peel; polygala root; schisandra fruit; liquorice.
*Tonic.*

**Kanebo Sairei-to** *Kanebo, Jpn.*
Jujube; scutellaria root; bupleurum root; poria sclerotium; cinnamon; polyporus sclerotium; liquorice; ginger; ginseng; pinellia tuber; alisma rhizome; atractylodes rhizome.
*Gastrointestinal disorders; oedema.*

**Kanebo Sho-saiko-to** *Kanebo, Jpn.*
Bupleurum root; pinellia tuber; scutellaria root; jujube; ginseng; liquorice; ginger.
*Gastrointestinal disorders; liver disorders.*

**Kanendos** *Fournier, Ital.†.*
Bekanamycin sulfate (p.162·2).
*Adjuvant in hyperammonaemia; intestinal infections.*

**Kanescin** *Torlan, Spain†.*
Kanamycin sulfate (p.225·1).
*Bacterial infections.*

**Kaneuron**
*SERB, Fr.; IFET (ΙΦΕΤ), Gr.*
Phenobarbital (p.367·3).
*Epilepsy.*

**Kangen** *General Drugs, Thai.*
Kanamycin acid sulfate (p.224·3).
*Bacterial infections.*

**Kanibel** *Willmar, Mex.†.*
Kanamycin (p.225·2).
*Bacterial infections.*

**Kanin** *LBS, Thai.*
Hyoscine butylbromide (p.483·3).
*Gastro-duodenitis; nausea and vomiting; peptic ulcer; smooth muscle spasm.*

**Kank-A**
*Note. This name is used for preparations of different composition.*
*Blistex, Canad.*
Benzocaine (p.1370·3); cetylpyridinium chloride (p.1173·1).
*Canker sores; mouth irritation.*

*Blistex, Israel.*
Benzocaine (p.1370·3); cetylpyridinium chloride (p.1173·1); siam benzoin (p.1744·1).
*Mouth irritation.*

*Blistex, USA.*
Benzocaine (p.1370·3); compound benzoin tincture.
*Mouth disorders.*

**Kank-Eze** *Rider, Chile.*
Benzocaine (p.1370·3); cetylpyridinium chloride (p.1173·1).
*Mouth disorders.*

**Kan-Mycin** *Olan-Kemed, Thai.*
Kanamycin sulfate (p.225·1).
*Bacterial infections.*

**Kanolone** *LBS, Thai.*
Triamcinolone acetonide (p.1110·2).
*Musculoskeletal and joint disorders; skin disorders.*

**Kan-Ophtal** *Winzer, Ger.*
Kanamycin sulfate (p.225·1).
*Bacterial eye infections.*

**Kanormal** *German Remedies, India.*
Sterculia (p.1290·2); frangula bark (p.1266·3).
*Constipation.*

**Kanrenol** *Abbott, Ital.*
Potassium canrenoate (p.984·2).
*Hyperaldosteronism; hypertension.*

**Kantrex**
*Bristol-Myers, Spain; Apothecon, USA.*
Kanamycin sulfate (p.225·1).
*Bacterial infections.*

**Kantrexil** *Opus, S.Afr.*
Kanamycin sulfate (p.225·1); dimevamide (p.481·3); pectin (p.1580·3); bismuth subcarbonate (p.1252·1); activated attapulgite (p.1251·1).
*Gastro-enteritis.*

**Kao** *Covan, S.Afr.*
Kaolin (p.1268·3); pectin (p.1580·3).
*Diarrhoea.*

**Kaobrol** *GlaxoSmithKline Sante, Fr.*
Magnesium carbonate (p.1272·1); calcium carbonate (p.1254·2); heavy kaolin (p.1268·3).
*Gastrointestinal disorders.*

**Kaochlor**
*Pharmacia Upjohn, Canad.†; Adria, USA†.*
Potassium chloride (p.1232·2).
*Hypokalaemia; potassium depletion.*

**Kaodene** *Sovereign, UK.*
Codeine phosphate (p.27·1); light kaolin (p.1268·3).
*Diarrhoea.*

**Kaodene Non-Narcotic** *Pfeiffer, USA.*
Kaolin (p.1268·3); pectin (p.1580·3); bismuth salicylate (p.1252·1).
*Diarrhoea.*

**Kaogel** *Sedabel, Braz.*
Aluminium hydroxide (p.1249·2); kaolin (p.1268·3); pectin (p.1580·3).
*Diarrhoea.*

**Kaologeais** *Chiesi, Fr.*
Magnesium oxide (p.1272·3); meprobamate (p.706·2); magnesium sulfate (p.1228·2); kaolin (p.1268·3); sterculia (p.1290·2).
*Gastrointestinal disorders.*

**Kaomagma**
*Note. This name is used for preparations of different composition.*
*Whitehall, Austral.†.*
Kaolin (p.1268·3); aluminium hydroxide (p.1249·2).
*Diarrhoea.*

*Sigma, Braz.*
Kaolin (p.1268·3); aluminium hydroxide (p.1249·2); pectin (p.1580·3).
*Diarrhoea.*

**Kaomagma with Pectin** *Whitehall, Austral.†.*
Kaolin (p.1268·3); aluminium hydroxide (p.1249·2); pectin (p.1580·3).
*Diarrhoea.*

**Kaomuth** *Bailly, Fr.*
Kaolin (p.1268·3); magnesium hydroxide (p.1272·2).
*Gastrointestinal disorders.*

**Kaomycin** *Armstrong, Mex.*
Neomycin sulfate (p.235·1); kaolin (p.1268·3); pectin (p.1580·3).
*Gastro-enteritis.*

**Kaon**
*Montpellier, Arg.; Pharmacia, Canad.; Savage, USA.*
Potassium gluconate (p.1232·2).
*Hypokalaemia; potassium depletion.*

**Kaon-Cl** *Savage, USA.*
Potassium chloride (p.1232·2).
*Hypokalaemia; potassium depletion.*

**Kao-Paverin** *Reese, USA.*
*Capsules:* Loperamide hydrochloride (p.1271·1).
*Oral liquid:* Kaolin (p.1268·3); pectin (p.1580·3); bismuth salicylate (p.1252·1).

**Kaopectal** *Silom, Thai.*
Kaolin (p.1268·3); pectin (p.1580·3).
*Diarrhoea; dysentery; food poisoning.*

**Kaopectal-N** *Silom, Thai.†.*
Neomycin sulfate (p.235·1); kaolin (p.1268·3); pectin (p.1580·3).
*Diarrhoea; dysentery; enterocolitis.*

**Kaopectate**
*Note. This name is used for preparations of different composition.*
*Pharmacia, Austral.†; Pharmacia Upjohn, Belg.†; Pharmacia Upjohn, Braz.†; Pharmacia-Upjohn, Gr.; Pharmacia, Irl.; Pharmacia, Malaysia; Pharmacia Upjohn, Mex.; Pharmacia, Singapore; Pharmacia, Switz.†; Pharmacia Upjohn, Thai.†.*
Kaolin (p.1268·3); pectin (p.1580·3).
*Diarrhoea.*

*Johnson & Johnson, Canad.*
Attapulgite (p.1251·1).
*Cramps; diarrhoea.*

*Pharmacia, USA.*
Bismuth salicylate (p.1252·1).
*Gastrointestinal disorders.*

**Kaopectate II** *Upjohn, USA.*
Loperamide hydrochloride (p.1271·1).
*Diarrhoea.*

**Kaopectate Advanced Formula** *Upjohn, USA.*
Attapulgite (p.1251·1).
*Diarrhoea.*

**Kaopectate Maximum Strength** *Upjohn, USA.*
Attapulgite (p.1251·1).
*Diarrhoea.*

**Kaopectin**
*Dinafarma, Braz.†; Vitamed, Israel; Adcock Ingram, S.Afr.*
Kaolin (p.1268·3); pectin (p.1580·3).
*Diarrhoea.*

**Kaoprompt-H** *Pharmacia, Ger.*
Kaolin (p.1268·3); pectin (p.1580·3).
*Diarrhoea.*

**Kao-Pront** *Lachifarma, Ital.†.*
Kaolin (p.1268·3).
*Diarrhoea.*

**Kao-Spen** *Century, USA.*
Kaolin (p.1268·3); pectin (p.1580·3).
*Diarrhoea.*

**Kaostase** *Sedar, Braz.†.*
Kaolin (p.1268·3); clioquinol (p.196·3); homatropine (p.483·2).
*Diarrhoea.*

**Kaostase Suspension** *Sedar, Braz.†.*
Kaolin (p.1268·3); pectin (p.1580·3); aluminium hydroxide (p.1249·2).
*Diarrhoea.*

**Kaostatex** *Garec, S.Afr.*
Light kaolin (p.1268·3); pectin (p.1580·3); sodium lactate; potassium chloride; sodium chloride (p.1222·2).
*Diarrhoea.*

**Kaosyl** *Anpharm (Ανφαρμ), Gr.*
Sodium cromoglicate (p.795·3).
*Allergic conjunctivitis; allergic rhinitis.*

**Kaotalil** *Tocogino, Mex.†.*
Phthalylsulfathiazole (p.242·3).

**Kapabloc** *Allen, Austria.*
Morphine sulfate (p.60·2).
*Opioid withdrawal syndrome.*

**Kapake**
*Galen, Irl.; Galen, UK.*
Paracetamol (p.76·2); codeine phosphate (p.27·1).
These ingredients can be described by the British Approved Name Co-codamol.
*Pain.*

**Kapanol**
*GlaxoSmithKline, Austral.; GlaxoSmithKline, Austria; GlaxoSmithKline, Belg.; Glaxo Wellcome, Denm.†; GlaxoSmithKline, Fr.; GlaxoSmithKline, Ger.; GlaxoSmithKline, Israel; Glaxo Wellcome, Mex.†; GlaxoSmithKline, Neth.; Glaxo Wellcome, Norw.†; GlaxoSmithKline, NZ; GlaxoSmithKline, Switz.*
Morphine sulfate (p.60·2).
*Pain.*

**Kaparlon-S** *Anpharm (Ανφαρμ), Gr.*
Enalapril maleate (p.909·2).
*Heart failure; hypertension.*

**Kapectin Forte** *Taro, Israel.*
Kaolin (p.1268·3); pectin (p.1580·3).
*Diarrhoea.*

**Kaplon** *Approved Prescription Services, UK.*
Captopril (p.879·2).
*Heart failure; hypertension.*

**Kapodin** *Efarmes, Spain†.*
Minoxidil (p.960·1).
*Alopecia.*

**Kaposalt** *Tecnofarma, Mex.*
Potassium bicarbonate (p.1223·1); potassium tartrate (p.1232·2); citric acid (p.1673·1).
*Hypokalaemia.*

**Kaptin** *Julphar, UAE.*
Light kaolin (p.1268·3); pectin (p.1580·3).
*Diarrhoea.*

**Kaptin II** *Julphar, UAE.*
Activated attapulgite (p.1251·1).
*Diarrhoea.*

**Kaput** *Maxfarma, Spain†.*
Povidone-iodine (p.1190·3).
*Skin and instrument disinfection; skin disorders.*

**Kara** *Polipharm, Thai.*
Ketoconazole (p.403·3).
*Scalp disorders.*

**Karacil** *ICN, Canad.†.*
Ispaghula (p.1268·1).

**Karaya Bismuth** *Sanofi Synthelabo, Ger.†.*
Bismuth subnitrate (p.1252·2); sterculia (p.1290·2).
*Diarrhoea; inflammatory bowel disease.*

**Karayal** *Chiesi, Fr.*
Magnesium oxide (p.1272·3); magnesium sulfate (p.1228·2); kaolin (p.1268·3); sterculia (p.1290·2).
*Gastrointestinal disorders.*

**Karbac** *Pharmus, Braz.†.*
Carbamazepine (p.353·3).
*Epilepsy; psychoses.*

**Karbaderm** *NM, Swed.*
Urea (p.1162·2).
*Dry skin.*

**Karbasal** *CCS, Swed.*
Urea (p.1162·2).
*Dry skin.*

**Karbasalin** *Laboratorios Chile, Chile.*
Benzathine benzylpenicillin (p.162·3); benzathine benzylpenicillin (p.162·3); procaine benzylpenicillin (p.246·1).
*Streptococcal sore throat.*

**Karbolytt**
*Fresenius Kabi, Denm.†; Fresenius Kabi, Norw.*
Electrolyte infusion with glucose (p.1217·1).
*Carbohydrate source; fluid and electrolyte disorders.*

**Karbons** *Eagle, Austral.†.*
Activated charcoal (p.1030·2).
*Digestive system disorders.*

**Kardegic**
*Sanofi Synthelabo, Braz.†; Sanofi Synthelabo, Fr.; Synthelabo, Switz.*
Lysine aspirin (p.54·3).
*Thrombosis prophylaxis.*

**Karden** *Novartis, Austria.*
Nicardipine hydrochloride (p.965·1).
*Angina pectoris; hypertension.*

**Kardiamed** *Medice, Ger.†.*
β-Acetyldigoxin (p.851·1).
*Arrhythmias; heart failure.*

**Kardil** *Orion, Norw.†.*
Diltiazem hydrochloride (p.900·1).
*Angina pectoris.*

**Kardion** *Lemery, Mex.*
Dobutamine (p.906·1).

**Kardioplex** *SAD, Denm.*
Electrolytes (p.1217·1); procaine hydrochloride (p.1383·2).
*Cardioplegia in open heart surgery.*

**Kardopal** *Orion, Fin.*
Levodopa (p.1205·2); carbidopa (p.1204·3).
*Parkinsonism.*

**Karelyne** *Urgo, Fr.†.*
Sweet almond oil peroxide (p.1651·1).
*Anorectal disorders.*

**Karex**
*Wolff, Ger.; Medika, Switz.*
Erythromycin stinoprate (p.210·3).
*Bacterial infections.*

**Kariax** *Koni-Cofarm, Chile.*
Triclosan (p.1195·2); sodium fluoride (p.1444·3).
*Caries prophylaxis; oral hygiene.*

**Karicare AR**
*Nutricia, Austral.†; Nutricia, NZ.*
Infant feed (p.1417·1).
*Gastro-oesophageal reflux.*

**Karicare Baby Bath Oil** *Karicare, NZ†.*
Hydrous wool fat (p.1483·1); light liquid paraffin (p.1479·1).
*Dry skin; pruritus.*

**Karicare Barrier Cream** *Nutricia, NZ.*
Dimethicone (p.1482·1); cetrimide (p.1172·1).
*Nappy rash; skin irritation.*

**Karicare Breast and Body Cream** *Nutricia, NZ.*
Glycerol (p.1694·3); light liquid paraffin (p.1479·1).
This preparation was formerly marketed as Karicare Breast Care.
*Moisturiser; nipple care during pregnancy and lactation.*

**Karicare De Lact Infant** *Nutricia, NZ.*
Infant feed (p.1417·1).
*Lactose intolerance.*

**Karicare Food Thickener**
*Nutricia, Austral.†; Nutricia, NZ.*
Pregelatinised maize starch (p.1449·1).
*Dysphagia; gastro-oesophageal reflux in infants.*

**Karicare Goat Milk**
*Nutricia, Austral.†; Nutricia, NZ.*
Infant feed (p.1417·1).
*Cow's milk intolerance.*

**Karicare Mother and Baby** *Karicare, NZ†.*
Hydrous wool fat (p.1483·1); light liquid paraffin (p.1479·1).
*Dry skin.*

**Karicare Nutrilon** *Nutricia, Austral.†.*
Infant feed (p.1417·1).
*Cow's milk, lactose, and disaccharide intolerance; galactosaemia.*

**Karicare Ointment** *Nutricia, NZ.*
Zinc oxide (p.1163·2); glycerol (p.1694·3).
*Nappy rash; skin irritation.*

**Karicare Soya**
*Nutricia, Austral.†; Nutricia, NZ.*
Infant feed (p.1417·1).
*Cow's milk intolerance; galactosaemia; lactose intolerance.*

**Karidina** *Kerifarm, Spain†.*
Cefazolin sodium (p.170·3).
*Bacterial infections.*

**Karidium**
*Note. This name is used for preparations of different composition.*
*Aventis, Arg.*
Clobazam (p.358·2).
*Anxiety; epilepsy.*

*Lorvic, Canad.; Lorvic, USA.*
Sodium fluoride (p.1444·3).
*Dental caries prophylaxis.*

**Karigel** *Lorvic, USA.*
Sodium fluoride (p.1444·3).
*Dental caries prophylaxis.*

**Karigel-N** *Lorvic, USA.*
Sodium fluoride (p.1444·3).
*Dental caries prophylaxis.*

**Karil** *Novartis, Ger.*
Calcitonin (salmon) acetate (p.769·2).
*Hypercalcaemia; osteolysis; osteoporosis; Paget's disease of bone; sympathetic pain syndromes.*

**Karile** *Phoenix, Arg.*
Nortriptyline hydrochloride (p.310·2); perphenazine (p.714·2).
*Depression.*

**Karilexina** *Reig Jofre, Spain†.*
Cefalexin (p.168·1).
*Bacterial infections.*

**Karin**
*Note. This name is used for preparations of different composition.*
*Gilton, Braz.†.*
Levonorgestrel (p.1563·2); ethinylestradiol (p.1553·2).
*Combined oral contraceptive.*

*Unipharm, Israel.*
Clarithromycin (p.192·2).
*Bacterial infections.*

**Karison** *Dermapharm, Ger.*
Clobetasol propionate (p.1095·2).
*Skin disorders.*

**Kariva** *Barr, USA.*
21 Tablets, desogestrel (p.1547·2); ethinylestradiol (p.1553·2); 5 tablets, ethinylestradiol; 2 tablets, inert.
*Sequential-type oral contraceptive.*

**Karlit** *Biotenk, Arg.*
Lithium carbonate (p.301·1).
*Bipolar disorder; schizophrenia.*

**Karoyan S** *Daiichi, Hong Kong†.*
Carpronium chloride; pantothenyl ethyl ether; tocoferil acetate (p.1465·1); salicylic acid (p.1157·1); diphenhydramine hydrochloride (p.431·3); asunaron; menthol (p.1711·3).
*Alopecia; dandruff.*

**Karrer** *Lisapharma, Ital.*
Levocarnitine (p.1423·3).
*Carnitine deficiency; myocardial ischaemia.*

**Kartal** *Phoinix Pharm (Φοινιξ Φαρμ), Gr.*
Nimesulide (p.67·1).
*Inflammation; musculoskeletal disorders; pain.*

**Karvea**
*Sanofi Synthelabo, Austral.; Bristol-Myers Squibb, Ger.; Sanofi Synthelabo, Gr.; Bristol-Myers Squibb, Ital.; Bristol-Myers, Spain.*
Irbesartan (p.940·1).
*Diabetic nephropathy; hypertension.*

**Karvezide**
*Sanofi Synthelabo, Austral.; Bristol-Myers Squibb, Ger.; Bristol-Myers Squibb, Ital.; Bristol-Myers, Spain.*
Irbesartan (p.940·1); hydrochlorothiazide (p.933·2).
*Hypertension.*

**Karvisin** *Synpharma, Austria.*
Fennel (p.1687·2); chamomile (p.1669·3); caraway (p.1667·2).
*Gastrointestinal disorders.*

**Karvol**
*Note. This name is used for preparations of different composition.*
*Boots, Austral.†.*
Menthol (p.1711·3); oleum pini sylvestris; pumilio pine oil (p.1737·1); terpineol (p.1752·2).
*Nasal congestion.*

*Boots Healthcare, Irl.; Crookes Healthcare, UK.*
Chlorobutanol (p.1176·3); menthol (p.1711·3); oleum pini sylvestris; pumilio pine oil (p.1737·1); terpineol (p.1752·2); thymol (p.1194·2).
*Cold symptoms; nasal congestion.*

*Boots, Israel.*
Menthol (p.1711·3); cinnamon oil (p.1672·2); terpineol (p.1752·2); chlorobutanol (p.1176·3); oleum pini sylvestris; thymol (p.1194·2); pumilio pine oil (p.1737·1).
*Cold symptoms.*

*Boots Healthcare, NZ.*
Menthol (p.1711·3); pine oil; cinnamon oil (p.1672·2).
*Nasal congestion.*

*Permark, S.Afr.; Boots, Singapore.*
Chlorobutanol (p.1176·3); menthol (p.1711·3); cinnamon oil (p.1672·2); pine oil; terpineol (p.1752·2); thymol (p.1194·2).
*Nasal congestion.*

**Karvol Plus** *Solvay, India.*
Menthol (p.1711·3); terpineol (p.1752·2); chlorothymol (p.1177·2); camphor (p.1665·3); cineole (p.1672·1).
*Cold symptoms; nasal congestion.*

**Kary Uni**
*Santen, Hong Kong; Santen, Singapore.*
Pirenoxine (p.1732·2).
*Cataract.*

**Kas** *Nutricia-Bago, Arg.*
Preparation for enteral nutrition (p.1417·1).
*Cow's milk protein allergy; diarrhoea; pancreatic insufficiency; soya allergy.*

**Ka-Sabona** *Sabona, Ger.*
Kava (p.1703·2).
*Anxiety disorders.*

**Kas-Bah** *Potter's, UK.*
Buchu (p.1663·1); clivers (p.1673·2); couch-grass (p.1676·2); equisetum (p.1684·1); bearberry (p.1659·2); senna (p.1288·2).
*Urinary and bladder discomfort.*

**Kasele** *Baxter, Mex.*
Potassium chloride (p.1232·2).

**Kaskadil** *Lab Francais du Fractionnement, Fr.*
A factor IX preparation (p.752·2).
*Haemorrhagic disorders.*

**Kasmal** *Silanes, Mex.*
Ketotifen fumarate (p.788·1).
*Asthma; bronchitis; rhinitis.*

**Kastipron** *YSP, Malaysia.*
Carbocisteine (p.1116·2).
*Respiratory-tract disorders associated with increased mucus.*

**Kata** *Ibirn, Ital.*
Verapamil hydrochloride (p.1019·1).
*Angina pectoris; arrhythmias; hypertension; myocardial infarction.*

**Katabios** *SIT, Ital.*
Multivitamin preparation (p.1417·1).

**Katadolon**
*Asta Medica, Braz.; AWD, Ger.; Procter & Gamble, Ger.*
Flupirtine gluconate (p.43·3) or flupirtine maleate (p.43·3).
*Pain.*

**Katagrip** *Lepori, Port.†.*
Ethenzamide (p.37·2); paracetamol (p.76·2).
*Cold symptoms.*

**Katalem** *Lemery, Mex.*
Ranitidine (p.1285·2).
*Peptic ulcer.*

**Katapekt** *Vitabalans, Fin.*
Codeine phosphate (p.27·1); guaifenesin (p.1122·1); ammonium chloride (p.1115·2); thyme (p.1755·2).
*Coughs.*

**Katar** *Berna, Ital.†.*
*Streptococcus pneumoniae*; *Staphylococcus aureus*; *Staphylococcus albus*; *Streptococcus*; *Klebsiella pneumoniae*; *Moraxella catarrhalis*; *Haemophilus influenzae*; *Corynebacterium pseudodiphtheriae*.
*Respiratory-tract congestion.*

**Katasma** *Bruschettini, Ital.*
Diprophylline (p.784·3).
*Obstructive airways disease.*

**Kataval** *Farmigea, Ital.*
Triamcinolone acetonide (p.1110·2); neomycin sulfate (p.235·1).
*Anorectal disorders; otitis externa; skin disorders.*

**Katifen** *General Drugs, Thai.*
Ketotifen (p.788·2).
*Asthma; hypersensitivity reactions.*

**Katin** *Instituto Sanitas, Chile.*
Menadione (p.1466·3); bile salts (p.1660·3).
*Biliary-tract and liver disorders; coumarin anticoagulant overdosage; hypoprothrombinaemia.*

**Kation** *Searle, Ital.†.*
Potassium citrate (p.1223·1).
*Hypokalaemia.*

**Kationen** *Fresenius Kabi, Austria.*
A trace element preparation (p.1417·1).
*Parenteral nutrition.*

**Katoderm** *Deverge, Ital.*
Emollient.
Formerly contained collagen and silver.
*Skin irritation.*

**Katogel** *Deverge, Ital.*
Emollient.
*Dry skin; skin irritation.*

**Katomed** *Deverge, Ital.*
Silver (p.1746·1).
*Burns; skin ulcers; wounds.*

**Katopril** *Delta, Singapore†.*
Captopril (p.879·2).
*Heart failure; hypertension.*

**Katosilver** *Deverge, Ital.*
Silver sucralfate.
*Prevention of decubitus ulcers; skin irritation.*

**Katovit** *Fher, Spain†.*
Prolintane hydrochloride (p.1592·3); vitamins.
*Tonic.*

**Katoxyn** *Deverge, Ital.*
Silver (p.1746·1); benzoyl peroxide (p.1143·2); kaolin (p.1268·3); calcium gluconate (p.1225·2).
*Disinfection of wounds and burns; skin irritation.*

**Katrim** *Kanda, Braz.†.*
Co-trimoxazole (p.199·3).
*Bacterial infections; Pneumocystis carinii pneumonia; protozoal infections.*

**Katrim Balsamico** *Kanda, Braz.†.*
Co-trimoxazole (p.199·3); guaifenesin (p.1122·1); ammonium chloride (p.1115·2).
*Bacterial infections.*

**Katrum** *Smaller, Spain.*
Capsaicin (p.24·2).
*Muscle and joint pain.*

**Katsin** *M & H, Thai.*
Ketoconazole (p.403·3).
*Fungal infections; seborrhoeic dermatitis.*

**Kattwiderm** *Kattwiga, Ger.*
Homoeopathic preparation.

**Kattwigast** *Kattwiga, Ger.*
Homoeopathic preparation.

**Kattwigripp** *Kattwiga, Ger.*
Homoeopathic preparation.

**Kattwilact** *Kattwiga, Ger.*
Lactulose (p.1269·1).
*Constipation; hepatic encephalopathy.*

**Kattwilon N** *Kattwiga, Ger.†.*
Isoprenaline sulfate (p.940·2).
*Allergic rashes; midge bites; pruritus; vaccination pocks; varicella.*

**Katulcin-R** *Kattwiga, Ger.*
Bismuth salicylate (p.1252·1).
*Gastritis; peptic ulcer.*

**Katulcin-Rupha** *Kattwiga, Ger.†.*
Bismuth subnitrate (p.1252·2); bismuth salicylate (p.1252·1).
*Gastritis; hyperchlorhydria; peptic ulcer.*

**Kavacur** *Biocur, Ger.†.*
Kava (p.1703·2).
*Anxiety disorders.*

**Kavaform** *Novartis Consumer, Austria.*
*Capsules:* Kawain (p.1703·2); magnesium orotate (p.1724·3); vitis vinifera rubra.
*Oral suspension:* Kawain (p.1703·2); magnesium orotate (p.1724·3).
*Tonic.*

**Kavaform N** *Klinge, Ger.†.*
Kawain (p.1703·2).
*Mental function disorders; psychiatric disorders.*

**Kavain Harras N** *Harras-Curarina, Ger.*
Kava (p.1703·2).
*Anxiety disorders.*

**Kavain Harras Plus** *Harras-Curarina, Ger.†.*
Kawain (p.1703·2); kava (p.1703·2).
*Anxiety disorders.*

**Kavakan** *Ativus, Braz.*
Kava (p.1703·2).
*Anxiety; insomnia; tension.*

**Kavalac** *Fontovit, Braz.*
Kava (p.1703·2).
*Anxiety.*

**Kava-Phyton** *Merckle, Ger.*
Kava (p.1703·2).
*Anxiety disorders.*

**Kavasedon**
*Sigma, Braz.; Harras-Curarina, Ger.†; HPC, Switz.†.*
Kava (p.1703·2).
*Anxiety disorders.*

**Kavasol** *Ecosol, Switz.†.*
Kava (p.1703·2).
*Anxiety disorders; insomnia.*

**Kavatino** *Bionorica, Ger.†.*
Kava (p.1703·2).
*Anxiety disorders.*

**Kavavit** *Novartis Consumer, Austria.*
Kawain (p.1703·2); vitamins (p.1417·1).
*Tonic.*

**Kavepenin**
*AstraZeneca, Norw.; Astra, Swed.*
Phenoxymethylpenicillin potassium (p.242·1).
*Bacterial infections.*

**Kaveri** *Lichtwer, Ger.*
Ginkgo biloba leaf (p.1692·3).
*Intermittent claudication; mental function impairment; vestibular disorders.*

**Kavetten** *Kneipp, Switz.†.*
Kava (p.1703·2).
*Agitation; anxiety.*

**Kavipen** *Maver, Mex.*
Phenoxymethylpenicillin potassium (p.242·1).
*Bacterial infections.*

**Kavit** *Cristalia, Braz.*
Phytomenadione (p.1467·1).

**Kavitol** *Lannacher, Austria.*
Menadione sodium bisulfite (p.1466·3).
*Haemorrhage; overdosage with coumarin anticoagulants.*

**Kavosan** *Oral-B, Ital.*
Sodium perborate (p.1192·2).
*Oral hygiene.*

**Kavosporal comp** *Muller Goppingen, Ger.*
Kava (p.1703·2); valerian (p.1762·2).
*Anxiety disorders.*

**Kavosporal forte** *Muller Goppingen, Ger.*
Kava (p.1703·2).
*Anxiety disorders.*

**Kawaform** *Klinge, Switz.*
Kawain (p.1703·2); magnesium orotate (p.1724·3); vitis vinifera.
*Insomnia; tension; tonic.*

**Kay Ciel** *Forest Pharmaceuticals, USA.*
Potassium chloride (p.1232·2).
*Hypokalaemia; potassium depletion.*

**Kay-Cee-L**
*Geistlich, Irl.; Geistlich, UK.*
Potassium chloride (p.1232·2).
*Hypokalaemia; potassium depletion.*

**Kayexalate**
*Sanofi Synthelabo, Canad.; Sanofi Synthelabo, Fr.; IFET (ΙΦΕΤ), Gr.; Sanofi Winthrop, Israel; Sanofi Synthelabo, Ital.; Sanofi Synthelabo, Thai.; Sanofi Winthrop, USA.*
Sodium polystyrene sulfonate (p.1053·1).
*Hyperkalaemia.*

**Kayexalate Calcium** *Sanofi Synthelabo, Belg.*
Calcium polystyrene sulfonate (p.1032·3).
*Hyperkalaemia.*

**Kayexalate Sodium** *Sanofi Synthelabo, Belg.*
Sodium polystyrene sulfonate (p.1053·1).
*Hyperkalaemia.*

**Kaytwo** *Eisai, Jpn.*
Menatetrenone (p.1467·1).
*Vitamin K deficiency.*

**Kazak** *Knoll, Austral.†.*
Cerivastatin sodium (p.881·3).
*Hypercholesterolaemia.*

**Kazinal** *Asian Pharm, Thai.*
Ketoconazole (p.403·3).
*Fungal infections.*

**K-Biofen** *Alpha, Mex.†.*
Chloramphenicol (p.185·1).
*Bacterial infections.*

**K-C** *Century, USA.*
Kaolin (p.1268·3); pectin (p.1580·3); bismuth subcarbonate (p.1252·1).
*Diarrhoea.*

**K-Cil** *TP, Thai.*
Cloxacillin sodium (p.198·2).
*Bacterial infections.*

**KCl-retard**
*Novartis Consumer, Austria; Novartis, Ger.*
Potassium chloride (p.1232·2).
*Hypokalaemia.*

**K.C.M.C** *Knop, Chile.*
Carmellose (p.1577·3); marine algae; cholic acid (p.1660·3).
*Obesity.*

**Kdiron** *Julphar, UAE.*
Ferrous sulfate (p.1428·2).
*Iron deficiency anaemia.*

**K-Dur**
*Key, Canad.; Schering-Plough, Mex.; Key, USA.*
Potassium chloride (p.1232·2).
*Hypokalaemia.*

**Keal** *EG, Fr.*
Sucralfate (p.1290·2).
*Peptic ulcer.*

**Kebir** *Aspen, Arg.*
Oxaliplatin (p.577·1).
*Malignant neoplasms.*

**Kebirtecan** *Aspen, Arg.*
Irinotecan hydrochloride (p.564·1).
*Colorectal cancer.*

**Keciflox** *Pfleger, Ger.*
Ciprofloxacin (p.188·2).
*Bacterial infections.*

**Kedacillin** *Hormona, Mex.*
Sulbenicillin sodium (p.257·2).
Mepivacaine hydrochloride (p.1381·2) is included in this preparation to alleviate the pain of injection.
*Bacterial infections.*

**Kedacillina** *Bracco, Ital.†.*
Sulbenicillin sodium (p.257·2).

Lidocaine hydrochloride (p.1377·3) is included in this preparation to alleviate the pain of injection.
*Bacterial infections.*

**Keduo** *Kampel Martian, Arg.*
Ketoconazole (p.403·3).
*Fungal skin and scalp infections.*

**Keduril**
*Rhodia, Braz.†.*
Ketoprofen (p.51·2).
*Gout; musculoskeletal, joint, and peri-articular disorders; pain.*

*Aventis, Mex.*
Ketoprofen sodium (p.51·3).
*Inflammation; musculoskeletal, joint, and peri-articular disorders; pain.*

**Keefloxin** *Helfarma, Port.*
Ciprofloxacin hydrochloride (p.188·2).

**Keep Alert** *Reese, USA.*
Caffeine (p.782·1).

**Keep Clear Anti-Dandruff Shampoo** *Avon, Canad.†.*
Pyrithione zinc (p.1156·2).

**Kefaclor** *LSP, Thai.*
Cefaclor (p.167·1).
*Bacterial infections.*

**Kefadim**
*Lilly, Belg.; Lilly, Braz.†; Lilly, Thai.†; Lilly, UK.*
Ceftazidime (p.180·2).
*Bacterial infections.*

**Kefadol**
*Lilly, Irl.; Lilly, UK†.*
Cefamandole nafate (p.169·3).
*Bacterial infections.*

**Kefalex** *Ratiopharm, Fin.*
Cefalexin (p.168·1).
*Bacterial infections.*

**Kefalexin** *Royton, Braz.*
Cefalexin (p.168·1).
*Bacterial infections.*

**Kefalotin** *Biochimico, Braz.*
Cefalotin (p.169·2).
*Bacterial infections.*

**Kefamin** *Elanco, Spain.*
Ceftazidime (p.180·2).
*Bacterial infections.*

**Kefandol** *Lilly, Fr.†.*
Cefamandole nafate (p.169·3).
*Bacterial infections.*

**Kefazim** *Lilly, Austria.*
Ceftazidime (p.180·2).
*Bacterial infections.*

**Kefazin** *Vitamed, Israel.*
Cefazolin sodium (p.170·3).
*Bacterial infections.*

**Kefazol** *Lilly, Braz.*
Cefazolin sodium (p.170·3).
*Bacterial infections.*

**Kefazon** *Esseti, Ital.†.*
Cefoperazone sodium (p.174·3).
Lidocaine hydrochloride (p.1377·3) is included in this preparation to alleviate the pain of injection.
*Bacterial infections.*

**Kefdole** *Aspen, S.Afr.*
Cefamandole nafate (p.169·3).
*Bacterial infections.*

**Kefen** *Pacific, NZ†.*
Ketoprofen (p.51·2).
*Gout; musculoskeletal, joint, and peri-articular disorders; pain.*

**Kefentech** *JE IL, Singapore.*
Ketoprofen (p.51·2).
*Inflammation; musculoskeletal, joint, and peri-articular disorders; pain.*

**Kefexin**
*Orion, Fin.; Orion, Irl.; Orion, Malaysia.*
Cefalexin (p.168·1).
*Bacterial infections.*

**Keflaxina** *Hexal, Braz.*
Cefalexin (p.168·1).
*Bacterial infections.*

**Keflex**
*Lilly, Austral.; Lilly, Austria; Lilly, Braz.; Lilly, Canad.†; Lilly, Denm.; Lilly, Hong Kong; Lilly, Irl.; Lilly, Israel; Lilly, Mex.; Lilly, Norw.; Lilly, NZ; Lilly, Port.; Aspen, S.Afr.; Lilly, Swed.; Lilly, Switz.†; Lilly, Thai.; Lilly, UK; Dista, USA.*
Cefalexin (p.168·1).
*Bacterial infections.*

**Keflin**
*Lilly, Arg.; Lilly, Austria†; Lilly, Braz.; Lilly, Canad.†; Lilly, Denm.; Lilly, Fin.; Lilly, Fr.†; Lilly, Israel; Lilly, Ital.; Lilly, Mex.; Lilly, Neth.; Lilly, Norw.; Lilly, NZ†; Aspen, S.Afr.; Lilly, Spain†; Lilly, Swed.†; Lilly, Thai.*
Cefalotin sodium (p.168·3).
*Bacterial infections.*

**Keflin Neutral** *Lilly, Austral.*
Cefalotin sodium (p.168·3).
*Bacterial infections.*

**Keflor**
*Alphapharm, Austral.; Lilly, Chile; Ranbaxy, India.*
Cefaclor (p.167·1).
*Bacterial infections.*

**Kefloridina** *Elanco, Spain.*
Cefalexin (p.168·1).
*Bacterial infections.*

**Kefloridina Mucolitico** *Lilly, Spain†.*
Bromhexine hydrochloride (p.1115·3); cefalexin (p.168·1).
*Respiratory-tract infections.*

**Kefol** *Irisfarma, Spain.*
Cefazolin sodium (p.170·3).
*Bacterial infections.*

**Kefolor**
*Lilly, Fin.; Lilly, Swed.†.*
Cefaclor (p.167·1).
*Bacterial infections.*

**Keforal**
*Lilly, Arg.; Lilly, Belg.; Lilly, Fr.; Lilly, Ital.; Lilly, Neth.*
Cefalexin (p.168·1).
*Bacterial infections.*

**Kefox** *CT, Ital.*
Cefuroxime sodium (p.184·1).
*Bacterial infections.*

**Kefoxin** *Biochimico, Braz.*
Cefotaxime sodium (p.175·3).
*Bacterial infections.*

**Kefoxina** *CT, Ital.†.*
Propylene glycol cefatrizine (p.170·3).
*Bacterial infections.*

**Kefspor** *Asta Medica, Ger.†.*
Cefaclor (p.167·1).
*Bacterial infections.*

**Keftab** *Biovail, USA.*
Cefalexin hydrochloride (p.168·1).
*Bacterial infections.*

**Keftid**
*Galen, Irl.; Galen, UK.*
Cefaclor (p.167·1).
*Bacterial infections.*

**Keftriaxon** *Vitamed, Israel.*
Ceftriaxone sodium (p.182·3).
*Bacterial infections.*

**Kefurim** *Vitamed, Israel.*
Cefuroxime sodium (p.184·1).
*Bacterial infections.*

**Kefurion** *Orion, Fin.†.*
Cefuroxime sodium (p.184·1).
*Bacterial infections.*

**Kefurox**
*Lilly, Belg.; Lilly, Canad.; Lilly, USA†.*
Cefuroxime sodium (p.184·1).
*Bacterial infections.*

**Kefzim**
*Lilly, Chile; Lilly, S.Afr.*
Ceftazidime (p.180·2).
*Bacterial infections.*

**Kefzol**
*Lilly, Austral.; Lilly, Austria; Lilly, Belg.; Lilly, Canad.; Lilly, Chile; Lilly, Israel; Lilly, Neth.; Lilly, NZ; Rolab, S.Afr.; Lilly, Switz.; Lilly, Thai.†; Lilly, UK†; Lilly, USA†.*
Cefazolin sodium (p.170·3).
*Bacterial infections.*

**Keimax** *Essex, Ger.*
Ceftibuten (p.182·1).
*Bacterial infections.*

**Keimicina** *Zambon, Ital.*
Kanamycin sulfate (p.225·1).
*Vulvovaginal bacterial infections.*

**Kela** *TO-Chemicals, Thai.*
Triamcinolone acetonide (p.1110·2).
*Skin disorders.*

**Kelac** *Richmond, Arg.*
Ketorolac (p.52·3).
*Inflammation; pain.*

**Kelaplus** *TO-Chemicals, Thai.*
Miconazole nitrate (p.405·3); triamcinolone acetonide (p.1110·2).
*Fungal skin infections.*

**Kelatin**
*Yamanouchi, Belg.; Yamanouchi, Neth.*
Penicillamine (p.1046·3).
*Cystinuria; heavy-metal poisoning; rheumatoid arthritis; Wilson's disease.*

**Kelatine** *Yabrofarma, Port.*
Penicillamine (p.1046·3).
*Heavy-metal poisoning; rheumatoid arthritis.*

**Kelavitam** *Iodo Suma, Braz.†.*
Buclizine (p.426·3); carnitine; vitamin B substances; gamma-aminobutyric acid (p.1417·1).
*Reduced appetite; tonic.*

**Kelbium** *Sankyo, Spain†.*
Cefpodoxime proxetil (p.178·3).
*Bacterial infections.*

**Kelefusin** *Pisa, Mex.*
Potassium chloride (p.1232·2).

**Kelfer** *Vianex (Βιανέξ), Gr.*
Deferiprone (p.1033·1).
*Iron overload.*

**Kelfiprim**
*Pharmacia Upjohn, Ital.†; Pharmacia Upjohn, Mex.†; Pharmacia Upjohn, Thai.†.*
Trimethoprim (p.272·2); sulfametopyrazine (p.263·1).
*Bacterial infections; Pneumocystis carinii pneumonia.*

**Kelfizina**
*Pharmacia Upjohn, Belg.†; Pharmacia Upjohn, Ital.†.*
Sulfametopyrazine (p.263·1).
*Bacterial infections; toxoplasmosis.*

**Kelfizine W**
*Pharmacia Upjohn, Irl.†; Pharmacia, UK†.*
Sulfametopyrazine (p.263·1).
*Bacterial infections.*

**Keli-med** *Permamed, Switz.*
Garlic (p.1691·1); hyoscyamus (p.485·2); allantoin (p.1141·3); heparin sodium (p.928·1); avobenzone (p.1142·3); enzacamene (p.1147·1).
*Scars.*

**Kelnac**
*Sankyo, Jpn; Sankyo, Thai.*
Plaunotol (p.1284·1).
*Gastritis; peptic ulcer.*

**Keloc** *Approved Prescription Services, UK.*
Felodipine (p.914·3).
*Hypertension.*

**Kelo-Cote** *Advanced Biotechnologies, Israel.*
Polysiloxane (p.1482·1); silicon dioxide (p.1581·3).
*Aid in skin healing.*

**Kelocyanor**
*SERB, Fr.; IFET (ΙΦΕΤ), Gr.; Lipha, Irl.†; Cambridge, UK†.*
Dicobalt edetate (p.1036·2).
Now known as Dicobalt Edetate Ampoules in the *UK.*
*Cyanide poisoning.*

**Kelofibrase** *Azupharma, Ger.*
Urea (p.1162·2); heparin sodium (p.928·1); camphor (p.1665·3).
*Keloids; scars.*

**Kelosal** *Quimifar, Spain.*
Cisapride (p.1259·2).
*Gastro-oesophageal reflux; gastroparesis.*

**Kelosoft**
*Chemomedica, Austria; Geistlich, Switz.*
Hyoscyamus oil (p.485·2).
*Nasal disorders; scars.*

**Kelp Plus 3** *Larkhall Laboratories, UK.*
Kelp (p.1742·3); vitamin $B_6$ (p.1456·3); soya lecithin (p.1706·1); cider vinegar.

**Kelsef** *Alpharma, Fr.*
Cefradine (p.179·3).
*Bacterial infections.*

**Kelsopen** *Reig Jofre, Spain.*
Amoxicillin trihydrate (p.155·3); potassium clavulanate (p.193·3).
*Bacterial infections.*

**Keltican N** *Trommsdorff, Ger.*
Trisodium uridine triphosphate (p.1760·3); disodium uridine diphosphate; disodium uridine phosphate; disodium cytidine phosphate.
Lidocaine hydrochloride (p.1377·3) is included in the injection to alleviate the pain of injection.
*Neuralgia; neuritis; neuropathy.*

**Kelual**
*Pierre Fabre, Arg.; Ducray, Fr.*
Keluamid (p.1151·2).
*Seborrhoeic dermatitis; skin disorders.*

**Kelual Zinc**
*Pierre Fabre, Arg.; Ducray, Fr.*
Keluamid (p.1151·2); zinc sulfate (p.1469·3).
*Seborrhoeic dermatitis; skin disorders.*

**Kemadren** *GlaxoSmithKline, Spain.*
Procyclidine hydrochloride (p.488·2).
*Drug-induced extrapyramidal disorders; parkinsonism.*

**Kemadrin**
*Glaxo Wellcome, Austral.†; GlaxoSmithKline, Austria; GlaxoSmithKline, Belg.; GlaxoSmithKline, Canad.; GlaxoSmithKline, Denm.; GlaxoSmithKline, India; Wellcome, Irl.; Wellcome, Israel; GlaxoSmithKline, Ital.; GlaxoSmithKline, Malaysia; Glaxo Wellcome, Neth.†; GlaxoSmithKline, NZ; Glaxo Wellcome, Swed.†; GlaxoSmithKline, Switz.; Auden McKenzie, UK; GlaxoSmithKline, UK; Glaxo Wellcome, USA.*
Procyclidine hydrochloride (p.488·2).
*Drug-induced extrapyramidal disorders; parkinsonism.*

**Kemanat** *Finadiet, Arg.*
Ketorolac trometamol (p.52·1).
*Pain.*

**Kemeol** *Interdelta, Switz.*
Ephedrine (p.1120·1); neroli oil (p.1719·2); eucalyptus oil (p.1686·2).
*Nasal congestion.*

**Kemerhine** *Interdelta, Switz.†.*
Ephedrine hydrochloride (p.1120·1); neroli oil (p.1719·2); eucalyptus oil (p.1686·2).
*Nasal congestion.*

**Kemerhinose** *Interdelta, Switz.*
Sodium chloride (p.1233·3); benzododecinium bromide (p.1170·2).
*Nasal congestion.*

**Kemicetin** *Pharmacia, Austria.*
Chloramphenicol (p.185·1).
*Bacterial eye infections.*

**Kemicetina** *Pharmacia, Belg.*
Chloramphenicol (p.185·1).
*Bacterial infections.*

**Kemicetine**
*Pharmacia, Hong Kong; Mac, India; Pharmacia, Singapore; Pharmacia, Thai.; Pharmacia, UK.*
Chloramphenicol (p.185·1) or chloramphenicol sodium succinate (p.185·1).
*Bacterial infections.*

**Kemicetine Antiozena** *Mac, India.*
Chloramphenicol (p.185·1); estradiol dipropionate (p.1550·1); colecalciferol (p.1461·3).
*Rhinitis; rhinopharyngitis.*

**Kemicetine Otological** *Mac, India.*
*Ear drops (1%):* Chloramphenicol (p.185·1).
*Ear drops (5%):* Chloramphenicol (p.185·1); lidocaine hydrochloride (p.1377·3).
*Ear infections.*

**Kemocarb**
*Dabur, India; Dabur, Thai.*
Carboplatin (p.533·3).
*Malignant neoplasms.*

**Kemodyn** *Esseti, Ital.*
Citicoline sodium (p.1672·3).
*Cerebrovascular disorders; parkinsonism.*

**Kemoplat**
*Dabur, India; Dabur, Thai.*
Cisplatin (p.538·1).
*Malignant neoplasms.*

**Kemphor** *Salusif, Port.*
Zinc chloride (p.1469·2); sumatra benzoin (p.1751·1); gualtheria oil; menthol (p.1711·3).
*Mouth disorders.*

**Kempi** *Pharmacia, Spain.*
Spectinomycin hydrochloride (p.255·2).
*Gonorrhoea.*

**Kemsol** *Carter Horner, Canad.*
Dimethyl sulfoxide (p.1473·2).
*Scleroderma.*

**Kemstro** *Schwarz, USA.*
Baclofen (p.1386·3).
*Skeletal muscle spasm and spasticity.*

**Kemzid**
*Unison, Hong Kong; Unison, Singapore; Unison, Thai.*
Triamcinolone acetonide (p.1110·2).
*Skin and scalp disorders.*

**Kenacomb**
*Bristol-Myers Squibb, Arg.; Bristol-Myers Squibb, Austral.; Westwood-Squibb, Canad.; Bristol-Myers Squibb, Hong Kong; Sarabhai Piramal, India; Bristol-Myers Squibb, Irl.; Bristol-Myers Squibb, Israel; Bristol-Myers Squibb, Malaysia; Bristol-Myers Squibb, Mex.; Bristol-Myers Squibb, NZ; Bristol-Myers Squibb, Port.; Bristol-Myers Squibb, S.Afr.; Bristol-Myers Squibb, Singapore; Bristol-Myers Squibb, Thai.*
Triamcinolone acetonide (p.1110·2); neomycin sulfate (p.235·1); gramicidin (p.220·2); nystatin (p.406·3).
*Infected skin disorders.*

**Kenacombin Novum** *Bristol-Myers Squibb, Swed.*
Triamcinolone acetonide (p.1110·2); nystatin (p.406·3).
*Fungal skin infections.*

**Kenacort**
*Bristol-Myers Squibb, Arg.; Bristol-Myers Squibb, Belg.; UPSA, Fr.; Sarabhai Piramal, India; Bristol-Myers Squibb, Ital.; Bristol-Myers Squibb, Mex.; Bristol-Myers Squibb, Switz.; Bristol-Myers Squibb, Thai.; Apothecon, USA†.*
Triamcinolone (p.1110·2) or triamcinolone acetonide (p.1110·2).
*Corticosteroid.*

**Kenacort Solubile** *Bristol-Myers Squibb, Belg.†.*
Triamcinolone acetonide dipotassium phosphate (p.1110·3).
*Corticosteroid.*

**Kenacort-A**
*Note. This name is used for preparations of different composition.*
*Bristol-Myers Squibb, Arg.; Bristol-Myers Squibb, Austral.; Bristol-Myers Squibb, Belg.; Bristol-Myers Squibb, Chile; Bristol-Myers Squibb, Hong Kong; Bristol-Myers Squibb, Malaysia; Bristol-Myers Squibb, Neth.; Bristol-Myers Squibb, NZ; Bristol-Myers Squibb, Singapore; Bristol-Myers Squibb, Switz.*
Triamcinolone acetonide (p.1110·2).
*Corticosteroid.*

*Bristol-Myers Squibb, Switz.*
*Tincture:* Triamcinolone acetonide (p.1110·2); salicylic acid (p.1157·1).
*Skin disorders.*

**Kenacort-A Solubile** *Bristol-Myers Squibb, Switz.*
Triamcinolone acetonide dipotassium phosphate (p.1110·3).
*Corticosteroid.*

**Kenacort-T**
*Bristol-Myers Squibb, Fin.; Bristol-Myers Squibb, Norw.; Bristol-Myers Squibb, Swed.*
Triamcinolone acetonide (p.1110·2).
*Corticosteroid.*

**Kenacort-T comp**
*Bristol-Myers Squibb, Fin.†; Bristol-Myers Squibb, Norw.; Bristol-Myers Squibb, Swed.*
Triamcinolone acetonide (p.1110·2); salicylic acid (p.1157·1).
*Otitis externa; skin disorders.*

**Kenacutan**
*Bristol-Myers Squibb, Denm.; Bristol-Myers Squibb, Norw.; Bristol-Myers Squibb, Swed.*
Triamcinolone acetonide (p.1110·2); halquinol (p.220·3).
*Infected skin disorders.*

**Kenaderm** *Raza, Malaysia; Pharmaniaga, Malaysia.*
Triamcinolone acetonide (p.1110·2).
*Skin disorders.*

**Kenadion** *Samarth, India.*
Phytomenadione (p.1467·1).
*Antidote to coumarin anticoagulants in hypoprothrombinaemia.*

**Kenaject** *Mayrand, USA†.*
Triamcinolone acetonide (p.1110·2).
*Corticosteroid.*

**Kenalcol** *Bristol-Myers Squibb, Fr.*
Triamcinolone acetonide (p.1110·2); salicylic acid (p.1157·1); benzalkonium chloride (p.1168·3).
*Skin disorders.*

**Kenalin** Kendrick, Mex.
Sulindac (p.91·2).
*Gout; musculoskeletal, joint, and peri-articular disorders.*

**Kenalog**
Note. This name is used for preparations of different composition.
Westwood-Squibb, Canad.; Bristol-Myers Squibb, Denm.; Bristol-Myers Squibb, Ger.; Bristol-Myers Squibb, Irl.; Bristol-Myers Squibb, Israel; Bristol-Myers Squibb, UK; Westwood-Squibb, USA.
Triamcinolone acetonide (p.1110·2).
*Corticosteroid.*

Bristol-Myers Squibb, Neth.
Triamcinolone acetonide (p.1110·2); salicylic acid (p.1157·1).
*Keratinisation disorders; psoriasis.*

**Kenalog Comp** Bristol-Myers Squibb, Denm.†.
Triamcinolone acetonide (p.1110·2); gramicidin (p.220·2); neomycin sulfate (p.235·1).
*Infected skin disorders.*

**Kenalog Comp med Mycostatin** Bristol-Myers Squibb, Denm.
Triamcinolone acetonide (p.1110·2); gramicidin (p.220·2); neomycin sulfate (p.235·1); nystatin (p.406·3).
*Infected skin disorders.*

**Kenalog Dental** Bristol-Myers Squibb, Mex.
Triamcinolone (p.1110·2).
*Mouth disorders.*

**Kenalog med Salicylsyre** Bristol-Myers Squibb, Denm.
Triamcinolone acetonide (p.1110·2); salicylic acid (p.1157·1).
*Skin disorders.*

**Kenalog in Orabase**
Bristol-Myers Squibb, Austral.; Westwood-Squibb, Canad.; Bristol-Myers Squibb, Hong Kong; Bristol-Myers Squibb, Israel; Bristol-Myers Squibb, Malaysia; Bristol-Myers Squibb, NZ; Bristol-Myers Squibb, S.Afr.; Bristol-Myers Squibb, Singapore; Squibb, Spain; Bristol-Myers Squibb, Thai.; Apothecon, USA.
Triamcinolone acetonide (p.1110·2).
*Oral lesions.*

**Kenalog-S** Sarabhai Piramal, India.
Triamcinolone acetonide (p.1110·2); gramicidin (p.220·2); neomycin sulfate (p.235·1).
*Inflammatory eye disorders.*

**Kenalone** Bristol-Myers Squibb, Austral.†.
Triamcinolone acetonide (p.1110·2).
*Skin disorders.*

**Kenalyn** Silom, Thai.
Ketoconazole (p.403·3).
*Fungal scalp infections.*

**Kenapril** Kener, Mex.†.
Captopril (p.879·2).

**Kenaprol** Kener, Mex.†.
Metoprolol tartrate (p.957·1).

**Kenaprox** Kener, Mex.†.
Naproxen (p.65·1).

**Kenazol**
Note. This name is used for preparations of different composition.
Kendrick, Mex.
Etoposide (p.551·3).
*Malignant neoplasms.*

Pharmasant, Thai.
Ketoconazole (p.403·3).
*Fungal infections.*

**Kenazole** Greater Pharma, Thai.
Ketoconazole (p.403·3).
*Fungal infections.*

**Kenciclen** Kener, Mex.†.
Doxycycline (p.206·2).
*Bacterial infections.*

**Kendazol** Kener, Mex.†.
Danazol (p.1545·2).

**Kendix** EG, Fr.
Aciclovir (p.626·1).
*Herpesvirus infections.*

**Kendural** Abbott, Switz.
Ferrous sulfate (p.1428·2).
Sodium ascorbate (p.1460·2) is included in this preparation to increase the absorption and availability of iron.
*Iron deficiency; iron-deficiency anaemia.*

**Kendural C** Abbott, Ger.
Ferrous sulfate (p.1428·2).
Ascorbic acid (p.1460·2) is included in this preparation to increase the absorption and availability of iron.
*Iron deficiency; iron-deficiency anaemias.*

**Kendural-Fol-500** Abbott, Ger.
Ferrous sulfate (p.1428·3); folic acid (p.1429·1).
Ascorbic acid (p.1460·2) is included in this preparation to increase the absorption and availability of iron.
*Iron and folic acid deficiency; iron-deficiency anaemias.*

**Kendural-Plus** Abbott, Ger.†.
Ferrous sulfate (p.1428·3); vitamins.
*Iron deficiency.*

**Kenedril** Biospray, Gr.
Azelaic acid (p.1142·3).
*Acne.*

**Kenefen** Pharmasant, Thai.
Ketotifen fumarate (p.788·1).
*Asthma; bronchitis; hypersensitivity reactions.*

**Kenergon** Magistra, Switz.
Lidocaine (p.1377·3).
*Premature ejaculation.*

**Kenesil** Cantabria, Spain.
Nimodipine (p.972·3).
*Mental function impairment; neurological deficit following subarachnoid haemorrhage.*

**Kenhancer**
Sang-A, Malaysia; Sang-A Pharm, Singapore.
Ketoprofen (p.51·2).
*Musculoskeletal, joint, peri-articular, and soft-tissue disorders.*

**Keno** TO-Chemicals, Thai.
Triamcinolone acetonide (p.1110·2).
*Oral lesions.*

**Kenoid** Bristol-Myers Squibb, NZ†.
Triamcinolone acetonide (p.1110·2); lidocaine hydrochloride (p.1377·3); nystatin (p.406·3).
*Anorectal disorders; skin disorders.*

**Kenoket** Kendrick, Mex.
Clonazepam (p.359·1).
*Epilepsy.*

**Kenolan** Kendrick, Mex.
Captopril (p.879·2).
*Heart failure; hypertension.*

**Kenona** Kener, Mex.†.
Propafenone (p.989·2).

**Kenonel** Marnel, USA.
Triamcinolone acetonide (p.1110·2).
*Skin disorders.*

**Kenopril** Kendrick, Mex.
Enalapril maleate (p.909·2).
*Heart failure; hypertension.*

**Kenoral** General Drugs, Thai.
Ketoconazole (p.403·3).
*Fungal infections.*

**Kensodic** Kendrick, Mex.
Roxithromycin (p.254·2).
*Bacterial infections.*

**Kenspa** Kenyaku, Thai.
Chlordiazepoxide (p.674·2); clidinium bromide (p.480·2).
*Gastrointestinal disorders; smooth muscle spasm.*

**Kenstatin** Kendrick, Mex.
Pravastatin sodium (p.984·3).
*Hypercholesterolaemia.*

**Kentacef** Bristol-Myers Squibb, Gr.
Propylene glycol cefatrizine (p.170·3).
*Bacterial infections.*

**Kentadin** Kendrick, Mex.
Pentoxifylline (p.979·3).
*Vascular disorders.*

**Kentamol** Ivax, UK.
Salbutamol (p.791·3).
*Asthma.*

**Kentosanil** Kener, Mex.†.
Oxolamine citrate (p.1126·1).

**Kentovase** Kent, UK.
Prazosin hydrochloride (p.985·1).
*Heart failure; hypertension.*

**Kenvestin** Kener, Mex.
Pravastatin (p.985·1).
*Hyperlipidaemias.*

**Kenwood Therapeutic Liquid** Kenwood, USA.
Multivitamin and mineral preparation (p.1417·1).

**Kenya-Mox** Kenyaku, Thai.
Amoxicillin trihydrate (p.155·3).
*Bacterial infections.*

**Kenzen** Takeda, Fr.
Candesartan cilexetil (p.878·3).
*Hypertension.*

**Kenzoflex** Collins, Mex.
Ciprofloxacin hydrochloride (p.188·2).
*Bacterial infections.*

**Kenzolol** Kendrick, Mex.
Nimodipine (p.972·3).
*Neurological deficit following subarachnoid haemorrhage.*

**Kenzomyl** Kendrick, Mex.
Mesalazine (p.1273·2).
*Inflammatory bowel disease.*

**Kephalodoron** Weleda, Austria.
Ferrous sulfate (p.1428·2); silicon dioxide (p.1581·3).
*Migraine; nervous disorders; vasomotor headache.*

**Kepinol** Pfleger, Ger.
Co-trimoxazole (p.199·3).
*Bacterial infections; Pneumocystis carinii pneumonia.*

**Keppra**
Rontag, Arg.; UCB, Austral.; UCB, Belg.; UCB, Denm.; UCB, Fin.; UCB, Fr.; UCB, Ger.; UCB, Hong Kong; UCB, Irl.; UCB, Ital.; UCB, Norw.; UCB, Port.; UCB, Singapore; UCB, Spain; UCB, Swed.; UCB, Switz.; UCB, Thai.; UCB, UK; UCB, USA.
Levetiracetam (p.366·1).
*Epilepsy.*

**Keppur** Drossapharm, Switz.
*Cream:* Heparin sodium (p.928·1); comfrey (p.1675·2); hypericum oil (p.299·2); calendula oil (p.1665·2).
*Topical gel:* Heparin sodium (p.928·1); comfrey (p.1675·2).
*Musculoskeletal, joint, peri-articular, and soft-tissue disorders; peripheral vascular disorders.*

**Kepra** UCB, Gr.
Levetiracetam (p.366·1).
*Epilepsy.*

**Keprobiozol** Columbia, Mex.
Ketoconazole (p.403·3).
*Fungal infections.*

**Keprodol** Ratiopharm, Austria.
Ketoprofen (p.51·2).
*Inflammation; musculoskeletal and joint disorders; pain.*

**Kepsidol** Kener, Mex.†.
Haloperidol (p.701·2).

**Keptan Compuesto** Sanofi Synthelabo, Arg.
Trospium chloride (p.491·2); dipyrone (p.35·3).
*Muscle spasm; pain.*

**Keracnyl**
Note. This name is used for preparations of different composition.
Pierre Fabre, Arg.; Ducray, Fr.
*Cream:* Poly hydroxy acids; alpha hydroxy acids; saw palmetto (p.1569·1); zinc salicylate (p.1157·2).
*Acne; seborrhoea.*

Pierre Fabre, Arg.; Ducray, Fr.
*Topical mousse:* Poly hydroxy acids; glycolic acid (p.1147·3); saw palmetto (p.1569·1); zinc salicylate (p.1157·2).
*Seborrhoea.*

Ducray, Fr.
*Face mask:* Glycolic acid (p.1147·3); zinc salicylate (p.1157·2); kaolin (p.1268·3).
*Seborrhoea.*

**Kerafilm** Pierre Fabre Sante, Fr.
Salicylic acid (p.1157·1); lactic acid (p.1704·1).
*Calluses; corns; verrucae.*

**Keraflex** Pergam, Ital.
Carbocisteine (p.1116·2); malic acid (p.1709·2); mucopolysaccharides; urea (p.1162·2); allantoin (p.1141·3).
*Cicatrisation.*

**Keral**
Menarini, Irl.; Menarini, UK.
Dexketoprofen trometamol (p.51·2).
*Pain.*

**Keralac Plus** LED, Fr.
Ammonium lactate (p.1142·3); salicylic acid (p.1157·1); zinc gluconate (p.1469·2).
*Acne.*

**Keralin** East India Pharma, India.
Hydrocortisone acetate (p.1103·3); salicylic acid (p.1157·1); benzoic acid (p.1169·3).
*Corns; fungal skin infections.*

**Keraliss 14** LED, Fr.†.
Ammonium lactate (p.1142·3); zinc gluconate (p.1469·2).
*Acne.*

**Keralyt**
Westwood-Squibb, Canad.†; Summers, USA.
Salicylic acid (p.1157·1).
*Hyperkeratosis.*

**Keranon** Pentamedical, Ital.
Salicylic acid (p.1157·1).
*Keratinisation disorders.*

**Kerapil**
Fouchard, Chile; LED, Fr.
Ammonium lactate (p.1142·3).
*Keratinisation disorders.*

**Kerarer** Kampel Martian, Arg.
Ketorolac trometamol (p.52·1).
*Pain.*

**Kerasal**
Optimapharma, Canad.; Spirig, Switz.
Salicylic acid (p.1157·1); urea (p.1162·2).
*Skin disorders.*

**Keratisdin** Isdin, Spain.
Lactic acid (p.1704·1).
*Skin disorders.*

**Kerato Biciron** S & K, Ger.
Calcium pantothenate (p.1442·3).
*Corneal injury.*

**Keratocynesine** Boiron, Canad.†.
Homoeopathic preparation.

**Keratolip** Ogna, Ital.
Betacarotene (p.1422·3); propolis (p.1735·2).
*Emollient for lips.*

**Keratosane** Biorga, Fr.†.
Urea (p.1162·2); pentosan polysulfate (p.979·2).
*Skin disorders.*

**Keratosis** Widmer, Austria.
Urea (p.1162·2); dexpanthenol (p.1727·2).
*Hyperkeratotic skin disorders.*

**Keratosis forte** Widmer, Austria.
Urea (p.1162·2); dexpanthenol (p.1727·2); tretinoin (p.1161·1).
*Skin disorders.*

**Keratospor** Agis, Israel.
Bifonazole (p.395·1); urea (p.1162·2).
*Fungal nail infections.*

**Keratotal** Collagen, Ital.†.
Ammonium lactate (p.1142·3).
*Dry skin; scalp disorders.*

**Keratyl**
Sidus, Arg.; Chauvin, Fr.; Chauvin ankerpharm, Ger.; Bausch & Lomb, Switz.; Chauvin, Thai.
Nandrolone sodium sulfate (p.1561·3).
*Eye disorders; eye injury and inflammation.*

**Keri**
Bristol-Myers Squibb, Canad.; Bristol-Myers Squibb, Hong Kong; Westwood, Singapore†; Bristol-Myers Squibb, UK; Westwood, USA.
A range of emollient and moisturiser preparations.
*Dry skin.*

**Keri Lotion** Bristol-Myers Squibb, Canad.
*SPF 15:* Octinoxate (p.1154·3); octisalate (p.1154·3); oxybenzone (p.1154·3).
*Sunscreen.*

**Keri Silky Smooth** Bristol-Myers, Austral.†.
Emollient.
*Dry skin disorders; pruritus; skin irritation.*

**Keri Soap** Bristol-Myers Squibb, Canad.†.
Emollient.

**Kerlocal** Pierre Fabre, Fr.†.
Tretinoin (p.1161·1).
*Keratinisation disorders.*

**Kerlofin** Chrispa (Χρισπα), Gr.
Omeprazole (p.1278·2).
*Acid aspiration; eradication of Helicobacter pylori in combination with antimicrobials; peptic ulcer; reflux oesophagitis; Zollinger-Ellison syndrome.*

**Kerlon**
Lorex, Denm.; Sanofi Synthelabo, Fin.; Sanofi Synthelabo, Ital.; Sanofi Synthelabo, Neth.; Pharmacia, Swed.; Synthelabo, Switz.
Betaxolol hydrochloride (p.873·1).
*Angina pectoris; hypertension.*

**Kerlone**
Sanofi Synthelabo, Austria; Sanofi Synthelabo, Belg.; Sanofi Synthelabo, Fr.; Sanofi Synthelabo, Ger.; Lavipharm, Gr.; Synthelabo, Hong Kong†; Synthelabo, Israel; Sanofi Synthelabo, Malaysia; Sanofi Synthelabo, Singapore; Sanofi Synthelabo, Thai.†; Sanofi Synthelabo, UK†; Sanofi, USA.
Betaxolol hydrochloride (p.873·1).
*Angina pectoris; hypertension.*

**Kernit** CT, Ital.
Levocarnitine (p.1423·3).
*Carnitine deficiency; myocardial ischaemia.*

**Kernosan Elixir** Kern, Switz.
Aniseed (p.1655·2); horseradish (p.1697·3); calamus (p.1664·1); fennel (p.1687·2); hedera helix; imperatoria root; Iceland moss; pimpinella root; plantain seed (p.1733·1); oak bark (p.1722·3); primula root (p.1735·1); liquorice (p.1270·2).
*Bronchitis; catarrh; coughs.*

**Kernosan Heidelberger Poudre** Kern, Switz.
Absinthium (p.1645·1); aniseed (p.1655·2); caraway (p.1667·2); fennel (p.1687·2); juniper (p.1703·1); achillea (p.1646·2); pimpinella root.
*Digestive system disorders.*

**Kernosan Huile de Massage** Kern, Switz.†.
Plum oil; camphor (p.1665·3); methyl salicylate (p.59·3); eucalyptus oil (p.1686·2); lavender oil (p.1705·2); mint oil (p.1715·2); rosemary oil (p.1740·2); sage oil (p.1741·2); thyme oil (p.1755·3); turpentine oil (p.1760·1); hyoscyamus oil (p.485·2).
*Musculoskeletal, joint, and peri-articular pain.*

**Keroderm** Turimed, Switz.
Linoleic acid ethyl ester; triclosan (p.1195·2); cholesterol; cod-liver oil (p.1425·2); zinc oxide (p.1163·2); titanium dioxide (p.1160·3).
*Eczema; inflammation; minor skin lesions.*

**Kerodex**
Miba, Ital.; Whitehall, USA.
Topical barrier preparation.

**Keromask** Network Health & Beauty, UK.
A covering cream.
*Concealment of birth marks, scars, and disfiguring skin disease.*

**Kerpet** Roux-Ocefa, Arg.
Budesonide (p.1094·2).

**Kertyol**
Pierre Fabre, Arg.; Ducray, Fr.
Salicylic acid (p.1157·1).
*Dandruff.*

**Kertyol-S** Ducray, Fr.
Kertyol; salicylic acid (p.1157·1); zinc thiosalicylate.
*Scalp disorders.*

**Kesan** Baliarda, Arg.
Ibuprofen (p.45·3).
*Pain.*

**Kesint** Copernico, Ital.
Cefuroxime sodium (p.184·1).
*Gram-negative bacterial infections.*

**Kess** Filaxis, Arg.
Lamivudine (p.648·2).
*HIV infection.*

**Kess Complex** Filaxis, Arg.
Lamivudine (p.648·2); zidovudine (p.658·2).
*HIV infecion.*

**Kessar**
Pharmacia Upjohn, Austral.†; Pharmacia, Austria; Pharmacia, Braz.; Pharmacia, Chile; Pharmacia, Fr.; Pharmacia, Ger.; Pharmacia-Upjohn, Gr.; Pharmacia Upjohn, Ital.; Pharmacia Upjohn, Mex.; Pharmacia, S.Afr.; Pharmacia, Switz.
Tamoxifen citrate (p.584·1).
*Breast cancer; endometrial cancer.*

**Kest** Torbet Laboratories, UK.
Magnesium sulfate (p.1228·2).
Formerly contained magnesium sulfate and phenolphthalein.
*Constipation.*

**Kestin** Pharmafarm, Fr.
Ebastine (p.433·1).
*Allergic rhinitis; urticaria.*

**Kestine**
Nycomed, Denm.; Nycomed, Fin.; Rhone-Poulenc Rorer, Hong Kong; Rhone-Poulenc Rorer, Israel†; Almirall, Neth.; Nycomed, Norw.; Probi-

os, Port.; Aspen, S.Afr.; Almirall, Singapore; Ranbaxy, Singapore; Nycomed, Swed.
Ebastine (p.433·1).
*Allergic conjunctivitis; allergic rhinitis; pruritus; urticaria.*

**Kestomatine** Sanofi Synthelabo, Belg.
Algeldrate (p.1249·2); simeticone (p.1289·2).
*Gastrointestinal disorders.*

**Kestomatine Baby** Sanofi Synthelabo, Belg.
Simeticone (p.1289·2); ceratonia (p.1579·1).
*Abdominal distension; flatulence; vomiting.*

**Kestomatine Bebe** Synthelabo, Switz.†.
Dimethicone (p.1289·2); carob fruit and seed (p.1579·1).
*Gastrointestinal disorders.*

**Kestomicol** Farmaco, Mex.
Ketoconazole (p.403·3).
*Fungal infections.*

**Kestrone** Hyrex, USA.
Estrone (p.1553·1).
*Abnormal uterine bleeding; breast cancer; female castration; female hypogonadism; menopausal vulval and vaginal atrophy; primary ovarian failure; prostatic cancer.*

**Keta** Astrapin, Ger.; Curasan, Ger.; Hameln, Ger.
Ketamine hydrochloride (p.1302·1).
*General anaesthesia; status asthmaticus.*

**Keta-Hameln** Hameln, Thai.; TTN, Thai.
Ketamine hydrochloride (p.1302·1).
*General anaesthesia.*

**Ketalar**
Parke, Davis, Arg.; Pfizer, Austral.; Parke, Davis, Austria†; Pfizer, Belg.; Pfizer, Braz.; Pfizer, Canad.; Pfizer, Denm.; Pfizer, Fin.; Pfizer, Fr.†; Pfizer, Hong Kong; Parke, Davis, India; Pfizer, Irl.; Parke, Davis, Israel; Parke, Davis, Ital.†; Parke, Davis, Neth.; Pfizer, Norw.; Pfizer, NZ; Pfizer, Swed.; Pfizer, Switz.; Pfizer, Thai.; Pfizer, UK; Monarch, USA.
Ketamine hydrochloride (p.1302·1).
*General anaesthesia.*

**Ketalgesic** Max Farma, Ital.†.
Ketoprofen (p.51·2).
*Pain.*

**Ketalgine** Amino, Switz.
Methadone hydrochloride (p.57·2).
*Pain.*

**Ketalin** Galen, Mex.
Ketamine hydrochloride (p.1302·1).
*General anaesthesia.*

**Ketanest**
Scott-Cassara, Arg.; Pfizer, Austria; Pfizer, Fin.; Parke, Davis, Ger.; Pfizer, Ger.; Parke, Davis, Neth.
Ketamine hydrochloride (p.1302·1).
*General anaesthesia; regional anaesthesia; status asthmaticus.*

**Ketanine** Korea United, Singapore.
Captopril (p.879·2).
*Heart failure; hypertension.*

**Ketanov**
Ranbaxy, India; Ranbaxy, Malaysia.
Ketorolac trometamol (p.52·1).
*Pain; postoperative eye inflammation.*

**Ketartrium** Esseti, Ital.
Ketoprofen (p.51·2).
*Inflammation; musculoskeletal, joint, and peri-articular disorders.*

**Ketas** Kyorin, Jpn.
Ibudilast (p.786·3).
*Asthma; cerebrovascular disorders.*

**Ketasma**
Sun, India; Lesvi, Spain.
Ketotifen fumarate (p.788·1).
*Allergic conjunctivitis; allergic rhinitis; asthma.*

**Ketava** Atlantic, Malaysia.
Ketamine hydrochloride (p.1302·1).
*General anaesthesia.*

**Ketazol**
Aspen, S.Afr.; Shiwa, Thai.
Ketoconazole (p.403·3).
*Fungal infections.*

**Ketazon**
Note. This name is used for preparations of different composition.
Bristol-Myers Squibb, Arg.
Piroxicam (p.84·2).
*Gout; musculoskeletal and joint disorders; pain.*

Gerot, Austria; Medphano, Ger.†.
Kebuzone (p.51·1) or kebuzone sodium (p.51·1).
Trimecaine (p.1385·3) is included in the injection to alleviate the pain of injection.
*Gout; inflammation; musculoskeletal and joint disorders; neuralgia; neuritis; pain; thrombophlebitis.*

Siam Bheasach, Thai.
Ketoconazole (p.403·3).
*Fungal infections.*

**Ketazon Flex** Bristol-Myers Squibb, Arg.
Piroxicam (p.84·2); carisoprodol (p.1392·1).
*Musculoskeletal and joint disorders with muscle spasm.*

**Ketek**
Aventis, Arg.; Aventis, Belg.; Aventis, Braz.; Aventis, Chile; Aventis, Fr.; Aventis, Ger.; Aventis, Irl.; Lepetit, Ital.; Aventis, Norw.; Aventis, Spain; Aventis, Swed.; Aventis, UK; Aventis, USA.
Telithromycin (p.265·2).
*Bacterial infections of the respiratory tract.*

**Keten** Siam Bheasach, Thai.
Ketotifen (p.788·2).
*Asthma; hypersensitivity reactions.*

**Ketensin** Pharmacia, Neth.
Ketanserin tartrate (p.943·1).
*Hypertension.*

**Ketesse**
Lusofarmaco, Ital.; Menarini, Port.; Tecefarma, Spain; Menarini, Switz.
Dexketoprofen trometamol (p.51·2).
*Pain.*

**Ketidin** Montpellier, Arg.
Raloxifene hydrochloride (p.1568·3).
*Osteoporosis.*

**Ketifen**
Biolab, Hong Kong; Biopharm, Hong Kong; Biolab, Malaysia; Biolab, Thai.
Ketotifen fumarate (p.788·1).
*Asthma; bronchitis; hypersensitivity reactions.*

**Ketil** Tillomed, UK.
Ketoprofen (p.51·2).
*Dysmenorrhoea; musculoskeletal, joint, and peri-articular disorders.*

**Ketina** Piso, Mex.†.
Ketamine (p.1303·1).

**Ketlur** Milmet, India.
Ketorolac trometamol (p.52·1).
*Allergic conjunctivitis.*

**Ketmin** Themis Chemicals, India.
Ketamine hydrochloride (p.1302·1).
*General anaesthesia.*

**Keto**
Note. This name is used for preparations of different composition.
Vitabalans, Fin.
Ketoprofen (p.51·2).
*Fever; gout; inflammation; musculoskeletal and joint disorders; pain.*

YSP, Malaysia; Yung Shin, Singapore.
Ketorolac trometamol (p.52·1).
*Pain.*

Masa, Thai.
Ketotifen fumarate (p.788·1).
*Asthma; hypersensitivity reactions.*

**Ketocev** Cevallos, Arg.
Ketotifen (p.788·2).

**Ketocid** Trinity, UK.
Ketoprofen (p.51·2).
*Gout; musculoskeletal, joint, and peri-articular disorders; pain.*

**Ketocine** Progress, Thai.
Ketoconazole (p.403·3).
*Fungal infections.*

**Ketocon** Cibran, Braz.†.
Ketoconazole (p.403·3).
*Fungal infections.*

**Ketoderm** Janssen-Cilag, Fr.
Ketoconazole (p.403·3).
*Fungal skin infections.*

**Keto-Diabur Test** Roche Diagnostics, Irl.
Test for glucose and ketones in urine.

**Keto-Diabur Test 5000**
Roche, Arg.; Roche Diagnostics, Austral.; Roche Diagnostics, Fr.; Roche, Mex.; Roche Diagnostics, NZ; Roche Diagnostics, UK.
Test for glucose and ketones in urine.

**Ketodiaburtest 5000**
Roche, Chile; Roche Diagnostics, Ital.
Test for glucose and ketones in urine.

**Keto-Diastix**
Bayer, Arg.; Bayer, Austral.; Bayer, Canad.; Bayer Diagnostics, Fr.; Bayer Diagnostics, Irl.; Bayer Diagnostici, Ital.; Bayer Diagnostics, Mex.; Bayer, NZ; Bayer, Port.; Bayer Diagnostics, UK; Bayer, USA.
Test for glucose and ketones in urine.

**Ketodol** Wassermann, Ital.
Ketoprofen (p.51·2).
Sucralfate (p.1290·2) is included in this preparation in an attempt to limit adverse effects on the gastrointestinal mucosa.
*Pain.*

**Ketodur**
Pharmacia, Denm.; Pharmacia, Norw.; Pharmacia, Swed.
Ketobemidone hydrochloride (p.51·1).
*Pain.*

**Ketof** Hexal, Ger.
Ketotifen fumarate (p.788·1).
*Hypersensitivity reactions.*

**Ketofar** Farcoral, Mex.
Ketoconazole (p.403·3).
*Fungal infections.*

**Ketofen**
Note. This name is used for preparations of different composition.
Pharmacia Upjohn, Fin.†.
Ketoprofen (p.51·2).
*Fever; gout; inflammation; musculoskeletal and joint disorders; pain.*

Del Saz & Filippini, Ital.†.
Ketoprofen lysine (p.51·3).
*Musculoskeletal and joint pain.*

Asian Pharm, Thai.
Ketotifen fumarate (p.788·1).
*Asthma; hypersensitivity reactions.*

**Ketofene** Alter, Port.
Ketoprofen (p.51·2).

**Ketoflam** Parke-Med, S.Afr.
Ketoprofen (p.51·2).
*Gout; musculoskeletal, joint, and peri-articular disorders; pain.*

**Ketoftil** Farmigea, Ital.
Ketotifen fumarate (p.788·1).
*Allergic conjunctivitis.*

**Ketogan**
Pharmacia, Denm.; Pharmacia, Norw.; Pharmacia, Swed.
Ketobemidone hydrochloride (p.51·1); N,N-dimethyl-4,4-diphenyl-3-buten-2-amine hydrochloride.
*Pain.*

**Ketogan Novum** Pharmacia, Swed.
Ketobemidone hydrochloride (p.51·1).
*Adjunct in regional anaesthesia; pain.*

**Ketogel** Stiefel, Arg.
Ketoconazole (p.403·3).
*Dandruff; seborrhoeic dermatitis.*

**Ketohair** Euroderm, Arg.
Ketoconazole (p.403·3); collagen; coconut oil.
*Dandruff.*

**Ketohexal** Hexal, S.Afr.
Ketotifen fumarate (p.788·1).
*Allergic rhinitis; allergic skin disorders; asthma.*

**Ketoisdin** Isdin, Spain.
Ketoconazole (p.403·3).
*Fungal infections.*

**Ketokid** Hexal, Arg.
Ketotifen fumarate (p.788·1).
*Allergic rhinitis; allergic skin disorders; asthma; bronchospasm.*

**Ketolan** Olan-Kemed, Thai.
Ketoconazole (p.403·3).
*Fungal skin and scalp infections.*

**Ketolar** Pfizer, Spain.
Ketamine hydrochloride (p.1302·1).
*General anaesthesia.*

**Ketolist** Thiemann, Ger.
Ketoprofen (p.51·2).
*Gout; musculoskeletal, joint, and soft-tissue disorders.*

**Ketomed** Medifive, Thai.
Ketoconazole (p.403·3).
*Fungal infections.*

**Ketomex** Ratiopharm, Fin.
Ketoprofen (p.51·2).
*Fever; gout; inflammation; musculoskeletal and joint disorders; pain.*

**Ketomicol** Luper, Braz.
Ketoconazole (p.403·3).
*Fungal infections; seborrheoic dermatitis.*

**Ketomizol** Reuffer, Mex.†.
Ketoconazole (p.403·3).
*Fungal infections.*

**Ketonal** Agis, Israel.
Ketoprofen (p.51·2).
*Musculoskeletal and joint disorders; pain.*

**Ketonan** Marjan, Braz.
Ketoconazole (p.403·3).
*Fungal infections.*

**Ketonazol**
Lafedar, Arg.; Bunker, Braz.
Ketoconazole (p.403·3).
*Fungal infections; seborrheoic dermatitis.*

**Ketonazole** Polipharm, Thai.
Ketoconazole (p.403·3).
*Fungal infections.*

**Ketone** Wayne, Mex.†.
Ketoconazole (p.403·3).
*Fungal infections.*

**Ketonex**
Abbott, Austral.; Ross, USA.
A range of isoleucine-, leucine-, and valine-free preparations for enteral nutrition (p.1417·1).
*Beta-ketothiolase deficiency; maple syrup urine disease.*

**Ketonic** Nicholas Piramal, India.
Ketorolac trometamol (p.52·1).
*Pain.*

**Ketonil** Grunenthal, Chile.
Ketoconazole (p.403·3).
*Fungal infections; seborrheoic dermatitis.*

**Ketop** Biobras, Braz.
Ketoprofen (p.51·2).

**Ketopharm** ICN, Arg.
Ketorolac trometamol (p.52·1).
*Allergic conjunctivitis; postoperative eye inflammation.*

**Ketoplus** Pantafarm, Ital.
Ketoprofen (p.51·2).
*Gout; inflammation; musculoskeletal, joint, peri-articular, and soft-tissue disorders; pain; phlebitis.*

**Ketoral** Community Pharmacy, Thai.
Ketoconazole (p.403·3).
*Fungal infections.*

**Ketorax** Pharmacia, Norw.
Ketobemidone hydrochloride (p.51·1).
*Pain.*

**Ketorin** Orion, Fin.
Ketoprofen (p.51·2).
*Fever; gout; inflammation; musculoskeletal and joint disorders; pain.*

**Ketoselect** Menarini, Ital.
Ketoprofen (p.51·2).
*Gout; musculoskeletal, joint, and peri-articular disorders; thrombophlebitis.*

**Ketosil** Silom, Thai.
Ketoconazole (p.403·3).
*Fungal infections.*

**Ketosolan** Spyfarma, Spain.
Ketoprofen (p.51·2).
*Gout; musculoskeletal, joint, and peri-articular disorders; pain.*

**Ketoson** CCS, Swed.
Ketoconazole (p.403·3).
*Seborrhoeic dermatitis.*

**Ketosteril**
Fresenius Kabi, Austria; Fresenius Kabi, Fr.†; Fresenius Kabi, Ger.; Fresenius Kabi, Hong Kong; Fresenius Kabi, Malaysia; Fresenius Kabi, Mex.; Fresenius Kabi, Port.; Fresenius Kabi, Singapore; Fresenius Kabi, Switz.; Fresenius Kabi, Thai.
Amino-acid preparation (p.1417·1).
*Nutritional supplement in renal failure.*

**Ketostix**
Bayer, Austral.; Bayer, Canad.; Bayer Diagnostics, Irl.; Bayer Diagnostici, Ital.; Bayer, NZ; Bayer Diagnostics, UK; Bayer, USA.
Test for ketones in urine, plasma, and serum.

**Ketotab** Nakorn, Thai.†.
Ketotifen fumarate (p.788·1).
*Asthma; hypersensitivity reactions.*

**Ketotard** Galen, UK†.
Ketoprofen (p.51·2).
*Dysmenorrhoea; gout; musculoskeletal, joint, and peri-articular pain; sciatica.*

**Ketotisin** Chemopharma, Chile.
Ketotifen (p.788·2).
*Hypersensitivity reactions.*

**Ketotop** Pacific, Singapore.
Ketoprofen (p.51·2).
*Musculoskeletal, joint, peri-articular, and soft-tissue disorders.*

**Ketovail** Approved Prescription Services, UK.
Ketoprofen (p.51·2).
*Inflammation; musculoskeletal and joint disorders; pain.*

**Ketovite**
Paines & Byrne, Irl.
*Oral liquid:* Vitamin A, choline chloride, vitamin D, and cyanocobalamin (p.1417·1).
*Dietary supplement.*

Paines & Byrne, Irl.; Paines & Byrne, NZ; Paines & Byrne, UK.
Multivitamin preparation (p.1417·1).

**Ketozal** Pond's, Thai.
Ketoconazole (p.403·3).
*Fungal infections.*

**Ketozip** Ashbourne, UK.
Ketoprofen (p.51·2).
*Dysmenorrhoea; gout; musculoskeletal, joint, and peri-articular disorders; sciatica.*

**Ketozol**
Galderma, Arg.; Mepha, Switz.
Ketoconazole (p.403·3).
*Fungal infections.*

**Ketozole** DHA, Singapore.
Ketoconazole (p.403·3).
*Fungal infections.*

**Ketrax**
AstraZeneca, Irl.; IDIS, UK.
Levamisole hydrochloride (p.107·2).
*Worm infections.*

**Ketrel**
Biorga, Fr.; Saninter, Port.
Tretinoin (p.1161·1).
*Acne; keratinisation disorders.*

**Ketrizin** Esseti, Ital.
Propylene glycol cefatrizine (p.170·3).
*Bacterial infections.*

**Ketum** Menarini, Fr.
Ketoprofen (p.51·2).
*Musculoskeletal, joint, and soft-tissue disorders.*

**Ketur-Test**
Roche Diagnostics, Irl.; Roche Diagnostics, Ital.; Roche Diagnostics, NZ; Roche Diagnostics, UK.
Test for ketones in urine.

**Keval** Pharmacos Abug, Mex.
Lansoprazole (p.1269·3).
*Acid aspiration; gastro-oesophageal reflux; peptic ulcer; Zollinger-Ellison syndrome.*

**Kevatril** Roche, Ger.
Granisetron hydrochloride (p.1267·1).
*Nausea and vomiting associated with cytotoxic chemotherapy or radiotherapy.*

**Kevis** Pfizer Consumer, Ital.
Pyrithione magnesium (p.1156·2); iceland moss.
*Seborrhoeic dermatitis.*

**Kevopril** Rhone-Poulenc Rorer, Austria†.
Quinupramine (p.316·3).
*Depression.*

**Kexelate** Adcock Ingram, S.Afr.
Sodium polystyrene sulfonate (p.1053·1).
*Hyperkalaemia.*

**Kexidil** Kener, Mex.†.
Trihexyphenidyl hydrochloride (p.490·2).

**K-Exit** Omega, Canad.
Sodium polystyrene sulfonate (p.1053·1).
*Hyperkalemia.*

**Keyerpril** Keyerson, Mex.
Captopril (p.879·2).
*Hypertension.*

**Keylyte** Wallace, India.
Potassium chloride (p.1232·2).
*Hypokalaemia.*

**Key-Plex** *Hyrex, USA.*
Vitamin B substances and vitamin C (p.1417·1).
*Parenteral nutrition.*

**Key-Pred** *Hyrex, USA.*
Prednisolone acetate (p.1108·1).
*Corticosteroid.*

**Key-Pred-SP** *Hyrex, USA.*
Prednisolone sodium phosphate (p.1108·1).
*Corticosteroid.*

**Kezepin** *Wayne, Mex.†.*
Carbamazepine (p.353·3).

**Kezer** *Zerboni, Mex.†.*
Ketoprofen (p.51·2).

**Kezon** *Osoth, Thai.*
Ketoconazole (p.403·3).
*Fungal skin infections.*

**Kezoral** *Upha, Malaysia.*
Ketoconazole (p.403·3).
*Fungal infections.*

**K-Flebo** *Nuovo ISM, Ital.*
Potassium aspartate (p.1233·1).
*Hyperammonaemia; hypokalaemia.*

**K-Fosfosteril** *Orion, Fin.*
Dibasic potassium phosphate (p.1230·3).
*Potassium deficiency.*

**K-G Elixir** *Geneva, USA.*
Potassium gluconate (p.1232·2).
*Hypokalaemia; potassium depletion.*

**KGS-PE** *Cypress, USA.*
Phenylephrine hydrochloride (p.1126·3); sulfogaiacol (p.1131·1).
*Coughs; upper respiratory-tract congestion.*

**KH3**
*Note. This name is used for preparations of different composition.*
*Raffo, Arg.*
Procaine; ginseng; alfa tocoferol (p.1417·1).
*Tonic.*
*Schwarzhaupt, Austria; Schwarzhaupt, Hong Kong; Neo-Farmaceutica, Port.†; Torbet Laboratories, UK†.*
Procaine hydrochloride (p.1383·2); haematoporphyrin (p.1696·2).
*Tonic.*
*Deutsche, Chile.*
Procaine (p.1383·2); haematoporphyrin (p.1696·2).
*Tonic.*
*Schwarzhaupt, Ger.; Bamford, NZ; Schwarzhaupt, Thai.*
Procaine hydrochloride (p.1383·2); haematoporphyrin (p.1696·2); magnesium carbonate; magnesium phosphate; potassium chloride; sodium phosphate (p.1417·1).
*Tonic.*

**KH3 Powel** *Kenfarma, Spain†.*
Procaine hydrochloride (p.1383·2); haematoporphyrin (p.1696·2).
*Tonic.*

**Khellangan N** *Ardeypharm, Ger.*
Ammi visnaga fruit (p.1653·3).
*Cardiac disorders; obstructive airways disease.*

**KH3-Vit** *Deutsche, Chile.*
Procaine hydrochloride (p.1383·2); haematoporphyrin (p.1696·2); vitamins.
*Tonic.*

**Kiadon**
*Merck, Braz.; Merck, Chile.*
Ginkgo biloba (p.1692·3).
*Cerebral and peripheral vascular disorders; ear disorders; eye disorders; vestibular disorders.*

**Kiatrium** *Gross, Braz.*
Diazepam (p.690·1).
*Alcohol withdrawal syndrome; anxiety; epilepsy; insomnia; premedication; sedative; skeletal muscle spasm.*

**Kid Kare Childrens Cough/Cold** *Rugby, USA.*
Chlorphenamine maleate (p.427·3); dextromethorphan hydrobromide (p.1117·3); pseudoephedrine hydrochloride (p.1129·2).
*Coughs and cold symptoms.*

**Kid Kare Pediatric Nasal Decongestant** *Rugby, USA.*
Pseudoephedrine hydrochloride (p.1129·2).
*Nasal congestion.*

**Kidbar** *Piam, Ital.*
Food for special diets (p.1417·1).
*Phenylketonuria.*

**Kiddi**
*Boehringer Ingelheim, Arg.; Pharmaton, Israel; Pharmaton, S.Afr.*
Lysine hydrochloride; vitamins; minerals (p.1417·1).
*Nutritional supplement.*
*Pharmaton, Switz.*
Multivitamin and mineral preparation (p.1417·1).
Formerly known as Kiddi Nouvelle formule.

**Kiddi Choo** *Boehringer Ingelheim, S.Afr.*
Multivitamin and mineral preparation (p.1417·1).

**Kiddi Pharmaton**
*Boehringer Ingelheim, Hong Kong; Boehringer Ingelheim, Irl.; Pharmaton, Malaysia; Boehringer Ingelheim Promeco, Mex.; Pharmaton, Singapore; Pharmaton, Thai.*
Multivitamin and mineral preparation with lysine (p.1417·1).
*Tonic.*

**Kiddicrom** *Boehringer Ingelheim, S.Afr.†.*
Sodium cromoglicate (p.795·3).
*Asthma.*

**Kiddie Vite** *Covan, S.Afr.*
Ferrous gluconate (p.1428·1); vitamin $B_1$ (p.1455·2).
*Iron-deficiency anaemia.*

**Kiddiekof** *Covan, S.Afr.†.*
Codeine phosphate (p.27·1); mepyramine maleate (p.437·1); ephedrine hydrochloride (p.1120·1).
*Coughs.*

**Kiddyflu** *Caps, S.Afr.*
Paracetamol (p.76·2); dextromethorphan hydrobromide (p.1117·3); phenylephrine hydrochloride (p.1126·3); chlorphenamine maleate (p.427·3).
*Cold and influenza symptoms.*

**Kid-Eeze** *Pharmachoice, S.Afr.*
Paracetamol (p.76·2); codeine phosphate (p.27·1); promethazine hydrochloride (p.439·1).
*Fever; pain.*

**Kidmin**
*Otsuka, Jpn; Thai Otsuka, Thai.*
Amino-acid infusion (p.1417·1).
*Parenteral nutrition in renal failure.*

**Kidrolase**
*Aventis, Arg.; Aventis, Canad.; Aventis, Fr.; Aventis, Israel.*
Asparaginase (p.528·3).
*Malignant neoplasms.*

**Kid's Bumps** *Homeocan, Canad.*
Homoeopathic preparation.

**Kid's Colic** *Homeocan, Canad.*
Homoeopathic preparation.

**Kids' Earache** *Homeocan, Canad.*
Homoeopathic preparation.

**Kids Sunblock** *Tanning Research, Canad.*
*SPF 30:* Homosalate (p.1148·1); octinoxate (p.1154·3); octisalate (p.1154·3); oxybenzone (p.1154·3).
*Sunscreen.*

**Kids' Teething** *Homeocan, Canad.*
Homoeopathic preparation.

**KIE** *Laser, USA.*
Ephedrine hydrochloride (p.1120·1); potassium iodide (p.1598·1).
*Coughs.*

**KI-Expectorante** *Cimed, Braz.*
Oxomemazine hydrochloride (p.438·2); potassium iodide (p.1598·1); guaifenesin (p.1122·1); sodium benzoate (p.1169·3); ipecacuanha (p.1122·3).
*Respiratory-tract congestion.*

**Kikelaio EF 3** *Norma (Νορμα), Gr.*
Castor oil (p.1668·2).
*Bowel evacuation.*

**Kilios**
*Note. This name is used for preparations of different composition.*
*Pharmacia, Chile.*
18 Tablets, estradiol (p.1550·1); 13 tablets, medroxyprogesterone acetate (p.1557·2).
*Menopausal disorders; osteoporosis.*
*Pharmacia Upjohn, Ital.*
Aspirin (p.15·1).
*Fever; pain.*

**Kilkof** *Bell, UK.*
Cetylpyridinium chloride (p.1173·1); benzoin tincture (p.1751·1); ipecacuanha tincture (p.1122·3); capsicum tincture (p.1667·1).
*Cold symptoms; coughs; sore throat.*

**Killgrip** *Sedabel, Braz.*
Dipyrone (p.35·3); sodium camsilate; guaifenesin (p.1122·1); cineole (p.1672·1); niaouli oil (p.1719·3); lidocaine hydrochloride (p.1377·3); ascorbic acid (p.1460·2); mepyramine maleate (p.437·1).
*Cold and influenza symptoms.*

**Killit** *Biosintetica, Braz.*
Fluorouracil (p.554·2).
*Malignant neoplasms.*

**Killpan** *Labitec, Spain†.*
Camphor (p.1665·3); arnica (p.1656·3); capsicum (p.1667·1); aesculus (p.1648·2); scrophularia aquatica; menthol (p.1711·3); rosemary (p.1740·2); turpentine oil (p.1760·1).
*Rheumatic and muscle pain.*

**Kilmicen** *Pharmacia Upjohn, Mex.†.*
Tolciclate (p.410·1).
*Fungal skin infections.*

**Kilnits** *Andromaco, Chile.*
Permethrin (p.1508·3).
*Pediculosis.*

**Kilor** *Guidotti, Spain.*
Ferritin (p.1427·2).
*Iron-deficiency anaemia.*

**Kilovit** *Italmex, Mex.*
Vitamin and mineral preparation (p.1417·1).

**Kilpane** *GlaxoSmithKline, India.*
Eucalyptus oil (p.1686·2); methyl salicylate (p.59·3); menthol (p.1711·3).
*Musculoskeletal disorders.*

**Kimafan** *Duopharma, Hong Kong.*
Captopril (p.879·2).
*Diabetic nephropathy; heart failure; hypertension; myocardial infarction.*

**Kiminto** *Rhone-Poulenc Rorer, UK†.*
Peppermint oil (p.1283·2).

**Kin** *Andromaco, Chile.*
Ibuprofen (p.45·3).
*Inflammation; pain.*

**Kin Soff** *Kanion, Israel.*
Pyrethrum (p.1509·3); piperonyl butoxide (p.1509·2).
*Pediculosis.*

**Kinabide** *Bago, Arg.*
Selegiline hydrochloride (p.1214·1).
*Parkinsonism.*

**Kinasten** *Kinder, Braz.*
Clotrimazole (p.396·2).
*Fungal infections.*

**Kincare** *Moraz, UK†.*
Parsley (p.1728·3); garlic (p.1691·1).
*Pediculosis.*

**Kinciclina** *Kin, Spain†.*
Tetracycline megallate (p.268·1).
*Bacterial infections.*

**Kindaren** *Kinder, Braz.*
Diclofenac sodium (p.32·1).

**Kindcalcio** *Kinder, Braz.*
Calcium phosphate; cyanocobalamin; ergocalciferol; sodium fluoride (p.1417·1).

**Kindcetin** *Kinder, Braz.*
Neomycin sulfate (p.235·1); bacitracin zinc (p.161·3).

**Kindelmin** *Kinder, Braz.*
Mebendazole (p.108·2).
*Worm infections.*

**Kinder Em-eukal Hustensaft** *Soldan, Ger.*
Thyme (p.1755·2); primula root (p.1735·1).
*Catarrh; respiratory-tract congestion.*

**Kinder Erkaltungsbalsam**
*Note. This name is used for preparations of different composition.*
*Genericon, Austria.*
Menthol (p.1711·3); camphor (p.1665·3); eucalyptus oil (p.1686·2).
*Catarrh; cold symptoms.*
*Ratiopharm, Austria.*
Camphor (p.1665·3); turpentine oil (p.1760·1); eucalyptus oil (p.1686·2).
*Cold symptoms.*

**Kinder Finimal** *Roche Consumer, Neth.*
Paracetamol (p.76·2).
*Fever; pain.*

**Kinder Luuf** *Apomedica, Austria.*
Camphor (p.1665·3); menthol (p.1711·3); eucalyptus oil (p.1686·2); turpentine oil (p.1760·1); thymol (p.1194·2).
*Catarrh; coughs and cold symptoms.*

**Kindercal** *Mead Johnson Nutritionals, USA.*
Preparation for enteral nutrition (p.1417·1).

**Kindergen**
*Scientific Hospital Supplies, Austral.; Scientific Hospital Supplies, Irl.†; Nutricia, NZ; Scientific Hospital Supplies, NZ; Scientific Hospital Supplies, UK.*
Preparation for enteral nutrition (p.1417·1).
*Renal failure.*

**Kinderval** *Bago, Arg.*
Permethrin (p.1508·3).
*Pediculosis.*

**Kindomet** *Kinder, Braz.*
Methyldopa (p.953·2).
*Hypertension.*

**Kindpasm** *Kinder, Braz.*
Dipyrone (p.35·3); hyoscine butylbromide (p.483·3).
*Pain; skeletal muscle spasm.*

**Kinedak** *Ono, Jpn.*
Epalrestat (p.331·1).
*Diabetic neuropathy.*

**Kinerase**
*ICN, Arg.; ICN, Hong Kong; ICN, Malaysia; ICN, Mex.; ICN, Singapore; ICN, USA.*
$N^6$-furfuryladenine.
*Photodamaged skin; skin hyperpigmentation.*

**Kineret**
*Amgen, Fr.; Amgen, Irl.; Amgen, Port.; Amgen, UK; Amgen, USA.*
Anakinra (p.14·3).
*Rheumatoid arthritis.*

**Kinestase** *Liomont, Mex.*
Cisapride (p.1259·2).
*Dyspepsia; gastro-oesophageal reflux; gastroparesis; impaired gastric motility.*

**Kinet** *Solvay, Spain†.*
Cisapride (p.1259·2).
*Gastro-oesophageal reflux; gastroparesis.*

**Kinetizine** *Cetus, Arg.*
Cisapride (p.1259·2).

**Kineto** *Systopic, India.*
Serrapeptase (p.1743·2).
*Inflammation; pain.*

**Kinetone** *Knoll, India.*
Multivitamin and mineral preparation (p.1417·1).

**Kinevac**
*Bracco, Canad.; Bracco, USA.*
Sincalide (p.1746·2).
*Diagnosis of biliary-tract and pancreatic disorders.*

**Kinex** *Psicofarma, Mex.*
Biperiden hydrochloride (p.479·3).
*Extrapyramidal disorders; parkinsonism.*

**Kinfil** *Bristol-Myers Squibb, Arg.*
Enalapril (p.909·2).
*Heart failure; hypertension.*

**Kinidin**
*AstraZeneca, Austral.; Durascan, Denm.; AstraZeneca, Fin.†; AstraZeneca, Hong Kong; AstraZeneca, Irl.; Astra, Norw.†; AstraZeneca, NZ†; Hassle, Swed.; AstraZeneca, Switz.; AstraZeneca, Thai.†; AstraZeneca, UK.*
Quinidine bisulfate (p.991·3).
*Arrhythmias.*
*Nycomed, Denm.†.*
Quinidine sulfate (p.991·3).
*Arrhythmias.*

**Kinidin durules** *IFET (ΙΦΕΤ), Gr.*
Quinidine (p.991·3).
*Arrythmias.*

**Kinidine**
*AstraZeneca, Belg.; AstraZeneca, Neth.*
Quinidine bisulfate (p.991·3).
*Arrhythmias.*

**Kiniduron** *Orion, Fin.*
Quinidine bisulfate (p.991·3).
*Arrhythmias.*

**Kinin**
*Nycomed, Denm.; NM, Swed.*
Quinine hydrochloride (p.460·2).
*Malaria; myotonia.*

**Kinline** *Siam Bheasach, Thai.*
Selegiline hydrochloride (p.1214·1).
*Parkinsonism.*

**Kinogen** *Geymonat, Ital.*
Tyrothricin (p.275·1); hydrocortisone sodium succinate (p.1104·1).
*Vulvovaginal infections.*

**Kinolymphat** *PGM, Ger.*
Homoeopathic preparation.

**Kinot** *Farex, Canad.†.*
Camphor (p.1665·3); expressed mustard oil (p.1718·2).

**Kinson** *Alphapharm, Austral.*
Levodopa (p.1205·2); carbidopa (p.1204·3).
*Parkinsonism.*

**Kintavit** *Synthelabo, Switz.*
Multivitamin and mineral preparation with ginseng (p.1417·1).

**Kinupril** *Rhone-Poulenc Rorer, Fr.†.*
Quinupramine (p.316·3).
*Depression.*

**Kinurea H** *Fuca, Fr.*
Quinine and urea hydrochloride (p.1737·2).
*Anorectal disorders.*

**Kionex** *Paddock, USA.*
Sodium polystyrene sulfonate (p.1053·1).
*Hyperkalaemia.*

**Kiper** *Monserrat, Arg.*
Paracetamol (p.76·2); butetamate citrate (p.1116·2); phenylephrine hydrochloride (p.1126·3); caffeine (p.782·1).
*Cold and influenza symptoms.*

**Kipress** *Kyorin, Jpn.*
Montelukast sodium (p.788·3).
*Asthma.*

**Kir Richter** *Lepetit, Ital.†.*
Aprotinin (p.742·3).
*Antidote to thrombolytics; haemorrhage; shock.*

**Kira**
*Kwizda, Austria; Lichtwer, Canad.; Riemser, Ger.; Lichtwer, UK.*
Hypericum (p.299·1).
*Depression; nervous disorders.*

**Kiri** *Lampugnani, Ital.*
Lactic-acid-producing organisms (p.1704·2); vitamin B substances (p.1417·1).
*Disturbances of the gastrointestinal flora.*

**kirim** *Hormosan, Ger.*
Bromocriptine mesilate (p.1200·3).
*Parkinsonism.*

**kirim gyn** *Taurus, Ger.*
Bromocriptine mesilate (p.1200·3).
*Hyperprolactinaemia; lactation inhibition.*

**Kirin**
*Medochemie, Hong Kong; Medochemie, Malaysia.*
Spectinomycin hydrochloride (p.255·2).
*Gonorrhoea.*

**Kiro Rub** *Prodemdis, Canad.*
Methyl salicylate (p.59·3); camphor (p.1665·3); menthol (p.1711·3); eucalyptus oil (p.1686·2).

**Kirsan** *Ativus, Braz.*
Ginkgo biloba (p.1692·3).
*Cerebral and peripheral vascular disorders.*

**Kisolv** *Ecupharma, Ital.*
Urokinase (p.1018·2).
*Thromboembolic disorders.*

**Kitacne** *Fortbenton, Arg.*
Erythromycin (p.208·1).
*Acne.*

**Kitacne AR** *Fortbenton, Arg.*
Erythromycin (p.208·1); tretinoin (p.1161·1).
*Acne.*

**Kitacne PB** *Fortbenton, Arg.*
Erythromycin (p.208·1); benzoyl peroxide (p.1143·2).
*Acne.*

**Kitadol** *Laboratorios Chile, Chile.*
Paracetamol (p.76·2).
*Fever; pain.*

**Kitadol Flu** *Laboratorios Chile, Chile.*
Paracetamol (p.76·2); caffeine (p.782·1); noscapine hydrochloride (p.1125·3); sodium ascorbate (p.1460·2).
*Cold and influenza symptoms.*

**Kitadol Flu Noche** *Laboratorios Chile, Chile.*
Paracetamol (p.76·2); caffeine (p.782·1); noscapine hydrochloride (p.1125·3); sodium ascorbate (p.1460·2); chlorphenamine maleate (p.427·3).
*Allergic rhinitis; cold and influenza symptoms.*

**Kitadol Max** *Laboratorios Chile, Chile.*
Paracetamol (p.76·2); caffeine (p.782·1).
*Fever; pain.*

**Kitadol Periodo Menstrual** *Laboratorios Chile, Chile.*
Paracetamol (p.76·2); pamabrom (p.978·2); mepyramine (p.437·1).
*Menstrual disorders.*

**Kitapen** *Dansk-Flama, Braz.†.*
Benzathine benzylpenicillin (p.162·3); bacterial antigens.
*Bacterial infections.*

**Kitnos**
*Pharmacia, Braz.; Pharmacia Upjohn, Mex.*
Etofamide (p.605·2).
*Amoebiasis.*

**Kiton** *Pulitzer, Ital.*
Isosorbide mononitrate (p.942·1).
*Angina pectoris; cardiac stenosis; heart failure; myocardial infarction.*

**Kit-Syrup** *Continental Pharma, Thai.*
Paracetamol (p.76·2).
*Fever; pain.*

**kivat** *Hormosan, Ger.*
Fluspirilene (p.701·1).
*Anxiety disorders.*

**Klacid**
*Abbott, Austral.; Abbott, Austria; Abbott, Denm.; Abbott, Fin.; Abbott, Ger.; Abbott, Hong Kong; Abbott, Irl.; Abbott, Israel; Abbott, Ital.; Abbott, Malaysia; Abbott, Neth.; Abbott, Norw.; Abbott, NZ; Abbott, Port.; Abbott, S.Afr.; Abbott, Singapore; Abbott, Spain; Abbott, Swed.; Abbott, Switz.; Abbott, Thai.*
Clarithromycin (p.192·2) or clarithromycin lactobionate (p.193·2).
*Bacterial infections.*

**Klacid HP 7**
*Note. This name is used for preparations of different composition.*
*Abbott, Austral.*
Capsules, omeprazole (Losec) (p.1278·2); capsules, amoxicillin trihydrate (Amoxil) (p.155·3); tablets, clarithromycin (Klacid) (p.192·2).
*Helicobacter pylori-associated peptic ulcer.*

*Abbott, Malaysia; Biochemie, Malaysia; Altana, Malaysia.*
Tablets, pantoprazole (Controloc) (p.1283·1); tablets, amoxicillin (Ospamox) (p.155·3); tablets, clarithromycin (Klacid) (p.192·2).
*Helicobacter pylori-associated peptic ulcer.*

*Abbott, NZ.*
Tablets, clarithromycin (p.192·2); capsules, amoxicillin trihydrate (p.155·3); capsules, omeprazole (p.1278·2).
*Helicobacter pylori-associated peptic ulcer.*

**Klaciped** *Abbott, Switz.*
Clarithromycin (p.192·2).
*Bacterial infections.*

**Klafotaxim** *Be-Tabs, S.Afr.*
Cefotaxime sodium (p.175·3).
*Bacterial infections.*

**Klamacin** *Hua, Thai.*
Clotrimazole (p.396·2).
*Trichomoniasis.*

**Klaricid**
*Abbott, Arg.; Abbott, Braz.; Abbott, Chile; Abbott, Gr.; Abbott, Mex.; Abbott, UK.*
Clarithromycin (p.192·2) or clarithromycin lactobionate (p.193·2).
*Bacterial infections.*

**Klariderm** *Clariana, Spain.*
Fluocinonide (p.1101·3).
*Skin disorders.*

**Klaridex** *Dexcel, Israel.*
Clarithromycin (p.192·2).
*Bacterial infections.*

**Klarivitina** *Clariana, Spain.*
Cyproheptadine hydrochloride (p.430·1).
*Allergic rhinitis; reduced appetite; urticaria.*

**Klaron**
*Dermik, Israel; Dermik, USA.*
Sulfacetamide sodium (p.257·3).
*Acne.*

**Klaryl** *Labocean, Fr.*
Sambucus; black currant; cynara; spiraea ulmaria; bladderwrack (p.1417·1).
*Tonic.*

**KLB6** *Nature's Bounty, USA.*
Pyridoxine hydrochloride (p.1456·3); soya lecithin (p.1706·1); kelp (p.1742·3); cider vinegar.

**KLB6 Fruit Diet** *Natural Life, Arg.*
Kelp (p.1742·3); lecithin (p.1706·1); vitamin $B_6$ (p.1457·2); glucomannan (p.1693·3); grapefruit; bearberry (p.1659·2); cider vinegar; phenylalanine (p.1443·1).
*Obesity.*

**Klean-Prep**
*Norgine, Austria; Norgine, Belg.; Rivex, Canad.; Norgine, Denm.; Sabora, Fin.; Norgine, Fr.; Norgine, Ger.; Kite (Κιτε), Gr.; Norgine, Hong Kong; Helsinn Birex, Irl.; Norgine, Ital.; Norgine, Neth.; Norgine, Norw.; Norgine, NZ; Zuellig, NZ; Helsinn, Port.; Norgine, S.Afr.; Norgine, Singapore; UCB, Spain; Biolac, Swed.; Norgine, Switz.; Norgine, UK.*
Macrogol 3350 (p.1709·1); electrolytes (p.1217·1).
*Bowel evacuation.*

**K-Lease** *Adria, USA.*
Potassium chloride (p.1232·2).
*Potassium deficiency.*

**Kleen-Handz** *American Medical, USA.*
Alcohol (p.1166·1).
*Hand disinfection.*

**Kleenocid** *Agepha, Austria.*
Chlorhexidine acetate (p.1173·2).
*Skin disinfection.*

**Kleenosept** *Agepha, Austria.*
Hexetidine (p.1182·1).
*Skin disinfection.*

**Kleer** *Modern Health Products, UK†.*
Echinacea (p.1683·2); urtica (p.1762·1); lappa root (p.1704·3).
*Skin disorders.*

**Kleer Cream** *Lane, UK†.*
Hamamelis (p.1696·3); eucalyptus oil (p.1686·2); methyl salicylate (p.59·3); camphor (p.1665·3); ti-tree oil (p.1710·2); zinc oxide (p.1163·2).
Formerly known as Soothene.
*Minor skin disorders.*

**Klenac** *Klonal, Arg.*
Ketorolac (p.52·3).
*Eye disorders.*

**Kleotrat** *Kleva, Gr.*
Cefadroxil (p.167·2).
*Bacterial infections.*

**Klerist-D** *Nutripharm, USA.*
Pseudoephedrine hydrochloride (p.1129·2); chlorphenamine maleate (p.427·3).
*Upper respiratory-tract symptoms.*

**Klestran** *Rayere, Mex.*
Bezafibrate (p.873·2).
*Hyperlipidaemias.*

**Klevasin** *Kleva, Gr.*
Propylene glycol cefatrizine (p.170·3).
*Bacterial infections.*

**Klevistamin** *Kleva, Gr.*
Ketotifen fumarate (p.788·1).
*Allergic rhinitis; asthma.*

**Klexane**
*Aventis, Denm.; Aventis, Fin.; Aventis, Norw.; Aventis, Swed.*
Enoxaparin sodium (p.910·3).
*Thromboembolic disorders.*

**KLGH 3** *Faria, Braz.†.*
Procaine hydrochloride (p.1383·2); magnesium aspartate; potassium aspartate; calcium fluoride; calcium phosphate; ferrous sulfate; zinc oxide; magnesium sulfate; sodium molybdate; adenosine; etofylline; linoleic acid; gamolenic acid; tartaric acid (p.1417·1).
*Tonic.*

**Kliacef** *Fonten, Ital.*
Cefaclor (p.167·1).
*Bacterial infections.*

**Klifem** *Pekana, Ger.*
Homoeopathic preparation.

**Klimadynon**
*Bionorica, Ger.; Bionorica, Hong Kong; Bionorica, Singapore.*
Cimicifuga (p.1671·3).
*Menopausal disorders.*

**Klimaktoplant**
*Peithner, Austria; Omida, Switz.*
Homoeopathic preparation.

**Klimaktoplant H** *DHU, Ger.*
Homoeopathic preparation.

**Klimaktosin** *Meckel, Ger.*
Homoeopathic preparation.

**Klimalet** *Organon, Denm.*
11 Tablets, estradiol valerate (p.1550·2); 10 tablets, estradiol valerate; medroxyprogesterone acetate (p.1557·2).
*Menopausal disorders; osteoporosis.*

**Klimapur** *Kwizda, Austria.*
Estradiol (p.1550·1).
*Menopausal disorders; osteoporosis.*

**Klimareduct** *Solvay, Austria.*
Estradiol (p.1550·1).
*Menopausal disorders; osteoporosis.*

**Klimasyx** *Syxyl, Ger.*
Homoeopathic preparation.

**Klimax-Gastreu S R10** *Reckeweg, Ger.*
Homoeopathic preparation.

**Klimaxil** *Leo, Denm.*
12 Tablets, estradiol (p.1550·1); 10 tablets, estradiol; medroxyprogesterone acetate (p.1557·2).
*Menopausal disorders; osteoporosis.*

**Klimicin** *Lek, Thai.*
Clindamycin hydrochloride (p.194·2) or clindamycin phosphate (p.194·2).
*Bacterial infections.*

**Klimofol** *Ivamed, Ger.†.*
Propofol (p.1305·3).
*General anaesthesia.*

**Klimonorm**
*Jenapharm, Ger.; Jenapharm, Hong Kong; Jenapharm, Malaysia; Jenapharm, Thai.†.*
9 Tablets, estradiol valerate (p.1550·2); 12 tablets, estradiol valerate; levonorgestrel (p.1563·2).
*Menopausal disorders; osteoporosis.*

**Klinna** *Greater Pharma, Thai.*
Clindamycin phosphate (p.194·2).
*Acne.*

**Klinoc** *Wyeth Lederle, Austria.*
Minocycline hydrochloride (p.231·3).
*Bacterial infections.*

**Klinomycin** *Lederle, Ger.*
Minocycline hydrochloride (p.231·3).
*Bacterial infections.*

**Klinotab** *Wyeth Lederle, Belg.*
Minocycline hydrochloride (p.231·3).
*Acne.*

**Klinoxid** *Lederle, Ger.*
Benzoyl peroxide (p.1143·2).
*Acne.*

**Kliofem** *Novo Nordisk, UK.*
Estradiol (p.1550·1); norethisterone acetate (p.1562·2).
*Oestrogen deficiency; postmenopausal osteoporosis.*

**Kliogest**
*Elea, Arg.; Novo Nordisk, Austral.; Novo Nordisk, Austria; Novo Nordisk, Belg.; Medley, Braz.; Silesia, Chile; Novo Nordisk, Denm.; Novo Nordisk, Fin.; Novo Nordisk, Fr.; Novo Nordisk, Gr.; Novo Nordisk, Hong Kong; Novo Nordisk, Irl.; Novo Nordisk, Israel; Novo Nordisk, Ital.; Novo Nordisk, Malaysia; Novo Nordisk, Neth.; Novo Nordisk, Norw.; Novo Nordisk, NZ; Isdin, Port.; Novo Nordisk, S.Afr.; Novo Nordisk, Singapore; Novo Nordisk, Swed.; Novo Nordisk, Thai.†.*
Estradiol (p.1550·1); norethisterone acetate (p.1562·2).
*Menopausal disorders; osteoporosis.*

**Kliogest N**
*Novo Nordisk, Ger.; Novo Nordisk, Switz.*
Estradiol (p.1550·1); norethisterone acetate (p.1562·2).
Formerly contained estradiol, estriol, and norethisterone acetate in *Switz.*
*Menopausal disorders; osteoporosis.*

**Klion** *Gedeon Richter, Thai.†.*
Metronidazole (p.607·2).
*Anaerobic bacterial infections.*

**Kliovance**
*Novo Nordisk, Austral.; Novo Nordisk, NZ; Novo Nordisk, UK.*
Estradiol (p.1550·1); norethisterone acetate (p.1562·2).
*Menopausal disorders; osteoporosis.*

**Klipal**
*Pharmacia, Arg.*
Paracetamol (p.76·2); codeine (p.27·1).
*Pain.*

*Pierre Fabre, Fr.*
Paracetamol (p.76·2); codeine phosphate (p.27·1).
*Pain.*

**Klipal Codeine** *Pierre Fabre, Fr.†.*
Paracetamol (p.76·2); codeine phosphate (p.27·1).
Formerly known as Oralgan Codeine.
*Fever; pain.*

**Klismacort** *Bene, Ger.; Novartis Consumer, Ger.*
Prednisolone (p.1108·1).
*Rectal corticosteroid.*

**Klispel** *Ativus, Braz.*
Omeprazole (p.1278·2).
*Peptic ulcer.*

**Klistier** *Fresenius Kabi, Ger.*
Dibasic sodium phosphate (p.1231·1); monobasic sodium phosphate (p.1230·3).
*Bowel evacuation; constipation.*

**Klizin** *Cimed, Braz.*
Buclizine (p.426·3); vitamin B substances (p.1417·1).
*Reduced appetite; tonic.*

**KLN** *Roche Consumer, UK.*
Kaolin (p.1268·3); pectin (p.1580·3); sodium citrate (p.1223·2); peppermint oil (p.1283·2).
*Diarrhoea.*

**Kloclor** *Adcock Ingram, S.Afr.†.*
Cefaclor (p.167·1).
*Bacterial infections.*

**Klodin** *Savio, Ital.*
Ticlopidine hydrochloride (p.1011·2).
*Thrombosis prophylaxis.*

**Klodipin** *APS, Port.*
Ticlopidine hydrochloride (p.1011·2).
*Thrombosis prophylaxis.*

**Klomazole** *Klonal, Arg.*
Clotrimazole (p.396·2).
*Fungal infections.*

**Klomeprax** *Klonal, Arg.*
Omeprazole (p.1278·2).
*Peptic ulcer.*

**Klomicina** *Klonal, Arg.*
Roxithromycin (p.254·2).
*Bacterial infections.*

**Klonacid** *Klonal, Arg.*
Clarithromycin (p.192·2).
*Bacterial infections.*

**Klonadroxil** *Klonal, Arg.*
Cefadroxil (p.167·2).
*Bacterial infections.*

**Klonadryl** *Klonal, Arg.*
Diphenhydramine (p.431·3).

**Klonadryl Antitusivo** *Klonal, Arg.*
Diphenhydramine (p.431·3) ammonium chloride (p.1115·2).
*Coughs.*

**Klonafenac** *Klonal, Arg.*
Diclofenac (p.32·1).
*Inflammation; pain.*

**Klonalfenicol** *Klonal, Arg.*
Chloramphenicol (p.185·1).
*Bacterial infections.*

**Klonalmox** *Klonal, Arg.*
Amoxicillin (p.155·3); clavulanic acid (p.193·3).
*Bacterial infections.*

**Klonalol** *Klonal, Arg.*
Timolol (p.1012·3).
*Ocular hypertension.*

**Klonam** *Klonal, Arg.*
Imipenem (p.221·1); cilastatin sodium (p.188·1).
*Bacterial infections.*

**Klonametacina** *Klonal, Arg.*
Indometacin (p.47·3).
*Inflammation; pain.*

**Klonamicin** *Klonal, Arg.*
Tobramycin (p.271·2).
*Bacterial eye infections.*

**Klonatropina** *Klonal, Arg.*
Atropine (p.476·3).
*Production of mydriasis.*

**Klonazol** *Klonal, Arg.*
Fluconazole (p.398·1).
*Fungal infections.*

**Klonocarpina** *Klonal, Arg.*
Pilocarpine (p.1494·3).
*Glaucoma.*

**Klonopin** *Roche, USA.*
Clonazepam (p.359·1).
*Epilepsy; panic attacks.*

**Klont** *Medochemie, Thai.†.*
Metronidazole (p.607·2).
*Amoebiasis; anaerobic bacterial infections; giardiasis; trichomoniasis.*

**Klopoxid** *Nycomed, Denm.*
Chlordiazepoxide (p.674·2).
*Alcohol withdrawal syndrome; anxiety.*

**K-Lor**
*Abbott, Canad.; Abbott, USA.*
Potassium chloride (p.1232·2).
*Hypokalaemia; potassium depletion.*

**Kloraetyl** *Apodan, Denm.†.*
Ethyl chloride (p.1376·2).
*Local anaesthesia.*

**Klor-Con** *Upsher-Smith, USA.*
Potassium chloride (p.1232·2).
*Hypokalaemia.*

**Klor-Con/EF** *Upsher-Smith, USA.*
Potassium bicarbonate (p.1223·1); potassium citrate (p.1223·1).
*Hypokalaemia.*

**Klor-De** *Medentech, Israel.*
Sodium dichloroisocyanurate (p.1191·3).
*Surface and instrument disinfection.*

**Kloref**
*Adelco, Gr.*
Betaine hydrochloride (p.1660·2); potassium bicarbonate (p.1223·1).
*Hypokalaemia; potassium depletion.*

*Knoll, S.Afr.; Alpharma, UK.*
Betaine hydrochloride (p.1660·2); potassium bicarbonate (p.1223·1); potassium chloride (p.1232·2); potassium benzoate (p.1233·1).
*Hypokalaemia; potassium depletion.*

**Kloren** *Enila, Braz.†.*
Potassium chloride (p.1232·2).
*Hypokalaemia.*

**Klorhexol** *Leiras, Fin.*
Chlorhexidine gluconate (p.1173·2).
*Hand and skin disinfection.*

**Klor-Kleen** *Medentech, Irl.†.*
Sodium dichloroisocyanurate (p.1191·3); sodium dodecylbenzenesulphonate.
*Surface disinfection.*

**Klorokin** *Zerboni, Mex.†.*
Chloroquine (p.448·2).

**Klorpo**
*Upha, Malaysia.*
Chlordiazepoxide (p.674·2).
*Anxiety disorders.*

*Beacons, Singapore.*
Chlordiazepoxide hydrochloride (p.674·2).
*Alcohol withdrawal syndrome; anxiety; skeletal muscle spasm.*

**Klorproman** *Orion, Fin.*
Chlorpromazine hydrochloride (p.675·2).
*Alcohol withdrawal syndrome; nausea and vomiting; pain; psychoses; sedative.*

**Klorsept**
*Medentech, Irl.†; Medentech, Israel.*
Sodium dichloroisocyanurate (p.1191·3).
*Skin and wound disinfection; surface disinfection.*

**Klorvess** *Novartis, USA.*
*Effervescent tablets:* Potassium chloride (p.1232·2); potassium bicarbonate (p.1223·1); lysine hydrochloride (p.1439·2).
*Oral effervescent granules:* Potassium chloride (p.1232·2); potassium bicarbonate (p.1223·1); potassium citrate (p.1223·1); lysine hydrochloride (p.1439·2).
*Oral liquid:* Potassium chloride (p.1232·2).
*Hypokalaemic-hypochloraemic alkalosis; potassium depletion.*

**Klosartan** *Klonal, Arg.*
Losartan (p.948·2).
*Hypertension.*

**Klosidol** *Bago, Arg.*
Dextropropoxyphene hydrochloride (p.28·3) or dextropropoxyphene napsilate (p.28·3); dipyrone (p.35·3).
*Pain.*

**Klosidol B1 B6 B12** *Bago, Arg.*
Dextropropoxyphene hydrochloride (p.28·3) or dextropropoxyphene napsilate (p.28·3); dipyrone (p.35·3); cyanocobalamin (p.1458·2) or hydroxocobalamin (p.1458·2); thiamine hydrochloride (p.1455·1); pyridoxine hydrochloride (p.1456·3).
*Joint pain; neuralgia.*

**Klosterfrau Aktiv** *Klosterfrau, Ger.*
Garlic; vitamin A; alpha tocoferil acetate (p.1417·1).
*Tonic.*

**Klosterfrau Franzbranntwein** *Klosterfrau, Ger.*
Menthol (p.1711·3); camphor (p.1665·3); alcohol (p.1166·1).
*Musculoskeletal, joint, and soft-tissue disorders.*

**Klosterfrau Franzbranntwein Latschenkiefer** *Klosterfrau, Ger.*
*Topical gel†:* Camphor (p.1665·3); pumilio pine oil (p.1737·1).
*Topical lotion:* Camphor (p.1665·3); pumilio pine oil (p.1737·1); alcohol (p.1166·1).
*Musculoskeletal, joint, and soft-tissue disorders.*

**Klosterfrau Melissengeist** *Klosterfrau, Ger.*
Melissa; elecampane; angelica; ginger; clove; gentian; fruct. piperis nigri; galanga; nutmeg; dried bitter-orange peel; cinnamon bark; senna; cardamom; alcohol.
*Tonic.*

**Klosterfrau-Beruhigungskapseln** *Klosterfrau, Austria.*
Valerian (p.1762·2); lupulus (p.1708·1).
*Nervous disorders; sleep disorders.*

**Klotricid** *Pharmacia Upjohn, Fin.†.*
Clotrimazole (p.396·2).
*Fungal skin infections.*

**Klotriptyl** *Orion, Fin.*
Amitriptyline hydrochloride (p.280·3).
*Depression; insomnia.*

**Klotrix** *Apothecon, USA.*
Potassium chloride (p.1232·2).
*Hypokalaemia; potassium depletion.*

**Klyndaken** *Kendrick, Mex.*
Clindamycin phosphate (p.194·2).
*Bacterial infections.*

**Klysma Salinisch** *Baxter, Ger.*
Monobasic sodium phosphate (p.1230·3); dibasic sodium phosphate (p.1231·1).
*Bowel evacuation.*

**Klysma Sorbit** *Baxter, Ger.*
Sorbitol (p.1446·3); potassium sorbate (p.1192·3).
*Bowel evacuation; constipation.*

**Klysmol** *Demo, Gr.*
Dibasic sodium phosphate (p.1231·1); monobasic sodium phosphate (p.1230·3).
*Bowel evacuation; constipation.*

**K-Lyte**
*Wellspring, Canad.*
Potassium citrate (p.1223·1).
*Potassium depletion.*

*Apothecon, USA.*
Potassium bicarbonate (p.1223·1).
*Potassium deficiency.*

**K-Lyte DS** *Apothecon, USA.*
Potassium bicarbonate (p.1223·1); potassium citrate (p.1223·1).
*Potassium deficiency.*

**K-Lyte/Cl**
*Wellspring, Canad.*
Potassium chloride (p.1232·2).
*Potassium depletion.*

*Apothecon, USA.*
*Effervescent powder:* Potassium chloride (p.1232·2).
*Effervescent tablets:* Potassium chloride (p.1232·2); potassium bicarbonate (p.1223·1).
*Potassium deficiency.*

**Klyx**
*Ferring, Denm.; Ferring, Fin.; Ferring, Norw.; Ferring, Swed.*
Docusate sodium (p.1262·2); sorbitol (p.1446·3).
*Bowel evacuation; constipation.*

**Klyx Magnum** *Ferring, Switz.*
Docusate sodium (p.1262·2); dried magnesium sulfate (p.1229·1); urea (p.1162·2).
*Bowel evacuation; constipation.*

**KMA** *Berlin-Chemie, Ger.†.*
Potassium hydroxide (p.1734·2); magnesium oxide (p.1272·3).
*Cardiac disorders.*

**K-Mag** *Blackmores, Austral.*
Potassium aspartate (p.1233·1); magnesium aspartate (p.1227·3).
*Potassium and magnesium supplement.*

**K-Med** *Riva, Canad.†.*
Potassium chloride (p.1232·2); magnesium gluconate (p.1228·1).
*Potassium supplement.*

**KMG Plus** *Seroyal, Canad.†.*
Vitamin $B_6$ with magnesium and potassium (p.1417·1).

**KMH** *M & H, Thai.*
Kanamycin sulfate (p.225·1).
*Bacterial infections.*

**K-Mizol** *Arlex, Mex.†.*
Miconazole (p.405·2) or miconazole nitrate (p.405·3).

**KN Solution** *Otsuka, Jpn.*
Range of electrolyte infusions with glucose (p.1217·1).

**Kneipp Abfuhr Herbagran** *Kneipp, Ger.†.*
Ispaghula (p.1268·1).
*Constipation.*

**Kneipp Abfuhr Tee N** *Kneipp, Ger.†.*
Senna (p.1288·2).
*Constipation.*

**Kneipp Baldrian** *Kneipp, Ger.†.*
Valerian (p.1762·2).
*Anxiety disorders; sleep disorders.*

**Kneipp Baldrian + Hopfen** *Kneipp, Ger.†.*
Valerian (p.1762·2); lupulus (p.1708·1).
*Anxiety; sleep disorders.*

**Kneipp Baldrian Pflanzensaft Nerventrost** *Kneipp, Ger.†.*
Valerian (p.1762·2).
*Nervousness; sleep disorders.*

**Kneipp Balsamo** *Fher, Spain†.*
Camphor (p.1665·3); peru balsam (p.1730·2); cineole (p.1672·1); oleum pini sylvestris; thymol (p.1194·2); menthol (p.1711·3).
*Upper-respiratory-tract disorders.*

**Kneipp Beruhigungs-Bad spezial** *Kneipp, Ger.†.*
Citronella oil (p.1673·2).
*Anxiety; bath additive; tension.*

**Kneipp Birkenblatter Pflanzensaft** *Kneipp, Ger.†.*
Birch leaf (p.1660·3).
*Urinary-tract disorders.*

**Kneipp Blasen- und Nieren-Tee** *Kneipp, Ger.†.*
Equisetum (p.1684·1); solidago virgaurea (p.1748·3); birch leaf (p.1660·3); ononis (p.1723·3).
*Urinary-tract disorders.*

**Kneipp Brennesselkraut Pflanzensaft Kneippianum** *Kneipp, Ger.†.*
Urtica (p.1762·1).
*Rheumatic disorders; urinary-tract disorders.*

**Kneipp Brunnenkresse-Pflanzensaft** *Kneipp, Ger.†.*
Nasturtium.
*Diuretic.*

**Kneipp Calcium compositum N** *Kneipp, Ger.†.*
Multivitamin and mineral preparation (p.1417·1).
*Calcium deficiency.*

**Kneipp Drei-Pflanzen-Dragees N** *Kneipp, Ger.†.*
*Combination pack:* Tablets, Crataegus (p.1677·1); tablets, garlic (p.1691·1); tablets, mistletoe (p.1715·3).
*Arteriosclerosis.*

**Kneipp Entschlackungs-Tee** *Kneipp, Ger.†.*
Juniper (p.1703·1); peppermint leaf (p.1283·2); birch leaf (p.1660·3).
*Diuretic.*

**Kneipp Entwasserungstee** *Kneipp, Austria.*
Juniper (p.1703·1); peppermint leaf (p.1283·2); birch leaf (p.1660·3).
*Diuretic.*

**Kneipp Erkaltungs-Bad** *Kneipp, Ger.†.*
Thyme oil (p.1755·3).
*Bath additive; cold symptoms.*

**Kneipp Erkaltungsbad Spezial** *Kneipp, Ger.†.*
Eucalyptus oil (p.1686·2); camphor (p.1665·3).
*Bath additive; catarrh.*

**Kneipp Erkaltungs-Balsam N** *Kneipp, Ger.†.*
Eucalyptus oil (p.1686·2); siberian fir oil; rosemary oil (p.1740·2); pumilio pine oil (p.1737·1); thyme oil (p.1755·3); turpentine oil (p.1760·1).
*Coughs and associated respiratory-tract disorders.*

**Kneipp Erkaltungs-Tee** *Kneipp, Ger.†.*
Tilia (p.1756·2); sambucus (p.1741·3); thyme (p.1755·2).
*Cold symptoms.*

**Kneipp Fichtennadel Franzbranntwein** *Kneipp, Ger.†.*
Menthol (p.1711·3); alcohol (p.1166·1).
*Musculoskeletal, joint, and soft-tissue disorders; peripheral circulatory disorders.*

**Kneipp Flatuol** *Kneipp, Ger.†.*
Fennel (p.1687·2); caraway (p.1667·2); peppermint leaf (p.1283·2); gentian (p.1692·2).
*Flatulence; meteorism.*

**Kneipp Galle- und Leber-Tee** *Kneipp, Austria.*
Peppermint leaf (p.1283·2); turmeric (p.1058·3); taraxacum (p.1751·3).
*Gallbladder and liver disorders.*

**Kneipp Galle- und Leber-Tee N** *Kneipp, Ger.†.*
Peppermint leaf (p.1283·2); turmeric (p.1058·3); taraxacum (p.1751·3).
*Biliary and liver disorders; herbal tea.*

**Kneipp Ginsenetten** *Kneipp, Ger.†.*
Ginseng (p.1693·1).
*Tonic.*

**Kneipp Grippe-Tee** *Kneipp, Austria.*
Tilia (p.1756·2); salix purpurea (p.87·3); plantago lanceolata (p.1738·2); thyme (p.1755·2); chamomile (p.1669·3).
*Cold symptoms.*

**Kneipp Herz- und Kreislauf-Tee** *Kneipp, Ger.†.*
Rosemary (p.1740·2); crataegus (p.1677·1); motherwort (p.1717·1); hypericum (p.299·1); Paraguay tea.
*Cardiovascular disorders.*

**Kneipp Herz- und Kreislauf-Unterstutzungs-Tee** *Kneipp, Austria.*
Rosemary leaf (p.1740·2); crataegus (p.1677·1); maté leaf (p.1765·3).
*Cardiovascular disorders.*

**Kneipp Herzsalbe Unguentum Cardiacum Kneipp** *Kneipp, Ger.†.*
Rosemary oil (p.1740·2); camphor (p.1665·3); menthol (p.1711·3).
*Cardiac disorders.*

**Kneipp Heupack Herbatherm N** *Kneipp, Ger.†.*
Cut grasses and flowers.
*Biliary-tract, kidney, and bladder disorders; rheumatic and arthritic disorders.*

**Kneipp Husten- und Bronchial-Tee**
*Kneipp, Austria; Kneipp, Ger.†.*
Fennel (p.1687·2); cowslip flowers and calyx (p.1735·1); thyme (p.1755·2); plantago lanceolata (p.1738·2).
*Bronchitis; catarrh; coughs.*

**Kneipp Hustensaft Spitzwegerich** *Kneipp, Ger.†.*
Plantago lanceolata (p.1738·2).
*Catarrh.*

**Kneipp Knoblauch Dragees N** *Kneipp, Ger.†.*
Garlic (p.1691·1).
*Arteriosclerosis.*

**Kneipp Knoblauch-Pflanzensaft** *Kneipp, Ger.†.*
Garlic (p.1691·1).
*Arteriosclerosis; digestive system disorders; hypertension.*

**Kneipp Krauter Hustensaft N Kneipp Tannolsaft** *Kneipp, Ger.†.*
Norway spruce oil; pumilio pine oil (p.1737·1); cowslip flower (p.1735·1); thyme (p.1755·2).
*Coughs and associated respiratory-tract disorders.*

**Kneipp Krauter Taschenkur Nerven und Schlaf N** *Kneipp, Ger.†.*
*Combination pack:* Tablets, valerian (p.1762·2); tablets, hypericum (p.299·1); tablets, melissa leaves (p.1711·1); citronella oil (p.1673·2); lemon grass oil (p.1706·3).
*Nervous disorders.*

**Kneipp Kreislauf-Bad Rosmarin-Aquasan** *Kneipp, Ger.†.*
Camphor (p.1665·3); rosemary oil (p.1740·2).
*Bath additive; circulatory disorders.*

**Kneipp Latschenkiefer Franzbranntwein** *Kneipp, Ger.†.*
Camphor (p.1665·3); oleum pini sylvestris; alcohol (p.1166·1).
*Musculoskeletal and joint disorders; peripheral vascular disorders; soft-tissue disorders.*

**Kneipp Lowenzahn-Pflanzensaft** *Kneipp, Ger.†.*
Taraxacum (p.1751·3).
*Gall bladder and liver disorders.*

**Kneipp Magen-Tee** *Kneipp, Ger.†.*
Aniseed (p.1655·2); fennel (p.1687·2); caraway (p.1667·2).
*Gastrointestinal disorders.*

**Kneipp Melisse Pflanzensaft** *Kneipp, Ger.†.*
Melissa (p.1711·1).
*Nervous disorders.*

**Kneipp Milch-Molke-Bad** *Kneipp, Ger.†.*
Skimmed milk; whey; lactic acid (p.1704·1).
*Bath additive; burns; skin disorders.*

**Kneipp Minzol Trost Tropfen** *Kneipp, Ger.†.*
Mint oil (p.1715·2).
*Cold symptoms; gastrointestinal disorders; myalgia; neuralgia.*

**Kneipp Mistel-Pflanzensaft** *Kneipp, Ger.†.*
Mistletoe (p.1715·3).
*Circulatory disorders.*

**Kneipp Nerven- und Schlaf-Tee** *Kneipp, Austria.*
Melissa (p.1711·1); valerian (p.1762·2); sweet orange (p.1724·1).
*Nervous disorders; sleep disorders.*

**Kneipp Nerven- und Schlaf-Tee N** *Kneipp, Ger.†.*
Melissa (p.1711·1); valerian (p.1762·2); sweet orange peel.
*Nervous disorders.*

**Kneipp Neurodermatitis-Bad** *Kneipp, Ger.†.*
Soya oil (p.1447·2).
*Bath additive; dry skin; pruritus.*

**Kneipp Nieren- und Blasen-Tee** *Kneipp, Austria.*
Silver birch (p.1660·3); equisetum (p.1684·1); solidago virgaurea (p.1748·3); ononis (p.1723·3); peppermint leaf (p.1283·2); calendula (p.1665·2).
*Urinary-tract disorders.*

**Kneipp Petersilie N** *Kneipp, Ger.†.*
Parsley (p.1728·3).
*Diuretic.*

**Kneipp Pflanzen-Dragees Brennessel** *Kneipp, Ger.†.*
Urtica (p.1762·1).
*Urinary-tract disorders.*

**Kneipp Pflanzen-Dragees Mistel** *Kneipp, Ger.†.*
Mistletoe (p.1715·3).
*Circulatory disorders.*

**Kneipp Pflanzen-Dragees Weissdorn** *Kneipp, Ger.†.*
Crataegus leaves, flowers, and fruit (p.1677·1).
*Cardiac disorders.*

**Kneipp Rettich-Pflanzensaft** *Kneipp, Ger.†.*
Raphanus.
*Gall bladder and liver disorders.*

**Kneipp Rheuma Salbe** *Kneipp, Ger.†.*
Cayenne pepper (p.1667·1).
*Musculoskeletal and joint disorders; neuralgia; sciatica.*

**Kneipp Rheuma Stoffwechsel-Bad Heublumen-Aquasan** *Kneipp, Ger.†.*
Coumarin (p.1676·2); peppermint oil (p.1283·2); caraway oil (p.1667·3); sage oil (p.1741·2); thyme oil (p.1755·3).
*Bath additive; tonic bath.*

**Kneipp Rheuma Tee N** *Kneipp, Ger.†.*
Dulcamara stalk (p.1683·1); salix bark (p.87·3); sambucus leaf (p.1741·3); juniper berry (p.1703·1); red sandalwood.
*Rheumatic disorders.*

**Kneipp Rheuma-Bad** *Kneipp, Ger.†.*
Juniper oil (p.1703·1); sweet birch oil (p.60·1).
*Bath additive; rheumatism and spinal disorders.*

**Kneipp Rosmarin-Pflanzensaft** *Kneipp, Ger.†.*
Rosemary leaf (p.1740·2).
*Circulatory disorders.*

**Kneipp Schafgarbe-Pflanzensaft Frauentost N** *Kneipp, Ger.†.*
Achillea (p.1646·2).
*Anorexia; digestive system disorders.*

**Kneipp Spitzwegerich-Pflanzensaft Hustentrost** *Kneipp, Ger.†.*
Plantago lanceolata (p.1738·2).
*Catarrh; mouth and throat disorders.*

**Kneipp Stoffwechsel-Unterstutzungs-Tee** *Kneipp, Austria.*
Prunus spinosa; taraxacum (p.1751·3); peppermint leaf (p.1283·2); lovage (p.1708·1); hibiscus.
*Stimulation of metabolic activity.*

**Kneipp Tonikum-Bad Fichtennadel-Aquasan** *Kneipp, Ger.†.*
Norway spruce oil; eucalyptus oil (p.1686·2); turpentine oil (p.1760·1).
*Bath additive; tonic bath.*

**Kneipp Verdauungs-Tee** *Kneipp, Austria.*
Prunus spinosa; chamomile (p.1669·3); fennel (p.1687·2); centaury (p.1669·2).
*Gastrointestinal disorders.*

**Kneipp Verdauungs-Tee N** *Kneipp, Ger.†.*
Chamomile (p.1669·3); fennel (p.1687·2); centaury (p.1669·2).
*Gastrointestinal disorders.*

**Kneipp Wacholderbeer-Pflanzensaft** *Kneipp, Ger.†.*
Juniper (p.1703·1).
*Diuretic; gastrointestinal disorders.*

**Kneipp Weissdorn-Pflanzensaft Sebastianeum** *Kneipp, Ger.†.*
Crataegus (p.1677·1).
*Cardiac disorders.*

**Kneipp Weissdorn-Tee** *Kneipp, Ger.†.*
Crataegus (p.1677·1).
*Cardiac disorders.*

**Kneipp Woerisettes** *Roche, Switz.†.*
Aloes (p.1248·2); plant extracts.
*Constipation.*

**Kneipp Worisetten S** *Kneipp, Ger.†.*
Senna (p.1288·2).
*Constipation.*

**Kneipp Zinnkraut-Pflanzensaft** *Kneipp, Ger.†.*
Equisetum (p.1684·1).
*Urinary-tract disorders.*

**Kneipplax N** *Kneipp, Ger.†.*
Ispaghula (p.1268·1); senna (p.1288·2).
*Constipation.*

**Knoblauch-Vital** *Rosch & Handel, Austria.*
Garlic; vitamin E (p.1417·1).
*Tonic.*

**Knochenzement** *Synthes, Austria†.*
Methylmethacrylate/polymethylmethacrylate (p.1714·3).
*Bone cement in orthopaedic surgery.*

**Kno-Paine** *Continental Pharma, Thai.*
Dipyrone (p.35·3).
*Pain.*

**K-Norm** *Fisons, USA.*
Potassium chloride (p.1232·2).
*Hypokalaemia; potassium depletion.*

**Knowful** *YSP, Malaysia.*
Piracetam (p.1732·1).
*Mental function disorders.*

**Koal** *Ethicus, Arg.*
Salicylic acid (p.1157·1).
*Scalp disorders.*

**Koate** *Sintofarma, Braz.*
A factor VIII preparation (p.751·1).
*Haemorrhagic disorders.*

**Koate-DVI**
*Gador, Arg.; Bayer, Chile; Bayer Biological, Hong Kong; Bayer, Malaysia; Probifasa, Mex.; Bayer, Singapore; Bayer, USA.*
A factor VIII preparation (p.751·1).
*Haemorrhagic disorders.*

**Koate-HP**
*Bayer, Canad.†; Bayer, Israel; Probifasa, Mex.†; Bayer, USA†.*
A factor VIII preparation (p.751·1).
*Haemophilia A.*

**Koate-HS** *Sclavo, Ital.†.*
A factor VIII preparation (p.751·1).
*Haemorrhagic disorders.*

**Ko-Cap** *Sriprasit, Thai.*
Co-trimoxazole (p.199·3).
*Bacterial infections.*

**Kochsalz mit Glucose** *Braun, Ger.*
Sodium chloride (p.1233·3); glucose (p.1432·2).
*Fluid and electrolyte disorders.*

**Kodakon** *Loren, Mex.*
Dexamethasone (p.1097·1); neomycin (p.235·1).
*Bacterial eye infections.*

**Kodamid** *Nycomed, Denm.*
Codeine phosphate (p.27·1); caffeine (p.782·1); propyphenazone (p.85·3); salicylamide (p.87·3).
Magnesium hydroxide (p.1272·2) is included in this preparation in an attempt to limit adverse effects on the gastrointestinal mucosa.
*Pain.*

**Kodan Tinktur Forte** *Schulke & Mayr, Ger.*
Isopropyl alcohol (p.1184·3); propyl alcohol (p.1191·2); orthophenylphenol (p.1187·2).
*Skin disinfection.*

**Kodimagnyl** *Nycomed, Denm.*
Aspirin (p.15·1); codeine phosphate (p.27·1).

Magnesium hydroxide (p.1272·2) is included in some dosage forms in an attempt to limit adverse effects on the gastrointestinal mucosa.
*Pain.*

**Kodipar** *Nycomed, Denm.*
Codeine phosphate (p.27·1); paracetamol (p.76·2).
*Pain.*

**Kofarest** *Centaur, India.*
Salbutamol sulfate (p.791·3); ambroxol hydrochloride (p.1114·3); guaifenesin (p.1122·1); menthol (p.1711·3).
*Respiratory-tract disorders.*

**Kof-Eze** *Roberts, USA.*
Menthol (p.1711·3).
*Coughs; sore throats.*

**Koffazon** *Recip, Swed.*
Caffeine (p.782·1); phenazone (p.82·3).
*Pain.*

**Koffex** *Rougier, Canad.†.*
Dextromethorphan hydrobromide (p.1117·3).

**Koffex DM** *Technilab, Canad.*
Dextromethorphan hydrobromide (p.1117·3).
*Coughs.*

**Koffex DM-D** *Technilab, Canad.*
Dextromethorphan hydrobromide (p.1117·3); pseudoephedrine hydrochloride (p.1129·2).

**Koffex DM-D-E** *Technilab, Canad.*
Dextromethorphan hydrobromide (p.1117·3); pseudoephedrine hydrochloride (p.1129·2); guaifenesin (p.1122·1).
*Coughs; respiratory-tract congestion.*

**Koffex DM-E** *Technilab, Canad.*
Dextromethorphan hydrobromide (p.1117·3); guaifenesin (p.1122·1).
*Coughs.*

**Koffex Expectorant** *Technilab, Canad.*
Guaifenesin (p.1122·1).

**Koffisal** *Nycomed, Denm.*
Caffeine (p.782·1); phenazone salicylate (p.82·3); salicylamide (p.87·3).
*Pain.*

**Kofron** *Guidotti, Spain.*
Clarithromycin (p.192·2).
*Bacterial infections.*

**Kogenate**
*Bayer, Austral.; Bayer, Austria; Bayer, Belg.†; Bayer, Canad.; Bayer, Denm.; Bayer, Fr.; Bayer, Ger.; Bayer, Gr.; Bayer, Irl.; Bayer, Ital.; Bayer, Neth.; Bayer, Norw.; Bayer, NZ; Bayer, Port.†; Bayer, Spain; Bayer, Swed.; Bayer, Switz.; Bayer, UK; Bayer, USA.*
Octocog alfa (p.751·2).
*Haemorrhagic disorders.*

**Kohle-Compretten** *Merck, Ger.*
Activated charcoal (p.1030·2).
*Acute poisoning; diarrhoea.*

**Kohle-Hevert** *Hevert, Ger.*
Activated charcoal (p.1030·2).
*Acute poisoning; diarrhoea.*

**Kohlensaurebad Bastian** *Bastian, Ger.*
Sodium bicarbonate (p.1223·2).
*Bath additive; cardiac and circulatory disorders.*

**Kohle-Pulvis** *Kohler, Ger.*
Activated charcoal (p.1030·2).
*Acute poisoning; diarrhoea.*

**Kohle-Tabletten** *Cheplapharm, Ger.*
Activated charcoal (p.1030·2).
*Acute poisoning; diarrhoea.*

**Kohrsolin** *Bode, Ger.*
Glutaral (p.1180·3); 1,6-dihydroxy-2,5-dioxahexan; polymethylolurea derivative.
*Surface and instrument disinfection.*

**Kohrsolin FF** *Bode, Ger.*
Glutaral (p.1180·3); benzalkonium chloride (p.1168·3); didecyldimethylammonium chloride (p.1178·3).
*Surface disinfection.*

**Kohrsolin iD** *Bode, Ger.†.*
Glutaral (p.1180·3); 1,6-dihydroxy-2,5-dioxahexan; polymethylolurea derivative.
*Instrument disinfection.*

**Ko-Kure** *Sriprasit, Thai.*
Co-trimoxazole (p.199·3).
*Bacterial infections.*

**Kola Astier** *URPAC, Fr.†.*
Kola (p.1765·3); caffeine (p.782·1).
*Asthenia.*

**Kola Fosfatada Soel** *Regius, Braz.†.*
Kola (p.1765·3); nux vomica (p.1722·3); sodium glycerophosphate; calcium glycerophosphate (p.1417·1).
*Tonic.*

**Kola-Dallmann** *Dallmann, Ger.†.*
Kola (p.1765·3); caffeine (p.782·1).
*Fatigue.*

**Kola-Dallmann mit Lecithin** *Dallmann, Ger.†.*
Kola (p.1765·3); caffeine (p.782·1); egg lecithin (p.1706·1).
*Fatigue.*

**Koladex** *Laboratories for Applied Biology, UK†.*
Caffeine (p.782·1); kola nut (p.1765·3).
*Tonic.*

**Kolampept** *Teuto, Braz.*
Aluminium hydroxide (p.1249·2); magnesium hydroxide (p.1272·2); dimeticone (p.1289·2).
*Flatulence; gastrointestinal hyperacidity.*

**Kolanticon**
*Peckforton, Irl.†; Peckforton, UK.*
Aluminium hydroxide (p.1249·2); dicycloverine hydrochloride (p.481·2); light magnesium oxide (p.1272·3); simeticone (p.1289·2).
*Dyspepsia; gastritis; gastro-oesophageal reflux; peptic ulcer.*

**Kolantyl**
*Note. This name is used for preparations of different composition.*
*Medley, Braz.*
Aluminium hydroxide (p.1249·2); magnesium hydroxide (p.1272·2); methylcellulose (p.1580·2); magnesium trisilicate (p.1272·3).
Formerly contained dicycloverine hydrochloride, aluminium hydroxide, magnesium hydroxide, methylcellulose, and magnesium trisilicate.
*Gastrointestinal hyperacidity.*

*Adcock Ingram, S.Afr.*
*Oral gel:* Dicycloverine hydrochloride (p.481·2); aluminium hydroxide (p.1249·2); magnesium oxide (p.1272·3); methylcellulose (p.1580·2).
*Wafers:* Dicycloverine hydrochloride (p.481·2); aluminium hydroxide (p.1249·2); magnesium hydroxide (p.1272·2); methylcellulose (p.1580·2); magnesium trisilicate (p.1272·3).
*Gastrointestinal disorders.*

**Kolantyl DMP** *Medley, Braz.*
Aluminium hydroxide (p.1249·2); magnesium hydroxide (p.1272·2); methylcellulose (p.1580·2); dimeticone (p.1289·2).
*Flatulence; gastrointestinal hyperacidity.*

**Kolemed** *Rosch & Handel, Austria.*
Activated charcoal (p.1030·2).
*Diarrhoea; flatulence.*

**Kolephrin** *Pfeiffer, USA.*
Pseudoephedrine hydrochloride (p.1129·2); paracetamol (p.76·2); chlorphenamine maleate (p.427·3).
*Upper respiratory-tract symptoms.*

**Kolephrin GG/DM** *Pfeiffer, USA.*
Dextromethorphan hydrobromide (p.1117·3); guaifenesin (p.1122·1).
*Coughs.*

**Kolephrin/DM** *Pfeiffer, USA.*
Chlorphenamine maleate (p.427·3); dextromethorphan hydrobromide (p.1117·3); paracetamol (p.76·2); pseudoephedrine hydrochloride (p.1129·2).
*Coughs and cold symptoms.*

**Kolestop** *Omni, UK.*
Sitosterol (p.982·3); beta sitostanol (p.1448·3).
*Nutritional supplement to reduce serum cholesterol.*

**Kolibel** *Instituto Sanitas, Chile.*
Clofedanol hydrochloride (p.1117·1); pseudoephedrine sulfate (p.1129·2); chlorphenamine maleate (p.427·3).
*Cold and influenza symptoms; coughs.*

**Kolkin** *Duncan, Arg.*
Furosemide (p.919·3).
*Hypertension.*

**Kollagenase** *Cristalia, Braz.*
Collagenase (p.1675·1).
*Skin ulcers; wounds.*

**Kollagenase com cloranfenicol** *Cristalia, Braz.*
Collagenase (p.1675·1); chloramphenicol (p.185·1).
*Skin ulcers; wounds.*

**Kollaps-Gastreu N R67** *Reckeweg, Ger.*
Homoeopathic preparation.

**Kollateral** *Ursapharm, Ger.*
Moxaverine hydrochloride (p.1717·2).
*Cerebral, coronary, and peripheral vascular disorders.*

**Kollateral A + E** *Ursapharm, Ger.†.*
Moxaverine hydrochloride (p.1717·2); vitamin A acetate (p.1453·1); alpha tocoferil acetate (p.1465·1).
*Cerebral, coronary, and ocular vascular disorders.*

**Kolplex** *Collins, Mex.*
Multivitamin preparation (p.1417·1).

**Kolpovent** *Grunenthal, Chile.*
Salmeterol xinafoate (p.795·1).
*Asthma.*

**Kolsan** *Bittner, Austria.*
Homoeopathic preparation.

**Kolsuspension** *Abigo, Swed.*
Activated charcoal (p.1030·2).
*Diarrhoea; poisoning.*

**Kolton bronchiale Erkaltungssaft** *Promonta, Ger.†.*
Thyme (p.1755·2).
*Bronchitis; catarrh; coughs.*

**Kolton grippale N** *Byk Gulden, Ger.*
Piprinhydrinate (p.439·1); paracetamol (p.76·2); ethenzamide (p.37·2).
*Cold and influenza symptoms.*

**Komasin** *Medinova (Μενινοβα), Gr.*
Buspirone hydrochloride (p.672·2).
*Generalised anxiety.*

**Kombetin**
*Boehringer Mannheim, Ger.†; Roche, Ital.†.*
Strophanthin-K (p.1009·1).
*Cardiac disorders.*

**Komb-H-Insulin** *Hoechst, Ger.†.*
Mixture of insulin injection (human) 50% and isophane insulin (human) 50% (p.333·3).
*Diabetes mellitus.*

**Kombicrom** *Fisons, Denm.†.*
Sodium cromoglicate (p.795·3); xylometazoline hydrochloride (p.1132·2).
*Allergic rhinitis.*

**Kombinax** *Brocco, Ital.†.*
Sulfadiazine (p.258·2); trimethoprim (p.272·2).
*Bacterial infections.*

**Komb-Insulin**
*Aventis, Austria.*
Insulin injection (porcine) (p.333·3).
*Diabetes mellitus.*

*Aventis, Ger.*
Insulin (chromatographically purified, bovine), comprising a mixture of Insulin and Depot-Insulin *(Hoechst, Ger.)* (p.333·3).
*Diabetes mellitus.*

**Komb-Insulin S** *Aventis, Ger.*
Insulin (chromatographically purified, porcine), comprising a mixture of Insulin S and Depot-Insulin S *(Hoechst, Ger.)* (p.333·3).
*Diabetes mellitus.*

**Kombi-Stulln N** *Stulln, Ger.*
Polymyxin B sulfate (p.245·1); neomycin sulfate (p.235·1).
Kombi-Stulln formerly contained polymyxin B sulfate, neomycin sulfate, and gramicidin.
*Eye infections.*

**Komil** *Goldshield, UK.*
Furosemide (p.919·3); amiloride hydrochloride (p.858·2).
These ingredients can be described by the British Approved Name Co-amilofruse.
*Liver cirrhosis with ascites; oedema.*

**Kompensan**
*Pfizer, Ger.; Pfizer, Port.; Pfizer, Switz.*
Dihydroxyaluminum sodium carbonate (p.1261·2).
*Gastrointestinal disorders associated with hyperacidity.*

**Kompensan Dimeticon** *Pfizer, Ger.*
Dimeticone 350 (p.1289·2).
*Adjunct in gastrointestinal radiography; gastrointestinal disorders with excess gas.*

**Kompensan-S**
*Pfizer, Ger.; Pfizer, Port.*
Dihydroxyaluminum sodium carbonate (p.1261·2); dimethicone (p.1289·2).
*Gastrointestinal disorders.*

**Kona** *M & H, Thai.*
Dextromethorphan hydrobromide (p.1117·3); diphenhydramine hydrochloride (p.431·3); pseudoephedrine hydrochloride (p.1129·2).
*Cold symptoms; coughs; nasal congestion.*

**Konaderm** *ICN, Mex.*
Ketoconazole (p.403·3).
*Fungal skin infections.*

**Konakion**
*Roche, Arg.; Roche, Austral.; Roche, Austria; Roche, Belg.; Roche, Denm.; Roche, Fin.; Roche, Ger.; Roche, Gr.; Roche, Hong Kong; Roche, Irl.; Roche, Israel; Roche, Ital.; Roche, Mex.; Roche, Neth.; Roche, NZ; Roche, S.Afr.; Roche, Singapore†; Roche, Spain; Roche, Swed.; Roche, Switz.; Roche, Thai.; Roche, UK.*
Phytomenadione (p.1467·1).
*Anticoagulant antidote; hypoprothrombinaemia; vitamin K deficiency; vitamin K deficiency bleeding.*

**Konakion MM** *Roche, Chile.*
Phytomenadione (p.1467·1).
*Coumarin overdose; haemorrhagic disease of the newborn; hypoprothrombinaemia; phenylbutazone overdose; salicylate overdose; vitamin K deficiency.*

**Konakion Novum** *Roche, Norw.*
Phytomenadione (p.1467·1).
*Haemorrhage in neonates; hypoprothrombinaemia; warfarin overdose.*

**Konaturil** *IQFA, Mex.*
Ketoconazole (p.403·3).
*Fungal infections.*

**Konazil** *Sintofarma, Braz.†.*
Ketoconazole (p.403·3).
*Fungal infections.*

**Konazol** *PP Lab, Thai.*
Ketoconazole (p.403·3).
*Fungal infections.*

**Kondon's Nasal** *Kondon, USA.*
Ephedrine (p.1120·1).
*Nasal congestion.*

**Kondremul** *Fisons, USA.*
Liquid paraffin (p.1479·1).
*Constipation.*

**Konicortil** *Koni-Cofarm, Chile.*
Betamethasone (p.1093·1).
*Skin disorders.*

**Koniderm** *Koni-Cofarm, Chile.*
Clobetasol (p.1095·3).
*Skin disorders.*

**Konifungil** *Koni-Cofarm, Chile.*
Clotrimazole (p.396·2).
*Fungal skin infections.*

**Konirub** *Koni-Cofarm, Chile.*
Methyl nicotinate (p.59·2); methyl salicylate (p.59·3); benzocaine (p.1370·3).
*Musculoskeletal and joint disorders.*

**Konjax** *Murat, Fr.†.*
Glucomannan (p.1693·3).
*Obesity.*

**Konjunktival** *Alcon, Hong Kong.*
Naphazoline hydrochloride (p.1124·3); pheniramine maleate (p.438·3).
*Conjunctivitis.*

**Konjunktival Thilo** *Alcon, Ger.*
Naphazoline hydrochloride (p.1124·3); pheniramine maleate (p.438·3).
*Eye disorders.*

**Konlax**
*Shinyaku, Hong Kong; Shinyaku, Thai.†.*
Pridinol mesilate (p.1395·2).
*Skeletal muscle spasm.*

**Konor** *Italzama, Ital.*
Tar (p.1159·3).
*Seborrhoeic dermatitis.*

**Konorderm** *Italzama, Ital.*
Inositol, vitamin PP, vitamin E, betacarotene, selenium, L-cystine (p.1417·1).
*Antoxidant nutritional supplement.*

**Konovid** *TO-Chemicals, Thai.*
Ofloxacin (p.239·3).
*Bacterial infections.*

**Konstitutin** *CytoChemia, Ger.*
Eleutherococcus senticosis (p.1744·1).
*Tonic.*

**Konsyl**
*GlaxoSmithKline, Arg.; Konsyl, Israel; Glaxo Wellcome, Mex.; Pacific, NZ†; Mepha, Switz.†; Eastern Pharmaceuticals, UK; Konsyl, USA.*
Ispaghula (p.1268·1).
*Constipation; diarrhoea; irritable bowel syndrome.*

**Konsyl-D** *Konsyl, USA.*
Psyllium hydrophilic mucilloid (p.1268·1).
*Constipation.*

**Kontagripp Mono** *Azupharma, Ger.*
Ibuprofen (p.45·3).
*Fever; pain.*

**Kontakto Derm** *Combe, Ger.*
Benzocaine (p.1370·3).
Formerly contained benzocaine and benzyl benzoate.
*Eczema; pruritus.*

**Kontal** *Pharmia, Fin.*
Niclosamide (p.110·1).
*Worm infections.*

**Kontexin** *Pharmacia, Switz.*
Phenylpropanolamine hydrochloride (p.1127·3).
*Urinary incontinence.*

**Kontic** *Coup, Gr.*
Enalapril maleate (p.909·2).
*Heart failure; hypertension.*

**Konyne**
*Sintofarma, Braz.†; Cutter, Israel†.*
A factor IX preparation (p.752·2).
*Haemorrhagic disorders.*

**Konyne 80**
*Bayer Biological, Hong Kong†; Probifasa, Mex.; Bayer, USA†.*
Factor IX complex (p.752·2).
*Haemorrhagic disorders.*

**Kop Alerge Vacina** *Kopkins, Braz.†.*
An oral anticatarrh vaccine.
*Active immunisation.*

**Kop Hepar** *Kopkins, Braz.†.*
Solanum paniculatum; boldo (p.1661·2); cynara (p.1678·3).
*Liver disorders.*

**Kopen** *Athlone, Irl.*
Phenoxymethylpenicillin (p.242·1).
*Gram-positive bacterial infections.*

**Kophane Cough and Cold Formula** *Pfeiffer, USA†.*
Phenylpropanolamine hydrochloride (p.1127·3); chlorphenamine maleate (p.427·3); dextromethorphan hydrobromide (p.1117·3).
*Coughs and cold symptoms.*

**Korandil**
*Remedica, Singapore; Remedica, Thai.*
Enalapril maleate (p.909·2).
*Heart failure; hypertension.*

**Kordinol Compuesto** *Laboratorios Chile, Chile.*
Diiodohydroxyquinoline (p.603·3); phthalylsulfacetamide; vegetable carbon (p.1058·3); hyoscine butylbromide (p.483·3).
*Diarrhoea.*

**Koreberon** *Asta Medica, Ger.†.*
Sodium fluoride (p.1444·3).
*Osteoporosis.*

**Korec** *Sanofi Synthelabo, Fr.*
Quinapril hydrochloride (p.991·1).
*Heart failure; hypertension.*

**Koretic** *Sanofi Synthelabo, Fr.*
Quinapril hydrochloride (p.991·1); hydrochlorothiazide (p.933·2).
*Hypertension.*

**Korifen** *Collins, Mex.*
Citric acid (p.1673·1); dipyrone (p.35·3).
*Cold and influenza symptoms.*

**Koro** *M & H, Thai.*
Chloramphenicol (p.185·1).
*Bacterial eye infections.*

**Korodin**
*Note. This name is used for preparations of different composition.*
*Robugen, Ger.*
Camphor (p.1665·3); crataegus (p.1677·1).
*Cardiac disorders; circulatory disorders.*

*Medipharm, Switz.†.*
Chamomile (p.1669·3); crataegus (p.1677·1).
*Cardiac disorders.*

**Koromex** *QHP, USA†.*
*Vaginal cream:* Octoxinol (p.1414·1).

*Vaginal gel:* Nonoxinol 9 (p.1413·3).
*Contraceptive.*

**Koro-Nyhadin** *Robugen, Ger.*
Crataegus (p.1677·1).
*Heart failure.*

**Korseng** *Self-Care Products, UK.*
Ginseng (p.1693·1).

**Korsolex AF** *Bode, Ger.*
Laurylpropylenediamine; dodecylbispropylenetriamine.
*Instrument disinfection.*

**Korsolex basic** *Bode, Ger.*
Glutaral (p.1180·3); dihydroxydioxahexan.
*Instrument disinfection.*

**Korsolex Extra** *Bode, Ger.*
Dihydroxydioxahexan; glutaral (p.1180·3); benzalkonium chloride (p.1168·3); didecyldimethylammonium chloride (p.1178·3).
*Instrument disinfection.*

**Korsolex FF** *Bode, Ger.*
Glutaral (p.1180·3); benzalkonium chloride (p.1168·3); didecyldimethylammonium chloride (p.1178·3).
Formerly contained glutaral, succindialdehyde, and polyoxyethylene cocosamine.
*Instrument disinfection.*

**Korsolex Plus** *Bode, Ger.*
Dodecylbispropylenetriamine; didecyldimethylammonium chloride (p.1178·3).
*Instrument infection.*

**Korsolex-Endo-Disinfectant** *Bode, Ger.*
Glutaral (p.1180·3).
*Disinfection of endoscopes.*

**Korticoid** *Cophar, Switz.†.*
Fluocinonide (p.1101·3).
*Skin disorders.*

**Korticoid polyvalent** *Cophar, Switz.†.*
Fluocinonide (p.1101·3); gramicidin (p.220·2); neomycin sulfate (p.235·1); nystatin (p.406·3).
*Infected skin disorders.*

**Kortikoid-ratiopharm** *Ratiopharm, Ger.*
Triamcinolone acetonide (p.1110·2).
*Burns; skin disorders.*

**Korynase** *Kyorin, Thai.*
Promelase (p.1735·2).
*Inflammation; oedema.*

**Korzen** *Korean Drug, Singapore.*
Serrapeptase (p.1743·2).
*Inflammation; respiratory-tract congestion.*

**Kos** *Crinos, Ital.†.*
Ibuprofen pyridoxine (p.46·3).
*Musculoskeletal and joint disorders; pain.*

**Kosteo** *Arrow, Austral.*
Calcitriol (p.1461·2).
*Hypocalcaemia; osteoporosis.*

**Kovan** *Laboratorios Chile, Chile.*
Vancomycin (p.275·2).
*Gram-positive bacterial infections.*

**Kovilen** *Mediolanum, Ital.*
Nedocromil sodium (p.789·3).
*Ocular hypersensitivity reactions.*

**Kovinal** *Mediolanum, Ital.*
Nedocromil sodium (p.789·3).
*Allergic rhinitis.*

**Kovitonic** *Freeda, USA†.*
Ferric pyrophosphate (p.1427·2); folic acid (p.1429·1); vitamin B substances with L-lysine (p.1417·1).
*Iron-deficiency anaemias.*

**KP** *PP Lab, Thai.*
Phytomenadione (p.1467·1).
*Haemorrhagic disorders.*

**K-Pek** *Rugby, USA.*
Attapulgite (p.1251·1).
*Diarrhoea.*

**K-Pek II** *Rugby, USA.*
Loperamide hydrochloride (p.1271·1).
*Diarrhoea.*

**K-Phos MF** *Beach, USA.*
Monobasic potassium phosphate (p.1230·3); monobasic sodium phosphate (p.1230·3).
*Urinary acidification.*

**K-Phos Neutral** *Beach, USA.*
Dibasic sodium phosphate (p.1231·1); monobasic potassium phosphate (p.1230·3); monobasic sodium phosphate (p.1230·3).
*Phosphorus supplement.*

**K-Phos No.2** *Beach, USA.*
Monobasic potassium phosphate (p.1230·3); monobasic sodium phosphate (p.1230·3).
*Urinary acidification.*

**K-Phos Original** *Beach, USA.*
Monobasic potassium phosphate (p.1230·3).
*Urinary acidification.*

**Kpl** *Fouchard, Chile.*
Ketoconazole (p.403·3); piroctone; ammonium lactate (p.1142·3).
*Dandruff; seborrhoeic dermatitis.*

**KPN** *Freeda, USA.*
Multivitamin and mineral preparation with iron and folic acid (p.1417·1).

**KPP** *Novartis Consumer, S.Afr.*
Aspirin (p.15·1); paracetamol (p.76·2); caffeine citrate (p.782·1); caffeine (p.782·1).

**K-Profen** *Medix, Mex.*
Ketoprofen (p.51·2).
*Musculoskeletal, joint, and peri-articular disorders.*

**Kraftol** *Profarb, Braz.†.*
Vitamin and mineral preparation (p.1417·1).

**Krallendorn** *Immodal, Austria.*
Uncaria tomentosa.
*Rheumatoid arthritis.*

**Krama**
Note. This name is used for preparations of different composition.
*Duncan, Arg.*
Alprazolam (p.668·3).
*Anxiety.*

*Mibo, Ital.*
Barrier cream.

**Kranit Nova** *Codali, Belg.*
Caffeine (p.782·1); paracetamol (p.76·2); propyphenazone (p.85·3).
*Headache.*

**Kratalgin** *Kwizda, Austria.*
Ibuprofen (p.45·3).
*Pain.*

**Kratium** *Medochemie, Hong Kong.*
Diazepam (p.690·1).
*Alcohol withdrawal syndrome; anxiety; febrile convulsions; premedication; skeletal muscle spasm; sleep disorders; status epilepticus.*

**Kratofin simplex** *Kwizda, Austria.*
Paracetamol (p.76·2).
*Fever; pain.*

**Krauter Hustensaft** *Apomedica, Austria.*
Thyme (p.1755·2); ononis (p.1723·3); primula root (p.1735·1); liquorice (p.1270·2); castanea vulgaris; sambucus (p.1741·3).
*Catarrh; coughs.*

**Krauterdoktor Beruhigungstropfen** *Kollerics, Austria.*
Lupulus (p.1708·1); melissa (p.1711·1); orange flower (p.1723·3).
*Anxiety; nervous disorders.*

**Krauterdoktor Entschlackungs-Elixier** *Kollerics, Austria.*
Taraxacum (p.1751·3); viola tricolor; manna (p.1273·1); bitter-orange peel (p.1723·3); rose fruit (p.1740·1).
*Tonic.*

**Krauterdoktor Entspannungs- und Einschlaftropfen** *Kollerics, Austria.*
Valerian (p.1762·2); lupulus (p.1708·1); melissa (p.1711·1).
*Anxiety disorders; sleep disorders.*

**Krauterdoktor Entwasserungs-Elixier** *Kollerics, Austria.*
Birch leaf (p.1660·3); equisetum (p.1684·1); urtica (p.1762·1).
*Urinary-tract disorders.*

**Krauterdoktor Erkaltungstropfen** *Kollerics, Austria.*
Sambucus (p.1741·3); tilia (p.1756·2); centaury (p.1669·2).
*Cold symptoms.*

**Krauterdoktor Gallentreibende Tropfen** *Kollerics, Austria.*
Taraxacum (p.1751·3); achillea (p.1646·2); absinthium (p.1645·1).
*Biliary-tract disorders.*

**Krauterdoktor Harnstein- und Nierengriesstropfen** *Kollerics, Austria.*
Ononis (p.1723·3); taraxacum (p.1751·3); centaury (p.1669·2).
*Urinary-tract disorders.*

**Krauterdoktor Hustentropfen** *Kollerics, Austria.*
Fennel (p.1687·2); primula root (p.1735·1); thyme (p.1755·2).
*Catarrh; coughs.*

**Krauterdoktor Krampf- und Reizhustensirup** *Kollerics, Austria.*
Aniseed (p.1655·2); drosera (p.1683·1); thyme (p.1755·2).
*Coughs.*

**Krauterdoktor Magen-Darmtropfen** *Kollerics, Austria.*
Valerian (p.1762·2); caraway (p.1667·2); melissa (p.1711·1).
*Gastrointestinal disorders.*

**Krauterdoktor Nerven-Tonikum** *Kollerics, Austria.*
Valerian (p.1762·2); lupulus (p.1708·1); melissa (p.1711·1).
*Anxiety; nervousness; sleep disorders.*

**Krauterdoktor Rosmarin-Wein** *Kollerics, Austria.*
Rosemary (p.1740·2); melissa (p.1711·1).
*Circulatory disorders.*

**Krauterdoktor Verdauungsfordernde Tropfen** *Kollerics, Austria.*
Angelica (p.1655·1); centaury (p.1669·2); absinthium (p.1645·1).
*Gastrointestinal disorders.*

**Krauterelixier** *Bittner, Austria.*
Gentian (p.1692·2); chamomile (p.1669·3); peppermint oil (p.1283·2).
*Gastrointestinal disorders.*

**Krautergeist S** *Jukunda, Ger.†.*
Melissa; sloe; ginger; melissa oil; rosemary oil; lavender oil; capsicum oil; cinnamon oil; clove oil (p.1417·1).
*Tonic.*

**Krauterhaus Mag Kottas Babytee** *Kottas-Heldenberg, Austria.*
Chamomile (p.1669·3); mallow leaf (p.1709·3); melissa (p.1711·1); caraway (p.1667·2); fennel (p.1687·2).
*Gastrointestinal disorders.*

**Krauterhaus Mag Kottas Blasentee** *Kottas-Heldenberg, Austria.*
Birch leaf (p.1660·3); java tea (p.1702·3); herniaria (p.1697·1); couch-grass (p.1676·2); ononis (p.1723·3); peppermint leaf (p.1283·2).
*Urinary-tract disorders.*

**Krauterhaus Mag Kottas Entschlackungstee** *Kottas-Heldenberg, Austria.*
Birch leaf (p.1660·3); peppermint leaf (p.1283·2); taraxacum (p.1751·3); urtica (p.1762·1); ononis (p.1723·3); chamomile (p.1669·3).
*Diuretic.*

**Krauterhaus Mag Kottas Entwasserungstee** *Kottas-Heldenberg, Austria.*
Equisetum (p.1684·1); parsley root (p.1728·3); couch-grass (p.1676·2); solidago virgaurea (p.1748·3); urtica (p.1762·1); peppermint leaf (p.1283·2); calendula (p.1665·2).
*Urinary-tract disorders.*

**Krauterhaus Mag Kottas Fruhjahrs- und Herbstkurtee** *Kottas-Heldenberg, Austria.*
Peppermint leaf (p.1283·2); equisetum (p.1684·1); achillea (p.1646·2); urtica (p.1762·1); viola tricolor; calendula (p.1665·2); mallow flower (p.1709·3).
*Tonic.*

**Krauterhaus Mag Kottas Gallen- und Lebertee** *Kottas-Heldenberg, Austria.*
Mallow leaf (p.1709·3); peppermint leaf (p.1283·2); menyanthes (p.1712·1); agrimony (p.1649·1); taraxacum (p.1751·3); calendula (p.1665·2).
*Biliary-tract disorders.*

**Krauterhaus Mag Kottas Grippetee** *Kottas-Heldenberg, Austria.*
Sambucus (p.1741·3); tilia (p.1756·2); plantago lanceolata (p.1738·2); rose fruit (p.1740·1).
*Cold symptoms.*

**Krauterhaus Mag Kottas Husten- und Bronchialtee** *Kottas-Heldenberg, Austria.*
Verbascum flower (p.1764·1); althaea (p.1651·3); plantago lanceolata (p.1738·2); thyme (p.1755·2); mallow flower (p.1709·3).
*Catarrh; coughs; sore throat.*

**Krauterhaus Mag Kottas Magen- und Darmtee** *Kottas-Heldenberg, Austria.*
Chamomile (p.1669·3); mallow leaf (p.1709·3); melissa (p.1711·1); peppermint leaf (p.1283·2); achillea (p.1646·2); calendula (p.1665·2).
*Gastrointestinal disorders.*

**Krauterhaus Mag Kottas milder Abfuhrtee** *Kottas-Heldenberg, Austria.*
Prunus spinosa; fennel (p.1687·2); mallow leaf (p.1709·3); peppermint leaf (p.1283·2); rose fruit (p.1740·1).
*Constipation.*

**Krauterhaus Mag Kottas Nerven- und Schlaftee** *Kottas-Heldenberg, Austria.*
Bitter orange (p.1723·3); melissa (p.1711·1); peppermint leaf (p.1283·2); valerian (p.1762·2); lupulus (p.1708·1); calendula (p.1665·2).
*Anxiety disorders; sleep disorders.*

**Krauterhaus Mag Kottas Nierentee** *Kottas-Heldenberg, Austria.*
Java tea (p.1702·3); equisetum (p.1684·1); herniaria (p.1697·1); ononis (p.1723·3); rose fruit (p.1740·1); peppermint leaf (p.1283·2).
*Urinary-tract disorders.*

**Krauterhaus Mag Kottas Tee fur die Verdauung** *Kottas-Heldenberg, Austria.*
Mallow leaf (p.1709·3); peppermint leaf (p.1283·2); caraway (p.1667·2); absinthium (p.1645·1); bitter-orange peel (p.1723·3); calendula (p.1665·2).
*Gastrointestinal disorders.*

**Krauterhaus Mag Kottas Tee gegen Blahungen** *Kottas-Heldenberg, Austria.*
Mallow leaf (p.1709·3); peppermint leaf (p.1283·2); caraway (p.1667·2); fennel (p.1687·2); achillea (p.1646·2); calendula (p.1665·2).
*Flatulence.*

**Krauterhaus Mag Kottas Tee gegen Durchfall** *Kottas-Heldenberg, Austria.*
*Erwachsene Tee:* Tormentil (p.1757·2); chamomile (p.1669·3); mallow leaf (p.1709·3); myrtillus (p.1718·3); bitter-orange peel (p.1723·3); mallow flower (p.1709·3).
*Kinder Tee:* Chamomile (p.1669·3); mallow leaf (p.1709·3); myrtillus (p.1718·3); rubus fruticosus; aniseed (p.1655·2).
*Diarrhoea.*

**Krauterhaus Mag Kottas Wechseltee** *Kottas-Heldenberg, Austria.*
Melissa (p.1711·1); peppermint leaf (p.1283·2); achillea (p.1646·2); sage (p.1741·2); valerian (p.1762·2); chamomile (p.1669·3); calendula (p.1665·2).
*Menopausal disorders.*

**Krauterlax A** *Dolorgiet, Ger.*
Aloes (p.1248·2).
*Constipation.*

**Krauterlax-S** *Henk, Ger.†.*
Sennoside (p.1288·2).
*Constipation.*

**Krauterpfarrer Weidinger Rheumatee** *Kottas-Heldenberg, Austria.*
Urtica (p.1762·1); ononis (p.1723·3); birch leaf (p.1660·3); salix (p.87·3); valerian (p.1762·2).
*Musculoskeletal and joint disorders.*

**Krauterpfarrer Weidinger Tee bei Darmtragheit** *Kottas-Heldenberg, Austria.*
Angelica (p.1655·1); flos bellidis; althaea (p.1651·3); prunus spinosa; centaurea cyanus.
*Constipation.*

**Krauterpfarrer Weidinger Tee bei Fruhjahrsmudigkeit** *Kottas-Heldenberg, Austria.*
Vervain (p.1764·1); cowslip (p.1735·1); herba majoranae; peppermint leaf (p.1283·2); rosemary (p.1740·2).
*Circulatory disorders.*

**Krauterpfarrer Weidinger Tee bei Husten und Heiserkeit** *Kottas-Heldenberg, Austria.*
Wild thyme; eucalyptus leaf (p.1686·1); cowslip (p.1735·1); iceland moss; verbascum flower (p.1764·1).
*Catarrh; coughs.*

**Krauterpfarrer Weidinger Tee bei Nieren- und Blasenbeschwerden** *Kottas-Heldenberg, Austria.*
Equisetum (p.1684·1); solidago virgaurea (p.1748·3); rose fruit (p.1740·1); chamomile (p.1669·3); sweet basil.
*Kidney and bladder disorders.*

**Krauterpfarrer Weidinger Tee bei Schlafstorungen** *Kottas-Heldenberg, Austria.*
Apple; melissa (p.1711·1); lupulus (p.1708·1); orange flower (p.1724·1); agrimony (p.1649·1); hibiscus flower.
*Sleep disorders.*

**Krauterpfarrer Weidinger Tee bei Sodbrennen** *Kottas-Heldenberg, Austria.*
Coriander (p.1676·1); achillea (p.1646·2); chamomile (p.1669·3); asperula; centaury (p.1669·2).
*Gastrointestinal disorders.*

**Krauterpfarrer Weidinger Tee bei Verstimmungen und Erregungszustanden** *Kottas-Heldenberg, Austria.*
Wild thyme; melissa (p.1711·1); origanum vulgaris; orange flower (p.1724·1); viola odorata.
*Nervous disorders.*

**Krauterpfarrer Weidinger Tee bei Vollegefuhl und Blahungen** *Kottas-Heldenberg, Austria.*
Angelica (p.1655·1); fragaria leaf; melissa (p.1711·1); calamus (p.1664·1); fennel (p.1687·2).
*Gastrointestinal disorders.*

**Krauterpfarrer Weidinger Tee bei Wetterfuhligkeit und Kreislaufstorungen** *Kottas-Heldenberg, Austria.*
Melissa (p.1711·1); cowslip (p.1735·1); asperula; vervain (p.1764·1); sweet basil.
*Circulatory disorders.*

**Krauterpfarrer Weidinger Tee fur das Altersherz** *Kottas-Heldenberg, Austria.*
Crataegus (p.1677·1); melissa (p.1711·1); angelica (p.1655·1); rosemary (p.1740·2).
*Cardiac disorders.*

**Krauterpfarrer Weidinger Tee fur Leber und Galle** *Kottas-Heldenberg, Austria.*
Agrimony (p.1649·1); achillea (p.1646·2); rose fruit (p.1740·1); fennel (p.1687·2).
*Liver and biliary-tract disorders.*

**Krauterpfarrer Weidinger Tee zur Entschlackung** *Kottas-Heldenberg, Austria.*
Viola tricolor; solidago virgaurea (p.1748·3); taraxacum (p.1751·3); urtica (p.1762·1); sambucus (p.1741·3).
*Tonic.*

**Krauterpfarrer Weidinger Tee zur Entwasserung** *Kottas-Heldenberg, Austria.*
Parsley root (p.1728·3); ononis (p.1723·3); tormentil root (p.1757·2); birch leaf (p.1660·2); rosemary (p.1740·2).
*Urinary-tract disorders.*

**Krauterpfarrer Weidinger Tee zur Starkung der Abwehrkrafte** *Kottas-Heldenberg, Austria.*
Rose fruit (p.1740·1); satureja montana; cichorium intybus; juglans regia.
*Tonic.*

**Krebsilasi** *Wyeth Lederle, Ital.*
Pancrelipase (p.1725·3).
*Cystic fibrosis; malabsorption syndromes.*

**Kredex**
*Roche, Austral.; Roche, Belg.; Roche, Fr.; SmithKline Beecham, Ital.†; Roche, Norw.; Lusofarmaco, Port.†; Roche, Spain†; Roche, Swed.*
Carvedilol (p.881·1).
*Angina pectoris; heart failure; hypertension.*

**Kreislauf Katovit** *Boehringer Ingelheim, Ger.†.*
Etilefrine hydrochloride (p.914·1).
*Hypotension.*

**Kreislaufja** *OTW, Ger.*
Homoeopathic preparation.

**Kreislauftropen** *APS, Ger.†.*
Crataegus (p.1677·1); camphor (p.1665·3).
Formerly known as Cardiagen.
*Cardiovascular disorders.*

**Kremil** *Therapharma, Thai.; Great Eastern, Thai.*
Aluminium hydroxide-magnesium carbonate co-dried gel (p.1250·1); simeticone (p.1289·2).
*Gastrointestinal hyperacidity; peptic ulcer.*

**Kremil-S** *Great Eastern, Thai.; Therapharma, Thai.*
Aluminium hydroxide-magnesium carbonate co-dried gel (p.1250·1); simeticone (p.1289·2); dicycloverine hydrochloride (p.481·2).
*Gastrointestinal disorders.*

**Krenosin**
*Sanofi Synthelabo, Fr.; Sanofi Synthelabo, Ital.; Sanofi Synthelabo, Mex.*
Adenosine (p.851·2).
*Diagnosis of arrhythmias; paroxysmal supraventricular tachycardia.*

**Krenosine** Sanofi Synthelabo, Switz.
Adenosine (p.851·2).
*Supraventricular tachycardia.*

**Kreon**
Solvay, Austria; Solvay, Ger.; Solvay, Port.; Solvay, Spain.
Pancreatin (p.1725·3).
*Pancreatic insufficiency.*

**Kresse** Pharmacia Upjohn, Spain†.
Minoxidil (p.960·1).
*Alopecia.*

**Kreuzlinger Klosterliniment** Luond, Switz.
Salicylic acid (p.1157·1); camphor (p.1665·3); plant extracts.
*Musculoskeletal, joint, and soft-tissue disorders.*

**Kriadex** Psicofarma, Mex.
Clonazepam (p.359·1).
*Anxiety; epilepsy; mania; obsessive-compulsive disorder; panic disorders.*

**Kriolen** Rafarm, Gr.
Ambroxol hydrochloride (p.1114·3).
*Respiratory disorders associated with viscous mucus.*

**Kriptiser** Serral, Mex.
Bromocriptine (p.1202·3).

**Kripton** Alphapharm, Austral.
Bromocriptine mesilate (p.1200·3).
*Acromegaly; hyperprolactinaemia; lactation inhibition; parkinsonism.*

**Kriptonal** Chemopharma, Chile.
Bromocriptine (p.1202·3).
*Acromegaly; benign breast disorders; female infertility; hyperprolactinaemia; lactation inhibition; menstrual disorders; parkinsonism; prolactinomas.*

**Krisovin**
Upha, Malaysia; Beacons, Singapore.
Griseofulvin (p.400·3).
*Fungal skin, hair, and nail infections.*

**Kristalose** Bertek, USA.
Lactulose (p.1269·1).
*Constipation.*

**Kritel** Monserrat, Arg.
Sodium picosulfate (p.1289·3).
*Bowel evacuation; constipation.*

**Krol** Benitol, Arg.
Ketoconazole (p.403·3).
*Dandruff; fungal skin infections.*

**Kronel** Hebron, Braz.
Pistacia lentiscus.
*Wounds.*

**Kronofed-A** Ferndale, USA.
Pseudoephedrine hydrochloride (p.1129·2); chlorphenamine maleate (p.427·3).
*Respiratory-tract congestion.*

**Krophan N** Repha, Ger.
Bladderwrack (p.1742·3); potassium iodide (p.1598·1); thyreoidinum.
*Iodine-deficiency disorders.*

**Krucef** Krugher, Ital.
Cefonicid sodium (p.174·2).
Lidocaine hydrochloride (p.1377·3) is included in this preparation to alleviate the pain of injection.
*Gram-negative bacterial infections.*

**Kruschels** Pharmethic, Belg.†.
Dried magnesium sulfate (p.1229·1); sodium chloride (p.1233·3); anhydrous sodium sulfate (p.1290·1); potassium sulfate (p.1232·2); potassium chloride (p.1232·2).
*Constipation.*

**Kruses Fluid Magnesia** Felton, Austral.†.
Magnesium bicarbonate.
*Gastrointestinal hyperacidity.*

**Kryobulin** Immuno, Braz.†.
A factor VIII preparation (p.751·1).
*Haemorrhagic disorders.*

**Kryobulin TIM 3** Immuno, Spain†.
A factor VIII preparation (p.751·1).
*Factor VIII deficiency.*

**Kryobulin TIM 3-I** Immuno, Ital.†.
A factor VIII preparation (p.751·1).
*Haemorrhagic disorders.*

**Kryobuline S-TIM 3** Immuno, Switz.†.
A factor VIII preparation (p.751·1).
*Haemophilia A; von Willebrand's disease.*

**Kryptocur**
Aventis, Austria; Aventis, Belg.†; Aventis, Ger.; Aventis, Ital.
Gonadorelin (p.1325·1).
*Cryptorchidism.*

Aventis, Switz.
Gonadorelin acetate (p.1325·2).
*Cryptorchidism.*

**KSR**
Alphapharm, Austral.; Alphapharm, Hong Kong; Alphapharm, Malaysia; Merck, Malaysia; Alphapharm, Singapore; Merck, Singapore.
Potassium chloride (p.1232·2).
*Hypokalaemia.*

**K-SR** Pacific, NZ.
Potassium chloride (p.1232·2).
*Potassium supplement.*

**K-Tab** Abbott, USA.
Potassium chloride (p.1232·2).
*Hypokalaemia; potassium depletion.*

**K-Thrombin** Sigma, NZ.
Menadione sodium bisulfite (p.1466·3).
*Prothrombin deficiency; vitamin K deficiency.*

**Kudona** Synmosa, Singapore.
Glucosamine sulfate (p.1694·1).
*Maintenance of healthy joints and cartilage.*

**Kudrox Double Strength** Schwarz, USA†.
Aluminium hydroxide (p.1249·2); magnesium hydroxide (p.1272·2); simeticone (p.1289·2).
*Hyperacidity.*

**Kuhlprednon** Gerot, Austria.
Prednisolone (p.1108·1).
*Skin disorders.*

**Kupa** M & H, Thai.
Bromhexine hydrochloride (p.1115·3); guaifenesin (p.1122·1).
*Respiratory-tract disorders associated with increased or viscous mucus.*

**Kuracid** Gea, Denm.
Ranitidine hydrochloride (p.1285·2).
*Acid aspiration; gastro-oesophageal reflux; peptic ulcer; Zollinger-Ellison syndrome.*

**Kurapel** Elvetium, Arg.
Silicone oil (p.1482·1).
*Barrier preparation.*

**Kurgan**
APS, Port.; Normon, Spain.
Cefazolin sodium (p.170·3).
Lidocaine hydrochloride (p.1377·3) may be included in the intramuscular injection to alleviate the pain of injection.
*Bacterial infections.*

**Kurom** Grunenthal, Chile.
Codeine phosphate (p.27·1); pseudoephedrine hydrochloride (p.1129·2); chlorphenamine maleate (p.427·3).
*Coughs; nasal congestion.*

**Kuson** Labitec, Spain†.
Potassium hydroxide (p.1734·2).
*Verrucas; warts.*

**Kutapressin** Schwarz, USA†.
Liver-derivative complex.
*Skin disorders.*

**Kutesan** Plurisystem, Ital.
Emollient.

**Kutrase** Schwarz, USA.
Lipase; amylase (p.1654·2); protease.
Formerly contained lipase, amylase, protease, cellulase, hyoscyamine sulfate, and phenyltoloxamine citrate.
*Functional dyspepsia devoid of organic pathology (nervous dyspepsia).*

**Ku-Zyme** Schwarz, USA.
Lipase; amylase (p.1654·2); protease.
*Functional dyspepsia due to enzyme deficiency or imbalance.*

**Ku-Zyme HP** Schwarz, USA.
Pancrelipase (p.1725·3).
*Pancreatic insufficiency.*

**Kvilla** Pharmacia, Fin.
Quillaia (p.1416·1); ammonium chloride (p.1115·2).
*Coughs.*

**KW** Lagos, Arg.
Aloe vera (p.1141·3); camphor (p.1665·3); mallow (p.1709·3); chamomile (p.1669·3); ethyl linoleate.
*Pruritus.*

**Kwai**
Kwizda, Austria; Lichtwer, Canad.; Lichtwer, Ger.; Solvay, Ital.; Lichtwer, Switz.; Lichtwer, UK.
Garlic (p.1691·1).
*Atherosclerosis; dietary supplement.*

**Kwan Loong Oil** Haw Par, Canad.
Methyl salicylate (p.59·3); menthol (p.1711·3); eucalyptus oil (p.1686·2).

**Kwelcof** Ascher, USA.
Hydrocodone tartrate (p.45·1); guaifenesin (p.1122·1).
*Coughs.*

**Kwell**
Note. A similar name is used for preparations of different composition (see Kwells, below).
GlaxoSmithKline, Arg.; GlaxoSmithKline, Braz.
Permethrin (p.1508·3).
*Pediculosis.*

**Kwellada** Reed & Carnrick, Canad.†.
Lindane (p.1506·3).
*Pediculosis; scabies.*

**Kwellada-P** Reed & Carnrick, Canad.
Permethrin (p.1508·3).
*Pediculosis; scabies.*

**Kwells**
Note. A similar name is used for preparations of different composition (see Kwell, above).
Roche Consumer, Austral.; Roche Consumer, Irl.; Roche Consumer, UK.
Hyoscine hydrobromide (p.483·3).
*Motion sickness.*

**Kwicap** Cevallos, Arg.
Cefaclor (p.167·1).
*Bacterial infections.*

**Kwikprep** Dendy, Austral.†.
Monobasic sodium phosphate (p.1230·3); dibasic sodium phosphate (p.1231·1).
*Bowel evacuation; constipation.*

**Kwim** Duopharm, Ger.
Vitamin A palmitate (p.1453·1); riboflavin sodium phosphate (p.1456·1).
*Eye disorders.*

**K-Y**
Johnson & Johnson Medical, Fr.; Ethnor, India; Johnson & Johnson, Israel; Ethicon, Ital.; Johnson & Johnson, NZ; Johnson & Johnson, Switz.†; Johnson & Johnson, UK; Johnson & Johnson, USA.
Lubricating gel.
*Aid in ultrasound scanning; lubrication of mucous membranes and instruments.*

**K-Y Plus Spermicidal Lubricant** Johnson & Johnson, Canad.
Nonoxinol 9 (p.1413·3).
Formerly known as K-Y Personal Lubricant.
*Contraceptive; vaginal lubricant.*

**Kyaugutt** Krewel, Ger.†.
Crataegus (p.1677·1).
*Heart failure.*

**Kybernin**
Aventis Behring, Braz.; Aventis Behring, Ger.; Aventis Behring, Switz.
An antithrombin III preparation (p.742·2).
*Antithrombin III deficiency.*

**Kybernin P**
Aventis Behring, Austria; Gerolimatos (Γερολυματος), Gr.; Aventis Behring, Ital.; Aventis Behring, Spain.
Antithrombin III (p.742·2).
*Antithrombin III deficiency.*

**Kymazol** Rafarm, Gr.
Simvastatin (p.997·1).
*Primary hypercholesterolaemia.*

**Kyolarte** Kyorin, Thai.
Electrolyte infusion with glucose (p.1217·1).
*Fluid and electrolyte disorders.*

**Kyolic**
Quest, Canad.; Quest, UK.
Garlic (p.1691·1).

**Kyolic 101** Quest, Canad.
Garlic (p.1691·1); brewers yeast; kelp (p.1742·3).

**Kyolic 102** Quest, Canad.
Garlic (p.1691·1); enzyme complex; rice protein complex.

**Kyolic 103** Quest, Canad.
Garlic (p.1691·1); vitamin C; astragulus (p.1417·1).

**Kyolic 104** Quest, Canad.
Garlic (p.1691·1); lecithin (p.1706·1).

**Kyolic 106** Quest, Canad.
Garlic (p.1691·1); vitamin E; crataegus; cayenne (p.1417·1).

**Kyolic Formula 103** Quest, Canad.
Calcium ascorbate (p.1460·2).
*Dietary supplement.*

**Kyolic Formula 105** Quest, Canad.
Betacarotene, selenium, vitamin C, and vitamin E (p.1417·1).

**Kyolic Formula 106** Quest, Canad.
*d*-Alpha tocoferil acid succinate (p.1465·1).

**Kyolic Super Formula** Primula, Arg.
Garlic (p.1691·1).
*Hyperlipidaemias; hypertension.*

**Kytinon** Asmopul, Arg.
Porcine skin (p.1158·1); mucopolysaccharides; chloroxylenol (p.1177·2).
*Wounds.*

**Kytinon ABC** Asmopul, Arg.
Lidocaine (p.1377·3); porcine skin (p.1158·1); polysaccharides.
*Mouth disorders.*

**Kytril**
Roche, Arg.; Mayne, Austral.; Roche, Austria; Roche, Belg.; Roche, Braz.; Roche, Canad.; Roche, Chile; Roche, Denm.; Roche, Fin.; Roche, Fr.; Roche, Gr.; Roche, Hong Kong; Roche, Irl.; SmithKline Beecham, Israel; Roche, Ital.; SmithKline Beecham, Mex.; SmithKline Beecham, Neth.; Roche, Norw.; Roche, Port.; Roche, S.Afr.; Roche, Singapore; Roche, Spain; Roche, Swed.; Roche, Switz.; SmithKline Beecham, Thai.; Roche, UK; SmithKline Beecham, USA.
Granisetron hydrochloride (p.1267·1).
*Nausea and vomiting.*

**Kytta** Merck, Ger.
Glycol salicylate (p.44·3).
*Inflammation; pain; superficial vascular disorders.*

**Kytta Baume** Melisana, Switz.
Comfrey (p.1675·2); methyl nicotinate (p.59·2).
*Musculoskeletal pain.*

**Kytta Pommade** Melisana, Switz.
Comfrey (p.1675·2); pine-needle oil; lavender oil (p.1705·2).
*Musculoskeletal pain; soft-tissue injury; wounds.*

**Kytta-Balsam f** Merck, Ger.
Comfrey (p.1675·2); methyl nicotinate (p.59·2).
*Local circulatory disorders; musculoskeletal, joint, and soft-tissue disorders.*

**Kytta-Cor** Merck, Ger.
Crataegus (p.1677·1).
*Cardiac disorders.*

**Kytta-Femin** Merck, Ger.
Agnus castus (p.1649·1).
*Mastalgia; menstrual disorders.*

**Kytta-Kava** Merck, Ger.†.
Kava (p.1703·2).
*Anxiety disorders.*

**Kytta-Kliman** Merck, Ger.†.
Cimicifuga (p.1671·3).
*Menopausal disorders.*

**Kytta-Modal** Merck, Ger.
Hypericum (p.299·1).
*Depression.*

**Kytta-Plasma f** Merck, Ger.
Comfrey (p.1675·2).
*Soft-tissue disorders.*

**Kytta-Rheumabad N** Merck, Ger.
Norway spruce oil.
*Bath additive; rheumatism.*

**Kytta-Salbe f** Merck, Ger.
Comfrey (p.1675·2).
*Soft-tissue disorders.*

**Kytta-Sedativum f** Merck, Ger.
Valerian (p.1762·2); lupulus (p.1708·1); passion flower (p.1729·1).
*Agitation; sleep disorders.*

**Kytta-Thermopack** Merck, Ger.
Peat; medicinal mud.
*Hemiplegia; musculoskeletal, joint, and soft-tissue disorders; myelitis.*

**Kyypakkaus** Orion, Fin.
Hydrocortisone (p.1103·3).
*Bee and wasp stings; snake bites.*

**L 25** Lehning, Fr.
Homoeopathic preparation.

**L 28** Lehning, Fr.
Homoeopathic preparation.

**L 52** Lehning, Fr.
Homoeopathic preparation.

**L 72** Lehning, Fr.
Homoeopathic preparation.

**L 114** Lehning, Fr.
Homoeopathic preparation.

**LA-12** Hyrex, USA.
Hydroxocobalamin (p.1458·2).
*Schilling test; vitamin $B_{12}$ deficiency.*

**LA Morph** Pharmacia, NZ.
Morphine sulfate (p.60·2).
*Pain.*

**Lab/A** Tosi, Ital.
*Lactobacillus* (p.1704·2).
*Vulvovaginal candidiasis.*

**Labdiazina** Lab, Port.
Sulfadiazine (p.258·2).
*Bacterial infections.*

**Label** Asta Medica, Braz.
Ranitidine hydrochloride (p.1285·2).
*Acid aspiration; gastro-oesophageal reflux; gastrointestinal haemorrhage; peptic ulcer; Zollinger-Ellison syndrome.*

**Labello Active** Beiersdorf, Canad.†.
*SPF 15:* Octinoxate (p.1154·3); oxybenzone (p.1154·3).
*Sunscreen.*

**Labello UV** Beiersdorf, Canad.
*SPF 30:* Octocrilene (p.1154·3); octinoxate (p.1154·3); oxybenzone (p.1154·3); titanium dioxide (p.1160·3).
*Sunscreen.*

**Labelphen** Chrispa (Χρισπα), Gr.
Ketotifen fumarate (p.788·1).
*Allergic rhinitis; asthma.*

**Labenda** Progress, Thai.
Albendazole (p.101·2).
*Worm infections.*

**Labentrol** Chrispa (Χρισπα), Gr.
Ciprofloxacin hydrochloride (p.188·2).
*Bacterial infections.*

**Labfcilina** Faria, Braz.†.
Ampicillin trihydrate (p.157·2); bromelains (p.1662·2).
*Bacterial infections.*

**Labigeron** Teuto, Braz.
Cinnarizine (p.428·3).

**Labileno** Faes, Spain.
Lamotrigine (p.363·3).
*Epilepsy.*

**Labilex** Pharmaten (Φαρματεν), Gr.
Ceftriaxone sodium (p.182·3).
*Bacterial infections.*

**Labimion** Labinca, Arg.
Etoposide (p.551·3).
*Malignant neoplasms.*

**Labiosan** Schoenenberger, Ger.
Zinc oxide (p.1163·2).
*Lip disorders.*

**Labirin** Apsen, Braz.
Betahistine hydrochloride (p.1660·1).
*Vestibular disorders.*

**Labisan** Schutz, Austria.
Phenol (p.1188·1); zinc oxide (p.1163·2); precipitated sulfur (p.1158·2).
*Herpes labialis.*

**Labistatin** Labinca, Arg.
Simvastatin (p.997·1).
*Hyperlipidaemias.*

**Labiton** Laboratories for Applied Biology, UK.
Thiamine (p.1455·2); caffeine (p.782·1); kola nuts (p.1765·3); alcohol.
*Tonic.*

**Labitrix** Bioquimico, Mex.†.
Metronidazole (p.607·2).

**Labocaina** Combe, Ital.
Benzocaine (p.1370·3); resorcinol (p.1156·3); chlorothymol (p.1177·2).
*Pruritus.*

**Labocane** Combe, Ger.
Benzocaine (p.1370·3).
Formerly contained benzocaine, benzyl cinnamate, and benzyl benzoate.
*Eczema; pruritus.*

**Labocne** *Labomed, Chile.*
Erythromycin (p.208·1).
*Acne.*

**Labocton** *Viofar, Gr.*
Pefloxacin mesilate (p.241·3).
*Bacterial infections.*

**Labopal** *GlaxoSmithKline, Spain.*
Benazepril hydrochloride (p.867·2).
*Heart failure; hypertension; renal failure.*

**Labosalic** *Labomed, Chile.*
Betamethasone dipropionate (p.1093·1); salicylic acid (p.1157·1).
*Skin disorders.*

**Labosept**
*Laboratories for Applied Biology, Irl.†; Laboratories for Applied Biology, UK.*
Dequalinium chloride (p.1178·1).
*Mouth and throat infections.*

**Labosona** *Labomed, Chile.*
Betamethasone dipropionate (p.1093·1).
*Skin disorders.*

**Labosona G** *Labomed, Chile.*
Betamethasone dipropionate (p.1093·1); gentamicin sulfate (p.217·1).
*Infected skin disorders.*

**Labosona N** *Labomed, Chile.*
Betamethasone dipropionate (p.1093·1); neomycin sulfate (p.235·1).
*Infected skin disorders.*

**Labotensil** *Labomed, Chile.*
Atenolol (p.865·2).
*Angina pectoris; arrhythmias; hypertension.*

**Laboterol** *Labomed, Chile.*
Clotrimazole (p.396·2).
*Fungal skin and nail infections.*

**Laboxantryl** *Chrispa (Χρισπα), Gr.*
Mesalazine (p.1273·2).
*Inflammatory bowel disease.*

**Labrocol** *Lagap, UK†.*
Labetalol hydrochloride (p.943·3).
*Angina pectoris; hypertension.*

**Labstix**
*Bayer, Austral.†; Bayer, Canad.†; Bayer Diagnostics, Irl.; Bayer Diagnostici, Ital.; Bayer Diagnostics, UK; Bayer, USA.*
Test for pH, protein, glucose, ketones, and blood in urine.

**Labstix SG**
*Bayer, Canad.†; Bayer Diagnostics, UK.*
Test for pH, protein, glucose, ketones, blood, and specific gravity in urine.

**Laburide** *Wolfs, Belg.*
Pheneturide (p.367·3).
*Epilepsy.*

**Labycarbol** *Arlex, Mex.†.*
Methocarbamol (p.1395·1).

**Labydon** *Arlex, Mex.†.*
Nalidixic acid (p.234·1).

**Labymetacyn** *Arlex, Mex.†.*
Indometacin (p.47·3).

**Labypurol** *Arlex, Mex.†.*
Allopurinol (p.412·2).

**Labysal** *Arlex, Mex.†.*
Aspirin (p.15·1).

**Lac 4 n** *Parke, Davis, Ger.†.*
Almasilate (p.1248·2).
*Gastrointestinal disorders.*

**Lacalut** *Pietrasanta, Ital.*
Aluminium lactate (p.1653·1); aluminium fluoride (p.1445·3); aluminium hydroxide (p.1249·2); silicon dioxide (p.1581·3).
*Gum disorders; oral hygiene; sensitive teeth.*

**Lacbon** *Sankyo, Thai.*
*Lactobacillus* spp. (p.1704·2).
*Constipation; restoration of intestinal flora.*

**Laccoderme a l'huile de cade** *Pierre Fabre, Fr.*
Rectified cade oil (p.1159·2); hyoscyamus oil (p.485·2); salicylic acid (p.1157·1).
*Psoriasis; seborrhoeic dermatitis.*

**Lacdigest** *Grogg, Switz.*
Tilactase (p.1756·2).
*Lactase deficiency.*

**Lac-Dol** *Douglas, Austral.*
Lactulose (p.1269·1).
*Constipation; hepatic encephalopathy.*

**Laceran**
*Beiersdorf, Ger.†; Beiersdorf, Port.†.*
Urea (p.1162·2).
*Dry skin disorders.*

**Laceran Piel Seca** *Beiersdorf, Chile.*
A range of emollients.
*Dry skin.*

**Lacerdermol** *Lacer, Spain.*
Biotin (p.1423·2); calcium pantothenate (p.1442·3); vitamin A (p.1451·2).
*Blepharitis; fragile nails; glossitis; skin disorders.*

**Lacerdermol Complex** *Lacer, Spain.*
Vitamin B substances (p.1417·1); vitamin A (p.1451·2).
*Seborrhoeic blepharitis; skin disorders.*

**Lacermucin** *Lacer, Spain†.*
Tyloxapol (p.1416·3).
*Respiratory-tract disorders.*

**Lacerol** *Lacer, Spain.*
Diltiazem hydrochloride (p.900·1).
*Angina pectoris; hypertension.*

**Lacgel** *Lyka, India.*
Lactic acid (p.1704·1); glycogen.
*Vaginal disorders.*

**Lachemistol**
*Richter, Austria; Wiedemann, Ger.*
Homoeopathic preparation.

**Lachess** *Knop, Chile.*
Homoeopathic preparation.

**Lac-Hydrin**
*Bristol-Myers Squibb, Braz.; Westwood-Squibb, Canad.; Bristol-Myers Squibb, Mex.†; Bristol-Myers Squibb, NZ; Westwood-Squibb, USA.*
Ammonium lactate (p.1142·3).
*Dry skin disorders.*

**Lachydrin** *Bristol-Myers Squibb, Singapore.*
Lactic acid (p.1704·1).
*Dry skin.*

**Laciken** *Kendrick, Mex.*
Aciclovir (p.626·1).
*Viral infections.*

**Lacimen** *Menarini, Spain.*
Lacidipine (p.944·2).
*Hypertension.*

**Lacin** *Vana, Thai.*
Clindamycin hydrochloride (p.194·2).
*Bacterial infections.*

**Lacipil**
*GlaxoSmithKline, Arg.; GlaxoSmithKline, Braz.; Glaxo Wellcome, Gr.; GlaxoSmithKline, Hong Kong; GlaxoSmithKline, Ital.; GlaxoSmithKline, Malaysia; Glaxo Wellcome, Mex.; Glaxo Wellcome, Port.; GlaxoSmithKline, Singapore; GlaxoSmithKline, Spain.*
Lacidipine (p.944·2).
*Hypertension.*

**Lacirex** *Guidotti, Ital.*
Lacidipine (p.944·2).
*Hypertension.*

**Laclorene** *Spedrog, Arg.*
Arginine aspartate (p.1421·1).

**Laclorhex** *Sertex, Arg.*
Chlorhexidine gluconate (p.1173·2).
*Skin disinfection.*

**LAC-Lotion** *Paddock, USA.*
Ammonium lactate (p.1142·3).
*Emollient.*

**Lacoerdin Mg Plus** *Weber & Weber, Ger.*
Crataegus (p.1677·1); magnesium aspartate (p.1227·3); magnesium phosphate (p.1228·1); magnesium sulfate (p.1228·2).
*Cardiovascular disorders.*

**Lacoerdin-N** *Weber & Weber, Ger.†.*
Convallaria (p.1675·3); potassium aspartate (p.1233·1); magnesium aspartate (p.1227·3); magnesium phosphate trihydrate (p.1228·1); magnesium sulfate (p.1228·2); crataegus (p.1677·1).
*Cardiovascular disorders.*

**Lac-Oph** *Seng, Thai.*
Hypromellose (p.1579·3) (p.1164·2).
*Dry eyes; wetting solution for contact lenses.*

**Lacophtal** *Winzer, Ger.*
Povidone (p.1581·2).
*Dry eye disorders.*

**Lacovin** *Galderma, Spain.*
Minoxidil (p.960·1).
*Alopecia androgenetica.*

**Lacribase** *Tubilux, Ital.*
Benzalkonium chloride (p.1168·3).
*Eye disinfection.*

**Lacrifluid** *Europhta, Mon.*
Carbomer 940 (p.1577·2).
*Dry eyes.*

**Lacrigel**
*Note. This name is used for preparations of different composition.*
*Winzer, Ger.*
Hyetellose (p.1579·2).
*Dry eyes.*

*Farmigea, Ital.; Europhta, Mon.*
Carbomer 940 (p.1577·2).
*Dry eyes.*

**Lacri-Gel** *Medical Ophthalmics, USA.*
Soft paraffin (p.1479·3); liquid paraffin (p.1479·1); wool fat (p.1483·1).
*Dry eyes.*

**Lacrigel A** *Novartis Ophthalmics, Braz.*
Vitamin A (p.1451·2).
*Dry eyes.*

**Lacril**
*Note. This name is used for preparations of different composition.*
*Allergan, Braz.; Allergan, Denm.*
Polyvinyl alcohol (p.1581·1).
*Dry eyes.*

*Allergan, Canad.; Allergan, USA.*
Hypromellose (p.1579·3).
Formerly contained methylcellulose in *Canad.*
*Dry eyes.*

**Lacri-Lube**
*Allergan, Austral.; Allergan, Canad.; Allergan, Chile; Allergan, Irl.; Allergan, Israel†; Allergan, UK; Allergan, USA.*
White soft paraffin (p.1479·3); liquid paraffin (p.1479·1); wool alcohol (p.1482·3) or wool fat (p.1483·1).
*Dry eyes.*

**Lacrilube**
*Note. This name is used for preparations of different composition.*
*Allergan, Ital.; Allergan, Malaysia; Allergan, NZ; Allergan, S.Afr.†; Allergan, Singapore.*
White soft paraffin (p.1479·3); liquid paraffin (p.1479·1); wool alcohol (p.1482·3) or wool fat (p.1483·1).
*Dry eyes.*

*Allergan, Spain.*
Soft paraffin (p.1479·3).
*Dry eyes.*

**Lacrilux** *Tubilux, Ital.*
Polyvinyl alcohol (p.1581·1).
*Dry eyes.*

**Lacrima** *Alcon, Braz.*
Dextran 70 (p.746·2); hypromellose (p.1579·3).
*Dry eyes.*

**Lacrima Plus** *Alcon, Braz.*
Dextran 70 (p.746·2); hypromellose (p.1579·3).
*Dry eyes.*

**Lacrimal** *Allergan, Ger.*
Polyvinyl alcohol (p.1581·1).
*Dry eyes.*

**Lacrimal OK** *Allergan, Ger.*
Polyvinyl alcohol (p.1581·1); povidone (p.1581·2).
*Dry eyes.*

**Lacrimalfa** *INTES, Ital.*
Sodium chloride; sodium bicarbonate; sodium acid phosphate; magnesium sulfate.
*Dry eyes.*

**Lacrimart** *Baif, Ital.*
Methylcellulose (p.1580·2).
*Dry eyes; eye disinfection.*

**Lacrime** *Ogna, Ital.†.*
*Elixir:* Oleum pini sylvestris; storax (p.1749·3); cineole (p.1672·1).
*Pastilles:* Oleum pini sylvestris; storax (p.1749·3); cineole (p.1672·1); menthol (p.1711·3).
*Bronchial catarrh; coughs; sore throat.*

**Lacrimill** *Ottolenghi, Ital.*
Hypromellose (p.1579·3).
*Dry eyes; eye disinfection; eye irritation.*

**Lacrimol** *Fischer, Israel.*
*Eye drops:* Povidone (p.1581·2).
*Eye ointment:* White soft paraffin (p.1479·3); liquid paraffin (p.1479·1); wool fat (p.1483·1).
*Dry eyes.*

**Lacrinorm**
*Ophtapharma, Canad.; Chauvin, Fr.; Farmigea, Ital.; Bausch & Lomb, Switz.*
Carbomer 980 (p.1577·2).
*Dry eyes.*

**Lacripharma** *ICN, Arg.*
Sodium hyaluronate (p.1697·3).
*Dry eyes; keratitis.*

**Lacrisert**
*Sigma, Austral.; Merck Frosst, Canad.; Merck Sharp & Dohme, Denm.†; Merck Sharp & Dohme, Fin.; Merck Sharp & Dohme-Chibret, Fr.; Merck Sharp & Dohme, Ital.†; Merck Sharp & Dohme, Neth.; Merck Sharp & Dohme, Norw.; Merck Sharp & Dohme, S.Afr.†; Merck Sharp & Dohme, Swed.; Merck, USA.*
Hyprolose (p.1579·2).
*Dry eyes.*

**Lacrisic** *Alcon, Ger.*
Hypromellose (p.1579·3); povidone (p.1581·2); glycerol (p.1694·3).
*Dry eyes.*

**Lacrisifi**
*Craveri, Arg.; SIFI, Ital.; SIFI, Singapore.*
Hypromellose (p.1579·3).
*Dry eyes; eye irritation.*

**Lacrisol** *Bruschettini, Ital.*
Hypromellose (p.1579·3).
*Dry eyes; eye disinfection.*

**Lacri-Stulln** *Stulln, Ger.*
Povidone (p.1581·2).
*Dry eyes.*

**Lacri-Tears** *Medical Ophthalmics, USA.*
Hypromellose (p.1579·3); dextran (p.746·2).
*Dry eyes.*

**Lacromycin** *Fischer, Israel.*
Gentamicin sulfate (p.217·1).
*Eye infections.*

**Lacrycon** *Pharmacia, Switz.*
Sodium hyaluronate (p.1697·3); carbomer 981 (p.1577·2); glycerol (p.1694·3).
*Dry eyes.*

**Lacrypos** *Alcon, Fr.*
Chondroitin sulfate sodium (p.1670·2).
*Eye disorders.*

**Lacrystat** *Viatris, Belg.*
Hypromellose (p.1579·3); dextran 70 (p.746·2).
*Dry eyes.*

**Lacrytube** *Viatris, Belg.*
Liquid paraffin (p.1479·1); white soft paraffin (p.1479·3); wool fat (p.1483·1).
*Corneal protection in comatose or anaesthetised patients; keratoconjunctivitis sicca.*

**Lacryvisc**
*Alcon, Arg.; Alcon, Chile; Alcon, Fr.; Alcon, Hong Kong; Alcon, Port.; Alcon, Singapore; Alcon Cusi, Spain; Alcon, Swed.†; Alcon, Switz.; Alcon, Thai.*
Carbomer (p.1577·2).
*Dry eyes.*

**Lacson** *Aspen, S.Afr.*
Lactulose (p.1269·1).
*Constipation; hepatic encephalopathy.*

**Lactacyd**
*Rider, Chile; Sanofi Synthelabo, Hong Kong; Sanofi Synthelabo, Malaysia; GlaxoSmithKline Consumer, Port.; Sanofi Synthelabo, Singapore; Sanofi Synthelabo, Thai.*
Milk serum; lactic acid (p.1704·1).
*Skin disorders; vulvovaginal disorders.*

**Lactacyd Antibatterico** *GlaxoSmithKline Consumer, Ital.*
Triclosan (p.1195·2).
*Skin disinfection.*

**Lactacyd Derma**
*GlaxoSmithKline Sante, Fr.; GlaxoSmithKline Consumer, Ital.*
Milk serum; lactic acid (p.1704·1).
*Skin disorders.*

**Lactacyd Femina** *GlaxoSmithKline Sante, Fr.*
*Topical emulsion:* Milk serum; lactic acid (p.1704·1).
*Wipes:* Lactic acid (p.1704·1).
*Genital hygiene in females.*

**Lactacyd Intimo** *GlaxoSmithKline Consumer, Ital.*
Milk serum; lactic acid (p.1704·1).
*Genital hygiene.*

**Lactagel** *Creme d'Orient, Fr.†.*
Ammonium lactate (p.1142·3).
*Skin disorders.*

**Lacta-Gynecogel** *Medgenix, Belg.*
Lactic acid (p.1704·1).
*Anogenital infections.*

**Lactaid**
*Sunrise, Austral.†; McNeil Consumer, Canad.; Clonmel, Irl.†; Iketon, Ital.†; Myplan, UK†; McNeil Consumer, USA.*
Tilactase (p.1756·2) (derived from *Kluyveromyces lactis* or *Aspergillus oryzae*).
*Lactose intolerance.*

**Lactal** *Kabi, Swed.†.*
Lactic acid (p.1704·1); glycogen.
*Bacterial vaginosis.*

**Lactamax** *Beta, Arg.*
Cabergoline (p.1203·3).
*Hyperprolactinaemia; lactation inhibition; prolactinomas.*

**Lactar** *Creme d'Orient, Fr.†.*
Ammonium lactate (p.1142·3); cade oil (p.1159·2).
*Seborrhoeic dermatitis.*

**Lac-Tas** *Dominguez, Arg.*
Tilactase (p.1756·2).
*Lactose intolerance.*

**Lact-Easy** *Sunrise, Austral.†.*
Tilactase (p.1756·2).
*Lactose intolerance.*

**Lactec** *Otsuka, Jpn.*
Electrolyte infusion (p.1217·1).
*Fluid and electrolyte disorders.*

**Lactec D** *Otsuka, Jpn.*
Electrolyte infusion with glucose (p.1217·1).
*Carbohydrate source; fluid and electrolyte disorders.*

**Lactec G** *Otsuka, Jpn.*
Electrolyte infusion with d-sorbitol (p.1217·1).
*Carbohydrate source; fluid and electrolyte disorders.*

**Lactel** *Lactel, Fr.†.*
Nutritional supplement (p.1417·1).
*Lactose intolerance.*

**Lacteol**
*Menarini, Belg.; Lacteol, Fr.; Pohl, Ger.; Lacteol, Hong Kong; Bruschettini, Ital.; Biosaude, Port.; Lacteol, Singapore; Ramon Sala, Spain; Lacteol, Switz.; Lacteol, Thai.; Merck, Thai.*
*Lactobacillus acidophilus* (p.1704·2).
*Colopathy; diarrhoea; enterocolitis.*

**Lacteol Fort** *Carnot, Mex.*
*Lactobacillus acidophilus (Boucardii)* (p.1704·2).
*Diarrhoea; restoration of gastrointestinal flora.*

**Lacteol Forte** *Master, Chile.*
Lactobacillus acidophilus (p.1704·2).
*Diarrhoea.*

**Lactess** *Protein, Mex.†.*
Bromocriptine (p.1202·3).

**Lacticare**
*Note. This name is used for preparations of different composition.*
*Stiefel, Arg.; Stiefel, Braz.; Stiefel, Canad.; Stiefel, Chile; Stiefel, Fr.; Stiefel, Hong Kong; Stiefel, Irl.; Stiefel, Malaysia; Stiefel, Mex.; Stiefel, Singapore; Stiefel, Thai.; Stiefel, UK.*
Lactic acid (p.1704·1); sodium pidolate (p.1158·1).
*Dry skin disorders.*

*Stiefel, USA.*
Lactic acid (p.1704·1); liquid paraffin (p.1479·1).
*Emollient and moisturiser.*

**Lacticare-HC**
*Stiefel, Chile; Stiefel, Hong Kong; Stiefel, Mex.; Stiefel, USA.*
Hydrocortisone (p.1103·3).
*Skin disorders.*

**Lactiderm** *Cassara, Arg.*
Ammonium lactate (p.1142·3); urea (p.1162·2).
*Dry skin.*

**Lactiderm HC** *Cassara, Arg.*
Hydrocortisone (p.1103·3); ammonium lactate (p.1142·3); urea (p.1162·2).
*Skin disorders.*

**Lactidorm** *Galactopharm, Ger.*
Lupulus (p.1708·1).
*Anxiety.*

**Lactifero** *Bergamo, Braz.†.*
Urtica (p.1762·1); gentian (p.1692·2); calcium phosphate; sodium glycerophosphate; citric acid; lactic acid (p.1417·1).

**Lactigriet** Isdin, Port.
Dexpanthenol (p.1727·2); chlorhexidine (p.1173·2).
*Sore nipples.*

**Lactinex** Becton Dickinson, USA.
*Lactobacillus acidophilus* (p.1704·2); *Lactobacillus bulgaricus* (p.1704·2).
*Dietary supplement.*

**Lactinol** Pedinol, USA.
Lactic acid (p.1704·1).
*Dry skin.*

**Lactinol-E** Pedinol, USA.
Lactic acid (p.1704·1); vitamin E (p.1464·3).
*Dry skin.*

**Lactipan**
Byk, Braz.†; Ibi, Ital.
*Streptococcus lactis*; *Lactobacillus acidophilus* (p.1704·2); *Lactobacillus bulgaricus* (p.1704·2).
*Diarrhoea; maintenance of normal gastrointestinal flora.*

**Lactisan** Galactopharm, Ger.
Sour milk whey concentrate (p.1704·1).
*Gynaecological disorders; skin disinfection.*

**Lactisol** Galactopharm, Ger.
Lactic acid (p.1704·1).
*Coughs; gastrointestinal disorders; skin disorders; wounds.*

**Lactisona**
Stiefel, Port.; Stiefel, Spain.
Hydrocortisone (p.1103·3).
*Skin disorders.*

**Lactisporin** Medisint, Ital.
Lactic-acid-producing organisms (p.1704·2); dried yeast (p.1469·1); vitamin B substances (p.1417·1).
*Restoration of normal gastrointestinal flora.*

**Lactisyn** Franco-Indian, India.
*Lactobacillus lactis* (p.1704·2); *Lactobacillus acidophilus* (p.1704·2); *Streptococcus thermophilus* (p.1704·2); *Streptococcus lactis*.
*Aphthous stomatitis; diarrhoea.*

**Lactivis** Fitobucaneve, Ital.
*Capsules:* Vitamins (p.1417·1); *Lactobacillus acidophilus* (p.1704·2); dried yeast (p.1469·1); dried yogurt.
*Powder for oral liquid:* Vitamins (p.1417·1); lactic-acid-producing organisms (p.1704·2).
*Nutritional supplement.*

**Lacto Calamine**
Note. This name is used for preparations of different composition.
CSL, NZ.
Calamine (p.1144·1); hamamelis (p.1696·3).
*Insect bites; sunburn.*
Rolfe, S.Afr.
Calamine (p.1144·1); hamamelis water (p.1696·3); phenol (p.1188·1); zinc oxide (p.1163·2).
*Skin disorders.*
Schering-Plough, UK.
*Cream:* Calamine (p.1144·1); zinc oxide (p.1163·2); hamamelis (p.1696·3).
*Dry skin; sunburn.*
*Lotion:* Calamine (p.1144·1); zinc oxide (p.1163·2); hamamelis (p.1696·3); phenol (p.1188·1).
*Skin irritation; sunburn.*

**Lacto Pregomine** Milupa, Fr.
Infant feed (p.1417·1).
*Cow's milk intolerance.*

**Lacto Vagin** UCI, Braz.
Tyrothricin (p.275·1); hydroxyquinoline (p.1700·1); tannic acid (p.1751·2); lactic acid (p.1704·1); acetic acid (p.1645·2); camphor (p.1665·3).
*Vulvovaginal disorders.*

**Lactobac** Nutrition Care, Austral.†.
*Lactobacillus acidophilus* (p.1704·2); *Bifidobacterium bifidum* (p.1704·2).
*Dietary supplement.*

**Lactocal-F** Laser, USA.
Multivitamin and mineral preparation with iron and folic acid (p.1417·1).
*Supplement for pregnant or lactating women.*

**Lacto-Cev Zn** Cevallos, Arg.
Ammonium lactate (p.1142·3); zinc gluconate (p.1469·2).
*Skin disorders.*

**Lactocol** Ogna, Ital.
Guaiacol (p.1122·1); lactic acid (p.1704·1); calcium phosphate (p.1225·3); calcium lactate (p.1225·3); codeine hydrochloride (p.27·1); aconite (p.1646·3).
*Coughs.*

**Lactocol Expectorante** Alcala, Spain†.
Guaifenesin (p.1122·1).
*Coughs.*

**Lactocrem** Giscard, Arg.
Urea (p.1162·2) alfa hydroxyacids.
*Dry skin.*

**Lactocrem Bebe** Giscard, Arg.
Allantoin (p.1141·3); zinc (p.1469·2); vegetable extracts.
*Barrier preparation.*

**Lactocur** Biocur, Ger.
Lactulose (p.1269·1).
*Constipation; hepatic encephalopathy.*

**Lactofalk** Falk, Ger.†.
Lactulose (p.1269·1).
*Constipation; liver disorders; salmonella enteritis.*

**Lactoferment** Novartis Consumer, Switz.†.
*Lactobacillus acidophilus* (p.1704·2).
*Gastrointestinal disorders.*

**Lactoferrina** Chiesi, Spain.
Iron succinyl-protein complex (p.1438·1).
*Iron deficiency anaemia.*

**Lactofilus** Llorente, Spain.
*Lactobacillus acidophilus* (p.1704·2).
*Restoration of the gastrointestinal flora.*

**Lactofit** Germania, Austria.
*Lactobacillus rhamnosus* (p.1704·2).
*Diarrhoea.*

**Lactofree** Mead Johnson Nutritionals, USA.
Lactose-free infant feed (p.1417·1).

**Lactoger** Schwarz, Ital.
Lactulose (p.1269·1).
*Hepatic cirrhosis; hepatic encephalopathy.*

**Lactogermine** Humana, Ital.
Lactic-acid-producing organisms (p.1704·2); vitamins (p.1417·1).
*Nutritional supplement.*

**Lacto-Gin** Preciframa, Braz.†.
Tyrothricin (p.275·1); hydroxyquinoline (p.1700·1); acetic acid (p.1645·2); lactic acid (p.1704·1); tannic acid (p.1751·2); camphor (p.1665·3).
*Vulvovaginal disorders.*

**Lactolas** Infosint, Ital.
Lactulose (p.1269·1); inulin (p.1702·1); rhubarb (p.1287·3); frangula (p.1266·3); senna (p.1288·2); vitamin B substances (p.1417·1).
*Nutritional supplement.*

**Lactolavol** Rosch & Handel, Austria.
Calcium lactate (p.1225·3); tartaric acid (p.1752·1); atropine sulfate (p.477·1).
*Vaginal disorders.*

**Lactolife** Fitolife, Ital.
Dried yeast (p.1469·1); lactic-acid-producing organisms (p.1704·2).
*Gastrointestinal disorders; nutritional supplement.*

**Lactoliofil** Belmac, Spain†.
*Lactobacillus acidophilus* (p.1704·2).
*Restoration of the gastrointestinal flora.*

**Lactomannan** CaDiGroup, Ital.
Glucomannan (p.1693·3); lactulose (p.1269·1).
*Constipation; obesity.*

**Lactomina** Ibefar, Braz.†.
Calcium lactophosphate; manganese hypophosphite; vitamin B substances (p.1417·1).
*Nutritional supplement.*

**Lactonico** Dermoteca, Port.
Ammonium lactate (p.1142·3); squalane (p.1482·2); levomenol (p.1707·1); vitamin E.
*Barrier preparation; dry skin disorders.*

**Lactonorm** Geymonat, Ital.
*Lactobacillus acidophilus* (p.1704·2).
*Disturbances in vaginal flora.*

**Lactopectin** Sanofi Synthelabo, Mex.
Kaolin (p.1268·3); pectin (p.1580·3).
*Diarrhoea.*

**Lactophilus** Organon, Fin.
*Lactobacillus rhamnosus* (p.1704·2).
*Restoration of gastrointestinal flora.*

**Lactopregomine** Milupa, Fr.
Infant feed (p.1417·1).
*Milk protein intolerance.*

**Lacto-Purga** DM, Braz.†.
Phenolphthalein (p.1284·1); lactose (p.1438·3).
*Constipation.*

**Lactopurum** Pfluger, Ger.
Homoeopathic preparation.

**Lactored** Fides, Spain†.
Tilactase (p.1756·2); lipase; silicone (p.1289·2).
*Milk intolerance.*

**Lactosec** Aspen, S.Afr.
Pyridoxine hydrochloride (p.1456·3).
*Vitamin deficiency.*

**Lactovit** Herbaline, Ital.†.
Dried yeast (p.1469·1); myrtillus (p.1718·3); *Lactobacillus acidophilus* (p.1704·2).
*Nutritional supplement.*

**Lactrase**
Rivex, Canad.; Schwarz, USA.
Tilactase (p.1756·2).
*Lactase insufficiency; lactose intolerance.*

**Lactrex**
Note. This name is used for preparations of different composition.
Galderma, Arg.
Ammonium lactate (p.1142·3).
*Dry skin disorders.*
Galderma, Braz.
Allantoin (p.1141·3); ammonia (p.1653·3).
*Cicatrisation.*
Galderma, Chile.
Ammonium lactate (p.1142·3); allantoin (p.1141·3).
*Dry skin.*
SDR, USA.
Lactic acid (p.1704·1).
*Emollient.*

**Lactucol** Distriframa, Port.†.
Sodium benzoate (p.1169·3); bromoform (p.1663·1); ephedrine hydrochloride (p.1120·1); cherry-laurel water; balsamic syrup; maidenhair; peca; aconite (p.1646·3); belladonna (p.479·1); drosera (p.1683·1); grindelia (p.1696·1); lobelia (p.1589·1).
*Coughs.*

**Lactuflor** MIP, Ger.
Lactulose (p.1269·1).
*Constipation; hepatic encephalopathy.*

**Lactugal** Intrapharm, UK.
Lactulose (p.1269·1).
*Constipation; hepatic encephalopathy.*

**Lactul** YSP, Malaysia.
Lactulose (p.1269·1).
*Constipation; hepatic encephalopathy.*

**Lactulax**
Rougier, Canad.†; Sam-On, Israel; Senosiain, Mex.
Lactulose (p.1269·1).
*Constipation; hepatic encephalopathy.*

**Lactulon** Lazar, Arg.
Lactulose (p.1269·1).
*Constipation; hepatic encephalopathy.*

**Lactulona** Sankyo, Braz.
Lactulose (p.1269·1).
*Constipation; hepatic encephalopathy.*

**Lactumed** Medochemie, Malaysia.
Lactulose (p.1269·1).
*Constipation; hepatic encephalopathy.*

**Lactuverlan** Verla, Ger.
Lactulose (p.1269·1).
*Constipation; hepatic encephalopathy.*

**Lactyl** Ibirn, Ital.†.
Lactulose (p.1269·1).
*Cirrhosis; hepatic encephalopathy.*

**Ladazol** Mer-National, S.Afr.
Danazol (p.1545·2).
*Endometriosis; hereditary angioedema; mastalgia.*

**Ladinin** Pharmaten (Φαρματεν), Gr.
Ciprofloxacin hydrochloride (p.188·2) or ciprofloxacin lactate (p.188·3).
*Bacterial infections.*

**Ladip** Valda, Ital.
Lacidipine (p.944·2).
*Hypertension.*

**Ladiwin** Zydus, India.
Lamivudine (p.648·2).
*HIV infection.*

**Ladocort** LBS, Thai.
Miconazole nitrate (p.405·3); hydrocortisone (p.1103·3).
*Infected skin disorders.*

**Ladogal**
Sanofi Synthelabo, Arg.; Sanofi Synthelabo, Braz.; Sanofi Synthelabo, Malaysia; Sanofi Synthelabo, Mex.; Sanofi Synthelabo, Singapore; Sanofi Synthelabo, Thai.
Danazol (p.1545·2).
*Benign breast disorders; endometriosis; gynaecomastia; hereditary angioedema; menorrhagia; precocious puberty.*

**Ladose** Pharmaserve Lilly (Φαρμασερβ Λιλλυ), Gr.
Fluoxetine hydrochloride (p.292·1).
*Depression; obsessive-compulsive disorder; panic disorder.*

**Ladropen** Berk, UK.
Flucloxacillin sodium (p.213·3).
*Bacterial infections.*

**Lady-35** Masa, Thai.
Cyproterone acetate (p.1544·1); ethinylestradiol (p.1553·2).
*Oral contraceptive in women with androgenic symptoms.*

**Lady Fittig** Andromaco, Chile.
Undecenoic acid (p.410·3); zinc undecenoate (p.411·1); hexylresorcinol (p.1182·1); aluminium chlorohydrate (p.1142·1).
*Fungal skin infections.*

**Ladylen** Mertens, Arg.
Miconazole nitrate (p.405·3); tinidazole (p.617·1).
*Vaginal infections.*

**Ladylen Duo** Mertens, Arg.
Tinidazole (p.617·1).
*Bacterial infections; candidiasis; trichomoniasis.*

**Ladymega** Cantassium Co., UK.
Multivitamin and mineral preparation (p.1417·1).

**Lady-Ten 35** Laboratorios Chile, Chile.
Cyproterone acetate (p.1544·1); ethinylestradiol (p.1553·2).
*Androgen-dependent acne, hirsutism, and menstrual disorders.*

**Ladytone** Vitabiotics, UK.
Multivitamin and mineral preparation (p.1417·1).

**Ladyvital** Pharmadass, UK.
Multivitamin, mineral, and nutritional preparation (p.1417·1).

**Laevadosin** Fresenius Kabi, Austria†.
*Buccal tablets:* Adenosine (p.851·2); guanosine; adenosine phosphate disodium (p.1647·3); disodium cytidine phosphate; guanosine monophosphate, disodium salt; disodium uridine monophosphate.
*Injection:* Adenosine triphosphate, disodium salt (p.1648·1); adenosine phosphate disodium (p.1647·3); guanosine monophosphate, disodium salt; adenosine (p.851·2); inosine (p.1701·2); guanosine; uridine (p.1760·3).
*Myopathies; peripheral, cerebral, and coronary vascular disorders.*

**Laev-Amin** Laevosan, Austria†.
Amino-acid infusion (p.1417·1).
*Parenteral nutrition.*

**Laevilac S** Fresenius Kabi, Ger.
Lactulose (p.1269·1).
*Constipation; hepatic encephalopathy.*

**Laevodex** Laevosan, Austria†.
Dextran 40 (p.745·3) or dextran 60 (p.746·1) in sodium chloride infusion.
*Plasma volume expansion; thrombosis prophylaxis.*

**Laevofusin Isoton** Fresenius Kabi, Austria.
Electrolyte infusion (p.1217·1).
*Fluid and electrolyte disorders.*

**Laevofusin-Starter** Laevosan, Austria†.
Sodium, chloride, lactate, and acetate infusion (p.1217·1).
*Fluid and electrolyte disorders.*

**Laevolac**
Calea, Austria; Roche, Ital.; Douglas, NZ; Ferraz, Lynce, Port.; Byk Madaus, S.Afr.†; Medichemie Bioline, Switz.†.
Lactulose (p.1269·1).
*Constipation; gastrointestinal microflora disturbances; gum disorders; hepatic encephalopathy.*

**Laevoral** Fresenius Kabi, Austria.
Fructose (p.1431·3).
*Carbohydrate source; gastrointestinal disorders; glucose substitute; liver disorders.*

**Laevosan**
Laevosan, Austria†; Roche, Ital.
Fructose (p.1431·3).
*Alcohol poisoning; asthenia; cardiac disorders; glucose substitute; liver disorders.*

**Laevostrophan** Fresenius Kabi, Austria†.
Strophanthin-K (p.1009·1).
*Angina; arrhythmias; heart failure.*

**Laevostrophan compositum** Laevosan, Austria†.
Strophanthin-K (p.1009·1); diprophylline (p.784·3).
*Heart failure.*

**Laevovit $D_3$** Calea, Austria.
Colecalciferol (p.1461·3).
*Osteomalacia; rickets; vitamin D supplementation.*

**Lafarclor** Lafare, Ital.
Cefaclor (p.167·1).
*Bacterial infections.*

**Lafarin** Lafare, Ital.
Cefalexin (p.168·1).
*Bacterial infections.*

**Lafedam** Elvetium, Arg.
Alendronate sodium (p.765·3).
*Osteoporosis.*

**Lafena** Cinfa, Spain†.
Aspirin (p.15·1).
*Fever; inflammation; pain.*

**Lafigesic** Lafi, Chile.
Clonixin lysine (p.26·3).
*Inflammation; pain.*

**Lafigin** Drugtech, Chile.
Lamotrigine (p.363·3).
*Epilepsy.*

**Lafol** ICN, Ger.
Folic acid (p.1429·1).
*Folic acid supplement.*

**Lafurex** Lafare, Ital.
Cefuroxime sodium (p.184·1).
*Bacterial infections.*

**Lagarmicin** Bohm, Spain.
Erythromycin stearate (p.208·2).
*Bacterial infections.*

**Lagatrim**
Alliance, S.Afr.; Lagap, Switz.
Co-trimoxazole (p.199·3).
*Bacterial infections; Pneumocystis carinii pneumonia.*

**Lagenbach** Remexa, Mex.
Senna (p.1288·2).
*Constipation.*

**Lagin** Epifarma, Ital.
Benzydamine hydrochloride (p.21·1).
*Gynaecological disorders.*

**Lagricel** Sophia, Mex.
Sodium hyaluronate (p.1697·3).
*Dry eyes.*

**Lagricel Ofteno** SMB, Chile.
Sodium hyaluronate (p.1697·3).
*Dry eyes; eye irritation.*

**Lagrifilm Plus** Allergan, Mex.
Polyvinyl alcohol (p.1581·1); povidone (p.1581·2).
*Dry eyes.*

**Lagrima Artificial** Poen, Arg.
Polyvinyl alcohol (p.1581·1).
*Dry eyes.*

**Lagrima Humectante** Inmunolab, Arg.
Polyvinyl alcohol (p.1581·1).
*Dry eyes.*

**Lagrimas Artificiales** Biosano, Chile; Laboratorios Chile, Chile.
Polyvinyl alcohol (p.1581·1).
*Dry eyes.*

**Lagrimas de Santa Lucia** Ferro, Arg.
*Eye drops:* Zinc sulfate (p.1469·3); boric acid (p.1662·1); methylthioninium chloride (p.1042·2).
*Powder:* Mercuric oxycyanide (p.1713·3).
*Dry eyes.*

**Lagun** Pharmacal, Fin.
Dextromethorphan hydrobromide (p.1117·3).
*Coughs.*

**Lagur** Boehringer de Angeli, Braz.†.
Clarithromycin (p.192·2).
*Bacterial infections.*

**Lagylan** Alpha, Mex.†.
Metronidazole (p.607·2).

**Laidor** *Esseti, Ital.*
Nimesulide (p.67·1).
*Fever; inflammation; pain.*

**Laif** *Steigerwald, Ger.*
Hypericum (p.299·1).
*Depression.*

**Laikan 100** *Grunenthal, Chile.*
Kava (p.1703·2).
*Anxiety.*

**Laiken** *Farmasa, Mex.*
Kava extract (p.1703·2).
*Anxiety.*

**Lait Auto-Bronzant** *Clarins, Canad.*
*SPF 6:* Octinoxate (p.1154·3); avobenzone (p.1142·3).
Formerly contained octinoxate, oxybenzone, and titanium dioxide.
*Sunscreen.*

**Lait Bronzage** *Clarins, Canad.†.*
*SPF 19:* Octinoxate (p.1154·3); oxybenzone (p.1154·3); ensulizole (p.1147·1); titanium dioxide (p.1160·3).
*SPF 6; SPF 10:* Octinoxate (p.1154·3); oxybenzone (p.1154·3); titanium dioxide (p.1160·3).
*Sunscreen.*

**Lait Ecran Total** *Vichy, Canad.*
*SPF 25; SPF 30:* Avobenzone (p.1142·3); octocrilene (p.1154·3); ecamsule (p.1146·3); titanium dioxide (p.1160·3).
*Sunscreen.*

**Lait Hydratant Bronzage** *Vichy, Canad.†.*
*SPF 8:* Avobenzone (p.1142·3); enzacamene (p.1147·1); ecamsule (p.1146·3); titanium dioxide (p.1160·3).
*Sunscreen.*

**Lait Protecteur** *Lancome, Canad.†; Vichy, Canad.†.*
*SPF 8; SPF 15:* Avobenzone (p.1142·3); octocrilene (p.1154·3); ecamsule (p.1146·3); titanium dioxide (p.1160·3).
Formerly contained avobenzone, enzacamene, ecamsule, and titanium dioxide.
*Sunscreen.*

**Lait Solaire Ecran Total** *Lancome, Canad.*
*SPF 25:* Avobenzone (p.1142·3); enzacamene (p.1147·1); ecamsule (p.1146·3); titanium dioxide (p.1160·3).
*Sunscreen.*

**Lait Solaire Haute Protection** *Lancome, Canad.*
*SPF 15:* Avobenzone (p.1142·3); enzacamene (p.1147·1); octocrilene (p.1154·3); ecamsule (p.1146·3); titanium dioxide (p.1160·3).
*Sunscreen.*

**Laitan**
*Schwabe, Austria†; Altana, Braz.; Schwabe, Ger.†; Spitzner, Ger.†; Schwabe, Switz.†.*
Kava (p.1703·2).
*Anxiety disorders; sleep disorders.*

**Lake** *Faes, Spain.*
Ranitidine hydrochloride (p.1285·2).
*Acid aspiration; gastro-oesophageal reflux; peptic ulcer; Zollinger-Ellison syndrome.*

**Lakrima** *Bittner, Austria.*
Homoeopathic preparation.

**Lakriment Neu** *Dolorgiet, Ger.*
Liquorice (p.1270·2).
*Catarrh.*

**Laktipex** *Selena, Swed.*
Lactulose (p.1269·1).
*Constipation; hepatic encephalopathy.*

**Lalax** *Orion, Fin.*
Lactitol (p.1269·1).
*Constipation; hepatic encephalopathy.*

**Lama**
*Note. This name is used for preparations of different composition.*
*Stadmed, India.*
Amlodipine besilate (p.862·1).
*Angina pectoris; hypertension.*
*Pharmaland, Thai.*
Ketoconazole (p.403·3).
*Fungal skin infections.*

**Lamaline** *Solvay, Fr.*
Paracetamol (p.76·2); opium (p.74·2); caffeine (p.782·1).
Formerly contained paracetamol, belladonna, opium, and caffeine.
*Pain.*

**Lambda** *Isdin, Port.*
*Cream:* Triclosan (p.1195·2); aluminium hydroxide (p.1249·2).
*Roll-on:* Aluminium chlorohydrate (p.1142·1).
*Hyperhidrosis.*

**Lamblit** *Novag, Mex.*
Metronidazole (p.607·2).
*Amoebiasis; giardiasis; trichomoniasis.*

**Lambutol**
*Atlantic, Hong Kong†; Atlantic, Thai.*
Ethambutol hydrochloride (p.211·3).
*Tuberculosis.*

**Lamcoin** *Pond's, Thai.*
Clofazimine (p.197·1).
*Leprosy.*

**Lametec** *Cipla, India.*
Lamotrigine (p.363·3).
*Epilepsy.*

**Lamictal**
*GlaxoSmithKline, Arg.; GlaxoSmithKline, Austral.; GlaxoSmithKline, Austria; GlaxoSmithKline, Belg.; GlaxoSmithKline, Braz.; GlaxoSmithKline, Canad.; GlaxoSmithKline, Chile; GlaxoSmithKline, Denm.; GlaxoSmithKline, Fin.; GlaxoSmithKline, Fr.; GlaxoSmithKline, Ger.; Glaxo Wellcome, Gr.; GlaxoSmithKline, Hong Kong; GlaxoSmithKline, Irl.; Wellcome, Israel; GlaxoSmithKline, Ital.; GlaxoSmithKline, Malaysia; Glaxo Wellcome, Mex.; GlaxoSmithKline, Neth.; GlaxoSmithKline, Norw.; GlaxoSmithKline, NZ; Wellcome, Port.; GlaxoSmithKline, Singapore; GlaxoSmithKline, Spain; GlaxoSmithKline, Swed.; GlaxoSmithKline, Switz.; GlaxoSmithKline, Thai.; GlaxoSmithKline, UK; Glaxo Wellcome, USA.*
Lamotrigine (p.363·3).
*Bipolar disorder; epilepsy.*

**Lamictin** *GlaxoSmithKline, S.Afr.*
Lamotrigine (p.363·3).
*Epilepsy.*

**Lamidac** *Zydus, India.*
Lamivudine (p.648·2).
*Chronic hepatitis B.*

**Lamiden** *Eurofarma, Braz.†.*
Lamivudine (p.648·2).
*HIV infection.*

**Lamiderm** *Gifrer Barbezat, Fr.*
Trolamine (p.1758·2).

**Lamilea** *Elea, Arg.*
Lamivudine (p.648·2).
*HIV infection.*

**Lamisil**
*Novartis, Arg.; Novartis, Austral.; Novartis Consumer, Austral.; Novartis, Austria; Novartis, Belg.; Novartis, Braz.; Novartis, Canad.; Novartis, Chile; Novartis, Denm.; Novartis, Fin.; Novartis, Fr.; Novartis, Ger.; Novartis, Gr.; Novartis, Hong Kong; Novartis, India; Novartis, Irl.; Novartis, Israel; Novartis, Ital.; Novartis, Malaysia; Novartis, Mex.; Novartis, Neth.; Novartis, Norw.; Novartis, NZ; Novartis, Port.; Novartis, S.Afr.; Novartis, Singapore; Novartis, Spain; Novartis, Swed.; Novartis, Switz.; Novartis, Thai.; Novartis, UK; Novartis, USA.*
Terbinafine (p.408·2) or terbinafine hydrochloride (p.408·2).
*Fungal skin and nail infections.*

**Lamnotyl** *Farmasur, Spain.*
Boric acid (p.1662·1); hamamelis (p.1696·3); ichthammol (p.1148·2); zinc oxide (p.1163·2).
*Burns; grazes; skin disorders.*

**Lamoryl** *Leo, Norw.†.*
Griseofulvin (p.400·3).
*Fungal infections.*

**Lampicin** *Lakeside, Mex.†.*
Ampicillin (p.157·1), ampicillin sodium (p.157·1), or ampicillin trihydrate (p.157·2).
*Bacterial infections.*

**Lampocef** *Lampugnani, Ital.*
Cefonicid sodium (p.174·2).
Lidocaine hydrochloride (p.1377·3) is included in this preparation to alleviate the pain of injection.
*Gram-negative bacterial infections.*

**Lampocillina** *Salus, Ital.†.*
Ampicillin sodium (p.157·1).
*Bacterial infections.*

**Lampoflex** *Lampugnani, Ital.*
Piroxicam (p.84·2).
*Musculoskeletal, joint, and peri-articular disorders.*

**Lampomandol** *AGIPS, Ital.*
Cefamandole nafate (p.169·3).
Lidocaine hydrochloride (p.1377·3) is included in this preparation to alleviate the pain of injection.
*Bacterial infections.*

**Lampren**
*Ciba-Geigy, Jpn; Novartis, Neth.; Padro, Spain.*
Clofazimine (p.197·1).
*Leprosy.*

**Lamprene**
*Novartis, Austral.; Novartis, Fr.; IFET (ΙΦΕΤ), Gr.; Novartis, Hong Kong; Novartis, Malaysia; Novartis, NZ; Novartis, S.Afr.; Novartis, Switz.; Alliance, UK†; Geigy, USA.*
Clofazimine (p.197·1).
Available from WHO for the treatment of leprosy in the UK.
*Leprosy.*

**Lamra** *Merckle, Ger.*
Diazepam (p.690·1).
*Anxiety; premedication; skeletal muscle spasm.*

**Lamuna** *Hexal, Ger.*
Desogestrel (p.1547·2); ethinylestradiol (p.1553·2).
*Combined oral contraceptive.*

**Lamuran**
*Roche, Austria†; SIT, Ital.*
Raubasine (p.994·3).
*Peripheral and cerebral vascular disorders.*

**Lamuzid** *Zydus, India.*
Lamivudine (p.648·2); zidovudine (p.658·2).
*HIV infection.*

**Lanabiotic**
*Note. This name is used for preparations of different composition.*
*Combe, Canad.†.*
Bacitracin (p.161·3); polymyxin B sulfate (p.245·1).
*Wounds.*
*Combe, USA.*
Polymyxin B sulfate (p.245·1); neomycin sulfate (p.235·1); bacitracin (p.161·3); lidocaine (p.1377·3).
*Bacterial skin infections.*

**Lanacaina** *Combe, Arg.*
Benzocaine (p.1370·3).
*Pruritus.*

**Lanacane**
*Note. This name is used for preparations of different composition.*
*Combe, Israel; Combe, Spain; Combe, UK; Combe, USA.*
Benzocaine (p.1370·3).
*Skin irritation.*
*Formula, NZ.*
Benzocaine (p.1370·3); resorcinol (p.1156·3).
*Skin irritation.*

**Lanacane Medicated Cream** *Combe, Canad.*
Benzocaine (p.1370·3); resorcinol (p.1156·3).
*Skin disorders.*

**Lanacane Medicated Powder** *Combe, UK.*
Menthol (p.1711·3); zinc oxide (p.1163·2).
*Skin irritation.*

**Lanacef** *Lannacher, Austria.*
Cefaclor (p.167·1).
*Bacterial infections.*

**Lanacine** *Lannacher, Austria.*
Clindamycin hydrochloride (p.194·2) or clindamycin phosphate (p.194·2).
*Bacterial infections.*

**Lanacordin** *Kern, Spain.*
Digoxin (p.895·2).
*Arrhythmias; heart failure.*

**Lanacort**
*Combe, Canad.†; Combe, Israel; Combe, Ital.; Combe, UK; Combe, USA.*
Hydrocortisone acetate (p.1103·3).
*Skin disorders.*

**Lanacrist** *Tika, Swed.*
Digoxin (p.895·2).
*Arrhythmias; heart failure.*

**Lanalget** *Lannacher, Austria.*
Tramadol hydrochloride (p.94·3).
*Pain.*

**Lanamont** *Chrispa (Χρισπα), Gr.*
Buspirone hydrochloride (p.672·2).
*Generalised anxiety.*

**Lanaphilic**
*Medco, USA.*
Vehicle for topical preparations.
*Medco, USA.*
Urea (p.1162·2).
*Dry skin; hyperkeratosis.*

**Lanate** *Douglas, NZ.*
Ammonium lactate (p.1142·3).
*Dry skin disorders.*

**Lanatilin** *Nycomed, Austria.*
α-Acetyldigoxin (p.851·1).
*Heart failure.*

**Lanatin** *Nycomed, Denm.*
Lisinopril (p.946·3).
*Heart failure; hypertension.*

**Lancome-Creme Solaire** *Lancome, Canad.*
*SPF 15:* Avobenzone (p.1142·3); enzacamene (p.1147·1); ecamsule (p.1146·3); titanium dioxide (p.1160·3).
*Sunscreen.*

**Lancome-Gelee Fraicheur** *Lancome, Canad.*
*SPF 8:* Enzacamene (p.1147·1); octinoxate (p.1154·3); ecamsule (p.1146·3); titanium dioxide (p.1160·3).
Formerly known as Lancome-Creme Gelee.
*Sunscreen.*

**Lancome-Nutrisource Mains** *Lancome, Canad.*
*SPF 15:* Octinoxate (p.1154·3); titanium dioxide (p.1160·3).
*Sunscreen.*

**Lancome-UV Expert** *Lancome, Canad.*
*SPF 15:* Avobenzone (p.1142·3) octinoxate (p.1154·3); octisalate (p.1154·3).
*Sunscreen.*

**Lander Dandruff Control** *Lander, Canad.*
Pyrithione zinc (p.1156·2).
*Dandruff.*

**Lanex** *Lavipharm, Gr.*
Omeprazole (p.1278·2).
*Acid aspiration; eradication of Helicobacter pylori in combination with antimicrobials; peptic ulcer; reflux oesophagitis; Zollinger-Ellison syndrome.*

**Lanexat**
*Roche, Arg.; Roche, Braz.; Roche, Chile; Roche, Denm.; Roche, Fin.; Roche, Mex.; Roche, Swed.*
Flumazenil (p.1038·3).
*Benzodiazepine overdosage; reversal of benzodiazepine-induced sedation.*

**Lanfast** *Julphar, UAE.*
Lansoprazole (p.1269·3).
Formerly known as Lanso.
*Gastro-oesophageal reflux; peptic ulcer; Zollinger-Ellison syndrome.*

**Langoran** *Aventis, Fr.*
Isosorbide dinitrate (p.941·1).
*Angina pectoris; heart failure.*

**Laniazid** *Lannett, USA.*
Isoniazid (p.222·2).
*Tuberculosis.*

**Lanicor**
*Roche, Arg.; Roche, Austria; Teofarma, Ger.*
Digoxin (p.895·2).
*Heart failure; tachycardia.*

**Lanirapid** *Kern, Spain.*
Metildigoxin (p.955·2).
*Arrhythmias; heart failure.*

**Lanitop**
*Roche, Austria; Roche, Belg.; Asta Medica, Braz.; Roche, Ger.; Roche, Gr.; Roche, Hong Kong; Roche, Ital.; Roche, Port.; Roche, Switz.*
Metildigoxin (p.955·2).
*Arrhythmias; heart failure.*

**Lanoc** *Lannacher, Austria.*
Metoprolol tartrate (p.957·1).
*Angina pectoris; arrhythmias; hypertension; migraine; myocardial infarction.*

**Lanoclav** *Lannacher, Austria.*
Amoxicillin trihydrate (p.155·3); potassium clavulanate (p.193·3).
*Bacterial infections.*

**Lanofene** *Augot, Fr.†.*
Zinc oxide (p.1163·2).
*Eczema; nappy rash.*

**Lanogastro** *Teuto, Braz.*
Lansoprazole (p.1269·3).
*Peptic ulcer.*

**Lanohex**
*Rougier, Canad.†; Rougier, Hong Kong†.*
Phenoxyethanol (p.1189·1).
*Scalp disorders; skin cleansing.*

**Lanol** *Nakornpatana, Thai.*
Calamine (p.1144·1); zinc oxide (p.1163·2); phenol (p.1188·1); camphor (p.1665·3); menthol (p.1711·3).
*Skin disorders.*

**Lanolept** *Lannacher, Austria.*
Clozapine (p.685·3).
*Schizophrenia.*

**Lanolor** *Squibb, USA.*
Emollient and moisturiser.

**Lanomycin** *Pharmaten (Φαρματεν), Gr.*
Amikacin sulfate (p.154·1).
*Bacterial infections.*

**Lanorinal** *Lannett, USA†.*
Aspirin (p.15·1); caffeine (p.782·1); butalbital (p.673·3).
*Pain.*

**Lanoxicaps** *Cardinal Health, USA.*
Digoxin (p.895·2).
*Atrial fibrillation; heart failure.*

**Lanoxin**
*GlaxoSmithKline, Arg.; Sigma, Austral.; GlaxoSmithKline, Belg.; GlaxoSmithKline, Braz.; Virco, Canad.; Sigma, Hong Kong; GlaxoSmithKline, India; Wellcome, Irl.; Wellcome, Israel; GlaxoSmithKline, Ital.; GlaxoSmithKline, Malaysia; Glaxo Wellcome, Mex.; GlaxoSmithKline, Neth.; GlaxoSmithKline, Norw.; GlaxoSmithKline, NZ; Wellcome, Port.; GlaxoSmithKline, S.Afr.; GlaxoSmithKline, Singapore; GlaxoSmithKline, Swed.; Wellcome, Switz.†; GlaxoSmithKline, Thai.; GlaxoSmithKline, UK; Glaxo Wellcome, USA.*
Digoxin (p.895·2).
*Arrhythmias; heart failure.*

**Lanseka** *Hexal, Arg.*
Loperamide hydrochloride (p.1271·1).
*Diarrhoea.*

**Lansinoh** *Key, Austral.*
Wool fat (p.1483·1).
*Nipple care.*

**Lansox**
*Takeda, Ital.; Faribercia, Port.*
Lansoprazole (p.1269·3).
*Gastro-oesophageal reflux; peptic ulcer; Zollinger-Ellison syndrome.*

**Lansoyl**
*Armstrong, Arg.; Pfizer Consumer, Belg.; Axcan, Canad.; Pfizer Sante, Fr.; Parke, Davis, Switz.†.*
Liquid paraffin (p.1479·1).
*Constipation.*

**Lantadin** *Aventis, Austria.*
Deflazacort (p.1096·2).
*Corticosteroid.*

**Lantanon**
*Organon, Ital.; Donmed, S.Afr.; Organon, Spain.*
Mianserin hydrochloride (p.306·3).
*Depression.*

**Lantarel** *Wyeth, Ger.*
Methotrexate sodium (p.568·3).
*Psoriasis; psoriatic arthritis; rheumatoid arthritis.*

**Lantigen B**
*COB, Belg.†; Bruschettini, Ital.; Seber, Port.; Bruschettini, Switz.†.*
Antigen extracts of: *Streptococcus pneumoniae*; *Streptococcus pyogenes*; *Moraxella catarrhalis*; *Staphylococcus aureus*; *Klebsiella pneumoniae*; *Haemophilus influenzae* type b.
*Upper respiratory-tract infections.*

**Lantogent** *Bio Terapico Ralay, Spain†.*
Gentamicin sulfate (p.217·1).
*Bacterial infections.*

**Lantus**
*Aventis, Austral.; Aventis, Fr.; Aventis, Ger.; Aventis, Irl.; Aventis, Norw.; Aventis, UK; Aventis, USA.*
Insulin glargine (p.333·3).
*Diabetes mellitus.*

**Lanuretic** *Lannacher, Austria.*
Hydrochlorothiazide (p.933·2); amiloride hydrochloride (p.858·2).
*Hypertension; oedema.*

**Lanvis**
*GlaxoSmithKline, Arg.; GlaxoSmithKline, Austral.; GlaxoSmithKline, Belg.; GlaxoSmithKline, Braz.; GlaxoSmithKline, Canad.; GlaxoSmithKline, Chile; GlaxoSmithKline, Fr.; Glaxo Wellcome, Gr.; GlaxoSmithKline, Hong Kong; Wellcome, Irl.; Wellcome, Israel; GlaxoSmithKline, Malaysia; GlaxoSmithKline, Neth.; GlaxoSmithKline, NZ; GlaxoSmithKline, S.Afr.; GlaxoSmithKline, Singapore; GlaxoSmithKline, Swed.; GlaxoSmithKline, Switz.; GlaxoSmithKline, Thai.; GlaxoSmithKline, UK.*
Tioguanine (p.588·2).
*Leukaemias.*

**Lanz** *Sigma, Braz.*
Lansoprazole (p.1269·3).
*Peptic ulcer.*

**Lanzo** Wyeth Lederle, Denm.; Wyeth Lederle, Fin.; Orion, Fin.; Wyeth Lederle, Norw.; Wyeth Lederle, Swed.
Lansoprazole (p.1269·3).
*Gastro-oesophageal reflux; peptic ulcer; Zollinger-Ellison syndrome.*

**Lanzogastro** Biosaude, Port.
Lansoprazole (p.1269·3).
*Gastro-oesophageal reflux; peptic ulcer.*

**Lanzol** Ache, Braz.; Cipla, India.
Lansoprazole (p.1269·3).
*Dyspepsia; gastro-oesophageal reflux; peptic ulcer.*

**Lanzopral** Roemmers, Arg.; Pharma Investi, Chile.
Lansoprazole (p.1269·3).
*Gastro-oesophageal reflux; peptic ulcer; Zollinger-Ellison syndrome.*

**Lanzor** Aventis, Fr.; Aventis, Ger.; Aventis, S.Afr.
Lansoprazole (p.1269·3).
*Gastro-oesophageal reflux; gastrointestinal hyperacidity; peptic ulcer; Zollinger-Ellison syndrome.*

**Lao-Dal** Synthelabo, Fr.†.
Camphor (p.1665·3); menthol (p.1711·3); lidocaine hydrochloride (p.1377·3); chloroform (p.1296·3); methyl salicylate (p.59·3); turpentine oil (p.1760·1); glycol salicylate (p.44·3).
*Soft-tissue disorders.*

**Lapenax** Novartis, Arg.
Clozapine (p.685·3).
*Schizophrenia.*

**Lapices Epiderm Metadier** Prats, Spain.
Dithranol (p.1146·1); salicylic acid (p.1157·1).
*Skin disorders.*

**Lapidar** Swiss Herbal, Canad.†.
Cascara (p.1255·1); frangula (p.1266·3); senna (p.1288·2).

**Lapidar 10** Kunzle, Switz.
Frangula bark (p.1266·3); senna (p.1288·2); liquorice (p.1270·2).
*Constipation.*

**Laprazol** Vianex (Βιανεξ), Gr.
Lansoprazole (p.1269·3).
*Gastro-oesophageal reflux; peptic ulcer; Zollinger-Ellison syndrome.*

**Lapril** Pharmasant, Thai.
Enalapril maleate (p.909·2).
*Heart failure; hypertension.*

**Laprilen** Baldacci, Port.
Enalapril maleate (p.909·2); hydrochlorothiazide (p.933·2).
*Hypertension.*

**Lapsus** Klonal, Arg.
Fluoxetine (p.296·3).
*Depression.*

**Laracit** Laboratorios Chile, Chile; Lemery, Mex.
Cytarabine (p.543·1).
*Leukaemias; lymphomas.*

**Laractone** Lagap, UK†.
Spironolactone (p.1003·1).
*Ascites; heart failure; hyperaldosteronism; oedema.*

**Larafen** Sandoz, UK.
Ketoprofen (p.51·2).
*Musculoskeletal and joint disorders; pain.*

**Laraflex** Lagap, UK†.
Naproxen (p.65·1).
*Gout; inflammation; musculoskeletal disorders; pain.*

**Laragon** Roemmers, Arg.
Silymarin (p.1043·3).
*Liver disorders.*

**Larapam** Lagap, UK†.
Piroxicam (p.84·2).
*Gout; inflammation; musculoskeletal disorders; pain.*

**Laratrim** Lagap, UK†.
Co-trimoxazole (p.199·3).
*Bacterial infections.*

**Larch Resin comp.** Weleda, UK.
Ananassa fruit; lavender oil (p.1705·2); larch resin.
*Sore eyes.*

**Larcooral** Disprovent, Arg.
Staphylococcus; Micrococcus; Pneumococcus; Streptococcus; Klebsiella; *Moraxella catarrhalis*; *Haemophilus influenzae*.
*Respiratory-tract infections.*

**Largactil** Aventis, Austral.; Rhone-Poulenc Rorer, Austria†; Rhone-Poulenc Rorer, Belg.†; Aventis, Canad.; Aventis, Chile; Aventis, Denm.; Aventis, Fr.; Aventis, Gr.; Aventis, Hong Kong; Aventis, Irl.; Aventis, Ital.; Aventis, Mex.; Aventis, Neth.; Aventis, Norw.; Aventis, NZ; Vitoria, Port.; Aventis, S.Afr.; Aventis, Spain; Rhone-Poulenc Rorer, Switz.†; Hawgreen, UK.
Chlorpromazine (p.675·1), chlorpromazine embonate (p.675·1), or chlorpromazine hydrochloride (p.675·2).
*Alcohol or opioid withdrawal syndrome; anxiety; autism; induction of hypothermia; intractable hiccup; nausea and vomiting; pain; premedication; psychoses.*

**Largal ultra** Septodont, Switz.†.
Edetate sodium; cetrimonium bromide (p.1173·1).
*Adjunct in dental surgery.*

**Largatrex**
Note. This name is used for preparations of different composition.
Vitoria, Port.
Chlorpromazine hydrochloride (p.675·2).

Aventis, Spain.
Chlorpromazine (p.675·1); heptaminol (p.1697·1); trihexyphenidyl (p.490·3).
*Aggression; anxiety; psychoses.*

**Largitor** Italfarmaco, Spain†.
Myrtillus (p.1718·3).
*Vascular disorders.*

**Largon**
Note. This name is used for preparations of different composition.
Klinge, Austria.
Kawain (p.1703·2).
*Nervous disorders.*

Wyeth-Ayerst, USA†.
Propiomazine hydrochloride (p.440·3).
*Sedative.*

**Lariago** Ipca, India.
Chloroquine phosphate (p.448·2).
*Amoebiasis; lupus erythematosus; malaria; rheumatoid arthritis.*

**Lariam** Roche, Austral.; Roche, Austria; Roche, Belg.; Roche, Canad.; Roche, Chile; Roche, Denm.; Roche, Fin.; Roche, Fr.; Roche, Ger.; Roche, Gr.; Roche, Hong Kong; Roche, Irl.; Roche, Israel; Roche, Ital.; Roche, Neth.; Roche, Norw.; Roche, NZ; Roche, S.Afr.; Roche, Singapore; Roche, Swed.; Roche, Switz.; Roche, UK; Roche, USA.
Mefloquine hydrochloride (p.453·3).
*Malaria.*

**Lariamar** Roche, Braz.†.
Mefloquine (p.455·3).
*Malaria.*

**Laridal** Elfar, Spain†.
Astemizole (p.424·2).
*Hypersensitivity reactions.*

**Laridox** Ipca, India.
Sulfadoxine (p.259·3); pyrimethamine (p.458·1).
*Malaria.*

**Larifikehl** Sanum-Kehlbeck, Ger.
Homoeopathic preparation.

**Larilon** Bioprogress, Ital.†.
Chlorhexidine gluconate (p.1173·2); benzododecinium chloride (p.1170·2).
*Disinfection of wounds and burns.*

**Larimicina** Igefarma, Braz.†.
Diphenhydramine hydrochloride (p.431·3); ammonium chloride (p.1115·2); sodium citrate (p.1223·2).
*Coughs.*

**Laringex** Cazi, Braz.
Tyrothricin (p.275·1); cetrimonium bromide (p.1173·1); vitamin C (p.1460·2); lidocaine (p.1377·3).
*Mouth and throat disorders.*

**Larintil** Brasmedica, Braz.†.
Tyrothricin (p.275·1); neomycin sulfate (p.235·1); benzocaine (p.1370·3).
*Mouth and throat disorders.*

**Larither** Ipca, India.
Artemether (p.447·2).
*Malaria.*

**Larjancaina** Veinfar, Arg.
Lidocaine (p.1377·3).
Adrenaline (p.852·2) is included in some injections as a vasoconstrictor to diminish absorption and localise the effect of the local anaesthetic.
*Local anaesthesia.*

**Larjanfilina** Veinfar, Arg.
Aminophylline (p.780·2).
*Obstructive airways disease.*

**Larmabak** Andromaco, Chile; Thea, Fr.; Thea, Hong Kong; Pharmacia, Singapore.
Sodium chloride (p.1233·3).
*Dry eyes.*

**Larmadex** Schering, Arg.
Goserelin acetate (p.1326·3).
*Breast cancer; endometriosis; prostatic cancer; uterine fibroids.*

**Larmax** Andromaco, Chile.
Loratadine (p.436·1).
*Allergic skin disorders; rhinitis.*

**Larmecran** Thea, Fr.
Povidone (p.1581·2) (p.1164·2).
*Contact lens lubricant; dry eyes.*

**Larmes Artificielles** Novartis Ophthalmics, Fr.
Sodium chloride (p.1233·3).
*Dry eyes.*

**Larodopa** Roche, USA.
Levodopa (p.1205·2).
*Parkinsonism.*

**Laroferon** Roche, Fr.†.
Interferon alfa-2a (p.640·3).
*Hepatitis C.*

**Laroscorbine** Roche Nicholas, Fr.
Ascorbic acid (p.1460·2).
*Asthenia; vitamin C deficiency.*

**Larotabe**
Roche, Arg.
Betacarotene; vitamin C; vitamin E (p.1417·1).
*Antioxidant preparation.*

Roche, Chile.
Betacarotene; vitamin C; vitamin E; zinc; copper; selenium; manganese (p.1417·1).
*Antioxidant preparation.*

**Laroxyl** Roche, Fr.; Roche, Ital.
Amitriptyline hydrochloride (p.280·3).
*Depression; nocturnal enuresis; pain.*

**Larpose** Cipla, India.
Lorazepam (p.704·1).
*Anxiety; insomnia; sedative.*

**Larry** Unison, Thai.
Ketoconazole (p.403·3).
*Dandruff; pityriasis versicolor.*

**Lars** Duncan, Arg.
Cefalexin (p.168·1).
*Bacterial infections.*

**Larsen** Hexa-Medinova, Arg.
Tobramycin (p.271·2); dexamethasone (p.1097·1).
*Infected eye disorders.*

**Larsimal** Poen, Arg.
Fluorometholone (p.1102·2); tetryzoline (p.1131·2).
*Inflammatory eye disorders.*

**LarvE** SMTL, UK.
Sterile larvae of *Lucilia sericata* (p.1151·3).
*Infected or necrotic wounds.*

**Larvitan** Cimed, Braz.
Amino-acid, vitamin, and mineral preparation (p.1417·1).

**Larydol** Dolisos, Canad.
Homoeopathic preparation.

**Larylin** Andromaco, Chile.
Dequalinium chloride (p.1178·1).
*Mouth and throat infections.*

**Larylin Heissgetrank gegen Schmerzen und Fieber** Bayer, Ger.†.
Paracetamol (p.76·2).
*Fever; pain.*

**Larylin Husten-Heissgetrank** Bayer, Ger.†.
Ambroxol hydrochloride (p.1114·3).
*Respiratory disorders associated with viscid or excessive mucus.*

**Larylin Husten-Loser Pastillen** Merck, Ger.
Ambroxol hydrochloride (p.1114·3).
*Respiratory disorders associated with viscid or excessive mucus.*

**Larylin Husten-Loser Saft** Merck, Ger.
Ambroxol hydrochloride (p.1114·3).
*Respiratory disorders associated with viscid or excessive mucus.*

**Larylin Hustensirup N** Bayer, Ger.†.
Dropropizine (p.1119·3).
*Catarrh; coughs.*

**Larylin Husten-Stiller** Merck, Ger.
Dropropizine (p.1119·3).
*Coughs.*

**Larylin NAC Husten-Loser** Merck, Ger.†.
Acetylcysteine (p.1112·3).
*Respiratory-tract disorders associated with viscid or excessive mucus.*

**Larylin Nasenspray N** Bayer, Ger.†.
Oxymetazoline hydrochloride (p.1126·1).
A similar preparation formerly contained naphazoline nitrate and pheniramine maleate.
*Colds; middle ear inflammation; nasal congestion.*

**Laryngarsol** Sanofi Synthelabo, Belg.
Dequalinium chloride (p.1178·1).
*Mouth and throat disorders.*

**Laryng-O-Jet** Celltech, UK.
Lidocaine hydrochloride (p.1377·3).
*Local anaesthesia.*

**Laryngomedin N** Nattermann, Ger.
Hexamidine isetionate (p.1181·3).
*Mouth and throat disorders.*

**Laryngsan** Opfermann, Ger.
Camphor (p.1665·3); peppermint oil (p.1283·2).
Formerly contained camphor, caffeine and sodium benzoate, ammonia solution, and peppermint oil.
*Cold and influenza symptoms; laryngitis; pharyngitis.*

**Lary-Phary** Dr P, Ger.
Carmellose (p.1577·3); sodium chloride; magnesium chloride (p.1217·1).
*Dry mouth; mouth and throat lubricant.*

**Lasa** Euro-Labor, Port.; Grunenthal, Port.
Famotidine (p.1265·2).

**Lasa Antiasmatico** Lasa, Spain†.
Aminophylline (p.780·2); potassium iodide (p.1598·1).
*Obstructive airways disease.*

**Lasa Con Codeina** Ipsen, Spain.
Chlorphenamine maleate (p.427·3); codeine phosphate (p.27·1); pseudoephedrine hydrochloride (p.1129·2).
*Coughs; nasal congestion.*

**Lasain** Inibsa, Spain.
Metamizole magnesium (p.36·1).
*Fever; pain.*

**Lasalar-Y** Alpharma, Mex.
Fluocinolone acetonide (p.1101·2); clioquinol (p.196·3).
*Skin disorders.*

**Lasalar-Y Simple** Alpharma, Mex.
Clioquinol (p.196·3).
*Skin disorders.*

**Lasar** Biocur, Ger.†.
*dl*-Alpha tocoferil acetate (p.1465·1); magnesium oxide (p.1272·3).
*Vitamin E or magnesium deficiency.*

**Laser** Tosi, Ital.
Naproxen (p.65·1).
*Gout; musculoskeletal and joint disorders; neuralgia.*

**Laservis** Chemedica, Ger.; Chemedica, Switz.
Sodium hyaluronate (p.1697·3).
*Adjunct in ocular procedures.*

**Lasikal** Borg, UK.
Furosemide (p.919·3); potassium chloride (p.1232·2).
*Oedema.*

**Lasilacton** Aventis, Arg.; Aventis, Austria; Aventis, Mex.
Furosemide (p.919·3); spironolactone (p.1003·1).
*Ascites; hyperaldosteronism; oedema.*

**Lasilactona** Aventis, Braz.
Furosemide (p.919·3); spironolactone (p.1003·1).
*Hypertension; oedema.*

**Lasilactone** Aventis, India; Aventis, Switz.; Borg, UK.
Furosemide (p.919·3); spironolactone (p.1003·1).
*Hypertension; oedema.*

**Lasiletten** Aventis, Neth.
Furosemide (p.919·3).
*Hypertension; oedema.*

**Lasilix** Aventis, Fr.
Furosemide (p.919·3).
*Hypertension; oedema.*

**Lasiride** Aventis, Arg.
Furosemide (p.919·3); amiloride hydrochloride (p.858·2).
*Hypertension; oedema.*

**Lasitace** Aventis, Austria.
Furosemide (p.919·3); ramipril (p.994·1).
*Heart failure.*

**Lasitone** Aventis, Ital.
Furosemide (p.919·3); spironolactone (p.1003·1).
*Oedema.*

**Lasix** Aventis, Arg.; Aventis, Austral.; Aventis, Austria; Aventis, Belg.; Aventis, Braz.; Aventis, Canad.; Aventis, Chile; Aventis, Denm.; Aventis, Fin.; Aventis, Ger.; Hoechst Marion Roussel, Gr.; IFET (ΙΦΕΤ), Gr.; Aventis, Hong Kong; Aventis, India; Aventis, Irl.; Aventis, Israel; Aventis, Ital.; Aventis, Malaysia; Aventis, Mex.; Aventis, Neth.; Aventis, Norw.; Aventis, NZ; Aventis, Port.; Aventis, S.Afr.; Aventis, Singapore; Aventis, Swed.; Aventis, Switz.; Aventis, Thai.; Borg, UK; Aventis, USA.
Furosemide (p.919·3) or furosemide sodium (p.921·2).
*Forced diuresis; heart failure; hypertension; nephrotic syndrome; oedema; renal failure.*

**Lasma** Pharmax, Irl.†; Pharmax, UK†.
Theophylline (p.798·3).
*Obstructive airways disease.*

**Lasonil**
Note. This name is used for preparations of different composition.
Bayer Consumer, Austral.; Bayer, Austria; Bayer, Belg.; Bayer, Ital.; Bayer, Neth.; Bayer, Port.; Bayer Consumer, UK.
A heparinoid (p.931·1).
Formerly contained a heparinoid and hyaluronidase.
*Soft-tissue injury; thrombophlebitis; varicose ulcers.*

Bayer, Fr.†; Bayer, Israel†; Bayer, NZ; Bayer, Spain.
A heparinoid (p.931·1); hyaluronidase (p.1698·2).
*Bruising; haematomas; thrombophlebitis; varicose ulcers.*

**Lasonil H** Bayer, Ital.†.
A heparinoid (p.931·1); hyaluronidase (p.1698·2); vitamin A palmitate (p.1453·1); calcium pantothenate (p.1442·3); menthol (p.1711·3).
*Anorectal disorders.*

**Lasonil N** Bayer, Ger.
A heparinoid (p.931·1).
Lasonil formerly contained a heparinoid and hyaluronidase.
*Soft-tissue injury; superficial venous disorders.*

**Lasoproct** Bayer, Ital.†.
A heparinoid (p.931·1); hyaluronidase (p.1698·2); vitamin A palmitate (p.1453·1); calcium pantothenate (p.1442·3); dexamethasone (p.1097·1); tetracaine hydrochloride (p.1385·1); menthol (p.1711·3).
*Anorectal disorders.*

**Lasoreuma** Bayer, Ital.†.
A heparinoid (p.931·1); glycol salicylate (p.44·3); benzyl nicotinate (p.21·2).
*Inflammation; pain.*

**Lasoride** Aventis, Irl.; Borg, UK.
Furosemide (p.919·3); amiloride hydrochloride (p.858·2).
These ingredients can be described by the British Approved Name Co-amilofruse.
*Oedema.*

**Lasoven** Bayer, Ital.
A heparinoid (p.931·1).
*Venous insufficiency.*

**L-Asp** Pharmacia, Arg.
Asparaginase (p.528·3).
*Acute leukaemias.*

**Laspar** Bodene, S.Afr.
Asparaginase (p.528·3).
*Lymphoblastic leukaemias.*

**Lassadermil** Edol, Port.
Zinc oxide (p.1163·2).
*Minor burns and wounds; skin disorders.*

**Lassarmex** Precimex, Mex.†.
Zinc oxide (p.1163·2).

**Lassatina** Kedrion, Ital.
Senna (p.1288·2); cascara (p.1255·1); rhubarb (p.1287·3); liquorice (p.1270·2); belladonna (p.479·1); nux vomica (p.1722·3); aniseed (p.1655·2).
*Constipation.*

**Lassativi Vegetali** AFOM, Ital.; Farmatre, Ital.; Nova Argentia, Ital.; Ogna, Ital.; Ottolenghi, Ital.; Sella, Ital.; Zeta, Ital.
Aloes (p.1248·2); rhubarb (p.1287·3).
*Constipation.*

**Lassifar** *Lafare, Ital.*
Lactulose (p.1269·1).
*Disturbance of gastrointestinal bacterial flora; hyperammonaemia.*

**Lasten/Barn** *Ferrosan, Fin.†.*
Multivitamin preparation with manganese (p.1417·1).

**Lastet**
*Pharmacia, Chile; Khandelwal, India; Pharmacia, Ital.; Kayaku, Jpn; Sanfer, Mex.; Probios, Port.†; Prasfarma, Spain.*
Etoposide (p.551·3).
*Malignant neoplasms.*

**Lasticom**
*Asta Medica, Austria; Asta Medica, Ital.*
Azelastine hydrochloride (p.425·2).
*Allergic conjunctivitis; asthma; bronchitis.*

**Lastin**
*Santen, Fin.; Santen, Norw.; Santen, Swed.*
Azelastine hydrochloride (p.425·2).
*Allergic conjunctivitis; allergic rhinitis.*

**Lastrim** *Chew, Thai.*
Co-trimoxazole (p.199·3).
*Bacterial infections.*

**Lastuss** *FDC, India.*
Dextromethorphan (p.1117·3) or dextromethorphan hydrobromide (p.1117·3).
*Cough.*

**Latensin** *Sanum-Kehlbeck, Ger.*
*Bacillus cereus.*
*Immunotherapy.*

**Latesil** *Solvay, Port.*
Flufenamic acid (p.43·2); diethylamine salicylate (p.34·1); myrtecaine (p.1381·3).
*Musculoskeletal, joint, peri-articular, and soft-tissue disorders.*

**Latesyl** *Roth, Austria.*
Diethylamine salicylate (p.34·1); myrtecaine (p.1381·3).
*Musculoskeletal, joint, peri-articular, and soft-tissue disorders; neuralgia.*

**Laticort** *Medphano, Ger.*
Hydrocortisone butyrate (p.1104·1).
*Skin disorders.*

**Latimit** *Medphano, Ger.†.*
Hydrocortisone acetate (p.1103·3).
*Skin disorders.*

**Latof** *Saval, Chile.*
Latanoprost (p.1519·1).
*Glaucoma; ocular hypertension.*

**Latof-T** *Saval, Chile.*
Latanoprost (p.1519·1); timolol maleate (p.1012·2).
*Glaucoma; ocular hypertension.*

**Latonid** *Abbott, Swed.*
Meloxicam (p.56·1).
*Osteoarthritis.*

**Latonina** *Faran, Gr.*
Calcitonin (p.768·2).
*Hypercalcaemia; osteoporosis; Paget's disease of bone.*

**Latoren** *Anpharm (Ανφαρμ), Gr.*
Loratadine (p.436·1).
*Allergic rhinitis; pruritus.*

**Latotryd** *Atlantis, Mex.*
Erythromycin (p.208·1) or erythromycin stearate (p.208·2).
*Bacterial infections.*

**Lattubio** *Bioprogress, Ital.*
Lactulose (p.1269·1).
*Constipation.*

**Lattulac** *Sofar, Ital.*
Lactulose (p.1269·1).
*Cirrhosis; constipation; hepatic encephalopathy.*

**Latycin**
*Boucher & Muir, Austral.; Biochemie, Austria; Biochemie, Singapore†.*
Tetracycline hydrochloride (p.266·2).
*Bacterial eye infections.*

**Latycyn** *Biochemie, Malaysia.*
Tetracycline hydrochloride (p.266·2).
*Bacterial eye infections.*

**Laubeel** *Desitin, Ger.*
Lorazepam (p.704·1).
*Anxiety disorders.*

**Laudamonium** *Henkel, Ger.*
Benzalkonium chloride (p.1168·3).
*Skin and surface disinfection.*

**Laudefen** *Wayne, Mex.†.*
Difenidol (p.1261·1).

**Laudil** *Lafi, Chile.*
Pinaverium bromide (p.1732·1).

**Launol** *Laboratorios Chile, Chile.*
Deltamethrin (p.1503·1); piperonyl butoxide (p.1509·2).
*Pediculosis; scabies.*

**Laur** *Sons, Mex.*
Tetracycline (p.266·2).
*Bacterial infections.*

**Laurak** *Vita, Spain.*
Atracurium besilate (p.1399·1).
*Competitive neuromuscular blocker.*

**Lauricin** *Sons, Mex.*
Erythromycin estolate (p.208·1) or erythromycin stearate (p.208·2).
*Bacterial infections.*

**Laurimic** *Effik, Spain.*
Fenticonazole nitrate (p.397·3).
*Fungal skin and nail infections; vulvovaginal candidiasis.*

**Laurimicina** *Mavi, Mex.*
Erythromycin (p.208·1).
*Bacterial infections.*

**Laurina** *Organon, Austria.*
Desogestrel (p.1547·2); ethinylestradiol (p.1553·2).
28-Day packs also contain 7 inert tablets.
*Triphasic oral contraceptive.*

**Laurinol Plus** *Szama, Arg.*
Undecenoic acid diethanolamide; cade oil (p.1159·2); vitamin $B_6$.
*Psoriasis; scalp disorders.*

**Lauritran** *Chinoin, Mex.*
Erythromycin estolate (p.208·1).
*Bacterial infections.*

**Lauroderme** *Baldacci, Port.*
Salicylic acid (p.1157·1); zinc oxide (p.1163·2).
*Skin inflammation and irritation.*

**Lauroderme Po** *Baldacci, Port.*
Salicylic acid (p.1157·1); zinc oxide (p.1163·2); titanium dioxide (p.1160·3).
*Skin disorders.*

**Lauromentol** *Lepori, Port.*
Menthol (p.1711·3); methyl salicylate (p.59·3); salicylic acid (p.1157·1); laurel oil; turpentine oil (p.1760·1).
*Musculoskeletal, joint, peri-articular, and soft-tissue disorders.*

**Lauromicina** *Lafare, Ital.*
*Ointment:* Fluocinolone acetonide (p.1101·2); erythromycin stearate (p.208·2).
*Infected skin disorders.*
*Tablets:* Laurilsulfate salt of erythromycin stearate (p.208·2).
*Bacterial infections.*

**Lavaflac** *Antibioticos, Spain†.*
Sodium chloride (p.1233·3).
*Fluid and electrolyte disorders.*

**Lavagin** *Mayrhofer, Austria.*
Lactic acid (p.1704·1); sodium lactate (p.1223·2).
*Vaginal disorders.*

**Lavanda Sofar** *Sofar, Ital.*
Anhydrous citric acid (p.1673·1); sodium citrate (p.1223·2); alum (p.1652·1); phenol (p.1188·1).
*Vaginal disinfection.*

**Lavasept** *Fresenius Kabi, Switz.*
Polihexanide (p.1190·1).
*Bone and soft-tissue infections; wounds.*

**Lavement au Phosphate** *Norgine, Belg.*
Monobasic sodium phosphate (p.1230·3); dibasic sodium phosphate (p.1231·1).
*Bowel evacuation.*

**Laver** *Neopharm, Thai.*
Triamcinolone acetonide (p.1110·2).
*Skin disorders.*

**Laveran**
*Note. This name is used for preparations of different composition.*
*Brasmedica, Braz.†.*
Cimetidine (p.1255·3).
*Gastro-oesophageal reflux; gstro-intestinal haemorrhage; peptic ulcer; Zollinger-Ellison syndrome.*

*Unicure, India.*
Proguanil hydrochloride (p.457·1).
*Malaria.*

**Lavichthol** *Ichthyol, Austria.*
Ictasol (p.1148·3).
*Skin disorders.*

**Laviest** *Franco-Indian, India.*
*Saccharomyces cerevisiae* (p.1469·1).
*Moniliasis; vitamin B deficiency.*

**Lavisa** *Lesvi, Spain.*
Fluconazole (p.398·1).
*Fungal infections.*

**Lavolen** *Lacer, Spain.*
Trisodium polysaccharide sulfate; a nonoxinol (p.1413·2).
*Contraceptive.*

**Lavolho** *Regius, Braz.†.*
Boric acid (p.1662·1); chlorobutanol (p.1176·3).
*Eye disorders.*

**Lawefluor N** *Dental-Kosmetik, Ger.*
Olaflur (p.1442·3); dectaflur (p.1427·1); sodium fluoride (p.1444·3).
*Dental caries prophylaxis; hypersensitive teeth.*

**Lax Pills** *G & W, USA.*
Sennosides (p.1288·2).
*Constipation.*

**Laxa** *Nobel, Canad.†.*
Aloin (p.1248·3); cascara (p.1255·1); phenolphthalein (p.1284·1); bile salts (p.1660·3).

**Laxabon**
*AstraZeneca, Norw.; Hassle, Swed.*
Macrogol 3350 (p.1709·1); electrolytes (p.1217·1).
*Bowel evacuation.*

**Laxaco** *Jamieson, Canad.*
Cascara sagrada (p.1255·1); senna (p.1288·2).
*Constipation.*

**Laxadin** *Teva, Israel.*
Bisacodyl (p.1251·3).
*Constipation.*

**Laxadoron** *Weleda, UK.*
Homoeopathic preparation.

**Laxagel** *Everest, Canad.†.*
*Capsules:* Docusate sodium (p.1262·2).
*Constipation.*
*Oral powder:* Ispaghula (p.1268·1).

**Laxagetten** *CT, Ger.*
Bisacodyl (p.1251·3).
*Constipation.*

**Laxal** *Julphar, UAE.*
Senna (p.1288·2).
*Bowel evacuation; constipation.*

**Laxalpin** *Kwizda, Austria.*
Senna (p.1288·2); frangula bark (p.1266·3); fennel (p.1687·2); chamomile (p.1669·3); guaiacum wood; liquorice (p.1270·2); sambucus (p.1741·3); adiantum capillus veneris; potassium sodium tartrate (p.1284·3).
*Constipation.*

**Laxamalt**
*Bouchara-Recordati, Fr.; Bouchara, Switz.†.*
Liquid paraffin (p.1479·1).
*Constipation.*

**Laxamin** *Temis, Arg.*
*Oral drops:* Sodium picosulfate (p.1289·3).
*Tablets:* Bisacodyl (p.1251·3).
*Constipation.*

**Laxamucil** *Orion, Fin.*
Ispaghula (p.1268·1).
*Constipation.*

**Laxan**
*Note. This name is used for preparations of different composition.*
*QIF, Braz.†.*
Senna (p.1288·2); tamarind (p.1293·2); cassia pulp (p.1255·2).
*Constipation.*

*Chew, Thai.*
Methocarbamol (p.1395·1).
*Musculoskeletal pain.*

**Laxanin N** *Schwarzhaupt, Ger.*
Bisacodyl (p.1251·3).
*Constipation.*

**Laxans** *Schulke & Mayr, Austria.*
Ispaghula (p.1268·1).
*Constipation.*

**Laxans-ratiopharm** *Ratiopharm, Ger.*
Bisacodyl (p.1251·3).
*Constipation.*

**Laxans-ratiopharm Pico** *Ratiopharm, Ger.*
Sodium picosulfate (p.1289·3).
*Constipation.*

**Laxante Bescansa** *Bescansa, Spain†.*
Carrageenan mucilage (p.1578·2); phenolphthalein (p.1284·1).
*Constipation.*

**Laxante Bescansa Aloico** *Bescansa, Spain.*
Aloin (p.1248·3); belladonna (p.479·1); phenolphthalein (p.1284·1); rhubarb (p.1287·3).
*Constipation.*

**Laxante Bescansa Normal** *Bescansa, Spain.*
Senna (p.1288·2).
*Constipation.*

**Laxante Derly** *Derly, Spain†.*
Cascara (p.1255·1); senna (p.1288·2).
*Constipation.*

**Laxante Olan** *Puerto Galiano, Spain.*
Senna (p.1288·2).
Formerly contained ipomoea, phenolphthalein, sodium bicarbonate, and tartaric acid.
*Constipation.*

**Laxante Salud** *Boots Healthcare, Spain.*
Senna (p.1288·2).
Formerly contained aloes and phenolphthalein.
*Constipation.*

**Laxante Sanatorium** *Santiveri, Spain.*
Aloes (p.1248·2); aniseed (p.1655·2); sulfur (p.1158·2); senna (p.1288·2); chamomile (p.1669·3).
*Constipation.*

**Laxantil**
*Note. This name is used for preparations of different composition.*
*Teuto, Braz.†.*
Liquid paraffin (p.1479·1); phenolphthalein (p.1284·1); agar (p.1576·3).
*Constipation.*

*Chemopharma, Chile.*
Sodium picosulfate (p.1289·3).
*Bowel evacuation; constipation.*

**Laxarine** *Farmion, Braz.*
Senna (p.1288·2); cassia pulp (p.1255·2); tamarind (p.1293·2); coriander (p.1676·1); liquorice (p.1270·2).
*Constipation.*

**Laxarol** *Therapex, Canad.†.*
Phenolphthalein (p.1284·1); liquid paraffin (p.1479·1).

**Laxaron**
*Note. This name is used for preparations of different composition.*
*Merck Medication Familiale, Fr.*
Lactulose (p.1269·1).
*Constipation.*

*Strand, Malaysia.*
Liquid paraffin (p.1479·1).
*Constipation.*

**Laxasan**
*Note. This name is used for preparations of different composition.*
*Dolisos, Canad.†.*
Homoeopathic preparation.

*Dolisos, Fr.†.*
Senna (p.1288·2); tamarind (p.1293·2).
*Constipation.*

*Gebro, Switz.*
Sodium picosulfate (p.1289·3); fennel oil (p.1687·3); peppermint oil (p.1283·2).
*Constipation.*

**Laxative**
*Note. This name is used for preparations of different composition.*
*Lalco, Canad.*
Aloes (p.1248·2); cascara sagrada (p.1255·1); bile salts (p.1660·3).
*Constipation.*

*Trima, Israel.*
Aloin (p.1248·3); phenolphthalein (p.1284·1); belladonna (p.479·1).
*Constipation.*

**Laxative Comp** *Teva, Israel.*
Aloin (p.1248·3); phenolphthalein (p.1284·1); aloes (p.1248·2); ipecacuanha (p.1122·3); belladonna (p.479·1).
*Constipation.*

**Laxative Pills** *Stanley, Canad.*
Sennosides (p.1288·2).
Formerly contained phenolphthalein.

**Laxative & Stool Softener** *Rugby, USA.*
Docusate sodium (p.1262·2); casanthranol (p.1255·1).
*Constipation.*

**Laxative Tablets** *Herbal Concepts, UK.*
Aloes (p.1248·2); cascara (p.1255·1); senna (p.1288·2); valerian (p.1762·2).
*Constipation.*

**Laxativum Nouvelle Formule** *Giuliani, Switz.†.*
Cascara (p.1255·1); boldo (p.1661·2); senna (p.1288·2).
*Constipation.*

**Laxatol** *Santa, Gr.*
Sodium picosulfate (p.1289·3).
*Bowel evacuation; constipation.*

**Laxavit** *Wolfs, Belg.*
Docusate sodium (p.1262·2); glycerol (p.1694·3).
*Constipation.*

**Laxbene**
*Note. This name is used for preparations of different composition.*
*Ratiopharm, Austria.*
*Suppositories:* Bisacodyl (p.1251·3).
*Tablets:* Bisacodyl (p.1251·3); dimethicone (p.1289·2).
*Bowel evacuation; constipation.*

*Merckle, Ger.*
Bisacodyl (p.1251·3).
*Constipation.*

**Laxcodyl**
*Tanta, Canad.; Pharmasant, Thai.*
Bisacodyl (p.1251·3).
*Constipation.*

**Laxen** *Farmasa, Mex.†.*
Ispaghula (p.1268·1).

**Laxen Busto** *Salvat, Spain†.*
Phenolphthalein (p.1284·1).
*Constipation.*

**Laxette** *Medpro, S.Afr.*
Lactulose (p.1269·1).
*Constipation; hepatic encephalopathy.*

**Laxettes** *Mentholatum, Austral.*
*Chocolate†:* Phenolphthalein (p.1284·1).
*Tablets:* Calcium sennoside A (p.1288·3); calcium sennoside B (p.1288·3).
*Constipation.*

**Laxicaps P** *Propan, S.Afr.*
Phenolphthalein (p.1284·1).
*Constipation.*

**Laxicon** *Stadmed, India.*
Docusate sodium (p.1262·2).
*Constipation.*

**Laxicona** *Baliarda, Arg.*
Bisacodyl (p.1251·3); simeticone (p.1289·2).
*Constipation; flatulence.*

**Laxikal Forte** *Teva, Israel.*
Senna (p.1288·2).
*Constipation.*

**Laxilose** *Technilab, Canad.*
Lactulose (p.1269·1).
*Constipation.*

**Laxiplant** *Schwabe, Spain†.*
Ispaghula (p.1268·1); senna (p.1288·2).
*Constipation.*

**Laxiplant cum Senna** *Wander OTC, Switz.†.*
Ispaghula (p.1268·1); senna (p.1288·2).
*Constipation.*

**Laxiplant Soft**
*Schwabe, Ger.; Schwabe, Switz.*
Ispaghula (p.1268·1).
*Constipation; diarrhoea.*

**Laxisoft** *Schwabe, Spain.*
Ispaghula (p.1268·1).
*Constipation; diarrhoea.*

**Laxitab** *Ranbaxy, Thai.*
Bisacodyl (p.1251·3).
*Constipation.*

**Laxo Vian** *Alcala, Spain†.*
Atropine sulfate (p.477·1); hyoscyamus (p.485·2); cascara (p.1255·1); phenolphthalein (p.1284·1); podophyllum (p.1155·2); sodium bicarbonate.
*Constipation.*

**Laxoberal**
*Boehringer Ingelheim, Chile; Boehringer Ingelheim, Denm.; Boehringer Ingelheim, Ger.; Boehringer Ingelheim, Irl.; Boehringer Ingelheim,*

*Norw.; Boehringer Ingelheim, Swed.; Boehringer Ingelheim Self Medication, UK.*
Sodium picosulfate (p.1289·3).
*Bowel evacuation; constipation.*

**Laxoberal Bisa** *Boehringer Ingelheim, Ger.*
Bisacodyl (p.1251·3).
*Constipation.*

**Laxoberon**
*Boehringer Ingelheim, Belg.; Boehringer Ingelheim, Fin.; Teijin, Jpn; Boehringer Ingelheim Promeco, Mex.; Boehringer Ingelheim, Switz.*
Sodium picosulfate (p.1289·3).
*Bowel evacuation; constipation.*

**Laxocodyl** *Julphar, UAE.*
Bisacodyl (p.1251·3).
*Bowel evacuation; constipation.*

**Laxodal** *Baldacci, Port.*
Sodium picosulfate (p.1289·3).

**Laxofalk** *Falk, Ger.*
Macrogol 4000 (p.1709·1).
*Constipation.*

**Laxogeno** *Grunenthal, Chile.*
Oral solution, magnesium citrate (p.1272·1); oral powder, sodium bicarbonate (p.1223·2); tablets, bisacodyl (p.1251·3); suppositories, bisacodyl.
*Bowel evacuation.*

**Laxol** *Daudt, Braz.*
Castor oil (p.1668·2).
*Constipation.*

**Laxolen** *Basi, Port.*
Cascara (p.1255·1).
*Constipation.*

**Laxolind** *Metochem, Austria†.*
Senna (p.1288·2); frangula (p.1266·3); chamomile (p.1669·3).
*Bowel regulation.*

**Laxolyne** *Julphar, UAE.*
Glycerol (p.1694·3).
*Constipation.*

**Laxomax** *Soria Natural, Spain.*
Senna (p.1288·2); peppermint leaf (p.1283·2); liquorice (p.1270·2); aniseed (p.1655·2).
*Constipation.*

**Laxomild** *Renapharm, Switz.†.*
Calcium sennoside A (p.1288·3); calcium sennoside B (p.1288·3).
*Constipation.*

**Laxomundin** *Mundipharma, Ger.†.*
Lactulose (p.1269·1).
*Constipation.*

**Laxonol** *Madaus, Spain†.*
Sodium picosulfate (p.1289·3).
*Constipation.*

**Laxopol**
*Pohl, Ger.; Pohl, Israel.*
Castor oil (p.1668·2).
*Constipation.*

**Laxose** *Pinewood, Irl.*
Lactulose (p.1269·1).
*Constipation; hepatic encephalopathy.*

**Laxsol** *Sigma, NZ.*
Docusate sodium (p.1262·2); sennosides (p.1288·2).
*Constipation.*

**Laxtam** *Merck, Braz.*
Senna (p.1288·2); cassia pulp (p.1255·2); tamarind (p.1293·2); coriander (p.1676·1); liquorice (p.1270·2).
*Constipation.*

**Laxuave Enteral** *Elea, Arg.*
Liquid paraffin (p.1479·1).
*Constipation.*

**Laxucil** *Novopharm, Canad.*
Ispaghula (p.1268·1).

**Laxvital** *Maxfarma, Spain.*
Carmellose (p.1577·3); docusate sodium (p.1262·2); casanthranol (p.1255·1).
*Constipation.*

**Laxyl** *Solfran, Mex.*
Diazepam (p.690·1).

**Laxysat Burger** *Ysatfabrik, Ger.*
Bisacodyl (p.1251·3).
*Constipation.*

**Laxysat mono** *Ysatfabrik, Ger.†.*
Buckthorn (p.1254·1).
*Constipation.*

**Lazercreme** *Pedinol, USA.*
Vitamin E (p.1464·3); vitamin A (p.1451·2).
*Minor skin irritation.*

**Lazerformaldehyde** *Pedinol, USA.*
Formaldehyde (p.1179·3).
*Bromhidrosis (feet); hyperhidrosis; warts.*

**LazerSporin-C** *Pedinol, USA.*
Neomycin sulfate (p.235·1); polymyxin B sulfate (p.245·1); hydrocortisone (p.1103·3).
*Bacterial ear infections.*

**LB Jabon con Purcelin** *Billiet, Arg.*
Triclocarban (p.1195·1); purcelin oil.
*Skin cleansing.*

**LC-65**
*Allergan, Austral.†; Allergan, Canad.; Allergan, Israel†; Advanced Medical Optics, NZ; Allergan, Port.†; Allergan, USA.*
Range of solutions for contact lenses (p.1164·2).

**L-Carn** *Sigma-Tau, Ger.*
Levocarnitine (p.1423·3).
*Carnitine deficiency.*

**L-Cimexyl** *Cimex, Switz.*
Acetylcysteine (p.1112·3).
*Respiratory-tract disorders.*

**L-Combur-5-Test** *Roche Diagnostics, Austral.*
Test for pH, protein, glucose, ketones, and blood in urine.

**LCP** *Nutricia, Ital.*
Fish oil; borage oil; vegetable oil; vitamin E (p.1417·1).
*Amino-acid disorders; phenylketonuria.*

**Le 100 B** *Pharmalab, Canad.†.*
Cascara (p.1255·1); phenolphthalein (p.1284·1).

**Le 500 D** *Pharmalab, Canad.†.*
Cascara (p.1255·1).

**Le Face Protection** *Creative Brands, Austral.†.*
*SPF 15+:* Octinoxate (p.1154·3); avobenzone (p.1142·3).
*Sunscreen.*

**Le Fibre** *Or-Dov, Austral.†.*
Wheat fibre.
*Dietary fibre supplement; obesity.*

**Le Pont Tratamiento Ungueal Formula 405** *Dermaclin, Mex.*
Phospholipids; vitamin A; vitamin E (p.1417·1).
*Nail disorders.*

**Le Stick a Levres** *Duchesnay, Canad.*
Cinoxate (p.1145·1); allantoin (p.1141·3); vitamin A palmitate (p.1453·1).
*Sunscreen.*

**Le Tan Broad Spectrum** *Creative Brands, Austral.†.*
*SPF15+:* Octinoxate (p.1154·3); avobenzone (p.1142·3).
*Sunscreen.*

**Le Tan Fast Extra Dark** *Creative Brands, Austral.†.*
Dihydroxyacetone (p.1145·2).
*Artificial suntan.*

**Le Tan Fast Plus** *Creative Brands, Austral.†.*
*SPF 15:* Octinoxate (p.1154·3); avobenzone (p.1142·3); dihydroxyacetone (p.1145·2).
*Artificial suntan; sunscreen.*

**Le Tan Fast Self Tan** *Creative Brands, Austral.†.*
Dihydroxyacetone (p.1145·2).
*Artificial suntan.*

**Le Tan Gel** *Creative Brands, Austral.†.*
*SPF 8:* Octinoxate (p.1154·3); benzophenone (p.1143·1).
*SPF 15:* Octinoxate (p.1154·3); benzophenone (p.1143·1); avobenzone (p.1142·3).
*Sunscreen.*

**Le Tan Natural** *Creative Brands, Austral.†.*
*SPF 15:* Titanium dioxide (p.1160·3); zinc oxide (p.1163·2).
*Sunscreen.*

**Le Tan Roll On Lotion** *Creative Brands, Austral.†.*
*SPF 15:* Octinoxate (p.1154·3); avobenzone (p.1142·3).
*Sunscreen.*

**Le Tan Sensitive** *Creative Brands, Austral.†.*
*SPF 30+:* Octinoxate (p.1154·3); amiloxate (p.1142·2); octisalate (p.1154·3); zinc oxide (p.1163·2).
*Sunscreen.*

**Le Tan Sport Dry Lotion** *Creative Brands, Austral.†.*
*SPF 15:* Octinoxate (p.1154·3); oxybenzone (p.1154·3); avobenzone (p.1142·3).
*Sunscreen.*

**Le Tan Sport & Surf** *Creative Brands, Austral.†.*
*SPF 30+:* Octinoxate (p.1154·3); amiloxate (p.1142·2); octisalate (p.1154·3); zinc oxide (p.1163·2).
*Sunscreen.*

**Le Tan Sunblock Stick** *Creative Brands, Austral.†.*
*SPF 15:* Octinoxate (p.1154·3); avobenzone (p.1142·3).
*Sunscreen.*

**Le Tan Sunscreen Lotion** *Creative Brands, Austral.†.*
*SPF15:* Octinoxate (p.1154·3); avobenzone (p.1142·3).
*SPF 30+:* Octinoxate (p.1154·3); enzacamene (p.1147·1); avobenzone (p.1142·3).
*SPF4; SPF8:* Octinoxate (p.1154·3).
*Sunscreen.*

**Le Tan Sunscreen Lotion Broad Spectrum** *Creative Brands, Austral.†.*
*SPF 15+:* Octinoxate (p.1154·3); avobenzone (p.1142·3).
*Sunscreen.*

**Le Tan Ultimate** *Creative Brands, Austral.†.*
*SPF 8:* Octinoxate (p.1154·3); benzophenone (p.1143·1).
*SPF 15+:* Octinoxate (p.1154·3); avobenzone (p.1142·3); benzophenone (p.1143·1).
*Sunscreen.*

**Le Thermogene** *Tradiphar, Fr.*
Capsicum oleoresin (p.1667·1); glycol salicylate (p.44·3).
*Musculoskeletal and peri-articular pain; respiratory-tract congestion.*

**Le Trim-BM** *Or-Dov, Austral.†.*
Benzocaine (p.1370·3); methylcellulose (p.1580·2); ferrous gluconate; vitamins (p.1417·1).
*Obesity.*

**Lealgin** *Janssen-Cilag, Swed.†.*
Phenoperidine hydrochloride (p.83·2).
*Adjunct in neuroleptanalgesia; pain in surgical procedures; respiratory depressant in intensive care.*

**LEAN Formula w/ Advantra** *Usana, Hong Kong.*
Sour orange (p.1723·3); green tea (p.1765·3); guarana (p.1765·3); cayenne (p.1667·1).
*Obesity.*

**Leanor** *Aspen, S.Afr.*
Cathine hydrochloride (p.1585·2).
*Obesity.*

**Leaton fur Erwachsene** *Pharmacia, Austria.*
Multivitamins (p.1417·1) with caffeine (p.782·1).
*Tonic.*

**Leaton fur Kinder** *Pharmacia, Austria.*
Multivitamins (p.1417·1).
*Tonic.*

**Lebensenergie-Kapseln** *Twardy, Ger.*
Eleutherococcus (p.1744·1).
*Tonic.*

**Leberetic** *Ern, Spain.*
Potassium sulfate (p.1232·2); sodium bicarbonate (p.1223·2); sodium sulfate (p.1290·1).
*Liver disorders.*

**Leber-Galle-Tropfen 83** *Bio-Diat, Ger.*
Sage (p.1741·2); absinthium (p.1645·1); gentian (p.1692·2); fennel (p.1687·2); centaury (p.1669·2); elecampane (p.1119·3); anise oil (p.1655·2); peppermint oil (p.1283·2); calamus oil; lavender oil (p.1705·2).
*Biliary disorders; dyspepsia.*

**Leber-Galletropfen SN** *Cosmochema, Ger.*
Homoeopathic preparation.

**Leberinfusion** *Fresenius Kabi, Austria.*
Arginine (p.1421·1); malic acid (p.1709·2); sodium hydroxide (p.1747·3); potassium hydroxide (p.1734·2).
*Liver disorders.*

**Lebersal** *Ern, Spain.*
Magnesium sulfate (p.1228·2); sodium bicarbonate (p.1223·2); dibasic sodium phosphate (p.1231·1); sodium sulfate (p.1290·1).
*Gastrointestinal disorders; hepatic insufficiency.*

**Leberschutz** *Bregenzer, Austria.*
Silybum marianum (p.1043·3).
*Liver and biliary-tract disorders.*

**Lebic** *Alpharma-Isis, Ger.*
Baclofen (p.1386·3).
*Skeletal muscle spasm or spasticity.*

**Lebilon** *Pharmaten (Φαρματεν), Gr.*
Buspirone hydrochloride (p.672·2).
*Generalised anxiety.*

**Lebocar** *Pharmacia, Arg.*
Levodopa (p.1205·2); carbidopa (p.1204·3).
*Parkinsonism.*

**Lebopride** *Spyfarma, Spain.*
Sulpiride (p.722·2).
*Anxiety disorders; psychoses; vertigo.*

**Lebriton N** *Zeppenfeldt, Ger.†.*
Homoeopathic preparation.

**Lebrocetin** *Liferpal, Mex.*
Chloramphenicol (p.185·1).
*Bacterial infections.*

**Lecarge** *Klonal, Arg.*
Levodopa (p.1205·2); carbidopa (p.1204·3).
*Parkinsonism.*

**Leche Autobronceadora** *Pierre Fabre Dermo-Cosmetique, Arg.*
Dihydroxyacetone (p.1145·2).
*Artificial tanning.*

**Leche Autobronceadora Cara Y Cuerpo** *Silesia, Chile.*
Dihydroxyacetone (p.1145·2).
*Artificial suntan.*

**Leche de Magnesia Phillips**
*GlaxoSmithKline, Arg.; GlaxoSmithKline, Chile.*
Magnesium hydroxide (p.1272·2).
*Antacid; constipation.*

**Leche de Proteccion Total** *Pierre Fabre Dermo-Cosmetique, Arg.*
Titanium dioxide (p.1160·3); cinnamate.
*Sunscreen.*

**Lecia** *Caldeira & Marques, Port.*
Lactic acid (p.1704·1); salicylic acid (p.1157·1); collodion.
Formerly contained ortho-oxybenzoic acid, lactic acid, phenol, glacial acetic acid, and turpentine oil.
*Corns; verrucas.*

**Lecibral** *Solvay, Spain.*
Nicardipine hydrochloride (p.965·1).
*Angina pectoris; cerebrovascular disorders; hypertension.*

**Lecicarbon**
*Note. This name is used for preparations of different composition.*
*Brady, Austria.*
Sodium bicarbonate (p.1223·2); potassium acid tartrate (p.1284·3).
*Constipation.*
*Athenstaedt, Ger.; Athenstaedt, Switz.*
Sodium bicarbonate (p.1223·2); monobasic sodium phosphate (p.1230·3).
*Bowel evacuation; constipation.*

**Leciderm** *Darier, Mex.*
Lecithin (p.1706·1).
*Dry skin disorders.*

**Lecifar-K** *Farcoral, Mex.*
Lecithin (p.1706·1); kelp (p.1742·3); vitamin $B_6$ (p.1457·2); apple.
*Obesity.*

**Lecikur** *Agepha, Austria.*
Lecithin (p.1706·1); caffeine (p.782·1).
*Tonic.*

**Lecimar** *Spyfarma, Spain.*
Fluoxetine hydrochloride (p.292·1).
*Bulimia; depression; mixed anxiety depressive disorder; obsessive-compulsive disorder.*

**Lecinova** *Novartis Consumer, Ital.*
Nutritional supplement containing phospholipids and vitamins (p.1417·1).

**Leciplus** *Novartis Consumer, Ital.*
Nutritional supplement containing phospholipids and vitamins (p.1417·1).

**Lecithin ACE** *YSP, Malaysia.*
Lecithin; vitamin A; vitamin C; vitamin E (p.1417·1).
*Dietary supplement.*

**Lecithin AE** *YSP, Malaysia.*
Lecithin; vitamin A; vitamin E (p.1417·1).
*Dietary supplement.*

**Lecitone**
*Yves Ponroy, Fr.*
A range of nutritional supplements containing phospholipids (p.1417·1).
*Tonic.*
*Yves Ponroy, Singapore.*
Dietary supplement (p.1417·1).

**Lecivital** *Agepha, Austria.*
*Oral solution:* Lecithin (p.1706·1); caffeine (p.782·1); tocoferil acetate (p.1465·1).
*Tablets:* Lecithin (p.1706·1); vitamin E acetate (p.1465·1).
*Tonic.*

**Leclor A** *Provit, Mex.*
Chloramphenicol (p.185·1).
*Bacterial infections.*

**Leclyte** *David, India.*
Calcium lactate; potassium chloride; magnesium sulfate; sodium chloride; sodium acid phosphate; glucose (p.1222·2).
*Oral rehydration therapy.*
A range of electrolyte infusions with glucose (p.1217·1).
*Fluid and electrolyte imbalance.*

**Lecrolyn**
*Santen, Denm.; Santen, Fin.; Santen, Norw.; Santen, Swed.; Santen, Thai.*
Sodium cromoglicate (p.795·3).
*Allergic conjunctivitis.*

**Lectil** *Bouchara-Recordati, Fr.*
Betahistine hydrochloride (p.1660·1).
*Vertigo.*

**Lectopam** *Roche, Canad.*
Bromazepam (p.671·3).
*Anxiety; sedative.*

**Lectrum** *Labinca, Arg.*
Leuprorelin acetate (p.1331·1).

**Ledclair**
*IFET (IΦET), Gr.; Sinclair, Irl.; Durbin, UK.*
Sodium calcium edetate (p.1051·3).
*Heavy metal poisoning; hypercalcaemia.*

**Ledercillin VK** *Wyeth-Ayerst, Canad.†.*
Phenoxymethylpenicillin potassium (p.242·1).
*Bacterial infections.*

**Ledercort**
*Wyeth, Arg.; Wyeth Lederle, Belg.; Wyeth Lederle, India; Wyeth Lederle, Ital.; Lederle, Neth.†; Wyeth, S.Afr.†; Wyeth, Spain†; ICN, Switz.; Lederle, UK†.*
Triamcinolone (p.1110·2), triamcinolone acetonide (p.1110·2), or triamcinolone diacetate (p.1110·2).
*Corticosteroid.*

**Ledercort con Neomicina** *Wyeth, Arg.*
Triamcinolone acetonide (p.1110·2); neomycin sulfate (p.235·1).
*Ear and eye disorders.*

**Ledercort-N** *Wyeth Lederle, India.*
Triamcinolone acetonide (p.1110·2); neomycin sulfate (p.235·1).
*Infected skin disorders.*

**Lederderm** *Lederle, Ger.*
Minocycline hydrochloride (p.231·3).
*Bacterial infections.*

**Lederfen**
*Wyeth Lederle, Austria; Wyeth, Irl.; Lederle, Israel†; Goldshield, UK.*
Fenbufen (p.39·1).
*Musculoskeletal and joint disorders.*

**Lederfolat** *Lederle, Ger.*
Calcium folinate (p.1431·1).
*Folate deficiency.*

**Lederfolin**
*Wyeth, Irl.; Wyeth Lederle, Ital.; Wyeth, Spain; Wyeth, UK.*
Calcium folinate (p.1431·1).
*Adjunct to fluorouracil in colorectal cancer; folate deficiency; reduction of folic acid antagonist toxicity.*

**Lederfoline**
*Wyeth Lederle, Fr.; Teofarma, Port.*
Calcium folinate (p.1431·1).
*Drug-induced megaloblastic anaemia; folic acid deficiency; prevention of methotrexate toxicity.*

**Lederlind** *Lederle, Ger.*
Nystatin (p.406·3).
*Fungal infections of the skin and mucous membranes.*

**Lederlon** *Lederle, Ger.*
Triamcinolone hexacetonide (p.1110·2).
*Parenteral corticosteroid.*

**Ledermicina** *Cyanamid, Ital.†.*
Demeclocycline hydrochloride (p.204·3).
*Bacterial infections.*

**Ledermix**
Wyeth Lederle, Austria; Wyeth, Irl.†; Wyeth, S.Afr.†; ICN, Switz.; Blackwell, UK.
Paste, triamcinolone acetonide (p.1110·2); demeclocycline calcium (p.205·1); cement, triamcinolone acetonide; demeclocycline hydrochloride (p.204·3); solution, eugenol (p.1686·2).
*Bacterial infection and inflammatory disorders in dentistry.*

Wyeth Lederle, Denm.
Paste, triamcinolone acetonide (p.1110·2); demeclocycline calcium (p.205·1); cement, triamcinolone acetonide; demeclocycline calcium; hardener N, macrogol 400 (p.1709·1); hardener S, eugenol (p.1686·2).
*Bacterial infection and inflammatory disorders in dentistry.*

Lederle, Israel.
Triamcinolone acetonide (p.1110·2); demeclocycline calcium (p.205·1).
*Bacterial infection and inflammatory disorders in dentistry.*

**Ledermycin**
Wyeth, Austral.; Wyeth Lederle, Austria†; Wyeth Lederle, India; Wyeth, Irl.†; Lederle, Neth.; Lederle, NZ†; Goldshield, UK.
Demeclocycline hydrochloride (p.204·3).
*Amoebiasis; bacterial infections; hyponatraemia.*

**Lederpaediat** Lederle, Ger.†.
Erythromycin ethyl succinate (p.208·1).
*Bacterial infections.*

**Lederpax**
Wyeth, Arg.; Wyeth, Mex.; Wyeth, Spain.
Erythromycin (p.208·1).
*Acne.*

**Lederplatin** Pharmachemie, Denm.
Cisplatin (p.538·1).
*Malignant neoplasms.*

**Lederscon** Lederle, Hong Kong†.
Aluminium hydroxide (p.1249·2); magnesium hydroxide (p.1272·2); mannitol (p.950·2); simeticone (p.1289·2).
*Flatulence; meteorism.*

**Lederspan**
Wyeth Lederle, Austria†; Wyeth Lederle, Belg.†; Wyeth Lederle, Denm.†; Wyeth Lederle, Fin.†; Wyeth, Irl.†; Lederle, Neth.†; Wyeth Lederle, Norw.; Wyeth, S.Afr.†; Wyeth Lederle, Swed.†; Wyeth, UK†.
Triamcinolone hexacetonide (p.1110·2).
*Corticosteroid.*

**Ledertam** Wyeth Lederle, Ital.
Tamoxifen citrate (p.584·1).
*Breast cancer.*

**Ledertepa**
Wyeth Lederle, Belg.†; IFET (IΦET), Gr.; Lederle, Neth.
Thiotepa (p.588·1).
*Malignant neoplasms.*

**Ledertrexate**
Wyeth, Austral.; Wyeth Lederle, Belg.; Wyeth Lederle, Fr.; Wyeth, Mex.; Wyeth, Neth.; Lederle, NZ.
Methotrexate (p.568·2) or methotrexate sodium (p.568·3).
*Malignant neoplasms; mycosis fungoides; psoriasis; rheumatoid arthritis.*

**Ledervorin**
Wyeth Lederle, Belg.; Lederle, Neth.†.
Calcium folinate (p.1431·1).
*Adjunct to fluorouracil in colorectal cancer; adjunct to high-dose methotrexate therapy; overdosage with folic acid antagonists.*

**Ledion** Help, Gr.
Buspirone hydrochloride (p.672·2).
*Generalised anxiety.*

**Ledolid** Pulitzer, Ital.
Nimesulide (p.67·1).
*Fever; inflammation; pain.*

**Ledoren** Boniscontro & Gazzone, Ital.
Nimesulide (p.67·1).
*Fever; inflammation; pain.*

**Ledovit C** Bama, Spain†.
Ascorbic acid (p.1460·2).
*Adjunct in treatment of iron supplementation; vitamin C deficiency.*

**Ledox** Weifa, Norw.
Naproxen (p.65·1).
*Gout; musculoskeletal and joint disorders; pain.*

**Ledoxid Acne** Lederle, Switz.†.
Benzoyl peroxide (p.1143·2).
*Acne.*

**Ledoxina**
Laboratorios Chile, Chile; Lemery, Mex.
Cyclophosphamide (p.540·2).
*Malignant neoplasms.*

**Ledum Med Complex** Dynamit, Austria.
Homoeopathic preparation.

**Lefaenteril** Fecofar, Arg.
Neomycin (p.235·1); activated charcoal (p.1030·2); phthalylsulfathiazole (p.242·3).
*Diarrhoea.*

**Lefax**
Bayer, Ger.; Synpharma, Switz.
Simeticone (p.1289·2).
*Anti-foaming agent in radiography of the gastrointestinal tract; detergent intoxication; gastrointestinal disorders associated with excess gas.*

**Lefaxin** Lannacher, Austria.
Simeticone (p.1289·2).
*Flatulence.*

**Lefcar** GlaxoSmithKline, Ital.
Levocarnitine (p.1423·3).
*Carnitine deficiency; myocardial ischaemia.*

**Leferdivin** Hotz, Ger.†.
Vitamin B substances; lecithin; ferrous citrate; glutamic acid (p.1417·1).
*Tonic.*

**Lefkacid** Knop, Chile.
Calcium carbonate (p.1254·2); aluminium hydroxide (p.1249·2); magnesium hydroxide (p.1272·2).
*Gastric hyperacidity; gastritis; gastro-oesophageal reflux; peptic ulcer.*

**Lefkaflam** Knop, Chile.
Arnica (p.1656·3); menthol (p.1711·3); eucalyptus oil (p.1686·2); rosemary oil (p.1740·2).
*Musculoskeletal, joint, and peri-articular disorders; oedema.*

**Lefkur** Knop, Chile.
Cucurbita oil (p.1677·3).
*Benign prostatic hyperplasia.*

**Lefrine** Grin, Mex.
Phenylephrine hydrochloride (p.1126·3).
*Nasal congestion.*

**Leftose**
Shinyaku, Jpn; Shinyaku, Malaysia; Shinyaku, Singapore; Shinyaku, Thai.
Muramidase hydrochloride (p.1717·2).
*Haemorrhage; infections; inflammation.*

**Leg Cramps with Quinine** Hylands, Canad.
Homoeopathic preparation.

**Legalon**
Note. This name is used for preparations of different composition.
Madaus, Austria; Madaus, Fr.; Madaus, Ger.
Silybum marianum (p.1043·3).
*Liver disorders.*

Madaus, Belg.; Altana, Braz.; Roche, Chile; Madaus, Hong Kong; Madaus, Ital.; Byk Gulden, Mex.; Neo-Farmaceutica, Port.; Byk Madaus, S.Afr.; Madaus, Spain; Biomed, Switz.; Madaus, Thai.
Silymarin (p.1043·3).
*Liver disorders.*

IFET (IΦET), Gr.
Silibinin (p.1043·3).
*Mushroom poisoning.*

**Legalon SIL**
Madaus, Belg.; Madaus, Ger.; Biomed, Switz.
Disodium silibinin dihemisuccinate (p.1043·3).
*Mushroom poisoning.*

Madaus, Spain.
Silibinin dihemisuccinate (p.1043·3).
*Mushroom poisoning.*

**Legapas**
Pascoe, Ger.; Ebi, Switz.†.
Cascara (p.1255·1).
Formerly known as Legapas mono in *Ger.*
*Constipation.*

**Legapas comp** Pascoe, Ger.†.
Cascara (p.1255·1); silybum marianum (p.1043·3); greater celandine (p.1695·3); taraxacum (p.1751·3).
Formerly known as Legapas N.
*Liver disorders.*

**Legatrin PM** Columbia, USA.
Paracetamol (p.76·2); diphenhydramine hydrochloride (p.431·3).
*Insomnia.*

**Legatrin Rub** Columbia, USA.
Menthol (p.1711·3); benzocaine (p.1370·3).

**Legederm**
Schering-Plough, Denm.; Schering-Plough, Fin.; Schering-Plough, Ital.; Schering-Plough, Swed.
Alclometasone dipropionate (p.1090·3).
*Skin disorders.*

**Legendal**
Zambon, Neth.; Inpharzam, Switz.
Lactulose (p.1269·1).
*Constipation; hepatic encephalopathy.*

**Legifol CS** Pharmacia, Braz.
Calcium folinate (p.1431·1).

**Legil** Millet Roux, Braz.†.
Tenoxicam (p.93·1).
*Musculoskeletal, joint, and peri-articular disorders.*

**Legofer**
ITF, Chile; Elpen (Ελπεν), Gr.; Asta Medica, Ital.; ITF, Port.
Iron succinyl-protein complex (p.1438·1).
*Iron deficiency; iron-deficiency anaemia.*

**Lehydan** Abigo, Swed.
Phenytoin (p.370·2).
*Epilepsy.*

**Leiba** Uniao Quimica, Braz.
*Lactobacillus acidophilus* (p.1704·2).
*Diarrhoea; restoration of intestinal flora.*

**Leicester Retard** Polifarma, Ital.
Isosorbide mononitrate (p.942·1).
*Angina pectoris.*

**Leiguar** Labatec, Switz.
Guar gum (p.333·2).
*Diabetes mellitus; hyperlipidaemias.*

**Leioderm** Riemser, Ger.
Hydroxyquinoline sulfate (p.1700·1).
*Impetigo.*

**Leioderm P** Riemser, Ger.
Hydroxyquinoline sulfate (p.1700·1); prednisolone (p.1108·1).
*Infected skin disorders.*

**Leios** Wyeth, Ger.
Levonorgestrel (p.1563·2); ethinylestradiol (p.1553·2).
*Combined oral contraceptive.*

**Leite de Magnesia**
Hertz, Braz.†; Teuto, Braz.†; GlaxoSmithKline Consumer, Port.
Magnesium hydroxide (p.1272·2).
*Constipation.*

**Leite de Magnesia de Phillips** GlaxoSmithKline, Braz.
Magnesium hydroxide (p.1272·2).
*Constipation.*

**Lejguar** Meta Fackler, Ger.†.
Guar gum (p.333·2).
*Diabetes mellitus; hyperlipidaemias.*

**Lektinol** Madaus, Ger.
Mistletoe (p.1715·3).
*Malignant neoplasms.*

**Lelco 23** Defuen, Arg.
*SPF 23:* Amiloxate (p.1142·2); titanium dioxide (p.1160·3).
*Sunscreen.*

**Lelco Bebe** Defuen, Arg.
*SPF 15:* Titanium dioxide (p.1160·3).
*Sunscreen.*

**Lelco F** Defuen, Arg.
*SPF 6:* Amiloxate (p.1142·2).
*Sunscreen.*

**Lelco Labial** Defuen, Arg.
*p*-Methoxycinnamate; titanium dioxide (p.1160·3).
*Sunscreen for lips.*

**Lelco Locion Bronceadora** Defuen, Arg.
Avobenzone (p.1142·3); amiloxate (p.1142·2); octocrilene (p.1154·3).
*Sunscreen.*

**Lelco P** Defuen, Arg.
*SPF 15: p*-Methoxycinnamate; titanium dioxide (p.1160·3).
*Sunscreen.*

**Lelco P Ultra** Defuen, Arg.
*SPF 34: p*-Methoxycinnamate; octisalate (p.1154·3); oxybenzone (p.1154·3); avobenzone (p.1142·3); titanium dioxide (p.1160·3).
*Sunscreen.*

**Lelco sin Sol** Defuen, Arg.
Dihydroxyacetone (p.1145·2).
*Artificial tanning.*

**Lelco Spray** Defuen, Arg.
Amiloxate (p.1142·2); avobenzone (p.1142·3).
*Sunscreen.*

**Lelco Ultrablock** Defuen, Arg.
*SPF 65:* Amiloxate (p.1142·2); ensulizole (p.1147·1); titanium dioxide (p.1160·3); avobenzone (p.1142·3); oxybenzone (p.1154·3); octocrilene (p.1154·3).
*Sunscreen.*

**Lelong Contusions** Zambon, Fr.
Arnica (p.1656·3); tamus communis.
*Soft-tissue disorders.*

**Lelong Irritations** SmithKline Beecham Sante, Fr.†.
Enoxolone (p.36·2); propanocaine hydrochloride (p.1383·3).
*Inflammatory and pruritic skin disorders.*

**Lema C** Ern, Spain.
Ascorbic acid (p.1460·2); sodium perborate (p.1192·2).
*Halitosis; mouth and throat inflammation; pyorrhoea.*

**Lemazol** Petrasch, Austria.
Ascorbic acid (p.1460·2); potassium orotate (p.1724·3); inositol (p.1701·2); sorbitol (p.1446·3).
*Liver disorders.*

**Lemblastine**
Laboratorios Chile, Chile; Lemery, Mex.
Vinblastine sulfate (p.591·2).
*Malignant neoplasms.*

**Lembrol** Sanofi Synthelabo, Arg.
Diazepam (p.690·1).
*Anxiety; muscle spasm.*

**Lemdopa** Lemery, Mex.
Levodopa (p.1205·2); carbidopa (p.1204·3).
*Parkinsonism.*

**L-Emental** Nutrition Medical, Israel.
A range of preparations for enteral nutrition (p.1417·1).

**Lemeron** Lemery, Mex.
Interferon alfa-2b (p.640·3).
*Immunostimulant.*

**Lemesil** Anpharm (Ανφαρμ), Gr.
Nimesulide (p.67·1).
*Inflammation; musculoskeletal disorders; pain.*

**Lemgrip** Reckitt & Colman, Belg.†.
Paracetamol (p.76·2).
*Fever; pain.*

**Lemivit** Kemiprogress, Ital.†.
Vitamins (p.1417·1); lecithin (p.1706·1).
*Fatigue.*

**Lemlax** Co-Pharma, UK.
Lactulose (p.1269·1).
*Constipation.*

**Lemnis Fatty Cream** CSL, NZ; Yamanouchi, NZ.
Emollient.
*Barrier cream; emollient.*

**Lemnis Fatty Cream HC** Yamanouchi, NZ.
Hydrocortisone (p.1103·3).
*Skin disorders.*

**Lemocin**
Note. This name is used for preparations of different composition.
Novartis Consumer, Austria; Novartis Consumer, Belg.
Tyrothricin (p.275·1); cetrimide (p.1172·1); lidocaine (p.1377·3).
*Mouth and throat disorders.*

Novartis Consumer, Ger.; Novartis Consumer, Israel; Novartis Consumer, Switz.
Tyrothricin (p.275·1); cetrimonium bromide (p.1173·1); lidocaine (p.1377·3) or lidocaine hydrochloride (p.1377·3).
*Mouth and throat disorders.*

**Lemocin CX** Novartis Consumer, Ger.
Chlorhexidine gluconate (p.1173·2).
*Mouth and throat disorders.*

**Lemocin Flexibels** Novartis Consumer, Ger.†.
Benzoxonium chloride (p.1170·2); lidocaine hydrochloride (p.1377·3).
*Mouth and throat disorders.*

**Lemon Time** Buckley, Canad.
Paracetamol (p.76·2); phenylephrine hydrochloride (p.1126·3); mepyramine maleate (p.437·1); ascorbic acid (p.1460·2).
*Cold symptoms.*

**Lemonvit** Molteni, Ital.†.
Ascorbic acid (p.1460·2).
*Vitamin C deficiency.*

**Lemophar** Alpharma, Mex.
Hyoscine butylbromide (p.483·3).

**Lemotussin-DM** Seneca, USA.
Dextromethorphan hydrobromide (p.1117·3); guaifenesin (p.1122·1); sulfogaiacol (p.1131·1); pseudoephedrine hydrochloride (p.1129·2); chlorphenamine maleate (p.427·3).

**Lemoxin** Lemery, Mex.
Cefuroxime (p.184·1).
*Bacterial infections.*

**Lemoxol** Demo, Gr.
Ceftazidime (p.180·2).
*Bacterial infections.*

**Lem-Plus** Adcock Ingram, UK†.
*Capsules:* Paracetamol (p.76·2); caffeine (p.782·1); phenylephrine (p.1126·3).
*Oral powder:* Paracetamol (p.76·2); ascorbic acid (p.1460·2).
*Cold symptoms.*

**Lemsip**
Note. This name is used for preparations of different composition.
Reckitt & Colman, Austral.†; Meda, Swed.†.
Paracetamol (p.76·2).
*Cold and influenza symptoms.*

Reckitt Benckiser, Hong Kong.
Paracetamol (p.76·2); sodium citrate (p.1223·2); vitamin C (p.1460·2).
*Cold and influenza symptoms.*

Reckitt & Colman, S.Afr.†.
Paracetamol (p.76·2); phenylephrine hydrochloride (p.1126·3); sodium citrate (p.1223·2).
*Cold and influenza symptoms.*

**Lemsip Chesty Cough**
Reckitt Benckiser, Austral.†; Reckitt Benckiser, NZ.
Guaifenesin (p.1122·1).
*Coughs.*

**Lemsip Childrens Six+ Cold & Flu Relief**
Reckitt Benckiser, UK.
Paracetamol (p.76·2); phenylephrine hydrochloride (p.1126·3).
*Cold and influenza symptoms.*

**Lemsip Cold & Flu** Reckitt Benckiser, Irl.
Paracetamol (p.76·2); ascorbic acid (p.1460·2).
*Cold and influenza symptoms.*

**Lemsip Cold & Flu Breathe Easy** Reckitt Benckiser, UK.
Paracetamol (p.76·2); phenylephrine hydrochloride (p.1126·3); ascorbic acid (p.1460·2).
*Cold and influenza symptoms.*

**Lemsip Cold & Flu Combined Relief** Reckitt & Colman, UK†.
Paracetamol (p.76·2); phenylephrine hydrochloride (p.1126·3); caffeine (p.782·1).
*Cold and influenza symptoms.*

**Lemsip Cold & Flu Headcold** Reckitt Benckiser, NZ.
Paracetamol (p.76·2); menthol (p.1711·3).
*Cold and influenza symptoms.*

**Lemsip Cold & Flu Max Strength** Reckitt Benckiser, UK.
Paracetamol (p.76·2); phenylephrine hydrochloride (p.1126·3); ascorbic acid (p.1460·2).
*Cold and influenza symptoms.*

**Lemsip Cold & Flu Max Strength Capsules**
Reckitt Benckiser, UK.
Paracetamol (p.76·2); phenylephrine hydrochloride (p.1126·3); caffeine (p.782·1).
*Cold and influenza symptoms.*

**Lemsip Cold & Flu Original** Reckitt Benckiser, UK.
Paracetamol (p.76·2); ascorbic acid (p.1460·2); phenylephrine hydrochloride (p.1126·3).
*Cold and influenza symptoms.*

**Lemsip Cold & Flu Original, Cold & Flu Max**
Reckitt Benckiser, NZ.
Paracetamol (p.76·2).
*Cold and influenza symptoms.*

**Lemsip Cough & Cold Chesty Cough** Reckitt Benckiser, UK.
Guaifenesin (p.1122·1).
*Coughs.*

**Lemsip Cough & Cold Dry Cough** Reckitt Benckiser, UK.
Honey (p.1434·2); terpeneless lemon oil (p.1706·3); glycerol (p.1694·3); citric acid (p.1673·1).
*Coughs; sore throat.*

**Lemsip Dry Cough** *Reckitt Benckiser, NZ.*
Citric acid (p.1673·1); glycerol (p.1694·3); honey (p.1434·2); lemon oil (p.1706·2).
*Coughs.*

**Lemsip Flu** *Reckitt & Colman, Austral.†.*
Paracetamol (p.76·2); pseudoephedrine hydrochloride (p.1129·2); dextromethorphan hydrobromide (p.1117·3); chlorphenamine maleate (p.427·3).
*Cold and influenza symptoms; coughs.*

**Lemsip Flu 12Hr** *Reckitt Benckiser, UK.*
Ibuprofen (p.45·3); pseudoephedrine hydrochloride (p.1129·2).
*Cold and influenza symptoms.*

**Lemsip Flu Strength**
*Reckitt & Colman, Hong Kong†; Reckitt Benckiser, NZ.*
Paracetamol (p.76·2); pseudoephedrine hydrochloride (p.1129·2); ascorbic acid (p.1460·2).
*Cold and influenza symptoms.*

**Lemsip Headcold** *Reckitt Benckiser, Austral.†.*
Paracetamol (p.76·2).
*Fever; pain.*

**Lemsip Lozenges** *Reckitt & Colman, Austral.†.*
Cetylpyridinium chloride (p.1173·1).
*Sore throat.*

**Lemsip Max** *Reckitt Benckiser, Austral.†.*
Paracetamol (p.76·2).
*Fever; pain.*

**Lemsip Max Day & Night** *Reckitt Benckiser, NZ.*
Day, dextromethorphan hydrobromide (p.1117·3); paracetamol (p.76·2); pseudoephedrine hydrochloride (p.1129·2); night, dextromethorphan hydrobromide; paracetamol; chlorphenamine maleate (p.427·3).
*Cold and influenza symptoms.*

**Lemsip Max Strength Sinus Relief** *Reckitt Benckiser, UK.*
Paracetamol (p.76·2); phenylephrine hydrochloride (p.1126·3); caffeine (p.782·1).
*Cold symptoms; sinusitis.*

**Lemsip Non-Decongestant** *Reckitt Benckiser, UK†.*
Paracetamol (p.76·2); ascorbic acid (p.1460·2).
*Cold and influenza symptoms.*

**Lemsip Pharmacy Flu Strength**
*Note. This name is used for preparations of different composition.*
*Reckitt Benckiser, Irl.*
Ascorbic acid (p.1460·2); paracetamol (p.76·2); pseudoephedrine hydrochloride (p.1129·2).
*Cold and influenza symptoms.*

*Reckitt Benckiser, UK.*
Paracetamol (p.76·2); pseudoephedrine hydrochloride (p.1129·2).
*Cold and influenza symptoms; sinusitis.*

**Lemsip Pharmacy Power+** *Reckitt & Colman, UK†.*
Paracetamol (p.76·2); pseudoephedrine hydrochloride (p.1129·2); ascorbic acid (p.1460·2).
*Cold and influenza symptoms.*

**Lemsip Pharmacy Powercaps** *Reckitt Benckiser, UK.*
Ibuprofen (p.45·3); pseudoephedrine hydrochloride (p.1129·2).
*Cold and influenza symptoms.*

**Lemsip with Phenylephrine** *Reckitt Benckiser, Irl.*
Paracetamol (p.76·2); phenylephrine hydrochloride (p.1126·3); ascorbic acid (p.1460·2).
*Cold and influenza symptoms.*

**Lemsip Sore Throat** *Reckitt Benckiser, UK.*
Hexylresorcinol (p.1182·1).
*Sore throat.*

**Lemsip Throat Lozenges** *Reckitt Benckiser, NZ.*
Cetylpyridinium chloride (p.1173·1).
*Sore throat.*

**Lemsip Vapo-Patches** *Reckitt Benckiser, UK.*
Camphor (p.1665·3); eucalyptus oil (p.1686·2).
*Respiratory-tract congestion.*

**Lemtosid** *Lemery, Mex.*
Benzonatate (p.1115·3).
*Coughs.*

**Lemuval** *Bayer, Austria.*
A heparinoid (p.931·1); hyaluronidase (p.1698·2); vitamin A palmitate (p.1453·1); calcium pantothenate (p.1442·3); menthol (p.1711·3).
*Anorectal disorders.*

**Lemyflox** *Lemery, Mex.*
Ciprofloxacin hydrochloride (p.188·2).
*Bacterial infections.*

**Lemytriol** *Lemery, Mex.*
Calcitriol (p.1461·2).
*Hypoparathyroidism; osteoporosis; pseudohypoparathyroidism; renal osteodystrophy; rickets.*

**Len V.K.** *Aspen, S.Afr.*
Phenoxymethylpenicillin potassium (p.242·1).
*Bacterial infections.*

**Lenactin** *Roche, NZ†.*
Dextromethorphan hydrobromide (p.1117·3); cetylpyridinium chloride (p.1173·1); benzocaine (p.1370·3); menthol (p.1711·3).
*Coughs.*

**Lenadol** *Aspen, S.Afr.*
Paracetamol (p.76·2); codeine phosphate (p.27·1); diphenhydramine hydrochloride (p.431·3); caffeine (p.782·1).
*Fever; pain and associated tension.*

**Lenafen** *Aspen, S.Afr.*
Ibuprofen (p.45·3).
*Fever; pain.*

**Lenamet** *Aspen, S.Afr.*
Cimetidine (p.1255·3).
*Dyspepsia; gastric hypersecretion; gastro-oesophageal reflux; peptic ulcer.*

**Lenapain** *Aspen, S.Afr.*
Doxylamine succinate (p.432·3); codeine phosphate (p.27·1); caffeine (p.782·1); paracetamol (p.76·2).
*Pain and associated tension.*

**Lenar** *Biomedica-Chemica, Gr.*
Omeprazole (p.1278·2).
*Acid aspiration; eradication of Helicobacter pylori in combination with antimicrobials; peptic ulcer; reflux oesophagitis; Zollinger-Ellison syndrome.*

**Lenasone** *Aspen, S.Afr.*
Betamethasone sodium phosphate (p.1093·1).
*Corticosteroid.*

**Lenazine** *Aspen, S.Afr.*
Promethazine hydrochloride (p.439·1).
*Hypersensitivity reactions.*

**Lenazine Forte** *Aspen, S.Afr.*
Promethazine hydrochloride (p.439·1); codeine phosphate (p.27·1); ephedrine hydrochloride (p.1120·1).
*Coughs.*

**Lendianon** *QIF, Braz.†.*
Lindane (p.1506·3).
*Pediculosis; scabies.*

**Lenditro** *Aspen, S.Afr.*
Oxybutynin (p.487·1).
*Neurogenic bladder; nocturnal enuresis.*

**Lendorm**
*Boehringer Ingelheim, Austria; Roche, Denm.*
Brotizolam (p.672·1).
*Insomnia.*

**Lendormin**
*Boehringer Ingelheim, Belg.; Boehringer Ingelheim, Ger.; Boehringer Ingelheim, Ital.; Boehringer Ingelheim, Jpn; Boehringer Ingelheim, Neth.; Boehringer Ingelheim, Port.; Boehringer Ingelheim, S.Afr.*
Brotizolam (p.672·1).
*Insomnia; premedication.*

**Lendormine** *Boehringer Ingelheim, Switz.*
Brotizolam (p.672·1).
*Sleep disorders.*

**Lendrex** *Sidepal, Braz.*
Permethrin (p.1508·3).
*Pediculosis; scabies.*

**Lenen** *Scherax, Ger.†.*
Fluocortin butyl (p.1102·1).
*Rhinitis.*

**Leniartril** *San Carlo, Ital.†.*
Naproxen (p.65·1).
*Musculoskeletal and joint disorders; neuritis.*

**Lenicalm**
*Dolisos, Fr.; Dolisos, Ital.*
Asperula odorata; crataegus (p.1677·1); tilia (p.1756·2).
*Insomnia; nervous disorders.*

**Lenicet** *Athenstaedt, Ger.*
Aluminium diacetate hydroxide; aluminium hydroxide (p.1249·2).
*Skin disorders.*

**Lenident** *Zeta, Ital.*
Procaine hydrochloride (p.1383·2).
*Local anaesthesia.*

**Leniderm** *Inpharzam, Switz.*
Vitamin A (p.1451·2); alpha tocopherol (p.1464·3); dexpanthenol (p.1727·2); allantoin (p.1141·3); titanium dioxide (p.1160·3).
*Skin disorders.*

**Lenidermyl** *Oberlin, Fr.†.*
Palmitoyl collagen acid (p.1674·3).
*Skin disorders.*

**Lenide-T** *Aspen, S.Afr.*
Loperamide hydrochloride (p.1271·1).
*Diarrhoea; ostomy management.*

**Lenidolor** *Menarini, Ital.*
Meclofenamic acid (p.55·1) or meclofenamate sodium (p.55·1).
*Musculoskeletal and joint disorders; pain.*

**Lenidor** *Simoes, Braz.*
Thymol (p.1194·2); methyl salicylate (p.59·3); menthol (p.1711·3); camphor (p.1665·3).
*Musculoskeletal and joint disorders.*

**Lenifren** *DermoDuemila, Ital.*
Magnesium; kava; hypericum; rhodiola; vitamins (p.1417·1).
*Nutritional supplement.*

**Lenil** *Zeta, Ital.*
Chlorhexidine hydrochloride (p.1173·3).
*Disinfection of wounds and burns.*

**Leniline** *Erredici, Ital.†.*
Vitamin E; vitamin C; ginkgo biloba; melilotus; bioflavonoids (p.1417·1).
*Nutritional supplement.*

**Lenipasta** *Novogaleno, Ital.*
Zinc oxide (p.1163·2); rice starch (p.1449·1); enoxolone (p.36·2).
*Skin irritation; wounds.*

**Lenirit** *EG, Ital.*
Hydrocortisone acetate (p.1103·3).
*Skin disorders.*

**Lenirose** *Novogaleno, Ital.*
Sulfur (p.1158·2); titanium dioxide (p.1160·3); panthenol (p.1727·2); rusco; calendula (p.1665·2); oryzanol (p.1725·1); enoxolone (p.36·2).
*Rosacea; seborrhoeic dermatitis; skin irritation.*

**Lenisan** *Bittner, Austria.*
Homoeopathic preparation.

**Lenisolone** *Aspen, S.Afr.*
Prednisolone (p.1108·1).
*Corticosteroid.*

**Lenistar** *Pulitzer, Ital.*
Butamirate citrate (p.1116·2).
*Coughs.*

**Lenitil** *Mertens, Arg.*
Diclofenac sodium (p.32·1).
*Inflammation; pain.*

**Lenitin** *Teva, Israel.*
Bromazepam (p.671·3).
*Anxiety; premedication; sedative.*

**Lenitral**
*Besins, Fr.; Besins, Hong Kong; Besins-Iscovesco, Singapore†.*
Glyceryl trinitrate (p.923·2).
*Angina pectoris; heart failure; production of controlled hypotension.*

**Lenium**
*SmithKline Beecham, Irl.†; Johnson & Johnson MSD Consumer, UK†.*
Selenium sulfide (p.1157·3).
*Dandruff; scalp seborrhoea.*

**Lenixil** *Eurospital, Ital.†.*
Chlorhexidine gluconate (p.1173·2).
*Disinfection of minor wounds and burns.*

**Lenocef** *Aspen, S.Afr.*
Cefalexin (p.168·1).
*Bacterial infections.*

**Lenocin** *General Drugs, Thai.*
Tetracycline hydrochloride (p.266·2).
*Bacterial infections.*

**Lenolax** *Aspen, S.Afr.*
Dibasic sodium phosphate (p.1231·1); monobasic sodium phosphate (p.1230·3).
*Bowel evacuation; constipation.*

**Lenoltec No 4** *Technilab, Canad.*
Paracetamol (p.76·2); codeine phosphate (p.27·1).
Formerly known as Lenoltec with Codeine No 4.
*Pain.*

**Lenoltec No 1, No 2, or No 3** *Technilab, Canad.*
Paracetamol (p.76·2); caffeine (p.782·1); codeine phosphate (p.27·1).
*Cold symptoms; pain.*

**Lenovate** *Aspen, S.Afr.*
Betamethasone valerate (p.1093·2).
*Corticosteroid.*

**Lenovor** *Serono, Mex.†.*
Folinic acid (p.1431·1).

**Lenoxin** *GlaxoSmithKline, Ger.*
Digoxin (p.895·2).
*Heart failure; tachycardia.*

**Lenpryl** *Galen, Mex.*
Captopril (p.879·2).
*Heart failure; hypertension.*

**Lens Fresh** *Allergan, Ger.†.*
Macrogol 300 (p.1709·1); macrogol stearate 2000.
*Comfort drops for contact lenses.*

**Lens Lubricant** *Bausch & Lomb, USA.*
Wetting solution for hard contact lenses (p.1164·2).

**Lens Plus**
*Allergan, Austral.†; Allergan-Frumtost, Braz.†; Advanced Medical Optics, NZ; Allergan, USA.*
Range of solutions for contact lenses (p.1164·2).

**Lens Plus Buffered Saline Solution** *Allergan, Canad.*
Buffered sodium chloride (p.1233·3)(p.1164·2).
*Rinsing solution for contact lenses.*

**Lens Plus Rewetting Drops** *Allergan, Canad.†.*
Wetting solution for soft contact lenses (p.1164·2).

**Lens Tears** *Agepha, Austria.*
Wetting solution for contact lenses (p.1164·2).

**Lens Wet** *Agepha, Austria.*
Wetting solution for contact lenses (p.1164·2).

**Lensan A** *Ciba Vision, Austria†.*
Hydrogen peroxide (p.1182·2) (p.1164·2).
*Disinfecting solution for contact lenses.*

**Lensan B** *Ciba Vision, Austria†.*
Catalase (p.1668·3) (p.1164·2).
*Neutralising solution for contact lenses.*

**Lensept** *Ciba Vision, Austria†.*
Hydrogen peroxide (p.1182·2) (p.1164·2).
*Disinfecting solution for soft contact lenses.*

**Lensrins NT** *Ciba Vision, Austria†.*
Storage and rinsing solution for soft contact lenses (p.1164·2).

**Lenta** *Pentafarma, Chile.*
Insulin zinc suspension (amorphous 30%, crystalline 70%) (bovine and porcine) (p.333·3).
*Diabetes mellitus.*

**Lentard** *Knoll, India.*
Insulin zinc suspension (porcine, highly purified) (amorphous 30%, crystalline 70%) (p.333·3).
*Diabetes mellitus.*

**Lentard MC** *Novo Nordisk, UK†.*
Insulin zinc suspension (amorphous porcine 30%, crystalline bovine 70%, monocomponent) (p.333·3).
*Diabetes mellitus.*

**Lentare** *Novartis, S.Afr.*
Formestane (p.557·1).
*Breast cancer.*

**Lentaron**
*Novartis, Arg.; Novartis, Austria; Ciba-Geigy, Belg.†; Novartis, Braz.; Novartis, Chile; Novartis, Denm.; Novartis, Fr.†; Novartis, Ger.; Novartis, Gr.; Novartis, Hong Kong; Novartis, Irl.†; Novartis, Israel†; Novartis, Ital.; Novartis, Malaysia; Novartis, Neth.; Novartis, Port.†; Novartis, Spain; Novartis, Switz.†; Novartis, UK†.*
Formestane (p.557·1).
*Breast cancer.*

**Lente**
*Novo Nordisk, Ger.†; Novo Nordisk, USA.*
Insulin zinc suspension (bovine or porcine) (p.333·3).
*Diabetes mellitus.*

**Lente Iletin I** *Lilly, USA†.*
Insulin zinc suspension (bovine and porcine) (p.333·3).
*Diabetes mellitus.*

**Lente Iletin II** *Lilly, USA.*
Insulin zinc suspension (porcine) (p.333·3).
*Diabetes mellitus.*

**Lente L** *Novo Nordisk, USA†.*
Insulin zinc suspension (porcine) (p.333·3).
*Diabetes mellitus.*

**Lente MC**
*Novo Nordisk, Austral.†; Novo Nordisk, Austria†; Novo Nordisk, Belg.†; Novo Nordisk, Spain†; Novo Nordisk, Switz.*
Insulin zinc suspension (amorphous 30%, crystalline 70%) (bovine with porcine, monocomponent) (p.333·3).
*Diabetes mellitus.*

**Lentisol** *Barnes Hind, Arg.*
Polyvinyl alcohol (p.1581·1) (p.1164·2).
*Wetting solution for hard contact lenses.*

**Lentizol**
*Pfizer, Irl.; Pfizer, UK†.*
Amitriptyline hydrochloride (p.280·3).
*Depression.*

**Lento C** *Eurofarma, Braz.†.*
Ascorbic acid (p.1460·2).
*Vitamin C deficiency; vitamin C supplement.*

**Lentocilin-S** *Atral, Port.*
Benzathine benzylpenicillin (p.162·3).
*Bacterial infections.*

**Lentogesic** *Mer-National, S.Afr.*
*Capsules:* Dextropropoxyphene hydrochloride (p.28·3); paracetamol (p.76·2); pemoline (p.1591·2); glutamine (p.1433·2).
*Pain.*
*Syrup:* Paracetamol (p.76·2); codeine phosphate (p.27·1); promethazine hydrochloride (p.439·1).
*Fever; pain.*

**Lentogest** *Amsa, Ital.*
Hydroxyprogesterone caproate (p.1556·3).
*Infertility; menstrual and menopausal disorders; threatened or recurrent miscarriage.*

**Lento-Kalium** *Roche, Ital.*
Potassium chloride (p.1232·2).
*Hypokalaemia.*

**Lentolith** *Mer-National, S.Afr.*
Lithium carbonate (p.301·1).
*Bipolar disorder; depression.*

**Lentopenil** *Grossman, Mex.*
Benzathine benzylpenicillin (p.162·3).
*Bacterial infections.*

**Lentoquine** *Sanofi Synthelabo, Spain.*
Hydroquinidine hydrochloride (p.937·3).
*Arrhythmias.*

**Lentorem** *Remir, Mex.†.*
Hydroxocobalamin (p.1458·2).

**Lentorsil** *Italfarmaco, Ital.*
Ursodeoxycholic acid (p.1760·3).
*Biliary disorders; cholesterol gallstones.*

**Lentusin** *Chobet, Arg.*
Dihydrocodeine resinate; phenyltoloxamine resinate.

**Leo-400** *Charoen, Thai.*
Albendazole (p.101·2).
*Worm infections.*

**Leo-Doce** *Solfran, Mex.*
Hydroxocobalamin (p.1458·2).

**Leodrin** *Osteolab, Chile.*
Alendronate sodium (p.765·3).
*Osteoporosis.*

**Leogumil** *Leovan, Gr.*
Butamirate citrate (p.1116·2).
*Cough.*

**Leonal** *Byk Leo, Spain†.*
Ibuprofen (p.45·3).
*Fever; pain.*

**Leonitren** *Medinova (Μεντινοβα), Gr.*
Nitrendipine (p.973·3).
*Hypertension.*

**Leopin** *Quest, Canad.*
Vitamin B substances (p.1417·1).
*Dietary supplement.*

**Leotrim** *Leofarma, Braz.†.*
Co-trimoxazole (p.199·3).
*Bacterial infections; Pneumocystis carinii pneumonia; protozoal infections.*

**Leovinezal** *Medinova (Μεντινοβα), Gr.*
Enalapril maleate (p.909·2).
*Heart failure; hypertension.*

**Leparan** *Italfarmaco, Ital.*
Suleparoid (p.1009·1).
*Thrombosis prophylaxis.*

**Lepheton** *Ipex, Swed.*
Ethylmorphine hydrochloride (p.37·3); ephedrine hydrochloride (p.1120·1).
*Bronchitis; coughs.*

**Lephin** *Pharmadica, Thai.*
Ceftriaxone sodium (p.182·3).
*Bacterial infections.*

**Lepicortinolo** *Decomed, Port.*
Prednisolone (p.1108·1) or prednisolone sodium succinate (p.1108·2).
*Corticosteroid.*

**Lepinal** Desitin, Ger.†.
Phenobarbital (p.367·3).
*Epilepsy.*

**Lepinaletten** Desitin, Ger.†.
Phenobarbital (p.367·3).
*Epilepsy.*

**Lepisor** Soria Natural, Spain.
Lepidium latifolium; java tea (p.1702·3).
*Prostatitis; renal calculi.*

**Lepobron** Lepori, Port.
Theophylline (p.798·3).
*Asthma.*

**Leponex**
Novartis, Austria; Novartis, Belg.; Novartis, Braz.; Novartis, Chile; Novartis, Denm.; Novartis, Fin.; Novartis, Fr.; Novartis, Ger.; Novartis, Gr.; Novartis, Israel; Novartis, Ital.; Novartis, Mex.; Novartis, Neth.; Novartis, Norw.; Novartis, Port.; Novartis, S.Afr.; Novartis, Spain; Novartis, Swed.; Novartis, Switz.
Clozapine (p.685·3).
*Parkinsonism; schizophrenia.*

**Leptanal**
Janssen-Cilag, Norw.; Janssen-Cilag, Swed.
Fentanyl citrate (p.40·1).
*Adjunct in neuroleptanalgesia; pain.*

**Lepticur** Aventis, Fr.
Tropatepine hydrochloride (p.491·1).
*Extrapyramidal disorders; parkinsonism.*

**Leptilan**
Novartis, Chile; Novartis, Denm.†; Novartis, Ger.; Novartis, Mex.
Sodium valproate (p.380·1).
*Epilepsy.*

**Leptilanil** Novartis, Austria.
Sodium valproate (p.380·1).
*Epilepsy; febrile convulsions.*

**Leptofen** Pharmacia Upjohn, Ital.
Fentanyl (p.40·1); droperidol (p.697·2).
*Neuroleptanalgesia; premedication.*

**Leptoprol** Mavi, Mex.†.
Metoprolol (p.956·3).

**Leptopsique** Psicofarma, Mex.
Perphenazine (p.714·2).
*Anxiety disorders; nausea and vomiting; pain; psychoses.*

**Lepur** Kleva, Gr.
Simvastatin (p.997·1).
*Primary hypercholesterolaemia.*

**Lercadip**
Gador, Arg.; Innova, Ital.; Biohorm, Spain.
Lercanidipine hydrochloride (p.946·1).
*Hypertension.*

**Lercan** Pierre Fabre, Fr.
Lercanidipine hydrochloride (p.946·1).
*Hypertension.*

**Lerdip** Byk, Neth.
Lercanidipine hydrochloride (p.946·1).
*Hypertension.*

**Lergigan** Recip, Swed.
Promethazine hydrochloride (p.439·1).
*Alcoholism; anxiety; croup; hypersensitivity reactions; nausea; premedication; sedative; sleep disorders; tension; vertigo.*

**Lergigan comp** Recip, Swed.
Promethazine hydrochloride (p.439·1); caffeine (p.782·1); ephedrine sulfate (p.1120·1).
*Alcoholism; anxiety; croup; hypersensitivity reactions; nausea; premedication; sedative; sleep disorders; tension; vertigo.*

**Lergocil** Juste, Spain.
Azatadine maleate (p.425·1).
*Hypersensitivity reactions.*

**Lerin** Allergan, Braz.
Naphazoline hydrochloride (p.1124·3); zinc phenolsulfonate (p.1163·3); berberine sulfate (p.1659·3).
*Ocular congestion.*

**Leritine** Merck Frosst, Canad.†.
Anileridine hydrochloride (p.15·1) or anileridine phosphate (p.15·1).
*Adjunct in general anaesthesia; anxiety; pain.*

**Lerivon**
Organon, Arg.; Organon, Austral.†; Organon, Belg.
Mianserin hydrochloride (p.306·3).
*Depression.*

**Lermex** Sriprasit, Thai.
Aciclovir (p.626·1).
*Herpesvirus infections.*

**Lerogin** Recalcine, Chile.
Chlordiazepoxide (p.674·2); clidinium bromide (p.480·2).
*Gastrointestinal disorders; urinary-tract disorders.*

**Leroid** Geminis, Arg.
Phenazone (p.82·3); benzocaine (p.1370·3); sulfathiazole (p.264·1).
*Ear disorders.*

**Lertamine**
Note. This name is used for preparations of different composition.
White, Arg.; Undra, Mex.
Loratadine (p.436·1).
*Allergic rhinitis; urticaria.*

Schering-Plough, Chile.
Loratadine (p.436·1); pseudoephedrine sulfate (p.1129·2).
*Allergic rhinitis; cold symptoms.*

**Lertamine D**
White, Arg.; Undra, Mex.
Loratadine (p.436·1); pseudoephedrine sulfate (p.1129·2).
*Allergic rhinitis; nasal congestion.*

**Lertamine Extra** Schering-Plough, Chile.
Loratadine (p.436·1); pseudoephedrine sulfate (p.1129·2).
*Allergic rhinitis; cold symptoms.*

**Lertus**
Note. This name is used for preparations of different composition.
Gunther, Braz.†.
Fluconazole (p.398·1).
*Fungal infections.*

Tecnofarma, Chile.
Diclofenac (p.32·1), diclofenac diethylamine (p.32·1) or diclofenac sodium (p.32·1).
*Fever; gout; inflammation; musculoskeletal, joint, peri-articular, and soft-tissue disorders; pain.*

**Lertus Biotic** Elvetium, Arg.
Diclofenac potassium (p.32·1); amoxicillin trihydrate (p.155·3).
*Respiratory-tract infections.*

**Leruze** Rafarm, Gr.
Lisinopril (p.946·3).
*Heart failure; hypertension; myocardial infarction.*

**Lervipan** Emilio, Spain†.
Pivampicillin (p.244·1).
*Bacterial infections.*

**Lerzam** Pharmazam, Spain.
Lercanidipine hydrochloride (p.946·1).
*Hypertension.*

**Les Yeux 1** Bilosa, Austria†.
Hydrogen peroxide (p.1182·2) (p.1164·2).
*Disinfecting solution for gas-permeable contact lenses.*

**Les Yeux 2** Bilosa, Austria†.
Catalase (p.1668·3) (p.1164·2).
*Neutralising solution for gas-permeable contact lenses.*

**Lescol**
Novartis, Arg.; Novartis, Austral.; Novartis, Austria; Novartis, Belg.; Novartis, Braz.; Novartis, Canad.; Novartis, Denm.; Novartis, Fin.; Novartis, Fr.; Novartis, Gr.; Novartis, Hong Kong; Novartis, Irl.; Novartis, Israel; Novartis, Ital.; Novartis, Malaysia; Novartis, Mex.; Novartis, Neth.; Novartis, Norw.; Novartis, NZ; Novartis, Port.; Novartis, S.Afr.; Novartis, Singapore; Novartis, Spain; Novartis, Swed.; Novartis, Switz.; Novartis, Thai.; Novartis, UK; Novartis, USA.
Fluvastatin sodium (p.918·2).
*Atherosclerosis; hypercholesterolaemia; prevention of coronary events following percutaneous coronary intervention.*

**Leshcutan**
Biosintetica, Braz.†; Teva, Israel.
Paromomycin (p.613·1); methylbenzethonium chloride (p.1186·1).
*Cutaneous leishmaniasis.*

**Lesil** Farmatrading, Port.†.
Tolu balsam (p.1131·3); sulfogaiacol (p.1131·1); pine oil.
*Coughs.*

**Lespenefril**
Produfarma, Port.; Aventis, Spain†.
Lespedeza capitata.
*Diuretic.*

**Lespenephryl**
UCB, Austria; UCB, Fr.
Lespedeza capitata.
*Diuresis.*

**Lessina** Barr, USA.
Levonorgestrel (p.1563·2); ethinylestradiol (p.1553·2). 28-Day packs also contain 7 inert tablets.
*Combined oral contraceptive.*

**Lessmusec** Brunel, S.Afr.
Carbocisteine (p.1116·2).
*Respiratory-tract disorders with increased or viscous mucus.*

**Lesspain** Adcock Ingram, S.Afr.
Paracetamol (p.76·2); codeine phosphate (p.27·1); promethazine hydrochloride (p.439·1).
*Fever; pain.*

**Lesterol**
Aventis, Braz.†; Hoechst Marion Roussel, Mex.†.
Probucol (p.986·3).
*Hyperlipidaemias.*

**Lestid**
Pharmacia, Denm.; Pharmacia, Fin.; Pharmacia, Norw.; Pharmacia, Swed.
Colestipol hydrochloride (p.889·2).
*Hyperlipidaemias.*

**Lestric** Ranbaxy, Malaysia.
Lovastatin (p.949·1).
*Hypercholesterolaemia.*

**Lestrin** Cedar Health, UK.
Sitosterol (p.982·3); beta sitostanol (p.1448·3).
*Food supplement.*

**Letansil** IQB, Braz.†.
Diazepam (p.690·1).
*Anxiety.*

**Letequatro** Upsifarma, Port.
Levothyroxine sodium (p.1600·1).
*Hypothyroidism.*

**Lethyl** Aspen, S.Afr.
Phenobarbital (p.367·3).
*Anxiety; insomnia; migraine.*

**Letigen** Nycomed, Denm.
Caffeine (p.782·1); ephedrine hydrochloride (p.1120·1).
*Obesity.*

**Letofort** Salus, Ital.†.
Letosteine (p.1123·3).
*Respiratory-tract disorders associated with increased or viscous mucus.*

**Letondal** Finadiet, Arg.
Ambroxol hydrochloride (p.1114·3); paracetamol (p.76·2); oxatomide (p.438·1).

**Letoprol** Mavi, Mex.†.
Metoprolol (p.956·3).

**Letter** Aventis, Port.
Levothyroxine sodium (p.1600·1).
*Hypothyroidism.*

**Letus**
Unison, Hong Kong; Unison, Thai.
Co-trimoxazole (p.199·3).
*Bacterial infections.*

**Letynol** Norma (Νορμα), Gr.
Cefotaxime sodium (p.175·3).
*Bacterial infections.*

**LeucinAde** Taranis, Fr.
Food for special diets (p.1417·1).
*Leucinosis.*

**Leuco-4** Pharmascience, Fr.
Adenine (p.1647·3).
*Asthenia.*

**Leuco Hubber**
Rhone-Poulenc Rorer, Port.; Teofarma, Spain.
Hydrocortisone acetate (p.1103·3); neomycin sulfate (p.235·1).
*Vulvovaginal inflammatory disorders.*

**Leucobasal**
Germania, Austria; Biobasal, Switz.†.
Mequinol (p.1151·3).
*Hyperpigmentation.*

**Leucocalcin** Kampel Martian, Arg.
Calcium levofolinate (p.1431·1).

**Leucocida** Simoes, Braz.
Hydroxyquinoline sulfate (p.1700·1); borax (p.1661·3); cetrimonium bromide (p.1173·1).
*Vulvovaginal disorders.*

**Leucocitim** Blausiegel, Braz.
Molgramostim (p.756·1).
*Neutropenia.*

**Leucodin** Darrow, Braz.
Mequinol (p.1151·3).
*Vitiligo.*

**Leucodinine B** Chiesi, Fr.
Mequinol (p.1151·3).
*Hyperpigmentation.*

**Leucodinin-M** Unipharma, Gr.
Mequinol (p.1151·3).
*Hyperpigmentation.*

**Leucogen** Ache, Braz.
Thymomodulin (p.1756·1).
*Diabetes mellitus; immunodeficiencies; malignant neoplasms; rheumatoid arthritis; skin disorders.*

**Leucomax**
Essex, Arg.; Aesca, Austria; Novartis, Austria; Novartis, Belg.; Novartis, Braz.; Schering-Plough, Chile; Novartis, Denm.; Schering-Plough, Denm.; Schering-Plough, Fin.; Novartis, Fin.; Novartis, Fr.†; Schering-Plough, Fr.†; Novartis, Ger.; Essex, Ger.; Novartis, Gr.; Novartis, Hong Kong; Schering-Plough, Hong Kong; Schering-Plough, Irl.; Novartis, Israel; Novartis, Ital.; Novartis, Malaysia; Schering-Plough, Malaysia; Novartis, Mex.; Novartis, Neth.; Schering-Plough, Norw.; Novartis, NZ; Novartis, Port.†; Schering-Plough, S.Afr.; Novartis, Singapore†; Schering-Plough, Singapore†; Novartis, Spain; Schering-Plough, Swed.; Novartis, Swed.; Essex, Switz.; Novartis, Switz.; Novartis, Thai.; Schering-Plough, Thai.; Schering-Plough, UK.
Molgramostim (p.756·1).
*Neutropenia induced by antineoplastic agents, bone marrow transplantation, or ganciclovir.*

**Leucorsan** Zilliken, Ital.†.
*Vaginal capsules:* Benzydamine hydrochloride (p.21·1); hydroxyquinoline sulfate (p.1700·1); hydroxyquinoline benzoate (p.1700·1).
*Vaginal douche:* Benzydamine hydrochloride (p.21·1); hydroxyquinoline sulfate (p.1700·1); hydroxyquinoline benzoate (p.1700·1); cetrimonium tosilate (p.1173·1).
*Vaginal and cervical inflammation.*

**Leucotrofina**
Bago, Arg.; Pharmacia Upjohn, Mex.†.
Thymomodulin (p.1756·1).
*Hypersensitivity; infections; leucopenia.*

**Leukase** Merck, Austria.
Framycetin sulfate (p.215·1); trypsin (p.1758·3).
*Infected burns and wounds; infected skin disorders.*

**Leukase N** Dermapharm, Ger.
*Topical gel:* Framycetin sulfate (p.215·1); lidocaine hydrochloride (p.1377·3).
*Topical powder; ointment:* Framycetin sulfate (p.215·1).
*Infected skin disorders; infected wounds.*

**Leukase-Kegel** Merck, Austria.
Framycetin sulfate (p.215·1); trypsin (p.1758·3); lidocaine hydrochloride (p.1377·3).
*Infected skin and mouth disorders.*

**Leukeran**
GlaxoSmithKline, Arg.; GlaxoSmithKline, Austral.; GlaxoSmithKline, Austria; GlaxoSmithKline, Belg.; GlaxoSmithKline, Braz.; GlaxoSmithKline, Canad.; GlaxoSmithKline, Chile; GlaxoSmithKline, Denm.; GlaxoSmithKline, Fin.; GlaxoSmithKline, Ger.; Glaxo Wellcome, Gr.; IFET (ΙΦΕΤ), Gr.; GlaxoSmithKline, Hong Kong; GlaxoSmithKline, India; Wellcome, Irl.; Wellcome, Israel; GlaxoSmithKline, Ital.; GlaxoSmithKline, Malaysia; Glaxo Wellcome, Mex.; GlaxoSmithKline, Neth.; GlaxoSmithKline, Norw.; GlaxoSmithKline, NZ; Wellcome, Port.; GlaxoSmithKline, S.Afr.; GlaxoSmithKline, Singapore; Wellcome, Spain; GlaxoSmithKline, Swed.; GlaxoSmithKline, Switz.; GlaxoSmithKline, Thai.; GlaxoSmithKline, UK; Glaxo Wellcome, USA†.
Chlorambucil (p.536·1).
*Malignant neoplasms.*

**Leukichtan**
Ichthyol, Austria.
Ictasol (p.1148·3); cod-liver oil (p.1425·2).
*Burns; skin disorders; wounds.*

Ichthyol, Ger.
Ictasol (p.1148·3).
*Ulcers; wounds.*

**Leukine** Berlex, USA.
Sargramostim (p.760·1).
*Mobilisation of autologous peripheral blood progenitor cells; neutropenia.*

**leukominerase** Biosyn, Ger.
Lithium carbonate (p.301·1).
*Bipolar disorder; depression; mania.*

**Leukona-Beruhigungsbad** Atzinger, Ger.
Valerian (p.1762·2); lupulus (p.1708·1).
*Bath additive; nervous disorders.*

**Leukona-Eukalpin-Bad** Atzinger, Ger.
Norway spruce oil; eucalyptus oil (p.1686·2).
*Bath additive; respiratory-tract disorders.*

**Leukona-Jod-Bad**
Richter, Austria; Atzinger, Ger.
Iodine (p.1598·1).
*Arteriosclerosis; bath additive; circulatory disorders; iodine-deficiency goitre; neuralgia; spinal disorders.*

**Leukona-Kreislauf-Bad** Atzinger, Ger.
Rosemary oil (p.1740·2); camphor (p.1665·3); eucalyptus oil (p.1686·2).
*Bath additive; circulatory disorders.*

**Leukona-Mintol** Atzinger, Ger.†.
Peppermint oil (p.1283·2).
*Gastrointestinal disorders; respiratory-tract disorders.*

**Leukona-Rheuma-Bad** Richter, Austria.
Pumilio pine oil (p.1737·1); turpentine oil (p.1760·1); methyl salicylate (p.59·3).
*Musculoskeletal, joint, peri-articular, and soft-tissue disorders.*

**Leukona-Rheuma-Bad N** Atzinger, Ger.
Methyl salicylate (p.59·3); turpentine oil (p.1760·1); Norway spruce oil.
*Bath additive; rheumatic disorders.*

**Leukona-Rheumasalbe** Atzinger, Ger.
Camphor (p.1665·3); turpentine oil (p.1760·1); rosemary oil (p.1740·2).
*Cold symptoms; frostbite; rheumatism; soft-tissue injury.*

**Leukona-Sedativ-Bad** Atzinger, Ger.†.
Cloral hydrate (p.684·1); lupulus (p.1708·1); valerian (p.1762·2).
*Bath additive; nervous disorders; sleep disorders; spasmophilia.*

**Leukona-Sedativ-Bad sine Chloralhydrat** Atzinger, Ger.†.
Valerian (p.1762·2); lupulus (p.1708·1).
*Bath additive; nervous disorders; sleep disorders.*

**Leukona-Stoffwechsel-Bad** Atzinger, Ger.
Juniper oil (p.1703·1).
*Allergic skin disorders; bath additive; metabolic disorders.*

**Leukona-Sulfomoor-Bad** Richter, Austria.
Sulfurated potash (p.1158·3); colloidal sulfur (p.1158·2); sodium humate; peat.
*Musculoskeletal and joint disorders; skin disorders.*

**Leukona-Sulfomoor-Bad F** Atzinger, Ger.
Sodium humate.
Formerly contained sulfurated potash, peat, and sodium humate.
*Bath additive; musculoskeletal and joint disorders.*

**Leukona-Wundsalbe** Atzinger, Ger.
Cod-liver oil (p.1425·2); hamamelis water (p.1696·3); allantoin (p.1141·3).
*Wounds.*

**LeukoNorm** CytoChemia, Ger.
Leucocytes (p.756·1).
*Immunological disorders.*

**LeukoScan** Byk Gulden, Ital.
Technetium-99m (p.1525·2) sulesomab.
*Bone scanning in osteomyelitis.*

**Leumostin** Pharmacia, Arg.
Lenograstim (p.755·3).
*Neutropenia.*

**Leunase**
Aventis, Austral.; Kyowa, Hong Kong; Biochem, India; Kyowa, Jpn; Kyowa, Malaysia; Sanfer, Mex.; Aventis, NZ; Kyowa, Singapore; Kyowa, Thai.
Asparaginase (p.528·3).
*Acute leukaemias; malignant lymphomas.*

**Leuplin** Takeda, Jpn.
Leuprorelin acetate (p.1331·1).
*Breast cancer; endometriosis; precocious puberty; prostatic cancer; uterine myoma.*

**Leustat**
Janssen-Cilag, Arg.; Janssen-Cilag, UK.
Cladribine (p.539·3).
*Chronic lymphocytic leukaemia; hairy-cell leukaemia.*

**Leustatin**
Janssen-Cilag, Austral.; Janssen-Cilag, Austria; Janssen-Cilag, Braz.; Janssen-Ortho, Canad.; Janssen-Cilag, Denm.; Janssen-Cilag, Fin.;

*Janssen-Cilag, Ger.; Janssen-Cilag, Gr.; Cilag, Hong Kong; Janssen-Cilag, Israel; Janssen-Cilag, Ital.; Janssen-Cilag, Neth.; Janssen-Cilag, Norw.; Janssen-Cilag, NZ; Janssen-Cilag, S.Afr.; Janssen-Cilag, Spain; Janssen-Cilag, Swed.; Janssen-Cilag, Switz.; Janssen-Cilag, Thai.; Ortho Biotech, USA.*
Cladribine (p.539·3).
*Chronic lymphocytic leukaemia; hairy-cell leukaemia.*

**Leustatine** *Janssen-Cilag, Fr.*
Cladribine (p.539·3).
*Hairy-cell leukaemia.*

**Leutrol**
*Abbott, Braz.; Abbott, Ital.*
Meloxicam (p.56·1).
*Ankylosing spondylitis; osteoarthritis; rheumatoid arthritis.*

**Levadin** *Wiener, Mex.†.*
Yeast (p.1469·1).

**Levadol** *Italfar, Ital.*
Paracetamol (p.76·2).
*Fever; pain.*

**Levaknel** *Crinos, Ital.†.*
Zinc oxide (p.1163·2); chlorhexidine (p.1173·2); triclosan (Irgasan DP 300) (p.1195·2).
*Seborrhoea.*

**Levaliver** *Byk Elmu, Spain†.*
Aceglutamide (p.1645·2); amino acids (p.1417·1); betaine hydrochloride (p.1660·2); cyclobutyrol sodium (p.1678·2); pyridoxal phosphate (p.1456·3); sorbitol (p.1446·3).
*Liver disorders.*

**Levall** *CTEX, USA.*
Phenylephrine hydrochloride (p.1126·3); hydrocodone tartrate (p.45·1); guaifenesin (p.1122·1).
*Coughs.*

**Levamin** *Pisa, Mex.*
Amino-acid infusion (p.1417·1).
*Parenteral nutrition.*

**Levantol Procaina** *Mertens, Arg.*
Calcium phosphate; methionine; pyritinol hydrochloride; procaine; vitamin B substances (p.1417·1).
*Asthenia; mental function impairment.*

**Levanxol**
*Strallhofer, Austria; Pharmacia Upjohn, Belg.†.*
Temazepam (p.723·2).
*Anxiety disorders; sleep disorders.*

**Levaquin**
*Janssen-Cilag, Arg.; Janssen-Cilag, Braz.; Janssen-Ortho, Canad.; Ortho McNeil, USA.*
Levofloxacin (p.225·3).
*Bacterial infections.*

**Levate** *ICN, Canad.†.*
Amitriptyline hydrochloride (p.280·3).
*Depression.*

**Levatol** *Schwarz, USA.*
Penbutolol sulfate (p.979·1).
*Hypertension.*

**Levaxin**
*Nycomed, Norw.; Nycomed, Swed.*
Levothyroxine sodium (p.1600·1).
*Hypothyroidism; thyroid cancer.*

**Levbid** *Schwarz, USA.*
Hyoscyamine sulfate (p.485·1).
*Biliary and renal colic; gastrointestinal disorders; parkinsonism; rhinitis; urinary-tract disorders.*

**Levedad** *ICN, Arg.*
Diclofenac sodium (p.32·1).
*Postoperative eye inflammation.*

**Leveglutan** *Bunker, Braz.*
Dried yeast; vitamin B substances (p.1417·1).
*Dietary supplement.*

**Level Up** *Garden House, Arg.*
Ginseng; minerals (p.1417·1).
*Dietary supplement.*

**Levelina** *Ern, Spain.*
Bifonazole (p.395·1).
*Fungal skin and nail infections.*

**Leviax** *Aventis, Norw.*
Telithromycin (p.265·2).
*Bacterial infections.*

**Levicor** *Bioindustria, Ital.†.*
Metaraminol tartrate (p.952·2).
*Hypotension.*

**Leviden** *Toho, Hong Kong.*
Liver hydrolysate.
*Liver disorders.*

**Levifusa** *Ifusa, Mex.*
Yeast (p.1469·1).
*Dietary supplement.*

**Levitra**
*Bayer, UK; Bayer, USA; GlaxoSmithKline, USA.*
Vardenafil hydrochloride (p.1763·1).
*Erectile dysfunction.*

**Levium** *Hexal, Ger.*
Levomepromazine maleate (p.703·2).
*Pain; psychoses.*

**Levlen**
*Schering, Austria†; Berlex, USA.*
Levonorgestrel (p.1563·2); ethinylestradiol (p.1553·2).
28-Day packs also contain 7 inert tablets.
*Combined oral contraceptive.*

**Levlen ED**
*Schering, Austral.; Schering, NZ.*
21 Tablets, Levonorgestrel (p.1563·2); ethinylestradiol (p.1553·2); 7 tablets, inert.
*Combined oral contraceptive.*

**Levlite**
*Barr, USA; Berlex, USA.*
Levonorgestrel (p.1563·2); ethinylestradiol (p.1553·2).
28-Day packs also contain 7 inert tablets.
*Combined oral contraceptive.*

**Levobens** *Asta Medica, Austria.*
Levodopa (p.1205·2); benserazide hydrochloride (p.1200·2).
*Parkinsonism.*

**Levobeta C** *Betapharm, Ger.*
Levodopa (p.1205·2); carbidopa (p.1204·3).
*Parkinsonism.*

**Levobren** *GiEnne, Ital.*
Levosulpiride (p.722·2).
*Gastrointestinal disorders; headache; migraine; vertigo.*

**Levo-C** *Aliud, Ger.*
Levodopa (p.1205·2); carbidopa (p.1204·3).
*Parkinsonism.*

**Levocarb**
*Biolab Sanus, Braz.; Teva, Ger.*
Levodopa (p.1205·2); carbidopa (p.1204·3).
*Parkinsonism.*

**Levocarnil** *Sigma-Tau, Fr.*
Carnitine (p.1423·3).
*Carnitine deficiency.*

**Levocarnin** *Sintofarma, Braz.*
Carnitine (p.1423·3).
*Nutritional supplement.*

**Levocarvit** *Mitim, Ital.*
Levocarnitine (p.1423·3).
*Carnitine deficiency; myocardial ischaemia.*

**Levocina** *Cryopharma, Mex.*
Levomepromazine maleate (p.703·2).
*Psychoses.*

**Levocomp** *Hexal, Ger.*
Levodopa (p.1205·2); carbidopa (p.1204·3).
*Parkinsonism.*

**Levodex** *Dexxon, Israel.*
Diltiazem hydrochloride (p.900·1).
*Angina pectoris.*

**Levodexan** *Grin, Mex.*
Dexamethasone sodium phosphate (p.1097·2); chloramphenicol (p.185·1).
*Infected eye disorders.*

**Levodop** *Neuraxpharm, Ger.*
Levodopa (p.1205·2); carbidopa (p.1204·3).
*Parkinsonism.*

**Levodopa Comp** *CT, Ger.; Ratiopharm, Ger.*
Levodopa (p.1205·2); carbidopa (p.1204·3).
*Parkinsonism.*

**Levodopa comp B** *Stada, Ger.*
Levodopa (p.1205·2); benserazide hydrochloride (p.1200·2).
*Drug-induced extrapyramidal disorders; parkinsonism.*

**Levodopa comp C** *Stada, Ger.*
Levodopa (p.1205·2); carbidopa (p.1204·3).
*Parkinsonism.*

**Levodopa-Carbi** *Azupharma, Ger.*
Levodopa (p.1205·2); carbidopa (p.1204·3).
*Parkinsonism.*

**Levo-Dromoran** *ICN, USA.*
Levorphanol tartrate (p.54·1).
*Pain.*

**Levofamil** *Andromaco, Chile.*
Levodopa (p.1205·2); carbidopa (p.1204·3).
*Parkinsonism.*

**Levofenil** *Grin, Mex.*
Dexamethasone sodium phosphate (p.1097·2); chloramphenicol (p.185·1); phenylephrine hydrochloride (p.1126·3).
*Inflammatory eye infections.*

**Levofolene** *Farmades, Ital.*
Calcium levofolinate (p.1431·1).
*Antidote to folic acid antagonists; folate deficiency anaemia.*

**Levoglutil Vitaminado** *Spedrog, Arg.*
Glutamine; vitamin $B_6$; vitamin $B_{12}$; calcium lactate; magnesium gluconate (p.1417·1).
*Dietary supplement.*

**Levograf** *Juste, Spain.*
Galactose (p.1063·1).
*Ultrasound contrast medium.*

**Levolac**
*Leiras, Fin.; Fresenius Kabi, Norw.*
Lactulose (p.1269·1).
*Constipation; hepatic encephalopathy.*

**Levomed**
*Medochemie, Hong Kong; Medochemie, Malaysia; Medochemie, Thai.*
Levodopa (p.1205·2); carbidopa (p.1204·3).
*Parkinsonism.*

**Levomet**
*Note. This name is used for preparations of different composition.*
*Unison, Hong Kong; Unison, Singapore.*
Levodopa (p.1205·2); carbidopa (p.1204·3).
*Parkinsonism.*

*Chiesi, Ital.*
Levodopa methyl hydrochloride (p.1209·1).
*Parkinsonism.*

**Levomycetin** *Chew, Thai.*
Chloramphenicol (p.185·1).
*Bacterial infections.*

**Levonelle**
*Schering, Ital.; Schering, NZ; Schering, Port.; Schering, UK.*
Levonorgestrel (p.1563·2).
*Postcoital oral contraceptive.*

**Levonova**
*Leiras, Denm.; Schering, Norw.*
Levonorgestrel (p.1563·2).
*Menorrhagia; progestogen-only oral contraceptive.*

*Leiras, Fin.; Schering, Swed.*
Levonorgestrel (p.1563·2).
*Menorrhagia; progestogen-releasing intra-uterine contraceptive device.*

**Levopa** *Wallace, India.*
Levodopa (p.1205·2).
*Parkinsonism.*

**Levopa-C** *Wallace, India.*
Levodopa (p.1205·2); carbidopa (p.1204·3).
*Parkinsonism.*

**Levopar** *Hexal, Ger.*
Levodopa (p.1205·2); benserazide (p.1200·2).
*Drug-induced extrapyramidal disorders; parkinsonism.*

**Levopar Plus** *Teva, Israel.*
Levodopa (p.1205·2); benserazide hydrochloride (p.1200·2).
*Parkinsonism.*

**Levophed**
*Abbott, Austral.; Abbott, Belg.; Abbott, Braz.; Abbott, Canad.; IFET (ΙΦΕΤ), Gr.; Abbott, Hong Kong; Abbott, Irl.; Abbott, Israel; Abbott, Malaysia; Abbott, NZ; Abbott, Singapore; Abbott, UK†; Abbott, USA.*
Noradrenaline acid tartrate (p.974·3).
Now known as Noradrenaline (Norepinephrine) 1:1000 in the *UK*.
*Cardiac arrest; hypotensive states.*

**Levophta**
*Chauvin, Fr.; Novartis Ophthalmics, Ger.; Winzer, Ger.*
Levocabastine hydrochloride (p.435·2).
*Allergic conjunctivitis.*

**Levoplus** *Montefarmaco, Ital.*
Dietary fibre (p.1253·2); lactulose (p.1269·1); lactitol (p.1269·1); mannitol (p.950·2).

**Levopraid**
*Therabel, Belg.; Abbott, Ital.*
Levosulpiride (p.722·2).
*Depression; gastrointestinal disorders; headache; psychoses; vertigo.*

**Levoprome** *Lederle, USA†.*
Levomepromazine hydrochloride (p.703·2).
*Pain; premedication.*

**Levopront**
*Mack, Singapore; Mack, Thai.*
Levodropropizine (p.1119·3).
*Coughs.*

**Levoptin** *Archifar, Thai.*
Chloramphenicol (p.185·1); prednisolone sodium phosphate (p.1108·1); naphazoline hydrochloride (p.1124·3).
*Eye disorders.*

**Levora** *Watson, USA.*
Levonorgestrel (p.1563·2); ethinylestradiol (p.1553·2).
28-Day packs also contain 7 inert tablets.
*Combined oral contraceptive.*

**Levordiol** *Sigma, Braz.*
21 Tablets, levonorgestrel (p.1563·2); ethinylestradiol (p.1553·2); pyridoxine hydrochloride (p.1456·3); 7 tablets, pyridoxine hydrochloride.
*Triphasic oral contraceptive.*

**Levorin**
*Wyeth Lederle, Austria†; Blausiegel, Braz.*
Calcium levofolinate (p.1431·1).
*Anaemias; antidote to folic acid antagonists; enhancement of fluorouracil activity; methotrexate toxicity.*

**Levostab** *Formenti, Ital.*
Levocabastine hydrochloride (p.435·2).
*Allergic conjunctivitis; allergic rhinitis.*

**Levo-T**
*Pharmascience, Canad.†; Lederle, USA†.*
Levothyroxine sodium (p.1600·1).
*Hypothyroidism; TSH suppression.*

**Levotec** *Technilab, Canad.†.*
Levothyroxine sodium (p.1600·1).
*Hypothyroidism.*

**Levothroid**
*Aventis, Spain; Forest Laboratories, USA.*
Levothyroxine sodium (p.1600·1).
*Hypercholesterolaemia; hypothyroidism; TSH suppression.*

**Levothym** *Lundbeck, Ger.*
Oxitriptan (p.311·1).
*Neurological disorders.*

**Levothyrox** *Lipha Sante, Fr.*
Levothyroxine sodium (p.1600·1).
*Hypothyroidism.*

**Levotiroxina** *Farmedica, Braz.†.*
Levothyroxine sodium (p.1600·1); liothyronine sodium (p.1602·2).
*Hypothyroidism.*

**Levotonine** *Panpharma, Fr.*
Oxitriptan (p.311·1).
*Myoclonus.*

**Levotrin** *GlaxoSmithKline, Arg.*
Liothyronine sodium (p.1602·2); levothyroxine sodium (p.1600·1).
*Hypothyroidism.*

**Levotuss**
*Janssen-Cilag, Belg.†; Boehringer Ingelheim, Gr.; Dompe, Ital.; Almirall, Spain.*
Levodropropizine (p.1119·3).
*Coughs.*

**Levovist**
*Schering, Arg.; Schering, Austral.; Schering, Austria; Schering, Braz.†; Berlex, Canad.; Schering, Denm.; Schering, Fin.; Schering, Fr.; Schering, Ger.; Schering, Israel†; Schering, Ital.; Schering, Neth.; Schering, Norw.; Schering, NZ†; Schering, Port.; Schering, Spain; Schering, Swed.; Schering, Switz.; Schering, UK.*
Galactose (p.1063·1).
*Ultrasound contrast medium.*

**Levoxacin** *GlaxoSmithKline, Ital.*
Levofloxacin (p.225·3).
*Bacterial infections.*

**Levoxyl** *Jones, USA.*
Levothyroxine sodium (p.1600·1).
Formerly known as Levoxine.
*Hypothyroidism; TSH suppression.*

**Levozin** *Orion, Fin.*
Levomepromazine maleate (p.703·2).
*Agitation; insomnia; pain; psychoses.*

**Levozine** *Cristalia, Braz.*
Levomepromazine maleate (p.703·2).
*Adjunct in general anaesthesia; pain in obstetrics; premedication; psychoses.*

**Levsin**
*Rivex, Canad.; Schwarz, Hong Kong; Schwarz, USA.*
Hyoscyamine sulfate (p.485·1).
*Adjunct to hypotonic duodenography; anticholinesterase poisoning; biliary and renal colic; gastrointestinal disorders; improvement of radiological visibility of the kidneys; neurogenic bladder; pancreatitis; parkinsonism; partial heart block associated with vagal activity; premedication; rhinitis.*

**Levsinex** *Schwarz, USA.*
Hyoscyamine sulfate (p.485·1).
*Biliary and renal colic; gastrointestinal disorders; parkinsonism; rhinitis; urinary-tract disorders.*

**Levucal** *Pasteur, Chile.*
Calcium carbonate (p.1254·2).
*Calcium deficiency; osteomalacia; osteoporosis; rickets; tetany.*

**Levucal D** *Pasteur, Chile.*
Calcium carbonate (p.1254·2); colecalciferol (p.1461·3).
*Calcium deficiency; osteoporosis.*

**Levudin** *GD, Ital.*
Yeast (p.1469·1); betacarotene (p.1422·3).

**Levugen** *Travenol, UK†.*
Fructose (p.1431·3).

**Levulan Kerastick** *DUSA, USA.*
Aminolevulinic acid hydrochloride (p.527·2).
*Actinic keratoses.*

**Levulosado** *Bieffe, Spain.*
Fructose (p.1431·3).
*Fluid and electrolyte disorders; liver disorders.*

**Levulosalino Isot** *Braun, Spain†.*
Sodium chloride (p.1233·3); fructose (p.1431·3).
*Carbohydrate source; fluid and electrolyte disorders.*

**Levunolol** *Luar, Arg.*
Levobunolol (p.946·2).
*Ocular hypertension.*

**Levuplex** *Apsen, Braz.†.*
Multivitamin preparation with fructose (p.1417·1).

**Levure Or** *Grimberg, Fr.*
Potassium bromoaurate; dried yeast (p.1469·1).
*Rheumatic disorders.*

**Levurinetten** *Novartis Consumer, Austria.*
Dried yeast (p.1469·1); vitamin B substances (p.1417·1).
*Skin disorders.*

**Levurinetten N** *Teofarma, Ger.*
Dried yeast (p.1469·1).
*Appetite loss; skin disorders.*

**Levusalino** *Ern, Spain†.*
Fructose (p.1431·3); sodium chloride (p.1233·3).
*Carbohydrate source; fluid and electrolyte disorders.*

**Levviax** *Aventis, Spain.*
Telithromycin (p.265·2).
*Bacterial respiratory-tract infections.*

**Lexapro**
*Abbott, Chile.*
Escitalopram (p.292·1).
*Depression.*

*Lundbeck, Austral.; Lundbeck, Irl.; Forest Pharmaceuticals, USA.*
Escitalopram oxalate (p.292·1).
*Depression; panic attacks.*

**Lexat** *Eagle, Austral.†.*
Bile salts (p.1660·3); pancreatin (p.1725·3); boldo (p.1661·2); greater celandine (p.1695·3); aloes (p.1248·2); agar (p.1576·3); sanguinaria (p.1741·3).
*Constipation; digestive system disorders.*

**Lexatin** *Roche, Spain.*
Bromazepam (p.671·3).
*Anxiety.*

**Lexavite** *Bajer, Arg.*
Liquid paraffin (p.1479·1).
*Bowel evacuation.*

**Lexemin**
*Unison, Hong Kong; Unison, Singapore; Unison, Thai.*
Fenofibrate (p.915·2).
*Hyperlipidaemias.*

**Lexfor** *Nakorn, Thai.*
Norfloxacin (p.238·3).
*Bacterial infections.*

**Lexibiotico** *Llano, Spain†.*
Cefalexin (p.168·1).
*Bacterial infections.*

**Lexiflox** *Duopharma, Hong Kong.*
Norfloxacin (p.238·3).
*Bacterial infections.*

**Lexil** *Roche, Ital.*
Bromazepam (p.671·3); propantheline bromide (p.489·1).
*Gastrointestinal disorders.*

**Lexilium** *Remedica, Hong Kong.*
Bromazepam (p.671·3).
*Anxiety.*

**Lexin**
*Biotenk, Arg.; Teuto, Braz.*
Cefalexin (p.168·1).
*Bacterial infections.*

**Lexincef** *Serra Pamies, Spain.*
Cefalexin (p.168·1).
*Bacterial infections.*

**Lexinor**
*AstraZeneca, Fin.; AstraZeneca, Hong Kong; AstraZeneca, Malaysia; AstraZeneca, Singapore†; Astra, Swed.; AstraZeneca, Thai.*
Norfloxacin (p.238·3).
*Bacterial infections.*

**Lexis** *Mintlab, Chile.*
Clindamycin phosphate (p.194·2).
*Bacterial skin infections.*

**Lexiva** *GlaxoSmithKline, USA.*
Fosamprenavir calcium (p.634·1).
*HIV infection.*

**Lexobene** *Merckle, Ger.*
Diclofenac sodium (p.32·1).
Lidocaine hydrochloride (p.1377·3) is included in this preparation to alleviate the pain of injection.
*Gout; inflammation; musculoskeletal, joint, and soft-tissue disorders; neuralgia; neuritis; pain.*

**Lexomil** *Roche, Fr.*
Bromazepam (p.671·3).
*Alcohol withdrawal syndrome; anxiety.*

**Lexostad** *Stada, Ger.*
Bromazepam (p.671·3).
*Anxiety disorders; insomnia.*

**Lexotan**
*Roche, Austral.; Roche, Belg.; Roche, Braz.; Roche, Denm.; Roche, Hong Kong; Roche, Irl.; Roche, Ital.; Roche, Mex.; Roche, Port.; Roche, S.Afr.; Roche, Singapore; Roche, Thai.; Roche, UK†.*
Bromazepam (p.671·3).
*Anxiety; psychosomatic disorders.*

**Lexotanil**
*Roche, Arg.; Roche, Austria; Roche, Chile; Roche, Ger.; Roche, Gr.; Roche, Neth.; Roche, Switz.*
Bromazepam (p.671·3).
*Anxiety disorders; psychosomatic symptoms.*

**Lexpec** *Rosemont, UK.*
Folic acid (p.1429·1).
*Anaemias.*

**Lexpec with Iron** *Rosemont, UK.*
Ferric ammonium citrate (p.1427·2); folic acid (p.1429·1).
*Iron and folic acid deficiency.*

**Lexpec with Iron-M** *Rosemont, UK.*
Ferric ammonium citrate (p.1427·2); folic acid (p.1429·1).
*Iron and folic acid deficiency.*

**Lextarol** *Biomedica-Chemica, Gr.*
Ambroxol hydrochloride (p.1114·3).
*Respiratory disorders associated with viscous mucus.*

**Lextrasa** *Valeas, Ital.*
Mesalazine (p.1273·2).
*Crohn's disease; ulcerative colitis.*

**Lexxel** *Astra, USA.*
Enalapril maleate (p.909·2); felodipine (p.914·3).
*Hypertension.*

**Lexxema** *Italfarmaco, Spain.*
Methylprednisolone aceponate (p.1106·3).
*Skin disorders.*

**Leza** *Bioclon, Mex.†.*
Yeast (p.1469·1).
*Modification of gastrointestinal flora.*

**Lezidim** *Lemery, Mex.*
Ceftazidime (p.180·2).
*Bacterial infections.*

**Lezole** *Kampel Martian, Arg.*
Anastrozole (p.528·1).
*Malignant neoplasms.*

**L-G Vita** *Mertens, Arg.*
Calcium phosphate; methionine; pyritinol hydrochloride; vitamin B substances (p.1417·1).
*Asthenia; mental function impairment.*

**L-Gel** *Medical Industries, Austral.*
Lubricating gel.

**LH Predict** *Aptus, NZ.*
Fertility test (p.1734·3).

**Li 450** *Ziethen, Ger.*
Lithium carbonate (p.301·1).
*Bipolar disorder; depression; mania.*

**Liaderyl** *Kleva, Gr.*
Tenoxicam (p.93·1).
*Dysmenorrhoea; gout; inflammation; osteoarthritis; pain; rheumatoid arthritis; spondyloarthropathies.*

**Liamycin** *Coup, Gr.*
Propylene glycol cefatrizine (p.170·3).
*Bacterial infections.*

**Liatriz** *Solfran, Mex.*
Meclozine (p.436·3); pyridoxine (p.1457·2).
*Nausea and vomiting.*

**Libeeda** *Nutravite, Canad.*
Bee pollen; damiana; ginseng; tribulus terrestris (p.1417·1).

**Libenar**
*GlaxoSmithKline Consumer, Ital.; GlaxoSmithKline Consumer, Port.; Sterling Health, Spain†.*
Sodium chloride (p.1233·3).
*Nasal dryness; nasal hygiene.*

**Liberal** *Asian Pharm, Thai.*
Flunarizine hydrochloride (p.434·1).
*Cerebrovascular disorders; vestibular disorders.*

**Liberalgium** *Diviser Aquilea, Spain†.*
Diclofenac sodium (p.32·1).
*Gout; inflammation; musculoskeletal, joint, and periarticular disorders; pain; renal colic.*

**Liberan**
*Note. This name is used for preparations of different composition.*
*Apsen, Braz.*
Bethanechol (p.1488·1).
*Urinary retention.*

*AF, Mex.*
Simeticone (p.1289·2).
*Flatulence.*

**Liberanas** *OTC, Spain†.*
Sodium chloride (p.1233·3).
*Nasal congestion.*

**Liberate** *SNBTS, UK.*
A factor VIII preparation (p.751·1).
*Haemorrhagic disorders.*

**Liberbil** *Ferrer, Spain†.*
Cyclobutyrol sodium (p.1678·2); theophylline dehydrocholinate; metoclopramide hydrochloride (p.1274·3).
*Hepatobiliary disorders.*

**Liberen** *Lisapharma, Ital.*
Dextropropoxyphene hydrochloride (p.28·3).
*Pain; renal and hepatic colic.*

**Liberim T** *SNBTS, UK.*
A tetanus immunoglobulin (p.1640·3).
*Passive immunisation.*

**Liberol** *Galactina, Switz.†.*
Camphor (p.1665·3); methyl salicylate (p.59·3); guaiacol (p.1122·1); mustard spirit (p.1718·2); pumilio pine oil (p.1737·1); thyme oil (p.1755·3); eucalyptus oil (p.1686·2); turpentine oil (p.1760·1); hyoscyamus oil (p.485·2).
*Chilblains; cold symptoms; muscle and joint pain.*

**Liberol Baby N** *Mavena, Switz.*
Eucalyptus oil (p.1686·2); pumilio pine oil (p.1737·1); anise oil (p.1655·2); juniper oil (p.1703·1).
*Cold symptoms.*

**Liberol Bain** *Mavena, Switz.*
Thyme oil (p.1755·3); pumilio pine oil (p.1737·1); eucalyptus oil (p.1686·2); rosemary oil (p.1740·2); lavender oil (p.1705·2); niaouli oil (p.1719·3).
*Coughs and cold symptoms.*

**Liberol Dragees contre la toux** *Mavena, Switz.*
Thyme (p.1755·2); hedera helix.
*Coughs.*

**Liberol N** *Mavena, Switz.*
Camphor (p.1665·3); pumilio pine oil (p.1737·1); thyme oil (p.1755·3); eucalyptus oil (p.1686·2).
*Cold symptoms.*

**Liberol Pastilles contre la toux** *Mavena, Switz.*
Thyme (p.1755·2); senega root (p.1130·2).
*Coughs.*

**Liberol Sirop contre la toux** *Mavena, Switz.*
Thyme (p.1755·2); hedera helix; senega root (p.1130·2); liquorice (p.1270·2).
*Coughs.*

**Liberprost** *Kampel Martian, Arg.*
Bicalutamide (p.530·1).

**Libertin** *Robugen, Ger.*
Hypericum (p.299·1).
*Depression.*

**Libertrim** *AF, Mex.*
Trimebutine (p.1758·1).
*Gastrointestinal motility disorders; irritable bowel syndrome.*

**Libexin** *Khandelwal, India.*
Prenoxdiazine hydrochloride (p.1129·1).
*Cough.*

**Libexin Mucolitico** *Teofarma, Ital.*
Prenoxdiazine hibenzate (p.1129·1); carbocisteine (p.1116·2).
*Coughs.*

**Libexine** *Labatec, Switz.†.*
Prenoxdiazine hibenzate (p.1129·1) or prenoxdiazine hydrochloride (p.1129·1).
*Coughs.*

**Libexine Compositum** *Labatec, Switz.†.*
Prenoxdiazine hydrochloride (p.1129·1); guaifenesin (p.1122·1); terpin hydrate (p.1131·1).
*Coughs.*

**Libiam** *Libbs, Braz.*
Tibolone (p.1572·3).
*Anabolic.*

**Libidomega** *Cantassium Co., UK.*
Amino-acid, vitamin, and mineral preparation (p.1417·1).

**Libiocid** *Rayere, Mex.*
Lincomycin hydrochloride (p.226·2).
*Bacterial infections.*

**Libiplus** *Delta, Braz.*
Vitamins; yohimbine hydrochloride (p.1766·2); glutamic acid; phytin (p.1417·1).
*Tonic.*

**Liblan**
*YSP, Malaysia; Yung Shin, Thai.†.*
Chlordiazepoxide (p.674·2); clidinium bromide (p.480·2).
*Dysmenorrhoea; gastric hyperacidity; gastroduodenitis; gastrointestinal motility disorders; irritable bowel syndrome; peptic ulcer; ureteric spasm and dyskinesia.*

**Libradin** *Andromaco, Spain.*
Barnidipine hydrochloride (p.866·3).
*Hypertension.*

**Librax**
*ICN, Arg.; Roche, Belg.†; ICN, Fin.; CSP, Fr.; ICN, Hong Kong; Roche, Israel†; ICN, Ital.; ICN, Port.; Pharmaco, S.Afr.; ICN, Singapore; ICN, Switz.; ICN, Thai.*
Chlordiazepoxide (p.674·2); clidinium bromide (p.480·2).
*Dysmenorrhoea; irritable bowel syndrome; nocturnal enuresis; peptic ulcer; smooth muscle spasm.*

*ICN, Canad.; Roche, USA.*
Chlordiazepoxide hydrochloride (p.674·2); clidinium bromide (p.480·2).
*Irritable bowel syndrome; peptic ulcer (adjunct).*

**Libraxin** *Roche, Chile.*
Chlordiazepoxide (p.674·2); clidinium bromide (p.480·2).
*Colitis; irritable colon; nocturnal enuresis; peptic ulcer; smooth muscle spasm.*

**Libritabs** *Roche Products, USA†.*
Chlordiazepoxide (p.674·2).
*Anxiety.*

**Librium**
*ICN, Ger.; ICN, Hong Kong; Piramal, India; ICN, Irl.; Pharmaco, S.Afr.*
Chlordiazepoxide (p.674·2).
*Alcohol withdrawal syndrome; anxiety; insomnia; skeletal muscle spasm.*

*ICN, Ital.; ICN, UK; ICN, USA.*
Chlordiazepoxide hydrochloride (p.674·2).
*Alcohol withdrawal syndrome; anxiety; insomnia; premedication; skeletal muscle spasm.*

**Librofem** *Eastern Pharmaceuticals, UK.*
Ibuprofen (p.45·3).
*Fever; pain.*

**Libronchin** *Altana, Neth.*
Acetylcysteine (p.1112·3).
*Respiratory-tract disorders with increased or viscous mucus.*

**Libronchin Prikkelhoest** *Byk, Neth.*
Noscapine hydrochloride (p.1125·3).
*Coughs.*

**Licab**
*Torrent, India; Torrent, Thai.†.*
Lithium carbonate (p.301·1).
*Bipolar disorder; depression; mania.*

**Licain** *Curasan, Ger.*
Lidocaine hydrochloride (p.1377·3).
*Local anaesthesia.*

**Licarb** *RX, Thai.*
Lithium carbonate (p.301·1).
*Bipolar disorder; depression; mania.*

**Licarbium** *Rekah, Israel.*
Lithium carbonate (p.301·1).
*Bipolar disorder.*

**Licarpin** *Allergan, Swed.†.*
Pilocarpine nitrate (p.1495·1).
*Glaucoma.*

**Lice Blaster** *Douglas, NZ.*
Adhatoda vasica; echinacea (p.1683·2); melaleuca oil (p.1710·2); stemona sessifolia root.
*Pediculosis.*

**Lice Rid** *Florafaun, Austral.*
Malathion (Maldison) (p.1507·1).
*Pediculosis.*

**Licetrol** *Stanley, Canad.*
Pyrethrins (p.1509·3); piperonyl butoxide (p.1509·2).
*Pediculosis.*

**Lichtena** *UCB, Singapore.*
Emollient.
*Dry skin.*

**Licide** *Reese, USA.*
Pyrethrum (p.1509·3); piperonyl butoxide (p.1509·2).
*Pediculosis.*

**Licilon** *Sanval, Braz.*
Amoxicillin trihydrate (p.155·3).
*Bacterial infections.*

**Liconar**
*Biolab, Singapore; Biolab, Thai.*
Miconazole nitrate (p.405·3).
*Fungal and Gram-positive bacterial skin infections.*

**Licor Amoniacal** *Asens, Spain†.*
Alcohol (p.1166·1); ammonia (p.1653·3); ammonium carbonate (p.1115·1).
*Exhaustion; nausea; shock.*

**Licor de Cacau** *Virtus, Braz.†.*
Piperazine (p.111·2); citric acid (p.1673·1); theobroma (p.1754·3); cinnamon (p.1672·2); cascara (p.1255·1).
*Intestinal nematode infections.*

**Licor de Tayuya** *Dansk-Flama, Braz.†.*
Sarsaparilla (p.1742·1); tayuya; ceratonia (p.1579·1).

**Licostrata** *Cantabria, Spain.*
Hydroquinone (p.1148·1).
*Hyperpigmentation.*

**Licovit** *Ativus, Braz.*
Vitamin A (p.1451·2); vitamin E (p.1464·3); lycopene.
*Skin disorders.*

**Licrease** *Laphal, Fr.*
Pancreatin (p.1725·3).
*Pancreatic insufficiency.*

**Licuamon** *Merck, Arg.*
Aspirin (p.15·1); dipyridamole (p.903·1).
*Atherosclerosis; thromboembolic disorders.*

**Lidaflan** *Biochimico, Braz.†.*
Nimesulide (p.67·1).

**Lidaltrin** *Lacer, Spain.*
Quinapril hydrochloride (p.991·1).
*Heart failure; hypertension.*

**Lidaltrin Diu** *Lacer, Spain.*
Quinapril hydrochloride (p.991·1); hydrochlorothiazide (p.933·2).
*Hypertension.*

**LidaMantle** *Doak, USA.*
Lidocaine hydrochloride (p.1377·3).
*Local anaesthesia.*

**LidaMantle HC** *Doak, USA.*
Hydrocortisone acetate (p.1103·3); lidocaine hydrochloride (p.1377·3).
*Skin disorders.*

**Lidaprim**
*Note. This name is used for preparations of different composition.*
*Nycomed, Austria; Nycomed, Gr.; Nycomed, Hong Kong; Lisapharma, Ital.; Nycomed, Thai.*
Sulfametrole (p.263·2); trimethoprim (p.272·2).
*Bacterial infections; Pneumocystis carinii pneumonia; toxoplasmosis.*

*Hormona, Mex.†.*
Co-trimoxazole (p.199·3).
*Bacterial infections.*

**Lidazon** *Democal, Switz.*
Cetylpyridinium chloride (p.1173·1); dichlorobenzyl alcohol (p.1178·3); lidocaine (p.1377·3) or lidocaine hydrochloride (p.1377·3).
Lidazon lozenges formerly contained cetylpyridinium chloride, dichlorobenzyl alcohol, lidocaine, and chlorquinaldol.
*Mouth and throat disorders.*

**Lid-Care**
*Novartis Ophthalmics, Austral.; Novartis Ophthalmics, Canad.; Novartis, NZ; Novartis Ophthalmics, UK.*
Eyelid cleanser.

**Lidemol** *Medicis, Canad.*
Fluocinonide (p.1101·3).
*Skin disorders.*

**Lidene** *Cooperation Pharmaceutique, Fr.*
Doxylamine succinate (p.432·3).
*Insomnia.*

**Lidenix** *Nobel, Ital.*
Nimesulide (p.67·1).
*Fever; inflammation; pain.*

**Lident Adrenalina** *Warner-Lambert, Ital.*
Lidocaine hydrochloride (p.1377·3).
Adrenaline acid tartrate (p.852·2) is included in this preparation as a vasoconstrictor to diminish absorption and localise the effect of the local anaesthetic.
*Local anaesthesia in dentistry.*

**Lident Andrenor** *Warner-Lambert, Ital.*
Lidocaine hydrochloride (p.1377·3).
Adrenaline acid tartrate (p.852·2) and noradrenaline acid tartrate (p.974·3) are included in this preparation as vasoconstrictors to diminish absorption and localise the effect of the local anaesthetic.
*Local anaesthesia in dentistry.*

**Liderclox** *Levofarma, Ital.*
Flucloxacillin sodium (p.213·3).
*Bacterial infections.*

**Liderflex** *Farmalider, Spain†.*
Camphor (p.1665·3); methyl salicylate (p.59·3); menthol (p.1711·3).
*Muscular and joint pain.*

**Liderma** *Medika, Switz.*
Isotretinoin (p.1148·3).
*Acne.*

**Liderman** *Jacoby, Austria.*
Oxiconazole nitrate (p.407·3).
*Fungal and Gram-positive bacterial skin infections.*

**Liderplus** *Farmalider, Spain†.*
Paracetamol (p.76·2); pseudoephedrine sulfate (p.1129·2); chlorphenamine maleate (p.427·3).
*Cold and influenza symptoms; respiratory-tract congestion.*

**Lidesthesin** *Ritsert, Ger.*
Lidocaine hydrochloride (p.1377·3).
*Local anaesthesia.*

**Lidex**
*Yamanouchi, Belg.; Medicis, Canad.; Minerva (Μινερβα), Gr.; MD, Singapore; Medicis, USA.*
Fluocinonide (p.1101·3).
*Skin disorders.*

**Lidial** *Bunker, Braz.*
Lidocaine (p.1377·3).
*Local anaesthesia.*

**Lidifen** *Berk, UK†.*
Ibuprofen (p.45·3).
*Fever; inflammation; musculoskeletal and joint disorders; pain.*

**Lidinal** Fustery, Mex.†.
Nalidixic acid (p.234·1).

**Lidixin** Ofimex, Mex.†.
Nalidixic acid (p.234·1).

**Lidl** Roemmers, Arg.
Oxymetazoline hydrochloride (p.1126·1).
*Nasal congestion.*

**Lido Spray** Ritter, Thai.
Lidocaine hydrochloride (p.1377·3).
*Local anaesthesia.*

**Lido Tea** Trima, Israel.
Senna (p.1288·2); caraway (p.1667·2); liquorice (p.1270·2); chamomile (p.1669·3); peppermint leaf (p.1283·2).
*Constipation.*

**Lidobama Complex** Bama, Spain†.
Cellulase (p.1669·1); cyclobutyrol (p.1678·2); dimethicone (p.1289·2); lidocaine hydrochloride (p.1377·3); pancreatin (p.1725·3).
*Digestive-system disorders.*

**Lidocabbott** Abbott, Braz.
Lidocaine hydrochloride (p.1377·3).
Adrenaline (p.852·2) is included in some injections as a vasoconstrictor to diminish absorption and localise the effect of the local anaesthetic.
*Arrhythmias; local anaesthesia.*

**Lidocadren** Teva, Israel.
Lidocaine hydrochloride (p.1377·3).
Adrenaline (p.852·2) is included in this preparation as a vasoconstrictor to diminish absorption and localise the effect of the local anaesthetic.
*Local anaesthesia.*

**Lidocalm** Teuto, Braz.
Lidocaine hydrochloride (p.1377·3).
*Local anaesthesia.*

**Lidocard**
Orion, Fin.; Braun, Ger.
Lidocaine hydrochloride (p.1377·3).
*Arrhythmias.*

**Lidocation** Weimer, Thai.
Lidocaine hydrochloride (p.1377·3).
Adrenaline (p.852·2) is included in this preparation as a vasoconstrictor to diminish absorption and localise the effect of the local anaesthetic.
*Local anaesthesia.*

**Lidocaton**
Weimer, Ger.†; Weimer, Switz.†; Weimer, Thai.
Lidocaine hydrochloride (p.1377·3).
Adrenaline (p.852·2) is included in this preparation as a vasoconstrictor to diminish absorption and localise the effect of the local anaesthetic.
*Local anaesthesia.*

**Lidocord** Apsen, Braz.†.
Lidocaine hydrochloride (p.1377·3).
*Arrhythmias.*

**Lidocorit** Gebro, Austria.
Lidocaine hydrochloride (p.1377·3).
*Arrhythmias.*

**Lidodan** Odan, Canad.
Lidocaine (p.1377·3) or lidocaine hydrochloride (p.1377·3).
*Local anaesthesia.*

**Lidoderm** Endo, USA.
Lidocaine (p.1377·3).
*Postherpetic neuralgia.*

**Lidogel** Neo Quimica, Braz.
Lidocaine hydrochloride (p.1377·3).
*Local anaesthesia.*

**Lidogeyer** Geyer, Braz.
Lidocaine hydrochloride (p.1377·3).
Adrenaline (p.852·2) is included in this preparation as a vasoconstrictor to diminish absorption and localise the effect of the local anaesthetic.
*Local anaesthesia.*

**Lidohex** Bichsel, Switz.
Lidocaine hydrochloride (p.1377·3); chlorhexidine gluconate (p.1173·2).
*Catheterisation; endoscopy.*

**Lido-Hyal**
Ogna, Ital.; Wild, Switz.
Hyaluronidase (p.1698·2); lidocaine hydrochloride (p.1377·3).
*Local anaesthesia; prophylaxis of soft-tissue disorders.*

**Lidoject**
Hexal, Ger.; Mayrand, USA†.
Lidocaine hydrochloride (p.1377·3).
*Local anaesthesia.*

**Lidojet** Uniao Quimica, Braz.
Lidocaine hydrochloride (p.1377·3).
*Local anaesthesia.*

**Lidomol** Molteni, Ital.
Lidocaine hydrochloride (p.1377·3).
Adrenaline acid tartrate (p.852·2) is included in the injection as a vasoconstrictors to diminish absorption and localise the effect of the local anaesthetic.
*Local anaesthesia.*

**Lidomyxin** Sabex, Canad.
Polymyxin B sulfate (p.245·1); lidocaine hydrochloride (p.1377·3).
*Ear infections, pain, and pruritus.*

**Lidonostrum** Nostrum, Port.
Lidocaine (p.1377·3).
Adrenaline (p.852·2) is included in some injections as a vasoconstrictor to diminish absorption and localise the effect of the local anaesthetic.
*Catheterisation; endoscopy; local anaesthesia; tracheal entubation.*

**LidoPen**
Meridian, Israel; Survival Technology, USA.
Lidocaine hydrochloride (p.1377·3).
*Arrhythmias.*

**LidoPosterine** Kade, Ger.
Lidocaine (p.1377·3).
*Anorectal disorders.*

**Lidosen** Senese, Ital.
Lidocaine hydrochloride (p.1377·3).
*Local anaesthesia.*

**Lidosporin**
Note. This name is used for preparations of different composition.
Zest, Braz.
Polymyxin B sulfate (p.245·1); lidocaine (p.1377·3).
*Ear infections.*

Pfizer Consumer, Canad.
*Ear drops:* Polymyxin B sulfate (p.245·1); lidocaine hydrochloride (p.1377·3).
*Ear infections.*

Warner-Lambert, Canad.†.
*Cream:* Polymyxin B sulfate (p.245·1); gramicidin (p.220·2); lidocaine hydrochloride (p.1377·3).
*Skin disorders.*

**Lidospray** Apsen, Braz.
Lidocaine (p.1377·3).
*Local anaesthesia.*

**Lidoston** Ariston, Braz.
Lidocaine (p.1377·3).
*Local anaesthesia.*

**Lidoxin**
Unison, Hong Kong; Unison, Singapore; Unison, Thai.
Cloxacillin sodium (p.198·2).
*Bacterial infections.*

**Lid-Pack** Ciba Vision, Canad.†.
Polymyxin B sulfate (p.245·1); bacitracin zinc (p.161·3).

**Lidrian** Baxter, Ital.
Lidocaine hydrochloride (p.1377·3).
*Local anaesthesia.*

**Lidrone** Serra Pamies, Spain†.
Phenylephrine hydrochloride (p.1126·3); naphazoline nitrate (p.1124·3); prednisolone (p.1108·1); cetrimide (p.1172·1).
*Cold symptoms; rhinitis; sinusitis.*

**Lievistar** Skills, Ital.†.
Dried yeast (p.1469·1); cynara (p.1678·3).
*Nutritional supplement.*

**Lievitosohn** Antonetto, Ital.
*Saccharomyces cerevisiae* (p.1469·1); vitamin B substances (p.1417·1).
*Restoration of normal gastrointestinal flora.*

**Lievitovit** Novartis Consumer, Ital.
Dried yeast (p.1469·1); vitamin B substances (p.1417·1).
*Restoration of normal gastrointestinal flora.*

**Lievitovit 300** Gazzoni, Ital.†.
Dried yeast (p.1469·1).

**Lifar** Grunenthal, Chile.
Tibolone (p.1572·3).
*Menopausal disorders.*

**Lifaton B12** Sabater, Spain†.
Cyanocobalamin (p.1458·2).
*Vitamin B12 deficiency.*

**Life Brand Baby Sunblock and Kids Sunblock** Tanning Research, Canad.
*SPF 30:* Octinoxate (p.1154·3); octisalate (p.1154·3); titanium dioxide (p.1160·3).
*Sunscreen.*

**Life Brand Cough Lozenges** Sutton, Canad.†.
Menthol (p.1711·3).

**Life Brand Natural Source** Tanning Research, Canad.†.
*SPF 25:* Titanium dioxide (p.1160·3).
*Sunscreen.*

**Life Brand Sport Sunblock** Tanning Research, Canad.
*SPF 15; SPF 30:* Octinoxate (p.1154·3); octisalate (p.1154·3); oxybenzone (p.1154·3).
*Sunscreen.*

**Life Brand Sunblock** Tanning Research, Canad.
*SPF 15:* Octinoxate (p.1154·3); oxybenzone (p.1154·3).
*SPF 30:* Octinoxate (p.1154·3); homosalate (p.1148·1); octisalate (p.1154·3); oxybenzone (p.1154·3).
Formerly contained octinoxate, avobenzone, and homosalate.
*Sunscreen.*

**Life Drops** Potter's, UK.
Capsicum (p.1667·1); sambucus (p.1741·3); peppermint oil (p.1283·2).
*Cold symptoms; sore throat.*

**Lifechange Circulation Aid** Cenovis, Austral.†.
Fish oil (p.976·2); *dl*-alpha tocoferil acetate (p.1465·1); ginkgo biloba (p.1692·3); crataegus (p.1677·1).
*Peripheral circulatory disorders; wounds.*

**Lifechange Menopause Formula** Cenovis, Austral.†.
Soya bean (p.1447·2); red clover (p.1737·3).
*Menopausal disorders.*

**Lifechange Mens Complex with Saw Palmetto** Cenovis, Austral.†.
Zinc amino acid chelate (p.1469·3); cucurbita (p.1677·3); saw palmetto (p.1569·1).
*Tonic.*

**Lifechange Multi Plus Antioxidant** Cenovis, Austral.†.
Vitamins and minerals (p.1417·1); vitis vinifera; ginkgo biloba (p.1692·3).
*Peripheral circulatory disorders; vitamin and mineral deficiencies.*

**Lifedrops** Lifeplan, UK†.
Sambucus (p.1741·3); peppermint (p.1283·2).
*Coughs and cold symptoms; flatulence.*

**Lifenac** Liferpal, Mex.
Diclofenac sodium (p.32·1).
*Musculoskeletal, joint, and peri-articular disorders.*

**Lifermycin** Leovan, Gr.
Amikacin sulfate (p.154·1).
*Bacterial infections.*

**Liferost** Leovan, Gr.
Propylene glycol cefatrizine (p.170·3).
*Bacterial infections.*

**Liferxina** Liferpal, Mex.
Ciprofloxacin (p.188·2).
*Bacterial infections.*

**Liferzit** Leovan, Gr.
Lovastatin (p.949·1).
*Primary hypercholesterolaemia.*

**Lifestyle** Ansell, NZ.
Contraceptive; lubricating gel.

**Lifestyles** Ansell, Canad.
Nonoxinol 9 (p.1413·3).
*Contraceptive.*

**Lifesystem Herbal Formula 1 Arthritic Aid** Cenovis, Austral.†.
Celery (p.1669·1); juniper (p.1703·1); devil's claw root (p.28·2); salix (p.87·3).
*Arthritic and rheumatic pain.*

**Lifesystem Herbal Formula 7 Liver Tonic** Cenovis, Austral.†.
Silybum marianum (p.1043·3); taraxacum (p.1751·3); cynara (p.1678·3); garlic (p.1691·1).
*Digestive disorders; liver tonic.*

**Lifesystem Herbal Formula 6 For Peripheral Circulation** Cenovis, Austral.†.
Ginkgo biloba (p.1692·3); crataegus (p.1677·1); zanthoxylum (p.1766·3); capsicum (p.1667·1); rutoside (p.1688·2); hesperidin (p.1688·2).
*Peripheral circulatory disorders.*

**Lifesystem Herbal Formula 12 Willowbark** Cenovis, Austral.†.
Skullcap (p.1746·3); devil's claw root (p.28·2); salix (p.87·3).
*Headache.*

**Lifesystem Herbal Formula 4 Women's Formula** Cenovis, Austral.†.
Angelica (p.1655·1); cimicifuga (p.1671·3); blue cohosh (p.1661·2); pulsatilla (p.1737·1); agnus castus (p.1649·1).
*Menstrual disorders.*

**Lifesystem Herbal Plus Formula 8 Echinacea** Cenovis, Austral.†.
Echinacea (p.1683·2); *d*-alpha tocoferil acid succinate (p.1465·1); betacarotene (p.1422·3); ascorbic acid (p.1460·2); sodium ascorbate (p.1460·2); zinc amino acid chelate (p.1469·3).
*Minor upper respiratory-tract disorders; skin disorders; wounds.*

**Lifesystem Herbal Plus Formula 5 Eye Relief** Cenovis, Austral.†.
Euphrasia officinalis (p.1686·3); ginkgo biloba (p.1692·3); betacarotene (p.1422·3); *d*-alpha tocoferil acid succinate (p.1465·1); ascorbic acid (p.1460·2); rutoside (p.1688·2); hesperidin (p.1688·2).
*Eye strain; tired eyes.*

**Lifesystem Herbal Plus Formula 9 Fatty Acids And Vitamin E** Cenovis, Austral.†.
*d*-Alpha tocopherol (p.1464·3); evening primrose oil (p.1686·3); omega-3 marine triglycerides (p.976·2).
*Dietary supplement.*

**Lifesystem Herbal Plus Formula 11 Ginkgo** Cenovis, Austral.†.
Ginkgo biloba (p.1692·3); ginger (p.1267·1); dibasic potassium phosphate (p.1230·3); magnesium oxide (p.1272·3).
*Peripheral circulatory disorders; tonic.*

**Lifesystem Herbal Plus Formula 3 Male Formula** Cenovis, Austral.†.
Eleutherococcus senticosis; equisetum; sarsaparilla; liquorice; damiana; zinc amino acid chelate; betacarotene; pyridoxine hydrochloride; *d*-alpha tocoferil acid succinate; magnesium oxide (p.1417·1).
*Tonic.*

**Lifesystem Herbal Plus Formula 2 Valerian** Cenovis, Austral.†.
Valerian (p.1762·2); passion flower (p.1729·1); dibasic potassium phosphate (p.1230·3); magnesium oxide (p.1272·3).
*Nervous tension; sleep disorders.*

**Lifesystem Mineral Plus Formula 10 Osteoporosis** Cenovis, Austral.†.
Calcium carbonate (p.1254·2); colecalciferol (p.1461·3).
*Calcium deficiency; osteoporosis.*

**Lifo-Scrub** Braun, Switz.
Chlorhexidine gluconate (p.1173·2).
*Skin and hand disinfection.*

**Lifril** Casen Fleet, Spain†.
Pirlindole (p.316·2).
*Depression.*

**Lifurom** Lilly, S.Afr.
Cefuroxime sodium (p.184·1).
*Bacterial infections.*

**Lifurox**
Lilly, Denm.†; Lilly, Fin.†; Lilly, Norw.†; Elanco, Spain; Lilly, Swed.†.
Cefuroxime sodium (p.184·1).
*Bacterial infections.*

**Liga** Jacobs, UK†.
Gluten-free food for special diets (p.1417·1).

**Lightening** Mac, Ital.
Glycolic acid (p.1147·3); fytic acid (p.1052·3).
*Hyperpigmentation disorders.*

**Lightning Cough Remedy** Potter's, UK.
Liquorice (p.1270·2); anise oil (p.1655·2).
*Coughs.*

**Lignaform** Lignaform, Mon.
Preparation for enteral nutrition (p.1417·1).

**Lignospan**
Dentsply, Austral.; Septodont, Switz.
Lidocaine hydrochloride (p.1377·3).
Adrenaline acid tartrate (p.852·2) is included in this preparation as a vasoconstrictor to diminish absorption and localise the effect of the local anaesthetic.
*Local anaesthesia.*

**Lignospan Special** Dental Warehouse, S.Afr.
Lidocaine (p.1377·3).
Adrenaline (p.852·2) is included in this preparation as a vasoconstrictor to diminish absorption and localise the effect of the local anaesthetic.
*Local anaesthesia.*

**Lignosporin** Glaxo Wellcome, Singapore†.
Polymyxin B sulfate (p.245·1); lidocaine hydrochloride (p.1377·3).
*Ear infections.*

**Lignostab-A** Dentsply, UK.
Lidocaine hydrochloride (p.1377·3).
Adrenaline (p.852·2) is included in this preparation as a vasoconstrictor to diminish absorption and localise the effect of the local anaesthetic.
*Local anaesthesia.*

**Ligofragmin** Gador, Arg.
Dalteparin sodium (p.891·1).
*Thromboembolic disorders.*

**Ligramex** Fada, Arg.
Cefuroxime (p.184·1).
*Bacterial infections.*

**Li-iL Rheuma-Bad** Li-il, Ger.†.
Glycol salicylate (p.44·3); methyl salicylate (p.59·3).
*Bath additive; musculoskeletal, joint, and soft-tissue disorders.*

**Likacin**
Lisapharm, Israel.
Amikacin (p.154·1).
*Gram-negative bacterial infections.*

Lisapharma, Ital.
Amikacin sulfate (p.154·1).
*Gram-negative bacterial infections.*

**Likenil** Antibioticos, Spain.
Lisinopril (p.946·3).
*Diabetic nephropathy; heart failure; hypertension; myocardial infarction.*

**Likuden M** Aventis, Ger.
Griseofulvin (microfine) (p.400·3).
*Fungal infections.*

**Lilacillin** Takeda, Jpn.
Sulbenicillin sodium (p.257·2).
Mepivacaine hydrochloride (p.1381·2) is included in the intramuscular injection to alleviate the pain of injection.
*Bacterial infections.*

**Liliam** Columbia, Mex.
Hyoscine butylbromide (p.483·3).

**Li-Liquid** Rosemont, UK.
Lithium citrate (p.301·1).
*Depression; mania; psychoses.*

**Lilium Med Complex** Dynamit, Austria.
Homoeopathic preparation.

**Lillypen Profil 10, 20, 30, and 40** Lilly, Fr.†.
Mixtures of insulin injection (human, prb) 10%, 20%, 30%, and 40% and isophane insulin injection (human, prb) 90%, 80%, 70%, and 60% respectively (p.333·3).
*Diabetes mellitus.*

**Lillypen Protamine Isophane** Lilly, Fr.†.
Isophane insulin injection (human, prb) (p.333·3).
*Diabetes mellitus.*

**Lillypen Rapide** Lilly, Fr.
Insulin injection (human, prb) (p.333·3).
*Diabetes mellitus.*

**Liman**
Solvay, Austria†; Solvay, Ger.†.
Tenoxicam (p.93·1).
*Gout; musculoskeletal and joint disorders.*

**Limao Bravo**
Note. This name is used for preparations of different composition.
Catarinense, Braz.†.
Siparuna guyanensis; aconite (p.1646·3); grindelia (p.1696·1); senega (p.1130·2); sodium benzoate (p.1169·3).
*Respiratory-tract congestion.*

Farmedica, Braz.†.
Siparuna guyanensis; sodium benzoate (p.1169·3); aconite (p.1646·3); bromoform (p.1663·1); grindelia (p.1696·1); menthol (p.1711·3).
*Coughs.*

*Heralds, Braz.†.*
Siparuna guyanensis; rorippa nasturtium aquaticum; mikania; fig (p.1266·3).
*Respiratory-tract congestion.*

*Legrand, Braz.†.*
Siparuna guyanensis; bromoform (p.1663·1); althaea (p.1651·3); aconite (p.1646·3); sodium benzoate (p.1169·3); guaifenesin (p.1122·1).
*Coughs.*

*Simoes, Braz.*
Siparuna apiosyce; ascorbic acid (p.1460·2); cetylpyridinium chloride (p.1173·1).

**Limao Bravo com Vitamina C** *Cazi, Braz.*
Cetylpyridinium chloride (p.1173·1); vitamin C (p.1460·2); siparuna guyanensis.
*Mouth and throat disorders.*

**Limarin** *Serum Institute, India.*
Silymarin (p.1043·3).
*Liver disorders.*

**Limbao** *Kanoldt, Ger.†.*
Kava (p.1703·2).
*Anxiety disorders.*

**Limbatril** *ICN, Ger.†.*
Amitriptyline hydrochloride (p.280·3); chlordiazepoxide (p.674·2).
*Dystonias; non-psychotic mental disorders.*

**Limbial** *Chiesi, Ital.*
Oxazepam (p.712·2).
*Anxiety; insomnia; nervous disorders.*

**Limbitrol**
*ICN, Austria; Roche, Belg.†; ICN, Braz.; ICN, Fin.; Pharmaco, S.Afr.; ICN, Switz.; ICN, USA.*
Amitriptyline hydrochloride (p.280·3); chlordiazepoxide (p.674·2).
*Mixed anxiety depressive states.*

**Limbitryl** *ICN, Ital.*
Amitriptyline hydrochloride (p.280·3); chlordiazepoxide (p.674·2).
*Mixed anxiety depressive states.*

**Limcee** *Sarabhai Piramal, India.*
Vitamin C (p.1460·2).
*Infections; scurvy; wounds.*

**Limclair**
*Sinclair, Irl.; Durbin, UK.*
Trisodium edetate (p.1037·3).
*Calcareous corneal opacities; digitalis-induced arrhythmias; hypercalcaemia; parathyroidism.*

**Limectant** *Maurino, Arg.*
Sodium laurilsulfate (p.1574·2)(p.1164·2).
*Cleansing solution for soft contact lenses.*

**Limed** *Medifive, Thai.*
Lithium carbonate (p.301·1).
*Bipolar disorder.*

**Limethason**
*Green Cross, Hong Kong†; Mitsubishi, Jpn; Yoshitomi, Malaysia; Welfide, Singapore; Mitsubishi, Thai.*
Dexamethasone palmitate (p.1097·3).
*Rheumatoid arthritis.*

**Limexx** *Agepha, Austria.*
Tyrothricin (p.275·1); benzalkonium chloride (p.1168·3).
*Mouth and throat disorders.*

**Limican** *Sanofi Synthelabo, Ital.*
Alizapride hydrochloride (p.1248·1).
*Nausea and vomiting.*

**Limifen** *Janssen-Cilag, Spain.*
Alfentanil hydrochloride (p.12·2).
*General anaesthesia.*

**Liminate** *Modern Health Products, UK†.*
Turkey rhubarb (p.1287·3); senna leaf (p.1288·2); chondrus (p.1578·2).
*Constipation.*

**Liminos** *Glaxo Wellcome, Mex.*
Alosetron hydrochloride (p.1248·3).
*Irritable bowel syndrome.*

**Limit-X** *UB Interpharm, Switz.*
Cathine hydrochloride (p.1585·2).
*Obesity.*

**Limonal** *Falqui, Ital.†.*
Light magnesium carbonate (p.1272·1); anhydrous citric acid (p.1673·1).
*Constipation.*

**Limone** *CliniMed, UK.*
A deodorant spray for stoma care.

**Limovan** *Aventis, Spain.*
Zopiclone (p.729·3).
*Insomnia.*

**Limoxin** *Liferpal, Mex.*
Amoxicillin (p.155·3).
*Bacterial infections.*

**Limpacid** *Bajer, Arg.*
Bioallethrin (p.1500·3); piperonyl butoxide (p.1509·2).
*Pediculosis.*

**Limpele** *Dovalle, Braz.†.*
Econazole nitrate (p.397·2).
*Fungal skin infections.*

**Limpidex** *Sigma-Tau, Ital.*
Lansoprazole (p.1269·3).
*Gastro-oesophageal reflux; peptic ulcer; Zollinger-Ellison syndrome.*

**Limptar**
*Aventis, Austria; Cassella-med, Ger.*
Quinine sulfate (p.460·2); aminophylline (p.780·2).
*Night cramp.*

**Limptar N** *Cassella-med, Ger.*
Quinine sulfate (p.460·2).
*Night cramp.*

**Linadin** *Sedabel, Braz.†.*
Attapulgite (p.1251·1); pectin (p.1580·3); homatropine (p.483·2).
*Diarrhoea.*

**Linamin Plus** *Seber, Port.*
Fursultiamine (p.1454·3); cyanocobalamin (p.1458·2) or hydroxocobalamin (p.1458·2); pyridoxine hydrochloride (p.1456·3).
Mepivacaine hydrochloride (p.1381·2) is included in the intramuscular injection to alleviate the pain of injection.
*Neuralgia; neuritis; neuropathy; rheumatoid arthritis.*

**Lin-Amox** *Linson, Canad.*
Amoxicillin trihydrate (p.155·3).
*Bacterial infections.*

**Linapen** *Welfer, Mex.†.*
Ampicillin (p.157·1).
*Bacterial infections.*

**Linaris** *RAN, Ger.†.*
Co-trimoxazole (p.199·3).
*Bacterial infections.*

**Linatil**
*Gea, Fin.; Gea, Norw.; Gea, Swed.*
Enalapril maleate (p.909·2).
*Heart failure; hypertension.*

**Linatil Comp** *Gea, Fin.*
Enalapril maleate (p.909·2); hydrochlorothiazide (p.933·2).
*Hypertension.*

**Linazine** *Asian Pharm, Thai.*
Cinnarizine (p.428·3).
*Cerebrovascular disorders; migraine; motion sickness; peripheral vascular disorders; vestibular disorders.*

**Lincaina** *Braun, Port.*
Lidocaine hydrochloride (p.1377·3).
Adrenaline hydrochloride (p.852·3) is included in some injections as a vasoconstrictor to diminish absorption and localise the effect of the local anaesthetic.
*Local anaesthesia.*

**Lincil** *Almirall, Spain.*
Nicardipine hydrochloride (p.965·1).
*Angina pectoris; cerebrovascular disorders; hypertension.*

**Linco**
*Atlantic, Malaysia.*
Lincomycin hydrochloride (p.226·2).
*Gram-positive bacterial infections.*

*ANB, Thai.; General Drugs, Thai.*
Lincomycin (p.226·2).
*Gram-positive bacterial infections.*

**Lincocin**
*Pharmacia, Austral.; Pharmacia, Belg.; Pharmacia, Canad.; Pharmacia, Chile; IFET (ΙΦΕΤ), Gr.; Pharmacia, Hong Kong; Pharmacia Upjohn, Ital.; Pharmacia Upjohn, Mex.; Pharmacia, Neth.; Pharmacia, S.Afr.; Pharmacia, Singapore; Pharmacia, Spain; Pharmacia Upjohn, Swed.†; Pharmacia Upjohn, Switz.†; Pharmacia, Thai.; Upjohn, USA.*
Lincomycin hydrochloride (p.226·2).
*Bacterial infections.*

**Lincocina** *Pharmacia, Port.*
Lincomycin hydrochloride (p.226·2).
*Bacterial infections.*

**Lincocine** *Pharmacia, Fr.*
Lincomycin hydrochloride (p.226·2).
*Bacterial infections.*

**Lincoflan** *Bunker, Braz.*
Lincomycin hydrochloride (p.226·2).
*Bacterial infections.*

**Lincogin** *Samakeephaesaj, Thai.*
Lincomycin hydrochloride (p.226·2).
*Gram-positive bacterial infections.*

**Lincolan** *Olan-Kemed, Thai.*
Lincomycin hydrochloride (p.226·2).
*Gram-positive bacterial infections.*

**Lincomiral** *Ducto, Braz.*
Lincomycin hydrochloride (p.226·2).
*Bacterial infections.*

**Lincomy** *Nakorn, Thai.*
Lincomycin hydrochloride (p.226·2).
*Gram-positive bacterial infections.*

**Lincomyn** *Teuto, Braz.*
Lincomycin hydrochloride (p.226·2).
*Bacterial infections.*

**Lincono** *Milano, Thai.*
Lincomycin (p.226·2).
*Bacterial infections.*

**Linco-Ped** *Stiefel, Braz.†.*
Lincomycin (p.226·2).
*Bacterial infections.*

**Lincoplax** *Royton, Braz.*
Lincomycin hydrochloride (p.226·2).
*Bacterial infections.*

**Linco-Plus** *Cibran, Braz.†.*
Lincomycin hydrochloride (p.226·2).
*Bacterial infections.*

**Lincorex** *Hyrex, USA.*
Lincomycin hydrochloride (p.226·2).
*Bacterial infections.*

**Lincotax** *Luper, Braz.*
Lincomycin hydrochloride (p.226·2).
*Bacterial infections.*

**Linctifed** *GlaxoSmithKline, S.Afr.*
Triprolidine hydrochloride (p.442·3); pseudoephedrine hydrochloride (p.1129·2); codeine phosphate (p.27·1); guaifenesin (p.1122·1).
*Coughs.*

**Linctodyl** *Pharmaceutical Enterprises, S.Afr.*
Dextromethorphan hydrobromide (p.1117·3); ephedrine hydrochloride (p.1120·1); ammonium chloride (p.1115·2).
*Coughs.*

**Linctosan** *Garec, S.Afr.*
Diphenhydramine hydrochloride (p.431·3); ammonium chloride (p.1115·2); sodium citrate (p.1223·2); menthol (p.1711·3).
*Coughs.*

**Linctus Tussi Infans** *Propan, S.Afr.*
Ipecacuanha (p.1122·3); squill (p.1130·3); tolu (p.1131·3).
*Coughs.*

**Lindanoxil** *Dakota, Braz.†.*
*Ointment; topical liquid:* Lindane (p.1506·3).
*Pediculosis; scabies.*

*Soap:* Lindane (p.1506·3); hexachlorophene (p.1181·2).
*Skin disinfection.*

**Lindasol** *Kleva, Gr.*
Clindamycin phosphate (p.194·2).
*Acne.*

**Lindemil** *Abbott, Spain.*
Alum (p.1652·1); benzalkonium chloride (p.1168·3).
*Vaginal antiseptic; vulvovaginal trichomoniasis (adjuvant).*

**Lindigoa S** *Riemser, Ger.*
Aesculus (p.1648·2); troxerutin (p.1688·3).
*Haemorrhoids; thrombophlebitis; venous insufficiency.*

**Lindilane** *Grunenthal, Fr.*
Paracetamol (p.76·2); codeine phosphate (p.27·1).
*Pain.*

**Lindiol** *Organon, Arg.*
Lynestrenol (p.1557·1); ethinylestradiol (p.1553·2).
*Combined oral contraceptive.*

**Lindisc**
*Schering, Arg.; Berlimed, Braz.*
Estradiol (p.1550·1).
*Menopausal disorders; osteoporosis.*

**Lindisc Duo** *Berlimed, Braz.*
Patch 1, estradiol (p.1550·1); patch 2, estradiol; levonorgestrel (p.1563·2).

**Lindofluid N** *Lindopharm, Ger.*
Bornyl acetate (p.1662·2); α-pinene; arnica (p.1656·3); melissa (p.1711·1).
*Musculoskeletal, joint, and soft-tissue disorders.*

**Lindormin** *Boehringer Ingelheim, Mex.*
Brotizolam (p.672·1).
*Insomnia.*

**Lindotab** *Lindopharm, Ger.†.*
Tiaprofenic acid (p.93·3).
*Inflammation; musculoskeletal, joint, and soft-tissue disorders.*

**Lindoxyl** *Brahms, Ger.*
Ambroxol hydrochloride (p.1114·3).
*Respiratory-tract disorders associated with increased or viscous mucus.*

**Linea** *Valeas, Ital.†.*
Diethylpropion hydrochloride (p.1587·1).
*Obesity.*

**Linea F** *Angelini, Ital.*
Benzalkonium chloride (p.1168·3); benzydamine hydrochloride (p.21·1).
*Disinfection of wounds and burns.*

**Lineafarm** *Wyeth, Spain†.*
Nonoxinol 9 (p.1413·3).
*Contraceptive.*

**Linervidol** *Interdelta, Switz.*
Paracetamol (p.76·2); pyridoxine hydrochloride (p.1456·3); promethazine hydrochloride (p.439·1).
*Agitation; fever; pain.*

**Linfocilin** *Climax, Braz.*
Benzylpenicillin potassium (p.163·2); procaine benzylpenicillin (p.246·1).
*Bacterial infections.*

**Linfogex** *Climax, Braz.*
Vitamin B substances (p.1417·1).
*Vitamin B deficiency.*

**Linfoglobulina**
*Aventis Pasteur, Arg.; Aventis Pasteur, Chile; Imtix, Spain.*
Antilymphocyte immunoglobulin (horse) (p.1348·3).
*Aplastic anaemia; graft-versus-host disease; transplant rejection.*

**Linfol** *Omega, Arg.*
*Pessaries:* Metronidazole (p.607·2); nystatin (p.406·3); neomycin sulfate (p.235·1); dexamethasone (p.1097·1); lidocaine (p.1377·3).
*Vulvovaginal infections.*

*Tablets:* Metronidazole (p.607·2); nystatin (p.406·3).
*Anaerobic bacterial infections; protozoal infections.*

**Linfolysin** *Nuovo ISM, Ital.†.*
Chlorambucil (p.536·1).
*Chronic lymphoid leukaemia; Hodgkin's disease; lymphoma.*

**Lingo** *Siam Bheasach, Thai.*
Lincomycin hydrochloride (p.226·2).
*Gram-positive bacterial infections.*

**Lingopen** *Viofar, Gr.*
Propylene glycol cefatrizine (p.170·3).
*Bacterial infections.*

**Lingraine**
*Sanofi Winthrop, Irl.†; Sanofi Synthelabo, UK†.*
Ergotamine tartrate (p.467·2).
*Migraine and other vascular headaches.*

**Linibon** *G Gam, Fr.†.*
Veratrol; menthol (p.1711·3); salicylic acid (p.1157·1).
Formerly known as Lini-Bombe and contained veratrol, menthol, salicylic acid, and cloral hydrate.
*Musculoskeletal and joint disorders.*

**Liniderm** *Remexa, Mex.*
Almond oil (p.1651·1); calcium hydroxide (p.1664·3).
*Skin disorders.*

**Liniment Balm** *Greenridge, Austral.†.*
Sweet birch oil (p.60·1); menthol (p.1711·3).
*Musculoskeletal, joint, and soft-tissue pain.*

**Linimento de Sloan** *Warner-Lambert Consumer, Port.†.*
Turpentine oil (p.1760·1); capsicum oil; pine oil; camphor oil; methyl salicylate (p.59·3).
*Musculoskeletal pain.*

**Linimento Klari** *Clariana, Spain.*
Camphor (p.1665·3); amyl salicylate (p.14·3); rosemary oil (p.1740·2); sassafras oil (p.1742·1); turpentine oil (p.1760·1).
Formerly contained camphor, capsicum, amyl salicylate, rosemary oil, sassafras oil, and turpentine oil.
*Rheumatic and muscle pain.*

**Linimento Naion** *Puerto Galiano, Spain.*
Camphor (p.1665·3); alcohol (p.1166·1); salicylic acid (p.1157·1); turpentine; menthol (p.1711·3); soft soap (p.1575·2); capsicum (p.1667·1); methyl salicylate (p.59·3); rosemary (p.1740·2); lavender (p.1705·1).
*Rheumatic and muscle pain.*

**Linimento Sloan** *Warner-Lambert, Spain†.*
Ammonia (p.1653·3); capsicum (p.1667·1); methyl salicylate (p.59·3); oleum pini sylvestris; sassafras (p.1742·1); turpentine oil (p.1760·1); camphor (p.1665·3).
*Rheumatic and muscle pain.*

**Liniplant** *Spitzner, Ger.*
Eucalyptus oil (p.1686·2); cajuput oil (p.1664·1).
*Upper respiratory-tract disorders.*

**Linisol** *Braun, Belg.*
Lidocaine hydrochloride (p.1377·3).
*Local anaesthesia.*

**Linitul** *Bama, Spain.*
Peru balsam (p.1730·2); castor oil.
*Burns; wounds.*

**Linitul Antibiotico** *Bama, Spain†.*
Acexamic acid (p.1646·2); bacitracin (p.161·3); neomycin sulfate (p.235·1); polymyxin B sulfate (p.245·1).
*Burns; infected skin disorders; ulcers; wounds.*

**Link**
*Note. This name is used for preparations of different composition.*
*Alpharma, Denm.; Alpharma, Fin.; Alpharma, Norw.; Alpharma, Swed.*
Aluminium hydroxide-magnesium carbonate co-dried gel (p.1250·1).
*Dyspepsia; gastric hyperacidity; gastritis; heartburn; peptic ulcer.*

*Savio, Ital.*
Citicoline sodium (p.1672·3).
*Cerebrovascular disorders.*

**Links-Glaukosan** *Teclapharm, Ger.*
Adrenaline acid tartrate (p.852·2); adrenalone hydrochloride (p.1648·2).
*Glaucoma; inflammatory eye disorders.*

**Linmycin** *Vana, Thai.*
Lincomycin hydrochloride (p.226·2).
*Gram-positive bacterial infections.*

**Linna-Oil** *Knop, Chile.*
Linseed oil (p.1707·2).
*Essential fatty acid supplement.*

**Linobion-Globuli** *Linobion, Austria†.*
Fatty acids; cod-liver oil (p.1425·2); thymol (p.1194·2).
*Vaginal disorders.*

**Linobion-Heilsalbe** *Linobion, Austria†.*
Fatty acids.
*Skin disorders.*

**Linobion-Kapseln** *Linobion, Austria†.*
Fatty acids.
*Skin disorders.*

**Linobion-Salbenstift** *Linobion, Austria†.*
Fatty acids; thymol (p.1194·2).
*Skin disorders.*

**Linobion-Sulfonamid** *Linobion, Austria†.*
Fatty acids; sulfathiazole (p.264·1).
*Infected skin disorders.*

**Linobion-Zinksalbe** *Linobion, Austria†.*
Fatty acids; zinc oxide (p.1163·2).
*Skin disorders.*

**Linoforce** *Bioforce, Switz.*
Linseed (p.1707·2); senna (p.1288·2); frangula bark (p.1266·3).
*Constipation.*

**Linola**
*Wolff, Ger.; Medika, Switz.*
Linoleic acid (p.1690·2); 9,11-octadecadienoic acid.
*Skin disorders.*

**Linola gamma** *Wolff, Ger.*
Evening primrose oil (p.1686·3).
*Skin disorders.*

**Linola gras** *Medika, Switz.*
Linoleic acid (p.1690·2); 9,11-octadecadienoic acid; betacarotene (p.1422·3); colecalciferol (p.1461·3); tocoferil acetate (p.1465·1).
*Skin disorders.*

**Linola mi-gras** *Medika, Switz.*
Linoleic acid (p.1690·2); 9,11-octadecadienoic acid.
*Skin disorders.*

**Linola Urea**
*Wolff, Ger.; Medika, Switz.*
Urea (p.1162·2).
*Skin disorders.*

**Linoladiol**
*Note. This name is used for preparations of different composition.*
*Montavit, Austria.*
Estradiol (p.1550·1).
*Vaginal disorders.*

*Medika, Switz.*
Estradiol (p.1550·1); linoleic acid (p.1690·2); 9,11-octadecadienoic acid.
*Vulvovaginal disorders.*

**Linoladiol N** *Wolff, Ger.*
Estradiol (p.1550·1).
*Oestrogen deficiency; skin disorders; vaginal disorders.*

**Linoladiol-H N** *Wolff, Ger.*
Estradiol (p.1550·1); prednisolone (p.1108·1).
*Acne; ulcus cruris; vaginal disorders.*

**Linola-Fett**
*Note. This name is used for preparations of different composition.*
*Montavit, Austria.*
Fatty acids, betacarotene, and vitamin E (p.1417·1).
*Skin disorders.*

*Wolff, Ger.*
Linoleic acid (p.1690·2); 9,11-octadecadienoic acid.
*Skin disorders.*

**Linola-Fett 2000** *Wolff, Ger.*
Linoleic acid (p.1690·2).
*Skin disorders.*

**Linola-Fett-N Olbad** *Wolff, Ger.*
Bath additive; emollient.

**Linola-H N** *Wolff, Ger.*
Prednisolone (p.1108·1).
*Skin disorders.*

**Linola-H-compositum N** *Wolff, Ger.*
Prednisolone (p.1108·1); neomycin sulfate (p.235·1).
*Burns; infected skin disorders; skin ulcers.*

**Linola-H-Fett N** *Wolff, Ger.*
Prednisolone (p.1108·1).
*Skin disorders.*

**Linola-sept** *Wolff, Ger.*
Clioquinol (p.196·3).
*Infected skin disorders.*

**Linopril** *Klinger, Braz.†.*
Lisinopril (p.946·3).
*Hypertension.*

**Linoril** *Stadmed, India.*
Lisinopril (p.946·3).
*Heart failure; hypertension.*

**Linosun** *Silesia, Chile.*
Lynestrenol (p.1557·1).
*Progestogen only oral contraceptive.*

**Linotar**
*Trans Dermal, Austral.; Rolab, S.Afr.*
Coal tar (p.1159·2).
*Skin and scalp disorders.*

**Linox** *Unichem, India.*
Linezolid (p.226·3).
*Bacterial infections.*

**Linsal** *Sigma, Austral.*
Methyl salicylate (p.59·3).
*Rubefacient and topical analgesic.*

**L-Insulin** *Berlin-Chemie, Ger.†.*
Neutral insulin suspension (porcine) (p.333·3).
*Diabetes mellitus.*

**L-Insulin SNC** *Berlin-Chemie, Ger.†.*
Neutral insulin suspension (porcine) (p.333·3).
*Diabetes mellitus.*

**Lintia** *Protina, Ger.*
Salix (p.87·3).
*Fever; headache; rheumatic disorders.*

**Linurin** *Dovalle, Braz.*
Co-trimoxazole (p.199·3).
*Bacterial infections.*

**Linusit Creola** *Fink, Ger.†.*
Linseed (p.1707·2).
*Gastrointestinal disorders.*

**Linusit Darmaktiv Leinsamen** *Fink, Ger.†.*
Linseed (p.1707·2).
*Gastrointestinal disorders.*

**Linusit Gold** *Drogenhansa, Austria†.*
Linseed (p.1707·2).
*Gastrointestinal disorders.*

**Linvas** *Cadila Pharma, India.*
Lisinopril (p.946·3).
*Heart failure; hypertension.*

**Linvite** *Linton, S.Afr.†.*
Multivitamin and mineral preparation (p.1417·1).

**Liobifar** *Italfarmaco, Ital.*
Lactic acid producing organisms; vitamin B substances (p.1417·1).

**Liocarpina** *SIFI, Ital.†.*
Pilocarpine hydrochloride (p.1495·1).
*Glaucoma; ocular hypertension.*

**Liofindol** *ICN, Mex.†.*
Mazindol (p.1589·1).

**Liogynon** *Schering, Austria†.*
Levonorgestrel (p.1563·2); ethinylestradiol (p.1553·2).
*Triphasic oral contraceptive.*

**Lio-Levedura** *Vitoria, Port.*
*Saccharomyces cerevisiae* (p.1469·1).

**Liomagen** *Chrispa (Χρισπα), Gr.*
Trimetazidine (p.1018·1).
*Angina.*

**Liometacen**
*Gerot, Austria; Promedica, Ital.; Chiesi, Thai.†.*
Meglumine indometacin (p.48·3).
*Gout; musculoskeletal, joint, and peri-articular disorders; pain; renal and biliary colic; thrombophlebitis.*

**Lio-Morbillo** *Nuovo ISM, Ital.†.*
A measles vaccine (Schwarz strain) (p.1623·1).
*Active immunisation.*

**Lion** *Filaxis, Arg.*
Stavudine (p.654·2).
*Viral infections.*

**Lion Cleansing Herbs** *Potter's, UK.*
Buckthorn (p.1254·1); psyllium seed (p.1268·1); senna (p.1288·2); sambucus (p.1741·3); fennel (p.1687·2); maté (p.1765·3).
*Constipation.*

**Lioram** *Schering-Plough, Braz.*
Zolpidem tartrate (p.728·3).
*Insomnia.*

**Lioresal**
*Novartis, Arg.; Novartis, Austral.; Novartis, Austria; Novartis, Belg.; Novartis, Braz.; Novartis, Canad.; Novartis, Denm.; Novartis, Fin.; Novartis, Fr.; Novartis, Ger.; Novartis, Hong Kong; Novartis, India; Novartis, Irl.; Novartis, Israel; Novartis, Ital.; Novartis, Malaysia; Novartis, Neth.; Novartis, Norw.; Novartis, NZ†; Novartis, Port.; Novartis, S.Afr.; Novartis, Singapore; Novartis, Spain; Novartis, Swed.; Novartis, Switz.; Novartis, Thai.; Novartis, UK; Geigy, USA.*
Baclofen (p.1386·3).
*Skeletal muscle spasm or spasticity.*

**Lioresyl** *Novartis, Chile.*
Baclofen (p.1386·3).
*Skeletal muscle spasm or spasticity.*

**Liosiero** *Nuovo ISM, Ital.†.*
A botulism antitoxin (types A, B, and E) (p.1610·3).
*Botulism.*

**Liotec** *Technilab, Canad.*
Baclofen (p.1386·3).

**Lioton**
*Menarini, Hong Kong; Sanofi Synthelabo, Ital.; Menarini, Switz.*
Heparin sodium (p.928·1).
*Peripheral vascular disorders; soft-tissue disorders.*

**Liotrex** *Raffo, Chile.*
Sumatriptan succinate (p.471·2).
*Migraine.*

**Liotropina** *SIFI, Ital.†.*
Atropine sulfate (p.477·1).
*Eye disorders.*

**Liozim** *Farmanova, Ital.*
Fructose (p.1431·3); acacia honey (p.1434·2); lactic-acid-producing organisms (p.1704·2).
*Nutritional supplement.*

**Lip Block Sunscreen** *Norwood, Canad.*
*SPF 15:* Octinoxate (p.1154·3); oxybenzone (p.1154·3); titanium dioxide (p.1160·3).
*Sunscreen.*

**Lip Medex**
*Note. This name is used for preparations of different composition.*
*Blistex, Canad.*
Camphor (p.1665·3); phenol (p.1188·1); menthol (p.1711·3).
*Dry, cracked lips; herpes labialis.*

*Blistex, USA.*
Camphor (p.1665·3); phenol (p.1188·1).
*Oral lesions.*

**Lip Tone**
*Note. This name is used for preparations of different composition.*
*Rider, Chile.*
*SPF 15:* Octinoxate (p.1154·3); oxybenzone (p.1154·3).
*Sunscreen.*

*Blistex, USA.*
*SPF 15:* Octinoxate (p.1154·3); meradimate (p.1151·3).
*Sunscreen.*

**Lip Treatment** *Shaklee, Canad.*
*SPF 15:* Octinoxate (p.1154·3); oxybenzone (p.1154·3).
*Sunscreen.*

**Lipactin**
*Novartis Consumer, Canad.; Widmer, Ger.; Widmer, Switz.*
Heparin sodium (p.928·1); zinc sulfate (p.1469·3).
*Herpes labialis.*

**Lipanon** *Allergan-Frumtost, Braz.†.*
Fenofibrate (p.915·2).
*Hyperlipidaemias.*

**Lipanor**
*Sanofi Synthelabo, Fr.; CTI, Israel; Sanofi Synthelabo, Port.*
Ciprofibrate (p.884·2).
*Hyperlipidaemias.*

**Lipanthyl**
*Fournier, Belg.; Fournier, Fr.; Fournier, Ger.; Fournier, Gr.; Fournier, Hong Kong; Formenti, Ital.; Fournier, Malaysia; Fournier, Port.; Fournier, Singapore; Selena, Swed.; Fournier, Switz.; Fournier, Thai.*
Fenofibrate (p.915·2).
*Hyperlipidaemias.*

**Lipantil**
*Fournier, Irl.; Fournier, UK.*
Fenofibrate (p.915·2).
*Hyperlipidaemias.*

**Liparison** *Novartis, Spain.*
Fenofibrate (p.915·2).
*Hyperlipidaemias.*

**Liparol** *Ashbourne, UK†.*
Bezafibrate (p.873·2).
*Hyperlipidaemias.*

**Lipaten** *Merck, S.Afr.†.*
Clofibrate (p.884·3); nicotinyl alcohol tartrate (p.966·2).
*Hyperlipidaemias.*

**Lipaxan** *Italfarmaco, Ital.*
Fluvastatin sodium (p.918·2).
*Hypercholesterolaemia.*

**Lipaz** *Baldacci, Port.*
Simvastatin (p.997·1).
*Hyperlipidaemias.*

**Lipazil** *Douglas, Austral.*
Gemfibrozil (p.923·1).
*Hyperlipdaemias.*

**Lipazym** *Bittermedizin, Ger.*
Pancreatin (p.1725·3).
*Pancreatic insufficiency.*

**Lipbalm with Sunscreen** *Hyde, Canad.*
Padimate O (p.1155·1).
*Sunscreen.*

**Lipcor**
*Note. This name is used for preparations of different composition.*
*Nycomed, Austria.*
Fenofibrate (p.915·2).
*Hyperlipidaemias.*

*Pharmacia, Braz.*
Eicosapentaenoic acid (p.976·2); docosahexaenoic acid (p.976·1).
*Hyperlipidaemias; nutritional supplement.*

**Lipcut** *Gea, Fin.*
Simvastatin (p.997·1).
*Atherosclerosis; hypercholesterolaemia.*

**Lipdaune** *Sofex, Port.*
Lovastatin (p.949·1).
*Hypercholesterolaemia.*

**Lipei** *Steiner, Ger.*
Cynara (p.1678·3).
*Dyspepsia.*

**Lipemol** *Squibb, Spain.*
Pravastatin sodium (p.984·3).
*Hypercholesterolaemia.*

**Lipenan** *Klinger, Braz.*
Poliglusam.
*Obesity.*

**Liperol** *Spirig, Fr.*
Urea (p.1162·2); piroctone olamine (p.1155·2).
*Scalp disorders.*

**Lipex**
*Note. This name is used for preparations of different composition.*
*Elea, Arg.*
Policosanol (p.984·2).
*Hypercholesterolaemia.*

*Amrad, Austral.; Merck Sharp & Dohme, NZ.*
Simvastatin (p.997·1).
*Coronary atherosclerosis; hyperlipidaemias.*

**Lip-Eze** *SmithKline Beecham Consumer, Austral.†.*
*SPF 15+:* Octinoxate (p.1154·3); avobenzone (p.1142·3).
*Dry, cracked, and chapped lips; sunscreen.*

**Lipibec** *Armstrong, Arg.*
Atorvastatin calcium (p.866·1).
*Hypercholesterolaemia.*

**Lipicard** *USV, India.*
Fenofibrate (p.915·2).
*Hyperlipidaemias.*

**Lipidal** *Bristol-Myers Squibb, Israel.*
Pravastatin sodium (p.984·3).
*Hypercholesterolaemia.*

**Lipidavit** *Rodisma, Ger.*
Garlic (p.1691·1); alpha tocoferil acetate (p.1465·1); lecithin (p.1706·1).
*Hyperlipidaemias.*

**Lipidax** *UCB, Ital.†.*
Fenofibrate (p.915·2).
*Hyperlipidaemias.*

**Lipidem** *Braun, Switz.†.*
Soya oil (p.1447·2).
Contains egg lecithin.
*Lipid infusion for parenteral nutrition.*

**Lipiderm** *Chauvin, Fr.*
Moisturiser.
*Dry skin disorders.*

**Lipidil**
*Craveri, Arg.; Allergan-Frumtost, Braz.†; Fournier, Canad.; Andromaco, Chile; Fournier, Ger.; Fournier, Gr.; Schering-Plough, Mex.*
Fenofibrate (p.915·2).
*Hyperlipidaemias.*

**Lipidless** *Faran, Gr.*
Lovastatin (p.949·1).
*Primary hypercholesterolaemia.*

**Lipidos** *Abbott, Arg.*
Cartamo oil (p.1443·3).
Contains egg phospholipids.
*Lipid infusion for parenteral nutrition.*

**Lipidys** *Medifive, Thai.*
Gemfibrozil (p.923·1).
*Hyperlipidaemias.*

**Lipifen** *Raffo, Arg.*
Atorvastatin (p.866·2).
*Hyperlipidaemias.*

**Lipikar**
*Roche-Posay, Arg.; Roche-Posay, Braz.; Roche-Posay, Irl.*
Emollient.
*Dry skin; psoriasis.*

**Lipilim** *Atlantic, Hong Kong.*
Clofibrate (p.884·3).
*Hyperlipidaemias.*

**Lipiodol**
*Temis, Arg.; Aspen, Austral.; Guerbet, Austria; Codali, Belg.; Guerbet, Braz.†; Rider, Chile; Guerbet, Denm.; Guerbet, Fr.; Guerbet, Ger.; R+N, Gr.; Guerbet, Israel; Guerbet, Ital.; Guerbet, Neth.†; Guerbet, Norw.; Biotek, NZ; Guerbet, Port.; May & Baker, UK.*
Iodised oil (p.1063·2).
*Radiographic contrast medium.*

**Lipirex** *Irex, Fr.*
Fenofibrate (p.915·2).
*Hyperlipidaemias.*

**Lipiscor** *Sanum-Kehlbeck, Ger.*
Marine fish oil (p.976·2).
*Hyperlipidaemias.*

**Lipison**
*Unison, Hong Kong; Unison, Singapore; Unison, Thai.*
Gemfibrozil (p.923·1).
*Hyperlipidaemias.*

**Lipisorb**
*Mead Johnson, Austral.; Mead Johnson Nutritionals, Canad.†; Mead Johnson Nutritionals, Thai.†; Mead Johnson Nutritionals, USA.*
Food for special diets (p.1417·1).
*Fat malabsorption.*

**Lipistorol**
*Hovid, Hong Kong; Hovid, Malaysia.*
Gemfibrozil (p.923·1).
*Hyperlipidaemias.*

**Lipitor**
*Parke, Davis, Arg.; Pfizer, Austral.; Pfizer, Belg.; Pfizer, Braz.; Pfizer, Canad.; Parke, Davis, Chile; Pfizer, Fin.; Pfizer, Gr.; Pfizer, Hong Kong; Pfizer, Irl.; Parke, Davis, Israel; Warner-Lambert, Ital.; Pfizer, Malaysia; Parke, Davis, Mex.; Parke, Davis, Neth.; Pfizer, Norw.; Pfizer, NZ; Pfizer, S.Afr.; Pfizer, Singapore; Pfizer, Swed.; Pfizer, Thai.; Pfizer, UK; Parke, Davis, USA; Pfizer, USA.*
Atorvastatin calcium (p.866·1).
*Atherosclerosis; hypercholesterolaemia.*

**Lipitrol** *Julphar, UAE.*
Bezafibrate (p.873·2).
*Hyperlipidaemias.*

**Lipivas** *Merck Sharp & Dohme, Denm.†.*
Lovastatin (p.949·1).
*Hypercholesterolaemia.*

**Liplat** *Esteve, Spain.*
Pravastatin sodium (p.984·3).
*Hypercholesterolaemia.*

**Liple** *Mitsubishi, Jpn.*
Alprostadil (p.1512·3).
*Maintenance of patent ductus arteriosus; mesenteric arterial portography; peripheral vascular disorders; skin ulcers.*

**Lipmagik** *Reese, USA.*
Benzocaine (p.1370·3); phenol (p.1188·1); alcohol (p.1166·1).

**Lipo Cordes** *Ichthyol, Ger.*
Allantoin (p.1141·3); dexpanthenol (p.1727·2); ethyl linoleate.
*Skin disorders.*

**Lipo Sol** *Widmer, Switz.*
Triclosan (p.1195·2).
*Acne; seborrhoea.*

**Lipoabsorver** *Neves, Port.*
Poliglusam; vitamin C.
*Hypercholesterolaemia; slimming aid.*

**Lipobalsamo** *Teofarma, Ital.*
Cineole (p.1672·1); guaiacol (p.1122·1).
*Respiratory-tract disorders.*

**Lipobase**
*Yamanouchi, Irl.; CSL, NZ; Yamanouchi, NZ; Yamanouchi, UK.*
Emollient.
*Diluent for Locoid Lipocream; dry skin; pruritus.*

**Lipobay**
*Bayer, Austral.†; Bayer, Austria†; Bayer, Belg.†; Bayer, Braz.†; Bayer, Denm.†; Bayer, Fin.†; Bayer, Ger.†; Bayer, Irl.†; Bayer, Ital.†; Bayer, Neth.†; Bayer, Norw.†; Bayer, Port.†; Bayer, Singapore†; Bayer, Spain†; Bayer, Swed.†; Bayer, Switz.†; Bayer, Thai.†; Bayer, UK†.*
Cerivastatin sodium (p.881·3).
*Hypercholesterolaemia.*

**Lipocal** *Remexa, Mex.†.*
Calcium hydroxide (p.1664·3).

**Lipocambi** *Microsules Bernabo, Arg.*
Atorvastatin calcium (p.866·1).
*Hypercholesterolaemia.*

**Lipochol**
*Note. This name is used for preparations of different composition.*
*Takeda, Hong Kong.*
Orotic acid (p.1724·3); thioctic acid amide (p.1754·3); turmeric (p.1058·3); methionine (p.1042·1); vitamin B substances; vitamin C (p.1417·1); inositol (p.1701·2).
*Liver disorders.*

*Takeda, Thai.*
Orotic acid (p.1724·3); thioctic acid amide (p.1754·3); methionine (p.1042·1); vitamin B substances; vitamin C (p.1417·1); inositol (p.1701·2).
*Liver disorders.*

**Lipociden** *Vita, Spain.*
Simvastatin (p.997·1).
*Hyperlipidaemias; secondary prophylaxis of ischaemic heart disease.*

**Lipocin** *Kener, Mex.*
Bezafibrate (p.873·2).
*Hypercholesterolaemia.*

**Lipoclar** *Crinos, Ital.*†.
Fenofibrate (p.915·2).
*Hyperlipidaemias.*

**Lipoclin** *Sumitomo, Jpn.*
Clinofibrate (p.884·3).
*Hyperlipidaemias.*

**Lipocol** *Merz, Ger.*
Colestyramine (p.889·3).
*Hypercholesterolaemia.*

**Lipodel** *Synthelabo, Ital.*†.
Pantethine (p.978·3).
*Lipid disorders.*

**Lipoenergy** *Farma Energy, Ital.*
Choline; inositol; methionine; carnitine; vitamin $B_6$ (p.1417·1).
*Nutritional supplement.*

**Lipofacton** *Organon, Braz.*
Clofibrate (p.884·3); nicotinyl alcohol tartrate (p.966·2).
*Hyperlipidaemias.*

**Lipofen** *Vitoria, Port.*
Fenofibrate (p.915·2).
*Hyperlipidaemias.*

**Lipofene** *Teofarma, Ital.*
Fenofibrate (p.915·2).
*Hyperlipidaemias.*

**Lipoflavonoid** *Numark, USA.*
Multivitamin preparation with lemon bioflavonoids (p.1688·2)(p.1417·1).

**Lipofor**
*Remedica, Hong Kong; Remedica, Malaysia; Remedica, Singapore.*
Gemfibrozil (p.923·1).
*Hyperlipidaemias.*

**Lipoforte** *Neves, Port.*
Poliglusam; ascorbic acid (p.1460·2); green tea (p.1765·3).
*Obesity.*

**Lipofren** *Abello, Spain.*
Lovastatin (p.949·1).
*Atherosclerosis; hypercholesterolaemia.*

**Lipofundin**
*Braun, Austria; Braun, Chile; Braun, Denm.*†*; Braun, UK.*
Soya oil (p.1447·2).
*Lipid infusion for parenteral nutrition.*

**Lipofundin MCT**
*Braun, Ger.; Braun, Ital.; Braun, Switz.*
Soya oil (p.1447·2); medium-chain triglycerides (p.1440·3).
Contains egg phospholipids.
*Lipid infusion for parenteral nutrition.*

**Lipofundin MCT/LCT**
*Braun, Arg.; Braun, Chile; Bioser (Βιοσερ), Gr.; Braun, Hong Kong; Braun, Israel; Braun, S.Afr.; Braun, Singapore; Braun, Thai.; Braun, UK.*
Soya oil (p.1447·2); medium-chain triglycerides (p.1440·3).
Contains egg lecithin or egg phospholipids.
*Lipid infusion for parenteral nutrition.*

**Lipofundin MCT/LCT-E** *Braun, Arg.*
Soya oil (p.1447·2); medium-chain triglycerides (p.1440·3); alpha-tocopherol (p.1464·3).
Contains egg lecithin.
*Lipid infusion for parenteral nutrition.*

**Lipofundin mit MCT** *Braun, Austria.*
Soya oil (p.1447·2); medium-chain triglycerides (p.1440·3).
Contains egg phospholipid.
*Lipid infusion for parenteral nutrition.*

**Lipofundin N**
*Braun, Arg.; Braun, Ger.; Braun, Hong Kong.*
Soya oil (p.1447·2).
Contains egg lecithin or egg phospholipid.
*Lipid infusion for parenteral nutrition.*

**Lipofundin S**
*Braun, Braz.*†*; Braun, Irl.*†*; Braun, Ital.; Braun, Thai.*
Soya oil (p.1447·2).
*Lipid infusion for parenteral nutrition.*

**Lipofundina MCT/LCT**
*Braun, Port.; Braun, Spain.*
Soya oil (p.1447·2); medium-chain triglycerides (p.1440·3).
Contains egg lecithin.
*Lipid infusion for parenteral nutrition.*

**Lipogen**
*Note. This name is used for preparations of different composition.*
*Biores, Ital.*
Gemfibrozil (p.923·1).
*Hyperlipidaemias.*

*Goldline, USA.*
Vitamin B substances (p.1417·1).
It may also contain vitamin C.

**Lipogis** *Agis, Israel*†.
Cerivastatin sodium (p.881·3).
*Hypercholesterolaemia.*

**Lipograsil** *Uriach, Spain.*
Cynara (p.1678·3); cascara (p.1255·1); bladderwrack (p.1742·3).
Formerly contained cynara, cascara, phenolphthalein, and bladderwrack.
*Obesity.*

**Lipoicin**
*Takeda, Hong Kong*†*; Takeda, Thai.*
Thioctic acid (p.1754·3).
*Liver disorders.*

**Lipoite** *Helfarma, Port.*
Gemfibrozil (p.923·1).
*Hyperlipidaemias.*

**Lipolan** *Orion, Fin.*
Emollient.
*Dry skin disorders.*

**Lipolest** *Ardern, UK*†.
Ispaghula (p.1268·1); guar gum (p.333·2).
*Hypercholesterolaemia.*

**Lipoleum** *SFD, Port.*
Emollient.
*Barrier preparation; skin disorders.*

**Lipolo** *Macrophar, Thai.*
Gemfibrozil (p.923·1).
*Hyperlipidaemias.*

**Lipolotion** *Pacific Biosciences, Singapore; Spirig, Singapore.*
Emollient and moisturiser.
*Dry skin disorders.*

**Lipomax** *Makros, Braz.*†.
Fenproporex hydrochloride (p.1588·3).
*Obesity.*

**Lipomega** *Nutri-Well, Hong Kong.*
Omega-3 marine triglycerides (p.976·2).
*Hypercholesterolaemia.*

**Lipo-Merz**
*Kolassa, Austria; Grunenthal, Chile; Merz, Ger.; Merz, Hong Kong; Merz, Malaysia; Medinfar, Port.; Merz, Singapore; Merz, Switz.*
Etofibrate (p.914·2).
*Hyperlipidaemias.*

**Lipomul** *Roberts, USA.*
High calorie preparation containing maize oil for enteral nutrition (p.1417·1)(p.1439·2).

**Liponet** *Vedim, Spain.*
Pantethine (p.978·3).
*Hyperlipidaemias.*

**Liponol** *Rugby, USA.*
Vitamin B substances with methionine (p.1417·1).

**Liponorm**
*Note. This name is used for preparations of different composition.*
*Lazar, Arg.*
Atorvastatin calcium (p.866·1).
*Hypercholesterolaemia.*

*Gentili, Ital.*
Simvastatin (p.997·1).
*Atherosclerosis; hypercholesterolaemia.*

**Lipopharm** *Spreewald, Ger.*
Soya phospholipid (p.1447·2).
*Hypercholesterolaemia.*

**Lipoplasmin** *Elvetium, Arg.*
Fenofibrate (p.915·2).
*Hyperlipidaemias.*

**Liporex** *Genepharm, Gr.*
Simvastatin (p.997·1).
*Primary hypercholesterolaemia.*

**Liporon** *General Drugs, Thai.*
Choline bitartrate (p.1424·3); inositol (p.1701·2); methionine (p.1042·1); vitamin B substances (p.1417·1).
*Liver disorders.*

**Liposcler** *CEPA, Spain.*
Lovastatin (p.949·1).
*Atherosclerosis; hypercholesterolaemia.*

**Liposel** *Wassen, Ital.*
Vitamin A; vitamin C; vitamin E; selenium; lipoic acid; astaxanthin (p.1417·1).
*Nutritional supplement.*

**Liposic**
*Bausch & Lomb, Arg.; Chauvin, Fr.; Mann, Ger.; Mann, Irl.; Bausch & Lomb, UK.*
Carbomer 980 (p.1577·2).
*Dry eyes.*

**Liposit** *Merz, Ger.*†.
Sitosterol (p.982·3).
*Hyperlipidaemias.*

**Liposom** *Fidia, Ital.*
Hypothalamic phospholipids (p.1709·3).
*Neuroendocrine disorders.*

**Liposperse** *Summit, Port.*†.
Vegetable lipids.
*Adjunct in cholecystography.*

**Lipostabil**
*Note. This name is used for preparations of different composition.*
*Nattermann, Ger.*
Essential phospholipids.
*Lipid disorders.*

*Rhone-Poulenc Rorer, Hong Kong*†.
Essential phospholipids; vitamins (p.1417·1); theophylline (p.798·3).
*Hyperlipidaemias; thromboembolic disorders; vascular disorders.*

*Aventis, Ital.*
Phosphatidyl choline (p.1731·1).
*Fat emboli; hyperlipidaemias.*

*Aventis, S.Afr.*
*Capsules*†: Essential phospholipids; multivitamins (p.1417·1); theophylline (p.798·3).
*Injection:* Essential phospholipids; multivitamins (p.1417·1); adenosine phosphate (p.1647·3).
*Atherosclerosis; diabetic angiopathies; hyperlipidaemias; thromboembolism prophylaxis.*

**Lipostat**
*Bristol-Myers Squibb, Irl.; Bristol-Myers Squibb, Israel*†*; Bristol-Myers Squibb, NZ; Bristol-Myers Squibb, UK.*
Pravastatin sodium (p.984·3).
*Atherosclerosis; hypercholesterolaemia; myocardial infarction.*

**Liposterol**
*Bayer, Austria*†*; Vita, Spain*†.
Cerivastatin sodium (p.881·3).
*Hypercholesterolaemia.*

**Lipostop** *Francia, Ital.*†.
A heparinoid (p.931·1).
*Thrombosis prophylaxis.*

**Liposyn**
*Abbott, Chile; Abbott, Denm.; Abbott, Fin.; Abbott, Israel; Abbott, Ital.; Abbott, Mex.; Abbott, Swed.*
Fractionated safflower oil (p.1443·3); fractionated soya oil (p.1447·2).
Contains fractionated egg lecithin or egg phospholipids.
*Lipid infusion for parenteral nutrition.*

**Liposyn II** *Abbott, USA.*
Safflower oil (p.1443·3); soya oil (p.1447·2).
Contains egg phospholipids.
*Lipid infusion for parenteral nutrition.*

**Liposyn III** *Abbott, USA.*
Soya oil (p.1447·2).
Contains egg phospholipids.
*Lipid infusion for parenteral nutrition.*

**Lipotalon** *Merckle, Ger.*
Dexamethasone palmitate (p.1097·3).
*Rheumatic disorders.*

**Lipoton** *Basi, Port.*
Choline; inositol; methionine (p.1417·1).

**Lipotop** *Spirig, Fr.*
A range of skin care and barrier preparations.

**Lipotrend Cholesterol** *Roche Diagnostics, Ital.*
Test for cholesterol in blood.

**Lipotriad** *Numark, USA.*
Multivitamin and mineral preparation (p.1417·1).

**Lipotril** *Instituto Sanitas, Chile.*
Gemfibrozil (p.923·1).
*Hyperlipidaemias.*

**Lipotropic** *Drugtech, Chile.*
Atorvastatin (p.866·2).
*Hypercholesterolaemia.*

**Lipotropic Factors** *Solgar, UK.*
Choline bitartrate (p.1424·3); inositol (p.1701·2); methionine (p.1042·1).
*Dietary supplement.*

**Lipovastinklonal** *Klonal, Arg.*
Atorvastatin (p.866·2).
*Hyperlipidaemias.*

**Lipoven** *Fresenius Kabi, Fr.*†.
Soya oil (p.1447·2).
Contains egg lecithin.
*Lipid infusion for parenteral nutrition.*

**Lipovenoes**
*Fresenius, Belg.*†*; Bioser (Βιοσερ), Gr.; Fresenius Kabi, Mex.; Fresenius Kabi, Port.; Fresenius Kabi, S.Afr.*†*; Fresenius Kabi, Thai.*
Soya oil (p.1447·2).
Contains egg lecithin or egg phospholipids.
*Lipid infusion for parenteral nutrition.*

**Lipovenoes MCT** *Fresenius Kabi, Mex.*
Soya oil (p.1447·2); medium-chain triglycerides (p.1440·3).
Contains egg lecithin.
*Lipid infusion for parenteral nutrition.*

**Lipovenos**
*Roux-Ocefa, Arg.; Fresenius Kabi, Austria; Fresenius, Braz.*†*; Fresenius Kabi, Denm.*†*; Fresenius Kabi, Ger.; Fresenius Kabi, Ital.; Fresenius Kabi, Norw.*†*; Fresenius Kabi, Spain; Fresenius Kabi, Swed.; Fresenius Kabi, Switz.; Fresenius Kabi, UK*†.
Fractionated soya oil (p.1447·2).
Contains egg lecithin or egg phospholipids.
*Lipid infusion for parenteral nutrition.*

**Lipovenos MCT** *Fresenius Kabi, Ger.*
Soya oil (p.1447·2); medium-chain triglycerides (p.1440·3).
Contains egg phospholipid.
*Lipid infusion for parenteral nutrition.*

**Lipovit** *Brunel, S.Afr.*†.
Multivitamin preparation (p.1417·1).

**Lipovitan** *Medphano, Ger.*
Choline bitartrate (p.1424·3); dexpanthenol (p.1727·2); myo-inositol (p.1701·2); methionine (p.1042·1); vitamin B substances (p.1417·1); alpha tocoferil acetate (p.1465·1).
*Liver disorders.*

**Lipovitasi-Or** *Atlantis, Mex.*
Carnitine orotate (p.1724·3); thiamine nitrate (p.1455·1); DL-methionine (p.1042·1).
*Liver disorders.*

**Lipox**
*Note. This name is used for preparations of different composition.*
*Laboratorios Chile, Chile.*
Atorvastatin (p.866·2).
*Hypercholesterolaemia.*

*TAD, Ger.*
Bezafibrate (p.873·2).
*Hyperlipidaemias.*

**Lipozid** *Monsanto, Ital.*
Gemfibrozil (p.923·1).
*Hyperlipidaemias.*

**Lipozil** *M & H, Thai.*
Gemfibrozil (p.923·1).
*Hyperlipidaemias.*

**Liprace** *Douglas, Austral.*
Lisinopril (p.946·3).

**Lipraken** *Kener, Mex.*
Enalapril (p.909·2).
*Hypertension.*

**Lipram** *Global, USA.*
Pancrelipase (p.1725·3).
*Pancreatic insufficiency.*

**Lipreren** *Labomed, Chile.*
Lisinopril (p.946·3).
*Heart failure; hypertension.*

**Liprevil** *Schwarz, Ger.*†*; Sanol, Ger.*†.
Pravastatin sodium (p.984·3).
*Hyperlipidaemias.*

**Lipril**
*Lupin, India; Merck, Port.*
Lisinopril (p.946·3).
*Heart failure; hypertension.*

**Liprocil** *Nestle, Fr.*
Medium-chain triglycerides (p.1440·3); vitamins (p.1417·1).
*Nutritional supplement.*

**Lip-Sed**
*Parke, Davis, Austral.*†*; Pfizer, NZ.*
Avobenzone (p.1142·3); octinoxate (p.1154·3); oxybenzone (p.1154·3).
*Sunscreen.*

**Lipshield Lipbalm** *Mentholatum, Canad.*
*SPF 21:* Padimate O (p.1155·1); octinoxate (p.1154·3); oxybenzone (p.1154·3).
*Sunscreen.*

**Lipsin**
*Nycomed, Austria; Caber, Ital.; Aventis, S.Afr.*
Fenofibrate (p.915·2).
*Hyperlipidaemias.*

**Lipsorex** *Canderm, Canad.*
Benzethonium chloride (p.1169·2); menthol (p.1711·3); thymol (p.1194·2).

**Lipur** *Pfizer, Fr.*
Gemfibrozil (p.923·1).
*Hyperlipidaemias.*

**Lipus** *BA Farma, Port.*
Lovastatin (p.949·1).
*Hypercholesterolaemia.*

**Liqiprin** *SmithKline Beecham, Israel*†.
Paracetamol (p.76·2).
*Fever; pain.*

**Liquemin**
*Roche, Austria.*
Heparin (p.927·3).
*Thromboembolic disorders.*

*Roche, Ital.*
Heparin sodium (p.928·1).
*Thromboembolic disorders.*

**Liquemin N** *Roche, Ger.*
Heparin sodium (p.928·1).
*Thromboembolic disorders.*

**Liquemine**
*Roche, Belg.; Roche, Braz.; Roche, Switz.*
Heparin sodium (p.928·1).
*Hyperlipidaemias; thromboembolic disorders.*

**Liqufruta Garlic Cough Medicine** *Pfizer Consumer, UK.*
Garlic oil (p.1691·2); guaifenesin (p.1122·1).
*Coughs.*

**LiquiBand** *Medlogic, UK.*
Enbucrilate (p.1678·1).
*Tissue adhesive for wound closure.*

**Liquibid** *Capellon, USA.*
Guaifenesin (p.1122·1).

**Liquibid-D** *Capellon, USA.*
Guaifenesin (p.1122·1); phenylephrine hydrochloride (p.1126·3).
*Upper respiratory-tract symptoms.*

**Liquibid-PD** *Capellon, USA.*
Phenylephrine hydrochloride (p.1126·3); guaifenesin (p.1122·1).
*Upper respiratory-tract disorders.*

**Liquicard** *Duopharm, Ger.*†.
Crataegus (p.1677·1).
*Circulatory disorders; heart failure.*

**Liqui-Char**
*Oxford Pharmaceuticals, UK*†*; Jones, USA.*
Activated charcoal (p.1030·2).
*Emergency treatment of poisoning.*

**Liquid Antacid** *Pennex, Israel.*
Magnesium hydroxide (p.1272·2); aluminium hydroxide (p.1249·2).
*Gastrointestinal hyperacidity; heartburn.*

**Liquid Antacid Plus Simethicon** *Pennex, Israel.*
Magnesium hydroxide (p.1272·2); aluminium hydroxide (p.1249·2); simeticone (p.1289·2).
*Flatulence; gastrointestinal hyperacidity; heartburn.*

**Liquid B Complex** *Jamieson, Canad.*†.
Vitamin B substances (p.1417·1).

**Liquid Pred** *Muro, USA.*
Prednisone (p.1109·3).
*Corticosteroid.*

**Liquid Soap Pre-Op**
*Orion, Austral.; Orion, NZ.*
Triclosan (p.1195·2).
*Skin cleansing.*

**Liquidepur** *Woelm, Ger.*
Senna (p.1288·2).
*Constipation.*

**Liquido de Dakin** *Granado, Braz.*
Sodium hypochlorite (p.1192·1).
*Disinfection.*

**Liquidorm N** *Hanosan, Ger.*
Homoeopathic preparation.

**Liqui-Doss** *Ferndale, USA.*
Liquid paraffin (p.1479·1).
*Constipation.*

**Liquifer**
*Note. This name is used for preparations of different composition.*
*Abbott, Austria; Abbott, Ital.; Abbott, Switz.†.*
Ferrous polystyrene sulfonate (p.1436·1).
Ascorbic acid (p.1460·2) or sodium ascorbate (p.1460·2) is included in this preparation to increase the absorption and availability of iron.
*Iron-deficiency anaemias.*

*Abbott, Neth.*
Ferrous sulfate (p.1428·2).
*Iron-deficiency anaemia.*

**Liquifilm**
*Allergan, Austral.; Allergan, Austria†; Allergan, Belg.; Allergan, Canad.; Allergan, Fin.; Allergan, Fr.†; Allergan, Ger.; Allergan, Hong Kong; Allergan, Irl.; Allergan, Malaysia; Allergan, NZ; Allergan, Port.; Allergan, Switz.; Allergan, USA.*
Polyvinyl alcohol (p.1581·1) (p.1164·2).
*Dry eyes; eye irritation; wetting solution for hard contact lenses.*

**Liquifilm Lagrimas**
*Allergan, Arg.; Allergan, Chile; Allergan, Spain.*
Polyvinyl alcohol (p.1581·1) (p.1164·2).
*Dry eyes; lubricating solution for contact lenses.*

**Liquifilm OK** *Allergan, Ger.*
Polyvinyl alcohol (p.1581·1); povidone (p.1581·2).
*Dry eyes.*

**Liquifilm Tears**
*Alvia (Αλβια), Gr.; Allergan, Israel; Allergan, S.Afr.; Allergan, Singapore; Allergan, Thai.; Allergan, UK.*
Polyvinyl alcohol (p.1581·1) (p.1164·2).
*Dry eyes; lubricant for hard contact lenses.*

**Liquifilm Wetting**
*Allergan, Israel†; Allergan, USA.*
Wetting solution for hard contact lenses (p.1164·2).

**Liquifresh** *Allergan, Spain.*
Polyvinyl alcohol (p.1581·1); povidone (p.1581·2) (p.1164·2).
*Contact lens discomfort; dry eyes.*

**Liquigel** *Allergan, Ger.*
Carbomer 974P (p.1577·2).
*Dry eyes.*

**Liquigen**
*Scientific Hospital Supplies, Austral.; Nutricia, Fin.; SHS, Fr.; Scientific Hospital Supplies, Irl.; Nutricia, NZ; Scientific Hospital Supplies, NZ; SHS, Singapore†; Scientific Hospital Supplies, UK.*
Medium-chain triglycerides (p.1440·3).
*Impaired fat absorption; nutritional supplement.*

**Liquigesic Co** *Paedpharm, Austral.*
Paracetamol (p.76·2); codeine phosphate (p.27·1).
*Pain.*

**Liqui-Histine DM** *Liquipharm, USA†.*
Dextromethorphan hydrobromide (p.1117·3); phenylpropanolamine hydrochloride (p.1127·3); brompheniramine maleate (p.426·1).
*Upper respiratory-tract symptoms.*

**Liquimat** *Summers, USA.*
Sulfur (p.1158·2).
*Acne; oily skin.*

**Liquipake** *Lafayette, USA.*
Barium sulfate (p.1061·1).
*Contrast medium for gastrointestinal radiography.*

**Liquipom Dexa Antib** *Iquinosa, Spain.*
Dexamethasone sodium phosphate (p.1097·2); neomycin sulfate (p.235·1); polymyxin B sulfate (p.245·1).
*Infected eye and ear disorders.*

**Liquipom Dexa Const** *Iquinosa, Spain†.*
Dexamethasone sodium phosphate (p.1097·2); phenylephrine hydrochloride (p.1126·3).
*Eye disorders.*

**Liquipom Dexamida** *Iquinosa, Spain†.*
Dexamethasone sodium phosphate (p.1097·2); phenylephrine hydrochloride (p.1126·3); sulfacetamide sodium (p.257·3).
*Infected eye disorders.*

**Liquipom Medrisone** *Iquinosa, Spain†.*
Medrysone (p.1106·1).
*Eye disorders.*

**Liquiprin** *Menley & James, USA.*
Paracetamol (p.76·2).
*Fever; pain.*

**Liquirit N** *Loges, Ger.†.*
Algeldrate (p.1249·2); magnesium carbonate (p.1272·1); liquorice (p.1270·2).
*Gastrointestinal disorders.*

**Liquisorbon MCT** *Nutricia, Irl.†.*
Gluten-free, fructose-free, low-lactose food for special diets (p.1417·1).

**LiquiVent** *Alliance, USA.*
Perflubron (p.1730·1).
*Acute respiratory distress syndrome.*

**Liquivisc** *Allergan, UK.*
Carbomer 974P (p.1577·2).
*Dry eyes.*

**Liracol** *Medipharm, Chile.*
Nifuroxazide (p.237·2); phthalylsulfathiazole (p.242·3).
*Gastrointestinal infections.*

**Liroken** *Kendrick, Mex.*
Diclofenac sodium (p.32·1).
*Gout; musculoskeletal and joint disorders.*

**Lironex** *Master, Chile.*
Chlordiazepoxide (p.674·2); clidinium bromide (p.480·2).

**Lirugen** *Aventis Pasteur, Arg.*
A measles vaccine (Schwarz strain) (p.1623·1).
*Active immunisation.*

**Lis** *Lisapharma, Ital.*
Lactulose (p.1269·1).
*Constipation; disturbances of the gastrointestinal flora; hepatic cirrhosis; hepatic encephalopathy.*

**Lisa**
*Lisapharma, Israel; Lisapharma, Ital.*
Cefonicid sodium (p.174·2).
Lidocaine hydrochloride (p.1377·3) may be included in the intramuscular injection to alleviate the pain of injection.
*Gram-negative bacterial infections.*

**Lisac** *Microsules Bernabo, Arg.*
Simvastatin (p.997·1).
*Coronary insufficiency; hypercholesterolaemia.*

**Lisacef** *Lisapharma, Ital.*
Cefradine (p.179·3).
Lidocaine hydrochloride (p.1377·3) is included in the intramuscular injection to alleviate the pain of injection.
*Bacterial infections.*

**Lisacne** *Andromaco, Chile.*
Isotretinoin (p.1148·3).
*Acne.*

**Lisacol** *Hebron, Braz.*
Eicosapentaenoic acid (p.976·2); docosahexaenoic acid (p.976·1).
*Hyperlipidaemias.*

**Lisador** *Farmasa, Braz.*
Dipyrone (p.35·3); promethazine (p.439·1); adiphenine hydrochloride (p.1648·1).
*Smooth muscle spasm.*

**Lisaglucon** *Farmasa, Braz.*
Glibenclamide (p.331·2).
*Diabetes mellitus.*

**Lisaler** *Fortbenton, Arg.*
Loratadine (p.436·1).

**Lisaler Beta** *Fortbenton, Arg.*
Loratadine (p.436·1); betamethasone (p.1093·1).

**Lisalgil** *Boehringer Ingelheim, Arg.*
Metamizole magnesium (p.36·1).
*Pain.*

**Lisalgil Compuesto** *Boehringer Ingelheim, Arg.*
Metamizole magnesium (p.36·1); hyoscine butylbromide (p.483·3).
*Painful gastrointestinal spasm.*

**Lisan** *Hebron, Braz.*
Liver extract; vitamin $B_1$ (p.1454·3); vitamin $B_{12}$ (p.1458·2).
*Anaemias.*

**Lisanirc** *Lisapharma, Ital.*
Nicardipine hydrochloride (p.965·1).
*Angina pectoris; heart failure; hypertension.*

**Lisapres** *Libbs, Braz.*
Guanabenz acetate (p.926·2).
*Hypertension.*

**Lisaspin** *Euro-Labor, Port.; Grunenthal, Port.*
Lysine aspirin (p.54·3).
*Fever; pain; thromboembolism prophylaxis.*

**Lisba** *Rafarm, Gr.*
Nitrendipine (p.973·3).
*Hypertension.*

**Lisbak** *Savio, Ital.*
A *Bacillus subtilis* preparation.
*Gastrointestinal disorders.*

**Lisedema** *Climax, Braz.*
Piroxicam (p.84·2).
*Dysmenorrhoea; gout; musculoskeletal, joint, and peri-articular disorders.*

**Lisenteral** *Lisapharma, Ital.*
Lysates of various *Escherichia coli* strains and other coliform bacteria.
*Colibacilliary gastrointestinal and genito-urinary infections.*

**Liserdol**
*Teofarma, Ger.; Pharmacia, Hong Kong; Teofarma, Ital.; Pharmacia Upjohn, S.Afr.†; Pharmacia, Singapore; Wyeth, Switz.*
Metergoline (p.1211·2).
*Gastric motility disorders; hyperprolactinaemia; lactation inhibition; menstrual disorders; migraine and vascular headache.*

**Liseta** *Organon, Austria.*
12 Tablets, estradiol (p.1550·1); 12 tablets, estradiol; desogestrel (p.1547·2); 4 tablets, inert.
*Menopausal disorders; osteoporosis.*

**Lisi** *ABZ, Ger.; Hennig, Ger.*
Lisinopril (p.946·3).
*Heart failure; hypertension.*

**Lisi Lich** *Lichtenstein, Ger.*
Lisinopril (p.946·3).
*Heart failure; hypertension.*

**Lisibeta** *Betapharm, Ger.*
Lisinopril (p.946·3).
*Heart failure; hypertension; myocardial infarction.*

**Lisiflen** *De Salute, Ital.*
Diclofenac sodium (p.32·1).
*Inflammation; musculoskeletal and joint disorders; pain.*

**Lisigamma** *Worwag, Ger.*
Lisinopril (p.946·3).
*Heart failure; hypertension.*

**Lisigon** *Ofimex, Mex.†.*
Danazol (p.1545·2).

**Lisihexal** *Hexal, Ger.*
Lisinopril (p.946·3).
*Heart failure; hypertension.*

**Lisiken** *Kendrick, Mex.*
Clindamycin hydrochloride (p.194·2).
*Bacterial infections.*

**Lisil** *KBR, Ital.†.*
Carbocisteine (p.1116·2).
*Respiratory-tract disorders associated with increased or viscous mucus.*

**Lisin Sorb** *Nikkho, Braz.*
Lysine hydrochloride; vitamin B substances; gastric mucosa extract (p.1417·1).
*Tonic.*

**Lisinal** *Beta, Arg.*
Lisinopril (p.946·3).
*Heart failure; hypertension.*

**Lisinfos** *Fabra, Arg.*
Vitamin B substances (p.1417·1).

**Lisino** *Essex, Ger.*
Loratadine (p.436·1).
*Allergic rhinitis; atopic eczema; urticaria.*

**Lisinospes** *Specifar (Σπεσιφαρ), Gr.*
Lisinopril (p.946·3).
*Heart failure; hypertension; myocardial infarction.*

**Lisinotyrol** *Tyrol, Austria.*
Lisinopril (p.946·3).
*Heart failure; hypertension; myocardial infarction.*

**Lisinvitan** *Quimioterapica, Braz.†.*
Buclizine (p.426·3); lysine; tryptophan; vitamin $B_6$; vitamin $B_{12}$ (p.1417·1).
*Reduced appetite; tonic.*

**Lisiofer** *Garant, Ital.†.*
Sodium ferric gluconate complex (p.1444·3).
*Anaemia.*

**Lisipril** *Orion, Fin.*
Lisinopril (p.946·3).
*Heart failure; hypertension; myocardial infarction.*

**Lisipril Comp** *Orion, Fin.*
Lisinopril (p.946·3); hydrochlorothiazide (p.933·2).
*Hypertension.*

**Lisi-Puren** *Alpharma-Isis, Ger.*
Lisinopril (p.946·3).
*Heart failure; hypertension; myocardial infarction.*

**Liskantin** *Desitin, Ger.*
Primidone (p.376·3).
*Epilepsy.*

**Liskonum** *GlaxoSmithKline, UK.*
Lithium carbonate (p.301·1).
*Bipolar disorder; mania.*

**Lismol** *Lesvi, Spain.*
Colestyramine (p.889·3).
*Hyperlipidaemias.*

**Lisoder** *Laboratorios Chile, Chile.*
Mometasone furoate (p.1107·2).
*Skin disorders.*

**Lisoderma** *Armstrong, Arg.*
Acexamic acid (p.1646·2); gentamicin sulfate (p.217·1).
*Burns; ulcers; wounds.*

**Lisodren** *Bristol-Myers Squibb, Braz.*
Mitotane (p.575·1).
*Adrenal cortex cancer; Cushing's syndrome.*

**Lisodur** *Alphapharm, Austral.*
Lisinopril (p.946·3).
*Heart failure; hypertension; myocardial infarction.*

**Lisodura** *Merck dura, Ger.*
Lisinopril (p.946·3).
*Heart failure; hypertension; myocardial infarction.*

**Lisofenicol** *IMA, Braz.†.*
Chloramphenicol (p.185·1); muramidase hydrochloride (p.1717·2); hydroxyquinoline sulfate (p.1700·1); boric acid (p.1662·1); glucose (p.1432·2).
*Vulvovaginal disorders.*

**Lisoflu** *Sanofi Synthelabo, Ital.†.*
Paracetamol(p.76·2); ascorbic acid (p.1460·2); pseudoephedrine hydrochloride (p.1129·2); dextromethorphan hydrobromide (p.1117·3).
*Cold symptoms.*

**Lisolac** *Tecnimede, Port.*
Tilactase (p.1756·2).

**Lisolip** *Gap, Gr.*
Gemfibrozil (p.923·1).
*Hyperlipidaemias.*

**Lisomuc** *Elofar, Braz.†.*
Carbocisteine (p.1116·2).
*Respiratory-tract congestion.*

**Lisomucil** *Sanofi Synthelabo OTC, Ital.*
Carbocisteine (p.1116·2).
*Respiratory-tract disorders.*

**Lisomucil Gola** *Sanofi Synthelabo OTC, Ital.*
Dequalinium chloride (p.1178·1); enoxolone (p.36·2).
*Mouth and throat disorders.*

**Lisomucil Tosse Sedativo** *Sanofi Synthelabo OTC, Ital.*
Dextromethorphan hydrobromide (p.1117·3).
*Coughs.*

**Lisomucin** *Cipan, Port.*
Bromhexine hydrochloride (p.1115·3).
*Respiratory-tract disorders associated with increased or viscous mucus.*

**Lisoneurin B12** *Dupomar, Arg.*
Hydroxocobalamin (p.1458·2).
*Megaloblastic anaemia; peripheral neuropathy.*

**Lisonotec** *Teuto, Braz.*
Lisinopril (p.946·3); hydrochlorothiazide (p.933·2).
*Hypertension.*

**Lisopress** *Niche, Irl.*
Lisinopril (p.946·3).
*Heart failure; hypertension; myocardial infarction.*

**Lisopride** *Sanofi Synthelabo, Port.*
Sulpiride (p.722·2).

**Lisopulm** *Esseti, Ital.*
Ambroxol hydrochloride (p.1114·3).
*Respiratory-tract disorders.*

**Lisoquinol** *IMA, Braz.†.*
Muramidase hydrochloride (p.1717·2); furazolidone (p.605·2); hydroxyquinoline sulfate (p.1700·1); boric acid (p.1662·1).
*Vulvovaginal disorders.*

**Lisorane** *Zeneca, Mex.†.*
Isoflurane (p.1301·1).
*General anaesthesia.*

**Lisoril**
*Ipca, India; IPCA, Singapore.*
Lisinopril (p.946·3).
*Heart failure; hypertension.*

**Lisoril-5HT** *Ipca, India.*
Lisinopril (p.946·3); hydrochlorothiazide (p.933·2).
*Hypertension.*

**Lisosmalen** *Varos, Braz.†.*
Magnesium oxide (p.1272·3); vitamin $B_6$ (p.1456·3).
*Renal calculi.*

**Lisotox** *Cifarma, Braz.†.*
Cynara (p.1678·3); liver extract; choline citrate (p.1424·3); cyanocobalamin (p.1458·2).
*Liver disorders.*

**Lisotran** *Dovalle, Braz.*
Erythromycin (p.208·1).
*Bacterial infections.*

**Lisotrex** *Profarb, Braz.†.*
Erythromycin (p.208·1).
*Bacterial infections.*

**Lisovyr**
*Elea, Arg.; Mintlab, Chile.*
Aciclovir (p.626·1).
*Herpesvirus infections.*

**Lispor** *Medipharm, Chile.*
Lovastatin (p.949·1).
*Hypercholesterolaemia.*

**Lispril** *Siam Bheasach, Thai.*
Lisinopril (p.946·3).
*Hypertension.*

**Listaflex** *Finadiet, Arg.*
Carisoprodol (p.1392·1).
*Muscle spasm.*

**Listerfluor** *Parke, Davis, S.Afr.†.*
Sodium fluoride (p.1444·3).
*Dental caries prophylaxis.*

**Listerine**
*Note. This name is used for preparations of different composition.*
*Warner-Lambert, Braz.†; Warner-Lambert, Irl.†; Pfizer Consumer, Port.; Warner-Lambert, USA.*
Thymol (p.1194·2); cineole (p.1672·1); methyl salicylate (p.59·3); menthol (p.1711·3).
*Dental plaque prophylaxis; oral hygiene.*

*Pfizer Consumer, Canad.*
*Mouthwash:* Cineole (p.1672·1); thymol (p.1194·2); menthol (p.1711·3).
*Dental plaque prophylaxis; oral hygiene.*

*Parke, Davis, Chile.*
Alcohol (p.1166·1); thymol (p.1194·2); cineole (p.1672·1); methyl salicylate (p.59·3); menthol (p.1711·3); benzoic acid (p.1169·3).
*Oral hygiene.*

*Pfizer, NZ.*
Benzoic acid (p.1169·3); cineole (p.1672·1); thymol (p.1194·2).
*Oral hygiene.*

**Listerine Antiseptic Mouthwash** *Pfizer Consumer, UK.*
Cineole (p.1672·1); menthol (p.1711·3); methyl salicylate (p.59·3); thymol (p.1194·2).
*Oral hygiene.*

**Listerine Antisptic Tartar Control** *Pfizer Consumer, Canad.*
Cineole (p.1672·1); menthol (p.1711·3); thymol (p.1194·2); zinc chloride (p.1469·2).
*Dental plaque; oral hygiene.*

**Listerine Clasico** *Interbelle, Arg.*
Cineole (p.1672·1); menthol (p.1711·3); methyl salicylate (p.59·3); thymol (p.1194·2).
*Oral hygiene.*

**Listerine Cool Mint** *Interbelle, Arg.*
Thymol (p.1194·2); cineole (p.1672·1); methyl salicylate (p.59·3).
*Oral hygiene.*

**Listerine Fresh Burst** *Interbelle, Arg.*
Cineole (p.1672·1); menthol (p.1711·3); methyl salicylate (p.59·3); thymol (p.1194·2).
*Oral hygiene.*

**Listerine Tartar Control** *Pfizer, NZ.*
Benzoic acid (p.1169·3); cineole (p.1672·1); thymol (p.1194·2); zinc chloride (p.1469·2).
*Oral hygiene.*

**Listermint** *Pfizer Consumer, UK.*
Cetylpyridinium chloride (p.1173·1).
*Oral hygiene.*

**Listermint Arctic Mint Mouthwash** *Warner-Wellcome, USA.*
Glycerol (p.1694·3).

**Listermint Con Fluor** *Parke, Davis, Chile.*
Sodium fluoride (p.1444·3); alcohol (p.1166·1); thymol (p.1194·2); methyl salicylate (p.59·3); eugenol (p.1686·2).
*Dental caries prophylaxis; oral hygiene.*

**Listermint with Fluoride**
*Warner-Lambert, Irl.†; Pfizer Consumer, UK.*
Sodium fluoride (p.1444·3); cetylpyridinium chloride (p.1173·1).
*Dental plaque prophylaxis; oral hygiene.*

**Listran** *Uriach, Spain.*
Nabumetone (p.63·3).
*Osteoarthritis; rheumatoid arthritis.*

**Lisvifar** *Farcoral, Mex.*
Multivitamin preparation (p.1417·1).

**Lit-300** *Hua, Thai.*
Lithium carbonate (p.301·1).
*Bipolar disorder.*

**Litak**
*Lipomed, Israel; Lipomed, Switz.*
Cladribine (p.539·3).
*Chronic lymphocytic leukaemia; hairy-cell leukaemia; non-Hodgkin's lymphoma.*

**Litalgin** *Leiras, Fin.*
Dipyrone (p.35·3); pitofenone hydrochloride (p.1732·3).
*Gastrointestinal, biliary, and renal colic.*

**Litalir**
*Bristol-Myers Squibb, Austria; Bristol-Myers Squibb, Ger.; Bristol-Myers Squibb, Switz.*
Hydroxycarbamide (p.559·1).
*Malignant neoplasms.*

**Litarek** *Ipsen, Spain†.*
Gemfibrozil (p.923·1).
*Hyperlipidaemias.*

**Litarex**
*Alpharma, Denm.; Astra, Norw.†; Alpharma, Switz.; Dumex, UK†.*
Lithium citrate (p.301·1).
*Bipolar disorder; mania.*

**Lithane** *Pfizer, Canad.*
Lithium carbonate (p.301·1).
*Bipolar disorder.*

**Litheum** *Valdecasas, Mex.*
Lithium carbonate (p.301·1).
*Bipolar disorder.*

**Lithiagel** *Cochon, Fr.†.*
Basic aluminium carbonate (p.1249·1).
*Diagnosis of hyperparathyroidism; hyperphosphataemia.*

**Lithias-cyl N Ho-Len-Complex** *Liebermann, Ger.*
Homoeopathic preparation.

**Lithicarb**
*Aspen, Austral.; Pacific, Hong Kong; Pacific, NZ.*
Lithium carbonate (p.301·1).
*Bipolar disorder; depression; schizophrenia.*

**Lithimole** *Cooper (Κοπερ), Gr.*
Timolol maleate (p.1012·2).
*Glaucoma.*

**Lithioderm** *Labcatal, Fr.*
Lithium.
*Seborrhoeic dermatitis.*

**Lithiofor**
*Nikolakopoulos (Νικολακοπουλος), Gr.; Vifor, Hong Kong; Vifor, Switz.*
Lithium sulfate (p.305·1).
*Bipolar disorder; mania.*

**Lithionit**
*AstraZeneca, Norw.; Astra, Swed.*
Lithium sulfate (p.305·1).
*Bipolar disorder; mania.*

**Lithiumeel** *Peithner, Austria†.*
Homoeopathic preparation.

**Lithiun** *Elisium, Arg.*
Lithium carbonate (p.301·1).
*Bipolar disorder.*

**Lithizine** *Technilab, Canad.†.*
Lithium carbonate (p.301·1).
*Bipolar disorder.*

**Lithobid** *Solvay, USA.*
Lithium carbonate (p.301·1).
*Bipolar disorder.*

**Lithofalk**
*Merck, Austria; Falk, Ger.; Phardi, Switz.†.*
Chenodeoxycholic acid (p.1670·1); ursodeoxycholic acid (p.1760·3).
*Cholesterol gallstones.*

**Lithonate** *Approved Prescription Services, UK.*
Lithium carbonate (p.301·1).
*Bipolar disorder; depression; mania.*

**Lithostat** *Mission Pharmacal, USA.*
Acetohydroxamic acid (p.1645·3).
*Adjunct in urinary-tract infection with urea-splitting organisms.*

**Lithosun** *Sun, Singapore†.*
Lithium carbonate (p.301·1).
*Bipolar disorder.*

**Lithurex S** *Phonix, Ger.*
Magnesium citrate (p.1272·1); citric acid (p.1673·1); sodium citrate (p.1223·2); potassium citrate (p.1223·1).
*Urinary-tract disorders.*

**Litiax** *Novag, Spain.*
Gall (p.1690·2).
*Renal calculi.*

**Litican**
*Sanofi Synthelabo, Belg.; Lorex Synthelabo, Neth.†.*
Alizapride hydrochloride (p.1248·1).
*Nausea; vomiting.*

**Litiocar** *Biosintetica, Braz.*
Lithium carbonate (p.301·1).
*Bipolar disorder; depression; migraine and other vascular headaches; neutropenia; schizophrenia.*

**Litiofarm** *ICN, Arg.*
Lithium succinate (p.1151·2); zinc sulfate (p.1469·3).
*Seborrhoeic dermatitis.*

**Lito** *Orion, Fin.*
Lithium carbonate (p.301·1).
*Bipolar disorder.*

**Litobile** *Poli, Ital.†.*
Magnesium trihydrate salt of chenodeoxycholic (p.1670·1) and ursodeoxycholic acids (p.1760·3).
*Biliary dyspepsia; gallstones.*

**Litocit** *Apsen, Braz.*
Potassium citrate (p.1223·1).
*Renal calculi.*

**Litoff** *Caber, Ital.*
Ursodeoxycholic acid (p.1760·3).
*Biliary-tract disorders.*

**Litosmil** *Evans, Fr.†.*
Diosmin (p.1688·2).
*Peripheral vascular disorders.*

**Litoxol** *Centrapharm, Fr.†.*
Sulfaguanidine (p.260·3); aluminium salicylate.
*Infective diarrhoea.*

**Litrison**
*Note. This name is used for preparations of different composition.*
*Klinger, Braz.†.*
Cynara (p.1678·3); solanum paniculatum; boldo (p.1661·2); choline bitartrate (p.1424·3); magnesium sulfate (p.1228·2).
*Liver disorders.*

*Roche, Ital.†.*
Alpha tocoferil acetate; vitamin B substances (p.1417·1).
Formerly contained choline bitartrate, DL-methionine, and vitamin B substances.

**Litursol** *Crinos, Ital.*
Ursodeoxycholic acid (p.1760·3).
*Biliary-tract disorders.*

**Liv 52** *Ebi, Switz.*
Capparis spinosa; cichorium intybus; solanum nigrum; cassia occidentalis; terminalia arjuna; achillea millefolium; tamarix gallica; ferrum bhasma.
*Gastrointestinal disorders; tonic.*

**Livadex** *Rolab, S.Afr.*
Vitamin B substances; liver extracts; caffeine (p.1417·1).
*Tonic.*

**Livamine** *Bioceuticals, UK.*
Multivitamin and mineral preparation (p.1417·1).

**Liv-Detox** *Blackmores, Austral.†.*
DL-Methionine (p.1042·1); choline bitartrate (p.1424·3); inositol (p.1701·2); glutamine (p.1433·2); pyridoxine hydrochloride (p.1456·3); riboflavin (p.1456·1); sodium sulfate (p.1290·1).
*Liver disorders.*

**Liver Tonic Capsules** *Vitaglow, Austral.†.*
Silybum marianum (p.1043·3).
*Dyspepsia; stress.*

**Liver Tonic Herbal Formula 6** *Vitelle, Austral.†.*
Silybum marianum (p.1043·3); taraxacum (p.1751·3); cynara (p.1678·3); garlic (p.1691·1).
*Digestive disorders; liver tonic.*

**Liverall** *Sankyo, Hong Kong.*
Di-isopropylammonium dichloroacetate (p.900·1); calcium gluconate (p.1225·2).
*Liver disorders.*

**Liverasi** *Francia, Ital.*
Cogalactoisomerase sodium (p.1674·3).
*Liver disorders.*

**Livercrom** *Byk Elmu, Spain†.*
Arginine timonacicate (p.1421·2).
*Liver disorders.*

**Livesan** *Bouchara-Recordati, Fr.†.*
Fenofibrate (p.915·2).
*Hyperlipidaemias.*

**Livial**
*Organon, Austral.; Organon, Belg.; Organon, Braz.; Organon, Chile; Organon, Denm.; Organon, Fin.; Organon, Fr.; Organon (Οργανον), Gr.; Organon, Hong Kong; Infar, India; Organon, Irl.; Organon, Ital.; Organon, Malaysia; Organon, Mex.; Organon, Neth.; Organon, Norw.; Organon, NZ; Organon, Port.; Organon, Singapore; Organon, Swed.; Organon, Switz.; Organon, Thai.; Organon, UK.*
Tibolone (p.1572·3).
*Menopausal disorders; osteoporosis.*

**Liviane Compuesto** *Knoll, Spain†.*
Aescin (p.1648·2); thiocolchicoside (p.1395·2).
*Musculoskeletal lesions; peripheral vascular disorders.*

**Liviel** *Organon, Austria.*
Tibolone (p.1572·3).
*Menopausal disorders; osteoporosis.*

**Liviella** *Organon, Ger.; Nourypharma, Ger.*
Tibolone (p.1572·3).
*Menopausal disorders.*

**Livifem** *Donmed, S.Afr.*
Tibolone (p.1572·3).
*Menopausal disorders; osteoporosis.*

**Liviton** *Restan, S.Afr.*
Vitamins; minerals; caffeine; liver extracts (p.1417·1).
*Tonic.*

**Livitrinsic-f** *Goldline, USA.*
Ferrous fumarate (p.1427·3); folic acid (p.1429·1); intrinsic factor; vitamin $B_{12}$ substances (p.1458·2).
Vitamin C (p.1460·2) is included in this preparation to increase the absorption and availability of iron.
*Anaemias.*

**Livo Luk** *Panacea, India.*
Lactulose (p.1269·1).
*Constipation; hepatic encephalopathy.*

**Livocab**
*Janssen-Cilag, Ger.; Janssen-Cilag, Ital.; Janssen-Cilag, Neth.; Janssen-Cilag, Spain.*
Levocabastine hydrochloride (p.435·2).
*Allergic conjunctivitis; allergic rhinitis.*

**Livogen** *Merck, India.*
*Capsules:* Liver; dried yeast (p.1469·1); vitamin B substances (p.1454·3); folic acid (p.1429·1); vitamin C (p.1460·2); ferrous fumarate (p.1427·3).
*Anaemias.*
*Oral liquid:* Liver; dried yeast; vitamin $B_{12}$; nicotinic acid (p.1417·1).
*Tonic.*

**Livolon** *Biolab Sanus, Braz.*
Tibolone (p.1572·3).
*Menopausal disorders.*

**Livomarin** *Varifarma, Arg.*
Conjugated oestrogens (p.1543·2).

**Livomedrox** *Varifarma, Arg.*
Medroxyprogesterone (p.1557·3).

**Livomonil** *Varifarma, Arg.*
Clotrimazole (p.396·2).
*Fungal vaginal infections.*

**Livostin**
*Janssen-Cilag, Austral.; Janssen-Cilag, Austria; Janssen-Cilag, Belg.; Janssen-Cilag, Braz.; Novartis Ophthalmics, Braz.; Janssen-Ortho, Canad.; Janssen-Cilag, Chile; Janssen-Cilag, Denm.; Janssen-Cilag, Fin.; Janssen-Cilag, Gr.; Janssen-Cilag, Israel; Janssen-Cilag, Ital.; Shinyaku, Jpn; Janssen, Mex.; Janssen-Cilag, Norw.; Janssen-Cilag, NZ; Janssen-Cilag, S.Afr.; Janssen-Cilag, Swed.; Janssen-Cilag, Switz.; Janssen-Cilag, Thai.; Janssen, Thai.; Novartis, UK; Novartis Ophthalmics, USA.*
Levocabastine hydrochloride (p.435·2).
*Allergic conjunctivitis; allergic rhinitis.*

**Livten** *Ativus, Braz.*
Polyunsaturated fatty acids.
*Dietary supplement.*

**Lixacol** *Schering-Plough, Spain.*
Mesalazine (p.1273·2).
*Crohn's disease; ulcerative colitis.*

**Lixamide** *Xeragen, S.Afr.*
Indapamide (p.938·2).
*Hypertension.*

**Lixidol** *Roche, Ital.*
Ketorolac trometamol (p.52·1).
*Pain.*

**Lixir** *Abigo, Swed.*
Multivitamins (p.1417·1); caffeine.

**Lixogan** *Tocogino, Mex.†.*
Naproxen (p.65·1).

**Lizarona** *Northia, Arg.*
Metoclopramide (p.1274·3).
*Nausea and vomiting.*

**Lizepat** *Cosmopharm, Gr.*
Nimesulide (p.67·1).
*Inflammation; musculoskeletal disorders; pain.*

**Lizipaina** *Fher, Spain.*
Bacitracin (p.161·3); muramidase (p.1717·2); papain (p.1727·3).
*Mouth and throat inflammation.*

**Lizovag** *Novag, Mex.*
Ketoconazole (p.403·3).
*Fungal infections.*

**Lizul** *Baldacci, Port.*
Lansoprazole (p.1269·3).
*Gastro-oesophageal reflux; peptic ulcer; Zollinger-Ellison syndrome.*

**Llantusil** *Soria Natural, Spain.*
Eucalyptus (p.1686·1); satureja montana; wild thyme; althaea (p.1651·3); coltsfoot (p.1117·2); plantago lanceolata (p.1738·2).
*Respiratory-tract infections.*

**Llorentecaina Noradrenal** *Llorente, Spain†.*
Lidocaine hydrochloride (p.1377·3).
Noradrenaline acid tartrate (p.974·3) is included in this preparation as a vasoconstrictor to diminish absorption and localise the effect of the local anaesthetic.
*Local anaesthesia.*

**Lloyd's Cream** *Thornton & Ross, UK.*
Diethylamine salicylate (p.34·1).
*Musculoskeletal and soft-tissue disorders.*

**LM6** *AF, Mex.*
*Oral solution:* Chlorphenamine maleate (p.427·3); paracetamol (p.76·2).
*Fever; hypersensitivity; pain.*
*Tablets:* Paracetamol (p.76·2); mepyramine maleate (p.437·1); phenylephrine hydrochloride (p.1126·3); caffeine (p.782·1).
*Cold symptoms.*

**L-M-X4** *Ferndale, USA.*
Lidocaine (p.1377·3).
Formerly known as ELA-Max.
*Anorectal disorders; topical anaesthesia.*

**Lo-Acid** *Be-Tabs, S.Afr.*
Simeticone (p.1289·2); magnesium hydroxide (p.1272·2); aluminium hydroxide (p.1249·2).
*Antacid; flatulence.*

**Lobac** *Seatrace, USA.*
Salicylamide (p.87·3); phenyltoloxamine (p.439·1); paracetamol (p.76·2).
*Musculoskeletal pain.*

**Lobacin** *TO-Chemicals, Thai.†.*
Neomycin sulfate (p.235·1); bacitracin (p.161·3); amylocaine hydrochloride (p.1370·2).
*Mouth and throat disorders.*

**Lobak** *Zurich, S.Afr.†.*
Chlormezanone (p.675·1); paracetamol (p.76·2).
*Pain; skeletal muscle spasm.*

**Lobamine-Cysteine**
*Pierre Fabre, Fr.; Actipharm, Switz.†.*
Methionine (p.1042·1); cysteine hydrochloride (p.1426·3).
*Hair and nail disorders.*

**Lobana** *Ulmer, USA.*
Soap-free skin cleanser.

**Lobana Body** *Ulmer, USA.*
Emollient and moisturiser.

**Lobana Derm-Aide** *Ulmer, USA.*
Vitamin A (p.1451·2); vitamin D (p.1461·2); vitamin E (p.1464·3).
*Skin disorders.*

**Lobana Peri-Garde** *Ulmer, USA.*
Vitamin A (p.1451·2); vitamin D (p.1461·2); vitamin E (p.1464·3); chloroxylenol (p.1177·2).
*Skin disorders.*

**Lobate** *Boots Piramal, India.*
Clobetasol propionate (p.1095·2).
*Skin disorders.*

**Lobate-G** *Boots Piramal, India.*
Clobetasol propionate (p.1095·2); gentamicin sulfate (p.217·1).
*Infected skin disorders.*

**Lobate-GM** *Boots Piramal, India.*
Clobetasol propionate (p.1095·2); gentamicin sulfate (p.217·1); miconazole nitrate (p.405·3).
*Infected skin disorders.*

**Lobate-M** *Boots Piramal, India.*
Clobetasol propionate (p.1095·2); miconazole nitrate (p.405·3).
*Infected skin disorders.*

**Lobelia Composta** *Simoes, Braz.†.*
Grindelia (p.1696·1); lobelia (p.1589·1); mephitis putorius.
*Coughs.*

**Lobelia Compound** *Gerard House, UK†.*
Lobelia (p.1589·1); gum ammoniacum; squill (p.1130·3).
*Cough and cold symptoms.*

**Lobelia Med Complex** *Dynamit, Austria.*
Homoeopathic preparation.

**Lobesol** *Sunward, Malaysia.*
Clobetasol propionate (p.1095·2).
*Skin disorders.*

**Lobeta** *Betapharm, Ger.*
Loratadine (p.436·1).
*Allergic conjunctivitis; allergic rhinitis; atopic eczema; urticaria.*

**Lobevat**
*Stiefel, Chile; Stiefel, Mex.*
Clobetasol propionate (p.1095·2).
*Skin disorders.*

**Lobione** *Aventis, Belg.†.*
Betahistine mesilate (p.1660·1).
*Vertigo.*

**Lobivon**
*Menarini, Gr.; Menarini, Ital.; Menarini, Spain.*
Nebivolol hydrochloride (p.964·3).
*Hypertension.*

**Lobu** *Ohara, Jpn.*
Loxoprofen sodium (p.54·3).
*Inflammation; pain.*

**Locabase** *Pierre Fabre, Fr.*
Basis for topical preparations.

**Locabiosol**
*Servier, Austria; Grunenthal, Chile; Servier, Ger.; Servier, Port.*
Fusafungine (p.215·2).
*Upper respiratory-tract infections and inflammation.*

**Locabiotal**
*Servier, Belg.; Servier, Braz.; Therval, Fr.; Servier, Hong Kong; Servier, Irl.; Stroder, Ital.; Servier, Malaysia; AF, Mex.†; Servier, S.Afr.; Servier, Switz.; Servier, UK.*
Fusafungine (p.215·2).
*Upper respiratory-tract infection and inflammation.*

**Locacid**
Pierre Fabre, Fr.; Primal, Hong Kong; Pierre Fabre, Israel; Pierre Fabre, Port.
Tretinoin (p.1161·1).
*Acne; psoriasis.*

**Locacorten**
Ciba, Canad.†; Bioglan, Ger.; Novartis, Israel†; Novartis, Neth.; Novartis, Switz.
Flumetasone pivalate (p.1101·1).
*Skin disorders.*

**Locacorten med Salicylsyre** Novartis, Denm.†.
Flumetasone pivalate (p.1101·1); salicylic acid (p.1157·1).
*Skin disorders.*

**Locacorten mit Neomycin** Novartis, Austria.
Flumetasone pivalate (p.1101·1); neomycin sulfate (p.235·1).
*Infected skin disorders.*

**Locacorten with Neomycin** Novartis, Israel.
Flumetasone pivalate (p.1101·1); neomycin sulfate (p.235·1).
*Skin disorders.*

**Locacorten Tar**
Novartis, Austria; Novartis, Hong Kong; Novartis, Israel†; Max Ritter, Switz.†.
Flumetasone pivalate (p.1101·1); coal tar (p.1159·2); salicylic acid (p.1157·1).
*Skin disorders.*

**Locacorten Triclosan** Max Ritter, Switz.†.
Flumetasone pivalate (p.1101·1); triclosan (p.1195·2).
*Infected skin disorders.*

**Locacorten Vioform**
Novartis, Austral.; Novartis, Austria; Novartis, Canad.; Novartis, Denm.; Novartis, Fin.; Bioglan, Ger.; Novartis, Neth.; Novartis, Norw.†; Novartis, S.Afr.; Novartis, Swed.
Flumetasone pivalate (p.1101·1); clioquinol (p.196·3).
*External ear disorders; infected skin disorders.*

**Locacortene**
Novartis Consumer, Belg.†.
Flumetasone pivalate (p.1101·1).
*Skin disorders.*

Medifa, Fr.†.
Flumetasone pivalate (p.1101·1); neomycin sulfate (p.235·1).
*Infected skin disorders.*

**Locacortene Tar** Novartis Consumer, Belg.†.
Flumetasone pivalate (p.1101·1); coal tar (p.1159·2); salicylic acid (p.1157·1).
*Skin disorders.*

**Locacortene Vioforme**
Novartis Consumer, Belg.†; Medifa, Fr.†.
Flumetasone pivalate (p.1101·1); clioquinol (p.196·3).
*External ear disorders; skin disorders.*

**Localin** Fischer, Israel.
Oxybuprocaine hydrochloride (p.1382·1).
*Local anaesthesia.*

**Localone**
Pierre Fabre, Fr.; Pierre Fabre, Port.
Triamcinolone acetonide (p.1110·2); salicylic acid (p.1157·1).
*Skin disorders.*

**Localyn** Recordati, Ital.
*Ear drops:* Fluocinolone acetonide (p.1101·2); neomycin sulfate (p.235·1).
*Ear disorders.*
*Lotion; ointment; topical solution:* Fluocinolone acetonide (p.1101·2).
*Skin disorders.*
*Nasal spray:* Fluocinolone acetonide (p.1101·2); clonazoline hydrochloride (p.1117·1).
*Nasal inflammation and hypersensitivity.*

**Localyn SV** Recordati, Ital.
Fluocinolone acetonide (p.1101·2).
*Nasal inflammation and hypersensitivity.*

**Localyn-Neomicina** Recordati, Ital.
Fluocinolone acetonide (p.1101·2); neomycin sulfate (p.235·1).
*Infected skin disorders.*

**Locao Mancha Branca** Stevia, Braz.†.
Benzoic acid (p.1169·3); iodine (p.1598·1); licor de Hoffman (alcohol, solvent ether).
*Fungal skin infections.*

**Locapred**
Pierre Fabre, Fr.; Pierre Fabre, Port.; Pierre Fabre, Switz.
Desonide (p.1096·3).
*Skin disorders.*

**Locasalen**
Novartis, Austria; Novartis Consumer, Belg.†; Bioglan, Ger.; Novartis, Hong Kong; Novartis, Israel†; Novartis, Neth.; Novartis, Singapore†; Novartis, Switz.; Novartis, Thai.
Flumetasone pivalate (p.1101·1); salicylic acid (p.1157·1).
*Skin disorders.*

**Locasalene**
Medifa, Fr.†; Novartis, Gr.
Salicylic acid (p.1157·1); flumetasone pivalate (p.1101·1).
*Skin disorders.*

**Locaseptil-Neo** Drossapharm, Switz.
Prednisolone acetate (p.1108·1); cinchocaine (p.1373·2).
*Nasal and buccal lesions.*

**Locasil** Locatelli, Ital.†.
Silymarin (p.1043·3).
*Liver disorders.*

**Locasol**
Nutricia, Austral.; Baxter, NZ; Nutricia, NZ; Scientific Hospital Supplies, UK.
Low-calcium milk substitute (p.1417·1).
*Calcium and vitamin D restriction; calcium intolerance.*

**Locasol New Formula** Scientific Hospital Supplies, Irl.
Low-calcium food for special diets (p.1417·1).

**Locason** Proel, Gr.
Betamethasone valerate (p.1093·2).
*Topical corticosteroid.*

**Locasyn** Roche, Denm.
Flunisolide (p.1101·1).
*Rhinitis.*

**Locatop**
Pierre Fabre, Arg.; Pierre Fabre, Fr.; Pierre Fabre, Switz.
Desonide (p.1096·3).
*Skin disorders.*

**Locemix** Euroderm, Arg.
Minoxidil (p.960·1).
*Alopecia androgenetica.*

**Loceptin** Nycomed, Swed.†.
Morphine sulfate (p.60·2).
*Pain.*

**Loceryl**
Galderma, Austral.; AB-Consult, Austria; Galderma, Belg.; Galderma, Braz.; Galderma, Chile; Galderma, Denm.; Galderma, Fin.; Galderma, Fr.; Galderma, Ger.; Lavipharm, Gr.; Galderma, Hong Kong; Galderma, Irl.; Galderma, Malaysia; Galderma, Mex.; Galderma, Norw.; Galderma, NZ; Galderma, S.Afr.; Galderma, Singapore; Galderma, Swed.; Galderma, Switz.; Galderma, UK.
Amorolfine hydrochloride (p.391·1).
*Fungal skin and nail infections.*

**Locetar**
Galderma, Arg.; Galderma, Ital.; Galderma, Port.; Galderma, Spain.
Amorolfine hydrochloride (p.391·1).
*Fungal skin and nail infections.*

**Lochol** Novartis, Jpn.
Fluvastatin sodium (p.918·2).
*Hyperlipidaemias.*

**Locholes** TO-Chemicals, Thai.
Gemfibrozil (p.923·1).
*Hyperlipidaemias.*

**Locholest** Warner Chilcott, USA.
Colestyramine (p.889·3).
*Hypercholesterolaemia; pruritus associated with biliary obstruction.*

**Lociherp** Maigal, Arg.
Urea (p.1162·2).
*Skin disorders.*

**Locilan** Pharmacia, Austral.
Norethisterone (p.1562·2).
*Progestogen-only contraceptive.*

**Locion Axel** Grisi, Mex.
Sulfur (p.1158·2); sulfacetamide (p.257·3).
*Acne.*

**Locion Corporal Suavizante AHA Formula 405** Dermaclin, Mex.
*SPF 15:* Octinoxate (p.1154·3); oxybenzone (p.1154·3).
*Skin disorders; sunscreen.*

**Locion Limpiadora AHA Formula 405** Dermaclin, Mex.
Soap substitute.
*Acne; xerosis.*

**Lockesol** Dzwon, India.
Solution 1, sodium chloride; potassium chloride; sodium phosphate; sodium bicarbonate; solution 2, calcium chloride; magnesium chloride; glucose; glutathione disulfate (p.1217·1).
*Eye irrigation.*

**Lockets** Mars, UK.
Menthol (p.1711·3); cineole (p.1672·1); honey (p.1434·2); glycerol (p.1694·3).
*Nasal congestion; sore throat.*

**Lockets Medicated Linctus** Thornton & Ross, UK.
Ipecacuanha (p.1122·3); honey (p.1434·2); glucose (p.1432·2); glycerol (p.1694·3); menthol (p.1711·3).
*Coughs; sore throats.*

**Locko** General Drugs, Thai.†.
Dextromethorphan hydrobromide (p.1117·3); chlorphenamine maleate (p.427·3); phenylpropanolamine hydrochloride (p.1127·3); paracetamol (p.76·2).
*Cold and influenza symptoms.*

**Lockolys**
Fresenius Medical, Denm.†; Fresenius Medical, Fin.†.
Range of solutions containing glucose; sodium chloride; sodium lactate; calcium chloride; magnesium chloride (p.1221·1).
*Peritoneal dialysis.*

**Locobase**
Yamanouchi, Fin.
Vehicle for topical preparations.

Yamanouchi, Ital.; Yamanouchi, Switz.
Emollient.

**Locoid**
Yamanouchi, Belg.; Eurofarma, Braz.; Labomed, Chile; Yamanouchi, Denm.; Yamanouchi, Fin.; Yamanouchi, Fr.; Yamanouchi, Irl.; Sanofi Synthelabo, Mex.; Yamanouchi, Neth.; Yamanouchi, Norw.; CSL, NZ; Yamanouchi, NZ; Yamanouchi, Port.; Pharmaplan, S.Afr.; Yamanouchi, Swed.; Yamanouchi, Switz.; Yamanouchi, UK; Ferndale, USA.
Hydrocortisone butyrate (p.1104·1).
*Skin disorders.*

**Locoid C**
Yamanouchi, Irl.; CSL, NZ; Yamanouchi, NZ; Yabrofarma, Port.; Yamanouchi, UK.
Hydrocortisone butyrate (p.1104·1); chlorquinaldol (p.187·3).
*Skin disorders with bacterial or fungal infection.*

**Locoid Crelo** Yamanouchi, Swed.
Hydrocortisone butyrate (p.1104·1).
*Eczema; otitis externa; psoriasis.*

**Locoide N** Yamanouchi, Fr.†.
Hydrocortisone butyrate (p.1104·1); neomycin sulfate (p.235·1).
*Infected skin disorders.*

**Locoidol**
Yamanouchi, Denm.; Yamanouchi, Fin.; Yamanouchi, Norw.
Hydrocortisone butyrate (p.1104·1); chlorquinaldol (p.187·3).
*Infected skin disorders.*

**Locoidon**
CSC, Austria; Yamanouchi, Ital.
Hydrocortisone butyrate (p.1104·1).
*Skin disorders.*

**LOCOL** Novartis, Ger.
Fluvastatin sodium (p.918·2).
*Hypercholesterolaemia.*

**Locomin** UCB, Switz.
Aceclofenac (p.11·2).
*Musculoskeletal and joint disorders.*

**Locomucil** Pharmazam, Spain.
Acetylcysteine (p.1112·3).
*Respiratory-tract disorders.*

**Locorten** Novartis, Ital.
*Cream; ointment:* Flumetasone pivalate (p.1101·1); neomycin sulfate (p.235·1).
*Otitis externa; skin disorders.*
*Ear drops; oral drops:* Flumetasone pivalate (p.1101·1); clioquinol (p.196·3).
*Gingivitis; oral inflammatory lesions; otitis.*
*Lotion:* Flumetasone pivalate (p.1101·1).
*Otitis externa; skin disorders.*

**Locorten Neomicina** Novartis, Braz.
Flumetasone pivalate (p.1101·1); neomycin sulfate (p.235·1).
*Skin disorders.*

**Locorten Vioform**
Novartis, NZ; Novartis Consumer, UK.
Flumetasone pivalate (p.1101·1); clioquinol (p.196·3).
*Inflammatory disorders of the ear with bacterial or fungal infection; otorrhoea.*

**Locorten Vioformio**
Novartis, Braz.; Novartis, Ital.; Novartis Consumer, Port.
Flumetasone pivalate (p.1101·1); clioquinol (p.196·3).
*Infected skin disorders.*

**Locorten Vioformo** Novartis, Arg.
Flumetasone pivalate (p.1101·1); clioquinol (p.196·3).
*Infected skin disorders.*

**Locortene** Novartis, Spain†.
Flumetasone pivalate (p.1101·1).
*Skin disorders.*

**Locortene Vioformo** Novartis, Spain†.
Clioquinol (p.196·3); flumetasone pivalate (p.1101·1).
*Infected skin disorders.*

**Locose** T Man, Thai.
Glibenclamide (p.331·2).
*Diabetes mellitus.*

**Locrim** Pharma Investi, Chile.
Betamethasone dipropionate (p.1093·1); clotrimazole (p.396·2).
*Fungal skin infections with inflammation.*

**Loctenk** Biotenk, Arg.
Losartan potassium (p.947·2).
*Heart failure; hypertension.*

**Locula** East India Pharma, India.
Sulfacetamide sodium (p.257·3).
*Bacterial eye infections.*

**Lodales** Sanofi Synthelabo, Fr.
Simvastatin (p.997·1).
*Hypercholesterolaemia.*

**Loderix** EGIS, Hung.
Setastine hydrochloride (p.441·1).
*Hypersensitivity reactions.*

**Loderm** Vinas, Spain.
Erythromycin (p.208·1) or erythromycin laurilsulfate.
*Acne.*

**Loderm Retinoico** Vinas, Spain.
Erythromycin laurilsulfate; tretinoin (p.1161·1).
*Acne.*

**Lodiarid** Clement, Fr.†.
Loperamide hydrochloride (p.1271·1).
*Diarrhoea.*

**Lodimol** Kener, Mex.†.
Dipyridamole (p.903·1).

**Lodine**
Wyeth Lederle, Austria; Algol, Fin.; Fornet, Fr.; Wyeth, Hong Kong; Wyeth Lederle, Ital.; Wyeth, Mex.; Wyeth Lederle, Port.; Sigma-Tau, Switz.; Shire, UK; Wyeth-Ayerst, USA.
Etodolac (p.37·3).
*Gout; inflammation; musculoskeletal, joint, and peri-articular disorders; pain.*

**Lodipen** Royton, Braz.
Amlodipine besilate (p.862·1).
*Hypertension.*

**Lodipres** Laboratorios Chile, Chile.
Carvedilol (p.881·1).
*Angina pectoris; heart failure; hypertension.*

**Lodis** Eugal, Ital.†.
Loperamide hydrochloride (p.1271·1).
*Diarrhoea.*

**Lodixal** Knoll, Belg.
Verapamil hydrochloride (p.1019·1).
*Hypertension.*

**Lodoc** Disprovent, Arg.
Benzocaine (p.1370·3).
*Obesity.*

**Lodopin** Fujisawa, Jpn.
Zotepine (p.730·2).
*Schizophrenia.*

**Lodosyn** Bristol-Myers Squibb, USA.
Carbidopa (p.1204·3).
*Parkinsonism.*

**Lodot** BA Farma, Port.
Etodolac (p.37·3).
*Gout; musculoskeletal, joint, and peri-articular disorders; pain.*

**Lodoz**
Lipha Sante, Fr.; Merck, Hong Kong.
Bisoprolol fumarate (p.875·1); hydrochlorothiazide (p.933·2).
*Hypertension.*

**Lodrane** ECR, USA.
Pseudoephedrine hydrochloride (p.1129·2); brompheniramine maleate (p.426·1).
*Allergic rhinitis; nasal congestion.*

**Lodrane 12** ECR, USA.
Brompheniramine maleate (p.426·1).
Formerly known as Lodrane Allergy.
*Allergic rhinitis.*

**Lodrane 12D** ECR, USA.
Pseudoephedrine hydrochloride (p.1129·2); brompheniramine maleate (p.426·1).
*Allergic rhinitis; nasal congestion.*

**Lodronat**
Roche, Austria; Roche, Chile.
Disodium clodronate (p.770·2).
*Hypercalcaemia of malignancy; osteolysis of malignancy.*

**Lodyfen** Grin, Mex.
Diclofenac sodium (p.32·1).
*Inflammatory eye disorders; prevention of miosis and cystoid macular oedema in ocular surgery.*

**Loesfer** Pharmacia, Switz.
Ferrous gluconate (p.1428·1).
Ascorbic acid (p.1460·2) is included in this preparation to increase the absorption and availability of iron.
*Iron deficiency; iron-deficiency anaemia.*

**Loesfer + acide folique** Searle, Switz.†.
Ferrous gluconate (p.1428·1); folic acid (p.1429·1).
Ascorbic acid (p.1460·2) is included in this preparation to increase the absorption and availability of iron.
*Folic acid deficiency; iron deficiency; iron-deficiency anaemia.*

**Loestrin**
Galen, UK; Warner Chilcott, USA.
Norethisterone acetate (p.1562·2); ethinylestradiol (p.1553·2).
*Combined oral contraceptive.*

**Loestrin 1.5/30** Pfizer, Canad.
Norethisterone acetate (p.1562·2); ethinylestradiol (p.1553·2).
*Combined oral contraceptive.*

**Loestrin Fe** Warner Chilcott, USA.
21 Tablets, norethisterone acetate (p.1562·2); ethinylestradiol (p.1553·2); 7 tablets, ferrous fumarate (p.1427·3).
*Combined oral contraceptive.*

**Loette**
Wyeth, Austral.; Wyeth Lederle, Austria; Wyeth, Chile; Wyeth Lederle, Ital.; Wyeth, Malaysia; Wyeth, NZ; Wyeth, S.Afr.; Wyeth, Singapore; Wyeth, Spain.
Levonorgestrel (p.1563·2); ethinylestradiol (p.1553·2).
28-Day packs also contain 7 inert tablets.
*Combined oral contraceptive.*

**Loexom** IQFA, Mex.
Ambroxol (p.1114·3).
*Respiratory-tract congestion.*

**Lofacol** Dexa, Hong Kong.
Lovastatin (p.949·1).
*Hypercholesterolaemia.*

**Lofenac** Chew, Thai.
Diclofenac diethylamine (p.32·1).
*Musculoskeletal, joint, and peri-articular disorders.*

**Lofenalac**
Mead Johnson, Austral.; Bristol-Myers Squibb, Belg.†; Mead Johnson Nutritionals, Canad.; Mead Johnson, Fr.; Mead Johnson, Irl.; Mead Johnson, Israel; Mead Johnson, Ital.; Mead Johnson, NZ†; Mead Johnson, Port.†; Mead Johnson Nutritionals, Thai.; Mead Johnson Nutritionals, UK†.
Food for special diets (p.1417·1).
*Phenylketonuria.*

**Lofenoxal** Pharmacia, Austral.
Diphenoxylate hydrochloride (p.1261·3).
Atropine sulfate (p.477·1) is included in this preparation to discourage abuse.
*Diarrhoea.*

**Lofensaid** Trinity, UK.
Diclofenac sodium (p.32·1).
*Inflammation; musculoskeletal, joint, and peri-articular disorders; pain.*

**Lofibra** Gate, USA.
Fenofibrate (p.915·2).
*Hyperlipidaemias.*

**Lofoxin** *Locatelli, Ital.†*
Fosfomycin calcium (p.214·2).
*Bacterial infections.*

**Loftan** *GlaxoSmithKline, Ger.*
Salbutamol sulfate (p.791·3).
*Obstructive airways disease.*

**Lofton**
*Abbott, Arg.; Abbott, Spain.*
Buflomedil hydrochloride (p.877·2).
*Cerebral and peripheral vascular disorders.*

**Loftyl**
*Abbott, Austria; Abbott, Belg.; Abbott, Chile; Abbott, Fr.; Abbott, Ital.; Abbott, Mex.; Abbott, Neth.; Abbott, Port.; Abbott, S.Afr.; Abbott, Switz.*
Buflomedil hydrochloride (p.877·2).
*Cerebral and peripheral vascular disorders.*

**Logacron** *Inexfa, Spain†.*
Merbromin (p.1185·3).
*Wound disinfection.*

**Logan** *Ist. Chim. Inter., Ital.*
Citicoline sodium (p.1672·3).
*Arteriosclerosis; cerebral vascular disorders; parkinsonism.*

**Logascid** *AstraZeneca, India.*
Aluminium hydroxide (p.1249·2); magnesium hydroxide (p.1272·2); simeticone (p.1289·2).
*Gastrointestinal hyperacidity; peptic ulcer.*

**Logastin** *Osoth, Thai.*
Simeticone (p.1289·2).
*Flatulence.*

**Logastric** *AstraZeneca, Belg.*
Omeprazole (p.1278·2) or omeprazole magnesium (p.1278·2).
*Gastro-oesophageal reflux; peptic ulcer; Zollinger-Ellison syndrome.*

**Logat** *Libbs, Braz.*
Ranitidine hydrochloride (p.1285·2).
*Acid aspiration; gastro-oesophageal reflux; gastrointestinal haemorrhage; peptic ulcer; Zollinger-Ellison syndrome.*

**Logecine** *Genopharm, Fr.†.*
Erythromycin (p.208·1).
*Bacterial infections.*

**Logen** *Goldline, USA.*
Diphenoxylate hydrochloride (p.1261·3).
Atropine sulfate (p.477·1) is included in this preparation to discourage abuse.
*Diarrhoea.*

**Logesic** *Carter-Wallace, Mex.†.*
Diclofenac sodium (p.32·1).
*Gout; inflammation; musculoskeletal, joint, and soft-tissue disorders; pain.*

**Logical**
*Note. This name is used for preparations of different composition.*
*Armstrong, Arg.*
Magnesium valproate (p.382·2) or sodium valproate (p.380·1).
*Epilepsy.*

*Recalcine, Chile.*
Vitamin E; ascorbic acid; ubidecarenone (p.1417·1).
*Antioxidant preparation.*

*Serum Institute, India.*
Calcium carbonate (p.1254·2); lysine hydrochloride (p.1439·2); vitamin D (p.1461·2).
*Calcium supplement.*

*Armstrong, Mex.*
Crospovidone (p.1581·2).
*Diarrhoea.*

**Logican** *Win-Medicare, India.*
Fluconazole (p.398·1).
*Fungal infections.*

**Logicin Chest Rub** *Sigma, Austral.*
Menthol (p.1711·3); camphor (p.1665·3); eucalyptus oil (p.1686·2).
*Nasal congestion.*

**Logicin Cough & Cold** *Sigma, Austral.†.*
Codeine phosphate (p.27·1); paracetamol (p.76·2); pseudoephedrine hydrochloride (p.1129·2).
*Cold and influenza symptoms.*

**Logicin Cough Mixture for Congested Chesty Coughs**
*Sigma, Austral.; Sigma, Hong Kong.*
Guaifenesin (p.1122·1); pseudoephedrine hydrochloride (p.1129·2).
*Coughs; nasal congestion.*

**Logicin Cough Mixture for Dry Coughs**
*Sigma, Austral.; Sigma, Hong Kong.*
Dextromethorphan hydrobromide (p.1117·3); pseudoephedrine hydrochloride (p.1129·2).
*Coughs; nasal congestion.*

**Logicin Cough Suppressant** *Sigma, Austral.†.*
Pholcodine (p.1128·3).
*Coughs.*

**Logicin Expectorant** *Sigma, Austral.*
Bromhexine bromide (p.1115·3); guaifenesin (p.1122·1).
*Coughs and cold symptoms.*

**Logicin Flu Strength**
*Sigma, Austral.; Sigma, Hong Kong.*
Paracetamol (p.76·2); pseudoephedrine hydrochloride (p.1129·2); dextromethorphan hydrobromide (p.1117·3).
*Cold and influenza symptoms.*

**Logicin Flu Strength Day & Night**
*Sigma, Austral.; Sigma, Hong Kong.*
Day-time tablets, paracetamol (p.76·2); pseudoephedrine hydrochloride (p.1129·2); dextromethorphan hydrobromide (p.1117·3); night-time tablets, paracetamol; pseudoephedrine hydrochloride; chlorphenamine maleate (p.427·3).
*Cold and influenza symptoms.*

**Logicin Hay Fever** *Sigma, Austral.*
Paracetamol (p.76·2); pseudoephedrine hydrochloride (p.1129·2); chlorphenamine maleate (p.427·3).
*Hay fever.*

**Logicin Junior Childrens Cough Mixture**
*Sigma, Austral.; Sigma, Hong Kong.*
Dextromethorphan hydrobromide (p.1117·3); pseudoephedrine hydrochloride (p.1129·2).
*Coughs; nasal congestion.*

**Logicin Natural Lozenges** *Sigma, Austral.*
Zinc gluconate (p.1469·2); echinacea (p.1683·2); vitamin C (p.1460·2); honey (p.1434·2).

**Logicin Rapid Relief**
*Note. This name is used for preparations of different composition.*
*Sigma, Austral.; Sigma, Hong Kong.*
*Lozenges:* Lidocaine hydrochloride (p.1377·3); benzydamine hydrochloride (p.21·1); dichlorobenzyl alcohol (p.1178·3).
*Mouth and throat disorders.*

*Sigma, Austral.; Sigma, Hong Kong.*
*Nasal spray:* Oxymetazoline hydrochloride (p.1126·1).
*Nasal congestion.*

**Logicin Sinus**
*Sigma, Austral.; Sigma, Hong Kong.*
Pseudoephedrine hydrochloride (p.1129·2).
*Upper respiratory-tract congestion.*

**Logicin Sore Throat** *Sigma, Austral.*
Povidone-iodine (p.1190·3).
*Sore throat.*

**Logiflox** *Pharmacia, Fr.*
Lomefloxacin hydrochloride (p.227·2).
*Cystitis in women.*

**Logimat** *AstraZeneca, Belg.*
Felodipine (p.914·3); metoprolol succinate (p.957·1).
*Hypertension.*

**Logimax**
*AstraZeneca, Austria; AstraZeneca, Denm.; AstraZeneca, Fin.; Astra-Zeneca, Fr.; Astra, Israel; Astra, Mex.; AstraZeneca, Neth.; Astra, Norw.†; Lailan, Spain; Hassle, Swed.; AstraZeneca, Switz.*
Felodipine (p.914·3); metoprolol succinate (p.957·1).
*Hypertension.*

*AstraZeneca, Hong Kong.*
Felodipine (p.914·3); metoprolol tartrate (p.957·1).
*Hypertension.*

**Logiparin** *Novo Nordisk, Austria†.*
Tinzaparin sodium (p.1013·1).
*Thrombosis prophylaxis.*

**Logirene** *Pharmacia, Fr.*
Furosemide (p.919·3); amiloride hydrochloride (p.858·2).
*Heart failure.*

**Logoderm**
*Schering-Plough, Austral.; Essex, Chile; Schering-Plough, Mex.; Schering-Plough, NZ.*
Alclometasone dipropionate (p.1090·3).
*Skin disorders.*

**Logradin** *SP, Spain†.*
Loratadine (p.436·1); pseudoephedrine sulfate (p.1129·2).
*Allergic rhinitis.*

**Logrosal** *Silesia, Chile.*
Triflusal (p.1017·3).
*Thromboembolic disorders.*

**Logroton**
*Novartis, Belg.; Novartis, Fr.; Novartis, Malaysia; Novartis, Neth.†; Novartis, Switz.*
Metoprolol tartrate (p.957·1); chlortalidone (p.882·3).
*Hypertension.*

**Logryx** *Wyeth Lederle, Fr.†.*
Minocycline hydrochloride (p.231·3).
*Bacterial infections.*

**Logynon**
*Schering, Irl.; Schering, Israel; Schering, UK.*
Levonorgestrel (p.1563·2); ethinylestradiol (p.1553·2).
28-Day packs also contain 7 inert tablets.
*Triphasic oral contraceptive.*

**Logynon ED**
*Schering, Austral.; Schering, S.Afr.*
21 Tablets, levonorgestrel (p.1563·2); ethinylestradiol (p.1553·2); 7 tablets, inert.
*Menstrual disorders; triphasic oral contraceptive.*

**Lohp** *Ingens, Arg.*
Cystine (p.1426·3); pyridoxine hydrochloride (p.1456·3).
*Skin, nail, and eye disorders.*

**Loisan** *Baliarda, Arg.*
Loratadine (p.436·1).
*Allergic disorders of the respiratory tract; allergic skin disorders; conjunctivitis.*

**Loisan-D** *Baliarda, Arg.*
Loratadine (p.436·1); pseudoephedrine (p.1129·2).
*Conjunctivitis; respiratory-tract disorders.*

**Loitin** *Vita, Spain.*
Fluconazole (p.398·1).
*Fungal infections.*

**Lokalicid** *Dermapharm, Ger.†.*
Clotrimazole (p.396·2).
*Fungal skin infections.*

**Lokalison-antimikrobiell Creme N** *Dermapharm, Ger.*
Dexamethasone (p.1097·1); neomycin sulfate (p.235·1); nystatin (p.406·3).
*Infected skin disorders.*

**LoKara** *PharmaDerm, USA.*
Desonide (p.1096·3).
*Skin disorders.*

**Lokilan** *Roche, Norw.*
Flunisolide (p.1101·1).
*Rhinitis.*

**Lokilan Nasal** *Roche, Swed.†.*
Flunisolide (p.1101·1).
*Allergic rhinitis.*

**Lomabronchin N** *Lomapharm, Ger.*
Homoeopathic preparation.

**Lomac**
*Cipla, India; Cipla, Thai.*
Omeprazole (p.1278·2).
*Gastro-oesophageal reflux; peptic ulcer; Zollinger-Ellison syndrome.*

**Lomacin** *Novartis, Mex.*
Lomefloxacin hydrochloride (p.227·2).
*Bacterial eye infections.*

**Lomadryl** *Chrispa (Χρισπα), Gr.*
Ranitidine hydrochloride (p.1285·2).
*Conditions where gastric acid reduction is beneficial; gastric hypersecretion including Zollinger-Ellison syndrome; peptic ulcer.*

**Lomaherpan**
*Madaus, Austria; Lomapharm, Ger.*
Melissa (p.1711·1).
*Herpesvirus infections of the skin and mucous membranes.*

**Lomahypericum**
*Lomapharm, Ger.; Lomapharm, Singapore†.*
Hypericum (p.299·1).
Formerly known as Lophakomp-Hypericum in *Ger.*
*Anxiety; depression.*

**Lomal** *Lomapharm, Ger.*
Thyme (p.1755·2); drosera (p.1683·1).
*Coughs and cold symptoms.*

**Lomar** *Aegis, Hong Kong.*
Lovastatin (p.949·1).
*Atherosclerosis; hypercholesterolaemia.*

**Lomarheumin N** *Lomapharm, Ger.*
Homoeopathic preparation.

**Lomarin** *Geymonat, Ital.*
Dimenhydrinate (p.431·1).
*Nausea; vertigo; vomiting.*

**Lomasatin M** *Lomapharm, Ger.†.*
Myrrh (p.1718·3).
*Mouth and throat inflammation.*

**Lomasleep** *Lomapharm, Ger.*
Valerian (p.1762·2); lupulus (p.1708·1).
*Agitation; sleep disorders.*

**Lomatol** *Lomapharm, Ger.*
*Oral drops:* Peppermint leaf (p.1283·2); fennel (p.1687·2); caraway (p.1667·2); absinthium (p.1645·1).
*Tablets:* Absinthium (p.1645·1); caraway (p.1667·2); peppermint leaf (p.1283·2); caraway oil (p.1667·3); peppermint oil (p.1283·2).
*Gastrointestinal disorders.*

**Lomatuell H** *Lohmann, Ital.*
White soft paraffin (p.1479·3).
*Wound dressing.*

**Lomax** *Julphar, UAE.*
Lomefloxacin hydrochloride (p.227·2).
*Bacterial infections.*

**Lomazell forte N** *Lomapharm, Ger.*
Benzyl nicotinate (p.21·2); nonivamide (p.67·2); bovine placental extract.
*Circulatory disorders of the skin.*

**Lombalgina** *Neo Quimica, Braz.*
Ibuprofen (p.45·3).
*Fever; inflammation; pain.*

**Lombriareu** *Areu, Spain.*
Pyrantel embonate (p.113·2).
*Worm infections.*

**Lombrimade** *Esfar, Port.*
Piperazine (p.111·2).

**Lomef** *Torrent, India.*
Lomefloxacin hydrochloride (p.227·2).
*Bacterial infections.*

**Lomeflon** *Senju, Jpn.*
Lomefloxacin hydrochloride (p.227·2).
*Bacterial eye and ear infections.*

**Lomepral** *Pharmacia, Braz.*
Omeprazole (p.1278·2).
*Peptic ulcer.*

**Lomesone** *Schering-Plough, Gr.*
Alclometasone dipropionate (p.1090·3).
*Topical corticosteroid.*

**Lomex** *Saval, Chile.*
Omeprazole (p.1278·2) or omeprazole sodium (p.1278·2).
*Acid aspiration; gastro-oesophageal reflux; gastrointestinal haemorrhage; peptic ulcer; Zollinger-Ellison syndrome.*

**Lomexin**
*Elea, Arg.; Gerot, Austria; Altana, Braz.; Effik, Fr.; S & K, Ger.; Organon Teknika (Οργανον Τεχνικα), Gr.; Recordati, Ital.; Aspen, S.Afr.; MD, Singapore; Recordati, Spain; Akita, UK.*
Fenticonazole nitrate (p.397·3).
*Fungal skin and nail infections; vulvovaginal candidiasis.*

**Lomfer** *Osorio de Moraes, Braz.*
Ferrous sulfate (p.1428·2).
*Iron-deficiency anaemia.*

**Lomflox**
*Ipca, India; IPCA, Singapore.*
Lomefloxacin hydrochloride (p.227·2).
*Bacterial infections.*

**Lomide**
*Note. This name is used for preparations of different composition.*
*Alcon, Austral.; Alcon, Austria; Alcon, NZ.*
Lodoxamide trometamol (p.1707·3).
*Allergic conjunctivitis; vernal keratoconjunctivitis.*

*Siam Bheasach, Thai.*
Loperamide hydrochloride (p.1271·1).
*Diarrhoea.*

**Lomine** *Riva, Canad.*
Dicycloverine hydrochloride (p.481·2).
*Smooth muscle spasm.*

**Lomir**
*Novartis, Austria; Novartis, Belg.; Novartis, Braz.; Novartis, Denm.; Novartis, Fin.; Novartis, Ger.; Novartis, Gr.; Novartis, Ital.; Novartis, Neth.; Novartis, Norw.; Novartis, Port.; Mizar, Spain; Novartis, Swed.; Novartis, Switz.*
Isradipine (p.942·2).
*Hypertension.*

**Lomofen** *RPG, India.*
Diphenoxylate hydrochloride (p.1261·3); furazolidone (p.605·2).
Atropine sulfate (p.477·1) is included in this preparation to discourage abuse.
*Bacterial diarrhoea.*

**Lomont** *Rosemont, UK†.*
Lofepramine hydrochloride (p.305·3).
*Depression.*

**Lomotil**
*Pharmacia, Austral.; Pharmacia, Braz.; Pharmacia, Canad.; Pharmacia, Hong Kong; RPG, India; Goldshield, Irl.; Pharmacia, Malaysia; Searle, Mex.; Pharmacia, NZ; Monsanto, Port.; Pharmacia, S.Afr.; Pharmacia, Singapore; Pharmacia, Thai.; Goldshield, UK; Searle, USA.*
Diphenoxylate hydrochloride (p.1261·3).
Atropine sulfate (p.477·1) is included in this preparation to discourage abuse.
These ingredients can be described by the British Approved Name Co-phenotrope.
*Diarrhoea; ostomy management; ulcerative colitis.*

**Lomper** *Esteve, Spain.*
Mebendazole (p.108·2).
*Worm infections.*

**Lomprax** *Mintlab, Chile.*
Dimeticones (p.1482·1).
*Flatulence.*

**Lomudal**
*Aventis, Belg.; Aventis, Denm.; Aventis, Fin.; Aventis, Fr.; Aventis, Gr.; Fisons, Israel; Aventis, Ital.; Aventis, Neth.; Aventis, Norw.; Aventis, S.Afr.†; Aventis, Swed.; Aventis, Switz.*
Sodium cromoglicate (p.795·3).
*Allergic conjunctivitis; allergic rhinitis; asthma; bronchial hypersensitivity; food hypersensitivity; inflammatory bowel disease.*

**Lomupren** *Aventis, Ger.*
Sodium cromoglicate (p.795·3).
*Allergic rhinitis.*

**Lomupren compositum** *Aventis, Ger.*
Sodium cromoglicate (p.795·3); xylometazoline hydrochloride (p.1132·2).
*Allergic rhinitis.*

**Lomusol**
*Sigmapharm, Austria; Aventis, Belg.; Aventis, Fr.; Aventis, Neth.; Aventis, Switz.*
Sodium cromoglicate (p.795·3).
*Allergic conjunctivitis; allergic rhinitis.*

**Lomusol plus Xylometazoline** *Aventis, Belg.†.*
Sodium cromoglicate (p.795·3); xylometazoline hydrochloride (p.1132·2).
*Allergic rhinitis; nasal congestion.*

**Lomusol-X** *Aventis, Switz.*
Sodium cromoglicate (p.795·3); xylometazoline hydrochloride (p.1132·2).
*Allergic rhinitis; nasal congestion.*

**Lomuspray** *Aventis, Ital.*
Sodium cromoglicate (p.795·3).
*Asthma.*

**Lomy** *Masa, Thai.*
Loperamide hydrochloride (p.1271·1).
*Diarrhoea.*

**Lonactene** *Ferring, UK†.*
Carbetocin (p.1320·2).
*Postpartum haemorrhage; postpartum uterine atony.*

**Lonaflam** *Merck, Braz.*
Meloxicam (p.56·1).
*Inflammation; musculoskeletal and joint disorders; pain.*

**Lonalac** *Mead Johnson Nutritionals, USA.*
Preparation for enteral nutrition (p.1417·1).

**Lonalgal** *Boehringer Ingelheim, Gr.*
Codeine phosphate (p.27·1); paracetamol (p.76·2).
*Pain.*

**Lonarid**
*Boehringer Ingelheim, Ger.; Boehringer Ingelheim, Ital.*
Paracetamol (p.76·2); codeine phosphate (p.27·1).
*Pain.*

**Lonarid Aplo** *Boehringer Ingelheim, Gr.*
Paracetamol (p.76·2).
*Fever; pain.*

**Lonarid Mono** *Boehringer Ingelheim, Belg.†.*
Paracetamol (p.76·2).
*Fever; pain.*

**Lonarid N**
*Note. A similar name is used for preparations of different composition*

(see below).
Boehringer Ingelheim, Belg.
Paracetamol (p.76·2); caffeine (p.782·1).
Formerly contained paracetamol, caffeine, and codeine phosphate.
*Pain.*

**Lonarid-N**
Note. A similar name is used for preparations of different composition (see above).
Boehringer Ingelheim, Gr.
Codeine phosphate (p.27·1); paracetamol (p.76·2); caffeine (p.1417·1).
*Pain.*

**Lonavar** CSL, Austral.†; Biotechnology, Israel.
Oxandrolone (p.1565·1).
*Anabolic; growth failure in boys.*

**Loncord** Diffucap, Braz.
Nifedipine (p.966·2).
*Angina pectoris; hypertension.*

**Londerm-N** Kinder, Braz.
Triamcinolone acetonide (p.1110·2); gramicidin (p.220·2); nystatin (p.406·3); neomycin sulfate (p.235·1).
*Infected skin disorders.*

**London Drugs Dark Tanning** Tanning Research, Canad.†.
*SPF 4:* Meradimate (p.1151·3); octinoxate (p.1154·3).
*Sunscreen.*

**London Drugs Kids Sunblock** Tanning Research, Canad.†.
*SPF 30:* Octinoxate (p.1154·3); homosalate (p.1148·1); octisalate (p.1154·3); oxybenzone (p.1154·3).
Formerly known as London Drugs Baby Sunblock.
*Sunscreen.*

**London Drugs Sport** Tanning Research, Canad.†.
*SPF 15:* Octinoxate (p.1154·3); oxybenzone (p.1154·3).
*SPF 30:* Octinoxate (p.1154·3); octisalate (p.1154·3); oxybenzone (p.1154·3).
*Sunscreen.*

**London Drugs Sunblock** Tanning Research, Canad.†.
*SPF 15:* Octinoxate (p.1154·3); oxybenzone (p.1154·3).
*SPF 30:* Octinoxate (p.1154·3); homosalate (p.1148·1); octisalate (p.1154·3); oxybenzone (p.1154·3).
*Sunscreen.*

**London Drugs Sunscreen** Tanning Research, Canad.†.
*SPF 8:* Octinoxate (p.1154·3); oxybenzone (p.1154·3).
*Sunscreen.*

**Lonestin** Rayere, Mex.
Clotrimazole (p.396·2).
*Fungal skin infections.*

**Long Lasting Nasal Mist** Stanley, Canad.
Oxymetazoline hydrochloride (p.1126·1).

**Longachin** Teofarma, Ital.
Quinidine arabogalactane sulfate (p.993·2).
*Arrhythmias.*

**Longacilin** Biolab Sanus, Braz.
Benzathine benzylpenicillin (p.162·3).
*Bacterial infections.*

**Longacor**
Procter & Gamble, Fr.†; Rovi, Spain; Elaiapharm, Switz.
Quinidine arabogalactane sulfate (p.993·2).
*Arrhythmias.*

**Longactil** Cristalia, Braz.
Chlorpromazine hydrochloride (p.675·2).
*Psychoses.*

**Longalgic** Evans, Fr.†.
Benorilate (p.20·3).
*Pain.*

**Longastatina** Italfarmaco, Ital.
Octreotide (p.1333·3).
*Acromegaly; diarrhoea associated with immunodeficiency; gastrointestinal endocrine tumours; gastrointestinal haemorrhage; pancreatic disorders.*

**Longasteril 40** Fresenius Kabi, Ger.
Dextran 40 (p.745·3) in glucose or sodium chloride.
*Plasma volume expansion; thrombosis prophylaxis; vascular disorders.*

**Longasteril 70** Fresenius Kabi, Ger.
Dextran 70 (p.746·2) with electrolytes.
*Plasma volume expansion; thrombosis prophylaxis.*

**Longatren** Bayer, Austria.
Azidocillin sodium (p.159·1).
*Bacterial infections.*

**Longazem** De Salute, Ital.
Diltiazem hydrochloride (p.900·1).
*Angina pectoris; hypertension.*

**Longbalsem** Wolfs, Belg.
Ethylmorphine hydrochloride (p.37·3); guaifenesin (p.1122·1).
*Coughs.*

**Longevit** Hexal, Braz.
Vitamin B substances; vitamin E; arginine aspartate (p.1417·1).

**Longevit Plus** Hexal, Braz.
Ginseng; erythroxylon catuaba; ptychopetalum uncinatum; vitamins (p.1417·1).

**Longevital**
Note. This name is used for preparations of different composition.
Bago, Arg.
Procaine; vitamin B substances; prasterone (p.1417·1).
*Mental function impairment.*

Sanitalia, Ital.
Pollen; royal jelly (p.1740·3); rose fruit (p.1740·1); selenium (p.1444·1).
*Nutritional supplement.*

**Longifene**
UCB, Belg.; UCB, Hong Kong; UCB, Malaysia; Covan, S.Afr.; UCB, Singapore.
Buclizine hydrochloride (p.426·3).
*Appetite loss; hypersensitivity reactions; motion sickness; nausea and vomiting.*

**Longimin** Raza, Malaysia; Pharmaniaga, Malaysia.
Buclizine hydrochloride (p.426·3).
*Hypersensitivity reactions; motion sickness; nausea and vomiting.*

**Longivol** Medical, Spain†.
Embryo extract; methyltestosterone; vitamins (p.1417·1); caffeine; calcium magnesium fytate; ethinylestradiol.
*Tonic.*

**Longtussin Duplex Tag und Nacht N** Tussin, Ger.
Day capsules, guaifenesin (p.1122·1); night capsules, codeine (p.27·1).
*Bronchitis; coughs.*

**Longum**
Pharmacia Upjohn, Belg.†; Pharmacia, Ger.
Sulfametopyrazine (p.263·1).
*Bacterial infections; malaria; toxoplasmosis.*

**Lonikan** Merck, Arg.
Fludrocortisone (p.1100·2).
*Corticosteroid.*

**Lonine** Wyeth, Gr.
Etodolac (p.37·3).
*Inflammation; osteoarthritis; pain; rheumatoid arthritis.*

**Loniten**
Pharmacia, Austral.; Pharmacia, Austria; Pharmacia, Braz.; Pharmacia, Canad.; IFET (ΙΦΕΤ), Gr.; Pharmacia, Hong Kong; Pharmacia, Irl.; Pharmacia Upjohn, Ital.; Pharmacia Upjohn, NZ†; Pharmacia, Port.; Pharmacia, S.Afr.; Pharmacia Upjohn, Singapore†; Pharmacia, Spain; Pharmacia, Switz.; Pharmacia, Thai.; Pharmacia, UK; Upjohn, USA.
Minoxidil (p.960·1).
*Alopecia androgenetica; hypertension.*

**Lonnoten**
Pharmacia Upjohn, Belg.†; Pharmacia, Neth.
Minoxidil (p.960·1).
*Hypertension.*

**Lonol**
Note. This name is used for preparations of different composition.
Khandelwal, India.
Atenolol (p.865·2).
*Angina pectoris; hypertension.*

Boehringer Ingelheim Promeco, Mex.
Benzydamine hydrochloride (p.21·1).
*Musculoskeletal, joint and peri-articular disorders.*

Garec, S.Afr.
Allopurinol (p.412·2).
*Gout; hyperuricaemia.*

**Lonol Sport** Boehringer Ingelheim Promeco, Mex.
Benzydamine hydrochloride (p.21·1); methyl salicylate (p.59·3); menthol (p.1711·3).
*Musculoskeletal, joint, peri-articular and soft-tissue disorders.*

**Lonolox** Pharmacia, Ger.
Minoxidil (p.960·1).
*Hypertension.*

**Lonoten** Pharmacia, Fr.
Minoxidil (p.960·1).
*Hypertension.*

**Lonox** Geneva, USA.
Diphenoxylate hydrochloride (p.1261·3).
Atropine sulfate (p.477·1) is included in this preparation to discourage abuse.
*Diarrhoea.*

**Lonseren** Aventis, Spain.
Pipotiazine palmitate (p.716·1).
*Anxiety; psychoses.*

**Lontadex** Lafi, Chile.
Loratadine (p.436·1).
*Hypersensitivity disorders.*

**Lontadex D** Lafi, Chile.
Loratadine (p.436·1); pseudoephedrine (p.1129·2).

**Lonza** Progress, Thai.
Lorazepam (p.704·1).
*Anxiety.*

**Loortan** Therabel, Belg.
Losartan potassium (p.947·2).
*Hypertension.*

**Loortan Plus** Therabel, Belg.
Losartan potassium (p.947·2); hydrochlorothiazide (p.933·2).
*Hypertension.*

**Lo/Ovral** Wyeth-Ayerst, USA.
Norgestrel (p.1563·2); ethinylestradiol (p.1553·2).
28-Day packs also contain 7 inert tablets.
*Combined oral contraceptive.*

**Lopalind** Lindopharm, Ger.
Loperamide hydrochloride (p.1271·1).
*Diarrhoea.*

**Lopamide** Torrent, India.
Loperamide hydrochloride (p.1271·1).
*Diarrhoea.*

**Lopamine** Shiwa, Thai.
Loperamide hydrochloride (p.1271·1).
*Diarrhoea.*

**Lo-P-Caps** ST, Thai.
Calcium acetate (p.1225·1).
*Hyperphosphataemia.*

**Lop-Dia** Philopharm, Ger.
Loperamide hydrochloride (p.1271·1).
*Diarrhoea.*

**Lopediar** Pasteur, Chile.
Loperamide hydrochloride (p.1271·1).
*Diarrhoea.*

**Lopedium**
Hexal, Ger.; Hexal, S.Afr.
Loperamide hydrochloride (p.1271·1).
*Diarrhoea; ileostomy management.*

**Lopela** Pharmasant, Thai.
Loperamide hydrochloride (p.1271·1).
*Diarrhoea.*

**Lopelin** Fumouze, Fr.†.
Loperamide hydrochloride (p.1271·1).
*Diarrhoea.*

**Lopemid** Gentili, Ital.
Loperamide hydrochloride (p.1271·1).
*Diarrhoea; ileostomy management.*

**Lopepham** Phamos, Ger.
Loperamide hydrochloride (p.1271·1).
*Diarrhoea.*

**Loperacap** ICN, Canad.
Loperamide hydrochloride (p.1271·1).

**LoperaGen** Goldshield, UK†.
Loperamide hydrochloride (p.1271·1).
*Diarrhoea.*

**Loperamerck** Merck, Ger.†.
Loperamide hydrochloride (p.1271·1).
*Diarrhoea.*

**Loperamil** DHA, Singapore.
Loperamide hydrochloride (p.1271·1).
*Diarrhoea.*

**Loperan** Chiesi, Spain.
Loperamide hydrochloride (p.1271·1).
*Diarrhoea.*

**Loperastat** Be-Tabs, S.Afr.
Loperamide hydrochloride (p.1271·1).
*Diarrhoea; ostomy management.*

**Loperax** Xepa-Soul Pattinson, Hong Kong.
Loperamide hydrochloride (p.1271·1).
*Diarrhoea.*

**Lopercin** Polipharm, Thai.
Loperamide hydrochloride (p.1271·1).
*Diarrhoea.*

**Loperdium** General Drugs, Thai.
Loperamide hydrochloride (p.1271·1).
*Diarrhoea.*

**Loperhoe** Betapharm, Ger.
Loperamide hydrochloride (p.1271·1).
*Diarrhoea.*

**Loperia** Great Eastern, Thai.; Therapharma, Thai.
Loperamide hydrochloride (p.1271·1).
*Diarrhoea.*

**Loperid** Vitamed, Israel.
Loperamide hydrochloride (p.1271·1).
*Diarrhoea.*

**Loperidol** Medley, Braz.
Haloperidol (p.701·2).
*Autism; Huntington's chorea; nausea and vomiting; psychoses; Tourette's syndrome.*

**Loperium**
Remedica, Hong Kong; Pharbita, Israel; Remedica, Malaysia.
Loperamide hydrochloride (p.1271·1).
*Diarrhoea.*

**Loperkey** Inkeysa, Spain.
Loperamide hydrochloride (p.1271·1).
*Diarrhoea.*

**Lopermide**
Atlantic, Hong Kong; Atlantic, Malaysia; Atlantic, Singapore; Vana, Thai.
Loperamide hydrochloride (p.1271·1).
*Diarrhoea.*

**Loperyl** SmithKline Beecham, Ital.†.
Loperamide hydrochloride (p.1271·1).
*Diarrhoea.*

**Lopetrans** Fresenius-Praxis, Ger.†.
Loperamide hydrochloride (p.1271·1).
*Diarrhoea.*

**Lopex** Leiras, Fin.
Loperamide hydrochloride (p.1271·1).
*Diarrhoea; ileostomy management.*

**Lophakomp-B1** Lomapharm, Ger.†.
Thiamine hydrochloride (p.1455·1).
*Vitamin $B_1$ deficiency.*

**Lophakomp-B6** Lomapharm, Ger.†.
Pyridoxine hydrochloride (p.1456·3).
*Vitamin $B_6$ deficiency.*

**Lophakomp-B 12** Lomapharm, Ger.
Cyanocobalamin (p.1458·2).
*Vitamin $B_{12}$ deficiency.*

**Lophakomp-B 12 Depot** Lomapharm, Ger.
Hydroxocobalamin acetate (p.1458·2).
*Vitamin $B_{12}$ deficiency.*

**Lophakomp-Echinacea H** Lomapharm, Ger.†.
Homoeopathic preparation.

**Lophakomp-Hamamelis H** Lomapharm, Ger.†.
Homoeopathic preparation.

**Lophakomp-Procain N** Lomapharm, Ger.
Procaine hydrochloride (p.1383·2).
*Nervous system disorders.*

**Lopid**
Parke, Davis, Arg.; Pfizer, Austral.; Parke, Davis, Belg.†; Ache, Braz.; Pfizer, Canad.; Parke, Davis, Chile; Pfizer, Denm.; Pfizer, Fin.; Pfizer, Gr.; Warner-Lambert, Gr.; Pfizer, Hong Kong; Parke, Davis, India; Parke, Davis, Irl.; Parke, Davis, Ital.; Pfizer, Malaysia; Parke, Davis, Mex.; Parke, Davis, Neth.; Parke, Davis, NZ†; Pfizer, Port.; Pfizer, S.Afr.; Pfizer, Singapore; Parke, Davis, Spain; Pfizer, Swed.; Pfizer, Thai.; Pfizer, UK; Parke, Davis, USA.
Gemfibrozil (p.923·1).
*Hyperlipidaemias.*

**Lopiden** Royton, Braz.†.
Amlodipine besilate (p.862·1).
*Hypertension.*

**Lopimed** Ecosol, Switz.
Loperamide hydrochloride (p.1271·1).
*Diarrhoea.*

**Lopiretic** Bristol-Myers Squibb, Port.
Captopril (p.879·2); hydrochlorothiazide (p.933·2).
*Hypertension.*

**Lopirin**
Bristol-Myers Squibb, Austria; Bristol-Myers Squibb, Ger.; Bristol-Myers Squibb, Switz.
Captopril (p.879·2).
*Diabetic nephropathy; heart failure; hypertension; myocardial infarction.*

**Lopitrex** Bristol-Myers Squibb, Hong Kong†.
Cefapirin sodium (p.170·2).
*Bacterial infections.*

**Loporic** M & H, Thai.
Allopurinol (p.412·2).
*Gout; hyperuricaemia; renal calculi; uric acid nephropathy.*

**Loprazol** Teuto, Braz.
Omeprazole (p.1278·2).
*Peptic ulcer.*

**Lopresor**
Novartis, Arg.
Metoprolol (p.956·3).
*Hypertension.*

Novartis, Austral.; AstraZeneca, Austria; Novartis, Belg.; Novartis, Canad.; Novartis, Ger.; Novartis, Gr.; Novartis, Irl.; Novartis, Israel; Novartis, Ital.; Novartis, Mex.; Novartis, Neth.; Novartis, NZ.; Novartis, Port.; Novartis, S.Afr.; Novartis, Spain; Novartis, Switz.; Novartis, UK.
Metoprolol fumarate (p.956·3) or metoprolol tartrate (p.957·1).
*Angina pectoris; arrhythmias; hypertension; hyperthyroidism; migraine; myocardial infarction.*

**Lopress** Siam Bheasach, Thai.
Prazosin hydrochloride (p.985·1).
*Hypertension.*

**Lopressor**
Novartis, Braz.; Novartis, Fr.; Novartis, USA.
Metoprolol tartrate (p.957·1).
*Angina pectoris; arrhythmias; cardiomyopathies; hypertension; migraine and other vascular headache; myocardial infarction; neuroleptic-induced akathisia; prolapsed mitral valve; tremor.*

**Lopressor HCT** Novartis, USA.
Metoprolol tartrate (p.957·1); hydrochlorothiazide (p.933·2).
*Hypertension.*

**Lopril**
Note. This name is used for preparations of different composition.
Bristol-Myers Squibb, Braz.
Captopril (p.879·2); hydrochlorothiazide (p.933·2).
*Heart failure; hypertension.*

Orion, Fin.; Bristol-Myers Squibb, Fr.
Captopril (p.879·2).
*Diabetic nephropathy; heart failure; hypertension; myocardial infarction.*

**Loproc** Norma (Νορμα), Gr.
Omeprazole (p.1278·2).
*Acid aspiration; eradication of Helicobacter pylori in combination with antimicrobials; peptic ulcer; reflux oesophagitis; Zollinger-Ellison syndrome.*

**Loprofin**
SHS, Fr.; Scientific Hospital Supplies, Irl.; Nutricia, Ital.; Nutricia, NZScientific Hospital Supplies, UK.
A range of gluten-free, low protein foods for special diets (p.1417·1).
*Phenylketonuria; protein restriction.*

**Loprox**
Aventis, Arg.; Aventis, Braz.; Dermik, Canad.; Aventis, Mex.; Biphar-ma, Neth.; Aventis, Thai.; Medicis, USA.
Ciclopirox (p.396·1) or ciclopirox olamine (p.396·1).
*Fungal skin and nail infections.*

**Loptomit** Bournonville, Neth.†.
Timolol maleate (p.1012·2).
*Glaucoma; raised intra-ocular pressure.*

**Lopurax** Sanval, Braz.
Allopurinol (p.412·2).
*Gout.*

**Lora**
Note. This name is used for preparations of different composition.
Basics, Ger.; Phoinix Pharm (Φοινιξ Φαρμ), Gr.
Loratadine (p.436·1).
*Allergic conjunctivitis; allergic rhinitis; atopic eczema; urticaria.*

Atlantic, Thai.; PP Lab, Thai.
Lorazepam (p.704·1).
*Anxiety; insomnia.*

**Lorabenz** Norton Healthcare, Denm.
Lorazepam (p.704·1).
*Anxiety.*

**Lorabid**
Lilly, Austria†; Lilly, Hong Kong†; Lilly, Mex.; Lilly, S.Afr.; Lilly, Swed.; Monarch, USA.
Loracarbef (p.228·1).
*Bacterial infections.*

**Loraclar** Krewel, Ger.
Loratadine (p.436·1).
*Allergic conjunctivitis; allergic rhinitis; atopic eczema; urticaria.*

**Loradine** Teuto, Braz.
Loratadine (p.436·1).
*Hypersensitivity reactions.*

**Loradur** Ratiopharm, Austria.
Amiloride hydrochloride (p.858·2); hydrochlorothiazide (p.933·2).
*Ascites; hypertension; oedema.*

**Lorafem** Zambon, Ger.
Loracarbef (p.228·1).
*Bacterial infections.*

**Loraga**
Note. This name is used for preparations of different composition.
Parke, Davis, Braz.†.
Psyllium (p.1268·1).
*Constipation.*

Pfizer, Fin.; Parke, Davis, Swed.
Lactulose (p.1269·1).
*Constipation; hepatic encephalopathy.*

**Loragalen** Galen, Ger.
Loratadine (p.436·1).
*Allergic conjunctivitis; allergic rhinitis; atopic eczema; urticaria.*

**Loragamma** Worwag, Ger.
Loratadine (p.436·1).
*Allergic conjunctivitis; allergic rhinitis; urticaria.*

**Loralerg** Farmasa, Braz.
Loratadine (p.436·1).
*Hypersensitivity reactions.*

**Loralerg-D** Farmasa, Braz.
Loratadine (p.436·1); pseudoephedrine hydrochloride (p.1129·2).
*Nasal congestion.*

**Lora-Lich** Lichtenstein, Ger.
Loratadine (p.436·1).
*Allergic conjunctivitis; allergic rhinitis; urticaria.*

**Loramed** Medifive, Thai.
Lorazepam (p.704·1).
*Anxiety; insomnia.*

**Loramet**
Wyeth Lederle, Belg.; Wyeth, Gr.; Wyeth, Hong Kong; Wyeth, Irl.†; Wyeth, Neth.; Akromed, S.Afr.; Wyeth, Singapore; Wyeth, Spain; ICN, Switz.; Wyeth-Ayerst, Thai.
Lormetazepam (p.705·2).
*Insomnia; premedication.*

**Loramide**
YSP, Malaysia; Yung Shin, Singapore.
Loperamide hydrochloride (p.1271·1).
*Diarrhoea.*

**Loranil** Libbs, Braz.
Loratadine (p.436·1).
*Hypersensitivity reactions.*

**Loranil D** Libbs, Braz.
Loratadine (p.436·1); pseudoephedrine sulfate (p.1129·2).
*Nasal congestion.*

**Lorano** Hexal, Ger.
Loratadine (p.436·1).
*Allergic conjunctivitis; allergic rhinitis; urticaria.*

**Loranox** Charoen, Thai.
Loratadine (p.436·1).
*Allergic rhinitis; allergic skin disorders.*

**Lorans**
Medochemie, Hong Kong; Schwarz, Ital.; Medochemie, Malaysia; Medochemie, Singapore†.
Lorazepam (p.704·1).
*Anxiety; insomnia.*

**Lorapam**
Pacific, NZ; Siam Bheasach, Thai.
Lorazepam (p.704·1).
*Anxiety; insomnia; premedication.*

**Lora-Puren** Alpharma-Isis, Ger.
Loratadine (p.436·1).
*Allergic conjunctivitis; allergic rhinitis; atopic eczema; urticaria.*

**Lorasifar** Siphar, Switz.
Lorazepam (p.704·1).
*Anxiety; sedative; sleep disorders.*

**Lorastine** Schering-Plough, Israel.
Loratadine (p.436·1).
*Allergic rhinitis; urticaria.*

**Lorastyne**
Schering-Plough, Austral.; Schering-Plough, Malaysia.
Loratadine (p.436·1).
*Allergic rhinitis; allergic skin disorders; urticaria.*

**Loratab** Zekides, Gr.
Loratadine (p.436·1).
*Allergic rhinitis; pruritus.*

**Lora-Tabs** Pacific, NZ.
Loratadine (p.436·1).
*Allergic rhinitis; allergic skin disorders; urticaria.*

**Loratadura** Merck dura, Ger.
Loratadine (p.436·1).
*Allergic conjunctivitis; allergic rhinitis; atopic eczema; urticaria.*

**Loratamed** Cimed, Braz.
Loratadine (p.436·1).
*Hypersensitivity reactions.*

**Loratin** Julphar, UAE.
Loratadine (p.436·1).
*Allergic conjunctivitis; allergic rhinitis; pruritus; urticaria.*

**Loratyn** Aesca, Austria.
Loratadine (p.436·1).
*Allergic rhinitis; urticaria.*

**Loratyne** Schering-Plough, S.Afr.
Loratadine (p.436·1).
*Allergic rhinitis; urticaria.*

**Lorax**
Note. This name is used for preparations of different composition.
Lilly, Austria†; Lilly, Neth.
Loracarbef (p.228·1).
*Bacterial infections.*

Wyeth, Braz.
Lorazepam (p.704·1).
*Anxiety; premedication.*

**Lorazene** Berlin Pharm, Thai.
Lorazepam (p.704·1).
*Anxiety; epilepsy; muscle relaxation.*

**Lorazep** Asian Pharm, Thai.
Lorazepam (p.704·1).
*Anxiety.*

**Lorazepan** Dovalle, Braz.
Lorazepam (p.704·1).
*Anxiety.*

**Lorbef** Pharmaserve Lilly (Φαρμασερβ Λιλλυ), Gr.
Loracarbef (p.228·1).
*Bacterial infections.*

**Lorbi** Bioquimico, Arg.
Bromhexine (p.1115·3) or bromhexine hydrochloride (p.1115·3).
*Respiratory-tract disorders.*

**Lorcet 10/650** Forest Pharmaceuticals, USA.
Hydrocodone tartrate (p.45·1); paracetamol (p.76·2).
*Pain.*

**Lorcet Plus** Forest Pharmaceuticals, USA.
Hydrocodone tartrate (p.45·1); paracetamol (p.76·2).
*Pain.*

**Lorcet-HD** Forest Pharmaceuticals, USA.
Hydrocodone tartrate (p.45·1); paracetamol (p.76·2).
*Pain.*

**Loremex** Phoenix, Arg.
Loratadine (p.436·1); pseudoephedrine hydrochloride (p.1129·2) or pseudoephedrine sulfate (p.1129·2).
*Allergic rhinitis; cold symptoms; otitis.*

**Loremix** Ativus, Braz.
Loratadine (p.436·1).
*Hypersensitivity reactions.*

**Loremix D** Ativus, Braz.
Loratadine (p.436·1); pseudoephedrine (p.1129·2).
*Nasal congestion.*

**Lorenin** Wyeth Lederle, Port.
Lorazepam (p.704·1).

**Lorentin** Hexal, Austral.
Methylphenidate hydrochloride (p.1590·2).

**Lorenzo's Oil** Scientific Hospital Supplies, UK.
Glycerol trioleate; glycerol trierucate (p.1707·3).
*Adrenoleucodystrophy.*

**Loretam** ICN, Ger.
Lormetazepam (p.705·2).
*Insomnia; premedication.*

**Loretic** Xixia, S.Afr.†.
Triamterene (p.1016·2); hydrochlorothiazide (p.933·2).
*Hypertension; oedema.*

**Lorexen** Loren, Mex.
Naproxen (p.65·1).
*Fever; inflammation; pain.*

**Lorfast** Cadila Pharma, India.
Loratadine (p.436·1).
*Hypersensitivity reactions.*

**Lorfenil** Loren, Mex.
Phenylbutazone (p.83·2).
*Inflammation.*

**Loricin** Sigma-Tau, Ital.
Sulbactam sodium (p.257·2); ampicillin sodium (p.157·1).
Lidocaine hydrochloride (p.1377·3) is included in the intramuscular injection to alleviate the pain of injection.
*Bacterial infections.*

**Loride** Medinfar, Port.
Loperamide hydrochloride (p.1271·1).
*Diarrhoea.*

**Loridem** Sandipro, Belg.
Lorazepam (p.704·1).
*Anxiety; insomnia; premedication.*

**Loriderm** Raza, Malaysia; Pharmaniaga, Malaysia.
Clotrimazole (p.396·2).
*Fungal skin infections.*

**Loridin** Cadila, India.
Loratadine (p.436·1).
*Hypersensitivity reactions.*

**Loridin-D** Cadila, India.
Loratadine (p.436·1); pseudoephedrine (p.1129·2).
*Allergic rhinitis.*

**Lorien** Aspen, S.Afr.
Fluoxetine hydrochloride (p.292·1).
*Bulimia nervosa; depression; obsessive-compulsive disorder.*

**Lorinden T** Medphano, Ger.
Flumetasone pivalate (p.1101·1); coal tar (p.1159·2); salicylic acid (p.1157·1).
*Skin disorders.*

**Lorita** Farmaline, Thai.
Loratadine (p.436·1).
*Allergic skin disorders.*

**Loriter** Elvetium, Arg.
Lovastatin (p.949·1).
*Atherosclerosis; hypercholesterolaemia.*

**Lorityne** LSP, Thai.
Loratadine (p.436·1).
*Allergic rhinitis; allergic skin disorders.*

**Lorium** Ache, Braz.†.
Lorazepam (p.704·1).
*Alcohol withdrawal syndrome; anxiety; epilepsy; insomnia; nausea and vomiting; premedication.*

**Lorivan**
Remedica, Hong Kong; Dexxon, Israel.
Lorazepam (p.704·1).
*Anxiety; insomnia; premedication.*

**Lormine** Northia, Arg.
Dexamethasone (p.1097·1).
*Corticosteroid.*

**Lornazol** Loren, Mex.
Ketoconazole (p.403·3).
*Fungal infections.*

**Lornox** Nycomed, Austria.
Lornoxicam (p.54·2).
*Inflammation; pain.*

**Loron**
Ercopharm, Denm.†; Roche, Irl.; Roche, UK.
Disodium clodronate (p.770·2).
*Hypercalcaemia of malignancy; tumour-induced osteolysis and bone pain.*

**Lorophyn**
Note. This name is used for preparations of different composition.
Key, Arg.
Nonoxinol 9 (p.1413·3); methylbenzethonium chloride (p.1186·1).
*Bacterial vaginal infections; contraceptive.*

Columbia, Mex.
Nonoxinol 9 (p.1413·3).
*Contraception.*

**Loroxide**
Dermik, Canad.†; Summers, USA†.
Benzoyl peroxide (p.1143·2).
*Acne.*

**Lorpa** Beacons, Singapore.
Loperamide (p.1271·2).
*Diarrhoea.*

**Lorsacor** Hexal, Braz.
Losartan potassium (p.947·2).
*Hypertension.*

**Lorsedal** Prospa, Port.
Lorazepam (p.704·1).

**Lorsedin** Siam Bheasach, Thai.
Loratadine (p.436·1).
*Allergic conjunctivitis; allergic rhinitis; allergic skin disorders.*

**Lortaan**
Merck Sharp & Dohme, Ital.; Medinfar, Port.
Losartan potassium (p.947·2).
*Heart failure; hypertension.*

**Lortaan Plus** Medinfar, Port.
Losartan potassium (p.947·2); hydrochlorothiazide (p.933·2).
*Hypertension.*

**Lortab** UCB, USA.
Hydrocodone tartrate (p.45·1); paracetamol (p.76·2).
*Pain.*

**Lortab ASA** UCB, USA.
Hydrocodone tartrate (p.45·1); aspirin (p.15·1).
*Pain.*

**Lortadine** Olan-Kemed, Thai.
Loratadine (p.436·1).
*Allergic rhinitis; allergic skin disorders.*

**Lortuss DM** Proethic, USA.
Brompheniramine maleate (p.426·1); phenylephrine hydrochloride (p.1126·3); dextromethorphan hydrobromide (p.1117·3).
*Upper respiratory-tract disorders.*

**Lortuss HC** Proethic, USA.
Hydrocodone tartrate (p.45·1); phenylephrine hydrochloride (p.1126·3).
*Upper respiratory-tract disorders.*

**Lorvas**
Torrent, India; Torrent, Thai.†.
Indapamide (p.938·2).
*Hypertension.*

**Lorzaar** MSD Chibropharm, Ger.
Losartan potassium (p.947·2).
*Heart failure; hypertension.*

**Lorzaar plus** MSD Chibropharm, Ger.
Losartan potassium (p.947·2); hydrochlorothiazide (p.933·2).
*Hypertension.*

**Lorzem** Douglas, NZ†.
Lorazepam (p.704·1).
*Anxiety.*

**Losacar** Zydus, India.
Losartan potassium (p.947·2).
*Hypertension.*

**Losacar-H** Zydus, India.
Losartan potassium (p.947·2); hydrochlorothiazide (p.933·2).
*Hypertension.*

**Losacor** Roemmers, Arg.
Losartan potassium (p.947·2).
*Hypertension.*

**Losacor D** Roemmers, Arg.
Losartan potassium (p.947·2); hydrochlorothiazide (p.933·2).
*Hypertension.*

**Losalen**
Novartis, Braz.; Novartis, Ital.; Novartis Consumer, Port.; Geminis, Spain.
Flumetasone pivalate (p.1101·1); salicylic acid (p.1157·1).
*Skin disorders.*

**Losamel** Clonmel, Irl.
Omeprazole (p.1278·2).
*Gastro-oesophageal reflux; peptic ulcer; Zollinger-Ellison syndrome.*

**Losan Fe** Hexal, Ger.†.
Ferrous gluconate (p.1428·1).
*Iron deficiency.*

**Losapan** Duopharm, Ger.
Cynara (p.1678·3).
*Dyspepsia.*

**Losapres** Pharma Investi, Chile.
Losartan potassium (p.947·2).
*Heart failure; hypertension.*

**Losapres-D** Pharma Investi, Chile.
Losartan potassium (p.947·2); hydrochlorothiazide (p.933·2).
*Hypertension.*

**Losaprex** Sigma-Tau, Ital.
Losartan potassium (p.947·2).
*Hypertension.*

**Losaprol** Luper, Braz.
Omeprazole (p.1278·2).
*Peptic ulcer.*

**Losar** Biochimico, Braz.; Aurantis, Braz.
Omeprazole (p.1278·2).
*Peptic ulcer.*

**Losartec** Marjan, Braz.
Losartan potassium (p.947·2).
*Hypertension.*

**Losatal** Hebron, Braz.
Losartan potassium (p.947·2).
*Hypertension.*

**Losazid** Sigma-Tau, Ital.
Losartan potassium (p.947·2); hydrochlorothiazide (p.933·2).
*Hypertension.*

**Loscalcon** Lilly, Ger.
Calcium carbonate (p.1254·2).
*Calcium deficiency.*

**Loscon** Galderma, Ger.
Tioxolone (p.1160·3); benzoxonium chloride (p.1170·2).
*Scalp disorders.*

**Losec**
AstraZeneca, Arg.; AstraZeneca, Austral.; AstraZeneca, Austria; AstraZeneca, Belg.; AstraZeneca, Braz.; AstraZeneca, Canad.; AstraZeneca, Chile; AstraZeneca, Denm.; AstraZeneca, Fin.; AstraZeneca, Gr.; AstraZeneca, Hong Kong; AstraZeneca, Irl.; Abic, Israel; AstraZeneca, Ital.; AstraZeneca, Malaysia; AstraZeneca, Mex.; AstraZeneca, Neth.; AstraZeneca, Norw.; AstraZeneca, NZ; AstraZeneca, Port.; AstraZeneca, S.Afr.; AstraZeneca, Singapore; Astra, Spain; Hassle, Swed.; AstraZeneca, Thai.; AstraZeneca, UK.
Omeprazole (p.1278·2), omeprazole magnesium (p.1278·2), or omeprazole sodium (p.1278·2).
*Acid aspiration; dyspepsia; gastro-oesophageal reflux; peptic ulcer; Zollinger-Ellison syndrome.*

**Losec 1-2-3 A** AstraZeneca, Canad.
Omeprazole magnesium (p.1278·2); amoxicillin (p.155·3); clarithromycin (p.192·2).
*Helicobacter pylori-associated peptic ulcer.*

**Losec Helicopak** AstraZeneca, Austral.†.
Tablets, omeprazole magnesium (Losec) (p.1278·2); capsules, amoxicillin trihydrate (Amoxil) (p.155·3); tablets, metronidazole (Flagyl) (p.607·2).
*Peptic ulcer associated with Helicobacter pylori infection.*

**Losec Helira** AstraZeneca, Fin.
Tablets I, metronidazole (p.607·2); tablets II, omeprazole magnesium (Losec) (p.1278·2); tablets III, amoxicillin trihydrate (p.155·3).
*Helicobacter pylori-associated peptic ulcer.*

**Losec Hp 7**
AstraZeneca, Austral.
Tablets, omeprazole magnesium (Losec) (p.1278·2); capsules, amoxicillin trihydrate (Amoxil) (p.155·3); tablets, clarithromycin (Klacid) (p.192·2).
*Helicobacter pylori-associated peptic ulcer.*

AstraZeneca, NZ.
Capsules, omeprazole (p.1278·2); capsules, amoxicillin trihydrate (p.155·3); tablets, clarithromycin (p.192·2).
*Helicobacter pylori-associated peptic ulcer.*

**Losec 1-2-3 M** AstraZeneca, Canad.
Omeprazole magnesium (p.1278·2); metronidazole (p.607·2); clarithromycin (p.192·2).
*Helicobacter pylori-associated peptic ulcer.*

**Losec 20 Triple** *AstraZeneca, S.Afr.*
Capsules, omeprazole (Losec) (p.1278·2); tablets, clarithromycin (Klacid) (p.192·2); capsules, amoxicillin (Moxan) (p.155·3).
*Peptic ulcer associated with Helicobacter pylori infection.*

**Lose.Lax** *Strallhofer, Austria.*
Lactulose (p.1269·1).
*Constipation.*

**Losferron**
*Asta Medica, Austria; Grunenthal, Belg.; Lilly, Ger.; SPA, Ital.; Will-Pharma, Neth.; Prospa, Port.*
Ferrous gluconate (p.1428·1).
Ascorbic acid (p.1460·2) may be included in this preparation to increase the absorption and availability of iron.
*Iron-deficiency; iron-deficiency anaemias.*

**Losferron-Fol** *Asta Medica, Austria.*
Ferrous gluconate (p.1428·1); folic acid (p.1429·1).
Ascorbic acid (p.1460·2) is included in this preparation to increase the absorption and availability of iron.
*Iron and folic acid deficiency anaemias.*

**Losnesium** *Lilly, Ger.*
Magnesium carbonate (p.1272·1); magnesium oxide (p.1272·3).
*Magnesium deficiency.*

**Losopil** *Medipharm, Chile.*
Zopiclone (p.729·3).
*Insomnia.*

**Lostapres** *Temis, Arg.*
Ramipril (p.994·1).
*Hypertension.*

**Lostatin** *Reddy, Singapore.*
Lovastatin (p.949·1).
*Hypercholesterolaemia.*

**Lostradyl** *Chrispa (Χρισπα), Gr.*
Nitrendipine (p.973·3).
*Hypertension.*

**Lotadine** *Jean-Marie, Hong Kong.*
Loratadine (p.436·1).
*Hypersensitivity reactions.*

**Lotem** *Adcock Ingram, S.Afr.*
Ibuprofen (p.45·3); paracetamol (p.76·2).
*Fever; pain.*

**Lotemax**
*Bausch & Lomb, Arg.; Bausch & Lomb, USA.*
Loteprednol etabonate (p.1105·3).
*Eye disorders.*

**Lotemp** *Biolab, Thai.*
Paracetamol (p.76·2).
*Fever; pain.*

**Loten** *Alphapharm, Malaysia; Merck, Malaysia.*
Atenolol (p.865·2).
*Angina pectoris; arrhythmias; hypertension.*

**Lo-Ten**
*Pacific, Hong Kong; Pacific, NZ.*
Atenolol (p.865·2).
*Angina pectoris; arrhythmias; hypertension; myocardial infarction.*

**Lotensin**
*Novartis, Braz.; Novartis, Canad.; Novartis, Mex.; Novartis, USA.*
Benazepril hydrochloride (p.867·2).
*Heart failure; hypertension; renal failure.*

**Lotensin H** *Novartis, Braz.*
Benazepril hydrochloride (p.867·2); hydrochlorothiazide (p.933·2).
*Hypertension.*

**Lotensin HCT** *Novartis, USA.*
Benazepril hydrochloride (p.867·2); hydrochlorothiazide (p.933·2).
*Hypertension.*

**Loteprol** *BL, Braz.†.*
Loteprednol etabonate (p.1105·3).
*Inflammatory eye disorders.*

**Lotesoft** *Poen, Arg.*
Loteprednol etabonate (p.1105·3).
*Inflammatory eye disorders.*

**Lotharin** *Berk, UK†.*
Diphenoxylate hydrochloride (p.1261·3).
Atropine sulfate (p.477·1) is included in this preparation to discourage abuse.
The ingredients in this preparation can be described by the British Approved Name Co-phenotrope.
*Diarrhoea.*

**Lotil** *Fenton, UK.*
Emollient.
*Dry skin.*

**Lotin** *Fustery, Mex.*
Cefalotin (p.169·2).
*Bacterial infections.*

**Lotio decapans** *Widmer, Switz.*
Resorcinol (p.1156·3); salicylic acid (p.1157·1).
*Scalp disorders.*

**Lotio Zinc** *Sam-On, Israel.*
Zinc oxide (p.1163·2).
*Skin irritation.*

**Lotio Zinci** *Floris, Israel.*
Zinc oxide (p.1163·2).
*Skin irritation.*

**Lotioblanc** *Panalab, Arg.*
Tretinoin (p.1161·1).
*Dry skin.*

**Lotion Ecran Solaire Extreme** *Prodemdis, Canad.*
*SPF 30:* Avobenzone (p.1142·3); octinoxate (p.1154·3); oxybenzone (p.1154·3); titanium dioxide (p.1160·3).
*Sunscreen.*

**Lotion pour Feux Sauvages**
*Note. This name is used for preparations of different composition.*
*Atlas, Canad.*
Camphor (p.1665·3); zinc salicylate (p.1157·2).

*Sabex, Canad.*
Benzoin (p.1751·1); camphor (p.1665·3); menthol (p.1711·3); myrrh (p.1718·3).

*Valmo, Canad.†.*
Benzoin (p.1751·1); camphor (p.1665·3); menthol (p.1711·3).

**Lotoquis** *Beta, Arg.*
Phenytoin calcium (p.375·2); phenobarbital (p.367·3).
*Epilepsy.*

**Lotoquis Simple** *Beta, Arg.*
Phenytoin calcium (p.375·2).
*Epilepsy.*

**Lotrel** *Novartis, USA.*
Amlodipine besilate (p.862·1); benazepril hydrochloride (p.867·2).
*Hypertension.*

**Lotremin**
*Schering-Plough, Hong Kong; Schering-Plough, Malaysia; Schering-Plough, Singapore.*
Clotrimazole (p.396·2).
*Fungal skin infections.*

**Lotremine** *Plough, Port.*
Clotrimazole (p.396·2).

**Lotrial**
*Roemmers, Arg.; Pharma Investi, Chile.*
Enalapril (p.909·2) or enalaprilat (p.909·3).
*Heart failure; hypertension.*

**Lotrial D**
*Roemmers, Arg.; Pharma Investi, Chile.*
Enalapril maleate (p.909·2); hydrochlorothiazide (p.933·2).
*Hypertension.*

**Lotricomb**
*Key, Arg.; Essex, Ger.; Schering-Plough, NZ.*
Betamethasone dipropionate (p.1093·1); clotrimazole (p.396·2).
*Skin disorders with fungal infection.*

**Lotriderm**
*Schering-Plough, Belg.; Schering, Canad.; Schering-Plough, Chile; Pliva, Irl.; Schering-Plough, S.Afr.; Dominion, UK†.*
Betamethasone dipropionate (p.1093·1); clotrimazole (p.396·2).
*Skin disorders with fungal infection.*

**Lotrimin**
*Schering-Plough, Mex.; Schering, USA.*
Clotrimazole (p.396·2).
*Fungal skin infections.*

**Lotrimin AF**
*Note. This name is used for preparations of different composition.*
*Schering-Plough, Mex.*
Miconazole nitrate (p.405·3).
*Fungal skin infections.*

*Schering-Plough, USA.*
*Cream; lotion; topical solution:* Clotrimazole (p.396·2).
*Fungal skin infections.*
*Powder; spray:* Miconazole nitrate (p.405·3).

**Lotrimin Ultra** *Schering-Plough, USA.*
Butenafine hydrochloride (p.395·2).
*Fungal skin infections.*

**Lotrisone** *Schering, USA.*
Betamethasone dipropionate (p.1093·1); clotrimazole (p.396·2).
*Fungal skin infections.*

**Lotrix** *Roemmers, Arg.*
Enalapril maleate (p.909·2); diltiazem hydrochloride (p.900·1).
*Hypertension.*

**Lotronex**
*GlaxoSmithKline, Arg.; GlaxoSmithKline, USA.*
Alosetron hydrochloride (p.1248·3).
*Irritable bowel disease in women.*

**Lotusix** *Torlan, Spain†.*
Phenylephrine hydrochloride (p.1126·3); guaifenesin (p.1122·1); co-trimoxazole (p.199·3).
*Respiratory-tract infections.*

**Lotussin** *Pharmacia, S.Afr.*
Diphenhydramine hydrochloride (p.431·3); dextromethorphan hydrobromide (p.1117·3); ephedrine hydrochloride (p.1120·1); guaifenesin (p.1122·1).
*Coughs.*

**Lotussin Expectorant** *Pharmacia, S.Afr.*
Diphenhydramine (p.431·3); aminophylline (p.780·2); ammonium chloride (p.1115·2).
*Coughs.*

**Louten**
*Poen, Arg.; Poen, Chile.*
Latanoprost (p.1519·1).
*Glaucoma; ocular hypertension.*

**Lovacol**
*Saval, Chile; Orion, Fin.*
Lovastatin (p.949·1).
*Hyperlipidaemias.*

**Lovacor** *Farmasa, Braz.*
Simvastatin (p.997·1).
*Hyperlipidaemias.*

**Lovalip** *Merck Sharp & Dohme, Israel.*
Lovastatin (p.949·1).
*Hypercholesterolaemia.*

**Lovamine** *MVM, Fr.†.*
Nutritional supplement (p.1417·1).

**Lovan**
*Alphapharm, Austral.; Lilly, NZ†.*
Fluoxetine hydrochloride (p.292·1).
*Bulimia; depression; obsessive-compulsive disorder; premenstrual dysphoric disorder.*

**Lovarin** *Collins, Mex.*
Loratadine (p.436·1).
*Hypersensitivity.*

**Lovarin P** *Collins, Mex.*
Loratadine (p.436·1); pseudoephedrine (p.1129·2).
*Hypersensitivity; nasal congestion.*

**Lovasc** *Klinger, Braz.†.*
Lovastatin (p.949·1).
*Hyperlipidaemias.*

**Lovast** *Teuto, Braz.*
Lovastatin (p.949·1).
*Hyperlipidaemias.*

**Lovastin** *YSP, Malaysia.*
Lovastatin (p.949·1).
*Hypercholesterolaemia.*

**Lovatex** *Gap, Gr.*
Lovastatin (p.949·1).
*Primary hypercholesterolaemia.*

**Lovaton** *Royton, Braz.*
Lovastatin (p.949·1).
*Hyperlipidaemias.*

**Lovatop** *Phoinix Pharm (Φοινιξ Φαρμ), Gr.*
Lovastatin (p.949·1).
*Primary hypercholesterolaemia.*

**Lovelle**
*Note. This name is used for preparations of different composition.*
*Biolab Sanus, Braz.*
Levonorgestrel (p.1563·2); ethinylestradiol (p.1553·2).
*Combined oral contraceptive.*

*Organon, Ger.*
Desogestrel (p.1547·2); ethinylestradiol (p.1553·2).
*Combined oral contraceptive.*

**Lovenox**
*Gerot, Austria; Aventis, Canad.; Aventis, Fr.; Aventis, Port.; Roche, Switz.†; Aventis, USA.*
Enoxaparin sodium (p.910·3).
*Prevention of coagulation during haemodialysis; thromboembolic disorders.*

**Loveral** *Rayere, Mex.*
Albendazole (p.101·2).
*Worm infections.*

**Lovilia** *ICN, Arg.*
Piroctone olamine (p.1155·2).
*Seborrhoeic dermatitis.*

**Lovina** *Hexal, Ger.†.*
Desogestrel (p.1547·2); ethinylestradiol (p.1553·2).
*Combined oral contraceptive.*

**Lovir**
*Douglas, Austral.; Ranbaxy, Malaysia; Douglas, NZ; Ranbaxy, Singapore.*
Aciclovir (p.626·1).
*Herpesvirus infections.*

**Lovire** *Ranbaxy, S.Afr.*
Aciclovir (p.626·1).
*Herpesvirus infections.*

**Loviscol** *Wyeth, Mex.†.*
Carbocisteine (p.1116·2).

**Lovrak** *Julphar, UAE.*
Aciclovir (p.626·1).
*Herpes simplex skin infections; varicella-zoster skin infections.*

**Low Centyl K** *Leo, Irl.*
Bendroflumethiazide (p.867·3); potassium chloride (p.1232·2).
*Hypertension.*

**Low Liquemine** *Roche, Switz.†.*
Dalteparin sodium (p.891·1).
*Anticoagulant during haemodialysis or haemofiltration; thromboembolic disorders.*

**Lowadina** *Wayne, Mex.†.*
Loratadine (p.436·1).

**Lowasa** *Central, Irl.*
Aspirin (p.15·1).
*Thromboembolism prophylaxis.*

**Lowden** *Saval, Chile.*
Atorvastatin (p.866·2).
*Hypercholesterolaemia.*

**Lowe-Komplex** *Infirmarius-Rovit, Ger.*
A range of homoeopathic preparations.

**Lowfin** *Mintlab, Chile.*
Sertraline hydrochloride (p.317·2).
*Depression.*

**Lowila Cake**
*Bristol-Myers Squibb, Hong Kong.*
Sodium lauril sulfoacetate (p.1574·3).
*Soap substitute.*

*Westwood-Squibb, USA.*
Skin cleanser.

**Lowin** *Duopharma, Hong Kong.*
Gemfibrozil (p.923·1).
*Hyperlipidaemias.*

**Lowlipid** *Biomedica-Chemica, Gr.*
Lovastatin (p.949·1).
*Primary hypercholesterolaemia.*

**Lowpre** *Ehlinger, Mex.†.*
Captopril (p.879·2).

**Lowpress** *Sanval, Braz.*
Enalapril maleate (p.909·2).
*Hyperension.*

**Lowsium Plus** *Rugby, USA.*
Magaldrate (p.1271·3); simeticone (p.1289·2).
*Hyperacidity.*

**Loxam** *Neo Quimica, Braz.*
Meloxicam (p.56·1).

**Loxapac**
*Wyeth Lederle, Belg.†; Wyeth-Ayerst, Canad.†; Wyeth Lederle, Denm.†; Biodim, Fr.; Wyeth, Gr.; Wyeth Lederle, India; Wyeth, Irl.†; Wyeth, NZ†; Wyeth, UK.*
Loxapine (p.705·2), loxapine hydrochloride (p.705·2), or loxapine succinate (p.705·2).
*Psychoses.*

**Loxapin** *Norma (Νορμα), Gr.*
Buspirone hydrochloride (p.672·2).
*Generalised anxiety.*

**Loxavit** *Vitamed, Israel.*
Cloxacillin sodium (p.198·2).
*Bacterial infections.*

**Loxazol**
*Warner-Lambert, Neth.; Pfizer, Switz.*
Permethrin (p.1508·3).
*Pediculosis.*

**Loxen** *Novartis, Fr.*
Nicardipine hydrochloride (p.965·1).
*Hypertension.*

**Loxetine** *March, Thai.*
Fluoxetine hydrochloride (p.292·1).
*Mixed anxiety depressive states.*

**Loxibest** *Best, Mex.*
Meloxicam (p.56·1).
*Gout; inflammation; pain.*

**Loxifen** *Gador, Arg.*
Raloxifene hydrochloride (p.1568·3).
*Osteoporosis.*

**Loxiflan** *Farmasa, Braz.*
Meloxicam (p.56·1).
*Inflammation; pain.*

**Loxin** *Mann, Ger.*
Azelastine hydrochloride (p.425·2).
*Allergic conjunctivitis.*

**Loxina** *Neves, Port.*
Lomefloxacin hydrochloride (p.227·2).
*Bacterial infections.*

**Loxitan** *Vianex (Βιανεξ), Gr.*
Meloxicam (p.56·1).
*Ankylosing spondylitis; inflammation; osteoarthritis; pain; rheumatoid arthritis.*

**Loxitane** *Watson, USA.*
Loxapine succinate (p.705·2).
*Psychoses.*

**Loxitenk** *Biotenk, Arg.*
Meloxicam (p.56·1).
*Musculoskeletal and joint disorders.*

**Loxonin**
*Sankyo, Braz.; Sankyo, Jpn; Sankyo, Thai.*
Loxoprofen sodium (p.54·3).
*Inflammation; musculoskeletal, joint, and peri-articular disorders; pain.*

**Loxyn** *Anglo-French Drugs, India.*
Amoxicillin trihydrate (p.155·3).
*Bacterial infections.*

**Lozan** *Teuto, Braz.*
Ketoconazole (p.403·3).
*Fungal infections.*

**Lozap** *Farmoquimica, Braz.*
Omeprazole (p.1278·2).
*Peptic ulcer.*

**Lozapin** *Torrent, India.*
Clozapine (p.685·3).
*Schizophrenia.*

**Lozapine** *Taro, Israel.*
Clozapine (p.685·3).
*Schizophrenia.*

**Lozaprin** *Coup, Gr.*
Omeprazole (p.1278·2).
*Acid aspiration; eradication of Helicobacter pylori in combination with antimicrobials; peptic ulcer; reflux oesophagitis; Zollinger-Ellison syndrome.*

**Lozide** *Servier, Canad.*
Indapamide (p.938·2).
*Hypertension.*

**Lozione Same AS** *Savoma, Ital.†.*
Methionine (p.1042·1); zinc sulfate (p.1469·3); pyridoxine (p.1457·2).
*Seborrhoea.*

**Lozione Same Urto** *Savoma, Ital.*
Coltsfoot (p.1117·2); achillea (p.1646·2); china; ginger oil (p.1267·1).
*Hair loss.*

**Lozione Vittoria** *Ottolenghi, Ital.*
Benzalkonium chloride (p.1168·3).
*Disinfection of burns, skin, and wounds.*

**Lozitan** *Wockhardt, India.*
Losartan potassium (p.947·2).
*Hypertension.*

**Lozol** *Rhone-Poulenc Rorer, USA.*
Indapamide (p.938·2).
*Heart failure; hypertension.*

**Lozopin** *Merck, Hong Kong.*
Betamethasone dipropionate (p.1093·1); clotrimazole (p.396·2); neomycin sulfate (p.235·1).
*Infected skin disorders.*

**LP Drink** *Support, Braz.*
Preparation for enteral nutrition (p.1417·1).

**LP Mix** *Braun, Fr.*
Amino-acid and lipid infusion (p.1417·1).
*Parenteral nutrition.*

**L-Polamidon** *Aventis, Ger.*
Levomethadone (p.58·3) or levomethadone hydrochloride (p.54·1).
*Opioid withdrawal syndrome; pain.*

**LP-Truw mono** *Truw, Ger.†.*
Sitosterol (p.982·3).
*Hyperlipidaemias.*

**LPV** *CSL, Austral.*
Phenoxymethylpenicillin potassium (p.242·1).
*Bacterial infections.*

**LSP** *Seroyal, Canad.†.*
Calcium aspartate (p.1226·1); magnesium aspartate (p.1227·3).

**Luan** *Molteni, Ital.*
Lidocaine hydrochloride (p.1377·3).
*Local anaesthesia.*

**Luar-G** *Klonal, Arg.*
Hyoscine (p.483·3).

**Luar-G Compositum** *Klonal, Arg.*
Hyoscine (p.483·3); dipyrone (p.35·3).

**Luarprofeno** *Luar, Arg.*
Flurbiprofen (p.43·3).
*Eye disorders.*

**Luase** *Sankyo, Spain.*
Diclofenac sodium (p.32·1).
*Gout; inflammation; musculoskeletal, joint, and periarticular disorders; pain; renal colic.*

**Lubafax** *Douglas, Austral.*
Lubricant for skin or for medical instruments.

**Lubalix** *Drossapharm, Switz.*
Cloxazolam (p.685·3).
*Anxiety disorders; insomnia.*

**Lubarol** *Biovital, Austral.*
Nonoxinol 9 (p.1413·3).
*Contraceptive.*

**Lubentyl** *Sanofi Synthelabo OTC, Fr.*
Liquid paraffin (p.1479·1).
*Constipation.*

**Lubentyl a la Magnesie** *Sanofi Synthelabo OTC, Fr.*
Liquid paraffin (p.1479·1); magnesium hydroxide (p.1272·2).
*Constipation.*

**Lubex** *Permamed, Switz.*
Sodium sulfosuccinated undecenoic acid monoethanolamide (p.411·1).
*Skin disorders.*

**Lubexyl** *Permamed, Switz.*
Benzoyl peroxide (p.1143·2).
*Acne.*

**Lubical** *Lisapharma, Ital.*
Calcium carbonate (p.1254·2).
Formerly known as Calciomed.
*Calcium deficiency; calcium supplement.*

**Lubo** *Synthelabo, Switz.†.*
Guar mucilage (p.333·2).
*Lubricant.*

**Lubogliss** *Streuli, Switz.†.*
Lidocaine hydrochloride (p.1377·3).
*Catheterisation; endoscopy.*

**Luborant**
*Note. This name is used for preparations of different composition.*
*Antigen, Irl.†; Antigen, UK.*
Electrolytes (p.1217·1); carmellose sodium (p.1577·3); sorbitol (p.1446·3).
*Saliva substitute.*

*Antigen, NZ†; Baxter, NZ†.*
Electrolytes (p.1217·1); sodium fluoride (p.1444·3).
*Saliva substitute.*

**LubraSol** *Pharmaceutical Specialties, USA†.*
Emollient.

**Lubricans** *Vitamed, Israel.*
Emollient.
*Dry skin.*

**Lubriderm**
*Note. This name is used for preparations of different composition.*
*Fortbenton, Arg.*
Vitamin A; progesterone (p.1566·2); estradiol (p.1550·1).
*Skin disorders.*

*Pfizer Consumer, Canad.*
Wool fat (p.1483·1); liquid paraffin (p.1479·1).
*Skin disorders.*

*Parke, Davis, Chile.*
A range of emollients.
*Dry skin.*

*Warner-Lambert, USA.*
Emollient and moisturiser.

**Lubriderm AHA** *Pfizer Consumer, Canad.*
Lactic acid (p.1704·1).

**Lubriderm Daily UV**
*Pfizer Consumer, Canad.*
*SPF 15:* Octinoxate (p.1154·3); octisalate (p.1154·3); oxybenzone (p.1154·3).
Formerly contained avobenzone, octinoxate, and ensulizole.
*Sunscreen.*

*Warner-Lambert, USA.*
Octinoxate (p.1154·3); octisalate (p.1154·3); oxybenzone (p.1154·3).
*Dry skin; sunscreen.*

**Lubriderm UV 15** *Parke, Davis, Chile.*
Octinoxate (p.1154·3); octisalate (p.1154·3); oxybenzone (p.1154·3).
*Sunscreen.*

**Lubrificante Anestesico** *Braun, Port.*
Tetracaine hydrochloride (p.1385·1); glycerol (p.1694·3).
*Local anaesthesia and lubricant for catheterisation and endoscopy.*

**Lubrifilm**
*Cusi, Singapore†; Alcon Cusi, Spain.*
White soft paraffin (p.1479·3); liquid paraffin (p.1479·1); wool fat (p.1483·1).
*Dry eyes; eye irritation.*

**Lubrigel** *Rudefsa, Mex.†.*
Carbomers (p.1577·2).

**Lubrik**
*Note. This name is used for preparations of different composition.*
*Alcon, Braz.*
Hypromellose (p.1579·3).
*Eye irritation.*

*Grin, Mex.*
Polyvinyl alcohol (p.1581·1).
*Dry eyes.*

**Lubrikano** *Farco, Ger.*
Glycerol (p.1694·3); hyetellose (p.1579·2).
*Adjunct in radiography; catheterisation; endoscopy.*

**Lubrilax** *Normon, Spain.*
Sodium picosulfate (p.1289·3).
*Constipation.*

**Lubrilent** *SIFI, Ital.†.*
Wetting solution for hard contact lenses (p.1164·2).

**Lubrilin** *Grin, Mex.†.*
White soft paraffin (p.1479·3).

**Lubrin**
*Aurora, Austral.; Upsher Smith, Israel; Torbet Laboratories, UK; Kenwood, USA.*
Vaginal lubricant.

**Lubrirhin** *Alcon, Ger.†.*
Bromhexine (p.1115·3).
*Rhinitis.*

**Lubrisec** *Poen, Arg.*
Acetylcysteine (p.1112·3).
*Eye disorders.*

**Lubri-Tears** *Alcon, UK.*
Liquid paraffin (p.1479·1); white soft paraffin (p.1479·3); wool fat (p.1483·1).
*Eye lubrication and protection.*

**LubriTears** *Bausch & Lomb, USA.*
*Eye drops:* Hypromellose (p.1579·3); dextran 70 (p.746·2).
*Eye ointment:* White soft paraffin (p.1479·3); liquid paraffin (p.1479·1); wool fat (p.1483·1).
*Dry eyes.*

**Lubritina Franklin** *GlaxoSmithKline, Arg.*
Liquid paraffin (p.1479·1).
*Constipation.*

**Lubrizal** *Columbia, Mex.*
Benzalkonium chloride (p.1168·3).
*Vaginal lubricant.*

**Lucebanol** *Hormona, Mex.*
Idebenone (p.1700·3).
*Cerebrovascular disorders; mental function disorders.*

**Lucen** *Malesci, Ital.*
Esomeprazole magnesium (p.1265·1).
*Gastro-oesophageal reflux; peptic ulcer.*

**Lucenfal** *Farma Lepori, Spain.*
Nicardipine hydrochloride (p.965·1).
*Angina pectoris; cerebrovascular disorders; hypertension.*

**Luci** *Rexcel, India.*
Fluocinolone acetonide (p.1101·2).
*Skin disorders.*

**Lucibran** *Bracco, Ital.†.*
Alfoscerate olamine.
*Anxiety; confusion.*

**Lucidex** *Xanodyne, USA.*
Caffeine (p.782·1).

**Lucidril**
*Kolassa, Austria; Lipha Sante, Fr.†.*
Meclofenoxate hydrochloride (p.1710·1).
*Mental function disorders.*

**Lucilium** *Ecosol, Switz.*
Hypericum (p.299·1).
*Insomnia; tension.*

**Lucisan** *Pfizer Consumer, Ital.†.*
Naphazoline nitrate (p.1124·3).
*Eye irritation.*

**Lucitan** *Pharmus, Braz.†.*
Bromazepam (p.671·3).
*Anxiety.*

**Luckyhepa** *YSP, Malaysia.*
Silymarin (p.1043·3); vitamin B substances (p.1454·3).
*Liver disease.*

**Luco-Oph** *Seng, Thai.*
Sulfamethizole (p.260·3).
*Eye and ear infections.*

**Lucopenin** *Durascan, Denm.†.*
Meticillin sodium (p.230·3).
*Staphylococcal infections.*

**Lucosil**
*Rosco, Denm.; Rosco, Norw.*
Sulfamethizole (p.260·3).
*Bacterial infections.*

**Lucretin** *Farmasa, Braz.*
Boric acid (p.1662·1); salicylic acid (p.1157·1); ammonium alum (p.1652·1).
*Vulvovaginal disorders.*

**Lucrin**
*Abbott, Austral.; Abbott, Belg.; Abbott, Fr.; Abbott, Hong Kong; Takeda, Israel; Abbott, Israel; Abbott, Malaysia; Abbott, Mex.; Abbott, Neth.; Abbott, NZ; Abbott, Port.; Abbott, S.Afr.; Abbott, Singapore; Abbott, Switz.*
Leuprorelin (p.1331·1) or leuprorelin acetate (p.1331·1).
*Endometriosis; precocious puberty; prostatic cancer; uterine fibroids.*

**Luctor** *Sanofi Synthelabo, Ger.†.*
Naftidrofuryl oxalate (p.964·1).
*Peripheral vascular disorders.*

**Ludeal** *Pierre Fabre Sante, Fr.*
Ethinylestradiol (p.1553·2); levonorgestrel (p.1563·2).
*Combined oral contraceptive.*

**Ludilat** *Organon, Austria.*
Bencyclane fumarate (p.867·3).
*Peripheral and cerebral vascular disorders.*

**Ludiomil**
*Novartis, Austria; Novartis, Belg.; Novartis, Braz.; Novartis, Canad.; Novartis, Denm.; Novartis, Fr.; Novartis, Ger.; Novartis, Gr.; Novartis, Hong Kong; Novartis, Israel†; Novartis, Ital.; Novartis, Malaysia; Novartis, Mex.; Novartis, Neth.; Novartis, NZ.; Novartis, Port.; Novartis, S.Afr.; Novartis, Singapore; Novartis, Spain; Novartis, Swed.; Novartis, Switz.; Novartis, Thai.; Novartis, UK; Novartis, USA†.*
Maprotiline hydrochloride (p.306·1) or maprotiline mesilate (p.306·2).
*Depression.*

**Luditec** *Collins, Mex.*
Glipizide (p.332·2).
*Diabetes mellitus.*

**Luffa comp-Heel Nasentropfen** *Heel, Ger.†.*
Homoeopathic preparation.

**Luffa compositum** *Heel, Ger.†.*
Homoeopathic preparation.

**Luffa compositum-Heel** *Peithner, Austria.*
Homoeopathic preparation.

**Luffa comp.-Tropfen-Pascoe N** *Pascoe, Ger.†.*
Homoeopathic preparation.

**Luffa Med Complex** *Dynamit, Austria.*
Homoeopathic preparation.

**Luffa Nasentropfen** *DHU, Ger.*
Homoeopathic preparation.

**luffa-loges** *Loges, Ger.†.*
Homoeopathic preparation.

**Luffasan** *Sanum-Kehlbeck, Ger.*
Homoeopathic preparation.

**Luffeel Comp** *Heel, Ger.*
Homoeopathic preparation.

**Luforan** *Serono, Spain.*
Gonadorelin (p.1325·1).
*Hypothalamic-pituitary dysfunction.*

**Luftal** *Bristol-Myers Squibb, Braz.*
Dimeticone (p.1289·2).
*Flatulence.*

**Luftgaz** *Gilton, Braz.†.*
Dimethicone (p.1289·2); calcium pantothenate (p.1442·3).
*Flatulence.*

**Lufyllin** *Wallace, USA.*
Diprophylline (p.784·3).
*Asthma; reversible bronchospasm.*

**Lufyllin-EPG** *Wallace, USA.*
Diprophylline (p.784·3); ephedrine hydrochloride (p.1120·1); guaifenesin (p.1122·1); phenobarbital (p.367·3).
*Bronchospasm.*

**Lufyllin-GG** *Wallace, USA.*
Diprophylline (p.784·3); guaifenesin (p.1122·1).
*Asthma; reversible bronchospasm.*

**Lugesteron** *Leiras, Fin.*
Progesterone (p.1566·2).
*Female infertility; menstrual and menopausal disorders; progesterone deficiency.*

**Luiflex**
*Sankyo, Austria; Sankyo, Belg.*
Indometacin (p.47·3).
*Musculoskeletal, joint, peri-articular and soft-tissue disorders.*

**Luitase** *Euderma, Ital.*
Pancrelipase (p.1725·3).
*Cystic fibrosis; malabsorption.*

**Luivac**
*Rontag, Arg.; Sankyo, Austria; Sankyo, Ger.; Byk Gulden, Mex.; Sankyo, Switz.*
Lysate of *Staphylococcus aureus*; *Streptococcus mitis*; *Streptococcus pyogenes*; *Streptococcus pneumoniae*; *Klebsiella pneumoniae*; *Moraxella catarrhalis*; *Haemophilus influenzae*.
*Respiratory-tract infections.*

**Luizym**
*Note. This name is used for preparations of different composition.*
*Luitpold, Ger.†.*
Enzyme extract from *Aspergillus oryzae*.
*Digestive system disorders.*

*Luitpold, Ital.†.*
Protease; cellulase (p.1669·1); amylase (p.1654·2).
*Digestive disorders.*

*Sankyo, Port.†.*
Amylase (p.1654·2); protease.

**Lukadin** *San Carlo, Ital.*
Amikacin sulfate (p.154·1).
*Gram-negative bacterial infections.*

**Lukair** *Sidus, Arg.*
Montelukast sodium (p.788·3).
*Asthma.*

**Lukasm** *Addenda, Ital.*
Montelukast sodium (p.788·3).
*Asthma.*

**Lullan** *Sumitomo, Jpn.*
Perospirone hydrochloride (p.714·1).
*Schizophrenia.*

**Lumaren**
*Elpen (Ελπεν), Gr.; Elpen, Singapore.*
Ranitidine hydrochloride (p.1285·2).
*Acid aspiration; peptic ulcer; Zollinger-Ellison syndrome.*

**Lumat** *Casasco, Arg.*
Permethrin (p.1508·3).
*Pediculosis.*

**Lumbago-Gastreu S R11** *Reckeweg, Ger.*
Homoeopathic preparation.

**Lumbalgine** *Cooperation Pharmaceutique, Fr.*
Glycol salicylate (p.44·3); menthol (p.1711·3); camphor (p.1665·3); turpentine oil (p.1760·1); benzyl nicotinate (p.21·2).
*Muscular disorders.*

**Lumbicid** *Offenbach, Mex.*
Mebendazole (p.108·2).
*Amoebiasis.*

**Lumbinon** *Lichtenstein, Ger.*
Glycol salicylate (p.44·3).
*Migraine; musculoskeletal, joint, peri-articular, and soft-tissue disorders; neuralgia.*

**Lumbriquil** *Regius, Braz.†.*
Piperazine (p.111·2); prune (p.1285·1).
*Intestinal nematode infections.*

**Lumiactiv** *Vichy, Canad.*
Avobenzone (p.1142·3); octocrilene (p.1154·3); ecamsule (p.1146·3).
*Sunscreen.*

**Lumiclar** *ICN, Arg.*
Disodium inosinate (p.1681·3).
*Eye disorders.*

**Lumidrops** *Unipharma, Gr.*
Phenobarbital (p.367·3).
*Epilepsy.*

**Lumifurex** *Irex, Fr.*
Nifuroxazide (p.237·2).
*Diarrhoea.*

**Lumigan**
*Allergan, Arg.; Allergan, Austral.; Allergan, Braz.; Allergan, Chile; Allergan, Ger.; Allergan, Irl.; Allergan, Ital.; Allergan, Norw.; Allergan, Spain; Allergan, Thai.; Allergan, UK; Allergan, USA.*
Bimatoprost (p.1514·1).
*Glaucoma; ocular hypertension.*

**Lumin** *Alphapharm, Austral.*
Mianserin hydrochloride (p.306·3).
*Depression.*

**Luminal**
*Bayer, Arg.; Desitin, Ger.; Bayer, India; Abbott, Israel; Bayer, Port.; Bayer, Spain; Merck, Switz.; Sanofi Winthrop, USA.*
Phenobarbital (p.367·3) or phenobarbital sodium (p.367·3).
*Epilepsy; insomnia; sedative.*

**Luminale** *Bracco, Ital.*
Phenobarbital (p.367·3) or phenobarbital sodium (p.367·3).
*Barbiturate withdrawal; epilepsy; sedative.*

**Luminaletas**
*Bayer, Arg.; Bayer, Port.; Bayer, Spain.*
Phenobarbital (p.367·3).
*Anxiety; convulsive disorders; depression; insomnia; smooth muscle spasm.*

**Luminalette** *Bracco, Ital.*
Phenobarbital (p.367·3).
*Barbiturate withdrawal; epilepsy; sedative.*

**Luminaletten** *Desitin, Ger.*
Phenobarbital (p.367·3).
*Epilepsy.*

**Luminalettes** *Bayer, India.*
Phenobarbital (p.367·3).
*Epilepsy; sedative.*

**Luminovag** *Novag, Mex.*
Quinfamide (p.615·2).
Formerly contained ketoconazole.
*Amoebiasis.*

**Lumirelax** *Alpharma, Fr.*
*Cream; tablets:* Methocarbamol (p.1395·1).
*Musculoskeletal and joint disorders.*

**Lumirem**
*Sanova, Austria; Guerbet, Denm.; Guerbet, Fin.; Guerbet, Fr.; Guer-*

bet, Ger.; Guerbet, Ital.; Guerbet, Neth.†; Guerbet, Port.; Gothia, Swed.; Guerbet, Switz.†.
Ferumoxsil (p.1061·3).
*Contrast medium for magnetic resonance imaging of the gastrointestinal tract.*

**Lumitens** Solvay, Fr.
Xipamide (p.1029·2).
*Hypertension; oedema.*

**Lumix** Bago, Arg.
Sildenafil citrate (p.1744·2).
*Erectile dysfunction.*

**Lumox** IQFA, Mex.
Amoxicillin (p.155·3).
*Bacterial infections.*

**Lunadon** Singer, Switz.
Tolazoline hydrochloride (p.1015·1); drofenine hydrochloride (p.482·1); diphenhydramine hydrochloride (p.431·3).
*Nervous disorders; sleep disorders.*

**Lundiran** Vir, Spain.
Naproxen (p.65·1).
*Fever; gout; musculoskeletal and joint disorders; pain.*

**Lunelax**
AstraZeneca, Norw.; Tika, Swed.
Ispaghula (p.1268·1).
*Adjunct in treatment of diarrhoea; bowel evacuation; constipation; irritable bowel syndrome.*

**Lunelax comp** Tika, Swed.†.
Ispaghula (p.1268·1); sennosides (p.1288·2).
*Constipation.*

**Lunelle** Pharmacia Upjohn, USA.
Medroxyprogesterone acetate (p.1557·2); estradiol cipionate (p.1550·1).
*Injectable contraceptive.*

**Lunerin**
AstraZeneca, Fin.†; Tika, Swed.†.
Brompheniramine maleate (p.426·1); phenylpropanolamine hydrochloride (p.1127·3).
*Rhinitis.*

**Lunibron** Valeas, Ital.
Flunisolide (p.1101·1).
*Hypersensitivity disorders of the respiratory tract.*

**Lunis** Valeas, Ital.
Flunisolide (p.1101·1).
*Allergic rhinitis.*

**Luparen** Luper, Braz.
Diclofenac sodium (p.32·1).

**Lupectrim** Luper, Braz.
Co-trimoxazole (p.199·3).
*Bacterial infections; Pneumocystis carinii pneumonia; protozoal infections.*

**Lupectrim Balsamico** Luper, Braz.†.
Co-trimoxazole (p.199·3); guaifenesin (p.1122·1); ammonium chloride (p.1115·2).
*Bacterial infections.*

**Lu-Peracina** Reuffer, Mex.†.
Piperazine (p.111·2).

**Lupercaina** Luper, Braz.†.
Yohimbine hydrochloride (p.1766·2); vitamin B substances; vitamin E (p.1417·1); ptychopetalum uncinatum; erythroxylon catuaba.
*Erectile dysfunction.*

**Luperzol** Quimica y Farmacia, Mex.†.
Ketoconazole (p.403·3).

**Lupidon** Seid, Spain.
Calcium pantothenate (p.1442·3); dimethicone (p.1289·2); magnesium polygalacturonate.
*Flatulence.*

**Lupidon G**
Bruschettini, Hong Kong†; Bruschettini, Ital.†.
A herpes simplex type 2 vaccine (p.1620·1).
*Active immunisation.*

**Lupidon H** Bruschettini, Ital.†.
A herpes simplex type 1 vaccine (p.1620·1).
*Active immunisation.*

**Lupidon H+G** Boots Healthcare, Switz.†.
Lupidon H, a herpes simplex vaccine (type I); Lupidon G, a herpes simplex vaccine (type II) (p.1620·1).
*Herpes simplex infections.*

**Lupihist** Lupin, India.
Diphenhydramine hydrochloride (p.431·3); ammonium chloride (p.1115·2); sodium citrate (p.1223·2).
*Cough; hypersensitivity reactions.*

**Lupizyme** Lupin, India.
Pepsin (p.1729·3); amylase (p.1654·2); vitamin B substances (p.1454·3).
*Dyspepsia; flatulence.*

**Lupovalin** Selz, Ger.†.
Diphenhydramine hydrochloride (p.431·3).
*Insomnia.*

**Luprac** Toyama, Jpn.
Torasemide (p.1015·3).
*Oedema.*

**Lupride** Sun, India.
Leuprorelin acetate (p.1331·1).
*Prostatic cancer.*

**Lupron**
Abbott, Arg.; Abbott, Braz.; Abbott, Canad.; Abbott, Chile; TAP, USA.
Leuprorelin (p.1331·1) or leuprorelin acetate (p.1331·1).
*Endometriosis; fibroids; precocious puberty; prostatic cancer.*

**Lurdex** Liferpal, Mex.
Albendazole (p.101·2).
*Worm infections.*

**Luret** Sanofi Synthelabo, Ger.†.
Azosemide (p.866·3).
*Oedema.*

**Luride** Colgate-Palmolive, USA.
Sodium fluoride (p.1444·3).
*Dental caries prophylaxis.*

**Lurline PMS** Fielding, USA.
Paracetamol (p.76·2); pamabrom (p.978·2); pyridoxine (p.1457·2).
*Premenstrual syndrome.*

**Lurselle**
Aventis, Austral.†; Hoechst, Ger.†; Hoechst Marion Roussel, Hong Kong†; Mer-National, S.Afr.; Aventis, Thai.
Probucol (p.986·3).
*Hypercholesterolaemia.*

**Lusap** Interdelta, Switz.
Malathion (p.1507·1).
*Pediculosis.*

**Lusemin** Best, Mex.
Nimesulide (p.67·1).
*Fever; inflammation; pain.*

**Lustra**
Medicis, Canad.; Medicis, USA.
Hydroquinone (p.1148·1).
*Hyperpigmentation.*

**Lustra-AF** Medicis, Canad.
Hydroquinone (p.1148·1); octinoxate (p.1154·3); avobenzone (p.1142·3).
*Hyperpigmentation.*

**Lustral**
Invicta, Irl.; Pfizer, Israel; Pfizer, UK.
Sertraline hydrochloride (p.317·2).
*Depression; mixed anxiety depressive states; obsessive-compulsive disorder; post-traumatic stress disorder.*

**Lustys Herbalene** Lane, UK.
Senna leaf (p.1288·2); frangula bark (p.1266·3); sambucus (p.1741·3); fennel (p.1687·2).
*Constipation.*

**Lutalmin** Offenbach, Mex.
Dydrogesterone (p.1549·2); estradiol (p.1550·1).
*Injectable contraceptive.*

**Lutamidal** Tecnofarma, Chile.
Bicalutamide (p.530·1).
*Prostatic cancer.*

**Lutebiol** Euro Bio, Fr.
Lutein.
*Prevention of eye disorders.*

**Lutene** Herbarium, Braz.
Agnus castus (p.1649·1).
*Female infertility; hyperprolactinaemia; mastodynia; menstrual disorders.*

**Lutenil** Merck, Braz.
Nomegestrol acetate (p.1562·1).
*Menstrual disorders.*

**Lutenyl**
Temis, Arg.; Merck, Belg.; Merck, Chile; Merck-Theramex, Hong Kong; Theramex, Ital.; Theramex, Mon.; Sanofi Synthelabo, Port.
Nomegestrol acetate (p.1562·1).
*Endometriosis; menopausal disorders; menstrual disorders.*

**Luteoliberina** Elea, Arg.
Gonadorelin (p.1325·1).
*Amenorrhoea; male and female infertility.*

**Luteran** Aventis, Fr.
Chlormadinone acetate (p.1542·1).
*Endometriosis; fibromas; menstrual disorders.*

**Lutionex** Roussel, Fr.†.
Demegestone (p.1547·2).
*Endometriosis; fibromas; menstrual disorders.*

**Lutogin** Farmigea, Ital.
Progesterone (p.1566·2).
*Female infertility; menopausal disorders; menstrual disorders; threatened or habitual miscarriage.*

**Lutoginestryl F** Aventis, Mex.
Progesterone (p.1566·2); estradiol benzoate (p.1550·1).
*Menstrual disorders.*

**Lutogynestryl** Aventis, Arg.
Ethisterone; ethinylestradiol (p.1553·2).

**Lutometrodiol** Monsanto, Fr.†.
Etynodiol diacetate (p.1554·2).
*Endometriosis; fibromas; mastopathy; menstrual disorders; progestogen-only oral contraceptive.*

**Lutopolar** Orion, Fin.
Medroxyprogesterone acetate (p.1557·2).
*Dysfunctional uterine bleeding; endometriosis; malignant neoplasms; menstrual disorders.*

**Lutoral**
Note. This name is used for preparations of different composition.
Sanofi Winthrop, Ital.†.
Medroxyprogesterone acetate (p.1557·2).
*Menstrual disorders; premature labour; prostatic hyperplasia; threatened miscarriage.*

Searle, Mex.
Chlormadinone acetate (p.1542·1).
*Menstrual disorders; uterine cancer; uterine fibroids.*

**Lutoral E** Searle, Mex.
Chlormadinone acetate (p.1542·1); mestranol (p.1559·2).
*Endometriosis; menstrual disorders.*

**Lutrax** Alcon, Mex.
Azapentacene.
*Cataracts.*

**Lutrelef**
Ferring, Austria; Ferring, Fr.; Ferring, Ger.; Ferring, Israel; Ferring, Ital.; Ferring, Neth.; Ferring, Swed.; Ferring, Switz.
Gonadorelin acetate (p.1325·2).
*Delayed puberty; hypogonadism; maintenance of luteal function; male and female infertility.*

**Lutrepulse**
Ferring, Canad.; Ferring, USA†.
Gonadorelin acetate (p.1325·2).
*Infertility.*

**Luuf Balsam** Apomedica, Austria.
Camphor (p.1665·3); menthol (p.1711·3); eucalyptus oil (p.1686·2); turpentine oil (p.1760·1); pumilio pine oil (p.1737·1); oleum pini sylvestris; thymol (p.1194·2).
*Respiratory-tract disorders.*

**Luuf Bronchial** Apomedica, Austria.
Eucalyptus oil (p.1686·2).
*Catarrh; coughs.*

**Luuf Krauter-Hustensaft** Apomedica, Austria.
Thyme (p.1755·2); Iceland moss; senega root (p.1130·2); bitter-orange peel (p.1723·3).
*Coughs.*

**Luuf-Erkaltungsol** Apomedica, Austria.
Oleum pini sylvestris; eucalyptus oil (p.1686·2); pumilio pine oil (p.1737·1).
*Respiratory-tract disorders.*

**Luuf-Halspastillen** Apomedica, Austria.
Sage (p.1741·2); plantago lanceolata (p.1738·2); chlorhexidine hydrochloride (p.1173·3).
*Mouth and throat disorders.*

**Luuf-Halspastillen fur Kinder** Apomedica, Austria.
Althaea (p.1651·3); myrtillus (p.1718·3); chlorhexidine hydrochloride (p.1173·3).
*Mouth and throat disorders.*

**Luuf-Heilpflanzenol** Apomedica, Austria.
Eucalyptus oil (p.1686·2); peppermint oil (p.1283·2); cajuput oil (p.1664·1).
*Digestive disorders; flatulence; migraine; pain; respiratory tract disorders; soft-tissue injury.*

**Luuf-Hustentee** Apomedica, Austria.
Thyme (p.1755·2); guaifenesin (p.1122·1); menthol (p.1711·3); camphor (p.1665·3); fennel oil (p.1687·3); anise oil (p.1655·2); eucalyptus oil (p.1686·2); thyme oil (p.1755·3).
*Coughs and cold symptoms.*

**Luuf-Nasenspray** Apomedica, Austria.
Naphazoline hydrochloride (p.1124·3); diphenhydramine hydrochloride (p.431·3).
*Colds; hay fever; sinusitis.*

**Luva Invisivel** Dermoteca, Port.†.
Barrier preparation.

**Luvased**
Wyeth Lederle, Austria; Biocur, Ger.
Valerian (p.1762·2); lupulus (p.1708·1).
*Anxiety disorders; sleep disorders.*

**Luvased-Tropfen N** Biocur, Ger.†.
Valerian (p.1762·2); lupulus (p.1708·1); melissa (p.1711·1); passion flower (p.1729·1).
*Nervous disorders; sleep disorders.*

**Luveris**
Serono, Arg.; Serono, Denm.; Serono, Fin.; Serono, Fr.; Serono, Ger.; Serono, Neth.; Serono, Norw.; Serono, Port.; Serono, Spain; Serono, Swed.; Serono, UK.
Lutropin alfa (p.1332·1).
*Female infertility.*

**Luvier** Casasco, Arg.
Ranitidine (p.1285·2).
*Gastritis; gastro-oesophageal reflux; peptic ulcer.*

**Luvion** GiEnne, Ital.
Canrenone (p.879·1) or potassium canrenoate (p.984·2).
*Hyperaldosteronism; hypertension.*

**Luvos Heilerde** Luvos, Ger.†.
Natural loess.
*Gastrointestinal disorders; skin disorders.*

**Luvox**
Pharmacia, Arg.; Solvay, Austral.; Pharmacia, Braz.; Solvay, Canad.; Pharmacia, Chile; Solvay, Malaysia; Pharmacia Upjohn, Mex.; Solvay, S.Afr.; Solvay, USA.
Fluvoxamine maleate (p.298·2).
*Depression; obsessive-compulsive disorder.*

**Luxazone** Allergan, Ital.
Dexamethasone (p.1097·1).
*Eye disorders.*

**Luxazone Eparina** Tubilux, Ital.
Dexamethasone (p.1097·1); heparin sodium (p.928·1).
*Eye disorders.*

**Luxiq** Connetics, USA.
Betamethasone valerate (p.1093·2).
*Skin disorders.*

**Luxiva** Norman, Canad.
*SPF 15:* Octinoxate (p.1154·3); titanium dioxide (p.1160·3).
*Sunscreen.*

**Luxiva Changing** Norman, Canad.
*SPF 15:* Octinoxate (p.1154·3); zinc oxide (p.1163·2).
*Sunscreen.*

**Luxivia Ultra** Norman, Canad.†.
*SPF 15:* Octinoxate (p.1154·3); oxybenzone (p.1154·3).
*Sunscreen.*

**Luxoben** Asta Medica, Ital.†.
Tiapride hydrochloride (p.725·1).
*Anxiety; dyskinesia.*

**Luxofort** Solfran, Mex.
Vitamin B substances (p.1417·1).

**Luxomicina** Tubilux, Ital.
Micronomicin sulfate (p.231·3).
*Eye infections.*

**Luzolona Simple** IQFA, Mex.
Clioquinol (p.196·3).

**Luzolona Y** IQFA, Mex.
Clioquinol (p.196·3); fluocinolone (p.1101·2).

**Luzone** Sigma-Tau, Spain.
Sulodexide (p.1009·2).
*Atherosclerosis; hyperlipidaemias; thromboembolic disorders.*

**L-Vist** Shepa, Gr.
Palmitic acid; galactose (p.1063·1).
*Adjunct to ultrasound.*

**Lyasin** MC, Ital.†.
Chlorhexidine gluconate (p.1173·2).
*Hand disinfection.*

**Lyban** Rhone-Poulenc Rorer, Austral.†.
Pyrethrins (p.1509·3); piperonyl butoxide (p.1509·2).
*Pediculosis.*

**Lybovit** Frankin, Hong Kong†.
Cyproheptadine (p.430·2); vitamins; lysine (p.1417·1).
*Appetite loss; vitamin supplement.*

**Lycazid** Jagson, India.
Gliclazide (p.332·1).
*Diabetes mellitus.*

**Lyceft** Lyka, India.
Ceftriaxone sodium (p.182·3).
*Bacterial infections.*

**Lycia Luminique** Artsana, Ital.
Benzalkonium chloride (p.1168·3); hamamelis (p.1696·3); chamomile (p.1669·3).
*Eye disinfection; eye irritation.*

**Lycitrope** Cooper (Κοπερ), Gr.
Suxamethonium chloride (p.1406·2).
*Depolarising neuromuscular blocker.*

**Lyclear**
Pfizer Consumer, Austral.; Warner-Lambert, Irl.; Glaxo Wellcome, Irl.; Wellcome, Israel; Glaxo Wellcome, NZ†; GlaxoSmithKline, S.Afr.; Pfizer Consumer, UK.
Permethrin (p.1508·3).
*Pediculosis; scabies.*

**Lycoaktin** Steigerwald, Ger.
Homoeopathic preparation.

**Lycoaktin M** Steigerwald, Ger.†.
Lycopus virginicus.
*Hyperthyroidism with nervous disorders.*

**Lycobiol** Euro Bio, Fr.
Tomato extract.
*Antoxidant dietary supplement.*

**Lycovowen-N** Weber & Weber, Ger.
Homoeopathic preparation.

**Lyderm**
Note. This name is used for preparations of different composition.
Optimapharma, Canad.
Fluocinonide (p.1101·3).
*Skin disorders.*

PSM, NZ.
Permethrin (p.1508·3).
*Scabies.*

**Lydonide** Technilab, Canad.
Fluocinonide (p.1101·3).
*Skin disorders.*

**Lydroxil** Lyka, India.
Cefadroxil (p.167·2).
*Bacterial infections.*

**Lyflex** Chemidex, UK.
Baclofen (p.1386·3).
*Spasticity.*

**Lyforan** Lyka, India.
Cefotaxime sodium (p.175·3).
*Bacterial infections.*

**Lygal E Creme** Taurus, Ger.†.
Betamethasone benzoate (p.1093·1).
*Skin disorders.*

**Lygal E Tinktur** Taurus, Ger.
Betamethasone benzoate (p.1093·1); salicylic acid (p.1157·1).
*Skin disorders.*

**Lygal Kopfsalbe N** Taurus, Ger.
Salicylic acid (p.1157·1).
*Scalp disorders.*

**Lygal Kopftinktur N** Taurus, Ger.
Prednisolone (p.1108·1).
Lygal Kopftinktur formerly contained prednisolone, salicylic acid, and dexpanthenol.
*Scalp disorders.*

**Lygal Wundsalbe** Taurus, Ger.†.
Wheat-germ oil.
*Burns; wounds.*

**Lyman** Drossapharm, Switz.
Heparin sodium (p.928·1); allantoin (p.1141·3); dexpanthenol (p.1727·2).
*Peripheral vascular disorders; soft-tissue disorders.*

**LYMErix**
GlaxoSmithKline, Canad.†; SmithKline Beecham, USA†.
A lyme disease vaccine (recombinant) (p.1622·2).
*Active immunisation.*

**Lymetel** Andromaco, Spain.
Fluvastatin sodium (p.918·2).
*Atherosclerosis; hyperlipidaemias.*

**Lymphaden N** Hevert, Ger.
Homoeopathic preparation.

**Lymphaden PE** *Hevert, Ger.*
Homoeopathic preparation.

**Lymphadenomtropfen N** *Syxyl, Ger.*
Homoeopathic preparation.

**Lymphazurin** *US Surgical, USA.*
Sulphan blue (p.1750·3).
*Adjunct to lymphography.*

**Lymphdiaral** *Pascoe, Ger.*
Homoeopathic preparation.

**Lymphdiaral Aktiv** *Pascoe, Ger.*
Homoeopathic preparation.

**Lymphex** *Drossapharm, Switz.†.*
Coumarin (p.1676·2).
*Lymphoedema.*

**Lymphoglobulin**
*Imtix, Ger.; IFET (ΙΦΕΤ), Gr.*
An antilymphocyte immunoglobulin (horse) (p.1348·3).
*Aplastic anaemia; graft-versus-host disease; transplant rejection.*

**Lymphoglobuline**
*Imtix, Belg.†; Aventis Pasteur, Braz.; Imtix, Fr.; Pasteur Merieux, Hong Kong†; Pasteur Merieux, Israel; Imtix, Ital.; Sangstat, Neth.; Aventis, S.Afr.; Sangstat, Singapore; Pacific Biosciences, Singapore; Imtix, Switz.; Aventis Pasteur, Thai.*
An antilymphocyte immunoglobulin (horse) (p.1348·3).
Formerly known as Lymfoglobuline in *Neth.*
*Aplastic anaemia; graft-versus-host disease; transplant rejection.*

**Lymphomyosot**
*Peithner, Austria; Heel, Ger.; Heel, S.Afr.*
Homoeopathic preparation.

**Lymphozil** *Cesra, Ger.*
Echinaceae pallida (p.1683·2).
*Tonic.*

**Lymphtropfen S** *Cosmochema, Ger.*
Homoeopathic preparation.

**Lyndak** *Eurofarmaco, Ital.†.*
Sulindac (p.91·2).
*Gout; musculoskeletal and joint disorders; neuritis; soft-tissue injury.*

**Lyndiol**
*Organon, Austria†; Organon, Belg.†; Organon, Denm.†; Organon, Ger.†; Organon, Hong Kong†; Organon, Thai.*
Lynestrenol (p.1557·1); ethinylestradiol (p.1553·2).
*Combined oral contraceptive.*

**Lyndiolett** *Organon, Swed.†.*
Lynestrenol (p.1557·1); ethinylestradiol (p.1553·2).
*Combined oral contraceptive.*

**Lynoral**
*Infar, India; Organon, Neth.*
Ethinylestradiol (p.1553·2).
*Breast cancer; menstrual disorders; oestrogen deficiency; postcoital contraceptive; prostatic cancer.*

**Lyn-ratiopharm** *Ratiopharm, Ger.†.*
Lynestrenol (p.1557·1); ethinylestradiol (p.1553·2).
*Combined oral contraceptive; menstrual disorders.*

**Lyn-ratiopharm-Sequenz** *Ratiopharm, Ger.*
7 Capsules, ethinylestradiol (p.1553·2); 15 capsules, lynestrenol (p.1557·1); ethinylestradiol.
*Sequential-type oral contraceptive.*

**Lynx** *Wallace, India.*
Lincomycin hydrochloride (p.226·2).
*Bacterial infections.*

**Lyobalsam** *Truw, Ger.†.*
Camphor (p.1665·3); eucalyptus oil (p.1686·2).
*Respiratory-tract disorders.*

**Lyo-Bifidus** *Alpharma, Fr.*
*Bifidobacterium bifidus* (*Bacillus bifidus*) (p.1704·2).
*Diarrhoea.*

**Lyofoam** *SSL, UK.*
Polyurethane foam dressing.
*Ulcers; wounds.*

**Lyofoam C** *SSL, UK.*
Activated charcoal (p.1030·2).
*Malodorous wounds.*

**Lyogen** *Lundbeck, Ger.*
Fluphenazine decanoate (p.699·3) or fluphenazine hydrochloride (p.699·3).
*Psychoses.*

**Lyomer** *Jaba, Port.*
Sea water (p.1233·3).
*Nasal hygiene.*

**Lyorodin** *Rodleben, Ger.; UCB, Ger.*
Fluphenazine decanoate (p.699·3) or fluphenazine hydrochloride (p.699·3).
*Psychoses.*

**Lyostypt**
*Braun Surgical, Switz.†; Davis & Geck, UK†.*
Collagen (p.1674·3).
*Haemorrhage.*

**Lyovac Cosmegen**
*Merck Sharp & Dohme, Belg.; Merck Sharp & Dohme, Ger.; Merck Sharp & Dohme, Neth.*
Dactinomycin (p.545·1).
*Malignant neoplasms.*

**Lyphocin**
*APP, Hong Kong; American Pharmaceutical, USA.*
Vancomycin hydrochloride (p.275·2).
*Bacterial infections.*

**Lypholyte** *American Pharmaceutical, USA.*
A range of electrolyte preparations (p.1217·1).
*Fluid and electrolyte disorders.*

**Lyprinol** *Life Plus, UK.*
Green-lipped mussel lipid extract (p.1696·1).

**Lypsyl Cold Sore Gel** *Novartis Consumer, UK.*
Lidocaine hydrochloride (p.1377·3); zinc sulfate (p.1469·3); cetrimide (p.1172·1).
*Herpes labialis.*

**Lyrica** *Pfizer, UK.*
Pregabalin (p.376·2).
*Epilepsy; neuropathic pain.*

**Lyrinel XL** *Janssen-Cilag, UK.*
Oxybutynin hydrochloride (p.486·3).
Formerly known as Ditropan XL.
*Urinary incontinence.*

**Lysalgo** *SIT, Ital.*
Mefenamic acid (p.55·2).
*Inflammation; pain.*

**Lysantin** *Gea, Denm.*
Orphenadrine hydrochloride (p.486·1).
*Drug-induced extrapyramidal disorders; parkinsonism.*

**Lysanxia**
*Pfizer, Belg.; Pfizer, Fr.*
Prazepam (p.716·2).
*Alcohol withdrawal syndrome; anxiety.*

**Lysbex** *Provita, Austria.*
Bibenzonium bromide (p.1115·3).
*Coughs.*

**Lysedem** *Knoll, Fr.†.*
Coumarin (p.1676·2).
*Post-mastectomy lymphoedema.*

**Lysedil** *Vifor, Switz.*
Promethazine hydrochloride (p.439·1); belladonna (p.479·1).
*Coughs; gastrointestinal disorders; hypersensitivity reactions; sedative.*

**Lysedil compositum** *Vifor, Switz.†.*
Promethazine hydrochloride (p.439·1); belladonna (p.479·1); paracetamol (p.76·2).
*Coughs; fever; gastrointestinal disorders; hypersensitivity reactions; pain; sedative.*

**Lyseen** *Novartis Consumer, Ital.*
Pridinol mesilate (p.1395·2).
*Skeletal muscle spasm.*

**Lysetol V** *Schulke & Mayr, Ger.†.*
Formaldehyde (p.1179·3); glutaral (p.1180·3); didecyldimethylammonium chloride (p.1178·3).
Formerly contained formaldehyde, glutaral, and ethylhexanal.
*Instrument disinfection.*

**Lysetol FF** *Schulke & Mayr, Ger.*
Glutaral (p.1180·3); ethylhexanal.
*Instrument disinfection.*

**Lysetol Med** *Schulke & Mayr, Ger.*
Cocospropylendiguanidinacetat; phenoxypropanol (p.1189·1); benzalkonium chloride (p.1168·3).
*Instrument disinfection.*

**Lysinotol** *Viatris, Spain.*
Lysine aspirin (p.54·3).
*Fever; musculoskeletal, joint, and peri-articular disorders; pain; thromboembolism prophylaxis.*

**Lysivit $B_{12}$ a l'inositol** *Sarget, Fr.†.*
Lysine hydrochloride; inositol; cyanocobalamin (p.1417·1).
*Tonic.*

**Lyso-6**
*UCB, Fr.; UCB, Switz.*
Muramidase hydrochloride (p.1717·2); pyridoxine hydrochloride (p.1456·3).
*Mouth disorders.*

**Lysocalm** *UCB, Fr.†.*
Muramidase hydrochloride (p.1717·2); menthol (p.1711·3).
*Mouth and throat infections.*

**Lysocline** *Pfizer, Fr.*
Methacycline hydrochloride (p.230·1).
*Bacterial infections.*

**Lysodren**
*Bristol, Canad.; IFET (ΙΦΕΤ), Gr.; Bristol-Myers Squibb Oncology, USA.*
Mitotane (p.575·1).
*Adrenal cortical cancer.*

**Lysodrop** *Viatris, Belg.*
Acetylcysteine (p.1112·3).
*Dry eyes.*

**Lysofon** *Lafon, Fr.†.*
*Lozenges:* Chlorhexidine acetate (p.1173·2); tetracaine hydrochloride (p.1385·1).
Formerly contained tricarbaurinium and tetracaine hydrochloride.
*Mouth and throat pain.*
*Throat spray:* Chlorhexidine gluconate (p.1173·2).
Formerly contained tricarbaurinium.
*Mouth and throat disorders.*

**Lysoform** *Lysoform, Ger.*
Formaldehyde (p.1179·3).
*Skin disorders; surface and linen disinfection.*

**Lysoform Killavon** *Lysoform, Ger.*
Benzalkonium chloride (p.1168·3).
*Disinfection of skin, mucous membranes, and surfaces; skin disorders.*

**Lysoformin** *Lysoform, Ger.*
Formaldehyde (p.1179·3); glutaral (p.1180·3).
*Surface disinfection.*

**Lysoformin 3000** *Lysoform, Ger.*
Glyoxal (p.1181·1); glutaral (p.1180·3); didecyldimethylammonium chloride (p.1178·3).
*Disinfection of instruments and surfaces.*

**Lysoformin spezial** *Lysoform, Ger.*
Guanidine derivative; didecyldimethylammonium chloride (p.1178·3).
*Disinfection of surfaces.*

**Lysomucil**
*Strallhofer, Austria; Zambon, Belg.*
Acetylcysteine (p.1112·3).
*Paracetamol overdose; respiratory-tract disorders associated with viscous mucus.*

**Lysopaine**
*Boehringer Ingelheim, Fr.*
Muramidase hydrochloride (p.1717·2); papaya sap; bacitracin (p.161·3).
*Mouth and throat infections.*

*Boehringer Ingelheim, Switz.*
Muramidase hydrochloride (p.1717·2); papain (p.1727·3); bacitracin (p.161·3).
*Mouth and throat disorders.*

**Lysoprin** *Rafa, Israel.*
Lysine aspirin (p.54·3).
Glycine (p.1433·3) is included in this preparation in an attempt to limit adverse effects on the gastrointestinal mucosa.
*Fever; pain.*

**Lysovir** *Alliance, UK.*
Amantadine hydrochloride (p.1197·2).
*Influenza A.*

**Lysox** *Menarini, Belg.*
Acetylcysteine (p.1112·3).
*Respiratory-tract disorders associated with viscous secretions.*

**Lyssavac N**
*Berna, Hong Kong†; Berna, Ital.; Berna, Switz.; Berna, Thai.†.*
A rabies vaccine (duck embryo) (p.1635·3).
*Active immunisation.*

**Lyssuman** *Berna, Spain†.*
A rabies immunoglobulin (p.1635·3).
*Passive immunisation.*

**Lysthenon**
*Nycomed, Austria; Nycomed, Ger.; Nycomed, Switz.*
Suxamethonium chloride (p.1406·2).
*Depolarising neuromuscular blocker.*

**Lystin**
*Biolab, Hong Kong; Biolab, Thai.*
Nystatin (p.406·3).
*Vaginal candidiasis.*

**Lysuron** *Roche, Switz.†.*
Allopurinol (p.412·2).
*Gout; hyperuricaemia; renal calculi.*

**Lyteers** *Fischer, Israel.*
Sodium chloride (p.1233·3); potassium chloride (p.1232·2).
*Dry eyes.*

**Lyteprep** *E-Z-EM, Canad.*
Electrolyte solution (p.1217·1).
*Gastrointestinal lavage.*

**Lytos** *Roche, Fr.*
Disodium clodronate (p.770·2).
*Malignant hypercalcaemia; malignant osteolysis.*

**Lytren**
*Mead Johnson Nutritionals, Canad.*
Glucose; potassium citrate; sodium chloride; sodium citrate; citric acid (p.1222·2).
*Diarrhoea; oral rehydration therapy.*

*Mead Johnson, Fr.*
Maltodextrin; glucose; potassium citrate; sodium chloride; citric acid; sodium citrate; calcium gluconate; magnesium phosphate (p.1222·2).
*Diarrhoea; oral rehydration therapy.*

**Lytren RHS** *Mead Johnson Nutritionals, Canad.†.*
Citric acid; potassium citrate; sodium chloride; sodium citrate (p.1222·2).

**Lyzyme** *Shin Poong, Singapore.*
Muramidase hydrochloride (p.1717·2).
*Haemorrhage; respiratory-tract congestion; sinusitis.*

**M & M** *Malam, UK.*
*Dressing:* Cod-liver oil (p.1425·2); purified honey (p.1434·2).

**Ma Ma Sustagen** *Mead Johnson, Hong Kong†.*
Preparation for enteral nutrition (p.1417·1).
*Pregnancy and lactation.*

**Maalox**
*Note. This name is used for preparations of different composition.*
*Raffo, Arg.; Novartis Consumer, Canad.; Aventis, Chile; Theraplix, Fr.; Nattermann, Ger.; Aventis, Gr.; Aventis, Hong Kong; Aventis, Irl.; Aventis, Israel; Aventis, Ital.; Aventis, S.Afr.; Aventis, Spain; Aventis, UK; Novartis Consumer, USA.*
Aluminium hydroxide (p.1249·2); magnesium hydroxide (p.1272·2).
These ingredients can be described by the British Approved Name Co-magaldrox.
*Gastric hyperacidity; gastritis; heartburn; peptic ulcer.*

*Gerot, Austria.*
Algeldrate or aluminium hydroxide (p.1249·2); magnesium hydroxide (p.1272·2).
*Gastrointestinal disorders associated with hyperacidity.*

*Aventis, Belg.; Aventis, Neth.*
Algeldrate (p.1249·2); magnesium hydroxide (p.1272·2).
*Gastritis; gastro-oesophageal reflux; heartburn; peptic ulcer.*

*Aventis, Chile.*
*Oral suspension:* Aluminium magnesium hydroxide.
*Antacid.*

**Maalox Antacid/Calcium** *Novartis, USA.*
Calcium carbonate (p.1254·2).
*Calcium supplement; hyperacidity.*

**Maalox Anti-Diarrheal** *Rhone-Poulenc Rorer, USA†.*
Loperamide hydrochloride (p.1271·1).
*Diarrhoea.*

**Maalox Anti-Gas** *Rhone-Poulenc Rorer, USA.*
Simeticone (p.1289·2).
*Flatulence.*

**Maalox Anti-Gas Extra Strength** *Novartis, USA.*
Aluminium hydroxide (p.1249·2); magnesium hydroxide (p.1272·2); simeticone (p.1289·2).
*Antacid; flatulence.*

**Maalox Ballonnements** *Theraplix, Fr.*
Aluminium hydroxide (p.1249·2); magnesium hydroxide (p.1272·2); dimeticone (p.1289·2).
*Flatulence; gastric hyperacidity.*

**Maalox Daily Fiber** *Rhone-Poulenc Rorer, USA†.*
Psyllium hydrophilic mucilloid (p.1268·1).

**Maalox Extra Strength Anti-Gas** *Novartis, USA.*
Simeticone (p.1289·2).
*Excess gastrointestinal gas.*

**Maalox GRF** *Novartis Consumer, Canad.†.*
Simeticone (p.1289·2).
*Dyspepsia; flatulence.*

**Maalox $H_2$ Acid Controller** *Novartis Consumer, Canad.*
Famotidine (p.1265·2).
*Gastrointestinal hyperacidity.*

**Maalox Heartburn Relief** *Rhone-Poulenc Rorer, USA†.*
Aluminium hydroxide-magnesium carbonate co-dried gel (p.1250·1); magnesium carbonate (p.1272·1).
*Hyperacidity.*

**Maalox HRF** *Novartis Consumer, Canad.*
Calcium carbonate (p.1254·2); sodium alginate (p.1577·1); magnesium carbonate (p.1272·1).
Formerly contained aluminium hydroxide-magnesium carbonate co-dried gel, magnesium alginate,and magnesium carbonate.
*Dyspepsia; gastro-oesophageal reflux; heartburn.*

**Maalox Plus**
*Aventis, Braz.; Novartis Consumer, Canad.; Aventis, Chile; Aventis, Gr.; Aventis, Hong Kong; Aventis, Irl.; Aventis, Israel; Aventis, Ital.; Aventis, Malaysia; Aventis, Neth.; Aventis, Port.; Aventis, S.Afr.; Aventis, UK; Rhone-Poulenc Rorer, USA.*
Aluminium hydroxide (p.1249·2); magnesium hydroxide (p.1272·2); simeticone (p.1289·2).
*Dyspepsia; flatulence; gastritis; gastro-oesophageal reflux; heartburn; peptic ulcer.*

**Maalox Quick Dissolve**
*Novartis Consumer, Canad.; Novartis, USA.*
Calcium carbonate (p.1254·2).
*Antacid.*

**Maalox Quick Dissolve with Antigas** *Novartis Consumer, Canad.*
Calcium carbonate (p.1254·2); simeticone (p.1289·2).
*Antacid; flatulence.*

**Maalox TC**
*Rhodia, Braz.†; Novartis Consumer, Canad.; Aventis, Ital.; Aventis, UK†.*
Aluminium hydroxide (p.1249·2); magnesium hydroxide (p.1272·2).
Formerly known as Maalox Concentrate in the *UK.* These ingredients can be described by the British Approved Name Co-magaldrox.
*Gastrointestinal hyperacidity; peptic ulcer.*

**Maaloxan**
*Nattermann, Ger.; Piraud, Switz.†.*
Aluminium hydroxide (p.1249·2); magnesium hydroxide (p.1272·2).
*Gastric hyperacidity; peptic ulcer.*

**Maaloxan Ca** *Rhone-Poulenc Rorer, Switz.†.*
Aluminium hydroxide (p.1249·2); magnesium hydroxide (p.1272·2); calcium carbonate (p.1254·2).
Formerly known as Camalox.
*Gastric hyperacidity.*

**Mab** *Whitehall, Fr.*
Magnesium carbonate (p.1272·1); calcium carbonate (p.1254·2); sodium bicarbonate (p.1223·2).
*Gastrointestinal disorders.*

**MabCampath**
*Schering, Denm.; Schering, Fin.; Schering, Fr.; MSO, Ger.; Schering, Ger.; Schering, Irl.; Schering, Ital.; Schering, Port.; Schering, Spain; Schering, Swed.; Schering, UK.*
Alemtuzumab (p.526·1).
*Chronic lymphocytic leukaemia.*

**Mabicrol** *Promeco, Mex.*
Clarithromycin (p.192·2).
*Bacterial infections.*

**Mabis** *Lacefa, Arg.*
Aluminium hydroxide (p.1249·2); magnesium hydroxide (p.1272·2); bismuth subnitrate (p.1252·2).
*Gastrointestinal hyperacidity.*

**Mabogastrol** *Merck, Spain.*
Aluminium hydroxide (p.1249·2); magnesium carbonate (p.1272·1); sodium bicarbonate (p.1223·2).
Formerly contained anethole, aluminium hydroxide, magnesium carbonate, and sodium bicarbonate.
*Dyspepsia.*

**Mabosil** *Mabo, Spain†.*
Magnesium trisilicate (p.1272·3).
*Gastrointestinal hyperacidity.*

**Maboterpen**
*Mabo, Spain†.*
*Suppositories:* Camphor (p.1665·3); cineole (p.1672·1); dextromethorphan (p.1117·3); niaouli oil (p.1719·3); guaiacol (p.1122·1).
*Respiratory-tract disorders.*

Tedec Meiji, Spain†.
*Syrup:* Tolu balsam (p.1131·3); diphenhydramine hydrochloride (p.431·3); ephedrine hydrochloride (p.1120·1); niaouli oil (p.1719·3); oleum pini sylvestris; sodium benzoate (p.1169·3); bitter orange; sulfogaiacol (p.1131·1).
*Upper-respiratory-tract disorders.*

**Mabron** Medochemie, Hong Kong; Medochemie, Malaysia; Medochemie, Singapore; Medochemie, Thai.
Tramadol hydrochloride (p.94·3).
*Pain.*

**Mabthera** Roche, Arg.; Roche, Austral.; Roche, Austria; Roche, Belg.; Roche, Braz.; Roche, Chile; Roche, Denm.; Roche, Fin.; Roche, Fr.; Roche, Ger.; Roche, Gr.; Roche, Hong Kong; Roche, Irl.; Roche, Israel; Roche, Ital.; Roche, Mex.; Roche, Neth.; Roche, Norw.; Roche, NZ; Roche, Port.; Roche, S.Afr.; Roche, Singapore; Roche, Spain; Roche, Swed.; Roche, Switz.; Roche, Thai.; Roche, UK.
Rituximab (p.582·3).
*Follicular lymphoma; non-Hodgkin's lymphoma.*

**Mac** Ernest Jackson, UK†.
Amylmetacresol (p.1168·2); menthol (p.1711·3).
*Sore throat.*

**Mac Dual Action** Ernest Jackson, UK†.
Hexylresorcinol (p.1182·1).
Formerly known as Mac Extra.
*Sore throat.*

**Mac Sugar Free** Ernest Jackson, UK†.
Dequalinium chloride (p.1178·1).
*Mouth and throat infections.*

**Macaine** Adcock Ingram, S.Afr.
Bupivacaine hydrochloride (p.1371·1).
Adrenaline acid tartrate (p.852·2) is included in some injections as a vasoconstrictor to diminish absorption and localise the effect of the local anaesthetic.
*Local anaesthesia.*

**Macalvit**
Note. This name is used for preparations of different composition.
Novartis Consumer, Austria; Novartis, Swed.
Calcium lactate gluconate (p.1225·3); calcium carbonate (p.1254·2); ascorbic acid (p.1460·2).
*Calcium and vitamin C deficiency.*

Novartis Consumer, Ger.
Ascorbic acid (p.1460·2); calcium lactate gluconate (p.1225·3); calcium phosphinate.
*Cold and influenza symptoms; tonic.*

Novartis, India.
Calcium glubionate (p.1225·1); calcium lactobionate (p.1225·3); colecalciferol (p.1461·3); vitamin $B_{12}$ (p.1458·2).
*Calcium supplement; tonic.*

**Macbirs** Maigal, Arg.
Sulfur (p.1158·2).
*Seborrhoeic dermatitis.*

**Macbirs Minoxidil** Maigal, Arg.
Minoxidil (p.960·1).
*Alopecia.*

**Macgel** YSP, Malaysia; Yung Shin, Singapore.
Magnesium hydroxide (p.1272·2); aluminium hydroxide (p.1249·2); simeticone (p.1289·2).
*Flatulence; gastric hyperacidity; gastritis; peptic ulcer.*

**Mach-2** Tocogino, Mex.†.
Dipyrone (p.35·3).

**Machlor** Eagle, Austral.†.
Magnesium chloride (p.1228·1); magnesium oxide (p.1272·3); magnesium amino acid chelate (p.1229·1).
*Magnesium supplement.*

**Machto** Nakornpatana, Thai.
*Oral gel:* Aluminium hydroxide-magnesium carbonate co-dried gel (p.1250·1); magnesium hydroxide (p.1272·2); simeticone (p.1289·2).
*Tablets:* Aluminium hydroxide (p.1249·2); magnesium trisilicate (p.1272·3); magnesium hydroxide (p.1272·2); peppermint oil (p.1283·2).
*Flatulence; gastric hyperacidity; heartburn; peptic ulcer.*

**Mackenzies Menthoids** BML, Austral.†.
Phenolphthalein (p.1284·1); potassium nitrate (p.1190·1); methylthioninium chloride (p.1042·2).
*Backache; rheumatic pain.*

**Mackenzies Smelling Salts** Alpharma, UK.
Ammonia (p.1653·3); eucalyptus oil (p.1686·2).
*Catarrh; colds.*

**Macladin** Guidotti, Ital.
Clarithromycin (p.192·2).
*Bacterial infections.*

**Maclar** Abbott, Austria; Abbott, Belg.; Abbott, Port.†.
Clarithromycin (p.192·2).
*Opportunistic mycobacterial infections.*

**Maclean Indigestion Tablets** SmithKline Beecham Consumer, UK†.
Calcium carbonate (p.1254·2); light magnesium carbonate (p.1272·1); aluminium hydroxide (p.1249·2).
*Gastrointestinal disorders.*

**Macleans Mouthguard** GlaxoSmithKline Consumer, UK.
Cetylpyridinium chloride (p.1173·1); sodium fluoride (p.1444·3).
*Oral hygiene.*

**Macleans Sensitive** SmithKline Beecham Consumer, Austral.†.
Sodium fluoride (p.1444·3); strontium acetate.
*Dental caries prophylaxis; pain associated with sensitive teeth.*

**Maclov** Mavi, Mex.
Aciclovir (p.626·1).
*Herpesvirus infections.*

**Macmiror** Sanova, Austria; Poli, Hong Kong†; Monsanto, Ital.; Italmex, Mex.; Farma Lepori, Spain†; Poli, Switz.†.
Nifuratel (p.611·2).
*Bacterial genito-urinary-tract infections; gastrointestinal amoebiasis; trichomoniasis.*

**Macmiror Complex** Poli, Hong Kong†; Monsanto, Ital.
Nifuratel (p.611·2); nystatin (p.406·3).
*Vulvovaginal infections.*

**Macmiror Complex V** Italmex, Mex.
Nifuratel (p.611·2); nystatin (p.406·3).
*Vulvovaginal infections.*

**Macobal** Gramon, Arg.
Nimodipine (p.972·3).
*Cerebrovascular disorders.*

**Macoderm** LDA, Arg.
Zinc oxide (p.1163·2); acetylated wool alcohols (p.1483·1).
*Skin disorders.*

**Macodin** Parggon, Mex.
Dipyrone (p.35·3).
*Fever; pain.*

**Macorel** Elpen (Ελπεν), Gr.
Nifedipine (p.966·2).
*Angina; hypertension.*

**Macosil** Vifor, Switz.†.
Aluminium hydroxide (p.1249·2); magnesium hydroxide (p.1272·2); simeticone (p.1289·2).
*Gastrointestinal disorders.*

**Macril** Andromaco, Arg.
Betamethasone valerate (p.1093·2); gentamicin sulfate (p.217·1); miconazole nitrate (p.405·3).
*Infected skin disorders.*

**Macro Antioxidant** Whitehall, Austral.†.
Vitamin and mineral preparation (p.1417·1).
*Dietary supplement.*

**Macro Anti-Stress** Whitehall, Austral.†.
Vitamin B substances, ascorbic acid, and valerian (p.1762·2)(p.1417·1).
*Dietary supplement; stress.*

**Macro B** Whitehall, Austral.†.
Vitamin B substances and ascorbic acid (p.1417·1).
*Dietary supplement.*

**Macro C** Whitehall Consumer, Austral.
Ascorbic acid (p.1460·2); calcium ascorbate (p.1460·2); citrus bioflavonoids (p.1688·2); rutoside (p.1688·2); hesperidin (p.1688·2).
*Vitamin C supplement.*

**Macro E** Whitehall, Austral.†.
*d*-Alpha tocopherol (p.1464·3).
*Vitamin E deficiency; vitamin E supplement.*

**Macro Garlic** Whitehall, Austral.†.
Odourless Arizona garlic (p.1691·1).
*Cold and influenza symptoms.*

**Macro Maxepa** Whitehall, Austral.†.
Eicosapentaenoic acid (p.976·2); docosahexaenoic acid (p.976·1); *d*-alpha tocoferil acetate.
*Omega-3 fatty acid supplement.*

**Macro Multi M** Whitehall Consumer, Austral.
Multivitamin and mineral preparation (p.1417·1).
*Dietary supplement.*

**Macro Natural Vitamin E Cream** Whitehall Consumer, Austral.
*d*-Alpha tocoferil acetate (p.1465·1); vitamin A palmitate (p.1453·1); panthenol (p.1727·2); allantoin (p.1141·3); avocado oil.
*Dry skin; minor skin disorders.*

**Macrobid** Alza, Canad.; Goldshield, Irl.; Goldshield, UK; Procter & Gamble, USA.
Nitrofurantoin (p.237·2).
*Urinary-tract infections.*

**Macrocilin** Ofimex, Mex.†.
Tetracycline (p.266·2).

**Macrodantin** Pharmacia, Austral.; Alza, Canad.; Goldshield, Irl.; Procter & Gamble, Israel; Geymonat, Ital.; GlaxoSmithKline, S.Afr.; Goldshield, UK; Procter & Gamble, USA.
Nitrofurantoin (macrocrystalline) (p.237·2).
*Urinary-tract infections.*

**Macrodantina** Schering-Plough, Braz.; Boehringer Ingelheim, Chile; Boehringer Ingelheim, Mex.
Nitrofurantoin (p.237·2).
*Urinary-tract infections.*

**Macrodex** Pharmacia, Austral.†; Pharmacia Upjohn, Canad.†; Pharmalink, Denm.; Pharmacia Upjohn, Israel; Pisa, Mex.; Pharmalink, Norw.; Alliance, S.Afr.; Pharmacia, Spain†; Pharmalink, Swed.; Braun, Switz.; Pharmacia, UK†; Pharmacia, USA.
Dextran 70 (p.746·2) in glucose or sodium chloride.
*Plasma volume expansion; thromboembolism prophylaxis.*

Torrex, Austria; Pharmalink, Ger.
Dextran 60 (p.746·1) in sodium chloride.
*Plasma volume expansion; thrombosis prophylaxis.*

**Macrodexin** Braun, Braz.†.
Dextran in glucose.
*Plasma volume expansion.*

**Macrofurin** Mavi, Mex.†.
Nitrofurantoin (p.237·2).

**Macrolax** Carlo Erba OTC, Ital.
Docusate sodium (p.1262·2); sorbitol (p.1446·3).
*Constipation.*

**Macrolin**
Note. This name is used for preparations of different composition.
Haller, Braz.†.
Lincomycin (p.226·2).
*Bacterial infections.*

Chiron, Fr.†.
Aldesleukin (p.562·3).
*HIV infection.*

**Macromax** ICN, Arg.
Azithromycin (p.159·1).
*Bacterial infections.*

**Macromicina** Frasca, Arg.
Clarithromycin (p.192·2).
*Bacterial infections.*

**Macromin** Macrophar, Thai.
Metformin hydrochloride (p.342·3).
*Diabetes mellitus.*

**Macro-P** Promefarm, Ital.
Macrogol 4000 (p.1709·1); electrolytes (p.1217·1).
*Bowel evacuation.*

**Macropen**
Note. This name is used for preparations of different composition.
Menarini, Port.
Cefatrizine (p.170·3).
*Bacterial infections.*

Xixia, S.Afr.
Amoxicillin (p.155·3); flucloxacillin (p.213·3).
*Bacterial infections.*

**Macroral** Malesci, Ital.
Midecamycin (p.231·3).
*Bacterial infections.*

**Macrosan** Instituto Sanitas, Chile.
Nitrofurantoin (p.237·2).
*Bacterial urinary-tract infections.*

**Macrosil** Faes, Spain.
Roxithromycin (p.254·2).
*Bacterial infections.*

**Macroten** Bergamo, Braz.†.
Phenolphthalein (p.1284·1); bladderwrack (p.1742·3); thyroid (p.1604·2); bile salts (p.1660·3).
*Constipation.*

**Macsoralen** Mac, India.
Methoxsalen (p.1152·1).
*Vitiligo.*

**Mactam** Coli, Ital.†.
Latamoxef disodium (p.225·3).
*Gram-negative bacterial infections.*

**Mactex** Osteolab, Chile.
Norgestimate (p.1563·2); ethinylestradiol (p.1553·2).
*Combined oral contraceptive.*

**Madar** Ravizza, Ital.
Nordazepam (p.710·3).
*Sleep disorders.*

**Made B12** Esfar, Port.†.
Vitamin $B_{12}$ (p.1458·2).

**Madecassol** Roche, Austria; Roche, Belg.; Roche, Chile; Roche Nicholas, Fr.; Sanofi Synthelabo, Mex.; Serdex, Port.; Syntex, Switz.†; Serdex, Thai.
Centella (p.1144·3).
*Burns; keloids; ulcers; venous insufficiency; wounds.*

**Madecassol C** Sanofi Synthelabo, Mex.
Centella (p.1144·3); metronidazole (p.607·2); nitrofurazone (p.238·2).
*Bacterial vaginosis; trichomoniasis.*

**Madecassol N** Sanofi Synthelabo, Mex.
Centella (p.1144·3); nitrofurazone (p.238·2).
*Vaginosis.*

**Madecassol Neomicina** Roche, Chile.
Centella (p.1144·3); neomycin sulfate (p.235·1).
*Infected skin disorders; wounds.*

**Madecassol Neomycine Hydrocortisone** Nicholas, Fr.
Centella (p.1144·3); neomycin sulfate (p.235·1); hydrocortisone acetate (p.1103·3).
*Infected skin disorders.*

**Madecassol Tulgras** Roche Nicholas, Fr.
Centella (p.1144·3).
*Ulcers; wounds.*

**Maderan** Nycomed, Switz.†.
Sulfametrole (p.263·2); trimethoprim (p.272·2).
*Bacterial infections.*

**Maderil** Medifarma, Mex.†.
Oxyphenbutazone (p.76·1).

**Madicure** Taxandria, Neth.
Mebendazole (p.108·2).
*Enterobiasis.*

**Madiplot** Takeda, Thai.
Manidipine hydrochloride (p.950·2).
*Hypertension.*

**Madiprazole** Pharmadica, Thai.
Omeprazole (p.1278·2).
*Gastro-oesophageal reflux; peptic ulcer; Zollinger-Ellison syndrome.*

**Maditez** Medipharma, Arg.
Terbinafine (p.408·2) or terbinafine hydrochloride (p.408·2).
*Fungal infections.*

**Madol** Masa, Thai.
Tramadol hydrochloride (p.94·3).
*Pain.*

**Madola** Pharmaland, Thai.
Tramadol hydrochloride (p.94·3).
*Pain.*

**Madomine** Atlantic, Malaysia; Atlantic, Singapore.
Sulfadoxine (p.259·3); pyrimethamine (p.458·1).
*Malaria.*

**Madonna** Biolab, Thai.
Levonorgestrel (p.1563·2).
*Postcoital oral contraceptive.*

**Madopar** Roche, Arg.; Roche, Austral.; Roche, Austria; Roche, Denm.; Roche, Fin.; Roche, Ger.; Roche, Gr.; Roche, Hong Kong; Roche, Irl.; Roche, Ital.; Roche, Mex.; Roche, Neth.; Roche, Norw.; Roche, NZ; Roche, Port.; Roche, S.Afr.; Roche, Singapore; Roche, Spain; Roche, Switz.; Roche, Thai.; Roche, UK.
Levodopa (p.1205·2); benserazide hydrochloride (p.1200·2).
These ingredients can be described by the British Approved Name Co-beneldopa.
*Parkinsonism.*

**Madopark** Roche, Swed.
Levodopa (p.1205·2); benserazide hydrochloride (p.1200·2).
*Parkinsonism.*

**Madoxy** Pharmadica, Thai.
Doxycycline (p.206·2).
*Bacterial infections.*

**Madurase** Tecnobio, Spain†.
Clebopride malate (p.1260·3).
*Adjunct in gastrointestinal radiography and intubation; gastro-oesophageal reflux; gastroparesis; nausea and vomiting.*

**Mafel** Raymos, Arg.
Progesterone (p.1566·2).

**Mafen** Osotspa, Thai.†.
Ibuprofen (p.45·3).
*Fever; inflammation; pain.*

**Mafena** Maver, Mex.
Diclofenac sodium (p.32·1).
*Gout; inflammation; musculoskeletal, joint, and periarticular disorders; pain.*

**Maflurell** Sanorell, Ger.
Homoeopathic preparation.

**Maformin** Pharmadica, Thai.
Metformin hydrochloride (p.342·3).
*Diabetes mellitus.*

**Mafu** Bayer, Ital.†.
Tetramethrin (p.1510·2); piperonyl butoxide (p.1509·2).
*Insecticide.*

**Mag-200** Optimox, USA.
Magnesium oxide (p.1272·3).
*Magnesium deficiency.*

**Mag 2** Charton, Canad.†; Cooperation Pharmaceutique, Fr.; Galenica, Gr.; Sanofi Synthelabo, Ital.; Casen Fisons, Spain†; Aventis, Switz.
Magnesium carbonate (p.1272·1) or magnesium pidolate (p.1228·2).
*Magnesium deficiency; magnesium supplement.*

**Mag 50** Vitaplex, Austral.†.
Magnesium amino acid chelate (p.1229·1).
*Magnesium supplement.*

**Mag 77** Osotspa, Thai.
Aluminium hydroxide (p.1249·2); magnesium hydroxide (p.1272·2); simeticone (p.1289·2).
*Flatulence; gastric hyperacidity; gastritis; gastro-oesophageal reflux; peptic ulcer.*

**Mag Cit Prep** Medefield, Austral.
Magnesium citrate (p.1272·1).
*Bowel evacuation.*

**Mag Doskar's Leber-Galletonikum** Doskar, Austria.
Cynara (p.1678·3); taraxacum (p.1751·3); peppermint leaf (p.1283·2).
*Liver and biliary-tract disorders.*

**Mag Doskar's Magentonikum** Doskar, Austria.
Chamomile (p.1669·3); peppermint leaf (p.1283·2); melissa (p.1711·1).
*Gastrointestinal disorders.*

**Mag Doskar's Nerventonikum** Doskar, Austria.
Valerian (p.1762·2); lupulus (p.1708·1); melissa (p.1711·1); chamomile (p.1669·3).
*Nervous disorders.*

**Mag Doskar's Nieren- und Blasentonikum** Doskar, Austria.
Urtica (p.1762·1); equisetum (p.1684·1); birch leaf (p.1660·3).
*Renal and bladder disorders.*

**Mag Kottas Baby-Tee** Kottas-Heldenberg, Austria.
Chamomile (p.1669·3); mallow leaves (p.1709·3); spearmint (p.1749·1); caraway (p.1667·2); fennel (p.1687·2).
*Gastrointestinal disorders.*

**Mag Kottas Beruhigungstee** Kottas-Heldenberg, Austria.
Melissa (p.1711·1); spearmint (p.1749·1); valerian (p.1762·2); flos aurantii (p.1723·3); mallow leaves (p.1709·3); rose fruit (p.1740·1); mallow flowers (p.1709·3).
*Nervous disorders.*

**Mag Kottas Blahungs-Verdauungstee** Kottas-Heldenberg, Austria.
Mallow leaves (p.1709·3); peppermint leaf (p.1283·2); caraway (p.1667·2); fennel (p.1687·2); centaury (p.1669·2); calendula (p.1665·2).
*Gastrointestinal disorders.*

**Mag Kottas Entschlackungstee** *Kottas-Heldenberg, Austria.*
Birch leaf (p.1660·3); peppermint leaf (p.1283·2); urtica (p.1762·1); violae tricoloris; taraxacum (p.1751·3); calendula (p.1665·2).
*Tonic.*

**Mag Kottas Entwasserungstee** *Kottas-Heldenberg, Austria.*
Java tea (p.1702·3); equisetum (p.1684·1); herniaria (p.1697·1); taraxacum (p.1751·3); peppermint leaf (p.1283·2); calendula (p.1665·2).
*Renal and bladder disorders.*

**Mag Kottas Grippe-Tee** *Kottas-Heldenberg, Austria.*
Sambucus (p.1741·3); tilia (p.1756·2); plantago lanceolata (p.1738·2); rose fruit (p.1740·1).
*Cold symptoms.*

**Mag Kottas Herz- und Kreislauftee** *Kottas-Heldenberg, Austria.*
Orange flower (p.1723·3); crataegus (p.1677·1); maté leaves (p.1765·3); peppermint leaf (p.1283·2); rosemary (p.1740·2).
*Cardiovascular disorders.*

**Mag Kottas Husten-Bronchialtee** *Kottas-Heldenberg, Austria.*
Althaea leaves and root (p.1651·3); plantago lanceolata (p.1738·2); thyme (p.1755·2); aniseed (p.1655·2); verbascum flowers (p.1764·1).
*Respiratory-tract disorders.*

**Mag Kottas Krauterexpress-Beruhigungstee** *Kottas-Heldenberg, Austria.*
Melissa (p.1711·1); spearmint (p.1749·1); valerian (p.1762·2); flos aurantii (p.1723·3); mallow leaves (p.1709·3); rose fruit (p.1740·1).
*Nervous disorders.*

**Mag Kottas Krauterexpress-Blahungs-Verdauungstee** *Kottas-Heldenberg, Austria.*
Mallow leaves (p.1709·3); peppermint leaf (p.1283·2); caraway (p.1667·2); fennel (p.1687·2); centaury (p.1669·2).
*Gastrointestinal disorders.*

**Mag Kottas Krauterexpress-Entschlackungstee** *Kottas-Heldenberg, Austria.*
Birch leaf (p.1660·3); peppermint leaf (p.1283·2); urtica (p.1762·1); violae tricoloris; taraxacum (p.1751·3).
*Tonic.*

**Mag Kottas Krauterexpress-Entwasserungstee** *Kottas-Heldenberg, Austria.*
Java tea (p.1702·3); equisetum (p.1684·1); herniaria (p.1697·1); taraxacum (p.1751·3); peppermint leaf (p.1283·2).
*Renal and bladder disorders.*

**Mag Kottas Krauterexpress-Grippe-Tee** *Kottas-Heldenberg, Austria.*
Sambucus (p.1741·3); tilia (p.1756·2); plantago lanceolata (p.1738·2); orris; rose fruit (p.1740·1).
*Cold symptoms.*

**Mag Kottas Krauterexpress-Husten-Bronchialtee** *Kottas-Heldenberg, Austria.*
Plantago lanceolata (p.1738·2); thyme (p.1755·2); aniseed (p.1655·2); althaea root (p.1651·3); iceland moss.
*Catarrh; cough.*

**Mag Kottas Krauterexpress-Leber-Gallentee** *Kottas-Heldenberg, Austria.*
Chamomile (p.1669·3); peppermint leaf (p.1283·2); menyanthes (p.1712·1); herba teucrii; taraxacum (p.1751·3).
*Biliary disorders.*

**Mag Kottas Krauterexpress-Magen-Darm-Tee** *Kottas-Heldenberg, Austria.*
Chamomile (p.1669·3); mallow leaves (p.1709·3); peppermint leaf (p.1283·2); centaury (p.1669·2); calamus (p.1664·1); fennel (p.1687·2).
*Gastrointestinal disorders.*

**Mag Kottas Krauterexpress-Nerven-Schlaf-Tee** *Kottas-Heldenberg, Austria.*
Lupulus (p.1708·1); flos aurantii (p.1723·3); melissa (p.1711·1); peppermint leaf (p.1283·2); valerian (p.1762·2).
*Nervous disorders.*

**Mag Kottas Krauterexpress-Nieren-Blasentee** *Kottas-Heldenberg, Austria.*
Peppermint leaf (p.1283·2); java tea (p.1702·3); equisetum (p.1684·1); herniaria (p.1697·1); ononis (p.1723·3).
*Renal and bladder disorders.*

**Mag Kottas Krauterexpress-Tee fur stillende Mutter** *Kottas-Heldenberg, Austria.*
Melissa (p.1711·1); mallow leaves (p.1709·3); peppermint leaf (p.1283·2); caraway (p.1667·2); fennel (p.1687·2).
*Gastrointestinal disorders during lactation.*

**Mag Kottas Krauterexpress-Wechseltee** *Kottas-Heldenberg, Austria.*
Melissa (p.1711·1); peppermint leaf (p.1283·2); chamomile (p.1669·3); achillea (p.1646·2); valerian (p.1762·2).
*Menopausal disorders.*

**Mag Kottas Leber-Gallentee** *Kottas-Heldenberg, Austria.*
Mallow leaves (p.1709·3); peppermint leaf (p.1283·2); menyanthes (p.1712·1); cnicus benedictus (p.1673·3); taraxacum (p.1751·3); calendula (p.1665·2).
*Biliary disorders; gastrointestinal disorders.*

**Mag Kottas Magen- und Darmtee** *Kottas-Heldenberg, Austria.*
Mallow leaves (p.1709·3); melissa (p.1711·1); peppermint leaf (p.1283·2); chamomile (p.1669·3); calamus (p.1664·1); calendula (p.1665·2).
*Gastrointestinal disorders.*

**Mag Kottas May-Cur-Tee** *Kottas-Heldenberg, Austria.*
Frangula bark (p.1266·3); senna (p.1288·2); fennel (p.1687·2); chamomile (p.1669·3); magnesium sulfate (p.1228·2).
*Bowel evacuation; constipation.*

**Mag Kottas Nerven-Beruhigungstee** *Kottas-Heldenberg, Austria.*
Melissa (p.1711·1); peppermint leaf (p.1283·2); valerian (p.1762·2); flos aurantii (p.1723·3); mistletoe (p.1715·3); calendula (p.1665·2).
*Nervous disorders.*

**Mag Kottas Nieren-Blasentee** *Kottas-Heldenberg, Austria.*
Peppermint leaf (p.1283·2); java tea (p.1702·3); equisetum (p.1684·1); herniaria (p.1697·1); bearberry (p.1659·2); calendula (p.1665·2).
*Renal and bladder disorders.*

**Mag Kottas Schlaftee** *Kottas-Heldenberg, Austria.*
Lupulus (p.1708·1); flos aurantii (p.1723·3); melissa (p.1711·1); peppermint leaf (p.1283·2); valerian (p.1762·2).
*Nervous disorders.*

**Mag Kottas Tee fur stillende Mutter** *Kottas-Heldenberg, Austria.*
Melissa (p.1711·1); mallow leaves (p.1709·3); peppermint leaf (p.1283·2); caraway (p.1667·2); fennel (p.1687·2); calendula (p.1665·2).
*Gastrointestinal disorders during lactation.*

**Mag Kottas Wechseltee** *Kottas-Heldenberg, Austria.*
*Tea:* Melissa (p.1711·1); peppermint leaf (p.1283·2); chamomile (p.1669·3); potentilla anserina; valerian (p.1762·2).
*Menopausal disorders.*

**Magagel** *Genpharm, S.Afr.†.*
Aluminium oxide (p.1140·1); magnesium trisilicate (p.1272·3).
*Gastro-oesophageal reflux; peptic ulcer.*

**Magalba** *Salters, S.Afr.†.*
Magnesium sulfate (p.1228·2); magnesium carbonate (p.1272·1).
*Constipation.*

**Magalite** *Codifra, Fr.*
Cod-liver oil (p.1425·2); minerals; vitamins (p.1417·1).
*Nutritional supplement.*

**Magalphil** *Philopharm, Ger.†.*
Magaldrate (p.1271·3).
*Gastrointestinal disorders associated with hyperacidity.*

**Magan** *Savage, USA.*
Magnesium salicylate (p.55·1).
*Fever; osteoarthritis; pain; rheumatoid arthritis.*

**Magasan** *Gastropharm, Ger.†.*
Magaldrate (p.1271·3).
*Gastric hyperacidity.*

**Magastron** *1A, Ger.*
Magaldrate (p.1271·3).
*Gastric hyperacidity; peptic ulcer.*

**Mag-Cal Mega** *Freeda, USA.*
Magnesium (p.1227·3); calcium (p.1225·1).
*Dietary supplement.*

**Mag-Carb** *R&D, USA.*
Magnesium carbonate (p.1272·1).
*Nutritional supplement.*

**Magcol** *Pharmasant, Thai.*
Aluminium hydroxide (p.1249·2); magnesium hydroxide (p.1272·2); simeticone (p.1289·2).
*Flatulence; gastric hyperacidity; peptic ulcer.*

**Magel** *Vitamed, Israel†.*
Aluminium hydroxide (p.1249·2); magnesium hydroxide (p.1272·2).
*Gastritis; gastrointestinal hyperacidity; peptic ulcer.*

**Magen-700** *Wassen, Ital.*
Magnesium; potassium; sodium; taurine (p.1417·1).
*Nutritional supplementarcinia.*

**Magen-Darmtropfen S** *Cosmochema, Ger.*
Homoeopathic preparation.

**Magenpulver Hafter** *Streuli, Switz.*
Bismuth subnitrate (p.1252·2); calcium carbonate (p.1254·2); magnesium peroxide (p.1185·2).
*Gastric hyperacidity.*

**Magentabletten Hafter** *Streuli, Switz.*
Bismuth subnitrate (p.1252·2); calcium carbonate (p.1254·2); magnesium carbonate (p.1272·1).
*Gastric hyperacidity.*

**Magentee**
*Note. This name is used for preparations of different composition.*
*Weleda, Austria†.*
Angelica (p.1655·1); gentian (p.1692·2); menyanthes (p.1712·1); caraway (p.1667·2); parsley (p.1728·3); achillea (p.1646·2).
*Gastrointestinal disorders.*

*Bad Heilbrunner, Ger.†.*
Chamomile (p.1669·3); fennel (p.1687·2); peppermint leaf (p.1283·2).
*Dyspepsia; flatulence.*

**Magentee EF-EM-ES** *Smetana, Austria.*
Absinthium (p.1645·1); centaury (p.1669·2); taraxacum (p.1751·3); sweet orange peel (p.1724·1); hypericum (p.299·1).
*Gastrointestinal disorders.*

**Magen-Tee Stada N** *Stada, Ger.†.*
Chamomile (p.1669·3); peppermint leaf (p.1283·2); achillea (p.1646·2).
*Gastrointestinal disorders.*

**Magentropen N Legastol** *Twardy, Austria†.*
Peppermint leaf (p.1283·2); cynara (p.1678·3); taraxacum (p.1751·3).
*Gastrointestinal and biliary-tract disorders.*

**Magesto**
*Takeda, Hong Kong.*
Calcium carbonate (p.1254·2); sodium bicarbonate (p.1223·2); amylase (p.1654·2); thiamine (p.1455·2); scopolia; clove oil (p.1673·3); fennel oil (p.1687·3); ginger oil (p.1267·1); cinnamon oil (p.1672·2); orange oil (p.1724·1); aluminium hydroxide (p.1249·2); menthol (p.1711·3).
*Digestive-system disorders.*

*Takeda, Thai.*
Mamylase; amylase (p.1654·2); vitamin $B_1$; scopolia; sodium bicarbonate (p.1223·2); calcium carbonate (p.1254·2); cinnamon oil (p.1672·2); clove oil (p.1673·3); fennel oil (p.1687·3); ginger oil (p.1267·1); orange peel oil (p.1724·1); menthol (p.1711·3); aluminium hydroxide gel (p.1249·2).
*Gastrointestinal tract disorders.*

**Mag-G** *Cypress, USA.*
Magnesium gluconate (p.1228·1).
*Dietary supplement.*

**Magic Mix** *Taranis, Fr.*
Maize starch (p.1449·1).
*Dietary aid; gastro-oesophageal reflux in infants.*

**Magicul** *Alphapharm, Austral.*
Cimetidine (p.1255·3).
*Gastro-oesophageal reflux; peptic ulcer; Zollinger-Ellison syndrome.*

**Magion** *Ern, Spain.*
Magaldrate (p.1271·3).
*Dyspepsia; gastro-oesophageal reflux; gastrointestinal hyperacidity.*

**Magisbile** *Magis, Ital.*
Fencibutirol (p.1687·1); boldo (p.1661·2); rhubarb (p.1287·3); cascara (p.1255·1); sorbitol (p.1446·3).
*Constipation; dyspepsia; haemorrhoids.*

**Magium**
*Hexal, Austria; Hexal, Ger.*
Magnesium aspartate (p.1227·3) or magnesium oxide (p.1272·3).
*Magnesium deficiency.*

**Magium E** *Hexal, Ger.†.*
*dl*-Alpha tocoferil acetate (p.1465·1); magnesium oxide (p.1272·3).
*Vitamin E and magnesium deficiency.*

**Magium K** *Hexal, Ger.*
Potassium aspartate (p.1233·1); magnesium aspartate (p.1227·3).
*Potassium and magnesium deficiency.*

**Maglid** *Aventis, Belg.*
Aluminium hydroxide (p.1249·2); magnesium hydroxide (p.1272·2).
*Gastrointestinal disorders associated with hyperacidity.*

**Maglucate** *Pharmascience, Canad.*
Magnesium gluconate (p.1228·1).
*Hypomagnesaemia.*

**Magluphen** *Tyrol, Austria.*
Diclofenac sodium (p.32·1).
*Gout; inflammation; musculoskeletal, joint, and periarticular disorders; pain; renal and biliary colic.*

**Maglut** *Magis, Ital.*
Glutathione (p.1040·3).
*Alcohol and drug poisoning; radiation trauma.*

**Magmed** *Lichtenstein, Ger.†.*
Magaldrate (p.1271·3).
*Gastric hyperacidity; peptic ulcer.*

**Magmin** *Vitaglow, Austral.†.*
Magnesium aspartate (p.1227·3).
*Magnesium deficiency; magnesium supplement.*

**Mag-Min** *Selmag, Switz.*
Magnesium aspartate (p.1227·3).
*Magnesium deficiency; magnesium supplement.*

**Magnacal** *Sherwood, USA.*
Lactose-free preparation for enteral nutrition (p.1417·1).

**Magnalox** *Schein, USA†.*
Aluminium hydroxide (p.1249·2); magnesium hydroxide (p.1272·2).
*Hyperacidity.*

**Magnalum** *Protein, Mex.†.*
Aluminium hydroxide (p.1249·2).

**Magnamycin** *Pfizer, India.*
Cefoperazone sodium (p.174·3).
*Bacterial infections.*

**Magnapen** *CP Pharmaceuticals, UK.*
*Capsules:* Ampicillin trihydrate (p.157·2); flucloxacillin sodium (p.213·3).
*Injection:* Ampicillin sodium (p.157·1); flucloxacillin sodium (p.213·3).
*Syrup:* Ampicillin trihydrate (p.157·2); flucloxacillin magnesium (p.213·3).
These ingredients can be described by the British Approved Name Co-fluampicil.
*Bacterial infections.*

**Magnaprin** *Rugby, USA.*
Aspirin (p.15·1).
Aluminium hydroxide (p.1249·2), calcium carbonate (p.1254·2), and magnesium hydroxide (p.1272·2) are included in this preparation in an attempt to limit adverse effects on the gastrointestinal mucosa.
*Fever; inflammation; myocardial infarction; pain; transient ischaemic attacks.*

**Magnaspart** *Rosen, Ger.*
Magnesium aspartate (p.1227·3).
*Magnesium deficiency.*

**Magnaspor** *Ranbaxy, Thai.*
Cefuroxime axetil (p.184·1).
*Bacterial infections.*

**Magnatil** *Tecnofarma, Chile.*
Magnesium; vitamin C (p.1417·1).
*Dietary supplement.*

**Magnatil Calcico** *Tecnofarma, Chile.*
Ascorbic acid; magnesium; calcium (p.1417·1).
*Dietary supplement.*

**Magne-$B_6$** *Sanofi Synthelabo, Fr.*
*Oral solution:* Magnesium lactate (p.1228·1); magnesium pidolate (p.1228·2); pyridoxine hydrochloride (p.1456·3).
*Tablets:* Magnesium lactate (p.1228·1); pyridoxine hydrochloride (p.1456·3).
*Magnesium deficiency.*

**Magnebe** *Dominguez, Arg.*
*Injection:* Magnesium pidolate (p.1228·2).
*Tablets:* Magnesium citrate (p.1272·1); pyridoxine hydrochloride (p.1456·3).
*Magnesium supplement.*

**MagneBind** *Nephro-Tech, USA.*
Magnesium carbonate (p.1272·1); calcium carbonate (p.1254·2).
*Dietary phosphate binder.*

**Magnecyl** *Pharmacia, Swed.*
Aspirin (p.15·1).
*Fever; inflammation; pain.*

**Magnecyl-koffein** *Pharmacia, Swed.*
Aspirin (p.15·1); caffeine (p.782·1).
*Fever; inflammation; pain.*

**Magneforte** *Hexal, Arg.*
Magnesium oxide (p.1272·3).
*Magnesium supplement.*

**Magnefusin** *Pisa, Mex.*
Magnesium sulfate (p.1228·2).

**Magnerot** *Worwag, Ger.*
Magnesium gluconate (p.1228·1).
*Magnesium deficiency.*

**Magnerot A** *Worwag, Ger.*
Magnesium aspartate (p.1227·3).
*Magnesium deficiency.*

**magnerot Classic** *Worwag, Ger.*
Magnesium orotate (p.1724·3).
*Magnesium deficiency.*

**Magnerot N** *Worwag, Ger.*
Magnesium phosphate (p.1228·1); magnesium citrate (p.1272·1).
*Magnesium deficiency.*

**Magnesia**
*Nycomed, Denm.; Cinfa, Spain.*
Magnesium hydroxide (p.1272·2).
*Constipation; gastritis; gastro-oesophageal reflux; peptic ulcer.*

**Magnesia Bisurada** *Whitehall, Braz.*
Magnesium carbonate (p.1272·1); bismuth subcarbonate (p.1252·1); calcium carbonate (p.1254·2); sodium bicarbonate (p.1223·2).
*Gastrointestinal hyperacidity.*

**Magnesia Bisurata** *Wyeth Lederle, Ital.†.*
Magnesium carbonate (p.1272·1); sodium bicarbonate (p.1223·2); kaolin (p.1268·3).
*Gastrointestinal disorders associated with hyperacidity.*

**Magnesia Bisurata Aromatic** *Wyeth Lederle, Ital.*
Magnesium carbonate (p.1272·1); sodium bicarbonate (p.1223·2); calcium carbonate (p.1254·2).
*Gastrointestinal hyperacidity.*

**Magnesia Bisurata Aromatic Plus** *Wyeth Lederle, Ital.†.*
Oxetacaine (p.1382·1); aluminium hydroxide (p.1249·2); magnesium carbonate (p.1272·1) or magnesium oxide (p.1272·3).
*Gastrointestinal disorders associated with hyperacidity.*

**Magnesia Effervescente Sella** *Sella, Ital.*
Magnesium hydroxide (p.1272·2); tartaric acid (p.1752·1); sodium bicarbonate (p.1223·2).
*Constipation; gastrointestinal hyperacidity.*

**Magnesia Fluida** *Virtus, Braz.†.*
Magnesium hydroxide (p.1272·2).
*Gastrointestinal hyperacidity.*

**Magnesia Pasteur** *Pasteur, Chile.*
Magnesium hydroxide (p.1272·2).
*Antacid; constipation.*

**Magnesia Phosphorica I Oligoplex** *Madaus, Arg.*
Magnesium phosphate (p.1228·1); sodium sulfate (p.1290·1); lycopodium.
*Biliary-tract disorders.*

**Magnesia S Pellegrino**
*Saprochi, Israel†; Sanofi Synthelabo OTC, Ital.; Saprochi, Switz.*
Magnesium hydroxide (p.1272·2).
*Constipation; gastrointestinal hyperacidity.*

**Magnesia San Pellegrino**
*Welt, Arg.; Seid, Spain.*
Magnesium hydroxide (p.1272·2).
*Constipation; dyspepsia.*

**Magnesia Volta** *Edmond Pharma, Ital.*
Magnesium hydroxide (p.1272·2).
*Constipation; gastrointestinal hyperacidity.*

**Magnesiamaito** *Orion, Fin.*
Magnesium hydroxide (p.1272·2).
*Gastrointestinal disorders.*

**Magnesie Plus** *Whitehall, Belg.†.*
Magnesium carbonate (p.1272·1); sodium bicarbonate (p.1223·2); calcium carbonate (p.1254·2).
*Gastrointestinal disorders associated with hyperacidity.*

**Magnesie S Pellegrino** *Zambon, Fr.*
Magnesium hydroxide (p.1272·2).
*Constipation.*

**Magnesin** *Neckerman, Braz.†.*
Aluminium hydroxide (p.1249·2); magnesium hydroxide (p.1272·2); dimeticone (p.1289·2).
*Flatulence; gastrointestinal hyperacidity.*

**Magnesio + C/Mag-CE** *Asofarma, Arg.*
Magnesium; ascorbic acid (p.1417·1).
*Dietary supplement.*

**Magnesioboi** *BOI, Spain.*
Magnesium lactate (p.1228·1).
*Magnesium depletion.*

**Magnesiocard**
*Verla, Ger.; Tecnimede, Port.; Biomed, Switz.*
Magnesium aspartate hydrochloride (p.1229·1).
*Magnesium deficiency; magnesium supplement.*

**Magnesiol** *Teuto, Braz.*
Magnesium hydroxide (p.1272·2).
*Antacid.*

**Magnesiomix** *Provita, Ital.†.*
Multivitamin preparation with magnesium (p.1417·1).

**Magnesit** *Byk Madaus, S.Afr.*
Magnesium l-aspartate hydrochloride (p.1229·1).
*Hypomagnesaemia.*

**Magnesium Biomed** *Biomed, Switz.*
*Effervescent tablets; granules for oral liquid:* Magnesium aspartate (p.1227·3).
*Tablets:* Magnesium glutamate (p.1229·1); magnesium citrate (p.1272·1).
*Magnesium deficiency; magnesium supplement.*

**Magnesium Complexe** *Golaz, Switz.*
Magnesium chloride (p.1228·1); magnesium glutamate (p.1229·1); magnesium glycerophosphate (p.1228·1); magnesium orotate (p.1724·3); magnesium aspartate (p.1227·3).
*Magnesium deficiency; magnesium supplement.*

**Magnesium compositum** *OPW, Ger.*
Magnesium adipate (p.1229·1); magnesium nicotinate.
*Circulatory disorders.*

**Magnesium Diasporal**
*Austroplant, Austria; Nycomed, Austria; Protina, Ger.; Protina, Switz.*
Magnesium citrate (p.1272·1), magnesium levulinate (p.1229·1), magnesium oxide (p.1272·3), or magnesium sulfate (p.1228·2).
*Magnesium deficiency.*

**Magnesium Glycocolle Lafarge** *SERP, Mon.*
Magnesium lactate (p.1228·1); glycine (p.1433·3).
*Magnesium deficiency.*

**Magnesium Plus** *Cenovis, Austral.†; Vitelle, Austral.†.*
Magnesium orotate (p.1724·3); magnesium oxide (p.1272·3); magnesium amino acid chelate (p.1229·1); monobasic potassium phosphate (p.1230·3); calcium hydrogen phosphate (p.1225·2).
*Mineral supplement.*

**Magnesium Pyre** *Salvat, Spain.*
Magnesium bromide (p.1229·1); magnesium chloride (p.1228·1); magnesium fluoride; magnesium iodide (p.1229·1).
*Magnesium depletion.*

**Magnesium Tonil** *APS, Ger.*
*Capsules:* Heavy magnesium oxide (p.1272·3); *dl*-alpha tocoferil acetate (p.1465·1).
*Magnesium or vitamin E deficiency.*
*Injection†:* Magnesium sulfate (p.1228·2).
*Magnesium deficiency.*

**Magnesium Tonil N** *APS, Ger.†.*
Magnesium citrate (p.1272·1).
*Magnesium deficiency.*

**Magnesium Tonil Vitamin E** *Richter, Austria.*
Magnesium oxide (p.1272·3); *dl*-alpha tocoferil acetate (p.1465·1).
*Vitamin E and magnesium deficiency.*

**Magnesium Verla** *Verla, Ger.*
Magnesium citrate (p.1272·1); magnesium glutamate (p.1229·1); magnesium aspartate (p.1227·3); magnesium sulfate (p.1228·2).
*Magnesium deficiency.*

**Magnesium Vital** *Golaz, Switz.*
Magnesium aspartate (p.1227·3).
*Magnesium deficiency; magnesium supplement.*

**Magnesium-B** *Wassen, UK.*
Magnesium; vitamin $B_6$; betaine hydrochloride (p.1417·1).

**Magnesium-Eufidol** *Medopharm, Ger.†.*
Potassium aspartate (p.1233·1); magnesium aspartate (p.1227·3).
*Cardiac disorders; magnesium or potassium deficiency.*

**Magnesium-OK**
*Wassen, Ital.; Helsinn, Port.; Wassen, UK†.*
Magnesium; vitamins; minerals (p.1417·1).
*Nutritional supplement.*

**Magnesium-Plus-Hevert** *Hevert, Ger.*
Magnesium oxide (p.1272·3); *d*-alpha tocopherol (p.1464·3).
*Magnesium or vitamin E deficiency.*

**Magnesoide** *Argenfarma, Arg.*
Magnesium (p.1227·3).
*Magnesium supplement.*

**Magnesona** *Vitoria, Port.*
Magnesium pidolate (p.1228·2).
*Magnesium deficiency.*

**Magnesorot** *Worwag, Ger.*
Magnesium orotate (p.1724·3).
*Magnesium deficiency.*

**Magnespasmil** *Euro-Labor, Port.; Grunenthal, Port.*
Magnesium lactate (p.1228·1).
*Magnesium deficiency.*

**Magnespasmyl**
*Meuse, Belg.; Cooperation Pharmaceutique, Fr.; Sanofi Synthelabo, Switz.*
Magnesium lactate (p.1228·1).
*Magnesium deficiency; magnesium supplement.*

**Magnesplus** *Chemedica, Switz.†.*
Magnesium carbonate (p.1272·1); vitamin $B_6$ (p.1456·3).
*Magnesium deficiency.*

**Magnetop** *Grunenthal, Belg.*
Magnesium citrate (p.1272·1).

**Magnetrans forte** *Niddapharm, Ger.*
Magnesium oxide (p.1272·3).
*Magnesium deficiency.*

**Magnevist**
*Schering, Arg.; Schering, Austral.; Schering, Austria; Schering, Belg.; Berlex, Canad.; Schering, Denm.; Schering, Fin.; Schering, Fr.; Schering, Ger.; Shepa, Gr.; Schering, Ital.; Schering, Neth.; Schering, Norw.; Schering, NZ; Schering, Port.; Schering, S.Afr.; Schering, Spain; Schering, Swed.; Schering, Switz.; Schering, UK; Berlex, USA.*
Meglumine gadopentetate (p.1062·2).
*Contrast medium for magnetic resonance imaging.*

**Magnevistan**
*Schering, Braz.†; Schering, Chile.*
Meglumine gadopentetate (p.1062·2).
*Contrast medium for magnetic resonance imaging.*

**Magnezie** *Lifeplan, UK†.*
Vitamin and mineral preparation (p.1417·1).

**Magnezyme** *Reckitt & Colman, Belg.†.*
Magnesium carbonate (p.1272·1).
*Fatigue.*

**Magnidol-Plus** *Streger, Mex.*
Paracetamol (p.76·2).
*Fever; pain.*

**Magnihexal** *Hexal, Austria.*
Magnesium oxide (p.1272·3).
*Magnesium deficiency.*

**Magnil** *Sons, Mex.*
Dipyrone (p.35·3).
*Pain.*

**Magniton-R** *Coup, Gr.*
Indapamide (p.938·2).
*Hypertension.*

**Magno Sanol** *Sanol, Ger.; Schwarz, Ger.*
Magnesium oxide (p.1272·3).
*Magnesium deficiency.*

**Magnodor** *Teuto, Braz.*
Metamizole magnesium (p.36·1).
*Fever; pain.*

**Magnofit**
*Asta Medica, Austria.*
*Chewable tablets:* Magnesium citrate (p.1272·1); magnesium carbonate (p.1272·1).
*Effervescent tablets:* Magnesium oxide (p.1272·3).
*Magnesium deficiency.*
*Asta Medica, Ital.*
Magnesium carbonate (p.1272·1).
*Magnesium deficiency.*

**Magnogen** *Baliarda, Arg.*
Buprenorphine hydrochloride (p.21·3).
*Pain.*

**Magnogene**
*Note. This name is used for preparations of different composition.*
*Novartis Sante, Fr.; Interdelta, Switz.*
Magnesium chloride (p.1228·1).
*Magnesium deficiency; magnesium supplement.*
*Diviser Aquilea, Spain.*
Magnesium bromide (p.1229·1); magnesium chloride (p.1228·1); magnesium fluoride; magnesium iodide (p.1229·1).
*Magnesium depletion.*

**Magnograf** *Juste, Spain.*
Meglumine gadopentetate (p.1062·2).
*Contrast medium for magnetic resonance imaging.*

**Magnol** *Atlantis, Mex.*
Dipyrone (p.35·3).
*Fever; pain.*

**Magnolat** *Daudt, Braz.*
Magnesium pidolate (p.1228·2).
*Manesium supplement.*

**Magnolax** *Wampole, Canad.*
Magnesium hydroxide (p.1272·2); liquid paraffin (p.1479·1).
*Constipation.*

**Magnolex** *Sante Naturelle, Canad.*
Magnesium chloride (p.1228·1) or magnesium gluceptate (p.1228·1).

**Magnonorm** *Genericon, Austria.*
Magnesium oxide (p.1272·3).
*Magnesium deficiency.*

**Magnoplasm** *Faulding, Austral.*
Glycerol (p.1694·3); magnesium sulfate (p.1228·2).
*Poultice for abscesses, boils, and carbuncles.*

**Magnopyrol**
*Farmasa, Braz.; Rhein, Mex.*
Metamizole magnesium (p.36·1).
*Fever; pain.*

**Magnoral** *Medinfar, Port.*
Magnesium chloride (p.1228·1).
*Magnesium deficiency.*

**Magnorbin** *Merck, Ger.†.*
Magnesium ascorbate (p.1227·3).
*Magnesium deficiency.*

**Magnorell** *Sanorell, Ger.†.*
Magnesium citrate (p.1272·1).
*Magnesium deficiency.*

**Magnorol** *Rolmex, Canad.*
Magnesium gluceptate (p.1228·1).

**Magnoscorbol** *Roche Nicholas, Fr.†.*
Magnesium chloride (p.1228·1); ascorbic acid (p.1460·2).
*Anxiety attacks; magnesium deficiency.*

**Magnosol**
*Sarget, Fr.; Asta Medica, Ital.*
Magnesium carbonate (p.1272·1); magnesium oxide (p.1272·3).
*Magnesium deficiency; magnesium supplement.*

**Magnosolv** *Asta Medica, Austria.*
Precipitated magnesium carbonate (p.1272·1); magnesium oxide (p.1272·3).
*Magnesium deficiency.*

**Magnostase** *Neo Quimica, Braz.†.*
Furazolidone (p.605·2); diphenoxylate hydrochloride (p.1261·3); attapulgite (p.1251·1); pectin (p.1580·3).
*Diarrhoea.*

**Magnoston** *Ariston, Braz.*
Magnesium sulfate (p.1228·2).

**Magnotab** *Genericon, Austria.*
Magnesium oxide (p.1272·3).
*Magnesium deficiency.*

**Magnovit** *Igefarma, Braz.†.*
Rutosides; vitamins; minerals (p.1417·1).

**Magnox** *Lennod, USA.*
Aluminium hydroxide (p.1249·2); magnesium hydroxide (p.1272·2).
*Hyperacidity.*

**Magnurol** *Esteve, Spain.*
Terazosin hydrochloride (p.1010·3).
*Benign prostatic hyperplasia; hypertension.*

**Magnus** *Sidus, Arg.*
Sildenafil citrate (p.1744·2).
*Erectile dysfunction.*

**Magnyl** *Nycomed, Denm.*
Aspirin (p.15·1).
Magnesium hydroxide (p.1272·2) is included in this preparation in an attempt to limit adverse effects on the gastrointestinal mucosa.
*Fever; inflammation; ischaemic heart disease; pain; thromboembolism prophylaxis.*

**Magocean** *Proceane, Fr.*
Magnesium oxide (p.1272·3).
*Magnesium supplement.*

**Magonate** *Fleming, USA.*
Magnesium gluconate (p.1228·1); calcium hydrogen phosphate (p.1225·2).
Formerly contained magnesium gluconate.
*Dietary supplement.*

**Magopsor** *Strathmann, Ger.†.*
Dexamethasone (p.1097·1); allantoin (p.1141·3); vitamin A palmitate (p.1453·1); alpha tocoferil acetate (p.1465·1).
*Skin disorders.*

**Magoral** *ST, Thai.*
Magnesium oxide (p.1272·3).
*Gastric hyperacidity; magnesium deficiency.*

**Mag-Oro** *Eagle, Austral.†.*
Magnesium orotate (p.1724·3); magnesium aspartate (p.1227·3); magnesium amino acid chelate (p.1229·1); potassium aspartate (p.1233·1); pyridoxine hydrochloride (p.1456·3).
*Magnesium, potassium, and vitamin $B_6$ supplement.*

**Mag-Ox** *Blaine, USA.*
Magnesium oxide (p.1272·3).
*Hyperacidity; magnesium deficiency.*

**Magralibi** *Ibi, Ital.*
Magaldrate (p.1271·3).
*Gastritis; gastro-oesophageal reflux; gastroduodenitis; peptic ulcer.*

**Magrilan**
*Medochemie, Hong Kong; Medochemie, Singapore; Medochemie, Thai.*
Fluoxetine hydrochloride (p.292·1).
*Depression; mixed anxiety depressive states.*

**Magrinex** *Heralds, Braz.†.*
Mazindol (p.1589·1).
*Obesity.*

**Magroton** *Sanval, Braz.†.*
Phenolphthalein (p.1284·1); thyroid (p.1604·2); bladderwrack (p.1742·3); bile salts (p.1660·3).
*Constipation; obesity.*

**Magsal** *US Pharmaceutical, USA†.*
Magnesium salicylate (p.55·1); phenyltoloxamine citrate (p.439·1).
*Pain.*

**Magsil** *Fortune, Hong Kong.*
Aluminium hydroxide (p.1249·2); magnesium hydroxide (p.1272·2); dimethicone (p.1289·2).
*Gastrointestinal hyperacidity; meteorism.*

**Magsons** *Sons, Mex.*
Dipyrone (p.35·3).
*Fever; pain.*

**Mag-SR** *Cypress, USA.*
Magnesium chloride (p.1228·1).
*Magnesium supplement.*

**Mag-SR plus Calcium** *Cypress, USA.*
Magnesium chloride (p.1228·1); calcium carbonate (p.1254·2).
*Magnesium and calcium supplement.*

**Mag-Tab** *Rider, Chile.*
Magnesium lactate (p.1228·1).
*Magnesium supplement.*

**Mag-Tab SR** *Niche, USA.*
Magnesium lactate (p.1228·1).
*Magnesium deficiency.*

**Magto** *Polipharm, Thai.*
Aluminium hydroxide (p.1249·2); magnesium hydroxide (p.1272·2).
*Gastrointestinal hyperacidity.*

**Magtrate** *Mission Pharmacal, USA.*
Magnesium gluconate (p.1228·1).
*Dietary supplement.*

**Magvital**
*Panderma, Austria; Vifor, Switz.†.*
Magnesium aspartate (p.1227·3) or magnesium sulfate (p.1228·2).
*Eclampsia; magnesium deficiency; premature labour.*

**Mahiou** *Vectem, Spain.*
Phenolphthalein (p.1284·1); vitamin F.
*Chilblains; haematomas; haemorrhoids; insect bites and stings; varices.*

**Mainnox** *Charoen, Thai.*
Mefenamic acid (p.55·2); dicycloverine hydrochloride (p.481·2).
*Smooth muscle spasm.*

**Maintain**
*Note. A similar name is used for preparations of different composition (see below).*
*Schmid, Israel.*
Benzocaine (p.1370·3).
*Local anaesthesia.*

**Maintane**
*Note. A similar name is used for preparations of different composition (see above).*
*Jagson, India.*
*Injection:* Hydroxyprogesterone caproate (p.1556·3).
*Tablets:* Allylestrenol (p.1541·3).
*Premature labour; threatened miscarriage.*

**Maiorad**
*Rotta, Ital.; Delta, Port.; Rotta, Thai.*
Tiropramide hydrochloride (p.1757·1).
*Smooth muscle spasm.*

**Maizar** *Vitoria, Port.*
Salmeterol xinafoate (p.795·1); fluticasone propionate (p.1102·3).
*Asthma.*

**Majeptil**
*Aventis, Belg.†; Aventis, Canad.; Aventis, Fr.†; Aventis, Gr.; Aventis, Mex.; Aventis, Spain.*
Thioproperazine mesilate (p.724·1).
*Anxiety; psychoses.*

**Majocarmin forte** *Hevert, Ger.*
Caraway oil (p.1667·3); fennel oil (p.1687·3); peppermint oil (p.1283·2); absinthium (p.1645·1); cinnamon (p.1672·2); gentian (p.1692·2); pimpinella; ginger (p.1267·1); sweet orange (p.1724·1); cinchona bark (p.1671·3); condurango (p.1675·3).
*Gastrointestinal disorders.*

**Majocarmin mite** *Hevert, Ger.*
Absinthium (p.1645·1); calamus (p.1664·1); cinchona bark (p.1671·3); gentian (p.1692·2); valerian (p.1762·2); peppermint leaf (p.1283·2).
*Dyspepsia; hypochlorhydria; loss of appetite.*

**Majocarmin-Tee** *Hevert, Ger.*
Aniseed (p.1655·2); fennel (p.1687·2); caraway (p.1667·2); chamomile (p.1669·3); peppermint leaf (p.1283·2).
*Gastrointestinal disorders.*

**Majolat** *Klinge, Austria.*
Nifedipine (p.966·2).
*Angina pectoris; hypertension.*

**Major-Con** *Major, USA.*
Simeticone (p.1289·2).
*Flatulence.*

**Major-gesic** *Major, USA.*
Phenyltoloxamine citrate (p.439·1); paracetamol (p.76·2).
*Upper respiratory-tract symptoms.*

**Majorpen** *Ipso, Ital.*
Amoxicillin trihydrate (p.155·3).
*Bacterial infections.*

**Makatussin** *Gebro, Switz.†.*
*Ointment:* Camphor (p.1665·3); menthol (p.1711·3); cypress oil; eucalyptus oil (p.1686·2); pumilio pine oil (p.1737·1); oleum pini sylvestris; turpentine oil (p.1760·1); thyme oil (p.1755·3).
*Respiratory-tract disorders.*
*Oral drops:* Drosera (p.1683·1); liquorice (p.1270·2); pimpinella; senega root (p.1130·2); thyme (p.1755·2); anise oil (p.1655·2); eucalyptus oil (p.1686·2); camphor (p.1665·3); menthol (p.1711·3).
*Catarrh; coughs.*

*Syrup:* Drosera (p.1683·1); liquorice (p.1270·2); senega root (p.1130·2); thyme (p.1755·2).
*Bronchitis.*

**Makatussin Balsam mit Menthol** *Roland, Ger.†.*
Eucalyptus oil (p.1686·2); menthol (p.1711·3); thyme oil (p.1755·3).
*Bronchitis; catarrh.*

**Makatussin Codein** *Roland, Ger.*
Codeine phosphate (p.27·1).
*Coughs.*

**Makatussin Comp** *Gebro, Switz.*
Dihydrocodeine hydrochloride (p.35·2); diphenhydramine hydrochloride (p.431·3).
*Respiratory-tract disorders.*

**Makatussin forte** *Gebro, Switz.†.*
Dihydrocodeine hydrochloride (p.35·2); drosera (p.1683·1); liquorice (p.1270·2); pimpinella; senega root (p.1130·2); thyme (p.1755·2); anise oil (p.1655·2); eucalyptus oil (p.1686·2); camphor (p.1665·3); menthol (p.1711·3).
*Bronchitis; coughs.*

**Makatussin nouvelle formule** *Gebro, Switz.*
Codeine phosphate (p.27·1).
*Coughs.*

**Makatussin Saft** *Altana, Ger.*
Thyme (p.1755·2).
*Bronchitis; catarrh.*

**Makatussin Saft Drosera** *Altana, Ger.*
Drosera (p.1683·1).
*Coughs.*

**Makatussin Tropfen** *Altana, Ger.*
Thyme (p.1755·2); star anise oil.
*Bronchitis; catarrh.*

**Makatussin Tropfen Drosera** *Altana, Ger.*
Drosera (p.1683·1).
*Coughs.*

**Makatussin Tropfen forte** *Altana, Ger.*
Dihydrocodeine hydrochloride (p.35·2); drosera (p.1683·1).
*Coughs.*

**Makovan** *Crocus, Gr.*
Cefaclor (p.167·1).
*Bacterial infections.*

**Makrocilin** *Makros, Braz.†.*
Ampicillin (p.157·1).
*Bacterial infections.*

**Maladin** *Unicure, India.*
Mepacrine hydrochloride (p.606·3).
*Malaria.*

**Malafene** *Knoll, Belg.*
Ibuprofen (p.45·3).
*Fever; inflammation; pain.*

**Malandil** *Bohm, Spain.*
Carnitine hydrochloride (p.1424·1); cobamamide (p.1459·1); lysine hydrochloride (p.1439·2).
*Anaemias; tonic.*

**Malarex** *Alpharma, Denm.*
Chloroquine phosphate (p.448·2).
*Amoebiasis; lupus erythematosus; malaria; photosensitivity; rheumatoid arthritis.*

**Malarone**
*GlaxoSmithKline, Austral.; GlaxoSmithKline, Austria; GlaxoSmithKline, Belg.; Glaxo Wellcome, Braz.†; GlaxoSmithKline, Canad.; GlaxoSmithKline, Denm.; GlaxoSmithKline, Fr.; GlaxoSmithKline, Ger.; GlaxoSmithKline, Norw.; GlaxoSmithKline, NZ; GlaxoSmithKline, Singapore; GlaxoSmithKline, Spain; GlaxoSmithKline, Swed.; GlaxoSmithKline, Switz.; GlaxoSmithKline, UK; Glaxo Wellcome, USA.*
Atovaquone (p.601·3); proguanil hydrochloride (p.457·1).
*Malaria.*

**Malastop** *Sterop, Belg.*
Pyrimethamine (p.458·1); sulfadoxine (p.259·3).
*Malaria.*

**Malaviron** *Wallace Mfg Chem., UK.*
Chloroquine phosphate (p.448·2).
*Malaria.*

**Male +** *Homeocan, Canad.*
Homoeopathic preparation.

**Male Formula Herbal Plus Formula 2** *Vitelle, Austral.†.*
Eleutherococcus senticosis; equisetum; sarsaparilla; liquorice; damiana; zinc amino acid chelate; betacarotene; pyridoxine hydrochloride; *d*-alpha tocoferil acid succinate; magnesium oxide (p.1417·1).
*Tonic.*

**Maleapril** *Gallia, Braz.†.*
Enalapril maleate (p.909·2).
*Hypertension.*

**Malen** *BA Farma, Port.*
Enalapril maleate (p.909·2).
*Heart failure; hypertension.*

**Malexin** *BASF, Ger.†.*
Naproxen (p.65·1).
*Gout; inflammation; musculoskeletal, joint, and soft-tissue disorders; pain.*

**Malfin** *Nettopharma, Denm.†.*
Morphine sulfate (p.60·2).
*Pain.*

**Maliasin**
*Ebewe, Austria; Abbott, Braz.; BASF, Ger.†; Abbott, Ital.; Knoll, Switz.*
Barbexaclone (p.353·3).
*Epilepsy.*

**Malidens** *Nicholas Piramal, India.*
Paracetamol (p.76·2).
*Fever; pain.*

**Malimed** *Ecosol, Switz.*
Cimetidine (p.1255·3).
*Gastric hyperacidity; gastro-oesophageal reflux; gastrointestinal haemorrhage; peptic ulcer; Zollinger-Ellison syndrome.*

**Malinert** *Strathmann, Ger.†.*
Aspirin (p.15·1); paracetamol (p.76·2).
*Inflammation; pain.*

**Malipuran** *Pharmacia, Ger.*
Bufexamac (p.21·3).
*Skin disorders.*

**Malirid** *Ipca, India.*
Primaquine phosphate (p.456·2).
*Malaria.*

**Malival** *Silanes, Mex.*
Indometacin (p.47·3).
*Gout; musculoskeletal, joint and peri-articular disorders.*

**Malival Compuesto** *Silanes, Mex.*
Methocarbamol (p.1395·1); indometacin (p.47·3).
*Musculoskeletal, joint and peri-articular disorders; skeletal muscle spasm.*

**Malix** *Lagap, UK†.*
Glibenclamide (p.331·2).
*Diabetes mellitus.*

**Mallamint** *Roberts, USA.*
Calcium carbonate (p.1254·2).
*Hyperacidity.*

**Mallazine** *Roberts, USA; Hauck, USA.*
Tetryzoline hydrochloride (p.1131·2).
*Minor eye irritation.*

**Mallebrin** *Krewel, Ger.*
Hexaurea aluminium chloride.
Formerly known as Mallebrinetten.
*Mouth and throat disorders.*

**Mallebrin Konzentrat** *Krewel, Ger.*
Aluminium chloride (p.1142·1).
*Mouth and throat inflammation.*

**Mallorol** *Novartis, Swed.*
Thioridazine (p.724·2) or thioridazine hydrochloride (p.724·2).
*Pain; psychoses.*

**Malocide** *Aventis, Fr.*
Pyrimethamine (p.458·1).
*Toxoplasmosis.*

**Malocin** *M & H, Thai.*
Erythromycin stearate (p.208·2).
*Bacterial infections.*

**Malogen Aqueous** *Germiphene, Canad.†.*
Testosterone (p.1569·3).
*Androgenic.*

**Malogen in Oil** *Germiphene, Canad.†.*
Testosterone propionate (p.1570·1).
*Androgenic.*

**Malogex** *Germiphene, Canad.†.*
Testosterone enantate (p.1570·1).
*Androgenic.*

**Maloprim**
*Wellcome, Irl.; GlaxoSmithKline, S.Afr.; Wellcome, UK†.*
Pyrimethamine (p.458·1); dapsone (p.202·2).
*Malaria.*

**Malortil** *Specifar (Σπεσφαρ), Gr.*
Omeprazole (p.1278·2).
*Acid aspiration; eradication of Helicobacter pylori in combination with antimicrobials; peptic ulcer; reflux oesophagitis; Zollinger-Ellison syndrome.*

**Maltlevol** *Carter Horner, Canad.*
Multivitamin preparation (p.1417·1) with ferric ammonium citrate (p.1427·2).
*Food supplement; iron-deficiency anaemia.*

**Maltlevol-M** *Carter Horner, Canad.*
Multivitamin and mineral preparation (p.1417·1).

**Maltofer**
*Andromaco, Chile; Meda, Fin.; Therabel, Fr.; Vifor, Malaysia; Vifor International, Switz.*
Iron polymaltose (p.1437·3).
*Iron deficiency; iron-deficiency anaemia.*

**Maltofer Fol**
*Andromaco, Chile; Vifor International, Switz.*
Iron polymaltose (p.1437·3); folic acid (p.1429·1).
*Iron and folic acid deficiency.*

**Maltofer Vitaminado** *Andromaco, Chile.*
Multivitamin and mineral preparation (p.1417·1).
*Dietary supplement.*

**Maltogen** *Nestle, Austral.†.*
Infant feed supplement (p.1417·1).
*Anorexia; constipation.*

**Malton E** *Riemser, Ger.*
*d*-Alpha tocopherol (p.1464·3).
*Vitamin E deficiency.*

**Maltovis** *Volchem, Ital.*
Maltodextrin (p.1439·3).
*Carbohydrate source.*

**Maltsupex** *Wallace, USA.*
Malt extract (p.1439·2).
*Constipation.*

**Maltyl** *Merckle, Ger.*
Dequalinium chloride (p.1178·1).
*Mouth and throat disorders.*

**Maludil** *Durascan, Denm.*
Maprotiline hydrochloride (p.306·1).
*Depression.*

**Malugel** *Charoen, Thai.*
Calcium carbonate (p.1254·2); simeticone (p.1289·2).
*Flatulence; gastric hyperacidity; heartburn; peptic ulcer.*

**Malva Composta** *Windson, Braz.†.*
Mallow (p.1709·3); benzocaine (p.1370·3); menthol (p.1711·3).
*Mouth and throat disorders.*

**Malvaliz** *Soria Natural, Spain.*
Althaea (p.1651·3); liquorice (p.1270·2); clay.
*Gastrointestinal disorders.*

**Malvatricin** *Daudt, Braz.*
Sodium fluoride (p.1444·3); tyrothricin (p.275·1).
*Dental caries prophylaxis.*

**Malvedrin** *Adroka, Switz.*
*Ointment:* Mallow leaves (p.1709·3); vitamin A (p.1451·2); vitamin D (p.1461·2); chamomile oil (p.1669·3); hypericum oil (p.299·2); linseed oil (p.1707·2).
*Skin irritation; superficial wounds.*
*Topical liquid:* Mallow leaves (p.1709·3).
*Mouth and throat disorders; superficial wounds.*

**Malveol** *Magistra, Switz.*
Althaea leaves (p.1651·3); mallow leaves (p.1709·3); salicylic acid (p.1157·1); mint oil (p.1715·2).
*Mouth and throat disorders.*

**Malvitona**
*Leo, Fin.; Leo, Swed.*
Vitamin B substances (p.1417·1); caffeine (p.782·1).
*Tonic.*

**Malvodon** *IMA, Braz.*
Mallow (p.1709·3); poppy (p.1129·1).
*Mouth disorders.*

**Malvol** *Hearst, Braz.†.*
Cetylpyridinium chloride (p.1173·1); benzocaine (p.1370·3); phenosalyl; menthol (p.1711·3); mallow (p.1709·3); eucalyptus oil (p.1686·2).
*Mouth and throat disorders.*

**Malvona** *Prima, Braz.*
*Mouthwash; pastilles:* Benzocaine (p.1370·3); cetylpyridinium chloride (p.1173·1); borax (p.1661·3).
Formerly contained phenosalyl, menthol, benzocaine, mallow, and cetylpyridinium chloride.
*Mouth and throat disorders.*
*Toothpaste:* Borax (p.1661·3); sodium chloride (p.1233·3); benzocaine (p.1370·3).

**Malvosulfam** *Hearst, Braz.†.*
Sulfanilamide (p.263·2); phenosalyl; salol (p.88·1); procaine hydrochloride (p.1383·2); myrrh (p.1718·3); mallow (p.1709·3); peppermint oil (p.1283·2).
*Mouth and throat disorders.*

**Mamellin** *Calea, Austria.*
Vitamin F; peru balsam (p.1730·2); alpha tocoferil acetate (p.1465·1).
*Skin damage.*

**Mammol** *Abbott, USA.*
Bismuth subnitrate (p.1252·2); castor oil (p.1668·2); peru balsam (p.1730·2).
*Nipple care.*

**Mamofen** *Khandelwal, India.*
Tamoxifen (p.585·3).
*Breast cancer.*

**Mamograf** *Temis, Arg.*
Activated charcoal (p.1030·2).
*Adjunct in breast examination.*

**Man Formula** *Avon, Canad.*
Multivitamin and mineral preparation (p.1417·1).

**Manaderm** *Wyeth, India.*
Psoralen (p.1153·1).
*Skin disorders.*

**Manceau** *SmithKline Beecham Consumer, Belg.†.*
Senna (p.1288·2); mali comm. syrup.
*Constipation.*

**Mancef** *Lafare, Ital.*
Cefamandole nafate (p.169·3).
Lidocaine hydrochloride (p.1377·3) is included in this preparation to alleviate the pain of injection.
*Gram-negative bacterial infections.*

**Mandafen** *Pharmachem, UK.*
Ibuprofen (p.45·3).
*Cold and influenza symptoms; fever; pain.*

**Mandal 425** *Golaz, Switz.†.*
Hypericum (p.299·1).
*Insomnia; nervous disorders.*

**Mandalyn Expectorant** *Pharmachem, UK.*
Diphenhydramine hydrochloride (p.431·3); ammonium chloride (p.1115·2).
*Coughs and cold symptoms.*

**Mandalyn Paediatric** *Pharmachem, UK.*
Diphenhydramine hydrochloride (p.431·3).
*Coughs and cold symptoms.*

**Mandanol** *Pharmachem, UK.*
Paracetamol (p.76·2).
*Fever; pain.*

**Mandarine** *Boiron, Canad.*
Homoeopathic preparation.

**Mandelamine**
*Pfizer, Canad.; Parke, Davis, Ger.†; Aspen, S.Afr.; Warner Chilcott, USA.*
Methenamine mandelate (p.230·2).
*Urinary-tract infections.*

**Mandelan** *Sydenham, Mex.†.*
Methenamine (p.230·1).

**Mandelip** *Dermoteca, Port.*
Mandelic acid (p.228·3) with sunscreens.
*Chapped lips.*

**Mandelo-katt** *Kattwiga, Ger.*
Homoeopathic preparation.

**Mandepiril** *Tegur, Mex.†.*
Methenamine (p.230·1).

**Mandokef**
*Lilly, Austria; Lilly, Ger.†; Pharmaserve Lilly (Φαρμασερβ Λιλλυ), Gr.; Lilly, Ital.; Lilly, Port.; Aspen, S.Afr.; Lilly, Spain†; Lilly, Switz.*
Cefamandole nafate (p.169·3).
Lidocaine hydrochloride (p.1377·3) may be included in the intramuscular injection to alleviate the pain of injection.
*Bacterial infections.*

**Mandol**
*Lilly, Austral.; Lilly, Belg.; Lilly, Canad.†; Lilly, Hong Kong; Lilly, Neth.; Lilly, NZ; Lilly, Thai.; Lilly, USA†.*
Cefamandole nafate (p.169·3).
*Bacterial infections.*

**Mandolgin** *Durascan, Denm.*
Tramadol hydrochloride (p.94·3).
*Pain.*

**Mandolsan** *San Carlo, Ital.*
Cefamandole nafate (p.169·3).
Lidocaine hydrochloride (p.1377·3) is included in the intramuscular injection to alleviate the pain of injection.
*Bacterial infections.*

**Mandragora comp** *Weleda, Ger.*
Homoeopathic preparation.

**Mandragora Med Complex** *Dynamit, Austria.*
Homoeopathic preparation.

**Mandrogripp** *Dolorgiet, Ger.†.*
Paracetamol (p.76·2).
*Fever; pain.*

**Mandrolax** *Dolorgiet, Ger.†.*
Bisacodyl (p.1251·3).
*Constipation.*

**Mandrolax Lactu** *Dolorgiet, Ger.†.*
Lactulose (p.1269·1).
*Constipation; hepatic encephalopathy; salmonella enteritis.*

**Mandrolax Pico** *Dolorgiet, Ger.†.*
Sodium picosulfate (p.1289·3).
*Constipation.*

**Mandros Diarstop** *Dolorgiet, Ger.†.*
Loperamide hydrochloride (p.1271·1).
*Diarrhoea.*

**Mandros Reise** *Dolorgiet, Ger.†.*
Dimenhydrinate (p.431·1).
*Motion sickness; nausea; vertigo; vomiting.*

**Maneon** *Poli, Ital.†.*
Amineptine hydrochloride (p.280·3).
*Depression.*

**Manerix**
*Roche, Canad.; Roche, Irl.; Roche, Spain; Roche, UK.*
Moclobemide (p.308·2).
*Depression.*

**Manevac** *Galen, UK.*
Ispaghula (p.1268·1); senna fruit (p.1288·2).
A similar product was formerly marketed in the *UK* under the name Agiolax.
*Bowel evacuation; constipation.*

**Mangaplexe** *Lehning, Fr.*
Manganese gluconate (p.1440·1).
*Hypersensitivity.*

**Manibee Complejo** *Rhone-Poulenc Rorer, Mex.†.*
Vitamin B substances (p.1417·1).

**Manibee-C** *Aventis, Mex.*
Vitamin B substances; vitamin C (p.1417·1).

**Manic** *Medifive, Thai.*
Mefenamic acid (p.55·2).
*Pain.*

**Manicol** *Martin, Fr.†.*
Mannitol (p.950·2).
*Bowel evacuation; constipation; dyspepsia.*

**Manidon** *Abbott, Spain.*
Verapamil hydrochloride (p.1019·1).
*Angina pectoris; arrhythmias; hypertension; myocardial infarction.*

**Manimon** *Asta Medica, Ger.†.*
Propranolol hydrochloride (p.989·3); triamterene (p.1016·2); hydrochlorothiazide (p.933·2).
*Hypertension.*

**Maninil** *Berlin-Chemie, Ger.*
Glibenclamide (p.331·2).
*Diabetes mellitus.*

**Maniprex** *Wolfs, Belg.*
Lithium carbonate (p.301·1).
*Bipolar disorder; depression.*

**Maniton** *Kyorin, Thai.*
Mannitol (p.950·2).
*Anuria; oliguria; raised intracranial pressure.*

**Manivasc** *Farmalab, Braz.*
Manidipine hydrochloride (p.950·2).
*Hypertension.*

**Manmox** *T Man, Thai.*
Amoxicillin trihydrate (p.155·3).
*Bacterial infections.*

**Mann** *SMB, Belg.*
Paracetamol (p.76·2); caffeine (p.782·1).
*Fever; pain.*

**Mannex** *Bioceuticals, UK.*
Multivitamin and mineral preparation (p.1417·1).

**Mannistol** *Bieffe, Ital.*
Mannitol (p.950·2).
*Cranial and ocular hypertension.*

**Mannite** *Soprochi, Switz.*
Mannitol (p.950·2).
*Constipation.*

**Mannit-Losung** *Serag-Wiessner, Ger.*
Mannitol (p.950·2).
*Forced diuresis; oedema; renal failure.*

**Mano** *March, Thai.*
Tetryzoline hydrochloride (p.1131·2); boric acid (p.1662·1); sodium chloride (p.1233·3).
*Allergic eye disorders.*

**Manobrozil** *March, Thai.*
Gemfibrozil (p.923·1).
*Hyperlipidaemias.*

**Manodepo** *March, Thai.*
Medroxyprogesterone acetate (p.1557·2).
*Menopausal disorders; menstrual disorders; threatened or recurrent miscarriage.*

**Manoflox** *March, Thai.*
Norfloxacin (p.238·3).
*Bacterial infections.*

**Manoglucon** *March, Thai.*
Glibenclamide (p.331·2).
*Diabetes mellitus.*

**Manoketo** *March, Thai.*
Ketoconazole (p.403·3).
*Scalp disorders.*

**Manolio** *Brasmedica, Braz.†.*
Hamamelis (p.1696·3); yeast (p.1469·1); rutoside (p.1688·2); phenolphthalein (p.1284·1).

**Manolone** *Lam Thong, Thai.*
Triamcinolone acetonide (p.1110·2).
*Skin disorders.*

**Manomet** *March, Thai.*
Cimetidine (p.1255·3).
*Peptic ulcer; Zollinger-Ellison syndrome.*

**Manon** *Igefarma, Braz.†.*
Agar (p.1576·3); phenolphthalein (p.1284·1); light liquid paraffin (p.1479·1).
*Constipation.*

**Manorfen** *Manor, UK.*
Ibuprofen (p.45·3).

**Manorifcin** *March, Thai.*
Rifampicin (p.250·2).
*Gonorrhoea; tuberculosis.*

**Manoron** *March, Thai.*
Cinnarizine (p.428·3).
*Cerebral and peripheral vascular disorders; migraine; motion sickness; vestibular disorders.*

**Manotran** *March, Thai.*
Dipotassium clorazepate (p.685·1).
*Anxiety; insomnia.*

**Manovon** *March, Thai.*
Bromhexine hydrochloride (p.1115·3).
*Obstructive airways disease.*

**Mansal** *Vita, Spain.*
Cimetidine (p.1255·3).
*Acid aspiration; gastro-oesophageal reflux; gastrointestinal haemorrhage; gastrointestinal hyperacidity; peptic ulcer; short-bowel syndrome; Zollinger-Ellison syndrome.*

**Mansil** *Pfizer, Braz.*
Oxamniquine (p.110·3).
*Schistosomiasis.*

**Mantadan** *Boehringer Ingelheim, Ital.*
Amantadine hydrochloride (p.1197·2).
*Influenza A; mental function impairment; parkinsonism.*

**Mantadix**
*Du Pont, Belg.†; Bristol-Myers Squibb, Fr.*
Amantadine hydrochloride (p.1197·2).
*Influenza A; parkinsonism.*

**Mantai** *Tecnimede, Port.†.*
Minoxidil (p.960·1).

**Mantidan** *Eurofarma, Braz.*
Amantadine hydrochloride (p.1197·2).
*Drug-induced extrapyramidal disorders; fatigue associated with multiple sclerosis; influenza A; parkinsonism.*

**Mantus** *Labinca, Arg.*
A heparinoid (p.931·1); triamcinolone acetonide (p.1110·2); hexetidine (p.1182·1); lidocaine (p.1377·3).
*Haemorrhoids.*

**Manugel** *Anios, Fr.*
Isopropyl alcohol (p.1184·3); phenoxyethanol (p.1189·1).
*Skin disinfection.*

**Manusept**
*Note. This name is used for preparations of different composition.*
*Bode, Ger.†; Beiersdorf, Switz.*
Orthophenylphenol (p.1187·2).
*Hand disinfection.*

*SSL, UK.*
Triclosan (p.1195·2); isopropyl alcohol (p.1184·3).
*Skin disinfection.*

**Manusept HD** *Bode, Ger.*
Alcohol (p.1166·1).
*Hand disinfection.*

**Manzan** *Gezzi, Arg.*
Camphor (p.1665·3); phenol (p.1188·1); thymol (p.1194·2); hamamelis (p.1696·3); eucalyptus oil (p.1686·2).
*Haemorrhoids.*

**Manzan Plus** *Gezzi, Arg.*
Zinc oxide (p.1163·2); lidocaine hydrochloride (p.1377·3).
*Haemorrhoids.*

**Maolate** *Upjohn, USA.*
Chlorphenesin carbamate (p.1392·2).
*Musculoskeletal pain.*

**Maoni** *Lichtwer, Ger.*
Kava (p.1703·2).
*Nervous disorders.*

**Maosig** *Sigma, Austral.*
Moclobemide (p.308·2).
*Depression.*

**MAOtil** *Acis, Ger.*
Selegiline hydrochloride (p.1214·1).
*Parkinsonism.*

**Maox** *Manne, USA.*
Magnesium oxide (p.1272·3).
*Hyperacidity.*

**Map An** *Pharmacia, Arg.*
Medroxyprogesterone stearate (p.1557·3).
*Malignant neoplasms.*

**Mapap** *Major, USA.*
Paracetamol (p.76·2).
*Fever; pain.*

**Mapap Cold Formula** *Major, USA.*
Paracetamol (p.76·2); chlorphenamine maleate (p.427·3); pseudoephedrine hydrochloride (p.1129·2); dextromethorphan hydrobromide (p.1117·3).

**Mapezine** *Siam Bheasach, Thai.*
Carbamazepine (p.353·3).
*Epilepsy; trigeminal neuralgia.*

**Mapin** *Duopharma, Hong Kong.*
Naloxone hydrochloride (p.1044·3).
*Opioid overdosage; reversal of opioid depression.*

**Maple Melts** *Green Turtle Bay Vitamin Co., USA.*
Vitamin and mineral preparation (p.1417·1).
*Tonic.*

**Mapluxin** *Novartis, Mex.*
Digoxin (p.895·2).
*Heart failure; paroxysmal supraventricular tachycardia.*

**Mapox** *Niddapharm, Ger.*
Aciclovir (p.626·1).
*Herpesvirus infections.*

**Mapro-GRY** *Gry, Ger.†.*
Maprotiline hydrochloride (p.306·1).
*Depression.*

**Maprolu** *Hexal, Ger.*
Maprotiline hydrochloride (p.306·1).
*Depression.*

**Mapurit** *Sanum-Kehlbeck, Ger.*
*dl*-Alpha tocoferil acetate (p.1465·1); magnesium oxide (p.1272·3).
*Magnesium or vitamin E deficiency.*

**Maquil** *Pharmaton, Ger.†.*
Cynara (p.1678·3).
*Dyspepsia.*

**Maqui-Libre** *Lancome, Canad.*
*SPF 15:* Octinoxate (p.1154·3).
*Sunscreen.*

**Mar** *Masa, Thai.*
Dried aluminium hydroxide gel (p.1249·2); magnesium hydroxide (p.1272·2); simeticone (p.1289·2).
*Flatulence; gastric hyperacidity; peptic ulcer.*

**Mar Plus**
*Stada, Austria.*
Dexpanthenol (p.1727·2); sea water.
*Nasal congestion.*

*Stada, Ger.*
Dexpanthenol (p.1727·2); sodium chloride (p.1233·3).
*Nasal congestion.*

**Maracugina** *Virtus, Braz.†.*
Passion flower (p.1729·1); erythrina mulungu (p.1717·2); crataegus (p.1677·1).
*Sedative.*

**Marament Balsam W** *Wider, Ger.†.*
Camphor (p.1665·3); methyl salicylate (p.59·3); benzyl nicotinate (p.21·2).
*Neuralgia; rheumatism; sciatica; sprains.*

**Marament-N** *Amino, Switz.*
Camphor (p.1665·3); methyl salicylate (p.59·3); benzyl nicotinate (p.21·2); oleum pini sylvestris.
*Musculoskeletal, joint, and soft-tissue disorders.*

**Maranon H** *Henkel, Ger.*
Sodium hypochlorite (p.1192·1).
*Instrument disinfection.*

**Maranox** *Dent, USA.*
Paracetamol (p.76·2).
*Fever; pain.*

**Marathon**
*Armstrong, Arg.; Laboratorios Chile, Chile.*
Vitamins; minerals; ubidecarenone; ginseng (p.1417·1).
*Dietary supplement.*

**Marathon Antioxidante** *Armstrong, Arg.*
Ubidecarenone; vitamin E; betacarotene; selenium (p.1417·1).
*Antioxidant preparation.*

**Marax**
*Note. This name is used for preparations of different composition.*
*Pfizer, Braz.; Pfizer, USA.*
Ephedrine sulfate (p.1120·1); theophylline (p.798·3); hydroxyzine hydrochloride (p.434·3).
*Bronchospasm.*

*Asche, Ger.*
Magaldrate (p.1271·3).
*Gastrointestinal hyperacidity; peptic ulcer.*

*Unimed, India.*
Hydroxyzine hydrochloride (p.434·3); ephedrine hydrochloride (p.1120·1); theophylline (p.798·3).
*Asthma; bronchospasm.*

**Marben** *Medifarma, Mex.†.*
Mebendazole (p.108·2).

**Marblen** *Fleming, USA.*
Calcium carbonate (p.1254·2); magnesium carbonate (p.1272·1).
*Hyperacidity.*

**Marcain**
*AstraZeneca, Austral.; Dentsply, Austral.; AstraZeneca, Denm.; AstraZeneca, Fin.; Sarabhai Piramal, India; AstraZeneca, Irl.; AstraZeneca, Malaysia; AstraZeneca, Norw.; AstraZeneca, NZ; AstraZeneca, Singapore; AstraZeneca, Swed.; AstraZeneca, UK.*
Bupivacaine hydrochloride (p.1371·1).
Adrenaline (p.852·2) or adrenaline acid tartrate (p.852·2) is included in some injections as a vasoconstrictor to diminish absorption and localise the effect of the local anaesthetic.
*Local anaesthesia.*

**Marcain with Fentanyl**
*AstraZeneca, Austral.; AstraZeneca, NZ.*
Bupivacaine hydrochloride (p.1371·1); fentanyl citrate (p.40·1).
*Epidural analgesia.*

**Marcain with Pethidine**
*AstraZeneca, Austral.; AstraZeneca, NZ†.*
Bupivacaine hydrochloride (p.1371·1); pethidine hydrochloride (p.80·2).
*Epidural analgesia.*

**Marcaina**
*AstraZeneca, Braz.; AstraZeneca, Ital.; AstraZeneca, Port.*
Bupivacaine hydrochloride (p.1371·1).
Adrenaline acid tartrate (p.852·2) is included in some injections as a vasoconstrictor to diminish absorption and localise the effect of the local anaesthetic.
*Local anaesthesia.*

**Marcaine**
*AstraZeneca, Belg.; Abbott, Canad.; AstraZeneca, Fr.; IFET (IΦET), Gr.; AstraZeneca, Hong Kong; Astra, Israel; AstraZeneca, Neth.; AstraZeneca, Thai.; Sanofi Winthrop, USA.*
Bupivacaine hydrochloride (p.1371·1).
Adrenaline (p.852·2) or adrenaline acid tartrate (p.852·2) is included in some injections as a vasoconstrictor to diminish absorption and localise the effect of the local anaesthetic.
*Analgesia; local anaesthesia.*

**Marcelle Moisture Eye Cream** *Prof. Pharm. Corp., Canad.*
*SPF 15:* Titanium dioxide (p.1160·3); zinc oxide (p.1163·2).
*Sunscreen.*

**Marcelle Multi-Defense** *Prof. Pharm. Corp., Canad.*
*SPF 15:* Meradimate (p.1151·3); octinoxate (p.1154·3); ensulizole (p.1147·1).
*Sunscreen.*

**Marcelle Protective Block** *Prof. Pharm. Corp., Canad.*
*SPF 15:* Titanium dioxide (p.1160·3).
*SPF 25:* Titanium dioxide (p.1160·3); zinc oxide (p.1163·2).
*Sunscreen.*

**Marcelle Sunblock** *Prof. Pharm. Corp., Canad.*
*SPF 8:* Octinoxate (p.1154·3); oxybenzone (p.1154·3).
*SPF 15; SPF 20:* Octinoxate (p.1154·3); octisalate (p.1154·3); oxybenzone (p.1154·3).
*Sunscreen.*

**Marcen** *Pharmacia, Spain.*
Ketazolam (p.703·1).
*Anxiety; insomnia; skeletal muscle spasm.*

**Marcillin** *Marnel, USA†.*
Ampicillin trihydrate (p.157·2).

**Marclorhex** *Cristalia, Braz.*
Chlorhexidine gluconate (p.1173·2).
*Skin disinfection.*

**Marco Rub Camphorated** *Marc-O, Canad.†.*
Camphor (p.1665·3); menthol (p.1711·3); cineole (p.1672·1).

**Marco Sweet Light** *Laboratorios Chile, Chile.*
Aspartame (p.1422·1); acesulfame potassium (p.1420·3).
*Sugar substitute.*

**Marco Sweett** *Laboratorios Chile, Chile.*
Aspartame (p.1422·1).
*Sugar substitute.*

**Marcocid** *Willvonseder, Austria.*
Propyl alcohol (p.1191·2); isopropyl alcohol (p.1184·3).
*Skin disinfection.*

**Marcodine** *Cristalia, Braz.*
Povidone-iodine (p.1190·3).
*Skin disinfection.*

**Marcof** *Marnel, USA.*
Hydrocodone tartrate (p.45·1); sulfogaiacol (p.1131·1).
*Coughs.*

**Marcoumar**
*Roche, Austria; Roche, Belg.; Roche, Braz.; Roche, Denm.; Roche, Neth.; Roche, Switz.*
Phenprocoumon (p.981·3).
*Thromboembolic disorders.*

**Marcumar** *Roche, Ger.*
Phenprocoumon (p.981·3).
*Thromboembolic disorders.*

**marcuphen** *CT, Ger.*
Phenprocoumon (p.981·3).
*Thromboembolic disorders.*

**Marduk** *S & K, Ger.*
Benzoyl peroxide (p.1143·2).
*Acne.*

**Mareamin** *Volta, Chile.*
Dimenhydrinate (p.431·1).
*Motion sickness.*

**Mareen** *Krewel, Ger.*
Doxepin hydrochloride (p.291·2).
*Anxiety disorders; depression; sleep disorders; withdrawal syndromes.*

**Marespin** *Abiogen, Ital.*
Sulfamazone sodium (p.260·3).
*Respiratory-tract infections.*

**Marevan**
*Boots Healthcare, Austral.; Therabel, Belg.; Zest, Braz.; Nycomed, Denm.; Orion, Fin.; IFET (IΦET), Gr.; Nycomed, Norw.; GlaxoSmithKline, NZ; GlaxoSmithKline, Singapore; Goldshield, UK.*
Warfarin sodium (p.1022·2).
*Thromboembolic disorders.*

**Marevit** *Pensa, Spain†.*
Meclozine hydrochloride (p.436·3).
*Motion sickness.*

**Marezine** *Himmel, USA.*
Cyclizine hydrochloride (p.429·3).
*Motion sickness.*

**Margesic** *Marnel, USA.*
Butalbital (p.673·3); paracetamol (p.76·2); caffeine (p.782·1).
*Tension headache.*

**Margesic H** *Marnel, USA.*
Hydrocodone tartrate (p.45·1); paracetamol (p.76·2).
*Pain.*

**Marianon** *Klein, Ger.*
Silybum marianum (p.1043·3); greater celandine (p.1695·3); achillea (p.1646·2); absinthium (p.1645·1); hypericum (p.299·1).
*Biliary disorders.*

**Mariazeller** *Apotheke Gnadenmutter, Austria.*
Cinnamon (p.1672·2); cinchona bark (p.1671·3); dried bitter-orange peel (p.1723·3); clove (p.1673·2); flos aurantii (p.1723·3); chamomile (p.1669·3); folium aurantium; melissa (p.1711·1); menyanthes (p.1712·1); cardamom fruit (p.1667·3); fructus aurantii immat (p.1723·3); coriander (p.1676·1); absinthium (p.1645·1); cnicus benedictus (p.1673·3); centaury (p.1669·2); achillea moschata; achillea (p.1646·2); guaiacum wood; juniper (p.1703·1); galanga; gentian (p.1692·2); ginger (p.1267·1); nutmeg (p.1722·2).
*Gastrointestinal disorders.*

**Marienbader Pillen N** *Riemser, Ger.*
Bisacodyl (p.1251·3).
*Constipation.*

**Mariendistel Curarina** *Harras-Curarina, Ger.*
Silybum marianum (p.1043·3).
*Liver disorders.*

**Maril**
*Atlantic, Malaysia; Atlantic, Singapore; Atlantic, Thai.*
Metoclopramide hydrochloride (p.1274·3).
*Gastrointestinal motility disorders; nausea and vomiting.*

**Marimer** *Gilbert, Fr.*
Sea water.
*Nasal hygiene.*

**Marine** *Hexal, Arg.*
Dimenhydrinate (p.431·1).
*Motion sickness.*

**Marine Lipid Concentrate** *Vitaline, USA.*
Omega-3 marine triglycerides with vitamin E (p.976·2).
*Dietary supplement.*

**Marinepa** *Lifeplan, UK†.*
Omega-3 marine triglycerides (p.976·2).
*Nutritional supplement.*

**MarinEx** *MarinEx, Hong Kong.*
Glucosamine sulfate (p.1694·1).
*Degenerative joint disorders.*

**Marinol**
*Note. This name is used for preparations of different composition.*
*Sanofi Synthelabo, Canad.; Unimed, USA.*
Dronabinol (p.1264·2).
*AIDS related anorexia; nausea and vomiting associated with cancer chemotherapy.*

*Pharmadeveloppement, Fr.*
Iodine (p.1598·1); marine algae; calcium dihydrogen phosphate (p.1664·2); tannic acid (p.1751·2); phosphoric acid (p.1731·2); sea water.
*Tonic.*

**Mariston**
*Codal Synto, Malaysia; Codal Synto, Thai.*
Gemfibrozil (p.923·1).
*Hyperlipidaemias.*

**Markalakt**
*Koch, Austria; Pascoe, Ger.*
Chamomile (p.1669·3).
*Allergic disorders; gastrointestinal disorders; skin disorders.*

**Marks-Losung** *Serag-Wiessner, Ger.†.*
Electrolyte infusion with glucose (p.1217·1).
*Fluid and electrolyte disorders.*

**Marlidan** *Vinas, Spain†.*
Liver extract.
*Tonic.*

**Marlin Salt System** *Marlin, USA.*
Sodium chloride (p.1233·3)(p.1164·2).
*Rinsing and storage solution for soft contact lenses.*

**Marlyn Formula 50** *Marlyn, USA.*
Amino acids; pyridoxine hydrochloride (p.1456·3).
*Nail disorders; postnatal hair-loss.*

**Marly-Skin** *Sandoz, Ital.†.*
Barrier preparation.

**Marnatal-F** *Marnel, USA.*
Multivitamin and mineral preparation with iron and folic acid (p.1417·1).

**Marolderm** *Dermapharm, Ger.†.*
Dexpanthenol (p.1727·2).
*Burns; skin ulceration; sunburn; wounds.*

**Maronil** *Unipharm, Israel.*
Clomipramine hydrochloride (p.289·3).
*Depression; obsessive-compulsive disorder.*

**Marovil** *Medipharm, Chile.*
Cisapride (p.1259·2).
*Gastroparesis; gastro-oesophageal reflux; dyspepsia; gastrointestinal pseudo-obstruction.*

**Marovilina** *Atlantis, Mex.*
Ampicillin trihydrate (p.157·2).
*Bacterial infections.*

**Marplan**
*Royal, Chile; Medilink, Denm.; Roche, USA.*
Isocarboxazid (p.300·3).
*Depression.*

**Marpres** *Marnel, USA.*
Hydrochlorothiazide (p.933·2); reserpine (p.995·1); hydralazine hydrochloride (p.931·2).
*Hypertension.*

**Marrubene Codethyline** *Lemoine, Fr.†.*
Elecampane (p.1119·3); marrubium (p.1124·1); terpin (p.1131·1); sodium benzoate (p.1169·3); ethylmorphine hydrochloride (p.37·3).
*Respiratory-tract congestion.*

**Marsil** *Crosara, Ital.†.*
Silybum marianum (p.1043·3).
*Liver disorders.*

**Marsilid** *Laphal, Fr.*
Iproniazid phosphate (p.300·3).
*Depression.*

**Marsonil** *Makros, Braz.†.*
Ephedrine hydrochloride (p.1120·1); homatropine methylbromide (p.483·2).
*Obstructive airways disease.*

**Marten-Tab** *Marnel, USA.*
Butalbital (p.673·3); paracetamol (p.76·2).
*Tension headache.*

**Marthritic** *Marnel, USA.*
Salsalate (p.88·1).

**Martigene** *Novartis Ophthalmics, Fr.*
Phenylephrine hydrochloride (p.1126·3); brompheniramine maleate (p.426·1).
*Allergic conjunctivitis.*

**Martimil** *Synthelabo, Spain†.*
Nortriptyline hydrochloride (p.310·2).
*Depression.*

**Martindale Methadone Mixture DTF** *Martindale Pharmaceuticals, UK.*
Methadone hydrochloride (p.57·2).
It contains hydroxybenzoate esters as preservatives.
NOTE. There is no connection between Martindale, The Complete Drug Reference and Martindale Pharmaceuticals.
*Opioid withdrawal.*

**Martispasmol** *Martin & Harris, India.*
Cyclandelate (p.890·3).
*Peripheral vascular disorders.*

**Martos-10** *Otsuka, Jpn.*
Maltose (p.1440·1).
*Carbohydrate source; diabetes mellitus.*

**Mar-V** *Dupomar, Arg.*
Electrolytes (p.1217·1).
*Respiratory-tract congestion.*

**Marvelon**
*Organon, Arg.; Organon, Austral.; Organon, Austria; Organon, Belg.; Organon, Canad.; Organon, Chile; Organon, Denm.; Organon, Fin.; Organon, Ger.; Organon (Οργανον), Gr.; Organon, Hong Kong; Organon, Malaysia; Organon, Mex.; Organon, Neth.; Organon, Norw.; Organon, NZ; Organon, Port.; Donmed, S.Afr.; Organon, Singapore; Organon, Switz.; Organon, Thai.; Organon, UK.*
Desogestrel (p.1547·2); ethinylestradiol (p.1553·2).
28-Day packs also contain 7 inert tablets.
*Combined oral contraceptive.*

**Marvil** *Elisium, Arg.*
Alendronate sodium (p.765·3).
*Osteoporosis.*

**Marviol** *Organon, Irl.*
Desogestrel (p.1547·2); ethinylestradiol (p.1553·2).
*Combined oral contraceptive.*

**Marzine**
*Glaxo Wellcome, Canad.†.*
Cyclizine lactate (p.429·3).
*Nausea and vomiting; vertigo.*

*Pfizer, Denm.; Pfizer, Fin.; GlaxoSmithKline, Fin.; GlaxoSmithKline, Hong Kong; Pfizer, Norw.; Pfizer, NZ; GlaxoSmithKline, Singapore; GlaxoSmithKline, Swed.; Pfizer, Switz.*
Cyclizine hydrochloride (p.429·3).
*Motion sickness; nausea and vomiting; vestibular disorders.*

**Marzolam** *March, Thai.*
Alprazolam (p.668·3).
*Anxiety; mixed anxiety depressive states.*

**Masa Balm**
*Note. This name is used for preparations of different composition.*
*British Dispensary, Thai.†.*
Methyl salicylate (p.59·3); menthol (p.1711·3); camphor (p.1665·3); eucalyptus oil (p.1686·2).
*Musculoskeletal and joint pain.*

*Masa, Thai.†.*
Methyl salicylate (p.59·3); menthol (p.1711·3); eugenol (p.1686·2).
*Musculoskeletal and joint pain; sprains; strains.*

**Masaga** *Nakornpatana, Thai.*
Methyl salicylate (p.59·3); menthol (p.1711·3); camphor (p.1665·3); eucalyptus oil (p.1686·2); clove oil (p.1673·3).
*Musculoskeletal pain; neuralgia; sciatica.*

**Masagil** *Perez Gimenez, Spain.*
*Liniment:* Camphor (p.1665·3); ammonia (p.1653·3); methyl salicylate (p.59·3); rosemary oil (p.1740·2); turpentine oil (p.1760·1).
*Topical Spray:* Camphor (p.1665·3); methyl salicylate (p.59·3); turpentine oil (p.1760·1); menthol (p.1711·3).
*Rheumatic and muscle pain.*

**Masarax** *Masa, Thai.*
Hydroxyzine hydrochloride (p.434·3).
*Hypersensitivity reactions; sedative.*

**Masaren** *Masa, Thai.*
Diclofenac diethylamine (p.32·1).
*Musculoskeletal, joint, and peri-articular disorders.*

**Masarol** *Masa, Thai.*
Ketoconazole (p.403·3).
*Fungal infections.*

**Masaworm** *Masa, Thai.*
Albendazole (p.101·2).
*Worm infections.*

**Masaworm-1** *Masa, Thai.*
Mebendazole (p.108·2).
*Worm infections.*

**Masculine Herbal Complex** *GNLD, Austral.†.*
Saw palmetto; avena; celery; damiana; achillea; hypericum; skullcap; astragalus; chillies.
*Tonic.*

**Masdil** *Esteve, Spain.*
Diltiazem hydrochloride (p.900·1).
*Angina pectoris; arrhythmias; hypertension.*

**Masern-Impfstoff Merieux** *Aventis Pasteur, Ger.*
A live measles vaccine (attenuated Schwarz strain) (p.1623·1).
*Active immunisation.*

**Masern-Lebend-Impfstoff** *Chiron Behring, Ger.†.*
A live measles vaccine (more attenuated Enders strain) (p.1623·1).
*Active immunisation.*

**Masern-Vaccinol** *Procter & Gamble, Ger.†.*
A live measles vaccine (attenuated Schwarz strain) (p.1623·1).
*Active immunisation.*

**Masern-Virus-Impfstoff** *Chiron Behring, Ger.†.*
A live measles vaccine (more attenuated Enders strain) (p.1623·1).
*Active immunisation.*

**Masferol** *Quimica y Farmacia, Mex.*
Paracetamol (p.76·2).
*Fever; pain.*

**Masflex** *Abbott, Mex.*
Meloxicam (p.56·1).
*Gout; inflammation; musculoskeletal, joint, and peri-articular disorders; pain.*

**Masigel K** *Boehringer Ingelheim, Ger.†.*
Dimagnesium aluminium trisilicate.
*Gastrointestinal disorders.*

**Masivol** *ICN, Arg.*
Vitamin A (p.1451·2).
*Skin disorders.*

**Masivol Urea** *ICN, Arg.*
Hydrocortisone acetate (p.1103·3); vitamin A palmitate (p.1453·1); urea (p.1162·2).
*Skin disorders.*

**Maskam Krauter-Tee** *Duopharm, Ger.†.*
Senna (p.1288·2).
*Constipation; exogenous obesity.*

**Masnoderm** *Dominion, UK†.*
Clotrimazole (p.396·2).
*Fungal skin infections.*

**Masor** *Formenti, Ital.†.*
Stepronin lysine (p.1130·3).
*Respiratory-tract disorders.*

**Massage Balm with Calendula** *Weleda, UK.*
Calendula (p.1665·2); betula alba (p.1660·3); lavender oil (p.1705·2).
*Muscle tension.*

**Massageol** *Neo Quimica, Braz.*
Camphor (p.1665·3); turpentine oil (p.1760·1); menthol (p.1711·3); methyl salicylate (p.59·3); chlorophyll (p.1057·1).
*Musculoskeletal and joint disorders.*

**Massagim** *Vitoria, Port.*
Diethylamine salicylate (p.34·1).

**Masse**
*Note. This name is used for preparations of different composition.*
*Johnson & Johnson, Braz.†; Janssen-Cilag, Chile; Janssen-Cilag, Irl.†; Advanced Care, USA.*
Emollient and moisturiser.
*Nipple care.*

*Janssen-Cilag, S.Afr.†.*
Allantoin (p.1141·3); aminoacridine (p.1165·3).
*Napkin rash; nipple care.*

**Masse Cream** *Ethnor, India.*
Allantoin (p.1141·3).
*Nipple disorders.*

**Massengill** *SmithKline Beecham Consumer, USA.*
*Concentrated solution:* Lactic acid (p.1704·1); sodium lactate (p.1223·2); sodium bicarbonate (p.1223·2); alcohol (p.1166·1); octoxinol 9 (p.1414·1).
*Powder:* Ammonium alum (p.1652·1); phenol (p.1188·1); methyl salicylate (p.59·3); eucalyptus oil (p.1686·2); menthol (p.1711·3); thymol (p.1194·2); sodium chloride (p.1233·3).
*Vaginal disorders.*

**Massengill Disposable**
*Note. This name is used for preparations of different composition.*
*SmithKline Beecham Consumer, USA.*
Alcohol (p.1166·1); lactic acid (p.1704·1); sodium lactate (p.1223·2); octoxinol 9 (p.1414·1); propylene glycol (p.1735·2); cetylpyridinium chloride (p.1173·1); diazolidinyl urea.
*Vaginal disorders.*

*SmithKline Beecham Consumer, USA.*
Vinegar (p.1645·2).
*Vaginal disorders.*

**Massengill Feminine Cleansing Wash** *SmithKline Beecham Consumer, USA.*
Vaginal cleanser.

**Massengill Medicated**
*Note. This name is used for preparations of different composition.*
*SmithKline Beecham Consumer, Canad.†; SmithKline Beecham, Israel; SmithKline Beecham Consumer, USA.*
Povidone-iodine (p.1190·3).
*Vaginal disorders.*

*SmithKline Beecham Consumer, USA.*
*Soft cloth towelette:* Hydrocortisone (p.1103·3).
*Corticosteroid.*

**Massorax** *RTA, Switz.*
Methyl salicylate (p.59·3); isopropyl nicotinate; capsicum (p.1667·1); camphor (p.1665·3); turpentine oil (p.1760·1); eucalyptus oil (p.1686·2); lavender oil (p.1705·2).
*Musculoskeletal, joint, and soft-tissue disorders.*

**Massubal** *Dermopen, Braz.†.*
Methyl salicylate (p.59·3); turpentine oil (p.1760·1); guaiacol (p.1122·1).
*Musculoskeletal and joint disorders.*

**Mastaflu** *Solvay, UK.*
An influenza vaccine (surface antigen) (p.1620·2).
*Active immunisation.*

**Master-Aid** *Pietrasanta, Ital.*
Chlorhexidine gluconate (p.1173·2).
*Disinfection of skin, burns, and wounds.*

**Masterelax** *Master, Chile.*
Cyclobenzaprine hydrochloride (p.1393·1).
*Skeletal muscle spasm.*

**Master-Gel** *Master, Chile.*
Etofenamate (p.38·1).
*Inflammation.*

**Mastia** *Inexfa, Spain†.*
Aspirin (p.15·1); caffeine (p.782·1).
Contains thiamine.
*Fever; pain.*

**Mastical** *Altana, Spain.*
Calcium carbonate (p.1254·2).
*Hypocalcaemia; osteoporosis.*

**Mastika** *Goldshield, UK.*
Mastic gum (p.1710·1).
*Peptic ulcer.*

**Mastiol** *Reig Jofre, Spain.*
Chlorhexidine acetate (p.1173·2); benzocaine (p.1370·3); vitamin A (p.1451·2).
*Mastitis.*

**Mastodanatrol** *Sanofi Synthelabo, Port.*
Danazol (p.1545·2).
*Benign breast disorders.*

**Mastodynon**
*Bionorica, Ger.; Bionorica, Thai.*
Homoeopathic preparation.

**Mastu S**
*Stada, Ger.; Stada, Hong Kong; Stada, Thai.*
Bufexamac (p.21·3); bismuth subgallate (p.1252·2); titanium dioxide (p.1160·3); lidocaine hydrochloride (p.1377·3).
*Anorectal disorders.*

**Masvitalin Ginseng** *Spedrog, Arg.*
Ginseng; magnesium glycerophosphate; vitamins (p.1417·1).
*Tonic.*

**Maswin** *Masa, Thai.*
Piroxicam (p.84·2).
*Gout; musculoskeletal and joint disorders.*

**Matai** *Engelhard, Ger.*
Devil's claw root (p.28·2).
*Degenerative joint disorders.*

**Matcine**
*Atlantic, Malaysia; Atlantic, Singapore; Atlantic, Thai.*
Chlorpromazine hydrochloride (p.675·2).
*Affective disorders; controlled hypotension; hypothermia induction; nausea and vomiting; premedication; schizophrenia; sedative.*

**Matenol** *Unison, Thai.*
Trimetazidine hydrochloride (p.1018·1).
*Angina pectoris.*

**Mater Test** *Ofar, Arg.*
Pregnancy test (p.1734·3).

**Matergam** *Aventis Behring, Braz.*
An anti-D immunoglobulin (p.1608·1).
*Prevention of rhesus sensitisation.*

**Matergam-P** *Zydus, India.*
An anti-D immunoglobulin (p.1608·1).
*Prevention of rhesus sensitisation.*

**Materlac** *Andromaco, Chile.*
Ritodrine hydrochloride (p.1739·2).
*Fetal distress; premature labour; threatened abortion.*

**Materna**
*Wyeth, Braz.; Wyeth-Ayerst, Canad.; Wyeth, Chile; Wyeth, Hong Kong; Wyeth-Ayerst, Israel; Wyeth, Mex.; Lederle, USA†.*
Multivitamin and mineral preparation (p.1417·1).
*Dietary supplement during pregnancy and lactation.*

**Materna Nova** *Lederle, Switz.*
Multivitamin and mineral preparation (p.1417·1).

**Materna Tsimchit** *Maabarot, Israel.*
Infant feed (p.1417·1).
*Milk intolerance.*

**MaternAid** *Gerber, Mex.*
Preparation for enteral nutrition (p.1417·1).
*Pregnancy and lactation.*

**Maternity One** *Swiss Herbal, Canad.*
Multivitamin and mineral preparation (p.1417·1).

**Matersupre** *Teuto, Braz.*
Multivitamin and mineral preparation (p.1417·1).

**Matervit** *Farmoquimica, Braz.*
Multivitamin and mineral preparation (p.1417·1).

**Mathieu Cough Syrup** *Mathieu, Canad.†.*
Ammonium chloride (p.1115·2); potassium iodide (p.1598·1).

**Mathoine** *Wolfs, Belg.†.*
Phenytoin (p.370·2); methylphenobarbital (p.366·3).
*Epilepsy.*

**Matico Compuesto** *Knop, Chile.*
Homoeopathic preparation.

**Matidan** *Mintlab, Chile.*
Nitrofurantoin (p.237·2).
*Urinary-tract infections.*

**Matiga** *Pierre Fabre, Fr.†.*
Arachis oil (p.1656·1); menthol (p.1711·3).
*Musculoskeletal, joint, peri-articular, and soft-tissue disorders.*

**Matikomp** *Knop, Chile.*
Matico; calendula (p.1665·2); arnica (p.1656·3).
*Soft-tissue injury; ulcers; wounds.*

**Matmille** *Ritsert, Ger.*
*Bath additive:* Chamomile (p.1669·3); chamomile oil (p.1669·3).
*Skin and mucous-membrane disorders.*
*Ointment; oral liquid:* Chamomile (p.1669·3).
*Gastrointestinal disorders; skin and mucous-membrane disorders.*

**Mato** *Hevert, Ger.*
Homoeopathic preparation.

**Matrabec** *Warner-Lambert, Spain†.*
Multivitamin and mineral preparation (p.1417·1).

**Matricaria C/Vit AED2 Composta** *Dansk-Flama, Braz.*
Vitamin A; ergocalciferol; matricaria; calcium lactate; tribasic calcium phosphate (p.1417·1).

**Matricaria Vitam AED** *Dansk-Flama, Braz.†.*
Chamomile (p.1669·3); vitamin A; vitamin D; calcium phosphate; calcium carbonate; pepsin (p.1417·1).

**Matrifolin** *Orion, Fin.*
Ferrous fumarate (p.1427·3); vitamin B substances; alfa tocoferil acetate (p.1417·1).
*Iron-deficiency anaemia; vitamin supplement.*

**Matrix**
*Note. This name is used for preparations of different composition.*
*Beta, Arg.*
Diacerein (p.30·1).
*Musculoskeletal and joint disorders.*

*Wyeth Lederle, Ital.*
A heparinoid (p.931·1).
*Osteoarthritis.*

**Matulane** *Roche, USA.*
Procarbazine hydrochloride (p.581·2).
*Malignant neoplasms.*

**Mature Balance** *Pharmavite, Canad.†.*
Multivitamin and mineral preparation (p.1417·1).

**Maturity Test** *Blausiegel, Braz.*
Test for the menopause.

**Maux de gorge** *Pharmacard, Switz.*
Cetylpyridinium chloride (p.1173·1); lidocaine hydrochloride (p.1377·3); menthol (p.1711·3).
*Throat disorders.*

**Maveral** *Farmades, Ital.*
Fluvoxamine maleate (p.298·2).
*Depression; obsessive-compulsive disorder.*

**Mavid** *Abbott, Ger.*
Clarithromycin (p.192·2).
*Mycobacterial infections.*

**Mavigen Sebo** *Mavi, Ital.*
Cystine (p.1426·3).
*Seborrhoea.*

**Mavik**
*Abbott, Canad.; Abbott, USA.*
Trandolapril (p.1016·1).
*Heart failure following myocardial infarction; hypertension.*

**Mavipiu** *Mavi, Ital.*
Calamine (p.1144·1); zinc oxide (p.1163·2); oryzanol (p.1725·1).
*Barrier preparation; nappy rash.*

**Mavitalon** *Help, Gr.*
Diltiazem (p.901·3).
*Angina; hypertension.*

**Mavixan** *Pharmaten (Φαρματεν), Gr.*
Ambroxol hydrochloride (p.1114·3).
*Respiratory disorders associated with viscous mucus.*

**Max**
*Unison, Hong Kong; Unison, Singapore; Unison, Thai.*
Ambroxol hydrochloride (p.1114·3).
*Respiratory-tract disorders associated with increased or viscous mucus.*

**Max Uric** *Labinca, Arg.*
Benzbromarone (p.414·3).
*Hyperuricaemia.*

**Maxadol** *Restan, S.Afr.*
*Capsules:* Paracetamol (p.76·2); codeine phosphate (p.27·1).
*Syrup†:* Paracetamol (p.76·2); codeine phosphate (p.27·1); promethazine hydrochloride (p.439·1).
*Fever; pain.*

**Maxadol Forte** *Restan, S.Afr.†.*
Paracetamol (p.76·2); codeine phosphate (p.27·1); caffeine (p.782·1); meprobamate (p.706·2).
*Pain.*

**Maxadol-P** *Restan, S.Afr.†.*
Paracetamol (p.76·2).
*Fever; pain.*

**Maxair**
*3M, Canad.†; Jouveinal, Canad.†; 3M, Fr.; 3M, Switz.; 3M, USA.*
Pirbuterol acetate (p.790·3).
*Obstructive airways disease.*

**Maxalt**
*Merck Sharp & Dohme, Arg.; Merck Sharp & Dohme, Austria; Merck Sharp & Dohme, Belg.; Merck Sharp & Dohme, Braz.; Merck Frosst, Canad.; Merck Sharp & Dohme, Chile; Merck Sharp & Dohme, Denm.; Merck Sharp & Dohme, Fin.; Merck Sharp & Dohme, Ger.; Vianex (Βιανεξ), Gr.; Merck Sharp & Dohme, Ital.; Merck Sharp & Dohme, Mex.; Merck Sharp & Dohme, Neth.; Merck Sharp & Dohme, Norw.; Merck Sharp & Dohme, NZ; Merck Sharp & Dohme, Port.; Merck Sharp & Dohme, S.Afr.; Merck Sharp & Dohme, Spain; Merck Sharp & Dohme, Swed.; Merck Sharp & Dohme, Switz.; Merck Sharp & Dohme, UK; Merck, USA.*
Rizatriptan benzoate (p.471·1).
*Migraine.*

**Maxamaid MSUD** *SHS, Fr.*
Food for special diets (p.1417·1).
*Leucinosis.*

**Maxamaid RVHB** *Nutricia, NZ†; Scientific Hospital Supplies, NZ†.*
Methionine-free food for special diets (p.1417·1).
*Homocystinuria; hypermethioninaemia.*

**Maxamaid XLEU** *SHS, Fr.*
Food for special diets (p.1417·1).
*Isovaleric acidaemia.*

**Maxamaid XLYS, Low Try** *SHS, Fr.*
Food for special diets (p.1417·1).
*Glutaric aciduria.*

**Maxamaid XMET** *SHS, Fr.*
Food for special diets (p.1417·1).
*Homocystinuria.*

**Maxamaid XMET, Cys** *SHS, Fr.*
Food for special diets (p.1417·1).
*Sulfite oxidase deficiency.*

**Maxamaid XMTVI** *SHS, Fr.*
Food for special diets (p.1417·1).
*Methylmalonic or propionic acidaemia.*

**Maxamaid XP**
*Scientific Hospital Supplies, Israel†; Nutricia, Ital.*
Food for special diets (p.1417·1).
*Phenylketonuria.*

**Maxamaid XPTM** *SHS, Fr.*
Food for special diets (p.1417·1).
*Tyrosinaemia.*

**Maxamin Forte** *Anglo-French Drugs, India.*
Multivitamin and mineral preparation (p.1417·1).

**Maxamox** *Biochemie, Austral.*
Amoxicillin trihydrate (p.155·3).
*Bacterial infections.*

**Maxamum MSUD**
*SHS, Fr.; Nutricia, NZ†; Scientific Hospital Supplies, NZ†.*
Food for special diets (p.1417·1).
*Maple syrup urine disease.*

**Maxamum XLYS, Low Try** *SHS, Fr.*
Food for special diets (p.1417·1).
*Glutaric aciduria.*

**Maxamum XMET** *SHS, Fr.*
Food for special diets (p.1417·1).
*Homocystinuria.*

**Maxamum XMTVI** *SHS, Fr.*
Food for special diets (p.1417·1).
*Methylmalonic or propionic acidaemia.*

**Maxamum XP**
*Scientific Hospital Supplies, Israel†; Nutricia, Ital.*
Food for special diets (p.1417·1).
*Phenylketonuria.*

**Maxamum XPhen, Tyr** *SHS, Fr.*
Food for special diets (p.1417·1).
*Tyrosinaemia.*

**Maxaquin**
*Pharmacia, Braz.; Pharmacia, Hong Kong; Searle, Israel†; Monsanto, Ital.; Searle, Mex.; Pharmacia, Port.; Aspen, S.Afr.; Pharmacia, Switz.; Pharmacia, Thai.; Searle, USA.*
Lomefloxacin hydrochloride (p.227·2).
*Bacterial infections.*

**Maxcef**
*Bristol-Myers Squibb, Arg.; Bristol-Myers Squibb, Braz.; Bristol-Myers Squibb, Israel.*
Cefepime hydrochloride (p.172·1).
*Bacterial infections.*

**Maxcil** *Triomed, S.Afr.*
Amoxicillin trihydrate (p.155·3).
*Bacterial infections.*

**Maxenal** *McNeil Consumer, Canad.†.*
Pseudoephedrine hydrochloride (p.1129·2).
*Nasal congestion.*

**Maxepa**
*Cenovis, Austral.†; Vitelle, Austral.†; Pierre Fabre, Fr.; Scherer, Hong Kong†; Novartis Consumer, Ital.; Seven Seas, UK; Solgar, USA.*
Omega-3 marine triglycerides (p.976·2).
*Dietary supplement; lipid disorders.*
*Merck, India.*
Eicosapentaenoic acid (p.976·2); docosahexaenoic acid (p.976·1).
*Hypertriglyceridaemia.*

**Maxepa & EPO** *Vitaplex, Austral.†.*
Marine fish oil (p.976·2); evening primrose oil (p.1686·3).
*Dietary supplement.*

**Maxepa Plus** *Vitaglow, Austral.†.*
Marine fish oil (p.976·2); magnesium phosphate (p.1228·1).
*Psoriasis; rheumatoid arthritis.*

**Maxeran** *Hoechst Marion Roussel, Canad.†.*
Metoclopramide hydrochloride (p.1274·3).
*Adjunct in gastrointestinal radiography; delayed gastric emptying; facilitation of small bowel intubation; postoperative vomiting.*

**Maxeron** *Wallace, India.*
Metoclopramide hydrochloride (p.1274·3).
*Dyspepsia; gastritis; gastro-oesophageal reflux; gastrointestinal hyperacidity; hiatus hernia; hiccups; nausea and vomiting.*

**Maxi-6** *Desbergers, Canad.†.*
Multivitamin preparation (p.1417·1).

**Maxi-10** *Desbergers, Canad.†.*
Multivitamin preparation (p.1417·1).

**Maxi Force Energy Cocktail** *Homeocan, Canad.*
Homoeopathic preparation.

**Maxi-B**
*Sanofi Synthelabo, Belg.†; Sanofi Winthrop, Neth.†.*
Vitamin B substances (p.1417·1).
*Neurological or rheumatic pain.*

**Maxibol** *Aventis, Mex.*
Cobamamide (p.1459·1).
*Tonic.*

**Maxibone** *Unipharm, Israel.*
Alendronate sodium (p.765·3).
*Osteoporosis.*

**Maxicaine** *Sanofi Synthelabo OTC, Fr.†.*
Parethoxycaine hydrochloride (p.1382·2).
*Throat disorders.*

**Maxi-calc** *Pharmacia, Switz.*
Calcium carbonate (p.1254·2).
*Calcium deficiency; calcium supplement.*

**Maxi-Calsor** *Orion, Fin.†.*
Calcium carbonate (p.1254·2).
*Calcium deficiency; calcium supplement.*

**Maxicardil** *Northia, Arg.*
Dipyridamole (p.903·1).

**Maxicilina** *Antibioticos, Spain.*
Ampicillin sodium (p.157·1); ampicillin benzathine (p.158·1).
*Bacterial infections.*

**Maxicrom**
*Alcon, Braz.; Alcon, Mex.*
Sodium cromoglicate (p.795·3).
*Allergic conjunctivitis.*

**Maxid** *Fonten, Ital.*
Cefonicid sodium (p.174·2).
Lidocaine hydrochloride (p.1377·3) is included in this preparation to alleviate the pain of injection.
*Gram-negative bacterial infections.*

**Maxidauno** *Varifarma, Arg.*
Daunorubicin (p.546·1).
*Malignant neoplasms.*

**Maxidex**
*Alcon, Austral.; Alcon, Belg.; Alcon, Braz.; Alcon, Canad.; Alcon, Chile; Alcon, Denm.; Alcon, Fr.; Alkon (Αλκον), Gr.; Alcon, Hong Kong; Alcon, Irl.; Alcon, Israel; Alcon, Malaysia; Alcon, NZ; Alcon, S.Afr.; Alcon, Singapore; Alcon Cusi, Spain; Alcon, Switz.; Alcon, UK; Alcon, USA.*
Dexamethasone (p.1097·1) or dexamethasone sodium phosphate (p.1097·2).
*Inflammatory external ear disorders; inflammatory eye disorders.*

**Maxidon** *Astra, Swed.†.*
Morphine sulfate (p.60·2).
*Pain.*

**Maxidone** *Watson, USA.*
Hydrocodone tartrate (p.45·1); paracetamol (p.76·2).
*Pain.*

**Maxidraine** *Bio2, Fr.*
Black currant (p.1661·1); taraxacum (p.1751·3); bladderwrack (p.1742·3); green tea (p.1765·3).
*Water retention.*

**Maxidrol** *Alcon, Fr.*
Dexamethasone (p.1097·1); neomycin sulfate (p.235·1); polymyxin B sulfate (p.245·1).
*Infected eye disorders.*

**Maxifed** *MCR, USA.*
Guaifenesin (p.1122·1); pseudoephedrine hydrochloride (p.1129·2).
*Nasal Congestion.*

**Maxifed DM** *MCR, USA.*
Guaifenesin (p.1122·1); pseudoephedrine hydrochloride (p.1129·2); dextromethorphan hydrobromide (p.1117·3).
*Coughs; nasal congestion.*

**Maxifed DMX** *MCR, USA.*
Dextromethorphan hydrobromide (p.1117·3); guaifenesin (p.1122·1); pseudoephedrine hydrochloride (p.1129·2).
*Coughs; respiratory-tract congestion.*

**Maxifed G** *MCR, USA.*
Guaifenesin (p.1122·1); pseudoephedrine hydrochloride (p.1129·2).
*Coughs; nasal Congestion.*

**Maxifem** *Ecosol, Switz.*
Cimicifuga (p.1671·3).
*Menopausal disorders.*

**Maxiflor** *Allergan, USA.*
Diflorasone diacetate (p.1099·3).
*Skin disorders.*

**Maxijul**
*Note. This name is used for preparations of different composition.*
*Scientific Hospital Supplies, Austral.†; Scientific Hospital Supplies, Israel†.*
Maltodextrin (p.1439·3).
*Carbohydrate food supplement.*
*SHS, Fr.; Scientific Hospital Supplies, Irl.; Scientific Hospital Supplies, UK.*
Food for special diets. (p.1417·1).

**Maxi-Kalz** *Asta Medica, Austria.*
Calcium monocitrate (p.1225·1); calcium dicitrate (p.1225·1).
*Calcium supplementation.*

**Maxi-Kalz Vit D3** *Asta Medica, Austria.*
Calcium carbonate (p.1254·2); colecalciferol (p.1461·3).
*Osteoporosis.*

**Maxilase**
*Sanofi Synthelabo, Fr.; Sanofi Synthelabo, Port.*
Alpha-amylase (p.1654·2).
*Oedema; upper respiratory-tract congestion.*

**Maxilase-Bacitracine** *Sanofi Winthrop, Fr.†.*
Alpha-amylase (p.1654·2); bacitracin (p.161·3).
*Bacterial infections of the mouth and throat.*

**Maxilief** *Clonmel, Irl.*
Caffeine (p.782·1); codeine phosphate (p.27·1); paracetamol (p.76·2).
*Pain.*

**Maxiliv** *Ache, Braz.*
Dipyrone (p.35·3).
*Fever; pain.*

**Maxilube** *Mission Pharmacal, USA.*
Dimethicone (p.1482·1); glycerol (p.1694·3); carbomer 934 (p.1577·2); trolamine (p.1758·2); sodium laurilsulfate (p.1574·2).
*Vaginal lubricant.*

**Maxim Hp** *Dabur, India.*
Preparation for enteral nutrition (p.1417·1).

**Maximiton** *Varifarma, Arg.*
Mitomycin (p.573·3).
*Malignant neoplasms.*

**Maximum Blue Label** *Vitaline, USA.*
Multivitamin and mineral preparation (p.1417·1).

**Maximum Green Label** *Vitaline, USA.*
Multivitamin and mineral preparation (p.1417·1).

**Maximum Once A Day** *Quest, Canad.*
Multivitamin and mineral preparation (p.1417·1).

**Maximum Potential for Men** *Natural Life, Arg.*
Vitamins; minerals; royal jelly; pollen; ginseng; kola; saw palmetto; damiana (p.1417·1).

**Maximum Red Label** *Vitaline, USA.*
Multivitamin and mineral preparation with iron and folic acid (p.1417·1).

**Maximum Relief Ex-Lax** *Novartis Consumer, USA.*
Senna (p.1288·2).
Formerly contained phenolphthalein.
*Constipation.*

**Maximum Strength Allergy Drops** *Bausch & Lomb, USA.*
Naphazoline hydrochloride (p.1124·3); hypromellose (p.1579·3).
*Minor eye irritation.*

**Maximum Strength Anbesol** *Whitehall, USA.*
Benzocaine (p.1370·3); alcohol (p.1166·1).
*Local anaesthesia.*

**Maximum Strength Aqua-Ban** *Thompson, USA.*
Pamabrom (p.978·2).
*Premenstrual water retention.*

**Maximum Strength Arthriten** *Alva, USA†.*
Paracetamol (p.76·2); magnesium salicylate (p.55·1); caffeine (p.782·1).

**Maximum Strength Desenex Antifungal** *Ciba, USA.*
Miconazole nitrate (p.405·3).

**Maximum Strength Dristan Cold** *Whitehall, USA.*
Paracetamol (p.76·2); pseudoephedrine hydrochloride (p.1129·2); brompheniramine maleate (p.426·1).
*Cold symptoms; nasal congestion.*

**Maximum Strength Flexall 454** *Chattem, USA.*
Menthol (p.1711·3); aloe vera (p.1141·3); eucalyptus oil (p.1686·2); methyl salicylate (p.59·3); thyme oil (p.1755·3).
*Musculoskeletal disorders; pain.*

**Maximum Strength Ornex** *Menley & James, USA.*
Pseudoephedrine hydrochloride (p.1129·2); paracetamol (p.76·2).
*Upper respiratory-tract symptoms.*

**Maximum Strength Sine-Aid** *McNeil Consumer, USA.*
Pseudoephedrine hydrochloride (p.1129·2); paracetamol (p.76·2).
*Upper respiratory-tract symptoms.*

**Maximum Strength Sinutab Without Drowsiness** *Warner-Lambert, USA.*
Pseudoephedrine hydrochloride (p.1129·2); paracetamol (p.76·2).
*Upper respiratory-tract symptoms.*

**Maximum Strength Sleepinal** *Thompson, USA.*
Diphenhydramine hydrochloride (p.431·3).
*Insomnia.*

**Maximum Strength Sudogest Sinus** *Major, USA.*
Paracetamol (p.76·2); pseudoephedrine hydrochloride (p.1129·2).
*Upper respiratory-tract congestion.*

**Maximum Strength TheraFlu Non-Drowsy** *Novartis, USA.*
Paracetamol (p.76·2); dextromethorphan hydrobromide (p.1117·3); pseudoephedrine hydrochloride (p.1129·2).
*Coughs and cold symptoms.*

**Maximum Strength Tylenol Allergy Sinus** *McNeil Consumer, USA.*
Pseudoephedrine hydrochloride (p.1129·2); chlorphenamine maleate (p.427·3); paracetamol (p.76·2).
*Upper respiratory-tract symptoms.*

**Maximum Strength Tylenol Allergy Sinus NightTime** *McNeil Consumer, USA.*
Pseudoephedrine hydrochloride (p.1129·2); diphenhydramine hydrochloride (p.431·3); paracetamol (p.76·2).

**Maximum Strength Tylenol Sinus** *McNeil Consumer, USA.*
Pseudoephedrine hydrochloride (p.1129·2); paracetamol (p.76·2).
*Upper respiratory-tract symptoms.*

**Maximum Strength Unisom SleepGels** *Pfizer Consumer, USA.*
Diphenhydramine hydrochloride (p.431·3).
*Insomnia.*

**Maxiphen DM** *AMBI, USA.*
Dextromethorphan hydrobromide (p.1117·3); guaifenesin (p.1122·1); phenylephrine hydrochloride (p.1126·3).
*Coughs.*

**Maxipime**
*Bristol-Myers Squibb, Austral.; Bristol-Myers Squibb, Austria; Bristol-Myers Squibb, Belg.; Bristol-Myers Squibb, Canad.; Bristol-Myers Squibb, Chile; Bristol-Myers Squibb, Denm.; Bristol-Myers Squibb, Fin.; Bristol-Myers Squibb, Ger.; Bristol-Myers Squibb, Gr.; Bristol-Myers Squibb, Hong Kong; Bristol-Myers Squibb, Irl.; Bristol-Myers Squibb, Ital.; Bristol-Myers Squibb, Malaysia; Bristol-Myers Squibb, Mex.; Bristol-Myers Squibb, Neth.†; Bristol-Myers Squibb, NZ; Bristol-Myers Squibb, Port.; Bristol-Myers Squibb, S.Afr.; Bristol-Myers Squibb, Singapore; Bristol-Myers, Spain; Bristol-Myers Squibb, Swed.; Bristol-Myers Squibb, Switz.; Bristol-Myers Squibb, Thai.; Bristol-Myers Squibb, USA.*
Cefepime hydrochloride (p.172·1).
*Bacterial infections.*

**Maxipro** *Scientific Hospital Supplies, UK.*
Food for special diets (p.1417·1).
*Hypoproteinaemia.*

**Maxipro HBV** *Scientific Hospital Supplies, Irl.†.*
Food for special diets (p.1417·1).

**Maxiquin** *Sterop, Belg.*
Quinine-resorcinol.
*Malaria.*

**Maxisalic** *ICN, Arg.*
Betamethasone dipropionate (p.1093·1); salicylic acid (p.1157·1).
*Skin disorders.*

**Maxisona** *ICN, Arg.*
Betamethasone dipropionate (p.1093·1).
*Skin disorders.*

**Maxisorb**
*Scientific Hospital Supplies, Irl.; Scientific Hospital Supplies, UK.*
Preparation for enteral nutrition (p.1417·1).

**Maxisporin** *Yamanouchi, Neth.*
Cefradine (p.179·3).
*Bacterial infections.*

**Maxitone** *Brunel, S.Afr.*
Haematoporphyrin; cyanocobalamin; caffeine; rose hip; yeast (p.1417·1).
*Tonic.*

**Maxitratobes** *Disprovent, Arg.*
Mazindol (p.1589·1); dipotassium clorazepate (p.685·1).
*Obesity.*

**Maxitrol**
*Alcon, Belg.; Alcon, Braz.; Alcon, Canad.; Alcon, Chile; Alcon, Fin.; Alcon, Hong Kong; Alcon, Irl.; Alcon, Israel; Alcon, Malaysia; Alcon,*

Mex.; Alcon, Norw.; Alcon, NZ.; Alcon, S.Afr.; Alcon, Singapore; Alcon Cusi, Spain; Alcon, Switz.; Alcon, Thai.; Alcon, UK; Alcon, USA.
Dexamethasone (p.1097·1); neomycin sulfate (p.235·1); polymyxin B sulfate (p.245·1).
*Inflammatory eye infections.*

**Maxi-Tuss HCG** *MCR, USA.*
Hydrocodone tartrate (p.45·1); guaifenesin (p.1122·1).
*Coughs.*

**Maxi-Tuss HCX** *MCR, USA.*
Hydrocodone tartrate (p.45·1); chlorphenamine maleate (p.427·3); phenylephrine hydrochloride (p.1126·3).
*Coughs.*

**Maxius** *OM, Port.*
Tibezonium iodide (p.1756·2).
*Mouth and throat disorders.*

**Maxivalet** *Demo, Gr.*
Amitriptyline hydrochloride (p.280·3).
*Depression.*

**Maxivate** *Westwood-Squibb, USA.*
Betamethasone dipropionate (p.1093·1).
*Skin disorders.*

**Maxivent** *Ashbourne, UK†.*
Salbutamol (p.791·3).
*Asthma; bronchospasm.*

**Maxivision** *Medical Ophthalmics, USA.*
Vitamin, mineral, and nutrient preparation (p.1417·1).

**Maxivit** *Pfizer, Switz.*
Multivitamin and mineral preparation (p.1417·1).

**Maxi-Vite** *Goldline, USA.*
Multivitamin, mineral, and amino-acid preparation (p.1417·1).

**Maxolon**
*ICN, Austral.; ICN, Hong Kong; Shire, Irl.; ICN, Malaysia; ICN, NZ; Pharmaco, S.Afr.; ICN, Singapore; Monmouth, UK; SmithKline Beecham, USA.*
Metoclopramide hydrochloride (p.1274·3).
*Aid in gastrointestinal investigations; gastrointestinal disorders; migraine; nausea and vomiting.*

**Maxomat** *Sanofi Synthelabo, Fr.*
Somatropin (p.1327·2).
*Growth-hormone deficiency; Turner's syndrome.*

**Maxor** *Alphapharm, Austral.*
Omeprazole (p.1278·2).
*Gastro-oesophageal reflux; peptic ulcer; Zollinger-Ellison syndrome.*

**Maxoral** *Armstrong, Mex.*
Tibezonium iodide (p.1756·2).
*Mouth and throat disorders.*

**Maxovite** *Tyson, USA.*
Multivitamin and mineral preparation (p.1417·1).
*Premenstrual syndrome.*

**Max-Pax** *Biolab Sanus, Braz.*
Lorazepam (p.704·1).
*Alcohol withdrawal syndrome; anxiety; epilepsy; insomnia; nausea and vomiting; premedication.*

**Maxsoten** *Wyeth Lederle, Belg.*
Bisoprolol fumarate (p.875·1); hydrochlorothiazide (p.933·2).
*Hypertension.*

**Maxsulid** *Farmasa, Braz.†.*
Nimesulide betadex (p.67·1).

**Maxtral** *Baliarda, Arg.*
Alendronate sodium (p.765·3).
*Osteoporosis.*

**Maxtrex** *Pharmacia, UK.*
Methotrexate (p.568·2).
*Malignant neoplasms; psoriasis; rheumatoid arthritis.*

**Maxtrim** *Bristol-Myers Squibb, Mex.*
Co-trimoxazole (p.199·3).
*Bacterial infections; Pneumocystis carinii pneumonia.*

**Maxudin** *Menarini, Gr.*
Pravastatin sodium (p.984·3).
*Primary hypercholesterolaemia.*

**Maxum Multi-vite** *Seroyal, Canad.†.*
Multivitamin and mineral preparation (p.1417·1).

**Maxus** *Biocumed, Arg.*
Chondroitin sulfate; aprotinin (p.742·3); sodium hyaluronate (p.1697·3).
*Dry eyes.*

**Maxzide**
*Wyeth Lederle, Belg.†; Bertek, USA.*
Triamterene (p.1016·2); hydrochlorothiazide (p.933·2).
*Hypertension; oedema.*

**Maycor**
*Parke, Davis, Ger.; Godecke, Ger.; Parke, Davis, Spain†.*
Isosorbide dinitrate (p.941·1).
*Angina pectoris; heart failure; myocardial infarction; peripheral vascular disorders.*

**Mayfung** *Mayrhofer, Austria.*
*Bath additive:* Disodium sulfosuccinated undecenoic acid monoethanolamide (p.411·1).
*Fungal infections.*
*Topical solution:* Undecenoic acid monoethanolamide (p.411·1).
*Fungal skin infections.*

**Maygace** *Bristol-Myers, Spain.*
Megestrol acetate (p.1558·2).
*AIDS-associated cachexia; breast cancer; endometrial cancer.*

**Maylox** *Nicholas Piramal, India.*
Aluminium hydroxide (p.1249·2); magnesium hydroxide (p.1272·2); dimethicone (p.1289·2).
*Dyspepsia; flatulence; gastro-oesophageal relux; gastrointestinal hyperacidity; peptic ulcer.*

**Maylyt** *Mayrhofer, Austria.*
A range of electrolyte infusions with or without glucose (p.1217·1).
*Fluid and electrolyte disorders.*

**Maynar** *Novag, Spain.*
Aciclovir (p.626·1).
*Herpesvirus infections.*

**Mayogel** *Propan, S.Afr.*
Aluminium hydroxide (p.1249·2); magnesium oxide (p.1272·3).
*Gastrointestinal disorders.*

**Mayopirina** *Mayo, Mex.†.*
Dipyrone (p.35·3).

**May-Vita** *Merz, USA†.*
Vitamin B substances with minerals (p.1417·1).

**Mazanor** *Wyeth-Ayerst, USA†.*
Mazindol (p.1589·1).
*Obesity.*

**Mazetol** *Sarabhai Piramal, India.*
Carbamazepine (p.353·3).
*Bipolar disorder; epilepsy; trigeminal neuralgia.*

**Mazitrom** *Uniao Quimica, Braz.*
Azithromycin (p.159·1).
*Bacterial infections.*

**Mazon Medicated Cream** *Nasmark, Canad.*
Coal tar (p.1159·2); resorcinol (p.1156·3); salicylic acid (p.1157·1).
*Skin disorders.*

**Mazon Medicated Shampoo** *Nasmark, Canad.*
Coal tar (p.1159·2); salicylic acid (p.1157·1); sulfur (p.1158·2).
*Scalp disorders.*

**Mazon Medicated Soap** *Nasmark, Canad.*
Coal tar (p.1159·2).
*Skin disorders.*

**M&B Cough Syrup** *Nicholas Piramal, India.*
Dextromethorphan hydrobromide (p.1117·3); pseudoephedrine hydrochloride (p.1129·2); guaifenesin (p.1122·1).
*Coughs.*

**M-Bentabs** *Allen, Mex.*
Mebendazole (p.108·2).
*Worm infections.*

**M-beta** *Betapharm, Ger.*
Morphine sulfate (p.60·2).
*Pain.*

**MC Modulo Calorico** *Braun, Arg.*
Maltodextrin (p.1439·3).
*Nutritional supplement.*

**M-Caps** *Pal-Pak, USA.*
Methionine (p.1042·1).
*Odour, dermatitis, and ulceration in incontinent adults.*

**MCP** *Acis, Ger.; Alpharma-Isis, Ger.; Aliud, Ger.; Betapharm, Ger.; CT, Ger.; Hexal, Ger.; Ratiopharm, Ger.; Stada, Ger.*
Metoclopramide (p.1274·3) or metoclopramide hydrochloride (p.1274·3).
*Gastrointestinal disorders.*

**MCPham** *Phamos, Ger.*
Metoclopramide hydrochloride (p.1274·3).
*Gastrointestinal motility disorders.*

**MCR**
*Note. A similar name is used for preparations of different composition (see below).*
*Rafa, Israel.*
Morphine sulfate (p.60·2).
*Pain.*

**MCR-50**
*Note. A similar name is used for preparations of different composition (see above).*
*Pharmacia, UK.*
Isosorbide mononitrate (p.942·1).
*Angina pectoris.*

**MCT**
*Mead Johnson, Israel; Milk Industries, Israel; Nutricia, Ital.; Mead Johnson, Singapore; Mead Johnson Nutritionals, USA.*
Medium-chain triglycerides (p.1440·3).
*Adjunct in the management of disorders of fat absorption and transport.*

**MCT Duocal**
*Scientific Hospital Supplies, Irl.; Scientific Hospital Supplies, UK.*
Protein-, lactose-, gluten-, fructose-, and sucrose-free food with medium-chain triglycerides (p.1440·3) (p.1417·1).
*Fat malabsorption.*

**MCT Oil**
*Scientific Hospital Supplies, Austral.; Mead Johnson Nutritionals, Canad.; Mead Johnson, Malaysia; Nutricia, NZ; Baxter, NZ; Nutricia, Port.; Mead Johnson, Port.; Mead Johnson Nutritionals, Thai.†; Mead Johnson Nutritionals, UK; Scientific Hospital Supplies, UK.*
Medium-chain triglycerides (p.1440·3).
*Ketogenic diets; malabsorption syndromes; type I hyperlipoproteinaemia.*

**MCT Oljy** *Nutricia, Fin.*
Medium-chain triglycerides (p.1440·3).
*Fat malabsorption.*

**MCT Pepdite**
*Scientific Hospital Supplies, Irl.; Scientific Hospital Supplies, UK.*
Infant feed (p.1417·1).
*Disorders of fat absorption; protein intolerance.*

**MCT Peptide** *Nutricia, NZ; Scientific Hospital Supplies, NZ.*
Infant feed (p.1417·1).
*Cystic fibrosis; gastrointestinal disorders; lymphatic disorders.*

**mct Psycho Dragees N** *Eurim, Ger.†.*
Hypericum (p.299·1).
*Anxiety disorders; depression.*

**M-D** *Milano, Thai.*
Diphenhydramine hydrochloride (p.431·3); calamine (p.1144·1).
*Contact dermatitis; urticaria.*

**MD-60** *Mallinckrodt, Austral.*
Meglumine amidotrizoate (p.1060·2); sodium amidotrizoate (p.1060·2).
*Radiographic contrast medium.*

**MD-76**
*Mallinckrodt, Arg.; Mallinckrodt, Austral.; Mallinckrodt, Canad.; Mallinckrodt, USA.*
Meglumine amidotrizoate (p.1060·2); sodium amidotrizoate (p.1060·2).
*Radiographic contrast medium.*

**MD Complejo** *Liferpal, Mex.*
Vitamin B substances (p.1417·1).

**MD-Gastroview**
*Mallinckrodt, Arg.; Mallinckrodt, Austral.; Mallinckrodt, USA.*
Meglumine amidotrizoate (p.1060·2); sodium amidotrizoate (p.1060·2).
*Contrast medium for gastrointestinal radiography.*

**Mdiltiwas** *Wasserman, Spain†.*
Diltiazem hydrochloride (p.900·1).
*Angina pectoris; hypertension.*

**M-Dolor**
*Ethypharm, Austria; Hexal, Ger.*
Morphine sulfate (p.60·2).
*Pain.*

**MDR Fitness Tabs** *MDR, USA.*
Multivitamin and mineral preparation (p.1417·1).

**MDS Quick** *MDS Diagnostics, NZ.*
Pregnancy test (p.1734·3).

**Mealin** *Pharmasant, Thai.*
Mianserin hydrochloride (p.306·3).
*Depression.*

**Measlegam** *NBI, S.Afr.†.*
Measles immunoglobulin (p.1623·1).
*Passive immunisation.*

**Meaverin** *Aventis, Ger.*
*Injection:* Mepivacaine hydrochloride (p.1381·2).
*Local anaesthesia.*
*Topical gel:* Mepivacaine hydrochloride (p.1381·2); lauromacrogol 400 (p.1412·3).
*Catheterisation; intubation; local anaesthesia.*

**Meaverin "A" mit Adrenalin** *Rhone-Poulenc Rorer, Ger.†.*
Mepivacaine hydrochloride (p.1381·2).
Adrenaline acid tartrate (p.852·2) is included in this preparation as a vasoconstrictor to diminish absorption and localise the effect of the local anaesthetic.
*Local anaesthesia.*

**Meaverin hyperbar** *Rhone-Poulenc Rorer, Ger.†.*
Mepivacaine hydrochloride (p.1381·2).
*Local anaesthesia.*

**Meaverin "N" mit Noradrenaline** *Rhone-Poulenc Rorer, Ger.†.*
Mepivacaine hydrochloride (p.1381·2).
Noradrenaline acid tartrate (p.974·3) is include in this preparation as a vasoconstrictor to diminish absorption and localise the effect of the local anaesthetic.
*Local anaesthesia.*

**Meba** *Polipharm, Thai.†.*
Mebendazole (p.108·2).
*Worm infections.*

**Meban** *Kener, Mex.†.*
Mebendazole (p.108·2).

**Mebandozer** *Zerboni, Mex.†.*
Mebendazole (p.108·2).

**Mebaral** *Ovation, USA.*
Methylphenobarbital (p.366·3).
*Anxiety; epilepsy.*

**Mebaxin** *Milano, Thai.†.*
Methocarbamol (p.1395·1).
*Musculoskeletal pain.*

**Mebaxol** *Richmond, Arg.*
Ornidazole (p.612·2).

**Mebeciclol** *Sanofi Synthelabo, Mex.*
Mebendazole (p.108·2); tinidazole (p.617·1).
*Nematode infections; protozoal infections.*

**Mebelmin** *Jofrain, Mex.†.*
Mebendazole (p.108·2).

**Mebemerck** *Merck dura, Ger.*
Mebeverine hydrochloride (p.1273·1).
*Irritable bowel syndrome.*

**Meben**
*UCI, Braz.†; General Drugs, Thai.*
Mebendazole (p.108·2).
*Worm infections.*

**Mebendan** *Tedec Meiji, Spain.*
Mebendazole (p.108·2).
*Worm infections.*

**Mebenda-P** *PP Lab, Thai.*
Mebendazole (p.108·2).
*Worm infections.*

**Mebendazotil** *Iodo Suma, Braz.†.*
Mebendazole (p.108·2).
*Worm infections.*

**Mebendil** *Uniao Quimica, Braz.†.*
Mebendazole (p.108·2).
*Worm infections.*

**Mebenix** *Cimed, Braz.*
Albendazole (p.101·2).
*Worm infections.*

**Mebenlax** *British Dispensary, Thai.†.*
Mebendazole (p.108·2).
*Worm infections.*

**Mebensole** *Sanofi Synthelabo, Mex.*
Mebendazole (p.108·2).
*Worm infections.*

**Mebental** *Royton, Braz.*
Mebendazole (p.108·2).
*Worm infections.*

**Mebentiasis** *Keton, Mex.†.*
Mebendazole (p.108·2).

**Mebentine** *Vitae, Mex.†.*
Mebendazole (p.108·2).
*Worm infections.*

**Mebentral** *Berman, Mex.*
Mebendazole (p.108·2).
*Worm infections.*

**Mebetin** *Sam Chun Dang, Singapore.*
Mebeverine hydrochloride (p.1273·1).
*Gastrointestinal spasm; irritable bowel syndrome.*

**Mebex** *Cipla, India.*
Mebendazole (p.108·2).
*Worm infections.*

**Mebo**
*Mebo, Thai.; Julphar, UAE.*
Sitosterol (p.982·3).
*Burns; haemorrhoids; ulcers; wounds.*

**Mebocaina** *Novartis Consumer, Port.*
Tyrothricin (p.275·1); cetylpyridinium chloride (p.1173·1); oxybuprocaine hydrochloride (p.1382·1).
*Mouth and throat disorders.*

**Mebonat** *Roche, Spain.*
Disodium clodronate (p.770·2).
*Hypercalcaemia of malignancy; osteolytic bone metastases.*

**Meb-Overoid** *Valdecasas, Mex.*
Mebendazole (p.108·2).
*Worm infections.*

**Mebran** *Willmar, Mex.†.*
Dextromethorphan (p.1117·3).

**Mebron**
*Nikkho, Braz.; Daiichi, Jpn.*
Epirizole (p.36·3).
*Fever; inflammation; pain.*

**Mebryl** *GlaxoSmithKline, India.*
Embramine hydrochloride (p.433·2).
*Angioedema; eczema; hypersensitivity reactions; urticaria.*

**Mebucaine** *Novartis Consumer, Switz.*
Cetylpyridinium chloride (p.1173·1); oxybuprocaine hydrochloride (p.1382·1); tyrothricin (p.275·1).
*Mouth and throat disorders.*

**Mebucalets f** *Novartis Consumer, Switz.*
Benzoxonium chloride (p.1170·2); lidocaine (p.1377·3).
*Mouth and throat disorders.*

**Mebucasol f** *Novartis Consumer, Switz.*
Lidocaine hydrochloride (p.1377·3); muramidase hydrochloride (p.1717·2); tyrothricin (p.275·1).
*Mouth and throat disorders.*

**Mebutan** *GlaxoSmithKline, Neth.*
Nabumetone (p.63·3).
*Osteoarthritis; rheumatoid arthritis.*

**Mebutar** *Andromaco, Arg.*
Mebendazole (p.108·2).
*Worm infections.*

**Mebutar Compuesto** *Andromaco, Arg.*
Mebendazole (p.108·2); tinidazole (p.617·1).

**Mebutol** *Igefarma, Braz.†.*
Salbutamol sulfate (p.791·3).
*Obstructive airways disease.*

**Mebzol** *Julphar, UAE.*
Mebendazole (p.108·2).
*Worm infections.*

**Mecain** *Curasan, Ger.*
Mepivacaine hydrochloride (p.1381·2).
*Local anaesthesia.*

**Mecanyl** *Beta, Arg.*
Glucosamine sulfate (p.1694·1).
Lidocaine hydrochloride (p.1377·3) is included in the intramuscular injection to alleviate the pain of injection.
*Musculoskeletal and joint disorders.*

**Mecca** *Mentholatum, Canad.*
Camphor (p.1665·3); phenol (p.1188·1); zinc oxide (p.1163·2).

**Mecholyl** *Gordon, USA.*
Methacholine chloride (p.1492·1).
*Iontophoresis.*

**Mechovit** *Streuli, Switz.*
DL-methionine (p.1042·1); vitamins (p.1417·1).
*Liver disorders.*

**Meclan** *Ortho Dermatological, USA†.*
Meclocycline sulfosalicylate (p.229·1).
*Acne.*

**Meclifar** *Farcoral, Mex.*
Meclozine (p.436·3); vitamin $B_6$ (p.1457·2).
*Nausea and vomiting; vertigo.*

**Mecloderm** *Shire, Ital.*
Meclocycline sulfosalicylate (p.229·1).
*Bacterial skin infections.*

**Mecloderm Antiacne** *Shire, Ital.*
Meclocycline sulfosalicylate (p.229·1).
*Acne; seborrhoeic dermatitis.*

**Mecloderm F** *Shire, Ital.*
Meclocycline sulfosalicylate (p.229·1); fluocinolone acetonide (p.1101·2).
*Infected skin disorders.*

**Mecloderm Ovuli** *Shire, Ital.*
Meclocycline sulfosalicylate (p.229·1).
*Vulvovaginal and cervical infections.*

**Mecloderm Polvere Aspersoria** *Shire, Ital.*
Meclocycline sulfosalicylate (p.229·1).
*Bacterial skin infections.*

**Meclodol** *Parke, Davis, Ital.*
Meclofenamate sodium (p.55·1).
*Musculoskeletal and joint disorders; pain.*

**Meclomen**
*Parke, Davis, Austria†; Parke, Davis, Chile; Parke, Davis, Hong Kong†; Parke-Med, S.Afr.†; Parke, Davis, Spain.*
Meclofenamate sodium (p.55·1).
*Menorrhagia; musculoskeletal, joint, and peri-articular disorders; pain.*

**Meclomid** *Randall, Mex.*
Metoclopramide hydrochloride (p.1274·3).
*Gastrointestinal motility disorders; nausea and vomiting.*

**Meclon** *Farmigea, Ital.*
Clotrimazole (p.396·2); metronidazole (p.607·2).
*Vulvovaginal and cervical infections.*

**Meclosil** *Sunward, Singapore.*
Aluminium hydroxide-magnesium carbonate co-dried gel (p.1250·1); simeticone (p.1289·2); dicycloverine hydrochloride (p.481·2).
*Dyspepsia; flatulence; gastric hyperacidity; heartburn.*

**Meclosorb** *S & K, Ger.*
Meclocycline sulfosalicylate (p.229·1).
*Bacterial skin infections.*

**Meclutin** *ABC, Ital.*
Meclocycline sulfosalicylate (p.229·1); fluocinolone acetonide (p.1101·2).
*Infected skin disorders.*

**Meclutin Semplice** *ABC, Ital.*
Meclocycline sulfosalicylate (p.229·1).
*Bacterial skin infections.*

**Mecolin** *Stadmed, India.*
Tricholine citrate (p.1424·3); sorbitol (p.1446·3).
*Biliary hypotonia; constipation; fatty infiltration of liver.*

**Mecoten** *Promeco, Mex.*
Dipyrone (p.35·3).
*Pain.*

**Mectizan**
*Merck Sharp & Dohme-Chibret, Fr.; Merck, USA.*
Ivermectin (p.105·3).
Veterinary names include: Eqvalan; Ivomec; Oramec.
*Lymphatic filariasis; onchocerciasis.*

**Meda** *Circle, USA.*
Paracetamol (p.76·2).
*Fever; pain.*

**Medacaps N** *Palmicol, Ger.†.*
Deanol hydrogen tartrate (p.1585·3).
Medacaps formerly contained inositol nicotinate, deanol hydrogen tartrate, crataegus, procaine hydrochloride, haematoporphyrin, hesperidin, and alpha tocoferil acetate.
*Tonic.*

**Medacter** *Faran, Gr.*
Miconazole nitrate (p.405·3).
*Fungal skin infections.*

**Med-Actigen** *Medical Supply, Thai.*
Triprolidine hydrochloride (p.442·3); pseudoephedrine hydrochloride (p.1129·2).
*Cold symptoms; hay fever; rhinitis; upper respiratory-tract congestion.*

**Medalgin** *Medical Supply, Thai.*
Dipyrone (p.35·3).
*Pain.*

**Medalginan** *Medinfar, Port.*
Benzyl nicotinate (p.21·2); capsicum (p.1667·1); camphor (p.1665·3); diethylamine salicylate (p.34·1).
*Musculoskeletal and joint disorders; neuritis.*

**Medamet** *Caps, S.Afr.*
Metronidazole (p.607·2).
*Anaerobic bacterial infections; protozoal infections.*

**Medamol Co** *Medical Supply, Thai.†.*
Paracetamol (p.76·2); chlorphenamine maleate (p.427·3); phenylpropanolamine hydrochloride (p.1127·3).
*Cold and influenza symptoms; hay fever; sinusitis.*

**Medamor** *Merck Sharp & Dohme, Fin.*
Amiloride hydrochloride (p.858·2).
*Hypertension; liver cirrhosis with ascites; oedema.*

**Med-Anspasmic** *Medical Supply, Thai.*
Mefenamic acid (p.55·2); dicycloverine hydrochloride (p.481·2).
*Smooth muscle spasm.*

**Medapur** *Rentschler, Ger.†.*
Diphenhydramine hydrochloride (p.431·3).
*Pruritus; skin irritation.*

**Medaren** *Medical Supply, Thai.*
Diclofenac sodium (p.32·1).
*Musculoskeletal, joint, and peri-articular disorders; pain.*

**Medarex** *Medipharm, Chile.*
Cyclobenzaprine (p.1393·2).
*Skeletal muscle spasm.*

**Medaspor** *Medpro, S.Afr.*
Clotrimazole (p.396·2).
*Fungal infections.*

**Medazine** *Medpro, S.Afr.*
Cyclizine hydrochloride (p.429·3).
*Motion sickness; nausea and vomiting; vestibular disorders.*

**Medazol** *Offenbach, Mex.*
Metronidazole (p.607·2).
*Amoebiasis.*

**Medazol Gel** *Medipharm, Chile.*
Metronidazole (p.607·2).
*Anaerobic bacterial infections; rosacea.*

**Medazole** *Asian Pharm, Thai.*
Mebendazole (p.108·2).
*Worm infections.*

**Medazyl** *M & H, Thai.*
Metronidazole (p.607·2).
*Anaerobic bacterial infections.*

**Med-Broncodil** *Medical Supply, Thai.*
Terbutaline sulfate (p.797·2).
*Obstructive airways disease.*

**Med-Broncodil Expectorant** *Medical Supply, Thai.*
Terbutaline sulfate (p.797·2); guaifenesin (p.1122·1).
*Obstructive airways disease.*

**Med-Circuron** *Medical Supply, Thai.*
Cinnarizine (p.428·3).
*Cerebrovascular disorders; migraine; motion sickness; peripheral vascular disorders; vestibular disorders.*

**Medebar**
*Medefield, Austral.; Regional Health, NZ.*
Barium sulfate (p.1061·1).
*Contrast medium for gastrointestinal radiography.*

**Medebiotin** *Medea, Spain.*
Biotin sodium (p.1423·2).
*Biotin deficiency.*

**Medecitral** *Medea, Spain†.*
Belladonna alkaloids (p.479·1); sodium bromide (p.1663·1); sodium citrate (p.1223·2).
*Vomiting.*

**Medefizz**
*Medefield, Austral.; Regional Health, NZ.*
Potassium bicarbonate; citric acid.
*Effervescent system for double-contrast radiography.*

**Medefoam**
*Medefield, Austral.; Regional Health, NZ.*
Simeticone (p.1289·2).
*Antifoaming agent for barium radiography.*

**Medefungin** *Reig Jofre, Spain†.*
Miconazole nitrate (p.405·3).
*Fungal skin and nail infections.*

**Medemycin** *Meiji, Jpn.*
Midecamycin (p.231·3).
*Bacterial infections.*

**Medenorex** *Medea, Spain.*
Cyproheptadine hydrochloride (p.430·1); amino acids and vitamins (p.1417·1).
*Tonic.*

**Medent-DM** *Stewart Jackson, USA.*
Guaifenesin (p.1122·1); pseudoephedrine hydrochloride (p.1129·2); dextromethorphan hydrobromide (p.1117·3).
*Coughs.*

**Mede-Prep**
*Medefield, Austral.; Regional Health, NZ.*
Mannitol (p.950·2).
*Bowel evacuation.*

**Mederebro** *Medea, Spain.*
Cyanocobalamin (p.1458·2); thiamine (p.1455·2); pyridoxine hydrochloride (p.1456·3).
*Vitamin B deficiency.*

**Mederebro Compuesto** *Medea, Spain†.*
Cyanocobalamin (p.1458·2); cerebral medullary neuropeptides; pyridoxine hydrochloride (p.1456·3); phosphoserine; thiamine nitrate (p.1455·1); glutamie (p.1433·2).
*Neurological disorders.*

**Mederma**
*Sigma, Austral.; Merz, Malaysia; Merz, Singapore; Merz, USA.*
Onion (p.1723·2).
*Scars.*

**Mederreumol** *Medea, Spain.*
Indometacin (p.47·3).
*Gout; inflammation; musculoskeletal, joint, and periarticular disorders; pain.*

**Medescan** *Medefield, Austral.*
Barium sulfate (p.1061·1).
*Radiographic contrast medium.*

**Medeserpine Co** *Medical Supply, Thai.*
Reserpine (p.995·1); hydrochlorothiazide (p.933·2).
*Hypertension.*

**Medesup** *Medea, Spain†.*
Bisacodyl (p.1251·3).
*Bowel evacuation; constipation.*

**Medeton** *TP, Thai.*
Medroxyprogesterone acetate (p.1557·2).
*Endometriosis; progestogen-only injectable contraceptive.*

**Medevac**
*Medefield, Austral.; Regional Health, NZ.*
Arachis oil (p.1656·1); sorbitol (p.1446·3).
*Gallbladder evacuant for oral cholecystography.*

**Medex Rub** *Sidus, Arg.*
*Adult rub:* Sulfogaiacol (p.1131·1); methyl nicotinate (p.59·2); camphor (p.1665·3); menthol (p.1711·3); pine oil; eucalyptus oil (p.1686·2).
*Infant rub:* Eucalyptus oil (p.1686·2); pine oil; niaouli oil (p.1719·3).
*Catarrh; cold symptoms.*

**Med-Gastramet** *Medical Supply, Thai.*
Cimetidine (p.1255·3).
*Gastric hyperacidity; gastro-oesophageal reflux; peptic ulcer.*

**Medgesic** *Medifive, Thai.*
Orphenadrine citrate (p.486·1); paracetamol (p.76·2).
*Musculoskeletal disorders; pain.*

**Med-Glionil** *Medical Supply, Thai.*
Glibenclamide (p.331·2).
*Diabetes mellitus.*

**Med-Guaiphan** *Medical Supply, Thai.*
Dextromethorphan hydrobromide (p.1117·3); guaifenesin (p.1122·1); terpin hydrate (p.1131·1).
*Coughs.*

**Medi Creme** *Warner-Lambert, Austral.†.*
Chlorhexidine acetate (p.1173·2); cetrimide (p.1172·1); hexamidine isetionate (p.1181·3); allantoin (p.1141·3); lidocaine (p.1377·3).
*Abrasions; cuts; insect bites and stings; minor burns; skin irritation.*

**Medi Pulv** *Warner-Lambert, Austral.†.*
Hexamidine isetionate (p.1181·3); chlorhexidine hydrochloride (p.1173·3); allantoin (p.1141·3).
*Cuts; minor burns and scalds.*

**Mediabet** *Medice, Ger.*
Metformin hydrochloride (p.342·3).
*Diabetes mellitus.*

**Medialipide**
*Braun, Belg.; Braun, Fr.*
Soya oil (p.1447·2); medium-chain triglycerides (p.1440·3).
Contains egg lecithin.
*Lipid infusion for parenteral nutrition.*

**Mediamik** *Medisint, Ital.*
Amikacin sulfate (p.154·1).
*Bacterial infections.*

**Mediamox** *Biohorm, Spain†.*
Amoxicillin trihydrate (p.155·3).
*Bacterial infections.*

**Medianox** *Grossmann, Switz.*
Cloral hydrate (p.684·1).
*Nervousness; sleep disorders.*

**Medianut** *Braun, Fr.*
Amino-acid and lipid infusion (p.1417·1).
*Parenteral nutrition.*

**Mediatensyl** *Fournier, Fr.*
Urapidil (p.1018·1).
*Hypertension.*

**Mediator**
*Biopharma, Fr.; Servier, Port.*
Benfluorex hydrochloride (p.868·1).
*Adjunct in asymptomatic diabetes; hyperlipidaemias.*

**Mediaven**
*Will-Pharma, Belg.; Drossapharm, Switz.*
Naftazone (p.757·1).
*Diabetic retinopathy; venous insufficiency.*

**Mediaxal**
*Servier, Hong Kong; Servier, Ital.; Servier, Malaysia; Servier, Singapore.*
Benfluorex hydrochloride (p.868·1).
*Diabetes mellitus; hyperlipidaemias.*

**Medibronc** *Monot, Fr.†.*
Carbocisteine (p.1116·2).
*Respiratory-tract congestion.*

**Medic** *DNR, Arg.*
Salicylic acid (p.1157·1); allantoin (p.1141·3); coal tar (p.1159·2).
*Skin and scalp disorders.*

**Medica** *Qualiphar, Belg.*
Chlorhexidine gluconate (p.1173·2); lidocaine hydrochloride (p.1377·3).
*Throat disorders.*

**Medicaid** *Eastern Pharmaceuticals, UK.*
Cetrimide (p.1172·1).
*Nappy rash.*

**Medicaina** *Cristalia, Braz.†.*
Lidocaine (p.1377·3); prilocaine (p.1382·3).
*Local anaesthesia.*

**Medical Pic** *Artsana, Ital.†.*
Chlorhexidine gluconate (p.1173·2); undebenzophene (p.1195·3).
*Wound and burn disinfection.*

**Medicament Sinus** *Prodemdis, Canad.*
Pseudoephedrine hydrochloride (p.1129·2); paracetamol (p.76·2).

**Medicap** *Xepa-Soul Pattinson, Hong Kong.*
Mefenamic acid (p.55·2).
*Pain; soft-tissue injuries.*

**Medicated Analgesic Cream** *Prodemdis, Canad.*
Methyl salicylate (p.59·3); camphor (p.1665·3); menthol (p.1711·3); eucalyptus oil (p.1686·2).

**Medicated Chest Rub** *Hyde, Canad.†.*
Camphor (p.1665·3); eucalyptus oil (p.1686·2); menthol (p.1711·3).

**Medicated Extract of Rosemary** *Potter's, UK.*
Geranium oil (p.1692·2); rosemary oil (p.1740·2); methyl salicylate (p.59·3); bay oil (p.1659·1).
*Scalp disorders.*

**Medichrom** *Qualiphar, Belg.*
Merbromin (p.1185·3).
*Disinfection of minor wounds.*

**Medicillin** *Ratiopharm, Fin.*
Phenoxymethylpenicillin potassium (p.242·1).
*Bacterial infections.*

**Medicinal Gargle** *Weleda, UK.*
Homoeopathic preparation.

**Mediclear** *Boots, UK†.*
Benzoyl peroxide (p.1143·2).
*Acne.*

**Medicoal** *Concord, UK†.*
Activated charcoal (p.1030·2).
*Acute poisoning; drug overdosage.*

**Medicone** *Dickinson, USA.*
Yeast extract (p.1469·1); shark-liver oil.

**Medicone Derma** *Medicone, USA.*
Benzocaine (p.1370·3); zinc oxide (p.1163·2); hydroxyquinoline sulfate (p.1700·1); ichthammol (p.1148·2); menthol (p.1711·3).
*Skin disorders.*

**Medicone Rectal** *Medicone, USA.*
*Ointment:* Benzocaine (p.1370·3); hydroxyquinoline sulfate (p.1700·1); zinc oxide (p.1163·2); menthol (p.1711·3); castor oil (p.1668·2); peru balsam (p.1730·2).
*Suppositories:* Benzocaine (p.1370·3); hydroxyquinoline sulfate (p.1700·1); zinc oxide (p.1163·2); menthol (p.1711·3); peru balsam (p.1730·2).
*Anorectal disorders.*

**Medicreme**
*Note. This name is used for preparations of different composition.*
*Bajer, Arg.*
Vitamin A palmitate (p.1453·1); collagen (p.1674·3).
*Skin disorders.*

*Pharmacare, Hong Kong.*
Chlorhexidine acetate (p.1173·2); cetrimide (p.1172·1); hexamidine isetionate (p.1181·3); lidocaine (p.1377·3); allantoin (p.1141·3).
*Burns; cuts and abrasions; skin irritation.*

*Amadeus, India.*
Methyl nicotinate (p.59·2); mephenesin (p.1394·3); methyl salicylate (p.59·3); menthol (p.1711·3).
*Musculoskeletal, joint, and soft-tissue disorders.*

*Pharmabroker, NZ.*
Chlorhexidine acetate (p.1173·2); cetrimide (p.1172·1); hexamidine isetionate (p.1181·3); lidocaine (p.1377·3).
*Bites; burns; insect stings; wounds.*

**Medicyclomine** *Brunel, S.Afr.*
Dicycloverine hydrochloride (p.481·2).
*Gastrointestinal spasm; urinary-tract spasm.*

**Medi-Dan** *Mahdeen, Canad.*
Coal tar (p.1159·2); benzalkonium chloride (p.1168·3); salicylic acid (p.1157·1).

**Medident** *Medibrands, Israel.*
Chlorhexidine gluconate (p.1173·2).
*Mouth disinfection.*

**Medifed** *Medpro, S.Afr.*
Triprolidine hydrochloride (p.442·3); pseudoephedrine hydrochloride (p.1129·2); dextromethorphan hydrobromide (p.1117·3).
*Coughs.*

**Medifen**
*Note. This name is used for preparations of different composition.*
*Medipharma, Hong Kong.*
Chlorphenamine maleate (p.427·3).

*Grisi, Mex.*
Ibuprofen (p.45·3).
*Pain.*

**Medifer** *Medimport, Mex.*
Ferrous fumarate (p.1427·3).
*Iron-deficiency anaemia.*

**Medi-First Sinus Decongestant** *Textilease, USA.*
Pseudoephedrine hydrochloride (p.1129·2).
*Nasal congestion.*

**Mediflex** *Crown, S.Afr.*
Indometacin (p.47·3).
*Musculoskeletal and joint disorders.*

**Mediflor no 11 Draineur Renal et Digestif**
*Merck Medication Familiale, Fr.*
Boldo (p.1661·2); birch leaf (p.1660·3); black currant (p.1661·1).
*Digestive disorders; kidney disorders.*

**Mediflor Tisane Antirhumatismale No 2** *Merck Medication Familiale, Fr.*
Birch leaf (p.1660·3); ash; meadowsweet (p.1710·1); strawberry plant; parietaria; couch-grass (p.1676·2); asparagus; juniper (p.1703·1); bearberry (p.1659·2); black currant (p.1661·1); tilia (p.1756·2); frangula bark (p.1266·3).
*Muscular pain; rheumatic pain.*

**Mediflor Tisane Calmante Troubles du Sommeil No 14** *Merck Medication Familiale, Fr.*
Passion flower (p.1729·1); bitter orange (p.1723·3); crataegus (p.1677·1); melissa (p.1711·1); tilia (p.1756·2); valerian (p.1762·2).
*Insomnia; nervous disorders.*

**Mediflor Tisane Circulation du Sang No 12**
*Merck Medication Familiale, Fr.*
Aesculus (p.1648·2); red vine; hyssop; valerian (p.1762·2); hamamelis (p.1696·3); cypress nut; mistletoe (p.1715·3); willow leaf (p.87·3); melissa (p.1711·1); crataegus (p.1677·1); frangula bark (p.1266·3).
*Peripheral vascular disorders.*

**Mediflor Tisane Contre la Constipation Passagere No 7** *Merck Medication Familiale, Fr.*
Senna (p.1288·2); ash; fennel (p.1687·2); liquorice (p.1270·2); rosemary (p.1740·2).
*Constipation.*

**Mediflor Tisane Digestive No 3** *Merck Medication Familiale, Fr.*
Aniseed (p.1655·2); mint (p.1749·1); angelica (p.1655·1); lavender (p.1705·1); orange leaf; rosemary (p.1740·2); elecampane (p.1119·3); fennel (p.1687·2); coriander (p.1676·1); hyssop.
*Digestive disorders.*

**Mediflor Tisane Hepatique No 5** *Merck Medication Familiale, Fr.*
Boldo (p.1661·2); kinkeliba (p.1703·3); elecampane root (p.1119·3); rosemary (p.1740·2); liquorice (p.1270·2); berberis; mercury herb; mallow leaves (p.1709·3); senna leaves (p.1288·2).
*Digestive disorders; liver disorders.*

**Mediflor Tisane No 4 Diuretique** *Merck Medication Familiale, Fr.*
Asparagus; fennel (p.1687·2); couch-grass (p.1676·2); bearberry (p.1659·2); ash; meadowsweet (p.1710·1); strawberry root; althaea leaf (p.1651·3); liquorice (p.1270·2).
*Diuresis; renal calculi.*

**Mediflor Tisane Pectorale d'Alsace** *Monot, Fr.†.*
Mallow (p.1709·3); althaea flowers (p.1651·3); poppy (p.1129·1); coltsfoot flowers and leaves (p.1117·2); verbascum flowers and leaves (p.1764·1); gnaphalium dioicum; althaea herb and root (p.1651·3); calendula (p.1665·2); wild thyme; ground ivy (p.1696·1); liquorice (p.1270·2); melissa (p.1711·1); meadowsweet (p.1710·1); couch-grass (p.1676·2).
*Respiratory-tract disorders.*

**Medifolin** *Medinfar, Port.*
Calcium folinate (p.1431·1).
*Folate deficiency; megaloblastic anaemia; toxicity due to folic acid antagonists.*

**Medifome** *MBP, Ger.; Medimex, Ger.*
Collagen (porcine) (p.1674·3).
*Haemorrhage.*

**Medifon** *Medinfar, Port.*
Tyrothricin (p.275·1); benzocaine (p.1370·3); dequalinium chloride (p.1178·1); vitamin C (p.1460·2); menthol (p.1711·3).
*Mouth and throat disorders.*

**Medifungol** *Hexa-Medinova, Arg.*
Clotrimazole (p.396·2).
*Fungal skin infections.*

**Medigel**
*Note. This name is used for preparations of different composition.*
*Medice, Ger.*
Bamethan sulfate (p.866·3); ephedrine sulfate (p.1120·1); lauromacrogol 400 (p.1412·3).
*Soft-tissue injury; venous insufficiency.*

*Medifood, Ital.*
Nutritional supplement (p.1417·1).
*Vomiting.*

*Propan, S.Afr.; Premier, S.Afr.*
Dicycloverine hydrochloride (p.481·2); aluminium hydroxide gel (p.1249·2); magnesium oxide (p.1272·3); simeticone (p.1289·2); sodium laurilsulfate (p.1574·2); methylcellulose (p.1580·2).
*Gastrointestinal disorders.*

**Medigesic**
*Note. This name is used for preparations of different composition.*
*Maver, Chile.*
Clonixin lysine (p.26·3).
*Pain.*

*US Pharmaceutical, USA.*
Butalbital (p.673·3); paracetamol (p.76·2); caffeine (p.782·1).
*Tension headache.*

**Medihaler** *3M, Arg.*
Salbutamol (p.791·3).
*Obstructive airways disease.*

**Medihaler-Epi** *3M, Switz.†.*
Adrenaline acid tartrate (p.852·2).
*Hypersensitivity reactions.*

**Medihaler-Iso**
*3M, Belg.†; 3M, Neth.†; 3M, Port.†; 3M, USA.*
Isoprenaline sulfate (p.940·2).
*Bronchospasm.*

**Medijel**
*Key, Austral.; DDD, Hong Kong; DDD, Israel; DDD, Malaysia; Wilson, NZ; DDD, Singapore; DDD, UK.*
Lidocaine hydrochloride (p.1377·3); aminoacridine hydrochloride (p.1165·3).
*Mouth ulcers; sore gums.*

**Medi-Kain** *Parke-Med, S.Afr.*
Cetylpyridinium chloride (p.1173·1); benzocaine (p.1370·3).
*Sore throat.*

**Medi-Keel A** *Restan, S.Afr.*
*Lozenges:* Cetylpyridinium chloride (p.1173·1); benzocaine (p.1370·3).
*Sore throat.*
*Throat spray:* Phenol (p.1188·1).
*Mouth and throat infections.*

**Medikem** *Maver, Chile.*
Benzocaine (p.1370·3); benzyl alcohol (p.1170·2).

**Mediker** *SIT, Ital.*
Phenothrin (p.1509·1).
*Pediculosis.*

**Mediklin** *Maver, Chile.*
Salicylic acid (p.1157·1).
*Acne.*

**Medikol** *Selena, Swed.*
Activated charcoal (p.1030·2).
*Diarrhoea; poisoning.*

**Medi-Kord** *Medirel, Switz.†.*
Adrenaline hydrochloride (p.852·3); zinc phenolsulfonate octahydrate (p.1163·3).
*Adjunct in dental procedures.*

**Medil** *Crosara, Ital.†.*
Buflomedil hydrochloride (p.877·2).
*Cerebral and peripheral vascular disorders.*

**Medilar** *Fidia, Ital.*
Multivitamin and mineral preparation with gamolenic acid (p.1417·1).
*Nutritional supplement.*

**Medilax** *Medic, Denm.*
Lactulose (p.1269·1).
*Constipation; hepatic encephalopathy.*

**Medilaxan** *Beta, Arg.*
Ispaghula (p.1268·1); sennosides (p.1288·2).
*Constipation.*

**Medilet**
*Madaus, Austria; Medice, Ger.*
Lactulose (p.1269·1).
*Constipation; hepatic encephalopathy; salmonella enteritis.*

**Medilium** *Medifive, Thai.*
Flunarizine (p.434·2).
*Cerebrovascular disorders; migraine.*

**Medilyn** *Medpro, S.Afr.*
Diphenhydramine hydrochloride (p.431·3); ammonium chloride (p.1115·2); sodium citrate (p.1223·2).
*Coughs.*

**Medimegen** *Medical Supply, Thai.†.*
Brompheniramine maleate (p.426·1); phenylephrine hydrochloride (p.1126·3); phenylpropanolamine hydrochloride (p.1127·3).
*Hypersensitivity reactions; nasal congestion.*

**Medin G** *Grisi, Mex.*
Paracetamol (p.76·2); chlorphenamine (p.428·1).
*Cold and influenza symptoms.*

**Medinat Esten** *Bioglan, Austral.†.*
Vitamins; minerals (p.1417·1); equisetum (p.1684·1); eleutherococcus senticosis (p.1744·1); damiana (p.1679·1); cimicifuga (p.1671·3); angelica (p.1655·1).
*Menopausal disorders.*

**Medinat PMT-Eze** *Bioglan, Austral.†.*
Pyridoxine hydrochloride (p.1456·3); cyanocobalamin (p.1458·2); ferrous fumarate (p.1427·3); buchu (p.1663·1); bearberry (p.1659·2); parsley (p.1728·3); juniper oil (p.1703·1); evening primrose oil (p.1686·3).
*Premenstrual syndrome.*

**Medinol** *SSL, UK.*
Paracetamol (p.76·2).
Formerly known as Cupanol.
*Fever; pain.*

**Mediocin** *Medical Supply, Thai.*
Diiodohydroxyquinoline (p.603·3); furazolidone (p.605·2); phthalylsulfathiazole (p.242·3).
*Diarrhoea; dysentery; food poisoning.*

**Mediolax** *Medice, Ger.*
Bisacodyl (p.1251·3).
*Constipation.*

**Medipam** *Ratiopharm, Fin.*
Diazepam (p.690·1).
*Anxiety disorders; insomnia; neuroses; pain; premedication; psychosomatic disorders; skeletal muscle spasm.*

**Medipax** *Tecnifar, Port.*
Dipotassium clorazepate (p.685·1).
*Anxiety.*

**Medipe** *Sam-On, Israel†.*
Chlorhexidine gluconate (p.1173·2).
*Mouth disinfection.*

**Medipekt** *Orion, Fin.*
Bromhexine hydrochloride (p.1115·3).
*Respiratory-tract congestion.*

**Medipina** *Medinfar, Port.*
Nifedipine (p.966·2).
*Angina pectoris; hypertension.*

**Medipirol** *Medimport, Mex.*
Metamizole magnesium (p.36·1).
*Pain.*

**Mediplant** *Roche, Austria.*
*Ointment:* Menthol (p.1711·3); camphor (p.1665·3); eucalyptus oil (p.1686·2).
*Pastilles:* Menthol (p.1711·3); eucalyptus oil (p.1686·2).
*Respiratory-tract disorders.*

**Mediplant Inhalations** *Roche, Austria.*
Menthol (p.1711·3); camphor (p.1665·3); eucalyptus oil (p.1686·2).
*Respiratory-tract disorders.*

**Mediplant Krauter** *Roche, Austria.*
Althaea (p.1651·3); thyme (p.1755·2); ammonium chloride (p.1115·2).
*Respiratory-tract disorders.*

**Mediplast** *Beiersdorf, USA.*
Salicylic acid (p.1157·1).
*Hyperkeratosis.*

**Mediplaster** *Montefarmaco, Ital.*
Menthol (p.1711·3); camphor (p.1665·3); methyl salicylate (p.59·3).
*Musculoskeletal pain.*

**Mediplex** *US Pharmaceutical, USA†.*
Multivitamin and mineral preparation (p.1417·1).

**Mediplus** *Angelini, Ital.*
Benzalkonium chloride (p.1168·3); benzydamine hydrochloride (p.21·1).
*Disinfection of skin, wounds, and burns.*

**Medipo** *Mediolanum, Ital.*
Simvastatin (p.997·1).
*Atherosclerosis; hypercholesterolaemia.*

**Medi-Prep** *SSL, UK.*
Cetrimide (p.1172·1).
*Skin disinfection.*

**Mediprim** *Medika, Switz.*
Co-trimoxazole (p.199·3).
*Bacterial infections.*

**Medipulv**
*Rosken, Hong Kong; Pharmabroker, NZ.*
Chlorhexidine hydrochloride (p.1173·3); hexamidine isetionate (p.1181·3); allantoin (p.1141·3).
*Burns; wounds.*

**Medi-Quik**
*Note. This name is used for preparations of different composition.*
*Mentholatum, Canad.†.*
*Aerosol:* Benzalkonium chloride (p.1168·3); camphor (p.1665·3); lidocaine (p.1377·3).
*Mentholatum, Canad.†; Mentholatum, USA.*
*Topical spray:* Lidocaine (p.1377·3); benzalkonium chloride (p.1168·3).
*Skin disorders.*

**Medised** *SSL, UK†.*
Paracetamol (p.76·2); promethazine hydrochloride (p.439·1).
*Fever; pain.*

**Medised Infant** *SSL, UK.*
Diphenhydramine hydrochloride (p.431·3); paracetamol (p.76·2).
*Cold symptoms; fever; pain.*

**Medisense** *Abbott, Irl.*
Test for glucose and ketones in blood (p.1694·2).

**Medisense G2** *Medisense, UK.*
Test for glucose in blood (p.1694·2).

**MediSense Sof-Tact** *Medisense, Austral.*
Test for glucose in blood (p.1694·2).

**Medisept** *Laboratorios Chile, Chile.*
Chlorhexidine gluconate (p.1173·2); benzalkonium chloride (p.1168·3); benzyl alcohol (p.1170·2).
*Burns; disinfection of instruments and skin; wounds.*

**Medisepta** *Medgenix, Belg.*
Chlorhexidine acetate (p.1173·2) or chlorhexidine gluconate (p.1173·2).
*Burns; skin disinfection; skin infections; wounds.*

**Medismon** *Medice, Ger.†.*
Erythromycin stinoprate (p.210·3).
*Bacterial infections.*

**Medi-Sol** *Mykol, UK†.*
Adhesive remover.

**Medisport Athlete's Foot** *Medisport, UK†.*
Clotrimazole (p.396·2).
*Tinea pedis.*

**Medi-Swab** *SSL, UK.*
Isopropyl alcohol (p.1184·3).
*Pre-injection swab.*

**Medi-Swab H** *SSL, UK.*
Isopropyl alcohol (p.1184·3); chlorhexidine acetate (p.1173·2).
*Pre-injection swab.*

**Meditapp** *Medifive, Thai.*
Brompheniramine maleate (p.426·1); phenylephrine hydrochloride (p.1126·3).
Formerly contained brompheniramine maleate, phenylephrine hydrochloride, and phenylpropanolamine hydrochloride.
*Coughs; hypersensitivity reactions.*

**Meditapp Expectorant** *Medifive, Thai.*
Guaifenesin (p.1122·1); brompheniramine maleate (p.426·1); phenylephrine hydrochloride (p.1126·3).
Formerly contained guaifenesin, brompheniramine maleate, phenylephrine hydrochloride, and phenylpropanolamine hydrochloride.
*Coughs; hypersensitivity reactions.*

**Meditar** *Yamanouchi, Ital.†.*
Coal tar (Stantar) (p.1159·2).
*Seborrhoeic dermatitis of the scalp.*

**Medi-Test Combi 2** *BHR, UK.*
Test for glucose and protein in urine.

**Medi-Test Combi 5** *Dutec, Austral.*
Test for glucose, blood, ascorbic acid, protein, and pH in urine.

**Medi-Test Combi 7** *Dutec, Austral.*
Test for glucose, blood, ketones, ascorbic acid, nitrite, protein, and pH in urine.

**Medi-Test Combi 9**
*Dutec, Austral.; BHR, UK.*
Test for glucose, ascorbic acid, ketones, blood, protein, nitrite, pH, bilirubin, and urobilinogen in urine.

**Medi-Test Combi 3A** *Dutec, Austral.*
Test for glucose, protein, pH, and ascorbic acid in urine.

**Medi-Test Combi 4A** *Dutec, Austral.*
Test for nitrite, blood, protein, pH, and ascorbic acid in urine.

**Medi-Test Combi 6A** *Dutec, Austral.*
Test for blood, bilirubin, protein, ascorbic acid, glucose, and pH in urine.

**Medi-Test Combi 5N** *Dutec, Austral.*
Test for pH, glucose, blood, ascorbic acid, protein, and nitrite in urine.

**Medi-Test Glucose**
*Dutec, Austral.; BHR, UK.*
Test for glucose in urine (p.1694·2).

**Medi-Test Glucose 2** *Dutec, Austral.*
Test for glucose and ascorbic acid in urine.

**Medi-Test Glucose 3** *Dutec, Austral.*
Test for glucose, ketones, and ascorbic acid in urine.

**Medi-Test Glycaemie C** *BHR, UK.*
Test for glucose in blood (p.1694·2).

**Medi-Test Keton** *Dutec, Austral.*
Test for ketones in urine.

**Medi-Test Nitrit** *Dutec, Austral.*
Test for nitrite in urine.

**Medi-Test Protein 2** *Dutec, Austral.*
Test for protein and pH in urine.

**Medi-Test Urbi** *Dutec, Austral.*
Test for urobilinogen and bilirubin in urine.

**Medithane** *Wyeth, India.*
Hydrocortisone acetate (p.1103·3); skin respiratory factor derived from yeast cells (p.1469·1); shark-liver oil; vitamin A (p.1451·2).
*Anorectal disorders.*

**Medi-Tissue** *SSL, UK†.*
Alcohol (p.1166·1); benzalkonium chloride (p.1168·3).
*Skin and instrument disinfection.*

**Meditoina** *Medipharm, Chile.*
Mebeverine hydrochloride (p.1273·1).
*Gastrointestinal spasm.*

**Meditonsin**
*Europharm, Austria; Medice, Ger.*
Homoeopathic preparation.

**Medituss** *Crown, S.Afr.*
Mepyramine maleate (p.437·1); ammonium chloride (p.1115·2); sodium citrate (p.1223·2); cetrimide (p.1172·1); menthol (p.1711·3); ephedrine hydrochloride (p.1120·1).
*Respiratory-tract congestion.*

**Mediuresix** *Medical Supply, Thai.*
Furosemide (p.919·3).
*Ascites; oedema.*

**Mediveine** *Elerte, Fr.*
Diosmin (p.1688·2).
*Haemorrhoids; peripheral vascular disorders.*

**Medivitan N** *Medice, Ger.*
Hydroxocobalamin (p.1458·2); sodium folate (p.1429·3); pyridoxine hydrochloride (p.1456·3).
Lidocaine hydrochloride (p.1377·3) is included in this preparation to alleviate the pain of injection.
*Vitamin deficiency.*

**Medivitan N Neuro** *Medice, Ger.*
Thiamine hydrochloride (p.1455·1); pyridoxine hydrochloride (p.1456·3).
*Neuralgia; neuritis; polyneuropathies.*

**Medi-Wipe** *SSL, UK.*
Chlorhexidine gluconate (p.1173·2); alcohol (p.1166·1).
*Hard surface disinfection.*

**Medixel** *Taro, Israel.*
Paclitaxel (p.577·3).
*Breast cancer; Kaposi's sarcoma; non-small-cell lung cancer; ovarian cancer.*

**Medixil** *Rider, Chile.*
Sibutramine hydrochloride (p.1593·1).
*Obesity.*

**Medixin** *Pierrel, Ital.†.*
Co-trimoxazole (p.199·3).
*Bacterial infections.*

**Medizol**
*Note. This name is used for preparations of different composition.*
*Ratiopharm, Fin.*
Miconazole nitrate (p.405·3).
*Fungal skin infections.*

*Medimport, Mex.*
Metronidazole (p.607·2).
*Trichomoniasis.*

**Medizyme** *Utopian, Thai.*
Serrapeptase (p.1743·2).
*Inflammation; respiratory-tract congestion.*

**Med-Kafuzone** *Medical Supply, Thai.*
Furazolidone (p.605·2); kaolin (p.1268·3); pectin (p.1580·3).
*Bacterial gastro-enteritis; diarrhoea.*

**Medkofen** *Medifive, Thai.*
Ketotifen fumarate (p.788·1).
*Asthma; hypersensitivity reactions.*

**Med-Mucolo** *Medical Supply, Thai.*
Bromhexine hydrochloride (p.1115·3); sulfogaiacol (p.1131·1).
*Respiratory-tract disorders associated with increased or viscous mucus.*

**Med-Myolax** *Medical Supply, Thai.*
Orphenadrine citrate (p.486·1); paracetamol (p.76·2).
*Musculoskeletal and joint pain; neuralgia.*

**Mednil** *Pharmaland, Thai.*
Mefenamic acid (p.55·2).
*Pain.*

**Medobeta** *Medochemie, Singapore†.*
Betamethasone (p.1093·1).
*Skin disorders.*

**Medobiotin**
*Apotheke Raten Krebs, Austria; Medopharm, Ger.*
Biotin (p.1423·2).
*Biotin deficiency; hair and nail disorders.*

**Medocalum**
Medochemie, Hong Kong; Medochemie, Singapore.
Chlordiazepoxide (p.674·2); clidinium bromide (p.480·2).
*Gastrointestinal disorders; nocturnal enuresis; smooth muscle spasm.*

**Medocarnitin** Medosan, Ital.
Levocarnitine (p.1423·3).
*Carnitine deficiency.*

**Medocef**
Medochemie, Singapore†; Medochemie, Thai.
Cefoperazone sodium (p.174·3).
*Bacterial infections.*

**Medociprin** Medochemie, Thai.†.
Ciprofloxacin (p.188·2).
*Bacterial infections.*

**Medoclazide**
Medochemie, Singapore†; Medochemie, Thai.
Gliclazide (p.332·1).
*Diabetes mellitus.*

**Medoclor** Medochemie, Hong Kong.
Cefaclor (p.167·1).
*Bacterial infections.*

**Medocodene** Schwarz, UK†.
Paracetamol (p.76·2); codeine phosphate (p.27·1).
These ingredients can be described by the British Approved Name Co-codamol.
*Fever; pain.*

**Medocor** Roemmers, Arg.
Isosorbide mononitrate (p.942·1).
*Ischaemic heart disease.*

**Medocriptine**
Medochemie, Hong Kong; Medochemie, Malaysia.
Bromocriptine mesilate (p.1200·3).
*Acromegaly; benign breast disorders; galactorrhoea; hypogonadism; infertility; lactation inhibition; menstrual disorders; parkinsonism; prolactinomas.*

**Medocycline** Medochemie, Hong Kong.
Tetracycline hydrochloride (p.266·2).
*Bacterial infections.*

**Medodermone**
Medochemie, Hong Kong; Medochemie, Singapore†; Medochemie, Thai.
Clobetasol propionate (p.1095·2).
*Skin disorders.*

**Medoenzym** Medicopharm, Austria.
Mucosal stomach extract.
*Gastrointestinal disorders.*

**Medofloxine** Medochemie, Malaysia.
Ofloxacin (p.239·3).
*Bacterial infections.*

**Medofulvin**
Medochemie, Malaysia; Medochemie, Singapore†.
Griseofulvin (p.400·3).
*Fungal infections.*

**Medoglycin**
Medochemie, Hong Kong; Medochemie, Malaysia.
Lincomycin hydrochloride (p.226·2).
*Bacterial infections.*

**Medolexin**
Medochemie, Hong Kong; Medochemie, Malaysia.
Cefalexin (p.168·1).
*Bacterial infections.*

**Medolin**
Medochemie, Singapore†; Medochemie, Thai.†.
Salbutamol sulfate (p.791·3).
*Obstructive airways disease.*

**Medomet** DDSA Pharmaceuticals, UK†.
Methyldopa (p.953·2).

**Medomycin**
Medochemie, Hong Kong; Medochemie, Malaysia; Medochemie, Singapore†; Medochemie, Thai.
Doxycycline hyclate (p.206·2).
*Bacterial infections.*

**Medonol** Medochemie, Hong Kong.
Paracetamol (p.76·2); dextropropoxyphene hydrochloride (p.28·3).
*Fever; pain.*

**Medopa**
Note. This name is used for preparations of different composition.
Medinfar, Port.
Dopamine hydrochloride (p.907·1).
*Shock.*

Atlantic, Thai.
Methyldopa (p.953·2).
*Hypertension.*

**Medopal** Fustery, Mex.†.
Methyldopa (p.953·2).

**Medopam** Schwulst, S.Afr.†.
Oxazepam (p.712·2).
*Alcohol withdrawal syndrome; anxiety.*

**Medopate** Atlantic, Thai.†.
Methyldopa (p.953·2).
*Hypertension.*

**Medophyll** Li-il, Ger.
Thymol (p.1194·2).
*Skin ulceration; superficial skin disorders; wounds.*

**Medopren** Malesci, Ital.
Methyldopa (p.953·2).
*Hypertension.*

**Medoric** Medifive, Thai.
Allopurinol (p.412·2).
*Gout; hyperuricaemia.*

**Medostatin**
Medochemie, Hong Kong; Medochemie, Malaysia; Medochemie, Singapore.
Lovastatin (p.949·1).
*Atherosclerosis; hypercholesterolaemia.*

**Medotar** Medco, USA.
Coal tar (p.1159·2); zinc oxide (p.1163·2).
*Skin disorders.*

**Medotifen** Medical Supply, Thai.
Ketotifen fumarate (p.788·1).
*Asthma; hypersensitivity reactions.*

**Medovascin** Pharmacypria, Gr.
Lovastatin (p.949·1).
*Primary hypercholesterolaemia.*

**Medovent**
Medochemie, Hong Kong; Medochemie, Thai.
Ambroxol hydrochloride (p.1114·3).
*Respiratory-tract disorders associated with increased or viscous mucus.*

**Medovir**
Medochemie, Hong Kong; Medochemie, Malaysia; Medochemie, Singapore; Medochemie, Thai.†.
Aciclovir (p.626·1).
*Herpesvirus infections.*

**Medoxem** Pharmacypria, Gr.
Cefuroxime sodium (p.184·1).
*Bacterial infections.*

**Medoxim** Medici, Ital.†.
Cefuroxime sodium (p.184·1).
*Bacterial infections.*

**Medoxin** Milano, Thai.
Doxycycline hyclate (p.206·2).
*Bacterial infections.*

**Medozem** Medochemie, Thai.
Diltiazem hydrochloride (p.900·1).
*Angina pectoris; hypertension.*

**Medozide** Malesci, Ital.
Methyldopa (p.953·2); hydrochlorothiazide (p.933·2).
*Hypertension.*

**Medozine**
Medochemie, Hong Kong; Medochemie, Thai.
Cinnarizine (p.428·3).
*Cerebrovascular disorders; migraine; peripheral vascular disorders.*

**Medphlem** Medpro, S.Afr.†.
Carbocisteine (p.1116·2).
*Respiratory-tract disorders.*

**Med-Phylline** Medical Supply, Thai.
Theophylline (p.798·3).
*Obstructive airways disease.*

**Medpramol** Schwulst, S.Afr.†.
Paracetamol (p.76·2).
*Fever; pain.*

**Medral** Offenbach, Mex.
Omeprazole (p.1278·2).
*Acid aspiration; gastro-oesophageal reflux; gastrointestinal hyperacidity; peptic ulcer; Zollinger-Ellison syndrome.*

**Medralone** Keene, USA†.
Methylprednisolone acetate (p.1106·1).
*Corticosteroid.*

**Medramil** Farmigea, Ital.†.
Medrysone (p.1106·1); tetryzoline hydrochloride (p.1131·2); pheniramine maleate (p.438·3).
*Eye disorders.*

**Medramine retard** Mepha, Switz.†.
Dimenhydrinate (p.431·1); pyridoxine hydrochloride (p.1456·3).
*Nausea; vomiting.*

**Medramine-B$_6$ Rectocaps** Mepha, Switz.†.
Dimenhydrinate (p.431·1); pyridoxine hydrochloride (p.1456·3); caffeine (p.782·1).
*Nausea; vomiting.*

**Medrate** Pharmacia, Ger.
Methylprednisolone (p.1106·1) or methylprednisolone sodium succinate (p.1106·2).
*Corticosteroid.*

**Medrocis** Schering, UK.
Technetium-99m medronate (p.1525·2).
*Bone scintigraphy.*

**Medricol** Alcon Cusi, Spain†.
Chloramphenicol (p.185·1); medroxyprogesterone acetate (p.1557·2).
*Eye disorders.*

**Medrisocil** Oftalder, Port.
Medrysone (p.1106·1).
*Eye disorders.*

**Medrivas**
Alcon, Port.†; Alcon Cusi, Spain.
Medroxyprogesterone acetate (p.1557·2); tetryzoline hydrochloride (p.1131·2).
*Eye disorders.*

**Medrivas Antib** Alcon Cusi, Spain.
Chloramphenicol succinate (p.186·3); medroxyprogesterone acetate (p.1557·2); tetryzoline hydrochloride (p.1131·2).
*Infected eye disorders.*

**Medrivas Antibiotico** Alcon, Port.
Chloramphenicol (p.185·1); medroxyprogesterone acetate (p.1557·2); tetryzoline hydrochloride (p.1131·2).
*Eye disorders.*

**Medrocil** Fortbenton, Arg.
Hydrocortisone (p.1103·3).
*Skin disorders.*

**Medrocis** Schering, UK.
Technetium-99m medronate (p.1525·2).
*Bone scintigraphy.*

**Medrol**
Pharmacia, Austral.; Pharmacia, Belg.; Pharmacia, Canad.; Pharmacia, Chile; Pharmacia, Denm.; Pharmacia, Fin.; Pharmacia, Fr.; Pharmacia-Upjohn, Gr.; Pharmacia, Hong Kong; Pharmacia Upjohn, Israel; Pharmacia Upjohn, Ital.; Pharmacia, Neth.; Pharmacia, Norw.; Pharmacia, NZ; Pharmacia, Port.; Pharmacia, S.Afr.; Pharmacia, Swed.; Pharmacia, Switz.; Pharmacia Upjohn, USA.
Methylprednisolone (p.1106·1).
*Corticosteroid.*

**Medrol Acne Lotion** Pharmacia, Canad.
Methylprednisolone acetate (p.1106·1); aluminium chlorohydrate complex (p.1142·1); sulfur (p.1158·2).
*Acne; seborrhoeic dermatitis.*

**Medrol Lozione Antiacne** Pharmacia Upjohn, Ital.
Methylprednisolone acetate (p.1106·1); aluminium chlorohydrate (p.1142·1); colloidal sulfur (p.1158·2).
*Acne.*

**Medrol Veriderm** Pharmacia Upjohn, Canad.†.
Methylprednisolone acetate (p.1106·1).
Formerly called Medrol Topical.
*Skin disorders.*

**Medronate** Activa, Braz.†.
Disodium medronate (p.773·2).
*Radiographic contrast medium.*

**Medrone**
Pharmacia Upjohn, Irl.†; Pharmacia, UK.
Methylprednisolone (p.1106·1).
*Corticosteroid.*

**Medrosterona** Gador, Arg.
Medroxyprogesterone acetate (p.1557·2).
*Endometrial cancer; renal cancer.*

**Medroxitest** Delta, Braz.
Medroxyprogesterone acetate (p.1557·2).

**Medroxyhexal** Hexal, Austral.
Medroxyprogesterone acetate (p.1557·2).
*Endometriosis; menopausal disorders; menstrual disorders.*

**Medroxyurea** Medac, Gr.
Hydroxycarbamide (p.559·1).
*Chronic myeloid leukaemia; myelodysplastic syndromes; polycythaemia vera; primary thrombocythaemia.*

**MED-Rx** Iomed, USA.
Blue tablets, pseudoephedrine hydrochloride (p.1129·2); guaifenesin (p.1122·1); white tablets, guaifenesin.
*Upper respiratory-tract symptoms.*

**MED-Rx DM** Iopharm, USA.
Blue tablets, pseudoephedrine hydrochloride (p.1129·2); guaifenesin (p.1122·1); green tablets, guaifenesin; dextromethorphan hydrobromide (p.1117·3).
*Upper respiratory-tract symptoms.*

**Medsara** Asofarma, Mex.
Cytarabine (p.543·1).
*Malignant neoplasms.*

**Medsatrexate** Asofarma, Mex.
Methotrexate (p.568·2).
*Malignant neoplasms.*

**Medsavorina** Asofarma, Mex.
Calcium folinate (p.1431·1).
*Megaloblastic anaemia; reduction of methotrexate toxicity.*

**Med-Spastic** Medical Supply, Thai.
Oxyphencyclimine hydrochloride (p.487·2).
*Gastrointestinal disorders; genito-urinary disorders.*

**Med-Sultrim** Medical Supply, Thai.
Co-trimoxazole (p.199·3).
*Bacterial infections.*

**Med-Tricocide** Medical Supply, Thai.
Metronidazole (p.607·2).
*Amoebiasis; anaerobic bacterial infections; giardiasis; trichomoniasis.*

**Med-Tussin** Medical Supply, Thai.
Diphenhydramine hydrochloride (p.431·3); ammonium chloride (p.1115·2); sodium citrate (p.1223·2).
*Coughs.*

**Medusit** Grunenthal, Port.
Sodium fluoride (p.1444·3).
*Osteoporosis.*

**Med-Xyzarax** Medical Supply, Thai.
Hydroxyzine hydrochloride (p.434·3).
*Allergic skin disorders; anxiety.*

**Medyn** Medice, Ger.
Pyridoxine hydrochloride (p.1456·3); folic acid (p.1429·1); cyanocobalamin (p.1458·2).
*Prevention of elevated homocysteine concentration.*

**ME-F** Nakorn, Thai.
Metformin hydrochloride (p.342·3).
*Diabetes mellitus.*

**Mefa** Macrophar, Thai.
Mefenamic acid (p.55·2).
*Inflammation; pain.*

**Mefac** Rowex, Irl.
Mefenamic acid (p.55·2).
*Musculoskeletal and joint disorders; pain.*

**Mefacap**
Malayan, Hong Kong†; Malayan, Singapore.
Mefenamic acid (p.55·2).
*Menstrual disorders; musculoskeletal and joint disorders; pain.*

**Mefamic** Merck, Hong Kong.
Mefenamic acid (p.55·2).
*Pain; peri-articular and soft-tissue disorders.*

**Mefazil** Mayo, Mex.†.
Indometacin (p.47·3).

**mefe-basan** Schonenberger, Switz.
Mefenamic acid (p.55·2).
*Fever; pain.*

**Mefedra-N** Medipharma, Hong Kong.
Noscapine hydrochloride (p.1125·3); ephedrine hydrochloride (p.1120·1); chlorphenamine maleate (p.427·3); cocillana (p.1117·2); euphorbia (p.1686·3); adhatoda; senega (p.1130·2); squill (p.1130·3).
*Cold and influenza symptoms.*

**Mefen**
Strand, Malaysia; Milano, Thai.
Mefenamic acid (p.55·2).
*Pain.*

**Mefenacide** Streuli, Switz.
Mefenamic acid (p.55·2).
*Influenza symptoms; pain.*

**Mefenan** Greater Pharma, Thai.
Mefenamic acid (p.55·2).
*Pain.*

**Mefenix**
Note. This name is used for preparations of different composition.
Phoenix, Arg.
Tenoxicam (p.93·1).
*Inflammation; pain.*

Ranbaxy, Singapore; Ranbaxy, Thai.†.
Mefenamic acid (p.55·2).
*Pain.*

**Mefenix Relax** Phoenix, Arg.
Tenoxicam (p.93·1); carisoprodol (p.1392·1); dexamethasone (p.1097·1).
*Musculoskeletal, joint, and peri-articular disorders; pain.*

**Mefic**
Pfizer, Austral.; Alphapharm, Hong Kong; Alphapharm, Malaysia; Merck, Malaysia.
Mefenamic acid (p.55·2).
*Dysmenorrhoea; menorrhagia; pain.*

**Mefiron** Chew, Thai.
Metronidazole (p.607·2).
*Trichomoniasis.*

**Mefliam** Cipla-Medpro, S.Afr.
Mefloquine hydrochloride (p.453·3).
*Malaria.*

**Meflotas** Intas, India.
Mefloquine (p.455·3).
*Malaria.*

**Meflox** Klinger, Braz.
Lomefloxacin (p.227·3).
*Bacterial infections.*

**Meformed** Medifive, Thai.
Metformin hydrochloride (p.342·3).
*Diabetes mellitus.*

**Mefoxil** Vianex (Βιανεξ), Gr.
Cefoxitin sodium (p.177·2).
*Bacterial infections.*

**Mefoxin**
Merck Sharp & Dohme, Arg.; Merck Sharp & Dohme, Austral.; Merck Sharp & Dohme, Belg.; Merck Sharp & Dohme, Braz.; Merck Frosst, Canad.; Merck Sharp & Dohme, Fin.; Merck Sharp & Dohme-Chibret, Fr.; Merck Sharp & Dohme, Hong Kong; Merck Sharp & Dohme, Irl.†; Merck Sharp & Dohme, Ital.; Merck Sharp & Dohme, Neth.; Merck Sharp & Dohme, NZ; Merck Sharp & Dohme, Port.; Merck Sharp & Dohme, S.Afr.; Merck Sharp & Dohme, UK; Merck, USA.
Cefoxitin sodium (p.177·2).
Lidocaine hydrochloride (p.1377·3) may be included in the intramuscular injection to alleviate the pain of injection.
*Bacterial infections.*

**Mefoxitin**
Merck Sharp & Dohme, Austria; Merck Sharp & Dohme, Ger.; Merck Sharp & Dohme, Norw.; Merck Sharp & Dohme, Spain; Merck Sharp & Dohme, Swed.; Merck Sharp & Dohme, Switz.
Cefoxitin sodium (p.177·2).
Lidocaine hydrochloride (p.1377·3) may be included in the intramuscular injection to alleviate the pain of injection.
*Bacterial infections.*

**Mefpa** Pharmasant, Thai.
Methyldopa (p.953·2).
*Hypertension.*

**Mefren Incolore** Novartis Consumer, Belg.
Chlorhexidine gluconate (p.1173·2).
*Disinfection of minor wounds; disinfection of the skin.*

**Mefren Pastilles** Novartis Consumer, Belg.
Chlorhexidine hydrochloride (p.1173·3).
*Mouth and throat infections.*

**Mega 65** Arkopharma, Fr.†.
Fish oil (p.976·2).
*Nutritional supplement.*

**Mega Acidophilus** Bullivants, Austral.†.
Lactic-acid-producing organisms (p.1704·2).
*Maintenance of normal gastrointestinal flora.*

**Mega AO** Usana, Canad.
Multivitamin preparation with ubidecarenone (p.1760·2) (p.1417·1).

**Mega B**
Sisu, Canad.; Quest, Canad.; Quest, UK; Arco, USA.
Vitamin B substances (p.1417·1).
*Vitamin B deficiency.*

**Mega B Extra Strength** *Cenovis, Austral.†.*
Vitamin B substances; ascorbic acid (p.1417·1).
*Vitamin B deficiency.*

**Mega B Slow Release** *Vitaglow, Austral.†.*
Vitamin B substances; ascorbic acid (p.1417·1).
*Dietary supplement; premenstrual syndrome.*

**Mega Balance** *Pharmavite, Canad.*
Multivitamin and mineral preparation (p.1417·1).

**Mega Cal Calcium** *Jamieson, Canad.*
Calcium carbonate; calcium citrate; calcium fumarate; calcium glutamate; calcium malate; calcium succinate (p.1225·1); vitamin D (p.1461·2).

**Mega Capsule** *Quest, Canad.†.*
Multivitamin and mineral preparation (p.1417·1).

**Mega E** *Cenovis, Austral.†.*
*dl*-Alpha tocoferil acetate (p.1465·1).
*Vitamin E supplement.*

**Mega Men** *General Nutrition, Canad.†.*
Multivitamin and mineral preparation (p.1417·1).

**Mega Multi** *Cenovis, Austral.†.*
Vitamin and mineral preparation (p.1417·1).

**Mega Stress Vitamins** *Vita Pharm, Canad.*
Multivitamin and mineral preparation (p.1417·1).

**Mega Swiss One** *Swiss Herbal, Canad.*
Multivitamin and mineral preparation (p.1417·1).

**Mega Vim** *Jamieson, Canad.*
Multivitamin and mineral preparation (p.1417·1).

**Mega VM** *Nature's Bounty, USA.*
Multivitamin and mineral preparation (p.1417·1).

**Mega-Antioxidant** *Usana, Hong Kong.*
Multivitamin preparation with inositol, rutoside, hesperidin, green tea, bilberry, choline bitartrate, L-cysteine hydrochloride, cabbage, broccoli (p.1417·1).

**Megabrain** *Hebron, Braz.*
Multivitamin and mineral preparation (p.1417·1).

**Megabron** *Sidus, Arg.*
*Streptococcus pneumoniae*; *Staphylococcus aureus*; *Streptococcus viridans*; *Haemophilus influenzae*; *Klebsiella.*
*Respiratory-tract infections.*

**Megabyl** *Martin, Fr.†.*
Diisopromine hydrochloride (p.1261·2); sorbitol (p.1446·3).
*Constipation; dyspepsia.*

**Mega-Cal** *Jamieson, Hong Kong.*
Calcium (p.1225·1).
*Calcium deficiency; calcium supplement.*

**Mega-Cal with Vit D** *Jamieson, Hong Kong.*
Calcium (p.1225·1); vitamin D (p.1461·2).
*Calcium deficiency; calcium supplement.*

**Mega-Calcium**
*Novartis Consumer, Austria; Novartis, Fin.*
Calcium lactate gluconate (p.1225·3); calcium carbonate (p.1254·2).
*Calcium deficiency.*

**Mega-calcium Sandoz** *Novartis, Gr.*
Calcium carbonate (p.1254·2); calcium gluconate (p.1417·1); calcium lactate (p.1225·3).
*Prevention and treatment of calcium deficiency.*

**Megace**
*Bristol-Myers Squibb, Arg.; Bristol-Myers Squibb, Austral.; Bristol-Myers Squibb, Austria; Bristol-Myers Squibb, Belg.; Bristol, Canad.; Bristol-Myers Squibb, Chile; Bristol-Myers Squibb, Denm.; Bristol-Myers Squibb, Fin.; Bristol-Myers Squibb, Fr.; Bristol-Myers Squibb, Gr.; Bristol-Myers Squibb, Hong Kong; Bristol-Myers Squibb, Irl.; Bristol-Myers Squibb, Israel; Bristol-Myers Squibb, Ital.; Bristol-Myers Squibb, Malaysia; Bristol-Myers Squibb, Mex.; Bristol-Myers Squibb, Neth.; Bristol-Myers Squibb, Norw.; Bristol-Myers Squibb, NZ; Bristol-Myers Squibb, Port.; Bristol-Myers Squibb, Singapore; Bristol-Myers Squibb, Swed.; Bristol-Myers Squibb, Thai.; Bristol-Myers Squibb, UK; Bristol-Myers Squibb Oncology, USA.*
Megestrol acetate (p.1558·2).
*AIDS-associated and cancer-associated cachexia; breast cancer; endometrial cancer; prostatic cancer.*

**Megacillin**
*Note. This name is used for preparations of different composition.*
*Grunenthal, Austria.*
Phenoxymethylpenicillin potassium (p.242·1).
*Bacterial infections.*

*Frosst, Canad.†.*
Benzathine benzylpenicillin (p.162·3) or benzylpenicillin potassium (p.163·2).
*Bacterial infections.*

**Megacillin oral** *Grunenthal, Ger.*
Phenoxymethylpenicillin potassium (p.242·1).
*Bacterial infections.*

**Megacilline** *Grunenthal, Switz.*
*Injection:* Clemizole penicillin (p.194·1).
*Syrup; tablets:* Phenoxymethylpenicillin potassium (p.242·1).
*Bacterial infections.*

**Megacina** *Reprefar, Port.†.*
Ofloxacin (p.239·3).
*Bacterial infections.*

**Megacistin** *ICN, Arg.*
Cystine (p.1426·3); vitamin $B_6$ (p.1456·3).
*Eye disorders; skin, hair, and nail disorders.*

**Megacistin G** *ICN, Arg.*
Piroctone olamine (p.1155·2).
*Seborrhoeic dermatitis.*

**Megacort** *Uno, Ital.*
Dexamethasone sodium phosphate (p.1097·2).
*Musculoskeletal and joint disorders.*

**Megadin** *Medipharma, Hong Kong†.*
Cimetidine (p.1255·3).
*Dyspepsia; gastritis; gastro-oesophageal reflux; peptic ulcer.*

**Megadose**
*Note. This name is used for preparations of different composition.*
*Fada, Arg.*
Dopamine (p.907·3).

*Arco, USA.*
Multivitamin and mineral preparation (p.1417·1).

**Megadoxa** *Restan, S.Afr.*
Vitamin B substances (p.1417·1).

**Megafer** *Pulitzer, Ital.*
Ferrous gluconate (p.1428·1).
Ascorbic acid (p.1460·2) is included in this preparation to increase the absorption and availability of iron.
*Iron-deficiency anaemia.*

**Megaflox** *Baldacci, Port.*
Ciprofloxacin hydrochloride (p.188·2).
*Bacterial infections.*

**Megafol** *Alphapharm, Austral.*
Folic acid (p.1429·1).
*Folic acid deficiency; megaloblastic anaemia.*

**Megagrisevit** *Pharmacia, Ger.*
Clostebol acetate (p.1543·2).
*Anabolic; fractures; osteoporosis.*

**Megal Simple** *Andromaco, Mex.*
Dextromethorphan hydrobromide (p.1117·3).
*Coughs.*

**Megalac** *Krewel, Ger.*
Almasilate (p.1248·2) or hydrotalcite (p.1267·3).
*Gastrointestinal hyperacidity.*

**Megalat** *Agis, Israel.*
Nifedipine (p.966·2).
*Angina pectoris; hypertension; Raynaud's syndrome.*

**Megalax** *Propan, S.Afr.*
Bisacodyl (p.1251·3).
*Bowel evacuation; constipation.*

**Megalex** *Phoenix, Arg.*
Ranitidine hydrochloride (p.1285·2); domperidone (p.1263·2).
*Gastritis; gastro-oesophageal reflux; peptic ulcer.*

**Megalocin** *Kyorin, Jpn.*
Fleroxacin (p.213·2).
*Bacterial infections.*

**Megalotect**
*Biogam, Arg.; Biotest, Fin.†; Ionios (Ιονιος), Gr.; Intra Pharma, Irl.; Biotest, Israel; Boehringer Ingelheim, Port.; Mednostica, S.Afr.; Leo, Swed.†; Biotest, Thai.*
A cytomegalovirus immunoglobulin (p.1612·1).
*Passive immunisation.*

**Megamag** *Mayoly-Spindler, Fr.*
Magnesium aspartate (p.1227·3).
*Magnesium deficiency.*

**Megamilbedoce** *Andromaco, Spain.*
Hydroxocobalamin (p.1458·2).
*Vitamin B12 deficiency.*

**Megamox** *Garec, S.Afr.*
Ampicillin (p.157·1); cloxacillin (p.198·2).
*Bacterial infections.*

**Megamylase** *Leurquin, Fr.*
Alpha-amylase (p.1654·2).
*Upper respiratory-tract congestion.*

**Meganest** *Clarben, Spain.*
Articaine.
Adrenaline (p.852·2) is included in this preparation as a vasoconstrictor to diminish absorption and localise the effect of the local anaesthetic.
*Local anaesthesia in dentistry.*

**Megapen**
*Note. This name is used for preparations of different composition.*
*Euroforma, Braz.*
Benzylpenicillin potassium (p.163·2).
*Bacterial infections.*

*Garec, S.Afr.*
Amoxicillin (p.155·3); flucloxacillin (p.213·3).
*Bacterial infections.*

**Megapenil** *Lakeside, Mex.*
*Injection:* Clemizole penicillin (p.194·1).
*Tablets:* Phenoxymethylpenicillin potassium (p.242·1).
*Bacterial infections.*

**Megapenil Forte** *Lakeside, Mex.*
Clemizole penicillin (p.194·1); benzylpenicillin sodium (p.163·2).
Lidocaine hydrochloride (p.1377·3) is included in this preparation to alleviate the pain of injection.
*Bacterial infections.*

**Megaplatin** *Genepharm, Gr.*
Carboplatin (p.533·3).
*Ovarian cancer; small-cell lung cancer.*

**Megaplus** *ICN, Arg.*
Cystine (p.1426·3); pyridoxine hydrochloride (p.1456·3); biotin (p.1423·2); calcium pantothenate (p.1442·3); zinc sulfate (p.1469·3); gelatin (p.754·3).
*Hair and nail disorders; seborrhoea.*

**Megapress** *Genepharm, Gr.*
Enalapril maleate (p.909·2).
*Heart failure; hypertension.*

**Mega-Prim** *Hua, Thai.*
Co-trimoxazole (p.199·3).
*Bacterial infections.*

**Megapyn** *Aspen, S.Afr.*
*Syrup:* Paracetamol (p.76·2); codeine phosphate (p.27·1); promethazine hydrochloride (p.439·1).
*Fever; pain.*

*Tablets:* Paracetamol (p.76·2); codeine phosphate (p.27·1); caffeine (p.782·1); meprobamate (p.706·2).
*Pain and associated tension.*

**Megareal** *Novartis Nutrition, Fr.*
Preparation for enteral nutrition (p.1417·1).

**Megasin** *Pierre Fabre, Port.*
Ofloxacin (p.239·3).
*Bacterial infections.*

**Megastene** *Servier, Arg.*
Sulbutiamine (p.1455·1).
*Asthenia.*

**Megastrol** *Libra, Braz.†.*
Megestrol (p.1558·3).
*Malignant neoplasms.*

**Megatears** *ICN, Arg.*
Povidone (p.1581·2).
*Dry eyes.*

**Megaton** *Hyrex, USA.*
Vitamin B substances with minerals (p.1417·1).

**Megaval** *Lafi, Chile.*
Fenfluramine hydrochloride (p.1588·2).
*Obesity.*

**Megavir** *Gador, Arg.*
Didanosine (p.630·3).
*HIV infection.*

**Megavis** *Volchem, Ital.*
Levocarnitine (p.1423·3).
*Asthenia.*

**Megavit** *Laboratorios Chile, Chile.*
Vitamins; minerals; ginseng; procaine hydrochloride (p.1383·2) (p.1417·1).
*Dietary supplement.*

**Megavit Natal** *Laboratorios Chile, Chile.*
Vitamin and mineral preparation (p.1417·1).

**Megavites** *ICN, Canad.*
Vitamin B substances and vitamin C(p.1417·1).

**Megavix** *Irex, Fr.*
Tetrazepam (p.724·1).
*Skeletal muscle spasm.*

**Megaxin** *Agis, Israel.*
Moxifloxacin (p.233·1).
*Bacterial infections.*

**Megefren** *Prasfarma, Spain.*
Megestrol acetate (p.1558·2).
*Breast cancer; endometrial cancer.*

**Megestat**
*Bristol-Myers Squibb, Braz.; Bristol-Myers Squibb, Ger.; Bristol-Myers Squibb, Switz.*
Megestrol acetate (p.1558·2).
*Breast cancer; endometrial cancer.*

**Megestil** *Roche, Ital.*
Megestrol acetate (p.1558·2).
*AIDS-associated and cancer-associated cachexia; breast cancer; endometrial cancer.*

**Megestin**
*Nettopharma, Denm.†; Leiras, Fin.*
Megestrol acetate (p.1558·2).
*Breast cancer; menopausal disorders; menstrual disorders.*

**Megestran** *Sigma, Braz.*
21 Tablets, norethisterone (p.1562·2); mestranol (p.1559·2); 7 tablets, pyridoxine hydrochloride (p.1456·3).
*Combined oral contraceptive.*

**Meggezones**
*Schering-Plough, Canad.; Schering-Plough, UK.*
Menthol (p.1711·3).
*Catarrh; coughs; nasal congestion; sore throats.*

**Meglucon**
*Hexal, Austria; Hexal, Ger.*
Metformin hydrochloride (p.342·3).
*Diabetes mellitus.*

**Meglum** *Bago, Arg.*
Levamisole (p.107·1).
*Immunostimulant.*

**Megostat**
*Bristol-Myers Squibb, Austral.†; Bristol-Myers Squibb, NZ†; Squibb, Spain.*
Megestrol acetate (p.1558·2).
*AIDS-associated cachexia; breast cancer; endometrial cancer.*

**Megral** *Glaxo Wellcome, Canad.†.*
Ergotamine tartrate (p.467·2); cyclizine hydrochloride (p.429·3); caffeine hydrate (p.782·1).
*Migraine and other vascular headaches.*

**Meiact** *Meiji, Jpn.*
Cefditoren pivoxil (p.172·1).
*Bacterial infections.*

**Meibi** *Kampel Martian, Arg.*
Minocycline (p.231·3).
*Bacterial infections.*

**Meicelin**
*Meiji, Jpn; Meiji, Thai.*
Cefminox sodium (p.174·1).
*Bacterial infections.*

**Meiceral** *Tedec-Meiji, Thai.*
Omeprazole (p.1278·2).
*Gastro-oesophageal reflux; peptic ulcer; Zollinger-Ellison syndrome.*

**Meiclox** *Meiji, Thai.*
Cloxacillin sodium (p.198·2).
*Bacterial infections.*

**Meilax** *Meiji, Jpn.*
Ethyl loflazepate (p.698·1).
*Anxiety; sleep disorders.*

**Meinfusona** *Mein, Spain†.*
Electrolyte infusion with vitamin B substances (p.1217·1)(p.1417·1).
*Electrolyte depletion; vitamin B deficiency.*

**Meinvenil Fisiologico** *Fresenius Kabi, Spain.*
Sodium chloride (p.1233·3).
*Fluid and electrolyte disorders.*

**Meinvenil Glucosalina** *Fresenius Kabi, Spain.*
Glucose (p.1432·2); sodium chloride (p.1233·3).
*Carbohydrate source; fluid and electrolyte disorders.*

**Meixil** *Meiji, Thai.*
Amoxicillin trihydrate (p.155·3).
*Bacterial infections.*

**Mejoral**
*Note. This name is used for preparations of different composition.*
*Elisium, Arg.*
Paracetamol (p.76·2).
*Fever; pain.*

*SmithKline Beecham, Mex.†; SmithKline Beecham, Spain.*
Aspirin (p.15·1).
*Fever; musculoskeletal and joint disorders; pain; periarticular disorders; thromboembolism prophylaxis.*

**Mejoral Cafeina**
*Note. This name is used for preparations of different composition.*
*Elisium, Arg.*
Paracetamol (p.76·2); caffeine (p.782·1).
*Pain.*

*SmithKline Beecham, Spain.*
Aspirin (p.15·1); caffeine (p.782·1).
*Fever; pain.*

**Mejoralito** *SmithKline Beecham, Mex.*
Paracetamol (p.76·2).
*Fever; pain; post-vaccination reactions.*

**Mejorultra** *SmithKline Beecham, Mex.†.*
Ibuprofen (p.45·3).

**Mekan** *Biomedica-Chemica, Gr.*
Propylene glycol cefatrizine (p.170·3).
*Bacterial infections.*

**Mel de Jatahy** *Legrand, Braz.†.*
Sulfogaiacol (p.1131·1); sodium benzoate (p.1169·3); senega (p.1130·2); tolu balsam (p.1131·3); honey (p.1434·2); hymenaea courbarie.
*Respiratory-tract congestion.*

**Melablock** *Forder, Arg.*
Octinoxate (p.1154·3); zinc oxide (p.1163·2).
*Sunscreen.*

**Melabon**
*Provita, Austria.*
Paracetamol (p.76·2); propyphenazone (p.85·3); caffeine citrate (p.782·1).
*Fever; pain.*

*Lacer, Spain.*
Paracetamol (p.76·2); propyphenazone (p.85·3); caffeine (p.782·1).
*Fever; pain.*

**Melabon Infantil** *Lacer, Spain.*
Paracetamol (p.76·2).
*Fever; pain.*

**Melabon K** *Oramon, Ger.†.*
Aspirin (p.15·1); paracetamol (p.76·2); caffeine (p.782·1).
*Fever; pain.*

**Melabon N** *Adroka, Switz.*
Aspirin (p.15·1); paracetamol (p.76·2); caffeine (p.782·1).
*Pain.*

**Melabon plus C** *Oramon, Ger.†.*
Aspirin (p.15·1); ascorbic acid.
*Cold symptoms; fever; pain.*

**Melac** *Collins, Mex.*
Multivitamins with folic acid (p.1417·1).

**Melacine** *Schering, Canad.*
Melanoma theraccine.
*Malignant melanoma.*

**Melacler** *Forder, Arg.*
Hydroquinone (p.1148·1); glycolic acid (p.1147·3).
*Skin lightener.*

**Melactone** *Clonmel, Irl.†.*
Spironolactone (p.1003·1).
*Heart failure; hepatic cirrhosis; hypertension; idiopathic oedema; nephrotic syndrome.*

**Meladinina** *Chinoin, Mex.*
Methoxsalen (p.1152·1).
*Psoriasis; vitiligo.*

**Meladinine**
*Chiesi, Fr.; Galderma, Ger.; Promedica, Malaysia; Galderma, Neth.; Galderma, Switz.; Promedica, Thai.*
Methoxsalen (p.1152·1).
*Mycosis fungoides; psoriasis; vitiligo.*

**Melagel** *Giscard, Arg.*
Ascorbic acid (p.1460·2); placenta extract.
*Skin disorders.*

**Melagesic PM** *Ascher, USA.*
Paracetamol (p.76·2); melatonin (p.1710·2).
*Pain; sleep disorders.*

**Melagriao** *Catarinense, Braz.†.*
Nasturtium officinale; aconite (p.1646·3); mikania glomerata; ipecacuanha (p.1122·3); senega (p.1130·2); tolu balsam (p.1131·3); honey (p.1434·2).
*Respiratory-tract congestion.*

**Melanasa** *Vinas, Spain.*
Hydroquinone (p.1148·1).
*Skin hyperpigmentation.*

**Melanex**
*Note. This name is used for preparations of different composition.*
*Cilag, Mex.; Paraphar, Singapore†; Neutrogena, USA†.*
Hydroquinone (p.1148·1).
*Skin hyperpigmentation.*

*Boehringer Mannheim, S.Afr.†.*
Raubasine (p.994·3).
*Vascular disorders.*

**Melanex Duo** *Paraphar, Fr.†; Sofex, Port.†.*
Hydroquinone (p.1148·1); alpha hydroxy acids.
*Skin hyperpigmentation.*

**Melanocyl** *Franco-Indian, India.*
*Ointment:* Methoxsalen (p.1152·1); aminobenzoic acid (p.1142·2).
*Psoriasis.*
*Tablets; solution:* Methoxsalen (p.1152·1).
*Psoriasis; skin depigmentation.*

**Melanox** *Surya, Singapore†.*
Hydroquinone (p.1148·1).
*Skin hyperpigmentation.*

**Melaoline** *Unipharma, Gr.*
Methoxsalen (p.1152·1).
*Atopic dermatitis; psoriasis; vitiligo.*

**Melaprugna** *Lampugnani, Ital.†.*
Dietary fibre supplement (p.1253·2).

**Melapure** *Genzyme, Hong Kong.*
Melatonin (p.1710·2).
*Insomnia associated with melatonin deficiency; jet lag.*

**Melasmax** *Dominguez, Arg.*
Hydroquinone (p.1148·1); tretinoin (p.1161·1); dexamethasone phosphate (p.1097·2).
*Skin hyperpigmentation.*

**Melasoft** *Forder, Arg.*
Kojic acid (p.1151·2); arbutin.
*Skin lightener.*

**Melatol** *Elisium, Arg.*
Melatonin (p.1710·2).
*Sleep disorders.*

**Melatouch** *Forder, Arg.*
Saxifraga sarmentosa; aminoethylphosphinic acid.
*Skin lightener.*

**Melavir** *Australian Bodycare, UK.*
Melaleuca oil (p.1710·2).
*Herpes labialis.*

**Melaxose** *Boehringer Ingelheim, Fr.*
Lactulose (p.1269·1); liquid paraffin (p.1479·1).
*Constipation.*

**Melbetese** *Clonmel, Irl.†.*
Glibenclamide (p.331·2).
*Diabetes mellitus.*

**Melbin**
*Sumitomo, Hong Kong; Sumitomo, Jpn.*
Metformin hydrochloride (p.342·3).
*Diabetes mellitus.*

**Mel-C** *Fresenius Kabi, Austria.*
Sodium ascorbate (p.1460·2).
*Vitamin C deficiency.*

**Meldopa** *Clonmel, Irl.*
Methyldopa (p.953·2).
*Hypertension.*

**Meleril**
*Novartis, Arg.; Novartis, Chile; Novartis, Spain.*
Thioridazine (p.724·2) or thioridazine hydrochloride (p.724·2).
*Anxiety; behaviour disorders; mixed anxiety depressive states; psychoses; sleep disorders.*

**Melfen** *Clonmel, Irl.*
Ibuprofen (p.45·3).
*Musculoskeletal, joint, and peri-articular disorders; pain.*

**Melfiat** *Numark, USA.*
Phendimetrazine tartrate (p.1592·1).
*Obesity.*

**Melgar** *Hexa-Medinova, Arg.*
Naproxen (p.65·1).
*Gout; musculoskeletal and joint disorders; pain.*

**Melgisorb**
*SSL, Austral.*
Calcium alginate (p.745·1).
*Wounds.*

*Molnlycke, Fr.*
Calcium alginate (p.745·1); carmellose (p.1577·3).
*Exudative wounds.*

**Mel-H**
*Fresenius Kabi, Austria; Nycomed, Thai.*
Multivitamin and amino-acid preparation (p.1417·1).

**Melhoral**
*DM, Braz.; GlaxoSmithKline Consumer, Port.*
Aspirin (p.15·1); caffeine (p.782·1).
*Fever; pain.*

**Melhoral C** *DM, Braz.*
Aspirin (p.15·1); ascorbic acid (p.1460·2).
*Fever; pain.*

**Melhoral Infantil**
*SmithKline Beecham, Braz.†; GlaxoSmithKline Consumer, Port.*
Aspirin (p.15·1).
*Fever; pain.*

**Meli Rephastasan** *Repha, Ger.*
Melilotus officinalis.
*Haemorrhoids; thrombophlebitis; venous insufficiency.*

**Meliane**
*Schering, Austria; Schering, Belg.; Schering, Fin.; Schering, Fr.; Shepa, Gr.; Schering, Hong Kong; Schering, Israel; Schering, Malaysia; Schering, Neth.; Schering, Singapore; Schering, Spain; Schering, Thai.*
Gestodene (p.1556·1); ethinylestradiol (p.1553·2).
*Combined oral contraceptive; menstrual disorders.*

**Melic** *Pharmasant, Thai.*
Methandienone (p.1559·3).
*Osteoporosis.*

**Melicat** *Coup, Gr.*
Nimesulide (p.67·1).
*Inflammation; musculoskeletal disorders; pain.*

**Melicron**
*Xepa-Soul Pattinson, Malaysia; Xepa-Soul Pattinson, Singapore.*
Gliclazide (p.332·1).
*Diabetes mellitus.*

**Melipass** *Knop, Chile.*
Melissa (p.1711·1); passiflora coerulea.
*Anxiety; gastrointestinal disorders; sedative.*

**Melipramine** *Boucher & Muir, Austral.*
Imipramine hydrochloride (p.300·1).
*Depression.*

**Meliseptol** *Braun, Ger.*
Propyl alcohol (p.1191·2); glyoxal (p.1181·1).
*Surface disinfection.*

**Meliseptol Rapid** *Braun, Ger.*
Propyl alcohol (p.1191·2); didecyldimethylammonium chloride (p.1178·3).
*Surface disinfection.*

**Melisol** *Max Ritter, Switz.†.*
Soya oil (p.1447·2); liquid paraffin (p.1479·1).
*Dry skin.*

**Melissa Comp.** *Weleda, UK.*
Angelica root (p.1655·1); cinnamon (p.1672·2); melissa leaf (p.1711·1); nutmeg (p.1722·2); lemon oil (p.1706·2); coriander (p.1676·1); clove (p.1673·2).
*Diarrhoea; dyspepsia; nausea; stomach pain.*

**Melissa (Specie Composta)** *Dynacren, Ital.*
Valerian (p.1762·2); melissa (p.1711·1); lupulus (p.1708·1); peppermint leaf (p.1283·2).

**Melissa Tonic** *Geistlich, Switz.†.*
Melissa (p.1711·1); monarda; rosemary (p.1740·2); red-poppy petal (p.1058·1); hibiscus; valerian (p.1762·2); passion flower (p.1729·1).
*Agitation; nervousness; sleep disorders.*

**Melissengeist**
*Note. This name is used for preparations of different composition.*
*Pharmonta, Austria.*
Nutmeg oil (p.1722·3); clove oil (p.1673·3); cinnamon oil (p.1672·2); citronella oil (p.1673·2).
*Digestive disorders; nausea; sleep disorders.*

*Hofmann & Sommer, Ger.*
Melissa (p.1711·1); sage (p.1741·2); rosemary (p.1740·2); thyme (p.1755·2); angelica (p.1655·1); nutmeg (p.1722·2); cinnamon (p.1672·2); clove (p.1673·2); lemon oil (p.1706·2); menthol (p.1711·3); citronella oil (p.1673·2); clove oil (p.1673·3); cinnamon oil (p.1672·2).
*Gastrointestinal disorders; headache; neuralgia.*

**Melissin** *Surf Ski International, UK†.*
Guaifenesin (p.1122·1); menthol (p.1711·3); glycerol (p.1694·3); melissa (p.1711·1); benzoic acid (p.1169·3); citric acid (p.1673·1).
*Colds; coughs.*

**Melitase** *Tecnofarma, Chile.*
Levodopa (p.1205·2); benserazide (p.1200·2).
*Parkinsonism.*

**Melitrast** *Kohler, Ger.*
Iosarcol.
*Radiographic contrast medium.*

**Melival** *Hofmann & Sommer, Ger.†.*
Valerian (p.1762·2).
*Agitation; sleep disorders.*

**Melix**
*Lagap, Hong Kong†; Lagap, Switz.*
Glibenclamide (p.331·2).
*Diabetes mellitus.*

**Melizid** *Leiras, Fin.*
Glipizide (p.332·2).
*Diabetes mellitus.*

**Melizide**
*Alphapharm, Austral.; Alphapharm, Malaysia; Merck, Malaysia; Alphapharm, Singapore; Merck, Singapore; Merck, Thai.*
Glipizide (p.332·2).
*Diabetes mellitus.*

**Mellaril**
*Novartis, Canad.†; Novartis, USA.*
Thioridazine (p.724·2) or thioridazine hydrochloride (p.724·2).
*Behaviour disorders; insomnia; mixed anxiety depressive states; psychoses.*

**Mellerette** *Novartis, Ital.†.*
Thioridazine (p.724·2) or thioridazine hydrochloride (p.724·2).
*Anxiety; behaviour disorders.*

**Melleretten**
*Novartis, Austria†; AWD, Ger.; Sandoz, Ger.†; Novartis, Neth.*
Thioridazine (p.724·2) or thioridazine hydrochloride (p.724·2).
*Behaviour disorders; insomnia; mixed anxiety depressive states; psychoses.*

**Mellerettes** *Novartis, Switz.*
Thioridazine hydrochloride (p.724·2).
*Schizophrenia.*

**Melleril**
*Novartis, Austral.; Novartis, Austria; Novartis, Belg.; Novartis, Braz.; Novartis, Denm.; Novartis, Fin.; Novartis, Fr.; AWD, Ger.; Novartis, Gr.; Novartis, Hong Kong; Novartis, Irl.; Novartis, Israel†; Novartis, Ital.; Novartis, Malaysia; Novartis, Mex.; Novartis, Neth.; Novartis, Norw.; Novartis, NZ; Novartis, Port.; Novartis, S.Afr.; Novartis, Switz.; Novartis, UK.*
Thioridazine (p.724·2) or thioridazine hydrochloride (p.724·2).
*Alcohol withdrawal syndrome; anxiety; behavioural disorders; depression; psychoses.*

**Mellin** *Mellin, Ital.*
Infant feed (p.1417·1).
*Diarrhoea.*

**Mellin AR** *Mellin, Ital.*
Infant feed (p.1417·1).
*Gastro-oesophageal reflux.*

**Mellin HA** *Mellin, Ital.*
Infant feed (p.1417·1).
*Food intolerance.*

**Mellin Polilat** *Mellin, Ital.*
Infant feed (p.1417·1).
*Cow's milk intolerance.*

**Mellitron** *Cilag, Mex.*
Metformin (p.342·3); chlorpropamide (p.330·3).
*Diabetes mellitus.*

**Melneurin** *Hexal, Ger.*
Melperone hydrochloride (p.706·1).
*Alcoholism; anxiety disorders; psychoses.*

**Melocin** *Curasan, Ger.†.*
Mezlocillin sodium (p.231·1).
*Bacterial infections.*

**Mel-OD** *Cadila, India.*
Meloxicam (p.56·1).
*Ankylosing spondylitis; osteoarthritis; rheumatoid arthritis.*

**Meloden**
*Schering, Denm.; Schering, Switz.*
Gestodene (p.1556·1); ethinylestradiol (p.1553·2).
*Combined oral contraceptive.*

**Melodene**
*Schering, NZ; Schering, S.Afr.*
21 Tablets, gestodene (p.1556·1); ethinylestradiol (p.1553·2); 7 tablets, inert.
*Combined oral contraceptive.*

**Melodene 15** *Schering, Spain.*
24 Tablets, gestodene (p.1556·1); ethinylestradiol (p.1553·2); 4 tablets, inert.
*Combined oral contraceptive; menstrual disorders.*

**Melodia** *Schering, Fr.*
24 Tablets, gestodene (p.1556·1); ethinylestradiol (p.1553·2); 4 tablets, inert.
*Combined oral contraceptive.*

**Melodil** *Unipharm, Israel.*
Maprotiline hydrochloride (p.306·1).
*Depression; mixed anxiety depressive states.*

**Melodol** *Raffo, Chile.*
Meloxicam (p.56·1).
*Musculoskeletal, joint, and peri-articular disorders.*

**Meloids** *Boots, Thai.*
Liquorice (p.1270·2); menthol (p.1711·3); cinnamon (p.1672·2); capsicum (p.1667·1).
*Throat disorders.*

**Meloka** *Lacer, Spain.*
Benfotiamine (p.1454·3); caffeine (p.782·1); codeine phosphate (p.27·1); paracetamol (p.76·2); propyphenazone (p.85·3).
*Fever; pain.*

**Melol** *Pharmasant, Thai.*
Metoprolol tartrate (p.957·1).
*Angina pectoris; hypertension; myocardial infarction.*

**Melopat** *Medopharm, Ger.*
Betahistine mesilate (p.1660·1).
*Ménière's syndrome; vestibular disorders.*

**Melosteral** *Silanes, Mex.*
Meloxicam (p.56·1).
*Gout; inflammation; musculoskeletal, joint, and soft-tissue disorders; pain.*

**Melotec** *EMS, Braz.*
Meloxicam (p.56·1).
*Fever; inflammation; pain.*

**Melox Plus** *Aventis, Mex.*
Aluminium hydroxide (p.1249·2); magnesium hydroxide (p.1272·2); dimeticone (p.1289·2).
*Flatulence; gastrointestinal hyperacidity.*

**Meloxat** *Clonmel, Irl.*
Paroxetine mesilate (p.311·2).
*Depression; obsessive-compulsive disorder; panic attacks.*

**Meloxigran** *Legrand, Braz.*
Meloxicam (p.56·1).
*Fever; inflammation; pain.*

**Meloxil** *Ativus, Braz.*
Meloxicam (p.56·1).

**Melpax** *Orion, Fin.*
Melperone hydrochloride (p.706·1).
*Alcohol withdrawal syndrome; anxiety disorders; pain; psychoses.*

**Melpaz** *Profarb, Braz.†.*
Dipyrone (p.35·3); papaverine hydrochloride (p.1728·1).
*Smooth muscle spasm.*

**Melperomerck** *Merck dura, Ger.*
Melperone hydrochloride (p.706·1).
*Alcoholism; anxiety disorders; psychoses.*

**Mel-Puren** *Alpharma-Isis, Ger.*
Melperone hydrochloride (p.706·1).
*Alcoholism; anxiety disorders; psychoses.*

**Melrose** *Roberts & Sheppey, UK.*
Hydrous wool fat (p.1483·2); yellow soft paraffin (p.1479·3); hard paraffin (p.1479·1).
*Emollient.*

**Melrosum** *Aventis, Neth.*
Honey (p.1434·2).
*Coughs.*

**Melrosum Codein Hustensirup** *Nattermann, Ger.*
Codeine phosphate (p.27·1).
*Coughs and catarrh.*

**Melrosum Extra Sterk** *Aventis, Neth.*
Codeine phosphate (p.27·1); vegetable extracts.
*Coughs.*

**Melrosum Hustensirup** *Nattermann, Ger.*
Thyme (p.1755·2).
*Bronchitis; catarrh; cough.*

**Melrosum Hustensirup N** *Rhone-Poulenc Rorer, Ger.†.*
Grindelia (p.1696·1); pimpinella; primula root (p.1735·1); rose petals (p.1058·1); thyme (p.1755·2).
*Catarrh.*

**Melrosum Medizinalbad** *Nattermann, Ger.*
Thyme oil (p.1755·3); oleum pini sylvestris.
*Bath additive; respiratory-tract disorders.*

**Melsept**
*Braun, Ger.; Braun, Ital.*
Formaldehyde (p.1179·3); glutaral (p.1180·3); glyoxal (p.1181·1).
*Surface disinfection.*

**Melsept SF**
*Braun, Ger.; Braun, Ital.*
Glutaral (p.1180·3); glyoxal (p.1181·1); didecyldimethylammonium chloride (p.1178·3).
*Surface disinfection.*

**Melsept Spray** *Braun, Ital.*
Alcohol (p.1166·1); glyoxal (p.1181·1).
*Disinfection of minor wounds and surfaces.*

**Melsitt** *Braun, Ger.*
Formaldehyde (p.1179·3); glutaral (p.1180·3); didecyldimethylammonium chloride (p.1178·3).
*Surface disinfection.*

**Meltonar** *Teva Tuteur, Arg.*
Megestrol (p.1558·3).

**Meltus Baby** *SSL, UK.*
Dilute acetic acid (p.1645·2).
*Coughs.*

**Meltus Decongestant** *Cupal, UK.*
Pseudoephedrine hydrochloride (p.1129·2).
*Catarrh; sinusitis.*

**Meltus Dry Cough** *SSL, UK.*
Dextromethorphan hydrobromide (p.1117·3); pseudoephedrine hydrochloride (p.1129·2).
*Coughs.*

**Meltus Expectorant** *SSL, UK.*
Guaifenesin (p.1122·1); cetylpyridinium chloride (p.1173·1); honey (p.1434·2).
*Coughs.*

**Meltus Expectorant with Decongestant** *SSL, UK.*
Guaifenesin (p.1122·1); pseudoephedrine hydrochloride (p.1129·2).
*Coughs; nasal and sinus congestion.*

**Meltus Honey & Lemon** *SSL, UK.*
Guaifenesin (p.1122·1); honey (p.1434·2); glycerol (p.1694·3); terpeneless lemon oil (p.1706·3).
*Coughs.*

**Meltus Junior Expectorant** *SSL, UK.*
Guaifenesin (p.1122·1); cetylpyridinium chloride (p.1173·1).
*Catarrh; coughs.*

**Meltus Junior Night Time** *SSL, UK.*
Diphenhydramine hydrochloride (p.431·3); sodium citrate (p.1223·2).
*Cold symptoms; coughs.*

**Meltus Night Time** *SSL, UK.*
Diphenhydramine hydrochloride (p.431·3); ammonium chloride (p.1115·2); sodium citrate (p.1223·2).
*Cold symptoms; coughs.*

**Melubrin** *Solus, India.*
Chloroquine phosphate (p.448·2).
*Amoebiasis; lupus erythematosus; malaria; rheumatoid arthritis.*

**Melur** *Medika, Switz.*
Mefenamic acid (p.55·2).
*Fever; pain.*

**Melvit** *Beta, Ital.*
Multivitamin and mineral preparation (p.1417·1).

**Melxi** *Hebron, Braz.*
Pineapple; honey (p.1434·2).
*Respiratory-tract congestion.*

**Melzine** *Clonmel, Irl.*
Thioridazine hydrochloride (p.724·2).
*Agitation; anxiety disorders; childhood behaviour disorders; psychoses; senile confusion; tension.*

**Memac** *Bracco, Ital.*
Donepezil hydrochloride (p.1489·2).
*Alzheimer's disease.*

**Membracel** *Celina, Arg.*
Collagen (p.1674·3).
*Medicated dressing.*

**MembraneBlue** *DORC, Neth.*
Trypan blue (p.1758·3).
*Ophthalmic stain.*

**Memento** *Merck, Arg.*
Pipemidic acid (p.243·1).
*Skin infections; urinary-tract infections.*

**Memento NF** *Merck, Arg.*
Norfloxacin (p.238·3).
*Bacterial infections of the urinary tract.*

**Memfit** *Boehringer Ingelheim, Belg.*
Ginkgo biloba (p.1692·3).
*Mental function disorders.*

**Memoactive** *Farmila, Ital.*
Omega-3 triglycerides (p.976·1); phospholipids (p.1417·1); ginkgo biloba (p.1692·3).
*Mental function disorders.*

**Memocap** *Kotra, Malaysia.*
Ginkgo biloba (p.1692·3).
*Peripheral circulatory disorders.*

**Memoloba** *Goldshield, Singapore.*
Ginkgo biloba (p.1692·3); vitamin C (p.1460·2); iron (p.1434·3); phosphatidyl choline (p.1731·1).
*Maintenance of mental function.*

**Memonol** *Utopian, Thai.*
Pyritinol hydrochloride (p.1737·2).
*Mental function disorders.*

**Memo-Puren** *Alpharma-Isis, Ger.*
Piracetam (p.1732·1).
*Mental function disorders.*

**Memoq** *Parke, Davis, Ger.*†.
Nicergoline (p.1719·3).
*Mental function disorders.*

**Memorandum** *Lampugnani, Ital.*
Ginkgo biloba (p.1692·3); guarana (p.1765·3); levocarnitine (p.1423·3).
*Mental function disorders.*

**Memorex** *Provita, Ital.*†.
Amino-acid preparation with vitamins and minerals (p.1417·1).
*Mental function disorders.*

**Memorex Compuesto** *Montpellier, Arg.*
Vitamin B substances; amino acids (p.1417·1).
*Tonic.*

**Memorfix** *Heralds, Braz.*†.
Vitamin B substances, amino acids, and minerals (p.1417·1).

**Memoria** *Bittner, Austria.*
Homoeopathic preparation.

**Memoril** *Recordati, Ital.*
Glutamine (p.1433·2).
*Mental function impairment.*

**Memorino** *Vita, Spain*†.
Piracetam (p.1732·1); pyritinol hydrochloride (p.1737·2).
*Cerebrovascular disorders; mental function impairment.*

**Memorioglutan** *Bunker, Braz.*
Multivitamin, mineral, and amino-acid preparation (p.1417·1).

**Memoriol B6** *Baldacci, Braz.*
Glutamine; calcium glutamate; ditetraethylammonium phosphate; pyridoxine hydrochloride (p.1417·1).
*Nutritional supplement.*

**Memorisan** *Loprofar, Braz.*
Phosphoric acid; saw palmetto; turnera aphrodisiaca; calcium phosphate; selenium (p.1417·1).
*Tonic.*

**Memorit** *Unipharm, Israel.*
Donepezil.
*Alzheimer's disease.*

**Memory Booster** *Natural Life, Arg.*
Glutamine; ribonucleic acid; phenylalanine; choline; kola; lecithin (p.1417·1).
*Tonic.*

**Memory Plus** *Life Essence, UK.*
Becopa.
*Memory impairment.*

**Memoserina S** *Aventis, Ital.*†.
DL-Phosphoserine; glutamine (p.1433·2); cyanocobalamin (p.1458·2); protein hydrolysate (p.1417·1).
*Tonic.*

**Memosprint** *Monsanto, Ital.*
Pyridoxine phosphoserinate (p.1457·2).
*Mental function impairment; tonic.*

**Memovigor** *Euro-Pharma, Ital.*
Multivitamin and mineral preparation with phospholipids, acetylcarnitine, myrtillus, and ginkgo biloba (p.1417·1).
*Mental function disorders.*

**Memovisus** *Carlo Erba OTC, Ital.*
Myrtillus (p.1718·3); cobamamide (p.1459·1); DL-phosphoserine; aceglutamide (p.1645·2).
*Tonic.*

**Memovit B12** *Magis, Ital.*
Glutamine (p.1433·2); DL-phosphoserine; cyanocobalamin (p.1458·2).
*Tonic.*

**Mempil** *General Drugs, Thai.*
Piracetam (p.1732·1).
Formerly known as Memphil.
*Cerebrovascular disorders; mental function disorders.*

**Memzotil** *Pharmasant, Thai.*
Tenoxicam (p.93·1).
*Musculoskeletal and joint disorders.*

**Men Hormone** *TP, Thai.*
Methyltestosterone (p.1559·3); vitamin E (p.1464·3).
*Hypogonadism.*

**Menabil Complex** *Menarini, Spain.*
Cynara (p.1678·3); boldine (p.1661·2); cyclobutyrol (p.1678·2); methionine phenylbutyrate; rhubarb (p.1287·3); bile salts (p.1660·3); fenipentol sodium hemisuccinate (p.1687·2); belladonna (p.479·1); cascara (p.1255·1).
*Constipation; hepatobiliary disorders.*

**Menabol** *CFL, India.*
Stanozolol (p.1569·2).
*Anabolic; aplastic anaemia; osteoporosis.*

**Menaderm** *Menarini, Ital.*
Beclometasone dipropionate (p.1091·1); neomycin sulfate (p.235·1).
*Infected skin disorders.*

**Menaderm Clio** *Menarini, Spain.*
Beclometasone dipropionate (p.1091·1); clioquinol (p.196·3).
*Infected skin disorders.*

**Menaderm Neomicina** *Menarini, Spain.*
Beclometasone dipropionate (p.1091·1); neomycin sulfate (p.235·1).
*Infected skin disorders.*

**Menaderm Otologico** *Menarini, Spain.*
Beclometasone dipropionate (p.1091·1); clioquinol (p.196·3).
*External ear disorders.*

**Menaderm Simple**
*Menarini, Arg.; Menarini, Spain.*
Beclometasone dipropionate (p.1091·1).
*Skin disorders.*

**Menaderm Simplex** *Menarini, Ital.*
Beclometasone dipropionate (p.1091·1).
*Skin disorders.*

**Menadol** *Rugby, USA.*
Ibuprofen (p.45·3).

**Menalation** *McGloin, Austral.*†.
Menthol (p.1711·3); pumilio pine oil (p.1737·1).
*Cold symptoms.*

**Menalcol** *Orravan, Spain.*
Alcohol (p.1166·1); chlorhexidine gluconate (p.1173·2).
*Skin and wound disinfection.*

**Menalgil B6** *Menarini, Spain.*
Cyanocobalamin (p.1458·2); thiamine hydrochloride (p.1455·1) pyridoxine hydrochloride (p.1456·3).
Lidocaine (p.1377·3) is included in the injection to alleviate the pain of injection.
Formerly contained cyanocobalamin, di-isopropylammonium dichloroacetate, monophosphothiamine, and pyridoxine hydrochloride.
*Vitamin B deficiency.*

**Menalgon** *Fidia, Ital.*†.
Monophosphothiamine (p.1455·2); cyanocobalamin (p.1458·2).
*Neuritis.*

**Menalgon B6** *Fidia, Ital.*†.
Monophosphothiamine (p.1455·2); pyridoxine hydrochloride (p.1456·3); cyanocobalamin (p.1458·2).
*Nerve and muscle pain and inflammation.*

**Menalmina** *Orravan, Spain.*
Chlorhexidine gluconate (p.1173·2).
*Skin and wound disinfection.*

**Menamin** *PP Lab, Thai.*
Prosultiamine (p.1455·1).
*Beri-beri; thiamine deficiency.*

**Menarini-Metforal** *EciFarma, Chile.*
Metformin (p.342·3).
*Diabetes mellitus.*

**Menaven** *Menarini, Spain.*
Heparin sodium (p.928·1).
*Peripheral vascular disorders.*

**Mencalisvit** *Menarini, Spain.*
Calcium lactate (p.1225·3); colecalciferol (p.1461·3).
*Vitamin D and calcium deficiency.*

**Mencevax** *GlaxoSmithKline, S.Afr.*
A meningococcal vaccine (p.1626·1).
*Active immunisation.*

**Mencevax AC**
*SmithKline Beecham, Israel; GlaxoSmithKline, Norw.; SmithKline Beecham, Singapore*†*; GlaxoSmithKline, Spain.*
A meningococcal vaccine (groups A and C) (p.1626·1).
*Active immunisation.*

**Mencevax ACWY**
*GlaxoSmithKline, Austral.; GlaxoSmithKline, Austria; GlaxoSmithKline, Belg.; GlaxoSmithKline, Fin.; GlaxoSmithKline, Ger.; GlaxoSmithKline, Hong Kong; GlaxoSmithKline, Ital.; GlaxoSmithKline, NZ; GlaxoSmithKline, Singapore.*
A meningococcal vaccine (groups A, C, W$_{135}$, and Y) (p.1626·1).
*Active immunisation.*

**Mencirax** *Ativus, Braz.*
Cimicifuga (p.1671·3).
*Menopausal disorders; menstrual disorders.*

**Mencogrin** *Defuen, Arg.*
*Cream:* Coal tar (p.1159·2); allantoin (p.1141·3); betamethasone valerate (p.1093·2).
*Skin and scalp disorders.*
*Shampoo:* Salicylic acid (p.1157·1); climbazole (p.396·2) coconut fatty acids; allantoin (p.1141·3).
*Scalp disorders.*
*Topical gel:* Salicylic acid (p.1157·1); allantoin (p.1141·3).
*Skin disorders.*
*Topical solution:* Coal tar (p.1159·2); salicylic acid (p.1157·1); betamethasone valerate (p.1093·2).
*Skin and scalp disorders.*

**Mencogrin AP** *Defuen, Arg.*
Coal tar (p.1159·2); salicylic acid (p.1157·1); cade oil (p.1159·2); allantoin (p.1141·3).
*Scalp disorders.*

**Menegradil** *Fada, Arg.*
Etilefrine (p.914·1).
*Hypotension.*

**Meneparol** *Menarini, Spain*†.
Amino acids (p.1417·1); cyanocobalamin (p.1458·2); liver extract.
*Liver disorders.*

**Menest**
*Raffo, Arg.; Monarch, USA.*
Esterified oestrogens (p.1549·3).
*Breast cancer; female castration; female hypogonadism; menopausal vasomotor symptoms; primary ovarian failure; prostatic cancer; vulval and vaginal atrophy.*

**Menfazona** *Menarini, Spain*†.
Nefazodone hydrochloride (p.309·2).
*Depression.*

**Mengivac (A+C)**
*Aventis, Irl.; Aventis Pasteur, UK*†.
A meningococcal vaccine (groups A and C) (p.1626·1).
*Active immunisation.*

**Meni-D** *Seatrace, USA.*
Meclozine hydrochloride (p.436·3).
*Motion sickness; vertigo.*

**Meniero** *Jean-Marie, Hong Kong.*
Betahistine hydrochloride (p.1660·1).
*Menière's disease.*

**Meniex** *Fortbenton, Arg.*
Betahistine hydrochloride (p.1660·1).
*Ménière's disease.*

**Meningitec**
*Wyeth, Arg.; Wyeth, Austral.; Wyeth Lederle, Belg.; Wyeth Lederle, Fr.; Wyeth, Ger.; Wyeth, Gr.; Wyeth, Irl.; Wyeth Lederle, Ital.; Wyeth Lederle, Port.; Wyeth, Spain; Lederle, Switz.; Wyeth, UK.*
A meningococcal C conjugate vaccine (diphtheria CRM$_{197}$ protein conjugate) (p.1626·1).
*Active immunisation.*

**Meningo A+C** *Aventis Pasteur, Braz.*†.
A meningococcal vaccine (groups A and C) (p.1626·1).
*Active immunisation.*

**Meningococcal A+C**
*Aventis Pasteur, Hong Kong; Aventis Pasteur, Thai.*
A meningococcal vaccine (groups A and C) (p.1626·1).
*Active immunisation.*

**Meningokokken-Impfstoff A + C** *Aventis Pasteur, Ger.*
A meningococcal vaccine (groups A and C) (p.1626·1).
*Active immunisation.*

**Meningovax A+C**
*Aventis Pasteur, Belg.; Aventis Pasteur, Denm.; Aventis Pasteur, Fin.; Aventis Pasteur, Neth.; Aventis Pasteur, Norw.; Aventis Pasteur, Swed.*
A meningococcal vaccine (groups A and C) (p.1626·1).
*Active immunisation.*

**Meninvact**
*Aventis Pasteur, Fr.; Aventis Pasteur, Spain.*
A meningococcal C conjugate vaccine (diphtheria CRM$_{197}$ protein conjugate) (p.1626·1).
*Active immunisation.*

**Menisole** *Atlantic, Thai.*
Metronidazole (p.607·2).
*Anaerobic bacterial infections.*

**Menjugate**
*CSL, Austral.; Aventis Pasteur, Belg.; Socopharm, Fr.; Aventis Pasteur, Irl.; Chiron, Irl.; Chiron, Ital.; Esteve, Port.; Esteve, Spain; Chiron, UK.*
A meningococcal C conjugate vaccine (diphtheria CRM$_{197}$ protein conjugate) (p.1626·1).
*Active immunisation.*

**Menobarb** *Milano, Thai.*
Phenobarbital sodium (p.367·3).
*Epilepsy; insomnia; sedative.*

**Menobiol** *Yves Ponroy, Fr.*†.
Multivitamin and mineral preparation with fatty acids (p.1417·1).
*Menopausal disorders.*

**Menocal**
*Welfide, Malaysia; Welfide, Singapore.*
Calcitonin (salmon) (p.768·2).
*Bone pain due to osteolysis; hypercalcaemia; osteoporosis; Paget's disease of bone; pancreatitis.*

**Menoconfort** *Yves Ponroy, Fr.*
Nutritional supplement (p.1417·1).
*Menopausal disorders.*

**Meno-cyl Ho-Len-Complex** *Liebermann, Ger.*
Homoeopathic preparation.

**Menodoron**
*Note. This name is used for preparations of different composition.*
*Weleda, Austria.*
Shepherd's purse (p.1744·1); majorana fructus; achillea (p.1646·2); oak bark (p.1722·3); urtica (p.1762·1).
*Menstrual disorders.*
*Weleda, UK.*
Homoeopathic preparation.

**Menofem**
*Boehringer Ingelheim, Arg.; Boehringer de Angeli, Braz.*†*; Pharmaton, Switz.*†.
Cimicifuga (p.1671·3).
*Menopausal disorders.*

**Menoflavon** *Cedar Health, UK.*
Red clover (p.1737·3).
*Menopausal disorders.*

**Menoflush** *Pharmaceutical Enterprises, S.Afr.*
Ethinylestradiol (p.1553·2); multivitamins (p.1417·1).
*Menopausal disorders.*

**Menoflush + $^1/_4$** *Pharmaceutical Enterprises, S.Afr.*†.
Ethinylestradiol (p.1553·2); multivitamins (p.1417·1); phenobarbital (p.367·3).
Formerly known as Menoflush-Menogloed + $^1/_4$.
*Menopausal disorders.*

**Menogen** *Breckenridge, USA*†.
Esterified oestrogens (p.1549·3); methyltestosterone (p.1559·3).
*Menopausal disorders.*

**Menogon**
*Ferring, Belg.*†*; Ferring, Braz.*†*; Ferring, Denm.; Ferring, Fin.; Ferring, Fr.*†*; Ferring, Ger.; Chemipharma, Gr.; Ferring, Hong Kong; Ferring, Irl.; Ferring, Israel; Ferring, Ital.; Ferring, Neth.; Ferring, Singapore; Ferring, Spain*†*; Ferring, Switz.; Ferring, UK.*
Menotrophin (p.1330·1).
*Male and female infertility.*

**Menograine** *Aspen, S.Afr.*
Clonidine hydrochloride (p.885·2).
*Menopausal flushing; migraine.*

**Meno-Implant**
*Organon, Belg.; Organon, Neth.*
Estradiol (p.1550·1).
*Oestrogen deficiency.*

**Menolistica** *Holistica, Fr.*
Nutritional supplement (p.1417·1).
*Menopausal disorders.*

**Meno-MPA** *Antigen, Israel.*
16 Tablets, estradiol (p.1550·1); 12 tablets, estradiol; medroxyprogesterone acetate (p.1557·2).
*Menopausal disorders; osteoporosis.*

**Menomune**
*Aventis Pasteur, Austral.; Aventis Pasteur, Canad.; Aventis Pasteur, Fr.; Vianex (Βιανέξ), Gr.; Aventis Pasteur, Ital.; Aventis Pasteur, Malaysia; CSL, NZ; Aventis Pasteur, Singapore; Pasteur Merieux, USA.*
A meningococcal vaccine (groups A, C, Y and W-135) (p.1626·1).
*Active immunisation.*

**Menomune ACYW** *Aventis Pasteur, Austria.*
A meningococcal polysaccharide vaccine (groups A, C, W, and Y)(p.1626·1).
*Active immunisation.*

**Meno-Net** *Antigen, Israel.*
16 Tablets, estradiol (p.1550·1); 12 tablets, estradiol; norethisterone (p.1562·2).
*Menopausal disorders; osteoporosis.*

**Menopace**
*Vitabiotics, Hong Kong; Vitabiotics, UK.*
Multivitamin and mineral preparation (p.1417·1).
*Menopausal disorders.*

**Meno-Patch** *Hexal, Israel.*
Estradiol (p.1550·1).
*Menopausal disorders.*

**Menopause** *Homeocan, Canad.*
Homoeopathic preparation.

**Menopause L122** *Homeocan, Canad.*
Homoeopathic preparation.

**Menopause Test** *Electramed, Irl.*
Test for raised FSH in urine.

**Menopax** *Ache, Braz.*
Cyclofenil (p.1544·1).
*Anovulatory infertility.*

**Menophase** *Searle, Irl.*†.
15 Tablets, mestranol (p.1559·2); 13 tablets, mestranol; norethisterone (p.1562·2).
*Menopausal disorders; osteoporosis.*

**Menoplex** *Fiske, USA*†.
Paracetamol (p.76·2); phenyltoloxamine citrate (p.439·1).
*Pain.*

**Menoprem**
*Wyeth, Austral.*
Maroon tablets, conjugated oestrogens (Premarin) (p.1543·2); blue tablets, medroxyprogesterone acetate (Provera) (p.1557·2).
*Menopausal disorders; osteoporosis.*
*Wyeth, NZ.*
28 Tablets, conjugated oestrogens (p.1543·2); 14 tablets, medroxyprogesterone acetate (p.1557·2).
*Menopausal disorders; osteoporosis.*

**Menopur**
*Ferring, Austria; Ferring, Belg.; Ferring, Denm.; Ferring, Fr.; Ferring, Irl.; Ferring, Israel; Ferring, Neth.; Ferring, Spain; Ferring, UK.*
Menotrophin (p.1330·1).
*Male and female infertility.*

**Menorest**
*Novartis, Austral.; Novartis, Austria; Novartis, Braz.; Rhone-Poulenc Rorer, Denm.*†*; Novartis, Fin.; Novartis, Fr.; Novartis, Ger.; Novartis, Gr.; Novartis, Irl.; Zambon, Ital.; Novartis, Neth.; Novartis, Norw.*†*; Novartis, Port.; Novartis, Spain; Novartis, Swed.; Novartis, Switz.; Novartis, UK*†.
Estradiol (p.1550·1).
*Menopausal disorders; osteoporosis.*

**Menoring** *Galen, UK.*
Estradiol acetate (p.1551·1).
*Menopausal disorders.*

**Menosan** *Bioforce, Switz.*
Homoeopathic preparation.

**Menosedan** *Haller, Braz.*
Conjugated oestrogens (p.1543·2).
*Menopausal disorders.*

**Menosedan Ciclo** *Haller, Braz.*
14 Tablets, conjugated oestrogens (p.1543·2); 14 tablets, conjugated oestrogens; medroxyprogesterone acetate (p.1557·2).
*Menopausal disorders.*

**Menosedan Fase** *Haller, Braz.*
Conjugated oestrogens (p.1543·2); medroxyprogesterone acetate (p.1557·2).
*Menopausal disorders.*

**Menosedan MPA** *Haller, Braz.*
Conjugated oestrogens (p.1543·2); medroxyprogesterone acetate (p.1557·2).
*Menopausal disorders.*

**Menoselect** *Dreluso, Ger.†.*
Homoeopathic preparation.

**Menosor** *TP, Thai.*
Mebeverine hydrochloride (p.1273·1).
*Smooth muscle spasm.*

**Menostress** *Dansk-Flama, Braz.†.*
Chlordiazepoxide (p.674·2); conjugated oestrogens (p.1543·2).
*Menopausal disorders.*

**Menotensil** *Sintofarma, Braz.*
Chlordiazepoxide (p.674·2); conjugated oestrogens (p.1543·2).
*Menopausal disorders.*

**Menotime** *Matara, Fr.*
Test for menopause.

**Menovis** *Teofarma, Ital.*
Estradiol benzoate (p.1550·1); progesterone (p.1566·2).
*Menstrual disorders.*

**Menoxicor** *Guidotti, Spain†.*
Cloridarol (p.889·1).
*Ischaemic heart disease.*

**Menpovax 4**
*Chiron Vaccines, Ital.†; Chiron, Thai.†.*
A meningococcal vaccine (groups A, C, W, and Y) (p.1626·1).
*Active immunisation.*

**Menpovax A+C**
*Chiron Vaccines, Ital.†; Chiron, Thai.†.*
A meningococcal vaccine (groups A and C) (p.1626·1).
*Active immunisation.*

**Menpros** *Continental, Spain†.*
Misoprostol (p.1519·2).
*Peptic ulcer.*

**Mensalgin** *Chobet, Arg.*
Ibuprofen (p.45·3); codeine phosphate (p.27·1).
*Pain.*

**Mensana** *Darrow, Braz.*
Ginkgo biloba (p.1692·3).
*Peripheral vascular disorders.*

**Mensifem**
*Boehringer Ingelheim, Chile; Boehringer Ingelheim Promeco, Mex.*
Cimicifuga (p.1671·3).
*Menopausal disorders.*

**Mensiso** *Menarini, Ital.*
Sisomicin sulfate (p.254·3).
*Bacterial infections.*

**Mensoma** *Baldacci, Port.*
Famotidine (p.1265·2).
*Gastric hypersecretion; peptic ulcer.*

**Mensoton** *Berlin-Chemie, Ger.*
Ibuprofen (p.45·3).
*Pain.*

**Menstrogen** *Organon, Arg.*
Estradiol benzoate (p.1550·1); progesterone (p.1566·2).
*Amenorrhoea.*

**Menstruasan** *Bioforce, Switz.*
Homoeopathic preparation.

**Menstrunat** *Soria Natural, Spain.*
Artemisia vulgaris; calendula (p.1665·2); greater celandine (p.1695·3); achillea (p.1646·2); sage (p.1741·2).
*Menstrual disorders.*

**Ment Vital** *Andromaco, Chile.*
Ginkgo biloba (p.1692·3).
*Cerebral and peripheral vascular disorders; cerebral trauma; diabetic retinopathy.*

**Mentacur** *Asche, Ger.*
Peppermint oil (p.1283·2).
*Irritable bowel syndrome.*

**Mental Alertness** *Homeocan, Canad.*
Homoeopathic preparation.

**Mentalgina** *Novartis, Mex.*
Cetylpyridinium chloride (p.1173·1); oxybuprocaine hydrochloride (p.1382·1).
*Mouth and throat disorders.*

**Mentalol** *Neckerman, Braz.†.*
Menthol (p.1711·3); terpineol (p.1752·2); camphor (p.1665·3); cineole (p.1672·1); niaouli oil (p.1719·3); turpentine oil (p.1760·1); lavender oil (p.1705·2); cedar oil.
*Musculoskeletal and joint disorders.*

**Mentamida** *Kin, Spain.*
Benzydamine hydrochloride (p.21·1); hexetidine (p.1182·1).
*Mouth and throat inflammation.*

**Mentania** *Saval, Chile.*
Ginkgo biloba (p.1692·3); ginseng (p.1693·1).
*Mental function impairment.*

**Mentax**
*Allergan-Frumtost, Braz.†; Agis, Israel; Kaken, Jpn; Bertek, USA.*
Butenafine hydrochloride (p.395·2).
*Fungal skin infections.*

**Menthacin** *Mentholatum, USA.*
Capsaicin (p.24·2); menthol (p.1711·3).
*Arthritis.*

**Menthodex** *Bell, UK.*
Ammonium chloride (p.1115·2); sodium citrate (p.1223·2); menthol (p.1711·3).
*Coughs.*

**Mentholatum Balm** *Mentholatum, Israel.*
Menthol (p.1711·3); camphor (p.1665·3); eucalyptus oil (p.1686·2); pumilio pine oil (p.1737·1); methyl salicylate (p.59·3).
*Cold and hay fever symptoms.*

**Mentholatum Cherry Chest Rub** *Mentholatum, USA.*
Camphor (p.1665·3); menthol (p.1711·3); eucalyptus oil (p.1686·2).
*Coughs and cold symptoms.*

**Mentholatum Cherry Ice** *Mentholatum, USA.*
*SPF 11:* Padimate O (p.1155·1); dimethicone (p.1482·1).
*Dry lips; sunscreen.*

**Mentholatum Cough Drops** *Mentholatum, Canad.*
Eucalyptus oil (p.1686·2); menthol (p.1711·3).

**Mentholatum Extra Strength Ointment** *Mentholatum, Canad.†.*
Camphor (p.1665·3); eucalyptus oil (p.1686·2); menthol (p.1711·3).

**Mentholatum Ibuprofen** *Mentholatum, UK.*
Ibuprofen (p.45·3).
*Musculoskeletal, joint, and soft-tissue disorders.*

**Mentholatum Nasal Inhaler**
*Mentholatum, Israel†; Mentholatum, UK†.*
Menthol (p.1711·3); camphor (p.1665·3); methyl salicylate (p.59·3).
*Cold and hay fever symptoms; nasal congestion.*

**Mentholatum Natural Ice** *Mentholatum, USA.*
*SPF 14:* Padimate O (p.1155·1); dimethicone (p.1482·1).
*Dry lips; sunscreen.*

**Mentholatum Natural Ice Lip Protectant**
*Mentholatum, USA.*
Menthol (p.1711·3); camphor (p.1665·3).
*Dry lips.*

**Mentholatum Ointment**
*Note. This name is used for preparations of different composition.*
*Mentholatum, Canad.; Mentholatum, Singapore.*
Camphor (p.1665·3); menthol (p.1711·3).
*Cold symptoms; skin disorders.*

*Mentholatum, USA.*
Camphor (p.1665·3); menthol (p.1711·3); eucalyptus oil (p.1686·2).
*Coughs and cold symptoms.*

**Mentholatum Rub** *Mentholatum, UK.*
Menthol (p.1711·3); camphor (p.1665·3); eucalyptus oil (p.1686·2); pumilio pine oil (p.1737·1); methyl salicylate (p.59·3).
*Catarrh; cold symptoms; hay fever; minor skin disorders; musculoskeletal and joint disorders.*

**Mentholatum Softlips** *Mentholatum, USA.*
Dimethicone (p.1482·1).
*Dry lips.*

**Mentholatum Softlips Lipbalm** *Mentholatum, USA.*
Dimethicone (p.1482·1); padimate O (p.1155·1).
*Dry lips.*

**Mentholatum Softlips Lipbalm (UV)** *Mentholatum, USA.*
Octinoxate (p.1154·3); padimate O (p.1155·1); oxybenzone (p.1154·3); dimethicone (p.1482·1).
*Dry lips; sunscreen.*

**Mentholatum Vapour Rub** *Mentholatum, UK.*
Menthol (p.1711·3); camphor (p.1665·3); methyl salicylate (p.59·3).
*Musculoskeletal, joint, and soft-tissue pain; nasal congestion; skin irritation.*

**Mentholease** *Warner-Lambert, UK†.*
Menthol (p.1711·3); eucalyptus oil (p.1686·2).
*Hay fever.*

**Mentholon Original N** *Schoning-Berlin, Ger.*
Menthol (p.1711·3); camphor (p.1665·3); eucalyptus oil (p.1686·2).
*Catarrh.*

**Menthoneurin**
*Note. This name is used for preparations of different composition.*
*Byk, Austria; Byk, Neth.†.*
*Liniment:* Glycol salicylate (p.44·3); benzyl nicotinate (p.21·2).
*Musculoskeletal, joint, peri-articular, and soft-tissue disorders; neuralgia.*

*Byk, Austria.*
*Ointment:* Glycol salicylate (p.44·3); menthol (p.1711·3).
*Headache; musculoskeletal, joint, peri-articular, and soft-tissue disorders; neuralgia.*

*Byk, Neth.†.*
*Cream:* Glycol salicylate (p.44·3); menthol (p.1711·3).
*Muscle and joint pain.*

**Menthoneurin-Salbe** *Altana, Ger.; Byk Gulden, Ger.*
Glycol salicylate (p.44·3); menthol (p.1711·3).
*Musculoskeletal, joint, peri-articular, and soft-tissue disorders; neuralgia; neuritis.*

**Menthoneurin-Vollbad N** *Tosse, Ger.†.*
Glycol salicylate (p.44·3); benzyl nicotinate (p.21·2); methyl nicotinate (p.59·2).
*Bath additive; musculoskeletal and joint disorders.*

**MenthoRub** *Schein, USA†.*
Menthol (p.1711·3); camphor (p.1665·3).
*Muscle, joint, and soft-tissue pain; neuralgia.*

**Menthose** *Pasteur, Chile.*
Menthol (p.1711·3); camphor (p.1665·3); eucalyptus oil (p.1686·2); pine oil; methyl salicylate (p.59·3).
*Mucous membrane inflammation; musculoskeletal pain; soft-tissue injury.*

**Menthymin mono** *Chauvin ankerpharm, Ger.*
Thyme (p.1755·2).
*Bronchitis; catarrh.*

**Mentis** *Menarini, Spain.*
Pirisudanol maleate (p.1732·3).
*Cerebrovascular impairment; senile dementia.*

**Mentium** *Guidotti, Ital.*
Pirisudanol maleate (p.1732·3).
*Mental function disorders.*

**Mentobox** *Edigen, Spain.*
*Ointment:* Camphor (p.1665·3); Cedrus deodora oil; cineole (p.1672·1); methyl salicylate (p.59·3); thymol (p.1194·2); turpentine; menthol (p.1711·3).
*Tablets†:* Camphor (p.1665·3); tolu balsam (p.1131·3); cineole (p.1672·1); drosera (p.1683·1); thyme (p.1755·2); menthol (p.1711·3); sodium benzoate (p.1169·3).
*Upper respiratory-tract disorders.*

**Mentobox Antitusivo** *Alcala, Spain†.*
Dextromethorphan hydrobromide (p.1117·3); benzocaine (p.1370·3); guaifenesin (p.1122·1); menthol (p.1711·3).
*Respiratory-tract disorders.*

**Mentocaina R** *Azevedos, Port.*
Tyrothricin (p.275·1); benzocaine (p.1370·3).
*Mouth and throat disorders.*

**Mentodrin** *Ibefar, Braz.†.*
Diphenhydramine hydrochloride (p.431·3); neomycin sulfate (p.235·1); naphazoline hydrochloride (p.1124·3).
*Nasal congestion.*

**Mentofenol** *Distrifarma, Port.†.*
Zinc chloride (p.1469·2); menthol (p.1711·3).
*Mouth disorders.*

**Mentolatun** *EMS, Braz.†.*
Menthol (p.1711·3); cineole (p.1672·1); thymol (p.1194·2); terpineol (p.1752·2); chlorophyll (p.1057·1).
*Mouth and throat disorders.*

**Mento-O-Cap** *Rekah, Israel.*
Turpentine oil (p.1760·1); eucalyptus oil (p.1686·2); pine oil; capsicum (p.1667·1); methyl salicylate (p.59·3); menthol (p.1711·3); camphor (p.1665·3).
*Cold symptoms; musculoskeletal and joint disorders.*

**Mentopin**
*Note. This name is used for preparations of different composition.*
*Brady, Austria.*
Lavender flower (p.1705·1); sage (p.1741·2); peppermint leaf (p.1283·2); paprika (p.1667·1); urtica (p.1762·1); pine; camphor (p.1665·3); menthol (p.1711·3); pumilio pine oil (p.1737·1); peppermint oil (p.1283·2).
*Musculoskeletal and joint disorders; neuralgia.*

*Hermes, Ger.†.*
Acetylcysteine (p.1112·3).
*Coughs; respiratory disorders associated with viscid or excessive mucus.*

**Mentopin Echinacea** *Hermes, Ger.†.*
Echinacea purpura (p.1683·2).
*Respiratory- and urinary-tract infections.*

**Mentopin Erkaltungsbalsam** *Hermes, Ger.†.*
Eucalyptus oil (p.1686·2); pine needle oil.
*Cold symptoms.*

**Mentopin Gurgellosung** *Hermes, Ger.†.*
Chlorhexidine gluconate (p.1173·2).
*Inflammation and infection of the mouth and throat.*

**Mentopin Hustenstiller** *Hermes, Ger.†.*
Clobutinol hydrochloride (p.1117·1).
*Catarrh; coughs.*

**Mentopin Nasenspray** *Hermes, Ger.*
Xylometazoline hydrochloride (p.1132·2).
*Nasal congestion; sinusitis.*

**Mentopin Vitamin C + ASS** *Hermes, Ger.†.*
Aspirin (p.15·1); ascorbic acid (p.1460·2).
*Fever; pain.*

**Mentor** *Lifeplan, UK†.*
Ginkgo biloba (p.1692·3).

**Mentoval** *Canonne, Braz.†.*
Benzoic acid (p.1169·3); glycerol (p.1694·3); xylitol (p.1469·1); menthol (p.1711·3).
*Oral hygiene.*

**Mentozil** *Ibefar, Braz.†.*
Tyrothricin (p.275·1); sulfathiazole (p.264·1); chlorophyll (p.1057·1); menthol (p.1711·3); benzocaine (p.1370·3).
*Mouth and throat disorders.*

**Menutil** *Hoechst Marion Roussel, Belg.†.*
Diethylpropion hydrochloride (p.1587·1).
*Obesity.*

**Menzotil** *Pharmasant, Thai.†.*
Tenoxicam (p.93·1).
*Musculoskeletal, joint, and peri-articular disorders.*

**Meocil** *Edol, Port.*
Prednisolone acetate (p.1108·1); neomycin sulfate (p.235·1); sulfacetamide sodium (p.257·3).
*Infected eye disorders.*

**282 Mep** *Lioh, Canad.*
Aspirin (p.15·1); caffeine citrate (p.782·1); codeine phosphate (p.27·1); meprobamate (p.706·2).
*Anxiety; pain; skeletal muscle spasm.*

**Mepagyl** *Nakorn, Thai.*
Metronidazole (p.607·2).
*Amoebiasis; anaerobic bacterial infections; trichomoniasis.*

**Mepalax** *ABC, Ital.*
Boldo (p.1661·2); rhubarb (p.1287·3); cascara (p.1255·1).
*Constipation.*

**Mepastat** *Orion, Fin.*
Medroxyprogesterone acetate (p.1557·2).
*Malignant neoplasms.*

**Mepergan** *Wyeth-Ayerst, USA†.*
Pethidine hydrochloride (p.80·2); promethazine hydrochloride (p.439·1).
*Premedication.*

**Meperol** *Kampel Martian, Arg.*
Pethidine (p.81·3).
*Pain.*

**Mephadolor** *Mepha, Switz.*
Mefenamic acid (p.55·2).
*Fever; pain.*

**Mephamesone** *Mepha, Switz.*
Dexamethasone sodium phosphate (p.1097·2).
*Corticosteroid.*

**Mephanol**
*Mepha, Hong Kong; Mepha, Switz.; Mepha, Thai.†.*
Allopurinol (p.412·2).
*Gout; hyperuricaemia; renal calculi.*

**Mephaquin**
*Mepha, Braz.; Mepha, Hong Kong; Mepha, Israel; Mepha, Malaysia; Mepha, Port.; Mepha, Singapore; Mepha, Thai.*
Mefloquine hydrochloride (p.453·3).
*Malaria.*

**Mephaquine** *Mepha, Switz.*
Mefloquine hydrochloride (p.453·3).
*Malaria.*

**Mephathiol** *Mepha, Switz.*
Carbocisteine (p.1116·2).
*Respiratory-tract disorders associated with increased mucus.*

**Mephatussine** *Mepha, Switz.†.*
Prenoxdiazine hydrochloride (p.1129·1).
*Coughs.*

**Mephatussine Compositum** *Mepha, Switz.†.*
Prenoxdiazine hydrochloride (p.1129·1); guaifenesin (p.1122·1); terpin hydrate (p.1131·1).
*Coughs.*

**Mephaxine** *Mepha, Switz.†.*
Prenoxdiazine hydrochloride (p.1129·1) or prenoxdiazine hibenzate (p.1129·1).
*Coughs.*

**Mephaxine Compositum** *Mepha, Switz.†.*
Prenoxdiazine hydrochloride (p.1129·1); guaifenesin (p.1122·1); terpin hydrate (p.1131·1).
*Coughs.*

**Mephentine** *Wyeth, India.*
Mephentermine sulfate (p.952·1).
*Hypotension; shock.*

**Mephyton** *Merck, USA.*
Phytomenadione (p.1467·1).
*Coagulation disorders due to faulty formation of factors II, VII, IX, and X.*

**Mepibil** *Biologici Italia, Ital.*
Mepivacaine hydrochloride (p.1381·2).
*Local anaesthesia.*

**Mepicain** *Monico, Ital.*
Mepivacaine hydrochloride (p.1381·2).
Adrenaline acid tartrate (p.852·2) is included in some injections as a vasoconstrictor to diminish absorption and localise the effect of the local anaesthetic.
*Local anaesthesia.*

**Mepicaton**
*Weimer, Ger.†; Weimer, Switz.†; Weimer, Thai.*
Mepivacaine hydrochloride (p.1381·2).
*Local anaesthesia.*

**Mepident** *Warner-Lambert, Ital.*
Mepivacaine hydrochloride (p.1381·2).
Adrenaline acid tartrate (p.852·2) is included in some injections as a vasoconstrictor to diminish absorption and localise the effect of the local anaesthetic.
*Local anaesthesia in dentistry.*

**Mepiforan** *Baxter, Ital.*
Mepivacaine hydrochloride (p.1381·2).
Adrenaline acid tartrate (p.852·2) is included in some injections as a vasoconstrictor to diminish absorption and localise the effect of the local anaesthetic.
*Local anaesthesia.*

**Mepiform** *Molnlycke, Ital.*
Silicone (p.1482·1).
*Hypertrophic and keloid scars.*

**Mepihexal** *Hexal, Ger.*
Mepivacaine hydrochloride (p.1381·2).
*Local anaesthesia.*

**Mepi-Mynol** *Molteni, Ital.†.*
Mepivacaine hydrochloride (p.1381·2).
Adrenaline acid tartrate (p.852·2) is included in some injections as a vasoconstrictor to diminish absorption and localise the effect of the local anaesthetic.
*Local anaesthesia.*

**Mepinaest** *Gebro, Austria.*
Mepivacaine hydrochloride (p.1381·2).
*Local anaesthesia.*

**Mepisolver** *Solver, Ital.*
Mepivacaine hydrochloride (p.1381·2).
Adrenaline acid tartrate (p.852·2) is included in some injections as a vasoconstrictor to diminish absorption and localise the effect of the local anaesthetic.
*Local anaesthesia.*

**Mepitel** *Molnlycke, Ital.*
Silicone (p.1482·1).
*Wounds.*

**Mepivamol** *Molteni, Ital.*
Mepivacaine hydrochloride (p.1381·2).

Adrenaline acid tartrate (p.852·2) is included in some injections as a vasoconstrictor to diminish absorption and localise the effect of the local anaesthetic.
*Local anaesthetic.*

**Mepivastesin** *Espe, Ger.; 3M, Hong Kong.*
Mepivacaine hydrochloride (p.1381·2).
*Local anaesthesia.*

**Mepivirgi** *Keryos, Ital.*
Mepivacaine hydrochloride (p.1381·2).
*Local anaesthetic.*

**Mepotin** *Mepha, Braz.*
Epoetin (p.747·1).
*Anaemias.*

**Mepral** *Bracco, Ital.*
Omeprazole (p.1278·2) or omeprazole sodium (p.1278·2).
*Gastro-oesophageal reflux; peptic ulcer; Zollinger-Ellison syndrome.*

**Meprate**
*Note. This name is used for preparations of different composition.*
*Serum Institute, India.*
Medroxyprogesterone acetate (p.1557·2).
*Endometriosis; menstrual disorders.*

*DDSA Pharmaceuticals, UK†.*
Meprobamate (p.706·2).

**Mepraz** *Baldacci, Port.*
Omeprazole (p.1278·2).
*Gastro-oesophageal reflux; peptic ulcer; Zollinger-Ellison syndrome.*

**Meprazan** *Cazi, Braz.*
Omeprazole (p.1278·2).
*Peptic ulcer.*

**Mepril** *Kwizda, Austria.*
Enalapril maleate (p.909·2).
*Heart failure; hypertension.*

**Meprizina** *Pisa, Mex.*
Ampicillin (p.157·1).
*Bacterial infections.*

**Mepro** *Rekah, Israel.*
Meprobamate (p.706·2).
*Anxiety; insomnia.*

**Meprodil** *Streuli, Switz.*
Meprobamate (p.706·2).
*Anxiety; muscle relaxant; sedative.*

**Meprofen** *AGIPS, Ital.*
Ketoprofen (p.51·2).
*Musculoskeletal, joint, peri-articular, and soft-tissue disorders.*

**Meprogesic** *Propan, S.Afr.*
Paracetamol (p.76·2); codeine phosphate (p.27·1); meprobamate (p.706·2).
*Pain and associated tension.*

**Meprogest** *Infosint, Ital.*
Megestrol acetate (p.1558·2).
*Breast cancer; endometrial cancer.*

**Meprolol** *TAD, Ger.*
Metoprolol tartrate (p.957·1).
*Arrhythmias; hypertension; ischaemic heart disease; migraine; myocardial infarction.*

**Meprolol Comp** *TAD, Ger.*
Metoprolol tartrate (p.957·1); hydrochlorothiazide (p.933·2).
*Hypertension.*

**Mepromol** *Rolab, S.Afr.*
*Syrup:* Paracetamol (p.76·2); codeine phosphate (p.27·1); promethazine hydrochloride (p.439·1).
*Fever; pain.*
*Tablets:* Paracetamol (p.76·2); codeine phosphate (p.27·1); caffeine (p.782·1); meprobamate (p.706·2).
*Pain and associated tension.*

**Mepron**
*GlaxoSmithKline, Canad.; Glaxo Wellcome, USA.*
Atovaquone (p.601·3).
*Pneumocystis carinii pneumonia.*

**Mepronet** *Nettopharma, Denm.*
Metoprolol tartrate (p.957·1).
*Angina pectoris; arrhythmias; hypertension; hyperthyroidism; migraine; myocardial infarction.*

**Mepronizine** *Sanofi Synthelabo, Fr.*
Meprobamate (p.706·2); aceprometazine maleate (p.668·3).
*Insomnia.*

**Meprosona-F** *Sons, Mex.*
Prednisone (p.1109·3).
*Corticosteroid.*

**Meptid**
*Riemser, Ger.; Shire, Irl.; Monmouth, UK.*
Meptazinol (p.57·2) or meptazinol hydrochloride (p.56·3).
*Pain.*

**Meptidol** *Wyeth Lederle, Austria.*
Meptazinol hydrochloride (p.56·3).
*Pain.*

**Meptin**
*Otsuka, Hong Kong; Otsuka, Jpn; Otsuka, Malaysia; Otsuka, Singapore; Otsuka, Thai.*
Procaterol hydrochloride (p.791·1).
*Obstructive airways disease.*

**Mepyl** *Molteni, Ital.†.*
Mepivacaine hydrochloride (p.1381·2).
Adrenaline acid tartrate (p.852·2) is included in this preparation as a vasoconstrictor to diminish absorption and localise the effect of the local anaesthetic.
*Local anaesthesia.*

**Mepyraderm** *Be-Tabs, S.Afr.*
Mepyramine maleate (p.437·1).
*Allergic and pruritic skin disorders.*

**Mepyrimal** *Propan, S.Afr.*
Mepyramine maleate (p.437·1).
*Hypersensitivity reactions.*

**Mequin** *Atlantic, Thai.*
Mefloquine hydrochloride (p.453·3).
*Malaria.*

**Meracilina** *Asta Medica, Braz.*
Phenoxymethylpenicillin potassium (p.242·1).
*Bacterial infections.*

**Meracote** *Sigma, Austral.*
Alginic acid (p.1576·3); aluminium hydroxide (p.1249·2); magnesium trisilicate (p.1272·3); sodium bicarbonate (p.1223·2).
*Gastric reflux; heartburn.*

**Meralop**
*Thea, Ital.; Thea, Spain.*
Keracyanin (p.1703·2).
*Disorders of vision.*

**Meralops** *Thea, Fr.†.*
Keracyanin (p.1703·2).
*Visual impairment.*

**Meramide** *Hua, Thai.*
Metoclopramide hydrochloride (p.1274·3).
*Gastrointestinal motility disorders; nausea and vomiting; peptic ulcer.*

**Merankol Pastiglie** *Bruno, Ital.*
Dicycloverine hydrochloride (p.481·2); methylcellulose; sodium laurilsulfate; magnesium hydroxide (p.1272·2); dried aluminium hydroxide (p.1249·2); magnesium trisilicate (p.1272·3).
*Gastrointestinal disorders.*

**Merapiran** *Finadiet, Arg.*
Meloxicam (p.56·1).
*Inflammation; musculoskeletal and joint disorders.*

**Merapril** *CT, Ital.*
Captopril (p.879·2).
*Diabetic nephropathy; heart failure; hypertension; myocardial infarction.*

**Merasyn** *Adcock Ingram, S.Afr.*
Aluminium hydroxide gel (p.1249·2); magnesium hydroxide (p.1272·2); simeticone (p.1289·2); methylcellulose (p.1580·2).
*Flatulence; hyperchlorhydria.*

**Merbenloc** *Maigal, Arg.*
Sulfur (p.1158·2).
*Acne; seborrhoea.*

**Merbentyl**
*Sigma, Austral.; Aventis, Irl.; Sigma, NZ; Adcock Ingram, S.Afr.; Florizel, UK.*
Dicycloverine hydrochloride (p.481·2).
*Gastrointestinal spasm; irritable bowel syndrome.*

**Mercalm** *Pfizer Sante, Fr.*
Caffeine (p.782·1); dimenhydrinate (p.431·1).
*Motion sickness.*

**Mercap** *Medac, Ger.†.*
Mercaptopurine (p.567·2).
*Acute lymphatic leukaemia; non-Hodgkin's lymphoma.*

**Mercaptina** *Zambon, Braz.†.*
Mercaptopurine (p.567·2).
*Inflammatory bowel disease; leukaemias; non-Hodgkin's lymphomas; polycythaemia vera; psoriatic arthritis.*

**Mercaptizol** *Taro, Israel.*
Thiamazole (p.1603·3).
*Hyperthyroidism; toxic adenoma.*

**Mercaptyl** *Knoll, Switz.*
Penicillamine (p.1046·3).
*Biliary cirrhosis; cystinuria; heavy-metal poisoning; hepatitis; pulmonary fibrosis; rheumatoid arthritis; scleroderma.*

**Merced** *Menarini, Belg.*
Midecamycin acetate (p.231·3).
*Bacterial infections.*

**Mercilon**
*Organon, Arg.; Organon, Austria; Organon, Belg.; Organon, Braz.; Organon, Denm.; Organon, Fin.; Organon, Fr.; Organon (Οργανον), Gr.; Organon, Hong Kong; Organon, Irl.; Organon, Israel; Organon, Ital.; Organon, Malaysia; Organon, Mex.; Organon, Neth.; Organon, NZ; Organon, Port.; Donmed, S.Afr.; Organon, Singapore; Organon, Swed.; Organon, Switz.; Organon, Thai.; Organon, UK.*
Desogestrel (p.1547·2); ethinylestradiol (p.1553·2).
28-Day packs also contain 7 inert tablets.
*Combined oral contraceptive.*

**Mercina** *Merck, Chile.*
Erythromycin ethyl succinate (p.208·1).
*Bacterial infections.*

**Merck-Cough Linctus** *Xixia, S.Afr.*
Triprolidine hydrochloride (p.442·3); pseudoephedrine hydrochloride (p.1129·2); codeine phosphate (p.27·1).
*Coughs.*

**Merckenzyme** *Merck, India.*
Bromelains (p.1662·2); pancreatin (p.1725·3); ox bile (p.1660·3).
*Pancreatic insufficiency.*

**Merck-Expectorant** *Xixia, S.Afr.*
Triprolidine hydrochloride (p.442·3); pseudoephedrine hydrochloride (p.1129·2); codeine phosphate (p.27·1); guaifenesin (p.1122·1).
*Coughs.*

**Merck-Fed** *Xixia, S.Afr.*
Triprolidine hydrochloride (p.442·3); pseudoephedrine hydrochloride (p.1129·2).
*Cold and influenza symptoms.*

**Merck-Flu** *Xixia, S.Afr.*
Paracetamol (p.76·2); vitamin C (p.1460·2); phenylephrine hydrochloride (p.1126·3); chlorphenamine maleate (p.427·3); caffeine (p.782·1).
*Cold and influenza symptoms.*

**Merck-Gesic** *Xixia, S.Afr.*
Paracetamol (p.76·2).
*Fever; pain.*

**Mercodol with Decapryn** *Hoechst Marion Roussel, Canad.†.*
Hydrocodone tartrate (p.45·1); etafedrine hydrochloride (p.1121·2); sodium citrate (p.1223·2); doxylamine succinate (p.432·3).
*Coughs.*

**Mercromina** *Lainco, Spain.*
Merbromin (p.1185·3).
*Wound disinfection.*

**Mercrotona** *Orravan, Spain.*
Merbromin sodium (p.1185·3); alcohol (p.1166·1).
*Wound disinfection.*

**Mercryl** *Menarini, Fr.*
Chlorhexidine gluconate (p.1173·2); benzalkonium chloride (p.1168·3).
Formerly known as Mercryl Lauryle and contained mercurobutol.
*Bacterial infections of the skin and mucous membranes.*

**Mercryl Lauryle** *Sanofi Synthelabo, Spain†.*
Mercurobutol (p.1185·3).
*Skin and mucous membrane disinfection.*

**Mercryl Plus** *Sanofi Synthelabo, Spain.*
Chlorhexidine gluconate (p.1173·2); benzalkonium chloride (p.1168·3).
*Burns; skin disinfection; wounds.*

**Mercuchrom** *Krewel, Ger.*
Merbromin (p.1185·3).
*Burns; skin disinfection; skin ulceration; wounds.*

**Mercural** *Berman, Mex.†.*
Thiomersal (p.1194·1).

**Mercurin** *Monik, Spain.*
Merbromin sodium (p.1185·3).
*Wound disinfection.*

**Mercurio Cromo**
*Note. This name is used for preparations of different composition.*
*Phos-Kola, Braz.†.*
Merbromin (p.1185·3).
*Skin disinfection.*

*Sobral, Braz.†.*
Thiomersal (p.1194·1).
*Disinfection.*

**Mercurobromo** *Spyfarma, Spain.*
Merbromin (p.1185·3).
*Wound disinfection.*

**Mercutina Brota** *Escaned, Spain.*
Merbromin (p.1185·3).
*Wound disinfection.*

**Mercuval** *Biosyn, Ger.*
Unithiol (p.1055·3).
*Lead poisoning; mercury poisoning.*

**Merebral** *Byk, Arg.*
Amino acids; cyanocobalamin; ginseng (p.1417·1).
*Mental function impairment.*

**Meredazol** *Wayne, Mex.†.*
Metronidazole (p.607·2).

**Mereprine**
*Note. This name is used for preparations of different composition.*
*Aventis, Fr.†; Cassella-med, Ger.*
Doxylamine succinate (p.432·3).
*Allergic disorders; restlessness and excitement in children; sleep disorders.*

*Inibsa, Port.*
Captopril (p.879·2).
*Heart failure; hypertension.*

**Meresa**
*Sanova, Austria; Dolorgiet, Ger.*
Sulpiride (p.722·2).
*Depression; schizophrenia; vestibular disorders.*

**Meretek UBT** *Meretek, USA.*
Carbon-13 (p.1667·3) labelled urea (Pranactin).
*Diagnosis of Helicobacter pylori infection.*

**Merex** *Tentan, Switz.*
Phenylpropanolamine hydrochloride (p.1127·3).
*Obesity.*

**Merfen** *Novartis Consumer, Switz.*
Chlorhexidine gluconate (p.1173·2) or chlorhexidine hydrochloride (p.1173·3); benzoxonium chloride (p.1170·2).
*Skin and wound disinfection.*

**Merfene** *Novartis Sante, Fr.*
Chlorhexidine gluconate (p.1173·2).
Formerly contained phenylmercuric borate.
*Wound disinfection.*

**Merfluan Sali Dentali** *Colgate-Palmolive, Ital.†.*
Sodium fluoride (p.1444·3); minerals.
*Dental caries prophylaxis.*

**Mericomb**
*Novartis, Austria; Novartis, Braz.; Novartis, Fin.; Novartis, Ger.; Pierre Fabre, Ger.; Novartis, Switz.*
16 Tablets, estradiol valerate (p.1550·2); 12 tablets, estradiol valerate; norethisterone (p.1562·2).
*Menopausal disorders; osteoporosis.*

**Meridia**
*Ebewe, Austria; Abbott, Canad.; Abbott, USA.*
Sibutramine hydrochloride (p.1593·1).
*Obesity.*

**Meridol**
*GABA, Fr.; Teva, Israel; Inibsa, Port.†.*
Olaflur (p.1442·3); stannous fluoride (p.1448·3).
*Dental caries prophylaxis; gingivitis.*

**Meridol-D** *Pharmaceutical Enterprises, S.Afr.†.*
Paracetamol (p.76·2); codeine phosphate (p.27·1); diphenhydramine (p.431·3).
*Fever; pain.*

**Meriestra** *Novartis, Spain.*
Estradiol valerate (p.1550·2).
*Menopausal disorders.*

**Merigest**
*Novartis, Austria; Novartis, Braz.; Novartis, Fin.; Novartis, Ger.; Pierre Fabre, Ger.; Novartis, Spain; Novartis, Switz.*
Estradiol valerate (p.1550·2); norethisterone (p.1562·2).
*Menopausal disorders; osteoporosis.*

**Merigest Sequi** *Novartis, Spain.*
16 Tablets, estradiol valerate (p.1550·2); 12 tablets, estradiol valerate; norethisterone (p.1562·2).
Formerly known as Merigest Combi.
*Menopausal disorders.*

**Merimono**
*Novartis, Austria; Novartis, Braz.; Novartis, Fin.; Novartis, Ger.; Pierre Fabre, Ger.*
Estradiol valerate (p.1550·2).
*Menopausal disorders.*

**Merional**
*IBSA, Hong Kong; IBSA, Switz.; Denfleet, UK.*
Menotrophin (p.1330·1).
*Male and female infertility.*

**Merional-HMG** *BPL-Meizler, Braz.*
Gonadotrophin (p.1330·1).
*Female infertility.*

**Merislon**
*Eisai, Hong Kong; Eisai, Jpn; Eisai, Singapore; Eisai, Thai.*
Betahistine mesilate (p.1660·1).
*Ménière's disease; vertigo.*

**Meristel** *Aqualab, Fr.†.*
Sea-water.
*Nasal and skin irrigation.*

**Meritene**
*Novartis, Arg.; Novartis, Braz.; Sandoz Nutrition, Canad.†; Novartis, Norw.†; Novartis Consumer, Port.; Novartis, Swed.†; Wander Health Care, Switz.†; Novartis Nutrition, USA.*
Preparation for enteral nutrition (p.1417·1).

**Merlin** *TO-Chemicals, Thai.*
Betahistine mesilate (p.1660·1).
*Ménière's disease; vertigo.*

**Merlit** *Ebewe, Austria.*
Lorazepam (p.704·1).
*Anxiety disorders; sleep disorders.*

**Mermid** *Merck, Mex.*
Dipyrone (p.35·3).
*Fever; pain.*

**Merocaine**
*SSL, Irl.; SSL, UK.*
Benzocaine (p.1370·3); cetylpyridinium chloride (p.1173·1).
*Adjunct in dental procedures; mouth and throat disorders.*

**Merocets**
*SSL, Irl.; SSL, UK.*
Cetylpyridinium chloride (p.1173·1).
*Throat infections.*

**Merocets Plus** *SSL, UK.*
Cetylpyridinium chloride (p.1173·1); menthol (p.1711·3); eucalyptus oil (p.1686·2).
Formerly known as Merothol.
*Nasal congestion; sore mouth and throat.*

**Meroken New** *Taro, Israel.*
Macrogol 3350 (p.1709·1); electrolytes (p.1217·1).
*Bowel evacuation.*

**Merol** *Medecine Vegetale, Fr.†.*
Pentoxyverine citrate (p.1126·2).
*Coughs.*

**Meromycin** *Ratiopharm, Austria.*
Erythromycin (p.208·1), erythromycin ethyl succinate (p.208·1), or erythromycin stearate (p.208·2).
*Bacterial infections.*

**Meronem**
*AstraZeneca, Belg.; AstraZeneca, Braz.; AstraZeneca, Chile; AstraZeneca, Denm.; AstraZeneca, Fin.; AstraZeneca, Ger.; Grunenthal, Ger.; Cana, Gr.; AstraZeneca, Hong Kong; AstraZeneca, Irl.; AstraZeneca, Israel; AstraZeneca, Malaysia; AstraZeneca, Neth.; AstraZeneca, Norw.; AstraZeneca, Port.; Zeneca, S.Afr.; AstraZeneca, Singapore; AstraZeneca, Spain; AstraZeneca, Swed.; AstraZeneca, Switz.; AstraZeneca, Thai.; AstraZeneca, UK.*
Meropenem (p.229·1).
*Bacterial infections.*

**Meropen** *Sumitomo, Jpn.*
Meropenem (p.229·1).
*Bacterial infections.*

**Merozen** *AstraZeneca, Arg.*
Meropenem (p.229·1).
*Bacterial infections.*

**Merpal** *Prater, Chile.*
Diclofenac (p.32·1), diclofenac diethylamine (p.32·1), diclofenac resinate (p.33·1), or diclofenac sodium (p.32·1).
*Inflammation; pain.*

**Merphen** *Novartis Consumer, Israel.*
Chlorhexidine gluconate (p.1173·2); benzoxonium chloride (p.1170·2).
*Burns; insect bites; wounds.*

**Merrem**
AstraZeneca, Austral.; AstraZeneca, Canad.; AstraZeneca, Ital.; AstraZeneca, Mex.; AstraZeneca, NZ; Zeneca, USA.
Meropenem (p.229·1).
*Bacterial infections.*

**MerSol**
Note. A similar name is used for preparations of different composition (see below).
Ratiopharm, Ger.
Nicotinamide (p.1441·2); folic acid (p.1429·1).
*Photosensitivity.*

**Mersol**
Note. A similar name is used for preparations of different composition (see above).
Century, USA.
Thiomersal (p.1194·1).
*Skin disinfection.*

**Mersyndol**
Aventis, Austral.; Aventis, NZ.
Paracetamol (p.76·2); codeine phosphate (p.27·1); doxylamine succinate (p.432·3).
*Fever; pain.*

**Mersyndol with Codeine** Aventis, Canad.
Paracetamol (p.76·2); codeine phosphate (p.27·1); doxylamine succinate (p.432·3).
*Cold symptoms; pain.*

**Mersyndol Daystrength** Aventis, Austral.
Paracetamol (p.76·2); codeine phosphate (p.27·1).
*Fever; pain.*

**Merthiolate**
Note. This name is used for preparations of different composition.
Gramon, Arg.; Lilly, Arg.; Aspen, S.Afr.; Lilly, Thai.
Thiomersal (p.1194·1).
*Skin disinfection; wounds.*
Lilly, Braz.†; Lilly, Mex.
Benzalkonium chloride (p.1168·3).
*Skin disinfection.*

**Meruvax**
Aventis Pasteur, Denm.; Aventis Pasteur, Swed.
A rubella vaccine (Wistar RA 27/3 strain) (p.1637·3).
*Active immunisation.*

**Meruvax II**
Merck Sharp & Dohme, Austral.; Prodome, Braz.†; Merck Sharp & Dohme, Hong Kong†; Pro Vaccine, Switz.; Merck, USA.
A rubella vaccine (Wistar RA 27/3 strain) (p.1637·3).
*Active immunisation.*

**Merxil** Merck, Mex.
Diclofenac sodium (p.32·1).
*Inflammation; musculoskeletal, joint and peri-articular disorders; pain.*

**Merz Spezial** Medra, Austria.
Multivitamin and mineral preparation (p.1417·1).

**Merz Spezial Dragees N** Merz, Ger.
Multivitamin preparation with iron and acetylmethionine (p.1417·1).

**Merzbiotin** Medra, Austria.
Biotin (p.1423·2).
*Biotin deficiency; hair and nail disorders.*

**Mesacol**
Sun, India; Sun, Singapore†; Sun, Thai.
Mesalazine (p.1273·2).
*Inflammatory bowel disease.*

**Mesactol** Labinca, Arg.
Lansoprazole (p.1269·3).
*Peptic ulcer.*

**Mesaflor** Fonten, Ital.
Mesalazine (p.1273·2).
*Crohn's disease; ulcerative colitis.*

**Mesagin** Kleva, Gr.
Mesalazine (p.1273·2).
*Inflammatory bowel disease.*

**Mesantoin** Novartis, USA†.
Mephenytoin (p.366·2).
*Epilepsy.*

**Mesasal**
GlaxoSmithKline, Austral.; GlaxoSmithKline, Canad.; Sanofi Winthrop, Denm.; Sanofi Synthelabo, Norw.; Sanofi Synthelabo, Swed.
Mesalazine (p.1273·2).
*Inflammatory bowel disease.*

**Mesatil** Soria Natural, Spain.
Melissa (p.1711·1); salix (p.87·3); tilia (p.1756·2); rosemary (p.1740·2).
*Migraine.*

**Mescolor** Horizon, USA.
Chlorphenamine maleate (p.427·3); pseudoephedrine hydrochloride (p.1129·2); hyoscine methonitrate (p.483·3).
*Upper respiratory-tract symptoms.*

**Mescorit** Roche, Ger.
Metformin hydrochloride (p.342·3).
*Diabetes mellitus.*

**Mesid** Janssen-Cilag, Ital.†.
Nimesulide (p.67·1).
*Fever; inflammation; pain.*

**Mesigyna**
Schering, Arg.; Berlimed, Braz.; Schering, Chile; Schering, Mex.
Norethisterone enantate (p.1562·2); estradiol valerate (p.1550·2).
*Combined injectable contraceptive.*

**Mesiken** Kener, Mex.†.
Bromocriptine (p.1202·3).

**Mesin** Unison, Thai.
Albendazole (p.101·2).
*Worm infections.*

**Mesitol** Laborsil, Braz.†.
Methionine (p.1042·1); choline (p.1424·3); betaine (p.1660·1).
*Liver disorders.*

**M-Eslon**
Aventis, Canad.; Grunenthal, Chile.
Morphine sulfate (p.60·2).
*Pain.*

**Mesmerin** Sigma, Braz.
Lorazepam (p.704·1).
*Alcohol withdrawal syndrome; anxiety; epilepsy; insomnia; nausea and vomiting; premedication.*

**Mesnex**
Kampel Martian, Arg.; Bristol-Myers Squibb Oncology, USA.
Mesna (p.1041·2).
*Prevention of oxazophosphorine-induced urinary-tract toxicity.*

**Mesnil**
Zodiac, Braz.†; Asofarma, Mex.
Mesna (p.1041·2).
*Prevention of urotoxicity due to antineoplastic therapy.*

**Mesocaine** Pharmy, Fr.
Lidocaine hydrochloride (p.1377·3).
*Local anaesthesia.*

**Mesodal** Helber, Mex.
Mesna (p.1041·2).
*Prevention of ifosfamide and cyclophosphamide-induced haemorrhagic cystitis.*

**Mesolex** Shiwa, Thai.
Metronidazole (p.607·2).
*Amoebiasis; giardiasis; trichomoniasis.*

**Mesolona** Laboratorios Chile, Chile.
Chlormezanone (p.675·1); diazepam (p.690·1).
*Anxiety; insomnia; skeletal muscle spasm.*

**Mesonex** Adelco, Gr.
Atenolol (p.865·2).
*Angina; arrythmias; hypertension.*

**Mesopran** Royton, Braz.
Omeprazole (p.1278·2).
*Peptic ulcer.*

**Mesorfan** Collins, Mex.
Pseudoephedrine (p.1129·2); chlorphenamine (p.428·1); dextromethorphan (p.1117·3).
*Coughs.*

**Mesotina** Rivero, Arg.
Papaverine hydrochloride (p.1728·1).
*Vascular spasm.*

**Mespafin** Merckle, Ger.
Doxycycline hyclate (p.206·2).
*Bacterial infections.*

**Mesporan** Mepha, Braz.
Ceftriaxone (p.183·3).
*Bacterial infections.*

**Mesporin**
Mepha, Hong Kong; Mepha, Port.
Ceftriaxone sodium (p.182·3).
*Bacterial infections.*

**Mesren** Ivax, UK.
Mesalazine (p.1273·2).
*Crohn's disease; ulcerative colitis.*

**Mestacine** Wyeth Lederle, Fr.
Minocycline hydrochloride (p.231·3).
*Bacterial infections.*

**Mestian** Kampel Martian, Arg.
Mesna (p.1041·2).

**Mestil-Ka** Fada, Arg.
Menadione (p.1466·3).
*Vitamin K supplement.*

**Mestinon**
ICN, Arg.; ICN, Austral.; ICN, Austria; Sanico, Belg.†; ICN, Braz.; ICN, Canad.; Roche, Chile; ICN, Denm.; ICN, Fin.; CSP, Fr.; ICN, Ger.; IFET (ΙΦΕΤ), Gr.; ICN, Hong Kong; ICN, Irl.; ICN, Israel; ICN, Ital.; ICN, Malaysia; ICN, Mex.; ICN, Neth.; ICN, Norw.; ICN, NZ; Pacific, NZ; ICN, Port.; Pharmaco, S.Afr.; ICN, Singapore; ICN, Spain; Medilink, Swed.; ICN, Switz.; ICN, Thai.; ICN, UK; ICN, USA.
Pyridostigmine bromide (p.1496·1).
*Atonic constipation; intestinal atony; myasthenia gravis; postoperative urinary retention; reversal of competitive neuromuscular blockade.*

**Mesto-Of** Pond's, Thai.
Amylase (p.1654·2); sodium bicarbonate (p.1223·2); calcium carbonate (p.1254·2); thiamine nitrate (p.1455·1); menthol (p.1711·3); ginger oil (p.1267·1); anise oil (p.1655·2); cinnamon oil (p.1672·2); clove oil (p.1673·3); scopolia.
*Dyspepsia; gastritis; gastrointestinal motility disorders; heartburn; hyperacidity.*

**Mestoranum**
Schering, Denm.; Schering, Norw.†; Schering, Swed.†.
Mesterolone (p.1559·1).
*Breast cancer; hypogonadism; metrorrhagia.*

**Mestrel**
Laboratorios Chile, Chile; Lemery, Mex.; Lemery, Thai.
Megestrol acetate (p.1558·2).
*Breast cancer; endometrial cancer.*

**Mesulid**
CSC, Austria; Therabel, Belg.; Boehringer Ingelheim, Gr.; Helsinn, Hong Kong; Schering-Plough, Hong Kong; Stadmed, India; Ergha, Irl.; Rafa, Israel; Novartis, Ital.; Roche, Mex.
Nimesulide (p.67·1) or nimesulide betadex (p.67·1).
*Fever; inflammation; musculoskeletal, joint, peri-articular, and soft-tissue disorders; pain.*

**Mesupon** Cooper (Κοπερ), Gr.
Nimesulide (p.67·1).
*Inflammation; musculoskeletal disorders; pain.*

**Mesura** Andromaco, Chile.
Sibutramine (p.1593·2).
*Obesity.*

**Met** Betapharm, Ger.
Metformin hydrochloride (p.342·3).
*Diabetes mellitus.*

**Meta Framan** Oftalmiso, Spain†.
Metampicillin sodium (p.229·3).
*Bacterial infections.*

**metabiarex** Meta Fackler, Ger.
Homoeopathic preparation.

**Metabol** Jagson, India.
Nandrolone phenylpropionate (p.1561·3).
*Adjuvant to steroid therapy; debility; osteoporosis; uraemia.*

**Metabolic Mineral Mixture**
Scientific Hospital Supplies, Austral.; Nutricia, NZ; Scientific Hospital Supplies, NZ; Scientific Hospital Supplies, UK.
Mineral and trace element preparation (p.1417·1).
*Mineral supplementation for enteral diets.*

**Metabolicum** Novag, Spain†.
Sodium cytidine monophosphate; cobamamide (p.1459·1); hydroxocobalamin (p.1458·2).
*Megaloblastic anaemias; neuritis; tonic.*

**Metabolite-A** Forder, Arg.
Retinol (p.1451·2).
*Skin disorders.*

**Metabyn** Byk Gulden, Mex.†.
Ispaghula (p.1268·1).

**Metacaf** Chong Kun Dang, Ital.
Cefmetazole sodium (p.173·3).
Lidocaine hydrochloride (p.1377·3) is included in the intramuscular injection to alleviate the pain of injection.
*Gram-negative bacterial infections.*

**Metacard** Ipca, India.
Trimetazidine hydrochloride (p.1018·1).
*Ischaemic heart disease.*

**Metacen** Promedica, Ital.
Indometacin (p.47·3).
*Musculoskeletal and joint disorders.*

**Metacidil** Teuto, Braz.
Indometacin (p.47·3).

**Metacuprol** Lemoine, Fr.
Copper sulfate (p.1426·1).
*Skin and mucous membrane infections.*

**Metadate**
Medeva, Israel; Celltech, USA.
Methylphenidate hydrochloride (p.1590·2).
*Attention deficit hyperactivity disorder; narcoleptic syndrome.*

**Metadec** Jagson, India.
Nandrolone decanoate (p.1561·2).
*Anabolic; anaemia; osteoporosis.*

**Metadol** Pharmascience, Canad.
Methadone hydrochloride (p.57·2).
*Opioid dependence.*

**Metadon** Cristalia, Braz.
Methadone hydrochloride (p.57·2).
*Opioid withdrawal syndrome; pain.*

**Metadoxil**
Silesia, Chile; Baldacci, Ital.; Baldacci, Port.; Eurodrug, Thai.
Metadoxine (p.1456·3).
*Liver disorders.*

**Metadyne** Pharmavite, Canad.†.
Povidone-iodine (p.1190·3).

**Metafar** Lafare, Ital.
Cefmetazole sodium (p.173·3).
Lidocaine hydrochloride (p.1377·3) is included in the intramuscular injection to alleviate the pain of injection.
*Gram-negative bacterial infections.*

**Metaflex** Montpellier, Arg.
Nimesulide (p.67·1).
*Fever; inflammation; musculoskeletal and joint disorders; pain.*

**Metaflex NF** Montpellier, Arg.
Diclofenac potassium (p.32·1) or diclofenac sodium (p.32·1).
*Musculoskeletal and joint disorders; pain.*

**Metaflex Plus** Montpellier, Arg.
Nimesulide (p.67·1); orphenadrine citrate (p.486·1).
*Musculoskeletal and joint disorders.*

**Metaflex Plus NF** Montpellier, Arg.
Diclofenac sodium (p.32·1); pridinol mesilate (p.1395·2).
*Musculoskeletal, joint, and peri-articular disorders.*

**metaginkgo** Meta Fackler, Ger.
Homoeopathic preparation.

**Metaglip** Bristol-Myers Squibb, USA.
Glipizide (p.332·2); metformin hydrochloride (p.342·3).
*Diabetes mellitus.*

**Metagliz** Almirall, Spain.
Metoclopramide glycyrrhizinate (p.1276·1).
*Aid in gastrointestinal examination; gastro-oesophageal reflux; gastroparesis; nausea and vomiting.*

**Metagliz Bismutico** Prodes, Spain†.
Bismuth subnitrate (p.1252·2); metoclopramide glycyrrhizinate (p.1276·1).
*Gastritis; peptic ulcer; vomiting.*

**Metagyl** Ranbaxy, S.Afr.
Metronidazole (p.607·2).
*Anaerobic bacterial infections; protozoal infections.*

**Metahydrin** Hoechst Marion Roussel, USA.
Trichlormethiazide (p.1017·2).
*Hypertension; oedema.*

**Meta-K** Reuffer, Mex.†.
Cefalexin (p.168·1).
*Bacterial infections.*

**metakaveron** Meta Fackler, Ger.
Homoeopathic preparation.

**Metakelfin** Pharmacia Upjohn, Ital.
Sulfametopyrazine (p.263·1); pyrimethamine (p.458·1).
*Malaria.*

**Metakes** Inexfa, Spain†.
Metampicillin sodium (p.229·3).
*Bacterial infections.*

**Metalax** Leiras, Fin.
Bisacodyl (p.1251·3).
*Constipation.*

**Metalcaptase**
Heyl, Ger.; Knoll, S.Afr.
Penicillamine (p.1046·3).
*Cystine calculi; cystinuria; heavy-metal poisoning; rheumatoid arthritis; scleroderma; Wilson's disease.*

**Metalgin** Hexal, Ger.
Dipyrone (p.35·3).
*Pain.*

**Metalon** Caps, S.Afr.
Metoclopramide hydrochloride (p.1274·3).
*Gastrointestinal motility disorders; vomiting.*

**Metalpha** Ashbourne, UK†.
Methyldopa (p.953·2).

**Metalyse**
Boehringer Ingelheim, Austral.; Boehringer Ingelheim, Braz.; Boehringer Ingelheim, Denm.; Boehringer Ingelheim, Fin.; Boehringer Ingelheim, Fr.; Boehringer Ingelheim, Ger.; Boehringer Ingelheim, Gr.; Boehringer Ingelheim, Irl.; Boehringer Ingelheim, Norw.; Boehringer Ingelheim, NZ; Boehringer Ingelheim, Port.; Boehringer Ingelheim, S.Afr.; Boehringer Ingelheim, Spain; Boehringer Ingelheim, Swed.; Boehringer Ingelheim, Switz.; Boehringer Ingelheim, UK.
Tenecteplase (p.1010·2).
*Myocardial infarction.*

**metamagnesol** Meta Fackler, Ger.
Magnesium aspartate (p.1227·3).
*Magnesium deficiency.*

**Metamide** Pacific, NZ.
Metoclopramide hydrochloride (p.1274·3).
*Gastrointestinal motility disorders; nausea and vomiting.*

**Metamidol** Irex, Port.
Diazepam (p.690·1).
*Anxiety; febrile convulsions; insomnia; skeletal muscle spasm.*

**Metamucil**
Temis, Arg.; Procter & Gamble, Austral.†; Procter & Gamble, Austria; Procter & Gamble, Belg.†; Procter & Gamble, Braz.; Procter & Gamble, Canad.; Gynopharm, Chile; Wick, Ger.; Pharmacia, Hong Kong; Searle, Israel†; Procter & Gamble, Mex.; Pharmacia, Neth.; Procter & Gamble, NZ.; Monsanto, Port.†; Searle, S.Afr.; Searle, Singapore†; Procter & Gamble, Spain; Procter & Gamble, Switz.; Pharmacia, Thai.; Procter & Gamble, USA.
Ispaghula (p.1268·1).
*Constipation; diverticular disease; irritable bowel syndrome; ostomy management.*

**Metandren** Novartis, Canad.†.
Methyltestosterone (p.1559·3).
*Androgen replacement therapy; breast cancer.*

**Metanium**
Bengue, Irl.†; Ransom, UK.
Titanium dioxide (p.1160·3); titanium peroxide (p.1160·3); titanium salicylate (p.1160·3).
*Macerated skin; nappy rash.*

**Metanor** Viatris, Port.
Flupirtine maleate (p.43·3).
*Pain.*

**metaossylen** Meta Fackler, Ger.†.
Homoeopathic preparation.

**Metapio** Master, Chile.
Phenol (p.1188·1).
*Disinfection.*

**Metapirona** Allen, Mex.
Dipyrone (p.35·3).
*Fever; pain.*

**Metaplatin** Teva Tuteur, Arg.
Oxaliplatin (p.577·1).
*Malignant neoplasms.*

**Metaplex**
Takeda, Hong Kong; Takeda, Thai.
Vitamin B substances (p.1417·1).
*Vitamin deficiency.*

**Metaplexan**
Rhone-Poulenc Rorer, Austria†; Pierre Fabre, Ger.
Mequitazine (p.437·2).
*Hypersensitivity disorders.*

**Metargen Pediatrico** Farmaco, Mex.
Vitamin preparation (p.1417·1).

**Metasal** Salus, Ital.
Cefmetazole sodium (p.173·3).
Lidocaine hydrochloride (p.1377·3) is included in the intramuscular injection to alleviate the pain of injection.
*Gram-negative bacterial infections.*

**Metasedin** Esteve, Spain.
Methadone hydrochloride (p.57·2).
*Opioid withdrawal; pain.*

**Metasin** Fustery, Mex.
Metadoxine (p.1456·3).
*Alcohol withdrawal syndrome; liver disorders.*

**metasolidago S** Meta Fackler, Ger.
Homoeopathic preparation.

**Metasolvens** Hogapharm, Switz.†.
Bromhexine hydrochloride (p.1115·3).
*Respiratory-tract disorders associated with increased mucus.*

**Metason** Fortbenton, Arg.
Mometasone furoate (p.1107·2).
*Allergic rhinitis; skin disorders.*

**Metaspirine** GlaxoSmithKline Sante, Fr.
Aspirin (p.15·1); caffeine (p.782·1).
*Fever; pain.*

**Metaspray** Cipla, India.
Mometasone furoate (p.1107·2).
*Allergic rhinitis.*

**Metastron**
Amersham, Austral.; Nycomed, Austria; Amersham, Canad.†; Amersham, Fr.; Amersham, Ital.; Amersham, Spain; Amersham, UK; Medi-Physics, USA; Amersham, USA.
Strontium-89 chloride (p.1525·2).
*Metastatic bone pain.*

**Metatensin** Hoechst Marion Roussel, USA.
Trichlormethiazide (p.1017·2); reserpine (p.995·1).
*Hypertension.*

**Metatone**
Pfizer Consumer, Irl.; Pfizer Consumer, UK.
Calcium glycerophosphate; manganese glycerophosphate; potassium glycerophosphate; sodium glycerophosphate; thiamine hydrochloride (p.1417·1).
*Tonic.*

**metavirulent** Meta Fackler, Ger.
Homoeopathic preparation.

**Metax** Sons, Mex.; Solfran, Mex.
Dexamethasone (p.1097·1).
*Corticosteroid.*

**Metaxol** Propan, S.Afr.; Covan, S.Afr.
Theophylline (p.798·3); codeine phosphate (p.27·1); mepyramine maleate (p.437·1).
*Coughs.*

**Metazem**
Bioglan, Hong Kong†; Bioglan, Irl.†; Clonmel, Irl.†; Bioglan, Singapore†; Bioglan, Thai.†; Bioglan, UK†.
Diltiazem hydrochloride (p.900·1).
*Angina pectoris.*

**Metazin** Clintex, Port.
Etodolac (p.37·3).
*Gout; musculoskeletal and joint disorders; pain.*

**Metazinc** 20th Century, Mex.†.
Zinc sulfate (p.1469·3).

**Metazol**
Note. This name is used for preparations of different composition.
CT, Ital.
Cefmetazole sodium (p.173·3).
Lidocaine hydrochloride (p.1377·3) is included in this preparation to alleviate the pain of injection.
*Bacterial infections.*

Alliance, S.Afr.
Metronidazole (p.607·2).
*Anaerobic bacterial infections; protozoal infections.*

**Metbay** Bayer, Ital.
Metformin hydrochloride (p.342·3).
*Diabetes mellitus.*

**Metblock** Pharmacia, Fin.
Metoprolol tartrate (p.957·1).
*Angina pectoris; arrhythmias; hypertension; hyperthyroidism; migraine; myocardial infarction.*

**Metcon** Docmed, S.Afr.†.
Metoclopramide hydrochloride (p.1274·3).
*Gastrointestinal disorders; nausea and vomiting.*

**Metcort** Delta, Braz.
Dexamethasone phosphate (p.1097·2); neomycin sulfate (p.235·1).
*Infected skin disorders.*

**Meted**
Medicis, Canad.; Dermapharm, Irl.; Dermapharm, UK; GenDerm, USA.
Salicylic acid (p.1157·1); sulfur (p.1158·2).
*Scalp disorders.*

**Metenan** Apsen, Braz.†.
Monobasic sodium phosphate (p.1230·3); methenamine (p.230·1).
*Urinary-tract pain.*

**Metenix 5** Borg, UK.
Metolazone (p.956·2).
*Ascites; hypertension; oedema.*

**Meteophyt forte** OTW, Ger.
Pancreatin (p.1725·3).
*Pancreatic disorders.*

**Meteophyt N** OTW, Ger.†.
Turmeric (p.1058·3).
*Dyspepsia.*

**Meteophyt S** OTW, Ger.†.
Chamomile (p.1669·3); peppermint leaf (p.1283·2); dried bitter-orange peel (p.1723·3); caraway (p.1667·2).
*Dyspepsia; loss of appetite.*

**Meteoril** Salvat, Spain.
Simeticone (p.1289·2); magnesium trisilicate (p.1272·3); aluminium glycinate (p.1249·1).
Formerly contained simeticone, magnesium trisilicate, aluminium glycinate, and metoclopramide hydrochloride.
*Flatulence; gastrointestinal hyperacidity.*

**Meteosan** Novartis Consumer, Ger.
Dimethicone (p.1289·2).
*Gastrointestinal disorders associated with excess gas.*

**Meteosim** Ibi, Ital.
Simeticone (p.1289·2).
*Aerophagia; meteorism.*

**Meteospasmyl**
Mayoly-Spindler, Fr.; Mayoly-Spindler, Hong Kong†; Mayoly-Spindler, Malaysia; Mayoly-Spindler, Singapore; Mayoly-Spindler, Thai.
Alverine citrate (p.1250·2); simeticone (p.1289·2).
*Dyspepsia; flatulence; gastrointestinal spasm; irritable bowel syndrome.*

**Meteoxane** Tonipharm, Fr.
Simeticone (p.1289·2); phloroglucinol (p.1731·1).
*Gastrointestinal disorders.*

**Meteozym** Novartis Consumer, Ger.
Pancreatin (p.1725·3); simeticone (p.1289·2).
*Digestive-system disorders.*

**Meterfolic** Durbin, UK.
Ferrous fumarate (p.1427·3); folic acid (p.1429·1).
*Iron and folic acid deficiency in pregnancy; neural tube defect prophylaxis.*

**Metex** Medac, Ger.
Methotrexate sodium (p.568·3).
*Arthritis; psoriasis.*

**Metfin** Ecosol, Switz.
Metformin hydrochloride (p.342·3).
*Diabetes mellitus.*

**Metfirex** Irex, Fr.†.
Metformin hydrochloride (p.342·3).
*Diabetes mellitus.*

**Metfogamma** Worwag, Ger.
Metformin hydrochloride (p.342·3).
*Diabetes mellitus.*

**Metfor** Acis, Ger.
Metformin hydrochloride (p.342·3).
*Diabetes mellitus.*

**Metfor-500** Masa, Thai.
Metformin hydrochloride (p.342·3).
*Diabetes mellitus.*

**Metforal**
Guidotti, Ital.; Menarini, Singapore.
Metformin hydrochloride (p.342·3).
*Diabetes mellitus.*

**Metforem** Orion, Fin.
Metformin hydrochloride (p.342·3).
*Diabetes mellitus.*

**Metfori** Hexal, Arg.
Metformin hydrochloride (p.342·3).
*Diabetes mellitus.*

**Metform** ABZ, Ger.
Metformin hydrochloride (p.342·3).
*Diabetes mellitus.*

**Metformax** Menarini, Belg.
Metformin hydrochloride (p.342·3).
*Diabetes mellitus.*

**Metfron** Asian Pharm, Thai.
Metformin hydrochloride (p.342·3).
*Diabetes mellitus.*

**Methacin**
Note. This name is used for preparations of different composition.
Mentholatum, Canad.
Menthol (p.1711·3); capsaicin (p.24·2).

Hovid, Singapore†.
Indometacin (p.47·3).
*Gout; musculoskeletal and joint disorders.*

**Methaddict** Addicare, Ger.†.
Methadone hydrochloride (p.57·2).
*Opioid withdrawal.*

**Methadose**
Rosemont, UK; Mallinckrodt, USA.
Methadone hydrochloride (p.57·2).
*Opioid withdrawal; pain.*

**Methagual** Gordon, USA.
Methyl salicylate (p.59·3); guaiacol (p.1122·1).
*Muscle, joint, and soft-tissue pain; neuralgia.*

**Methalgen** Alra, USA.
Methyl salicylate (p.59·3); menthol (p.1711·3); camphor (p.1665·3); mustard oil (p.1718·2).
*Musculoskeletal and joint pain.*

**Metharmon-F** Zoki, Thai.
Pregnenolone; androstenedione (p.1542·1); androstenediol; testosterone (p.1569·3); estrone (p.1553·1); thyroid (p.1604·2).
*Menopausal disorders; ovarian disorders.*

**Methatabs** PSM, NZ.
Methadone hydrochloride (p.57·2).
*Coughs; opioid withdrawal syndrome; pain.*

**Methatropic** Goldline, USA.
Vitamin B substances with methionine (p.1417·1).

**Methazil** Bell, India.
Methyl alcohol (p.1475·2); salicylic acid (p.1157·1).
*Fungal ear infections.*

**Methergin**
Novartis, Austria; Novartis, Belg.; Novartis, Braz.; Novartis, Chile; Novartis, Denm.; Novartis, Fin.; Novartis, Fr.; Novartis, Ger.; Novartis, Gr.; Novartis, Hong Kong; Novartis, India; Novartis, Israel; Novartis, Ital.; Novartis, Malaysia; Novartis, Mex.; Novartis, Neth.; Novartis, Port.; Novartis, Spain; Novartis, Swed.; Novartis, Switz.
Methylergometrine maleate (p.1714·2).
*Menorrhagia; postpartum haemorrhage; postpartum uterine atony or subinvolution.*

**Methergine** Novartis, USA.
Methylergometrine maleate (p.1714·2).
*Postpartum atony; postpartum haemorrhage.*

**Methex** Generics, UK†.
Methadone hydrochloride (p.57·2).
*Opioid withdrawal.*

**Methiotrans** Abbott, Ger.
Methionine (p.1042·1).
*Phosphate calculi; urinary acidification.*

**Methnine** Medical Research, Austral.
Methionine (p.1042·1).
*Liver disorders; paracetamol overdosage.*

**Methoblastin**
Pharmacia, Austral.
Methotrexate sodium (p.568·3).
*Malignant neoplasms; psoriasis; rheumatoid arthritis.*

Pharmacia Upjohn, Mex.†; Pharmacia, NZ; Pharmacia Upjohn, S.Afr.†.
Methotrexate (p.568·2).
*Malignant neoplasms; psoriasis.*

**Methoblastine** Pharmacia Upjohn, Belg.†.
Methotrexate (p.568·2).
*Malignant neoplasms.*

**Methocaps** Caps, S.Afr.
Indometacin (p.47·3).
*Gout; musculoskeletal and joint disorders.*

**Methocel**
Note. This name is used for preparations of different composition.
Novartis Ophthalmics, Ger.; Novartis Ophthalmics, Hong Kong; Ciba Vision, Ital.†; Restan, S.Afr.; Novartis Ophthalmics, Singapore.
Hypromellose (p.1579·3) (p.1164·2).
*Aid in eye examination; lubricating and disinfecting drops for use with contact lenses.*

Novartis Ophthalmics, Malaysia.
Methylcellulose (p.1580·2).
*Aid in eye examination.*

**Method M** Baxter, Thai.
A factor VIII preparation (p.751·1).
*Haemorrhagic disorders.*

**Methopt**
Sigma, Austral.; Sigma, NZ.
Hypromellose (p.1579·3).
*Dry eyes.*

**Methorcon** YF Chem, Thai.
Chlorphenamine maleate (p.427·3); dextromethorphan hydrobromide (p.1117·3); *dl*-methylephedrine hydrochloride (p.1124·2).
*Coughs.*

**Methoxacet** Technilab, Canad.
Methocarbamol (p.1395·1); paracetamol (p.76·2).
*Musculoskeletal, joint, peri-articular and soft-tissue disorders.*

**Methoxacet-C** Technilab, Canad.
Methocarbamol (p.1395·1); paracetamol (p.76·2); codeine phosphate (p.27·1).
*Pain associated with skeletal muscle spasm.*

**Methoxisal** Technilab, Canad.
Methocarbamol (p.1395·1); aspirin (p.15·1).
*Pain associated with skeletal muscle spasm.*

**Methoxisal-C** Technilab, Canad.
Methocarbamol (p.1395·1); aspirin (p.15·1); codeine phosphate (p.27·1).
*Pain associated with skeletal muscle spasm.*

**Methozane** Taro, Israel.
Levomepromazine maleate (p.703·2).
*Anxiety; bipolar disorder; pain; premedication; psychoses.*

**Methycobal**
TRB, Arg.; TRB, Braz.†; Eisai, Hong Kong; Wockhardt, India; Eisai, Jpn; Eisai, Malaysia; Eisai, Singapore; Eisai, Thai.
Mecobalamin (p.1459·1).
*Megaloblastic anaemia; peripheral neuropathies.*

**Methyl Salicylate Compound Liniment** McGloin, Austral.†.
Methyl salicylate (p.59·3); menthol (p.1711·3); eucalyptus oil (p.1686·2).
*Muscle pain.*

**Methyl Salicylate Ointment Compound** McGloin, Austral.†.
Methyl salicylate (p.59·3); menthol (p.1711·3); cineole (p.1672·1); cajuput oil (p.1664·1).
*Muscle pain.*

**Methylergobrevin** Wernigerode, Ger.
Methylergometrine maleate (p.1714·2).
*Postpartum haemorrhage; third-stage labour; uterine atony.*

**Methylin**
Rontag, Arg.; Mallinckrodt, USA.
Methylphenidate hydrochloride (p.1590·2).
*Attention deficit hyperactivity disorder; minimal brain dysfunction; narcoleptic syndrome.*

**Methyment** Pharmonta, Austria.
Aluminium acetotartrate (p.1652·3); aluminium formate; methylthioninium chloride (p.1042·2).
*Inflammation and infection of the mouth and throat.*

**Metibasol** Sanobia, Port.
Thiamazole (p.1603·3).
*Hyperthyroidism.*

**Meticel**
Note. This name is used for preparations of different composition.
Sophia, Mex.
Hypromellose (p.1579·3).
*Eye irritation.*

Alter, Spain.
Ranitidine hydrochloride (p.1285·2).
*Acid aspiration; gastro-oesophageal reflux; peptic ulcer; Zollinger-Ellison syndrome.*

**Meticil** Elvetium, Arg.
Ampicillin (p.157·1); diclofenac sodium (p.32·1).
*Mouth and throat infections.*

**Meticortelone**
Schering-Plough, Ital.; Schering-Plough, S.Afr.
Prednisolone (p.1108·1).
*Corticosteroid.*

**Meticorten**
White, Arg.; Schering-Plough, Braz.; Essex, Chile; Schering-Plough, Mex.; Schering-Plough, Port.; Schering-Plough, S.Afr.; Schering, USA.
Prednisone (p.1109·3).
*Corticosteroid.*

**Metifarma** Merck, Spain†.
Amoxicillin trihydrate (p.155·3).
*Bacterial infections.*

**Metifarma Mucolit** Merck, Spain†.
Amoxicillin trihydrate (p.155·3); bromhexine hydrochloride (p.1115·3); guaifenesin (p.1122·1).
*Respiratory-tract infections.*

**Metifex** Cassella-med, Ger.
Ethacridine lactate (p.1165·3).
*Diarrhoea; gastro-enteritis.*

**Metifex-L** Cassella-med, Ger.†.
Loperamide hydrochloride (p.1271·1).
*Diarrhoea.*

**Metiguanide** Pharmacia Upjohn, Ital.
Metformin hydrochloride (p.342·3).
*Diabetes mellitus.*

**Metilbetasone Solubile** SoSe, Ital.
Methylprednisolone acetate (p.1106·1).
*Injectable corticosteroid.*

**Metilcord** Luper, Braz.
Methyldopa (p.953·2).
*Hypertension.*

**Metilon** Daiichi, Hong Kong.
Dipyrone (p.35·3).
*Fever.*

**Metilpren** Faulding, Port.
Methylprednisolone (p.1106·1).

**Metilsedor** Elofar, Braz.†.
Dipyrone (p.35·3); papaverine (p.1728·1).
*Smooth muscle spasm.*

**Metimyd**
Schering, Canad.†; Schering-Plough, Mex.; Schering-Plough, Swed.†; Schering, USA.
Prednisolone acetate (p.1108·1); sulfacetamide sodium (p.257·3).
*Ear infections; eye infections.*

**Metina** Fournier, Ital.
Levocarnitine hydrochloride (p.1424·1).
*Carnitine deficiency; myocardial ischaemia.*

**Metinal-Idantoina** Bayer, Ital.
Phenytoin (p.370·2); methylphenobarbital (p.366·3).
*Epilepsy.*

**Metinal-Idantoina L** Bayer, Ital.
Phenytoin (p.370·2); methylphenobarbital (p.366·3); phenobarbital (p.367·3).
*Epilepsy.*

**Metindo** Kenyaku, Thai.
Indometacin (p.47·3).
*Gout; musculoskeletal, joint, and peri-articular disorders; polyneuritis; sciatic pain.*

**Metinet** Nettopharma, Denm.†.
Cimetidine (p.1255·3).
*Acid aspiration; gastro-oesophageal reflux; peptic ulcer; Zollinger-Ellison syndrome.*

**Metiocolin B12** Farmasa, Braz.
Methionine (p.1042·1); choline chloride (p.1424·3); inositol (p.1701·2); vitamin $B_{12}$ (p.1458·2).
*Liver disorders.*

**Metiocolin Composto** Farmasa, Braz.
Methionine (p.1042·1); choline citrate (p.1424·3); betaine (p.1660·1); cyanocobalamin (p.1458·2).
*Liver disorders.*

**Metionina** Esfar, Port.†.
Choline (p.1424·3); inositol (p.1701·2); methionine (p.1042·1).

**Metionina Composta** Kanda, Braz.†.
Methionine (p.1042·1); choline (p.1424·3); inositol (p.1701·2); cynara (p.1678·3); boldo (p.1661·2); cascara (p.1255·1); carqueja amarga.
*Liver disorders.*

**Metirel** Pharmacia, Arg.
Hydroxychloroquine sulfate (p.452·3).
*Lupus erythematosus; rheumatoid arthritis.*

**Metison** Unison, Thai.
Cisapride (p.1259·2).
*Constipation; dyspepsia; gastro-oesophageal reflux; gastroparesis.*

**Metisona** Precimex, Mex.†.
Methylprednisolone (p.1106·1).

**Metivirol** Ripari-Gero, Ital.†.
Inosine pranobex (p.640·2).
*Viral infections.*

**Metixen** Berlin-Chemie, Ger.†.
Metixene hydrochloride (p.485·3).
*Drug-induced extrapyramidal disorders; parkinsonism.*

**Meto** ABZ, Ger.; Alpharma-Isis, Ger.; APS, Ger.; Phamos, Ger.
Metoprolol tartrate (p.957·1).
*Arrhythmias; hypertension; ischaemic heart disease; migraine; myocardial infarction.*

**Meto comp** ABZ, Ger.
Metoprolol tartrate (p.957·1); hydrochlorothiazide (p.933·2).
*Hypertension.*

**Metobeta** Betapharm, Ger.
Metoprolol tartrate (p.957·1).
*Arrhythmias; hypertension; ischaemic heart disease; migraine; myocardial infarction.*

**Metobeta comp** Betapharm, Ger.
Metoprolol tartrate (p.957·1); hydrochlorothiazide (p.933·2).
*Hypertension.*

**Metoblock** Silom, Thai.
Metoprolol tartrate (p.957·1).
*Angina pectoris; arrhythmias; hypertension; myocardial infarction.*

**Metoc** Oriental, Arg.
Metoclopramide (p.1274·3).
*Gastrointestinal disorders.*

**Metocal** Rottapharm, Ital.
Calcium carbonate (p.1254·2).
*Calcium deficiency; calcium supplement.*

**Metocal Vitamina D** Rottapharm, Ital.
Calcium carbonate (p.1254·2); colecalciferol (p.1461·3).
*Calcium and vitamin D deficiency; osteoporosis.*

**Metocalcium** Rottapharm, Fr.
Calcium carbonate (p.1254·2); colecalciferol (p.1461·3).
*Calcium and vitamin D supplement.*

**Metocar** Pharmacodane, Denm.
Metoprolol (p.956·3).
*Angina pectoris; arrhythmias; hypertension; hyperthyroidism; migraine; myocardial infarction.*

**Metoclan** Medinfar, Port.
Metoclopramide hydrochloride (p.1274·3).
*Dyspepsia; gastritis; nausea and vomiting.*

**Metoclor** Pharmaland, Thai.
Metoclopramide hydrochloride (p.1274·3).
*Gastrointestinal motility disorders; nausea and vomiting.*

**Metoclosan** Sanval, Braz.
Metoclopramide hydrochloride (p.1274·3).
*Nausea and vomiting.*

**Meto-comp** Ratiopharm, Ger.†.
Metoprolol tartrate (p.957·1); hydrochlorothiazide (p.933·2).
*Hypertension.*

**Metocontin** Modi-Mundipharma, India.
Metoclopramide hydrochloride (p.1274·3).
*Duodenitis; dyspepsia; gastritis; gastro-oesophageal reflux; nausea and vomiting.*

**Metocor** Rowex, Irl.
Metoprolol tartrate (p.957·1).
*Angina pectoris; arrhythmias; hypertension; hyperthyroidism; migraine; myocardial infarction.*

**Metocyl**
Rowa, Hong Kong; Rowa, Irl.; Rowa, Malaysia; Rowa, Singapore.
Metoclopramide hydrochloride (p.1274·3).
*Gastrointestinal disorders.*

**Metodine** Searle, Mex.
Diiodohydroxyquinoline (p.603·3); metronidazole (p.607·2) or metronidazole benzoate (p.607·2).

**Metodoc** Docpharm, Ger.
Metoprolol tartrate (p.957·1).
*Angina pectoris; arrhythmias; heart failure; hypertension; migraine; myocardial infarction.*

**Metodura** Merck dura, Ger.
Metoprolol tartrate (p.957·1).
*Arrhythmias; hypertension; ischaemic heart disease; migraine; myocardial infarction.*

**Metodura comp** Merck dura, Ger.
Metoprolol tartrate (p.957·1); hydrochlorothiazide (p.933·2).
*Hypertension.*

**Metofen Compound** Raza, Malaysia; Pharmaniaga, Malaysia.
Dextromethorphan hydrobromide (p.1117·3); promethazine hydrochloride (p.439·1).
*Coughs.*

**Metofen Forte** Raza, Malaysia; Pharmaniaga, Malaysia.
Dextromethorphan hydrobromide (p.1117·3).
*Coughs.*

**Metogastron** Hexal, Austria.
Metoclopramide hydrochloride (p.1274·3).
*Nausea and vomiting; upper gastrointestinal motility disorders.*

**Metohexal**
Hexal, Austral.; Hexal, Austria; Hexal, Ger.
Metoprolol tartrate (p.957·1).
*Angina pectoris; arrhythmias; hypertension; hyperthyroidism; migraine; myocardial infarction.*

**Metohexal comp** Hexal, Ger.
Metoprolol tartrate (p.957·1); hydrochlorothiazide (p.933·2).
*Hypertension.*

**Metolar** Cipla, India.
Metoprolol tartrate (p.957·1).
*Angina pectoris; arrhythmias; myocardial infarction.*

**Metole** Merck, Hong Kong.
Metronidazole (p.607·2).
*Amoebiasis; giardiasis; ulcerative gingivitis.*

**Metolol**
Douglas, Austral.; Ratiopharm, Austria†; Pharmaland, Thai.
Metoprolol tartrate (p.957·1).
*Angina pectoris; arrhythmias; hypertension; hyperthyroidism; migraine; myocardial infarction.*

**Metolol compositum** Ratiopharm, Austria†.
Metoprolol tartrate (p.957·1); hydrochlorothiazide (p.933·2).
*Hypertension.*

**Metolon** Malaysia Chemist, Singapore.
Metoclopramide hydrochloride (p.1274·3).
*Nausea and vomiting.*

**MetoMed** S Med, Austria.
Metoprolol tartrate (p.957·1).
*Angina pectoris; arrhythmias; hypertension; migraine; myocardial infarction.*

**Metomerck** Merck dura, Ger.
Metoprolol tartrate (p.957·1).
*Arrhythmias; hypertension; ischaemic heart disease; migraine; myocardial infarction.*

**Metomide** Grunenthal, Port.
Co-trimoxazole (p.199·3).
*Bacterial infections.*

**Metomin** Pacific, NZ.
Metformin hydrochloride (p.342·3).
*Diabetes mellitus.*

**Metomit** Laboratorios Chile, Chile.
Mitomycin (p.573·3).
*Malignant neoplasms.*

**Metono** Milano, Thai.†.
Metoclopramide hydrochloride (p.1274·3).
*Nausea and vomiting.*

**Metop** Gerard, Irl.
Metoprolol tartrate (p.957·1).
*Angina pectoris; arrhythmias; hypertension; hyperthyroidism; migraine; myocardial infarction.*

**Metopal** Aliud, Austria.
Metoprolol tartrate (p.957·1).
*Angina pectoris; arrhythmias; hypertension; hyperthyroidism; migraine; myocardial infarction.*

**Metopiron**
Novartis, Neth.; Novartis, Swed.
Metyrapone (p.1715·1).
*Cushing's syndrome; diagnosis of ACTH deficiencies or adrenocortical hyperfunction; hyperaldosteronism; oedema.*

**Metopirone**
Novartis, Austral.; Novartis, Fr.; Novartis, Irl.; Novartis, NZ†; Novartis, Switz.; Alliance, UK; Ciba-Geigy, USA.
Metyrapone (p.1715·1).
*Cushing's syndrome; diagnosis of ACTH deficiencies or adrenocortical hyperfunction; hyperaldosteronism.*

**Metoplex** Jean-Marie, Hong Kong.
Dextromethorphan hydrobromide (p.1117·3); carbinoxamine maleate (p.426·3); bromhexine hydrochloride (p.1115·3); ephedrine hydrochloride (p.1120·1); caffeine (p.782·1); papaverine hydrochloride (p.1728·1).
*Coughs; viscous bronchial secretions.*

**Metopram** Leiras, Fin.
Metoclopramide hydrochloride (p.1274·3).
*Adjunct in gastrointestinal investigations; gastro-oesophageal reflux; gastrointestinal motility disorders; nausea and vomiting.*

**Metopresol** Tecnofarma, Mex.
Metoprolol (p.956·3).
*Hypertension.*

**Metopress**
Agis, Israel; Ecosol, Switz.
Metoprolol tartrate (p.957·1).
*Angina pectoris; arrhythmias; hypertension; hyperthyroidism; migraine; myocardial infarction.*

**Metoprin** Bunker, Braz.
Co-trimoxazole (p.199·3).
*Bacterial infections; Pneumocystis carinii pneumonia; protozoal infections.*

**Metoprin Balsamico** Bunker, Braz.†.
Co-trimoxazole (p.199·3); guaifenesin (p.1122·1); ammonium chloride (p.1115·2).
*Bacterial infections.*

**Metoprogamma** Worwag, Ger.
Metoprolol tartrate (p.957·1).
*Arrhythmias; hypertension; ischaemic heart disease; migraine; myocardial infarction.*

**Metoprolin** Ratiopharm, Fin.
Metoprolol tartrate (p.957·1).
*Angina pectoris; arrhythmias; hypertension; hyperthyroidism; migraine; myocardial infarction.*

**Metoral** Unison, Thai.
Triamcinolone acetonide (p.1110·2).
*Mouth disorders.*

**Metorene** Sanofi Synthelabo, Spain†.
Naftazone (p.757·1).
*Peripheral vascular disorders.*

**Metorfan** Fonten, Ital.
Dextromethorphan hydrobromide (p.1117·3).
*Coughs.*

**Metoros** Novartis, Austria†.
Metoprolol fumarate (p.956·3).
*Angina pectoris; hypertension.*

**Metosan** Lannacher, Austria.
Beclometasone dipropionate (p.1091·1).
*Obstructive airways disease.*

**Metosix** Igefarma, Braz.†.
Metoclopramide hydrochloride (p.1274·3).
*Nausea and vomiting.*

**Metostad Comp** Stada, Ger.
Metoprolol tartrate (p.957·1); hydrochlorothiazide (p.933·2).
*Hypertension.*

**Metosyn**
Bioglan, Denm.; Zeneca, Irl.†; Bioglan, Norw.; Bioglan, Singapore†; GP, UK.
Fluocinonide (p.1101·3).
*Skin disorders.*

**Meto-Tablinen** Lichtenstein, Ger.
Metoprolol tartrate (p.957·1).
*Arrhythmias; hypertension; ischaemic heart disease; migraine; myocardial infarction.*

**meto-thiazid** CT, Ger.
Metoprolol tartrate (p.957·1); hydrochlorothiazide (p.933·2).
*Hypertension.*

**Metotyrol** Tyrol, Austria.
Metoprolol tartrate (p.957·1).
*Angina pectoris; arrhythmias; hypertension; hyperthyroidism; migraine; myocardial infarction.*

**Metovit** Brasmedica, Braz.†.
Metoclopramide hydrochloride (p.1274·3).
*Nausea and vomiting.*

**Metoxiprim** Rhein, Mex.
Co-trimoxazole (p.199·3).
*Bacterial infections.*

**Metozoc**
Gea, Denm.; Gea, Fin.; Gea, Norw.
Metoprolol tartrate (p.957·1).
*Angina pectoris; arrhythmias; hypertension; hyperthyroidism; migraine; myocardial infarction.*

**Metozzard** Pizzard, Mex.†.
Metoprolol (p.956·3).

**Metral** Sanitas, Arg.
Metronidazole (p.607·2).
*Anaerobic bacterial infections; protozoal infections.*

**Metram** Merck, Hong Kong.
Metoclopramide hydrochloride (p.1274·3).
*Duodenitis; dyspepsia; flatulence; gastritis; gastro-oesophageal reflux; nausea and vomiting; peptic ulcer.*

**Metran** Aventis, Spain†.
Cefpirome sulfate (p.178·2).
*Bacterial infections.*

**Metrazole**
MDI, S.Afr.; General Drugs, Thai.
Metronidazole (p.607·2).
*Anaerobic bacterial infections; protozoal infections.*

**Metrazone** Boehringer de Angeli, Braz.†.
Feprazone (p.43·1).
*Fever; musculoskeletal and joint disorders.*

**Metrecina** Liferpal, Mex.
Oxytetracycline (p.241·1).
*Bacterial infections.*

**Metrergina** Biol, Arg.
Ergometrine maleate (p.1684·1).
*Postpartum haemorrhage.*

**Metreton** Schering, Canad.†.
Prednisone acetate (p.1109·3); chlorphenamine maleate (p.427·3); ascorbic acid (p.1460·2).
*Hypersensitivity disorders.*

**Metrexato** Blausiegel, Braz.
Methotrexate sodium (p.568·3).

**Metricom** Protein, Mex.†.
Metronidazole (p.607·2).

**Metrigen Fuerte** Organon, Mex.
Estradiol benzoate (p.1550·1); progesterone (p.1566·2).
*Menstrual disorders.*

**Metrim** Siam Bheasach, Thai.
Co-trimoxazole (p.199·3).
*Bacterial infections.*

**Metrine** TP, Thai.
Methylergometrine maleate (p.1714·2).
*Postpartum haemorrhage; postpartum uterine atony.*

**Metrizol** Liferpal, Mex.
Metronidazole (p.607·2).
*Protozoal infections.*

**Metro** McGaw, USA†.
Metronidazole (p.607·2).
*Amoebiasis; anaerobic bacterial infections; trichomoniasis.*

**Metrocide** Pharmaland, Thai.
Metronidazole (p.607·2).
*Amoebiasis; trichomoniasis.*

**Metrocream**
Galderma, Canad.; Galderma, Chile; Galderma, Mex.; Galderma, USA.
Metronidazole (p.607·2).
*Rosacea.*

**Metrodax** Rayton, Braz.
Metronidazole (p.607·2) or metronidazole benzoate (p.607·2).

**Metroderme** Galderma, Port.
Metronidazole (p.607·2).
*Rosacea.*

**Metrodin**
Serono, Austral.; Serono, Braz.; Serono, Canad.†; Serono, Gr.; Serono, Hong Kong; Serum Institute, India; Serono, Irl.; Teva, Israel; Serono, Israel; Serono, Ital.; Serono, Neth.†; Serono, NZ†; Serono, Port.; Serono, S.Afr.; Serono, Singapore; Serono, Switz.; Serono, Thai.†; Serono, UK†; Serono, USA.
Urofollitropin (p.1342·1).
*Male and female infertility.*

**Metrodine** Serono, Fr.†.
Urofollitropin (p.1342·1).
*Female infertility; ovarian stimulation for fertilisation in vitro.*

**Metrodiyod** Serral, Mex.
Diiodohydroxyquinoline (p.603·3); metronidazole (p.607·2).
*Amoebiasis; giardiasis; trichomoniasis.*

**Metrofur** Sanofi Synthelabo, Mex.
Metronidazole (p.607·2); nystatin (p.406·3).
*Trichomoniasis.*

**Metrogel**
Galderma, Canad.; Galderma, Chile; Galderma, Denm.; Galderma, Ger.; Bioglan, Irl.†; Galderma, Mex.; Galderma, Neth.; Novartis, UK; Galderma, USA.
Metronidazole (p.607·2).
*Fungating malodorous tumours; rosacea.*

**Metrogel Vaginal** 3M, USA.
Metronidazole (p.607·2).
*Bacterial vaginosis.*

**Metrogyl**
Alphapharm, Austral.; Cooper (Κοπερ), Gr.; Alphapharm, Hong Kong; Unique, India; Teva, Israel; Unique, Thai.
Metronidazole (p.607·2) or metronidazole benzoate (p.607·2).
*Anaerobic bacterial infections; protozoal infections.*

**Metrogyl-F** Unique, India.
Metronidazole (p.607·2) or metronidazole benzoate (p.607·2); furazolidone (p.605·2).
*Amoebiasis; giardiasis.*

**Metrolex** Siam Bheasach, Thai.
Metronidazole (p.607·2).
*Amoebiasis; anaerobic bacterial infections; giardiasis; trichomoniasis.*

**Metrolyl** Sandoz, UK.
Metronidazole (p.607·2).
*Anaerobic bacterial infections.*

**Metronib** Ibfarma, Braz.†.
Metronidazole (p.607·2).
*Bacterial infections; protozoal infections.*

**Metronide**
Aventis, Austral.; Prodotti, Braz.†; Clonmel, Irl.
Metronidazole (p.607·2).
*Anaerobic bacterial infections; protozoal infections.*

**Metronid-Puren** Alpharma-Isis, Ger.
Metronidazole (p.607·2).
*Anaerobic bacterial infections; protozoal infections.*

**Metronil**
Cazi, Braz.; Sydenham, Mex.†.
Metronidazole benzoate (p.607·2).

**Metronimerck** Merck dura, Ger.
Metronidazole (p.607·2).
*Anaerobic bacterial infections; protozoal infections.*

**Metronix** Cristalia, Braz.
Metronidazole (p.607·2).
*Anaerobic bacterial infections; protozoal infections.*

**Metronour** Nourypharma, Ger.
Metronidazole (p.607·2).
*Anaerobic bacterial infections; protozoal infections.*

**Metront** Hexal, Ger.
Metronidazole (p.607·2).
*Anaerobic bacterial infections; protozoal infections.*

**Metropast** Pasteur, Chile.
Metronidazole (p.607·2).
*Anaerobic bacterial infections; protozoal infections.*

**Metrosa** Linderma, UK.
Metronidazole (p.607·2).
*Rosacea.*

**Metroson** Sons, Mex.
Metronidazole (p.607·2).
*Amoebiasis; trichomoniasis.*

**Metrostat** Propan, S.Afr.
Metronidazole (p.607·2).
*Anaerobic bacterial infections; protozoal infections.*

**Metrotex** Aventis, Braz.†.
Methotrexate (p.568·2).
*Malignant neoplasms.*

**Metrotop**
SSL, Irl.; SSL, UK.
Metronidazole (p.607·2).
*Malodorous fungating tumours; malodorous skin ulcers; rosacea.*

**Metroval** Sanval, Braz.
Metronidazole (p.607·2) or metronidazole benzoate (p.607·2).

**Metrozine** Searle, Hong Kong†.
Metronidazole (p.607·2).
*Anaerobic bacterial infections.*

**Metrozol**
Elofar, Braz.†; Parkfields, UK.
Metronidazole (p.607·2).
*Bacterial infections; protozoal infections.*

**Metrozole** Malayan, Singapore.
Metronidazole (p.607·2).
*Anaerobic bacterial infections; protozoal infections.*

**Met-Rx** Met-Rx, USA.
Preparations for enteral nutrition (p.1417·1).

**Metsal**
3M, Austral.; 3M, Hong Kong; 3M, Malaysia; 3M, NZ; 3M, Singapore.
Menthol (p.1711·3); eucalyptus oil (p.1686·2); methyl salicylate (p.59·3).
*Musculoskeletal, joint, peri-articular, and soft-tissue disorders.*

**Metsal Analgesic** 3M, Austral.†.
Trolamine salicylate (p.95·3); menthol (p.1711·3).
*Muscle pain.*

**Metsal AR Analgesic** 3M, Austral.
Trolamine salicylate (p.95·3).
*Musculoskeletal and joint pain.*

**Metsal AR Heat Rub** 3M, Austral.†.
Methyl salicylate (p.59·3); eucalyptus oil (p.1686·2); menthol (p.1711·3).
*Musculoskeletal and joint pain.*

**Metsal Heat Rub** 3M, Austral.†.
Methyl salicylate (p.59·3); eucalyptus oil (p.1686·2); menthol (p.1711·3).
*Musculoskeletal and joint pain.*

**Metsal Liniment** 3M, Austral.†.
Methyl salicylate (p.59·3).
*Musculoskeletal and joint disorders.*

**Metsec** TP, Thai.
Omeprazole (p.1278·2).
*Gastro-oesophageal reflux; peptic ulcer; Zollinger-Ellison syndrome.*

**Met-Sil** TP, Thai.
Metoclopramide hydrochloride (p.1274·3).
*Gastrointestinal motility disorders; nausea and vomiting.*

**Metubine**
Lilly, Canad.†; Dista, USA†.
Metocurine iodide (p.1403·3).
*Competitive neuromuscular blocker.*

**Metussa** Jean-Marie, Singapore†.
Carbinoxamine maleate (p.426·3); dextromethorphan hydrobromide (p.1117·3).
*Coughs.*

**Metussan** Biomedis, Thai.; Great Eastern, Thai.
Dextromethorphan hydrobromide (p.1117·3); chlorphenamine maleate (p.427·3); guaifenesin (p.1122·1); sodium citrate (p.1223·2).
*Coughs.*

**Metvix**
Photocure, Swed.; Galderma, UK.
Methyl aminolevulinate hydrochloride (p.527·2).
*Actinic keratoses; basal cell carcinoma.*

**Metxaprim** General Drugs, Thai.
Co-trimoxazole (p.199·3).
*Bacterial infections.*

**Metypred** Galen, Ger.
Methylprednisolone (p.1106·1) or methylprednisolone sodium succinate (p.1106·2).
*Corticosteroid.*

**Metypresol** Intramed, S.Afr.†.
Methylprednisolone sodium succinate (p.1106·2).
*Corticosteroid.*

**Metysolon** Dermapharm, Ger.
Methylprednisolone (p.1106·1).
*Corticosteroid.*

**Mevacor**
Merck Sharp & Dohme, Austria; Merck Sharp & Dohme, Braz.; Merck Frosst, Canad.; Merck Sharp & Dohme, Denm.; Merck Sharp & Dohme, Fin.; Vianex (Βιανεξ), Gr.; Merck Sharp & Dohme, Hong Kong; Merck Sharp & Dohme, Malaysia; Merck Sharp & Dohme, Mex.; Merck Sharp & Dohme, Norw.; Merck Sharp & Dohme, Spain; Merck, USA.
Lovastatin (p.949·1).
*Atherosclerosis; hypercholesterolaemia.*

**Mevalon** Guidotti, Ital.
Meglutol (p.952·1).
*Hyperlipidaemias.*

**Mevalotin**
Sankyo, Braz.; Sankyo, Ger.; Bristol-Myers Squibb, Jpn; Sankyo, Switz.; Sankyo, Thai.
Pravastatin sodium (p.984·3).
*Hypercholesterolaemia.*

**Mevamox** Teuto, Braz.
Meloxicam (p.56·1).

**Mevaren** Juste, Spain.
Estradiol valerate (p.1550·2); dienogest (p.1548·1).
*Menopausal disorders.*

**Mevasterol** Cantabria, Spain.
Lovastatin (p.949·1).
*Atherosclerosis; hypercholesterolaemia.*

**Mevastin** Genepharm, Gr.
Lovastatin (p.949·1).
*Primary hypercholesterolaemia.*

**Mevedal** Help, Gr.
Nabumetone (p.63·3).
*Inflammation; musculoskeletal and joint disorders; pain.*

**Mevilin-L**
Evans Medical, Israel†; Medeva, UK†.
A measles vaccine (Schwarz strain) (p.1623·1).
*Active immunisation.*

**Mevinacor**
Merck Sharp & Dohme, Ger.; Merck Sharp & Dohme, Port.
Lovastatin (p.949·1).
*Hypercholesterolaemia.*

**Mevinol** Vianex (Βιανεξ), Gr.
Lovastatin (p.949·1).
*Primary hypercholesterolaemia.*

**Mevlor**
Merck Sharp & Dohme, Arg.; Pharmacia, Port.
Lovastatin (p.949·1).
*Atherosclerosis; hypercholesterolaemia.*

**Mex** Phoenix, Arg.
Pseudoephedrine hydrochloride (p.1129·2).
*Nasal congestion.*

**Mexalen** Ratiopharm, Austria.
Paracetamol (p.76·2).
*Fever; pain.*

**Mexan** Teva, Israel.
Mesna (p.1041·2).
*Prevention of ifosfamide or cyclophosphamide urothelial toxicity.*

**Mexasone** Malayan, Singapore.
Dexamethasone (p.1097·1).
*Corticosteroid.*

**Mexa-Vit C** Ratiopharm, Austria.
Paracetamol (p.76·2); ascorbic acid (p.1460·2).
*Cold symptoms.*

**Mexcyn** Ofimex, Mex.†.
Erythromycin (p.208·1).

**Mexe N** Merckle, Ger.
Codeine phosphate (p.27·1); paracetamol (p.76·2).
*Pain.*

**Mexilen** Rafa, Israel.
Mexiletine hydrochloride (p.958·1).
*Ventricular arrhythmias.*

**Mexitil**
Boehringer Ingelheim, Austral.; Boehringer Ingelheim, Austria; Boehringer Ingelheim, Belg.; Boehringer de Angeli, Braz.; Boehringer Ingelheim, Canad.; Boehringer Ingelheim, Denm.†; Boehringer Ingelheim, Fin.; Boehringer Ingelheim, Fr.†; Boehringer Ingelheim, Ger.; Boehringer Ingelheim, Gr.; Boehringer Ingelheim, Hong Kong; German Remedies, India; Boehringer Ingelheim, Irl.; Boehringer Ingelheim, Ital.; Boehringer Ingelheim, Mex.; Boehringer Ingelheim, Neth.†; Boehringer Ingelheim, Norw.†; Boehringer Ingelheim, NZ; Boehringer Ingelheim, S.Afr.; Boehringer Ingelheim, Spain; Boehringer Ingelheim, Swed.; Boehringer Ingelheim, Switz.†; Boehringer Ingelheim, Thai.; Boehringer Ingelheim, UK; Boehringer Ingelheim, USA.
Mexiletine hydrochloride (p.958·1).
*Ventricular arrhythmias.*

**Mexitilen** Boehringer Ingelheim, Arg.
Mexiletine hydrochloride (p.958·1).
*Arrhythmias.*

**Mexona** Orthos, Mex.†.
Dexamethasone (p.1097·1).
*Corticosteroid.*

**Mexsana** Schering-Plough, USA.
Kaolin (p.1268·3); eucalyptus oil (p.1686·2); camphor (p.1665·3); corn starch (p.1449·1); lemon oil (p.1706·2); zinc oxide (p.1163·2).
*Nappy rash.*

**Meylon** Otsuka, Jpn.
Sodium bicarbonate (p.1223·2).
*Drug intoxication; metabolic acidosis; nausea; vomiting.*

**Mezabox** Sriprasit, Thai.
Dipyrone (p.35·3).
*Pain.*

**Mezen** Errekappa, Ital.
Promelase (p.1735·2).
*Inflammation; oedema.*

**Mezenol** Aspen, S.Afr.
Co-trimoxazole (p.199·3).
*Bacterial infections.*

**Mezinc** Abigo, Swed.
Zinc oxide (p.1163·2); zinc resin (p.1469·2).
*Wound dressing.*

**Meziv** Euroderm, Ital.
Methionine (p.1042·1); vitamin B substances (p.1417·1); zinc sulfate (p.1469·3).
*Hair loss.*

**Mezlin** Bayer, USA†.
Mezlocillin sodium (p.231·1).
*Bacterial infections.*

**Mezolitan** Pharmaten (Φαρματεν), Gr.
Miconazole nitrate (p.405·3).
*Fungal skin infections.*

**Mezym F** Berlin-Chemie, Ger.
Pancreatin (p.1725·3).
*Pancreatic disorders.*

**MF 110** Max Farma, Ital.†.
Nimesulide (p.67·1).
*Fever; inflammation; pain.*

**MFV-Ject** Pasteur Merieux, UK†.
An inactivated influenza vaccine (split virion) (p.1620·2).
*Active immunisation.*

**MG400** Triton, USA.
Salicylic acid (p.1157·1); sulfur (p.1158·2).
*Seborrhoea.*

**MG 50** Terapeutico, Ital.
Magnesium proteinate (p.1227·3).
*Magnesium deficiency; magnesium supplement.*

**MG Cold Sore Formula** Outdoor Recreations, USA.
Menthol (p.1711·3); lidocaine (p.1377·3).

**Mg 5-Granoral** Vifor, Switz.
Magnesium aspartate (p.1227·3).
*Magnesium deficiency; magnesium supplement.*

**Mg 5-Granulat** Artesan, Ger.; Cassella-med, Ger.
Magnesium aspartate (p.1227·3).
*Magnesium deficiency.*

**Mg 5-Longoral**
Kolassa, Austria; Artesan, Ger.; Cassella-med, Ger.; Vifor, Switz.
Magnesium aspartate (p.1227·3).
*Magnesium deficiency; magnesium supplement.*

**MG217 Medicated** Triton, USA.
Coal tar (p.1159·2).
MG217 Medicated shampoo and ointment formerly contained coal tar, salicylic acid, and colloidal sulfur.
*Skin disorders.*

**MG217 Medicated Tar-Free** Triton, USA.
Sulfur (p.1158·2); salicylic acid (p.1157·1).
*Dandruff.*

**Mg 5-Oraleff** Vifor, Switz.
Magnesium aspartate (p.1227·3).
*Magnesium deficiency; magnesium supplement.*

**MG217 Sal-Acid** Triton, USA.
Salicylic acid (p.1157·1).
*Psoriasis.*

**Mg 5-Sulfat**
Artesan, Ger.; Cassella-med, Ger.; Vifor, Switz.
Magnesium sulfate (p.1228·2).
*Arrhythmias; eclampsia; fetal hypotrophy; magnesium deficiency; myocardial infarction; pre-eclampsia; premature labour.*

**Mg-nor** Teofarma, Ger.
Magnesium aspartate (p.1227·3).
*Magnesium deficiency.*

**MHP-A** Cypress, USA.
Hyoscyamine sulfate (p.485·1); methenamine (p.230·1); salol (p.88·1); atropine sulfate (p.477·1); methylthioninium chloride (p.1042·2); benzoic acid (p.1169·3).
*Lower urinary-tract disorders.*

**Miabene** Ratiopharm, Austria.
Mianserin hydrochloride (p.306·3).
*Depression.*

**Miacalcic**
Novartis, Austral.; Novartis, Austria; Novartis, Belg.; Novartis, Braz.; Novartis, Chile; Novartis, Denm.; Novartis, Fin.; Novartis, Fr.; Novartis, Gr.; Novartis, Hong Kong; Novartis, Israel; LPB, Ital.; Novartis, Malaysia; Novartis, Mex.; Novartis, Norw.; Novartis, NZ; Novartis, Port.; Novartis, S.Afr.; Novartis, Singapore; Novartis, Spain; Novartis, Swed.; Novartis, Switz.; Novartis, Thai.; Novartis, UK.
Calcitonin (salmon) (p.768·2).
*Acute pancreatitis; hypercalcaemia; hyperparathyroidism; osteolytic or osteopenic bone pain; osteoporosis; Paget's disease of bone; reflex sympathetic dystrophy; vitamin D intoxication.*

**Miacalcin**
Novartis, Canad.; Novartis, USA.
Calcitonin (salmon) (p.768·2).
*Hypercalcaemia; osteoporosis; Paget's disease of bone.*

**Mi-Acid** Major, USA.
Aluminium hydroxide (p.1249·2); magnesium hydroxide (p.1272·2); simeticone (p.1289·2).
*Hyperacidity.*

**Mi-Acid Gelcaps** Major, USA.
Calcium carbonate (p.1254·2); magnesium carbonate (p.1272·1).
*Hyperacidity.*

**Miadenil**
Anpharm (Ανφαρμ), Gr.; Francia, Ital.
Calcitonin (salmon) (p.768·2).
*Hypercalcaemia; osteoporosis; Paget's disease of bone; reflex sympathetic dystrophy.*

**Mialgex** Cazi, Braz.
Methyl salicylate (p.59·3); turpentine oil (p.1760·1); camphor (p.1665·3); mustard oil (p.1718·2); rosemary oil (p.1740·2); lavender oil (p.1705·2).
*Musculoskeletal and joint disorders.*

**Mialin** Biomedica, Ital.
Alprazolam (p.668·3).
*Anxiety disorders.*

**Miambutol** Wyeth Lederle, Ital.
Ethambutol hydrochloride (p.211·3).
*Tuberculosis.*

**Mianeurin** Hexal, Ger.
Mianserin hydrochloride (p.306·3).
*Depression.*

**Miantor** Pharmacia Upjohn, Mex.†.
Etomidoline.

**Miantrex** Pharmacia, Braz.
Methotrexate (p.568·2).
*Malignant neoplasms.*

**Miaxan** Orion, Fin.
Mianserin hydrochloride (p.306·3).
*Depression; insomnia.*

**Miazide** Cyanamid, Ital.†.
Ethambutol hydrochloride (p.211·3); isoniazid (p.222·2).
*Tuberculosis.*

**Miazide B6** Wyeth Lederle, Ital.
Ethambutol hydrochloride (p.211·3); isoniazid (p.222·2); pyridoxine hydrochloride (p.1456·3).
*Tuberculosis.*

**Mibazol** Precimex, Mex.†.
Metronidazole (p.607·2).

**Mibrox** Orion, Ger.†.
Ambroxol hydrochloride (p.1114·3).
*Respiratory disorders associated with viscid or excessive mucus.*

**Miburell** Sanorell, Ger.
Homoeopathic preparation.

**Mica** Epifarma, Ital.
Heparin calcium (p.927·3).
*Thromboembolic disorders.*

**Mical** Sam-On, Israel.
Carbocisteine (p.1116·2).
*Respiratory-tract disorders associated with viscous mucus.*

**Micalpha** Chrispa (Χρισπα), Gr.
Amikacin sulfate (p.154·1).
*Bacterial infections.*

**Micane** Edol, Port.
Miconazole nitrate (p.405·3).
*Fungal and Gram-positive bacterial skin infections.*

**Micanol**
Link, Austral.; Schering, Austria; Tramedico, Belg.; Canderm, Canad.; Bioglan, Denm.; Bioglan, Fin.; Bioglan, Ger.; Bioglan, Hong Kong; Celltech, Irl.; Bioglan, Israel; Bioglan, Norw.; AFT, NZ; CS, Port.†; Bioglan, Singapore†; Vinas, Spain; Bioglan, Swed.; Bioglan, Thai.; Bioglan, UK.
Dithranol (p.1146·1).
*Psoriasis.*

**Micar** Microsules, Arg.
Piroxicam (p.84·2).
*Fever; inflammation; pain.*

**Micardis**
Boehringer Ingelheim, Arg.; Boehringer Ingelheim, Austral.; Boehringer Ingelheim, Belg.; Boehringer de Angeli, Braz.; Boehringer Ingelheim, Canad.; Boehringer Ingelheim, Chile; Boehringer Ingelheim, Denm.; Boehringer Ingelheim, Fin.; Boehringer Ingelheim, Fr.; Boehringer Ingelheim, Ger.; Boehringer Ingelheim, Gr.; Boehringer Ingelheim, Hong Kong; Boehringer Ingelheim, Irl.; Boehringer Ingelheim, Ital.; Boehringer Ingelheim, Malaysia; Boehringer Ingelheim, Mex.; Boehringer Ingelheim, Neth.; Boehringer Ingelheim, Norw.; Boehringer Ingelheim, Port.; Boehringer Ingelheim, S.Afr.; Boehringer Ingelheim, Singapore; Boehringer Ingelheim, Spain; Boehringer Ingelheim, Swed.; Boehringer Ingelheim, Switz.; Boehringer Ingelheim, Thai.; Boehringer Ingelheim, UK; Boehringer Ingelheim, USA.
Telmisartan (p.1010·1).
*Hypertension.*

**Micardis HCT** Boehringer Ingelheim, USA.
Telmisartan (p.1010·1); hydrochlorothiazide (p.933·2).
*Hypertension.*

**Micardis Plus**
Boehringer Ingelheim, Austral.; Boehringer Ingelheim, Canad.; Boehringer Ingelheim, Chile; Boehringer Ingelheim, Port.; Boehringer Ingelheim, Spain.
Telmisartan (p.1010·1); hydrochlorothiazide (p.933·2).
*Hypertension.*

**MicardisPlus**
Boehringer Ingelheim, Fr.; Boehringer Ingelheim, Irl.; Boehringer Ingelheim, UK.
Telmisartan (p.1010·1); hydrochlorothiazide (p.933·2).
*Hypertension.*

**Micarzin** AF, Mex.†.
Ibuprofen (p.45·3).
*Inflammation; musculoskeletal and joint disorders; pain.*

**Micatin**
McNeil Consumer, Canad.; Advanced Care, USA.
Miconazole nitrate (p.405·3).
*Fungal skin infections.*

**Micaveen**
Note. This name is used for preparations of different composition.
Rydelle, Fr.†.
Avena (p.1658·2); undecenoic acid (p.410·3).
*Fungal skin infections.*
Johnson & Johnson, Ital.
Avena (p.1658·2).
*Soap substitute.*
Dermoteca, Port.†.
Avena (p.1658·2); undecenoic acid (p.410·3); benzoic acid (p.1169·3).
*Fungal skin infections.*

**Micazin** Chew, Thai.
Miconazole (p.405·2).
*Fungal skin and nail infections.*

**Miccil** Senosiain, Mex.
Bumetanide (p.877·2).
*Hypertension; oedema.*

**Micebrina** Sanofi Synthelabo, Spain.
A range of multivitamin preparations with or without minerals (p.1417·1).

**Micelle E** HSL, NZ.
*d*-Alpha tocoferil acetate (p.1465·1).
*Vitamin E supplement.*

**Micerfin** Kampel Martian, Arg.
Lomifylline; dihydroergocristine (p.1680·1).
*Cerebrovascular disorders.*

**Micetal**
Silesia, Chile; Uriach, Spain.
Flutrimazole (p.400·3).
*Fungal skin infections.*

**Micetinoftalmina** Davi, Port.
Chloramphenicol (p.185·1).
*Bacterial eye infections.*

**Miciclin** Reuffer, Mex.†.
Tetracycline (p.266·2).
*Bacterial infections.*

**Micifrona** Iquinosa, Spain.
Lespedeza capitata.
*Uraemia.*

**Miclast** Pierre Fabre, Ital.
Ciclopirox olamine (p.396·1).
*Fungal skin and vaginal infections.*

**Miclobet** Rayere, Mex.
Betamethasone (p.1093·1); clotrimazole (p.396·2); gentamicin (p.219·1).
*Infected skin disorders.*

**Miclonazol** Cazi, Braz.
Clotrimazole (p.396·2).
*Fungal infections.*

**Micoban** Genepharm, Gr.
Mupirocin (p.233·1).
*Bacterial skin infections.*

**Micocert** Sidus, Arg.
Piroctone olamine (p.1155·2); climbazole (p.396·2).
*Scalp disorders.*

**Micocid** Windson, Braz.†.
Salicylic acid (p.1157·1); benzoic acid (p.1169·3); iodine (p.1598·1).
*Fungal skin infections.*

**Micocide** Bago, Arg.
Econazole nitrate (p.397·2).
*Fungal skin, nail, and vaginal infections.*

**Micoderm** Kemyos, Ital.†.
Miconazole nitrate (p.405·3).
*Fungal and bacterial infections.*

**Micoespec** Centrum, Spain.
Econazole nitrate (p.397·2).
*Fungal skin and nail infections.*

**Micoffen** Offenbach, Mex.
Miconazole nitrate (p.405·3).
*Fungal skin infections.*

**Micofim** Elofar, Braz.
Miconazole nitrate (p.405·3).
Formerly contained benzoic acid, salicylic acid, and iodine.
*Fungal skin infections.*

**Micofin** Andromaco, Chile.
Fluconazole (p.398·1).
*Fungal infections.*

**Micofitex** Pharmacia, Arg.
Econazole nitrate (p.397·2).
*Fungal skin infections.*

**Micofoot** Zeta, Ital.
Undecenoic acid (p.410·3); usnic acid (p.1762·1); salicylic acid (p.1157·1); aluminium acetate (p.1652·3).
*Disinfection of skin, burns, and wounds; fungal skin infections.*

**Micofulvin** Cantabria, Spain.
Fenticonazole nitrate (p.397·3).
*Fungal infections.*

**Micogal** Galen, Mex.†.
Ketoconazole (p.403·3).
*Fungal infections.*

**Micogel** Cipla, India.
Miconazole nitrate (p.405·3).
*Fungal infections of the skin and nails; Gram-positive bacterial skin infections.*

**Micogen** Genepharm, Gr.
Fluprednidene (p.1102·2); miconazole (p.405·2).
*Fungal skin infections with inflammation.*

**Micogin** Crosara, Ital.†.
Econazole nitrate (p.397·2).
*Fungal and bacterial infections.*

**Micogyn** Elofar, Braz.
Miconazole nitrate (p.405·3).
*Vulvovaginal candidiasis.*

**Micoisdin** Isdin, Spain.
Tolnaftate (p.410·1).
*Fungal skin infections.*

**Micoless** Sigma, Braz.†.
Miconazole nitrate (p.405·3).
*Fungal skin infections.*

**Micolette**
Dominion, Irl.; Pinewood, UK.
Sodium citrate (p.1223·2); sodium lauril sulfoacetate (p.1574·3); glycerol (p.1694·3).
*Bowel evacuation; constipation.*

**Micolis**
ICN, Arg.; Pharma Investi, Chile.
Econazole nitrate (p.397·2).
*Fungal infections.*

**Micolis Novo** ICN, Arg.
Fluconazole (p.398·1).
*Fungal infections.*

**Micoliv** Farmalab, Braz.
Ciclopirox olamine (p.396·1).
*Fungal vulvovaginal infections.*

**Micomax** Max Farma, Ital.†.
Miconazole pivoxil chloride (p.406·1).
*Fungal infections; Gram-positive bacterial superinfections.*

**Micomazol** ICN, Arg.
Clotrimazole (p.396·2).
*Fungal skin infections.*

**Micomazol B** ICN, Arg.
Clotrimazole (p.396·2); betamethasone dipropionate (p.1093·1).
*Infected skin disorders.*

**Micomazol Deo** ICN, Arg.
Clotrimazole (p.396·2).
*Fungal skin infections.*

**Micomicen** Sanofi Synthelabo, Ital.
Ciclopirox olamine (p.396·1).
*Vulvovaginal candidiasis.*

**Micomisan** Restan, S.Afr.
Clotrimazole (p.396·2).
*Fungal skin infections; vaginal candidiasis.*

**Miconacina** Grin, Mex.
Natamycin (p.406·2).
*Bacterial eye infections.*

**Miconal** Ecobi, Ital.
Miconazole (p.405·2) or miconazole nitrate (p.405·3).
*Fungal infections; secondary Gram-positive bacterial infections.*

**Miconan** Ativus, Braz.
Ketoconazole (p.403·3).
*Fungal infections.*

**Miconax** Teuto, Braz.†.
Miconazole nitrate (p.405·3).
*Fungal infections.*

**Miconol** Lafedar, Arg.
Miconazole (p.405·2).
*Fungal skin infections.*

**Micopirox** Cassara, Arg.
Ciclopirox (p.396·1).
*Fungal skin infections.*

**Micoplex** Cazi, Braz.
Tiabendazole (p.114·2); neomycin sulfate (p.235·1).
*Skin infections.*

**Micoral**
ICN, Arg.; Elofar, Braz.
Ketoconazole (p.403·3).
*Fungal infections.*

**Micoren** Novartis Consumer, Ital.
Prethcamide (p.1592·3).
*Respiratory insufficiency.*

**Micos** AGIPS, Ital.
Econazole (p.397·1) or econazole nitrate (p.397·2).
*Fungal infections; Gram-positive bacterial infections.*

**Micosan** Brasmedica, Braz.†.
Undecenoic acid (p.410·3); triacetin (p.410·2); hexachlorophene (p.1181·2).
*Skin disinfection.*

**Micoser** Serral, Mex.
Ketoconazole (p.403·3).
*Fungal infections.*

**Micoset** Bago, Chile.
Terbinafine hydrochloride (p.408·2).
*Fungal skin and nail infections.*

**Micosid** Wayne, Mex.†.
Miconazole (p.405·2).

**Micosil** Teuto, Braz.
Terbinafine hydrochloride (p.408·2).
*Fungal skin infections.*

**Micosol** Cassara, Arg.
Bifonazole (p.395·1).
*Fungal skin infections.*

**Micosona** Schering, Spain.
Naftifine hydrochloride (p.406·2).
*Fungal skin infections.*

**Micostatin**
Bristol-Myers Squibb, Arg.; Bristol-Myers Squibb, Braz.; Bristol-Myers Squibb, Chile; Bristol-Myers Squibb, Mex.†.
Nystatin (p.406·3).
*Candidiasis.*

**Micosten** Hexal, Braz.
Clotrimazole (p.396·2).
*Fungal infections.*

**Micostop** Andromaco, Chile.
Terbinafine hydrochloride (p.408·2).
*Fungal skin and nail infections.*

**Micostyl**
Stiefel, Braz.; Stiefel, Mex.
Econazole nitrate (p.397·2).
*Fungal skin, scalp, and nail infections.*

**Micotar** Dermapharm, Ger.
Miconazole (p.405·2) or miconazole nitrate (p.405·3).
*Fungal infections of the skin and mucous membranes.*

**Micotarin** Uniao Quimica, Braz.†.
Miconazole (p.405·2).
*Fungal infections.*

**Micotef** LPB, Ital.
Miconazole (p.405·2) or miconazole nitrate (p.405·3).
*Fungal infections; Gram-positive bacterial infections.*

**Micotenk** Biotenk, Arg.
Itraconazole (p.401·3).
*Fungal infections.*

**Micotiazol** Cazi, Braz.
Benzoic acid (p.1169·3); salicylic acid (p.1157·1); iodine (p.1598·1).
*Fungal skin infections.*

**Micoticum** Vita, Spain.
Ketoconazole (p.403·3).
*Fungal infections.*

**Micotissim** Stevia, Braz.†.
Salicylic acid (p.1157·1); benzoic acid (p.1169·3); iodine (p.1598·1); sumatra benzoin (p.1751·1).
*Fungal skin infections.*

**Micotopic** Recalcine, Chile.
Bifonazole (p.395·1).
*Fungal skin infections.*

**Micotox** Ibefar, Braz.†.
Undecenoic acid (p.410·3); sodium propionate (p.408·1); benzoic acid (p.1169·3); copper sulfate (p.1426·1); menthol (p.1711·3); coumarin (p.1676·2).
*Disinfection.*

**Micotral** LA, Arg.
Miconazole (p.405·2).
*Fungal skin infections.*

**Micotrat** Delta, Braz.
Clotrimazole (p.396·2).
*Fungal infections.*

**Micotrim** Key, Arg.
Clotrimazole (p.396·2).
*Fungal skin infections.*

**Micotrim P** Key, Arg.
Miconazole nitrate (p.405·3).
*Fungal skin infections.*

**Micotrim S** Key, Arg.
Miconazole nitrate (p.405·3).
*Fungal skin infections.*

**Micotrizol** Eurofarma, Braz.†.
Clotrimazole (p.396·2).
*Fungal skin infections.*

**Micoxolamina** Mastelli, Ital.
Ciclopirox olamine (p.396·1).
*Fungal infections.*

**Micoz** Hexal, Braz.
Undecenoic acid (p.410·3); sodium undecenoate (p.411·1); salicylic acid (p.1157·1); benzoic acid (p.1169·3); hexylresorcinol (p.1182·1); sumatra benzoin (p.1751·1).
*Skin infections.*

**Micozen** Teuto, Braz.
Miconazole nitrate (p.405·3).
*Fungal infections.*

**Micozol Compuesto** Klonal, Arg.
Ketoconazole (p.403·3); hydrocortisone (p.1103·3); gentamicin (p.219·1).
*Infected skin disorders.*

**Micozole**
Taro, Canad.
Miconazole nitrate (p.405·3).
*Vaginal fungal infections.*

AFT, NZ†.
Miconazole (p.405·2).
*Vulvovaginal candidiasis.*

**Micrainin** Wallace, USA.
Aspirin (p.15·1); meprobamate (p.706·2).
*Pain.*

**Micral Test** Roche Diagnostics, Irl.
Test for microalbuminuria.

**Micral Test II**
Roche Diagnostics, Austral.; Roche, Mex.; Roche Diagnostics, UK.
Test for microalbuminuria in diagnosis of diabetic nephropathy.

**Micral Test S** Lakeside, Mex.†.
Test for microalbuminuria.

**Micralax**
Pharmacia, Spain; Celltech, UK.
Sodium citrate (p.1223·2); sodium alkylsulfoacetate (p.1574·3).
*Bowel evacuation; constipation.*

**Micraleve** Elvetium, Arg.
Mitoxantrone hydrochloride (p.575·2).
*Malignant neoplasms.*

**Micraltest II** Roche, Chile.
Test for microalbuminuria.

**Micranet** Ogna, Ital.
Propyphenazone (p.85·3); paracetamol (p.76·2); caffeine (p.782·1).
*Migraine; toothache.*

**Micranil** Phoenix, Arg.
Sumatriptan succinate (p.471·2).
*Migraine.*

**Micreme** Pacific, NZ.
Miconazole nitrate (p.405·3).
*Fungal and Gram-positive bacterial infections of skin and vulvovagina.*

**Micreme H** Pacific, NZ.
Miconazole nitrate (p.405·3); hydrocortisone (p.1103·3).
*Infected skin disorders.*

**MICRhoGAM** Ortho Diagnostic, USA.
An anti-D immunoglobulin (p.1608·1).
*Prevention of rhesus sensitisation.*

**Micristin** OPW, Ger.†.
Aspirin (p.15·1).
*Myocardial infarction; thrombosis prophylaxis; vascular disorders.*

**Micro +** Sabex, Canad.†.
A range of trace element preparations (p.1417·1).

**Micro I** Sabex, Canad.†.
Sodium iodide (p.1598·1).
*Trace element additive.*

**Micro Cr** Sabex, Canad.†.
Chromium trichloride (p.1425·1).
*Trace element additive.*

**Micro Cu** Sabex, Canad.†.
Copper sulfate (p.1426·1).
*Trace element additive.*

**Micro Mn** Sabex, Canad.†.
Manganese sulfate (p.1440·1).
*Trace element additive.*

**Micro Se** Sabex, Canad.†.
Selenious acid (p.1444·1).
*Trace element additive.*

**Micro Zn** Sabex, Canad.†.
Zinc sulfate (p.1469·3).
*Trace element additive.*

**Microalbustix** Bayer Diagnostics, Irl.
Test for albumin and creatinine in urine.

**Microbactim** Pharmacos, Mex.
Co-trimoxazole (p.199·3).
*Bacterial infections.*

**Microbamat** Sanochemia, Austria.
Meprobamate (p.706·2).
*Anxiety disorders; sleep disorders.*

**Microbar-Colon** Bracco, Switz.†.
Barium sulfate (p.1061·1).
*Contrast medium for gastrointestinal radiography.*

**Microbar-HD (E-Z-HD)** Bracco, Switz.
Barium sulfate (p.1061·1).
*Contrast medium for gastrointestinal double-contrast radiography.*

**Microbiogen** Brasmedica, Braz.†.
Betamethasone dipropionate (p.1093·1); gentamicin sulfate (p.217·1).
*Infected skin disorders.*

**Microbumintest** Bayer Diagnostici, Ital.†.
Test for albumin in urine.

**Microcasen** Casen Fleet, Spain†.
Sodium lauril sulfoacetate (p.1574·3); sodium citrate (p.1223·2).
*Bowel evacuation; constipation; painful defaecation.*

**Microcid**
Note. This name is used for preparations of different composition.
Bioglan, Denm.; Bioglan, Swed.
Hydrogen peroxide (p.1182·2).
*Bacterial skin infections.*

Boniscontro & Gazzone, Ital.
Cefonicid sodium (p.174·2).
Lidocaine hydrochloride (p.1377·3) is included in this preparation to alleviate the pain of injection.
*Gram-negative bacterial infections.*

**Microcidal** Aspen, S.Afr.
Griseofulvin (p.400·3).
*Fungal infections of the skin and nails.*

**Microclisma Evacuante AD-BB** Sofar, Ital.†.
Glycerol (p.1694·3); chamomile (p.1669·3); mallow (p.1709·3).

**Microclismi Marco Viti** Marco Viti, Ital.
Glycerol (p.1694·3); chamomile (p.1669·3); mallow (p.1709·3).
*Bowel evacuation; constipation.*

**Microclismi Sella** Sella, Ital.
Glycerol (p.1694·3); chamomile (p.1669·3); mallow (p.1709·3).
*Bowel evacuation; constipation.*

**Microdiol**
Organon, Braz.; Organon, Israel; Organon, Spain.
Desogestrel (p.1547·2); ethinylestradiol (p.1553·2).
*Combined oral contraceptive; menstrual disorders.*

**Microdit** Kener, Mex.†.
Ranitidine (p.1285·2).

**Microdoine** Gomenol, Fr.
Nitrofurantoin (p.237·2).
*Cystitis.*

**Microfemin** Grunenthal, Chile.
21 Tablets ethinylestradiol (p.1553·2); levonorgestrel (p.1563·2); 7 tablets, ferrous fumarate (p.1427·3).
*Combined oral contraceptive.*

**Microfer** Vianex (Βιανεξ), Gr.
Ferrous sulfate (p.1428·2).
*Iron-deficiency anaemia.*

**Microgel** Restan, S.Afr.
*Oral suspension:* Dicycloverine hydrochloride (p.481·2); aluminium hydroxide (p.1249·2); magnesium oxide (p.1272·3); simeticone (p.1289·2).
*Tablets:* Calcium carbonate (p.1254·2); magnesium carbonate (p.1272·1); magnesium trisilicate (p.1272·3); simeticone (p.1289·2).
*Gastrointestinal disorders.*

**Microgen** Silesia, Chile.
Gestodene (p.1556·1); ethinylestradiol (p.1553·2).
*Combined oral contraceptive.*

**Microgest** Schering, Thai.
21 Tablets, levonorgestrel (p.1563·2); ethinylestradiol (p.1553·2); 7 tablets, inert.
*Combined oral contraceptive.*

**Microgeste** Schering, Port.
Gestodene (p.1556·1); ethinylestradiol (p.1553·2).
*Combined oral contraceptive.*

**Microginon** Schering, Port.
Levonorgestrel (p.1563·2); ethinylestradiol (p.1553·2).
*Combined oral contraceptive.*

**Microgyn** Schering, Denm.
Levonorgestrel (p.1563·2); ethinylestradiol (p.1553·2).
*Combined oral contraceptive.*

**Microgynon**
Schering, Arg.; Schering, Austral.; Schering, Austria; Schering, Belg.; Schering, Chile; Schering, Fin.; Schering, Ger.; Schering, Hong Kong; Schering, Israel; Schering, Ital.; Schering, Mex.; Schering, Neth.; Schering, Norw.; Schering, NZ; Schering, Singapore; Schering, Spain; Schering, Switz.; Schering, Thai.
Levonorgestrel (p.1563·2); ethinylestradiol (p.1553·2).
28-Day packs also contain 7 inert tablets.
*Combined oral contraceptive.*

**Microgynon 30**
Schering, Irl.; Schering, Malaysia; Schering, UK.
Levonorgestrel (p.1563·2); ethinylestradiol (p.1553·2).
28-Day packs also contain 7 inert tablets.
*Combined oral contraceptive.*

**Micro-K**
Wyeth-Ayerst, Canad.; Ther-Rx, USA.
Potassium chloride (p.1232·2).
*Hypokalaemia; potassium depletion.*

**Microka** ICN, Mex.
Vitamin A (p.1451·2); phytomenadione (p.1467·1).
*Bruising; periorbital hyperpigmentation; purpuric or petechial discharge; telangiectasia.*

**Micro-Kalium** Lannacher, Austria.
Potassium chloride (p.1232·2).
*Potassium deficiency.*

**Microklist**
Pharmacia, Austria; Pharmacia Upjohn, Ger.; Pharmacia, Switz.
Sodium citrate (p.1223·2); sodium lauril sulfoacetate (p.1574·3); sorbitol (p.1446·3).
*Bowel evacuation; constipation.*

**Microlax**
Note. This name is used for preparations of different composition.
Pharmacia, Austral.; Pharmacia, Belg.; Pharmacia, Canad.; Pharmacia, Fin.; Pharmacia, Fr.; Pharmacia, Hong Kong; Pharmacia, Malaysia; Pharmacia, Norw.; Pharmacia, NZ; Pharmacia, S.Afr.; Pharmacia, Swed.; Pharmacia, Switz.†.
Sodium citrate (p.1223·2); sodium lauril sulfoacetate (p.1574·3); sorbitol (p.1446·3).
*Bowel evacuation; constipation.*

Pharmacia, Denm.; Pharmacia, Irl.; Sanofi Synthelabo, Mex.; Bonafarma, Port.; Pharmacia, Singapore.
Sodium citrate (p.1223·2); sodium lauril sulfoacetate (p.1574·3).
*Bowel evacuation; constipation.*

Pharmacia, Neth.
Sodium lauril sulfoacetate (p.1574·3); sorbitol (p.1446·3).
*Bowel evacuation; constipation.*

**Microlet** Dexxon, Israel.
Sodium citrate (p.1223·2); sodium lauril sulfoacetate (p.1574·3); glycerol (p.1694·3).
*Constipation.*

**Microlev** Ido, Fr.
Dried yeast (p.1469·1).
*Vitamin B deficiency.*

**Microlevlen ED** Schering, Austral.
21 Tablets, levonorgestrel (p.1563·2); ethinylestradiol (p.1553·2); 7 tablets, inert.
*Combined oral contraceptive.*

**Microlipid**
Mead Johnson Nutritionals, Canad.; Sherwood, USA.
Preparation for enteral nutrition containing safflower oil (p.1443·3) (p.1417·1).

**Microlite** Schering, Irl.
Ethinylestradiol (p.1553·2); levonorgestrel (p.1563·2).
*Combined oral contraceptive.*

**Microlut**
Schering, Arg.; Schering, Austral.; Schering, Belg.; Schering, Chile; Schering, Ger.; Schering, Ital.†; Schering, Mex.; Schering, NZ; Schering, Switz.
Levonorgestrel (p.1563·2).
*Progestogen-only oral contraceptive.*

**Microluton**
Schering, Denm.; Schering, Fin.; Schering, Norw.
Levonorgestrel (p.1563·2).
*Progestogen-only oral contraceptive.*

**Micromex** Recalcine, Chile.
Omeprazole (p.1278·2).
*Gastric hyperacidity.*

**Micromycin** Darier, Mex.
Minocycline hydrochloride (p.231·3).
*Bacterial infections.*

**Micronase** Pharmacia Upjohn, USA.
Glibenclamide (p.331·2).
*Diabetes mellitus.*

**microNefrin** Bird, USA.
Racepinefrine hydrochloride (p.854·1).
*Bronchospasm.*

**Micronema** Gador, Arg.
Glycerol (p.1694·3).
*Constipation.*

**Micronoan** Abbott, Ital.
Diazepam (p.690·1).
*Epilepsy; sedative.*

**Micronor**
Janssen-Cilag, Austral.; Janssen-Cilag, Braz.; Janssen-Ortho, Canad.; Janssen-Cilag, Irl.†; Janssen-Cilag, UK.
Norethisterone (p.1562·2).
*Progestogen-only oral contraceptive.*

**Micronor HRT** Janssen-Cilag, UK.
Norethisterone (p.1562·2).
*Menopausal disorders.*

**Micronovum**
Janssen-Cilag, Austria; Janssen-Cilag, Ger.†; Janssen-Cilag, S.Afr.; Janssen-Cilag, Switz.
Norethisterone (p.1562·2).
*Progestogen-only oral contraceptive.*

**Micropaque**
Codali, Belg.; Guerbet, Denm.; Guerbet, Fr.; Guerbet, Ger.; R+N, Gr.; Guerbet, Neth.†; Guerbet, Port.; Pan Quimica, Spain; Guerbet, Switz.
Barium sulfate (p.1061·1).
*Contrast medium for gastrointestinal radiography.*

**Microphta** Europhta, Mon.
Micronomicin sulfate (p.231·3).
*Bacterial eye infections.*

**Microphyllin** Aventis, S.Afr.
Theophylline (p.798·3).
*Asthma; bronchospasm.*

**Micropil** Sigma, Braz.
Gestodene (p.1556·1); ethinylestradiol (p.1553·2).
*Combined oral contraceptive.*

**Micropirin**
Dexcel, Israel; Ratiopharm, UK.
Aspirin (p.15·1).
*Thrombosis prophylaxis.*

**Micropur**
Sirmeta, Austral.†; Voyage, Fr.
Silver chloride complex (p.1746·1).
*Water disinfection.*

**Micropyrin** Nicholas Piramal, India.
Aspirin (p.15·1); caffeine (p.782·1).
*Fever; inflammation; pain.*

**Microrgan** Liomont, Mex.
Ciprofloxacin hydrochloride (p.188·2).
*Bacterial infections.*

**Microsan N** Biosyn, Ger.
Multivitamin and magnesium preparation (p.1417·1).

**Microser**
Grunenthal, Arg.; Grunenthal, Chile; Formenti, Ital.
Betahistine hydrochloride (p.1660·1).
*Vestibular disorders.*

**Microshield 2, 4 and 5** Johnson & Johnson, Austral.
Chlorhexidine gluconate (p.1173·2).
*Skin, wound, and instrument disinfection.*

**Microshield Antimicrobial Hand Gel** Johnson & Johnson, Austral.
Alcohol (p.1166·1).
*Skin disinfection.*

**Microshield Antiseptic** Johnson & Johnson, Austral.
Cetrimide (p.1172·1); chlorhexidine gluconate (p.1173·2).
*Skin, wound, burn, and instrument disinfection.*

**Microshield Handrub** Johnson & Johnson, Austral.
Chlorhexidine gluconate (p.1173·2); alcohol (p.1166·1).
*Skin disinfection.*

**Microshield PVP** Johnson & Johnson, Austral.
Povidone-iodine (p.1190·3).
*Skin disinfection.*

**Microshield PVP Plus** Johnson & Johnson, Austral.†.
Povidone-iodine (p.1190·3); triclosan (p.1195·2).
*Skin disinfection.*

**Microshield PVP-S** Johnson & Johnson, Austral.
Povidone-iodine (p.1190·3).
*Bacterial or fungal skin and mucous membrane infections; skin, wound, and burn disinfection.*

**Microshield T** Johnson & Johnson, Austral.
Triclosan (p.1195·2).
*Skin disinfection.*

**Microshield Tincture** Johnson & Johnson, Austral.
Chlorhexidine gluconate (p.1173·2); alcohol (p.1166·1).
*Skin, surface, and instrument disinfection.*

**Microsol** Herbaxt, Fr.
A range of trace element and mineral preparations (p.1417·1).

**Microsona** ICN, Arg.
Hydrocortisone (p.1103·3).
*Skin disorders.*

**Microsona C** ICN, Arg.
Hydrocortisone acetate (p.1103·3); ketoconazole (p.403·3); gentamicin sulfate (p.217·1).
*Infected skin disorders.*

**Microsona Otica** ICN, Arg.
Hydrocortisone (p.1103·3); acetic acid (p.1645·2).
*Ear disorders.*

**Microstix-3**
Ames, Israel; Bayer, USA.
Test for nitrite in urine and for bacterial growth.

**Microstix Candida** Ames, Israel.
Test for *Candida albicans* in vaginal flora.

**Microsulf** Microsules, Arg.
Ciprofloxacin hydrochloride (p.188·2).
*Bacterial infections.*

**Microterol** Microsules, Arg.
Salbutamol sulfate (p.791·3).
*Obstructive airways disease.*

**Microtid** Kener, Mex.†.
Ranitidine (p.1285·2).

**Microtrast**
Guerbet, Denm.; Guerbet, Fr.; Guerbet, Ger.; Guerbet, Port.
Barium sulfate (p.1061·1).
*Contrast medium for gastrointestinal radiography.*

**Microtrim** Rosen, Ger.
Co-trimoxazole (p.199·3).
*Bacterial infections.*

**Microvacin** Asta Medica, Braz.
Bacterial antigens.
*Allergen immunotherapy.*

**Microval**
Wyeth, Austral.; Wyeth Lederle, Belg.; Wyeth, Chile; Wyeth Lederle, Denm.†; Wyeth Lederle, Fr.; Wyeth, NZ; Akromed, S.Afr.; Wyeth, UK.
Levonorgestrel (p.1563·2).
*Progestogen-only oral contraceptive.*

**Microvibrate** Lavipharm, Gr.
Doxycycline hyclate (p.206·2).
*Bacterial infections.*

**Microvita** ICN, Mex.
Vitamin A (p.1451·2).
*Acne; cellulitis; keratinisation disorders; sun-induced skin damage.*

**Microvlar**
Schering, Arg.; Schering, Braz.
Levonorgestrel (p.1563·2); ethinylestradiol (p.1553·2).
*Combined oral contraceptive.*

**Microxin** Rayere, Mex.
Norfloxacin (p.238·3).
*Bacterial infections.*

**Microzepam** Microsules, Arg.
Lorazepam (p.704·1).
*Anxiety.*

**Microzide** Watson, USA.
Hydrochlorothiazide (p.933·2).
*Hypertension; oedema.*

**Mictarin** Sedabel, Braz.†.
Sodium benzoate (p.1169·3); methenamine (p.230·1).
*Urinary-tract infections.*

**Mictasol**
Note. This name is used for preparations of different composition.
Medgenix, Belg.
Camphor monobromide; methenamine (p.230·1); mallow fruit (p.1709·3).
Formerly contained camphor monobromide, methenamine, mallow fruit, esculoside, and rutoside.
*Anorectal disorders; urogenital disorders.*

Millet Roux, Braz.
Mallow (p.1709·3).
Formerly contained mallow and camphor monobromide.
*Urinary-tract infections.*

Martin, Fr.
Mallow (p.1709·3); methenamine (p.230·1).
Formerly contained mallow, camphor monobromide, and methenamine.
*Urinary-tract disorders.*

**Mictasol Azul** GlaxoSmithKline, Arg.
Mallow (p.1709·3); camphor monobromide; methylthioninium chloride (p.1042·2).
*Genito-urinary tract disorders.*

**Mictasol Bleu**
Note. This name is used for preparations of different composition.
Martin, Fr.†.
Mallow (p.1709·3); camphor monobromide; methylthioninium chloride (p.1042·2).
*Urinary-tract infections.*

Formenti, Ital.
Mallow (p.1709·3); methylthioninium chloride (p.1042·2).
*Genito-urinary tract disorders; haemorrhoids.*

**Mictasol com Sulfa** Millet Roux, Braz.
Mallow (p.1709·3); sulfachlorpyridazine (p.258·1); camphor (p.1665·3).
*Urinary-tract infections.*

**Mictasone** Formenti, Ital.
Hydrocortisone acetate (p.1103·3); tetracycline hydrochloride (p.266·2); mallow (p.1709·3).
*Genito-urinary tract infections; haemorrhoids.*

**Mictonetten** Apogepha, Ger.
Propiverine hydrochloride (p.489·1).
*Bladder disorders; urinary incontinence.*

**Mictonorm** Apogepha, Ger.
Propiverine hydrochloride (p.489·1).
*Bladder disorders; urinary incontinence.*

**Mictral**
Sanofi Synthelabo, Irl.; Sanofi Synthelabo, UK†.
Nalidixic acid (p.234·1); sodium citrate (p.1223·2); citric acid (p.1673·1); sodium bicarbonate (p.1223·2).
*Urinary-tract infections.*

**Mictrex** Heralds, Braz.†.
Co-trimoxazole (p.199·3); phenazopyridine (p.83·2).
*Urinary-tract infections.*

**Mictrin** Econo Med, USA.
Hydrochlorothiazide (p.933·2).
*Hypertension; oedema.*

**Micturol Sedante** Bioresearch, Spain.
Phenazopyridine hydrochloride (p.83·1); sulfamethizole (p.260·3).
*Urinary-tract infections.*

**Micutrin** Monsanto, Ital.
Pyrrolnitrin (p.408·1).
*Fungal skin infections.*

**Micutrin Beta** Monsanto, Ital.
Pyrrolnitrin (p.408·1); betamethasone valerate (p.1093·2).
*Inflammatory fungal skin infections; onychomycosis.*

**Midacina** Lensa, Spain.
Fluocinolone acetonide (p.1101·2); gramicidin (p.220·2); neomycin (p.235·1).
*Infected skin disorders.*

**Midalet** Silesia, Chile.
Desogestrel (p.1547·2); ethinylestradiol (p.1553·2).
*Combined oral contraceptive.*

**Midalgan**
Note. This name is used for preparations of different composition.
Welcker-Lyster, Canad.
Histamine hydrochloride (p.1697·1); methyl nicotinate (p.59·2); glycol salicylate (p.44·3); capsaicin (p.24·2).
*Musculoskeletal and joint disorders.*

Sanofi Synthelabo, Port.
Histamine hydrochloride (p.1697·1); methyl nicotinate (p.59·2); glycol salicylate (p.44·3).
*Musculoskeletal and joint disorders.*

Qualicare, Switz.
Histamine hydrochloride (p.1697·1); methyl nicotinate (p.59·2); glycol salicylate (p.44·3); capsicum (p.1667·1).
*Musculoskeletal and joint disorders.*

**Midamor**
Merck Sharp & Dohme, Austral.; Merck Sharp & Dohme, Austria; Merck Frosst, Canad.; Merck Sharp & Dohme, Hong Kong†; Merck Sharp & Dohme, Neth.†; Merck Sharp & Dohme, Norw.†; Merck Sharp & Dohme, NZ; Merck Sharp & Dohme, Swed.; Merck Sharp & Dohme, Switz.; Merck, USA.
Amiloride hydrochloride (p.858·2).
*Heart failure; hepatic cirrhosis with ascites; hypertension; oedema.*

**Midarine**
GlaxoSmithKline, India; GlaxoSmithKline, Ital.; GlaxoSmithKline, Switz.
Suxamethonium chloride (p.1406·2).
*Depolarising neuromuscular blocker.*

**Midaselect** Curasan, Ger.
Midazolam hydrochloride (p.707·2).
*Premedication; sedative.*

**Midatenk** Biotenk, Arg.
Metoclopramide (p.1274·3).
*Gastrointestinal disorders.*

**Midax** Gador, Arg.
Olanzapine (p.710·3).
*Psychoses.*

**Midazol**
Taro, Israel; Hameln, Thai.; TTN, Thai.
Midazolam (p.707·1).
*General anaesthesia; premedication; status epilepticus.*

**Midchlor** Schein, USA†.
Isometheptene mucate (p.1702·1); dichloralphenazone (p.697·1); paracetamol (p.76·2).
*Tension and vascular headaches.*

**Midecamin**
Merck, Braz.†.
Midecamycin (p.231·3).
*Respiratory-tract infections.*

Merck, Mex.
Midecamycin acetate (p.231·3).
*Upper respiratory-tract infections.*

**Midecin** Farmaka, Ital.
Midecamycin (p.231·3).
*Bacterial infections.*

**Midelin** Quimica y Farmacia, Mex.
Dipyrone (p.35·3).
*Fever; pain.*

**Miderm** Mendelejeff, Ital.
Miconazole (p.405·2) or miconazole nitrate (p.405·3).
*Fungal and Gram-positive bacterial infections.*

**Midermus** Ofar, Arg.
Vitamin A (p.1451·2).
*Skin disorders.*

**Midetol** Precimex, Mex.
Metoclopramide (p.1274·3).
*Nausea and vomiting.*

**Midium** Teofarma, Ital.
Vitamin A palmitate (p.1453·1); tocoferil acetate (p.1465·1); pyridoxine hydrochloride (p.1456·3).
*Metabolic disorders.*

**Midol**
Note. This name is used for preparations of different composition.
Andromaco, Chile.
Paracetamol (p.76·2); ibuprofen (p.45·3).
*Fever; inflammation; musculoskeletal, joint, peri-articular, and soft-tissue disorders; pain.*

ICN, Hong Kong†.
Aspirin (p.15·1); caffeine (p.782·1); cinnamedrine hydrochloride (p.1672·2).
*Pain.*

**Midol Cramp & Body Aches** Bayer Consumer, USA.
Ibuprofen (p.45·3).
*Dysmenorrhoea; musculoskeletal and joint disorders.*

**Midol Douche** Bayer, Canad.†.
Acetic acid (p.1645·2).
*Vaginal cleansing.*

**Midol Extra Strength** Bayer Consumer, Canad.
Paracetamol (p.76·2); caffeine (p.782·1); mepyramine maleate (p.437·1).
Formerly contained paracetamol, pamabrom, mepyramine maleate.
*Dysmenorrhoea.*

**Midol Maximum Strength Multi-Symptom Menstrual** Sterling Health, USA.
Paracetamol (p.76·2); mepyramine maleate (p.437·1).
*Pain.*

**Midol Multi-Symptom** Bayer, Canad.†.
Paracetamol (p.76·2); caffeine (p.782·1); mepyramine maleate (p.437·1).
*Backache; bloating; dysmenorrhoea; headache.*

**Midol Original** Bayer, Canad.†.
Aspirin (p.15·1); cinnamedrine (p.1672·2); caffeine (p.782·1).
*Pain.*

**Midol PM** Sterling Health, USA.
Paracetamol (p.76·2); diphenhydramine (p.431·3).

**Midol PMS Extra Strength** Bayer Consumer, Canad.
Paracetamol (p.76·2); pamabrom (p.978·2); mepyramine maleate (p.437·1).
*Premenstrual syndrome.*

**Midol Pre-Menstrual Syndrome** Bayer Consumer, USA.
Paracetamol (p.76·2); pamabrom (p.978·2); mepyramine maleate (p.437·1).
*Menstrual disorders.*

**Midol Regular** Bayer Consumer, Canad.
Aspirin (p.15·1); caffeine (p.782·1).
*Pain.*

**Midol Teen Formula** Bayer Consumer, USA.
Paracetamol (p.76·2); pamabrom (p.978·2).
*Menstrual disorders.*

**Midol Traditional** Bayer Consumer, Canad.
Aspirin (p.15·1); caffeine (p.782·1).
*Dysmenorrhoea.*

**Midolam** Rafa, Israel.
Midazolam (p.707·1).
*General anaesthesia; premedication.*

**Midolen** Degorts, Mex.
Aspirin (p.15·1).
*Fever; inflammation; pain.*

**Midon** Shire, Irl.
Midodrine hydrochloride (p.959·2).
*Orthostatic hypotension.*

**Midoride** Amrad, Austral.†.
Amiloride hydrochloride (p.858·2).
*Ascites; hypertension; oedema.*

**Midotens**
Boehringer Ingelheim, Arg.; Boehringer de Angeli, Braz.; Boehringer

*Ingelheim, Denm.; Boehringer Ingelheim, Mex.; Boehringer Ingelheim, Swed.†.*
Lacidipine (p.944·2).
*Hypertension.*

**Midrat** *Novartis, Mex.*
Captopril (p.879·2).
*Diabetic nephropathy; heart failure; hypertension; myocardial infarction.*

**Midriati** *Llorens, Spain.*
Atropine sulfate (p.477·1); hyoscine hydrobromide (p.483·3); phenylephrine hydrochloride (p.1126·3).
*Eye disorders; production of mydriasis.*

**Midriaticum** *Allergan, Arg.*
Tropicamide (p.491·1).
*Production of mydriasis.*

**Midrid**
*Shire, Hong Kong; Manx, UK.*
Isometheptene mucate (p.1702·1); paracetamol (p.76·2).
*Migraine and other vascular headaches.*

**Midrin** *Women First, USA.*
Isometheptene mucate (p.1702·1); dichloralphenazone (p.697·1); paracetamol (p.76·2).
*Tension and vascular headaches.*

**Midriodavi** *Davi, Port.*
Cyclopentolate hydrochloride (p.480·3).
*Production of mydriasis.*

**Midro**
*Note. This name is used for preparations of different composition.*
*Wolfs, Belg.; Midro, Switz.*
Senna (p.1288·2).
*Constipation.*

*Vaillant, Ital.*
Senna (p.1288·2); liquorice (p.1270·2); peppermint leaf (p.1283·2); caraway (p.1667·2).
*Constipation.*

*Crefar, Port.*
Senna (p.1288·2); liquorice (p.1270·2); peppermint leaf (p.1283·2); clove (p.1673·2); calcatrippae; mallow (p.1709·3).
*Constipation.*

**Midro Abfuhr** *Midro, Ger.*
Senna (p.1288·2).
*Constipation.*

**Midro Pico** *Midro, Ger.*
Sodium picosulfate (p.1289·3).
*Constipation.*

**Midro Tee**
*Note. This name is used for preparations of different composition.*
*Sanova, Austria.*
Senna (p.1288·2); peppermint leaf (p.1283·2); caraway (p.1667·2); liquorice (p.1270·2); delphinium consolida; mallow flowers (p.1709·3).
*Constipation.*

*Midro, Ger.*
Senna (p.1288·2).
*Constipation.*

**Midro-Tea** *Midro, Israel.*
Senna (p.1288·2); peppermint leaf (p.1283·2); caraway (p.1667·2); liquorice (p.1270·2); delphinium consolida flower; mallow flower (p.1709·3).
*Constipation.*

**Miduret** *PP Lab, Thai.*
Amiloride hydrochloride (p.858·2); hydrochlorothiazide (p.933·2).
*Hepatic cirrhosis with ascites; hypertension; oedema.*

**Midy Vitamine C** *GlaxoSmithKline Sante, Fr.*
Ascorbic acid (p.1460·2).
*Asthenia; vitamin C deficiency.*

**Midysalb** *Sanofi Winthrop, Ger.†.*
Glycol salicylate (p.44·3); methyl nicotinate (p.59·2); histamine hydrochloride (p.1697·1).
*Musculoskeletal and joint disorders; neuralgia.*

**Miegel** *SAN, Ital.†.*
Honey (p.1434·2); royal jelly (p.1740·3).

**Mielocol** *Herbes Universelles, Canad.*
Guaifenesin (p.1122·1); aralia racemosa; cineole (p.1672·1); honey (p.1434·2); poplar buds (p.1733·3); sanguinaria (p.1741·3); white pine; wild cherry (p.1765·2).

**Mielogen**
*Schering-Plough, Gr.; Schering-Plough, Ital.*
Molgramostim (p.756·1).
*Neutropenia induced by antineoplastics, or bone marrow transplant.*

**Mielomade** *Esfar, Port.*
Gamma-aminobutyric acid (p.1690·2).
*Hypertension; mental function disorders.*

**Mielucin** *Zambon, Braz.†.*
Busulfan (p.532·2).
*Malignant neoplasms.*

**Mifegest** *Zydus, India.*
Mifepristone (p.1560·2).
*Termination of pregnancy.*

**Mifegyne**
*Femagen, Austria; Exelgyn, Denm.; Exelgyn, Fin.; Exelgyn, Fr.; Exelgyn, Israel; Exelgyn, Norw.; Exelgyn, Spain; Exelgyn, Swed.; Cosan, Switz.; Exelgyn, UK.*
Mifepristone (p.1560·2).
*Termination of pregnancy.*

**Mifeprex** *Danco, USA.*
Mifepristone (p.1560·2).
*Termination of pregnancy.*

**Miferen** *Sterling Health, Spain.*
Aspirin (p.15·1); chlorphenamine maleate (p.427·3); phenylpropanolamine hydrochloride (p.1127·3).
*Cold and influenza symptoms.*

**Miflasona** *Novartis, Braz.*
Beclometasone dipropionate (p.1091·1).
*Asthma.*

**Miflasone**
*Novartis, Fr.; Novartis, NZ.*
Beclometasone dipropionate (p.1091·1).
*Asthma.*

**Miflonide**
*Novartis, Austria; Novartis, Belg.; Novartis, Braz.; Novartis, Denm.; Novartis, Ger.; Novartis, Ital.; Novartis, Port.; Novartis, Spain; Novartis, Switz.*
Budesonide (p.1094·2).
*Asthma.*

**Miformin** *Greater Pharma, Thai.*
Metformin hydrochloride (p.342·3).
*Diabetes mellitus.*

**Migard** *Menarini, UK.*
Frovatriptan succinate (p.469·2).
*Migraine.*

**Migea**
*Gea, Denm.; Gea, Fin.; Gea, Norw.; Gea, Swed.*
Tolfenamic acid (p.94·2).
*Migraine.*

**Migent** *Wayne, Mex.†.*
Gentamicin (p.219·1).
*Bacterial infections.*

**Miglucan** *Roche, Fr.*
Glibenclamide (p.331·2).
*Diabetes mellitus.*

**Migpriv**
*Sanofi Synthelabo, Belg.; Sanofi Winthrop, Denm.; Sanofi Synthelabo, Fin.; Sanofi Synthelabo, Fr.; Sanofi Synthelabo, Ital.; Sanofi Synthelabo, Norw.; Sanofi Synthelabo, Swed.; Synthelabo, Switz.*
Lysine aspirin (p.54·3); metoclopramide hydrochloride (p.1274·3).
*Migraine.*

**Migra Dioxadol** *Bago, Arg.*
Metamizole magnesium (p.36·1); ergotamine tartrate (p.467·2); caffeine (p.782·1).
*Migraine.*

**Migra Dorixina** *Roemmers, Arg.*
Clonixin lysine (p.26·3); ergotamine tartrate (p.467·2).
*Migraine.*

**Migracin** *Max Farma, Ital.*
Amikacin sulfate (p.154·1).
*Bacterial infections.*

**Migradon** *Schmidgall, Austria.*
Propyphenazone (p.85·3); paracetamol (p.76·2); caffeine (p.782·1).
*Fever; pain.*

**Migraeflux MCP** *Hennig, Ger.*
Paracetamol (p.76·2); metoclopramide hydrochloride (p.1274·3).
*Migraine.*

**Migraeflux N** *Hennig, Ger.*
Orange tablets, dimenhydrinate (p.431·1); paracetamol (p.76·2); green tablets, paracetamol; codeine phosphate (p.27·1).
*Migraine and other vascular headaches.*

**Migraeflux orange N** *Hennig, Ger.*
Dimenhydrinate (p.431·1); paracetamol (p.76·2).
*Migraine and other vascular headaches.*

**Migrafen** *Chatfield Laboratories, UK.*
Ibuprofen (p.45·3).

**Migrafin** *Sanofi Synthelabo, Neth.*
Lysine aspirin (p.54·3); metoclopramide (p.1274·3).
*Migraine.*

**Migragesic** *Andromaco, Chile.*
Ergotamine tartrate (p.467·2); dipyrone (p.35·3); caffeine (p.782·1); chlorphenamine maleate (p.427·3).
*Migraine and other vascular headaches.*

**Migraine Ice** *Mentholatum, UK.*
Water-based gel compress.
*Migraine and other severe headache.*

**Migraine-Kranit** *Krewel, Switz.*
Paracetamol (p.76·2); caffeine (p.782·1); chlorphenamine maleate (p.427·3).
*Migraine and other vascular headaches.*

**Migraine-Kranit Nova** *Codali, Belg.†.*
Caffeine (p.782·1); paracetamol (p.76·2); propyphenazone (p.85·3).
*Migraine.*

**Migral**
*Note. This name is used for preparations of different composition.*
*Montpellier, Arg.*
Ergotamine tartrate (p.467·2); caffeine (p.782·1); dipyrone (p.35·3).
*Cluster headache; migraine; tension headache.*

*Glaxo Wellcome, Austral.†.*
Ergotamine tartrate (p.467·2); cyclizine hydrochloride (p.429·3); caffeine (p.782·1).
*Migraine.*

*QIF, Braz.†.*
Phenylephrine hydrochloride (p.1126·3); caffeine (p.782·1); dexbrompheniramine (p.426·2).
*Migraine.*

**Migral II** *Montpellier, Arg.*
Ibuprofen (p.45·3); caffeine (p.782·1); ergotamine tartrate (p.467·2).
*Cluster headache; migraine; tension headache.*

**Migral Compositum** *Montpellier, Arg.*
Ergotamine tartrate (p.467·2); caffeine (p.782·1); dipyrone (p.35·3); metoclopramide hydrochloride (p.1274·3).
*Cluster headache; migraine; tension headache.*

**Migralave N** *Temmler, Ger.*
Buclizine hydrochloride (p.426·3); paracetamol (p.76·2).
*Migraine and other vascular headaches.*

**Migraleve**
*Note. This name is used for preparations of different composition.*
*Pfizer Consumer, Irl.; Charwell, Singapore†; Pfizer Consumer, UK.*
Pink tablets, buclizine hydrochloride (p.426·3); paracetamol (p.76·2); codeine phosphate (p.27·1); yellow tablets, paracetamol; codeine phosphate.
*Migraine and other vascular headaches.*

*Charwell, Israel; Llorens, Spain.*
Buclizine hydrochloride (p.426·3); paracetamol (p.76·2); codeine phosphate (p.27·1); docusate sodium (p.1262·2).
*Migraine and other vascular headaches.*

*Pfizer Consumer, Port.; Simco, Switz.*
Buclizine hydrochloride (p.426·3); paracetamol (p.76·2); codeine phosphate (p.27·1).
*Migraine and other vascular headaches.*

**Migralgine** *Martin, Fr.*
Paracetamol (p.76·2); codeine phosphate (p.27·1); caffeine (p.782·1).
*Pain.*

**Migraliv** *Sigma, Braz.*
Caffeine (p.782·1); dipyrone (p.35·3); dihydroergotamine mesilate (p.465·3).
*Migraine.*

**Migramax** *Elan, UK.*
Lysine aspirin (p.54·3); metoclopramide hydrochloride (p.1274·3).
*Migraine.*

**Migranal**
*Novartis, Austria; Novartis, Canad.; Novartis, Ital.; Novartis, Swed.; Novartis, UK†; Xcel, USA.*
Dihydroergotamine mesilate (p.465·3).
*Migraine.*

**Migranat** *Rowa, Irl.*
Caffeine (p.782·1); ergotamine tartrate (p.467·2); pipoxolan hydrochloride (p.1732·1).
*Migraine and other vascular headaches.*

**Migrane** *Sigma, Braz.*
Aspirin (p.15·1); ergotamine tartrate (p.467·2); homatropine methylbromide (p.483·2); caffeine (p.782·1).
*Migraine.*

**Migra-Nefersil** *Pharma Investi, Chile.*
Clonixin lysine (p.26·3); ergotamine tartrate (p.467·2).
*Migraine and other vascular headaches.*

**Migrane-Gastreu R16** *Reckeweg, Ger.*
Homoeopathic preparation.

**Migrane-Kranit Duo** *Krewel, Ger.*
Paracetamol (p.76·2); propyphenazone (p.85·3).
*Dysmenorrhoea; headache including migraine.*

**Migrane-Kranit Kombi** *Krewel, Ger.†.*
Ethaverine hydrochloride (p.1685·2); paracetamol (p.76·2); propyphenazone (p.85·3).
*Headache including migraine.*

**Migrane-Kranit mono** *Krewel, Ger.*
Phenazone (p.82·3).
*Pain.*

**Migrane-Kranit N** *Krewel, Ger.*
Paracetamol (p.76·2); propyphenazone (p.85·3); codeine phosphate (p.27·1).
*Headache including migraine.*

**Migrane-Neuridal** *Krewel, Ger.*
Paracetamol (p.76·2); metoclopramide hydrochloride (p.1274·3).
*Migraine and other vascular headaches.*

**Migranerton** *Dolorgiet, Ger.*
Paracetamol (p.76·2); metoclopramide hydrochloride (p.1274·3).
*Migraine and other vascular headaches.*

**Migranil** *Inga, India.*
*Injection:* Dihydroergotamine mesilate (p.465·3).
*Tablets:* Ergotamine tartrate (p.467·2); caffeine (p.782·1).
*Migraine.*

**Migranin** *Boots Healthcare, Ger.*
Phenazone (p.82·3); caffeine (p.782·1).
*Migraine; pain.*

**Migranin Ibuprofen** *Boots Healthcare, Ger.*
Ibuprofen (p.45·3).
*Headache including migraine.*

**Migranol** *Bago, Chile.*
Ergotamine tartrate (p.467·2); dipyrone (p.35·3); caffeine (p.782·1).
*Migraine and other vascular headaches.*

**Migraprim** *Inverni della Beffa, Ital.*
Lysine aspirin (p.54·3); metoclopramide hydrochloride (p.1274·3).
*Migraine.*

**Migraspirina** *Bayer, Port.*
Aspirin (p.15·1).

**Migrastick** *Arkopharma, UK.*
Lavender oil (p.1705·2); peppermint oil (p.1283·2).
*Migraine.*

**Migratam** *Laboratorios Chile, Chile.*
Ergotamine tartrate (p.467·2); caffeine (p.782·1); dipyrone (p.35·3).
*Migraine and other vascular headaches.*

**Migratan S** *Berlin-Chemie, Ger.*
Ergotamine tartrate (p.467·2); propyphenazone (p.85·3).
*Migraine and other vascular headaches.*

**Migratapsin** *Maver, Chile.*
Paracetamol (p.76·2); caffeine (p.782·1); dihydroergotamine mesilate (p.465·3).
*Migraine.*

**Migratine** *Major, USA.*
Isometheptene mucate (p.1702·1); dichloralphenazone (p.697·1); paracetamol (p.76·2).
*Tension and vascular headaches.*

**Migravess** *Bayer Consumer, UK†.*
Aspirin (p.15·1); metoclopramide hydrochloride (p.1274·3).
*Migraine.*

**Migrax** *Saval, Chile.*
Paracetamol (p.76·2); caffeine (p.782·1); dihydroergotamine mesilate (p.465·3).
*Vascular headache.*

**Migretil** *Bial, Port.*
Belladonna (p.479·1); caffeine (p.782·1); ergotamine (p.468·3); paracetamol (p.76·2).
*Migraine.*

**Migrexa**
*Note. This name is used for preparations of different composition.*
*Lichtenstein, Ger.*
Ergotamine tartrate (p.467·2).
*Cluster headache; migraine.*

*Sanorania, Switz.†.*
Ergotamine tartrate (p.467·2); caffeine (p.782·1).
*Dysmenorrhoea; migraine and other vascular headaches.*

**Migril**
*Note. This name is used for preparations of different composition.*
*GlaxoSmithKline, Austria; GlaxoSmithKline, Hong Kong; Wellcome, Irl.; Glaxo Wellcome, NZ†; GlaxoSmithKline, S.Afr.; Glaxo Wellcome, Singapore†; Wellcome, Switz.†; CP Pharmaceuticals, UK.*
Ergotamine tartrate (p.467·2); cyclizine hydrochloride (p.429·3); caffeine hydrate (p.782·1).
*Migraine.*

*Sintofarma, Braz.†.*
Sumatriptan succinate (p.471·2).
*Migraine.*

**Migristene**
*Aventis, Mex.; Rhone-Poulenc Rorer, Spain†.*
Dimetiotazine mesilate (p.431·3).
*Migraine.*

**Migwell** *GlaxoSmithKline, Fr.†.*
Ergotamine tartrate (p.467·2); caffeine (p.782·1); cyclizine hydrochloride (p.429·3).
*Migraine.*

**Mihexine** *Milano, Thai.*
Bromhexine hydrochloride (p.1115·3).
*Respiratory-tract disorders associated with increased or viscous mucus.*

**Mijal** *Juste, Spain†.*
Butibufen (p.23·3).
*Musculoskeletal, joint, and peri-articular disorders; pain.*

**Mijex** *Pickles, UK.*
Diethyltoluamide (p.1503·3).
*Insect repellent.*

**Mijex Extra** *Pickles, UK.*
Butylacetylamino propionate.
*Insect repellent.*

**Mikacin** *Julphar, UAE.*
Amikacin sulfate (p.154·1).
*Bacterial infections.*

**Mikan** *Boniscontro & Gazzone, Ital.*
Amikacin sulfate (p.154·1).
*Gram-negative bacterial infections.*

**mikanil** *Mickan, Ger.*
Glycol salicylate (p.44·3); benzyl nicotinate (p.21·2).
*Musculoskeletal, joint, and soft-tissue disorders; superficial vascular disorders.*

**Mikavir** *Salus, Ital.*
Amikacin sulfate (p.154·1).
*Gram-negative bacterial infections.*

**Mikazul** *Ederka, Mex.†.*
Amikacin (p.154·1).
*Bacterial infections.*

**Mikelan**
*Lipha Sante, Fr.; Otsuka, Jpn; Aventis, S.Afr.†; Otsuka, Spain.*
Carteolol hydrochloride (p.880·3).
*Angina pectoris; arrhythmias; glaucoma; hypertension; ocular hypertension.*

**Mikesan** *Baliarda, Arg.*
Ergotamine tartrate (p.467·2); cyproheptadine hydrochloride (p.430·1); clonixin (p.26·3).
*Migraine.*

**Mi-Ke-Sons** *Sons, Mex.*
Ketoconazole (p.403·3).
*Fungal infections.*

**Miketos** *Chinoin, Mex.†.*
Ketoconazole (p.403·3).

**Mikium** *Grunenthal, Chile.*
Ciclopirox (p.396·1).
*Nail, skin, and vulvovaginal infections.*

**Miklogen** *Klonal, Arg.*
Miconazole (p.405·2); betamethasone (p.1093·1); gentamicin (p.219·1).
*Infected skin disorders.*

**Mikostat** *Julphar, UAE.*
Nystatin (p.406·3).
*Candidiasis.*

**Mikostat Baby Ointment** *Julphar, UAE.*
Nystatin (p.406·3); zinc oxide (p.1163·2).
*Fungal skin infections; nappy rash.*

**Mikozal** *Julphar, UAE.*
Miconazole nitrate (p.405·3).
*Fungal skin infections.*

**Mikro-30** *Wyeth, Ger.*
Levonorgestrel (p.1563·2).
*Progestogen-only oral contraceptive.*

**Mikrobac** *Bode, Ger.*
Benzalkonium chloride (p.1168·3); dodecylbispropylenetriamine.
*Surface disinfection.*

**Mikrozid** *Schulke & Mayr, Ger.†.*
Alcohol (p.1166·1); propyl alcohol (p.1191·2).
*Surface disinfection.*

**Mikutan N** *Streuli, Switz.*
Aluminium acetate (p.1652·3); zinc oxide (p.1163·2).
*Skin disorders.*

**Mil Cobalin Nueva Formula** *Richet, Arg.*
Hydroxocobalamin; thiamine; pyridoxine (p.1417·1).
*Neuritis; vitamin supplement.*

**Mila-Asma** *Milano, Thai.*
Theophylline (p.798·3); guaifenesin (p.1122·1).
*Obstructive airways disease.*

**Mila-Cono** *Milano, Thai.*
Codeine phosphate (p.27·1); guaifenesin (p.1122·1).
*Coughs.*

**Milafed** *Milano, Thai.*
Triprolidine hydrochloride (p.442·3); pseudoephedrine hydrochloride (p.1129·2).
*Allergic rhinitis; cold symptoms; hay fever; nasal congestion.*

**Milagin** *Milano, Thai.*
Paracetamol (p.76·2); dextromethorphan hydrobromide (p.1117·3); chlorphenamine maleate (p.427·3).
Formerly contained paracetamol, phenylpropanolamine hydrochloride, dextromethorphan hydrobromide, and chlorphenamine maleate.
*Cold symptoms.*

**Milamet** *Milano, Thai.*
Cimetidine (p.1255·3).
*Peptic ulcer.*

**Milamox** *Milano, Thai.*
Amoxicillin trihydrate (p.155·3).
*Bacterial infections.*

**Milanidazole** *Milano, Thai.*
Metronidazole (p.607·2).
*Anaerobic bacterial infections.*

**Milanolone** *Milano, Thai.*
Triamcinolone acetonide (p.1110·2).
*Mouth disorders.*

**Mila-Tercon** *Milano, Thai.*
Codeine phosphate (p.27·1); guaifenesin (p.1122·1); terpin hydrate (p.1131·1).
*Coughs.*

**Milavir** *Novartis Consumer, Spain.*
Aciclovir (p.626·1).
*Herpes simplex infections.*

**Milax** *Berlin-Chemie, Ger.*
Glycerol (p.1694·3).
*Bowel evacuation; constipation.*

**Milbedoce Anabolico** *Andromaco, Spain†.*
Cobamamide (p.1459·1); hydroxocobalamin acetate (p.1458·2).
*Tonic.*

**Milbeta** *Offenbach, Mex.*
Cyanocobalamin (p.1458·2); hydroxocobalamin (p.1458·2).

**Milbron** *Silesia, Chile.*
Ambroxol hydrochloride (p.1114·3).
*Respiratory-tract congestion.*

**Milco** *Piam, Ital.*
Preparation for enteral nutrition (p.1417·1).
*Phenylketonuria.*

**Milcopen** *Leiras, Fin.*
Phenoxymethylpenicillin potassium (p.242·1).
*Bacterial infections.*

**Mildison**
*Yamanouchi, Denm.; Yamanouchi, Fin.†; Yamanouchi, Irl.; Yamanouchi, Neth.; Yamanouchi, Norw.; CSL, NZ; Yamanouchi, NZ; Yamanouchi, Swed.; Yamanouchi, UK.*
Hydrocortisone (p.1103·3).
*Skin disorders.*

**Miles Nervine** *Miles, USA.*
Diphenhydramine hydrochloride (p.431·3).
*Insomnia.*

**Milfarin** *Milupa, Port.*
Nutritional supplement (p.1417·1).

**milgamma** *Worwag, Ger.*
Benfotiamine (p.1454·3); pyridoxine hydrochloride (p.1456·3).
*Neurological symptoms associated with vitamin B deficiency.*

**milgamma mono** *Worwag, Ger.*
Benfotiamine (p.1454·3).
*Vitamin $B_1$ deficiency.*

**milgamma N** *Worwag, Ger.*
Thiamine hydrochloride (p.1455·1); pyridoxine hydrochloride (p.1456·3); cyanocobalamin (p.1458·2).
*Myalgia; neuralgia; neuritis; polyneuropathy.*

**milgamma-NA** *Worwag, Ger.*
Benfotiamine (p.1454·3); pyridoxine hydrochloride (p.1456·3).
*Neurological symptoms associated with vitamin B deficiency.*

**Milgex** *Klinger, Braz.*
Aluminium hydroxide (p.1249·2); magnesium hydroxide (p.1272·2); dimeticone (p.1289·2).
*Flatulence; gastrointestinal hyperacidity.*

**Milical** *Recalcine, Chile.*
Sibutramine hydrochloride (p.1593·1).
*Obesity.*

**Milice** *Mipharm, Ital.*
Piperonyl butoxide (p.1509·2); pyrethrin (p.1509·3).
*Pediculosis.*

**Milid**
*Sanochemia, Austria; Opfermann, Ger.†; Rotta, Hong Kong†; Rottapharm, Ital.; Delta, Port.; Rotta, Thai.†.*
Proglumide (p.1284·3).
*Gastrointestinal disorders.*

**Milidon** *Malayan, Singapore.*
Paracetamol (p.76·2).
*Cold and influenza symptoms; fever; pain.*

**Milidon CF** *Malayan, Singapore.*
Chlorphenamine maleate (p.427·3); paracetamol (p.76·2); pseudoephedrine hydrochloride (p.1129·2).
*Nasal and sinus congestion; rhinitis.*

**Milidon Compound** *MPF, Singapore†.*
Chlorphenamine maleate (p.427·3); paracetamol (p.76·2); phenylpropanolamine hydrochloride (p.1127·3).
*Nasal and sinus congestion; rhinitis.*

**Miliken Mucol Med Retard** *Teofarma, Spain†.*
Ampicillin sodium (p.157·1); ampicillin benzathine (p.158·1); bromhexine hydrochloride (p.1115·3).
Lidocaine hydrochloride (p.1377·3) is included in this preparation to alleviate the pain of injection.
*Respiratory-tract infections.*

**Miliken Mucol Retard** *Teofarma, Spain†.*
Ampicillin sodium (p.157·1); ampicillin benzathine (p.158·1); bromhexine hydrochloride (p.1115·3); guaifenesin hydrochloride (p.1122·1).
Lidocaine hydrochloride (p.1377·3) is included in this preparation to alleviate the pain of injection.
*Respiratory-tract infections.*

**Miliken Mucolitico** *Teofarma, Spain†.*
Ampicillin sodium (p.157·1); bromhexine hydrochloride (p.1115·3); guaifenesin (p.1122·1).
Lidocaine hydrochloride (p.1377·3) is included in this preparation to alleviate the pain of injection.
*Respiratory-tract infections.*

**Milithin** *Minerva (Μινερβα), Gr.*
Lithium carbonate (p.301·1).
*Bipolar disorder; mania.*

**Milk of Magnesia**
*SmithKline Beecham, Gr.; SmithKline Beecham Consumer, Irl.; GlaxoSmithKline Consumer, UK; Cypress, USA.*
Magnesium hydroxide (p.1272·2).
*Constipation; dyspepsia; heartburn.*

**Milk Thistle** *Nutravite, Canad.*
Cynara flower (p.1678·3); silybum marianum (p.1043·3); turmeric rhizome (p.1058·3).

**Milk Thistle Formula** *Nutravite, Canad.*
Butternut root; taraxacum root (p.1751·3); liquorice root (p.1270·2); silybum marianum (p.1043·3); wild yam root.

**Milkinol** *Schwarz, USA†.*
Liquid paraffin (p.1479·1).
*Constipation.*

**Milla** *SIT, Ital.*
Chamomile (p.1669·3).

**Millerspas** *Aspen, S.Afr.*
Hyoscyamine sulfate (p.485·1); atropine sulfate (p.477·1); hyoscine hydrobromide (p.483·3); phenobarbital (p.367·3).
*Peptic ulcer; reduction of respiratory and gastrointestinal secretions; renal and biliary colic.*

**Milli Anovlar** *Schering, Fr.†.*
Norethisterone acetate (p.1562·2); ethinylestradiol (p.1553·2).
*Combined oral contraceptive.*

**Millibar**
*Lisapharma, Hong Kong; Lisapharma, Ital.; Lisapharma, Singapore.*
Indapamide (p.938·2).
*Hypertension.*

**Millicortene** *Novartis, Switz.*
Dexamethasone (p.1097·1).
*Corticosteroid.*

**Millicortenol** *Novartis, India.*
Dexamethasone (p.1097·1).
*Skin disorders.*

**Millicorten-Vioform**
*Novartis, Ger.†; Novartis, India.*
Dexamethasone pivalate (p.1097·3); clioquinol (p.196·3).
*Infected skin disorders.*

**Milligynon** *Schering, Fr.*
Norethisterone acetate (p.1562·2).
*Progestogen-only oral contraceptive.*

**Millisrol**
*Khandelwal, India; Kayaku, Jpn.*
Glyceryl trinitrate (p.923·2).
*Angina pectoris; heart failure; hypertension during surgery; maintenance of hypotension during surgery.*

**Millypar** *Adcock Ingram Self Medication, S.Afr.†.*
Magnesium hydroxide (p.1272·2); liquid paraffin (p.1479·1).
*Constipation.*

**Milneuron NA** *Worwag, Ger.*
Benfotiamine (p.1454·3); pyridoxine hydrochloride (p.1456·3).
*Neuralgia; neuritis; neurological symptoms associated with vitamin B deficiency.*

**Milneuron Plus** *Worwag, Ger.†.*
Benfotiamine; cyanocobalamin; pyridoxine hydrochloride (p.1417·1); propyphenazone (p.85·3).
*Neuralgia; neuritis; neurological symptoms associated with vitamin B deficiency.*

**Miloderme** *Schering-Plough, Port.*
Alclometasone dipropionate (p.1090·3).
*Skin disorders.*

**Milorex** *Remedica, Thai.*
Amiloride hydrochloride (p.858·2); hydrochlorothiazide (p.933·2).
*Hepatic cirrhosis with ascites; hypertension; oedema.*

**Miloride** *Pharmacia, Fin.*
Amiloride hydrochloride (p.858·2); hydrochlorothiazide (p.933·2).
*Hypertension; liver cirrhosis with ascites; oedema.*

**Mil-Par**
*Gramon, Arg.; Merck Consumer, UK.*
Magnesium hydroxide (p.1272·2); liquid paraffin (p.1479·1).
*Constipation.*

**Milpar** *Sanofi Synthelabo, Mex.*
Magnesium hydroxide (p.1272·2); liquid paraffin (p.1479·1).
*Constipation.*

**Milrila** *Yamanouchi, Jpn.*
Milrinone (p.959·2).

**Milrosina** *Biogalenica, Spain.*
Resorcinol (p.1156·3); borax (p.1661·3).
*Mouth ulcers.*

**Milrosina Nistatina** *Biogalenica, Spain.*
Hydrocortisone hydrogen succinate (p.1104·1); nystatin (p.406·3).
*Oral candidiasis.*

**Milsan** *Merck, Mex.*
Preparation for enteral nutrition (p.1417·1).
*Gastro-enteritis.*

**Milsana** *Milte, Ital.*
Zinc oxide (p.1163·2).
*Barrier cream; nappy rash.*

**Miltaun** *Byk, Austria.*
Meprobamate (p.706·2).
*Anxiety disorders; premedication; skeletal muscle spasticity; sleep disorders.*

**Miltex**
*Asta Medica, Austria; Asta Oncologia, Braz.; Asta Médica, Chile; Baxter, Chile; Asta Medica, Fin.; Baxter Oncology, Fr.; Baxter Oncology, Ger.; Asta Medica, Israel; Baxter Oncology, Singapore; Prasfarma, Spain; Asta Medica, Swed.; IDIS, UK.*
Miltefosine (p.573·2).
*Skin metastases of breast cancer.*

**Miltina HA** *Milte, Port.†.*
Infant feed (p.1417·1).
*Food hypersensitivity.*

**Miltina IPO** *Milte, Ital.*
Infant feed (p.1417·1).
*Food intolerance.*

**Milton**
*Note. This name is used for preparations of different composition.*
*Procter & Gamble, Braz.†; Lachartre, Fr.†; Procter & Gamble, Irl.†; SIT, Ital.; Ceuta, UK.*
*Liquid:* Sodium hypochlorite (p.1192·1).
*Decontamination of fruit and vegetables; sterilisation of feeding bottles; water purification.*

*Lachartre, Fr.†; Procter & Gamble, Irl.†; Ceuta, UK.*
*Sterilising tablets:* Sodium dichloroisocyanurate (p.1191·3).
*Disinfection.*

**Milton Anti-Bacterial** *Procter & Gamble, Austral.†.*
Sodium dichloroisocyanurate (p.1191·3) or sodium hypochlorite (p.1192·1).
*Disinfection of infant feeding equipment; disinfection of surfaces and equipment.*

**Miltown** *Wallace, USA.*
Meprobamate (p.706·2).
*Anxiety.*

**Milumel AR** *Milupa, Fr.*
Infant feed (p.1417·1).
*Regurgitation.*

**Milumel HA** *Milupa, Fr.*
Infant feed (p.1417·1).
*Milk-protein allergy.*

**Milumil**
*Milupa, Ital.; Milupa, Port.†.*
Infant feed (p.1417·1).
*Gastro-oesophageal reflux.*

**Milupa** *Wyeth-Ayerst, Canad.†.*
A range of foods for special diets (p.1417·1).

**Milupa Aptamil HA** *Milupa, Ital.*
Infant feed (p.1417·1).
*Food intolerance.*

**Milupa basic** *Milupa, Ital.*
A range of foods for special diets (p.1417·1).

**Milupa Biber-C** *Milupa, Ital.*
Carbohydrate, amino-acid, lipid, and mineral preparation with vitamin C (p.1417·1).
*Nutritional supplement.*

**Milupa Biberfrutta** *Milupa, Ital.*
Carbohydrate, amino-acid, and lipid preparation with vitamin C and iron (p.1417·1).
*Nutritional supplement.*

**Milupa GES**
*Milupa, Austria; Milupa, Ital.*
Glucose; electrolytes (p.1222·2).
*Diarrhoea; oral rehydration therapy.*

**Milupa HIST** *Milupa, Ital.†.*
Food for special diets (p.1417·1).
*Histidinaemia.*

**Milupa Hn 25**
*Milupa, Ital.; Byk Gulden, Mex.*
Food for special diets (p.1417·1).
*Diarrhoea; gluten intolerance.*

**Milupa HOM** *Milupa, Ital.*
Food for special diets (p.1417·1).
*Homocystinuria.*

**Milupa Low Protein Drink** *Milupa, UK.*
Food for special diets (p.1417·1).
*Inherited disorders of amino-acid metabolism in childhood.*

**Milupa lpd** *Milupa, Irl.†.*
Low-protein drink (p.1417·1).
*Disorders of amino-acid metabolism in childhood.*

**Milupa Lpf** *Milupa, Ital.*
Food for special diets (p.1417·1).
*Protein metabolism disorders; renal impairment.*

**Milupa LYS** *Milupa, Ital.*
Food for special diets (p.1417·1).
*Hyperlysinaemia.*

**Milupa MSUD** *Milupa, Ital.*
Food for special diets (p.1417·1).
*Maple syrup urine disease.*

**Milupa OS** *Milupa, Ital.*
Food for special diets (p.1417·1).
*Methylmalonic aciduria; propionic acidaemia.*

**Milupa PKU**
*Milupa, Irl.†; Milupa, Ital.*
Food for special diets (p.1417·1).
*Hyperphenylalaninaemia; phenylketonuria.*

**Milupa Pregomin** *Milupa, Ital.*
Preparation for enteral nutrition (p.1417·1).
*Diarrhoea; disorders of fructose and galactose metabolism; food hypersensitivity; gastrointestinal resection; milk and soya intolerance.*

**Milupa Som** *Milupa, Ital.*
Food for special diets (p.1417·1).
*Disaccharide deficiency; fructosaemia; galactosaemia; milk intolerance.*

**Milupa TYR** *Milupa, Ital.*
Food for special diets (p.1417·1).
*Hypertyrosinaemia.*

**Milupa UCD** *Milupa, Ital.*
Food for special diets (p.1417·1).
*Argininosuccinic aciduria; citrullinaemia; hyperammonaemia; hyperargininaemia; ornithinaemia.*

**Milurit**
*Thiemann, Ger.; Egis, Hong Kong.*
Allopurinol (p.412·2).
*Gout; hyperuricaemia; renal calculi; uric acid nephropathy.*

**Milvane**
*Schering, Denm.; Schering, Ital.; Schering, Switz.*
Gestodene (p.1556·1); ethinylestradiol (p.1553·2).
*Triphasic oral contraceptive.*

**Milyzer** *Mitsui, Jpn.*
Nateplase (p.964·2).

**Milzine** *Vickmans, Hong Kong.*
*Oral suspension:* Oxetacaine (p.1382·1); magnesium hydroxide (p.1272·2); aluminium hydroxide (p.1249·2).
*Tablets:* Oxetacaine (p.1382·1); magnesium carbonate (p.1272·1); aluminium hydroxide (p.1249·2).
*Dyspepsia; gastritis; gastro-oesophageal reflux; heartburn; peptic ulcer.*

**Mimedran** *Esteve, Spain.*
Piperazine sultamate (p.112·1).
*Hyperlipidaemias.*

**Mimixin** *Merck, Arg.*
Buflomedil (p.877·2); diosmin (p.1688·2).
*Peripheral vascular disorders; thromboses; venous insufficiency.*

**Min Huil** *Neo Dermos, Arg.*
Pyrithione zinc (p.1156·2).
*Pityriasis.*

**Min O** *Biol, Arg.*
Nystatin (p.406·3); neomycin sulfate (p.235·1); polymyxin B sulfate (p.245·1).
*Vaginal infections.*

**Minac 50** *Spirig, Switz.*
Minocycline hydrochloride (p.231·3).
*Acne.*

**Minachlor** *Esoform, Ital.*
Tosylchloramide sodium (p.1194·3).
*Disinfection of wounds, burns, and external genitalia.*

**Minadex** *Seven Seas, UK.*
Multivitamin preparation with or without minerals (p.1417·1).

**Minadex Mix** *Grifols, Spain†.*
Multivitamin and mineral preparation (p.1417·1).

**Minadex Mix Ginseng** *Grifols, Spain†.*
Multivitamins and minerals (p.1417·1); ginseng (p.1693·1).

**Minakne** *Bioglan, Ger.*
Minocycline hydrochloride (p.231·3).
*Skin disorders.*

**Minalfene** Bouchara-Recordati, Fr.
Alminoprofen (p.14·1).
*Inflammation; pain.*

**Minalgin** Streuli, Switz.
Dipyrone (p.35·3).
*Colic; fever; pain.*

**Minalka** Cedar Health, UK.
Mineral preparation with vitamin D (p.1417·1).
*Musculoskeletal and joint disorders.*

**Minamino**
MPS, Austral.†.
Vitamins, minerals, and amino acids with liver, spleen, and gastric mucosa (p.1417·1).
*Dietary supplement.*

Aspen, S.Afr.
Amino acids; vitamin B substances; minerals; organ extracts (p.1417·1).
*Tonic.*

Ayrton, UK.
Vitamin B substances; amino acids; minerals (p.1417·1).

**Minaphlex**
Scientific Hospital Supplies, Austral.; SHS, UK.
Food for special diets (p.1417·1).
*Phenylketonuria.*

**Min-A-Pon** Minerva (Μινερβα), Gr.
Nimesulide (p.67·1).
*Inflammation; musculoskeletal disorders; pain.*

**Minard's Liniment** Stella, Canad.
Camphor (p.1665·3); ammonium hydroxide; turpentine.

**Minax**
Alphapharm, Austral.; Alphapharm, Hong Kong; Merck, Thai.
Metoprolol tartrate (p.957·1).
*Angina pectoris; hypertension; migraine; myocardial infarction.*

**Minaxen** Aegis, Hong Kong.
Minocycline hydrochloride (p.231·3).
*Bacterial infections.*

**Minaza** British Dispensary, Thai.†.
Miconazole nitrate (p.405·3).
*Fungal skin, hair, and nail infections; Gram-positive bacterial skin infections.*

**Minazol** Cimed, Braz.
Phenazopyridine (p.83·2); nitroxoline (p.238·3).
*Urinary-tract infections.*

**Mincifit** Arkopharma, Fr.
Black currant leaves (p.1661·1); green tea (p.1765·3).
*Obesity.*

**Mindac** Eagle, Austral.†.
Bacopa monnieri; ginkgo biloba; centella asiatica; withania somnifera; schizandra chinensis; capsicum; glutamine; calcium glycerophosphate; nux vomica.
*Tonic.*

**Mindiab**
Pharmacia, Denm.; Pharmacia, Fin.; Pharmacia, Norw.; Pharmacia, Swed.
Glipizide (p.332·2).
*Diabetes mellitus.*

**Mindol** Pacific, NZ.
Mebendazole (p.108·2).
*Worm infections.*

**Mindol-Merck** Bracco, Ital.
Propyphenazone (p.85·3); caffeine (p.782·1); ethylmorphine hydrochloride (dionina) (p.37·3).
*Pain.*

**Mindosan V** Loren, Mex.
Miconazole nitrate (p.405·3).
*Fungal vaginal infections.*

**Minegyl** Luper, Braz.
Metronidazole (p.607·2) or metronidazole benzoate (p.607·2).

**Minegyl C/Nistatina** Luper, Braz.
Metronidazole (p.607·2); nystatin (p.406·3).
*Vaginal infections.*

**Mineral** Volchem, Ital.
Mineral preparation (p.1417·1).

**Minerasol** Pharno-Wedropharm, Ger.
Emser salts.
*Nasal congestion.*

**Minerell** Sanorell, Ger.†.
Vitamin and mineral preparation (p.1417·1).

**Minerva**
Schering, Austria; Berlipharm, Fr.; Schering, S.Afr.
Cyproterone acetate (p.1544·1); ethinylestradiol (p.1553·2).
28-Day packs also contain 7 inert tablets.
*Androgen-associated acne, seborrhoea, alopecia, or hirsutism in women; oral contraceptive in women with androgenisation.*

**Minervicomplex** Provita, Ital.†.
Multivitamin and mineral preparation (p.1417·1).

**Minervit** Medisint, Ital.
Multivitamin and mineral preparation (p.1417·1).

**Minervit Plus** Viternat, Braz.
Vitamin and mineral preparation (p.1417·1).

**Minesol** Janssen-Cilag, Braz.
Titanium; zinc; beta glucan; ginkgo biloba (p.1417·1).
*Tonic.*

**Minesse**
Wyeth, Arg.; Wyeth Lederle, Austria; Wyeth, Braz.; Wyeth, Chile; Wyeth Lederle, Fr.; Wyeth, Irl.†; Wyeth, Israel; Wyeth Lederle, Ital.; Wyeth, S.Afr.; Wyeth, Spain; Wyeth, Switz.
24 Tablets, gestodene (p.1556·1); ethinylestradiol (p.1553·2); 4 tablets, inert.
*Combined oral contraceptive.*

**Minestril** Parke, Davis, Belg.
Norethisterone acetate (p.1562·2); ethinylestradiol (p.1553·2).
*Combined oral contraceptive; gynaecological disorders.*

**Minestrin** Pfizer, Canad.
Norethisterone acetate (p.1562·2); ethinylestradiol (p.1553·2).
28-Day packs also contain 7 inert tablets.
*Combined oral contraceptive.*

**Minfaden** Mintlab, Chile.
Paracetamol (p.76·2); pamabrom (p.978·2); mepyramine maleate (p.437·1).

**Minha** Vifor, Switz.
Naphazoline nitrate (p.1124·3).
*Eye disorders.*

**28 mini** Jenapharm, Ger.
Levonorgestrel (p.1563·2).
*Progestogen-only oral contraceptive.*

**Mini New Gen** Roche, Ital.†.
Vitamin, mineral, and carbohydrate preparation (p.1417·1).
*Nutritional supplement.*

**Mini Ovulo Lanzas** Ipsen, Spain.
Benzalkonium chloride (p.1168·3).
*Contraceptive.*

**Mini Pregnon** Nourypharma, Neth.
22 Tablets, lynestrenol (p.1557·1); ethinylestradiol (p.1553·2); 6 tablets, inert.
*Combined oral contraceptive.*

**Mini Pseudo** BDI, USA.
Pseudoephedrine hydrochloride (p.1129·2).
Formerly known as Mini Thin Pseudo.
*Nasal congestion.*

**Mini Two-Way Action** BDI, USA.
Ephedrine hydrochloride (p.1120·1); guaifenesin (p.1122·1).
Formerly known as Mini Thin Asthma Relief.

**Minian** Libbs, Braz.
Desogestrel (p.1547·2); ethinylestradiol (p.1553·2).
*Combined oral contraceptive.*

**Minias** Farmades, Ital.
Lormetazepam (p.705·2).
*Insomnia.*

**Miniasal** OPW, Ger.
Aspirin (p.15·1).
*Thromboembolism prophylaxis.*

**Minibit** Polipharm, Thai.
Glipizide (p.332·2).
*Diabetes mellitus.*

**Miniblock** USV, India.
Esmolol hydrochloride (p.913·1).
*Arrhythmias; hypertension during surgery.*

**Minidalton** Hoechst Marion Roussel, Ital.†.
Parnaparin sodium (p.978·3).
*Thrombosis prophylaxis.*

**Miniderm** ACO Hud, Swed.
Glycerol (p.1694·3).
*Dry skin.*

**Minidex** Alcon, Braz.
Dexamethasone (p.1097·1).
*Eye disorders.*

**Minidiab**
Pharmacia, Austral.; Pharmacia, Austria; Pharmacia, Belg.; Pharmacia, Braz.; Pharmacia, Chile; Pharmacia, Fr.; Pharmacia, Hong Kong; Pharmacia Upjohn, Ital.; Pharmacia, Neth.; Pharmacia, NZ; Pharmacia, Port.; Pharmacia, S.Afr.; Pharmacia, Singapore; Pharmacia, Thai.
Glipizide (p.332·2).
*Diabetes mellitus.*

**Minidine** Sigma, Austral.
Povidone-iodine (p.1190·3).
*Herpes labialis; sore throat; wounds.*

**Minidol** Andromaco, Chile.
Tramadol hydrochloride (p.94·3).
*Pain.*

**Minidril** Wyeth Lederle, Fr.
Levonorgestrel (p.1563·2); ethinylestradiol (p.1553·2).
*Combined oral contraceptive.*

**Minidyne** Pedinol, USA.
Povidone-iodine (p.1190·3).
*Skin disinfection.*

**Minifom**
Astra, Denm.†; AstraZeneca, Fin.; AstraZeneca, Norw.; Draco, Swed.
Dimeticone (p.1289·2) (Antifoam M).
*Adjunct to gastrointestinal radiography and endoscopy; colic; flatulence.*

**Mini-Gamulin Rh** Armour, USA†.
An anti-D immunoglobulin (p.1608·1).
*Prevention of rhesus sensitisation.*

**Minigeste** Schering, Port.
Gestodene (p.1556·1); ethinylestradiol (p.1553·2).
*Combined oral contraceptive.*

**Mini-Glynase** Julphar, UAE.
Glibenclamide (p.331·2).
*Diabetes mellitus.*

**Mini-Gravigard** SPA, Ital.†.
Copper (p.1425·3).
*Intra-uterine contraceptive device.*

**Minihep**
Leo, Irl.; Leo, Neth.†; CSL, NZ†; Leo, NZ†; Leo, UK†.
Heparin sodium (p.928·1).
*Thromboembolic disorders.*

**Minilax**
Note. This name is used for preparations of different composition.
Eurofarma, Braz.
Sorbitol (p.1446·3).
*Constipation.*

Sam-On, Israel.
Glycerol (p.1694·3).
*Constipation.*

**Minima** Yung Shin, Thai.†.
Prazosin hydrochloride (p.985·1).
*Hypertension.*

**Minims Artificial Tears**
Smith & Nephew, Austral.; Chauvin, Irl.; Bausch & Lomb, UK.
Hyetellose (p.1579·2); sodium chloride (p.1233·3).
*Dry eyes.*

**Mini-Pe**
Pharmacia, Denm.; Pharmacia, Swed.
Norethisterone (p.1562·2).
*Progestogen-only oral contraceptive.*

**Miniphase** Schering, Fr.
Norethisterone acetate (p.1562·2); ethinylestradiol (p.1553·2).
*Biphasic oral contraceptive.*

**Minipil** Sigma, Braz.
Levonorgestrel (p.1563·2).
*Progestogen-only oral contraceptive.*

**Mini-Pill** Pharmacia, Fin.
Norethisterone (p.1562·2).
*Progestogen-only oral contraceptive.*

**Minipres**
Pfizer, Arg.; Pfizer, Mex.; Nostrum, Spain.
Prazosin hydrochloride (p.985·1).
*Benign prostatic hyperplasia; heart failure; hypertension; Raynaud's syndrome.*

**Minipress**
Pfizer, Austral.; Pfizer, Austria; Pfizer, Belg.; Pfizer, Braz.; Pfizer, Canad.; Pfizer, Fr.; Pfizer, Ger.; Pfizer, Hong Kong; Pfizer, India; Pfizer, Jpn; Pfizer, Malaysia; Pfizer, Neth.; Pfizer, S.Afr.; Pfizer, Singapore; Pfizer, Switz.; Pfizer, Thai.; Pfizer, USA.
Prazosin hydrochloride (p.985·1).
*Benign prostatic hyperplasia; heart failure; hypertension; Raynaud's syndrome.*

**Minirin**
Ferring, Austral.; Ferring, Austria; Ferring, Belg.; Ferring, Denm.; Ferring, Fin.; Ferring, Fr.; Ferring, Ger.; Chemipharma, Gr.; Ferring, Hong Kong; Ferring, Israel; Ferring, Malaysia; IQFA, Mex.; Ferring, Norw.; Ferring, NZ; Pharmaco, NZ; Ferring, Port.; Ferring, Singapore; Ferring, Swed.; Ferring, Switz.; Ferring, Thai.; Ferring, USA.
Desmopressin acetate (p.1322·3).
*Diabetes insipidus; haemophilia A; nocturnal enuresis; test of renal concentrating capacity; von Willebrand's disease.*

**Minirin/DDAVP** Ferring, Ital.
Desmopressin acetate (p.1322·3).
*Diabetes insipidus; haemophilia A; nocturnal enuresis; polydipsia; polyuria; renal function tests.*

**Miniscap** Vifor, Switz.
Cathine hydrochloride (p.1585·2).
*Obesity.*

**Mini-sintrom** Novartis, Fr.
Acenocoumarol (p.848·3).
*Thromboembolic disorders.*

**Minisiston** Jenapharm, Ger.
Ethinylestradiol (p.1553·2); levonorgestrel (p.1563·2).
*Combined oral contraceptive; menstrual disorders.*

**Minisol** Ederka, Mex.†.
Ambroxol (p.1114·3).

**Minison** YSP, Malaysia.
Prazosin hydrochloride (p.985·1).
*Hypertension.*

**Ministat**
Organon, Belg.†; Organon, Neth.
Lynestrenol (p.1557·1); ethinylestradiol (p.1553·2).
*Combined oral contraceptive.*

**Miniten** Utopian, Thai.
Nitrendipine (p.973·3).
*Hypertension.*

**Minitran**
Note. This name is used for preparations of different composition.
3M, Arg.; 3M, Austral.; Byk, Austria; 3M, Belg.; 3M, Canad.; 3M, Fin.; 3M, Hong Kong†; 3M, Ital.; 3M, Mex.; 3M, Neth.; 3M, Norw.; 3M, NZ; 3M, Spain; 3M, Swed.; 3M, Switz.; 3M, Thai.†; 3M, UK; 3M, USA.
Glyceryl trinitrate (p.923·2).
*Angina pectoris; maintenance of venous patency at peripheral infusion sites.*

Adelco, Gr.
Perphenazine (p.714·2); amitriptyline hydrochloride (p.280·3).
*Depression accompanied by psychosis.*

**MinitranS** 3M, Ger.
Glyceryl trinitrate (p.923·2).
*Angina pectoris.*

**Minit-Rub** Bristol-Myers Products, USA.
Methyl salicylate (p.59·3); menthol (p.1711·3); camphor (p.1665·3).
*Muscle, joint, and soft-tissue pain; neuralgia.*

**Minizide** Pfizer, USA.
Prazosin hydrochloride (p.985·1); polythiazide (p.984·2).
*Hypertension.*

**Mino-50** Wyeth Lederle, Belg.
Minocycline hydrochloride (p.231·3).
*Acne.*

**Mino T** Wyeth, S.Afr.†.
Minocycline hydrochloride (p.231·3).
*Acne; bacterial infections.*

**Minobese** Restan, S.Afr.†.
Phentermine hydrochloride (p.1592·2).
*Obesity.*

**Minocalve** Pharmacia, Port.
Minoxidil (p.960·1).
*Alopecia androgenetica.*

**Minocin**
Wyeth, Arg.; Wyeth Lederle, Austria; Wyeth Lederle, Belg.; Wyeth-Ayerst, Canad.; Wyeth, Chile; Wyeth, Gr.; Wyeth, Hong Kong; Wyeth, Irl.; Lederle, Israel; Wyeth Lederle, Ital.; Wyeth, Malaysia; Wyeth, Mex.; Wyeth, Neth.; Wyeth Lederle, Port.; Wyeth, Singapore; Wyeth, Spain; Lederle, Switz.; Wyeth-Ayerst, Thai.; Wyeth, UK; Lederle, USA.
Minocycline hydrochloride (p.231·3).
*Bacterial infections; intestinal amoebiasis.*

**Minoclin** Vitamed, Israel.
Minocycline hydrochloride (p.231·3).
*Bacterial infections.*

**Minoclir** Jenapharm, Ger.
Minocycline hydrochloride (p.231·3).
*Bacterial infections.*

**Minoderm** Stiefel, Braz.
Minocycline hydrochloride (p.231·3).
*Bacterial infections.*

**Minodiab**
Pharmacia, Arg.; Pharmacia-Upjohn, Gr.; Pharmacia Upjohn, Mex.; Kenfarma, Spain; Pharmacia, UK.
Glipizide (p.332·2).
*Diabetes mellitus.*

**Minofen** Liomont, Mex.†.
Paracetamol (p.76·2).
*Fever; pain.*

**Minogal** Galen, UK†.
Minocycline (p.231·3).

**Minogalen** Galen, Ger.†.
Minocycline hydrochloride (p.231·3).
*Acne.*

**Minolis** Pharmascience, Fr.
Minocycline hydrochloride (p.231·3).
*Bacterial infections.*

**Minomax** Wyeth, Braz.
Minocycline hydrochloride (p.231·3).
*Bacterial infections.*

**Minomex** Liferpal, Mex.†.
Paracetamol (p.76·2).
*Fever; pain.*

**Minomycin**
Sigma, Austral.; Sigma, NZ; Wyeth, S.Afr.†.
Minocycline hydrochloride (p.231·3).
*Amoebiasis; bacterial infections; trachoma.*

**Minona** Orion, Fin.†.
Minoxidil (p.960·1).
*Hypertension.*

**Minoplus** Rosen, Ger.
Minocycline hydrochloride (p.231·3).
*Bacterial infections.*

**Minopres** Precimex, Mex.†.
Pancuronium bromide (p.1404·3).
*Competitive neuromuscular blocker.*

**Minor** Biosintetica, Braz.
Lovastatin (p.949·1).
*Hyperlipidaemias.*

**Minoral** Liferpal, Mex.
Dipyrone (p.35·3).
*Fever; pain.*

**Minorplex** Abigo, Swed.
Multivitamin preparation (p.1417·1).

**Minostad** Stada, Austria.
Minocycline hydrochloride (p.231·3).
*Bacterial infections.*

**Minot** Roemmers, Arg.
Sulconazole nitrate (p.408·2).
*Fungal skin infections.*

**Minotab**
Wyeth Lederle, Belg.; Wyeth, Neth.†.
Minocycline hydrochloride (p.231·3).
*Bacterial infections.*

**Minotabs**
Wyeth, NZ; Hexal, S.Afr.
Minocycline hydrochloride (p.231·3).
*Bacterial infections.*

**Minoton**
Note. This name is used for preparations of different composition.
Ariston, Braz.
Aminophylline (p.780·2).
*Obstructive airways disease.*

Madaus, Spain.
Magaldrate (p.1271·3).
*Dyspepsia; gastro-oesophageal reflux; peptic ulcer.*

**Minotrex** Medinfar, Port.
Minocycline hydrochloride (p.231·3).
*Bacterial infections.*

**Minotyrol** Tyrol, Austria.
Minocycline hydrochloride (p.231·3).
*Bacterial infections.*

**Minovag** Novag, Mex.
Secnidazole (p.615·3).
*Amoebiasis; giardiasis; trichomoniasis.*

**Minovital** *Terapeutico, Ital.*
Minoxidil (p.960·1).
*Alopecia.*

**Min-Ovral** *Wyeth-Ayerst, Canad.*
Levonorgestrel (p.1563·2); ethinylestradiol (p.1553·2). 28-Day packs also contain 7 inert tablets.
*Combined oral contraceptive.*

**Mino-Wolff** *Wolff, Ger.*
Minocycline hydrochloride (p.231·3).
*Acne.*

**Minox**
*Note. This name is used for preparations of different composition.*
*Riva, Canad.; Edol, Port.*
Minoxidil (p.960·1).
*Alopecia androgenetica.*

*Rowex, Irl.*
Minocycline (p.231·3).
*Bacterial infections.*

**Minoxi** *Trima, Israel.*
Minoxidil (p.960·1).
*Alopecia androgenetica.*

**Minoxidine** *Sanval, Braz.†.*
Minoxidil (p.960·1).
*Alopecia androgenetica.*

**Minoxigaine** *Kenral, Canad.†.*
Minoxidil (p.960·1).
*Alopecia androgenetica.*

**Minoximen** *Menarini, Ital.*
Minoxidil (p.960·1).
*Alopecia.*

**Minoxitrim**
*Trima, Singapore; Unipharm, Singapore; Trima, Thai.*
Minoxidil (p.960·1).
*Alopecia androgenetica.*

**Minozinan** *Rhone-Poulenc Rorer, Switz.†.*
Levomepromazine maleate (p.703·2).
*Anxiety; asthma; excitement; hypersensitivity reactions; insomnia; psychoses.*

**Minprog**
*Pharmacia, Austria; Pharmacia, Ger.*
Alprostadil (p.1512·3).
*Maintenance of ductus arteriosus patency.*

**Minprostin**
*Pharmacia, Denm.; Pharmacia, Fin.; Pharmacia, Norw.; Pharmacia, Swed.*
Dinoprostone (p.1515·1).
*Labour induction.*

**Minprostin $E_2$** *Pharmacia, Ger.*
Dinoprostone (p.1515·1).
*Labour induction; production of cervical dilatation.*

**Minprostin $F_2\alpha$** *Pharmacia, Ger.*
Dinoprost trometamol (p.1514·3).
*Uterine bleeding.*

**Minra** *Nakorn, Thai.*
Brompheniramine maleate (p.426·1); phenylephrine hydrochloride (p.1126·3).
Formerly contained brompheniramine maleate, phenylephrine hydrochloride, and phenylpropanolamine hydrochloride.
*Hay fever; rhinitis.*

**Minrin** *Ferring, Neth.*
Desmopressin acetate (p.1322·3).
*Diabetes insipidus; haemorrhagic disorders; nocturnal enuresis; polyuria; test of renal concentrating capacity; uraemia.*

**Mintaglos** *Mintlab, Chile.*
Halibut oil (p.1434·1); vitamin A; vitamin D; zinc oxide (p.1163·2).
*Skin disorders; wounds.*

**Mintamox** *Mintlab, Chile.*
Ambroxol (p.1114·3).
*Respiratory-tract congestion.*

**Mintavit-C** *Mintlab, Chile.*
Ascorbic acid (p.1460·2).
*Vitamin C supplement.*

**Mintec**
*Key, Austral.†; Wilson, NZ; Monmouth, UK.*
Peppermint oil (p.1283·2).
*Irritable bowel syndrome; spastic colon syndrome.*

**Mintetten Truw** *Truw, Ger.†.*
Cowslip rhizome (p.1735·1); drosera (p.1683·1); thyme (p.1755·2).
*Catarrh; cough.*

**Mintezol**
*Merck Sharp & Dohme, Austral.; Merck Frosst, Canad.†; IFET (IΦET), Gr.; Merck Sharp & Dohme, Irl.†; Merck Sharp & Dohme, UK†; Merck, USA.*
Tiabendazole (p.114·2).
*Worm infections.*

**Mint-Lysoform** *Lysoform, Ger.*
Myrrh tincture (p.1718·3); peppermint oil (p.1283·2).
Formerly known as Fluomint and contained potassium fluoride, myrrh tincture, and peppermint oil.
*Mouth and throat disorders.*

**Mintox** *Major, USA.*
Aluminium hydroxide (p.1249·2); magnesium hydroxide (p.1272·2).
*Hyperacidity.*

**Mintox Plus** *Major, USA.*
Aluminium hydroxide (p.1249·2); magnesium hydroxide (p.1272·2); simeticone (p.1289·2).
*Hyperacidity.*

**Minulet**
*Wyeth, Arg.; Wyeth, Austral.; Wyeth Lederle, Austria; Wyeth Lederle, Belg.; Wyeth, Braz.; Wyeth, Chile; Wyeth Lederle, Denm.; Wyeth Lederle, Fin.; Wyeth Lederle, Fr.; Wyeth, Ger.; Wyeth, Gr.; Wyeth, Hong Kong; Wyeth, Irl.; Wyeth-Ayerst, Israel; Wyeth Lederle, Ital.; Wyeth, Malaysia; Wyeth, Mex.; Wyeth, Neth.; Wyeth, NZ; Wyeth Lederle, Port.; Wyeth, Singapore; Wyeth, Spain; Wyeth, Switz.; Wyeth-Ayerst, Thai.; Wyeth, UK.*
Gestodene (p.1556·1); ethinylestradiol (p.1553·2). 28-Day packs also contain 7 inert tablets.
*Combined oral contraceptive.*

**Minulette** *Wyeth, S.Afr.*
21 Tablets, gestodene (p.1556·1); ethinylestradiol (p.1553·2); 7 tablets, inert.
*Combined oral contraceptive.*

**Minuric** *Sanofi Synthelabo, S.Afr.*
Benzbromarone (p.414·3).
*Gout; hyperuricaemia.*

**Minurin** *Ferring, Spain.*
Desmopressin (p.1322·3) or desmopressin acetate (p.1322·3).
*Diabetes insipidus; haemorrhage; nocturnal enuresis; test of renal concentrating capacity.*

**Minus Fat** *Ocean Health, Singapore†.*
L112 Absorbitol.
*Reduction of fat and bile acid absorption.*

**Minus Fat Extra** *Ocean Health, Singapore†.*
Gymnema silvestre; chromium polynicotinate.
*Dietary aid.*

**Minuslip** *Armstrong, Arg.*
Fenofibrate (p.915·2).
*Hyperlipidaemias.*

**Minusorb** *UCI, Braz.*
Alendronate sodium (p.765·3).
*Osteoporosis.*

**Minute-Gel** *Oral-B, USA.*
Acidulated phosphate fluoride (p.1444·3).
*Dental caries prophylaxis.*

**Minutil** *Henkel, Ger.*
Formaldehyde (p.1179·3); glyoxal (p.1181·1); glutaral (p.1180·3).
*Surface disinfection.*

**MinVitin** *Wander Health Care, Switz.*
Food for special diets (p.1417·1).
*Obesity.*

**Mio Aldoron** *Armstrong, Arg.*
Nimesulide (p.67·1); orphenadrine citrate (p.486·1).
*Musculoskeletal disorders.*

**Mio Relax** *Belmac, Spain.*
Carisoprodol (p.1392·1).
*Skeletal muscle spasm.*

**Miocacin**
*Faran, Gr.; Aventis, Port.*
Midecamycin acetate (p.231·3).
*Bacterial infections.*

**Miocalven** *Farmalab, Braz.*
Calcium citrate (p.1225·1).
*Calcium supplement.*

**Miocalven D** *Farmalab, Braz.*
Calcium citrate (p.1225·1); colecalciferol (p.1461·3).
*Calcium deficiency; osteoporosis.*

**Miocamen**
*Menarini, Gr.; Menarini, Ital.*
Midecamycin acetate (p.231·3).
*Bacterial infections.*

**Miocamycin** *Meiji, Jpn.*
Midecamycin acetate (p.231·3).
*Bacterial infections.*

**Miocardin** *Magis, Ital.*
Levocarnitine (p.1423·3).
*Carnitine deficiency; myocardial ischaemia.*

**Miocarpine** *Novartis Ophthalmics, Canad.*
Pilocarpine hydrochloride (p.1495·1).
*Open-angle glaucoma.*

**Miochol**
*Novartis, Austral.; Bournonville, Belg.†; Ciba Vision, Canad.; Novartis, Irl.; Iolab, Israel; Novartis, NZ; Restan, S.Afr.; Ciba Vision, Swed.†; Novartis Ophthalmics, Switz.; General Drugs, Thai.; Novartis, UK; Novartis Ophthalmics, USA.*
Acetylcholine chloride (p.1487·1).
*Production of miosis in eye surgery.*

**Miochol-E**
*Ciba Vision, Braz.†; Novartis Ophthalmics, Canad.; Novartis, Chile; Novartis, Fin.; Novartis Ophthalmics, Ger.; Novartis, Gr.; OMJ, Hong Kong; Novartis Ophthalmics, Hong Kong; Ciba Vision, Israel; Ciba Vision, Ital.; Novartis Ophthalmics, Singapore.*
Acetylcholine chloride (p.1487·1).
*Production of miosis in eye surgery.*

**Miochole** *Novartis Ophthalmics, Fr.*
Acetylcholine chloride (p.1487·1).
*Production of miosis in eye surgery.*

**Miociclin** *QIF, Braz.†.*
Tetracycline hydrochloride (p.266·2).
*Bacterial infections.*

**Mio-Citalgan** *Merck, Braz.*
Carisoprodol (p.1392·1); caffeine (p.782·1); vitamin B substances (p.1417·1); paracetamol (p.76·2).
Formerly contained carisoprodol, caffeine, vitamin B substances, and metamizole calcium.
*Skeletal muscle spasm.*

**Miocor** *Ecobi, Ital.*
Levocarnitine (p.1423·3).
*Carnitine deficiency; myocardial ischaemia.*

**Miocoron** *Cristalia, Braz.*
Amiodarone hydrochloride (p.859·2).
*Arrhythmias.*

**Miocrin**
*Rubio, Singapore; Rubio, Spain.*
Sodium aurothiomalate (p.88·2).
*Lupus erythematosus; rheumatoid arthritis.*

**Miocuril** *Terapeutico, Ital.*
Sodium uridine triphosphate (p.1760·3).
*Heart failure; muscular disorders.*

**Miodarid** *Neo Quimica, Braz.*
Amiodarone hydrochloride (p.859·2).
*Arrhythmias.*

**Miodaron** *Biosintetica, Braz.*
Amiodarone hydrochloride (p.859·2).
*Arrhythmias.*

**Miodene** *Bioprogress, Ital.*
Ubidecarenone (p.1760·2).
*Cardiac disorders.*

**Miodom** *Dominguez, Arg.*
Tolperisone hydrochloride (p.1396·3).
*Muscle relaxant.*

**Miodrina** *Apsen, Braz.*
Ritodrine hydrochloride (p.1739·2).
*Premature labour.*

**Miodrone** *Alter, Port.*
Amiodarone hydrochloride (p.859·2).
*Arrhythmias.*

**Mioflex**
*Note. This name is used for preparations of different composition.*
*Farmasa, Braz.*
Carisoprodol (p.1392·1); paracetamol (p.76·2); phenylbutazone (p.83·2).
*Skeletal muscle spasm.*

*Braun, Port.; Braun, Spain.*
Suxamethonium chloride (p.1406·2).
*Depolarising neuromuscular blocker.*

**Miogesil** *GlaxoSmithKline, Arg.*
Meloxicam (p.56·1).
*Musculoskeletal and joint disorders.*

**Miokacin** *FIRMA, Ital.*
Midecamycin (p.231·3).
*Bacterial infections.*

**Miokalium** *Bama, Spain†.*
Magnesium chloride (p.1228·1); potassium aspartate (p.1233·1); potassium chloride (p.1232·2).
*Potassium depletion.*

**Miol** *Robert, Spain.*
Omeprazole (p.1278·2).
*Gastro-oesophageal reflux; peptic ulcer; Zollinger-Ellison syndrome.*

**Miolastan** *Sanofi Synthelabo, Mex.*
Tetrazepam (p.724·1).

**Miolene** *Lusofarmaco, Ital.*
Ritodrine hydrochloride (p.1739·2).
*Premature labour; threatened miscarriage.*

**Mionevrasi** *Roche, Ital.*
Cyanocobalamin (p.1458·2); pyridoxine hydrochloride (p.1456·3); cocarboxylase (p.1455·2).
Lidocaine hydrochloride (p.1377·3) is included in this preparation to alleviate the pain of injection.
*Neuralgia; neuritis; vitamin B deficiencies.*

**Mionevrix** *Ache, Braz.*
Carisoprodol (p.1392·1); dipyrone (p.35·3); vitamin B substances (p.1417·1).
*Skeletal muscle spasm.*

**Miopat** *Polifarma, Ital.†.*
Metildigoxin (p.955·2).
*Heart failure.*

**Miopropan** *Microsules Bernabo, Arg.*
Trimebutine (p.1758·1) or trimebutine maleate (p.1758·1).
*Gastrointestinal spasm.*

**Miopropan Proctologico** *Microsules Bernabo, Arg.*
Ruscogenin (p.1741·1); trimebutine (p.1758·1).
*Haemorrhoids.*

**Miopropan-T** *Microsules Bernabo, Arg.*
Trimebutine maleate (p.1758·1); bromazepam (p.671·3).

**Miorel**
*Note. This name is used for preparations of different composition.*
*Fornet, Fr.*
Thiocolchicoside (p.1395·2).
*Skeletal muscle spasm.*

*Kleva, Gr.*
Baclofen (p.1386·3).
*Spasticity.*

**Miorrelax** *Ducto, Braz.*
Dipyrone (p.35·3); orphenadrine citrate (p.486·1); caffeine (p.782·1).
*Skeletal muscle spasm.*

**Mios** *INTES, Ital.*
Pilocarpine hydrochloride (p.1495·1); carbachol (p.1488·1); paraoxon (p.1494·1); procaine hydrochloride (p.1383·2).
*Raised intra-ocular pressure.*

**Miosal** *Technilab, Canad.†.*
Trolamine salicylate (p.95·3).
*Pain.*

**Miosan** *Apsen, Braz.*
Cyclobenzaprine hydrochloride (p.1393·1).
*Skeletal muscle spasm.*

**Miosen** *Belmac, Spain†.*
Dipyridamole (p.903·1).
*Thromboembolism prophylaxis.*

**Miostat**
*Alcon, Arg.; Alcon, Austral.; Alcon, Belg.; Alcon, Canad.; Alcon, Hong Kong; Alcon, Israel; Alcon, Malaysia; Pacific, NZ†; Alcon, Singapore; Alcon, Switz.; Alcon, Thai.; Alcon, USA.*
Carbachol (p.1488·1).
*Production of miosis.*

**Miostenil** *Bial, Port.*
Magnesium aspartate (p.1227·3); potassium aspartate (p.1233·1).

**Miosys** *Alcon, S.Afr.*
Carbachol (p.1488·1).
*Production of miosis.*

**Miotenk** *Biotenk, Arg.*
Amiodarone hydrochloride (p.859·2).
*Arrhythmias.*

**Miotens** *Dompe, Ital.*
Thiocolchicoside (p.1395·2).
*Neuromuscular pain; parkinsonism; spasticity.*

**Miotic Double** *Asta Medica, Belg.†.*
Physostigmine salicylate (p.1494·1); pilocarpine hydrochloride (p.1495·1).
*Glaucoma; herniated iris.*

**Mioticol** *Farmigea, Ital.*
Carbachol (p.1488·1).
*Production of miosis in eye surgery.*

**Miotin** *Meiji, Thai.*
Midecamycin acetate (p.231·3).
*Bacterial infections.*

**Miotonachol** *Fortbenton, Arg.*
Bethanechol chloride (p.1487·3).
*Prostate disorders.*

**Miotonal** *Caber, Ital.*
Levocarnitine (p.1423·3).
*Carnitine deficiency; myocardial ischaemia.*

**Miotyn** *Ibirn, Ital.*
Ubidecarenone (p.1760·2).
*Cardiac disorders.*

**Mio-Virobron** *Temis, Arg.*
Nimesulide (p.67·1); orphenadrine citrate (p.486·1).
*Musculoskeletal inflammation.*

**Miovisin** *Farmigea, Ital.*
Acetylcholine chloride (p.1487·1).
*Production of miosis in eye surgery.*

**Miowas G** *Wasserman, Spain†.*
Gallamine triethiodide (p.1403·2).
*Competitive neuromuscular blocker.*

**Miozac** *Fisiopharma, Ital.*
Dobutamine hydrochloride (p.905·3).
*Cardiac inotropic.*

**Miozets** *Dermofarm, Spain.*
Benzocaine (p.1370·3); tyrothricin (p.275·1).
*Mouth and throat disorders.*

**Miphar** *Pharbita, Israel.*
Furosemide (p.919·3).
*Hypertension; oedema.*

**Mi-Pilo** *Fischer, Israel.*
Pilocarpine hydrochloride (p.1495·1).
*Glaucoma; production of miosis.*

**Mipramid** *IQFA, Mex.*
Metoclopramide (p.1274·3).
*Nausea and vomiting.*

**Mipraz** *Amrad, Austral.†.*
Prazosin hydrochloride (p.985·1).
*Benign prostatic hyperplasia; heart failure; hypertension; Raynaud's syndrome.*

**MIR** *Rafa, Israel.*
Morphine sulfate (p.60·2).
*Pain.*

**Mira Klonal** *Klonal, Arg.*
Naphazoline (p.1124·3); pheniramine (p.438·3).
*Eye disorders.*

**Mirabel** *Allergan, Braz.*
Tetryzoline hydrochloride (p.1131·2); zinc sulfate (p.1469·3).
*Ocular congestion.*

**Mirabol** *Volchem, Ital.*
Preparations for enteral nutrition (p.1417·1).

**Miracef** *Tosi, Ital.*
Propylene glycol cefatrizine (p.170·3).
*Bacterial infections.*

**Miracid** *Berlin Pharm, Thai.*
Omeprazole (p.1278·2).
*Gastro-oesophageal reflux; peptic ulcer; Zollinger-Ellison syndrome.*

**Miraclar** *Iquinosa, Spain.*
Naphazoline hydrochloride (p.1124·3).
*Eye disorders.*

**Miraclid** *Mochida, Jpn.*
Ulinastatin (p.1760·2).
*Pancreatitis.*

**Miraclin** *Farmacologico Milanese, Ital.*
Doxycycline hyclate (p.206·2).
*Bacterial infections.*

**Miracorten**
*Novartis Consumer, Austria†; Max Ritter, Switz.†.*
Ulobetasol propionate (p.1111·3).
*Skin disorders.*

**Miradol** *Durbin, UK.*
Paracetamol (p.76·2).

**Miradon** *Schering, USA†.*
Anisindione (p.863·3).
*Thromboembolic disorders.*

**Miraflow**
*Ciba Vision, Austral.†; Ciba Vision, Canad.; Novartis, NZ; Ciba Vision, USA.*
Range of solutions for contact lenses (p.1164·2).

**Mirafur** *Orion, Fin.*
Carmofur (p.535·1).
*Breast cancer; ovarian cancer.*

**Miral**
Note. This name is used for preparations of different composition.
Laboratorios Chile, Chile.
Pheniramine maleate (p.438·3); naphazoline hydrochloride (p.1124·3).
*Eye disorders.*

Leiras, Fin.
Potassium chloride (p.1232·2); magnesium hydroxide (p.1272·2).
*Potassium and magnesium deficiency.*

**MiraLax** Braintree, USA.
Macrogol 3350 (p.1709·1).
*Bowel evacuation.*

**Miralis** Ativus, Braz.
Myrtillus (p.1718·3).
*Retinopathy.*

**Miraluma** Du Pont, USA.
Technetium-99m sestamibi (p.1525·2).
*Breast imaging.*

**Miramycin**
Atlantic, Hong Kong; Atlantic, Malaysia; Atlantic, Singapore; Atlantic, Thai.
Gentamicin sulfate (p.217·1).
*Bacterial infections.*

**Miranax**
Grunenthal, Austria; Roche, Denm.; Roche, Fin.; Syntex, Swed.†.
Naproxen sodium (p.65·1).
*Gout; inflammation; musculoskeletal, joint, and peri-articular disorders; pain.*

**Miranova**
Schering, Arg.; Schering, Ger.; Farmades, Ital.; Schering, Port.
Ethinylestradiol (p.1553·2); levonorgestrel (p.1563·2).
*Combined oral contraceptive.*

**Mirantal** Ciba Vision, Spain†.
Phenylephrine hydrochloride (p.1126·3); medrysone (p.1106·1); neomycin sulfate (p.235·1); zinc sulfate (p.1469·3).
*Infected eye disorders.*

**Mirapex**
Pharmacia, Arg.; Pharmacia, Braz.; Boehringer Ingelheim, Canad.; Boehringer Ingelheim, USA.
Pramipexole hydrochloride (p.1212·2).
*Parkinsonism.*

**Mirapexin**
Pharmacia, Belg.; Pharmacia, Irl.; Pharmacia Upjohn, Ital.; Pharmacia, Spain.
Pramipexole (p.1212·3).
*Parkinsonism.*

Pharmacia-Upjohn, Gr.; Pharmacia, UK.
Pramipexole hydrochloride (p.1212·2).
*Parkinsonism.*

**Mirapront N**
Mack, Illert., Ger.†.
Cathine polystyroldivinylbenzol-sulfonic acid (p.1585·2).
*Obesity.*

Mack, Hong Kong†; Mack, Singapore†; Mack, Thai.
Cathine (p.1585·2).
*Obesity.*

**Mirasan** Allergan, Arg.
Naphazoline hydrochloride (p.1124·3).
*Eye disorders.*

**MiraSept** Alcon, USA.
Hydrogen peroxide (p.1182·2) (p.1164·2).
*Disinfecting solution for soft contact lenses.*

**Miraton** Codal Synto, Malaysia.
Loperamide hydrochloride (p.1271·1).
*Diarrhoea.*

**Mirax**
Berlin Pharm, Singapore; Berlin Pharm, Thai.
Domperidone (p.1263·2) or domperidone maleate (p.1263·2).
*Delayed gastric emptying; dyspepsia; nausea and vomiting.*

**Miraxid** Leo, Austria†.
Pivampicillin (p.244·1); pivmecillinam (p.244·2) or pivmecillinam hydrochloride (p.244·2).
*Bacterial infections.*

**Miraxx** Neopharmed, Ital.
Rofecoxib (p.86·3).
*Pain.*

**Mirazul** Fardi, Spain.
Phenylephrine hydrochloride (p.1126·3).
*Eye irritation.*

**Mircette** Organon, USA.
21 Tablets, desogestrel (p.1547·2); ethinylestradiol (p.1553·2); 5 tablets, ethinylestradiol; 2 tablets, placebo.
*Sequential oral contraceptive.*

**Mircol**
Rhone-Poulenc Rorer, Belg.†; Recalcine, Chile; Italfarmaco, Spain.
Mequitazine (p.437·2).
*Hypersensitivity reactions.*

**Mirelle**
Schering, Arg.; Schering, Austria; Schering, Belg.; Schering, Braz.; Schering, Chile; Schering, Fin.; Schering, S.Afr.; Schering, Switz.
24 Tablets, gestodene (p.1556·1); ethinylestradiol (p.1553·2); 4 tablets, inert.
24-Day packs contain no inert tablets.
*Combined oral contraceptive.*

**Mirena**
Schering, Arg.; Schering, Austral.; Schering, Austria; Schering, Belg.; Berlimed, Braz.; Berlex, Canad.; Schering, Chile; Schering, Fr.; Schering, Ger.; Schering, Hong Kong; Schering, Irl.; Leiras, Israel; Schering, Israel; Schering, Ital.; Schering, Malaysia; Schering, Neth.; Schering, NZ; Schering, Port.; Schering, S.Afr.; Schering, Singapore; Schering, Spain; Schering, Switz.; Schering, Thai.; Schering, UK; Berlex, USA.
Levonorgestrel (p.1563·2).
*Menorrhagia; progestogen-releasing intra-uterine contraceptive device.*

**Miretic** Utopian, Thai.
Amiloride hydrochloride (p.858·2); hydrochlorothiazide (p.933·2).
*Hypertension; oedema.*

**Mireze** Allergan, Canad.†.
Nedocromil sodium (p.789·3).
*Allergic conjunctivitis.*

**Mirfat** Merckle, Ger.
Clonidine hydrochloride (p.885·2).
*Hypertension.*

**Mirfudorm** Merckle, Ger.
Oxazepam (p.712·2).
*Anxiety; sleep disorders.*

**Mirfulan**
Ratiopharm, Austria; Merckle, Ger.
Cod-liver oil (p.1425·2); zinc oxide (p.1163·2); hamamelis (p.1696·3); urea (p.1162·2).
*Burns; skin disorders; wounds.*

**Mirfulan Spray N** Merckle, Ger.
Cod-liver oil (p.1425·2); zinc oxide (p.1163·2); levomenol (p.1707·1).
*Burns; skin disorders; wounds.*

**Mirfusot** Merckle, Ger.
Thyme (p.1755·2).
*Coughs and associated respiratory-tract disorders.*

**Mirion** Pharmacia, Chile.
Estradiol valerate (p.1550·2).

**Mirorroidin** Sedabel, Braz.
Rutoside (p.1688·2); hamamelis (p.1696·3); aesculus (p.1648·2); zinc (p.1469·2); menthol (p.1711·3); benzocaine (p.1370·3).
*Haemorrhoids.*

**Miroton** Knoll, Ger.
Squill (p.1130·3); convallaria (p.1675·3); oleander (p.1723·1); adonis vernalis (p.1648·1).
*Cardiovascular disorders.*

**Miroton N** Knoll, Ger.
Adonis vernalis (p.1648·1); convallaria (p.1675·3); squill (p.1130·3).
*Cardiac disorders.*

**Mirpan** Dolorgiet, Ger.†.
Maprotiline hydrochloride (p.306·1).
*Depression.*

**Mirquin** Mirren, S.Afr.
Chloroquine sulfate (p.448·2).
*Malaria.*

**Mirsol** Permamed, Switz.†.
Zipeprol hydrochloride (p.1132·3).
*Adjunct in bronchial examination; coughs.*

**Mirtaz** Sun, India.
Mirtazapine (p.307·3).
*Depression.*

**Mirtazon** Arrow, Austral.
Mirtazapine (p.307·3).
*Depression.*

**Mirtex P** DMG, Ital.
Vitamin, mineral, and lipid preparation with myrtillus (p.1417·1).
*Nutritional supplement.*

**Mirtilene** SIFI, Ital.
Myrtillus (p.1718·3); betacarotene (p.1422·3); *dl*-alpha tocoferil acetate (p.1465·1).
*Capillary disorders; eye disorders.*

**Mirtilene Forte**
Craveri, Arg.; SIFI, Ital.
Myrtillus (p.1718·3).
*Eye disorders.*

**Mirtilus** Llorens, Spain.
Betacarotene (p.1422·3); myrtillus (p.1718·3).
*Eye disorders.*

**Mirtilvedo C** Fitobucaneve, Ital.
Vitamin preparation with betacarotene, myrtillus, carrot, and rose fruit (p.1417·1).
*Nutritional supplement.*

**Mirtiros** Pharmafar, Ital.†.
Hamamelis (p.1696·3); myrtillus (p.1718·3); crataegus (p.1677·1).
*Skin disorders.*

**Mirtivit** SIFI, Singapore.
Food supplement (p.1417·1).

**Mirus**
Alcon, Arg.; Alcon, Chile.
Pheniramine maleate (p.438·3); naphazoline hydrochloride (p.1124·3).
*Eye disorders.*

**Mirus-S** Alcon, Arg.
Naphazoline hydrochloride (p.1124·3).
*Eye irritation.*

**Miscidon** Torlan, Spain.
Spironolactone (p.1003·1); hydrochlorothiazide (p.933·2).
*Hypertension; oedema.*

**Misodex** Sefarma, Ital.
Misoprostol (p.1519·2).
*NSAID-induced peptic ulcer.*

**Misodomin** Kleva, Gr.
Lovastatin (p.949·1).
*Primary hypercholesterolaemia.*

**Misofenac** Sefarma, Ital.
Diclofenac sodium (p.32·1).
Misoprostol (p.1519·2) is included in this preparation in an attempt to limit adverse effects on the gastrointestinal mucosa.
*Musculoskeletal and joint disorders.*

**Misone** PD, Thai.
Miconazole nitrate (p.405·3).
*Fungal skin, hair, and nail infections.*

**Misordil** Wyeth, Arg.
Isosorbide mononitrate (p.942·1).
*Angina pectoris.*

**Misostol** Zodiac, Braz.
Mitoxantrone hydrochloride (p.575·2).
*Malignant neoplasms.*

**Misotrol** Sanofi Synthelabo, Chile.
Misoprostol (p.1519·2).
*Peptic ulcer.*

**Misovan** TO-Chemicals, Thai.
Ambroxol hydrochloride (p.1114·3).
*Respiratory-tract disorders associated with increased or viscous mucus.*

**Mission Prenatal** Mission Pharmacal, USA.
A range of multivitamin and mineral preparations with iron and folic acid (p.1417·1).
*Iron-deficiency anaemias; prenatal and postpartum supplement.*

**Mission Surgical Supplement** Mission Pharmacal, USA.
Ferrous gluconate (p.1428·1); multivitamins and minerals (p.1417·1).
*Dietary supplement for pre- and postsurgical patients; iron-deficiency anaemias.*

**Mist Expect Stim** Vida, Hong Kong.
Ammonium bicarbonate (p.1115·1); ammonium chloride (p.1115·2); sodium citrate (p.1223·2); squill (p.1130·3); senega (p.1130·2); liquorice (p.1270·2).
*Cold symptoms; coughs.*

**Mistabron**
UCB, Austria; UCB, Belg.; UCB, Hong Kong; UCB, Malaysia; UCB, Neth.; UCB, S.Afr.; UCB, Singapore; UCB, Switz.; UCB, Thai.
Mesna (p.1041·2).
*Respiratory-tract disorders associated with increased or viscous mucus.*

**Mistabronco** UCB, Ger.
Mesna (p.1041·2).
*Respiratory-tract disorders.*

**Mistalin** Galderma, Neth.
Mizolastine (p.437·3).
*Allergic rhinoconjunctivitis; urticaria.*

**Mistaline** Galderma, Fr.†.
Mizolastine (p.437·3).
*Allergic rhinoconjunctivitis; urticaria.*

**Mistamin** AB-Consult, Austria.
Mizolastine (p.437·3).
*Allergic rhinoconjunctivitis; urticaria.*

**Mistamine**
Galderma, Arg.; Galderma, Belg.; Galderma, Chile; Galderma, Denm.†; Galderma, Irl.; Galderma, Mex.; Galderma, Port.; Galderma, Spain; Galderma, Swed.†; Galderma, Switz.; Galderma, UK†.
Mizolastine (p.437·3).
*Allergic conjunctivitis; allergic rhinitis; urticaria.*

**Mistel Curarina** Harras-Curarina, Ger.
Mistletoe (p.1715·3).
*Circulatory disorders.*

**Mistel-Krautertabletten** Salushaus, Ger.
Mistletoe (p.1715·3).
*Circulatory disorders.*

**Mistelol-Kapseln** Twardy, Ger.
Mistletoe (p.1715·3).
*Cardiovascular disorders.*

**Misteltropfen** Bio-Diat, Ger.
Mistletoe (p.1715·3).
*Circulatory disorders.*

**Misteltropfen Hofmanns** Hofmann & Sommer, Ger.
Mistletoe (p.1715·3).
*Circulatory disorders.*

**Mistick Verde** Marco Viti, Ital.
Geranium oil (p.1692·2); citronella oil (p.1673·2); lavender oil (p.1705·2).
*Insect repellent.*

**Mistral** Mediolanum, Ital.
Dermatan sulfate sodium (p.892·2).
*Thrombosis prophylaxis.*

**Misubar** Farmachimici, Ital.
Barrier preparation.
*Nappy rash.*

**Misulban** Nuovo ISM, Ital.†.
Busulfan (p.532·2).
*Chronic myeloid leukaemia.*

**Misultina** Microsules Bernabo, Arg.
Azithromycin (p.159·1).
*Bacterial infections.*

**Misura** Searle, Ital.†.
Soya lecithin (p.1706·1).

**Misurid** Farmachimici, Ital.
Sulfur (p.1158·2).
*Skin disorders.*

**Misurid Plus** Farmachimici, Ital.
Barrier cream.

**Mita-c** Milano, Thai.
Ascorbic acid (p.1460·2).
*Vitamin C deficiency.*

**Mitan** Toyo, Hong Kong†.
Vitamin B substances (p.1417·1).
*Neuralgias; vitamin B deficiencies.*

**Mitchell Expel Anti Lice Spray** Mitchell, UK†.
Carbaryl (p.1501·2).
*Pediculosis.*

**Miten** CEPA, Spain.
Valsartan (p.1018·3).
*Hypertension.*

**Miten Plus** CEPA, Spain.
Valsartan (p.1018·3); hydrochlorothiazide (p.933·2).
*Hypertension.*

**Mitex** Kampel Martian, Arg.
Miltefosine (p.573·2).
*Skin metastases.*

**Mite-X** Fischer, Israel.
Permethrin (p.1508·3).
*Scabies.*

**Mitexan** Asta Oncologia, Braz.
Mesna (p.1041·2).
*Prevention of urotoxicity due to oxazaphosphorine antineoplastics.*

**Mithen** Fidia, Ital.
Amino acids; vitamins; minerals (p.1417·1); hypericum (p.299·1).
*Nutritional supplement.*

**Mithracin**
IFET (ΙΦΕΤ), Gr.; Pfizer, Norw.†; Bayer, USA†.
Plicamycin (p.580·2).
*Hypercalcaemia of malignancy; hypercalciuria of malignancy; testicular cancer.*

**Mithracine** Pfizer, Fr.†.
Plicamycin (p.580·2).
*Hypercalcaemia of malignancy; malignant neoplasms.*

**Miticocan** Asta Medica, Braz.
Benzyl benzoate (p.1500·2).
*Pediculosis; scabies.*

**Mitiderma** Milo, Spain.
Camphor (p.1665·3); eucalyptus oil (p.1686·2); methyl salicylate (p.59·3); oleum pini sylvestris; menthol (p.1711·3).
*Coughs; muscular pain; nasal congestion.*

**Mitil** Aspen, S.Afr.
Prochlorperazine maleate (p.716·3).
*Migraine; nausea and vomiting; nonpsychotic mental disorders; vestibular disorders.*

**Mitilase** Spedrog, Arg.
Fluoxetine hydrochloride (p.292·1).
*Depression.*

**Mitituss** Magis, Ital.
Cloperastine fendizoate (p.1117·2).
*Coughs.*

**Mitocin** Bristol-Myers Squibb, Braz.
Mitomycin (p.573·3).
*Malignant neoplasms.*

**Mitocin-C** Bristol-Myers Squibb, Mex.
Mitomycin (p.573·3).
*Malignant neoplasms.*

**Mitocor** Zambon, Ital.
Ubidecarenone (p.1760·2).
*Cardiac disorders; co-enzyme $Q_{10}$ deficiency.*

**Mitocortyl** Sanofi Synthelabo OTC, Fr.
Hydrocortisone (p.1103·3).
*Insect and nettle stings; sunburn.*

**Mitocyna** Richmond, Arg.
Mitomycin (p.573·3).
*Malignant neoplasms.*

**Mitog** Microsules, Arg.
Oxaliplatin (p.577·1).
*Malignant neoplasms.*

**Mitokebir** Aspen, Arg.
Mitomycin (p.573·3).
*Malignant neoplasms.*

**Mitokor** Biotenk, Arg.
Amlodipine (p.862·2).
*Angina pectoris; hypertension.*

**Mitolem** Lemery, Mex.
Mitomycin (p.573·3).
*Malignant neoplasms.*

**Mito-medac** Medac, Ger.
Mitomycin (p.573·3).
*Malignant neoplasms.*

**Mitonovag** Gobbi, Arg.
Mitomycin (p.573·3).
*Malignant neoplasms.*

**Mitostat** Orion, Fin.
Mitomycin (p.573·3).
*Malignant neoplasms.*

**Mitosyl**
Note. This name is used for preparations of different composition.
Sanofi Synthelabo, Belg.; Sanofi Synthelabo, Ger.
Cod-liver oil (p.1425·2); zinc oxide (p.1163·2); methyl salicylate (p.59·3).
*Burns; skin disorders; wounds.*

Sanofi Synthelabo OTC, Fr.; Sanofi Synthelabo, Port.
Fish-liver oil; zinc oxide (p.1163·2).
*Burns; skin disorders; wounds.*

Sanofi Synthelabo, Spain.
Colecalciferol (p.1461·3); vitamin A (p.1451·2); zinc oxide (p.1163·2).
*Burns; skin disorders; wounds.*

**Mitotie** Gautier, Arg.
Mitomycin (p.573·3).
*Malignant neoplasms.*

**Mitoxal** Asta Oncologia, Braz.
Mitoxantrone hydrochloride (p.575·2).
*Malignant neoplasms.*

**Mitoxana** *Asta Medica, Irl.; Baxter Oncology, UK.*
Ifosfamide (p.561·1).
*Malignant neoplasms.*

**Mitoxgen** *Gautier, Arg.*
Mitoxantrone hydrochloride (p.575·2).
*Malignant neoplasms.*

**Mitoxmar** *Kampel Martian, Arg.*
Mitoxantrone (p.576·1).
*Malignant neoplasms.*

**Mitozytrex** *SuperGen, USA.*
Mitomycin (p.573·3).
*Adenocarcinoma of the stomach or pancreas.*

**Mitran** *Hauck, USA†.*
Chlordiazepoxide hydrochloride (p.674·2).
*Alcohol withdrawal syndrome; anxiety.*

**Mitranax** *Polipharm, Thai.*
Alprazolam (p.668·3).
*Anxiety.*

**Mitroken** *Kendrick, Mex.*
Ciprofloxacin hydrochloride (p.188·2).
*Bacterial infections.*

**Mitrolan** *Robins, USA†.*
Polycarbophil calcium (p.1284·2).
*Constipation; diarrhoea.*

**Mitrotan** *Gap, Gr.*
Ergometrine maleate (p.1684·1).
*Postpartum haemorrhage.*

**Mitrotil** *Recalcine, Chile.*
Tenoxicam (p.93·1).
*Gout; inflammation; musculoskeletal, joint, and periarticular disorders.*

**Mitroxone** *Columbia, Mex.†.*
Mitoxantrone hydrochloride (p.575·2).
*Malignant neoplasms.*

**Mit's Linctus Codeinae Co** *AstraZeneca, India.*
Codeine phosphate (p.27·1); chlorphenamine maleate (p.427·3).
*Coughs.*

**Mittavin** *Nicholas Piramal, India.*
Multivitamin preparation (p.1417·1).

**Mittoval** *Inverni della Beffa, Ital.*
Alfuzosin hydrochloride (p.856·2).
*Benign prostatic hyperplasia.*

**Mivacron**
*GlaxoSmithKline, Arg.; GlaxoSmithKline, Austral.; GlaxoSmithKline, Austria; GlaxoSmithKline, Belg.; GlaxoSmithKline, Braz.; Abbott, Canad.; GlaxoSmithKline, Chile; GlaxoSmithKline, Denm.; GlaxoSmithKline, Fin.; GlaxoSmithKline, Fr.; GlaxoSmithKline, Ger.; Glaxo Wellcome, Gr.; GlaxoSmithKline, Hong Kong; Wellcome, Irl.; Wellcome, Israel; GlaxoSmithKline, Ital.; GlaxoSmithKline, Malaysia; Glaxo Wellcome, Mex.†; GlaxoSmithKline, Neth.; GlaxoSmithKline, Norw.; GlaxoSmithKline, NZ; Wellcome, Port.†; GlaxoSmithKline, S.Afr.; GlaxoSmithKline, Singapore; GlaxoSmithKline, Spain; GlaxoSmithKline, Swed.; GlaxoSmithKline, Switz.; Glaxo Wellcome, Thai.†; GlaxoSmithKline, UK; Abbott, USA.*
Mivacurium chloride (p.1403·3).
*Competitive neuromuscular blocker.*

**Mivalen** *Ativus, Braz.*
Simvastatin (p.997·1).
*Hyperlipidaemias.*

**mivitase 2000** *Biosyn, Ger.*
Multivitamin and mineral preparation (p.1417·1).

**Mixandex** *Pisa, Mex.*
Mitomycin (p.573·3).
*Malignant neoplasms.*

**Mixavit** *Julphar, UAE.*
Multivitamin preparation (p.1417·1).

**Mixavit-M** *Julphar, UAE.*
Multivitamin and mineral preparation (p.1417·1).

**Mixed Vegetable Tablets** *Dorwest, UK.*
Rorippa nasturtium aquaticum; celery seed and plant (p.1669·1); horseradish (p.1697·3); parsley (p.1728·3).
*Cystitis; minor bladder disorders; musculoskeletal and joint disorders.*

**Mixer** *Biomedica, Ital.*
Atenolol (p.865·2); nifedipine (p.966·2).
*Angina pectoris; hypertension.*

**Mixgen** *Laboratorios Chile, Chile.*
Betamethasone (p.1093·1) or betamethasone dipropionate (p.1093·1); gentamicin (p.219·1) or gentamicin sulfate (p.217·1).
*Infected eye disorders; infected skin disorders.*

**Mixobar**
*Astra Tech, Denm.; Astra Tech, Fin.; Byk Gulden, Ital.; Astra Tech, Norw.; Astra Tech, Swed.*
Barium sulfate (p.1061·1).
*Contrast medium for gastrointestinal radiography.*

**Mixogen**
*Note. This name is used for preparations of different composition.*
*Infar, India; Donmed, S.Afr.*
*Injection:* Estradiol benzoate (p.1550·1); estradiol phenylpropionate (p.1550·2); testosterone propionate (p.1570·1); testosterone phenylpropionate (p.1570·1); testosterone isocaproate (p.1570·1).
*Menopausal disorders.*

*Infar, India.*
*Tablets:* Ethinylestradiol (p.1553·2); methyltestosterone (p.1559·3).
*Menopausal disorders.*

**Mixotone** *Teofarma, Ital.*
Polymyxin B sulfate (p.245·1); neomycin sulfate (p.235·1); hydrocortisone sodium succinate (p.1104·1); lidocaine hydrochloride (p.1377·3).
*Bacterial infections of the ear.*

**Mixtard** *Novo Nordisk, Ger.†.*
Mixture of insulin injection (porcine, highly-purified) 30% and isophane insulin (porcine, highly-purified) 70% (p.333·3).
A 50:50 mixture may be known as Initard.
*Diabetes mellitus.*

**Mixtard 10, 20, 30, 40, and 50**
*Novo Nordisk, Irl.; Novo Nordisk, Spain; Novo Nordisk, UK.*
Mixtures of insulin injection (human) 10%, 20%, 30%, 40%, and 50% and isophane insulin injection (human) 90%, 80%, 70%, 60%, and 50% respectively (p.333·3).
Formerly known as Human Mixtard in the *UK*.
*Diabetes mellitus.*

**Mixtard 10/90, 20/80, 30/70, 40/60, and 50/50**
*Novo Nordisk, Denm.; Novo Nordisk, Fin.; Novo Nordisk, Neth.; Novo Nordisk, Norw.; Novo Nordisk, Swed.*
Mixtures of insulin injection (human) and isophane insulin injection (human) respectively in the proportions indicated (p.333·3).
*Diabetes mellitus.*

**Mixtard 20/80** *Novo Nordisk, S.Afr.*
A mixture of soluble insulin injection (human) 80% and isophane insulin injection (human) 20% respectively (p.333·3).
*Diabetes mellitus.*

**Mixtard 20/80, 30/70, 50/50** *Novo Nordisk, Austral.*
Mixtures of neutral insulin injection (human, pyr, monocomponent) and isophane insulin injection (human, pyr, monocomponent) respectively in the proportions indicated (p.333·3).
*Diabetes mellitus.*

**Mixtard 30/70** *Novo Nordisk, Spain.*
Mixture of insulin injection (human, emp) 30% and isophane insulin injection (human, emp) 70% (p.333·3).
*Diabetes mellitus.*

**Mixtard HM** *Pentafarma, Chile.*
Mixture of insulin injection (human) 20% and 30% and isophane insulin injection (human) 80% and 70%, respectively (p.333·3).
*Diabetes mellitus.*

**Mixtard 10, 20, 30, 40, and 50 HM**
*Novo Nordisk, Arg.; Novo Nordisk, Fr.; Novo Nordisk, Hong Kong; Novo Nordisk, Port.*
Mixtures of insulin injection (human, monocomponent) 10%, 20%, 30%, 40%, and 50% and isophane insulin injection (human, monocomponent) 90%, 80%, 70%, 60%, and 50%, respectively (p.333·3).
*Diabetes mellitus.*

**Mixtard 20, 30, 50 HM**
*Novo Nordisk, Singapore; Novo Nordisk, Thai.*
Mixtures of insulin injection (human, monocomponent) 20%, 30%, and 50% and isophane insulin injection (human, monocomponent) 80%, 70%, and 50%, respectively (p.333·3).
*Diabetes mellitus.*

**Mixtard 30 HM** *Novo Nordisk, Malaysia.*
Mixture of insulin injection (human, monocomponent) 30% and isophane insulin injection (human, monocomponent) 70% (p.333·3).
*Diabetes mellitus.*

**Mixtard HM 10, 20, 30, 40, 50** *Novo Nordisk, Switz.*
Mixtures of insulin injection (human, monocomponent) 10%, 20%, 30%, 40%, and 50% and isophane insulin injection (human, monocomponent) 90%, 80%, 70%, 60%, and 50%, respectively (p.333·3).
*Diabetes mellitus.*

**Mixtard HM 10/90, 20/80, 30/70, 40/60, and 50/50**
*Novo Nordisk, Austria; Novo Nordisk, Belg.*
Mixtures of insulin injection (human, monocomponent) and isophane insulin suspension (human, monocomponent) respectively in the proportions indicated (p.333·3).
*Diabetes mellitus.*

**Mixtard 30 MC** *Novo Nordisk, Switz.*
Mixture of insulin injection (porcine, monocomponent) 30% and isophane insulin injection (porcine, monocomponent) 70% (p.333·3).
*Diabetes mellitus.*

**Mixtard 30/70 or 50/50** *Novo Nordisk, NZ.*
Mixtures of insulin injection (human) 30% or 50% and isophane insulin (human) 70% or 50% (p.333·3).
*Diabetes mellitus.*

**Mixtus** *Orion, Fin.*
Clobutinol hydrochloride (p.1117·1).
*Coughs.*

**Miya-BM** *Miyarisan, Jpn.*
*Clostridium butyricum.*
*Restoration of gastrointestinal flora.*

**Mizar** *Monsanto, Ital.*
Flurithromycin ethyl succinate (p.214·2).
*Bacterial infections.*

**Mizolen**
*Sanofi Synthelabo, Braz.†; Sanofi Synthelabo, Spain.*
Mizolastine (p.437·3).
*Hypersensitivity reactions.*

**Mizollen**
*Sanofi Synthelabo, Austria; Sanofi Synthelabo, Belg.; Sanofi Winthrop, Denm.; Sanofi Synthelabo, Fin.; Sanofi Synthelabo, Fr.; Sanofi Synthelabo, Ger.; Sanofi Synthelabo, Gr.; Sanofi Synthelabo, Israel; Sanofi Synthelabo, Ital.; Sanofi Synthelabo, Neth.; Sanofi Synthelabo, Port.; Sanofi Synthelabo, S.Afr.; Sanofi Synthelabo, Swed.; Synthelabo, Switz.; Schwarz, UK.*
Mizolastine (p.437·3).
*Allergic rhinoconjunctivitis; urticaria.*

**Mizolmex** *Ofimex, Mex.†.*
Mebendazole (p.108·2).

**Mizoltec** *Tecnofarma, Mex.*
Dipyrone (p.35·3).
*Fever; pain.*

**Mizonase** *Osteolab, Chile.*
Miconazole (p.405·2); tinidazole (p.617·1).
*Fungal balanitis; trichomoniasis; vulvovaginal infections.*

**Mizoron** *Milano, Thai.*
Ketoconazole (p.403·3).
*Fungal infections.*

**Mizosin** *Duopharma, Hong Kong.*
Prazosin hydrochloride (p.985·1).
*Benign prostatic hyperplasia; heart failure; hypertension; Raynaud's disease.*

**ML 20** *Blackmores, Austral.†.*
Magnesium phosphate (p.1228·1); dibasic potassium phosphate (p.1230·3); dried yeast (p.1469·1); lecithin (p.1706·1); *d*-alpha tocoferil acid succinate (p.1465·1).
*Magnesium deficiency.*

**ML Cu 250** *CCD, Fr.†.*
Copper-wound plastic (p.1425·3).
*Intra-uterine contraceptive device.*

**ML Cu 375** *CCD, Fr.†.*
Copper-wound plastic (p.1425·3).
*Intra-uterine contraceptive device.*

**M-long**
*Grunenthal, Austria; Grunenthal, Ger.*
Morphine sulfate (p.60·2).
*Pain.*

**MM Diplovax** *Pasteur Merieux, Ger.†.*
A measles and mumps vaccine (more attenuated Enders' and Jeryl Lynn strains, respectively) (p.1624·3).
*Active immunisation.*

**MM Expectorante** *Farmasa, Braz.*
Potassium iodide (p.1598·1); lobelia (p.1589·1); hyoscyamus (p.485·2).
*Respiratory-tract congestion.*

**M-M Vax**
*Chiron Behring, Ger.; Pro Vaccine, Switz.†.*
A measles and mumps vaccine (Enders' attenuated Edmonston and Jeryl Lynn (level B) strains respectively) (p.1624·3).
*Active immunisation.*

**MMR** *Aventis Pasteur, Denm.*
A measles, mumps, and rubella vaccine (Enders Edmonston, Jeryl Lynn, and Wistar RA 27/3 strains, respectively) (p.1625·1).
*Active immunisation.*

**MMR II**
*Merck Sharp & Dohme, Arg.; Merck Sharp & Dohme, Austral.; Merck Sharp & Dohme, Braz.; Merck Frosst, Canad.; Aventis Pasteur, Fin.; Vianex (Βιανέξ), Gr.; Merck Sharp & Dohme, Hong Kong; Aventis Pasteur, Irl.; Merck Sharp & Dohme, Israel; Aventis Pasteur, Ital.; Merck Sharp & Dohme, Malaysia; Merck Sharp & Dohme, Mex.; Merck Sharp & Dohme, NZ; Merck Sharp & Dohme, S.Afr.†; Merck Sharp & Dohme, Singapore; Aventis Pasteur, Swed.; Pro Vaccine, Switz.; Merck Sharp & Dohme, Thai.; Aventis Pasteur, UK; Merck, USA.*
A measles, mumps, and rubella vaccine (Enders' attenuated Edmonston, Jeryl Lynn (B level), and Wistar RA 27/3 strains respectively) (p.1625·1).
*Active immunisation.*

**MMR Triplovax** *Aventis Pasteur, Ger.*
A measles, mumps, and rubella vaccine (More attenuated Enders', Jeryl Lynn, and Wistar RA 27/3 strains, respectively) (p.1625·1).
*Active immunisation.*

**MMR Vax**
*Aventis Pasteur, Austria; Aventis Pasteur, Belg.; Chiron Behring, Ger.*
A measles, mumps, and rubella vaccine (Enders' attenuated Edmonston, Jeryl Lynn B, and Wistar RA 27/3 strains, respectively) (p.1625·1).
*Active immunisation.*

**MND** *Malaysia Chemist, Singapore.*
Metronidazole (p.607·2).
*Amoebiasis; trichomoniasis.*

**Mnesis** *Takeda, Ital.*
Idebenone (p.1700·3).
*Cerebrovascular disorders.*

**MN-Fusin** *Pisa, Mex.*
Manganese sulfate (p.1440·1).

**Moban**
*Du Pont, Hong Kong†; Endo, USA.*
Molindone hydrochloride (p.709·3).
*Psychoses.*

**Mobec** *Boehringer Ingelheim, Ger.*
Meloxicam (p.56·1).
*Ankylosing spondylitis; rheumatoid arthritis.*

**Mobemide** *Unipharm, Israel.*
Moclobemide (p.308·2).
*Depression.*

**Moben** *Elofar, Braz.*
Mebendazole (p.108·2).
*Worm infections.*

**Mobex** *Boehringer Ingelheim, Chile.*
Meloxicam (p.56·1).
*Alkylosing spondylitis; osteoarthritis; rheumatoid arthritis.*

**Mobic**
*Boehringer Ingelheim, Arg.; Boehringer Ingelheim, Austral.; Boehringer Ingelheim, Austria; Boehringer Ingelheim, Belg.; Boehringer Ingelheim, Denm.; Boehringer Ingelheim, Fin.; Boehringer Ingelheim, Fr.; Boehringer Ingelheim, Hong Kong; Boehringer Ingelheim, Irl.; Boehringer Ingelheim, Ital.; Boehringer Ingelheim, Malaysia; Boehringer Ingelheim, Norw.; Boehringer Ingelheim, NZ; Boehringer Ingelheim, S.Afr.; Boehringer Ingelheim, Singapore; Boehringer Ingelheim, Swed.; Boehringer Ingelheim, Thai.; Boehringer Ingelheim, UK; Abbott, USA; Boehringer Ingelheim, USA.*
Meloxicam (p.56·1).
*Musculoskeletal and joint disorders.*

**Mobicox**
*Boehringer Ingelheim, Canad.; Promeco, Mex.; Boehringer Ingelheim, Switz.*
Meloxicam (p.56·1).
*Gout; inflammation; musculoskeletal, joint and periarticular disorders; pain.*

**Mobidin** *Ascher, USA.*
Magnesium salicylate (p.55·1).
*Fever; inflammation; pain.*

**Mobiflex**
*Roche, Canad.†; Roche, Irl.; Roche, UK.*
Tenoxicam (p.93·1).
*Musculoskeletal, joint, peri-articular, and soft-tissue disorders.*

**Mobiforton** *Lichtenstein, Ger.*
Tetrazepam (p.724·1).
*Skeletal muscle spasm; spasticity.*

**Mobigesic** *Ascher, USA.*
Magnesium salicylate (p.55·1); phenyltoloxamine citrate (p.439·1).
*Pain.*

**Mobilat**
*Note. This name is used for preparations of different composition.*
*Sankyo, Austria; Sankyo, Belg.; Sankyo, Braz.; Sanofi Synthelabo, Chile; Sankyo, Fin.; Sankyo, Ger.; Sankyo, Hong Kong; Sankyo, Singapore; Sankyo, Switz.†; Sankyo, Thai.*
Suprarenal extract (p.1110·1); a heparinoid (p.931·1); salicylic acid (p.1157·1).
*Musculoskeletal, joint, and soft-tissue disorders.*

*Luitpold, Ger.†.*
*Tablets:* Ibuprofen (p.45·3).
*Fever; pain.*

*Sankyo, Ital.*
Hydrocortisone (p.1103·3); a heparinoid (p.931·1); salicylic acid (p.1157·1).
*Musculoskeletal and joint trauma; peri-articular and soft-tissue disorders.*

*Byk Gulden, Mex.; Sankyo, Neth.*
A heparinoid (p.931·1); salicylic acid (p.1157·1).
*Peri-articular and soft-tissue disorders.*

*Sankyo, Port.*
Prednisolone (p.1108·1); a heparinoid (p.931·1); salicylic acid (p.1157·1).
*Peri-articular and soft-tissue disorders.*

*Byk Madaus, S.Afr.†.*
Adrenal gland extract; a heparinoid (p.931·1); salicylic acid (p.1157·1).
*Musculoskeletal and joint disorders.*

**Mobilat Aktiv** *Sankyo, Ger.*
A heparinoid (p.931·1); salicylic acid (p.1157·1).
*Soft-tissue injury.*

**Mobilat Akut HES** *Sankyo, Ger.*
Glycol salicylate (p.44·3).
*Soft-tissue injury.*

**Mobilat Akut Indo** *Sankyo, Ger.*
Indometacin (p.47·3).
*Musculoskeletal, joint, and soft-tissue disorders.*

**Mobilat Akut Piroxicam** *Sankyo, Ger.*
Piroxicam (p.84·2).
*Soft-tissue injury.*

**Mobilat N** *Sankyo, Switz.*
A heparinoid (p.931·1); salicylic acid (p.1157·1).
*Joint and soft-tissue disorders.*

**Mobilis**
*Alphapharm, Austral.; Alphapharm, Singapore†; Merck, Singapore†.*
Piroxicam (p.84·2).
*Musculoskeletal and joint disorders.*

**Mobilisin**
*Note. This name is used for preparations of different composition.*
*Sankyo, Austria; Sankyo, Belg.; Sankyo, Ger.†; Sankyo, Ital.; Sankyo, Port.; Sankyo, Switz.*
Flufenamic acid (p.43·2); glycol salicylate (p.44·3) or salicylic acid (p.1157·1); a heparinoid (p.931·1).
*Musculoskeletal, joint, peri-articular, and soft-tissue disorders; neuralgias.*

*Sankyo, Port.*
*Cream:* Flufenamic acid (p.43·2); a heparinoid (p.931·1).
*Musculoskeletal, joint, and peri-articular disorders.*

**Mobilisin Composto** *Sankyo, Braz.*
Flufenamic acid (p.43·2); a heparinoid (p.931·1); glycol salicylate (p.44·3).
*Musculoskeletal and joint disorders.*

**Mobilisin plus** *Sankyo, Austria.*
Flufenamic acid (p.43·2); a heparinoid (p.931·1); benzyl nicotinate (p.21·2).
Formerly contained flufenamic acid, a heparinoid, benzyl nicotinate, and glycol salicylate.
*Musculoskeletal and joint disorders.*

**Mobilyzer** *Omni, UK.*
Green-lipped mussel (p.1696·1).
*Nutritional supplement for joint care.*

**Mobisyl** *Ascher, USA.*
Trolamine salicylate (p.95·3).
*Muscle, joint, and soft-tissue pain; neuralgia.*

**Mobloc** *AstraZeneca, Ger.; Promed, Ger.*
Felodipine (p.914·3); metoprolol succinate (p.957·1).
*Hypertension.*

**Moclamine** *Roche, Fr.*
Moclobemide (p.308·2).
*Depression.*

**Moclix** *Hexal, Ger.*
Moclobemide (p.308·2).
*Depression.*

**Moclo A** *Ecosol, Switz.*
Moclobemide (p.308·2).
*Depression; social phobia.*

**Moclodura** *Merck dura, Ger.*
Moclobemide (p.308·2).
*Depression.*

**Moctanin** *Ethitek, USA.*
Monoctanoin (p.1715·3).
*Gallstones.*

**Mocydone** *Pharmasant, Thai.*
Domperidone (p.1263·2).
*Digestive disorders; dyspepsia; nausea and vomiting.*

**Mod** *IRBI, Ital.†.*
Domperidone (p.1263·2).
*Gastrointestinal disorders.*

**Modal** *Rafa, Israel.*
Sulpiride (p.722·2).
*Gastrointestinal disorders; peptic ulcer; psychiatric disorders; vertigo.*

**Modalim**
*Sanofi Synthelabo, Malaysia; Sanofi Synthelabo, Neth.; Sanofi Synthelabo, Singapore; Sanofi Synthelabo, UK.*
Ciprofibrate (p.884·2).
*Hyperlipidaemias.*

**Modalina** *Sanofi Synthelabo, Ital.*
Trifluoperazine hydrochloride (p.726·3).
*Psychiatric disorders.*

**Modamide** *Merck Sharp & Dohme-Chibret, Fr.*
Amiloride hydrochloride (p.858·2).
*Ascites; hypertension; oedema.*

**Modane**
*Note. This name is used for preparations of different composition.*
*Bago, Chile.*
Dantron (p.1261·1); calcium pantothenate (p.1442·3).
*Constipation.*
*Cooperation Pharmaceutique, Fr.*
Calcium pantothenate (p.1442·3); senna (p.1288·2).
*Constipation.*
*Reig Jofre, Spain.*
Calcium sennoside A (p.1288·3); calcium sennoside B (p.1288·3).
*Constipation.*
*Savage, USA.*
Bisacodyl (p.1251·3).
*Constipation.*

**Modane Bulk** *Adria, USA†.*
Psyllium hydrophilic mucilloid (p.1268·1).
*Constipation.*

**Modane Soft** *Adria, USA†.*
Docusate sodium (p.1262·2).
*Constipation.*

**Modantis** *Surf Ski International, UK†.*
Antazoline hydrochloride (p.424·2); titanium dioxide (p.1160·3); allantoin (p.1141·3); cetrimide (p.1172·1).
*Minor burns and scalds; sunburn.*

**Modasomil**
*Ratiopharm, Austria; Mepha, Switz.*
Modafinil (p.1591·1).
*Narcoleptic syndrome.*

**Modaton**
*Note. This name is used for preparations of different composition.*
*Montpellier, Arg.*
*Oral drops:* Sodium picosulfate (p.1289·3).
*Tablets:* Bisacodyl (p.1251·3).
*Constipation.*
*Armstrong, Mex.*
Calcium pantothenate (p.1442·3); dantron (p.1261·1).
*Constipation.*

**Modaton NI** *Montpellier, Arg.*
Liquid paraffin (p.1479·1).
*Constipation.*

**Modavigil**
*CSL, Austral.; CSL, NZ.*
Modafinil (p.1591·1).
*Narcoleptic syndrome.*

**Modecate**
*Bristol-Myers Squibb, Austral.; Squibb, Canad.; Bristol-Myers Squibb, Chile; Sanofi Synthelabo, Fr.; Bristol-Myers Squibb, Hong Kong; Bristol-Myers Squibb, Irl.; Bristol-Myers Squibb, Israel†; Bristol-Myers Squibb, NZ; Bristol-Myers Squibb, S.Afr.; Bristol-Myers Squibb, Singapore; Squibb, Spain; Bristol-Myers Squibb, Thai.†; Sanofi Synthelabo, UK.*
Fluphenazine decanoate (p.699·3).
*Psychoses.*

**Modecate Acutum** *Bristol-Myers Squibb, S.Afr.†.*
Fluphenazine hydrochloride (p.699·3).
*Psychoses.*

**Modekal** *Crealko, Arg.*
Glucomannan (p.1693·3).
*Dietary fibre supplement.*

**Modellsweet** *Mintlab, Chile.*
Aspartame (p.1422·1).
*Sugar substitute.*

**Modenol** *Roche, Ger.*
Butizide (p.878·2); reserpine (p.995·1).
*Hypertension.*

**Moderil** *Klinger, Braz.†.*
Garcinia cambogia.
*Obesity.*

**Moderin Acne** *Pharmacia, Spain.*
Aluminium chlorohydrate (p.1142·1); sulfur (p.1158·2); methylprednisolone acetate (p.1106·1).
*Acne.*

**Moderine** *Uniao Quimica, Braz.*
Mazindol (p.1589·1); diazepam (p.690·1).
*Obesity.*

**Moderlax** *Atral, Port.*
Bisacodyl (p.1251·3).
*Bowel evacuation; constipation.*

**Modern Herbals Cold & Catarrh** *Lane, UK.*
Althaea (p.1651·3); echinacea (p.1683·2); sambucus (p.1741·3).
*Catarrh; sinus congestion.*

**Modern Herbals Cold & Congestion** *Lane, UK.*
Lobelia (p.1589·1); tolu solution (p.1131·3).
*Catarrh; cold symptoms; congestion; hay fever; rhinitis.*

**Modern Herbals Cough Mixture** *Lane, UK.*
Ipecacuanha (p.1122·3); marrubium (p.1124·1); squill vinegar (p.1130·3).
*Catarrh; cold symptoms; coughs; sore throat.*

**Modern Herbals Laxative** *Lane, UK.*
Senna (p.1288·2); aloin (p.1248·3); cascara (p.1255·1).
*Constipation.*

**Modern Herbals Menopause** *Lane, UK.*
Parsley (p.1728·3); vervain (p.1764·1); clivers (p.1673·2); senna (p.1288·2).
*Menopausal disorders.*

**Modern Herbals Muscular Pain** *Lane, UK.*
Camphor (p.1665·3); menthol (p.1711·3); eucalyptus oil (p.1686·2); methyl salicylate (p.59·3); turpentine oil (p.1760·1).
*Muscle pain.*

**Modern Herbals Pile** *Lane, UK.*
*Ointment:* Hamamelis (p.1696·3); compound benzoin tincture; zinc oxide (p.1163·2).
*Tablets:* Cascara (p.1255·1); slippery elm (p.1747·1).
*Haemorrhoids.*

**Modern Herbals Rheumatic Pain** *Lane, UK.*
Celery leaf (p.1669·1); menyanthes (p.1712·1); cimicifuga (p.1671·3).
*Musculoskeletal and joint pain.*

**Modern Herbals Sleep Aid** *Lane, UK.*
Passion flower (p.1729·1).
*Insomnia.*

**Modern Herbals Stress** *Lane, UK.*
Motherwort (p.1717·1); valerian (p.1762·2); vervain (p.1764·1); passion flower (p.1729·1).
*Irritability; stresses and strains.*

**Modern Herbals Trapped Wind & Indigestion** *Lane, UK.*
Activated charcoal (p.1030·2).
*Diarrhoea; dyspepsia; flatulence; heartburn.*

**Modern Herbals Water Retention** *Lane, UK.*
Bearberry (p.1659·2); clivers (p.1673·2); lappa (p.1704·3).
*Water retention.*

**Modernel** *Phoenix, Arg.*
Sodium picosulfate (p.1289·3).
*Bowel evacuation; constipation.*

**Modicef** *Ipso, Ital.*
Cefonicid sodium (p.174·2).
Lidocaine hydrochloride (p.1377·3) is included in this preparation to alleviate the pain of injection.
*Gram-negative bacterial infections.*

**Modicon**
*Janssen-Cilag, Neth.; Ortho McNeil, USA.*
Norethisterone (p.1562·2); ethinylestradiol (p.1553·2).
28-Day packs also contain 7 inert tablets.
*Combined oral contraceptive.*

**Modiem** *Piam, Ital.*
Cefonicid sodium (p.174·2).
Lidocaine hydrochloride (p.1377·3) is included in this preparation to alleviate the pain of injection.
*Gram-negative bacterial infections.*

**Modifast**
*Novartis Consumer, Austral.†; Wander Health Care, Switz.*
Food for special diets (p.1417·1).
*Obesity.*

**Modifenac**
*Alpharma, Denm.; Alpharma, Norw.; Alpharma, Swed.*
Diclofenac sodium (p.32·1).
*Dysmenorrhoea; musculoskeletal and joint disorders.*

**Modifical** *Zodiac, Braz.*
Ondansetron hydrochloride (p.1281·1).
*Nausea and vomiting induced by cytotoxics or radiotherapy.*

**Modil** *General Drugs, Thai.*
Minoxidil (p.960·1).
*Hypertension.*

**Modilac AR** *Sodilac, Fr.†.*
Infant feed (p.1417·1).
*Regurgitation in infants.*

**Modilac HA** *Sodilac, Fr.*
Infant feed (p.1417·1).
*Milk-protein allergy.*

**Modilac sans Lactose** *Sodilac, Fr.*
Infant feed (p.1417·1).
*Diarrhoea; lactose intolerance.*

**ModimMunal** *Medice, Ger.*
*Escherichia coli* antigens.
*Arthritis.*

**Modina** *Neves, Port.*
Nimodipine (p.972·3).
*Neurological deficit following subarachnoid haemorrhage.*

**Modiodal**
*Lafon, Denm.; Lafon, Fr.; Genesis, Gr.; Nourypharma, Neth.; Aneid, Port.; CEPA, Spain; Organon, Swed.*
Modafinil (p.1591·1).
*Narcoleptic syndrome.*

**Modip** *Promed, Ger.; AstraZeneca, Ger.*
Felodipine (p.914·3).
*Hypertension.*

**Modisal** *Sandoz, UK.*
Isosorbide mononitrate (p.942·1).
*Angina pectoris.*

**Modiscop** *Brady, Austria.*
Morphine hydrochloride (p.60·1); ethylmorphine hydrochloride (p.37·3); hyoscine hydrobromide (p.483·3).
*Pain.*

**Moditen**
*Squibb, Canad.; Sanofi Synthelabo, Fr.; Sanofi Synthelabo, UK.*
Fluphenazine enantate (p.699·3) or fluphenazine hydrochloride (p.699·3).
*Anxiety; disturbed behaviour; psychoses.*

**Moditen Depot** *Bristol-Myers Squibb, Ital.*
Fluphenazine decanoate (p.699·3).
*Psychoses.*

**Modium** *Pharmaten (Φαρματεν), Gr.*
Lorazepam (p.704·1).
*Anxiety disorders; insomnia; status epilepticus.*

**Modival** *Saval, Chile.*
Dipotassium clorazepate (p.685·1).
*Anxiety disorders; insomnia; premedication.*

**Modivid**
*Hoechst Marion Roussel, Irl.†; Aventis, Ital.; Aventis, Mex.; Aventis, Port.; Hoechst Marion Roussel, Thai.†.*
Cefodizime sodium (p.174·1).
Lidocaine (p.1377·3) or lidocaine hydrochloride (p.1377·3) may be included in the intramuscular injection to alleviate the pain of injection.
*Bacterial infections.*

**Modizide** *Amrad, Austral.†.*
Amiloride hydrochloride (p.858·2); hydrochlorothiazide (p.933·2).
*Ascites; hypertension; oedema.*

**Modomed** *Medifive, Thai.*
Domperidone (p.1263·2).
*Digestive disorders; dyspepsia; heartburn; nausea and vomiting.*

**Modopar** *Roche, Fr.*
Levodopa (p.1205·2); benserazide hydrochloride (p.1200·2).
*Parkinsonism.*

**Modrasone**
*Pliva, Irl.; Pliva, UK.*
Alclometasone dipropionate (p.1090·3).
*Skin disorders.*

**Modrenal** *Wanskerne, UK.*
Trilostane (p.1757·3).
*Breast cancer; Cushing's syndrome; hyperaldosteronism.*

**Moducal**
*Mead Johnson, Austral.†; Mead Johnson Nutritionals, Canad.; Mead Johnson, NZ; Mead Johnson, Port.; Mead Johnson Nutritionals, USA.*
Maltodextrin (p.1439·3).
*Carbohydrate supplement.*

**Moducren**
*Sidus, Arg.; Merck Sharp & Dohme-Chibret, Fr.; Merck Sharp & Dohme, Hong Kong; Merck Sharp & Dohme, Irl.; Merck Sharp & Dohme, Mex.†; Merck Sharp & Dohme, Neth.†; Merck Sharp & Dohme, Port.; Merck Sharp & Dohme, S.Afr.; Merck Sharp & Dohme, Switz.; Merck Sharp & Dohme, UK.*
Amiloride hydrochloride (p.858·2); hydrochlorothiazide (p.933·2); timolol maleate (p.1012·2).
*Hypertension.*

**Moducrin**
*Merck Sharp & Dohme, Austria; Merck Sharp & Dohme, Ger.*
Amiloride hydrochloride (p.858·2); hydrochlorothiazide (p.933·2); timolol maleate (p.1012·2).
*Hypertension.*

**Modula** *Antonetto, Ital.*
Polycarbophil calcium (p.1284·2).
*Constipation; diarrhoea.*

**Modul'Aid** *Voyage, Fr.*
Permethrin (p.1508·3).
*Mosquito repellent.*

**Modulamin** *Braun, Switz.*
Amino-acid infusion with or without electrolytes (p.1417·1).
*Parenteral nutrition.*

**Modulan** *Macrophar, Thai.*
Amiloride hydrochloride (p.858·2); hydrochlorothiazide (p.933·2).
*Hepatic cirrhosis with ascites; hypertension; oedema.*

**Modulanzime** *Andromaco, Port.; Grunenthal, Port.*
Bromopride (p.1254·1); dimethicone (p.1289·2); pepsin (p.1729·3); amylase (p.1654·2); fungal lipase.
*Gastrointestinal disorders.*

**Modulator** *Servier, Spain.*
Benfluorex hydrochloride (p.868·1).
*Diabetes mellitus; hyperlipidaemias.*

**Modulen IBD**
*Nestle, Austral.; Nestle, Fr.; Nestle Clinical, Irl.; Nestle, Ital.*
Preparation for enteral nutrition (p.1417·1).
*Inflammatory bowel disease.*

**Modulo Calorico** *Braun, Chile.*
Maltodextrin (p.1439·3).
*Nutritional supplement.*

**Modulon**
*Axcan, Canad.; Pfizer, Fr.*
Trimebutine maleate (p.1758·1).
*Gastrointestinal disorders.*

**Modu-Puren** *Isis Puren, Ger.†.*
Amiloride hydrochloride (p.858·2); hydrochlorothiazide (p.933·2).
*Hypertension; oedema.*

**Moduret**
*Merck Frosst, Canad.; Du Pont, Irl.; Merck Sharp & Dohme, UK.*
Amiloride hydrochloride (p.858·2); hydrochlorothiazide (p.933·2).
These ingredients can be described by the British Approved Name Co-amilozide.
*Ascites; heart failure; hypertension; oedema.*

**Moduretic**
*Sidus, Arg.; Merck Sharp & Dohme, Austral.; Merck Sharp & Dohme, Austria; Merck Sharp & Dohme, Belg.; Prodome, Braz.; Merck Sharp & Dohme, Denm.; Merck Sharp & Dohme, Fin.; Bristol-Myers Squibb, Fr.; Vianex (Βιανεξ), Gr.; Merck Sharp & Dohme, Hong Kong; Du Pont, Irl.†; Merck Sharp & Dohme, Ital.; Merck Sharp & Dohme, Malaysia; Merck Sharp & Dohme, Mex.; Merck Sharp & Dohme, Neth.; Merck Sharp & Dohme, NZ†; Merck Sharp & Dohme, Port.; Merck Sharp & Dohme, S.Afr.; Merck Sharp & Dohme, Swed.; Merck Sharp & Dohme, Switz.; Merck Sharp & Dohme, Thai.; Merck Sharp & Dohme, UK; Merck, USA.*
Amiloride hydrochloride (p.858·2); hydrochlorothiazide (p.933·2).
These ingredients can be described by the British Approved Name Co-amilozide.
*Ascites; heart failure; hypertension; oedema.*

**Moduretic Mite** *Merck Sharp & Dohme, Norw.*
Amiloride hydrochloride (p.858·2); hydrochlorothiazide (p.933·2).
*Hypertension; oedema.*

**Moduretik** *Bristol-Myers Squibb, Ger.*
Amiloride hydrochloride (p.858·2); hydrochlorothiazide (p.933·2).
*Ascites; hypertension; oedema.*

**Modus** *Almirall, Spain.*
Nimodipine (p.972·3).
*Mental function impairment; neurological deficit following subarachnoid haemorrhage.*

**Modustatina** *Sanofi Synthelabo, Ital.*
Somatostatin acetate (p.1339·3).
*Adjunct in gastrointestinal radiography; diabetic ketoacidosis; gastrointestinal haemorrhage; pancreatic disorders.*

**Modustatine**
*Sanofi Synthelabo, Belg.; Sanofi Synthelabo, Fr.*
Somatostatin acetate (p.1339·3).
*Gastrointestinal haemorrhage; postoperative gastrointestinal fistulae.*

**Modutrol** *Osteolab, Chile.*
Ethinylestradiol (p.1553·2); levonorgestrel (p.1563·2).
*Triphasic oral contraceptive.*

**Moex**
*Ercopharm, Denm.†; Schwarz, Fr.; Schwarz, Hong Kong.*
Moexipril hydrochloride (p.961·2).
*Hypertension.*

**Mofesal** *Medice, Ger.†.*
Mofebutazone (p.60·1).
*Rheumatism; superficial thrombophlebitis.*

**Mofesal N** *Medice, Ger.*
Mofebutazone sodium (p.60·1).
Lidocaine hydrochloride (p.1377·3) is included in this preparation to alleviate the pain of injection.
*Rheumatism; superficial thrombophlebitis.*

**Mogadan** *ICN, Ger.*
Nitrazepam (p.710·1).
*Sleep disorders.*

**Mogadon**
*ICN, Austral.; ICN, Austria; Sanico, Belg.†; ICN, Canad.; ICN, Denm.; CSP, Fr.; Roche, Hong Kong; ICN, Irl.; ICN, Ital.; ICN, Malaysia; ICN, Neth.; ICN, Norw.; Pharmaco, S.Afr.; Medilink, Swed.; ICN, Switz.; ICN, UK.*
Nitrazepam (p.710·1).
*Epilepsy; insomnia.*

**Mogasinte** *CPH, Port.*
Domperidone (p.1263·2).
*Adjunct in gastrointestinal examinations; dyspepsia; nausea and vomiting.*

**Mogetic** *Azupharma, Ger.*
Morphine sulfate (p.60·2).
*Pain.*

**Mohexal** *Hexal, Austral.*
Moclobemide (p.308·2).
*Depression.*

**Mohrus** *Hisamitsu, Jpn.*
Ketoprofen (p.51·2).
*Inflammation; musculoskeletal, joint, and peri-articular disorders; pain.*

**Moisol** *FDC, India.*
Hypromellose (p.1579·3).
*Dry eyes; eye irritation.*

**Moist Again** *Lake, USA.*
Vaginal lubricant.

**Moi-Stir**
*Paladin, Canad.; Kingswood, USA.*
Carmellose sodium (p.1577·3); electrolytes (p.1217·1); sorbitol (p.1446·3).
*Dry mouth.*

**Moisture Drops**
*Note. This name is used for preparations of different composition.*
*Bausch & Lomb, Canad.; Bausch & Lomb, S.Afr.*
Hypromellose (p.1579·3); glycerol (p.1694·3); povidone (p.1581·2).
*Dry eye; eye irritation.*
*Bausch & Lomb, USA.*
Hypromellose (p.1579·3); dextran 70 (p.746·2); glycerol (p.1694·3).
*Dry eyes.*

**Moisture Eyes** *Co-Pharma, UK†.*
Hypromellose (p.1579·3).
*Keratoconjunctivitis sicca; lubrication of artificial eyes and hard contact lenses.*

**Moisture Lift Protective** *Avon, Canad.*
*SPF 15:* Octinoxate (p.1154·3); octisalate (p.1154·3); oxybenzone (p.1154·3).
*Sunscreen.*

**Moisture Shield** *Avon, Canad.*
*SPF 15:* Octinoxate (p.1154·3); oxybenzone (p.1154·3).
*Sunscreen.*

**Moisture Therapy** *Avon, Canad.*
*SPF 15:* Octinoxate (p.1154·3); oxybenzone (p.1154·3).
*Sunscreen.*

**Moisturel**
*Westwood-Squibb, Canad.*
White soft paraffin (p.1479·3); dimethicone (p.1482·1).
*Dry skin disorders.*
*Westwood-Squibb, USA.*
Emollient.
*Dry skin disorders.*

**Molagar** *Finadiet, Arg.*
Leflunomide (p.53·2).

**Molax** *Siam Bheasach, Thai.*
Domperidone (p.1263·2) or domperidone maleate (p.1263·2).
*Gastrointestinal disorders.*

**Molca** *Andromaco, Chile.*
Benzethonium chloride (p.1169·2); proflavine hydrochloride (p.1165·3).
*Disinfection of instruments; mucous membranes, and skin.*

**Molcain** *Molteni, Ital.*
Mepivacaine hydrochloride (p.1381·2).
Adrenaline acid tartrate (p.852·2) is included in some injections as a vasoconstrictor to diminish absorption and localise the effect of the local anaesthetic.
*Local anaesthesia.*

**Molcer** *Wallace Mfg Chem., UK.*
Docusate sodium (p.1262·2).
*Ear wax removal.*

**Moldina** *Juventus, Spain.*
Bifonazole (p.395·1).
*Fungal skin infections.*

**Molelant** *Chrispa (Χρισπα), Gr.*
Cefotaxime sodium (p.175·3).
*Bacterial infections.*

**Molevac**
*Pfizer, Austria; Parke, Davis, Ger.; Parke, Davis, Switz.†.*
Pyrvinium embonate (p.113·3).
*Enterobiasis.*

**Molfenac** *Amsa, Ital.*
Diclofenac epolamine (p.33·1).
*Inflammation; musculoskeletal and joint disorders; pain.*

**Molipaxin**
*Aventis, Irl.; Aventis, S.Afr.; Aventis, UK.*
Trazodone hydrochloride (p.319·1).
*Depression.*

**Molival** *Temis, Arg.*
Bromazepam (p.671·3).
*Anxiety.*

**Mollifene** *Pfeiffer, USA.*
Urea hydrogen peroxide (p.1195·3).
*Ear wax removal.*

**Mollipect** *Draco, Swed.*
Bromhexine hydrochloride (p.1115·3); ephedrine hydrochloride (p.1120·1).
*Coughs.*

**Molnia** *Maigal, Arg.*
Sulfur (p.1158·2); pyrithione zinc (p.1156·2).
*Seborrhoea.*

**Molsi-Azu** *Azupharma, Ger.*
Molsidomine (p.961·3).
*Ischaemic heart disease.*

**Molsicor**
*Hexal, Arg.; Hexal, Austria; Betapharm, Ger.*
Molsidomine (p.961·3).
*Angina pectoris.*

**Molsidain** *Aventis, Spain.*
Molsidomine (p.961·3).
*Angina pectoris.*

**Molsidaine** *Aventis, Arg.*
Molsidomine (p.961·3).
*Angina pectoris.*

**Molsidirex** *Irex, Fr.†.*
Molsidomine (p.961·3).

**Molsidolat** *Aventis, Austria.*
Molsidomine (p.961·3).
*Angina pectoris.*

**Molsihexal**
*Hexal, Austria; Hexal, Ger.*
Molsidomine (p.961·3).
*Angina pectoris.*

**molsiket** *Schwarz, Ger.*
Molsidomine (p.961·3).
*Ischaemic heart disease.*

**Molsi-Puren** *Alpharma-Isis, Ger.*
Molsidomine (p.961·3).
*Ischaemic heart disease.*

**Molybdene Injectable** *Aguettant, Fr.*
Ammonium molybdate (p.1440·3).
*Parenteral nutrition.*

**Molypen** *American Pharmaceutical, USA.*
Ammonium molybdate (p.1440·3).
*Parenteral nutrition.*

**Molzyme** *FDC, India.*
Papain (p.1727·3); amylase (p.1654·2); cumin oil; ajowan oil; activated charcoal (p.1030·2); simeticone (p.1289·2); belladonna (p.479·1).
*Anorexia; dyspepsia.*

**Mom** *Nestle, Mex.*
Nutritional supplement during pregnancy and lactation (p.1417·1).

**Mom Gel** *Candioli, Ital.*
Phenothrin (p.1509·1).
*Pediculosis.*

**Mom Lozione Preventiva** *Candioli, Ital.*
Benzyl benzoate (p.1500·2).
*Insect repellent.*

**Mom Piretro Emulsione** *Candioli, Ital.*
Tetramethrin (p.1510·2); piperonyl butoxide (p.1509·2).
*Pediculosis.*

**Mom Shampoo Antiparassitario** *Candioli, Ital.*
Tetramethrin (p.1510·2); phenothrin (p.1509·1).
*Pediculosis.*

**Mom Shampoo Schiuma** *Candioli, Ital.*
Phenothrin (p.1509·1).
*Pediculosis.*

**Mom Zanzara** *Candioli, Ital.†.*
Benzyl benzoate (p.1500·2); ethyl hexanediol.
*Insect repellent.*

**Momendol**
*Angelini, Ital.; Lepori, Port.*
Naproxen sodium (p.65·1).
*Fever; inflammation; musculoskeletal and joint disorders; pain.*

**Moment**
*Note. This name is used for preparations of different composition.*
*Apsen, Braz.*
Capsaicin (p.24·2).
*Neuralgia.*
*Angelini, Ital.; Lepori, Port.*
Ibuprofen (p.45·3).
*Fever; influenza symptoms; pain.*

**Momentol** *Squibb, Spain.*
Co-trimoxazole (p.199·3).
*Bacterial infections; Pneumocystis carinii pneumonia.*

**Momentum**
*Note. This name is used for preparations of different composition.*
*Wyeth Lederle, Austria; Wyeth Consumer, Neth.*
Paracetamol (p.76·2).
*Fever; pain.*
*Whitehall, USA.*
Aspirin (p.15·1); phenyltoloxamine citrate (p.439·1).
*Backache.*

**Momentum Analgetikum** *Much, Ger.†.*
Paracetamol (p.76·2).
*Fever; pain.*

**Momentum Muscular Backache Formula**
*Whitehall, USA.*
Magnesium salicylate (p.55·1).
*Pain.*

**Momicine** *Farmacusi, Spain.*
Midecamycin acetate (p.231·3).
*Bacterial infections.*

**Monafed** *Monarch, USA†.*
Guaifenesin (p.1122·1).
*Coughs.*

**Monafed DM** *Monarch, USA.*
Guaifenesin (p.1122·1); dextromethorphan hydrobromide (p.1117·3).
*Coughs.*

**Mona-Lisa** *Mona Lisa, Israel†.*
Copper-wound plastic (p.1425·3).
*Intra-uterine contraceptive device.*

**Monapax** *Nattermann, Ger.*
Homoeopathic preparation.

**Monarc-M**
*Teva Tuteur, Arg.; Kamada, Israel; American Red Cross, USA.*
A factor VIII preparation (p.751·1).
*Haemorrhagic disorders.*

**Monarit** *Rontag, Arg.*
Naproxen sodium (p.65·1).
*Pain.*

**Monaspor** *Grunenthal, Austria†.*
Cefsulodin sodium (p.180·2).
*Pseudomonas aeruginosa infections.*

**Monaxin** *Therabel, Belg.*
Clarithromycin (p.192·2).
*Bacterial infections.*

**Monazol** *Theramex, Mon.*
Sertaconazole nitrate (p.408·1).
*Vaginal candidiasis.*

**Monazole** *Technilab, Canad.*
Miconazole nitrate (p.405·3).
*Fungal vaginal infections.*

**Mondrian** *Andromaco, Chile.*
Bupropion hydrochloride (p.287·2).
*Aid to smoking withdrawal; depression.*

**Mondus** *Labinca, Arg.*
Flunarizine hydrochloride (p.434·1).
*Cerebral and peripheral vascular disorders; motion sickness.*

**Moneva** *Schering, Fr.*
Gestodene (p.1556·1); ethinylestradiol (p.1553·2).
*Combined oral contraceptive.*

**Moni** *Lichtenstein, Ger.*
Isosorbide mononitrate (p.942·1).
*Angina pectoris; heart failure; pulmonary hypertension.*

**Monicil** *Sanval, Braz.*
Rifampicin (p.250·2).
*Tuberculosis.*

**Monicor**
*Pierre Fabre, Fr.; Wallace, India.*
Isosorbide mononitrate (p.942·1).
*Angina pectoris; heart failure.*

**Monilac** *Chugai, Jpn.*
Lactulose (p.1269·1).
*Constipation; hyperammonaemia.*

**Monilen** *Recip, Swed.*
Urea (p.1162·2).
*Dry skin.*

**Monipax** *Haller, Braz.*
Fluconazole (p.398·1).
*Fungal infections.*

**Monistat**
*Janssen-Cilag, Austral.; McNeil Consumer, Canad.; Janssen-Cilag, Switz.; Advanced Care, USA.*
Miconazole nitrate (p.405·3).
*Fungal skin infections; vulvovaginal candidiasis.*

**Monit** *Sanofi Synthelabo, UK.*
Isosorbide mononitrate (p.942·1).
*Angina pectoris; heart failure.*

**Monitan** *Wyeth-Ayerst, Canad.*
Acebutolol hydrochloride (p.848·1).
*Angina pectoris; hypertension.*

**Monit-Puren** *Alpharma-Isis, Ger.*
Isosorbide mononitrate (p.942·1).
*Angina pectoris; heart failure; pulmonary hypertension.*

**Monizole** *Pharmaceutical Co, India.*
Metronidazole (p.607·2).
*Amoebiasis; giardiasis.*

**Mono Acis** *Acis, Ger.*
Isosorbide mononitrate (p.942·1).
*Angina pectoris; heart failure; pulmonary hypertension.*

**mono corax** *corax, Ger.*
Isosorbide mononitrate (p.942·1).
*Angina pectoris.*

**Mono Demetrin** *Parke, Davis, Ger.*
Prazepam (p.716·2).
*Anxiety disorders; sleep disorders.*

**Mono & Disaccharide Free Diet Powder (Product 3232A)** *Mead Johnson, Austral.*
Preparation for enteral nutrition (p.1417·1).
*Impaired glucose transport; intractable diarrhoea; lactase, sucrase, or maltase deficiency; test for fructose utilisation.*

**Mono Mack**
*Pfizer, Austria; Bago, Chile; Mack, Illert., Ger.; Mack, Hong Kong; Armstrong, Mex.; AstraZeneca, Neth.; Mack, Singapore†; Mack, Thai.*
Isosorbide mononitrate (p.942·1).
*Angina pectoris; heart failure; myocardial infarction; pulmonary hypertension.*

**Mono Maycor** *Parke, Davis, Ger.†; Godecke, Ger.†.*
Isosorbide mononitrate (p.942·1).
*Heart failure; ischaemic heart disease; myocardial infarction.*

**Mono Praecimed** *Molimin, Ger.*
Paracetamol (p.76·2).
*Fever; pain.*

**Mono Wolff** *Wolff, Ger.*
Isosorbide mononitrate (p.942·1).
*Angina pectoris; heart failure.*

**Mono-A** *Troikaa, India.*
Isosorbide mononitrate (p.942·1); aspirin (p.15·1).
*Angina pectoris; myocardial infarction.*

**Monobac** *Bristol-Myers Squibb, Mex.*
Aztreonam (p.160·3).
*Gram-negative bacterial infections.*

**Monobeta** *Betapharm, Ger.*
Isosorbide mononitrate (p.942·1).
*Angina pectoris.*

**Monobios** *CT, Ital.*
Cefonicid sodium (p.174·2).
Lidocaine hydrochloride (p.1377·3) is included in this preparation to alleviate the pain of injection.
*Gram-negative bacterial infections.*

**Monobiotic** *Ecobi, Ital.*
Cefonicid sodium (p.174·2).
Lidocaine hydrochloride (p.1377·3) is included in this preparation to alleviate the pain of injection.
*Gram-negative bacterial infections.*

**Monocal** *Mericon, USA.*
Calcium carbonate (p.1254·2); monofluorophosphate.
*Nutritional supplement.*

**Monocaps** *Freeda, USA.*
Multivitamin and mineral preparation with iron and folic acid (p.1417·1).

**Mono-Cedocard**
*Byk, Neth.; Pharmacia Upjohn, UK†.*
Isosorbide mononitrate (p.942·1).
*Angina pectoris.*

**Monocef**
*Note. This name is used for preparations of different composition.*
*Aristo, India.*
Ceftriaxone sodium (p.182·3).
*Bacterial infections.*
*Goldshield, Israel.*
Cefonicid (p.174·2).
*Bacterial infections.*

**Monocetin** *Novaquimica, Braz.†.*
Tetracycline hydrochloride (p.266·2); bromelains (p.1662·2).
*Bacterial infections.*

**Monocid**
*Note. This name is used for preparations of different composition.*
*Abbott, Austria.*
Clarithromycin (p.192·2).
*Bacterial infections.*
*GlaxoSmithKline, Belg.; SmithKline Beecham, Hong Kong†; Shire, Ital.; Decomed, Port.; Rottapharm, Spain; SmithKline Beecham, USA†.*
Cefonicid sodium (p.174·2).
Lidocaine hydrochloride (p.1377·3) may be included in the intramuscular injection to alleviate the pain of injection.
*Bacterial infections.*

**Monocide** *Fischer, Israel†.*
Carbophos; bioallethrin (p.1500·3).
*Pediculosis.*

**Monocinque**
*Menarini, Hong Kong; Lusofarmaco, Ital.*
Isosorbide mononitrate (p.942·1).
*Angina pectoris; heart failure; myocardial infarction.*

**Monoclair** *Hennig, Ger.*
Isosorbide mononitrate (p.942·1).
*Angina pectoris.*

**Monoclate-P**
*Aventis Behring, Austria; Aventis Behring, Braz.; Aventis Behring, Denm.; Aventis Behring, Fr.; Aventis Behring, Ger.; Aventis Behring, Irl.; Centeon, Israel; Centeon, Mex.†; Aventis Behring, Spain; Aventis Behring, Swed.; Aventis Behring, UK; Centeon, USA.*
A factor VIII preparation (p.751·1).
*Haemorrhagic disorders.*

**Monocline** *Bouchara-Recordati, Fr.†.*
Doxycycline hyclate (p.206·2).
*Bacterial infections.*

**Monoclox**
*Medochemie, Hong Kong; Medochemie, Malaysia; Medochemie, Singapore†; Medochemie, Thai.†.*
Cloxacillin sodium (p.198·2).
*Bacterial infections.*

**Monocontin** *Win-Medicare, India.*
Isosorbide mononitrate (p.942·1).
*Angina pectoris.*

**Monocor**
*Biovail, Canad.; Wyeth Lederle, Denm.†; Wyeth, UK.*
Bisoprolol fumarate (p.875·1).
*Angina pectoris; hypertension.*

**Monocord** *Dexxon, Israel.*
Isosorbide mononitrate (p.942·1).
*Angina pectoris; heart failure.*

**Monocordil** *Baldacci, Braz.*
Isosorbide mononitrate (p.942·1).
*Angina pectoris.*

**Monodox** *Oclassen, USA.*
Doxycycline (p.206·2).
*Bacterial infections; intestinal amoebiasis.*

**Monodoxin** *Crosara, Ital.†.*
Doxycycline hyclate (p.206·2).
*Bacterial infections.*

**Monodur** *PMC, Austral.*
Isosorbide mononitrate (p.942·1).
*Angina pectoris.*

**Mono-Embolex** *Novartis, Ger.*
Certoparin sodium (p.882·1).
*Postoperative thrombosis prophylaxis.*

**Monofed** *Garec, S.Afr.*
Pseudoephedrine hydrochloride (p.1129·2).
*Upper respiratory-tract congestion.*

**Monofeme**
*Wyeth, Austral.; Wyeth, NZ.*
21 Tablets, ethinylestradiol (p.1553·2); levonorgestrel (p.1563·2); 7 tablets, inert.
*Combined oral contraceptive.*

**Monoferro** *Ganassini, Ital.*
Ferrous gluconate (p.1428·1).
Ascorbic acid (p.1460·2) is included in this preparation to increase the absorption and availablitiy of iron.
*Iron-deficiency anaemia.*

**Monofix** *CSL, NZ.*
A factor IX preparation (p.752·2).
*Haemophilia B.*

**Monofix-VF** *CSL, Austral.*
A factor IX preparation (p.752·2).
*Haemophilia B.*

**Monoflam** *Lichtenstein, Ger.*
Diclofenac sodium (p.32·1).
*Gout; inflammation; musculoskeletal, joint, and soft-tissue disorders; pain.*

**Monoflocet** *Aventis, Fr.*
Ofloxacin (p.239·3).
*Bacterial infections.*

**Monofoscin** *CEPA, Spain†.*
Fosfomycin trometamol (p.214·3).
*Urinary-tract infections.*

**Monogen**
*Scientific Hospital Supplies, Austral.; Nutricia, NZ; Scientific Hospital Supplies, NZ; Scientific Hospital Supplies, UK.*
Preparation for enteral nutrition (p.1417·1).
*Lipid and lymphatic disorders.*

**Mono-Gesic** *Schwarz, USA†.*
Salsalate (p.88·1).
*Fever; osteoarthritis; pain; rheumatoid arthritis.*

**Monogestin** *Wyeth Lederle, Austria†.*
Gestodene (p.1556·1); ethinylestradiol (p.1553·2).
*Combined oral contraceptive.*

**Monoginal** *Novartis, Gr.*
Isosorbide mononitrate (p.942·1).
*Angina; heart failure.*

**Mono-Jod** *Philopharm, Ger.*
Potassium iodide (p.1598·1).
*Iodine deficiency.*

**Monoket**
*Sidus, Arg.; Gebro, Austria; Lavipharm, Gr.; Chiesi, Ital.; Pharmacia, Norw.; Neo-Farmaceutica, Port.; Pharmacia, Swed.; Schwarz, USA.*
Isosorbide mononitrate (p.942·1).
*Angina pectoris; heart failure; myocardial infarction; pulmonary hypertension.*

**Mono-Latex** *Wampole, USA.*
Test for infectious mononucleosis.

**Monolin** *Berlin Pharm, Thai.*
Isosorbide mononitrate (p.942·1).
*Angina pectoris; heart failure; pulmonary hypertension.*

**Monolin NPH** *Biobras, Braz.†.*
Isophane insulin injection (porcine, monocomponent) (p.333·3).
*Diabetes mellitus.*

**Monolin Regular** *Biobras, Braz.†.*
Neutral insulin injection (porcine, monocomponent) (p.333·3).
*Diabetes mellitus.*

**Monolitum**
*Lepori, Port.; Salvat, Spain.*
Lansoprazole (p.1269·3).
*Gastro-oesophageal reflux; peptic ulcer; Zollinger-Ellison syndrome.*

**Monolong**
*Alpharma-Isis, Ger.; CTI, Israel.*
Isosorbide mononitrate (p.942·1).
*Angina pectoris; heart failure; pulmonary hypertension.*

**Monomax** *Trinity, UK.*
Isosorbide mononitrate (p.942·1).
*Angina pectoris.*

**Monomycin**
*Grunenthal, Austria; Grunenthal, Ger.*
Erythromycin (p.208·1) or erythromycin ethyl succinate (p.208·1).
*Bacterial infections.*

**Monomycine** *Grunenthal, Switz.†.*
Erythromycin ethyl succinate (p.208·1).
*Bacterial infections.*

**Mononine**
*Aventis Behring, Braz.; Aventis Behring, Denm.; Aventis Behring, Fr.; Aventis Behring, Ger.; Aventis Behring, Irl.; Aventis Behring, Ital.; Aventis, Neth.; Aventis Behring, Spain; Aventis Behring, Swed.; Aventis Behring, UK; Centeon, USA.*
A factor IX preparation (p.752·2).
*Haemophilia B.*

**Mononit** *Medis, Israel.*
Isosorbide mononitrate (p.942·1).
*Angina pectoris; heart failure.*

**Mononitrat** *Verla, Ger.*
Isosorbide mononitrate (p.942·1).
*Angina pectoris.*

**Mononitril** *Baldacci, Port.*
Isosorbide mononitrate (p.942·1).
*Heart failure; ischaemic heart disease.*

**Monoparin**
*CP Pharmaceuticals, Irl.; Artex, NZ; CP Pharmaceuticals, UK.*
Heparin calcium (p.927·3) or heparin sodium (p.928·1).
*Thromboembolic disorders.*

**Monopina** *Bioindustria, Ital.*
Amlodipine besilate (p.862·1).
*Angina pectoris; hypertension.*

**Monoplus**
*Bristol-Myers Squibb, Austral.; Bristol-Myers Squibb, Braz.*
Fosinopril sodium (p.919·1); hydrochlorothiazide (p.933·2).
*Hypertension.*

**Monopress** *Bayer, Spain†.*
Nitrendipine (p.973·3).
*Angina pectoris; hypertension; Raynaud's syndrome.*

**Monopril**
*Bristol-Myers Squibb, Austral.; Bristol-Myers Squibb, Braz.; Bristol-Myers Squibb, Canad.; Bristol-Myers Squibb, Chile; Bristol-Myers Squibb, Denm.; Bristol-Myers Squibb, Gr.; Bristol-Myers Squibb, Hong Kong; Bristol-Myers Squibb, Malaysia; Bristol-Myers Squibb, Mex.; Bristol-Myers Squibb, Norw.†; Bristol-Myers Squibb, S.Afr.; Bristol-Myers Squibb, Singapore; Bristol-Myers Squibb, Swed.; Bristol-Myers Squibb, Thai.; Bristol-Myers Squibb, USA.*
Fosinopril sodium (p.919·1).
*Heart failure; hypertension.*

**Monopril comp** *Bristol-Myers Squibb, Swed.*
Fosinopril sodium (p.919·1); hydrochlorothiazide (p.933·2).
*Hypertension.*

**Monopril-HCT** *Bristol-Myers Squibb, USA.*
Fosinopril sodium (p.919·1); hydrochlorothiazide (p.933·2).
*Hypertension.*

**Monoprim** *Nycomed, Austria†.*
Trimethoprim (p.272·2).
*Urinary and respiratory-tract bacterial infections.*

**Monopront** *Ferraz, Lynce, Port.*
Isosorbide mononitrate (p.942·1).
*Angina pectoris; heart failure; pulmonary hypertension.*

**Monopur** *Pohl, Ger.*
Isosorbide mononitrate (p.942·1).
*Angina pectoris; heart failure; pulmonary hypertension.*

**Monoquin** *Zambon, Port.*
Lomefloxacin hydrochloride (p.227·2).
*Bacterial infections.*

**Monores** *Valeas, Ital.*
Clenbuterol hydrochloride (p.784·2).
*Obstructive airways disease.*

**Monorythm** *Gerolimatos (Γερολυματος), Gr.*
Isosorbide mononitrate (p.942·1).
*Angina; heart failure.*

**Monos** *Selvi, Ital.*
Rufloxacin hydrochloride (p.254·3).
*Bacterial infections.*

**Monosol** *Baxter, Austria.*
Glucose; electrolytes (p.1221·1).
*Haemodialysis; haemofiltration.*

**Monosorbitrate** *Nicholas Piramal, India.*
Isosorbide mononitrate (p.942·1).
*Angina pectoris.*

**Monosordil** *Elpen (Ελπεν), Gr.*
Isosorbide mononitrate (p.942·1).
*Angina; heart failure.*

**Monostenase** *Azupharma, Ger.*
Isosorbide mononitrate (p.942·1).
*Angina pectoris.*

**MonoStep** *Asche, Ger.*
Ethinylestradiol (p.1553·2); levonorgestrel (p.1563·2).
*Combined oral contraceptive.*

**Monostop** *Synthelabo, Spain†.*
Bifonazole (p.395·1).
*Fungal skin and nail infections.*

**Monotard**
*Novo Nordisk, Austral.; Novo Nordisk, Denm.; Novo Nordisk, Fin.; Novo Nordisk, Fr.; Novo Nordisk, Irl.; Novo Nordisk, Jpn; Novo Nordisk, Neth.; Novo Nordisk, Norw.; Novo Nordisk, NZ; Novo Nordisk, Port.; Novo Nordisk, Spain; Novo Nordisk, Swed.; Novo Nordisk, UK.*
Insulin zinc suspension (amorphous 30%, crystalline 70%) (human, pyr) (p.333·3).
Formerly known as Human Monotard in the *UK.*
*Diabetes mellitus.*

**Monotard HM**
*Novo Nordisk, Arg.; Novo Nordisk, Austria; Novo Nordisk, Belg.; Pentafarma, Chile; Novo Nordisk, Ger.; Novo Nordisk, Gr.; Novo Nordisk, Hong Kong; Novo Nordisk, Ital.; Novo Nordisk, Malaysia; Novo Nordisk, S.Afr.; Novo Nordisk, Singapore; Novo Nordisk, Switz.; Novo Nordisk, Thai.*
Insulin zinc suspension (amorphous 30%, crystalline 70%) (human, monocomponent) (p.333·3).
*Diabetes mellitus.*

**Monotard MC**
*Novo Nordisk, Arg.; Novo Nordisk, Braz.; Novo Nordisk, Hong Kong.*
Insulin zinc suspension (amorphous 30%, crystalline 70%) (porcine) (p.333·3).
*Diabetes mellitus.*

**Monotest**
*Aventis Pasteur, Austria; Aventis Pasteur, Fr.; Aventis Pasteur, Ital.; CSL, NZ; Aventis, S.Afr.; Aventis Pasteur, Swed.*
Tuberculin PPD (p.1759·1).
*Sensitivity test.*

**Mono-Tildiem**
*Sanofi Synthelabo, Fr.; Sanofi Synthelabo, Malaysia; Sanofi Synthelabo, Singapore; Sanofi Synthelabo, Thai.†.*
Diltiazem hydrochloride (p.900·1).
*Angina pectoris; hypertension.*

**Monotrate**
*Sun, India; Sun, Singapore†; Sun, Thai.*
Isosorbide mononitrate (p.942·1).
*Angina pectoris; heart failure.*

**Monotrean**
*Note. This name is used for preparations of different composition.*
*Sankyo, Braz.; Sankyo, Ital.*
Papaverine (p.1728·1); quinine hydrochloride (p.460·2).
*Vertigo.*

*Luitpold, Ger.†.*
Dimenhydrinate (p.431·1).
*Dizziness; nausea; vomiting.*

**Monotrean B6** *Sankyo Luitpold, Braz.†.*
Papaverine (p.1728·1); quinine hydrochloride (p.460·2); pyridoxine (p.1457·2).
*Vertigo.*

**Mono-Tridin** *Opfermann, Ger.*
Sodium monofluorophosphate (p.1446·2).
*Osteoporosis.*

**Monotrim**
*Gea, Denm.; Solvay, Irl.; Gea, Switz.; Solvay, UK.*
Trimethoprim (p.272·2).
*Bacterial infections.*

**Monotrin** *Bago, Arg.*
Isosorbide mononitrate (p.942·1).
*Angina pectoris; heart failure; pulmonary hypertension.*

**Monotussin** *Beige, S.Afr.†.*
Codeine phosphate (p.27·1); mepyramine maleate (p.437·1); ephedrine hydrochloride (p.1120·1).
*Coughs.*

**Mono-Vacc Test (O.T.)** *Pasteur Merieux, USA†.*
Old tuberculin (p.1759·1).
*Diagnosis of tuberculosis.*

**Monovacc-Test** *Aventis Pasteur, Belg.*
Old tuberculin (p.1759·1).
*Test for tuberculin sensitivity.*

**Monovax** *Aventis Pasteur, Fr.*
A BCG vaccine (p.1609·2).
*Active immunisation.*

**Monovent** *Sandoz, UK.*
Terbutaline sulfate (p.797·2).
*Obstructive airways disease; premature labour.*

**Monozide**
*Note. This name is used for preparations of different composition.*
*Bristol-Myers Squibb, S.Afr.*
Fosinopril sodium (p.919·1); hydrochlorothiazide (p.933·2).
*Hypertension.*

*Wyeth, UK†.*
Bisoprolol fumarate (p.875·1); hydrochlorothiazide (p.933·2).
*Hypertension.*

**Monozol** *Legrand, Braz.*
Albendazole (p.101·2).
*Worm infections.*

**Monphytol** *Laboratories for Applied Biology, UK.*
Methyl undecenoate (p.411·1); propyl undecenoate (p.411·1); salicylic acid (p.1157·1); methyl salicylate (p.59·3); propyl salicylate (p.1157·2); chlorobutanol (p.1176·3).
*Fungal skin and nail infections.*

**Montair** *Cipla, India.*
Montelukast (p.789·1).
*Asthma.*

**Montalen** *Pharmonta, Austria.*
Magnesium trisilicate (p.1272·3); aluminium hydroxide (p.1249·2); peppermint oil (p.1283·2).
*Gastrointestinal disorders associated with hyperacidity.*

**Montamed** *Montavit, Austria.*
Salverine hydrochloride (p.1741·3); propyphenazone (p.85·3); caffeine (p.782·1).
*Pain.*

**Montana** *Pharmonta, Austria.*
Lupulus (p.1708·1); gentian (p.1692·2); cinnamon (p.1672·2); bitter-orange peel (p.1723·3); caraway (p.1667·2); taraxacum (p.1751·3); peppermint oil (p.1283·2); pterocarpus santalinus.
*Gastrointestinal disorders.*

**Montana N** *EGS, Ger.*
Cardamom (p.1667·3); cinnamon (p.1672·2); centaury (p.1669·2); caraway (p.1667·2); bitter-orange peel (p.1723·3); peppermint leaf (p.1283·2); gentian (p.1692·2).
Montana formerly contained cardamom, cinnamon, centaury, caraway, bitter-orange peel, peppermint oil, gentian, senna, juniper, menyanthes, pterocarpus santalinus, sassafras, absinthium, calamus, valerian, rhubarb, sarsaparilla, aloes.
*Gastrointestinal disorders.*

**Montavon** *Aerocid, Fr.†.*
Pilocarpine nitrate (p.1495·1); antimony potassium tartrate (p.103·1).
*Alcohol withdrawal syndrome.*

**Montegen** *Gentili, Ital.*
Montelukast sodium (p.788·3).
*Asthma.*

**Monticina** *Mintlab, Chile.*
Bacitracin (p.161·3); neomycin sulfate (p.235·1).
*Skin infections.*

**Montricin**
*Asta Medica, Braz.; SPA, Ital.†.*
Mepartricin sodium laurilsulfate (p.405·2).
*Vulvovaginal candidiasis and trichomoniasis.*

**Monuril**
*Zambon, Austria; Zambon, Belg.; Zambon, Braz.; Zambon, Fr.; Apogepha, Ger.; Pharmax, Irl.†; Zambon, Ital.; Zambon, Neth.; Zambon, Port.; Inpharzam, Switz.*
Fosfomycin trometamol (p.214·3).
*Urinary-tract infections.*

**Monurol**
*Purdue, Canad.; Labomed, Chile; Orion, Fin.; Gerolimatos (Γερολυματος), Gr.; Inpharzam, Hong Kong; Rafa, Israel; Sanofi Synthelabo, Mex.; Pharmazam, Spain; Orion, Swed.; Forest Pharmaceuticals, USA.*
Fosfomycin trometamol (p.214·3).
*Bacterial infections of the urinary tract.*

**Monydrin**
*Tika, Norw.†; Tika, Swed.†.*
Phenylpropanolamine hydrochloride (p.1127·3).
*Rhinitis.*

**MoodLift** *Naturopathica, Austral.*
Ademetionine (p.1647·2).
*Tonic.*

**Moorbad-Saar N** *CPF, Ger.†.*
Salicylic acid (p.1157·1); sodium humate.
*Bath additive; gynaecological disorders; musculoskeletal and joint disorders; neuralgia.*

**Moorland** *Torbet Laboratories, UK.*
Bismuth aluminate (p.1252·1); magnesium trisilicate (p.1272·3); dried aluminium hydroxide gel (p.1249·2); heavy magnesium carbonate (p.1272·1); light kaolin (p.1268·3); calcium carbonate (p.1254·2).
*Dyspepsia; flatulence; heartburn.*

**Moorlauge Bastian** *Bastian, Ger.†.*
Medicinal mud.
*Bath additive; rheumatic disorders.*

**Mopen** *FIRMA, Ital.*
Amoxicillin trihydrate (p.155·3).
*Bacterial infections.*

**Moperidona** *Sidus, Arg.*
Domperidone (p.1263·2).
*Gastrointestinal disorders.*

**Moperidona AF** *Sidus, Arg.*
Domperidone (p.1263·2); simeticone (p.1289·2).
*Gastrointestinal disorders with excess gas.*

**Moperidona Enzimatica** *Sidus, Arg.*
Domperidone (p.1263·2); pancreatin (p.1725·3); simeticone (p.1289·2).
*Gastrointestinal disorders with excess gas; pancreatic insufficiency.*

**Mopral**
*AstraZeneca, Fr.; AstraZeneca, Mex.; AstraZeneca, Spain.*
Omeprazole (p.1278·2), omeprazole magnesium (p.1278·2), or omeprazole sodium (p.1278·2).
*Acid aspiration; dyspepsia; gastro-oesophageal reflux; peptic ulcer; Zollinger-Ellison syndrome.*

**Mopsoralen** *Wolfs, Belg.*
Methoxsalen (p.1152·1).
*Mycosis fungoides; psoriasis; vitiligo.*

**Moradorm** *Bouhon, Ger.*
Valerian (p.1762·2); passion flower (p.1729·1); diphenhydramine hydrochloride (p.431·3).
*Nervous disorders; sleep disorders.*

**Moradorm S** *Bouhon, Ger.*
Valerian (p.1762·2); passion flower (p.1729·1); lupulus (p.1708·1).
*Nervous disorders; sleep disorders.*

**Morapid** *Mundipharma, Austria.*
Morphine sulfate (p.60·2).
*Pain.*

**Moraten**
*Berna, Hong Kong†; Berna, Ital.†; Pharmabroker, NZ†; Berna, Port.†; Byk Madaus, S.Afr.†; Berna, Singapore†; Berna, Switz.; Berna, Thai.†.*
A measles vaccine (attenuated Edmonston-Zagreb strain) (p.1623·1).
*Active immunisation.*

**Moraxen** *Schwarz, UK†.*
Morphine sulfate (p.60·2).
*Pain.*

**Morbil** *Biagini, Ital.†.*
A measles immunoglobulin (p.1623·1).
*Passive immunisation.*

**Morbilvax**
*Chiron Vaccines, Ital.; Biovac, S.Afr.; Chiron, Thai.*
A measles vaccine (attenuated Schwarz strain) (p.1623·1).
*Active immunisation.*

**Morcap** *Mayne, UK.*
Morphine sulfate (p.60·2).
*Pain.*

**Morcontin** *Modi-Mundipharma, India.*
Morphine sulfate (p.60·2).
*Pain.*

**Morde X** *Vitafarma, Spain.*
Alcohol (p.1166·1); sucrose octa-acetate (p.1750·2).
*Nail biting deterrent.*

**MoreDophilus** *Freeda, USA.*
Acidophilus-carrot derivative (p.1704·2).
*Dietary supplement.*

**Morelin** *Laboratorios Chile, Chile.*
Amitriptyline (p.280·3); chlordiazepoxide (p.674·2).
*Mixed anxiety depressive states.*

**Morera Compuesta** *Hochstetter, Chile.*
Homoeopathic preparation.

**Morfex** *Tecnifar, Port.*
Flurazepam hydrochloride (p.700·3).
*Insomnia.*

**Morgenxil** *Llorente, Spain.*
Amoxicillin trihydrate (p.155·3).
*Bacterial infections.*

**Morhulin**
*Thornton & Ross, Irl.; Thornton & Ross, UK.*
Cod-liver oil (p.1425·2); zinc oxide (p.1163·2).
*Skin disorders.*

**Moriamin** *Ajinomoto, Thai.*
Multivitamin and amino-acid preparation (p.1417·1).

**Morlan FB 25** *Andromaco, Mex.*
Indometacin (p.47·3); methocarbamol (p.1395·1).
*Musculoskeletal and joint disorders.*

**Morniflu** *Master Pharma, Ital.*
Morniflumate (p.60·1).
*Fever; inflammation; pain.*

**Moronal** *Bristol-Myers Squibb, Ger.*
Nystatin (p.406·3).
*Fungal infections.*

**Moronal V** *Bristol-Myers Squibb, Ger.*
Nystatin (p.406·3); triamcinolone acetonide (p.1110·2).
*Skin disorders with fungal infection.*

**Morphalgin** *Fawns & McAllan, Austral.*
Morphine hydrochloride (p.60·1); aspirin (p.15·1).
*Pain.*

**Morphex** *Lannacher, Israel.*
Morphine hydrochloride (p.60·1).
*Pain.*

**Morphgesic** *Amdipharm, UK.*
Morphine sulfate (p.60·2).
*Pain.*

**Morphitec** *Technilab, Canad.*
Morphine hydrochloride (p.60·1).
*Pain.*

**Morrhulan** *Streuli, Switz.*
Cod-liver oil (p.1425·2).
*Minor skin lesions.*

**Morruetil** *Quimioterapica, Braz.†.*
Vitamin A; vitamin D; cineole; benzyl cinnamate; camphor (p.1417·1).
*Nutritional supplement.*

**Morrugripe** *Quimioterapica, Braz.†.*
Benzyl cinnamate; vitamin A; vitamin D (p.1417·1); cineole (p.1672·1).
*Cold and influenza symptoms.*

**Morstel** *Clonmel, Irl.*
Morphine sulfate (p.60·2).
*Pain.*

**Morton Salt Substitute** *Morton Salt, USA.*
Low sodium dietary salt substitute (p.1417·1).

**Morubel** *Chiron Vaccines, Ital.†.*
A measles and rubella vaccine (Schwarz and Wistar RA 27/3 strains respectively) (p.1624·3).
*Active immunisation.*

**Moruman** *Berna, Ital.†.*
A measles immunoglobulin (p.1623·1).
*Passive immunisation.*

**Morupar**
*Chiron Vaccines, Ital.; Fustery, Mex.; Biovac, S.Afr.*
A measles, mumps, and rubella vaccine (Schwarz, Urabe AM9, and Wistar RA 27/3 strains, respectively) (p.1625·1).
*Active immunisation.*

**MoRu-Viraten**
*Berna, Canad.†; Berna, Switz.†.*
A measles (Edmonston-Zagreb strain) and rubella (Wistar RA 27/3 strain) vaccine (p.1624·3).
*Active immunisation.*

**MOS** *ICN, Canad.*
Morphine hydrochloride (p.60·1) or morphine sulfate (p.60·2).
*Pain.*

**Mosalan** *Chrispa (Χρισπα), Gr.*
Cefuroxime sodium (p.184·1).
*Bacterial infections.*

**Mosar** *Phoenix, Arg.*
Mosapride citrate (p.1276·3).
*Dyspepsia; gastritis.*

**Mosco**
*Medtech, Canad.†; Medtech, USA.*
Salicylic acid (p.1157·1).
*Hyperkeratosis.*

**Moscontin** *Viatris, Fr.*
Morphine sulfate (p.60·2).
*Pain.*

**Mosegor**
*Novartis, Ger.; Novartis, Gr.; Novartis, Spain; Novartis, Switz.; Novartis, Thai.*
Pizotifen (p.470·3) or pizotifen malate (p.470·3).
*Anorexia; migraine.*

**Moselar** *Milano, Thai.*
Pizotifen malate (p.470·3).
*Migraine.*

**Mosil** *Menarini, Fr.*
Midecamycin acetate (p.231·3).
*Bacterial infections.*

**Moskizol** *Moskizol, Fr.†.*
*Solution:* Permethrin (p.1508·3).
*Topical gel:* Diethyltoluamide (p.1503·3).
*Insect repellent.*

**Mostardina** *Ibefar, Braz.†.*
Methyl salicylate (p.59·3); camphor (p.1665·3); salicylic acid (p.1157·1); menthol (p.1711·3); mustard oil (p.1718·2).
*Musculoskeletal and joint disorders.*

**Mostrelan** *Chrispa (Χρισπα), Gr.*
Famotidine (p.1265·2).
*Conditions where gastric acid reduction is beneficial; gastric hypersecretion including Zollinger-Ellison syndrome; peptic ulcer.*

**Motens**
*Boehringer Ingelheim, Belg.; Boehringer Ingelheim, Ger.; Glaxo Wellcome, Ger.; Boehringer Ingelheim, Gr.; Boehringer Ingelheim, Neth.; Boehringer Ingelheim, Spain; Boehringer Ingelheim, Switz.; Boehringer Ingelheim, Thai.; Boehringer Ingelheim, UK.*
Lacidipine (p.944·2).
*Hypertension.*

**Mother and Child Vitamin Drops** *SSL, UK.*
Vitamins A, C, and D (p.1417·1).

**Motiax** *Neopharmed, Ital.*
Famotidine (p.1265·2).
*Gastro-oesophageal reflux; peptic ulcer; Zollinger-Ellison syndrome.*

**Moticlod** *Lisapharma, Ital.*
Disodium clodronate (p.770·2).
*Hyperparathyroidism; multiple myeloma; osteolysis of malignancy; osteoporosis.*

**Moticon** *Condrugs, Thai.*
Domperidone (p.1263·2).
*Dyspepsia; nausea and vomiting.*

**Motidine**
*Unison, Hong Kong; Unison, Singapore; Unison, Thai.*
Famotidine (p.1265·2).
*Gastro-oesophageal reflux; multiple endocrine adenoma; peptic ulcer; systemic mastocytosis; Zollinger-Ellison syndrome.*

**Motidom** *TO-Chemicals, Thai.*
Domperidone (p.1263·2).
*Gastrointestinal motility disorders; nausea and vomiting.*

**Motifene**
*Sankyo, Belg.; Sankyo, Fin.; Sankyo, UK.*
Diclofenac sodium (p.32·1).
*Gout; inflammation; musculoskeletal, joint, peri-articular and soft-tissue disorders; pain.*

**Motilex** *Guidotti, Ital.*
Clebopride malate (p.1260·3).
*Gastrointestinal disorders.*

**Motilidone** *Technilab, Canad.†.*
Domperidone maleate (p.1263·2).

**Motilium**
*Janssen-Cilag, Arg.; Janssen-Cilag, Austral.; Janssen-Cilag, Austria; Janssen-Cilag, Belg.; Janssen-Cilag, Braz.; Janssen-Ortho, Canad.; Janssen-Cilag, Denm.; Janssen-Cilag, Fr.; Byk Gulden, Ger.; Janssen, Hong Kong; Janssen-Cilag, Irl.; Janssen-Cilag, Israel; Janssen-Cilag, Ital.; Janssen-Cilag, Malaysia; Janssen, Mex.; Janssen-Cilag, Neth.; Janssen-Cilag, NZ; Janssen-Cilag, Port.; Janssen-Cilag, S.Afr.; Janssen-Cilag, Singapore; Esteve, Spain; Janssen-Cilag, Switz.; Janssen, Thai.; Sanofi Synthelabo, UK.*
Domperidone (p.1263·2) or domperidone maleate (p.1263·2).
*Abdominal discomfort; delayed gastric emptying; dyspepsia; gastro-oesophageal reflux; hiccup; nausea and vomiting.*

**Motilyo** *Janssen-Cilag, Fr.*
Domperidone (p.1263·2).
*Abdominal distension; gastro-oesophageal reflux; nausea and vomiting.*

**Motional** *Beta, Arg.*
Ispaghula (p.1268·1).
*Constipation; diverticular disease; irritable bowel syndrome.*

**Motipress** *Sanofi Synthelabo, UK†.*
Fluphenazine hydrochloride (p.699·3); nortriptyline hydrochloride (p.310·2).
*Mixed anxiety depressive states.*

**Motitrel** *Bristol-Myers Squibb, Chile.*
Fluphenazine hydrochloride (p.699·3); nortriptyline hydrochloride (p.310·2).
*Mixed anxiety depressive states.*

**Motival**
*Bristol-Myers Squibb, Hong Kong†; Bristol-Myers Squibb, Irl.; Bristol-Myers Squibb, S.Afr.; Bristol-Myers Squibb, Thai.†; Sanofi Synthelabo, UK.*
Fluphenazine hydrochloride (p.699·3); nortriptyline hydrochloride (p.310·2).
*Mixed anxiety depressive states.*

**Motivan**
*Note. This name is used for preparations of different composition.*
*Faes, Spain.*
Paroxetine hydrochloride (p.311·2).
*Anxiety disorders; depression.*

*Samakeephaesaj, Thai.*
Dimenhydrinate (p.431·1).
*Motion sickness; nausea and vomiting; vestibular disorders.*

**Motiven** *Fontovit, Braz.*
Hypericum (p.299·1).
*Depression.*

**Motivone** *BASF, Ger.†.*
Fluoxetine (p.296·3).
*Depression.*

**Motofen** *Carnrick, USA.*
Difenoxin hydrochloride (p.1261·2).
Atropine sulfate (p.477·1) is included in this preparation to discourage abuse.
*Diarrhoea.*

**Motosol** *Boehringer Ingelheim, Spain.*
Ambroxol hydrochloride (p.1114·3).
*Respiratory-tract disorders.*

**Motozina** *Biomedica, Ital.*
Dimenhydrinate (p.431·1).
*Motion sickness.*

**Motrax** *Labinca, Arg.*
Ibuprofen (p.45·3).
*Inflammation; pain.*

**Motrim** *Lannacher, Austria.*
Trimethoprim (p.272·2).
*Bacterial infections.*

**Motrin**
*Pharmacia Upjohn, Belg.†; Pharmacia, Braz.; McNeil Consumer, Canad.; Pharmacia, Chile; Pharmacia Upjohn, Mex.; Pharmacia Upjohn, Port.; Pharmacia, UK; McNeil Consumer, USA.*
Ibuprofen (p.45·3).
Formerly known as Pediaprofen in the *USA*.
*Fever; gout; inflammation; musculoskeletal, joint, peri-articular and soft-tissue disorders; pain.*

**Motrin IB Sinus** *McNeil Consumer, USA.*
Pseudoephedrine hydrochloride (p.1129·2); ibuprofen (p.45·3).
*Cold symptoms; sinusitis.*

**Mouth Kote** *Alcon, Canad.*
Eriodictyon (p.1121·2).
*Dry mouth.*

**MouthKote**
*Parnell, Irl.; Parnell, USA.*
Artificial saliva.
*Dry mouth.*

**MouthKote F/R** *Parnell, USA†.*
Sodium fluoride (p.1444·3).

**MouthKote O/R** *Unimed, USA.*
*Oral rinse:* Benzyl alcohol (p.1170·2); menthol (p.1711·3).
*Minor mouth or throat irritation.*
*Topical solution:* Cetylpyridinium chloride (p.1173·1); diphenhydramine (p.431·3).
*Sore throat.*

**MouthKote P/R** *Unimed, USA.*
*Ointment:* Diphenhydramine hydrochloride (p.431·3).
*Oral lesions.*
*Topical solution:* Diphenhydramine (p.431·3); cetylpyridinium chloride (p.1173·1).
*Minor mouth or throat irritation.*

**Mouthrinse** *Arjo, Canad.†.*
Cetylpyridinium chloride (p.1173·1); sodium benzoate (p.1169·3).
*Mouth and throat disorders; oral hygiene.*

**Mouthwash** *National Care, Canad.*
Cetylpyridinium chloride (p.1173·1).

**Mouthwash Antiseptic & Gargle** *Lander, Canad.*
Alcohol (p.1166·1); eucalyptus oil (p.1686·2); menthol (p.1711·3); thymol (p.1194·2).
*Oral hygiene.*

**Mouthwash & Gargle** *Scott, Canad.†.*
Cetylpyridinium chloride (p.1173·1); domiphen bromide (p.1179·1).

**Mouthwash Mint/Peppermint** *Lander, Canad.†.*
Cetylpyridinium chloride (p.1173·1); domiphen bromide (p.1179·1).

**Mova Nitrat** *Lindopharm, Ger.*
Silver nitrate (p.1746·1).
*Eye disorders.*

**Movacox** *Hexal, Braz.*
Meloxicam (p.56·1).
*Inflammation; musculoskeletal and joint disorders; pain.*

**Movalis**
*Boehringer Ingelheim, Austria; Boehringer Ingelheim, Port.; Boehringer Ingelheim, Spain.*
Meloxicam (p.56·1).
*Ankylosing spondylitis; osteoarthritis; rheumatoid arthritis.*

**Movana** *Quest, Canad.*
Hypericum (p.299·1).

**Movatec**
*Boehringer de Angeli, Braz.; Boehringer Ingelheim, Gr.*
Meloxicam (p.56·1).
*Ankylosing spondylitis; inflammation; osteoarthritis; pain; rheumatoid arthritis.*

**Movelat**
*Note. This name is used for preparations of different composition.*
*Key, Austral.; Sankyo, Thai.; Sankyo, UK.*
A heparinoid (p.931·1); salicylic acid (p.1157·1).
*Musculoskeletal, joint, and soft-tissue disorders.*

*Wilson, NZ.*
Adrenal extract; a heparinoid (p.931·1); salicylic acid (p.1157·1).
*Musculoskeletal and joint disorders.*

**Movelium** *Progress, Thai.*
Domperidone (p.1263·2) or domperidone maleate (p.1263·2).
*Delayed gastric emptying; nausea and vomiting.*

**Movens** *Pharmafar, Ital.*
Meclofenamate sodium (p.55·1) or meclofenamic acid (p.55·1).
*Musculoskeletal and joint disorders; pain.*

**Movent** *Community Pharmacy, Thai.*
Ambroxol hydrochloride (p.1114·3).
*Respiratory-tract disorders associated with increased or viscous mucus.*

**Mover** *Mitsubishi, Jpn.*
Actarit (p.12·1).
*Rheumatoid arthritis.*

**Movergan** *Orion, Ger.*
Selegiline hydrochloride (p.1214·1).
*Parkinsonism.*

**Movex** *Vitamed, Israel.*
Bromhexine hydrochloride (p.1115·3).
*Bronchitis.*

**Movicard** *Ravensberg, Ger.*
Magnesium aspartate (p.1227·3); potassium aspartate (p.1233·1); troxerutin (p.1688·3).
*Cardiac disorders.*

**Movicol**
*Norgine, Austral.; Norgine, Austria; Norgine, Belg.; Norgine, Denm.; Sabora, Fin.; Norgine, Fr.; Norgine, Ger.; Norgine, Hong Kong; Norgine, Irl.; Norgine, Ital.; Norgine, Norw.; Norgine, NZ; Norgine, S.Afr.; Norgine, Singapore; Norgine, Spain; Biolac, Swed.; Norgine, Switz.; Norgine, UK.*
Macrogol 3350 (p.1709·1); electrolytes (p.1217·1).
*Constipation; faecal impaction.*

**Movicolon** *Norgine, Neth.*
Macrogol 3350 (p.1709·1); electrolytes (p.1217·1).
*Constipation.*

**Movicox** *Boehringer Ingelheim, Neth.*
Meloxicam (p.56·1).
*Ankylosing spondylitis; osteoarthritis; rheumatoid arthritis.*

**Movidone** *Milano, Thai.*
Povidone-iodine (p.1190·3).
*Skin disinfection.*

**Moviflex**
*Note. This name is used for preparations of different composition.*
*Sankyo, Austria; Sankyo, Fin.*
Phenylephrine hydrochloride (p.1126·3); a heparinoid (p.931·1); glycol salicylate (p.44·3).
*Musculoskeletal, joint, peri-articular, and soft-tissue disorders.*

*Sanofi Synthelabo, Chile.*
Indometacin (p.47·3).
*Musculoskeletal, joint, peri-articular, and soft-tissue disorders.*

**Movilat** *Sankyo, Spain.*
A heparinoid (p.931·1); salicylic acid (p.1157·1).
*Rheumatic and muscular pain.*

**Movilisin**
*Sankyo, Hong Kong†; Sankyo, Spain.*
Flufenamic acid (p.43·2); a heparinoid (p.931·1); glycol salicylate (p.44·3) or salicylic acid (p.1157·1).
*Musculoskeletal, joint, peri-articular, and soft-tissue disorders.*

**Movin** *Neo-Farmaceutica, Port.*
Ticlopidine hydrochloride (p.1011·2).
*Thromboembolic disorders.*

**Movina** *Pharmaton, Switz.†.*
Hypericum (p.299·1).
*Depression.*

**Movistal** *SMB, Belg.*
Metoclopramide hydrochloride (p.1274·3).
*Gastro-oesophageal reflux; gastrointestinal motility disorders; nausea and vomiting.*

**Movithiol** *Pharmanik (Φαρμανικ), Gr.*
Betamethasone valerate (p.1093·2).
*Topical corticosteroid.*

**Movon** *Ipca, India.*
Piroxicam (p.84·2).
*Dysmenorrhoea; gout; musculoskeletal, joint, and soft-tissue disorders disorders.*

**Movone** *Gebro, Austria.*
Dexibuprofen (p.46·1).
*Musculoskeletal, joint, and peri-articular disorders; pain.*

**Movox** *Alphapharm, Austral.*
Fluvoxamine maleate (p.298·2).
*Depression.*

**Movoxicam** *Bunker, Braz.*
Meloxicam (p.56·1).

**Mowineuron** *Rodisma, Ger.*
Vitamin B substances; vitamin E (p.1417·1).
*Tonic.*

**Mowivit** *Rodisma, Ger.*
*d*-Alpha tocopherol (p.1464·3).
*Vitamin E deficiency.*

**Mox** *Ranbaxy, India.*
Amoxicillin (p.155·3).
*Bacterial infections.*

**Moxacef**
*Bristol-Myers Squibb, Belg.; Mead Johnson, Gr.*
Cefadroxil (p.167·2).
*Bacterial infections.*

**Moxacil** *Raza, Malaysia; Pharmaniaga, Malaysia.*
Amoxicillin trihydrate (p.155·3).
*Bacterial infections.*

**Moxacin** *CSL, Austral.*
Amoxicillin sodium (p.155·3) or amoxicillin trihydrate (p.155·3).
*Bacterial infections.*

**Moxadent** *Vitoria, Port.*
Amoxicillin (p.155·3).
*Bacterial infections.*

**Moxal** *Julphar, UAE.*
Dried aluminium hydroxide (p.1249·2); magnesium hydroxide (p.1272·2).
*Gastritis; gastrointestinal hyperacidity; peptic ulcer.*

**Moxal II** *Julphar, UAE.*
Aluminium hydroxide (p.1249·2); magnesium hydroxide (p.1272·2).
*Gastritis; gastrointestinal hyperacidity; peptic ulcer.*

**Moxal Plus** *Julphar, UAE.*
Aluminium hydroxide (p.1249·2); magnesium hydroxide (p.1272·2); simeticone (p.1289·2).
*Flatulence; gastro-oesophageal reflux; gastrointestinal hyperacidity.*

**Moxaline** *Bristol-Myers Squibb, Belg.*
Amoxicillin trihydrate (p.155·3).
*Bacterial infections.*

**Moxan** *Garec, S.Afr.*
Amoxicillin (p.155·3).
*Bacterial infections.*

**Moxapen** *Olan-Kemed, Thai.*
Amoxicillin trihydrate (p.155·3).
*Bacterial infections.*

**Moxcil** *TP, Thai.*
Amoxicillin sodium (p.155·3) or amoxicillin trihydrate (p.155·3).
*Bacterial infections.*

**Moxcin** *General Drugs, Thai.*
Amoxicillin trihydrate (p.155·3).
*Bacterial infections.*

**Moxicam** *Milano, Thai.*
Piroxicam (p.84·2).
*Gout; musculoskeletal and joint disorders.*

**Moxicel** *Welfer, Mex.†.*
Amoxicillin (p.155·3).
*Bacterial infections.*

**Moxiclav** *Medochemie, Hong Kong; Medochemie, Malaysia; Medochemie, Singapore.*
Amoxicillin trihydrate (p.155·3); potassium clavulanate (p.193·3).
*Bacterial infections.*

**Moxif** *Torrent, India.*
Moxifloxacin (p.233·1).
*Bacterial infections.*

**Moxilcap** *Masa, Thai.*
Amoxicillin trihydrate (p.155·3).
*Bacterial infections.*

**Moxilen** *Medochemie, Hong Kong; Medochemie, Malaysia; Medochemie, Singapore†; Medochemie, Thai.†.*
Amoxicillin trihydrate (p.155·3).
*Bacterial infections.*

**Moxilin** *The Forty-Two, Thai.*
Amoxicillin trihydrate (p.155·3).
*Bacterial infections.*

**Moximed** *Unison, Thai.*
Amoxicillin trihydrate (p.155·3).
*Bacterial infections.*

**Moxina** *Richmond, Arg.*
Rifampicin (p.250·2).
*Bacterial infections including tuberculosis.*

**Moxipan** *Nakorn, Thai.*
Amoxicillin trihydrate (p.155·3).
*Bacterial infections.*

**Moxipen**
*Xepa-Soul Pattinson, Malaysia; Sanofi Synthelabo, Port.; Xepa-Soul Pattinson, Singapore.*
Amoxicillin (p.155·3).
*Bacterial infections.*

**Moxiplus** *Medley, Braz.†.*
Amoxicillin (p.155·3).
*Bacterial infections.*

**Moxiral** *Pharmacia, Austria.*
Minoxidil (p.960·1).
*Alopecia androgenetica.*

**Moxiren** *Ist. Chim. Inter., Ital.*
Amoxicillin trihydrate (p.155·3).
*Bacterial infections.*

**Moxitral** *LA, Arg.*
Amoxicillin (p.155·3).
*Bacterial infections.*

**Moxlin**
*Pacific, Hong Kong; Merck, Mex.†; Pacific, NZ†.*
Amoxicillin trihydrate (p.155·3).
*Bacterial infections.*

**Moxon**
*Solvay, Belg.; Solvay, Spain.*
Moxonidine (p.962·3).
*Hypertension.*

**Moxycarb** *Nicholas Piramal, India.*
Amoxicillin (p.155·3); carbocisteine (p.1116·2).
*Otitis media; respiratory-tract disorders.*

**Moxyclav** *Garec, S.Afr.*
Amoxicillin (p.155·3); clavulanic acid (p.193·3).
*Bacterial infections.*

**Moxydar** *Grimberg, Fr.*
Aluminium hydroxide (p.1249·2); magnesium hydroxide (p.1272·2); aluminium phosphate (p.1250·1); guar gum (p.333·2).
*Gastrointestinal disorders.*

**Moxymax** *Parke-Med, S.Afr.†.*
Amoxicillin (p.155·3).
*Bacterial infections.*

**Moxypen**
*Biogal, Israel; Aspen, S.Afr.*
Amoxicillin trihydrate (p.155·3).
*Bacterial infections.*

**Moxyvit** *Vitamed, Israel.*
Amoxicillin trihydrate (p.155·3).
*Bacterial infections.*

**Moz-Bite**
*Hoe, Malaysia; Hoe, Singapore.*
Crotamiton (p.1145·1).
*Insect bites; stings.*

**Mozzie Patch** *Bioconcepts, UK.*
Citronella oil (p.1673·2).
*Insect repellent.*

**MPA** *Hexal, Ger.*
Medroxyprogesterone acetate (p.1557·2).
*Breast cancer; endometrial cancer.*

**MPA Gyn** *Hexal, Ger.*
Medroxyprogesterone acetate (p.1557·2).
*Menopausal disorders; menstrual disorders.*

**MPA-beta** *Betapharm, Ger.*
Medroxyprogesterone acetate (p.1557·2).
*Breast cancer; endometrial cancer.*

**MPA-Noury** *Nourypharma, Ger.*
Medroxyprogesterone acetate (p.1557·2).
*Breast cancer; endometrial cancer.*

**M-Prednisol** *Pasadena, USA†.*
Methylprednisolone acetate (p.1106·1).
*Corticosteroid.*

**Mr. Multy** *Ideal Health, UK.*
Multivitamin and mineral preparation (p.1417·1).

**Mr Nits** *Pacific, NZ.*
Avocado; azadirachta (p.1658·2); borage (p.1661·3); canola oil (p.1666·3); coconut oil (p.1481·1); evening primrose oil (p.1686·3); geranium oil (p.1692·2); hemp; jojoba oil; melissa (p.1711·1).
*Pediculosis.*

**Mrs Cullen's Powders** *Cullen & Davison, UK.*
Aspirin (p.15·1); caffeine (p.782·1).
*Fever; pain.*

**M-R-Vax II** *Merck, USA†.*
A measles and rubella vaccine (more attenuated Enders' attenuated Edmonston, and Wistar RA 27/3 strains respectively) (p.1624·3).
*Active immunisation.*

**MRX** *Mahdeen, Canad.*
Benzethonium chloride (p.1169·2); camphor (p.1665·3); alcohol (p.1166·1); benzoic acid (p.1169·3).

**MS Contin**
*Mundipharma, Austral.; Viatris, Belg.; Purdue, Canad.; Asta Medica, Ital.; Viatris, Neth.; Purdue Frederick, USA.*
Morphine sulfate (p.60·2).
*Pain.*

**MS Direct** *Viatris, Belg.*
Morphine sulfate (p.60·2).
*Pain.*

**MS Mono** *Mundipharma, Austral.*
Morphine sulfate (p.60·2).
*Pain.*

**MSI** *Mundipharma, Ger.*
Morphine sulfate (p.60·2).
*Pain.*

**MSIR**
*Purdue, Canad.; Purdue Frederick, USA.*
Morphine sulfate (p.60·2).
*Pain.*

**MS-Long** *Janssen-Cilag, Braz.*
Morphine sulfate (p.60·2).
*Pain.*

**MSP** *Rafa, Israel.*
Morphine sulfate (p.60·2).
*Pain; sedative.*

**MSP-Blu** *Cypress, USA.*
Methenamine (p.230·1); monobasic sodium phosphate (p.1230·3); salol (p.88·1); methylthioninium chloride (p.1042·2); hyoscyamine sulfate (p.485·1).
*Urinary-tract disorders.*

**MSPD** *Seroyal, Canad.†.*
Mineral preparation with vitamin C (p.1417·1).

**MSR** *Mundipharma, Ger.*
Morphine sulfate (p.60·2).
*Pain.*

**MST**
*Mundipharma, Ger.; Viatris, Port.*
Morphine sulfate (p.60·2) or morphine polistirex.
*Pain.*

**MST Continus**
*Raffo, Arg.; Asta Medica, Braz.; Mundipharma, Hong Kong; Napp, Irl.; Columbia, Mex.†; Douglas, NZ; Adcock Ingram, S.Afr.; Asta Medica, Singapore†; Viatris, Spain; Mundipharma, Switz.; Napp, UK.*
Morphine sulfate (p.60·2).
*Pain.*

**MST Unicontinus** *Viatris, Spain.*
Morphine sulfate (p.60·2).
*Dyspnoea; pain; premedication.*

**MSTA**
*Aventis Pasteur, Canad.†; Pasteur Merieux, USA†.*
Mumps skin test (p.1717·2).
*Assessment of cell-mediated immunity; detection of delayed hypersensitivity to mumps.*

**M-Stada** *Stada, Ger.*
Morphine hydrochloride (p.60·1).
*Pain.*

**MSUD** *Nutricia, NZ; Scientific Hospital Supplies, NZ.*
Food for special diets (p.1417·1).
*Maple syrup urine disease.*

**MSUD 1** *Support, Braz.*
Food for special diets (p.1417·1).

**MSUD 2** *Support, Braz.*
Food for special diets (p.1417·1).

**MSUD III** *Scientific Hospital Supplies, Irl.*
Food for special diets (p.1417·1).
*Maple syrup urine disease.*

**MSUD Aid**
*Scientific Hospital Supplies, Austral.; Scientific Hospital Supplies, UK.*
Food for special diets (p.1417·1).
*Disorders of branched-chain amino acid metabolism; maple syrup urine disease.*

**MSUD Analog** *Scientific Hospital Supplies, Austral.*
Food for special diets (p.1417·1).
*Maple syrup urine disease.*

**MSUD Diet** *Mead Johnson, Hong Kong.*
Food for special diets (p.1417·1).
*Disorders of branched-chain amino-acid metabolism; maple syrup urine disease.*

**MSUD Maxamaid**
*Scientific Hospital Supplies, Austral.; Support, Braz.; Scientific Hospital Supplies, Irl.; Scientific Hospital Supplies, UK.*
Food for special diets (p.1417·1).
*Maple syrup urine disease.*

**MSUD Maxamum** *Scientific Hospital Supplies, Austral.*
Food for special diets (p.1417·1).
*Maple syrup urine disease.*

**MTE**
*Fujisawa, Hong Kong†; Baxter, NZ; American Pharmaceutical, USA.*
A range of trace element preparations (p.1417·1).
*Additive for intravenous total parenteral nutrition solutions.*

**M-Trim** *Milano, Thai.*
Cotrimoxazole (p.199·3).
*Bacterial infections.*

**MTX**
*Hexal, Ger.*
Methotrexate sodium (p.568·3).
*Arthritis; malignant neoplasms; psoriasis.*

*Choongwae, Singapore†.*
Methotrexate (p.568·2).
*Malignant neoplasms.*

**Mucabrox** *Streuli, Switz.*
Ambroxol hydrochloride (p.1114·3).
*Respiratory-tract disorders associated with increased or viscous mucus.*

**Mucaderma S** *Merz, Ger.*
Zinc oxide (p.1163·2); titanium dioxide (p.1160·3).
*Wounds.*

**Mucaine**
*Note. This name is used for preparations of different composition.*
*Bago, Arg.; Whitehall, Austral.; Axcan, Canad.; Wyeth Consumer, Chile; Wyeth-Ayerst, Hong Kong†; Wyeth, India; Wyeth, Irl.†; Whitehall, NZ; Akromed, S.Afr.; Wyeth Consumer, Singapore; Whitehall, Thai.; Wyeth, UK†.*
Aluminium hydroxide (p.1249·2); magnesium hydroxide (p.1272·2); oxetacaine (p.1382·1).
*Gastritis; gastro-oesophageal reflux; peptic ulcer.*

*Wyeth, Hong Kong; Wyeth Consumer, Singapore; Whitehall, Thai.*
*Tablets:* Aluminium hydroxide (p.1249·2); magnesium carbonate (p.1272·1); oxetacaine (p.1382·1).
*Gastritis; gastro-oesophageal reflux; peptic ulcer.*

**Mucaine 2 in 1** *Whitehall, Austral.*
Aluminium hydroxide (p.1249·2); magnesium hydroxide (p.1272·2); simeticone (p.1289·2).
*Dyspepsia; flatulence.*

**Mucal**
*Note. This name is used for preparations of different composition.*
*Bournonville, Belg.†; OM, Port.*
Aluminium silicate (p.1250·2); magnesium silicate (p.1580·2); calcium silicate (p.1226·1).
*Gastrointestinal disorders.*

*OM, Ger.†.*
Aluminium magnesium silicate (p.1577·1); aluminium calcium silicate (p.1250·2).
*Gastrointestinal disorders.*

**Mucalan** *Microsules Bernabo, Arg.*
Aluminium hydroxide (p.1249·2); magnesium hydroxide (p.1272·2); simeticone (p.1289·2).
*Gastrointestinal disorders.*

**Mucantil** *Serpero, Ital.†.*
*Aerosol; elixir; oral drops:* Iodinated glycerol (p.1122·3); phenylpropanolamine hydrochloride (p.1127·3).
*Capsules:* Iodinated glycerol (p.1122·3); phenylpropanolamine hydrochloride (p.1127·3); peppermint oil (p.1283·2).
*Respiratory-tract disorders.*

**Mucasept-A** *Merz, Ger.*
Isopropyl alcohol (p.1184·3); alcohol (p.1166·1).
*Hand disinfection.*

**Mucedokehl** *Sanum-Kehlbeck, Ger.*
Homoeopathic preparation.

**Muchan** *Fada, Arg.*
Ephedrine (p.1120·1).

**Mucibron**
*Medley, Braz.; Normon, Spain.*
Ambroxol hydrochloride (p.1114·3).
*Respiratory-tract congestion.*

*Novag, Mex.*
Ambroxol (p.1114·3).

**Muciclar**
*Note. This name is used for preparations of different composition.*
*Pfizer, Fr.*
Carbocisteine (p.1116·2).
*Respiratory-tract congestion.*

*Piam, Ital.*
Ambroxol hydrochloride (p.1114·3).
*Respiratory-tract disorders.*

**Mucil** *TO-Chemicals, Thai.*
Acetylcysteine (p.1112·3).
*Respiratory-tract disorders associated with increased or viscous mucus.*

**Mucilar** *Spirig, Switz.*
Ispaghula (p.1268·1).
*Gastrointestinal disorders; obesity.*

**Mucilar Avena** *Spirig, Switz.*
Ispaghula (p.1268·1); avena (p.1658·2).
*Constipation; obesity.*

**Mucilax**
*Douglas, Austral.; Douglas, NZ.*
Ispaghula (p.1268·1).
*Constipation.*

**Mucilin**
*Berlin Pharm, Singapore; Berlin Pharm, Thai.*
Ispaghula (p.1268·1).
*Constipation; dietary fibre supplement.*

**Mucilloid** *Lalco, Canad.†.*
Ispaghula (p.1268·1).

**Mucine** *Silom, Thai.*
Bromhexine hydrochloride (p.1115·3).
*Respiratory-tract disorders associated with increased or viscous mucus.*

**Mucinex** *Adams, USA.*
Guaifenesin (p.1122·1).
*Coughs.*

**Mucinol** *Sanofi Synthelabo, Ger.*
Anethole trithione (p.1655·1).
*Dry mouth.*

**Mucinum**
*Note. This name is used for preparations of different composition.*
*Pharmethic, Belg.†.*
Bisacodyl (p.1251·3).
Formerly contained phenolphthalein, senna, cascara, boldo, aniseed, pancreas extract, erepsin, enterokinase, ox bile extract, belladonna, ipomoea resin, and dried magnesium sulfate.
*Constipation.*

*Sabex, Canad.*
Cascara (p.1255·1); senna (p.1288·2).
Formerly contained phenolphthalein and senna.
*Constipation.*

*Innothera, Fr.†.*
Phenolphthalein (p.1284·1); whole bile (p.1660·3); belladonna leaf (p.479·1); senna leaf (p.1288·2); frangula bark (p.1266·3); boldo (p.1661·2); ipomoea (p.1267·3); aniseed (p.1655·2).
*Constipation.*

*Innotech, Port.*
Cascara (p.1255·1).
*Constipation.*

**Mucinum a l'Extrait de Cascara** *Innotech, Fr.*
Cascara (p.1255·1); senna leaf (p.1288·2); boldo (p.1661·2); aniseed (p.1655·2).
*Constipation.*

**Mucinum Cascara** *Innotech, Hong Kong.*
Senna (p.1288·2); boldo (p.1661·2); cascara (p.1255·1); aniseed (p.1655·2).
*Constipation.*

**Muciplasma** *Edigen, Spain.*
Methylcellulose (p.1580·2).
*Constipation.*

**Mucipulgite**
*Ipsen, Belg.†; Dexo, Fr.; Beaufour, Switz.*
Activated attapulgite (p.1251·1); guar gum (p.333·2).
*Gastrointestinal disorders.*

**Mucisol** *Deca, Ital.*
Acetylcysteine (p.1112·3).
*Respiratory-tract disorders.*

**Muciteran** *Farmasan, Ger.*
Acetylcysteine (p.1112·3).
*Respiratory-tract disorders associated with increased or viscous mucus.*

**Mucitux** *E Pharma, Fr.†.*
Eprazinone hydrochloride (p.1121·1).
*Respiratory-tract congestion.*

**Mucivital**
*Frere, Belg.†; Arkopharma, Fr.; Arkopharma, Israel; Arkofarm, Ital.†.*
Ispaghula (p.1268·1).
*Constipation; diarrhoea; stool softener.*

**Muclox** *Sigma-Tau, Spain†.*
Famotidine (p.1265·2).
*Gastro-oesophageal reflux; peptic ulcer; Zollinger-Ellison syndrome.*

**Muco4** *Sanofi Synthelabo, Ital.*
Neltenexine (p.1125·2).
*Respiratory-tract disorders.*

**Muco Cortos** *Raffo, Arg.*
Ambroxol hydrochloride (p.1114·3); astemizole (p.424·2); butetamate citrate (p.1116·2); phenylephrine hydrochloride (p.1126·3).

**Muco Dosodos** *Beta, Arg.*
Ambroxol hydrochloride (p.1114·3); butamirate citrate (p.1116·2); chlorphenamine maleate (p.427·3).
*Coughs.*

**Muco Dosodos Biotic** *Beta, Arg.*
Amoxicillin (p.155·3); ambroxol hydrochloride (p.1114·3); butamirate citrate (p.1116·2); chlorphenamine maleate (p.427·3).
*Respiratory-tract infections.*

**Muco Panoral** *Lilly, Ger.†.*
Bromhexine hydrochloride (p.1115·3); cefaclor (p.167·1).
*Bacterial infections of the respiratory tract.*

**Muco Rhinathiol** *Sanofi Synthelabo, Belg.*
Carbocisteine (p.1116·2).
Formerly known as Rhinathiol Mucolyticum.
*Respiratory-tract disorders associated with abnormal mucus production.*

**Muco Sanigen** *Thiemann, Ger.*
Acetylcysteine (p.1112·3).
*Respiratory-tract disorders associated with increased or viscous mucus.*

**Muco-Anestyl** *Preston, Arg.*
Lidocaine (p.1377·3); benzocaine (p.1370·3); procaine (p.1383·2).
*Local anaesthesia.*

**Muco-Aspecton** *Krewel, Ger.*
Ambroxol hydrochloride (p.1114·3).
*Respiratory-tract disorders associated with increased or viscous mucus.*

**Mucobase** *Defuen, Arg.*
Plastibase; dexpanthenol (p.1727·2); aloe vera (p.1141·3).
*Aphthous ulcers.*

**Mucobene** *Ratiopharm, Austria.*
Acetylcysteine (p.1112·3).
*Respiratory-tract disorders associated with viscous mucus.*

**Mucobrol** *Pharmafina, Chile.*
Bromhexine (p.1115·3); clofedanol (p.1117·1); ammonium citrate (p.1654·1).
*Coughs.*

**Mucobron** *OFF, Ital.*
Ambroxol hydrochloride (p.1114·3).
*Respiratory-tract disorders.*

**Mucobronchyl** *Pharmacal, Switz.†.*
Isoprenaline sulfate (p.940·2); phenylephrine hydrochloride (p.1126·3).
*Bronchitis.*

**Mucobroxol** *Mundipharma, Ger.*
Ambroxol hydrochloride (p.1114·3).
*Respiratory-tract disorders associated with increased or viscous mucus.*

**Mucocaps** *Roche, S.Afr.*
Carbocisteine (p.1116·2).
*Respiratory-tract disorders with increased, viscous mucus.*

**Mucocedyl** *3M, Ger.*
Acetylcysteine (p.1112·3).
*Respiratory-tract disorders associated with increased or viscous mucus.*

**Mucocef** *Lilly, Mex.*
Cefalexin (p.168·1); bromhexine hydrochloride (p.1115·3).
*Respiratory-tract infections with excessive mucus.*

**Mucocil**
*Note. This name is used for preparations of different composition.*
*Farmion, Braz.†.*
Carbocisteine (p.1116·2).
*Respiratory-tract congestion.*

*Novartis, Neth.; Utopian, Thai.*
Acetylcysteine (p.1112·3).
*Respiratory-tract disorders associated with increased or viscous mucus.*

**Mucocis** *Fonten, Ital.*
Carbocisteine (p.1116·2).
*Respiratory-tract disorders.*

**Mucocistein** *Neo Quimica, Braz.*
Carbocisteine (p.1116·2).
*Respiratory-tract congestion.*

**Mucoclean** *Royton, Braz.*
Ambroxol hydrochloride (p.1114·3).
*Respiratory-tract congestion.*

**Muco-cyl Ho-Len-Complex** *Liebermann, Ger.*
Homoeopathic preparation.

**Muco-Dest** *Klus, Switz.*
Peppermint oil (p.1283·2); camphor oil.
*Nasal disorders.*

**Mucodestrol** *Eurofarma, Braz.†.*
Carbocisteine (p.1116·2).
*Respiratory-tract congestion.*

**Mucodex** *Dexcel, Israel†.*
Acetylcysteine (p.1112·3).
*Respiratory-tract disorders associated with viscous mucus.*

**Mucodic** *Progress, Thai.*
Ambroxol hydrochloride (p.1114·3).
*Respiratory-tract disorders associated with increased or viscous mucus.*

**Mucodil** *Valeas, Ital.†.*
Stepronin lysine (p.1130·3).
*Respiratory-tract disorders.*

**Mucodox** *Delta, Port.*
Sobrerol (p.1130·2).
*Respiratory-tract congestion.*

**Mucodrenol** *Medinfar, Port.*
Ambroxol (p.1114·3).
*Respiratory-tract congestion.*

**Mucodyne**
*Rhone-Poulenc Rorer, Hong Kong†; Aventis, Irl.; Kyorin, Jpn; Aventis, Neth.; Beacon, UK.*
Carbocisteine (p.1116·2).
*Respiratory-tract disorders with excess or viscous mucus.*

**Mucofalk**
*Abbott, Arg.; Falk, Ger.; Falk, Hong Kong; Falk, Malaysia; Falk, Port.; Falk, Singapore; Falk, Thai.*
Ispaghula (p.1268·1).
*Constipation; diarrhoea; diverticular disease; hypercholesterolaemia; inflammatory bowel disease; irritable bowel syndrome; stool softener.*

**Mucofan** *Whitehall, Braz.*
Carbocisteine (p.1116·2).
*Respiratory-tract congestion.*

**Muco-Fen** *Ivax, USA.*
Guaifenesin (p.1122·1).
*Coughs.*

**Muco-Fen DM** *Ivax, USA; Wakefield, USA.*
Dextromethorphan hydrobromide (p.1117·3); guaifenesin (p.1122·1).
*Coughs.*

**Muco-Fen-LA** *Wakefield, USA†.*
Guaifenesin (p.1122·1).
*Coughs.*

**Mucofial** *SoSe, Ital.*
Acetylcysteine (p.1112·3).
*Cyclophosphamide-induced uropathy; paracetamol poisoning; respiratory-tract disorders.*

**Muco-Fips** *Lichtenstein, Ger.†.*
Ambroxol hydrochloride (p.1114·3).
*Respiratory-tract disorders associated with increased or viscous mucus.*

**Mucoflem** *Xixia, S.Afr.*
Carbocisteine (p.1116·2).
*Respiratory-tract disorders with increased, viscous mucus.*

**Mucofluid**
*Note. This name is used for preparations of different composition.*
*Aventis Pasteur, Chile; UCB, Fr.; UCB, Ital.; UCB, Spain.*
Mesna (p.1041·2).
*Respiratory-tract disorders.*

*Spirig, Switz.*
Acetylcysteine (p.1112·3).
*Respiratory-tract disorders.*

**Mucoflux**
*Note. This name is used for preparations of different composition.*
*Merck, Braz.*
Carbocisteine (p.1116·2).
*Respiratory-tract congestion.*

*Rotta, Hong Kong; Rotta, Malaysia; Rotta, Singapore; Rotta, Thai.*
Sobrerol (p.1130·2).
*Respiratory-tract disorders associated with increased or viscous mucus.*

**Mucofor** *Vifor, Switz.*
Erdosteine (p.1121·1).
*Respiratory-tract disorders associated with excess mucus.*

**Mucogel** *Forest Laboratories, UK.*
Aluminium hydroxide (p.1249·2); magnesium hydroxide (p.1272·2).
These ingredients can be described by the British Approved Name Co-magaldrox.
*Dyspepsia; gastro-oesophageal reflux; heartburn.*

**Mucogen** *Antigen, Irl.*
Carbocisteine (p.1116·2).
*Lower respiratory-tract disorders with excessive or viscous mucus.*

**Mucogeran** *Ogera, Switz.*
Carbocisteine (p.1116·2).
*Respiratory-tract congestion.*

**Mucogyne** *Biogyne, Fr.*
Mallow (p.1709·3); chamomile (p.1669·3); sodium hyaluronate (p.1697·3).
*Menopausal vaginal disorders.*

**Mucojet** *Segix, Ital.*
Carbocisteine (p.1116·2).
*Respiratory-tract disorders.*

**Mucokehl** *Sanum-Kehlbeck, Ger.*
Homoeopathic preparation.

**Mucola** *Samakeephaesaj, Thai.*
Bromhexine hydrochloride (p.1115·3).
*Respiratory-tract disorders associated with increased or viscous mucus.*

**Mucolair** *3M, Belg.†.*
Acetylcysteine (p.1112·3).
*Adjuvant in respiratory-tract infections.*

**Mucolan** *Milano, Thai.*
Ambroxol hydrochloride (p.1114·3).
*Asthma; bronchitis.*

**Mucolase** *Lampugnani, Ital.*
Carbocisteine (p.1116·2).
*Respiratory-tract disorders.*

**Mucolator**
*Labima, Belg.†; Abbott, Fr.; Abbott, Hong Kong; Abbott, Malaysia.*
Acetylcysteine (p.1112·3).
*Paracetamol poisoning; respiratory-tract disorders associated with increased or viscous mucus.*

**Mucolavi** *Vitoria, Port.*
Sobrerol (p.1130·2).

**Mucolene** *Formenti, Ital.*
Mesna (p.1041·2).
*Respiratory-tract disorders associated with excess or viscous mucus.*

**Mucoless** *Parke-Med, S.Afr.*
Carbocisteine (p.1116·2).
*Respiratory-tract disorders with increased, viscous mucus.*

**Mucolex**
*Warner-Lambert, Irl.; Pfizer Consumer, Port.; Osoth, Thai.*
Carbocisteine (p.1116·2).
*Respiratory-tract disorders associated with increased or viscous mucus.*

**Mucolexin**
*Pediatrica, Malaysia; Pediatrica, Singapore.*
Dextromethorphan hydrobromide (p.1117·3); guaifenesin (p.1122·1); sodium citrate (p.1223·2).
*Coughs.*

**Mucolid** *Greater Pharma, Thai.*
Ambroxol hydrochloride (p.1114·3).
*Asthma; bronchitis.*

**Mucolin**
*Note. This name is used for preparations of different composition.*
*Abbott, Braz.; Cooper (Κοπερ), Gr.*
Ambroxol hydrochloride (p.1114·3).
*Respiratory disorders associated with viscous mucus.*

*Sanofi Synthelabo, Mex.*
Carbocisteine (p.1116·2).

**Mucolin A** *Sanofi Synthelabo, Mex.*
Ampicillin (p.157·1); carbocisteine (p.1116·2).
*Respiratory-tract infections.*

**Mucolinc** *Cipla, India.*
Bromhexine hydrochloride (p.1115·3); salbutamol (p.791·3).
*Obstructive airways disease.*

**Mucolinct** *Propan, S.Afr.†.*
Carbocisteine (p.1116·2).
*Respiratory-tract disorders.*

**Mucolisil** *Sanofi Synthelabo, Braz.*
Carbocisteine (p.1116·2).
*Respiratory-tract congestion.*

**Mucolit** *CTI, Israel.*
Carbocisteine (p.1116·2).
*Respiratory-tract disorders associated with abnormal or viscous mucus.*

**Mucolitic**
*Bristol-Myers Squibb, Arg.; Altana, Braz.*
Carbocisteine (p.1116·2).
*Respiratory-tract congestion.*

**Mucolitic Antitusivo** *Bristol-Myers Squibb, Arg.*
Carbocisteine (p.1116·2); dextromethorphan hydrobromide (p.1117·3).
*Coughs.*

**Mucolitico** *Instituto Sanitas, Chile.*
Acetylcysteine (p.1112·3).
*Respiratory-tract congestion.*

**Mucolitico Maggioni** *Sanofi Winthrop, Ital.†.*
Domiodol (p.1119·1).
*Respiratory-tract congestion.*

**Mucolix**
*Note. This name is used for preparations of different composition.*
*Cifarma, Braz.†.*
Carbocisteine (p.1116·2).
*Respiratory-tract congestion.*

*Xepa-Soul Pattinson, Hong Kong†.*
Bromhexine hydrochloride (p.1115·3).
*Obstructive airways disease.*

**Mucolysin**
*Note. This name is used for preparations of different composition.*
*Durascan, Denm.*
Acetylcysteine (p.1112·3).
*Respiratory-tract congestion.*

*Farmila, Ital.; Interdelta, Switz.*
Tiopronin (p.1054·3).
*Respiratory-tract disorders.*

**Mucolyt**
*Note. A similar name is used for preparations of different composition (see below).*
*Hamilton, Austral.*
Sodium chloride (p.1233·3).
*Viscous mucus in the throat.*

**Mucolyte**
*Note. A similar name is used for preparations of different composition (see above).*
*Julphar, UAE.*
Bromhexine hydrochloride (p.1115·3).
*Respiratory-tract disorders associated with viscous mucus.*

**Mucomax** *Hexal, Braz.†.*
Carbocisteine (p.1116·2).
*Respiratory-tract congestion.*

**Mucomed**
*Note. This name is used for preparations of different composition.*
*Medibrands, Israel.*
Carbocisteine (p.1116·2).
*Respiratory-tract disorders associated with viscous mucus.*

*Medifive, Thai.*
Ambroxol hydrochloride (p.1114·3).
*Respiratory-tract disorders associated with increased or viscous mucus.*

**Muco-Mepha** *Mepha, Switz.*
Acetylcysteine (p.1112·3).
*Respiratory-tract disorders associated with increased or viscous mucus.*

**Mucomex** *Phoenix, Arg.*
Ambroxol acefyllinate (p.1114·3).
*Obstructive airways disease.*

**Mucomix** *Samarth, India.*
Acetylcysteine (p.1112·3).
*Paracetamol poisoning; respiratory-tract disorders.*

**Mucomyst**
*Bristol-Myers Squibb, Austral.; Bristol-Myers Squibb, Austria; Bristol-Myers Squibb, Belg.; Wellspring, Canad.; AstraZeneca, Denm.; AstraZeneca, Fin.; UPSA, Fr.; Bristol-Myers Squibb, Gr.; Bristol-Myers Squibb, Israel; Bristol-Myers Squibb, Neth.; AstraZeneca, Norw.; Draco, Swed.; Apothecon, USA.*
Acetylcysteine (p.1112·3) or acetylcysteine sodium (p.1113·1).
*Paracetamol poisoning; respiratory-tract disorders associated with viscous mucus.*

**Muconorm** *Prospa, Ital.*
Telmesteine (p.1131·1).
*Respiratory-tract disorders.*

**Mucopec** *Macrophar, Thai.*
Ambroxol hydrochloride (p.1114·3).
*Respiratory-tract disorders associated with increased or viscous mucus.*

**Mucophlogat** *Azupharma, Ger.*
Ambroxol hydrochloride (p.1114·3).
*Respiratory-tract disorders associated with increased or viscous mucus.*

**Mucoporetta** *Pharmacia, Fin.*
Acetylcysteine (p.1112·3).
*Respiratory-tract congestion.*

**Mucoprednibron** *Pharmacia, Arg.*
Ambroxol (p.1114·3); astemizole (p.424·2); butetamate (p.1116·2); phenylephrine hydrochloride (p.1126·3).
*Respiratory-tract disorders.*

**Mucopront**
*Mack, Illert., Ger.; Mack, Malaysia; Mack, Singapore; Mack, Thai.*
Carbocisteine (p.1116·2) or carbocisteine sodium (p.1116·3).
*Respiratory-tract disorders associated with increased or viscous mucus.*

**Mucorama** *Roche, Spain†.*
Phenylpropanolamine hydrochloride (p.1127·3); iodinated glycerol (p.1122·3).
*Obstructive airways disease.*

**Mucorama TS** *Boehringer Mannheim Roche, Spain†.*
Iodinated glycerol (p.1122·3); co-trimoxazole (p.199·3).
*Respiratory-tract infections.*

**Mucorem** *Remek, Gr.*
Carbocisteine (p.1116·2).
*Respiratory disorders associated with viscous mucus.*

**Mucorex** *Almirall, Spain.*
Citiolone (p.1672·3).
*Respiratory-tract disorders.*

**Mucorex Ampicilina**
*Almirall, Spain†.*
*Capsules; tablets:* Ampicillin (p.157·1); citiolone (p.1672·3).
*Respiratory-tract infections.*

*Berenguer Infale, Spain†.*
*Injection:* Ampicillin sodium (p.157·1); ampicillin benzathine (p.158·1); citiolone (p.1672·3).
Lidocaine hydrochloride (p.1377·3) is included in this preparation to alleviate the pain of injection.
*Respiratory-tract infections.*

**Mucorex Ciclin** *Almirall, Spain†.*
Citiolone (p.1672·3); tartaric acid (p.1752·1); tetracycline hydrochloride (p.266·2).
*Respiratory-tract infections.*

**Mucorhinathiol Mucoral** *Sanofi Synthelabo, Port.*
Carbocisteine (p.1116·2).
Formerly known as Mucoral.
*Respiratory-tract disorders.*

**Mucorhinyl** *Synthelabo, Belg.†.*
Phenylephrine hydrochloride (p.1126·3); chlorphenamine maleate (p.427·3); sulfanilamide (p.263·2).
*Rhinitis; rhinopharyngitis; sinusitis.*

**Mucosa compositum** *Heel, Ger.*
Homoeopathic preparation.

**Mucosan** *Boehringer Ingelheim, Spain.*
Ambroxol hydrochloride (p.1114·3).
*Respiratory-tract disorders.*

**Muco-Sana** *Klus, Switz.*
Peppermint oil (p.1283·2); camphor oil; lavender oil (p.1705·2).
*Nasal disorders.*

**Mucoseptal** *Actipharm, Switz.†.*
Carbocisteine (p.1116·2).
*Respiratory-tract disorders.*

**Mucosil** *Dey, USA.*
Acetylcysteine sodium (p.1113·1).
*Mucolytic in bronchopulmonary disorders.*

**Mucosirop** *Roche, S.Afr.*
Carbocisteine (p.1116·2).
*Respiratory-tract disorders with increased, viscous mucus.*

**Mucosol**
*Note. This name is used for preparations of different composition.*
*AstraZeneca, India.*
Terbutaline sulfate (p.797·2); bromhexine (p.1115·3).
*Respiratory-tract disorders.*

*Malaysia Chemist, Singapore.*
Bromhexine hydrochloride (p.1115·3).
*Respiratory-tract disorders associated with increased or viscous mucus.*

**Mucosolvan**
*Boehringer Ingelheim, Austria; Boehringer de Angeli, Braz.; Boehringer Ingelheim, Chile; Boehringer Ingelheim, Ger.; Boehringer Ingelheim, Gr.; Boehringer Ingelheim, Hong Kong; Boehringer Ingelheim, Ital.; Teijin, Jpn; Boehringer Ingelheim, Malaysia; Boehringer Ingelheim Promeco, Mex.; Boehringer Ingelheim, Port.; Boehringer Ingelheim, Singapore; Boehringer Ingelheim, Thai.*
Ambroxol hydrochloride (p.1114·3).
*Neonatal respiratory distress syndrome; respiratory-tract disorders associated with increased or viscous mucus.*

**Mucosolvan Compositum** *Boehringer Ingelheim Promeco, Mex.*
Ambroxol hydrochloride (p.1114·3); clenbuterol hydrochloride (p.784·2).
*Respiratory-tract congestion.*

**Mucosolvon**
*Boehringer Ingelheim, Arg.; Boehringer Ingelheim, Switz.*
Ambroxol hydrochloride (p.1114·3).
*Respiratory-tract congestion.*

**Mucosolvon Compositum** *Boehringer Ingelheim, Arg.*
Ambroxol hydrochloride (p.1114·3); clenbuterol hydrochloride (p.784·2).
*Respiratory-tract congestion.*

**Mucospas**
*Boehringer Ingelheim, Austria; Boehringer Ingelheim, Port.*
Ambroxol hydrochloride (p.1114·3); clenbuterol hydrochloride (p.784·2).
*Respiratory-tract disorders.*

**Mucospect**
*Universal, Hong Kong; Triomed, S.Afr.*
Carbocisteine (p.1116·2).
*Respiratory-tract disorders associated with increased or viscous mucus.*

**Mucospire** *Rosa-Phytopharma, Fr.*
Acetylcysteine (p.1112·3).
*Respiratory-tract disorders.*

**Mucosta** *Otsuka, Jpn.*
Rebamipide (p.1287·3).
*Gastritis; peptic ulcer.*

**Mucostar** *Krugher, Ital.*
Carbocisteine (p.1116·2).
*Respiratory-tract congestion.*

**Mucosteine** *Medgenix, Belg.*
Carbocisteine (p.1116·2).
*Respiratory-tract disorders associated with viscous mucus.*

**Mucostop** *Mepha, Switz.*
Acetylcysteine (p.1112·3).
*Respiratory-tract disorders associated with viscous mucus.*

**Mucosyt** *Bioprogress, Ital.*
Tiopronin (p.1054·3).
*Respiratory-tract disorders associated with increased or viscous mucus.*

**Mucotablin** *Lichtenstein, Ger.†.*
Ambroxol hydrochloride (p.1114·3).
*Respiratory-tract disorders associated with increased or viscous mucus.*

**Muco-Tablinen** *Sanorania, Ger.†.*
Ambroxol hydrochloride (p.1114·3).
*Respiratory-tract disorders associated with increased or viscous mucus.*

**Mucotectan**
*Boehringer Ingelheim, Austria†; Boehringer Ingelheim, Ger.†.*
Ambroxol hydrochloride (p.1114·3); doxycycline hyclate (p.206·2).
*Bacterial infections of the respiratory tract.*

**Mucothera** *Therabel, Belg.*
Erdosteine (p.1121·1).
*Respiratory-tract disorders.*

**Mucotherm** *Lannacher, Austria.*
Ethyl nicotinate (p.37·2).
*Anorectal disorders; prostatitis.*

**Mucothiol**
*Note. This name is used for preparations of different composition.*
*Theratech, Fr.; Geymonat, Ital.*
Methyl dacisteine (p.1124·2).
*Respiratory-tract congestion.*

*Sanofi Synthelabo, Gr.*
Carbocisteine (p.1116·2).
*Respiratory disorders associated with viscous mucus.*

**Mucotic** *Hua, Thai.*
Acetylcysteine (p.1112·3).
*Bronchitis associated with increased or viscous mucus.*

**Mucotoss** *Sigma, Braz.*
Carbocisteine (p.1116·2).
*Respiratory-tract congestion.*

**Mucotreis** *Ecobi, Ital.*
Carbocisteine (p.1116·2).
*Respiratory-tract disorders.*

**Muco-Trin** *Klus, Switz.*
Xylometazoline hydrochloride (p.1132·2); peppermint oil (p.1283·2); camphor oil.
*Nasal congestion.*

**Mucotrophir** *Sanofi Synthelabo, Fr.†.*
Carbocisteine (p.1116·2).
*Respiratory-tract disorders.*

**Mucovibrol** *Liomont, Mex.*
Ambroxol hydrochloride (p.1114·3).
*Respiratory-tract congestion.*

**Mucovibrol C** *Liomont, Mex.*
Ambroxol hydrochloride (p.1114·3); clenbuterol hydrochloride (p.784·2).
*Respiratory-tract congestion.*

**Mucovibrol T** *Liomont, Mex.*
Ambroxol hydrochloride (p.1114·3).
*Respiratory-tract congestion.*

**Mucovin** *Leiras, Fin.*
Bromhexine hydrochloride (p.1115·3).
*Respiratory-tract congestion.*

**Mucovital** *Almirall, Spain.*
Carbocisteine lysine (p.1116·3).
*Respiratory-tract congestion.*

**Mucoxan** *IBSA, Ital.*
Acetylcysteine (p.1112·3).
*Respiratory-tract congestion.*

**Mucoxin**
*Note. This name is used for preparations of different composition.*
*Wyeth Lederle, Ital.†.*
*Oral suspension:* Oxetacaine (p.1382·1); aluminium hydroxide (p.1249·2); magnesium oxide (p.1272·3).
*Tablets:* Oxetacaine (p.1382·1); algeldrate (p.1249·2); magnesium carbonate (p.1272·1).
*Gastrointestinal disorders associated with hyperacidity.*

*Pharmasant, Thai.*
Bromhexine hydrochloride (p.1115·3).
*Respiratory-tract disorders associated with increased or viscous mucus.*

**Mucoxine-F** *Pharmasant, Thai.*
Ambroxol hydrochloride (p.1114·3).
*Respiratory-tract disorders.*

**Mucoxol** *Serral, Mex.*
Ambroxol (p.1114·3).
*Respiratory-tract congestion.*

**Mucoxolan** *Teuto, Braz.*
Ambroxol hydrochloride (p.1114·3).
*Respiratory-tract congestion.*

**Mucoza**
*Pond's Chemical, Singapore; Pond's, Thai.*
Acetylcysteine (p.1112·3).
*Respiratory-tract disorders with increased or viscous mucus.*

**Mucozan** *Pond's, Thai.*
Ambroxol hydrochloride (p.1114·3).
*Asthma; bronchitis.*

**Mucozym** *Mucos, Ger.*
Bromelains (p.1662·2).
*Nasal inflammation.*

**Mucret** *AstraZeneca, Ger.; Stern, Ger.*
Acetylcysteine (p.1112·3).
*Respiratory-tract disorders associated with increased or viscous mucus.*

**Mu-Cron**
*Novartis Consumer, Irl.†; Novartis Consumer, UK†.*
Paracetamol (p.76·2); phenylpropanolamine hydrochloride (p.1127·3).
*Nasal congestion; sinus pain.*

**Muc-Sabona** *Sabona, Ger.*
Hedera helix; liquorice (p.1270·2); thyme (p.1755·2).
*Respiratory-tract disorders with viscous mucus.*

**Mudagrip** *Geminis, Arg.*
Aspirin (p.15·1); ascorbic acid (p.1460·2); caffeine (p.782·1).
*Fever; pain.*

**Mudantil** *Geminis, Arg.*
Astemizole (p.424·2).
*Hypersensitivity reactions.*

**Mudantos H** *Geminis, Arg.*
Diphenhydramine (p.431·3).

**Mudapenil** *Geminis, Arg.*
Procaine benzylpenicillin (p.246·1).
*Bacterial infections.*

**Mudd Acne** *Chattem, Canad.†.*
Salicylic acid (p.1157·1).
*Acne.*

**Mudrane** *ECR, USA†.*
Potassium iodide (p.1598·1); aminophylline (p.780·2); phenobarbital (p.367·3); ephedrine hydrochloride (p.1120·1).
*Bronchospasm.*

**Mudrane GG** *ECR, USA†.*
Guaifenesin (p.1122·1); aminophylline (p.780·2); phenobarbital (p.367·3); ephedrine hydrochloride (p.1120·1).
*Bronchospasm.*

**Mudrane GG-2** *ECR, USA†.*
Guaifenesin (p.1122·1); aminophylline (p.780·2).
*Bronchospasm.*

**Muelita** *Cabuchi, Arg.*
Benzocaine (p.1370·3); benzalkonium chloride (p.1168·3); peppermint oil (p.1283·2); methylthioninium chloride (p.1042·2).

**Muflex** *TO-Chemicals, Thai.*
Carbocisteine (p.1116·2).
*Respiratory-tract disorders associated with increased or viscous mucus.*

**Muforan** *Pharmacia, Arg.*
Fotemustine (p.557·2).
*Cerebral cancer; malignant melanoma.*

**Mulcatel** *Maver, Chile.*
Sucralfate (p.1290·2).
*Peptic ulcer.*

**Mulimen**
*Peithner, Austria; Fides, Ger.*
Homoeopathic preparation.

**Mulkine** *Dexo, Fr.*
Montmorillonite; guar gum (p.333·2).
*Constipation.*

**Mulmicor** *Scheffler, Ger.*
Camphor (p.1665·3).
*Hypotension.*

**Mulsal A Megadosis** *Vitafarma, Spain†.*
Vitamin A (p.1451·2).
*Vitamin A deficiency.*

**Mulsal N** *Mucos, Ger.*
Trypsin (p.1758·3); papain (p.1727·3); bromelains (p.1662·2).
*Inflammation; musculoskeletal and joint disorders; oedema.*

**Mul-Tab** *British Dispensary, Thai.†.*
Multivitamin preparation (p.1417·1).

**Multene** *Baxter, Fr.†.*
Amino-acid preparation (p.1417·1).
*Parenteral nutrition.*

**Multe-Pak** *SoloPak, USA.*
A range of trace element preparations (p.1417·1).
*Parenteral nutrition.*

**Multi-12** *Sabex, Canad.*
A multivitamin preparation (p.1417·1).
*Parenteral nutrition.*

**Multi II** *Solgar, UK.*
Amino-acid, multivitamin, and mineral preparation (p.1417·1).

**Multi II IV VI** *Sisu, Canad.*
Multivitamin and mineral preparation (p.1417·1).

**Multi 75** *Fibertone, USA.*
Multivitamin and mineral preparation (p.1417·1).

**Multi 1000** *Sabex, Canad.†.*
Multivitamin preparation (p.1417·1).
*Parenteral nutrition.*

**Multi B** *Seroyal, Canad.†.*
Vitamin B substances (p.1417·1).

**Multi B Complex** *Quest, UK.*
Vitamin B and C preparation (p.1417·1).

**Multi Cal-Mag** *Seroyal, Canad.†.*
Vitamin and mineral preparation (p.1417·1).

**Multi Formula for Men 50+** *Jamieson, Canad.†.*
Multivitamin and mineral preparation (p.1417·1).

**Multi Forte 29** *Stanley, Canad.*
Multivitamin and mineral preparation (p.1417·1).

**Multi Hance** *Gerolimatos (Γερολυματος), Gr.*
Gadobenate dimeglumine (p.1062·1).
*Contrast medium for magnetic resonance imaging.*

**Multi Up** *Fher, Ital.*
Multivitamin and mineral preparation with ginseng (p.1417·1).
*Tonic.*

**Multi Vit Drops with Iron** *Barre-National, USA.*
Multivitamin preparation with iron (p.1417·1).

**Multi for Women** *Jamieson, Canad.†.*
Multivitamin and mineral preparation (p.1417·1).

**Multi-Action Actifed** *Pfizer Consumer, UK.*
Triprolidine hydrochloride (p.442·3); pseudoephedrine hydrochloride (p.1129·2).
Formerly known as Actifed.
*Cold and influenza symptoms; rhinitis.*

**Multi-Action Actifed Chesty Coughs Expectorant** *Pfizer Consumer, UK.*
Triprolidine hydrochloride (p.442·3); pseudoephedrine hydrochloride (p.1129·2); guaifenesin (p.1122·1).
Formerly known as Actifed Expectorant.
*Coughs; upper respiratory-tract congestion.*

**Multi-Action Actifed Dry Coughs** *Pfizer Consumer, UK.*
Triprolidine hydrochloride (p.442·3); pseudoephedrine hydrochloride (p.1129·2); dextromethorphan hydrobromide (p.1117·3).
Formerly known as Actifed Compound.
*Coughs; upper respiratory-tract congestion.*

**Multi-B Forte** *Pfizer Consumer, Austral.*
Vitamin B substances and vitamin C (p.1417·1).

**Multi-B Strong** *Vitabalans, Fin.*
Vitamin B substances (p.1417·1).

**Multibay** *Bayer, India.*
Multivitamin preparation (p.1417·1).

**Multibionta**
*Merck, Austria; Merck, Ger.; Merck, Spain; Merck, Switz.*
Multivitamin preparation (p.1417·1).

*Merck, Chile.*
Vitamin and mineral preparation (p.1417·1).
*Dietary supplement.*

*Merck, Irl.; E. Merck, UK†.*
Multivitamins for infusion (p.1417·1).
*Parenteral nutrition.*

**Multibionta Complex Gins** *Merck, Spain.*
Multivitamin and mineral preparation with ginseng (p.1417·1).

**Multibionta Junior** *Merck, Austria†.*
Multivitamin preparation with calcium (p.1417·1).

**Multibionta Mineral** *Merck, Spain.*
Multivitamin and mineral preparation (p.1417·1).

**Multibionta plus Mineral** *Merck, Ger.*
Multivitamin and mineral preparation (p.1417·1).

**Multibionta plus Mineralien** *Merck, Austria.*
Multivitamin and mineral preparation (p.1417·1).

**Multibionta Probiotic** *Seven Seas, Irl.*
Vitamins; minerals; *Lactobacillus acidophilus*; *Bifidobacterium longum* (p.1417·1).

**Multicap** *Sriprasit, Thai.*
Multivitamin and mineral preparation (p.1417·1).

**Multicebrina Efevit** *Sanofi Synthelabo, Spain.*
Multivitamin and mineral preparation (p.1417·1).

**Multicentrum**
*Wyeth Consumer, Chile; Whitehall, Ital.*
Vitamin, mineral, and trace-element preparations (p.1417·1).
*Nutritional supplement.*

**Multichew** *Chew, Thai.*
Multivitamin preparation (p.1417·1).

**Multicrom** *Menarini, Fr.*
Sodium cromoglicate (p.795·3).
*Allergic eye disorders.*

**Multi-Day** *Nature's Bounty, USA.*
A range of vitamin preparations (p.1417·1).

**Multiderm** *Agis, Israel.*
Diflucortolone valerate (p.1099·3); chlorquinaldol (p.187·3).
*Skin disorders.*

**Multielmin** *Osorio de Moraes, Braz.*
Mebendazole (p.108·2).
*Worm infections.*

**Multifebrin** *Bajer, Arg.*
Paracetamol (p.76·2).
*Fever; pain.*

**Multiferon** *Viranative, Swed.*
Interferon alfa (leucocyte) (p.640·3).
Formerly known as Interferon Alfanative.
*Chronic myeloid leukaemia; hairy-cell leukaemia.*

**Multifluorid** *DMG, Ger.*
Sodium fluoride (p.1444·3); olaflur (p.1442·3); dectaflur (p.1427·1).
*Dental caries prophylaxis; hypersensitive teeth.*

**Multiformil** *Pharmedia (Φαρμεντια), Gr.*
Nimesulide (p.67·1).
*Inflammation; musculoskeletal disorders; pain.*

**Multifung** *Rider, Chile.*
Bifonazole (p.395·1).
*Fungal and Gram-positive bacterial skin infections.*

**Multifungin**
*Note. This name is used for preparations of different composition.*
*Ebewe, Austria.*
*Topical powder:* Bromochlorosalicylanilide (p.395·2).
*Topical solution; ointment:* Bromochlorosalicylanilide (p.395·2); bamipine lactate (p.425·3) or bamipine salicylate (p.425·3).
*Fungal skin and nail infections.*

*Nicholas Piramal, India.*
*Topical powder:* Bromochlorosalicylanilide (p.395·2); salicylic acid (p.1157·1).
*Topical solution; cream:* Bromochlorosalicylanilide (p.395·2); bamipine salicylate (p.425·3).
*Fungal skin infections.*

**Multifungin H** *Nicholas Piramal, India.*
Bromochlorosalicylanilide (p.395·2); bamipine (p.425·3); hydrocortisone acetate (p.1103·3).
*Inflamed fungal skin infections.*

**Multigen AL** *Asta Medica, Braz.*
Allergen extracts of dust, pneumococcus, neisseria, streptococcus, *Haemophilus influenzae*, *Staphylococcus aureus*, and *Klebsiella pneumoniae* (p.1650·1).
*Allergen immunotherapy.*

**Multi-gesic**
*Note. A similar name is used for preparations of different composition (see below).*
*Multi-Pro, Canad.*
Paracetamol (p.76·2).
*Pain.*

**Multigesic**
*Note. A similar name is used for preparations of different composition (see above).*
*Nicholas Piramal, India.*
Diethylamine salicylate (p.34·1).
*Fibrositis; lumbago; sciatica; sprains.*

**Multiglyco** *Seroyal, Canad.†.*
Vitamin B substances, vitamin C, and minerals (p.1417·1).

**Multigotas** *Gobbi, Arg.*
Multivitamin preparation (p.1417·1).

**Multi-Gyn** *Farmalight, Port.†.*
Preparations for vaginal hygiene and lubrication.

**MultiHance**
*Gerot, Austria; Byk, Belg.; Bracco, Denm.; Astra Tech, Fin.; Byk, Fr.; Byk Gulden, Ger.; Merck, Irl.; Bracco, Ital.; Byk, Neth.; Bracco, Port.; Astra Tech, Swed.; Bracco, UK.*
Meglumine gadobenate (p.1062·1).
*Contrast medium for magnetic resonance imaging.*

**Multi-12/K1** *Sabex, Canad.*
Multivitamin preparation for infusion (p.1417·1).

**Multilase** *Sigma-Tau, Ital.†.*
Anistreplase (p.863·3).
*Myocardial infarction.*

**Multilens Solution** *Agepha, Austria.*
Disinfection and storage solution for hard contact lenses (p.1164·2).

**Multilex** *Rugby, USA.*
A range of vitamin preparations (p.1417·1).

**Multilim**
*Atlantic, Hong Kong; Atlantic, Thai.*
Multivitamin preparation (p.1417·1).
*Tonic; vitamin supplement.*

**Multilim RG** *Atlantic, Thai.*
Ginseng (p.1693·1); royal jelly (p.1740·3); vitamins; minerals (p.1417·1).

**Multilind**
*Bristol-Myers Squibb, Chile; Niddapharm, Ger.; Bristol-Myers Squibb, Switz.*
Nystatin (p.406·3); zinc oxide (p.1163·2).
*Fungal skin infections.*

**Multiload**
*Organon, Austral.; Organon, Braz.; Organon, Chile; Organon, Denm.; Organon, Fr.; Nourypharma, Ger.; Organon, Hong Kong; Organon, Irl.†; Multilan, Israel; Organon, Ital.; Organon, Malaysia; Organon, Mex.; Organon, Neth.; Organon, NZ; Organon, Port.; Donmed, S.Afr.; Organon, Singapore; Organon, Switz.; Organon, Thai.; Organon, UK.*
Copper-wound plastic (p.1425·3).
*Intra-uterine contraceptive device.*

**Multilyte** *American Pharmaceutical, USA.*
A range of electrolyte preparations (p.1217·1).
*Fluid and electrolyte disorders.*

**Multi-Mam Compressas** *Farmalight, Port.*
Aloe (p.1141·3); glycerol (p.1694·3).
*Nipple care during breastfeeding.*

**Multi-Mam Lanolina** *Farmalight, Port.*
Wool fat (p.1483·1).
*Nipple care during breastfeeding.*

**Multi-Mega** *Natural Life, Arg.*
Multivitamin, mineral, and nutritional preparation (p.1417·1).

**Multi-Min** *GNLD, Austral.†.*
Mineral and trace element preparation with vitamin D (p.1417·1).

**Multi-Min Electro** *Quest, Canad.†.*
Mineral preparation with vitamins $B_2$ and C (p.1417·1).

**MultiMineral** *Usana, Canad.*
Mineral preparation (p.1417·1).

**Multi-Mins** *Seroyal, Canad.†.*
Mineral preparation (p.1417·1).

**Multi-Mulsin N** *Mucos, Ger.*
Multivitamin preparation (p.1417·1).

**Multin** *Lazar, Arg.*
Paracetamol (p.76·2); dipyrone (p.35·3).
*Fever; pain.*

**Multiparin**
*CP Pharmaceuticals, Irl.; Artex, NZ; CP Pharmaceuticals, UK.*
Heparin sodium (p.928·1).
*Thromboembolic disorders.*

**Multipax** *Rhone-Poulenc Rorer, Canad.†.*
Hydroxyzine hydrochloride (p.434·3).
*Anxiety.*

**Multi-Phyto** *Pharmavite, Canad.†.*
Multivitamin and mineral preparation (p.1417·1).

**Multipore** *Orion, Fin.*
Multivitamin and mineral preparation (p.1417·1).

**Multi-Pro** *Alpharma, Malaysia.*
Multivitamin preparation (p.1417·1).

**Multi-Purpose Lens Drops** *Bausch & Lomb, Canad.*
Wetting solution for contact lenses (p.1164·2).

**Multiron** *Vitabiotics, UK.*
Multivitamin and mineral preparation with ginseng (p.1417·1).

**Multi-Sanasol** *Vifor, Switz.*
Multivitamin and mineral preparation (p.1417·1).

**Multi-Sanostol**
*Altana, Ger.*
Multivitamin and mineral preparation (p.1417·1).
*Byk Gulden, Hong Kong†.*
Multivitamin preparation (p.1417·1).
*Altana, Malaysia.*
Multivitamin preparation with calcium (p.1417·1).

**Multi-Sanosvit mit Eisen** *Altana, Ger.*
Multivitamin preparation with minerals including iron (p.1417·1).

**Multisedil** *Andromaco, Chile.*
Diazepam (p.690·1); chlormezanone (p.675·1).
*Anxiety; skeletal muscle spasm; sleep disorders.*

**Multiselect 29** *Stanley, Canad.*
Multivitamin and mineral preparation (p.1417·1).

**Multisoy** *Dieterba, Ital.*
Infant feed (p.1417·1).
*Milk intolerance.*

**Multistix**
*Bayer, Austral.; Bayer, Canad.†; Bayer Diagnostici, Ital.; Bayer, USA.*
Test for glucose, protein, blood, ketones, bilirubin, urobilinogen, and pH in urine.

**Multistix 2**
*Bayer, Canad.†; Miles, Ital.; Bayer, USA.*
Test for nitrites and leucocytes in urine.

**Multistix 5**
*Bayer, Austral.; Bayer, Canad.†.*
Test for glucose, blood, protein, nitrites, and leucocytes in urine.

**Multistix 7**
*Bayer, Austral.†; Bayer, USA.*
Test for glucose, protein, blood, ketones, nitrites, leucocytes, and pH in urine.

**Multistix 9**
*Bayer, Austral.; Bayer, USA.*
Test for pH, protein, glucose, ketones, bilirubin, blood, urobilinogen, nitrites, and leucocytes in urine.

**Multistix GP** *Bayer Diagnostics, UK.*
Test for specific gravity, pH, protein, glucose, ketones, blood, nitrites, and leucocytes in urine.

**Multistix SG**
*Bayer, Austral.†; Bayer, Canad.†; Bayer Diagnostics, Irl.; Bayer Diagnostics, UK; Bayer, USA.*
Test for pH, protein, glucose, ketones, bilirubin, blood, urobilinogen, and specific gravity in urine.

**Multistix 8 SG**
*Bayer, Austral.; Bayer, Canad.†; Bayer Diagnostics, Fr.; Bayer Diagnostics, UK; Bayer, USA.*
Test for glucose, protein, blood, ketones, nitrites, leucocytes, pH, and specific gravity in urine.

**Multistix 9 SG** *Bayer, USA.*
Test for glucose, protein, blood, ketones, bilirubin, nitrites, leucocytes, pH, and specific gravity in urine.

**Multistix 10 SG**
*Bayer, Austral.; Bayer, Canad.†; Bayer Diagnostics, Fr.; Bayer Diagnostics, Irl.; Bayer Diagnostici, Ital.; Bayer Diagnostics, Mex.; Bayer, Port.; Bayer Diagnostics, UK; Bayer, USA.*
Test for pH, protein, glucose, ketones, bilirubin, blood, urobilinogen, nitrites, leucocytes, and specific gravity in urine.

**Multi-Symptom Tylenol Cold** *McNeil Consumer, USA.*
Chlorphenamine maleate (p.427·3); dextromethorphan hydrobromide (p.1117·3); paracetamol (p.76·2); pseudoephedrine hydrochloride (p.1129·2).
*Coughs and cold symptoms.*

**Multi-Symptom Tylenol Cough** *McNeil Consumer, USA.*
Dextromethorphan hydrobromide (p.1117·3); paracetamol (p.76·2).
Formerly known as Maximum Strength Tylenol Cough.
*Coughs.*

**Multi-Symptom Tylenol Cough with Decongestant** *McNeil Consumer, USA.*
Pseudoephedrine hydrochloride (p.1129·2); dextromethorphan hydrobromide (p.1117·3); paracetamol (p.76·2).
Formerly known as Maximum Strength Tylenol Cough with Decongestant.
*Coughs and cold symptoms.*

**Multi-Tabs Neo** *Ferrosan, Fin.*
Multivitamin and mineral preparation (p.1417·1).

**Multi-Tar** *ICN, Hong Kong.*
Pyrithione zinc (p.1156·2); tar (p.1159·3); cade oil (p.1159·2); coal tar (p.1159·2).
*Scalp disorders.*

**Multi-Tar Plus** *ICN, Canad.*
Cade oil (p.1159·2); tar (p.1159·3); coal tar (p.1159·2); pyrithione zinc (p.1156·2).
*Seborrhoeic dermatitis.*

**Multitest**
*Serotherapeutisches, Austria; Richter, Austria; Pasteur Merieux, Belg.†; Aventis Pasteur, Braz.†; Biosyn, Ger.*
Tetanus antigen; diphtheria antigen; streptococcus antigen; tuberculin antigen (p.1759·1); candida albicans antigen; trichophyton antigen; proteus mirabilis antigen.
*Assessment of cell-mediated immunity.*

**Multitest CMI**
*CSL, Austral.; Connaught, Canad.†; Pasteur Merieux, Israel; Imtix, Neth.†; CSL, NZ; Aventis, S.Afr.; Pasteur Merieux, USA†.*
Tetanus antigen; diphtheria antigen; streptococcus antigen; tuberculin antigen (p.1759·1); candida albicans antigen; trichophyton antigen; proteus mirabilis antigen.
*Assessment of cell-mediated immunity.*

**Multitest IMC**
*Aventis Pasteur, Fr.†; Imtix, Ital.†; Rhone-Poulenc Rorer, Spain†.*
Tetanus antigen; diphtheria antigen; streptococcus antigen; tuberculin antigen (p.1759·1); candida albicans antigen; trichophyton antigen; proteus mirabilis antigen.
*Assessment of cell-mediated immunity.*

**Multiton** *Biochimici, Ital.*
Multivitamin and mineral preparation (p.1417·1).

**Multivac VR** *Nikkho, Braz.*
*Staphylococcus aureus*; *Streptococcus pyogenes*; *Streptococcus viridans*; group D Streptococcus; *Moraxella catarrhalis*; *Corynebacterium diphtheroides*; *Streptococcus pneumoniae*; *Listeria monocytogenes*; *Klebsiella pneumoniae*; *Pseudomonas aeruginosa*; *Serratia marcesens* (p.1650·1); *Haemophilus influenzae*; *Candida albicans*; *Penicillium* sp.; *Alternaria* sp.; *Rhodotorula mucilaginosa*; *Mucor racemosus*; *Hormodendrum*; *Aspergillus niger*.
*Allergen immunotherapy.*

**Multi-Vi-Min** *Sisu, Canad.*
Multivitamin and mineral preparation (p.1417·1).

**Multivit** *Garden House, Arg.*
Multivitamin preparation (p.1417·1).

**Multi-Vit** *Lafarmen, Arg.*
Multivitamin preparation (p.1417·1).

**Multivit Biovital** *Roche, Switz.†.*
Multivitamin and mineral preparation with plant extracts (p.1417·1).

**Multi-Vitamin Day & Night** *Cenovis, Austral.†.*
Day tablets, vitamins and minerals (p.1417·1); night tablets, valerian (p.1762·2); passion flower (p.1729·1); chamomile (p.1669·3); crataegus (p.1677·1); vitamins and minerals.
*Dietary supplement; insomnia; tonic.*

**Multivitamin Phytopharma V** *OTW, Ger.*
Multivitamin preparation (p.1417·1).

**Multivitamin-Aufbau-Kapseln** *Wiedemann, Ger.*
Multivitamin and mineral preparation (p.1417·1).

**Multivitamin-Dragees-Pascoe** *Pascoe, Ger.†.*
Multivitamin preparation (p.1417·1).

**Multivitamines** *Gisand, Switz.*
Multivitamin and mineral preparation (p.1417·1).

**Multivitaplex**
*Alpharma, Malaysia; Alpharma, Singapore.*
Multivitamin preparation (p.1417·1).

**Multivit-B** *Lannacher, Austria.*
Vitamin B substances (p.1417·1).

**Multi-Vite** *Seroyal, Canad.†.*
Multivitamin and mineral preparation (p.1417·1).

**Multivite Six** *Boots Healthcare, NZ.*
Multivitamin preparation (p.1417·1).

**Multivitol** *Hermes, Ger.†.*
Multivitamin and mineral preparation (p.1417·1).

**Multodrin** *Montavit, Austria.*
Dexamethasone (p.1097·1); diphenhydramine hydrochloride (p.431·3).
*Skin disorders.*

**Multojod-Gastreu N R12** *Reckeweg, Ger.*
Homoeopathic preparation.

**Multosin** *Takeda, Ger.*
Estramustine meglumine phosphate (p.551·2) or estramustine sodium phosphate (p.551·1).
*Prostatic cancer.*

**Multovitan** *Worwag, Ger.†.*
Vitamin B substances; ascorbic acid (p.1417·1).

**Multum**
*Note. This name is used for preparations of different composition.*
*Rosen, Ger.*
Chlordiazepoxide (p.674·2).
*Anxiety disorders; sleep disorders.*
*Lampugnani, Ital.*
Benzydamine hydrochloride (p.21·1).
*Gynaecological disorders; mouth and throat disorders; musculoskeletal, joint, peri-articular, and soft-tissue disorders.*

**Mulvidren-F Softab** *Stuart, USA.*
Sodium fluoride (p.1444·3) with multivitamins (p.1417·1).
*Dental caries prophylaxis in children.*

**Mulvitin** *Silom, Thai.†.*
Multivitamin preparation (p.1417·1).

**Mumaten**
*Berna, Hong Kong†; Berna, Ital.†; Byk Madaus, S.Afr.†; Berna, Switz.†; Berna, Thai.†.*
A mumps vaccine (attenuated Rubini strain) (p.1626·3).
*Active immunisation.*

**Mumpsvax**
*Prodome, Braz.†; Merck Frosst, Canad.; Aventis Pasteur, Denm.; Chiron Behring, Ger.; Pasteur Merieux, Irl.†; Pasteur Merieux, Ital.†; Pro Vaccine, Switz.; Pasteur Merieux, UK†; Merck, USA.*
A mumps vaccine (Jeryl Lynn (B level) strain) (p.1626·3).
*Active immunisation.*

**Mundidol** *Mundipharma, Austria.*
Morphine sulfate (p.60·2).
*Pain.*

**Mundil** *Mundipharma, Ger.*
Captopril (p.879·2).
*Heart failure; hypertension.*

**Mundiphyllin** *Mundipharma, Austria.*
Aminophylline (p.780·2).
*Heart failure; oedema; respiratory-tract disorders.*

**Mundisal**
*Mundipharma, Austria; Mundipharma, Ger.; Mundipharma, Switz.*
Choline salicylate (p.26·2); cetalkonium chloride (p.1172·1).
*Mouth and throat disorders.*

**Mundisept** *Mundipharma, Switz.†.*
Isopropyl alcohol (p.1184·3).
*Hand disinfection.*

**Mundra** *Zilly, Ger.†.*
Tormentil (p.1757·2); peppermint leaf (p.1283·2).
*Mouth and throat disorders.*

**Municaps** *Schwarzhaupt, Ger.*
Multivitamin preparation (p.1417·1).
*Tonic.*

**Munit-E** *Holista, Canad.*
Vitamins; echinacea; garlic; ginger; zinc gluconate (p.1417·1).

**Munitren H** *Robugen, Ger.*
Hydrocortisone (p.1103·3).
*Anogenital pruritus; skin disorders.*

**Munleit** *Hommel, Ger.*
Doxylamine succinate (p.432·3).
*Insomnia.*

**Munobal**
*Aventis, Arg.; Aventis, Austria; Aventis, Ger.; Aventis, Mex.; Aventis, Switz.*
Felodipine (p.914·3).
*Angina pectoris; hypertension.*

**Munolan** *Allergan-Frumtost, Braz.†.*
Bacterial and fungal antigens (p.1650·1); muramidase hydrochloride (p.1717·2).
*Immunostimulant.*

**Munostin** *Atlantis, Mex.*
Lysates of *Streptococcus pneumoniae*; *Moraxella catarrhalis*; *Streptococcus pyogenes*; *Haemophilus influenzae*(p.0·0); *Staphylococcus aureus*; *Klebsiella pneumoniae*.
*Respiratory-tract infections.*

**Munti-Vim** *Hua, Thai.*
Multivitamin preparation (p.1417·1).

**Mupaten** *Schering, Arg.*
Isoconazole (p.401·3) or isoconazole nitrate (p.401·3).
*Fungal or Gram-positive bacterial vaginal infections; fungal skin infections.*

**Mupax** *Lazar, Arg.*
Mupirocin (p.233·1).
*Bacterial skin infections.*

**Muphoran**
*Servier, Austral.; Servier, Austria; Servier, Braz.; Servier, Fr.; Servier, Gr.; Servier, Hong Kong†; Servier, Israel; Italfarmaco, Ital.*
Fotemustine (p.557·2).
*Cerebral cancer; disseminated malignant melanoma.*

**Mupiderm** *Pharmafarm, Fr.*
Mupirocin (p.233·1).
*Bacterial skin infections.*

**Mupirox** *Fortbenton, Arg.*
Mupirocin (p.233·1).
*Bacterial skin infections; elimination of nasal staphylococci.*

**Muporin** *TO-Chemicals, Thai.*
Mupirocin (p.233·1).
*Bacterial skin infections.*

**Muraligne** *Shire, Fr.*
Glucomannan (p.1693·3).
*Obesity.*

**Muramyl** *Master, Chile.*
Hexetidine (p.1182·1).
*Mouth and throat disorders.*

**Murazyme**
*Grunenthal, Belg.; Asta Medica, Braz.*
Muramidase hydrochloride (p.1717·2).
*Viral skin infections.*

**Murelax** *Sigma, Austral.*
Oxazepam (p.712·2).
*Alcohol withdrawal syndrome; anxiety.*

**Muricalm** *Novartis, Braz.*
Pimethixene (p.439·1).
*Respiratory-tract disorders in children.*

**Murine**
*Note. This name is used for preparations of different composition.*
*Abbott, Austral.†; Abbott, NZ†.*
Berberine chloride (p.1659·3).
*Eye irritation.*
*Abbott, Canad.; Ross, USA.*
*Ear drops:* Urea hydrogen peroxide (p.1195·3).
*Removal of ear wax.*
*Abbott, Canad.; Ross, USA.*
*Eye drops:* Polyvinyl alcohol (p.1581·1); povidone (p.1581·2).
*Dry eyes.*
*Abbott, Port.†; Prestige, UK.*
Naphazoline hydrochloride (p.1124·3).
*Eye irritation.*

**Murine Allergy** *Abbott, Austral.†.*
Antazoline sulfate (p.424·2); xylometazoline hydrochloride (p.1132·2).
*Allergic eye disorders.*

**Murine Clear Eyes** *Abbott, S.Afr.*
Naphazoline hydrochloride (p.1124·3).
*Eye irritation.*

**Murine Contact** *Abbott, Austral.†.*
Hypromellose (p.1579·3); glycerol (p.1694·3).
*Comfort drops for contact lenses.*

**Murine NTF** *Abbott, Malaysia.*
Polyvinyl alcohol (p.1581·1); povidone (p.1581·2).
*Dry eyes.*

**Murine Plus**
*Note. This name is used for preparations of different composition.*
*Abbott, Chile.*
Tetryzoline hydrochloride (p.1131·2).
*Eye irritation.*
*Abbott, Malaysia; Ross, USA.*
Polyvinyl alcohol (p.1581·1); povidone (p.1581·2); tetryzoline hydrochloride (p.1131·2).
*Minor eye irritation.*

**Murine Revital Eyes** *Abbott, Austral.*
Polyvinyl alcohol (p.1581·1); povidone (p.1581·2).
*Dry eyes; eye cleansing; eye irritation.*

**Murine Sore Eyes** *Abbott, Austral.*
Tetryzoline hydrochloride (p.1131·2).
*Eye irritation.*

**Murine Supplemental Tears** *Abbott, Canad.*
Artificial tears.

**Murine Tears for Eyes** *Abbott, Austral.*
Polyvinyl alcohol (p.1581·1); povidone (p.1581·2).
*Dry eyes; eye irritation.*

**Muro 128**
*Bausch & Lomb, Arg.; Bausch & Lomb, Canad.; Bausch & Lomb, USA.*
Sodium chloride (p.1233·3).
*Corneal oedema.*

**Murocel**
*Bausch & Lomb, Canad.†; Bausch & Lomb, USA.*
Methylcellulose (p.1580·2).
*Dry eyes.*

**Murocoll-2** *Bausch & Lomb, USA.*
Hyoscine hydrobromide (p.483·3); phenylephrine hydrochloride (p.1126·3).
*Induction of mydriasis and cycloplegia; uveitis.*

**Murode** *Teofarma, Spain.*
Diflorasone diacetate (p.1099·3).
*Skin disorders.*

**Muroptic** *Optopics, USA.*
Sodium chloride (p.1233·3).
*Corneal oedema.*

**Murri Antidolorifico** *Bracco, Ital.*
Aspirin (p.15·1); paracetamol (p.76·2); caffeine (p.782·1).
*Fever; pain.*

**Mus** *Grunenthal, Chile.*
Clarithromycin (p.192·2).
*Bacterial infections.*

**Musapam** *Krewel, Ger.*
Tetrazepam (p.724·1).
*Skeletal muscle tension and spasm.*

**Musaril** *Sanofi Synthelabo, Ger.*
Tetrazepam (p.724·1).
*Skeletal muscle spasm.*

**Musashi** *Sidus, Arg.*
Amino-acid preparation (p.1417·1).
*Dietary supplement.*

**Musashi Barras Growling Dog** *Sidus, Arg.*
Preparation for enteral nutrition (p.1417·1).

**Musashi Creatina** *Sidus, Arg.*
Creatine (p.1677·2).
*Muscular fatigue.*

**Muscadol** *Julphar, UAE.*
Orphenadrine citrate (p.486·1); paracetamol (p.76·2).
*Musculoskeletal pain.*

**Muscalax** *Polipharm, Thai.*
Methyl salicylate (p.59·3); menthol (p.1711·3); eugenol (p.1686·2).
*Musculoskeletal and joint pain; sprains; strains.*

**Muscaran** *Christiaens, Belg.†.*
Bethanechol chloride (p.1487·3).
*Urinary bladder atony; urinary retention.*

**Muscarsan** *Sanum-Kehlbeck, Ger.*
Homoeopathic preparation.

**Muscelax** *Hua, Thai.*
Carisoprodol (p.1392·1); paracetamol (p.76·2).
*Musculoskeletal and joint disorders; skeletal muscle spasm.*

**Muscinil** *Opus, UK.*
Procyclidine hydrochloride (p.488·2).
*Drug-induced extrapyramidal disorders; parkinsonism.*

**Muscle & Back Pain Relief** *Stanley, Canad.; Technilab, Canad.*
Paracetamol (p.76·2); methocarbamol (p.1395·1).

**Muscle & Back Pain Relief-8** *Stanley, Canad.*
Paracetamol (p.76·2); codeine phosphate (p.27·1); methocarbamol (p.1395·1).

**Muscle Relaxant and Analgesic** *Technilab, Canad.*
Aspirin (p.15·1); methocarbamol (p.1395·1).

**Muscle Rub** *Schein, USA†.*
Methyl salicylate (p.59·3); menthol (p.1711·3).
*Muscle, joint, and soft-tissue pain; neuralgia.*

**Muscoflex** *Epifarma, Ital.*
Thiocolchicoside (p.1395·2).
*Neuromuscular pain; parkinsonism; spasticity.*

**Muscol**
*Teva, Israel; Teva, Thai.*
Orphenadrine citrate (p.486·1); paracetamol (p.76·2).
*Headache; musculoskeletal and joint disorders; neuralgia.*

**Musco-ril** *Sanofi Synthelabo, Gr.*
Thiocolchicoside (p.1395·2).
*Muscle spasm.*

**Muscoril** *Inverni della Beffa, Ital.*
Thiocolchicoside (p.1395·2).
*Muscle spasticity; neuromuscular pain; oedema; parkinsonism; soft-tissue disorders.*

**Muscunor** *Fada, Arg.*
Vitamin B substances (p.1417·1).

**Muse**
*Abbott, Austral.; Vivus, Austria; Abbott, Braz.; Paladin, Canad.; Meda, Denm.; Abbott, Fin.; Abbott, Fr.; Abbott, Ger.; Janssen, Hong Kong†; Abbott, Irl.; Janssen-Cilag, Israel; Janssen, Mex.; Abbott, NZ; Abbott, S.Afr.; Janssen-Cilag, Singapore†; Astra, Spain†; Abbott, Switz.; Janssen, Thai.; Meda, UK; Vivus, USA.*
Alprostadil (p.1512·3).
*Erectile dysfunction.*

**Muskelat** *Azupharma, Ger.*
Tetrazepam (p.724·1).
*Skeletal muscle tension and spasm.*

**Muskol** *Schering-Plough, Canad.*
*SPF 6:* Diethyltoluamide (p.1503·3); homosalate (p.1148·1); octinoxate (p.1154·3); octisalate (p.1154·3); oxybenzone (p.1154·3).
*Insect repellent; sunscreen.*

**Muslax** *Biological E, India.*
Methyl salicylate (p.59·3); menthol (p.1711·3).
*Musculoskeletal, joint, and soft-tissue disorders.*

**Musocalm** *Progress, Thai.*
Tolperisone hydrochloride (p.1396·3).
*Skeletal muscle spasm.*

**Musocan** *Sriprasit, Thai.*
Ambroxol hydrochloride (p.1114·3).
*Respiratory-tract disorders associated with increased or viscous mucus.*

**Musside** *Cosmofarma, Port.*
Lindane (p.1506·3).
*Pediculosis.*

**Mustargen**
*Merck Frosst, Canad.; Merck Sharp & Dohme, Israel; Merck Sharp & Dohme, Switz.; Merck, USA.*
Chlormethine hydrochloride (p.537·1).
*Malignant neoplasms; mycosis fungoides; polycythaemia vera.*

**Musterole** *Schering-Plough, USA.*
Methyl salicylate (p.59·3); menthol (p.1711·3); methyl nicotinate (p.59·2).
*Muscle, joint, and soft-tissue pain; neuralgia.*

**Musterole Extra** *Schering-Plough, USA.*
Methyl salicylate (p.59·3); camphor (p.1665·3); menthol (p.1711·3); mustard oil (p.1718·2).
*Muscle, joint, and soft-tissue pain; neuralgia.*

**Mustoforan** *Servier, Spain.*
Fotemustine (p.557·2).
*Malignant melanoma.*

**Musxan** *Pharmasant, Thai.*
Methocarbamol (p.1395·1).
*Skeletal muscle spasm.*

**Mutabase** *Schering-Plough, Spain.*
Perphenazine (p.714·2); amitriptyline hydrochloride (p.280·3).
*Depression.*

**Mutabon**
*Schering-Plough, Ital.; Schering-Plough, Port.*
Perphenazine (p.714·2); amitriptyline hydrochloride (p.280·3).
*Psychiatric disorders.*

**Mutabon D**
*Kirby, Arg.*
Perphenazine (p.714·2); amitriptyline (p.280·3).
*Mixed anxiety depressive states.*

*Essex, Chile.*
Perphenazine (p.714·2); amitriptyline hydrochloride (p.280·3).
*Agitation; anxiety; mixed anxiety depressive states; schizophrenia.*

**Mutacol** *Berna, Canad.*
A live oral attenuated cholera vaccine (CVD 103-HgR) (p.1611·2).
*Active immunisation.*

**Mutaflor**
*Emonta, Austria; Ardeypharm, Ger.*
*Escherichia coli.*
*Gastrointestinal disorders.*

**Mutagrip**
*Sanofi Synthelabo, Belg.; Pasteur Vaccins, Fr.; Aventis Pasteur, Ger.; Aventis Pasteur, Ital.; Aventis, Spain; Pro Vaccine, Switz.*
An inactivated influenza vaccine (split virion) (p.1620·2).
*Active immunisation.*

**Mutamycin**
*Bristol, Canad.; Bristol-Myers Squibb, Fin.; Bristol-Myers Squibb, Norw.; Bristol-Myers Squibb, Swed.; Bristol-Myers Squibb Oncology, USA.*
Mitomycin (p.573·3).
*Malignant neoplasms.*

**Mutamycine** *Bristol-Myers Squibb, Switz.*
Mitomycin (p.573·3).
*Malignant neoplasms.*

**Mutan** *Lannacher, Austria.*
Fluoxetine hydrochloride (p.292·1).
*Bulimia nervosa; depression; obsessive-compulsive disorder.*

**Mutellon** *Klein, Ger.*
Lycopus europaeus; motherwort (p.1717·1); valerian (p.1762·2).
*Hyperthyroidism.*

**Mutesa** *Wyeth Lederle, Fr.*
Aluminium hydroxide (p.1249·2); magnesium oxide (p.1272·3); oxetacaine (p.1382·1).
*Gastro-oesophageal pain.*

**Muthesa**
*Whitehall, Belg.†; ICN, Switz.*
Aluminium hydroxide (p.1249·2); magnesium carbonate (p.1272·1) or magnesium oxide (p.1272·3); oxetacaine (p.1382·1).
*Gastrointestinal disorders.*

**Muthesa N** *Wyeth Consumer, Neth.*
Aluminium hydroxide (p.1249·2); magnesium hydroxide (p.1272·2).
*Eructation; heartburn.*

**Mutum** *Raffo, Arg.*
Fluconazole (p.398·1).
*Fungal infections.*

**Muvial** *AGIPS, Ital.*
Timonacic methyl hydrochloride (p.1756·3).
*Otorhinolaryngeal disorders; respiratory-tract disorders.*

**Muvidina** *Kampel Martian, Arg.*
Zidovudine (p.658·2); lamivudine (p.648·2).
*HIV infection.*

**Muxol**
*Note. This name is used for preparations of different composition.*
*Saval, Chile.*
Ambroxol (p.1114·3).
*Respiratory-tract disorders.*

*Leurquin, Fr.; Andromaco, Mex.*
Ambroxol hydrochloride (p.1114·3).
*Respiratory-tract congestion.*

*Vifor, Switz.*
Bisacodyl (p.1251·3).
*Constipation.*

**M-Vac** *Serum Institute, India.*
A measles vaccine (attenuated Edmonston Zagreb strain) (p.1623·1).
*Active immunisation.*

**MVI**
*Aventis, Canad.; USV, India; Grossman, Mex.; Aventis, NZ†; Astra, USA.*
Multivitamin infusion (p.1417·1).
*Parenteral nutrition.*

**MVI-12**
*Rhone-Poulenc Rorer, Austral.†; Rhone-Poulenc Rorer, Hong Kong†; Armour, Israel†.*
Multivitamin preparation (p.1417·1).
*Parenteral nutrition.*

**MVI Paediatric** *Rhone-Poulenc Rorer, Austral.†.*
Multivitamin preparation (p.1417·1).
*Parenteral nutrition.*

**MVI-Ped** *Armour, Israel†.*
Multivitamin preparation (p.1417·1).
*Parenteral nutrition.*

**MVM** *Tyson, USA.*
Multivitamin and mineral preparation (p.1417·1).

**MXL**
*Napp, Irl.; Viatris, Port.; Napp, UK.*
Morphine sulfate (p.60·2).
*Pain.*

**Myacyne** *Schur, Ger.*
*Ointment:* Neomycin sulfate (p.235·1).
*Infected skin disorders; infected wounds.*

*Topical powder spray†:* Neomycin sulfate (p.235·1); tyrothricin (p.275·1).
*Infected skin disorders.*

**Myadec**
*Warner-Lambert, Austral.†; Warner-Lambert, NZ†; Parke, Davis, USA.*
Multivitamin and mineral preparation (p.1417·1).

**Myalgesic** *Wolfs, Belg.†.*
Salicylamide (p.87·3); benzocaine (p.1370·3).
*Musculoskeletal, joint, peri-articular, and joint disorders.*

**Myalgol N** *Robugen, Ger.†.*
Glycol salicylate (p.44·3); benzyl nicotinate (p.21·2).
Formerly contained salicylic acid, camphor, glycol salicylate, benzyl nicotinate, and capsicum.
*Circulatory disorders of the skin; muscle and joint pain; soft-tissue disorders.*

**Myambutol**
*Sigma, Austral.; Wyeth Lederle, Austria; Wyeth Lederle, Belg.; Wyeth-Ayerst, Canad.†; Meda, Denm.; Wyeth Lederle, Fr.; Lederle, Ger.; Wyeth, Gr.; Wyeth, Hong Kong; Wyeth Lederle, India; Wyeth, Irl.†; Lederle, Israel; Wyeth, Mex.; Teofarma, Neth.; Sigma, NZ; Wyeth, S.Afr.†; Teofarma, Spain; Meda, Swed.; Lederle, Switz.; Wyeth-Ayerst, Thai.; Lederle, USA.*
Ethambutol hydrochloride (p.211·3).
*Opportunistic mycobacterial infections; tuberculosis.*

**Myambutol-INH**
*Wyeth Lederle, Austria; Lederle, Ger.; Wyeth, Mex.; Lederle, Switz.*
Ethambutol hydrochloride (p.211·3); isoniazid (p.222·2).
*Tuberculosis.*

**Mybacin** *Greater Pharma, Thai.*
Neomycin sulfate (p.235·1); bacitracin (p.161·3); amylocaine hydrochloride (p.1370·2).
*Mouth and throat disorders.*

**Mybacin Dermic** *Greater Pharma, Thai.*
Bacitracin (p.161·3); neomycin (p.235·1).
*Infected skin disorders.*

**Mybulen** *Aspen, S.Afr.*
Ibuprofen (p.45·3); paracetamol (p.76·2); codeine phosphate (p.27·1).
*Pain.*

**Mycardol** *Sanofi Winthrop, Irl.†.*
Pentaerithrityl tetranitrate (p.979·1).
*Angina pectoris.*

**Mycatox** *Riemser, Ger.*
Dequalinium chloride (p.1178·1); hexylresorcinol (p.1182·1); sage (p.1741·2).
*Bath additive; fungal infections.*

**Mycel** *Biolab Sanus, Braz.*
Isoconazole nitrate (p.401·3).
*Fungal skin infections.*

**Mycelex** *Bayer, USA.*
Clotrimazole (p.396·2).
*Oral candidiasis.*

**Mycelex-3** *Bayer, USA.*
Butoconazole nitrate (p.395·2).
*Vaginal candidiasis.*

**Mycelex-7** *Bayer, USA.*
Clotrimazole (p.396·2).
*Vulvovaginal candidiasis.*

**Mycelex-G** *Bayer, USA†.*
Clotrimazole (p.396·2).
*Vulvovaginal candidiasis.*

**Mycella** *Silom, Thai.*
Ketoconazole (p.403·3).
*Fungal infections.*

**Mycetin** *Farmigea, Ital.*
Chloramphenicol (p.185·1).
*Bacterial eye infections.*

**Myciclid** *Wayne, Mex.†.*
Carbenicillin (p.166·3).
*Bacterial infections.*

**Mycidal** *Greater Pharma, Thai.†.*
Glutaral (p.1180·3).
*Instrument disinfection.*

**Mycidex** *Mac, India.*
Dexamethasone phosphate (p.1097·2); neomycin sulfate (p.235·1).
*Eye disorders.*

**Mycifradin**
*Pharmacia Upjohn, Canad.†; Pharmacia Upjohn, Hong Kong†; Pharmacia Upjohn, Irl.†; Pharmacia Upjohn, S.Afr.†; Pharmacia Upjohn, UK†; Upjohn, USA.*
Neomycin sulfate (p.235·1).
*Bacterial infections; hepatic coma; pre-operative bowel preparation.*

**Myciguent**
*Pharmacia Upjohn, Canad.†; Upjohn, USA†.*
Neomycin sulfate (p.235·1).
*Bacterial skin infections.*

**Mycil**
*Note. This name is used for preparations of different composition.*
*Wellspring, Canad.*
Chlorphenesin (p.396·1).
*Fungal and bacterial skin infections.*

*Boots, Hong Kong.*
Tolnaftate (p.410·1); benzalkonium chloride (p.1168·3); chlorhexidine hydrochloride (p.1173·3).
*Fungal skin infections.*

*Boots Healthcare, Irl.; Crookes Healthcare, UK.*
*Ointment:* Tolnaftate (p.410·1); benzalkonium chloride (p.1168·3).
*Fungal skin infections.*

*Boots Healthcare, Irl.; Crookes Healthcare, UK.*
*Topical powder:* Tolnaftate (p.410·1); chlorhexidine hydrochloride (p.1173·3).
*Fungal skin infections.*

*Boots Healthcare, Irl.; Crookes Healthcare, UK.*
*Topical spray:* Tolnaftate (p.410·1).
*Fungal skin infections.*

**Mycil Gold** *Crookes Healthcare, UK†.*
Clotrimazole (p.396·2).
*Fungal skin infections.*

**Mycil Healthy Feet** *Boots, Austral.*
*Cream:* Tolnaftate (p.410·1); benzalkonium chloride (p.1168·3).
*Topical powder:* Tolnaftate (p.410·1); chlorhexidine hydrochloride (p.1173·3).
*Fungal skin infections.*

**Mycinette** *Pfeiffer, USA.*
Phenol (p.1188·1); alum (p.1652·1).
*Sore throat.*

**Mycinettes** *Pfeiffer, USA.*
Benzocaine (p.1370·3).
*Sore throat.*

**Mycinopred** *Allergan, Switz.*
Prednisolone acetate (p.1108·1); polymyxin B sulfate (p.245·1); neomycin sulfate (p.235·1).
*Infected eye disorders.*

**Myci-Spray** *Misemer, USA.*
Phenylephrine hydrochloride (p.1126·3); mepyramine maleate (p.437·1).
*Nasal congestion.*

**Mycitracin** *Upjohn, USA.*
Bacitracin (p.161·3); neomycin sulfate (p.235·1); polymyxin B sulfate (p.245·1).
*Bacterial skin infections.*

**Mycitracin Plus** *Upjohn, USA†.*
Bacitracin (p.161·3); neomycin sulfate (p.235·1); polymyxin B sulfate (p.245·1); lidocaine (p.1377·3).
*Bacterial skin infections.*

**Myclo-Derm** *Boehringer Ingelheim, Canad.†.*
Clotrimazole (p.396·2).
*Fungal skin infections.*

**Myclo-Gyne** *Boehringer Ingelheim, Canad.†.*
Clotrimazole (p.396·2).
*Vaginal candidiasis.*

**Myco-Aid** *Raza, Malaysia; Pharmaniaga, Malaysia.*
Tolnaftate (p.410·1).
*Fungal skin infections.*

**Mycoapaisyl** *Merck Medication Familiale, Fr.*
Econazole nitrate (p.397·2).
Formerly known as Furazanol.
*Fungal skin infections.*

**Mycobacter** *Zekides, Gr.*
Econazole nitrate (p.397·2).
*Fungal skin and vaginal infections.*

**Mycoban** *Rolab, S.Afr.*
Clotrimazole (p.396·2).
*Fungal skin infections; vulvovaginal candidiasis.*

**Myco-Biotic II** *Moore, USA.*
Triamcinolone acetonide (p.1110·2); nystatin (p.406·3).
*Skin disorders.*

**Mycobutin**
*Pharmacia, Austral.; Pharmacia, Austria; Pharmacia, Belg.; Pharmacia, Canad.; Pharmacia, Ger.; Pharmacia-Upjohn, Gr.; Pharmacia, Hong Kong; Pharmacia Upjohn, Israel; Pharmacia Upjohn, Ital.; Pharmacia, Neth.; Pharmacia, NZ; Pharmacia, Port.; Pharmacia, S.Afr.; Pharmacia, Switz.; Pharmacia, UK; Pharmacia Upjohn, USA.*
Rifabutin (p.249·1).
*Opportunistic mycobacterial infections; tuberculosis.*

**Mycobutol** *Cadila Pharma, India.*
Ethambutol (p.212·2).
*Tuberculosis.*

**Mycochlorin** *Sermmitr, Thai.*
Chloramphenicol palmitate (p.185·1).
*Bacterial infections.*

**Mycocid** *Chemo-Pharma, India.*
Clotrimazole (p.396·2).
*Fungal skin and nail infections.*

**Mycocide NS** *Woodward, USA.*
Benzalkonium chloride (p.1168·3).
*Skin disinfection.*

**Mycodecyl** *Diepharmex, Fr.*
*Cream:* Undecenoic acid (p.410·3); zinc undecenoate (p.411·1).
*Topical powder:* Undecenoic acid (p.410·3); zinc undecenoate (p.411·1); calcium undecenoate (p.410·3).
*Topical solution:* Undecenoic acid (p.410·3).
*Fungal skin infections.*

**Mycoderm**
*Note. This name is used for preparations of different composition.*
*Ego, Austral.; Ego, Hong Kong.*
*Cream:* Salicylic acid (p.1157·1); undecenoic acid monoethanolamide (p.411·1); sodium propionate (p.408·1); butyl hydroxybenzoate (p.1183·2).
*Fungal skin infections.*

*Ego, Austral.; Ego, Hong Kong; Ego, Malaysia.*
*Dusting powder:* Salicylic acid (p.1157·1); sodium propionate (p.408·1); butyl hydroxybenzoate (p.1183·2).
*Fungal skin infections.*

*FDC, India.*
Salicylic acid (p.1157·1); benzoic acid (p.1169·3); menthol (p.1711·3).
*Bromhidrosis; fungal skin infections; hyperhidrosis; seborrhoeic dermatitis.*

**Mycoderm-C** *FDC, India.*
Clotrimazole (p.396·2).
*Fungal skin infections.*

**Mycodermil** *Vifor, Switz.*
Fenticonazole nitrate (p.397·3).
*Fungal skin infections.*

**Mycodib** *Diba, Mex.*
Ketoconazole (p.403·3).
*Fungal infections.*

**Mycofebrin** *Coup, Gr.*
Ketoconazole (p.403·3).
*Fungal infections.*

**Mycofen** *Nycomed, Denm.*
Ciclopirox (p.396·1) or ciclopirox olamine (p.396·1).
*Fungal skin and nail infections.*

**Myco-flusemidon** *Anpharm (Ανφαρμ), Gr.*
Bifonazole (p.395·1).
*Fungal skin infections.*

**Mycofug** *Hermal, Ger.*
Clotrimazole (p.396·2).
*Fungal skin infections.*

**Mycogel**
*Biorga, Fr.; Saninter, Port.†.*
Copper pidolate; zinc pidolate; melaleuca oil (p.1710·2).
*Fungal skin infections; scalp disorders.*

**Mycogen II** *Goldline, USA.*
Triamcinolone acetonide (p.1110·2); nystatin (p.406·3).
*Skin disorders.*

**Mycohaug C** *Betapharm, Ger.†.*
Clotrimazole (p.396·2).
*Fungal skin infections.*

**Myco-Hermal**
*Hermal, Israel; Hermal, Singapore.*
Clotrimazole (p.396·2).
*Fungal skin infections.*

**Mycohexal** *Hexal, S.Afr.*
Clotrimazole (p.396·2).
*Vaginal candidiasis.*

**Mycol** *Greater Pharma, Thai.*
Paracetamol (p.76·2); chlorphenamine maleate (p.427·3).
Formerly contained paracetamol, chlorphenamine maleate, and phenylpropanolamine hydrochloride.
*Cold symptoms.*

**Mycolog**
*Note. This name is used for preparations of different composition.*
*Sanofi Synthelabo, Belg.; Sanofi Synthelabo, Neth.; Sanofi Synthelabo, Switz.*
Triamcinolone acetonide (p.1110·2); gramicidin (p.220·2); neomycin sulfate (p.235·1); nystatin (p.406·3).
*Infected skin disorders.*

*Bristol-Myers Squibb, Fr.*
Triamcinolone acetonide (p.1110·2); neomycin sulfate (p.235·1); nystatin (p.406·3).
*Infected skin disorders.*

**Mycolog-II** *Westwood-Squibb, USA.*
Triamcinolone acetonide (p.1110·2); nystatin (p.406·3).
*Cutaneous candidiasis.*

**Myconel** *Marnel, USA.*
Triamcinolone acetonide (p.1110·2); nystatin (p.406·3).
*Skin disorders.*

**Myconex** *Cadila Pharma, India.*
Ethambutol (p.212·2); isoniazid (p.222·2).
*Tuberculosis.*

**Myconil** *Raza, Malaysia; Pharmaniaga, Malaysia.*
Griseofulvin (p.400·3).
*Fungal skin and nail infections.*

**Myconip** *Uni-Sankyo, India.*
*Lactobacillus sporogenes* (p.1704·2).
*Leucorrhoea; vaginitis.*

**Mycopol** *Nycomed, Austria.*
Undecenoic acid (p.410·3); benzoic acid (p.1169·3); isopropyl alcohol (p.1184·3).
*Fungal skin and nail infections.*

**Mycoral** *Kalbe, Singapore†.*
Ketoconazole (p.403·3).
*Dandruff; fungal infections; seborrhoeic dermatitis.*

**Mycoril**
*Remedica, Hong Kong; Remedica, Singapore.*
Clotrimazole (p.396·2).
*Fungal skin infections.*

**Mycosamthong** *Sermmitr, Thai.*
Co-trimoxazole (p.199·3).
*Bacterial infections.*

**Mycosin** *Prodotti, Braz.*
Miconazole nitrate (p.405·3).
*Fungal skin infections.*

**Mycospor**
*Note. This name is used for preparations of different composition.*
*Bayer, Arg.; Bayer, Austral.; Bayer, Belg.; Bayer, Braz.; Bayer, Denm.†; Bayer, Ger.; Bayer, Gr.; Bayer, Hong Kong; Bayer, Mex.; Bayer, Neth.; Bayer, Norw.†; Bayer, Port.; Bayer, S.Afr.; Bayer, Spain; Bayer, Thai.†.*
Bifonazole (p.395·1).
*Fungal skin infections.*

*Bayer, Port.*
*Ointment:* Bifonazole (p.395·1); urea (p.1162·2).
*Fungal nail infections.*

**Mycospor Carbamid**
*Bayer, Denm.†; Bayer, Norw.†.*
Bifonazole (p.395·1); urea (p.1162·2).
*Fungal nail infections.*

**Mycospor Nagelset** *Bayer, Ger.*
Bifonazole (p.395·1); urea (p.1162·2).
*Fungal nail infections.*

**Mycospor Onicoset**
*Bayer, Mex.; Bayer, Spain.*
Bifonazole (p.395·1); urea (p.1162·2).
*Fungal nail infections.*

**Mycosporan**
*Bayer, Chile; Bayer, Swed.*
Bifonazole (p.395·1).
*Fungal skin infections.*

**Mycosporan Karbamid** *Bayer, Swed.†.*
Bifonazole (p.395·1); urea (p.1162·2).
*Fungal nail infections.*

**Mycosporan Onycoset** *Bayer, Chile.*
Bifonazole (p.395·1); urea (p.1162·2).
*Fungal nail infections.*

**Mycosquam** *Pierre Fabre, Fr.*
Ciclopirox olamine (p.396·1).
*Scalp disorders.*

**Mycostatin**
*Bristol-Myers Squibb, Austral.; Bristol-Myers Squibb, Austria; Squibb, Canad.; Convatec, Canad.; Bristol-Myers Squibb, Denm.; Bristol-Myers Squibb, Fin.; Bristol-Myers Squibb, Hong Kong; Sarabhai Piramal, India; Bristol-Myers Squibb, Irl.; Bristol-Myers Squibb, Ital.; Bristol-Myers Squibb, Malaysia; Bristol-Myers Squibb, Norw.; Bristol-Myers Squibb, NZ; Bristol-Myers Squibb, Port.; Bristol-Myers Squibb, S.Afr.; Bristol-Myers Squibb, Singapore; Squibb, Spain; Bristol-Myers Squibb, Swed.; Bristol-Myers Squibb, Thai.; Apothecon, USA; Bristol-Myers Squibb Oncology, USA; Mead Johnson Laboratories, USA; Westwood-Squibb, USA.*
Nystatin (p.406·3).
*Candidiasis.*

**Mycostatin V** *Bristol-Myers Squibb, Austria.*
Triamcinolone acetonide (p.1110·2); neomycin sulfate (p.235·1); gramicidin (p.220·2); nystatin (p.406·3).
*Infected skin disorders.*

**Mycostatine**
*Bristol-Myers Squibb, Fr.; Sanofi Synthelabo, Switz.*
Nystatin (p.406·3).
*Candidiasis.*

**Mycostatin-Zinkoxid** *Bristol-Myers Squibb, Austria.*
Nystatin (p.406·3); zinc oxide (p.1163·2).
*Candidiasis.*

**Mycoster**
*Pierre Fabre, Fr.; Pierre Fabre, Port.*
Ciclopirox (p.396·1) or ciclopirox olamine (p.396·1).
*Fungal and bacterial skin infections; fungal nail infections.*

**Myco-Synalar**
*Note. This name is used for preparations of different composition.*
*Grunenthal, Austria; Grunenthal, Switz.*
*Cream:* Fluocinolone acetonide (p.1101·2); chlormidazole hydrochloride (p.396·1).
*Fungal skin infections.*

*Grunenthal, Austria; Yamanouchi, Spain†; Grunenthal, Switz.*
*Topical solution:* Fluocinolone acetonide (p.1101·2); chlormidazole hydrochloride (p.396·1); salicylic acid (p.1157·1).
*Fungal skin infections.*

**Mycota**
*Note. This name is used for preparations of different composition.*
*Boots, Hong Kong†; Reckitt Benckiser, S.Afr.; Thornton & Ross, UK.*
*Cream; topical powder:* Undecenoic acid (p.410·3); zinc undecenoate (p.411·1).
*Fungal skin infections.*

*Reckitt Benckiser, S.Afr.; Thornton & Ross, UK.*
*Topical spray:* Undecenoic acid (p.410·3); dichlorophen (p.104·1).
*Fungal skin infections.*

**Mycotel** *SM, Thai.*
Albendazole (p.101·2).
*Worm infections.*

**Myco-Triacet II** *Lemmon, USA.*
Triamcinolone acetonide (p.1110·2); nystatin (p.406·3).
*Skin disorders.*

**Mycotricide** *SM, Thai.*
Praziquantel (p.112·2).
*Schistosomiasis.*

**Myco-Ultralan** *Schering, Fr.†.*
Fluocortolone (p.1102·1); fluocortolone caproate (p.1102·1); nystatin (p.406·3); neomycin sulfate (p.235·1).
*Infected skin disorders.*

**Mycozole** *Osoth, Thai.*
Clotrimazole (p.396·2).
*Fungal skin infections.*

**Mycurium** *Taro, Israel.*
Atracurium besilate (p.1399·1).
*Competitive neuromuscular blocker.*

**Mydfrin**
*Alcon, Arg.; Alcon, Canad.; Alcon, Chile; Alcon, Hong Kong; Alcon, Malaysia; Alcon, Singapore; Alcon, USA.*
Phenylephrine hydrochloride (p.1126·3).
*Funduscopy; open-angle glaucoma; ophthalmic examination; pupil dilatation during surgery; refraction without cycloplegia; uveitis.*

**Mydocalm**
*Strathmann, Ger.; Gedeon Richter, Hong Kong; Labatec, Switz.; Gedeon Richter, Thai.*
Tolperisone hydrochloride (p.1396·3).
*Skeletal muscle spasm.*

**Mydocalm-A** *Chinoin, Mex.*
Tolperisone hydrochloride (p.1396·3); paracetamol (p.76·2).
*Skeletal muscle spasm and pain.*

**Mydosone** *Condrugs, Thai.*
Tolperisone hydrochloride (p.1396·3).
*Skeletal muscle spasm.*

**Mydral**
*Agepha, Austria; Ocusoft, USA.*
Tropicamide (p.491·1).
*Production of mydriasis.*

**Mydramide** *Fischer, Israel.*
Tropicamide (p.491·1).
*Production of mydriasis.*

**Mydriacil** *Alcon, Irl.*
Tropicamide (p.491·1).
*Production of mydriasis and cycloplegia.*

**Mydriacyl**
*Alcon, Austral.; Alcon, Braz.; Alcon, Canad.; Alcon, Chile; Alcon, Denm.; Alcon, Hong Kong; Alcon, Malaysia; Alcon, NZ; Alcon, S.Afr.; Alcon, Singapore; Alcon, Swed.; Alcon, Thai.; Alcon, UK; Alcon, USA.*
Tropicamide (p.491·1).
*Production of mydriasis and cycloplegia.*

**Mydrial-Atropin** *Winzer, Ger.*
Tyramine hydrochloride (p.1760·1); atropine borate (p.478·1); adrenaline acid tartrate (p.852·2).
*Production of mydriasis.*

**Mydrian** *Novartis, Norw.*
Tropicamide (p.491·1).
*Production of mydriasis.*

**Mydriasert** *Ioltech, Fr.*
Phenylephrine hydrochloride (p.1126·3); tropicamide (p.491·1).
*Production of mydriasis.*

**Mydriaticum**
*Agepha, Austria; Bournonville, Belg.†; Merck Sharp & Dohme-Chibret, Fr.; Stulln, Ger.; Novartis Ophthalmics, Hong Kong; Restan, S.Afr.; Novartis Ophthalmics, Switz.*
Tropicamide (p.491·1).
*Production of mydriasis and cycloplegia.*

**Mydril** *Alcon, Arg.*
Tropicamide (p.491·1).
*Production of mydriasis and cycloplegia.*

**Mydrilate**
*Intrapharm, Irl.; Intrapharm, UK.*
Cyclopentolate hydrochloride (p.480·3).
*Production of mydriasis and cycloplegia.*

**Mydrin-P** *Santen, Hong Kong.*
Tropicamide (p.491·1); phenylephrine hydrochloride (p.1126·3).
*Production of mydriasis and cycloplegia.*

**Mydrum** *Chauvin ankerpharm, Ger.*
Tropicamide (p.491·1).
*Aid in eye examination; production of mydriasis.*

**Myelobromol**
*Enzypharm, Austria; Durbin, UK.*
Mitobronitol (p.573·2).
*Chronic myeloid leukaemia.*

**Myelostim** *Italfarmaco, Ital.*
Lenograstim (p.755·3).
*Mobilisation of autologous peripheral blood progenitor cells; neutropenia induced by bone-marrow transplantation or cytotoxic chemotherapy.*

**Myfortic**
*Novartis, Switz.; Novartis, USA.*
Mycophenolate sodium.
*Renal transplant rejection.*

**Myfungar**
*Riemser, Ger.; Rhein, Mex.; Klinge, Switz.†.*
Oxiconazole nitrate (p.407·3).
*Fungal and Gram-positive bacterial infections.*

**Mygale compositum** *Weleda, Austria.*
Homoeopathic preparation.

**Mygdalon** *DDSA Pharmaceuticals, UK†.*
Metoclopramide hydrochloride (p.1274·3).

**Mygel** *Geneva, USA.*
Aluminium hydroxide (p.1249·2); magnesium hydroxide (p.1272·2); simeticone (p.1289·2).
*Hyperacidity.*

**Mygesal** *Greater Pharma, Thai.†.*
Methyl salicylate (p.59·3).
*Musculoskeletal and joint pain; sprains; strains.*

**Myk** *Cassenne, Fr.†.*
Sulconazole nitrate (p.408·2).
*Fungal skin infections.*

**Myk-1**
*Will-Pharma, Belg.; Will-Pharma, Neth.*
Sulconazole nitrate (p.408·2).
*Fungal skin infections.*

**Myko Cordes**
*Note. This name is used for preparations of different composition.*
*Ichthyol, Austria; Ichthyol, Ger.*
*Cream:* Clotrimazole (p.396·2).
*Fungal skin infections.*

*Ichthyol, Austria.*
*Paste:* Clotrimazole (p.396·2); zinc oxide (p.1163·2).
*Fungal skin infections.*

**Myko Cordes Plus** *Ichthyol, Ger.*
Clotrimazole (p.396·2); zinc oxide (p.1163·2).
*Fungal skin infections.*

**Mykoderm Heilsalbe** *Engelhard, Ger.*
Nystatin (p.406·3).
*Fungal skin infections.*

**Mykoderm Mund-Gel** *Engelhard, Ger.*
Miconazole (p.405·2).
*Fungal mouth infections.*

**Mykofungin** *Riemser, Ger.*
Clotrimazole (p.396·2).
*Fungal and bacterial infections of skin and genito-urinary tract.*

**Mykohaug** *Betapharm, Ger.*
Clotrimazole (p.396·2).
*Fungal and bacterial infections of skin and vagina; vaginal trichomoniasis.*

**Mykontral** *Riemser, Ger.*
Tioconazole (p.409·3).
*Fungal skin infections.*

**MykoPosterine N** *Kade, Ger.*
Nystatin (p.406·3).
*Anorectal fungal infections.*

**mykoproct sine** *Stegropharm, Ger.*
Nystatin (p.406·3); triamcinolone acetonide (p.1110·2).
*Fungal skin infections.*

**Mykosert** *Pfleger, Ger.*
Sertaconazole nitrate (p.408·1).
*Fungal skin infections.*

**Mykotin** *Ardeypharm, Ger.*
Miconazole (p.405·2) or miconazole nitrate (p.405·3).
*Fungal skin infections.*

**Mykrox** *Celltech, USA.*
Metolazone (p.956·2).
Formerly known as Microx.
*Hypertension.*

**Mykundex** *Bioglan, Ger.*
Nystatin (p.406·3).
*Fungal infections.*

**Mykundex Heilsalbe** *Bioglan, Ger.*
Nystatin (p.406·3); zinc oxide (p.1163·2).
*Fungal infections.*

**Mykundex mono** *Bioglan, Ger.*
Nystatin (p.406·3).
*Fungal infections.*

**Mylagen** *Goldline, USA.*
*Capsules:* Calcium carbonate (p.1254·2); magnesium carbonate (p.1272·1).
*Oral liquid:* Aluminium hydroxide (p.1249·2); magnesium hydroxide (p.1272·2); simeticone (p.1289·2).
*Hyperacidity.*

**Mylanta**
*Note. This name is used for preparations of different composition.*
*Pfizer Consumer, Austral.; Pfizer Consumer, Canad.; Parke, Davis, Chile; Johnson & Johnson, Hong Kong; Janssen-Cilag, Malaysia; Pfizer, NZ; Janssen-Cilag, Singapore; J&J-Merck, USA.*
*Oral suspension:* Aluminium hydroxide (p.1249·2); magnesium hydroxide (p.1272·2); simeticone (p.1289·2).
*Dyspepsia; flatulence; heartburn.*

*Janssen-Cilag, Belg.†.*
Algeldrate (p.1249·2); magnesium hydroxide (p.1272·2); simeticone (p.1289·2).
*Peptic ulcer.*

*Johnson & Johnson, Hong Kong; Janssen-Cilag, Malaysia; Janssen-Cilag, Singapore.*
*Tablets:* Calcium carbonate (p.1254·2); magnesium hydroxide (p.1272·2).
*Dyspepsia; heartburn.*

*J&J-Merck, USA.*
*Lozenges:* Calcium carbonate (p.1254·2).
*Hyperacidity.*

**Mylanta II** *Parke, Davis, Arg.*
Aluminium hydroxide (p.1249·2); magnesium hydroxide (p.1272·2); simeticone (p.1289·2).
*Flatulence; gastrointestinal hyperacidity.*

**Mylanta AR Acid Reducer** *J&J-Merck, USA.*
Famotidine (p.1265·2).
*Dyspepsia; heartburn.*

**Mylanta Effervescent** *Pfizer, NZ.*
Magnesium oxide (p.1272·3).
*Antacid.*

**Mylanta Gas**
*Parke, Davis, Arg.; J&J-Merck, USA.*
Simeticone (p.1289·2).
*Gastrointestinal disorders with excess gas.*

**Mylanta Gelcaps** *J&J-Merck, USA.*
Calcium carbonate (p.1254·2); magnesium carbonate (p.1272·1).
*Hyperacidity.*

**Mylanta Heartburn Relief**
*Note. This name is used for preparations of different composition.*
*Pfizer Consumer, Austral.*
*Oral liquid:* Aluminium hydroxide (p.1249·2); magnesium hydroxide (p.1272·2); calcium carbonate (p.1254·2); sodium bicarbonate (p.1223·2); alginic acid (p.1576·3).
Formerly known as Mylanta Plus.
*Tablets:* Magaldrate (p.1271·3); alginic acid (p.1576·3); sodium bicarbonate (p.1223·2).
Formerly known as Mylanta Plus.
*Dyspepsia; gastro-oesophageal reflux.*

*Pfizer, NZ.*
Alginic acid (p.1576·3); calcium carbonate (p.1254·2); aluminium hydroxide (p.1249·2); magnesium hydroxide (p.1272·2); sodium bicarbonate (p.1223·2).
*Antacid; gastro-oesophageal reflux.*

**Mylanta Max** *Parke, Davis, Arg.*
Aluminium hydroxide (p.1249·2); magnesium hydroxide (p.1272·2); simeticone (p.1289·2).
*Flatulence; gastrointestinal hyperacidity.*

**Mylanta Natural Fiber** *J&J-Merck, USA.*
Psyllium hydrophilic mucilloid (p.1268·1).

**Mylanta Plain** *Pfizer Consumer, Canad.*
Aluminium hydroxide (p.1249·2); magnesium hydroxide (p.1272·2).
*Gastrointestinal disorders associated with hyperacidity.*

**Mylanta Plus**
*Parke, Davis, Arg.; Ache, Braz.*
Aluminium hydroxide (p.1249·2); magnesium hydroxide (p.1272·2); simeticone (p.1289·2).
*Flatulence; gastrointestinal hyperacidity.*

**Mylanta Pocket** *Parke, Davis, Arg.*
Calcium carbonate (p.1254·2).
*Gastrointestinal hyperacidity.*

**Mylanta Reflux** *Parke, Davis, Arg.*
*Oral liquid:* Aluminium hydroxide (p.1249·2); magnesium hydroxide (p.1272·2); alginic acid (p.1576·3); sodium carbonate (p.1747·1).
*Tablets:* Aluminium hydroxide (p.1249·2); magnesium trisilicate (p.1272·3); alginic acid (p.1576·3).
*Gastro-oesophageal reflux; gastrointestinal hyperacidity.*

**Mylanta Rolltabs**
*Pfizer Consumer, Austral.; Pfizer, NZ.*
Calcium carbonate (p.1254·2); magnesium hydroxide (p.1272·2).
*Antacid.*

**Mylanta Simple** *Parke, Davis, Arg.*
Aluminium hydroxide (p.1249·2); magnesium hydroxide (p.1272·2).
*Gastrointestinal hyperacidity.*

**Mylepsinum** *AstraZeneca, Ger.*
Primidone (p.376·3).
*Epilepsy.*

**Myleran**
*GlaxoSmithKline, Arg.; GlaxoSmithKline, Austral.; GlaxoSmithKline, Austria; GlaxoSmithKline, Belg.; GlaxoSmithKline, Braz.; GlaxoSmithKline, Canad.; GlaxoSmithKline, Chile; GlaxoSmithKline, Fr.; GlaxoSmithKline, Ger.; IFET (ΙΦΕΤ), Gr.; GlaxoSmithKline, Hong Kong; GlaxoSmithKline, India; Wellcome, Irl.; Wellcome, Israel; GlaxoSmithKline, Ital.; GlaxoSmithKline, Malaysia; Glaxo Wellcome, Mex.; GlaxoSmithKline, Neth.; Glaxo Wellcome, Norw.†; GlaxoSmithKline, NZ; Wellcome, Port.; GlaxoSmithKline, S.Afr.; GlaxoSmithKline, Singapore; GlaxoSmithKline, Swed.; GlaxoSmithKline, Switz.; GlaxoSmithKline, Thai.; GlaxoSmithKline, UK; Glaxo Wellcome, USA.*
Busulfan (p.532·2).
*Bone-marrow transplantation; chronic myeloid leukaemia; essential thrombocythaemia; myelofibrosis; polycythaemia vera.*

**Myleuca** *IPRAD, Fr.*
Melaleuca oil (p.1710·2).
*Adjunct in fungal skin infections; skin cleansing.*

**Mylicon**
*Pfizer, Denm.; Warner-Lambert, Ital.; J&J-Merck, USA.*
Simeticone (p.1289·2).
*Adjunct in gastrointestinal investigations; infant colic; meteorism.*

**Mylocel** *MGI, USA.*
Hydroxycarbamide (p.559·1).
*Malignant neoplasms.*

**Mylocort** *Triomed, S.Afr.*
Hydrocortisone acetate (p.1103·3).
*Skin disorders.*

**Mylol** *Rolfe, S.Afr.*
*Topical liquid:* Diethyltoluamide (p.1503·3); dimethyl phthalate (p.1504·1); dibutyl phthalate (p.1503·1).
*Topical spray:* Diethyltoluamide (p.1503·3).
*Insect repellent.*

**Mylom** *Ranbaxy, Thai.*
Simeticone (p.1289·2).
*Flatulence.*

**Mylotarg**
*Wyeth, Arg.; Wyeth-Ayerst, USA.*
Gemtuzumab ozogamicin (p.558·3).
*Acute myeloid leukaemia.*

**Mylproin** *Desitin, Ger.†.*
Valproic acid (p.380·1).
*Epilepsy.*

**Mymin C** *Greater Pharma, Thai.†.*
Vitamin C (p.1460·2).
*Vitamin C deficiency.*

**Myminic Expectorant** *Morton Grove, USA†.*
Phenylpropanolamine hydrochloride (p.1127·3); guaifenesin (p.1122·1).
*Coughs.*

**Myminic Syrup** *Morton Grove, USA†.*
Phenylpropanolamine hydrochloride (p.1127·3); chlorphenamine maleate (p.427·3).

**Myminicol** *Morton Grove, USA†.*
Phenylpropanolamine hydrochloride (p.1127·3); chlorphenamine maleate (p.427·3); dextromethorphan hydrobromide (p.1117·3).
*Coughs and cold symptoms.*

**Mynah** *Wyeth, S.Afr.†.*
Ethambutol hydrochloride (p.211·3); isoniazid (p.222·2).
*Tuberculosis.*

**Mynatal** *ME Pharmaceuticals, USA.*
Multivitamin and mineral preparation with iron and folic acid (p.1417·1).

**Mynate 90 Plus** *ME Pharmaceuticals, USA.*
Multivitamin and mineral preparation (p.1417·1).

**Mynocine** *Wyeth Lederle, Fr.*
Minocycline hydrochloride (p.231·3).
*Bacterial infections.*

**Myo Hermes** *Organon, Spain†.*
Bethanechol chloride (p.1487·3).
*Gastrointestinal motility disorders; urinary retention.*

**Myobid** *Panacea, India.*
Ethionamide (p.212·3).
*Tuberculosis.*

**Myobloc** *Elan, USA.*
Botulinum B toxin (p.1388·3).
*Spasmodic torticollis.*

**Myocardon** *Byk, Austria.*
Aminophylline hydrochloride (p.780·3); papaverine hydrochloride (p.1728·1); atropine methonitrate (p.477·1); glyceryl trinitrate (p.923·2).
*Angina pectoris; heart failure; myocardial infarction.*

**Myocardon mono** *Byk, Austria.*
Isosorbide mononitrate (p.942·1).
*Angina pectoris; heart failure; myocardial infarction.*

**Myocardon N** *Byk Gulden, Ger.†.*
Theophylline (p.798·3).
Formerly contained aminophylline hydrate, phenobarbital, papaverine hydrochloride, atropine methonitrate, and glyceryl trinitrate.
*Cardiac disorders.*

**Myocet**
*Elan, Fr.; Elan, Ger.; Elan, Irl.; Segix, Ital.; Esteve, Port.; Elan, Spain; Elan, UK.*
Liposomal doxorubicin citrate (p.549·3) (p.547·3) or liposomal doxorubicin hydrochloride (p.547·3) (p.547·3).
*Breast cancer.*

**Myocholine**
*Croma, Austria; Glenwood, Ger.; Vifor, Switz.*
Bethanechol chloride (p.1487·3).
*Antimuscarinic effects of tricyclic antidepressants; dysphagia; gastro-oesophageal reflux; urinary retention.*

**Myochrysine**
*Prodome, Braz.†; Aventis, Canad.; Taylor, USA.*
Sodium aurothiomalate (p.88·2).
*Rheumatoid arthritis.*

**Myocin** *Shiwa, Thai.*
Methocarbamol (p.1395·1).
*Cramps; skeletal muscle spasm.*

**Myocord** *Elvetium, Arg.*
Atenolol (p.865·2).
*Arrhythmias; hypertension.*

**Myocrisin**
*Aventis, Austral.; Aventis, Denm.; Aventis, Fin.; Rhone-Poulenc Rorer, Hong Kong†; Aventis, Irl.; Aventis, Norw.; Aventis, NZ; Aventis, S.Afr.; Aventis, Swed.; Aventis, Thai.; JHC Healthcare, UK.*
Sodium aurothiomalate (p.88·2).
*Juvenile idiopathic arthritis; rheumatoid arthritis.*

**Myodipine** *Help, Gr.*
Nimodipine (p.972·3).
*Neurological deficit following subarachnoid haemorrhage.*

**Myodrine** *Charoen, Thai.*
Orphenadrine citrate (p.486·1); paracetamol (p.76·2).
*Muscle pain; tension headache.*

**Myodura** *Wockhardt, India.*
Amlodipine besilate (p.862·1).
*Angina pectoris; hypertension.*

**Myo-Echinacin** *Madaus, Austria.*
Echinaceae purpureae (p.1683·2).
*Urinary and respiratory-tract infections.*

**Myofedrin** *Apogepha, Ger.*
Oxyfedrine hydrochloride (p.978·2).
*Heart failure; ischaemic heart disease; myocardial infarction.*

**Myoflex**
*Note. This name is used for preparations of different composition.*
*Bayer Consumer, Canad.; Armstrong, Mex.; Fisons, USA.*
Trolamine salicylate (p.95·3).
*Muscle, joint, and soft-tissue pain; neuralgia.*

*Aspen Consumer, S.Afr.†.*
Paracetamol (p.76·2); chlormezanone (p.675·1).
*Pain and associated tension.*

*Siam Bheasach, Thai.*
Orphenadrine citrate (p.486·1); paracetamol (p.76·2).
*Musculoskeletal and joint pain; neuralgia.*

**Myoflex Ice** *Bayer, Canad.†.*
Menthol (p.1711·3).
*Pain.*

**Myoflex Ice Plus** *Bayer Consumer, Canad.*
Trolamine salicylate (p.95·3); menthol (p.1711·3).
*Muscle pain.*

**Myogard** *RPG, India.*
Nifedipine (p.966·2).
*Angina pectoris; hypertension.*

**Myogeloticum N** *Hanosan, Ger.*
Homoeopathic preparation.

**Myogit** *Pfleger, Ger.*
Diclofenac sodium (p.32·1).
*Inflammation; rheumatism.*

**Myolastan**
*Sanofi Synthelabo, Austria; Sanofi Synthelabo, Belg.; Sanofi Synthelabo, Fr.; Sanofi Synthelabo, Spain.*
Tetrazepam (p.724·1).
*Skeletal muscle spasm.*

**Myolax**
*Note. This name is used for preparations of different composition.*
*Shiwa, Thai.†.*
Tolperisone hydrochloride (p.1396·3).
*Parkinsonism; skeletal muscle spasm.*

*Siam Bheasach, Thai.*
Carisoprodol (p.1392·1).
*Skeletal muscle spasm.*

**Myolosyx** *Syxyl, Ger.*
Homoeopathic preparation.

**Myomethol** *Abic-Teva, Thai.*
Methocarbamol (p.1395·1).
*Cramps; skeletal muscle spasm.*

**Myonac** *M & H, Thai.*
Diclofenac diethylamine (p.32·1) or diclofenac sodium (p.32·1).
*Gout; inflammation; musculoskeletal, joint, and peri-articular disorders.*

**Myonal**
*Eisai, Jpn; Eisai, Malaysia; Eisai, Singapore; Eisai, Thai.*
Eperisone hydrochloride (p.1394·3).
*Myotonias; skeletal muscle spasm; spasticity.*

**Myonil** *Nycomed, Denm.*
Diltiazem hydrochloride (p.900·1).
*Angina pectoris; hypertension.*

**Myonit** *Troikaa, India.*
Glyceryl trinitrate (p.923·2).
*Angina pectoris; heart failure; hypertension and controlled hypotension during surgery.*

**Myopar** *Ranbaxy, Thai.†.*
Orphenadrine citrate (p.486·1); paracetamol (p.76·2).
*Musculoskeletal and joint pain; tension headache.*

**Myopax** *Orion, Denm.†.*
Atenolol (p.865·2).
*Angina pectoris; arrhythmias; hypertension; myocardial infarction.*

**Myophen** *Charoen, Thai.*
Carisoprodol (p.1392·1); phenylbutazone (p.83·2).
*Musculoskeletal, joint, and peri-articular disorders.*

**Myoplege** *Genevrier, Fr.*
Thiocolchicoside (p.1395·2).
*Skeletal muscle spasm.*

**Myoplegine** *Christiaens, Belg.*
Suxamethonium chloride (p.1406·2).
*Depolarising neuromuscular blocker.*

**Myoprin** *Desatnik, S.Afr.*
Aspirin (p.15·1).
*Fever; pain; thromboembolism prophylaxis.*

**Myoquin** *Fawns & McAllan, Austral.*
Quinine bisulfate (p.460·1).
*Malaria; nocturnal cramps.*

**Myoscain** *Sanochemia, Austria.*
Guaifenesin (p.1122·1).
*Coughs.*

**Myoscint** *Byk Gulden, Ital.†.*
Indium-111 imciromab pentetate (p.1523·3).
*Diagnosis of myocardial infarction.*

**Myosic** *M & H, Thai.*
Orphenadrine citrate (p.486·1); paracetamol (p.76·2).
*Musculoskeletal pain.*

**Myoson** *IPG, Ger.*
Pridinol mesilate (p.1395·2).
*Skeletal muscle spasm.*

**Myospasmal** *TAD, Ger.*
Tetrazepam (p.724·1).
*Skeletal muscle tension and spasm.*

**Myospaz** *Win-Medicare, India.*
Paracetamol (p.76·2); chlorzoxazone (p.1392·3).
*Muscle spasm; pain.*

**Myospaz Forte** *Win-Medicare, India.*
Diclofenac potassium (p.32·1); paracetamol (p.76·2); chlorzoxazone (p.1392·3).
*Muscle spasm; pain.*

**Myotenlis** *Pharmacia Upjohn, Ital.*
Suxamethonium chloride (p.1406·2).
*Depolarising neuromuscular blocker.*

**Myotonachol**
*Glenwood, Canad.; Glenwood, USA.*
Bethanechol chloride (p.1487·3).
*Gastro-oesophageal reflux; neurogenic bladder; urinary retention.*

**Myotonine** *Glenwood, UK.*
Bethanechol chloride (p.1487·3).
*Gastro-oesophageal reflux; urinary retention.*

**Myovek** *Faran, Gr.*
Mexiletine hydrochloride (p.958·1).
*Arrythmias.*

**Myoview**
*Amersham, Austral.; Amersham, Fr.; Nycomed, Ital.; Amersham, Spain; Nycomed Amersham, UK.*
Technetium-99m tetrofosmin (p.1525·2).
*Myocardial perfusion imaging.*

**Myovin** *Cadila Pharma, India.*
Glyceryl trinitrate (p.923·2).
*Angina pectoris.*

**Myoviton** *Therabel, Fr.†.*
Adenosine triphosphate, disodium salt (p.1648·1).
Formerly contained pyridoxine hydrochloride and adenosine triphosphate, disodium salt.
*Pain.*

**Myoxam**
*Menarini, Arg.; Menarini, Spain.*
Midecamycin acetate (p.231·3).
*Bacterial infections.*

**Myoxan** *TO-Chemicals, Thai.*
Tolperisone hydrochloride (p.1396·3).
*Parkinsonism; skeletal muscle spasm.*

**Mypaid** *Restan, S.Afr.*
Ibuprofen (p.45·3); paracetamol (p.76·2).
*Fever; pain.*

**Myphetane DC** *Morton Grove, USA†.*
Phenylpropanolamine hydrochloride (p.1127·3); codeine phosphate (p.27·1); brompheniramine maleate (p.426·1).
*Coughs and cold symptoms.*

**Myphetane DX** *Morton Grove, USA.*
Pseudoephedrine hydrochloride (p.1129·2); brompheniramine maleate (p.426·1); dextromethorphan hydrobromide (p.1117·3).
*Coughs and cold symptoms.*

**Myprodol** *Adcock Ingram, S.Afr.*
Ibuprofen (p.45·3); paracetamol (p.76·2); codeine phosphate (p.27·1).
*Inflammation; pain.*

**Myproflam** *Adcock Ingram, S.Afr.*
Ketoprofen (p.51·2).
*Musculoskeletal, joint, and peri-articular disorders.*

**Myra 300-E**
*Scherer, Hong Kong; Myra, Singapore.*
Vitamin E (p.1464·3).
*Vitamin E deficiency.*

**Myriacyl** *Alcon, Mex.*
Tropicamide (p.491·1).
*Production of mydriasis and cycloplegia.*

**Myrin**
*Wyeth, S.Afr.†; Wyeth-Ayerst, Thai.*
Ethambutol hydrochloride (p.211·3); isoniazid (p.222·2); rifampicin (p.250·2).
*Tuberculosis.*

**Myrin Plus** *Wyeth, S.Afr.*
Ethambutol hydrochloride (p.211·3); isoniazid (p.222·2); rifampicin (p.250·2); pyrazinamide (p.246·3).
*Tuberculosis.*

**Myrin-P** *Wyeth-Ayerst, Thai.*
Ethambutol hydrochloride (p.211·3); isoniazid (p.222·2); rifampicin (p.250·2); pyrazinamide (p.246·3).
*Tuberculosis.*

**Myristoll** *Eagle, Austral.†.*
Cetyl myristoleate.
*Dietary supplement.*

**Myrol** *Dorom, Ital.†.*
Dihydroergocryptine mesilate (p.1680·1).
*Dementia; hyperprolactinaemia; lactation inhibition; parkinsonism; vascular headache.*

**Myrrhinil-Intest** *Repha, Ger.*
Myrrh (p.1718·3); carbo coffeae (p.1765·3); chamomile (p.1669·3).
*Gastrointestinal disorders.*

**Myrtaven** *IBSA, Switz.*
Myrtillus (p.1718·3).
*Peripheral vascular disorders.*

**Myrtilen** *Synpharma, Austria.*
Myrtillus (p.1718·3); caraway (p.1667·2); rice starch (p.1449·1).
*Diarrhoea.*

**Myser** *Mitsubishi, Jpn.*
Difluprednate (p.1100·1).
*Skin disorders.*

**Mysial** *Douglas, Thai.†; TTN, Thai.†.*
Prazosin hydrochloride (p.985·1).
*Hypertension.*

**Myslee** *Fujisawa, Jpn.*
Zolpidem tartrate (p.728·3).
*Insomnia.*

**Mysocort** *Greater Pharma, Thai.*
Miconazole nitrate (p.405·3).
*Fungal and Gram-positive bacterial skin infections.*

**Mysoline**
*AstraZeneca, Arg.; AstraZeneca, Austral.; AstraZeneca, Austria; AstraZeneca, Belg.; AstraZeneca, Braz.; Draxis, Canad.; AstraZeneca, Chile; AstraZeneca, Denm.; AstraZeneca, Fin.; AstraZeneca, Fr.; Cona, Gr.; Zeneca, Hong Kong†; ICI, India; AstraZeneca, Irl.; SIT, Ital.; Zeneca, Mex.; AstraZeneca, Neth.†; AstraZeneca, Norw.; AstraZeneca, NZ†; Zeneca, Port.; Zeneca, S.Afr.; AstraZeneca, Singapore†; AstraZeneca, Spain; Astra, Swed.; AstraZeneca, Switz.; AstraZeneca, UK; Athena Neurosciences, USA.*
Primidone (p.376·3).
*Epilepsy; essential tremor.*

**Mysolone-N** *Greater Pharma, Thai.*
Prednisolone (p.1108·1); neomycin sulfate (p.235·1).
*Burns; skin disorders; wounds.*

**Mysoven** *Greater Pharma, Thai.*
Acetylcysteine (p.1112·3).
*Respiratory-tract disorders associated with increased or viscous mucus.*

**Mysteclin**
*Note. This name is used for preparations of different composition.*
*Bristol-Myers Squibb, Austral.†.*
Tetracycline hydrochloride (p.266·2).
*Bacterial infections.*

*Bristol-Myers Squibb, Austria; Bristol-Myers Squibb, Ger.*
Tetracycline (p.266·2); amphotericin B (p.391·2).
*Vaginal infections.*

**Mysteclin-V** *Bristol-Myers Squibb, Austral.†.*
Tetracycline (p.266·2); nystatin (p.406·3).
*Bacterial infections.*

**Mytancid** *Synco, Hong Kong.*
Aluminium hydroxide (p.1249·2); magnesium hydroxide (p.1272·2); dimethicone (p.1289·2).
*Flatulence; gastrointestinal hyperacidity.*

**Mytelase**
*Sanofi Synthelabo, Fr.; IFET (ΙΦΕΤ), Gr.; Sanofi Synthelabo, Swed.; Sanofi Winthrop, USA.*
Ambenonium chloride (p.1487·3).
*Myasthenia gravis.*

**Mytex** *Morton Grove, USA†.*
Phenylephrine hydrochloride (p.1126·3); phenylpropanolamine hydrochloride (p.1127·3); guaifenesin (p.1122·1).

**Mytic 810** *Piam, Ital.*
Medium-chain triglycerides (p.1440·3).
*Obesity.*

**Mytobrin** *Intramed, S.Afr.†.*
Tobramycin sulfate (p.271·3).
*Bacterial infections.*

**Mytrex** *Savage, USA†.*
Triamcinolone acetonide (p.1110·2); nystatin (p.406·3).
*Skin disorders.*

**Mytussin** *Morton Grove, USA†.*
Guaifenesin (p.1122·1).
*Coughs.*

**Mytussin AC** *Morton Grove, USA.*
Codeine phosphate (p.27·1); guaifenesin (p.1122·1).
*Coughs.*

**Mytussin CF** *Morton Grove, USA†.*
Guaifenesin (p.1122·1); phenylpropanolamine hydrochloride (p.1127·3); dextromethorphan hydrobromide (p.1117·3).

**Mytussin DAC** *Morton Grove, USA.*
Pseudoephedrine hydrochloride (p.1129·2); guaifenesin (p.1122·1); codeine phosphate (p.27·1).
*Coughs.*

**Mytussin DM** *Morton Grove, USA.*
Dextromethorphan hydrobromide (p.1117·3); guaifenesin (p.1122·1).
*Coughs.*

**Mytussin PE** *Morton Grove, USA.*
Guaifenesin (p.1122·1); pseudoephedrine hydrochloride (p.1129·2).

**My-Vitalife** *ME Pharmaceuticals, USA.*
Multivitamin and mineral preparation (p.1417·1).

**Myvlar** *Schering, Austria†.*
Gestodene (p.1556·1); ethinylestradiol (p.1553·2).
*Combined oral contraceptive.*

**Myxina** *Norma (Νορμα), Gr.*
Nimesulide (p.67·1).
*Inflammation; musculoskeletal disorders; pain.*

**Myxofat** *Fatol, Ger.*
Acetylcysteine (p.1112·3).
*Respiratory-tract disorders associated with increased or viscous mucus.*

**MZM** *Ciba Vision, USA.*
Methazolamide (p.953·1).

**M-Zole** *Alpharma, USA.*
Miconazole nitrate (p.405·3).
*Vulvovaginal candidiasis.*

**N32 Collutorio** *Esoform, Ital.†.*
Chlorhexidine gluconate (p.1173·2).
*Oral disinfection.*

**N D Clear** *Seatrace, USA.*
Pseudoephedrine hydrochloride (p.1129·2); chlorphenamine maleate (p.427·3).
*Upper respiratory-tract symptoms.*

**Naabak**
*Allergan, Braz.; Thea, Fr.; Pharmacia, Singapore.*
Sodium isospaglumate (p.1702·2).
*Allergic eye disorders.*

**Naaprep**
*GlaxoSmithKline Consumer, Belg.; SmithKline Beecham Consumer, Switz.*
Sodium chloride (p.1233·3).
*Cleansing of eyelids; nasal irrigation; rinsing solution for contact lenses.*

**Naaxia**
*Allergan, Braz.; Thea, Fr.; Novartis, Spain.*
Sodium isospaglumate (p.1702·2).
*Allergic conjunctivitis.*

*Novartis, Gr.; Restan, S.Afr.*
Spaglumic acid; isospaglumic acid (p.1702·2).
*Allergic conjunctivitis.*

*Thea, Hong Kong.*
Isospaglumic acid (p.1702·2).
*Allergic conjunctivitis.*

*Ciba Vision, Ital.; Ciba Vision, Port.*
Sodium spaglumate.
*Allergic conjunctivitis.*

*Novartis Ophthalmics, Switz.*
Sodium isospaglumate (p.1702·2); spaglumate decahydrate.
*Allergic keratoconjunctivitis.*

**Nabicortin** *Help, Gr.*
Lovastatin (p.949·1).
*Primary hypercholesterolaemia.*

**Nabi-HB** *Nabi, USA.*
A hepatitis B immunoglobulin (p.1617·2).
*Passive immunisation.*

**Nabone** *TO-Chemicals, Thai.*
Nabumetone (p.63·3).
*Osteoarthritis; rheumatoid arthritis.*

**Nabonet** *M & H, Thai.*
Nabumetone (p.63·3).
*Osteoarthritis; rheumatoid arthritis.*

**Nabuco** *Trima, Israel.*
Nabumetone (p.63·3).
*Osteoarthritis; rheumatoid arthritis.*

**Nabucox** *Mayoly-Spindler, Fr.*
Nabumetone (p.63·3).
*Musculoskeletal and joint disorders.*

**Nabuser** *Geymonat, Ital.*
Nabumetone (p.63·3).
*Musculoskeletal, joint, and peri-articular disorders.*

**Nabutil** *Oberlin, Fr.*
Loperamide hydrochloride (p.1271·1).
*Diarrhoea.*

**Nabuton** *Medichrom, Gr.*
Nabumetone (p.63·3).
*Inflammation; musculoskeletal and joint disorders; pain.*

**Nac**
*Note. A similar name is used for preparations of different composition (see below).*
*Klonal, Arg.*
Piroxicam (p.84·2).
*Inflammation; pain.*

*Systopic, India.*
Diclofenac sodium (p.32·1).
*Gout; musculoskeletal and joint disorders.*

**NAC**
*Note. A similar name is used for preparations of different composition (see above).*
*1A, Ger.; ABZ, Ger.; Aliud, Ger.; CT, Ger.; Hemopharm, Ger.; Ratiopharm, Ger.; Stada, Ger.; Asta Medica, Thai.; Temmler, Thai.*
Acetylcysteine (p.1112·3).
*Paracetamol poisoning; respiratory-tract disorders associated with increased or viscous mucus.*

**Nacgel** *Systopic, India.*
Diclofenac diethylamine (p.32·1).
*Soft-tissue disorders.*

**Nacha** *Lineafarm, Spain.*
A nonoxinol (p.1413·2).
*Contraceptive.*

**Naclof**
*Novartis, Neth.; Restan, S.Afr.†; Ciba Vision, Thai.*
Diclofenac sodium (p.32·1).
*Eye inflammation; inhibition of intra-operative miosis; prevention of cystoid macular oedema following eye surgery.*

**Naclon** *Teofarma, Ital.†.*
Sodium hypochlorite (p.1192·1).
*Disinfection of skin, wounds, external genitalia, and drinking water.*

**Nacom** *Du Pont, Ger.†.*
Carbidopa (p.1204·3); levodopa (p.1205·2).
*Parkinsonism.*

**Nacor** *Merck, Spain.*
Enalapril maleate (p.909·2).
*Heart failure; hypertension.*

**Nacozil** *TO-Chemicals, Thai.*
Isoconazole nitrate (p.401·3).
*Fungal skin infections.*

**Nacro** *Investigaciones Filosoficas y Cientificas, Mex.†.*
Nicotinamide (p.1441·2).

**Nactol** *Offenbach, Mex.*
Benzonatate (p.1115·3).
*Coughs.*

**Nad** *Medical, Spain.*
Nadide (p.1719·1).
*Vertigo.*

**Nadamen**
*Medochemie, Hong Kong; Medochemie, Malaysia; Medochemie, Singapore†; Medochemie, Thai.*
Tenoxicam (p.93·1).
*Gout; inflammation; musculoskeletal, joint, peri-articular, and soft-tissue disorders.*

**Nadem** *Armstrong, Arg.*
Aesculus (p.1648·2).
*Haemorrhoids; venous insufficiency.*

**Nadem Forte** *Armstrong, Arg.*
Bamethan succinate (p.866·3); aesculus (p.1648·2).
*Haemorrhoids; venous insufficiency.*

**Nadetos** *Raymos, Arg.*
Oxeladin (p.1126·1).
*Coughs.*

**Nadex**
*Zyma, Belg.†; Novartis, Switz.†.*
Pirisudanol maleate (p.1732·3).
*Asthenia; depression; mental function impairment.*

**Nadib** *Diba, Mex.*
Glibenclamide (p.331·2).
*Diabetes mellitus.*

**Nadinola** *Nadinola, Canad.*
Hydroquinone (p.1148·1).

**Nadione** *DMG, Ital.*
Bioflavonoids; vitamin C; phytomenadione (p.1417·1).
*Nutritional supplement.*

**Nadipinia** *Scherer, Hong Kong.*
Nifedipine (p.966·2).
*Heart failure; hypertension.*

**Naditone** *Kleva, Gr.*
Nabumetone (p.63·3).
*Inflammation; musculoskeletal and joint disorders; pain.*

**Nadiwil** *Willmar, Mex.†.*
Nalidixic acid (p.234·1).

**Nadixa**
*Galderma, Braz.†; Galderma, Mex.*
Nadifloxacin (p.233·3).
*Bacterial infections.*

**Nadona** *Medea, Spain.*
Hydroquinone (p.1148·1).
*Skin hyperpigmentation.*

**Nadopen-V** *Lioh, Canad.*
Phenoxymethylpenicillin potassium (p.242·1).
*Bacterial infections.*

**Nadostine**
*Nadeau, Canad.; Rougier, Hong Kong†.*
Nystatin (p.406·3).
*Candidiasis.*

**Nadrifor** *Kleva, Gr.*
Buspirone hydrochloride (p.672·2).
*Generalised anxiety.*

**Naetene** *Novartis, Braz.*
Multivitamin and mineral preparation (p.1417·1).

**Naf Buches** *Naf, Arg.*
Sodium fluoride (p.1444·3).
*Dental caries prophylaxis.*

**Nafacil** *Tecnofarma, Mex.*
Cefalexin (p.168·1).
*Bacterial infections.*

**Nafasol** *Aspen, S.Afr.*
Naproxen (p.65·1).
*Dysmenorrhoea; gout; musculoskeletal and joint disorders.*

**Nafazair** *Bausch & Lomb, USA.*
Naphazoline hydrochloride (p.1124·3).
*Minor eye irritation.*

**Nafazair A** *Bausch & Lomb, USA.*
Naphazoline hydrochloride (p.1124·3); pheniramine maleate (p.438·3).
*Eye irritation.*

**Nafcon A** *Alcon, Ital.*
Naphazoline hydrochloride (p.1124·3); pheniramine maleate (p.438·3).
*Conjunctivitis.*

**Naferon** *Sclavo, Ital.†.*
Interferon beta (p.645·3).
*Malignant neoplasms; viral infections.*

**Naflapen** *Collins, Mex.*
Naproxen (p.65·1).
*Fever; inflammation; pain.*

**Naflex** *Seven Stars, Thai.*
Nabumetone (p.63·3).
*Osteoarthritis; rheumatoid arthritis.*

**Nafloxin** *Cooper (Κοπερ), Gr.*
Ciprofloxacin lactate (p.188·3).
*Bacterial infections.*

**Nafluor** *Naf, Arg.*
Sodium fluoride (p.1444·3).
*Dental caries prophylaxis.*

**Nafluryl** *Atlantis, Mex.*
Flunarizine (p.434·2).
*Migraine; peripheral vascular disorders.*

**Nafluvent** *Fada, Arg.*
Fentanyl (p.40·1).
*Pain.*

**Nafordyl** *Kleva, Gr.*
Lisinopril (p.946·3).
*Heart failure; hypertension; myocardial infarction.*

**NaFril** *Merckle, Ger.*
Sodium fluoride (p.1444·3).
*Osteoporosis.*

**Nafrine** *Schering, Canad.*
Oxymetazoline hydrochloride (p.1126·1).

**Naftazolina** *Bruschettini, Ital.*
Naphazoline hydrochloride (p.1124·3).
*Eye congestion; eye irritation.*

**Nafti** *CT, Ger.; Alpharma-Isis, Ger.; Ratiopharm, Ger.*
Naftidrofuryl oxalate (p.964·1).
*Peripheral vascular disorders.*

**Naftilong** *Hexal, Ger.*
Naftidrofuryl oxalate (p.964·1).
*Peripheral vascular disorders.*

**Naftilux** *Therabel, Fr.*
Naftidrofuryl oxalate (p.964·1).
*Mental function impairment in the elderly; peripheral vascular and cerebrovascular disorders.*

**Naftin**
*Allergan, Canad.; Allergan, USA; Merz, USA.*
Naftifine hydrochloride (p.406·2).
*Fungal skin infections.*

**Naftodril** *Arcana, Austria.*
Naftidrofuryl oxalate (p.964·1).
*Peripheral and cerebral vascular disorders.*

**Nagel Batrafen** *Aventis, Ger.*
Ciclopirox (p.396·1).
*Fungal nail infections.*

**Nagun** *Dosa, Arg.*
Doxorubicin (p.547·3).
*Malignant neoplasms.*

**Nahora** *Hearst, Braz.†.*
Procaine hydrochloride (p.1383·2); phenol (p.1188·1).
*Local anaesthesia.*

**Nail Nutrition** *Cantassium Co., UK.*
Multivitamins; minerals; amino acids (p.1417·1).

**4 Nails** *Marlyn, USA.*
Multivitamin, mineral, and amino-acid preparation (p.1417·1).

**NailVit** *Pharmadass, UK.*
Multivitamin, mineral, and amino-acid preparation (p.1417·1).

**Nalador**
*Schering, Austria; Schering, Fin.; Schering, Fr.; Schering, Ger.; Schering, Hong Kong; Schering, Ital.; Schering, Neth.; Schering, Port.; Schering, Singapore†; Schering, Switz.; Schering, Thai.*
Sulprostone (p.1520·3).
*Labour induction in case of fetal death; postpartum haemorrhage; termination of pregnancy.*

**Nalapres** *Mediolanum, Ital.*
Lisinopril (p.946·3); hydrochlorothiazide (p.933·2).
*Hypertension.*

**Nalapril** *Klonal, Arg.*
Enalapril (p.909·2).
*Hypertension.*

**Nalaprix** *Royton, Braz.*
Enalapril maleate (p.909·2).
*Hypertension.*

**Nalbu** *20th Century, Mex.†.*
Nalbuphine (p.64·3).

**Nalcrom**
*Aventis, Canad.; Aventis, Irl.; Fisons, Israel†; Aventis, Ital.; Aventis, Neth.; Aventis, NZ; Rhone-Poulenc Rorer, S.Afr.†; Rhone-Poulenc Rorer, Spain†; Aventis, Switz.; Pantheon, UK.*
Sodium cromoglicate (p.795·3).
*Food allergies; inflammatory bowel disease.*

**Nalcron** *Aventis, Fr.*
Sodium cromoglicate (p.795·3).
*Food hypersensitivity.*

**Nalcryn** *Cryopharma, Mex.*
Nalbuphine (p.64·3).
*Pain.*

**Naldecol NF** *Bristol-Myers Squibb, Chile.*
*Oral drops; syrup:* Pseudoephedrine hydrochloride (p.1129·2); paracetamol (p.76·2).
*Tablets:* Pseudoephedrine hydrochloride (p.1129·2); chlorphenamine maleate (p.427·3); paracetamol (p.76·2).
*Cold symptoms.*

**Naldecol-D** *Bristol-Myers Squibb, Chile.*
Pseudoephedrine sulfate (p.1129·2); chlorphenamine maleate (p.427·3).

**Naldecon**
*Note. This name is used for preparations of different composition.*
*Bristol-Myers Squibb, Braz.*
*Oral solution:* Paracetamol (p.76·2); phenylephrine hydrochloride (p.1126·3); carbinoxamine maleate (p.426·3).
*Tablets:* Yellow tablets, paracetamol (p.76·2); phenylephrine hydrochloride (p.1126·3); orange tablets, paracetamol; carbinoxamine maleate (p.426·3).

*Apothecon, USA†.*
Phenylpropanolamine hydrochloride (p.1127·3); phenylephrine hydrochloride (p.1126·3); phenyltoloxamine citrate (p.439·1); chlorphenamine maleate (p.427·3).
*Nasal congestion.*

**Naldecon CX** *Apothecon, USA†.*
Phenylpropanolamine hydrochloride (p.1127·3); guaifenesin (p.1122·1); codeine phosphate (p.27·1).
*Coughs and cold symptoms.*

**Naldecon DX** *Apothecon, USA†.*
Phenylpropanolamine hydrochloride (p.1127·3); guaifenesin (p.1122·1); dextromethorphan hydrobromide (p.1117·3).
*Coughs.*

**Naldecon EX** *Apothecon, USA†.*
Phenylpropanolamine hydrochloride (p.1127·3); guaifenesin (p.1122·1).
*Coughs and cold symptoms.*

**Naldecon Pediatrico** *Bristol-Myers Squibb, Braz.*
Paracetamol (p.76·2); carbinoxamine maleate (p.426·3).

**Naldecon Senior DX** *Apothecon, USA†.*
Guaifenesin (p.1122·1); dextromethorphan hydrobromide (p.1117·3).
*Coughs.*

**Naldecon Senior EX** *Apothecon, USA†.*
Guaifenesin (p.1122·1).
*Coughs and cold symptoms.*

**Naldelate DX Adult** *Barre-National, USA†.*
Phenylpropanolamine hydrochloride (p.1127·3); dextromethorphan hydrobromide (p.1117·3); guaifenesin (p.1122·1).
*Coughs.*

**Nalerona** *Silesia, Chile.*
Naltrexone hydrochloride (p.1046·1).
*Alcohol withdrawal syndrome; opioid withdrawal.*

**Nalex** *Blansett, USA.*
Pseudoephedrine hydrochloride (p.1129·2); guaifenesin (p.1122·1).

**Nalex DH** *Blansett, USA.*
Hydrocodone tartrate (p.45·1); phenylephrine hydrochloride (p.1126·3).

**Nalex-A** *Blansett, USA.*
Chlorphenamine maleate (p.427·3); phenyltoloxamine citrate (p.439·1); phenylephrine hydrochloride (p.1126·3).

**Nalfan** *Novaquimica, Braz.†.*
Vitamin A (p.1451·2).
*Vitamin A deficiency.*

**Nalfon**
*Lilly, Austria†; Lilly, Canad.; Lilly, Denm.; Lilly, Mex.; Lilly, Spain†; Dista, USA.*
Fenoprofen calcium (p.39·2).
*Fever; gout; musculoskeletal and joint disorders; pain.*

**Nalgesic**
*Note. This name is used for preparations of different composition.*
*Hexo-Medinova, Arg.*
Piroxicam (p.84·2).
*Dysmenorrhoea; gout; musculoskeletal and joint disorders.*

*Lilly, Fr.†.*
Fenoprofen calcium (p.39·2).
*Pain.*

**Nalgest** Major, USA†.
Phenylpropanolamine hydrochloride (p.1127·3); phenylephrine hydrochloride (p.1126·3); chlorphenamine maleate (p.427·3); phenyltoloxamine citrate (p.439·1).
*Upper respiratory-tract symptoms.*

**Nalidin** TAD, Ger.
Tilidine hydrochloride (p.94·1).
Naloxone hydrochloride (p.1044·3) is included in this preparation to discourage abuse.
*Pain.*

**Nalidix** Lacefa, Arg.
Nalidixic acid (p.234·1).
*Urinary-tract infections.*

**Nalidixan** Bioquimico, Mex.†.
Nalidixic acid (p.234·1).

**Nalidixin** NCSN, Ital.
Nalidixic acid (p.234·1).
*Gram-negative genito-urinary tract infections.*

**Nalidoid** Valdecasas, Mex.†.
Nalidixic acid (p.234·1).

**Naligram** Geymonat, Ital.
Nalidixic acid (p.234·1).
*Gram-negative genito-urinary tract infections.*

**Naline** Pharmaland, Thai.
Co-dergocrine mesilate (p.1674·1).
*Cerebral and peripheral vascular disorders.*

**Nalion** Elan, Spain.
Norfloxacin (p.238·3).
*Bacterial infections.*

**Nalissina** Aventis, Ital.†.
Nalidixic acid (p.234·1).
*Gram-negative urinary-tract infections.*

**Nalix** Reuffer, Mex.†.
Nalidixic acid (p.234·1).

**Nalixone** Sons, Mex.
Nalidixic acid (p.234·1); phenazopyridine hydrochloride (p.83·1).
*Urinary-tract infections and pain.*

**Nallpen** SmithKline Beecham, USA†.
Nafcillin sodium (p.233·3).
*Bacterial infections.*

**Nalone** SERB, Fr.
Naloxone hydrochloride (p.1044·3).
*Diagnosis of opioid dependence; diagnosis of toxic coma; opioid overdosage; opioid-induced respiratory depression.*

**Nalopril** Siam Bheasach, Thai.
Enalapril maleate (p.909·2).
*Heart failure; hypertension.*

**Nalorex**
Schering-Plough, Fr.; Vianex (Βιανέξ), Gr.; Du Pont, Irl.; Bristol-Myers Squibb, Ital.; Vitoria, Port.; Bristol-Myers Squibb, UK.
Naltrexone hydrochloride (p.1046·1).
*Alcohol withdrawal syndrome; opioid withdrawal.*

**Nalox** Omega, Arg.
Metronidazole (p.607·2).
*Bacterial infections; trichomoniasis.*

**Naltrox** Richmond, Arg.
Nalbuphine (p.64·3).
*Pain.*

**Naluril** Cazi, Braz.
Nalidixic acid (p.234·1).
*Bacterial infections.*

**Nalvir** Richmond, Arg.
Nelfinavir (p.650·1).
*HIV infection.*

**Namenda** Forest Laboratories, USA.
Memantine hydrochloride (p.1711·2).
*Alzheimer's disease.*

**Nametone** Pharmasant, Thai.
Nabumetone (p.63·3).
*Osteoarthritis; rheumatoid arthritis.*

**Namic**
Atlantic, Malaysia; Atlantic, Thai.
Mefenamic acid (p.55·2).
*Fever; pain.*

**Namifen** Novag, Mex.
Mefenamic acid (p.55·2).
*Pain.*

**Namir** Duncan, Arg.
Bromhexine (p.1115·3).
*Respiratory-tract congestion.*

**Nan** Nestle, Braz.
A range of infant feeds (p.1417·1).

**Nan AR**
Nestle, Arg.; Nestle, Mex.
Infant feed (p.1417·1).
*Gastro-oesophageal reflux.*

**Nan HA**
Nestle, Arg.; Nestle, Hong Kong; Nestle, Malaysia; Nestle, Mex.; Nestle, Port.; Nestle, Singapore; Nestle, Thai.
Infant feed (p.1417·1).
*Cow's milk allergy.*

**Nan HA/AR** Nestle, Port.
Infant feed (p.1417·1).
*Gastro-oesophageal reflux.*

**Nan sin Lactosa**
Nestle, Arg.; Nestle, Mex.
Infant feed (p.1417·1).
*Gastro-enteritis; lactose intolerance.*

**Nan Soya**
Nestle, Arg.; Nestle, Mex.
Infant feed (p.1417·1).
*Cow's milk allergy; lactose intolerance.*

**Nanafed** PD, Thai.
Triprolidine hydrochloride (p.442·3); pseudoephedrine hydrochloride (p.1129·2).
*Coughs; nasal congestion.*

**Nanalan** Merck, Austria.
Bisoprolol fumarate (p.875·1).
*Angina pectoris; hypertension.*

**Nanalan Plus** Merck, Austria.
Bisoprolol fumarate (p.875·1); hydrochlorothiazide (p.933·2).
*Hypertension.*

**Nanbacine** Rhone-Poulenc Rorer, Fr.†.
Xibornol (p.277·3).
*Respiratory-tract disorders.*

**Nandain** Ciba Vision, Port.
Nandrolone sodium sulfate (p.1561·3).
*Corneal disorders.*

**Nandrol**
Allergan-Frumtost, Braz.†.
Nandrolone sulfate (p.1561·3).
*Eye disorders.*

Novartis, Spain†.
Nandrolone sodium sulfate (p.1561·3).
*Corneal transplants; eye disorders.*

**Nandrosande** Sanderson, Chile.
Nandrolone (p.1561·2).
*Anabolic.*

**Nani Pre Dental** Alter, Spain.
Benzocaine (p.1370·3).
Formerly contained saffron, guaiazulene, lidocaine hydrochloride, myrrh, and menthol.
*Toothache.*

**Nanocoll** Nycomed Amersham, UK.
Technetium-99m (p.1525·2) labelled albumin colloid.
*Imaging of bone marrow and lymphatic system; scanning for inflammation.*

**Nanotiv**
Pharmacia Upjohn, Norw.†; Biovitrum, Swed.
A factor IX preparation (p.752·2).
*Haemorrhagic disorders.*

**Nansius** Almirall, Spain†.
Dipotassium clorazepate (p.685·1).
*Anxiety; insomnia.*

**Naox** Eurofarma, Braz.
Oxytocin (p.1336·1).

**Napa** Beximco, Singapore.
Paracetamol (p.76·2).
*Fever; pain.*

**Napacod** Propan, S.Afr.
Paracetamol (p.76·2); codeine phosphate (p.27·1).
*Fever; pain.*

**Napamide**
Douglas, Austral.; Douglas, Hong Kong†; Douglas, NZ†; Douglas, Singapore; Douglas, Thai.; TTN, Thai.
Indapamide (p.938·2).
*Hypertension.*

**Napamol** Propan, S.Afr.
Paracetamol (p.76·2).
*Fever; pain.*

**Napan**
DHA, Hong Kong; DHA, Malaysia.
Mefenamic acid (p.55·2).
*Fever; musculoskeletal, joint, and soft-tissue disorders; pain.*

**Napflam** Quatromed, S.Afr.
Naproxen (p.65·1).
*Dysmenorrhoea; gout; musculoskeletal and joint disorders.*

**Napha Forte** Medical Ophthalmics, USA.
Naphazoline hydrochloride (p.1124·3).

**Naphacel** Sophia, Mex.
Naphazoline hydrochloride (p.1124·3); hypromellose (p.1579·3).
*Eye irritation.*

**Naphasal** Sam-On, Israel.
Naphazoline hydrochloride (p.1124·3).
*Nasal congestion; rhinitis; sinusitis.*

**Naphazoline Plus** Parmed, USA.
Naphazoline hydrochloride (p.1124·3); pheniramine maleate (p.438·3).
*Minor eye irritation.*

**Naphcon**
Alcon, Austral.; Alcon, NZ; Alcon, Thai.; Alcon, USA.
Naphazoline hydrochloride (p.1124·3).
*Eye irritation.*

**Naphcon Forte**
Alcon, Canad.; Alcon, Israel.
Naphazoline hydrochloride (p.1124·3).
*Eye irritation; nasal congestion.*

**Naphcon-A**
Alcon, Austral.; Alcon, Canad.; Alcon, Chile; Alcon, Hong Kong; Alcon, Malaysia; Alcon, NZ†; Alcon, Singapore; Alcon, Thai.; Alcon, USA.
Naphazoline hydrochloride (p.1124·3); pheniramine maleate (p.438·3).
*Allergic or inflammatory eye disorders.*

**Naphensyl** Propan, S.Afr.
Phenylephrine hydrochloride (p.1126·3).
*Respiratory-tract congestion.*

**Naphoptic-A** Optopics, USA.
Naphazoline hydrochloride (p.1124·3); pheniramine maleate (p.438·3).
*Eye irritation.*

**Naphtears** Alcon, Chile.
Naphazoline hydrochloride (p.1124·3); dextran 70 (p.746·2).
*Eye disorders.*

**Napilene** Chinta, Thai.
Benzalkonium chloride (p.1168·3); cetrimide (p.1172·1).
*Minor burns and wounds; napkin rash.*

**Napiro** Brasmedica, Braz.†.
Chlorphenamine (p.428·1); vitamin C (p.1460·2); guaifenesin (p.1122·1); dipyrone (p.35·3); cineole (p.1672·1); terpineol (p.1752·2); chlorophyll (p.1057·1).
*Cold and influenza symptoms.*

**Naplin** Pacific, NZ.
Indapamide (p.938·2).
*Hypertension.*

**Napmel** Clonmel, Irl.
Naproxen (p.65·1).
*Dysmenorrhoea; gout; musculoskeletal and joint disorders.*

**Nappy Rash Powder** Sigma, Austral.†.
Chlorphenesin (p.396·1).
*Chafing; nappy rash; prickly heat.*

**Nappy Rash Relief Cream** Brauer, Austral.†.
Calendula (p.1665·2); clematis recta; hypericum (p.299·1); chamomile (p.1669·3); mezereum.
*Nappy rash.*

**Nappy-Hippo** Sriprasit, Thai.
Zinc oxide (p.1163·2).
*Nappy rash.*

**Nappy-Mate** Ethicare, Austral.†.
Aluminium chlorohydrate (p.1142·1); zinc oxide (p.1163·2); benzoin tincture (p.1751·1); silicone (p.1482·1).
*Nappy rash.*

**Napratec** Pharmacia, UK.
Naproxen (p.65·1).
Misoprostol (p.1519·2) is included in this preparation in an attempt to limit adverse effects on the gastrointestinal mucosa.
*Ankylosing spondylitis; osteoarthritis; rheumatoid arthritis.*

**Napreben** Fulton, Ital.
Naproxen betainate sodium (p.65·3).
*Musculoskeletal, joint, peri-articular, and soft-tissue disorders.*

**Naprel** Brunel, S.Afr.
Naproxen (p.65·1).
*Dysmenorrhoea; gout; musculoskeletal and joint disorders.*

**Naprelan** Wyeth-Ayerst, USA.
Naproxen sodium (p.65·1).
*Gout; musculoskeletal, joint, and peri-articular disorders; pain.*

**Napren** Nycomed, Norw.; AFI, Norw.
Naproxen (p.65·1).
*Gout; musculoskeletal and joint disorders; pain.*

**Naprex**
Note. This name is used for preparations of different composition.
Pinewood, Irl.
Naproxen (p.65·1).
*Dysmenorrhoea; gout; musculoskeletal and joint disorders.*

Curex, Israel†.
Naproxen sodium (p.65·1).
*Gout; musculoskeletal and joint disorders; pain.*

Pediatrica, Malaysia; Pediatrica, Singapore.
Paracetamol (p.76·2).
*Fever; pain.*

**Naprilene**
Sigma-Tau, Ital.; Sigma-Tau, Spain.
Enalapril maleate (p.909·2).
*Angina pectoris; heart failure; hypertension.*

**Naprina** Pisa, Mex.†.
Noradrenaline (p.974·3).

**Naprius** Aesculapius, Ital.
Naproxen (p.65·1).
*Fever; inflammation; musculoskeletal, joint, peri-articular, and soft-tissue disorders; pain.*

**Naprix** Libbs, Braz.
Ramipril (p.994·1).
*Heart failure; hypertension; myocardial infarction; primary prophylaxis of atherosclerotic complications.*

**Naprix D** Libbs, Braz.
Ramipril (p.994·1); hydrochlorothiazide (p.933·2).
*Hypertension.*

**Naprizide** Taro, Israel.
Enalapril maleate (p.909·2); hydrochlorothiazide (p.933·2).
*Hypertension.*

**Naprobene** Ratiopharm, Austria.
Naproxen (p.65·1).
*Gout; inflammation; musculoskeletal and joint disorders; pain.*

**Naprocet** Boniscontro & Gazzone, Ital.
Naproxen cetrimonium (p.65·3).
*Mouth and throat disorders.*

**Naprocoat** Roche, Neth.
Naproxen (p.65·1).
*Musculoskeletal and joint disorders.*

**Naprodil** Diba, Mex.
Naproxen (p.65·1) or naproxen sodium (p.65·1).
*Inflammation; musculoskeletal, joint, and peri-articular disorders; pain.*

**Naprodol** Upsamedica, Ital.†.
Naproxen sodium (p.65·1).
*Pain.*

**Napro-Dorsch** Orion, Ger.†.
Naproxen (p.65·1).
*Inflammation; pain.*

**Naprofidex** Fidex, Arg.
Naproxen (p.65·1).
*Inflammation; pain.*

**Naprogen** Klonal, Arg.
Naproxen (p.65·1).
*Fever; pain.*

**Naprogesic**
Roche Consumer, Austral.; Roche, Chile; Roche, NZ.
Naproxen sodium (p.65·1).
*Inflammation; musculoskeletal and joint disorders; pain.*

**Naprokes** Inexfa, Spain†.
Naproxen (p.65·1).
*Fever; gout; musculoskeletal and joint disorders; pain.*

**Naprometin** Roche, Fin.
Naproxen (p.65·1).
*Fever; gout; inflammation; musculoskeletal and joint disorders; pain.*

**Napromex** Ratiopharm, Fin.
Naproxen (p.65·1).
*Gout; inflammation; musculoskeletal and joint disorders; pain.*

**Napronet** Nettopharma, Denm.†.
Naproxen (p.65·1).
*Musculoskeletal and joint disorders; pain.*

**Naprontag** Pharmacia, Arg.
Naproxen (p.65·1).
*Fever; gout; inflammation; musculoskeletal, joint, and peri-articular disorders; pain.*

**Naprontag Flex** Pharmacia, Arg.
Naproxen (p.65·1); carisoprodol (p.1392·1).
*Inflammation; musculoskeletal spasm.*

**Naprorex**
Aegis, Hong Kong.
Naproxen (p.65·1).
*Gout; musculoskeletal and joint disorders; pain.*

Lampugnani, Ital.
Naproxen sodium (p.65·1).
*Inflammation; musculoskeletal and joint disorders; pain.*

**Naproscript** Ranbaxy, S.Afr.
Naproxen (p.65·1).
*Dysmenorrhoea; gout; musculoskeletal and joint disorders.*

**Naprosian** Asian Pharm, Thai.
Naproxen (p.65·1).
*Musculoskeletal and joint disorders.*

**Naproso** M & H, Thai.†.
Naproxen sodium (p.65·1).
*Gout; musculoskeletal, joint, and peri-articular disorders; pain.*

**Naprosyn**
Roche, Austral.; Aventis, Braz.†; Roche, Canad.; Roche, Denm.; Roche, Fin.; Minerva (Μινέρβα), Gr.; Roche, Hong Kong; RPG, India; Roche, Irl.; Recordati, Ital.; Roche, Norw.; Roche, NZ; Roche, Port.; Roche, S.Afr.; Roche, Singapore†; Roche, Spain; Roche, Swed.; Roche, Switz.; Roche, Thai.; Roche, UK; Roche, USA.
Naproxen (p.65·1) or naproxen sodium (p.65·1).
*Fever; gout; musculoskeletal, joint, peri-articular, and soft-tissue disorders; pain.*

**Naprosyne**
Roche, Belg.; Grunenthal, Fr.; Roche, Neth.†.
Naproxen (p.65·1).
*Fever; gout; inflammation; musculoskeletal and joint disorders; pain.*

**Naproval** Reig Jofre, Spain.
Naproxen (p.65·1).
*Fever; gout; musculoskeletal and joint disorders; pain.*

**Naprovite** Roche, Neth.
Naproxen sodium (p.65·1).
*Fever; gout; inflammation; musculoskeletal and joint disorders; pain.*

**Naprox** Teuto, Braz.
Naproxen (p.65·1).
*Inflammation; pain.*

**Naproxi** Gerard, Israel.
Naproxen (p.65·1).
*Musculoskeletal and joint disorders; pain.*

**Naprux** Andromaco, Arg.
Naproxen (p.65·1) or naproxen sodium (p.65·1).
*Fever; inflammation; musculoskeletal and joint disorders; pain.*

**Napsen** Sriprasit, Thai.
Naproxen (p.65·1).
*Gout; musculoskeletal, joint, and soft-tissue disorders.*

**Napxen**
Merck, Hong Kong; Berlin Pharm, Thai.
Naproxen (p.65·1).
*Gout; musculoskeletal and joint disorders.*

**Naqua**
Note. This name is used for preparations of different composition.
Bial, Port.
Furosemide (p.919·3).
*Forced diuresis; nephrotic syndrome; oedema; renal failure.*

Schering, USA.
Trichlormethiazide (p.1017·2).
*Hypertension; oedema.*

**Naquinto** Makros, Braz.†.
Sodium dibunate (p.1130·2); homatropine (p.483·2); bromoform (p.1663·1).
*Coughs.*

**Naragran** GlaxoSmithKline, Denm.
Naratriptan hydrochloride (p.470·1).
*Migraine.*

**Naramig**
*GlaxoSmithKline, Arg.; GlaxoSmithKline, Austral.; GlaxoSmithKline, Austria; GlaxoSmithKline, Belg.; GlaxoSmithKline, Braz.; GlaxoSmithKline, Chile; GlaxoSmithKline, Fin.; GlaxoSmithKline, Fr.; GlaxoSmithKline, Ger.; Schwarz, Ger.; Glaxo Wellcome, Gr.; GlaxoSmithKline, Israel; Glaxo Wellcome, Mex.; GlaxoSmithKline, Neth.; GlaxoSmithKline, Norw.; Glaxo Wellcome, Port.; GlaxoSmithKline, S.Afr.; GlaxoSmithKline, Singapore; GlaxoSmithKline, Spain; GlaxoSmithKline, Swed.; GlaxoSmithKline, Switz.; GlaxoSmithKline, Thai.; GlaxoSmithKline, UK.*
Naratriptan hydrochloride (p.470·1).
*Migraine.*

**Naranocor** *Pfluger, Ger.†.*
Crataegus (p.1677·1).
*Arrhythmias; heart failure.*

**Naranocut H** *Pfluger, Ger.*
Homoeopathic preparation.

**Naranofem** *Pfluger, Ger.*
Homoeopathic preparation.

**Naranopect P** *Pfluger, Ger.*
Hedera helix.
*Respiratory-tract disorders.*

**Naranotox** *Pfluger, Ger.*
Homoeopathic preparation.

**Naranotox Plus** *Pfluger, Ger.*
Homoeopathic preparation.

**Narapril** *Julphar, UAE.*
Enalapril maleate (p.909·2).
*Heart failure; hypertension.*

**Narcan**
*Boots Healthcare, Austral.; Bristol-Myers Squibb, Belg.; Cristalia, Braz.; Du Pont, Canad.; SERB, Fr.; Vianex (Βιανέξ), Gr.; Du Pont, Hong Kong; Boots, Hong Kong; Du Pont, Irl.; Du Pont, Israel; Crinos, Ital.; Bristol-Myers Squibb, Malaysia; Boots Healthcare, NZ; Vitoria, Port.; Sanofi Synthelabo, S.Afr.; Bristol-Myers Squibb, Singapore; Du Pont, Switz.; Boots, Thai.; Bristol-Myers Squibb, Thai.; Bristol-Myers Squibb, UK; Endo, USA.*
Naloxone hydrochloride (p.1044·3).
*Opioid overdosage; reversal of opioid depression.*

**Narcanti**
*AstraZeneca, Arg.; Torrex, Austria; Bristol-Myers Squibb, Denm.; Meda, Fin.; Bristol-Myers Squibb, Ger.; Aventis, Mex.; Du Pont, Norw.; Bristol-Myers Squibb, Swed.*
Naloxone hydrochloride (p.1044·3).
*Opioid overdosage; reversal of opioid depression.*

**Narcaricin**
*Heumann, Ger.; Heumann, Hong Kong†; Ludwig, Singapore; Heumann, Thai.*
Benzbromarone (p.414·3).
*Gout; hyperuricaemia; renal calculi.*

**Narcaricina** *Asta Medica, Braz.*
Benzbromarone (p.414·3).
*Gout; hyperuricaemia.*

**Narcoral** *Crinos, Ital.*
Naltrexone hydrochloride (p.1046·1).
*Opioid overdosage; opioid withdrawal.*

**Narcotan** *Troikaa, India.*
Naloxone hydrochloride (p.1044·3).
*Opioid overdosage; reversal of opioid depression.*

**Narcotuss** *Legrand, Braz.*
Guaifenesin (p.1122·1); ammonium chloride (p.1115·2).
*Respiratory-tract disorders.*

**Narcozep** *Roche, Fr.*
Flunitrazepam (p.698·2).
*General anaesthesia; premedication.*

**Nardelzine** *Parke, Davis, Belg.*
Phenelzine sulfate (p.312·1).
*Depression.*

**Nardil**
*Link, Austral.; Pfizer, Canad.; Hansam, Irl.; Warner-Lambert, Israel†; Parke, Davis, NZ†; Hansam, UK; Parke, Davis, USA.*
Phenelzine sulfate (p.312·1).
*Depression; mixed anxiety depressive states.*

**Nardyl** *Vifor, Switz.*
Promethazine hydrochloride (p.439·1); hyoscyamine sulfate (p.485·1); atropine sulfate (p.477·1); hyoscine hydrobromide (p.483·3).
*Anxiety; neuroses; sleep disorders; tension.*

**Narfen** *Alter, Spain†.*
Ibuprofen (p.45·3).
*Fever; musculoskeletal, joint, and peri-articular disorders; pain.*

**Narial** *Sinterapico, Braz.†.*
Naphazoline hydrochloride (p.1124·3).
*Nasal congestion.*

**Naribel** *Sanofi Synthelabo, Ital.*
Sodium chloride (p.1233·3).
*Nasal disorders.*

**Naricin** *Sintofarma, Braz.†.*
Naphazoline hydrochloride (p.1124·3); mepyramine maleate (p.437·1).
*Nasal congestion.*

**Naride** *Amrad, Austral.†.*
Indapamide (p.938·2).
*Hypertension.*

**Naridex** *Sibras, Braz.†.*
Naphazoline hydrochloride (p.1124·3).
*Nasal congestion.*

**Naridrin** *EMS, Braz.*
Naphazoline hydrochloride (p.1124·3); mepyramine maleate (p.437·1); dexpanthenol (p.1727·2).
*Nasal congestion.*

**Narifont** *Rappai, Switz.*
Electrolytes (p.1217·1).
*Nasal dryness; nasal irrigation.*

**Narifresh** *Rappai, Switz.*
Sea salt (p.1233·3); chamomile (p.1669·3).
*Nasal disorders.*

**Narigen** *Vocate, Gr.*
Ranitidine hydrochloride (p.1285·2).
*Conditions where gastric acid reduction is beneficial; gastric hypersecretion including Zollinger-Ellison syndrome; peptic ulcer.*

**Narilet** *Fher, Spain†.*
Ipratropium bromide (p.787·1).
*Rhinorrhoea.*

**Narine** *Schering-Plough, Spain.*
Pseudoephedrine sulfate (p.1129·2); loratadine (p.436·1).
*Allergic rhinitis.*

**Narisoro** *Legrand, Braz.*
Sodium chloride (p.1233·3).
*Nasal congestion.*

**Naristar**
*UCB, Ital.; UCB, Spain.*
Cetirizine hydrochloride (p.427·1); pseudoephedrine hydrochloride (p.1129·2).
*Conjunctivitis; rhinitis.*

**Naritec** *TO-Chemicals, Thai.*
Enalapril maleate (p.909·2).
*Heart failure; hypertension.*

**Narium**
*Hamilton, Austral.†; Hamilton, NZ.*
Sodium chloride (p.1233·3).
*Nasal irritation and inflammation.*

**Narix** *Cimed, Braz.*
Naphazoline (p.1124·3).
*Nasal congestion.*

**Narixan** *Wassermann, Ital.*
Pseudoephedrine hydrochloride (p.1129·2).
*Rhinitis; upper respiratory-tract congestion.*

**Narizima** *Baldacci, Port.*
Muramidase hydrochloride (p.1717·2); thonzylamine hydrochloride (p.442·2); isobenzidrine iodide.
*Rhinitis; sinusitis.*

**Narizima Adulto** *Baldacci, Braz.†.*
Muramidase hydrochloride (p.1717·2); ethylenediamine hydrochloride (p.1686·1); methylethylamine hydrochloride; oxymetazoline (p.1126·2); glycerol (p.1694·3).
*Nasal congestion.*

**Narizima Pediatrico** *Baldacci, Braz.†.*
Muramidase hydrochloride (p.1717·2); dimethylethylenediamine hydrochloride; oxyphenylmethylamine hydrochloride; glycerol (p.1694·3).
*Nasal congestion.*

**Narizine** *Beacons, Singapore.*
Flunarizine hydrochloride (p.434·1).
*Epilepsy; migraine; peripheral vascular disorders; vestibular disorders.*

**Narlisim** *Baldacci, Ital.*
Muramidase hydrochloride (p.1717·2); phenolpropamine iodide; thonzylamine hydrochloride (p.442·2).
*Nasal congestion.*

**Narobic** *Alliance, S.Afr.*
Metronidazole (p.607·2).
*Anaerobic bacterial infections; protozoal infections.*

**Narocin** *Teva, Israel.*
Naproxen sodium (p.65·1).
*Fever; musculoskeletal and joint disorders; pain.*

**Narol** *Almirall, Spain†.*
Buspirone hydrochloride (p.672·2).
*Anxiety.*

**Narop**
*Astra, Israel; AstraZeneca, Swed.*
Ropivacaine hydrochloride (p.1384·2).
*Local anaesthesia.*

**Naropeine**
*AstraZeneca, Fr.; Cana, Gr.; AstraZeneca, Port.*
Ropivacaine hydrochloride (p.1384·2).
*Local anaesthesia.*

**Naropin**
*AstraZeneca, Arg.; AstraZeneca, Austral.; AstraZeneca, Austria; AstraZeneca, Belg.; AstraZeneca, Braz.; AstraZeneca, Canad.; AstraZeneca, Chile; AstraZeneca, Denm.; AstraZeneca, Fin.; AstraZeneca, Ger.; AstraZeneca, Hong Kong; AstraZeneca, Irl.; AstraZeneca, Malaysia; Astra, Mex.; AstraZeneca, Neth.; AstraZeneca, Norw.; AstraZeneca, NZ; Astra, S.Afr.; AstraZeneca, Singapore; AstraZeneca, Spain; AstraZeneca, Switz.; AstraZeneca, Thai.; AstraZeneca, UK; Astra, USA.*
Ropivacaine hydrochloride (p.1384·2).
*Local anaesthesia.*

**Naropin with Fentanyl**
*AstraZeneca, Austral.; AstraZeneca, NZ.*
Ropivacaine hydrochloride (p.1384·2); fentanyl citrate (p.40·1).
*Epidural analgesia.*

**Naropina** *AstraZeneca, Ital.*
Ropivacaine hydrochloride (p.1384·2).
*Epidural anaesthesia; local anaesthesia; pain.*

**Narphen** *Napp, UK†.*
Phenazocine hydrobromide (p.82·2).
*Pain.*

**Nartap** *Condrugs, Thai.*
Brompheniramine maleate (p.426·1); phenylephrine hydrochloride (p.1126·3).
Formerly contained brompheniramine maleate, phenylephrine hydrochloride, and phenylpropanolamine hydrochloride.
*Nasal congestion; respiratory-tract disorders.*

**Narvizol** *Narval, Spain.*
Astemizole (p.424·2).
*Allergic conjunctivitis; allergic rhinitis; urticaria.*

**Narzen** *Shiwa, Thai.*
Naproxen (p.65·1).
*Musculoskeletal and joint disorders.*

**Nasa-12** *Glaxo Wellcome, Belg.†.*
Pseudoephedrine hydrochloride (p.1129·2).
*Rhinitis.*

**Nasa Rhinathiol** *Sanofi Synthelabo, Belg.*
Xylometazoline hydrochloride (p.1132·2).
*Nasal congestion.*

**Nasabid** *Jones, USA.*
Pseudoephedrine hydrochloride (p.1129·2); guaifenesin (p.1122·1).
*Cough; nasal congestion.*

**Nasacor** *Aventis, S.Afr.*
Triamcinolone acetonide (p.1110·2).
*Allergic rhinitis.*

**Nasacort**
*Aventis, Arg.; Aventis, Austria; Aventis, Braz.; Aventis, Canad.; Aventis, Chile; Aventis, Denm.; Aventis, Fin.; Aventis, Fr.; Aventis, Ger.; Aventis, Hong Kong; Aventis, Irl.; Aventis, Ital.; Aventis, Mex.; Rhone-Poulenc Rorer, Neth.; Aventis, Norw.; Aventis, NZ†; Aventis, Singapore; Aventis, Spain; Aventis, Swed.; Aventis, Switz.; Aventis, Thai.; Aventis, UK; Aventis, USA.*
Triamcinolone acetonide (p.1110·2).
*Allergic rhinitis.*

**Nasacort AQ**
*Rhone-Poulenc Rorer, Austral.†; Aventis, Malaysia.*
Triamcinolone acetonide (p.1110·2).
*Allergic rhinitis.*

**NaSal** *Sterling Health, USA.*
Sodium chloride (p.1233·3).
*Nasal congestion.*

**Nasal Decongestant** *Prodemdis, Canad.*
Xylometazoline hydrochloride (p.1132·2).

**Nasal Inhaler** *Pickles, UK†.*
Eucalyptus (p.1686·1); menthol (p.1711·3); methyl salicylate (p.59·3); pumilio pine oil (p.1737·1).
*Nasal congestion.*

**Nasal Jelly**
Note. This name is used for preparations of different composition.
*Thuna, Canad.*
Ephedrine hydrochloride (p.1120·1); methyl salicylate (p.59·3); thymol (p.1194·2).

*Kondon, USA.*
Phenol (p.1188·1); camphor (p.1665·3); menthol (p.1711·3); eucalyptus oil (p.1686·2); lavender oil (p.1705·2).
*Nasal congestion.*

**Nasal Moist** *Blairex, USA.*
Sodium chloride (p.1233·3).
*Inflammation and dryness of nasal membranes.*

**Nasal Relief** *Rugby, USA.*
Oxymetazoline hydrochloride (p.1126·1).
*Nasal congestion.*

**Nasal & Sinus Cold Formula** *Stanley, Canad.*
Phenylephrine hydrochloride (p.1126·3); chlorphenamine maleate (p.427·3); paracetamol (p.76·2).

**Nasal & Sinus Relief** *Stanley, Canad.*
Pseudoephedrine hydrochloride (p.1129·2).

**Nasal Spray** *Reese, USA.*
Oxymetazoline hydrochloride (p.1126·1).

**Nasal Spray for Hayfever** *Unichem, UK†.*
Beclometasone dipropionate (p.1091·1).
*Hay fever.*

**Nasalate** *Paedpharm, Austral.*
Chlorhexidine (p.1173·2); phenylephrine hydrochloride (p.1126·3).
*Epistaxis; nasal surgery; nasal vestibulitis.*

**Nasal-Bec** *Ivax, UK.*
Beclometasone dipropionate (p.1091·1).
*Rhinitis.*

**Nasalcrom** *Pharmacia, USA.*
Sodium cromoglicate (p.795·3).
*Allergic rhinitis.*

**Nasal-Ease** *Health Care Products, USA.*
*Nasal gel:* Zinc acetate (p.1469·2); aloe vera (p.1141·3); calendula (p.1665·2).

*Nasal spray:* Zinc gluconate (p.1469·2); sodium chloride (p.1233·3).

*Inflammation and dryness of nasal membranes.*

**Nasalemed** *SmithKline Beecham, Ital.†.*
Xylometazoline hydrochloride (p.1132·2); domiphen bromide (p.1179·1).
*Nasal congestion.*

**Nasaleze** *Dendron, UK.*
Cellulose (p.1578·3).
*Allergic rhinitis.*

**Nasalflu** *Berna, Switz.*
An influenza vaccine (p.1620·2).
*Active immunisation.*

**Nasalgen** *Kenyaku, Thai.†.*
*Syrup:* Phenylpropanolamine hydrochloride (p.1127·3); carbinoxamine maleate (p.426·3).

*Tablets:* Phenylpropanolamine hydrochloride (p.1127·3); phenylephrine hydrochloride (p.1126·3); carbinoxamine maleate (p.426·3).

*Hay fever; nasal congestion; rhinitis.*

**Nasalide**
*Aventis, Fr.; Ivax, USA†.*
Flunisolide (p.1101·1).
*Rhinitis.*

**Nasamine** *Maxi, Thai.*
Dexchlorpheniramine maleate (p.427·3).
*Hypersensitivity reactions.*

**Nasan** *Hexal, Ger.*
Xylometazoline hydrochloride (p.1132·2).
*Nasal congestion.*

**Nasanal** *Brady, Austria.*
Aluminium acetotartrate (p.1652·3); pumilio pine oil (p.1737·1).
*Nasal disorders.*

**Nasapert** *Searle, Belg.†.*
Brompheniramine maleate (p.426·1); phenylpropanolamine hydrochloride (p.1127·3).
*Rhinitis.*

**Nasarel**
Note. This name is used for preparations of different composition.
*Dabur, India.*
Nafarelin acetate (p.1332·3).
*Endometriosis; pituitary desensitisation in controlled ovarian stimulation.*

*Ivax, USA.*
Flunisolide (p.1101·1).
*Rhinitis.*

**Nasarox** *Plough, Port.*
Oxymetazoline hydrochloride (p.1126·1).
*Nasal congestion.*

**Nasasinutab** *Pfizer Consumer, Belg.*
Xylometazoline hydrochloride (p.1132·2).
*Nasal congestion.*

**Nasatab LA** *ECR, USA.*
Guaifenesin (p.1122·1); pseudoephedrine hydrochloride (p.1129·2).
*Coughs.*

**Nasben** *Democal, Switz.*
Xylometazoline hydrochloride (p.1132·2).
*Nasal congestion.*

**Nasben Soft** *Democal, Switz.†.*
Sodium chloride (p.1233·3).
*Nasal disorders.*

**Nasciodine** *Pharmadass, UK.*
Iodine (p.1598·1); menthol (p.1711·3); methyl salicylate (p.59·3); turpentine oil (p.1760·1); rectified camphor oil.
*Musculoskeletal, joint, and soft-tissue disorders.*

**Nascobal**
*Nastech, Israel; Questcor, USA.*
Cyanocobalamin (p.1458·2).
*Vitamin $B_{12}$ deficiency.*

**Nasdro** *Adcock Ingram, S.Afr.*
Phenylephrine hydrochloride (p.1126·3); naphazoline nitrate (p.1124·3).
*Nasal congestion.*

**Nasea**
*Yamanouchi, Jpn; Yamanouchi, Thai.*
Ramosetron hydrochloride (p.1285·2).
*Nausea and vomiting induced by cytotoxic chemotherapy.*

**Nasengel** *Ratiopharm, Ger.*
Xylometazoline hydrochloride (p.1132·2).
*Catarrh; nasal congestion; sinusitis.*

**Nasengel AL** *Aliud, Ger.*
Xylometazoline hydrochloride (p.1132·2).
*Rhinitis.*

**Nasenspray AL** *Aliud, Ger.*
Xylometazoline hydrochloride (p.1132·2).
*Rhinitis.*

**Nasenspray E** *Ratiopharm, Ger.*
Xylometazoline hydrochloride (p.1132·2).
*Catarrh; nasal congestion; sinusitis.*

**Nasenspray K** *Ratiopharm, Ger.*
Xylometazoline hydrochloride (p.1132·2).
*Catarrh; nasal congestion; sinusitis.*

**Nasentropfen AL** *Aliud, Ger.*
Xylometazoline hydrochloride (p.1132·2).
*Rhinitis.*

**Nasentropfen E** *Ratiopharm, Ger.*
Xylometazoline hydrochloride (p.1132·2).
*Nasal congestion.*

**Nasentropfen K** *Ratiopharm, Ger.*
Xylometazoline hydrochloride (p.1132·2).
*Nasal congestion.*

**Nasentropfen-ratiopharm** *Ratiopharm, Ger.*
Pine needle oil; peppermint oil (p.1283·2); pumilio pine oil (p.1737·1); eucalyptus oil (p.1686·2); thymol (p.1194·2).
*Cold symptoms; nasal congestion.*

**Naseptin**
*Alliance, Irl.; Genop, S.Afr.†; Alliance, UK.*
Chlorhexidine hydrochloride (p.1173·3); neomycin sulfate (p.235·1).
*Nasal carriage of staphylococci; staphylococcal infections.*

**Nasex**
Note. This name is used for preparations of different composition.
*Felton, Austral.†.*
Oxymetazoline hydrochloride (p.1126·1); cineole (p.1672·1); menthol (p.1711·3).
*Nasal congestion.*

*Janssen-Cilag, Port.*
Oxymetazoline hydrochloride (p.1126·1).

*DP-Medica, Switz.*
Phenylephrine hydrochloride (p.1126·3); cetylpyridinium chloride (p.1173·1).
*Nasal disorders.*

**Nasic** *Cassella-med, Ger.; Artesan, Ger.*
Xylometazoline hydrochloride (p.1132·2); dexpanthenol (p.1727·2).
*Nasal congestion.*

**Nasicortin** *Bracco, Ital.†.*
Dexamethasone tebutate (p.1097·3); oxymetazoline hydrochloride (p.1126·1).
*Nasal polyps; rhinitis; rhinopharyngitis; sinusitis.*

**Nasicur** *Cassella-med, Ger.; Artesan, Ger.*
Dexpanthenol (p.1727·2).
*Rhinitis sicca.*

**Nasil** *Silom, Thai.†.*
Oxymetazoline hydrochloride (p.1126·1).
*Nasal congestion.*

**Nasilex** *Recalcine, Chile.*
Pseudoephedrine hydrochloride (p.1129·2) or pseudoephedrine sulfate (p.1129·2); chlorphenamine maleate (p.427·3).

**Nasimild** *Merck, Austria†.*
Benzalkonium chloride (p.1168·3); polysorbate 80 (p.1415·2).
*Nasal disorders.*

**Nasin** *Tika, Swed.*
Oxymetazoline hydrochloride (p.1126·1).
*Rhinitis; sinusitis.*

**Nasivin**
*Merck, Austria; Merck, Braz.; Merck, Israel; Bracco, Ital.†; Merck, Neth.; Julphar, UAE; Merck, UK.*
Oxymetazoline hydrochloride (p.1126·1).
*Nasal congestion; rhinitis; sinus disorders.*

**Nasivin gegen Erkaltung Kinderbad** *Merck, Ger.†.*
Eucalyptus oil (p.1686·2).
*Respiratory-tract congestion.*

**Nasivin gegen Erkaltung N** *Merck, Ger.†.*
Eucalyptus oil (p.1686·2); thyme oil (p.1755·3); camphor (p.1665·3).
*Bath additive; catarrh.*

**Nasivin gegen Schnupfen** *Merck, Ger.*
Oxymetazoline hydrochloride (p.1126·1).
*Catarrh; otitis media; rhinitis; sinusitis.*

**Nasivin Intensiv-Bad N** *Merck, Ger.†.*
Eucalyptus oil (p.1686·2); thyme oil (p.1755·3); camphor (p.1665·3).
*Respiratory-tract congestion.*

**Nasivin Sanft** *Merck, Ger.*
Oxymetazoline hydrochloride (p.1126·1).
*Catarrh; nasal congestion; otitis media; rhinitis; sinusitis.*

**Nasivine** *Asta Medica, Switz.*
Oxymetazoline hydrochloride (p.1126·1).
*Catarrh; rhinitis; sinusitis.*

**Nasivinetten gegen Schnupfen** *Merck, Ger.*
Oxymetazoline hydrochloride (p.1126·1).
*Catarrh; otitis media; rhinitis; sinusitis.*

**Nasivinettes** *Asta Medica, Switz.*
Oxymetazoline hydrochloride (p.1126·1).
Formerly known as Nasivinetten.
*Catarrh; rhinitis; sinusitis.*

**Nasivion** *Merck, India.*
Oxymetazoline (p.1126·2) or oxymetazoline hydrochloride (p.1126·1).
*Nasal congestion.*

**nasmer** *Democal, Switz.*
Dead Sea salt (p.1233·3).
*Nasal dryness.*

**Naso Instil** *Dinafarma, Braz.†.*
Tyrothricin (p.275·1); naphazoline hydrochloride (p.1124·3).
*Nasal congestion.*

**Naso Pekamin** *Medical, Spain.*
Phenylephrine hydrochloride (p.1126·3); kanamycin sulfate (p.225·1); trypsin (p.1758·3).
*Nose and throat disorders.*

**Nasobec**
*Baker Norton, Hong Kong†; Ivax, Irl.; Ivax, UK.*
Beclometasone dipropionate (p.1091·1).
*Rhinitis.*

**Nasobol** *Sanofi, Switz.*
Benzoic acid (p.1169·3); peru balsam (p.1730·2); verbena oil; eucalyptus oil (p.1686·2); lavender oil (p.1705·2); wild thyme oil.
*Respiratory-tract disorders.*

**Naso-Calma** *Salusif, Port.*
Ephedrine hydrochloride (p.1120·1); silver protein (p.1746·2).
*Cold and influenza symptoms.*

**Nasocan** *Protein, Mex.†.*
Naproxen sodium (p.65·1).

**Nasoclean** *Terme di Tabiano, Ital.*
Thermal water.
*Nasal cleansing.*

**Nasocort** *Teva, Israel.*
Budesonide (p.1094·2).
*Rhinitis.*

**Nasoferm** *Nordic, Swed.*
Xylometazoline hydrochloride (p.1132·2).
*Rhinitis; sinusitis.*

**Nasoflux** *IQB, Braz.†.*
Sodium chloride (p.1233·3).
*Nasal congestion.*

**Nasogrip** *Cazi, Braz.*
Phenylephrine hydrochloride (p.1126·3); paracetamol (p.76·2); mepyramine maleate (p.437·1); caffeine (p.782·1).
*Cold and influenza symptoms.*

**Nasojol** *Geminis, Arg.*
Naphazoline (p.1124·3); neomycin (p.235·1).
*Nasal congestion.*

**Nasolac** *Hebron, Braz.*
Sodium chloride (p.1233·3).
*Nasal congestion.*

**Nasolin**
*Note. This name is used for preparations of different composition.*
*Orion, Fin.*
Xylometazoline hydrochloride (p.1132·2).
*Allergic rhinitis.*

*Nakorn, Thai.*
Triprolidine hydrochloride (p.442·3); pseudoephedrine hydrochloride (p.1129·2).
*Allergic rhinitis; cold symptoms; hay fever; nasal congestion.*

**Nasolina** *Salvat, Spain†.*
Oxymetazoline hydrochloride (p.1126·1).
*Nasal congestion.*

**Nasomet** *Schering-Plough, Port.*
Mometasone furoate (p.1107·2).
*Rhinitis.*

**Nasomicina** *Northia, Arg.*
Naphazoline (p.1124·3); neomycin (p.235·1); gramicidin (p.220·2).
*Nasal disorders.*

**Nasomicina Salina** *Northia, Arg.*
Sodium chloride (p.1233·3).
*Nasal congestion.*

**Nasomin** *Medipharm, Chile.*
Bacitracin zinc (p.161·3); neomycin sulfate (p.235·1); xylometazoline hydrochloride (p.1132·2); antazoline phosphate (p.424·2).
*Upper resiratory-tract disorders.*

**Nasomixin**
*Note. This name is used for preparations of different composition.*
*Teofarma, Ital.*
Phenylpropanolamine hydrochloride (p.1127·3); hydrocortisone (p.1103·3).
*Cold symptoms; rhinitis; sinusitis.*

*Aventis, S.Afr.*
Phenylephrine hydrochloride (p.1126·3); phenylpropanolamine hydrochloride (p.1127·3); hydrocortisone (p.1103·3); neomycin sulfate (p.235·1).
*Rhinitis; sinusitis.*

**Nasonex**
*Kirby, Arg.; Schering-Plough, Austral.; Aesca, Austria; Schering-Plough, Belg.; Schering-Plough, Braz.; Schering, Canad.; Schering-Plough, Chile; Schering-Plough, Denm.; Schering-Plough, Fin.; Schering-Plough, Fr.; Essex, Ger.; Schering-Plough, Hong Kong; Schering-Plough, Irl.; Schering-Plough, Israel; Schering-Plough, Ital.; Schering-Plough, Malaysia; Schering-Plough, Neth.; Schering-Plough, Norw.; Schering-Plough, S.Afr.; Schering-Plough, Singapore; Schering-Plough, Spain; Schering-Plough, Swed.; Essex, Switz.; Schering-Plough, Thai.; Schering-Plough, UK; Schering, USA.*
Mometasone furoate (p.1107·2).
*Allergic rhinitis.*

**Nasopan** *Heralds, Braz.†.*
Naphazoline hydrochloride (p.1124·3); mepyramine maleate (p.437·1); dexpanthenol (p.1727·2).
*Nasal congestion.*

**Nasopomada** *Medical, Spain.*
Bismuth subgallate (p.1252·2); prednisolone (p.1108·1); rutoside (p.1688·2); sulfanilamide (p.263·2); tetracycline hydrochloride (p.266·2); urea; benzocaine (p.1370·3).
*Nasal furunculosis; sinusitis.*

**Naso-Prieulina** *Medical, Port.*
Naphazoline hydrochloride (p.1124·3); ephedrine hydrochloride (p.1120·1); mepyramine maleate (p.437·1).
*Rhinitis; sinusitis.*

**Nasorest** *Community Pharmacy, Thai.*
*Expectorant:* Brompheniramine maleate (p.426·1); pseudoephedrine hydrochloride (p.1129·2); bromhexine hydrochloride (p.1115·3).
*Coughs; respiratory-tract disorders.*

*Syrup; tablets:* Brompheniramine maleate (p.426·1); pseudoephedrine hydrochloride (p.1129·2).
*Allergic rhinitis; cold symptoms; hay fever; nasal congestion.*

**Nasosil** *Silom, Thai.†.*
Brompheniramine maleate (p.426·1); phenylephrine hydrochloride (p.1126·3); phenylpropanolamine hydrochloride (p.1127·3).
*Nasal congestion.*

**Nasotic Oto** *Juventus, Spain†.*
Betamethasone valerate (p.1093·2); neomycin sulfate (p.235·1); papain (p.1727·3); polymyxin B sulfate (p.245·1).
*Ear disorders; rhinitis.*

**Nasovalda** *Sterling Health, Spain†.*
Oxymetazoline hydrochloride (p.1126·1).
*Nasal congestion.*

**Naspor** *Genepharm, Gr.*
Cefotaxime sodium (p.175·3).
*Bacterial infections.*

**Nasterid** *Ativus, Braz.*
Finasteride (p.1554·2).
*Benign prostatic hyperplasia.*

**Nasteril** *Raffo, Arg.*
Finasteride (p.1554·2).
*Prostate disorders.*

**Nastifrin** *Laboratorios Chile, Chile.*
Chlorphenamine maleate (p.427·3); pseudoephedrine sulfate (p.1129·2).
*Upper respiratory-tract disorders.*

**Nastifrin Compuesto** *Laboratorios Chile, Chile.*
Paracetamol (p.76·2); pseudoephedrine (p.1129·2); chlorphenamine maleate (p.427·3).
*Allergic rhinitis; cold symptoms.*

**Nastifrin DN Compuesto** *Laboratorios Chile, Chile.*
Day tablets, paracetamol (p.76·2); pseudoephedrine sulfate (p.1129·2); night tablets, paracetamol; pseudoephedrine sulfate; chlorphenamine maleate (p.427·3).
*Cold and influenza symptoms.*

**Nastil** *Best, Mex.*
Ketoconazole (p.403·3).
*Fungal infections.*

**Nastizol**
*Note. This name is used for preparations of different composition.*
*Bago, Arg.*
*Nose drops:* Xylometazoline hydrochloride (p.1132·2).
*Oral drops; syrup; tablets:* Pseudoephedrine sulfate (p.1129·2); chlorphenamine maleate (p.427·3).
*Nasal congestion.*

*Bago, Chile.*
Pseudoephedrine sulfate (p.1129·2); chlorphenamine maleate (p.427·3).
*Rhinitis; upper respiratory-tract disorders.*

**Nastizol Antialergico** *Bago, Arg.*
Loratadine (p.436·1).
*Hypersensitivity reactions.*

**Nastizol Compositum**
*Note. This name is used for preparations of different composition.*
*Bago, Arg.*
Pseudoephedrine sulfate (p.1129·2); chlorphenamine maleate (p.427·3); bromhexine hydrochloride (p.1115·3); paracetamol (p.76·2).
*Influenza symptoms.*

*Bago, Chile.*
Pseudoephedrine sulfate (p.1129·2); chlorphenamine maleate (p.427·3); paracetamol (p.76·2).
*Coughs and cold symptoms; rhinitis; sinusitis.*

**Nastizol Expectorante** *Bago, Arg.*
Bromhexine hydrochloride (p.1115·3).
*Respiratory-tract disorders with excess or viscous mucus.*

**Nastizol Hidrospray** *Bago, Arg.*
Budesonide (p.1094·2).
*Rhinitis.*

**Nastizol-L** *Bago, Arg.*
Loratadine (p.436·1); pseudoephedrine sulfate (p.1129·2).
*Allergic rhinitis; cold symptoms.*

**Nastop** *Democal, Switz.†.*
Dexpanthenol (p.1727·2); peppermint oil (p.1283·2); camphor (p.1665·3).
*Nasal disorders.*

**Nastoren** *Lepetit, Ital.*
Somatostatin acetate (p.1339·3).
*Gastrointestinal haemorrhage; prevention of postoperative complications following pancreatic surgery.*

**Nastul** *Chemopharma, Chile.*
Pseudoephedrine sulfate (p.1129·2); chlorphenamine maleate (p.427·3).
*Upper respiratory-tract disorders.*

**Nastul Compuesto** *Chemopharma, Chile.*
Pseudoephedrine sulfate (p.1129·2); chlorphenamine maleate (p.427·3); paracetamol (p.76·2).
*Upper respiratory-tract disorders.*

**Nasulind** *Steierl, Ger.*
Peppermint oil (p.1283·2); thyme oil (p.1755·3).
*Nasal congestion.*

**Natabec**
*Pfizer, Austria; Parke, Davis, Chile; Pfizer Consumer, Ger.; Warner-Lambert, Hong Kong†; Pfizer, Switz.*
Multivitamin and mineral preparation (p.1417·1).

**Natabec F** *Pfizer Consumer, Ger.*
Multivitamin and mineral preparation (p.1417·1) with sodium fluoride (p.1444·3).

**NataChew** *Warner Chilcott, USA.*
A multivitamin preparation with iron (p.1417·1).

**Natacyn**
*Alcon, Arg.; Alcon, S.Afr.; Alcon, Singapore; Alcon, Thai.; Alcon, USA.*
Natamycin (p.406·2).
*Fungal eye infections.*

**Natafort** *Warner Chilcott, USA.*
Multivitamin and mineral preparation (p.1417·1).

**Natafucin** *Yamanouchi, Ital.*
Natamycin (p.406·2).
*Fungal skin infections.*

**Natal** *Diepharmex, Fr.*
Multivitamin and mineral preparation (p.1417·1).
*Nutritional supplement during pregnancy.*

**Natal Extra** *Cypress, USA.*
Multivitamin and mineral preparation (p.1417·1).
Docusate sodium (p.1262·2) is included in this preparation to reduce the constipating effects of iron.

**NatalCare** *Ethex, USA.*
A range of multivitamin and multivitamin and mineral preparations (p.1417·1).

**Natalin** *Mead Johnson Nutritionals, USA.*
Multivitamin and mineral preparation with iron and folic acid (p.1417·1).
*Dietary supplement during pregnancy and lactation.*

**Natalins** *Mead Johnson, Hong Kong†.*
Multivitamin and mineral preparation (p.1417·1).
*Dietary supplement in pregnancy and lactation.*

**Natalins com Fluor** *Mead Johnson, Braz.*
Multivitamin and mineral preparation with iron, folic acid, and fluoride (p.1417·1).

**Natalins Folico** *Mead Johnson, Braz.*
Multivitamin and mineral preparation (p.1417·1).

**Nataral** *Kenyaku, Thai.*
Multivitamin and mineral preparation (p.1417·1).

**Natarex Prenatal** *Major, USA.*
Multivitamin and mineral preparation with iron and folic acid (p.1417·1).

**NataTab** *Ethex, USA.*
Multivitamin and mineral preparation (p.1417·1).

**Natavite** *Schein, Canad.*
Multivitamin preparation with iron and folic acid (p.1417·1).

**Natead** *Lab Francais du Fractionnement, Fr.*
An anti-D immunoglobulin (p.1608·1).
*Prevention of rhesus incompatibility.*

**Natecal**
*Note. This name is used for preparations of different composition.*
*Eurofarma, Braz.; ITF, Chile; Italfarmaco, Spain.*
Calcium carbonate (p.1254·2).
*Hypocalcaemia; osteoporosis.*

*Italfarmaco, Ital.*
Calcium carbonate (p.1254·2); colecalciferol (p.1461·3).
*Calcium and vitamin D deficiency; osteoporosis.*

**Natecal D**
*Eurofarma, Braz.; ITF, Chile; Italfarmaco, Spain.*
Calcium carbonate (p.1254·2); colecalciferol (p.1461·3).
*Calcium and vitamin D supplement; osteoporosis.*

**Nateglin** *Phoenix, Arg.*
Nateglinide (p.343·3).
*Diabetes mellitus.*

**Nathergen** *PD, Thai.*
Methylergometrine maleate (p.1714·2).
*Functional uterine bleeding; management of third stage of labour; postpartum haemorrhage; puerperal haemorrhage.*

**Naticardina** *Viatris, Ital.*
Quinidine polygalacturonate (p.991·3).
*Arrhythmias.*

**Natigesta** *Farmalab, Braz.*
Multivitamin and mineral preparation (p.1417·1).

**Nati-K** *Centropharm, Fr.†.*
Potassium tartrate (p.1232·2).
*Hypokalaemia.*

**Natiken** *Kener, Mex.†.*
Ibuprofen (p.45·3).

**Natil** *3M, Ger.*
Cyclandelate (p.890·3).
*Cerebral metabolic and vascular disorders; migraine; retinopathy; vestibular disorders.*

**Natinate** *Atlantic, Thai.†.*
Nicotinic acid (p.1441·1).
*Pellagra.*

**Natisedina** *Teofarma, Ital.*
Quinidine phenylethylbarbiturate (p.993·2).
*Arrhythmias.*

**Natisedine**
*Note. This name is used for preparations of different composition.*
*Barrenne, Braz.†.*
Quinidine (p.991·3).
*Arrhythmias.*

*Sabex, Canad.†.*
Quinidine phenylethylbarbiturate (p.993·2).
*Nervous disorders with arrhythmia.*

*Procter & Gamble, Fr.†.*
Phenobarbital (p.367·3); passion flower (p.1729·1).
Formerly contained quinidine phenylethylbarbiturate.
*Anxiety; insomnia; palpitations.*

**Natispray**
*Procter & Gamble, Fr.; Teofarma, Ital.; Nativelle, Switz.†.*
Glyceryl trinitrate (p.923·2).
*Angina pectoris; pulmonary oedema.*

**Nativa HA** *Guigoz, Ital.*
Infant feed (p.1417·1).
*Milk intolerance.*

**Nativit** *Sigma, Braz.*
Multivitamin and mineral preparation with iron (p.1417·1).

**Nativit Fluor** *Sigma, Braz.*
A multivitamin and mineral preparation with fluoride (p.1417·1).

**Na-To-Caps** *SIT, Ital.†.*
Mixed tocopherols (p.1464·3).
*Vitamin E deficiency.*

**Natopherol**
*Abbott, Hong Kong; Abbott, Malaysia; Abbott, Singapore.*
Vitamin E (p.1464·3).
*Vitamin E supplement.*

**Natopherol Dermal-Day** *Scherer, Malaysia.*
*SPF 30: d*-Alpha tocopherol (p.1464·3); octinoxate (p.1154·3); titanium dioxide (p.1160·3).
*Dry skin disorders; sunscreen.*

**Natoss** *Biologia, Braz.†.*
Sodium dibunate (p.1130·2); sodium benzoate (p.1169·3).
*Coughs.*

**Natovit** *Bruno, Ital.*
Tocoferil acetate (p.1465·1).
*Vitamin E deficiency.*

**Natracalm** *Chefaro, UK.*
Passion flower (p.1729·1).
*Tension.*

**NatraFlex** *Nutralife, UK.*
Capsaicin (p.24·2); dimethyl sulfone; boswellia serrata (p.1690·1).
*Joint pain.*

**Natraleze** *English Grains, UK†.*
Slippery elm bark (p.1747·1); meadowsweet (p.1710·1); liquorice (p.1270·2).
*Dyspepsia; flatulence; heartburn.*

**Natrapel** *Ardern, UK.*
Citronella oil (p.1673·2).
*Insect repellent.*

**Natrasleep** *Chefaro, UK.*
Lupulus (p.1708·1); valerian (p.1762·2).
*Insomnia.*

**Natrecor** *Scios, USA.*
Nesiritide citrate (p.964·3).
*Heart failure.*

**Natriclo** *Sterop, Belg.*
Sodium chloride (p.1233·3).
*Hyponatraemia.*

**Natrilix**
*Servier, Arg.; Servier, Austral.; Servier, Braz.; Servier, Denm.; Servier, Fin.; Servier, Ger.; Servier, Hong Kong; Serdia, India; Servier, Irl.; Servier, Ital.; Servier, Malaysia; Servier, NZ; Servier, S.Afr.; Servier, Singapore; Servier, Thai.; Servier, UK.*
Indapamide (p.938·2).
*Hypertension.*

**Natrioxen** *Benedetti, Ital.†.*
Naproxen sodium (p.65·1).
Lidocaine hydrochloride (p.1377·3) is included in the intramuscular injection to alleviate the pain of injection.
*Inflammation; musculoskeletal and joint disorders; pain.*

**Natrium-Homaccord** *Peithner, Austria.*
Homoeopathic preparation.

**Natrocitral** *Tarbis, Spain.*
Oxetacaine (p.1382·1); sodium citrate (p.1223·2); aluminium glycinate (p.1249·1).
*Gastrointestinal disorders.*

**Natropas** *Finadiet, Arg.*
Cinnarizine (p.428·3).
*Cerebral and peripheral vascular disorders.*

**Natrosteril** *Orion, Fin.*
A range of sodium chloride infusions with or without glucose (p.1233·3).
*Fluid and electrolyte disorders.*

**Natsurf** *Pharmacia, Arg.*
Pulmonary surfactant (p.1736·1).
*Neonatal respiratory distress syndrome.*

**Natucor** *Rodisma, Ger.*
Crataegus (p.1677·1).
*Heart failure.*

**Natuderm** *Rodisma, Ger.*
Biotin (p.1423·2).
*Biotin deficiency.*

**Natudolor** *Duopharm, Ger.*
Potentilla anserina.
*Dysmenorrhoea.*

**Natudophilus** *Cantassium Co., UK.*
*Lactobacillus acidophilus* (p.1704·2); *Bifidobacterium bifidum* (p.1704·2).

**Natudor**
*Note. This name is used for preparations of different composition.*
*Dolisos, Belg.*
Valerian (p.1762·2); crataegus (p.1677·1); tilia (p.1756·2).
*Anxiety; insomnia.*

*Plantes et Medecines, Fr.*
Crataegus (p.1677·1); passion flower (p.1729·1).
*Anxiety; insomnia; palpitations.*

**Natu-fem** *Rodisma, Ger.*
Cimicifuga (p.1671·3).
*Menopausal disorders.*

**Natulan**
*Link, Austral.; Roche, Belg.†; Sigma-Tau, Canad.; Sigma-Tau, Fr.; Sigma-Tau, Ger.; IFET (ΙΦΕΤ), Gr.; Roche, Israel†; Sigma-Tau, Ital.; Roche, Mex.†; Sigma-Tau, Neth.; AFT, NZ; Roche, S.Afr.†; Sigma-Tau, Spain; Roche, Switz.†.*
Procarbazine hydrochloride (p.581·2).
*Malignant neoplasms.*

**Natulanar** *Eurofarma, Braz.†.*
Procarbazine hydrochloride (p.581·2).
*Malignant neoplasms.*

**Natulax**
*Note. This name is used for preparations of different composition.*
*Natufarma, Arg.*
Cascara (p.1255·1).
*Constipation.*

*Lichtenstein, Ger.†.*
Lactulose (p.1269·1).
*Constipation; hepatic encephalopathy; salmonella enteritis.*

**Natura Asep** *Maurino, Arg.*
Solutions for soft contact lens care (p.1164·2).

**Natura Fenac** *Amhof, Arg.*
Diclofenac sodium (p.32·1).
*Eye disorders.*

**Natura Fresh** *Maurino, Arg.*
Carmellose sodium (p.1577·3).
*Dry eyes.*

**Natura Lagrimas** *Amhof, Arg.*
Hypromellose (p.1579·3).
*Dry eyes.*

**Natura Medica** *Dolisos, Fr.†.*
A range of herbal extracts.

**Natura Perflex** *Maurino, Arg.*
Ethoxylated propylene glycol.
*Cleansing solution for flexible and gas permeable contact lenses.*

**Natura Plus** *Maurino, Arg.*
Poloxamine (p.1164·2).
*Cleansing, disinfecting, storage, and wetting solution for soft contact lenses.*

**Natura Viva** *Novartis Consumer, Ital.†.*
Royal jelly (p.1740·3).
*Nutritional supplement.*

**Natura Wet** *Maurino, Arg.*
Polyvinyl alcohol (p.1581·1) (p.1164·2).
*Wetting solution for flexible and gas permeable contact lenses.*

**Naturaform Fruchtewurfel mit Manna** *Bregenzer, Austria.*
Manna (p.1273·1); fig (p.1266·3); tamarind (p.1293·2); sorbitol (p.1446·3).
*Constipation.*

**Natural Defense** *Maybelline, Canad.†.*
Titanium dioxide (p.1160·3).
*Sunscreen.*

**Natural Diet** *AM, Arg.*
Bladderwrack; centella; equisetum; carnitine; vitamin E (p.1417·1).
*Dietary supplement.*

**Natural Fibre** *Cenovis, Austral.†; Vitelle, Austral.†.*
Psyllium seed (p.1268·1).
*Constipation; dietary fibre supplement.*

**Natural Herb Tablets** *Dorwest, UK.*
Senna (p.1288·2); aloes (p.1248·2); cascara (p.1255·1); valerian (p.1762·2); taraxacum (p.1751·3).
*Constipation.*

**Natural Horizons Solar Block Extreme** *Mentholatum, Austral.†.*
*SPF 30+:* Octinoxate (p.1154·3); zinc oxide (p.1163·2).
*Sunscreen.*

**Natural Horizons Solar Block Lotion** *Mentholatum, Austral.†.*
*SPF 15:* Octinoxate (p.1154·3); avobenzone (p.1142·3); octil triazone (p.1154·3); titanium dioxide (p.1160·3).
*SPF 30+:* Octinoxate (p.1154·3); zinc oxide (p.1163·2).
*Sunscreen.*

**Natural Horizons Solar Block Toddler** *Mentholatum, Austral.†.*
*SPF 30+:* Octinoxate (p.1154·3); zinc oxide (p.1163·2).
*Sunscreen.*

**Natural Ice Extreme** *Mentholatum, Canad.*
*SPF 30:* Avobenzone (p.1142·3); octinoxate (p.1154·3); octisalate (p.1154·3).
*Sunscreen.*

**Natural Ice Lipbalm** *Mentholatum, Canad.*
Octinoxate (p.1154·3); octisalate (p.1154·3).
*SPF 15:* Padimate O (p.1155·1).
*Sunscreen.*

**Natural Source Laxative** *Adams, Canad.*
Ispaghula (p.1268·1).
*Constipation; fibre supplementation.*

**Natural Wealth Beta** *Transcontinental, Braz.†.*
Vitamin A (p.1451·2); vitamin D (p.1461·2).

**Natural Zanzy** *Montefarmaco, Ital.†.*
Geranium oil (p.1692·2); lavender oil (p.1705·2); citronella oil (p.1673·2).
*Insect repellent.*

**Naturalag** *Alcon, Mex.*
Hypromellose (p.1579·3).
*Dry eyes.*

**Naturalass** *Naturmed, Ital.*
Lactulose (p.1269·1); mannitol (p.950·2); glycerol (p.1694·3); inulin (p.1702·1); plant fibre; minerals (p.1417·1).
*Gastrointestinal disorders.*

**Naturalist** *Prater, Chile.*
Aspartame (p.1422·1).
*Sugar substitute.*

**Naturalyte** *Unico, USA.*
Glucose; electrolytes (p.1222·2).
*Diarrhoea; oral rehydration therapy.*

**Naturcil** *London Drugs, Canad.†.*
Ispaghula (p.1268·1).

**Nature Throid** *Western Research, USA.*
Thyroid (p.1604·2).
*Hypothyroidism.*

**Nature's Choice** *New Vision, Canad.*
Multivitamin and mineral preparation (p.1417·1).

**Natures Own Acidophilus Plus** *Bullivants, Austral.†.*
*Lactobacillus acidophilus* (p.1704·2); *Lactobacillus bulgaricus* (p.1704·2); apple pectin (p.1580·3).
*Maintenance of normal gastrointestinal flora.*

**Natures Own Colds & Flu** *Bullivants, Austral.†.*
Ferrous phosphate; potassium chloride (p.1232·2).
*Cold and influenza symptoms.*

**Natures Own Digestive Enzymes** *Bullivants, Austral.†.*
Pepsin (p.1729·3); bromelains (p.1662·2); peppermint oil (p.1283·2); pancreatin (p.1725·3); papain (p.1727·3).
*Digestive disorders; dyspepsia; flatulence.*

**Natures Own Maxepa** *Bullivants, Austral.†.*
Fish oil (p.976·2).
*Dietary fatty acid supplement.*

**Natures Own Maxi B** *Bullivants, Austral.†.*
Vitamin B substances (p.1417·1).
*Vitamin B supplement.*

**Natures Own Mega-B + L-Tryptophan** *Bullivants, Austral.†.*
Vitamin B substances; tryptophan; ginseng; fo-ti-tieng; rosehips; alfalfa (p.1417·1).
*Tonic; vitamin B supplement.*

**Natures Own Super B Complex** *Bullivants, Austral.†.*
Vitamin B substances; vitamin C; methionine; wheatgerm; lecithin (p.1417·1).
*Tonic; vitamin B supplement.*

**Natures Remedy**
*Note. This name is used for preparations of different composition.*
*Block, Canad.*
Senna (p.1288·2).
Formerly contained aloes and cascara.

*SmithKline Beecham Consumer, USA†.*
Aloes (p.1248·2); cascara (p.1255·1).
*Constipation.*

**Nature's Tears** *Rugby, USA.*
Hypromellose (p.1579·3); dextran 70 (p.746·2).
*Dry eyes.*

**Natures Way Acidophilus Plus** *Roche Consumer, Austral.†.*
*Lactobacillus acidophilus* (p.1704·2); *Bifidobacterium bifidum* (p.1704·2).
*Maintenance of normal gastrointestinal flora.*

**Natures Way All-in-One** *Roche Consumer, Austral.†.*
Multivitamin and mineral preparation with ginseng (p.1417·1).

**Natures Way Executive Formula** *Roche Consumer, Austral.†.*
Vitamins; minerals; valerian; passion flower; chamomile (p.1417·1).
*Stress; vitamin B supplement.*

**Natures Way Hi B Plus C** *Roche Consumer, Austral.†.*
Vitamin B substances; ascorbic acid; minerals (p.1417·1).
*Vitamin B and C deficiency.*

**Natures Way Lifespan Antioxidant** *Roche Consumer, Austral.†.*
Multivitamin and mineral preparation (p.1417·1).

**Natures Way Mega B** *Roche Consumer, Austral.†.*
Vitamin B substances; ascorbic acid; minerals (p.1417·1).
*Vitamin B supplement.*

**Natures Way Mega Multi** *Roche Consumer, Austral.†.*
Multivitamin, mineral, and herbal preparation (p.1417·1).
*Dietary supplement; tonic.*

**Natures Way Omega 3** *Roche Consumer, Austral.†.*
Omega-3 marine triglycerides (p.976·2).
*Dietary fatty acid supplement.*

**Natures Way Omega 3 Complex** *Roche Consumer, Austral.†.*
Omega-3 marine triglycerides; lecithin; garlic oil (p.1417·1).
*Dietary supplement.*

**Natures Way Total C** *Roche Consumer, Austral.†.*
Ascorbic acid (p.1460·2); hesperidin (p.1688·2); rutoside (p.1688·2); bioflavonoids (p.1688·2).
*Cold and influenza symptoms.*

**Natures Way Total Calcium Plus** *Roche Consumer, Austral.†.*
Calcium carbonate (p.1254·2); colecalciferol (p.1461·3).
*Calcium and vitamin D supplement; osteoporosis.*

**Natures Way Total Zinc** *Roche Consumer, Austral.†.*
Zinc amino acid chelate (p.1469·3); vitamin A palmitate (p.1453·1); pyridoxine hydrochloride (p.1456·3); magnesium phosphate (p.1228·1); manganese amino acid chelate (p.1440·2).
*Skin disorders; wounds.*

**Natures Way Womens All-in-One** *Roche Consumer, Austral.†.*
Multivitamin and mineral preparation (p.1417·1).

**Naturest**
*Note. This name is used for preparations of different composition.*
*Vitaglow, Austral.†.*
Valerian (p.1762·2); passion flower (p.1729·1); skullcap (p.1746·3); vervain (p.1764·1); magnesium oxide (p.1272·3); calcium phosphate (p.1225·3).
*Insomnia.*

*Lane, UK.*
Passion flower (p.1729·1).
*Insomnia.*

**Naturetin**
*Squibb, Canad.†; Apothecon, USA.*
Bendroflumethiazide (p.867·3).
*Hypertension; oedema.*

**Naturetti** *Aventis, Mex.*
Senna (p.1288·2); cassia (p.1255·2); tamarind (p.1293·2); coriander (p.1676·1); liquorice (p.1270·2).
*Constipation.*

**Naturgen terre silice** *Marbot, Switz.†.*
Medicinal mud.
*Bronchitis; coughs; musculoskeletal and joint disorders; phlebitis.*

**Naturgen terre volcanique** *Marbot, Switz.†.*
Medicinal volcanic mud.
*Digestive-system disorders.*

**Naturine** *Leo, Fr.†.*
Bendroflumethiazide (p.867·3).
*Hypertension; oedema.*

**Naturland Entschlackungstee** *Strallhofer, Austria.*
Solidago virgaurea (p.1748·3); couch-grass (p.1676·2); taraxacum (p.1751·3); urtica (p.1762·1); hibiscus.
*Diuretic.*

**Naturland Entschlackungstonikum** *Strallhofer, Austria.*
Parsley (p.1728·3); birch leaf (p.1660·3); ononis (p.1723·3).
*Urinary-tract disorders.*

**Naturland Heilkrautermundwasser** *Strallhofer, Austria.*
Agrimony (p.1649·1); calendula (p.1665·2); clove (p.1673·2); cinnamon (p.1672·2); thyme (p.1755·2).
*Mouth and throat disorders; mouth hygiene.*

**Naturland Herz-Kreislauf** *Naturland, Austria.*
Crataegus (p.1677·1); rosemary (p.1740·2).
*Cardiovascular disorders.*

**Naturland Magentonikum** *Strallhofer, Austria.*
Angelica (p.1655·1); zedoary; gentian (p.1692·2); myrrh; manna; chamomile; peppermint leaf; menyanthes; cinnamon; agrimony; basil; origano; valerian; ginger; star anise; cardamom; cardo benedict; solidago virgaurea; galangal; bitter-orange peel; clove; mullen; cubeb; rosemary.
*Gastrointestinal disorders.*

**Naturland Rheuma Tee** *Strallhofer, Austria.*
Rosemary (p.1740·2); urtica (p.1762·1); equisetum (p.1684·1); taraxacum (p.1751·3); salix (p.87·3).
*Inflammation; pain.*

**Naturland Sportcreme** *Strallhofer, Austria.*
Camphor (p.1665·3); menthol (p.1711·3); rosemary oil (p.1740·2).
*Musculoskeletal, joint, and soft-tissue disorders.*

**Naturland Sportmassageol** *Strallhofer, Austria.*
Rosemary oil (p.1740·2); lavender oil (p.1705·2); menthol (p.1711·3).
*Musculoskeletal, joint, and soft-tissue disorders.*

**Naturland Verdauungs** *Strallhofer, Austria.*
Peppermint leaf (p.1283·2); gentian (p.1692·2); caraway (p.1667·2).
*Gastrointestinal disorders.*

**Naturlax** *Maver, Chile.*
*Jelly:* Senna (p.1288·2); liquorice (p.1270·2); plum.
*Tea:* Senna (p.1288·2).
*Constipation.*

**Naturogest** *German Remedies, India.*
Progesterone (p.1566·2).
*Premenstrual syndrome; puerperal depression.*

**Naturvite** *Solgar, UK†.*
Multivitamin and mineral preparation (p.1417·1).

**Natus Gerin** *Legrand, Braz.*
Multivitamin, mineral, and amino-acid preparation with ginseng (p.1417·1).

**Natusan** *Johnson & Johnson, Spain.*
Glyceroborate complex; boric acid (p.1662·1); borax (p.1661·3).
*Skin irritation.*

**Natuscap retard** *Vifor, Switz.*
Chlorphenamine maleate (p.427·3); codeine phosphate (p.27·1); phenylephrine hydrochloride (p.1126·3).
*Coughs and associated respiratory-tract disorders.*

**Natuscilin** *Natus, Braz.†.*
Ampicillin (p.157·1).
*Bacterial infections.*

**Natusgel** *Natus, Braz.†.*
*Oral suspension:* Aluminium hydroxide (p.1249·2).
*Tablets:* Aluminium hydroxide (p.1249·2); magnesium hydroxide (p.1272·2); calcium carbonate (p.1254·2).
*Gastrointestinal hyperacidity.*

**Natusor Aerofane** *Soria Natural, Spain.*
Pimpinella; fennel (p.1687·2); peppermint leaf (p.1283·2); caraway (p.1667·2); melissa (p.1711·1).
*Aerophagia; gastrointestinal spasm.*

**Natusor Artilane** *Soria Natural, Spain.*
Ash; urtica (p.1762·1); solidago (p.1748·3); equisetum (p.1684·1); betula alba (p.1660·3).
*Musculoskeletal and joint disorders.*

**Natusor Asmaten** *Soria Natural, Spain.*
Elecampane (p.1119·3); satureja montana; thyme (p.1755·2); hyssopus officinalis; marrubium (p.1124·1).
*Asthma.*

**Natusor Astringel** *Soria Natural, Spain.*
Lythrum salicaria; satureja hortensis; oak bark (p.1722·3); agrimony (p.1649·1); pimpinella; liquorice (p.1270·2).
*Diarrhoea.*

**Natusor Broncopul** *Soria Natural, Spain.*
Eucalyptus (p.1686·1); verbascum flower (p.1764·1); althaea (p.1651·3); elecampane (p.1119·3); marrubium (p.1124·1).
*Lower respiratory-tract infections.*

**Natusor Circusil** *Soria Natural, Spain.*
Cupressus sempervirens; juglans regia; achillea (p.1646·2).
*Haemorrhoids; phlebitis; varices.*

**Natusor Farinol** *Soria Natural, Spain.*
Agrimony (p.1649·1); althaea (p.1651·3); sage (p.1741·2); thyme (p.1755·2); plantago lanceolata (p.1738·2).
*Mouth and throat disorders.*

**Natusor Gastrolen** *Soria Natural, Spain.*
Liquorice (p.1270·2); plantago lanceolata (p.1738·2); althaea (p.1651·3); hypericum (p.299·1); achillea (p.1646·2).
*Gastritis; peptic ulcer.*

**Natusor Gripotul** *Soria Natural, Spain.*
Thyme (p.1755·2); tilia (p.1756·2); eucalyptus (p.1686·1); sambucus (p.1741·3).
*Catarrh; influenza symptoms; sore throat.*

**Natusor Harpagosinol** *Soria Natural, Spain.*
Devil's claw root (p.28·2); salix (p.87·3); equisetum (p.1684·1); meadowsweet (p.1710·1); peppermint flower (p.1283·2).
*Musculoskeletal and joint disorders.*

**Natusor Hepavesical** *Soria Natural, Spain.*
Cichorium intybus; rosemary (p.1740·2); fumitory (p.1690·1); centaury (p.1669·2); boldo (p.1661·2); greater celandine (p.1695·3); peppermint leaf (p.1283·2).
*Gallstones; liver disorders.*

**Natusor High Blood Pressure** *Soria Natural, Spain.*
Olive oil (p.1723·2); betula alba (p.1660·3); crataegus (p.1677·1).
*Hypertension.*

**Natusor Infenol** *Soria Natural, Spain.*
Red-rose petal (p.1058·1); equisetum (p.1684·1); juglans regia; thyme (p.1755·2); plantago lanceolata (p.1738·2).
*Vaginal irrigation; wounds.*

**Natusor Jaquesan** *Soria Natural, Spain.*
Salix (p.87·3); bitter orange (p.1723·3); melissa (p.1711·1); achillea (p.1646·2); tilia (p.1756·2).
*Headache; migraine.*

**Natusor Low Blood Pressure** *Soria Natural, Spain.*
Eleutherococcus senticosis (p.1744·1); rosemary (p.1740·2); satureja hortensis; liquorice (p.1270·2); sage (p.1741·2).
*Hypotension.*

**Natusor Malvasen** *Soria Natural, Spain.*
Senna (p.1288·2); althaea (p.1651·3); fennel (p.1687·2).
*Constipation.*

**Natusor Renal** *Soria Natural, Spain.*
Thyme (p.1755·2); meadowsweet (p.1710·1); equisetum (p.1684·1); betula alba (p.1660·3); solidago (p.1748·3); peppermint leaf (p.1283·2).
*Urinary-tract infections.*

**Natusor Sinulan** *Soria Natural, Spain.*
Thyme (p.1755·2); rosemary (p.1740·2); sambucus (p.1741·3); origanum majorana; tilia (p.1756·2).
*Catarrh.*

**Natusor Somnisedan** *Soria Natural, Spain.*
Valerian (p.1762·2); hypericum (p.299·1); tilia (p.1756·2); spike lavender (p.1749·2); crataegus (p.1677·1).
*Depression; insomnia; nervous disorders.*

**Natuvit**
*Roche Nicholas, Fr.†.*
Dietary fibre supplement (p.1417·1).

*Asta Medica, Neth.†.*
Nutritional supplement (p.1417·1).

**Natuzilium** *Teuto, Braz.*
Kava (p.1703·2).
*Anxiety.*

**Natyl** *Interdelta, Switz.†.*
Dipyridamole (p.903·1).
*Thromboembolism prophylaxis.*

**Naudicelle**
*Key, Austral.†; Swiss Herbal, Canad.†; Bio-Oil Research, Irl.; Bio-Oil Research, UK†.*
Evening primrose oil (p.1686·3).
*Dietary supplement.*

**Naudicelle Forte** *Bio-Oil Research, UK†.*
Borage oil (p.1661·3); marine fish oil (p.976·2).

**Naudicelle Marine** *Key, Austral.†.*
Evening primrose oil (p.1686·3); marine fish oil (p.976·2).
*Dietary supplement.*

**Naudicelle Plus** *Bio-Oil Research, UK†.*
Evening primrose oil (p.1686·3); marine fish oil (p.976·2).

**Naudicelle SL** *Bio-Oil Research, UK†.*
Salmon oil (p.976·1); lecithin (p.1706·1).

**Naudivite** *Bio-Oil Research, UK†.*
A range of vitamin, mineral, and nutritional supplements (p.1417·1).

**Naupathon** *Staufen, Ger.†.*
Homoeopathic preparation.

**Nausamine** *Sriprasit, Thai.*
Dimenhydrinate (p.431·1).
*Nausea; vomiting.*

**Nausea Relief** *Brauer, Austral.†.*
Homoeopathic preparation.

**Nauseatol** *Sabex, Canad.*
Dimenhydrinate (p.431·1).
*Nausea and vomiting.*

**Nausedron** *Cristalia, Braz.*
Ondansetron hydrochloride (p.1281·1).
*Nausea and vomiting.*

**Nausefe** *Inibsa, Port.*
Dicycloverine hydrochloride (p.481·2); doxylamine succinate (p.432·3); pyridoxine hydrochloride (p.1456·3).
*Nausea; vomiting.*

**Nausetum** *Ferrier, Fr.*
Homoeopathic preparation.

**Nausex**
*Asta Medica, Austria; Nobel, Canad.†.*
Dimenhydrinate (p.431·1).
*Ménière's disease; motion sickness; nausea and vomiting; vestibular disorders.*

**Nausicalm**
*Note. This name is used for preparations of different composition.*
*Uniao Quimica, Braz.*
Dimenhydrinate (p.431·1); pyridoxine hydrochloride (p.1456·3).
*Nausea and vomiting; vertigo.*

*Brothier, Fr.*
Dimenhydrinate (p.431·1).
*Motion sickness; vertigo.*

**Nausigon** *Mundipharma, Austria†.*
Metoclopramide hydrochloride (p.1274·3).
*Gastrointestinal ulcers; intractable hiccups; nausea and vomiting; upper gastrointestinal motility disorders.*

**Nausil**
*Hertz, Braz.†.*
Metoclopramide (p.1274·3).
*Nausea and vomiting.*

*Siam Bheasach, Thai.*
Metoclopramide hydrochloride (p.1274·3).
*Dyspepsia; flatulence; gastro-oesophageal reflux; nausea and vomiting; peptic ulcer.*

**Nausilen** *Baldacci, Ital.†.*
Alizapride hydrochloride (p.1248·1).
*Nausea and vomiting.*

**Nausilon B6** *Cifarma, Braz.†.*
Dimenhydrinate (p.431·1); pyridoxine hydrochloride (p.1456·3).
*Nausea and vomiting; vertigo.*

**Nausyn**
*Weleda, Austria; Weleda, UK.*
Homoeopathic preparation.

**Nautamine** *Sanofi Synthelabo OTC, Fr.*
Diphenhydramine di(acefyllinate) (p.431·3).
*Motion sickness.*

**Nautigo** *Bell, India.*
Domperidone (p.1263·2).
*Dyspepsia; nausea; vomiting.*

**Nautisol** *Medochemie, Malaysia.*
Prochlorperazine mesilate (p.716·3).
*Anxiety; mania; nausea and vomiting; psychoses; vertigo.*

**Nautrol** *Precimex, Mex.†.*
Difenidol (p.1261·1).

**Nauzelin** *Janssen-Cilag, Spain†.*
Domperidone (p.1263·2).
*Gastroparesis; nausea and vomiting.*

**Nauzine** *Be-Tabs, S.Afr.*
Cyclizine hydrochloride (p.429·3).
*Motion sickness; nausea and vomiting; vestibular disorders.*

**Navamed** *Greater Pharma, Thai.†.*
Dimenhydrinate (p.431·1).
*Motion sickness; nausea and vomiting.*

**Navamin** *Greater Pharma, Thai.*
Dimenhydrinate (p.431·1).
Formerly known as Navamine.
*Motion sickness; nausea and vomiting.*

**Navane**
*Pfizer, Austral.; Pfizer, Braz.†; Pfizer, Canad.; Pfizer, Hong Kong; Pfizer, Neth.; Pfizer, Thai.†; Pfizer, USA.*
Tiotixene (p.725·2) or tiotixene hydrochloride (p.725·2).
*Psychoses.*

**Navasprin** *Ache, Braz.†.*
Aspirin (p.15·1); ascorbic acid (p.1460·2).
*Fever; pain.*

**Navelbine**
*Pharmacia, Arg.; Pierre Fabre, Austral.; Boehringer Ingelheim, Austria; Pierre Fabre, Belg.; Asta Oncologia, Braz.; GlaxoSmithKline, Canad.; Asta Médica, Chile; Baxter, Chile; Pierre Fabre, Denm.; Pierre Fabre, Fin.; Pierre Fabre, Fr.; Pierre Fabre, Ger.; Pierre Fabre, Gr.; Pierre Fabre, Hong Kong; Orient, Hong Kong; Pierre Fabre, Israel; Pierre Fabre, Ital.; Pierre Fabre, Malaysia; Schering-Plough, Mex.; Pierre Fabre, Norw.; Asta Medica, NZ; NZ Medical & Scientific, NZ; Pierre Fabre, Port.; Tema, S.Afr.; Pierre Fabre, Singapore; Pierre Fabre, Spain; Pierre Fabre, Swed.; Robapharm, Switz.; Baxter, Thai.; Pierre Fabre, UK; Glaxo Wellcome, USA.*
Vinorelbine tartrate (p.594·1).
*Breast cancer; non-small cell lung cancer.*

**Navicalm**
*Note. This name is used for preparations of different composition.*
*UCB, Neth.*
Hydroxyzine hydrochloride (p.434·3).
*Anxiety; pruritus; urticaria.*

*Confar, Port.*
Meclozine (p.436·3).

*UCB, Spain.*
Meclozine hydrochloride (p.436·3).
*Motion sickness.*

**Navidoxine**
*UCB, Hong Kong; UCB, Malaysia; UCB, Singapore.*
Meclozine hydrochloride (p.436·3); pyridoxine hydrochloride (p.1456·3).
*Nausea and vomiting.*

**Navidrex**
*Novartis, NZ; Goldshield, UK.*
Cyclopenthiazide (p.890·3).
*Heart failure; hypertension; oedema.*

**Naviga** *Bittner, Austria.*
Homoeopathic preparation.

**Navispare**
*Novartis, Hong Kong; Novartis, Irl.†; Novartis, UK.*
Cyclopenthiazide (p.890·3); amiloride hydrochloride (p.858·2).
*Hypertension.*

**Navixen**
*Note. This name is used for preparations of different composition.*
*Mavi, Mex.†.*
Naproxen (p.65·1).

*Ferrer, Spain.*
Eprosartan mesilate (p.912·1).
*Hypertension.*

**Navoban**
*Novartis, Arg.; Novartis, Austral.; Novartis, Austria; Novartis, Braz.; Novartis, Chile; Novartis, Denm.; Novartis, Fin.; Novartis, Fr.; Novartis, Ger.; Novartis, Gr.; Novartis, Hong Kong; Novartis, Irl.†; Novartis, Israel; Novartis, Ital.; Novartis, Jpn; Novartis, Malaysia; Novartis, Mex.; Novartis, Norw.; Novartis, NZ; Novartis, Port.; Novartis, S.Afr.; Novartis, Spain; Novartis, Swed.; Novartis, Switz.; Novartis, Thai.; Novartis, UK.*
Tropisetron (p.1293·3) or tropisetron hydrochloride (p.1293·3).
*Nausea and vomiting induced by cytotoxic therapy; postoperative nausea and vomiting.*

**Naxan** *Hikma, Port.*
Naloxone hydrochloride (p.1044·3).

**Naxen**
*Altimed, Canad.; Syntex, Mex.; Douglas, NZ.*
Naproxen (p.65·1).
*Gout; musculoskeletal, joint, peri-articular, and soft-tissue disorders; pain.*

**Naxidine** *Lilly, Neth.†.*
Nizatidine (p.1277·2).
*Gastro-oesophageal reflux; peptic ulcer.*

**Naxil** *Galen, Mex.†.*
Naproxen (p.65·1).

**Naxilan-Plus** *Rayere, Mex.*
Nalidixic acid (p.234·1); phenazopyridine (p.83·2).
*Urinary-tract infections.*

**Naxo** *Sons, Mex.*
Chloramphenicol (p.185·1).
*Bacterial infections.*

**Naxo C** *Rontag, Arg.*
Fluconazole (p.398·1).
*Fungal infections.*

**Naxo TV** *Rontag, Arg.*
Metronidazole (p.607·2); nystatin (p.406·3); dexamethasone (p.1097·1); lidocaine (p.1377·3); neomycin sulfate (p.235·1).
*Vaginal infections.*

**Naxocina** *Rontag, Arg.*
Azithromycin (p.159·1).
*Bacterial infections.*

**Naxoclinda** *Rontag, Arg.*
Clindamycin phosphate (p.194·2).
*Vaginal infections.*

**Naxodol** *Syntex, Mex.*
Naproxen (p.65·1); carisoprodol (p.1392·1).
*Musculoskeletal, joint, and peri-articular disorders.*

**Naxogil** *Pharmacia Upjohn, Mex.†.*
Nimorazole (p.611·3).

**Naxogin**
*Rontag, Arg.; Pharmacia, Austria; Pharmacia, Belg.; Pharmacia, Braz.; Pharmacia, Chile; Pharmacia Upjohn, Hong Kong†; Pharmacia Upjohn, Thai.†.*
Nimorazole (p.611·3).
*Acute ulcerative gingivitis; amoebiasis; giardiasis; vaginal trichomoniasis.*

**Naxogin Compositum** *Pharmacia, Chile.*
Nimorazole (p.611·3); nystatin (p.406·3); chloramphenicol (p.185·1).
*Vaginal infections.*

**Naxogin Composto** *Pharmacia, Braz.*
Nimorazole (p.611·3); chloramphenicol (p.185·1); nystatin (p.406·3).
*Vulvovaginal infections.*

**Naxogin Dos** *Pharmacia, Chile.*
Nimorazole (p.611·3); nystatin (p.406·3).
*Vaginal infections.*

**Naxogyn** *Pharmacia, Fr.†.*
Nimorazole (p.611·3).
*Trichomoniasis.*

**Naxolan** *Faulding, Port.*
Naloxone hydrochloride (p.1044·3).

**Naxopren** *Pharmacia, Fin.*
Naproxen (p.65·1).
*Fever; gout; inflammation; musculoskeletal and joint disorders; pain.*

**Naxpa** *Novag, Spain.*
Ambroxol hydrochloride (p.1114·3).
*Respiratory-tract disorders.*

**Naxy** *Sanofi Synthelabo, Fr.*
Clarithromycin (p.192·2).
*Bacterial infections.*

**Naxyn** *Teva, Israel.*
Naproxen (p.65·1).
*Dysmenorrhoea; gout; musculoskeletal, joint, and peri-articular disorders.*

**Nazalet** *Stanley, Israel.*
Xylometazoline hydrochloride (p.1132·2).
*Nasal congestion.*

**Nazalin** *Bell, India.*
Naphazoline hydrochloride (p.1124·3); phenylephrine hydrochloride (p.1126·3); sulfacetamide sodium (p.257·3).
*Nasal congestion.*

**Nazamit** *Mintlab, Chile.*
Phenazopyridine hydrochloride (p.83·1).
*Urinary-tract pain.*

**Nazene** *Restan, S.Afr.*
Oxymetazoline hydrochloride (p.1126·1); zinc sulfate (p.1469·3).
*Allergic rhinitis; nasal congestion; sinusitis.*

**Nazicol** *Kinder, Braz.*
Naphazoline hydrochloride (p.1124·3).
*Nasal congestion.*

**Nazobel** *Sedabel, Braz.*
Naphazoline (p.1124·3); neomycin (p.235·1).
*Nasal disorders.*

**Nazobio** *Luper, Braz.*
Naphazoline hydrochloride (p.1124·3); panthenol (p.1727·2).
*Nasal congestion.*

**Nazodin** *Vitamed, Israel.*
Naphazoline hydrochloride (p.1124·3); diphenhydramine hydrochloride (p.431·3); neomycin sulfate (p.235·1).
*Allergic rhinitis; nasal congestion.*

**Nazolfarm** *Continentales, Mex.†.*
Ketoconazole (p.403·3).

**Nazolin** *Beximco, Singapore.*
Oxymetazoline hydrochloride (p.1126·1).
*Nasal congestion.*

**Nazophyl** *Medecine Vegetale, Fr.†.*
Eucalyptus oil (p.1686·2); pine oil.
*Nose and throat infections.*

**Nazosoro** *Sedabel, Braz.*
Sodium chloride (p.1233·3).
*Nasal Congestion.*

**Nazotiran** *Gilton, Braz.†.*
Naphazoline (p.1124·3); thiomersal (p.1194·1).
*Nasal congestion.*

**N-Combur Test** *Roche Diagnostics, Austral.*
Test for nitrite, protein, glucose, and pH in urine.

**ND-Gesic** *Hyrex, USA.*
Phenylephrine hydrochloride (p.1126·3); paracetamol (p.76·2); chlorphenamine maleate (p.427·3); mepyramine maleate (p.437·1).
*Upper respiratory-tract symptoms.*

**Nealorin**
*Probios, Port.†; Prasfarma, Spain.*
Carboplatin (p.533·3).
*Malignant neoplasms.*

**Neat Effect** *Neat Feat, NZ.*
Aluminium chlorohydrate (p.1142·1).
*Hyperhidrosis.*

**Neat Feat** *Neat Feat, NZ.*
Aluminium chlorohydrate (p.1142·1).
*Hyperhidrosis.*

**Neat One** *Neat Feat, NZ.*
Aluminium-zirconium tetrachlorohydrex glycine (p.1142·1).
*Hyperhidrosis.*

**Neat Touch** *Neat Feat, NZ.*
Aluminium chlorohydrate (p.1142·1).
*Hyperhidrosis.*

**Neatenol** *Fides Ecopharma, Spain.*
Atenolol (p.865·2).
*Angina pectoris; arrhythmias; hypertension; myocardial infarction.*

**Neatenol Diu** *Fides Ecopharma, Spain.*
Bendroflumethiazide (p.867·3); atenolol (p.865·2).
*Hypertension.*

**Neatenol Diuvas** *Fides Ecopharma, Spain.*
Bendroflumethiazide (p.867·3); hydralazine hydrochloride (p.931·2); atenolol (p.865·2).
*Hypertension.*

**Nebacetin**
*Tyrol, Austria; Altana, Braz.; Yamanouchi, Ger.; Altana, Hong Kong; Eumedica, Switz.*
Neomycin sulfate (p.235·1); bacitracin (p.161·3) or bacitracin zinc (p.161·3).
*Bacterial infections.*

**Nebacetin N** *Yamanouchi, Ger.*
Neomycin sulfate (p.235·1).
*Burns; skin infections; wounds.*

**Nebacetina** *Byk Gulden, Mex.*
Neomycin sulfate (p.235·1); bacitracin (p.161·3).
*Bacterial skin infections; infected burns, wounds, and ulcers.*

**Nebacina** *Neovita, Braz.†.*
Neomycin sulfate (p.235·1); bacitracin (p.161·3).
*Bacterial skin infections.*

**Nebacitrin** *Neo Quimica, Braz.*
Bacitracin zinc (p.161·3); neomycin sulfate (p.235·1).
*Skin infections.*

**Nebal** *Reuffer, Mex.†.*
Hydroxocobalamin (p.1458·2).

**Nebalon** *Sinterapico, Braz.†.*
Neomycin sulfate (p.235·1); bacitracin (p.161·3).
*Bacterial skin infections.*

**Nebapol B** *Galderma, Arg.*
Neomycin sulfate (p.235·1); bacitracin zinc (p.161·3); polymyxin B sulfate (p.245·1).
*Burns; skin, nose, and ear infections; wounds.*

**Nebapul** *Royal, Chile.*
Methylphenidate hydrochloride (p.1590·2).
*Attention-deficit hyperactivity disorder; narcoleptic syndrome.*

**Nebasulf** *Omni-Protech, India.*
Neomycin sulfate (p.235·1); bacitracin (p.161·3); sulfacetamide (p.257·3) or sulfacetamide sodium (p.257·3).
*Bacterial skin infections.*

**Nebcin**
*Lilly, Austral.; Lilly, Canad.; Pharmaserve Lilly (Φαρμασερβ Λιλλυ), Gr.; Lilly, Hong Kong; Lilly, Irl.; Lilly, Israel; Lilly, NZ; Aspen Consumer, S.Afr.; King, UK; Lilly, USA.*
Tobramycin sulfate (p.271·3).
*Bacterial infections.*

**Nebcina**
*Lilly, Denm.; Lilly, Fin.; Lilly, Norw.; Lilly, Swed.*
Tobramycin sulfate (p.271·3).
*Bacterial infections.*

**Nebcine** *Lilly, Fr.*
Tobramycin sulfate (p.271·3).
*Bacterial infections.*

**Nebicina** *Lilly, Ital.*
Tobramycin sulfate (p.271·3).
*Bacterial infections.*

**Nebilet**
*Menarini, Arg.; Berlin-Chemie, Ger.; Menarini, Irl.; Menarini, Neth.; Menarini, Port.; Menarini, Singapore; Menarini, Switz.; Menarini, UK.*
Nebivolol hydrochloride (p.964·3).
*Hypertension.*

**Nebilox** *Lusofarmaco, Ital.*
Nebivolol hydrochloride (p.964·3).
*Hypertension.*

**Nebiotin** *CGM, Ital.*
Biotin (p.1423·2).
*Biotin deficiency.*

**Neblic** *Lazar, Arg.*
Azithromycin (p.159·1).
*Bacterial infections.*

**Neblik** *Yamanouchi, Spain.*
Formoterol fumarate (p.786·1).
*Obstructive airways disease.*

**Nebril** *Montpellier, Arg.*
Desipramine dibudinate (p.290·2) or desipramine hydrochloride (p.290·2).
*Depression; pain.*

**Nebris** *Celafar, Ital.†.*
Olax dissitiflora; chamomile (p.1669·3).
*Dry skin.*

**Nebufur** *Fabra, Arg.*
Bezafibrate (p.873·2).
*Hyperlipidaemias.*

**Nebulasma** *Urbion, Spain.*
Sodium cromoglicate (p.795·3).
*Asthma; bronchospasm.*

**Nebulcort** *Italchimici, Ital.*
Flunisolide (p.1101·1).
*Allergic rhinitis; asthma; bronchitis.*

**Nebulcrom** *Aventis, Spain.*
Sodium cromoglicate (p.795·3).
*Asthma; bronchospasm.*

**Nebulicina**
*Note. This name is used for preparations of different composition.*
*Boehringer Ingelheim, Arg.*
Fenoxazoline hydrochloride (p.1121·3).
*Nasal congestion.*

*Fher, Spain.*
Oxymetazoline hydrochloride (p.1126·1).
Formerly contained fenoxazoline hydrochloride.
*Nasal congestion.*

**NebuPent** *American Pharmaceutical, USA.*
Pentamidine isetionate (p.613·2).
*Pneumocystis carinii pneumonia.*

**NEC** *Piam, Ital.*
Protein-free preparation for enteral nutrition (p.1417·1).
*Renal disease.*

**Necamin** *Ache, Braz.*
Mebendazole (p.108·2).
*Worm infections.*

**Necid** *New Research, Ital.*
Cefonicid sodium (p.174·2).
Lidocaine hydrochloride (p.1377·3) is included in this preparation to alleviate the pain of injection.
*Gram-negative bacterial infections.*

**Necloral** *New Research, Ital.*
Cefaclor (p.167·1).
*Bacterial infections.*

**Neclovir** *New Research, Ital.*
Aciclovir (p.626·1).
*Herpesvirus infections.*

**Necon 0.5/35, 1/35** *Watson, USA.*
Norethisterone (p.1562·2); ethinylestradiol (p.1553·2).
28-Day packs also contain 7 inert tablets.
*Combined oral contraceptive.*

**Necon 1/50** *Watson, USA.*
Norethisterone (p.1562·2); mestranol (p.1559·2).
28-Day packs also contain 7 inert tablets.
*Combined oral contraceptive.*

**Necon 10/11** *Watson, USA.*
Norethisterone (p.1562·2); ethinylestradiol (p.1553·2).
28-Day packs also contain 7 inert tablets.
*Biphasic oral contraceptive.*

**Necopen** *Esteve, Spain.*
Cefixime (p.172·3).
*Bacterial infections.*

**Necro B-6** *Bunker, Braz.*
Adenosine (p.851·2); methionine (p.1042·1); betaine (p.1660·1); choline citrate (p.1424·3); pyridoxine hydrochloride (p.1456·3).
*Liver disorders.*

**Necrohepat** *Heralds, Braz.†.*
Methionine (p.1042·1); betaine tartrate (p.1660·2); choline (p.1424·3); inositol (p.1701·2); nicotinamide (p.1441·2); cynara (p.1678·3); liver extract.
*Liver disorders.*

**Necroplex** *Heralds, Braz.†.*
Citrulline (p.1425·2); ornithine (p.1442·3); arginine (p.1421·1); oxypurines.
*Liver disorders.*

**Necta C** *Maver, Chile.*
Sodium ascorbate (p.1460·2).
*Vitamin C supplement.*

**Necyrane** *Celltech, Fr.*
Ritiometan magnesium (p.1191·3).
*Nose and throat infections.*

**Neda Fruchtewurfel**
*Note. This name is used for preparations of different composition.*
*Novartis Consumer, Austria.*
Senna (p.1288·2); fig (p.1266·3); tamarind (p.1293·2).
*Constipation.*

*Novartis Consumer, Ger.*
Senna (p.1288·2).
*Constipation.*

**Neda Lactiv Importal** *Novartis Consumer, Ger.†.*
Lactitol (p.1269·1).
*Constipation.*

**Nedax** *Stiefel, Braz.*
Permethrin (p.1508·3).
*Pediculosis; scabies.*

**Nedax Plus** *Stiefel, Braz.*
Permethrin (p.1508·3).
*Pediculosis; scabies.*

**Nedeltran** *Aventis, Neth.*
Alimemazine tartrate (p.423·3).
*Hypersensitivity reactions; psychoses.*

**Nedios** *Byk, Neth.*
Acipimox (p.851·1).
*Hyperlipidaemias.*

**Nedis** *Omega, Arg.*
Miconazole nitrate (p.405·3).
*Vulvovaginal infections.*

**Nedolon P** *Merck, Ger.*
Paracetamol (p.76·2); codeine phosphate (p.27·1).
*Pain.*

**NEE 1/35** *Lexis, USA.*
Ethinylestradiol (p.1553·2); norethisterone (p.1562·2).
28-Day packs also contain 7 inert tablets.
*Combined oral contraceptive.*

**Nefadar**
*Bristol-Myers Squibb, Denm.†; Bristol-Myers Squibb, Fin.†; Bristol-Myers Squibb, Ger.†; Hormosan, Ger.†; Bristol-Myers Squibb, Norw.†; Bristol-Myers Squibb, Swed.†; Bristol-Myers Squibb, Switz.†.*
Nefazodone hydrochloride (p.309·2).
*Depression.*

**Nefadol** *Zilliken, Ital.†.*
Nefopam hydrochloride (p.66·2).
*Pain.*

**Nefam** *Kedrion, Ital.*
Nefopam hydrochloride (p.66·2).
*Pain.*

**Nefazan** *Phoenix, Arg.*
Clopidogrel bisulfate (p.888·3).
*Atherosclerosis.*

**Nefazol** *New Research, Ital.*
Cefazolin sodium (p.170·3).
Lidocaine hydrochloride (p.1377·3) is included in this preparation to alleviate the pain of injection.
*Bacterial infections.*

**Nefelid** *Vilco, Gr.*
Nifedipine (p.966·2).
*Angina; hypertension.*

**Nefersil** *Pharma Investi, Chile.*
Clonixin lysine (p.26·3).
*Pain.*

**Nefersil B** *Pharma Investi, Chile.*
Clonixin lysine (p.26·3); thiamine hydrochloride (p.1455·1) or thiamine nitrate (p.1455·1); pyridoxine hydrochloride (p.1456·3); cyanocobalamin (p.1458·2) or hydroxocobalamin acetate (p.1458·2).
*Musculoskeletal, joint, and peri-articular disorders; neuralgia; neuritis.*

**Nefirel** *Bristol-Myers Squibb, Gr.†.*
Nefazodone hydrochloride (p.309·2).
*Depression.*

**Nefluan** *Molteni, Ital.*
Lidocaine hydrochloride (p.1377·3); neomycin sulfate (p.235·1); fluocinolone acetonide (p.1101·2).
*Endoscopy.*

**Nefoben** *Armstrong, Arg.*
Theophylline (p.798·3).
*Obstructive airways disease.*

**Nefrin** *Geyer, Braz.*
Adrenaline (p.852·2).

**Nefro Diet** *Support, Braz.*
Preparation for enteral nutrition in renal disease (p.1417·1).

**Nefroamino** *Braun, Chile.*
Amino-acid infusion (p.1417·1).
*Parenteral nutrition in renal failure.*

**Nefrocarnit** *Medice, Ger.*
Levocarnitine (p.1423·3).
*Carnitine deficiency.*

**Nefrodial** *Abbott, Braz.*
Preparation for enteral nutrition (p.1417·1).

**Nefrolactona** *Vedim, Port.*
Spironolactone (p.1003·1).
*Hepatic cirrhosis; hyperaldosteronism; hypertension of pregnancy; hypokalaemia; hypomagnesaemia; oedema.*

**Nefroplasmal** *Braun, Port.*
Amino-acid infusion (p.1417·1).
*Parenteral nutrition in renal failure.*

**Nefrosol** *Glicolabor, Braz.†.*
Sodium chloride (p.1233·3).
*Haemodialysis.*

**Nefro-Zinc** *Medice, Ger.*
Zinc chloride (p.1469·2).
*Zinc deficiency in dialysis patients.*

**Nefryl** *Armstrong, Mex.*
Oxybutynin hydrochloride (p.486·3).
*Bladder instability.*

**Negaban** *Bournonville, Belg.*
Temocillin sodium (p.266·1).
*Gram-negative bacterial infections.*

**Negacef** *Julphar, UAE.*
Ceftazidime (p.180·2).
*Bacterial infections.*

**Negacne** *Wierhom, Arg.*
Salicylic acid (p.1157·1); glycolic acid (p.1147·3); zinc sulfate (p.1469·3); coltsfoot (p.1117·2); aloe vera (p.1141·3).
*Acne.*

**Negadix** *CFL, India.*
Nalidixic acid (p.234·1).
*Urinary-tract infections.*

**Negalerg** *ICN, Arg.*
Betamethasone (p.1093·1); loratadine (p.436·1).
*Hypersensitivity reactions.*

**Negalerg L** *ICN, Arg.*
Loratadine (p.436·1).
*Allergic rhinitis; urticaria.*

**Negaporosis** *Bajer, Arg.*
Calcium carbonate (p.1254·2); sodium monofluorophosphate (p.1446·2).
*Osteoporosis.*

**Negatol**
*Byk, Fr.; Byk Gulden, Ital.; Juventus, Spain†; Altana, Switz.*
Metacresolsulfonic acid-formaldehyde (p.756·1).
*Burns; chilblains; furunculosis; gynaecological disorders; minor haemorrhage; ulcers; vaginitis; wounds.*

**Negatol Dental** *Wild, Switz.*
Metacresolsulfonic acid-formaldehyde (p.756·1).
*Aphthous stomatitis; gingival haemorrhage.*

**Negazole** *Julphar, UAE.*
Metronidazole (p.607·2) or metronidazole benzoate (p.607·2).
*Anaerobic bacterial infections; bacterial vaginosis; dracunculiasis; inflammatory bowel disease; protozoal infections.*

**NegGram**
*Sanofi Synthelabo, Canad.; Sanofi Winthrop, Israel; Sanofi Synthelabo, Ital.; Sanofi Winthrop, USA.*
Nalidixic acid (p.234·1).
*Gram-negative urinary-tract infections.*

**Negram**
*Sanofi Synthelabo, Austral.†; Sanofi Winthrop, Denm.†; Sanofi Synthelabo, Fr.; Sanofi Synthelabo, Irl.; Sanofi Winthrop, Norw.†; Sanofi Winthrop, NZ†; Sanofi Synthelabo, UK.*
Nalidixic acid (p.234·1).
*Gram-negative urinary- and gastrointestinal-tract infections.*

**Nehydrin** *Sanochemia, Austria.*
Dihydroergocristine mesilate (p.1680·1).
*Cerebrovascular disorders.*

**Nehydrin N** *TAD, Ger.†.*
Co-dergocrine mesilate (p.1674·1).
*Mental function disorders.*

**NeisVac** *Baxter, Fr.*
A meningococcal group C conjugate vaccine (p.1626·1).
*Active immunisation.*

**NeisVac-C**
*Baxter, Austral.; Baxter, Denm.; Baxter, Fin.; Baxter, Ger.; Baxter, Gr.; Baxter, Ital.; Baxter, Spain; Baxter, Swed.; Baxter BioScience, UK.*
A meningococcal group C conjugate vaccine (tetanus toxoid protein conjugate) (p.1626·1).
*Active immunisation.*

**Nekacin** *New Research, Ital.*
Amikacin sulfate (p.154·1).
*Gram-negative bacterial infections.*

**Nelapine** *Berlin Pharm, Thai.*
Nifedipine (p.966·2).
*Cardiac disorders; hypertension.*

**Nelbinex** *Pharmaten (Φαρματεν), Gr.*
Nimodipine (p.972·3).
*Neurological deficit following subarachnoid haemorrhage.*

**Nelconil** *Pharmaten (Φαρματεν), Gr.*
Nitrendipine (p.973·3).
*Hypertension.*

**Nelex**
*Byk Gulden, Denm.†; Meda, Fin.†; Byk, Port.; Byk Madaus, S.Afr.; Pharmacia Upjohn, Swed.†.*
Metacresolsulfonic acid-formaldehyde (p.756·1).
*Anogenital warts; burns; gynaecological disorders; haemorrhage.*

**Nelfilea** *Elea, Arg.*
Nelfinavir (p.650·1).
*HIV infection.*

**Nelfir** *Eurofarma, Braz.†.*
Nelfinavir mesilate (p.650·1).
*HIV infection.*

**Nelin** *Biolab, Thai.*
Netilmicin sulfate (p.236·3).
*Bacterial infections.*

**Nelova 10/11** *Warner Chilcott, USA†.*
Norethisterone (p.1562·2); ethinylestradiol (p.1553·2).
28-Day packs also contain 7 inert tablets.
*Biphasic oral contraceptive.*

**Nelova 0.5/35E and 1/35E** *Warner Chilcott, USA†.*
Norethisterone (p.1562·2); ethinylestradiol (p.1553·2).
28-Day packs also contain 7 inert tablets.
*Combined oral contraceptive.*

**Nelova 1/50M** *Warner Chilcott, USA†.*
Norethisterone (p.1562·2); mestranol (p.1559·2).
28-Day packs also contain 7 inert tablets.
*Combined oral contraceptive.*

**Nelsons Clikpak Series** *Nelson, UK.*
A range of homoeopathic remedies.

**Nemactil** *Aventis, Spain.*
Pericyazine (p.714·1).
*Anxiety; behaviour disorders; psychoses.*

**Nemapres** *Precimex, Mex.†.*
Mebendazole (p.108·2).

**Nemasol** *ICN, Canad.*
Sodium aminosalicylate (p.155·1).
*Tuberculosis.*

**Nemasole** *Janssen-Cilag, Arg.*
Mebendazole (p.108·2).
*Worm infections.*

**Nembutal**
*Abbott, Canad.; Abbott, Hong Kong; Abbott, Thai.; Ovation, USA.*
Pentobarbital sodium (p.713·3).
*Epilepsy; insomnia; premedication; sedative.*

**Nemdyn** *Hamilton, Austral.*
Neomycin undecylenate (p.235·2); bacitracin zinc (p.161·3).
*Fungal or bacterial ear infections.*

**Nemegel** *Medica, Arg.*
Sulfur (p.1158·2); resorcinol (p.1156·3); zinc oxide (p.1163·2); vitamin A palmitate (p.1453·1).
*Acne.*

**Nemesil** *Sanofi Synthelabo, Braz.†.*
Ketotifen fumarate (p.788·1).
*Allergic conjunctivitis; allergic rhinitis; asthma; urticaria.*

**Nemestran**
*Aventis, Arg.; Aventis, Mex.; Aventis, Neth.; Aventis, Spain; Aventis, Switz.*
Gestrinone (p.1556·2).
*Endometriosis.*

**Nemexin**
*Torrex, Austria; Bristol-Myers Squibb, Ger.; Du Pont, Switz.*
Naltrexone hydrochloride (p.1046·1).
*Opioid withdrawal.*

**Nemicina** *Bunker, Braz.*
Neomycin sulfate (p.235·1).
*Bacterial skin infections.*

**Nemocebral** *Armstrong, Arg.*
Idebenone (p.1700·3).
*Alzheimer's disease.*

**Nemocid** *Mexin, India.*
Pyrantel embonate (p.113·2).
*Worm infections.*

**Nemodine**
*Note. This name is used for preparations of different composition.*
*Diffucap, Braz.*
Amlodipine besilate (p.862·1).
*Angina pectoris; hypertension.*

*Kener, Mex.†.*
Ketotifen (p.788·2).

**Nemozole** *Ipca, India.*
Albendazole (p.101·2).
*Hydatid cyst; worm infections.*

**Nene Dent**
*Note. This name is used for preparations of different composition.*
*Byk, Arg.*
Benzocaine (p.1370·3); ethacridine lactate (p.1165·3); acriflavinium chloride (p.1165·3).
*Mouth disorders.*

*Byk Gulden, Mex.*
Lidocaine (p.1377·3); lauromacrogol 400 (p.1412·3).
*Local anaesthesia.*

**Nene Dent N** *Altana, Braz.*
Lidocaine hydrochloride (p.1377·3); lauromacrogol 400 (p.1412·3); chamomile (p.1669·3).
Nene Dent contained butoxycaine hydrochloride, benzocaine, ethacridine lactate, acriflavinium chloride, myrrh, chamomile, and menthol.
*Teething disorders.*

**Nene-Lax** *Dentinox, Ger.*
Glycerol (p.1694·3).
*Bowel evacuation; constipation.*

**Neo Analsona** *Casen Fleet, Spain.*
Benzocaine (p.1370·3); fluocinolone acetonide (p.1101·2); neomycin (p.235·1); ruscogenin (p.1741·1).
*Anorectal disorders.*

**Neo Aritmina** *Solvay, Ital.†.*
Prajmalium bitartrate (p.984·3).
*Arrhythmias.*

**Neo Artrol** *Recordati, Spain.*
Flurbiprofen (p.43·3).
*Inflammation; musculoskeletal, joint, and peri-articular disorders; pain.*

**Neo Atromid** *Zeneca, Spain†.*
Clofibrate (p.884·3).
*Hyperlipidaemias.*

**Neo A-V** *Neo Dermos, Arg.*
Salicylic acid (p.1157·1).
*Astringent.*

**Neo Axedil** *Norma (Νορμα), Gr.*
Piroxicam (p.84·2).
*Dysmenorrhoea; gout; inflammation; musculoskeletal and joint disorders; pain.*

**Neo Baby Cream** *Neo Laboratories, UK.*
Cetrimide (p.1172·1); benzalkonium chloride (p.1168·3).
*Nappy rash; skin irritation.*

**Neo Bace** *Pharmavite, Canad.†.*
Bacitracin (p.161·3); polymyxin B sulfate (p.245·1).

**Neo Bacitrin** *Fides Ecopharma, Spain.*
*Ointment:* Bacitracin (p.161·3); neomycin sulfate (p.235·1); zinc oxide (p.1163·2).
*Topical powder:* Bacitracin (p.161·3); neomycin sulfate (p.235·1).
*Burns; skin infections; ulcers; wounds.*

**Neo Bacitrin Hidrocortis** *Fides Ecopharma, Spain†.*
Bacitracin (p.161·3); hydrocortisone acetate (p.1103·3); neomycin sulfate (p.235·1); zinc oxide (p.1163·2).
*Infected skin disorders.*

**Neo Bendazol** *Neo Quimica, Braz.*
Albendazole (p.101·2).

**Neo Benzil** *Neo Quimica, Braz.*
Benzathine benzylpenicillin (p.162·3).
*Bacterial infections.*

**Neo Borocillina** *Wassermann, Ital.*
Dichlorobenzyl alcohol (p.1178·3); sodium benzoate (p.1169·3).
*Mouth and throat disinfection.*

**Neo Borocillina Balsamica** *Wassermann, Ital.*
Dichlorobenzyl alcohol (p.1178·3); terpin hydrate (p.1131·1); menglytate (p.1124·2).
*Mouth and throat disinfection; respiratory-tract infections.*

**Neo Borocillina C** *Wassermann, Ital.*
Dichlorobenzyl alcohol (p.1178·3); ascorbic acid (p.1460·2).
*Mouth and throat disinfection.*

**Neo Borocillina Collutorio** *Wassermann, Ital.*
Dichlorobenzyl alcohol (p.1178·3).
*Mouth and throat disinfection.*

**Neo Borocillina Spray** *Wassermann, Ital.*
Dichlorobenzyl alcohol (p.1178·3).
*Mouth and throat disinfection.*

**Neo Borocillina Tosse Compresse** *Wassermann, Ital.*
Dextromethorphan hydrobromide (p.1117·3); dichlorobenzyl alcohol (p.1178·3).
Formerly contained dextromethorphan hydrobromide, guaifenesin, menglytate, and dichlorobenzyl alcohol.
*Coughs; mouth and throat disinfection.*

**Neo Borocillina Tosse Sciroppo** *Wassermann, Ital.*
Dextromethorphan hydrobromide (p.1117·3).
Formerly contained dextromethorphan hydrobromide, guaifenesin, and menglytate.
*Coughs.*

**Neo Butartrol** *Instituto Sanitas, Chile.*
Ibuprofen (p.45·3); dipyrone (p.35·3); chlormezanone (p.675·1).
*Headache; musculoskeletal and joint disorders.*

**Neo Butazol** *Neo Quimica, Braz.*
Phenylbutazone calcium (p.84·1).

**Neo Cal** *Neolab, Canad.*
Calcium carbonate (p.1254·2).

**Neo Cal D** *Neolab, Canad.*
Calcium carbonate (p.1254·2); vitamin D (p.1461·2).

**Neo Carbone Belloc** *Vaillant, Ital.†.*
Activated charcoal (p.1030·2).
*Diarrhoea; flatulence.*

**Neo Cardiol** *Francia, Ital.*
Levocarnitine (p.1423·3).
*Carnitine deficiency; myocardial ischaemia.*

**Neo Cebetil** *Uniao Quimica, Braz.*
Vitamin B substances with vitamin C and fructose (p.1417·1).

**Neo Cefadril** *Neo Quimica, Braz.*
Cefadroxil (p.167·2).
*Bacterial infections.*

**Neo Cefix** *Neo Quimica, Braz.*
Cefixime (p.172·3).
*Bacterial infections.*

**Neo Ceflex** *Neo Quimica, Braz.*
Cefalexin (p.168·1).
*Bacterial infections.*

**Neo Cepacol Collutorio** *Lepetit, Ital.†.*
Cetylpyridinium chloride (p.1173·1); sodium phosphate; sodium diphosphate; disodium edetate; methyl salicylate; cineole; cinnamon oil; mint oil; menthol.
*Dental plaque prevention; mouth and throat disinfection.*

**Neo Cepacol Pastiglie** *Aventis, Ital.*
Cetylpyridinium chloride (p.1173·1).
*Mouth and throat disinfection.*

**Neo Citran**
*Novartis, Austria; Novartis Consumer, Canad.*
Paracetamol (p.76·2); pheniramine maleate (p.438·3); phenylephrine hydrochloride (p.1126·3); ascorbic acid (p.1460·2).
*Cold and influenza symptoms.*

**Neo Citran A** *Novartis Consumer, Canad.*
Phenylephrine hydrochloride (p.1126·3); pheniramine maleate (p.438·3); ascorbic acid (p.1460·2).

**Neo Citran Calorie Reduced** *Novartis Consumer, Canad.*
Phenylephrine hydrochloride (p.1126·3); pheniramine maleate (p.438·3); paracetamol (p.76·2).
Formerly known as Neo Citran Nutrasweet.

**Neo Citran Chest Congestion & Cough** *Novartis Consumer, Canad.*
Pseudoephedrine hydrochloride (p.1129·2); dextromethorphan hydrobromide (p.1117·3); guaifenesin (p.1122·1); paracetamol (p.76·2).

**Neo Citran Cough Cold & Flu** *Novartis Consumer, Canad.*
Pseudoephedrine hydrochloride (p.1129·2); chlorphenamine maleate (p.427·3); dextromethorphan hydrobromide (p.1117·3); paracetamol (p.76·2).

**Neo Citran Daycaps** *Sandoz, Canad.†.*
Pseudoephedrine hydrochloride (p.1129·2); dextromethorphan hydrobromide (p.1117·3); paracetamol (p.76·2).

**Neo Citran DM** *Novartis Consumer, Canad.*
Phenylephrine hydrochloride (p.1126·3); pheniramine maleate (p.438·3); dextromethorphan hydrobromide (p.1117·3).

**Neo Citran Extra Strength** *Novartis Consumer, Canad.*
Phenylephrine hydrochloride (p.1126·3); pheniramine maleate (p.438·3); paracetamol (p.76·2).

**Neo Citran Grippe/refroidissement** *Novartis Consumer, Switz.*
Paracetamol (p.76·2); pheniramine maleate (p.438·3); phenylephrine hydrochloride (p.1126·3); ascorbic acid (p.1460·2).
*Cold symptoms.*

**Neo Citran Sinus** *Novartis Consumer, Canad.*
Phenylephrine hydrochloride (p.1126·3); paracetamol (p.76·2).

**Neo Citran Sore Throat & Cough** *Novartis Consumer, Canad.*
Pseudoephedrine hydrochloride (p.1129·2); chlorphenamine maleate (p.427·3); dextromethorphan hydrobromide (p.1117·3); paracetamol (p.76·2).

**Neo Clodil** *Neo Quimica, Braz.*
Clonidine hydrochloride (p.885·2).
*Hypertension.*

**Neo Clotrimazyl** *Neo Quimica, Braz.*
Clotrimazole (p.396·2).
*Fungal infections.*

**Neo Coltirot** *Roux-Ocefa, Arg.*
*Lozenges:* Neomycin sulfate (p.235·1); gramicidin (p.220·2); benzocaine (p.1370·3).
*Topical spray:* Neomycin sulfate (p.235·1); gramicidin (p.220·2); benzalkonium chloride (p.1168·3); benzocaine (p.1370·3).
*Mouth and throat disorders.*

**Neo Coricidin** *Schering-Plough, Ital.*
Chlorphenamine maleate (p.427·3); aspirin (p.15·1); caffeine (p.782·1).
*Cold symptoms.*

**Neo Coricidin Gola** *Schering-Plough, Ital.*
Cetylpyridinium chloride (p.1173·1).
*Mouth and throat disinfection.*

**Neo Cortofen** *Biodue, Ital.*
Dexamethasone (p.1097·1); neomycin sulfate (p.235·1).
*Eczema; nasal mucosal inflammation; otitis externa; rhinitis.*

**Neo Decabutin** *Inkeysa, Spain.*
Indometacin (p.47·3).
*Gout; inflammation; musculoskeletal, joint, and peri-articular disorders; pain.*

**Neo Decapeptyl** *Ache, Braz.*
Triptorelin (p.1341·2).
*Prostatic cancer.*

**Neo Dohyfral** *Solvay, Neth.†.*
Colecalciferol (p.1461·3).
*Vitamin D deficiency.*

**Neo Dulceril** *Codilab, Port.†.*
Aspartame (p.1422·1).
*Sugar substitute.*

**Neo Duplofer** *Hexal, Braz.*
Vitamins; minerals; liver extract; gastric mucosa (p.1417·1).

**Neo Eblimon** *Guidotti, Ital.*
Naproxen (p.65·1).
*Inflammation; musculoskeletal and joint disorders; pain.*

**Neo Elixifilin** *Morrith, Spain†.*
Theophylline (p.798·3).
*Heart failure; obstructive airways disease.*

**Neo Emocicatrol** *Bouty, Ital.*
Tannic acid (p.1751·2); benzalkonium chloride (p.1168·3).

**Neo Emoform** *Byk Gulden, Ital.*
Sodium monofluorophosphate (p.1446·2).
*Gingivitis; oral hygiene.*

**Neo Esoformolo** *Esoform, Ital.*
Sodium *o*-phenylphenol (p.1187·2).
*Disinfection of waste materials.*

**Neo Expectan** *Wander OTC, Switz.†.*
Acetylcysteine (p.1112·3).
*Respiratory-tract disorders associated with increased or viscous mucus.*

**Neo Fedipina** *Neo Quimica, Braz.*
Nifedipine (p.966·2).
*Hypertension.*

**Neo Fenicol** *Neo Quimica, Braz.*
Chloramphenicol (p.185·1) or chloramphenicol sodium succinate (p.185·1).
*Bacterial infections.*

**Neo Fertinorm** *Serono, Spain.*
Urofollitropin (p.1342·1).
*Female infertility; male infertility.*

**Neo Fluostomygen** *Stomygen, Ital.*
Sodium monofluorophosphate (p.1446·2).
*Dental caries prophylaxis.*

**Neo Folico** *Neo Quimica, Braz.*
Folic acid (p.1429·1).
*Anaemias.*

**Neo Formitrol** *Mipharm, Ital.*
Cetylpyridinium chloride (p.1173·1).
*Mouth disinfection.*

**Neo Fulvigal** *Anpharm (Ανφαρμ), Gr.*
Ticlopidine (p.1012·1).
*Thromboembolic disorders.*

**Neo Furasil** *Neo Quimica, Braz.*
Furazolidone (p.605·2).

**Neo Gastrausil** *Searle, Ital.†.*
Cimetidine (p.1255·3).
*Gastrointestinal disorders associated with hyperacidity.*

**Neo Genyl** *Meuse, Belg.†.*
*Injection:* Liver extract.
*Vitamin $B_{12}$ deficiency.*

**Neo Gripe Mixture** *Neo Laboratories, UK.*
Dill oil (p.1680·2); ginger (p.1267·1); sodium bicarbonate (p.1223·2).
*Colic; teething.*

**Neo H2** *Boniscontro & Gazzone, Ital.*
Roxatidine acetate hydrochloride (p.1288·1).
*Gastro-oesophageal reflux; peptic ulcer.*

**Neo Hidroclor** *Neo Quimica, Braz.*
Hydrochlorothiazide (p.933·2).
*Diuretic.*

**Neo Hubber** *Teofarma, Spain.*
Hydrocortisone acetate (p.1103·3); neomycin sulfate (p.235·1).
*Ear disorders; rhinitis.*

**Neo Iloticina** *Dista, Spain.*
Erythromycin estolate (p.208·1).
*Bacterial infections.*

**Neo Isocaden** *Neo Quimica, Braz.*
Isoconazole nitrate (p.401·3).
*Vaginal infections.*

**Neo Itrax** *Neo Quimica, Braz.*
Itraconazole (p.401·3).
*Fungal infections.*

**Neo Kef** *Phoenix, Arg.*
Loperamide hydrochloride (p.1271·1); neomycin sulfate (p.235·1).
*Diarrhoea.*

**Neo Kodan** *Schulke & Mayr, Ger.*
Octenidine hydrochloride (p.1187·2); propyl alcohol (p.1191·2); isopropyl alcohol (p.1184·3).
*Skin disinfection.*

**Neo Lacrim** *Alcon Cusi, Spain†.*
Phenylephrine hydrochloride (p.1126·3).
*Eye irritation.*

**Neo Lactoflorene** *Montefarmaco, Ital.*
Lactic-acid-producing organisms (p.1704·2); vitamins (p.1417·1).
*Nutritional supplement.*

**Neo Linco** *Neo Quimica, Braz.*
Lincomycin hydrochloride (p.226·2).
*Bacterial infections.*

**Neo Loratadin** *Neo Quimica, Braz.*
Loratadine (p.436·1).
*Hypersensitivity reactions.*

**Neo Lyndiol** *Organon, Spain†.*
Ethinylestradiol (p.1553·2); lynestrenol (p.1557·1).
*Combined oral contraceptive; menstrual disorders.*

**Neo Makatussin N** *Gebro, Switz.†.*
Dihydrocodeine hydrochloride (p.35·2); diphenhydramine hydrochloride (p.431·3).
*Bronchitis; coughs.*

**Neo Mebend** *Neo Quimica, Braz.*
Mebendazole (p.108·2).
*Worm infections.*

**Neo Melubrina** *Aventis, Spain.*
Dipyrone (p.35·3).
*Fever; pain.*

**Neo Metrodazol** *Neo Quimica, Braz.*
Metronidazole (p.607·2).

**Neo Mistatin** *Neo Quimica, Braz.*
Nystatin (p.406·3).
*Fungal infections.*

**Neo Moderin** *Pharmacia Upjohn, Spain†.*
Methylprednisolone acetate (p.1106·1); neomycin sulfate (p.235·1).
*Infected skin disorders.*

**Neo Moldava** *ICN, Arg.*
Salicylic acid (p.1157·1); pyrithione zinc (p.1156·2).
*Skin disorders.*

**Neo Mom** *Candioli, Ital.*
Tetramethrin (p.1510·2); phenothrin (p.1509·1).
*Pediculosis.*

**Neo Moxicilin** *Neo Quimica, Braz.*
Amoxicillin trihydrate (p.155·3).
*Bacterial infections.*

**Neo Nifalium** *Pharmanik (Φαρμανικ), Gr.*
Flunitrazepam (p.698·2).
*Insomnia.*

**Neo Nisidina C-Fher** *Boehringer Ingelheim, Ital.†.*
Aspirin (p.15·1); paracetamol (p.76·2); ascorbic acid (p.1460·2).
*Cold symptoms; pain.*

**Neo Nisidina-Fher** *Boehringer Ingelheim, Ital.*
Aspirin (p.15·1); paracetamol (p.76·2); caffeine (p.782·1).
*Cold symptoms; fever; pain.*

**neo OPT** *Optimed, Ger.*
Bromazepam (p.671·3).
*Anxiety; sleep disorders.*

**Neo Pelvicillin** *Temis, Arg.*
Neomycin undecenoate (p.235·2); neomycin sulfate (p.235·1); gramicidin (p.220·2); hydrocortisone (p.1103·3); nitrofurazone (p.238·2); chlorphenamine maleate (p.427·3).
*Vaginal infections.*

**Neo Perginol** *Gambar, Ital.*
Chlorhexidine gluconate (p.1173·2).
*Genital hygiene.*

**Neo POM** *Uniao Quimica, Braz.*
Neomycin sulfate (p.235·1).
*Skin infections.*

**Neo Propranol** *Neo Quimica, Braz.*
Propranolol hydrochloride (p.989·3).
*Hypertension.*

**Neo Quimica Colirio** *Neo Quimica, Braz.*
Naphazoline hydrochloride (p.1124·3); zinc phenolsulfonate (p.1163·3); berberine sulfate (p.1659·3).
*Eye congestion.*

**Neo Rhinovit** *Menarini, Gr.*
Ephedrine hydrochloride (p.1120·1).
*Nasal congestion.*

**Neo Rinactive** *Alcon Cusi, Spain.*
Budesonide (p.1094·2).
*Rhinitis.*

**Neo Rinoleina** *Sanofi Synthelabo OTC, Ital.*
Xylometazoline hydrochloride (p.1132·2).
*Nasal congestion.*

**Neo Sampoon**
*Eisai, Hong Kong; Eisai, Malaysia; Eisai, Singapore.*
Menfegol (p.1413·2).
*Spermicidal contraceptive.*

**Neo Sativan** *Cibran, Braz.†.*
Salicylamide (p.87·3); ephedrine hydrochloride (p.1120·1); ascorbic acid (p.1460·2); garlic (p.1691·1).
*Cold and influenza symptoms.*

**Neo Silvikrin** *Doetsch, Grether, Switz.†.*
Wheat-germ oil; millet extract; keratin; L-cysteine; vitamins (p.1417·1).
*Hair disorders.*

**Neo-Sintrom** *Novartis, Chile.*
Acenocoumarol (p.848·3).
*Thromboembolic disorders.*

**Neo Soluzione Sulfo Balsamica** *Deca, Ital.†.*
Sodium sulfide; sodium bromide (p.1663·1); cineole (p.1672·1).
*Catarrhal sore throat; rhinitis.*

**Neo Sulfazina** *Neo Quimica, Braz.*
Sulfadiazine (p.258·2).
*Bacterial infections.*

**Neo Tionazol** *Neo Quimica, Braz.*
Tioconazole (p.409·3).
*Fungal infections.*

**Neo Tomizol** *Tarbis, Spain.*
Carbimazole (p.1596·2).
*Hyperthyroidism.*

**Neo Topico Giusto** *Milupa, Ital.†.*
Benzethonium chloride (p.1169·2); hamamelis (p.1696·3).
*Nipple care during breast feeding; wound disinfection.*

**Neo Uniplus** *Angelini, Ital.*
Aspirin (p.15·1); paracetamol (p.76·2).
*Cold symptoms; pain.*

**Neo Uniplus C** *Angelini, Ital.*
Aspirin (p.15·1); paracetamol (p.76·2); ascorbic acid (p.1460·2).
*Cold symptoms; pain.*

**Neo Urgenin**
*Neo-Farmaceutica, Port.†; Madaus, Spain.*
Echinacea angustifolia (p.1683·2); pygeum africanum (p.1568·2); saw palmetto (p.1569·1).
*Prostatic disorders.*

**Neo Vastrictol** Allergan-Frumtost, Braz.†.
Antazoline mesilate (p.424·2); ephedrine hydrochloride (p.1120·1); ascorbic acid (p.1460·2); zinc sulfate (p.1469·3).
*Nasal congestion.*

**Neo Verpamil** Neo Quimica, Braz.
Verapamil hydrochloride (p.1019·1).
*Arrhythmias; hypertension.*

**Neo Visage** Otsuka, Spain†.
Sulfur (p.1158·2); dexpanthenol (p.1727·2); hexachlorophene (p.1181·2); hydrocortisone acetate (p.1103·3); placenta extract; basic zinc carbonate (p.1163·2).
*Acne.*

**Neo Vitalisan** Zeller, Port.†.
Ginseng (p.1693·1).
*Tonic.*

**Neo Zeta-Foot** Zeta, Ital.†.
*Cream:* Usnic acid (p.1762·1); salicylic acid (p.1157·1); undecenoic acid (p.410·3); aluminium acetate (p.1652·3).
*Topical powder:* Usnic acid (p.1762·1); undecenoic acid (p.410·3); aluminium oxide (p.1140·1); zinc stearate (p.1575·3); zinc oxide (p.1163·2); kaolin (p.1268·3); magnesium carbonate (p.1272·1); thyme oil (p.1755·3).
*Foot infections.*

**Neo-Acarina** Upsifarma, Port.
Benzyl benzoate (p.1500·2).
*Pediculosis.*

**Neo-adlibamin** Norma (Νορμα), Gr.
Tenoxicam (p.93·1).
*Dysmenorrhoea; gout; inflammation; osteoarthritis; pain; rheumatoid arthritis; spondyloarthropathies.*

**Neo-Alcos-Anal** Will-Pharma, Belg.†.
Sodium oleate (p.1574·3); lauromacrogol 400 (p.1412·3).
*Haemorrhoids.*

**Neo-Ampiplus** Menarini, Ital.
Amoxicillin trihydrate (p.155·3).
*Bacterial infections.*

**Neo-Angin**
Note. This name is used for preparations of different composition.
Klosterfrau, Austria.
*Gargle:* Hexetidine (p.1182·1); anise oil (p.1655·2); clove oil (p.1673·3); peppermint oil (p.1283·2).
*Pastilles:* Dichlorobenzyl alcohol (p.1178·3); amylmetacresol (p.1168·2); anise oil (p.1655·2); peppermint oil (p.1283·2); menthol (p.1711·3).
*Mouth and throat disorders.*
Divapharma, Ger.†.
Hexetidine (p.1182·1); benzalkonium chloride (p.1168·3).
*Mouth and throat infection and inflammation.*

**Neo-Angin au miel et citron** Doetsch, Grether, Switz.
Dichlorobenzyl alcohol (p.1178·3); amylmetacresol (p.1168·2); honey (p.1434·2); lemon oil (p.1706·2); mint oil (p.1715·2).
*Sore throat.*

**Neo-Angin avec vitamin C exempt de sucre**
Doetsch, Grether, Switz.
Dichlorobenzyl alcohol (p.1178·3); amylmetacresol (p.1168·2); menthol (p.1711·3); ascorbic acid (p.1460·2).
*Sore throat.*

**Neo-Angin exempt de sucre** Doetsch, Grether, Switz.
Dichlorobenzyl alcohol (p.1178·3); amylmetacresol (p.1168·2); menthol (p.1711·3); anethole (p.1654·3); mint oil (p.1715·2); rectified camphor oil.
*Sore throat.*

**Neo-Angin Lido** Doetsch, Grether, Switz.
Cetylpyridinium chloride (p.1173·1); lidocaine hydrochloride (p.1377·3); menthol (p.1711·3).
*Mouth and throat disorders.*

**Neo-Angin N** Divapharma, Ger.
Dichlorobenzyl alcohol (p.1178·3); menthol (p.1711·3); amylmetacresol (p.1168·2).
*Mouth and throat disorders.*

**Neo-antiperstam** Biostam (Βιοσταμ), Gr.
Tenoxicam (p.93·1).
*Dysmenorrhoea; gout; inflammation; osteoarthritis; pain; rheumatoid arthritis; spondyloarthropathies.*

**Neo-Audiocort** Teofarma, Ital.†.
Triamcinolone acetonide hemisuccinate (p.1110·3); neomycin sulfate (p.235·1).
*Ear disorders.*

**Neobac** Dermapharm, Ger.
Neomycin sulfate (p.235·1); bacitracin (p.161·3).
*Burns; skin and nose infections; wounds.*

**Neobacigrin** Grin, Mex.
Polymyxin B sulfate (p.245·1); neomycin sulfate (p.235·1); dexamethasone sodium phosphate (p.1097·2).
*Infected eye disorders.*

**Neobacina** Hexal, Braz.
Neomycin sulfate (p.235·1); bacitracin (p.161·3).
*Skin infections.*

**Neobacipan** Royton, Braz.
Neomycin (p.235·1); bacitracin zinc (p.161·3).
*Skin infections.*

**Neobacitracina** Virtus, Braz.†.
Neomycin sulfate (p.235·1); bacitracin (p.161·3).
*Bacterial skin infections.*

**Neobacitracine** Erfa, Belg.
Bacitracin (p.161·3); neomycin sulfate (p.235·1).
*Bacterial infections.*

**Neo-Ballistol** Klever, Ger.
*Capsules:* Potassium oleate (p.1574·3); peppermint oil (p.1283·2); anise oil (p.1655·2); caraway oil (p.1667·3).
*Oral liquid:* Potassium oleate (p.1574·3); ammonium oleate; peppermint oil (p.1283·2); anise oil (p.1655·2).
*Gastrointestinal disorders.*

**Neobar** Merck, Braz.†.
Barium sulfate (p.1061·1).
*Contrast medium for gastrointestinal radiography.*

**Neobes** Medix, Mex.
Diethylpropion hydrochloride (p.1587·1).
*Obesity.*

**Neo-Bex** Neolab, Canad.
Vitamin B substances (p.1417·1).

**Neo-Bex Forte** Neolab, Canad.
Vitamin B substances with ascorbic acid and zinc (p.1417·1).

**Neo-Biphyllin** Zyma, Switz.†.
Diprophylline (p.784·3); proxyphylline (p.791·2); theophylline (p.798·3).
*Obstructive airways disease.*

**Neobitiol Compuesto** Fortbenton, Arg.
Aluminium chlorohydrate (p.1142·1); neomycin (p.235·1).
*Hyperhidrosis.*

**Neobloc** Unipharm, Israel.
Metoprolol tartrate (p.957·1).
*Angina pectoris; hypertension; migraine; myocardial infarction; reduction of paroxysmal tachycardia before cardiac catheterisation.*

**Neo-Boldolaxine** GNR, Fr.†.
Senna (p.1288·2); docusate sodium (p.1262·2); boldo (p.1661·2).
Formerly contained bisacodyl, docusate sodium, boldo, aloin, and belladonna.
*Constipation.*

**Neobonsen** Duopharm, Ger.
Evening primrose oil (p.1686·3).
*Eczema.*

**Neo-botacreme** Norma (Νορμα), Gr.
Ciclopirox olamine (p.396·1).
*Fungal skin infections.*

**Neobradoral** Novartis Consumer, Port.
Domiphen bromide (p.1179·1).
*Mouth and throat infections.*

**Neobron** Pfizer, Switz.
Multivitamin and mineral preparation (p.1417·1).

**Neo-Bronchol**
Note. This name is used for preparations of different composition.
Divapharma, Ger.
Ambroxol hydrochloride (p.1114·3).
*Respiratory-tract disorders associated with increased or viscous mucus.*
DP-Medica, Switz.
Guaifenesin (p.1122·1); cineole (p.1672·1); anise oil (p.1655·2).
*Coughs.*

**Neobrontyl** Collins, Mex.
Guaifenesin (p.1122·1); sodium dibunate (p.1130·2); dipyrone (p.35·3).
*Coughs.*

**NeoBros** Fidia, Ital.
Phosphatidyl serine (p.1731·2); vitamin E (p.1417·1).
*Mental function disorders.*

**NeoBros 10** Fidia, Ital.
Phosphatidyl serine (p.1731·2); vitamins; minerals (p.1417·1).
*Mental function disorders.*

**NeoBros C** Fidia, Ital.
Phosphatidyl serine (p.1731·2); creatine; vitamins; minerals (p.1417·1).
*Nutritional supplement.*

**Neobrufen** Abbott, Spain.
Ibuprofen (p.45·3).
*Fever; musculoskeletal, joint, peri-articular, and soft-tissue disorders; pain.*

**Neo-Bucosin** Synpharma, Switz.†.
Dequalinium chloride (p.1178·1); lidocaine hydrochloride (p.1377·3).
*Mouth and throat disorders.*

**Neo-C** GNLD, Austral.†.
Ascorbic acid (p.1460·2); Neo-Plex Concentrate (dried whole citrus juice; flavedo; mesocarp; endocarp; citrus protopectin; flavonoid complex); rutoside; hesperidin; lemon bioflavonoid complex.
*Vitamin C deficiency.*

**Neocaina** Cristalia, Braz.
Bupivacaine hydrochloride (p.1371·1).
Adrenaline acid tartrate (p.852·2) is included in some injections as a vasoconstrictor to diminish absorption and localise the effect of the local anaesthetic.
*Local anaesthesia.*

**Neocalcit** Biospray, Gr.
Calcium phosphate (p.1225·3).
*Prevention and treatment of calcium deficiency.*

**Neo-Calglucon** Novartis, USA†.
Calcium glubionate (p.1225·1).
*Calcium deficiency; inadequate dietary calcium intake.*

**Neocalmans** Chobet, Arg.
Morphine hydrochloride (p.60·1).
*Pain.*

**Neocapil** Spirig, Switz.
Minoxidil (p.960·1).
*Androgenic alopecia.*

**Neocarbo** Neocorp, Ger.
Carboplatin (p.533·3).
*Malignant neoplasms.*

**Neocarbon** Galenogal, Braz.†.
Charcoal (p.1030·2).
*Diarrhoea.*

**Neocardon** Gap, Gr.
Atenolol (p.865·2).
*Angina; arrythmias; hypertension.*

**Neocate**
Scientific Hospital Supplies, Austral.; Support, Braz.; Nutricia, Fin.; SHS, Fr.; Scientific Hospital Supplies, Irl.; SHS, Israel; Nutricia, Ital.; Nutricia, NZ; Scientific Hospital Supplies, NZ; Nutricia, Port.; SHS, Singapore; Scientific Hospital Supplies, UK.
Infant feed (p.1417·1).
*Cow's milk protein intolerance; gastrointestinal disorders; whole protein intolerance.*

**Neocate One +** SHS, USA.
Preparation for enteral nutrition (p.1417·1).

**Neocef** Atral, Port.
Cefixime (p.172·3).
*Bacterial infections.*

**Neocefal** Metapharma, Ital.†.
Cefamandole nafate sodium (p.169·3).
Lidocaine (p.1377·3) is included in this preparation to alleviate the pain of injection.
*Bacterial infections.*

**Neoceflex** Neo Quimica, Braz.
Cefalexin (p.168·1).
*Bacterial infections.*

**Neoceftriona** Neo Quimica, Braz.
Ceftriaxone sodium (p.182·3).
Lidocaine hydrochloride (p.1377·3) is included in the intramuscular injection to alleviate the pain of injection.
*Bacterial infections.*

**Neocel** Pharmacia, Arg.
Docetaxel (p.547·1).
*Breast cancer; non-small cell lung cancer.*

**Neocepacilina** CEPA, Spain†.
Benzylpenicillin sodium (p.163·2); procaine benzylpenicillin (p.246·1); benzathine benzylpenicillin (p.162·3).
*Bacterial infections; rheumatic fever.*

**Neoceptin-R** Beximco, Singapore.
Ranitidine (p.1285·2).
*Gastric hyperacidity; gastro-oesophageal reflux; peptic ulcer; Zollinger-Ellison syndrome.*

**Neocetrin** Bunker, Braz.
Neomycin sulfate (p.235·1); bacitracin (p.161·3).
*Bacterial skin infections.*

**NeoCeuticals Clear Skin** Nuova ICT, Ital.
Salicylic acid (p.1157·1); acetyl mandelic acid (p.228·3).
*Acne.*

**Neoceuticals Clear Skin Solution** Hamilton, Austral.†.
Salicylic acid (p.1157·1); alpha hydroxy acids.
*Oily skin.*

**Neoceuticals Crema Despigmentante de Dia** Ingens, Arg.
Hydroquinone (p.1148·1); gluconolactone; sunscreens.
*Skin hyperpigmentation.*

**Neoceuticals Gel de Limpieza Facial** Ingens, Arg.
Gluconolactone; triclosan (p.1195·2).
*Seborrhoea; skin cleanser.*

**Neoceuticals PDS** Hamilton, Austral.†.
Barrier cream.
*Dry skin.*

**NeoCeuticals Spot Treatment** Nuova ICT, Ital.
Glycolic acid (p.1147·3); acetyl mandelic acid (p.228·3); vitamin A (p.1451·2).
*Acne.*

**Neoceuticals Therapeutic Shampoo** Hamilton, Austral.†.
Piroctone olamine (p.1155·2).
*Dandruff.*

**Neochinosol** Chinosolfabrik, Ger.
Ethacridine lactate (p.1165·3).
*Mouth and throat disorders.*

**Neocibalena** Novartis Consumer, Spain.
Aspirin (p.15·1); caffeine (p.782·1); paracetamol (p.76·2).
*Fever; pain.*

**Neo-Cibalgin** Novartis Consumer, Switz.†.
Aspirin (p.15·1); paracetamol (p.76·2); caffeine (p.782·1).
*Fever; pain.*

**Neo-Cibalgina** Novartis Consumer, Ital.
Aspirin (p.15·1); paracetamol (p.76·2); caffeine (p.782·1).
*Fever; pain.*

**Neociclina** Upsifarma, Port.
Tetracycline hydrochloride (p.266·2).
*Bacterial infections.*

**Neociclina Vitaminada** Upsifarma, Port.†.
Tetracycline hydrochloride (p.266·2); vitamin B substances (p.1417·1).
*Bacterial infections.*

**Neo-Cimexon** Cimex, Switz.
Multivitamin and mineral preparation (p.1417·1).

**Neo-Cimexon G** Cimex, Switz.
Multivitamin and mineral preparation with ginseng (p.1417·1).

**Neocin**
Note. This name is used for preparations of different composition.
Fischer, Israel.
Neomycin sulfate (p.235·1).
*Bacterial eye infections.*
Ocusoft, USA.
Polymyxin B (p.245·2); neomycin (p.235·1); bacitracin (p.161·3).
*Bacterial eye infections.*

**Neocina**
Note. This name is used for preparations of different composition.
Elofar, Braz.
Neomycin sulfate (p.235·1).
Hexal, Braz.
Neomycin sulfate (p.235·1); zinc oxide (p.1163·2).

**Neocinolon** Teuto, Braz.
Neomycin sulfate (p.235·1); fluocinolone acetonide (p.1101·2).
*Infected skin disorders.*

**Neocitec** Labinca, Arg.
Vinorelbine tartrate (p.594·1).
*Malignant neoplasms.*

**Neocitran** Novartis Sante, Fr.†.
Paracetamol (p.76·2); pseudoephedrine hydrochloride (p.1129·2).
*Rhinitis.*

**NeoCitran** Sandoz, Ger.†.
Paracetamol (p.76·2).
*Fever; pain.*

**NeoCitran Antitussif** Novartis Consumer, Switz.
Butamirate citrate (p.1116·2).
*Coughs.*

**NeoCitran Expectorant** Novartis Consumer, Switz.
Acetylcysteine (p.1112·3).
*Coughs.*

**Neoclaritine** Essex, Chile.
Desloratadine (p.431·1).
*Allergic rhinitis.*

**Neoclarityn**
Schering-Plough, Irl.; Schering-Plough, UK.
Desloratadine (p.431·1).
*Allergic rhinitis; urticaria.*

**Neo-Cleanse** GNLD, Austral.†.
Senna leaf (p.1288·2); buckthorn bark (p.1254·1); liquorice root (p.1270·2); prune (p.1285·1); alfalfa leaf (p.1649·1); rhubarb root (p.1287·3); leptandra virginica root; blue malva flowers (p.1709·3); asparagus; aniseed (p.1655·2).
*Constipation.*

**Neoclym** Monsanto, Ital.
Cyclofenil (p.1544·1).
*Anovulatory infertility; menopausal disorders; menstrual disorders.*

**Neo-Codion**
Note. This name is used for preparations of different composition.
Therabel, Belg.†.
Codeine camsilate (p.27·3); sulfogaiacol (p.1131·1).
Formerly contained codeine camsilate, ethylmorphine camsilate, and sulfogaiacol.
*Coughs.*
Bouchara-Recordati, Fr.
*Infant syrup:* Sodium benzoate (p.1169·3); grindelia (p.1696·1); senega (p.1130·2).
*Respiratory-tract congestion.*
*Paediatric syrup:* Codeine camsilate (p.27·3); sodium benzoate (p.1169·3).
*Suppositories; paediatric suppositories:* Codeine camsilate (p.27·3); cineole (p.1672·1).
*Syrup:* Codeine camsilate (p.27·3).
*Tablets:* Codeine camsilate (p.27·3); sulfogaiacol (p.1131·1); grindelia (p.1696·1).
*Coughs.*

**Neo-Codion N** Bouchara, Switz.
*Syrup:* Codeine camsilate (p.27·3); ascorbic acid (p.1460·2); ipecacuanha (p.1122·3); tolu balsam (p.1131·3).
*Tablets:* Codeine camsilate (p.27·3); sulfogaiacol (p.1131·1); grindelia (p.1696·1).
*Coughs.*

**Neo-Codion NN** Fatol, Ger.
Codeine camsilate (p.27·3).
*Coughs.*

**Neocof** Masa, Thai.
Codeine phosphate (p.27·1); guaifenesin (p.1122·1).
*Coughs.*

**Neocoflan** Neo Quimica, Braz.
Diclofenac diethylamine (p.32·1).
*Inflammation.*

**Neocolan** Seid, Spain.
Dicycloverine hydrochloride (p.481·2); metochalcone (p.1714·3); procaine hydrochloride (p.1383·2).
*Hepatobiliary disorders.*

**Neocon** Janssen-Cilag, Neth.
Norethisterone (p.1562·2); ethinylestradiol (p.1553·2).
*Combined oral contraceptive.*

**Neocones**
Note. This name is used for preparations of different composition.
Austrodent, Austria.
Tetracaine hydrochloride (p.1385·1); neomycin sulfate (p.235·1); polymyxin B sulfate (p.245·1); tyrothricin (p.275·1).
*Temporary dental filling.*

Prats, Spain.
Tetracaine hydrochloride (p.1385·1); neomycin (p.235·1); polymyxin B sulfate (p.245·1); tyrothricin (p.275·1).
*Dental disorders.*

Septodont, Switz.
Neomycin sulfate (p.235·1); benzocaine (p.1370·3). Formerly contained tetracaine hydrochloride, neomycin sulfate, polymyxin B sulfate, and tyrothricin.
*Dental disorders.*

**Neocontrast** *Bama, Spain†.*
Iopanoic acid (p.1065·1).
*Contrast medium for biliary-tract radiography.*

**Neocopan** *Ducto, Braz.*
Hyoscine butylbromide (p.483·3); dipyrone (p.35·3).
*Pain; skeletal muscle spasm.*

**Neo-Cortef**
*Pharmacia, Canad.; Pharmacia Upjohn, Irl.†; Dominion, UK†.*
Hydrocortisone acetate (p.1103·3); neomycin sulfate (p.235·1).
*Infected skin, ear, or eye disorders.*

**Neocortin** *Legrand, Braz.*
Dexamethasone sodium phosphate (p.1097·2); neomycin sulfate (p.235·1).
*Infected eye and ear disorders.*

**Neocortizul** *Lersan, Arg.*
Chloramphenicol succinate (p.186·3); prednisolone (p.1108·1); phenylephrine hydrochloride (p.1126·3).

**Neo-Cratylen**
*Madaus, Austria; Madaus, Ger.†.*
Crataegus (p.1677·1).
*Cardiac disorders.*

**Neocristin** *GlaxoSmithKline, India.*
Vincristine sulfate (p.592·2).
*Leukaemias; lymphomas.*

**Neo-Cromaton Bicomplesso** *Menarini, Ital.*
Vitamin B substances (p.1417·1).
*Deficiency states; macrocytic anaemias.*

**Neo-Currino** *Fabra, Arg.*
Naphazoline (p.1124·3); neomycin (p.235·1).
*Nasal congestion.*

**Neo-Cutigenol** *Centrapharm, Belg.*
Chlorhexidine acetate (p.1173·2); vitamin A palmitate (p.1453·1).
Formerly contained hydroxyquinoline sulfate, vitamin A palmitate, titanium dioxide, zinc oxide, and cod-liver oil.
*Burns; skin disorders; wounds.*

**Neocutis** *Pentaderm, Ital.*
Azelaic acid (p.1142·3); jaluramina.
*Acne; seborrhoea.*

**Neo-Cystine** *Sofex, Port.*
Cystine; vitamin A (p.1417·1).
*Hair and nail disorders.*

**Neo-Cytamen**
*Mayne, Austral.; Celltech, Irl.; Teofarma, Ital.; GlaxoSmithKline, NZ; Celltech, UK.*
Hydroxocobalamin (p.1458·2).
*Leber's optic atrophy; macrocytic anaemias; tobacco amblyopia.*

**Neo-Dagracycline** *Viatris, Neth.*
Doxycycline fosfatex (p.206·2).
*Bacterial infections.*

**Neo-Davisolona** *Davi, Port.*
Neomycin sulfate (p.235·1); prednisolone metasulfobenzoate sodium (p.1108·1).
*Infected eye disorders.*

**Neodazol** *Neo Quimica, Braz.*
Secnidazole (p.615·3).
*Amoebiasis; trichomoniasis.*

**Neo-Debiol AD3** *Meuse, Belg.†.*
Vitamin A acetate (p.1453·1); colecalciferol (p.1461·3).
*Vitamin A and D deficiency.*

**Neo-Deca**
*Upha, Malaysia; Beacons, Singapore†.*
Dexamethasone sodium phosphate (p.1097·2); neomycin sulfate (p.235·1).
*Allergic and inflammatory eye and ear disorders.*

**NeoDecadron**
*Merck Sharp & Dohme, Canad.†; Merck, USA.*
Dexamethasone sodium phosphate (p.1097·2); neomycin sulfate (p.235·1).
*Inflammatory eye or ear disorders with bacterial infection; inflammatory skin disorders with secondary infection.*

**Neo-Decongestine** *Sanopharm, Switz.*
Kaolin (p.1268·3); glycerol (p.1694·3); guaiacol salicylate; methyl salicylate (p.59·3).
*Soft-tissue disorders.*

**Neo-Delphicort** *Wyeth Lederle, Austria.*
Triamcinolone acetonide (p.1110·2); neomycin sulfate (p.235·1).
*Ear or eye infection and inflammation.*

**Neo-Dentocain** *Taro, Israel†.*
Phenylephrine hydrochloride (p.1126·3); benzocaine (p.1370·3); menthol (p.1711·3).
*Gingivitis; local anaesthesia; stomatitis.*

**Neoderm**
*Note. This name is used for preparations of different composition.*
Desbergers, Canad.†.
Zinc oxide (p.1163·2); zinc peroxide (p.1195·3).
*Minor abrasions, wounds, and burns.*

Propan, S.Afr.
Hydrocortisone acetate (p.1103·3); neomycin sulfate (p.235·1).
*Skin disorders.*

Tai Guk, Singapore.
Betamethasone dipropionate (p.1093·1); clotrimazole (p.396·2); gentamicin sulfate (p.217·1).
*Infected skin disorders.*

**Neoderm Ginecologico** *Crosara, Ital.†.*
Fluocinolone acetonide (p.1101·2).
*Vulvovaginitis.*

**Neodesfila** *Kin, Spain†.*
Cresol (p.1177·3); eugenol (p.1686·2); hydroxyquinoline sulfate (p.1700·1); lidocaine hydrochloride (p.1377·3).
*Toothache.*

**Neo-Desogen** *Rusch, Ital.*
Benzalkonium chloride (p.1168·3).
*Instrument disinfection; skin, burn, and wound disinfection.*

**Neo-Destomygen** *Stomygen, Ital.*
Chlorhexidine gluconate (p.1173·2).
*Oral hygiene.*

**Neodetoxergon** *Baldacci, Ital.*
Amino-acid, vitamin, and mineral preparation (p.1417·1).
*Nutritional supplement.*

**Neodex**
*Note. This name is used for preparations of different composition.*
Neo Quimica, Braz.
*Cream:* Dexamethasone acetate (p.1097·1); neomycin sulfate (p.235·1).
*Infected skin disorders.*
*Tablets:* Dexamethasone acetate (p.1097·1).
*Corticosteroid.*

Osoth, Thai.
Dexamethasone (p.1097·1); neomycin sulfate (p.235·1).
*Infected skin disorders.*

**Neo-Dex (Improved)**
*Jean-Marie, Hong Kong.*
Dexamethasone sodium phosphate (p.1097·2); chloramphenicol (p.185·1).
*Inflammatory eye infections.*

Jean-Marie, Singapore†.
Dexamethasone (p.1097·1); chloramphenicol (p.185·1).
*Inflammatory eye infections.*

**Neodexa** *Llorens, Spain.*
Dexamethasone phosphate (p.1097·2); neomycin sulfate (p.235·1).
*Infected eye disorders.*

**Neodexa Plus** *Novartis Ophthalmics, Arg.*
Dexamethasone sodium phosphate (p.1097·2); neomycin sulfate (p.235·1); naphazoline hydrochloride (p.1124·3).

**Neo-Dexameth** *Major, USA.*
Dexamethasone sodium phosphate (p.1097·2); neomycin sulfate (p.235·1).
*Eye inflammation with bacterial infection.*

**Neodexasone** *Medical Ophthalmics, USA.*
Dexamethasone phosphate (p.1097·2); neomycin (p.235·1).
*Infected eye disorders.*

**Neodexon** *Bournonville, Belg.†.*
Dexamethasone sodium phosphate (p.1097·2); neomycin sulfate (p.235·1).
*Infected inflammatory eye disorders.*

**Neodextril 40** *Fresenius Kabi, Port.†.*
Dextran 40 (p.745·3) in glucose or sodium chloride.
*Plasma volume expansion; thromboembolism prophylaxis.*

**Neodextril 70** *Fresenius Kabi, Port.*
Dextran 70 (p.746·2) in glucose or sodium chloride.
*Plasma volume expansion; thromboembolism prophylaxis.*

**Neo-Diaral** *Roberts, USA.*
Loperamide (p.1271·2).
*Diarrhoea.*

**Neo-Diophen** *Hamilton, Austral.†.*
Mepyramine maleate (p.437·1); phenylpropanolamine hydrochloride (p.1127·3); dextromethorphan hydrobromide (p.1117·3); atropine sulfate (p.477·1).
*Asthma; bronchitis; coughs and cold symptoms; hay fever.*

**Neo-Disterin** *Norma (Νορμα), Gr.*
Fenofibrate (p.915·2).
*Hyperlipidaemias.*

**Neodol** *Diba, Mex.*
Paracetamol (p.76·2).
*Fever; pain.*

**Neodolito** *Diba, Mex.*
Paracetamol (p.76·2).
*Fever; pain.*

**Neodolpasse** *Fresenius Kabi, Austria.*
Diclofenac sodium (p.32·1); orphenadrine citrate (p.486·1).
*Inflammation; musculoskeletal and joint disorders; pain.*

**Neodone** *Biochem, Ital.†.*
Paracetamol (p.76·2); aspirin (p.15·1); caffeine (p.782·1).
*Fever; pain.*

**Neodox** *Rosen, Ger.*
Doxycycline hyclate (p.206·2).
*Bacterial infections.*

**Neo-DP** *DP-Medica, Switz.*
Guaifenesin (p.1122·1); sodium benzoate (p.1169·3); althaea (p.1651·3); tolu balsam (p.1131·3); plantago lanceolata (p.1738·2); thyme (p.1755·2); pini turionum; spesierum pectoralium.
*Coughs.*

**Neodrea** *VHB, India.*
Hydroxycarbamide (p.559·1).
*Malignant neoplasms.*

**Neoduplamox** *Procter & Gamble, Ital.*
Amoxicillin trihydrate (p.155·3); potassium clavulanate (p.193·3).
*Bacterial infections.*

**Neo-Durabolic** *Hauck, USA.*
Nandrolone decanoate (p.1561·2).
*Anaemia in renal disease.*

**Neodyn**
*Carlo Erba OTC, Ital.*
*Sachets:* Vitamin, mineral, and carbohydrate preparation with creatine (p.1417·1).
*Nutritional supplement.*

Sepharma, Ital.†.
*Tablets:* Carbohydrate, amino-acid, and fatty-acid preparation with creatine (p.1417·1).
*Nutritional supplement.*

**Neoefodil** *Lafage, Arg.*
Naphazoline (p.1124·3); sodium citrate (p.1223·2); ephedrine (p.1120·1).
*Nasal congestion.*

**Neo-egmol** *Norma (Νορμα), Gr.*
Ketoconazole (p.403·3).
*Fungal scalp infections.*

**Neo-Emedyl** *Montavit, Austria.*
Dimenhydrinate (p.431·1); caffeine (p.782·1).
*Motion sickness; nausea and vomiting; vestibular disorders.*

**Neo-endusix** *Anpharm (Ανφαρμ), Gr.*
Tenoxicam (p.93·1).
*Dysmenorrhoea; gout; inflammation; osteoarthritis; pain; rheumatoid arthritis; spondyloarthropathies.*

**Neo-enteroseptol** *Specifar (Σπεσιφαρ), Gr.*
Loperamide (p.1271·2).
*Diarrhoea.*

**Neo-Eparbiol** *Ecobi, Ital.*
Inosine (p.1701·2); cyanocobalamin (p.1458·2).
*Anaemias; tonic.*

**Neo-Eunomin** *Grunenthal, Ger.*
Ethinylestradiol (p.1553·2); chlormadinone acetate (p.1542·1).
*Acne; alopecia; biphasic oral contraceptive; hirsutism; seborrhoea.*

**Neo-Eunomine** *Janssen-Cilag, Switz.†.*
Ethinylestradiol (p.1553·2); chlormadinone acetate (p.1542·1).
*Biphasic oral contraceptive.*

**Neofam** *Silesia, Chile.*
Norgestimate (p.1563·2); ethinylestradiol (p.1553·2).
*Combined oral contraceptive.*

**Neofarmotox** *Brasmedica, Braz.†.*
Xanthine; methionine (p.1042·1); choline (p.1424·3).
*Liver disorders.*

**Neofazol** *Rubio, Spain.*
Cefazolin sodium (p.170·3).
Lidocaine hydrochloride (p.1377·3) is included in this preparation to alleviate the pain of injection.
*Bacterial infections.*

**Neofed** *Propan, S.Afr.*
Triprolidine hydrochloride (p.442·3); pseudoephedrine hydrochloride (p.1129·2); guaifenesin (p.1122·1); codeine phosphate (p.27·1).
*Coughs.*

**Neofenox** *Boots Healthcare, Belg.*
Phenylephrine hydrochloride (p.1126·3); dichlorobenzyl alcohol (p.1178·3); naphazoline nitrate (p.1124·3).
*Adjuvant in sinusitis; nasal congestion.*

**Neo-Fepramol** *Istoria, Ital.†.*
Paracetamol (p.76·2).
*Fever; pain.*

**Neo-Fer** *Neolab, Canad.*
Ferrous fumarate (p.1427·3).
*Iron deficiency.*

**Neoflogin** *Neo Quimica, Braz.*
Benzydamine hydrochloride (p.21·1).
*Fever; inflammation; pain.*

**Neofloxin**
*Note. This name is used for preparations of different composition.*
Neo Quimica, Braz.
Norfloxacin (p.238·3).
*Bacterial infections.*

Beximco, Singapore.
Ciprofloxacin (p.188·2).
*Bacterial infections.*

**Neofolin** *Neocorp, Ger.*
Calcium folinate (p.1431·1).
*Folic acid deficiency; prevention of methotrexate toxicity.*

**Neofomiral** *Silanes, Mex.*
Fluconazole (p.398·1).
*Fungal infections.*

**Neo-fradin** *Pharma Tek, USA.*
Neomycin sulfate (p.235·1).

**Neofrin** *Ocusoft, USA.*
Phenylephrine hydrochloride (p.1126·3).

**Neoftalm** *ICN, Arg.*
Trimethoprim (p.272·2); polymyxin B sulfate (p.245·1).
*Eye infections.*

**Neoftalm Dexa** *ICN, Arg.*
Trimethoprim (p.272·2); polymyxin B sulfate (p.245·1); dexamethasone sodium phosphate (p.1097·2).
*Eye infections.*

**Neofulvin** *Chew, Thai.*
Griseofulvin (p.400·3).
*Fungal infections.*

**Neo-Furadantin** *Formenti, Ital.*
Nitrofurantoin (p.237·2).
*Bacterial infections of the genito-urinary tract.*

**Neofyllin** *Abigo, Denm.†.*
Proxyphylline (p.791·2).
*Obstructive airways disease.*

**Neogadine** *Raptakos, India.*
Iodised peptone; magnesium chloride; manganese sulfate; zinc sulfate; sodium metavanadate; vitamin $B_6$; vitamin $B_{12}$; nicotinamide (p.1417·1).
*Asthenia; tonic.*

**Neogadine SG** *Raptakos, India.*
Iodised peptone; sulfogaiacol (p.1131·1); magnesium chloride; manganese sulfate; zinc sulfate; vitamin $B_6$; vitamin $B_{12}$; nicotinamide (p.1417·1).
*Chronic bronchitis.*

**neogama** *Hormosan, Ger.*
Sulpiride (p.722·2).
*Psychiatric disorders; vestibular disorders.*

**neogama D novo** *Hormosan, Ger.*
Sulpiride (p.722·2).
*Depression.*

**Neogasol** *Pharmafina, Chile.*
Dimeticones (p.1482·1).
*Aerophagia.*

**Neogecim** *Gemballa, Braz.*
Neomycin (p.235·1).

**Neogel** *Masa, Thai.*
Piroxicam (p.84·2).
*Musculoskeletal and joint disorders.*

**Neogentrol** *Wyeth Lederle, Denm.*
Ethinylestradiol (p.1553·2); levonorgestrel (p.1563·2).
*Combined oral contraceptive.*

**Neogest** *Schering, UK.*
Norgestrel (p.1563·2).
*Progestogen-only oral contraceptive.*

**Neo-Geynevral** *Geymonat, Ital.†.*
Thiamine diphosphate hydrochloride; pyridoxine hydrochloride (p.1456·3); cyanocobalamin (p.1458·2).
*Neuritis.*

**Neo-Gilurythmal** *Giulini, Israel.*
Prajmalium bitartrate (p.984·3).
*Arrhythmias.*

**Neo-Gilurytmal**
*Solvay, Austria; Solvay, Ger.; Lacer, Spain†.*
Prajmalium bitartrate (p.984·3).
*Arrhythmias.*

**Neogluconin** *Sanochemia, Austria†.*
Glibenclamide (p.331·2).
*Diabetes mellitus.*

**Neogobion** *Pharos, Singapore.*
Ferrous gluconate (p.1428·1); manganese sulfate (p.1440·1); folic acid (p.1429·1); copper sulfate (p.1426·1); vitamin $B_{12}$ (p.1458·2).
Vitamin C (p.1460·2) is included in this preparation to increase the absorption and availability of iron.
*Anaemias.*

**Neo-Golaseptine** *SMB, Belg.*
Chlorhexidine (p.1173·2); benzethonium chloride (p.1169·2).
*Mouth and throat disorders.*

**Neogram** *SIFI, Ital.†.*
Neomycin sulfate (p.235·1); gramicidin (p.220·2).
*Eye infections.*

**Neogrip** *Rider, Chile.*
Paracetamol (p.76·2); pseudoephedrine hydrochloride (p.1129·2); chlorphenamine maleate (p.427·3).
*Cold and influenza symptoms; rhinitis.*

**Neogynon**
*Schering, Arg.; Schering, Austria; Schering, Belg.; Schering, Denm.; Schering, Ger.; Shepa, Gr.; Schering, Hong Kong; Schering, Israel; Schering, Mex.; Schering, Neth.; Schering, Switz.*
Levonorgestrel (p.1563·2); ethinylestradiol (p.1553·2). 28-Day packs contain 7 inert tablets.
*Combined oral contraceptive.*

**Neogynona** *Schering, Spain.*
Levonorgestrel (p.1563·2); ethinylestradiol (p.1553·2).
*Combined oral contraceptive; menstrual disorders.*

**Neo-Healar** *Arab, Malaysia.*
Lupinus albus; vateria indica; peppermint (p.1283·2); aloe vera (p.1141·3).
*Haemorrhoids.*

**Neo-Heparbil** *Montefarmaco, Ital.†.*
Fencibutirol (p.1687·1); frangula (p.1266·3); rhubarb (p.1287·3); cascara sagrada (p.1255·1); belladonna (p.479·1).
*Constipation.*

**Neo-Hesna** *Takeda, Thai.*
Carbazochrome sodium sulfonate (p.745·1).
*Haemorrhagic disorders.*

**Neohexal** *Riedel-Zabinka, Braz.†.*
Methenamine (p.230·1).
*Bacterial urinary-tract infections.*

**Neo-Hydro**
*Upha, Malaysia; Streuli, Switz.*
Hydrocortisone acetate (p.1103·3); neomycin sulfate (p.235·1).
*Inflammation and infection of the eye, nose, or ear; skin disorders with bacterial infection.*

**Neo-Hytisone** *Atlantic, Thai.†.*
Neomycin sulfate (p.235·1); hydrocortisone acetate (p.1103·3).
*Bacterial skin infections.*

**Neo-Intol** *Carlo Erba OTC, Ital.†.*
Cetrimonium tosilate (p.1173·1).
*External genital disinfection.*

**Neoiodarsolo** *Baldacci, Ital.*
Amino-acid preparation with vitamin B substances (p.1417·1).
*Tonic.*

**Neo-Ipertas** *Norma (Νορμα), Gr.*
Captopril (p.879·2).
*Heart failure; hypertension; myocardial infarction.*

**Neo-Kap** *Degorts, Mex.*
Furazolidone (p.605·2); kaolin (p.1268·3); pectin (p.1580·3).
*Gastrointestinal infections.*

**Neokratin** *Fresenius Kabi, Austria.*
Paracetamol (p.76·2); propyphenazone (p.85·3); caffeine (p.782·1).
*Fever; pain.*

**Neo-Lapitrypsin** *Truw, Ger.†.*
Oleum pini sylvestris; pumilio pine oil (p.1737·1); melissa oil (p.1711·2); spike lavender oil (p.1749·2); juniper oil (p.1703·1); fennel oil (p.1687·3); peppermint oil (p.1283·2).
*Biliary disorders; gallstones; renal calculi.*

**Neolapril** *Biobras, Braz.*
Enalapril maleate (p.909·2).
*Hypertension.*

**Neo-Laryngobis** *Technilab, Canad.*
Bismuth dipropylacetate (p.1253·1).
*Sore throat.*

**Neolasil** *Neo Quimica, Braz.*
Metoclopramide hydrochloride (p.1274·3).
*Nausea and vomiting.*

**Neolette** *Silesia, Chile.*
21 Tablets, desogestrel (p.1547·2); ethinylestradiol (p.1553·2); 5 tablets, ethinylestradiol; 2 tablets, placebo.
*Sequential oral contraceptive.*

**Neo-Lidocaton**
*Weimer, Ger.†.*
Lidocaine hydrochloride (p.1377·3).
Lypressin (p.1342·3) and noradrenaline (p.974·3) are included in this preparation as vasoconstrictors to diminish absorption and localise the effect of the local anaesthetic.
*Local anaesthesia.*

*Weimer, Thai.*
Lidocaine hydrochloride (p.1377·3).
Vasopressin (p.1342·2) and noradrenaline (p.974·3) are included in this preparation as vasoconstrictors to diminish absorption and localise the effect of the local anaesthetic.
*Local anaesthesia.*

**Neolidona** *Neo Quimica, Braz.*
Chlortalidone (p.882·3).
*Hypertension.*

**Neolipid** *Biobras, Braz.*
Lovastatin (p.949·1).
*Hyperlipidaemias.*

**Neoloid**
*Bradley, Canad.; Kenwood, USA.*
Castor oil (p.1668·2).
*Bowel evacuation; constipation; diarrhoea.*

**Neolon-D** *Neo Quimica, Braz.*
Gramicidin (p.220·2); neomycin sulfate (p.235·1); nystatin (p.406·3); triamcinolone acetonide (p.1110·2).
*Infected skin disorders.*

**Neo-Lotan** *Neopharmed, Ital.*
Losartan potassium (p.947·2).
*Hypertension.*

**Neo-Lotan Plus** *Neopharmed, Ital.*
Losartan potassium (p.947·2); hydrochlorothiazide (p.933·2).
*Hypertension.*

**Neomas** *Temis, Arg.*
Neomycin sulfate (p.235·1).
*Gastrointestinal infections.*

**Neomas L** *Temis, Arg.*
Neomycin sulfate (p.235·1); loperamide hydrochloride (p.1271·1).
*Diarrhoea.*

**Neomed** *Cimed, Braz.*
Neomycin (p.235·1).

**Neomedil** *Farmec, Ital.*
Benzalkonium chloride (p.1168·3); alcohol (p.1166·1).
*Skin and wound disinfection.*

**Neo-Medrol**
*Note. This name is used for preparations of different composition.*
*Pharmacia, Austral.; Pharmacia Upjohn, Israel; Pharmacia, S.Afr.*
Methylprednisolone acetate (p.1106·1); neomycin sulfate (p.235·1); aluminium chlorohydrate (p.1142·1); sulfur (p.1158·2).
*Acne.*

*Pharmacia, Malaysia; Pharmacia, Singapore; Pharmacia, Thai.*
Methylprednisolone acetate (p.1106·1); neomycin sulfate (p.235·1); alcloxa (p.1141·2); sulfur (p.1158·2).
*Acne; rosacea; seborrhoeic dermatitis.*

**Neo-Medrol Acne**
*Pharmacia, Canad.; Pharmacia, Hong Kong.*
Methylprednisolone acetate (p.1106·1); neomycin sulfate (p.235·1); aluminium chlorohydrate (p.1142·1); colloidal sulfur (p.1158·2).
*Acne; seborrhoeic dermatitis.*

**Neo-Medrol comp** *Pharmacia, Fin.*
Methylprednisolone acetate (p.1106·1); neomycin sulfate (p.235·1); aluminium chlorohydrate (p.1142·1); sulfur (p.1158·2).
*Acne.*

**Neo-Medrol Veriderm**
*Pharmacia, Canad.; Pharmacia Upjohn, Ital.*
Methylprednisolone acetate (p.1106·1); neomycin sulfate (p.235·1).
*Infected skin disorders.*

**Neo-Medrone** *Pharmacia Upjohn, Irl.†.*
*Cream:* Methylprednisolone acetate (p.1106·1); neomycin sulfate (p.235·1).
*Inflamed skin infections.*

*Topical lotion:* Methylprednisolone acetate (p.1106·1); neomycin sulfate (p.235·1); aluminium chlorohydrate (p.1142·1); sulfur (p.1158·2).
*Acne; rosacea; seborrhoeic dermatitis.*

**Neomelin** *Collins, Mex.*
Dipyrone (p.35·3).
*Fever; pain.*

**Neo-Melubrina** *Aventis, Mex.*
Dipyrone (p.35·3).
*Fever; pain.*

**Neo-Mercazole**
*Roche, Austral.; Roche, Denm.; Roche, Fr.; Roche, Hong Kong†; Nicholas Piramal, India; Roche, Irl.; Roche, Norw.; Roche, NZ; Aspen, S.Afr.; Roche, Singapore†; Roche, Switz.; Roche, UK.*
Carbimazole (p.1596·2).
*Hyperthyroidism.*

**Neomercurocromo** *SIT, Ital.*
*Ointment; topical powder:* Chlorhexidine gluconate (p.1173·2).

*Topical solution:* Chloroxylenol (p.1177·2).
*Wound disinfection.*

**Neomeritine** *Janssen-Cilag, Belg.†.*
Ambucetamide hydrochloride (p.1653·2); aspirin (p.15·1); paracetamol (p.76·2); codeine phosphate (p.27·1); caffeine (p.782·1).
*Gynaecological pain.*

**Neo-Meton** *Jean-Marie, Singapore†.*
Brompheniramine maleate (p.426·1).
*Hypersensitivity reactions.*

**Neomicina Composta** *Uniao Quimica, Braz.†.*
Neomycin (p.235·1); tyrothricin (p.275·1).
*Mouth and throat infections.*

**Neomicol** *Medix, Mex.*
Miconazole nitrate (p.405·3).
*Fungal infections.*

**Neomigran** *Hexal, Braz.*
Isometheptene mucate (p.1702·1); dipyrone (p.35·3); caffeine (p.782·1).
*Pain.*

**Neo-Mindol** *Bracco, Ital.†.*
Ibuprofen (p.45·3).
*Pain.*

**Neomite** *M & H, Thai.†.*
Miconazole nitrate (p.405·3).
*Fungal skin infections.*

**Neomixen** *Pisa, Mex.*
Neomycin (p.235·1).

**Neomixin** *Hauck, USA†.*
Polymyxin B sulfate (p.245·1); neomycin sulfate (p.235·1); bacitracin (p.161·3).
*Bacterial skin infections.*

**Neomonovar** *Wyeth Lederle, Port.*
Levonorgestrel (p.1563·2); ethinylestradiol (p.1553·2).
*Combined oral contraceptive.*

**Neo-Mudapenil** *Geminis, Arg.*
Betamethasone valerate (p.1093·2); neomycin sulfate (p.235·1).
*Infected skin disorders.*

**Neo-Mune**
*Otsuka, Hong Kong†; Thai Otsuka, Thai.*
Preparation for enteral nutrition (p.1417·1).

**Neo-mycodermol** *Adelco, Gr.*
Ciclopirox olamine (p.396·1).
*Fungal skin infections.*

**Neo-Mydrial** *Winzer, Ger.*
Phenylephrine hydrochloride (p.1126·3).
Formerly known as Mydrial.
*Production of mydriasis.*

**Neomyrt Plus** *Baif, Ital.*
Myrtillus (p.1718·3); bioflavonoids (p.1688·2); centella (p.1144·3); selenium (p.1444·1); vitamin C (p.1460·2); rutoside (p.1688·2).
*Nutritional supplement.*

**Neo-NaClex**
*GlaxoSmithKline, NZ; Goldshield, UK.*
Bendroflumethiazide (p.867·3).
*Hypertension; oedema.*

**Neo-NaClex-K** *Goldshield, UK.*
Bendroflumethiazide (p.867·3); potassium chloride (p.1232·2).
*Hypertension; oedema.*

**Neonaxil** *Galen, Mex.*
Naproxen (p.65·1).
*Gout; musculoskeletal, joint, and peri-articular disorders; pain.*

**Neo-Nevral** *Aventis, Ital.*
Paracetamol (p.76·2); aspirin (p.15·1); caffeine (p.782·1).
*Fever; pain.*

**Neoniagar** *Sintesa, Belg.†.*
Mebutizide (p.951·2).
*Hypertension; oedema.*

**Neo-omnipen** *Norma (Νορμα), Gr.*
Ticlopidine (p.1012·1).
*Thrombosis prophylaxis.*

**Neo-Optal** *Olan-Kemed, Thai.*
Dexamethasone sodium phosphate (p.1097·2); neomycin sulfate (p.235·1).
*Infected eye and ear disorders.*

**Neo-Optalidon** *Novartis Consumer, Ital.*
Paracetamol (p.76·2); propyphenazone (p.85·3); caffeine (p.782·1).
*Fever; pain.*

**NeoOstrogynal** *Asche, Ger.*
Estradiol valerate (p.1550·2); estriol (p.1552·3).
*Menopausal disorders; oestrogenic.*

**Neopam** *Troikaa, India.*
Pralidoxime iodide (p.1050·1).
*Organophosphorus poisoning.*

**Neopan** *Propan, S.Afr.*
Neomycin sulfate (p.235·1); sodium propionate (p.408·1).
*Ear infections.*

**Neopankreoflat** *Grunenthal, Chile.*
Pancreatin (p.1725·3); dimeticones (p.1482·1).
*Digestive disorders; flatulence.*

**Neo-Panlacticos** *Italmex, Mex.*
Lactic-acid-producing organisms (p.1704·2); vitamin B substances (p.1417·1).
*Restoration of normal gastrointestinal flora.*

**Neo-Panlacticos Plus** *Italmex, Mex.*
Lactic-acid-producing organisms (p.1704·2); vitamin B substances (p.1417·1); dimeticone (p.1289·2).
*Flatulence; restoration of normal gastrointestinal flora.*

**Neoparyl Framycetine** *Ciba Vision, Fr.†.*
Phenylephrine and meglumine heparinate; framycetin sulfate (p.215·1).
*Eye infections and burns.*

**Neopect** *Masa, Thai.†.*
Codeine phosphate (p.27·1); guaifenesin (p.1122·1); phenylpropanolamine hydrochloride (p.1127·3).
*Cold symptoms; coughs; nasal congestion.*

**Neopelle** *Also, Ital.*
Collagen (p.1674·3).
*Wound dressing.*

**Neo-Penotran** *Embil, Singapore.*
Metronidazole (p.607·2); miconazole nitrate (p.405·3).
*Bacterial and trichomonal vaginitis; vaginal candidiasis.*

**Neopenyl** *Grunenthal, Spain.*
Benzylpenicillin sodium (p.163·2); clemizole penicillin (p.194·1).
Lidocaine hydrochloride (p.1377·3) is included in this preparation to alleviate the pain of injection.
*Bacterial infections.*

**Neopeptine** *Raptakos, India.*
*Capsules:* Amylase (p.1654·2); papain (p.1727·3); simeticone (p.1289·2).

*Oral drops:* Amylase (p.1654·2); papain (p.1727·3); dill oil (p.1680·2); anise oil (p.1655·2); caraway oil (p.1667·3).

*Oral liquid:* Amylase (p.1654·2); papain (p.1727·3).

*Anorexia; dyspepsia; flatulence; meteorism.*

**Neoperazona** *Neo Quimica, Braz.*
Cefoperazone sodium (p.174·3).
*Bacterial infections.*

**Neo-Pergonal** *Serono, Fr.†.*
Menotrophin (p.1330·1).
*Male and female infertility.*

**Neopermease** *Novartis, Austria†.*
Hyaluronidase (p.1698·2).
*Adjunct with chemotherapy for malignant neoplasms.*

**Neophedan** *Bodene, S.Afr.*
Tamoxifen citrate (p.584·1).
*Breast cancer.*

**Neo-Phlogicid** *Sanochemia, Austria†.*
Aluminium acetotartrate (p.1652·3); camphor (p.1665·3); methyl salicylate (p.59·3); salicylic acid (p.1157·1); menthol (p.1711·3); eucalyptus oil (p.1686·2).
*Frostbite; inflammation; musculoskeletal and joint disorders; sciatica.*

**Neophyllin** *Eisai, Jpn.*
Aminophylline (p.780·2).
*Congestive heart failure; obstructive airways disease.*

**Neopiridin** *Neo Quimica, Braz.*
Benzocaine (p.1370·3); cetylpyridinium chloride (p.1173·1).

**Neo-Planotest** *Bio Merieux, UK.*
Pregnancy test (p.1734·3).

**Neoplatin** *Bristol-Myers, Spain.*
Cisplatin (p.538·1).
*Malignant neoplasms.*

**Neoplaxol** *Richmond, Arg.*
Etoposide (p.551·3).
*Malignant neoplasms.*

**Neoplex** *Austroplant, Austria.*
Albumin tannate (p.1248·1); liquorice (p.1270·2); magnesium trisilicate (p.1272·3).
*Gastrointestinal disorders.*

**Neoplex B** *Neo Quimica, Braz.*
Vitamin B substances (p.1417·1).

**Neoplex B+C** *Neo Quimica, Braz.*
Vitamin B substances; ascorbic acid (p.1417·1).

**Neoplus** *Terapeutico, Ital.*
Royal jelly (p.1740·3); pollen; ginseng (p.1693·1).
*Nutritional supplement.*

**Neopolydex** *Medical Ophthalmics, USA.*
Dexamethasone (p.1097·1); neomycin (p.235·1); polymyxin B (p.245·2).
*Infected eye disorders.*

**Neoprazol** *Neo Quimica, Braz.*
Omeprazole (p.1278·2).
*Peptic ulcer.*

**Neopred** *PD, Thai.*
Neomycin sulfate (p.235·1); prednisolone (p.1108·1).
*Allergic and inflammatory skin disorders.*

**Neo-Preocil** *Edol, Port.*
Fluorometholone (p.1102·2); neomycin (p.235·1).
*Infected eye disorders.*

**Neopress** *Neo Quimica, Braz.*
Losartan potassium (p.947·2); hydrochlorothiazide (p.933·2).
*Hypertension.*

**Neoprex** *Sigma-Tau, Ital.*
Enalapril maleate (p.909·2); hydrochlorothiazide (p.933·2).
*Hypertension.*

**Neo-Primovlar** *Schering, Fin.*
Levonorgestrel (p.1563·2); ethinylestradiol (p.1553·2).
*Combined oral contraceptive.*

**Neoproct** *Schering, Fin.*
Fluocortolone pivalate (p.1102·1); lidocaine hydrochloride (p.1377·3).
*Anorectal disorders.*

**Neo-Prunex** *Neolab, Canad.†.*
Phenolphthalein (p.1284·1).
*Constipation.*

**Neopulmonier** *Quimica y Farmacia, Mex.*
Dextromethorphan hydrobromide (p.1117·3).
*Coughs.*

**Neo-Pyodron** *Cassella-med, Ger.*
Zinc oxide (p.1163·2); almasilate (p.1248·2); dequalinium chloride (p.1178·1).
*Infected skin disorders; pyoderma.*

**Neo-Pyrazol** *Bonapace, Thai.*
Phenylbutazone sodium (p.84·1); lidocaine (p.1377·3).
*Musculoskeletal, joint, and soft-tissue disorders.*

**Neo-Pyrazon**
*United American, Malaysia; United American, Singapore.*
Diclofenac sodium (p.32·1).
*Musculoskeletal and joint disorders; pain.*

**Neopyrin** *Riemser, Ger.*
Paracetamol (p.76·2); caffeine (p.782·1).
*Pain.*

**Neoquin** *Cassara, Arg.*
Hydroquinone (p.1148·1); glycolic acid (p.1147·3); kojic acid (p.1151·2) titanium dioxide (p.1160·3).
*Skin hyperpigmentation.*

**Neoquin Forte** *Cassara, Arg.*
Hydroquinone (p.1148·1); glycolic acid (p.1147·3).
*Skin hyperpigmentation.*

**Neoral**
*Novartis, Austral.; Novartis, Canad.; Novartis, Fr.; Novartis, Irl.; Novartis, Neth.; Novartis, NZ; Novartis, Switz.; Novartis, UK; Novartis, USA.*
Ciclosporin (p.1351·2).
*Atopic dermatitis; graft-versus-host disease; nephrotic syndrome; psoriasis; rheumatoid arthritis; transplant rejection.*

**Neoral-Sandimmun** *Novartis, Belg.*
Ciclosporin (p.1351·2).
*Auto-immune disorders; transplant rejection.*

**NeoRecormon**
*Roche, Austria; Roche, Belg.; Roche, Denm.; Roche, Fin.; Roche, Fr.; Roche, Ger.; Roche, Gr.; Roche, Irl.; Roche, Ital.; Roche, Norw.; Roche, Port.; Roche, Spain; Roche, Swed.; Roche, UK.*
Epoetin beta (p.747·2).
Formerly known as Recormon in *Swed.*
*Anaemias; autologous blood transfusion.*

**Neorinol** *Silesia, Chile.*
Ipratropium bromide (p.787·1).
*Rhinitis; rhinorrhoea.*

**Neorlest** *Parke, Davis, Ger.†.*
Ethinylestradiol (p.1553·2); norethisterone acetate (p.1562·2).
*Combined oral contraceptive.*

**Neo-Rowachol** *Rowa Wagner, Hong Kong.*
Menthol (p.1711·3); menthone; α-pinene; β-pinene; borneol; camphene; cineole (p.1672·1).
*Biliary disorders; gallstones; liver disorders.*

**Neo-Rowatinex** *Rowa Wagner, Hong Kong.*
Camphene; borneol; fenchone; cineole (p.1672·1); α-pinene; β-pinene; anethole (p.1654·3).
*Urinary-tract disorders.*

**Neorutin** *Helvepharm, Switz.*
Rutoside (p.1688·2).
*Venous insufficiency.*

**Neorythmin** *Unipharm, Israel†.*
Prajmalium bitartrate (p.984·3).
*Arrhythmias.*

**neos nitro OPT** *Optimed, Ger.*
Glyceryl trinitrate (p.923·2).
*Angina pectoris.*

**Neo-Sabenyl** *Qualiphar, Belg.*
Clorophene (p.1177·3); trolamine laurilsulfate (p.1574·3).
*Disinfection of skin, hands, mucous membranes, instruments, and materials; irrigation in ear, nose, and throat procedures; skin disorders; wound irrigation.*

**Neosac** *Neo Quimica, Braz.*
Ranitidine hydrochloride (p.1285·2).
*Peptic ulcer.*

**Neosaldina** *Abbott, Braz.*
Dipyrone (p.35·3); isometheptene mucate (p.1702·1); caffeine (p.782·1).
*Smooth muscle spasm.*

**Neosar** *Gensia, USA.*
Cyclophosphamide (p.540·2).
*Malignant neoplasms.*

**Neosayomol** *Cinfa, Spain.*
Diphenhydramine hydrochloride (p.431·3).
*Allergic skin reactions.*

**Neosec** *Masa, Thai.*
Paracetamol (p.76·2); orphenadrine citrate (p.486·1).
*Pain.*

**Neosed** *Advance, Hong Kong†.*
Salicylamide (p.87·3); phenylephrine hydrochloride (p.1126·3); paracetamol (p.76·2); caffeine (p.782·1); brompheniramine maleate (p.426·1).
*Cold and influenza symptoms.*

**Neosemid** *Neo Quimica, Braz.*
Furosemide (p.919·3).
*Hypertension.*

**Neoseptil** *Dinafarma, Braz.†.*
Bismuth subgallate (p.1252·2); zinc oxide (p.1163·2).
*Barrier preparation; skin disorders.*

**Neosidantoina** *Squibb, Spain.*
Phenytoin sodium (p.370·2).
*Epilepsy.*

**Neo-Sinedol** *Wild, Switz.*
Lidocaine hydrochloride (p.1377·3).
*Local anaesthesia.*

**Neo-Sinefrina**
*Sanofi Synthelabo, Braz.†.*
Phenylephrine hydrochloride (p.1126·3).
*Nasal congestion.*

*GlaxoSmithKline Consumer, Port.*
Phenylephrine (p.1126·3).

**Neosol** *Breckenridge, USA.*
Hyoscyamine sulfate (p.485·1).

**Neosolets** *SMB, Chile.*
Glycolic acid (p.1147·3).
*Acne; keratinisation disorders.*

**Neosona** *Amhof, Arg.*
Dexamethasone sodium phosphate (p.1097·2); neomycin sulfate (p.235·1); naphazoline hydrochloride (p.1124·3).
*No indications.*

**Neosoralen** *Mac, India.*
Trioxysalen (p.1162·2).
*Vitiligo.*

**Neosoro** *Neo Quimica, Braz.*
Naphazoline hydrochloride (p.1124·3).
*Nasal congestion.*

**Neo-Soyal** *Nutricia, Ital.†.*
Infant feed (p.1417·1).
*Galactosaemia; milk intolerance.*

**Neospect** *Amersham, Spain.*
Technetium 99-m depreotide (p.1525·2).
*Pulmonary radiography.*

**Neosporin**
*Note. This name is used for preparations of different composition.*
*Pfizer Consumer, Austral.; GlaxoSmithKline, Canad.; GlaxoSmithKline, Hong Kong; GlaxoSmithKline, India; Glaxo Wellcome, Irl.; Glaxo Wellcome, Mex.; Glaxo Wellcome, S.Afr.; Glaxo Wellcome, Singapore†; GlaxoSmithKline, Switz.; GlaxoSmithKline, Thai.; Pliva, UK; Monarch, USA.*
*Cream; eye and ear drops:* Neomycin sulfate (p.235·1); polymyxin B sulfate (p.245·1); gramicidin (p.220·2).
*Bacterial eye and ear infections; bacterial skin infections.*

*Pfizer Consumer, Austral.; GlaxoSmithKline, Canad.; GlaxoSmithKline, Hong Kong; GlaxoSmithKline, India; Glaxo Wellcome, Mex.; GlaxoSmithKline, S.Afr.; Warner-Lambert, USA; Monarch, USA.*
*Eye ointment; ointment:* Neomycin sulfate (p.235·1); polymyxin B sulfate (p.245·1); bacitracin (p.161·3) or bacitracin zinc (p.161·3).
*Bacterial eye infections; bacterial skin infections.*

*GlaxoSmithKline, Canad.*
*Bladder irrigation:* Neomycin sulfate (p.235·1); polymyxin B sulfate (p.245·1).
*Bacterial urinary-tract infections.*

*Glaxo Wellcome, USA†.*
*Cream:* Neomycin sulfate (p.235·1); polymyxin B sulfate (p.245·1).
*Skin infections.*

**Neosporin GU** *Glaxo Wellcome, USA.*
Neomycin sulfate (p.235·1); polymyxin B sulfate (p.245·1).
*Prevention of catheter-associated urinary-tract infections.*

**Neosporin + Pain Relief** *Warner-Lambert, USA.*
*Cream:* Neomycin (p.235·1); polymyxin B sulfate (p.245·1); pramocaine hydrochloride (p.1382·2).
*Ointment:* Neomycin (p.235·1); polymyxin B sulfate (p.245·1); bacitracin zinc (p.161·3); pramocaine hydrochloride (p.1382·2).

**Neosporin Plus** *Glaxo Wellcome, USA†.*
*Cream:* Neomycin (p.235·1); polymyxin B sulfate (p.245·1); lidocaine (p.1377·3).
*Ointment:* Neomycin (p.235·1); polymyxin B sulfate (p.245·1); lidocaine (p.1377·3); bacitracin zinc (p.161·3).

**Neosporin-H** *GlaxoSmithKline, India.*
*Ear drops:* Polymyxin B sulfate (p.245·1); neomycin sulfate (p.235·1); hydrocortisone (p.1103·3).
*Otitis externa.*
*Ointment:* Polymyxin B sulfate (p.245·1); neomycin sulfate (p.235·1); bacitracin zinc (p.161·3); hydrocortisone (p.1103·3).
*Infected skin disorders.*

**Neossolvan** *Neo Quimica, Braz.*
Ambroxol hydrochloride (p.1114·3).
*Respiratory-tract congestion.*

**Neostatin** *Delta, Braz.*
Nystatin (p.406·3).
*Fungal infections.*

**Neo-Stediril**
*Wyeth Lederle, Austria; Wyeth Lederle, Belg.; Wyeth, Ger.; Wyeth, Neth.†; Wyeth, Switz.†.*
Levonorgestrel (p.1563·2); ethinylestradiol (p.1553·2).
*Combined oral contraceptive.*

**Neostesin** *Nycomed, Gr.; Neiadas (Νειαδας), Gr.*
Calcitonin (p.768·2).
*Hypercalcaemia; osteoporosis; Paget's disease of bone.*

**Neostigmine Min-I-Mix** *IMS, USA.*
Neostigmine metilsulfate (p.1492·2).
Atropine sulfate (p.477·1) is included in this preparation to protect against muscarinic actions.
*Reversal of competitive neuromuscular blockade.*

**Neostig-Reu** *Reusch, Ger.†.*
Neostigmine metilsulfate (p.1492·2).
*Myasthenia gravis; reversal of competitive neuromuscular blockade.*

**Neostil** *Novartis Consumer, Port.*
Dimetindene maleate (p.431·2).
*Hypersensitivity reactions.*

**Neostix-N** *Bayer, Austral.*
Test for protein, glucose, blood, and nitrite in urine.

**Neo-Stomygen** *Stomygen, Ital.*
*Mouthwash:* Chlorhexidine gluconate (p.1173·2); cetylpyridinium chloride (p.1173·1).
Formerly contained sodium monofluorophosphate, cetylpyridinium chloride, enoxolone, and xylitol.
*Toothpaste:* Sodium monofluorophosphate (p.1446·2); propolis (p.1735·2); enoxolone (p.36·2); cetylpyridinium chloride (p.1173·1).
*Oral disinfection; oral hygiene.*

**Neostrata**
*Note. This name is used for preparations of different composition.*
*Ingens, Arg.; Hamilton, Austral.†; Canderm, Canad.; Finn Vita, Chile; Nuova ICT, Ital.*
A range of preparations containing glycolic acid (p.1147·3) or gluconolactone with emollients and humectants.
*Skin care.*

*Finn Vita, Chile.*
*Cream SPF 15:* Glycolic acid (p.1147·3); gluconolactone; octinoxate (p.1154·3); titanium dioxide (p.1160·3).
*Sunscreen.*
*Depigmenting cream SPF 15:* Octinoxate (p.1154·3); hydroquinone (p.1148·1); titanium dioxide (p.1160·3); gluconolactone.
*Skin pigmentation disorders; sunscreen.*
*Depigmenting gel:* Glycolic acid (p.1147·3); hydroquinone (p.1148·1).
*Skin pigmentation disorders.*
*Depigmenting gel forte:* Gluconolactone; lactobionic acid; kojic acid (p.1151·2); hydroquinone (p.1148·1); liquorice (p.1270·2).
*Skin pigmentation disorders.*
*Lip conditioner:* Glucurolactone; octinoxate (p.1154·3); octisalate (p.1154·3); titanium dioxide (p.1160·3).
*Chapped lips; sunscreen.*
*Shampoo:* Gluconolactone; mandelic acid (p.228·3); piroctone olamine (p.1155·2).
*Dandruff.*

**Neostrata AHA Astringent Acne** *Canderm, Canad.*
Salicylic acid (p.1157·1).

**Neostrata AHA Blemish** *Canderm, Canad.*
Salicylic acid (p.1157·1); glycolic acid (p.1147·3).

**Neostrata AHA Daytime** *Canderm, Canad.*
*SPF 15:* Octinoxate (p.1154·3); oxybenzone (p.1154·3); glycolic acid (p.1147·3).

**Neostrata AHA HQ** *Canderm, Canad.*
Hydroquinone (p.1148·1).
*Skin hyperpigmentation.*

**Neostrata AHA Light** *Canderm, Canad.*
*SPF 15:* Octinoxate (p.1154·3); oxybenzone (p.1154·3); gluconolactone.

**Neostrata AHA Smoothing and Moisturizing** *Canderm, Canad.*
*SPF 15:* Octinoxate (p.1154·3); oxybenzone (p.1154·3); glycolic acid (p.1147·3).

**Neostrata Astringent Acne Treatment** *Canderm, Canad.*
Benzoyl peroxide (p.1143·2).
*Acne.*

**Neostrata Blemish Spot** *Canderm, Canad.*
Benzoyl peroxide (p.1143·2).
*Acne.*

**Neostrata Daytime Protection Cream** *Hamilton, Austral.†.*
Octinoxate (p.1154·3); oxybenzone (p.1154·3); titanium dioxide (p.1160·3).
*Emollient; sunscreen.*

**Neostrata Gel Despigmentante** *Ingens, Arg.*
Hydroquinone (p.1148·1); glycolic acid (p.1147·3).
*Skin hyperpigmentation.*

**Neostrata Lip Conditioner** *Hamilton, Austral.†.*
*SPF 15:* Octinoxate (p.1154·3); octisalate (p.1154·3).
*Dry lips; sunscreen.*

**Neosulf**
*Alphapharm, Austral.; Pacific, NZ.*
Neomycin sulfate (p.235·1).
*Bowel sterilisation before surgery; hepatic encephalopathy.*

**Neosulida** *Neo Quimica, Braz.*
Nimesulide (p.67·1).

**Neosulin Lenta** *Biobras, Braz.†.*
Insulin zinc suspension (porcine, monocomponent) (p.333·3).
*Diabetes mellitus.*

**Neosulin NPH** *Biobras, Braz.†.*
Isophane insulin injection (porcine, monocomponent) (p.333·3).
*Diabetes mellitus.*

**Neosulin Regular** *Biobras, Braz.†.*
Insulin injection (porcine, monocomponent) (p.333·3).
*Diabetes mellitus.*

**Neo-Suxigal** *Anpharm (Ανφαρμ), Gr.*
Roxithromycin (p.254·2).
*Bacterial infections.*

**Neo-Synalar** *Yamanouchi, Spain†.*
Fluocinolone acetonide (p.1101·2); neomycin sulfate (p.235·1).
*Infected skin disorders.*

**Neo-Synephrine**
*Abbott, Austral.; Sanofi Synthelabo, Austral.; Sanofi Synthelabo, Belg.†; Abbott, Canad.; Sanofi Winthrop, Israel; Teofarma, Ital.; Sanofi Winthrop, Swed.†; Sanofi Winthrop, USA.*
Phenylephrine hydrochloride (p.1126·3).
*Maintenance of blood pressure during surgery; paroxysmal supraventricular tachycardia; production of mydriasis; spinal and regional analgesia; vascular failure in shock or drug-induced hypotension or hypersensitivity.*

**Neosynephrine**
*Merck Sharp & Dohme-Chibret, Fr.; Novartis Ophthalmics, Fr.; Abbott, NZ.*
Phenylephrine hydrochloride (p.1126·3).
*Production of mydriasis.*

**Neo-Synephrine 12 Hour** *Sterling Health, USA.*
Oxymetazoline hydrochloride (p.1126·1).
*Nasal congestion.*

**Neosynephrin-POS** *Ursapharm, Ger.*
Phenylephrine hydrochloride (p.1126·3).
*Eye disorders.*

**Neo-Synodorm** *Synpharma, Switz.†.*
Diphenhydramine (p.431·3).
*Agitation; nervousness; sleep disorders.*

**Neotaflan** *Neo Quimica, Braz.*
Diclofenac (p.32·1).

**Neotalem**
*Laboratorios Chile, Chile; Lemery, Mex.*
Mitoxantrone hydrochloride (p.575·2).
*Malignant neoplasms.*

**Neotaren** *Neo Quimica, Braz.*
Diclofenac sodium (p.32·1).

**NeoTect** *Diatide, USA.*
Technetium-99m depreotide (p.1525·2).
*Scintigraphic imaging for pulmonary malignancy.*

**Neotenol** *Biobras, Braz.*
Atenolol (p.865·2).
*Angina pectoris; arrhythmias; hypertension; myocardial infarction.*

**Neotensin** *CEPA, Spain.*
Enalapril maleate (p.909·2).
*Heart failure; hypertension.*

**Neotensin Diu** *CEPA, Spain.*
Hydrochlorothiazide (p.933·2); enalapril maleate (p.909·2).
*Hypertension.*

**Neotest** *Merieux, Fr.†.*
Tuberculin PPD (p.1759·1).
*Sensitivity testing.*

**Neotetranase** *Rottapharm, Ital.*
Amoxicillin trihydrate (p.155·3).
*Bacterial infections.*

**Neo-Thyreostat** *Herbrand, Ger.; Berlin-Chemie, Ger.*
Carbimazole (p.1596·2).
*Hyperthyroidism.*

**Neotica** *Nakorn, Thai.*
*Balm:* Methyl salicylate (p.59·3); camphor (p.1665·3); menthol (p.1711·3); eucalyptus oil (p.1686·2); eugenol (p.1686·2).
*Insect bites; muscle pain and inflammation; sports injuries; sprains.*
*Capsules:* Piroxicam (p.84·2).
*Gout; musculoskeletal and joint disorders.*

**Neotigason**
*Roche, Arg.; Roche, Austral.; Roche, Austria; Roche, Belg.; Roche, Braz.; Roche, Chile; Roche, Denm.; Roche, Fin.; Roche, Ger.; Roche, Gr.; Roche, Hong Kong; Roche, Irl.; Roche, Israel; Roche, Ital.; Roche, Mex.; Roche, Neth.; Roche, Norw.; Roche, NZ; Roche, Port.; Roche, S.Afr.; Roche, Singapore; Roche, Spain; Roche, Swed.; Roche, Switz.; Roche, Thai.; Roche, UK.*
Acitretin (p.1140·2).
*Keratinisation disorders; psoriasis.*

**Neo-Tinic** *Neolab, Canad.*
Multivitamins and iron (p.1417·1).

**Neo-Tiroimade** *Esfar, Port.*
Liothyronine sodium (p.1602·2).

**Neo-Tizide** *Pharmacia, Austria.*
Methaniazide calcium (p.230·1).
*Tuberculosis.*

**Neotomic** *NBZ, India.*
Glycerol (p.1694·3); sodium chloride (p.1233·3).
*Bowel evacuation; constipation.*

**Neoton** *Monsanto, Ital.*
Fosfocreatine sodium.
*Cardiac disorders.*

**Neotonico** *Hertz, Braz.†.*
Phosphoric acid; vitamin B substances; cinchona (p.1417·1).
*Nutritional supplement.*

**Neotop** *Medley, Braz.*
Neomycin sulfate (p.235·1); bacitracin zinc (p.161·3).
*Bacterial skin infections.*

**Neotopic**
*Technilab, Canad.*
Polymyxin B sulfate (p.245·1); bacitracin zinc (p.161·3); neomycin sulfate (p.235·1).
*Bacterial skin infections.*

*Technilab, Hong Kong†.*
Polymyxin B sulfate (p.245·1); bacitracin (p.161·3); neomycin sulfate (p.235·1).
*Skin disorders.*

**Neo-Tosel** *Geminis, Arg.*
Bromhexine (p.1115·3); clofedanol (p.1117·1).
*Coughs.*

**Neotoss** *Neo Quimica, Braz.*
Dropropizine (p.1119·3).
*Coughs.*

**Neotrace** *American Pharmaceutical, USA.*
Trace element preparation (p.1417·1).
*Additive for intravenous total parenteral nutrition solutions.*

**Neotracin**
*Ciba Vision, Ger.†; Novartis Ophthalmics, Switz.*
Neomycin sulfate (p.235·1); bacitracin (p.161·3).
*Bacterial eye infections.*

**Neotretin** *Cassara, Arg.*
Tretinoin (p.1161·1).
*Acne; keratinisation disorders.*

**Neotrexate** *GlaxoSmithKline, India.*
Methotrexate (p.568·2).
*Malignant neoplasms; psoriasis; rheumatoid arthritis.*

**Neotri** *Lilly, Ger.*
Xipamide (p.1029·2); triamterene (p.1016·2).
*Hypertension; oedema.*

**Neotricin** *Legrand, Braz.*
Neomycin sulfate (p.235·1); bacitracin zinc (p.161·3).
*Eye infections.*

**Neotricin HC** *Bausch & Lomb, USA.*
Neomycin sulfate (p.235·1); bacitracin zinc (p.161·3); polymyxin B sulfate (p.245·1); hydrocortisone acetate (p.1103·3).
*Eye inflammation with bacterial infection.*

**Neo-Trim Fibre** *GNLD, Austral.†.*
Fibre blend (from oat bran, barley bran, soy bran, orange gibre, acacia, ispaghula husk) (p.1253·2); methylcellulose (p.1580·2).
*Obesity.*

**Neo-Trim Meal Replacement** *GNLD, Austral.†.*
Food for special diets (p.1417·1).
*Obesity.*

**Neotrin** *Neo Quimica, Braz.*
Co-trimoxazole (p.199·3).
*Bacterial infections; Pneumocystis carinii pneumonia; protozoal infections.*

**Neotrin Balsamico** *Neo Quimica, Braz.†.*
Co-trimoxazole (p.199·3); guaifenesin (p.1122·1); ammonium chloride (p.1115·2).
*Bacterial infections.*

**Neotroparin** *Chinoin, Hung.*
Drotaverine hydrochloride (p.1683·1); homatropine methylbromide (p.483·2).
*Smooth muscle spasm.*

**Neo-Tuss** *Neolab, Canad.*
Dextromethorphan hydrobromide (p.1117·3); chlorphenamine maleate (p.427·3); phenylephrine hydrochloride (p.1126·3); sodium citrate (p.1223·2); guaifenesin (p.1122·1).
*Coughs; respiratory-tract congestion.*

**NeoTussan** *Novartis Consumer, Ger.*
Dextromethorphan polistirex (p.1118·1).
*Coughs.*

**Neotyf** *Chiron Vaccines, Ital.†.*
A typhoid vaccine (p.1642·2).
*Active immunisation.*

**Neo-Ulcoid** *Valdecasas, Mex.*
Dextromethorphan hydrobromide (p.1117·3).
*Coughs.*

**Neo-Uridixico** *Rimsa, Mex.†.*
Nalidixic acid (p.234·1).

**Neo-Ustiol** *INTES, Ital.*
Sodium citrate (p.1223·2); sodium aminobenzoate (p.1747·1); procaine (p.1383·2); cod-liver oil (p.1425·2).
*Ophthalmic burns.*

**Neovermin** *Neo Quimica, Braz.*
Mebendazole (p.108·2); tiabendazole (p.114·2).
*Worm infections.*

**Neovis** *Pharmacia, Ital.*
Vitamin, carbohydrate, and mineral preparation with creatine (p.1417·1).
*Nutritional supplement.*

**NeoVisc** *Stellar, Canad.*
Sodium hyaluronate (p.1697·3).
*Replacement of synovial fluid following arthrocentesis.*

**Neovita**
*Savoy, Singapore; Wallace Mfg Chem., UK.*
Multivitamin and ginseng preparation with or without minerals and lecithin (p.1417·1).

**Neo-Vites** *Neolab, Canad.†.*
Multivitamins or multivitamins and minerals (p.1417·1).

**Neo-Vivactil** *Sanofi Winthrop, Switz.†.*
Amino-acid, mineral, and vitamin C preparation (p.1417·1).

**Neovlar** *Schering, Braz.*
Ethinylestradiol (p.1553·2); levonorgestrel (p.1563·2).
*Combined oral contraceptive.*

**Neovletta** *Schering, Swed.*
Levonorgestrel (p.1563·2); ethinylestradiol (p.1553·2).
*Combined oral contraceptive.*

**Neoxane** *Asta Oncologia, Braz.*
Doxorubicin hydrochloride (p.547·3).
*Malignant neoplasms.*

**Neoxene** *Ecobi, Ital.*
Chlorhexidine gluconate (p.1173·2).
*Disinfection of skin, wounds, burns, and vagina.*

**Neoxidil**
*Galderma, Belg.; Galderma, Braz.; Galderma, Fr.†; Galderma, Hong Kong; Galderma, Israel; Galderma, Singapore; Galderma, Thai.†.*
Minoxidil (p.960·1).
*Alopecia androgenetica.*

**Neoxil**
*Note. This name is used for preparations of different composition.*
*Galderma, Mex.†.*
Minoxidil (p.960·1).

*Offenbach, Mex.*
Neomycin (p.235·1); kaolin (p.1268·3); pectin (p.1580·3); homatropine (p.483·2).
*Diarrhoea.*

**Neoxinal** *Farmec, Ital.*
Chlorhexidine gluconate (p.1173·2).
*Disinfection of skin, wounds, and burns.*

**Neo-Xylestesin** *Espe, Austria.*
Lidocaine hydrochloride (p.1377·3).
Adrenaline hydrochloride (p.852·3) is included in this preparation as a vasoconstrictor to diminish absorption and localise the effect of the local anaesthetic.
*Local anaesthesia in dentistry.*

**Neo-Xylestesin forte and Neo-Xylestesin special** *Espe, Austria.*
Lidocaine hydrochloride (p.1377·3).
Adrenaline hydrochloride (p.852·3) and noradrenaline hydrochloride (p.975·1) are included in this preparation as vasoconstrictors to diminish absorption and localise the effect of the local anaesthetic.
*Local anaesthesia in dentistry.*

**Neoyod** *Grunenthal, Chile.*
Povidone-iodine (p.1190·3).
*Disinfection of mucous membranes, skin, and wounds; vaginal infections.*

**Neozep**
*Note. This name is used for preparations of different composition.*
*United American, Hong Kong.*
Phenylpropanolamine hydrochloride (p.1127·3); paracetamol (p.76·2); salicylamide (p.87·3); chlorphenamine maleate (p.427·3); vitamin C (p.1460·2).
*Cold and influenza symptoms; nasopharyngeal disorders.*

*Great Eastern, Thai.; Myra, Thai.*
Paracetamol (p.76·2); chlorphenamine maleate (p.427·3).
Formerly contained paracetamol, phenylpropanolamine hydrochloride, and chlorphenamine maleate.
*Allergic rhinitis; cold symptoms; hay fever; sinusitis.*

**Neozimina** *Neo Quimica, Braz.*
Clofazimine (p.197·1).
*Leprosy.*

**Neozine**
*Note. This name is used for preparations of different composition.*
*Aventis, Braz.*
Levomepromazine hydrochloride (p.703·2).
*Adjunct in general anaesthesia; pain; premedication; psychoses.*

*Sanofi Synthelabo, Port.*
Oxymetazoline hydrochloride (p.1126·1).
*Nasal congestion.*

**Neo-Zol** *Neolab, Canad.*
Clotrimazole (p.396·2).

**Neozolone** *British Dispensary, Thai.*
Prednisolone (p.1108·1); neomycin (p.235·1).
*Eczema; infected skin disorders; seborrhoeic dermatitis.*

**Nepenic** *New Research, Ital.*
Flucloxacillin sodium (p.213·3).
*Bacterial infections.*

**Neper** *Elvetium, Arg.*
Mesna (p.1041·2).
*Prevention of urotoxicity due to oxazaphosphorine antineoplastics.*

**NephPlex RX** *Nephro-Tech, USA.*
Multivitamin preparation for dialysis patients (p.1417·1).

**Nephral** *Pfleger, Ger.*
Triamterene (p.1016·2); hydrochlorothiazide (p.933·2).
*Hypertension; oedema.*

**Nephramine**
*Fresenius Kabi, Fr.; Braun McGaw, Hong Kong†; Pisa, Mex.; McGaw, NZ†; Braun, Spain; R&D, USA.*
Amino-acid infusion (p.1417·1).
*Parenteral nutrition in renal impairment.*

**Nephrex**
*Rhone-Poulenc Rorer, Austral.†; Fisons, Hong Kong†.*
Calcium acetate (p.1225·1).
*Hyperphosphataemia.*

**Nephril**
*Pfizer, Irl.†; Pfizer, UK†.*
Polythiazide (p.984·2).
*Hypertension; oedema.*

**Nephrisan P** *Ziethen, Ger.*
Squill (p.1130·3); crataegus (p.1677·1).
*Heart failure.*

**Nephrisol mono** *Cesra, Ger.*
Solidago virgaurea (p.1748·3).
*Urinary-tract disorders.*

**Nephritin** *Tentan, Switz.*
Homoeopathic preparation.

**Nephro-Calci** *R&D, USA.*
Calcium carbonate (p.1254·2).
*Calcium deficiency; dietary supplement.*

**Nephrocaps** *Fleming, USA.*
Vitamin B substances with vitamin C (p.1417·1).
*Vitamin deficiency in renal dialysis.*

**Nephrocare** *Ross, Israel; Abbott, Israel.*
Preparation for enteral nutrition (p.1417·1).
*Complete nutrition or food supplement in renal disease.*

**Nephro-Fer** *R&D, USA.*
Ferrous fumarate (p.1427·3).
*Iron-deficiency anaemias.*

**Nephro-Fer Rx** *R&D, USA.*
Ferrous fumarate (p.1427·3); folic acid (p.1429·1).
*Iron deficiency.*

**Nephrogesic** *Ethnor, India.*
Phenazopyridine hydrochloride (p.83·1); nitrofurantoin (p.237·2).
*Urinary-tract infections.*

**Nephrolith mono** *Biomo, Ger.*
Solidago virgaurea (p.1748·3).
*Renal calculi.*

**Nephrolithol N** *Pfluger, Ger.†.*
Homoeopathic preparation.

**nephro-loges** *Loges, Ger.*
Equisetum (p.1684·1); solidago virgaurea (p.1748·3); ononis (p.1723·3); parsley root (p.1728·3).
*Urinary-tract disorders.*

**Nephron** *Nephron, USA.*
Racepinefrine hydrochloride (p.854·1).
*Bronchospasm.*

**Nephron FA** *Nephro-Tech, USA.*
Multivitamin preparation with iron and folic acid (p.1417·1).
Docusate sodium (p.1262·2) is included in this preparation to reduce the constipating effects of iron.

**Nephronorm med**
*Note. This name is used for preparations of different composition.*
*APS, Ger.*
*Tablets:* Java tea (p.1702·3).
*Urinary-tract disorders.*

*Mauermann, Ger.*
*Tea:* Silver birch (p.1660·3); solidago virgaurea (p.1748·3); java tea (p.1702·3); ononis (p.1723·3); rose fruit (p.1740·1); centaurea cyanus; calendula (p.1665·2).
*Urinary-tract disorders.*

**Nephro-Pasc** *Pascoe, Ger.*
Solidago virgaurea (p.1748·3); birch leaf (p.1660·3); java tea (p.1702·3).
*Urinary-tract disorders.*

**Nephroplasmal N** *Braun, Ger.†.*
Amino-acid and glycerol infusion (p.1417·1).
*Parenteral nutrition in renal disease.*

**Nephropur tri** *Repha, Ger.*
Solidago virgaurea (p.1748·3); birch leaf (p.1660·3); java tea (p.1702·3).
*Urinary-tract disorders.*

**Nephroselect M** *Dreluso, Ger.*
Solidago virgaurea (p.1748·3); equisetum (p.1684·1); birch leaf (p.1660·3); ononis (p.1723·3); lovage (p.1708·1); tropaeolum majus (p.1659·3); saw palmetto (p.1569·1).
*Urinary-tract disorders.*

**Nephrosolid** *Bioforce, Switz.*
Solidago virgaurea (p.1748·3); silver birch (p.1660·3); ononis (p.1723·3); equisetum (p.1684·1).
*Urinary-tract disorders.*

**Nephrosteril**
*Roux-Ocefa, Arg.; Fresenius, Belg.†; Fresenius Kabi, Hong Kong; Fresenius Kabi, Ital.; Fresenius Kabi, Singapore; Fresenius Kabi, Switz.; Fresenius Kabi, Thai.*
Amino-acid infusion (p.1417·1).
*Parenteral nutrition in renal disease.*

**Nephrotect** *Fresenius Kabi, Ger.*
Amino-acid infusion (p.1417·1).
*Parenteral nutrition in renal failure.*

**Nephrotrans**
*Medice, Ger.; Salmon, Switz.*
Sodium bicarbonate (p.1223·2).
*Metabolic acidosis.*

**Nephro-Vite** *R&D, USA.*
Multivitamin preparations (p.1417·1).

**Nephro-Vite +Fe** *R&D, USA.*
Multivitamin preparation with iron (p.1417·1).

**Nephrox** *Fleming, USA.*
Aluminium hydroxide (p.1249·2).
*Hyperacidity.*

**Nephrubin-N** *Weber & Weber, Ger.*
*Herbal tea:* Birch leaf (p.1660·3); ononis (p.1723·3); java tea (p.1702·3); solidago (p.1748·3).
*Tablets:* Birch leaf (p.1660·3); java tea (p.1702·3).
*Urinary-tract disorders.*

**Nephur 4**
*Roche Diagnostics, Austral.†; Roche Diagnostics, Irl.†.*
Test for pH, protein, glucose, and nitrite in urine.

**Nephur 6**
*Roche Diagnostics, Austral.; Roche Diagnostics, Irl.*
Test for pH, protein, glucose, nitrite, blood, and leucocytes in urine.

**Nephur 7**
*Roche Diagnostics, Austral.†; Roche Diagnostics, Fr.; Roche Diagnostics, Irl.*
Test for pH, protein, glucose, nitrite, blood, leucocytes, and ketones in urine.

**Nephur-Test + Leucocytes**
*Roche Diagnostics, Austral.; Roche Diagnostics, UK†.*
Test for leucocytes, nitrites, pH, protein, glucose, and blood in urine.

**Nepituss** *Bioindustria, Ital.*
Nepinalone hydrochloride (p.1125·2).
*Coughs.*

**Nepresol**
*Note. This name is used for preparations of different composition.*
*Novartis, Austria; Novartis, Belg.; Novartis, Denm.†; Teofarma, Ger.; Novartis, Gr.; IFET (ΙΦΕΤ), Gr.; Novartis, Hong Kong; Novartis, India; Novartis, Israel†; Novartis, Malaysia; Novartis, Neth.†; Novartis, Norw.†; Novartis, S.Afr.; Novartis, Swed.; Novartis, Switz.; Novartis, Thai.*
Dihydralazine (p.900·1), dihydralazine mesilate (p.900·1), or dihydralazine sulfate (p.899·3).
*Hypertension.*

*Cristalia, Braz.*
Hydralazine hydrochloride (p.931·2).
*Heart failure; hypertension.*

**Nepressol** *Novartis, Fr.*
Dihydralazine mesilate (p.900·1).
*Pre-eclampsia.*

**Nepro**
*Abbott, Arg.; Abbott, Austral.; Abbott, Canad.†; Abbott, Fin.; Abbott, Hong Kong; Abbott, Irl.; Abbott, Mex.; Abbott, NZ; Abbott, Thai.; Abbott Nutrition, UK; Ross, USA.*
Preparation for enteral nutrition in renal dialysis patients (p.1417·1).

**Neptal** *Procter & Gamble, Ger.†.*
Acebutolol hydrochloride (p.848·1).
*Cardiac disorders; hypertension.*

**Neptazane**
*Lederle, Austral.†; Wyeth-Ayerst, Canad.; Lederle, Israel; Wyeth-Ayerst, Thai.; Lederle, USA†.*
Methazolamide (p.953·1).
*Glaucoma.*

**Nerapin** *Kampel Martian, Arg.*
Nevirapine (p.650·2).
*HIV infection.*

**Nerdipina**
*OM, Port.; Ferrer, Spain.*
Nicardipine hydrochloride (p.965·1).
*Angina pectoris; cerebrovascular disorders; hypertension.*

**Nerdipine** *Medochemie, Thai.*
Nicardipine (p.965·2).
*Angina pectoris; hypertension.*

**Nereflun** *New Research, Ital.*
Flunisolide (p.1101·1).
*Allergic rhinitis; asthma; bronchostenosis.*

**Nerelid** *New Research, Ital.*
Nimesulide (p.67·1).
*Fever; inflammation; pain.*

**Nerex** *Farmanova, Ital.*
Royal jelly (p.1740·3); honey (p.1434·2); myrtillus (p.1718·3); fructose.
*Nutritional supplement.*

**Nergadan** *Uriach, Spain.*
Lovastatin (p.949·1).
*Atherosclerosis; hypercholesterolaemia.*

**Neribas**
*Schering, Ger.†; Asche, Ger.†; Schering, Switz.*
Emollient.
*Skin disorders.*

**Neribase**
*Schering, Denm.; Schering, Fin.; Schering, Fr.; Schering, Ital.; Schering, Port.*
Basis for topical preparations; emollient.
*Skin disorders.*

**Neribax** *Baxter, Mex.*
Hydroxocobalamin (p.1458·2).

**Nericur** *Schering, UK†.*
Benzoyl peroxide (p.1143·2).
*Acne.*

**Neriderm** *Pharma Clal, Israel.*
Diflucortolone valerate (p.1099·3).
*Skin disorders.*

**Neriforte** *Schering, Austria.*
Diflucortolone valerate (p.1099·3).
*Skin disorders.*

**Neriquinol** *Schering, Austria†.*
Diflucortolone valerate (p.1099·3); chlorquinaldol (p.187·3).
*Infected skin disorders.*

**Nerisalic**
*Stiefel, Canad.; Schering, Fr.*
Diflucortolone valerate (p.1099·3); salicylic acid (p.1157·1).
*Skin disorders.*

**Nerisona**
*Schering, Arg.; Schering, Austria; Schering, Belg.; Schering, Braz.; Schering, Denm.; Schering, Ger.; Asche, Ger.; Schering, Ital.; Schering, Mex.; Schering, Neth.; Schering, Port.; Schering, Switz.*
Diflucortolone valerate (p.1099·3).
*Skin disorders.*

**Nerisona C**
*Schering, Arg.; Schering, Ger.; Asche, Ger.; Schering, Ital.; Schering, Port.*
Diflucortolone valerate (p.1099·3); chlorquinaldol (p.187·3).
*Infected skin disorders.*

**Nerisone**
*Stiefel, Canad.; Schering, Fr.; Schering, Hong Kong; Schering, Malaysia; Schering, NZ; Schering, S.Afr.; Schering, Singapore; Meadow, UK.*
Diflucortolone valerate (p.1099·3).
*Skin disorders.*

**Nerisone C**
*Schering, Fr.; Schering, Hong Kong; Schering, NZ; Schering, Singapore.*
Diflucortolone valerate (p.1099·3); chlorquinaldol (p.187·3).
*Infected skin disorders.*

**Nerixia** *Abiogen, Ital.*
Neridronate sodium (p.773·2).
*Osteogenesis imperfecta.*

**Nerizina** *Neckerman, Braz.†.*
Cinnarizine (p.428·3).
*Vertigo.*

**Nero** *Elea, Arg.*
Phloroglucinol (p.1731·1); trimethylphloroglucinol (p.1731·1).
*Smooth muscle spasm.*

**Nerolid** *Sydenham, Mex.†.*
Diazepam (p.690·1).

**Nerpemide** *Morrith, Spain†.*
Proteolytic enzymes.
*Herpesvirus infections; neuritis.*

**Nervade** *Covan, S.Afr.†.*
Caffeine (p.782·1); sodium glycerophosphate (p.1695·2); magnesium glycerophosphate (p.1228·1); potassium glycerophosphate (p.1695·2); glycerophosphoric acid (p.1695·2); potassium citrate (p.1223·1); yeast extract.
*Tonic.*

**Nervan** *Rosch & Handel, Austria.*
Paracetamol (p.76·2); propyphenazone (p.85·3); caffeine citrate (p.782·1).
*Fever; pain.*

**Nervatona** *Brauer, Austral.†.*
*Oral liquid:* Anamirta cocculus; helonias (p.1696·3); passion flower (p.1729·1); ignatia; nux vomica; phosphoricum acidum; sepia; zincum metallicum.
*Anxiety.*
*Oral spray:* Homoeopathic preparation.

**Nervatona Plus**
*Brauer, Austral.†.*
*Oral liquid:* Anamirta cocculus; helonias (p.1696·3); ginseng (p.1693·1); passion flower (p.1729·1); ignatia; kali phosphoricum; magnesia phosphorica; nux vomica; phosphoricum acidum; sepia; valeriana; zincum metallicum.
*Anxiety; stress.*

*Hamilton, Austral.†.*
*Oral spray; Tablets:* Homoeopathic preparation.

**Nervaxon** *Fidia, Ital.*
Hypericum (p.299·1).
*Depression.*

**Nerve Tonic** *Hylands, Canad.*
Homoeopathic preparation.

**Nervei** *Rodisma, Ger.*
Hypericum (p.299·1).
*Depression.*

**Nervencreme S** *Fides, Ger.*
Peppermint oil (p.1283·2); eucalyptus oil (p.1686·2).
*Pain.*

**Nervendragees**
*Note. This name is used for preparations of different composition.*
*Rosch & Handel, Austria.*
Valerian (p.1762·2); lupulus (p.1708·1); melissa (p.1711·1).
*Nervous disorders; sleep disorders.*

*Ratiopharm, Ger.*
Valerian root (p.1762·2); passion flower (p.1729·1); lupulus (p.1708·1).
*Anxiety disorders; insomnia.*

**Nerven-Dragees** *Zeller, Israel.*
Crataegus (p.1677·1); passion flower (p.1729·1); lupulus (p.1708·1); valerian (p.1762·2).
*Insomnia; nervous disorders.*

**Nervenja** *OTW, Ger.*
Homoeopathic preparation.

**Nervenruh** *Klosterfrau, Austria.*
Valerian (p.1762·2); passion flower (p.1729·1); lupulus (p.1708·1).
*Anxiety disorders; sleep disorders.*

**Nerventee EF-EM-ES** Smetana, Austria.
Valerian (p.1762·2); lupulus (p.1708·1); hypericum (p.299·1); peppermint leaf (p.1283·2); calluna vulgaris; delphinium consolida.
*Anxiety disorders; sleep disorders.*

**Nerven-Tee Stada N** Stada, Ger.†.
Passion flower (p.1729·1); peppermint leaf (p.1283·2); melissa (p.1711·1); valerian (p.1762·2).
*Sedative; sleep disorders.*

**Nervfluid S** Fides, Ger.†.
Camphor (p.1665·3); eucalyptus oil (p.1686·2); pumilio pine oil (p.1737·1).
*Nerve, muscle, and joint pain.*

**Nervifene** Interdelta, Switz.
Cloral hydrate (p.684·1).
*Agitation; insomnia.*

**Nervifloran** Bioflora, Austria.
Valerian (p.1762·2); lupulus (p.1708·1); melissa (p.1711·1); orange flower (p.1723·3); rosemary (p.1740·2).
*Nervous disorders; sleep disorders.*

**Nervigenol Magnesio** Labinca, Arg.
Vitamin C (p.1460·2); magnesium aspartate (p.1227·3).
*Dietary supplement.*

**Nervikan** Schwabe, Spain.
Valerian (p.1762·2); melissa (p.1711·1).
*Anxiety; insomnia.*

**Nervine** Mathieu, Canad.†.
Aspirin (p.15·1); caffeine (p.782·1).

**Nervinetten**
Eurim, Ger.†; Zellaforte, Switz.
Valerian (p.1762·2); lupulus (p.1708·1).
*Agitation; sleep disorders.*

**Nervinfant N** Rubiepharm, Ger.
Lupulus (p.1708·1); passion flower (p.1729·1).
*Agitation; sleep disorders.*

**Nervipan** Medopharm, Ger.†.
Valerian (p.1762·2).
*Anxiety.*

**Nervistop L** Lacefa, Arg.
Lorazepam (p.704·1).
*Anxiety; muscle spasm.*

**Nervita** Boiron, Canad.
Homoeopathic preparation.

**Nervitone** Alembic, India.
Peptone; calcium gluconate; magnesium chloride; manganese sulfate; yeast extract (p.1417·1).
*Tonic.*

**Nervium** De Mayo, Braz.
Bromazepam (p.671·3).
*Anxiety; insomnia.*

**nervo OPT N** Optimed, Ger.
Diphenhydramine hydrochloride (p.431·3).
*Sleep disorders.*

**Nervobion** Merck, Spain.
Cyanocobalamin (p.1458·2); pyridoxine hydrochloride (p.1456·3); thiamine hydrochloride (p.1455·1) or thiamine nitrate (p.1455·1).
*Vitamin B deficiency.*

**Nervobion Fuerte** Merck, Arg.
Cyanocobalamin (p.1458·2); pyridoxine hydrochloride (p.1456·3); thiamine hydrochloride (p.1455·1) or thiamine nitrate (p.1455·1).
*Neuralgia; neuritis; neuropathy; vitamin B deficiency.*

**Nervocaine** Keene, USA.
Lidocaine hydrochloride (p.1377·3).
*Local anaesthesia.*

**Nervocalm** Garden House, Arg.
Passion flower (p.1729·1); melissa (p.1711·1); valerian (p.1762·2); tilia (p.1756·2).
*Nervous disorders.*

**Nervocur** Fabra, Arg.
Levodopa (p.1205·2); carbidopa (p.1204·3).
*Parkinsonism.*

**Nervoforcan** INQ, Braz.†.
Iron (p.1434·3); sodium glycerophosphate; magnesium glycerophosphate; vitamin B substances (p.1417·1).
*Iron deficiency; iron-deficiency anaemias.*

**Nervogastrol N** Sanofi Synthelabo, Ger.
Bismuth subnitrate (p.1252·2); bismuth subgallate (p.1252·2); heavy magnesium carbonate (p.1272·1); calcium carbonate (p.1254·2); sodium bicarbonate (p.1223·2); greater celandine (p.1695·3); condurango (p.1675·3).
*Gastrointestinal disorders.*

**Nervoheel** Peithner, Austria.
Homoeopathic preparation.

**Nervoject N** Syxyl, Ger.
Homoeopathic preparation.

**Nervolta** Volta, Chile.
Calcium bromolactobionate (p.674·1).
*Sedative.*

**Nervomax TB12** TRB, Arg.
Thiamine hydrochloride (p.1455·1); pyridoxine hydrochloride (p.1456·3); cyanocobalamin (p.1458·2); thioctic acid (p.1754·3).
*Alcoholism; antoxidant; neuritis; tonic.*

**Nervonocton N** Pfluger, Ger.
Kava (p.1703·2).
*Nervous disorders.*

**Nervopax** Lehning, Fr.
Homoeopathic preparation.

**Nervoregin forte** Pfluger, Ger.
Valerian (p.1762·2); lupulus (p.1708·1); passion flower (p.1729·1).
*Nervous disorders.*

**Nervoregin H** Pfluger, Ger.
Homoeopathic preparation.

**Nervosal** Neuropharma, Arg.
Fluoxetine (p.296·3).
*Depression.*

**Nervosana** Riemser, Ger.
Achillea (p.1646·2); liquorice (p.1270·2); melissa (p.1711·1); peppermint leaf (p.1283·2); rubus fruticosus; chamomile (p.1669·3); tilia (p.1756·2); valerian (p.1762·2); absinthium (p.1645·1).
*Nervous disorders; sleep disorders.*

**Nervostal** Pharmanik (Φαρμανικ), Gr.
Buspirone hydrochloride (p.672·2).
*Generalised anxiety.*

**Nervpin N** Schoning-Berlin, Ger.
Menthol (p.1711·3); noble fir oil.
*Musculoskeletal, joint, and soft-tissue disorders; neuralgia; superficial vascular disorders.*

**Nervuton N** Cesra, Ger.
Homoeopathic preparation.

**Nesacain** AstraZeneca, Switz.
Chloroprocaine hydrochloride (p.1373·1).
*Local anaesthesia.*

**Nesacaine**
AstraZeneca, Canad.; Astra, USA.
Chloroprocaine hydrochloride (p.1373·1).
*Local anaesthesia.*

**Nesdonal**
Rhone-Poulenc Rorer, Belg.†; Rhone-Poulenc Rorer, Neth.†.
Thiopental sodium (p.1309·1).
*General anaesthesia.*

**Nesfare** Madaus, Spain.
Framycetin sulfate (p.215·1); triamcinolone acetonide (p.1110·2); centella (p.1144·3).
*Infected skin disorders.*

**Nesivine** Merck, Belg.
Oxymetazoline hydrochloride (p.1126·1).
*Eustachian-tube inflammation; nasal congestion; otitis media; sinusitis.*

**Nesol** Orthos, Mex.†.
Dipyrone (p.35·3).

**Nesoro** Novaquimica, Braz.†.
Sodium chloride (p.1233·3).
*Nasal congestion.*

**Nespo** Dompe Biotec, Ital.
Darbepoetin alfa (p.745·2).
*Anaemia in renal failure.*

**Nestabs** Fielding, USA.
Multivitamin and mineral preparation with iron and folic acid (p.1417·1).
*Multivitamin and mineral supplement for pregnancy and lactation.*

**Nestargel**
Nestle, Switz.; Nestle, UK.
Ceratonia (p.1579·1).
*Infant feed thickener.*

**Nesthakchen** Schulke & Mayr, Austria.
Fennel (p.1687·2); aniseed (p.1655·2); caraway (p.1667·2); chamomile (p.1669·3); liquorice (p.1270·2); fennel oil (p.1687·3); anise oil (p.1655·2); caraway oil (p.1667·3); chamomile oil (p.1669·3).
*Gastrointestinal disorders.*

**Nestic** Asian Pharm, Thai.
Clotrimazole (p.396·2).
*Trichomoniasis; vaginal fungal infections.*

**Nestle VHC** Nestle, USA.
Preparation for enteral nutrition (p.1417·1).

**Nestosyl**
Note. This name is used for preparations of different composition.
Pharmethic, Belg.†.
Pramocaine (p.1382·2); chlorhexidine hydrochloride (p.1173·3); zinc oxide (p.1163·2).
Formerly contained benzocaine, butyl aminobenzoate, resorcinol, and zinc oxide.
*Minor wounds; skin disorders.*

Sanofi Synthelabo, Braz.†.
Benzocaine (p.1370·3); butyl aminobenzoate (p.1373·1); benzalkonium chloride (p.1168·3); zinc oxide (p.1163·2); hydroxyquinoline (p.1700·1).
*Skin disorders.*

Alpharma, Fr.
*Ointment:* Benzocaine (p.1370·3); butyl aminobenzoate (p.1373·1); resorcinol (p.1156·3); hydroxyquinoline (p.1700·1); zinc oxide (p.1163·2).
*Insect stings.*
*Topical solution:* Benzocaine (p.1370·3); butyl aminobenzoate (p.1373·1); hydroxyquinoline (p.1700·1).
*Catheterisation; local anaesthesia.*

**Nestum** Nestle, Port.
Gluten-free food (p.1417·1).

**Nesvital** Nestle, Fr.
A range of foods for special diets (p.1417·1).
*Obesity.*

**Netaf** Chemopharma, Chile.
Ketorolac (p.52·3).
*Pain.*

**Nethaprin Dospan** Mer-National, S.Afr.
Bufylline (p.781·3); doxylamine succinate (p.432·3); etafedrine hydrochloride (p.1121·2); phenylephrine hydrochloride (p.1126·3).
*Coughs; obstructive airways disease.*

**Nethaprin Expectorant** Mer-National, S.Afr.
Bufylline (p.781·3); doxylamine succinate (p.432·3); etafedrine hydrochloride (p.1121·2); guaifenesin (p.1122·1).
*Obstructive airways disease.*

**Neticin** Undra, Mex.
Netilmicin sulfate (p.236·3).
*Bacterial infections.*

**Netillin**
Schering-Plough, Irl.; Schering-Plough, UK.
Netilmicin sulfate (p.236·3).
*Bacterial infections.*

**Netilyn**
Schering-Plough, Denm.; Schering-Plough, Fin.; Schering-Plough, Norw.; Schering-Plough, Swed.
Netilmicin sulfate (p.236·3).
*Bacterial infections.*

**Netira** Craveri, Arg.
Netilmicin sulfate (p.236·3).
*Bacterial eye infections.*

**Netocur** Duncan, Arg.
Co-trimoxazole (p.199·3).
*Bacterial infections.*

**Netocur Balsamico** Duncan, Arg.
Co-trimoxazole (p.199·3); guaifenesin (p.1122·1).
*Bacterial infections.*

**Netra** Sam-On, Israel.
Calcium carbonate (p.1254·2); magnesium carbonate (p.1272·1).
*Calcium supplement; gastrointestinal hyperacidity; heartburn.*

**Netrocin** Schering-Plough, Spain.
Netilmicin sulfate (p.236·3).
*Bacterial infections.*

**Netromicina**
Schering-Plough, Braz.; Schering-Plough, Mex.; Schering-Plough, Port.
Netilmicin sulfate (p.236·3).
*Bacterial infections.*

**Netromicine** Schering-Plough, Fr.
Netilmicin sulfate (p.236·3).
*Bacterial infections.*

**Netromycin**
Schering-Plough, Austral.; Schering, Canad.; Schering-Plough, Gr.; Schering-Plough, Hong Kong; Fulford, India; Schering-Plough, NZ; Schering-Plough, S.Afr.; Schering-Plough, Thai.; Schering, USA†.
Netilmicin sulfate (p.236·3).
*Bacterial infections.*

**Netromycine**
Schering-Plough, Belg.; Schering-Plough, Neth.; Essex, Switz.
Netilmicin sulfate (p.236·3).
*Bacterial infections.*

**Nettacin** Schering-Plough, Ital.
Netilmicin sulfate (p.236·3).
*Bacterial infections.*

**Nettinerv S** Iso, Ger.
Homoeopathic preparation.

**Nettle Rash L88** Homeocan, Canad.
Homoeopathic preparation.

**Netunal** Merck, Arg.
Sucralfate (p.1290·2).
*Gastro-oesophageal reflux; peptic ulcer.*

**Netux** Roche Nicholas, Fr.
Codeine (p.27·1); phenyltoloxamine (p.439·1).
*Coughs.*

**Neu Viplex** Siam Bheasach, Thai.
Vitamin B substances (p.1417·1).
*Vitamin deficiency.*

**Neuart** Mitsubishi, Jpn.
Antithrombin III (p.742·2).
*Antithrombin III deficiency.*

**Neubee** Medifive, Thai.
Vitamin $B_1$ (p.1455·2); vitamin $B_6$ (p.1457·2); vitamin $B_{12}$ (p.1458·2).
*Neuritis; neuropathy; vitamin B deficiency.*

**Neucare** Hoe, Singapore.
Topical barrier preparation.

**Neucor** CT, Ital.
Nicardipine hydrochloride (p.965·1).
*Angina pectoris; heart failure; hypertension.*

**Neuer**
Daiichi, Hong Kong†; Daiichi, Jpn.
Cetraxate hydrochloride (p.1255·2).
*Gastritis; peptic ulcer.*

**Neufil** Bial, Port.
Diprophylline (p.784·3).
*Obstructive airways disease.*

**Neuflo** Yung Shin, Singapore.
Muramidase hydrochloride (p.1717·2).
*Haemorrhage; sinusitis.*

**Neugal** Diba, Mex.
Ranitidine hydrochloride (p.1285·2).
*Gastro-oesophageal reflux; peptic ulcer; Zollinger-Ellison syndrome.*

**Neugen** Bioprogress, Ital.†.
Nicergoline (p.1719·3).
*Cerebrovascular disorders.*

**Neugeron** Armstrong, Mex.
Carbamazepine (p.353·3).
*Epilepsy; neuralgias.*

**Neugra N** Hermes, Ger.†.
Multivitamin and mineral preparation (p.1417·1).

**Neulactil**
Aventis, Austral.; Aventis, Denm.; Aventis, Fin.; Aventis, Hong Kong; Aventis, Irl.; Rhone-Poulenc Rorer, Norw.†; Aventis, NZ; Aventis, S.Afr.; JHC Healthcare, UK.
Pericyazine (p.714·1).
*Anxiety disorders; behaviour disorders in children; psychoses.*

**Neulasta**
Amgen, Austral.; Amgen, Fr.; Amgen, Port.; Amgen, UK; Amgen, USA.
Pegfilgrastim (p.753·3).
*Neutropenia.*

**Neuleptil**
Aventis, Arg.; Rhone-Poulenc Rorer, Austria; Rhone-Poulenc Rorer, Belg.†; Aventis, Braz.; Aventis, Canad.; Aventis, Chile; Aventis, Fr.; Aventis, Israel; Aventis, Ital.; Aventis, Neth.; Rhone-Poulenc Rorer, Switz.†.
Pericyazine (p.714·1) or pericyazine mesilate (p.714·1).
*Behaviour disorders in childhood; psychoses.*

**Neumak** Biotenk, Arg.
A pneumococcal vaccine (14-valent) (p.1633·1).
*Active immunisation.*

**Neumega**
Wyeth, Arg.; Wyeth, Braz.; Wyeth, Chile; Wyeth, Mex.; Genetics Institute, USA.
Oprelvekin (p.757·1).
*Thrombocytopenia.*

**Neumobacticel** Bago, Arg.
Co-trimoxazole (p.199·3); bromhexine hydrochloride (p.1115·3).
*Bacterial infections.*

**Neumopectolina** Inkeysa, Spain.
Guaifenesin (p.1122·1); sodium benzoate (p.1169·3); co-trimoxazole (p.199·3).
*Respiratory-tract infections.*

**Neumoral** Medestea, Ital.†.
Hypericum (p.299·1); magnesium oxide (p.1272·3).
*Tonic.*

**Neumoterol** Phoenix, Arg.
Budesonide (p.1094·2); formoterol fumarate (p.786·1).
*Asthma.*

**Neumotex** Phoenix, Arg.
Budesonide (p.1094·2).
*Allergic rhinitis; obstructive airways disease.*

**Neuners Krautertee Nr 16 - Beruhigungstee bei Wechselbeschwerden** Neuners, Austria.
Sage (p.1741·2); orange flowers (p.1723·3); achillea (p.1646·2); melissa (p.1711·1); lupulus (p.1708·1); calendula (p.1665·2).
*Menopausal disorders.*

**Neuners Krautertee Nr 107 - Blahungstee**
Neuners, Austria.
Angelica (p.1655·1); sage (p.1741·2); caraway (p.1667·2); peppermint leaf (p.1283·2); aniseed (p.1655·2); sweet basil.
*Gastrointestinal disorders.*

**Neuners Krautertee Nr 3 - Blasentee** Neuners, Austria.
Bearberry (p.1659·2); parsley (p.1728·3); veronica; solidago virgaurea (p.1748·3); equisetum (p.1684·1); rosemary (p.1740·2).
*Urinary-tract disorders.*

**Neuners Krautertee Nr 7 - Bronchial- und Lungentee** Neuners, Austria.
Althaea (p.1651·3); plantago lanceolata (p.1738·2); thyme (p.1755·2); aniseed (p.1655·2); marrubium vulgare (p.1124·1).
*Catarrh; coughs.*

**Neuners Krautertee Nr 311 - Bronchialtee zur Inhalation** Neuners, Austria.
Peppermint leaf (p.1283·2); thyme (p.1755·2); chamomile (p.1669·3); sage (p.1741·2).
*Catarrh; coughs.*

**Neuners Krautertee Nr 25 - Entschlackungstee** Neuners, Austria.
Parsley (p.1728·3); birch leaf (p.1660·3); ononis (p.1723·3); taraxacum (p.1751·3); rubus fruticosus; rose fruit (p.1740·1).
*Tonic.*

**Neuners Krautertee Nr 2 - Fruhjahrskurtee**
Neuners, Austria.
Birch leaf (p.1660·3); lovage root (p.1708·1); solidago virgaurea (p.1748·3); couch-grass (p.1676·2); prunus spinosa; sambucus (p.1741·3); calendula (p.1665·2).
*Urinary-tract disorders.*

**Neuners Krautertee Nr 10 - Grippetee** Neuners, Austria.
Tilia (p.1756·2); thyme (p.1755·2); sage (p.1741·2); sambucus (p.1741·3); aniseed (p.1655·2); fennel (p.1687·2).
*Cold and influenza symptoms.*

**Neuners Krautertee Nr 19 - Harntreibender Stoffwechseltee** Neuners, Austria.
Silver birch (p.1660·3); urtica (p.1762·1); juniper (p.1703·1); lovage root (p.1708·1); viola tricoloris.
*Diuresis.*

**Neuners Krautertee Nr 31 - Harnwegstee**
Neuners, Austria.
Bearberry (p.1659·2); java tea (p.1702·3); lovage root (p.1708·1).
*Diuresis.*

**Neuners Krautertee Nr 210 - Krauterhexlein Kinder-Schweisstreibender Tee** Neuners, Austria.
Tilia (p.1756·2); sambucus (p.1741·3); peppermint leaf (p.1283·2); bitter-orange peel (p.1723·3).
*Cold symptoms.*

**Neuners Krautertee Nr 204 - Krauterhexlein Kinder Nieren- und Blasentee** *Neuners, Austria.*
Birch leaf (p.1660·3); ononis (p.1723·3); solidago virgaurea (p.1748·3); bearberry (p.1659·2); peppermint leaf (p.1283·2).
*Urinary-tract disorders.*

**Neuners Krautertee Nr 201 - Krauterhexlein Kinder-Beruhigungstee** *Neuners, Austria.*
Melissa (p.1711·1); lavender flower (p.1705·1); lupulus (p.1708·1); peppermint leaf (p.1283·2); orange flower (p.1723·3).
*Nervous disorders.*

**Neuners Krautertee Nr 217 - Krauterhexlein Kinder-Blahungstee** *Neuners, Austria.*
Chamomile (p.1669·3); fennel (p.1687·2); caraway (p.1667·2); peppermint leaf (p.1283·2); bitter-orange peel (p.1723·3).
*Gastrointestinal disorders.*

**Neuners Krautertee Nr 207 - Krauterhexlein Kinder-Brusttee** *Neuners, Austria.*
Galeopsis ochroleuca; wild thyme; rose fruit (p.1740·1); calendula (p.1665·2).
*Catarrh; coughs.*

**Neuners Krautertee Nr 211 - Krauterhexlein Kinder-Hustentee** *Neuners, Austria.*
Thyme (p.1755·2); drosera (p.1683·1); aniseed (p.1655·2); verbascum flowers (p.1764·1).
*Catarrh; coughs.*

**Neuners Krautertee Nr 209 - Krauterhexlein Kinder-Magentee** *Neuners, Austria.*
Chamomile (p.1669·3); peppermint leaf (p.1283·2); melissa (p.1711·1); orange flower (p.1723·3).
*Gastrointestinal disorders.*

**Neuners Krautertee Nr 32 - Kreislafregulierungstee** *Neuners, Austria.*
Mistletoe (p.1715·3); crataegus (p.1677·1); equisetum (p.1684·1); prunus spinosa.
*Circulatory and metabolic disorders.*

**Neuners Krautertee Nr 44 - Kreislaufanregender Tee** *Neuners, Austria.*
Crataegus (p.1677·1); juglans leaf; achillea (p.1646·2); linaria vulgaris; angelica (p.1655·1); calendula flower (p.1665·2).
*Circulatory disorders; gastrointestinal disorders.*

**Neuners Krautertee Nr 20 - Kreislauftee** *Neuners, Austria.*
Crataegus (p.1677·1); taraxacum (p.1751·3); gentian (p.1692·2); centaury (p.1669·2); mistletoe (p.1715·3); rosemary (p.1740·2).
*Cardiovascular disorders.*

**Neuners Krautertee Nr 17 - Lebertee** *Neuners, Austria.*
Taraxacum (p.1751·3); turmeric (p.1058·3); centaury (p.1669·2); absinthium (p.1645·1); chamomile (p.1669·3); caraway (p.1667·2).
*Liver and biliary disorders.*

**Neuners Krautertee Nr 9 - Magentee** *Neuners, Austria.*
Centaury (p.1669·2); menyanthes (p.1712·1); valerian (p.1762·2); melissa (p.1711·1); chamomile (p.1669·3); fennel (p.1687·2).
*Gastrointestinal disorders.*

**Neuners Krautertee Nr 8 - Magentee gegen Ubersauerung** *Neuners, Austria.*
Urtica (p.1762·1); sage (p.1741·2); fennel (p.1687·2); peppermint leaf (p.1283·2); chamomile (p.1669·3).
*Gastrointestinal disorders.*

**Neuners Krautertee Nr 1 - Nerventee** *Neuners, Austria.*
Valerian (p.1762·2); lupulus (p.1708·1); melissa (p.1711·1); lavender flower (p.1705·1); chamomile (p.1669·3).
*Nervous disorders.*

**Neuners Krautertee Nr 4 - Nierentee** *Neuners, Austria.*
Equisetum (p.1684·1); juniper (p.1703·1); solidago virgaurea (p.1748·3); parsley (p.1728·3); rose fruit (p.1740·1); peppermint leaf (p.1283·2).
*Urinary-tract disorders.*

**Neuners Krautertee Nr 141 - Schlaftee** *Neuners, Austria.*
Lupulus (p.1708·1); valerian (p.1762·2); melissa (p.1711·1); lavender flower (p.1705·1); peppermint leaf (p.1283·2).
*Nervous disorders.*

**Neuners Krautertee Nr 126 - Starkungstee fur stillende Mutter** *Neuners, Austria.*
Caraway (p.1667·2); aniseed (p.1655·2); fennel (p.1687·2); parsley (p.1728·3); thyme (p.1755·2).
*Breast feeding.*

**Neuners Krautertee Nr 18 - Stoffwechseltee** *Neuners, Austria.*
Juniper (p.1703·1); parsley (p.1728·3); ononis (p.1723·3).
*Urinary-tract disorders.*

**Neuners Krautertee Nr 29 - Stoffwechseltee mild** *Neuners, Austria.*
Birch leaf (p.1660·3); taraxacum (p.1751·3); juniper (p.1703·1); rosemary (p.1740·2); flos bellidis.
*Diuresis.*

**Neuners Krautertee Nr 30 - Stoffwechseltee stark** *Neuners, Austria.*
Juniper (p.1703·1); ononis (p.1723·3); birch leaf (p.1660·3); rosemary (p.1740·2); absinthium (p.1645·1); herba majoranae.
*Diuresis.*

**Neuners Krautertee Nr 14 - Verdauungstee** *Neuners, Austria.*
Prunus spinosa; linaria vulgaris; fennel (p.1687·2); caraway (p.1667·2); centaury (p.1669·2); peppermint leaf (p.1283·2).
*Gastrointestinal disorders.*

**Neuners Krautertee Nr 124 - zur Entspannung vor der Geburt** *Neuners, Austria.*
Valerian (p.1762·2); achillea (p.1646·2); chamomile (p.1669·3); plantago lanceolata (p.1738·2); peppermint leaf (p.1283·2).
*Labour.*

**Neuners Krautertee Nr 11 - zur Unterstutzung der Tatigkeit der Bronchien und Atemwege** *Neuners, Austria.*
Althaea (p.1651·3); plantago lanceolata (p.1738·2); aniseed (p.1655·2); fennel (p.1687·2); galeopsis ochroleuca.
*Upper respiratory-tract disorders.*

**Neuners Krautertee Nr 28 - zur Unterstutzung der Tatigkeit der Galle** *Neuners, Austria.*
Marrubium vulgare (p.1124·1); agrimony herb (p.1649·1); absinthium (p.1645·1); cichorium intybus; angelica (p.1655·1); peppermint leaf (p.1283·2).
*Biliary disorders.*

**Neupax**
*Note. This name is used for preparations of different composition.*
*Bago, Arg.*
Fluoxetine hydrochloride (p.292·1).
*Bulimia; depression; obsessive-compulsive disorder; panic attacks.*
*Armstrong, Mex.*
Alprazolam (p.668·3).
*Anxiety; mixed anxiety depressive states.*

**Neupogen**
*Roche, Arg.; Amgen, Austral.; Roche, Austria; Amgen, Belg.; Amgen, Canad.; Roche, Chile; Amgen, Denm.; Amgen, Fin.; Amgen, Fr.; Amgen, Ger.; Roche, Ger.; Roche, Hong Kong; Amgen, Irl.; Roche, Israel; Dompe Biotec, Ital.; Roche, Mex.; Amgen, Neth.; Roche, Norw.; Roche, NZ; Amgen, Port.; Roche, S.Afr.; Roche, Singapore; Amgen, Spain; Amgen, Swed.; Roche, Switz.; Roche, Thai.; Amgen, UK; Amgen, USA.*
Filgrastim (p.753·3).
*Mobilisation of autologous peripheral blood progenitor cells; neutropenia.*

**Neupram** *Neuropharma, Arg.*
Haloperidol (p.701·2).

**Neupramir** *Lusofarmaco, Ital.*
Pramiracetam sulfate (p.1734·3).
*Mental function impairment.*

**Neuquinon**
*Eisai, Jpn; Eisai, Malaysia.*
Ubidecarenone (p.1760·2).
*Heart failure.*

**Neuraben** *Pfizer, Ital.*
Thiamine bezomil (p.1455·2); pyridoxine hydrochloride (p.1456·3); cyanocobalamin (p.1458·2).
*Neuritis.*

**Neurabol** *Cadila, India.*
*Capsules:* Stanozolol (p.1569·2).
*Injection:* Nandrolone phenylpropionate (p.1561·3).
*Anabolic; osteoporosis.*

**Neuractin** *Drugtech, Chile.*
Valproate semisodium (p.380·1).
*Epilepsy.*

**Neuractiv** *Novartis, Ital.†.*
Oxiracetam (p.1725·2).
*Mental function impairment.*

**Neuragon** *Sriprasit, Thai.*
Perphenazine (p.714·2); amitriptyline hydrochloride (p.280·3).
*Mixed anxiety depressive states.*

**Neuralgietabletten N** *Cosmochema, Ger.*
Homoeopathic preparation.

**Neuralgietropfen CM** *Cosmochema, Ger.*
Homoeopathic preparation.

**Neuralgin** *Pfleger, Ger.*
Aspirin (p.15·1); paracetamol (p.76·2); caffeine (p.782·1).
*Pain.*

**Neuralgin ASS** *Pfleger, Ger.†.*
Aspirin (p.15·1).
*Fever; pain.*

**Neuralin** *Chinoin, Mex.*
1 Ampoule, thiamine hydrochloride (p.1455·1); pyridoxine hydrochloride (p.1456·3); hydroxocobalamin (p.1458·2); 1 ampoule, dexamethasone sodium phosphate (p.1097·2); lidocaine hydrochloride (p.1377·3).
*Inflammation; neuralgias; neuritis; rheumatism.*

**Neuralprona** *Bioquimico, Arg.*
Naproxen (p.65·1).
*Fever; inflammation; pain.*

**Neuralysan S** *Steigerwald, Ger.*
Thiamine hydrochloride (p.1455·1); pyridoxine hydrochloride (p.1456·3).
*Neuralgia; neuritis.*

**Neuramag P** *CT, Ger.†.*
Paracetamol (p.76·2); caffeine (p.782·1).
*Pain.*

**Neuramate** *Halsey, USA.*
Meprobamate (p.706·2).
*Anxiety.*

**Neuramide Sherman** *Difa, Ital.*
Neuramide.
*Herpesvirus infections.*

**Neuramin** *Orion, Fin.*
Thiamine hydrochloride (p.1455·1).
*Thiamine deficiency; wernicke-Korsakoff syndrome.*

**Neuramizone** *Sriprasit, Thai.*
Belladonna alkaloids (p.479·1); ergotamine tartrate (p.467·2); phenobarbital (p.367·3).
*Sedative.*

**Neur-Amyl** *Sigma, Austral.*
Amobarbital (p.670·1).
*Hypnotic; sedative.*

**Neuranidal** *Stada, Ger.*
Aspirin (p.15·1); paracetamol (p.76·2); caffeine (p.782·1).
*Pain.*

**Neuranidal Duo** *LAW, Ger.†.*
Aspirin (p.15·1); caffeine (p.782·1).
*Fever; pain.*

**Neurapas** *Pascoe, Ger.*
Hypericum (p.299·1); valerian (p.1762·2); passion flower (p.1729·1).
Formerly contained hypericum, valerian, passion flower, larkspur, and eschscholtzia.
*Psychiatric disorders.*

**Neurax** *Agepha, Austria.*
Vitamin B substances (p.1417·1).

**NeuRecover** *NeuroGenesis, USA.*
A range of multivitamin, mineral, and amino-acid preparations (p.1417·1).

**Neurex**
*Note. This name is used for preparations of different composition.*
*Beta, Arg.*
Acetylcarnitine hydrochloride (p.1646·1).
*Cerebral vasculopathy; peripheral neuropathy.*
*Euro-Pharma, Ital.*
Citicoline sodium (p.1672·3).
*Cerebrovascular disorders; parkinsonism.*

**Neuri B6** *Cazi, Braz.*
Pyridoxine hydrochloride (p.1456·3).
*Neuritis.*

**Neuriberi** *Haller, Braz.*
Vitamin $B_1$; vitamin $B_6$; vitamin $B_{12}$ (p.1417·1).
*Vitamin B deficiency.*

**Neuriclor** *Sanofi Synthelabo, Arg.*
Citicoline (p.1672·3).
*Cerebrovascular disorders.*

**Neuriclor Vascular** *Sanofi Synthelabo, Arg.*
Citicoline (p.1672·3); co-dergocrine mesilate (p.1674·1).
*Cerebrovascular disorders; neurological disorders.*

**Neuri-cyl N Ho-Len-Complex** *Liebermann, Ger.*
Homoeopathic preparation.

**Neuridon** *Synthelabo, Belg.†.*
Paracetamol (p.76·2).
*Fever; pain.*

**Neuridon Forte** *Sanofi Synthelabo, Belg.†.*
Paracetamol (p.76·2); propyphenazone (p.85·3); codeine phosphate (p.27·1).
*Fever; pain.*

**Neuril** *Sanova, Austria.*
Melperone hydrochloride (p.706·1).
*Anxiety disorders; drug and alcohol withdrawal syndrome; psychoses; senile dementia; sleep disorders.*

**Neurilan** *Gross, Braz.*
Bromazepam (p.671·3).
*Anxiety.*

**Neurinase** *Rudefsa, Mex.†.*
Barbital sodium (p.671·2).
*Sedative; sleep disorders.*

**Neuriplege** *Genevrier, Fr.*
*Cream:* Chlorproethazine hydrochloride (p.675·1).
*Ointment†:* Chlorproethazine hydrochloride (p.675·1); cymene (p.28·2).
*Painful skeletal muscle spasm.*

**Neurium**
*Note. This name is used for preparations of different composition.*
*Sintofarma, Braz.*
Lamotrigine (p.363·3).
*Epilepsy.*
*Hexal, Ger.*
Ethylenediamine thioctate (p.1754·3).
*Diabetic polyneuropathy.*

**Neuro** *Stada, Ger.*
Thiamine hydrochloride (p.1455·1); pyridoxine hydrochloride (p.1456·3).
*Nervous-system disorders.*

**Neuro B** *Raza, Malaysia; Pharmaniaga, Malaysia.*
Vitamin $B_1$ (p.1455·2); vitamin $B_6$ (p.1457·2); vitamin $B_{12}$ (p.1458·2).
*Diabetic neuropathy; neuralgia; neuritis; vitamin B deficiency.*

**Neuro B1-6-12** *Jean-Marie, Hong Kong.*
Vitamin $B_1$ (p.1455·2); vitamin $B_6$ (p.1457·2); vitamin $B_{12}$ (p.1458·2).
*Neuralgias; neuritis; vitamin B deficiencies.*

**Neuro Calme** *Geistlich, Switz.*
Vitamin B substances and mineral preparation (p.1417·1).
*Tonic.*

**Neuro Nutrients** *Solgar, UK.*
Amino-acid preparation with vitamin B substances, vitamin C, and ginkgo biloba (p.1417·1).

**Neuro uno** *Stada, Ger.*
Benfotiamine (p.1454·3); pyridoxine hydrochloride (p.1456·3).
*Nervous-system disorders.*

**Neuroactil** *Bago, Arg.*
Acetylcarnitine hydrochloride (p.1646·1).

**Neuro-AS N** *Teva, Ger.*
Thiamine hydrochloride (p.1455·1); pyridoxine hydrochloride (p.1456·3).
*Vitamin B deficiency.*

**neuro-B forte** *Biomo, Ger.*
Thiamine hydrochloride (p.1455·1); pyridoxine hydrochloride (p.1456·3).
*Neurological system disorders.*

**Neurobex** *British Dispensary, Thai.*
Vitamin $B_1$ (p.1455·2); vitamin $B_6$ (p.1457·2); vitamin $B_{12}$ (p.1458·2).
Lidocaine hydrochloride (p.1377·3) is included in the injection to alleviate the pain of injection.
*Anaemias; neurological disorders.*

**Neurobiol** *Teofarma, Ital.*
Phenobarbital (p.367·3).
*Epilepsy; insomnia; sedative.*

**Neurobion**
*Merck, Austria; Merck, Belg.; Merck, Fin.; Merck, Ger.; Merck, Hong Kong; Merck, Malaysia; Merck, Mex.; Merck, Port.; Merck, S.Afr.; Merck, Singapore; Merck, Swed.; Merck, Thai.*
Thiamine disulfide (p.1455·2) or thiamine hydrochloride (p.1455·1); pyridoxine hydrochloride (p.1456·3); cyanocobalamin (p.1458·2).
*Neuralgia; neuritis; neuropathies; vitamin B deficiency.*
*Merck, India.*
Vitamin $B_1$; vitamin $B_6$; vitamin $B_{12}$; nicotinamide; calcium pantothenate (p.1417·1).
*Vitamin B deficiency.*
*E. Merck, Irl.†; Merck, Neth.*
Vitamin B substances (p.1417·1).
*Peripheral neuropathy; vitamin B deficiency.*

**Neurobion N** *Merck, Ger.*
Thiamine nitrate (p.1455·1) or thiamine disulfide (p.1455·2); pyridoxine hydrochloride (p.1456·3).
*Neuralgia; neuritis.*

**Neurobionta**
*Merck, Chile; Bracco, Ital.†.*
Thiamine hydrochloride (p.1455·1); pyridoxine hydrochloride (p.1456·3); cyanocobalamin (p.1458·2).
Lidocaine (p.1377·3) is included in some injections to alleviate the pain of injection.
*Musculoskeletal and joint pain; neuralgia; neuritis; vitamin B deficiency.*

**NeuroBloc**
*Elan, Fr.; Elan, Ger.; Elan, Irl.; Elan, Ital.; Esteve, Port.; Elan, Spain; Elan, UK.*
Botulinum B toxin (p.1388·3).
*Spasmodic torticollis.*

**Neurocalcium**
*Biologiques de l'Ile-de-France, Fr.†.*
*Syrup:* Calcium bromide (p.1663·1); calcium chloride (p.1225·1); calcium gluconogluceptate.
*Anxiety; insomnia.*
*Medix, Fr.†.*
*Tablets:* Calcium gluconate (p.1225·2); calcium bromide (p.1663·1).
Formerly contained calcium gluconate, calcium bromide, and phenobarbital.
*Anxiety; insomnia; palpitations.*

**Neurocam** *Pharmafina, Chile.*
Clonixin lysine (p.26·3); thiamine hydrochloride (p.1455·1); pyridoxine hydrochloride (p.1456·3); vitamin $B_{12}$ (p.1458·2).
*Pain.*

**Neurocardol** *Cavalheiro, Port.*
Passion flower (p.1729·1); crataegus (p.1677·1); salix (p.87·3); valerian (p.1762·2).

**Neurocatavin Dexa** *Llorente, Spain.*
Vitamin B substances (p.1417·1); dexamethasone sodium phosphate (p.1097·2); suprarenal cortex (p.1110·1).
Lidocaine (p.1377·3) is included in this preparation to alleviate the pain of injection.
*Myalgia; neuralgia; neuritis; rheumatism.*

**Neurochol C** *Merck, Ger.*
Greater celandine (p.1695·3); taraxacum (p.1751·3); absinthium (p.1645·1).
*Biliary disorders; dyspepsia.*

**Neurocil** *Bayer, Ger.*
Levomepromazine hydrochloride (p.703·2) or levomepromazine maleate (p.703·2).
*Bipolar disorder; pain; psychoses.*

**Neurocine** *Armstrong, Arg.*
Bifemelane hydrochloride (p.1660·2).
*Cerebrovascular disorders; mental function impairment.*

**Neurodavur** *Belmac, Spain.*
Vitamin B substances (p.1417·1).
*Vitamin B deficiency.*

**Neurodavur Plus** *Belmac, Spain.*
Vitamin B substances (p.1417·1); dexamethasone sodium phosphate (p.1097·2).
Lidocaine hydrochloride (p.1377·3) is included in this preparation to alleviate the pain of injection.
*Myalgia; neuralgia; neuritis.*

**Neurodep** *Med. Prod. Panam., USA.*
*Capsules:* Vitamin B substances (p.1417·1).
*Injection:* Vitamin B substances and vitamin C (p.1417·1).

**Neurodex** *Dexa, Singapore.*
Vitamin $B_1$ (p.1455·2); vitamin $B_6$ (p.1457·2); vitamin $B_{12}$ (p.1458·2).
*Anaemias; nausea; neurological disorders; tonic; vitamin B deficiency.*

**Neurodif** *Vinas, Spain†.*
Lysine aspirin (p.54·3); vitamin B substances (p.1417·1).
Lidocaine hydrochloride (p.1377·3) is included in the intramuscular injection to alleviate the pain of injection.
*Musculoskeletal and joint disorders; neuritis.*

**Neuro-Do** *Grasler, Ger.*
Homoeopathic preparation.

**Neurodol Tissugel** *IBSA, Switz.*
Lidocaine (p.1377·3).
*Post-herpetic neuralgia.*

**Neuro-Effekton B** *Teofarma, Ger.*
Thiamine hydrochloride (p.1455·1); pyridoxine hydrochloride (p.1456·3).
*Nervous-system disorders.*

**Neurofenac**
*Merck, Austria; Merck, Hong Kong.*
Diclofenac sodium (p.32·1); vitamin B substances (p.1417·1).
*Gout; musculoskeletal and joint disorders; neuralgia; neuritis; pain.*

**Neurofitol** *Heralds, Braz.†.*
Methyltestosterone (p.1559·3); vitamin E (p.1464·3); calcium magnesium fytate.
*Erectile dysfunction.*

**Neuroflax** *Aventis, Mex.*
Cobamamide (p.1459·1); thiocolchicoside (p.1395·2).
*Musculoskeletal and joint disorders.*

**Neuroflorine** *Fuca, Fr.*
Passion flower (p.1729·1); crataegus (p.1677·1); valerian (p.1762·2).
*Anxiety; insomnia; palpitations.*

**Neurofor** *Aventis, Mex.*
Cobamamide (p.1459·1).
*Anaemias; neuralgias; neuritis.*

**Neuroforte** *Beacons, Singapore.*
Vitamin $B_1$ (p.1455·2); vitamin $B_6$ (p.1457·2); vitamin $B_{12}$ (p.1458·2).
*Diabetic neuropathy; neuralgia; poluneuritis.*

**Neuroftal** *INTES, Ital.*
*Injection:* Thiamine hydrochloride (p.1455·1); nicotinamide (p.1441·2); strychnine glycerophosphate. Procaine hydrochloride (p.1383·2) is included in this preparation to alleviate the pain of injection.
*Tablets:* Thiamine hydrochloride (p.1455·1); riboflavin (p.1456·1); nicotinamide (p.1441·2); strychnine nitrate (p.1750·1); sodium glycerophosphate (p.1695·2).
*Optic nerve atrophy.*

**Neurogamma** *Worwag, Ger.†.*
Cyanocobalamin; pyridoxine hydrochloride; thiamine nitrate (p.1417·1).
*Neuralgia; neuritis.*

**Neurogen-E**
*Imperial, Malaysia; Imperial, Singapore.*
Vitamin $B_1$; vitamin $B_6$; vitamin $B_{12}$; vitamin E (p.1417·1).
*Vitamin supplement.*

**Neurogeron** *Andromaco, Chile.*
Nimodipine (p.972·3).
*Cerebrovascular disorders; migraine; neurological deficit following neurosugery or subarachnoid haemorrhage.*

**Neuroglutamin** *Pharmonta, Austria.*
Glutamic acid (p.1433·2).
*Memory and concentration disorders.*

**Neurogrisevit N** *Pharmacia Upjohn, Ger.†.*
Thiamine nitrate (p.1455·1); pyridoxine hydrochloride (p.1456·3).
*Nervous-system disorders.*

**Neurol**
*Note. This name is used for preparations of different composition.*
*SIT, Ital.*
Sodium valerate; sodium glycerophosphate (p.1695·2).
Lidocaine hydrochloride (p.1377·3) is included in this preparation to alleviate the pain of injection.
*Tonic.*

*Abigo, Swed.*
Valerian (p.1762·2).
*Insomnia; nervous disorders.*

**Neurolea** *Elea, Arg.*
Bifemelane hydrochloride (p.1660·2).
*Cerebrovascular disorders; mental function impairment.*

**Neurolep** *Promeco, Mex.†.*
Carbamazepine (p.353·3).

**Neurolepsin** *Kwizda, Austria.*
Lithium carbonate (p.301·1).
*Depression; mania.*

**Neuro-Lichtenstein** *Lichtenstein, Ger.*
Thiamine hydrochloride (p.1455·1); pyridoxine hydrochloride (p.1456·3); cyanocobalamin (p.1458·2).
*Vitamin B deficiency.*

**Neuro-Lichtenstein N** *Lichtenstein, Ger.*
Thiamine hydrochloride (p.1455·1); pyridoxine hydrochloride (p.1456·3).
*Nervous-system disorders.*

**Neurolil** *Sigma, Braz.*
Zopiclone (p.729·3).
*Insomnia.*

**Neurolite**
*Bristol-Myers Squibb, Belg.; Du Pont, Fr.; Bristol-Myers Squibb, Spain.*
Technetium-99m bicisate (p.1525·2).
*Cerebral perfusion imaging.*

**Neurolithium**
*Cristalia, Braz.*
Lithium carbonate (p.301·1).
*Alcoholism; bipolar disorder; depression; headache; mania; psychoses.*

*Labcatal, Fr.; Labcatal, Switz.*
Lithium gluconate (p.305·1).
*Bipolar disorder; hypomania; mania.*

**Neuromade** *Teofarma, Spain.*
Cyanocobalamin (p.1458·2); thiamine hydrochloride (p.1455·1); pyridoxine hydrochloride (p.1456·3).
Lidocaine hydrochloride (p.1377·3) is included in the intramuscular injection to alleviate the pain of injection.
*Vitamin B deficiency.*

**Neuromax** *Vitabalans, Fin.*
Vitamin B substances (p.1417·1).
*Vitamin B deficiency.*

**Neuromerck** *Merck, Austria.*
Thiamine disulfide (p.1455·2); pyridoxine hydrochloride (p.1456·3); cyanocobalamin (p.1458·2).
*Neuralgias; neuritis.*

**Neuromet**
*Note. This name is used for preparations of different composition.*
*GlaxoSmithKline, Ital.†.*
Oxiracetam (p.1725·2).
*Mental function impairment.*

*Merck, Thai.*
Mecobalamin (p.1459·1).
*Peripheral neuropathies; vitamin $B_{12}$ deficiency.*

**Neuromethyn** *Sam Chun Dang, Singapore.*
Mecobalamin (p.1459·1).
*Megaloblastic anaemia; peripheral neuropathies.*

**Neuromins** *Andromaco, Chile.*
Docosahexaenoic acid (p.976·1).
*Dietary supplement.*

**Neuromultivit** *Lannacher, Austria.*
Thiamine hydrochloride (p.1455·1); pyridoxine hydrochloride (p.1456·3); cyanocobalamin (p.1458·2).
*Neuropathy.*

**Neuronal Vascular** *Elvetium, Arg.*
Pyridoxine phosphoserinate (p.1457·2); co-dergocrine mesilate (p.1674·1).
*Cerebrovascular disorders.*

**Neuronika** *Fujisawa, Ger.*
Kawain (p.1703·2).
*Alcohol withdrawal syndrome; psychiatric disorders.*

**Neurontin**
*Parke, Davis, Arg.; Pfizer, Austral.; Pfizer, Austria; Pfizer, Belg.; Pfizer, Braz.; Pfizer, Canad.; Pfizer, Fin.; Pfizer, Fr.; Parke, Davis, Ger.; Pfizer, Ger.; Pfizer, Gr.; Pfizer, Hong Kong; Parke, Davis, India; Pfizer, Irl.; Parke, Davis, Israel; Parke, Davis, Ital.; Pfizer, Malaysia; Parke, Davis, Mex.; Parke, Davis, Neth.; Pfizer, Norw.; Pfizer, NZ; Pfizer, Port.; Pfizer, S.Afr.; Pfizer, Singapore; Pfizer, Spain; Pfizer, Swed.; Pfizer, Switz.; Pfizer, Thai.; Pfizer, UK; Pfizer, USA.*
Gabapentin (p.362·2).
*Epilepsy; neuropathic pain.*

**Neuropax** *SERP, Mon.*
Passion flower (p.1729·1); crataegus (p.1677·1).
Formerly contained passion flower, crataegus, and phenobarbital.
*Anxiety; insomnia.*

**Neurophosphates** *GlaxoSmithKline, India.*
Vitamin $B_1$; vitamin $B_2$; vitamin $B_6$; vitamin $B_{12}$; nicotinamide (p.1417·1).
*Tonic; vitamin B supplement.*

**Neuroplant** *Schwabe, Ger.*
Hypericum (p.299·1).
*Anxiety; depression.*

**Neuroplus** *Baliarda, Arg.*
Memantine (p.1711·2).
*Mental function impairment; parkinsonism; spasticity.*

**Neuro-ratiopharm** *Ratiopharm, Ger.*
Thiamine hydrochloride (p.1455·1); pyridoxine hydrochloride (p.1456·3); cyanocobalamin (p.1458·2).
*Nervous-system disorders.*

**Neuro-ratiopharm N** *Ratiopharm, Ger.*
Thiamine hydrochloride (p.1455·1); pyridoxine hydrochloride (p.1456·3).
*Nervous-system disorders.*

**Neurorestol** *Bros, Gr.*
Buspirone hydrochloride (p.672·2).
*Generalised anxiety.*

**Neurorubin** *Mepha, Switz.*
Vitamin B substances (p.1417·1).
*Neuralgias; neuritis; neuropathy.*

**Neurorubine**
*Mepha, Hong Kong; Mepha, Malaysia; Mepha, Singapore.*
Vitamin $B_1$ (p.1455·2); vitamin $B_6$ (p.1457·2); vitamin $B_{12}$ (p.1458·2).
Lidocaine hydrochloride (p.1377·3) is included in the injection to alleviate the pain of injection.
*Neuralgia; neuritis; neuropathy.*

**Neurosande** *Sanderson, Chile.*
Pyridoxine; cyanocobalamin; thiamine (p.1417·1).
*Vitamin B supplement.*

**Neurosedol** *Hearst, Braz.†.*
Passion flower (p.1729·1); crataegus (p.1677·1); erythrina mulungu (p.1717·2).

**Neuroselect** *Dreluso, Ger.*
Homoeopathic preparation.

**Neurosine** *Armstrong, Mex.†.*
Buspirone hydrochloride (p.672·2).
*Anxiety disorders.*

**NeuroSlim** *NeuroGenesis, USA; Matrix, USA.*
Multivitamin, mineral, and amino-acid preparation (p.1417·1).

**Neurosthenol** *Richard, Fr.*
Glutamic acid; phosphoric acid; electrolytes (p.1417·1).
*Tonic.*

**Neurostil** *Ivax, Irl.*
Gabapentin (p.362·2).
*Epilepsy; seizures.*

**Neurostop** *Lacer, Spain.*
Benfotiamine (p.1454·3).
*Vitamin B1 deficiency.*

**Neurostop Complex** *Lacer, Spain.*
Benfotiamine (p.1454·3); hydroxocobalamin acetate (p.1458·2); pyridoxine hydrochloride (p.1456·3).
*Vitamin B deficiency.*

**Neurotensyl** *Sciencex, Fr.†.*
Crataegus (p.1677·1); passion flower (p.1729·1); valerian (p.1762·2).
*Anxiety; insomnia; palpitations.*

**Neurothioct** *Knoll, Ger.†.*
Thioctic acid (p.1754·3).
*Diabetic polyneuropathy.*

**Neurotioct** *TRB, Arg.*
Thioctic acid (p.1754·3).
*Neuropathy.*

**Neurotisan** *Hanosan, Ger.†.*
Hypericum (p.299·1).
*Psychiatric disorders.*

**Neurotol** *Orion, Fin.*
Carbamazepine (p.353·3).
*Alcohol withdrawal syndrome; bipolar disorder; epilepsy; trigeminal neuralgia.*

**Neuroton** *NCSN, Ital.*
Citicoline sodium (p.1672·3).
*Cerebrovascular disorders; parkinsonism.*

**Neurotonico** *EMS, Braz.*
Minerals with vitamin B substances (p.1417·1).

**Neurotop**
*Gerot, Austria; Gerot, Singapore.*
Carbamazepine (p.353·3).
*Alcohol withdrawal syndrome; bipolar disorder; diabetes insipidus; diabetic neuropathy; epilepsy; trigeminal neuralgia.*

**Neurotrat**
*Note. This name is used for preparations of different composition.*
*Knoll, Ger.†.*
Thiamine hydrochloride (p.1455·1); pyridoxine hydrochloride (p.1456·3); cyanocobalamin (p.1458·2).
*Neuralgias; neuritis; neuropathies.*

*German Remedies, India.*
*Capsules:* Vitamin $B_1$; vitamin $B_6$; vitamin $B_{12}$; vitamin C; folic acid; nicotinamide; calcium pantothenate; zinc sulfate; chromium tripicolinate (p.1417·1).
*Injection:* 1 Vial, vitamin C; 1 vial, vitamin $B_{12}$; folic acid; nicotinamide (p.1417·1).
*Vitamin B and C deficiency.*

*Knoll, Switz.†.*
Thiamine nitrate (p.1455·1); pyridoxine hydrochloride (p.1456·3); cyanocobalamin (p.1458·2).
*Neuralgias; neuritis; neuropathy.*

**Neurotrat $B_{12}$** *Knoll, Ger.†.*
Cyanocobalamin (p.1458·2).
*Vitamin $B_{12}$ deficiency.*

**Neurotrat S** *Abbott, Ger.*
Thiamine nitrate (p.1455·1); pyridoxine hydrochloride (p.1456·3).
*Nervous-system disorders.*

**neurotropan** *Phonix, Ger.*
Choline citrate (p.1424·3).
*Liver disorders.*

**Neurovegetalin** *Verla, Ger.*
Hypericum (p.299·1).
*Depression.*

**Neuro-Vibolex** *Chephasaar, Ger.*
*Injection:* Thiamine hydrochloride (p.1455·1); pyridoxine hydrochloride (p.1456·3); cyanocobalamin (p.1458·2).
*Tablets:* Thiamine hydrochloride (p.1455·1); pyridoxine hydrochloride (p.1456·3).
*Neuralgia; neuritis; neuropathy.*

**Neurovit**
*Hovid, Malaysia.*
Vitamin $B_1$ (p.1455·2); vitamin $B_6$ (p.1457·2); vitamin $B_{12}$ (p.1458·2).
*Neuritis; vitamin B deficiency.*

*Hovid, Singapore.*
Thiamine nitrate (p.1455·1); pyridoxine hydrochloride (p.1456·3); cyanocobalamin (p.1458·2).
*Neuralgia; peripheral neuropathy.*

**Neurovitan**
*Orion, Fin.*
Thiamine nitrate (p.1455·1); pyridoxine hydrochloride (p.1456·3); nicotinamide (p.1441·2); cyanocobalamin (p.1458·2).
*Vitamin B deficiency.*

*Fujisawa, Jpn.*
Octotiamine (p.1455·1); riboflavin (p.1456·1); pyridoxine hydrochloride (p.1456·3); cyanocobalamin (p.1458·2).
*Vitamin B deficiency; vitamin B supplement.*

**Neuro-Wied** *Wiedemann, Ger.*
Vitamin B substances (p.1417·1); di-isopropylammonium dichloroacetate (p.900·1); magnesium orotate (p.1724·3).
*Memory and concentration disorders in children; migraine; nerve pain; sleep disorders.*

**Neurozan** *Vitabiotics, UK.*
Phosphatidyl serine; ubidecarenone; glutathione; omega-3 docosahexaenoic acid; arginine; folic acid; vitamin $B_6$; vitamin $B_{12}$ (p.1417·1).

**Neurozepam** *Labinca, Arg.*
Bromazepam (p.671·3).
*Anxiety.*

**Neuryl**
*Bago, Arg.; Bago, Chile.*
Clonazepam (p.359·1).
*Anxiety; epilepsy; panic attacks.*

**Neusinol** *Labima, Belg.*
Naphazoline nitrate (p.1124·3).
*Nasal congestion.*

**Neut** *Abbott, USA.*
Sodium bicarbonate (p.1223·2).
*Neutralising additive solution for acidic intravenous infusions.*

**Neutracido** *Medquimica, Braz.†.*
Sodium bicarbonate (p.1223·2); bismuth subcarbonate (p.1252·1); kaolin (p.1268·3); magnesium hydroxide (p.1272·2); calcium carbonate (p.1254·2); belladonna (p.479·1).
*Gastrointestinal hyperacidity.*

**Neutracol** *Beta, Arg.*
Thioctic acid (p.1754·3).
*Diabetic neuropathy.*

**Neutrafluor** *Colgate-Palmolive, Austral.*
Sodium fluoride (p.1444·3).
*Fluoride supplement; sensitive teeth.*

**Neutraforte** *Ariston, Braz.*
Magnesium hydroxide (p.1272·2); aluminium hydroxide (p.1249·2); simeticone (p.1289·2).
*Flatulence; gastrointestinal hyperacidity.*

**NeutraGard Advanced** *Pascal, USA.*
Sodium fluoride (p.1444·3).
*Dental caries prophylaxis.*

**Neutragel** *Propan, S.Afr.*
Dicycloverine hydrochloride (p.481·2); dried aluminium hydroxide (p.1249·2); light magnesium oxide (p.1272·3).
*Gastrointestinal hyperacidity.*

**Neutralca-S** *Desbergers, Canad.†.*
Aluminium hydroxide (p.1249·2); magnesium hydroxide (p.1272·2).
*Gastric hyperacidity; peptic ulcer.*

**Neutralice** *Key, Austral.†.*
Melaleuca oil (p.1710·2); lavender oil (p.1705·2).
*Pediculosis.*

**Neutramine** *YSP, Malaysia.*
Terfenadine (p.441·1).
*Hypersensitivity reactions.*

**Neutran** *Prodotti, Braz.*
Aluminium hydroxide (p.1249·2); magnesium hydroxide (p.1272·2).
*Gastrointestinal hyperacidity.*

**Neutra-Phos** *Alza, USA.*
Monobasic and dibasic sodium and potassium phosphates (p.1230·3) (p.1231·1) (p.1230·3) (p.1230·3).
*Phosphorus supplement.*

**Neutra-Phos-K** *Alza, USA.*
Monobasic and dibasic potassium phosphates (p.1230·3) (p.1230·3).
*Phosphorus supplement.*

**Neutrexin**
*Lilly, Canad.†; US Bioscience, Denm.†; Ipsen Biotech, Fr.†; Schering-Plough, Hong Kong; Ipsen, Irl.; Ipsen, Ital.†; Ipsen, Spain; Swedish Orphan, Swed.†; Schering-Plough, Thai.; Ipsen, UK†; Medimmune, USA.*
Trimetrexate glucuronate (p.410·2).
*Pneumocystis carinii pneumonia.*

**Neutro Bar** *Darier, Mex.*
Glycerol (p.1694·3).

**Neutrodor** *ICN, Arg.*
Methionine (p.1042·1).
*Urinary acidification.*

**Neutrofer** *Sigma, Braz.*
Ferrous glycinate (p.1428·2).
*Anaemias.*

**Neutrofer Folico** *Sigma, Braz.*
Ferrous glycinate (p.1428·2); folic acid (p.1429·1).
*Anaemias.*

**Neutrogen TGel** *Johnson & Johnson, Braz.†.*
Coal tar (p.1159·2).
*Skin disorders.*

**Neutrogena**
*Note. This name is used for preparations of different composition.*
*Faulding, Austral.†.*
Trolamine (p.1758·2).
*Soap substitute.*

*Johnson & Johnson, Braz.; Key, Chile; Johnson & Johnson, NZ; Neutrogena Dermatologics, USA.*
A range of soap substitutes, shampoos, and skin care preparations.

*Neutrogena, Fr.†.*
*SPF 18.5:* Octinoxate (p.1154·3); avobenzone (p.1142·3); enzacamene (p.1147·1).
*Sunscreen.*

*Neutrogena, USA.*
*SPF 8:* Octinoxate (p.1154·3); methyl anthranilate (p.1154·1); titanium dioxide (p.1160·3).
*SPF 15:* Octinoxate (p.1154·3); octisalate (p.1154·3); methyl anthranilate (p.1154·1); titanium dioxide (p.1160·3).
*SPF 25:* Octinoxate (p.1154·3); oxybenzone (p.1154·3); octisalate (p.1154·3).

*SPF 30:* Octinoxate (p.1154·3); octocrilene (p.1154·3); methyl anthranilate (p.1154·1); zinc oxide (p.1163·2).
*Sunscreen.*

**Neutrogena Acne Mask** *Faulding, Austral.†; Johnson & Johnson, Canad.; Neutrogena Dermatologics, USA†.*
Benzoyl peroxide (p.1143·2).
*Acne.*

**Neutrogena Acne Skin Cleanser** *Faulding, Austral.†.*
Triclosan (p.1195·2).
*Acne; oily skin.*

**Neutrogena Acne Wash** *Johnson & Johnson, Canad.*
Salicylic acid (p.1157·1).
*Acne.*

**Neutrogena Acondicionador Neutar Gel** *Key, Chile.*
Salicylic acid (p.1157·1).
*Scalp disorders.*

**Neutrogena Antiacne** *Johnson & Johnson, Braz.*
Salicylic acid (p.1157·1).
*Acne.*

**Neutrogena Anti-Acne** *Johnson & Johnson, Ital.†.*
*Topical gel:* Salicylic acid (p.1157·1).
*Topical solution:* Chamomile (p.1669·3); aloe (p.1248·2).
*Acne.*

**Neutrogena Antiseptic** *Neutrogena, USA.*
Skin cleanser.

**Neutrogena Anti-Wrinkle** *Johnson & Johnson, Canad.*
*SPF 15:* Octinoxate (p.1154·3); ensulizole (p.1147·1).
*Sunscreen.*

**Neutrogena Barra** *Key, Chile.*
*SPF 15:* Octinoxate (p.1154·3); octyl palmitate.
*Chapped lips; sunscreen.*

**Neutrogena Bloqueador Solar** *Key, Chile.*
*SPF 30, SPF 45:* Methoxycinnamic acid esters; benzimidazole; homosalate (p.1148·1).
*Sunscreen.*

**Neutrogena Bloqueador Solar Piel Sensible** *Key, Chile.*
*SPF 30:* Titanium dioxide (p.1160·3).
*Sunscreen.*

**Neutrogena Bronceador** *Key, Chile.*
Dihydroxyacetone (p.1145·2).
*Suntanning agent.*

**Neutrogena Chemical-Free** *Neutrogena, USA.*
*SPF 17:* Titanium dioxide (p.1160·3).
*Sunscreen.*

**Neutrogena Clear Pore** *Johnson & Johnson, Canad.*
Salicylic acid (p.1157·1).
*Acne.*

**Neutrogena Crema Humectante** *Key, Chile.*
*SPF 15:* Octinoxate (p.1154·3); titanium dioxide (p.1160·3).
*Sunscreen.*

**Neutrogena Drying** *Neutrogena Dermatologics, USA.*
Hamamelis (p.1696·3).

**Neutrogena Gel Control Brillo** *Key, Chile.*
Salicylic acid (p.1157·1).
*Seborrhoea.*

**Neutrogena Glow** *Neutrogena, USA.*
*SPF 8:* Octinoxate (p.1154·3).
*Sunscreen.*

**Neutrogena Healthy Scalp Anti-Dandruff** *Johnson & Johnson, Canad.*
Salicylic acid (p.1157·1).

**Neutrogena Healthy Skin**
*Note. This name is used for preparations of different composition.*
*Johnson & Johnson, Braz.*
Octinoxate (p.1154·3); oxybenzone (p.1154·3).
*Sunscreen.*

*Johnson & Johnson, Canad.*
*SPF 15:* Octinoxate (p.1154·3); oxybenzone (p.1154·3).
*Sunscreen.*

*Key, Chile.*
*SPF 15:* Octinoxate (p.1154·3); oxybenzone (p.1154·3); glycolic acid (p.1147·3).
*Skin pigmentation disorders; sunscreen.*

**Neutrogena Healthy Skin Anti-rugas** *Johnson & Johnson, Braz.*
*SPF 15:* Octinoxate (p.1154·3); ensulizole (p.1147·1).
*Sunscreen.*

**Neutrogena Intensified** *Johnson & Johnson, Canad.; Neutrogena, USA.*
*SPF 15:* Octinoxate (p.1154·3); ensulizole (p.1147·1); titanium dioxide (p.1160·3).
*Sunscreen.*

**Neutrogena Kids Sunblock** *Johnson & Johnson, Canad.*
*SPF 30:* Homosalate (p.1148·1); octinoxate (p.1154·3); octisalate (p.1154·3); oxybenzone (p.1154·3).
*Sunscreen.*

**Neutrogena Limpiadora** *Key, Chile.*
Glycolic acid (p.1147·3); salicylic acid (p.1157·1).
*Skin cleansing.*

**Neutrogena Linea Acne** *Key, Chile.*
Salicylic acid (p.1157·1).
*Acne; seborrhoea.*

**Neutrogena Lip** *Neutrogena, USA.*
*SPF 15:* Octinoxate (p.1154·3); oxybenzone (p.1154·3).
*Sunscreen.*

**Neutrogena Locion Humectante** *Key, Chile.*
*SPF 15:* Octinoxate (p.1154·3); octisalate (p.1154·3).
*Sunscreen.*

**Neutrogena Moisture**
*Note. This name is used for preparations of different composition.*
*Johnson & Johnson, Canad.*
*SPF 15:* Octinoxate (p.1154·3); octisalate (p.1154·3); oxybenzone (p.1154·3).
*Sunscreen.*

*Neutrogena, USA.*
*SPF 5:* Octinoxate (p.1154·3).
*SPF 15:* Octinoxate (p.1154·3); oxybenzone (p.1154·3).
*Sunscreen.*

**Neutrogena New Hands** *Johnson & Johnson, Braz.*
*SPF 15:* Octinoxate (p.1154·3); oxybenzone (p.1154·3).
*Sunscreen.*

**Neutrogena Norwegian Formula Dermatological Cream** *Neutrogena, UK.*
Glycerol (p.1694·3).
*Dry skin.*

**Neutrogena No-Stick** *Neutrogena, USA.*
Octinoxate (p.1154·3); homosalate (p.1148·1); oxybenzone (p.1154·3); octisalate (p.1154·3).
*Sunscreen.*

**Neutrogena No-Stick Sunblock** *Johnson & Johnson, Canad.†.*
*SPF 30:* Octinoxate (p.1154·3); homosalate (p.1148·1); octisalate (p.1154·3); oxybenzone (p.1154·3).
*Sunscreen.*

**Neutrogena Oil-Free Sunblock** *Johnson & Johnson, Canad.*
*SPF 30:* Homosalate (p.1148·1); octinoxate (p.1154·3); octisalate (p.1154·3); oxybenzone (p.1154·3).
*Sunscreen.*

**Neutrogena On The Spot Acne Treatment** *Johnson & Johnson, Canad.*
Benzoyl peroxide (p.1143·2).
*Acne.*

**Neutrogena Sensitive Skin** *Johnson & Johnson, Canad.*
*SPF 30:* Titanium dioxide (p.1160·3).
*Sunscreen.*

**Neutrogena Shampoo Neutar** *Key, Chile.*
Coal tar (p.1159·2).
*Scalp disorders.*

**Neutrogena Skin Cleaning** *Johnson & Johnson, Canad.*
Salicylic acid (p.1157·1).
*Acne.*

**Neutrogena SPF 15** *Johnson & Johnson, Canad.*
*SPF 15:* Avobenzone (p.1142·3); octinoxate (p.1154·3); oxybenzone (p.1154·3).
*Sunscreen.*

**Neutrogena SPF 30** *Johnson & Johnson, Canad.*
*SPF 30:* Avobenzone (p.1142·3); homosalate (p.1148·1); octinoxate (p.1154·3); octisalate (p.1154·3); oxybenzone (p.1154·3).
*Sunscreen.*

**Neutrogena SPF 45** *Johnson & Johnson, Canad.*
*SPF 45:* Avobenzone (p.1142·3); homosalate (p.1148·1); octinoxate (p.1154·3); octisalate (p.1154·3); oxybenzone (p.1154·3).
*Sunscreen.*

**Neutrogena Sunblock** *Johnson & Johnson, Canad.*
*SPF 20:* Homosalate (p.1148·1); meradimate (p.1151·3); octinoxate (p.1154·3); octisalate (p.1154·3).
*SPF 30:* Meradimate (p.1151·3); octocrilene (p.1154·3); octinoxate (p.1154·3); octisalate (p.1154·3).
*Sunscreen.*

**Neutrogena Sunblocker** *Professional Health, Canad.†.*
*SPF 17:* Titanium dioxide (p.1160·3).
*Sunscreen.*

**Neutrogena T/Derm** *Neutrogena, USA†.*
Coal tar (p.1159·2).
*Skin disorders.*

**Neutrogena T/Gel** *Faulding, Austral.†; Johnson & Johnson, Canad.; Neutrogena, USA.*
Coal tar (p.1159·2).
*Scalp disorders.*

**Neutrogena T/Gel Therapeutic** *Johnson & Johnson, Canad.*
Salicylic acid (p.1157·1).
*Scalp disorders.*

**Neutrogena T/Sal** *Faulding, Austral.†; Neutrogena Dermatologics, USA.*
Salicylic acid (p.1157·1); coal tar (p.1159·2).
*Scalp disorders; seborrhoeic dermatitis.*

**Neutrogena T/Scalp** *Neutrogena Dermatologics, USA.*
Hydrocortisone (p.1103·3).
*Pruritus of the scalp.*

**Neutrogerm** *Hertz, Braz.†.*
Triclosan (p.1195·2).
*Skin infections.*

**Neutrogin** *Chugai, Jpn.*
Lenograstim (p.755·3).
*Mobilisation of peripheral blood progenitor cells; neutropenia.*

**Neutrolac** *SIT, Ital.*
Aluminium hydroxide (p.1249·2); calcium carbonate (p.1254·2); magnesium trisilicate (p.1272·3).
*Gastrointestinal hyperacidity.*

**Neutromax** *Sidus, Arg.; Biolatina, Chile; Bio Sidus, Thai.*
Filgrastim (p.753·3).
*Neutropenia.*

**Neutromed** *Kwizda, Austria.*
Cimetidine (p.1255·3).
*Acid aspiration; gastro-oesophageal reflux; gastrointestinal erosions; gastrointestinal haemorrhage; peptic ulcer; Zollinger-Ellison syndrome.*

**Neutronorm** *Ebewe, Austria; Ebewe, Hong Kong†.*
Cimetidine (p.1255·3).
*Gastro-oesophageal reflux; gastrointestinal erosions; gastrointestinal haemorrhage; peptic ulcer; Zollinger-Ellison syndrome.*

**Neutrose S Pellegrino** *Sanofi Synthelabo OTC, Ital.*
Calcium carbonate (p.1254·2); magnesium carbonate (p.1272·1); kaolin (p.1268·3); magnesium trisilicate (p.1272·3).
*Gastrointestinal hyperacidity.*

**Neutroses** *Pharmethic, Belg.†; DB, Fr.; DB, Switz.*
Calcium carbonate (p.1254·2); light magnesium carbonate (p.1272·1); heavy kaolin (p.1268·3); magnesium trisilicate (p.1272·3).
*Bloating; flatulence; gastric hyperacidity; gastritis; gastro-oesophageal reflux; peptic ulcer.*

**Neuvita** *Fujisawa, Jpn.*
Octotiamine (p.1455·1).
*Vitamin $B_1$ deficiency; vitamin $B_1$ supplement.*

**Neuzym** *Eisai, Hong Kong; Eisai, Jpn; Eisai, Malaysia.*
Muramidase hydrochloride (p.1717·2).
*Chronic sinusitis; haemorrhage; respiratory-tract congestion and inflammation.*

**Neuzyme** *Eisai, Singapore.*
Muramidase hydrochloride (p.1717·2).
*Haemorrhage; respiratory-tract congestion and inflammation; sinusitis.*

**Nevacort** *Finderm, Ital.*
Hydrocortisone (p.1103·3); neomycin sulfate (p.235·1).
*Bacterial vaginal infections.*

**Nevimune** *Cipla, India.*
Nevirapine (p.650·2).
*HIV infection.*

**Neviralea** *Elea, Arg.*
Nevirapine (p.650·2).
*HIV infection.*

**Neviran** *Fonten, Ital.*
Aciclovir (p.626·1).
*Herpesvirus infections.*

**Nevralgex** *Cimed, Braz.*
Dipyrone (p.35·3); orphenadrine (p.486·2).
*Pain; smooth muscle spasm.*

**Nevralgina** *Climax, Braz.†.*
Dipyrone (p.35·3).
*Fever; pain.*

**Nevramin**
*Note. This name is used for preparations of different composition.*
*Takeda, Hong Kong; Takeda, Malaysia; Takeda, Singapore; Takeda, Thai.*
Fursultiamine (p.1454·3) or fursultiamine hydrochloride (p.1455·2); vitamin $B_6$ (p.1457·2); vitamin $B_{12}$ (p.1458·2).
Mepivacaine hydrochloride (p.1381·2) is included in the intramuscular injection to alleviate the pain of injection.
*Anaemias; diabetic neuropathy; myelitis; neuralgia; neuritis; paresis; rheumatic disorders.*

*Takeda, Malaysia.*
*Tablets:* Fursultiamine (p.1454·3); pyridoxine hydrochloride (p.1456·3); cyanocobalamin (p.1458·2).
*Anaemias; neuralgia; rheumatic disorders.*

**Nevril**
*Note. This name is used for preparations of different composition.*
*Amnol, Ital.*
*Cream:* Hamamelis (p.1696·3); devil's claw root (p.28·2); chamomile (p.1669·3); mallow (p.1709·3); calendula (p.1665·2); salix (p.87·3); copper; zinc; menthol (p.1711·3).
*Musculoskeletal and joint disorders.*

*Tosi, Ital.†.*
*Injection:* Thiamine phosphate monochloride (p.1455·2); hydroxocobalamin (p.1458·2).
*Megaloblastic anaemia; neuralgias; neuritis.*

**Nevril Crono** *Amnol, Ital.*
Multivitamin and mineral preparation with plant extracts (p.1417·1).
*Musculoskeletal and joint disorders; nutritional supplement.*

**Nevrine Codeine** *Pharmacobel, Belg.†.*
Paracetamol (p.76·2); caffeine hydrate (p.782·1); codeine phosphate (p.27·1).
*Fever; pain.*

**Nevrol** *Prodotti, Braz.*
Camphor (p.1665·3); menthol (p.1711·3); methyl salicylate (p.59·3); turpentine oil (p.1760·1); lavender oil (p.1705·2); rosemary oil (p.1740·2); mustard oil (p.1718·2).
*Musculoskeletal and joint disorders.*

**Nevrosthenine Glycocolle Freyssinge** *3M, Belg.†; 3M, Fr.†.*
Glycine; sodium glycerophosphate; potassium glycerophosphate; magnesium glycerophosphate (p.1417·1).
*Tonic.*

**New B-Cool** *Julphar, UAE.*
Cetylpyridinium chloride (p.1173·1); lidocaine hydrochloride (p.1377·3).
*Mouth and throat disorders.*

**New Daigaku** *Santen, Singapore.*
Boric acid (p.1662·1); d-borneol; menthol (p.1711·3); zinc sulfate (p.1469·3).
*Eye irritation.*

**New Decongestant Pediatric** *Goldline, USA†.*
Phenylpropanolamine hydrochloride (p.1127·3); phenylephrine hydrochloride (p.1126·3); chlorphenamine maleate (p.427·3); phenyltoloxamine citrate (p.439·1).
*Upper respiratory-tract symptoms.*

**New Era Biochemic Tissue Salts** *Seven Seas, UK.*
Homoeopathic preparation.

**New Era Calm & Clear** *Seven Seas, UK†.*
Dibasic potassium phosphate (p.1230·3).

**New Era Combination Remedy** *Seven Seas, UK.*
Homoeopathic preparation.

**New Era Elasto** *Seven Seas, UK.*
Homoeopathic preparation.

**New Era Nervone** *Seven Seas, UK.*
Homoeopathic preparation.

**New Era Zief** *Seven Seas, UK†.*
Iron phosphate; silica (p.1581·3); sodium phosphate; sodium sulfate (p.1290·1).
*Rheumatic pain.*

**New Eye Lotion** *Optrex, India.*
Boric acid (p.1662·1); borax (p.1661·3); allantoin (p.1141·3); salicylic acid (p.1157·1); zinc sulfate (p.1469·3).
*Eye irritation; tired eyes.*

**New Gen** *Roche, Ital.*
Multivitamin and mineral preparation (p.1417·1).
*Nutritional supplement.*

**New Hands** *Johnson & Johnson, Canad.*
*SPF 15:* Octinoxate (p.1154·3); oxybenzone (p.1154·3).
*Sunscreen.*

**New Mixavit** *Julphar, UAE.*
Multivitamin preparation (p.1417·1).

**New Patecs A** *Daiichi, Hong Kong.*
Arnica (p.1656·3); glycol salicylate (p.44·3).
*Musculoskeletal and joint disorders.*

**NewAce** *Bristol-Myers Squibb, Neth.*
Fosinopril sodium (p.919·1).
*Heart failure; hypertension.*

**Newderm** *Wolfs, Belg.*
Zinc oxide (p.1163·2); vitamin A (p.1451·2); vitamin D (p.1461·2); cod-liver oil (p.1425·2).
*Skin irritation.*

**Newrelax** *Potter's, UK.*
Lupulus (p.1708·1); skullcap (p.1746·3); valerian (p.1762·2); vervain (p.1764·1).
*Tension.*

**New-Skin** *Medtech, USA.*
Topical barrier preparation.

**Nexadron** *Klonal, Arg.*
Dexamethasone (p.1097·1).
*Corticosteroid.*

**Nexadron Compuesto** *Klonal, Arg.*
Dexamethasone (p.1097·1); naphazoline (p.1124·3); neomycin (p.235·1).

**Nexen** *Therabel, Fr.*
Nimesulide (p.67·1).
*Musculoskeletal and joint disorders.*

**Nexiam** *AstraZeneca, Belg.; Astra, S.Afr.*
Esomeprazole magnesium (p.1265·1).
*Gastro-oesophageal reflux; peptic ulcer.*

**Nexit** *Grunenthal, Chile.*
Hydroxyzine hydrochloride (p.434·3).
*Anxiety; pruritus; sedative.*

**Nexium** *AstraZeneca, Arg.; AstraZeneca, Austral.; AstraZeneca, Austria; AstraZeneca, Braz.; AstraZeneca, Canad.; AstraZeneca, Chile; AstraZeneca, Denm.; AstraZeneca, Fin.; AstraZeneca, Ger.; Promed, Ger.; Stern, Ger.; AstraZeneca, Hong Kong; AstraZeneca, Irl.; AstraZeneca, Israel; AstraZeneca, Ital.; AstraZeneca, Malaysia; AstraZeneca, Neth.; AstraZeneca, Norw.; AstraZeneca, Port.; AstraZeneca, Singapore; Astra, Spain; Hassle, Swed.; AstraZeneca, Switz.; AstraZeneca, Thai.; AstraZeneca, UK; AstraZeneca, USA.*
Esomeprazole magnesium (p.1265·1) or esomeprazole sodium (p.1265·1).
*Gastro-oesophageal reflux; peptic ulcer.*

**Nexium Hp** *Hassle, Swed.*
Tablets, esomeprazole magnesium (Nexium) (p.1265·1); tablets, amoxicillin trihydrate (Imacillin) (p.155·3); tablets, clarithromycin (Klacid) (p.192·2).
*Peptic ulcer.*

**Nexvep** *Bristol-Myers Squibb, Braz.*
Etoposide (p.551·3).
*Malignant neoplasms.*

**Nexxair** *Schwarz, Fr.*
Beclometasone dipropionate (p.1091·1).
*Asthma.*

**NeyArthros (Revitorgan-Dilutionen Nr 43)** *Vitorgan, Ger.*
Articuli fet.; cartilago; synovia.
*Inflammatory and degenerative joint disorders.*

**NeyArthros-Liposome (Revitorgan Lp Nr 83)** *Vitorgan, Ger.*
Cartilago articuli; synovia; articuli fet.; thymus fet.; funicul. umbilical.; metenolone acetate; prednisolone acetate; lipid extract of cartilago articuli/synovia/articuli fet.; zinc sulfate manganese sulfate; magnesium chlo-

ride; potassium chloride; calcium chloride; columna vertebralis fet.; capsula articuli fet.; musculi fet.; gland. suprarenal.
*Inflammatory and degenerative joint disorders.*

**NeyCalm (Revitorgan-Dilutionen Nr 98, Revitorgan-Lingual Nr 98)** *Vitorgan, Ger.*
Animal tissue extract: cortex cerebri; diencephalon; epiphysis; placenta mat.
*Nervous disorders.*

**NeyChondrin N (Revitorgan-Dilutionen N Nr 68)** *Vitorgan, Ger.*
Animal tissue extracts (NeyChondrin) (p.1709·3); metenolone acetate (p.1559·2); prednisolone acetate (p.1108·1); alpha tocoferil acetate (p.1465·1); procaine hydrochloride (p.1383·2).
*Muscular, neuromuscular, and joint disorders.*

**NeyChondrin (Revitorgan-Dilutionen Nr 68)** *Vitorgan, Ger.*
Thymus fet.; hypophysis; diencephalon; medulla spinal; gland. suprarenal.; testes juv.; hepar; pancreas; musculi; columna vertebral. fet.; articuli fet.; ren; placenta; nucleus pulp.
*Muscular, neuromuscular, and joint disorders.*

**NeyChondrin (Revitorgan-Lingual Nr. 68)** *Vitorgan, Ger.*
Animal tissue extracts (NeyChondrin); metenolone acetate; prednisolone acetate; alpha tocoferil acetate; procaine hydrochloride.
*Muscular, neuromuscular, and joint disorders.*

**NeyCorenar (Revitorgan-Dilutionen Nr 6)** *Vitorgan, Ger.*
Cor fet.
*Cardiovascular disorders.*

**NeyDesib (Revitorgan-Dilutionen Nr 78)** *Vitorgan, Ger.*
Thymus fet.; lien fet.; lymphonodi; gland. suprarenal.
*Allergies; auto-immune disorders.*

**Neydin-F** *Vitorgan, Ger.*
Homoeopathic preparation.

**Neydin-M** *Vitorgan, Ger.*
Homoeopathic preparation.

**NeyDop N (Revitorgan-Dilutionen N Nr 97)** *Vitorgan, Ger.*
Cortex cerebri; diencephalon; cerebellum; placenta fet.; ascorbic acid (p.1460·2); lithium chloride (p.305·1); levodopa (p.1205·2).
*Central nervous system disorders.*

**NeyDop (Revitorgan-Dilutionen Nr 97)** *Vitorgan, Ger.*
Cortex cerebri; diencephalon; cerebellum; placenat fet.
*Central nervous system disorders.*

**NeyDop (Revitorgan-Lingual Nr. 97)** *Vitorgan, Ger.*
Animal tissue extracts (NeyDop N); ascorbic acid; lithium chloride; levodopa.
*Central nervous system disorders.*

**NeyFaexan (Revitorgan-Dilutionen Nr 55)** *Vitorgan, Ger.*
Mucosa intestinal.; muc. vesicae urinar.; mucosa vesicae felleae; muc. nasopharyngea.
*Gastrointestinal disorders.*

**NeyFegan (Revitorgan-Dilutionen Nr 26)** *Vitorgan, Ger.*
Liver extract.
*Liver disorders.*

**NeyGeront N (Revitorgan-Dilutionen N Nr 64)** *Vitorgan, Ger.*
Animal tissue extracts (NeyGeront); heparin (p.927·3); metenolone acetate (p.1559·2); liothyronine hydrochloride; vitamins (p.1417·1); procaine hydrochloride.
*Tonic.*

**NeyGeront (Revitorgan-Dilutionen Nr 64)** *Vitorgan, Ger.*
Embryo tot.; placenta; amnion; funiculus umbilical.; cor; ren; pancreas; mucosa intestinal.; lien; thymus juv.; gland. suprarenal.; gland. parathyreoid.; testes juv.; hypophysis; diencephalon; cort. cerebri.
*Tonic.*

**NeyGeront (Revitorgan-Lingual Nr 64)** *Vitorgan, Ger.*
Animal tissue extracts (NeyGeront); heparin; metenolone acetate; liothyronine hydrochloride; vitamins; procaine hydrochloride.
*Tonic.*

**NeyGeront-Vitalkapseln** *Vitorgan, Ger.*
Animal tissue extracts; heparin; metenolone acetate; liothyronine hydrochloride; procaine hydrochloride; lecithin; trace elements and vitamins.
*Tonic.*

**NeyImmun (Revitorgan-Dilutionen Nr 73)** *Vitorgan, Ger.*
Placenta mat.; funiculus umbilical.; thymus juv.
*Tonic.*

**NeyNormin N (Revitorgan-Dilutionen N Nr 65)** *Vitorgan, Ger.*
Animal tissue extracts (NeyNormin); prednisolone acetate (p.1108·1); liothyronine hydrochloride (p.1602·2); estradiol benzoate (p.1550·1); chorionic gonadotrophin (p.1320·3); alpha tocoferil acetate (p.1465·1); cyanocobalamin (p.1458·2).
*Allergic diathesis; insufficiency of the diencephalon-pituitary-adrenal system; rheumatism; vegetative dystonias; virus infection.*

**NeyNormin (Revitorgan-Dilutionen Nr 65)** *Vitorgan, Ger.*
Thymus fet.; gland. suprarenal.; lymphonodi; gland. parathyreoidea; hepar; ren; pancreas; lien; vasa fet.; funiculus umbilical.; hypophysis; diencephalon; mucosae miscae; cutis; medulla ossium.
*Allergic diathesis; insufficiency of the diencephalon-pituitary-adrenal system; rheumatism; vegetative dystonias; virus infection.*

**NeyNormin (Revitorgan-Lingual Nr 65)** *Vitorgan, Ger.*
Animal tissue extracts (NeyNormin); prednisolone acetate; liothyronine hydrochloride; estradiol benzoate; chorionic gonadotrophin; alpha tocoferil acetate; cyanocobalamin.
*Allergic diathesis; insufficiency of the diencephalon-pituitary-adrenal system; rheumatism; vegetative dystonias; viral infections.*

**NeyParadent-Liposome** *Vitorgan, Ger.*
Protein extracts from crista dentalis, placenta, and diencephalon; metenolone acetate; alpha tocoferil acetate; procaine hydrochloride; lipid extract from crista dentalis; sodium salicylate; ascorbic acid; chamomile; arnica; myrrh; sea salt.
*Mouth disorders.*

**NeyPsorin (Revitorgan-Dilutionen Nr 5)** *Vitorgan, Ger.*
Bovine skin extract.
*Skin disorders.*

**NeyPulpin N (Revitorgan-Dilutionen N Nr 10)** *Vitorgan, Ger.*
Crista dentalis; placenta; diencephalon; metenolone acetate (p.1559·2); alpha tocoferil acetate (p.1465·1); ascorbic acid (p.1460·2); procaine hydrochloride (p.1383·2).
*Dental disorders.*

**NeyPulpin (Revitorgan-Dilutionen Nr 10)** *Vitorgan, Ger.*
Crista dental. fet.; placenta; diencephalon.
*Dental disorders.*

**Neythymun** *Vitorgan, Ger.*
Thymus extract (p.1756·1).
*Allergic disorders; immunosuppressant in rheumatic disorders; immunotherapy.*

**NeyTroph (Revitorgan-Dilutionen Nr 96)** *Vitorgan, Ger.*
Musculi juv.; musculi fet.; cor fet.; thymus; medulla spinal.; cort. cerebri; epiphysis; diencephalon.
*Muscular and nervous disorders.*

**NeyTroph (Revitorgan-Lingual Nr 96)** *Vitorgan, Ger.*
Musculi juv.; musculi fet.; cor fet.; thymus; medulla spinal.; cort. cerebri; epiphysis; diencephalon.
*Muscular and nervous disorders.*

**NeyTumorin N (Revitorgan-Dilutionen N Nr 66)** *Vitorgan, Ger.*
Animal tissue extracts (NeyTumorin) (p.1709·3); metenolone acetate (p.1559·2); prednisolone acetate (p.1108·1); liothyronine hydrochloride (p.1602·2); alpha tocoferil acetate (p.1465·1); cyanocobalamin (p.1458·2).
*Neoplasms.*

**NeyTumorin (Revitorgan-Dilutionen Nr 66)** *Vitorgan, Ger.*
Diencephalon; placenta mat.; funiculus umbilical.; thymus juv.; epiphysis; testes juv.; gland. suprarenal.; gland. thyreoidea; medulla ossium; pulmo; hepar; pancreas; ren; lien; mucosa intestinal.
*Neoplasms.*

**NeyTumorin (Revitorgan-Lingual Nr 66)** *Vitorgan, Ger.*
Animal tissue extracts (NeyTumorin) (p.1709·3); metenolone acetate; prednisolone acetate; liothyronine hydrochloride; alpha tocoferil acetate; cyanocobalamin.
*Neoplasms.*

**Nezeril**
*Astra, Denm.†; AstraZeneca, Fin.†; AstraZeneca, Hong Kong; Draco, Swed.*
Oxymetazoline hydrochloride (p.1126·1).
*Nasal congestion; rhinitis; sinusitis.*

**NF Cough Syrup with Codeine** *Technilab, Canad.*
Pseudoephedrine hydrochloride (p.1129·2); codeine phosphate (p.27·1); guaifenesin (p.1122·1).

**NGT** *Geneva, USA.*
Triamcinolone acetonide (p.1110·2); nystatin (p.406·3).
*Skin disorders.*

**Nia** *Novo Nordisk, Austria†.*
Megestrol acetate (p.1558·2).
*Breast cancer; endometrial cancer.*

**Niacel** *Medifarma, Mex.†.*
Metronidazole (p.607·2).

**Niacex** *Andromaco, Chile.*
Nicotinamide (p.1441·2).
*Acne.*

**Niacor** *Upsher-Smith, USA†.*
Nicotinic acid (p.1441·1).
*Hyperlipidaemia (adjunct); nicotinic acid deficiency; pellagra.*

**Nialen** *Novag, Spain.*
Ibuproxam (p.47·2).
*Peri-articular and soft-tissue disorders.*

**Niar**
*Abbott, Braz.; Knoll, Mex.*
Selegiline hydrochloride (p.1214·1).
*Parkinsonism.*

**Niaspan**
*Merck, UK; KOS, USA.*
Nicotinic acid (p.1441·1).
*Hyperlipidaemias.*

**NiaStase** *Novo Nordisk, Canad.*
Eptacog alfa (activated) (p.750·3).
*Haemophilia.*

**Niberan** *Medhel, Gr.*
Nimesulide (p.67·1).
*Inflammation; musculoskeletal disorders; pain.*

**Nibiol** *Fournier, Fr.*
Nitroxoline (p.238·3).
*Bacterial infections of the urinary tract.*

**Nibocin** *Zekides, Gr.*
Propylene glycol cefatrizine (p.170·3).
*Bacterial infections.*

**Nibren** *Coup, Gr.*
Ambroxol hydrochloride (p.1114·3).
*Respiratory disorders associated with viscous mucus.*

**Nicabate**
*GlaxoSmithKline Consumer, Austral.; GlaxoSmithKline, NZ.*
Nicotine (p.1720·1) or nicotine polacrilex (p.1720·1).
*Aid to smoking withdrawal.*

**Nicam** *Dermal Laboratories, UK.*
Nicotinamide (p.1441·2).
*Acne.*

**Nican** *Uhlmann-Eyraud, Switz.*
Codeine (p.27·1); belladonna (p.479·1); drosera (p.1683·1); grindelia (p.1696·1); plantaginis (p.1738·2); thyme (p.1755·2); sodium benzoate (p.1169·3).
*Coughs.*

**Nicangin** *Hassle, Swed.*
Nicotinic acid (p.1441·1).
*Hyperlipidaemias.*

**Nicant** *Piam, Ital.*
Nicardipine hydrochloride (p.965·1).
*Angina pectoris; heart failure; hypertension.*

**Nicaphlogyl** *Vifor, Switz.*
Propyphenazone (p.85·3); ethenzamide (p.37·2).
*Inflammation; pain.*

**Nicapress** *Benedetti, Ital.*
Nicardipine hydrochloride (p.965·1).
*Angina pectoris; heart failure; hypertension.*

**Nicardal** *Italfarmaco, Ital.*
Nicardipine hydrochloride (p.965·1).
*Angina pectoris; heart failure; hypertension.*

**Nicardia** *Unique, India.*
Nifedipine (p.966·2).
*Angina pectoris; hypertension.*

**Nicardium** *Drug Research, Ital.†.*
Nicardipine hydrochloride (p.965·1).
*Angina pectoris; heart failure; hypertension.*

**Nicarpin** *San Carlo, Ital.*
Nicardipine hydrochloride (p.965·1).
*Angina pectoris; hypertension.*

**Nicaven** *Uno, Ital.*
Nicardipine hydrochloride (p.965·1).
*Angina pectoris; heart failure; hypertension.*

**N'ice** *SmithKline Beecham Consumer, USA.*
*Lozenges:* Menthol (p.1711·3).
*Throat spray:* Menthol (p.1711·3); glycerol (p.1694·3).
*Sore throat.*

**N'ice 'n Clear** *SmithKline Beecham Consumer, USA.*
Menthol (p.1711·3).

**N'ice Vitamin C** *SmithKline Beecham Consumer, USA.*
Ascorbic acid (p.1460·2).
*Scurvy; vitamin C deficiency.*

**Nicef** *Galen, UK.*
Cefradine (p.179·3).
*Bacterial infections.*

**Nicene** *Adcock Ingram, S.Afr.†.*
Nitroxoline (p.238·3); sulfamethizole (p.260·3); pyridoxine hydrochloride (p.1456·3).
*Urinary-tract infections.*

**Nicene N** *Adcock Ingram, S.Afr.*
Nitroxoline (p.238·3).
*Urinary-tract infections.*

**Nicer** *Ist. Chim. Inter., Ital.*
Nicergoline (p.1719·3).
*Cerebrovascular disorders.*

**Nicergobeta** *Betapharm, Ger.*
Nicergoline (p.1719·3).
*Mental function disorders.*

**Nicergolent** *Sanofi Synthelabo, Arg.*
Nicergoline (p.1719·3).
*Vascular disorders.*

**Nicerium** *Hexal, Ger.*
Nicergoline (p.1719·3).
*Mental function impairment.*

**Nicetile** *Sigma-Tau, Ital.*
Acetylcarnitine hydrochloride (p.1646·1).
*Cerebrovascular disorders; nerve disorders.*

**Nicholin**
*Wyeth Lederle, Ital.; Takeda, Jpn.*
Citicoline (p.1672·3).
*Cerebrovascular disorders; pancreatitis; parkinsonism.*

**Nicizina** *Pharmacia Upjohn, Ital.*
Isoniazid (p.222·2).
*Tuberculosis.*

**Niclosan**
*GlaxoSmithKline, India; Pharmasant, Thai.*
Niclosamide (p.110·1).
*Diphyllobothriasis; hymenolepiasis; taeniasis.*

**Nico Hepatocyn** *Uriach, Spain.*
Cynara (p.1678·3); aloes (p.1248·2); boldo (p.1661·2); cascara (p.1255·1).
*Constipation.*

**Nicobid** *Rhone-Poulenc Rorer, Hong Kong†.*
Nicotinic acid (p.1441·1).
*Hyperlipidaemias; nicotinic acid supplement.*

**Nicobio** *Columbia, Mex.*
Polymyxin B (p.245·2); neomycin (p.235·1); gramicidin (p.220·2).
*Bacterial infections.*

**Nicobion**
*AstraZeneca, Fr.; Merck, Ger.*
Nicotinamide (p.1441·2).
*Nicotinamide deficiency.*

**NicoBloc** *Galpharm, UK.*
Aid to smoking withdrawal.

**Nicobrevin**
*Pro-Health, NZ; Cedar Health, UK.*
Menthyl valerate; quinine (p.460·1); camphor (p.1665·3); eucalyptus oil (p.1686·2).
*Aid to smoking withdrawal.*

**Nicodan** *Wernigerode, Ger.*
Propyl nicotinate (p.85·3).
*Musculoskeletal and joint pain; neuralgia; peripheral vascular disorders.*

**Nicodan N** *Wernigerode, Ger.*
Propyl nicotinate (p.85·3).
*Musculoskeletal and joint pain; neuralgia; peripheral vascular disorders.*

**Nicoderm**
*Pharmacia Consumer, Canad.; SmithKline Beecham Consumer, USA.*
Nicotine (p.1720·1).
*Aid to smoking withdrawal.*

**Nicodisc** *Lacer, Spain†.*
Nicotine (p.1720·1).
*Aid to smoking withdrawal.*

**Nicogum** *Pierre Fabre, Fr.*
Nicotine (p.1720·1).
*Aid to smoking withdrawal.*

**Nicojuvel** *Basi, Port.*
Tocoferil nicotinate (p.1015·1).

**Nicol** *Upha, Malaysia.*
Chloramphenicol (p.185·1).
*Bacterial eye and ear infections.*

**Nicolan**
*Pharmacia Upjohn, Austria†; Biosintetica, Braz.†; Meda, Swed.†.*
Nicotine (p.1720·1).
*Aid to smoking withdrawal.*

**Nicolip** *Hennig, Ger.*
Inositol nicotinate (p.939·3).
*Hyperlipidaemias.*

**Nicolmycetin** *Unison, Thai.*
Chloramphenicol (p.185·1).
*Bacterial infections.*

**Nicolsint** *Epifarma, Ital.*
Citicoline (p.1672·3).
*Cerebrovascular disorders; parkinsonism.*

**Nicomax** *Pensa, Spain.*
Nicotine (p.1720·1) or nicotine polacrilex (p.1720·1).
*Aid to smoking withdrawal.*

**Nicomide** *Sirius, USA.*
Nicotinamide; zinc oxide; copper oxide; folic acid (p.1417·1).

**Niconil** *Elan, Irl.†.*
Nicotine (p.1720·1).
*Aid to smoking withdrawal.*

**Nicopatch** *Pierre Fabre Sante, Fr.*
Nicotine (p.1720·1).
*Aid to smoking withdrawal.*

**Nicopaverina** *Enila, Braz.*
Nicotinic acid (p.1441·1); papaverine hydrochloride (p.1728·1).
*Atherosclerosis.*

**Nicopaverina B6** *Enila, Braz.*
Nicotinic acid (p.1441·1); papaverine hydrochloride (p.1728·1); pyridoxine hydrochloride (p.1456·3).
*Atherosclerosis.*

**Nicoprive**
*Note. This name is used for preparations of different composition.*
*DB, Fr.*
Ascorbic acid (p.1460·2); crataegus (p.1677·1); vitamin B substances (p.1417·1).
Formerly contained quinine ascorbate, crataegus, and vitamins.
*Aid to smoking withdrawal.*
*IFI, Ital.†.*
Quinine ascorbate (p.1737·2); vitamins (p.1417·1); crataegus (p.1677·1).
*Aid to smoking withdrawal.*

**Nicord** *Marjan, Braz.*
Amlodipine besilate (p.862·1).
*Hypertension.*

**Nicorette**
*Sidus, Arg.; Pharmacia, Austral.; Pharmacia, Austria; Pharmacia, Belg.; Pharmacia, Braz.†; Pharmacia Consumer, Canad.; Pharmacia, Chile; Pharmacia, Denm.; Pharmacia, Fin.; Pharmacia, Fr.; Pharmacia, Ger.; Pharmacia, Hong Kong; Pharmacia, Irl.; Pharmacia Upjohn, Israel; Pharmacia Upjohn, Ital.; Pharmacia, Malaysia; Hoechst Marion Roussel, Mex.†; Pharmacia, Neth.; Pharmacia, Norw.; Pharmacia, NZ; Pharmacia, Port.; Pharmacia, S.Afr.; Pharmacia, Singapore; Pharmacia, Spain; Pharmacia, Swed.; Pharmacia, Switz.; Pharmacia, Thai.; Pfizer Consumer, UK; SmithKline Beecham Consumer, USA.*
Nicotine (p.1720·1), nicotine betadex (p.1721·1), or nicotine resin complex (p.1720·1).
*Aid to smoking withdrawal.*

**Nicostop TTS** *Drossapharm, Switz.†.*
Nicotine (p.1720·1).
*Aid to smoking withdrawal.*

**Nicosyn** *Sirius, USA.*
Sulfur (p.1158·2); sulfacetamide sodium (p.257·3).
*Acne.*

**Nicotabs** *Thaipharmed, Thai.*
Nicotinic acid (p.1441·1).
*Hyperlipidaemias; nicotinic acid deficiency; vascular disorders.*

**Nicotears** *Saval, Chile.*
*Eye drops:* Hypromellose (p.1579·3); dextran 70 (p.746·2).
*Eye gel:* Carbomer 940 (p.1577·2).
*Dry eyes.*

**Nicotibine** *Aventis, Belg.*
Isoniazid (p.222·2).
*Tuberculosis.*

**Nicotinell**
*Novartis Consumer, Austral.; Novartis Consumer, Austria; Novartis Consumer, Belg.; Novartis, Chile; Novartis, Denm.; Novartis, Fin.; Novartis Sante, Fr.; Novartis Consumer, Ger.; Novartis, Hong Kong; Novartis Consumer, Irl.; Novartis, Israel; Novartis, Malaysia; Novartis Consumer, Neth.; Novartis, Norw.; Novartis, NZ; Novartis Nutrition, Singapore; Novartis Consumer, Spain; Novartis, Swed.; Novartis, Switz.; Novartis, Thai.; Novartis Consumer, UK.*
Nicotine (p.1720·1), nicotine resin complex (p.1720·1), or nicotine tartrate (p.1720·1).
*Aid to smoking withdrawal.*

**Nicotinell TTS**
*Novartis, Arg.; Novartis, Braz.; Novartis, India; Novartis Consumer, Ital.; Novartis, Mex.; Novartis Consumer, Port.; Novartis Consumer, S.Afr.†.*
Nicotine (p.1720·1).
*Aid to smoking withdrawal.*

**Nicotinex** *Fleming, USA†.*
Nicotinic acid (p.1441·1).
*Hyperlipidaemia (adjunct); nicotinic acid deficiency; pellagra.*

**Nicotinoid** *Valdecasas, Mex.†.*
Nicotinamide (p.1441·2).

**Nicotrans**
*Recordati, Ital.†; Pharmacia Upjohn, Spain†.*
Nicotine (p.1720·1).
*Aid to smoking withdrawal.*

**Nicotrol**
*Pharmacia, Austria; Johnson & Johnson, Canad.; Pharmacia, NZ; Pharmacia, Spain; Pharmacia, USA.*
Nicotine (p.1720·1).
*Aid to smoking withdrawal.*

**Nicovitol** *Lannacher, Austria.*
Nicotinamide (p.1441·2).
*Nicotinamide deficiency.*

**Nicozid**
*IFET (ΙΦΕΤ), Gr.; Piam, Ital.*
Isoniazid (p.222·2).
*Tuberculosis.*

**Nicozinc** *Chobet, Arg.*
*Tablets:* Zinc nicotinamide.
*Peripheral vascular disorders.*
*Topical solution:* Zinc nicotinamide; lincomycin hydrochloride (p.226·2).
*Skin infections.*

**NidaGel** *3M, Canad.*
Metronidazole (p.607·2).
*Bacterial vaginosis.*

**Nidal** *Zerboni, Mex.†.*
Chlormadinone (p.1542·1).

**Nidal AR** *Nestle, Fr.*
Infant feed (p.1417·1).
*Regurgitation in infants.*

**Nidal HA** *Nestle, Fr.*
Infant feed (p.1417·1).
*Potential hypersensitivity to cows milk.*

**Nidazolem** *Lemery, Mex.†.*
Metronidazole (p.607·2).

**Nidazolin** *Bunker, Braz.*
Nystatin (p.406·3).
*Fungal infections.*

**Nide** *Ibirn, Ital.*
Nimesulide (p.67·1).
*Fever; inflammation; pain.*

**Nidem** *Arrow, Austral.*
Gliclazide (p.332·1).
*Diabetes mellitus.*

**Nidex**
*Nestle, Braz.; Nestle, Ital.*
Maltodextrin (p.1439·3).
*Nutritional supplement.*

**Nidina Confort** *Nestle, Ital.*
Infant feed (p.1417·1).
*Regurgitation.*

**Nidina HA**
*Nestle, Ital.; Nestle, Port.*
Infant feed (p.1417·1).
*Protein intolerance.*

**Nidina probiotico** *Nestle, Ital.*
Infant feed (p.1417·1).
*Gastrointestinal disorders.*

**Nidol**
*Eurodrug, Hong Kong; Damor, Ital.†; Eurodrug, Malaysia; Eurodrug, Singapore; Eurodrug, Thai.*
Nimesulide (p.67·1).
*Fever; inflammation; pain.*

**Nidralon** *Liferpal, Mex.*
Metronidazole (p.607·2).
*Protozoal infections.*

**Nidran** *Sankyo, Jpn.*
Nimustine hydrochloride (p.576·3).
*Malignant neoplasms.*

**Nidrel** *Schwarz, Fr.*
Nitrendipine (p.973·3).
*Hypertension.*

**Nidrozol** *Fustery, Mex.*
Metronidazole (p.607·2) or metronidazole benzoate (p.607·2).
*Amoebiasis; giardiasis; trichomoniasis.*

**Nieral** *Schuck, Ger.*
Solidago virgaurea (p.1748·3).
*Urinary-tract disorders.*

**Nierano HM** *Pfluger, Ger.*
Homoeopathic preparation.

**Nieren-Elixier ST** *Cosmochema, Ger.*
Homoeopathic preparation.

**Nierentee 2000** *Sanofi Synthelabo, Ger.*
Birch leaf (p.1660·3); java tea (p.1702·3); juniper berry oil (p.1703·1); fennel oil (p.1687·3).
*Urinary-tract disorders.*

**Nierentee EF-EM-ES** *Smetana, Austria.*
Ononis (p.1723·3); equisetum (p.1684·1); herb. polygonii.
*Urinary-tract disorders.*

**Nieron Blasen- und Nieren-Tee VI** *Hoyer, Ger.*
Birch leaf (p.1660·3); java tea (p.1702·3); solidago virgaurea (p.1748·3); peppermint leaf (p.1283·2); liquorice root (p.1270·2); ononis (p.1723·3).
*Urinary-tract disorders.*

**Nieron S** *Hoyer, Ger.*
Solidago virgaurea (p.1748·3); taraxacum (p.1751·3).
*Urinary-tract disorders.*

**Nieron-Tee N** *Hoyer, Ger.*
Birch leaf (p.1660·3); equisetum (p.1684·1); taraxacum (p.1751·3); ononis (p.1723·3).
*Urinary-tract disorders.*

**Nieroxin N** *Hoyer, Ger.*
Maté leaf (p.1765·3); solidago virgaurea (p.1748·3); juniper oil (p.1703·1).
*Urinary-tract disorders.*

**Nifadil** *Sanval, Braz.*
Nifedipine (p.966·2).
*Angina pectoris.*

**Nifal** *Aliud, Austria.*
Nifedipine (p.966·2).
*Angina pectoris; hypertension; Raynaud's syndrome.*

**Nifalin** *Pharmanik (Φαρμανικ), Gr.*
Lorazepam (p.704·1).
*Anxiety disorders; insomnia; status epilepticus.*

**Nifangin** *Orion, Fin.*
Nifedipine (p.966·2).
*Angina pectoris; hypertension; Raynaud's syndrome.*

**Nif-Atenil** *Ecosol, Switz.*
Atenolol (p.865·2); nifedipine (p.966·2).
*Hypertension.*

**Nifatenol** *Hexal, Ger.*
Atenolol (p.865·2); nifedipine (p.966·2).
*Hypertension.*

**Nifdemin** *Ratiopharm, Fin.*
Nifedipine (p.966·2).
*Angina pectoris; hypertension; Raynaud's syndrome.*

**Nife** *1A, Ger.; ABZ, Ger.; CT, Ger.; Alpharma-Isis, Ger.; Wolff, Ger.*
Nifedipine (p.966·2).
*Angina pectoris; hypertension; Raynaud's syndrome.*

**nife uno** *CT, Ger.*
Nifedipine (p.966·2).
*Hypertension.*

**nife-basan** *Schonenberger, Switz.*
Nifedipine (p.966·2).
*Hypertension; ischaemic heart disease.*

**Nifebene** *Ratiopharm, Austria.*
Nifedipine (p.966·2).
*Angina pectoris; hypertension; Raynaud's syndrome.*

**Nifecard**
*Note. This name is used for preparations of different composition.*
*Sigma, Austral.; Asta Medica, Austria; Lek, Hong Kong; Lek, Singapore; Lek, Thai.*
Nifedipine (p.966·2).
*Angina pectoris; cardiomyopathy; hypertension; pulmonary hypertension; Raynaud's syndrome.*

*Bros, Gr.*
Nitrendipine (p.973·3).
*Hypertension.*

**Nifeclair** *Hennig, Ger.*
Nifedipine (p.966·2).
*Angina pectoris; hypertension; Raynaud's syndrome.*

**Nifecodan** *Pharmacodane, Denm.*
Nifedipine (p.966·2).
*Angina pectoris; hypertension; Raynaud's syndrome.*

**Nifecor**
*Hexal, Arg.; Pharmacia, Fin.; Betapharm, Ger.*
Nifedipine (p.966·2).
*Angina pectoris; hypertension; hypertrophic cardiomyopathy; Raynaud's syndrome.*

**Nifed** *Rowex, Irl.*
Nifedipine (p.966·2).
*Angina pectoris; hypertension.*

**Nifed Sol** *Phoenix, Arg.*
Nifedipine (p.966·2).
*Angina pectoris; hypertension.*

**Nifedalat** *Hexal, S.Afr.*
Nifedipine (p.966·2).
*Angina pectoris; hypertension; Raynaud's syndrome.*

**Nifedate** *Euro-Labor, Port.; Grunenthal, Port.*
Nifedipine (p.966·2).
*Hypertension; ischaemic heart disease; Raynaud's syndrome.*

**Nifedax** *Royton, Braz.*
Nifedipine (p.966·2).
*Angina pectoris; hypertension.*

**Nifedel** *Klonal, Arg.*
Nifedipine (p.966·2).
*Angina pectoris.*

**Nifediac** *Teva, USA.*
Nifedipine (p.966·2).
*Hypertension.*

**Nifedical** *Teva, USA.*
Nifedipine (p.966·2).
*Hypertension.*

**Nifedicor**
*Nikolakopoulos (Νικολακοπουλος), Gr.; Monsanto, Ital.; Streuli, Switz.*
Nifedipine (p.966·2).
*Angina pectoris; hypertension; Raynaud's syndrome.*

**Nifedicron** *Monsanto, Ital.*
Nifedipine (p.966·2).
*Angina pectoris; hypertension.*

**Nifedi-Denk** *Denk, Singapore.*
Nifedipine (p.966·2).
*Hypertension; ischaemic heart disease; Raynaud's syndrome.*

**Nifedigel** *Pharmacaps, Mex.†.*
Nifedipine (p.966·2).

**Nifedin**
*Cristalia, Braz.; Benedetti, Ital.*
Nifedipine (p.966·2).
*Angina pectoris; hypertension; Raynaud's syndrome.*

**Nifedine** *Sarabhai Piramal, India.*
Nifedipine (p.966·2).
*Angina pectoris; hypertension.*

**Nifedipat** *Azupharma, Ger.*
Nifedipine (p.966·2).
*Angina pectoris; hypertension.*

**Nifedipres** *Cryopharma, Mex.*
Nifedipine (p.966·2).
*Angina pectoris; heart failure; hypertension.*

**Nifedipress** *Dexcel, UK.*
Nifedipine (p.966·2).
*Angina pectoris; hypertension.*

**Nifehexal**
*Hexal, Austral.; Hexal, Austria; Hexal, Braz.; Hexal, Ger.*
Nifedipine (p.966·2).
*Angina pectoris; hypertension; Raynaud's syndrome.*

**Nifehexal Sali** *Hexal, Ger.†.*
Nifedipine (p.966·2); mefruside (p.951·3).
*Hypertension.*

**Nifelat**
*Note. This name is used for preparations of different composition.*
*Sidus, Arg.; TAD, Ger.; Cipla, India; Remedica, Singapore; Remedica, Thai.*
Nifedipine (p.966·2).
*Angina pectoris; hypertension; hypertrophic cardiomyopathy; Raynaud's syndrome.*

*Biosintetica, Braz.*
Nifedipine (p.966·2); atenolol (p.865·2).
*Angina pectoris; hypertension.*

**Nifelease** *Pinewood, Irl.*
Nifedipine (p.966·2).
*Angina pectoris.*

**Niferex**
*Landmark, Canad.†; Raffo, Chile; Schwarz, Hong Kong; Tillomed, UK; Ther-Rx, USA.*
Polysaccharide-iron complex (p.1443·2).
*Iron-deficiency anaemia.*

*Erol, Swed.*
Ferrous glycine sulfate (p.1428·2).
*Iron deficiency; iron-deficiency anaemia.*

**Niferex Forte** *Ther-Rx, USA.*
Polysaccharide-iron complex (p.1443·2); folic acid (p.1429·1); cyanocobalamin (p.1458·2).
*Iron-deficiency anaemia; megaloblastic anaemia.*

**Niferex Prenatal** *Raffo, Chile.*
Multivitamin and mineral preparation with iron and folic acid (p.1417·1).

**Niferex-PN** *Ther-Rx, USA.*
Multivitamin and mineral preparation with iron and folic acid (p.1417·1).

**Nifesal** *Salus, Ital.*
Nifedipine (p.966·2).
*Angina pectoris; hypertension.*

**Nifetex** *BPRL, Singapore.*
Atenolol (p.865·2); nifedipine (p.966·2).
*Angina pectoris; hypertension.*

**Nifetolol** *Anglo-French Drugs, India.*
Atenolol (p.865·2); nifedipine (p.966·2).
*Hypertension.*

**Nifezzard** *Pizzard, Mex.*
Nifedipine (p.966·2).
*Angina pectoris; hypertension.*

**Nifical** *Lichtenstein, Ger.*
Nifedipine (p.966·2).
*Angina pectoris; hypertension.*

**Nificard** *Ranbaxy, Thai.†.*
Nifedipine (p.966·2).
*Angina pectoris; hypertension; myocardial infarction.*

**Nifint**
*Ratiopharm, Austria; Merckle, Ger.*
Menthol (p.1711·3).
*Upper respiratory-tract catarrh.*

**Nifiran** *Ranbaxy, Thai.*
Nifedipine (p.966·2).
*Angina pectoris; heart failure; hypertension; myocardial infarction.*

**Niflactol** *Upsamedica, Spain.*
Morniflumate (p.60·1) or niflumic acid (p.67·1).
*Musculoskeletal, joint, peri-articular, and soft-tissue disorders; pain.*

**Niflam**
*Note. This name is used for preparations of different composition.*
*Roemmers, Arg.*
Celecoxib (p.25·2).
*Osteoarthritis; rheumatoid arthritis.*

*Upsa, Ital.*
*Capsules; cream; topical gel:* Niflumic acid (p.67·1).
*Suppositories:* Morniflumate (p.60·1).
*Inflammation; pain.*

**Niflamol** *Bristol-Myers Squibb, Gr.*
Niflumic acid (p.67·1).
*Inflammatory joint disorders; spondyloarthropathies.*

**Niflan** *Yoshitomi, Jpn; Senju, Jpn.*
Pranoprofen (p.85·2).
*Inflammatory eye disorders.*

**Niflucan** *Duncan, Arg.*
Flunarizine (p.434·2).
*Cerebral and peripheral vascular disorders.*

**Niflugel**
*Bristol-Myers Squibb, Belg.; UPSA, Fr.; Upsamedica, Switz.†.*
Niflumic acid (p.67·1).
*Musculoskeletal, joint, peri-articular and soft-tissue disorders.*

**Nifluril**
*Note. This name is used for preparations of different composition.*
*Bristol-Myers Squibb, Belg.; UPSA, Fr.; UPSA, Hong Kong†; Bristol-Myers Squibb, Port.; Upsamedica, Switz.†.*
*Capsules; ointment:* Niflumic acid (p.67·1).
*Gout; inflammation; musculoskeletal, joint, peri-articular, and soft-tissue disorders; pain; phlebitis.*

*UPSA, Fr.†; Bristol-Myers Squibb, Port.†.*
*Dental gel:* Niflumic acid glycinamide (p.67·1); hexetidine (p.1182·1).
*Gingivitis; inflammatory mouth disorders.*

*UPSA, Fr.; Upsamedica, Switz.†.*
*Suppositories:* Morniflumate (p.60·1).
*Inflammation; musculoskeletal, joint, and peri-articular disorders; pain.*

**Niflux** *Alter, Port.*
Carbocisteine (p.1116·2); sobrerol (p.1130·2).
*Respiratory-tract congestion.*

**Nifopress** *Goldshield, UK.*
Nifedipine (p.966·2).
*Angina pectoris; hypertension; Raynaud's syndrome.*

**Nifostin** *Richmond, Arg.*
Azithromycin (p.159·1).
*Bacterial infections.*

**Nifreal** *Realpharma, Ger.†.*
Nifedipine (p.966·2).
*Hypertension; ischaemic heart disease; Raynaud's syndrome.*

**Nif-Ten**
*AstraZeneca, Austria; AstraZeneca, Fin.; AstraZeneca, Ger.; AstraZeneca, Hong Kong; AstraZeneca, Irl.; AstraZeneca, Ital.; Zeneca, Neth.; AstraZeneca, Singapore; AstraZeneca, Switz.*
Atenolol (p.865·2); nifedipine (p.966·2).
*Angina pectoris; hypertension.*

**Nifucin** *Apogepha, Ger.†.*
*Topical gel:* Nitrofurazone (p.238·2).
*Burns; wounds.*
*Topical liquid:* Nitrofurazone (p.238·2); propipocaine hydrochloride (p.1383·3).
*Bacterial skin infections; burns.*

**Nifur** *Lafon, Fr.†.*
Nifuroxazide (p.237·2).
Now known as Nifuroxazide-Ratiopharm.
*Diarrhoea.*

**Nifuran**
*Note. This name is used for preparations of different composition.*
*Jenapharm, Ger.*
Furazolidone (p.605·2).
*Vaginal infections.*

*Bamford, NZ.*
Nitrofurantoin (p.237·2).
*Urinary-tract infections.*

**Nifurantin** *Apogepha, Ger.*
Nitrofurantoin (p.237·2).
*Urinary-tract infections.*

**Nifurantin B 6** *Apogepha, Ger.*
Nitrofurantoin (p.237·2); pyridoxine hydrochloride (p.1456·3).
*Urinary-tract infections.*

**Nifurat** *Bago, Chile.*
Nifuroxazide (p.237·2); activated attapulgite (p.1251·1).
*Diarrhoea.*

**Nifuretten** *Apogepha, Ger.*
Nitrofurantoin (p.237·2).
*Urinary-tract infections.*

**Nifurol** *Reuffer, Mex.†.*
Nitrofurazone (p.238·2).

**Nifurtox** *Richmond, Arg.*
Fluconazole (p.398·1).
*Fungal infections.*

**Nigalax** *Sanofi Synthelabo, Arg.*
*Suppositories:* Bisacodyl (p.1251·3); docusate sodium (p.1262·2); sodium lauril sulphoacetate (p.1574·3).
*Tablets:* Bisacodyl (p.1251·3); docusate sodium (p.1262·2).
*Bowel evacuation.*

**Nigersan** *Sanum-Kehlbeck, Ger.*
Homoeopathic preparation.

**Night Cold Comfort** *Boots, UK†.*
Paracetamol (p.76·2); pseudoephedrine hydrochloride (p.1129·2); diphenhydramine hydrochloride (p.431·3); pholcodine (p.1128·3).
*Cold symptoms.*

**Night Nurse**
*SmithKline Beecham Consumer, Irl.; GlaxoSmithKline Consumer, UK.*
Paracetamol (p.76·2); promethazine hydrochloride (p.439·1); dextromethorphan hydrobromide (p.1117·3).
*Cold and influenza symptoms.*

**Night Time** *Peter Black, UK†.*
Valerian (p.1762·2); lupulus (p.1708·1); passion flower (p.1729·1).
*Sleep disturbances.*

**Night Time Cold/Flu Relief** *Prometic, USA.*
Doxylamine succinate (p.432·3); dextromethorphan hydrobromide (p.1117·3); paracetamol (p.76·2); pseudoephedrine hydrochloride (p.1129·2).
*Coughs and cold symptoms.*

**Night Time Liquigels** *Scherer, Braz.†.*
Doxylamine (p.433·1); paracetamol (p.76·2); pseudoephedrine (p.1129·2).
*Cold and influenza symptoms.*

**Nightcalm** *Galpharm, UK.*
Diphenhydramine hydrochloride (p.431·3).
*Insomnia.*

**Night-Care** *CT, Ger.†.*
Pumilio pine oil (p.1737·1); thyme oil (p.1755·3); eucalyptus oil (p.1686·2); menthol (p.1711·3).
*Catarrh.*

**Nightpeel** *Lierac, Fr.*
Salicylic acid (p.1157·1); glycolic acid (p.1147·3); urea (p.1162·2); enoxolone (p.36·2).
*Sun-induced skin damage.*

**Night-Time** *WestCan, Canad.*
Pseudoephedrine hydrochloride (p.1129·2); doxylamine succinate (p.432·3); dextromethorphan hydrobromide (p.1117·3); paracetamol (p.76·2).
Formerly contained pseudoephedrine hydrochloride and menthol.

**Nighttime Cold & Flu** *Stanley, Canad.*
Pseudoephedrine hydrochloride (p.1129·2); doxylamine succinate (p.432·3); dextromethorphan hydrobromide (p.1117·3); paracetamol (p.76·2).

**Night-Time Effervescent Cold** *Goldline, USA†.*
Phenylpropanolamine hydrochloride (p.1127·3); diphenhydramine citrate (p.431·3); aspirin (p.15·1).
*Upper respiratory-tract symptoms.*

**Nighttime Pamprin** *Chattem, USA.*
Diphenhydramine hydrochloride (p.431·3); paracetamol (p.76·2).
*Insomnia.*

**NightTime Theraflu** *Novartis, USA.*
Paracetamol (p.76·2); dextromethorphan hydrobromide (p.1117·3); pseudoephedrine hydrochloride (p.1129·2); chlorphenamine maleate (p.427·3).
*Coughs and cold symptoms.*

**Niglinar** *Rivero, Arg.*
Glyceryl trinitrate (p.923·2).

**Nigrantyl** *Lacteol, Fr.†.*
Black currant (p.1661·1); sodium citrate (p.1223·2).
*Capillary fragility.*

**Nigroids** *Ernest Jackson, UK.*
Liquorice (p.1270·2); menthol (p.1711·3).

**Nij-Terol** *Deutsche, Chile.*
Lovastatin (p.949·1).
*Hypercholesterolaemia.*

**Nikableomicina** *Pharmacia, Chile.*
Bleomycin hydrochloride (p.531·2).
*Malignant neoplasms.*

**Nikarin** *TO-Chemicals, Thai.*
Miconazole nitrate (p.405·3).
*Candidiasis.*

**Nikion** *Roux-Ocefa, Arg.*
Enalapril maleate (p.909·2); felodipine (p.914·3).
*Hypertension.*

**Nikkho Vac** *Nikkho, Braz.*
Allergen extracts (airborne proteins, food proteins, and respiratory-tract bacterial antigens) (p.1650·1).
*Allergen immunotherapy.*

**Niklod** *Savio, Ital.*
Disodium clodronate (p.770·2).
*Hyperparathyroidism; multiple myeloma; osteolysis of malignancy; osteoporosis.*

**nikofrenon** *Hefa, Ger.*
Nicotine (p.1720·1).
*Aid to smoking withdrawal.*

**Nikorazol** *Mavi, Mex.†.*
Ketoconazole (p.403·3).

**Nikoril** *Medinfar, Port.*
Nicorandil (p.965·3).
*Angina pectoris.*

**Nikotugg** *ACO, Swed.*
Nicotine resin (p.1720·1).
*Aid to smoking withdrawal.*

**Nilandron** *Hoechst Marion Roussel, USA.*
Nilutamide (p.576·2).
*Prostatic cancer.*

**Nilcid** *Abbott, Mex.*
Magaldrate (p.1271·3); simeticone (p.1289·2).
*Gastrointestinal disorders.*

**Nilcid-MPS** *Abbott, Hong Kong.*
Magaldrate (p.1271·3); simeticone (p.1289·2).
*Flatulence; gastrointestinal hyperacidity; heartburn.*

**Nilevar** *Laphal, Fr.*
Norethandrolone (p.1562·2).
*Medullary aplasia.*

**Nilflux** *Biol, Arg.*
*Staphylococcus aureus*; haemolytic Streptococcus; *Streptococcus pyogenes*; non-haemolytic Streptococcus; *Enterococcus faecalis* (p.1704·2); *Streptococcus pneumoniae*; *Klebsiella pneumoniae*; *Micrococcus roseus*; *Moraxella catarrhalis*; *Haemophilus influenzae*; hyaluronidase (p.1698·2); ox bile (p.1660·3); ascorbic acid (p.1460·2).
*Respiratory-tract infections.*

**Nilgrip** *Biol, Arg.*
An influenza vaccine (p.1620·2).
*Active immunisation.*

**Nilken** *Kener, Mex.†.*
Buphenine hydrochloride (p.1663·2).

**NilnOcen** *Zeppenfeldt, Ger.†.*
Paracetamol (p.76·2).
*Fever; pain.*

**Nilodor** *Cussons, UK†.*
A deodorant liquid for use with colostomies and ileostomies.

**Nilperidol** *Cristalia, Braz.*
Fentanyl citrate (p.40·1); droperidol (p.697·2).

**Nilstat**
*Sigma, Austral.; Wyeth Lederle, Belg.; Technilab, Canad.; Zuellig, NZ; Lederle, USA.*
Nystatin (p.406·3).
*Candidiasis.*

**Nim** *Hexal, Ger.*
Nimodipine (p.972·3).
*Cerebral disorders in the elderly; neurological deficit following cerebral vasospasm.*

**Nimadorm** *Durascan, Denm.*
Zolpidem tartrate (p.728·3).
*Insomnia.*

**Nimalgex** *Hexal, Braz.*
Nimesulide (p.67·1).

**Nimaz** *EG, Fr.†.*
Loperamide hydrochloride (p.1271·1).
*Diarrhoea.*

**Nimbex**
*GlaxoSmithKline, Arg.; GlaxoSmithKline, Austral.; GlaxoSmithKline, Austria; GlaxoSmithKline, Belg.; Abbott, Canad.; GlaxoSmithKline, Chile; GlaxoSmithKline, Denm.; GlaxoSmithKline, Fin.; GlaxoSmithKline, Fr.; GlaxoSmithKline, Ger.; Glaxo Wellcome, Gr.; GlaxoSmithKline, Hong Kong; Wellcome, Irl.; GlaxoSmithKline, Ital.; GlaxoSmithKline, Malaysia; Glaxo Wellcome, Mex.; GlaxoSmithKline, Neth.; GlaxoSmithKline, Norw.; Wellcome, Port.; GlaxoSmithKline, S.Afr.; GlaxoSmithKline, Singapore; GlaxoSmithKline, Spain; GlaxoSmithKline, Swed.; GlaxoSmithKline, Switz.; GlaxoSmithKline, Thai.; GlaxoSmithKline, UK; Glaxo Wellcome, USA.*
Cisatracurium besilate (p.1399·1).
*Competitive neuromuscular blocker.*

**Nimbisan** *De Angeli, Ital.†.*
Brotizolam (p.672·1).
*Insomnia.*

**Nimbium** *GlaxoSmithKline, Braz.*
Cisatracurium besilate (p.1399·1).
*Competitive neuromuscular blocker.*

**Nimbus**
*Marco, Austral.; Biomerica, USA.*
Pregnancy test (p.1734·3).

**Nimed**
*Aventis, Fin.; Aventis, Port.*
Nimesulide (p.67·1).
*Fever; inflammation; pain.*

**Nimedex** *Italfarmaco, Ital.*
Nimesulide betadex (p.67·1).
*Fever; inflammation; pain.*

**Nimeflan** *Infabra, Braz.†.*
Nimesulide (p.67·1).

**Nimegen** *Medica Korea, Singapore.*
Isotretinoin (p.1148·3).
*Acne.*

**Nimelide** *Genepharm, Gr.*
Nimesulide (p.67·1).
*Inflammation; musculoskeletal disorders; pain.*

**Nimenol** *Krugher, Ital.*
Nimesulide (p.67·1).
*Fever; inflammation; pain.*

**Nimepast** *Pasteur, Chile.*
Nimesulide (p.67·1).
*Fever; inflammation; pain.*

**Nimesil** *Lusofarmaco, Ital.*
Nimesulide (p.67·1).
*Fever; inflammation; pain.*

**Nimesilam** *Sigma, Braz.*
Nimesulide (p.67·1).

**Nimesul** *Medichrom, Gr.*
Nimesulide (p.67·1).
*Inflammation; musculoskeletal disorders; pain.*

**Nimesulene** *Guidotti, Ital.*
Nimesulide (p.67·1).
*Fever; inflammation; pain.*

**Nimesulin** *Cifarma, Braz.†.*
Nimesulide (p.67·1).

**Nimesulix** *Teuto, Braz.*
Nimesulide (p.67·1).

**Nimesulon** *Sanval, Braz.*
Nimesulide (p.67·1).
*Inflammation.*

**Nimesyl** *Rider, Chile.*
Nimesulide (p.67·1).
*Fever; inflammation; pain.*

**Nimesyl Gel** *Rider, Chile.*
Nimesulide (p.67·1).
*Inflammation; pain.*

**Nimex** *Andromaco, Chile.*
Nimesulide (p.67·1).
*Inflammation; pain.*

**Nimexan** *Angelini, Ital.*
Nimesulide (p.67·1).
*Fever; inflammation; pain.*

**Nimfast** *Cadila, India.*
Nimesulide (p.67·1).
*Inflammation; musculoskeletal, joint, and peri-articular disorders; pain.*

**Nimicon** *Precimex, Mex.†.*
Miconazole (p.405·2).

**Nimicor**
*Note. This name is used for preparations of different composition.*
*Drugtech, Chile.*
Simvastatin (p.997·1).
*Hyperlipidaemias.*
*Formenti, Ital.*
Nicardipine hydrochloride (p.965·1).
*Angina pectoris; heart failure; hypertension.*

**Nimodil** *Remedina, Gr.*
Nimodipine (p.972·3).
*Neurological deficit following subarachnoid haemorrhage.*

**Nimodilat** *Lazar, Arg.*
Nimodipine (p.972·3).
*Neurological deficit following subarachnoid haemorrhage.*

**Nimodilat Plus** *Lazar, Arg.*
Nimodipine (p.972·3); citicoline sodium (p.1672·3).
*Cerebrovascular disorders.*

**Nimodrel** *Opus, UK†.*
Nifedipine (p.966·2).
*Angina pectoris; hypertension.*

**Nimopect** *Hevert, Ger.*
Thyme (p.1755·2).
*Bronchitis; catarrh; coughs.*

**Nimoreagin** *Baliarda, Arg.*
Nimodipine (p.972·3); citicoline (p.1672·3).
*Cerebrovascular disorders.*

**Nimotop**
*Bayer, Arg.; Bayer, Austral.; Bayer, Austria; Bayer, Belg.; Bayer, Braz.; Bayer, Canad.; Bayer, Chile; Bayer, Denm.; Bayer, Fin.; Bayer, Fr.; Bayer, Ger.; Bayer, Gr.; Bayer, Hong Kong; Bayer, Irl.; Bayer, Israel; Bayer, Ital.; Bayer, Malaysia; Bayer, Mex.; Bayer, Neth.; Bayer, Norw.; Bayer, NZ; Bayer, Port.; Bayer, S.Afr.; Bayer, Singapore; Bayer, Spain; Bayer, Swed.; Bayer, Switz.; Bayer, Thai.; Bayer, UK; Bayer, USA.*
Nimodipine (p.972·3).
*Mental function disorders in the elderly; neurological deficit following subarachnoid haemorrhage.*

**Nimovas** *Diffucap, Braz.*
Nimodipine (p.972·3).

**Nims** *Caber, Ital.*
Nimesulide (p.67·1).
*Fever; inflammation; pain.*

**Nimulid** *Panacea, India.*
Nimesulide (p.67·1).
*Inflammation; musculoskeletal, joint, and peri-articular disorders; pain.*

**Nimulid Nugel** *Panacea, India.*
Nimesulide (p.67·1); menthol (p.1711·3); methyl salicylate (p.59·3); capsaicin (p.24·2); linseed oil (p.1707·2).
*Musculoskeletal, joint, and peri-articular disorders.*

**Nimus** *Tecnofarma, Chile.*
Bezafibrate (p.873·2).
*Atherosclerosis; hyperlipidaemias.*

**Nimusyp** *Centaur, India.*
Nimesulide (p.67·1).
*Inflammation; musculoskeletal, joint, and peri-articular disorders; pain.*

**Nimutab** *Centaur, India.*
Nimesulide (p.67·1).
*Inflammation; musculoskeletal, joint, and peri-articular disorders; pain.*

**Nina** *Medichemie, Switz.*
Paracetamol (p.76·2).
*Fever; pain.*

**Nina cum Diphenhydramino** *Medichemie, Switz.†.*
Paracetamol (p.76·2); diphenhydramine hydrochloride (p.431·3).
*Fever; pain.*

**Ninazol** *TO-Chemicals, Thai.*
Ketoconazole (p.403·3).
*Fungal infections.*

**Nindaxa** *Ashbourne, UK.*
Indapamide (p.938·2).

**Ninderm** *Maigal, Arg.*
Wool fat (p.1483·1); azulene (p.1658·3); zinc (p.1469·2).

**Nine Rubbing Oils** *Potter's, UK.*
Amber oil; clove oil (p.1673·3); eucalyptus oil (p.1686·2); linseed oil (p.1707·2); methyl salicylate (p.59·3); volatile mustard oil (p.1718·2); turpentine oil (p.1760·1); thyme oil (p.1755·3); peppermint oil (p.1283·2).
*Musculoskeletal, joint, and soft-tissue disorders.*

**Ninlium** *Chinta, Thai.*
Domperidone (p.1263·2).
*Delayed gastric emptying; dyspepsia; nausea and vomiting.*

**Ni-No-Fluid N** *Hotz, Ger.†.*
Peppermint oil (p.1283·2).
*Cold symptoms; gastrointestinal disorders.*

**Niocitran** *Novartis Consumer, Belg.*
Paracetamol (p.76·2); pseudoephedrine hydrochloride (p.1129·2).
*Cold symptoms.*

**Niofen** *Recalcine, Chile.*
Ibuprofen (p.45·3).
*Fever.*

**Niofen Flu** *Recalcine, Chile.*
Ibuprofen (p.45·3); pseudoephedrine (p.1129·2).
*Influenza symptoms.*

**Niong retard** *Rhone-Poulenc Rorer, Switz.†.*
Glyceryl trinitrate (p.923·2).
*Angina pectoris; heart failure.*

**Niopam**
*Merck, Irl.; Bracco, UK.*
Iopamidol (p.1064·3).
*Radiographic contrast medium.*

**Niotal** *Sanofi Synthelabo, Ital.*
Zolpidem tartrate (p.728·3).
*Insomnia.*

**Nipactrin** *Heralds, Braz.†.*
Sulfamethoxypyridazine (p.263·1); nitrofurantoin (p.237·2); pyridine.
*Urinary-tract infections.*

**Nipaxon** *Pharmacia, Swed.*
Noscapine (p.1125·3).
*Coughs.*

**Nipent**
*SuperGen, Canad.; Wyeth Lederle, Fr.; Wyeth, Ger.; Pfizer, Gr.; Parke, Davis, Ital.; Wyeth Lederle, Port.†; Parke, Davis, Spain†; Wyeth, UK; SuperGen, USA.*
Pentostatin (p.579·2).
*Hairy-cell leukaemia.*

**Nipin** *Lisapharma, Ital.*
Nifedipine (p.966·2).
*Angina pectoris; hypertension.*

**Nipiol** *Billiet, Arg.*
Cyproheptadine (p.430·2); dexamethasone (p.1097·1).

**Nipodur** *Anpharm (Ανφαρμ), Gr.*
Ranitidine hydrochloride (p.1285·2).
*Conditions where gastric acid reduction is beneficial; gastric hypersecretion including Zollinger-Ellison syndrome; peptic ulcer.*

**Nipogalin** *Anpharm (Ανφαρμ), Gr.*
Cefuroxime sodium (p.184·1).
*Bacterial infections.*

**Nipolept**
*Ebewe, Austria; Aventis, Ger.*
Zotepine (p.730·2).
*Schizophrenia.*

**Nipress** *Rider, Chile.*
Nifedipine (p.966·2).
*Angina pectoris; hypertension; Raynaud's syndrome.*

**Nipride**
*Biolab Sanus, Braz.; Roche, Canad.†; Roche, Irl.; Roche, Israel†.*
Sodium nitroprusside (p.1000·2).
*Controlled hypotension; ergot intoxication; heart failure; hypertensive crisis.*

**Niprina** *Pensa, Spain.*
Nitrendipine (p.973·3).
*Angina pectoris; hypertension; Raynaud's syndrome.*

**Niprus** *Medis, Israel.*
Sodium nitroprusside (p.1000·2).
*Hypertensive crisis.*

**Niprusodio** *Fada, Arg.*
Sodium nitroprusside (p.1000·2).

**Nipruss** *Schwarz, Ger.*
Sodium nitroprusside (p.1000·2).
*Controlled hypotension; hypertension.*

**NiQuitin**
*GlaxoSmithKline Consumer, Belg.; SmithKline Beecham, Braz.†; SmithKline Beecham, Denm.; GlaxoSmithKline Sante, Fr.; GlaxoSmithKline Consumer, Ger.; GlaxoSmithKline, Irl.; GlaxoSmithKline, Israel; SmithKline Beecham, Mex.; GlaxoSmithKline Consumer, Swed.; GlaxoSmithKline Consumer, UK.*
Nicotine (p.1720·1) or nicotine polacrilex (p.1720·1).
*Aid to smoking withdrawal.*

**Niraben** *Samchully, Singapore.*
Nifuroxazide (p.237·2).
*Bacterial diarrhoea.*

**Nirapel** *Armstrong, Arg.*
Nitrendipine (p.973·3).
*Hypertension.*

**Nirason N** *Ravensberg, Ger.*
Pentaerithrityl tetranitrate (p.979·1).
*Ischaemic heart disease; myocardial infarction.*

**Nirolex for Chesty Coughs** *Boots, UK†.*
Guaifenesin (p.1122·1); ephedrine hydrochloride (p.1120·1); menthol (p.1711·3).
*Coughs.*

**Nirolex Chesty Coughs with Decongestant** Boots, UK.
Guaifenesin (p.1122·1); pseudoephedrine hydrochloride (p.1129·2).
*Coughs.*

**Nirolex Day Cold & Flu** Boots, UK.
Paracetamol (p.76·2); pholcodine (p.1128·3); pseudoephedrine hydrochloride (p.1129·2).
*Cold and influenza symptoms.*

**Nirolex Dry Cough** Boots, UK.
Glycerol (p.1694·3).
*Coughs.*

**Nirolex for Dry Coughs** Boots, UK†.
Dextromethorphan hydrobromide (p.1117·3).
*Coughs.*

**Nirolex Dry Coughs with Decongestant** Boots, UK.
Dextromethorphan hydrobromide (p.1117·3); pseudoephedrine hydrochloride (p.1129·2).
*Coughs.*

**Nirolex Night Cold & Flu** Boots, UK.
Paracetamol (p.76·2); pholcodine (p.1128·3); pseudoephedrine hydrochloride (p.1129·2); diphenhydramine hydrochloride (p.431·3).
*Cold and influenza symptoms.*

**Nirox** Medici, Ital.†.
Piroxicam (p.84·2).
*Musculoskeletal and joint disorders.*

**Nirulid** Merck Sharp & Dohme, Denm.
Amiloride hydrochloride (p.858·2).
*Hypertension; oedema.*

**Nirvaxal** Teva, Israel.
Chlordiazepoxide (p.674·2); clidinium bromide (p.480·2).
*Nervous gastrointestinal disorders.*

**Nisaid** Alliance, S.Afr.
Indometacin (p.47·3).
*Gout; inflammation; musculoskeletal and joint disorders; pain.*

**Nisal** Epifarma, Ital.†.
Nimesulide (p.67·1).
*Fever; inflammation; pain.*

**Nisalgen** UCI, Braz.
Nimesulide (p.67·1).

**Nisapulvol**
Mayoly-Spindler, Fr.; Mayoly-Spindler, Malaysia.
Benzyl hydroxybenzoate (p.1183·2).
*Pruritus.*

**Nisaseptol** Mayoly-Spindler, Fr.
Benzyl hydroxybenzoate (p.1183·2).
Formerly contained propyl hydroxybenzoate and benzyl hydroxybenzoate.
*Intertrigo; pruritus.*

**Nisasol** Mayoly-Spindler, Fr.
Benzyl hydroxybenzoate (p.1183·2).
Formerly contained methyl hydroxybenzoate, ethyl hydroxybenzoate, and propyl hydroxybenzoate.
*Burn and wound disinfection.*

**Nise**
Reddy's, India; Reddy, Singapore.
Nimesulide (p.67·1).
*Fever; inflammation; musculoskeletal, joint, and periarticular disorders; pain.*

**Nisicur** Apomedica, Austria.
Ethenzamide (p.37·2); diphenhydramine hydrochloride (p.431·3); caffeine (p.782·1); ascorbic acid (p.1460·2).
*Cold and influenza symptoms.*

**Nisis** Aventis, Fr.
Valsartan (p.1018·3).
*Hypertension.*

**Nisisco** Aventis, Fr.
Valsartan (p.1018·3); hydrochlorothiazide (p.933·2).
*Hypertension.*

**Nisita**
Note. This name is used for preparations of different composition.
Engelhard, Ger.
Sodium chloride (p.1233·3); sodium bicarbonate (p.1223·2).
*Dry mouth; nasal dryness.*

Engelhard, Hong Kong.
Sodium iodide; sodium bromide; sodium chloride; lithium chloride; sodium bicarbonate; sodium sulfate; sodium phosphate; potassium sulfate (p.1217·1).
*Nasal dryness.*

Engelhard, Switz.†.
Sal ems.
*Nasal disorders.*

**Nisodipen** Roemmers, Arg.
Nisoldipine (p.973·2).
*Angina pectoris; hypertension.*

**Nisolid** Chiesi, Ital.
Flunisolide (p.1101·1).
*Obstructive airways disease; rhinitis.*

**Nistaglos** Andromaco, Chile.
Halibut-liver oil (p.1434·1); nystatin (p.406·3); zinc oxide (p.1163·2).
*Fungal skin infections; nappy rash.*

**Nistagrand** Ahimsa, Arg.
Nystatin (p.406·3).
*Fungal infections.*

**Nistagyn** Medley, Braz.
Nystatin (p.406·3).
*Vaginal candidiasis.*

**Nistaken** Kendrick, Mex.
Propafenone hydrochloride (p.988·3).
*Arrhythmias.*

**Nistan** Protein, Mex.†.
Nystatin (p.406·3).

**Nistanil** Ducto, Braz.
Nystatin (p.406·3).
*Fungal infections.*

**Nistaquim** Quimica y Farmacia, Mex.
Nystatin (p.406·3).
*Fungal infections.*

**Nistat** Cevallos, Arg.
Nystatin (p.406·3).
*Bacterial and fungal infections.*

**Nistaval** Sanval, Braz.
Nystatin (p.406·3).
*Fungal infections.*

**Nistax** Luper, Braz.
Nystatin (p.406·3).
*Fungal infections.*

**Nistazol** Hebron, Braz.
Metronidazole benzoate (p.607·2); nystatin (p.406·3).
*Vaginal infections.*

**Nistoral** Laboratorios Chile, Chile.
Nystatin (p.406·3).
*Candidiasis.*

**Nisuflex** Cazi, Braz.
Nimesulide (p.67·1).
*Inflammation; pain.*

**Nisulid**
Asta Medica, Braz.; Grunenthal, Chile; Robapharm, Switz.
Nimesulide (p.67·1).
*Fever; inflammation; musculoskeletal, joint, and periarticular disorders; pain.*

**Nisural** Laboratorios Chile, Chile.
Nimesulide (p.67·1).
*Fever; inflammation; pain.*

**Nisylen**
Peithner, Austria; DHU, Ger.
Homoeopathic preparation.

**Nitagon** Medpro, S.Afr.
Permethrin (p.1508·3); piperonyl butoxide (p.1509·2).
*Pediculosis.*

**Nitan**
Note. This name is used for preparations of different composition.
Rekah, Israel.
Pemoline (p.1591·2).
*Attention deficit hyperactivity disorder; depression; fatigue.*

Abbott, Mex.
Sodium nitroprusside (p.1000·2).
*Controlled hypotension during surgery; heart failure; hypertension.*

**Nitavan** Stadmed, India.
Nitrazepam (p.710·1).
*Insomnia.*

**Nite Time Cold Formula** Barre-National, USA.
Pseudoephedrine hydrochloride (p.1129·2); dextromethorphan hydrobromide (p.1117·3); doxylamine succinate (p.432·3); paracetamol (p.76·2).
*Coughs and cold symptoms.*

**Nite Time Diet** Natural Life, Arg.
Lysine; ornithine; arginine (p.1417·1).
*Slimming aid.*

**Nitecall** Restan, S.Afr.
Paracetamol (p.76·2); dextromethorphan hydrobromide (p.1117·3); chlorphenamine maleate (p.427·3); phenylpropanolamine hydrochloride (p.1127·3).
*Cold and influenza symptoms.*

**Niten** Armstrong, Arg.
Losartan potassium (p.947·2).
*Hypertension.*

**Niten D** Armstrong, Arg.
Losartan potassium (p.947·2); hydrochlorothiazide (p.933·2).
*Hypertension.*

**Nitens** Pulitzer, Ital.
Naproxen cetrimonium (p.65·3).
*Gynaecological disorders; mouth and throat disorders.*

**Nitepax** Aspen, S.Afr.
Noscapine resin complex (p.1125·3).
*Coughs.*

**Niterey** Lagos, Arg.
Tretinoin (p.1161·1).
*Light-induced skin damage.*

**Nitesco Smagliature** Pharmafar, Ital.†.
Ruscus aculeatus; hedera helix; aesculus (p.1648·2); aescin (p.1648·2).
*Stretch marks.*

**Nitised** Petsiavas (Πετσιαβας), Gr.
Ranitidine hydrochloride (p.1285·2).
*Conditions where gastric acid reduction is beneficial; gastric hypersecretion including Zollinger-Ellison syndrome; peptic ulcer.*

**Nitlotion** Shantys, UK.
Coconut oil (p.1481·1).
*Pediculosis.*

**Nitoman**
Virgo Healthcare, Austral.†; Shire, Canad.; Medilink, Denm.
Tetrabenazine (p.1752·2).
*Drug-induced extrapyramidal disorders; hyperkinesis.*

**Nitopro** Maruishi, Jpn.
Sodium nitroprusside (p.1000·2).
*Hypertension.*

**Nitorol**
Eisai, Hong Kong†; Eisai, Jpn; Eisai, Malaysia.
Isosorbide dinitrate (p.941·1).
*Angina pectoris; coronary sclerosis; myocardial infarction.*

**Nitossil** Novartis Consumer, Ital.
Cloperastine fendizoate (p.1117·2) or cloperastine hydrochloride (p.1117·2).
*Coughs.*

**Nitradisc**
Pharmacia, Arg.; Pharmacia, Austral.†; Searle, Braz.†; Heumann, Ger.†; Searle, Mex.; Pharmacia, Port.; Searle, S.Afr.†; Pharmacia, Spain; Searle, Thai.†.
Glyceryl trinitrate (p.923·2).
*Angina pectoris; heart failure; myocardial infarction.*

**Nitrados**
Douglas, NZ; Douglas, Singapore; Douglas, Thai.; TTN, Thai.
Nitrazepam (p.710·1).
*Epilepsy; infantile spasm; insomnia.*

**Nitramin** Coup, Gr.
Isosorbide mononitrate (p.942·1).
*Angina; heart failure.*

**Nitrangin** Alpharma-Isis, Ger.
Glyceryl trinitrate (p.923·2).
*Angina pectoris; coronary spasm; heart failure; myocardial infarction.*

**Nitrangin compositum** Alpharma-Isis, Ger.
Glyceryl trinitrate (p.923·2); valerian (p.1762·2).
*Angina pectoris; myocardial infarction.*

**Nitrangin forte** Wernigerode, Ger.†.
Glyceryl trinitrate (p.923·2).
*Angina pectoris; coronary spasm; myocardial infarction.*

**Nitrapamil** Orion, Fin.†.
Diazepam (p.690·1); methylpropylpropanediol dinitrate.
*Angina pectoris.*

**Nitrapan** Cristalia, Braz.
Nitrazepam (p.710·1).
*Epilepsy; insomnia.*

**Nitravet** Anglo-French Drugs, India.
Nitrazepam (p.710·1).
*Insomnia.*

**Nitrazadon** ICN, Canad.
Nitrazepam (p.710·1).

**Nitrazep** CT, Ger.†.
Nitrazepam (p.710·1).
*Insomnia.*

**Nitrazepan**
Cristalia, Braz.†; Prodes, Spain†.
Nitrazepam (p.710·1).
*Epilepsy; insomnia.*

**Nitrazepol** Farmasa, Braz.
Nitrazepam (p.710·1).
*Epilepsy; insomnia.*

**Nitrazine Paper** Apothecon, USA†.
Test for pH in urine.

**Nitre** ABZ, Ger.
Nitrendipine (p.973·3).
*Hypertension.*

**Nitregamma** Worwag, Ger.
Nitrendipine (p.973·3).
*Hypertension.*

**Nitrek** Bertek, USA.
Glyceryl trinitrate (p.923·2).
*Angina pectoris.*

**Nitren** 1A, Ger.; Acis, Ger.
Nitrendipine (p.973·3).
*Hypertension.*

**Nitren Lich** Lichtenstein, Ger.
Nitrendipine (p.973·3).
*Hypertension.*

**Nitrencord** Biosintetica, Braz.
Nitrendipine (p.973·3).
*Hypertension.*

**Nitrendepat** Azupharma, Ger.
Nitrendipine (p.973·3).
*Hypertension.*

**Nitrendicor** Labomed, Chile.
Nitrendipine (p.973·3).
*Hypertension.*

**Nitrendidoc** Docpharm, Ger.
Nitrendipine (p.973·3).
*Hypertension.*

**Nitrendil** Bago, Arg.
Nitrendipine (p.973·3).
*Hypertension.*

**Nitrendimerck** Merck dura, Ger.
Nitrendipine (p.973·3).
*Hypertension.*

**Nitrenpress** Sintofarma, Braz.†.
Nitrendipine (p.973·3).
*Hypertension.*

**Nitrensal** TAD, Ger.
Nitrendipine (p.973·3).
*Hypertension.*

**Nitrepress** Hexal, Ger.
Nitrendipine (p.973·3).
*Hypertension.*

**Nitre-Puren** Alpharma-Isis, Ger.
Nitrendipine (p.973·3).
*Hypertension.*

**Nitrex** Essex, Ital.
Isosorbide mononitrate (p.942·1).
*Angina pectoris.*

**Nitriate**
SERB, Fr.; IFET (ΙΦΕΤ), Gr.
Sodium nitroprusside (p.1000·2).
*Controlled hypotension; heart failure; hypertensive crisis.*

**Nitridazol** Ingens, Arg.
Itraconazole (p.401·3).
*Fungal infections.*

**Nitriderm TTS** Novartis, Fr.
Glyceryl trinitrate (p.923·2).
*Angina pectoris.*

**Nitrilan** Biomedica-Chemica, Gr.
Isosorbide mononitrate (p.942·1).
*Angina; heart failure.*

**Nitrileno** Libbs, Braz.
Nitrofurazone (p.238·2); naphazoline hydrochloride (p.1124·3).
*Nasal disorders.*

**Nitro**
Genericon, Austria; Orion, Fin.
Glyceryl trinitrate (p.923·2).
*Angina pectoris; controlled hypotension; heart failure; hypertension during cardiac surgery; myocardial infarction; prophylaxis of phlebitis and peripheral extravasation..*

**Nitro Mack**
Pfizer, Austria; Mack, Illert., Ger.; Galenica, Gr.; Mack, Hong Kong; Mack, Singapore; Mack, Switz.; Mack, Thai.
Glyceryl trinitrate (p.923·2).
*Angina pectoris; controlled hypotension; heart failure; myocardial infarction; pulmonary hypertension.*

**Nitro Pohl**
Sanova, Austria; Pohl, Hong Kong; Pohl, Neth.†.
Glyceryl trinitrate (p.923·2).
*Angina pectoris; heart failure; hypertension during coronary bypass; myocardial infarction pain.*

**Nitro Solvay** Solvay, Ger.
Glyceryl trinitrate (p.923·2).
*Angina pectoris; heart failure; myocardial infarction.*

**Nitro-Bid**
Aventis, Austral.†; Hoechst Marion Roussel, USA.
Glyceryl trinitrate (p.923·2).
*Angina pectoris; controlled hypotension; heart failure; perioperative hypertension.*

**Nitrobid** Zambon, Braz.†.
Nitrofurantoin (p.237·2).
*Urinary-tract infections.*

**Nitrocine**
Schwarz, Hong Kong; Schwarz, Irl.; Medis, Israel; Schwarz, Malaysia; Omnimed, S.Afr.; Schwarz, Singapore; Schwarz, Thai.; Schwarz, UK.
Glyceryl trinitrate (p.923·2).
*Angina pectoris; controlled hypotension; heart failure; hypertension during cardiac surgery; myocardial ischaemia during and after cardiovascular surgery; pulmonary oedema.*

**Nitrocit** Genpharm, S.Afr.†.
Potassium citrate (p.1223·1).
*Urinary alkalinisation.*

**Nitrocod** Adcock Ingram, S.Afr.
Paracetamol (p.76·2); codeine phosphate (p.27·1).
*Fever; pain.*

**Nitrocontin** Modi-Mundipharma, India.
Glyceryl trinitrate (p.923·2).
*Angina pectoris.*

**Nitrocor** 3M, Chile.
Glyceryl trinitrate (p.923·2).
*Angina pectoris.*

**Nitro-Crataegutt** Schwabe, Ger.
Pentaerithrityl tetranitrate (p.979·1); crataegus (p.1677·1).
*Heart failure.*

**Nitro-cum** Eu Rho, Ger.†.
Glyceryl trinitrate (p.923·2); crataegus (p.1677·1); valerian (p.1762·2).
*Angina pectoris; heart failure.*

**Nitroder** Keton, Mex.†.
Glyceryl trinitrate (p.923·2).

**Nitroderm**
Novartis, Austria; Novartis, Belg.; Novartis, Chile; Novartis, Malaysia; Novartis, NZ; Novartis, Spain; Novartis, Thai.
Glyceryl trinitrate (p.923·2).
*Angina pectoris; heart failure; prophylaxis of phlebitis and extravasation.*

**Nitro-Derm** Reuabuen, USA.
Glyceryl trinitrate (p.923·2).
*Angina pectoris.*

**Nitroderm TTS**
Novartis, Arg.; Novartis, Braz.; Novartis, Ger.; Novartis, Hong Kong; Novartis, India; Novartis, Israel; Novartis, Ital.; Novartis, Mex.; Novartis, Port.; Novartis, S.Afr.†; Novartis, Switz.
Glyceryl trinitrate (p.923·2).
*Angina pectoris; heart failure; prophylaxis of phlebitis and extravasation during cannulation.*

**Nitrodex**
Dexo, Fr.; Dexo, Switz.
Pentaerithrityl tetranitrate (p.979·1).
*Angina pectoris; heart failure.*

**Nitrodisc** Roberts, USA.
Glyceryl trinitrate (p.923·2).
*Angina pectoris.*

**Nitro-Dur**
Schering-Plough, Austral.; Ebewe, Austria; Key, Canad.; Schering-Plough, Hong Kong; Schering-Plough, Irl.; Sigma-Tau, Ital.; Schering-Plough, Mex.; Schering-Plough, Neth.; Schering-Plough, Norw.; Scher-

*ing-Plough, Port.; Schering-Plough, Spain; Essex, Switz.; Schering-Plough, UK; Key, USA.*
Glyceryl trinitrate (p.923·2).
*Angina pectoris.*

**Nitrodyl**
*Therabel, Belg.; Lavipharm, Gr.*
Glyceryl trinitrate (p.923·2).
*Angina pectoris; heart failure.*

**Nitroflu** *Beige, S.Afr.*
Aspirin (p.15·1); caffeine (p.782·1); ascorbic acid (p.1460·2); chlorphenamine maleate (p.427·3).
*Cold and influenza symptoms.*

**Nitrofur-C** *Leiras, Fin.*
Nitrofurantoin (p.237·2).
*Urinary-tract infections.*

**Nitrogard** *Forest Pharmaceuticals, USA.*
Glyceryl trinitrate (p.923·2).
*Angina pectoris.*

**Nitrogesic** *Troikaa, India.*
Glyceryl trinitrate (p.923·2).
*Anal fissures.*

**Nitroglyn**
*Kenwood, Hong Kong†; Kenwood, USA.*
Glyceryl trinitrate (p.923·2).
*Angina pectoris.*

**Nitrogray** *Gray, Arg.*
Glyceryl trinitrate (p.923·2).

**Nitroina** *Teofarma, Spain.*
Acetic acid (p.1645·2); greater celandine (p.1695·3); salicylic acid (p.1157·1); iodine tincture (p.1598·1); thuja occidentalis (p.1755·1).
*Warts.*

**Nitroject**
*Omega, Canad.; Sun, Thai.*
Glyceryl trinitrate (p.923·2).
*Angina pectoris; controlled hypotension; heart failure; hypertension; myocardial infarction.*

**Nitrokapseln-ratiopharm** *Ratiopharm, Ger.†.*
Glyceryl trinitrate (p.923·2).
*Angina pectoris.*

**Nitrokor** *Robugen, Ger.*
Glyceryl trinitrate (p.923·2).
*Angina pectoris; heart failure; myocardial infarction.*

**Nitrol**
*Note. This name is used for preparations of different composition.*
*Paladin, Canad.; Savage, USA†.*
Glyceryl trinitrate (p.923·2).
*Angina pectoris.*

*GlaxoSmithKline Sante, Fr.*
Celandine (p.1695·3); thuja (p.1755·1); iodine (p.1598·1); salicylic acid (p.1157·1); glacial acetic acid (p.1645·2).
*Warts.*

**Nitrolerg** *Sedabel, Braz.*
Hydrocortisone (p.1103·3); nitrofurazone (p.238·2).
*Infected skin disorders.*

**Nitrolingual**
*Aventis, Austral.; Sanova, Austria; Tramedico, Belg.; Aventis, Canad.; Pohl, Denm.†; Pohl, Ger.; Lavipharm, Gr.; Pohl, Hong Kong; Lipha, Irl.; Pohl, Israel; Pohl, Neth.; Pohl, Norw.; Douglas, NZ; Mer-National, S.Afr.; Meda, Swed.; Pohl, Switz.; Merck, UK; Rhone-Poulenc Rorer, USA; Horizon, USA.*
Glyceryl trinitrate (p.923·2).
*Angina pectoris; catheter-induced spasms during coronary angiography; heart failure; myocardial infarction; pulmonary oedema.*

**Nitromed** *Omedir, Arg.*
Nitrofurazone (p.238·2).
*Bacterial infections.*

**Nitromex**
*Alpharma, Denm.; Alpharma, Fin.; Alpharma, Norw.; Alpharma, Swed.*
Glyceryl trinitrate (p.923·2).
*Angina pectoris.*

**Nitromidager** *Streger, Mex.†.*
Metronidazole (p.607·2).
*Amoebiasis; giardiasis; trichomoniasis.*

**Nitromin**
*Servier, Irl.; Egis, UK.*
Glyceryl trinitrate (p.923·2).
*Angina pectoris.*

**Nitromint**
*Aventis, Port.; Rhone-Poulenc Rorer, Switz.†.*
Glyceryl trinitrate (p.923·2).
*Angina pectoris; atherosclerosis; coronary artery spasm.*

**Nitronal**
*Sanova, Austria†; Biobras, Braz.; Royal, Chile; Pohl, Ger.†; Pohl, Hong Kong†; Lipha, Irl.; Pohl, Israel; Douglas, NZ; Pohl, Switz.; Merck, UK.*
Glyceryl trinitrate (p.923·2).
*Angina pectoris; controlled hypotension; heart failure; hypertension and myocardial ischaemia during and after cardiac surgery.*

**Nitronasal** *Eversil, Braz.†.*
Naphazoline hydrochloride (p.1124·3); nitrofurazone (p.238·2); panthenol (p.1727·2).
*Nasal disorders.*

**Nitrong**
*Chemomedica, Austria†; Rhone-Poulenc Rorer, Belg.†; Aventis, Canad.; Ethicals, Denm.†; Lavipharm, Gr.; Orion, Swed.†; Rhone-Poulenc Rorer, USA.*
Glyceryl trinitrate (p.923·2).
*Angina pectoris; heart failure.*

**Nitro-Obsidan** *Alpharma-Isis, Ger.*
Pentaerithrityl tetranitrate (p.979·1); propranolol hydrochloride (p.989·3).
*Angina pectoris; hypertension.*

**Nitropacin** *Juste, Spain†.*
Glyceryl trinitrate (p.923·2).
*Angina pectoris; heart failure; myocardial infarction.*

**Nitro-Pflaster-ratiopharm TL** *Ratiopharm, Ger.*
Glyceryl trinitrate (p.923·2).
*Angina pectoris.*

**Nitroplast** *Lacer, Spain.*
Glyceryl trinitrate (p.923·2).
*Angina pectoris.*

**Nitro-Praecordin N** *Roland, Ger.†.*
Glyceryl trinitrate (p.923·2); benzyl nicotinate (p.21·2).
*Angina pectoris; coronary vascular disorders.*

**Nitropresabbott** *Abbott, Braz.*
Sodium nitroprusside (p.1000·2).
*Hypertension.*

**Nitropress** *Abbott, USA.*
Sodium nitroprusside (p.1000·2).
*Controlled hypotension; hypertensive crisis.*

**Nitro-pro** *Elan, USA.*
Lactose-free, gluten-free preparation for enteral nutrition (p.1417·1).
Formerly known as Nitrolan.

**Nitroprus**
*Scott-Cassara, Arg.; Cristalia, Braz.*
Sodium nitroprusside (p.1000·2).

**Nitroprussiat** *Fides Ecopharma, Spain.*
Sodium nitroprusside (p.1000·2).
*Controlled hypotension; heart failure; hypertension; myocardial infarction; phaeochromocytoma.*

**Nitropulse** *KV, Hong Kong†.*
Glyceryl trinitrate (p.923·2).
*Angina pectoris.*

**NitroQuick** *Ethex, USA.*
Glyceryl trinitrate (p.923·2).
*Angina pectoris.*

**Nitroretard-Faran** *Faran, Gr.*
Glyceryl trinitrate (p.923·2).
*Angina; heart failure.*

**Nitrosid** *Pharmacal, Fin.*
Isosorbide dinitrate (p.941·1).
*Angina pectoris; heart failure; myocardial infarction.*

**Nitrosorbide**
*Lusofarmaco, Ital.; Menarini, Singapore†.*
Isosorbide dinitrate (p.941·1).
*Angina pectoris; cardiac disorders; ischaemic heart disease.*

**Nitrosorbon** *Pohl, Ger.*
Isosorbide dinitrate (p.941·1).
*Heart failure; ischaemic heart disease; myocardial infarction; pulmonary hypertension.*

**Nitrostat**
*Pfizer, Canad.; Parke, Davis, Hong Kong†; Parke, Davis, Neth.; Parke, Davis, USA.*
Glyceryl trinitrate (p.923·2).
*Angina pectoris.*

**Nitrosylon** *Abbott, Ital.*
Glyceryl trinitrate (p.923·2).
*Angina pectoris.*

**NitroTab** *Able, USA.*
Glyceryl trinitrate (p.923·2).
*Angina pectoris.*

**Nitro-Tablinen** *Sanorania, Ger.†.*
Isosorbide dinitrate (p.941·1).
*Cardiac disorders.*

**Nitrotard** *Berenguer Infale, Spain†.*
Glyceryl trinitrate (p.923·2).
*Angina pectoris; heart failure; myocardial infarction.*

**Nitro-Time** *Time-Cap, USA.*
Glyceryl trinitrate (p.923·2).
*Angina pectoris.*

**Nitrourean** *Prasfarma, Spain†.*
Carmustine (p.535·1).
*Malignant neoplasms.*

**Nitroven** *Pohl, Norw.*
Glyceryl trinitrate (p.923·2).
*Angina pectoris; blood pressure control during cardiac surgery; heart failure.*

**Nitrovis** *CTI, Israel†.*
Glyceryl trinitrate (p.923·2).
*Angina pectoris; cardiac stenosis; myocardial infarction.*

**Nitrumon**
*Almirall, Belg.; IFET (ΙΦΕΤ), Gr.*
Carmustine (p.535·1).
*Malignant neoplasms.*

**Nitux** *Inpharzam, Switz.*
Morclofone (p.1124·3).
*Coughs.*

**Nivabetol** *Alpharma, Fr.*
Betaine (p.1660·1); acetylmethionine; sorbitol (p.1446·3).
*Constipation; dyspepsia.*

**Nivadil**
*Dolorgiet, Ger.; Klinge, Irl.; Fujisawa, Jpn; Menarini, Port.; Klinge, Switz.*
Nilvadipine (p.972·2).
*Hypertension.*

**Nivador** *Menarini, Spain.*
Cefuroxime axetil (p.184·1).
*Bacterial infections.*

**Nivagin** *TP, Thai.*
Dipyrone (p.35·3).
Lidocaine hydrochloride (p.1377·3) is included in the injection to alleviate the pain of injection.
*Fever; pain.*

**Nivalin** *Sanochemia, Austria†.*
Galantamine hydrobromide (p.1491·2).
*Alzheimer's disease; cerebrovascular disorders; glaucoma; myasthenia gravis; myelitis; neuritis; poliomyelitis; reversal of competitive neuromuscular blockade; smooth muscle atony.*

**Nivaquine**
*Aventis, Arg.; Aventis, Belg.; Aventis, Fr.; Aventis, Neth.; Aventis, NZ; Aventis, S.Afr.; Aventis, Switz.; Beacon, UK.*
Chloroquine sulfate (p.448·2).
*Giardiasis; hepatic amoebiasis; light-sensitive skin conditions; lupus erythematosus; malaria; rheumatoid arthritis.*

**Nivaquine-P** *Nicholas Piramal, India.*
Chloroquine phosphate (p.448·2).
*Amoebiasis; lupus erythematosus; malaria; rheumatoid arthritis.*

**Nivas**
*Note. This name is used for preparations of different composition.*
*Raffo, Arg.*
Nimodipine (p.972·3).
*Cerebrovascular disorders; neurological deficit following subarachnoid haemorrhage.*

*Tecnofarma, Chile.*
Nisoldipine (p.973·2).
*Angina pectoris; hypertension.*

**Nivas Plus** *Raffo, Arg.*
Nimodipine (p.972·3); citicoline (p.1672·3).
*Cerebrovascular disorders.*

**Nivea** *Beiersdorf, USA.*
A range of emollient, cleansing, and moisturising preparations.

**Nivea Sun** *Beiersdorf, USA.*
*SPF 15:* Octinoxate (p.1154·3); octisalate (p.1154·3); oxybenzone (p.1154·3); ensulizole (p.1147·1).
*Sunscreen.*

**Nivea Visage** *Beiersdorf, Canad.*
*SPF 4:* Octinoxate (p.1154·3); oxybenzone (p.1154·3).
*SPF 15:* Octinoxate (p.1154·3); oxybenzone (p.1154·3); ensulizole (p.1147·1).
*Sunscreen.*

**Nivelan** *Lacefa, Arg.*
Sulpiride (p.722·2).
*Sedative.*

**Nivelipol** *Temis, Arg.*
Simvastatin (p.997·1).
*Hypercholesterolaemia.*

**Nivelon** *Essex, Chile.*
Diphemanil metilsulfate (p.481·3).
*Peptic ulcer.*

**Nivemycin**
*IFET (ΙΦΕΤ), Gr.; Sovereign, UK.*
Neomycin sulfate (p.235·1).
*Bacterial infections; bowel preparation; hepatic coma.*

**Niven** *Pulitzer, Ital.*
Nicardipine hydrochloride (p.965·1).
*Angina pectoris; heart failure; hypertension.*

**Niver** *Medeva, Fr.†.*
Codeine phosphate (p.27·1); grindelia (p.1696·1); thyme (p.1755·2); mallow (p.1709·3).
*Coughs.*

**Nivoflox**
*Andromaco, Mex.; Euro-Labor, Port.; Grunenthal, Port.*
Ciprofloxacin hydrochloride (p.188·2).
*Bacterial infections.*

**Nix**
*Warner-Lambert, Austral.†; Pfizer Consumer, Belg.; Pfizer Consumer, Canad.; GlaxoSmithKline, Canad.; Pfizer, Denm.; Pfizer, Fin.; Pfizer Sante, Fr.; Pfizer, Gr.; Warner-Lambert, Ital.; Pfizer, Norw.; Pfizer Consumer, Port.; GlaxoSmithKline, Swed.; Warner-Lambert, Swed.; Warner-Lambert, USA.*
Permethrin (p.1508·3).
*Pediculosis; scabies.*

**Nixal** *Columbia, Mex.*
Naproxen sodium (p.65·1).
*Fever; inflammation; pain.*

**Nixin**
*Mepha, Braz.; Mepha, Port.*
Ciprofloxacin hydrochloride (p.188·2).
*Bacterial infections.*

**Nixoderm**
*Note. This name is used for preparations of different composition.*
*Galenogal, Braz.†.*
Benzoyl peroxide (p.1143·2); triclosan (p.1195·2); allantoin (p.1141·3).
*Acne.*

*Asia Pharma, Malaysia.*
Benzoic acid (p.1169·3); salicylic acid (p.1157·1); sulfur (p.1158·2).
*Skin disorders.*

**Nixyn** *Teofarma, Spain.*
*Capsules; suppositories:* Isonixin (p.51·1).
*Gout; musculoskeletal, joint, and peri-articular disorders; pain.*
*Cream:* Isonixin (p.51·1); methyl salicylate (p.59·3).
*Peri-articular and soft-tissue disorders.*

**Niyaplat** *Precimex, Mex.†.*
Cisplatin (p.538·1).

**Nizacol** *PS, Ital.*
Miconazole (p.405·2) or miconazole nitrate (p.405·3).
*Fungal infections; Gram-positive bacterial infections.*

**Nizale** *Janssen-Cilag, Port.*
Ketoconazole (p.403·3).
*Fungal infections.*

**Nizax**
*Whitehall, Braz.†; Lilly, Denm.; Lilly, Fin.; Lilly, Ger.; Lilly, Ital.; Lilly, Swed.*
Nizatidine (p.1277·2).
*Gastro-oesophageal reflux; peptic ulcer.*

**Nizaxid**
*Lafi, Chile; Norgine, Fr.; Lilly, Port.*
Nizatidine (p.1277·2).
*Gastro-oesophageal reflux; peptic ulcer.*

**Nizcreme** *Janssen-Cilag, S.Afr.*
Ketoconazole (p.403·3).
*Fungal skin infections.*

**Nizole** *Hovid, Singapore.*
Metronidazole (p.607·2).
*Anaerobic bacterial infections; protozoal infections.*

**Nizoral**
*Janssen-Cilag, Austral.; Janssen-Cilag, Austria; Janssen-Cilag, Belg.; Janssen-Cilag, Braz.; McNeil Consumer, Canad.; Janssen-Cilag, Denm.; Janssen-Cilag, Fin.; Orion, Fin.; Janssen-Cilag, Fr.; Janssen-Cilag, Ger.; Janssen, Hong Kong; Janssen-Cilag, Irl.; Janssen-Cilag, Israel; Janssen-Cilag, Ital.; Janssen-Cilag, Malaysia; Janssen, Mex.; Janssen-Cilag, Neth.; Janssen-Cilag, NZ; Janssen-Cilag, Port.; Janssen-Cilag, S.Afr.; Janssen-Cilag, Singapore; Janssen-Cilag, Switz.; Janssen-Cilag, Thai.; Janssen-Cilag, UK; Johnson & Johnson MSD Consumer, UK; Janssen, USA; McNeil Consumer, USA.*
Ketoconazole (p.403·3).
*Dandruff; fungal infections; seborrhoeic dermatitis.*

**Nizorelle** *Janssen-Cilag, S.Afr.*
Ketoconazole (p.403·3).
*Dandruff.*

**Nizoretic** *Kinder, Braz.*
Ketoconazole (p.403·3).
*Fungal infections.*

**Nizovules** *Janssen-Cilag, S.Afr.*
Ketoconazole (p.403·3).
*Vaginal candidiasis.*

**Nizshampoo** *Janssen-Cilag, S.Afr.*
Ketoconazole (p.403·3).
*Fungal scalp infections.*

**N-Labstix**
*Bayer Diagnostics, Irl.; Bayer Diagnostics, UK.*
Test for glucose, protein, pH, ketones, blood, and nitrites in urine.

**N-Multistix**
*Bayer, Austral.†; Ames, Israel; Bayer, USA.*
Test for glucose, protein, blood, ketones, bilirubin, urobilinogen, nitrites, and pH in urine.

**N-Multistix SG**
*Bayer, Austral.†; Bayer, Canad.†; Bayer Diagnostics, Irl.; Bayer Diagnostici, Ital.; Bayer Diagnostics, UK; Bayer, USA.*
Test for specific gravity, glucose, protein, blood, ketones, bilirubin, urobilinogen, nitrite, and pH in urine.

**No 440** *Herbes Universelles, Canad.*
Vitamins A, C, and D (p.1417·1).

**No Doz** *Key, Austral.†.*
Caffeine (p.782·1).
*Fatigue.*

**No Doz Plus** *Key, Austral.†.*
Caffeine (p.782·1); vitamin B substances (p.1417·1); glucose (p.1432·2).
*Fatigue.*

**No Drowsiness Sinarest** *Ciba, USA.*
Pseudoephedrine hydrochloride (p.1129·2); paracetamol (p.76·2).
*Upper respiratory-tract symptoms.*

**No Gas** *Key, Austral.†.*
Activated charcoal (p.1030·2); simeticone (p.1289·2).
*Diarrhoea; drug poisoning; excess gastrointestinal gas.*

**No Grip** *Vifor, Switz.†.*
Salicylamide (p.87·3); noscapine hydrochloride (p.1125·3); mepyramine maleate (p.437·1); ascorbic acid (p.1460·2); hesperidin methyl chalcone (p.1688·3).
*Cold symptoms.*

**No Grip C** *Vifor, Switz.*
Paracetamol (p.76·2); ascorbic acid (p.1460·2).
*Cold symptoms.*

**No Name Cough Lozenge** *Sutton, Canad.†.*
Menthol (p.1711·3).

**No Pain-HP** *Young Again Nutrients, USA.*
Capsaicin (p.24·2).
*Pain.*

**No-Acid** *Infabra, Braz.†.*
Aluminium hydroxide (p.1249·2).
*Gastrointestinal hyperacidity.*

**Noacid** *OBA, Denm.*
Dihydroxyaluminum sodium carbonate (p.1261·2).
*Gastritis; gastro-oesophageal reflux; peptic ulcer.*

**NO-AD Babies** *Solar, Canad.*
*SPF 30; SPF 45:* Octinoxate (p.1154·3); octisalate (p.1154·3); oxybenzone (p.1154·3) with or without zinc oxide (p.1163·2).
*Sunscreen.*

**NO-AD Easy Block** *Solar, Canad.*
*SPF 30:* Octinoxate (p.1154·3); octisalate (p.1154·3); oxybenzone (p.1154·3).
*Sunscreen.*

**NO-AD Kids** *Solar, Canad.*
*SPF 30:* Octinoxate (p.1154·3); octisalate (p.1154·3); oxybenzone (p.1154·3)with or without zinc oxide (p.1163·2).
*Sunscreen.*

**NO-AD Sport** *Solar, Canad.*
*SPF 15; SPF 30:* Octinoxate (p.1154·3); octisalate (p.1154·3); oxybenzone (p.1154·3).
*Sunscreen.*

**NO-AD Sunblock** *Solar, Canad.*
*SPF 15; SPF 30; SPF 45:* Octinoxate (p.1154·3); octisalate (p.1154·3); oxybenzone (p.1154·3).
*Sunscreen.*

**NO-AD Sunscreen** *Solar, Canad.*
*SPF 8:* Octinoxate (p.1154·3); oxybenzone (p.1154·3).
*Sunscreen.*

**Noalgil** *Pharmacia Upjohn, Spain†.*
Ibuprofen (p.45·3).
*Fever; inflammation; musculoskeletal, joint, and peri-articular disorders; pain.*

**Noalgos** *Levofarma, Ital.*
Nimesulide (p.67·1).
*Fever; inflammation; pain.*

**Noameba-DS** *Ipca, India.*
Secnidazole (p.615·3).
*Amoebiasis; giardiasis.*

**Noan**
*Farmasa, Braz.; Abbott, Ital.*
Diazepam (p.690·1).
*Alcohol withdrawal syndrome; anxiety; epilepsy; insomnia; premedication; sedative; skeletal muscle spasm.*

**Nobactam** *Microsules, Arg.*
Amoxicillin trihydrate (p.155·3).
*Bacterial infections.*

**Nobactam Bronquial** *Microsules, Arg.*
Amoxicillin trihydrate (p.155·3); ambroxol hydrochloride (p.1114·3).
*Respiratory-tract infections.*

**Nobacter** *Eucerin, Fr.*
Triclocarban (p.1195·1).
*Skin cleansing and disinfection.*

**Nobec** *MDI, S.Afr.*
Beclometasone dipropionate (p.1091·1).
*Allergic rhinitis.*

**Nobecutan** *Astra, Ger.†.*
Thiram (p.1755·1).
*Burns; wounds.*

**Nobecutane** *Astra, Belg.†.*
Thiram (p.1755·1).
*Antiseptic aerosol dressing.*

**Nobese** *Farmedica, Braz.†.*
Fenproporex hydrochloride (p.1588·3).
*Obesity.*

**Nobese No. 1** *Restan, S.Afr.*
Cathine hydrochloride (p.1585·2).
*Obesity.*

**No-Bite** *Brunel, S.Afr.*
Diethyltoluamide (p.1503·3); citronella oil (p.1673·2).
*Mosquito bites.*

**Nobiten** *Menarini, Belg.*
Nebivolol hydrochloride (p.964·3).
*Hypertension.*

**Nobligan**
*Grunenthal, Denm.; Janssen, Mex.; Grunenthal, Norw.; Pharmacia, Swed.*
Tramadol hydrochloride (p.94·3).
*Pain.*

**Nobliten** *Lacer, Spain†.*
A nonoxinol (p.1413·2).
*Contraceptive.*

**Nobritol** *Kern, Spain.*
Amitriptyline hydrochloride (p.280·3); medazepam (p.706·1).
*Depression.*

**Noc** *Recalcine, Chile.*
Apomorphine hydrochloride (p.1199·1).

**Noceptin** *Christiaens, Neth.*
Morphine sulfate (p.60·2).
*Pain.*

**Nocertone**
*Sanofi Synthelabo, Belg.; Sanofi Synthelabo, Fr.*
Oxetorone fumarate (p.470·2).
*Cluster headache; migraine.*

**Nociclin** *EMS, Braz.*
Levonorgestrel (p.1563·2); ethinylestradiol (p.1553·2).
*Combined oral contraceptive.*

**Nocid** *Farmaline, Thai.*
Omeprazole (p.1278·2).
*Gastro-oesophageal reflux; peptic ulcer; Zollinger-Ellison syndrome.*

**Nocpaz** *Instituto Sanitas, Chile.*
Doxylamine succinate (p.432·3).
*Insomnia.*

**Noctal**
*Note. This name is used for preparations of different composition.*
*UCB, Austria.*
Amantadine sulfate (p.1197·2).
*Influenza A; parkinsonism.*

*Abbott, Braz.*
Estazolam (p.697·3).
*Insomnia.*

**Noctamid**
*Schering, Austria; Schering, Belg.; Schering, Ger.; Asche, Ger.; Schering, Irl.; Schering, Neth.; Schering, NZ; Schering, Port.; Schering, S.Afr.; Schering, Spain; Schering, Switz.*
Lormetazepam (p.705·2).
*Premedication; sleep disorders.*

**Noctamide** *Schering, Fr.*
Lormetazepam (p.705·2).
*Insomnia.*

**Noctazepam** *Hexal, Ger.*
Oxazepam (p.712·2).
*Anxiety; sleep disorders.*

**Noctilan** *Boehringer Ingelheim, Chile.*
Brotizolam (p.672·1).
*Insomnia.*

**Noctiplon** *Medipharm, Chile.*
Zaleplon (p.727·3).
*Insomnia.*

**Noctirex** *Irex, Fr.†.*
Zopiclone (p.729·3).
*Insomnia.*

**Noctis** *Bouty, Ital.*
Valerian (p.1762·2); passion flower (p.1729·1); crataegus (p.1677·1).
*Sleep disorders.*

**Noctisan** *Dolisos, Fr.†.*
Crataegus (p.1677·1); tilia (p.1756·2); valerian (p.1762·2).
*Insomnia.*

**Noctium** *Ferrier, Fr.*
Homoeopathic preparation.

**Nocton** *Saval, Chile.*
Lormetazepam (p.705·2).
*Sleep disorders.*

**Noctor** *Montavit, Austria.*
Diphenhydramine hydrochloride (p.431·3).
*Hypersensitivity reactions; sedative.*

**Noctran** *Menarini, Fr.*
Dipotassium clorazepate (p.685·1); acepromazine (p.668·3); aceprometazine (p.668·3).
*Insomnia.*

**Noctura**
*Note. This name is used for preparations of different composition.*
*Recalcine, Chile.*
Midazolam (p.707·1).
*Hypnotic.*

*Nelson, UK.*
Homoeopathic preparation.

**Nocturne** *Wyeth, Austral.*
Temazepam (p.723·2).
*Insomnia.*

**Nocturno** *Unipharm, Israel.*
Zopiclone (p.729·3).
*Insomnia.*

**Noctyl** *Merck Medication Familiale, Fr.*
Doxylamine succinate (p.432·3).
*Insomnia.*

**Nocutil**
*Gebro, Austria; Hoyer, Ger.; Gebro, Switz.; Norgine, UK.*
Desmopressin acetate (p.1322·3).
*Diabetes insipidus; nocturnal enuresis.*

**Nocvalene** *Arkopharma, Fr.*
Crataegus (p.1677·1); red-poppy petal (p.1058·1); passion flower (p.1729·1).
*Insomnia.*

**Node DS** *Bioderma, Fr.*
Ichthammol (p.1148·2); cade oil (p.1159·2); salicylic acid (p.1157·1); climbazole (p.396·2); pyrithione zinc (p.1156·2); piroctone olamine (p.1155·2).
*Scalp disorders.*

**Node G** *Bioderma, Fr.*
Sage oil (p.1741·2).
*Scalp disorders.*

**Node P** *Bioderma, Fr.*
Cade oil (p.1159·2); salicylic acid (p.1157·1); climbazole (p.396·2); pyrithione zinc (p.1156·2); piroctone olamine (p.1155·2).
*Scalp disorders.*

**Node Tar** *Piam, Ital.†.*
Coal tar (p.1159·2); cade oil (p.1159·2); selenium sulfide (p.1157·3); salicylic acid (p.1157·1).
*Scalp disorders.*

**Nodepe**
*Euro-Labor, Port.; Grunenthal, Port.; Andromaco, Spain.*
Fluoxetine hydrochloride (p.292·1).
*Bulimia; depression; mixed anxiety depressive states; obsessive-compulsive disorder.*

**Nodex** *Brothier, Fr.*
Dextromethorphan hydrobromide (p.1117·3).
*Coughs.*

**Nodict** *Sun, India.*
Naltrexone hydrochloride (p.1046·1).
*Alcohol withdrawal syndrome; opioid withdrawal syndrome.*

**Nodipir** *Klonal, Arg.*
Paracetamol (p.76·2).
*Fever; pain.*

**Nodoff** *Potter's, UK.*
*Oral liquid:* Passion flower (p.1729·1); skullcap (p.1746·3); lupulus (p.1708·1); valerian (p.1762·2); Jamaica dogwood (p.1702·3).
*Tablets:* Passion flower (p.1729·1).
*Insomnia.*

**Nodolex** *Bago, Arg.*
Paracetamol (p.76·2).
*Fever; pain.*

**Nodolfen** *Lacer, Spain.*
Ibuprofen (p.45·3).
*Fever; pain.*

**Nodor** *Pharmus, Braz.†.*
Nimesulide (p.67·1).

**NoDoz** *Bristol-Myers Products, USA.*
Caffeine (p.782·1).
*Fatigue.*

**No-Drowsiness Allerest** *Ciba, USA.*
Pseudoephedrine hydrochloride (p.1129·2); paracetamol (p.76·2).
*Upper respiratory-tract symptoms.*

**Nodryl** *Teva, Israel.*
Diphenhydramine hydrochloride (p.431·3); naphazoline hydrochloride (p.1124·3); neomycin sulfate (p.235·1).
*Allergic rhinitis; nasal congestion.*

**Noducil** *Silesia, Chile.*
Sibutramine (p.1593·2).
*Obesity.*

**Noemin N** *Trommsdorff, Ger.†.*
Bismuth aluminate (p.1252·1).
*Gastrointestinal disorders.*

**Nofagus** *Biolab Sanus, Braz.†.*
Mazindol (p.1589·1); diazepam (p.690·1).
*Obesity.*

**Nofebrin** *Legrand, Braz.*
Dipyrone (p.35·3).
*Fever; pain.*

**Nofedol** *Aventis, Spain†.*
Paracetamol (p.76·2).
*Fever; pain.*

**Noflam** *Pacific, NZ†.*
Naproxen (p.65·1) or naproxen sodium (p.65·1).
*Gout; musculoskeletal, joint, and peri-articular disorders; pain.*

**Noflam-N**
*Pacific, Hong Kong; Merck, Singapore; Pacific, Singapore.*
Naproxen sodium (p.65·1).
*Gout; musculoskeletal and joint disorders; pain.*

**No-Flu** *Klinge, Switz.*
Paracetamol (p.76·2); dextromethorphan hydrobromide (p.1117·3); phenylephrine hydrochloride (p.1126·3).
*Cold symptoms.*

**Noflux** *YSP, Malaysia.*
Muramidase hydrochloride (p.1717·2).
*Haemorrhage; sinusitis.*

**No-Gas** *Giuliani, Ital.*
Dimeticone (p.1289·2); activated charcoal (p.1030·2).
*Aerophagia; meteorism.*

**Nogastra** *Silesia, Chile.*
*Oral suspension:* Simeticone (p.1289·2); aluminium hydroxide (p.1249·2); magnesium hydroxide (p.1272·2).
*Tablets:* Simeticone (p.1289·2); magnesium carbonate (p.1272·1); magnesium hydroxide (p.1272·2); aluminium hydroxide (p.1249·2).
*Antacid; flatulence.*

**No-Gravid** *Irmed, Ital.*
Copper (p.1425·3).
*Intra-uterine contraceptive device.*

**No-Hist** *Dunhall, USA†.*
Phenylephrine hydrochloride (p.1126·3); phenylpropanolamine hydrochloride (p.1127·3); pseudoephedrine hydrochloride (p.1129·2).
*Nasal congestion.*

**Noiafren** *Aventis, Spain.*
Clobazam (p.358·2).
*Alcohol withdrawal syndrome; anxiety; epilepsy.*

**Noivy** *Hilarys, Canad.†.*
Calamine (p.1144·1); camphor (p.1665·3); menthol (p.1711·3); benzocaine (p.1370·3).

**Nok** *CTS, Israel.*
Permethrin (p.1508·3).
*Pediculosis.*

**Nokatar** *Prater, Chile.*
Ginkgo biloba (p.1692·3).

**Nokid** *Benedetti, Ital.*
Cefonicid sodium (p.174·2).
Lidocaine hydrochloride (p.1377·3) is included in this preparation to alleviate the pain of injection.
*Gram-negative bacterial infections.*

**Noklot** *Zydus, India.*
Clopidogrel bisulfate (p.888·3).
*Atherosclerosis; myocardial infarction; peripheral arterial disease.*

**Noktone** *Gea, Norw.†.*
Ranitidine hydrochloride (p.1285·2).
*Aspiration syndrome; gastro-oesophageal reflux; peptic ulcer; Zollinger-Ellison syndrome.*

**Nolac** *Nestle, Ital.*
Infant feed (p.1417·1).
*Intolerance to cow's milk, soya, egg, and gluten.*

**Nolahist** *Carnrick, USA.*
Phenindamine tartrate (p.438·2).
*Allergic rhinitis.*

**Nolamine** *Carnrick, USA†.*
Phenindamine tartrate (p.438·2); chlorphenamine maleate (p.427·3); phenylpropanolamine hydrochloride (p.1127·3).
*Nasal congestion.*

**Nolarac** *Fada, Arg.*
Ketorolac (p.52·3).
*Inflammation; pain.*

**Nolder** *Pharmacia, Ital.*
Amino-acid, carbohydrate, and phospholipid preparation with vitamins and selenium (p.1417·1).
*Nutritional supplement.*

**Noleptan** *Promeco, Mex.*
Fominoben (p.1121·3) or fominoben hydrochloride (p.1121·3).
*Coughs.*

**Nolgen** *Antigen, Irl.*
Tamoxifen citrate (p.584·1).
*Breast cancer.*

**Nolil** *Offenbach, Mex.*
Clioquinol (p.196·3).
*Fungal skin infections.*

**Nolipax** *Salus, Ital.*
Fenofibrate (p.915·2).
*Diabetic retinopathy; hyperlipidaemias; xanthomatosis.*

**Nolipid** *Samil, Ital.†.*
Colextran hydrochloride (p.890·3).
*Hyperlipidaemia.*

**Nolol** *Docmed, S.Afr.†.*
Propranolol hydrochloride (p.989·3).
*Angina pectoris; anxiety; arrhythmias; hypertension; hyperthyroidism; phaeochromocytoma.*

**Nolotil**
*Boehringer Ingelheim, Port.; Boehringer Ingelheim, Spain.*
Metamizole magnesium (p.36·1).
*Fever; pain.*

**Nolotil Compositum** *Europharma, Spain.*
Metamizole magnesium (p.36·1); hyoscine butylbromide (p.483·3).
*Gastrointestinal spasm; pain.*

**Nolvadex**
*AstraZeneca, Arg.; AstraZeneca, Austral.; AstraZeneca, Austria; AstraZeneca, Belg.; AstraZeneca, Braz.; AstraZeneca, Canad.; AstraZeneca, Chile; AstraZeneca, Fin.; AstraZeneca, Fr.; AstraZeneca, Ger.; Astra-Zeneca, Gr.; AstraZeneca, Hong Kong; ICI, India; AstraZeneca, Irl.; AstraZeneca, Israel; AstraZeneca, Ital.; AstraZeneca, Malaysia; Zeneca, Mex.; AstraZeneca, Neth.; AstraZeneca, Norw.; AstraZeneca, NZ; AstraZeneca, Port.; Zeneca, S.Afr.; AstraZeneca, Singapore; AstraZeneca, Spain; AstraZeneca, Swed.; AstraZeneca, Switz.; AstraZeneca, Thai.; AstraZeneca, UK; AstraZeneca, USA.*
Tamoxifen citrate (p.584·1).
*Anovulatory infertility; breast cancer; endometrial cancer.*

**Nomafen** *Fidia, Ital.*
Tamoxifen citrate (p.584·1).
*Breast cancer.*

**Nomapam** *Amrad, Austral.†.*
Temazepam (p.723·2).
*Insomnia.*

**Nomigrain** *Torrent, India.*
Flunarizine hydrochloride (p.434·1).
*Migraine.*

**Nominfone** *Atlantic, Thai.†.*
Dipyrone (p.35·3).
*Fever; pain.*

**Nomon mono** *Hoyer, Ger.*
Cucurbita (p.1677·3).
*Urinary-tract disorders.*

**Nomopain** *Aventis, S.Afr.*
Paracetamol (p.76·2); caffeine (p.782·1); doxylamine succinate (p.432·3); codeine phosphate (p.27·1).
*Pain and associated tension.*

**Nomotec** *Tecnofarma, Mex.*
Ketotifen (p.788·2).
*Asthma; hypersensitivity.*

**Non Acid** *FIRMA, Ital.†.*
*Oral granules:* Sodium citrate (p.1223·2); potassium citrate (p.1223·1); tribasic sodium phosphate (p.1231·1); tartaric acid (p.1752·1); sodium bicarbonate (p.1223·2).
*Tablets:* Sodium citrate (p.1223·2); potassium citrate (p.1223·1); tribasic sodium phosphate (p.1231·1).
*Gastrointestinal disorders.*

**Nonak** *Pentamedical, Ital.*
Azeloyl glycinate; sulfosalicylic acid; piroctone olamine (p.1155·2).
*Skin disorders.*

**No-Name Dandruff Treatment** *Sutton, Canad.†.*
Pyrithione zinc (p.1156·2).

**Nonan**
*Baxter, Belg.†; Aguettant, Fr.*
Mineral preparation (p.1417·1).
*Parenteral nutrition.*

**Nonavit** *De Mayo, Braz.*
Multivitamin, amino-acid, and mineral preparation (p.1417·1).

**Non-Drowsy Sinutab** *Pfizer Consumer, UK.*
Paracetamol (p.76·2); pseudoephedrine hydrochloride (p.1129·2).
Formerly known as Sinutab and contained paracetamol and phenylpropanolamine hydrochloride.
*Nasal and sinus congestion.*

**Non-Drowsy Sudafed Congestion Cold & Flu** *Pfizer Consumer, UK.*
Pseudoephedrine hydrochloride (p.1129·2); paracetamol (p.76·2).
Formerly known as Sudafed Co.
*Cold and influenza symptoms.*

**Non-Drowsy Sudafed Congestion Relief** *Pfizer Consumer, UK.*
Phenylephrine hydrochloride (p.1126·3).
*Nasal congestion.*

**Non-Drowsy Sudafed Decongestant** *Pfizer Consumer, UK.*
Pseudoephedrine hydrochloride (p.1129·2).
Formerly known as Sudafed.
*Cold and influenza symptoms; hay fever.*

**Non-Drowsy Sudafed Decongestant Nasal Spray** *Pfizer Consumer, UK.*
Xylometazoline hydrochloride (p.1132·2).
Formerly known as Sudafed Nasal Spray and contained oxymetazoline hydrochloride.
*Nasal congestion.*

**Non-Drowsy Sudafed Dual Relief** *Pfizer Consumer, UK.*
Paracetamol (p.76·2); phenylephrine hydrochloride (p.1126·3); caffeine (p.782·1).
Formerly known as Sudafed Dual Relief.
*Cold and influenza symptoms.*

**Non-Drowsy Sudafed Dual Relief Max** *Pfizer Consumer, UK.*
Ibuprofen (p.45·3); pseudoephedrine hydrochloride (p.1129·2).
*Nasal and sinus congestion.*

**Non-Drowsy Sudafed Expectorant** *Pfizer Consumer, UK.*
Pseudoephedrine hydrochloride (p.1129·2); guaifenesin (p.1122·1).
Formerly known as Sudafed Expectorant.
*Coughs; upper respiratory-tract congestion.*

**Non-Drowsy Sudafed Linctus** *Pfizer Consumer, UK.*
Pseudoephedrine hydrochloride (p.1129·2); dextromethorphan hydrobromide (p.1117·3).
Formerly known as Sudafed Linctus.
*Coughs; upper respiratory-tract congestion.*

**No-Nerviol** *Higate, Arg.*
Chamomile (p.1669·3); tilia (p.1756·2); passion flower (p.1729·1).
*Sedative.*

**Non-Ovlon** *Jenapharm, Ger.*
Ethinylestradiol (p.1553·2); norethisterone acetate (p.1562·2).
*Combined oral contraceptive; menstrual disorders.*

**Noocetam** *Pharmasant, Thai.*
Piracetam (p.1732·1).
*Cerebral trauma; cerebrovascular disorders; chronic alcoholism; mental function impairment.*

**Noodipina** *Apsen, Braz.*
Nimodipine (p.972·3).
*Neurological deficit following subarachnoid haemorrhage.*

**Noodis** *UCB, Belg.*
Piracetam (p.1732·1).
*Childhood learning difficulties.*

**Noostan**
*Rontag, Arg.; UCB, Port.*
Piracetam (p.1732·1).
*Alcohol withdrawal syndrome; cerebrovascular disorders; dyslexia in children; mental function disorders; vertigo.*

**Nootrofic** *Cristalia, Braz.*
Piracetam (p.1732·1).

**Nootron** *Biosintetica, Braz.*
Piracetam (p.1732·1).
*Alcoholism; behaviour disorders in children; cerebrovascular disorders; senile dementia; vertigo.*

**Nootrop** *UCB, Ger.*
Piracetam (p.1732·1).
*Mental function disorders.*

**Nootropil**
*UCB, Austria; UCB, Belg.; Aventis, Braz.†; UCB, Fin.; UCB, Hong Kong; UCB, Ital.; UCB, Malaysia; UCB, Mex.; UCB, Neth.; UCB, Norw.; Vedim, Port.; UCB, S.Afr.; UCB, Singapore; UCB, Spain; UCB, Swed.; UCB, Switz.; UCB, Thai.; UCB, UK.*
Piracetam (p.1732·1).
*Cerebrovascular disorders; chronic alcoholism; dyslexia; mental function impairment; myoclonus.*

**Nootropyl**
*Aventis Pasteur, Chile; UCB, Fr.*
Piracetam (p.1732·1).
*Alcoholism; cerebrovascular disorders; dyslexia in children; mental function impairment in the elderly; myoclonus; stroke; vertigo.*

**Nopain** *Krewel, Ger.*
Dipyrone (p.35·3).
*Fever; pain.*

**Nopan** *CTI, Israel.*
Buprenorphine (p.21·3) or buprenorphine hydrochloride (p.21·3).
*Pain.*

**Nopar**
*Note. This name is used for preparations of different composition.*
*Unipharma, Gr.*
Homatropine (p.483·2).
*Gastrointestinal disorders characterised by smooth muscle spasm.*

*Lilly, Ital.*
Pergolide mesilate (p.1211·2).
*Parkinsonism.*

**Nopil** *Mepha, Switz.*
Co-trimoxazole (p.199·3).
*Bacterial infections; Pneumocystis carinii pneumonia.*

**Noplak** *Daudt, Braz.*
Chlorhexidine gluconate (p.1173·2).
*Oral hygeine.*

**Nopres** *Dexa, Hong Kong.*
Fluoxetine hydrochloride (p.292·1).
*Bulimia; depression; obsessive-compulsive disorder.*

**Nopriken** *Kendrick, Mex.*
Pefloxacin mesilate (p.241·3).
*Bacterial infections.*

**Nopron**
*Genopharm, Fr.†; Sanofi Synthelabo, Ital.*
Niaprazine (p.438·1).
*Insomnia.*

**Noprop** *Farmasa, Braz.*
Pantoprazole (p.1283·1).
*Gastro-oesophageal reflux; gastrointestinal hyperacidity; peptic ulcer.*

**Nopucid** *Interbelle, Arg.*
Permethrin (p.1508·3).
*Pediculosis.*

**Nopucid Composto** *Aventis, Braz.†.*
Deltamethrin (p.1503·1); piperonyl butoxide (p.1509·2).
*Pediculosis; scabies.*

**Nopucid Compuesto** *Interbelle, Arg.*
Deltamethrin (p.1503·1); piperonyl butoxide (p.1509·2).
*Pediculosis.*

**Nopucid MC** *Interbelle, Arg.*
Phenothrin (p.1509·1).
*Pediculosis.*

**Nopyn** *Rolab, S.Afr.*
Paracetamol (p.76·2); codeine phosphate (p.27·1); caffeine (p.782·1); meprobamate (p.706·2).
*Pain associated with tension.*

**Noquerat** *ICN, Arg.*
Calcium dimethylfumarate; calcium ethylfumarate; magnesium ethylfumarate; zinc ethylfumarate.
*Psoriasis.*

**Nor 2** *Raffo, Arg.*
Norfloxacin (p.238·3); phenazopyridine (p.83·2).
*Urinary-tract infections.*

**Nora** *Nakorn, Thai.*
Ketoconazole (p.403·3).
*Fungal infections; seborrhoeic dermatitis.*

**Norabromol N** *Michallik, Ger.*
Sodium 3,5-dibromo-4-hydroxybenzenesulphonate.
*Wounds.*

**Norace** *Hormona, Mex.*
14 Tablets, mestranol (p.1559·2); 7 tablets, mestranol; norethisterone (p.1562·2).
*Menopausal disorders; menstrual disorders; sequential oral contraceptive.*

**Noracin**
*Cibran, Braz.†; Chew, Thai.*
Norfloxacin (p.238·3).
*Bacterial infections.*

**Noradran** *Norma, UK.*
Diphenhydramine hydrochloride (p.431·3); diprophylline (p.784·3); ephedrine hydrochloride (p.1120·1); guaifenesin (p.1122·1).
*Coughs.*

**Norakin N** *Hexal, Ger.*
Biperiden hydrochloride (p.479·3).
*Blepharospasm; drug-induced extrapyramidal disorders; dystonias; parkinsonism; torticollis.*

**Noralget** *Quatromed, S.Afr.*
Paracetamol (p.76·2); codeine phosphate (p.27·1); caffeine (p.782·1); meprobamate (p.706·2).
*Pain and associated tension.*

**Noralone** *Taro, Israel†.*
Nandrolone phenylpropionate (p.1561·3).
*Anabolic breast cancer; osteoporosis.*

**Nor-Anaesthol** *Merz, Ger.†.*
Lidocaine hydrochloride (p.1377·3).
Noradrenaline (p.974·3) is included in this preparation as a vasoconstrictor to diminish absorption and localise the effect of the local anaesthetic.
*Local anaesthesia.*

**Noranat** *Labinca, Arg.*
Indapamide (p.938·2).
*Hypertension.*

**Nora-ratiopharm** *Ratiopharm, Ger.*
Ethinylestradiol (p.1553·2); norethisterone (p.1562·2).
*Combined oral contraceptive.*

**Noravid** *Aventis, Ital.*
Defibrotide (p.892·1).
*Thromboembolic disorders.*

**Noraxin** *TP, Thai.†.*
Norfloxacin (p.238·3).
*Bacterial infections.*

**Norbactin**
*Solus, India; Ranbaxy, Malaysia; Ranbaxy, Singapore; Ranbaxy, Thai.*
Norfloxacin (p.238·3).
*Bacterial infections.*

**Norbal** *Relyo, Gr.*
Buspirone hydrochloride (p.672·2).
*Generalised anxiety.*

**Norbiline**
*Aventis, Fr.†; Aventis, Ital.†.*
Prozapine hydrochloride (p.1736·1); sorbitol (p.1446·3).
*Biliary-tract disorders; gastrointestinal disorders.*

**Norboral** *Silanes, Mex.*
Glibenclamide (p.331·2).
*Diabetes mellitus.*

**Norcalcin** *Biomedica-Chemica, Gr.*
Calcitonin (p.768·2).
*Osteoporosis.*

**Norciden** *Kendrick, Mex.†.*
Danazol (p.1545·2).
*Breast cancer; endometriosis; hereditary angioedema; hypogonadism; hypopituitarism; mastalgia; osteoporosis; precocious puberty; suppression of lactation.*

**Norcin** *The Forty-Two, Thai.; Utopian, Thai.*
Norfloxacin (p.238·3).
*Bacterial infections.*

**Norco** *Watson, USA.*
Hydrocodone tartrate (p.45·1); paracetamol (p.76·2).
*Pain.*

**Norcolut**
*Gedeon Richter, Hong Kong; Gedeon Richter, Malaysia; Gedeon Richter, Singapore.*
Norethisterone (p.1562·2).
*Dysfunctional uterine bleeding; endometriosis; female infertility; lactation inhibition; menopausal disorders; menstrual disorders.*

**Norcuron**
*Organon, Arg.; Organon, Austral.; Organon, Austria; Organon, Belg.; Organon, Braz.; Organon, Canad.; Organon, Chile; Organon Teknika, Denm.†; Organon, Fin.; Organon, Fr.; Organon, Ger.; Organon (Οργανον), Gr.; Organon Teknika, Hong Kong; Infar, India; Organon Teknika, Irl.; Organon Teknika, Israel; Organon, Ital.; Organon, Malaysia; Organon Teknika, Mex.†; Organon Teknika, Neth.; Organon, Norw.; Organon, NZ; Organon, Port.; Sanofi Synthelabo, S.Afr.; Organon, Singapore; Organon, Spain; Organon, Swed.; Organon, Switz.; Organon, Thai.; Organon, UK; Organon, USA.*
Vecuronium bromide (p.1409·3).
*Competitive neuromuscular blocker.*

**Nordapanin N** *Michallik, Ger.*
Benzocaine (p.1370·3); acriflavinium chloride (p.1165·3).
*Mouth and throat disorders.*

**Nordathricin N** *Michallik, Ger.*
Tyrothricin (p.275·1); cetylpyridinium chloride (p.1173·1); benzocaine (p.1370·3).
*Mouth and throat disorders.*

**Nordaz**
*Bouchara-Recordati, Fr.; Bouchara, Singapore.*
Nordazepam (p.710·3).
*Alcohol withdrawal syndrome; anxiety.*

**Norden** *Akzo, Braz.†.*
Multivitamins (p.1417·1); iron (p.1434·3).
*Iron deficiency; iron-deficiency anaemias.*

**Nordet** *Wyeth, Mex.*
Levonorgestrel (p.1563·2); ethinylestradiol (p.1553·2).
*Combined oral contraceptive.*

**Nordette**
*Wyeth, Arg.; Wyeth, Austral.; Wyeth, Braz.; Wyeth, Chile; Wyeth, Gr.; Wyeth, Hong Kong; Wyeth-Ayerst, Israel; Wyeth, Malaysia; Wyeth, NZ; Akromed, S.Afr.; Wyeth, Singapore; Wyeth-Ayerst, Thai.; Wyeth-Ayerst, USA.*
Levonorgestrel (p.1563·2); ethinylestradiol (p.1553·2).
28-Day packs also contain 7 inert tablets.
*Combined oral contraceptive.*

**Nordiate** *Hemasure, Denm.†.*
A factor VIII preparation (p.751·1).
*Haemorrhagic disorders.*

**Nordicort** *Ascot, Austral.†.*
Hydrocortisone sodium succinate (p.1104·1).
*Corticosteroid.*

**Nordimmun**
*Hemasure, Denm.†; Hemasure, Swed.†.*
A normal immunoglobulin (p.1627·2).
*Hypogammaglobulinaemia; idiopathic thrombocytopenic purpura.*

**Nordiol**
*Wyeth, Arg.; Wyeth, Austral.; Wyeth, Chile; Wyeth-Ayerst, Hong Kong†; Wyeth, Mex.; Wyeth, NZ; Akromed, S.Afr.; Wyeth-Ayerst, Thai.†.*
Levonorgestrel (p.1563·2); ethinylestradiol (p.1553·2).
28-Day packs also contain 7 inert tablets.
*Combined oral contraceptive; menstrual disorders.*

**Nordiol-21** *Wyeth, Gr.*
Ethinylestradiol (p.1553·2); levonorgestrel (p.1563·2).
*Combined oral contraceptive.*

**Norditropin**
*Novo Nordisk, Arg.; Novo Nordisk, Austral.; Novo Nordisk, Austria; Novo Nordisk, Belg.; Novo Nordisk, Braz.†; Pentafarma, Chile; Novo Nordisk, Denm.; Novo Nordisk, Fin.; Novo Nordisk, Ger.; Novo Nordisk, Gr.; Novo Nordisk, Hong Kong; Novo Nordisk, Irl.; Novo Nordisk, Israel; Novo Nordisk, Ital.; Novo Nordisk, Jpn; Novo Nordisk, Malaysia; Pisa, Mex.; Novo Nordisk, Neth.; Novo Nordisk, Norw.; Novo Nordisk, NZ; Novo Nordisk, Port.; Novo Nordisk, S.Afr.; Novo Nordisk, Singapore; Novo Nordisk, Spain; Novo Nordisk, Swed.; Novo Nordisk, UK; Novo Nordisk, USA.*
Somatropin (p.1327·2).
*Growth disorders in renal failure; growth hormone deficiency; Turner's syndrome.*

**Norditropine**
*Novo Nordisk, Fr.; Novo Nordisk, Switz.*
Somatropin (p.1327·2).
*Growth disorders in renal failure; growth hormone deficiency; Turner's syndrome.*

**Nordolce** *Vegetal, Ital.*
Acero canadese.
*Nutritional supplement.*

**Nordonil** *Medinfar, Port.*
Domperidone (p.1263·2).
*Dyspepsia; nausea; vomiting.*

**Nordotol** *Orion, Denm.*
Carbamazepine (p.353·3).
*Alcohol withdrawal syndrome; benzodiazepine withdrawal syndrome; diabetes insipidus; epilepsy; neuralgias.*

**Nordox** *Tecnofarma, Chile.*
Phenazopyridine hydrochloride (p.83·1).
*Urinary-tract pain and irritation.*

**Nordyl** *Rosemont, Thai.*
Promethazine hydrochloride (p.439·1); codeine phosphate (p.27·1).
*Coughs.*

**Norebox** *Pharmacia, Spain.*
Reboxetine mesilate (p.316·3).
*Depression.*

**Norecil** *Maver, Mex.*
Metronidazole (p.607·2); diiodohydroxyquinoline (p.603·3).
*Amoebiasis.*

**No-Ref** *Instituto Sanitas, Chile.*
Simeticone (p.1289·2); metoclopramide (p.1274·3); chlordiazepoxide (p.674·2).
*Gastrointestinal disorders.*

**Norel** *US Pharmaceutical, USA†.*
Phenylephrine hydrochloride (p.1126·3); phenylpropanolamine hydrochloride (p.1127·3); guaifenesin (p.1122·1).
*Upper respiratory-tract symptoms.*

**Norel DM** *US Pharmaceutical, USA.*
Chlorphenamine maleate (p.427·3); phenylephrine hydrochloride (p.1126·3); hyoscine methonitrate (p.483·3).
*Upper respiratory-tract disorders.*

**Norel Plus** *US Pharmaceutical, USA†.*
Phenylpropanolamine hydrochloride (p.1127·3); paracetamol (p.76·2); chlorphenamine maleate (p.427·3); phenyltoloxamine citrate (p.439·1).
*Upper respiratory-tract symptoms.*

**Norel SD** *US Pharmaceutical, USA.*
Dextromethorphan hydrobromide (p.1117·3); chlorphenamine maleate (p.427·3); phenylephrine hydrochloride (p.1126·3).
Formerly known as Norel DM.

**Norelbin** *Eurofarma, Braz.*
Vinorelbine tartrate (p.594·1).
*Malignant neoplasms.*

**Norepine** *Sterop, Belg.*
Noradrenaline (p.974·3).

**Noreskin** *Genepharm, Gr.*
Azelaic acid (p.1142·3).
*Acne.*

**Norestin** *Biolab Sanus, Braz.*
Norethisterone (p.1562·2).
*Progestogen-only oral contraceptive.*

**Norethin 1/35E** *Schiapparelli Searle, USA†.*
Norethisterone (p.1562·2); ethinylestradiol (p.1553·2).
28-Day packs also contain 7 inert tablets.
*Combined oral contraceptive.*

**Norethin 1/50M** *Schiapparelli Searle, USA†.*
Norethisterone (p.1562·2); mestranol (p.1559·2).
28-Day packs also contain 7 inert tablets.
*Combined oral contraceptive.*

**Norfcin** *SM, Thai.*
Norfloxacin (p.238·3).
*Bacterial infections.*

**Norfemac** *Hoechst Marion Roussel, Canad.†.*
Bufexamac (p.21·3).
*Anorectal disorders; inflammatory skin disorders; phlebitis; vulval disorders.*

**Norfenazin** *Reig Jofre, Spain.*
Nortriptyline hydrochloride (p.310·2).
Formerly contained nortriptyline hydrochloride and perphenazine.
*Depression.*

**Norfenon** *Knoll, Mex.*
Propafenone hydrochloride (p.988·3).
*Arrhythmias.*

**Norfisar** *Typen, Arg.*
Chondroitin sulfate A.

**Norflam T** *3M, S.Afr.*
Ibuprofen (p.45·3).
*Fever; pain.*

**Norflamin** *Royton, Braz.*
Norfloxacin (p.238·3).
*Bacterial infections.*

**Norflex**
*3M, Austral.; 3M, Belg.†; 3M, Canad.; 3M, Denm.; 3M, Fin.; 3M, Ger.; Cana, Gr.; 3M, Malaysia; 3M, Mex.; 3M, NZ; 3M, Port.; 3M, S.Afr.; 3M, Singapore†; 3M, Swed.; 3M, Switz.†; 3M, Thai.; 3M, USA.*
Orphenadrine citrate (p.486·1).
*Drug-induced extrapyramidal disorders; hiccups; parkinsonism; skeletal muscle spasm; tension headache.*

**Norflex Co** *3M, S.Afr.*
Orphenadrine citrate (p.486·1); paracetamol (p.76·2).
*Fever; pain; skeletal muscle spasm.*

**Norflex Plus** *3M, Mex.*
Orphenadrine citrate (p.486·1); paracetamol (p.76·2).
*Skeletal muscle spasm.*

**Norflo** *Medifive, Thai.*
Norfloxacin (p.238·3).
*Bacterial infections.*

**Norflocin** *Polipharm, Thai.*
Norfloxacin (p.238·3).
*Bacterial infections.*

**Norflocine** *Mepha, Switz.*
Norfloxacin (p.238·3).
*Bacterial infections.*

**Norflohexal**
*Hexal, Austral.; Hexal, Ger.*
Norfloxacin (p.238·3).
*Bacterial infections.*

**Norflok** *Inkeysa, Spain.*
Norfloxacin (p.238·3).
*Bacterial infections.*

**Norflol** *Oriental, Arg.*
Norfloxacin (p.238·3).
*Bacterial infections.*

**Norflosal** TAD, Ger.
Norfloxacin (p.238·3).
*Urinary-tract infections.*

**Norflox**
1A, Ger.; CT, Ger.; Cipla, India.
Norfloxacin (p.238·3).
*Bacterial infections.*

Infosint, Ital.
Norfloxacin pivoxil (p.239·1).
*Urinary-tract infections.*

**Norfloxasan** Sanval, Braz.
Norfloxacin (p.238·3).
*Bacterial infections.*

**Norflox-Azu** Azupharma, Ger.
Norfloxacin (p.238·3).
*Bacterial infections of the urinary tract.*

**Norfloxbeta** Betapharm, Ger.
Norfloxacin (p.238·3).
*Bacterial infections.*

**Norfloxin** TO-Chemicals, Thai.
Norfloxacin (p.238·3).
*Bacterial infections.*

**Norfloxinor** Upha, Malaysia.
Norfloxacin (p.238·3).
*Bacterial infections.*

**Norflox-Puren** Alpharma-Isis, Ger.
Norfloxacin (p.238·3).
*Bacterial infections.*

**Norforms** Fleet, USA.
*Pessaries:* Vaginal deodorant.
*Topical powder:* Corn starch (p.1449·1); zinc oxide (p.1163·2).
*Vaginal irritation.*

**Norgagil** Norgine, Fr.†.
Sterculia (p.1290·2); attapulgite (p.1251·1); meprobamate (p.706·2).
*Gastrointestinal disorders.*

**Norgalax**
Norgine, Belg.; Norgine, Fr.; Norgine, Ger.†; Norgine, Hong Kong; Norgine, Irl.; Norgine, Neth.; Norgine, Singapore; Norgine, Switz.; Norgine, UK.
Docusate sodium (p.1262·2).
*Bowel evacuation; constipation.*

**Norgalax Miniklistier** Norgine, Ger.
Docusate sodium (p.1262·2); glycerol (p.1694·3).
*Bowel evacuation; constipation.*

**Norgeal** Wyeth, Arg.
Levonorgestrel (p.1563·2).
*Progestogen-only oral contraceptive.*

**Norgesic**
Note. This name is used for preparations of different composition.
3M, Austral.; Sanova, Austria; 3M, Chile; 3M, Fin.; 3M, Hong Kong; 3M, Irl.; 3M, Israel; 3M, Malaysia; 3M, NZ†; 3M, Port.; 3M, Singapore; 3M, Swed.; 3M, Switz.†; 3M, Thai.
Orphenadrine citrate (p.486·1); paracetamol (p.76·2).
*Musculoskeletal pain; skeletal muscle spasm; tension headache.*

3M, Canad.; 3M, USA.
Orphenadrine citrate (p.486·1); aspirin (p.15·1); caffeine (p.782·1).
*Musculoskeletal pain.*

**Norgesic N** 3M, Ger.
Orphenadrine citrate (p.486·1); propyphenazone (p.85·3).
*Dysmenorrhoea; headache; musculoskeletal pain.*

**Norgeston** Schering, UK.
Levonorgestrel (p.1563·2).
*Progestogen-only oral contraceptive.*

**Norgestrel Max** Biotenk, Arg.
Levonorgestrel (p.1563·2).
*Progestogen-only oral contraceptive.*

**Norgestrel Plus** Biotenk, Arg.
Levonorgestrel (p.1563·2); ethinylestradiol (p.1553·2).
*Combined oral contraceptive; menstrual disorders.*

**Norgic** Pond's, Thai.
Orphenadrine citrate (p.486·1); paracetamol (p.76·2).
*Skeletal muscle spasm.*

**Norglicem** Rottapharm, Spain.
Glibenclamide (p.331·2).
*Diabetes mellitus.*

**Norgotin** Helsinn Birex, Hong Kong†.
Chlorhexidine acetate (p.1173·2); ephedrine hydrochloride (p.1120·1); tetracaine hydrochloride (p.1385·1).
*Otitis.*

**Norica** Ottolenghi, Ital.
*Solution:* Benzalkonium chloride (p.1168·3).
*Room disinfection and deodorization.*
*Spray:* Orthophenylphenol (p.1187·2); benzalkonium chloride (p.1168·3).
*Surface disinfection.*

**Noricaven** Bionorica, Singapore.
Asperula odorata; silybum marianum (p.1043·3); crataegus (p.1677·1); rue (p.1741·1); echinacea (p.1683·2).
*Haemorrhoids; venous insufficiency.*

**Noricaven novo** Bionorica, Ger.
Aesculus (p.1648·2).
*Venous insufficiency.*

**Noriclan** Lilly, Spain†.
Dirithromycin (p.206·1).
*Bacterial infections.*

**Noriday**
Pharmacia, Austral.; Pharmacia, Irl.; Pharmacia, Malaysia; Pharmacia, NZ; Pharmacia, UK.
Norethisterone (p.1562·2).
*Progestogen-only oral contraceptive.*

**Noriderm** EMS, Braz.
Ketoconazole (p.403·3).
*Fungal infections.*

**Norifortan** Hoechst Marion Roussel, S.Afr.†.
Avapyrazone; dipyrone (p.35·3).
*Painful smooth muscle spasm.*

**Norimin**
Pharmacia, Austral.; Pharmacia, Hong Kong; Pharmacia, NZ; Pharmacia, UK.
Norethisterone (p.1562·2); ethinylestradiol (p.1553·2).
28-Day packs also contain 7 inert tablets.
*Combined oral contraceptive.*

**Norimode**
Quatromed, S.Afr.; Tillomed, UK.
Loperamide hydrochloride (p.1271·1).
*Diarrhoea; ostomy management.*

**Norincol** Volchem, Ital.
Carbohydrate, lipid, amino-acid, and dietary fibre preparation (p.1417·1).
*Nutritional supplement.*

**Norinyl** Searle, Mex.
Norethisterone (p.1562·2); mestranol (p.1559·2).
28-Day packs also contain 7 inert tablets.
*Combined oral contraceptive; menopausal disorders.*

**Norinyl-1**
Pharmacia, Austral.; Pharmacia, Hong Kong; Searle, Irl.†; Pharmacia, NZ; Pharmacia, UK.
Norethisterone (p.1562·2); mestranol (p.1559·2).
28-Day packs also contain 7 inert tablets.
*Combined oral contraceptive.*

**Norinyl-1/28** Pharmacia, S.Afr.
21 Tablets, norethisterone (p.1562·2); mestranol (p.1559·2); 7 tablets, inert.
*Combined oral contraceptive.*

**Norinyl 1 + 35** Searle, USA.
Norethisterone (p.1562·2); ethinylestradiol (p.1553·2).
28-Day packs also contain 7 inert tablets.
*Combined oral contraceptive.*

**Norinyl 1 + 50** Searle, USA.
Norethisterone (p.1562·2); mestranol (p.1559·2).
28-Day packs also contain 7 inert tablets.
*Combined oral contraceptive.*

**Norinyl 1/50** Searle, Canad.†.
Norethisterone (p.1562·2); mestranol (p.1559·2).
28-Day packs also contain 7 inert tablets.
*Combined oral contraceptive.*

**Noripam** Aspen, S.Afr.
Oxazepam (p.712·2).
*Alcohol withdrawal syndrome; anxiety disorders.*

**Noripurum** Altana, Braz.
Iron polymaltose (p.1437·3).
*Iron deficiency; iron-deficiency anaemias.*

**Noripurum Folico** Altana, Braz.
Folic acid (p.1429·1); iron polymaltose (p.1437·3).
*Iron deficiency; iron-deficiency anaemias.*

**Noripurum Vitaminado** Altana, Braz.
Iron polymaltose (p.1437·3); vitamins (p.1417·1).
*Iron-deficiency anaemia.*

**Norisodrine with Calcium Iodide** Abbott, USA.
Isoprenaline sulfate (p.940·2); calcium iodide (p.1116·2).
*Coughs.*

**Noristerat**
Schering, Fr.†; Schering, Ger.; German Remedies, India; Schering, Malaysia; Schering, Mex.; Schering, Singapore; Schering, Thai.; Schering, UK.
Norethisterone enantate (p.1562·2).
*Progestogen-only injectable contraceptive.*

**Norit**
Norit, Austria; Wolfs, Belg.; Norit, Gr.; Norit, Israel; Vemedia, Neth.
Activated charcoal (p.1030·2).
*Acute diarrhoea; flatulence; poisoning.*

**Noritate**
Ingens, Arg.; Dermik, Canad.; Finn Vita, Chile; Dermik, Hong Kong; Pangeo, Israel; Aventis, UK; Dermik, USA.
Metronidazole (p.607·2).
*Acne; rosacea.*

**Norit-Carbomix**
Norit, Austria; Wolfs, Belg.
Activated charcoal (p.1030·2).
*Diarrhoea; treatment of poisoning.*

**Noritet** Quatromed, S.Afr.†.
Doxycycline hyclate (p.206·2).
*Bacterial infections.*

**Noritren**
Lundbeck, Denm.; Lundbeck, Fin.; Lundbeck, Ital.; Lundbeck, Norw.
Nortriptyline hydrochloride (p.310·2).
*Depression.*

**Norivite** Aventis, S.Afr.†.
Vitamin B substances (p.1417·1).

**Norivite-12** Aventis, S.Afr.†.
Cyanocobalamin (p.1458·2).
*Anaemias; tonic.*

**Norizal** EMS, Braz.†.
Ketoconazole (p.403·3).
*Fungal infections.*

**Norizine** Aspen, S.Afr.
Cyclizine hydrochloride (p.429·3).
*Nausea and vomiting; vestibular disorders.*

**Norkotral Tema** Desitin, Ger.
Temazepam (p.723·2).
*Sleep disorders.*

**Norlevo**
Besins, Belg.; BPL-Meizler, Braz.; HRA, Denm.; Nycomed, Fin.; HRA, Fr.; Gerolimatos (Γερολυματος), Gr.; Angelini, Ital.; HRA, Norw.; Fargin, Port.; Medi Challenge, S.Afr.; Alcala, Spain; Nycomed, Swed.
Levonorgestrel (p.1563·2).
*Postcoital oral contraceptive.*

**Norline** Pharmaland, Thai.
Nortriptyline hydrochloride (p.310·2).
*Depression.*

**Norlip** Unipharm, Israel.
Bezafibrate (p.873·2).
*Hyperlipidaemias.*

**Norlutate** Pfizer, Canad.
Norethisterone acetate (p.1562·2).
*Abnormal uterine bleeding; amenorrhoea; endometriosis.*

**Norluten** SmithKline Beecham, Fr.†.
Norethisterone (p.1562·2).
*Endometriosis; fibromas; menstrual disorders.*

**Normabenzil** Farmoquimica, Braz.†.
Benzathine benzylpenicillin (p.162·3).
*Bacterial infections.*

**Normabrain** UCB, Ger.
Piracetam (p.1732·1).
*Mental function disorders.*

**Normacidine** Synthelabo, Belg.†.
Calcium carbonate (p.1254·2); aluminium glycinate (p.1249·1).
*Gastrointestinal disorders associated with hyperacidity.*

**Normacol**
Note. This name is used for preparations of different composition.
Norgine, Belg.; Rivex, Canad.; Norgine, Fr.; Norgine, Hong Kong; Norgine, Irl.; Norgine, Ital.; Norgine, Malaysia; Norgine, Neth.; Norgine, NZ; Zuellig, NZ; Norgine, S.Afr.; Norgine, Singapore; Norgine, Switz.; Norgine, Thai.; Norgine, UK.
Sterculia (p.1290·2).
Formerly known as Normacol Special in the *UK*.
*Constipation; diverticular disease; ingestion of foreign bodies; ostomy management.*

Schering, Mex.†.
Bassorin; frangula bark (p.1266·3).
*Constipation.*

**Normacol a la Bourdaine** Norgine, Fr.
Sterculia (p.1290·2); frangula bark (p.1266·3).
*Constipation.*

**Normacol Antispasmodique** Norgine, Belg.
Sterculia (p.1290·2); alverine citrate (p.1250·2).
*Constipation.*

**Normacol (avec bourdaine)** Norgine, Switz.
Sterculia (p.1290·2); frangula (p.1266·3).
*Constipation.*

**Normacol Forte** Rubio, Spain.
Sterculia (p.1290·2); frangula bark (p.1266·3).
*Constipation.*

**Normacol Lavement** Norgine, Fr.
Monobasic sodium phosphate (p.1230·3); dibasic sodium phosphate (p.1231·1).
*Bowel evacuation.*

**Normacol Plus**
Norgine, Austral.; Norgine, Belg.; Norgine, Hong Kong; Norgine, Irl.; Norgine, Neth.; Norgine, NZ; Zuellig, NZ; Helsinn, Port.; Norgine, S.Afr.; Norgine, Singapore; Norgine, UK.
Sterculia (p.1290·2); frangula (p.1266·3).
Formerly known as Normacol Standard in the *UK*.
*Constipation; diverticular disease; ostomy management.*

**Normafenac** Norma (Νορμα), Gr.
Cefuroxime sodium (p.184·1).
*Bacterial infections.*

**Normafibe** Norgine, Austral.
Sterculia (p.1290·2).
*Constipation; fibre supplement.*

**Normaflu** Wassermann, Ital.
Paracetamol (p.76·2).
*Cold and influenza symptoms; fever; pain.*

**Normaform** Sodip, Switz.†.
Phentermine resin (as an ion-exchange resin complex) (p.1592·2).
*Obesity.*

**Normagit** Sanofi Synthelabo, Port.
Tiapride hydrochloride (p.725·1).

**Normagrin** Hexal, Braz.†.
Phenolphthalein (p.1284·1); bladderwrack (p.1742·3); thyroid (p.1604·2); colecalciferol (p.1461·3); bile salts (p.1660·3).
*Constipation; obesity.*

**Normalac** Osteolab, Chile.
Lynestrenol (p.1557·1).
*Progestogen-only oral contraceptive.*

**Normalax** Herbaline, Ital.†.
Rhamnus alpinus; globularia vulgaris; chamomile (p.1669·3); red-poppy petal (p.1058·1); liquorice (p.1270·2); fennel (p.1687·2).
*Constipation.*

**Normalene** Montefarmaco, Ital.
Bisacodyl (p.1251·3).
*Constipation.*

**NormaLine**
Note. A similar name is used for preparations of different composition (see below).
Antonetto, Ital.
Glucomannan (p.1693·3).
*Dietary supplement in diabetes mellitus and hyperlipidaemias; obesity.*

**Normaline**
Note. A similar name is used for preparations of different composition (see above).
Julphar, UAE; Apothecary, USA.
Sodium chloride (p.1233·3).
*Nasal congestion; sodium depletion.*

**Normalip** Quesada, Arg.
Atorvastatin (p.866·2).
*Hypercholesterolaemia.*

**Normalip pro** Abbott, Ger.
Fenofibrate (p.915·2).
*Hyperlipidaemias.*

**Normalite** Codifra, Fr.
Multivitamin and mineral preparation with ginseng (p.1417·1).

**Normaloe** Tillomed, UK.
Loperamide hydrochloride (p.1271·1).
*Diarrhoea.*

**Normalol** Dexxon, Israel.
Atenolol (p.865·2).
*Angina pectoris; hypertension; migraine; myocardial infarction.*

**Normamor** Uniao Quimica, Braz.
Ethinylestradiol (p.1553·2); levonorgestrel (p.1563·2).
*Combined oral contraceptive.*

**Normapril** Cazi, Braz.
Captopril (p.879·2).
*Hypertension.*

**Normase** Molteni, Ital.
Lactulose (p.1269·1).
*Constipation; gastrointestinal disorders; hepatic cirrhosis; hepatic encephalopathy.*

**Normasol**
Seton, Israel; SSL, UK.
Sodium chloride (p.1233·3).
*Irrigation solution.*

**Normastigmin** Sigmapharm, Austria.
Neostigmine metilsulfate (p.1492·2).
*Gastrointestinal atony; myasthenia gravis; reversal of competitive neuromuscular blockade; urinary retention.*

**Normastigmin mit Pilocarpin** Sigmapharm, Austria.
Neostigmine bromide (p.1492·2); pilocarpine hydrochloride (p.1495·1).
*Glaucoma; pre- and post-operative lowering of intraocular pressure; reversal of mydriasis and cycloplegia.*

**Normaten**
Note. This name is used for preparations of different composition.
Bago, Chile.
Enalapril maleate (p.909·2); hydrochlorothiazide (p.933·2).
*Hypertension.*

Xepa-Soul Pattinson, Hong Kong; Xepa-Soul Pattinson, Malaysia; Xepa-Soul Pattinson, Singapore.
Atenolol (p.865·2).
*Angina pectoris; arrhythmias; hypertension; myocardial infarction.*

**Normaten Plus** Bago, Chile.
Enalapril maleate (p.909·2); hydrochlorothiazide (p.933·2).
*Hypertension.*

**Normatens** Solvay, Neth.
Moxonidine (p.962·3).
*Hypertension.*

**Normatensil** Phoenix, Arg.
Methyldopa (p.953·2); guanethidine sulfate (p.926·3); hydrochlorothiazide (p.933·2); reserpine (p.995·1).
*Hypertension.*

**Normatol** Parke, Davis, Chile.
Gabapentin (p.362·2).
*Epilepsy.*

**Normavom** Cryopharma, Mex.
Difenidol hydrochloride (p.1261·1).
*Nausea and vomiting; vertigo.*

**Normax**
Note. This name is used for preparations of different composition.
Ipca, India.
Norfloxacin (p.238·3).
*Bacterial infections.*

Celltech, UK.
Dantron (p.1261·1); docusate sodium (p.1262·2).
These ingredients can be described by the British Approved Name Co-danthrusate.
*Constipation.*

**Normaxin** Systopic, India.
Clidinium bromide (p.480·2); chlordiazepoxide (p.674·2); dicycloverine hydrochloride (p.481·2).
*Diarrhoea; gastritis; irritable bowel syndrome; peptic ulcer.*

**Normell** Hoechst Marion Roussel, Gr.
Glibenclamide (p.331·2); metformin (p.342·3).
*Diabetes mellitus.*

**Normensan** Disperga, Austria†.
Papaverine hydrochloride (p.1728·1); hyoscyamine (p.485·1); propyphenazone (p.85·3).
*Dysmenorrhoea; migraine; smooth muscle spasm.*

**Normex** Heralds, Braz.†.
Etynodiol (p.1554·2); ethinylestradiol (p.1553·2).
*Combined oral contraceptive.*

**Normhydral** *Gebro, Austria.*
Anhydrous glucose; sodium chloride; sodium citrate; potassium chloride (p.1222·2).
*Diarrhoea; oral rehydration therapy.*

**Normicina** *Tedec Meiji, Spain.*
Midecamycin acetate (p.231·3).
*Bacterial infections.*

**Normiflo** *Wyeth-Ayerst, USA†.*
Ardeparin sodium (p.864·3).
*Thrombosis prophylaxis.*

**Normin** *Searle, Irl.†.*
Norethisterone (p.1562·2); ethinylestradiol (p.1553·2).
*Combined oral contraceptive.*

**Normison**
*Sigma, Austral.; Wyeth Lederle, Belg.; Wyeth Lederle, Denm.†; Wyeth Lederle, Fin.; Wyeth Lederle, Fr.; Wyeth, Gr.; Wyeth, Irl.; Wyeth Lederle, Ital.; Eurocept, Neth.; Wyeth, NZ†; Teofarma, Port.; Akromed, S.Afr.; Wyeth, Switz.; Wyeth, UK†.*
Temazepam (p.723·2).
*Insomnia; premedication.*

**Normiten** *Abic, Israel.*
Atenolol (p.865·2).
*Angina pectoris; hypertension; myocardial infarction.*

**Normitrol** *Searle, Mex.†.*
Difenidol (p.1261·1).

**Normix** *Wassermann, Ital.*
Rifaximin (p.254·1).
*Gastrointestinal bacterial infections; hyperammonaemia.*

**Normlgel** *Molnlycke, Fr.*
Sodium chloride (p.1233·3).
*Ulcers; wounds.*

**Normo Gastryl** *Sabex, Canad.*
Sodium bicarbonate (p.1223·2); sodium sulfate (p.1290·1); sodium phosphate (p.1231·1).
*Gastric hyperacidity.*

**Normo Nar** *Zambon, Spain.*
Muramidase hydrochloride (p.1717·2); thonzylamine hydrochloride (p.442·2); methylethylaminophenol hydriodide.
*Nasal congestion; sinus congestion.*

**Normobren** *Medosan, Ital.*
Acetylcarnitine hydrochloride (p.1646·1).
*Cerebrovascular disorders.*

**Normoc** *Merckle, Ger.*
Bromazepam (p.671·3).
*Anxiety; insomnia.*

**Normocir** *Inkeysa, Spain.*
Ginkgo biloba (p.1692·3).
*Cerebral and peripheral vascular disorders.*

**Normodiar** *Hoechst Marion Roussel, Mex.†.*
Nifurzide (p.237·2).

**Normodyne** *Schering, USA.*
Labetalol hydrochloride (p.943·3).
*Hypertension.*

**Normofenicol** *Normon, Spain.*
Chloramphenicol sodium succinate (p.185·1).
Lidocaine hydrochloride (p.1377·3) is included in the injection to alleviate the pain of injection.
*Bacterial infections.*

**Normofer** *Magis, Ital.†.*
Iron acetylaspartilate-protein complex (p.1436·1).
*Anaemias; iron deficiency.*

**Normoflex** *Degorts, Mex.*
Bromhexine (p.1115·3).
*Respiratory-tract congestion.*

**Normofundin** *Braun, Fin.*
Electrolyte infusion with glucose (p.1217·1).
*Carbohydrate source; fluid and electrolyte disorders.*

**Normofundin X** *Braun, Ger.†.*
Electrolyte infusion with xylitol (p.1217·1).
*Carbohydrate source; fluid and electrolyte disorders.*

**Normofundin G-5** *Braun, Ger.*
Electrolyte infusion with glucose (p.1217·1).
*Carbohydrate source; fluid and electrolyte disorders.*

**Normofundin OP** *Braun, Ger.*
Electrolyte infusion (p.1217·1).
*Fluid and electrolyte disorders.*

**Normofundin sKG** *Braun, Ger.†.*
Potassium-free electrolyte infusion with glucose (p.1217·1).
*Carbohydrate source; fluid and electrolyte disorders.*

**Normofusin** *Fresenius Kabi, Fin.*
Electrolyte infusion with glucose (p.1217·1).
*Carbohydrate source; fluid and electrolyte disorders.*

**Normogam** *ICT, Ital.*
Gamolenic acid (p.1690·2).
*Gamolenic acid deficiency; nutritional supplement.*

**Normogamma** *Nuovo ISM, Ital.†.*
A normal immunoglobulin (p.1627·2).
*Passive immunisation.*

**Normogastryl**
*Note. This name is used for preparations of different composition.*
*Upsamedica, Belg.†.*
Sodium bicarbonate (p.1223·2); sodium sulfate (p.1290·1); sodium phosphate (p.1231·1); sodium bromide (p.1663·1); sodium benzoate (p.1169·3); sodium citrate (p.1223·2).
*Gastrointestinal disorders.*

*UPSA Conseil, Fr.; Upsamedica, Spain†; Upsamedica, Switz.†.*
Sodium bicarbonate (p.1223·2); sodium sulfate (p.1290·1); sodium phosphate (p.1230·3).
*Gastrointestinal disorders.*

**Normogin** *Baldacci, Ital.*
*Bacilli vaginalis* culture.
*Vaginal bacterial infections.*

**Normoglaucon**
*Tramedico, Belg.; Mann, Ger.; Mann, Malaysia; Tramedico, Neth.; Lepori, Port.; Mann, Singapore; Bausch & Lomb, Thai.; Mann, Thai.*
Metipranolol hydrochloride (p.956·1); pilocarpine hydrochloride (p.1495·1).
*Glaucoma.*

**Normoglucon** *Klinge, Austria.*
Glibenclamide (p.331·2).
*Diabetes mellitus.*

**Normolaxil** *Trenker, Belg.*
Lactitol (p.1269·1).
*Constipation.*

**Normolip** *Sun, India.*
Gemfibrozil (p.923·1).
*Hyperlipidaemias.*

**Normo-Loges** *Loges, Ger.*
Homoeopathic preparation.

**Normolose** *Adelco, Gr.*
Captopril (p.879·2).
*Heart failure; hypertension; myocardial infarction.*

**Normolyt** *Gebro, Austria.*
Anhydrous glucose; sodium chloride; sodium citrate; potassium chloride (p.1222·2).
*Diarrhoea; oral rehydration therapy.*

**Normolytoral** *Gebro, Switz.*
Anhydrous glucose; sodium chloride; sodium citrate; potassium chloride (p.1222·2).
*Diarrhoea; oral rehydration therapy.*

**Normomensil** *Sedabel, Braz.*
Progesterone (p.1566·2); estradiol (p.1550·1).
*Menopausal disorders; menstrual disorders.*

**Normonal** *Eisai, Thai.*
Tripamide (p.1018·1).
*Hypertension.*

**Normoparin** *Caber, Ital.*
Heparin sodium (p.928·1).
*Thromboembolic disorders.*

**Normophasic** *Nourypharma, Switz.†.*
7 Tablets, ethinylestradiol (p.1553·2); 15 tablets, ethinylestradiol; lynestrenol (p.1557·1).
*Sequential-type oral contraceptive.*

**Normopres** *Delta, Braz.*
Nifedipine (p.966·2).
*Hypertension.*

**Normopresan** *Rafa, Israel.*
Clonidine hydrochloride (p.885·2).
*Hypertension.*

**Normopresil** *Sanofi Synthelabo, Spain.*
Chlortalidone (p.882·3); atenolol (p.865·2).
*Hypertension.*

**Normopress**
*Note. This name is used for preparations of different composition.*
*Caber, Ital.*
Atenolol (p.865·2); indapamide (p.938·2).
*Hypertension.*

*Alliance, S.Afr.*
Methyldopa (p.953·2).
*Hypertension.*

**Normopride Enzimatico** *Sanofi Synthelabo, Braz.†.*
Bromopride (p.1254·1); dimethicone (p.1289·2); lipase; cellulase (p.1669·1); amylase (p.1654·2).
*Digestive-system disorders; nausea and vomiting.*

**Normoprost** *Silesia, Chile.*
Mepartricin (p.405·2).
*Benign prostatic hypertrophy.*

**Normoprost Compuesto** *Temis, Arg.*
Pygeum africanum (p.1568·2); glutamic acid (p.1433·2); alanine (p.1421·1); glycine (p.1433·3).
*Prostate disorders.*

**Normoprost Plus** *Temis, Arg.*
Pygeum africanum (p.1568·2); saw palmetto (p.1569·1).
*Prostate disorders.*

**Normo-real** *Novartis Nutrition, Fr.†.*
A range of preparations for enteral nutrition (p.1417·1).

**Normorix**
*Nycomed, Norw.; Nycomed, Swed.*
Hydrochlorothiazide (p.933·2); amiloride hydrochloride (p.858·2).
*Hypertension; liver cirrhosis with ascites; oedema.*

**Normorytmin** *Abbott, Arg.*
Propafenone hydrochloride (p.988·3).
*Arrhythmias.*

**Normosang**
*Leiras, Fin.; Orphan, Fr.; Orphan, Ger.†; Orphan, Ital.; Orphan, Spain; Schering, Swed.; Stauffacher, Switz.; Orphan, UK.*
Haem arginate (p.1040·3).
*Porphyria.*

**Normoskin** *Hautel, Arg.*
Aluminium chlorohydrate (p.1142·1).

**Normosol**
*Abbott, Hong Kong; Abbott, USA.*
A range of electrolyte infusions with or without glucose (p.1217·1).
*Fluid and electrolyte disorders.*

**Normosol M 900 Cal** *Abbott, Ital.*
Electrolyte infusion with glucose and fructose (p.1217·1).
*Carbohydrate source; fluid and electrolyte disorders.*

**Normosol M Con Glucosio 5%** *Abbott, Ital.*
Electrolyte infusion with glucose (p.1217·1).
*Fluid and electrolyte disorders.*

**Normosol R** *Abbott, Ital.*
Electrolyte infusion (p.1217·1).
*Fluid and electrolyte disorders.*

**Normosol R Con Glucosio 5%** *Abbott, Ital.*
Electrolyte infusion with glucose (p.1217·1).
*Carbohydrate source; fluid and electrolyte disorders.*

**Normosol R/K Con Glucosio 5%** *Abbott, Ital.*
Electrolyte infusion with glucose (p.1217·1).
*Carbohydrate source; fluid and electrolyte disorders.*

**Normospor** *Propan, S.Afr.*
Clotrimazole (p.396·2).
*Fungal skin infections; vulvovaginal fungal infections.*

**Normosteril** *Baxter, Fin.*
Electrolyte infusion with glucose (p.1217·1).
*Carbohydrate source; fluid and electrolyte disorders.*

**Normotensin** *Hoechst Marion Roussel, Austria†.*
Penbutolol sulfate (p.979·1); furosemide (p.919·3).
*Hypertension.*

**Normotensor** *Geyer, Braz.*
Furosemide (p.919·3).

**Normothen** *Bioindustria, Ital.*
Doxazosin mesilate (p.908·3).
*Hypertension.*

**Normotherin** *Unipharma, Gr.*
Simvastatin (p.997·1).
*Primary hypercholesterolaemia.*

**Normotil** *APS, Port.*
Captopril (p.879·2); hydrochlorothiazide (p.933·2).
*Hypertension.*

**Normotin VI** *OTW, Ger.†.*
Crataegus (p.1677·1).
*Cardiac disorders.*

**Normotin-R** *OTW, Ger.*
Etamivan (p.1588·1); norfenefrine hydrochloride (p.975·3); heptaminol hydrochloride (p.1697·1).
*Hypotension.*

**Normovite Antianemico** *Normon, Spain.*
Folic acid (p.1429·1); ferrous gluceptate (p.1428·1).
*Iron and folic acid deficiency.*

**Normovlar ED** *Schering, S.Afr.†.*
21 Tablets, levonorgestrel (p.1563·2); ethinylestradiol (p.1553·2); 7 tablets, inert.
*Biphasic oral contraceptive; menstrual disorders.*

**Normoxidil** *Medosan, Ital.*
Minoxidil (p.960·1).
*Alopecia.*

**Normoxin** *Asta Medica, Austria.*
Moxonidine (p.962·3).
*Hypertension.*

**Normpress** *Greater Pharma, Thai.*
Propranolol hydrochloride (p.989·3).
*Angina pectoris; hypertension; myocardial infarction.*

**Normulen** *Grunenthal, Spain.*
Diclofenac sodium (p.32·1).
Misoprostol (p.1519·2) is included in this preparation in an attempt to limit adverse effects on the gastrointestinal mucosa.
*Osteoarthritis; rheumatoid arthritis.*

**Normum** *Serpero, Ital.†.*
Sulpiride (p.722·2).
*Dysthymia; psychoses.*

**Norocin** *Vianex (Βιανέξ), Gr.*
Norfloxacin (p.238·3).
*Urinary tract infections.*

**Norogil** *Aventis, Braz.*
Dihydroergocristine mesilate (p.1680·1); lomifylline.
*Impaired mental function; migraine and other vascular headaches; orthostatic hypotension; thrombosis prophylaxis.*

**No-Roma** *Salts Healthcare, UK†.*
A deodorant liquid for use with colostomies and ileostomies.

**Noronal** *Ducto, Braz.*
Ketoconazole (p.403·3).
*Fungal infections.*

**Noroxin**
*Merck Sharp & Dohme, Arg.; Merck Sharp & Dohme, Austral.; Merck Frosst, Canad.; Merck Sharp & Dohme, Chile; Merck Sharp & Dohme, Fin.; Merck Sharp & Dohme, Ital.; Merck Sharp & Dohme, Mex.; Merck Sharp & Dohme, Neth.; Merck Sharp & Dohme, NZ; Merck Sharp & Dohme, Port.; Merck Sharp & Dohme, S.Afr.; Merck Sharp & Dohme, Spain; Merck Sharp & Dohme, Switz.; Merck, USA; Roberts, USA.*
Norfloxacin (p.238·3).
*Bacterial infections.*

**Noroxine** *Merck Sharp & Dohme-Chibret, Fr.*
Norfloxacin (p.238·3).
*Bacterial infections of the urinary tract; gonococcal cervicitis; gonococcal urethritis.*

**Nor-Pa** *Salus, Ital.*
Atenolol (p.865·2); indapamide (p.938·2).
*Hypertension.*

**Norpace**
*Pharmacia, Austral.†; Roberts, Canad.†; Searle, Denm.†; Heumann, Ger.; Searle, Hong Kong†; RPG, India; Pharmacia, S.Afr.; Pharmacia, Switz.; Searle, Thai.†; Searle, USA.*
Disopyramide phosphate (p.903·3).
*Arrhythmias.*

**Norphen**
*Atlantic, Singapore; Atlantic, Thai.*
Orphenadrine citrate (p.486·1); paracetamol (p.76·2).
*Dysmenorrhoea; musculoskeletal pain; tension headache.*

**Norphin** *Unichem, India.*
Buprenorphine hydrochloride (p.21·3).
*Pain; premedication.*

**Norphyllin** *Norton, UK†.*
Aminophylline (p.780·2).
*Bronchospasm.*

**Norpid** *Greater Pharma, Thai.*
Gemfibrozil (p.923·1).
*Hyperlipidaemias.*

**Norpilen** *Andromaco, Chile.*
Venlafaxine (p.322·3).
*Depression.*

**Norplant**
*Wyeth-Ayerst, Canad.; Discotrade, Israel†; Schering, Malaysia; Sanofi Winthrop, Mex.†; Schering, Singapore; Schering, Swed.; Schering, Thai.; Wyeth-Ayerst, USA†.*
Levonorgestrel (p.1563·2).
*Progestogen-only implantable contraceptive.*

**Norpramin**
*Note. This name is used for preparations of different composition.*
*Aventis, Canad.; Aventis, Mex.; Hoechst Marion Roussel, USA.*
Desipramine hydrochloride (p.290·2).
*Depression.*

*CEPA, Spain.*
Omeprazole (p.1278·2).
*Gastro-oesophageal reflux; peptic ulcer; Zollinger-Ellison syndrome.*

**Norpress** *Pacific, NZ.*
Nortriptyline hydrochloride (p.310·2).
*Depression.*

**Norpril** *Fustery, Mex.*
Enalapril maleate (p.909·2).
*Heart failure; hypertension.*

**Norprolac**
*Novartis, Austria; Novartis, Fin.; Novartis, Fr.; Novartis, Ger.; Novartis, Gr.; Novartis, Hong Kong; Novartis, Israel; Novartis, Mex.; Novartis, Neth.; Novartis, Norw.; Novartis, S.Afr.; Novartis, Spain; Novartis, Swed.; Novartis, Switz.; Novartis, UK.*
Quinagolide hydrochloride (p.1213·1).
*Acromegaly; hyperprolactinaemia; lactation inhibition.*

**Nor-QD** *Watson, USA.*
Norethisterone (p.1562·2).
*Progestogen-only oral contraceptive.*

**Norsa** *Shiwa, Thai.*
Norfloxacin (p.238·3).
*Bacterial infections.*

**Norset** *Organon, Fr.*
Mirtazapine (p.307·3).
*Depression.*

**Norsic** *Andromaco, Chile.*
Quetiapine (p.719·1).

**Norsol**
*Finadiet, Arg.; Ecosol, Switz.*
Norfloxacin (p.238·3).
*Bacterial infections.*

**Norspor** *Pond's, Thai.*
Itraconazole (p.401·3).
*Fungal infections.*

**Nortase** *Asche, Ger.*
Rizolipase; protease and amylase from *Aspergillus oryzae*.
*Pancreatic insufficiency.*

**Nortec** *Ativus, Braz.*
Fluoxetine hydrochloride (p.292·1).
*Depression.*

**Nortem** *Ivax, Irl.*
Temazepam (p.723·2).
*Insomnia.*

**Norterol** *Tecnifar, Port.*
Nortriptyline hydrochloride (p.310·2).
*Anxiety; depression; excitable states; insomnia.*

**Northiron** *Norma (Νορμα), Gr.*
Propylene glycol cefatrizine (p.170·3).
*Bacterial infections.*

**Nortimil** *Chiesi, Ital.*
Desipramine hydrochloride (p.290·2).
*Depression; psychoses.*

**Nortolan** *Anpharm (Ανφαρμ), Gr.*
Nimodipine (p.972·3).
*Neurological deficit following subarachnoid haemorrhage.*

**Norton** *Farmasa, Braz.*
Nimodipine (p.972·3).
*Neurological deficit following subarachnoid haemorrhage.*

**Nortrel** *Wyeth, Braz.*
Levonorgestrel (p.1563·2).
*Progestogen-only oral contraceptive.*

**Nortrilen**
*Lundbeck, Austria; Lundbeck, Belg.; Lundbeck, Ger.; Lundbeck, Gr.; Lundbeck, Hong Kong; Lundbeck, Neth.; Lundbeck, Switz.; Lundbeck, Thai.*
Nortriptyline hydrochloride (p.310·2).
*Depression.*

**Nortrix** *Tecnifar, Port.*
Nortriptyline hydrochloride (p.310·2).
*Anxiety disorders; depression.*

**Nortron** *Dista, Spain†.*
Dirithromycin (p.206·1).
*Bacterial infections.*

**Nortuss** *Rosemont, Thai.*
Promethazine hydrochloride (p.439·1); codeine phosphate (p.27·1).
*Coughs.*

**Nortussine**
*Note. This name is used for preparations of different composition.*
*Norgine, Belg.*
Dextromethorphan hydrobromide (p.1117·3); mepyramine maleate (p.437·1); phenylephrine hydrochloride (p.1126·3); guaifenesin (p.1122·1).
*Coughs.*

*Norgine, Fr.*
*Paediatric syrup:* Dextromethorphan hydrobromide (p.1117·3); mepyramine maleate (p.437·1); guaifenesin (p.1122·1).
*Syrup:* Dextromethorphan hydrobromide (p.1117·3); mepyramine maleate (p.437·1).
*Coughs.*

**Nortussine Mono** *Norgine, Belg.*
Dextromethorphan hydrobromide (p.1117·3).
*Coughs.*

**Nortylin** *Rekah, Israel.*
Nortriptyline hydrochloride (p.310·2).
*Depression.*

**Nortyline** *Condrugs, Thai.*
Nortriptyline hydrochloride (p.310·2).
*Depression.*

**Norum** *Chew, Thai.*
Aciclovir (p.626·1).
*Herpes simplex infections of the skin and mucous membranes.*

**Noruxol** *Smith & Nephew, Ital.*
Collagenase (p.1675·1).
*Necrotic wounds and ulcers.*

**Norvas**
*Pfizer, Mex.; Pfizer, Spain.*
Amlodipine besilate (p.862·1).
*Angina pectoris; hypertension.*

**Norvasc**
*Pfizer, Austral.; Pfizer, Austria; Pfizer, Braz.; Pfizer, Canad.; Pfizer, Chile; Pfizer, Denm.; Pfizer, Fin.; Godecke, Ger.; Mack, Illert., Ger.; Parke, Davis, Ger.; Pfizer, Ger.; Pfizer, Gr.; Pfizer, Hong Kong; Pfizer, Israel; Pfizer, Ital.; Pfizer, Jpn; Pfizer, Malaysia; Pfizer, Neth.; Pfizer, Norw.; Pfizer, NZ; Pfizer, Port.; Pfizer, S.Afr.; Pfizer, Singapore; Pfizer, Swed.; Pfizer, Switz.; Pfizer, Thai.; Pfizer, USA.*
Amlodipine besilate (p.862·1).
*Angina pectoris; hypertension.*

**Norvectan** *Fardi, Spain.*
Ibuprofen lysine (p.46·3).
*Fever; musculoskeletal and joint disorders; pain.*

**Norvedan**
*Roche, Austria†; Helsinn, Port.*
Fentiazac (p.43·1) or fentiazac calcium (p.43·1).
*Fever; inflammation; musculoskeletal and joint disorders; pain.*

**Norventyl** *ICN, Canad.*
Nortriptyline hydrochloride (p.310·2).
*Depression.*

**Norvetal** *Gynopharm, Chile.*
Levonorgestrel (p.1563·2); ethinylestradiol (p.1553·2).
*Combined oral contraceptive.*

**Norvic** *Libbs, Braz.†.*
Alendronic acid (p.765·3).
*Osteoporosis.*

**Norvil** *Libbs, Braz.†.*
Verapamil (p.1021·1).
*Arrhythmias; hypertension.*

**Norvir**
*Abbott, Austral.; Abbott, Belg.; Abbott, Canad.; Abbott, Chile; Abbott, Denm.; Abbott, Fin.; Abbott, Fr.; Abbott, Ger.; Abbott, Gr.; Abbott, Hong Kong; Abbott, Irl.; Abbott, Israel; Abbott, Ital.; Dainabot, Jpn; Abbott, Malaysia; Abbott, Mex.; Abbott, Neth.; Abbott, Norw.; Abbott, NZ; Abbott, Port.†; Abbott, S.Afr.; Abbott, Spain; Abbott, Swed.; Abbott, Switz.; Abbott, Thai.; Abbott, UK; Abbott, USA.*
Ritonavir (p.653·2).
*HIV infection.*

**Norwich Extra Strength** *Procter & Gamble, USA.*
Aspirin (p.15·1).
*Fever; inflammation; myocardial infarction; pain; transient ischaemic attacks.*

**Norxacin** *Siam Bheasach, Thai.*
Norfloxacin (p.238·3).
*Bacterial infections.*

**Norxia** *Asian Pharm, Thai.*
Norfloxacin (p.238·3).
*Bacterial infections.*

**Norxin** *Cazi, Braz.*
Norfloxacin (p.238·3).
*Urinary-tract infections.*

**Norzac** *Ivax, Irl.*
Fluoxetine hydrochloride (p.292·1).
*Bulimia; depression.*

**Norzetam** *IPFI, Ital.*
Piracetam (p.1732·1).
*Mental function impairment.*

**Norzol** *Rosemont, UK.*
Metronidazole benzoate (p.607·2).
*Bacterial infections.*

**Nos** *Dermofarm, Spain.*
Famotidine (p.1265·2).
*Dyspepsia; gastro-oesophageal reflux; peptic ulcer; Zollinger-Ellison syndrome.*

**Nosatel** *Guidotti, Gr.*
Dexketoprofen trometamol (p.51·2).
*Pain.*

**Noscaflex** *Wolfs, Belg.*
*Paediatric syrup:* Noscapine camsilate (p.1125·3).
*Syrup:* Noscapine hydrochloride (p.1125·3); guaifenesin (p.1122·1).
*Tablets:* Noscapine (p.1125·3).
*Coughs.*

**Noscal** *Sankyo, Jpn†.*
Troglitazone (p.348·2).
*Diabetes mellitus.*

**Nosca-Mereprine** *Novum, Belg.*
Noscapine hydrochloride (p.1125·3).
*Coughs.*

**Noscorex** *Interdelta, Switz.*
Noscapine hydrochloride (p.1125·3); guaifenesin (p.1122·1).
*Coughs; upper respiratory-tract inflammation.*

**Nose Fresh** *Rappai, Switz.*
Sea salt (p.1233·3).
*Nasal disorders.*

**Nosebo** *Ottolenghi, Ital.†.*
Sulfur (p.1158·2).
*Acne; skin cleansing.*

**NoseEase** *Impharm, UK†.*
Jojoba oil; hyssop oil; artemisia oil; eucalyptus oil (p.1686·2); peppermint oil (p.1283·2).
*Nasal congestion.*

**Nosenil** *Farbo, Ital.†.*
Ginkgo biloba (p.1692·3); eleutherococcus (p.1744·1); kola (p.1765·3); equisetum (p.1684·1); urtica (p.1762·1).

**Nosipren** *Collins, Mex.*
Prednisone (p.1109·3).
*Corticosteroid.*

**Nositrol** *Cryopharma, Mex.*
Hydrocortisone sodium succinate (p.1104·1).
*Corticosteroid.*

**No-Sor Nose Balm** *Pickles, UK.*
Dibrompropamidine isetionate (p.1178·2); wheat-germ oil; menthol (p.1711·3); eucalyptus (p.1686·1).

**No-Sor Vapour Rub** *Pickles, UK.*
Camphor (p.1665·3); turpentine; menthol (p.1711·3); eucalyptus oil (p.1686·2); nutmeg oil (p.1722·3); cedar wood oil; thymol (p.1194·2).
*Upper respiratory-tract congestion.*

**No-Spa**
*Chinoin, Hung.; Sanofi Synthelabo, Thai.*
Drotaverine hydrochloride (p.1683·1).
*Pain; peptic ulcer; smooth muscle spasm.*

**Nospan**
*YSP, Malaysia; Yung Shin, Singapore.*
Dextromethorphan hydrobromide (p.1117·3).
*Coughs.*

**Nospasmin** *Instituto Sanitas, Chile.*
Pipethanate (p.487·3).
*Smooth muscle spasm.*

**Nospasmin Compuesto** *Instituto Sanitas, Chile.*
Metamizole magnesium (p.36·1); pipethanate hydrochloride (p.487·3).
*Nausea and vomiting; smooth muscle spasm.*

**Nossacin** *Benedetti, Ital.*
Cinoxacin (p.188·1).
*Bacterial infections of the urinary tract.*

**Nostaden** *Mintlab, Chile.*
Cyclobenzaprine hydrochloride (p.1393·1).
*Skeletal muscle spasm.*

**Nostimex** *Rafarm, Gr.*
Ketotifen fumarate (p.788·1).
*Allergic rhinitis; asthma.*

**Nostress** *Schwartz, Fr.*
Juglans regia; lupulus (p.1708·1); ginseng (p.1693·1).
*Tonic.*

**Nostril**
*Note. This name is used for preparations of different composition.*
*Boehringer Ingelheim, Fr.*
Chlorhexidine gluconate (p.1173·2); cetrimonium bromide (p.1173·1).
*Nose and throat infections.*

*Ciba, USA.*
Phenylephrine hydrochloride (p.1126·3).
*Nasal congestion.*

**Nostrilet** *Osoth, Thai.*
Triprolidine hydrochloride (p.442·3); pseudoephedrine hydrochloride (p.1129·2).
*Allergic rhinitis; cold symptoms; hay fever; nasal congestion.*

**Nostrilla** *Ciba Consumer, USA.*
Oxymetazoline hydrochloride (p.1126·1).
*Nasal congestion.*

**Nostroline** *Co-Pharma, UK.*
Menthol (p.1711·3); cineole (p.1672·1); geranium oil (p.1692·2).
*Nasal congestion.*

**Nosweat** *Madaus, Austria.*
Sage (p.1741·2).
*Hyperhidrosis.*

**Notacilin** *Ortoquimica, Braz.†.*
Ampicillin (p.157·1).
*Bacterial infections.*

**Notagol** *Grunenthal, Chile.*
Piroxicam (p.84·2).
*Gout; musculoskeletal and joint disorders; pain.*

**Notakehl** *Sanum-Kehlbeck, Ger.*
Homoeopathic preparation.

**Notem** *Fustery, Mex.*
Paracetamol (p.76·2).
*Fever; pain.*

**Noten**
*Alphapharm, Austral.; Alphapharm, Malaysia; Merck, Malaysia; Alphapharm, Singapore; Merck, Thai.†.*
Atenolol (p.865·2).
*Angina pectoris; arrhythmias; hypertension; myocardial infarction.*

**Notensyl** *CTI, Israel.*
Dicycloverine hydrochloride (p.481·2).
*Irritable bowel syndrome.*

**Notezine** *Aventis, Fr.*
Diethylcarbamazine citrate (p.104·1).
*Filariasis.*

**Nothav** *Chiron Vaccines, Ital.*
A hepatitis A vaccine (p.1617·1).
*Active immunisation.*

**Notorium** *Adelco, Gr.*
Bromazepam (p.671·3).
*Anxiety disorders.*

**No-Tos Adultos** *Gramon, Arg.*
*Lozenges:* Hexylresorcinol (p.1182·1); senega (p.1130·2); liquorice (p.1270·2); tolu balsam (p.1131·3); cineole (p.1672·1).
*Syrup:* Sodium benzoate (p.1169·3); ammonium chloride (p.1115·2); ephedrine hydrochloride (p.1120·1); senega (p.1130·2); aconite (p.1646·3); niaouli oil (p.1719·3); tolu (p.1131·3); liquorice (p.1270·2).
*Coughs.*

**No-Tos Biotic** *Gramon, Arg.*
Amoxicillin trihydrate (p.155·3); ambroxol hydrochloride (p.1114·3).
*Respiratory-tract infections.*

**No-Tos Infantil** *Gramon, Arg.*
*Lozenges:* Sodium benzoate (p.1169·3); sulfogaiacol (p.1131·1); senega (p.1130·2); liquorice (p.1270·2); ipecacuanha (p.1122·3); tolu balsam (p.1131·3).
*Syrup:* Sodium benzoate (p.1169·3); ammonium chloride (p.1115·2); sulfogaiacol (p.1131·1); liquorice (p.1270·2); tolu balsam (p.1131·3); Desessartz syrup.
*Coughs.*

**No-Tos Mucolitico** *Gramon, Arg.*
Bromhexine hydrochloride (p.1115·3).
*Coughs.*

**Notosil** *Grunenthal, Chile.*
Drosera (p.1683·1); quillaia (p.1416·1); pectoral; tolu balsam (p.1131·3).
*Coughs.*

**Notoxid** *Zambon, Braz.†.*
Acetylcysteine (p.1112·3).
*Respiratory-tract congestion.*

**Notoxin** *Szama, Arg.*
Cholesterol; chlorophyll (p.1057·1); turpentine oil (p.1760·1); zinc oxide (p.1163·2).
*Burns; skin cleansing; skin infections; ulcers; wounds.*

**Notozen** *Bouzen, Arg.*
Bromhexine (p.1115·3); clofedanol (p.1117·1).
*Coughs.*

**Notrab** *Microsules, Arg.*
Ranitidine (p.1285·2).
*Peptic ulcer.*

**Notta** *Bittner, Austria.*
Homoeopathic preparation.

**Nottem** *Angelini, Ital.*
Zolpidem tartrate (p.728·3).
*Insomnia.*

**Notul** *Mendelejeff, Ital.*
Cimetidine hydrochloride (p.1255·3).
*Gastritis; gastroduodenitis; gastrointestinal haemorrhage; peptic ulcer; Zollinger-Ellison syndrome.*

**Notuss** *Ache, Braz.*
Paracetamol (p.76·2); diphenhydramine hydrochloride (p.431·3); pseudoephedrine hydrochloride (p.1129·2); dropropizine (p.1119·3).
*Coughs.*

**Notuss PD** *Stewart Jackson, USA.*
Hydrocodone tartrate (p.45·1); dexchlorpheniramine maleate (p.427·3); phenylephrine hydrochloride (p.1126·3).
*Upper respiratory-tract disorders.*

**Nourilax** *Chefaro, Neth.†.*
Bisacodyl (p.1251·3).
*Constipation.*

**Nourishake** *GNLD, Austral.†.*
Nutritional supplement (p.1417·1).

**Noury Hoofdlotion** *Alfaco, Neth.†.*
Malathion (p.1507·1).
*Pediculosis.*

**Nourymag** *Nourypharma, Ger.*
Magnesium aspartate (p.1227·3).
*Magnesium deficiency.*

**Nourytam** *Nourypharma, Ger.*
Tamoxifen citrate (p.584·1).
*Breast cancer.*

**Nova Derm** *Darier, Mex.*
*Cream; lotion; topical solution:* Glycolic acid (p.1147·3).
*Acne; dry skin disorders.*
*Topical gel:* Glycolic acid (p.1147·3); hydroquinone (p.1148·1).
*Hyperpigmentation disorders.*

**Nova Paratopina** *Lazar, Arg.*
Pargeverine hydrochloride (p.487·3).
*Smooth muscle spasm.*

**Nova Paratropina Compositum** *Lazar, Arg.*
Pargeverine hydrochloride (p.487·3); clonixin lysine (p.26·3).
*Colic; dyskinesia; menstrual disorders.*

**Nova Perfecting Lotion** *Avon, Canad.†.*
Salicylic acid (p.1157·1).
*Acne.*

**Nova Rectal** *Sabex, Canad.†.*
Pentobarbital sodium (p.713·3).
*Insomnia; sedative.*

**Nova Vizol** *Bell, India.*
Hypromellose (p.1579·3).
*Dry eyes.*

**Novaban**
*Novartis, Belg.; Novartis, Neth.*
Tropisetron hydrochloride (p.1293·3).
*Nausea and vomiting.*

**Novaboin** *Dermopen, Braz.†.*
Aesculus (p.1648·2); menthol (p.1711·3); boric acid (p.1662·1); rutoside (p.1688·2); lidocaine (p.1377·3); adrenaline (p.852·2).
*Haemorrhoids.*

**Novabritine** *GlaxoSmithKline, Belg.*
Amoxicillin sodium (p.155·3) or amoxicillin trihydrate (p.155·3).
*Bacterial infections.*

**Novabupi** *Cristalia, Braz.*
Levobupivacaine hydrochloride (p.1377·1).
Adrenaline acid tartrate (p.852·2) is included in some injections as a vasoconstrictor to diminish absorption and localise the effect of the local anaesthetic.
*Local anaesthesia.*

**NovaCare** *Fielding, USA.*
Vitamin and mineral preparation with iron and folic acid (p.1417·1).

**Novacef**
*Note. This name is used for preparations of different composition.*
*Gador, Arg.; Promeco, Mex.*
Cefixime (p.172·3).
*Bacterial infections.*

*IFI, Ital.*
Propylene glycol cefatrizine (p.170·3).
*Bacterial infections.*

**Novacefrex** *Sanofi Synthelabo, Port.†.*
Cefradine (p.179·3).
*Bacterial infections.*

**Novacet** *Medicis, USA.*
Sulfacetamide sodium (p.257·3); sulfur (p.1158·2).
*Acne; seborrhoeic dermatitis.*

**Novacetol**
*Note. This name is used for preparations of different composition.*
*Prater, Chile.*
Clotrimazole (p.396·2).
*Fungal skin infections; trichomoniasis.*

*Pharmastra, Fr.*
Aspirin (p.15·1); paracetamol (p.76·2); codeine hydrochloride (p.27·1).
*Fever; pain.*

**Novacil** *Dovalle, Braz.*
Amoxicillin (p.155·3).
*Bacterial infections.*

**Novacilina** *Tecnofarma, Chile.*
Levofloxacin (p.225·3).
*Bacterial infections.*

**Novacler** *Monserrat, Arg.*
Dipyrone (p.35·3).
*Colic; fever; pain.*

**Novaclox** *Cipla, India.*
Amoxicillin sodium (p.155·3) or amoxicillin trihydrate (p.155·3); cloxacillin sodium (p.198·2).
*Bacterial infections.*

**Novacloxab** *Relyo, Gr.*
Loratadine (p.436·1).
*Allergic rhinitis; pruritus.*

**Novacnyl** *Esseti, Ital.†.*
Meclocycline sulfosalicylate (p.229·1).
*Skin infections.*

**Novacort**
*Note. This name is used for preparations of different composition.*
*Ache, Braz.*
Ketoconazole (p.403·3); neomycin sulfate (p.235·1); betamethasone (p.1093·1).
*Infected skin disorders.*

*Syntex, Mex.†.*
Cloprednol (p.1096·1).
*Corticosteroid.*

**Novacrium** *Allen, Austria.*
Mivacurium chloride (p.1403·3).
*Competitive neuromuscular blocker.*

**Nova-Dec** *Rugby, USA.*
Multivitamin and mineral preparation with iron and folic acid (p.1417·1).

**Novaderm** *Farmasa, Braz.*
Clostebol acetate (p.1543·2); neomycin sulfate (p.235·1).
*Infected wounds.*

**Novadex** *Novag, Mex.†.*
Naproxen (p.65·1).

**Novador** *Novartis, Mex.*
Cefuroxime axetil (p.184·1) or cefuroxime sodium (p.184·1).
*Bacterial infections.*

**Novadral**
*Pfizer, Austria; Godecke, Ger.; Pfizer, Switz.*
Norfenefrine hydrochloride (p.975·3).
*Hypotension.*

**Novadrel** *Prater, Chile.*
Betamethasone (p.1093·1); clotrimazole (p.396·2).
*Fungal skin infections with inflammation.*

**Novafac** *Silesia, Chile.*
10 Tablets, conjugated oestrogens (p.1543·2); 11 tablets conjugated oestrogens; medroxyprogesterone acetate (p.1557·2).
*Menopausal disorders; osteoporosis.*

**Novafac 30** *Silesia, Chile.*
17 Tablets, conjugated oestrogens (p.1543·2); 13 tablets conjugated oestrogens; medroxyprogesterone acetate (p.1557·2).
*Menopausal disorders; osteoporosis.*

**Novafac CC** *Silesia, Chile.*
Conjugated oestrogens (p.1543·2); medroxyprogesterone acetate (p.1557·2).
*Menopausal disorders; osteoporosis.*

**Novafed A** *Hoechst Marion Roussel, USA.*
Pseudoephedrine hydrochloride (p.1129·2); chlorphenamine maleate (p.427·3).
*Upper respiratory-tract symptoms.*

**Novafem** *Silesia, Chile.*
Medroxyprogesterone acetate (p.1557·2); estradiol cipionate (p.1550·1).
*Combined injectable contraceptive.*

**Novafix** *EciFarma, Chile.*
Cleanser for removable dental appliances.

**Novafix Extra Fuerte** *EciFarma, Chile.*
Vinyl copolymer; carmellose (p.1577·3).
*Dental fixative.*

**Novafur** *Novag, Mex.†.*
Furazolidone (p.605·2).

**Novag Grip** *Novag, Spain.*
Chlorphenamine maleate (p.427·3); pseudoephedrine hydrochloride (p.1129·2); paracetamol (p.76·2).
Formerly contained chlorphenamine maleate, phenylpropanolamine hydrochloride, and paracetamol.
*Cold and influenza symptoms; fever; pain.*

**Novagcilina** *Novag, Spain†.*
Amoxicillin sodium (p.155·3) or amoxicillin trihydrate (p.155·3).
*Bacterial infections.*

**Novagest Expectorant with Codeine** *Major, USA.*
Guaifenesin (p.1122·1); pseudoephedrine hydrochloride (p.1129·2); codeine phosphate (p.27·1).
*Coughs.*

**Novagon** *Novag, Mex.*
Ispaghula (p.1268·1).
*Constipation.*

**Novahaler** *3M, Spain†.*
Beclometasone dipropionate (p.1091·1).
*Asthma.*

**Novahistex C** *Hoechst Marion Roussel, Canad.†.*
Codeine phosphate (p.27·1); phenylephrine hydrochloride (p.1126·3).
*Coughs.*

**Novahistex DH** *Aventis, Canad.*
Hydrocodone tartrate (p.45·1); phenylephrine hydrochloride (p.1126·3).
*Coughs.*

**Novahistex DH Expectorant** *Hoechst Marion Roussel, Canad.†.*
Phenylephrine hydrochloride (p.1126·3); hydrocodone tartrate (p.45·1); guaifenesin (p.1122·1).
*Coughs.*

**Novahistex DM** *Buckley, Canad.†.*
Dextromethorphan hydrobromide (p.1117·3).
Formerly contained dextromethorphan hydrobromide and pseudoephedrine hydrochloride.
*Coughs.*

**Novahistex DM Decongestant** *Buckley, Canad.†.*
Dextromethorphan hydrobromide (p.1117·3); pseudoephedrine hydrochloride (p.1129·2).
*Coughs; respiratory-tract congestion.*

**Novahistex DM Decongestant Expectorant** *Buckley, Canad.†.*
Dextromethorphan hydrobromide (p.1117·3); pseudoephedrine hydrochloride (p.1129·2); guaifenesin (p.1122·1).
*Coughs; respiratory-tract congestion.*

**Novahistex DM Expectorant** *Hoechst Marion Roussel, Canad.†.*
Dextromethorphan hydrobromide (p.1117·3); guaifenesin (p.1122·1); pseudoephedrine hydrochloride (p.1129·2).
Formerly contained dextromethorphan hydrobromide, phenylephrine hydrochloride, and guaifenesin.
*Coughs; nasal/sinus congestion.*

**Novahistex Expectorant** *Hoechst Marion Roussel, Canad.†.*
Guaifenesin (p.1122·1); pseudoephedrine hydrochloride (p.1129·2).
Formerly contained phenylephrine hydrochloride and guaifenesin.
*Respiratory-tract congestion.*

**Novahistine** *Buckley, Canad.†.*
Phenylephrine hydrochloride (p.1126·3).
*Nasal/sinus congestion.*

**Novahistine DH**
*Note. This name is used for preparations of different composition.*
*Aventis, Canad.*
Hydrocodone tartrate (p.45·1); phenylephrine hydrochloride (p.1126·3).
*Coughs.*

*SmithKline Beecham Consumer, USA.*
Codeine phosphate (p.27·1); pseudoephedrine hydrochloride (p.1129·2); chlorphenamine maleate (p.427·3).
*Coughs and cold symptoms; respiratory allergies.*

**Novahistine DM** *Buckley, Canad.†.*
Dextromethorphan hydrobromide (p.1117·3).
Formerly contained dextromethorphan hydrobromide and pseudoephedrine hydrochloride.
*Coughs.*

**Novahistine DM Decongestant** *Buckley, Canad.†.*
Dextromethorphan hydrobromide (p.1117·3); pseudoephedrine hydrochloride (p.1129·2).
*Coughs; respiratory-tract congestion.*

**Novahistine DM Decongestant Expectorant** *Buckley, Canad.†.*
Dextromethorphan hydrobromide (p.1117·3); pseudoephedrine hydrochloride (p.1129·2); guaifenesin (p.1122·1).
*Coughs; respiratory-tract congestion.*

**Novahistine DM Expectorant** *Hoechst Marion Roussel, Canad.†.*
Dextromethorphan hydrobromide (p.1117·3); guaifenesin (p.1122·1); pseudoephedrine hydrochloride (p.1129·2).
Formerly contained dextromethorphan hydrobromide, phenylephrine hydrochloride, and guaifenesin.
*Coughs; nasal/sinus congestion.*

**Novahistine DMX** *SmithKline Beecham Consumer, USA.*
Pseudoephedrine hydrochloride (p.1129·2); dextromethorphan hydrobromide (p.1117·3); guaifenesin (p.1122·1).
*Coughs; nasal congestion.*

**Novain** *Agepha, Austria.*
Oxybuprocaine hydrochloride (p.1382·1).
*Local anaesthesia.*

**Novalac AC**
*Menarini, Fr.; Neo-Farmaceutica, Port.*
Infant feed (p.1417·1).
*Colic; digestive disorders.*

**Novalac AD** *Novalac, Fr.*
Infant feed (p.1417·1).
*Diarrhoea.*

**Novalac AR** *Menarini, Fr.*
Infant feed (p.1417·1).
*Gastro-oesophageal reflux in infants.*

**Novalac HA** *Menarini, Fr.*
Infant feed (p.1417·1).
*Infants with a family history of allergy.*

**Novalan** *Orion, Fin.*
Emollient.
*Skin disorders; vehicle for topical drugs.*

**Novalexin** *Hexa-Medinova, Arg.*
Cefalexin (p.168·1).
*Bacterial infections.*

**Novalgin**
*Aventis, Austria; Aventis, Ger.; Aventis, India; Aventis, Israel; Aventis, Neth.; Hoechst Marion Roussel, Swed.†; Aventis, Thai.*
Dipyrone (p.35·3).
*Fever; pain.*

**Novalgina**
*Aventis, Arg.; Aventis, Braz.; Aventis, Chile; Aventis, Ital.; Hoeport, Port.†.*
Dipyrone (p.35·3).
*Fever; pain.*

**Novalgine**
*Aventis, Belg.; Aventis, Fr.; Aventis, Switz.*
Dipyrone (p.35·3).
*Fever; pain.*

**Novalgrip** *Hexal, Braz.†.*
Dipyrone (p.35·3); ascorbic acid (p.1460·2); sodium camsilate; guaifenesin (p.1122·1); cineole (p.1672·1).
*Cold and influenza symptoms.*

**Novalm** *LDM, Fr.†.*
Meprobamate (p.706·2).
*Anxiety.*

**Novalona** *Andromaco, Chile.*
Hyoscine (p.483·3); oxazepam (p.712·2).
*Smooth muscle spasm.*

**Novalox** *Santa, Gr.*
Aluminium glycinate (p.1249·1); magnesium oxide (p.1272·3).
*Antacid.*

**Novalucol** *Hassle, Swed.*
Calcium carbonate (p.1254·2); magnesium hydroxide (p.1272·2).
*Heartburn.*

**Novaluzid**
*AstraZeneca, Denm.; AstraZeneca, Fin.; AstraZeneca, Malaysia; AstraZeneca, Norw.; Hassle, Swed.*
Aluminium hydroxide (p.1249·2); magnesium hydroxide (p.1272·2); magnesium carbonate (p.1272·1).
*Dyspepsia; gastritis; heartburn; hyperacidity; peptic ulcer.*

**Novamet**
*GlaxoSmithKline, Denm.; SmithKline Beecham, Mex.†.*
Cimetidine (p.1255·3).
*Acid aspiration; gastro-oesophageal reflux; peptic ulcer; Zollinger-Ellison syndrome.*

**Novamilor** *Novopharm, Canad.*
Amiloride hydrochloride (p.858·2); hydrochlorothiazide (p.933·2).
*Hypertension; oedema.*

**Novamin** *Bristol-Myers Squibb, Braz.*
Amikacin sulfate (p.154·1).
*Bacterial infections.*

**Novamina** *PQS, Spain†.*
Benzalkonium chloride (p.1168·3).
*Skin, mucous membrane, and wound disinfection.*

**Novamine** *Clintec, USA.*
Amino-acid infusion (p.1417·1).
*Parenteral nutrition.*

**Novaminsulfon**
*Lichtenstein, Ger.; Ratiopharm, Ger.; Weimer, Hong Kong†.*
Dipyrone (p.35·3).
*Fever; pain.*

**Novamir** *Medinova (Μεντνοβα), Gr.*
Butamirate citrate (p.1116·2).
*Cough.*

**Novamix**
*Orion, Fin.†; Pharmalink, Swed.†.*
Amino-acid, electrolyte, carbohydrate, and lipid (from safflower oil (p.1443·3) and soya oil (p.1447·2)) infusion (p.1417·1).
*Parenteral nutrition.*

**Novamox**
*Note. This name is used for preparations of different composition.*
*Ache, Braz.*
Amoxicillin trihydrate (p.155·3); potassium clavulanate (p.193·3).
*Bacterial infections.*

*Cipla, India.*
Amoxicillin (p.155·3) or amoxicillin trihydrate (p.155·3).
*Bacterial infections.*

**Novamoxin** *Novopharm, Canad.*
Amoxicillin trihydrate (p.155·3).
*Bacterial infections.*

**Novanaest** *Gebro, Austria.*
Procaine hydrochloride (p.1383·2).
*Local anaesthesia.*

**Novaneurina B12** *Kedrion, Ital.†.*
Monophosphothiamine monochloride (p.1455·2); cyanocobalamin (p.1458·2).
*Neuritis; vitamin supplement.*

**Novanox** *Pfleger, Ger.*
Nitrazepam (p.710·1).
*Sleep disorders.*

**Novantron**
*Wyeth Lederle, Austria; Wyeth, Ger.; Lederle, Switz.*
Mitoxantrone hydrochloride (p.575·2).
*Malignant neoplasms.*

**Novantrone**
*Sigma, Austral.; Wyeth Lederle, Belg.; Wyeth, Braz.†; Wyeth-Ayerst, Canad.; Wyeth Lederle, Denm.; Wyeth Lederle, Fin.; Wyeth Lederle, Fr.; Wyeth, Gr.; Wyeth, Hong Kong; Wyeth, Irl.; Lederle, Israel; Wyeth Lederle, Ital.; Wyeth, Malaysia; Wyeth, Mex.†; Wyeth, Neth.; Wyeth Lederle, Norw.; Zuellig, NZ; Wyeth Lederle, Port.†; Wyeth, S.Afr.; Wyeth, Singapore; Wyeth, Spain; Wyeth Lederle, Swed.; Wyeth-Ayerst, Thai.; Wyeth, UK; Serono, USA.*
Mitoxantrone hydrochloride (p.575·2).
*Malignant neoplasms.*

**Novapam**
*Note. This name is used for preparations of different composition.*
*Douglas, NZ†.*
Chlordiazepoxide hydrochloride (p.674·2).
*Anxiety; premedication; skeletal muscle spasm.*

*Asian Pharm, Thai.*
Dipyrone (p.35·3); paracetamol (p.76·2).
*Fever; pain.*

**Novapamyl** *Novalis, Fr.†.*
Verapamil hydrochloride (p.1019·1).
*Hypertension.*

**Novapen** *Pinewood, Irl.*
Ampicillin (p.157·1).
*Bacterial infections.*

**Novaphylline** *Cooper (Κοπερ), Gr.*
Theophylline (p.798·3).
*Asthma; chronic obstructive pulmonary disease; neonatal apnoea and bradycardia.*

**Novapirina** *Novartis Consumer, Ital.*
Diclofenac sodium (p.32·1).
*Fever; pain.*

**Novapres** *Novag, Mex.*
Captopril (p.879·2).
*Hypertension.*

**Novaprin** *Pharmexco, UK.*
Ibuprofen (p.45·3).

**Novapsyl** *Novag, Mex.*
Benzonatate (p.1115·3).
*Coughs.*

**Novarel** *Ferring, USA.*
Chorionic gonadotrophin (p.1320·3).
*Male and female infertility.*

**Novarnela** *Andromaco, Chile.*
Clotrimazole (p.396·2); betamethasone (p.1093·1).
*Fungal skin infections with inflammation.*

**Novarok** *Schering, Jpn.*
Imidapril hydrochloride (p.938·2).
*Hypertension.*

**Novarrutina** *Zurita, Braz.*
Rutoside (p.1688·2); aesculus (p.1648·2); polygonum punctatum; smilax japicanga.
Formerly contained rutoside and aesculus.
*Venous insufficiency.*

**Novartril** *Andromaco, Mex.*
Ibuprofen (p.45·3).
*Fever; inflammation; pain.*

**Novasal** *US Pharmaceutical, USA.*
Magnesium salicylate (p.55·1).
Formerly contained magnesium salicylate and phenyltoloxamine citrate.
*Inflammation; pain.*

**Novasen** *Novopharm, Canad.*
Aspirin (p.15·1).
*Inflammation; pain.*

**Novasone**
*Kirby, Arg.; Essex, Austral.*
Mometasone furoate (p.1107·2).
*Skin disorders.*

**Novasource**
*Novartis Consumer, Austral.; Novartis Consumer, Ital.; Novartis Consumer, Port.*
A range of preparations for enteral nutrition (p.1417·1).

**Novasource 2.0** *Novartis, Braz.*
Preparation for enteral nutrition (p.1417·1).

**Novasource Diabet** *Novartis Nutrition, Fr.*
Preparation for enteral nutrition (p.1417·1).
*Hyperglycaemia.*

**Novasource GI Control**
*Novartis, Fin.; Novartis Nutrition, Fr.*
Preparation for enteral nutrition (p.1417·1).
Formerly known as Sandosource GI Control in *Fin.*
*Diarrhoea.*

**Novasource Megareal** *Novartis Nutrition, Fr.*
Preparation for enteral nutrition (p.1417·1).

**Novasource Peptide** *Novartis Nutrition, Fr.*
Preparation for enteral nutrition (p.1417·1).

**Novasource Pulmonary com Nutrishield** *Novartis, Braz.*
Preparation for enteral nutrition (p.1417·1).
*Respiratory-tract disorders.*

**Novasource Renal**
*Novartis, Arg.; Novartis, Braz.; Novartis Nutrition, Canad.†; Novartis Nutrition, Hong Kong; Novartis Nutrition, USA.*
Preparation for enteral nutrition in renal failure (p.1417·1).

**Novastan** *Mitsubishi, Jpn.*
Argatroban (p.864·3).
*Thromboembolic disorders.*

**Novasten** *Novag, Mex.*
Astemizole (p.424·2).
*Hypersensitivity.*

**NovaStep** *Asche, Ger.*
Levonorgestrel (p.1563·2); ethinylestradiol (p.1553·2).
*Triphasic oral contraceptive.*

**Novasulfon** *Terrier, Mex.*
Dapsone (p.202·2).
*Kaposi's sarcoma; leprosy; Pneumocystis carinii pneumonia; rheumatoid arthritis; skin disorders.*

**Nova-T**
*Berlex, Canad.; Schering, Chile; Schering, Fr.; Schering, Ger.; Schering, Hong Kong; Schering, Israel; Schering, Ital.; Schering, Malaysia; Schering, Mex.; Schering, Neth.; Schering, NZ; Schering, S.Afr.; Schering, Singapore; Schering, Switz.; Schering, Thai.; Schering, UK†.*
Copper-wound plastic (p.1425·3) with a silver core (p.1746·1).
*Intra-uterine contraceptive device.*

**Novatec**
*Merck Sharp & Dohme, Belg.; Merck Sharp & Dohme, Neth.*
Lisinopril (p.946·3).
*Heart failure; hypertension; myocardial infarction.*

**Novativ** *Ativus, Braz.*
Sertraline hydrochloride (p.317·2).
*Depression.*

**Novatox** *Pulitzer, Ital.†.*
Glutathione (p.1040·3).
*Alcohol and drug poisoning; radiation trauma.*

**Novatrex**
*Note. This name is used for preparations of different composition.*
*Ache, Braz.*
Azithromycin (p.159·1).
*Bacterial infections.*

*Wyeth Lederle, Fr.*
Methotrexate (p.568·2).
*Psoriasis; rheumatoid arthritis.*

**Novatrim** *Promeco, Mex.*
Brodimoprim (p.165·3).
*Bacterial infections.*

**Novatropina** *Biolab Sanus, Braz.*
Homatropine methylbromide (p.483·2).
*Smooth muscle spasm.*

**Novavir** *Novag, Mex.†.*
Zidovudine (p.658·2).
*HIV infection.*

**Novaxen** *Novag, Mex.*
Naproxen (p.65·1).
*Inflammation; musculoskeletal and joint disorders; pain.*

**Novazam** *Pharmy, Fr.*
Diazepam (p.690·1).
*Alcohol withdrawal syndrome; anxiety.*

**Novazepam** *Sigma, Braz.*
Bromazepam (p.671·3).
*Anxiety.*

**Novazyd**
*Merck Sharp & Dohme, Belg.; Merck Sharp & Dohme, Neth.*
Lisinopril (p.946·3); hydrochlorothiazide (p.933·2).
*Hypertension.*

**Novegam** *Chinoin, Mex.*
Clenbuterol hydrochloride (p.784·2).
*Obstructive airways disease.*

**Novel** *Maver, Chile.*
Melatonin (p.1710·2).
*Sleep disorders.*

**Novel 1000** *Novel, Ital.†.*
Ginseng (p.1693·1).

**Novel Ginkgo** *Skills, Ital.*
Ginkgo biloba (p.1692·3).

**Novel Jelly** *Novel, Ital.*
Royal jelly (p.1740·3).
*Nutritional supplement.*

**Novelciclina** *Sabater, Spain†.*
Doxycycline hyclate (p.206·2).
*Bacterial infections.*

**Noveldexis** *Pisa, Mex.*
Cisplatin (p.538·1).
*Bladder cancer; ovarian cancer; testicular cancer.*

**Novelian** *Knoll, Spain†.*
Sumatriptan succinate (p.471·2).
*Cluster headache; migraine.*

**Novelmin** *Bunker, Braz.*
Mebendazole (p.108·2).
*Worm infections.*

**Novelon** *Infar, India.*
Desogestrel (p.1547·2); ethinylestradiol (p.1553·2).
*Combined oral contraceptive.*

**Novemina** *Lazar, Arg.*
Dipyrone (p.35·3).
*Fever; pain.*

**Noveril**
*Novartis, Austria; Novartis, Ger.; Novartis, Israel; Novartis, Switz.*
Dibenzepin hydrochloride (p.290·3).
*Depression; nocturnal enuresis.*

**Novesin**
*Novartis Ophthalmics, Hong Kong; Novartis Ophthalmics, Malaysia; Restan, S.Afr.; Novartis Ophthalmics, Singapore; Novartis Ophthalmics, Switz.; Novartis, Thai.*
Oxybuprocaine hydrochloride (p.1382·1).
*Local anaesthesia.*

**Novesina** *Novartis, Ital.*
Oxybuprocaine hydrochloride (p.1382·1).
*Local anaesthesia.*

**Novesine**
*Bournonville, Belg.†; Merck Sharp & Dohme-Chibret, Fr.; Novartis Ophthalmics, Ger.*
Oxybuprocaine hydrochloride (p.1382·1).
*Local anaesthesia.*

**Novhepar** *Coup, Gr.*
Lorazepam (p.704·1).
*Anxiety disorders; insomnia; status epilepticus.*

**Novial** *Organon, Ger.*
Desogestrel (p.1547·2); ethinylestradiol (p.1553·2).
*Triphasic oral contraceptive.*

**Novicarbon** *CTI, Israel.*
Activated charcoal (p.1030·2); senna (p.1288·2); rhubarb (p.1287·3); fennel oil (p.1687·3).
*Constipation; dyspepsia; flatulence.*

**Novid** *Nycomed, Norw.†.*
Aspirin (p.15·1).
*Fever; pain.*

**Novidat** *Temis, Arg.*
Ciprofloxacin hydrochloride (p.188·2).
*Bacterial infections.*

**Novidol** *Sympharma, Switz.†.*
Salicylamide (p.87·3); propyphenazone (p.85·3); caffeine (p.782·1).
*Fever; pain.*

**Novidrine** *Northia, Arg.*
Co-trimoxazole (p.199·3).
*Bacterial infections.*

**Novidroxin** *Fatol, Ger.*
Hydroxocobalamin acetate (p.1458·2).
*Arteritis; arthritic and rheumatic pain; neuralgia; neuritis.*

**Noviform**
*Novartis Ophthalmics, Ger.; Meda, Swed.; Novartis Ophthalmics, Switz.*
Bibrocathol (p.1660·2).
*Eye disorders.*

**Noviforme-Blache** *Chauvin Novopharma, Switz.†.*
Bibrocathol (p.1660·2).
*Eye disorders.*

**Novifort** *Novartis Ophthalmics, Ger.*
Bibrocathol (p.1660·2); hydrocortisone acetate (p.1103·3).
*Allergic and inflammatory disorders of the eye.*

**Novilax** *Eurospital, Ital.*
Sodium lauril sulfoacetate (p.1574·3); sodium citrate (p.1223·2); glycerol (p.1694·3); sorbitol (p.1446·3).
*Constipation.*

**Novim** *Laico, Canad.†.*
Multivitamin and mineral preparation (p.1417·1).

**Novimax** *Anpharm (Ανφαρμ), Gr.*
Doxycycline hyclate (p.206·2).
*Bacterial infections.*

**Novipec** *Montavit, Austria.*
Salverine (p.1741·3); ephedrine (p.1120·1); spike lavender oil (p.1749·2).
*Respiratory-tract disorders.*

**Novirasin** *CTI, Israel.*
Phentermine resinate (p.1592·2).
*Obesity.*

**Novirell B** *Sanorell, Ger.†.*
Thiamine hydrochloride (p.1455·1); pyridoxine hydrochloride (p.1456·3); cyanocobalamin (p.1458·2).
Lidocaine hydrochloride (p.1377·3) is included in this preparation to alleviate the pain of injection.
*Dermatoses; neuralgia; neuritis; rheumatic disorders; spinal disorders.*

**Novirell B Duo** *Sanorell, Ger.*
Thiamine hydrochloride (p.1455·1); pyridoxine hydrochloride (p.1456·3).
Lidocaine hydrochloride (p.1377·3) is included in this preparation to alleviate the pain of injection.
*Dermatoses; neuralgia; neuritis; rheumatic disorders; spinal disorders.*

**Novirell B Mono** *Sanorell, Ger.*
Cyanocobalamin (p.1458·2).
*Megaloblastic anaemia; vitamin $B_{12}$ deficiency.*

**Novital** *Inpharzam, Switz.*
Eucalyptus oil (p.1686·2); japanese mint oil (p.1715·2); pine cone oil; citronella oil (p.1673·2); rosemary oil (p.1740·2); cajuput oil (p.1664·1); pine oil; cypress oil.
*Coughs and colds.*

**Novitan** *Theranol-Deglaude, Fr.†.*
Procaine hydrochloride (p.1383·2); haematoporphyrin (p.1696·2).
*Tonic.*

**Novitropan** *CTI, Israel.*
Oxybutynin hydrochloride (p.486·3).
*Neurogenic bladder; nocturnal enuresis.*

**Novo AC and C** *Novopharm, Canad.*
Aspirin (p.15·1); caffeine (p.782·1); codeine phosphate (p.27·1).
*Pain.*

**Novo Aerofil Sedante** *Reig Jofre, Spain.*
Dimethicone (p.1289·2); metoclopramide hydrochloride (p.1274·3); oxazepam (p.712·2).
*Aerophagia; gastrointestinal dystonias; meteorism.*

**Novo B** *Novopharm, Canad.*
Vitamin B substances and vitamin C (p.1417·1).

**Novo Bacticort** *Montpellier, Arg.*
Diflorasone diacetate (p.1099·3); gentamicin sulfate (p.217·1).
*Infected skin disorders.*

**Novo Bacticort Complex** *Montpellier, Arg.*
Diflorasone diacetate (p.1099·3); gentamicin sulfate (p.217·1); econazole nitrate (p.397·2).
*Infected skin disorders.*

**Novo Dermoquinona** *Llorente, Spain†.*
Mequinol (p.1151·3).
*Hyperpigmentation.*

**Novo E** *Novopharm, Canad.*
*d*-Alpha tocoferil acetate (p.1465·1) or *dl*-alpha tocoferil acetate (p.1465·1).

**Novo V-K** *Novo Nordisk, S.Afr.*
Phenoxymethylpenicillin potassium (p.242·1).
*Bacterial infections.*

**Novo Mandrogallan N** *Dolorgiet, Ger.†.*
Greater celandine (p.1695·3); taraxacum (p.1751·3); absinthium (p.1645·1).
*Biliary-tract disorders; dyspepsia.*

**Novo Melanidina** *Llorente, Spain†.*
Psoralen (p.1153·1).
*Suntanning; vitiligo.*

**Novo Paramicon** *Northia, Arg.*
Econazole (p.397·1).
*Fungal infections.*

**Novo Petrin** *OTW, Ger.*
Paracetamol (p.76·2); propyphenazone (p.85·3); caffeine (p.782·1).
*Fever; pain.*

**Novo Rino** *Bunker, Braz.*
Naphazoline hydrochloride (p.1124·3); sodium chloride (p.1233·3).
*Nasal congestion.*

**Novo Rino-S** *Bunker, Braz.*
Sodium chloride (p.1233·3).
*Nasal congestion.*

**Novo Vagran** *Finadiet, Arg.*
Loratadine (p.436·1).
*Hypersensitivity reactions.*

**Novo Vagran D** *Finadiet, Arg.*
Loratadine (p.436·1); pseudoephedrine sulfate (p.1129·2).

**Novo Vegestabil** *Labinca, Arg.*
Alprazolam (p.668·3); sulpiride (p.722·2).
*Anxiety; depression.*

**Novo Wilpan** *Microsules Bernabo, Arg.*
Ibuprofen (p.45·3); phenylephrine (p.1126·3).
*Cold symptoms; sinusitis.*

**Novo-Alprazol** *Novopharm, Canad.*
Alprazolam (p.668·3).
*Anxiety; sedative.*

**Novo-Atenol** *Novopharm, Canad.*
Atenolol (p.865·2).
*Angina pectoris; hypertension.*

**Novo-AZT** *Novopharm, Canad.*
Zidovudine (p.658·2).
*HIV infection.*

**Novobedouze** *Therabel, Belg.†.*
Hydroxocobalamin acetate (p.1458·2).
*Neuralgia; vitamin $B_{12}$ deficiency.*

**Novobiocyl** *Francia, Ital.*
Cefoperazone sodium (p.174·3).
Lidocaine hydrochloride (p.1377·3) is included in this preparation to alleviate the pain of injection.
*Gram-negative bacterial infections.*

**Novobroncol** *Lafage, Arg.*
Camphor (p.1665·3); menthol (p.1711·3); pine oil; thymol (p.1194·2).
*Respiratory-tract disorders.*

**Novo-Butamide** *Novopharm, Canad.†.*
Tolbutamide (p.348·1).
*Diabetes mellitus.*

**Novo-Butazone** *Novopharm, Canad.†.*
Phenylbutazone (p.83·2).
*Arthritis; inflammation.*

**Novocain**
*Abbott, Canad.; Aventis, Ger.; Abbott, USA.*
Procaine hydrochloride (p.1383·2).
*Local anaesthesia.*

**Novocalm** *Vitamed, Israel.*
Paracetamol (p.76·2); salicylamide (p.87·3); caffeine (p.782·1); codeine phosphate (p.27·1).
*Fever; pain.*

**Novo-Captoril**
*Novopharm, Canad.; Novopharm, Hong Kong.*
Captopril (p.879·2).
*Heart failure; hypertension.*

**Novo-Carbamaz** *Novopharm, Canad.*
Carbamazepine (p.353·3).
*Epilepsy.*

**Novocephal** *Fresenius Kabi, Austria.*
Piracetam (p.1732·1).
*Alcohol or opioid withdrawal syndrome; mental function disorders.*

**Novo-Cerusol** *Bausch & Lomb, Switz.*
Xylene (p.1478·2).
*Ear wax removal.*

**Novocetam** *Lilly, Ger.†.*
Piracetam (p.1732·1).
*Mental function disorders.*

**Novo-Chlorocap** *Novopharm, Canad.†.*
Chloramphenicol (p.185·1).
*Bacterial infections.*

**Novo-Cholamine** *Novopharm, Canad.*
Colestyramine (p.889·3).
*Bile-acid induced diarrhoea; hypercholesterolaemia; pruritus associated with partial biliary obstruction.*

**Novocholin** *Adler, Austria.*
Herba teucrii; agrimony herb (p.1649·1); rhubarb (p.1287·3); peppermint oil (p.1283·2).
*Biliary disorders.*

**Novocilin** *Ache, Braz.*
Amoxicillin trihydrate (p.155·3).
*Bacterial infections.*

**Novocilin Balsamico** *Ache, Braz.†.*
Amoxicillin (p.155·3); bromhexine hydrochloride (p.1115·3).
*Respiratory-tract infections.*

**Novocillin** *Novo Nordisk, S.Afr.*
Procaine benzylpenicillin (p.246·1).
*Bacterial infections.*

**Novo-Cimetine** *Novopharm, Canad.*
Cimetidine (p.1255·3).
*Histamine $H_2$ receptor antagonist.*

**Novo-Clopamine** *Novopharm, Canad.*
Clomipramine hydrochloride (p.289·3).
*Depression; obsessive-compulsive disorder.*

**Novo-Clopate** *Novopharm, Canad.*
Dipotassium clorazepate (p.685·1).
*Anxiety; sedative.*

**Novo-Cloxin** *Novopharm, Canad.*
Cloxacillin sodium (p.198·2).
*Bacterial infections.*

**Novocortal** *Novel, Ital.†.*
Hydrocortisone acetate (p.1103·3).
*Skin disorders.*

**Novo-Cromolyn** *Novopharm, Canad.†.*
Sodium cromoglicate (p.795·3).
*Asthma.*

**Novo-Cycloprine** *Novopharm, Canad.*
Cyclobenzaprine hydrochloride (p.1393·1).
*Skeletal muscle spasm.*

**Novodentin** *Faria, Braz.†.*
Sodium fluoride (p.1444·3).
*Dental caries prophylaxis.*

**Novo-Difenac**
*Novopharm, Canad.; Novopharm, Hong Kong.*
Diclofenac potassium (p.32·1) or diclofenac sodium (p.32·1).
*Inflammation; osteoarthritis; pain; rheumatoid arthritis.*

**Novodig** *Casasco, Arg.*
Pancreatin (p.1725·3); dehydrocholic acid (p.1679·2); simeticone (p.1289·2).

**Novodigal**
*Asta Medica, Austria; Asta Medica, Belg.†; Lilly, Ger.*
Acetyldigoxin (p.851·1) or digoxin (p.895·2).
*Arrhythmias; heart failure.*

**Novodil**
*Note. This name is used for preparations of different composition.*
*Augot, Fr.†.*
Cyclandelate (p.890·3).
*Mental function impairment in the elderly.*
*OFF, Ital.†.*
Dipyridamole (p.903·1).
*Thromboembolic disorders.*

**Novo-Diltazem** *Novopharm, Canad.*
Diltiazem hydrochloride (p.900·1).
*Angina pectoris; hypertension.*

**Novo-Dimenate** *Novopharm, Canad.*
Dimenhydrinate (p.431·1).
*Nausea and vomiting; vertigo.*

**Novo-Dipam** *Novopharm, Canad.†.*
Diazepam (p.690·1).

**Novo-Dipiradol** *Novopharm, Canad.*
Dipyridamole (p.903·1).
*Cardiac disorders.*

**Novo-Doparil** *Novopharm, Canad.†.*
Methyldopa (p.953·2); hydrochlorothiazide (p.933·2).
*Hypertension.*

**Novo-Doxylin** *Novopharm, Canad.*
Doxycycline hyclate (p.206·2).
*Bacterial infections.*

**Novofarma Champu** *Novofarma, Arg.*
Undecenoic acid (p.410·3); menthol (p.1711·3).
*Dandruff; seborrhoea.*

**Novofem**
*Novo Nordisk, Ger.*
Red tablets, estradiol (p.1550·1); white tablets, estradiol; norethisterone acetate (p.1562·2).
*Menopausal disorders; osteoporosis.*
*Novo Nordisk, Irl.; Novo Nordisk, Norw.; Novo Nordisk, UK.*
12 Tablets, estradiol (p.1550·1); norethisterone acetate (p.1562·2); 16 tablets, estradiol.
*Menopausal disorders; osteoporosis.*

**Novofemme** *Novo Nordisk, Fr.*
16 Tablets, estradiol (p.1550·1); 12 tablets, estradiol; norethisterone acetate (p.1562·2).
*Menopausal disorders.*

**Novofen**
*Remedica, Malaysia; Remedica, Thai.*
Tamoxifen citrate (p.584·1).
*Anovulatory infertility; breast cancer.*

**Novofer** *Ache, Braz.*
Ferrous sulfate (p.1428·2); vitamin B substances (p.1417·1).
Ascorbic acid (p.1460·2) is included in this preparation to increase the absorption and availability of iron.
*Iron deficiency; iron-deficiency anaemias.*

**Novo-Ferrogluc** *Novopharm, Canad.*
Ferrous gluconate (p.1428·1).
*Iron-deficiency anaemia.*

**Novo-Ferrosulfate** *Novopharm, Canad.†.*
Ferrous sulfate (p.1428·2).
*Iron-deficiency anaemia.*

**Novo-Fibrate** *Novopharm, Canad.†.*
Clofibrate (p.884·3).
*Hyperlipidaemias.*

**Novo-Fibre** *Novopharm, Canad.*
Grain and citrus fibre (p.1417·1).
*Bowel disorders; constipation; fibre supplement.*

**Novofilin** *Ferrer, Spain.*
Diprophylline (p.784·3); proxyphylline (p.791·2); theophylline (p.798·3).
*Obstructive airways disease.*

**Novo-Flupam** *Novopharm, Canad.†.*
Flurazepam hydrochloride (p.700·3).
*Insomnia.*

**Novo-Flurazine** *Novopharm, Canad.†.*
Trifluoperazine hydrochloride (p.726·3).

**Novo-Flurprofen** *Novopharm, Canad.*
Flurbiprofen (p.43·3).
*Inflammation; pain.*

**Novo-Folacid** *Novopharm, Canad.†.*
Folic acid (p.1429·1).
*Anaemias.*

**Novo-Fumar** *Novopharm, Canad.†.*
Ferrous fumarate (p.1427·3).
*Iron deficiency anaemias.*

**Novo-Furantoin** *Novopharm, Canad.*
Nitrofurantoin (p.237·2).
*Bacterial infections of the urinary tract.*

**Novogel**
*Note. This name is used for preparations of different composition.*
*Morado, Ital.†.*
Royal jelly (p.1740·3); liver extract.
*Nutritional supplement.*
*Ford Medical, UK.*
Hydrogel dressing.
*Wounds.*

**Novogent** *Temmler, Ger.*
Ibuprofen (p.45·3).
*Musculoskeletal and joint disorders.*

**Novo-Gesic** *Novopharm, Canad.*
Paracetamol (p.76·2).
*Fever; pain.*

**Novo-Gesic C** *Novopharm, Canad.*
Paracetamol (p.76·2); caffeine (p.782·1); codeine phosphate (p.27·1).
*Fever; pain.*

**Novogyn** *Schering, Ital.*
Levonorgestrel (p.1563·2); ethinylestradiol (p.1553·2).
*Combined oral contraceptive.*

**Novo-Helisen**
*Allergopharma, Ger.; Allergopharma, Switz.*
Allergen extracts (p.1650·1).
*Allergen immunotherapy.*

**Novo-Herklin 2000** *Armstrong, Mex.*
Permethrin (p.1508·3).
*Pediculosis; scabies.*

**Novo-Hexidyl** *Novopharm, Canad.†.*
Trihexyphenidyl hydrochloride (p.490·2).

**Novo-Hydrazide** *Novopharm, Canad.†.*
Hydrochlorothiazide (p.933·2).
*Hypertension; oedema.*

**Novo-Hydrocort** *Novopharm, Canad.*
Hydrocortisone (p.1103·3).
*Skin disorders.*

**Novo-Hylazin** *Novopharm, Canad.*
Hydralazine hydrochloride (p.931·2).
*Hypertension.*

**Novo-Ipramide** *Novopharm, Canad.*
Ipratropium bromide (p.787·1).
*Bronchodilator.*

**Novo-Keto** *Novopharm, Canad.*
Ketoprofen (p.51·2).
*Fever; pain.*

**Novolax**
*Note. This name is used for preparations of different composition.*
*Medley, Braz.†.*
Liquorice (p.1270·2); cassia pulp (p.1255·2); coriander (p.1676·1); senna (p.1288·2); tamarind (p.1293·2).
*Constipation.*

*Trima, Israel.*
Lactitol (p.1269·1).
*Constipation; hepatic encephalopathy.*

**NovoLet N** *Novo Nordisk, Jpn.*
Isophane insulin injection (human, recombinant) (p.333·3).
*Diabetes mellitus.*

**NovoLet R** *Novo Nordisk, Jpn.*
Insulin injection (human, recombinant) (p.333·3).
*Diabetes mellitus.*

**NovoLet 10R,20R, 30R, 40R, 50R** *Novo Nordisk, Jpn.*
Mixtures of insulin injection (human, recombinant) 10%, 20%, 30%, 40%, and 50% and isophane insulin injection (human, recombinant) 90%, 80%, 70%, 60%, and 50% respectively (p.333·3).
*Diabetes mellitus.*

**Novo-Lexin** *Novopharm, Canad.*
Cefalexin (p.168·1).
*Bacterial infections.*

**Novolin 10/90, 20/80, 30/70, 40/60, 50/50** *Novo Nordisk, Canad.*
Mixtures of insulin injection (human, pyr) and isophane insulin injection (human) in the proportions indicated (p.333·3).
*Diabetes mellitus.*

**Novolin 30/70** *Pisa, Mex.*
Mixture of insulin injection (human) and isophane insulin injection (human) respectively in the proportions indicated (p.333·3).
*Diabetes mellitus.*

**Novolin 70/30** *Novo Nordisk, USA.*
Mixture of isophane insulin suspension (human, crb) 70% and insulin injection (human, crb) 30% (p.333·3).
*Diabetes mellitus.*

**Novolin 90/10, 80/20, 70/30, and 60/40** *Novo Nordisk, Braz.*
Mixtures of isophane insulin injection (human) and insulin injection (human) (p.333·3), respectively, in the proportions indicated.
*Diabetes mellitus.*

**Novolin L**
*Novo Nordisk, Braz.; Pisa, Mex.; Novo Nordisk, USA†.*
Insulin zinc suspension (human) (p.333·3).
*Diabetes mellitus.*

**Novolin Lente** *Novo Nordisk, Canad.*
Insulin zinc suspension (crystalline 70%) (human, pyr) (p.333·3).
*Diabetes mellitus.*

**Novolin N**
*Novo Nordisk, Braz.; Novo Nordisk, Jpn; Pisa, Mex.; Novo Nordisk, USA.*
Isophane insulin suspension (human) (p.333·3).
*Diabetes mellitus.*

**Novolin NPH** *Novo Nordisk, Canad.*
Isophane insulin injection (human, pyr) (p.333·3).
*Diabetes mellitus.*

**Novolin R**
*Novo Nordisk, Braz.; Novo Nordisk, Jpn; Pisa, Mex.; Novo Nordisk, USA.*
Insulin injection (human) (p.333·3).
*Diabetes mellitus.*

**Novolin 30R** *Novo Nordisk, Jpn.*
Mixture of insulin injection (human, recombinant) 30% and isophane insulin (human, recombinant) 70% (p.333·3).
*Diabetes mellitus.*

**Novolin Toronto** *Novo Nordisk, Canad.*
Neutral insulin injection (human, pyr) (p.333·3).
*Diabetes mellitus.*

**Novolin U**
*Novo Nordisk, Braz.; Novo Nordisk, Jpn.*
Insulin zinc suspension (crystalline) (human, recombinant) (p.333·3).
*Diabetes mellitus.*

**Novolin Ultralente** *Novo Nordisk, Canad.*
Insulin zinc suspension (crystalline) (human, pyr) (p.333·3).
*Diabetes mellitus.*

**NovoLog** *Novo Nordisk, USA.*
Insulin aspart (p.339·2).
*Diabetes mellitus.*

**NovoLog Mix 70/30** *Novo Nordisk, USA.*
A mixture of protamine insulin aspart 70% and insulin aspart 30% (p.339·2).
*Diabetes mellitus.*

**Novo-Lorazem** *Novopharm, Canad.*
Lorazepam (p.704·1).
*Anxiety; sedative.*

**Novo-Medopa** *Novopharm, Canad.†.*
Methyldopa (p.953·2).
*Hypertension.*

**Novo-Medrone** *Novopharm, Canad.*
Medroxyprogesterone acetate (p.1557·2).

**Novo-Meprazine** *Novopharm, Canad.*
Levomepromazine maleate (p.703·2).
*Insomnia; nausea; pain; psychoses; vomiting.*

**Novo-Mepro** *Novopharm, Canad.†.*
Meprobamate (p.706·2).
*Anxiety.*

**Novomet** *Novo Nordisk, Austral.*
Metformin hydrochloride (p.342·3).
*Diabetes mellitus.*

**Novo-Methacin** *Novopharm, Canad.*
Indometacin (p.47·3).
*Inflammation; pain.*

**Novo-Metoprol**
*Novopharm, Canad.; Novopharm, Hong Kong.*
Metoprolol tartrate (p.957·1).
*Angina pectoris; hypertension.*

**Novomin**
*Xepa-Soul Pattinson, Hong Kong; Xepa-Soul Pattinson, Malaysia; Xepa-Soul Pattinson, Singapore†.*
Dimenhydrinate (p.431·1).
*Ménière's disease; motion sickness; nausea and vomiting.*

**Novomint N** *Demopharm, Switz.†.*
Cetylpyridinium chloride (p.1173·1); lidocaine hydrochloride (p.1377·3); menthol (p.1711·3).
*Mouth and throat disorders.*

**Novomit** *Klonal, Arg.*
Metoclopramide (p.1274·3).
*Dyspepsia; nausea and vomiting.*

**No-Vomit** *IMA, Braz.*
Metoclopramide (p.1274·3).
*Gastrointestinal motility disorders; nausea and vomiting.*

**NovoMix 30**
*Novo Nordisk, Austral.; Novo Nordisk, Fr.; Novo Nordisk, Ger.; Novo Nordisk, Irl.; Novo Nordisk, Spain; Novo Nordisk, UK.*
A mixture of insulin aspart 30% and protamine insulin aspart 70% (p.339·2).
*Diabetes mellitus.*

**Novo-Mucilax** *Novopharm, Canad.*
Ispaghula (p.1268·1).
*Constipation.*

**Novomyxine** *Thea, Fr.*
Framycetin sulfate (p.215·1); polymyxin B sulfate (p.245·1).
*Bacterial eye infections.*

**Novo-Naprox** *Novopharm, Canad.*
Naproxen (p.65·1) or naproxen sodium (p.65·1).
*Inflammation; pain.*

**Novo-Nastizol** *Bago, Arg.*
Astemizole (p.424·2); pseudoephedrine sulfate (p.1129·2).

**Novonausin** *Camps, Spain.*
Sodium citrate (p.1223·2); cerium oxalate (p.1255·2).
*Nausea and vomiting.*

**Novo-Nidazol** *Novopharm, Canad.*
Metronidazole (p.607·2).
*Trichomoniasis.*

**Novo-Nifedin** *Novopharm, Canad.*
Nifedipine (p.966·2).
*Angina pectoris.*

**NovoNorm**
*Novo Nordisk, Arg.; Novo Nordisk, Austral.; Novo Nordisk, Austria; Novo Nordisk, Belg.; Novo Nordisk, Braz.; Pentafarma, Chile; Novo Nordisk, Denm.; Novo Nordisk, Fin.; Novo Nordisk, Fr.; Novo Nordisk, Ger.; Novo Nordisk, Gr.; Novo Nordisk, Hong Kong; Novo Nordisk, Irl.; Novo Nordisk, Israel; Novo Nordisk, Ital.; Novo Nordisk, Malaysia; Novo Nordisk, Neth.; Novo Nordisk, Norw.; Novo Nordisk, NZ; Novo Nordisk, S.Afr.; Novo Nordisk, Singapore; Novo Nordisk, Spain; Novo Nordisk, Swed.; Novo Nordisk, Switz.; Novo Nordisk, Thai.; Novo Nordisk, UK.*
Repaglinide (p.344·3).
*Diabetes mellitus.*

**Novopac** *Lacefa, Arg.*
Barium sulfate (p.1061·1).
*Radiographic contrast medium.*

**Novopasmil Compuesto** *Lacefa, Arg.*
Hyoscine (p.483·3); dipyrone (p.35·3).

**Novopen** *Novo Nordisk, S.Afr.*
Benzylpenicillin sodium (p.163·2).
*Bacterial infections.*

**Novo-Pen-G** *Novopharm, Canad.†.*
Benzylpenicillin potassium (p.163·2).
*Bacterial infections.*

**Novo-Pen-VK** *Novopharm, Canad.*
Phenoxymethylpenicillin potassium (p.242·1).
*Bacterial infections.*

**Novo-Peridol** *Novopharm, Canad.*
Haloperidol (p.701·2).
*Nausea and vomiting; psychoses.*

**Novo-Pheniram** *Novopharm, Canad.*
Chlorphenamine maleate (p.427·3).

**Novopin MIG** *Schoning-Berlin, Ger.*
Menthol (p.1711·3).
*Headache; migraine.*

**Novo-Pindol** *Novopharm, Canad.*
Pindolol (p.983·2).
*Angina pectoris; hypertension.*

**Novo-Pirocam** *Novopharm, Canad.*
Piroxicam (p.84·2).
*Inflammation; pain.*

**Novoplat** *Pharmacia Upjohn, Mex.†.*
Carboplatin (p.533·3).

**Novoplatinum** *Faulding, Port.*
Carboplatin (p.533·3).

**Novo-Plus** *Novopharm, Canad.†.*
Lactose (p.1438·3).
*Placebo.*

**Novo-Poxide** *Novopharm, Canad.†.*
Chlordiazepoxide hydrochloride (p.674·2).

**Novo-Pramine** *Novopharm, Canad.†.*
Imipramine hydrochloride (p.300·1).
*Depression.*

**Novo-Pranol** *Novopharm, Canad.†.*
Propranolol hydrochloride (p.989·3).
*Cardiac disorders; hypertension; migraine headache; phaeochromocytoma.*

**Novo-Prazin** *Novopharm, Canad.*
Prazosin hydrochloride (p.985·1).
*Hypertension.*

**Novo-Profen** *Novopharm, Canad.*
Ibuprofen (p.45·3).
*Inflammation; pain.*

**Novo-Propamide** *Novopharm, Canad.†.*
Chlorpropamide (p.330·3).
*Diabetes mellitus.*

**Novo-Propoxyn** *Novopharm, Canad.†.*
Dextropropoxyphene hydrochloride (p.28·3).
*Pain.*

**Novoprotect** *Merck dura, Ger.*
Amitriptyline hydrochloride (p.280·3).
*Depression.*

**Novoptine** *Thea, Fr.*
Cetylpyridinium chloride (p.1173·1).
*Eye infections.*

**Novopulmon** *Viatris, Ger.*
Budesonide (p.1094·2).
*Obstructive airways disease.*

**Novo-Purol** *Novopharm, Canad.†.*
Allopurinol (p.412·2).

**Novo-Pyrazone** *Novopharm, Canad.†.*
Sulfinpyrazone (p.417·3).

**Novoquin** *Rayere, Mex.*
Ciprofloxacin hydrochloride (p.188·2).
*Bacterial infections.*

**Novo-Ranidine**
*Novopharm, Canad.; Novopharm, Hong Kong.*
Ranitidine hydrochloride (p.1285·2).
*Gastro-oesophageal reflux; peptic ulcer.*

**NovoRapid**
*Novo Nordisk, Austral.; Novo Nordisk, Denm.; Novo Nordisk, Fin.; Novo Nordisk, Fr.; Novo Nordisk, Ger.; Novo Nordisk, Hong Kong; Novo Nordisk, Irl.; Novo Nordisk, Israel; Novo Nordisk, Ital.; Novo Nordisk, Jpn; Novo Nordisk, Neth.; Novo Nordisk, Norw.; Novo Nordisk, NZ; Novo Nordisk, S.Afr.; Novo Nordisk, Singapore; Novo Nordisk, Spain; Novo Nordisk, Swed.; Novo Nordisk, Switz.; Novo Nordisk, UK.*
Insulin aspart (p.339·2).
*Diabetes mellitus.*

**Novo-Renal** *Novopharm, Canad.†.*
Multivitamin and mineral preparation for dialysis patients (p.1417·1).

**Novo-Ridazine** *Novopharm, Canad.†.*
Thioridazine hydrochloride (p.724·2).
*Psychiatric disorders.*

**Novorutin** *Negma, Israel†.*
Troxerutin (p.1688·3).
*Peripheral vascular disorders.*

**Novo-Rythro** *Novopharm, Canad.†.*
Erythromycin (p.208·1).
*Bacterial infections.*

**Novosal** *Novartis Consumer, Ital.*
Low sodium dietary salt substitute (p.1417·1).

**Novo-Salmol** *Novopharm, Canad.*
Salbutamol (p.791·3) or salbutamol sulfate (p.791·3).
*Obstructive airways disease.*

**Novo-Semide** *Novopharm, Canad.†.*
Furosemide (p.919·3).
*Oedema.*

**NovoSeven**
*Novo Nordisk, Arg.; Novo Nordisk, Austral.; Novo Nordisk, Austria; Novo Nordisk, Belg.; Novo Nordisk, Braz.; Novo Nordisk, Denm.; Novo Nordisk, Fin.; Novo Nordisk, Fr.; Novo Nordisk, Ger.; Novo Nordisk, Hong Kong; Novo Nordisk, Irl.; Novo Nordisk, Israel; Novo Nordisk, Ital.; Novo Nordisk, Jpn; Novo Nordisk, Malaysia; Novo Nordisk, Neth.; Novo Nordisk, Norw.; Novo Nordisk, NZ; Novo Nordisk, S.Afr.; Novo Nordisk, Singapore; Novo Nordisk, Spain; Novo Nordisk, Swed.; Novo Nordisk, Switz.; Novo Nordisk, Thai.; Novo Nordisk, UK; Novo Nordisk, USA.*
Eptacog alfa (activated) (p.750·3).
*Haemorrhagic disorders.*

**Novo-Sorbide** *Novopharm, Canad.†.*
Isosorbide dinitrate (p.941·1).
*Angina pectoris.*

**Novo-Soxazole** *Novopharm, Canad.†.*
Sulfafurazole (p.260·1).

**Novo-Spiroton** *Novopharm, Canad.*
Spironolactone (p.1003·1).
*Hyperaldosteronism.*

**Novo-Spirozine** *Novopharm, Canad.*
Hydrochlorothiazide (p.933·2); spironolactone (p.1003·1).
*Hypertension; oedema.*

**Novospray** *Peters, Fr.†.*
Mixed amphoteric and quaternary ammonium salts; polihexanide (p.1190·1); alcohol (p.1166·1); isopropyl alcohol (p.1184·3).
*Disinfection.*

**Novostrep** *Novo Nordisk, S.Afr.*
Streptomycin sulfate (p.256·2).
*Bacterial infections.*

**Novo-Sucralate** *Novopharm, Canad.*
Sucralfate (p.1290·2).
*Peptic ulcer.*

**Novo-Sundac** *Novopharm, Canad.*
Sulindac (p.91·2).
*Inflammation; pain.*

**Novo-Tears** *Saval, Chile.*
Naphazoline hydrochloride (p.1124·3); hypromellose (p.1579·3); dextran.
*Eye congestion; eye irritation.*

**Novoter**
*Cusi, Hong Kong†; Teofarma, Spain.*
Fluocinonide (p.1101·3).
*Skin disorders.*

**Novoter Gentamicin** *Cusi, Hong Kong†.*
Fluocinonide (p.1101·3); gentamicin sulfate (p.217·1).
*Infected skin disorders.*

**Novoter Gentamicina** *Teofarma, Spain.*
Fluocinonide (p.1101·3); gentamicin sulfate (p.217·1).
*Infected skin disorders.*

**Novo-Tetra** *Novopharm, Canad.*
Tetracycline hydrochloride (p.266·2).
*Bacterial infections.*

**Novo-Thalidone** *Novopharm, Canad.†.*
Chlortalidone (p.882·3).
*Hypertension; oedema.*

**Novo-Theophyl**
*Novopharm, Canad.; Novopharm, Hong Kong.*
Theophylline (p.798·3).
*Bronchospasm.*

**Novothyral**
*Merck, Austria; Merck, Belg.; Merck, Chile; Merck, Ger.; Merck, Switz.*
Liothyronine sodium (p.1602·2); levothyroxine sodium (p.1600·1).
*Adjunct to antithyroid therapy; euthyroid goitre; hypothyroidism; thyroiditis.*

**Novothyrox** *Genpharm, USA.*
Levothyroxine sodium (p.1600·1).
*Hypothyroidism.*

**Novo-Timol** *Novopharm, Canad.*
Timolol maleate (p.1012·2).
*Angina pectoris; hypertension.*

**Novotiral** *Merck, Mex.*
Liothyronine sodium (p.1602·2); levothyroxine sodium (p.1600·1).
*Adjunct to antithyroid therapy; euthyroid goitre; hypothyroidism.*

**Novotossil** *Zambon, Belg.*
Cloperastine fendizoate (p.1117·2) or cloperastine hydrochloride (p.1117·2).
*Coughs.*

**Novo-Triamzide** *Novopharm, Canad.*
Triamterene (p.1016·2); hydrochlorothiazide (p.933·2).
*Hypertension; oedema.*

**Novo-Trimel** *Novopharm, Canad.*
Co-trimoxazole (p.199·3).
*Bacterial infections.*

**Novo-Triolam** *Novopharm, Canad.†.*
Triazolam (p.725·3).
*Insomnia; sedative.*

**Novo-Triphyl** *Novopharm, Canad.†.*
Choline theophyllinate (p.784·2).

**Novo-Tripramine** *Novopharm, Canad.*
Trimipramine maleate (p.320·2).
*Depression.*

**Novo-Triptyn** *Novopharm, Canad.†.*
Amitriptyline hydrochloride (p.280·3).
*Depression.*

**Novotussan** *Gemballa, Braz.*
Oxeladin (p.1126·1); diphenhydramine (p.431·3); ephedrine (p.1120·1); butamirate citrate (p.1116·2).
*Coughs.*

**Novo-Veramil** *Novopharm, Canad.*
Verapamil hydrochloride (p.1019·1).
*Angina pectoris; arrhythmias; hypertension.*

**Novo-Vites** *Novopharm, Canad.*
Multivitamin preparation with or without iron (p.1417·1).

**Novoxapam** *Novopharm, Canad.†.*
Oxazepam (p.712·2).

**Novoxil** *Luper, Braz.*
Amoxicillin (p.155·3).
*Bacterial infections.*

**Novozitron** *Hexa-Medinova, Arg.*
Azithromycin (p.159·1).
*Bacterial infections.*

**Novo-Zolamide** *Novopharm, Canad.†.*
Acetazolamide (p.849·1).

**Novral** *Sintofarma, Braz.†.*
Lisinopril (p.946·3).
*Heart failure; hypertension.*

**Novutrax** *Pisa, Mex.*
Cytarabine (p.543·1).
*Leukaemias; non-Hodgkin's lymphoma.*

**Novuxol**
*Note. This name is used for preparations of different composition.*
*Knoll, Ger.†.*
Enzymes from *Clostridium histolyticum*.
*Cleansing of skin ulcers.*

Smith & Nephew, Neth.
Collagenase (p.1675·1).
*Wound debridement.*

**Novynette** Durascan, Denm.; Gedeon Richter, Hong Kong; Gedeon Richter, Malaysia.
Desogestrel (p.1547·2); ethinylestradiol (p.1553·2).
*Combined oral contraceptive.*

**Nowax** Bell, UK.
Cineole (p.1672·1); nutmeg oil (p.1722·3); terpineol (p.1752·2); arachis oil (p.1656·1).
*Ear wax removal.*

**Noxacorn**
Note. This name is used for preparations of different composition.
Dexxon, Israel.
Salicylic acid (p.1157·1); benzocaine (p.1370·3).
*Corns; warts.*

Roche, Neth.†.
Lidocaine (p.1377·3); salicylic acid (p.1157·1).
*Calluses; corns; warts.*

**Noxalide** Lampugnani, Ital.
Nimesulide (p.67·1).
*Fever; inflammation; pain.*

**Noxema 2-in-1** Procter & Gamble, Canad.
Salicylic acid (p.1157·1).
*Acne.*

**Noxenur** Disperga, Austria†.
Atropine sulfate (p.477·1); ephedrine hydrochloride (p.1120·1); thiamine hydrochloride (p.1455·1).
*Nocturnal enuresis.*

**Noxenur S** Galenika, Ger.†.
Atropine sulfate (p.477·1).
*Nocturnal enuresis.*

**Noxidil** TO-Chemicals, Thai.
Minoxidil (p.960·1).
*Hypertension.*

**Noxiflex** Bago, Chile.
Diclofenac epolamine (p.33·1).
*Musculoskeletal, joint, peri-articular, and soft-tissue disorders.*

**Noxigram** FIRMA, Ital.
Cinoxacin (p.188·1).
*Bacterial infections of the urinary tract.*

**Noxigur** Tegur, Mex.†.
Nitroxoline (p.238·3).

**Noxine** Sriprasit, Thai.
Norfloxacin (p.238·3).
*Bacterial infections.*

**Noxinor** Masa, Thai.
Norfloxacin (p.238·3).
*Bacterial infections.*

**Noxobran** Biomedica-Chemica, Gr.
Gemfibrozil (p.923·1).
*Hyperlipidaemias.*

**Noxom S** Fides, Ger.†.
Homoeopathic preparation.

**Noxotab** Fides, Ger.†.
Homoeopathic preparation.

**Nox-Pain** T Man, Thai.
Methyl salicylate (p.59·3); eugenol (p.1686·2); menthol (p.1711·3).
*Musculoskeletal and joint pain.*

**Noxraxin** Osoth, Thai.
Miconazole nitrate (p.405·3).
*Fungal skin infections.*

**Noxworm** Pond's, Thai.
Mebendazole (p.108·2).
*Worm infections.*

**Noxyflex** Innotech, Fr.
Noxytiolin (p.1187·1).
*Intraperitoneal infections.*

**Noxyflex S**
Geistlich, Irl.; Geistlich, UK.
Noxytiolin (p.1187·1).
*Fungal and bacterial infections.*

**Nozid** Vitalpharma, Belg.
Aluminium hydroxide-magnesium carbonate co-dried gel (p.1250·1); magnesium hydroxide (p.1272·2) or magnesium oxide (p.1272·3).
*Digestive disorders associated with hyperacidity.*

**Nozinan**
Aventis, Arg.; Gerot, Austria; Aventis, Belg.; Aventis, Canad.; Aventis, Denm.; Aventis, Fin.; Aventis, Fr.; IFET (ΙΦΕΤ), Gr.; Aventis, Irl.; Aventis, Israel; Aventis, Ital.; Aventis, Neth.; Pharmacia, Norw.; Aventis, NZ; Vitoria, Port.; Aventis, Swed.; Aventis, Switz.; Link, UK.
Levomepromazine (p.703·2), levomepromazine embonate (p.703·3), levomepromazine hydrochloride (p.703·2), or levomepromazine maleate (p.703·2).
Tablets were formerly known as Veractil in the *UK*.
*Alcohol withdrawal syndrome; anxiety disorders; insomnia; nausea and vomiting; pain; premedication; psychoses.*

**Nozolon** ICN, Mex.†.
Gentamicin (p.219·1).
*Bacterial infections.*

**NPH Iletin I** Lilly, USA†.
Isophane insulin suspension (bovine and porcine) (p.333·3).
*Diabetes mellitus.*

**NPH Iletin II** Lilly, USA.
Isophane insulin suspension (porcine) (p.333·3).
*Diabetes mellitus.*

**N-Statin** Cipla, Austral.
Nystatin (p.406·3).
*Oral candidiasis.*

**NTR** Teofarma, Ital.
Phenylephrine hydrochloride (p.1126·3); thenyldiamine hydrochloride (p.442·1).
*Cold symptoms.*

**NTZ Long Acting Nasal** Sterling Health, USA.
Oxymetazoline hydrochloride (p.1126·1).
*Nasal congestion.*

**Nu-Alpraz** Nu-Pharm, Canad.
Alprazolam (p.668·3).
*Anxiety; sedative.*

**Nu-Amilzide** Nu-Pharm, Canad.
Hydrochlorothiazide (p.933·2); amiloride hydrochloride (p.858·2).
*Hypertension; oedema.*

**Nu-Amoxi** Nu-Pharm, Canad.
Amoxicillin trihydrate (p.155·3).
*Bacterial infections.*

**Nu-Ampi** Nu-Pharm, Canad.
Ampicillin trihydrate (p.157·2).
*Bacterial infections.*

**Nuardin** Tramedico, Belg.
Cimetidine (p.1255·3).
*Gastrointestinal disorders associated with hyperacidity.*

**Nu-Atenol** Nu-Pharm, Canad.
Atenolol (p.865·2).
*Angina pectoris; hypertension.*

**Nu-Baclo** Nu-Pharm, Canad.
Baclofen (p.1386·3).
*Muscle relaxation; skeletal muscle spasticity.*

**Nubain**
Torrex, Austria; Cristalia, Braz.; Du Pont, Canad.; SERB, Fr.; Bristol-Myers Squibb, Ger.; Vianex (Βιανέξ), Gr.; Du Pont, Hong Kong; Boots, Hong Kong; Du Pont, Israel; Bristol-Myers Squibb, Malaysia; Aventis, Mex.; Boots Healthcare, NZ†; Sanofi Omnimed, S.Afr.; Bristol-Myers Squibb, Singapore; Du Pont, Switz.; Bristol-Myers Squibb, Thai.; Boots, Thai.; Bristol-Myers Squibb, UK; Endo, USA.
Nalbuphine hydrochloride (p.64·2).
*Adjunct to anaesthesia; pain; premedication.*

**Nubaina** AstraZeneca, Arg.
Nalbuphine hydrochloride (p.64·2).
*Pain.*

**Nubak** Kampel Martian, Arg.
Nalbuphine (p.64·3).
*Pain.*

**Nubevital BB** Stiefel, Arg.
*SPF 24:* Oxybenzone (p.1154·3); sulisobenzone (p.1158·3); octinoxate (p.1154·3); titanium dioxide (p.1160·3).
*Sunscreen.*

**Nubevital P** Stiefel, Arg.
Oxybenzone (p.1154·3); octinoxate (p.1154·3); titanium dioxide (p.1160·3).
*Sunscreen.*

**Nubevital Sunblock Ultra** Stiefel, Arg.
*SPF 55:* Oxybenzone (p.1154·3); sulisobenzone (p.1158·3); octinoxate (p.1154·3); titanium dioxide (p.1160·3).
*Sunscreen.*

**Nubral**
AB-Consult, Austria; Galderma, Ger.
Urea (p.1162·2).
*Dry skin.*

**Nubral 4** Galderma, Ger.
Urea (p.1162·2); sodium chloride (p.1233·3).
*Dry skin.*

**Nubral Forte** Galderma, Ger.
Urea (p.1162·2); sodium chloride (p.1233·3).
*Skin disorders.*

**Nubral 4 HC** Galderma, Ger.†.
Hydrocortisone (p.1103·3); urea (p.1162·2); sodium chloride (p.1233·3).
*Skin disorders.*

**Nu-Cal** Odan, Canad.
Calcium carbonate (p.1254·2).
*Calcium deficiency.*

**Nu-Capto** Nu-Pharm, Canad.
Captopril (p.879·2).
*ACE inhibitor.*

**Nu-Cephalex** Nu-Pharm, Canad.
Cefalexin (p.168·1).
*Bacterial infections.*

**Nu-Cidex** Johnson & Johnson, Fr.
Peracetic acid (p.1187·3).
*Instrument disinfection.*

**Nu-Cimet** Nu-Pharm, Canad.
Cimetidine (p.1255·3).
*Histamine $H_2$-receptor inhibitor.*

**Nuclav** Knoll, India.
Amoxicillin trihydrate (p.155·3); potassium clavulanate (p.193·3).
*Bacterial infections.*

**Nucleo CMP**
Note. This name is used for preparations of different composition.
Gobbi, Arg.; Gross, Braz.
Disodium cytidine phosphate; trisodium uridine triphosphate (p.1760·3); hydroxocobalamin (p.1458·2).
*Neuralgia; neuritis.*

Ferrer, Spain.
Sodium cytidine monophosphate; disodium uridine diphosphate; disodium uridilic acid; sodium uridine triphosphate (p.1760·3).
*Neuralgias; neuritis.*

**Nucleodoxina** Baldacci, Port.†.
Taurine; adenosine monophosphate potassium; uridine monophosphate potassium; vitamin $B_6$; vitamin $B_{12}$ (p.1417·1).
*Neuromuscular disorders.*

**Nucleserina** Medea, Spain.
Pyridoxine hydrochloride (p.1456·3); ribonucleic acid (p.1738·2); phosphoserine; glutamine (p.1433·2).
*Mental function disorders; tonic.*

**Nuclevit $B_{12}$** Synthelabo, Fr.†.
Nucleotide preparation with cyanocobalamin (p.1458·2) (p.1417·1).
*Tonic.*

**Nuclosina**
ICN, Port.; ICN, Spain.
Omeprazole (p.1278·2).
*Gastro-oesophageal reflux; peptic ulcer; Zollinger-Ellison syndrome.*

**Nu-Cloxi** Nu-Pharm, Canad.
Cloxacillin sodium (p.198·2).
*Bacterial infections.*

**Nucoa** Llorente, Spain†.
Isopropyl myristate (p.1481·2).
*Skin irritation; ulcers; wounds.*

**Nucobrox** Bangkok Lab & Cosmetic, Thai.
Ambroxol hydrochloride (p.1114·3).
*Respiratory-tract disorders associated with increased or viscous mucus.*

**Nucofed** Roberts, USA.
Codeine phosphate (p.27·1); pseudoephedrine hydrochloride (p.1129·2).
*Coughs and cold symptoms.*

**Nucofed Expectorant** Roberts, USA.
Codeine phosphate (p.27·1); pseudoephedrine hydrochloride (p.1129·2); guaifenesin (p.1122·1).
*Coughs and cold symptoms.*

**Nucolox**
Sigma, Austral.; Sigma, NZ.
Ispaghula (p.1268·1); starch (p.1449·1).
*Constipation; hypercholesterolaemia.*

**Nucosef** Pfizer Consumer, Austral.
Codeine phosphate (p.27·1); pseudoephedrine hydrochloride (p.1129·2).
*Coughs; upper respiratory-tract congestion.*

**Nucosef DM** Pfizer Consumer, Austral.
Dextromethorphan hydrobromide (p.1117·3).
*Coughs.*

**Nu-Cotrimox** Nu-Pharm, Canad.
Co-trimoxazole (p.199·3).
*Bacterial infections.*

**Nucotuss Expectorant** Barre-National, USA.
Pseudoephedrine hydrochloride (p.1129·2); guaifenesin (p.1122·1); codeine phosphate (p.27·1).
*Coughs.*

**Nuctalon** Takeda, Fr.
Estazolam (p.697·3).
*Insomnia.*

**Nuctane**
Note. This name is used for preparations of different composition.
Bago, Chile.
Zopiclone (p.729·3).
*Insomnia.*

Armstrong, Mex.
Phenytoin sodium (p.370·2).
*Epilepsy.*

**Nu-Diclo** Nu-Pharm, Canad.
Diclofenac sodium (p.32·1).
*Inflammation; pain.*

**Nu-Diltiaz** Nu-Pharm, Canad.
Diltiazem hydrochloride (p.900·1).
*Angina pectoris; hypertension.*

**Nudopa** Douglas, Austral.†.
Methyldopa (p.953·2).
*Hypertension.*

**Nuelin**
3M, Austral.; 3M, Denm.; 3M, Fin.; 3M, Hong Kong; 3M, Irl.; 3M, Malaysia; 3M, Norw.; 3M, NZ; 3M, S.Afr.; 3M, Singapore; 3M, Thai; 3M, UK.
Theophylline (p.798·3) or theophylline sodium glycinate (p.804·3).
*Obstructive airways disease.*

**Nuevapina** Fabop, Arg.
Aspirin (p.15·1).
*Fever; pain.*

**Nueve Lunas** Hexa-Medinova, Arg.
Pregnancy test (p.1734·3).

**Nufarol** Rafarm, Gr.
Sulpiride (p.722·2).
*Psychoses.*

**Nufex** RPG, India.
Cefalexin (p.168·1).
*Bacterial infections.*

**Nu-Gel**
Note. This name is used for preparations of different composition.
Johnson & Johnson Medical, Fr.; Ethicon, Ital.
*Dressing:* Povidone (p.1581·2).
*Burns; wounds.*

Johnson & Johnson Medical, Fr.; Johnson & Johnson, Israel; Ethicon, Ital.
*Topical gel:* Sodium alginate (p.1577·1).
*Wounds.*

Johnson & Johnson, Ger.
Sodium alginate (p.1577·1); carmellose (p.1577·3); hyetellose (p.1579·2).
*Burns; skin ulcers; wounds.*

Quatromed, S.Afr.†.
Dicycloverine hydrochloride (p.481·2); aluminium hydroxide (p.1249·2); light magnesium oxide (p.1272·3).
*Gastrointestinal disorders.*

**Nuhair** Polipharm, Thai.
Minoxidil (p.960·1).
*Alopecia androgenetica.*

**Nuhist** Dayton, USA.
Phenylephrine tannate (p.1127·2); chlorphenamine tannate (p.428·1).
*Upper respiratory-tract disorders.*

**Nu-Hydral** Nu-Pharm, Canad.
Hydralazine hydrochloride (p.931·2).
*Hypertension.*

**Nuicalm** GlaxoSmithKline Consumer, Belg.
Diphenhydramine hydrochloride (p.431·3).
*Insomnia.*

**Nuidor** Monot, Fr.†.
Phenobarbital (p.367·3); passion flower (p.1729·1); crataegus (p.1677·1).
*Anxiety; insomnia.*

**Nu-Indo** Nu-Pharm, Canad.
Indometacin (p.47·3).
*Inflammation; pain.*

**Nu-Iron** Merz, USA.
Polysaccharide-iron complex (p.1443·2).
*Iron-deficiency anaemia.*

**Nu-Iron V** Merz, USA.
Polysaccharide-iron complex (p.1443·2); folic acid (p.1429·1); vitamins and calcium (p.1417·1).
*Iron-deficiency anaemias.*

**Nu-Iron Plus** Merz, USA†.
Polysaccharide-iron complex (p.1443·2); cyanocobalamin (p.1458·2); folic acid (p.1429·1).
*Iron-deficiency anaemia.*

**Nujol**
Schering-Plough, Braz.; Schering-Plough, Canad.; Fumouze, Fr.†; Schering-Plough, Gr.
Liquid paraffin (p.1479·1).
*Constipation.*

**Nulacin** Goldshield, UK.
Magnesium trisilicate (p.1272·3); heavy magnesium oxide (p.1272·3); calcium carbonate (p.1254·2); heavy magnesium carbonate (p.1272·1); peppermint oil (p.1283·2).
*Gastrointestinal hyperacidity.*

**Nulacin Fermentos** Seid, Spain.
Amylolytic enzymes; proteolytic enzymes; lipolytic enzymes (p.1725·3); dehydrocholic acid (p.1679·2); procaine (p.1383·2).
*Digestive enzyme deficiency.*

**Nulagrip C** Medical, Arg.
Ascorbic acid (p.1460·2); salicylic acid (p.1157·1); caffeine (p.782·1).
*Influenza symptoms.*

**Nularef** Poen, Arg.
Loratadine (p.436·1).
*Hypersensitivity reactions.*

**Nularef Cort** Poen, Arg.
Loratadine (p.436·1); betamethasone (p.1093·1).
*Allergic rhinitis; allergic skin disorders.*

**Nularef-D** Poen, Arg.
Loratadine (p.436·1); pseudoephedrine sulfate (p.1129·2).
*Cold and influenza symptoms; otitis; rhinitis; sinusitis.*

**Nulastres** Duncan, Arg.
Bromazepam (p.671·3).
*Anxiety.*

**Nulceran** Euro-Labor, Port.; Grunenthal, Port.
Famotidine (p.1265·2).
*Gastro-oesophageal reflux; gastrointestinal bleeding; peptic ulcer; Zollinger-Ellison syndrome.*

**Nulcerin** Andromaco, Spain.
Famotidine (p.1265·2).
*Gastro-oesophageal reflux; peptic ulcer; Zollinger-Ellison syndrome.*

**Nuleron** Teofarma, Ital.
Magnesium polygalacturonate; calcium pantothenate (p.1442·3); promethazine hydrochloride (p.439·1); dimeticone (p.1289·2).
*Gastrointestinal disorders associated with excess gas.*

**NuLev** Schwarz, USA.
Hyoscyamine sulfate (p.485·1).

**Nu-Levocarb** Nu-Pharm, Canad.
Levodopa (p.1205·2); carbidopa (p.1204·3).
*Parkinsonism.*

**Nulip** Gufic, India.
Nucleic acid (p.1722·2).
*Viral infections.*

**Nullatuss** Hofmann & Sommer, Ger.
Clobutinol hydrochloride (p.1117·1).
*Coughs.*

**Nulobes** Disprovent, Arg.
Tiratricol (p.1604·3).
*Obesity.*

**Nu-Loraz** Nu-Pharm, Canad.
Lorazepam (p.704·1).
*Anxiety; sedative.*

**Nu-Lotan** Banyu, Jpn.
Losartan potassium (p.947·2).
*Hypertension.*

**NuLytely**
Zodiac, Braz.†; Asofarma, Mex.; Braintree, USA.
Macrogol 3350 (p.1709·1); electrolytes (p.1217·1).
*Bowel evacuation.*

**Numalin** *Raza, Malaysia; Pharmaniaga, Malaysia.*
Theophylline (p.798·3).
*Obstructive airways disease.*

**Numark** *Boehringer Ingelheim, Mex.*
Budesonide (p.1094·2).
*Obstructive airways disease.*

**Numatol** *Spyfarma, Spain.*
Citicoline sodium (p.1672·3).
*Cerebrovascular disorders; tonic.*

**Numbon** *Teva, Israel.*
Nitrazepam (p.710·1).
*Insomnia.*

**Nu-Medopa** *Nu-Pharm, Canad.*
Methyldopa (p.953·2).
*Hypertension.*

**Numencial**
*Note. This name is used for preparations of different composition.*
*Armstrong, Arg.*
Galantamine hydrobromide (p.1491·2).
*Alzheimer's disease.*

*Armstrong, Mex.*
Sulpiride (p.722·2); diazepam (p.690·1).
*Mixed anxiety depressive states.*

**Nu-Metop** *Nu-Pharm, Canad.*
Metoprolol tartrate (p.957·1).
*Angina pectoris; hypertension.*

**Numidan** *Therabel, Ital.†.*
Naproxen piperazine (p.65·3).
*Musculoskeletal, joint, peri-articular, and soft-tissue disorders.*

**Numonyl** *Sanofi Synthelabo, Mex.*
Cineole (p.1672·1); menthol (p.1711·3); camphor (p.1665·3).
*Nasal congestion.*

**Numonyl C** *Sanofi Synthelabo, Mex.*
Chlorphenamine (p.428·1); paracetamol (p.76·2); caffeine (p.782·1).
*Pain.*

**Numonyl D** *Sanofi Synthelabo, Mex.*
Dextromethorphan (p.1117·3).
*Coughs.*

**Numonyl T** *Sanofi Synthelabo, Mex.*
Paracetamol (p.76·2); chlorphenamine (p.428·1); pseudoephedrine (p.1129·2).
*Cold symptoms.*

**Numonyl Tex** *Sanofi Synthelabo, Mex.*
Paracetamol (p.76·2); chlorphenamine (p.428·1); pseudoephedrine (p.1129·2); dextromethorphan (p.1117·3).
*Cold symptoms.*

**Numorphan**
*Du Pont, Canad.; Endo, USA.*
Oxymorphone hydrochloride (p.76·1).
*Adjunct to general anaesthesia; pain; premedication.*

**Numosol** *Medipharm, Chile.*
Oxolamine citrate (p.1126·1).
*Respiratory-tract disorders.*

**Numzident** *Goodys, USA.*
Benzocaine (p.1370·3).
*Oral lesions.*

**Num-Zit**
*Note. A similar name is used for preparations of different composition (see below).*
*Master, Chile.*
Zinc sulfate (p.1469·3).
*Dietary supplement.*

**Numzit**
*Note. A similar name is used for preparations of different composition (see above).*
*Beige, S.Afr.†.*
Benzocaine (p.1370·3); menthol (p.1711·3).
*Teething pain.*

*Goodys, USA.*
*Lotion:* Benzocaine (p.1370·3); glycerol (p.1694·3).
*Topical gel:* Benzocaine (p.1370·3); clove oil (p.1673·3).
*Oral lesions.*

**Nu-Naprox** *Nu-Pharm, Canad.*
Naproxen (p.65·1).
*Inflammation; pain.*

**Nu-Nifed** *Nu-Pharm, Canad.*
Nifedipine (p.966·2).
*Angina pectoris.*

**Nuomin** *Masa, Thai.†.*
Multivitamin and mineral preparation (p.1417·1).

**Nu-Oxybutyn** *Nu-Pharm, Canad.*
Oxybutynin hydrochloride (p.486·3).

**Nu-Pen-VK** *Nu-Pharm, Canad.*
Phenoxymethylpenicillin potassium (p.242·1).
*Bacterial infections.*

**Nupercainal**
*Note. This name is used for preparations of different composition.*
*Novartis, Braz.; Novartis Consumer, Canad.; Novartis, India; Zyma, Switz.†; Eastern Pharmaceuticals, UK; Ciba, USA.*
Cinchocaine (p.1373·2) or cinchocaine hydrochloride (p.1373·2).
*Anorectal disorders; pain; pruritus.*

*Novartis Consumer, Canad.*
*Cream:* Cinchocaine (p.1373·2); domiphen bromide (p.1179·1).
*Pain; pruritus.*

*Ciba, USA.*
*Suppositories:* Zinc oxide (p.1163·2).
*Anorectal disorders.*

**Nupercaine Heavy** *AstraZeneca, Austral.†.*
Cinchocaine hydrochloride (p.1373·2).
*Spinal anaesthesia.*

**Nu-Pindol** *Nu-Pharm, Canad.*
Pindolol (p.983·2).
*Angina pectoris; hypertension.*

**Nu-Pirox** *Nu-Pharm, Canad.*
Piroxicam (p.84·2).
*Inflammation; pain.*

**Nupra** *Grunenthal, Chile.*
Pipemidic acid (p.243·1).
*Urinary-tract infections.*

**Nuprafen** *Beximco, Singapore.*
Naproxen (p.65·1).
*Gout; musculoskeletal and joint disorders; pain.*

**Nu-Prazo** *Nu-Pharm, Canad.*
Prazosin hydrochloride (p.985·1).
*Hypertension.*

**Nuprilan** *Medinfar, Port.*
Ibuprofen (p.45·3).
*Fever; musculoskeletal, joint, peri-articular, and soft-tissue disorders; pain.*

**Nuprin** *Bristol-Myers Products, USA.*
Ibuprofen (p.45·3).
*Fever; osteoarthritis; pain; rheumatoid arthritis.*

**Nuprin Backache** *Bristol-Myers Products, USA.*
Magnesium salicylate (p.55·1).
*Pain.*

**Nu-Prochlor** *Nu-Pharm, Canad.*
Prochlorperazine maleate (p.716·3).
*Psychoses; vomiting.*

**Nur 1 Tropfen Chlorhexidin** *One Drop Only, Ger.*
Chlorhexidine gluconate (p.1173·2).
*Mouth and throat disorders.*

**Nur 1 Tropfen medizinisches Mundwasser**
*One Drop Only, Ger.*
Peppermint oil (p.1283·2); clove oil (p.1673·3); menthol (p.1711·3); sumatra benzoin (p.1751·1).
*Mouth and throat disorders.*

**Nu-Ranit** *Nu-Pharm, Canad.*
Ranitidine hydrochloride (p.1285·2).
*Histamine $H_2$-receptor antagonist.*

**Nurasic** *TO-Chemicals, Thai.*
Orphenadrine citrate (p.486·1); paracetamol (p.76·2).
*Musculoskeletal pain.*

**Nureflex**
*Boots Healthcare, Fr.; Boots Healthcare, Ital.; Boots Healthcare, Spain†.*
Ibuprofen (p.45·3).
*Fever; musculoskeletal, joint, and peri-articular disorders; pain.*

**Nuriban** *Roux-Ocefa, Arg.*
Furosemide diethylaminoethanol (p.921·2).
*Diuretic.*

**Nuriban A** *Roux-Ocefa, Arg.*
Furosemide (p.919·3) amiloride hydrochloride (p.858·2).
*Oedema.*

**Nuri-Kapseln** *Sanochemia, Austria.*
Halibut-liver oil (p.1434·1); cod-liver oil (p.1425·2).
*Vitamin A and D deficiency.*

**Nuril**
*Note. This name is used for preparations of different composition.*
*USV, India.*
Enalapril maleate (p.909·2).
*Heart failure; hypertension; myocardial infarction.*

*Almirall, Spain.*
Pipemidic acid (p.243·1).
*Urinary-tract infections.*

**Nuriphasic** *Nouryphanna, Ger.†.*
7 Tablets, ethinylestradiol (p.1553·2); 15 tablets, lynestrenol (p.1557·1); ethinylestradiol.
*Menorrhagia; menstrual disorders.*

**Nur-Isterate** *Schering, S.Afr.*
Norethisterone enantate (p.1562·2).
*Injectable contraceptive.*

**Nurocain**
*Dentsply, Austral.; AstraZeneca, NZ†.*
Lidocaine (p.1377·3) or lidocaine hydrochloride (p.1377·3).
Adrenaline (p.852·2) is included in this preparation as a vasoconstrictor to diminish absorption and localise the effect of the local anaesthetic.
*Local anaesthesia.*

**Nurocain with Sympathin** *Astra, Austral.†.*
Lidocaine hydrochloride (p.1377·3).
Adrenaline (p.852·2) and noradrenaline (p.974·3) are included in this preparation as vasoconstrictors to diminish absorption and localise the effect of the local anaesthetic.
*Local anaesthesia.*

**Nurofen**
*Boots Healthcare, Austral.; Boots Healthcare, Austria; Boots Healthcare, Belg.; Boots, Denm.†; Boots Healthcare, Fr.; Boots, Ger.; Boots, Hong Kong; Boots Healthcare, Irl.; Boots, Israel; Boots Healthcare, Ital.; Boots Healthcare, Malaysia; Boots Healthcare, Neth.; Boots Healthcare, NZ; Boots Healthcare, S.Afr.; Boots, Singapore; Boots Healthcare, Spain; Astra, Swed.†; Boots, Switz.; Boots, Thai.; Crookes Healthcare, UK.*
Ibuprofen (p.45·3) or ibuprofen lysine (p.46·3).
*Fever; inflammation; musculoskeletal, joint, peri-articular, and soft-tissue disorders; pain.*

**Nurofen Advance** *Crookes Healthcare, UK†.*
Ibuprofen lysine (p.46·3).
*Fever; pain.*

**Nurofen + Codeine** *Boots Healthcare, Belg.†.*
Ibuprofen (p.45·3); codeine phosphate (p.27·1).
*Fever; pain.*

**Nurofen Cold & Flu**
*Boots Healthcare, Austral.; Boots Healthcare, Irl.; Boots Healthcare, NZ; Boots Healthcare, S.Afr.; Crookes Healthcare, UK.*
Ibuprofen (p.45·3); pseudoephedrine hydrochloride (p.1129·2).
*Cold and influenza symptoms.*

**Nurofen Complex** *Boots Healthcare, Spain.*
Ibuprofen (p.45·3); pseudoephedrine hydrochloride (p.1129·2).
*Cold symptoms.*

**Nurofen Migraine** *Crookes Healthcare, UK.*
Ibuprofen lysine (p.46·3).
*Headache; migraine.*

**Nurofen Plus**
*Boots Healthcare, Austral.; Boots Healthcare, Irl.; Boots Healthcare, NZ; Crookes Healthcare, UK.*
Ibuprofen (p.45·3); codeine phosphate (p.27·1).
*Pain.*

**Nurofen Rhume** *Boots Healthcare, Fr.*
Ibuprofen (p.45·3); pseudoephedrine hydrochloride (p.1129·2).
*Cold symptoms.*

**Nurofen Sinus** *Crookes Healthcare, UK.*
Ibuprofen (p.45·3); pseudoephedrine hydrochloride (p.1129·2).
*Cold and influenza symptoms.*

**Nurogrip** *Boots Healthcare, Spain†.*
Ibuprofen (p.45·3); pseudoephedrine hydrochloride (p.1129·2).
*Cold and influenza symptoms.*

**Nurolasts** *Boots Healthcare, Austral.*
Naproxen sodium (p.65·1).

**Nuromax**
*Abbott, Canad.; Glaxo Wellcome, USA.*
Doxacurium chloride (p.1403·1).
*Competitive neuromuscular blocker.*

**Nurse Harvey's Gripe Mixture**
*Note. This name is used for preparations of different composition.*
*Harvey Scruton, Israel.*
Dill oil (p.1680·2); sodium bicarbonate (p.1223·2).
*Infant colic.*

*Harvey-Scruton, UK.*
Dill oil (p.1680·2); caraway oil (p.1667·3); sodium bicarbonate (p.1223·2).
*Infant colic.*

**Nurse Sykes Balsam** *Anglian, UK†.*
Guaifenesin (p.1122·1).
*Coughs.*

**Nurse Sykes Powders** *Anglian, UK.*
Aspirin (p.15·1); paracetamol (p.76·2); caffeine (p.782·1).
*Cold and influenza symptoms; fever; pain.*

**Nursoy**
*Wyeth, Arg.; Wyeth, Braz.; Nestle, Canad.; Wyeth, Chile; Wyeth, Malaysia; Wyeth, Mex.; Wyeth, Singapore.*
Soy protein infant feed (p.1417·1).
*Cow's milk intolerance; galactokinase deficiency; lactose intolerance.*

**Nurture Nourishing** *Heinz-Wattie, NZ.*
Preparation for enteral nutrition in pregnancy and lactation (p.1417·1).

**Nu-Salt** *Cumberland, USA.*
Low sodium dietary salt substitute (p.1417·1).

**Nu-Seals**
*Alliance, Irl.; Alliance, UK.*
Aspirin (p.15·1).
*Fever; inflammation; pain; thromboembolic disorders.*

**Nussidex** *Teva, Israel.*
Dexchlorpheniramine maleate (p.427·3); pseudoephedrine hydrochloride (p.1129·2).
*Allergic rhinitis; cold symptoms.*

**Nustasium** *Labima, Belg.*
Diphenhydramine hydrochloride (p.431·3).
*Insomnia.*

**Nuta** *Osotspa, Thai.*
Paracetamol (p.76·2); chlorphenamine maleate (p.427·3).
Formerly contained paracetamol, chlorphenamine maleate, and phenylpropanolamine hydrochloride.
*Cold symptoms; fever; pain.*

**Nutacough** *Osotspa, Thai.*
Dextromethorphan hydrobromide (p.1117·3); ammonium chloride (p.1115·2); chlorphenamine maleate (p.427·3).
*Coughs.*

**Nutamol** *Osotspa, Thai.*
Paracetamol (p.76·2).
*Fever; pain.*

**Nu-Tears** *Optopics, USA.*
Polyvinyl alcohol (p.1581·1).
*Dry eyes.*

**Nu-Tears II** *Optopics, USA.*
Polyvinyl alcohol (p.1581·1); macrogol 400 (p.1709·1).
*Dry eyes.*

**Nutegen A** *Grisi, Mex.*
Triclocarban (p.1195·1).
*Acne.*

**Nutegen G** *Grisi, Mex.*
Coconut oil (p.1481·1); castor oil (p.1668·2); glycerol (p.1694·3).
*Seborrhoea.*

**Nutegen H** *Grisi, Mex.*
Hypericum (p.299·1).
*Skin hypersensitivity.*

**Nu-Tetra** *Nu-Pharm, Canad.*
Tetracycline hydrochloride (p.266·2).
*Bacterial infections.*

**Nutilis**
*Nutricia, Austral.; Nutricia, Fr.†; Nutricia, Irl.; Baxter, NZ; Nutricia, NZ; Nutricia, Port.; Nutricia Clinical, UK.*
Food thickener (p.1417·1).
*Dysphagia.*

**Nutra Fibra** *Investigacion, Mex.*
Multivitamin and mineral preparation with fibre (p.1417·1).

**Nutra Nutrabain** *Galderma, Fr.†.*
Soap substitute.
*Dry skin.*

**Nutra Nutraderme** *Galderma, Fr.†.*
Liquid paraffin (p.1479·1).
*Dry skin.*

**Nutrabase** *Filorga, Fr.*
Fructo-oligosaccharides; lactic-acid producing organisms; vitamins; magnesium (p.1417·1).
*Restoration of normal gastrointestinal flora.*

**Nutrabeaute** *Filorga, Fr.†.*
Fructo-oligosaccharides; lactic-acid producing organisms; vitamins; minerals; yeast; lappa; borage (p.1417·1).
*Skin disorders.*

**Nutrabiotique** *Filorga, Fr.*
Nutritional supplement (p.1417·1).

**Nutracel**
*Note. This name is used for preparations of different composition.*
*Isdin, Spain.*
Guanosine; inosine (p.1701·2); miconazole nitrate (p.405·3); vitamin F.
*Skin disorders.*

*Baxter, UK.*
Glucose and electrolyte infusion (p.1417·1).
*Parenteral nutrition.*

**Nutracort**
*Galderma, Braz.; Lavipharm, Gr.; Galderma, Mex.; Healthpoint, USA.*
Hydrocortisone (p.1103·3).
*Skin disorders.*

*Orion, Fin.*
Hydrocortisone acetate (p.1103·3).
*Skin disorders.*

**Nutra-D** *Galderma, Austral.*
Emollient.

**Nutraderm**
*Galderma, Arg.; Galderma, Braz.; Galderma, Canad..; Galderma, Chile; Orion, Fin.; Galderma, Mex.; Healthpoint, USA.*
Emollient and moisturiser; pharmaceutical vehicle.

*Galderma, Singapore; Galderma, Thai.†.*
Liquid paraffin (p.1479·1).
*Dry skin; emollient.*

**Nutraderme** *Filorga, Fr.*
Fructo-oligosaccharides; lactic-acid producing organisms; vitamins; minerals; yeast; citrus; lappa; borage (p.1417·1).
*Skin care.*

**Nutradex** *Fresenius Kabi, Swed.*
Carbohydrate and electrolyte infusion (p.1417·1).
*Parenteral nutrition.*

**Nutrafilm** *Giscard, Arg.*
Lactic acid (p.1704·1); silanols.
*Dry skin.*

**Nutraflow** *Alcon, Fr.†.*
Rinsing, neutralising, and storage solution for soft contact lenses (p.1164·2).

**Nutraforme** *Filorga, Fr.*
Fructo-oligosaccharides; lactic-acid producing organisms; vitamins; minerals; yeast; guarana (p.1417·1).
*Tonic.*

**Nutraisdin**
*Note. This name is used for preparations of different composition.*
*Ingens, Arg.*
*Cream:* Dexpanthenol (p.1727·2); zinc oxide (p.1163·2).
*Nappy rash.*
*Lotion:* Dexpanthenol (p.1727·2).
*Moisturiser.*

*Isdin, Port.*
*Cream:* Dexpanthenol (p.1727·2); zinc oxide (p.1163·2); borage oil (p.1661·3); vitamin E (p.1464·3).
*Lotion:* Dexpanthenol (p.1727·2); glycerol (p.1694·3); borage oil (p.1661·3); avocado oil.
*Nappy rash.*

**Nutralcon** *Galderma, Arg.*
Urea (p.1162·2).
*Dry skin disorders.*

**Nutralona** *Galderma, Chile.*
Hydrocortisone (p.1103·3).
*Skin disorders.*

**Nutraloric** *Nutraloric, USA.*
Preparation for enteral nutrition (p.1417·1).

**Nutrament** *Mead Johnson Nutritionals, USA.*
Preparation for enteral nutrition (p.1417·1).

**Nutramigen**
*Mead Johnson, Austral.; Mead Johnson Nutritionals, Fin.; Mead Johnson, Fr.; Mead Johnson, Hong Kong; Mead Johnson, Irl.; Mead Johnson, Israel; Mead Johnson, Ital.; Mead Johnson, NZ†; Mead Johnson,*

*Port.; Mead Johnson Nutritionals, Thai.; Mead Johnson Nutritionals, UK; Mead Johnson Nutritionals, USA.*
Protein hydrolysate preparation for special diets (p.1417·1).
*Galactokinase deficiency; galactosaemia; lactose or sucrose intolerance; protein sensitivity.*

**Nutramince** *Filorga, Fr.*
Fructo-oligosaccharides; lactic-acid producing organisms; vitamins; magnesium; pineapple; citrus; bladderwrack; guarana; black currant; red vine (p.1417·1).
*Obesity.*

**Nutra'Mix** *Beaubour Nutrition, Fr.*
Preparation for enteral nutrition (p.1417·1).

**NutraMX** *Vita Health, Singapore.*
Multivitamin and mineral preparation with ginkgo biloba, ginseng, glutamine, inositol, and lysine (p.1417·1).

**Nutraplus**
*Galderma, Austral.; Galderma, Braz.; Galderma, Chile; Galderma, Fr.; Galderma, Hong Kong; Galderma, Irl.; Galderma, Malaysia; Galderma, Mex.; Galderma, NZ; Pacific, NZ; Galderma, Singapore; Galderma, Spain; Galderma, Switz.; Galderma, UK; Healthpoint, USA.*
Urea (p.1162·2).
*Dry skin; hyperkeratosis.*

**Nutrapurete** *Filorga, Fr.*
Fructo-oligosaccharides; lactic-acid producing organisms; vitamins; magnesium; sorbitol; black currant; black radish; cynara; heather; birch leaf; parsley (p.1417·1).
*Tonic.*

**Nutrarepos** *Filorga, Fr.*
Fructo-oligosaccharides; lactic-acid producing organisms; vitamins; magnesium; calcium; passion flower; valerian; melissa (p.1417·1).
*Sleep disorders; stress.*

**Nutrasoothe** *Brimms, Israel.*
Avena (p.1658·2).
*Skin disorders.*

**Nutra-Soothe** *Pertussin, USA.*
Emollient.

**Nutrasorb**
*Note. This name is used for preparations of different composition.*
*Galderma, Austral.†.*
Acrylate copolymer; glycerol (p.1694·3); menthol (p.1711·3).
*Acne; oily skin.*

*Galderma, Mex.*
Acrylate copolymer; glycerol (p.1694·3).
*Acne; seborrhoea.*

**Nutrasweet**
*Note. This name is used for preparations of different composition.*
*Merisant, Arg.*
Aspartame (p.1422·1).
*Sugar substitute.*

*Rider, Chile.*
Aspartame (p.1422·1); maltodextrin (p.1439·3).
*Sugar substitute.*

**Nutravit Light** *Investigacion, Mex.*
Protein, multivitamin and mineral supplement (p.1417·1).
*Obesity.*

**Nutren**
*Nestle, Braz.; Nestle, Hong Kong; Nestle, Israel; Nestle, Malaysia; Nestle, Thai.; Clintec, USA.*
Range of preparations for enteral nutrition (p.1417·1).

**Nutren IBD** *Nestle, Austral.†.*
Preparation for enteral nutrition (p.1417·1).
*Crohn's disease.*

**Nutr-E-Sol** *Advanced Nutritional Technology, USA.*
Tocofersolan (p.1465·3).
*Vitamin E supplement.*

**Nutrex** *Beta, Ital.†.*
Royal jelly (p.1740·3); pollen; ginkgo biloba (p.1692·3); eleutherococcus (p.1744·1).
*Nutritional supplement.*

**Nutri Concentrated** *Nutricia, Austral.†.*
Preparation for enteral nutrition (p.1417·1).

**Nutri 2000 (Nutrinaut)** *Nutricia, Ital.†.*
Preparation for enteral nutrition (p.1417·1).

**Nutri Twin** *Baxter, Ger.*
Amino-acid, electrolyte, and carbohydrate solution (p.1417·1).
*Parenteral nutrition.*

**Nutri Yin-Nutri Yang** *Neom, Fr.†.*
Nutritional supplement (p.1417·1).
*Tonic.*

**Nu-Triazide** *Nu-Pharm, Canad.*
Triamterene (p.1016·2); hydrochlorothiazide (p.933·2).
*Hypertension; oedema.*

**Nutribraun** *Braun, Port.*
Amino-acid, electrolyte, and lipid (from soya oil (p.1447·2) and medium-chain triglycerides (p.1440·3)) (p.1417·1).
*Parenteral nutrition.*

**Nutrical**
*Nutricia, Ital.*
Preparation for enteral nutrition (p.1417·1).

*Baxter, NZ†; Nutricia, NZ†.*
Nutritional supplement in renal and liver impairment (p.1417·1).

**Nutricalcio** *Nutrilab, Braz.*
Calcium carbonate (p.1254·2).
*Calcium supplement.*

**Nutricap** *Yves Ponroy, Fr.*
Amino-acid, fatty-acid, vitamin, and mineral preparation (p.1417·1).
*Hair and nail disorders.*

**Nutricomp**
*Braun, Irl.†; Braun, Ital.†; Braun, UK†.*
Preparations for enteral nutrition (p.1417·1).

**Nutricon** *Pasadena, USA.*
Multivitamin and mineral preparation with iron and folic acid (p.1417·1).

**Nutricremal** *Novartis Nutrition, Fr.*
High-protein nutritional supplement (p.1417·1).

**Nutrideen** *Bioceuticals, UK.*
Marine protein extract with vitamin C and zinc (p.1417·1).

**Nutridoral** *Novartis Nutrition, Fr.*
High-protein nutritional supplement (p.1417·1).

**Nutridrink**
*Nutricia, Austral.; Support, Braz.; Nutricia, Fin.; Nutricia, Fr.†; Nutricia, Ital.; Baxter, NZ†; Nutricia, NZ†; Nutricia, Port.*
Preparation for enteral nutrition (p.1417·1).

**Nutrifac** *Rising Pharmaceuticals, USA.*
Vitamin and mineral preparation (p.1417·1).

**Nutriflex**
*Braun, Arg.; Braun, Austria; Braun, Belg.†; Braun, Chile; Braun, Fin.; Braun, Fr.; Braun, Ger.; Braun, Hong Kong; Braun, Norw.; Braun, Port.; Braun, Swed.; Braun, Switz.; Braun, UK.*
A range of amino acid, glucose, and electrolyte infusions (p.1417·1).
*Parenteral nutrition.*

**Nutriflex Lipid**
*Note. This name is used for preparations of different composition.*
*Braun, Arg.; Braun, Austria; Braun, Denm.; Braun, Ger.; Bioser (Βιοσερ), Gr.; Braun, Port.*
A range of amino-acid, glucose, and lipid (from soya oil (p.1447·2)) infusions, with or without electrolytes (p.1417·1).
*Parenteral nutrition.*

*Braun, Fin.; Braun, Norw.*
A range of amino-acid, glucose, lipid (from soya oil (p.1447·2) and medium-chain triglycerides (p.1440·3)), and electrolyte infusions (p.1417·1).
*Parenteral nutrition.*

**Nutriflex Lipid N** *Braun, Swed.*
Amino-acid, carbohydrate, electrolyte, and lipid (from soya oil (p.1447·2)) infusion (p.1417·1).
*Parenteral nutrition.*

**Nutriflex Lipide** *Braun, Fr.*
Amino-acid, carbohydrate, electrolyte, and lipid (from soya oil (p.1447·2)) infusion (p.1417·1).
*Parenteral nutrition.*

**NutriFocus** *Ross, USA.*
Preparation for enteral nutrition (p.1417·1).

**Nutrifol** *Pentamedical, Ital.*
Multivitamin and amino-acid preparation (p.1417·1).
*Prevention of hair loss.*

**Nutrigel** *Farbo, Ital.*
Fructose; soya lecithin (p.1706·1); honey (p.1434·2); royal jelly (p.1740·3).

**Nutrigene** *GNR, Fr.†.*
Yellow tablets, deoxyribonucleic acid (p.1679·2); vitamin B substances (p.1417·1); alpha tocopherol acetate; blue tablets, ribonucleic acid (p.1738·2).
The yellow tablets were formerly brown, and the blue tablets formerly contained adenosine triphosphate, ribonucleic acid, magnesium iodide, and horse muscle extract.
*Painful arthritic disorders.*

**Nutrigil** *Novartis Nutrition, Fr.*
A range of preparations for enteral nutrition (p.1417·1).

**NutriHeal** *Nestle, USA.*
Preparation for enteral nutrition (p.1417·1).

**Nutri-Junior**
*Nutricia, Fin.; Nutricia, Ital.*
Infant feed (p.1417·1).
*Hypersensitivity disorders.*

**Nutrilac** *Mellin, Ital.†.*
Infant feed (p.1417·1).
*Lactose intolerance.*

**Nutrilamine** *Braun, Fr.*
Amino-acid infusion (p.1417·1).
*Parenteral nutrition.*

**Nutrilan** *Galagen, USA.*
Lactose-free preparation for enteral nutrition (p.1417·1).

**Nutrilife Pro** *Nutrimed, Fr.*
Nutritional supplement (p.1417·1).

**Nutrilin** *Great Eastern, Thai.; Pediatrica, Thai.*
Multivitamin preparation with iron (p.1417·1).

**Nutrilon AR**
*Nutricia, Fr.; Nutricia, Ital.; Nutricia, Port.*
Infant feed (p.1417·1).
*Gastro-oesophageal reflux.*

**Nutrilon Lactomin** *Nutricia, Port.*
Infant feed (p.1417·1).
*Lactose intolerance.*

**Nutrilon L-K** *Nutricia-Bago, Arg.*
Infant feed (p.1417·1).
*Diarrhoea; lactose intolerance.*

**Nutrilon Pepti**
*Cow & Gate, Irl.; Nutricia, Ital.; Nutricia, Port.*
Infant feed (p.1417·1).
*Cow's milk intolerance.*

**Nutrilon Soja** *Nutricia, Fr.†.*
Infant feed (p.1417·1).
*Diarrhoea.*

**Nutrilon Soya**
*Nutricia-Bago, Arg.; Cow & Gate, Israel; Nutricia, Ital.*
Infant feed (p.1417·1).
*Cow's milk intolerance; galactosaemia; lactose intolerance.*

**Nutrilyte** *American Regent, USA.*
A range of electrolyte preparations (p.1217·1).
*Fluid and electrolyte disorders.*

**Nutrimaiz SM** *Uniao Quimica, Braz.*
Vitamin B substances; glutamic acid; ferric ammonium citrate or ferrous sulfate; magnesium chloride or magnesium sulfate; calcium phosphate (p.1417·1); buclizine hydrochloride (p.426·3); carnitine hydrochloride.
*Reduced appetite; tonic.*

**Nutrimed** *Nutrimed, Fr.*
Preparation for enteral nutrition (p.1417·1).

**Nutri-Mega** *American Health, Hong Kong†.*
Multivitamin and mineral preparation (p.1417·1).

**Nutri-Min** *Chlorella, UK†.*
Mineral and trace element preparation (p.1417·1).

**Nutrineal**
*Baxter, Braz.†; Baxter, Port.†.*
Peritoneal dialysis solution (p.1221·1).

**Nutrineal PD4**
*Baxter, Austria; Baxter, Canad.†; Baxter, Denm.; Baxter, Ger.; Baxter, Israel; Baxter, Spain; Baxter, Swed.; Baxter, Switz.; Baxter, UK.*
Electrolytes; amino acids (p.1221·1).
*Peritoneal dialysis.*

**Nutrineal PD2 and PD4** *Baxter, Ital.*
Calcium chloride; magnesium chloride; sodium lactate; sodium chloride; amino acids (p.1221·1).
*Peritoneal dialysis solution.*

**Nutrini**
*Nutricia, Austral.; Support, Braz.; Nutricia, Fr.; Nutricia, Irl.; Baxter, NZ; Nutricia, NZ; Nutricia, Port.; Nutricia Clinical, UK.*
A range of preparations for enteral nutrition (p.1417·1).

**Nutri-Ped** *Stiefel, Braz.*
Vitamins B substances; minerals; glutamic acid; buclizine hydrochloride (p.426·3); levocarnitine (p.1417·1).
*Nutritional supplement.*

**Nutriperi Lipid** *Braun, Ital.*
An amino-acid, glucose, lipid (from soya oil (p.1447·2) and medium-chain triglycerides (p.1440·3)), and electrolyte infusion (p.1417·1).
*Parenteral nutrition.*

**Nutriplasmal** *Braun, Spain.*
Amino-acid, glucose, and lipid (from soya oil (p.1447·2)) infusion (p.1417·1).
*Parenteral nutrition.*

**NutriPlus** *Nutricia Clinical, UK.*
Preparation for enteral nutrition (p.1417·1).

**Nutriplus Lipid** *Braun, Ital.*
An amino-acid, glucose, and lipid (from soya oil (p.1447·2) and medium-chain triglycerides (p.1440·3)) infusion with or without electrolytes (p.1417·1).

**Nutrisan** *Novartis, India.*
Multivitamin and mineral preparation (p.1417·1).

**NutriScience** *Wassen, UK.*
Selenium; antoxidant vitamins; ubidecarenone; plant extracts (p.1417·1).

**Nutri-Soija** *Nutricia, Fin.*
Infant feed (p.1417·1).
*Cow's milk allergy; lactose intolerance.*

**Nutrisol** *Green Cross Guangzhou, Singapore.*
Amino-acid infusion (p.1417·1).
*Parenteral nutrition.*

**Nutrisol-S** *Green Cross, Malaysia.*
Amino-acid infusion (p.1417·1).
*Parenteral nutrition.*

**Nutrison**
*Nutricia-Bago, Arg.; Nutricia, Austral.; Nutricia, Fin.; Nutricia, Fr.; Nutricia, Irl.; Nutricia, Ital.; Baxter, NZ; Nutricia, NZ; Nutricia, Port.; Nutricia Clinical, UK.*
A range of preparations for enteral nutrition (p.1417·1).
Formerly known as Fortison in the *UK*.

**Nutrison MCT** *Nutricia Clinical, UK.*
Gluten- and fructose-free, low-lactose preparation for enteral nutrition (p.1417·1).
Formerly known as Liquisorbon MCT.
*Fat malabsorption.*

**Nutrison Pepti** *Nutricia Clinical, UK†.*
Gluten-free preparation for enteral nutrition (p.1417·1).

**Nutrisource**
*Novartis Nutrition, Canad.†; Novartis Nutrition, Port.†.*
Preparation for enteral nutrition (p.1417·1).

**Nutrispecial Lipid** *Braun, Ital.*
An amino-acid, glucose, and lipid (from soya oil (p.1447·2) and medium-chain triglycerides (p.1440·3)) infusion with or without electrolytes (p.1417·1).
*Parenteral nutrition.*

**Nutrisun Lait Solaire Insectifuge 16** *Charton, Canad.†.*
*SPF 16:* Avobenzone (p.1142·3); octinoxate (p.1154·3); oxybenzone (p.1154·3).
*Sunscreen.*

**Nutrisun Lait Solaire Insectifuge 30** *Charton, Canad.†.*
*SPF 30:* Avobenzone (p.1142·3); octinoxate (p.1154·3); oxybenzone (p.1154·3); octisalate (p.1154·3).
*Sunscreen.*

**Nutrisun Lotion Solaire Insectifuge 8** *Charton, Canad.†.*
*SPF 8:* Avobenzone (p.1142·3); octinoxate (p.1154·3); oxybenzone (p.1154·3).
*Sunscreen.*

**Nutritrace** *Braun, Fin.*
Trace element preparation (p.1417·1).
*Parenteral nutrition.*

**NutriTwin G** *Fresenius Kabi, Austria.*
Amino-acid, carbohydrate, and electrolyte infusion (p.1417·1).
*Parenteral nutrition.*

**Nutrivisc** *Novartis Ophthalmics, Fr.*
Povidone (p.1581·2).
*Dry eyes.*

**Nutrivit**
*Note. This name is used for preparations of different composition.*
*Makros, Braz.†.*
Multivitamin and mineral preparation with lysine (p.1417·1).

*Dynacren, Ital.*
Brewer's yeast (p.1469·1).

*Medifarma, Mex.*
Vitamin or vitamin and mineral preparation (p.1417·1).
*Anaemias; vitamin deficiency.*

**Nutrizim** *Merck, Braz.*
Pancreatin (p.1725·3); bromelains (p.1662·2); dimethicone (p.1289·2); ox bile (p.1660·3).
*Digestive disorders.*

**Nutrizima** *Merck, Chile.*
Pancreatin (p.1725·3); dimeticone (p.1289·2).
*Digestive disorders.*

**Nutrizym**
*Note. This name is used for preparations of different composition.*
*Merck, Austria†.*
Pancreatin (p.1725·3); bromelains (p.1662·2); ox bile (p.1660·3).
*Digestive disorders.*

*Merck, Irl.; Merck, UK.*
Pancreatin (p.1725·3).
*Pancreatic insufficiency.*

*Merck, Port.†.*
Pancreatin (p.1725·3); bromelains (p.1662·2); ox bile (p.1660·3); dimethicone (p.1289·2).
*Digestive disorders.*

**Nutrizym N** *Cascan, Ger.; GlaxoSmithKline, Ger.*
Pancreatin (p.1725·3).
*Pancreatic insufficiency.*

**Nutrocal** *Wockhardt, India.*
Preparation for enteral nutrition (p.1417·1).

**Nutrocal DM** *Wockhardt, India.*
Preparation for enteral nutrition (p.1417·1).

**Nutrodrip**
*Novartis, Fin.†; Novartis Nutrition, Fr.†; Novartis, Irl.; Novartis Consumer, Ital.†; Novartis, UK.*
A range of preparations for enteral nutrition (p.1417·1).

**Nutrol V** *Rolmex, Canad.*
Betacarotene, selenium, vitamin C, and vitamin E (p.1417·1).

**Nutrol A** *Rolmex, Canad.*
Halibut-liver oil (p.1434·1).

**Nutrol A D** *Rolmex, Canad.*
Vitamin A (p.1451·2); vitamin D (p.1461·2).

**Nutrol B Complex** *Rolmex, Canad.*
A vitamin B preparation (p.1417·1).

**Nutrol C** *Rolmex, Canad.*
Ascorbic acid (p.1460·2).

**Nutrol E** *Rolmex, Canad.*
*d*-Alpha tocoferil acetate (p.1465·1).

**Nutrol E plus Zinc & Selenium** *Rolmex, Canad.*
Vitamin E, zinc, and selenium (p.1417·1).

**Nutrol No 1** *Rolmex, Canad.*
Multivitamin and mineral preparation (p.1417·1).

**Nutrolin-B** *Cipla, India.*
Lactobacillus (p.1704·2); vitamin B substances (p.1417·1).
*Adjunct to antibiotic therapy; aphthous ulcers.*

**Nutropin**
*Roche, Canad.; Ipsen, UK; Genentech, USA.*
Somatropin (p.1327·2).
*Growth failure associated with renal insufficiency; growth hormone deficiency; Turner's syndrome.*

**Nutroplex**
*United American, Hong Kong; United American, Malaysia; United American, Singapore; Great Eastern, Thai.; United American, Thai.*
Ferric ammonium citrate (p.1427·2); vitamins; minerals (p.1417·1).
*Iron-deficiency anaemia; nutritional supplement.*

**Nutroplex with Iron & Lysine**
*United American, Hong Kong; United American, Malaysia; United American, Singapore.*
Multivitamin and mineral preparation with iron and lysine (p.1417·1).
*Tonic.*

**Nutroplex Lysine** *Great Eastern, Thai.; United American, Thai.*
Multivitamin and mineral preparation with iron and lysine (p.1417·1).
*Iron-deficiency anaemia; nutritional supplement.*

**Nutrosa** *Nutricia-Bago, Arg.*
Glucose (p.1432·2).
*Dietary supplement.*

**Nutrox** *Tyson, USA.*
Multivitamin, mineral, and amino-acid preparation (p.1417·1).

**Nuvacthen Depot** *Novartis, Spain.*
Tetracosactide hexa-acetate (p.1340·3).
*Adrenocorticotrophic hormone.*

**Nuvapen** *Reig Jofre, Spain.*
Ampicillin sodium (p.157·1).
*Bacterial infections.*

**NuvaRing**
*Organon, Denm.; Organon, Irl.; Organon, USA.*
Etonogestrel (p.1554·1); ethinylestradiol (p.1553·2).
*Contraceptive vaginal ring.*

**Nuvelle**
*Schering, Denm.; Schering, Irl.; Farmades, Ital.; Schering, NZ; Schering, Port.; Schering, Spain; Schering, UK.*
16 Tablets, estradiol valerate (p.1550·2); 12 tablets, estradiol valerate; levonorgestrel (p.1563·2).
*Menopausal disorders; osteoporosis.*

**Nuvelle Continuous** *Schering, UK.*
Estradiol (p.1550·1); norethisterone acetate (p.1562·2).
*Menopausal disorders; osteoporosis.*

**Nuvelle TS**
*Farmades, Ital.; Schering, UK†.*
Phase I patches, estradiol (p.1550·1); phase II patches, estradiol; levonorgestrel (p.1563·2).
*Menopausal disorders.*

**Nu-Verap** *Nu-Pharm, Canad.*
Verapamil hydrochloride (p.1019·1).
*Angina pectoris; arrhythmias; hypertension.*

**Nuvir** *Infar, India.*
Testosterone undecylate (p.1570·1).
*Male hypogonadism; osteoporosis.*

**Nuvit** *Pharmaland, Thai.*
Vitamin $B_1$ (p.1455·2); vitamin $B_6$ (p.1457·2); vitamin $B_{12}$ (p.1458·2).
*Anorexia; neurasthenia; neurological disorders; neuropathy; toxaemia of pregnancy.*

**Nuvorell** *Sanorell, Ger.*
Homoeopathic preparation.

**Nux ISO** *Iso, Ger.†.*
Homoeopathic preparation.

**Nux Med Complex** *Dynamit, Austria.*
Homoeopathic preparation.

**Nux Vomica Oligoplex** *Madaus, Ger.*
Homoeopathic preparation.

**Nux Vomica-Homaccord** *Peithner, Austria.*
Homoeopathic preparation.

**Nux Vomica-Injeel** *Peithner, Austria.*
Homoeopathic preparation.

**Nuxil** *Dolisos, Canad.*
Homoeopathic preparation.

**Nuzak** *Cipla-Medpro, S.Afr.*
Fluoxetine hydrochloride (p.292·1).
*Bulimia nervosa; depression; obsessive-compulsive disorder.*

**Nyaderm** *Taro, Canad.*
Nystatin (p.406·3).
*Fungal and bacterial infections.*

**Nyal Bronchitis** *ICN, Austral.*
Ammonium chloride (p.1115·2).
Formerly contained ammonium chloride, squill, liquorice, and senega.

**Nyal Chesty Cough** *ICN, Austral.*
Guaifenesin (p.1122·1); glucose (p.1432·2); treacle.
*Coughs; upper respiratory-tract congestion.*

**Nyal Cold Sore** *SmithKline Beecham Consumer, Austral.†.*
*Cream:* Menthol (p.1711·3); camphor (p.1665·3).
*Cracked lips; herpes labialis.*
*Topical lotion:* Benzoin (p.1751·1); menthol (p.1711·3); camphor (p.1665·3).
*Herpes labialis.*

**Nyal Decongestant** *ICN, Austral.*
Phenylephrine hydrochloride (p.1126·3).
*Nasal congestion.*

**Nyal Dry Cough** *ICN, Austral.*
Pentoxyverine citrate (p.1126·2).
*Coughs.*

**Nyal Medithroat Anaesthetic Lozenges** *SmithKline Beecham Consumer, Austral.†.*
Hexylresorcinol (p.1182·1).
*Sore mouth and throat.*

**Nyal Medithroat Gargle** *SmithKline Beecham Consumer, Austral.†.*
Povidone-iodine (p.1190·3).
*Sore throat.*

**Nyal Plus+ Allergy Relief** *ICN, Austral.*
Promethazine hydrochloride (p.439·1).

**Nyal Plus+ Chesty Cough** *ICN, Austral.*
Guaifenesin (p.1122·1); pseudoephedrine hydrochloride (p.1129·2).
*Coughs; nasal congestion.*

**Nyal Plus+ Cold & Flu** *ICN, Austral.*
Codeine phosphate (p.27·1); paracetamol (p.76·2); pseudoephedrine hydrochloride (p.1129·2).
*Cold and influenza symptoms.*

**Nyal Plus+ Day & Night Cold & Flu** *ICN, Austral.*
Day tablets, paracetamol (p.76·2); codeine phosphate (p.27·1); pseudoephedrine hydrochloride (p.1129·2); night tablets, paracetamol; pseudoephedrine hydrochloride; chlorphenamine maleate (p.427·3).
*Cold and influenza symptoms.*

**Nyal Plus+ Day Night Sinus Relief** *ICN, Austral.*
Day tablets, paracetamol (p.76·2); pseudoephedrine hydrochloride (p.1129·2); night tablets, paracetamol; pseudoephedrine hydrochloride; chlorphenamine maleate (p.427·3).
*Upper respiratory-tract congestion.*

**Nyal Plus+ Decongestant** *ICN, Austral.*
Pseudoephedrine hydrochloride (p.1129·2).
*Nasal congestion.*

**Nyal Plus+ Decongestant Antihistamine** *ICN, Austral.*
Chlorphenamine maleate (p.427·3); phenylephrine hydrochloride (p.1126·3).

**Nyal Plus+ Dry Cough** *ICN, Austral.*
Pholcodine (p.1128·3).
*Coughs.*

**Nyal Plus+ Sinus Relief with Antihistamine** *ICN, Austral.*
Chlorphenamine maleate (p.427·3); paracetamol (p.76·2); pseudoephedrine hydrochloride (p.1129·2).

**Nyal Sinus Relief** *ICN, Austral.*
Phenylephrine hydrochloride (p.1126·3).
*Upper respiratory-tract congestion.*

**Nyal Toothache Drops** *ICN, Austral.*
Benzocaine (p.1370·3); phenol (p.1188·1).
*Toothache.*

**Nycodol** *Nycomed, Austria.*
Tramadol hydrochloride (p.94·3).
*Pain.*

**Nycoflox**
*Nycomed, Denm.†; Nycomed, Norw.†.*
Fluoxetine hydrochloride (p.292·1).
*Bulimia nervosa; depression.*

**Nycoheparin** *Leo, Norw.†.*
Heparin sodium (p.928·1).
*Thromboembolic disorders.*

**Nycopin**
*Nycomed, Denm.†; Nycomed, Norw.†.*
Nifedipine (p.966·2).
*Angina pectoris; hypertension.*

**Nycoplus Neo-Fer** *Nycomed, Norw.*
Ferrous fumarate (p.1427·3).
*Iron deficiency; iron-deficiency anaemia.*

**Nycopren**
*Nycomed, Austria; Nycomed, Denm.†; Nycomed, Fin.†; Nycomed, Gr.; Sanofi Synthelabo, Neth.; Nycomed, Switz.; Ardern, UK.*
Naproxen (p.65·1).
*Fever; gout; inflammation; musculoskeletal and joint disorders; pain.*

**Nycovir** *Nycomed, Austria.*
Aciclovir (p.626·1) or aciclovir sodium (p.626·1).
*Herpes simplex infections; varicella-zoster infections.*

**Nydrazid** *Apothecon, USA.*
Isoniazid (p.222·2).
*Tuberculosis.*

**Nyefax**
*Douglas, Austral.; Douglas, NZ; Douglas, Thai.; TTN, Thai.*
Nifedipine (p.966·2).
*Angina pectoris; hypertension.*

**Nylax with Senna** *Crookes Healthcare, UK.*
Senna (p.1288·2).
*Constipation.*

**Nylex** *Proel, Gr.*
Calcitonin (p.768·2).
*Hypercalcaemia; osteoporosis; Paget's disease of bone.*

**Nylipark** *Pharmanik (Φαρμανικ), Gr.*
Sulpiride (p.722·2).
*Psychoses.*

**Nymix Mucolytikum** *Dolorgiet, Ger.†.*
Ambroxol hydrochloride (p.1114·3).
*Respiratory-tract disorders associated with increased or viscous mucus.*

**Nyogel**
*Novartis Ophthalmics, Fr.; Novartis Ophthalmics, Ger.; Novartis Ophthalmics, Irl.; Novartis, Ital.; Novartis Ophthalmics, Port.; Novartis, UK.*
Timolol maleate (p.1012·2).
*Glaucoma; ocular hypertension.*

**Nyolol**
*Novartis Ophthalmics, Braz.; Novartis, Chile; Novartis Ophthalmics, Fr.; Novartis, Gr.; Novartis Ophthalmics, Hong Kong; Ciba Vision, Israel; Novartis Ophthalmics, Malaysia; Novartis, Mex.; Novartis Ophthalmics, Port.; Novartis Ophthalmics, Singapore; Novartis, Spain; Novartis Ophthalmics, Switz.; Novartis, Thai.*
Timolol maleate (p.1012·2).
*Glaucoma; ocular hypertension.*

**NyQuil** *Procter & Gamble, Canad.*
Dextromethorphan hydrobromide (p.1117·3); doxylamine succinate (p.432·3); pseudoephedrine hydrochloride (p.1129·2); paracetamol (p.76·2).
*Coughs and cold symptoms.*

**NyQuil Hot Therapy** *Richardson-Vicks, USA.*
Paracetamol (p.76·2); pseudoephedrine hydrochloride (p.1129·2); dextromethorphan hydrobromide (p.1117·3); doxylamine succinate (p.432·3).
*Coughs and cold symptoms.*

**NyQuil Nighttime Cold/Flu** *Richardson-Vicks, USA.*
Pseudoephedrine hydrochloride (p.1129·2); doxylamine succinate (p.432·3); dextromethorphan hydrobromide (p.1117·3); paracetamol (p.76·2).
*Coughs and cold symptoms.*

**Nyrene** *Planta, Canad.†.*
Melissa (p.1711·1); valerian (p.1762·2).
*Insomnia.*

**Nyrin**
*BPL-Meizler, Braz.*
Calcium levofolinate (p.1431·1).
*Adjuvant to chemotherapy; anaemia; antidote to folic acid antagonists.*
*Korean United, Malaysia.*
Calcium folinate (p.1431·1).
*Adjunct to fluorouracil in colorectal cancer; megaloblastic anaemia; rescue after high-dose methotrexate.*

**Nysconitrine** *Therabel, Belg.*
Glyceryl trinitrate (p.923·2).
*Angina pectoris; heart failure.*

**Nyspes** *DDSA Pharmaceuticals, UK†.*
Nystatin (p.406·3).
*Vaginal candidiasis.*

**Nystacid** *Aspen, S.Afr.*
Nystatin (p.406·3).
*Candidiasis.*

**Nystacortone** *Spirig, Switz.*
Prednisolone acetate (p.1108·1); nystatin (p.406·3); chlorhexidine hydrochloride (p.1173·3).
*Infected skin disorders.*

**Nystaderm** *Dermapharm, Ger.*
Nystatin (p.406·3).
*Fungal infections.*

**Nystaderm comp** *Dermapharm, Ger.*
Nystatin (p.406·3); hydrocortisone acetate (p.1103·3).
*Infected skin disorders.*

**Nystadermal** *Squibb, UK†.*
Nystatin (p.406·3); triamcinolone acetonide (p.1110·2).
*Inflammatory candidiasis.*

**Nystaform**
*Bayer, Irl.; Typharm, UK.*
Nystatin (p.406·3); chlorhexidine hydrochloride (p.1173·3).
*Fungal and bacterial skin infections.*

**Nystaform-HC**
*Bayer, Irl.; Typharm, UK.*
Nystatin (p.406·3); chlorhexidine acetate (p.1173·2) or chlorhexidine hydrochloride (p.1173·3); hydrocortisone (p.1103·3).
*Infected skin disorders.*

**Nystalocal**
*Nourypharma, Ger.; Medinova, Switz.*
Dexamethasone (p.1097·1); chlorhexidine hydrochloride (p.1173·3); nystatin (p.406·3).
*Infected skin disorders.*

**Nystamont**
*IFET (ΙΦΕΤ), Gr.; Rosemont, UK.*
Nystatin (p.406·3).
*Candidiasis.*

**Nystan** *Bristol-Myers Squibb, UK.*
Nystatin (p.406·3).
*Fungal infections.*

**Nystasan** *Bioquimico, Mex.†.*
Nystatin (p.406·3).

**Nystatin-Dome** *Lagap, UK†.*
Nystatin (p.406·3).
*Candidiasis.*

**Nystex** *Savage, USA†.*
Nystatin (p.406·3).
*Candidiasis.*

**Nystin** *Polipharm, Thai.*
Nystatin (p.406·3); diiodohydroxyquinoline (p.603·3); benzalkonium chloride (p.1168·3).
*Vaginal infections.*

**Nystop** *Paddock, USA.*
Nystatin (p.406·3).
*Candidiasis.*

**Nytamel** *Clonmel, Irl.*
Zolpidem tartrate (p.728·3).
*Insomnia.*

**Nytcold Medicine** *Rugby, USA.*
Pseudoephedrine hydrochloride (p.1129·2); dextromethorphan hydrobromide (p.1117·3); doxylamine succinate (p.432·3); paracetamol (p.76·2).
*Coughs and cold symptoms.*

**Nytol**
*Stafford-Miller, Austral.†; Block, Canad.; Block, Ger.†; Stafford-Miller, Ital.; Stafford-Miller, Mex.; Searle, S.Afr.†; Stafford-Miller, Spain; GlaxoSmithKline Consumer, UK; Block, USA.*
Diphenhydramine hydrochloride (p.431·3).
*Insomnia.*

**Nytol Herbal** *GlaxoSmithKline Consumer, UK.*
Lupulus (p.1708·1); Jamaica dogwood (p.1702·3); passion flower (p.1729·1); pulsatilla (p.1737·1); wild lettuce (p.1765·2).
*Insomnia.*

**Nytol Natural Source** *Block, Canad.*
Valerian (p.1762·2).
*Insomnia.*

**O A R** *Colgate Oral Care, Austral.†.*
Sodium nitrite (p.1052·3).
*Rust prevention in disinfecting solutions. Not for use on human skin.*

**O-4 Cycline** *Garec, S.Afr.*
Oxytetracycline hydrochloride (p.241·1).
*Bacterial infections.*

**Oasil** *Gap, Gr.*
Chlordiazepoxide hydrochloride (p.674·2).
*Anxiety disorders.*

**Oasil Simes** *Daker Farmasimes, Spain†.*
Meprobamate (p.706·2).
*Anxiety; insomnia; skeletal muscle spasm.*

**Oat Milk Treatment Cream** *Pierre Fabre, Hong Kong†.*
Avena (p.1658·2); levomenol (p.1707·1).
*Chapped skin; herpes labialis; skin irritation.*

**Oaxen** *Rafarm, Gr.*
Butamirate citrate (p.1116·2).
*Cough.*

**Obaron** *Mepha, Switz.*
Benzbromarone (p.414·3).
*Gout; hyperuricaemia.*

**Obbekjaers** *Bennett, UK.*
Peppermint oil (p.1283·2).
*Irritable bowel syndrome.*

**Obecirol** *Pharmedia (Φαρμεντια), Gr.*
Budesonide (p.1094·2).
*Topical corticosteroid.*

**Obeflorine** *Lehning, Fr.*
Bladderwrack (p.1742·3); cichorium intybus; couchgrass (p.1676·2); equisetum (p.1684·1); ash leaves.
Formerly contained bladderwrack, senna leaflets, liquorice root, and ash leaves.
*Obesity.*

**Obegyn Prenatal** *Fleming, USA.*
Multivitamin preparation (p.1417·1).

**Obelin** *Bergamo, Braz.†.*
Tiratricol (p.1604·3).
*Lipolytic.*

**Obe-Nix** *Holloway, USA†.*
Phentermine hydrochloride (p.1592·2).
*Obesity.*

**Obesan-X** *Technikon, S.Afr.*
Phendimetrazine tartrate (p.1592·1).
*Obesity.*

**Obesidex** *Bunker, Braz.*
Phenolphthalein (p.1284·1); bladderwrack (p.1742·3); thyroid (p.1604·2).
*Obesity.*

**Obesifran** *Faria, Braz.*
Phenolphthalein (p.1284·1); bladderwrack (p.1742·3); thyroid (p.1604·2).
*Obesity.*

**Obestat** *Cipla, India.*
Sibutramine (p.1593·2).
*Obesity.*

**Obetine** *Alpro, Spain.*
Almagate (p.1248·2).
*Dyspepsia; gastritis; gastro-oesophageal reflux; peptic ulcer.*

**Obex-LA** *Adcock Ingram, S.Afr.*
Phendimetrazine tartrate (p.1592·1).
*Obesity.*

**Obifen** *Ayrton, UK.*
Ibuprofen (p.45·3).

**Obimin**
*Westmont, Hong Kong; Westmont, Malaysia; Westmont, Singapore.*
Multivitamin and mineral preparation (p.1417·1).
*Dietary supplement during pregnancy and lactation.*

**Obimin-AF** *Great Eastern, Thai.; Westmont, Thai.*
Multivitamin and mineral preparation (p.1417·1).
*Nutritional supplement.*

**Obimin-AZ** *Great Eastern, Thai.; Westmont, Thai.*
Ferrous fumarate (p.1427·3); vitamins; minerals (p.1417·1).

**Obimol** *Ayrton, UK.*
Paracetamol (p.76·2).

**Obinese** *Pfizer, Mex.*
Chlorpropamide (p.330·3); metformin hydrochloride (p.342·3).
*Diabetes mellitus.*

**O-Biol** *Biol, Arg.*
Nystatin (p.406·3); neomycin sulfate (p.235·1); nitrofurazone (p.238·2); vitamin A (p.1451·2).
*Vaginal infections.*

**O-Biol P** *Biol, Arg.*
Nystatin (p.406·3); neomycin sulfate (p.235·1); polymyxin B sulfate (p.245·1).
*Vaginal infections.*

**Obiron Extra** *Pfizer Consumer, Austral.*
Multivitamin and iron preparation (p.1417·1).

**Obisin** *Casmar, Mex.†.*
Fenproporex (p.1588·3).

**Oblax A-I-I** *Knop, Chile.*
Phenolphthalein (p.1284·1); magnesium oxide (p.1272·3); marine algae.
*Bowel evacuation; constipation.*

**Obleas Chinas** *Maver, Chile.*
Aspirin (p.15·1); caffeine (p.782·1).
*Cold symptoms.*

**Oblioser** *Serono, Spain†.*
Morphine sulfate (p.60·2).
*Pain.*

**Obliterol** *Faes, Spain.*
Pantethine (p.978·3).
*Hyperlipidaemias.*

**Oboliz** *Rafarm, Gr.*
Isoniazid (p.222·2); rifampicin (p.250·2).
*Tuberculosis.*

**Obracin**
*Lilly, Belg.; Lilly, Neth.; Lilly, Switz.*
Tobramycin sulfate (p.271·3).
*Bacterial infections.*

**Obry** Grin, Mex.
Tobramycin (p.271·2).
*Bacterial eye infections.*

**Obrydex** Grin, Mex.
Tobramycin (p.271·2); dexamethasone phosphate (p.1097·2).
*Bacterial eye infections with inflammation.*

**Obrypre** Grin, Mex.
Tobramycin (p.271·2); prednisolone acetate (p.1108·1).
*Bacterial eye infections with inflammation.*

**Obsidan**
Note. This name is used for preparations of different composition.
Verman, Fin.
Ferrous glycine sulfate (p.1428·2).
*Iron deficiency; iron-deficiency anaemia.*

Alpharma-Isis, Ger.
Propranolol hydrochloride (p.989·3).
*Angina pectoris; anxiety; arrhythmias; hypertension; hyperthyroidism; migraine; myocardial infarction; tremor.*

**Obsidan comp** Verman, Fin.
Ferrous glycine sulfate (p.1428·2); folic acid (p.1429·1).
*Iron and folic acid deficiency.*

**Obsilazin N** Alpharma-Isis, Ger.
Propranolol hydrochloride (p.989·3); dihydralazine sulfate (p.899·3).
*Hypertension.*

**Obstar** Johnson & Johnson, Braz.†.
Loperamide hydrochloride (p.1271·1).
*Diarrhoea.*

**Obstetrix** Seyer, USA.
Vitamin and mineral preparation with iron and folic acid (p.1417·1).
Docusate sodium (p.1262·2) is included in this preparation to reduce the constipating effects of iron.

**Obstilax** Sanico, Belg.†.
Sodium picosulfate (p.1289·3).
*Constipation.*

**Obstinol M** Thiemann, Ger.
Liquid paraffin (p.1479·1).
Formerly known as Obstinol mild.
*Bowel regulation.*

**Obtrex** Pronova, USA.
Multivitamin and mineral preparation (p.1417·1).

**Obus Form Therapeutic Heat** Mentholatum, Canad.†.
Methyl salicylate (p.59·3); menthol (p.1711·3).

**Obus Form Therapeutic Ice** Mentholatum, Canad.†.
Menthol (p.1711·3).

**Obusforme**
Note. This name is used for preparations of different composition.
Wampole, Canad.
Paracetamol (p.76·2); methocarbamol (p.1395·1).

Wampole, Canad.
Aspirin (p.15·1); methocarbamol (p.1395·1).

**Obusonid** Velka, Gr.
Budesonide (p.1094·2).
*Allergic rhinitis; topical corticosteroid.*

**Ocacin** Novartis, Spain.
Lomefloxacin hydrochloride (p.227·2).
*Bacterial eye infections.*

**Ocadrik** Aventis, Fr.
Verapamil (p.1021·1); trandolapril (p.1016·1).
*Hypertension.*

**O-Cal** Pharmics, USA.
A range of vitamin and mineral preparations with iron and folic acid (p.1417·1).

**O-Cal Prenatal** Pharmics, USA.
Vitamin and mineral preparation (p.1417·1).

**Occhivit** Giuliani, Ital.
Multivitamin and mineral preparation with myrtillus (p.1417·1).
*Nutritional supplement.*

**Occidal** Ranbaxy, Thai.
Ofloxacin (p.239·3).
*Bacterial infections.*

**Occlucort** GenDerm, Canad.†.
Betamethasone dipropionate (p.1093·1).
*Skin disorders.*

**Occlusal**
Medicis, Canad.; Dermapharm, Irl.; Dermapharm, UK; GenDerm, USA.
Salicylic acid (p.1157·1).
*Warts.*

**Occodem** Pharno-Wedropharm, Ger.
Homoeopathic preparation.

**Occu System** Jagson, India.
Hypromellose (p.1579·3).
*Dry eyes.*

**Ocean** Fleming, USA.
Sodium chloride (p.1233·3).
*Nasal irritation.*

**Oceantone** Cantassium Co., UK.
Green-lipped mussel (p.1696·1).

**Ocefax** Roux-Ocefa, Arg.
Ciprofloxacin (p.188·2).
*Bacterial infections.*

**Oceral**
Asta Medica, Austria; Roche, Braz.; Medika, Switz.
Oxiconazole nitrate (p.407·3).
*Fungal infections; mixed fungal and Gram-positive bacterial infections.*

**Oceral GB** Yamanouchi, Ger.
Oxiconazole nitrate (p.407·3).
*Fungal infections.*

**Ochozim** Italmex, Mex.
Pepsin (p.1729·3); trypsin (p.1758·3); chymotrypsin (p.1671·2); amylase (p.1654·2); lipase; cellulase (p.1669·1); rennet; ox bile extract (p.1660·3); dimeticone (p.1289·2).
*Gastrointestinal disorders.*

**Ocid** Cadila, India.
Omeprazole (p.1278·2).
*Gastro-oesophageal reflux; peptic ulcer; Zollinger-Ellison syndrome.*

**OCL** Abbott, USA.
Macrogol 3350 (p.1709·1); electrolytes (p.1217·1).
*Bowel evacuation.*

**Oclovir** Roux-Ocefa, Arg.
Rimantadine hydrochloride (p.653·1).
*Influenza.*

**OCM** Gobbi, Arg.
Chlordiazepoxide hydrochloride (p.674·2).

**Ocsaar** Merck Sharp & Dohme, Israel.
Losartan potassium (p.947·2).
*Heart failure; hypertension.*

**Ocsaar Plus** Merck Sharp & Dohme, Israel.
Losartan potassium (p.947·2); hydrochlorothiazide (p.933·2).
*Hypertension.*

**Octacosanol** Cantassium Co., UK.
Vitamin E (p.1464·3); octacosanol.

**Octadon P** Thiemann, Ger.
Paracetamol (p.76·2); caffeine (p.782·1).
*Pain.*

**Octagam**
Octapharma, Austria; Bago, Chile; Octapharma, Fr.; Octapharma, Ger.; Octapharma, Hong Kong†; Octapharma, Norw.; Octapharma, Swed.; Octapharma, Switz.; Octapharma, UK.
A normal immunoglobulin (p.1627·2).
*Bone marrow transplantation; Guillain-Barré syndrome; hypogammaglobulinaemia; idiopathic thrombocytopenic purpura; immunodeficiency; Kawasaki disease; passive immunisation.*

**Octamide** Adria, USA.
Metoclopramide hydrochloride (p.1274·3).
*Nausea and vomiting.*

**Octanate**
Octapharma, Austria; Bago, Chile; Octapharma, Ger.
A factor VIII preparation (p.751·1).
*Haemorrhagic disorders.*

**Octanine**
Octapharma, Austria; Octapharma, Ger.
A factor IX preparation (p.752·2).
Formerly known as Octanyne in *Ger.*
*Haemorrhagic disorders.*

**Octanyl** Bago, Arg.
Bromazepam (p.671·3).
*Anxiety.*

**Octanyne**
Bago, Chile; Octapharma, Norw.†.
A factor IX preparation (p.752·2).
*Haemorrhagic disorders.*

**Octaplas**
Octapharma, Austria; Octapharma, Ger.; Kedrion, Ital.; Octapharma, Norw.; Octapharma, Switz.; Octapharma, UK.
Plasma (p.757·3).
*Haemorrhagic disorders; reversal of oral anticoagulant effects; thrombocytopenic purpura.*

**Octatron** VAAS, Ital.
Amino-acid, vitamin, and mineral preparation (p.1417·1).

**Octavi** Octapharma, Norw.†.
A factor VIII preparation (p.751·1).
*Haemorrhagic disorders.*

**Octegra**
Bago, Arg.; Bayer, Austria; Bago, Chile; Elpen (Ελπεν), Gr.; Lilly, Ital.; Vita, Spain.
Moxifloxacin hydrochloride (p.233·1).
*Bacterial infections.*

**Octelmin** Schering-Plough, Braz.
Mebendazole (p.108·2); tiabendazole (p.114·2).
*Worm infections.*

**Octenisept**
Schulke & Mayr, Austria; Schulke & Mayr, Ger.; Schulke & Mayr, Switz.
Octenidine hydrochloride (p.1187·2); phenoxyethanol (p.1189·1).
*Skin and mucous membrane disinfection.*

**Octex** Degorts, Mex.
Co-trimoxazole (p.199·3); guaifenesin (p.1122·1).
*Respiratory-tract infections.*

**Octiban** Degorts, Mex.
Co-trimoxazole (p.199·3).
*Bacterial infections.*

**Octicair** Bausch & Lomb, USA.
Hydrocortisone (p.1103·3); neomycin sulfate (p.235·1); polymyxin B (p.245·2).
*Bacterial ear infections.*

**Octil** Genpharm, Israel.
Timolol maleate (p.1012·2).
*Glaucoma; ocular hypertension.*

**Octilia**
Craveri, Arg.; Bouty, Ital.; SIFI, Singapore.
Tetryzoline hydrochloride (p.1131·2).
*Eye irritation and congestion.*

**Octim** Ferring, Fr.
Desmopressin acetate (p.1322·3).
*Haemorrhage.*

**Octinum** Knoll, Switz.†.
Isometheptene hydrochloride (p.1702·1).
*Migraine; smooth muscle spasm; vegetative dystonia.*

**Octinum-D** Pharmalex (Φαρμαλεξ), Gr.
Octamylamine.
*Smooth muscle spasm.*

**Octiveran** Rafarm, Gr.
Tenoxicam (p.93·1).
*Dysmenorrhoea; gout; inflammation; osteoarthritis; pain; rheumatoid arthritis; spondyloarthropathies.*

**Octocaine**
Clarben, Spain†.
Lidocaine (p.1377·3).
*Local anaesthesia.*

Novocol, USA.
Lidocaine hydrochloride (p.1377·3).
Adrenaline (p.852·2) is included in this preparation as a vasoconstrictor to diminish absorption and localise the effect of the local anaesthetic.
*Local anaesthesia.*

**Octofene**
Fournier, Fr.; Fournier, Ital.; Fournier, Port.
Clofoctol (p.198·1).
*Ear, nose, and throat infections; respiratory-tract infections.*

**Octonativ-M**
Pharmacia Upjohn, Norw.†; Biovitrum, Swed.
A factor VIII preparation (p.751·1).
*Haemorrhagic disorders.*

**Octonox** Pharmacobel, Belg.
Lormetazepam (p.705·2).
*Insomnia.*

**Octopil** Talcris, Arg.
Piroctone.
*Dandruff.*

**Octorax** Demo, Gr.
Enalapril maleate (p.909·2).
*Heart failure; hypertension.*

**Octostim**
Ferring, Arg.; Ferring, Austral.; Ferring, Austria; Ferring, Braz.†; Ferring, Canad.; Ferring, Chile; Ferring, Denm.; Ferring, Fin.; Ferring, Ger.; Ferring, Hong Kong; Ferring, Israel; Ferring, Neth.; Ferring, Norw.; Ferring, NZ; Pharmaco, NZ; Ferring, Singapore; Ferring, Swed.; Ferring, Switz.
Desmopressin acetate (p.1322·3).
*Diabetes insipidus; haemophilia A; platelet dysfunction; test of renal concentrating capacity; von Willebrand's disease.*

**Octotensina** Bioquimico, Mex.†.
Civanetidine.

**Octovit** Goldshield, UK†.
Multivitamin and mineral preparation (p.1417·1).

**Octreoscan**
BSM, Austria; Byk Gulden, Ital.; Mallinckrodt, USA.
Indium-111 pentetreotide (p.1523·3).
*Diagnosis and location of neuroendocrine and carcinoid tumours.*

**Ocubrax**
Alcon, Belg.; Alcon Cusi, Spain.
Diclofenac sodium (p.32·1); tobramycin (p.271·2).
*Ocular inflammation and infection following cataract surgery.*

**Ocu-Caine** Ocumed, USA.
Proxymetacaine hydrochloride (p.1384·1).
*Local anaesthesia.*

**OcuCaps** Akorn, USA.
Antoxidant, vitamin, and mineral supplement (p.1417·1).

**Ocu-Carpine** Ocumed, USA.
Pilocarpine hydrochloride (p.1495·1).
*Glaucoma; raised intra-ocular pressure; reversal of mydriasis.*

**Ocuclear**
Schering, Canad.†; Schering-Plough, Mex.; Schering-Plough, USA.
Oxymetazoline hydrochloride (p.1126·1).
*Minor eye irritation.*

**Ocucoat**
Note. This name is used for preparations of different composition.
Bausch & Lomb, Belg.†; Storz, Israel; Storz, UK†; Bausch & Lomb, USA.
Hypromellose (p.1579·3).
*Adjunct in ocular surgery.*

Bausch & Lomb, USA.
*Eye drops:* Dextran 70 (p.746·2); hypromellose (p.1579·3).
*Dry eyes.*

**Ocudiafan** Eczane, Arg.
Tetryzoline (p.1131·2).
*Eye congestion.*

**Ocufen**
Allergan, Austral.; Allergan, Braz.; Allergan, Canad.; Allergan, Chile; Allergan, Denm.†; Allergan, Fr.; Allergan, Hong Kong; Allergan, Irl.; Allergan, Ital.; Allergan, Mex.; Allergan, NZ; Allergan, S.Afr.; Allergan, Singapore; Allergan, Thai.†; Allergan, UK; Allergan, USA.
Flurbiprofen sodium (p.44·1).
*Intra-operative miosis inhibition; postoperative anterior eye inflammation; prevention of postoperative cystoid macular oedema.*

**Ocuflox**
Allergan, Austral.; Allergan, Canad.; Allergan, Mex.; Allergan, USA.
Ofloxacin (p.239·3).
*Bacterial eye infections.*

**Ocuflur**
Allergan, Austria; Allergan, Belg.; Allergan, Ger.; Alvia (Αλβια), Gr.; FDC, India; Allergan, Port.; Allergan, Spain; Allergan, Switz.
Flurbiprofen sodium (p.44·1).
*Intra-operative miosis inhibition; postoperative eye inflammation and pain; prevention of cystoid macular oedema following cataract surgery.*

**Ocufort** Farmila, Ital.
Multivitamin and mineral preparation (p.1417·1).
*Eye disorders; nutritional supplement.*

**Ocufri** Allergan, Norw.
Polyvinyl alcohol (p.1581·1).
*Dry eyes.*

**Ocugel** Viatris, Belg.
Carbomer 974P (p.1577·2).
*Dry eyes.*

**Ocugram** Charton, Canad.†.
Gentamicin sulfate (p.217·1).
*Bacterial infections.*

**Ocuhist** Pfizer Consumer, USA.
Naphazoline hydrochloride (p.1124·3); pheniramine maleate (p.438·3).
*Eye irritation and pruritus.*

**Oculac**
Novartis, Denm.; Novartis, Fin.; Novartis, Norw.; Novartis Ophthalmics, Swed.; Novartis Ophthalmics, Switz.
Povidone (p.1581·2) (p.1164·2).
*Contact lens wetting solution; dry eyes.*

**Oculastin** Asta Medica, Austria.
Azelastine hydrochloride (p.425·2).
*Allergic conjunctivitis.*

**Oculoforte** Restan, S.Afr.
Zinc sulfate (p.1469·3); phenylephrine hydrochloride (p.1126·3); tetryzoline hydrochloride (p.1131·2).
*Eye irritation.*

**Oculoheel** Peithner, Austria.
Homoeopathic preparation.

**Oculosan**
Note. This name is used for preparations of different composition.
Novartis, Chile; Novartis, Gr.; Novartis Ophthalmics, Hong Kong; Novartis Ophthalmics, Malaysia; Restan, S.Afr.; Novartis, Thai.
Zinc sulfate (p.1469·3); naphazoline nitrate (p.1124·3).
*Eye irritation.*

Novartis Ophthalmics, Switz.
Zinc sulfate (p.1469·3); naphazoline nitrate (p.1124·3); hamamelis (p.1696·3); euphrasia (p.1686·3); neroli oil (p.1719·2); lavender oil (p.1705·2).
*Eye irritation.*

**Oculosan forte** Ciba Vision, Switz.†.
Zinc sulfate (p.1469·3); phenylephrine hydrochloride (p.1126·3); tetryzoline hydrochloride (p.1131·2); hamamelis (p.1696·3).
*Eye irritation.*

**Oculosan N** Novartis Ophthalmics, Ger.
Zinc sulfate (p.1469·3); naphazoline nitrate (p.1124·3).
*Inflammatory and allergic disorders of the eye.*

**Oculotec** Novartis, Chile.
Povidone (p.1581·2).
*Dry eyes.*

**Oculotect**
Note. This name is used for preparations of different composition.
Novartis, Austria; Novartis, Gr.; Novartis Ophthalmics, Malaysia; Ciba Vision, Neth.; Novartis Ophthalmics, Port.; Novartis Ophthalmics, Singapore; Novartis, Spain; Novartis, UK.
Povidone (p.1581·2) (p.1164·2).
*Dry eyes; wetting solution for contact lenses.*

Novartis Ophthalmics, Ger.
*Eye drops:* Vitamin A palmitate (p.1453·1); hypromellose (p.1579·3).
*Dry eyes.*

Novartis Ophthalmics, Ger.; Novartis Ophthalmics, Switz.
Vitamin A palmitate (p.1453·1).
*Corneal damage; dry eyes.*

**Oculotect Fluid** Novartis Ophthalmics, Ger.
Povidone (p.1581·2).
*Dry eyes.*

**Oculotect sine** Novartis Ophthalmics, Ger.
Vitamin A palmitate (p.1453·1).
*Eye disorders.*

**Oculube** Charton, Canad.†.
White soft paraffin (p.1479·3); liquid paraffin (p.1479·1).
*Dry eyes.*

**Ocu-Lube** Ocumed, USA.
White soft paraffin (p.1479·3).
*Dry eyes.*

**Ocu-Mycin** Ocumed, USA.
Gentamicin sulfate (p.217·1).
*Bacterial eye infections.*

**Ocu-Pentolate** Ocumed, USA.
Cyclopentolate hydrochloride (p.480·3).

**Ocu-Phrin** Ocumed, USA.
Phenylephrine hydrochloride (p.1126·3).

**Ocupol** Centaur, India.
Polymyxin B sulfate (p.245·1); chloramphenicol (p.185·1).
*Bacterial ear or eye infections.*

**Ocupol-D** Centaur, India.
Polymyxin B sulfate (p.245·1); chloramphenicol (p.185·1); dexamethasone sodium phosphate (p.1097·2).
*Infected inflammatory ear or eye disorders.*

**Ocupres**
Note. A similar name is used for preparations of different composition

(see below).
Cadila Pharma, India.
Timolol (p.1012·3).
*Glaucoma; ocular hypertension.*

**Ocupress**
Note. A similar name is used for preparations of different composition (see above).
Novartis Ophthalmics, USA.
Carteolol hydrochloride (p.880·3).
*Glaucoma; ocular hypertension.*

**Ocuprost** Biocumed, Arg.
Latanoprost (p.1519·1).
*Ocular hypertension.*

**Ocurest** Centaur, India.
Phenylephrine hydrochloride (p.1126·3); naphazoline hydrochloride (p.1124·3); menthol (p.1711·3); camphor (p.1665·3).
*Eye irritation.*

**Ocurest-AH** Centaur, India.
Phenylephrine hydrochloride (p.1126·3); naphazoline hydrochloride (p.1124·3); menthol (p.1711·3); camphor (p.1665·3); chlorphenamine maleate (p.427·3).
*Conjunctivitis.*

**Ocurest-Z** Centaur, India.
Phenylephrine hydrochloride (p.1126·3); naphazoline hydrochloride (p.1124·3); zinc sulfate (p.1469·3); menthol (p.1711·3); camphor (p.1665·3).
*Eye irritation.*

**Ocusert**
Allergan, Austral.†; Allergan, NZ†; Dominion, UK†; Alza, USA.
Pilocarpine (p.1494·3).
*Glaucoma; ocular hypertension.*

**Ocusoft Pads** Poen, Arg.
Eyelid cleanser.

**Ocusoft VMS**
Poen, Arg.; Ocusoft, USA.
Multivitamin and mineral preparation (p.1417·1).

**Ocusol**
ANB, Malaysia; ANB, Thai.
Calcium chloride; magnesium chloride; potassium chloride; sodium acetate; sodium chloride; sodium citrate (p.1217·1).
*Irrigation during eye surgery.*

**Ocu-Spor-B** Ocumed, USA.
Polymyxin B sulfate (p.245·1); neomycin sulfate (p.235·1); bacitracin zinc (p.161·3).
*Eye infections.*

**Ocu-Spor-G** Ocumed, USA.
Polymyxin B sulfate (p.245·1); neomycin sulfate (p.235·1); gramicidin (p.220·2).
*Eye infections.*

**Ocustil** SIFI, Ital.
Sodium hyaluronate (p.1697·3).
*Eye protection.*

**Ocustress** Farmila, Ital.
Multivitamin preparation with ubidecarenone and ginseng (p.1417·1).
*Nutritional supplement.*

**Ocusulf-10** Optopics, USA.
Sulfacetamide sodium (p.257·3).
*Eye infections.*

**Ocutears**
Note. A similar name is used for preparations of different composition (see below).
Charton, Canad.†.
Hypromellose (p.1579·3); dextran 40 (p.745·3).
*Dry eyes.*

**Ocu-Tears**
Note. A similar name is used for preparations of different composition (see above).
Ocumed, USA.
Polyvinyl alcohol (p.1581·1).
*Dry eyes.*

**Ocuton** Ritter, Hong Kong.
Oxedrine hydrochloride (p.977·3).
*Eye irritation.*

**Ocutricin** Bausch & Lomb, USA.
*Eye drops:* Polymyxin B sulfate (p.245·1); neomycin sulfate (p.235·1); gramicidin (p.220·2).
*Eye ointment:* Polymyxin B sulfate (p.245·1); neomycin sulfate (p.235·1); bacitracin zinc (p.161·3).
*Eye infections.*

**Ocutrien** Cantassium Co., UK.
Multivitamin and mineral preparation (p.1417·1).

**Ocu-Trol** Ocumed, USA.
Polymyxin B sulfate (p.245·1); neomycin sulfate (p.235·1); dexamethasone (p.1097·1).
*Infected eye disorders.*

**Ocu-Tropic** Ocumed, USA.
Tropicamide (p.491·1).

**Ocu-Tropine** Ocumed, USA.
Atropine sulfate (p.477·1).

**Ocutrulan** Truw, Ger.†.
Homoeopathic preparation.

**Ocuvite**
Bausch & Lomb, Arg.; Bausch & Lomb, Canad.; Lederle, Israel; Lepori, Port.; Intrapharm, UK; Bausch & Lomb, USA.
A range of multivitamin and mineral preparations (p.1417·1).

**Odaban**
Petrus, Austral.; Bracey, UK.
Aluminium chloride (p.1142·1).
*Hyperhidrosis.*

**Odala wern** Wernigerode, Ger.†.
Chamomile (p.1669·3); sage (p.1741·2); benzocaine (p.1370·3).
*Inflammatory mouth disorders.*

**Odamesol** Pharmanik (Φαρμανικ), Gr.
Omeprazole (p.1278·2).
*Acid aspiration; eradication of Helicobacter pylori in combination with antimicrobials; peptic ulcer; reflux oesophagitis; Zollinger-Ellison syndrome.*

**Odamida** Pelayo, Spain.
Benzalkonium chloride (p.1168·3); zinc chloride (p.1469·2).
Formerly contained alum, sulfanilamide, and zinc chloride.
*Mouth disorders.*

**Odanet** Pharmanik (Φαρμανικ), Gr.
Ranitidine hydrochloride (p.1285·2).
*Conditions where gastric acid reduction is beneficial; gastric hypersecretion including Zollinger-Ellison syndrome; peptic ulcer.*

**Odanex** Saval, Chile.
Ondansetron (p.1281·1).
*Nausea and vomiting.*

**Odasol** Genepharm, Gr.
Omeprazole (p.1278·2).
*Acid aspiration; eradication of Helicobacter pylori in combination with antimicrobials; peptic ulcer; reflux oesophagitis; Zollinger-Ellison syndrome.*

**Oddibil**
Gerot, Austria; Aventis, Braz.; Cooperation Pharmaceutique, Fr.; Nattermann, Ger.; Rhone-Poulenc Rorer, Mex.†.
Fumitory (p.1690·1).
*Biliary-tract disorders; digestive and renal disorders.*

**Oddispasmol** Ratiopharm, Austria.
Fumitory (p.1690·1); ethaverine hydrochloride (p.1685·2).
Formerly contained fumitory.
*Biliary disorders.*

**Odemase** Azupharma, Ger.
Furosemide (p.919·3).
*Hypertension; oedema.*

**Odemin** Santen, Fin.
Acetazolamide (p.849·1).
*Epilepsy; glaucoma; oedema.*

**Odenil Unas** Isdin, Spain.
Amorolfine hydrochloride (p.391·1).
*Fungal nail infections.*

**Odiron-C**
Medichem, Malaysia; Medichem, Singapore.
Ferrous fumarate (p.1427·3); vitamin B substances (p.1417·1); vitamin E.
Vitamin C (p.1460·2) is included in this preparation to increase the absorption and availability of iron.
*Anaemias.*

**Odisor** Soria Natural, Spain.
Chamomile (p.1669·3); fumitory (p.1690·1); centaury (p.1669·2); boldo (p.1661·2).
*Digestive disorders.*

**Odo-fre** Self-Care Products, UK.
Parsley seed oil.

**Odol Control Sarro** Colgate, Arg.
Sodium fluoride (p.1444·3); sodium pyrophosphate; sodium bicarbonate.
*Dental caries prophylaxis.*

**Odol Med Antiplaca** Colgate, Arg.
Sodium fluoride (p.1444·3); sodium monofluorophosphate (p.1446·2); triclosan (p.1195·2); allantoin; guaiazulene.
*Dental caries prophylaxis.*

**Odol Med Dental** SmithKline Beecham, Spain†.
Chlorhexidine gluconate (p.1173·2).
*Bacterial mouth infections.*

**Odol Tratamiento de Encias** Colgate, Arg.
Sodium fluoride (p.1444·3); triclosan (p.1195·2); sodium bicarbonate.
*Dental caries prophylaxis.*

**Odongi** Candioli, Ital.
Benzalkonium chloride (p.1168·3); eugenol (p.1686·2); tetracaine (p.1385·1).
*Dental caries.*

**Odon-Pyr** Jofrain, Mex.†.
Dipyrone (p.35·3).

**Odontalg** Giovanardi, Ital.
Lidocaine hydrochloride (p.1377·3).
*Local anaesthesia.*

**Odontalgiche (Dentali)** AFOM, Ital.; Farmatre, Ital.; Nova Argentia, Ital.; Ogna, Ital.; Sella, Ital.
Eugenol (p.1686·2); chlorobutanol (p.1176·3).
*Dental pain.*

**Odontalgico Dr. Knapp con Vit. B1** Montefarmaco, Ital.
Paracetamol (p.76·2); propyphenazone (p.85·3); thiamine hydrochloride (p.1455·1); caffeine (p.782·1).
*Pain.*

**Odontocromil c Sulfamida** Kin, Spain.
Ascorbic acid (p.1460·2); chlorophyllin copper complex sodium (p.1057·1); phenol (p.1188·1); sulfanilamide sodium (p.263·3); zinc chloride (p.1469·2); methyl salicylate (p.59·3); peppermint oil (p.1283·2); anise oil (p.1655·2).
*Mouth inflammation; mouth wounds.*

**Odonton-Echtroplex** Weber & Weber, Ger.
Homoeopathic preparation.

**Odontovac** Nikkho, Braz.
Procaine benzylpenicillin (p.246·1); benzylpenicillin potassium (p.163·2); bacterial antigens.
*Bacterial infections.*

**Odontoxina** Molteni, Ital.†.
Chlorhexidine gluconate (p.1173·2); melissa oil; geranium oil; carnation oil; peppermint oil; spearmint oil.
*Oral disinfection.*

**Odor Eze** Novartis, NZ.
Aloe vera (p.1141·3); aluminium starch octenylsuccinate; corn starch (p.1449·1); silicon dioxide (p.1581·3); talc (p.1159·1).
*Foot odour.*

**Odourless Garlic**
Note. This name is used for preparations of different composition.
Blackmores, Austral.†.
Garlic (p.1691·1); parsley (p.1728·3).
*Cold and influenza symptoms.*

Vitaplex, Austral.†.
Garlic (p.1691·1); echinacea purpurea (p.1683·2); zinc gluconate (p.1469·2); betacarotene (p.1422·3).
*Upper respiratory-tract congestion.*

**Odoxil** Lupin, India.
Cefadroxil (p.167·2).
*Bacterial infections.*

**Odranal**
Note. This name is used for preparations of different composition.
Raffo, Arg.
Bupropion (p.288·2).
*Depression.*

Raffo, Chile.
Oxybutynin (p.487·1).
*Neurogenic bladder.*

**Odric** Hoechst Marion Roussel, Jpn.
Trandolapril (p.1016·1).
*Hypertension.*

**Odrik**
Aventis, Austral.; Asta Medica, Braz.; Aventis, Denm.; Aventis, Fr.; Hoechst Marion Roussel, Gr.; Aventis, Irl.; Aventis, NZ; Vitoria, Port.; Alter, Spain; Aventis, UK.
Trandolapril (p.1016·1).
*Hypertension; left ventricular dysfunction following myocardial infarction.*

**O-Due** Teofarma, Ital.
Taurine (p.1752·1).
*Vascular disorders.*

**Odupril** Pharmanik (Φαρμανικ), Gr.
Captopril (p.879·2).
*Heart failure; hypertension; myocardial infarction.*

**Oecotrim** Fresenius Kabi, Austria.
Co-trimoxazole (p.199·3).
*Bacterial infections; Pneumocystis carinii pneumonia.*

**Oecozol** Fresenius Kabi, Austria†.
Metronidazole (p.607·2).
*Anaerobic bacterial infections.*

**Oedemex** Mepha, Switz.
Furosemide (p.919·3).
*Forced diuresis; hypertension; oedema.*

**OeKolp** Kade, Ger.
Estriol (p.1552·3).
*Menopausal disorders; vaginal disorders.*

**Oemine** Kappa, Fr.
A range of nutritional supplements (p.1417·1).

**Oenobiol** Oenobiol, Fr.
A range of nutritional supplements (p.1417·1).

**Oesclim**
Fournier, Austria; Allergan-Frumtost, Braz.†; Paladin, Canad.; Andromaco, Chile; Fournier, Fr.; Selena, Swed.
Estradiol (p.1550·1).
*Menopausal disorders; osteoporosis.*

**Oesto-Mins** Tyson, USA.
Multivitamin and mineral preparation (p.1417·1).

**Oestraclin** Seid, Spain.
Estradiol (p.1550·1).
*Menopausal disorders; osteoporosis.*

**Oestrifen** Ashbourne, UK†.
Tamoxifen citrate (p.584·1).
*Anovulatory infertility; breast cancer.*

**Oestrilin** Desbergers, Canad.†.
Estrone (p.1553·1).
*Kraurosis vulvae; pruritus vulvae; vaginitis.*

**Oestring** Pharmacia, Swed.
Estradiol (p.1550·1).
*Vaginal disorders due to oestrogen deficiency.*

**Oestrodose**
Besins, Fr.; Besins, Israel; Seid, Spain.
Estradiol (p.1550·1).
*Menopausal disorders; osteoporosis.*

**Oestro-Feminal**
Pfizer, Austria; Mack, Switz.
Conjugated oestrogens (p.1543·2).
*Menopausal disorders; osteoporosis.*

**Oestrofeminal** Mack, Illert., Ger.
Conjugated oestrogens (p.1543·2).
*Menopausal disorders; osteoporosis.*

**Oestrogel**
Besins, Belg.; Enila, Braz.; Besins, Fr.; Faran, Gr.; Besins, Hong Kong; Aventis, Irl.; Besins International, Israel; Besins-Iscovesco, Malaysia; Atlantis, Mex.; Besins-Iscovesco, Singapore; Golaz, Switz.; Piette, Thai.; Aventis, UK.
Estradiol (p.1550·1).
*Menopausal disorders; osteoporosis.*

**Oestro-Gynaedron M** Artesan, Ger.; Cassella-med, Ger.
Estriol (p.1552·3).
*Vaginal disorders.*

**Oestro-Gynaedron Nouveau** Artesan, Switz.
Estriol (p.1552·3).
*Adjunct in vaginal surgery; oestrogen deficiency.*

**OestroTabs Plus Cyclic** Golaz, Switz.
16 Tablets, estradiol (p.1550·1); 12 tablets, estradiol; medroxyprogesterone acetate (p.1557·2).
*Menopausal disorders; osteoporosis.*

**Oestrugol N** Atzinger, Ger.
Estriol (p.1552·3); urea (p.1162·2); thymol (p.1194·2).
*Vaginitis.*

**Ofal** Novartis Ophthalmics, Arg.
Timolol maleate (p.1012·2).
*Glaucoma; ocular hypertension.*

**Ofal P** Novartis Ophthalmics, Arg.
Timolol maleate (p.1012·2); pilocarpine hydrochloride (p.1495·1).
*Glaucoma.*

**Ofcin**
YSP, Malaysia; Yung Shin, Singapore.
Ofloxacin (p.239·3).
*Bacterial infections.*

**Off Skintastic** Johnson, Canad.
Octinoxate (p.1154·3); octisalate (p.1154·3); oxybenzone (p.1154·3).
*Sunscreen.*

**Offeno** Offenbach, Mex.
Ibuprofen (p.45·3).
*Inflammation; musculoskeletal and joint disorders.*

**Offentina** Offenbach, Mex.
Ranitidine (p.1285·2).
*Peptic ulcer.*

**Off-Ezy**
Del, Canad.; Del, USA.
Salicylic acid (p.1157·1).
*Calluses; corns; warts.*

**Ofil** Pharmazam, Spain†.
Pollen fractions.
*Prostatitis.*

**Ofisolona** Ofimex, Mex.
Prednisone (p.1109·3).
*Corticosteroid.*

**O-Flam** MDM, Ital.
Fentiazac (p.43·1).
*Inflammation; oedema.*

**Oflin** Cadila, India.
Ofloxacin (p.239·3).
*Bacterial infections.*

**Oflocee** Farmaline, Thai.
Ofloxacin (p.239·3).
*Bacterial infections.*

**Oflocet**
Aventis, Austral.†; Aventis, Fr.; Aventis, NZ†; Aventis, Port.
Ofloxacin (p.239·3) or ofloxacin hydrochloride (p.240·1).
*Bacterial infections.*

**Oflocin** GlaxoSmithKline, Ital.
Ofloxacin (p.239·3).
*Respiratory-tract infections; urinary-tract infections.*

**Oflodex** Dexcel, Israel.
Ofloxacin (p.239·3).
*Bacterial infections.*

**Oflodura** Merck dura, Ger.
Ofloxacin (p.239·3).
*Bacterial infections.*

**Oflohexal** Hexal, Ger.
Ofloxacin (p.239·3).
*Bacterial infections.*

**Oflono** SMB, Chile.
Ciprofloxacin hydrochloride (p.188·2).
*Bacterial infections.*

**Oflovir** Vir, Spain.
Ofloxacin (p.239·3).
*Bacterial infections.*

**Oflox**
Allergan, Arg.; Allergan, Braz.; Allergan, Chile; Azupharma, Ger.; CT, Ger.; Basics, Ger.; Wolff, Ger.; Allergan, Israel.
Ofloxacin (p.239·3).
*Bacterial eye infections.*

**O-Flox** Silom, Thai.
Ofloxacin (p.239·3).
*Bacterial infections.*

**Ofloxa** LBS, Thai.
Ofloxacin (p.239·3).
*Bacterial infections.*

**Ofloxan** Janssen-Cilag, Braz.
Ofloxacin (p.239·3).
*Bacterial infections.*

**Ofloxcin** Siam Bheasach, Thai.
Ofloxacin (p.239·3).
*Bacterial infections.*

**Ofloxin** BPL-Meizler, Braz.
Ofloxacin (p.239·3).
*Bacterial infections.*

**O-fluor** Onkoworks, Ger.
Fluorouracil (p.554·2).
*Malignant neoplasms.*

**Ofnifenil** Chrispa (Χρισπα), Gr.
Enalapril maleate (p.909·2).
*Heart failure; hypertension.*

**Ofnimarex** Zekides, Gr.
Omeprazole (p.1278·2).
*Acid aspiration; eradication of Helicobacter pylori in combination with antimicrobials; peptic ulcer; reflux oesophagitis; Zollinger-Ellison syndrome.*

**O-folin** Onkoworks, Ger.
Calcium folinate (p.1431·1).
*Antidote to folic acid antagonists; folic acid deficiency.*

**Ofoxin** *Zambon, Braz.*
Ciprofloxacin hydrochloride (p.188·2).
*Bacterial ear infections.*

**Oframax**
*Ranbaxy, India; Ranbaxy, Singapore; Ranbaxy, Thai.*
Ceftriaxone sodium (p.182·3).
*Bacterial infections.*

**Oftabiotico** *Saval, Chile.*
*Eye drops:* Polymyxin b sulfate (p.245·1); neomycin sulfate (p.235·1); gramicidin (p.220·2).
*Eye ointment:* Polymyxin b sulfate (p.245·1); neomycin sulfate (p.235·1); bacitracin (p.161·3).
*Bacterial eye infections.*

**Oftacilox**
*Alcon, Ital.; Alcon Cusi, Spain.*
Ciprofloxacin hydrochloride (p.188·2).
*Bacterial eye infections.*
*Alcon, Port.*
Ciprofloxacin (p.188·2).
*Bacterial eye infections.*

**Oftaciprox** *Laboratorios Chile, Chile.*
Ciprofloxacin hydrochloride (p.188·2).
*Bacterial eye infections.*

**Oftacon**
*Saval, Chile; Columbia, Mex.*
Sodium cromoglicate (p.795·3).
*Allergic eye disorders.*

**Oftadil** *Diba, Mex.*
Chloramphenicol (p.185·1).
*Bacterial eye infections.*

**Oftagel**
*Santen, Denm.; Santen, Fin.; Santen, Swed.*
Carbomer 974 P (p.1577·2).
*Dry eyes.*

**Oftagen**
*Saval, Chile.*
Gentamicin sulfate (p.217·1).
*Bacterial eye infections.*
*Novag, Mex.†.*
Gentamicin (p.219·1).
*Bacterial infections.*

**Oftagen Compuesto** *Saval, Chile.*
Gentamicin sulfate (p.217·1); betamethasone sodium phosphate (p.1093·1).
*Bacterial eye infections with inflammation.*

**Oftal** *Drawer, Arg.*
Neomycin (p.235·1); chloramphenicol (p.185·1); phenylephrine (p.1126·3).
*Eye infections.*

**Oftalar**
*Alcon, Ital.; Alcon, Port.; Alcon Cusi, Spain.*
Pranoprofen (p.85·2).
*Inflammatory eye disorders.*

**Oftalbrax** *Eczane, Arg.*
Tobramycin (p.271·2).
*Bacterial eye infections.*

**Oftaler** *Saval, Chile.*
Ketotifen (p.788·2).
*Allergic conjunctivitis.*

**Oftalirio**
*Saval, Chile.*
Naphazoline hydrochloride (p.1124·3); antazoline phosphate (p.424·2).
*Eye congestion.*
*Columbia, Mex.*
Naphazoline (p.1124·3); antazoline (p.424·2).

**Oftalmet** *Sophia, Mex.†.*
Hypromellose (p.1579·3).

**Oftalmil** *Bruschettini, Ital.*
Naphazoline hydrochloride (p.1124·3); zinc phenolsulfonate (p.1163·3).
*Eye irritation.*

**Oftalmo** *Medical, Spain†.*
Hydrocortisone acetate (p.1103·3); neomycin sulfate (p.235·1).
*Infected eye disorders.*

**Oftalmocaina** *Allergan, Arg.*
Oxybuprocaine hydrochloride (p.1382·1).
*Local anaesthesia.*

**Oftalmoflogol** *Poen, Arg.*
Prednisolone (p.1108·1); chloramphenicol (p.185·1).
*Infected eye disorders.*

**Oftalmol Dexa** *Reig Jofre, Spain†.*
Boric acid (p.1662·1); dexamethasone sodium metasulfobenzoate (p.1097·2); mercuric cyanide (p.1713·3); naphazoline nitrate (p.1124·3); trinitrophenol (p.1758·1); procaine hydrochloride (p.1383·2).
*Eye disorders.*

**Oftalmol Ocular** *Reig Jofre, Spain.*
Boric acid (p.1662·1); mercuric cyanide (p.1713·3); naphazoline nitrate (p.1124·3); trinitrophenol (p.1758·1); procaine hydrochloride (p.1383·2).
*Eye congestion; infected eye disorders.*

**Oftalmolets** *Alcon, Arg.*
Erythromycin estolate (p.208·1) or erythromycin lactobionate (p.208·2).
*Bacterial eye infections.*

**Oftalmolosa Cusi de Icol** *Cusi, Hong Kong†.*
Dexamethasone sodium phosphate (p.1097·2); chloramphenicol (p.185·1).
*Infected eye disorders.*

**Oftalmolosa Cusi Virucida** *Cusi, Hong Kong†.*
Idoxuridine (p.637·3).
*Viral eye infections.*

**Oftalmotonil** *Biocumed, Arg.*
Brimonidine (p.877·1).
*Glaucoma.*

**Oftalmotrim**
*Cusi, Hong Kong†; Alcon Cusi, Malaysia; Alcon, Port.; Cusi, Singapore†; Alcon Cusi, Spain.*
Polymyxin B sulfate (p.245·1); trimethoprim (p.272·2).
*Eye infections.*

**Oftalmotrim Dexa** *Alcon Cusi, Spain.*
Dexamethasone sodium (p.1097·3); polymyxin B sulfate (p.245·1); trimethoprim (p.272·2).
*Bacterial eye infections.*

**Oftalmowell** *Celltech, Spain.*
Gramicidin (p.220·2); neomycin sulfate (p.235·1); polymyxin B sulfate (p.245·1).
*Eye infections.*

**Oftalzina** *SIT, Ital.†.*
Procaine hydrochloride (p.1383·2); naphazoline nitrate (p.1124·3).
*Conjunctival congestion.*

**Oftamolol**
*Alcon, Denm.; Ophtha, Norw.*
Timolol maleate (p.1012·2).
*Glaucoma.*

**Oftan**
*Note. This name is used for preparations of different composition.*
*Santen, Fin.*
Polyvinyl alcohol (p.1581·1).
*Dry eyes.*
*Santen, Israel†; Santen, Norw.; Novartis Ophthalmics, Switz.; Santen, Thai.*
Timolol maleate (p.1012·2).
*Glaucoma; ocular hypertension.*

**Oftan Akvakol** *Santen, Fin.*
Chloramphenicol (p.185·1).
*Bacterial eye infections.*

**Oftan A-Pant** *Santen, Fin.*
Vitamin A palmitate (p.1453·1); dexpanthenol (p.1727·2).
*Eye disorders.*

**Oftan Atropin** *Santen, Fin.*
Atropine sulfate (p.477·1).
*Eye disorders.*

**Oftan C-C** *Santen, Fin.*
Hydrocortisone capronate; chloramphenicol (p.185·1).
*Eye disorders.*

**Oftan Chlora** *Santen, Fin.*
Chloramphenicol (p.185·1).
*Bacterial eye infections.*

**Oftan Dexa** *Santen, Fin.*
Dexamethasone (p.1097·1) or dexamethasone sodium phosphate (p.1097·2).
*Eye disorders.*

**Oftan Dexa-Chlora** *Santen, Fin.*
Dexamethasone (p.1097·1) or dexamethasone sodium phosphate (p.1097·2); chloramphenicol (p.185·1).
*Eye disorders.*

**Oftan Flurekain** *Santen, Fin.*
Oxybuprocaine hydrochloride (p.1382·1); fluorescein sodium (p.1689·1).
*Adjunct in eye examination.*

**Oftan Metaoksedrin** *Santen, Fin.*
Phenylephrine hydrochloride (p.1126·3).
*Production of mydriasis; uveitis.*

**Oftan Obucain** *Santen, Fin.*
Oxybuprocaine hydrochloride (p.1382·1).
*Local anaesthesia.*

**Oftan Starine** *Santen, Fin.*
Tetryzoline hydrochloride (p.1131·2).
*Eye disorders.*

**Oftan Syklo** *Santen, Fin.*
Cyclopentolate hydrochloride (p.480·3).
*Aid in eye examination.*

**Oftapinex**
*Santen, Denm.; Santen, Fin.; Santen, Norw.; Santen, Swed.*
Dipivefrine hydrochloride (p.1681·2).
*Glaucoma.*

**Oftaquin** *Columbia, Mex.*
Ciprofloxacin (p.188·2).
*Bacterial eye infections.*

**Oftaquix** *Santen, Swed.*
Levofloxacin (p.225·3).
*Bacterial infections.*

**Oftasona N** *Saval, Chile.*
Betamethasone sodium phosphate (p.1093·1); neomycin sulfate (p.235·1).
*Eye and ear infections with inflammation.*

**Oftasona P** *Saval, Chile.*
Betamethasone sodium phosphate (p.1093·1).
*Inflammatory eye disorders.*

**Oftasteril** *Alfa Intes, Ital.*
Povidone-iodine (p.1190·3).
*Eye irrigation; skin disinfection.*

**Oftavir** *Saval, Chile.*
Aciclovir (p.626·1).
*Herpesvirus eye infections.*

**Oftazil** *Wiener, Mex.†.*
Naphazoline (p.1124·3).

**Oftazul** *Heralds, Braz.†.*
Naphazoline hydrochloride (p.1124·3); methylthioninium chloride (p.1042·2).
*Ocular congestion.*

**Oftcor** *Allergan-Frumtost, Braz.†.*
Dexamethasone (p.1097·1); framycetin sulfate (p.215·1); polymyxin B (p.245·2).
*Infected eye disorders.*

**Oftic** *Saval, Chile.*
Diclofenac sodium (p.32·1).
*Cystoid macular oedema; eye disorders with inflammation; intra-operative miosis inhibition; pain, and pruritus.*

**Ofticlin** *Grin, Mex.*
Tetracycline hydrochloride (p.266·2).
*Bacterial eye infections.*

**Oftimolo** *Farmila, Ital.*
Timolol maleate (p.1012·2).
*Glaucoma; ocular hypertension.*

**Oftinal** *Schering-Plough, Spain.*
Oxymetazoline hydrochloride (p.1126·1).
*Eye irritation.*

**Oftrim** *Allergan-Frumtost, Braz.†.*
Polymyxin B sulfate (p.245·1); framycetin sulfate (p.215·1); gramicidin (p.220·2).
*Bacterial eye infections.*

**Oftyll Desoxydrop** *Omisan, Ital.†.*
Disinfecting solution for contact lens (p.1164·2).

**Ogamma** *Otsuka, Jpn.*
Interferon gamma-n1 (p.647·2).

**Ogast** *Takeda, Fr.*
Lansoprazole (p.1269·3).
*Gastro-oesophageal reflux; peptic ulcer; Zollinger-Ellison syndrome.*

**Ogasto**
*Abbott, Arg.; Abbott, Chile; Seber, Port.*
Lansoprazole (p.1269·3).
*Dyspepsia; gastro-oesophageal reflux; peptic ulcer; Zollinger-Ellison syndrome.*

**Ogastro**
*Abbott, Braz.; Abbott, Mex.*
Lansoprazole (p.1269·3).
*Gastro-oesophageal reflux; peptic ulcer; Zollinger-Ellison syndrome.*

**Ogen**
*Pharmacia, Austral.; Pharmacia, Canad.; Pharmacia Upjohn, Mex.†; Pharmacia Upjohn, USA.*
Estropipate (p.1553·1).
*Menopausal disorders; oestrogen deficiency; osteoporosis.*

**Ogenest** *Pharmacia, Braz.†.*
Estropipate (p.1553·1).
*Menopausal disorders.*

**Ogestane** *Besins-Iscovesco, Fr.†.*
A vitamin, mineral, and fish oil preparation (p.1417·1).

**Oglos** *Grunenthal, Spain.*
Morphine hydrochloride (p.60·1).
*Pain; premedication.*

**Ogyline** *Effik, Fr.†.*
Norgestrienone (p.1564·3).
*Progestogen-only oral contraceptive.*

**OH B12**
*Monsanto, Ital.; Jaba, Port.*
Hydroxocobalamin (p.1458·2).
*Anaemias; liver disorders; neuralgia; neuritis.*

**OH B12 B1** *Poli, Ital.†.*
Hydroxocobalamin (p.1458·2); monophosphothiamine chloride (p.1455·2).
*Anaemias; neuralgia; neuritis.*

**Ohexine** *Greater Pharma, Thai.*
Bromhexine hydrochloride (p.1115·3).
*Respiratory-tract disorders associated with increased or viscous mucus.*

**OIF** *Otsuka, Jpn.*
Interferon alfa (p.640·3).
*Chronic myeloid leukaemia; hepatitis; renal cancer.*

**Oil of Olay**
*Note. This name is used for preparations of different composition.*
*Procter & Gamble, Canad.*
Octinoxate (p.1154·3); zinc oxide (p.1163·2).
Formerly contained octinoxate and ensulizole.
*Sunscreen.*
*Procter & Gamble, USA.*
*SPF 15:* Octinoxate (p.1154·3); titanium dioxide (p.1160·3); ensulizole (p.1147·1).
*Sunscreen.*

**Oilalfo** *ICN, Arg.*
Coal tar (p.1159·2); salicylic acid (p.1157·1); benzalkonium chloride (p.1168·3).
*Seborrhoea.*

**Oilatum**
*Note. This name is used for preparations of different composition.*
*Stiefel, Arg.; Stiefel, Braz.†.*
Liquid paraffin (p.1479·1).
*Dry skin; soap substitute.*
*Stiefel, Canad.; Stiefel, Ital.; Stiefel, Spain†.*
Emollient.
*Stiefel, Chile; Stiefel, Mex.*
Arachis oil (p.1656·1).
*Dry skin disorders.*
*Stiefel, Israel.*
Soap substitute.
*Stiefel, Malaysia; Stiefel, NZ.*
Light liquid paraffin (p.1479·1).
*Dry skin.*

**Oilatum AD**
*Note. This name is used for preparations of different composition.*
*Stiefel, Fr.*
Sodium cocoyl isetionate; triclosan (p.1195·2).
*Dry skin; soap substitute.*
*Stiefel, Ital.*
Triclosan (p.1195·2).
*Atopic dermatitis.*

**Oilatum Bar**
*Stiefel, Austral.; Stiefel, Hong Kong; Stiefel, Singapore; Stiefel, Thai.*
Liquid paraffin (p.1479·1).
*Soap substitute.*

**Oilatum Bath Formula** *Stiefel, UK.*
Light liquid paraffin (p.1479·1).
*Dry skin disorders.*

**Oilatum Body Oil** *Stiefel, Fr.*
Liquid paraffin (p.1479·1); jojoba oil.
*Dry skin.*

**Oilatum Cream**
*Note. This name is used for preparations of different composition.*
*Stiefel, Fr.; Stiefel, Hong Kong; Stiefel, Thai.; Stiefel, UK.*
Light liquid paraffin (p.1479·1) or liquid paraffin (p.1479·1); white soft paraffin (p.1479·3).
Formerly contained arachis oil.
*Dry skin disorders.*
*Stiefel, Irl.†; Stiefel, Singapore.*
Arachis oil (p.1656·1).
*Dry skin disorders.*

**Oilatum Emollient**
*Note. This name is used for preparations of different composition.*
*Stiefel, Austral.; Stiefel, Fr.; Stiefel, Hong Kong; Stiefel, Singapore; Stiefel, Thai.*
Light liquid paraffin (p.1479·1).
Formerly contained light liquid paraffin and acetylated wool alcohols in *Austral.*
*Dry skin disorders.*
*Stiefel, Irl.; Stiefel, UK.*
Liquid paraffin (p.1479·1); acetylated wool alcohols (p.1483·1).
*Dry skin disorders.*

**Oilatum Fragrance Free** *Stiefel, UK.*
Light liquid paraffin (p.1479·1).
*Dry skin disorders.*

**Oilatum Gel**
*Stiefel, Hong Kong; Stiefel, Irl.†; Stiefel, Singapore; Stiefel, Thai.; Stiefel, UK.*
Light liquid paraffin (p.1479·1).
*Dry skin disorders.*

**Oilatum Junior** *Stiefel, UK.*
*Bath additive:* Light liquid paraffin (p.1479·1).
*Dry skin disorders.*
*Cream:* Light liquid paraffin (p.1479·1); white soft paraffin (p.1479·3).
*Dry skin; pruritus.*

**Oilatum Junior Flare-Up**
*Stiefel, Irl.†; Stiefel, UK.*
Light liquid paraffin (p.1479·1); triclosan (p.1195·2); benzalkonium chloride (p.1168·3).
*Dry skin disorders.*

**Oilatum Plus**
*Stiefel, Austral.; Stiefel, Hong Kong; Stiefel, Irl.; Stiefel, NZ; Stiefel, S.Afr.; Stiefel, Singapore; Stiefel, Thai.; Stiefel, UK.*
Light liquid paraffin (p.1479·1); triclosan (p.1195·2); benzalkonium chloride (p.1168·3).
*Eczema.*

**Oilatum Plus Antibacterial** *Stiefel, Malaysia.*
Light liquid paraffin (p.1479·1); triclosan (p.1195·2); benzalkonium chloride (p.1168·3).
*Eczema.*

**Oilatum Shampoo** *Stiefel, UK.*
Ciclopirox olamine (p.396·1).
*Scalp disorders.*

**Oilatum Shower Gel** *Stiefel, Austral.*
Light liquid paraffin (p.1479·1).
*Dry skin.*

**Oilatum Skin Therapy** *Stiefel, UK†.*
Light liquid paraffin (p.1479·1).
*Dry skin.*

**Oilatum Soap**
*Note. This name is used for preparations of different composition.*
*Stiefel, Fr.; Stiefel, UK.*
Liquid paraffin (p.1479·1).
*Dry skin disorders.*
*Stiefel, USA.*
Skin cleanser.

**Oil-Free Acne Wash** *Professional Health, Canad.†.*
Salicylic acid (p.1157·1).
*Acne.*

**Oil-Free Active Sunscreen** *Norwood, Canad.*
*SPF 15:* Octinoxate (p.1154·3); oxybenzone (p.1154·3).
*Sunscreen.*

**Oil-Free Sunblock** *Clinique, Canad.*
*SPF 15:* Octinoxate (p.1154·3); octocrilene (p.1154·3); octisalate (p.1154·3); oxybenzone (p.1154·3).
*Sunscreen.*

**Oil-Free Sunscreen**
*Note. This name is used for preparations of different composition.*
*Avon, Canad.*
*SPF 15:* Octinoxate (p.1154·3); octocrilene (p.1154·3); octisalate (p.1154·3).
*Sunscreen.*
*Norwood, Canad.*
*SPF 30:* Homosalate (p.1148·1); octinoxate (p.1154·3); octisalate (p.1154·3); oxybenzone (p.1154·3).
*Sunscreen.*

**Oil-Free Sunspray** Estee Lauder, Canad.
*SPF 15:* Octinoxate (p.1154·3); octisalate (p.1154·3); oxybenzone (p.1154·3).
*Sunscreen.*

**Ojensalve Neutral** Ophtha, Denm.†.
Liquid paraffin (p.1479·1); white soft paraffin (p.1479·3).
*Blepharitis; protection of eyelid and cornea.*

**Ojosbel** Dermofarm, Spain.
Hamamelis water (p.1696·3); naphazoline hydrochloride (p.1124·3).
*Eye irritation.*

**Ojosbel Azul** Dermofarm, Spain†.
Hamamelis water (p.1696·3); methylthioninium chloride (p.1042·2); naphazoline hydrochloride (p.1124·3).
*Eye irritation.*

**Okacin**
Novartis Ophthalmics, Arg.; Novartis, Austria; Novartis Ophthalmics, Braz.; Novartis, Chile; Novartis, Denm.; Novartis, Fin.; Novartis Ophthalmics, Ger.; Novartis Ophthalmics, Hong Kong; Ciba Vision, Israel; Ciba Vision, Ital.; Novartis Ophthalmics, Malaysia; Novartis Ophthalmics, Port.; Novartis Ophthalmics, Singapore; Novartis Ophthalmics, Switz.; Novartis, Thai.
Lomefloxacin hydrochloride (p.227·2).
*Bacterial eye infections.*

**Okacyn**
Restan, S.Afr.; Novartis Ophthalmics, UK†.
Lomefloxacin hydrochloride (p.227·2).
*Bacterial eye infections.*

**Okal** Puerto Galiano, Spain.
*Chewable tablets:* Aspirin (p.15·1); caffeine (p.782·1).
*Fever; pain.*
*Dispersible tablets; tablets:* Aspirin (p.15·1).
*Fever; musculoskeletal and joint disorders; pain; thrombosis prophylaxis.*

**Okalcin** Tenton, Switz.
Homoeopathic preparation.

**Okavax**
Aventis Pasteur, Malaysia; Aventis Pasteur, Thai.
An attenuated varicella-zoster vaccine (Oka strain) (p.1643·2).
*Active immunisation.*

**Oki** Dompe, Ital.
Ketoprofen lysine (p.51·3).
*Inflammation; pain.*

**Oklaricid** Abbott, Gr.
Clarithromycin (p.192·2).
*Adjunct in Helicobacter pylori eradication; bacterial infections.*

**Okokit II** Hughes & Hughes, UK†.
Test for faecal occult blood.

**Okoubarell** Sanorell, Ger.
Homoeopathic preparation.

**Okoubasan** Sanum-Kehlbeck, Ger.
Homoeopathic preparation.

**Oksibutin** Biochemie, Fin.
Oxybutynin hydrochloride (p.486·3).
*Bladder function disorders.*

**Okuzell** Pharmaselect, Austria.
Hypromellose (p.1579·3).
*Eye irritation.*

**O-Lac**
Bristol-Myers Squibb, Arg.; Mead Johnson, Austral.; Mead Johnson, Braz.; Mead Johnson, Fr.; Mead Johnson, Hong Kong; Mead Johnson, Ital.; Mead Johnson, Malaysia; Mead Johnson, NZ†; Mead Johnson, Port.; Mead Johnson, Singapore; Mead Johnson Nutritionals, Thai.
Infant feed (p.1417·1).
*Galactosaemia; lactose intolerance; sucrose intolerance.*

**Oladin** Collins, Mex.
Salbutamol (p.791·3).

**Olam** Valdecasas, Mex.
Kaolin (p.1268·3); pectin (p.1580·3).

**Olamin** Micro, India.
Ciclopirox olamine (p.396·1).
*Fungal skin infections.*

**Olamin P** Delta BKB, Ital.
Piroctone olamine (p.1155·2).
*Seborrhoeic dermatitis.*

**Ol-Amine** Meuse, Belg.
Multivitamin and mineral preparation (p.1417·1).

**Olamyc** Sanofi Synthelabo, Gr.
Salicylic acid (p.1157·1); triamcinolone acetonide (p.1110·2); benzalkonium chloride (p.1168·3).
*Skin disorders.*

**Olan-Gin** Olan-Kemed, Thai.
Dipyrone (p.35·3).
Lidocaine (p.1377·3) is included in some injections to alleviate the pain of injection.
*Fever; pain.*

**Olbad Cordes**
Ichthyol, Austria; Ichthyol, Ger.
Soya oil (p.1447·2).
*Bath additive; skin disorders.*

**Olbad Cordes comp** Ichthyol, Austria.
Soya oil (p.1447·2); shale oil.
*Bath additive; skin disorders.*

**Olbad Cordes F** Ichthyol, Ger.
Arachis oil (p.1656·1).
*Bath additive; skin disorders.*

**Olbas**
Note. This name is used for preparations of different composition.
Olbas, Ger.†.
*Pastilles:* Peppermint oil (p.1283·2); cajuput oil (p.1664·1); eucalyptus oil (p.1686·2); juniper oil (p.1703·1); sweet birch oil (p.60·1).
*Cold symptoms; mouth and throat disinfection.*
Schoenenberger, Ger.
*Drops:* Peppermint oil (p.1283·2); cajuput oil (p.1664·1); eucalyptus oil (p.1686·2); juniper oil (p.1703·1); sweet birch oil (p.60·1).
*Cold symptoms; gastrointestinal disorders; headache; neuralgia; pain; rheumatism.*
*Topical spray:* Ethyl chloride (p.1376·2); menthol (p.1711·3).
*Soft-tissue disorders; sports injuries.*
Synpharma, Switz.†.
*Inhaler:* Peppermint oil (p.1283·2); eucalyptus oil (p.1686·2); menthol (p.1711·3); cineole (p.1672·1).
*Nasal congestion.*
*Oil:* Peppermint oil (p.1283·2); eucalyptus oil (p.1686·2); cajuput oil (p.1664·1); sweet birch oil (p.60·1); juniper oil (p.1703·1); clove oil (p.1673·3).
*Cold symptoms; nasal congestion.*
*Ointment:* Peppermint oil (p.1283·2); eucalyptus oil (p.1686·2); cajuput oil (p.1664·1); sweet birch oil (p.60·1); turpentine oil (p.1760·1); clove oil (p.1673·3).
*Cold symptoms; nasal congestion.*
Lane, UK.
*Inhaler:* Cajuput oil (p.1664·1); menthol (p.1711·3); peppermint oil (p.1283·2); eucalyptus oil (p.1686·2).
*Nasal congestion.*
*Oil:* Cajuput oil (p.1664·1); eucalyptus oil (p.1686·2); sweet birch oil (p.60·1); clove oil (p.1673·3); juniper oil (p.1703·1); menthol (p.1711·3); dementholised mint oil (p.1715·2).
*Nasal congestion.*
*Pastilles:* Eucalyptus oil (p.1686·2); peppermint oil (p.1283·2); menthol (p.1711·3); juniper oil (p.1703·1); sweet birch oil (p.60·1); clove oil (p.1673·3).
*Cold symptoms; coughs.*

**Olbas for Children** Lane, UK.
Cajuput oil (p.1664·1); eucalyptus oil (p.1686·2); clove oil (p.1673·3); juniper oil (p.1703·1); menthol (p.1711·3); dementholised mint oil (p.1715·2); methyl salicylate (p.59·3).
*Respiratory-tract congestion.*

**Olbemox** Pharmacia, Ger.
Acipimox (p.851·1).
*Lipid disorders.*

**Olbenorm** Norma (Νορμα), Gr.
Ambroxol hydrochloride (p.1114·3).
*Respiratory disorders associated with viscous mucus.*

**Olbetam**
Pharmacia, Austria; Pharmacia, Belg.; Searle, Braz.; Pharmacia, Chile; Pharmacia, Denm.; Pharmacia-Upjohn, Gr.; Pharmacia, Hong Kong; Pharmacia, Irl.; Pharmacia Upjohn, Israel; Pharmacia Upjohn, Ital.; Pharmacia Upjohn, Mex.†; Pharmacia, Neth.; Pharmacia, NZ; Pharmacia, S.Afr.; Pharmacia, Singapore; Pharmacia, Switz.; Pharmacia, Thai.; Pharmacia, UK.
Acipimox (p.851·1).
*Hyperlipidaemias.*

**Ol-Bi** KG, Ital.
Vitamin B substances (p.1417·1).

**Olbiacor** Salus, Ital.†.
Fendiline hydrochloride (p.915·1).
*Ischaemic heart disease; myocardial infarction.*

**Olcadil**
Novartis, Braz.; Novartis, Port.
Cloxazolam (p.685·3).
*Anxiety disorders.*

**Olcam** Irex, Fr.†.
Piroxicam (p.84·2).
*Musculoskeletal and joint disorders.*

**Oldamin** Fuji, Jpn.
Monoethanolamine oleate (p.1716·1).
*Oesophageal varices.*

**Oldan** Europharma, Spain.
Acemetacin (p.11·3).
*Musculoskeletal, joint, and peri-articular disorders.*

**Oleatum**
Stiefel, Ger.†.
Light liquid paraffin (p.1479·1).
*Skin disorders.*
Stiefel, Ital.†.
Emollient.

**Oleatum Bar** Stiefel, Fr.†.
Liquid paraffin (p.1479·1).
*Dry skin.*

**Oleatum Emollient** Stiefel, Fr.†.
Liquid paraffin (p.1479·1).
*Dry skin.*

**Oleatum Gel** Stiefel, Fr.†.
Liquid paraffin (p.1479·1).
*Dry skin.*

**Oleo Calcarea** NewFaDem, Ital.; Nova Argentia, Ital.; Ogna, Ital.
Aluminium acetate (p.1652·3); glacial acetic acid (p.1645·2); zinc oxide (p.1163·2); calcium oxide (p.1664·3); menthol (p.1711·3).

**Oleo de Primula** Viternat, Braz.
Gamolenic acid (p.1690·2); linoleic acid (p.1690·2).

**Oleo Dermosina Simples** Davi, Port.
Zinc oxide (p.1163·2).
*Skin disorders.*

**Oleo Eletrico** CIF, Braz.
Camphor (p.1665·3); turpentine oil (p.1760·1); methyl salicylate (p.59·3).
*Musculoskeletal and joint disorders.*

**Oleobal** Pierre Fabre Dermo Kosmetik, Ger.
Soya oil (p.1447·2); light liquid paraffin (p.1479·1).
*Bath additive; skin disorders.*

**Oleoban** Medinfar, Port.
Sunflower oil (p.1451·1).
*Skin cleansing; skin disorders.*

**Oleoban Composto** Medinfar, Port.
Sunflower oil (p.1451·1); ichthammol (p.1148·2).
*Skin disorders.*

**Oleoban Gel** Medinfar, Port.
Sunflower oil (p.1451·1); liquid paraffin (p.1479·1).
*Dry skin disorders.*

**Oleocal** Remexa, Mex.†.
Calcium hydroxide (p.1664·3).

**Oleoderm** Remexa, Mex.
Calcium hydroxide (p.1664·3).
*Skin disorders.*

**Oleoderm Plus** Remexa, Mex.
Calcium hydroxide (p.1664·3); avobenzone (p.1142·3); octinoxate (p.1154·3).
*Sunscreen.*

**Oleo-Lax** Fada, Arg.
Propofol (p.1305·3).
*General anaesthesia.*

**Oleomycetin**
Agepha, Austria; Winzer, Ger.
Chloramphenicol (p.185·1).
*Bacterial eye infections.*

**Oleomycetin-Prednison**
Agepha, Austria; Winzer, Ger.
Chloramphenicol (p.185·1); prednisone (p.1109·3).
*Infected eye disorders.*

**Oleosint** Apomedica, Austria.
Diolamine oleate; soya oil (p.1447·2).
*Skin disorders.*

**Oleosorbate** Bournonville, Belg.†.
Polysorbate 80 (p.1415·2).
*Ear wax removal; rhinitis.*

**Oleovit** Calea, Austria.
Vitamin A palmitate (p.1453·1); dexpanthenol (p.1727·2).
*Eye disorders.*

**Oleovit A** Calea, Austria.
*Capsules:* Vitamin A palmitate (p.1453·1).
*Ear disorders; gastrointestinal disorders; hyperthyroidism; respiratory-tract disorders; skin disorders; urogenital disorders.*
*Oral drops:* Vitamin A (p.1451·2); betacarotene (p.1422·3).
*Vitamin A deficiency.*

**Oleovit A + D** Calea, Austria.
*Capsules:* Vitamin A palmitate (p.1453·1); colecalciferol (p.1461·3).
*Oral drops:* Vitamin A (p.1451·2); betacarotene (p.1422·3); colecalciferol (p.1461·3).
*Rickets; vitamin A and D supplementation.*

**Oleovit A + $D_3$** Vitamed, Israel.
Vitamin A (p.1451·2); colecalciferol (p.1461·3).
*Vitamin supplement.*

**Oleovit $D_3$** Calea, Austria.
Colecalciferol (p.1461·3).
*Hypoparathyroidism; rickets.*

**Oleum Rhinale** Weleda, UK.
Homoeopathic preparation.

**Olexa** Cipla, India.
Olanzapine (p.710·3).
*Bipolar disorder; psychoses.*

**Olexin** Rayere, Mex.
Omeprazole (p.1278·2).
*Gastro-oesophageal reflux; peptic ulcer; Zollinger-Ellison syndrome.*

**Olf** GNLD, Austral.†.
Reishi mushrooms; celery; avena; red sage; damiana; hypericum; astragalus; angelica; cinnamon; liquorice (p.1417·1).
*Tonic.*

**Olfen**
Mepha, Braz.; Mepha, Hong Kong; Mepha, Israel; Mepha, Malaysia; Mepha, Port.; Mepha, Singapore; Mepha, Switz.; Mepha, Thai.
Diclofenac sodium (p.32·1).
Lidocaine (p.1377·3) or lidocaine hydrochloride (p.1377·3) may be included in the intramuscular injection to alleviate the pain of injection.
*Gout; inflammation; musculoskeletal, joint, peri-articular, and soft-tissue disorders; pain; renal and biliary colic.*

**Olfex** Bial, Spain.
Budesonide (p.1094·2).
*Asthma; rhinitis.*

**Olfosonide** Iasis, Gr.
Budesonide (p.1094·2).
*Allergic rhinitis; topical corticosteroid.*

**Olibanum RA** Zilly, Ger.
Homoeopathic preparation.

**Olicard**
Solvay, Ger.; Solvay, Spain†.
Isosorbide mononitrate (p.942·1).
*Angina pectoris.*

**Olicardin** Solvay, Austria.
Isosorbide mononitrate (p.942·1).
*Angina pectoris; heart failure; myocardial infarction; pulmonary hypertension.*

**Olicide** Cosmofarma, Port.
Malathion (p.1507·1).
*Pediculosis.*

**Oliclinomel**
Baxter, Fr.
Amino-acid, carbohydrate, lipid (from soya oil (p.1447·2) and olive oil (p.1723·2)), and electrolyte infusion (p.1417·1).
Contains egg lecithin.
*Parenteral nutrition.*
Baxter, Spain.
Amino-acid, glucose, and lipid (from olive oil (p.1723·2) and soya oil (p.1447·2)) infusion (p.1417·1).
*Parenteral nutrition.*

**Olidermil** Edol, Port.
Zinc oxide (p.1163·2); almond oil (p.1651·1).
*Dry skin.*

**Oligobs** CCD, Fr.
A range of multivitamin and mineral preparations (p.1417·1).

**Oligocean** Ido, Fr.
Trace element and mineral preparation derived from shellfish (p.1417·1).
*Tonic.*

**Oligocean Minceur** Ido, Fr.
Marine algae preparation (p.1417·1).
*Obesity.*

**Oligocean Xtra** Ido, Fr.
Mineral preparation derived from shellfish (p.1417·1).

**Oligocomplesso** Chimicor, Fr.
Trace element preparation (p.1417·1).

**Oligocure** Labcatal, Fr.
Manganese gluconate; copper gluconate; colloidal gold (p.1417·1).
*Asthenia.*

**Oligoderm** Labcatal, Fr.
Manganese gluconate (p.1440·1); copper gluconate (p.1425·3).
*Cracked nipples.*

**Oligoelementos** Braun, Port.
Trace element preparation (p.1417·1).
*Parenteral nutrition.*

**Oligo-elements Aguettant** Aguettant, Fr.
Trace element preparation (p.1417·1).
*Parenteral nutrition.*

**Oligo-Essentials** Richelet, Fr.
A range of mineral and trace element preparations (p.1417·1).

**Oligofer** Sabex, Canad.†.
Mineral preparation with vitamin $B_{12}$ (p.1417·1).

**Oligoforme** Ido, Fr.
A range of nutritional supplements (p.1417·1).

**Oligogranul** Boiron, Fr.
A range of trace element and mineral preparations (p.1417·1).

**Oligophytum** Holistica, Fr.
A range of mineral-rich plant extracts.

**Oligoplex** Natural Touch, UK.
A range of homoeopathic remedies.

**Oligorhine** Monin, Fr.
Copper (p.1425·3); silver (p.1746·1).
*Nasal irrigation.*

**Oligosol**
Labcatal, Canad.†; Labcatal, Fr.; Labcatal, Switz.
A range of trace element and mineral preparations (p.1417·1).

**Oligossac** Support, Braz.
Maltodextrin (p.1439·3).
*Preparation for enteral nutrition.*

**Oligostim** Dolisos, Fr.
A range of trace element and mineral preparations (p.1417·1).

**Oligo-Yang** Ido, Fr.
Fish cartilage.
*Joint pain.*

**Olimag** Wassen, Ital.
Magnesium (p.1227·3).
*Nutritional supplement.*

**OlioClinomel** Baxter, UK.
An amino-acid, glucose and lipid (from olive oil (p.1723·2) and soya oil (p.1447·2)) infusion with or without electrolytes (p.1417·1).
Contains egg lecithin.
*Parenteral nutrition.*

**Oliviase** UPSA Conseil, Fr.
Olive leaves.
*Diuresis.*

**Olivysat** Ysatfabrik, Ger.
Olive leaves.
*Prevention of atherosclerosis.*

**Olmetec** Sankyo, UK.
Olmesartan medoxomil (p.975·3).
*Hypertension.*

**Olmifon** Lafon, Fr.
Adrafinil (p.1584·2).
*Mental function impairment in the elderly.*

**Olmoran** Novartis, Spain.
Zafirlukast (p.807·1).
*Asthma.*

**Olocynan** *Makros, Braz.†.*
Cynara (p.1678·3); choline (p.1424·3).
*Liver disorders.*

**Ologyn** *Labatec, Switz.*
Levonorgestrel (p.1563·2); ethinylestradiol (p.1553·2).
Formerly contained norgestrel and ethinylestradiol.
*Combined oral contraceptive.*

**Olohepat** *Makros, Braz.†.*
Liver extract; iron (p.1434·3); choline (p.1424·3).
*Liver disorders.*

**Oloprim** *Rudefsa, Mex.†.*
Allopurinol (p.412·2).

**Olren N** *Heumann, Ger.*
Scopolia carniolica.
*Urinary-tract disorders.*

**Oltens** *Biotherapie, Fr.†.*
Captopril (p.879·2).
*Diabetic nephropathy; heart failure; hypertension.*

**Olter** *Pharmacia, Arg.*
Flutamide (p.556·2).
*Prostatic cancer.*

**Olux** *Connetics, USA.*
Clobetasol propionate (p.1095·2).
*Psoriasis; scalp disorders.*

**Olympic Balm** *ANB, Thai.*
Methyl salicylate (p.59·3); menthol (p.1711·3); eugenol (p.1686·2); cineole (p.1672·1); cajuput oil (p.1664·1); peppermint oil (p.1283·2).
*Musculoskeletal, joint, and peri-articular disorders.*

**Olynth**
*Pfizer, Austria; Pfizer Consumer, Ger.; Pfizer, Switz.*
Xylometazoline hydrochloride (p.1132·2).
*Nasal congestion.*

**Olynth Erkaltungsbalsam** *Pfizer Consumer, Ger.*
Oleum pini sylvestris; eucalyptus oil (p.1686·2).
*Cold symptoms.*

**Olynth Kombi** *Warner-Lambert, Ger.†.*
Triprolidine hydrochloride (p.442·3); pseudoephedrine hydrochloride (p.1129·2).
*Rhinitis.*

**Olynth salin** *Pfizer Consumer, Ger.*
Sodium chloride (p.1233·3).
*Nasal congestion.*

**Olyspal** *Cosmopharm, Gr.*
Budesonide (p.1094·2).
*Asthma.*

**Olyster** *Cadila, India.*
Terazosin hydrochloride (p.1010·3).
*Benign prostatic hyperplasia; hypertension.*

**Omacor**
*Pharmacia, Norw.; Solvay, UK.*
Omega-3 acid ethyl esters (p.976·2).
*Hyperlipidaemias; myocardial infarction.*
*AstraZeneca, Thai.*
Omega-3 marine triglycerides (p.976·2).
*Hyperlipidaemias.*

**Omadine** *Erredici, Ital.†.*
Pyrithione disulfide (p.1156·2); urtica (p.1762·1).
*Seborrhoeic dermatitis.*

**Omaflaxina** *Eczane, Arg.*
Ciprofloxacin (p.188·2).
*Bacterial eye infections.*

**Omapren** *Vita, Spain.*
Omeprazole (p.1278·2).
*Gastro-oesophageal reflux; peptic ulcers; Zollinger-Ellison syndrome.*

**Ombolan** *Allergan-Frumtost, Braz.†.*
Droxicam (p.36·2).
*Fever; inflammation; pain.*

**Ombravist** *Schering, Austria.*
Galactose (p.1063·1).
*Contrast medium for Doppler sonography and echocardiography.*

**Ombrelle** *Dermtek, Canad.†.*
*SPF 30:* Avobenzone (p.1142·3); octinoxate (p.1154·3); oxybenzone (p.1154·3).
*Sunscreen.*

**Ombrelle Baume** *Cosmair, Canad.*
*SPF 30:* Avobenzone (p.1142·3); octocrilene (p.1154·3); ecamsule (p.1146·3); titanium dioxide (p.1160·3).
*Sunscreen.*

**Ombrelle Creme Ecran** *Cosmair, Canad.*
*SPF 60:* Avobenzone (p.1142·3); enzacamene (p.1147·1); ecamsule (p.1146·3); titanium dioxide (p.1160·3).
*Sunscreen.*

**Ombrelle Creme Kids** *Cosmair, Canad.*
*SPF 45:* Avobenzone (p.1142·3); octocrilene (p.1154·3); enzacamene (p.1147·1); ecamsule (p.1146·3); titanium dioxide.
*Sunscreen.*

**Ombrelle Extreme** *Cosmair, Canad.*
*SPF 30:* Avobenzone (p.1142·3); octocrilene (p.1154·3); ecamsule (p.1146·3); titanium dioxide (p.1160·3).
Formerly contained avobenzone, octinoxate, oxybenzone, and titanium dioxide.
*Sunscreen.*

**Ombrelle for Kids** *Cosmair, Canad.*
*SPF 30:* Avobenzone (p.1142·3); octinoxate (p.1154·3); ensulizole (p.1147·1); enzacamene (p.1147·1).
*Sunscreen.*

**Ombrelle Lotion** *Cosmair, Canad.*
*SPF 15:* Avobenzone (p.1142·3); octocrilene (p.1154·3); octisalate (p.1154·3).
*SPF 30:* Avobenzone (p.1142·3); enzacamene (p.1147·1); octocrilene (p.1154·3); ensulizole (p.1147·1); ecamsule (p.1146·3).
Formerly contained avobenzone, enzacamene, octinoxate and ensulizole.
*Sunscreen.*

**Ombrelle, Ombrelle Sport Spray** *Dermtek, Canad.†.*
*SPF 15:* Avobenzone (p.1142·3); octinoxate (p.1154·3); oxybenzone (p.1154·3).
*Sunscreen.*

**Ombrelle Vapo Sport** *Cosmair, Canad.*
*SPF 15:* Avobenzone (p.1142·3); octocrilene (p.1154·3); octisalate (p.1154·3).
*Sunscreen.*

**Omca** *Bristol-Myers Squibb, Ger.*
Fluphenazine hydrochloride (p.699·3).
*Psychoses.*

**Omcilon A** *Bristol-Myers Squibb, Braz.†.*
Triamcinolone acetonide (p.1110·2); salicylic acid (p.1157·1).
*Skin disorders.*

**Omcilon A M** *Bristol-Myers Squibb, Braz.*
Triamcinolone acetonide (p.1110·2); neomycin sulfate (p.235·1); gramicidin (p.220·2); nystatin (p.406·3).
*Infected skin disorders.*

**Omcilon A Orabase** *Bristol-Myers Squibb, Braz.*
Triamcinolone acetonide (p.1110·2).
*Mouth ulceration.*

**Om-Dicynone** *Labomed, Chile.*
Etamsylate (p.749·3).
*Haemorrhage.*

**Omebeta** *Betapharm, Ger.*
Omeprazole (p.1278·2).
*Gastro-oesophageal reflux; peptic ulcer; Zollinger-Ellison syndrome.*

**Omega** *Schmidgall, Austria.*
Proxyphylline (p.791·2); crataegus (p.1677·1); convallaria (p.1675·3).
*Cardiac disorders.*

**Omega-3** *Gisand, Switz.*
Omega-3 marine triglycerides (p.976·2).
*Dietary supplement; hyperlipidaemia.*

**Omega 3+** *Proceane, Fr.†.*
Omega-3 marine triglycerides (p.976·2).
*Dietary supplement.*

**Omega 7** *Pharma Nord, UK.*
Sea buckthorn oil (p.1742·3).
*Dietary supplement.*

**Omega 100** *Omega, Arg.*
Carbinoxamine maleate (p.426·3).
*Hypersensitivity reactions.*

**Omega 100 Bronquial** *Omega, Arg.*
Guaifenesin (p.1122·1).
*Coughs.*

**Omega 100 L** *Omega, Arg.*
Loratadine (p.436·1).
*Allergic rhinitis; conjunctivitis; urticaria.*

**Omegacoeur** *Holistica, Fr.*
Omega-3 triglycerides (p.976·1); herbs (p.1417·1).
*Circulatory disorders.*

**Omega-H3**
*Vitabiotics, Irl.*
Multivitamin and mineral preparation (p.1417·1).
*Vitabiotics, UK.*
Multivitamin, mineral, and nutritional preparation (p.1417·1).

**Omegaline** *Holistica, Fr.*
Borage oil (p.1661·3).
*Nutritional supplement.*

**Omegaven**
*Fresenius Kabi, Austria; Fresenius Kabi, Denm.; Fresenius Kabi, Fr.; Fresenius Kabi, Ger.; Fresenius Kabi, Ital.; Fresenius Kabi, Port.; Fresenius Kabi, Swed.; Fresenius Kabi, Switz.*
Omega-3 marine triglycerides (p.976·2).
*Lipid infusion for parenteral nutrition.*

**Omelind** *Lindopharm, Ger.*
Omeprazole (p.1278·2).
*Gastro-oesophageal reflux; peptic ulcer; Zollinger-Ellison syndrome.*

**Ome-nerton** *Dolorgiet, Ger.*
Omeprazole (p.1278·2).
*Gastro-oesophageal reflux; peptic ulcer; Zollinger-Ellison syndrome.*

**Omep**
*UCI, Braz.; Hexal, Ger.*
Omeprazole (p.1278·2).
*Gastro-oesophageal reflux; peptic ulcer; Zollinger-Ellison syndrome.*

**Omepra** *BA Farma, Port.*
Omeprazole (p.1278·2).
*Gastro-oesophageal reflux; peptic ulcer; Zollinger-Ellison syndrome.*

**Omepradex** *Dexcel, Israel.*
Omeprazole (p.1278·2).
*Gastro-oesophageal reflux; peptic ulcer; Zollinger-Ellison syndrome.*

**Omepral** *Astra, Jpn.*
Omeprazole (p.1278·2).
*Gastro-oesophageal reflux; peptic ulcer; Zollinger-Ellison syndrome.*

**Omeprasec**
*AstraZeneca, Arg.; Aventis, Braz.†.*
Omeprazole (p.1278·2), omeprazole magnesium (p.1278·2), or omeprazole sodium (p.1278·2).
*Acid aspiration; gastro-oesophageal reflux; peptic ulcer; Zollinger-Ellison syndrome.*

**Omeprax** *Instituto Sanitas, Chile.*
Omeprazole (p.1278·2).
*Gastro-oesophageal reflux; peptic ulcer; Zollinger-Ellison syndrome.*

**Omeprazen** *Malesci, Ital.*
Omeprazole (p.1278·2) or omeprazole sodium (p.1278·2).
*Gastro-oesophageal reflux; peptic ulcer; Zollinger-Ellison syndrome.*

**Omeprazin** *EMS, Braz.*
Omeprazole (p.1278·2) or omeprazole sodium (p.1278·2).

**Omeprol** *Medichrom, Gr.*
Omeprazole (p.1278·2).
*Acid aspiration; eradication of Helicobacter pylori in combination with antimicrobials; peptic ulcer; reflux oesophagitis; Zollinger-Ellison syndrome.*

**Omeprotec** *Hexal, Braz.*
Omeprazole (p.1278·2).
*Peptic ulcer.*

**Ome-Puren** *Alpharma-Isis, Ger.*
Omeprazole (p.1278·2).
*Gastro-oesophageal reflux; peptic ulcer; Zollinger-Ellison syndrome.*

**Omerol** *Helfarma, Port.*
Omeprazole (p.1278·2).
*Gastro-oesophageal reflux; peptic ulcer; Zollinger-Ellison syndrome.*

**Omesan** *Duomed, Switz.†.*
Omega-3 marine triglycerides (p.976·2).
*Hyperlipidaemias.*

**Omesec**
*CCM, Malaysia; CCM, Singapore.*
Omeprazole (p.1278·2).
*Gastro-oesophageal reflux; peptic ulcer; Zollinger-Ellison syndrome.*

**Ometon** *Clintex, Port.*
Omeprazole (p.1278·2).
*Gastro-oesophageal reflux; peptic ulcer; Zollinger-Ellison syndrome.*

**Omez** *Reddy, Thai.*
Omeprazole (p.1278·2).
*Gastro-oesophageal reflux; peptic ulcer; Zollinger-Ellison syndrome.*

**Omezol** *Alembic, India.*
Omeprazole (p.1278·2).
*Gastro-oesophageal reflux; peptic ulcer; Zollinger-Ellison syndrome.*

**Omezolan** *Euro-Labor, Port.; Grunenthal, Port.*
Omeprazole (p.1278·2).
*Gastro-oesophageal reflux; peptic ulcer; Zollinger-Ellison syndrome.*

**Omezole** *Hovid, Malaysia.*
Omeprazole (p.1278·2).
*Gastric hyperacidity; gastro-oesophageal reflux; peptic ulcer.*

**Omic** *Yamanouchi, Belg.*
Tamsulosin hydrochloride (p.1009·2).
*Benign prostatic hyperplasia.*

**Omicite** *Torrent, Thai.†.*
Clomifene citrate (p.1542·2).
*Anovulatory infertility; male infertility.*

**Omida Gel Antirhumatismal** *Omida, Switz.†.*
Homoeopathic preparation.

**Omida Granules Relaxants** *Omida, Switz.†.*
Homoeopathic preparation.

**Omida Spray Nasal** *Omida, Switz.†.*
Homoeopathic preparation.

**Omifin**
*Aventis, Mex.; Effik, Spain.*
Clomifene citrate (p.1542·2).
*Anovulatory infertility; male infertility.*

**Omilcal** *Franco-Indian, India.*
Calcium phosphate (p.1225·3); colecalciferol (p.1461·3); calcium lactate (p.1225·3).
*Calcium deficiency; osteoporosis.*

**Omilipis** *Richmond, Arg.*
Carboplatin (p.533·3).
*Malignant neoplasms.*

**Ominol** *Loren, Mex.*
Progesterone (p.1566·2); estradiol (p.1550·1).

**Omix**
*Yamanouchi, Austria; Yamanouchi, Fr.*
Tamsulosin hydrochloride (p.1009·2).
*Benign prostatic hyperplasia.*

**Ommunal** *Byk, Arg.*
Haemophilus influenzae Streptococcus pneumoniae; Klebsiella pneumoniae; Klebsiella ozaenae; Staphylococcus aureus; Streptococcus pyogenes; Streptococcus viridans; Moraxella catarrhalis.
*Respiratory-tract infections.*

**Omnalio** *Estedi, Spain.*
Chlordiazepoxide hydrochloride (p.674·2).
*Alcohol withdrawal syndrome; anxiety; insomnia; skeletal muscle spasm.*

**Omnatax** *Nicholas Piramal, India.*
Cefotaxime sodium (p.175·3).
*Bacterial infections.*

**Omneo** *Nutricia, Port.*
A range of infant feeds (p.1417·1).
*Gastrointestinal disorders.*

**Omnia** *Hochstetter, Chile.*
Camphor (p.1665·3); artemisia abrotanum.

**Omnia T** *Hochstetter, Chile.*
Vitamin and mineral preparation (p.1417·1).

**Omniadol** *Montefarmaco, Ital.†.*
Propyphenazone (p.85·3); paracetamol (p.76·2); caffeine (p.782·1).
*Cold symptoms; pain.*

**Omniapharm** *Merckle, Ger.*
Bromhexine hydrochloride (p.1115·3).
*Respiratory-tract disorders associated with increased or viscous mucus.*

**Omnibionta**
*Merck, Austria.*
Multivitamin infusion (p.1417·1).
*Merck-Belgolabo, Belg.†.*
Brown/red capsules, multivitamins (p.1417·1); yellow/ochre capsules, minerals.
*Merck, Spain.*
Multivitamin and trace element preparation (p.1417·1).
*Merck, Swed.*
Vitamin and mineral preparation (p.1417·1).

**Omnibionta Integral** *Merck, Belg.*
Multivitamin and mineral preparation (p.1417·1).

**Omnic**
*Temis, Arg.; Eurofarma, Braz.; Labomed, Chile; Yamanouchi, Denm.; Yamanouchi, Fin.; Yamanouchi, Ger.†; Gerolimatos (Γερολυματος), Gr.; Yamanouchi, Irl.; Yamanouchi, Israel; Yamanouchi, Ital.; Yamanouchi, Neth.; Yamanouchi, Norw.; Yamanouchi, Port.; Yamanouchi, Spain.*
Tamsulosin hydrochloride (p.1009·2).
*Benign prostatic hyperplasia.*

**Omnicare** *Allergan, Israel†.*
Solution, hydrogen peroxide (p.1182·2); tablets, catalase (p.1668·3) (p.1164·2).
*Disinfecting and neutralising system for soft contact lenses.*

**Omnicare Daily Cleaner**
*Allergan, Austral.†; Advanced Medical Optics, NZ.*
Cleansing solution for soft contact lenses (p.1164·2).

**Omnicare 1 Step**
*Allergan, Austral.†; Advanced Medical Optics, NZ.*
Solution, hydrogen peroxide (p.1182·2); tablets, catalase (p.1668·3) (p.1164·2).
*Disinfecting and neutralising system for soft contact lenses.*

**Omnicef**
*Pfizer, Austria; Pfizer, Thai.; Abbott, USA.*
Cefdinir (p.171·3).
*Bacterial infections.*

**Omniderm** *Face, Ital.*
Fluocinolone acetonide (p.1101·2).
*Inflammatory skin disorders.*

**Omniflora** *Novartis Consumer, Austria.*
*Lactobacillus gasseri; Bifidobacterium bifidum* (p.1704·2).
*Gastrointestinal disorders.*

**Omniflora Akut** *Novartis Consumer, Ger.*
*Saccharomyces boulardii* (p.1704·2).
*Diarrhoea.*

**Omniflora N** *Novartis Consumer, Ger.*
*Lactobacillus gasseri; Bifidobacterium longum.*
*Gastrointestinal disorders.*

**Omnigeriat** *Fabra, Arg.*
Cyproterone acetate (p.1544·1).

**Omnigraf** *Juste, Spain.*
Iohexol (p.1064·2).
*Radiographic contrast medium.*

**OmniHIB** *SmithKline Beecham, USA.*
A haemophilus influenzae conjugate vaccine (tetanus toxoid conjugate) (p.1616·1).
*Active immunisation.*

**Omnihist LA** *WE, USA.*
Phenylephrine hydrochloride (p.1126·3); chlorphenamine maleate (p.427·3); hyoscine methonitrate (p.483·3).
*Upper respiratory-tract symptoms.*

**Omnipaque**
*Nycomed, Arg.; Amersham, Austral.; Schering, Austria; Nycomed, Belg.†; Sanofi Synthelabo, Braz.; Nycomed Imaging, Canad.; Sanofi Synthelabo, Chile; Amersham, Denm.; Amersham, Fin.; Amersham, Fr.; Schering, Ger.; Nycomed, Gr.; Nycomed, Israel; Nycomed, Ital.; Nycomed Imaging, Norw.; Amersham, NZ; Amersham, Spain; Amersham, Swed.; Schering, Switz.; Nycomed Amersham, UK; Nycomed, USA.*
Iohexol (p.1064·2).
*Radiographic contrast medium.*

**Omnipen**
*Wyeth, Mex.; Wyeth-Ayerst, USA†.*
Ampicillin (p.157·1) or ampicillin sodium (p.157·1).
*Bacterial infections.*

**Omniplex** *Vitaplex, Austral.†.*
Multivitamin and mineral supplement with herbs (p.1417·1).
*Dietary supplement.*

**Omniscan**
*Nycomed, Arg.; Amersham, Austral.; Nycomed, Austria; Nycomed, Belg.†; Sanofi Synthelabo, Braz.; Nycomed Imaging, Canad.; Sanofi Synthelabo, Chile; Amersham, Denm.; Amersham, Fin.; Amersham, Fr.; Amersham, Ger.; Nycomed, Gr.; Nycomed, Israel; Nycomed, Ital.; Daiichi, Jpn; Nycomed Imaging, Norw.; Amersham, NZ; Amersham,*

*Spain; Amersham, Swed.; Nycomed Amersham, Switz.; Nycomed Amersham, UK; Sanofi Winthrop, USA.*
Gadodiamide (p.1062·1).
*Contrast medium for magnetic resonance imaging.*

**Omnisept** *Monchpharma, Ger.*
*Lactobacillus acidophilus* (p.1704·2).
*Diarrhoea.*

**Omnitest** *Braun, Austral.*
Test for glucose in blood (p.1694·2).

**Omnitrace** *Lifeplan, UK†.*
Trace element preparation (p.1417·1).

**Omnitrast** *Schering, Spain.*
Iohexol (p.1064·2).
*Radiographic contrast medium.*

**Omni-Tuss** *Aventis, Canad.*
Codeine resin (p.27·1); phenyltoloxamine resin (p.439·1); chlorphenamine resin (p.428·1); ephedrine resin (p.1120·1); guaiacol carbonate (p.1122·1).
*Coughs.*

**Omnival** *Knoll, Ger.†.*
Multivitamin and mineral preparation (p.1417·1).

**Omnopon** *Bodene, S.Afr.*
Papaveretum (p.74·3) (containing morphine hydrochloride, codeine hydrochloride, and papaverine hydrochloride).
*Pain.*

**OMP** *Chong Kun Dang, Thai.†.*
Omeprazole (p.1278·2).
*Gastro-oesophageal reflux; peptic ulcer; Zollinger-Ellison syndrome.*

**Ompranyt** *Bial, Spain.*
Omeprazole (p.1278·2).
*Gastro-oesophageal reflux; peptic ulcer; Zollinger-Ellison syndrome.*

**Omr-IgG** *Omrix, Israel.*
A normal immunoglobulin (p.1627·2).
*Idiopathic thrombocytopenic purpura; immunodeficiency; passive immunisation.*

**Omri-Hep-B** *Omrix, Israel.*
A hepatitis B immunoglobulin (p.1617·2).
*Passive immunisation.*

**Omrixate** *Omrix, Israel.*
A factor VIII preparation (p.751·1).
*Haemophilia A.*

**OMS Concentrate** *Upsher-Smith, USA†.*
Morphine sulfate (p.60·2).
*Pain.*

**Omycet** *Collins, Mex.*
Chloramphenicol (p.185·1).
*Bacterial infections.*

**Onagre** *Sante Naturelle, Canad.†.*
Evening primrose oil (p.1686·3).

**Onaka** *Max Farma, Ital.*
Pidotimod (p.1731·3).
*Immunostimulant.*

**Onapan** *Alpharma, Mex.*
Diazepam (p.690·1).

**Oncaspar**
*Aventis, Canad.; Medac, Ger.; Rhone-Poulenc Rorer, USA.*
Pegaspargase (p.528·3).
*Acute lymphoblastic leukaemia.*

**Once-a-Day**
*Quest, Canad.; Quest, UK†.*
Multivitamin and mineral preparation (p.1417·1).

**Oncet** *Wakefield, USA.*
Hydrocodone tartrate (p.45·1); paracetamol (p.76·2).
*Cough and cold symptoms.*

**Onciplus** *Prodotti, Braz.*
Gramicidin (p.220·2); neomycin sulfate (p.235·1); nystatin (p.406·3); triamcinolone acetonide (p.1110·2).
*Infected skin disorders.*

**Onclast** *Banyu, Jpn.*
Alendronate sodium (p.765·3).

**Onco Tiotepa**
*Zambon, Braz.†; Prasfarma, Spain.*
Thiotepa (p.588·1).
*Malignant neoplasms.*

**Oncocarb** *Asta Oncologia, Braz.*
Carboplatin (p.533·3).
*Malignant neoplasms.*

**Onco-Carbide** *Teofarma, Ital.*
Hydroxycarbamide (p.559·1).
*Chronic myeloid leukaemia; myelofibrosis; polycythaemia vera; thrombocythaemia.*

**Oncocarbil** *Kampel Martian, Arg.*
Dacarbazine (p.544·2).
*Malignant neoplasms.*

**Onco-Cloramin** *Zambon, Braz.†.*
Chlormethine (p.537·3).
*Malignant neoplasms; mycosis fungoides; polycythaemia vera.*

**Oncofu** *Pharmacia, Arg.*
Fluorouracil (p.554·2).
*Malignant neoplasms.*

**Oncosal** *Inibsa, Spain.*
Flutamide (p.556·2).
*Prostatic cancer.*

**OncoScint** *REM, Braz.†.*
Indium-111 satumomab pendetide (p.1523·3).
*Diagnosis of colorectal cancer.*

**OncoScint CR 103**
*Schering, Ital.†; CIS, Spain.*
Indium-111 satumomab pendetide (p.1523·3).
*Diagnosis of colorectal cancer.*

**OncoScint CR/OV** *Cytogen, USA.*
Indium-111 satumomab pendetide (p.1523·3).
*Detection of colorectal and ovarian metastases.*

**OncoSeeds** *Amersham, Austral.*
Iodine-125 (p.1524·2) titanium capsules.
*Prostatic cancer.*

**Oncotam** *Mayoly-Spindler, Fr.*
Tamoxifen citrate (p.584·1).
*Breast cancer.*

**Oncotaxina** *Pharmacia, Arg.*
Mitomycin (p.573·3).
*Malignant neoplasms.*

**OncoTICE**
*Organon, Austral.; Organon, Austria; Akzo, Braz.†; Organon Teknika, Canad.; Organon, Denm.; Organon, Fin.; Apogepha, Ger.; Organon (Οργανον), Gr.; Organon, Hong Kong; Organon Teknika, Israel; Organon, Ital.; Organon Teknika, Neth.; Organon, Norw.; Organon, NZ; Organon, Port.; Organon, Spain; Organon, Swed.; Organon, Switz.; Organon, UK.*
A BCG vaccine (p.1609·2).
*Bladder cancer.*

**Oncotron** *Sun, India.*
Mitoxantrone (p.576·1).
*Malignant neoplasms.*

**Oncovin**
*Lilly, Austral.; Lilly, Austria; Lilly, Belg.; Lilly, Braz.; Lilly, Canad.†; Lilly, Chile; Lilly, Denm.; Lilly, Fin.; Lilly, Fr.; Pharmaserve Lilly (Φαρμασερβ Λιλλυ), Gr.; Lilly, Irl.†; Lilly, Israel†; Lilly, Mex.; Lilly, Neth.†; Lilly, Norw.; Lilly, NZ†; Lilly, Port.; Lilly, S.Afr.; Lilly, Swed.; Lilly, Switz.; Clonmel, UK; Lilly, USA.*
Vincristine sulfate (p.592·2).
*Idiopathic thrombocytopenic purpura; malignant neoplasms.*

**Oncovite** *Mission Pharmacal, USA.*
Multivitamin preparation with zinc (p.1417·1).

**Onctose** *Monot, Fr.†.*
Diphenhydramine metilsulfate (p.432·2); lidocaine hydrochloride (p.1377·3).
*Pruritus.*

**Onctose a l'Hydrocortisone** *Denolin, Belg.†.*
Hydrocortisone acetate (p.1103·3); diphenhydramine metilsulfate (p.432·2); lidocaine hydrochloride (p.1377·3).
*Cutaneous hypersensitivity reactions; insect stings; pruritus.*

**Onctose Hydrocortisone** *Monot, Fr.†.*
Diphenhydramine metilsulfate (p.432·2); lidocaine hydrochloride (p.1377·3); hydrocortisone acetate (p.1103·3).
*Pruritus.*

**Ondax** *Saval, Chile.*
Cisapride (p.1259·2).
*Constipation; dyspepsia; gastro-oesophageal reflux; gastroparesis; pseudo-obstruction.*

**Ondolen** *Menarini, Port.*
Hydrochlorothiazide (p.933·2); spironolactone (p.1003·1).
*Ascites; hypertension; nephrotic syndrome; oedema.*

**Ondroly-A** *Boffi, Ital.*
Peppermint oil (p.1283·2); clove oil (p.1673·3); menthol (p.1711·3); benzoin tincture (p.1744·1); phenol (p.1188·1).
*Dentistry.*

**Ondrox** *LSI, USA.*
Multivitamin, mineral, and amino acid preparation (p.1417·1).

**One** *Natural Life, Arg.*
Multivitamin and mineral preparation (p.1417·1).

**One A Day**
*Bayer, Arg.; Bayer, Braz.; Bayer Consumer, Canad.; Bayer, Ital.†; Bayer Consumer, Singapore; Bayer, USA.*
Vitamin, multivitamin, or multivitamin and mineral preparations (p.1417·1).

**One Step** *Maurino, Arg.*
Hydrogen peroxide 3% (p.1182·2); catalase (p.1668·3) (p.1164·2).
*Disinfection and cleaning of contact lenses.*

**One Touch**
*Johnson & Johnson Medical, Arg.; Lifescan, Fr.; Lifescan, Irl.; Lifescan, Port.; Lifescan, USA.*
Test for glucose in blood (p.1694·2).

**Onealfa** *Teijin, Jpn.*
Alfacalcidol (p.1461·2).
*Disorders of vitamin D metabolism; osteoporosis.*

**One-Alpha**
*Leo, Canad.; Leo (Λεο), Gr.; Leo, Hong Kong; Leo, Irl.; Leo, Israel; Leo, Malaysia; CSL, NZ; Adcock Ingram, S.Afr.; Leo, Singapore; Leo, Thai.; Leo, UK.*
Alfacalcidol (p.1461·2).
*Hyperparathyroidism; hypocalcaemia; hypoparathyroidism; hypophosphataemia; osteomalacia; osteoporosis; renal osteodystrophy; rickets.*

**Onefin** *Kampel Martian, Arg.*
Donepezil (p.1490·1).

**Onelacne** *DNR, Arg.*
Amino acids; vitamin B substances (p.1417·1); sulfurated peptides (p.1158·2).
*Acne.*

**Onemer** *Piso, Mex.*
Ketorolac trometamol (p.52·1).
*Pain.*

**One-Tablet-Daily** *Goldline, USA.*
A range of vitamin preparations with or without minerals (p.1417·1).

**Onfor** *Fada, Arg.*
Nalbuphine (p.64·3).
*Pain.*

**Onglinex** *Medinfar, Port.*
Cystine; pyridoxine hydrochloride (p.1417·1).
*Hair and nail disorders.*

**Onguent Hemorrhoidal** *Prodemdis, Canad.*
Pramocaine hydrochloride (p.1382·2); zinc sulfate (p.1469·3).
*Haemorrhoids.*

**Onguent nasal Ruedi** *Spirig, Switz.*
Mint oil (p.1715·2); camphor oil.
*Nasal dryness.*

**Onico Fitex** *Belmac, Spain.*
Borogallic acid; salicylic acid (p.1157·1).
*Fungal nail infections.*

**Onixol** *Schering, Arg.*
Trolamine (p.1758·2); sodium sulfate; potassium acetate; urea (p.1162·2); lavender oil.
*Nail disorders.*

**Oniz** *Stadmed, India.*
Ornidazole (p.612·2).
*Amoebiasis; anaerobic bacterial infections; giardiasis; trichomoniasis.*

**Onkocristin** *Onkoworks, Ger.*
Vincristine sulfate (p.592·2).
*Malignant neoplasms.*

**Onkofluor** *Onkoworks, Ger.*
Fluorouracil (p.554·2).

**Onkomorphin** *Onkoworks, Ger.*
Morphine sulfate (p.60·2).
*Pain.*

**Onkoposid** *Onkoworks, Ger.*
Etoposide (p.551·3).
*Malignant neoplasms.*

**Onkotrone**
*Baxter, Austral.; Baxter Oncology, Ger.; Baxter Oncology, UK.*
Mitoxantrone hydrochloride (p.575·2).
*Malignant neoplasms.*

**Onkovertin**
*Braun, Austria†; Braun, Ger.†.*
Dextran 60 (p.746·1) in sodium chloride.
*Plasma volume expansion; pre-operative haemodilution; thromboembolism prophylaxis.*

*Braun, Thai.*
Dextran 40 (p.745·3) in sodium chloride.
*Plasma volume expansion.*

**Onkovertin N**
*Braun, Austria†; Braun, Ger.†.*
Dextran 40 (p.745·3) in sodium chloride.
*Circulatory disorders; thromboembolism prophylaxis.*

**Only One** *Sisu, Canad.*
Multivitamin and mineral preparation (p.1417·1).

**Onoact** *Ono, Jpn.*
Landiolol hydrochloride (p.945·1).
*Intra-operative tachyarrhythmias.*

**Onofin-K** *Rayere, Mex.*
Ketoconazole (p.403·3).
*Fungal infections.*

**Onon** *Ono, Jpn.*
Pranlukast (p.791·1).
*Allergic rhinitis; asthma.*

**Onopordon Comp B** *Weleda, UK.*
Onopordon; cowslip (p.1735·1); hyoscyamus (p.485·2).
*Cardiac disorders.*

**Onoprose** *Alter, Port.*
Promelase (p.1735·2).
*Inflammation.*

**Onoton**
*Sanofi Synthelabo, Chile; Sanofi Synthelabo, Mex.*
Pancreatin (p.1725·3); hemicellulase (p.1669·1); ox bile extract (p.1660·3); simeticone (p.1289·2).
*Adjunct in abdominal radiography; digestive disorders; pancreatic disorders.*

**Onrectal** *Herbes Universelles, Canad.*
Benzocaine (p.1370·3); bismuth subcarbonate (p.1252·1); bismuth subgallate (p.1252·2); hamamelis (p.1696·3); naphazoline hydrochloride (p.1124·3); zinc oxide (p.1163·2).
*Haemorrhoids.*

**Onsia** *Siam Bheasach, Thai.*
Ondansetron hydrochloride (p.1281·1).
*Nausea and vomiting induced by cytotoxics or radiotherapy; postoperative nausea and vomiting.*

**Onsudil** *Bonafarma, Port.*
Procaterol hydrochloride (p.791·1).
*Obstructive airways disease.*

**Onsukil** *Otsuka, Spain.*
Procaterol (p.791·1).
*Obstructive airways disease.*

**Ontak** *Ligand, USA.*
Denileukin diftitox (p.546·3).
*T-cell lymphoma.*

**Ontop** *Systopic, India.*
Lomefloxacin hydrochloride (p.227·2).
*Bacterial infections.*

**Ontosein** *Tedec Meiji, Spain.*
Orgotein (p.92·2).
*Arthropathies; cystitis; peri-articular disorders; secondary effects of radiotherapy.*

**Ontrax** *Blausiegel, Braz.*
Ondansetron hydrochloride (p.1281·1).
*Nausea and vomiting.*

**Onxol** *Zenith Goldline, USA.*
Paclitaxel (p.577·3).
*Malignant neoplasms.*

**Onycho Phytex**
*Note. This name is used for preparations of different composition.*
*Rupertus, Austria†.*
Sorbic acid (p.1192·3); tannic acid (p.1751·2); methyl salicylate (p.59·3); salicylic acid (p.1157·1); acetic acid (p.1645·2).
*Fungal nail infections.*

*UCB, Port.†.*
Boric acid (p.1662·1).

**Onychomal** *Hermal, Ger.*
Urea (p.1162·2).
*Nail disorders.*

**Ony-Clear** *Pedinol, USA.*
*Topical powder spray†:* Miconazole nitrate (p.405·3).
*Fungal skin infections.*
*Topical solution:* Benzalkonium chloride (p.1168·3). Formerly contained triacetin, cetylpyridinium chloride, and chloroxylenol.
*Fungal nail infections.*

**Opacist ER**
*Bracco, Ital.; Bracco, Switz.*
Meglumine iodamide (p.1063·2).
*Contrast medium for urinary-tract radiography.*

**Opacite** *Justesa Imagen, Arg.*
Meglumine gadopentetate (p.1062·2).
*Contrast medium for magnetic resonance imaging.*

**Opalgyne** *Innotech, Fr.*
Benzydamine hydrochloride (p.21·1).
*Vaginitis.*

**Opalia** *Ecobi, Ital.†.*
Royal jelly (p.1740·3).
*Nutritional supplement.*

**Opalino** *Weltrop, Arg.*
Sodium picosulfate (p.1289·3).
*Constipation.*

**Opalmon** *Ono, Jpn.*
Limaprost alfadex (p.1519·2).
*Intermittent claudication; thromboangiitis obliterans.*

**Opam** *Wockhardt, India.*
Pioglitazone (p.344·2).
*Diabetes mellitus.*

**Opamox** *Orion, Fin.*
Oxazepam (p.712·2).
*Anxiety disorders; depression; insomnia; psychoses.*

**Oparsan Con Lisina Y L-Glutamina** *Instituto Sanitas, Chile.*
Vitamins; minerals; amino acids (p.1417·1).
*Dietary supplement.*

**Opas** *Co-Pharma, UK.*
Sodium bicarbonate (p.1223·2); calcium carbonate (p.1254·2); magnesium carbonate (p.1272·1); magnesium trisilicate (p.1272·3).
*Dyspepsia; flatulence; gastric hyperacidity; heartburn.*

**Opatanol**
*Alcon, Denm.; Alcon, Fr.; Alcon, UK.*
Olopatadine (p.438·1).
*Allergic conjunctivitis.*

**Opazimes** *Co-Pharma, UK.*
Aluminium hydroxide (p.1249·2); light kaolin (p.1268·3); belladonna (p.479·1); morphine hydrochloride (p.60·1).
*Diarrhoea; dyspepsia; gastro-enteritis.*

**Opcon-A**
*Bausch & Lomb, Canad.; Bausch & Lomb, USA.*
Naphazoline hydrochloride (p.1124·3); pheniramine maleate (p.438·3).
*Eye irritation.*

**Operand** *Redi-Products, USA.*
Povidone-iodine (p.1190·3).
*Skin disinfection; vaginal disorders.*

**Operium** *PP Lab, Thai.*
Loperamide hydrochloride (p.1271·1).
*Diarrhoea.*

**Ophan** *Chew, Thai.*
Chlorphenamine maleate (p.427·3); ammonium chloride (p.1115·2).
*Coughs; nasal congestion.*

**Ophcillin N** *Medicopharm, Austria.*
Benzylpenicillin sodium (p.163·2); sulfadiazine (p.258·2).
*Bacterial eye infections.*

**Ophdilvas N** *Mann, Ger.*
Vincamine (p.1764·2).
*Cerebral and peripheral vascular disorders; circulatory disorders of the eye.*

**Ophidus** *Motima, Fr.*
Lactobacillus acidophilus (p.1704·2); bifidobacterium.
*Maintenance of intestinal flora.*

**Ophtacalm** *Chauvin, Fr.*
Sodium cromoglicate (p.795·3).
*Allergic eye disorders.*

**Ophtadil** *Chauvin, Fr.*
Buphenine hydrochloride (p.1663·2); ethoxazorutoside (p.1688·2); sodium ascorbate (p.1460·2); *d*-alpha tocoferil acetate (p.1465·1).
*Ocular vascular disorders.*

**Ophtagram**
*Chauvin, Fr.†; Chauvin ankerpharm, Ger.; Chauvin, Port.; Chauvin, Singapore†; Bausch & Lomb, Switz.*
Gentamicin sulfate (p.217·1).
*Bacterial eye infections.*

**Ophtaguttal** *Agepha, Austria.*
Naphazoline hydrochloride (p.1124·3); zinc sulfate (p.1469·3); boric acid (p.1662·1).
*Conjunctival irritation.*

**Ophtal** Winzer, Ger.†.
Idoxuridine (p.637·3).
*Herpes infections of the eye.*

**Ophtalin** Ciba Vision, Ital.
Sodium hyaluronate (p.1697·3).
*Eye surgery.*

**Ophtalmin** Winzer, Ger.†.
Oxedrine tartrate (p.977·3); naphazoline hydrochloride (p.1124·3); antazoline hydrochloride (p.424·2).
*Eye disorders.*

**Ophtalmin N** Winzer, Ger.
Tetryzoline hydrochloride (p.1131·2).
*Eye disorders.*

**Ophtalmine** Cooperation Pharmaceutique, Fr.
Boric acid (p.1662·1); borax (p.1661·3); red vine; rose water (p.1058·1); peppermint water (p.1283·2); hamamelis (p.1696·3).
*Eye irritation.*

**Ophtalmotrim** Viatris, Belg.
Trimethoprim (p.272·2); polymyxin B sulfate (p.245·1).
*Bacterial eye infections.*

**Ophtamedine** Bournonville, Belg.†.
Hexamidine isetionate (p.1181·3).
*Eye disorders; otitis; rhinitis.*

**Ophtasiloxane** Alcon, Fr.
Dimeticone (p.1482·1).
*Corneal burns; prevention of corneal adhesions.*

**Ophtasone** Bausch & Lomb, Switz.
Betamethasone sodium phosphate (p.1093·1); gentamicin sulfate (p.217·1).
*Infected eye disorders.*

**Ophtaxia** Chauvin, Fr.
Sodium chloride; potassium chloride; calcium chloride; magnesium chloride (p.1217·1).
*Eye irrigation.*

**Ophthalgan** Wyeth-Ayerst, USA†.
Glycerol (p.1694·3).
*Corneal oedema.*

**Ophthalin**
Ciba Vision, Austral.; Ciba Vision, Hong Kong†; Novartis, Irl.; Ciba Vision, Israel; Novartis, NZ; Ciba Vision, Singapore†; Ciba Vision, Thai.; Iocom, UK.
Sodium hyaluronate (p.1697·3).
*Adjunct in ocular surgery.*

**Ophthetic**
Allergan, Austral.; Allergan, Canad.; Allergan, NZ; Allergan, S.Afr.†; Allergan, USA.
Proxymetacaine hydrochloride (p.1384·1).
*Local anaesthesia.*

**Ophthifluor** Deklerht, USA.
Fluorescein sodium (p.1689·1).
*Ophthalmic diagnostic agent.*

**Ophtho-Bunolol** Altimed, Canad.
Levobunolol hydrochloride (p.946·2).
*Glaucoma.*

**Ophtho-Chloram** Altimed, Canad.†.
Chloramphenicol (p.185·1).
*Eye infections.*

**Ophthocort** Parke, Davis, Canad.†.
Chloramphenicol (p.185·1); hydrocortisone acetate (p.1103·3); polymyxin B sulfate (p.245·1).
*Infected eye disorders.*

**Ophtho-Sulf** Kenral, Canad.†.
Sulfacetamide sodium (p.257·3).
*Eye infections.*

**Ophtho-Tate** Altimed, Canad.
Prednisolone acetate (p.1108·1).
*Eye disorders.*

**Ophtilan** Lannacher, Austria.
Timolol maleate (p.1012·2).
*Glaucoma; ocular hypertension.*

**Ophtim** Thea, Fr.
Timolol maleate (p.1012·2).
*Glaucoma; ocular hypertension.*

**Ophtocain N** Winzer, Ger.
Tetracaine hydrochloride (p.1385·1).
Ophtocain formerly contained tetracaine hydrochloride and naphazoline hydrochloride.
*Local anaesthesia for ophthalmic procedures.*

**Ophtol-A** Winzer, Ger.†.
Vitamin A palmitate (p.1453·1).
*Eye disorders.*

**Ophtopur-N** Winzer, Ger.†.
Zinc borate (p.1662·1); naphazoline hydrochloride (p.1124·3).
*Eye disorders.*

**Ophtopur-Z** Winzer, Ger.
Zinc sulfate (p.1469·3).
*Eye disorders.*

**Ophtosan** Winzer, Ger.†.
Vitamin A palmitate (p.1453·1).
*Eye disorders.*

**Ophtrivin-A** Ciba Vision, Canad.†.
Xylometazoline hydrochloride (p.1132·2); antazoline sulfate (p.424·2).
*Eye disorders.*

**Opidina** BA Farma, Port.
Ticlopidine (p.1012·1).

**Opidol**
Norpharma, Denm.; Mundipharma, Fin.†; Mundipharma, Swed.; Mundipharma, Switz.
Hydromorphone hydrochloride (p.45·2).
*Pain.*

**Opilet** Rafarm, Gr.
Azelaic acid (p.1142·3).
*Acne.*

**Opilon**
Hansam, Irl.; Hansam, UK.
Moxisylyte hydrochloride (p.962·2).
*Menière's disease; peripheral vascular disorders; Raynaud's syndrome.*

**Opino**
Note. This name is used for preparations of different composition.
Kolassa, Austria.
*Tablets:* Buphenine hydrochloride (p.1663·2); aescin (p.1648·2).
*Topical gel:* Buphenine hydrochloride (p.1663·2); aescin (p.1648·2); rosemary oil (p.1740·2); pumilio pine oil (p.1737·1); melissa oil (p.1711·2).
*Vascular disorders.*

Biomo, Ger.
Aescin (p.1648·2).
*Soft-tissue injury; venous insufficiency.*

**opino N** Biomo, Ger.
Aescin (p.1648·2).
*Soft-tissue disorders; venous insufficiency.*

**opino N spezial** Gepepharm, Ger.
Buphenine hydrochloride (p.1663·2); aescin (p.1648·2).
*Soft-tissue disorders; venous insufficiency.*

**Opiren** Almirall, Spain.
Lansoprazole (p.1269·3).
*Gastro-oesophageal reflux; peptic ulcer.*

**O-Plat**
Raffo, Arg.; Zodiac, Braz.; Tecnofarma, Chile.
Oxaliplatin (p.577·1).
*Malignant neoplasms.*

**Opliphon** Fada, Arg.
Phenytoin (p.370·2).
*Epilepsy.*

**Opnol** Tika, Swed.
Dexamethasone sodium phosphate (p.1097·2).
*Inflammatory eye disorders.*

**Opobyl**
Note. This name is used for preparations of different composition.
Spedrog, Arg.
Bile salts (p.1660·3); boldo (p.1661·2); belladonna (p.479·1).

Bailly, Fr.; Uriach, Spain.
Aloes (p.1248·2); boldo (p.1661·2).
*Constipation.*

Interdelta, Switz.†.
Aloes (p.1248·2); boldo (p.1661·2); ox bile (p.1660·3).
*Constipation.*

**Opobyl-phyto** Medipharma, Ger.
Greater celandine (p.1695·3); turmeric (p.1058·3).
*Biliary-tract disorders.*

**Opocarbon** Monserrat, Arg.
Phthalylsulfathiazole (p.242·3); neomycin sulfate (p.235·1); activated charcoal (p.1030·2); kaolin (p.1268·3).
*Bowel sterilisation; diarrhoea; gastrointestinal infections.*

**Opocler** Monserrat, Arg.
Phthalylsulfathiazole (p.242·3); kaolin (p.1268·3); pectin (p.1580·3).
*Diarrhoea.*

**Opoenterol** Lafage, Arg.
Lactic acid (p.1704·1); homatropine (p.483·2); papain (p.1727·3); pepsin (p.1729·3).
*Muscle spasm.*

**Oponaf** Juste, Spain.
Lactitol (p.1269·1).
*Constipation; hepatic encephalopathy.*

**Opoplex** ICN, Braz.
Multivitamin, amino-acid, and mineral preparation (p.1417·1).

**Opo-Veinogene** Alpharma, Fr.
Red vine; aesculus (p.1648·2); esculoside (p.1648·2).
*Haemorrhoids; peripheral vascular disorders.*

**Opovital B12** Roux-Ocefa, Arg.
Vitamin B substances; minerals (p.1417·1).

**Opplin** Nakorn, Thai.
Boric acid (p.1662·1); borax (p.1661·3); allantoin (p.1141·3); chlorobutanol (p.1176·3); salicylic acid (p.1157·1); zinc sulfate (p.1469·3); hamamelis (p.1696·3).
*Eye irritation.*

**Oprad** Cryopharma, Mex.
Amikacin sulfate (p.154·1).
*Gram-negative bacterial infections.*

**Opragen** Lohmann, Ger.†.
Collagen (p.1674·3).
*Haemorrhage; skin ulcers; wounds.*

**Oprazole** Atlantic, Thai.
Omeprazole (p.1278·2).
*Gastro-oesophageal reflux; peptic ulcer; Zollinger-Ellison syndrome.*

**Oprazon** Ariston, Braz.
Omeprazole (p.1278·2).
*Peptic ulcer.*

**Opredsone** Greater Pharma, Thai.
Prednisolone (p.1108·1).
*Corticosteroid.*

**Opridan** Locatelli, Ital.†.
Bromopride hydrochloride (p.1254·1).
*Gastrointestinal disorders.*

**Oprimol** Taro, Israel.
Opipramol hydrochloride (p.311·1).
*Depression.*

**O'Prin** Dolisos, Canad.
Homoeopathic preparation.

**Oprisine** Opus, UK†.
Azathioprine (p.1349·1).
*Chronic active hepatitis; dermatomyositis; haemolytic anaemia; idiopathic thrombocytopenic purpura; immunosuppressant in organ and tissue transplantation; pemphigus; polyarteritis nodosa; pyoderma gangrenosa; rheumatoid arthritis; systemic lupus erythematosus.*

**Opsacin** PD, Thai.
Polymyxin B sulfate (p.245·1); neomycin sulfate (p.235·1); gramicidin (p.220·2).
*Bacterial eye infections.*

**Opsa-His** PD, Thai.
Antazoline hydrochloride (p.424·2); tetryzoline hydrochloride (p.1131·2).
*Allergic eye disorders; conjunctivitis.*

**Opsar** PD, Thai.
Sulfacetamide sodium (p.257·3).
*Bacterial eye infections.*

**Opsaram** PD, Thai.
Chloramphenicol (p.185·1).
*Bacterial eye infections.*

**Opsardex** PD, Thai.
Dexamethasone phosphate (p.1097·2); neomycin sulfate (p.235·1).
*Bacterial eye and ear infections.*

**Opsil** Silom, Thai.
Boric acid (p.1662·1); borax (p.1661·3); sodium chloride (p.1233·3).
*Eye irritation.*

**Opsil Tears** Silom, Thai.
Hypromellose (p.1579·3) (p.1164·2).
*Dry eye; wetting solution for hard contact lenses.*

**Opsil-A** Silom, Thai.
Tetryzoline hydrochloride (p.1131·2); antazoline hydrochloride (p.424·2).
Formerly contained tetryzoline hydrochloride.
*Allergic eye disorders.*

**Opsite**
Smith & Nephew, Austral.; Smith & Nephew, Fr.; Smith & Nephew, Ger.; Smith & Nephew, S.Afr.; Smith & Nephew Healthcare, UK.
Polyurethane dressing.
*Wounds.*

**Opsonat** Pekana, Ger.
Homoeopathic preparation.

**Optacilin** Altana, Braz.
Ampicillin benzathine (p.158·1); ampicillin sodium (p.157·1).
*Bacterial infections.*

**Optacilin Balsamico** Byk, Braz.†.
Ampicillin benzathine (p.158·1); ampicillin sodium (p.157·1); guaifenesin (p.1122·1); niaouli oil (p.1719·3); cineole (p.1672·1).
*Bacterial infections.*

**Optafen** Proge, Ital.†.
Chloramphenicol (p.185·1).
*Bacterial eye infections.*

**Optaflan** Gallia, Braz.†.
Nimesulide (p.67·1).

**Optal** Olan-Kemed, Thai.
*Eye drops:* Sulfacetamide sodium (p.257·3).
*Bacterial eye infections.*
*Eye lotion:* Boric acid (p.1662·1); borax (p.1661·3); chlorobutanol (p.1176·3); salicylic acid (p.1157·1).
*Eye irritation.*

**Optalgin**
Teva, Israel; Inibsa, Spain†.
Dipyrone (p.35·3).
*Fever; pain.*

**Optalia** Boiron, Canad.
Homoeopathic preparation.

**Optalidon**
Note. This name is used for preparations of different composition.
Novartis Consumer, Belg.; Novartis, Braz.†; Novartis Consumer, Port.; Novartis Consumer, Spain.
Propyphenazone (p.85·3); caffeine (p.782·1).
*Pain.*

Novartis Consumer, Ger.
Ibuprofen (p.45·3).
*Fever; pain.*

Novartis Consumer, Ital.
Propyphenazone (p.85·3); caffeine (p.782·1); butalbital (p.673·3).
*Pain.*

**Optalidon a la Noramidopyrine** Novartis Sante, Fr.†.
Caffeine (p.782·1); dipyrone (p.35·3).
*Pain.*

**Optalidon N** Novartis Consumer, Ger.
Propyphenazone (p.85·3); caffeine (p.782·1).
*Pain.*

**Optalidon special NOC** Novartis, Ger.
Dihydroergotamine mesilate (p.465·3); propyphenazone (p.85·3).
*Vascular headache.*

**Optamid** Proge, Ital.
Sulfacetamide sodium (p.257·3).
*Bacterial eye infections.*

**Optamide** McGloin, Austral.†.
Sulfacetamide sodium (p.257·3).
*Bacterial eye infections.*

**Optamine** Theraplix, Fr.†.
Co-dergocrine mesilate (p.1674·1).
*Cerebral vascular disorders; mental function impairment in the elderly.*

**Optamox**
Note. This name is used for preparations of different composition.
Roemmers, Arg.
Amoxicillin (p.155·3) or amoxicillin trihydrate (p.155·3); potassium clavulanate (p.193·3).
*Bacterial infections.*

Pharma Investi, Chile.
Amoxicillin trihydrate (p.155·3).
*Bacterial infections.*

**Optasid** Gador, Arg.
Etoposide (p.551·3).
*Lung cancer; testicular cancer.*

**Optavite** Dioptic, Canad.; Akorn, Canad.
Vitamin and mineral preparation (p.1417·1).

**Optazine**
Note. This name is used for preparations of different composition.
Whitehall Consumer, Austral.
Naphazoline hydrochloride (p.1124·3).
*Eye irritation.*

Uhlmann-Eyraud, Switz.†.
Naphazoline nitrate (p.1124·3); digitoxin (p.894·3); rutoside (p.1688·2); aesculus (p.1648·2); hamamelis (p.1696·3).
*Eye irritation.*

**Optazine Fresh** Whitehall Consumer, Austral.
Tetryzoline hydrochloride (p.1131·2).
*Eye irritation.*

**Optazol** Hormona, Mex.
Furazolidone (p.605·2); kaolin (p.1268·3); pectin (p.1580·3).
*Diarrhoea.*

**Opteron** GiEnne, Ital.
Ticlopidine hydrochloride (p.1011·2).
*Thrombosis prophylaxis.*

**Opthaflox** Grin, Mex.
Ciprofloxacin hydrochloride (p.188·2).
*Bacterial eye infections.*

**Opthavir** Grin, Mex.
Aciclovir (p.626·1).
*Herpes simplex keratitis.*

**Optibiol**
Yves Ponroy, Fr.
Nutritional supplement with fatty acids (p.1417·1).
*Visual disorders.*

Yves Ponroy, Singapore.
Protein; carbohydrate; lipids; phospholipids; anthocyanosides; betacarotene; vitamin E; zinc; chromium (p.1417·1).
*Nutritional supplement for maintenance of eye health.*

**Optical** Strallhofer, Austria.
Multivitamin preparation with calcium carbonate (p.1417·1).

**Optical mit Eisen** Strallhofer, Austria.
Multivitamin preparation with calcium carbonate and ferrous gluconate (p.1417·1).

**Opticare PMS** Standard Drug, USA.
Multivitamin and mineral preparation with iron and folic acid (p.1417·1).

**Opticef** Brahms, Ger.†.
Cefodizime sodium (p.174·1).
*Bacterial infections.*

**Opticide** Pharmaland, Thai.
Praziquantel (p.112·2).
*Trematode infections.*

**Opti-Clean**
Alcon, Braz.; Alcon, USA.
Range of solutions for contact lenses (p.1164·2).

**Opti-Clean II** Alcon, Canad.
Cleaning solution for hard and soft contact lenses (p.1164·2).

**Opticrom**
Aventis, Austral.; Rhone-Poulenc Rorer, Austria†; Aventis, Belg.; Fisons, Braz.†; Allergan, Canad.; Aventis, Ger.; Aventis, Hong Kong; Fisons, Irl.; Aventis, Israel; Aventis, Malaysia; Aventis, Mex.; Aventis, Neth.; Aventis, NZ; Aventis, Port.; Aventis, S.Afr.†; Aventis, Singapore; Aventis, Switz.; Aventis, Thai.; Aventis, UK; Allergan, USA.
Sodium cromoglicate (p.795·3).
*Allergic conjunctivitis; vernal keratoconjunctivitis.*

**Opticron** Cooperation Pharmaceutique, Fr.
Sodium cromoglicate (p.795·3).
*Allergic eye disorders.*

**Opticyl** Optopics, USA.
Tropicamide (p.491·1).
*Production of mydriasis and cycloplegia.*

**Optiderm**
Hermal, Austria†; Hermal, Ger.; Boots Healthcare, Ital.; Boots Healthcare, Switz.
Urea (p.1162·2); lauromacrogol 400 (p.1412·3).
*Dry skin disorders.*

**Optiderme** Hermal, Port.†.
Urea (p.1162·2); lauromacrogol 400 (p.1412·3).
*Dry skin disorders; pruritus.*

**Optidorm** Dolorgiet, Ger.
Zopiclone (p.729·3).
*Sleep disorders.*

**Optifast VLCD** Novartis Consumer, Austral.
Preparation for enteral nutrition (p.1417·1).
*Obesity.*

**Optifen** Spirig, Switz.
Ibuprofen (p.45·3).
*Fever; inflammation; musculoskeletal, joint, and periarticular disorders; pain.*

**Optifluor** Diba, Mex.
Fluorescein sodium (p.1689·1).
*Aid to eye examination.*

**Opti-Free**
Alcon, Austria†; Alcon, Braz.; Alcon, Canad.; Alcon, Fr.; Alcon, Israel†; Alcon, NZ; Alcon, USA.
A range of preparations for contact lens care (p.1164·2).

**Opti-Free Comfort** Alcon, Austral.†.
Cleansing and lubricating solution for contact lenses (p.1164·2).

**Opti-Free Daily** Alcon, Austral.†.
Cleansing solution for soft contact lenses (p.1164·2).

**Opti-Free Enzimatica** Alcon, Braz.
Pancreatin (p.1725·3) (p.1164·2).
*Cleansing and disinfecting of contact lenses.*

**Opti-Free Enzymatic** Alcon, Austral.†.
Pancreatin (p.1725·3) (p.1164·2).
*Cleansing and disinfecting of soft contact lenses.*

**Opti-Free Express**
Alcon, Austral.†; Alcon, Mex.; Alcon, UK.
A range of solutions for soft contact lens care (p.1164·2).

**Opti-Free Multi-Action** Alcon, Austral.†.
Cleaning, rinsing, disinfecting, storing, and lubricating solution for soft and disposable contact lenses (p.1164·2).

**Opti-free Supraclens** Alcon, Braz.
Pancreatin (p.1725·3) (p.1164·2).
*Cleansing of contact lenses.*

**Optigen** Xepa-Soul Pattinson, Hong Kong.
Gentamicin sulfate (p.217·1).
*Bacterial eye infections.*

**Optigene** Pfeiffer, USA.
Electrolytes (p.1217·1).
*Eye irrigation.*

**Optigene 3** Pfeiffer, USA.
Tetryzoline hydrochloride (p.1131·2).
*Minor eye irritation.*

**Opti-Genta** Vitamed, Israel.
Gentamicin sulfate (p.217·1).
*Bacterial eye infections.*

**Optiject**
Codali, Belg.; Guerbet, Fr.
Ioversol (p.1066·2).
*Radiographic contrast medium.*

**Optil** Opus, UK.
Diltiazem hydrochloride (p.900·1).
*Angina pectoris; hypertension.*

**Optilac** ICN, Arg.
Chondroitin sulfate sodium (p.1670·2); aprotinin (p.742·3).
*Dry eyes.*

**Optilast**
Asta Medica, Israel; Viatris, UK.
Azelastine hydrochloride (p.425·2).
*Allergic conjunctivitis.*

**Optilax** Phytomed, Switz.†.
Linseed (p.1707·2); senna (p.1288·2); frangula bark (p.1266·3); rhubarb (p.1287·3); malt extract (p.1439·2); chamomile (p.1669·3).
*Constipation.*

**Optilets**
Abbott, Hong Kong.
Multivitamin and mineral preparation (p.1417·1).

Abbott, USA.
Multivitamin preparation (p.1417·1).

**Optilets-M** Abbott, USA.
Multivitamin and mineral preparation with iron (p.1417·1).

**Optilube** Dioptic, Canad.
Wool fat (p.1483·1); liquid paraffin (p.1479·1); soft paraffin (p.1479·3).

**Optilube PVA** Dioptic, Canad.
Polyvinyl alcohol (p.1581·1).

**Optima**
Stanley, Canad.; Stanley, Israel.
Multivitamin and mineral preparation (p.1417·1).

**Optima 50 Plus** Unichem, UK†.
Multivitamin preparation with ginkgo and ginseng (p.1417·1).

**Opti-Mag** Dolisos, Ital.
Vitamin B substances; magnesium; zinc (p.1417·1).

**Optimal** Inibsa, Port.
Dicycloverine hydrochloride (p.481·2).
*Smooth muscle spasm.*

**Optimark**
Mallinckrodt, Austral.; Mallinckrodt, Braz.†.
Gadoversetamide (p.1063·1).
*Contrast medium for magnetic resonance imaging.*

**Optimax**
Note. This name is used for preparations of different composition.
E. Merck, Irl.†.
Tryptophan (p.320·3); pyridoxine hydrochloride (p.1456·3); ascorbic acid (p.1460·2).
*Depression.*

Merck, UK.
Tryptophan (p.320·3).
Formerly contained tryptophan, pyridoxine hydrochloride, and ascorbic acid.
*Depression.*

**Optimin**
Note. This name is used for preparations of different composition.
Abbott, Mex.
Multivitamin and mineral preparation (p.1417·1).

Essex, Spain.
Loratadine (p.436·1).
*Hypersensitivity reactions.*

**Optimina + Ginseng con Vit** Temis, Arg.
Pollen; ginseng; vitamins (p.1417·1).
*Tonic.*

**Optimina Plus** Temis, Arg.
Yohimbine hydrochloride (p.1766·2) pollen; ginseng (p.1693·1); vitamin E.
*Erectile dysfunction.*

**Optimine**
Schering-Plough, Belg.†; Schering, Canad.; Schering-Plough, Irl.†; Schering-Plough, S.Afr.†; Schering-Plough, UK†; Schering, USA†.
Azatadine maleate (p.425·1).
*Hypersensitivity reactions.*

**Optimoist** Colgate-Palmolive, USA.
Hyetellose (p.1579·2); electrolytes (p.1217·1); sodium monofluorophosphate (p.1446·2); xylitol (p.1469·1).
*Dry mouth.*

**Optimol**
Alphapharm, Austral.; Santen, Denm.; Duopharma, Hong Kong; Santen, Swed.
Timolol maleate (p.1012·2).
*Glaucoma; ocular hypertension.*

**Optimyxin** Sabex, Canad.
*Eye ointment:* Polymyxin B sulfate (p.245·1); bacitracin zinc (p.161·3).
*Eye infections.*
*Eye/ear drops:* Polymyxin B sulfate (p.245·1); gramicidin (p.220·2).
*Eye or ear infections.*

**Optimyxin Plus** Sabex, Canad.
Polymyxin B sulfate (p.245·1); gramicidin (p.220·2); neomycin sulfate (p.235·1).
*Eye or ear infections.*

**Optinate**
Aventis, Fin.; Lepetit, Ital.; Aventis, Norw.; Aventis, Swed.
Risedronate sodium (p.774·3).
*Osteoporosis; Paget's disease of bone.*

**Optinem** AstraZeneca, Austria.
Meropenem (p.229·1).
*Bacterial infections.*

**Optineuron** Lupin, India.
*Injection:* Vitamin B substances (p.1417·1); dexpanthenol (p.1727·2).
*Tablets:* Vitamin B substances (p.1417·1).
*Neuropathies.*

**Optipect** Thiemann, Ger.†.
Acetylcysteine (p.1112·3).
*Respiratory-tract disorders with excess mucus.*

**Optipect Kodein** Thiemann, Ger.
Codeine (p.27·1).
*Coughs.*

**Optipect N** Thiemann, Ger.
Camphor (p.1665·3); menthol (p.1711·3); peppermint oil (p.1283·2).
*Respiratory-tract disorders.*

**Optipect Neo** Thiemann, Ger.†.
Camphor (p.1665·3); menthol (p.1711·3); peppermint oil (p.1283·2).
*Respiratory-tract disorders.*

**Opti-Plus**
Alcon, Austral.†; Alcon, Fr.†.
Pancreatin (p.1725·3) (p.1164·2).
*Soft contact lens cleaner.*

Alcon, NZ.
Cleaning solution for soft contact lenses (p.1164·2).

**OptiPranolol** Bausch & Lomb, USA.
Metipranolol hydrochloride (p.956·1).
*Glaucoma; ocular hypertension.*

**Optipres** Cipla, India.
Betaxolol hydrochloride (p.873·1).
*Glaucoma; ocular hypertension.*

**Optipyrin** Pfleger, Ger.
Paracetamol (p.76·2); codeine phosphate (p.27·1).
*Pain.*

**Optiray**
Mallinckrodt, Arg.; Mallinckrodt, Austral.; Mallinckrodt, Austria; Codali, Belg.; Humana, Braz.†; Mallinckrodt, Canad.; Mallinckrodt, Denm.; MAP, Fin.; Guerbet, Fr.; Tyco, Ger.; Guerbet, Israel; Byk Gulden, Ital.; Tyco, Port.; Tyco, Spain; Tyco, Swed.; Guerbet, Switz.; Mallinckrodt, USA.
Ioversol (p.1066·2).
*Radiographic contrast medium.*

**Optisedine**
Pharmacobel, Belg.; Sterop, Belg.
Lorazepam (p.704·1).
*Anxiety.*

**Optisen** Allergan, Ital.†.
Carbohydrate, vitamin, and mineral preparation (p.1417·1).
*Antioxidant nutritional supplement.*

**Opti-Soak**
Alcon, Austral.†; Alcon, Austria†; Alcon, Braz.; Alcon, Canad.; Alcon, Fr.; Alcon, Israel†; Alcon, Mex.; Alcon, NZ.
Wetting, soaking, and disinfecting solution for hard and gas-permeable contact lenses (p.1164·2).

**Opti-Soft** Alcon, USA.
Rinsing and storage solution for soft contact lenses (p.1164·2).

**Optisol** Fischer, Israel.
Sulfacetamide sodium (p.257·3).
*Bacterial eye infections.*

**Optison**
Mallinckrodt, Arg.; Mallinckrodt, Austria†; Mallinckrodt, Denm.; Mallinckrodt, Ger.†; Mallinckrodt, Port.†; Amersham, Spain; Tyco, Swed.; Mallinckrodt, USA.
Perflutren-filled (p.1067·2) albumin microspheres.
*Contrast medium for echocardiography.*

**Opti-Tears**
Alcon, Austria†; Alcon, Braz.; Alcon, Canad.; Alcon, Israel†; Alcon, UK; Alcon, USA.
Rewetting drops for contact lenses (p.1164·2).

**Optium** Medisense, Austral.
Test for glucose in blood (p.1694·2).

**Opti-Up** Varifarma, Arg.
Barium sulfate (p.1061·1).
*Radiographic contrast medium.*

**Optivar** Medpointe, USA.
Azelastine hydrochloride (p.425·2).
*Allergic conjunctivitis.*

**Optivit** Leiras, Fin.
Multivitamin and mineral preparation (p.1417·1).

**Optivite PMT** Optimox, USA.
Multivitamin and mineral preparation (p.1417·1).
*Premenstrual syndrome.*

**Optizoline** Xepa-Soul Pattinson, Hong Kong.
Tetryzoline hydrochloride (p.1131·2).
*Eye irritation.*

**Optizor** Zicor, Fr.†.
Glyceryl trinitrate (p.923·2).
*Angina pectoris.*

**Opti-Zyme**
Alcon, Canad.; Alcon, USA.
Pancreatin (p.1725·3) (p.1164·2).
*Range of cleansing solutions for contact lenses.*

**Optobet** Vilco, Gr.
Diclofenac sodium (p.32·1).
*Prevention of miosis in ophthalmic surgery.*

**Optocain** Molteni, Ital.
Mepivacaine hydrochloride (p.1381·2).
Adrenaline acid tartrate (p.852·2) is included in some preparations as a vasoconstrictor to diminish absorption and localise the effect of the local anaesthetic.
*Local anaesthesia.*

**Optochinidin retard** Boehringer Mannheim, Ger.†.
Quinidine sulfate (p.991·3).
*Arrhythmias.*

**Optocillin**
Bayer, Austria†; Bayer, Ger.
Mezlocillin sodium (p.231·1); oxacillin sodium (p.240·2).
*Bacterial infections.*

**Optocor** Kanoldt, Ger.†.
Crataegus (p.1677·1).
*Heart failure.*

**Optomicin** Grin, Mex.
Erythromycin stearate (p.208·2).
*Bacterial eye infections.*

**Optovit**
Hermes, Ger.; Democal, Switz.
Alpha tocoferil acetate (p.1465·1).
*Vitamin E deficiency.*

**Optovit E**
Hermes, Austria; Qualiphar, Belg.
Alfa tocoferil acetate (p.1465·1).
*Vitamin E deficiency.*

**Optovite B12** Normon, Spain.
Cyanocobalamin (p.1458·2).
*Vitamin $B_{12}$ deficiency.*

**Optrelam** Boots Healthcare, Spain†.
Carmellose sodium (p.1577·3).
*Dry eyes.*

**Optrex**
Note. This name is used for preparations of different composition.
Boots Healthcare, Austral.
*Eye drops:* Hamamelis (p.1696·3); naphazoline hydrochloride (p.1124·3).
Formerly known as Optrex Medicated.
*Eye irritation.*

Boots Healthcare, Austral.; Schering-Plough, Canad.; Etris, Fr.; Boots Healthcare, Irl.†; Boots Healthcare, Ital.; Optrex, Malaysia; Boots Healthcare, NZ; Inibsa, Port.; Optrex, Singapore; Boots Healthcare, Spain; Boots Healthcare, Switz.; Boots, Thai.; Crookes Healthcare, UK.
Hamamelis (p.1696·3).
*Eye irritation.*

**Optrex Allergy** Crookes Healthcare, UK.
Sodium cromoglicate (p.795·3).
Formerly known as Optrex Hayfever Allergy.
*Allergic conjunctivitis.*

**Optrex Clear Eyes** Crookes Healthcare, UK.
Hamamelis (p.1696·3); naphazoline hydrochloride (p.1124·3).
Formerly known as Optrex Clearine.
*Eye irritation.*

**Optrex compresses** Boots Healthcare, Switz.
Hamamelis (p.1696·3); allantoin (p.1141·3).
*Eye irritation.*

**Optrex Hayfever Allergy** Boots Healthcare, NZ.
Sodium cromoglicate (p.795·3).
*Allergic conjunctivitis.*

**Optrex Red-Eye Relief** Boots Healthcare, NZ.
Hamamelis (p.1696·3); naphazoline hydrochloride (p.1124·3).
*Eye irritation.*

**Optrol** Amrad, Austral.†.
Salmeterol xinafoate (p.795·1).
*Obstructive airways disease.*

**Optruma**
Lilly, Austria; Robapharm, Fr.; Menarini, Ital.; Vitoria, Port.; Pensa, Spain.
Raloxifene hydrochloride (p.1568·3).
*Osteoporosis.*

**Optryl** Teva, Israel.
Naphazoline (p.1124·3); diphenhydramine hydrochloride (p.431·3).
*Eye disorders.*

**Opturem** Kade, Ger.
Ibuprofen (p.45·3).
*Gout; inflammation; musculoskeletal, joint, and soft-tissue disorders.*

**OPV** Aventis Pasteur, Braz.†.
Albumin (p.740·3).
*Plasma volume expansion.*

**OPV-Merieux** Aventis, S.Afr.
An oral poliomyelitis vaccine (p.1633·3).
*Active immunisation.*

**Ora** Masa, Thai.
Lorazepam (p.704·1).
*Anxiety.*

**ORA5** McHenry, USA.
Copper sulfate (p.1426·1); potassium iodide (p.1598·1); iodine (p.1598·1).
*Minor mouth or throat irritation.*

**Orabase**
Convatec, Austral.; Convatec, Canad.; Bristol-Myers Squibb, Irl.; Bristol-Myers Squibb, Israel; Bristol-Myers Squibb, NZ; Convatec, UK.
Carmellose sodium (p.1577·3); pectin (p.1580·3); gelatin (p.754·3).
*Oral and perioral lesions; stoma care.*

**Orabase Baby** Colgate-Hoyt, USA.
Benzocaine (p.1370·3).
*Mouth disorders.*

**Orabase Gel** Colgate Oral, USA.
Benzocaine (p.1370·3).

**Orabase HCA** Colgate-Hoyt, USA.
Hydrocortisone acetate (p.1103·3).
*Oral inflammatory and ulcerative lesions.*

**Orabase Lip** Colgate-Hoyt, USA.
Benzocaine (p.1370·3); allantoin (p.1141·3); menthol (p.1711·3); camphor (p.1665·3); phenol (p.1188·1).
*Minor irritation.*

**Orabase-B** Colgate-Palmolive, USA.
Benzocaine (p.1370·3).
*Oral lesions.*

**Orabet**
Note. This name is used for preparations of different composition.
Fresenius Kabi, Austria; Gea, Denm.; Gea, Norw.†; Lagap, UK†.
Metformin hydrochloride (p.342·3).
*Diabetes mellitus.*

Berlin-Chemie, Ger.
Tolbutamide (p.348·1).
*Diabetes mellitus.*

**Orabiot UD** Elvetium, Arg.
Clarithromycin (p.192·2).
*Bacterial infections.*

**Oracef** Lilly, Ger.
Cefalexin (p.168·1).
*Bacterial infections.*

**Oracefal** UPSA, Fr.
Cefadroxil (p.167·2).
*Bacterial infections.*

**Oracilin** Legrand, Braz.
Phenoxymethylpenicillin potassium (p.242·1).
*Bacterial infections.*

**Oracilline**
Aventis, Belg.†; Schwarz, Fr.
Phenoxymethylpenicillin (p.242·1) or benzathine phenoxymethylpenicillin (p.163·2).
*Bacterial infections.*

**Oracit** Carolina, USA.
Sodium citrate (p.1223·2); citric acid (p.1673·1).
*Chronic metabolic acidosis; urine alkalinising agent.*

**Oracort**
Taro, Canad.; Taro, Israel; AFT, NZ; Taro, Thai.†.
Triamcinolone acetonide (p.1110·2).
*Oral lesions.*

**Oracort E** Taro, Israel.
Triamcinolone acetonide (p.1110·2); lidocaine hydrochloride (p.1377·3).
*Oral lesions.*

**Oracyclin** Wyeth Lederle, Austria.
Minocycline hydrochloride (p.231·3).
*Acne.*

**Oraday**
Biolab, Malaysia; Biolab, Thai.
Atenolol (p.865·2).
*Hypertension.*

**Oradex** Raza, Malaysia; Pharmaniaga, Malaysia.
Chlorhexidine gluconate (p.1173·2).
*Gingivitis; mouth ulcers; oral hygiene.*

**Oradexon**
Organon, Belg.; Organon, Chile; Organon, Fin.; Organon (Οργανον),

*Gr.; Nourypharma, Neth.; Organon, Port.; Donmed, S.Afr.; Organon, Switz.†; Organon, Thai.*
Dexamethasone (p.1097·1) or dexamethasone sodium phosphate (p.1097·2).
*Corticosteroid.*

**Oradroxil** *Lampugnani, Ital.*
Cefadroxil (p.167·2).
*Bacterial infections.*

**Oradyne-Z** *Stafford-Miller, Ital.†.*
Benzalkonium saccharinate (p.1169·1); dodequinium bromide.
*Oral disinfection.*

**Orafen** *Technilab, Canad.*
Ketoprofen (p.51·2).
*Musculoskeletal and joint disorders; pain.*

**Orafer Comp** *Columbia, Mex.†.*
Ferrous sulfate (p.1428·2); cyanocobalamin (p.1458·2); folic acid (p.1429·1).
*Iron deficiency; iron-deficiency anaemia.*

**Oragalin Espasmolitico** *Lacer, Spain.*
Azintamide (p.1658·3); hyoscine methobromide (p.483·3).
*Hepatobiliary disorders.*

**Ora-Gallin** *Nycomed, Austria.*
Azintamide (p.1658·3); pancreatin (p.1725·3); cellulase (p.1669·1).
*Liver and biliary disorders.*

**Ora-Gallin compositum** *Nycomed, Austria.*
Azintamide (p.1658·3); papaverine hydrochloride (p.1728·1).
*Gastrointestinal disorders; liver and biliary disorders.*

**Ora-Gallin purum** *Nycomed, Austria.*
Azintamide (p.1658·3).
*Liver and biliary disorders.*

**Oragallin S** *Truw, Ger.†.*
Azintamide (p.1658·3); hyoscine methobromide (p.483·3).
*Biliary disorders; diarrhoea; spastic constipation.*

**Oragard**
*Note. This name is used for preparations of different composition.*
*Colgate-Palmolive, Ital.*
Hydrogen peroxide (p.1182·2).
*Mouth disorders.*

*Colgate-Palmolive, UK†.*
Lidocaine hydrochloride (p.1377·3); cetylpyridinium chloride (p.1173·1).
*Mouth disorders.*

**Oragard Baby** *Kolynos, Braz.†.*
Benzocaine (p.1370·3).
*Local anaesthesia.*

**Oragesic**
*Note. This name is used for preparations of different composition.*
*Jean-Marie, Hong Kong.*
Triamcinolone acetonide (p.1110·2); lidocaine hydrochloride (p.1377·3); chlorhexidine gluconate (p.1173·2).
*Mouth disorders.*

*Parnell, USA.*
Benzyl alcohol (p.1170·2); menthol (p.1711·3).
Formerly known as TiSol.
*Minor mouth or throat irritation.*

**Orageston** *Akzo, Braz.†.*
Allylestrenol (p.1541·3).
*Threatened miscarriage.*

**Oragrafin** *Squibb Diagnostics, USA†.*
Sodium iopodate (p.1065·2).
*Radiographic contrast medium for cholecystography.*

**Orahesive**
*Convatec, Austral.; Convatec, Canad.; Convatec, UK.*
Carmellose sodium (p.1577·3); pectin (p.1580·3); gelatin (p.754·3).
*Oral and perioral lesions; stoma care.*

**Oraica** *Esfor, Port.*
Orotic acid (p.1724·3); orazamide (p.1724·2).
*Gout; hyperuricaemia.*

**Orajel**
*Del, Canad.; Instituto Sanitas, Chile; Del, Switz.†; AHA, UK; Del, USA.*
Benzocaine (p.1370·3).
*Minor mouth or throat irritation; toothache.*

**Orajel Compuesto** *Instituto Sanitas, Chile.*
Benzocaine (p.1370·3); benzalkonium chloride (p.1168·3); zinc chloride (p.1469·2).
*Mouth disorders.*

**Orajel Mouth Aid**
*Note. This name is used for preparations of different composition.*
*Del, Canad.*
Benzocaine (p.1370·3); benzalkonium chloride (p.1168·3); zinc chloride (p.1469·2).

*Del, USA.*
*Topical gel:* Benzocaine (p.1370·3); benzalkonium chloride (p.1168·3); zinc chloride (p.1469·2).
*Mouth and lip sores.*
*Topical liquid:* Benzocaine (p.1370·3); cetylpyridinium chloride (p.1173·1).
*Mouth and throat disorders.*

**Orajel Perioseptic** *Del, USA.*
Urea hydrogen peroxide (p.1195·3).
*Oral hygiene; oral inflammation.*

**Orajel PM** *Del, USA.*
Benzocaine (p.1370·3); menthol (p.1711·3); methyl salicylate (p.59·3).
*Toothache.*

**Orakef** *Leiras, Fin.*
Cefalexin (p.168·1).
*Bacterial infections.*

**Orakit** *Fada, Arg.*
Potassium chloride (p.1232·2).
*Potassium supplement.*

**Oral Impact**
*Novartis Consumer, Austral.; Novartis, Fin.*
Preparation for enteral nutrition (p.1417·1).

**Oral Plan** *Abbott, Canad.*
Triclosan (p.1195·2); cetylpyridinium chloride (p.1173·1); sodium fluoride (p.1444·3).
*Oral hygiene.*

**Oral Rehidr Sal Farmasur** *Farmasur, Spain.*
Glucose; potassium iodide; sodium bicarbonate; sodium chloride (p.1222·2).
*Oral rehydration therapy.*

**Oral Spray** *Cabassi, Ital.*
Propolis (p.1735·2).

**Oral-Aid**
*Upha, Malaysia; Beacons, Singapore.*
Chlorhexidine hydrochloride (p.1173·3); triamcinolone acetonide (p.1110·2); lidocaine (p.1377·3).
*Mouth ulcers; sore gums; toothache.*

**Oralav** *Braun, Ger.*
Macrogol 4000 (p.1709·1); electrolytes (p.1217·1).
*Bowel evacuation.*

**Oral-B Anti-Bacterial with Fluoride** *Oral-B, Canad.*
Cetylpyridinium chloride (p.1173·1); sodium fluoride (p.1444·3).

**Oral-B Anti-Cavity Dental Rinse** *Oral-B, Canad.*
Sodium fluoride (p.1444·3).

**Oral-B Collutorio per la Protezione di Denti e Gengive** *Oral-B, Ital.*
Cetylpyridinium chloride (p.1173·1); sodium fluoride (p.1444·3).
*Prevention of dental disorders.*

**Oral-B Collutorio Protezione Anti-Carie Fluorinse** *Oral-B, Ital.*
Sodium fluoride (p.1444·3).
*Dental caries prophylaxis.*

**Oral-B Dientes Sensibles con Fluor** *Oral-B, Arg.*
Potassium nitrate (p.1190·1); sodium fluoride (p.1444·3).
*Dental caries prophylaxis; sensitive teeth.*

**Oral-B Enjuague Bucal** *Oral-B, Arg.*
Sodium fluoride (p.1444·3); cetylpyridinium chloride (p.1173·1).
*Dental caries prophylaxis; oral hygiene.*

**Oral-B Enjuague Bucal Amosan** *Oral-B, Arg.*
Sodium perborate (p.1192·2); sodium bitartrate (p.1290·1).
*Mouth disorders.*

**Oral-B Sensitive** *Oral-B, Austral.†.*
Potassium nitrate (p.1190·1); sodium fluoride (p.1444·3).
*Dental caries prophylaxis; sensitive teeth.*

**Oralbalance** *Ethical Research, Irl.†.*
Xylitol (p.1469·1).
*Saliva substitute.*

**Oralbiotico** *Sanofi Synthelabo, Port.*
*Oral liquid:* Tyrothricin (p.275·1); zinc chloride (p.1469·2).
*Tablets:* Tyrothricin (p.275·1); bacitracin zinc (p.161·3).
*Mouth and throat infections.*

**Oralcef** *Geymonat, Ital.*
Cefaclor (p.167·1).
*Bacterial infections.*

**Oralcer**
*Vitabiotics, Irl.†; Vitabiotics, UK†.*
Clioquinol (p.196·3); ascorbic acid.
*Mouth ulcers.*

**Oralcon**
*Alcon, Denm.†; Alcon, Swed.†.*
Diclofenamide (p.894·1).
*Glaucoma; preoperative control of intra-ocular pressure.*

**Oralcrom** *Monsanto, Spain†.*
Sodium cromoglicate (p.795·3).
*Gastrointestinal allergies; inflammatory bowel disease.*

**Oraldene**
*Pfizer Consumer, Irl.; Pfizer Consumer, UK.*
Hexetidine (p.1182·1).
*Mouth and throat infections.*

**Oraldine**
*Pfizer Consumer, S.Afr.; Warner-Lambert, Spain†.*
Hexetidine (p.1182·1).
*Mouth and throat infections.*

**Oralesper** *Pharmacia, Spain.*
Magnesium chloride hexahydrate; potassium chloride; monobasic potassium phosphate; sodium chloride; sodium phosphate dodecahydrate; sodium lactate; glucose (p.1222·2).
*Oral rehydration therapy.*

**Oralfene** *Pierre Fabre Sante, Fr.†.*
Ibuprofen (p.45·3).
*Fever; pain.*

**Oralgan** *Pierre Fabre, Fr.†.*
Paracetamol (p.76·2).
*Fever; pain.*

**Oralgar** *Marc-O, Canad.†.*
Benzocaine (p.1370·3); camphor (p.1665·3); chlorobutanol (p.1176·3).

**Oralgen** *Artu, Neth.*
Allergen extracts (p.1650·1).
*Allergen immunotherapy.*

**Oralgene** *Maver, Chile.*
*Dental gel:* Chlorhexidine gluconate (p.1173·2); sodium fluoride (p.1444·3).
*Mouthwash:* Chlorhexidine gluconate (p.1173·2).
*Tablets:* Chlorhexidine gluconate (p.1173·2); xylitol (p.1469·1).
*Oral hygiene.*

**Oralife Peppermint**
*Note. This name is used for preparations of different composition.*
*Pharmacia Upjohn, Austral.†.*
Peppermint oil (p.1283·2); chlorhexidine gluconate (p.1173·2).
*Dry lips and mouth.*

*Orion, NZ.*
Peppermint oil (p.1283·2); chlorhexidine gluconate (p.1173·2); wool fat (p.1483·1).
*Dry, cracked lips.*

**Oralipin** *Roche, Chile.*
Bezafibrate (p.873·2).
*Hyperlipidaemias.*

**Oral-K** *Sclavo, Ital.†.*
*dl*-Potassium aspartate (p.1233·1); *dl*-magnesium aspartate (p.1227·3).

**Oralmox** *Pulitzer, Ital.*
Amoxicillin trihydrate (p.155·3).
*Bacterial infections.*

**Oralmuv** *Kampel Martian, Arg.*
Lamivudine (p.648·2).
*HIV infection.*

**Oralone Dental** *Thames, USA.*
Triamcinolone acetonide (p.1110·2).
*Oral lesions.*

**Oralovite** *Meda, Swed.*
Vitamin B substances with vitamin C (p.1417·1).
*Alcoholism; polyneuropathy; vitamin deficiency.*

**Oralpadon**
*Stada, Austria.*
Glucose monohydrate; sodium chloride; potassium bicarbonate (p.1222·2).
*Gastrointestinal disorders; oral rehydration therapy.*

*Niddapharm, Ger.; Helvepharm, Switz.*
Glucose monohydrate; sodium chloride; potassium chloride; sodium acid citrate (p.1222·2).
*Diarrhoea; oral rehydration therapy.*

**Oralsan** *Bioprogress, Ital.†.*
Chlorhexidine hydrochloride (p.1173·3); sodium fluoride (p.1444·3); sodium monofluorophosphate (p.1446·2).
*Oral disinfection.*

**Oralsone**
*Gramon, Arg.; Vinas, Spain.*
Hydrocortisone hydrogen succinate (p.1104·1).
*Mouth ulcers.*

**Oralsone C** *Gramon, Arg.*
Tyrothricin (p.275·1); benzocaine (p.1370·3).
*Mouth and throat disorders.*

**Oralsone Topic** *Gramon, Arg.*
Rhubarb (p.1287·3); salicylic acid (p.1157·1).
*Mouth disorders.*

**Oralspray** *Pfizer Lambert, Spain†.*
Hexetidine (p.1182·1).
*Mouth and throat infections.*

**Oral-T** *Silom, Thai.*
Triamcinolone acetonide (p.1110·2).
*Oral lesions.*

**Oralten Troche** *Agis, Israel.*
Clotrimazole (p.396·2).
*Oropharyngeal candidiasis.*

**Oralube** *Orion, NZ.*
Electrolytes (p.1217·1).
*Saliva substitute.*

**Oralvac** *Bencard, Ger.*
Allergen extracts (p.1650·1).
*Allergen immunotherapy.*

**Oral-Virelon** *Chiron Behring, Ger.†.*
An oral poliomyelitis vaccine (p.1633·3).
*Active immunisation.*

**Oramedy** *Dong Kook, Singapore.*
Triamcinolone acetonide (p.1110·2).
*Oral lesions.*

**Oramet** *Gea, Fin.*
Metformin hydrochloride (p.342·3).
*Diabetes mellitus.*

**Oramil** *Ganassini, Ital.*
Rose honey (p.1434·2).
*Oral disinfection.*

**Oraminax** *BA Farma, Port.*
Amoxicillin (p.155·3).
*Bacterial infections.*

**Oraminic II** *Vortech, USA.*
Brompheniramine maleate (p.426·1).
*Hypersensitivity reactions.*

**Oramorph**
*Boehringer Ingelheim, Austria; Boehringer Ingelheim, Canad.; Boehringer Ingelheim, Irl.; Molteni, Ital.; Boehringer Ingelheim, Swed.†; Boehringer Ingelheim, UK; aai, USA.*
Morphine sulfate (p.60·2).
*Pain.*

**Oramox** *Antigen, Irl.*
Amoxicillin trihydrate (p.155·3).
*Bacterial infections.*

**Orangel** *Paraphar, Fr.†.*
Gelatin (p.754·3).
*Hair and nail tonic.*

**Oranol** *Roche, Switz.*
Multivitamin preparation (p.1417·1).

**Oranor** *AF, Mex.*
Norfloxacin (p.238·3).
*Bacterial infections.*

**Orap**
*Janssen-Cilag, Arg.; Janssen-Cilag, Austral.; Janssen-Cilag, Austria; Janssen-Cilag, Belg.; Janssen-Cilag, Braz.; Pharmascience, Canad.; Janssen-Cilag, Chile; Janssen-Cilag, Denm.; Janssen-Cilag, Fr.; Janssen-Cilag, Ger.; Janssen, Hong Kong; Ethnor, India; Janssen-Cilag, Irl.; Janssen-Cilag, Israel; Janssen-Cilag, Ital.; Fujisawa, Jpn; Janssen-Cilag, Neth.; Janssen-Cilag, Norw.†; Janssen-Cilag, NZ; Janssen-Cilag, S.Afr.; Janssen-Cilag, Singapore†; Janssen-Cilag, Spain; Janssen-Cilag, Swed.†; Janssen-Cilag, Switz.†; Janssen-Cilag, Thai.; Janssen-Cilag, UK; Gate, USA; Lemmon, USA.*
Pimozide (p.715·1).
*Behaviour disorders in children; psychoses; Tourette syndrome.*

**Oraphen-PD** *Great Southern, USA.*
Paracetamol (p.76·2).
*Fever; pain.*

**Orapred** *Ascent, USA.*
Prednisolone (p.1108·1).
*Corticosteroid.*

**Orascan** *Germiphene, Canad.†.*
Tolonium chloride (p.1757·1).
*Diagnosis of oral cancer.*

**Ora-Sed**
*Rosken, Hong Kong; Pfizer, NZ; Pfizer Consumer, Singapore.*
Choline salicylate (p.26·2).
*Mouth ulcers; sore gums; teething pain; toothache.*

**Ora-Sed Jel** *Warner-Lambert, Austral.*
Choline salicylate (p.26·2).
*Mouth lesions.*

**Orasept**
*Note. This name is used for preparations of different composition.*
*Silom, Thai.*
Cetylpyridinium chloride (p.1173·1).
*Mouth and throat disorders.*

*Pharmakon, USA.*
*Oral liquid:* Tannic acid (p.1751·2); methylbenzethonium chloride (p.1186·1).
*Throat spray:* Benzocaine (p.1370·3); methylbenzethonium chloride (p.1186·1); menthol (p.1711·3).
*Sore throat.*

**Oraseptic**
*Note. This name is used for preparations of different composition.*
*Prodemdis, Canad.†.*
Domiphen bromide (p.1179·1).

*Warner-Lambert, Ital.*
Hexetidine (p.1182·1).
*Mouth and throat disorders.*

**Oraseptic Gola** *Warner-Lambert, Ital.†.*
Cetylpyridinium chloride (p.1173·1); dichlorobenzyl alcohol (p.1178·3).
*Mouth and throat disorders.*

**Orasol** *Goldline, USA.*
Benzocaine (p.1370·3); phenol (p.1188·1); alcohol (p.1166·1); povidone-iodine (p.1190·3).

**Orasorbil**
*Exterius, Ger.; Rottapharm, Ital.†; Delta, Port.*
Isosorbide mononitrate (p.942·1).
*Angina pectoris.*

**Orastel** *Clintec, Fr.†.*
Preparations for enteral nutrition (p.1417·1).

**Orasthin** *Aventis, Ger.*
Oxytocin (p.1336·1).
*Induction and maintenance of labour; postpartum haemorrhage.*

**Orastina** *Aventis, Braz.*
Oxytocin (p.1336·1).
*Diagnosis of placental insufficiency or fetal distress; labour induction; lactation deficiency; postpartum haemorrhage.*

**Oratane**
*Douglas, Austral.; Douglas, Hong Kong; Douglas, NZ; Douglas, Singapore.*
Isotretinoin (p.1148·3).
*Acne.*

**Oratol** *Codilab, Port.*
Salicylic acid (p.1157·1); zinc chloride (p.1469·2).
*Mouth and throat disorders.*

**Oratol F** *Codilab, Port.*
Sodium fluoride (p.1444·3).
*Dental caries prophylaxis.*

**Oratrol**
*Alcon, Belg.; Alkon (Αλκον), Gr.; Alcon, Hong Kong†; Alcon Cusi, Spain†; Alcon, Switz.†.*
Diclofenamide (p.894·1).
*Glaucoma.*

**Oravil** *Streuli, Switz.*
Vitamin A acetate (p.1453·1); *d*-alpha tocoferil acetate (p.1465·1).
*Dietary supplement.*

**Oravir** *Novartis, Fr.*
Famciclovir (p.633·2).
*Varicella-zoster infections.*

**Oraxim** *Malesci, Ital.*
Cefuroxime axetil (p.184·1).
*Bacterial infections.*

**Orazinc** *Mericon, USA.*
Zinc sulfate (p.1469·3).
*Dietary supplement.*

**Orbenil** *Biogal, Israel.*
Cloxacillin sodium (p.198·2).
*Gram-positive bacterial infections.*

**Orbenin**
*Beecham, Belg.†; SmithKline Beecham, Gr.; SmithKline Beecham, Hong Kong†; SmithKline Beecham, Irl.†; SmithKline Beecham, Neth.; GlaxoSmithKline, S.Afr.; SmithKline Beecham, Singapore†; GlaxoSmithKline, Spain; GlaxoSmithKline, Thai.*
Cloxacillin sodium (p.198·2).
*Bacterial infections.*

**Orbenine** *Yamanouchi, Fr.*
Cloxacillin sodium (p.198·2).
*Bacterial infections.*

**Orbifen** *Orbis Consumer, UK.*
Ibuprofen (p.45·3).
*Fever; pain.*

**Orcel** *Ortec, USA.*
Bioengineered human skin equivalent (p.1158·1).
*Wounds.*

**Orchibion** *Bittermedizin, Ger.*
Bovine testicular extract (p.1569·3).
*Erectile dysfunction; male menopausal disorders.*

**Orcilone** *Chew, Thai.*
Triamcinolone acetonide (p.1110·2).
*Oral lesions.*

**Orcinol** *Julphar, UAE.*
Clobutinol hydrochloride (p.1117·1); orciprenaline sulfate (p.790·2); ammonium chloride (p.1115·2).
*Bronchitis; coughs.*

**Orcl** *Shinyaku, Jpn.*
Actarit (p.12·1).
*Musculoskeletal and joint disorders.*

**Orclor** *Willmar, Mex.†.*
Orasulon.

**Ordinal Forte** *Asche, Ger.*
Octodrine camsilate (p.975·3); norfenefrine hydrochloride (p.975·3).
*Circulatory disorders; hypotension.*

**Ordine** *Mundipharma, Austral.*
Morphine hydrochloride (p.60·1).
*Insomnia associated with pain; pain.*

**Ordov Chesty Cough** *Or-Dov, Austral.†.*
Guaifenesin (p.1122·1); bromhexine hydrochloride (p.1115·3).
*Coughs.*

**Ordov Congested Cough** *Or-Dov, Austral.†.*
Guaifenesin (p.1122·1); pseudoephedrine hydrochloride (p.1129·2).
*Respiratory-tract congestion.*

**Ordov Dry Tickly Cough** *Or-Dov, Austral.†.*
Pholcodine (p.1128·3).
*Coughs.*

**Ordov Extra Day & Night Cold and Flu** *Or-Dov, Austral.†.*
16 Daytime tablets, codeine phosphate (p.27·1); paracetamol (p.76·2); pseudoephedrine hydrochloride (p.1129·2); 8 night-time tablets, paracetamol; pseudoephedrine hydrochloride; chlorphenamine maleate (p.427·3).
*Cold and influenza symptoms.*

**Ordov Febrideine** *Or-Dov, Austral.†.*
Paracetamol (p.76·2); codeine phosphate (p.27·1).
*Fever; pain.*

**Ordov Febrigesic** *Or-Dov, Austral.†.*
Paracetamol (p.76·2).
*Pain.*

**Ordov Migradol** *Or-Dov, Austral.†.*
Paracetamol (p.76·2); codeine phosphate (p.27·1); doxylamine succinate (p.432·3).
*Pain.*

**Ordov Sinudec** *Or-Dov, Austral.†.*
Oxymetazoline hydrochloride (p.1126·1).
*Nasal congestion.*

**Ordov Sinus & Hayfever** *Or-Dov, Austral.†.*
Paracetamol (p.76·2); pseudoephedrine hydrochloride (p.1129·2); chlorphenamine maleate (p.427·3).
*Upper respiratory-tract disorders.*

**Ordrine AT Extended-Release** *Eon, USA†.*
Phenylpropanolamine hydrochloride (p.1127·3); caramiphen edisilate (p.1116·2).
*Coughs.*

**Oreda** *Hua, Thai.*
Glucose; sodium chloride; potassium chloride; sodium citrate (p.1222·2).
*Diarrhoea; oral rehydration therapy.*

**Orelox**
*Aventis, Austral.†; Aventis, Braz.; Hoechst Marion Roussel, Denm.†; Aventis, Fr.; Aventis, Ger.; Byk Gulden, Ital.; Aventis, Mex.; Aventis, Neth.; Aventis, S.Afr.; Roussel, Spain†; Aventis, Swed.; Aventis, Switz.; Aventis, UK.*
Cefpodoxime proxetil (p.178·3).
*Bacterial infections.*

**Oretic** *Abbott, USA.*
Hydrochlorothiazide (p.933·2).
*Hypertension; oedema.*

**Oreton Methyl** *Schering, USA†.*
Methyltestosterone (p.1559·3).
*Androgen replacement therapy; breast cancer; male hypogonadism; postpartum breast engorgement; postpubertal cryptorchidism.*

**Orexin** *Roberts, USA.*
Vitamin B preparation (p.1417·1).

**Orfarin**
*Orion, Malaysia; Orion, Thai.*
Warfarin sodium (p.1022·2).
*Thromboembolic disorders.*

**Orfen** *Wyeth, Spain†.*
Aluminium hydroxide (p.1249·2); magnesium oxide (p.1272·3).
*Hyperacidity.*

**Orfenace** *Kinsmor, Canad.†.*
Orphenadrine citrate (p.486·1).
*Skeletal muscle spasm.*

**Orfenal** *Remedica, Thai.*
Orphenadrine hydrochloride (p.486·1).
*Drug-induced extrapyramidal disorders; parkinsonism.*

**Orfidal** *Wyeth, Spain.*
Lorazepam (p.704·1).
*Alcohol withdrawal syndrome; anxiety; epilepsy; insomnia; nausea; vomiting.*

**Orfidora** *Wyeth, Spain†.*
Indoramin (p.939·3).
*Benign prostatic hyperplasia; hypertension.*

**Orfiril**
*Desitin, Denm.; Algol, Fin.; Desitin, Ger.; Desitin, Hong Kong†; Desitin, Israel; Desitin, Malaysia; Desitin, Norw.; Desitin, Singapore; Desitin, Swed.; Desitin, Switz.*
Sodium valproate (p.380·1).
Formerly known as Orfilept in *Swed.*
*Epilepsy; mania.*

**Orflex** *Chew, Thai.*
Orphenadrine citrate (p.486·1); paracetamol (p.76·2).
*Pain; skeletal muscle spasm.*

**Orgalutran**
*Organon, Arg.; Organon, Austral.; Organon, Braz.; Organon, Denm.; Organon, Fin.; Organon, Fr.; Organon, Ger.; Organon (Οργανον), Gr.; Organon, Irl.; Organon, Ital.; Organon, Norw.; Organon, Spain; Organon, Swed.; Organon, Switz.; Organon, UK.*
Ganirelix (p.1325·1) or ganirelix acetate (p.1325·1).
*Adjunct in ovarian stimulation for assisted reproduction.*

**Orgametril**
*Organon, Austria; Organon, Belg.; Organon, Denm.; Organon, Fin.; Organon, Fr.; Organon, Ger.; Organon (Οργανον), Gr.; Organon, Neth.; Organon, Port.; Organon, Spain; Organon, Swed.*
Lynestrenol (p.1557·1).
*Benign breast disorders; dysfunctional uterine bleeding; endometrial cancer; endometriosis; menstrual disorders; progestogen-only oral contraceptive.*

**Organex** *Sante Naturelle, Canad.*
*d*-Alpha tocoferil acetate (p.1465·1).

**Organidin NR** *Wallace, USA.*
Guaifenesin (p.1122·1).
Formerly contained iodinated glycerol.
*Coughs.*

**Organoneuro Cerebral** *Gross, Braz.*
Gamma-aminobutyric acid; glutamic acid; calcium phosphate; vitamin B substances (p.1417·1).
*Nutritional supplement.*

**Organoneuro Optico** *Gross, Braz.*
Tryptophan; vitamin A; thiamine; riboflavin; ascorbic acid; tocopherol (p.1417·1).
*Nutritional supplement.*

**Orgaplasma** *Ardeypharm, Ger.*
Ginseng (p.1693·1).
*Tonic.*

**Orgaran**
*Organon, Austral.; Organon, Austria; Organon, Belg.; Organon, Canad.; Organon, Fr.; Thiemann, Ger.; Nourypharma, Neth.; Organon, NZ; Organoid, Swed.; Organon, UK; Organon, USA.*
Danaparoid sodium (p.891·2).
*Thromboembolic disorders in patients with heparin-induced thrombocytopenia; thrombosis prophylaxis.*

**Orgasuline 30/70** *Organon, Fr.†.*
Mixture of insulin injection (human, emp, highly purified) 30% and isophane insulin injection (human, emp, highly purified) 70% (p.333·3).
*Diabetes mellitus.*

**Orgasuline NPH** *Organon, Fr.†.*
Isophane insulin injection (human, emp, highly purified) (p.333·3).
*Diabetes mellitus.*

**Orgasuline Rapide** *Organon, Fr.†.*
Insulin injection (human, emp, highly purified) (p.333·3).
*Diabetes mellitus.*

**Orgestriol** *Organon, Arg.*
Estriol (p.1552·3).
*Urogenital disorders in women associated with oestrogen deficiency.*

**Orgran** *Crombie, NZ.*
Gluten-free pasta (p.1417·1).
*Dermatitis herpetiformis; gluten-sensitive enteropathies.*

**Oribiox** *Bohm, Spain†.*
Oxolinic acid (p.240·3).
*Urinary-tract infections.*

**Oributol** *Orion, Fin.*
Ethambutol hydrochloride (p.211·3).
*Tuberculosis.*

**Oricant** *Luhr-Lehrs, Ger.†.*
Homoeopathic preparation.

**Oricitral** *TTK, India.*
Sodium acid citrate (p.1223·2).
*Urinary alkaliniser.*

**Oricyclin** *Orion, Fin.*
Tetracycline hydrochloride (p.266·2).
*Bacterial infections.*

**Oriens** *Galenica, Gr.*
Mizolastine (p.437·3).
*Allergic conjunctivitis; allergic rhinitis; pruritus.*

**Orifer F** *Aventis, Canad.*
Multivitamin and mineral preparation (p.1417·1).
*Prenatal supplement.*

**Orifungal** *Janssen-Cilag, Arg.*
Ketoconazole (p.403·3).
*Fungal infections.*

**Original** *Wassen, Ital.†.*
Multivitamin and mineral preparation (p.1417·1).
*Nutritional supplement.*

**Original Alka-Seltzer Effervescent Tablets** *Bayer, USA.*
Sodium bicarbonate (p.1223·2); citric acid (p.1673·1); aspirin (p.15·1).
*Hyperacidity.*

**Original Cabdrivers Expectorant** *Merck Consumer, UK.*
Dextromethorphan hydrobromide (p.1117·3); menthol (p.1711·3); terpin hydrate (p.1131·1); pumilio pine oil (p.1737·1); eucalyptus oil (p.1686·2).
*Coughs.*

**Original Schneckensirup** *Alsitan, Ger.*
Snail extract (p.1122·2); thyme (p.1755·2).
*Respiratory-tract disorders.*

**Original Sensodyne** *Block, USA.*
Potassium nitrate (p.1190·1).
*Hypersensitive teeth.*

**Original-Tinktur N Truw** *Truw, Ger.*
Homoeopathic preparation.

**Origlucon** *Orion, Fin.*
Glibenclamide (p.331·2).
*Diabetes mellitus.*

**Orimeten**
*Novartis, Arg.; Novartis, Austria; Novartis, Belg.; Novartis, Braz.; Novartis, Chile; Novartis, Ger.; Novartis, Irl.†; Novartis, Ital.; Novartis, Neth.; Novartis, S.Afr.; Novartis, Spain; Novartis, Swed.†; Novartis, UK.*
Aminoglutethimide (p.526·3).
*Breast cancer; Cushing's syndrome; prostatic cancer.*

**Orimetene**
*Novartis, Fr.; Novartis, Hong Kong; Novartis, Israel†; Novartis, Malaysia; Novartis, Switz.*
Aminoglutethimide (p.526·3).
*Breast cancer; Cushing's syndrome; hyperaldosteronism; prostatic cancer.*

**Orimune** *Lederle, USA†.*
An oral poliomyelitis vaccine (p.1633·3).
*Active immunisation.*

**Orinase**
*Hoechst Marion Roussel, Canad.†; Upjohn, USA.*
Tolbutamide (p.348·1).
*Diabetes mellitus.*

**Orinase Diagnostic** *Upjohn, USA.*
Tolbutamide sodium (p.348·2).
*Diagnosis of pancreatic adenoma.*

**Oriprim** *Cadila, India.*
Co-trimoxazole (p.199·3).
*Bacterial infections; Pneumocystis carinii pneumonia; toxoplasmosis.*

**Oris** *SM, Thai.*
Glucose; sodium chloride; potassium chloride; sodium citrate (p.1222·2).
*Diarrhoea; oral rehydration therapy.*

**Oritaxim** *Be-Tabs, S.Afr.†.*
Cefotaxime sodium (p.175·3).
*Bacterial infections.*

**Oritaxime** *Cadila, Thai.*
Cefotaxime sodium (p.175·3).
*Bacterial infections.*

**Orivan** *Orion, Fin.*
Vancomycin hydrochloride (p.275·2).
*Antibiotic-associated colitis; staphylococcal infections.*

**Orivir** *Orion, Denm.*
Aciclovir (p.626·1).
*Herpesvirus infections.*

**OrLAAM**
*Sipaco, Denm.†; Newport, Irl.†; Sipaco, Spain; Britannia Pharmaceuticals, UK†; Roxane, USA†.*
Levacetylmethadol hydrochloride (p.54·1).
*Opioid withdrawal syndrome.*

**Orlamix** *Alcon, Braz.†.*
Dexamethasone (p.1097·1); tobramycin (p.271·2).
*Infected eye disorders.*

**Orla-Wax** *Alcon, Arg.*
Trolamine (p.1758·2).
*Ear wax removal.*

**Orlaxyl** *Alcon, Braz.*
Xylometazoline hydrochloride (p.1132·2).
*Nasal congestion.*

**Orlept** *CP Pharmaceuticals, UK.*
Sodium valproate (p.380·1).
*Epilepsy.*

**Orlobin** *Help, Gr.*
Amikacin sulfate (p.154·1).
*Bacterial infections.*

**Orloc** *Orion, Fin.*
Bisoprolol fumarate (p.875·1).
*Angina pectoris; hypertension; migraine.*

**Orlon** *Osteolab, Chile.*
Blue tablets, norgestimate (p.1563·2); ethinylestradiol (p.1553·2); brown tablets, ferrous fumarate (p.1427·3).
*Combined oral contraceptive.*

**Ormigrein** *Organon, Braz.*
Paracetamol (p.76·2); ergotamine tartrate (p.467·2); caffeine (p.782·1); hyoscyamine sulfate (p.485·1); atropine sulfate (p.477·1).
Formerly contained paracetamol, ergotamine tartrate, caffeine, and belladonna.
*Migraine.*

**Ormir** *Neuropharma, Arg.*
Midazolam (p.707·1).

**Ormobyl CM** *Novartis Consumer, Ital.*
Calcium sennoside A (p.1288·3); calcium sennoside B (p.1288·3); polycarbophil calcium (p.1284·2).
*Constipation.*

**Ormodon** *Pharmaceutical Enterprises, S.Afr.*
Nitrazepam (p.710·1).
*Insomnia.*

**Ormox** *Orion, Fin.*
Isosorbide mononitrate (p.942·1).
*Angina pectoris; heart failure.*

**Ornade**
*Note. This name is used for preparations of different composition.*
*SmithKline Beecham, Belg.†; SmithKline Beecham Consumer, Canad.†; Biosaude, Port.†; SmithKline Beecham, USA†.*
Chlorphenamine maleate (p.427·3); phenylpropanolamine hydrochloride (p.1127·3).
*Cold symptoms; rhinitis; sinusitis.*

*Kern, Spain†.*
Cinnarizine (p.428·3); phenylpropanolamine hydrochloride (p.1127·3); isopropamide iodide (p.485·2).
*Nasal congestion.*

**Ornade Expectorant** *SmithKline Beecham Consumer, Canad.†.*
Chlorphenamine maleate (p.427·3); phenylpropanolamine hydrochloride (p.1127·3); guaifenesin (p.1122·1).
*Coughs and cold symptoms.*

**Ornade-DM** *SmithKline Beecham Consumer, Canad.†.*
Chlorphenamine maleate (p.427·3); phenylpropanolamine hydrochloride (p.1127·3); dextromethorphan hydrobromide (p.1117·3).
*Coughs and cold symptoms.*

**Ornatrol** *Enila, Braz.*
Diphenylpyraline hydrochloride (p.432·3); phenylpropanolamine hydrochloride (p.1127·3); isopropamide iodide (p.485·2).
*Nasal congestion.*

**Ornex**
*Note. This name is used for preparations of different composition.*
*ICN, Hong Kong†.*
Paracetamol (p.76·2); phenylpropanolamine hydrochloride (p.1127·3).
*Cold and influenza symptoms; sinusitis.*

*Ascher, USA.*
Paracetamol (p.76·2); pseudoephedrine hydrochloride (p.1129·2).
*Upper respiratory-tract symptoms.*

**Ornicetil**
*Ebewe, Austria; Chiesi, Fr.; Geymonat, Ital.; Sanofi Synthelabo, Spain†; Interdelta, Switz.†.*
Ornithine oxoglurate (p.1442·3).
*Hyperammonaemia; nausea induced by cancer chemotherapy; parenteral nutrition; pituitary function testing.*

**Ornicetil S** *Geymonat, Ital.†.*
Ornithine oxoglurate (p.1442·3).
*Mental function impairment.*

**Ornidyl** *Marion Merrell Dow, USA.*
Eflornithine hydrochloride (p.604·2).
*African trypanosomiasis.*

**Ornihepat** *Faria, Braz.*
Arginine (p.1421·1); citrulline (p.1425·2); ornithine (p.1442·3).
*Liver disorders.*

**Ornil** *Volchem, Ital.*
L-Ornithine (p.1442·3).
*Adjunct in dietary management of hypercholesterolaemia.*

**Ornil KGF** *Volchem, Ital.*
L-Ornithine oxoglurate (p.1442·3).
*Stress.*

**Ornitaine**
*Note. This name is used for preparations of different composition.*
*Microsules Bernabo, Arg.*
Amino-acid and vitamin B preparation (p.1417·1).
*Liver disorders.*

*Schwarz, Fr.*
Ornithine hydrochloride (p.1442·3); betaine (p.1660·1); sorbitol (p.1446·3); citric acid monohydrate (p.1673·1); magnesium oxide (p.1272·3).
*Dyspepsia.*

**Ornitargin** *Baldacci, Braz.*
Arginine (p.1421·1); ornithine (p.1442·3); citrulline (p.1425·2).
*Parenteral nutrition.*

**Oro B12** *Ripari-Gero, Ital.†.*
Orotic acid (p.1724·3); cyanocobalamin (p.1458·2); folic acid (p.1429·1).
*Nutritional supplement.*

**Oroacid** *Rosch & Handel, Austria.*
Betaine hydrochloride (p.1660·2); pepsin (p.1729·3).
*Hypochlorhydria; loss of appetite.*

**Orobicin** *Fulton, Ital.*
Bacitracin (p.161·3); neomycin sulfate (p.235·1).
*Gastrointestinal infections; pre-operative bowel preparation.*

**Orobiotic** *Fortbenton, Arg.*
Azithromycin (p.159·1).
*Bacterial infections.*

**Orocaine** *Beige, S.Afr.†.*
Cetrimide (p.1172·1); benzocaine (p.1370·3).
*Mouth and throat infections.*

**Orocal** Theramex, Mon.
Calcium carbonate (p.1254·2).
*Calcium deficiency; osteoporosis.*

**Orocal D$_3$** Theramex, Mon.
Calcium carbonate (p.1254·2); colecalciferol (p.1461·3).
*Calcium and vitamin D deficiency.*

**Orochlor** Triomed, S.Afr.
Benzocaine (p.1370·3); chlorhexidine gluconate (p.1173·2).
*Mouth and throat disorders.*

**Orochol**
Raffo, Arg.; CSL, Austral.; Pharmabroker, NZ†; Berna, Switz.
An oral cholera vaccine (p.1611·2).
*Active immunisation.*

**Orocholin** Rosch & Handel, Austria.
Choline dihydrogen citrate (p.1424·3); calcium citrate (p.1225·1).
*Adjuvant in surgery and radiotherapy; liver protection.*

**Orocil** Novartis, Gr.
Benzoxonium chloride (p.1170·2).
*Mouth infections.*

**Oro-Clense** Germiphene, Canad.†.
Chlorhexidine gluconate (p.1173·2).
*Gingivitis.*

**Or-O-Derm** Giuliani, Ital.†.
Vitamin and mineral preparation (p.1417·1).
*Antoxidant nutritional supplement.*

**Orodina** Laboratorios Chile, Chile.
Cyproheptadine hydrochloride (p.430·1); vitamins; lysine hydrochloride (p.1417·1).
*Reduced appetite.*

**Orofar**
Note. This name is used for preparations of different composition.
Novartis Consumer, Belg.
Benzoxonium chloride (p.1170·2).
*Mouth and throat disorders.*

Novartis Consumer, Port.; Novartis Consumer, Switz.; Novartis, Thai.†.
Benzoxonium chloride (p.1170·2); lidocaine hydrochloride (p.1377·3).
*Mouth and throat disorders.*

**Orofar Lidocaine** Novartis Consumer, Belg.
Benzoxonium chloride (p.1170·2); lidocaine hydrochloride (p.1377·3).
*Mouth and throat disorders.*

**Orofen** Durascan, Denm.
Ketoprofen (p.51·2).
*Dysmenorrhoea; gout; inflammation; musculoskeletal and joint disorders.*

**Orofluor** Colgate Oral Care, Austral.†.
Acidulated phosphate fluoride or sodium fluoride (p.1444·3).
*Dental caries prophylaxis; sensitive teeth.*

**Orofungin** Asta Medica, Braz.†.
Mepartricin (p.405·2).
*Vulvovaginal candidiasis and trichomoniasis.*

**Oroken** Aventis, Fr.
Cefixime (p.172·3).
*Otitis media; pyelonephritis; respiratory-tract infections; urinary-tract infections.*

**Oromag** Theramex, Mon.
Magnesium citrate (p.1272·1); magnesium lactate (p.1228·1).
*Magnesium deficiency.*

**Oromedine** Sanofi Synthelabo OTC, Fr.
Hexamidine isetionate (p.1181·3); tetracaine hydrochloride (p.1385·1).
*Mouth and throat disorders.*

**Oromone** Solvay, Fr.
Estradiol (p.1550·1).
*Menopausal disorders; osteoporosis.*

**Oro-NaF** Germiphene, Canad.
Sodium fluoride (p.1444·3).
*Dental caries prophylaxis.*

**Oro-Pivalone** Uhlmann-Eyraud, Switz.
Tixocortol pivalate (p.1110·1); bacitracin zinc (p.161·3).
*Mouth and throat disorders.*

**Oropivalone Bacitracine** Pfizer, Fr.
Tixocortol pivalate (p.1110·1); bacitracin zinc (p.161·3).
*Mouth and throat disorders.*

**Oropur** NHS, Fr.
Parsley oil; sunflower oil (p.1451·1).
*Halitosis.*

**Ororhinathiol** Sanofi Synthelabo, Belg.
Dequalinium chloride (p.1178·1); lidocaine hydrochloride (p.1377·3).
*Mouth and throat disorders.*

**Orosanyl** Berna, Ital.
Sodium monofluorophosphate (p.1446·2); cetylpyridinium chloride (p.1173·1).
*Gum disorders.*

**Orosept**
Note. This name is used for preparations of different composition.
Triomed, S.Afr.
Chlorhexidine gluconate (p.1173·2).
*Mouth disorders.*

OroClean, Switz.†.
Isopropyl alcohol (p.1184·3); propyl alcohol (p.1191·2); didecyldiammonium chloride.
*Hand disinfection.*

**Oroseptol Lysozyme** SmithKline Beecham Sante, Fr.†.
Dequalinium chloride (p.1178·1); tetracaine hydrochloride (p.1385·1); muramidase hydrochloride (p.1717·2).
*Mouth and throat disorders.*

**Orostat** Gingi-Pak, Switz.†.
Adrenaline hydrochloride (p.852·3).
*Dental haemorrhage and leakage of fluid from tissues.*

**Orostick** Ogna, Ital.†.
Propolis (p.1735·2); allantoin (p.1141·3).
*Emollient.*

**Orotre** Theramex, Ital.
Calcium carbonate (p.1254·2); colecalciferol (p.1461·3).
*Calcium and vitamin D deficiency; osteoporosis.*

**Orotrix** San Carlo, Ital.†.
Propylene glycol cefatrizine sulfate (p.170·3).
*Bacterial infections.*

**Orovite**
Thornton & Ross, Irl.; Thornton & Ross, UK.
Vitamin B substances with ascorbic acid (p.1417·1).

**Orovite '7'** Thornton & Ross, UK.
Multivitamin preparation (p.1417·1).

**Orovite Complorment B$_6$** Thornton & Ross, UK†.
Pyridoxine hydrochloride (p.1456·3).
*Isoniazid-induced peripheral neuritis; sideroblastic anaemia; vitamin B$_6$ deficiency.*

**Oroxadin**
Sanofi Synthelabo, Braz.; Sanofi Synthelabo, Mex.
Ciprofibrate (p.884·2).
*Hyperlipidaemias.*

**Oroxine**
Sigma, Austral.; GlaxoSmithKline, Malaysia; GlaxoSmithKline, Singapore.
Levothyroxine sodium (p.1600·1).
*Hypothyroidism; suppression of thyrotrophin; thyroiditis.*

**Orpar** Pharmasant, Thai.
Orphenadrine citrate (p.486·1); paracetamol (p.76·2).
*Muscle pain.*

**Orpec** Orion, Switz.†.
Ipecacuanha (p.1122·3).
*Poisoning.*

**Orphenadol** Yung Shin, Singapore.
Orphenadrine citrate (p.486·1); paracetamol (p.76·2).
*Musculoskeletal pain.*

**Orphengesic**
Note. This name is used for preparations of different composition.
Bangkok Lab & Cosmetic, Thai.
Orphenadrine citrate (p.486·1); paracetamol (p.76·2).
*Skeletal muscle pain; tension headache.*

Par, USA.
Orphenadrine citrate (p.486·1); aspirin (p.15·1); caffeine (p.782·1).
*Musculoskeletal pain.*

**Orphipal** GlaxoSmithKline, India.
Orphenadrine hydrochloride (p.486·1).
*Drug-induced extrapyramidal disorders; parkinsonism.*

**Orphol** Opfermann, Ger.
Co-dergocrine mesilate (p.1674·1).
*Mental function disorders.*

**Orpidix** Proel, Gr.
Ketotifen fumarate (p.788·1).
*Allergic rhinitis; asthma.*

**Orravina** Diviser Aquilea, Spain.
Aspirin (p.15·1).
*Fever; musculoskeletal, joint, and peri-articular disorders; pain; thromboembolism prophylaxis.*

**Orrepaste**
Hoe, Malaysia; Hoe, Singapore.
Triamcinolone acetonide (p.1110·2).
*Oral lesions.*

**ORS Bicarbonate** Raza, Malaysia; Pharmaniaga, Malaysia.
Sodium bicarbonate; sodium chloride; potassium chloride; glucose (p.1222·2).
*Diarrhoea; oral rehydration therapy.*

**Orsanil** Orion, Fin.
Thioridazine hydrochloride (p.724·2).
*Psychoses.*

**Orset** Servipharm, Israel.
Oral rehydration solution (p.1222·2).
*Diarrhoea; fluid and electrolyte depletion.*

**Orsinon** Rekah, Israel.
Tolbutamide (p.348·1).
*Diabetes mellitus.*

**Orstanorm**
Novartis, Fin.; Novartis, Swed.
Dihydroergotamine mesilate (p.465·3).
*Hypotension; migraine.*

**Ortenal** Specia, Fr.†.
Phenobarbital (p.367·3); amfetamine sulfate (p.1584·3).
*Epilepsy.*

**Ortensan** Cimex, Switz.†.
Paracetamol (p.76·2).
*Fever; pain.*

**Orthangin N** Roland, Ger.†.
Crataegus (p.1677·1).
*Cardiac disorders.*

**Orthangin novo** Altana, Ger.
Crataegus (p.1677·1).
*Heart failure.*

**Ortho** Janssen-Cilag, Irl.†.
Dienestrol (p.1547·3).
*Atrophic vaginitis; kraurosis vulvae.*

**Ortho 0.5/35** Janssen-Ortho, Canad.
Norethisterone (p.1562·2); ethinylestradiol (p.1553·2).
28-Day packs also contain 7 inert tablets.
*Combined oral contraceptive.*

**Ortho 1/35** Janssen-Ortho, Canad.
Norethisterone (p.1562·2); ethinylestradiol (p.1553·2).
28-Day packs also contain 7 inert tablets.
*Combined oral contraceptive.*

**Ortho 7/7/7** Janssen-Ortho, Canad.
Norethisterone (p.1562·2); ethinylestradiol (p.1553·2).
28-Day packs also contain 7 inert tablets.
*Triphasic oral contraceptive.*

**Ortho 10/11** Janssen-Ortho, Canad.†.
Norethisterone (p.1562·2); ethinylestradiol (p.1553·2).
28-Day packs also contain 7 inert tablets.
*Biphasic oral contraceptive.*

**Ortho Cyclen**
Janssen-Cilag, Israel; Ortho McNeil, USA.
Norgestimate (p.1563·2); ethinylestradiol (p.1553·2).
28-Day packs also contain 7 inert tablets.
*Combined oral contraceptive.*

**Ortho Evra** Ortho McNeil, USA.
Norelgestromin (p.1562·1); ethinylestradiol (p.1553·2).
*Combined transdermal contraceptive.*

**Ortho Gynest Depot** Janssen-Cilag, Ital.
Estriol (p.1552·3).
*Menopausal disorders.*

**Ortho Gyne-T** Janssen-Cilag, Irl.†.
Copper-wound plastic (p.1425·3).
*Intra-uterine contraceptive device.*

**Ortho Micronor** Ortho McNeil, USA.
Norethisterone (p.1562·2).
Formerly known as Micronor.
*Progestogen-only oral contraceptive.*

**Ortho Shields** Johnson & Johnson, Canad.†.
Nonoxinol 9 (p.1413·3).
*Contraceptive.*

**Ortho Tri-Cyclen** Ortho McNeil, USA.
Norgestimate (p.1563·2); ethinylestradiol (p.1553·2).
28-Day packs also contain 7 inert tablets.
*Triphasic oral contraceptive.*

**Orthocardon-N** Tosse, Ger.†.
Crataegus (p.1677·1).
*Cardiovascular disorders.*

**Ortho-Cept**
Janssen-Ortho, Canad.; Ortho McNeil, USA.
Desogestrel (p.1547·2); ethinylestradiol (p.1553·2).
28-Day packs also contain 7 inert tablets.
*Combined oral contraceptive.*

**Orthoclone OKT3**
Janssen-Cilag, Austral.; Janssen-Cilag, Belg.; Janssen-Cilag, Braz.; Janssen-Ortho, Canad.; Janssen-Cilag, Fin.; Janssen-Cilag, Fr.; Janssen-Cilag, Ger.; Cilag, Hong Kong; Janssen-Cilag, Israel; Janssen-Cilag, Ital.; Janssen-Cilag, Malaysia; Cilag, Mex.; Janssen-Cilag, Neth.; Janssen-Cilag, Norw.; Janssen-Cilag, NZ; Janssen-Cilag, Swed.; Janssen-Cilag, Switz.; Janssen-Cilag, Thai.; Ortho Biotech, USA.
Muromonab-CD3 (p.1360·3).
*Acute renal, cardiac, or hepatic allograft rejection.*

**Ortho-Creme**
Janssen-Cilag, Austral.†; Janssen-Cilag, Irl.; Janssen-Cilag, UK.
Nonoxinol 9 (p.1413·3).
*Contraceptive.*

**Ortho-Dienestrol** Ortho McNeil, USA.
Dienestrol (p.1547·3).
*Atrophic vaginitis; kraurosis vulvae.*

**Ortho-Dienoestrol**
Janssen-Cilag, Belg.†; Janssen-Cilag, Israel†; Janssen-Cilag, UK†.
Dienestrol (p.1547·3).
*Vulvovaginal disorders.*

**Ortho-Est**
Janssen-Cilag, S.Afr.; Women First, USA.
Estropipate (p.1553·1).
*Menopausal disorders; osteoporosis.*

**Orthoforms**
Janssen-Cilag, Irl.†; Janssen-Cilag, UK.
Nonoxinol 9 (p.1413·3).
*Contraceptive.*

**Ortho-Gel** Janssen-Cilag, Ger.†.
Nonoxinol 9 (p.1413·3).
*Contraceptive.*

**Ortho-Gynest**
Janssen-Cilag, Austria; Janssen-Cilag, Belg.; Janssen-Cilag, Ger.; Janssen-Cilag, Irl.; Janssen-Cilag, Israel; Cilag, Mex.; Janssen-Cilag, Switz.; Janssen-Cilag, UK.
Estriol (p.1552·3).
*Menopausal vulvovaginal disorders.*

**Ortho-Gynol**
Note. This name is used for preparations of different composition.
Janssen-Cilag, Austral.; Advanced Care, USA.
Octoxinol 9 (p.1414·1).
*Contraceptive.*

McNeil Consumer, Canad.†; Janssen-Cilag, NZ.
*p*-Di-isobutyl-phenoxypolyethoxyethanol (p.1411·2).
*Contraceptive.*

**Ortho-Gynol II** Johnson & Johnson, Canad.
Nonoxinol 9 (p.1413·3).
*Contraceptive.*

**Ortholan mit Salicylester** Medopharm, Ger.†.
Glycol salicylate (p.44·3); benzyl nicotinate (p.21·2).
*Musculoskeletal, joint, and soft-tissue disorders; peripheral vascular disorders.*

**Ortho-Maren retard** Lubapharm, Switz.
Pholedrine sulfate (p.982·3); norfenefrine hydrochloride (p.975·3).
*Hypotension.*

**Orthon** Remedina, Gr.
Fluoxetine hydrochloride (p.292·1).
*Depression; obsessive-compulsive disorder; panic disorder.*

**Orthonett Novum** Janssen-Cilag, Swed.
Norethisterone (p.1562·2); ethinylestradiol (p.1553·2).
*Combined oral contraceptive.*

**Ortho-Novin** Janssen-Cilag, Irl.†.
Norethisterone (p.1562·2); mestranol (p.1559·2).
*Combined oral contraceptive.*

**Ortho-Novum**
Janssen-Cilag, Austria; Cilag, Mex.
Norethisterone (p.1562·2); mestranol (p.1559·2).
*Combined oral contraceptive.*

**Ortho-Novum 1/35**
Janssen-Cilag, Fr.; Cilag, Mex.†; Ortho McNeil, USA.
Norethisterone (p.1562·2); ethinylestradiol (p.1553·2).
28-Day packs also contain 7 inert tablets.
*Combined oral contraceptive.*

**Ortho-Novum 1/50**
Janssen-Cilag, Belg.†; Janssen-Ortho, Canad.; Janssen-Cilag, Ger.†; Ortho McNeil, USA.
Norethisterone (p.1562·2); mestranol (p.1559·2).
28-Day packs also contain 7 inert tablets.
*Combined oral contraceptive; endometriosis; menstrual disorders.*

**Ortho-Novum 7/7/7** Ortho McNeil, USA.
Norethisterone (p.1562·2); ethinylestradiol (p.1553·2).
28-Day packs also contain 7 inert tablets.
*Triphasic oral contraceptive.*

**Ortho-Novum 10/11** Ortho McNeil, USA.
Norethisterone (p.1562·2); ethinylestradiol (p.1553·2).
28-Day packs also contain 7 inert tablets.
*Biphasic oral contraceptive.*

**Orthoplex SAD** Bioconcepts, Austral.
Vitamin B substances with trace elements and amino acids (p.1417·1).

**Orthosiphonblatter Indischer Nierentee**
Fides, Ger.
Java tea (p.1702·3).
*Urinary-tract disorders.*

**Orthovisc**
Zimmer, Ger.†; Anika, Israel; Surgicraft, UK; Ortho Biotech, USA.
Sodium hyaluronate (p.1697·3).
*Osteoarthritis of the knee and temporamandibular joint.*

**OrthoWash** Omnii, USA.
Sodium fluoride (p.1444·3).
*Dental caries prophylaxis.*

**Orthoxicol**
Note. This name is used for preparations of different composition.
Pharmacia Upjohn, Belg.†.
Dextromethorphan hydrobromide (p.1117·3); methoxyphenamine hydrochloride (p.1124·2).
*Coughs.*

Pharmacia Upjohn, S.Afr.†.
Codeine phosphate (p.27·1); methoxyphenamine hydrochloride (p.1124·2); sodium citrate (p.1223·2).
*Coughs.*

**Orthoxicol for Children Nightrest** Johnson & Johnson, Austral.†.
Chlorphenamine maleate (p.427·3); dextromethorphan hydrobromide (p.1117·3).
*Cold symptoms; coughs.*

**Orthoxicol Cold & Flu**
Johnson & Johnson, Austral.; Johnson & Johnson, NZ.
Paracetamol (p.76·2); pseudoephedrine hydrochloride (p.1129·2); dextromethorphan hydrobromide (p.1117·3).
*Cold and influenza symptoms.*

**Orthoxicol Congested Cough** Johnson & Johnson, Austral.†.
Guaifenesin (p.1122·1); pseudoephedrine hydrochloride (p.1129·2).
*Cold symptoms.*

**Orthoxicol Cough** Roberts, USA†.
Phenylpropanolamine hydrochloride (p.1127·3); chlorphenamine maleate (p.427·3); dextromethorphan hydrobromide (p.1117·3).
*Coughs and cold symptoms.*

**Orthoxicol Day & Night** Johnson & Johnson, NZ.
Day caplets, paracetamol (p.76·2); pseudoephedrine hydrochloride (p.1129·2); dextromethorphan hydrobromide (p.1117·3); night caplets, paracetamol; chlorphenamine maleate (p.427·3); dextromethorphan hydrobromide.
*Cold symptoms.*

**Orthoxicol Day & Night Cold & Flu** Johnson & Johnson, Austral.
Daytime caplets, paracetamol (p.76·2); pseudoephedrine hydrochloride (p.1129·2); dextromethorphan hydrobromide (p.1117·3); night-time caplets, paracetamol; dextromethorphan hydrobromide; chlorphenamine maleate (p.427·3).
*Cold and influenza symptoms.*

**Orthoxicol Dry Cough** Johnson & Johnson, Austral.†.
Paracetamol (p.76·2); dextromethorphan hydrobromide (p.1117·3).
*Cold symptoms.*

**Orthoxicol Headcold** Johnson & Johnson, Austral.†.
Paracetamol (p.76·2); pseudoephedrine hydrochloride (p.1129·2).
*Cold and influenza symptoms.*

**Orthoxicol Night Cold & Flu** *Johnson & Johnson, Austral.†.*
Paracetamol (p.76·2); chlorphenamine maleate (p.427·3); dextromethorphan hydrobromide (p.1117·3).
*Cold and influenza symptoms.*

**Orti B** *Seroyal, Canad.†.*
Vitamin B substances (p.1417·1).

**Ortic C** *Seroyal, Canad.†.*
Ascorbic acid (p.1460·2).

**Ortisan**
*Note. This name is used for preparations of different composition.*
*Cabassi, Ital.*
Senna (p.1288·2); tamarind (p.1293·2).
*Constipation.*

*Cedar Health, UK.*
Fruit and fibre preparation.
*Constipation.*

**Ortitruw** *Truw, Ger.*
Homoeopathic preparation.

**Orto Dermo P** *Normon, Spain.*
Povidone-iodine (p.1190·3).
*Burns; skin disinfection; wounds.*

**Orto Nasal** *Normon, Spain†.*
Cineole (p.1672·1); oxymetazoline hydrochloride (p.1126·1); menthol (p.1711·3).
*Nasal congestion.*

**Ortociclina** *Makros, Braz.†.*
Erythromycin (p.208·1).
*Bacterial infections.*

**Ortocilin** *Makros, Braz.†.*
Procaine benzylpenicillin (p.246·1); benzylpenicillin potassium (p.163·2); streptomycin (p.256·1); diphenhydramine (p.431·3).
*Bacterial infections.*

**Ortodermina** *Sofar, Ital.*
Lidocaine hydrochloride (p.1377·3).
*Surface anaesthesia of skin and mucous membranes.*

**Ortoflan** *Medley, Braz.*
Diclofenac sodium (p.32·1).
*Gout; inflammation; musculoskeletal, joint, and periarticular disorders.*

**Ortopsique** *Psicofarma, Mex.*
Diazepam (p.690·1).
*Alcohol withdrawal syndrome; anxiety disorders; epilepsy; insomnia; skeletal muscle spasm.*

**Ortoserpina** *Makros, Braz.†.*
Reserpine (p.995·1).
*Hypertension; Raynaud's syndrome.*

**Ortosol P** *Galderma, Braz.*
Piroctone olamine (p.1155·2); salicylic acid (p.1157·1).
*Scalp disorders.*

**Ortoton** *Bastian, Ger.*
Methocarbamol (p.1395·1).
*Skeletal muscle spasm and tension.*

**Ortoton Plus** *Bastian, Ger.*
Methocarbamol (p.1395·1); aspirin (p.15·1).
*Musculoskeletal, joint, and soft-tissue disorders.*

**Ortovermim** *Makros, Braz.†.*
Piperazine (p.111·2).
*Ascariasis; enterobiasis.*

**Ortoxine** *Volta, Chile.*
Chlorhexidine hydrochloride (p.1173·3).
*Oral hygiene.*

**Ortran** *Farmaco, Mex.*
Dipyrone (p.35·3); hyoscine butylbromide (p.483·3).
*Smooth muscle spasm.*

**Ortrip** *Pharmasant, Thai.*
Nortriptyline hydrochloride (p.310·2).
*Depression.*

**Ortrizol** *Forcoral, Mex.*
Metronidazole (p.607·2).
*Ascariasis; giardiasis; trichomoniasis.*

**Or-Tyl** *Ortega, USA.*
Dicycloverine hydrochloride (p.481·2).
*Functional bowel/irritable bowel syndrome.*

**Orucote** *Aventis, S.Afr.*
Ketoprofen (p.51·2).
*Dysmenorrhoea; gout; musculoskeletal, joint, and peri-articular disorders.*

**Orudis**
*Aventis, Arg.; Aventis, Austral.; Aventis, Canad.; Aventis, Denm.; Aventis, Fin.; Aventis, Ger.; Aventis, Hong Kong; Aventis, Irl.; Aventis, Ital.; Aventis, Malaysia; Aventis, Mex.; Aventis, Neth.; Aventis, Norw.; Aventis, NZ; Aventis, Spain; Aventis, Swed.; Rhone-Poulenc Rorer, Switz.†; Hawgreen, UK; Wyeth-Ayerst, USA.*
Ketoprofen (p.51·2).
*Gout; inflammation; musculoskeletal, joint, peri-articular, and soft-tissue disorders; oedema; pain.*

**Orugesic** *Aventis, Irl.*
Ketoprofen (p.51·2).
*Musculoskeletal, joint, peri-articular, and soft-tissue disorders.*

**Oruject** *Aventis, S.Afr.*
Ketoprofen (p.51·2).
*Gout; musculoskeletal, joint, and peri-articular disorders.*

**Orulop** *Llorente, Spain†.*
Loperamide hydrochloride (p.1271·1).
*Diarrhoea.*

**Oruvail**
*Aventis, Austral.; May & Baker, Canad.†; Aventis, Gr.; Aventis, Hong Kong; Aventis, Irl.; Aventis, Israel; Aventis, Malaysia; Aventis, NZ; Aventis, S.Afr.; Aventis, Singapore; Aventis, Thai.; Aventis, UK; Wyeth-Ayerst, USA.*
Ketoprofen (p.51·2).
*Gout; inflammation; musculoskeletal, joint, peri-articular, and soft-tissue disorders; pain.*

**Osa** *Piraud, Switz.†.*
Salicylamide (p.87·3); lidocaine hydrochloride (p.1377·3); calcium pantothenate (p.1442·3); calcium phosphate (p.1225·3).
*Gum pain.*

**Osa Gel de dentition aux plantes** *Piraud, Switz.†.*
Mint oil (p.1715·2); chamomile oil (p.1669·3); sage oil (p.1741·2); clove oil (p.1673·3); propolis (p.1735·2).
*Inflammatory dental disorders.*

**Osaline** *Hua, Thai.*
Glucose; sodium chloride; potassium chloride; sodium citrate (p.1222·2).
*Diarrhoea; oral rehydration therapy.*

**Osangin** *Antonetto, Ital.*
Dequalinium chloride (p.1178·1).
*Mouth and throat disinfection.*

**Osanit** *Zeppenfeldt, Ger.*
Homoeopathic preparation.

**Osaten** *Offenbach, Mex.*
Ketotifen (p.788·2).
*Hypersensitivity.*

**Os-Cal**
*Aventis, Braz.; Wyeth-Ayerst, Canad.; Aventis, Hong Kong; Marion Merrell Dow, Singapore; SmithKline Beecham Consumer, USA.*
Calcium carbonate (p.1254·2).
*Calcium deficiency; calcium supplement.*

**Oscal** *Aventis, NZ†.*
Calcium carbonate (p.1254·2).
*Calcium supplement.*

**Os-Cal D** *Wyeth-Ayerst, Canad.*
Calcium carbonate (p.1254·2); colecalciferol (p.1461·3).
*Calcium and vitamin D supplement.*

**Oscal D** *Aventis, NZ†.*
Calcium carbonate (p.1254·2); vitamin D (p.1461·2).
*Calcium supplement.*

**Os-Cal + D**
*Aventis, Braz.; Aventis, Hong Kong; Aventis, Malaysia; Marion Merrell Dow, Singapore; SmithKline Beecham Consumer, USA.*
Calcium carbonate (p.1254·2); vitamin D (p.1461·2).
*Calcium deficiency; calcium supplement.*

**Os-Cal Forte** *SmithKline Beecham Consumer, USA.*
Multivitamin and mineral preparation with iron (p.1417·1).

**Os-Cal Fortified** *SmithKline Beecham Consumer, USA.*
Multivitamin and mineral preparation with calcium and iron (p.1417·1).

**Os-Cal Plus** *SmithKline Beecham, USA.*
Multivitamin and mineral preparation with iron (p.1417·1).

**Oscalcio** *INQ, Braz.†.*
Vitamin $B_{12}$; vitamin D; calcium phosphate (p.1417·1).
*Nutritional supplement.*

**Oscevitin-A** *Grasler, Ger.*
Calcium phosphate (p.1225·3); vitamin A acetate; colecalciferol; ascorbic acid (p.1417·1).
*Calcium deficiency; vitamin deficiency.*

**Oscillococcinum**
*Boiron, Canad.; Silesia, Chile; Boiron, Fr.; Boiron, Port.; Boiron, Switz.*
Homoeopathic preparation.

**Oscorel** *Aventis, Neth.*
Ketoprofen (p.51·2).
*Musculoskeletal and joint disorders.*

**Osdron** *TRB, Braz.†.*
Alendronate sodium (p.765·3).
*Osteoporosis.*

**Osemin** *Degorts, Mex.*
Furosemide (p.919·3).

**Oseotal** *Chemopharma, Chile.*
Alendronic acid (p.765·3).
*Osteoporosis.*

**Oseototal** *Faes, Spain.*
Calcitonin (salmon) (p.768·2).
*Hypercalcaemia; metastatic bone pain; Paget's disease of bone; postmenopausal osteoporosis.*

**Oseum** *Grossman, Mex.*
Calcitonin (salmon) (p.768·2).
*Hypercalcaemia; osteolysis of malignancy; osteoporosis; Paget's disease of bone; reflex sympathetic dystrophy.*

**Osfolate**
*Asta Medica, Fr.†; Mayoly-Spindler, Switz.†.*
Calcium folinate (p.1431·1).
*Drug-induced megaloblastic anaemias; folate deficiency; prevention of folic-acid antagonist toxicity.*

**Osfolato** *Lusofarmaco, Ital.*
Calcium folinate (p.1431·1).
*Folate deficiency; reversal of methotrexate toxicity.*

**O-Sid** *Siam Bheasach, Thai.*
Omeprazole (p.1278·2).
*Gastro-oesophageal reflux; peptic ulcer; Zollinger-Ellison syndrome.*

**Osigraft** *Howmedica, Spain.*
Eptotermin alfa (p.768·2).
*Promotion of bone formation in fractures.*

**Osiren**
*Note. This name is used for preparations of different composition.*
*Lafedar, Arg.; Hoechst Marion Roussel, Austria†.*
Spironolactone (p.1003·1).
*Cardiac oedema; hyperaldosteronism; hypertension; liver cirrhosis with ascites; nephrotic syndrome.*

*Hoechst Marion Roussel, Austria†.*
*Injection:* Potassium canrenoate (p.984·2).
*Hyperaldosteronism.*

*Galen, Mex.*
Omeprazole (p.1278·2).
*Gastro-oesophageal reflux; peptic ulcer; Zollinger-Ellison syndrome.*

**Osmil**
*Note. This name is used for preparations of different composition.*
*Serono, Arg.*
Calcitonin (salmon) (p.768·2).
*Bone metastases; hypercalcaemia; osteolysis; osteoporosis; Paget's disease of bone; pancreatitis; sympathetic dystrophy.*

*Opfermann, Ger.*
16 Tablets, estradiol (p.1550·1); 12 tablets, estradiol; medroxyprogesterone acetate (p.1557·2).
*Menopausal disorders; osteoporosis.*

**Osmitrol**
*Baxter, Austral.; Baxter, Canad.; Baxter, USA.*
Mannitol (p.950·2).
*Acute renal failure; cerebral oedema; forced diuresis; raised intra-ocular pressure.*

**Osmo** *Nakorn, Thai.*
Multivitamin preparation with lysine (p.1417·1).

**Osmo-Adalat** *Pharma Clal, Israel.*
Nifedipine (p.966·2).
*Angina pectoris; hypertension.*

**Osmofundin 10%**
*Braun, Austria; Braun, Ger.†.*
Mannitol (p.950·2); sodium acetate (p.1223·1); sodium chloride (p.1233·3).
*Cataract surgery; cerebral oedema; forced diuresis; oliguria; renal failure.*

**Osmofundin 20%** *Braun, Austria.*
Mannitol (p.950·2).
*Cataract surgery; cerebral oedema; forced diuresis; oliguria; renal failure.*

**Osmofundin 15% N** *Braun, Ger.*
Mannitol (p.950·2).
*Fluid retention; renal failure.*

**Osmofundina**
*Note. This name is used for preparations of different composition.*
*Braun, Port.*
Mannitol (p.950·2).
*Forced diuresis; ocular hypertension; oedema; raised intracranial pressure; renal failure.*

*Braun, Spain†.*
Sodium bicarbonate (p.1223·2); sodium chloride (p.1233·3); mannitol (p.950·2).

**Osmofundina Concentrada** *Braun, Spain.*
Mannitol (p.950·2).
*Ascites; cranial hypertension; glaucoma; oedema; oliguria.*

**Osmogel**
*Note. This name is used for preparations of different composition.*
*Merck Medication Familiale, Fr.*
Magnesium sulfate (p.1228·2); lidocaine hydrochloride (p.1377·3).
*Soft-tissue disorders.*

*Alphrema, Ital.*
Suleparoid (p.1009·1); hyaluronic acid (p.1697·3); centella (p.1144·3); aescin (p.1648·2).
*Venous insufficiency.*

**Osmogenol** *INQ, Braz.†.*
Phenol (p.1188·1); tetracaine (p.1385·1); sodium bicarbonate (p.1223·2); sodium thiosulfate (p.1053·3).
*Ear infections.*

**Osmoglyn** *Alcon, USA.*
Glycerol (p.1694·3).
*Glaucoma; raised intra-ocular pressure before ophthalmic surgery.*

**Osmohes** *Laevosan, Austria.*
Pentastarch (p.750·1) in sodium chloride.
*Hypovolaemic shock.*

**Osmolac** *Sanofi Synthelabo OTC, Ital.*
Lactulose (p.1269·1).
*Constipation; hepatic cirrhosis; hepatic encephalopathy.*

**Osmoleine** *Pharmethic, Belg.†.*
Precipitated sulfur (p.1158·2); boric acid (p.1662·1).
*Rhinitis; sinusitis.*

**Osmolite**
*Abbott, Austral.; Abbott, Braz.; Abbott, Fin.; Abbott, Fr.; Abbott, Hong Kong; Abbott, Irl.; Abbott, Israel; Abbott, Ital.; Abbott, NZ; Abbott, Switz.†; Abbott Nutrition, UK; Ross, USA.*
A range of preparations for enteral nutrition (p.1417·1).

**Osmolite HN**
*Abbott, Arg.; Abbott, Canad.; Abbott, Mex.*
Preparation for enteral nutrition (p.1417·1).

**Osmopak-Plus** *Technilab, Canad.*
Hydrated magnesium sulfate (p.1228·2); benzocaine (p.1370·3).
*Superficial inflammatory conditions.*

**Osmoran** *Rafarm, Gr.*
Betamethasone valerate (p.1093·2).
*Topical corticosteroid.*

**Osmorich** *Abbott, Ital.*
Preparation for enteral nutrition (p.1417·1).

**Osmorol** *Pisa, Mex.*
Mannitol (p.950·2).

**Osmosal** *Leiras, Fin.*
Sodium chloride; potassium chloride; sodium citrate; glucose (p.1222·2).
*Diarrhoea; oral rehydration solution.*

**Osmosteril 10%** *Fresenius Kabi, Ger.*
Mannitol (p.950·2); sodium lactate (p.1223·2).
*Fluid retention; renal failure.*

**Osmosteril 20%** *Fresenius Kabi, Ger.*
Mannitol (p.950·2).
*Forced diuresis; renal failure.*

**Osmotan G** *Aguettant, Fr.*
Electrolyte infusion with glucose (p.1217·1).
*Carbohydrate source; fluid and electrolyte disorders.*

**Osmotil** *Hertz, Braz.†.*
Phenazone (p.82·3); lidocaine(p.1377·3).

**Osmotol** *Chauvin, Fr.*
Resorcinol (p.1156·3); ephedrine hydrochloride (p.1120·1).
*Otitis externa.*

**Osmovist** *Berlex, Canad.*
Iotrolan (p.1066·1).
*Radiographic contrast medium.*

**Osnervan** *GlaxoSmithKline, Ger.*
Procyclidine hydrochloride (p.488·2).
*Drug-induced extrapyramidal disorders; parkinsonism.*

**Ospamox**
*Biochemie, Austria; Biochemie, Hong Kong; Biochemie, Malaysia; Biochemie, NZ; Novartis, NZ; Normal, Port.; Biochemie, Singapore.*
Amoxicillin (p.155·3) or amoxicillin trihydrate (p.155·3).
*Bacterial infections.*

**Ospen**
*Biochemie, Austria; Novartis, Fr.; Novartis, Gr.; Biochemie, Hong Kong; Biochemie, Singapore; Medika, Switz.*
Benzathine phenoxymethylpenicillin (p.163·2), phenoxymethylpenicillin (p.242·1), or phenoxymethylpenicillin potassium (p.242·1).
*Bacterial infections.*

**Ospen KV** *Biochemie, Malaysia.*
Phenoxymethylpenicillin (p.242·1).
*Bacterial infections.*

**Ospexin**
*Biochemie, Austria; Biochemie, Hong Kong; Biochemie, Malaysia; Biochemie, Singapore.*
Cefalexin (p.168·1).
*Bacterial infections.*

**Ospocard** *Unipack, Austria.*
Nifedipine (p.966·2).
*Angina pectoris; hypertension; Raynaud's syndrome.*

**Ospolot**
*Pharmalab, Austral.; AOP Orphan, Austria; Desitin, Ger.; Desitin, Israel.*
Sultiame (p.377·3).
*Behavioural disorders; epilepsy.*

**Ospor** *Merck, Spain.*
Calcitonin (salmon) (p.768·2).
*Hypercalcaemia; metastatic bone pain; osteoporosis; Paget's disease of bone.*

**Osporin** *Hebron, Braz.*
Calcium carbonate (p.1254·2).
*Calcium supplement.*

**Ospronim** *Intramed, S.Afr.†.*
Pentazocine lactate (p.79·3).
*Pain.*

**Ospur Ca** *Henning, Ger.*
Calcium carbonate (p.1254·2).
*Calcium deficiency; osteoporosis.*

**Ospur $D_3$** *Henning, Ger.*
Colecalciferol (p.1461·3).
*Osteomalacia; osteoporosis; rickets; vitamin D deficiency.*

**Ospur F** *Henning, Ger.†.*
Sodium fluoride (p.1444·3).
*Osteolytic bone metastases; osteoporosis.*

**Osra** *Hua, Thai.*
Glucose; sodium chloride; sodium citrate; potassium chloride (p.1222·2).
*Diarrhoea; oral rehydration therapy.*

**Osseans D3** *Sciencex, Fr.*
Calcium (p.1225·1); colecalciferol (p.1461·3).
*Calcium and vitamin D deficiency; osteoporosis.*

**Osseocalcina** *Normal, Port.*
Calcitonin (salmon) (p.768·2).
*Osteoporosis.*

**Ossidal** *Truw, Ger.*
Homoeopathic preparation.

**Ossin**
*Note. This name is used for preparations of different composition.*
*Grunenthal, Ger.; Grunenthal, Switz.*
Sodium fluoride (p.1444·3).
*Osteoporosis.*

*Basi, Port.*
Chondroitin sulfate (p.1670·2).

**Ossiplex**
*Gebro, Austria; Henning, Ger.; Segix, Ital.; Aspen, S.Afr.*
Sodium fluoride (p.1444·3); ascorbic acid (p.1460·2).
*Osteoporosis.*

**Ossiten** *Roche, Ital.*
Disodium clodronate (p.770·2).
*Multiple myeloma; osteolytic tumours; postmenopausal osteoporosis; primary hyperparathyroidism.*

**Ossivite** *Wyeth, India.*
Vitamin A (p.1451·2); colecalciferol (p.1461·3); calcium carbonate (p.1254·2); calcium hydrogen phosphate (p.1225·2).
*Fractures; nutritional supplement; osteomalacia; osteoporosis; rickets.*

**Ossocal-D** *Delta, Braz.*
Calcium carbonate (p.1254·2); vitamin D (p.1461·2).
*Calcium and vitamin D supplement.*

**Ossofluor** *Streuli, Switz.*
Sodium fluoride (p.1444·3).
*Osteoporosis.*

**Ossofortin** *Strathmann, Ger.*
Calcium phosphate (p.1225·3); calcium gluconate (p.1225·2); colecalciferol (p.1461·3).
*Calcium and vitamin D deficiency; osteoporosis.*

**Ossofortin forte** *Strathmann, Ger.*
Calcium carbonate (p.1254·2); colecalciferol (p.1461·3).
*Calcium and vitamin $D_3$ deficiency; osteoporosis.*

**Ossomax** *Gallia, Braz.†.*
Alendronate sodium (p.765·3).
*Osteoporosis.*

**Ossopan**
*Germania, Austria; Asta Medica, Braz.; Robapharm, Fr.; Pierre Fabre, Ger.; TTK, India; Sanofi Synthelabo, Irl.; Byk Gulden, Mex.; Pierre Fabre, Port.; Pierre Fabre, Singapore; Berna, Spain; Robapharm, Switz.; Pierre Fabre, Thai.; Sanofi Synthelabo, UK†.*
Microcrystalline hydroxyapatite (p.1699·3).
*Calcium and phosphorus deficiency; dental caries prophylaxis; fractures; growth disorders in children; osteomalacia; osteoporosis; rickets.*

**Osspulvit S** *Madaus, Ger.*
Calcium phosphate (p.1225·3); colecalciferol (p.1461·3).
*Calcium deficiency.*

**Osspulvit S forte** *Madaus, Ger.*
Calcium phosphate (p.1225·3); vitamins (p.1417·1).

**Oss-regen** *Pekana, Ger.*
Homoeopathic preparation.

**OST Vit** *Greater Pharma, Thai.*
Vitamin $B_1$; vitamin $B_6$; vitamin $B_{12}$ (p.1417·1).

**Ostac**
*Roche, Belg.; Roche, Braz.; Roche, Canad.; Roche, Ger.; Roche, Gr.; Roche, Hong Kong; Boehringer Mannheim, Israel; Roche, Neth.; Roche, Norw.†; Roche, NZ†; Roche, Port.; Roche, S.Afr.; Roche, Singapore†; Roche, Swed.; Roche, Switz.*
Disodium clodronate (p.770·2).
*Hypercalcaemia of malignancy; osteolysis of malignancy.*

**Ostaren** *Utopian, Thai.*
Diclofenac sodium (p.32·1).
*Musculoskeletal and joint disorders.*

**Ostatac** *Spedrog, Arg.*
Glucosamine sulfate (p.1694·1).
*Osteoarthritis.*

**Ostedron** *Kleva, Gr.*
Disodium etidronate (p.771·2).
*Osteoporosis; Paget's disease of bone.*

**Ostelin**
*GlaxoSmithKline, Arg.; Boots Healthcare, Austral.; IFET (ΙΦΕΤ), Gr.; Teofarma, Ital.*
Ergocalciferol (p.1462·1).
*Vitamin D deficiency.*

**Osten** *Takeda, Jpn.*
Ipriflavone (p.773·2).
*Osteoporosis.*

**Ostenan** *Marjan, Braz.*
Alendronate sodium (p.765·3).
*Osteoporosis.*

**Ostenil**
*Chemedica, Fr.; Chemedica, Ger.; Chemedica, Switz.; Chemedica, UK.*
Sodium hyaluronate (p.1697·3).
*Osteoarthritis.*

**Osteo**
*Note. This name is used for preparations of different composition.*
*Quest, Canad.*
Calcium, magnesium, vitamin C, vitamin D, and silicon (p.1417·1).
*Healtheries, NZ.*
Calcium carbonate (p.1254·2).
*Calcium supplement.*

**Osteo Bi-Flex** *Bago, Chile.*
Glucosamine hydrochloride; chondroitin sulfate.
*Joint disorders.*

**Osteo Complex** *Peter, Ital.*
Calcium; vitamin D; boron; fluoride; zinc; copper; equisetum; lupulus (p.1417·1).
*Nutritional supplement for healthy bones.*

**Osteo D** *Teva, Israel†.*
Calcitriol (p.1461·2).
*Renal osteodystrophy in chronic haemodialysis.*

**Osteo Support** *Pharmagenics, UK.*
Hydroxyapatite (p.1699·3).
*Bone disorders.*

**Osteoapatite with Boron** *Nutrition Care, Austral.†.*
Calcium; manganese; zinc; copper; colecalciferol; boron (p.1417·1).
*Osteoporosis.*

**Osteobion** *Centrum, Spain.*
Calcitonin (salmon) (p.768·2).
*Hypercalcaemia; metastatic bone pain; osteoporosis; Paget's disease of bone.*

**Osteocal** *Medipha, Fr.*
Calcium carbonate (p.1254·2).
*Calcium deficiency; osteoporosis.*

**Osteocal D3** *Medipha, Fr.*
Calcium carbonate (p.1254·2); colecalciferol (p.1461·3).
*Calcium and vitamin D deficiency; osteoporosis.*

**Osteocalcic** *Biosintetica, Braz.*
Calcium citrate (p.1225·1).
*Calcium supplement.*

**Osteocalcil** *Dolisos, Canad.†.*
Homoeopathic preparation.

**Osteocalcin**
*Eurodrug, Hong Kong; Tosi, Ital.; Eurodrug, Malaysia; Eurodrug, Singapore†; Eurodrug, Thai.; Arcola, USA.*
Calcitonin (salmon) (p.768·2).
*Hypercalcaemia; osteolytic bone pain; osteoporosis; Paget's disease of bone; reflex sympathetic dystrophy.*

**Osteocalmine** *Oriental, Arg.*
Piroxicam (p.84·2).
*Inflammation; pain.*

**Osteocare**
*Vitabiotics, Hong Kong.*
Calcium (p.1225·1); magnesium (p.1227·3); zinc (p.1469·2); vitamin D (p.1461·2).
*Calcium deficiency; calcium supplement.*
*Vitabiotics, UK.*
Calcium carbonate (p.1254·2); calcium lactate (p.1225·3); calcium citrate (p.1225·1); magnesium hydroxide (p.1272·2); zinc sulfate (p.1469·3); colecalciferol (p.1461·3).

**Osteochondrin S** *Dyckerhoff, Ger.*
Ribonucleic acids from cattle and yeast (p.1738·2).
*Bone disorders.*

**Osteocis** *Schering, UK.*
Technetium-99m oxidronate (p.1525·2).
*Bone scintigraphy.*

**Osteocur** *Merck, Austria.*
Calcium phosphate (p.1225·3); colecalciferol (p.1461·3).
*Calcium and vitamin D deficiency; osteoporosis.*

**Osteocynesine**
*Boiron, Canad.†; Boiron, Fr.; Boiron, Port.*
Homoeopathic preparation.

**Osteodidronel** *Procter & Gamble, Belg.*
Disodium etidronate (p.771·2).
*Postmenopausal osteoporosis.*

**OsteoEze Bone & Joint Care** *Herron, Austral.*
Glucosamine hydrochloride; calcium carbonate (p.1254·2); vitamin D; vitamin $K_1$ (p.1417·1).
*Joint disorders.*

**Osteofem** *Grunenthal, Chile.*
Alendronate sodium (p.765·3).
*Osteoporosis.*

**Osteofix** *Promedica, Ital.*
Ipriflavone (p.773·2).
*Postmenopausal osteoporosis.*

**Osteoflam-MR** *Indoco, India.*
Diclofenac sodium (p.32·1); chlorzoxazone (p.1392·3); paracetamol (p.76·2).
*Painful muscle spasm.*

**Osteofluor**
*Merck, Austria†; Lipha Sante, Fr.†.*
Sodium fluoride (p.1444·3).
*Osteoporosis.*

**Osteoform** *Sigma, Braz.*
Alendronate sodium (p.765·3).
*Osteoporosis.*

**Osteofos D3**
*Menarini, Irl.; Menarini, Ital.*
Calcium phosphate (p.1225·3); colecalciferol (p.1461·3).
*Calcium and vitamin D deficiency; osteoporosis.*

**Osteogen** *Richard, Fr.†.*
Pyridoxine phosphate (p.1457·2); calcium ascorbate (p.1460·2); magnesium deoxyribonucleinate (p.1679·2); deoxyribonucleic acid (p.1679·2).
*Osteopathies; senile debility.*

**Osteogenon** *Germania, Austria.*
Hydroxyapatite (p.1699·3).
*Calcium deficiency; fractures; osteoporosis.*

**Osteomar** *Dupomar, Arg.*
Sodium monofluorophosphate (p.1446·2).
*Osteoporosis.*

**Osteomerck** *Merck, Spain.*
Calcium phosphate (p.1225·3); colecalciferol (p.1461·3).
*Hypocalcaemia; osteoporosis.*

**Osteomin** *Byk Gulden, Mex.*
Calcium carbonate (p.1254·2).
*Calcium supplement; osteoporosis.*

**Osteoplex** *Vitaplex, Austral.†.*
Mineral, vitamin, enzyme, and herb preparation (p.1417·1).
*Calcium deficiency; osteoporosis.*

**Osteoplus**
*Note. A similar name is used for preparations of different composition (see below).*
*Farmalab, Braz.*
Ipriflavone (p.773·2).
*Osteoporosis.*

**Osteo-Plus**
*Note. A similar name is used for preparations of different composition (see above).*
*Rolmex, Canad.*
Vitamin D and mineral preparation (p.1417·1).

**Osteopor** *Pierre Fabre, Spain.*
Hydroxyapatite (p.1699·3).
*Calcium deficiency; osteoporosis.*

**Osteoporosis Mineral Plus Formula 9** *Vitelle, Austral.†.*
Calcium carbonate (p.1254·2); colecalciferol (p.1461·3).
*Calcium deficiency; osteoporosis.*

**Osteopro**
*Note. This name is used for preparations of different composition.*
*Asta Medica, Austria.*
Sodium monofluorophosphate (p.1446·2).
*Osteoporosis.*
*Health Perception, UK.*
Ipriflavone (p.773·2); calcium (p.1225·1); vitamins; minerals (p.1417·1).
*Osteoporosis.*

**Osteoral** *Ache, Braz.*
Alendronate sodium (p.765·3).
*Osteoporosis.*

**Osteos** *TAD, Ger.*
Calcitonin (salmon) acetate (p.769·2).
*Hypercalcaemia; malignant osteolysis; osteoporosis; Paget's disease of bone; reflex sympathetic dystrophy.*

**Osteosan** *Silesia, Chile.*
Alendronate sodium (p.765·3).
*Osteoporosis.*

**Osteosil** *Ghimas, Ital.*
Equisetum (p.1684·1).
*Nutritional supplement.*

**Osteostab** *Rottapharm, Ital.*
Disodium clodronate (p.770·2).
*Hyperparathyroidism; multiple myeloma; osteolysis of malignancy; osteoporosis.*

**Osteostabil** *Jenapharm, Hong Kong†.*
Calcitonin (salmon) (p.768·2).
*Hypercalcaemia; osteoporosis; Paget's disease of bone; reflex sympathetic dystrophy; tumour-related bone pain.*

**Osteoton** *Herbaline, Ital.†.*
Food for special diets (p.1417·1).
*Bone disorders.*

**Osteotonina** *Menarini, Ital.*
Calcitonin (salmon) (p.768·2).
*Hypercalcaemia; osteoporosis; Paget's disease of bone; reflex sympathetic dystrophy.*

**Osteotop** *Silesia, Chile.*
Disodium etidronate (p.771·2).
*Ectopic ossification; osteoporosis; Paget's disease of bone.*

**Osteotrat** *Biosintetica, Braz.*
Alendronate sodium (p.765·3).
*Osteoporosis.*

**Osteotriol** *Gry, Ger.*
Calcitriol (p.1461·2).
*Osteoporosis; renal osteodystrophy.*

**Osteovis** *NCSN, Ital.*
Calcitonin (salmon) (p.768·2).
*Hypercalcaemia; osteoporosis; Paget's disease of bone; reflex sympathetic dystrophy.*

**Osteovit** *Pharmadass, UK.*
Multivitamin, mineral, and trace element preparation (p.1417·1).

**Ostepam** *Nordic, Fr.*
Disodium pamidronate (p.773·3).
*Hypercalcaemia of malignancy; myeloma; osteolytic bone lesions; Paget's disease of bone.*

**Osteral** *Silanes, Mex.*
Piroxicam (p.84·2).
*Gout; inflammation; musculoskeletal, joint, and periarticular disorders; pain.*

**Osteum** *Vinas, Spain.*
Disodium etidronate (p.771·2).
*Ectopic ossification; osteoporosis; Paget's disease of bone.*

**Osteus** *Iasis, Gr.*
Calcium phosphate (p.1225·3).
*Prevention and treatment of calcium deficiency.*

**Osticalcin** *Biomedica-Chemica, Gr.*
Calcitonin (p.768·2).
*Hypercalcaemia; osteoporosis; Paget's disease of bone.*

**Ostiderm** *Pedinol, USA.*
*Lotion:* Aluminium sulfate (p.1653·1); zinc oxide (p.1163·2).
Formerly contained aluminium sulfate and phenol.
*Roll-on:* Aluminium chlorohydrate (p.1142·1); camphor (p.1665·3).
*Foot odour; hyperhidrosis.*

**Ostidil-D3** *Garant, Ital.*
Alfacalcidol (p.1461·2).
*Hypoparathyroidism; osteomalacia; osteoporosis; renal osteodystrophy; rickets.*

**Ostifix** *Pharmedia (Φαρμεντια), Gr.*
Calcitonin (p.768·2).
*Hypercalcaemia; osteoporosis; Paget's disease of bone.*

**Ostine** *Farma Lepori, Spain.*
Calcium carbonate (p.1254·2); colecalciferol (p.1461·3).
*Calcium deficiency; osteoporosis.*

**Ostobon** *Coloplast, UK.*
A deodorant powder for use with ostomies.

**Ostocalcium** *GlaxoSmithKline, India.*
Calcium phosphate (p.1225·3); colecalciferol (p.1461·3).
*Calcium and vitamin D deficiency; rickets.*

**Ostocalcium B-12** *GlaxoSmithKline, India.*
Calcium phosphate (p.1225·3); colecalciferol (p.1461·3); vitamin $_{12}$ (p.1458·2).
*Calcium and vitamin D deficiency; rickets.*

**Ostochont** *Godecke, Ger.*
*Liniment:* Glycol salicylate (p.44·3); benzyl nicotinate (p.21·2); nonivamide (p.67·2).
*Musculoskeletal, joint, and soft-tissue disorders; neuralgia.*
*Ointment:* Heparin sodium (p.928·1); glycol salicylate (p.44·3); benzyl nicotinate (p.21·2).
*Musculoskeletal, joint, and soft-tissue disorders.*

**Ostofen** *Shiwa, Thai.*
Ibuprofen (p.45·3).
*Inflammation; pain.*

**Ostoforte** *Merck Frosst, Canad.*
Ergocalciferol (p.1462·1).
*Hypoparathyroidism; phosphataemia; rickets.*

**Ostogene** *Genepharm, Gr.*
Disodium etidronate (p.771·2).
*Osteoporosis; Paget's disease of bone.*

**Ostone-B12** *TP, Thai.*
Calcium (p.1225·1); ergocalciferol (p.1462·1); vitamin $B_{12}$ (p.1458·2).
*Megaloblastic anaemia; osteomalacia; rickets.*

**Ostopor** *Unipharma, Gr.*
Disodium etidronate (p.771·2).
*Osteoporosis; Paget's disease of bone.*

**Ostosalm**
*Pharmacia-Upjohn, Gr.; Pharmacia Upjohn, Port.*
Calcitonin (salmon) (p.768·2).
*Hypercalcaemia; osteoporosis; Paget's disease of bone.*

**Ostostabil**
*Jenapharm, Ger.; Jenapharm, Thai.†.*
Calcitonin (salmon) (p.768·2).
*Hypercalcaemia; osteolytic bone pain; osteoporosis; Paget's disease of bone; reflex sympathetic dystrophy.*

**Ostram**
*Merck, Arg.; Merck, Braz.†; Merck, Chile; Lipha Sante, Fr.; Merck, Mex.; Faes, Spain; Merck, Swed.†; Merck, UK†.*
Calcium phosphate (p.1225·3).
*Calcium deficiency; osteoporosis.*

**Ostram D3**
*Merck, Arg.; Merck, Chile.*
Calcium phosphate (p.1225·3); colecalciferol (p.1461·3).
*Calcium and vitamin D deficiency; osteoporosis.*

**Ostram $D_3$** *Bracco, Ital.*
Calcium phosphate (p.1225·3); colecalciferol (p.1461·3).
*Calcium and vitamin D deficiency; osteoporosis.*

**Ostram Vitamine $D_3$** *Lipha Sante, Fr.*
Calcium phosphate (p.1225·3); colecalciferol (p.1461·3).
*Calcium and vitamin D deficiencies; osteoporosis.*

**Ostram-Vit $D_3$**
*Merck, Austria; Merck, Fin.; Merck, Swed.†.*
Calcium phosphate (p.1225·3); colecalciferol (p.1461·3).
*Calcium and vitamin D deficiency; osteoporosis.*

**Ostranorm** *Nycomed, Denm.*
11 Tablets, estradiol (p.1550·1); 10 tablets, estradiol; norethisterone (p.1562·2).
*Menopausal disorders; osteoporosis.*

**Ostron** *Lifeplan, UK.*
Vitamin D; vitamin $B_6$; folic acid; calcium; magnesium; zinc; boron; copper; manganese (p.1417·1).
*Dietary supplement for healthy bones.*

**Ostronara** *Asche, Ger.*
16 Tablets, estradiol valerate (p.1550·2); 12 tablets, estradiol valerate; levonorgestrel (p.1563·2).
*Menopausal disorders; osteoporosis.*

**Ostro-Primolut** *Schering, Ger.*
Norethisterone acetate (p.1562·2); ethinylestradiol (p.1553·2).
*Menstrual disorders.*

**Osvical** *Alter, Spain†.*
Ascorbic acid (p.1460·2); calcium hypophosphite (p.1226·3); calcium levulinate (p.1225·3); colecalciferol (p.1461·3).
*Bone and dental disorders; calcium deficiency; osteomalacia; rickets.*

**Osvical D** *Alter, Spain.*
Calcium pidolate (p.1226·1); colecalciferol (p.1461·3).
*Calcium deficiency; osteoporosis.*

**Osyrol** *Aventis, Ger.*
Potassium canrenoate (p.984·2) or spironolactone (p.1003·1).
*Hyperaldosteronism; liver cirrhosis and ascites; oedema.*

**Osyrol Lasix** *Aventis, Ger.*
Spironolactone (p.1003·1); furosemide (p.919·3).
*Ascites; hyperaldosteronism; liver cirrhosis; oedema.*

**Otalex G** *Armstrong, Arg.*
Phenazone (p.82·3); gentamicin sulfate (p.217·1); procaine hydrochloride (p.1383·2).
*Otitis externa.*

**Otalgan**
*Note. This name is used for preparations of different composition.*
*Willvonseder, Austria; Wolfs, Belg.†.*
Lidocaine hydrochloride (p.1377·3); phenazone (p.82·3).
Formerly contained procaine hydrochloride and phenazone in *Belg.*
*Earache; otitis media.*

*Sudmedica, Ger.; Berna, Ital.; Jaba, Port.†; Berna, Spain; Medichemie, Switz.*
Procaine hydrochloride (p.1383·2); phenazone (p.82·3).
*Earache.*

*Vemedia, Neth.*
Lidocaine hydrochloride (p.1377·3).
*Earache.*

**Otalgicin** *Sudmedica, Ger.†.*
Xylometazoline hydrochloride (p.1132·2).
*Ear disorders; nasal congestion.*

**Otandrol** *Andromaco, Chile.*
Chloramphenicol (p.185·1); benzocaine (p.1370·3); betamethasone dipropionate (p.1093·1).
*Infected ear disorders.*

**Otarex** *Teva, Israel.*
Hydroxyzine hydrochloride (p.434·3).
*Anxiety; childhood behaviour disorders; premedication; pruritus.*

**Otauril** *Brasmedica, Braz.†.*
Neomycin sulfate (p.235·1); polymyxin B sulfate (p.245·1); fluocinolone acetonide (p.1101·2); lidocaine (p.1377·3).
*Ear disorders.*

**Otazol** *Bago, Chile.*
Polymyxin b sulfate (p.245·1); neomycin sulfate (p.235·1); betamethasone sodium phosphate (p.1093·1); lidocaine hydrochloride (p.1377·3).
*Infected ear disorders.*

**Otek-AC** *FDC, India.*
Prednisolone (p.1108·1); chloramphenicol (p.185·1); lidocaine hydrochloride (p.1377·3); acetic acid (p.1645·2).
*Ear disorders.*

**O-Tet** *Docmed, S.Afr.†.*
Oxytetracycline hydrochloride (p.241·1).
*Bacterial infections.*

**Otex** *Dendron, UK.*
Urea hydrogen peroxide (p.1195·3).
*Ear wax removal.*

**Otex HC** *Cassara, Arg.*
Ciprofloxacin hydrochloride (p.188·2); hydrocortisone (p.1103·3).
*Otitis externa.*

**Otiborin** *Santen, Fin.*
Boric acid (p.1662·1); alcohol (p.1166·1).
*Ear infections.*

**Otic Domeboro** *Bayer, USA.*
Acetic acid (p.1645·2); aluminium acetate (p.1652·3).
*Superficial infections of the external auditory canal.*

**Otic-Care** *Parmed, USA.*
Hydrocortisone (p.1103·3); neomycin sulfate (p.235·1); polymyxin B sulfate (p.245·1).
*Bacterial ear infections.*

**Oticerim** *Daudt, Braz.*
Sodium perborate (p.1192·2); urea (p.1162·2).
*Ear wax removal.*

**Oticum** *Saval, Chile.*
Polymyxin b sulfate (p.245·1); neomycin sulfate (p.235·1); betamethasone sodium phosphate (p.1093·1); lidocaine hydrochloride (p.1377·3).
*Infected ear disorders.*

**Otidin** *Teva, Israel.*
Phenazone (p.82·3); tetracaine hydrochloride (p.1385·1).
*Otitis externa; otitis media.*

**Otidrops** *Hexa-Medinova, Arg.*
Lidocaine hydrochloride (p.1377·3); cetrimide (p.1172·1); prednisolone (p.1108·1).
*Earache.*

**Otigent** *Allergan-Frumtost, Braz.†.*
Gentamicin sulfate (p.217·1); lidocaine hydrochloride (p.1377·3).
*Ear disorders.*

**Otilin** *Collins, Mex.*
Lidocaine (p.1377·3); neomycin (p.235·1).

**Oti-Med** *Hyrex, USA.*
Pramocaine hydrochloride (p.1382·2); hydrocortisone (p.1103·3).
*Ear disorders.*

**Otipax**
*Biodiphar, Belg.†; Biocodex, Fr.; Merck, Port.†; Inpharzam, Switz.*
Lidocaine hydrochloride (p.1377·3); phenazone (p.82·3).
*Earache.*

**Otised** *Propan, S.Afr.*
Phenazone (p.82·3); benzocaine (p.1370·3).
*Ear infections.*

**Otitex** *Sudmedica, Ger.*
Docusate sodium (p.1262·2).
*Removal of ear wax.*

**OtiTricin** *Bausch & Lomb, USA.*
Hydrocortisone (p.1103·3); neomycin sulfate (p.235·1); polymyxin B (p.245·2).
*Bacterial ear infections.*

**Otix** *Alcon Cusi, Spain.*
Dexamethasone phosphate (p.1097·2); polymyxin B sulfate (p.245·1); trimethoprim (p.272·2).
*Otitis externa.*

**Oto Betnovate** *Zest, Braz.*
Betamethasone valerate (p.1093·2); chlorphenesin (p.396·1); tetracaine hydrochloride (p.1385·1).
*Ear disorders.*

**Oto Biotaer** *Disprovent, Arg.*
Polymyxin B sulfate (p.245·1); neomycin sulfate (p.235·1); hydrocortisone acetate (p.1103·3); lidocaine hydrochloride (p.1377·3).
*Otitis externa; otitis media.*

**Oto Difusor** *Medical, Spain†.*
Benzocaine (p.1370·3); hyaluronidase (p.1698·2); hydrocortisone acetate (p.1103·3); neomycin sulfate (p.235·1); sulfanilamide sodium mesilate (p.263·3).
*Ear disorders.*

**Oto Neomicin Calm** *Ale, Spain†.*
Benzocaine (p.1370·3); hydrocortisone acetate (p.1103·3); neomycin sulfate (p.235·1); sulfacetamide sodium (p.257·3).
*Ear disorders.*

**Oto Vitna** *Quimifar, Spain.*
Dexamethasone (p.1097·1); benzocaine (p.1370·3); hydrocortisone acetate (p.1103·3); neomycin sulfate (p.235·1).
*External ear disorders.*

**Oto Xilodase** *Apsen, Braz.*
Lidocaine hydrochloride (p.1377·3); neomycin sulfate (p.235·1); hyaluronidase (p.1698·2).
*Ear disorders.*

**Otobacid N** *Asche, Ger.*
Dexamethasone (p.1097·1); cinchocaine hydrochloride (p.1373·2).
*Ear disorders.*

**Otobel** *Sedabel, Braz.*
Sulfathiazole (p.264·1); procaine hydrochloride (p.1383·2).
*Ear infections.*

**Oto-Biotic**
*Note. A similar name is used for preparations of different composition (see below).*
*Allergan, Braz.*
Sulfacetamide sodium (p.257·3); chloramphenicol (p.185·1); tetracaine hydrochloride (p.1385·1); boric acid (p.1662·1); urea (p.1162·2).
*Ear infections.*

**Otobiotic**
*Note. A similar name is used for preparations of different composition (see above).*
*Schering, USA.*
Polymyxin B sulfate (p.245·1); hydrocortisone (p.1103·3).
*Bacterial ear infections.*

**Otobrain** *Farmila, Ital.*
Multivitamin preparation with glycerophospholipids and ginkgo biloba (p.1417·1).
*Nutritional supplement; tinnitus; vertigo.*

**Otocain** *Abana, USA.*
Benzocaine (p.1370·3).
*Earache.*

**Otocalm** *Parmed, USA.*
Benzocaine (p.1370·3); phenazone (p.82·3).
*Earache.*

**Otocalma** *Salusif, Port.*
Procaine hydrochloride (p.1383·2); phenazone (p.82·3); sulfanilamide (p.263·2).
*Otitis.*

**Otocalmia** *Medical, Arg.*
Benzocaine (p.1370·3); chlorobutanol (p.1176·3); turpentine oil (p.1760·1); medium-chain triglycerides (p.1440·3).
*Ear wax removal; earache.*

**Otocalmine** *Pharmacobel, Belg.*
Phenazone (p.82·3); lidocaine (p.1377·3).
Formerly contained phenazone and procaine hydrochloride.
*Ear disorders.*

**Oto-Cer** *Allergan-Frumtost, Braz.†.*
Hydroxyquinoline borate (p.1700·1).
*Ear infections.*

**Otoceril** *Menarini, Port.*
Paradichlorobenzene (p.1728·3); benzocaine (p.1370·3); chlorobutanol (p.1176·3).
*Removal of ear wax.*

**Otocerum** *Reig Jofre, Spain.*
Phenol (p.1188·1); chlorobutanol (p.1176·3); benzocaine (p.1370·3); turpentine oil (p.1760·1); castor oil (p.1668·2).
*Removal of ear wax.*

**Otocipro** *Fortbenton, Arg.*
Hydrocortisone (p.1103·3); ciprofloxacin (p.188·2).
*Ear infections.*

**Otoclean Gotas Oticas** *Cassara, Arg.*
Sodium carbonate (p.1747·1); polysorbate 80 (p.1415·2); cetrimide (p.1172·1); phenazone (p.82·3); neomycin (p.235·1).
*Ear wax removal; earache.*

**Otoclean Solucion de Limpieza** *Cassara, Arg.*
Docusate sodium (p.1262·2).
*Ear wax removal.*

**Otocomb Otic** *Bristol-Myers Squibb, Austral.*
Triamcinolone acetonide (p.1110·2); neomycin sulfate (p.235·1); nystatin (p.406·3); gramicidin (p.220·2).
*Otitis externa.*

**Otocort**
*Note. This name is used for preparations of different composition.*
*Gemballa, Braz.*
Fluocinolone acetonide (p.1101·2); polymyxin B (p.245·2); neomycin (p.235·1); lidocaine (p.1377·3).
*Ear disorders.*

*Lemmon, USA.*
Hydrocortisone (p.1103·3); neomycin sulfate (p.235·1); polymyxin B (p.245·2).
*Bacterial ear infections.*

**Otocuril** *Fabra, Arg.*
Phenazone (p.82·3); sulfathiazole sodium (p.264·1); ethacridine lactate (p.1165·3).
*Ear disorders.*

**Oto-cyl Ho-Len-Complex** *Liebermann, Ger.*
Homoeopathic preparation.

**Otodex** *Aventis, Austral.*
Framycetin sulfate (p.215·1); gramicidin (p.220·2); dexamethasone (p.1097·1).
*Ear disorders.*

**Otodol** *Farmion, Braz.*
Nitrofurazone (p.238·2); neomycin sulfate (p.235·1); fludrocortisone acetate (p.1100·1); lidocaine hydrochloride (p.1377·3); dimethyl sulfoxide; menthol (p.1711·3).
*Ear disorders.*

**Otodolor** *Ursapharm, Ger.†.*
Phenazone (p.82·3); procaine hydrochloride (p.1383·2).
*Inflammatory ear disorders.*

**Otofa**
*Bouchara-Recordati, Fr.; Bouchara, Port.†; Bouchara, Switz.*
Rifamycin sodium (p.253·2).
*Otitis.*

**Otofenicol-D** *Allergan, Braz.*
Lidocaine hydrochloride (p.1377·3); dexamethasone (p.1097·1); chloramphenicol (p.185·1).
*Ear disorders.*

**Oto-Flexiole N** *Mann, Ger.†.*
Tetracaine hydrochloride (p.1385·1).
*Earache; otitis.*

**Otoflogin** *Heralds, Braz.†.*
Chloramphenicol (p.185·1); lidocaine (p.1377·3).
*Ear disorders.*

**Otoflour** *Bell, India.*
Sodium fluoride (p.1444·3).
*Conductive deafness; otosclerosis.*

**Otoflox** *Cassara, Arg.*
Ofloxacin (p.239·3).
*Otitis externa; otitis media.*

**Otofluor** *SIT, Ital.*
Sodium fluoride (p.1444·3); calcium gluconate (p.1225·2).
*Otosclerosis.*

**Otogen Calmante** *Belmac, Spain.*
Benzalkonium chloride (p.1168·3); clove oil (p.1673·3); phenol (p.1188·1); tetracaine hydrochloride (p.1385·1); menthol (p.1711·3).
*Ear disorders.*

**Otogesic** *Ethnor, India.*
Carboxymethylamino-4-aminodiphenylsulfone; dihydroxymethyl carbamide; cinchocaine (p.1373·2); glycerol (p.1694·3).
*Ear disorders.*

**Otoial** *Fidia, Ital.†.*
Sodium hyaluronate (p.1697·3).
*Tympanic membrane lesions.*

**Otolin** *Bergamo, Braz.†.*
Neomycin (p.235·1); nitrofurazone (p.238·2); lidocaine (p.1377·3).
*Ear infections.*

**Otolisan** *Pharma Investi, Chile.*
Polymyxin b sulfate (p.245·1); neomycin sulfate (p.235·1); betamethasone sodium phosphate (p.1093·1); lidocaine hydrochloride (p.1377·3).
*Infected ear disorders.*

**Otolitan N farblos** *3M, Ger.*
Dequalinium chloride (p.1178·1); lidocaine hydrochloride (p.1377·3).
*Earache; otitis.*

**Otolitan N mit Rivanol** *3M, Ger.*
Ethacridine lactate (p.1165·3); lidocaine hydrochloride (p.1377·3).
*Earache; otitis.*

**Otoloide** *Cimed, Braz.*
Phenol (p.1188·1); procaine hydrochloride (p.1383·2).
*Ear disorders.*

**Otolone**
*Note. This name is used for preparations of different composition.*
*Heralds, Braz.†.*
Polymyxin B sulfate (p.245·1); neomycin sulfate (p.235·1); fluocinolone (p.1101·2).
*Ear disorders.*

*Loren, Mex.*
Hydrocortisone (p.1103·3); chloramphenicol (p.185·1); benzocaine (p.1370·3).
*Ear infections.*

**Otolys** *Produfarma, Port.†.*
Hydrocortisone (p.1103·3); lidocaine (p.1377·3); neomycin (p.235·1); polymyxin B (p.245·2).

**Otolysine** *Chauvin, Fr.†.*
Trolamine caprylate.
*Removal of ear wax.*

**Otomar-HC** *Marnel, USA.*
Chloroxylenol (p.1177·2); hydrocortisone (p.1103·3); pramocaine hydrochloride (p.1382·2).
*Ear disorders.*

**Otomicetina** *Deca, Ital.†.*
Chloramphenicol (p.185·1); neomycin sulfate (p.235·1); tuaminoheptane sulfate (p.1132·1).
*Ear infections.*

**Otomicina** *Medley, Braz.*
Chloramphenicol (p.185·1); lidocaine hydrochloride (p.1377·3).
*Ear disorders.*

**Otomide** *SERB, Fr.*
Hexamidine isetionate (p.1181·3); lidocaine hydrochloride (p.1377·3).
*Otitis.*

**Otomidone** *SIT, Ital.*
Phenazone (p.82·3); procaine hydrochloride (p.1383·2).
*Earache.*

**Otomidrin** *Fardi, Spain.*
Fluocinolone acetonide (p.1101·2); framycetin sulfate (p.215·1); lidocaine hydrochloride (p.1377·3).
*Ear disorders.*

**Otomixyn** *EMS, Braz.*
Fluocinolone acetonide (p.1101·2); polymyxin B sulfate (p.245·1); neomycin sulfate (p.235·1); lidocaine hydrochloride (p.1377·3).
*Ear disorders.*

**Otomize**
*Stafford-Miller, Fin.†; Stafford-Miller, Irl.; Stafford-Miller, Israel; GlaxoSmithKline Consumer, UK.*
Dexamethasone (p.1097·1); neomycin sulfate (p.235·1).
*Otitis externa.*

**Otomycin** *Taro, Israel.*
Neomycin sulfate (p.235·1); phenylephrine hydrochloride (p.1126·3); sodium propionate (p.408·1); benzocaine (p.1370·3); benzyl alcohol (p.1170·2).
*Ear infections.*

**Otomycin-HPN** *Misemer, USA.*
Hydrocortisone (p.1103·3); neomycin sulfate (p.235·1); polymyxin B (p.245·2).
*Bacterial ear infections.*

**Otonal** *Biochimico, Braz.*
Paracetamol (p.76·2); zinc bromide; valeric acid.
*Vertigo.*

**Otonasal** *Diftersa, Spain†.*
Ephedrine hydrochloride (p.1120·1); procaine (p.1383·2); sulfanilamide (p.263·2).
*Congestion and infection of the nose and ear.*

**Otonax** *Sanval, Braz.†.*
Procaine hydrochloride (p.1383·2); phenol (p.1188·1).
*Ear infections.*

**Otonina** *Berna, Spain.*
Benzocaine (p.1370·3); neomycin sulfate (p.235·1); prednisolone (p.1108·1).
*Ear disorders.*

**Otonorthia** *Northia, Arg.*
Phenazone (p.82·3); procaine (p.1383·2); gentamicin (p.219·1).
*Ear disorders.*

**Otopax** *Vaillant, Ital.*
Procaine hydrochloride (p.1383·2); phenazone (p.82·3).
*Earache.*

**Oto-Ped** *Stiefel, Braz.†.*
Lidocaine hydrochloride (p.1377·3); neomycin sulfate (p.235·1); polymyxin B sulfate (p.245·1); nitrofurazone (p.238·2); fludrocortisone acetate (p.1100·1).
*Ear disorders.*

**Otopen** *Dinafarma, Braz.†.*
Chloramphenicol (p.185·1); lidocaine hydrochloride (p.1377·3).
*Ear disorders.*

**Oto-Phen** *Adcock Ingram, S.Afr.*
Phenazone (p.82·3).
*Earache; otitis.*

**Oto-Phen Forte** *Adcock Ingram, S.Afr.*
Benzocaine (p.1370·3); ephedrine hydrochloride (p.1120·1); phenazone (p.82·3); potassium hydroxyquinoline sulfate (p.1734·2).
*Earache; otitis.*

**Otoralgyl**
*Note. This name is used for preparations of different composition.*
*Aventis, Belg.†; Martin, Fr.†.*
Lidocaine hydrochloride (p.1377·3).
*Earache.*

*Martin, Switz.†.*
Sulfasuccinamide sodium (p.264·1); lidocaine hydrochloride (p.1377·3).
*Earache; otitis.*

**Otoralgyl a la phenylephrine** *Martin, Fr.*
Lidocaine hydrochloride (p.1377·3); phenylephrine hydrochloride (p.1126·3); sodium propionate (p.408·1).
*Otitis.*

**Otoralgyl sulfamide** *Martin, Fr.†.*
Sulfasuccinamide sodium (p.264·1); lidocaine hydrochloride (p.1377·3).
*Earache; otitis externa.*

**Otorinazol** *Montpellier, Arg.*
Sulfathiazole (p.264·1); atropine sulfate (p.477·1); niaouli oil (p.1719·3); cineole (p.1672·1).
*Cold and influenza symptoms; rhinitis.*

**Oto-Rinil** *Faria, Braz.†.*
Prednazoline (p.1129·1).
*Nasal disorders.*

**Otosal** *Coup, Gr.*
Doxycycline hyclate (p.206·2).
*Bacterial infections.*

**Otosamthong** *SM, Thai.*
Furaltadone hydrochloride (p.215·2); polymyxin B sulfate (p.245·1); neomycin sulfate (p.235·1); fludrocortisone acetate (p.1100·1); lidocaine hydrochloride (p.1377·3).
*Otitis externa; otitis media.*

**Otosan** *Streuli, Switz.*
Procaine hydrochloride (p.1383·2); phenazone (p.82·3).
*Ear disorders; earache.*

**Otosan Natural Ear Drops** *Otosan, Ital.*
Almond oil (p.1651·1); cajuput oil (p.1664·1); geranium oil (p.1692·2); juniper oil (p.1703·1); chamomile (p.1669·3); propolis (p.1735·2).
*Ear wax removal.*

**Otosedol** *Pensa, Spain.*
Phenazone (p.82·3); procaine hydrochloride (p.1383·2).
*Earache.*

**Otosedol Biotico** *Pensa, Spain.*
Chloramphenicol (p.185·1); benzocaine (p.1370·3); tyrothricin (p.275·1).
*Ear disorders.*

**Otoseptil**
*Note. This name is used for preparations of different composition.*
*Roux-Ocefa, Arg.*
Neomycin sulfate (p.235·1); hydrocortisone (p.1103·3); benzocaine (p.1370·3).
*Ear disorders.*

*Instituto Sanitas, Chile.*
Fluocinolone acetonide (p.1101·2); polymyxin B sulfate (p.245·1); neomycin sulfate (p.235·1); lidocaine hydrochloride (p.1377·3).
*Infected ear disorders.*

**Otosil** *Silom, Thai.†.*
Chloramphenicol (p.185·1); prednisolone (p.1108·1).
*Bacterial ear infections.*

**Otosporin**
*Note. This name is used for preparations of different composition.*
*GlaxoSmithKline, Arg.; GlaxoSmithKline, Austria; Pfizer Consumer, Belg.; Zest, Braz.; GlaxoSmithKline, Ger.†; GlaxoSmithKline, Hong Kong; Glaxo Wellcome, Irl.; GlaxoSmithKline, Israel†; GlaxoSmithKline, Neth.; Wellcome, Port.†; GlaxoSmithKline, S.Afr.; Glaxo Wellcome, Singapore†; GlaxoSmithKline, Spain; GlaxoSmithKline, Switz.; GlaxoSmithKline, Thai.; GlaxoSmithKline, UK; Calmic, USA.*
Hydrocortisone (p.1103·3); neomycin sulfate (p.235·1); polymyxin B sulfate (p.245·1).
*Bacterial ear infections.*

*Warner-Lambert, Ital.*
Neomycin sulfate (p.235·1); polymyxin B sulfate (p.245·1).
Formerly contained hydrocortisone, neomycin sulfate, and polymyxin B sulfate.
*Bacterial infections of the external ear.*

**Otosporin L** *GlaxoSmithKline, Arg.*
Hydrocortisone acetate (p.1103·3); neomycin sulfate (p.235·1); polymyxin B sulfate (p.245·1); lidocaine hydrochloride (p.1377·3).
*Bacterial ear infections.*

**Otospray** *Stafford-Miller, Switz.*
Neomycin sulfate (p.235·1); dexamethasone (p.1097·1).
*Ear disorders.*

**Otosulf** *Millet Roux, Braz.†.*
Sodium propionate (p.408·1); mafenide hydrochloride (p.228·2); benzethonium chloride (p.1169·2); benzocaine (p.1370·3).
*Ear disorders.*

**Otosynalar** *Roche, Braz.*
Fluocinolone acetonide (p.1101·2); polymyxin B sulfate (p.245·1); neomycin sulfate (p.235·1); lidocaine hydrochloride (p.1377·3).
*Ear disorders.*

**Oto-Synalar N** *Janssen-Cilag, Port.*
Fluocinolone acetonide (p.1101·2).

**Otothricinol** *Plan, Switz.*
Tyrothricin (p.275·1); phenazone (p.82·3); cetylpyridinium chloride (p.1173·1).
*Ear disorders.*

**Otovix** *Ibefar, Braz.†.*
Sulfanilamide (p.263·2); tyrothricin (p.275·1); benzocaine (p.1370·3); phenazone (p.82·3).
*Ear disorders.*

**Otovowen** *Weber & Weber, Ger.*
Homoeopathic preparation.

**Otowaxol** *Norgine, Ger.*
Docusate sodium (p.1262·2).
*Removal of ear wax.*

**Otradrops** *Manx, UK.*
Xylometazoline hydrochloride (p.1132·2).
*Nasal congestion.*

**Otrasel** *Cephalon, Fr.*
Selegiline hydrochloride (p.1214·1).
*Parkinsonism.*

**Otraspray** *Manx, UK.*
Xylometazoline hydrochloride (p.1132·2).
*Nasal congestion.*

**Otreon**
*Sankyo, Austria; Sankyo, Ital.; Sankyo, Spain.*
Cefpodoxime proxetil (p.178·3).
*Bacterial infections.*

**O-trexat** *Onkoworks, Ger.*
Methotrexate (p.568·2).
*Malignant neoplasms.*

**Otriflu** *Novartis, Norw.*
Diclofenac potassium (p.32·1).
*Fever; pain.*

**Otrinol**
*Novartis, Israel†; Novartis Consumer, Switz.*
Pseudoephedrine hydrochloride (p.1129·2).
*Nasal congestion.*

**Otrisal**
*Novartis Consumer, Austria; Novartis Consumer, Ger.*
Sodium chloride (p.1233·3).
*Nasal and pharyngeal dryness; nasal congestion.*

**Otrisalin** *Novartis, Gr.*
Sodium chloride (p.1233·3).
*Nasal congestion.*

**Otriven** *Novartis Ophthalmics, Ger.*
Xylometazoline hydrochloride (p.1132·2).
*Conjunctival disorders.*

**Otriven gegen Schnupfen** *Novartis Consumer, Ger.*
Xylometazoline hydrochloride (p.1132·2).
*Nasal congestion.*

**Otriven H** *Novartis Consumer, Ger.*
Sodium cromoglicate (p.795·3).
*Allergic rhinitis.*

**Otriven mit Dexpanthenol** *Novartis Consumer, Ger.*
Dexpanthenol (p.1727·2).
*Nasal disorders.*

**Otrivin**
*Novartis Consumer, Austral.; Novartis Consumer, Austria; Novartis Consumer, Canad.; Novartis, Denm.; Novartis, Fin.; Novartis, Gr.; Novartis, Hong Kong; Novartis, India; Novartis, Israel; Novartis Consumer, Ital.; Novartis, Malaysia; Novartis Consumer, Neth.; Novartis, Norw.; Novartis Consumer, S.Afr.; Novartis Nutrition, Singapore; Novartis Consumer, Spain; Novartis, Swed.; Novartis Consumer, Switz.; Novartis, Thai.; Ciba Consumer, USA.*
Xylometazoline hydrochloride (p.1132·2).
*Aid in rhinoscopy; nasal congestion; otitis media; sinus disorders.*

**Otrivin Menthol**
*Novartis, Denm.; Novartis, Fin.; Novartis Consumer, Neth.; Novartis, Swed.*
Xylometazoline hydrochloride (p.1132·2); menthol (p.1711·3); cineole (p.1672·1).
*Rhinitis; sinusitis; upper respiratory-tract congestion.*

**Otrivina**
*Novartis, Arg.; Novartis, Braz.; Novartis Consumer, Port.*
Xylometazoline hydrochloride (p.1132·2).
*Aid in rhinoscopy; nasal congestion; otitis media.*

**Otrivine**
*Novartis Consumer, Irl.; Novartis, NZ; Novartis Consumer, UK.*
Xylometazoline hydrochloride (p.1132·2).
*Nasal congestion; rhinitis; sinusitis.*

**Otrivine Anti-Allergic** *Novartis Consumer, Belg.*
Azelastine (p.425·2).

**Otrivine Anti-Rhinitis** *Novartis Consumer, Belg.*
Xylometazoline hydrochloride (p.1132·2).
*Nasal congestion; otitis; sinusitis.*

**Otrivine Menthol** *Novartis, NZ.*
Xylometazoline hydrochloride (p.1132·2); menthol (p.1711·3); eucalyptus (p.1686·1).
*Nasal congestion.*

**Otrivine Mu-Cron** *Novartis Consumer, UK.*
Pseudoephedrine hydrochloride (p.1129·2); paracetamol (p.76·2).
*Cold and influenza symptoms.*

**Otrivine-Antistin**
*Ciba Vision, Irl.; Novartis, NZ; Novartis Consumer, UK.*
Xylometazoline hydrochloride (p.1132·2); antazoline sulfate (p.424·2).
*Eye irritation.*

**Otrivini** *Novartis Consumer, Israel.*
Sodium chloride (p.1233·3).
*Nasal congestion.*

**Otrozol** *Pisa, Mex.*
Metronidazole (p.607·2).
*Amoebiasis; anaerobic bacterial infections.*

**Otsuka MV**
*Otsuka, Jpn; Otsuka, Thai.*
Multivitamin preparation (p.1417·1).
*Parenteral nutrition.*

**Ottocid** *Ottolenghi, Ital.*
Phenothrin (p.1509·1).
*Acaricide.*

**Ottoclor** *Ottolenghi, Ital.*
Tosylchloramide sodium (p.1194·3).
*Disinfection of skin, wounds, and burns.*

**Ottovis** *Fitolife, Ital.*
Royal jelly (p.1740·3); ginseng (p.1693·1); wheat-germ oil; soya lecithin (p.1706·1); pollen.
*Tonic.*

**Oturga** *Legrand, Braz.*
Tyrothricin (p.275·1); salicylic acid (p.1157·1); boric acid (p.1662·1); procaine hydrochloride (p.1383·2).
*Ear disorders.*

**Otylol** *Bridoux, Fr.†.*
Procaine hydrochloride (p.1383·2); tetracaine hydrochloride (p.1385·1); phenol (p.1188·1); ephedrine hydrochloride (p.1120·1); thyme oil (p.1755·3).
*Ear disorders.*

**Ouate Hemostatique** *Qualiphar, Belg.*
Ferric chloride (p.1688·1); phenazone (p.82·3).
*Haemorrhage.*

**Out of Africa** *Sutton, Canad.*
Pyrithione zinc (p.1156·2).

**Outgro**
*Note. This name is used for preparations of different composition.*
*Medtech, Canad.*
Benzocaine (p.1370·3).

*Whitehall-Robins, Canad.†; Whitehall, USA.*
Tannic acid (p.1751·2); chlorobutanol (p.1176·3).
*Ingrown toenails.*

**Outlook** *Lifeplan, UK.*
Hypericum; rosemary; avena; vitamin B substances (p.1417·1).

**Out-of-Sorts** *Potter's, UK.*
Senna (p.1288·2); aloes (p.1248·2); cascara (p.1255·1); taraxacum (p.1751·3); fennel (p.1687·2).
*Constipation.*

**Ouvidonal** *Neo Quimica, Braz.*
Chloramphenicol (p.185·1); lidocaine hydrochloride (p.1377·3).
*Ear disorders.*

**Ova** *Fada, Arg.*
Papaverine (p.1728·1).

**Ova-Mit**
*Remedica, Hong Kong; Remedica, Malaysia; Remedica, Singapore; Remedica, Thai.*
Clomifene citrate (p.1542·2).
*Anovulatory infertility.*

**Ovanon**
*Organon, Austria†; Aaciphar, Belg.†; Organon, Fr.†; Nourypharma, Ger.†; Nourypharma, Neth.; Ercopharm, Switz.†.*
7 Tablets, ethinylestradiol (p.1553·2); 15 tablets, ethinylestradiol; lynestrenol (p.1557·1).
*Sequential-type oral contraceptive.*

**Ovarell** *Sanorell, Ger.*
Homoeopathic preparation.

**Ovariusedan** *Labortecne, Braz.†.*
Plumeria; gossypium; cinnamon oil (p.1672·2); anise oil (p.1655·2).

**Ovariuteran** *Virtus, Braz.†.*
Cotton root bark; plumeria lancifolia; berberis laurina.
*Dysmenorrhoea.*

**Ovastat** *Medac, Ger.*
Treosulfan (p.590·2).
*Ovarian cancer.*

**Ovcon 35** *Bristol-Myers Squibb, USA.*
Norethisterone (p.1562·2); ethinylestradiol (p.1553·2).
28-Day packs also contain 7 inert tablets.
*Combined oral contraceptive.*

**Ovcon 50** *Bristol-Myers Squibb, USA.*
Norethisterone (p.1562·2); ethinylestradiol (p.1553·2).
28-Day packs also contain 7 inert tablets.
*Combined oral contraceptive.*

**Overal** *Lusofarmaco, Ital.*
Roxithromycin (p.254·2).
*Bacterial infections.*

**Overoid** *Valdecasas, Mex.*
Niclosamide (p.110·1).
Formerly contained chlorosalicylamide.
*Worm infections.*

**Overpon** *Valdecasas, Mex.*
Piperazine citrate (p.111·2).
*Worm infections.*

**Ovesterin**
*Organon, Norw.; Organon, Swed.*
Estriol (p.1552·3).
*Vulvovaginal disorders due to oestrogen deficiency.*

**Ovestin**
*Organon, Austral.; Organon, Austria; Organon, Chile; Organon, Denm.; Organon, Fin.; Organon, Ger.; Organon (Οργκανον), Gr.; Organon, Hong Kong; Organon, Irl.†; Organon, Israel; Organon, Ital.; Organon, Mex.; Organon, NZ; Organon, Port.; Organon, Singapore†; Organon, Switz.; Organon, Thai.; Organon, UK.*
Estriol (p.1552·3).
*Female infertility; vulvovaginal disorders due to oestrogen deficiency.*

**Ovestinon** *Organon, Spain.*
Estriol (p.1552·3).
*Oestrogen deficiency.*

**Ovestrion** *Organon, Braz.*
Estriol (p.1552·3).
*Menopausal disorders; osteoporosis.*

**Ovex** *Johnson & Johnson MSD Consumer, UK.*
Mebendazole (p.108·2).
*Enterobiasis.*

**Ovide** *Medicis, USA.*
Malathion (p.1507·1).
*Pediculosis.*

**Ovidol**
*Organon, Belg.; Nourypharma, Neth.; Nourypharma, Switz.†.*
7 Tablets, ethinylestradiol (p.1553·2); 15 tablets, ethinylestradiol; desogestrel (p.1547·2).
*Sequential-type oral contraceptive.*

**Ovidrel**
*Serono, Arg.; Serono, Hong Kong; Serono, USA.*
Choriogonadotropin alfa (p.1320·3).
*Female infertility.*

**Ovidrelle** *Serono, Spain.*
Choriogonadotropin alfa (p.1320·3).
*Female infertility.*

**Ovinol** *Norma (Νορμα), Gr.*
Norfloxacin (p.238·3).
*Urinary tract infections.*

**Ovinum**
*Biolab, Malaysia; Biolab, Singapore; Biolab, Thai.*
Clomifene citrate (p.1542·2).
*Anovulatory infertility; male infertility.*

**Oviol** *Nourypharma, Ger.*
7 Tablets, ethinylestradiol (p.1553·2); 15 tablets, ethinylestradiol; desogestrel (p.1547·2).
28-Day packs also contain 6 inert tablets.
*Sequential-type oral contraceptive.*

**Ovipreg** *Win-Medicare, India.*
Clomifene citrate (p.1542·2).
*Anovulatory infertility.*

**Ovis Neu** *Pfizer Consumer, Ger.*
Clotrimazole (p.396·2).
*Fungal skin infections.*

**Ovitrelle**
*Serono, Denm.; Serono, Fin.; Serono, Ger.; Serono, Neth.; Serono, Norw.; Serono, Port.; Serono, Swed.; Serono, UK.*
Choriogonadotropin alfa (p.1320·3).
Formerly known as Ovidrelle in the *UK*.
*Female infertility.*

**Ovofar** *Infar, India.*
Clomifene citrate (p.1542·2).
*Anovulatory infertility.*

**Ovol**
*Carter Horner, Canad.; Carter Horner, Hong Kong; Carter Horner, Thai.*
Simeticone (p.1289·2).
*Bloating; flatulence; infant colic.*

**Ovoplex** *Wyeth, Spain.*
Ethinylestradiol (p.1553·2); levonorgestrel (p.1563·2).
*Combined oral contraceptive; menstrual disorders.*

**Ovoresta**
*Organon, Braz.; Organon, Ger.†.*
Lynestrenol (p.1557·1); ethinylestradiol (p.1553·2).
*Combined oral contraceptive; menstrual disorders.*

**Ovoresta M** *Organon, Ger.*
Lynestrenol (p.1557·1); ethinylestradiol (p.1553·2).
*Combined oral contraceptive; menstrual disorders.*

**Ovosiston** *Jenapharm, Ger.*
Mestranol (p.1559·2); chlormadinone acetate (p.1542·1).
*Combined oral contraceptive; menstrual disorders.*

**Ovostat**
*Organon, Belg.†; Organon, Neth.; Donmed, S.Afr.†.*
Lynestrenol (p.1557·1); ethinylestradiol (p.1553·2).
28-Day packs also contain 7 inert tablets.
*Combined oral contraceptive.*

**Ovo-Vinces** *Wolff, Ger.†.*
Estriol (p.1552·3).
*Menopausal disorders.*

**Ovral**
*Note. This name is used for preparations of different composition.*
*Wyeth, Arg.; Wyeth-Ayerst, Canad.; Wyeth, Gr.; Wyeth-Ayerst, Hong Kong†; Wyeth, Mex.; Wyeth, NZ; Akromed, S.Afr.; Wyeth-Ayerst, Thai.†; Wyeth-Ayerst, USA.*
Norgestrel (p.1563·2); ethinylestradiol (p.1553·2).
28-Day packs also contain 7 inert tablets.
*Combined oral contraceptive; menstrual disorders.*

*Wyeth, India.*
Levonorgestrel (p.1563·2); ethinylestradiol (p.1553·2).
*Combined oral contraceptive; dysfunctional uterine bleeding; endometriosis; menstrual disorders.*

**Ovran**
*Wyeth, Irl.; Wyeth, UK†.*
Ethinylestradiol (p.1553·2); levonorgestrel (p.1563·2).
*Combined oral contraceptive; endometriosis; menstrual disorders.*

**Ovran 30**
*Wyeth, Irl.†; Wyeth, UK.*
Ethinylestradiol (p.1553·2); levonorgestrel (p.1563·2).
*Combined oral contraceptive.*

**Ovranet** *Wyeth Lederle, Ital.*
Ethinylestradiol (p.1553·2); levonorgestrel (p.1563·2).
*Combined oral contraceptive.*

**Ovranette**
*Wyeth Lederle, Austria; Wyeth, Irl.; Wyeth, UK.*
Ethinylestradiol (p.1553·2); levonorgestrel (p.1563·2).
*Combined oral contraceptive; endometriosis; menstrual disorders.*

**Ovrette** *Wyeth-Ayerst, USA.*
Norgestrel (p.1563·2).
*Progestogen-only oral contraceptive.*

**OvuGen** *BioGenex, USA.*
Fertility test (p.1734·3).

**Ovukalen** *Knop, Chile.*
Homoeopathic preparation.

**Ovukit**
*MediMar, UK†; Monoclonal Antibodies, USA.*
Fertility test (p.1734·3).

**Ovules Sedo-Hemostatiques du Docteur Jouve** *Gerda, Fr.†.*
Phenazone (p.82·3); calcium chloride (p.1225·1).
*Minor gynaecological surgery.*

**Ovuplan** *Key, Austral.*
Fertility test (p.1734·3).

**Ovuquick**
*MediMar, UK; Monoclonal Antibodies, USA.*
Fertility test (p.1734·3).

**Ovutest** *Scidia, Arg.*
Fertility test (p.1734·3).

**Ovysmen**
*Janssen-Cilag, Austria; Janssen-Cilag, Belg.; Janssen-Cilag, Ger.; Janssen-Cilag, Irl.†; Janssen-Cilag, Switz.; Janssen-Cilag, UK.*
Norethisterone (p.1562·2); ethinylestradiol (p.1553·2).
*Combined oral contraceptive.*

**Owbridges for Chesty Coughs** *Chefaro, UK†.*
Guaifenesin (p.1122·1).
*Coughs.*

**Owencet** *Galderma, Arg.*
Soap substitute.

**Oxa**
*Note. A similar name is used for preparations of different composition (see below).*
*Beta, Arg.*
Diclofenac diethylamine (p.32·1), diclofenac potassium (p.32·1), diclofenac resinate (p.33·1), or diclofenac sodium (p.32·1).
*Fever; musculoskeletal, joint, and peri-articular disorders; pain.*

**oxa**
Note. A similar name is used for preparations of different composition (see above).
CT, Ger.
Oxazepam (p.712·2).
*Anxiety disorders; sleep disorders.*

**Oxa B12** Beta, Arg.
Diclofenac potassium (p.32·1); betamethasone (p.1093·1) or betamethasone sodium phosphate (p.1093·1); cyanocobalamin (p.1458·2) or hydroxocobalamin (p.1458·2).
*Musculoskeletal, joint, and peri-articular disorders; neuritis.*

**Oxa Forte** Beta, Arg.
Diclofenac sodium (p.32·1); codeine phosphate (p.27·1).
*Pain.*

**Oxa Sport** Beta, Arg.
Diclofenac diethylamine (p.32·1); pridinol mesilate (p.1395·2); benzyl nicotinate (p.21·2); menthol (p.1711·3); lidocaine hydrochloride (p.1377·3); methyl salicylate (p.59·3).
*Musculoskeletal, joint, and peri-articular disorders with muscle spasm.*

**Oxabenal** Zerboni, Mex.†.
Oxyphenbutazone (p.76·1).

**Oxabenz** United Nordic, Denm.
Oxazepam (p.712·2).
*Anxiety.*

**Oxacant N** Klein, Ger.
Crataegus (p.1677·1); hypericum (p.299·1); convallaria (p.1675·3); adonis vernalis (p.1648·1); cereus (p.1669·2); scoparium (p.1742·2); melissa (p.1711·1); valerian (p.1762·2); motherwort (p.1717·1).
*Cardiac disorders.*

**Oxacant-forte N** Klein, Ger.
Crataegus (p.1677·1); convallaria (p.1675·3); adonis vernalis (p.1648·1); cereus (p.1669·2).
*Cardiac disorders.*

**Oxacant-Khella N** Klein, Ger.
Crataegus (p.1677·1); convallaria (p.1675·3); adonis vernalis (p.1648·1); cereus (p.1669·2); ammi visnaga (p.1653·3).
*Cardiac disorders.*

**Oxacant-mono** Klein, Ger.
Crataegus (p.1677·1).
*Heart failure.*

**Oxacant-sedativ** Klein, Ger.
Crataegus (p.1677·1); motherwort (p.1717·1); melissa (p.1711·1); valerian (p.1762·2).
*Nervous cardiac disorders.*

**Oxacatin** Taro, Israel.
Oxomemazine (p.438·2); sulfogaiacol (p.1131·1); sodium benzoate (p.1169·3).
*Coughs.*

**Oxacil**
Note. This name is used for preparations of different composition.
Biochimico, Braz.
Oxacillin sodium (p.240·2).
*Bacterial infections.*
Raza, Malaysia; Pharmaniaga, Malaysia.
Cloxacillin sodium (p.198·2).
*Staphylococcal infections.*

**Oxacycle-P** Specifar (Σπεσιφαρ), Gr.
Oxytetracycline hydrochloride (p.241·1); polymyxin B sulfate (p.245·1).
*Skin infections.*

**Oxadilene** Medeva, Fr.†.
Papaverine hydrochloride (p.1728·1).
Formerly contained butalamine hydrochloride and papaverine hydrochloride.
*Cerebrovascular disorders.*

**Oxadisten** Beta, Arg.
Diclofenac diethylamine (p.32·1) or diclofenac sodium (p.32·1); pridinol mesilate (p.1395·2).
*Inflammation; muscle spasm; pain.*

**Oxadol** Kedrion, Ital.
Nefopam hydrochloride (p.66·2).
*Pain.*

**Oxagesic** Beta, Arg.
Diclofenac potassium (p.32·1); paracetamol (p.76·2).
*Fever; pain.*

**Oxahexal** Hexal, Austria.
Oxazepam (p.712·2).
*Anxiety disorders; sleep disorders.*

**Oxaine-M** Wyeth, Gr.
Aluminium hydroxide (p.1249·2); magnesium oxide (p.1272·3); oxetacaine (p.1382·1).
*Antacid.*

**Oxalgin** Cadila, India.
Diclofenac sodium (p.32·1).
*Allergic conjunctivitis; corneal trauma; eye inflammation; prevention of intra-operative miosis.*

**Oxalgin-DP** Cadila, India.
Diclofenac sodium (p.32·1); paracetamol (p.76·2).
*Gout; inflammation; musculoskeletal, joint, and peri-articular disorders; pain.*

**Oxaltie** Gautier, Arg.
Oxaliplatin (p.577·1).
*Colorectal cancer.*

**Oxalyt** Madaus, Austria.
Potassium sodium hydrogen citrate (p.1224·1).
*Renal calculi.*

**Oxamin** Ratiopharm, Fin.
Oxazepam (p.712·2).
*Anxiety disorders; depression; insomnia.*

**Oxandrin**
CSL, Austral.; BTG, USA.
Oxandrolone (p.1565·1).
*Bone pain associated with osteoporosis; delayed puberty in boys; growth retardation in boys; protein catabolism; Turner's syndrome in girls; weight loss.*

**Oxanest** Leiras, Fin.
Oxycodone hydrochloride (p.75·2).
*Pain.*

**Oxapam** Lilly, Ital.†.
Oxazepam (p.712·2).
*Anxiety disorders.*

**Oxapax** Durascan, Denm.
Oxazepam (p.712·2).
*Anxiety.*

**Oxapen** Biolab Sanus, Braz.
Oxacillin sodium (p.240·2).
*Bacterial infections.*

**Oxaprost** Beta, Arg.
Diclofenac sodium (p.32·1).
Misoprostol (p.1519·2) is included in this preparation in an attempt to limit adverse effects on the gastrointestinal mucosa.
*Musculoskeletal, joint, and peri-articular disorders.*

**Oxarol** Chugai, Jpn.
Maxacalcitol (p.1462·1).
*Hyperparathyroidism.*

**Oxascand** Enapharm, Swed.
Oxazepam (p.712·2).
*Alcohol withdrawal syndrome; anxiety; sleep disorders.*

**Oxathos** Medix, Mex.
Oxolamine citrate (p.1126·1).
*Coughs.*

**Oxatokey** Inkeysa, Spain.
Oxatomide (p.438·1).
*Hypersensitivity reactions.*

**Oxbarukain** Chauvin ankerpharm, Ger.
Oxybuprocaine hydrochloride (p.1382·1).
*Local anaesthesia.*

**OxBipp** Masters, UK.
Bismuth subnitrate (p.1252·2); iodoform (p.1184·2).

**Oxcazen** Bouzen, Arg.
Oxcarbazepine (p.366·3).
*Epilepsy; neuralgia.*

**Oxcord** Biosintetica, Braz.
Nifedipine (p.966·2).
*Angina pectoris; hypertension; Raynaud's syndrome.*

**Oxelio** Jaldes, Fr.
Vitamin and mineral preparation (p.1417·1).

**Oxema Improved** Jean-Marie, Hong Kong.
Aluminium hydroxide (p.1249·2); magnesium hydroxide (p.1272·2) or magnesium trisilicate (p.1272·3); oxetacaine (p.1382·1).
*Gastrointestinal disorders.*

**Oxeno** Microsules Bernabo, Arg.
Loxoprofen sodium (p.54·3).
*Fever; inflammation; musculoskeletal and joint disorders; pain.*

**Oxeol** AstraZeneca, Fr.
Bambuterol hydrochloride (p.781·2).
*Asthma.*

**Oxepa**
Abbott, Arg.; Abbott, Hong Kong; Abbott, Ital.; Abbott Nutrition, UK.
Preparation for enteral nutrition (p.1417·1).

**Oxepam** Wyeth Lederle, Fin.
Oxazepam (p.712·2).
*Alcohol withdrawal syndrome; anxiety disorders.*

**Oxeprax** Wyeth, Spain†.
Tamoxifen citrate (p.584·1).
*Breast cancer.*

**Oxeron** Serono, Mex.†.
Hydroxycarbamide (p.559·1).

**Oxetine**
Note. This name is used for preparations of different composition.
Hexal, Austral.; Gea, Denm.
Paroxetine hydrochloride (p.311·2).
*Depression; obsessive-compulsive disorder; panic attacks.*
Pharmaland, Thai.
Fluoxetine hydrochloride (p.292·1).
*Depression; obsessive-compulsive disorder.*

**Oxez** Astra-Zeneca, Gr.
Formoterol fumarate (p.786·1).
*Asthma; chronic respiratory failure.*

**Oxeze** AstraZeneca, Canad.
Formoterol fumarate (p.786·1).
*Asthma.*

**Oxibran** Prospa, Port.
Piracetam (p.1732·1).

**Oxibron** Montpellier, Arg.
Clenbuterol hydrochloride (p.784·2).
*Obstructive airways disease.*

**Oxibron NF** Montpellier, Arg.
Clenbuterol hydrochloride (p.784·2); ambroxol hydrochloride (p.1114·3).
*Obstructive airways disease.*

**Oxibut** Microsules Bernabo, Arg.
Ibuprofen (p.45·3).
*Fever; gout; musculoskeletal, joint, and peri-articular disorders; pain.*

**Oxicam** Bioprogress, Ital.
Piroxicam (p.84·2).
*Musculoskeletal, joint, and peri-articular disorders.*

**Oxicanol** Fustery, Mex.
Piroxicam (p.84·2).
*Musculoskeletal, joint, peri-articular, and soft-tissue disorders; pain.*

**Oxicodal** Drugtech, Chile.
Oxcarbazepine (p.366·3).
*Epilepsy.*

**Oxiderma** Galderma, Spain.
Benzoyl peroxide (p.1143·2).
*Acne.*

**Oxidermiol Antihist** Farmasur, Spain†.
Benzocaine (p.1370·3); tyrothricin (p.275·1); tripelennamine hydrochloride (p.442·3).
*Cutaneous hypersensitivity reactions.*

**Oxidermiol Enzima** Farmasur, Spain.
Bacitracin (p.161·3); neomycin sulfate (p.235·1); trypsin (p.1758·3).
*Skin infections; wounds.*

**Oxidermiol Fuerte** Farmasur, Spain†.
Fluocinolone acetonide (p.1101·2).
*Skin disorders.*

**Oxidermiol Lassar** Farmasur, Spain.
Starch; salicylic acid (p.1157·1); soft paraffin; zinc oxide (p.1163·2).
*Skin disorders.*

**Oxidine** Labocean, Fr.
Antoxidant nutritional supplement (p.1417·1).

**Oxido Amari** Alcon Cusi, Spain†.
Mercuric chloride (p.1712·3); mercuric oxide (p.1712·3).
*Eye disorders.*

**Oxi-Freeda** Freeda, USA.
Multivitamin, mineral, and amino-acid preparation (p.1417·1).

**Oxifungol** Armstrong, Mex.
Fluconazole (p.398·1).
*Fungal infections.*

**Oxigen** Biosintetica, Braz.
Nimodipine (p.972·3).
*Neurological deficit following subarachnoid haemorrhage.*

**Oxiken** Kendrick, Mex.
Dobutamine hydrochloride (p.905·3).
*Heart failure; shock.*

**Oxiklorin** Orion, Fin.
Hydroxychloroquine sulfate (p.452·3).
*Light-sensitive skin disorders; lupus erythematosus; rheumatoid arthritis.*

**Oxilan** Tamustino, Braz.†.
Ioxilan (p.1066·3).
*Radiographic contrast medium.*

**Oxilin**
Allergan-Frumtost, Braz.†; Allergan, Ital.
Oxymetazoline hydrochloride (p.1126·1).
*Conjunctivitis; eye congestion.*

**Oxilium**
Labor, Austria; Oxo, Switz.
Tetrachlorodecaoxide (p.1752·3).
*Burns; skin disinfection; wounds.*

**Oximar** Dupomar, Arg.
Amoxicillin trihydrate (p.155·3).
*Bacterial infections.*

**Oximar Respiratorio** Dupomar, Arg.
Amoxicillin trihydrate (p.155·3); ambroxol hydrochloride (p.1114·3).
*Respiratory-tract infections.*

**Oximen** Orravan, Spain.
Hydrogen peroxide (p.1182·2); phosphoric acid (p.1731·2).
*Haemostasis; skin and mucous membrane disinfection.*

**5-Oxin** Torii, Hong Kong†.
5-Oxyanthranilic acid; anthranilic acid; vitamin B substances; vitamin C (p.1417·1).
*Constipation; diabetes; glaucoma.*

**Oxinovag** Gobbi, Arg.
Oxycodone hydrochloride (p.75·2).
*Pain.*

**Oxinovag Complex** Gobbi, Arg.
Oxycodone hydrochloride (p.75·2); paracetamol (p.76·2).
*Pain.*

**Oxipor** Medtech, Canad.
Coal tar (p.1159·2); salicylic acid (p.1157·1); benzocaine (p.1370·3).
*Skin disorders.*

**Oxipor VHC** Whitehall, USA.
Coal tar (p.1159·2).
Formerly contained coal tar, salicylic acid, and benzocaine.
*Psoriasis.*

**Oxis**
AstraZeneca, Arg.; AstraZeneca, Austral.; AstraZeneca, Austria; AstraZeneca, Belg.; AstraZeneca, Braz.; AstraZeneca, Denm.; AstraZeneca, Fin.; AstraZeneca, Ger.; Stern, Ger.; AstraZeneca, Hong Kong; AstraZeneca, Irl.; Teva, Israel; AstraZeneca, Ital.; AstraZeneca, Malaysia; Astra, Mex.; AstraZeneca, Neth.; AstraZeneca, Norw.; AstraZeneca, NZ; AstraZeneca, Port.; AstraZeneca, S.Afr.; AstraZeneca, Singapore; AstraZeneca, Spain; Draco, Swed.; AstraZeneca, Switz.; AstraZeneca, Thai.; AstraZeneca, UK.
Formoterol fumarate (p.786·1).
*Asthma.*

**Oxisept** Demo, Gr.
Povidone-iodine (p.1190·3).
*Mouth infections.*

**Oxistat**
GlaxoSmithKline, Arg.; Glaxo Wellcome, Mex.; Glaxo Wellcome, USA.
Oxiconazole nitrate (p.407·3).
*Fungal skin infections.*

**Oxi-T** Collins, Mex.
Tetracycline (p.266·2).
*Bacterial infections.*

**Oxi-Tabs C+E** Ferrosan, Fin.
*d*-Alpha tocoferil acetate; ascorbic acid; selenium (p.1417·1).
*Vitamins C and E and selenium deficiency.*

**Oxitina** Kampel Martian, Arg.
Oxybutynin (p.487·1).

**Oxiton** Uniao Quimica, Braz.
Oxytocin (p.1336·1).

**Oxitopisa** Pisa, Mex.
Oxytocin (p.1336·1).

**Oxitover** Llorente, Spain.
Mebendazole (p.108·2).
*Worm infections.*

**Oxitraklin** Atlantis, Mex.
Oxytetracycline (p.241·1).
*Bacterial infections.*

**Oxitrat** ICN, Braz.
Oxiconazole nitrate (p.407·3).
*Fungal infections.*

**Oxiurazina** UCI, Braz.†.
Piperazine (p.111·2).
*Ascariasis; enterobiasis.*

**Oxivel**
Zeller, Singapore†; Zeller, Switz.
Ginkgo biloba (p.1692·3).
*Tonic.*

**Oxivent**
Boehringer Ingelheim, Belg.; Boehringer Ingelheim, Denm.†; Boehringer Ingelheim, Irl.; Boehringer Ingelheim, Ital.; Boehringer Ingelheim, UK†.
Oxitropium bromide (p.790·3).
*Obstructive airways disease.*

**Oxivite** Neves, Port.†.
*dl*-Alpha tocoferil acetate (p.1465·1).
*Vitamin E deficiency.*

**Oxizole**
Note. This name is used for preparations of different composition.
Stiefel, Canad.
Oxiconazole nitrate (p.407·3).
*Tinea pedis.*
Orthos, Mex.†.
Mebendazole (p.108·2).

**Oxobron** Diba, Mex.
Oxolamine citrate (p.1126·1).
*Coughs.*

**Oxodal** Synthelabo, Spain†.
Betaxolol hydrochloride (p.873·1).
*Hypertension.*

**Oxoferin**
Note. This name is used for preparations of different composition.
Yamanouchi, Ger.
Reaction product of sodium chlorite, sodium hypochlorite, sulfuric acid, potassium chlorate, sodium carbonate-hydrogen peroxide, and sodium peroxide.
*Wounds.*
Oxo, Thai.
Tetrachlorodecaoxide (p.1752·3).
*Burns; ulcers; wounds.*

**Oxoinex** Inexfa, Spain.
Oxolinic acid (p.240·3).
*Urinary-tract infections.*

**Oxolam** Diba, Mex.†.
Oxolamine (p.1126·1).

**Oxomar** Offenbach, Mex.
Oxolamine (p.1126·1).
*Coughs.*

**Oxomifer** Reuffer, Mex.†.
Oxolamine (p.1126·1).

**Oxopurin** Dexxon, Israel.
Pentoxifylline (p.979·3).
*Vascular disorders.*

**Oxoquin** Protermex, Mex.†.
Oxolamine citrate (p.1126·1).

**Oxosint** Medivis, Ital.†.
Co-tetroxazine (p.199·3).
*Bacterial infections; Pneumocystis carinii pneumonia.*

**Oxo-Val** Saval, Chile.
Vitamin and mineral preparation (p.1417·1).
*Dietary supplement.*

**Oxoway** Wayne, Mex.†.
Ambroxol (p.1114·3).

**Ox-Pam** Douglas, NZ.
Oxazepam (p.712·2).
*Alcohol withdrawal syndrome; anxiety.*

**Oxrate** Merind, India.
Oxcarbazepine (p.366·3).
*Epilepsy.*

**Oxsac** Masa, Thai.
Fluoxetine hydrochloride (p.292·1).
*Depression; obsessive-compulsive disorder.*

**Oxsoralen**
ICN, Austral.; Gerot, Austria; ICN, Canad.; ICN, Hong Kong; ICN, Israel†; Italfarmaco, Ital.; ICN, Malaysia; ICN, Mex.; ICN, Neth.;

*ICN, NZ; Pharmaco, S.Afr.; ICN, Singapore; Galderma, Spain; ICN, USA.*
Methoxsalen (p.1152·1).
*Psoriasis; vitiligo.*

**Oxsoralon** *Wolfs, Belg.†.*
Methoxsalen (p.1152·1).
*Psoriasis.*

**Oxy**
*Note. This name is used for preparations of different composition.*
*GlaxoSmithKline Consumer, Austral.; GlaxoSmithKline Consumer, Canad.; SmithKline Beecham OTC, Ger.†; GlaxoSmithKline, Hong Kong; SmithKline Beecham, Israel; SmithKline Beecham, Mex.†; GlaxoSmithKline Consumer, UK; SmithKline Beecham Consumer, USA.*
Benzoyl peroxide (p.1143·2).
*Acne.*

*Triomed, S.Afr.†.*
Oxytetracycline hydrochloride (p.241·1).
*Bacterial infections.*

**Oxy Balance** *SmithKline Beecham, Hong Kong†.*
Salicylic acid (p.1157·1).
*Acne.*

**Oxy Biciron** *S & K, Ger.*
Oxytetracycline hydrochloride (p.241·1); tramazoline hydrochloride (p.1131·3).
*Bacterial eye infections.*

**Oxy Clean Facial Scrub** *GlaxoSmithKline Consumer, UK.*
Borax (p.1661·3); triclosan (p.1195·2).
*Acne.*

**Oxy Clean Medicated** *SmithKline Beecham, Israel.*
Salicylic acid (p.1157·1); alcohol (p.1166·1).
*Acne.*

**Oxy Clean Pore** *SmithKline Beecham Consumer, Canad.†.*
Salicylic acid (p.1157·1).
*Acne.*

**Oxy Cleanser** *GlaxoSmithKline Consumer, UK.*
*Regular:* Triclosan (p.1195·2); salicylic acid (p.1157·1); alcohol (p.1166·1).
Formerly called Oxy Clean Medicated Cleanser.
*Sensitive:* Salicylic acid (p.1157·1); alcohol (p.1166·1).
*Acne.*

**Oxy Control** *SmithKline Beecham Consumer, Canad.†.*
Salicylic acid (p.1157·1).
*Acne.*

**Oxy Daily Cleaning Pads** *GlaxoSmithKline Consumer, Canad.*
Salicylic acid (p.1157·1).
*Acne.*

**Oxy Daily Facial Cleanser Regular** *GlaxoSmithKline Consumer, Canad.*
Triclosan (p.1195·2).
*Acne.*

**Oxy Daily Skin Wash** *GlaxoSmithKline Consumer, NZ.*
Triclosan (p.1195·2).
*Acne.*

**Oxy Daily Wash** *GlaxoSmithKline, Hong Kong.*
Triclosan (p.1195·2).
*Skin disorders.*

**Oxy Deep Pore** *GlaxoSmithKline Consumer, Canad.*
Salicylic acid (p.1157·1).
*Acne.*

**Oxy Dots** *GlaxoSmithKline Consumer, UK.*
Salicylic acid (p.1157·1); triclosan (p.1195·2).
*Spots.*

**Oxy Duo Pads** *GlaxoSmithKline Consumer, UK.*
*Regular:* Triclosan (p.1195·2); salicylic acid (p.1157·1); alcohol (p.1166·1).
*Sensitive:* Salicylic acid (p.1157·1); alcohol (p.1166·1).
*Acne.*

**Oxy Facial Wash** *GlaxoSmithKline Consumer, UK.*
Triclosan (p.1195·2).
*Skin disorders.*

**Oxy Finishing Toner** *GlaxoSmithKline Consumer, Canad.*
Salicylic acid (p.1157·1).
*Acne.*

**Oxy Fissan** *Fink, Ger.†; Zyma, Ger.†.*
Benzoyl peroxide (p.1143·2).
*Acne.*

**Oxy Gentle** *SmithKline Beecham Consumer, Canad.†.*
Triclosan (p.1195·2).
*Acne.*

**Oxy Medicated Pads** *GlaxoSmithKline Consumer, Canad.*
Salicylic acid (p.1157·1).
Formerly known as Oxy Power Pads.
*Acne.*

**Oxy Medicated Soap**
*GlaxoSmithKline Consumer, Canad.; SmithKline Beecham, USA.*
Triclosan (p.1195·2).
*Acne.*

**Oxy Night Watch**
*SmithKline Beecham Consumer, Canad.†; SmithKline Beecham Consumer, USA.*
Salicylic acid (p.1157·1).
*Acne.*

**Oxy Sensitive** *SmithKline Beecham, Israel.*
Benzoyl peroxide (p.1143·2).
*Acne.*

**Oxy Skin Wash** *GlaxoSmithKline, Austral.*
Triclosan (p.1195·2).
*Acne; skin cleanser.*

**Oxyb** *ABZ, Ger.*
Oxybutynin hydrochloride (p.486·3).
*Bladder instability.*

**Oxybase**
*Hexal, Austria; Hexal, Ger.; Gea, Swed.*
Oxybutynin hydrochloride (p.486·3).
*Neurogenic bladder; urinary incontinence.*

**Oxyboldine** *Cooperation Pharmaceutique, Fr.*
Boldine (p.1661·2); anhydrous sodium sulfate (p.1290·1); monobasic sodium phosphate (p.1230·3).
*Dyspepsia.*

**Oxybubene** *Ratiopharm, Austria.*
Oxybutynin hydrochloride (p.486·3).
*Bladder instability; urinary incontinence.*

**Oxybugamma** *Worwag, Ger.*
Oxybutynin hydrochloride (p.486·3).
*Bladder instability; urinary incontinence.*

**Oxybutin** *Holsten, Ger.*
Oxybutynin hydrochloride (p.486·3).
*Bladder instability.*

**Oxybuton** *Abbott, Ger.*
Oxybutynin hydrochloride (p.486·3).
*Bladder instability; urinary incontinence.*

**Oxybutyn** *ICN, Canad.*
Oxybutynin hydrochloride (p.486·3).

**Oxy-Care** *Agepha, Austria.*
Hydrogen peroxide (p.1182·2); sodium chloride (p.1233·3) (p.1164·2).
*Disinfecting, cleaning, and storage solution for hard and soft contact lenses.*

**Oxycel**
*Associated Hospital Supply, UK; Becton Dickinson, USA.*
Oxidised cellulose (p.757·1).
*Bleeding in surgical procedures.*

**Oxycline** *General Drugs, Thai.*
Oxytetracycline hydrochloride (p.241·1).
*Bacterial infections.*

**Oxycocet** *Technilab, Canad.*
Oxycodone hydrochloride (p.75·2); paracetamol (p.76·2).
*Fever; pain.*

**Oxycod** *Rafa, Israel.*
Oxycodone hydrochloride (p.75·2).
*Pain.*

**Oxycodan** *Technilab, Canad.*
Oxycodone hydrochloride (p.75·2); aspirin (p.15·1).
*Fever; inflammation; pain.*

**Oxycontin**
*Raffo, Arg.; Mundipharma, Austral.; Zodiac, Braz.; Purdue, Canad.; Tecnofarma, Chile; Norpharma, Denm.; Mundipharma, Fin.; Mundipharma, Fr.; Napp, Irl.; Rafa, Israel; Asofarma, Mex.; Mundipharma, Norw.; Mundipharma, Swed.; Mundipharma, Switz.; Napp, UK; Purdue Frederick, USA.*
Oxycodone hydrochloride (p.75·2).
*Pain.*

**Oxyderm** *ICN, Canad.*
Benzoyl peroxide (p.1143·2).
*Acne.*

**Oxydermine** *Wild, Switz.*
Zinc oxide (p.1163·2); lauromacrogol 400 (p.1412·3).
*Burns; skin disorders; wounds.*

**Oxyfast** *Purdue Frederick, USA.*
Oxycodone hydrochloride (p.75·2).
*Pain.*

**Oxyflux** *Rayere, Mex.*
Clenbuterol hydrochloride (p.784·2).

**Oxygeron**
*Will-Pharma, Austria†; Drossapharm, Switz.; Willpharma, Thai.†.*
Vincamine (p.1764·2).
*Cerebrovascular disorders; circulatory eye disorders; dizziness; headache; migraine.*

**Oxygesic** *Mundipharma, Ger.*
Oxycodone hydrochloride (p.75·2).
*Pain.*

**Oxygirex** *Irex, Fr.†.*
Trimetazidine hydrochloride (p.1018·1).
*Angina pectoris; vascular eye disorders; vestibular disorders.*

**OxyIR** *Purdue Frederick, USA.*
Oxycodone hydrochloride (p.75·2).
*Pain.*

**Oxylim**
*Atlantic, Hong Kong; Atlantic, Thai.*
Oxytetracycline hydrochloride (p.241·1).
*Bacterial infections.*

*Atlantic, Malaysia; Atlantic, Singapore.*
Oxytetracycline (p.241·1).
*Bacterial infections.*

**Oxylin**
*Allergan, Hong Kong; Allergan, Israel†; Allergan, Mex.; Allergan, Port.; Allergan, S.Afr.; Allergan, Singapore†; Allergan, Thai.†.*
Oxymetazoline hydrochloride (p.1126·1).
*Conjunctivitis; eye irritation.*

**Oxymedin** *Kade, Ger.*
Oxybutynin hydrochloride (p.486·3).
*Neurogenic bladder; urinary incontinence.*

**Oxymet** *Greater Pharma, Thai.*
Oxymetazoline hydrochloride (p.1126·1).
*Nasal congestion; nasopharyngitis; rhinitis; sinusitis.*

**Oxymycin** *DDSA Pharmaceuticals, UK.*
Oxytetracycline (p.241·1).

**Oxyno** *Milano, Thai.*
Oxyphencyclimine hydrochloride (p.487·2).
*Gastrointestinal disorders; genito-urinary disorders.*

**Oxynorm**
*Mundipharma, Austral.; Norpharma, Denm.; Mundipharma, Fin.; Napp, Irl.; Mundipharma, Norw.; Mundipharma, Swed.; Napp, UK.*
Oxycodone hydrochloride (p.75·2).
*Pain.*

**Oxypan** *Propan, S.Afr.*
Oxytetracycline hydrochloride (p.241·1).
*Bacterial infections.*

**Oxypangam** *Lichtenstein, Ger.*
Di-isopropylammonium dichloroacetate (p.900·1).
*Hypoxia due to circulatory disorders.*

**Oxyperol** *Lemoine, Fr.*
Peru balsam (p.1730·2); zinc oxide (p.1163·2).
*Skin irritation.*

**Oxyplastine**
*Note. This name is used for preparations of different composition.*
*Bournonville, Belg.†.*
Zinc oxide (p.1163·2); peru balsam (p.1730·2); calcium hydroxide (p.1664·3).
*Barrier cream; skin disorders.*

*Pfizer, Fr.; Wild, Switz.*
Zinc oxide (p.1163·2).
*Skin disorders.*

**Oxysept**
*Note. This name is used for preparations of different composition.*
*Allergan, Austral.†; Allergan, Ger.†; Allergan, Israel†; Allergan, NZ†.*
Oxysept 1, hydrogen peroxide (p.1182·2); Oxysept 2, irrigating, neutralising, and storage solution (p.1164·2).
*Disinfecting, rinsing, and storage system for soft contact lenses.*

*Allergan, Braz.; Allergan, USA.*
Hydrogen peroxide (p.1182·2) (p.1164·2).
*Disinfecting solution for soft contact lenses.*

*Allergan, Canad.†.*
Cleaning and disinfecting solution for soft contact lenses (p.1164·2).

*Allergan, Port.†.*
Contact lens care solution (p.1164·2).

**Oxysept Comfort** *Allergan, Ger.†.*
Solution, hydrogen peroxide (p.1182·2); tablets, catalase (p.1668·3) (p.1164·2).
*Disinfection and neutralisation of soft contact lenses.*

**Oxyspas**
*Cipla, India; Cipla-Medpro, S.Afr.*
Oxybutynin hydrochloride (p.486·3).
*Neurogenic bladder; nocturnal enuresis; urinary incontinence.*

**Oxytel** *Coup, Gr.*
Tenoxicam (p.93·1).
*Dysmenorrhoea; gout; inflammation; osteoarthritis; pain; rheumatoid arthritis; spondyloarthropathies.*

**Oxytetral**
*Alpharma, Denm.†; Alpharma, Norw.; Alpharma, Swed.*
Oxytetracycline hydrochloride (p.241·1).
*Bacterial infections.*

**Oxytetramix** *Ashbourne, UK.*
Oxytetracycline (p.241·1).
*Bacterial infections.*

**Oxythyol** *Richard, Fr.*
Zinc oxide (p.1163·2); ichthammol (p.1148·2).
*Skin irritation.*

**Oxytrol** *Watson, USA.*
Oxybutynin (p.487·1).
*Bladder overactivity.*

**Oxyurin** *Klonal, Arg.*
Oxybutynin (p.487·1).
*Neurogenic bladder.*

**Oxyzal** *Gordon, USA.*
Hydroxyquinoline sulfate (p.1700·1); benzalkonium chloride (p.1168·3).
*Minor skin infections.*

**Oyo** *Polypharm, Ger.*
Sodium pangamate (p.1727·2).
*Cerebral and peripheral vascular disorders; ischaemic heart disease; migraine.*

**Oysco** *Rugby, USA.*
Calcium carbonate (p.1254·2).
*Calcium deficiency; dietary supplement.*

**Oysco D** *Rugby, USA.*
Calcium with vitamin D (p.1417·1).
*Calcium deficiency; dietary supplement.*

**Oyst-Cal** *Goldline, USA.*
Calcium carbonate (p.1254·2).
*Calcium deficiency; dietary supplement.*

**Oyst-Cal-D** *Goldline, USA.*
Calcium with vitamin D (p.1417·1).
*Calcium deficiency; dietary supplement.*

**Oyster Calcium**
*Note. This name is used for preparations of different composition.*
*Cypress, USA.*
Calcium (oyster shells) (p.1225·1).
*Calcium supplement.*

*Nature's Bounty, USA.*
Calcium with vitamins A and D (p.1417·1).
*Calcium deficiency; dietary supplement.*

**Oyster Calcium with Vitamin D**
*Cypress, USA.*
Calcium (oyster shells) (p.1225·1); colecalciferol (p.1461·3).
*Calcium and vitamin D supplement.*

*Nion, USA.*
Calcium with vitamin D (p.1417·1).
*Calcium deficiency; dietary supplement.*

**Oyster Shell Calcium** *Vangard, USA†.*
Calcium carbonate (p.1254·2).
*Calcium deficiency; dietary supplement.*

**Oyster Shell Calcium with Vitamin D** *Major, USA.*
Calcium with vitamin D (p.1417·1).
*Calcium deficiency; dietary supplement.*

**Oystercal** *Nature's Bounty, USA†.*
Calcium carbonate (p.1254·2).
*Calcium deficiency; dietary supplement.*

**Oystercal-D** *Nature's Bounty, USA.*
Calcium with vitamin D (p.1417·1).
*Calcium deficiency; dietary supplement.*

**Oz** *Aleph, Ital.*
Zinc oxide (p.1163·2).
*Skin disorders.*

**Ozex** *Toyama, Jpn.*
Tosufloxacin tosilate (p.272·2).
*Bacterial infections.*

**Ozidia** *Pfizer, Fr.*
Glipizide (p.332·2).
*Diabetes mellitus.*

**Ozoken** *Kener, Mex.*
Omeprazole (p.1278·2).
*Peptic ulcer.*

**Ozonol**
*Note. This name is used for preparations of different composition.*
*Bayer Consumer, Canad.*
Phenol (p.1188·1); zinc oxide (p.1163·2).
*Bites and stings; burns; cuts; skin irritation.*

*GlaxoSmithKline Consumer, Port.*
Ibuprofen (p.45·3).

**Ozonol Antibiotic Plus** *Bayer Consumer, Canad.*
Polymyxin B sulfate (p.245·1); bacitracin (p.161·3); lidocaine hydrochloride (p.1377·3).
*Minor cuts and burns; skin irritation.*

**Ozonosol** *Lagos, Arg.*
*SPF 40:* Titanium dioxide (p.1160·3); octinoxate (p.1154·3); oxybenzone (p.1154·3).
*Sunscreen.*

**Ozonyl** *Gross, Braz.*
Menthol (p.1711·3); guaiacol (p.1122·1); terpin hydrate (p.1131·1); cineole (p.1672·1); niaouli oil (p.1719·3); camphor (p.1665·3); benzyl cinnamate.
*Respiratory-tract congestion.*

**Ozonyl Aquoso** *Gross, Braz.*
Cineole (p.1672·1); niaouli oil (p.1719·3); guaifenesin (p.1122·1); sodium camsilate; lidocaine hydrochloride (p.1377·3).
*Respiratory-tract congestion.*

**Ozonyl Expectorante** *Gross, Braz.*
Diphenhydramine hydrochloride (p.431·3); ammonium chloride (p.1115·2); sodium camsilate; guaifenesin (p.1122·1); cineole (p.1672·1); niaouli oil (p.1719·3); menthol (p.1711·3).
*Respiratory-tract congestion.*

**Ozopulmin** *Geymonat, Ital.*
*Injection; nasal spray:* Verbenone.
*Suppositories:* Verbenone; pine oil.
*Respiratory-system disorders.*

**Ozopulmin G** *Geymonat, Ital.*
*Suppositories:* Verbenone; pine oil.
*Syrup:* Verbenone; dextromethorphan hydrobromide (p.1117·3).
*Topical gel:* Verbenone.
*Catarrh; coughs.*

**Ozothin**
*GlaxoSmithKline, Ger.*
*Injection; inhalation:* Oxidation product of turpentine oil Landes (p.1760·1); terpin hydrate (p.1131·1).
*Respiratory-tract disorders.*

*SmithKline Beecham, Ger.†.*
*Suppositories:* Paracetamol (p.76·2); oxidation product of turpentine oil Landes (p.1760·1); oleum pini sylvestris.
*Fever and pain associated with respiratory-tract disorders.*
*Tablets:* Diprophylline (p.784·3); oxidation products of turpentine oil Landes (p.1760·1).
*Respiratory-tract disorders.*

**Ozothine** *Laphal, Fr.*
*Suppositories:* Oxidation products of turpentine oil (p.1760·1).
*Syrup:* Oxidation products of turpentine oil (p.1760·1); sodium benzoate (p.1169·3).
*Respiratory-tract disorders.*

**Ozothine a la Diprophylline** *Laphal, Fr.*
Oxidation products of turpentine oil (p.1760·1); diprophylline (p.784·3).
*Respiratory-tract disorders.*

**Ozovit**
*Koch, Austria†; Pascoe, Ger.*
Magnesium peroxide (p.1185·2).
*Constipation; dyspepsia; meteorism.*

**Ozym** *Trommsdorff, Ger.*
Pancreatin (p.1725·3).
*Pancreatic insufficiency.*

**3P** *Beacons, Singapore.*
Pholcodine (p.1128·3); pseudoephedrine hydrochloride (p.1129·2); triprolidine hydrochloride (p.442·3).
*Coughs; upper respiratory-tract congestion.*

**P & S**
Note. This name is used for preparations of different composition.
Paladin, Canad.; Baker Cummins, USA.
*Scalp application:* Liquid phenol (p.1188·1).
*Psoriasis; seborrhoeic dermatitis.*

Paladin, Canad.; Baker Cummins, USA.
*Shampoo:* Salicylic acid (p.1157·1).
*Psoriasis; seborrhoea.*

**P & S Plus** Paladin, Canad.; Baker Cummins, USA†.
Coal tar (p.1159·2); salicylic acid (p.1157·1).
*Psoriasis; seborrhoeic dermatitis.*

**P. Veinos** Augot, Fr.†.
Aesculus (p.1648·2); cupressus sempervirens; hamamelis (p.1696·3).
*Peripheral vascular disorders.*

**Pabafilm**
Note. This name is used for preparations of different composition.
Alcon, Braz.†.
*SPF 10; SPF 15:* Padimate O (p.1155·1); benzophenone-6 (p.1143·1).
*Sunscreen.*

Galderma, Mex.†.
*SPF 10; SPF 15:* Padimate O (p.1155·1); oxybenzone (p.1154·3).
*Sunscreen.*

**Pabalat** Instituto Sanitas, Chile.
Nifedipine (p.966·2).
*Angina pectoris; hypertension; Raynaud's syndrome.*

**Pabalate** Robins, USA†.
Sodium salicylate (p.90·1); sodium aminobenzoate (p.1747·1).
*Pain.*

**Pabanox** Surya, Singapore†.
Oxybenzone (p.1154·3); dioxybenzone (p.1145·3); padimate O (p.1155·1); titanium dioxide (p.1160·3).
*Sunscreen.*

**Pabasol** Galderma, Mex.†.
Padimate O (p.1155·1); oxybenzone (p.1154·3).
*Sunscreen.*

**Pabasun** Alpharma, Fr.
Aminobenzoic acid (p.1142·2).
*Sunscreen.*

**Pabrinex** Link, Irl.; Link, UK.
Vitamin B substances; ascorbic acid (p.1417·1).
*Vitamin deficiencies; vitamin supplement.*

**P-A-C** Upjohn, USA.
Aspirin (p.15·1); caffeine (p.782·1).
*Pain.*

**Pac Merieux** Aventis Pasteur, Ger.
An acellular pertussis vaccine (p.1631·2).
*Active immunisation.*

**Pacaps** Lunsco, USA.
Butalbital (p.673·3); caffeine (p.782·1); paracetamol (p.76·2).

**Paceco** Malaysia Chemist, Singapore.
Codeine phosphate (p.27·1); paracetamol (p.76·2).
*Cold symptoms; fever; pain.*

**Paceflex** Gemballa, Braz.
Carisoprodol (p.1392·1); paracetamol (p.76·2); caffeine (p.782·1).
*Skeletal muscle spasm.*

**Pacemol** Gemballa, Braz.; Malaysia Chemist, Singapore.
Paracetamol (p.76·2).
*Fever; pain.*

**Pacerone** Upsher-Smith, USA.
Amiodarone hydrochloride (p.859·2).
*Ventricular arrhythmias.*

**Pacetal** Rekah, Israel.
Phenobarbital (p.367·3); paracetamol (p.76·2).
*Fever; pain.*

**Paceum** Orion, Switz.
Diazepam (p.690·1).
*Convulsions; non-psychotic mental disorders; premedication; skeletal muscle spasm; sleep disorders.*

**Pacifen** Pacific, NZ.
Baclofen (p.1386·3).
*Skeletal muscle spasm and spasticity.*

**Pacifene** Sussex, UK.
Ibuprofen (p.45·3).
*Fever; pain.*

**Pacifenity** Vitaplex, Austral.†.
Passion flower (p.1729·1); mistletoe (p.1715·3); avena (p.1658·2); valerian (p.1762·2); gentian (p.1692·2); lupulus (p.1708·1); skullcap (p.1746·3); motherwort (p.1717·1).
*Herbal relaxant.*

**Pacimol** Ipca, India; Multichem, NZ; Nat Druggists, S.Afr.
Paracetamol (p.76·2).
*Fever; pain.*

**Pacinax** Silesia, Chile.
Diazepam (p.690·1).
*Epilepsy.*

**Pacinol** Schering-Plough, Denm.; Schering-Plough, Fin.; Schering-Plough, Swed.
Fluphenazine hydrochloride (p.699·3).
*Hiccup; nausea and vomiting; psychoses.*

**Pacinone** Schering-Plough, Port.
Halazepam (p.701·2).

**Pacis** Filaxis, Arg.; Shire Biologics, Canad.; Urocor, USA.
A BCG vaccine (p.1609·2).
*Bladder cancer.*

**Pacisyn** Syntetic, Denm.
Nitrazepam (p.710·1).
*Epilepsy; insomnia.*

**Pacitane** Wyeth Lederle, India.
Trihexyphenidyl hydrochloride (p.490·2).
*Drug-induced extrapyramidal disorders; parkinsonism.*

**Pacium** Uriach, Spain.
Diazepam (p.690·1).
Contains pyridoxine hydrochloride.
*Alcohol withdrawal syndrome; anxiety; febrile convulsions; insomnia; skeletal muscle spasm.*

**Paclikebir** Aspen, Arg.
Paclitaxel (p.577·3).
*Malignant neoplasms.*

**Paclitax** Eurofarma, Braz.
Paclitaxel (p.577·3).
*Malignant neoplasms.*

**Pacliteva** Teva Tuteur, Arg.
Paclitaxel (p.577·3).
*Malignant neoplasms.*

**Pacofen** DHA, Singapore.
Codeine phosphate (p.27·1); paracetamol (p.76·2); caffeine (p.782·1).
*Pain.*

**Pacopan** Pharmasant, Thai.
Hyoscine butylbromide (p.483·3); paracetamol (p.76·2).
*Smooth muscle spasm.*

**Pactens**
Note. This name is used for preparations of different composition.
Galenica, Gr.
Bisoprolol fumarate (p.875·1).
*Angina; arrythmias; hypertension; hyperthyroidism; hypertrophic obstructive cardiomyopathy; myocardial infarction; phaechromocytoma.*

Merck, Mex.
Naproxen sodium (p.65·1).
*Inflammation; pain.*

**Pacyl** Jagson, India.
Alprazolam (p.668·3).
*Anxiety; mixed anxiety depressive states.*

**Padamin** Fresenius Kabi, Austria.
Amino-acid infusion (p.1417·1).
*Parenteral nutrition.*

**Paderyl** Gerda, Fr.
Codeine phosphate (p.27·1).
*Coughs.*

**Padet** Pharmatrix, Arg.
Metronidazole (p.607·2).
*Rosacea.*

**Padiacrom** Padia, Ger.
Sodium cromoglicate (p.795·3).
*Asthma.*

**Padiafusin** Fresenius Kabi, Austria; Baxter, Ger.
Electrolyte infusion with glucose (p.1217·1).
*Carbohydrate source; fluid and electrolyte disorders.*

**Padiafusin OP** Baxter, Ger.
Potassium-free electrolyte infusion with glucose (p.1217·1).
*Carbohydrate source; fluid and electrolyte disorders.*

**Padiamol** Padia, Ger.
Salbutamol sulfate (p.791·3).
*Obstructive airways disease.*

**Padiamuc** Padia, Ger.
Ambroxol hydrochloride (p.1114·3).
*Respiratory-tract disorders.*

**Padiatifen** Padia, Ger.
Ketotifen fumarate (p.788·1).
*Allergic rhinitis; allergic skin disorders; asthma; bronchitis.*

**Padiken** Kener, Mex.†.
Amantadine hydrochloride (p.1197·2).

**Padma 28** Padma, Switz.
Aegle sepiar fructus; amomi fructus; aquilegiae herba; calc. sulfas; calendulae flos.; cardamomi fructus; caryophylli flos.; costi amari radix; dextrocamphora; hedychii rhizoma; lactucae sativae folium; lichen islandicus; liquiritiae radix; meliae tousend fructus; myrobalani fructus; plantaginis herba; polygoni herba; potentillae aureae herba; santali rubri lignum; sidae cordifoliae herba; aconiti tuber; valerianae radix.
*Circulatory disorders.*

Cedar Health, UK.
Aegle sepiar fructus; amomi fructus; aquilegiae herba; calendula flos; cardamomi fructus; caryophylli flos; costi amari radix; hedychii rhizoma; lactucae sativae folium; lichen islandicus; liquiritiae radix; meliae tousend fructus; myrobalani fructus; plantaginis herba; polygoni herba; potentillae aureae herba; santali rubri lignum; sidae cordifoliae herba; aconiti tuber; valerianae radix; calcium sulfate; camphor.
*Circulatory disorders.*

**Padma-Lax** Padma, Switz.
Aloes (p.1248·2); kaolin (p.1268·3); calumba radix (p.1665·2); condurango (p.1675·3); enulae radix; gentian (p.1692·2); myrobalan; sodium bicarbonate (p.1223·2); anhydrous sodium sulfate (p.1290·1); piper longum; frangula bark (p.1266·3); cascara (p.1255·1); rhubarb (p.1287·3); nux vomica (p.1722·3); ginger (p.1267·1).
*Constipation.*

**Padmed Circosan** Padma, Switz.
Aegle sepiar fructus; amomi fructus; aquilegiae vulgaris herba; calcii sulfas pulv.; calendulae flos; cardamomi fructus; caryophylli flos; costi amari radix; dextrocamphora; hedychii rhizoma; lactucae sativae folium; lichen islandicus; liquiritiae radix; meliae tousend fructus; myrobalani fructus; plantaginis herba; polygoni herba; potentillae aureae herba; santali rubri lignum; sidae cordifoliae herba; aconiti tuber; valerianae radix.
*Circulatory disorders.*

**Padrin** Fujisawa, Jpn.
Prifinium bromide (p.488·2).
*Adjunct in gastrointestinal examination; pancreatitis; smooth muscle spasm.*

**Padutin** Wabosan, Austria; Bayer, Ger.†.
Kallidinogenase (Kallikrein) (p.1703·2).
*Male infertility.*

**Paedamin** Paedpharm, Austral.
Diphenhydramine hydrochloride (p.431·3); phenylephrine hydrochloride (p.1126·3).
*Upper respiratory-tract disorders.*

**Paedialgon** Chephasaar, Ger.
Paracetamol (p.76·2).
*Fever; pain.*

**Paediasure** Abbott, Irl.; Abbott Nutrition, UK.
A range of preparations for enteral nutrition (p.1417·1).

**Paediathrocin** Abbott, Ger.
Erythromycin ethyl succinate (p.208·1).
*Bacterial infections.*

**Paediatric Seravit** Scientific Hospital Supplies, Austral.; Nutricia, NZ; Scientific Hospital Supplies, NZ; Scientific Hospital Supplies, UK.
Multivitamin, mineral, and trace element preparation (p.1417·1).
*Dietary supplement.*

**Paedisup** Chephasaar, Ger.
Paracetamol (p.76·2); doxylamine succinate (p.432·3).
*Fever; pain.*

**Paf** Lofarma, Ital.
Bucarbetene.
*Scabies.*

**Paferxin** Liferpal, Mex.
Cefalexin (p.168·1).
*Bacterial infections.*

**Paftec** Boehringer Ingelheim, Port.†.
Flunisolide (p.1101·1).
*Asthma.*

**Pahtlisan** Bioquimico, Mex.†.
Chlorothiazide (p.882·1).

**Paididont** Metochem, Austria.
Chamomile (p.1669·3); cetylpyridinium chloride (p.1173·1); lauromacrogol 400 (p.1412·3).
*Teething pain.*

**Paidocin** Chiesi, Ital.
Rokitamycin (p.254·1).
*Bacterial infections.*

**Paidoflor** Ardeypharm, Ger.
*Lactobacillus acidophilus* (p.1704·2).
*Gastrointestinal disorders.*

**Paidolax** Casen Fleet, Spain.
Glycerol (p.1694·3).
*Constipation.*

**Paidomal** Malesci, Ital.
Lysine theophyllinate (p.804·3).
*Obstructive airways disease.*

**Paidorinovit** SIT, Ital.
Ephedrine (p.1120·1); cineole (p.1672·1); niaouli oil (p.1719·3).
*Nasal congestion.*

**Paidoterin Descongestivo NF** Aldo, Spain.
Chlorphenamine maleate (p.427·3); diphenhydramine hydrochloride (p.431·3); phenylephrine hydrochloride (p.1126·3).
Formerly known as Paidoterin Descongestivo and contained chlorphenamine maleate, diphenhydramine hydrochloride, phenylephrine hydrochloride, guaifenesin, choline salicylate, and sodium citrate.
*Upper-respiratory-tract congestion.*

**Paidovit** Andromaco, Chile.
Vitamin A palmitate; ergocalciferol; ascorbic acid.
*Vitamin A, D, and C deficiency.*

**Paidozim** Juventus, Spain.
Amylase (p.1654·2); cellulase (p.1669·1); lipase; metoclopramide (p.1274·3); protease.
*Digestive enzyme insufficiency; dyspepsia.*

**Paigastrol** Orravan, Spain†.
Pancreatin (p.1725·3); pepsin (p.1729·3).
*Digestive enzyme insufficiency.*

**Pain Aid** Zee, Canad.
Aspirin (p.15·1); caffeine (p.782·1).

**Pain Aid Free** Zee, Canad.
Paracetamol (p.76·2).

**Pain Buster** Prodemdis, Canad.
Methyl salicylate (p.59·3); camphor (p.1665·3); menthol (p.1711·3); eucalyptus oil (p.1686·2).

**Pain Bust-R II** Continental, USA.
Methyl salicylate (p.59·3); menthol (p.1711·3).
*Musculoskeletal and joint disorders.*

**Pain Doctor** Fougera, USA.
Capsaicin (p.24·2); methyl salicylate (p.59·3); menthol (p.1711·3).
*Pain.*

**Pain And Fever Relief** Brauer, Austral.†.
Homoeopathic preparation.

**Pain Relief Syrup for Children** Unichem, UK†.
Paracetamol (p.76·2).
*Fever; pain.*

**Pain Reliever** Rugby, USA†.
Paracetamol (p.76·2); aspirin (p.15·1); caffeine (p.782·1).
*Pain.*

**Pain Relieving Ointment** Jamieson, Canad.
Camphor (p.1665·3); menthol (p.1711·3); mentha arvensis; cajuput oil; cinnamon oil; clove oil.

**Painagon** Be-Tabs, S.Afr.
*Syrup:* Paracetamol (p.76·2); codeine phosphate (p.27·1); promethazine hydrochloride (p.439·1).
*Fever; pain.*
*Tablets:* Paracetamol (p.76·2); codeine phosphate (p.27·1); meprobamate (p.706·2); caffeine (p.782·1).
*Pain; pain associated with tension.*

**Painaid** Zee, USA.
Aspirin (p.15·1); salicylamide (p.87·3); paracetamol (p.76·2); caffeine (p.782·1).
*Pain.*

**Painaid BRF Back Relief Formula** Zee, USA.
Magnesium salicylate (p.55·1); paracetamol (p.76·2).
*Pain.*

**Painaid ESF Extra-Strength Formula** Zee, USA.
Paracetamol (p.76·2); aspirin (p.15·1); caffeine (p.782·1).
*Pain.*

**Painaid PMF Premenstrual Formula** Zee, USA.
Paracetamol (p.76·2); pamabrom (p.978·2).
*Pain.*

**Painamol** Be-Tabs, S.Afr.
Paracetamol (p.76·2).
*Fever; pain.*

**Painamol Plus** Be-Tabs, S.Afr.
Paracetamol (p.76·2); codeine phosphate (p.27·1).
Formerly known as Betacod.
*Fever; pain.*

**Paincod** Crown, S.Afr.
Aspirin (p.15·1); paracetamol (p.76·2); codeine phosphate (p.27·1).
*Fever; pain.*

**Paindol** Polipharm, Thai.
Tramadol hydrochloride (p.94·3).
*Pain.*

**Painex**
Note. This name is used for preparations of different composition.
Confar, Port.
Diclofenac sodium (p.32·1) or diclofenac diethylamine (p.32·1).
*Inflammation; musculoskeletal, joint, peri-articular, and soft-tissue disorders; pain.*

Lagap, UK.
Paracetamol (p.76·2); doxylamine succinate (p.432·3); caffeine (p.782·1); codeine phosphate (p.27·1).
*Pain.*

**Painil** Be-Tabs, S.Afr.
Ibuprofen (p.45·3).
*Fever; pain.*

**Painnox** Charoen, Thai.
Mefenamic acid (p.55·2).
*Inflammation; pain.*

**Painrite** Columbia, S.Afr.†.
Paracetamol (p.76·2); codeine phosphate (p.27·1); caffeine (p.782·1); meprobamate (p.706·2).
*Pain and associated tension.*

**Painrite SA** Columbia, S.Afr.†.
Paracetamol (p.76·2); codeine phosphate (p.27·1).
*Fever; pain.*

**Pains-of** Eagle, Austral.†.
Multivitamin and amino acid preparation (p.1417·1).
*Pain.*

**Painstop** Paedpharm, Austral.
Paracetamol (p.76·2); promethazine hydrochloride (p.439·1); codeine phosphate (p.27·1).
*Pain.*

**Painza** Siam Bheasach, Thai.
Methyl salicylate (p.59·3); menthol (p.1711·3); eugenol (p.1686·2).
*Musculoskeletal pain.*

**Pakinase** Finadiet, Arg.
Metoclopramide (p.1274·3); amylase (p.1654·2); papain (p.1727·3); cellulase (p.1669·1); pancreatin (p.1725·3); dehydrocholic acid (p.1679·2).
*Digestive disorders.*

**Paklitaxfil** Filaxis, Arg.
Paclitaxel (p.577·3).
*Malignant neoplasms.*

**Pakurat** Oriental, Arg.
Ibuprofen (p.45·3).
*Fever; inflammation; pain.*

**Palacos** Schering-Plough, Neth.; Essex, Switz.†.
Methylmethacrylate co-polymer (p.1714·3).
*Bone cement for orthopaedic surgery.*

**Palacos avec Garamycin** Essex, Switz.†.
Methylmethacrylate co-polymer (p.1714·3); gentamicin sulfate (p.217·1).
*Bone cement for orthopaedic surgery.*

**Palacos cum Gentamicin** *Schering-Plough, Denm.†; Schering-Plough, Norw.†; Schering-Plough, Swed.†.*
Polymethylmethacrylate (p.1714·3); gentamicin sulfate (p.217·1).
*Bone cement for orthopaedic surgery.*

**Palacos E** *Schering-Plough, Chile.*
Bone cement.
*Orthopaedic surgery.*

**Palacos E with Garamycin** *Schering-Plough, Austral.*
Methylmethacrylate/methyl acrylate copolymer (p.1714·3); gentamicin sulfate (p.217·1).
*Bone cement for orthopaedic surgery.*

**Palacos with Garamycin** *Schering-Plough, NZ.*
Methylmethacrylate/methylacrylate copolymer (p.1714·3); gentamicin sulfate (p.217·1).
*Bone cement for orthopaedic surgery.*

**Palacos LV avec Gentamicine** *Schering-Plough, Belg.; Schering-Plough, Fr.*
Methylmethacrylate/methacrylate copolymer (p.1714·3); gentamicin sulfate (p.217·1).
*Bone cement for orthopaedic surgery.*

**Palacos LV with Gentamicin** *Schering-Plough, UK.*
Methylmethacrylate/methylacrylate copolymer (p.1714·3); gentamicin sulfate (p.217·1).
*Bone cement for orthopaedic surgery.*

**Palacos met gentamicine** *Schering-Plough, Neth.*
Methylmethacrylate/methylacrylate copolymer (p.1714·3); gentamicin sulfate (p.217·1).
*Bone cement for orthopaedic surgery.*

**Palacos R** *Schering-Plough, Chile; Biomet Merck, Ger.; Schering-Plough, Port.†; Merck, Singapore; Merck, Thai.; Schering-Plough, UK.*
Methylmethacrylate/methylacrylate copolymer (p.1714·3).
*Bone cement for orthopaedic surgery.*

**Palacos R avec Gentamicine** *Schering-Plough, Belg.; Schering-Plough, Fr.*
Methylmethacrylate/methylacrylate copolymer (p.1714·3); gentamicin sulfate (p.217·1).
*Bone cement for orthopaedic surgery.*

**Palacos R com Gentamicina** *Schering-Plough, Port.†.*
Methylmethacrylate/methylacrylate copolymer (p.1714·3); gentamicin sulfate (p.217·1).
*Bone cement.*

**Palacos R con Gentamicina** *Schering-Plough, Chile.*
Methylmethacrylate-methylacrylate copolymer (p.1714·3); gentamicin sulfate (p.217·1).
*Bone cement for orthopaedic surgery.*

**Palacos R cum Gentamicin** *Schering-Plough, Fin.*
Methylmethacrylate/methylacrylate copolymer (p.1714·3); gentamicin sulfate (p.217·1).
*Bone cement for orthopaedic surgery.*

**Palacos R with Garamycin** *Schering-Plough, Austral.; Schering-Plough, S.Afr.*
Methylmethacrylate/methylacrylate copolymer (p.1714·3); gentamicin sulfate (p.217·1).
*Bone cement for orthopaedic surgery.*

**Palacos R with Gentamicin** *Schering-Plough, Irl.†; Schering-Plough, UK.*
Methylmethacrylate/methylacrylate copolymer (p.1714·3); gentamicin sulfate (p.217·1).
*Bone cement for orthopaedic surgery.*

**Palacos-R with Gentamycin** *Schering-Plough, Gr.*
Methylmethacrylate/methylacrylate copolymer (p.1714·3); gentamicin sulfate (p.217·1).
*Bacterial infections.*

**Palacril** *Pfizer Consumer, Ger.*
Diphenhydramine hydrochloride (p.431·3); zinc oxide (p.1163·2).
*Skin disorders.*

**Paladac** *Warner-Lambert, Mex.*
Vitamin preparation (p.1417·1).

**Palafer** *GlaxoSmithKline, Canad.*
Ferrous fumarate (p.1427·3).
*Iron deficiency; iron supplement; iron-deficiency anaemias.*

**Palafer CF** *GlaxoSmithKline, Canad.*
Ferrous fumarate (p.1427·3); folic acid (p.1429·1).
Ascorbic acid (p.1460·2) is included in this preparation to increase the absorption and availability of iron.
*Prenatal supplement.*

**Palamed** *Biomet Merck, Ger.*
Methylmethacrylate/methylacrylate copolymer (p.1714·3).
*Bone cement for orthopaedic surgery.*

**Palamed G** *Biomet Merck, Ger.*
Methylmethacrylate/methylacrylate copolymer (p.1714·3); gentamicin sulfate (p.217·1).
*Bone cement for orthopaedic surgery.*

**Palan** *Lacefa, Arg.*
Vitamin A (p.1451·2); neomycin (p.235·1); chlorophyll (p.1057·1).
*Wounds.*

**Palane** *Cryopharma, Mex.*
Enalapril maleate (p.909·2).
*Heart failure; hypertension.*

**Palaprin** *Roche, Austria†.*
Aloxiprin (p.14·1).
*Pain.*

**Palatol** *Pascoe, Ger.*
Peppermint oil (p.1283·2); niaouli oil (p.1719·3); cajuput oil (p.1664·1); eucalyptus oil (p.1686·2).
*Catarrh.*

**Palatol N** *Pascoe, Ger.†.*
Eucalyptus oil (p.1686·2); peppermint oil (p.1283·2); niaouli oil (p.1719·3); cajuput oil (p.1664·1); hamamelis (p.1696·3).
*Catarrh.*

**Palatrobil** *Monserrat, Arg.*
*Oral drops:* Cynara (p.1678·3); boldo (p.1661·2); wild carrot (p.1765·1); menthol (p.1711·3).
*Tablets:* Dehydrocholic acid (p.1679·2); cynara (p.1678·3).
*Digestive disorders.*

**Palcid** *Pharmadica, Thai.*
Cisapride (p.1259·2).
*Dyspepsia; gastro-oesophageal reflux; gastroparesis.*

**Palcol** *Jofrain, Mex.†.*
Chloramphenicol (p.185·1).
*Bacterial infections.*

**Paldar** *ICN, Arg.*
Mupirocin (p.233·1).
*Bacterial skin infections.*

**Paldesic** *Rosemont, UK.*
Paracetamol (p.76·2).
*Fever; pain.*

**Paleodina** *Liferpal, Mex.*
Dipyrone (p.35·3).
*Pain.*

**Palfium** *Faulding, Austral.†; Janssen-Cilag, Belg.†; Antigen, Irl.; Ace, Neth.; Roche, UK†.*
Dextromoramide tartrate (p.28·2).
*Pain.*

**Palgic DS** *Pan American, USA.*
Carbinoxamine maleate (p.426·3); pseudoephedrine hydrochloride (p.1129·2).
*Rhinitis.*

**Palgic-D** *Pan American, USA.*
Pseudoephedrine hydrochloride (p.1129·2); carbinoxamine maleate (p.426·3).
*Upper respiratory-tract disorders.*

**Paliatil** *Medifarma, Mex.*
Aminophylline (p.780·2); atropine (p.476·3); ephedrine (p.1120·1); phenobarbital (p.367·3).

**Palistop** *Gap, Gr.*
Flutamide (p.556·2).
*Prostatic cancer.*

**Paliuryl** *Richelet, Fr.*
Rhamnus paliurus.
*Stimulation of renal water excretion.*

**Palladon** *Mundipharma, Ger.*
Hydromorphone hydrochloride (p.45·2).
*Pain.*

**Palladone** *Napp, Irl.; Rafa, Israel; Napp, UK; Purdue Frederick, USA.*
Hydromorphone hydrochloride (p.45·2).
*Pain.*

**Pallia** *SmithKline Beecham, Hong Kong†.*
Cimetidine (p.1255·3).
*Gastro-oesophageal reflux; peptic ulcer.*

**Pallidone** *Douglas, NZ.*
Methadone hydrochloride (p.57·2).
*Opioid dependence; pain.*

**Palmer's Cocoa Butter Formula** *Propharm, Malaysia.*
Range of coconut oil (p.1481·1) preparations with vitamin E.
*Dry skin.*

**Palmer's Cocoa Butter Formula Nappy Rash** *Propharm, Malaysia.*
Coconut oil (p.1481·1); panthenol; soft paraffin; vitamin A.
*Nappy rash.*

**Palmer's Cocoa Butter Formula Nursing** *Propharm, Malaysia.*
Coconut oil (p.1481·1); panthenol; soft paraffin.
*Sore and cracked nipples.*

**Palmetto Plus** *Usana, Hong Kong.*
Saw palmetto (p.1569·1); lycopene; soya isoflavones (p.1447·2).
*Nutritional supplement.*

**Palmiclor** *Universales, Mex.†.*
Chloramphenicol (p.185·1).
*Bacterial infections.*

**Palmicol** *Riemser, Ger.*
Heavy magnesium carbonate (p.1272·1).
*Gastrointestinal disorders; magnesium deficiency.*

**Palmiffer** *Reuffer, Mex.†.*
Chloramphenicol (p.185·1).
*Bacterial infections.*

**Palmil** *Cantabria, Spain†.*
Castor oil (p.1668·2).
*Bowel evacuation.*

**Palmisan** *Riemser, Ger.*
Homoeopathic preparation.

**Palmisol** *Parggon, Mex.*
Chloramphenicol (p.185·1).
*Bacterial infections.*

**Palmitan** *Grunenthal, Chile.*
Palmidrol (p.1725·3).
*Respiratory-tract disorders.*

**Palmitate-A** *Akorn, USA.*
Vitamin A (p.1451·2).

**Palon** *Unison, Hong Kong; Unison, Thai.*
Propranolol hydrochloride (p.989·3).
*Angina pectoris; arrhythmias; hypertension; tremor.*

**Palpipax** *Pfizer, Fr.*
Meprobamate (p.706·2); valerian (p.1762·2).
*Nervous disorders.*

**Pals** *Glenwood, USA.*
Chlorophyllin copper complex (p.1057·1).
*Odour control in ostomy and incontinent patients.*

**Paltomiel** *Knop, Chile.*
*Adult syrup:* Eucalyptus (p.1686·1); avocado; aniseed (p.1655·2); honey (p.1434·2).
*Infant syrup:* Eucalyptus (p.1686·1); avocado; honey (p.1434·2).
*Respiratory-tract disorders.*

**Paltomiel Plus** *Knop, Chile.*
Eucalyptus (p.1686·1); avocado; honey (p.1434·2); lobelia (p.1589·1); echinacea (p.1683·2).
*Respiratory-tract disorders.*

**Paludil** *Farmoquimica, Braz.†.*
Quinine (p.460·1); methylthioninium chloride (p.1042·2).
*Babesiosis; leg cramps; malaria.*

**Paludrin** *Zeneca, Israel.*
Proguanil hydrochloride (p.457·1).
*Malaria.*

**Paludrine** *AstraZeneca, Austral.; AstraZeneca, Austria; AstraZeneca, Belg.; Wyeth-Ayerst, Canad.†; AstraZeneca, Denm.; AstraZeneca, Fin.; AstraZeneca, Fr.; AstraZeneca, Ger.; AstraZeneca, Irl.; AstraZeneca, Ital.; AstraZeneca, Malaysia; Zeneca, Neth.; AstraZeneca, Norw.; AstraZeneca, NZ†; AstraZeneca, Port.; AstraZeneca, S.Afr.; AstraZeneca, Singapore†; Astra, Swed.; AstraZeneca, Switz.; AstraZeneca, UK.*
Proguanil hydrochloride (p.457·1).
*Malaria.*

**Paluken** *Kener, Mex.†.*
Chloroquine (p.448·2).

**Palukin** *Kinder, Braz.*
Quinine hydrochloride (p.460·2) or quinine sulfate (p.460·2).
*Malaria.*

**Paluquina** *Quimioterapica, Braz.*
Quinine sulfate (p.460·2).
*Babesiosis; leg cramps; malaria.*

**Paluther** *Aventis, Braz.; Rhone-Poulenc Rorer, Fr.†.*
Artemether (p.447·2).
*Malaria.*

**Palux** *Biolab Sanus, Braz.†.*
Chloroquine hydrochloride (p.448·2) or chloroquine phosphate (p.448·2).
*Hepatic amoebiasis; juvenile arthritis; lupus erythematosus; malaria; rheumatoid arthritis; solar urticaria.*

**Pam** *Abbott, NZ.*
Pralidoxime iodide (p.1050·1).
*Anticholinesterase antagonist; organophosphorus insecticide poisoning.*

**Pamba** *OPW, Ger.*
Aminomethylbenzoic acid (p.742·1).
*Haemorrhage.*

**Pamecil** *Medochemie, Hong Kong.*
Ampicillin sodium (p.157·1).
*Bacterial infections.*

*Medochemie, Malaysia; Medochemie, Singapore†.*
Ampicillin (p.157·1).
*Bacterial infections.*

**Pamedox** *Medochemie, Hong Kong.*
Ampicillin trihydrate (p.157·2); cloxacillin sodium (p.198·2).
*Bacterial infections.*

**Pamelor** *Novartis, Braz.; Novartis, USA.*
Nortriptyline hydrochloride (p.310·2).
*Depression; narcoleptic syndrome; pain; panic disorder.*

**Pamergan** *Cristalia, Braz.*
Promethazine hydrochloride (p.439·1).
*Hypersensitivity reactions; insomnia; nausea and vomiting; pain; premedication; sedative.*

**Pamergan P100** *Martindale Pharmaceuticals, UK.*
Pethidine hydrochloride (p.80·2); promethazine hydrochloride (p.439·1).
NOTE. There is no connection between Martindale, The Complete Drug Reference and Martindale Pharmaceuticals.
*Pain; premedication.*

**Pamid** *CTI, Israel.*
Indapamide (p.938·2).
*Hypertension; oedema.*

**Pamidran** *Faulding, Port.*
Disodium pamidronate (p.773·3).

**Pamine** *Kenwood, USA.*
Hyoscine methobromide (p.483·3).
*Peptic ulcer (adjunct).*

**Pamisol** *Mayne, Austral.*
Disodium pamidronate (p.773·3).
*Hypercalcaemia of malignancy; osteolytic metastases in breast cancer and multiple myeloma; Paget's disease of bone.*

**Pamocil** *Uno, Ital.*
Amoxicillin trihydrate (p.155·3).
*Bacterial infections.*

**Pamol** *Nycomed, Denm.; Nycomed, Norw.; Pfizer, NZ; Docmed, S.Afr.†.*
Paracetamol (p.76·2).
*Fever; pain.*

**Pamoxan** *Uriach, Spain.*
Pyrvinium embonate (p.113·3).
*Worm infections.*

**Pamoxet** *Kampel Martian, Arg.*
Paroxetine (p.311·2).
*Depression.*

**Pampe** *Azevedos, Port.*
Lansoprazole (p.1269·3).
*Gastro-oesophageal reflux; peptic ulcer; Zollinger-Ellison syndrome.*

**Pamprin** *Chattem, Canad.; Chattem, USA.*
Paracetamol (p.76·2); pamabrom (p.978·2); mepyramine maleate (p.437·1).
*Pain; premenstrual syndrome.*

**Pan C** *Freeda, USA.*
Hesperidin (p.1688·2); citrus bioflavonoids complex (p.1688·2); vitamin C (p.1460·2).
*Capillary bleeding.*

**Pan Limpiador AL** *Pierre Fabre Dermo-Cosmetique, Arg.*
Soap substitute.

**Panac** *Bristol-Myers Squibb, Mex.*
Ampicillin (p.157·1); dicloxacillin (p.205·2).
*Bacterial infections.*

**Panac K** *Bristol-Myers Squibb, Mex.*
Ampicillin potassium (p.158·1); dicloxacillin sodium (p.205·2).
*Bacterial infections.*

**Panacef** *Lilly, Ital.*
Cefaclor (p.167·1).
*Bacterial infections.*

**Panacet** *ECR, USA†.*
Hydrocodone tartrate (p.45·1); paracetamol (p.76·2).

**Panacod** *Sanofi Synthelabo, Fin.*
Paracetamol (p.76·2); codeine phosphate (p.27·1).
*Pain.*

**Panacrearell** *Sanorell, Ger.*
Homoeopathic preparation.

**Panadeine**
Note. This name is used for preparations of different composition.
*Sanofi Synthelabo, Austral.; GlaxoSmithKline Consumer, Austral.; Sanofi Synthelabo, Hong Kong; GlaxoSmithKline, Irl.; GlaxoSmithKline, NZ; Sanofi Synthelabo, Singapore†.*
Paracetamol (p.76·2); codeine phosphate (p.27·1).
*Fever; pain.*

*SmithKline Beecham, Belg.†.*
Paracetamol (p.76·2); caffeine (p.782·1); codeine phosphate (p.27·1).
*Fever; pain.*

**Panadeine Plus** *SmithKline Beecham Consumer, Austral.†.*
Paracetamol (p.76·2); codeine phosphate (p.27·1); doxylamine succinate (p.432·3).
*Fever; pain.*

**Panado** *Restan, S.Afr.*
Paracetamol (p.76·2).
*Fever; pain.*

**Panado-Co** *Restan, S.Afr.*
Paracetamol (p.76·2); codeine phosphate (p.27·1).
*Fever; pain.*

**Panadol** *GlaxoSmithKline Consumer, Austral.; GlaxoSmithKline Consumer, Belg.; GlaxoSmithKline Consumer, Canad.; GlaxoSmithKline, Chile; GlaxoSmithKline, Fin.; GlaxoSmithKline Sante, Fr.; SmithKline Beecham, Gr.; GlaxoSmithKline, Hong Kong; GlaxoSmithKline, Irl.; GlaxoSmithKline Consumer, Ital.; GlaxoSmithKline Consumer, Malaysia; SmithKline Beecham, Mex.†; SmithKline Beecham Consumer, Neth.; GlaxoSmithKline, NZ; GlaxoSmithKline Consumer, Port.; GlaxoSmithKline, Singapore; SmithKline Beecham, Spain; SmithKline Beecham Consumer, Switz.; GlaxoSmithKline, Thai.; GlaxoSmithKline Consumer, UK; Glenbrook, USA; Sterling Health, USA.*
Paracetamol (p.76·2).
*Fever; pain.*

**Panadol Allergy Sinus** *GlaxoSmithKline Consumer, Austral.*
Paracetamol (p.76·2); pseudoephedrine hydrochloride (p.1129·2); chlorphenamine maleate (p.427·3).
*Allergic symptoms; pain; sinus congestion.*

**Panadol C** *GlaxoSmithKline Consumer, Malaysia.*
Paracetamol (p.76·2); pseudoephedrine hydrochloride (p.1129·2).
*Cold symptoms; rhinitis; sinus congestion.*

**Panadol CF** *GlaxoSmithKline Consumer, Malaysia.*
Paracetamol (p.76·2); pseudoephedrine hydrochloride (p.1129·2); chlorphenamine maleate (p.427·3).
*Allergic rhinitis; sinus congestion.*

**Panadol Codeine** *GlaxoSmithKline Consumer, Belg.*
Paracetamol (p.76·2); codeine phosphate (p.27·1).
*Pain.*

**Panadol Cold and Flu**
Note. This name is used for preparations of different composition.
*GlaxoSmithKline Consumer, Austral.*
Paracetamol (p.76·2); pseudoephedrine hydrochloride (p.1129·2); dextromethorphan hydrobromide (p.1117·3).
*Cold and influenza symptoms.*

*GlaxoSmithKline, Hong Kong.*
Paracetamol (p.76·2); vitamin C (p.1460·2); phenylephrine hydrochloride (p.1126·3); noscapine (p.1125·3); caffeine (p.782·1); terpin hydrate (p.1131·1).
*Cold and influenza symptoms.*

**Panadol for Cold & Flu** *GlaxoSmithKline, Singapore.*
Dextromethorphan hydrobromide (p.1117·3); pseudoephedrine hydrochloride (p.1129·2); paracetamol (p.76·2).
*Cold and influenza symptoms.*

**Panadol Cold & Flu Hot remedy** *GlaxoSmithKline, Hong Kong.*
Paracetamol (p.76·2); ascorbic acid (p.1460·2); phenylephrine hydrochloride (p.1126·3).
*Cold and influenza symptoms.*

**Panadol for Cold Relief** *GlaxoSmithKline, Singapore.*
Pseudoephedrine hydrochloride (p.1129·2); paracetamol (p.76·2).
*Cold and influenza symptoms.*

**Panadol Comp** *GlaxoSmithKline, Fin.*
Paracetamol (p.76·2); caffeine (p.782·1).
*Fever; pain.*

**Panadol Compuesto** *GlaxoSmithKline, Chile.*
Paracetamol (p.76·2); pseudoephedrine hydrochloride (p.1129·2).
*Cold and influenza symptoms.*

**Panadol Extra**
*GlaxoSmithKline, Hong Kong; GlaxoSmithKline, Irl.; GlaxoSmithKline, Singapore; GlaxoSmithKline Consumer, UK.*
Paracetamol (p.76·2); caffeine (p.782·1).
*Fever; pain.*

**Panadol Hot** *GlaxoSmithKline, Fin.*
Paracetamol (p.76·2); menthol (p.1711·3).
*Cold and influenza symptoms; fever; pain.*

**Panadol Menstrual**
*GlaxoSmithKline Consumer, Malaysia; GlaxoSmithKline, Singapore.*
Paracetamol (p.76·2); pamabrom (p.978·2).
*Menstrual disorders.*

**Panadol Night**
*GlaxoSmithKline Consumer, Austral.†; GlaxoSmithKline, Irl.; GlaxoSmithKline, NZ; GlaxoSmithKline Consumer, UK.*
Paracetamol (p.76·2); diphenhydramine hydrochloride (p.431·3).
*Insomnia; pain.*

**Panadol Plus**
*GlaxoSmithKline, Chile; SmithKline Beecham Consumer, Neth.*
Paracetamol (p.76·2); caffeine (p.782·1).
*Fever; pain.*

**Panadol Sinus** *GlaxoSmithKline Consumer, Austral.*
Paracetamol (p.76·2); pseudoephedrine hydrochloride (p.1129·2).
*Pain; sinus congestion.*

**Panadol Sinus Day/Night** *GlaxoSmithKline Consumer, Austral.*
Day caplets, paracetamol (p.76·2); pseudoephedrine hydrochloride (p.1129·2); night caplets, paracetamol; pseudoephedrine hydrochloride; chlorphenamine maleate (p.427·3).
*Cold symptoms; fever.*

**Panadol Ultra** *GlaxoSmithKline Consumer, UK.*
Paracetamol (p.76·2); codeine phosphate (p.27·1).
These ingredients can be described by the British Approved Name Co-codamol.
*Fever; pain.*

**Panadol-C** *SmithKline Beecham Consumer, Switz.*
Paracetamol (p.76·2); ascorbic acid (p.1460·2).
*Cold symptoms.*

**Panafcort**
*Aspen, Austral.; Propan, S.Afr.*
Prednisone (p.1109·3).
*Corticosteroid.*

**Panafcortelone**
*Aspen, Austral.; Aspen, Hong Kong.*
Prednisolone (p.1108·1).
*Corticosteroid.*

**Panafen** *GlaxoSmithKline, NZ.*
Ibuprofen (p.45·3).
*Musculoskeletal and joint disorders; pain.*

**Panafil** *Healthpoint, USA.*
Papain (p.1727·3); urea (p.1162·2); chlorophyllin copper complex sodium (p.1057·1).
*Burns; ulcers; wounds.*

**Panafil-White** *Rystan, USA.*
Papain (p.1727·3); urea (p.1162·2).
*Burns; ulcers; wounds.*

**Panaflu** *Malaysia Chemist, Singapore†.*
Chlorphenamine maleate (p.427·3); paracetamol (p.76·2); phenylpropanolamine hydrochloride (p.1127·3).
*Cold and influenza symptoms.*

**Panaflu Plus** *Malaysia Chemist, Singapore.*
Chlorphenamine maleate (p.427·3); paracetamol (p.76·2); pseudoephedrine hydrochloride (p.1129·2).
Formerly contained chlorphenamine maleate, paracetamol, phenylpropanolamine hydrochloride, and caffeine.
*Cold and influenza symptoms.*

**Panagesic** *Chemopharma, Chile.*
Paracetamol (p.76·2).
*Fever; pain.*

**Panagesic Con Cafeina** *Chemopharma, Chile.*
Paracetamol (p.76·2); caffeine (p.782·1).
*Pain.*

**Panalba** *Help, Gr.*
Famotidine (p.1265·2).
*Conditions where gastric acid reduction is beneficial; gastric hypersecretion including Zollinger-Ellison syndrome; peptic ulcer.*

**Panaleve** *Pinewood, UK.*
Paracetamol (p.76·2).
*Fever; pain.*

**Panalgesic** *Sanofi Synthelabo, Austral.*
Paracetamol (p.76·2); codeine phosphate (p.27·1); doxylamine succinate (p.432·3).
*Pain with tension.*

**Panalgesic Gold** *ECR, USA.*
*Cream:* Methyl salicylate (p.59·3); menthol (p.1711·3).
*Liniment:* Methyl salicylate (p.59·3); menthol (p.1711·3); camphor (p.1665·3).
*Muscle, joint, and soft-tissue pain; neuralgia.*

**Panaline** *Darier, Mex.*
Maize starch (p.1449·1).
*Napkin rash.*

**Panamax** *Sanofi Synthelabo, Austral.*
Paracetamol (p.76·2).
*Fever; pain.*

**Panamax Co** *Sanofi Synthelabo, Austral.*
Paracetamol (p.76·2); codeine phosphate (p.27·1).
*Fever; pain.*

**Panamic** *TO-Chemicals, Thai.*
Mefenamic acid (p.55·2).
*Pain.*

**Pan-Amin** *Thai Otsuka, Thai.*
Amino-acid infusion (p.1417·1).
*Parenteral nutrition.*

**Panamor** *Aspen, S.Afr.*
Diclofenac sodium (p.32·1).
*Gout; inflammation; musculoskeletal and joint disorders; pain.*

**Panasal** *ECR, USA†.*
Hydrocodone tartrate (p.45·1); aspirin (p.15·1).

**Panasol-S** *Seatrace, USA.*
Prednisone (p.1109·3).
*Corticosteroid.*

**Panasorbe** *Sanofi Synthelabo, Port.*
Paracetamol (p.76·2).
*Fever; pain.*

**Panataxel** *Gautier, Arg.*
Paclitaxel (p.577·3).
*Malignant neoplasms.*

**Panax** *Willvonseder, Austria†.*
Paracetamol (p.76·2); butetamate citrate (p.1116·2); caffeine (p.782·1).
*Fever; pain.*

**Panax Complex** *Blackmores, Austral.†.*
Avena (p.1658·2); fenugreek (p.1688·1); alfalfa (p.1649·1); ginseng (p.1693·1); multivitamins (p.1417·1).
*Tonic.*

**Panax N** *Medichemie, Switz.†.*
Ibuprofen (p.45·3).
*Fever; pain.*

**Panaxid** *Norgine, Belg.*
Nizatidine (p.1277·2).
*Gastrointestinal disorders associated with hyperacidity.*

**Panbesy**
*Eurodrug, Hong Kong; Eurodrug, Singapore; Eurodrug, Thai.*
Phentermine hydrochloride (p.1592·2).
*Obesity.*

**Pancardiol** *Almirall, Spain†.*
Isosorbide mononitrate (p.942·1).
*Angina pectoris; heart failure.*

**Pancebrin**
*Lilly, Hong Kong†; Aspen, S.Afr.; Lilly, Thai.*
Multivitamin preparation (p.1417·1).

**Pancenz** *Nutrition Care, Austral.†.*
Pancreatin (p.1725·3).
*Pancreatic insufficiency.*

**Panchelidon N** *Kanoldt, Ger.†.*
Greater celandine (p.1695·3).
*Smooth muscle spasms.*

**Pancholtruw N** *Truw, Ger.†.*
Pancreatin (p.1725·3).
Pancholtruw formerly contained pancreatin, bromelains, dehydrocholic acid, chelidonium, and silybum marianum.
*Digestive system disorders.*

**Pancillin** *Durascan, Denm.*
Phenoxymethylpenicillin potassium (p.242·1).
*Bacterial infections.*

**Panclasa** *Atlantis, Mex.*
Phloroglucinol (p.1731·1); trimethylphloroglucinol (p.1731·1).
*Smooth muscle spasm.*

**Panclor** *Elpen (Ελπεν), Gr.*
Cefaclor (p.167·1).
*Bacterial infections.*

**Pancof** *Pan American, USA.*
Dihydrocodeine tartrate (p.34·3); chlorphenamine maleate (p.427·3); pseudoephedrine hydrochloride (p.1129·2).
*Upper respiratory-tract disorders.*

**Pancof PD** *Pan American, USA.*
Dihydrocodeine tartrate (p.34·3); chlorphenamine maleate (p.427·3); phenylephrine hydrochloride (p.1126·3).
*Upper respiratory-tract disorders.*

**Pancof XP** *Pan American, USA.*
Hydrocodone tartrate (p.45·1); guaifenesin (p.1122·1); pseudoephedrine hydrochloride (p.1129·2).
*Coughs.*

**Pancof-EXP** *Pan American, USA.*
Dihydrocodeine tartrate (p.34·3); guaifenesin (p.1122·1); pseudoephedrine (p.1129·2).
*Coughs.*

**Pancof-HC** *Pan American, USA.*
Hydrocodone tartrate (p.45·1); chlorphenamine maleate (p.427·3); pseudoephedrine hydrochloride (p.1129·2).
*Coughs.*

**Pancof-XL** *Pan American, USA.*
Hydrocodone tartrate (p.45·1); guaifenesin (p.1122·1); pseudoephedrine hydrochloride (p.1129·2).
*Coughs.*

**Panconium** *Khandelwal, India.*
Pancuronium bromide (p.1404·3).
*Competitive neuromuscular blocker.*

**Pancoran** *Novartis, Gr.*
Glyceryl trinitrate (p.923·2).
*Angina; heart failure.*

**Pancreal Kirchner** *Gerda, Fr.†.*
Pancreatin (porcine) (p.1725·3).
*Dyspepsia.*

**Pancrease**
*Janssen-Cilag, Austral.; Janssen-Cilag, Belg.; Janssen-Cilag, Braz.; Janssen-Ortho, Canad.; Janssen-Cilag, Denm.; Janssen-Cilag, Fin.; Vianex (Βιανεξ), Gr.; Janssen-Cilag, Irl.; McNeil, Israel; Janssen-Cilag, Ital.; Cilag, Mex.; Janssen-Cilag, Neth.; Janssen-Cilag, Norw.; Janssen-Cilag, NZ; Janssen-Cilag, Spain; Janssen-Cilag, Swed.; Janssen-Cilag, UK; Ortho McNeil, USA.*
Pancreatic enzymes (p.1725·3).
*Pancreatic insufficiency.*

**Pancrease HL**
*Janssen-Cilag, Neth.; Janssen-Cilag, UK.*
Pancreatin (p.1725·3).
*Pancreatic insufficiency.*

**Pancrecura** *Abbott, Arg.*
Pancreatin (p.1725·3).
*Pancreatin insufficiency.*

**Pancrelase** *DB, Fr.†.*
Pancreatin (porcine) (p.1725·3); fungal cellulase (p.1669·1).
*Dyspepsia; pancreatic insufficiency.*

**Pancreoflat** *Solvay, Ital.*
Pancreatin (p.1725·3); dimeticone (p.1289·2).
*Digestive-system disorders.*

**Pancreolauryl** *Inibsa, Spain.*
Fluorescein dilaurate (p.1689·1); fluorescein sodium (p.1689·1).
*Evaluation of pancreatic function.*

**Pancreolauryl-Test**
*Note. This name is used for preparations of different composition.*
*Sanova, Austria; Pfizer Consumer, UK†.*
Blue capsules, fluorescein dilaurate (p.1689·1); red capsules, fluorescein sodium (p.1689·1).
*Evaluation of pancreatic function.*

*Geymonat, Ital.†.*
Fluorescein dilaurate (p.1689·1).
*Evaluation of pancreatic function.*

**Pancreolauryl-Test N** *Temmler, Ger.*
Blue capsules, fluorescein dilaurate (p.1689·1); red capsules, fluorescein sodium (p.1689·1).
*Evaluation of pancreatic function.*

**Pancreon** *Solvay, Ital.†.*
Pancreatin (p.1725·3).
*Cystic fibrosis; malabsorption syndromes.*

**Pancreon Compositum** *Solvay, Ital.†.*
Pancreatin (p.1725·3); ox bile extract (p.1660·3).
*Digestive system disorders.*

**Pancresil** *Edmond Pharma, Ital.*
Dimeticone (p.1289·2); pancreatin (p.1725·3).
*Digestive-system disorders.*

**Pancrex**
*Paines & Byrne, Irl.; LPB, Ital.; Paines & Byrne, NZ; Paines & Byrne, UK.*
Pancreatin (p.1725·3).
*Pancreatic insufficiency.*

**Pancrezyme 4X** *Vitaline, USA†.*
Pancreatin (p.1725·3); pancrelipase (p.1725·3).
*Pancreatic insufficiency.*

**Pancrin**
*Solvay, Austria; Solvay, Ital.†.*
Pancreatin (p.1725·3).
*Pancreatic insufficiency.*

**Pancrit** *Andromaco, Chile.*
Cetylpyridinium chloride (p.1173·1); allantoin (p.1141·3).
*Mouth and throat disorders.*

**Pancrotanon** *Geymonat, Ital.†.*
Pancreatin (p.1725·3).
*Digestive system disorders.*

**Pancuron**
*Scott-Cassara, Arg.; Cristalia, Braz.†.*
Pancuronium bromide (p.1404·3).
*Competitive neuromuscular blocker.*

**Pancurox** *Faulding, Port.*
Pancuronium bromide (p.1404·3).
*Competitive neuromuscular blocker.*

**Pancutan** *Purissimus, Arg.*
Halibut oil (p.1434·1); gentamicin embonate (p.219·1).
*Burns; skin infections; ulcers; wounds.*

**Pancutan Base** *Purissimus, Arg.*
Halibut oil (p.1434·1).
*Skin disorders.*

**Panda Baby Cream** *Thornton & Ross, UK†.*
Zinc oxide (p.1163·2); castor oil (p.1668·2).
*Dry skin; nappy rash.*

**Pandel**
*Silesia, Chile; Galderma, Ger.; Medinfar, Port.; CollaGenex, USA.*
Hydrocortisone buteprate (p.1104·1).
*Skin disorders.*

**Panderm** *Julphar, UAE.*
Nystatin (p.406·3); neomycin sulfate (p.235·1); gramicidin (p.220·2); triamcinolone acetonide (p.1110·2).
*Infected skin disorders.*

**Pandermil** *Edol, Port.*
Hydrocortisone (p.1103·3).
*Skin disorders.*

**Pandigal** *Zekides, Gr.*
Butamirate citrate (p.1116·2).
*Cough.*

**Panectyl** *Aventis, Canad.*
Alimemazine tartrate (p.423·3).
*Coughs; dyspnoea; pruritus.*

**Pan-Emecort** *Merck, Braz.*
Fluprednidene acetate (p.1102·2); gentamicin sulfate (p.217·1); hydroxyquinoline (p.1700·1).
*Skin disorders.*

**Pan-Enteral** *Thai Otsuka, Thai.*
Preparation for enteral nutrition (p.1417·1).

**Panfil G** *Pan American, USA.*
Diprophylline (p.784·3); guaifenesin (p.1122·1).
*Obstructive airways disease.*

**Panflavin** *Chinosolfabrik, Ger.†.*
Acriflavinium chloride (p.1165·3).
*Infections of the oropharynx.*

**Panflogin** *Farmion, Braz.†.*
Benzydamine hydrochloride (p.21·1).
*Fever; inflammation; pain.*

**Panfugan** *Altana, Braz.*
Mebendazole (p.108·2).
*Worm infections.*

**Pan-Fungex** *Irex, Port.*
Clotrimazole (p.396·2).
*Fungal vaginal infections; trichomoniasis.*

**Panfungol** *Esteve, Spain.*
Ketoconazole (p.403·3).
*Fungal infections.*

**Panfurex** *Bouchara-Recordati, Fr.*
Nifuroxazide (p.237·2).
*Diarrhoea.*

**Pangamox** *Sanofi Synthelabo, Spain†.*
Amoxicillin trihydrate (p.155·3); potassium clavulanate (p.193·3).
*Bacterial infections.*

**Pangastren** *Laboratorios Chile, Chile.*
Metoclopramide (p.1274·3); simeticone (p.1289·2).
*Dyspepsia; flatulence; gastro-oesophageal reflux.*

**Pangavit Hypak** *Carter-Wallace, Mex.*
Cyanocobalamin (p.1458·2); thiamine hydrochloride (p.1455·1); pyridoxine hydrochloride (p.1456·3).
*Neuralgias; neuritis; neuropathy; vitamin B deficiency.*

**Pangavit Pediatrico** *Carter-Wallace, Mex.*
Cyproheptadine hydrochloride (p.430·1); cyanocobalamin (p.1458·2); thiamine hydrochloride (p.1455·1); pyridoxine hydrochloride (p.1456·3); riboflavin sodium phosphate (p.1456·1).
*Appetite loss; megaloblastic anaemia; vitamin deficiency.*

**Pangel** *Pannoc, Belg.*
Benzoyl peroxide (p.1143·2).
*Acne.*

**Pangen**
*Urgo, Fr.; Urgo, Ger.*
Collagen (p.1674·3).
*Haemorrhagic disorders.*

**Pangest**
*Note. This name is used for preparations of different composition.*
*Beta, Arg.*
Pantoprazole sodium (p.1283·1).
*Gastritis; gastro-oesophageal reflux; peptic ulcer; Zollinger-Ellison syndrome.*

*Farmasa, Braz.*
Bromopride (p.1254·1).
*Gastro-oesophageal reflux; gastroparesis.*

**Panglobulin** *American Red Cross, USA.*
A normal immunoglobulin (p.1627·2).

**Pangon** *LBS, Thai.*
Pentazocine hydrochloride (p.79·3) or pentazocine lactate (p.79·3).
*Pain.*

**Pangrol** *Berlin-Chemie, Ger.*
Pancreatin (p.1725·3).
*Pancreatic insufficiency.*

**Panhematin**
*Abbott, Austral.†; Abbott, USA.*
Haematin (p.1040·3).
*Porphyria.*

**Panimun Bioral** *Panacea, India.*
Ciclosporin (p.1351·2).
*Graft-versus-host disease; psoriasis; rheumatoid arthritis; transplant rejection.*

**Panimycin** *Meiji, Jpn.*
Dibekacin sulfate (p.205·2).
*Bacterial infections.*

**Paniodal** *Adivar, Ital.*
Povidone-iodine (p.1190·3).
*Skin and wound disinfection.*

**Paniodine** *Angelini, Ital.*
Povidone-iodine (p.1190·3).
*Skin and wound disinfection.*

**Panitol**
*Note. This name is used for preparations of different composition.*
*Cryopharma, Mex.*
Propanidid (p.1305·3).
*General anaesthesia.*

*Pharmaland, Thai.*
Carbamazepine (p.353·3).
*Epilepsy; trigeminal neuralgia.*

**Panitone** Wesley, USA.
Paracetamol (p.76·2).
*Fever; pain.*

**Panix** Research Labs, S.Afr.†.
Alprazolam (p.668·3).
*Anxiety disorders; mixed anxiety depressive states; panic attacks.*

**Pankreaden** Knoll, Ital.†.
Pancrelipase (p.1725·3).
*Pancreatic insufficiency.*

**Pankreaplex Neu** Schaper & Brummer, Ger.
Silybum marianum (p.1043·3); syzygium jambolana; condurango (p.1675·3); sarsaparilla (p.1742·1).
*Gastrointestinal disorders.*

**Pankreas M Comp** Hanosan, Ger.
Homoeopathic preparation.

**Pankreas S Comp** Hanosan, Ger.
Homoeopathic preparation.

**Pankrease** Janssen-Cilag, S.Afr.
Pancrelipase (p.1725·3).
*Pancreatic disorders.*

**Pankreatan** Novartis Consumer, Ger.
Pancreatin (p.1725·3).
*Digestive system disorders.*

**Pankreaticum** Hevert, Ger.
Homoeopathic preparation.

**Pankreaticum N** Hevert, Ger.
Homoeopathic preparation.

**Pankreoflat**
Raffo, Arg.; Solvay, Austria; Sintofarma, Braz.; Solvay, Ger.; Solvay, Hong Kong; Solvay, India; Solvay, Israel; Byk Gulden, Mex.; Solvay, Port.; Solvay, S.Afr.; Solvay, Spain.
Pancreatin (p.1725·3); simeticone (p.1289·2).
*Excess gastrointestinal gas; pancreatic insufficiency; preparation for gastrointestinal examinations.*

**Pankreoflat Sedante** Raffo, Arg.
Oxazepam (p.712·2); pancreatin (p.1725·3); simeticone (p.1289·2).
*Digestive disorders.*

**Pankreon**
Byk, Braz.†; Solvay, Denm.; Solvay, Fin.; Solvay, Ger.; Solvay, Norw.; Solvay, Spain†; Solvay, Swed.
Pancreatin (p.1725·3).
*Cystic fibrosis; malabsorption; pancreatic insufficiency.*

**Pankreon compositum** Solvay, Austria†.
Pancreatin (p.1725·3); ox bile (p.1660·3).
*Digestive system disorders; pancreatic insufficiency.*

**Pankreon Compuesto** Raffo, Arg.
Pancreatin (p.1725·3); dehydrocholic acid (p.1679·2); deoxycholic acid (p.1660·3) vitamin B substances (p.1417·1).
*Digestive disorders; liver disorders.*

**Pankreon forte** Solvay, Austria.
Pancreatin (p.1725·3).
*Digestive system disorders; pancreatic insufficiency.*

**Pankreon Total** Raffo, Arg.
Pancreatin (p.1725·3); papain (p.1727·3); cellulase (p.1669·1); dehydrocholic acid (p.1679·2); simeticone (p.1289·2); metoclopramide hydrochloride (p.1274·3).
*Digestive disorders.*

**Pankreozym** Raffo, Arg.
Pancreatin (p.1725·3).
*Digestive disorders.*

**Pankrevowen** Weber & Weber, Ger.
Homoeopathic preparation.

**Panlem** Lemery, Mex.
Pancuronium bromide (p.1404·3).
*Competitive neuromuscular blocker.*

**Panlor DC** Pan American, USA.
Paracetamol (p.76·2); caffeine (p.782·1); dihydrocodeine tartrate (p.34·3).
*Pain.*

**Panmicol** Purissimus, Arg.
Clotrimazole (p.396·2).
*Fungal skin, mucous membrane, and nail infections.*

**Panmist JR** Pan American, USA.
Pseudoephedrine hydrochloride (p.1129·2); guaifenesin (p.1122·1).
*Coughs.*

**Panmist LA** Pan American, USA.
Pseudoephedrine hydrochloride (p.1129·2); guaifenesin (p.1122·1).
*Upper respiratory-tract disorders.*

**PanMist-DM** Pan American, USA.
Pseudoephedrine hydrochloride (p.1129·2); dextromethorphan hydrobromide (p.1117·3); guaifenesin (p.1122·1).
*Coughs.*

**Panmist-S** Pan American, USA.
Pseudoephedrine hydrochloride (p.1129·2); guaifenesin (p.1122·1).
*Upper respiratory-tract disorders.*

**Panmycin**
Pharmacia Upjohn, NZ†; Upjohn, USA†.
Tetracycline hydrochloride (p.266·2).
*Bacterial infections.*

**Pannaz** Pan American, USA.
Pseudoephedrine hydrochloride (p.1129·2); chlorphenamine maleate (p.427·3); hyoscine methonitrate (p.483·3).
Formerly contained phenylpropanolamine, chlorphenamine, and hyoscine.
*Upper respiratory-tract disorders.*

**Pannocort** Pannoc, Belg.
Hydrocortisone acetate (p.1103·3).
*Skin disorders.*

**Pannogel** CS, Fr.
Benzoyl peroxide (p.1143·2).
*Acne.*

**Panocaine** Hoechst Marion Roussel, Canad.†.
Benzocaine (p.1370·3); tetracaine hydrochloride (p.1385·1).
*Local anaesthesia in dentistry.*

**Panocod** Sanofi Synthelabo, Swed.
Paracetamol (p.76·2); codeine phosphate (p.27·1).
*Pain.*

**Panodil**
SmithKline Beecham, Denm.; GlaxoSmithKline, Norw.; GlaxoSmithKline Consumer, Swed.
Paracetamol (p.76·2).
*Fever; pain.*

**Panolase** Unichem, India.
Pancreatin (p.1725·3); hemicellulase (p.1669·1); ox bile (p.1660·3).
*Digestive disorders.*

**Pan-Ophtal** Winzer, Ger.
Dexpanthenol (p.1727·2).
*Eye disorders.*

**Panoptic** Biocumed, Arg.
Naphazoline hydrochloride (p.1124·3); diphenhydramine hydrochloride (p.431·3).
*Eye disorders.*

**Panoral** Lilly, Ger.
Cefaclor (p.167·1).
*Bacterial infections.*

**Panorex** Glaxo Wellcome, Ger.†.
Edrecolomab (p.550·2).
*Colorectal cancer.*

**Panos** Fornet, Fr.
Tetrazepam (p.724·1).
*Skeletal muscle spasm.*

**Panotil** Zambon, Braz.
Polymyxin B sulfate (p.245·1); neomycin sulfate (p.235·1); fludrocortisone acetate (p.1100·1); lidocaine hydrochloride (p.1377·3).
Formerly contained polymyxin B sulfate, neomycin sulfate, fludrocortisone acetate, lidocaine hydrochloride, and nitrofurazone.
*Ear disorders.*

**Panotile**
Note. This name is used for preparations of different composition.
Zambon, Belg.; Zambon, Fr.; Zambon, Neth.; Inpharzam, Switz.
Polymyxin B sulfate (p.245·1); neomycin sulfate (p.235·1); fludrocortisone acetate (p.1100·1); lidocaine hydrochloride (p.1377·3).
*Ear disorders.*

Zambon, Spain.
Polymyxin B sulfate (p.245·1); neomycin sulfate (p.235·1); fludrocortisone acetate (p.1100·1); furaltadone hydrochloride (p.215·2); lidocaine hydrochloride (p.1377·3).
*Ear disorders.*

**Panotile N** Zambon, Ger.
Polymyxin B sulfate (p.245·1); fludrocortisone acetate (p.1100·1); lidocaine hydrochloride (p.1377·3).
*Ear disorders.*

**Panotos** Armstrong, Arg.
Dextromethorphan hydrobromide (p.1117·3); bromhexine hydrochloride (p.1115·3); phenylephrine hydrochloride (p.1126·3); chlorphenamine maleate (p.427·3); paracetamol (p.76·2).
*Respiratory-tract disorders.*

**Panotos NF** Armstrong, Arg.
Bromhexine hydrochloride (p.1115·3); chlorphenamine maleate (p.427·3); paracetamol (p.76·2); pseudoephedrine sulfate (p.1129·2).
*Respiratory-tract disorders.*

**Panoxi** Biocumed, Arg.
Oxymetazoline hydrochloride (p.1126·1); vitamin A palmitate (p.1453·1); sodium hyaluronate (p.1697·3).
*Eye disorders.*

**PanOxyl**
Stiefel, Austral.; Sanova, Austria; Stiefel, Braz.; Stiefel, Canad.; Stiefel, Fin.†; Stiefel, Fr.; Stiefel, Ger.; Stiefel, Hong Kong; Stiefel, Irl.; Stiefel, Israel; Stiefel, Ital.; Stiefel, Malaysia; Stiefel, Mex.†; Stiefel, Norw.; Stiefel, NZ; Stiefel, Port.; Stiefel, S.Afr.; Stiefel, Singapore; Stiefel, Spain; Stiefel, Switz.; Stiefel, Thai.; Stiefel, UK; Stiefel, USA.
Benzoyl peroxide (p.1143·2).
*Acne.*

**PanOxyl Clear Acne** Stiefel, Canad.
Salicylic acid (p.1157·1); triclosan (p.1195·2).
*Acne.*

**Panpeptal N** Philopharm, Ger.
Pancreatin (p.1725·3).
*Pancreatic insufficiency.*

**Panpur** Abbott, Ger.
Porcine pancreatin (p.1725·3).
*Pancreatic insufficiency.*

**Panpurol**
Bioprogress, Ital.†; Shinyaku, Jpn; Shinyaku, Thai.†.
Pipethanate ethobromide (p.487·3).
Benzyl alcohol (p.1170·2) may be included in the injection to alleviate the pain of injection.
*Premedication for endoscopy and radiology; smooth muscle spasm.*

**Panquil** Warner-Lambert, Austral.
Promethazine hydrochloride (p.439·1); paracetamol (p.76·2).
*Fever; pain.*

**Panretin**
Ligand, Canad.†; Elan, Fr.; Ligand, USA.
Alitretinoin (p.526·2).
*Kaposi's sarcoma.*

**Pansan** Solvay, Austria†.
Stomach enzymes (p.1729·3); glutamic acid hydrochloride (p.1433·2).
*Gastrointestinal disorders.*

**Panscol** Baker Cummins, USA.
Salicylic acid (p.1157·1).
*Hyperkeratosis.*

**Pansebase** Sofex, Port.
Lecithin (p.1706·1); lactic acid (p.1704·1).
*Seborrhoeic dermatitis.*

**Pansebase Composto** Sofex, Port.
Lecithin (p.1706·1); lactic acid (p.1704·1); ichthammol (p.1148·2).
*Pruritus; psoriasis; seborrhoeic dermatitis.*

**Pansebase Solido** Sofex, Port.
Lecithin (p.1706·1).
*Seborrhoea; soap substitute.*

**Pansements Coricides** Seton Scholl, Fr.
Salicylic acid (p.1157·1).
*Corns.*

**Panseptil** Gedis, Ital.
Chlorhexidine gluconate (p.1173·2); cetrimide (p.1172·1); alcohol (p.1166·1); isopropyl alcohol (p.1184·3).
*Surface disinfection.*

**Pansoral**
Sidus, Arg.; Pierre Fabre Sante, Fr.; Pierre Fabre, Switz.†.
Choline salicylate (p.26·2); cetalkonium chloride (p.1172·1).
*Mouth disorders.*

**Pansporin** Takeda, Jpn.
Cefotiam hydrochloride (p.177·2) or cefotiam hexetil hydrochloride (p.177·2).
Mepivacaine hydrochloride (p.1381·2) is included in the intramuscular injection to alleviate the pain of injection.
*Bacterial infections.*

**Pansteryl** Sanofi Winthrop, Belg.†.
Benzalkonium chloride (p.1168·3).
*Disinfection of instruments, materials, and hands; storage of sterile materials.*

**Pan-Streptomycin** IFET (ΙΦΕΤ), Gr.
Streptomycin (p.256·1).
*Bacterial endocarditis; brucellosis; tuberculosis.*

**Pansulfox** Stiefel, Chile.
Benzoyl peroxide (p.1143·2).
*Acne.*

**Pan-Sun** Chauvin, Fr.
Dexpanthenol (p.1727·2).
*Sunburn.*

**Pantacid** Pantafarm, Ital.
Cefonicid sodium (p.174·2).
Lidocaine hydrochloride (p.1377·3) is included in this preparation to alleviate the pain of injection.
*Gram-negative bacterial infections.*

**Pantaflux** Pantafarm, Ital.
Flucloxacillin sodium (p.213·3).
*Bacterial infections.*

**Pantasol** Pantafarm, Ital.
Flunisolide (p.1101·1).
*Asthma; bronchitis; rhinitis.*

**Pantec** Cifarma, Braz.†.
Fluconazole (p.398·1).
*Fungal infections.*

**Pantecta**
Abbott, Ital.; Pharmacia, Spain.
Pantoprazole sodium (p.1283·1).
*Gastro-oesophageal reflux; peptic ulcer.*

**Pantederm** Hexal, Ger.
Zinc oxide (p.1163·2); dexpanthenol (p.1727·2).
*Burns; wounds.*

**Pantelmin**
Janssen-Cilag, Austria; Janssen-Cilag, Braz.; Janssen-Cilag, Port.
Mebendazole (p.108·2).
*Worm infections.*

**Pantenil** Quimica Medica, Spain.
Calcium pantothenate (p.1442·3); mercuric chloride (p.1712·3); aminobenzoic acid (p.1142·2).
*Hair, scalp, and skin disorders.*

**Panteston**
Organon, Fin.; Organon, NZ.
Testosterone undecylate (p.1570·1).
*Male hypogonadism; male infertility; osteoporosis in men; testosterone deficiency in men.*

**Pantestone**
Note. This name is used for preparations of different composition.
Filaxis, Arg.
Anastrozole (p.528·1).
*Malignant neoplasms.*

Organon, Fr.
Testosterone undecylate (p.1570·1).
*Male hypogonadism.*

**Pantetina** Sanofi Synthelabo, Ital.
Pantethine (p.978·3).
*Hypertriglyceridaemia.*

**Pantevit** EMS, Braz.
Pantothenic acid (p.1442·3); vitamin $B_6$ (p.1457·2); resorcinol (p.1156·3).
*Psoriasis.*

**Panthenol** Jenapharm, Ger.; Alcon, Ger.; Braun, Ger.; Ratiopharm, Ger.; Riemser, Ger.; Lichtenstein, Ger.; Chauvin ankerpharm, Ger.; CT, Ger.
Dexpanthenol (p.1727·2).
*Eye disorders; inflammatory disorders of the gastrointestinal tract; pantothenic acid deficiency; paraesthesias; paralytic ileus; postoperative gastrointestinal atony; wounds.*

**Panthisone** Rekah, Israel.
Panthenol (p.1727·2); hydrocortisone acetate (p.1103·3).
*Anorectal disorders; skin disorders; wounds.*

**Panthoderm** Jones, USA.
Dexpanthenol (p.1727·2).
*Skin disorders.*

**Panthoderm-A** Aventis Pasteur, Chile.
Vitamin a palmitate (p.1453·1); panthenol (p.1727·2).
*Skin disorders.*

**Panthogenat** Azupharma, Ger.
Dexpanthenol (p.1727·2).
*Wounds.*

**Pantiban** Alpes Chemie, Chile.
*Capsules:* Vitamins; minerals; rutoside; ginseng; procaine hydrochloride (p.1383·2) (p.1417·1).
*Syrup:* Amino acids; vitamins; minerals (p.1417·1).
*Dietary supplement.*

**Pantinol** Gerot, Austria.
Aprotinin (p.742·3).
*Hyperfibrinolytic haemorrhage.*

**Panto** Byk, Canad.
Pantoprazole sodium (p.1283·1).
*Gastrointestinal hyperacidity.*

**Panto Liquid** Nycomed, Austria.
Panthenol (p.1727·2); phenylmercuric borate (p.1189·2).
*Liver disorders; neuropathies; skin disorders; sweating; upper respiratory-tract inflammation.*

**Pantobamin** Medix, Spain.
Cyproheptadine (p.430·2); amino acids and vitamins (p.1417·1).
*Anorexia; tonic.*

**Pantobionta** Merck, Spain†.
Multivitamin and mineral preparation (p.1417·1).

**Pantobron** Abbott, Mex.
Erythromycin (p.208·1) or erythromycin ethyl succinate (p.208·1); bromhexine hydrochloride (p.1115·3).
*Respiratory-tract infections.*

**Pantoc** Byk, Port.
Pantoprazole sodium (p.1283·1).
*Gastro-oesophageal reflux; peptic ulcer.*

**Pantocal** Eurofarma, Braz.
Pantoprazole sodium (p.1283·1).
*Peptic ulcer.*

**Pantocarm** Byk Elmu, Spain.
Pantoprazole sodium (p.1283·1).
*Gastro-oesophageal reflux; peptic ulcer.*

**Pantocrinale** Simons, Ger.†.
Hydrocortisone sodium phosphate (p.1104·1); salicylic acid (p.1157·1).
*Scalp disorders.*

**Pantocycline** Chew, Thai.
Tetracycline hydrochloride (p.266·2).
*Bacterial infections.*

**Pantodac** Zydus, India.
Pantoprazole sodium (p.1283·1).
*Gastro-oesophageal reflux; peptic ulcer; Zollinger-Ellison syndrome.*

**Pantodrin** Abbott, Spain.
Erythromycin (p.208·1).
*Acne.*

**Pantogar**
Medra, Austria.
Calcium pantothenate; cystine (p.1417·1).
*Hair and nail disorders.*

Merz, Hong Kong; Cimex, Singapore†; Adroka, Switz.
Vitamins; medicinal yeast; keratin; aminobenzoic acid; cystine (p.1417·1).
*Hair and nail disorders.*

**Pantok** Lacer, Spain.
Simvastatin (p.997·1).
*Hypercholesterolaemia; ischaemic heart disease.*

**Pantolax** Curamed, Ger.
Suxamethonium chloride (p.1406·2).
*Depolarising neuromuscular blocker.*

**Pantoloc**
Byk, Austria; Solvay, Canad.; Byk, Canad.; Byk Gulden, Denm.; Altana, Hong Kong; Byk Madaus, S.Afr.; Nycomed, Swed.
Pantoprazole sodium (p.1283·1).
*Gastro-oesophageal reflux; peptic ulcer.*

**Pantometil** Lersan, Arg.
Polymyxin B sulfate (p.245·1); gramicidin (p.220·2); neomycin sulfate (p.235·1).
*Eye infections.*

**Pantomicina**
Abbott, Arg.; Abbott, Braz.; Abbott, Chile; Abbott, Mex.; Abbott, Spain.
Erythromycin (p.208·1), erythromycin ethyl succinate (p.208·1), erythromycin lactobionate (p.208·2), or erythromycin stearate (p.208·2).
*Bacterial infections.*

**Pantomin** Daiichi, Hong Kong.
Pantethine (p.978·3).
*Constipation; hyperlipidaemias; pantothenic acid deficiency.*

**Pantomucol** *Abbott, Arg.*
Erythromycin ethyl succinate (p.208·1) or erythromycin stearate (p.208·2); bromhexine (p.1115·3).
*Respiratory-tract infections.*

**Pantonate** *Eagle, Austral.*†.
Calcium pantothenate (p.1442·3).
*Vitamin $B_5$ supplement.*

**Pantop** *Byk, Arg.*
Pantoprazole sodium (p.1283·1).
*Gastro-oesophageal reflux; peptic ulcer.*

**PantoPAC** *Byk, Neth.*
Tablets, pantoprazole sodium (p.1283·1); tablets, clarithromycin (p.192·2); tablets, amoxicillin trihydrate (p.155·3).
*Peptic ulcer.*

**Pantopan** *Pharmacia Upjohn, Ital.*
Pantoprazole sodium (p.1283·1).
*Gastro-oesophageal reflux; peptic ulcer.*

**Pantopaz** *Hexal, Braz.*
Pantoprazole (p.1283·1).
*Peptic ulcer.*

**Pantopept** *Biosintetica, Braz.*
Pepsin (p.1729·3); amylase (p.1654·2).
*Digestive disorders.*

**Pantorc** *Byk Gulden, Ital.*
Pantoprazole sodium (p.1283·1).
*Gastro-oesophageal reflux; peptic ulcer.*

**Pantosin** *Daiichi, Jpn.*
Pantethine (p.978·3).
*Blood disorders; constipation; eczema; hyperlipidaemias; pantothenic acid deficiency; pantothenic acid supplement; streptomycin and kanamycin toxicity.*

**Pantostin** *Simons, Ger.*
Estradiol (p.1550·1).
*Alopecia androgenetica.*

**Pantothen**
*Note. This name is used for preparations of different composition.*
*Pharmaselect, Austria.*
Panthenol (p.1727·2).
*Anorectal disorders; skin disorders.*

*Streuli, Switz.*
Calcium pantothenate (p.1442·3).
*Intestinal atony; pantothenic acid deficiency; sensation of burning in feet.*

**Pantovigar N** *Simons, Ger.*
Thiamine nitrate (p.1455·1); calcium pantothenate (p.1442·3); medicinal yeast (p.1469·1); cystine (p.1426·3); keratin.
Pantovigar formerly contained thiamine nitrate, calcium pantothenate, medicinal yeast, cystine, keratin, and aminobenzoic acid.
*Disorders of the hair and nails.*

**Pantovit** *Sanova, Austria.*
Multivitamin preparation (p.1417·1).

**Pantovit Vital** *Sanova, Austria.*
Multivitamin, iron, and mineral preparation (p.1417·1).

**Pantozol**
*Byk, Belg.; Byk, Braz.; Byk Gulden, Ger.; Byk Gulden, Mex.; Byk, Neth.; Altana, Switz.*
Pantoprazole (p.1283·1) or pantoprazole sodium (p.1283·1).
*Gastro-oesophageal reflux; peptic ulcer; Zollinger-Ellison syndrome.*

**Pantozol-Rifun** *Byk Gulden, Ger.; Schwarz, Ger.*
Pantoprazole sodium (p.1283·1).
*Gastro-oesophageal reflux; peptic ulcer.*

**Pantricine** *Pharmacobel, Belg.*
Tyrothricin (p.275·1); lidocaine (p.1377·3).
*Sore throat.*

**Pantrop** *Lundbeck, Austria.*
Amitriptyline hydrochloride (p.280·3); chlordiazepoxide (p.674·2).
*Depression; sleep disorders.*

**Pantus** *Baliarda, Arg.*
Pantoprazole sodium (p.1283·1).
*Gastro-oesophageal reflux; peptic ulcer.*

**Pantyson** *Orion, Fin.*
Hydrocortisone (p.1103·3); dexpanthenol (p.1727·2).
*Skin disorders.*

**Panverm** *Teuto, Braz.*
Mebendazole (p.108·2).
*Worm infections.*

**Panvermin** *Andromaco, Mex.*
Mebendazole (p.108·2).
*Worm infections.*

**Panvit**
*Teuto, Braz.*
A range of multivitamin preparations with or without minerals (p.1417·1).

*Collins, Mex.*
Vitamin preparation (p.1417·1).

**Panvitan-M**
*Takeda, Hong Kong; Takeda, Singapore; Takeda, Thai.*
Multivitamin and mineral preparation (p.1417·1).

**Panvitina BC** *Neo Quimica, Braz.*
Multivitamin preparation (p.1417·1).

**Panvitrop** *Byk, Braz.*†.
Methionine (p.1042·1); choline tartrate (p.1424·3); sodium phenylethylacetate; liver extract; vitamin B substances; tocopherol (p.1417·1); rutoside (p.1688·2).
*Liver disorders.*

**Panwarfin** *Abbott, Gr.*
Warfarin sodium (p.1022·2).
*Thromboembolic disorders.*

**Panxeol** *IPRAD, Fr.*
Eschscholtzia californica; passion flower (p.1729·1).
*Insomnia; nervous disorders.*

**Panzid** *Valda, Ital.*
Ceftazidime (p.180·2).
*Bacterial infections.*

**Panzimine** *Malayan, Singapore.*
Buclizine hydrochloride (p.426·3).
*Hypersensitivity reactions; motion sickness; vertigo.*

**Panzynorm** *Pharmaselect, Austria.*
Pancreatin (p.1725·3).

**Panzynorm forte-N** *Abbott, Ger.*
Porcine pancreatin (p.1725·3).
*Pancreatic insufficiency.*

**Panzynorm-N** *German Remedies, India.*
Pancreatin (p.1725·3).
*Pancreatic insufficiency.*

**Panzytrat**
*Note. This name is used for preparations of different composition.*
*Technipro, Austral.; Pharmaco, NZ.*
Pancrelipase (p.1725·3).
Formerly contained pancreatin.
*Pancreatic insufficiency.*

*Abbott, Braz.; Abbott, Ger.; Vianex (Βιανεξ), Gr.; Knoll, Irl.*†*; Knoll, Neth.; Knoll, Switz.*
Pancreatin (p.1725·3).
*Pancreatic insufficiency.*

**Papaine** *DB, Fr.*
Carica papaya.
*Dyspepsia.*

**Papase** *Parke, Davis, Hong Kong*†.
Prolase.
*Inflammation; oedema.*

**Papasine** *Microsules Bernabo, Arg.*
Naproxen (p.65·1); tetracycline hydrochloride (p.266·2).
*Bacterial infections.*

**Papatropin** *Alpes Chemie, Chile.*
Atropine sulfate (p.477·1); papaverine hydrochloride (p.1728·1).
*Smooth muscle spasm.*

**Papaya Enzyme** *Nature's Bounty, USA.*
Papain (p.1727·3); amylase (p.1654·2).
*Gastrointestinal disorders.*

**Papaya Plus** *Gerard House, UK*†.
Charcoal (p.1030·3); papain (p.1727·3); slippery elm (p.1747·1); hydrastis (p.1698·3).
*Digestive disorders.*

**Papayasanit-N** *Weber & Weber, Ger.*†.
Homoeopathic preparation.

**Papenzima** *Parke, Davis, Chile.*
Papain (p.1727·3).
*Soft-tissue injury.*

**Papilo Lisin** *Remexa, Mex.*†.
Podophyllum (p.1155·2).

**Paps** *Richard, Fr.*
Sulfur (p.1158·2); zinc undecenoate (p.411·1); bismuth subgallate (p.1252·2); menthol (p.1711·3); camphor (p.1665·3); salicylic acid (p.1157·1); zinc oxide (p.1163·2); boric acid (p.1662·1); lavender oil (p.1705·2).
*Pruritus.*

**Papulex**
*Knoll, Austral.*†*; GenDerm, Canad.*†*; Helsinn Birex, Irl.*†*; Pharmagenix, UK*†.
Nicotinamide (p.1441·2).
*Acne.*

**Papytazyme**
*Anglo-French Drugs, India; Anglo-French Drugs, Thai.*
Papain (p.1727·3); pepsin (p.1729·3); amylase (p.1654·2); pancreatin (p.1725·3); ox bile extract (p.1660·3); ginger oleoresin (p.1267·1); activated charcoal (p.1030·2).
*Digestive disorders.*

**Par** *Daudt, Braz.*
Paracetamol (p.76·2); dipyrone (p.35·3).
*Fever; pain.*

**Par Glycerol** *Par, USA.*
Iodinated glycerol (p.1122·3).
*Coughs.*

**Para**
*Medgenix, Belg.; Medican, Canad.; SCAT, Denm.*†.
Bioallethrin (p.1500·3); piperonyl butoxide (p.1509·2).
*Pediculosis.*

**Para Lentes** *Pharmygiene, Fr.*
Acetic acid (p.1645·2).
*Pediculosis.*

**Para Piojicida** *Raymos, Arg.*
Bioallethrin (p.1500·3); piperonyl butoxide (p.1509·2).
*Pediculosis.*

**Para Plus**
*Raymos, Arg.; Medgenix, Belg.; Pharmygiene, Fr.; Rafa, Israel; Pacific, NZ.*
Malathion (p.1507·1); permethrin (p.1508·3); piperonyl butoxide (p.1509·2).
*Pediculosis.*

**Para Repulsif** *Pharmygiene, Fr.*
Piperonal (p.1509·1).
*Head lice repellent.*

**Para Special Poux** *Pharmygiene, Fr.*
Bioallethrin (p.1500·3); piperonyl butoxide (p.1509·2).
*Pediculosis.*

**Para Z Mol** *Cabuchi, Arg.*
Paracetamol (p.76·2).
*Fever; pain.*

**Parabowl** *Masa, Thai.*
Prazosin hydrochloride (p.985·1).
*Hypertension.*

**Paracap** *Masa, Thai.*
Paracetamol (p.76·2).
*Fever; pain.*

**Paracare** *PSM, NZ.*
Paracetamol (p.76·2).
*Fever; pain.*

**Paracefan** *Boehringer Ingelheim, Ger.*
Clonidine (p.885·2) or clonidine hydrochloride (p.885·2).
*Alcohol withdrawal syndrome; opioid withdrawal syndrome; tics.*

**Paracet**
*Weifa, Norw.; Osotspa, Thai.*
Paracetamol (p.76·2).
*Fever; pain.*

**paracet comp** *CT, Ger.*
Paracetamol (p.76·2); codeine phosphate (p.27·1).
*Pain.*

**Paracetacod**
*Note. This name is used for preparations of different composition.*
*Ratiopharm, Ger.*
Paracetamol (p.76·2); codeine phosphate (p.27·1).
*Pain.*

*Adcock Ingram, S.Afr.*
Paracetamol (p.76·2); codeine phosphate (p.27·1); ascorbic acid (p.1460·2).
*Pain.*

**Paracetamol comp** *Stada, Ger.; Aliud, Ger.*
Paracetamol (p.76·2); codeine phosphate (p.27·1).
*Pain.*

**Paracetamol plus**
*CT, Ger.; Ratiopharm, Ger.*
Paracetamol (p.76·2); caffeine (p.782·1).
*Cold symptoms; pain.*

**Paracets** *Sussex, UK.*
Paracetamol (p.76·2).
*Fever; pain.*

**Paracets Cold Relief** *Sussex, UK.*
Paracetamol (p.76·2); ascorbic acid (p.1460·2).
*Cold and influenza symptoms.*

**Paracets Plus** *Sussex, UK.*
Paracetamol (p.76·2); caffeine (p.782·1); phenylephrine hydrochloride (p.1126·3).
*Cold and influenza symptoms.*

**Parachoc** *Paedpharm, Austral.*
Methylcellulose (p.1580·2); liquid paraffin (p.1479·1).
*Constipation.*

**Paracin**
*Note. This name is used for preparations of different composition.*
*Stadmed, India.*
Paracetamol (p.76·2).
*Fever; pain.*

*Chinta, Thai.*†.
Paracetamol (p.76·2); potassium citrate (p.1223·1); chlorphenamine maleate (p.427·3); phenylephrine hydrochloride (p.1126·3).
*Cold and influenza symptoms; coughs.*

**Paraclear** *Roche Consumer, UK.*
Paracetamol (p.76·2).

**Paraclim** *Elea, Arg.*
Tibolone (p.1572·3).
*Menopausal disorders.*

**Paracne** *Panalab, Arg.*
Benzoyl peroxide (p.1143·2).
*Acne.*

**Paracod** *Sam-On, Israel.*
Paracetamol (p.76·2); codeine phosphate (p.27·1).
*Coughs; fever; pain.*

**Paracodin**
*Note. This name is used for preparations of different composition.*
*Knoll, Austral.; Ebewe, Austria; Abbott, Ger.; Abbott, Irl.; Knoll, S.Afr.; Knoll, Switz.*
Dihydrocodeine tartrate (p.34·3) or dihydrocodeine thiocyanate (p.35·2).
*Coughs; diarrhoea.*

*Ebewe, Austria.*
*Oral drops:* Dihydrocodeine thiocyanate (p.35·2); thyme (p.1755·2).
*Syrup:* Dihydrocodeine tartrate (p.34·3); althaea (p.1651·3); grindelia (p.1696·1).
*Coughs.*

**Paracodin N** *Abbott, Ger.*
Dihydrocodeine tartrate (p.34·3) or dihydrocodeine thiocyanate (p.35·2).
*Coughs.*

**Paracodin retard**
*Abbott, Ger.; Knoll, Switz.*
Dihydrocodeine tartrate (p.34·3); dihydrocodeine resin (p.35·2).
*Coughs; diarrhoea.*

**Paracodina**
*Note. This name is used for preparations of different composition.*
*Abbott, Ital.*
*Oral drops:* Dihydrocodeine thiocyanate (p.35·2).
*Syrup:* Dihydrocodeine tartrate (p.34·3); benzoic acid (p.1169·3).
*Coughs.*

*Knoll, Port.*†*; Abbott, Spain.*
Dihydrocodeine tartrate (p.34·3).
*Coughs; pain.*

**Paracodine** *Knoll, Belg.*
*Syrup:* Dihydrocodeine tartrate (p.34·3); grindelia (p.1696·1); althaea (p.1651·3).
*Tablets:* Dihydrocodeine tartrate (p.34·3).
*Coughs.*

**Paracodol**
*Roche Consumer, Irl.; Roche Consumer, UK.*
Paracetamol (p.76·2); codeine phosphate (p.27·1).
These ingredients can be described by the British Approved Name Co-codamol.
*Fever; pain.*

**Paractol**
*Note. This name is used for preparations of different composition.*
*Temmler, Ger.; German Remedies, India.*
*Tablets:* Simeticone (p.1289·2); aluminium hydroxide (p.1249·2).
*Gastrointestinal disorders with excess gas.*

*Temmler, Ger.; German Remedies, India.*
*Oral liquid:* Simeticone (p.1289·2); aluminium hydroxide (p.1249·2); magnesium hydroxide (p.1272·2).
*Gastrointestinal disorders with excess gas.*

**Paradenton** *Austroplant, Austria.*
Myrrh (p.1718·3); sage leaf (p.1741·2); chamomile flowers (p.1669·3); tannic acid (p.1751·2).
*Aphthous ulcers; bleeding gums; bruised gums; gingivitis; periodontitis.*

**Paraderm** *Whitehall Consumer, Austral.*
Bufexamac (p.21·3).
*Skin disorders.*

**Paraderm Plus**
*Whitehall Consumer, Austral.; Whitehall, NZ.*
Chlorhexidine gluconate (p.1173·2); lidocaine hydrochloride (p.1377·3); bufexamac (p.21·3).
*Insect bites; minor burns; minor skin lesions; stings; sunburn.*

**Paradex**
*Aspen, Austral.*
Dextropropoxyphene hydrochloride (p.28·3); paracetamol (p.76·2).
*Pain.*

*PSM, NZ.*
Dextropropoxyphene napsilate (p.28·3); paracetamol (p.76·2).
*Fever; pain.*

**Parador** *Boehringer de Angeli, Braz.*†.
Paracetamol (p.76·2).
*Fever; pain.*

**Paradote** *Penn, UK.*
Paracetamol (p.76·2); DL-methionine (p.1042·1).
These ingredients can be described by the British Approved Name Co-methiamol.
*Fever; pain.*

**Paradrine** *DHA, Singapore.*
Paracetamol (p.76·2); pseudoephedrine hydrochloride (p.1129·2); chlorphenamine maleate (p.427·3).
*Cold symptoms.*

**Paradroxil** *Gerolimatos (Γερολυματος), Gr.*
Amoxicillin trihydrate (p.155·3).
*Bacterial infections.*

**Paradryl med efedrin** *Ferrosan, Denm.*
Mefenidramium bromide; ephedrine hydrochloride (p.1120·1); ammonium chloride (p.1115·2).
*Coughs.*

**Paraflex**
*AstraZeneca, Denm.; Astra, Swed.; McNeil Pharmaceutical, USA.*
Chlorzoxazone (p.1392·3).
*Headache; premedication; skeletal muscle spasm.*

**Paraflex AN** *Janssen-Cilag, Arg.*
Chlorzoxazone (p.1392·3); paracetamol (p.76·2).
*Skeletal muscle pain and spasm.*

**Paraflex comp**
*AstraZeneca, Fin.; Astra, Swed.*
Chlorzoxazone (p.1392·3); aspirin (p.15·1); dextropropoxyphene napsilate (p.28·3).
*Headache; skeletal muscle spasm.*

**Paraflex Crema** *Janssen-Cilag, Arg.*
Ibuprofen (p.45·3).
*Musculoskeletal, joint, peri-articular, and soft-tissue disorders.*

**Paraflex Plus** *Janssen-Cilag, Arg.*
Chlorzoxazone (p.1392·3); paracetamol (p.76·2); dexamethasone (p.1097·1).
*Musculoskeletal, joint, peri-articular, and soft-tissue disorders.*

**Parafon**
*Janssen-Cilag, Austria; Ethnor, India; Janssen-Cilag, Thai.*
Chlorzoxazone (p.1392·3); paracetamol (p.76·2).
*Skeletal muscle pain and spasm.*

**Parafon DSC** *Ethnor, India.*
Chlorzoxazone (p.1392·3).
*Skeletal muscle spasm.*

**Parafon Forte**
*Johnson & Johnson, Canad.; Cilag, Mex.*
Chlorzoxazone (p.1392·3); paracetamol (p.76·2).
*Pain; skeletal muscle spasm.*

**Parafon Forte C8** *Johnson & Johnson, Canad.*†.
Chlorzoxazone (p.1392·3); paracetamol (p.76·2); codeine phosphate (p.27·1).
*Pain; skeletal muscle spasm.*

**Parafon Forte DSC** *Ortho McNeil, USA.*
Chlorzoxazone (p.1392·3).
*Musculoskeletal pain.*

**Paragar** *Spirig, Switz.*
Liquid paraffin (p.1479·1); agar (p.1576·3); phenolphthalein (p.1284·1).
*Constipation.*

**Paragard T380A** *Ortho McNeil, USA.*
Copper-wound plastic (p.1425·3).
*Intra-uterine contraceptive device.*

**Paragel** *Santa, Gr.*
Liquid paraffin (p.1479·1).
*Constipation.*

**Paraghurt** *Leo, Denm.*
*Enterococcus faecium* (p.1704·2).
*Diarrhoea.*

**Paragip** *Boiron, Canad.*
Homoeopathic preparation.

**Paragol N** *Streuli, Switz.*
Liquid paraffin (p.1479·1).
Paragol formerly contained liquid paraffin and phenolphthalein.
*Constipation.*

**Paragrippe**
*Boiron, Fr.; Boiron, Port.*
Homoeopathic preparation.

**Parahexal** *Hexal, Austral.*
Paracetamol (p.76·2).
*Fever; pain.*

**Para-Hist HD** *Pharmics, USA.*
Phenylephrine hydrochloride (p.1126·3); chlorphenamine maleate (p.427·3); hydrocodone tartrate (p.45·1).
*Coughs and cold symptoms.*

**Parahypon** *Calmic, Irl.†.*
Paracetamol (p.76·2); caffeine (p.782·1); codeine phosphate (p.27·1).
*Pain.*

**Parakapton** *Rosch & Handel, Austria.*
Paracetamol (p.76·2).
*Pain, fever.*

**Parake** *Galen, UK†.*
Paracetamol (p.76·2); codeine phosphate (p.27·1).
These ingredients can be described by the British Approved Name Co-codamol.
*Pain.*

**Paral** *Forest Pharmaceuticals, USA.*
Paraldehyde (p.713·1).
*Sedative.*

**Paralergin** *Vita, Spain†.*
Astemizole (p.424·2).
*Hypersensitivity reactions.*

**Paralgen** *Legrand, Braz.*
Paracetamol (p.76·2).
*Fever; pain.*

**Paralgesic** *ECR, USA.*
Methyl salicylate (p.59·3); menthol (p.1711·3); camphor (p.1665·3).

**Paralgin**
*Note. This name is used for preparations of different composition.*
*Fawns & McAllan, Austral.*
Paracetamol (p.76·2).
*Fever; pain.*

*Weifa, Norw.*
Codeine phosphate (p.27·1); paracetamol (p.76·2).
*Pain.*

**Paralice** *Fleet, Austral.*
Bioallethrin (p.1500·3); piperonyl butoxide (p.1509·2).
*Pediculosis.*

**Paralief** *Clonmel, Irl.*
Paracetamol (p.76·2).
*Fever; pain.*

**Paralink** *Rice Steele, Irl.*
Paracetamol (p.76·2).
*Fever; pain.*

**Paralon** *Janssen-Cilag, Braz.*
Chlorzoxazone (p.1392·3); paracetamol (p.76·2).
*Pain; smooth muscle spasm.*

**Paralymphine** *Andromaco, Chile.*
Iodine; manganese glycerophosphate; tannin; calcium phosphate; ferrous phosphate (p.1417·1).
*Tonic.*

**Paralyoc** *Lafon, Fr.*
Paracetamol (p.76·2).
*Fever; pain.*

**Paramax**
*Sanofi Synthelabo, Irl.; GlaxoSmithKline, NZ; Sanofi Synthelabo, UK.*
Paracetamol (p.76·2); metoclopramide hydrochloride (p.1274·3).
*Gastric stasis; migraine; nausea and vomiting.*

**Paramet** *Wallace, India.*
Paracetamol (p.76·2); metoclopramide (p.1274·3).
*Fever; nausea; pain.*

**Paramettes** *Whitehall-Robins, Canad.*
Multivitamin and mineral preparation (p.1417·1).

**Paramin** *Wallis, UK†.*
Paracetamol (p.76·2).
*Fever; pain.*

**Paraminan** *Alpharma, Fr.*
Aminobenzoic acid (p.1142·2).
*Skin disorders.*

**Paramine** *DHA, Singapore†.*
Chlorphenamine maleate (p.427·3); paracetamol (p.76·2); phenylpropanolamine hydrochloride (p.1127·3).
*Cold symptoms.*

**Paraminol** *Franco-Indian, India.*
Aminobenzoic acid (p.1142·2).
*Adjunct in vitiligo therapy.*

**Paramol**
*Note. This name is used for preparations of different composition.*
*Galen, Irl.; SSL, UK.*
Paracetamol (p.76·2); dihydrocodeine tartrate (p.34·3).
*Coughs; fever; pain.*

*General Drugs, Thai.*
Paracetamol (p.76·2).
*Fever; pain.*

**Paramol Forte** *Merck, Hong Kong.*
Paracetamol (p.76·2); caffeine (p.782·1).
*Fever; pain.*

**Paramol TP** *TP, Thai.*
Paracetamol (p.76·2).
Lidocaine hydrochloride (p.1377·3) is included in some injections to alleviate the pain of injection.
*Fever; pain.*

**Paramolan**
*Trima, Israel; Medinfar, Port.*
Paracetamol (p.76·2).
*Fever; pain.*

**Paramolan C** *Medinfar, Port.*
Paracetamol (p.76·2); ascorbic acid (p.1460·2).
*Fever; pain.*

**Paranal** *Siam Bheasach, Thai.*
Paracetamol (p.76·2).
*Fever; pain.*

**Paranal-L** *Siam Bheasach, Thai.*
Paracetamol (p.76·2).
Lidocaine hydrochloride (p.1377·3) is included in this preparation to alleviate the pain of injection.
*Fever; pain.*

**Paranorm** *Wallace Mfg Chem., UK.*
Dextromethorphan hydrobromide (p.1117·3); ephedrine hydrochloride (p.1120·1); guaifenesin (p.1122·1).
*Coughs.*

**Paranthil** *Xixia, S.Afr.†.*
Albendazole (p.101·2).
*Worm infections.*

**Paranzol** *Collins, Mex.*
Mebendazole (p.108·2).
*Worm infections.*

**Parapaed**
*Ritsert, Ger.; Pinewood, Irl.; Pinewood, UK.*
Paracetamol (p.76·2).
*Fever; pain.*

**Para-Pio** *Franco, Port.*
Pyrethrin (p.1509·3); piperonyl butoxide (p.1509·2).
*Pediculosis.*

**Paraplatin**
*Bristol-Myers Squibb, Arg.; Bristol-Myers Squibb, Austria; Bristol-Myers Squibb, Belg.; Bristol-Myers Squibb, Braz.; Bristol, Canad.; Bristol-Myers Squibb, Denm.; Bristol-Myers Squibb, Fin.; Bristol-Myers Squibb, Gr.; Bristol-Myers Squibb, Hong Kong; Bristol-Myers Squibb, Irl.; Bristol-Myers Squibb, Israel; Bristol-Myers Squibb, Ital.; Bristol-Myers Squibb, Malaysia; Bristol-Myers Squibb, Mex.; Bristol-Myers Squibb, Neth.; Bristol-Myers Squibb, Norw.; Bristol-Myers Squibb, NZ; Bristol-Myers Squibb, Port.; Bristol-Myers Squibb, S.Afr.; Bristol-Myers Squibb, Singapore; Bristol-Myers, Spain; Bristol-Myers Squibb, Swed.; Bristol-Myers Squibb, Switz.; Bristol-Myers Squibb, Thai.; Bristol-Myers Squibb, UK; Bristol-Myers Squibb Oncology, USA.*
Carboplatin (p.533·3).
*Malignant neoplasms.*

**Paraplatine** *Bristol-Myers Squibb, Fr.*
Carboplatin (p.533·3).
*Malignant neoplasms.*

**Para-plus** *Olvos, Gr.*
Permethrin (p.1508·3); piperonyl butoxide (p.1509·2); malathion (p.1507·1).
*Head lice.*

**Parapres** *Almirall, Spain.*
Candesartan cilexetil (p.878·3).
*Hypertension.*

**Parapres Plus** *Almirall, Spain.*
Candesartan cilexetil (p.878·3); hydrochlorothiazide (p.933·2).
*Hypertension.*

**Parapsyllium** *IPRAD, Fr.*
Ispaghula (p.1268·1); liquid paraffin (p.1479·1); sorbitol (p.1446·3).
*Constipation.*

**Paraqueimol** *Asta Medica, Braz.*
Sulfacetamide sodium (p.257·3); trolamine (p.1758·2).
*Skin infections.*

**Parartrin** *Cazi, Braz.*
Ibuprofen (p.45·3).
*Fever; inflammation; pain.*

**Paras** *YSP, Malaysia.*
Chlorzoxazone (p.1392·3); paracetamol (p.76·2).
*Skeletal muscle spasm and pain.*

**Parasidose**
*Gilbert, Fr.; Multichem, NZ.*
Phenothrin (p.1509·1).
*Pediculosis.*

**Parasimed** *Cimed, Braz.*
Benzyl benzoate (p.1500·2).

**Parasin** *Ache, Braz.*
Albendazole (p.101·2).
*Worm infections.*

**Parasone** *Vida, Hong Kong.*
Dexamethasone (p.1097·1); paracetamol (p.76·2); vitamin B substances (p.1417·1).
*Musculoskeletal, joint, and peri-articular disorders.*

**Para-Speciaal** *Byk, Neth.*
Bioallethrin (p.1500·3); piperonyl butoxide (p.1509·2).
*Pediculosis.*

**Para-Suppo** *Orion, Fin.*
Paracetamol (p.76·2).
*Fever; pain.*

**Parat** *Asian Pharm, Thai.*
Paracetamol (p.76·2).
*Fever; pain.*

**Para-Tabs** *Orion, Fin.*
Paracetamol (p.76·2).
*Fever; pain.*

**Paratabs** *PSM, NZ†.*
Paracetamol (p.76·2).
*Fever; pain.*

**Paratol** *Chew, Thai.*
Paracetamol (p.76·2).
*Fever; pain.*

**Paratosse** *Heralds, Braz.†.*
Diphenhydramine (p.431·3); ammonium chloride (p.1115·2); sodium citrate (p.1223·2); menthol (p.1711·3).
*Coughs.*

**Paratral** *LA, Arg.*
Paracetamol (p.76·2).
*Fever; pain.*

**Paratropina** *Lazar, Arg.*
Homatropine methylbromide (p.483·2).
*Habitual vomiting in infants; hyperchlorhydria; smooth muscle spasm.*

**Paratropina Compuesta** *Lazar, Arg.*
Homatropine methylbromide (p.483·2); metamizole magnesium (p.36·1).
*Colic; dysmenorrhoea.*

**Paratulle** *SSL, UK.*
Yellow soft paraffin (p.1479·3).
*Wounds.*

**Paraverm** *Hertz, Braz.†.*
Mebendazole (p.108·2).
*Worm infections.*

**Paravertebral LWS** *Infirmarius-Rovit, Ger.*
Homoeopathic preparation.

**Paraxin**
*Roche, Ger.*
Chloramphenicol sodium succinate (p.185·1).
*Bacterial infections.*

*Nicholas Piramal, India.*
Chloramphenicol (p.185·1) or chloramphenicol palmitate (p.185·1).
*Bacterial infections.*

**Paraxin Ear** *Nicholas Piramal, India.*
Chloramphenicol (p.185·1); benzocaine (p.1370·3).
*Otitis.*

**Parcaine** *Ocusoft, USA.*
Proxymetacaine hydrochloride (p.1384·1).

**Parcel** *Novartis, Braz.*
Paracetamol (p.76·2); dihydroergotamine mesilate (p.465·3); caffeine (p.782·1).
*Migraine.*

**Parche Leon Fortificante** *Beiersdorf, Chile.*
Capsicum (p.1667·1).
*Musculoskeletal and joint disorders.*

**Parcono** *Milano, Thai.*
Codeine phosphate (p.27·1); paracetamol (p.76·2).
*Pain.*

**Pardelprin** *Alpharma, UK.*
Indometacin (p.47·3).
*Dysmenorrhoea; musculoskeletal, joint, and peri-articular disorders.*

**Pa-Real** *Lampugnani, Ital.*
Royal jelly (p.1740·3).
*Nutritional supplement.*

**Parecid** *Proge, Ital.*
Cefonicid sodium (p.174·2).
Lidocaine hydrochloride (p.1377·3) is included in this preparation to alleviate the pain of injection.
*Gram-negative bacterial infections.*

**Paredrine** *Pharmics, USA.*
Hydroxyamfetamine hydrobromide (p.1699·3).
*Production of mydriasis.*

**Paregorique** *Lafran, Fr.*
Prepared opium (p.74·2); benzoic acid (p.1169·3); anise oil (p.1655·2); camphor (p.1665·3).
*Diarrhoea.*

**Parelmin** *Hexal, Braz.†.*
Mebendazole (p.108·2).
*Cestode infections; nematode infections.*

**Paremyd** *Akorn, USA.*
Hydroxyamfetamine hydrobromide (p.1699·3); tropicamide (p.491·1).
*Induction of mydriasis with partial cycloplegia.*

**Parencias** *Geminis, Arg.*
Ascorbic acid (p.1460·2); benzocaine (p.1370·3); borax (p.1661·3); nicotinic acid (p.1441·1).
*Mouth disorders.*

**Parenciclina** *Hoechst Marion Roussel, Mex.†.*
Tetracycline (p.266·2).
*Bacterial infections.*

**Parengesico** *Hoechst Marion Roussel, Mex.†.*
Paracetamol (p.76·2).
*Fever; pain.*

**Parentamin**
*Serag-Wiessner, Ger.; Fresenius Kabi, Ital.*
Amino-acid infusion (p.1417·1).
*Parenteral nutrition.*

**Parentamin E** *Serag-Wiessner, Ger.*
Amino-acid and electrolyte infusion (p.1417·1).
*Parenteral nutrition.*

**Parentamin X-E** *Serag-Wiessner, Ger.*
Amino-acid, electrolyte, and xylitol infusion (p.1417·1).
*Parenteral nutrition.*

**Parentamin EAS** *Serag-Wiessner, Ger.†.*
Amino-acid infusion (p.1417·1).
*Parenteral nutrition in renal impairment.*

**Parentamin G E** *Serag-Wiessner, Ger.*
Amino-acid, electrolyte, and glucose infusion (p.1417·1).
*Parenteral nutrition.*

**Parentamin GX E** *Serag-Wiessner, Ger.*
Amino-acid, electrolyte, glucose, and xylitol infusion (p.1417·1).
*Parenteral nutrition.*

**Parentamin-C-hepa** *Serag-Wiessner, Ger.†.*
Amino-acid, electrolyte, and xylitol infusion (p.1417·1).
*Parenteral nutrition in liver disease.*

**Parenteral** *Serag-Wiessner, Ger.*
Electrolyte infusion (p.1217·1).
*Fluid and electrolyte disorders.*

**Parenteral X** *Serag-Wiessner, Ger.†.*
Electrolyte infusion with xylitol (p.1217·1).
*Carbohydrate source; fluid and electrolyte disorders.*

**Parenteral BG** *Serag-Wiessner, Ger.*
Electrolyte infusion with glucose (p.1217·1).
*Carbohydrate source; fluid and electrolyte disorders.*

**Parenteral BX** *Serag-Wiessner, Ger.†.*
Electrolyte infusion with xylitol (p.1217·1).
*Carbohydrate source; fluid and electrolyte disorders.*

**Parenteral EK X** *Serag-Wiessner, Ger.†.*
Electrolyte infusion with xylitol (p.1217·1).
*Carbohydrate source; fluid and electrolyte disorders.*

**Parenteral EK Cal GX** *Serag-Wiessner, Ger.†.*
Electrolyte infusion with glucose and xylitol (p.1217·1).
*Carbohydrate source; fluid and electrolyte disorders.*

**Parenteral EK G** *Serag-Wiessner, Ger.*
Electrolyte infusion with glucose (p.1217·1).
*Carbohydrate source; fluid and electrolyte disorders.*

**Parenteral G** *Serag-Wiessner, Ger.*
Electrolyte infusion with glucose (p.1217·1).
*Carbohydrate source; fluid and electrolyte disorders.*

**Parenteral HG** *Serag-Wiessner, Ger.*
Electrolyte infusion with glucose (p.1217·1).
*Carbohydrate source; fluid and electrolyte disorders.*

**Parenteral HX** *Serag-Wiessner, Ger.†.*
Electrolyte infusion with xylitol (p.1217·1).
*Carbohydrate source; fluid and electrolyte disorders.*

**Parenteral K10** *Serag-Wiessner, Ger.†.*
Electrolyte infusion with glucose (p.1217·1).
*Fluid and electrolyte disorders.*

**Parenteral NS** *Serag-Wiessner, Ger.†.*
Electrolyte infusion with glucose (p.1217·1).
*Fluid and electrolyte disorders.*

**Parenteral OP** *Serag-Wiessner, Ger.*
Electrolyte infusion (p.1217·1).
*Fluid and electrolyte disorders.*

**Parenterin** *Legrand, Braz.*
Neomycin sulfate (p.235·1); phthalylsulfathiazole (p.242·3); aluminium hydroxide (p.1249·2); pectin (p.1580·3).
*Diarrhoea.*

**Parenzyme** *Medley, Braz.*
Trypsin (p.1758·3); chymotrypsin (p.1671·2).
*Inflammation.*

**Parenzyme Ampicilina** *Medley, Braz.*
Trypsin (p.1758·3); chymotrypsin (p.1671·2); ampicillin (p.157·1).
*Bacterial infections; inflammation.*

**Parenzyme Analgesico** *Medley, Braz.*
Trypsin (p.1758·3); chymotrypsin (p.1671·2); paracetamol (p.76·2).
*Inflammation; pain.*

**Parenzyme Tetraciclina** *Medley, Braz.*
Trypsin (p.1758·3); chymotrypsin (p.1671·2); tetracycline hydrochloride (p.266·2).
*Bacterial infections; inflammation.*

**Parexel** *Zodiac, Braz.*
Paclitaxel (p.577·3).
*Malignant neoplasms.*

**Par-F** *Pharmics, USA.*
Multivitamin and mineral preparation with iron and folic acid (p.1417·1).

**Parfenac**
*Wyeth-Whitehall, Arg.; Wyeth Lederle, Austria; Whitehall, Fr.; Lederle, Ger.; Chefaro, Neth.; Wyeth Consumer, Port.; Whitehall, S.Afr.†; Whitehall-Robins, Switz.*
Bufexamac (p.21·3).
*Burns; insect stings; skin disorders.*

**Parfenac Basisbad** *Lederle, Ger.*
Arachis oil (p.1656·1); light liquid paraffin (p.1479·1).
*Bath additive; dry, pruritic skin disorders.*

**Parfenal** *Wyeth Lederle, Ital.†.*
Bufexamac (p.21·3).
*Skin disorders.*

**Par-Gamma** *Biagini, Ital.†.*
A mumps immunoglobulin (p.1626·3).
*Passive immunisation.*

**Pargin** *Metapharma, Ital.†.*
Econazole nitrate (p.397·2).
*Fungal infections.*

**Pargine** *Viatris, Fr.*
Arginine aspartate (p.1421·1).
*Retarded growth.*

**Pargitan** *Abigo, Swed.*
Trihexyphenidyl hydrochloride (p.490·2).
*Drug-induced extrapyramidal disorders; parkinsonism; spasms in children.*

**Pargo** *Bio-Diät, Ger.*
Devil's claw root (p.28·2).
*Biliary disorders; degenerative joint disorders; gastrointestinal disorders.*

**Pariet**
*Janssen-Cilag, Arg.; Janssen-Cilag, Austral.; Janssen-Cilag, Austria; Janssen-Cilag, Belg.; Janssen-Cilag, Braz.; Janssen-Cilag, Denm.; Janssen-Cilag, Fin.; Janssen-Cilag, Fr.; Eisai, Ger.; Janssen-Cilag, Ger.; Solvay, Ger.; Janssen-Cilag, Gr.; Eisai, Hong Kong; Janssen-Cilag, Irl.; Janssen-Cilag, Ital.; Eisai, Jpn; Eisai, Malaysia; Janssen, Mex.; Janssen-Cilag, Neth.; Janssen-Cilag, Port.; Janssen-Cilag, S.Afr.; Eisai, Singapore; Janssen-Cilag, Spain; Janssen-Cilag, Swed.; Janssen-Cilag, Switz.; Eisai, Thai.; Eisai, UK.*
Rabeprazole sodium (p.1285·1).
*Gastro-oesophageal reflux; peptic ulcer; Zollinger-Ellison syndrome.*

**Parilac** *Teva, Israel.*
Bromocriptine mesilate (p.1200·3).
*Acromegaly; amenorrhoea; galactorrhoea; male and female infertility; parkinsonism; prolactinoma.*

**Parinix** *Richmond, Arg.*
Heparin (p.927·3).

**Paritrel** *Trima, Israel.*
Amantadine hydrochloride (p.1197·2).
*Drug-induced extrapyramidal disorders; influenza A; parkinsonism.*

**Parizac** *Lacer, Spain.*
Omeprazole (p.1278·2).
*Gastro-oesophageal reflux; peptic ulcers; Zollinger-Ellison syndrome.*

**Parkadina** *Basi, Port.*
Amantadine (p.1198·2).
*Parkinsonism.*

**Parkelase** *Parke, Davis, Spain†.*
Deoxyribonuclease (p.1119·1); fibrinolysin (p.916·2).
*Wound healing.*

**Parkelase Chloromycetin** *Parke, Davis, Spain†.*
Chloramphenicol (p.185·1); deoxyribonuclease (p.1119·1); fibrinolysin (p.916·2).
*Abscesses; burns; cervicitis; ulcers; vaginitis.*

**Parkemed**
*Pfizer, Austria; Parke, Davis, Ger.*
Mefenamic acid (p.55·2).
*Fever; inflammation; musculoskeletal and joint disorders; pain.*

**Parkexin** *Teuto, Braz.*
Selegiline hydrochloride (p.1214·1).
*Parkinsonism.*

**Parkinane** *Biodim, Fr.*
Trihexyphenidyl hydrochloride (p.490·2).
*Drug-induced extrapyramidal disorders; parkinsonism.*

**Parkinsan** *Lundbeck, Ger.*
Budipine hydrochloride (p.1203·3).
*Parkinsonism.*

**Parkinsol** *Teuto, Braz.*
Biperiden hydrochloride (p.479·3).
*Parkinsonism.*

**Parkipan**
*Bioes, Fr.*
*Ointment:* Trypan blue (p.1758·3); amylocaine hydrochloride (p.1370·2); titanium dioxide (p.1160·3).
*Herpes labialis.*

*L'Arguenon, Fr.†.*
*Topical solution:* Trypan blue (p.1758·3).
*Viral infections of the skin and mucous membranes.*

**Parkopan** *Hexal, Ger.*
Trihexyphenidyl hydrochloride (p.490·2).
*Parkinsonism.*

**Parkotil** *Lilly, Ger.*
Pergolide mesilate (p.1211·2).
*Parkinsonism.*

**Parks** *Hommel, Ger.*
Pridinol hydrochloride (p.1395·2).
*Extrapyramidal disorders; parkinsonism.*

**Parlax** *SERP, Mon.*
Liquid paraffin (p.1479·1).
*Constipation.*

**Parlib** *Enila, Braz.*
Gonadorelin (p.1325·1).
*Female infertility.*

**Parlide** *Pharmacia, Arg.*
Pergolide mesilate (p.1211·2).
*Parkinsonism.*

**Parlodel**
*Novartis, Arg.; Novartis, Austral.; Novartis, Austria; Novartis, Belg.; Novartis, Braz.; Novartis, Canad.; Novartis, Chile; Novartis, Denm.; Novartis, Fin.; Novartis, Fr.; Novartis, Gr.; Novartis, Hong Kong; Novartis, Irl.; Novartis, Israel; Novartis, Ital.; Novartis, Malaysia; Novartis, Mex.; Novartis, Neth.; Novartis, Norw.; Novartis, NZ†; Novartis, Port.; Novartis, S.Afr.; Novartis, Singapore; Novartis, Spain; Novartis, Switz.; Novartis, Thai.; Novartis, UK; Novartis, USA.*
Bromocriptine mesilate (p.1200·3).
*Acromegaly; benign breast disorders; female infertility; hyperprolactinaemia; lactation inhibition; menstrual disorders; parkinsonism; polycystic ovary syndrome; prolactinomas.*

**Parmecal**
*Geymonat, Ital.; Geymonat, Switz.*
Infant feed (p.1417·1).
*Colic; diarrhoea.*

**Parmentier** *Therabel, Belg.†.*
Caffeine (p.782·1); phenazone (p.82·3).
*Headache; migraine; pain.*

**Parmid** *Lagap, UK†.*
Metoclopramide hydrochloride (p.1274·3).
*Gastrointestinal disorders; migraine.*

**Parmodalin** *Sanofi Synthelabo, Ital.*
Tranylcypromine sulfate (p.318·3); trifluoperazine hydrochloride (p.726·3).
*Depression.*

**Parmol** *Hovid, Hong Kong; Merck, Hong Kong.*
Paracetamol (p.76·2).
*Fever; pain.*

**Par-Natal Plus 1 Improved** *Parmed, USA.*
Multivitamin and mineral preparation with iron and folic acid (p.1417·1).

**Parnate**
*Kirby, Arg.; Link, Austral.; GlaxoSmithKline, Braz.; GlaxoSmithKline, Canad.; Procter & Gamble, Ger.†; Goldshield, Irl.; Link, NZ; Pharmafrica, S.Afr.; SmithKline, Spain; Goldshield, UK†; SmithKline Beecham, USA.*
Tranylcypromine sulfate (p.318·3).
*Depression.*

**Parnoxil** *Zekides, Gr.*
Gemfibrozil (p.923·1).
*Hyperlipidaemias.*

**Paro** *Hoechst Marion Roussel, Ital.†.*
Hydrocortisone acetate (p.1103·3).
*Skin disorders.*

**Parocin** *Almirall, Spain.*
Meloxicam (p.56·1).
*Ankylosing spondylitis; osteoarthritis; rheumatoid arthritis.*

**Parodium**
*Sidus, Arg.; Pierre Fabre Sante, Fr.*
Chlorhexidine gluconate (p.1173·2); rhubarb (p.1287·3); formaldehyde (p.1179·3).
*Gum disorders.*

**Parodontal** *Serum-Werk Bernburg, Ger.*
Chamomile (p.1669·3); sage (p.1741·2); lidocaine (p.1377·3).
*Mouth inflammation.*

**Parodontal F5 med** *Wernigerode, Ger.†.*
Salol (p.88·1); thymol (p.1194·2); mint oil (p.1715·2); cineole (p.1672·1); clove oil (p.1673·3); sage oil (p.1741·2).
*Mouth inflammation.*

**Parodontax**
*Note. This name is used for preparations of different composition.*
*Block, Austria.*
*Mouthwash:* Echinacea purpurea (p.1683·2); chamomile (p.1669·3); myrrh (p.1718·3); menthol (p.1711·3); clove oil (p.1673·3); caraway oil (p.1667·3); sage oil (p.1741·2); peppermint oil (p.1283·2); mint oil (p.1715·2).
*Bleeding gums; inflammation of the mouth and gums; oral hygiene.*
*Toothpaste:* Echinacea purpurea (p.1683·2); sodium bicarbonate (p.1223·2); chamomile (p.1669·3); myrrh (p.1718·3); rhatany root (p.1738·1); sage oil (p.1741·2); peppermint oil (p.1283·2).
*Dental caries prophylaxis; oral hygiene.*

*Byk, Braz.†.*
Echinacea purpurea (p.1683·2); sodium bicarbonate (p.1223·2); chamomile (p.1669·3); myrrh (p.1718·3); rhatany root (p.1738·1).
*Oral hygiene.*

*Madaus, Israel.*
Echinacea (p.1683·2); sodium bicarbonate (p.1223·2); chamomile (p.1669·3); myrrh (p.1718·3); rhatany (p.1738·1); sage oil (p.1741·2); peppermint oil (p.1283·2).
*Dental disorders.*

*GlaxoSmithKline Consumer, Ital.*
Chlorhexidine (p.1173·2).
*Oral hygiene.*

**Paroex** *Pharmadent, Fr.*
Chlorhexidine gluconate (p.1173·2).
*Bacterial mouth infections.*

**Parogencyl** *Sanofi Synthelabo OTC, Ital.*
Metesculetol sodium (p.1714·1); provitamin B5.
*Gum disorders.*

**Parogencyl anti-age gencives** *Sanofi Synthelabo OTC, Fr.*
Sodium monofluorophosphate (p.1446·2); vitamin E (p.1464·3); chlorhexidine gluconate (p.1173·2); sodium fluoride (p.1444·3); ginkgo biloba (p.1692·3).
*Gum disorders.*

**Parogencyl Bi-Actif** *Rider, Chile.*
Metesculetol sodium (p.1714·1); provitamin B.
*Gum disorders.*

**Parogencyl gencives fragilisees** *Sanofi Synthelabo OTC, Fr.*
Metesculetol sodium (p.1714·1); provitamin $B_5$; alcohol (p.1166·1).
*Gum disorders.*

**Parogencyl sensibilite gencives** *Sanofi Synthelabo OTC, Fr.*
Chlorhexidine gluconate (p.1173·2); metesculetol sodium (p.1714·1).
*Gum disorders.*

**Parol** *Berman, Mex.†.*
Cyanocobalamin (p.1458·2).

**Paronal** *Christiaens, Belg.*
Asparaginase (p.528·3).
*Acute leukaemia.*

**Paroplak** *Sanofi Synthelabo OTC, Fr.*
Chlorhexidine gluconate (p.1173·2); polysorbate 20 (p.1415·1); sodium fluoride (p.1444·3).
*Dental caries prophylaxis.*

**Paroven**
*Novartis Consumer, Austral.; Novartis Consumer, Irl.†; Novartis, NZ†; Novartis Consumer, S.Afr.; Novartis Consumer, UK.*
Oxerutins (p.1688·2).
*Chronic venous insufficiency; haemorrhoids.*

**Parox** *Rowex, Irl.*
Paroxetine hydrochloride (p.311·2).
*Depression; obsessive-compulsive disorder; panic attacks.*

**Parox Meltab** *Saval, Chile.*
Paracetamol (p.76·2).
*Fever; pain.*

**Paroxat** *Hexal, Ger.*
Paroxetine hydrochloride (p.311·2).
*Anxiety; depression; obsessive-compulsive disorder; panic attacks.*

**Paroxedura** *Merck dura, Ger.*
Paroxetine hydrochloride (p.311·2).
*Depression; obsessive-compulsive disorder; panic attacks; social phobia.*

**Parsal** *Wyeth, Ger.*
Ibuprofen (p.45·3).
*Gout; inflammation; musculoskeletal, joint, and soft-tissue disorders; pain.*

**Parsel**
*Note. This name is used for preparations of different composition.*
*Novartis, Arg.; Novartis, Chile; Novartis, Mex.*
Dihydroergotamine mesilate (p.465·3); paracetamol (p.76·2); caffeine (p.782·1).
*Migraine and other vascular headaches.*

*Novartis Consumer, Port.*
Paracetamol (p.76·2).
*Fever; pain.*

**Parsilid** *Crinos, Ital.*
Ticlopidine hydrochloride (p.1011·2).
*Thrombosis prophylaxis.*

**Parsimonil** *Fabra, Arg.*
Flunitrazepam (p.698·2).

**Parsistene** *Boehringer Ingelheim, Chile.*
Fenoterol hydrobromide (p.785·2).
*Premature labour.*

**Parsitan** *Aventis, Canad.*
Profenamine hydrochloride (p.488·3).
*Drug-induced extrapyramidal disorders; parkinsonism.*

**Parstelin** *SmithKline Beecham, Irl.†.*
Tranylcypromine sulfate (p.318·3); trifluoperazine hydrochloride (p.726·3).
*Mixed anxiety depressive states.*

**Partamol**
*Atlantic, Malaysia; Atlantic, Thai.*
Paracetamol (p.76·2).
*Fever; pain.*

**Partane** *Taro, Israel.*
Trihexyphenidyl hydrochloride (p.490·2).
*Drug-induced extrapyramidal disorders; parkinsonism.*

**Partoben** *Purissimus, Arg.*
An anti-D immunoglobulin (p.1608·1).
*Prevention of rhesus sensitisation.*

**Partobulin**
*Immuno, Austria; Baxter, Ger.; Immuno, Hong Kong; Baxter, Ital.; Baxter, UK.*
An anti-D immunoglobulin (p.1608·1).
*Prevention of rhesus sensitisation.*

**Partocon**
*Ferring, Israel†; Ferring, Swed.†.*
Oxytocin (p.1336·1).
*Eclampsia; intra-uterine death; labour induction; pre-eclampsia; promotion of lactation.*

**Partogamma** *Immuno, Braz.†.*
An anti-D immunoglobulin (p.1608·1).
*Prevention of rhesus sensitisation.*

**Parto-Gamma** *Kedrion, Ital.*
An anti-D immunoglobulin (p.1608·1).
*Prevention of rhesus sensitisation.*

**Partogamma-T** *Baxter Immuno, Arg.*
An anti-D immunoglobulin (p.1608·1).
*Prevention of rhesus sensitisation.*

**Partusisten**
*Boehringer Ingelheim, Ger.; Promeco, Mex.; Boehringer Ingelheim, Neth.; Vifor, Switz.†.*
Fenoterol hydrobromide (p.785·2).
*Fetal distress; premature labour.*

**Partuss LA** *Parmed, USA†.*
Phenylpropanolamine hydrochloride (p.1127·3); guaifenesin (p.1122·1).
*Coughs.*

**Parulon** *Proveedora Teknimex, Mex.†.*
Pancuronium bromide (p.1404·3).
*Competitive neuromuscular blocker.*

**Paruman** *Berna, Ital.†.*
A mumps immunoglobulin (p.1626·3).
*Passive immunisation.*

**Parvisedil** *SIT, Ital.*
Aminohydroxybutyric acid (p.353·2); valerian (p.1762·2); passion flower (p.1729·1); chamomile (p.1669·3); crataegus (p.1677·1).
*Restlessness and insomnia in infants.*

**Parvlex** *Freeda, USA.*
Ferrous fumarate (p.1427·3); folic acid (p.1429·1); vitamin B substances with vitamin C (p.1417·1).
*Iron-deficiency anaemias.*

**Parvodex** *Jagson, India.*
Dextropropoxyphene hydrochloride (p.28·3).
*Pain.*

**Parvolex**
*Mayne, Austral.; Bioniche, Canad.; IFET (ΙΦΕΤ), Gr.; Mayne, Hong Kong; Celltech, Irl.; Faulding, Malaysia; Baxter, NZ; GlaxoSmithKline, S.Afr.; Celltech, UK.*
Acetylcysteine (p.1112·3).
*Paracetamol overdosage; respiratory-tract congestion.*

**Parvon** *Jagson, India.*
Dextropropoxyphene hydrochloride (p.28·3); paracetamol (p.76·2).
*Pain.*

**Parvon Forte** *Jagson, India.*
Dextropropoxyphene hydrochloride (p.28·3); ibuprofen (p.45·3).
*Inflammation; rheumatism.*

**Parvon-N** *Jagson, India.*
Dextropropoxyphene hydrochloride (p.28·3); paracetamol (p.76·2).
*Pain.*

**Parvon-Spas** *Jagson, India.*
Dextropropoxyphene hydrochloride (p.28·3); dicycloverine hydrochloride (p.481·2); paracetamol (p.76·2).
*Smooth muscle spasm.*

**Pas Hain** *Rudefsa, Mex.†.*
Isoniazid (p.222·2).

**Pasaden** *Farmades, Ital.*
Etizolam (p.698·1).
*Anxiety; insomnia.*

**Pasalen** *Pharmaland, Thai.*
Ketoconazole (p.403·3).
*Fungal infections.*

**Pasalix** *Marjan, Braz.*
Passion flower (p.1729·1); salix (p.87·3); crataegus (p.1677·1).
*Sedative.*

**Pascalium** *Pharmaten (Φαρματεν), Gr.*
Bromazepam (p.671·3).
*Anxiety disorders.*

**Pascallerg** *Pascoe, Ger.*
Homoeopathic preparation.

**Pascobilin novo** *Pascoe, Ger.*
Peppermint leaf (p.1283·2); taraxacum (p.1751·3); cynara (p.1678·3).
*Biliary-tract disorders.*

**Pascodolor Tropfen** *Pascoe, Ger.†.*
Homoeopathic preparation.

**Pascofemin** *Pascoe, Ger.*
Homoeopathic preparation.

**Pascohepan novo** *Pascoe, Ger.†.*
Greater celandine (p.1695·3); silybum marianum (p.1043·3); taraxacum (p.1751·3).
*Liver disorders.*

**Pascoletten N** *Pascoe, Ger.*
Aloes (p.1248·2); chamomile (p.1669·3).
*Constipation.*

**Pascoleucyn** *Pascoe, Ger.*
Homoeopathic preparation.

**Pascolibrin** *Pascoe, Ger.*
Homoeopathic preparation.

**Pascomag** *Pascoe, Ger.*
Bismuth subnitrate (p.1252·2); chamomile (p.1669·3); linseed (p.1707·2).
*Gastrointestinal disorders.*

**Pascomucil**
*Koch, Austria†; Pascoe, Ger.*
Ispaghula (p.1268·1).
*Constipation; diarrhoea.*

**Pasconal forte Nerventropfen** *Pascoe, Ger.*
Homoeopathic preparation.

**Pasconal Nerventropfen** *Pascoe, Ger.*
Homoeopathic preparation.

**Pasconeural-Injektopas** *Pascoe, Ger.*
Procaine hydrochloride (p.1383·2).
Formerly contained procaine hydrochloride and caffeine.
*Local anaesthesia.*

**Pasconeural-Injektopas 1%** *Pascoe, Ger.†.*
Procaine hydrochloride (p.1383·2).
*Local anaesthesia.*

**Pascopankreat**
*Note. This name is used for preparations of different composition.*
*Koch, Austria†.*
Condurango (p.1675·3); silybum marianum (p.1043·3); fennel fruit (p.1687·2); caraway oil (p.1667·3); chamomile oil (p.1669·3).
*Gastrointestinal disorders.*

*Pascoe, Ger.*
*Combination pack:* Yellow tablets, absinthium (p.1645·1); condurango (p.1675·3); red tablets, pancreatin (porcine) (p.1725·3).
*Digestive system disorders.*

**Pascopankreat novo** *Pascoe, Ger.*
Caraway oil (p.1667·3); chamomile oil (p.1669·3); condurango (p.1675·3); silybum marianum (p.1043·3); fennel (p.1687·2).
*Gastrointestinal disorders.*

**Pascopankreat S** Pascoe, Ger.†.
Pancreatin; caraway oil (p.1667·3); chamomile oil (p.1669·3); condurango; sarsaparilla; cholesterin.; menthol; ol. anisi; card. mar.; foenic.; syzyg. jamb.
*Digestive system disorders.*

**Pascorenal** Pascoe, Ger.
Homoeopathic preparation.

**Pascosabal** Pascoe, Ger.
Homoeopathic preparation.

**Pascosedon** Pascoe, Ger.
Valerian (p.1762·2); lupulus (p.1708·1); melissa (p.1711·1).
*Anxiety; sleep disorders.*

**Pascotox** Pascoe, Ger.†.
*Oral drops:* Echinacea (p.1683·2); baptisia; bryonia; eupator. perfol.; arnica; ferr. phosphoric.; thuja; china; lachesis; cupr. sulfuric.
*Tablets:* Echinacea (p.1683·2); baptisia; bryonia; eupatorium perfoliatum; thuja; lachesis.
*Tonic.*

**Pascotox forte-Injektopas** Pascoe, Ger.
Echinacea (p.1683·2).
*Tonic.*

**Pascotox mono** Pascoe, Ger.
Echinacea (p.1683·2).
*Tonic.*

**Pascovegeton** Pascoe, Ger.
Angelica (p.1655·1).
*Gastrointestinal disorders.*

**Pascovenol novo** Pascoe, Ger.†.
Aesculus (p.1648·2); melilotus; hamamelis (p.1696·3).
*Thromboembolic disorders; vascular disorders.*

**Pasedon** Lensa, Spain.
Miconazole nitrate (p.405·3).
*Fungal skin infections.*

**Pasem** Monserrat, Arg.
Salicylic acid (p.1157·1); lactic acid (p.1704·1).
*Callosities; verrucas; warts.*

**Paser** Jacobus, USA.
Aminosalicylic acid (p.154·3).
*Tuberculosis.*

**Pas-Fatol N** Fatol, Ger.
Sodium aminosalicylate (p.155·1).
*Tuberculosis.*

**Pasgensin** Pascoe, Ger.†.
Vitamins (p.1417·1); oxedrine tartrate (p.977·3).
*Hypotension; tonic.*

**Pasifen** Andromaco, Chile.
Diphenhydramine hydrochloride (p.431·3).
*Hypersensitivity reactions.*

**Pasil** Toyama, Jpn.
Pazufloxacin mesilate (p.241·3).
*Bacterial infections.*

**Pasisana** Riemser, Ger.
Herbal and homoeopathic preparation.

**Pasivital h** Riemser, Ger.
Homoeopathic preparation.

**Pasmalgin** Ibefar, Braz.†.
Dipyrone (p.35·3); papaverine hydrochloride (p.1728·1); homatropine methylbromide (p.483·2).
*Pain; smooth muscle spasm.*

**Pasminox** Beta, Arg.
Octilonium bromide (p.1725·1).
*Smooth muscle spasm.*

**Pasminox Somatico** Beta, Arg.
Octilonium bromide (p.1725·1); diazepam (p.690·1).
*Muscle spasm.*

**Pasmocalm** Bago, Chile.
Pargeverine hydrochloride (p.487·3).
*Smooth muscle spasm.*

**Pasmodil** Collins, Mex.
Dipyrone (p.35·3); butylhyoscine (p.484·2).
*Fever; pain.*

**Pasmodina** Drawer, Arg.
Hyoscine (p.483·3).
*Smooth muscle spasm.*

**Pasmolit** Jofrain, Mex.†.
Homatropine (p.483·2).

**Pasmosedan** Montpellier, Arg.
Pargeverine hydrochloride (p.487·3).
*Smooth muscle spasm.*

**Pasmosedan Compuesto** Montpellier, Arg.
Pargeverine hydrochloride (p.487·3); metamizole magnesium (p.36·1).
*Smooth muscle spasm.*

**Pasmovit** Finadiet, Arg.
Hyoscine (p.483·3).

**Paspat**
Note. This name is used for preparations of different composition.
Sankyo, Braz.
*Staphylococcus aureus*; *Staphylococcus epidermidis*; *Streptococcus viridans*; *Streptococcus haemolyticus*; *Streptococcus pneumoniae*; *Moraxella catarrhalis*; *Haemophilus influenzae*; *Candida albicans*.
*Immunotherapy.*

Sankyo, Ger.; Byk Gulden, Mex.; Sankyo, Thai.†.
Lysate of *Staphylococcus aureus*; *Staphylococcus albus*; *Streptococcus viridans*; *Streptococcus haemolyticus*; *Streptococcus pneumoniae*; *Moraxella catarrhalis*; *Haemophilus influenzae*; *Candida albicans*.
*Immunotherapy in respiratory-tract infections.*

Sankyo, Ital.
Lysate of *Staphylococcus aureus*; *Streptococcus mitis*; *Streptococcus pyogenes*; *Streptococcus pneumoniae*; *Klebsiella pneumoniae*; *Moraxella catarrhalis*; *Haemophilus influenzae*.
*Respiratory-tract infections.*

**Paspat Oral** Sankyo, Port.
*Staphylococcus aureus*; *Staphylococcus mitis*; *Streptococcus pyogenes*; *Streptococcus pneumoniae*; *Klebsiella pneumoniae*; *Moraxella catarrhalis*; *Haemophilus influenzae*.
*Respiratory-tract infections.*

**Paspertase**
Solvay, Austria; Solvay, Ger.
Metoclopramide hydrochloride (p.1274·3); pancreatin (p.1725·3).
*Gastrointestinal disorders.*

**Paspertin**
Solvay, Austria; Solvay, Ger.; Solvay, Switz.
Metoclopramide hydrochloride (p.1274·3).
*Adjunct in gastrointestinal radiography; gastrointestinal motility disorders; nausea and vomiting.*

**Pasrin** Aspen, S.Afr.
Buspirone hydrochloride (p.672·2).
*Anxiety disorders; mixed anxiety depressive states.*

**Passacanthine** Lafage, Arg.
Belladonna (p.479·1); convallaria (p.1675·3); crataegus (p.1677·1); passion flower (p.1729·1).
*Muscle spasm; nervous disorders.*

**Passagen** Durascan, Denm.
Xylometazoline hydrochloride (p.1132·2).
*Nasal congestion.*

**Passaja** Farmabraz, Braz.†.
Thymol (p.1194·2); menthol (p.1711·3); camphor (p.1665·3); eugenol (p.1686·2); procaine hydrochloride (p.1383·2).
*Oral hygiene.*

**Passaneuro** Bunker, Braz.
*Oral suspension:* Passion flower (p.1729·1); erythrina mulungu (p.1717·2); melissa (p.1711·1).
*Tablets:* Passion flower (p.1729·1); erythrina mulungu (p.1717·2); chamomile (p.1669·3).
*Sedative.*

**Passedan** Austroplant, Austria.
Passion flower (p.1729·1); melissa leaf (p.1711·1).
*Dystonias; menopausal disorders; sleep disorders.*

**Passedyl** Urgo, Fr.
Sodium benzoate (p.1169·3); sulfogaiacol (p.1131·1).
Formerly contained drosera, grindelia, sodium benzoate, potassium bromide, sulfogaiacol, orange-flower water, terpin, tolu balsam, and senega.
*Respiratory-tract congestion.*

**Passelyt** Smetana, Austria.
Passion flower (p.1729·1); melissa leaf (p.1711·1).
*Anxiety disorders; sleep disorders.*

**Passi Catha** Sedabel, Braz.†.
Passion flower (p.1729·1); crataegus (p.1677·1); salix (p.87·3).
*Sedative.*

**Passicalm** Gemballa, Braz.
Passion flower (p.1729·1); valerian (p.1762·2); erythrina mulungu (p.1717·2).

**Passicarbone** Millet Roux, Braz.†.
Vegetable charcoal (p.1030·3); passion flower (p.1729·1); crataegus (p.1677·1); salix alba (p.87·3).
*Diarrhoea.*

**Passiflora** Tamar, Israel.
Passion flower (p.1729·1); crataegus (p.1677·1); valerian (p.1762·2); orange flower (p.1723·3).
*Insomnia; nervousness; tension.*

**Passiflora Complex**
Note. This name is used for preparations of different composition.
Blackmores, Austral.†.
Passion flower (p.1729·1); lupulus (p.1708·1); skullcap (p.1746·3); valerian (p.1762·2); multivitamins (p.1417·1).
*Anxiety; insomnia; stress symptoms.*

Dolisos, Canad.
Homoeopathic preparation.

**Passiflora Compose** Boiron, Fr.
Homoeopathic preparation.

**Passiflora Composta**
Note. This name is used for preparations of different composition.
Infabra, Braz.†.
Crataegus (p.1677·1); erythrina mulungu (p.1717·2); passion flower (p.1729·1).
*Sedative.*

Luper, Braz.†.
Passion flower (p.1729·1); erythrina mulungu (p.1717·2); melissa (p.1711·1).
*Sedative.*

**Passiflora Compound** Vitamed, Israel.
Passion flower (p.1729·1); valerian (p.1762·2).
*Anxiety; insomnia; tension.*

**Passiflora Curarina** Harras-Curarina, Ger.
Passion flower (p.1729·1).
*Agitation.*

**Passiflora GHL** Lehning, Fr.
Homoeopathic preparation.

**Passiflorin** Austroplant, Austria.
Passion flower (p.1729·1).
*Nervous disorders; sleep disorders.*

**Passiflorine**
Note. This name is used for preparations of different composition.
Millet Roux, Braz.; Teofarma, Ital.
Passion flower (p.1729·1); crataegus (p.1677·1); salix alba (p.87·3).
*Insomnia.*

Theratech, Fr.; Chiesi, Spain†.
Passion flower (p.1729·1); crataegus (p.1677·1).
Formerly contained passion flower, crataegus, and salix alba in *Spain*.
*Anxiety; insomnia; menopausal disorders.*

**Passifuril** Millet Roux, Braz.
Nifuroxazide (p.237·2).
*Diarrhoea.*

**Passilex** Luper, Braz.
Passion flower (p.1729·1); erythrina mulungu (p.1717·2); melissa (p.1711·1).
*Anxiety.*

**Passilin** Galenogal, Braz.†.
Benzocaine (p.1370·3); tyrothricin (p.275·1).

**Passin** Simons, Ger.
Crataegus (p.1677·1); passion flower (p.1729·1).
*Nervous cardiovascular disorders.*

**Passinevryl** Clement Thionville, Fr.
Passion flower (p.1729·1); crataegus (p.1677·1); valerian (p.1762·2).
*Insomnia.*

**Passionflower Plus** Eagle, Austral.†.
Passion flower (p.1729·1); valerian (p.1762·2); skullcap (p.1746·3); lupulus (p.1708·1).
*Anxiety; insomnia.*

**Passiorin N** Simons, Ger.†.
Crataegus (p.1677·1); passion flower (p.1729·1).
*Nervous disorders; sleep disorders.*

**Past Ail** Medecine Vegetale, Fr.†.
Garlic (p.1691·1).
*Capillary fragility; circulatory disorders.*

**Pasta Arsenicale** Ogna, Ital.
Arsenic trioxide (p.1657·1); lidocaine (p.1377·3); ephedrine hydrochloride (p.1120·1).
*Dental disorders.*

**Pasta boli** Spirig, Switz.
Salicylic acid (p.1157·1); eucalyptus oil (p.1686·2); peppermint oil (p.1283·2); methyl salicylate (p.59·3).
*Musculoskeletal, joint, peri-articular, and soft-tissue disorders.*

**Pasta Cool** Apomedica, Austria.
Heparin sodium (p.928·1); salicylic acid (p.1157·1).
*Musculoskeletal and joint disorders; peri-articular disorders; soft-tissue injury.*

**Pasta d'Agua** Sedabel, Braz.
Zinc oxide (p.1163·2); purified talc (p.1159·1); glycerol (p.1694·3); agua de cal.
*Skin disorders.*

**Pasta De Lassar** Andromaco, Mex.; Columbia, Mex.
Zinc oxide (p.1163·2).
*Skin disorders.*

**Pasta Dermic** ICN, Arg.
Zinc oxide (p.1163·2).
*Skin disorders.*

**Pasta Devitalizzante** Ogna, Ital.
Paraformaldehyde (p.1187·3); lidocaine (p.1377·3).
*Dental disorders.*

**Pasta Dicofarm** Dicofarm, Ital.
Zinc oxide (p.1163·2); titanium dioxide (p.1160·3); vitamin E (p.1464·3); vitamin F.
*Skin irritation.*

**Pasta Lactisol** Galactopharm, Ger.†.
Sour milk whey concentrate.
*Skin disorders.*

**Pasta Lassar** Valma, Chile; Volta, Chile.
Zinc oxide (p.1163·2); wool fat (p.1483·1); white soft paraffin (p.1479·3).
*Skin disorders.*

**Pasta Lassar Imba** Perez Gimenez, Spain.
Almond oil (p.1651·1); lanolin; zinc oxide (p.1163·2).
*Burns; skin disorders; wounds.*

**Pasta Lassar Orravan** Orravan, Spain†.
Salicylic acid (p.1157·1); soft paraffin; zinc oxide (p.1163·2).
*Burns; skin disorders; wounds.*

**Pasta rubra salicylata** Apomedica, Austria.
Diethylamine salicylate (p.34·1); salicylic acid (p.1157·1); methyl salicylate (p.59·3).
*Gout; rheumatism; sciatica; soft-tissue injury; tendinitis.*

**Pastiglie Valda** Valda, Ital.
Cicliomenol (p.1177·3); enoxolone (p.36·2); menthol (p.1711·3); cineole (p.1672·1).
*Catarrh; mouth and throat irritation.*

**Pastilhas Valda** Canonne, Braz.†.
Menthol (p.1711·3); cineole (p.1672·1).
*Mouth disorders.*

**Pastillas Antisep Garg L** Procter & Gamble, Spain.
Ascorbic acid (p.1460·2); cetylpyridinium chloride (p.1173·1); citric acid (p.1673·1); menthol (p.1711·3).
*Throat irritation.*

**Pastillas Antisep Garg M** Procter & Gamble, Spain.
Camphor (p.1665·3); benzyl alcohol (p.1170·2); tolu balsam (p.1131·3); thymol (p.1194·2); menthol (p.1711·3); eucalyptus (p.1686·1); cetylpyridinium chloride (p.1173·1).
*Throat irritation.*

**Pastillas Dr Andreu** Roche, Spain.
Dextromethorphan hydrobromide (p.1117·3); sodium benzoate.
*Coughs.*

**Pastillas Juanola** Farma Lepori, Spain.
Cineole (p.1672·1); liquorice (p.1270·2); terpineol (p.1752·2); menthol (p.1711·3).
*Coughs; throat irritation.*

**Pastillas Koki Ment Tiro** Perez Gimenez, Spain.
Benzocaine (p.1370·3); tyrothricin (p.275·1); menthol (p.1711·3).
*Mouth and throat disorders.*

**Pastillas Lorbi** Bioquimico, Arg.
Allantoin (p.1141·3); benzocaine (p.1370·3); sulfadiazine (p.258·2).
*Mouth and throat disorders.*

**Pastillas Medex** Sidus, Arg.
Tolu balsam (p.1131·3); benzocaine (p.1370·3); hexylresorcinol (p.1182·1); allantoin (p.1141·3); eucalyptus oil (p.1686·2); menthol (p.1711·3).
*Coughs; sore throat.*

**Pastillas Pectoral Kely** Boots Healthcare, Spain.
Cineole (p.1672·1); niaouli oil (p.1719·3); senega (p.1130·2); liquorice (p.1270·2); sodium benzoate (p.1169·3); sulfogaiacol (p.1131·1); terpin monohydrate (p.1131·1).
*Respiratory-tract disorders.*

**Pastilles d'Ems** Siemens, Switz.†.
Sal ems.
*Cold symptoms; upper respiratory-tract inflammation.*

**Pastilles Medicinales Vicks** Lachartre, Fr.
Camphor (p.1665·3); menthol (p.1711·3); eucalyptus oil (p.1686·2); thymol (p.1194·2); tolu balsam (p.1131·3); benzyl alcohol (p.1170·2).
*Sore throats.*

**Pastilles Monleon** Toulade, Fr.
Methylthioninium chloride (p.1042·2); tolu balsam (p.1131·3); drosera (p.1683·1); hamamelis (p.1696·3).
*Mouth and throat disorders.*

**Pastilles pectorales Demo N** Democal, Switz.
Drosera (p.1683·1); hedera helix; ipecacuanha (p.1122·3); plantain (p.1733·1); tolu balsam (p.1131·3); anise oil (p.1655·2); orange peel (p.1723·3); eucalyptus oil (p.1686·2); mint oil (p.1715·2); menthol (p.1711·3).
*Coughs.*

**Pastilles pectorales formule 541** Renapharm, Switz.†.
Senega (p.1130·2); thyme (p.1755·2); drosera (p.1683·1); sage oil (p.1741·2); fennel oil (p.1687·3); star anise oil; menthol (p.1711·3); ephedrine hydrochloride (p.1120·1); eucalyptus oil (p.1686·2); liquorice (p.1270·2).
*Coughs.*

**Pastilles pour la gorge no 535** Iromedica, Switz.
Dequalinium salicylate (p.1178·1).
*Mouth and throat disorders.*

**Pastilles Valda** Valda, Canad.†.
Guaiacol (p.1122·1); cineole (p.1672·1); menthol (p.1711·3); terpin hydrate (p.1131·1); thymol (p.1194·2).

**Pastimmun** Pasteur Merieux, Belg.†.
A BCG vaccine (p.1609·2).
*Bladder cancer.*

**Pasuma-Dragees** Herchemie, Austria.
Methyltestosterone (p.1559·3); alpha tocoferil acetate (p.1465·1); yohimbine hydrochloride (p.1766·2); strychnine glycerophosphate; caffeine (p.782·1); oxedrine tartrate (p.977·3).

**Patanol**
Alcon, Arg.; Alcon, Austral.; Alcon, Braz.; Alcon, Canad.; Alcon, Chile; Alcon, Mex.; Alcon, Singapore; Alcon, Thai.; Alcon, USA.
Olopatadine hydrochloride (p.438·1).
*Allergic conjunctivitis.*

**Pat-Chobet** Chobet, Arg.
Animal tissue extracts (p.1709·3).
*Liver disorders.*

**Pate a l'Eau Roche-Posay** Roche-Posay, Fr.
Zinc oxide (p.1163·2); titanium dioxide (p.1160·3); borax (p.1661·3).
*Eczema.*

**Pate d'Unna** Rougier, Canad.†.
Zinc oxide (p.1163·2).

**Pate Iodoforme du Prof Dr Walkhoff** Haupt, Switz.†.
Iodoform (p.1184·2); parachlorophenol (p.1187·3); camphor (p.1665·3); menthol (p.1711·3).
*Dental inflammation.*

**Patector** AF, Mex.
Algestone acetophenide (p.1541·3); estradiol enantate (p.1550·1).
*Endometriosis; female infertility; injectable contraceptive; menstrual disorders.*

**Patentex**
Medra, Austria; Frere, Belg.†; Merz, Fin.; CCD, Fr.†; PCR, Ger.
Nonoxinol 9 (p.1413·3).
*Contraceptive.*

**Patentex Oval** Patentex, Ger.
Nonoxinol 9 (p.1413·3).
*Contraceptive.*

**Patentex Oval N** Patentex, Switz.
Nonoxinol 9 (p.1413·3).
*Contraceptive.*

**Pates Pectorales** Oberlin, Fr.†.
Codeine (p.27·1); tolu balsam (p.1131·3); cherry-laurel.
*Coughs.*

**Pathilon** Lederle, USA†.
Tridihexethyl chloride (p.490·2).
*Peptic ulcer (adjunct).*

**Pathocil** *Wyeth-Ayerst, USA†.*
Dicloxacillin sodium (p.205·2).
*Bacterial infections.*

**Patriot** *Agropharm, UK†.*
Pyrethrins (p.1509·3); piperonyl butoxide (p.1509·2).
*Insecticide and repellent.*

**Patropin** *Rekah, Israel.*
Papaverine hydrochloride (p.1728·1); atropine sulfate (p.477·1).
*Smooth muscle spasm.*

**Patsolin** *Leiras, Fin.†.*
Prazosin hydrochloride (p.985·1).
*Heart failure; hypertension.*

**Patuxan** *Collins, Mex.*
Vitamin preparation (p.1417·1).

**Patxen** *Ehlinger, Mex.†.*
Naproxen (p.65·1).

**Pausafren T** *Finadiet, Arg.*
Oxazepam (p.712·2).
*Anxiety.*

**Pausanol** *Leiras, Fin.*
Estriol (p.1552·3).
*Menopausal vaginal disorders; oestrogen deficiency.*

**Pausedal** *Alter, Spain.*
Levosulpiride (p.722·2).
*Dyspepsia.*

**Pausene** *Theramex, Ital.*
11 Tablets, estradiol valerate (p.1550·2); 10 tablets, estradiol valerate; cyproterone acetate (p.1544·1).
Formerly known as Pausal.
*Menopausal disorders.*

**Pausigin** *Lepori, Port.*
Estriol (p.1552·3).
*Vulvovaginal disorders.*

**Pavabid** *Hoechst Marion Roussel, USA.*
Papaverine hydrochloride (p.1728·1).
*Cerebral and peripheral ischaemia; smooth muscle spasm.*

**Pa-Vaccinol** *Procter & Gamble, Ger.†.*
A pertussis vaccine (p.1631·2).
*Active immunisation.*

**Pavacol-D** *Ransom, UK.*
Pholcodine (p.1128·3).
*Coughs.*

**Pavedal** *Pharma Investi, Chile.*
Metolazone (p.956·2).
*Ascites; heart failure; hypertension; nephrotic syndrome; oedema.*

**Paveriwern** *Wernigerode, Ger.*
Papaver somniferum.
*Gastrointestinal spasm.*

**Pavertrin** *Duncan, Arg.*
Idebenone (p.1700·3).
*Cerebrovascular disorders.*

**Paverysat forte N** *Ysatfabrik, Ger.*
Greater celandine (p.1695·3).
Paverysat forte formerly contained greater celandine and turmeric.
*Biliary-tract and gastrointestinal spasm.*

**Pavitron** *Alpha, Mex.†.*
Tetracycline (p.266·2).
*Bacterial infections.*

**Pavulon**
*Organon, Arg.; Organon, Austral.; Organon Teknika, Austria†; Organon, Braz.; Organon, Canad.†; Organon, Chile; Organon, Denm.; Organon, Fin.; Organon, Fr.; Organon (Οργανον), Gr.; Organon Teknika, Hong Kong; Organon Teknika, Irl.; Organon Teknika, Israel; Organon, Ital.; Organon, Malaysia; Organon Teknika, Mex.†; Organon, Neth.; Organon, Norw.; Organon, Port.; Sanofi Synthelabo, S.Afr.; Organon, Singapore; Organon, Spain; Organon, Swed.; Organon, Switz.; Organon, Thai.; Organon, UK†; Organon, USA.*
Pancuronium bromide (p.1404·3).
*Competitive neuromuscular blocker.*

**Pawa-Rutan** *Hanosan, Ger.*
Homoeopathic preparation.

**Pax** *Aspen, S.Afr.*
Diazepam (p.690·1).
*Alcohol withdrawal syndrome; anxiety; premedication.*

**Paxadorm** *Alliance, S.Afr.*
Nitrazepam (p.710·1).
*Insomnia.*

**Paxam** *Alphapharm, Austral.*
Clonazepam (p.359·1).
*Epilepsy.*

**Paxapride** *Labinca, Arg.*
Cinitapride acid tartrate (p.1259·2).
*Gastro-oesophageal reflux; gastrointestinal motility disorders.*

**Paxarel** *Circle, USA†.*
Acecarbromal (p.668·2).
*Anxiety; insomnia; sedative; spastic colitis.*

**Paxate** *Mead Johnson, Mex.†.*
Diazepam (p.690·1).

**Paxel** *Cristalia, Braz.*
Paclitaxel (p.577·3).
*Malignant neoplasms.*

**Paxeladine** *Beaufour, Fr.*
Oxeladin citrate (p.1126·1).
*Coughs.*

**Paxeladine Noctee** *Beaufour, Fr.†.*
Oxeladin citrate (p.1126·1); promethazine hydrochloride (p.439·1).
*Coughs.*

**Paxene** *Mayne, UK.*
Paclitaxel (p.577·3).
*Malignant neoplasms.*

**Paxetil** *Medibial, Port.*
Paroxetine hydrochloride (p.311·2).
*Anxiety disorders; depression; obsessive-compulsive disorder; panic disorder; post-traumatic stress disorder.*

**Paxical** *Intramed, S.Afr.†.*
Droperidol (p.697·2).
*Nausea and vomiting; neuroleptanalgesia; premedication.*

**Paxidal**
*Note. This name is used for preparations of different composition.*
*Propan, S.Afr.*
Paracetamol (p.76·2); doxylamine succinate (p.432·3); caffeine (p.782·1); codeine phosphate (p.27·1).
*Pain and associated tension.*

*Wallace Mfg Chem., UK.*
Caffeine (p.782·1); meprobamate (p.706·2); paracetamol (p.76·2).

**Paxidorm**
*Pharmaserve, Singapore; Norma, UK.*
Diphenhydramine hydrochloride (p.431·3).
*Insomnia.*

**Paxil**
*GlaxoSmithKline, Canad.; SmithKline Beecham, Mex.; GlaxoSmithKline, USA.*
Paroxetine hydrochloride (p.311·2).
*Anxiety; depression; obsessive-compulsive disorder; panic attacks; post-traumatic stress disorder; premenstrual dysphoric disorder; social phobia.*

**Paxilfar** *Tecnifar, Port.*
Tramadol hydrochloride (p.94·3).
*Pain.*

**Paxipam** *Schering-Plough, Ital.†.*
Halazepam (p.701·2).
*Anxiety.*

**Paxium** *Jaba, Port.*
Chlordiazepoxide (p.674·2).
*Alcohol withdrawal syndrome; anxiety; muscle spasm.*

**Paxon**
*Note. This name is used for preparations of different composition.*
*Gador, Arg.*
Losartan potassium (p.947·2).
*Hypertension.*

*Saval, Chile.*
Buspirone (p.673·1).
*Anxiety.*

**Paxon-D** *Gador, Arg.*
Losartan potassium (p.947·2); hydrochlorothiazide (p.933·2).
*Hypertension.*

**Paxtibi** *Dista, Spain.*
Nortriptyline hydrochloride (p.310·2).
*Depression.*

**Paxtine** *Alphapharm, Austral.*
Paroxetine hydrochloride (p.311·2).
*Depression; obsessive-compulsive disorder; panic disorder; social phobias.*

**Paxum** *East India Pharma, India.*
Diazepam (p.690·1).
*Alcohol withdrawal syndrome; anxiety; insomnia; muscle spasm; premedication.*

**Paxxet** *Unipharm, Israel.*
Paroxetine hydrochloride (p.311·2).
*Depression; obsessive-compulsive disorder; panic attacks.*

**Paxyl** *Faulding, Austral.*
Lidocaine (p.1377·3) or lidocaine hydrochloride (p.1377·3); benzalkonium chloride (p.1168·3); allantoin (p.1141·3).
*Burns; chapped skin; insect bites; skin abrasions; sunburn; windburn.*

**Payasanit gastro** *Weber & Weber, Ger.*
Homoeopathic preparation.

**Pazbronquial** *Cinfa, Spain.*
Codeine phosphate (p.27·1); ephedrine hydrochloride (p.1120·1); sodium benzoate (p.1169·3); sodium citrate (p.1223·2); sulfogaiacol (p.1131·1); thiamine hydrochloride (p.1455·1); pyridoxine hydrochloride (p.1456·3); menthol (p.1711·3); drosera (p.1683·1); lobelia inflata (p.1589·1); thyme (p.1755·2); origanum vulgare; grindelia (p.1696·1).
*Coughs.*

**Pazo** *Bristol-Myers Products, USA.*
Benzocaine (p.1370·3); ephedrine sulfate (p.1120·1); zinc oxide (p.1163·2); camphor (p.1665·3).
*Haemorrhoids.*

**Pazolam** *Atral, Port.*
Alprazolam (p.668·3).
*Anxiety disorders; mixed anxiety depressive states.*

**Pazolini** *Faria, Braz.*
Diazepam (p.690·1).
*Alcohol withdrawal syndrome; anxiety; epilepsy; insomnia; premedication; sedative; skeletal muscle spasm.*

**Pazucross** *Mitsubishi, Jpn.*
Pazufloxacin mesilate (p.241·3).
*Bacterial infections.*

**PB Gel** *Lagos, Arg.*
Benzoyl peroxide (p.1143·2).
*Acne.*

**PBZ** *Geigy, USA†.*
Tripelennamine citrate (p.442·3) or tripelennamine hydrochloride (p.442·3).
*Hypersensitivity reactions.*

**PC 30 V** *Terra-Bio, Ger.*
Aesculus (p.1648·2); dexpanthenol (p.1727·2); chamomile (p.1669·3).
*Skin disorders; ulcers; wounds.*

**PC Arthri-Spray** *Procare, Austral.†.*
Copper salicylate; methyl salicylate (p.59·3).
*Musculoskeletal, joint, and peri-articular disorders.*

**PC 30 N** *Terra-Bio, Ger.*
Chamomile (p.1669·3).
*Burns; skin disorders.*

**PC Regulax** *Procare, Austral.†.*
Peppermint leaf (p.1283·2); ispaghula (p.1268·1); slippery elm (p.1747·1); ginger (p.1267·1); pectin (p.1580·3).
*Gastrointestinal disorders; haemorrhoids; hyperlipidaemias; varicose veins.*

**PC Rei-shi** *Procare, Austral.†.*
Rei-shi; shi-taki.
*Nutritional supplement.*

**PC-Cap** *Alra, USA.*
Dextropropoxyphene hydrochloride (p.28·3); aspirin (p.15·1); caffeine (p.782·1).

**PCE**
*Abbott, Canad.; Abbott, Hong Kong; Abbott, USA.*
Erythromycin (p.208·1).
*Bacterial infections.*

**PCF N** *Ritsert, Ger.*
Homoeopathic preparation.

**PCL** *Hoe, Singapore.*
Codeine phosphate (p.27·1); promethazine (p.439·1).
*Coughs.*

**PCM**
*Note. This name is used for preparations of different composition.*
*Hemopharm, Ger.*
Paracetamol (p.76·2).
*Fever; pain.*

*Cypress, USA.*
Pseudoephedrine hydrochloride (p.1129·2); chlorphenamine maleate (p.427·3); hyoscine methonitrate (p.483·3).
*Rhinitis.*

**PD Cough** *PD, Thai.†.*
Dextromethorphan hydrobromide (p.1117·3); pentoxyverine citrate (p.1126·2); phenylpropanolamine hydrochloride (p.1127·3); guaifenesin (p.1122·1).
*Coughs.*

**PDF** *Pharmascience, Canad.*
Sodium fluoride (p.1444·3).
*Dental caries prophylaxis.*

**PDP Liquid Protein** *Wesley, USA.*
Tryptophan (p.320·3); hydrolysed animal collagen (p.1674·3).
*Dietary supplement.*

**Peace** *YSP, Malaysia.*
Triprolidine hydrochloride (p.442·3); pseudoephedrine hydrochloride (p.1129·2).
*Rhinitis.*

**Peacef** *Yung Shin, Singapore.*
Triprolidine hydrochloride (p.442·3); pseudoephedrine hydrochloride (p.1129·2).
*Rhinitis.*

**Peacetime** *Lifeplan, UK†.*
Nutritional supplement (p.1417·1).

**Pebegal** *Galen, Mex.*
Benzonatate (p.1115·3).
*Coughs.*

**PEC** *Universal, Hong Kong.*
Promethazine hydrochloride (p.439·1); ephedrine hydrochloride (p.1120·1); codeine phosphate (p.27·1).
*Coughs.*

**Pecasolin** *Rafarm, Gr.*
Lincomycin hydrochloride (p.226·2).
*Bacterial infections.*

**Pe-Ce** *Gebro, Austria.*
Turpentine oil (p.1760·1); eucalyptus oil (p.1686·2); nutmeg oil (p.1722·3); cedar leaf oil; camphor (p.1665·3); thymol (p.1194·2).
*Coughs and cold symptoms.*

**Pe-Ce Ven N** *Terra-Bio, Ger.*
Aescin (p.1648·2); heparin sodium (p.928·1).
*Vascular disorders.*

**Pect Hustenloser** *Rentschler, Ger.†.*
Ambroxol hydrochloride (p.1114·3).
*Respiratory-tract disorders associated with increased or viscous mucus.*

**Pectal** *Sedabel, Braz.*
Sodium dibunate (p.1130·2); aconite (p.1646·3); cineole (p.1672·1); grindelia (p.1696·1); mikania glomerata; senega (p.1130·2).
*Coughs.*

**Pectalin** *EMS, Braz.†.*
Kaolin (p.1268·3); aluminium hydroxide (p.1249·2); pectin (p.1580·3).
*Diarrhoea.*

**Pectamol** *Alpharma, Norw.†.*
Oxeladin citrate (p.1126·1).
*Coughs.*

**Pectapas** *Pascoe, Ger.*
Homoeopathic preparation.

**Pectimax** *Climax, Braz.†.*
Kaolin (p.1268·3); pectin (p.1580·3).
*Diarrhoea.*

**Pectin-K** *PD Pharm, S.Afr.*
Kaolin (p.1268·3); apple pectin (p.1580·3).
*Diarrhoea.*

**Pecto-Baby** *Democal, Switz.*
Guaifenesin (p.1122·1); pholcodine (p.1128·3); chlorphenamine maleate (p.427·3).
*Coughs.*

**Pectobal Dextro** *Clariana, Spain.*
Dextromethorphan hydrobromide (p.1117·3); mepyramine maleate (p.437·1).
*Respiratory-tract disorders.*

**Pectobron** *Sidus, Arg.*
Tiocol; sodium benzoate (p.1169·3); chlorphenamine maleate (p.427·3); senega (p.1130·2); tolu balsam (p.1131·3).
*Bronchitis.*

**Pectocalmine** *Democal, Switz.*
Codeine phosphate (p.27·1); guaifenesin (p.1122·1); ephedrine hydrochloride (p.1120·1); opium (p.74·2); senega (p.1130·2).
*Coughs and associated respiratory-tract disorders.*

**Pectocalmine Junior N** *Democal, Switz.*
Codeine phosphate (p.27·1); tolu balsam (p.1131·3); red-poppy; anethole (p.1654·3).
*Coughs and associated respiratory-tract disorders.*

**Pectocor N** *Riemser, Ger.*
Camphor (p.1665·3).
*Cardiac disorders.*

**Pectoderme** *Dolisos, Fr.*
α-Pinene; β-pinene; myrtol; lavender oil (p.1705·2); terpineol (p.1752·2); eugenol (p.1686·2); camphor (p.1665·3); cineole (p.1672·1).
*Respiratory-tract congestion.*

**Pectodrill** *Pierre Fabre, Spain.*
Carbocisteine (p.1116·2).
*Respiratory-tract disorders associated with viscous secretions.*

**Pectoids** *Medeva, Fr.†.*
Liquorice (p.1270·2); menthol (p.1711·3).
*Sore throat.*

**Pectojuvene** *Cooperation Pharmaceutique, Fr.†.*
Carbocisteine (p.1116·2).
*Respiratory-tract disorders.*

**Pectomucil** *Qualiphar, Belg.*
Acetylcysteine (p.1112·3).
*Paracetamol poisoning; respiratory-tract disorders associated with viscous secretions.*

**Pectoral**
*Note. This name is used for preparations of different composition.*
*Galenogal, Braz.†.*
Rorippa nasturtium aquaticum; pinus palustris oil; guaifenesin (p.1122·1); honey (p.1434·2).
*Coughs.*

*Mepha, Hong Kong.*
Ipecacuanha (p.1122·3); plantago lanceolata (p.1738·2); cowslip (p.1735·1); quillaia (p.1416·1); thyme (p.1755·2); senega (p.1130·2).
*Coughs.*

**Pectoral Brum** *Brum, Spain†.*
Aconite (p.1646·3); tolu balsam (p.1131·3); ipecacuanha (p.1122·3); orange; sodium benzoate (p.1169·3); sulfogaiacol (p.1131·1).
*Respiratory-tract disorders.*

**Pectoral Funk Antitus** *Funk, Spain†.*
Carbocisteine (p.1116·2); chlorphenamine maleate (p.427·3); phenylephrine hydrochloride (p.1126·3); oxolamine citrate (p.1126·1).
*Respiratory-tract disorders.*

**Pectoral Hebert** *Fecofar, Arg.*
Clofedanol (p.1117·1); bromhexine (p.1115·3).
*Coughs.*

**Pectoral N** *Mepha, Switz.*
Plantain (p.1733·1); cowslip (p.1735·1); senega (p.1130·2); thyme (p.1755·2).
Formerly contained ipecacuanha, plantain, primula, senega root, and thyme.
*Cold symptoms; coughs.*

**Pectoral Pagliano** *Lacefa, Arg.*
Sodium benzoate (p.1169·3); sulfogaiacol (p.1131·1).
*Coughs.*

**Pectoral Pasteur** *Pasteur, Chile.*
Sodium benzoate (p.1169·3); ammonium chloride (p.1115·2); drosera (p.1683·1); liquorice (p.1270·2).
*Respiratory-tract disorders.*

**Pectorina** *Fada, Arg.*
Cefalexin (p.168·1).
*Bacterial infections.*

**Pectosan** *Cooperation Pharmaceutique, Fr.†.*
Sulfogaiacol (p.1131·1); codeine (p.27·1); bromoform (p.1663·1); sodium camsilate.
Formerly contained sulfogaiacol, pholcodine, ethylmorphine hydrochloride, belladonna, senega, and sodium benzoate.
*Coughs.*

**Pectosan Ampicilina** *Roche, Spain†.*
Ampicillin trihydrate (p.157·2); ephedrine hydrochloride (p.1120·1).
*Respiratory-tract infections.*

**Pectosan Expectorant** *Cooperation Pharmaceutique, Fr.*
Carbocisteine (p.1116·2).
*Coughs.*

**Pectosan Toux Seche** *Cooperation Pharmaceutique, Fr.*
Pentoxyverine citrate (p.1126·2).
*Coughs.*

**Pectoserum** *Silesia, Chile.*
Codeine phosphate (p.27·1); noscapine hydrochloride (p.1125·3); ammonium chloride (p.1115·2); sodium benzoate (p.1169·3).
*Bronchitis; catarrh; coughs.*

**Pectosorin** *Richter, Austria.*
Sulfogaiacol (p.1131·1).
*Bronchitis; catarrh; coughs.*

**Pectoss** *Heralds, Braz.†.*
Ipecacuanha (p.1122·3); sodium benzoate (p.1169·3); thyme (p.1755·2); poppy (p.1129·1); grindelia (p.1696·1).
*Coughs.*

**Pectothymin** *Planta, Canad.†.*
Aniseed (p.1655·2); thyme (p.1755·2); cowslip (p.1735·1).
*Coughs.*

**Pectotussyl** *Medeva, Fr.†.*
Terpin hydrate (p.1131·1).
*Respiratory-tract disorders.*

**Pectover** *Maver, Chile.*
Diterbutyl napadisilate sodium; ammonium chloride (p.1115·2).
*Coughs.*

**Pectox**
*Italfarmaco, Spain; Piraud, Switz.†; Rhone-Poulenc Rorer, Thai.†.*
Carbocisteine (p.1116·2) or carbocisteine lysine (p.1116·3).
*Respiratory-tract disorders associated with increased or viscous mucus.*

**Pectox Ampicilina** *Italfarmaco, Spain†.*
Carbocisteine (p.1116·2); ampicillin (p.157·1).
*Respiratory-tract infections.*

**Pectramin** *Streuli, Switz.*
Diphenhydramine hydrochloride (p.431·3); ammonium chloride (p.1115·2); menthol (p.1711·3).
*Coughs.*

**Pectrolyte** *Restan, S.Afr.*
Kaolin (p.1268·3); pectin (p.1580·3); chloroform and morphine tincture (p.60·1); sodium lactate; potassium chloride; sodium chloride (p.1222·2).
*Diarrhoea.*

**Pectyl** *Nycomed, Denm.*
Opium (p.74·2); benzoic acid (p.1169·3); camphor (p.1665·3); glycerol (p.1694·3).
*Coughs.*

**Pedameth** *Forest Pharmaceuticals, USA.*
Methionine (p.1042·1).
*Control of odour, dermatitis, and ulceration in incontinent adults; nappy rash.*

**Ped-El**
*Baxter, NZ†; Kabi Pharmacia, NZ†; KabiVitrum, UK†.*
Electrolyte (p.1217·1) and trace element (p.1417·1) preparation.
*Parenteral nutrition.*

**Ped-Element** *Darrow, Braz.*
Electrolyte (p.1217·1) and trace element (p.1417·1) preparation.
*Parenteral nutrition.*

**PediaCare Allergy Formula** *McNeil Consumer, USA.*
Chlorphenamine maleate (p.427·3).

**PediaCare Childrens Multi-Symptom Cold**
*Pharmacia, USA.*
Pseudoephedrine hydrochloride (p.1129·2); chlorphenamine maleate (p.427·3); dextromethorphan hydrobromide (p.1117·3).
*Upper respiratory-tract disorders.*

**PediaCare Cough-Cold** *McNeil Consumer, USA.*
Pseudoephedrine hydrochloride (p.1129·2); chlorphenamine maleate (p.427·3); dextromethorphan hydrobromide (p.1117·3).
*Coughs and cold symptoms.*

**PediaCare Infant's Decongestant** *McNeil Consumer, USA.*
Pseudoephedrine hydrochloride (p.1129·2).
*Nasal congestion.*

**PediaCare NightRest Cough-Cold Formula**
*McNeil Consumer, USA.*
Pseudoephedrine hydrochloride (p.1129·2); chlorphenamine maleate (p.427·3); dextromethorphan hydrobromide (p.1117·3).
*Coughs and cold symptoms.*

**Pediacel** *Aventis Pasteur, UK.*
A diphtheria, tetanus, pertussis (acellular), poliomyelitis (inactivated), and haemophilus influenzae vaccine (p.1615·1).
*Active immunisation.*

**Pediacof** *Sanofi Winthrop, USA.*
Codeine phosphate (p.27·1); phenylephrine hydrochloride (p.1126·3); chlorphenamine maleate (p.427·3); potassium iodide (p.1598·1).
*Coughs.*

**Pedia-Col** *Greater Pharma, Thai.*
*Syrup:* Paracetamol (p.76·2); dextromethorphan hydrobromide (p.1117·3); chlorphenamine maleate (p.427·3).
Formerly contained paracetamol, phenylpropanolamine hydrochloride, dextromethorphan hydrobromide, and chlorphenamine maleate.
*Tablets:* Paracetamol (p.76·2); chlorphenamine maleate (p.427·3).
Formerly contained paracetamol, phenylpropanolamine hydrochloride, and chlorphenamine maleate.
*Cold symptoms.*

**Pediacon DX** *Goldline, USA†.*
Phenylpropanolamine hydrochloride (p.1127·3); guaifenesin (p.1122·1); dextromethorphan hydrobromide (p.1117·3).
*Coughs.*

**Pediacon EX** *Goldline, USA†.*
Phenylpropanolamine (p.1127·3); guaifenesin (p.1122·1).
*Coughs.*

**Pediaderm** *Andromaco, Chile.*
Cod-liver oil (p.1425·2); vitamin A (p.1451·2); vitamin D (p.1461·2); zinc oxide (p.1163·2).
*Burns; skin irritation; wounds.*

**Pediaflor** *Ross, USA.*
Sodium fluoride (p.1444·3).
*Dental caries prophylaxis in children.*

**Pedialyte**
*Abbott, Arg.*
Glucose; fructose; electrolytes (p.1222·2).
*Diarrhoea; oral rehydration therapy.*

*Abbott, Austral.†; Abbott, Braz.; Abbott, Canad.; Abbott, Chile; Abbott, Hong Kong; Abbott, Ital.; Abbott, NZ; Abbott, Singapore; Abbott, Thai.; Ross, USA.*
Glucose and electrolytes (p.1222·2).
*Diarrhoea; oral rehydration therapy.*

**Pediamino PLM** *Braun, Chile.*
Amino-acid infusion (p.1417·1).
*Parenteral nutrition.*

**Pediapirin** *Docta, Spain.*
Paracetamol (p.76·2).
*Fever; pain.*

**Pediapred**
*Aventis, Canad.; Celltech, USA.*
Prednisolone sodium phosphate (p.1108·1).
*Corticosteroid.*

**Pediaprofen** *Laboratorios Chile, Chile.*
Ibuprofen (p.45·3).
*Fever; inflammation; pain.*

**Pediarix** *SmithKline Beecham, USA.*
A diphtheria, tetanus, acellular pertussis, poliomyelitis, and recombinant hepatitis B vaccine (p.1615·2).
*Active immunisation.*

**PediaSure**
*Abbott, Arg.; Abbott, Austral.; Abbott, Braz.; Abbott, Canad.; Abbott, Chile; Abbott, Fin.; Abbott, Hong Kong; Abbott, Ital.; Abbott, Malaysia; Abbott, Mex.; Abbott, NZ; Abbott, Singapore; Abbott, Thai.; Ross, USA.*
Preparation for enteral nutrition in children (p.1417·1).

**Pediatex** *Zyber, USA.*
Carbinoxamine maleate (p.426·3).
*Allergic rhinitis.*

**Pediatex-D** *Zyber, USA.*
Pseudoephedrine hydrochloride (p.1129·2); carbinoxamine maleate (p.426·3).
*Upper respiratory-tract disorders.*

**Pediatex-DM** *Zyber, USA.*
Pseudoephedrine hydrochloride (p.1129·2); carbinoxamine maleate (p.426·3); dextromethorphan hydrobromide (p.1117·3).
*Coughs; upper respiratory-tract disorders.*

**Pedia-Tric** *Neckerman, Braz.†.*
Oral rehydration solution (p.1222·2).

**Pediatric** *Support, Braz.*
A range of preparations for enteral nutrition (p.1417·1).

**Pediatric Cough Syrup** *Technilab, Canad.†.*
Pseudoephedrine hydrochloride (p.1129·2); dextromethorphan hydrobromide (p.1117·3).

**Pediatric Electrolyte** *Pharmascience, Canad.*
Glucose; fructose; potassium citrate; sodium chloride; sodium citrate (p.1222·2).
*Diarrhoea; oral rehydration solution.*

**Pediatric Formula** *Reese, USA†.*
Phenylpropanolamine hydrochloride (p.1127·3); guaifenesin (p.1122·1); dextromethorphan hydrobromide (p.1117·3).

**Pediatrivite** *Seroyal, Canad.†.*
Multivitamin and mineral preparation (p.1417·1).

**Pediatrix** *Technilab, Canad.*
Paracetamol (p.76·2).
*Fever; pain.*

**Pediazole**
*Abbott, Arg.; Abbott, Canad.; Abbott, Chile; Abbott, Fr.; Abbott, Gr.; Abbott, Hong Kong; Abbott, Israel; Abbott, Mex.†; Abbott, S.Afr.†; Ross, USA.*
Erythromycin ethyl succinate (p.208·1); acetyl sulfafurazole (p.260·1).
*Otitis media.*

**Pedi-Bath** *Pedinol, USA†.*
Emollient.

**Pedi-Boro Soak Paks** *Pedinol, USA.*
Aluminium sulfate (p.1653·1); calcium acetate (p.1225·1).
*Skin irritation.*

**Pedic** *Stadmed, India.*
Multivitamin preparation with lysine and zinc (p.1417·1).

**Pedi-Cort V** *Pedinol, USA†.*
Hydrocortisone (p.1103·3); clioquinol (p.196·3).
*Skin disorders.*

**Pedicrem** *Prieto, Arg.*
Aloe vera (p.1141·3); permethrin (p.1508·3); wheat germ.
*Pediculosis.*

**Pedi-Dent** *Stanley, Canad.†.*
Sodium fluoride (p.1444·3).
*Dental caries prophylaxis.*

**Pedi-Dri** *Pedinol, USA.*
Nystatin (p.406·3).
*Candidiasis.*

**Pedifan** *Vilco, Gr.*
Piroxicam (p.84·2).
*Dysmenorrhoea; gout; inflammation; musculoskeletal and joint disorders; pain.*

**Pedigesic** *Parke-Med, S.Afr.†.*
Paracetamol (p.76·2); codeine phosphate (p.27·1); promethazine hydrochloride (p.439·1).
*Fever; pain.*

**Pedikurol** *Ratiopharm, Austria.*
Clotrimazole (p.396·2).
*Fungal skin and nail infections.*

**Pedil** *Salters, S.Afr.†.*
Zinc undecenoate (p.411·1); undecenoic acid (p.410·3).
*Fungal skin infections.*

**Pediletan** *Cimed, Braz.*
Lindane (p.1506·3).
*Pediculosis; scabies.*

**Pedimed** *Restan, S.Afr.*
Aluminium oxide (p.1140·1); magnesium oxide (p.1272·3); methylpolysiloxane (p.1289·2).
*Flatulence associated with hyperacidity.*

**Pediotic** *Monarch, USA.*
Hydrocortisone (p.1103·3); neomycin sulfate (p.235·1); polymyxin B sulfate (p.245·1).
*Bacterial ear infections.*

**Pediox** *Atley, USA.*
Pseudoephedrine hydrochloride (p.1129·2); chlorphenamine maleate (p.427·3).
*Upper respiratory-tract disorders.*

**Pedi-Pro** *Pedinol, USA.*
Aluminium chlorohydrate (p.1142·1); chloroxylenol (p.1177·2); menthol (p.1711·3); zinc undecenoate (p.411·1).
*Fungal skin infections; minor skin disorders.*

**Pediron** *ST, Thai.*
Ferrous sulfate (p.1428·2).
*Iron-deficiency anaemia.*

**Pedisafe** *BASF, Ger.†.*
Clotrimazole (p.396·2).
*Fungal infections.*

**Pedisol** *Fischer, Israel.*
*Cream:* Triclosan (p.1195·2); panthenol (p.1727·2); chamomile (p.1669·3); wool fat (p.1483·1).
*Dry skin; hard skin.*

*Topical spray:* Undecenoic acid (p.410·3); aluminium chlorohydrate (p.1142·1); menthol (p.1711·3); purified talc (p.1159·1).
*Foot odour.*

**Peditrace**
*Fresenius Kabi, Austria; Fresenius Kabi, Denm.; Fresenius Kabi, Fin.; Baxter, Ger.; Fresenius Kabi, Gr.; Fresenius Kabi, Hong Kong; Pharmacia Upjohn, Irl.†; Pharmacia Upjohn, Israel; Fresenius Kabi, Ital.; Fresenius Kabi, Neth.; Fresenius Kabi, Norw.; Baxter, NZ; Fresenius Kabi, NZ; Fresenius Kabi, Port.; Fresenius Kabi, S.Afr.†; Fresenius Kabi, Singapore; Fresenius Kabi, Swed.; Fresenius Kabi, Switz.; Fresenius Kabi, UK.*
Trace element preparation (p.1417·1).
*Parenteral nutrition.*

**Peditral** *RPG, India.*
Sodium chloride; potassium chloride; sodium citrate; anhydrous glucose (p.1222·2).
*Oral rehydration therapy.*

**Pedituss Cough** *Major, USA.*
Phenylephrine hydrochloride (p.1126·3); chlorphenamine maleate (p.427·3); codeine phosphate (p.27·1); potassium iodide (p.1598·1).
*Coughs.*

**Pedi-Vit-A** *Pedinol, USA.*
Vitamin A (p.1451·2).
*Irritated or dry skin.*

**Pedoc** *Ranbaxy, Thai.†.*
Docusate sodium (p.1262·2).
*Constipation.*

**Pedopur** *Jacoby, Austria.*
Vitis vinifera.
*Peripheral vascular disorders.*

**Pedoz** *Hamilton, Austral.*
Tetrabromocresol (p.1193·3); undecenoic acid (p.410·3); zinc undecenoate (p.411·1); zinc oxide (p.1163·2).
*Hyperhidrosis; skin irritation; tinea pedis.*

**Pedpain** *Aspen, S.Afr.*
Paracetamol (p.76·2); codeine phosphate (p.27·1); promethazine hydrochloride (p.439·1).
*Fever; pain.*

**Pedriachol** *Propan, S.Afr.†.*
Phenobarbital (p.367·3); pipenzolate bromide (p.487·3).
*Gastrointestinal disorders.*

**PedTE-PAK** *SoloPak, USA.*
Trace element preparation (p.1417·1).
*Parenteral nutrition.*

**Pedtrace** *American Pharmaceutical, USA.*
Trace element preparation (p.1417·1).
*Parenteral nutrition.*

**PedvaxHIB**
*Merck Sharp & Dohme, Arg.; Merck Sharp & Dohme, Austral.; Merck Sharp & Dohme, Braz.; Merck Frosst, Canad.; Chiron Behring, Ger.; Merck Sharp & Dohme, Hong Kong; Merck Sharp & Dohme, Israel; Merck Sharp & Dohme, Malaysia; Merck Sharp & Dohme, Mex.; Merck Sharp & Dohme, Singapore; Pasteur Merieux, Swed.†; Merck Sharp & Dohme, Thai.; Merck, USA.*
A haemophilus influenzae conjugate vaccine (meningococcal protein conjugate) (p.1616·1).
*Active immunisation.*

**Pedvitin** *Greater Pharma, Thai.*
Multivitamin preparation (p.1417·1).

**PeeHoo** *Orion, Fin.*
Aluminium hydroxide-magnesium carbonate co-dried gel (p.1250·1).
*Gastric hyperacidity.*

**Peerless Composition Essence** *Potter's, UK.*
Oak bark (p.1722·3); pinus canadensis; poplar bark (p.1733·3); prickly ash bark (p.1766·3); bayberry bark (p.1659·2).
*Colds.*

**Pefamic** *PP Lab, Thai.*
Mefenamic acid (p.55·2).
*Pain.*

**Pefbid** *Alembic, India.*
Pefloxacin (p.241·3).
*Bacterial infections.*

**Peflacin**
*Aventis, Braz.; Rhone-Poulenc Rorer, Ger.†; Aventis, Ital.*
Pefloxacin mesilate (p.241·3).
*Bacterial infections.*

**Peflacina** *Aventis, Mex.*
Pefloxacin mesilate (p.241·3).
*Bacterial infections.*

**Peflacine**
*Rhone-Poulenc Rorer, Austria†; Aventis, Belg.†; Aventis, Fr.; Aventis, Gr.; Rhone-Poulenc Rorer, Hong Kong†; Rhone-Poulenc Rorer, Israel†; Aventis, Malaysia; Aventis, Port.; Aventis, Spain; Aventis, Thai.*
Pefloxacin mesilate (p.241·3).
*Bacterial infections.*

**Peflox** *Formenti, Ital.*
Pefloxacin mesilate (p.241·3).
*Bacterial infections.*

**Pefloxidina** *Teuto, Braz.*
Pefloxacin mesilate (p.241·3).
*Bacterial infections.*

**Pefrakehl** *Sanum-Kehlbeck, Ger.*
Homoeopathic preparation.

**Pega** *Bailleul, Fr.*
Potassium and arginine phosphocitroglutamate.
*Asthenia.*

**Peganix** *Baliarda, Arg.*
Piroxicam (p.84·2); prednisone (p.1109·3).
*Inflammation.*

**Peganone** *Ovation, USA.*
Ethotoin (p.361·1).
*Epilepsy.*

**Pegasys**
*Roche, Braz.; Roche, Chile; Roche, Fr.; Roche, Irl.; Roche, NZ; Roche, Port.; Roche, Switz.; Roche, UK; Roche, USA.*
Peginterferon alfa-2a (p.643·1).
*Chronic hepatitis C.*

**Pegatron** *Schering-Plough, Austral.*
Capsules, ribavirin (Rebetol) (p.652·1); injection, peginterferon alfa-2b (PEG-Intron) (p.643·1).
*Chronic hepatitis C.*

**Pegina** *Potter's, UK.*
Calumba (p.1665·2); calamus (p.1664·1); compound cardamom tincture (p.1667·3); magnesium sulfate (p.1228·2); magnesium trisilicate (p.1272·3); rhubarb (p.1287·3).
*Dyspepsia; flatulence.*

**PegIntron**
*Schering-Plough, Austral.; Schering-Plough, Belg.; Schering-Plough, Braz.; Schering, Canad.; Schering-Plough, Chile; Schering-Plough, Denm.; Schering-Plough, Fin.; Essex, Ger.; Schering-Plough, Gr.; Schering-Plough, Hong Kong; Schering-Plough, Irl.; Schering-Plough, Israel; Schering-Plough, Ital.; Schering-Plough, Neth.; Schering-Plough, Norw.; Schering-Plough, Port.; Schering-Plough, Spain; Schering-Plough, Swed.; Schering-Plough, UK; Schering, USA.*
Peginterferon alfa-2b (rbe) (p.643·1).
*Chronic hepatitis C.*

**Peglyte**
Note. This name is used for preparations of different composition.
*Pharmascience, Canad.*
Macrogol 3350 (p.1709·1); electrolytes (p.1217·1).
*Bowel evacuation; constipation.*

*Pharmascience, Hong Kong.*
Electrolytes (p.1217·1).
*Gastrointestinal lavage.*

**Peinfort** *Ebewe, Austria.*
Paracetamol (p.76·2).
*Fever; pain.*

**Peitel** *Novag, Spain.*
Prednicarbate (p.1107·3).
*Skin disorders.*

**Peitoral Angico Pelotense** *CIF, Braz.*
Iceland moss; althaea (p.1651·3); cuscuta umbellata; mallow (p.1709·3); liquorice (p.1270·2); piptadenia colubrina; ammonium chloride (p.1115·2); tolu balsam (p.1131·3); sodium benzoate (p.1169·3).
*Respiratory-tract congestion.*

**Pekamin** *Medical, Spain†.*
Benzylpenicillin sodium (p.163·2).
*Bacterial infections.*

**Peking Ginseng Royal Jelly N** *Peking-Boell, Ger.*
Ginseng (p.1693·1); honey; royal jelly.
*Tonic.*

**Peking Royal Jelly N** *Peking-Boell, Ger.*
Royal jelly (p.1740·3); codonopsis pilosulae; honey.
*Tonic.*

**Pekiron** *Kyorin, Jpn.*
Amorolfine hydrochloride (p.391·1).
*Fungal skin infections.*

**Pel Cupron** *Asmopul, Arg.*
Porcine skin (p.1158·1).
*Burns.*

**Pelargon**
*Nestle, Fr.; Nestle, Ital.*
Infant feed (p.1417·1).
*Gastrointestinal disorders.*

**Peledox** *Novartis Consumer, Spain.*
Doxycycline hyclate (p.206·2).
*Bacterial infections; malaria.*

**Pelicrep** *Raffo, Arg.*
Finasteride (p.1554·2).
*Alopecia.*

**Pelina** *MIP, Ger.*
Dexpanthenol (p.1727·2).
*Skin and mucous membrane lesions.*

**Peliphane** *Saninter, Port.†.*
Piroctone olamine (p.1155·2); melaleuca oil (p.1710·2).
*Seborrhoeic dermatitis.*

**Pellexeme** *Coup, Gr.*
Ketotifen fumarate (p.788·1).
*Allergic rhinitis; asthma.*

**Pellit**
*Engelhard, Hong Kong; Asta Medica, Thai.*
Diphenhydramine hydrochloride (p.431·3); diethyltoluamide (p.1503·3); dimethyl phthalate (p.1504·1).
*Allergic skin reactions; insect bites; insect repellent.*

**Pellit dermal Wund- und Heilsalbe** *Engelhard, Ger.†.*
Tyrothricin (p.275·1); fomocaine hydrochloride (p.1376·3); diphenhydramine hydrochloride (p.431·3).
*Infected skin disorders.*

**Pellit Insektenstich, Pellit Sonnenallergie**
*Engelhard, Ger.†.*
Diphenhydramine hydrochloride (p.431·3).
*Allergic skin reactions; insect stings; minor burns.*

**Pellit Sonnenbrand** *Engelhard, Ger.†.*
Hamamelis (p.1696·3).
*Skin lesions and inflammation; sunburn.*

**Pelmec** *Casasco, Arg.*
Amlodipine besilate (p.862·1).
*Angina pectoris; hypertension.*

**Pelmec Duo** *Casasco, Arg.*
Amlodipine besilate (p.862·1); benazepril hydrochloride (p.867·2).
*Hypertension.*

**Pelmic** *Breves, Braz.†.*
Diphenylpyraline (p.432·3); methyl hydroxybenzoate (p.1183·3); propyl hydroxybenzoate (p.1183·3); alcohol (p.1166·1).
*Skin disinfection.*

**Pelo Libre**
Note. This name is used for preparations of different composition.
*GlaxoSmithKline, Arg.*
Acetic acid (p.1645·2).

*GlaxoSmithKline, Arg.*
Permethrin (p.1508·3).
*Pediculosis.*

**Pelox** *Wockhardt, India.*
Pefloxacin (p.241·3).
*Bacterial infections.*

**Pelsana Med** *Schmidgall, Austria.*
*Bath oil:* Sunflower oil (p.1451·1); undecenoic acid (p.410·3).
Formerly known as Pelsano.
*Ointment:* Sunflower oil (p.1451·1); dexpanthenol (p.1727·2).
Formerly known as Pelsano.
*Topical powder:* Zinc undecenoate (p.411·1).
Formerly known as Pelsano.
*Skin disorders.*

**Pelsano**
Note. This name is used for preparations of different composition.
*Wolfs, Belg.†.*
Undecenoic acid (p.410·3); zinc stearate (p.1575·3).
*Skin disorders.*

*Iromedica, Switz.*
*Bath additive:* Sunflower oil (p.1451·1); undecenoic acid (p.410·3).
*Ointment:* Sunflower oil (p.1451·1); dexpanthenol (p.1727·2).
*Skin disorders.*

**Pelson** *Berenguer Infale, Spain†.*
Nitrazepam (p.710·1).
*Insomnia.*

**Peltazon** *Grelan, Jpn.*
Pentazocine hydrochloride (p.79·3).
*Fever; inflammation; pain.*

**Pelvichthol** *Ichthyol, Austria†.*
Ictasol (p.1148·3); benzyl nicotinate (p.21·2); homofenazine hydrochloride (p.703·1).
*Urogenital disorders.*

**Pelvichthol N** *APS, Ger.*
Ictasol (p.1148·3); benzyl nicotinate (p.21·2).
*General pelvic symptoms.*

**Pelvo Magnesium** *3M, Belg.†.*
Onion (p.1723·2); magnesium carbonate (p.1272·1) or magnesium chloride (p.1228·1).
*Painful pelvic congestion in females; prostate and micturition disorders in men.*

**PemADD** *Mallinckrodt, USA.*
Pemoline (p.1591·2).
*Attention-deficit hyperactivity disorder.*

**Pemar** *Medipharm, Chile.*
Piroxicam (p.84·2).
*Inflammation; pain.*

**Pemine** *Lilly, Ital.*
Penicillamine hydrochloride (p.1049·1).
*Cystinuria; lead poisoning; rheumatoid arthritis; Wilson's disease.*

**PE-Mix** *Fresenius Kabi, Austria.*
Amino-acid, carbohydrate, electrolyte, and lipid (as soya oil (p.1447·2)) infusion (p.1417·1).
Contains egg lecithin.
*Parenteral nutrition.*

**Pemix** *Prodes, Spain†.*
Pirozadil (p.984·1).
*Hyperlipidaemias.*

**Pemol** *Chinta, Thai.*
Paracetamol (p.76·2).
*Fever; pain.*

**Pen** *ABZ, Ger.*
Phenoxymethylpenicillin potassium (p.242·1).
*Bacterial infections.*

**Pen di Ben** *Bago, Arg.*
Benzathine benzylpenicillin (p.162·3).
Lidocaine hydrochloride (p.1377·3) is included in this preparation to alleviate the pain of injection.
*Bacterial infections.*

**Pen Mega** *1A, Ger.*
Phenoxymethylpenicillin potassium (p.242·1).
*Bacterial infections.*

**Pen Oral** *Aventis, Arg.*
Phenoxymethylpenicillin (p.242·1).
*Bacterial infections.*

**Penaderm** *Johnson & Johnson, Ger.†.*
Urea (p.1162·2).
*Dry skin.*

**Penadur**
*Wyeth Lederle, Belg.; Wyeth, Gr.; Wyeth Lederle, Port.; Wyeth, Singapore†; Wyeth-Ayerst, Thai.*
Benzathine benzylpenicillin (p.162·3).
*Bacterial infections.*

**Penadur 6.3.3** *Wyeth Lederle, Port.*
Benzathine benzylpenicillin (p.162·3); benzylpenicillin potassium (p.163·2); procaine benzylpenicillin (p.246·1).
*Bacterial infections.*

**Penagrand** *Ahimsa, Arg.*
Phenoxymethylpenicillin (p.242·1).
*Bacterial infections.*

**Penalta** *Bristol-Myers Squibb, Fin.*
Amoxicillin trihydrate (p.155·3).
*Bacterial infections.*

**Penamox**
*SmithKline Beecham, Mex.; Douglas, NZ†; Tecnimede, Port.*
Amoxicillin sodium (p.155·3) or amoxicillin trihydrate (p.155·3).
*Bacterial infections.*

**Penamox M** *SmithKline Beecham, Mex.*
Amoxicillin trihydrate (p.155·3); bromhexine (p.1115·3).
*Respiratory-tract infections.*

**Penanyst** *PCR, Ger.*
Zinc oxide (p.1163·2); nystatin (p.406·3).
*Skin disorders with fungal infections.*

**Penaten**
Note. This name is used for preparations of different composition.
*Johnson & Johnson, Canad.*
Hamamelis (p.1696·3); zinc oxide (p.1163·2).

*Johnson & Johnson, Ger.*
Thyme oil (p.1755·3).
*Respiratory-tract disorders.*

**Penatoel** *PCR, Ger.*
Soya oil (p.1447·2).
*Dry skin; skin irritation.*

**Penbaccin** *Raza, Malaysia; Pharmaniaga, Malaysia.*
Bacampicillin hydrochloride (p.161·2).
*Bacterial infections.*

**Pen-BASF** *BASF, Ger.†.*
Phenoxymethylpenicillin potassium (p.242·1).
*Bacterial infections.*

**Penbene** *Ratiopharm, Austria.*
Phenoxymethylpenicillin potassium (p.242·1).
*Bacterial infections.*

**Penbeta** *Betapharm, Ger.*
Phenoxymethylpenicillin potassium (p.242·1).
*Bacterial infections.*

**Penbritin**
*Bencard, Belg.†; Wyeth-Ayerst, Canad.†; GlaxoSmithKline, Hong Kong; GlaxoSmithKline, Irl.; Hormona, Mex.; GlaxoSmithKline, S.Afr.; SmithKline Beecham, Singapore†; GlaxoSmithKline, Thai.; GlaxoSmithKline, UK.*
Ampicillin (p.157·1), ampicillin sodium (p.157·1), or ampicillin trihydrate (p.157·2).
*Bacterial infections.*

**Penclox** *Pisa, Mex.*
Dicloxacillin (p.205·2).
*Bacterial infections.*

**Pencom** *Alembic, India.*
Benzathine benzylpenicillin (p.162·3).
*Bacterial infections.*

**Pencor** *Unison, Thai.*
Doxazosin mesilate (p.908·3).
*Benign prostatic hyperplasia; hypertension.*

**Pencotrex** *Hua, Thai.*
Ampicillin trihydrate (p.157·2).
*Bacterial infections.*

**Pendiben Compuesto** *Pisa, Mex.*
Benzylpenicillin sodium (p.163·2); procaine benzylpenicillin (p.246·1); benzathine benzylpenicillin (p.162·3).
*Bacterial infections.*

**Pendine** *Alphapharm, Austral.*
Gabapentin (p.362·2).
*Epilepsy.*

**Pendium** *Zekides, Gr.*
Buspirone hydrochloride (p.672·2).
*Generalised anxiety.*

**Pendramine** *Asta Medica, UK†.*
Penicillamine (p.1046·3).
*Cystinuria; heavy-metal poisoning; hepatitis; rheumatoid arthritis; Wilson's disease.*

**Pendysin** *Jenapharm, Ger.*
Benzathine benzylpenicillin (p.162·3).
Lidocaine hydrochloride (p.1377·3) is included in this preparation to alleviate the pain of injection.
*Chronic streptococcal infections; syphilis.*

**Penecare**
*Penederm, Canad.†; Reed & Carnrick, USA.*
Emollient.

**Penecort** *Allergan, USA.*
Hydrocortisone (p.1103·3).
*Skin disorders.*

**Penederm** *Penederm, Canad.*
*Cream:* Lactic acid (p.1704·1); light liquid paraffin (p.1479·1).
*Lotion:* Lactic acid (p.1704·1).
*Dry skin.*

**Penedil** *Teva, Israel.*
Felodipine (p.914·3).
*Angina pectoris; hypertension.*

**Penegra** *Zydus, India.*
Sildenafil citrate (p.1744·2).
*Erectile dysfunction.*

**Pener** *Unison, Thai.*
Phenoxymethylpenicillin (p.242·1).
*Bacterial infections.*

**Penetran** *IMA, Braz.†.*
Naphazoline (p.1124·3); diphenhydramine (p.431·3); neomycin (p.235·1).
*Nasal congestion.*

**Penetrating Rub** *Golden Pride, Canad.†; Rawleigh, Canad.†.*
Methyl salicylate (p.59·3); menthol (p.1711·3); eucalyptus oil (p.1686·2); cajuput oil (p.1664·1); expressed mustard oil (p.1718·2).

**Penetrex** *Rhone-Poulenc Rorer, USA.*
Enoxacin (p.207·2).
*Gonorrhoea; urinary-tract infections.*

**Penetro** *Daudt, Braz.*
*Inhalation:* Terpineol (p.1752·2); cineole (p.1672·1); menthol (p.1711·3); benzoic acid (p.1169·3).
*Oral solution:* Ambroxol hydrochloride (p.1114·3); menthol (p.1711·3); cineole (p.1672·1).
*Respiratory-tract congestion.*

**Penfantil** *Klonal, Arg.*
Phenoxymethylpenicillin (p.242·1).
*Bacterial infections.*

**Penfill N** *Novo Nordisk, Jpn.*
Isophane insulin (human, recombinant) (p.333·3).
*Diabetes mellitus.*

**Penfill R** *Novo Nordisk, Jpn.*
Insulin injection (human, recombinant) (p.333·3).
*Diabetes mellitus.*

**Penfill 10R, 20R, 30R, 40R, 50R** *Novo Nordisk, Jpn.*
Mixtures of insulin injection (human, recombinant) 10%, 20%, 30%, 40%, and 50% and isophane insulin injection (human, recombinant) 90%, 80%, 70%, 60%, and 50% respectively (p.333·3).
*Diabetes mellitus.*

**Pengesic** *Hovid, Singapore.*
Tramadol hydrochloride (p.94·3).
*Pain.*

**Pengesod** *Lakeside, Mex.*
Benzylpenicillin sodium (p.163·2).
*Bacterial infections.*

**Penglobe**
*AstraZeneca, Austria; Astra, Belg.†; AstraZeneca, Canad.; Lundbeck, Denm.†; AstraZeneca, Fr.; Astra, Ger.†; AstraZeneca, Hong Kong; AstraZeneca, India; AstraZeneca, Ital.; AstraZeneca, Malaysia; Astra, Mex.; AstraZeneca, Singapore†; AstraZeneca, Spain; Astra, Swed.; AstraZeneca, Thai.*
Bacampicillin hydrochloride (p.161·2).
*Bacterial infections.*

**Penhexal** *Hexal, Ger.*
Phenoxymethylpenicillin potassium (p.242·1).
*Bacterial infections.*

**Penhexal VK** *Hexal, Austral.*
Phenoxymethylpenicillin potassium (p.242·1).
*Bacterial infections.*

**Penibiot** *Normon, Spain.*
Benzylpenicillin sodium (p.163·2).
*Bacterial infections.*

**Penibiot Lidocaina** *Normon, Spain†.*
Benzylpenicillin sodium (p.163·2).
Lidocaine hydrochloride (p.1377·3) is included in this preparation to alleviate the pain of injection.
*Bacterial infections.*

**Penibrin** *Biogal, Israel.*
Ampicillin (p.157·1).
*Bacterial infections.*

**Penicigran** *Legrand, Braz.*
Phenoxymethylpenicillin potassium (p.242·1).
*Bacterial infections.*

**Penicil** *Rimsa, Mex.*
Procaine benzylpenicillin (p.246·1); benzylpenicillin sodium (p.163·2).
*Bacterial infections.*

**Penicil Dermol** *Gador, Arg.*
Procaine benzylpenicillin (p.246·1).
*Bacterial skin infections.*

**Penicillat** *Azupharma, Ger.*
Phenoxymethylpenicillin potassium (p.242·1).
*Bacterial infections.*

**Penicillin Fortified** *Vitamed, Israel.*
Procaine benzylpenicillin (p.246·1); benzylpenicillin sodium (p.163·2).
*Bacterial infections.*

**Penicina** *Epicaris, Arg.*
Phenoxymethylpenicillin potassium (p.242·1).
*Bacterial infections.*

**Penidural** *Yamanouchi, Neth.*
Benzathine benzylpenicillin (p.162·3).
*Bacterial infections.*

**Penidural D/F** *Yamanouchi, Neth.*
Benzathine benzylpenicillin (p.162·3); procaine benzylpenicillin (p.246·1); benzylpenicillin potassium (p.163·2).
*Bacterial infections.*

**Penidure** *Wyeth, India.*
Benzathine benzylpenicillin (p.162·3).
*Bacterial infections.*

**Penilan** *Vitoria, Port.*
Amoxicillin trihydrate (p.155·3); potassium clavulanate (p.193·3).
*Bacterial infections.*

**Penilente Forte** *Novo Nordisk, S.Afr.*
Benzathine benzylpenicillin (p.162·3); procaine benzylpenicillin (p.246·1); benzylpenicillin sodium (p.163·2).
*Bacterial infections.*

**Penilente LA** *Novo Nordisk, S.Afr.*
Benzathine benzylpenicillin (p.162·3).
*Bacterial infections.*

**Penilevel** *Ern, Spain.*
*Capsules; oral sachets:* Phenoxymethylpenicillin potassium (p.242·1).
*Injection:* Benzylpenicillin sodium (p.163·2).
*Bacterial infections.*

**Penilevel Retard** *Ern, Spain.*
Benzylpenicillin sodium (p.163·2); benzathine benzylpenicillin (p.162·3); phenoxymethylpenicillin calcium (p.242·1).
*Bacterial infections; rheumatic fever.*

**Penilfedrin P** *Lerson, Arg.*
Benzylpenicillin potassium (p.163·2).
*Bacterial eye infections.*

**Penimox** *IBSA, Switz.*
Amoxicillin (p.155·3) or amoxicillin trihydrate (p.155·3).
*Bacterial infections.*

**Peni-Oral** *Wyeth Lederle, Belg.†.*
Phenoxymethylpenicillin potassium (p.242·1).
*Bacterial infections.*

**Penipot** *Antibioticos, Mex.*
Procaine benzylpenicillin (p.246·1); benzylpenicillin (p.163·2).
*Bacterial infections.*

**Peniroger** *UCB, Spain.*
Benzylpenicillin sodium (p.163·2).
*Bacterial infections.*

**Penisintex Bronquial** *Jorba, Spain.*
Ampicillin sodium (p.157·1); ampicillin benzathine (p.158·1); bromhexine (p.1115·3).
Lidocaine hydrochloride (p.1377·3) is included in this preparation to alleviate the pain of injection.
*Respiratory-tract infections.*

**Penisodina** *Pisa, Mex.*
Procaine benzylpenicillin (p.246·1); benzylpenicillin (p.163·2).
*Bacterial infections.*

**Penisol**
Note. This name is used for preparations of different composition.
*Fustery, Mex.*
Benzylpenicillin sodium (p.163·2).
*Bacterial infections.*

*Ecosol, Switz.*
Phenoxymethylpenicillin potassium (p.242·1).
*Bacterial infections.*

**Penkaron** *Ariston, Braz.*
Benzylpenicillin potassium (p.163·2); procaine benzylpenicillin (p.246·1).
*Bacterial infections.*

**Pen-Kera** *Ascher, USA.*
Emollient and moisturiser.

**Penlac** *Dermik, USA.*
Ciclopirox (p.396·1).
*Fungal nail infections.*

**Penles** *Wyeth Lederle, Jpn.*
Lidocaine (p.1377·3).
*Pain of inserting intravenous needles.*

**Penlol** *Pose, Thai.*
Pentoxifylline (p.979·3).
*Peripheral vascular disorders.*

**Penmix 10, 20, 30, 40, or 50**
*Novo Nordisk, Gr.; Novo Nordisk, NZ.*
Mixtures of insulin injection (human) 10%, 20%, 30%, 40%, or 50% and isophane insulin (human) 90%, 80%, 70%, 60% or 50% respectively (p.333·3).
*Diabetes mellitus.*

**Penmox** *Aspen, S.Afr.*
Amoxicillin (p.155·3).
*Bacterial infections.*

**Pennsaid** *Dimethaid, UK.*
Diclofenac sodium (p.32·1).
*Osteoarthritis.*

**Penntuss** *Rhone-Poulenc Rorer, Canad.†.*
Codeine polistirex (p.27·3); chlorphenamine polistirex (p.428·1).
*Allergic rhinitis; coughs and cold symptoms.*

**Pen-Os** *Biochemie, Austria.*
Benzathine phenoxymethylpenicillin (p.163·2).
*Bacterial infections.*

**Penotran** *Merck, Hong Kong.*
Hydrargaphen (p.1182·2); potassium dinaphthylmethanedisulfonate.
*Vaginal infections.*

**Penoxil V** *Raza, Malaysia; Pharmaniaga, Malaysia.*
Phenoxymethylpenicillin potassium (p.242·1).
*Bacterial infections.*

**Penprocilina** *Lakeside, Mex.*
Benzylpenicillin sodium (p.163·2); procaine benzylpenicillin (p.246·1).
*Bacterial infections.*

**Penrazol** *Elpen (Ελπεν), Gr.*
Omeprazole (p.1278·2).
*Acid aspiration; eradication of Helicobacter pylori in combination with antimicrobials; peptic ulcer; reflux oesophagitis; Zollinger-Ellison syndrome.*

**Penrazole** *Elpen, Singapore.*
Omeprazole (p.1278·2).
*Gastro-oesophageal reflux; gastrointestinal hypersecretion; peptic ulcer.*

**Penrite** *Columbia, S.Afr.†.*
Ampicillin trihydrate (p.157·2).
*Bacterial infections.*

**Pensodital** *Wayne, Mex.†.*
Thiopental (p.1310·1).

**Penstad** *Stada, Austria.*
Phenoxymethylpenicillin potassium (p.242·1).
*Bacterial infections.*

**Penstapho**
*Bristol-Myers Squibb, Belg.; Bristol-Myers Squibb, Ital.*
Oxacillin sodium (p.240·2).
*Gram-positive bacterial infections.*

**Penstaphon** *Bristol-Myers Squibb, Belg.*
Cloxacillin sodium (p.198·2).
Formerly known as Penstapho N.
*Staphylococcal infections.*

**Pensulan** *Andromaco, Chile.*
Bacitracin zinc (p.161·3); neomycin sulfate (p.235·1); zinc oxide (p.1163·2); aluminium hydroxide (p.1249·2).
*Skin infections.*

**Pensulvit** *SIFI, Ital.*
Tetracycline (p.266·2); sulfamethylthiazole (p.263·1).
*Bacterial eye infections.*

**Penta 500**
*Pediatrica, Malaysia; Pediatrica, Singapore.*
Vitamin B substances; lysine hydrochloride (p.1417·1).
*Tonic.*

**Penta-3B** *Sabex, Canad.*
Thiamine hydrochloride (p.1455·1); pyridoxine hydrochloride (p.1456·3); cyanocobalamin (p.1458·2).
*Alcoholism; neuritis; vitamin B supplement.*

**Penta-3B + C** *Sabex, Canad.*
Thiamine hydrochloride (p.1455·1); pyridoxine hydrochloride (p.1456·3); cyanocobalamin (p.1458·2); ascorbic acid (p.1460·2).
*Alcoholism; neuritis; vitamin supplement.*

**Penta-3B Plus** *Sabex, Canad.*
Multivitamin preparation (p.1417·1).

**Pentabil** *OFF, Ital.*
Fenipentol (p.1687·2).
*Hepatic and biliary-tract disorders.*

**Pentacard**
*Byk, Belg.†; Pacific, Thai.†.*
Isosorbide mononitrate (p.942·1).
*Angina pectoris.*

**Pentacarinat**
*Gerot, Austria; Aventis, Belg.; Aventis, Braz.; Aventis, Canad.; Aventis, Denm.; Aventis, Fin.; Aventis, Fr.; Aventis, Ger.; GlaxoSmithKline, Ger.; Rhone-Poulenc Rorer, Gr.; Aventis, Irl.; Aventis, Israel; Aventis, Ital.; Aventis, Neth.; Aventis, Norw.†; Aventis, NZ; Aventis, Port.; Aventis, S.Afr.†; Aventis, Spain; Aventis, Swed.; Aventis, Switz.; Aventis, Thai.; JHC Healthcare, UK; Armour, USA.*
Pentamidine isetionate (p.613·2).
*African trypanosomiasis; leishmaniasis; Pneumocystis carinii pneumonia.*

**Pentacel** *Aventis Pasteur, Canad.*
Vial, a haemophilus influenzae conjugate vaccine (tetanus toxoid conjugate)(Act-HIB); ampoule, a diphtheria, tetanus, pertussis, and poliomyelitis vaccine (Quadracel) (p.1615·1).
*Active immunisation.*

**Pentacine** *Via, Switz.†.*
Pentamycin (p.407·3).
*Vaginitis.*

**Pentacis** *Schering, UK.*
Technetium-99m pentetate (p.1525·2).
*Assessment of renal function; radionuclide imaging of the brain and lungs; studies of gastro-oesophageal reflux and gastric emptying.*

**Pentacol** *Sofar, Ital.*
Mesalazine (p.1273·2).
*Crohn's disease; ulcerative colitis.*

**Pentacoq** *Aventis Pasteur, Fr.*
Vial, a haemophilus influenzae conjugate vaccine (tetanus toxoid conjugate) (Act-HIB); syringe, a diphtheria, tetanus, pertussis, and poliomyelitis vaccine (Tetracoq) (p.1615·1).
*Active immunisation.*

**Pentacort** *Life, Ger.*
Betamethasone valerate (p.1093·2).
*Skin disorders.*

**Pentacrom** *Penta, Ger.*
Sodium cromoglicate (p.795·3).
*Allergic eye disorders.*

**Pentact** *Aventis Pasteur, Braz.*
A diphtheria, tetanus, pertussis, poliomyelitis, and haemophilus influenzae vaccine (p.1615·1).
*Active immunisation.*

**Pentact-HIB**
*Aventis Pasteur, Chile; Aventis Pasteur, Hong Kong; Pasteur Merieux, Israel; Aventis Pasteur, Thai.*
A diphtheria, tetanus, pertussis, poliomyelitis, and haemophilus influenzae conjugate vaccine (p.1615·1).
*Active immunisation.*

**Pentadecan** *Viatris, Ger.*
Pentadecanoic acid glyceride.
*Alopecia.*

**Pentadent** *Careiatrics, Arg.*
Hexetidine (p.1182·1); benzydamine (p.21·1).
*Mouth disorders.*

**Pentaderm** *Dermatech, Austral.*
Methoxsalen (p.1152·1).

**Pentafresh** *Careiatrics, Arg.*
Sodium fluoride (p.1444·3).
*Dental caries prophylaxis.*

**Pentagin** *Sankyo, Jpn.*
Pentazocine hydrochloride (p.79·3).
*Fever; inflammation; pain.*

**Pentaglobin**
*Biogam, Arg.; Biotest, Austria; Marcos Pedrilson, Braz.†; Pentafarma, Chile; Biotest, Ger.; Biotest, Hong Kong; Biotest, Ital.; Biotest, Malaysia; Precimex, Mex.†; Mednostica, S.Afr.; Biotest, Singapore; Biotest, Switz.; Biotest, Thai.*
Immunoglobulins (M, A, and G) (p.1627·2).
*Immunodeficiency; Kawasaki disease; thrombocytopenia.*

**Pentaglucano** *Biosan, Ital.†.*
Lactic-acid-producing organisms (p.1704·2); vitamin B substances (p.1417·1).
*Maintenance of normal gastrointestinal flora.*

**Pental Forte** *Cederroth, Spain.*
Benzalkonium chloride (p.1168·3); mafenide (p.228·2); sulfanilamide (p.263·2); zinc oxide (p.1163·2).
*Skin infections.*

**Pentalgina** *Pierrel, Ital.†.*
Pentazocine lactate (p.79·3).
*Pain.*

**Pentalmicina** *Cederroth, Spain†.*
Enoxolone (p.36·2); mafenide (p.228·2); neomycin sulfate (p.235·1); sulfanilamide (p.263·2).
*Skin infections.*

**Pentalong** *Alpharma-Isis, Ger.*
Pentaerithrityl tetranitrate (p.979·1).
*Angina pectoris.*

**Pentam**
*Pisa, Mex.†; American Pharmaceutical, USA.*
Pentamidine isetionate (p.613·2).
*Leishmaniasis; Pneumocystis carinii pneumonia; trypanosomiasis.*

**Pentamina** *Faulding, Port.*
Pentamidine isetionate (p.613·2).

**Pentamol** *Penta, Ger.*
Salbutamol sulfate (p.791·3).
*Obstructive airways disease.*

**Pentamycetin** *Sabex, Canad.*
Chloramphenicol (p.185·1).
*Eye infections.*

**Pentamycetin-HC** *Sabex, Canad.*
Chloramphenicol (p.185·1); hydrocortisone acetate (p.1103·3).
*Eye and ear infections.*

**Pentasa**
*Ferring, Arg.; Ferring, Austria; Ferring, Belg.; Ferring, Braz.†; Ferring, Canad.; Ferring, Chile; Ferring, Denm.; Ferring, Fin.; Ferring, Fr.; Ferring, Ger.; Gerolimatos (Γερολυματος), Gr.; Ferring, Hong Kong; Ferring, Irl.; Ferring, Israel; Ferring, Ital.; Kyorin, Jpn; Ferring, Malaysia; IQFA, Mex.; Ferring, Neth.; Ferring, Norw.; Ferring, NZ; Pharmaco, NZ; Ferring, Port.; Ferring, S.Afr.; Ferring, Singapore; Ferring, Spain; Ferring, Swed.; Ferring, Switz.; Ferring, UK; Roberts, USA.*
Mesalazine (p.1273·2).
*Inflammatory bowel disease.*

**Pentaspan**
*Aventis, Braz.; Du Pont, Canad.; Aventis, Mex.; Boots Healthcare, NZ; Geistlich, UK†; Du Pont, USA.*
Pentastarch (p.750·1) in sodium chloride.
*Leucopheresis; plasma volume expansion.*

**Penta-Thion** *Sabex, Canad.*
Ascorbic acid (p.1460·2); thiamine hydrochloride (p.1455·1).
*Vitamin supplement.*

**Pentatop** *Life, Ger.*
Sodium cromoglicate (p.795·3).
*Hypersensitivity reactions.*

**Pentavac**
*Aventis Pasteur, Fr.; Aventis Pasteur, Ger.; Aventis Pasteur, Irl.; Aventis Pasteur, Ital.; Aventis Pasteur, Spain; Aventis Pasteur, Swed.; Pro Vaccine, Switz.*
A diphtheria, tetanus, pertussis, poliomyelitis, and haemophilus influenzae vaccine (p.1615·1).
*Active immunisation.*

**Pentavite** *Nicholas Piramal, India.*
Ferrous gluconate (p.1428·1); vitamin B substances; calcium gluconate (p.1417·1).
*Anaemia.*

**Penta-Vite Chewable Multi Vitamins with Minerals** *Roche Consumer, Austral.†.*
Multivitamin and mineral preparation (p.1417·1).

**Penta-Vite Childrens Vitamins with Iron** *Roche Consumer, Austral.†.*
Multivitamin preparation with iron (p.1417·1).

**Penta-Vite Infant Vitamins** *Roche Consumer, Austral.†.*
Multivitamin preparation (p.1417·1).

**Pentavitol** *Nycomed, Austria†.*
Multivitamin preparation (p.1417·1).

**Pentawin** *Biochem, India.*
Pentazocine lactate (p.79·3).
*Pain; premedication.*

**Pentazine VC with Codeine** *Century, USA.*
Promethazine hydrochloride (p.439·1); codeine phosphate (p.27·1).
*Coughs and cold symptoms.*

**Pentazole** *Profarb, Braz.†.*
Mebendazole (p.108·2).
*Worm infections.*

**Pentcillin** *Toyama, Jpn.*
Piperacillin sodium (p.243·1).
Lidocaine (p.1377·3) is included in the intramuscular injection to alleviate the pain of injection.
*Bacterial infections.*

**Pent-HIBest** *Aventis Pasteur, Fr.†.*
Vial, a haemophilus influenzae conjugate vaccine (tetanus toxoid conjugate) (HIBest) (p.1616·1); syringe, a diphtheria, tetanus, pertussis, and poliomyelitis vaccine (DTCP) (p.1615·1).
*Active immunisation.*

**Penthotal** *Abbott, Chile.*
Thiopental sodium (p.1309·1).
*Convulsions; general anaesthesia; sedative.*

**Penthrox** *Medical Developments, Austral.*
Methoxyflurane (p.1304·1).
*Pain.*

**Pentibrom** *Maver, Mex.*
Ampicillin trihydrate (p.157·2); bromhexine hydrochloride (p.1115·3).
*Bacterial infections.*

**Pentibroxil** *Maver, Mex.*
Amoxicillin trihydrate (p.155·3); ambroxol hydrochloride (p.1114·3).
*Bacterial infections.*

**Penticlox** *Maver, Mex.*
Amoxicillin (p.155·3).
*Bacterial infections.*

**Penticort** *Wyeth Lederle, Fr.*
Amcinonide (p.1091·1).
*Skin disorders.*

**Penticort Neomycine** *Lederle, Fr.†.*
Amcinonide (p.1091·1); neomycin sulfate (p.235·1).
*Infected skin disorders.*

**Pentidix** *Maver, Mex.*
Ampicillin (p.157·1); dicloxacillin (p.205·2).
*Bacterial infections.*

**Pentids** *Sarabhai Piramal, India.*
Benzylpenicillin potassium (p.163·2).
*Bacterial infections.*

**Pentilzeno** *BA Farma, Port.†.*
Diltiazem hydrochloride (p.900·1).
*Angina pectoris; arrhythmias; heart failure; hypertension.*

**Pentiver** *Maver, Mex.*
Ampicillin (p.157·1).
*Bacterial infections.*

**Pento** *ABZ, Ger.*
Pentoxifylline (p.979·3).
*Peripheral vascular disorders.*

**Pentoclave** *Defuen, Arg.*
Erythromycin (p.208·1).
*Acne.*

**Pentoflux** *Bouchara-Recordati, Fr.*
Pentoxifylline (p.979·3).
*Intermittent claudication; mental function impairment in the elderly.*

**Pentohexal**
*Hexal, Austria; Hexal, Ger.*
Pentoxifylline (p.979·3).
*Peripheral vascular disorders.*

**Pentolab** *Frasca, Arg.*
Pentoxifylline (p.979·3).

**Pentolair** *Bausch & Lomb, USA.*
Cyclopentolate hydrochloride (p.480·3).

**Pentomer** *Ratiopharm, Austria.*
Pentoxifylline (p.979·3).
*Cerebral, ocular and peripheral vascular disorders; ear disorders.*

**Pento-Puren** *Alpharma-Isis, Ger.*
Pentoxifylline (p.979·3).
*Peripheral vascular disorders.*

**Pentorel** *Khandelwal, India.*
Buprenorphine hydrochloride (p.21·3).
*Pain; premedication.*

**Pentostam**
*Wellcome, Israel; GlaxoSmithKline, UK.*
Sodium stibogluconate (p.600·3).
*Leishmaniasis.*

**Pentothal**
*Abbott, Arg.; Abbott, Austral.; Abbott, Belg.; Abbott, Canad.; Abbott, Denm.; Abbott, Fin.; Abbott, Hong Kong; Abbott, Israel; Abbott, Ital.; Abbott, Mex.; Abbott, Norw.; Abbott, NZ†; Abbott, Singapore; Abbott, Spain; Abbott, Swed.; Abbott, Switz.; Abbott, Thai.; Abbott, USA.*
Thiopental sodium (p.1309·1).
*Convulsions; general anaesthesia; sedative.*

**Pentovena** *Iquinosa, Spain.*
Hidrosmin (p.1688·3).
*Peripheral vascular disorders.*

**Pentox**
*Farmasa, Braz.; CT, Ger.*
Pentoxifylline (p.979·3).
*Cerebral and peripheral vascular disorders.*

**Pentoxi**
*Genericon, Austria; Mepha, Switz.*
Pentoxifylline (p.979·3).
*Vascular disorders.*

**Pentoximed** *S Med, Austria.*
Pentoxifylline (p.979·3).
*Peripheral vascular disorders.*

**Pentoxin** *Ratiopharm, Fin.*
Pentoxifylline (p.979·3).
*Peripheral vascular disorders.*

**Pentoxy** *Heumann, Ger.*
Pentoxifylline (p.979·3).
*Peripheral vascular disorders.*

**Pentrax**
*Note. This name is used for preparations of different composition.*
*Medicis, Canad.; Dermapharm, Irl.; Dermapharm, UK; GenDerm, USA.*
Coal tar (Fractar) (p.1159·2).
*Scalp disorders.*

*Johnson & Johnson, Ital.†.*
Coal tar (Fractar) (p.1159·2); salicylic acid (p.1157·1).
*Seborrhoeic dermatitis.*

**Pentrax Gold** *GenDerm, USA†.*
Coal tar (p.1159·2).
*Scalp disorders.*

**Pentrexyl**
*Bristol-Myers Squibb, Belg.; Bristol-Myers Squibb, Denm.; Bristol-Myers Squibb, Gr.; Bristol-Myers Squibb, Hong Kong; Bristol-Myers Squibb, Israel†; Bristol-Myers Squibb, Ital.; Bristol-Myers Squibb, Mex.; Bristol-Myers Squibb, Neth.; Bristol-Myers Squibb, Norw.; Bristol-Myers Squibb, Swed.†; Bristol-Myers Squibb, Thai.*
Ampicillin (p.157·1), ampicillin sodium (p.157·1), or ampicillin trihydrate (p.157·2).
*Bacterial infections.*

**Pentrexyl Expec** *Bristol-Myers Squibb, Mex.*
Ampicillin trihydrate (p.157·2); ambroxol acefyllinate (p.1114·3).
*Bacterial infections of the respiratory tract.*

**Pen-V**
*Lannacher, Austria; Genericon, Austria.*
Phenoxymethylpenicillin potassium (p.242·1).
*Bacterial infections.*

*Atlantic, Hong Kong†; Atlantic, Thai.; General Drugs, Thai.*
Phenoxymethylpenicillin (p.242·1).
*Bacterial infections.*

**pen-V-basan** *Schonenberger, Switz.*
Phenoxymethylpenicillin potassium (p.242·1).
*Bacterial infections.*

**Pen-Vee** *Lioh, Canad.*
Benzathine phenoxymethylpenicillin (p.163·2) or phenoxymethylpenicillin (p.242·1).
*Bacterial infections.*

**Pen-Vee K** *Wyeth-Ayerst, USA.*
Phenoxymethylpenicillin potassium (p.242·1).
*Bacterial infections.*

**Penveno** *Milano, Thai.*
Phenoxymethylpenicillin (p.242·1).
*Bacterial infections.*

**Pen-Ve-Oral** *Eurofarma, Braz.*
Phenoxymethylpenicillin potassium (p.242·1).
*Bacterial infections.*

**Penvicilin** *Gemballa, Braz.*
Amoxicillin (p.155·3).
*Bacterial infections.*

**Pen-Vi-K** *Wyeth, Mex.*
Phenoxymethylpenicillin potassium (p.242·1).
*Bacterial infections.*

**Penvir** *Sigma, Braz.*
Famciclovir (p.633·2).
*HIV infection.*

**Pen-V-Merck** *Merck dura, Ger.†.*
Phenoxymethylpenicillin potassium (p.242·1).
*Bacterial infections.*

**PEP** *Galpharm, UK.*
Glucose (p.1432·2); caffeine (p.782·1).
*Fatigue.*

**Pepcid**
*Merck Sharp & Dohme, Austral.; Merck Sharp & Dohme, Austria; Merck Frosst, Canad.; Johnson & Johnson, Canad.; Pharmacia, Fin.; Woelm, Ger.; Merck Sharp & Dohme, Hong Kong†; Merck Sharp & Dohme, Irl.; Pharmacia, Neth.; Pharmacia, Norw.; Merck Sharp & Dohme, NZ; Merck Sharp & Dohme, S.Afr.†; Abello, Spain; Pharmacia, Swed.; Merck Sharp & Dohme, Switz.; Johnson & Johnson MSD Consumer, UK; J&J-Merck, USA; Merck, USA.*
Famotidine (p.1265·2).
*Dyspepsia; gastro-oesophageal reflux; heartburn; peptic ulcer; Zollinger-Ellison syndrome.*

**Pepcid Complete**
Johnson & Johnson, Canad.; Johnson & Johnson, USA.
Famotidine (p.1265·2); calcium carbonate (p.1254·2); magnesium hydroxide (p.1272·2).
*Dyspepsia; heartburn.*

**Pepcid Duo**
Pharmacia, Fin.; Pharmacia, Swed.
Famotidine (p.1265·2); magnesium hydroxide (p.1272·2); calcium carbonate (p.1254·2).
*Dyspepsia; heartburn.*

**Pepcidac** Martin, Fr.
Famotidine (p.1265·2).
*Gastro-oesophageal reflux.*

**Pepciddual**
Woelm, Ger.; Merck Sharp & Dohme, Ital.
Famotidine (p.1265·2); magnesium hydroxide (p.1272·2); calcium carbonate (p.1254·2).
*Gastrointestinal disorders associated with hyperacidity; gastro-oesophageal reflux.*

**Pepcidduo**
Martin-Johnson & Johnson, Fr.; Pharmacia, Norw.
Famotidine (p.1265·2); magnesium hydroxide (p.1272·2); calcium carbonate (p.1254·2).
*Gastro-oesophageal reflux; heartburn.*

**Pepcidin**
Merck Sharp & Dohme, Denm.; Merck Sharp & Dohme, Fin.; Merck Sharp & Dohme, Neth.; Merck Sharp & Dohme, Norw.; Merck Sharp & Dohme, Swed.
Famotidine (p.1265·2).
*Gastro-oesophageal reflux; peptic ulcer; Zollinger-Ellison syndrome.*

**Pepcidina** Frosst, Port.
Famotidine (p.1265·2).
*Gastric hyperacidity; gastro-oesophageal reflux; peptic ulcer; Zollinger-Ellison syndrome.*

**Pepcidine**
Merck Sharp & Dohme, Austral.; Merck Sharp & Dohme, Austria; Merck Sharp & Dohme, Belg.; Merck Sharp & Dohme, Hong Kong; Merck Sharp & Dohme, Malaysia; Merck Sharp & Dohme, Mex.; Merck Sharp & Dohme, NZ; Merck Sharp & Dohme, Singapore; Merck Sharp & Dohme, Switz.; Merck Sharp & Dohme, Thai.
Famotidine (p.1265·2).
*Gastro-oesophageal reflux; peptic ulcer; Zollinger-Ellison syndrome.*

**Pepcidtwo** Johnson & Johnson MSD Consumer, UK.
Calcium carbonate (p.1254·2); magnesium hydroxide (p.1272·2); famotidine (p.1265·2).
*Dyspepsia; heartburn.*

**Pepcine** Masa, Thai.
Famotidine (p.1265·2).
*Gastro-oesophageal reflux; peptic ulcer; Zollinger-Ellison syndrome.*

**Pepdenal** Macrophar, Thai.
Famotidine (p.1265·2).
*Gastro-oesophageal reflux; peptic ulcer; Zollinger-Ellison syndrome.*

**Pepdine** Merck Sharp & Dohme-Chibret, Fr.
Famotidine (p.1265·2).
*Gastro-oesophageal reflux; peptic ulcer; Zollinger-Ellison syndrome.*

**Pepdite**
Scientific Hospital Supplies, Irl.†; Scientific Hospital Supplies, UK.
Infant feed (p.1417·1).
*Bowel disorders; malabsorption syndromes; protein or lactose intolerance.*

**Pepdual** Abello, Spain.
Famotidine (p.1265·2); calcium carbonate (p.1254·2); magnesium hydroxide (p.1272·2).
*Gastric hyperacidity; gastro-oesophageal reflux.*

**Pepdul** MSD Chibropharm, Ger.
Famotidine (p.1265·2).
*Peptic ulcer; Zollinger-Ellison syndrome.*

**Pepevit** Diba, Mex.
Nicotinic acid (p.1441·1).
*Hypercholesterolaemia; pellagra.*

**Pepfamin** Siam Bheasach, Thai.
Famotidine (p.1265·2).
*Peptic ulcer; Zollinger-Ellison syndrome.*

**Pepp** Theranol-Deglaude, Fr.†.
Dimethicone (p.1289·2); aluminium hydroxide (p.1249·2); magnesium hydroxide (p.1272·2).
*Gastrointestinal disorders.*

**Pep-Rani** Medinfar, Port.
Ranitidine hydrochloride (p.1285·2).
*Gastric hyperacidity; gastro-oesophageal reflux; peptic ulcer; Zollinger-Ellison syndrome.*

**Peprazol** Libbs, Braz.
Omeprazole (p.1278·2).
*Gastro-oesophageal reflux; gastrointestinal hyperacidity; peptic ulcer.*

**Pepsaletten N** Riemser, Ger.
Glutamic acid hydrochloride (p.1433·2).
*Gastrointestinal disorders.*

**Pepsamar**
Gador, Arg.; Sanofi Synthelabo, Braz.; SmithKline Beecham, Gr.; Lepori, Port.; Sanofi Synthelabo, Spain.
Aluminium hydroxide (p.1249·2).
*Dyspepsia; gastro-oesophageal reflux; gastrointestinal hyperacidity; hyperphosphataemia.*

**Pepsamar Plus** Lepori, Port.
Aluminium hydroxide (p.1249·2); magnesium hydroxide (p.1272·2).
*Gastrointestinal disorders.*

**Pepsane** Rosa-Phytopharma, Fr.
Guaiazulene (p.1696·2); dimeticone (p.1289·2).
*Gastrointestinal disorders.*

**Pepsicaps** Hertz, Braz.†.
Omeprazole (p.1278·2).
*Peptic ulcer.*

**Pepsidol** Laboratorios Chile, Chile.
Simeticone (p.1289·2).
*Abdominal distension; flatulence.*

**Pepsitase** Hua, Thai.
Pepsin (p.1729·3); amylase (p.1654·2); papain (p.1727·3); gentian (p.1692·2); pancreatin (p.1725·3); activated charcoal (p.1030·2); vitamin $B_1$.
*Digestive disorders.*

**Pepsiton** Unipack, Austria.
Pepsin (p.1729·3); absinthium (p.1645·1).
*Gastrointestinal disorders.*

**Pepsivit** Gemballa, Braz.
Carnitine (p.1423·3); buclizine (p.426·3); vitamin B substances (p.1417·1).
*Reduced appetite; tonic.*

**Pepsogel** Legrand, Braz.
Aluminium hydroxide (p.1249·2); magnesium hydroxide (p.1272·2); simeticone (p.1289·2).
*Flatulence; gastrointestinal hyperacidity.*

**Pepsytoin** Pond's, Thai.
Phenytoin sodium (p.370·2).
*Epilepsy.*

**Peptab** Aventis, Port.
Ranitidine hydrochloride (p.1285·2).
*Gastro-oesophageal reflux; gastrointestinal haemorrhage; peptic ulcer; Zollinger-Ellison syndrome.*

**Peptac** Ivax, UK.
Sodium alginate (p.1577·1); sodium bicarbonate (p.1223·2); calcium carbonate (p.1254·2).
*Gastro-oesophageal reflux; heartburn; hiatus hernia.*

**Peptamen**
Nestle Clinical, Irl.; Nestle, Israel; Nestle, Ital.; Nestle, Malaysia; Nestle, Thai.; Nestle, UK; Carnation, USA.
Preparation for enteral nutrition (p.1417·1).
*Gastrointestinal disorders.*

**Peptan** Vianex (Βιανέξ), Gr.
Famotidine (p.1265·2).
*Conditions where gastric acid reduction is beneficial; gastric hypersecretion including Zollinger-Ellison syndrome; peptic ulcer.*

**Peptavlon**
Wyeth-Ayerst, Canad.†; Cambridge, Fr.†; Zeneca, Switz.†; Ayerst, USA†.
Pentagastrin (p.1729·3).
*Test of gastric secretory function.*

**Peptazol**
Montpellier, Arg.; Recordati, Ital.
Pantoprazole sodium (p.1283·1).
*Gastro-oesophageal reflux; peptic ulcer; Zollinger-Ellison syndrome.*

**Peptgel** Teuto, Braz.
Aluminium hydroxide (p.1249·2).
*Antacid.*

**Pepti-2000**
Nutricia, Austral.†; Nutricia, Port.†.
Preparation for enteral nutrition (p.1417·1).
*Malabsorption syndromes.*

**Pepti-2000 LF** Nutricia, Irl.†.
Preparation for enteral nutrition (p.1417·1).

**Peptic Guard** Genpharm, Canad.
Famotidine (p.1265·2).

**Peptic Relief**
Note. This name is used for preparations of different composition.
Genpharm, Canad.†.
Ranitidine hydrochloride (p.1285·2).

Rugby, USA.
Bismuth salicylate (p.1252·1).
*Gastrointestinal disorders.*

**Peptica** Unison, Thai.
Cimetidine (p.1255·3).
*Peptic ulcer; Zollinger-Ellison syndrome.*

**Pepticaine** Parke, Davis, India.
Oxetacaine (p.1382·1); magnesium hydroxide (p.1272·2); aluminium hydroxide (p.1249·2); simeticone (p.1289·2).
*Gastritis; gastro-oesophageal reflux; peptic ulcer.*

**Peptical** 3-OL, Israel.
Fructose (p.1431·3); glucose (p.1432·2); phosphoric acid (p.1731·2).
*Nausea and vomiting.*

**Peptichemio** Nuovo ISM, Ital.†.
Multialchilpeptide (p.576·2).
*Myeloproliferative disorders.*

**Pepticum**
Grunenthal, Chile; Andromaco, Spain.
Omeprazole (p.1278·2).
*Gastro-oesophageal reflux; peptic ulcer; Zollinger-Ellison syndrome.*

**Pepticus** Montpellier, Arg.
Omeprazole (p.1278·2).
*Acid aspiration; gastro-oesophageal reflux; peptic ulcer; Zollinger-Ellison syndrome.*

**Peptiditutteli** Valio, Fin.
Infant feed (p.1417·1).
*Cow's milk and soya protein intolerance.*

**Peptifar** Tecnimede, Port.
Ranitidine hydrochloride (p.1285·2).

**Pepti-Junior**
Nutricia, Austral.; Nutricia, Fin.; Nutricia, Fr.; Cow & Gate, Irl.; Cow & Gate, Israel; Nutricia, Ital.; Baxter, NZ; Nutricia, NZ; Nutricia, Port.; Cow & Gate, UK.
Food for special diets (p.1417·1).
*Diarrhoea; food intolerance; malabsorption.*

**Peptimax** Ashbourne, UK.
Cimetidine (p.1255·3).
*Gastrointestinal disorders.*

**Peptinal** Laboratorios Chile, Chile.
*Oral suspension:* Aluminium hydroxide (p.1249·2); magnesium hydroxide (p.1272·2); simeticone (p.1289·2).
*Tablets:* Aluminium hydroxide (p.1249·2); magnesium carbonate (p.1272·1); magnesium hydroxide (p.1272·2); simeticone (p.1289·2).
*Gastritis; gastro-oesophageal reflux; hyperphosphataemia; peptic ulcer.*

**Peptinal Forte** Laboratorios Chile, Chile.
Simeticone (p.1289·2); aluminium hydroxide (p.1249·2); magnesium hydroxide (p.1272·2); magnesium carbonate (p.1272·1).
*Flatulence; gastric hyperacidity; gastritis; gastro-oesophageal reflux.*

**Peptinaut** Nutricia, Ital.†.
Preparation for enteral nutrition (p.1417·1).

**Peptinex** Novartis Nutrition, USA.
Preparation for enteral nutrition (p.1417·1).

**Peptireal** Novartis Nutrition, Fr.†.
A range of preparations for enteral nutrition (p.1417·1).

**Peptison**
Support, Braz.; Nutricia, Ital.†; Nutricia, Port.†.
Preparation for enteral nutrition (p.1417·1).

**Peptisorb**
Nutricia, Austral.; Nutricia, Fin.; Nutricia, Ital.; Baxter, NZ; Nutricia, NZ; Nutricia, Port.; Pfrimmer Nutricia, Switz.†; Nutricia Clinical, UK.
Range of preparations for enteral nutrition (p.1417·1).

**Peptizole** LSP, Thai.†.
Omeprazole (p.1278·2).
*Gastro-oesophageal reflux; peptic ulcer; Zollinger-Ellison syndrome.*

**Pepto Diarrhea Control** Procter & Gamble, USA.
Loperamide hydrochloride (p.1271·1).
*Diarrhoea.*

**Pepto-Bismol**
Note. This name is used for preparations of different composition.
Procter & Gamble, Braz.; Procter & Gamble, Canad.; Procter & Gamble, Mex.; Procter & Gamble (H&B Care), UK; Procter & Gamble, USA.
Bismuth salicylate (p.1252·1).
*Diarrhoea; dyspepsia; heartburn; nausea; upset stomach.*

Procter & Gamble, Canad.
*Tablets:* Calcium carbonate (p.1254·2); bismuth salicylate (p.1252·1).
*Diarrhoea; dyspepsia; nausea; upset stomach.*

**Peptoci** Pharmasant, Thai.
Famotidine (p.1265·2).
*Peptic ulcer; Zollinger-Ellison syndrome.*

**Peptol** Carter Horner, Canad.†.
Cimetidine (p.1255·3).
*Gastric acid hypersecretion.*

**Peptomet** Remedica, Thai.
Domperidone (p.1263·2).
*Delayed gastric emptying; gastro-oesophageal reflux.*

**Peptonorm** Unipharma, Gr.
Sucralfate (p.1290·2).
*Peptic ulcer.*

**Peptonum** Linfar, Arg.
Bovine amino acids and polypeptides (p.1417·1).
*Dietary supplement.*

**Peptopancreasi** Dansk-Flama, Braz.
Pepsin (p.1729·3); pancreatin (p.1725·3).
*Digestive system disorders.*

**Pepto-Pancreasi** SIT, Ital.
Pepsin (p.1729·3); pancreatin (p.1725·3).
*Digestive system disorders.*

**Peptulan** Farmasa, Braz.
Bismuth citrate (p.1252·1).
*Gastritis; gastrointestinal hyperacidity; peptic ulcer.*

**Pepzan**
Douglas, Hong Kong†; Douglas, Malaysia; Douglas, NZ; Douglas, Singapore; Douglas, Thai.; TTN, Thai.
Famotidine (p.1265·2).
*Peptic ulcer; Zollinger-Ellison syndrome.*

**Pepzitrat** Berlin-Chemie, Ger.
Pepsin (p.1729·3); citric acid (p.1673·1).
*Gastrointestinal disorders.*

**Pepzol** APS, Port.
Lansoprazole (p.1269·3).
*Gastro-oesophageal reflux; peptic ulcer.*

**Peracel** Monot, Fr.†.
Loperamide hydrochloride (p.1271·1).
*Diarrhoea.*

**Peracil** Boniscontro & Gazzone, Ital.
Piperacillin sodium (p.243·1).
Lidocaine hydrochloride (p.1377·3) is included in this preparation to alleviate the pain of injection.
*Bacterial infections.*

**Peracon**
Note. This name is used for preparations of different composition.
Solvay, Austria†.
Isoaminile citrate (p.1123·3).
*Coughs.*

Recalcine, Chile.
Cyproheptadine hydrochloride (p.430·1); carnitine hydrochloride; lysine hydrochloride (p.1417·1).
*Reduced appetite.*

Solvay, Gr.
Isoaminile (p.1123·3).
*Cough.*

Aventis, S.Afr.
Isoaminile cyclamate (p.1123·3).
*Coughs.*

**Peracon Expectorant** Aventis, S.Afr.
Isoaminile cyclamate (p.1123·3); ammonium chloride (p.1115·2).
*Coughs.*

**Peragit** Gea, Denm.
Trihexyphenidyl hydrochloride (p.490·2).
*Drug-induced extrapyramidal disorders; parkinsonism.*

**Peralgin** Infabra, Braz.†.
Phenylbutazone calcium (p.84·1).
*Gout; musculoskeletal, joint, and peri-articular disorders.*

**Peran** BASF, Ger.†.
Acemetacin (p.11·3).
*Gout; inflammation; musculoskeletal, joint, and peri-articular disorders.*

**Perasian** Asian Pharm, Thai.
Loperamide hydrochloride (p.1271·1).
*Diarrhoea.*

**Perasthman N** CHR, Ger.†.
Theophylline (p.798·3).
*Obstructive airways disease.*

**Perative**
Note. This name is used for preparations of different composition.
Giscard, Arg.
Ketoconazole (p.403·3).
*Fungal infections.*

Abbott, Austral.; Abbott, Braz.; Abbott, Fr.; Abbott, Hong Kong; Abbott, Irl.; Ross, Israel; Abbott, Ital.; Abbott, Mex.; Abbott Nutrition, UK.
Preparation for enteral nutrition (p.1417·1).

**Peratsin** Orion, Fin.
Perphenazine (p.714·2), perphenazine decanoate (p.714·2), or perphenazine enantate (p.714·2).
*Psychoses.*

**Perbel** Medipharma, Arg.
Benzyl benzoate (p.1500·2); permethrin (p.1508·3).
*Pediculosis.*

**Perbilen** Aventis, Spain.
Piretanide (p.983·3).
*Hypertension; oedema.*

**Percapyl** GlaxoSmithKline, Arg.
Permethrin (p.1508·3).
*Pediculosis.*

**Percas** Elvetium, Arg.
Etoposide (p.551·3).
*Malignant neoplasms.*

**Perchloracap** Mallinckrodt, USA.
Potassium perchlorate (p.1602·3).
*To reduce accumulation of pertechnetate by the choroid plexus, salivary glands, and thyroid.*

**Perclar** Parke, Davis, Ital.
Mesoglycan sodium (p.1714·1).
*Thrombosis prophylaxis.*

**Perclusone** SERB, Fr.†.
Clofezone (p.26·3); clofexamide hydrochloride (p.26·3).
*Musculoskeletal, joint, peri-articular, and soft-tissue disorders; superficial phlebitis.*

**Percocet**
Du Pont, Canad.; Taro, Israel; Endo, USA.
Oxycodone hydrochloride (p.75·2); paracetamol (p.76·2).
*Pain.*

**Percodan**
Du Pont, Canad.
Oxycodone hydrochloride (p.75·2); aspirin (p.15·1).
*Fever; inflammation; pain.*

Taro, Israel; Endo, USA.
Oxycodone hydrochloride (p.75·2); oxycodone terephthalate (p.75·2); aspirin (p.15·1).
*Pain.*

**Percoffedrinol N** Passauer, Ger.
Caffeine (p.782·1).
*Fatigue.*

**Percogesic** Richardson-Vicks, USA.
Paracetamol (p.76·2); phenyltoloxamine citrate (p.439·1).
*Fever; pain.*

**Percolone** Endo, USA.
Oxycodone hydrochloride (p.75·2).
*Pain.*

**Percorina** Boehringer Ingelheim, Spain†.
Isosorbide mononitrate (p.942·1).
*Angina pectoris.*

**Percutafeine**
Pierre Fabre, Arg.; Asta Medica, Braz.; Pierre Fabre Sante, Fr.
Caffeine (p.782·1).
*Obesity.*

**Percutalgine**
Besins, Belg.; Besins, Fr.; Piette, Thai.
Dexamethasone (p.1097·1) or dexamethasone acetate (p.1097·1); salicylamide (p.87·3); glycol salicylate (p.44·3); methyl nicotinate (p.59·2).
*Musculoskeletal, joint, peri-articular, and soft-tissue disorders.*

**Percutalin** Almirall, Spain†.
Dexamethasone (p.1097·1) or dexamethasone acetate (p.1097·1); salicylamide (p.87·3); glycol salicylate (p.44·3); methyl nicotinate (p.59·2).
*Musculoskeletal, joint, peri-articular, and soft-tissue disorders.*

**Percutase N** *Godecke, Ger.†.*
Glycol salicylate (p.44·3); benzyl nicotinate (p.21·2).
Formerly contained glycol salicylate, heparin, benzyl nicotinate, and nonivamide.
*Musculoskeletal and joint disorders.*

**Percutol** *Pliva, UK.*
Glyceryl trinitrate (p.923·2).
*Angina pectoris.*

**Perderm**
*Schering-Plough, Hong Kong; Schering-Plough, Malaysia; Schering-Plough, Singapore.*
Alclometasone dipropionate (p.1090·3).
*Skin disorders.*

**Perdiem** *Novartis Consumer, USA.*
Ispaghula (p.1268·1); senna (p.1288·2).
*Constipation.*

**Perdiem Fiber** *Novartis Consumer, USA†.*
Ispaghula (p.1268·1).
*Constipation.*

**Perdiphen** *Spitzner, Ger.*
Ephedrine hydrochloride (p.1120·1); paracetamol (p.76·2); diphenylpyraline hydrochloride (p.432·3).
*Influenza symptoms.*

**Perdiphen phyto** *Spitzner, Ger.†; Schwabe, Ger.†.*
Cowslip rhizome (p.1735·1); thyme (p.1755·2).
*Cold symptoms.*

**Perdipina** *Yamanouchi, Ital.*
Nicardipine hydrochloride (p.965·1).
*Angina pectoris; heart failure; hypertension.*

**Perdipine** *Yamanouchi, Jpn.*
Nicardipine hydrochloride (p.965·1).
*Cerebrovascular disorders; heart failure; hypertension.*

**Perdix**
*Alpharma, Denm.†; Alpharma, Fin.†; Schwarz, Irl.; Medis, Israel; Omnimed, S.Afr.; Dumex-Alpharma, Swed.†; Schwarz, UK.*
Moexipril hydrochloride (p.961·2).
*Hypertension.*

**Perdogrip** *Janssen-Cilag, Belg.*
Paracetamol (p.76·2); vitamin C (p.1460·2).
*Cold symptoms.*

**Perdolan** *Janssen-Cilag, Belg.*
Paracetamol (p.76·2).
Formerly known as Perdolan Mono.
*Fever; pain.*

**Perdolan Codeine** *Janssen-Cilag, Belg.*
Paracetamol (p.76·2); codeine phosphate (p.27·1).
Formerly known as Perdolan Duo.
*Pain.*

**Perdolan Compositum** *Janssen-Cilag, Belg.*
*Suppositories (infant and child):* Aspirin (p.15·1); paracetamol (p.76·2); codeine phosphate (p.27·1).
*Tablets; Suppositories (adult):* Aspirin (p.15·1); paracetamol (p.76·2); caffeine (p.782·1); codeine phosphate (p.27·1).
*Fever; pain.*

**Perdolan Mono C** *Janssen-Cilag, Belg.*
Paracetamol (p.76·2); ascorbic acid (p.1460·2).
*Fever; pain.*

**Perduretas Codeina** *Medea, Spain.*
Codeine phosphate (p.27·1).
*Cough; diarrhoea; pain.*

**Perebron**
*Laboratorios Chile, Chile; Angelini, Ital.; Farma Lepori, Spain†.*
Oxolamine citrate (p.1126·1) or oxolamine phosphate (p.1126·1).
*Adjunct in obstructive airways disease; coughs.*

**Pereflat** *Solvay, Fr.†.*
Dimeticone (p.1289·2); pancreas extract (porcine).
*Dyspepsia; flatulence.*

**Peremesin**
*Bristol-Myers Squibb, Ger.; Meda, Norw.*
Meclozine hydrochloride (p.436·3).
Formerly contained meclozine hydrochloride and caffeine in *Norw.*
*Nausea; vertigo; vomiting.*

**Peremesin N** *Bristol-Myers Squibb, Ger.*
Meclozine hydrochloride (p.436·3).
Formerly contained meclozine hydrochloride and caffeine.
*Nausea; vertigo; vomiting.*

**Peremin** *Novartis, Austria†.*
Paracetamol (p.76·2); pheniramine maleate (p.438·3); phenylephrine hydrochloride (p.1126·3); ascorbic acid (p.1460·2).
*Cold and influenza symptom.*

**Perenal** *Medicus, Gr.*
Lisinopril (p.946·3).
*Heart failure; hypertension; myocardial infarction.*

**Perenan**
*Sanofi Synthelabo, Fr.†; Sanofi Synthelabo, Hong Kong; Sanofi Synthelabo, Singapore†; Sanofi Synthelabo, Thai.*
Co-dergocrine mesilate (p.1674·1).
*Behavioural and psychological disorders in the elderly.*

**Perennia** *Wyeth Lederle, Austria.*
Conjugated oestrogens (p.1543·2); medroxyprogesterone acetate (p.1557·2).
*Menopausal disorders; osteoporosis.*

**Perental** *BPL-Meizler, Braz.*
Pentoxyfylline (p.979·3).
*Cerebral and peripheral vascular disorders.*

**Perenterol**
*Biodiphor, Belg.†; Thiemann, Ger.; Biomed, Switz.*
*Saccharomyces boulardii* (p.1704·2).
*Diarrhoea; restoration of gastrointestinal flora; vitamin B deficiency-associated disorders.*

**Perenteryl** *Merck, Chile.*
Saccharomyces boulardii (p.1704·2).
*Diarrhoea.*

**Peresal**
*Henkel, Ger.; Henkel, Ital.*
Hydrogen peroxide (p.1182·2); peracetic acid (p.1187·3).
*Instrument disinfection.*

**Perfadex** *Vitrolife, Swed.*
Dextran 40 (p.745·3) in electrolytes.
*Organ perfusion before transplantation.*

**Perfalgan**
*UPSA, Fr.; Bristol-Myers Squibb, UK.*
Paracetamol (p.76·2).
*Fever; pain.*

**Perfan**
*Aventis, Belg.†; Carinopharm, Ger.; Hoechst Marion Roussel, Irl.†; Biomedica, Ital.; Aventis, Neth.; Aventis, UK.*
Enoximone (p.911·1).
*Heart failure.*

**Perfane** *OTL, Fr.*
Enoximone (p.911·1).
*Heart failure.*

**Perfarin** *Wayne, Mex.†.*
Piroxicam (p.84·2).

**Perfect Climate** *Estee Lauder, Canad.†.*
Octinoxate (p.1154·3).
*Sunscreen.*

**Perfectil**
*Vitabiotics, Hong Kong.*
Multivitamin and mineral preparation with echinacea and lappa (p.1417·1).
*Vitabiotics, UK.*
Multivitamin, amino-acid, mineral, and herbal preparation (p.1417·1).

**Perfluoron** *Alcon, USA.*
Perfluorooctane (p.1730·2).
*Ophthalmic tamponade.*

**Perflux** *Fresenius Kabi, Austria.*
Electrolyte infusion (p.1217·1).
*Forced diuresis.*

**Perfocyn** *Bell, India.*
Prednisolone (p.1108·1); chloramphenicol (p.185·1); benzocaine (p.1370·3); acetic acid (p.1645·2).
*Ear infections.*

**Perfolate** *Asta Medica, Fr.†.*
Calcium folinate (p.1431·1).
*Drug-induced megaloblastic anaemia; folate deficiency; prevention of methotrexate toxicity.*

**Perfolin** *Gambar, Ital.†.*
Calcium folinate (p.1431·1).
*Anaemias; antidote to folic acid antagonists; folate deficiency.*

**Perform** *Schulke & Mayr, Ger.†.*
Potassium peroxymonosulfate.
*Surface disinfection.*

**Performer** *Piam, Ital.*
Cefaclor (p.167·1).
*Bacterial infections.*

**Perfudal** *Odin, Spain.*
Felodipine (p.914·3).
*Angina pectoris; hypertension.*

**Perfudan** *Piam, Ital.*
Buflomedil hydrochloride (p.877·2).
*Cerebral and peripheral vascular disorders.*

**Perfungol**
*Note. This name is used for preparations of different composition.*
*Montpellier, Arg.*
Chlorocresol (p.1177·1); boric acid (p.1662·1); zinc oxide (p.1163·2).
*Fungal skin infections.*
*Bago, Chile.*
*Ointment:* Chlorocresol (p.1177·1); nicotinamide (p.1441·2); cholesterol (p.1480·3).
*Topical powder:* Chlorocresol (p.1177·1); zinc oxide (p.1163·2); boric acid (p.1662·1).
*Fungal skin infections.*

**Perfus Multivitaminico** *Almirall, Spain.*
Carbazochrome (p.745·1); vitamins (p.1417·1); electrolytes.
*Haemorrhage; skeletal muscle disorders.*

**Perfusion de PAS** *Bichsel, Switz.*
Sodium aminosalicylate (p.155·1).
*Tuberculosis.*

**Perfusion mixte** *Streuli, Switz.*
Sodium chloride (p.1233·3) infusion with glucose.
*Dehydration.*

**Pergalen**
*GlaxoSmithKline, Arg.; Aventis, Braz.†.*
Sodium apolate (p.1000·2); benzyl nicotinate (p.21·2).
*Soft-tissue injuries.*

**Pergamid** *Pharmacia, Arg.*
Aniracetam (p.1655·1).
*Mental function impairment.*

**Perganit** *AstraZeneca, Ital.*
Glyceryl trinitrate (p.923·2).
*Angina pectoris; hypertension; pulmonary oedema.*

**Pergastric** *Prodes, Spain†.*
Dimethicone (p.1289·2).
*Flatulence.*

**Pergidal** *Valeas, Ital.*
Macrogol 4000 (p.1709·1).
*Constipation.*

**Perginol** *Gambar, Ital.†.*
Sodium tetrachloroiodite.
*Gynaecological infections.*

**Pergogreen**
*Faran, Gr.; Serono, Ital.†; Serono, Switz.†.*
Menotrophin (p.1330·1).
*Male and female infertility.*

**Pergonal**
*Serono, Arg.; Serono, Braz.; Serono, Canad.; Novartis, Chile; Serono, Ger.†; Faran, Gr.; Serono, Hong Kong; Serum Institute, India; Serono, Irl.†; Teva, Israel; Serono, Mex.; Serono, Neth.†; Serono, S.Afr.†; Serono, Singapore†; Serono, Spain; Serono, Switz.; Serono, Thai.†; Serono, USA.*
Menotrophin (p.1330·1).
*Male and female infertility.*

**Pergotime**
*Serono, Denm.; Serono, Fr.; Serono, Norw.; Serono, Swed.*
Clomifene citrate (p.1542·2).
*Anovulatory infertility.*

**Periactin**
*Merck Sharp & Dohme, Austral.; Merck Sharp & Dohme, Austria; Merck Sharp & Dohme, Belg.; Johnson & Johnson, Canad.; Merck Sharp & Dohme, Denm.; Merck Sharp & Dohme, Hong Kong†; Merck Sharp & Dohme, Irl.; Sigma-Tau, Ital.; Merck Sharp & Dohme, Neth.; Merck Sharp & Dohme, NZ; Merck Sharp & Dohme, Port.†; Merck Sharp & Dohme, S.Afr.; Sigma-Tau, Spain; Merck Sharp & Dohme, Swed.; Merck Sharp & Dohme, Switz.; Merck Sharp & Dohme, Thai.; Merck Sharp & Dohme, UK; Merck, USA†.*
Cyproheptadine hydrochloride (p.430·1).
*Hypersensitivity reactions; migraine; reduced appetite.*

**Periactine** *Merck Sharp & Dohme-Chibret, Fr.*
Cyproheptadine hydrochloride (p.430·1).
*Hypersensitivity reactions.*

**Periamin** *Fresenius Kabi, Spain.*
Amino-acid, carbohydrate, and electrolyte infusion (p.1417·1).
*Parenteral nutrition.*

**Periamin X** *Baxter, Ger.*
Amino-acid, xylitol, and electrolyte infusion (p.1417·1).
*Parenteral nutrition.*

**Periamin G**
*Fresenius Kabi, Austria; Baxter, Ger.*
Amino-acid, glucose, and electrolyte infusion (p.1417·1).
*Parenteral nutrition.*

**Periatin** *Prodome, Braz.*
Cyproheptadine hydrochloride (p.430·1).
*Hypersensitivity reactions; migraine and other vascular headaches; reduced appetite.*

**Periatin BC** *Prodome, Braz.†.*
Cyproheptadine hydrochloride (p.430·1); vitamins (p.1417·1).
*Hypersensitivity reactions; migraine and other vascular headaches; reduced appetite.*

**Periavita** *Prodome, Braz.†.*
Cyproheptadine hydrochloride (p.430·1); multivitamins (p.1417·1).
*Hypersensitivity reactions; migraine and other vascular headaches; reduced appetite.*

**Peribilan** *Lannacher, Austria†.*
Ox bile (p.1660·3); pig bile (p.1660·3).
*Constipation; gastrointestinal disorders.*

**Periblastine** *Intramed, S.Afr.†.*
Vinblastine sulfate (p.591·2).
*Malignant neoplasms.*

**Pericaina** *Senese, Ital.*
Mepivacaine hydrochloride (p.1381·2).
*Local anaesthesia.*

**Perical** *Besins, Fr.*
Calcium carbonate (p.1254·2).
*Calcium deficiency; osteoporosis.*

**Pericam** *Clonmel, Irl.*
Piroxicam (p.84·2).
*Dysmenorrhoea; gout; musculoskeletal, joint, and peri-articular disorders.*

**Pericate** *Unipharm, Israel.*
Haloperidol decanoate (p.701·3).
*Psychoses.*

**Pericel** *Pharmafar, Ital.*
Flavodate sodium (p.1688·2).
*Vascular disorders.*

**Pericephal** *Arcana, Austria.*
Cinnarizine (p.428·3).
*Cerebral and peripheral vascular disorders; vestibular disorders.*

**Peri-Colace**
*Wellspring, Canad.; Roberts, USA†.*
Casanthranol (p.1255·1); docusate sodium (p.1262·2).
*Constipation.*

**Pericristine** *Teva, S.Afr.†.*
Vincristine sulfate (p.592·2).
*Malignant neoplasms.*

**Perida** *Codal Synto, Thai.*
Haloperidol (p.701·2).
*Behaviour disorders in children; psychoses; stuttering; tics.*

**Peridal** *Medley, Braz.†.*
Domperidone (p.1263·2).
*Gastrointestinal motility disorders; nausea and vomiting.*

**Peridane** *Columbia, Mex.*
Pentoxifylline (p.979·3).
*Cerebral and peripheral vascular disorders; thrombosis prophylaxis.*

**Perident** *Master, Chile.*
Chlorhexidine gluconate (p.1173·2).
*Oral hygiene.*

**Peridex**
*Zila, Canad.; Procter & Gamble, USA.*
Chlorhexidine gluconate (p.1173·2).
*Gingivitis.*

**Peridil** *Cryopharma, Mex.*
Azapetine phosphate (p.866·2).
*Peripheral vascular disorders.*

**Peridin-C** *Beutlich, USA.*
Hesperidin methyl chalcone (p.1688·3); hesperidin complex (p.1688·2); ascorbic acid (p.1460·2).
*Capillary bleeding.*

**Peridol** *Technilab, Canad.*
Haloperidol (p.701·2).
*Behaviour disorders; psychoses; Tourette syndrome.*

**Peridon** *Italchimici, Ital.*
Domperidone (p.1263·2).
*Gastrointestinal disorders.*

**Peridor** *Unipharm, Israel.*
Haloperidol (p.701·2).
*Hiccup; psychiatric disorders; Tourette syndrome; vomiting.*

**Peri-Dos Softgels** *Goldline, USA†.*
Docusate sodium (p.1262·2); casanthranol (p.1255·1).
*Constipation.*

**Peridys** *Pierre Fabre, Fr.*
Domperidone (p.1263·2).
*Dyspepsia; gastro-oesophageal reflux; nausea and vomiting.*

**Perifazo** *Pharmacia Upjohn, Fr.†.*
Amino-acid infusion (p.1417·1).
*Parenteral nutrition.*

**Perifem** *Organon, Spain.*
11 Tablets, estradiol valerate (p.1550·2); 10 tablets, estradiol valerate; medroxyprogesterone acetate (p.1557·2).
*Menopausal disorders.*

**Perifer H1** *BA Farma, Port.*
Astemizole (p.424·2).
*Allergic conjunctivitis; allergic rhinitis; urticaria.*

**Periflex** *Scientific Hospital Supplies, UK†.*
Preparation for enteral nutrition (p.1417·1).

**Perifusin** *Fresenius Kabi, Gr.*
Amino-acid infusion (p.1417·1).
*Parenteral nutrition.*

**Perikabiven** *Fresenius Kabi, Fr.*
Amino-acid, carbohydrate, lipid (from soya oil (p.1447·2)), and electrolyte infusion (p.1417·1).
Contains egg lecithin.
*Parenteral nutrition.*

**Perikan** *Austroplant, Austria.*
Hypericum (p.299·1).
*Depression.*

**Perikliman** *Kwizda, Austria.*
16 Tablets, estradiol (p.1550·1); 12 tablets, estradiol; norethisterone acetate (p.1562·2).
*Menopausal disorders; osteoporosis.*

**Perikursal**
*Wyeth Lederle, Austria; Wyeth, Ger.*
Levonorgestrel (p.1563·2); ethinylestradiol (p.1553·2).
*Biphasic oral contraceptive.*

**Perilax** *Nordic Drugs, Denm.*
Bisacodyl (p.1251·3).
*Bowel evacuation; constipation.*

**Perilox** *Drossapharm, Switz.*
Metronidazole (p.607·2).
*Rosacea.*

**Perinal**
*Dermal Laboratories, Irl.; Dermal, Israel; Dermal Laboratories, UK.*
Hydrocortisone (p.1103·3); lidocaine hydrochloride (p.1377·3).
*Anal and perianal pain and pruritus.*

**Perinorm**
*Ipca, India; Nat Druggists, S.Afr.*
Metoclopramide hydrochloride (p.1274·3).
*Gastrointestinal disorders; nausea and vomiting.*

**Perio-Aid** *Dentaid, Chile.*
Chlorhexidine gluconate (p.1173·2).
*Oral hygiene.*

**Perio-Aid c Cloruro de Cetilpiridinio** *Dentaid, Chile.*
Chlorhexidine gluconate (p.1173·2); cetylpyridinium chloride (p.1173·1).
*Oral hygiene.*

**Periobacter** *Naf, Arg.*
Chlorhexidine (p.1173·2); xylitol (p.1469·1).
*Mouth infections.*

**Periochip**
*AstraZeneca, Braz.†; Dexcel, Denm.; Dexcel, Israel; Vitaflo, Swed.; Procter & Gamble, UK†; Astra, USA.*
Chlorhexidine gluconate (p.1173·2).
*Periodontal disease.*

**Periocline** *Sunstar, Jpn.*
Minocycline hydrochloride (p.231·3).
*Periodontitis.*

**Period Pain Relief** *Herbal Concepts, UK.*
Alchemilla; motherwort (p.1717·1); valerian (p.1762·2); pulsatilla (p.1737·1); vervain (p.1764·1); helonias (p.1696·3).
*Dysmenorrhoea; premenstrual syndrome.*

**Periodent** *Grimberg, Arg.*
Chlorhexidine (p.1173·2); xylitol (p.1469·1).
*Mouth disorders.*

**Periodentix** *Germiphene, Israel†.*
Chlorhexidine gluconate (p.1173·2).
*Gingivitis; oral hygiene.*

**Periodentyl** *Glaxo Wellcome, Mex.*
*Mouthwash:* Triclosan (p.1195·2); zinc chloride (p.1469·2); vitamin E acetate (p.1465·1); xylitol (p.1469·1).
*Toothpaste:* Triclosan (p.1195·2); zinc citrate; enoxolone (p.36·2); sodium monofluorophosphate (p.1446·2).
*Oral hygiene.*

**Periodine Anti-Malarico** *Simoes, Braz.†.*
Sulfametopyrazine (p.263·1); pyrimethamine (p.458·1).
*Malaria.*

**Periodontil** *Aventis, Braz.*
Spiramycin (p.255·3); metronidazole (p.607·2).
*Bacterial infections; protozoal infections.*

**Periofem Ciclico** *Beta, Arg.*
14 Tablets, conjugated oestrogens (p.1543·2); 14 tablets, conjugated estrogens; medroxyprogesterone acetate (p.1557·2).
*Menopausal disorders; osteoporosis.*

**Periofem Continuo** *Beta, Arg.*
Conjugated oestrogens (p.1543·2); medroxyprogesterone acetate (p.1557·2).
*Menopausal disorders; osteoporosis.*

**Periogard**
*Note. This name is used for preparations of different composition.*
*Colgate-Palmolive, Ital.†; Asta Medica, Port.†.*
*Mouthwash; oral drops:* Sanguinaria (p.1741·3).
*Gum disorders; halitosis; oral hygiene.*
*Colgate-Palmolive, Ital.†; Asta Medica, Port.†.*
*Toothpaste:* Sanguinaria (p.1741·3); sodium monofluorophosphate (p.1446·2).
*Gingivitis; oral hygiene.*
*Colgate Oral, USA.*
Chlorhexidine gluconate (p.1173·2).
*Mouth disorders.*

**Periogard Chlorohex**
*Colgate Oral Care, Austral.†; Colgate-Palmolive, Ger.; Colgate-Palmolive, Ital.*
Chlorhexidine gluconate (p.1173·2).
*Mouth disorders; oral hygiene.*
*Asta Medica, Port.†.*
Chlorhexidine (p.1173·2).
*Oral hygiene.*

**Periogard Plus** *Colgate-Palmolive, Ital.*
*Oral drops:* Cetylpyridinium chloride (p.1173·1).
*Gum disorders.*
*Toothpaste:* Zinc citrate; sodium monofluorophosphate (p.1446·2).
*Gingivitis.*

**PerioMed** *Omnii, USA.*
Stannous fluoride (p.1448·3).
*Dental caries prophylaxis.*

**Periostat**
*CollaGenex, UK; CollaGenex, USA.*
Doxycycline hyclate (p.206·2).
*Bacterial infections.*

**Perioxidin**
*Note. This name is used for preparations of different composition.*
*Andromaco, Chile.*
Chlorhexidine gluconate (p.1173·2).
*Oral hygiene.*
*Glaxo Wellcome, Mex.*
*Dental gel:* Chlorhexidine gluconate (p.1173·2).
*Mouth infections.*
*Mouthwash:* Chlorhexidine gluconate (p.1173·2); xylitol (p.1469·1).
*Gingivitis; periodontitis.*

**Peripan** *Mepha, Braz.*
Pentoxyfylline (p.979·3).

**Periphramine** *Braun, Spain.*
Amino-acid and electrolyte infusion (p.1417·1).
*Parenteral nutrition.*

**Periplasmal**
*Braun, Austria; Braun, Ger.; Braun, Switz.†.*
Amino-acid, carbohydrate, and electrolyte infusion (p.1417·1).
*Parenteral nutrition.*

**Periplasmal G** *Braun, Spain.*
Amino-acid, carbohydrate, and electrolyte infusion (p.1417·1).
*Parenteral nutrition.*

**Periplasmal XE** *Braun, Ger.*
Amino-acid, xylitol, and electrolyte infusion (p.1417·1).
*Parenteral nutrition.*

**Periplum**
*Note. This name is used for preparations of different composition.*
*Fortbenton, Arg.*
Fluconazole (p.398·1).
*Fungal infections.*
*Italfarmaco, Ital.*
Nimodipine (p.972·3).
*Neurological deficit following cerebral vasospasm.*

**Peripress**
*Pfizer, Denm.; Pfizer, Fin.*
Prazosin hydrochloride (p.985·1).
*Benign prostatic hyperplasia; heart failure; hypertension; Raynaud's syndrome.*

**Peristaltine** *Novartis Sante, Fr.*
Cascara (p.1255·1).
*Constipation.*

**Peritoflex** *Fresenius Medical, Spain†.*
Calcium chloride; anhydrous glucose; magnesium chloride; sodium chloride; sodium lactate (p.1221·1).
*Peritoneal dialysis.*

**Peritofundin**
*Braun, Austria†; Braun, Braz.†.*
Electrolytes; glucose or sorbitol (p.1221·1).
*Peritoneal dialysis solution.*

**Peritofundinas** *Braun, Port.†.*
Glucose; sodium chloride; calcium chloride; magnesium chloride; potassium chloride; sodium lactate (p.1221·1).
*Peritoneal dialysis.*

**Peritol**
*Medphano, Ger.; Themis Chemicals, India.*
Cyproheptadine hydrochloride (p.430·1).
*Hypersensitivity disorders; migraine; pruritus; reduced appetite.*

**Peritone** *Blackmores, Austral.†.*
Aloes (p.1248·2); senna (p.1288·2); cascara (p.1255·1); ginger (p.1267·1); cardamom fruit (p.1667·3); peppermint oil (p.1283·2).
*Constipation.*

**Peritrast**
*Kohler, Austria†; Kohler, Ger.*
Lysine amidotrizoate (p.1061·1).
*Radiographic contrast medium.*

**Peritrast comp** *Kohler, Ger.*
Sodium amidotrizoate (p.1060·2); lysine amidotrizoate (p.1061·1).
*Radiographic contrast medium.*

**Peritrast-Infusio 160/32%** *Kohler, Ger.*
Lysine amidotrizoate (p.1061·1).
*Radiographic contrast medium.*

**Peritrast-Infusio 180/31%** *Kohler, Ger.*
Sodium amidotrizoate (p.1060·2); lysine amidotrizoate (p.1061·1).
*Radiographic contrast medium.*

**Peritrast-Oral CT** *Kohler, Ger.*
Lysine amidotrizoate (p.1061·1); sodium amidotrizoate (p.1060·2).
*Contrast medium for computer tomography of the abdominal cavity.*

**Peritrast-Oral-GI** *Kohler, Ger.*
Lysine amidotrizoate (p.1061·1).
*Contrast medium for gastrointestinal radiography.*

**Peritrast-RE** *Kohler, Ger.*
Lysine amidotrizoate (p.1061·1).
*Contrast medium for rectal radiography.*

**Peritrate**
*Parke, Davis, Canad.†; Parke, Davis, India; Teofarma, Ital.; Pfizer, Thai.*
Pentaerithrityl tetranitrate (p.979·1).
*Angina pectoris.*

**Perivar** *Intersan, Ger.*
Troxerutin (p.1688·3); heptaminol hydrochloride (p.1697·1); ginkgo biloba (p.1692·3).
*Haemorrhoids; venous insufficiency.*

**Perivar Rosskaven** *Intersan, Ger.*
Aesculus (p.1648·2).
*Venous insufficiency.*

**Perivar Venensalbe** *Intersan, Ger.*
Heparin sodium (p.928·1).
*Soft-tissue injury; vascular disorders.*

**Perkamillon**
*Note. This name is used for preparations of different composition.*
*Robugen, Ger.†; Medipharm, Switz.†.*
*Liquid:* Chamomile (p.1669·3).
*Inflammatory disorders of the skin or mucous membranes.*
*Medipharm, Switz.†.*
*Ointment:* Chamomile (p.1669·3); hamamelis (p.1696·3).
*Minor wounds.*

**Perketan** *Inverni della Beffa, Ital.†.*
Ketanserin tartrate (p.943·1).
*Hypertension.*

**Perkod** *Biogalenique, Fr.†.*
Dipyridamole (p.903·1).
*Thromboembolic disorders.*

**Perlas de PMMA con Gentamicina** *Merck, Chile.*
Methylmethacrylate methacrylate copolymer (p.1714·3); gentamicin sulfate (p.217·1).
*Bone and soft-tissue infections.*

**Perlatos** *Merck, Arg.*
Levodropropizine (p.1119·3).
*Coughs.*

**Perlax** *UCI, Braz.†.*
Dantron (p.1261·1); dexpanthenol (p.1727·2).
*Constipation.*

**Perlea** *Elea, Arg.*
Multivitamin and mineral preparation (p.1417·1).

**Perles d'huile de foie de morue du Dr Geistlich** *Geistlich, Switz.†.*
Cod-liver oil (p.1425·2); halibut-liver oil (p.1434·1).
*Vitamin A and D deficiency.*

**Perlice** *Galderma, India.*
Permethrin (p.1508·3).
*Pediculosis capitis.*

**Perlinganit**
*Nycomed, Austria; Orion, Fin.; Schwarz, Ger.; Orion, Swed.; Schwarz, Switz.*
Glyceryl trinitrate (p.923·2).
*Cardiovascular disorders; controlled hypotension.*

**Perlinsol Cutaneo** *Medea, Spain†.*
Acedoben sodium (p.1645·2); vitamin F.
*Skin disorders.*

**Perlol** *Asian Pharm, Thai.*
Propranolol hydrochloride (p.989·3).
*Angina pectoris; arrhythmias; hypertension.*

**Perludil** *Collins, Mex.*
Vitamin preparation (p.1417·1).
*Menstrual disorders.*

**Perlutal**
*Boehringer Ingelheim, Arg.; Promeco, Mex.*
Algestone acetophenide (p.1541·3); estradiol enantate (p.1550·1).
*Endometriosis; female infertility; injectable contraceptive; menstrual disorders.*

**Perlutan** *Boehringer de Angeli, Braz.*
Algestone acetophenide (p.1541·3); estradiol enantate (p.1550·1).
*Injectable contraceptive.*

**Perlutex**
*Leo, Denm.; Leo, Norw.*
Medroxyprogesterone acetate (p.1557·2).
*Endometriosis; menopausal disorders; test of ovarian function; uterine cancer.*

**Permadoze** *Alpharma, Port.*
Cyanocobalamin (p.1458·2).
*Neuralgia; vitamin $B_{12}$ deficiency.*

**Permapen** *Roerig, USA.*
Benzathine benzylpenicillin (p.162·3).
*Bacterial infections.*

**Permax**
*Lilly, Austral.; Lilly, Austria; Lilly, Belg.; Draxis, Canad.; Lilly, Denm.; Lilly, Fin.; Lilly, Mex.; Lilly, Neth.; Lilly, NZ; Lilly, Port.; Lilly, S.Afr.; Lilly, Switz.; Athena Neurosciences, USA.*
Pergolide mesilate (p.1211·2).
*Parkinsonism.*

**Permease** *Novartis, Austria†.*
Hyaluronidase (p.1698·2).
*Haematomas; increase absorption and reduce discomfort of injections; reduce viscosity of secretions and discharge.*

**Permecil** *Prieto, Arg.*
Benzyl benzoate (p.1500·2); permethrin (p.1508·3).
*Pediculosis.*

**Permetel** *Teuto, Braz.*
Permethrin (p.1508·3).
*Pediculosis.*

**Permetrix** *Galenogal, Braz.†.*
Permethrin (p.1508·3).

**Permicaps** *Bago, Arg.*
Saw palmetto (p.1569·1).
*Benign prostatic hyperplasia.*

**Permitabs** *Centrapharm, UK.*
Potassium permanganate (p.1190·2).
*Wound cleansing.*

**Permitil** *Schering, USA†.*
Fluphenazine hydrochloride (p.699·3).
*Psychoses.*

**Permixon**
*Pierre Fabre, Arg.; Germania, Austria; Asta Medica, Braz.; Pierre Fabre, Fr.; Pierre Fabre, Ital.; Schering-Plough, Mex.; Pierre Fabre, Port.; Pierre Fabre, Singapore; Pierre Fabre, Spain; Robapharm, Switz.; Pierre Fabre, Thai.*
Saw palmetto (p.1569·1).
*Benign prostatic hyperplasia.*

**Pernaemyl** *Biosyn, Ger.†.*
Bovine liver extract; cyanocobalamin (p.1458·2).
*Liver disorders; megaloblastic anaemia; vitamin $B_{12}$ deficiency.*

**Pernamed** *Medifive, Thai.*
Perphenazine (p.714·2).
*Nausea and vomiting; psychoses.*

**Pernazene** *Sanofi Synthelabo, Thai.*
Tymazoline hydrochloride (p.1132·1).
*Nasal congestion.*

**Pernazine** *Atlantic, Thai.*
Perphenazine (p.714·2).
*Nausea and vomiting; psychoses.*

**Pernexin** *Schering, Ital.*
Iron succinyl-protein complex (p.1438·1).
*Anaemias; iron deficiency.*

**Pernionin** *Krewel, Ger.†.*
Methyl salicylate (p.59·3); benzyl nicotinate (p.21·2); methyl nicotinate (p.59·2).
*Musculoskeletal and joint disorders; peripheral vascular disorders.*

**Pernionin N** *Krewel, Ger.*
Methyl salicylate (p.59·3); sage oil (p.1741·2).
*Circulatory disorders.*

**Pernionin Teil-Bad** *Krewel, Ger.*
Benzyl nicotinate (p.21·2).
Pernionin Teil-Bad N formerly contained methyl salicylate, benzyl nicotinate, and methyl nicotinate.
*Bath additive; musculoskeletal and joint disorders; peripheral vascular disorders.*

**Pernionin Voll-Bad N** *Krewel, Ger.*
Norway spruce oil; benzyl nicotinate (p.21·2); methyl nicotinate (p.59·2).
*Bath additive; musculoskeletal and joint disorders; peripheral vascular disorders.*

**Pernox**
*Westwood-Squibb, Canad.; Westwood, USA.*
Polyethylene granules (abrasive) (p.1140·1); sulfur (p.1158·2); salicylic acid (p.1157·1).
*Acne; oily skin.*

**Pernutrin** *Grifols, Spain†.*
Amino-acid, carbohydrate, electrolyte, and vitamin infusion (p.1417·1).
*Parenteral nutrition.*

**Pernyzol** *Recordati, Ital.†.*
Metronidazole benzoate (p.607·2).
*Bacterial mouth infections.*

**Pero** *Opfermann, Ger.†.*
Emollient.
*Skin disorders.*

**Perocef** *Pulitzer, Ital.†.*
Cefoperazone sodium (p.174·3).
Lidocaine hydrochloride (p.1377·3) is included in this preparation to alleviate the pain of injection.
*Bacterial infections.*

**Perocur**
*EciFarma, Chile; Biocur, Ger.*
*Saccharomyces boulardii* (p.1704·2).
*Diarrhoea.*

**Perofen**
*Remedica, Hong Kong; Remedica, Malaysia; Remedica, Thai.*
Ibuprofen (p.45·3).
*Musculoskeletal, joint, peri-articular, and soft-tissue disorders; pain.*

**Peroxacne** *Isdin, Spain.*
Benzoyl peroxide (p.1143·2).
*Acne.*

**Peroxiben** *Isdin, Spain.*
Benzoyl peroxide (p.1143·2).
*Acne.*

**Peroxiben Plus** *Andromaco, Chile.*
Benzoyl peroxide (p.1143·2).
*Acne; seborrhoea.*

**Peroximicina** *Kampel Martian, Arg.*
Benzoyl peroxide (p.1143·2); erythromycin (p.208·1).
*Acne.*

**Peroxin** *Dermol, USA†.*
Benzoyl peroxide (p.1143·2).
*Acne.*

**Peroxyl**
*Colgate-Palmolive, Austral.; Kolynos, Braz.†; Colgate-Palmolive, UK; Colgate-Palmolive, USA.*
Hydrogen peroxide (p.1182·2).
*Mouth disorders.*

**Perozon Erkaltungsbad** *Sanova, Austria.*
Eucalyptus oil (p.1686·2); camphor (p.1665·3); menthol (p.1711·3).
*Bath additive; cold symptoms; rheumatic disorders.*

**Perozon Heublumen** *Sanova, Austria.*
Thyme oil (p.1755·3); hay flowers.
*Bath additive.*

**Perozon Rosmarin-Olbad mono** *Spitzner, Ger.†.*
Rosemary oil (p.1740·2).
*Bath additive; peripheral vascular disorders.*

**Perpector** *Grossmann, Switz.*
Codeine phosphate (p.27·1); ephedrine hydrochloride (p.1120·1); potassium iodide (p.1598·1); primula root (p.1735·1); valerian (p.1762·2).
*Coughs.*

**Perphenan** *Taro, Israel.*
Perphenazine (p.714·2).
*Anxiety; nervous states; vomiting.*

**Perphyllon** *Asta Medica, Austria†.*
Etofylline (p.785·1); theophylline hydrate (p.798·3); papaverine hydrochloride (p.1728·1); atropine methonitrate (p.477·1).
*Asthma; bronchitis; emphysema.*

**Persa-Gel** *Ortho Dermatological, USA†.*
Benzoyl peroxide (p.1143·2).
*Acne.*

**Persantin**
*Boehringer Ingelheim, Arg.; Boehringer Ingelheim, Austral.; Boehringer Ingelheim, Austria; Boehringer de Angeli, Braz.; Boehringer Ingelheim, Chile; Boehringer Ingelheim, Denm.; Boehringer Ingelheim, Fin.; Boehringer Ingelheim, Ger.†; Boehringer Ingelheim, Gr.; IFET (ΙΦΕΤ), Gr.; Boehringer Ingelheim, Hong Kong; German Remedies, India; Boehringer Ingelheim, Irl.; Boehringer Ingelheim, Ital.; Boehringer Ingelheim, Malaysia; Boehringer Ingelheim, Mex.; Boehringer Ingelheim, Neth.; Boehringer Ingelheim, Norw.; Boehringer Ingelheim, NZ; Boehringer Ingelheim, Port.; Boehringer Ingelheim, S.Afr.; Boehringer Ingelheim, Singapore; Boehringer Ingelheim, Spain; Boehringer Ingelheim, Swed.; Boehringer Ingelheim, Thai.; Boehringer Ingelheim, UK.*
Dipyridamole (p.903·1) or dipyridamole hydrochloride (p.903·2).
*Adjunct in thallium scanning procedures; thromboembolic disorders.*

**Persantin Plus** *Boehringer Ingelheim, Hong Kong†.*
Dipyridamole (p.903·1); aspirin (p.15·1).
*Thromboembolic disorders.*

**Persantin S** *Boehringer de Angeli, Braz.†.*
Dipyridamole (p.903·1); aspirin (p.15·1).
*Thrombosis prophylaxis.*

**Persantine**
*Boehringer Ingelheim, Belg.; Boehringer Ingelheim, Canad.; Boehringer Ingelheim, Fr.; Boehringer Ingelheim, Switz.†; Boehringer Ingelheim, USA.*
Dipyridamole (p.903·1).
*Adjunct in myocardial thallium scanning; ischaemic heart disease; thromboembolism prophylaxis.*

**Persivate** *Aspen, S.Afr.*
Betamethasone valerate (p.1093·2).
*Skin disorders.*

**Perskindol**
*Singer, Hong Kong†; Singer, Switz.†.*
Menthol (p.1711·3).
*Muscle and joint pain.*

**Persol**
Note. This name is used for preparations of different composition.
Horner, Canad.†.
Benzoyl peroxide (p.1143·2); colloidal sulfur (p.1158·2).
*Acne; rosacea.*

Wallace, India.
Benzoyl peroxide (p.1143·2).
*Acne.*

**Persol Forte** Wallace, India.
Benzoyl peroxide (p.1143·2); sulfur (p.1158·2).
*Acne.*

**Persolv Richter** Lepetit, Ital.
Urokinase (p.1018·2).
*Thromboembolic disorders.*

**Personnel** Therapex, Canad.
Bismuth salicylate (p.1252·1).

**Personnelle Contre le Rhume** Therapex, Canad.
Pseudoephedrine hydrochloride (p.1129·2); dextromethorphan hydrobromide (p.1117·3); paracetamol (p.76·2).

**Personnelle DM** Therapex, Canad.†.
Pseudoephedrine hydrochloride (p.1129·2); dextromethorphan hydrobromide (p.1117·3).

**Persumbrax** Boehringer Ingelheim, Ital.†.
Dipyridamole (p.903·1); oxazepam (p.712·2).
*Cardiovascular disorders.*

**Pert Plus** Procter & Gamble, Canad.
Pyrithione zinc (p.1156·2).
*Seborrhoeic dermatitis.*

**Pertacel** Aventis Pasteur, Braz.
A diphtheria, tetanus, and pertussis vaccine (p.1613·3).
*Active immunisation.*

**Pertacilon**
Elpen (Ελπεν), Gr.; Elpen, Singapore.
Captopril (p.879·2).
*Diabetic nephropathy; heart failure; hypertension; myocardial infarction.*

**Pertamin** Yauquimia, Mex.†.
Vitamin A (p.1451·2).

**Pertaxol** Kleva, Gr.
Betaxolol hydrochloride (p.873·1).
*Glaucoma; hypertension; raised intra-ocular pressure.*

**Pertensal** Vinas, Spain.
Nifedipine (p.966·2).
*Angina pectoris; hypertension; Raynaud's syndrome.*

**Pertenso** Armstrong, Arg.
Clonidine (p.885·2); bendroflumethiazide (p.867·3).
*Hypertension.*

**Pertenso N** Fournier, Ger.
Propranolol hydrochloride (p.989·3); hydralazine hydrochloride (p.931·2); bendroflumethiazide (p.867·3).
*Hypertension.*

**Pertil** AstraZeneca, Spain.
Isosorbide mononitrate (p.942·1).
*Angina pectoris.*

**Pertiroid** Piam, Ital.
Potassium perchlorate (p.1602·3).
*Hyperthyroidism.*

**Pertix-Solo** Hommel, Ger.†.
Menadiol calcium diphosphate (p.1467·3).
*Coughs.*

**Pertix-Solo-N, Pertix-T, Pertix-Z, and Pertix-L** Hommel, Ger.
Pentoxyverine (p.1126·2) or pentoxyverine citrate (p.1126·2).
*Coughs and associated respiratory-tract disorders.*

**Pertofran**
Novartis, Austral.†; Novartis, Austria; Novartis, Belg.; Novartis, Fr.; Novartis, Ger.; Novartis, Neth.; Novartis, NZ.
Desipramine hydrochloride (p.290·2).
*Depression.*

**Pertoglobulin** Nuovo ISM, Ital.†.
A pertussis immunoglobulin (p.1631·2).
*Passive immunisation.*

**Pertranquil**
Note. This name is used for preparations of different composition.
Hoechst Marion Roussel, Austria†; Aventis, Belg.
Meprobamate (p.706·2).
*Anxiety; insomnia; neurodermatitis; premedication; sedative; skeletal muscle spasm.*

Llorente, Spain†.
Diazepam (p.690·1); aminohydroxybutyric acid (p.353·2).
*Anxiety; insomnia.*

**Pertrim** Allergan-Frumtost, Braz.†.
Polymyxin B sulfate (p.245·1); trimethoprim (p.272·2).
*Bacterial eye infections.*

**Pertriptyl** Orion, Fin.
Perphenazine (p.714·2); amitriptyline hydrochloride (p.280·3).
*Anxiety disorders; depression; schizophrenia.*

**Pertrombon** Gerot, Austria.
Sodium nicotinate (p.1442·1); heparin sodium (p.928·1).
*Decubitus ulcer; promote resorption of excess fluid; soft-tissue injury; thrombophlebitis; ulcus cruris; varices.*

**Pertudoron**
Weleda, Austria; Weleda, Fr.; Weleda, Ger.
Homoeopathic preparation.

**Pertusan** Argenfarma, Arg.
Centella (p.1144·3).
*Haemorrhoids; venous disorders.*

**Pertus-Gamma** Biagini, Ital.†.
A human pertussis immunoglobulin (p.1631·2).
*Passive immunisation.*

**Pertussex Compositum** Uhlmann-Eyraud, Switz.
Codeine phosphate (p.27·1); ephedrine hydrochloride (p.1120·1); drosera; galeopsis; thyme; Iceland moss; cowslip.
*Coughs and associated respiratory-tract disorders.*

**Pertussin**
Note. This name is used for preparations of different composition.
Knop, Chile.
Homoeopathic preparation.

Spreewald, Ger.
Thyme (p.1755·2).
*Coughs.*

Pertussin, USA†.
Dextromethorphan hydrobromide (p.1117·3).
*Coughs.*

**Pertuvac** Chiron Behring, Ger.†.
A pertussis vaccine (p.1631·2).
*Active immunisation.*

**Perubare** Mayoly-Spindler, Switz.
Peru balsam (p.1730·2); thymol (p.1194·2); thyme oil (p.1755·3); rosemary oil (p.1740·2); lavender oil (p.1705·2).
*Upper respiratory-tract disorders.*

**Perubore**
Note. This name is used for preparations of different composition.
ACP, Belg.
Peru balsam (p.1730·2); thyme oil (p.1755·3); rosemary oil (p.1740·2); thymol (p.1194·2).
*Rhinitis; sinusitis.*

Mayoly-Spindler, Fr.
Thyme oil (p.1755·3); rosemary oil (p.1740·2); lavender oil (p.1705·2); thymol (p.1194·2); peru balsam (p.1730·2).
*Upper respiratory-tract congestion.*

**Perudent** Dreveny, Austria†.
Peru balsam (p.1730·2).
*Dental preparation.*

**Peru-Lenicet** Athenstaedt, Ger.
Aluminium diacetate hydroxide; aluminium hydroxide gel (p.1249·2); peru balsam (p.1730·2).
*Skin disorders; wounds.*

**Perusliuos-K** Fresenius Kabi, Fin.
Electrolyte infusion with glucose (p.1217·1).
*Carbohydrate source; fluid and electrolyte disorders.*

**Pervasum** Lesvi, Spain†.
Cinnarizine (p.428·3).
*Migraine and other vascular headaches; motion sickness; vestibular disorders.*

**Perviam** Janssen-Cilag, Belg.
Ibuprofen lysine (p.46·3).
*Fever; pain.*

**Pervinox** Phoenix, Arg.
Povidone-iodine (p.1190·3).
*Skin, wound, and ulcer disinfection.*

**Pervinox D** Phoenix, Arg.
Povidone-iodine (p.1190·3); nonoxinol.
*Genital-tract infections.*

**Pervioral** Laboratorios Chile, Chile.
Valaciclovir hydrochloride (p.656·1).
*Herpesvirus infections.*

**Pervita** Lifeplan, UK†.
Betacarotene (p.1422·3).
*Nutritional supplement.*

**Pervivo** Bittner, Austria.
Manna, camphor; zedoary; angelica; myrrh; gentian; rowan; nutmeg; liquorice; helenin; centaury; clove; galanga; ginger; cnicus benedictus; ivae moschatae; theriac; iridus; verbascum; bitter orange peel; calamus; absinthium; aloes; cubeb; star anise; sweet orange peel; menyanthes.
*Gastrointestinal disorders; tonic.*

**Pervone** Sanofi Synthelabo, Gr.
Dihydroergotamine mesilate (p.465·3).
*Migraine; vascular headache.*

**Perycit** Astra, Swed.†.
Niceritrol (p.965·3).
*Hyperlipidaemias.*

**Perzine** PP Lab, Thai.
Perphenazine (p.714·2).
*Nausea and vomiting; psychoses.*

**Pesendorfer** Iso, Ger.
Homoeopathic preparation.

**Pesex-R** Zimaia, Port.†.
Fenproporex hydrochloride (p.1588·3).
*Obesity.*

**Pespir** Berman, Mex.
Vitamin preparation (p.1417·1).

**Pessarios Profilaticos Rendell** CIF, Braz.
Nonoxinol 10 (p.1413·3).
*Vulvovaginal infections.*

**Pestarin** Provit, Mex.
Rifampicin (p.250·2).
*Bacterial infections.*

**Petadolex** Weber & Weber, Ger.
Petasites officinalis (p.1663·3).
*Smooth muscle spasms.*

**Petadolor** Bioforce, Switz.
Petasites radix (p.1663·3).
*Migraine; smooth muscle spasm.*

**Petaforce V** Bioforce, Ger.
Petasites officinalis (p.1663·3).
*Migraine; urinary-tract spasm.*

**Pe-Tam** Qualiphar, Belg.†.
Paracetamol (p.76·2).
*Fever; pain.*

**Peteha**
Note. This name is used for preparations of different composition.
Fatol, Ger.
*Injection:* Protionamide (p.246·3); nicotinamide (p.1441·2).
*Tablets:* Protionamide (p.246·3).
*Tuberculosis.*

Fatol, Hong Kong.
Protionamide (p.246·3).
*Tuberculosis.*

**Petercillin** Aspen, S.Afr.
Ampicillin trihydrate (p.157·2).
*Bacterial infections.*

**Peterkaien** Intramed, S.Afr.†.
Lidocaine hydrochloride (p.1377·3).
*Arrhythmias; local anaesthesia.*

**Peterphyllin** Intramed, S.Afr.†.
Aminophylline (p.780·2).
*Heart failure; obstructive airways disease; oedema.*

**Peter's Sirop** Monot, Fr.†.
Ammoniated anise (p.1655·2); ethylmorphine hydrochloride (p.37·3); aconite (p.1646·3); belladonna (p.479·1); cherry laurel.
*Respiratory-tract disorders.*

**Petibelle** Jenapharm, Ger.
Drospirenone (p.1549·1); ethinylestradiol (p.1553·2).
*Combined oral contraceptive.*

**Petidion**
Gerot, Austria; Gerot, Switz.†.
Ethadione (p.360·1).
*Absence seizures; myoclonic seizures.*

**Petiflog** Biolab Sanus, Braz.†.
Benzydamine hydrochloride (p.21·1).
*Fever; inflammation; pain.*

**Petina Compound** Jean-Marie, Hong Kong.
Cyproheptadine hydrochloride (p.430·1); vitamins (p.1417·1).
*Appetite loss; tonic.*

**Petinimid**
Gerot, Austria; Gerot, Switz.
Ethosuximide (p.360·1).
*Absence seizures.*

**Petinutin**
Pfizer, Austria; Parke, Davis, Ger.; Pfizer, Switz.
Mesuximide (p.366·2).
*Epilepsy.*

**Petites Pilules Carters** Fumouze, Fr.
Boldine (p.1661·2); aloes (p.1248·2).
*Constipation.*

**Petnidan** Desitin, Ger.
Ethosuximide (p.360·1).
*Absence seizures.*

**Petogen**
Pharmacare, Malaysia; Medidata, Malaysia; Intramed, S.Afr.†.
Medroxyprogesterone acetate (p.1557·2).
*Progestogen-only injectable contraceptive.*

**Petrasch-Anthozym N** Reith & Petrasch, Ger.
Rote beete; ascorbic acid; lactic acid (p.1417·1).
*Tonic.*

**Petrolagar No. 2** Whitehall, Irl.†.
Liquid paraffin (p.1479·1); light liquid paraffin (p.1479·1); phenolphthalein (p.1284·1).
*Constipation.*

**Petrolagar with Phenolphthalein** Whitehall, Irl.†.
Light liquid paraffin (p.1479·1); liquid paraffin (p.1479·1); phenolphthalein (p.1284·1).
*Constipation.*

**Petroleum Med Complex** Dynamit, Austria.
Homoeopathic preparation.

**Petylyl** Temmler, Ger.
Desipramine hydrochloride (p.290·2).
*Depression.*

**Pevalip** Janssen-Cilag, Austria†.
Econazole (p.397·1).
*Fungal skin and nail infections.*

**Pevaryl**
Note. This name is used for preparations of different composition.
ICN, Austral.; Janssen-Cilag, Austria; Janssen-Cilag, Belg.; Janssen-Cilag, Denm.; Janssen-Cilag, Fin.; Janssen-Cilag, Fr.; Janssen-Cilag, Gr.; Cilag, Hong Kong; Janssen-Cilag, Irl.; Janssen-Cilag, Israel; Janssen-Cilag, Ital.; Janssen-Cilag, Malaysia; Cilag, Mex.; Janssen-Cilag, Neth.; Janssen-Cilag, Norw.; ICN, NZ; Janssen-Cilag, Port.; Janssen-Cilag, S.Afr.; Janssen-Cilag, Singapore; Pensa, Spain; Janssen-Cilag, Swed.; Janssen-Cilag, Switz.; Janssen-Cilag, UK.
Econazole (p.397·1) or econazole nitrate (p.397·2).
*Fungal and Gram-positive bacterial infections.*

Janssen-Cilag, Austria; Janssen-Cilag, Switz.
*Paste; topical powder:* Econazole nitrate (p.397·2); zinc oxide (p.1163·2).
*Fungal skin and nail infections; Gram-positive infections.*

**Pevaryl TC** Janssen-Cilag, UK†.
Econazole nitrate (p.397·2); triamcinolone acetonide (p.1110·2).
*Skin disorders with bacterial or fungal infection.*

**Pevidine** Rhone-Poulenc Rorer, Hong Kong†.
Povidone-iodine (p.1190·3).
*Burns; disinfection of skin and mucous membranes; wounds.*

**Pevison** Janssen-Cilag, Gr.
Triamcinolone acetonide (p.1110·2); econazole nitrate (p.397·2).
*Fungal skin infections with inflammation.*

**Pevisone**
Janssen-Cilag, Austria; Janssen-Cilag, Belg.; Janssen-Cilag, Denm.; Janssen-Cilag, Fin.; Janssen-Cilag, Fr.; Cilag, Hong Kong; Janssen-Cilag, Israel; Janssen-Cilag, Ital.; Janssen-Cilag, Malaysia; Janssen-Cilag, Norw.; Janssen-Cilag, Port.; Janssen-Cilag, S.Afr.; Janssen-Cilag, Singapore; Janssen-Cilag, Swed.; Janssen-Cilag, Switz.; Janssen-Cilag, Thai.
Econazole nitrate (p.397·2); triamcinolone acetonide (p.1110·2).
*Infected skin disorders.*

**Pexan E** Worwag, Ger.†.
*d*-Alpha tocopherol (p.1464·3) or alpha tocoferil acetate (p.1465·1).
*Vitamin E deficiency.*

**Pexeva** Synthon, USA.
Paroxetine hydrochloride (p.311·2).
*Depression; obsessive-compulsive disorder; panic attacks; post-traumatic stress disorder; premenstrual dysphoric disorder; social anxiety disorder.*

**Pexid** Sigma, Austral.†.
Perhexiline maleate (p.980·2).
*Angina pectoris.*

**Pexola** Boehringer Ingelheim, S.Afr.
Pramipexole (p.1212·3).
*Parkinsonism.*

**Pexsig**
Sigma, Austral.; Sigma, NZ.
Perhexiline maleate (p.980·2).
Formerly known as Pexid in *NZ*.
*Angina pectoris.*

**Pfeiffer's Cold Sore** Pfeiffer, USA.
Sumatra benzoin (p.1751·1); camphor (p.1665·3); menthol (p.1711·3); cineole (p.1672·1).
*Oral lesions.*

**Pfeil** Stada, Ger.
Ibuprofen (p.45·3).
*Pain.*

**P-Fen** Masa, Thai.
Ibuprofen (p.45·3).
*Gout; musculoskeletal and joint disorders.*

**Pfizerpen** Pfizer, USA.
Benzylpenicillin potassium (p.163·2).
*Bacterial infections.*

**PFT** Nicholas Piramal, India.
Simeticone (p.1289·2); magnesium hydroxide (p.1272·2); aluminium hydroxide (p.1249·2).
*Dyspepsia; flatulence; gastritis; gastrointestinal hyperacidity; hiatus hernia; peptic ulcer.*

**PG/53** Raymos, Arg.
Fertility test (p.1734·3).

**PG 53** Bouty, Ital.†.
Fertility test (p.1734·3).

**pH4** Biological E, India.
Magaldrate (p.1271·3); simeticone (p.1289·2).
*Flatulence; gastritis; gastrointestinal hyperacidity; peptic ulcer.*

**pH 550** Restan, S.Afr.
*Suspension:* Dicycloverine hydrochloride (p.481·2); aluminium hydroxide gel (p.1249·2); magnesium oxide (p.1272·3); calcium carbonate (p.1254·2); dimethicone (p.1289·2).
*Flatulence; gastric hyperacidity; hiatus hernia; peptic ulcer.*
*Tablets:* Calcium carbonate (p.1254·2); magnesium carbonate (p.1272·1); magnesium trisilicate (p.1272·3).
*Gastrointestinal disorders associated with hyperacidity.*

**PH maxi** Orion, Fin.†.
Aluminium hydroxide (p.1249·2); magnesium hydroxide (p.1272·2); aluminium hydroxide-magnesium carbonate co-dried gel (p.1250·1).
*Gastro-oesophageal reflux; hiatus hernia; peptic ulcer.*

**PH 4 Plus** Sintesina, Arg.
Paracetamol (p.76·2).
*Fever; pain.*

**Phacobiotic** Bros, Gr.
Propylene glycol cefatrizine (p.170·3).
*Bacterial infections.*

**Phacocef** Bros, Gr.
Cefotaxime sodium (p.175·3).
*Bacterial infections.*

**Phacotrex** Bros, Gr.
Cefaclor (p.167·1).
*Bacterial infections.*

**Phaeva** Schering, Fr.
Gestodene (p.1556·1); ethinylestradiol (p.1553·2).
*Triphasic oral contraceptive.*

**Phakan**
Chauvin, Fr.
*Combination pack:* Oral solution, glycine (p.1433·3); glutamic acid (p.1433·2); pyridoxine hydrochloride (p.1456·3); capsules, cysteine hydrochloride (p.1426·3); ascorbic acid (p.1460·2).
*Cataracts.*

Chauvin, Port.
White capsules, glycine (p.1433·3); glutamic acid (p.1433·2); pyridoxine (p.1457·2); blue capsules, cysteine (p.1426·3); vitamin C (p.1460·2).
*Cataracts.*

**Phakolen** Bausch & Lomb, Switz.
*Combination pack:* White capsules, glycine (p.1433·3); L-glutamic acid (p.1433·2); pyridoxine hydrochloride (p.1456·3); blue capsules, cysteine hydrochloride (p.1426·3); ascorbic acid (p.1460·2).
*Prevention of cataract formation.*

**Phamopril** Phamos, Ger.
Captopril (p.879·2).
*Heart failure; hypertension.*

**Phamoprofen** *Phamos, Ger.*
Ibuprofen (p.45·3).
*Inflammation; musculoskeletal and joint disorders; pain.*

**Phamoranit** *Phamos, Ger.*
Ranitidine hydrochloride (p.1285·2).
*Gastro-oesophageal reflux; peptic ulcer; Zollinger-Ellison syndrome.*

**Phamoxi** *Phamos, Ger.*
Amoxicillin trihydrate (p.155·3).
*Bacterial infections.*

**Phamuc** *Phamos, Ger.*
Acetylcysteine (p.1112·3).
*Respiratory-tract disorders with increased or viscous mucus.*

**Phanadex Cough** *Pharmakon, USA†.*
Phenylpropanolamine hydrochloride (p.1127·3); dextromethorphan hydrobromide (p.1117·3); mepyramine maleate (p.437·1); guaifenesin (p.1122·1).
*Coughs.*

**Phanalgin** *Trima, Israel.*
Dipyrone (p.35·3).
*Fever; pain.*

**Phanate** *Pharmaland, Thai.*
Lithium carbonate (p.301·1).
*Bipolar disorder.*

**Phanatuss Cough** *Pharmakon, USA.*
Dextromethorphan hydrobromide (p.1117·3); guaifenesin (p.1122·1).
*Coughs.*

**Phapax** *Lehning, Fr.*
Homoeopathic preparation.

**Pharcina** *Pharmacos, Mex.*
Ciprofloxacin hydrochloride (p.188·2).
*Bacterial eye infections.*

**Phardol mono** *Kreussler, Ger.*
Glycol salicylate (p.44·3).
*Musculoskeletal, joint, soft-tissue, and nerve disorders.*

**Phardol Rheuma** *Kreussler, Ger.*
Glycol salicylate (p.44·3); oleum pini sylvestris; benzyl nicotinate (p.21·2).
*Musculoskeletal, joint, soft-tissue, and nerve disorders.*

**Pharken** *Elanco, Spain.*
Pergolide mesilate (p.1211·2).
*Parkinsonism.*

**Pharma Plus** *Tanning Research, Canad.†.*
*SPF 15:* Octinoxate (p.1154·3); oxybenzone (p.1154·3).
*SPF 30:* Homosalate (p.1148·1); octinoxate (p.1154·3); octisalate (p.1154·3); oxybenzone (p.1154·3).
*Sunscreen.*

**Pharma Plus Oil Free** *Tanning Research, Canad.†.*
*SPF 30:* Octinoxate (p.1154·3); octisalate (p.1154·3); oxybenzone (p.1154·3).
*Sunscreen.*

**Pharma Plus Sport** *Tanning Research, Canad.†.*
*SPF 30:* Octinoxate (p.1154·3); octisalate (p.1154·3); oxybenzone (p.1154·3).
*Sunscreen.*

**Pharmacare Aspec** *PSM, NZ†.*
Aspirin (p.15·1).
*Thromboembolism prophylaxis.*

**Pharmacen** *Alpharma, Mex.*
Paracetamol (p.76·2).
*Fever; pain.*

**Pharmacetin** *Olan-Kemed, Thai.*
Chloramphenicol (p.185·1).
*Bacterial ear infections.*

**Pharmaceutix** *Medipharma, Arg.*
Rifampicin (p.250·2).
*Bacterial infections.*

**Pharmacilline** *Monot, Fr.†.*
Gramicidin (p.220·2).
*Infections of the mouth, nose, and throat.*

**Pharmacists Creme** *Reese, USA.*
Methyl salicylate (p.59·3); menthol (p.1711·3); capsicum oleoresin.

**Pharmacists Lotion** *Reese, USA.*
Methyl salicylate (p.59·3); menthol (p.1711·3); capsicum oleoresin.

**Pharmacol DM** *Therapex, Canad.†.*
Phenylpropanolamine hydrochloride (p.1127·3); pheniramine maleate (p.438·3); mepyramine maleate (p.437·1); dextromethorphan hydrobromide (p.1117·3).

**Pharma-Col Junior** *Pfizer Consumer, Austral.*
Dextromethorphan hydrobromide (p.1117·3); pseudoephedrine hydrochloride (p.1129·2); paracetamol (p.76·2).
*Coughs and cold symptoms.*

**Pharmacycare Barrier** *Douglas, NZ†.*
Dimethicone (p.1482·1).
*Barrier cream.*

**Pharmacycare Bath Oil** *Douglas, NZ†.*
Hydrous wool fat (p.1483·1); liquid paraffin (p.1479·1).
*Dry skin; pruritus.*

**Pharmacycare Cough** *Douglas, NZ†.*
Pholcodine (p.1128·3).
*Coughs.*

**Pharmacycare Cough Expectorant** *Douglas, NZ.*
Choline theophyllinate (p.784·2); guaifenesin (p.1122·1).
*Coughs.*

**Pharmacycare Hand & Body** *Douglas, NZ†.*
Hydrous wool fat (p.1483·1); liquid paraffin (p.1479·1).
*Dry skin; pruritus.*

**Pharma-Dentix** *Germiphene, Israel.*
Chlorhexidine gluconate (p.1173·2).
*Mouth disorders; oral hygiene.*

**Pharmadol** *Pharmaland, Thai.*
Tramadol hydrochloride (p.94·3).
*Pain.*

**Pharmadose alcool** *Gilbert, Fr.*
Alcohol (p.1166·1).
*Skin and wound disinfection.*

**Pharmadose mercuresceine** *Gilbert, Fr.*
Merbromin (p.1185·3).
*Wound and burn disinfection.*

**Pharmadose teinture d'arnica** *Gilbert, Fr.*
Arnica (p.1656·3).
*Ecchymoses.*

**Pharmaethyl** *Austrodent, Austria†.*
Cryofluorane (p.1235·3).
*Local anaesthesia in dentistry.*

**Pharmaflex** *Braun, Belg.*
Metronidazole (p.607·2).
*Anaerobic bacterial infections; protozoal infections.*

**Pharmaflur** *Pharmics, USA.*
Sodium fluoride (p.1444·3).
*Dental caries prophylaxis.*

**Pharmafort** *Boehringer Ingelheim, Arg.*
Ginseng; lecithin; rutoside; vitamins; minerals (p.1417·1).
*Tonic.*

**Pharmagrip** *Cinfa, Spain.*
Chlorphenamine maleate (p.427·3); phenylephrine hydrochloride (p.1126·3); paracetamol (p.76·2).
*Cold and influenza symptoms; fever; pain.*

**Pharmalgen**
*ALK, Belg.†; ALK, Denm.; ALK, Swed.†; Trimedal, Switz.; ALK, UK; ALK, USA.*
Venoms of bee (p.1650·2), wasp (p.1650·2), hornet, yellow jacket, and mixed vespids (p.1650·1).
*Allergen immunotherapy.*

**Pharmapress** *Aspen, S.Afr.*
Enalapril maleate (p.909·2).
*Heart failure; hypertension.*

**Pharmapress Co** *Aspen, S.Afr.*
Enalapril maleate (p.909·2); hydrochlorothiazide (p.933·2).
*Hypertension.*

**Pharmatex**
*Note. This name is used for preparations of different composition.*
*Raymos, Arg.; Innotech, Fr.; Agis, Israel; Sideforma, Port.*
Benzalkonium chloride (p.1168·3).
*Contraceptive.*

*Innotech, Fr.*
*Topical gel:* Hymetellose (p.1579·2); benzalkonium chloride (p.1168·3); glycerol (p.1694·3).
*Vaginal lubricant.*

**Pharmaton**
*Boehringer Ingelheim, Austral.; Boehringer Ingelheim, Hong Kong; Boehringer Ingelheim, NZ; Pharmaton, NZ; Boehringer Ingelheim, Port.; Boehringer Ingelheim Self Medication, UK.*
Multivitamins and minerals (p.1417·1); ginseng; lecithin.
*Tonic.*

*Boehringer de Angeli, Braz.; Boehringer Ingelheim, Chile.*
Ginseng; vitamins; minerals (p.1417·1).
*Tonic.*

*Boehringer Ingelheim, Fr.; Boehringer Ingelheim, Irl.*
Deanol bitartrate; ginseng; vitamins and minerals (p.1417·1).
*Tonic.*

*Pharmaton, Ger.*
Multivitamin and mineral preparation with ginseng and essential fatty acids (p.1417·1).

*Pharmaton, Malaysia.*
Vitamins; minerals; ginseng; lecithin; choline; linoleic acid; linolenic acid (p.1417·1).
*Tonic.*

*Boehringer Ingelheim Promeco, Mex.; Pharmaton, Singapore.*
Multivitamins; minerals; ginseng; lecithin; rutoside (p.1417·1).

*Pharmaton, Thai.*
Ginseng; deanol bitartrate; rutoside; lecithin; vitamins; minerals (p.1417·1).

**Pharmaton Complex**
*Boehringer Ingelheim, Arg.; Fher, Spain.*
Multivitamins and minerals (p.1417·1); ginseng; rutoside, lecithin; deanol bitartrate.
*Tonic.*

**Pharmaton Kiddi** *Boehringer de Angeli, Braz.†.*
Amino acids; vitamins; minerals (p.1417·1).

**Pharmaton SA** *Boehringer Ingelheim, S.Afr.*
Multivitamins and minerals (p.1417·1); ginseng; lecithin; rutoside.
*Tonic.*

**Pharmatovit**
*Boehringer Ingelheim, Austria; Pharmaton, Switz.*
Multivitamin and mineral preparation (p.1417·1).

*Pharmaton, Israel.*
Multivitamins and mineral preparation with lecithin and rutoside (p.1417·1).

**Pharmetapp** *Therapex, Canad.†.*
Phenylephrine hydrochloride (p.1126·3); phenylpropanolamine hydrochloride (p.1127·3); brompheniramine maleate (p.426·1).

**Pharmilin-DM** *Therapex, Canad.*
Dextromethorphan hydrobromide (p.1117·3).

**Pharminicol DM** *Therapex, Canad.†.*
Phenylpropanolamine hydrochloride (p.1127·3); pheniramine maleate (p.438·3); mepyramine maleate (p.437·1); dextromethorphan hydrobromide (p.1117·3).

**Pharminil DM** *Therapex, Canad.*
Dextromethorphan hydrobromide (p.1117·3).

**Pharmitussin DM** *Therapex, Canad.†.*
Dextromethorphan hydrobromide (p.1117·3); guaifenesin (p.1122·1).

**Pharmorubicin**
*Pharmacia, Austral.; Pharmacia, Canad.; Pharmacia, Hong Kong; Pharmacia, Irl.; Pharmacia, Malaysia; Pharmacia, NZ; Pharmacia, Singapore; Pharmacia, UK.*
Epirubicin hydrochloride (p.550·2).
*Malignant neoplasms.*

**Pharmotidine** *Community Pharmacy, Thai.*
Famotidine (p.1265·2).
*Gastro-oesophageal reflux; peptic ulcer; Zollinger-Ellison syndrome.*

**Pharnax** *Pharmaland, Thai.*
Alprazolam (p.668·3).
*Mixed anxiety depressive states.*

**Pharo-Tus** *Nakornpatana, Thai.†.*
Dextromethorphan hydrobromide (p.1117·3); phenylpropanolamine hydrochloride (p.1127·3); chlorphenamine maleate (p.427·3); guaifenesin (p.1122·1).
*Coughs.*

**Pharyngine a la Vitamine C** *Medeva, Fr.†.*
Tyrothricin (p.275·1); lidocaine hydrochloride (p.1377·3); ascorbic acid (p.1460·2).
Formerly contained tyrothricin, tetracaine hydrochloride, and ascorbic acid.
*Infections of the mouth and throat.*

**Pharyngor** *Rappai, Switz.*
Potassium chloride; sodium chloride; magnesium chloride; calcium chloride (p.1217·1).
*Dry mouth and throat.*

**Pharynx**
*DHA, Hong Kong; DHA, Malaysia; DHA, Singapore.*
Cetylpyridinium chloride (p.1173·1); benzocaine (p.1370·3).
*Mouth and throat infections.*

**Pharysyx N** *Syxyl, Ger.*
Homoeopathic preparation.

**Phase O** *Grunenthal, Chile.*
A range of sunscreen preparations.

**Phatropine** *Pharmaland, Thai.†.*
Benzatropine mesilate (p.479·2).
*Drug-induced extrapyramidal disorders; parkinsonism.*

**Phazyme**
*Reed & Carnrick, Canad.; Stafford-Miller, Spain†; Reed & Carnrick, USA.*
Simeticone (p.1289·2).
*Flatulence.*

**Phenadoz** *Paddock, USA.*
Promethazine hydrochloride (p.439·1).

**Phenaemal** *Desitin, Ger.†.*
Phenobarbital (p.367·3).
*Epilepsy.*

**Phenaemaletten** *Desitin, Ger.†.*
Phenobarbital (p.367·3).
*Epilepsy.*

**Phenahist-TR** *Williams, USA†.*
Phenylpropanolamine hydrochloride (p.1127·3); phenylephrine hydrochloride (p.1126·3); chlorphenamine maleate (p.427·3); hyoscyamine sulfate (p.485·1); hyoscine hydrobromide (p.483·3); atropine sulfate (p.477·1).
*Upper respiratory-tract symptoms.*

**Phenameth DM** *Major, USA.*
Promethazine hydrochloride (p.439·1); dextromethorphan hydrobromide (p.1117·3).
*Coughs and cold symptoms.*

**Phenamin** *Nycomed, Norw.*
Dexchlorpheniramine maleate (p.427·3).
*Hypersensitivity reactions; pruritus.*

**Phenapap** *Rugby, USA.*
Pseudoephedrine hydrochloride (p.1129·2); paracetamol (p.76·2).
*Upper respiratory-tract disorders.*

**Phenapap Sinus Headache & Congestion** *Rugby, USA.*
Pseudoephedrine hydrochloride (p.1129·2); paracetamol (p.76·2); chlorphenamine maleate (p.427·3).
*Upper respiratory-tract symptoms.*

**Phenaphen with Codeine**
*Note. This name is used for preparations of different composition.*
*Wyeth-Ayerst, Canad.†.*
Aspirin (p.15·1); phenobarbital (p.367·3); codeine phosphate (p.27·1).
*Pain.*

*Robins, USA†.*
Paracetamol (p.76·2); codeine phosphate (p.27·1).
*Pain.*

**Phenaseptic** *Rugby, USA.*
Phenol (p.1188·1).
*Minor mouth or throat irritation.*

**Phenate**
*Note. This name is used for preparations of different composition.*
*Alphapharm, Malaysia; Merck, Malaysia; Pacific, NZ; Alphapharm, Singapore; Merck, Singapore.*
Clomifene citrate (p.1542·2).
*Anovulatory infertility.*

*Roberts, USA†; Hauck, USA†.*
Phenylpropanolamine hydrochloride (p.1127·3); chlorphenamine maleate (p.427·3); paracetamol (p.76·2).
*Upper respiratory-tract symptoms.*

**PhenaVent** *Ethex, USA.*
Phenylephrine hydrochloride (p.1126·3); guaifenesin (p.1122·1).
*Upper respiratory-tract disorders.*

**Phenazin** *Faulding, Port.*
Fluphenazine hydrochloride (p.699·3).

**Phenazine** *Pharmaland, Thai.*
Fluphenazine decanoate (p.699·3).
*Psychoses.*

**Phenazo**
*ICN, Canad.; CPC, Hong Kong†.*
Phenazopyridine hydrochloride (p.83·1).
*Lower urinary-tract irritation; urinary-tract pain.*

**Phenchlor SHA** *Rugby, USA†.*
Phenylpropanolamine hydrochloride (p.1127·3); phenylephrine hydrochloride (p.1126·3); chlorphenamine maleate (p.427·3); hyoscyamine sulfate (p.485·1); hyoscine hydrobromide (p.483·3); atropine sulfate (p.477·1).
*Upper respiratory-tract symptoms.*

**Phencodin** *Medicap, Thai.*
Codeine phosphate (p.27·1); promethazine hydrochloride (p.439·1).
*Coughs.*

**Phendex** *Aspen Consumer, S.Afr.†.*
Triprolidine hydrochloride (p.442·3); pseudoephedrine hydrochloride (p.1129·2); guaifenesin (p.1122·1); codeine phosphate (p.27·1).
*Coughs.*

**Phendiridine** *TP, Thai.*
Phenazopyridine hydrochloride (p.83·1).
*Urinary-tract pain.*

**Phenedrine** *United American, Hong Kong†.*
Theophylline (p.798·3).
*Obstructive airways disease.*

**Phenerbel-S** *Rugby, USA.*
Phenobarbital (p.367·3); ergotamine tartrate (p.467·2); belladonna (p.479·1).

**Phenergan**
*Aventis, Austral.; Rhone-Poulenc Rorer, Austria†; Aventis, Belg.; Aventis, Canad.; Novartis Consumer, Canad.; Aventis, Denm.; Celltech, Fr.; Aventis, Gr.; IFET (ΙΦΕΤ), Gr.; Rhone-Poulenc Rorer, Hong Kong†; Nicholas Piramal, India; Aventis, Irl.; Rhone-Poulenc Rorer, Neth.†; Aventis, Norw.; Aventis, NZ; Aventis, S.Afr.; Rhone-Poulenc Rorer, Singapore†; Rhone-Poulenc Rorer, Switz.†; Aventis, Thai.; Aventis, UK; Wyeth-Ayerst, USA.*
Promethazine (p.439·1) or promethazine hydrochloride (p.439·1).
*Hypersensitivity reactions; insomnia; motion sickness; nausea and vomiting; parkinsonism; premedication; sedative.*

**Phenergan with Codeine** *Wyeth-Ayerst, USA†.*
Promethazine hydrochloride (p.439·1); codeine phosphate (p.27·1).
*Coughs and cold symptoms.*

**Phenergan with Dextromethorphan** *Wyeth-Ayerst, USA†.*
Promethazine hydrochloride (p.439·1); dextromethorphan hydrobromide (p.1117·3).
*Coughs and cold symptoms.*

**Phenergan Expectorant**
*Note. This name is used for preparations of different composition.*
*Rhone-Poulenc Rorer, Belg.†.*
Promethazine (p.439·1); sulfogaiacol (p.1131·1); ipecacuanha (p.1122·3).
*Coughs.*

*Novartis Consumer, Canad.†.*
Promethazine hydrochloride (p.439·1); sulfogaiacol (p.1131·1).
*Coughs.*

*Rhone-Poulenc Rorer, Switz.†.*
Promethazine hydrochloride (p.439·1); guaifenesin (p.1122·1); ipecacuanha (p.1122·3).
*Coughs.*

**Phenergan Expectorant with Codeine** *Novartis Consumer, Canad.†.*
Promethazine hydrochloride (p.439·1); sulfogaiacol (p.1131·1); codeine phosphate (p.27·1).
*Coughs.*

**Phenergan VC** *Wyeth-Ayerst, USA†.*
Promethazine hydrochloride (p.439·1); phenylephrine hydrochloride (p.1126·3).
*Cold symptoms; nasal congestion.*

**Phenergan VC with Codeine** *Wyeth-Ayerst, USA†.*
Promethazine hydrochloride (p.439·1); phenylephrine hydrochloride (p.1126·3); codeine phosphate (p.27·1).
*Cold symptoms; coughs; nasal congestion.*

**Phenergan VC Expectorant** *Novartis Consumer, Canad.†.*
Promethazine hydrochloride (p.439·1); phenylephrine hydrochloride (p.1126·3); sulfogaiacol (p.1131·1).
*Coughs.*

**Phenergan VC Expectorant with Codeine**
*Novartis Consumer, Canad.†.*
Promethazine hydrochloride (p.439·1); phenylephrine hydrochloride (p.1126·3); sulfogaiacol (p.1131·1); codeine phosphate (p.27·1).
*Coughs.*

**Phenex**
*Abbott, Austral.; Ross, USA.*
A range of phenylalanine-free preparations for enteral nutrition (p.1417·1).
*Hyperphenylalaninaemia; phenylketonuria.*

**Phenexpect**
*Note. This name is used for preparations of different composition.*
*DHA, Hong Kong.*
Diphenhydramine hydrochloride (p.431·3); ammonium chloride (p.1115·2); sodium citrate (p.1223·2).
*Coughs.*

*DHA, Malaysia; DHA, Singapore.*
Diphenhydramine hydrochloride (p.431·3); ammonium chloride (p.1115·2).
*Coughs.*

**Phenexpect CD** *DHA, Singapore.*
Diphenhydramine hydrochloride (p.431·3); codeine phosphate (p.27·1); ammonium chloride (p.1115·2).
*Coughs.*

**Phenhalal** *Halal, UK†.*
Promethazine hydrochloride (p.439·1).

**Phenhist DH with Codeine** *Rugby, USA.*
Pseudoephedrine hydrochloride (p.1129·2); chlorphenamine maleate (p.427·3); codeine phosphate (p.27·1).
*Coughs and cold symptoms.*

**Phenhist Expectorant** *Rugby, USA.*
Pseudoephedrine hydrochloride (p.1129·2); guaifenesin (p.1122·1); codeine phosphate (p.27·1).
*Coughs.*

**Phenhydan**
*Gerot, Austria; Desitin, Ger.; Desitin, Switz.*
Phenytoin (p.370·2) or phenytoin sodium (p.370·2).
*Arrhythmias; epilepsy; trigeminal neuralgia.*

**Phenicol** *Vitamed, Israel.*
Chloramphenicol (p.185·1).
*Bacterial eye infections.*

**Phenimixin** *Vitamed, Israel.*
Chloramphenicol (p.185·1); polymyxin B sulfate (p.245·1).
*Bacterial eye infections.*

**Phenobarb** *PP Lab, Thai.*
Phenobarbital (p.367·3).
*Epilepsy; insomnia; sedative.*

**Phenocillin** *Streuli, Switz.*
Benzathine phenoxymethylpenicillin (p.163·2) or phenoxymethylpenicillin (p.242·1).
*Bacterial infections.*

**Phenoptic** *Optopics, USA.*
Phenylephrine hydrochloride (p.1126·3).
*Funduscopy; open-angle glaucoma; ophthalmic examination; pupil dilatation during surgery; refraction without cycloplegia; uveitis.*

**Phenoris** *Germiphene, Canad.*
Clioquinol (p.196·3); allantoin (p.1141·3); phenol (p.1188·1).
*Topical antiseptic.*

**Phenoro** *Roche, Fr.†.*
Betacarotene (p.1422·3); canthaxanthin (p.1056·3).
*Lupus erythematosus; photosensitivity.*

**Phenotal** *Asian Pharm, Thai.*
Phenobarbital sodium (p.367·3).
*Epilepsy; insomnia; sedative.*

**Phenoxine** *Lannett, USA†.*
Phenylpropanolamine hydrochloride (p.1127·3).
*Obesity.*

**Phenpro** *Ratiopharm, Ger.*
Phenprocoumon (p.981·3).
*Thromboembolic disorders.*

**Phensedyl**
*Note. This name is used for preparations of different composition.*
*Aspen, Austral.*
Promethazine hydrochloride (p.439·1); pholcodine (p.1128·3); pseudoephedrine hydrochloride (p.1129·2).
*Coughs.*

*Nicholas Piramal, India.*
Chlorphenamine maleate (p.427·3); codeine phosphate (p.27·1).
*Coughs.*

*Aventis, Malaysia; Aventis, Singapore; Aventis, Thai.*
Promethazine hydrochloride (p.439·1); codeine phosphate (p.27·1).
*Cold symptoms; coughs.*

*Aventis, S.Afr.*
Promethazine hydrochloride (p.439·1); codeine phosphate (p.27·1); ephedrine hydrochloride (p.1120·1).
*Coughs.*

**Phensedyl Dry Family Cough** *Aventis, NZ.*
Promethazine hydrochloride (p.439·1); pholcodine (p.1128·3); pseudoephedrine hydrochloride (p.1129·2).
*Coughs.*

**Phensedyl Plus** *Rhone-Poulenc Rorer, UK†.*
Promethazine hydrochloride (p.439·1); pholcodine (p.1128·3); pseudoephedrine hydrochloride (p.1129·2).
*Congestion; coughs; sore throats.*

**Phensic** *Merck Consumer, UK.*
Aspirin (p.15·1); caffeine (p.782·1).
*Fever; pain.*

**Phensic Dual Action** *Merck Consumer, UK†.*
Paracetamol (p.76·2); codeine phosphate (p.27·1); caffeine (p.782·1).
*Cold and influenza symptoms; fever; pain.*

**Phensic Ibuprofen** *Merck Consumer, UK†.*
Ibuprofen (p.45·3).
*Fever; pain.*

**Phenylade** *Taranis, Fr.*
Food for special diets (p.1417·1).
*Phenylketonuria.*

**Phenyldrine** *Rugby, USA†.*
Phenylpropanolamine hydrochloride (p.1127·3).
*Obesity.*

**Phenylfenesin LA** *Goldline, USA†.*
Phenylpropanolamine hydrochloride (p.1127·3); guaifenesin (p.1122·1).
*Coughs.*

**Phenyl-Free**
*Mead Johnson, Hong Kong; Mead Johnson, Israel; Mead Johnson, Ital.; Mead Johnson, NZ; Mead Johnson Nutritionals, USA.*
Food for special diets (p.1417·1).
Formerly known as Lofenalac in the *USA*.
*Phenylketonuria.*

**Phenylgesic** *Goldline, USA.*
Phenyltoloxamine citrate (p.439·1); paracetamol (p.76·2).
*Upper respiratory-tract symptoms.*

**Phenyphrine-Azol** *Vitamed, Israel.*
Mepyramine maleate (p.437·1); naphazoline hydrochloride (p.1124·3); phenylephrine hydrochloride (p.1126·3).
*Nasal congestion.*

**Phenytek** *Bertek, USA.*
Phenytoin (p.370·2).
*Epilepsy.*

**Pheramin N** *Kanoldt, Ger.†.*
Diphenhydramine hydrochloride (p.431·3).
*Allergic disorders of the conjunctiva.*

**Pherarutin** *Kanoldt, Ger.†.*
Troxerutin (p.1688·3).
*Retinal disorders.*

**Pherazine with Codeine** *Halsey, USA.*
Promethazine hydrochloride (p.439·1); codeine phosphate (p.27·1).
*Coughs and cold symptoms.*

**Pherazine DM** *Halsey, USA.*
Promethazine hydrochloride (p.439·1); dextromethorphan hydrobromide (p.1117·3).
*Coughs and cold symptoms.*

**Pherazine VC** *Halsey, USA.*
Promethazine hydrochloride (p.439·1); phenylephrine hydrochloride (p.1126·3).
*Upper respiratory-tract symptoms.*

**Pherazine VC with Codeine** *Halsey, USA.*
Promethazine hydrochloride (p.439·1); phenylephrine hydrochloride (p.1126·3); codeine phosphate (p.27·1).
*Coughs and cold symptoms.*

**pH5-Eucerin**
*Beiersdorf, Chile; Beiersdorf, Ger.†; BDF, Mex.; Beiersdorf, Port.†; Beiersdorf, Thai.*
A range of skin cleansing and emollient preparations.

**pH5-Eucerin Solar** *Beiersdorf, Chile.*
*Gel SPF 16:* Octinoxate (p.1154·3); amiloxate (p.1142·2); avobenzone (p.1142·3); enzacamene (p.1147·1); titanium dioxide (p.1160·3).
*Gel SPF 8; Cream SPF 15; Cream SPF 25:* Octinoxate (p.1154·3); avobenzone (p.1142·3); enzacamene (p.1147·1).
*Lotion SPF 20; Lotion SPF 25:* Octinoxate (p.1154·3); avobenzone (p.1142·3); enzacamene (p.1147·1); titanium dioxide (p.1160·3).
*Sunscreen.*

**Phexin** *GlaxoSmithKline, India.*
Cefalexin (p.168·1).
*Bacterial infections.*

**Phicon** *Williams, USA.*
Pramocaine hydrochloride (p.1382·2); vitamin A (p.1451·2); vitamin E (p.1464·3).
*Local anaesthesia.*

**Phicon-F** *Williams, USA.*
Pramocaine hydrochloride (p.1382·2); undecenoic acid (p.410·3).
*Fungal skin infections.*

**Philinal** *Rekah, Israel.*
*Suppositories:* Diprophylline (p.784·3); phenobarbital (p.367·3).
*Tablets†:* Diprophylline (p.784·3); diphenhydramine hydrochloride (p.431·3).
*Obstructive airways disease.*

**Philinet** *Rekah, Israel.*
Diprophylline (p.784·3); phenobarbital (p.367·3).
*Obstructive airways disease.*

**Phillips' Chewable** *Sterling, USA.*
Magnesium hydroxide (p.1272·2).
*Hyperacidity.*

**Phillips Gelcaps** *Bayer, Canad.†.*
Docusate sodium (p.1262·2); phenolphthalein (p.1284·1).
*Constipation.*

**Phillips' Milk of Magnesia**
*Bayer, Canad.; Sterling Health, USA.*
Magnesium hydroxide (p.1272·2).
*Constipation; dyspepsia.*

**pHisoDerm**
*Note. This name is used for preparations of different composition.*
*SmithKline Beecham, Hong Kong†.*
Entsufon (p.1683·3).
*Skin, scalp, and hair cleanser.*

*Cilag, UK†; Chattem, USA.*
Skin cleanser.

**pHisoHex**
*Note. This name is used for preparations of different composition.*
*Sanofi Synthelabo, Canad.; Sanofi Winthrop, USA.*
Entsufon sodium (p.1683·3); hexachlorophene (p.1181·2).
*Skin cleansing; skin disinfection.*

*Sanofi Synthelabo, Malaysia.*
Triclosan (p.1195·2).
*Skin infections.*

**pHisoHex Face Wash** *GlaxoSmithKline Consumer, Austral.*
Triclosan (p.1195·2).
*Acne.*

**pHisoHex Reformulated**
*Note. This name is used for preparations of different composition.*
*Sanofi Synthelabo, Hong Kong.*
Triclosan (p.1195·2).
*Acne; skin infections.*

*Sanofi Synthelabo, Singapore.*
Triclosan (p.1195·2); pyrithione zinc (p.1156·2).
*Skin cleanser.*

**Phisomain** *Anios, Fr.*
Octenidine hydrochloride (p.1187·2).
*Hand disinfection.*

**pHiso-MED** *Sanofi Synthelabo, UK†.*
Chlorhexidine gluconate (p.1173·2).
Formerly contained hexachlorophene.
*Skin disinfection.*

**Phlebocreme** *Monot, Fr.†.*
Benzocaine (p.1370·3); dodeclonium bromide (p.1178·3); esculoside (p.1648·2); enoxolone (p.36·2).

**Phlebodril**
*Note. This name is used for preparations of different composition.*
*Germania, Austria; Robapharm, Switz.†.*
Ruscus aculeatus; hesperidin methyl chalcone (p.1688·3); ascorbic acid (p.1460·2).
*Venous insufficiency.*

*Pierre Fabre, Ger.*
Ruscus aculeatus; trimethylhesperidin chalcone (p.1688·3).
*Vascular disorders.*

*Robapharm, Switz.*
*Cream:* Petit houx root; melilotus officinalis.
*Venous insufficiency.*

**Phlebodril mono** *Pierre Fabre, Ger.*
Ruscus aculeatus.
*Haemorrhoids; venous insufficiency.*

**Phlebodril N**
*Note. This name is used for preparations of different composition.*
*Pierre Fabre, Ger.*
Ruscus aculeatus rhizome; melilotus officinalis; dextran sulfate (p.1679·2).
*Vascular disorders.*

*Robapharm, Switz.*
Ruscus aculeatus; hesperidin methyl chalcone (p.1688·3).
*Haemorrhoids; venous insufficiency.*

**Phlebogel** *Lipha Sante, Fr.*
Aescin (p.1648·2); buphenine hydrochloride (p.1663·2).
*Peripheral vascular disorders.*

**Phlebosedol** *Lehning, Fr.*
Aesculus (p.1648·2); hamamelis (p.1696·3); viburnum; alchemilla; red vine.
*Haemorrhoids; venous insufficiency.*

**Phlebostasin** *Klinge, Switz.*
Aesculus (p.1648·2).
*Peripheral vascular disorders.*

**Phlebostasin compositum** *Klinge, Switz.*
Aescin (p.1648·2); heparin sodium (p.928·1); glycol salicylate (p.44·3).
*Oedema; phlebitis; soft-tissue disorders; venous insufficiency.*

**Phlebosup** *Monot, Fr.†.*
Benzocaine (p.1370·3); dodeclonium bromide (p.1178·3); esculoside (p.1648·2); enoxolone (p.36·2).
*Anorectal disorders.*

**Phlexy**
*Scientific Hospital Supplies, Austral.; SHS, Fr.; Scientific Hospital Supplies, Irl.; Nutricia, Ital.; Nutricia, NZ; Scientific Hospital Supplies, NZ; SHS, UK.*
Food for special diets (p.1417·1).
*Phenylketonuria.*

**Phlexy Vits** *Scientific Hospital Supplies, Irl.*
Vitamin, mineral, and trace element preparation (p.1417·1).
*Inborn errors of metabolism.*

**Phlexyvits** *SHS, UK.*
Multivitamin and mineral preparation (p.1417·1).

**Phlogenzym**
*Enzimas, Arg.; Mucos, Austria; Khol, Braz.†; Mucos, Ger.; Romsa, Mex.*
Bromelains (p.1662·2); trypsin (p.1758·3); rutoside (p.1688·2).
*Inflammation; oedema; rheumatic disorders; soft-tissue disorders; thrombophlebitis.*

**Phlogidermil** *Vifor, Switz.†.*
Ichthammol (p.1148·2); hamamelis (p.1696·3); guaiazulene (p.1696·2); cod-liver oil (p.1425·2); lavender oil (p.1705·2); zinc oxide (p.1163·2).
*Inflammation; muscular pain.*

**Phlogont** *Azupharma, Ger.*
Glycol salicylate (p.44·3).
*Musculoskeletal, joint, and soft-tissue disorders.*

**Phlogont Rheuma** *Azupharma, Ger.*
Glycol salicylate (p.44·3).
*Musculoskeletal, joint, and soft-tissue disorders.*

**Phlogont-Thermal** *Azupharma, Ger.*
Glycol salicylate (p.44·3); benzyl nicotinate (p.21·2).
*Musculoskeletal and joint disorders; sports injuries.*

**Phocytan** *Aguettant, Fr.*
Glucose-1-phosphate disodium, tetrahydrate.
*Hypophosphataemia; parenteral nutrition.*

**Pholcodyl** *Medeva, Fr.†.*
Pholcodine (p.1128·3); erysimum.
*Coughs.*

**Pholcolin** *Antigen, Irl.*
Pholcodine (p.1128·3).
*Coughs.*

**Pholcolinct** *Propan, S.Afr.*
Pholcodine (p.1128·3).
*Cough.*

**Pholco-Mereprine** *Novum, Belg.*
Doxylamine succinate (p.432·3); pholcodine (p.1128·3); sulfogaiacol (p.1131·1); sodium benzoate (p.1169·3).
*Respiratory-tract disorders.*

**Pholcones** *Cooperation Pharmaceutique, Fr.†.*
Quinine sulfate (p.460·2); camphor (p.1665·3); cineole (p.1672·1); pholcodine (p.1128·3); amylocaine hydrochloride (p.1370·2).
*Coughs; respiratory disorders.*

**Pholcones Bismuth** *Cooperation Pharmaceutique, Fr.*
Guaifenesin (p.1122·1); bismuth succinate (p.1253·1); cineole (p.1672·1).
*Respiratory-tract congestion.*

**Pholtex** *3M, S.Afr.*
Pholcodine resin complex (p.1128·3); phenyltoloxamine resin complex (p.439·1).
*Coughs.*

**Pholtrate** *McGloin, Austral.†.*
Pholcodine (p.1128·3).
*Coughs.*

**Phol-Tussil** *Interdelta, Switz.*
Pholcodine (p.1128·3); sodium benzoate (p.1169·3); tolu balsam (p.1131·3).
*Coughs.*

**Phol-Tux** *Interdelta, Switz.*
Pholcodine (p.1128·3); ethylmorphine hydrochloride (p.37·3); sulfogaiacol (p.1131·1); belladonna (p.479·1); senega root (p.1130·2); sodium benzoate (p.1169·3).
*Coughs.*

**Phonal** *Reig Jofre, Spain.*
*Lozenges:* Bacitracin (p.161·3); benzocaine (p.1370·3); neomycin sulfate (p.235·1); polymyxin B sulfate (p.245·1).
*Throat spray:* Benzalkonium chloride (p.1168·3); dexamethasone sodium phosphate (p.1097·2).
*Mouth and throat disorders.*

**Phonix Antitox** *Phonix, Ger.†.*
Homoeopathic preparation.

**Phonix Arthrophon** *Phonix, Ger.†.*
Homoeopathic preparation.

**Phonix Aurum III/012B** *Phonix, Ger.†.*
Homoeopathic preparation.

**Phonix Bronchophon** *Phonix, Ger.†.*
Homoeopathic preparation.

**Phonix Ferrum 032 A** *Phonix, Ger.†.*
Homoeopathic preparation.

**Phonix Gastriphon** *Phonix, Ger.†.*
Artemisia abrotanum; absinthium (p.1645·1); centaury (p.1669·2); gentian (p.1692·2).
*Gastrointestinal disorders.*

**Phonix Hydrargyrum II/027A** *Phonix, Ger.†.*
Homoeopathic preparation.

**Phonix Lymphophon** *Phonix, Ger.†.*
Homoeopathic preparation.

**Phonix Phonohepan** *Phonix, Ger.†.*
Homoeopathic preparation.

**Phonix Plumbum 024 A** *Phonix, Ger.†.*
Homoeopathic preparation.

**Phonix Solidago II/035 B** *Phonix, Ger.†.*
Homoeopathic preparation.

**Phonix Tartarus III/020** *Phonix, Ger.†.*
Homoeopathic preparation.

**phono Arnica comp** *Phonix, Ger.*
Homoeopathic preparation.

**phono Chol** *Phonix, Ger.*
Homoeopathic preparation.

**phono Gripp** *Phonix, Ger.*
Homoeopathic preparation.

**phono Uren** *Phonix, Ger.*
Homoeopathic preparation.

**phono Ven** *Phonix, Ger.*
Homoeopathic preparation.

**Phor Pain** *Goldshield, UK.*
Ibuprofen (p.45·3).
*Muscle pain.*

**Phorpain** *Goldshield, Irl.*
Ibuprofen (p.45·3).
*Musculoskeletal, joint, and soft-tissue disorders; neuralgia.*

**Phos Kola** *Phos-Kola, Braz.†.*
Calcium; medicinal plants (p.1417·1).
*Nutritional supplement.*

**PhosChol** *American Lecithin, USA.*
Phosphatidyl choline (p.1731·1).
*Nutritional supplement.*

**Phoscortil** *Kolassa, Austria.*
Prednisolone metasulfobenzoate sodium (p.1108·1); aluminium phosphate (p.1250·1).

**Phosetamin** *Kohler-Pharma, Ger.*
Calcium, magnesium, and potassium salts of phosphorylcolamine.
*Electrolyte disorders.*

**Phos-Ex**
*Vitaline, Fin.; Gry, Ger.; Vitaline, Norw.; Vitaline, Swed.; Vitaline, UK.*
Calcium acetate (p.1225·1).
*Hyperphosphataemia.*

**Phos-Flur**
*Colgate Oral Care, Austral.†; Colgate-Hoyt, USA.*
Sodium fluoride (p.1444·3).
*Dental caries prophylaxis.*

**Phosfo Enema** *Cristalia, Braz.*
Monobasic sodium phosphate (p.1230·3); dibasic sodium phosphate (p.1231·1).
*Bowel evacuation; constipation.*

**Phosfomin** *Sarabhai Piramal, India.*
Vitamin B substances (p.1417·1).

**Phosfomin Iron** *Sarabhai Piramal, India.*
Iron polymaltose (p.1437·3).
*Iron-deficiency anaemia.*

**Phosfonema** *Cristalia, Braz.†.*
Calcium phosphate (p.1225·3).
*Constipation.*

**Phosforid** *Sun, India.*
Calcium acetate (p.1225·1).
*Hyperphosphataemia.*

**Phoslo** *Pasteur, Chile.*
Calcium acetate (p.1225·1).
*Hyperphosphataemia.*

**PhosLo** *Nabi, USA.*
Calcium acetate (p.1225·1).
*Hyperphosphataemia.*

**Phos-NaK** *Cypress, USA.*
Monobasic sodium phosphate (p.1230·3); dibasic sodium phosphate (p.1231·1); monobasic potassium phosphate (p.1230·3); dibasic potassium phosphate (p.1230·3).
*Nutritional supplement.*

**Phosoforme** *Monin, Fr.*
Phosphoric acid (p.1731·2).
*Urinary-tract disorders.*

**Phosphalugel**
*Kolassa, Austria; Yamanouchi, Belg.; Yamanouchi, Fr.; Yamanouchi, Ger.; Yamanouchi, Port.; Boehringer Ingelheim, Switz.*
Colloidal aluminium phosphate (p.1250·1).
*Gastrointestinal disorders associated with hyperacidity.*

**Phosphate-Novartis** *Novartis, Canad.*
Monobasic sodium phosphate (p.1230·3); potassium bicarbonate (p.1223·1).
Formerly known as Phosphate-Sandoz.
*Electrolyte supplement; hypercalciuria.*

**Phosphates** *Pharmascience, Canad.*
Monobasic sodium phosphate (p.1230·3); dibasic sodium phosphate (p.1231·1).
*Bowel evacuation; constipation.*

**Phosphate-Sandoz**
*Note. This name is used for preparations of different composition.*
*Novartis, Austral.*
Monobasic sodium phosphate (p.1230·3).
*Hypercalcaemia; rickets.*

*Novartis, NZ; Novartis, S.Afr.; HK Pharma, UK.*
Monobasic sodium phosphate (p.1230·3); sodium bicarbonate (p.1223·2); potassium bicarbonate (p.1223·1).
*Hypercalcaemia; hypophosphataemia.*

**Phosphocalcina Iodada** *CIF, Braz.*
Sodium carbonate; calcium hypophosphite; sodium hypophosphite; iodine; tannin (p.1222·2).
*Oral rehydration therapy.*

**Phosphocholine** *Yves Ponroy, Fr.†.*
Dibasic sodium phosphate (p.1231·1); choline citrate (p.1424·3); trisodium citrate (p.1223·2).
*Dyspepsia.*

**Phosphocol** *Mallinckrodt, USA.*
Phosphorus-32 (p.1525·1) in the form of chromic phosphate.
*Malignant neoplasms.*

**Phospho-Lax** *Sofar, Ital.*
Monobasic sodium phosphate (p.1230·3); dibasic sodium phosphate (p.1231·1).
*Constipation.*

**Phospholine Iodide**
*Wyeth, Austral.; Wyeth-Ayerst, Canad.†; Chiesi, Fr.†; Wyeth-Ayerst, Israel†; Dominion, UK†; Wyeth-Ayerst, USA.*
Ecothiopate iodide (p.1490·2).
Available on a named-patient basis only in the *UK*.
*Convergent strabismus; glaucoma.*

**Phosphoneuros** *Bouchara-Recordati, Fr.*
Phosphoric acid (p.1731·2); calcium dihydrogen phosphate (p.1664·2); dibasic sodium phosphate (p.1231·1); magnesium glycerophosphate (p.1228·1).
*Hypercalciuria; hypophosphataemic rickets.*

**Phosphonorm**
*Medice, Ger.; Salmon, Switz.*
Aluminium chlorohydrate (p.1142·1).
*Hyperphosphataemia.*

**Phosphoprep** *Pharmatel, Austral.*
Monobasic sodium phosphate (p.1230·3); dibasic sodium phosphate (p.1231·1).
*Bowel evacuation.*

**Phosphoral**
*De Witt, Denm.; Ferring, Fin.; De Witt, Norw.; Ferring, Swed.*
Monobasic sodium phosphate (p.1230·3); dibasic sodium phosphate (p.1231·1).
*Bowel evacuation; constipation.*

**Phosphore-Medifa** *Medipha, Fr.*
Monoammonium phosphate (p.1654·1); monobasic potassium phosphate (p.1230·3); manganese glycerophosphate (p.1695·2).
*Hypercalciuria; rickets.*

**Phosphor-Homaccord** *Peithner, Austria.*
Homoeopathic preparation.

**Phosphorus Med Complex** *Dynamit, Austria.*
Homoeopathic preparation.

**Phostal**
*Stallergenes, Ital.; Stallergenes, Switz.*
Allergan extracts (p.1650·1).
*Allergen immunotherapy.*

**Phostarac** *Pharmacia, Arg.*
Alendronate sodium (p.765·3).
*Osteolysis; osteoporosis.*

**Photoderm**
*Bioderma, Fr.†.*
*Capsules:* Betacarotene; tomato oleoresin; fish oil; rape-seed oil; soya lecithin; vitamin E (p.1417·1).

*Bioderma, Fr.†.*
*Tablets:* Lemon; tea; vitamin C; vitamin E (p.1417·1).

**Photoderm Latte** *Piam, Ital.†.*
Octinoxate (p.1154·3); avobenzone (p.1142·3).
*Sunscreen.*

**Photoderm Max** *Bioderma, Ital.*
*Cream:* Octinoxate (p.1154·3); titanium dioxide (p.1160·3); avobenzone (p.1142·3); enzacamene (p.1147·1).
*Topical milk:* Octil octanoate; octinoxate (p.1154·3); titanium dioxide (p.1160·3); avobenzone (p.1142·3); octocrilene (p.1154·3); zinc oxide (p.1163·2).
*Sunscreen.*

**Photoderm Mineral** *Bioderma, Ital.*
Octil octanoate; titanium dioxide (p.1160·3).
*Sunscreen.*

**Photoderm Special** *Polaris, Ital.†.*
Titanium dioxide (p.1160·3); octinoxate (p.1154·3); enzacamene (p.1147·1); avobenzone (p.1142·3); ensulizole (p.1147·1).
*Sunscreen.*

**Photofrin**
*Axcan, Canad.; Meduna, Ger.; Axcan, Israel; Ipsen, UK†; Sanofi Winthrop, USA.*
Porfimer sodium (p.580·3).
*Non-small-cell lung cancer; oesophageal cancer; papillary bladder cancer.*

**Photoplex** *Allergan, Canad.*
*SPF 15:* Avobenzone (p.1142·3); octisalate (p.1154·3); octocrilene (p.1154·3); oxybenzone (p.1154·3).
*Sunscreen.*

**Photoscreen**
*Note. This name is used for preparations of different composition.*
*Pierre Fabre, Arg.*
*SPF 60:* Octinoxate (p.1154·3); octocrilene (p.1154·3); titanium dioxide (p.1160·3); zinc oxide (p.1163·2).
*Sunscreen.*

*Ducray, Fr.*
*SPF 30; SPF 60:* Octinoxate (p.1154·3); octocrilene (p.1154·3); titanium dioxide (p.1160·3).
*Sunscreen.*

**Phrenilin** *Carnrick, USA.*
Butalbital (p.673·3); paracetamol (p.76·2).
*Tension headache.*

**Phycocyane** *Labocean, Fr.*
Spirulina (p.1749·2).
*Tonic.*

**Phylarm**
*Poen, Arg.; LCA, Fr.*
Sodium chloride (p.1233·3); borax (p.1661·3); boric acid (p.1662·1).
*Dry eyes; eye irritation.*

**Phyllocontin**
*Purdue, Canad.; Mundipharma, Hong Kong†; Napp, Irl.; Pharmafrica, S.Afr.; Napp, UK; Purdue Frederick, USA†.*
Aminophylline (p.780·2).
*Obstructive airways disease.*

**Phyllotemp**
*Mundipharma, Ger.; Mundipharma, Switz.*
Aminophylline (p.780·2).
*Obstructive airways disease.*

**Phylobid** *Wockhardt, India.*
Theophylline (p.798·3).
*Obstructive airways disease.*

**Phyloday** *Wockhardt, India.*
Theophylline (p.798·3).
*Obstructive airways disease.*

**Phylorinol** *Schaffer, USA.*
*Mouthwash:* Phenol (p.1188·1); methyl salicylate (p.59·3).
*Minor mouth or throat irritation.*
*Topical solution:* Phenol (p.1188·1); boric acid (p.1662·1); strong iodine solution (p.1598·1).
*Oral wounds and infections.*

**Phymet DTF** *Glaxo Wellcome, Irl.*
Methadone hydrochloride (p.57·2).
*Opioid addiction.*

**Phymorax** *Medica Korea, Singapore.*
Hydroxyzine hydrochloride (p.434·3).
*Alcohol withdrawal syndrome; anxiety; nausea and vomiting; premedication; skin disorders.*

**Phy-O** *Zekides, Gr.*
Sodium chloride (p.1233·3).
*Nasal congestion.*

**Physeptone**
*GlaxoSmithKline, Austral.; GlaxoSmithKline, Hong Kong; Wellcome, Irl.; GlaxoSmithKline, S.Afr.; GlaxoSmithKline, Singapore; Martindale, UK.*
Methadone hydrochloride (p.57·2).
NOTE. There is no connection between Martindale, The Complete Drug Reference and Martindale Pharmaceuticals.
*Cough; opioid withdrawal syndrome; pain.*

**Physex** *Byk Elmu, Spain†.*
Chorionic gonadotrophin (p.1320·3).
*Erectile dysfunction; male and female infertility; metrorrhagia; threatened or recurrent miscarriage.*

**Physiodose** *Geymonat, Ital.*
Sodium chloride (p.1233·3).
*Eye and nose cleansing.*

**Physiogel**
*Note. This name is used for preparations of different composition.*
*Stiefel, Fr.; Stiefel, Hong Kong; Stiefel, Ital.; Stiefel, Malaysia; Stiefel, Singapore.*
Sodium cocoyl isetionate.
*Soap substitute.*

*Braun, Switz.*
Modified gelatin (p.754·3) with electrolytes.
*Hypovolaemia.*

**Physiogesic** *Hebert, Canad.*
Diethylamine salicylate (p.34·1).

**Physiogine** *Organon, Fr.*
Estriol (p.1552·3).
*Oestrogen deficiency.*

**Physiolax** *Medipharm, Switz.†.*
Aloes (p.1248·2); belladonna (p.479·1).
*Constipation; stool softener.*

**Physiologic** *Democal, Switz.*
Sodium chloride (p.1233·3).
*Nasal irrigation.*

**Physiologica**
*Qualiphar, Belg.; Gifrer Barbezat, Fr.*
Sodium chloride (p.1233·3).
*Eye wash; nasal irrigation.*

**Physiolyte** *McGaw, USA.*
Electrolytes (p.1217·1).
*Irrigation solution.*

**Physiomenthol** *Hebert, Canad.*
Menthol (p.1711·3).

**Physiomer**
*Sanofi Winthrop, Fr.; Sanofi Synthelabo OTC, Ital.*
Sea water (p.1233·3).
*Nasal irrigation.*

**Physiomint** *Koch, Austria.*
Mint oil (p.1715·2).
*Gastrointestinal disorders; headache; migraine; respiratory-tract disorders; rheumatic disorders; soft-tissue and muscle injury.*

**Physiomycine** *Laphal, Fr.*
Methacycline hydrochloride (p.230·1).
*Bacterial infections.*

**Physioneal**
*Baxter, Austria; Baxter, Denm.; Baxter, Fin.; Baxter, Ger.; Baxter, Ital.; Baxter, Swed.; Baxter, Switz.; Baxter, UK.*
Anhydrous glucose; calcium chloride; magnesium chloride; sodium chloride; sodium bicarbonate; sodium lactate (p.1221·1).
*Peritoneal dialysis solution.*

**Physioneal Glucosa** *Baxter, Spain.*
Glucose monohydrate; calcium chloride; magnesium chloride; sodium chloride; sodium bicarbonate; sodium lactate (p.1221·1).
*Peritoneal dialysis.*

**Physiorhine** *Aventis, Belg.*
Sodium chloride (p.1233·3).
*Cleansing of nasal passages and eyelids.*

**Physio-Rub** *Hebert, Canad.*
Methyl salicylate (p.59·3); menthol (p.1711·3); cineole (p.1672·1).

**Physiosoin**
*Chauvin, Fr.; Bausch & Lomb, Switz.*
Sodium chloride (p.1233·3)(p.1164·2).
*Eye wash; nasal irrigation; rinsing solution for contact lens; wound irrigation.*

**PhysioSol** *Abbott, USA.*
Electrolytes (p.1217·1).
*Irrigation solution.*

**Physiostat** *Organon, Fr.†.*
7 Tablets, ethinylestradiol (p.1553·2); 15 tablets, ethinylestradiol; lynestrenol (p.1557·1).
*Sequential-type oral contraceptive.*

**Physiotens**
*Solvay, Denm.; Solvay, Fin.; Solvay, Fr.; Solvay, Ger.; Solvay, Norw.; Solvay, S.Afr.; Solvay, Singapore; Solvay, Swed.; Solvay, Switz.; Solvay, UK.*
Moxonidine (p.962·3).
*Hypertension.*

**Physiotherm** *Ferrier, Fr.*
Natural spring water of Berthemont-les-Bains (p.1217·1).
*Nasal irrigation.*

**Physiotulle**
*Coloplast, Fr.*
Carmellose (p.1577·3).
*Burns; ulcers; wounds.*

*Coloplast, UK.*
Carmellose sodium (p.1577·3).
*Wounds.*

**Physium** *Boiron, Canad.†.*
Sodium chloride (p.1233·3).
*Nasal congestion; nasal hygiene.*

**Phytat** *Cochon, Fr.†.*
Sodium fytate (p.1052·3).
*Hypercalciuria.*

**Phytemag** *Lesourd, Fr.*
Magnesium glycerophosphate; apium root; buchu leaf; equisetum; ginger (p.1417·1).
*Tonic.*

**Phytentielles** *Bionatec, Fr.†.*
A range of herbal preparations.

**Phytex**
*Rupertus, Austria†.*
Sorbic acid (p.1192·3); tannic acid (p.1751·2); methyl salicylate (p.59·3); salicylic acid (p.1157·1); acetic acid (p.1645·2).
*Fungal infections of the feet.*

*Pharmax, Irl.*
Tannic acid (p.1751·2); boric acid (p.1662·1); salicylic acid (p.1157·1); methyl salicylate (p.59·3); acetic acid (p.1645·2).
*Fungal skin and nail infections.*

*Forest Laboratories, UK.*
Borotannic complex (p.1751·2) (p.1662·1); salicylic acid (p.1157·1); methyl salicylate (p.59·3); acetic acid (p.1645·2).
*Fungal skin and nail infections.*

**Phytic Acid** *Mac, Ital.*
Fytic acid (p.1052·3); glycolic acid (p.1147·3).
*Hyperpigmentation disorders.*

**Phyto Corrective Gel** *Dispolab, Chile.*
Arbutin; pepino; thyme (p.1755·2); bioflavonoids (p.1688·2).
*Skin pigmentation disorders.*

**Phytoberidin** *Synpharma, Switz.†.*
Valerian (p.1762·2); hypericum (p.299·1); passion flower (p.1729·1); guaiazulene (p.1696·2); lupulus (p.1708·1); melissa (p.1711·1).
*Insomnia; nervous disorders.*

**Phytobronchin** *Steigerwald, Ger.*
Cowslip rhizome (p.1735·1); thyme (p.1755·2).
*Cold symptoms.*

**Phytocalm**
*Note. This name is used for preparations of different composition.*
*UPSA Conseil, Fr.*
Valerian (p.1762·2); ballota; crataegus (p.1677·1); passion flower (p.1729·1).
*Insomnia; nervous disorders.*

*Arkopharma, UK.*
Passion flower (p.1729·1).
*Insomnia; stress and strain.*

**Phyto-Care** *Panpharma, Hong Kong.*
Soya isoflavones (p.1447·2).
*Menopausal disorders; osteoporosis.*

**Phytocean** *Ido, Fr.*
Nutritional supplement (p.1417·1).

**Phytocold** *Arkopharma, UK.*
Echinacea (p.1683·2).
*Colds.*

**Phytocortal** *Steierl, Ger.*
Homoeopathic preparation.

**Phytoderm Compositum** *Teva, Israel.*
Tolnaftate (p.410·1); salicylic acid (p.1157·1); benzoic acid (p.1169·3).
*Fungal skin infections.*

**Phytodiet** *Phytodiet, Fr.*
High protein food for special diets (p.1417·1).

**Phytodolor**
*Madaus, Austria; Steigerwald, Ger.*
Populus tremula leaf and bark (p.1733·3); fraxinus excelsior bark; solidago virgaurea (p.1748·3).
*Musculoskeletal and joint disorders; neuralgia.*

**Phytodorma** *Hevert, Ger.*
Valerian (p.1762·2).
*Nervous disorders; sleep disorders.*

**Phyto-Embryonnaire** *Recherche Botanique, Fr.*
Crataegus; birch; black currant; rosa canina; ginkgo biloba; juglans regia (p.1417·1).
*Gastrointestinal disorders.*

**Phytoestrin** *Usana, Hong Kong.*
Soya isoflavones (p.1447·2); angelica sinensis (p.1655·1); cimicifuga (p.1671·3); agnus castus (p.1649·1); liquorice (p.1270·2).
*Menopausal disorders; menstrual disorders.*

**Phytoestrol N** *Muller Goppingen, Ger.*
Rhapontic rhubarb (p.1288·1).
*Endometritis; juvenile oligomenorrhoea and dysmenorrhoea; menopausal disorders; primary and secondary amenorrhoea.*

**Phytofibre** *Plantes et Medecines, Fr.†.*
Ispaghula (p.1268·1).
*Constipation.*

**Phytogran**
*Note. This name is used for preparations of different composition.*
*Synpharma, Austria.*
Valerian root (p.1762·2); lupulus (p.1708·1); melissa leaf (p.1711·1).
*Anxiety; sleep disorders.*

*Grandel-Synpharma, Ger.*
Lupulus (p.1708·1); hypericum (p.299·1).
*Nervous disorders.*

**Phytohepar** *Steigerwald, Ger.*
Silybum marianum (p.1043·3).
*Liver disorders.*

**Phytohustil** *Steigerwald, Ger.*
Althaea (p.1651·3).
Formerly known as Phytobronchin.
*Coughs.*

**Phyto-Hypophyson C** *Steierl, Ger.*
Homoeopathic preparation.

**Phyto-Hypophyson L** *Steierl, Ger.*
Homoeopathic preparation.

**Phytolax**
*Note. This name is used for preparations of different composition.*
*Sante Naturelle, Canad.†.*
Cascara (p.1255·1); phenolphthalein (p.1284·1); bile salts (p.1660·3); capsicum oleoresin (p.1667·1); papain (p.1727·3).
*Synpharma, Switz.†.*
Aloes (p.1248·2); frangula (p.1266·3); belladonna (p.479·1).
*Constipation.*

**Phyto-Laxia** *Phytopharma, Switz.*
Frangula bark (p.1266·3); senna (p.1288·2).
*Constipation.*

**PhytoLaxin** *Hanseler, Switz.*
Aloes (p.1248·2); frangula bark (p.1266·3); senna (p.1288·2).
Formerly known as Obducti laxativi vegetabiles S and contained aloes, belladonna, frangula bark, and senna.
*Constipation.*

**Phytolife** *Blackmores, Austral.†.*
Soya bean (p.1447·2); calcium (p.1225·1).
*Calcium deficiency; menopausal disorders.*

**Phytolife Plus** *Blackmores, UK.*
Calcium (p.1225·1); soya (p.1447·2).
*Menopausal disorders.*

**Phytolithe** *Phytosolba, Fr.*
Ichthammol (p.1148·2); cajuput oil (p.1664·1); cade oil (p.1159·2); storax (p.1749·3).
*Seborrhoeic dermatitis.*

**Phytomed Cardio** *Phytomed, Switz.*
Crataegus (p.1677·1); passion flower (p.1729·1); rosemary (p.1740·2).
*Cardiac disorders.*

**Phytomed Gastro** *Phytomed, Switz.†.*
Angelica (p.1655·1); centaury (p.1669·2); chamomile (p.1669·3); peppermint leaf (p.1283·2); caraway (p.1667·2); potato.
*Digestive disorders.*

**Phytomed Hepato** *Phytomed, Switz.*
Absinthium (p.1645·1); cynara (p.1678·3); peppermint leaf (p.1283·2); raphanus sativus var. nigra; silybum marianum (p.1043·3); taraxacum (p.1751·3).
*Digestive disorders.*

**Phytomed Nephro** *Phytomed, Switz.*
Silver birch (p.1660·3); solidago virgaurea (p.1748·3); java tea (p.1702·3); juniper (p.1703·1); ononis (p.1723·3); taraxacum (p.1751·3).
*Urinary-tract disorders.*

**Phytomed Nervo** *Phytomed, Switz.*
Melissa (p.1711·1); passion flower (p.1729·1); bitter orange (p.1723·3); lupulus (p.1708·1).
*Agitation; sleep disorders.*

**Phytomed Prosta** *Phytomed, Switz.*
Echinacea purpurea (p.1683·2); poplar buds (p.1733·3); saw palmetto (p.1569·1); solidago virgaurea (p.1748·3).
*Prostatic pain; urinary disorders.*

**Phytomed Rhino** *Phytomed, Switz.†.*
Cinchona bark (p.1671·3); echinacea purpurea (p.1683·2); salix (p.87·3); solidago virgaurea (p.1748·3).
*Cold symptoms; sinusitis.*

**Phytomed Somni** *Phytomed, Switz.*
Valerian (p.1762·2); passion flower (p.1729·1); lupulus (p.1708·1); lavandula angustifolia.
*Sleep disorders.*

**Phytomelis** *Lehning, Fr.*
Hamamelis (p.1696·3); aesculus (p.1648·2).
*Haemorrhoids; peripheral vascular disorders.*

**Phytonoctu** *Steigerwald, Ger.*
Melissa (p.1711·1); passion flower (p.1729·1); valerian (p.1762·2).
*Nervous disorders; sleep disorders.*

**Phytonoxon N** *Steigerwald, Ger.†.*
Corydalis cava; eschscholtzia californica.
*Sleep disorders.*

**Phytophanere** *Phytosolba, Fr.*
Wheat-germ oil; carrot oil; borage oil (p.1661·3); rice-bran oil; salmon oil (p.976·1); yeast (p.1469·1); antilles cherries; fish roe.
*Fragile hair and nails.*

**Phytopure** *Lalco, Canad.*
Multivitamin and mineral preparation (p.1417·1).

**Phytorelax** *Arkopharma, UK.*
Valerian (p.1762·2).
*Stress; tension.*

**Phytoslim** *Arkopharma, UK.*
Kelp (p.1742·3).
*Obesity.*

**Phytosyl Plus** *Vita Health, Singapore.*
Fibre; *Lactobacillus* species; aloe vera (p.1417·1).
*Dietary fibre supplement.*

**Phytotherapie Boribel no 8** *Dietetique et Sante, Fr.†.*
Tilia (p.1756·2); passion flower (p.1729·1); valerian (p.1762·2).
*Insomnia; nervous disorders.*

**Phytotherapie Boribel no 9** *Dietetique et Sante, Fr.†.*
Fraxinus excelsior; bladderwrack (p.1742·3).
*Obesity.*

**Phytotherapie Titree** *Boiron, Fr.*
A range of herbal preparations.

**Phytotux** *Lehning, Fr.*
Tolu balsam (p.1131·3); Desessartz syrup.
*Coughs.*

**Phytotux H** *Homeocan, Canad.*
Homoeopathic preparation.

**Phytovim** *Sante Naturelle, Canad.*
Multivitamin and mineral preparation (p.1417·1).

**PI Antiseptic Ointment** *Hexal, Austral.*
Povidone-iodine (p.1190·3).

**Piascledine**
*Sintofarma, Braz.; Pharmascience, Fr.; ABC, Ital.*
Avocado oil; soya oil (p.1447·2).
*Gum disorders; musculoskeletal and joint disorders; phlebitis; skin disorders; skin ulceration.*

**Piat** *Salus, Mex.*
Miconazole (p.405·2).
*Fungal infections.*

**Piazofolina** *Bracco, Ital.†.*
Morinamide hydrochloride (p.233·1).
*Tuberculosis.*

**Picalm** *Grunenthal, Port.*
Piketoprofen (p.84·1) or piketoprofen hydrochloride (p.84·1).
*Musculoskeletal, joint, peri-articular, and soft-tissue disorders.*

**Picapan** *DHA, Singapore.*
Paracetamol (p.76·2); caffeine (p.782·1).
*Fever; pain.*

**Picariz** *Picot, Fr.†.*
Food for special diets (p.1417·1).
*Diarrhoea.*

**Picibanil** *Chugai, Jpn.*
Lyophilised powder of *Streptococcus pyogenes.*
*Malignant neoplasms.*

**Picillin**
*Laboratorio Farm., Israel; CT, Ital.*
Piperacillin sodium (p.243·1).
Lidocaine hydrochloride (p.1377·3) may be included in this preparation to alleviate the pain of injection.
*Bacterial infections.*

**Pickles Antiseptic Cream** *Pickles, UK.*
Dibrompropamidine isetionate (p.1178·2).
*Burns; scalds; sunburn.*

**Pickles Chilblain Cream** *Pickles, UK.*
Methyl nicotinate (p.59·2).
*Chilblains.*

**Pickles Corn Caps** *Pickles, UK.*
Salicylic acid (p.1157·1); colophony (p.1675·1).
*Corns.*

**Pickles Foot Ointment** *Pickles, UK.*
Salicylic acid (p.1157·1).
*Calluses; corns.*

**Pickles Smelling Salts** *Pickles, UK.*
Strong ammonia solution (p.1653·3); eucalyptus oil (p.1686·2); pine oil.
*Headache; nasal congestion.*

**Picolax**
*Note. This name is used for preparations of different composition.*
*Dendy, Austral.*
Sodium picosulfate (p.1289·3); magnesium carbonate (p.1272·1); citric acid (p.1673·1).
*Bowel evacuation; constipation.*
*Ferring, Braz.†.*
Sodium picosulfate (p.1289·3).
*Constipation.*
*Ferring, Irl.; Ferring, UK.*
Sodium picosulfate (p.1289·3); magnesium citrate (p.1272·1).
*Bowel evacuation.*

**Picolaxine** *Pharmethic, Belg.†.*
Sodium picosulfate (p.1289·3).
*Constipation.*

**Picolite** *Picot, Fr.*
Maltodextrin; sucrose; sodium chloride; potassium citrate; citric acid (p.1222·2).
*Diarrhoea; oral rehydration therapy.*

**Picolon** *Medic, Denm.*
Sodium picosulfate (p.1289·3).
*Constipation.*

**Picoprep**
*Pharmatel, Austral.; Bamford, NZ.*
Sodium picosulfate (p.1289·3); magnesium oxide (p.1272·3); citric acid (p.1673·1).
*Bowel evacuation; constipation.*

**Pico-Salax**
*Ferring, Israel†; Ferring, Norw.†; Ferring, Swed.†; Ferring, Switz.†.*
Sodium picosulfate (p.1289·3); magnesium oxide (p.1272·3); citric acid (p.1673·1).
*Bowel evacuation.*

**Picosyl** *Synthelabo, Spain†.*
Hydrocortisone acetate (p.1103·3).
*Skin disorders.*

**Picot** *Picot, Fr.*
Dextrin (p.1427·1); maltose (p.1440·1).
*Sugar substitute.*

**Picot sans Gluten** *Picot, Fr.*
Food for special diets (p.1417·1).
*Coeliac disease.*

**Picot Sans Lactose** *Picot, Fr.*
Infant feed (p.1417·1).
*Lactose intolerance.*

**Picroprep** *Pharmatel, Malaysia.*
Sodium picosulfate (p.1289·3); magnesium oxide (p.1272·3); citric acid (p.1673·1).
*Bowel evacuation.*

**Pidilat** *Solvay, Ger.*
Nifedipine (p.966·2).
*Angina pectoris; hypertension; Raynaud's syndrome.*

**Pidocal** *Sanofi Synthelabo, Switz.*
Calcium pidolate (p.1226·1); calcium carbonate (p.1254·2).
*Calcium deficiency; osteoporosis.*

**Pidomag** *Baldacci, Braz.*
Magnesium pidolate (p.1228·2).
*Magnesium deficiency.*

**Piecidex** *Andromaco, Arg.*
*Cream; topical powder:* Undecenoic acid (p.410·3); zinc undecenoate (p.411·1); sodium propionate (p.408·1); salicylic acid (p.1157·1).
*Topical liquid; topical spray:* Undecenoic acid (p.410·3); sodium undecenoate (p.411·1); sodium propionate (p.408·1); propionic acid (p.407·3).
*Fungal skin, scalp, and nail infections.*

**Piel Vital** *AM, Arg.*
Betacarotene; vitamins; minerals; methionine (p.1417·1).
*Dietary supplement.*

**Pielograf**
*Justesa Imagem, Braz.†; Schering, Chile; Juste, Spain.*
Meglumine amidotrizoate (p.1060·2); sodium amidotrizoate (p.1060·2).
*Radiographic contrast medium.*

**Pierami** *Fournier, Ital.*
Amikacin sulfate (p.154·1).
*Bacterial infections.*

**Pifrol** *Arlex, Mex.†.*
Dipyrone (p.35·3).

**Pigenil** *Pharmafar, Ital.*
Pygeum africanum (p.1568·2).
*Prostatic hyperplasia.*

**Pigitil** *Dorom, Ital.*
Pidotimod (p.1731·3).
*Immunostimulant.*

**Pigmal** *Gramon, Arg.*
Pirolenoso acid.
*Pediculosis.*

**Pigmanorm**
*Note. This name is used for preparations of different composition.*
*Widmer, Ger.*
Hydroquinone (p.1148·1); tretinoin (p.1161·1); hydrocortisone (p.1103·3).
*Skin hyperpigmentation.*
*Widmer, Switz.*
Hydroquinone (p.1148·1); tretinoin (p.1161·1); dexamethasone (p.1097·1); dexpanthenol (p.1727·2); octinoxate (p.1154·3); avobenzone (p.1142·3).
*Skin hyperpigmentation.*

**Pigmentasa** *Vinas, Spain.*
Hydroquinone (p.1148·1).
*Skin hyperpigmentation.*

**Piketofen** *Reuffer, Mex.†.*
Ketoprofen (p.51·2).

**Pik-Gel** *Tetido, Ital.†.*
Centella asiatica (p.1144·3); ginkgo biloba (p.1692·3); peppermint (p.1283·2); devil's claw root (p.28·2).
*Skin disorders.*

**Pilagan** *Allergan, USA†.*
Pilocarpine nitrate (p.1495·1).
*Glaucoma; reversal of mydriasis.*

**Pilax** *Agepha, Austria.*
Pilocarpine hydrochloride (p.1495·1).
*Glaucoma; production of miosis.*

**Pilder** *Quimifar, Spain.*
Gemfibrozil (p.923·1).
*Hyperlipidaemias.*

**Pildoras Ferrug Sanatori** *Santiveri, Spain†.*
Sulfur (p.1158·2); ferrous sulfate (p.1428·2); cinchona (p.1671·3); rhubarb (p.1287·3).
*Anaemias.*

**Pildoras Zeninas** *Puerto Galiano, Spain.*
Aloes (p.1248·2); cascara (p.1255·1).
Formerly contained aloes, belladonna, cascara, jalap, podophyllum, phenolphthalein, and liquorice.
*Constipation.*

**Pileabs** *Lane, UK.*
Slippery elm bark (p.1747·1); cascara sagrada (p.1255·1).
*Haemorrhoids.*

**Pilem** *Uniao Quimica, Braz.*
Levonorgestrel (p.1563·2).
*Progestogen-only oral contraceptive.*

**Pilensar** *IMA, Braz.*
Lindane (p.1506·3).
*Pediculosis; scabies.*

**Piletabs** *Potter's, UK.*
Pilewort (p.1732·1); agrimony (p.1649·1); cascara (p.1255·1); stone root (p.1749·3).
*Haemorrhoids.*

**Pilewort Compound** *Gerard House, UK†.*
Pilewort (p.1732·1); senna leaf (p.1288·2); geum maculatum; cascara (p.1255·1).
*Constipation.*

**Pil-Food**
*Vifor, Port.†.*
Methionine; cystine; vitamins; millett (p.1417·1).
*Hair and nail disorders.*
*Serra Pamies, Spain.*
Vitamins; amino acids; panicum miliaceum (p.1417·1).
*Hair, scalp, and nail disorders.*
*Golaz, Switz.*
Multivitamins and amino acids (p.1417·1); protein hydrolysate; millet.
*Hair and nail disorders.*

**Pilfood** *Cedar Health, UK.*
Vitamin E; ribloflavin; vitamin $B_6$; biotin; panthothenic acid; methionine; cystine (p.1417·1).
*Dietary supplement for healthy hair.*

**Pilfor P** *BASF, Ger.†.*
Paracetamol (p.76·2); codeine phosphate (p.27·1).
*Pain.*

**Pil-G Uso** *Finadiet, Arg.*
Glacial acetic acid (p.1645·2).
*Pediculosis.*

**Pilison** *Schering, Austria.*
Fluocortolone pivalate (p.1102·1); salicylic acid (p.1157·1).
*Skin disorders.*

**Pilka**
*Novartis Consumer, Austria; Novartis, Israel; Ferrer, Spain.*
Drosera (p.1683·1); thyme (p.1755·2).
*Bronchitis; coughs; throat disorders.*
*Novartis Consumer, Switz.*
Drosera (p.1683·1); pinguiculae; thyme (p.1755·2).
*Coughs.*

**Pilka F** *Novartis Consumer, Port.*
Drosera (p.1683·1); wild thyme; pinguicula.
*Coughs.*

**Pilka Forte** *Novartis Consumer, Austria.*
Drosera (p.1683·1); thyme (p.1755·2); ephedrine hydrochloride (p.1120·1).
*Coughs.*

**Pillole Fattori** *Ogna, Ital.†.*
Cape aloes (p.1248·2); rhubarb (p.1287·3); cascara (p.1255·1).
*Constipation.*

**Pilmolite** *REM, Braz.†.*
Albumin (p.740·3).
*Diagnostic agent.*

**Pilo**
*Viatris, Belg.; Chauvin, Fr.; Upha, Malaysia; Grin, Mex.; Novartis, Norw.*
Pilocarpine hydrochloride (p.1495·1).
*Glaucoma; hernia of the iris; reversal of mydriasis and cycloplegia.*
*Chauvin Novopharma, Switz.†.*
Pilocarpine nitrate (p.1495·1).
*Glaucoma; ocular hypertension.*

**Pilobloc** *Farmila, Ital.*
Pilocarpine hydrochloride (p.1495·1); timolol maleate (p.1012·2).
*Glaucoma; ocular hypertension.*

**Pilocar**
*FDC, India.*
Pilocarpine nitrate (p.1495·1).
*Glaucoma; production of miosis.*
*Novartis Ophthalmics, USA.*
Pilocarpine hydrochloride (p.1495·1).
*Glaucoma; raised intra-ocular pressure; reversal of mydriasis.*

**Pilocarcil** *Edol, Port.*
Pilocarpine hydrochloride (p.1495·1).
*Ocular hypertension; production of miosis.*

**Pilocarpol**
*Lersan, Arg.*
Pilocarpine hydrochloride (p.1495·1).
*Glaucoma; production of miosis.*
*Winzer, Ger.*
Pilocarpine (p.1494·3).
*Glaucoma; production of miosis.*

**Pilocollyre** *Cooper (Κοπερ), Gr.*
Pilocarpine hydrochloride (p.1495·1).
*Glaucoma; production of mydriasis.*

**Pilodren** *Farmila, Ital.*
Pilocarpine hydrochloride (p.1495·1); adrenaline acid tartrate (p.852·2).
*Open-angle glaucoma.*

**Pilo-Eserin** *Ciba Vision, Ger.†.*
Pilocarpine hydrochloride (p.1495·1); physostigmine salicylate (p.1494·1).
*Glaucoma; reversal of drug-induced mydriasis.*

**Pilof Nicolich** *Novag, Mex.†.*
Pilocarpine (p.1494·3).

**Piloftal** *Agepha, Austria.*
Pilocarpine (p.1494·3).
*Glaucoma; ophthalmic surgery.*

**Pilogel**
*Alcon, Austria; Alcon, Chile; Alcon, Ger.†; Alcon, Irl.; Alcon, Israel; Alcon, Ital.; Alcon, S.Afr.; Alcon, Singapore; Alcon, Thai.†; Alcon, UK.*
Pilocarpine hydrochloride (p.1495·1).
*Glaucoma; ocular hypertension.*

**Pilogel HS**
*Alcon, Hong Kong; Alcon, Switz.†.*
Pilocarpine hydrochloride (p.1495·1).
*Glaucoma; ocular hypertension.*

**Pilomann**
*Mann, Ger.; Bausch & Lomb, Thai.†; Mann, Thai.†.*
Pilocarpine hydrochloride (p.1495·1).
*Glaucoma; reversal of drug-induced mydriasis.*

**Pilomann-Ol** *Mann, Ger.*
Pilocarpine (p.1494·3).
*Glaucoma; reversal of drug-induced mydriasis.*

**Pilomed**
*Note. This name is used for preparations of different composition.*
*Biocumed, Arg.*
Pilocarpine hydrochloride (p.1495·1).
*Glaucoma; production of miosis.*

*QIF, Braz.†.*
Jaborandi.
*Alopecia.*

**Pilopine HS** *Alcon, Canad.; Alcon, USA.*
Pilocarpine hydrochloride (p.1495·1).
*Glaucoma; raised intra-ocular pressure; reversal of mydriasis.*

**Piloplex** *Davi, Port.*
Pilocarpine (p.1494·3).
*Glaucoma; production of miosis.*

**Pilopos** *Ursapharm, Ger.*
Pilocarpine nitrate (p.1495·1).
*Glaucoma; reversal of drug-induced mydriasis.*

**Pilopt** *Allergan, Austral.; Sigma, NZ.*
Pilocarpine hydrochloride (p.1495·1).
*Glaucoma.*

**Piloptic** *Optopics, USA.*
Pilocarpine hydrochloride (p.1495·1).
*Glaucoma; reversal of mydriasis.*

**Pilopto-Carpine** *Lebeh, USA.*
Pilocarpine hydrochloride (p.1495·1).
*Glaucoma; raised intra-ocular pressure; reversal of mydriasis.*

**Pilostat** *Bausch & Lomb, USA.*
Pilocarpine hydrochloride (p.1495·1).
*Glaucoma; raised intra-ocular pressure; reversal of mydriasis.*

**Pilostigmin Puroptal** *Metochem, Austria.*
Neostigmine bromide (p.1492·2); pilocarpine hydrochloride (p.1495·1).
*Glaucoma; production of miosis.*

**Pilo-Stulln** *Stulln, Ger.*
Pilocarpine hydrochloride (p.1495·1).
*Glaucoma; reversal of drug-induced mydriasis.*

**Pilosuryl** *Pierre Fabre, Fr.†.*
Pilosella; phyllanthus.
*Water retention.*

**Pilotim** *Alcon, Arg.*
Timolol maleate (p.1012·2); pilocarpine hydrochloride (p.1495·1).
*Glaucoma; ocular hypertension.*

**Pilotina** *Genepharm, Gr.*
Pilocarpine nitrate (p.1495·1).
*Glaucoma; production of mydriasis.*

**Pilotonina** *Farmila, Ital.*
Pilocarpine hydrochloride (p.1495·1).
*Ocular hypertension; production of miosis.*

**Pilovital** *Lesvi, Spain†.*
Minoxidil (p.960·1).
*Alopecia androgenetica.*

**Piloxil** *Golaz, Switz.*
Minoxidil (p.960·1).
*Alopecia androgenetica.*

**Pilulas De Witt's** *CIF, Braz.*
Bearberry (p.1659·2); methylthioninium chloride (p.1042·2); fabiana imbricata; juniper (p.1703·1); potassium nitrate (p.1190·1); parapetalifera betulina; cascara (p.1255·1); sodium salicylate (p.90·1).
*Urinary-tract infections.*

**Pilulas Ross** *GlaxoSmithKline, Braz.*
Aloin (p.1248·3); capsicum (p.1667·1); ipecacuanha (p.1122·3); belladonna (p.479·1).
*Constipation.*

**Pilules de Vichy** *Spiphar, Belg.†.*
Sodium picosulfate (p.1289·3); electrolytes (p.1217·1).
Formerly contained dantron and electrolytes.
*Constipation.*

**Pilzcin**
*Kolassa, Austria; Merz, Ger.; Shionogi, Jpn.*
Croconazole hydrochloride (p.397·1).
*Fungal skin infections.*

**Pima** *Fleming, USA.*
Potassium iodide (p.1598·1).
*Respiratory-tract congestion.*

**Pima Biciron N** *S & K, Ger.*
Natamycin (p.406·2).
*Fungal eye infections.*

**Pimafucin**
*Yamanouchi, Belg.†; Yamanouchi, Fin.; Galderma, Ger.*
Natamycin (p.406·2).
*Fungal infections.*

**Pimafucort**
*Yamanouchi, Belg.†; Yamanouchi, Fin.; Yamanouchi, Ger.†; CSL, NZ; Yamanouchi, NZ; Yamanouchi, Port.*
Hydrocortisone (p.1103·3); natamycin (p.406·2); neomycin sulfate (p.235·1).
*Infected skin disorders.*

**Pimiken** *Kendrick, Mex.*
Magnesium valproate (p.382·2).
*Epilepsy.*

**Pinaclav** *Pinewood, Irl.*
Amoxycillin trihydrate (p.155·3); potassium clavulanate (p.193·3).
*Bacterial infections.*

**Pinaclor** *Pinewood, Irl.*
Cefaclor (p.167·1).
*Bacterial infections.*

**Pinadone DTF** *Pinewood, Irl.*
Methadone hydrochloride (p.57·2).
*Opioid addiction.*

**Pinadrina** *Pisa, Mex.*
Adrenaline (p.852·2).

**Pinal N** *Atzinger, Ger.†.*
Zinc oxide (p.1163·2); N-(2-hydroxyethyl)-10-undecenamide; salicylic acid (p.1157·1).
*Skin disorders.*

**Pinal S** *Atzinger, Ger.*
Zinc oxide (p.1163·2).
*Skin disorders.*

**Pin-Alcol** *Schoning-Berlin, Ger.*
Menthol (p.1711·3); pine oil.
*Neuromuscular and joint disorders; pruritus; soft-tissue injury.*

**Pinalgesic** *Pinewood, Irl.†.*
Mefenamic acid (p.55·2).
*Menorrhagia; pain.*

**Pinamet** *Pinewood, Irl.*
Cimetidine (p.1255·3).
*Gastric hyperacidity; peptic ulcer; Zollinger-Ellison syndrome.*

**Pinamox** *Pinewood, Irl.*
Amoxicillin (p.155·3).
*Bacterial infections.*

**Pindac** *Leo, Denm.†.*
Pinacidil (p.983·1).
*Hypertension.*

**Pinden** *Unipharm, Israel.*
Pindolol (p.983·2).
*Heart failure; hypertension.*

**Pindione** *Lipha Sante, Fr.†.*
Phenindione (p.981·1).
*Thromboembolic disorders.*

**Pindocor** *Pharmacia, Fin.*
Pindolol (p.983·2).
*Angina pectoris; arrhythmias; hypertension.*

**Pindol** *Pacific, NZ.*
Pindolol (p.983·2).
*Angina pectoris; arrhythmias; hypertension.*

**Pindoptan** *Kanoldt, Ger.†.*
Pindolol (p.983·2).
*Glaucoma.*

**Pindoreal** *Realpharma, Ger.†.*
Pindolol (p.983·2).
*Arrhythmias; hypertension; ischaemic heart disease.*

**Pine OPC** *Eagle, Austral.†.*
Pinus pinaster; myrtillus (p.1718·3).
*Peripheral circulatory disorders; tonic.*

**Pineal** *Laborest, Ital.*
Magnesium; nicotinic acid; tryptophan (p.1417·1).
*Depression.*

**Pinedrin** *Lisapharma, Ital.*
Pumilio pine oil (p.1737·1); thyme (p.1755·2).
*Respiratory system disorders.*

**Pinetarsol**
*Note. This name is used for preparations of different composition.*
*Ego, Austral.; Ego, Malaysia; Ego, NZ; Ego, Singapore.*
Pine tar (p.1159·3).
*Skin disorders.*

*Ego, Austral.*
*Bath oil:* Pine tar (p.1159·3); light liquid paraffin (p.1479·1).
*Solution:* Pine tar (p.1159·3); trolamine laurilsulfate (p.1574·3).
*Skin disorders.*

*Ego, Hong Kong.*
Tar (p.1159·3).
*Skin disorders.*

**Pinex**
*Alpharma, Denm.; Alpharma, Norw.*
Paracetamol (p.76·2).
*Fever; pain.*

**Pinex Comp** *Alpharma, Denm.*
Paracetamol (p.76·2); codeine phosphate (p.27·1).
*Pain.*

**Pinex Forte** *Alpharma, Norw.*
Paracetamol (p.76·2); codeine phosphate (p.27·1).
*Pain.*

**Pinex Major** *Alpharma, Norw.*
Paracetamol (p.76·2); codeine phosphate (p.27·1).
*Pain.*

**Pinifed** *Pinewood, Irl.*
Nifedipine (p.966·2).
*Hypertension; ischaemic heart disease.*

**Pinikehl** *Sanum-Kehlbeck, Ger.*
Homoeopathic preparation.

**Piniment** *Austroplant, Austria.*
*Balsam:* Camphor (p.1665·3); eucalyptus oil (p.1686·2); oleum pini sylvestris; pumilio pine oil (p.1737·1); turpentine oil (p.1760·1); guaiazulene (p.1696·2).
*Coughs; gastrointestinal spasm; musculoskeletal and joint disorders; respiratory-tract disorders.*
*Bath additive:* Camphor (p.1665·3); menthol (p.1711·3); eucalyptus oil (p.1686·2).
*Cold symptoms.*
*Nasal ointment:* Ephedrine hydrochloride (p.1120·1); camphor (p.1665·3); eucalyptus oil (p.1686·2); oleum pini sylvestris; pumilio pine oil (p.1737·1); turpentine oil (p.1760·1); sage oil (p.1741·2); sunflower oil (p.1451·1).
*Nasal congestion.*
*Ointment; topical solution:* Camphor (p.1665·3); menthol (p.1711·3); eucalyptus oil (p.1686·2); oleum pini sylvestris; pumilio pine oil (p.1737·1); turpentine oil (p.1760·1).
*Catarrh; cold and influenza symptoms; cough.*

**Pinimenthol** *Piniol, Switz.*
Camphor (p.1665·3); menthol (p.1711·3); orange oil (p.1724·1); pine cone oil; eucalyptus oil (p.1686·2); pumilio pine oil (p.1737·1); turpentine oil (p.1760·1); pine-needle oil.
*Influenza; muscle and joint pain; neuralgia.*

**Pinimenthol Erkaltungsbad** *Spitzner, Ger.*
Camphor (p.1665·3); eucalyptus oil (p.1686·2); menthol (p.1711·3).
*Bath additive; cold symptoms.*

**Pinimenthol Erkaltungsbad fur Kinder** *Spitzner, Ger.*
Eucalyptus oil (p.1686·2).
*Bath additive; cold symptoms.*

**Pinimenthol Erkaltungsinhalat** *Spitzner, Ger.*
Eucalyptus oil (p.1686·2); oleum pini sylvestris.
*Cold symptoms.*

**Pinimenthol Erkaltungskapseln** *Spitzner, Ger.*
Eucalyptus oil (p.1686·2).
*Cold symptoms.*

**Pinimenthol Erkaltungssalbe** *Spitzner, Ger.*
Eucalyptus oil (p.1686·2); pine needle oil; menthol (p.1711·3).
*Respiratory-tract disorders.*

**Pinimenthol Liquidum** *Spitzner, Ger.*
Eucalyptus oil (p.1686·2); pine needle oil; menthol (p.1711·3).
*Neuralgia; respiratory-tract disorders; rheumatic disorders; skin ulcer prophylaxis.*

**Pinimenthol N**
*Spitzner, Ger.†; Piniol, Switz.*
Eucalyptus oil (p.1686·2); pine needle oil; menthol (p.1711·3).
*Cold symptoms; muscle and joint pain.*

**Pinimenthol Nasensalbe** *Spitzner, Ger.*
Camphor (p.1665·3); eucalyptus oil (p.1686·2); oleum pini sylvestris.
*Nasal disorders.*

**Pinimenthol Oral N** *Spitzner, Ger.†.*
Anethole (p.1654·3); cineole (p.1672·1); pumilio pine oil (p.1737·1).
*Asthma; bronchitis.*

**Pinimenthol S** *Spitzner, Ger.*
Eucalyptus oil (p.1686·2); oleum pini sylvestris.
*Bronchitis; cold symptoms.*

**Piniol** *Spitzner, Ger.†.*
Naphazoline hydrochloride (p.1124·3).
*Rhinitis.*

**Piniol Erkaltungsbalsam** *Spitzner, Ger.*
Camphor (p.1665·3); eucalyptus oil (p.1686·2); oleum pini sylvestris.
*Neuritis; respiratory-tract disorders; rheumatic disorders.*

**Piniol Nasensalbe** *Spitzner, Ger.†.*
Camphor (p.1665·3); eucalyptus oil (p.1686·2); pine needle oil.
*Cold symptoms.*

**Piniol Nasenspray** *Spitzner, Ger.*
Naphazoline hydrochloride (p.1124·3).
*Nasal congestion; rhinitis.*

**Pink Bismuth Rose** *Technilab, Canad.†.*
Bismuth salicylate (p.1252·1).

**Pinklot** *Stiefel, Arg.*
Sulfur (p.1158·2); resorcinol (p.1156·3); salicylic acid (p.1157·1); calamine (p.1144·1).
*Acne.*

**Pinloc** *Orion, Fin.*
Pindolol (p.983·2).
*Angina pectoris; arrhythmias; hypertension.*

**Pino-Cort** *Bell, India.*
Atropine sulfate (p.477·1); hydrocortisone acetate (p.1103·3).
*Allergic conjunctivitis; corneal burns; pre- and post-medication in ocular surgery.*

**Pinorhinol** *Knoll, Fr.†.*
Menthol (p.1711·3); camphor (p.1665·3); cineole (p.1672·1).
*Nose and throat infections.*

**Pinosil** *Sedar, Braz.†.*
Sodium dibunate (p.1130·2); malt (p.1439·2); aconite (p.1646·3); lobelia (p.1589·1); pine oil; vitamin $B_1$; vitamin C; sulfogaiacol (p.1131·1); sodium benzoate (p.1169·3).
*Coughs.*

**Pin-Rid** *Apothecary, USA.*
Pyrantel embonate (p.113·2).

**Pinselina Knapp** *Montefarmaco, Ital.*
Benzocaine (p.1370·3); phenol (p.1188·1); thymol (p.1194·2); menthol (p.1711·3).
*Mouth disorders.*

**Pinsken** *TO-Chemicals, Thai.†.*
Pindolol (p.983·2).
*Angina pectoris; arrhythmias; hypertension.*

**Pintacrom** *Diafarm, Spain†.*
Merbromin (p.1185·3).
*Wound disinfection.*

**Pintal** *Specifar (Σπεσιφαρ), Gr.*
Butamirate citrate (p.1116·2).
*Cough.*

**Pin-X** *Effcon, USA.*
Pyrantel embonate (p.113·2).

**Piodermina** *Farmachimici, Ital.*
Sodium fusidate (p.215·2); thyme (p.1755·2); mallow (p.1709·3).
*Bacterial skin infections.*

**Piodrex** *Bunker, Braz.*
Lindane (p.1506·3).
*Pediculosis; scabies.*

**Pioglit** *Phoenix, Arg.*
Pioglitazone hydrochloride (p.344·1).
*Diabetes mellitus.*

**Pioletal** *Delta, Braz.*
Lindane (p.1506·3).
*Pediculosis; scabies.*

**Piolhol** *Simoes, Braz.*
Permethrin (p.1508·3); piperonyl butoxide (p.1509·2).
*Pediculosis; scabies.*

**Piolhol Plus** *Simoes, Braz.*
Permethrin (p.1508·3).
*Pediculosis.*

**Piolin** *Sibras, Braz.†.*
Juglans regia; artemisia; rue (p.1741·1).
*Pediculosis.*

**Pionax** *Sanval, Braz.†.*
Lindane (p.1506·3).
*Pediculosis; scabies.*

**Pioral Pasta** *Teofarma, Ital.*
Chlorothymol (p.1177·2).
*Oral disinfection.*

**Piorlis** *Diviser Aquilea, Spain.*
Cineole (p.1672·1); eugenol (p.1686·2); peppermint oil (p.1283·2); methyl salicylate (p.59·3); thymol (p.1194·2); tyrothricin (p.275·1).
*Gingivitis; gum disinfection; mouth ulcers; pyorrhoea.*

**Piosan** *Belfar, Braz.†.*
Permethrin (p.1508·3).

**Piosol** *Virtus, Braz.†.*
Permethrin (p.1508·3).

**Piostop** *Hexal, Braz.*
Permethrin (p.1508·3).

**Pipacid** *Iasis, Gr.*
Omeprazole (p.1278·2).
*Acid aspiration; eradication of Helicobacter pylori in combination with antimicrobials; peptic ulcer; reflux oesophagitis; Zollinger-Ellison syndrome.*

**Pipcil**
*Wyeth Lederle, Belg.; Lederle, Neth.†.*
Piperacillin sodium (p.243·1).
*Bacterial infections.*

**Pipeacid** *Del Saz & Filippini, Ital.*
Pipemidic acid (p.243·1).
*Urinary-tract infections.*

**Pipedac** *Teofarma, Ital.*
Pipemidic acid (p.243·1).
*Urinary-tract infections.*

**Pipedic** *Pharmasant, Thai.*
Pipemidic acid (p.243·1).
*Bacterial infections of the urinary tract.*

**Pipefort** *Lampugnani, Ital.*
Pipemidic acid (p.243·1).
*Urinary-tract infections.*

**Pipemed** *Tecnofarma, Mex.†.*
Piperazine (p.111·2).

**Pipemid** *Gentili, Ital.*
Pipemidic acid (p.243·1).
*Urinary-tract infections.*

**Pipemidol** *Quimica y Farmacia, Mex.†.*
Pipemidic acid (p.243·1).
*Urinary-tract infections.*

**Pipera** *Astrapin, Ger.; Hameln, Ger.*
Piperacillin sodium (p.243·1).
*Bacterial infections.*

**Piperac** *Klonal, Arg.*
Piperacillin (p.243·1).
*Bacterial infections.*

**Piperawitt DS** *Columbia, Mex.*
Piperazine (p.111·2).
*Worm infections.*

**Piperazil** *Allen, Mex.*
Piperazine (p.111·2).
*Ascariasis; enterobiasis.*

**Pipercream** *Usmed, Braz.†.*
Piperazine (p.111·2).
*Ascariasis; enterobiasis.*

**Piperilline** *Wyeth Lederle, Fr.†.*
Piperacillin sodium (p.243·1).
*Bacterial infections.*

**Piperital** *Ibi, Ital.*
Piperacillin sodium (p.243·1).
Lidocaine hydrochloride (p.1377·3) is included in this preparation to alleviate the pain of injection.
*Bacterial infections.*

**Pipermed** *Medimport, Mex.*
Piperazine citrate (p.111·2).
*Ascariasis; enterobiasis.*

**Pipermel** *Basi, Port.*
Piperazine (p.111·2).

**Piperonil** *Lusofarmaco, Ital.*
Pipamperone hydrochloride (p.716·1).
*Insomnia; psychiatric disorders.*

**Pipersal** *Uno, Ital.*
Piperacillin sodium (p.243·1).
Lidocaine hydrochloride (p.1377·3) is included in this preparation to alleviate the pain of injection.
*Bacterial infections.*

**Pipertex** *Pharmatex, Ital.*
Piperacillin sodium (p.243·1).
Lidocaine hydrochloride (p.1377·3) is included in this preparation to alleviate the pain of injection.
*Bacterial infections.*

**Pipertox** *Codilab, Port.*
Piperazine (p.111·2).
*Worm infections.*

**Pipervermin** *Heralds, Braz.†.*
Piperazine (p.111·2).
*Ascariasis; enterobiasis.*

**Pipetecan** *Richmond, Arg.*
Irinotecan (p.564·3).
*Malignant neoplasms.*

**Pipetexina** *Richmond, Arg.*
Piperacillin (p.243·1); tazobactam (p.264·3).
*Bacterial infections.*

**Pipiol** *Medeva, Fr.†.*
Menthol (p.1711·3); cloral hydrate (p.684·1); formaldehyde solution (p.1179·3).
*Insect stings.*

**Piplex** *Mediderm, Chile.*
Isotretinoin (p.1148·3); isotretinoin (p.1148·3).
*Acne.*

**Piportil**
*Aventis, Belg.†; Aventis, Braz.; Aventis, Fr.; Rhone-Poulenc Rorer, Hong Kong†; Aventis, Irl.; Aventis, Neth.; Aventis, NZ; Aventis, Singapore; Rhone-Poulenc Rorer, Switz.†; JHC Healthcare, UK.*
Pipotiazine (p.716·1) or pipotiazine palmitate (p.716·1).
*Psychoses.*

**Piportil L4**
*Aventis, Canad.; Aventis, Mex.*
Pipotiazine palmitate (p.716·1).
*Psychoses.*

**Piportyl** *Aventis, Chile.*
Pipotiazine palmitate (p.716·1).
*Psychoses.*

**Piportyl L4** *Aventis, Arg.*
Pipotiazine palmitate (p.716·1).
*Psychoses.*

**Pippen** *Pharmaland, Thai.*
Ibuprofen (p.45·3).
*Musculoskeletal and joint disorders.*

**Pipracil**
*Wyeth-Ayerst, Canad.; Wyeth, Hong Kong; Wyeth Lederle, India; Wyeth, Malaysia; Wyeth-Ayerst, Thai.; Lederle, USA†.*
Piperacillin sodium (p.243·1).
*Bacterial infections.*

**Pipracin** *IRBI, Ital.†.*
Piperacillin sodium (p.243·1).
Lidocaine hydrochloride (p.1377·3) is included in the intramuscular injection to alleviate the pain of injection.
*Bacterial infections.*

**Pipralen** *Lennon, S.Afr.†.*
Piperazine hydrate (p.111·2).
*Ascariasis; enterobiasis.*

**Pipram**
*Rhone-Poulenc Rorer, Belg.†; Aventis, Braz.; Aventis, Fr.; Aventis, Ital.; Aventis, Neth.*
Pipemidic acid (p.243·1).
*Urinary-tract infections.*

**Pipril**
*Wyeth, Austral.; Wyeth Lederle, Austria; Lederle, Ger.; Wyeth, Gr.; Wyeth, Irl.; Lederle, Israel; Lederle, NZ; Wyeth, S.Afr.†; Wyeth, Spain†; Lederle, Switz.; Wyeth, UK†.*
Piperacillin sodium (p.243·1).
Lidocaine (p.1377·3) may be included in the intramuscular injection to alleviate the pain of injection.
*Bacterial infections.*

**Piprine** *Be-Tabs, S.Afr.*
Piperazine citrate (p.111·2).
*Ascariasis; enterobiasis.*

**Piprol** *Elfar, Spain.*
Ciprofloxacin hydrochloride (p.188·2).
*Bacterial infections.*

**Piproxen** *Nuovo ISM, Ital.†.*
Naproxen piperazine (p.65·3).
*Gout; musculoskeletal, joint, and peri-articular disorders; neuralgia.*

**Piptalake P** *Hoechst Marion Roussel, Braz.†.*
Piperidyl benzilate; phenobarbital (p.367·3).
*Smooth muscle spasm.*

**Pipurin** *NCSN, Ital.*
Pipemidic acid (p.243·1).
*Genitourinary-tract infections.*

**Pipurol** *Zambon, Braz.*
Pipemidic acid (p.243·1).
*Urinary-tract infections.*

**Pira** *Omega, Arg.*
Glibenclamide (p.331·2).
*Diabetes mellitus.*

**Pirabene** *Ratiopharm, Austria.*
Piracetam (p.1732·1).
*Alcohol withdrawal syndrome; organic brain disorders.*

**Piracalamina** *Szama, Arg.*
Phenol (p.1188·1); mepyramine maleate (p.437·1); calamine (p.1144·1); zinc oxide (p.1163·2).
*Contact dermatitis; lichen; pruritus; sunburn.*

**Piracebral** *Hexal, Ger.*
Piracetam (p.1732·1).
*Mental function disorders.*

**Piracetam Complex** *Almirall, Spain.*
Co-dergocrine mesilate (p.1674·1); piracetam (p.1732·1).
*Cerebrovascular disorders.*

**Piracetrop** *Holsten, Ger.*
Piracetam (p.1732·1).
*Mental function disorders.*

**Pirafoid** *Valdecasas, Mex.†.*
Pyrazinamide (p.246·3).

**Pirafrin** *Diba, Mex.*
Paracetamol (p.76·2); caffeine (p.782·1); phenylephrine hydrochloride (p.1126·3); chlorphenamine maleate (p.427·3).
*Conjunctival congestion; fever; nasal congestion; pain; rhinitis.*

**Piraldin** *Vitae, Mex.†.*
Paracetamol (p.76·2).
*Fever; pain.*

**Piraldina** *Bracco, Ital.*
Pyrazinamide (p.246·3).
*Tuberculosis.*

**Piralgina** *Diba, Mex.*
Paracetamol (p.76·2); caffeine (p.782·1); ephedrine hydrochloride (p.1120·1).
*Congestion; fever; pain.*

**Piralone** *Ferrer, Spain†.*
Lorazepam pivalate (p.705·1).
*Alcohol withdrawal syndrome; anxiety; epilepsy; insomnia; nausea and vomiting.*

**Piram** *General Drugs, Thai.*
Piroxicam (p.84·2).
*Gout; musculoskeletal, joint, peri-articular, and soft-tissue disorders.*

**Piramagno** *Pharmacos, Mex.*
Dipyrone (p.35·3).
*Fever; pain.*

**Piram-D** *Pacific, NZ.*
Piroxicam (p.84·2).
*Dysmenorrhoea; gout; musculoskeletal and joint disorders; pain.*

**Piramin** *Elofar, Braz.*
Paracetamol (p.76·2).
*Fever; pain.*

**Pirandall** *Randall, Mex.*
Dipyrone (p.35·3).
*Fever; pain.*

**Pirantrim** *Keton, Mex.†.*
Pyrantel embonate (p.113·2).

**Piraside** *Upsifarma, Port.*
Pyrazinamide (p.246·3).
*Tuberculosis.*

**Piratam**
*GlaxoSmithKline, India; Beacons, Singapore.*
Piracetam (p.1732·1).
*Alcoholism; behaviour disorders in children; cerebral trauma; cerebrovascular disorders; mental function impairment; senile dementia; sickle-cell disease; vertigo.*

**Pirawil** *Willmar, Mex.†.*
Dipyrone (p.35·3).

**Pirax**
*Note. This name is used for preparations of different composition.*
*Ecosol, Switz.*
Piracetam (p.1732·1).
*Dyslexia; mental function impairment; myoclonus.*

*Pharmaland, Thai.*
Piroxicam (p.84·2).
*Musculoskeletal and joint disorders.*

**Pirazer** *Zerboni, Mex.†.*
Pyrazinamide (p.246·3).

**Pirazinon** *Sanval, Braz.*
Pyrazinamide (p.246·3).
*Tuberculosis.*

**Pirehexal** *Hexal, Ger.†.*
Pirenzepine hydrochloride (p.488·1).
*Gastrointestinal disorders.*

**piren-basan** *Schonenberger, Switz.*
Pirenzepine hydrochloride (p.488·1).
*Gastrointestinal disorders associated with hyperacidity.*

**Piretanyl** *Pasteur, Chile.*
*Syrup:* Chlorphenamine maleate (p.427·3); dipyrone (p.35·3).
*Tablets:* Chlorphenamine maleate (p.427·3); dipyrone (p.35·3); caffeine (p.782·1).
*Cold and influenza symptoms.*

**Pireuma** *Noos, Ital.†.*
Propyphenazone (p.85·3).
*Fever; pain.*

**Pirexyl** *Pasteur, Chile.*
Diclofenac sodium (p.32·1).
*Fever; musculoskeletal and joint disorders; pain.*

**Pirfalin** *Farmigea, Ital.*
Pirenoxine sodium (p.1732·2).
*Cataracts.*

**Piridasmin** *Astra, Spain†.*
Theophylline (p.798·3).
*Obstructive airways disease.*

**Pirifedrina** *Funk, Spain†.*
Codeine phosphate (p.27·1); ephedrine hydrochloride (p.1120·1); paracetamol (p.76·2).
*Influenza and cold symptoms.*

**Pirifur** *Sanofi Synthelabo, Mex.*
Phenazopyridine hydrochloride (p.83·1); nalidixic acid (p.234·1).
*Urinary-tract infections.*

**Piriject** *Link, UK†.*
Chlorphenamine maleate (p.427·3).
Formerly known as Piriton. Now known as Chlorphenamine Injection.
*Hypersensitivity reactions.*

**Pirilene** *Aventis, Fr.*
Pyrazinamide (p.246·3).
*Tuberculosis.*

**Pirimat** *Duopharma, Hong Kong.*
Chlorphenamine maleate (p.427·3).
*Hypersensitivity reactions.*

**Pirimetan** *Richmond, Arg.*
Propranolol (p.990·1).

**Pirimir** *Sanofi Synthelabo, Mex.*
Phenazopyridine (p.83·2).
*Urinary-tract infections.*

**Pirinace** *Sidus, Arg.*
Aspirin (p.15·1); ascorbic acid (p.1460·2).
*Influenza symptoms.*

**Pirinasol** *Bayer, Spain†.*
Paracetamol (p.76·2).
*Fever; pain.*

**Pirinovag** *Novag, Mex.*
Dipyrone (p.35·3).
*Fever; pain.*

**Piriteze** *GlaxoSmithKline Consumer, UK.*
Cetirizine hydrochloride (p.427·1).
*Allergic rhinitis.*

**Piriton**
*GlaxoSmithKline, Hong Kong; Stafford-Miller, Irl.; GlaxoSmithKline, Singapore; GlaxoSmithKline, Thai.; GlaxoSmithKline Consumer, UK.*
Chlorphenamine maleate (p.427·3).
*Hypersensitivity reactions.*

**Piriton Expectorant**
*GlaxoSmithKline, India; GlaxoSmithKline, Thai.*
Chlorphenamine maleate (p.427·3); ammonium chloride (p.1115·2); sodium citrate (p.1223·2).
*Cold symptoms; coughs.*

**Piritosse** *Bergamo, Braz.†.*
Diphenhydramine (p.431·3); ephedrine (p.1120·1); pentetrazol (p.1592·1); cineole (p.1672·1); Desessartz syrup.
*Cold and influenza symptoms.*

**Pirium** *Janssen-Cilag, Gr.*
Pimozide (p.715·1).
*Psychoses.*

**Pirkam** *Nycomed, Denm.†.*
Piroxicam (p.84·2).
*Inflammation; musculoskeletal and joint disorders; pain.*

**Piro** *ABZ, Ger.*
Piroxicam (p.84·2).
*Musculoskeletal, joint, and soft-tissue disorders.*

**Piro KD** *Kade, Ger.*
Piroxicam (p.84·2).
*Musculoskeletal, joint, and soft-tissue disorders.*

**Piroalgin** *Lafedar, Arg.*
Piroxicam (p.84·2).
*Inflammation; pain.*

**Pirobac** *Koni-Cofarm, Chile.*
Benzoyl peroxide (p.1143·2).
*Acne.*

**Pirobeta** *Betapharm, Ger.*
Piroxicam (p.84·2).
*Gout; musculoskeletal, joint, and soft-tissue disorders.*

**Pirobutil** *Degorts, Mex.*
Dipyrone (p.35·3); butylhyoscine (p.484·2).
*Muscle spasm; pain.*

**Pirocal** *Aliud, Austria.*
Piroxicam (p.84·2).
*Gout; inflammation; musculoskeletal joint, and peri-articular disorders; pain.*

**Pirocam**
*Ratiopharm, Austria; Spirig, Switz.*
Piroxicam (p.84·2).
*Gout; inflammation; musculoskeletal joint, and peri-articular disorders; pain.*

**Pirodax** *Lemery, Mex.*
Piroxicam (p.84·2).
*Musculoskeletal and joint disorders.*

**Pirofix** *Hexal, Arg.*
Piroxicam (p.84·2).
*Gout; musculoskeletal, joint, and soft-tissue disorders; pain.*

**Piroflam**
*Note. This name is used for preparations of different composition.*
*Medipharm, Chile.*
Diclofenac diethylamine (p.32·1) or diclofenac sodium (p.32·1).
*Inflammation; pain.*

*Lichtenstein, Ger.*
Piroxicam (p.84·2).
*Gout; musculoskeletal, joint, and soft-tissue disorders.*

**Piroflex** *Betapharm, Ger.*
Piroxicam (p.84·2).
*Musculoskeletal, peri-articular, and soft-tissue disorders.*

**Piroftal** *Bruschettini, Ital.*
Piroxicam (p.84·2).
*Eye inflammation; ocular oedema.*

**Pirogina** *Teuto, Braz.*
Dipyrone (p.35·3).
*Fever; pain.*

**Pirohexal-D** *Hexal, Austral.*
Piroxicam (p.84·2).
*Ankylosing spondylitis; osteoarthritis; rheumatoid arthritis.*

**Piroli-N** *Sibras, Braz.†.*
Deltamethrin (p.1503·1).

**Pirom**
*Note. This name is used for preparations of different composition.*
*Durascan, Denm.*
Piroxicam (p.84·2).
*Inflammation; musculoskeletal and joint disorders; pain.*

*Solmer, Switz.*
*Balm:* Camphor (p.1665·3); menthol (p.1711·3); methyl salicylate (p.59·3); eucalyptus oil (p.1686·2); cinnamon oil (p.1672·2).
*Headache; insect bites and stings; muscle and joint pain; sports injuries.*
*Embrocation:* Camphor (p.1665·3); menthol (p.1711·3); methyl salicylate (p.59·3); eucalyptus oil (p.1686·2); sweet birch oil (p.60·1); citrus oil.
*Cold symptoms; headache; insect bites and stings; muscle and joint pain; sports injuries.*

**Piromav** *Mavi, Mex.†.*
Piroxicam (p.84·2).

**Piromebrina** *Degorts, Mex.*
Dipyrone (p.35·3).
*Fever; pain.*

**Pironal**
*Note. This name is used for preparations of different composition.*
*Bago, Chile.*
Ibuprofen (p.45·3).
*Fever; musculoskeletal and joint disorders; pain.*

*Wiener, Mex.†.*
Dipyrone (p.35·3).

**Pironet** *Nettopharma, Denm.†.*
Piroxicam (p.84·2).
*Musculoskeletal and joint disorders; pain.*

**Pirongil** *Arlex, Mex.†.*
Dipyrone (p.35·3).

**Pirophen** *Pfizer, NZ.*
Aspirin (p.15·1); paracetamol (p.76·2); codeine phosphate (p.27·1).
*Fever; pain.*

**Piro-Phlogont** *Azupharma, Ger.*
Piroxicam (p.84·2).
*Gout; musculoskeletal, joint, and soft-tissue disorders.*

**Piro-Puren** *Isis Puren, Ger.†.*
Piroxicam (p.84·2).
*Musculoskeletal, joint, and soft-tissue disorders.*

**Pirorheum**
*Hexal, Austria; Hexal, Ger.*
Piroxicam (p.84·2).
*Gout; inflammation; musculoskeletal, joint, peri-articular, and soft-tissue disorders; pain.*

**PirorheumA** *Hexal, Ger.*
Piroxicam (p.84·2).
*Musculoskeletal, joint, peri-articular, and soft-tissue disorders.*

**Pirosol** *Ecosol, Switz.*
Piroxicam (p.84·2).
*Inflammation; musculoskeletal, joint, and peri-articular disorders; pain.*

**Pirox**
*Pfizer, Austral.†; Jacoby, Austria; CT, Ger.; Cipla, India; Alpharma, Norw.; Progress, Thai.*
Piroxicam (p.84·2).
*Gout; inflammation; musculoskeletal joint, peri-articular, and soft-tissue disorders; pain.*

**Piroxal** *Alpharma, Fin.*
Piroxicam (p.84·2).
*Dysmenorrhoea; musculoskeletal and joint disorders.*

**Piroxam** *PP Lab, Thai.*
Piroxicam (p.84·2).
*Gout; musculoskeletal and joint disorders.*

**Piroxan** *Diba, Mex.*
Piroxicam (p.84·2).
*Gout; inflammation; musculoskeletal, joint and peri-articular disorders; pain.*

**pirox-basan** *Schonenberger, Switz.*
Piroxicam (p.84·2).
*Gout; musculoskeletal and joint disorders; pain.*

**Piroxcin** *Polipharm, Thai.*
Piroxicam (p.84·2).
*Gout; musculoskeletal and joint disorders.*

**Piroxen**
*Ofimex, Mex.†; Codal Synto, Thai.*
Piroxicam (p.84·2).
*Gout; musculoskeletal and joint disorders.*

**Piroxene** *Sintofarma, Braz.*
Piroxicam (p.84·2).
*Dysmenorrhoea; gout; musculoskeletal, joint, and peri-articular disorders.*

**Piroxgel** *Barcino, Spain.*
Coal tar (p.1159·2).
*Dandruff; psoriasis; seborrhoeic dermatitis.*

**Piroxifen** *Dansk-Flama, Braz.*
Piroxicam (p.84·2).
*Dysmenorrhoea; gout; musculoskeletal, joint, and peri-articular disorders.*

**Piroxiflam** Sankyo, Braz.
Piroxicam (p.84·2).
*Dysmenorrhoea; gout; musculoskeletal, joint, and peri-articular disorders.*

**Piroxigea** Gea, Denm.
Piroxicam (p.84·2).
*Inflammation; musculoskeletal and joint disorders; pain.*

**Piroxil** Sanval, Braz.
Piroxicam (p.84·2).
*Dysmenorrhoea; gout; musculoskeletal, joint, and peri-articular disorders.*

**Piroximerck** Merck, Ger.†.
Piroxicam (p.84·2).
*Gout; musculoskeletal and joint disorders.*

**Piroxin** Medinovum, Fin.†.
Piroxicam (p.84·2).
*Inflammation; pain; peri-articular and soft-tissue disorders.*

**Piroxiplus** Hebron, Braz.
Piroxicam (p.84·2).
*Dysmenorrhoea; gout; musculoskeletal, joint, and peri-articular disorders.*

**Piroxistad** Stada, Austria.
Piroxicam (p.84·2).
*Gout; inflammation; musculoskeletal, joint, and peri-articular disorders; pain.*

**Piroxityrol** Tyrol, Austria.
Piroxicam (p.84·2).
*Gout; inflammation; musculoskeletal, joint, and peri-articular disorders; pain.*

**Piroxsil** Silom, Thai.
Piroxicam (p.84·2).
*Musculoskeletal and joint disorders.*

**Pirox-Spondyril** Orion, Ger.†.
Piroxicam (p.84·2).
*Gout; musculoskeletal, joint, and soft-tissue disorders.*

**Piroxy** Duopharma, Hong Kong.
Piroxicam (p.84·2).
*Ankylosing spondylitis; osteoarthritis; rheumatoid arthritis.*

**Pirozip** Ashbourne, UK†.
Piroxicam (p.84·2).
*Gout; musculoskeletal and joint disorders.*

**Pirrolfungin** Esfar, Port.
Pyrrolnitrin (p.408·1); salicylic acid (p.1157·1); diethyl sebacate (p.1157·3).
*Skin infections.*

**Pirxane** Lisapharma, Ital.
Buflomedil pyridoxal phosphate compound (p.877·2).
*Vascular disorders.*

**Pirzinol** Solfran, Mex.
Piperazine (p.111·2).

**Pisacaina** Pisa, Mex.
Lidocaine hydrochloride (p.1377·3).
Adrenaline (p.852·2) is included in some injections as a vasoconstrictor to diminish absorption and localise the effect of the local anaesthetic.
*Local anaesthesia; ventricular arrhythmias.*

**Pisatrina** Pisa, Mex.
Co-trimoxazole (p.199·3).
*Bacterial infections.*

**Pistofil** Rafarm, Gr.
Norfloxacin (p.238·3).
*Urinary tract infections.*

**Pitiriax** Cassara, Arg.
Salicylic acid (p.1157·1); piroctone olamine (p.1155·2).
*Dandruff.*

**Pitocin**
Parke, Davis, India; Warner-Lambert, Norw.†; Parke, Davis, USA.
Oxytocin (p.1336·1).
*Incomplete or inevitable abortion; induction of labour; postpartum haemorrhage; uterine inertia.*

**Pitressin**
Link, Austral.; Parke, Davis, Ger.; Goldshield, Irl.; Parke, Davis, NZ†; Goldshield, UK; Parke, Davis, USA.
Argipressin (p.1342·3).
*Aid in abdominal radiography; diabetes insipidus; postoperative abdominal distension; variceal haemorrhage.*

**Pitrex**
Taro, Canad.; Teva, Israel.
Tolnaftate (p.410·1).
*Fungal skin infections.*

**Pitrion** Rafa, Israel.
Miconazole nitrate (p.405·3).
*Fungal skin and nail infections.*

**Pitrisan** Rekah, Israel.
*Ointment:* Undecenoic acid (p.410·3); zinc undecenoate (p.411·1); allantoin (p.1141·3).
*Topical solution:* Undecenoic acid (p.410·3); salicylic acid (p.1157·1); benzoic acid (p.1169·3); chlorobutanol (p.1176·3); resorcinol (p.1156·3).
*Fungal skin infections.*

**Pityker** Roche-Posay, Fr.
Piroctone olamine (p.1155·2); salicylic acid (p.1157·1).
*Dandruff.*

**Pityval**
Note. This name is used for preparations of different composition.
Roche-Posay, Arg.
Piroctone olamine (p.1155·2); iodopropynyl butyl carbamate (Glicacil).
*Seborrhoeic dermatitis.*

Roche-Posay, Fr.
Piroctone olamine (p.1155·2); iodopropynyl butyl carbamate (Glycacil); thermal water.
*Skin irritation.*

Roche-Posay, Irl.
Emollient.

**Pivalone**
Pfizer, Fr.; Parke, Davis, Singapore; Uhlmann-Eyraud, Switz.
Tixocortol pivalate (p.1110·1).
*Nasal polyps; rhinitis.*

**Pivalone compositum** Uhlmann-Eyraud, Switz.
Tixocortol pivalate (p.1110·1); neomycin sulfate (p.235·1).
*Infected nasal disorders.*

**Pivalone Neomycin** Parke, Davis, Singapore.
Tixocortol pivalate (p.1110·1); neomycin sulfate (p.235·1).
*Infected nasal polyps; rhinitis; sinusitis.*

**Pivalone Neomycine** Pfizer, Fr.†.
Tixocortol pivalate (p.1110·1); neomycin sulfate (p.235·1).
*Rhinopharyngitis; sinusitis.*

**Pivaloxicam** Chiesi, Ital.†.
Piroxicam pivalate (p.85·1).
*Musculoskeletal and joint disorders.*

**Pivamiser** Serra Pamies, Spain†.
Pivampicillin hydrochloride (p.244·2).
*Bacterial infections.*

**Pivanozolo** Benedetti, Ital.
Miconazole pivoxil chloride (p.406·1).
*Fungal infections; Gram-positive bacterial superinfections.*

**Pixfix** Hoernecke, Ger.†.
Coal tar (p.1159·2).
*Skin disorders.*

**Pixicam** Hexal, S.Afr.
Piroxicam (p.84·2).
*Gout; musculoskeletal and joint disorders.*

**Pixidin** Sanico, Belg.†.
Chlorhexidine hydrochloride (p.1173·3).
Formerly contained tar, benzocaine, menthol, cineole, senna, and red-poppy petal.
*Mouth and throat disorders.*

**Pixor Stick Anti-acne N** Doetsch, Grether, Switz.
Salicylic acid (p.1157·1); triclosan (p.1195·2).
*Acne.*

**Piz Buin** Novartis Consumer, UK†.
*SPF 20:* Octinoxate (p.1154·3); avobenzone (p.1142·3); titanium dioxide (p.1160·3).
*Sunscreen.*

**Pizide** Pharmasant, Thai.
Pimozide (p.715·1).
*Psychoses.*

**Pizomed** Medifive, Thai.
Pizotifen malate (p.470·3).
*Anorexia; migraine.*

**PK Aid**
Scientific Hospital Supplies, Austral.; Scientific Hospital Supplies, Irl.†; Scientific Hospital Supplies, UK.
Amino-acid preparation without phenylalanine (p.1417·1).
*Phenylketonuria.*

**PK-Levo** Merz, Ger.
Levodopa (p.1205·2); benserazide hydrochloride (p.1200·2).
*Parkinsonism.*

**PK-Merz**
Kolassa, Austria; Grunenthal, Chile; Merz, Ger.; Merz, Hong Kong; Megapharm, Israel; Merz, Malaysia; Merz, Switz.
Amantadine sulfate (p.1197·2).
*Coma; influenza; parkinsonism; postherpetic neuralgia.*

**PKU** Support, Braz.
A range of foods for special diets (p.1417·1).
*Phenylketonuria.*

**PKU 2 and 3** Milupa, UK.
Food for special diets (p.1417·1).
*Phenylketonuria.*

**PKU 1 Mix** Milupa, Ital.
Food for special diets (p.1417·1).
*Hyperphenylalaninaemia; phenylketonuria.*

**Plac Out** Microsules Bernabo, Arg.
Chlorhexidine gluconate (p.1173·2).
*Mouth and throat infections; oral hygiene.*

**Placatus** Pfizer Consumer, Ital.
Nepinalone hydrochloride (p.1125·2).
*Coughs.*

**Placentex** Mastelli, Ital.
Polydeoxyribonucleotide (p.1679·2).
*Inflammatory and degenerative disorders.*

**Placentina** INTES, Ital.†.
Placenta extract.
*Inflammation; rheumatic disorders.*

**Placentrex** David, India.
*Injection; topical gel:* Placenta extract (human).
*Postphlebitic ulcer; scars; vitiligo.*
*Topical lotion:* Deoxyribonucleic acid (p.1679·2); ribonucleic acid (p.1738·2); tyrosine (p.1451·1).
*Vitiligo.*

**Placidox** Lupin, India.
Diazepam (p.690·1).
*Alcohol withdrawal syndrome; anxiety disorders; skeletal muscle spasm.*

**Placidyl** Abbott, USA†.
Ethchlorvynol (p.697·3).
*Insomnia.*

**Placil** Alphapharm, Austral.
Clomipramine hydrochloride (p.289·3).
*Depression; narcoleptic syndrome; obsessive-compulsive disorder; phobic states.*

**Placinoral** Robert, Spain.
Lorazepam pivalate (p.705·1).
*Alcohol withdrawal syndrome; anxiety; insomnia; nausea and vomiting; premedication.*

**Placis** Chiesi, Spain.
Cisplatin (p.538·1).
*Malignant neoplasms.*

**Plactidil** Novartis, Ital.
Picotamide (p.982·3).
*Thromboembolic disorders.*

**Plactosse** IMA, Braz.†.
Sodium dibunate (p.1130·2); sodium benzoate (p.1169·3); guaifenesin (p.1122·1).
*Coughs.*

**Plafonyl** Montpellier, Arg.
Chlordiazepoxide dibudinate (p.674·3); desipramine dibudinate (p.290·2).
*Anxiety; depression.*

**Plagex** Teuto, Braz.
Metoclopramide hydrochloride (p.1274·3).
*Nausea and vomiting.*

**Plagon** De Mayo, Braz.†.
Metoclopramide (p.1274·3); vitamin $B_6$ (p.1457·2).
*Nausea and vomiting.*

**Plak** Byk Gulden, Ital.
Chlorhexidine gluconate (p.1173·2).
*Oral hygiene.*

**Plak Out**
Byk, Austria; Byk Gulden, Ital.; Inibsa, Port.
Chlorhexidine gluconate (p.1173·2).
*Mouth infections.*

**Plaket** Biolab Sanus, Braz.†.
Ticlopidine hydrochloride (p.1011·2).
*Thromboembolism prophylaxis.*

**Plamet** Libbs, Braz.
Bromopride (p.1254·1).
*Aid in endoscopy; gastrointestinal disorders; nausea and vomiting.*

**Plamidasil** Delta, Braz.
Metoclopramide hydrochloride (p.1274·3).
*Nausea and vomiting.*

**Plamin** Apsen, Braz.†.
Metoclopramide hydrochloride (p.1274·3).
*Gastrointestinal motility disorders; nausea and vomiting.*

**Plamivon** Bunker, Braz.
Metoclopramide hydrochloride (p.1274·3).
*Nausea and vomiting.*

**Plan B**
Paladin, Canad.; Womens Capital, USA.
Levonorgestrel (p.1563·2).
*Progestogen-only postcoital contraceptive.*

**Plander** Fresenius Kabi, Ital.
Dextran 70 (p.746·2) in sodium chloride.
*Plasma volume expansion.*

**Plander R** Fresenius Kabi, Ital.
Dextran 40 (p.745·3) in sodium chloride.
*Extracorporeal perfusion; plasma volume expansion; thrombosis prophylaxis.*

**Planitrix** Bros, Gr.
Fenofibrate (p.915·2).
*Hyperlipidaemias.*

**Planizol** Solfran, Mex.
Metronidazole (p.607·2).
*Amoebiasis.*

**Planocid** Pulitzer, Ital.
Cefradine (p.179·3).
*Bacterial infections.*

**Planor** Effik, Fr.
Norgestrienone (p.1564·3); ethinylestradiol (p.1553·2).
*Combined oral contraceptive; endometriosis; mastalgia; menstrual disorders; polycystic ovary syndrome.*

**Planphylline** Asta Medica, Fr.†.
Aminophylline (p.780·2).
*Asthma; obstructive airways disease.*

**Plant Spray** Dolisos, Canad.
Homoeopathic preparation.

**Planta Lax** Hoeveler, Austria.
Senna leaf and pod (p.1288·2); frangula bark (p.1266·3); blackberry leaf; chamomile flowers (p.1669·3); coriander (p.1676·1); fennel (p.1687·2).
*Constipation.*

**Plantaben**
Byk, Arg.; Altana, Braz.; EciFarma, Chile; Madaus, Spain.
Ispaghula (p.1268·1).
*Constipation; diarrhoea; diverticular disease; hypercholesterolaemia; irritable colon.*

**Plantacard N** Madaus, Ger.
Homoeopathic preparation.

**Plantactiv** Hochstetter, Chile.
Marine algae.
*Obesity.*

**Plantaguar** Madaus, Spain.
Guar gum (p.333·2).
*Diabetes mellitus.*

**Plantax** Farmion, Braz.
Senna (p.1288·2); ispaghula (p.1268·1).
*Constipation.*

**Planten**
Whitehall, Israel; Whitehall, Ital.
Ispaghula (p.1268·1).
*Constipation; irritable bowel syndrome.*

**Plantiodine Plus** Blackmores, Austral.†.
Bladderwrack (p.1742·3); alfalfa (p.1649·1); protibel yeast (p.1469·1); rose fruit (p.1740·1); lecithin (p.1706·1).
*Tonic.*

**Plantival**
Note. This name is used for preparations of different composition.
Farmasa, Mex.
Valerian (p.1762·2); melissa (p.1711·1).
*Insomnia; nervous disorders.*

Schwabe, Switz.†.
Valerian (p.1762·2); passion flower (p.1729·1).
*Anxiety disorders.*

**Plantival novo** Schwabe, Ger.
Valerian (p.1762·2); melissa (p.1711·1).
*Agitation; sleep disorders.*

**Plantmobil** Plantina, Ger.†.
Camphor (p.1665·3); eucalyptus oil (p.1686·2); turpentine oil (p.1760·1).
*Cold symptoms; musculoskeletal and joint disorders.*

**Plantocur**
Hexal, Austria; Biocur, Ger.†.
Ispaghula (p.1268·1).
*Constipation.*

**Planum**
Note. This name is used for preparations of different composition.
Pharmacia, Ger.
Temazepam (p.723·2).
*Sleep disorders.*

Menarini, Ital.
Desogestrel (p.1547·2); ethinylestradiol (p.1553·2).
*Combined oral contraceptive.*

**Plaqacide** Oral-B, Austral.†.
Chlorhexidine gluconate (p.1173·2).
*Oral disorders; prevention of dental plaque.*

**Plaquenil**
Sanofi Synthelabo, Arg.; Sanofi Synthelabo, Austral.; Sanofi Synthelabo, Austria; Sanofi Synthelabo, Belg.; Sanofi Synthelabo, Canad.; Sanofi Winthrop, Denm.; Sanofi Synthelabo, Fin.; Sanofi Synthelabo, Fr.; IFET (ΙΦΕΤ), Gr.; Sanofi Synthelabo, Hong Kong; Sanofi Synthelabo, Irl.; Sanofi Winthrop, Israel; Sanofi Synthelabo, Ital.; Sanofi Synthelabo, Malaysia; Sanofi Synthelabo, Mex.; Sanofi Synthelabo, Neth.; Sanofi Synthelabo, Norw.; Sanofi Synthelabo, NZ; Sanofi Synthelabo, Singapore; Sanofi Synthelabo, Swed.; Sanofi Synthelabo, Switz.; Sanofi Synthelabo, Thai.; Sanofi Synthelabo, UK; Sanofi Winthrop, USA.
Hydroxychloroquine sulfate (p.452·3).
*Lupus erythematosus; malaria; photodermatoses; rheumatoid arthritis.*

**Plaquetal** Menarini, Port.
Ticlopidine hydrochloride (p.1011·2).
*Thrombosis prophylaxis.*

**Plaquetil** Rider, Chile.
Ticlopidine hydrochloride (p.1011·2).
*Thrombosis prophylaxis.*

**Plaquinol**
Sanofi Synthelabo, Braz.; Sanofi Synthelabo, Chile; Sanofi Synthelabo, Port.
Hydroxychloroquine sulfate (p.452·3).
*Amoebiasis; lupus erythematosus; malaria; photodermatoses; rheumatoid arthritis.*

**Plas-Amino** Otsuka, Jpn.
Amino-acid and carbohydrate infusion (p.1417·1).
*Parenteral nutrition.*

**Plasbumin**
Bayer, Canad.; Bayer, Chile; Bayer Biological, Hong Kong; Bayer, Israel.; Bayer, Malaysia; Bayer, Singapore; Bayer, Spain; Cutter, USA.
Albumin (p.740·3).
*Burns; cerebral oedema; hypoproteinaemia; shock.*

**Plasil**
Aventis, Braz.; Lepetit, Ital.; Aventis, Thai.
Metoclopramide hydrochloride (p.1274·3).
*Gastrointestinal motility disorders; nausea and vomiting.*

Aventis, Mex.
Metoclopramide (p.1274·3).
*Aid in gastrointestinal examination; disorders of gastrointestinal motility; nausea and vomiting.*

**Plasil Enzimatico**
Aventis, Braz.
Metoclopramide hydrochloride (p.1274·3); dimeticone (p.1289·2); pancreatin (p.1725·3); sodium dehydrocholate (p.1679·2); bromelains (p.1662·2).
*Digestive disorders.*

Aventis, Mex.
Metoclopramide (p.1274·3); bromelains (p.1662·2); pancreatin (p.1725·3); sodium dehydrocholate (p.1679·2); simeticone (p.1289·2).
*Gastrointestinal, biliary-tract and pancreatic disorders.*

**Plasimine** Isdin, Spain.
Mupirocin (p.233·1).
*Bacterial skin infections.*

**Plaskine Neomicina** Ipsen, Spain.
Lysine acexamate (p.1646·2); neomycin undecenoate (p.235·2).
*Burns; ulcers; wounds.*

**Plasma du Dr Quinton** Chimicor, Fr.
Sea water.

**Plasma Marin Hypertonique** Aqualab, Fr.†.
Mineral preparation (p.1417·1).

**Plasmacair** Clintec, Fr.†.
Dextran 40 (p.745·3) with electrolytes.
*Haemodilution; hypotension; shock.*

**Plasmaclar** *Lacer, Spain†.*
Xantinol nicotinate (p.1029·1); pentosan polysulfate sodium (p.979·2).
*Hyperlipidaemias.*

**Plasmafusin**
*Fresenius Kabi, Fin.; Baxter, Ger.*
Hetastarch (p.750·1) in sodium chloride.
*Plasma volume expansion; hypotension; hypovolaemia; shock.*

**Plasmagel** *Fresenius Kabi, Fr.†.*
Gelatin (p.754·3) with electrolytes or glucose.
*Hypotension; shock.*

**Plasma-Lyte**
*Baxter, Austral.; Baxter, Spain; Baxter, UK; Baxter, USA.*
A range of electrolyte infusions with or without glucose (p.1217·1).
*Fluid and electrolyte disorders.*

**Plasma-Lyte IV** *Baxter, NZ.*
A range of electrolyte infusions with or without glucose (p.1217·1).
*Fluid and electrolyte disorders.*

**Plasma-Lyte O** *Baxter, NZ.*
Electrolyte solution (p.1217·1).
*Diarrhoea; oral rehydration solution.*

**Plasmanate**
*Sintofarma, Braz.†; Bayer, Canad.†; Bayer Biological, Hong Kong†; Bayer, Israel; Bayer, Malaysia; Bayer, Singapore†; Cutter, USA.*
Plasma protein fraction (p.758·2).
*Hypoproteinaemia; hypovolaemia.*

**Plasma-Plex** *Armour, USA.*
Plasma protein fraction (p.758·2).
*Hypoproteinaemia; hypovolaemia.*

**Plasmarine** *Pharmadeveloppement, Fr.*
Mineral preparation (p.1417·1).
*Tonic.*

**Plasmasteril**
*Fresenius Kabi, Austria; Fresenius, Belg.†; Fresenius, Braz.†; Fresenius Kabi, Ger.; Fresenius Kabi, Switz.*
Hetastarch (p.750·1) in sodium chloride.
*Plasma volume expansion.*

**Plasmatein** *Alpha Therapeutic, USA†.*
Plasma protein fraction (p.758·2).
*Hypoproteinaemia; hypovolaemia.*

**Plasmaviral** *ISI, Ital.†.*
Plasma protein fraction (p.758·2).
*Hypoproteinaemia; shock.*

**Plasmion** *Fresenius Kabi, Fr.*
Gelatin (p.754·3) with electrolytes.
*Hypotension; shock.*

**Plasmocolit** *QIF, Braz.†.*
Furazolidone (p.605·2); homatropine methylbromide (p.483·2); pectin (p.1580·3).
*Diarrhoea.*

**Plasmodex**
*Pharmalink, Norw.; Pharmalink, Swed.*
Dextran 60 (p.746·1) with electrolytes.
*Plasma volume expansion.*

**Plasmonsoy** *Plasmon, Ital.†.*
Infant feed (p.1417·1).
*Cow's milk intolerance.*

**Plasmoquine** *Medchem, S.Afr.*
Chloroquine sulfate (p.448·2).
*Lupus; malaria; rheumatoid arthritis.*

**Plasmotrim**
*Mepha, Braz.; Mepha, Thai.*
Sodium artesunate (p.447·2).
*Malaria.*

**Plasonil** *Heralds, Braz.†.*
Metoclopramide hydrochloride (p.1274·3); pyridoxine hydrochloride (p.1456·3).
*Nausea and vomiting.*

**Plast Apyr Fisio Irrigac** *Mein, Spain†.*
Sodium chloride (p.1233·3).
*Urological irrigation.*

**Plast Apyr Fisiologico** *Fresenius Kabi, Spain.*
Sodium chloride (p.1233·3).
*Fluid and electrolyte disorders.*

**Plast Apyr Glucosado** *Fresenius Kabi, Spain.*
Glucose (p.1432·2).
*Carbohydrate source; fluid and electrolyte disorders.*

**Plast Apyr Glucosalino** *Fresenius Kabi, Spain.*
Glucose (p.1432·2); sodium chloride (p.1233·3).
*Carbohydrate source; fluid and electrolyte disorders.*

**Plastenan**
*Sanofi Synthelabo, Arg.; Bournonville, Belg.†; Kerapharm, Fr.*
Sodium acexamate (p.1646·2).
*Skin ulcers; wounds.*

*Sanofi Synthelabo, Braz.†.*
Acexamic acid (p.1646·2).
*Skin lesions; skin ulceration.*

**Plastenan con Neomicina** *Sanofi Synthelabo, Arg.*
Sodium acexamate (p.1646·2); neomycin sulfate (p.235·1).
*Wounds.*

**Plastenan Neomicina** *CPH, Port.; Choay, Port.*
Sodium acexamate (p.1646·2); neomycin sulfate (p.235·1).
*Burns; ulcers; wounds.*

**Plastesol** *CPH, Port.*
Acexamic acid (p.1646·2).
*Burns; wounds.*

**Plastistil** *Pharmacia Upjohn, Mex.†.*
Cisplatin (p.538·1).

**Plastranit** *Bonafarma, Port.*
Glyceryl trinitrate (p.923·2).
*Angina pectoris; heart failure.*

**Plastufer** *ICN, Ger.*
Ferrous sulfate (p.1428·2).
*Iron deficiency; iron-deficiency anaemia.*

**Plastulen N** *Niddapharm, Ger.*
Ferrous sulfate (p.1428·2); folic acid (p.1429·1).
*Iron and folic acid deficiency.*

**Plastules** *Wyeth, India.*
Dried ferrous sulfate (p.1428·3); dried yeast (p.1469·1); folic acid (p.1429·1); vitamin $B_{12}$ (p.1458·2); liver extract.
*Anaemias; iron deficiency.*

**Plasvit** *Collins, Mex.*
Vitamin and mineral preparation (p.1417·1).

**Platamine**
*Note. This name is used for preparations of different composition.*
*Pharmacia, Arg.; Pharmacia-Upjohn, Gr.; Pharmacia Upjohn, Ital.; Pharmacia Upjohn, NZ†; Pharmacia Upjohn, S.Afr.†.*
Cisplatin (p.538·1).
*Malignant neoplasms.*

*Pharmacia, Braz.*
Carboplatin (p.533·3).
*Malignant neoplasms.*

**Platenk** *Biotenk, Arg.*
Oxaliplatin (p.577·1).
*Malignant neoplasms.*

**Platiblastin**
*Pharmacia, Austria; Pharmacia Upjohn, Ger.†.*
Cisplatin (p.538·1).
*Malignant neoplasms.*

**Platiblastin-S** *Pharmacia, Switz.*
Cisplatin (p.538·1).
*Malignant neoplasms.*

**Platicarb** *Euroforma, Braz.*
Carboplatin (p.533·3).
*Malignant neoplasms.*

**Platin** *Wockhardt, India.*
Fluoxetine hydrochloride (p.292·1).
*Depression.*

**Platinex**
*Bristol-Myers Squibb, Ger.; Bristol-Myers Squibb, Israel†; Bristol-Myers Squibb, Ital.; Bristol-Myers Squibb, UK.*
Cisplatin (p.538·1).
*Malignant neoplasms.*

**Platino II** *Filaxis, Arg.*
Cisplatin (p.538·1).
*Malignant neoplasms.*

**Platinol**
*Bristol-Myers Squibb, Arg.; Bristol-Myers Squibb, Austria; Bristol-Myers Squibb, Belg.; Bristol, Canad.†; Bristol-Myers Squibb, Denm.; Bristol-Myers Squibb, Fin.; Bristol-Myers Squibb, Gr.; Bristol-Myers Squibb, Israel†; Bristol-Myers Squibb, Mex.; Bristol-Myers Squibb, Neth.†; Bristol-Myers Squibb, Norw.; Bristol-Myers Squibb, Swed.; Bristol-Myers Squibb, Switz.; Bristol-Myers Squibb, Thai.; Bristol-Myers Squibb Oncology, USA.*
Cisplatin (p.538·1).
*Malignant neoplasms.*

**Platinostyl** *Elvetium, Arg.*
Oxaliplatin (p.577·1).
*Malignant neoplasms.*

**Platinum Years** *General Nutrition, Canad.*
Multivitamin and mineral preparation (p.1417·1).

**Platinwas** *Chiesi, Spain.*
Carboplatin (p.533·3).
*Malignant neoplasms.*

**Platiran** *Bristol-Myers Squibb, Braz.*
Cisplatin (p.538·1).
*Malignant neoplasms.*

**Platistil** *Kenfarma, Spain.*
Cisplatin (p.538·1).
*Malignant neoplasms.*

**Platistin** *Pharmacia, Norw.*
Cisplatin (p.538·1).
*Malignant neoplasms.*

**Platistine**
*Pharmacia, Belg.; Pharmacia, Braz.*
Cisplatin (p.538·1).
*Malignant neoplasms.*

**Platium** *Rider, Chile.*
Vitamin and mineral preparations (p.1417·1).
*Dietary supplement.*

**Plato** *Aspen, S.Afr.*
Dipyridamole (p.903·1).
*Platelet function inhibition.*

**Platocillina** *Crosara, Ital.†.*
Ampicillin (p.157·1).
*Bacterial infections.*

**Platosin**
*Nycomed, Austria; Chemipharma, Gr.; Pharmachemie, Israel†; Pharmachemie, Malaysia; Pharmachemie, S.Afr.; Pharmachemie, Thai.; Teva, Thai.*
Cisplatin (p.538·1).
*Malignant neoplasms.*

**Platsul A**
*Note. A similar name is used for preparations of different composition (see below).*
*Grunenthal, Chile.*
Sulfadiazine silver (p.259·1); vitamin A (p.1451·2); vitamin D (p.1461·2).
*Infected burns and wounds.*

**Platsul-A**
*Note. A similar name is used for preparations of different composition (see above).*
*Chobet, Arg.*
Sulfadiazine silver (p.259·1); vitamin A (p.1451·2); lidocaine (p.1377·3).

**Plausital** *Pharmacia Upjohn, Mex.†.*
Morclofone (p.1124·3).

**Plausitin** *Carlo Erba OTC, Ital.*
Morclofone (p.1124·3).
*Coughs.*

**Plavix**
*Sanofi Synthelabo, Arg.; Sanofi Synthelabo, Austral.; Sanofi Winthrop, Austria; Sanofi Synthelabo, Belg.; Sanofi Synthelabo, Braz.; Sanofi Synthelabo, Canad.; Bristol-Myers Squibb, Canad.; Sanofi Synthelabo, Chile; Sanofi Synthelabo, Denm.; Sanofi Synthelabo, Fin.; Bristol-Myers Squibb, Fin.; Bristol-Myers Squibb, Fr.; Sanofi Synthelabo, Fr.; Sanofi Synthelabo, Ger.; Sanofi Synthelabo, Gr.; Sanofi Synthelabo, Hong Kong; Bristol-Myers Squibb, Hong Kong; Bristol-Myers Squibb, Irl.; Sanofi Synthelabo, Irl.; CTI, Israel; Sanofi Synthelabo, Ital.; Sanofi Synthelabo, Malaysia; Bristol-Myers Squibb, Malaysia; Sanofi Synthelabo, Mex.; Bristol-Myers Squibb, Neth.; Sanofi Synthelabo, Neth.; Sanofi Synthelabo, Norw.; Bristol-Myers Squibb, Norw.; Sanofi Synthelabo, NZ; Sanofi Synthelabo, Port.; Sanofi Synthelabo, S.Afr.; Bristol-Myers Squibb, Singapore; Sanofi Synthelabo, Singapore; Sanofi Synthelabo, Spain; Sanofi Synthelabo, Swed.; Bristol-Myers Squibb, Swed.; Bristol-Myers Squibb, Switz.; Sanofi, Switz.; Sanofi Synthelabo, Thai.; Sanofi Synthelabo, UK; Bristol-Myers Squibb, UK; Sanofi Winthrop, USA; Bristol-Myers Squibb, USA.*
Clopidogrel bisulfate (p.888·3).
*Atherosclerosis; unstable angina pectoris.*

**Plax**
*Note. This name is used for preparations of different composition.*
*Pfizer Consumer, Canad.*
Sodium benzoate (p.1169·3); sodium laurilsulfate (p.1574·2); sodium salicylate (p.90·1).

*Colgate-Palmolive, Ital.*
Triclosan (p.1195·2); sodium fluoride (p.1444·3).
*Dental plaque prevention.*

**Plazolit** *Fustery, Mex.†.*
Omeprazole (p.1278·2).

**Plebe** *Pharmadeveloppement, Fr.†.*
Vitamin and mineral preparation (p.1417·1).
*Tonic.*

**Plecor** *Teuto, Braz.*
Cefaclor (p.167·1).
*Bacterial infections.*

**Plegicil** *Pharmacia, Denm.*
Acepromazine maleate (p.668·3).
*Anxiety disorders; hiccup; nausea and vomiting.*

**Plegine**
*Wyeth Lederle, Ital.†; Wyeth-Ayerst, USA†.*
Phendimetrazine tartrate (p.1592·1).
*Obesity.*

**Plegisol**
*Abbott, Israel; Abbott, NZ; Abbott, USA.*
Electrolytes (p.1217·1).
*Cardioplegic solution.*

**Plegivex** *Ivex, UK†.*
Electrolyte solution for coronary instillation (p.1217·1).
*Induction of arrest during cardiothoracic surgery.*

**Pleiadon** *Zambon, Braz.†.*
Domperidone (p.1263·2).
*Gastrointestinal motility disorders; nausea and vomiting.*

**Pleiamide** *Sanofi Synthelabo, Ital.*
Chlorpropamide (p.330·3); metformin hydrochloride (p.342·3).
*Diabetes mellitus.*

**Plenacor**
*Note. This name is used for preparations of different composition.*
*Bago, Arg.; Merck Bago, Braz.*
Atenolol (p.865·2).
*Angina pectoris; hypertension.*

*Armstrong, Mex.*
Atenolol (p.865·2); nifedipine (p.966·2).
*Angina pectoris; hypertension.*

**Plenacor D** *Bago, Arg.*
Atenolol (p.865·2); hydrochlorothiazide (p.933·2); amiloride hydrochloride (p.858·2).
*Hypertension.*

**Plenactol** *3M, Chile.*
Orphenadrine citrate (p.486·1).
*Musculoskeletal pain.*

**Plenaer** *Valeas, Ital.*
Salbutamol sulfate (p.791·3); flunisolide (p.1101·1).
*Obstructive airways disease.*

**Plenax** *Merck, Braz.*
Cefixime (p.172·3).
*Bacterial infections.*

**Plenaxis** *Praecis, USA.*
Abarelix (p.1319·1).
*Prostatic cancer.*

**Plendil**
*AstraZeneca, Arg.; AstraZeneca, Austral.; AstraZeneca, Austria; AstraZeneca, Belg.; AstraZeneca, Canad.; AstraZeneca, Denm.; AstraZeneca, Fin.; Astra-Zeneca, Gr.; AstraZeneca, Hong Kong; AstraZeneca, Irl.; AstraZeneca, Ital.; AstraZeneca, Malaysia; Astra, Mex.; AstraZeneca, Neth.; AstraZeneca, Norw.; AstraZeneca, NZ; AstraZeneca, S.Afr.; AstraZeneca, Singapore; Beta, Spain; Hassle, Swed.; AstraZeneca, Switz.; AstraZeneca, Thai.; AstraZeneca, UK; Astra, USA.*
Felodipine (p.914·3).
*Angina pectoris; hypertension.*

**Plendur** *Durascan, Denm.*
Felodipine (p.914·3).
*Hypertension.*

**Plenidon** *Drugtech, Chile.*
Zaleplon (p.727·3).
*Insomnia.*

**Plenifem** *Schering, Arg.*
4 Patches, estradiol (p.1550·1); 4 patches, estradiol; levonorgestrel (p.1563·2).
*Menopausal disorders.*

**Plenigraf**
*Justesa Imagen, Arg.*
Meglumine amidotrizoate (p.1060·2); sodium amidotrizoate (p.1060·2).
*Radiographic contrast medium.*

*Justesa Imagem, Braz.†; Juste, Spain.*
Calcium amidotrizoate (p.1061·1); meglumine amidotrizoate (p.1060·2); sodium amidotrizoate (p.1060·2).
*Radiographic contrast medium.*

**Plenish-K** *Aspen, S.Afr.*
Potassium chloride (p.1232·2).
*Potassium deficiencies.*

**Plenitude Excell A-3** *L'Oreal, Canad.*
*SPF 8:* Octinoxate (p.1154·3).
*Sunscreen.*

**Plenocedan** *Makros, Braz.†.*
Dipyrone (p.35·3); papaverine hydrochloride (p.1728·1); homatropine methylbromide (p.483·2).
*Smooth muscle spasm.*

**Plenogripe** *Farmoquimica, Braz.†.*
Dipyrone (p.35·3); sodium camsilate; guaifenesin (p.1122·1); cineole (p.1672·1); niaouli oil (p.1719·3); lidocaine (p.1377·3); vitamin C (p.1460·2); mepyramine (p.437·1).
*Cold and influenza symptoms.*

**Plenolyt** *Madaus, Spain.*
Ciprofloxacin hydrochloride (p.188·2).
*Bacterial infections.*

**Plenomicina** *Cibran, Braz.†.*
Erythromycin stearate (p.208·2).
*Bacterial infections.*

**Plenosol N** *Madaus, Ger.†.*
Mistletoe (p.1715·3).
*Joint disorders.*

**Plenovit** *Dexter, Arg.*
A range of vitamin and mineral preparations (p.1417·1).

**Plentiva** *Wyeth, Malaysia.*
28 Tablets, conjugated oestrogens (p.1543·2); 28 tablets, medroxyprogesterone acetate (p.1557·2).
*Menopausal disorders; osteoporosis.*

**Plentiva Cycle 5** *Wyeth, Malaysia.*
28 Tablets, conjugated oestrogens (p.1543·2); 14 tablets, medroxyprogesterone acetate (p.1557·2).
*Menopausal disorders; osteoporosis.*

**Plenty** *Medley, Braz.*
Sibutramine hydrochloride (p.1593·1).
*Obesity.*

**Plenum** *Duncan, Arg.*
Guaifenesin (p.1122·1).
*Coughs.*

**Plenur** *Ipsen, Spain.*
Lithium carbonate (p.301·1).
*Bipolar disorder; depression; neutropenia.*

**Plenyl** *Oberlin, Fr.†.*
Vitamin and mineral preparation (p.1417·1).

**Pleo Vitamin** *Inibsa, Spain.*
Multivitamins and minerals (p.1417·1); orotic acid, diethylaminoethanol salt; adenosine phosphate.
*Tonic.*

**Pleocortex** *Retrain, Spain†.*
Suprarenal cortex (p.1110·1).
*Adrenal insufficiency; tonic.*

**Pleocortex B6** *Retrain, Spain†.*
Suprarenal cortex (p.1110·1); pyridoxine hydrochloride (p.1456·3).
*Vomiting.*

**Pleomix-Alpha** *Illa, Ger.*
Thioctic acid (p.1754·3) or trometamol thioctate (p.1754·3).
*Diabetic polyneuropathy.*

**Pleomix-B** *Trommsdorff, Ger.*
Thiamine hydrochloride (p.1455·1); pyridoxine hydrochloride (p.1456·3).
*Nervous-system disorders.*

**Pleon** *Lacer, Spain.*
Adenine; vitamin B substances; carnitine orotate; fructose diphosphate magnesium; potassium orotate; xanthine (p.1417·1).
*Tonic.*

**Pleon RA** *Henning, Ger.; Sanofi Synthelabo, Ger.*
Sulfasalazine (p.1291·1).
*Polyarthritis.*

**Plesmet**
*Link, Irl.; Link, UK.*
Ferrous glycine sulfate (p.1428·2).
*Iron-deficiency anaemia.*

**Pletaal**
*Janssen-Cilag, Arg.; Otsuka, Hong Kong; Otsuka, Jpn; Otsuka, Thai.*
Cilostazol (p.884·1).
*Intermittent claudication; ischaemic symptoms in arterial occlusion.*

**Pletal**
*Otsuka, UK; Otsuka, USA.*
Cilostazol (p.884·1).
*Intermittent claudication.*

**Pletil** *Pharmacia, Braz.*
Tinidazole (p.617·1).
*Anaerobic bacterial infections; protozoal infections.*

**Plex B** Delta, Braz.
Vitamin B substances (p.1454·3).

**Plex Ton** Auad, Braz.
Multivitamin and mineral preparation with lysine (p.1417·1).

**Plexion** Medicis, USA.
Sulfur (p.1158·2); sulfacetamide sodium (p.257·3).
*Acne.*

**Plexium** Lehning, Fr.
Selenium (p.1444·1).
*Muscular disorders; skin disorders.*

**Plexivita** Sedar, Braz.†.
Multivitamin and mineral preparation (p.1417·1).

**Plexo Enterin** Sanval, Braz.†.
Kaolin (p.1268·3); pectin (p.1580·3).
*Diarrhoea.*

**Plexoton B12** Fonten, Ital.
Vitamin B substances (p.1417·1).
*Anaemias; liver disorders; tonic.*

**Plexus** Lafi, Chile.
Betamethasone (p.1093·1); dexchlorpheniramine maleate (p.427·3).
*Hypersensitivity reactions.*

**Pliagel**
Alcon, Austral.; Alcon, Braz.†; Alcon, NZ†.
Poloxamer 407 (p.1414·2) (p.1164·2).
*Cleaning solution for soft contact lenses.*

**Plidan**
Note. This name is used for preparations of different composition.
Roemmers, Arg.
Diazepam (p.690·1).
*Anxiety; skeletal muscle spasm; spasticity.*

Rhein, Mex.
Pargeverine hydrochloride (p.487·3).
*Smooth muscle spasm.*

**Plidan Compuesto** Rhein, Mex.
Pargeverine hydrochloride (p.487·3); clonixin lysine (p.26·3).
*Smooth muscle pain and spasm.*

**Plidex** Roemmers, Arg.
Diazepam (p.690·1); isopropamide (p.485·2).
*Anxiety; muscle spasm.*

**Plinzene** Douglas, NZ.
Fluoxetine hydrochloride (p.292·1).
*Bulimia; depression; obsessive-compulsive disorder.*

**Plissamur** Ardeypharm, Ger.
Aesculus (p.1648·2).
*Venous insufficiency.*

**Plitican**
Sanofi Synthelabo, Fr.; Synthelabo, Hong Kong†; Synthelabo, Port.; Synthelabo, Switz.†.
Alizapride hydrochloride (p.1248·1).
*Nausea; vomiting.*

**Plokon**
Shinyaku, Hong Kong; Shinyaku, Thai.
Piprinhydrinate (p.439·1).
*Hypersensitivity reactions; Ménière's disease; motion sickness; urticaria.*

**Plomurol** Valma, Chile.
Lindane (p.1506·3).
*Pediculosis.*

**Plorinoc** Klonal, Arg.
Loperamide (p.1271·2).
*Diarrhoea.*

**Plostim** Alcon, Arg.
Timolol maleate (p.1012·2).
*Glaucoma.*

**Plovacal** Medipharma, Arg.
Paracetamol (p.76·2).
*Fever; pain.*

**Plumarol** Lacer, Spain.
Miglitol (p.343·2).
*Diabetes mellitus.*

**Plumger** Fada, Arg.
Pancuronium bromide (p.1404·3).
*Competitive neuromuscular blocker.*

**Pluravit**
Bayer, Austral.†; GlaxoSmithKline, NZ.
A range of multivitamin and mineral preparations (p.1417·1).

**Pluravit Super B** Sterling Health, Austral.†.
Vitamin B substances with ascorbic acid (p.1417·1).
*Vitamin B supplement.*

**Plurexid** Celltech, Fr.
Chlorhexidine gluconate (p.1173·2).
*Disinfection of skin and mucous membranes.*

**Pluribios** Madariaga, Spain.
Multivitamin preparation with cocarboxylase (p.1417·1).
*Eye disorders.*

**Pluricefo** Northia, Arg.
Cefoxitin sodium (p.177·2).
Lidocaine hydrochloride (p.1377·3) is included in the intramuscular injection to alleviate the pain of injection.
*Bacterial infections.*

**Pluriderm** Guieu, Ital.†.
Thyme (p.1755·2); carrot (p.1765·1); sage oil (p.1741·2); whey; lactic acid (p.1704·1).
*Skin disinfection.*

**Pluridoxina** Sidefarma, Port.
Doxycycline fosfatex (p.206·2).
*Bacterial infections.*

**Plurifactor** Gomenol, Fr.†.
Vitamin B substances; deoxyribonucleic acid; glycine (p.1417·1).
*Tonic.*

**Plurilac** Alphrema, Ital.
Acacia; inulin; lactulose; mannitol; dimethicone; fennel; mallow; peppermint (p.1253·2).
*Dietary fibre supplement; gastrointestinal disorders.*

**Plurimen** Viatris, Spain.
Selegiline hydrochloride (p.1214·1).
*Parkinsonism.*

**Plurimineral** Support, Braz.
Mineral preparation (p.1417·1).

**Plurisalina** Grifols, Spain.
Electrolyte injection (p.1217·1) with sodium lactate (p.1223·2).
*Fluid and electrolyte disorders.*

**Plurisan** Heralds, Braz.†.
Lindane (p.1506·3).
*Pediculosis; scabies.*

**Plurisemina** Northia, Arg.
Gentamicin (p.219·1).
*Bacterial infections.*

**Pluriverm** Medley, Braz.
Mebendazole (p.108·2).
*Worm infections.*

**Plurivermil** Ibefar, Braz.†.
Mebendazole (p.108·2).
*Worm infections.*

**Pluriviron mono** Stegropharm, Ger.
Yohimbine hydrochloride (p.1766·2).
*Erectile dysfunction.*

**Plurivitamin** Support, Braz.
Vitamin preparation (p.1417·1).

**30 Plus**
Note. This name is used for preparations of different composition.
Tanning Research, Canad.
*SPF 30:* Octinoxate (p.1154·3); octisalate (p.1154·3); titanium dioxide (p.1160·3).
*Sunscreen.*

Ajantha, Malaysia.
Ginseng (p.1693·1); ashwagandha.
*Tonic.*

**45 Plus** Tanning Research, Canad.
*SPF 45:* Octinoxate (p.1154·3); octisalate (p.1154·3); titanium dioxide (p.1160·3).
*Sunscreen.*

**50 Plus** Quest, Canad.
Multivitamin preparation (p.1417·1).

**Plus Kalium retard** Amino, Switz.
Potassium chloride (p.1232·2).
*Hypokalaemia.*

**Plus & Plus** Wierhom, Arg.
Copper oleate (p.1502·2); coconut diethanolamides; sodium laurilsulfate (p.1574·2).
*Pediculosis.*

**Plus Sinus** Pfizer Consumer, Canad.†.
Pseudoephedrine hydrochloride (p.1129·2).
*Nasal congestion.*

**30 Plus Sunblock** Tanning Research, Canad.
*SPF 30:* Homosalate (p.1148·1); octinoxate (p.1154·3); octisalate (p.1154·3); oxybenzone (p.1154·3).
*Sunscreen.*

**Plus & White** Wierhom, Arg.
Hydrogen peroxide (p.1182·2); phosphoric acid (p.1731·2); methyl salicylate (p.59·3).
*Dental whitener.*

**Plusapetit** IMA, Braz.†.
Lysine; vitamin $B_{12}$; calcium glycerophosphate (p.1417·1).
*Nutritional supplement.*

**Pluscal** Sanitas, Arg.
Calcium carbonate (p.1254·2).
*Calcium deficiency; calcium supplement; osteoporosis.*

**Pluscloran** Sintesina, Arg.
Chloramphenicol (p.185·1).
*Bacterial infections.*

**Plusderm** Bristol-Myers Squibb, Arg.
Zinc undecenoate (p.411·1); sodium propionate (p.408·1); diiodohydroxyquinoline (p.603·3); boric acid (p.1662·1); zinc oxide (p.1163·2).
*Eczema; ulcers; wounds.*

**Plusderm ATB** Bristol-Myers Squibb, Arg.
Rifamycin sodium (p.253·2).
*Infected wounds; skin infections.*

**Plusgel**
Note. This name is used for preparations of different composition.
Lagos, Arg.
Piroctone olamine (p.1155·2).
*Scalp disorders.*

Collins, Mex.
Aluminium hydroxide (p.1249·2); magnesium hydroxide (p.1272·2); dimeticone (p.1289·2).
*Gastrointestinal hyperacidity.*

**Plusgin**
Note. This name is used for preparations of different composition.
Asofarma, Arg.
Ciprofloxacin (p.188·2).
*Bacterial infections.*

Raffo, Chile.
Fluconazole (p.398·1).
*Fungal infections.*

**Plusplatin** Dosa, Arg.
Oxaliplatin (p.577·1).
*Malignant neoplasms.*

**Plustaxano** Dosa, Arg.
Docetaxel (p.547·1).
*Malignant neoplasms.*

**Plusvent** Almirall, Spain.
Salmeterol xinafoate (p.795·1); fluticasone propionate (p.1102·3).
*Asthma.*

**Plusvit** Ecofarm, Ital.
Octacosanol; yeasts rich in calcium, magnesium, zinc, and iron (p.1417·1).
*Tonic.*

**Pluviton** Sam-On, Israel.
Multivitamin and mineral preparation (p.1417·1).

**Pluviton B** Sam-On, Israel.
Vitamin B substances with lysine (p.1417·1).

**PM**
Note. A similar name is used for preparations of different composition (see below).
New Vision, Canad.
Multivitamin preparation (p.1417·1).

**pM**
Note. A similar name is used for preparations of different composition (see above).
Chiesi, Fr.
Aluminium chlorohydrate (p.1142·1).
*Hyperhidrosis.*

**P-Mega-Tablinen** Lichtenstein, Ger.
Phenoxymethylpenicillin potassium (p.242·1).
*Bacterial infections.*

**PML Crono**
SIFI, Ital.; SIFI, Singapore.
Nicotinamide; vitamin E; lutein (p.1417·1).
*Nutritional supplement.*

**PMQ-INGA** Inga, India.
Primaquine phosphate (p.456·2).
*Malaria.*

**PMS** Homeocan, Canad.
Homoeopathic preparation.

**PMS L21** Homeocan, Canad.
Homoeopathic preparation.

**PMS Support** Vitaplex, Austral.†.
Vitamins; minerals (p.1417·1); viburnum; buchu (p.1663·1); ginger (p.1267·1); evening primrose oil (p.1686·3).
*Muscular cramps; oedema.*

**PMS-Artificial Tears**
Pharmascience, Canad.; Pharmascience, Hong Kong; Pharmascience, Singapore†.
Polyvinyl alcohol (p.1581·1).
*Dry eyes.*

**PMS-Artificial Tears Extra** Pharmascience, Canad.
Polyvinyl alcohol (p.1581·1); povidone (p.1581·2).
*Dry eyes.*

**PMS-Baximycin** Pharmascience, Hong Kong.
Bacitracin (p.161·3); polymyxin B sulfate (p.245·1).
*Burns; wounds.*

**PMS-Dicitrate** Pharmascience, Canad.
Sodium citrate dihydrate (p.1223·2); citric acid monohydrate (p.1673·1).
*Neutralising buffer; systemic alkaliniser.*

**PMS-Egozinc** Pharmascience, Canad.†.
Zinc sulfate (p.1469·3).
*Zinc supplement.*

**PMS-Egozinc-HC** Pharmascience, Canad.
Zinc sulfate (p.1469·3); hydrocortisone acetate (p.1103·3).
*Anorectal disorders.*

**PMS-Enemol** Pharmascience, Hong Kong.
Monobasic sodium phosphate (p.1230·3); dibasic sodium phosphate (p.1231·1).
*Bowel evacuation; constipation.*

**PMS-Levazine** Pharmascience, Canad.†.
Perphenazine (p.714·2); amitriptyline hydrochloride (p.280·3).
*Depression; psychoses.*

**PMS-Phosphates** Pharmascience, Canad.†.
Monobasic sodium phosphate (p.1230·3); dibasic sodium phosphate (p.1231·1).
*Constipation.*

**PMS-Polytrimethoprim** Pharmascience, Canad.
Trimethoprim sulfate (p.272·2); polymyxin B sulfate (p.245·1).
*Bacterial eye infections.*

**PMT Complex**
Note. This name is used for preparations of different composition.
Brauer, Austral.†.
Homoeopathic preparation.

Cenovis, Austral.†; Vitelle, Austral.†.
Vitamins; minerals (p.1417·1); ginger (p.1267·1); viburnum; agnus castus (p.1649·1); cimicifuga (p.1671·3); bladderwrack (p.1742·3).
*Premenstrual syndrome.*

**PMT Formula** Vitalia, UK.
Evening primrose oil (p.1686·3); vitamins (p.1417·1); minerals; valerian (p.1762·2); passion flower (p.1729·1).
*Premenstrual syndrome.*

**PMT Oral Spray** Brauer, Austral.†.
Homoeopathic preparation.

**Pneucid** Scipharm, S.Afr.
Sodium citrate (p.1223·2); citric acid monohydrate (p.1673·1).
*Buffering agent for increasing gastric pH before anaesthesia.*

**Pneumaseptic** Cochon, Fr.†.
Sulfogaiacol (p.1131·1); sodium benzoate (p.1169·3).
*Respiratory-tract congestion.*

**Pneumo 23**
Aventis Pasteur, Arg.; Aventis Pasteur, Austria; Aventis Pasteur, Braz.; Aventis Pasteur, Canad.; Aventis Pasteur, Chile; Pasteur Vaccins, Fr.; Vianex (Βιανεξ), Gr.; Aventis Pasteur, Hong Kong; Aventis Pasteur, Ital.; Aventis Pasteur, Malaysia; CSL, NZ; Aventis Pasteur, Port.; Aventis Pasteur, Singapore; Aventis Pasteur, Spain; Aventis Pasteur, Thai.
A pneumococcal vaccine (23-valent) (p.1633·1).
*Active immunisation.*

**Pneumo 23 Imovax** Pasteur Merieux, Israel.
A pneumococcal vaccine (23-valent) (p.1633·1).
*Active immunisation.*

**Pneumoclar** Monot, Fr.†.
Carbocisteine (p.1116·2).

**Pneumodoron**
Weleda, Austria; Weleda, Ger.
A range of homoeopathic preparations.

**Pneumogeine** SERP, Mon.
Theophylline sodium acetate (p.804·3).
Formerly contained theophylline, caffeine, potassium iodide, and sodium benzoate.
*Asthma; obstructive airways disease.*

**Pneumogenol** Monot, Fr.†.
Codeine (p.27·1).

**Pneumolat** Farmion, Braz.†.
Salbutamol sulfate (p.791·3).
*Obstructive airways disease.*

**Pneumolat Expectorante** Farmion, Braz.†.
Salbutamol sulfate (p.791·3); guaifenesin (p.1122·1).
*Obstructive airways disease.*

**Pneumomist** ECR, USA†.
Guaifenesin (p.1122·1).

**Pneumopan**
Note. This name is used for preparations of different composition.
Gebro, Austria.
Thyme (p.1755·2); equisetum (p.1684·1); plantago lanceolata (p.1738·2); sulfogaiacol (p.1131·1).
*Coughs.*

GlaxoSmithKline Sante, Fr.
Codeine (p.27·1); chlorphenamine maleate (p.427·3).
Formerly contained codeine, chlorphenamine maleate, bromoform, and sodium benzoate.
*Coughs.*

**Pneumopect** Gebro, Austria†.
Noscapine (p.1125·3); thyme (p.1755·2); viola.
*Coughs.*

**Pneumopent** Aventis, Ital.†.
Pentamidine isetionate (p.613·2).
*Pneumocystis carinii pneumonia.*

**Pneumoplasme** Augot, Fr.†.
Black-mustard-flour paper (p.1718·2).
*Respiratory-tract congestion.*

**Pneumoplasme a l'Histamine** Augot, Fr.†.
Black-mustard-flour paper (p.1718·2); histamine hydrochloride (p.1697·1).
*Respiratory-tract congestion.*

**Pneumopur** Chiron Behring, Ger.
A pneumococcal vaccine (capsular polysaccharide, 23-valent) (p.1633·1).
*Active immunisation.*

**Pneumorel**
Eutherapie, Belg.†; Eutherapie, Fr.; Servier, Hong Kong; Stroder, Ital.; Servier, Port.
Fenspiride hydrochloride (p.786·1).
*Respiratory-tract disorders.*

**Pneumotussin** ECR, USA.
Hydrocodone tartrate (p.45·1); guaifenesin (p.1122·1).
*Coughs.*

**Pneumovax**
Aventis Pasteur, Denm.; Aventis Pasteur, Fin.; Aventis Pasteur, Ital.; Aventis Pasteur, Norw.; Aventis Pasteur, Swed.
A pneumococcal vaccine (23-valent) (p.1633·1).
*Active immunisation.*

**Pneumovax II**
Aventis Pasteur, Irl.; Aventis Pasteur, UK.
A pneumococcal vaccine (23-valent) (p.1633·1).
*Active immunisation.*

**Pneumovax 23**
Merck Sharp & Dohme, Arg.; Merck Sharp & Dohme, Austral.; Aventis Pasteur, Belg.; Merck Sharp & Dohme, Braz.; Merck Frosst, Canad.; Aventis Pasteur, Ger.; Merck Sharp & Dohme, Hong Kong; Merck Sharp & Dohme, Israel; Merck Sharp & Dohme, Malaysia; Aventis Pasteur, Neth.; Merck Sharp & Dohme, NZ; Merck Sharp & Dohme, S.Afr.; Merck Sharp & Dohme, Singapore; Pro Vaccine, Switz.; Merck Sharp & Dohme, Thai.; Merck, USA.
A pneumococcal vaccine (23-valent) (p.1633·1).
*Active immunisation.*

**Pneumune**
Wyeth Lederle, Belg.; Lederle, Neth.†.
A pneumococcal vaccine (23-valent) (p.1633·1).
*Active immunisation.*

**Pnu-Imune**
Wyeth Lederle, Austria; Wyeth, Irl.; Wyeth Lederle, Norw.; Wyeth Lederle, Port.; Wyeth Lederle, Swed.; Wyeth, UK†.
A pneumococcal vaccine (23 valent) (p.1633·1).
*Active immunisation.*

**Pnu-Imune 23** Wyeth-Ayerst, Canad.†; Wyeth Lederle, Fin.†; Wyeth, Gr.; Wyeth Lederle, Ital.; Wyeth, Mex.; Lederle, Switz.; Wyeth-Ayerst, USA†.
A pneumococcal vaccine (23-valent) (p.1633·1).
*Active immunisation.*

**Pnu-Inmune** Wyeth, Spain.
A pneumococcal vaccine (23-valent) (p.1633·1).
*Active immunisation.*

**P.O. 12** Boehringer Ingelheim, Fr.
Enoxolone (p.36·2).
*Skin irritation.*

**Po Antisseptico** Bunker, Braz.
Boric acid (p.1662·1); salicylic acid (p.1157·1); benzoic acid (p.1169·3).
*Skin disorders.*

**Pobrax** Pharmasant, Thai.
Chlordiazepoxide (p.674·2); clidinium bromide (p.480·2).
*Biliary dyskinesia; dysmenorrhoea; dyspepsia; irritable colon; peptic ulcer; ureteric spasm.*

**Pocin** Polipharm, Thai.†.
Erythromycin stearate (p.208·2).
*Bacterial infections.*

**Pocin G** Upha, Malaysia.
Polymyxin B sulfate (p.245·1); neomycin sulfate (p.235·1); gramicidin (p.220·2).
*Bacterial eye infections.*

**Pocin H** Upha, Malaysia.
Hydrocortisone (p.1103·3); neomycin sulfate (p.235·1); polymyxin B sulfate (p.245·1).
*Otitis.*

**PocketScan** Lifescan, Irl.
Test for glucose in blood (p.1694·2).

**Pockinal** Mauermann, Ger.†.
Hedera helix.
*Bronchitis.*

**Poconeol** Dolisos, Fr.
A range of homoeopathic preparations.

**Pocophage** Pharmasant, Thai.
Metformin hydrochloride (p.342·3).
*Diabetes mellitus.*

**Pocyl** Lacer, Spain.
Ibuprofen (p.45·3).
*Fever; pain.*

**Podactin** Reese, USA.
*Cream:* Miconazole nitrate (p.405·3).
*Topical powder:* Tolnaftate (p.410·1).

**Podase** Pose, Thai.
Serrapeptase (p.1743·2).
*Inflammation; oedema.*

**Pod-Ben-25** C & M, USA.
Podophyllum resin (p.1155·2).
*Warts.*

**Podertonic** Inkeysa, Spain.
Ferrocholinate (p.1427·3).
*Iron-deficiency anaemia.*

**Podine** Aspen, S.Afr.
Povidone-iodine (p.1190·3).
*Mouth and throat disinfection; mouth and throat infections; skin infections; wounds.*

**Podium** Torlan, Spain†.
Diazepam (p.690·1).
Contains pyridoxine hydrochloride.
*Alcohol withdrawal syndrome; anxiety; febrile convulsions; insomnia; skeletal muscle spasm.*

**Podocon** Paddock, USA.
Podophyllum resin (p.1155·2).
*Genital warts.*

**Podofilia** Bustillos, Mex.
Podophyllum resin (p.1155·2).
*Keratosis; veruccas; warts.*

**Podofilm**
Paladin, Canad.; Pharmascience, Hong Kong†; Pharmascience, Singapore†.
Podophyllum resin (p.1155·2).
*Warts.*

**Podofilox** Pharmalex (Φαρμαλεξ), Gr.
Podophyllotoxin (p.1155·3).
*Anogenital warts.*

**Podofin** Syosset, USA.
Podophyllum resin (p.1155·2).
*Epitheliomatosis; genital warts; keratoses.*

**Podomexef**
Sankyo, Ger.; Sankyo, Switz.
Cefpodoxime proxetil (p.178·3).
*Bacterial infections.*

**Podoxin** Cassara, Arg.
Podophyllotoxin (p.1155·3).
*Anogenital warts.*

**Poen Efrina** Poen, Arg.
Phenylephrine hydrochloride (p.1126·3).
*Production of mydriasis.*

**Poenbioptal** Poen, Arg.
Chloramphenicol (p.185·1); neomycin (p.235·1); phenylephrine (p.1126·3).
*Bacterial eye infections.*

**Poenbiotico** Poen, Arg.
Ampicillin sodium (p.157·1).
*Bacterial eye infections.*

**Poen-Caina NF** Poen, Arg.
Proxymetacaine (p.1384·1).
*Local anaesthesia.*

**Poenfenicol** Poen, Arg.
Chloramphenicol (p.185·1).
*Bacterial eye infections.*

**Poenflox** Poen, Chile.
Ofloxacin (p.239·3).
*Bacterial eye infections.*

**Poenglaucol** Poen, Arg.
Carteolol hydrochloride (p.880·3).
*Glaucoma; ocular hypertension.*

**Poenglausil** Poen, Arg.
Dorzolamide (p.908·3).
*Glaucoma.*

**Poenkerat**
Poen, Arg.; Poen, Chile.
Ketorolac trometamol (p.52·1).
*Cystoid macular oedema; eye inflammation; intra-operative miosis inhibition; uveitis.*

**Poentimol** Poen, Arg.
Timolol maleate (p.1012·2).
*Glaucoma; uveitis.*

**Poentobral Plus** Pharma Investi, Chile.
Dexamethasone (p.1097·1); tobramycin (p.271·2).
*Bacterial eye infections with inflammation.*

**Pofol**
Dong Kook, Singapore; Dong Kook, Thai.
Propofol (p.1305·3).
*General anaesthesia; sedative.*

**Poikicholan** Lomapharm, Ger.
Silybum marianum (p.1043·3).
*Liver disorders.*

**Poikigastran N** Lomapharm, Ger.†.
Algeldrate (p.1249·2); magnesium hydroxide (p.1272·2).
*Gastrointestinal disorders.*

**Poikigeron** Lomapharm, Ger.†.
Procaine hydrochloride; adenosine phosphate; haematoporphyrin; minerals; ginkgo biloba (p.1417·1).
*Tonic.*

**Poikilocard Mono** Lomapharm, Ger.
Crataegus (p.1677·1).
*Cardiac disorders.*

**Poikiven T** Lomapharm, Ger.
Homoeopathic preparation.

**Point** Trima, Israel.
Naproxen sodium (p.65·1).
*Musculoskeletal, joint, and soft-tissue disorders; pain.*

**Point-Two** Colgate-Hoyt, USA.
Sodium fluoride (p.1444·3).
*Dental caries prophylaxis.*

**Poison Antidote Kit** Bowman, USA.
*Combination pack:* Syrup, ipecacuanha (p.1122·3); suspension, charcoal (p.1030·2).
*Emergency treatment of poisoning.*

**Poison Ivy/Oak** Hylands, Canad.
Homoeopathic preparation.

**Polagen** Decomed, Port.
Grass pollen extract (p.1650·1).
*Allergen immunotherapy.*

**Polamin**
Teuto, Braz.; Schering-Plough, Ital.†.
Dexchlorpheniramine maleate (p.427·3).
*Hypersensitivity reactions.*

**Polamine** Strand, Malaysia.
Dexchlorpheniramine maleate (p.427·3).
*Hypersensitivity reactions.*

**Polar Ice** Scott, Canad.
Menthol (p.1711·3).
*Musculoskeletal and joint pain.*

**Polaramin**
Aesca, Austria; Schering-Plough, Denm.; Schering-Plough, Ital.; Schering-Plough, Norw.; Schering-Plough, Swed.
Dexchlorpheniramine maleate (p.427·3).
*Hypersensitivity reactions; pruritus.*

**Polaramin Espettorante** Schering-Plough, Ital.
Dexchlorpheniramine maleate (p.427·3); guaifenesin (p.1122·1); pseudoephedrine sulfate (p.1129·2).
*Colds; coughs.*

**Polaramine**
Schering-Plough, Austral.; Schering-Plough, Belg.; Schering-Plough, Braz.; Schering, Canad.†; Schering-Plough, Fr.; Schering-Plough, Gr.; Schering-Plough, Hong Kong; Schering-Plough, Malaysia; Schering-Plough, Mex.; Schering-Plough, Neth.; Schering-Plough, NZ; Schering-Plough, S.Afr.; Schering-Plough, Singapore; Schering-Plough, Spain; Essex, Switz.; Schering, USA†.
Dexchlorpheniramine maleate (p.427·3).
*Hypersensitivity reactions; pruritus.*

**Polaramine Expec** Schering-Plough, Mex.
Dexchlorpheniramine maleate (p.427·3); guaifenesin (p.1122·1); pseudoephedrine sulfate (p.1129·2).
*Coughs; rhinitis.*

**Polaramine Expectorant**
Schering-Plough, Belg.; Schering-Plough, Hong Kong; Schering-Plough, Malaysia; Schering-Plough, Singapore; Schering, USA.
Dexchlorpheniramine maleate (p.427·3); guaifenesin (p.1122·1); pseudoephedrine sulfate (p.1129·2).
*Asthma; cold symptoms; coughs; hay fever; rhinitis.*

**Polaramine Expectorante**
Schering-Plough, Braz.; Schering-Plough, Spain.
Dexchlorpheniramine maleate (p.427·3); guaifenesin (p.1122·1); pseudoephedrine sulfate (p.1129·2).
*Upper-respiratory-tract disorders.*

**Polaramine Pectoral** Schering-Plough, Fr.†.
Dexchlorpheniramine maleate (p.427·3); guaifenesin (p.1122·1).
Formerly contained dexchlorpheniramine maleate, pseudoephedrine sulfate, guaifenesin, and sodium benzoate.
*Coughs.*

**Polaramine Topico** Schering-Plough, Spain.
Allantoin (p.1141·3); dexchlorpheniramine maleate (p.427·3).
*Cutaneous hypersensitivity reactions.*

**Polaratyne** Schering-Plough, S.Afr.
Loratadine (p.436·1).
*Allergic rhinitis; urticaria.*

**Polaratyne D** Schering-Plough, S.Afr.
Loratadine (p.436·1); pseudoephedrine sulfate (p.1129·2).
*Upper respiratory-tract congestion.*

**Polaronil**
Note. This name is used for preparations of different composition.
Aesca, Austria†; Essex, Ger.
Dexchlorpheniramine maleate (p.427·3).
*Hypersensitivity reactions.*

Schering-Plough, Belg.†.
Dexamethasone (p.1097·1); dexchlorpheniramine maleate (p.427·3); ascorbic acid (p.1460·2).
*Hypersensitivity reactions.*

**Polase** Wyeth Lederle, Ital.
Potassium aspartate hemihydrate (p.1233·1); magnesium aspartate tetrahydrate (p.1227·3).
*Potassium and magnesium deficiency.*

**Polcortolon TC** Medphano, Ger.
Triamcinolone acetonide (p.1110·2); tetracycline hydrochloride (p.266·2).
*Infected skin disorders.*

**Poledin** Pfizer, Spain.
Sodium cromoglicate (p.795·3).
*Eye disorders.*

**Polenat** Natufarma, Arg.
Pollen.
*Dietary supplement.*

**Polendiamina** Fada, Arg.
Diphenhydramine (p.431·3); ephedrine (p.1120·1); guaifenesin (p.1122·1).
*Coughs.*

**Polery** Veyron-Froment, Fr.
*Paediatric syrup:* Pholcodine (p.1128·3); erysimin.
Formerly contained ethylmorphine hydrochloride, sodium bromide, sodium benzoate, codeine, belladonna, erysimin, and senega.
*Syrup:* Codeine (p.27·1); erysimin.
Formerly contained ethylmorphine hydrochloride, sodium bromide, sodium benzoate, codeine, aconite, belladonna, erysimin, senega, and cherry-laurel.
*Coughs.*

**Poli ABE** Vita, Spain†.
Pyridoxine hydrochloride (p.1456·3); placenta extract; vitamin A palmitate (p.1453·1); tocoferil acetate (p.1465·1).
*Deficiency of vitamins A and E.*

**Poli B Fuerte** Frasca, Arg.
Vitamin B substances (p.1417·1).

**Poli Miner Vit** QIF, Braz.†.
Multivitamin and mineral preparation (p.1417·1).

**Poliacel**
Aventis Pasteur, Arg.; Aventis Pasteur, Braz.
A diphtheria, tetanus, pertussis, poliomyelitis, and haemophilus influenzae vaccine (p.1615·1).
*Active immunisation.*

**Poliacel-Act-Hib** Pasteur Merieux, Israel.
A diphtheria, tetanus, pertussis, poliomyelitis, and haemophilus influenzae vaccine (p.1615·1).
*Active immunisation.*

**Polial**
Plasmon, Ital.†; Ultrapharm, UK.
Food for special diets (p.1417·1).
*Egg intolerance; gluten intolerance; milk intolerance.*

**Poliantib** Alcon Cusi, Spain†.
Chlortetracycline hydrochloride (p.187·3); polymyxin B sulfate (p.245·1).
*Bacterial eye infections.*

**Polibac** Hebron, Braz.
Amoxicillin (p.155·3).
*Bacterial infections.*

**Polibar**
E-Z-EM, Belg.; E-Z-EM, Port.; E-Z-EM, UK.
Barium sulfate (p.1061·1).
*Contrast medium for gastrointestinal radiography.*

**Polibar ACB**
E-Z-EM, Israel; Bracco, Switz.
Barium sulfate (p.1061·1).
*Contrast medium for gastrointestinal radiography.*

**Polibar Rapid** E-Z-EM, UK.
Barium sulfate (p.1061·1).
*Contrast medium for lower gastrointestinal radiography.*

**Polibar Viscous** E-Z-EM, UK†.
Barium sulfate (p.1061·1).
*Contrast medium for gastrointestinal radiography.*

**Polibatrin** Fustery, Mex.
Co-trimoxazole (p.199·3).
*Bacterial infections.*

**Poliben** Auad, Braz.
Mebendazole (p.108·2); tiabendazole (p.114·2).
*Worm infections.*

**Polibeta B12** Ceccarelli, Ital.
Vitamin B substances (p.1417·1).
*Vitamin B deficiency.*

**Polibimbi** Monsanto, Ital.
Electrolytes (p.1217·1).
*Nasal irrigation.*

**Polibiotic** Ecobi, Ital.
Bacampicillin hydrochloride (p.161·2).
*Bacterial infections.*

**Polibroxol** Polipharm, Thai.
Ambroxol hydrochloride (p.1114·3).
*Respiratory-tract disorders associated with increased or viscous mucus.*

**Polibutin** Juste, Spain.
Trimebutine (p.1758·1) or trimebutine maleate (p.1758·1).
*Gastrointestinal spasm; nausea and vomiting.*

**Poli-Cifloxin** Polipharm, Thai.
Ciprofloxacin (p.188·2).
*Bacterial infections.*

**Policol** Polipharm, Thai.
Pseudoephedrine hydrochloride (p.1129·2); triprolidine hydrochloride (p.442·3).
*Allergic rhinitis; cold symptoms; hay fever.*

**Policold** Polipharm, Thai.
Pseudoephedrine hydrochloride (p.1129·2); triprolidine hydrochloride (p.442·3).
*Cold symptoms; hay fever; hypersensitivity reactions; nasal congestion.*

**Policolinosil** Medea, Spain.
Amino acids (p.1417·1); liver extract; pangamic acid (p.1727·2); ribonucleic acid (p.1738·2); thioctic acid (p.1754·3); inositol (p.1701·2); vitamin B substances (p.1417·1).
*Liver disorders; tonic.*

**Poli-Cycline** Polipharm, Thai.
Doxycycline hyclate (p.206·2).
*Bacterial infections.*

**Polidasa** Almirall, Spain†.
Amylase (p.1654·2); cellulase (p.1669·1); dimethicone (p.1289·2); tilactase (p.1756·2); lipase.
*Digestive-system disorders.*

**Polideltaxin** Pharmacos, Mex.
Dexamethasone (p.1097·1).
*Infected eye disorders.*

**Poliderms** Uniao Quimica, Braz.
Betamethasone valerate (p.1093·2); gentamicin sulfate (p.217·1); tolnaftate (p.410·1); clioquinol (p.196·3).
*Infected skin disorders.*

**Polides** Farmigea, Ital.†.
Polydeoxyribonucleotide (p.1679·2).
*Gynaecological disorders.*

**Polienzim** Sanitas, Arg.
Lipase; protease; cellulase (p.1669·1); amylase (p.1654·2); simeticone (p.1289·2).
*Digestive disorders; flatulence.*

**Poli-Fibrozil** Polipharm, Thai.
Gemfibrozil (p.923·1).
*Hyperlipidaemias.*

**Polifluidil** Monsanto, Ital.
Carbocisteine (p.1116·2).
*Respiratory-tract congestion.*

**Poli-Flunarin** Polipharm, Thai.
Flunarizine (p.434·2).
*Cerebral and peripheral vascular disorders; irritability; memory impairment; migraine; sleep disorders.*

**Poli-Formin** Polipharm, Thai.
Metformin hydrochloride (p.342·3).
*Diabetes mellitus.*

**Poliginax** Sintofarma, Braz.
Neomycin sulfate (p.235·1); polymyxin B sulfate (p.245·1); nystatin (p.406·3); tinidazole (p.617·1).
*Vulvovaginal infections.*

**Poliglicol Anti Acne** Kin, Spain†.
Sulfur (p.1158·2); calamine (p.1144·1); resorcinol acetate (p.1156·3); triclosan (p.1195·2); zinc oxide (p.1163·2).
*Acne.*

**Poligot** Polipharm, Thai.†.
Dihydroergotamine mesilate (p.465·3).
*Hypotension; migraine and other vascular headache.*

**Poligot-CF** Polipharm, Thai.
Ergotamine tartrate (p.467·2); caffeine (p.782·1).
*Migraine and other vascular headaches.*

**Poligram** Puebla, Arg.
Polysaccharides from *Pseudomonas aeruginosa*.
*Immunostimulant.*

**Polijodurato** Farmigea, Ital.
Sodium iodide (p.1598·1); potassium iodide (p.1598·1); rubidium iodide (p.1741·1); calcium chloride (p.1225·1).
*Cataracts.*

**Polilevo** Monsanto, Ital.
Arginine hydrochloride (p.1421·1); ornithine hydrochloride (p.1442·3); citrulline (p.1425·2).
*Liver disorders.*

**Polilevo N** Taurus, Ger.
Arginine hydrochloride (p.1421·1); ornithine hydrochloride (p.1442·3); citrulline (p.1425·2).
*Liver disorders.*

**Polimerosa** Nutricia-Bago, Arg.
Carbohydrate supplement (p.1417·1).
*Nutritional supplement.*

**Polimixina B Composto** Delta, Braz.†.
Clioquinol butyl; polymyxin B sulfate (p.245·1); prednisolone (p.1108·1).
*Infected skin disorders.*

**Polimod** *Monsanto, Ital.*
Pidotimod (p.1731·3).
*Immunostimulant.*

**Polimoxil** *Legrand, Braz.*
Amoxicillin (p.155·3).
*Bacterial infections.*

**Polimucil**
*Note. This name is used for preparations of different composition.*
*Byk, Arg.*
Carbocisteine (p.1116·2); sobrerol (p.1130·2).
*Respiratory-tract disorders with excess mucus.*

*Monsanto, Ital.*
Carbocisteine (p.1116·2).
*Respiratory-tract disorders.*

**Polinazolo** *Rottapharm, Ital.*
Econazole nitrate (p.397·2).
*Fungal and Gram-positive bacterial skin infections; vulvovaginal candidiasis.*

**Polineural** *Biotekfarma, Ital.*†.
Citicoline sodium (p.1672·3).
*Mental function impairment; parkinsonism.*

**Polinorm** *AstraZeneca, Austria.*
Atenolol (p.865·2); chlortalidone (p.882·3); hydralazine hydrochloride (p.931·2).
*Hypertension.*

**Polio Sabin**
*GlaxoSmithKline, Ital.; SmithKline Beecham, Mex.; GlaxoSmithKline, Thai.*
An oral poliomyelitis vaccine (p.1633·3).
*Active immunisation.*

**Poliodine** *Gifrer Barbezat, Fr.*
Povidone-iodine (p.1190·3).
*Wound and skin disinfection.*

**Polioftal** *ICN, Arg.*
Tobramycin (p.271·2); dexamethasone sodium phosphate (p.1097·2).
*Infected eye disorders.*

**PolioHib** *SBL, Swed.*
A poliomyelitis and haemophilus influenzae vaccine (p.1616·3).
*Active immunisation.*

**poliomyelan** *Feldhoff, Ger.*
Bovine testicular extract (p.1569·3); bovine placental extract.
*Musculoskeletal and joint disorders.*

**Polioral**
*Sclavo, Israel; Chiron Vaccines, Ital.; Chiron Behring, Malaysia; Fustery, Mex.; Biovac, S.Afr.; Chiron, Thai.*
An oral poliomyelitis vaccine (p.1633·3).
*Active immunisation.*

**Polio-Vaccinol** *Procter & Gamble, Ger.*†.
An oral poliomyelitis vaccine (p.1633·3).
*Active immunisation.*

**Poliovax-IN** *Chiron Vaccines, Ital.*
An inactivated poliomyelitis vaccine (p.1633·3).
*Active immunisation.*

**Polipectol** *Fapromed, Arg.*
Mepyramine maleate (p.437·1); tiocol; caffeine (p.782·1); ammonium acetate (p.1115·1); tolu balsam (p.1131·3).
*Respiratory-tract disorders.*

**Polipirox** *Biologici Italia, Ital.*
Piroxicam (p.84·2).
*Musculoskeletal and joint disorders.*

**Poliplex** *Mead Johnson, Braz.*
Multivitamin and mineral preparation (p.1417·1).

**Polipred** *Allergan, Braz.*
Prednisolone acetate (p.1108·1); neomycin sulfate (p.235·1); polymyxin B sulfate (p.245·1); polyvinyl alcohol (p.1581·1).
*Infected eye disorders.*

**Poliptal** *Sydenham, Mex.*†.
Pipenzolate (p.487·3).

**Poli-Relaxane** *Polipharm, Thai.*
Orphenadrine citrate (p.486·1); paracetamol (p.76·2).
*Musculoskeletal pain; tension headache.*

**Polireumin** *TRB, Braz.*
Sodium hyaluronate (p.1697·3).
*Osteoarthritis.*

**Poliroxin** *Polipharm, Thai.*
Roxithromycin (p.254·2).
*Bacterial infections.*

**Polirreumin** *TRB, Arg.*
Hydroxychloroquine (p.453·1).
*Lupus erythematosus; malaria; rheumatoid arthritis.*

**Polisan** *Milano, Ital.*
Benzalkonium chloride (p.1168·3).
*Surface disinfection.*

**Polised** *Monsanto, Ital.*
Sulfogaiacol (p.1131·1); dextromethorphan hydrobromide (p.1117·3).
*Coughs.*

**Poliseng** *Teuto, Braz.*
Amino acids; mineral; vitamins; ginseng (p.1693·1) (p.1417·1).
*Tonic.*

**Polisep** *Drag, Chile.*
Menthol (p.1711·3); thymol (p.1194·2); salol (p.88·1).
*Mouth and throat disorders.*

**Polisilan Gel** *Upsamedica, Spain*†.
Aluminium hydroxide (p.1249·2); dimethicone (p.1289·2); sorbitol (p.1446·3).
*Gastrointestinal hyperacidity and flatulence.*

**Polisilon** *Upsa, Ital.*
Aluminium hydroxide (p.1249·2); dimeticone (p.1289·2).
*Aerophagia; gastrointestinal disorders associated with hyperacidity.*

**Polistin Pad** *Trommsdorff, Ger.*†.
Carbinoxamine maleate (p.426·3).
*Hypersensitivity reactions.*

**Polistin T-Caps** *Trommsdorff, Ger.*†.
Carbinoxamine maleate (p.426·3).
*Hypersensitivity reactions.*

**Polisulfade** *Sanobia, Port.*
Polymyxin B sulfate (p.245·1); bacitracin zinc (p.161·3).
*Skin infections.*

**Politelmin** *Gilton, Braz.*†.
Mebendazole (p.108·2).
*Worm infections.*

**Politifen** *Polipharm, Thai.*
Ketotifen fumarate (p.788·1).
*Asthma; bronchitis; hypersensitivity reactions.*

**Politosse** *Monsanto, Ital.*
Cloperastine fendizoate (p.1117·2).
*Coughs.*

**Poli-Uretic** *Polipharm, Thai.*
Amiloride hydrochloride (p.858·2); hydrochlorothiazide (p.933·2).
*Hepatic cirrhosis; hypertension; oedema.*

**Polivitaminico** *CPH, Port.*
Multivitamin preparation (p.1417·1).

**Poliwit** *Fisiopharma, Ital.*
Multivitamin and mineral preparation (p.1417·1).

**Polixan** *Polipharm, Thai.*
Carisoprodol (p.1392·1); paracetamol (p.76·2).
*Muscle pain and spasm.*

**Polixima** *Sifarma, Ital.*†.
Cefuroxime sodium (p.184·1).
*Bacterial infections.*

**Polixin** *Sophia, Mex.*
*Eye drops:* Polymyxin B sulfate (p.245·1); neomycin sulfate (p.235·1); gramicidin (p.220·2).
*Eye ointment:* Polymyxin B sulfate (p.245·1); neomycin sulfate (p.235·1); bacitracin zinc (p.161·3).
*Bacterial eye infections.*

**Polizep** *Polipharm, Thai.*
Dipotassium clorazepate (p.685·1).
*Anxiety; insomnia.*

**Polizine** *Polipharm, Thai.*
Hydroxyzine hydrochloride (p.434·3).
*Hypersensitivity reactions.*

**Pollcapsan M** *Alsitan, Ger.*†.
Pollen.
*Tonic.*

**Pollen Royal** *Ido, Fr.*
Pollen; propolis (p.1735·2); royal jelly (p.1740·3).
*Nutritional supplement.*

**Pollenase Allergy** *Peach, UK.*
Sodium cromoglicate (p.795·3).
*Allergic conjunctivitis.*

**Pollenase Antihistamine** *Peach, UK.*
Chlorphenamine (p.428·1).
*Hypersensitivity reactions.*

**Pollenase Nasal** *Peach, UK.*
Beclometasone dipropionate (p.1091·1).
Formerly known as Pollenase Hayfever.
*Hypersensitivity reactions.*

**Pollen-B** *Wassen, UK*†.
Pollen; dolomite.

**Pollenna** *Nelson, UK.*
Homoeopathic preparation.

**Pollergon** *Motima, Fr.*
Pollen.
*Nutritional supplement.*

**Pollinex**
*Stallergenes, Belg.; Artu, Neth.; Allergy Therapeutics, UK.*
Grass or tree pollen allergen extracts (p.1650·1).
*Allergen immunotherapy.*

**Pollinex Quattro** *Bencard, Ger.*
Pollen extracts(p.1650·1).
*Allergen immunotherapy.*

**Pollinex-R** *Allergy Therapeutics, Canad.*
Aqueous extract of short ragweed pollen(p.1650·1).
*Allergen immunotherapy of ragweed pollen.*

**Pollingel** *Bracco, Ital.*
Pollen; royal jelly (p.1740·3).
*Nutritional supplement.*

**Pollingel con Ginkgo Biloba** *Bracco, Ital.*
Pollen; ginkgo biloba (p.1692·3).
*Nutritional supplement.*

**Pollingel Ginseng** *Bracco, Ital.*
Pollen; ginseng (p.1693·1); honey (p.1434·2).
*Nutritional supplement.*

**Pollinil** *Dolisos, Canad.*
Homoeopathic preparation.

**Pollinosan**
*Bioforce, Ger.; Bioforce, Switz.*
Homoeopathic preparation.

**Pollinose S** *Alsitan, Ger.*
Pollen.
*Pollen hypersensitivity.*

**Pollstimol** *Strathmann, Ger.*†.
Grass pollen extracts.
*Benign prostatic hyperplasia.*

**Pollyferm** *Nordic, Swed.*
Sodium cromoglicate (p.795·3).
*Allergic conjunctivitis; allergic rhinitis.*

**Polmonin** *Pharmanik (Φαρμανικ), Gr.*
Tolfenamic acid (p.94·2).
*Dysmenorrhoea; inflammation; musculoskeletal and joint disorders; pain.*

**Polocaine**
*AstraZeneca, Canad.; AstraZeneca, USA.*
Mepivacaine hydrochloride (p.1381·2).
Corbadrine (p.1675·3) or corbadrine hydrochloride (p.1675·3) is included in some injections as a vasoconstrictor to diminish absorption and localise the effect of the local anaesthetic.
*Local anaesthesia.*

**Poloral** *Berna, Switz.*†.
An oral poliomyelitis vaccine (p.1633·3).
*Active immunisation.*

**Poloren** *Loren, Mex.*
Dipyrone (p.35·3).
*Fever; inflammation; pain.*

**Poloris** *GlaxoSmithKline Consumer, Ger.*†.
Coal tar (p.1159·2); allantoin (p.1141·3).
*Psoriasis.*

**Polper B12** *Casasco, Arg.*
Amino acids; vitamin $B_{12}$ (p.1417·1).
*Dietary supplement.*

**Polper Calcio-Magnesio** *Casasco, Arg.*
Vitamin B substances; vitamin C; calcium carbonate (p.1417·1).
*Tonic.*

**Polper Vascular** *Casasco, Arg.*
Dihydroergotamine mesilate (p.465·3); amino acids; vitamin $B_{12}$ (p.1417·1).
*Cerebrovascular disorders.*

**Polvac** *Teomed, Switz.*
Pollen allergen extracts (p.1650·1).
*Allergen immunotherapy.*

**Polviderm NF** *Bajer, Arg.*
Zinc oxide (p.1163·2); benzalkonium chloride (p.1168·3); phenoxyethanol (p.1189·1).
*Skin disorders.*

**Polvilho Antisseptico** *Granado, Braz.*
Salicylic acid (p.1157·1); sulfur (p.1158·2); boric acid (p.1662·1); zinc oxide (p.1163·2).

**Polvo Roge** *Casasco, Arg.*
Magnesium oxide (p.1272·3); magnesium carbonate (p.1272·1).
*Constipation.*

**Polvos Alcalinos** *Volta, Chile.*
Calcium carbonate (p.1254·2); magnesium oxide (p.1272·3); sodium bicarbonate (p.1223·2).
*Antacid.*

**Polvos Antibioticos** *Silesia, Chile.*
Bacitracin (p.161·3); neomycin (p.235·1); sulfathiazole (p.264·1).
*Burns; infected skin disorders; wounds.*

**Polvos Wilfe** *Perez Gimenez, Spain.*
Sulfanilamide (p.263·2); sulfathiazole (p.264·1).
*Skin infections.*

**Poly C** *Usana, Hong Kong.*
Vitamin C (p.1460·2); flavonoids (p.1688·2).
*Antioxidant; vitamin C supplement.*

**Poly Gel** *Alcon, Austral.*
Carbomer (p.1577·2).
*Dry eyes; eye irritation.*

**Poly Pred** *Allergan, Spain.*
Neomycin sulfate (p.235·1); polymyxin B sulfate (p.245·1); prednisolone acetate (p.1108·1).
*Infected eye disorders.*

**Poly Visc** *Ioquin, Austral.*
Paraffin (p.1479·3); wool fat (p.1483·1).
*Dry eyes.*

**Polyanion** *Sigmapharm, Austria.*
Pentosan polysulfate sodium (p.979·2).
*Hyperlipidaemias; thromboembolic disorders.*

**Poly-B con Vitamina C** *Grossman, Mex.*
Vitamin B substances; vitamin C (p.1417·1).

**Polybactrin** *Wellcome, Irl.*†.
Neomycin sulfate (p.235·1); polymyxin B sulfate (p.245·1); bacitracin zinc (p.161·3).
*Infected skin lesions.*

**Polybamycin** *Shin Poong, Singapore.*
Bacitracin (p.161·3); neomycin sulfate (p.235·1); polymyxin B sulfate (p.245·1).
*Bacterial skin infections.*

**Polybee** *Chew, Thai.*
Vitamin B substances with yeast (p.1417·1).

**Polybion**
*Merck, Fin.; Bracco, Ital.*†.
Vitamin B substances (p.1417·1).
*Nutritional supplement.*

*Merck, India.*
Vitamin B substances with or without vitamin C (p.1417·1).
*Vitamin B and C deficiency.*

**Polybion Forte** *Merck, Ger.*
Vitamin B substances (p.1417·1).
*Vitamin B deficiency.*

**Polybion N** *Merck, Ger.*
Vitamin B substances (p.1417·1).
*Vitamin B deficiency.*

**Polycal**
*Nutricia, Austral.; Nutricia, Irl.; Baxter, NZ; Nutricia, NZ; Nutricia Clinical, UK.*
Food for special diets (p.1417·1).
Formerly known as Fortical in the *UK*.

**Polycare** *Alcon, Fr.*†.
Sodium dichloroisocyanurate (p.1191·3)(p.1164·2).
*Soft contact-lens cleanser.*

**Polycidin** *Novartis Ophthalmics, Canad.*
*Eye ointment:* Bacitracin zinc (p.161·3); polymyxin B sulfate (p.245·1).
*Eye infections.*
*Eye/ear drops:* Gramicidin (p.220·2); polymyxin B sulfate (p.245·1).
*Eye and ear infections.*

**Polycin** *Nakornpatana, Thai.*
Nitrofurazone (p.238·2).
*Burns; skin ulcers; wound infections.*

**Polycin-B** *Ocusoft, USA.*
Bacitracin zinc (p.161·3); polymyxin B sulfate (p.245·1).
*Bacterial eye infections.*

**Polycitra** *Alza, USA.*
Potassium citrate (p.1223·1); sodium citrate (p.1223·2); citric acid monohydrate (p.1673·1).
*Chronic metabolic acidosis; urine alkalinising agent.*

**Polycitra-K**
*Alza, Canad.*
Potassium citrate (p.1223·1).
*Hypokalaemia.*

*Alza, USA.*
Potassium citrate (p.1223·1); citric acid monohydrate (p.1673·1).
*Chronic metabolic acidosis; urine alkalinising agent.*

**Polycitra-LC** *Alza, USA.*
Potassium citrate (p.1223·1); sodium citrate (p.1223·2); citric acid monohydrate (p.1673·1).
*Chronic metabolic acidosis; urine alkalinising agent.*

**Polyclean** *Alcon, Fr.*
Cleansing solution for contact lenses (p.1164·2).

**Polyclens**
*Alcon, Austral.*†*; Alcon, Braz.; Alcon, Mex.; Alcon, NZ.*
Cleaning solution for contact lenses (p.1164·2).

**Polyclox** *Siam Bheasach, Thai.*†.
Ampicillin (p.157·1); cloxacillin (p.198·2).
*Bacterial infections.*

**Polycolvit** *Pharmasant, Thai.*
Ferrous fumarate (p.1427·3); vitamin B substances; vitamin C; calcium phosphate (p.1417·1).
*Anaemias; vitamin B and C deficiency.*

**Polycose**
*Abbott, Austral.; Abbott, Braz.; Abbott, Canad.; Abbott, Fin.*†*; Abbott, Hong Kong; Ross, Israel; Abbott, Ital.; Abbott, NZ; Abbott, Singapore; Abbott Nutrition, UK; Ross, USA.*
Glucose polymers (p.1417·1).
*Nutritional carbohydrate supplement.*

**Polycrol** *Reckitt Piramal, India.*
Simeticone (p.1289·2); magnesium hydroxide (p.1272·2); aluminium hydroxide (p.1249·2).
*Gastrointestinal hyperacidity; peptic ulcer.*

**Polycutan** *Agis, Israel.*
Clotrimazole (p.396·2); dexamethasone acetate (p.1097·1); neomycin sulfate (p.235·1).
*Infected skin disorders.*

**Polyderm**
*Note. This name is used for preparations of different composition.*
*Taro, Canad.*
Bacitracin zinc (p.161·3); polymyxin B sulfate (p.245·1).
*Burns; minor wounds.*

*Chowgule, India.*
Prednisolone (p.1108·1); clioquinol (p.196·3); mesulphen (p.1152·1); salicylic acid (p.1157·1).
*Infected skin disorders.*

**Polydex**
*Note. A similar name is used for preparations of different composition (see below).*
*Pharmasant, Thai.*
Dextromethorphan hydrobromide (p.1117·3).
*Coughs.*

**Poly-Dex**
*Note. A similar name is used for preparations of different composition (see above).*
*Ocusoft, USA.*
Dexamethasone (p.1097·1); neomycin sulfate (p.235·1); polymyxin B sulfate (p.245·1).
*Infected eye disorders.*

**Polydexa**
*Therabel, Belg.; Bouchara-Recordati, Fr.; Neo-Farmaceutica, Port.; Bouchara, Singapore; Bouchara, Switz.*
Neomycin sulfate (p.235·1); polymyxin B sulfate (p.245·1); dexamethasone sodium metasulfobenzoate (p.1097·2).
*Infected eye and ear disorders.*

**Polydexa a la Phenylephrine** *Bouchara-Recordati, Fr.*†.
Neomycin sulfate (p.235·1); polymyxin B sulfate (p.245·1); dexamethasone sodium metasulfobenzoate (p.1097·2); phenylephrine hydrochloride (p.1126·3).
*Rhinitis; sinusitis.*

**Polydiet** *DHN, Fr.*
Preparation for enteral nutrition (p.1417·1).

**Polydine**
*Note. This name is used for preparations of different composition.*
*Fischer, Israel; Century, USA.*
Povidone-iodine (p.1190·3).
*Skin and vaginal infections; skin disinfection.*

Pharmasant, Thai.
Dextromethorphan hydrobromide (p.1117·3); brompheniramine maleate (p.426·1); phenylephrine hydrochloride (p.1126·3); ammonium chloride (p.1115·2).
*Coughs.*

**Polydol** Pharmasant, Thai.
Orphenadrine citrate (p.486·1); paracetamol (p.76·2).
*Dysmenorrhoea; muscle pain; tension headache.*

**Polydona** Bioglan, Ger.
Povidone-iodine (p.1190·3).
*Burns; skin ulcers; wounds.*

**Polyenzyme-I** Chew, Thai.
Amylase (p.1654·2); papain (p.1727·3); pancreatin (p.1725·3); vitamin B substances (p.1417·1); diphenhydramine hydrochloride (p.431·3); homatropine methylbromide (p.483·2); simeticone (p.1289·2); activated charcoal (p.1030·2).
*Digestive disorders.*

**Polyenzyme-N** Chew, Thai.
Pancreatin (p.1725·3); simeticone (p.1289·2).
*Digestive disorders.*

**Polyerga** Hor-Fer-Vit, Ger.
Polypeptides derived from spleen.
*Adjuvant tumour therapy.*

**Polyfax**
GlaxoSmithKline, Hong Kong; Intra Pharma, Irl.; Pliva, UK.
Polymyxin B sulfate (p.245·1); bacitracin zinc (p.161·3).
*Bacterial infections of the skin and eye.*

**Polyfra** Alcon, Fr.
*Eye drops:* Framycetin sulfate (p.215·1); polymyxin B sulfate (p.245·1); oxedrine hydrochloride (p.977·3).
*Eye ointment:* Framycetin sulfate (p.215·1); polymyxin B sulfate (p.245·1).
Formerly contained muramidase hydrochloride, framycetin sulfate, and polymyxin B sulfate.
*Bacterial eye infections.*

**Polygam**
NBI, S.Afr.; American Red Cross, USA.
A normal immunoglobulin (p.1627·2).
*Hypogammaglobulinaemia; idiopathic thrombocytopenic purpura; Kawasaki disease.*

**Polyglobin**
Bayer, Ger.; Bayer, Spain†; Bayer, Swed.
A normal immunoglobulin (p.1627·2).
*Guillain-Barré syndrome; hypogammaglobulinaemia; idiopathic thrombocytopenic purpura; Kawasaki syndrome; passive immunisation.*

**Polygot** Pharmasant, Thai.
Ergotamine tartrate (p.467·2); caffeine (p.782·1).
*Migraine and other vascular headaches.*

**Polygynax**
Raymos, Arg.; UCB, Ger.
Neomycin (p.235·1); nystatin (p.406·3); polymyxin B sulfate (p.245·1).
*Vulvovaginal infections.*

UCB, Belg.; Innotech, Fr.; Innotech, Hong Kong; UCB, Port.†; Innotech, Singapore.
Neomycin sulfate (p.235·1); nystatin (p.406·3); polymyxin B sulfate (p.245·1).
*Vulvovaginal and cervical infections.*

**Polygynax Virgo** Innotech, Fr.
Neomycin sulfate (p.235·1); nystatin (p.406·3); polymyxin B sulfate (p.245·1).
*Vulvovaginitis.*

**Polyhadol** Pharmasant, Thai.
Haloperidol (p.701·2).
*Alcoholism; schizophrenia.*

**Poly-Histine** Sanofi Synthelabo, USA.
Phenyltoloxamine citrate (p.439·1); mepyramine maleate (p.437·1); pheniramine maleate (p.438·3).
*Allergic rhinitis.*

**Poly-Histine CS** Sanofi Winthrop, USA†.
Codeine phosphate (p.27·1); phenylpropanolamine hydrochloride (p.1127·3); brompheniramine maleate (p.426·1).
*Coughs and cold symptoms.*

**Poly-Histine D** Sanofi Winthrop, USA†.
Phenylpropanolamine hydrochloride (p.1127·3); phenyltoloxamine citrate (p.439·1); mepyramine maleate (p.437·1); pheniramine maleate (p.438·3).
*Allergic rhinitis; nasal congestion.*

**Poly-Histine DM** Sanofi Winthrop, USA†.
Dextromethorphan hydrobromide (p.1117·3); phenylpropanolamine hydrochloride (p.1127·3); brompheniramine maleate (p.426·1).
*Coughs and cold symptoms.*

**Polyionique** Pharmacie Centrale des Hopitaux, Fr.
Electrolyte infusion with glucose (p.1217·1).
*Carbohydrate source; fluid and electrolyte disorders.*

**Poly-Iron** Cypress, USA.
Polysaccharide-iron complex (p.1443·2).
*Iron deficiency.*

**Poly-Iron Forte** Cypress, USA.
Polysaccharide-iron complex (p.1443·2); folic acid (p.1429·1); cyanocobalamin (p.1458·2).
*Iron-deficiency anaemia; megaloblastic anaemia.*

**Poly-Joule** Nutricia, Austral.
Dextrin (p.1427·1).
*Nutritional supplement.*

**Poly-Karaya**
Sanofi Synthelabo, Fr.; Kramer, Switz.†.
Sterculia (p.1290·2); povidone (p.1581·2).
*Constipation; diarrhoea; meteorism.*

**Polymox** Bristol-Myers Squibb, Mex.
Amoxicillin trihydrate (p.155·3).
*Bacterial infections.*

**Polymycin** Medical Ophthalmics, USA.
*Eye drops:* Neomycin (p.235·1); polymyxin B (p.245·2); gramicidin (p.220·2).
*Eye ointment:* Neomycin (p.235·1); polymyxin B (p.245·2); bacitracin (p.161·3).
*Eye infections.*

**Polynase** YSP, Malaysia.
Dexchlorpheniramine maleate (p.427·3); pseudoephedrine hydrochloride (p.1129·2).
*Allergic conjunctivitis; allergic skin disorders; rhinitis.*

**Polyoph**
Seng, Hong Kong; Seng, Thai.
Neomycin sulfate (p.235·1); polymyxin B sulfate (p.245·1); gramicidin (p.220·2).
*Bacterial eye infections.*

**Polyphed** Pharmasant, Thai.
Theophylline (p.798·3); guaifenesin (p.1122·1).
*Obstructive airways disease.*

**Polypirine** Lehning, Fr.
Aspirin (p.15·1); caffeine citrate (p.782·1); meadowsweet (p.1710·1).
Formerly contained propyphenazone, phenicarbazide, phenacetin, caffeine citrate, cinnamon, ipecacuanha, and squill.
*Fever; pain.*

**Polypred**
Note. A similar name is used for preparations of different composition (see below).
Pharmasant, Thai.
Prednisolone (p.1108·1).
*Skin disorders.*

**Poly-Pred**
Note. A similar name is used for preparations of different composition (see above).
Allergan, USA.
Prednisolone acetate (p.1108·1); neomycin sulfate (p.235·1); polymyxin B sulfate (p.245·1).
*Eye inflammation with bacterial infection.*

**Polypress**
Note. This name is used for preparations of different composition.
Pfizer, Ger.
Prazosin hydrochloride (p.985·1); polythiazide (p.984·2).
*Hypertension.*

Pharmasant, Thai.
Prazosin hydrochloride (p.985·1).
*Hypertension.*

**Polyquin** Tai Guk, Singapore.
Hydroquinone (p.1148·1).
*Skin hyperpigmentation.*

**Polyrhinium** Arkomedika, Fr.
Homoeopathic preparation.

**Polyrinse** Alcon, Fr.
Sodium chloride (p.1233·3) (p.1164·2).
*Rinsing and soaking solution for contact lenses.*

**Polyrinse Desinfektionssystem** Alcon, Austria†.
Sodium dichloroisocyanurate (p.1191·3)(p.1164·2).
*Disinfection and rinsing of soft contact lenses.*

**Polyrinse-Aufnahmelosung** Alcon, Austria†.
Sodium chloride (p.1233·3)(p.1164·2).
*Storage solution for soft contact lenses.*

**Polyrinse-Augenelement** Alcon, Austria†.
Sodium chloride (p.1233·3)(p.1164·2); boric acid (p.1662·1).
*Comfort drops for contact lenses.*

**Poly-Rivitin** Clinced, Austria†.
Multivitamin preparation (p.1417·1).

**Polysept**
Dermapharm, Ger.; Rekah, Israel.
Povidone-iodine (p.1190·3).
*Burns; skin and mucous membrane disinfection; skin ulcers; wounds.*

**Polyseptol** Qualiphar, Belg.
Filtrate from culture of: *Staphylococcus aureus*, *Streptococcus pyogenes*, *Pseudomonas aeruginosa*, and *Escherichia coli*; sulfanilamide (p.263·2); cod-liver oil (p.1425·2).
*Infected skin disorders.*

**Polysilane**
Note. This name is used for preparations of different composition.
Sanofi Synthelabo, Hong Kong; Sanofi Synthelabo, Malaysia; Sanofi Synthelabo, Singapore; Sanofi Synthelabo, Thai.
Aluminium hydroxide (p.1249·2); simeticone (p.1289·2).
*Dyspepsia; flatulence; gastritis; heartburn; pyrosis.*

Upsamedica, Switz.
Dimethicone (p.1289·2).
*Gastrointestinal disorders.*

**Polysilane Delalande** Sanofi Synthelabo OTC, Fr.
Aluminium hydroxide (p.1249·2); simeticone (p.1289·2).
*Gastrointestinal disorders.*

**Polysilane Joullie** Synthelabo, Fr.†.
*Chewable tablets/lozenges:* Simeticone (p.1289·2); aluminium hydroxide (p.1249·2).
*Gastrointestinal disorders.*
*Paediatric oral granules:* Simeticone (p.1289·2); ceratonia (p.1579·1).
*Gastro-oesophageal reflux.*

**Polysilic III** Beacons, Singapore.
Aluminium hydroxide (p.1249·2); magnesium trisilicate (p.1272·3); simeticone (p.1289·2).
*Dyspepsia; flatulence; gastritis; gastro-oesophageal reflux; meteorism; peptic ulcer.*

**Polysilon** Upsamedica, Belg.†.
Dimethicone (p.1289·2).
*Gastrointestinal disorders associated with hyperacidity.*

**Polysorb** Fougera, USA.
Emollient and moisturiser.

**Polyspectran**
Note. This name is used for preparations of different composition.
Alcon, Ger.; Thilo, Hong Kong†.
*Eye and ear drops:* Polymyxin B sulfate (p.245·1); neomycin sulfate (p.235·1); gramicidin (p.220·2).
*Bacterial infections of the eye and ear.*

Alcon-Thilo, Ger.; Thilo, Hong Kong†.
*Eye ointment; ointment:* Polymyxin B sulfate (p.245·1); bacitracin (p.161·3); neomycin sulfate (p.235·1).
*Bacterial infections of the eye, ear, and nose.*

**Polyspectran HC** Alcon, Ger.
Polymyxin B sulfate (p.245·1); bacitracin (p.161·3); hydrocortisone acetate (p.1103·3).
*Bacterial and inflammatory eye, ear and nose disorders; skin disorders.*

**Polysporin**
Note. This name is used for preparations of different composition.
Pfizer Consumer, Canad.
*Cream; eye/ear drops:* Polymyxin B sulfate (p.245·1); gramicidin (p.220·2).
*Bacterial contamination prophylaxis; eye and ear infections; infected skin disorders.*
*Eye ointment; ointment:* Polymyxin B sulfate (p.245·1); bacitracin (p.161·3).
*Eye and ear infections; infected lesions.*

GlaxoSmithKline, Fin.
Polymyxin B sulfate (p.245·1); neomycin sulfate (p.235·1); gramicidin (p.220·2).
*Eye infections.*

Glaxo Wellcome, S.Afr.†.
Polymyxin B sulfate (p.245·1); bacitracin zinc (p.161·3).
*Burns; skin infections; wounds.*

Warner-Lambert, USA; Monarch, USA.
Polymyxin B sulfate (p.245·1); bacitracin (p.161·3) or bacitracin zinc (p.161·3).
*Eye infections; skin infections.*

**Polysporin Plus Pain Relief** Pfizer Consumer, Canad.
Polymyxin B sulfate (p.245·1); gramicidin (p.220·2); lidocaine hydrochloride (p.1377·3).
Formerly known as Polysporin Burn Formula.
*Infected burns; skin pain.*

**Polysporin Triple Antibiotic** Pfizer Consumer, Canad.
Polymyxin B sulfate (p.245·1); bacitracin (p.161·3); gramicidin (p.220·2).
*Burns; minor wounds.*

**Polysporina** Wellcome, Port.†.
Polymyxin B sulfate (p.245·1); neomycin sulfate (p.235·1); gramicidin (p.220·2).
*Eye infections.*

**Polytab** Pharmasant, Thai.
Cyproheptadine hydrochloride (p.430·1).
*Hypersensitivity reactions; pruritus; reduced appetite.*

**Polytabs-F** Major, USA.
Multivitamin preparation with fluoride (p.1417·1)(p.1444·3).
*Dental caries prophylaxis; dietary supplement.*

**Polytamin** Brench, Ger.
Vitamins; rutoside; adenosine; aminobenzoic acid; linoleic acid; yeast; minerals; procaine hydrochloride (p.1383·2) (p.1417·1).
*Atherosclerosis; tonic.*

**Polytanol** Pharmasant, Thai.
Amitriptyline hydrochloride (p.280·3).
*Depression.*

**Polytar**
Note. This name is used for preparations of different composition.
Stiefel, Austral.; Stiefel, Braz.; Stiefel, Ger.†; Stiefel, Hong Kong; Stiefel, Irl.; Stiefel, Israel; Stiefel, Malaysia; Stiefel, Mex.; Stiefel, NZ; Stiefel, Port.; Stiefel, S.Afr.; Stiefel, Singapore; Stiefel, Thai.
Tar (p.1159·3); cade oil (p.1159·2); coal tar (p.1159·2).
*Skin and scalp disorders.*

Stiefel, Canad.
Wood tar (p.1159·3); mineral tar (p.1159·2).
*Seborrhoeic dermatitis.*

Stiefel, Ital.†.
Vegetable and mineral tars (p.1159·2).
*Cleansing of the scalp; seborrhoeic dermatitis.*

Stiefel, Spain.
Tar (p.1159·3); juniper oil (p.1703·1); coal tar (p.1159·2).
*Skin and scalp disorders.*

Stiefel, USA.
Coal tar solution; crude coal tar (p.1159·2).
*Scalp and skin disorders.*

**Polytar AF**
Note. This name is used for preparations of different composition.
Stiefel, Canad.
Coal tar (p.1159·2); pyrithione disulfide (p.1156·2); salicylic acid (p.1157·1); menthol (p.1711·3).
*Scalp disorders.*

Stiefel, UK.
Tar (p.1159·3); cade oil (p.1159·2); coal tar (p.1159·2); pyrithione zinc (p.1156·2).
*Scalp disorders.*

**Polytar Emollient**
Stiefel, Hong Kong; Stiefel, Irl.; Stiefel, NZ; Stiefel, UK.
Tar (p.1159·3); cade oil (p.1159·2); coal tar (p.1159·2); liquid paraffin (p.1479·1).
*Aid to ointment and paste removal in psoriasis; skin disorders.*

**Polytar Liquid** Stiefel, UK.
Tar (p.1159·3); cade oil (p.1159·2); coal tar (p.1159·2).
*Aid to ointment and paste removal in psoriasis; scalp disorders.*

**Polytar Plus**
Stiefel, Hong Kong†; Stiefel, Irl.†; Stiefel, NZ; Stiefel, UK.
Tar (p.1159·3); cade oil (p.1159·2); coal tar (p.1159·2).
*Aid to ointment removal in psoriasis; scalp disorders.*

**Poly-Tears**
Iquinn, Austral.; Alcon, NZ.
Hypromellose (p.1579·3); dextran 70 (p.746·2).
*Dry eyes.*

**Polytonyl**
Upsamedica, Belg.†; UPSA Conseil, Fr.; Upsamedica, Switz.†.
Vitamin, mineral, and amino-acid preparation (p.1417·1).

**Polytopic** Sabex, Canad.
*Cream:* Polymyxin B sulfate (p.245·1); gramicidin (p.220·2).
*Ointment:* Polymyxin B sulfate (p.245·1); bacitracin (p.161·3).
*Infected lesions.*

**Polytracin**
Metapharma, Canad.†.
Bacitracin zinc (p.161·3); polymyxin B sulfate (p.245·1).
*Bacterial infections.*

Medical Ophthalmics, USA.
Bacitracin (p.161·3); polymyxin B (p.245·2).
*Eye infections.*

**Polytrim**
GlaxoSmithKline, Austria; GlaxoSmithKline, Belg.; GlaxoSmithKline, Neth.; GlaxoSmithKline, S.Afr.; Pliva, UK; Allergan, USA.
Trimethoprim (p.272·2); polymyxin B sulfate (p.245·1).
*Bacterial eye infections.*

Allergan, Canad.
Trimethoprim sulfate (p.272·2); polymyxin B sulfate (p.245·1).
*Bacterial eye infections.*

**Poly-Tussin** Pharmakon, USA.
Hydrocodone tartrate (p.45·1); chlorphenamine maleate (p.427·3); phenylephrine hydrochloride (p.1126·3).
*Upper respiratory-tract disorders.*

**Polyvalent Snake Antivenom** CSL, Austral.
A snake antiserum of king brown snake, tiger snake, brown snake, death adder and taipan (p.1639·1).
*Passive immunisation.*

**Poly-Vi-Flor**
Mead Johnson Nutritionals, Canad.†; Mead Johnson Nutritionals, Thai.; Mead Johnson Nutritionals, USA.
A range of vitamin preparations with fluoride (p.1417·1)(p.1444·3).
*Dental caries prophylaxis; dietary supplement.*

**Poly-Vi-Fluor** Mead Johnson, Braz.
Multivitamin preparation (p.1417·1) with fluoride (p.1444·3).
*Dietary supplement.*

**Poly-Visc** Alcon, NZ.
Liquid paraffin (p.1479·1); white soft paraffin (p.1479·3).
*Eye lubrication and protection.*

**Poly-Vi-Sol**
Bristol-Myers Squibb, Arg.; Mead Johnson Nutritionals, Canad.; Mead Johnson, Hong Kong; Bristol-Myers Squibb, Mex.; Mead Johnson Nutritionals, Thai.; Mead Johnson Nutritionals, USA.
A range of vitamin preparations (p.1417·1).

**Polyvit**
Note. This name is used for preparations of different composition.
Taro, Israel.
*Oral drops:* Multivitamin preparation (p.1417·1).
*Tablets:* Multivitamin and mineral preparation with ginseng (p.1417·1).

Pharmasant, Thai.
Ferrous fumarate (p.1427·3); riboflavin; vitamin C; folic acid; citric acid (p.1417·1).
*Anaemias; vitamin supplement.*

**Polyvit 30 Plus** Taro, Israel.
Multivitamin and mineral preparation with ginseng and rutoside (p.1417·1).

**Polyvita** Piette, Belg.†.
Multivitamin, mineral, and amino-acid preparation (p.1417·1).

**Poly-Vitamin Plus** Chephasaar, Ger.†.
Multivitamin and mineral preparation (p.1417·1).

**Polyxan-Blau N** Ritsert, Ger.
Homoeopathic preparation.

**Polyxan-Blau N comp** Ritsert, Ger.
Homoeopathic preparation.

**Polyxan-Gelb N** Ritsert, Ger.
Homoeopathic preparation.

**Polyxan-Gelb N comp** Ritsert, Ger.
Homoeopathic preparation.

**Polyxan-Grun N** Ritsert, Ger.
Homoeopathic preparation.

**Polyxan-Grun N comp** Ritsert, Ger.
Homoeopathic preparation.

**Polyxen** Pharmasant, Thai.
Naproxen (p.65·1).
*Gout; musculoskeletal and joint disorders.*

**Polyxicam** Pharmasant, Thai.
Piroxicam (p.84·2).
*Gout; musculoskeletal and joint disorders.*

**Polyxit** Pharmasant, Thai.
Gemfibrozil (p.923·1).
*Hyperlipidaemias.*

**Polyzalip** Pharmasant, Thai.
Bezafibrate (p.873·2).
*Hyperlipidaemias.*

**Polyzym**
Note. This name is used for preparations of different composition.
Alcon, Austral.†; Alcon, Austria†; Alcon, Braz.; Alcon, Fr.; Alcon, Mex.†.
Pancreatin (p.1725·3)(p.1164·2).
*Contact lens cleanser.*

Alcon, NZ.
Cleaning of soft and gas-permeable contact lenses (p.1164·2).

**Pomada Antibiotica** Abbott, Spain.
Bacitracin (p.161·3); neomycin sulfate (p.235·1); polymyxin B sulfate (p.245·1).
*Burns; skin infections; ulcers; wounds.*

**Pomada Antihemorroidal** Drag, Chile.
Zinc (p.1469·2); lidocaine (p.1377·3).
*Haemorrhoids.*

**Pomada Balsamica** Alcala, Spain†.
Camphor (p.1665·3); cedrus deodora oil; cineole (p.1672·1); methyl salicylate (p.59·3); thymol (p.1194·2); turpentine.
*Cold symptoms.*

**Pomada Blumen** Luper, Braz.†.
Zinc (p.1469·2); boric acid (p.1662·1); zinc oxide (p.1163·2).
*Skin disorders.*

**Pomada Heridas** Asens, Spain.
Benzalkonium chloride (p.1168·3); phenazone (p.82·3); sulfanilamide (p.263·2); zinc oxide (p.1163·2).
*Skin infections.*

**Pomada Infantil Vera** Labitec, Spain.
Bismuth subnitrate (p.1252·2); boric acid (p.1662·1); talc (p.1159·1); zinc oxide (p.1163·2).
*Skin irritation.*

**Pomada Martel** Galenogal, Braz.†.
Merbromin (p.1185·3); Peru balsam (p.1730·2); camphor (p.1665·3); zinc (p.1469·2).

**Pomada Minancora** Minancora, Braz.
Benzalkonium chloride (p.1168·3); zinc oxide (p.1163·2); camphor (p.1665·3).
*Skin disorders.*

**Pomada Revulsiva** Orravan, Spain†.
Camphor (p.1665·3); capsicum oleoresin (p.1667·1); eugenol (p.1686·2); methyl salicylate (p.59·3); turpentine oil (p.1760·1).
*Musculoskeletal, joint, peri-articular, and soft-tissue disorders.*

**Pomada Vitaminica** Pasteur, Chile.
Vitamin A palmitate (p.1453·1); colecalciferol (p.1461·3); dexpanthenol (p.1727·2); zinc oxide (p.1163·2).
*Skin disorders.*

**Pomada Wilfe** Perez Gimenez, Spain.
Sulfanilamide (p.263·2); sulfathiazole (p.264·1).
*Skin infections.*

**Pomaderme** Legrand, Braz.
Theobroma oil; boric acid (p.1662·1); zinc oxide (p.1163·2); talc (p.1159·1).
*Skin disorders.*

**Pomadom** Pharmasant, Thai.
Dipotassium clorazepate (p.685·1).
*Anxiety; epilepsy.*

**Pomaglos** Merck, Port.†.
Vitamin A; vitamin D (p.1417·1); cod-liver oil (p.1425·2); zinc oxide (p.1163·2).
*Burns; skin irritation; wounds.*

**Pomaglos Pomada** EMS, Braz.†.
Zinc oxide (p.1163·2); boric acid (p.1662·1).
*Skin disorders.*

**Pomalgex** Uniao Quimica, Braz.†.
Methacholine chloride (p.1492·1); methyl salicylate (p.59·3); menthol (p.1711·3); thymol (p.1194·2).
*Musculoskeletal and joint disorders.*

**Pomata Midy HC** Maggioni, Ital.†.
Benzocaine (p.1370·3); hamamelis (p.1696·3); aesculus (p.1648·2); hydrocortisone acetate (p.1103·3).
*Anorectal disorders.*

**Pommade au The des Bois** Valmo, Canad.†.
Methyl salicylate (p.59·3); camphor (p.1665·3); menthol (p.1711·3); cineole (p.1672·1).

**Pommade Lelong** Zambon, Fr.
Peru balsam (p.1730·2); vitamin A (p.1451·2).
Formerly contained peru balsam, vitamin A, and sulfapyridine.
*Skin disorders.*

**Pommade Maurice** Cooperation Pharmaceutique, Fr.
Yellow mercuric oxide (p.1712·3).
*Eye infections.*

**Pommade Midy** Welcker-Lyster, Canad.†.
Amylocaine hydrochloride (p.1370·2); benzocaine (p.1370·3); hamamelis (p.1696·3); aesculus (p.1648·2).
*Haemorrhoids.*

**Pommade Mo Cochon** Tradiphar, Fr.
Salicylic acid (p.1157·1).
*Callus; corns; verrucae.*

**Pommade nasale Ruedi** Stotzer, Switz.†.
Camphorated oil; mint oil (p.1715·2).
*Nasal dryness.*

**Pommade Po-Ho N A Vogel** Bioforce, Switz.†.
Hypericum (p.299·1); peppermint oil (p.1283·2); hamamelis (p.1696·3); peppermint leaf (p.1283·2); calendula (p.1665·2); lemon oil (p.1706·2).
*Catarrh; cold and influenza symptoms; sinus disorders.*

**Ponac** Aspen, S.Afr.
Mefenamic acid (p.55·2).
*Musculoskeletal, joint, and soft-tissue disorders; pain.*

**Ponalar** Godecke, Ger.
Mefenamic acid (p.55·2).
*Inflammation; musculoskeletal, joint, and soft-tissue disorders; pain.*

**Ponalgic** Antigen, Irl.
Mefenamic acid (p.55·2).
*Menorrhagia; musculoskeletal and joint disorders; pain.*

**Ponaris** Panalab, Arg.
Fluconazole (p.398·1).
*Fungal infections.*

**Pondactil** Pond's, Thai.
Triprolidine hydrochloride (p.442·3); pseudoephedrine hydrochloride (p.1129·2).
*Allergic rhinitis; cold symptoms; hay fever; nasal congestion.*

**Pondactone** Pond's, Thai.
Spironolactone (p.1003·1).
*Aldosteronism; hypertension; oedema.*

**Pondarmett** Pond's, Thai.
Cimetidine (p.1255·3).
*Gastro-oesophageal reflux; peptic ulcer; Zollinger-Ellison syndrome.*

**Pondera** Euroforma, Braz.
Paroxetine hydrochloride (p.311·2).
*Depression.*

**Pondicilina** Altana, Braz.
Cetalkonium chloride (p.1172·1); cetylpyridinium chloride (p.1173·1).
*Mouth and throat disorders.*

**Pondnacef** Pond's, Thai.
Cefalexin (p.168·1).
*Bacterial infections.*

**Pondnadysmen** Pond's, Thai.
Mefenamic acid (p.55·2).
*Pain.*

**Pondnoxcill** Pond's, Thai.
Amoxicillin trihydrate (p.155·3).
*Bacterial infections.*

**Pondocillin**
Leo, Canad.; Leo, Denm.; Leo, Norw.; Adcock Ingram, S.Afr.†; Leo, Swed.
Pivampicillin (p.244·1).
*Bacterial infections.*

**Pondperdone** Pond's, Thai.
Domperidone (p.1263·2).
*Dyspepsia; gastrointestinal disorders; nausea and vomiting.*

**Ponds Prevent** Unilever, Canad.
*SPF 15 cream:* Octinoxate (p.1154·3); oxybenzone (p.1154·3).
*SPF 15 lotion:* Octinoxate (p.1154·3); ensulizole (p.1147·1).
*Sunscreen.*

**Pondtroxin** Pond's, Thai.
Levothyroxine sodium (p.1600·1).
*Hypothyroidism.*

**Pondusvitam** IQB, Braz.
Buclizine (p.426·3); vitamin B substances (p.1417·1).
*Reduced appetite; tonic.*

**Pongesic** Raza, Malaysia; Pharmaniaga, Malaysia.
Mefenamic acid (p.55·2).
*Pain.*

**Ponmel** Clonmel, Irl.
Mefenamic acid (p.55·2).
*Pain.*

**Ponnac** Sriprasit, Thai.†.
Mefenamic acid (p.55·2).
*Pain.*

**Ponnesia** Asian Pharm, Thai.
Mefenamic acid (p.55·2).
*Pain.*

**Ponoxylan** Aventis, NZ.
Polynoxylin (p.1190·1).
*Skin infections.*

**Ponsolit** Biomedica-Chemica, Gr.
Tenoxicam (p.93·1).
*Dysmenorrhoea; gout; inflammation; osteoarthritis; pain; rheumatoid arthritis; spondyloarthropathies.*

**Ponstan**
Pfizer Consumer, Austral.; Ache, Braz.; Pfizer, Canad.; Pfizer, Fin.; Pfizer, Gr.; Pfizer, Hong Kong; Parke, Davis, India; Elan, Irl.; Pfizer, Malaysia; Parke, Davis, Mex.; Pfizer, NZ; Parke, Davis, Port.; Pfizer, S.Afr.; Pfizer, Singapore; Pfizer, Switz.; Pfizer, Thai.; Chemidex, UK.
Mefenamic acid (p.55·2).
*Dysmenorrhoea; fever; inflammation; menorrhagia; musculoskeletal, joint, peri-articular, and soft-tissue disorders; pain.*

**Ponstel**
Parke-Med, S.Afr.; Parke, Davis, USA.
Mefenamic acid (p.55·2).
*Fever; menorrhagia; pain.*

**Ponstil** Parke, Davis, Arg.
Mefenamic acid (p.55·2).
*Fever; inflammation; menorrhagia; pain.*

**Ponstil Mujer** Parke, Davis, Arg.
Ibuprofen (p.45·3).
*Fever; musculoskeletal, joint, and peri-articular disorders; pain.*

**Ponstin** Parke, Davis, Arg.
Ibuprofen (p.45·3).
*Fever; musculoskeletal and joint disorders; pain.*

**Ponstyl** Pfizer, Fr.
Mefenamic acid (p.55·2).
*Pain.*

**Pontacid** Duopharma, Hong Kong.
Mefenamic acid (p.55·2).
*Pain.*

**Pontalon**
YSP, Malaysia; Yung Shin, Singapore; Yung Shin, Thai.†.
Mefenamic acid (p.55·2).
*Pain.*

**Pontefix** Fimo, Ital.
Zinc phosphate (p.1469·3).
*Cement in dentistry.*

**Pontin** Hexal, Braz.
Mefenamic acid (p.55·2).
*Fever; inflammation; pain.*

**Pontiride** Psicofarma, Mex.
Sulpiride (p.722·2).
*Anxiety disorders; obsessive-compulsive disorder; schizophrenia; vertigo.*

**Pontocaine**
Abbott, Canad.; Sanofi Winthrop, Israel; Sanofi Winthrop, USA.
Tetracaine (p.1385·1) or tetracaine hydrochloride (p.1385·1).
*Local anaesthesia.*

**Pontuc**
Novartis, Austria; Novartis, Ger.†.
Co-dergocrine mesilate (p.1674·1); nifedipine (p.966·2).
*Hypertension.*

**Pontyl** Malaysia Chemist, Singapore.
Mefenamic acid (p.55·2).
*Inflammation; pain.*

**Pool 8** Fiori, Ital.
Amino-acid preparation (p.1417·1).
*Nutritional supplement.*

**Po-Pon-S** Shionogi, USA.
Multivitamin and mineral preparation (p.1417·1).

**POR 8**
Ferring, Austral.; Ferring, Austria; Sandoz, Ger.†; Aventis, NZ†; Ferring, S.Afr.; Ferring, Switz.†.
Ornipressin (p.1335·3).
*Reduction of bleeding during surgery; variceal haemorrhage.*

**Porazine** Pharmasant, Thai.
Perphenazine (p.714·2).
*Anxiety; nausea and vomiting.*

**Porcelana Daytime Formula** Schwarzkopf, Canad.
Hydroquinone (p.1148·1); octinoxate (p.1154·3).
Formerly known as Porcelana with Sunscreen.

**Porcelana Nighttime Formula** Schwarzkopf, Canad.
Hydroquinone (p.1148·1).
Formerly known as Porcelana.

**Porcoll** MBP, Ger.
Collagen (p.1674·3).
*Haemorrhage.*

**Poremax-C** Orion, Fin.
Ascorbic acid (p.1460·2).
*Vitamin C deficiency; vitamin C supplement.*

**Porfirin 12** Teofarma, Ital.
Haematoporphyrin dihydrochloride (p.1696·2); cyanocobalamin (p.1458·2); inositol (p.1701·2).
*Tonic.*

**Pork Actrapid** Novo Nordisk, UK.
Insulin injection (porcine, highly purified) (p.333·3).
*Diabetes mellitus.*

**Pork Insulatard** Novo Nordisk, UK.
Isophane insulin injection (porcine, highly purified) (p.333·3).
*Diabetes mellitus.*

**Pork Mixtard 30** Novo Nordisk, UK.
Mixture of neutral insulin injection (porcine, highly purified) 30% and isophane insulin injection (porcine, highly purified) 70% (p.333·3).
Formerly known as Mixtard 30/70.
*Diabetes mellitus.*

**Poro**
YSP, Malaysia; Yung Shin, Singapore.
Paracetamol (p.76·2).
*Fever; pain.*

**Porosis D** Cedar Health, UK†.
Calcium citrate (p.1225·1); magnesium citrate (p.1272·1); boron; vitamin D (p.1461·2).

**Porostenina** Savio, Ital.†.
Calcitonin (salmon) (p.768·2).
*Hypercalcaemia; osteoporosis; Paget's disease of bone; reflex sympathetic dystrophy.*

**Porphin** Crawford, UK.
5-Aminolevulinic acid (p.527·2).
Available only on a named patient basis.
*Precancerous skin disorders; skin cancer.*

**Porphyrocin** Medochemie, Hong Kong.
Erythromycin stearate (p.208·2).
*Bacterial infections.*

**Porriver** Ogna, Ital.†.
Trichloroacetic acid (p.1162·1).
*Verrucae; warts.*

**Portagen**
Mead Johnson, Austral.; Mead Johnson Nutritionals, Canad.; Mead Johnson Nutritionals, Fin.; Mead Johnson, Hong Kong; Mead Johnson, Irl.; Mead Johnson, Ital.; Mead Johnson, Malaysia; Mead Johnson, NZ†; Mead Johnson, Port.; Bristol-Myers Squibb, S.Afr.; Mead Johnson, Singapore; Mead Johnson Nutritionals, USA.
Preparation for enteral nutrition (p.1417·1).
*Disorders of fat digestion and absorption.*

**Portamin** Darrow, Braz.
Amino-acid infusion (p.1417·1).
*Parenteral nutrition.*

**Portia** Barr, USA.
Ethinylestradiol (p.1553·2); levonorgestrel (p.1563·2).
28-Day packs also contain 7 inert tablets.
*Combined oral contraceptive.*

**Portolac**
Novartis Consumer, Austria; Novartis Consumer, Belg.; Novartis Consumer, Ital.; Shinyaku, Jpn.
Lactitol (p.1269·1).
*Constipation; hepatic encephalopathy; hyperammonaemia.*

**Posalfilin**
Norgine, Austral.; Norgine, Hong Kong; Norgine, Irl.; Norgine, Malaysia; Norgine, NZ; Norgine, S.Afr.; Norgine, Singapore; Norgine, UK.
Podophyllum resin (p.1155·2); salicylic acid (p.1157·1).
*Warts.*

**Posanin** Pose, Thai.
Dipyridamole (p.903·1).
*Ischaemic heart disease; thrombosis prophylaxis.*

**Posdrink** Catarinense, Braz.
Aspirin (p.15·1); mepyramine (p.437·1); caffeine (p.782·1).
Aluminium hydroxide (p.1249·2) is included in this preparation in an attempt to limit adverse effects on the gastrointestinal mucosa.
*Fever; pain.*

**Pose-Bac** Pose, Thai.
Benzalkonium chloride (p.1168·3).
*Disinfection.*

**Pose-CM** Pose, Thai.†.
Cimetidine (p.1255·3).
*Gastro-oesophageal reflux; hypersensitivity reactions; peptic ulcer; Zollinger-Ellison syndrome.*

**Posecus** Pose, Thai.†.
Ambroxol hydrochloride (p.1114·3).
*Respiratory-tract disorders associated with increased or viscous mucus.*

**Posedene** Pose, Thai.
Piroxicam (p.84·2).
*Musculoskeletal and joint disorders.*

**Pose-Dex** Pose, Thai.†.
Glutaral (p.1180·3).
*Instrument and surface disinfection.*

**Poselium** Pose, Thai.†.
Domperidone (p.1263·2).
*Dyspepsia; nausea and vomiting.*

**Posene** Pose, Thai.
Dipotassium clorazepate (p.685·1).
*Anxiety; insomnia.*

**Posicycline** Alcon, Fr.
Oxytetracycline hydrochloride (p.241·1).
*Bacterial eye infections.*

**Posidol** Pharmaland, Thai.
Mebhydrolin napadisilate (p.436·3).
*Hypersensitivity reactions.*

**Posifenicol** Ursapharm, Ger.
Azidamfenicol (p.159·1).
*Bacterial eye infections.*

**Posifenicol C** Ursapharm, Ger.
Chloramphenicol (p.185·1).
*Bacterial eye infections.*

**Posiformin** Ursapharm, Ger.
Bibrocathol (p.1660·2).
*Inflammatory eye disorders.*

**Posiject**
Boehringer Ingelheim, Irl.; Alliance, S.Afr.; Boehringer Ingelheim, UK.
Dobutamine hydrochloride (p.905·3).
*Agent for cardiac stress testing; heart failure.*

**Posilent** Ursapharm, Ger.†.
Cytidine.
*Muscular, accommodative, and nervous eye disorders.*

**Posine** Alcon, Fr.
Oxedrine tartrate (p.977·3); chlorhexidine gluconate (p.1173·2).
*Conjunctival irritation.*

**Posipen** Sanfer, Mex.
Dicloxacillin sodium (p.205·2).
*Bacterial infections.*

**Positivum** Sanova, Austria.
Fluoxetine hydrochloride (p.292·1).
*Bulimia nervosa; depression; obsessive-compulsive disorder.*

**Positon** Iquinosa, Spain.
Neomycin sulfate (p.235·1); nystatin (p.406·3); triamcinolone (p.1110·2) or triamcinolone acetonide (p.1110·2).
*Infected skin disorders.*

**Posivil** Orion, Fin.
Aspirin (p.15·1); caffeine (p.782·1); noscapine hydrochloride (p.1125·3); ascorbic acid (p.1460·2).
*Cold and influenza symptoms; coughs.*

**Posivyl** Laboratorios Chile, Chile.
Paroxetine hydrochloride (p.311·2).
*Depression.*

**Posmox** *Pose, Thai.*†.
Amoxicillin trihydrate (p.155·3).
*Bacterial infections.*

**Posnac** *Pose, Thai.*
Diclofenac sodium (p.32·1).
*Musculoskeletal and joint disorders.*

**Posorutin** *Ursapharm, Ger.*
Troxerutin (p.1688·3).
*Haemorrhoids; ophthalmic disorders; venous insufficiency.*

**Postacne** *Dermik, Canad.*
Colloidal sulfur (p.1158·2).
*Acne; oily skin.*

**Postadoxin N** *Rodleben, Ger.*
Meclozine hydrochloride (p.436·3).
*Motion sickness; nausea; vomiting.*

**Postadoxine** *UCB, Belg.*†.
Meclozine (p.436·3); vitamin $B_6$ (p.1456·3).
*Nausea and vomiting.*

**Postafen**
*Note. This name is used for preparations of different composition.*
*Aventis, Braz.*
Buclizine hydrochloride (p.426·3).
*Reduced appetite.*

*UCB, Denm.; UCB, Fin.; UCB, Ger.; UCB, Norw.; UCB, Swed.*
Meclozine (p.436·3) or meclozine hydrochloride (p.436·3).
*Hypersensitivity reactions; nausea; vomiting.*

**Postafene**
*UCB, Belg.; UCB, Gr.; UCB, Hong Kong.*
Meclozine hydrochloride (p.436·3).
*Motion sickness; nausea and vomiting; vertigo.*

**Postafeno** *UCB, Port.*
Buclizine (p.426·3).

**Postap** *Pose, Thai.*
Brompheniramine maleate (p.426·1); phenylephrine hydrochloride (p.1126·3).
Formerly contained brompheniramine maleate, phenylephrine hydrochloride, and phenylpropanolamine hydrochloride.
*Coughs; hypersensitivity reactions; nasal congestion.*

**Postap Expectorant** *Pose, Thai.*
Guaifenesin (p.1122·1); brompheniramine maleate (p.426·1); phenylephrine hydrochloride (p.1126·3).
Formerly contained guaifenesin, brompheniramine maleate, phenylephrine hydrochloride, and phenylpropanolamine hydrochloride.
*Coughs; hypersensitivity reactions; nasal congestion.*

**Postarax** *Pose, Thai.*
Hydroxyzine hydrochloride (p.434·3).
*Anxiety; nausea and vomiting; pruritus.*

**Postavit-B** *Riker, Mex.*†.
Buclizine (p.426·3).

**Posterine** *Kade, Ger.*
Hamamelis (p.1696·3).
*Anorectal disorders.*

**Posterine Corte** *Kade, Ger.*
Hydrocortisone acetate (p.1103·3).
*Anorectal disorders.*

**Posterisan**
*Mayrhofer, Austria; Kade, Ger.; Kade, Hong Kong; Knoll, S.Afr.*†.
Cell contents and metabolic products of *Escherichia coli*.
*Anorectal disorders.*

**Posterisan Forte**
*Kade, Ger.; Kade, Hong Kong.*
Cell components and metabolic products of *Escherichia coli*; hydrocortisone (p.1103·3).
*Anorectal disorders.*

**Posti N** *Kade, Ger.*
Rutoside (p.1688·2); esculoside (p.1648·2).
*Haemorrhoids; venous insufficiency.*

**Postinor**
*Ache, Braz.; Schering, Fin.; Gedeon Richter, Malaysia; Gedeon Richter, Singapore; Schering, Spain; Gedeon Richter, Thai.*
Levonorgestrel (p.1563·2).
*Postcoital oral contraceptive.*

**Postinor-2**
*Schering, Austral.; Grunenthal, Chile; Gedeon Richter, Hong Kong; Gedeon Richter, Israel; Schering, NZ; Medimpex, UK.*
Levonorgestrel (p.1563·2).
Available on a named-patient basis only in the *UK*.
*Postcoital oral contraception.*

**PostMI** *Ashbourne, UK*†.
Aspirin (p.15·1).
*Angina; ischaemic heart disease; myocardial infarction.*

**Postopyl** *LED, Fr.*
Oxidised glycerol triester.
*Minor skin damage.*

**Postoval**
*Note. This name is used for preparations of different composition.*
*Wyeth, Braz.*
White tablets, estradiol valerate (p.1550·2); orange tablets, estradiol valerate; levonorgestrel (p.1563·2).
*Menopausal disorders; menstrual disorders.*

*Wyeth, Chile.*
11 Tablets, estradiol valerate (p.1550·2); 10 tablets, estradiol valerate; levonorgestrel (p.1563·2).
*Menopausal disorders.*

*Akromed, S.Afr.*
11 Tablets, estradiol valerate (p.1550·2); 10 tablets, estradiol valerate; norgestrel (p.1563·2); 7 tablets, inert.
*Menopausal disorders; menstrual disorders.*

**Posture** *Whitehall, USA.*
Calcium phosphate (p.1225·3).
*Calcium supplement.*

**Posture D** *Wyeth, Mex.*
Tribasic calcium phosphate (p.1225·3); colecalciferol (p.1461·3).
*Calcium and vitamin D supplement; osteomalacia; osteoporosis; rickets; tetanus.*

**Posture-D** *Whitehall, USA.*
Calcium phosphate (p.1225·3); vitamin D (p.1461·2).
*Calcium supplement.*

**Potaba**
*Croma, Austria; Glenwood, Canad.; Glenwood, Ger.; Glenwood, Hong Kong*†*; Glenwood, Switz.*†*; Glenwood, UK; Glenwood, USA.*
Potassium aminobenzoate (p.1733·3).
*Dermatomyositis; linear scleroderma; morphoea; pemphigus; Peyronie's disease; scleroderma.*

**Potabex** *Tegur, Mex.*†.
Potassium aminobenzoate (p.1733·3).

**Potable Aqua**
*IBIS, UK; Wisconsin Pharmacal, USA.*
Tetraglycine hydroperiodide (p.1194·1).
*Disinfection of drinking water.*

**Potacol-R** *Otsuka, Jpn.*
Carbohydrate and electrolyte infusion (p.1417·1).
*Carbohydrate source; fluid and electrolyte disorders; metabolic acidosis.*

**Potasalan** *Lannett, USA.*
Potassium chloride (p.1232·2).
*Hypokalaemia; potassium depletion.*

**Potasi** *Eagle, Austral.*†.
Dibasic potassium phosphate (p.1230·3); potassium citrate (p.1223·1); potassium amino acid chelate (p.1233·1); potassium chloride (p.1232·2); potassium carbonate; potassium sulfate (p.1232·2).
*Potassium supplement.*

**Potasio C** *Dominguez, Arg.*
Potassium chloride (p.1232·2); sodium ascorbate (p.1460·2).
*Electrolyte supplement.*

**Potasion** *Sanofi Synthelabo, Spain.*
Potassium chloride (p.1232·2).
*Potassium depletion.*

**Potasion Solucion** *Sanofi Synthelabo, Spain.*
Potassium gluceptate (p.1233·1).
*Hypokalaemia.*

**Potasoral** *Armstrong, Mex.*
Potassium gluconate (p.1232·2).
*Hypokalaemia.*

**Potassion** *Miba, Ital.*
Potassium succinate (p.1233·1); potassium malate (p.1233·1); potassium citrate (p.1223·1); potassium acid tartrate (p.1284·3); potassium bicarbonate (p.1223·1).
*Acidosis; potassium deficiency.*

**Potassium Iodide and Stramonium Compound** *McGloin, Austral.*†.
Potassium iodide (p.1598·1); stramonium (p.489·2); lobelia (p.1589·1); liquorice (p.1270·2).
*Coughs; respiratory-tract congestion.*

**Potassium MG** *Miba, Ital.*
Potassium gluconate (p.1232·2); magnesium hydroxide (p.1272·2).
*Magnesium and potassium supplement.*

**Potassium-Rougier** *Rougier, Canad.*
Potassium gluconate (p.1232·2).
*Potassium supplement.*

**Potassride** *General Drugs, Thai.*
Potassium chloride (p.1232·2).
*Hypokalaemia.*

**Pota-Vi-Kin** *Collins, Mex.*
Phenoxymethylpenicillin potassium (p.242·1).
*Bacterial infections.*

**Potcit** *Upha, Malaysia.*
Potassium citrate (p.1223·1); citric acid (p.1673·1).
*Alkalinisation of urine; urinary-tract infections.*

**Potekam** *Dosa, Arg.*
Topotecan (p.589·1).
*Malignant neoplasms.*

**Potenciator** *Iquinosa, Spain.*
Arginine aspartate (p.1421·1).
*Tonic.*

**Potencil** *Sanitas, Arg.*
Cyproheptadine hydrochloride (p.430·1); arginine hydrochloride; cobamamide (p.1417·1).
*Anabolic; reduced appetite.*

**Potencort** *Julphar, UAE.*
Fluticasone propionate (p.1102·3).
*Skin disorders.*

**Potendal** *Allen, Spain*†.
Ceftazidime (p.180·2).
*Bacterial infections.*

**Potensone** *Pharmasant, Thai.*
Fluphenazine hydrochloride (p.699·3).
*Anxiety.*

**Potentol** *Orion, Fin.*
Methyltestosterone (p.1559·3); meprobamate (p.706·2); yohimbine hydrochloride (p.1766·2).
*Erectile dysfunction.*

**Potenzia** *Lifeplan, UK.*
Vitamins; minerals; saw palmetto; pygeum africanum; urticaria; bearberry; curcumin; tomato (p.1417·1).
*Dietary supplement for men.*

**Potional** *Kleva, Gr.*
Nitrendipine (p.973·3).
*Hypertension.*

**Potklor** *Martin & Harris, India.*
Potassium chloride (p.1232·2).
*Hepatic cirrhosis with ascites; potassium depletion.*

**Po-Trim** *Polipharm, Thai.*
Co-trimoxazole (p.199·3).
*Bacterial infections.*

**Potsilo N** *Stark, Ger.*
Bisacodyl (p.1251·3); calcium pantothenate (p.1442·3).
Potsilo formerly contained bisacodyl, calcium pantothenate, docusate sodium, and benzyl mandelate.
*Constipation.*

**Potter's Catarrh Pastilles** *Ernest Jackson, UK.*
Oleum pini sylvestris; pumilio pine oil (p.1737·1); eucalyptus oil (p.1686·2); creosote (p.1117·2); menthol (p.1711·3); thymol (p.1194·2); althaea (p.1651·3).
*Cough and cold symptoms.*

**Potters Children's Cough Pastilles** *Ernest Jackson, UK.*
Ipecacuanha (p.1122·3); squill (p.1130·3); citric acid (p.1673·1); honey (p.1434·2).
Formerly known as Jacksons Childrens Cough Pastilles.
*Coughs.*

**Potters Day & Night Cough Pastilles** *Ernest Jackson, UK*†.
Codeine phosphate (p.27·1); wild cherry bark (p.1765·2).
Formerly known as Night Cough Pastilles.
*Coughs.*

**Potters Decongestant Pastilles** *Ernest Jackson, UK.*
Menthol (p.1711·3); eucalyptus oil (p.1686·2).
*Coughs; nasal congestion.*

**Potters Gees Linctus** *Ernest Jackson, UK.*
Camphorated opium tincture; squill (p.1130·3); cinnamic acid (p.1177·3); benzoic acid (p.1169·3); glacial acetic acid (p.1645·2); honey (p.1434·2).
*Coughs.*

**Potters Strong Bronchial Catarrh Pastilles** *Ernest Jackson, UK.*
Menthol (p.1711·3); benzoin tincture (p.1751·1); creosote (p.1117·2); anise oil (p.1655·2); peppermint oil (p.1283·2); capsicum oleoresin (p.1667·1).
*Catarrh; coughs and cold symptoms.*

**Potters Sugar Free Cough Pastilles** *Ernest Jackson, UK.*
Liquorice (p.1270·2); menthol (p.1711·3); benzoin tincture (p.1751·1); anise oil (p.1655·2); clove oil (p.1673·3); peppermint oil (p.1283·2); capsicum oleoresin (p.1667·1).
*Catarrh; cold symptoms; coughs.*

**Povadine** *Hua, Thai.*
Povidone-iodine (p.1190·3).
*Burns; wound disinfection.*

**Povanyl** *Pfizer Sante, Fr.*
Pyrvinium embonate (p.113·3).
*Enterobiasis.*

**Povi Complex** *Hexa-Medinova, Arg.*
Povidone-iodine (p.1190·3).
*Skin, mucous membrane, and instrument disinfection.*

**Povibac** *Sertex, Arg.*
Povidone-iodine (p.1190·3).
*Skin infections; skin, mucous membrane, wound, and burn disinfection.*

**Povicler** *Monserrat, Arg.*
Povidone-iodine (p.1190·3).
*Disinfection.*

**Povid-Derme** *Kinder, Braz.*†.
Povidone-iodine (p.1190·3).
*Skin and wound disinfection.*

**Poviderm** *Farmec, Ital.*
Povidone-iodine (p.1190·3).
*Skin and wound disinfection.*

**Povidine** *Stadmed, India.*
Povidone-iodine (p.1190·3).
*Burns; mouth and throat inflammation; skin infections; wounds.*

**Povin** *Silesia, Chile.*
Vitamin A (p.1451·2); vitamin D (p.1461·2); pantothenic alcohol; zinc oxide (p.1163·2).
*Skin disorders.*

**Poviral** *Roemmers, Arg.*
Aciclovir (p.626·1).
*Herpesvirus infections.*

**Powdered C** *GNLD, Austral.*†.
Ascorbic acid and other vitamin C substances (p.1417·1).
*Vitamin C deficiency.*

**Power Orot** *Worwag, Ger.*
Magnesium orotate (p.1724·3).
*Magnesium deficiency.*

**Power Rub** *Pfizer, Mex.*†.
Methyl salicylate (p.59·3); menthol (p.1711·3); camphor (p.1665·3).
*Musculoskeletal and joint disorders.*

**Powercef** *Wockhardt, India.*
Ceftriaxone sodium (p.182·3).
*Bacterial infections.*

**Powergel** *Menarini, UK.*
Ketoprofen (p.51·2).
*Inflammation; pain.*

**PowerLean** *Matley, UK*†.
Conjugate linoleic acid (p.1690·2).
*Nutritional supplement.*

**PowerMate** *Green Turtle Bay Vitamin Co., USA.*
Vitamins; minerals; green tea extract; ginkgo biloba extract; glutathione; acetylcysteine; echinacea; golden seal root; pine bark extract (p.1417·1).
*Tonic.*

**PowerSleep** *Green Turtle Bay Vitamin Co., USA.*
Vitamins; minerals; passion flower; valerian; oxitriptan; melatonin (p.1417·1).
*Tonic.*

**PowerVites** *Green Turtle Bay Vitamin Co., USA.*
Vitamins; minerals; aminobenzoic acid; inositol; bioflavonoids; bee pollen; folic acid (p.1417·1).
*Tonic.*

**Poxider** *Martin, Spain*†.
Fluocinolone acetonide (p.1101·2); gramicidin (p.220·2); neomycin sulfate (p.235·1).
*Infected skin disorders.*

**Pozapam** *Pharmasant, Thai.*
Prazepam (p.716·2).
*Anxiety.*

**Pozato** *Libbs, Braz.*
Levonorgestrel (p.1563·2).
*Progestogen-only oral contraceptive.*

**Pozhexol** *Pharmasant, Thai.*
Trihexyphenidyl hydrochloride (p.490·2).
*Parkinsonism.*

**PPD Tine Test** *Wyeth, S.Afr.*†.
Tuberculin (p.1759·1).
*Diagnosis of tuberculosis.*

**PPG** *Bago, Chile.*
Policosanol (p.984·2).
*Hypercholesterolaemia.*

**PPG-5** *Fustery, Mex.*†.
Policosanol (p.984·2).
*Hypercholesterolaemia.*

**PPS** *Baxter, Ital.*
Plasma protein fraction (p.758·2).
*Burns; hypovolaemia; shock.*

**PPSB Konzentrat S-TIM** *Baxter, Ger.*
A factor IX preparation (p.752·2).
*Haemorrhagic disorders.*

**PR 100** *Farmacologico Milanese, Ital.*†.
Desonide pivalate (p.1096·3).
*Skin disorders.*

**PR 100-Cloressidina** *Farmacologico Milanese, Ital.*†.
Desonide pivalate (p.1096·3); chlorhexidine (p.1173·2).
*Skin disorders.*

**PR Freeze Spray** *Crookes Healthcare, UK.*
Dimethyl ether (p.1236·1); dimethoxymethane (p.1680·3).
Formerly contained trichlorofluoromethane and dichlorodifluoromethane.
*Muscular pain and stiffness.*

**PR Heat Spray** *Crookes Healthcare, UK.*
Methyl salicylate (p.59·3); ethyl nicotinate (p.37·2); camphor (p.1665·3).
*Bruises; muscular and rheumatic pain; sprains.*

**Prabioquim** *Bioquimico, Mex.*†.
Prazosin (p.986·1).

**Pra-Brexidol** *Pharmacia, Ger.*
Piroxicam (p.84·2).
*Gout; musculoskeletal, joint, and soft-tissue disorders.*

**Pracap** *Darrow, Braz.*
Finasteride (p.1554·2).
*Alopecia.*

**Pracem** *Novag, Mex.*
Dipyridamole (p.903·1).

**Pracne** *Grunenthal, Chile.*
Minocycline (p.231·3).
*Bacterial infections.*

**Practazin** *Cardel, Fr.*
Spironolactone (p.1003·1); altizide (p.858·1).
*Hypertension; oedema.*

**Practil** *Organon, Ital.*
Desogestrel (p.1547·2); ethinylestradiol (p.1553·2).
*Combined oral contraceptive.*

**Practin** *Merind, India.*
Cyproheptadine hydrochloride (p.430·1).
*Hypersensitivity disorders; migraine.*

**Practiser** *Serral, Mex.*
Diclofenac (p.32·1).
*Inflammation.*

**Practizol** *Collins, Mex.*
Astemizole (p.424·2).
*Hypersensitivity.*

**Practo-Clyss**
*Braun, Belg.; Fresenius Kabi, Ger.; Braun, Switz.*
Monobasic sodium phosphate (p.1230·3); dibasic sodium phosphate (p.1231·1).
*Bowel evacuation; constipation.*

**Practomil** *Braun, Switz.*
Glycerol (p.1694·3).
*Bowel evacuation; constipation.*

**Practon** *Cardel, Fr.*
Spironolactone (p.1003·1).
*Hyperaldosteronism; hypertension; myasthenia; oedema.*

**Pradente** *Dinafarma, Braz.*†.
Procaine hydrochloride (p.1383·2); phenol (p.1188·1).
*Mouth and throat disorders.*

**Pradif**
*Boehringer Ingelheim, Gr.; Boehringer Ingelheim, Ital.; Boehringer Ingelheim, Port.; Boehringer Ingelheim, Switz.*
Tamsulosin hydrochloride (p.1009·2).
*Benign prostatic hyperplasia.*

**Pradinolol** *Ducto, Braz.*
Propranolol hydrochloride (p.989·3).
*Arrhythmias; hypertension.*

**Praecicor** Molimin, Ger.†.
Verapamil hydrochloride (p.1019·1).
*Angina pectoris; arrhythmias; hypertension.*

**Praeciglucon** Pfleger, Ger.
Glibenclamide (p.331·2).
*Diabetes mellitus.*

**Praecineural** Pfleger, Ger.
Aspirin (p.15·1); codeine phosphate (p.27·1).
Glycine (p.1433·3) is included in the tablets in an attempt to limit adverse effects on the gastrointestinal mucosa.
*Pain; rheumatism.*

**Praecordin S** Altana, Ger.
Strong camphor oil; menthol (p.1711·3); benzyl nicotinate (p.21·2).
*Cardiac disorders.*

**Praedex** Fresenius Kabi, Austria.
Dextran 1 (p.745·2).
*Prevention of anaphylactic reactions to infusions of dextrans.*

**Praefeminon plus** Cesra, Ger.
Ferric ammonium citrate (p.1427·2); pulsatilla pratensis; valeriana officinalis.
*Gynaecological disorders.*

**Praesidin** Medopharm, Ger.†.
Lidocaine hydrochloride (p.1377·3); diphenhydramine metilsulfate (p.432·2); titanium dioxide (p.1160·3).
*Skin disorders.*

**Pragman** Hoechst Marion Roussel, Austria†.
Tolpropamine hydrochloride (p.442·2).
*Pruritus.*

**Pragmatar**
Note. This name is used for preparations of different composition.
GlaxoSmithKline, India.
Benzoic acid (p.1169·3); salicylic acid (p.1157·1); menthol (p.1711·3); camphor (p.1665·3).
*Dandruff; fungal skin infections; seborrhoeic dermatitis.*

Alliance, Irl.; Alliance, UK.
Coal tar (p.1159·2); sulfur (p.1158·2); salicylic acid (p.1157·1).
*Scalp disorders.*

**Pragmaten** Sanofi Synthelabo, Chile.
Fluoxetine (p.296·3).
*Depression; mixed anxiety depressive states.*

**Prairie Gold** Larkhall Laboratories, UK.
Vitamin E (p.1464·3).

**Pralenal** Opus, UK.
Enalapril maleate (p.909·2).
*Angina pectoris; heart failure; hypertension.*

**Pralifan** Inibsa, Spain.
Mitoxantrone hydrochloride (p.575·2).
*Malignant neoplasms.*

**Pralol** Pharmasant, Thai.
Propranolol hydrochloride (p.989·3).
*Angina pectoris; anxiety; hypertension; migraine; myocardial infarction; tremor.*

**Pramace** Hassle, Swed.
Ramipril (p.994·1).
*Atherosclerosis; diabetic nephropathy; heart failure; hypertension.*

**PrameGel**
Medicis, Canad.; GenDerm, USA.
Pramocaine hydrochloride (p.1382·2); menthol (p.1711·3).
*Pruritus.*

**Pramet** Abbott, Port.
Multivitamin and mineral preparation (p.1417·1).

**Pramet FA** Abbott, Hong Kong.
Multivitamin and mineral preparation with iron and folic acid (p.1417·1).

**Pramidal** Galen, Mex.
Loperamide hydrochloride (p.1271·1).
*Diarrhoea.*

**Pramide** Irex, Port.
Pyrazinamide (p.246·3).
*Tuberculosis.*

**Pramidin** Crinos, Ital.
Metoclopramide hydrochloride (p.1274·3).
*Gastrointestinal disorders.*

**Pramigel** Carnot, Mex.
Metoclopramide hydrochloride (p.1274·3); aluminium hydroxide (p.1249·2); magnesium hydroxide (p.1272·2); dimeticone (p.1289·2).
*Gastrointestinal disorders.*

**Pramilem** Lemery, Mex.
Metoclopramide (p.1274·3).
*Nausea and vomiting.*

**Pramilet FA**
Abbott, Malaysia; Abbott, Singapore; Abbott, Thai.; Ross, USA†.
Multivitamin and mineral preparation with iron and folic acid (p.1417·1).

**Pramin**
Alphapharm, Austral.; Rafa, Israel.
Metoclopramide hydrochloride (p.1274·3).
*Adjunct in gastrointestinal examination; dyspepsia; gastroparesis; hiccups; nausea and vomiting; peptic ulcer.*

**Praminan** Cazi, Braz.
Imipramine hydrochloride (p.300·1).
*Depression.*

**Pramino** Janssen-Cilag, Ger.
Norgestimate (p.1563·2); ethinylestradiol (p.1553·2).
*Triphasic oral contraceptive.*

**Pramistar** FIRMA, Ital.†.
Pramiracetam sulfate (p.1734·3).
*Anxiety disorders; mental function impairment.*

**Pramosone** Ferndale, USA.
Hydrocortisone acetate (p.1103·3); pramocaine hydrochloride (p.1382·2).
*Skin disorders.*

**PramOtic** Hawthorn, USA.
Chloroxylenol (p.1177·2); pramocaine hydrochloride (p.1382·2).
*Bacterial infections of the external ear.*

**Pramotil** Pisa, Mex.
Metoclopramide (p.1274·3).
*Nausea and vomiting.*

**Pramox** Isdin, Spain.
Pramocaine hydrochloride (p.1382·2).
*Pruritus.*

**Pramox HC** Dermtek, Canad.
Hydrocortisone acetate (p.1103·3); pramocaine hydrochloride (p.1382·2).
*Skin disorders.*

**Panadox** Pisa, Mex.
Zidovudine (p.658·2).
*HIV infection.*

**Prandase**
Bayer, Canad.; Pharma Clal, Israel.
Acarbose (p.328·3).
*Diabetes mellitus.*

**Prandin**
Medley, Braz.; Menarini, Spain; Novo Nordisk, USA.
Repaglinide (p.344·3).
*Diabetes mellitus.*

**Prandin $E_2$** Pharmacia, S.Afr.
Dinoprostone (p.1515·1).
*Labour induction.*

**Pranoflog** SIFI, Ital.
Pranoprofen (p.85·2).
*Anterior eye inflammation.*

**Pranolol** Alpharma, Norw.
Propranolol hydrochloride (p.989·3).
*Angina pectoris; arrhythmias; hypertension; hyperthyroidism; migraine; myocardial infarction; tremor.*

**Pranosine** Sanfer, Mex.
Inosine pranobex (p.640·2).
*Viral infections.*

**Pranox** Viatris, Belg.
Pranoprofen (p.85·2).
*Eye inflammation.*

**Pranoxen** Propan, S.Afr.†.
Naproxen (p.65·1).
*Dysmenorrhoea; gout; musculoskeletal and joint disorders.*

**Prantal**
Schering-Plough, Austral.; Schering-Plough, Ital.; Schering-Plough, NZ.
Diphemanil metilsulfate (p.481·3).
*Hyperhidrosis.*

**Pranzo** Vinas, Spain.
Cyproheptadine hydrochloride (p.430·1); carnitine hydrochloride (p.1424·1); lysine hydrochloride (p.1439·2).
*Anorexia; tonic.*

**Praquantel** Atlantic, Thai.
Praziquantel (p.112·2).
*Trematode infections.*

**Prareduct**
Sankyo, Belg.; Sankyo, Spain.
Pravastatin sodium (p.984·3).
*Atherosclerosis; hypercholesterolaemia.*

**Prascolend** Fustery, Mex.
Pravastatin sodium (p.984·3).
*Atherosclerosis; hypercholesterolaemia.*

**Prasepine** Pfizer, Thai.
Prazepam (p.716·2).
*Anxiety; skeletal muscle spasm.*

**Prasig** Sigma, Austral.
Prazosin hydrochloride (p.985·1).
*Benign prostatic hyperplasia; heart failure; hypertension; Raynaud's syndrome.*

**Prasikon** Polipharm, Thai.
Praziquantel (p.112·2).
*Trematode infections.*

**Prasterol** Malesci, Ital.
Pravastatin sodium (p.984·3).
*Cardiovascular disorders; hypercholesterolaemia.*

**Pratazine** Sedabel, Braz.†.
Sulfadiazine silver (p.259·1).
*Skin infections.*

**Praticef** Caber, Ital.
Cefonicid sodium (p.174·2).
Lidocaine hydrochloride (p.1377·3) is included in this preparation to alleviate the pain of injection.
*Gram-negative bacterial infections.*

**Pratsiol**
Douglas, Austral.; Orion, Fin.; Douglas, Hong Kong†; Douglas, NZ; Aspen, S.Afr.; Orion, Thai.
Prazosin hydrochloride (p.985·1).
*Benign prostatic hyperplasia; heart failure; hypertension; Raynaud's syndrome.*

**Prava**
Note. This name is used for preparations of different composition.
Bristol-Myers Squibb, S.Afr.
Pravastatin sodium (p.984·3).
*Hypercholesterolaemia.*

Bristol-Myers Squibb, Switz.
Lomustine (p.565·2).
*Malignant neoplasms.*

**Pravachol**
Bristol-Myers Squibb, Austral.; Bristol-Myers Squibb, Austria; Squibb, Canad.; Bristol-Myers Squibb, Denm.; Bristol-Myers Squibb, Fin.; Bristol-Myers Squibb, Gr.; Bristol-Myers Squibb, Hong Kong; Bristol-Myers Squibb, Malaysia; Bristol-Myers Squibb, Norw.; Bristol-Myers Squibb, Singapore; Bristol-Myers Squibb, Swed.; Bristol-Myers Squibb, USA.
Pravastatin sodium (p.984·3).
*Atherosclerosis; hypercholesterolaemia.*

**Pravacilin** Abbott, Braz.†.
Metampicillin (p.229·3).
*Bacterial infections.*

**Pravacol**
Bristol-Myers Squibb, Arg.; Bristol-Myers Squibb, Braz.; Bristol-Myers Squibb, Chile; Bristol-Myers Squibb, Mex.; Bristol-Myers Squibb, Port.
Pravastatin sodium (p.984·3).
*Coronary atherosclerosis; hypercholesterolaemia.*

**Pravaselect** Menarini, Ital.
Pravastatin sodium (p.984·3).
*Cardiovascular disorders; hypercholesterolaemia.*

**Pravasin** Bristol-Myers Squibb, Ger.
Pravastatin sodium (p.984·3).
*Hypercholesterolaemia.*

**Pravasine** Bristol-Myers Squibb, Belg.
Pravastatin sodium (p.984·3).
*Hypercholesterolaemia.*

**Pravator** Stancare, India.
Pravastatin (p.985·1).
*Angina pectoris; hypercholesterolaemia.*

**Pravidel**
Novartis, Ger.; Novartis, Swed.
Bromocriptine mesilate (p.1200·3).
*Acromegaly; amenorrhoea; breast disorders; galactorrhoea; hyperprolactinaemia; infertility; lactation inhibition; ovulation disorders; parkinsonism.*

**Pravigard PAC** Bristol-Myers Squibb, USA.
Tablets, aspirin (p.15·1); tablets, pravastatin sodium (p.984·3).

**Prax** Ferndale, USA.
Pramocaine hydrochloride (p.1382·2).
*Local anaesthesia.*

**Praxel**
Laboratorios Chile, Chile; Lemery, Mex.
Paclitaxel (p.577·3).
*Breast cancer; ovarian cancer.*

**Praxilene**
Merck, Belg.; Lipha Sante, Fr.; Merck-Lipha, Hong Kong; Lipha, Irl.; Formenti, Ital.; Merck, Port.; Merck, Singapore; Faes, Spain; Lipha, Switz.; Merck, Thai.; Merck, UK.
Naftidrofuryl oxalate (p.964·1).
*Cerebral and peripheral vascular disorders.*

**Praxinor** Lipha Sante, Fr.
Theodrenaline hydrochloride (p.1754·3); cafedrine hydrochloride (p.878·2).
*Hypotension.*

**Praxis** Armstrong, Arg.
Simeticone (p.1289·2); domperidone (p.1263·2); pancreatin (p.1725·3).
*Gastrointestinal disorders.*

**Praxiten**
Wyeth Lederle, Austria; Teofarma, Ger.
Oxazepam (p.712·2).
*Anxiety disorders; sleep disorders.*

**Prayanol** Instituto Sanitas, Chile.
Amantadine hydrochloride (p.1197·2).
*Influenza; parkinsonism.*

**Prazac** Orion, Denm.
Prazosin hydrochloride (p.985·1).
*Heart failure; hypertension; Raynaud's syndrome.*

**Prazam**
Royal, Chile; Euro-Labor, Port.; Grunenthal, Port.
Alprazolam (p.668·3).
*Anxiety disorders; depression; insomnia.*

**Prazen** Delta, Braz.
Hypericum (p.299·1).
*Depression.*

**Prazene** Parke, Davis, Ital.
Prazepam (p.716·2).
*Anxiety disorders; psychoneurotic disorders.*

**Prazentol** Ferring, Port.
Omeprazole (p.1278·2).
*Gastro-oesophageal reflux; peptic ulcer; Zollinger-Ellison syndrome.*

**Prazidec** Tecnofarma, Mex.
Omeprazole (p.1278·2).
*Gastro-oesophageal reflux; peptic ulcer; Zollinger-Ellison syndrome.*

**Prazine**
Note. This name is used for preparations of different composition.
Wyeth Lederle, Belg.; Wyeth, Switz.
Promazine hydrochloride (p.717·3).
*Behaviour disorders in children; hiccups; nausea; psychoses; sedative; tetany; vomiting.*

IFET (ΙΦΕΤ), Gr.
Levomepromazine hydrochloride (p.703·2).
*Severe anxiety and agitation.*

**Prazinil** Pierre Fabre, Fr.
Carpipramine hydrochloride (p.674·2).
*Anxiety; psychoses.*

**Prazite** Asian Pharm, Thai.
Praziquantel (p.112·2).
*Trematode infections.*

**Prazocor** Pharmacia Upjohn, Fin.†.
Prazosin hydrochloride (p.985·1).
*Heart failure; hypertension.*

**Prazohexal** Hexal, Austral.
Prazosin hydrochloride (p.985·1).
*Hypertension.*

**Prazoken** Kendrick, Mex.†.
Megestrol (p.1558·3).

**Prazol** Medley, Braz.
Lansoprazole (p.1269·3).
*Peptic ulcer.*

**Prazolene** Cipan, Port.
Omeprazole (p.1278·2).
*Acid aspiration; gastro-oesophageal reflux; peptic ulcer; Zollinger-Ellison syndrome.*

**Prazolit** Fustery, Mex.
Omeprazole (p.1278·2).
*Acid aspiration; gastro-oesophageal reflux; peptic ulcer; Zollinger-Ellison syndrome.*

**Prazolo** Mintlab, Chile.
Omeprazole (p.1278·2).
*Peptic ulcer.*

**Prazonil** Sanval, Braz.
Omeprazole (p.1278·2).
*Peptic ulcer.*

**Pre Clean Mom** Candioli, Ital.
Permethrin (p.1508·3).
*Pediculosis.*

**Pre Clor** Grin, Mex.
Chloramphenicol (p.185·1); prednisone (p.1109·3).
*Infected eye disorders.*

**Pre Natal** Cenovis, Austral.†.
Omega-3 marine triglycerides (p.976·2); folic acid (p.1429·1).
*Fatty-acid supplement; prevention of neural tube defects.*

**Pre Nutrison** Nutricia, Ital.
Preparation for enteral nutrition (p.1417·1).

**Preastig** Alfa Intes, Ital.
Multivitamin and mineral preparation with glutathione (p.1417·1).
*Nutritional supplement.*

**Pre-Attain** Sherwood, USA.
Lactose-free preparation for enteral nutrition (p.1417·1).

**PreCare** Ther-Rx, USA.
Multivitamin and mineral preparation (p.1417·1).

**Precedex**
Abbott, Arg.; Abbott, Austral.; Abbott, Braz.; Abbott, Israel; Abbott, Malaysia; Abbott, NZ; Abbott, Singapore; Abbott, USA.
Dexmedetomidine hydrochloride (p.689·3).
*Sedation in mechanically ventilated patients.*

**Precef** Bristol-Myers Squibb, Belg.
Ceforanide (p.175·2); L-lysine.
*Bacterial infections.*

**Precidona** Precimex, Mex.†.
Dipyrone (p.35·3).

**Precifen** Precimex, Mex.†.
Paracetamol (p.76·2).
*Fever; pain.*

**Precifenac** Precimex, Mex.†.
Diclofenac (p.32·1).

**Precileucin** Precimex, Mex.†.
Folic acid (p.1429·1).

**Precision**
Wander, Ital.†; Sandoz Nutrition, USA.
A range of preparations for enteral nutrition (p.1417·1).

**Precision Plus**
Abbott, Arg.; Medisense, Austral.; Medica, NZ.
Test for glucose in blood (p.1694·2).

**Precitene** Novartis Consumer, Port.†.
A range of preparations for enteral nutrition (p.1417·1).

**Precitene MCT 50** Wander Health Care, Switz.†.
Preparation for enteral nutrition (p.1417·1).

**Pre-Clar** Laboratorios Chile, Chile.
Clarithromycin (p.192·2).
*Bacterial infections; peptic ulcer.*

**Preconceive** Lane, UK.
Folic acid (p.1429·1).
*Prevention of neural tube defects in pregnancy.*

**Precopen** Fides Ecopharma, Spain†.
Amoxicillin trihydrate (p.155·3).
*Bacterial infections.*

**Precopen Mucolitico** Fides Ecopharma, Spain†.
Amoxicillin trihydrate (p.155·3); bromhexine hydrochloride (p.1115·3).
*Respiratory-tract infections.*

**Precortalon aquosum** Organon, Swed.
Prednisolone sodium succinate (p.1108·2).
*Corticosteroid.*

**Precortil** Cazi, Braz.
Prednisone (p.1109·3).
*Corticosteroid.*

**Precortisyl** Aventis, UK.
Prednisolone (p.1108·1).
*Corticosteroid.*

**Precosa**
Biocodex, Denm.; Biocodex, Fin.; AstraZeneca, Norw.†; Astra, Swed.
*Saccharomyces boulardii* (p.1704·2).
*AIDS-related diarrhoea; antibiotic-associated diarrhoea.*

**Precose** Bayer, USA.
Acarbose (p.328·3).
*Diabetes mellitus.*

**Precosol** Wolfs, Belg.
Macrogol 4000 (p.1709·1); electrolytes (p.1217·1).
*Bowel evacuation.*

**Prectal** Infectopharm, Ger.
Prednisolone acetate (p.1108·1).
*Bronchitis; hypersensitivity reactions; laryngotracheal stenosis.*

**Precurgen** Knoll, Spain†.
Cytosine inosinate.
*Liver disorders.*

**Precyclan** Lisapharm, Fr.
Meprobamate (p.706·2); bendroflumethiazide (p.867·3); medroxyprogesterone acetate (p.1557·2).
*Premenstrual syndrome.*

**Pred**
Grin, Mex.; Allergan, Singapore; Alcon, USA.
Prednisolone acetate (p.1108·1) or prednisolone sodium phosphate (p.1108·1).
*Inflammatory eye disorders.*

**Pred Fort** Allergan, Braz.
Prednisolone acetate (p.1108·1).
*Inflammatory eye disorders.*

**Pred Forte**
Allergan, Belg.; Allergan, Canad.; Allergan, Chile; Allergan, Fin.; Allergan, Hong Kong; Allergan, Irl.; Allergan, Israel; Allergan, Malaysia; Allergan, NZ; Allergan, Spain; Allergan, Switz.; Allergan, Thai.; Allergan, UK; Allergan, USA.
Prednisolone acetate (p.1108·1).
*Inflammatory eye disorders.*

**Pred G**
Allergan, Chile; Allergan, S.Afr.†; Allergan, Switz.†; Allergan, USA.
Prednisolone acetate (p.1108·1); gentamicin sulfate (p.217·1).
*Infected eye disorders.*

**Pred Mild**
Allergan, Braz.; Allergan, Canad.; Allergan, Chile; Allergan, Hong Kong; Allergan, Irl.; Allergan, Malaysia; Allergan, NZ; Allergan, S.Afr.; Allergan, Switz.; Allergan, Thai.; Allergan, USA.
Prednisolone acetate (p.1108·1).
*Allergic and inflammatory eye disorders; corneal burns.*

**Pred Oph** Seng, Thai.
Prednisolone sodium phosphate (p.1108·1); gentamicin sulfate (p.217·1).
*Infected eye and ear disorders.*

**Predalgic** Pharmascience, Fr.†.
Tramadol hydrochloride (p.94·3).
*Pain.*

**Predalon** Organon, Ger.
Chorionic gonadotrophin (p.1320·3).
*Cryptorchidism; delayed puberty; stimulation of gonadal function.*

**Predalone** Forest Laboratories, USA.
Prednisolone acetate (p.1108·1).
*Corticosteroid.*

**Pred-Clysma**
Leiras, Denm.; Schering, Norw.; Schering, Swed.
Prednisolone sodium phosphate (p.1108·1).
*Crohn's disease; proctosigmoiditis; ulcerative colitis.*

**Predcor** Hauck, USA.
Prednisolone acetate (p.1108·1).
*Corticosteroid.*

**Predeltin** Quatromed, S.Afr.
Prednisone (p.1109·3).
*Corticosteroid.*

**Predenema**
Pharmax, Hong Kong†; Pharmax, Irl.; Forest Laboratories, UK.
Prednisolone metasulfobenzoate sodium (p.1108·1).
*Ulcerative colitis.*

**Predermid** CSC, Austria.
Budesonide (p.1094·2).
*Skin disorders.*

**Predesic** Pred, Fr.
Articaine hydrochloride (p.1370·3).
Adrenaline acid tartrate (p.852·2) is included in this preparation as a vasoconstrictor to diminish absorption and localise the effect of the local anaesthetic.
*Local anaesthesia.*

**Predex** Takeda, Thai.
Neomycin sulfate (p.235·1); prednisolone (p.1108·1).
*Skin disorders.*

**Predfoam**
Pharmax, Hong Kong†; Pharmax, Irl.; Forest Laboratories, UK.
Prednisolone metasulfobenzoate sodium (p.1108·1).
*Proctitis; ulcerative colitis.*

**Predicor** Pisa, Mex.
Prednisone (p.1109·3).
*Corticosteroid.*

**Predicorten** Stiefel, Braz.
Prednisone (p.1109·3).
*Corticosteroid.*

**Predictor**
Organon, Austral.†; Organon, Braz.; Chefaro Ardeval, Fr.; Chefaro, Israel; Angelini, Ital.; Chefaro, UK.
Pregnancy test (p.1734·3).

**Predisole** PP Lab, Thai.
Prednisolone (p.1108·1).
*Corticosteroid.*

**Predmetil** Eurofarma, Braz.
Methylprednisolone sodium succinate (p.1106·2).
*Corticosteroid.*

**Predmicin** EMS, Braz.
Polymyxin B sulfate (p.245·1); prednisolone (p.1108·1); benzocaine (p.1370·3); clioquinol (p.196·3).
Formerly contained polymyxin B sulfate, prednisolone, butyl aminobenzoate, and hydroxyquinoline iodochloride.
*Skin disorders.*

**Predmix** Aspen, Austral.
Prednisolone sodium phosphate (p.1108·1).
*Corticosteroid.*

**Predmycin** Allergan, Thai.
Prednisolone acetate (p.1108·1); polymyxin B sulfate (p.245·1); neomycin sulfate (p.235·1).
*Bacterial eye infections.*

**Predmycin P** Allergan, Belg.
Prednisolone acetate (p.1108·1); polymyxin B sulfate (p.245·1); neomycin sulfate (p.235·1).
*Eye disorders.*

**Predmycin-P** Allergan, Singapore.
Prednisolone acetate (p.1108·1); polymyxin B sulfate (p.245·1); neomycin sulfate (p.235·1).
*Infected eye disorders.*

**Prednabene** Merckle, Ger.
Prednisolone sodium phosphate (p.1108·1).
*Musculoskeletal, joint, and peri-articular disorders.*

**Prednefrin**
Allergan, Arg.; Allergan, Austral.
Prednisolone acetate (p.1108·1); phenylephrine hydrochloride (p.1126·3).
*Eye inflammation.*

**Prednefrin SF** Allergan, Mex.
Prednisolone acetate (p.1108·1).
*Inflammatory eye disorders.*

**Prednersone** General Drugs, Thai.
Prednisolone (p.1108·1).
*Corticosteroid.*

**Prednesol**
GlaxoSmithKline, Irl.; Sovereign, UK†.
Prednisolone sodium phosphate (p.1108·1).
*Corticosteroid.*

**Predni** Lichtenstein, Ger.
Prednisolone acetate (p.1108·1).
*Parenteral corticosteroid.*

**Predni Azuleno** Lacer, Spain.
Chloramphenicol (p.185·1); guaiazulene (p.1696·2); prednisolone (p.1108·1).
*Infected skin disorders.*

**Predni H** Lichtenstein, Ger.
Prednisolone (p.1108·1) or prednisolone acetate (p.1108·1).
*Corticosteroid.*

**Predni M** Lichtenstein, Ger.
Methylprednisolone (p.1106·1).
*Oral corticosteroid.*

**Predni Tablinen** Lichtenstein, Ger.
Prednisone (p.1109·3).
*Oral corticosteroid.*

**Prednicort** Continental Pharma, Belg.
Prednisone (p.1109·3).
*Corticosteroid.*

**Prednicortelone** Continental Pharma, Belg.
Prednisolone (p.1108·1).
*Corticosteroid.*

**Predniderma** Caldeira & Marques, Port.
Prednisolone (p.1108·1); neomycin sulfate (p.235·1).
*Skin disorders.*

**Prednidib** Diba, Mex.
Prednisone (p.1109·3).
*Corticosteroid.*

**Prednifarma** ICN, Arg.
Prednisolone sodium phosphate (p.1108·1); phenylephrine hydrochloride (p.1126·3).
*Inflammatory eye disorders.*

**Predni-F-Tablinen** Sanorania, Ger.†.
Dexamethasone (p.1097·1).
*Oral corticosteroid.*

**Predniftalmina** Davi, Port.
Chloramphenicol (p.185·1); prednisolone (p.1108·1).
*Infected eye disorders.*

**Prednigalen** Galen, Ger.
Prednisolone acetate (p.1108·1).
*Corticosteroid.*

**Predni-Helvacort** Helvepharm, Switz.†.
Prednisolone (p.1108·1).
*Corticosteroid.*

**Prednihexal**
Hexal, Austria; Hexal, Ger.
Prednisolone (p.1108·1) or prednisolone acetate (p.1108·1).
*Corticosteroid.*

**Prednilem** Lemery, Mex.
Methylprednisolone sodium succinate (p.1106·2).
*Corticosteroid.*

**Predniment**
Ferring, Denm.†; Ferring, Fin.†.
Prednisolone sodium phosphate (p.1108·1).
*Proctitis; ulcerative colitis.*

**Predniocil** Edol, Port.
Prednisolone acetate (p.1108·1).
*Eye disorders.*

**Predni-Ophtal** Winzer, Ger.
Prednisolone acetate (p.1108·1).
*Inflammatory eye disorders.*

**Prednipirine** Lafage, Arg.
Prednisone (p.1109·3).
*Corticosteroid.*

**Predni-POS** Ursapharm, Ger.
Prednisolone acetate (p.1108·1).
*Inflammatory eye disorders.*

**Prednis Neomic** Alcon Cusi, Spain.
Neomycin sulfate (p.235·1); prednisone (p.1109·3).
*Infected eye disorders.*

**Prednisil** Silom, Thai.
*Cream:* Prednisolone (p.1108·1).
*Skin disorders.*
*Eye drops:* Prednisolone sodium phosphate (p.1108·1); neomycin sulfate (p.235·1).
*Infected eye disorders.*

**Prednisil-N** Silom, Thai.
Prednisolone (p.1108·1); neomycin sulfate (p.235·1).
*Infected skin disorders.*

**Prednisol** Pasadena, USA.
Prednisolone tebutate (p.1108·2).
*Corticosteroid.*

**Prednisolut** Jenapharm, Ger.
Prednisolone hydrogen succinate (p.1108·1).
*Parenteral corticosteroid.*

**Prednistyle** Fischer, Israel†.
Prednisolone ester (p.1108·1); sulfacetamide sodium (p.257·3).
*Infected eye disorders.*

**Prednitone** Vitamed, Israel.
Prednisone (p.1109·3).
*Corticosteroid.*

**Prednitop**
Aventis, Austria; Knoll, Switz.
Prednicarbate (p.1107·3).
*Inflammatory skin disorders.*

**Prednitracin**
Ciba Vision, Ger.†; Novartis Ophthalmics, Hong Kong; Novartis Ophthalmics, Switz.
Prednisolone acetate (p.1108·1); neomycin sulfate (p.235·1); bacitracin (p.161·3).
*Infected eye disorders.*

**Predonium**
Servier, Austria.
Perindopril erbumine (p.980·2); indapamide (p.938·2).
*Hypertension.*
Servier, Hong Kong.
Perindopril (p.980·2); indapamide (p.938·2).
*Hypertension.*

**Pred-Phosphate** Medical Ophthalmics, USA.
Prednisolone phosphate (p.1109·1).
*Eye disorders.*

**Predsim** Schering-Plough, Braz.
Prednisolone (p.1108·1) or prednisolone sodium phosphate (p.1108·1).
*Corticosteroid.*

**Predsol**
Sigma, Austral.; Celltech, Irl.; Glaxo Wellcome, NZ†; GlaxoSmithKline, S.Afr.; Celltech, UK.
Prednisolone sodium phosphate (p.1108·1).
*Crohn's disease; inflammatory disorders of the ear or eye; proctitis; ulcerative colitis.*

**Predsolets** SMB, Chile.
Prednisolone acetate (p.1108·1).
*Inflammatory eye disorders.*

**Predsol-N** Celltech, UK.
Prednisolone sodium phosphate (p.1108·1); neomycin sulfate (p.235·1).
*Inflammatory disorders of the ear or eye with bacterial infection.*

**Predual**
Note. This name is used for preparations of different composition.
Bristol-Myers Squibb, Arg.
Paracetamol (p.76·2); clofedanol hydrochloride (p.1117·1); pseudoephedrine sulfate (p.1129·2); astemizole (p.424·2).
*Respiratory-tract disorders.*
Andromaco, Chile.
Pamabrom (p.978·2); paracetamol (p.76·2); mepyramine maleate (p.437·1).
*Premenstrual syndrome.*

**Predual Descongestivo** Bristol-Myers Squibb, Arg.
*Oral drops; syrup:* Pseudoephedrine sulfate (p.1129·2); chlorphenamine maleate (p.427·3).
*Tablets:* Pseudoephedrine sulfate (p.1129·2); astemizole (p.424·2).
*Rhinitis; sinusitis.*

**Predual DI** Andromaco, Chile.
Paracetamol (p.76·2); ibuprofen (p.45·3).
*Fever; musculoskeletal, joint, peri-articular, and soft-tissue disorders; pain.*

**Predualito** Bristol-Myers Squibb, Arg.
Paracetamol (p.76·2).
*Fever; pain.*

**Predval** Sanval, Braz.
Prednisone (p.1109·3).
*Corticosteroid.*

**Prefagyl** Oberlin, Fr.
Magnesium chloride (p.1228·1); sodium bicarbonate (p.1223·2); anhydrous sodium sulfate (p.1290·1); dibasic sodium phosphate (p.1231·1).
*Gastrointestinal disorders.*

**Prefamone**
Asta Medica, Belg.†; Dexo, Switz.; Dexo, Thai.†.
Diethylpropion hydrochloride (p.1587·1).
*Obesity.*

**Prefem** Labomed, Chile.
Aspirin (p.15·1); paracetamol (p.76·2); caffeine (p.782·1).
*Premenstrual syndrome.*

**Prefemine** Zeller, Switz.
Agnus castus (p.1649·1).
*Premenstrual syndrome.*

**Preferid**
Yamanouchi, Belg.†; Yamanouchi, Irl.†; Yamanouchi, Ital.; Yamanouchi, Norw.†; Yamanouchi, Switz.†.
Budesonide (p.1094·2).
*Skin disorders.*

**Preferred Remedies** Reese, USA.
A range of homoeopathic preparations.

**Prefest**
Janssen-Cilag, Arg.; Monarch, USA.
15 Tablets, estradiol (p.1550·1); 15 tablets, estradiol; norgestimate (p.1563·2).
Formerly known as Ortho-Prefest in the *USA*.
*Menopausal disorders; osteoporosis.*
Janssen-Cilag, Braz.
Estradiol (p.1550·1); norgestimate (p.1563·2).
*Menopausal disorders.*

**Prefesta** Janssen-Cilag, S.Afr.
Pink tablets, estradiol (p.1550·1); white tablets, estradiol; norgestimate (p.1563·2).
*Menopausal disorders.*

**Prefin** Key, Spain.
Buprenorphine hydrochloride (p.21·3).
*Pain.*

**Prefine** Pierre Fabre Sante, Fr.†.
Sterculia (p.1290·2).
*Obesity.*

**Preflex Daily Cleaner** Alcon, USA.
Cleansing solution for soft contact lenses (p.1164·2).

**Prefolic** Abbott, Ital.
Calcium mefolinate (p.1431·2).
*Antidote to folic acid antagonists; folate deficiency; reduction of aminopterin and methotrexate toxicity.*

**Preforms** Terrier, Mex.†.
Nonoxinol (p.1413·2).

**Prefrin**
Allergan, Arg.; Allergan, Austral.; Allergan, Austria†; Allergan, Canad.; Allergan, Hong Kong; Allergan, Israel; Allergan, Malaysia; Allergan, NZ; Allergan, S.Afr.; Allergan, Singapore; Allergan, USA.
Phenylephrine hydrochloride (p.1126·3).
*Eye irritation.*

**Prefrin A**
Allergan, Austria†; Allergan, Canad.; Allergan, Malaysia; Allergan, Singapore.
Mepyramine maleate (p.437·1); phenylephrine hydrochloride (p.1126·3).
*Eye inflammation; eye irritation.*

**Prefrin Z**
Allergan, Austral.†; Allergan, NZ†.
Phenylephrine hydrochloride (p.1126·3); zinc sulfate (p.1469·3).
*Eye irritation.*

**Pregaday** Celltech, UK.
Ferrous fumarate (p.1427·3); folic acid (p.1429·1).
*Prophylaxis of iron and folic acid deficiency in pregnancy.*

**Pregamal** GlaxoSmithKline, S.Afr.
Folic acid (p.1429·1); ferrous fumarate (p.1427·3).
*Anaemias.*

**Pregestimil**
Bristol-Myers Squibb, Arg.; Mead Johnson, Austral.; Mead Johnson, Braz.; Mead Johnson, Chile; Mead Johnson Nutritionals, Fin.; Mead Johnson, Fr.; Mead Johnson, Hong Kong; Mead Johnson, Irl.; Mead Johnson, Israel; Mead Johnson, Ital.; Mead Johnson, Malaysia; Mead Johnson, NZ†; Mead Johnson, Port.; Mead Johnson, Singapore; Mead Johnson Nutritionals, Thai.; Mead Johnson Nutritionals, UK; Mead Johnson Nutritionals, USA.
Infant feed (p.1417·1).
*Galactokinase deficiency; galactosaemia; impaired fat absorption; lactose or sucrose and protein intolerance.*

**Preglandin** Ono, Jpn.
Gemeprost (p.1518·1).
*Termination of pregnancy.*

**Pregnacare**
Vitabiotics, Hong Kong; Vitabiotics, UK.
Multivitamin and mineral preparation (p.1417·1).
*Dietary supplement in pregnancy and lactation.*

**Pregna-Cert** Merlin, UK†.
Pregnancy test (p.1734·3).

**Pregnafort** Thompson, Austral.†.
Multivitamin and mineral preparation (p.1417·1).

**Pregnancy Formula** Eagle, Austral.†.
Multivitamin, mineral, and amino-acid preparation with bioflavonoids, ginger and lecithin (p.1417·1).
*Nutritional supplement.*

**Pregna-Sure HCG** Merlin, UK†.
Pregnancy test (p.1734·3).

**Pregnatal** Scanpharm, Hong Kong.
Multivitamin and mineral preparation (p.1417·1).
*Dietary supplement in pregnancy and lactation.*

**Pregnavit** Ratiopharm, Austria.
Multivitamin and iron preparation (p.1417·1).

**Pregnavit F** Merckle, Ger.
Multivitamin preparation (p.1417·1).

**Pregnavite Forte F** Goldshield, UK†.
Dried ferrous sulfate (p.1428·3); folic acid (p.1429·1); vitamins (p.1417·1); calcium phosphate.
*Prophylaxis of neural tube defects in pregnancy.*

**Pregnazon** Pharmadass, UK.
Multivitamin, mineral, and trace element preparation (p.1417·1).

**Pregnesin** Serono, Ger.
Chorionic gonadotrophin (p.1320·3).
*Delayed puberty in males; infertility in females and males.*

**Pregnidoxin** UCB, India.
Meclozine hydrochloride (p.436·3); caffeine (p.782·1).
*Ménière's syndrome; nausea and vomiting.*

**Pregnifer** Weifa, Norw.†.
Ferrous sulfate (p.1428·2); folic acid (p.1429·1).
*Iron and folic acid deficiency.*

**Pregnon L** Nourypharma, Ger.†.
Lynestrenol (p.1557·1); ethinylestradiol (p.1553·2).
*Combined oral contraceptive.*

**Pregnorm** Win-Medicare, India.
Menotrophin (p.1330·1).
*Male and female infertility.*

**Pregnosis**
Key, Austral.; Roche, USA.
Pregnancy test (p.1734·3).

**Pregnospia Duoclon** Bio Merieux, UK.
Pregnancy test (p.1734·3).

**Pregnosticon** Organon, Israel.
Pregnancy test (p.1734·3).

**Pregnyl**
Organon, Arg.; Organon, Austral.; Organon, Austria; Organon, Belg.; Organon, Braz.; Organon, Canad.; Organon, Chile; Organon, Denm.; Organon, Fin.; Organon (Οργκανον), Gr.; Organon, Hong Kong; Organon, Irl.; Organon, Israel; Organon, Ital.; Organon, Malaysia; Organon, Mex.; Organon, Neth.; Organon, Norw.; Organon, NZ†; Organon, Port.; Donmed, S.Afr.; Organon, Singapore; Organon, Spain†; Organon, Swed.; Organon, Switz.; Organon, Thai.; Organon, UK; Organon, USA.
Chorionic gonadotrophin (p.1320·3).
*Cryptorchidism; delayed puberty; hypogonadotrophic hypogonadism; male and female infertility; metrorrhagia.*

**Pregomin**
Support, Braz.; Milupa, Singapore†; Milupa, Switz.
Infant feed (p.1417·1).
*Carbohydrate malabsorption syndromes; cow's-milk-protein intolerance; digestive system disorders; soya-milk-protein intolerance.*

**Pregomine** Milupa, Fr.
Nutritional supplement (p.1417·1).
*Gastrointestinal disorders.*

**Prehist** Marnel, USA.
Phenylephrine hydrochloride (p.1126·3); chlorphenamine maleate (p.427·3).
*Upper respiratory-tract symptoms.*

**Prehist D** Marnel, USA.
Phenylephrine hydrochloride (p.1126·3); chlorphenamine maleate (p.427·3); hyoscine methonitrate (p.483·3).
*Upper respiratory-tract symptoms.*

**Prejomin**
Milupa, Irl.; Milupa, UK.
Gluten-free preparation for special diets (p.1417·1).
*Galactokinase deficiency; lactose, sucrose and fructose intolerance; protein sensitivity.*

**Prelac** Mead Johnson, Port.†.
Nutritional supplement for pregnant and lactating women (p.1417·1).

**Prelafel** Akromed, S.Afr.†.
Multivitamin and mineral preparation (p.1417·1).

**Prelectal** Stroder, Ital.
Perindopril erbumine (p.980·2); indapamide (p.938·2).
*Hypertension.*

**Prelertan** Asofarma, Arg.
Losartan (p.948·2).
*Hypertension.*

**Prelis** Novartis, Ger.
Metoprolol tartrate (p.957·1).
*Arrhythmias; hypertension; ischaemic heart disease; migraine; myocardial infarction.*

**Prelis comp** Novartis, Ger.
Metoprolol tartrate (p.957·1); chlortalidone (p.882·3).
*Hypertension.*

**Prelisin** Cosmopharm, Gr.
Gemfibrozil (p.923·1).
*Hyperlipidaemias.*

**Prelloran**
Novartis, Hong Kong; Novartis Consumer, Switz.
A heparinoid (p.931·1); glycol salicylate (p.44·3).
*Haematomas; musculoskeletal pain and inflammation; peripheral vascular disorders; phlebitis; soft-tissue disorders; sports injuries.*

**Prelone**
Asta Medica, Braz.; Asta Medica, Hong Kong; Muro, Israel; Adcock Ingram, S.Afr.; Aero, USA.
Prednisolone (p.1108·1) or prednisolone sodium phosphate (p.1108·1).
*Corticosteroid.*

**Prelu-2** Roxane, USA; Boehringer Ingelheim, USA.
Phendimetrazine tartrate (p.1592·1).
*Obesity.*

**Prelude** Rendell, UK.
Nonoxinol 9 (p.1413·3).
*Spermicidal contraceptive.*

**Prelus** Sanofi Synthelabo, Port.
Isoprenaline hydrochloride (p.940·2); phenobarbital (p.367·3); ephedrine sulfate (p.1120·1); theophylline (p.798·3); potassium iodide (p.1598·1).
*Asthma; bronchitis; coughs.*

**Premagnol** Allen, Mex.
Prednisone (p.1109·3).
*Inflammation; musculoskeletal and joint disorders.*

**Premandol** Spirig, Switz.
Prednisolone acetate (p.1108·1); almond oil (p.1651·1); zinc oxide (p.1163·2).
*Skin disorders.*

**Premaril** Dexxon, Israel.
Conjugated oestrogens (p.1543·2).
*Menopausal disorders; osteoporosis.*

**Premaril MP** Dexxon, Israel.
Conjugated oestrogens (p.1543·2); medroxyprogesterone acetate (p.1557·2).
*Menopausal disorders; oestrogen deficiency.*

**Premaril Plus MP** Dexxon, Israel.
28 Tablets, conjugated oestrogens (p.1543·2); 14 tablets, medroxyprogesterone acetate (p.1557·2).
*Menopausal disorders; osteoporosis.*

**Premarin**
Wyeth, Arg.; Wyeth, Austral.; Wyeth Lederle, Austria; Wyeth Lederle, Belg.; Wyeth, Braz.; Wyeth-Ayerst, Canad.; Wyeth Lederle, Denm.; Wyeth Lederle, Fin.; Wyeth Lederle, Fr.; Wyeth, Gr.; IFET (ΙΦΕΤ), Gr.; Wyeth, Hong Kong; Wyeth, India; Wyeth, Irl.; Wyeth Lederle, Ital.; Wyeth, Malaysia; Wyeth, Mex.; Wyeth, Neth.; Wyeth, NZ; Wyeth, S.Afr.; Wyeth, Singapore; Wyeth, Spain; Wyeth, Switz.; Wyeth-Ayerst, Thai.; Wyeth, UK; Wyeth-Ayerst, USA.
Conjugated oestrogens (p.1543·2).
*Breast cancer; dysfunctional uterine bleeding; menopausal disorders; oestrogen deficiency; osteoporosis.*

**Premarin compositum** Wyeth Lederle, Austria.
16 Tablets, conjugated oestrogens (p.1543·2); 12 tablets, conjugated oestrogens; medrogestone (p.1557·1).
*Oestrogen deficiency; osteoporosis.*

**Premarin with Methyltestosterone** Wyeth-Ayerst, USA†.
Conjugated oestrogens (p.1543·2); methyltestosterone (p.1559·3).
*Menopausal disorders; postpartum breast engorgement.*

**Premarin MPA**
Wyeth Lederle, Austria†; Wyeth, Braz.
Conjugated oestrogens (p.1543·2); medroxyprogesterone acetate (p.1557·2).
*Atrophic urethritis; atrophic vaginitis; menopausal disorders; oestrogen deficiency; osteoporosis.*

**Premarin Pak** Wyeth, Mex.†.
21 Tablets, conjugated oestrogens (p.1543·2); 10 tablets, medrogestone (p.1557·1).
*Menopausal disorders; osteoporosis.*

**Premarin Plus**
Wyeth Lederle, Austria; Wyeth, Neth.; Wyeth Lederle, Port.; Wyeth, Switz.
28 Tablets, conjugated oestrogens (p.1543·2); 12 tablets, medrogestone (p.1557·1).
*Adjunct in vaginitis and cystitis; menopausal disorders; osteoporosis; ovarian insufficiency.*

**Premarina** Wyeth Lederle, Swed.
Conjugated oestrogens (p.1543·2).
*Hypogenitalism; menopausal disorders; osteoporosis.*

**Premdoc** Alltracel, Irl.
Calcium oxidised cellulose (p.757·2); sodium oxidised cellulose (p.757·2).
*Capillary bleeding.*

**Preme** Nakorn, Thai.
Cyproterone acetate (p.1544·1); ethinylestradiol (p.1553·2).
*Androgen-dependent acne, seborrhoea, alopecia, and hirsutism in females; oral contraceptive in women with androgenic symptoms.*

**Premella** Wyeth, Switz.
Conjugated oestrogens (p.1543·2); medroxyprogesterone acetate (p.1557·2).
*Menopausal disorders; osteoporosis.*

**Premelle**
Wyeth Lederle, Belg.; Wyeth, Braz.; Wyeth, Gr.; Wyeth, Hong Kong; Wyeth, Malaysia; Wyeth, Mex.; Wyeth, Neth.; Wyeth Lederle, Port.; Wyeth, S.Afr.; Wyeth, Singapore; Wyeth, Spain; Wyeth Lederle, Swed.; Wyeth-Ayerst, Thai.
Conjugated oestrogens (p.1543·2); medroxyprogesterone acetate (p.1557·2).
*Menopausal disorders; oestrogen deficiency; osteoporosis.*

**Premelle C** Wyeth Lederle, Ital.
Conjugated oestrogens (p.1543·2); medroxyprogesterone acetate (p.1557·2).
*Menopausal disorders; osteoporosis.*

**Premelle Ciclico**
Wyeth, Arg.
14 Tablets, conjugated oestrogens (p.1543·2); 14 tablets, conjugated oestrogens; medroxyprogesterone acetate (p.1557·2).
*Menopausal disorders; osteoporosis.*

Wyeth, Spain.
28 Tablets, conjugated oestrogens (p.1543·2); 14 tablets, medroxyprogesterone acetate (p.1557·2).
*Menopausal disorders; osteoporosis.*

**Premelle Ciclo** Wyeth, Braz.
14 Tablets, conjugated oestrogens (p.1543·2); 14 tablets, conjugated oestrogens (p.1543·2); medroxyprogesterone acetate (p.1557·2).
*Menopausal disorders; osteoporosis; vaginal and vulval atrophy.*

**Premelle Continuo** Wyeth, Arg.
Conjugated oestrogens (p.1543·2); medroxyprogesterone acetate (p.1557·2).
*Menopausal disorders; osteoporosis.*

**Premelle Cycle**
Wyeth, Hong Kong; Wyeth Lederle, Port.; Wyeth, Singapore; Wyeth-Ayerst, Thai.
14 Tablets, conjugated oestrogens (p.1543·2); 14 tablets, conjugated oestrogens; medroxyprogesterone acetate (p.1557·2).
*Menopausal disorders; oestrogen deficiency; osteoporosis.*

Wyeth, Neth.
28 Tablets, conjugated oestrogens (p.1543·2); 14 tablets, medroxyprogesterone acetate (p.1557·2).
*Menopausal disorders; osteoporosis.*

**Premelle S** Wyeth Lederle, Ital.
14 Tablets, conjugated oestrogens (p.1543·2); 14 tablets, conjugated oestrogens; medroxyprogesterone acetate (p.1557·2).
*Menopausal disorders; osteoporosis.*

**Premelle Sekvens** Wyeth Lederle, Swed.
14 Tablets, conjugated oestrogens (p.1543·2); 14 tablets, conjugated oestrogens; medroxyprogesterone acetate (p.1557·2).
Formerly known as Prempac Sekvens.
*Oestrogen deficiency; osteoporosis.*

**Premelle Sequenziale** Wyeth Lederle, Ital.
14 Tablets, conjugated oestrogens (p.1543·2); 14 tablets conjugated oestrogens; medroxyprogesterone acetate (p.1557·2).
*Menopausal disorders; osteoporosis.*

**Premence**
Vitabiotics, Hong Kong; Vitabiotics, UK.
Multivitamin and mineral preparation (p.1417·1).
*Premenstrual syndrome.*

**PreMens** Zeller, Switz.
Agnus castus (p.1649·1).
*Premenstrual syndrome.*

**Prementaid** Potter's, UK.
Vervain (p.1764·1); motherwort (p.1717·1); pulsatilla (p.1737·1); bearberry (p.1659·2); valerian (p.1762·2).
*Premenstrual syndrome.*

**PremesisRx** Ther-Rx, USA.
Vitamin $B_6$ (p.1457·2); vitamin $B_{12}$ (p.1458·2); folic acid (p.1429·1); calcium (p.1225·1).
*Nausea.*

**Premia**
Wyeth, Austral.; Wyeth, NZ.
14 Tablets, conjugated oestrogens (p.1543·2); 14 tablets, conjugated oestrogens; medroxyprogesterone acetate (p.1557·2).
*Menopausal disorders; osteoporosis.*

**Premia Continuous**
Wyeth, Austral.; Wyeth, NZ.
Conjugated oestrogens (p.1543·2); medroxyprogesterone acetate (p.1557·2).
*Menopausal disorders; osteoporosis.*

**Premia Low** Wyeth, Austral.
Conjugated oestrogens (p.1543·2); medroxyprogesterone acetate (p.1557·2).
*Menopausal disorders.*

**Premicia** Therabel, Fr.
Hyetellose (p.1579·2); diethylene glycol monoethyl ether.
*Vaginal lubricant.*

**Premid**
Note. This name is used for preparations of different composition.
Shire, Denm.
Balsalazide sodium (p.1251·2).
*Ulcerative colitis.*

Grin, Mex.
Prednisolone acetate (p.1108·1); sulfacetamide sodium (p.257·3).
*Infected eye disorders.*

**Premique**
Wyeth, Irl.; Wyeth, UK.
Conjugated oestrogens (p.1543·2); medroxyprogesterone acetate (p.1557·2).
*Menopausal disorders; osteoporosis.*

**Premique Cycle**
Wyeth, Irl.; Wyeth, UK.
14 Tablets, conjugated oestrogens (p.1543·2); 14 tablets, conjugated oestrogens; medroxyprogesterone acetate (p.1557·2).
*Menopausal disorders; osteoporosis.*

**Premium** Quest, Canad.
A range of vitamin and mineral preparations (p.1417·1).

**Premjact** Pound International, UK.
Lidocaine (p.1377·3).
*Premature ejaculation.*

**Premofil M** ZLB, Switz.†.
A factor VIII preparation (p.751·1).
*Haemorrhagic disorders.*

**Premosan** Julphar, UAE.
Metoclopramide (p.1274·3) or metoclopramide hydrochloride (p.1274·3).
*Adjunct in gastrointestinal procedures; gastro-oesophageal reflux; gastrointestinal motility disorders; hiccup; nausea and vomiting.*

**Premox** Precimex, Mex.†.
Pyrazinamide (p.246·3).

**Prempak**
Note. This name is used for preparations of different composition.
Wyeth, Chile.
Conjugated oestrogens (p.1543·2); medroxyprogesterone acetate (p.1557·2).
*Menopausal disorders.*

Wyeth, Hong Kong; Wyeth, Malaysia; Wyeth-Ayerst, Thai.†.
21 Tablets, conjugated oestrogens (p.1543·2); 10 tablets, medrogestone (p.1557·1).
*Menopausal disorders; oestrogen deficiency; osteoporosis.*

Wyeth Lederle, Ital.
28 Tablets, conjugated oestrogens (p.1543·2); 12 tablets, medrogestone (p.1557·1).
*Atrophic urethritis; menopausal disorders; oestrogen deficiency; osteoporosis; vaginitis.*

**Prempak N** Wyeth, S.Afr.
21 Tablets, conjugated oestrogens (p.1543·2); 10 tablets, medrogestone (p.1557·1).
28-Day packs also contain 7 inert tablets.
*Menopausal disorders; osteoporosis.*

**Prempak-C**
Wyeth, Irl.; Wyeth, Neth.; Wyeth, NZ; Wyeth, Singapore; Wyeth, UK.
28 Tablets, conjugated oestrogens (p.1543·2); 12 tablets, norgestrel (p.1563·2).
*Menopausal disorders; oestrogen deficiency; osteoporosis.*

**Premphase** Wyeth-Ayerst, USA.
Maroon tablets, conjugated oestrogens (p.1543·2); blue tablets, conjugated oestrogens; medroxyprogesterone acetate (p.1557·2).
*Menopausal disorders; osteoporosis.*

**Premplus**
Note. This name is used for preparations of different composition.
Wyeth Lederle, Belg.
28 Tablets, conjugated oestrogens (p.1543·2); 12 tablets, medrogestone (p.1557·1).
*Oestrogen deficiency.*

Wyeth-Ayerst, Canad.
14 Tablets, conjugated oestrogens (Premarin) (p.1543·2); 14 tablets, medroxyprogesterone acetate (p.1557·2).
*Menopausal disorders; osteoporosis.*

**Prempro** Wyeth-Ayerst, USA.
Conjugated oestrogens (p.1543·2); medroxyprogesterone acetate (p.1557·2).
*Menopausal disorders; osteoporosis.*

**Prempro Bifasico** Sigma, Braz.
14 Blue tablets, conjugated oestrogens (p.1543·2); medroxyprogesterone acetate (p.1557·2); 14 red tablets, conjugated oestrogens.
*Menopausal disorders.*

**Prempro Monofasico** Sigma, Braz.
Conjugated oestrogens (p.1543·2); medroxyprogesterone acetate (p.1557·2).
*Menopausal disorders.*

**Premsyn PMS** Chattem, USA.
Paracetamol (p.76·2); pamabrom (p.978·2); mepyramine maleate (p.437·1).
*Pain.*

**Premular** Flordis, Austral.
Agnus castus (p.1649·1).
*Premenstrual syndrome.*

**Prenacid**
Craveri, Arg.; SIFI, Ital.
Desonide sodium phosphate (p.1096·3).
*Inflammatory eye disorders.*

**Prenadona** Ariston, Arg.
Alprazolam (p.668·3).
*Anxiety.*

**Prenafort** Cypress, USA.
Multivitamin preparation with iron (p.1417·1).

**Prenalex** Servier, Ger.†.
Tertatolol hydrochloride (p.1011·1).
*Hypertension.*

**Prenalon** Degorts, Mex.
Ketoconazole (p.403·3).
*Fungal infections.*

**Prenatabs** Cypress, USA.
A range of multivitamin and mineral preparations (p.1417·1).

**Prenatal**
Bio-Sante, Canad.; Jamieson, Canad.; Quest, Canad.; Stanley, Canad.; General Nutrition, Canad.; Wyeth Lederle, India; Stanley, Israel; Wyeth, Mex.; Teofarma, Port.; Be-Tabs, S.Afr.; Ethex, USA.
Multivitamin and mineral preparation (p.1417·1).
Formerly known as Be-Natal in *S.Afr.*

Cypress, USA.
A range of multivitamin and mineral preparations with iron and folic acid (p.1417·1).
Docusate sodium (p.1262·2) may be included in this preparation to reduce the constipating effects of iron.

**Prenatal with Folic Acid** Geneva, USA.
Multivitamin and mineral preparation with iron and folic acid (p.1417·1).

**Prenatal Nutrients** Solgar, UK.
Multivitamin and mineral preparation (p.1417·1).

**Prenatal PC** Integrity, USA.
Vitamin and mineral preparation with iron and folic acid (p.1417·1).

**Prenatal Plus** Zenith Goldline, USA.
Multivitamin and mineral preparation with calcium and iron (p.1417·1).

**Prenatal Plus Iron** Major, USA.
Multivitamin and mineral preparation with iron (p.1417·1).

**Prenatal Plus-Improved** Rugby, USA.
Multivitamin and mineral preparation with iron and folic acid (p.1417·1).

**Prenatal-S** Goldline, USA.
Multivitamin and mineral preparation with iron and folic acid (p.1417·1).

**Prenate** *First Horizon, USA.*
Multivitamin and mineral preparation with iron and folic acid (p.1417·1).

**Prenatex** *Medix, Mex.*
Multivitamin and mineral preparation (p.1417·1).

**Prenatol** *Wyeth-Ayerst, Hong Kong.*
Amino acids; proteins (p.1417·1).
*Prevention of stretch marks during pregnancy.*

**Prenavit** *Gynopharm, Chile.*
Vitamins; calcium phosphate; ferrous gluconate (p.1417·1).
*Dietary supplement.*

**Prenavite**
*Roberts, Canad.†; Rugby, USA.*
Multivitamin and mineral preparation (p.1417·1).
*Dietary supplement during pregnancy and lactation.*

**Prenefrin** *Breves, Braz.†.*
Prednisolone (p.1108·1); phenylephrine (p.1126·3); mepyramine (p.437·1); neomycin (p.235·1).
*Nasal disorders.*

**Prenilone** *British Dispensary, Thai.†.*
Prednisolone (p.1108·1).
*Corticosteroid.*

**Prenisonal** *Klonal, Arg.*
Prednisone (p.1109·3).
*Corticosteroid.*

**Prenolol**
*Berlin Pharm, Singapore; Berlin Pharm, Thai.*
Atenolol (p.865·2).
*Angina pectoris; arrhythmias; hypertension; myocardial infarction.*

**Prenomod** *AstraZeneca, Arg.*
Atenolol (p.865·2); hydrochlorothiazide (p.933·2); amiloride hydrochloride (p.858·2).
*Hypertension.*

**Prenoretic** *AstraZeneca, Arg.*
Atenolol (p.865·2); chlortalidone (p.882·3).
*Hypertension.*

**Prenormine** *AstraZeneca, Arg.*
Atenolol (p.865·2).
*Angina pectoris; arrhythmias; hypertension; myocardial infarction.*

**Prenoxan au phenobarbital** *Schering-Plough, Fr.†.*
Phenobarbital (p.367·3); aspirin (p.15·1).
*Fever; pain.*

**Prent**
*Bayer, Ger.; Gepepharm, Ger.; Bayer, Ital.; Bayer, Port.*
Acebutolol hydrochloride (p.848·1).
*Arrhythmias; hypertension; ischaemic heart disease.*

**Pre-Nutrison** *Nutricia, Port.*
Preparation for enteral nutrition (p.1417·1).

**Pre-Op**
*Nutricia, Austral.; Baxter, NZ; Nutricia, NZ.*
Preparation for pre-operative enteral nutrition (p.1417·1).

**Prep Kit-C** *Pharmatel, Austral.*
One sachet, macrogol 3350 (p.1709·1); electrolytes (p.1217·1) (Glycoprep-C); Two sachets, sodium picosulfate (p.1289·3) (PicoPrep).
*Bowel evacuation.*

**Prepacol**
*Guerbet, Austria; Codali, Belg.; Guerbet, Fr.; Guerbet, Ger.*
*Combination pack:* Tablets, bisacodyl (p.1251·3); oral solution, dibasic sodium phosphate (p.1231·1); monobasic sodium phosphate (p.1230·3).
*Bowel evacuation.*

**Prepacort H** *Whitehall, Ital.*
Hydrocortisone acetate (p.1103·3); benzocaine (p.1370·3).
*Haemorrhoids.*

**Prepadine** *Berk, UK.*
Dosulepin hydrochloride (p.291·1).
*Depression.*

**Pre-Par**
*Solvay, Belg.†; Solvay, Fr.†; Solvay, Ger.†; Solvay, Ital.†; Solvay, Neth.†; Solvay, Port.; Reig Jofre, Spain.*
Ritodrine hydrochloride (p.1739·2).
*Fetal asphyxia; premature labour; prevention of uterine contractions during surgery in pregnancy; prevention of uterine hypermotility in labour; production of uterine relaxation.*

**Preparacion H** *Wyeth, Spain.*
Yeast extract (p.1469·1); shark-liver oil.
*Haemorrhoids.*

**Preparado H** *Whitehall, Braz.†.*
Live yeast (p.1469·1); cod-liver oil (p.1425·2); vitamin A (p.1451·2).
*Haemorrhoids.*

**Preparation H**
*Note. This name is used for preparations of different composition.*
*Whitehall, Austral.†; Whitehall-Robins, Canad.; Wyeth Consumer, Irl.; Whitehall, Israel; Wyeth Consumer, Singapore; Wyeth Consumer, UK; Whitehall, USA.*
Live yeast cell derivative (p.1469·1); shark-liver oil.
*Haemorrhoids.*

*Whitehall, Fr.*
*Rectal cream:* Yeast (p.1469·1); halibut-liver oil (p.1434·1).
*Suppositories:* Butyl aminobenzoate (p.1373·1); yeast (p.1469·1); esculoside (p.1648·2); halibut-liver oil (p.1434·1).
*Haemorrhoids.*

*Whitehall, Hong Kong; Wyeth, Mex.; Whitehall, Thai.; Whitehall-Robins, USA.*
Shark-liver oil; phenylephrine hydrochloride (p.1126·3).
*Anorectal disorders.*

**Preparation H Cleansing Pads** *Whitehall-Robins, Canad.†.*
Hamamelis (p.1696·3).
*Anal and vaginal hygiene; anal irritation; haemorrhoids.*

**Preparation H Clear Gel** *Wyeth Consumer, UK.*
Hamamelis (p.1696·3).
*Haemorrhoids.*

**Preparation H Cooling Gel**
*Whitehall-Robins, Canad.; Whitehall-Robins, USA.*
Hamamelis (p.1696·3); phenylephrine hydrochloride (p.1126·3).
*Anorectal disorders.*

**Preparation H Sperti** *Whitehall, Belg.†.*
Dried yeast (p.1469·1).
*Haemorrhoids.*

**Preparation H Veinotonic** *Whitehall, Fr.*
Diosmin (p.1688·2).
*Haemorrhoids.*

**Preparazione Antiemorroidaria** *Giuliani, Ital.*
Hydrocortisone acetate (p.1103·3); benzocaine (p.1370·3).
*Haemorrhoids.*

**Preparazione H** *Whitehall, Ital.*
Yeast cell extract (p.1469·1); shark-liver oil.
*Haemorrhoids.*

**Prepcare** *Darrow, Braz.†.*
Povidone-iodine (p.1190·3).
*Skin and wound disinfection.*

**Prepcat** *Lafayette, USA.*
Barium sulfate (p.1061·1).
*Contrast medium for gastrointestinal radiography.*

**Pre-Pen**
*Rivex, Canad.†; Biolac, Swed.†; Bayer, USA.*
Penicilloyl-polylysine (p.1729·2).
*Diagnosis of penicillin hypersensitivity.*

**Prephen** *Orion, NZ.*
Substituted phenols.
*Disinfection.*

**Prepidil**
*Pharmacia, Austria; Pharmacia, Belg.; Pharmacia, Canad.; Pharmacia, Fr.; Pharmacia, Ger.; Pharmacia Upjohn, Hong Kong†; Pharmacia Upjohn, Irl.†; Pharmacia Upjohn, Israel; Pharmacia Upjohn, Ital.; Pharmacia Upjohn, Mex.; Pharmacia, Neth.; Pharmacia Upjohn, NZ†; Pharmacia, S.Afr.; Pharmacia, Spain; Pharmacia, Switz.; Pharmacia Upjohn, UK†; Pharmacia Upjohn, USA.*
Dinoprostone (p.1515·1).
*Labour induction.*

**Preptin** *Teuto, Braz.*
Cyproheptadine hydrochloride (p.430·1).
*Reduced appetite.*

**Prepulsid**
*Janssen-Cilag, Arg.; Janssen-Cilag, Austral.; Janssen-Cilag, Austria; Janssen-Cilag, Belg.; Janssen-Cilag, Braz.; Janssen-Ortho, Canad.†; Janssen-Cilag, Chile; Janssen-Cilag, Denm.; Janssen-Cilag, Fin.; Janssen-Cilag, Fr.; Janssen, Hong Kong; Janssen-Cilag, Irl.; Janssen-Cilag, Israel; Janssen-Cilag, Ital.†; Janssen, Mex.; Janssen-Cilag, Neth.; Janssen-Cilag, Norw.; Janssen-Cilag, NZ; Janssen-Cilag, Port.; Janssen-Cilag, S.Afr.; Janssen-Cilag, Singapore†; Janssen-Cilag, Spain; Janssen-Cilag, Swed.; Janssen-Cilag, Switz.; Janssen, Thai.; Janssen-Cilag, UK†.*
Cisapride (p.1259·2) or cisapride tartrate (p.1259·2).
*Dyspepsia; gastro-oesophageal reflux; gastrointestinal motility disorders; gastroparesis; regurgitation and vomiting in babies.*

**Prepurex**
*Wellcome, Israel; Wellcome Diagnostics, UK†.*
Pregnancy test (p.1734·3).

**Preran** *Hoechst Marion Roussel, Jpn.*
Trandolapril (p.1016·1).
*Hypertension.*

**Pres** *Boehringer Ingelheim, Ger.*
Enalapril maleate (p.909·2) or enalaprilat (p.909·3).
*Heart failure; hypertension.*

**Pres plus** *Boehringer Ingelheim, Ger.*
Enalapril maleate (p.909·2); hydrochlorothiazide (p.933·2).
*Hypertension.*

**Presabet** *Royal, Chile.*
Nitrendipine (p.973·3).
*Hypertension.*

**Prescaina** *Llorens, Spain.*
Oxybuprocaine hydrochloride (p.1382·1).
*Local anaesthesia.*

**Prescal** *Novartis, UK.*
Isradipine (p.942·2).
*Hypertension.*

**Presco** *Polipharm, Thai.*
Dextromethorphan hydrobromide (p.1117·3); bromhexine hydrochloride (p.1115·3).
*Respiratory-tract disorders.*

**Prescol** *Atlantis, Mex.*
Trimebutine (p.1758·1).
*Gastrointestinal motility disorders.*

**Presept**
*Ethicon, Ital.†; Johnson & Johnson Medical, UK.*
Sodium dichloroisocyanurate (p.1191·3).
*Instrument and surface disinfection.*

**Preservex** *UCB, UK.*
Aceclofenac (p.11·2).
*Musculoskeletal and joint disorders.*

**Presi Regul** *Fabra, Arg.*
Enalapril (p.909·2).
*Hypertension.*

**Presi Regul D** *Fabra, Arg.*
Enalapril (p.909·2); hydrochlorothiazide (p.933·2).
*Hypertension.*

**President's Choice Sport Sunblock** *Fruit of the Earth, Canad.*
*SPF 15:* Octinoxate (p.1154·3); oxybenzone (p.1154·3).
*SPF 30:* Octinoxate (p.1154·3); octisalate (p.1154·3); oxybenzone (p.1154·3).
*Sunscreen.*

**President's Choice Sunblock** *Fruit of the Earth, Canad.*
*SPF 15:* Octinoxate (p.1154·3); oxybenzone (p.1154·3).
*SPF 30:* Octocrilene (p.1154·3); octinoxate (p.1154·3); octisalate (p.1154·3); oxybenzone (p.1154·3); titanium dioxide (p.1160·3).
*Sunscreen.*

**President's Choice Sunblock for Babies** *Fruit of the Earth, Canad.*
*SPF 45:* Octocrilene (p.1154·3); octinoxate (p.1154·3); octisalate (p.1154·3); oxybenzone (p.1154·3); titanium dioxide (p.1160·3).
*Sunscreen.*

**President's Choice Sunblock for Children**
*Fruit of the Earth, Canad.*
*SPF 30:* Octocrilene (p.1154·3); octinoxate (p.1154·3); octisalate (p.1154·3); oxybenzone (p.1154·3); titanium dioxide (p.1160·3).
*Sunscreen.*

**President's Choice Sunscreen** *Fruit of the Earth, Canad.*
*SPF 8:* Octinoxate (p.1154·3); oxybenzone (p.1154·3).
*Sunscreen.*

**Presilam** *Pasteur, Chile.*
Amlodipine besilate (p.862·1).
*Angina pectoris; hypertension.*

**Presinex** *Pliva, UK.*
Desmopressin acetate (p.1322·3).
*Diabetes insipidus; nocturnal enuresis; test of renal concentrating capacity.*

**Presinol**
*Bayer, Austria†; Teofarma, Ger.*
Methyldopa (p.953·2).
*Hypertension.*

**Presistin** *Maver, Mex.*
Cisapride (p.1259·2).
*Gastro-oesophageal reflux; gastrointestinal motility disorders.*

**Preslow**
*AstraZeneca, Port.; Astra, Spain†.*
Felodipine (p.914·3).
*Angina pectoris; hypertension.*

**Presocor** *Rider, Chile.*
Verapamil hydrochloride (p.1019·1).
*Angina pectoris; arrhythmias; hypertension.*

**Presoken** *Kener, Mex.†.*
Diltiazem (p.901·3).

**Presokin** *Chemopharma, Chile.*
Lisinopril (p.946·3).
*Heart failure; hypertension.*

**Presol** *Cesam, Port.†.*
*SPF 20:* Titanium dioxide (p.1160·3); zinc oxide (p.1163·2).
*Sunscreen.*

**Presolar** *Cipla, India.*
Atenolol (p.865·2); nifedipine (p.966·2).
*Angina pectoris; hypertension.*

**Presolol** *Alphapharm, Austral.*
Labetalol hydrochloride (p.943·3).
*Hypertension.*

**Presomen** *Solvay, Ger.*
Extract from pregnant mare's urine.
*Menopausal disorders; osteoporosis.*

**Presomen compositum** *Solvay, Ger.*
*Combination pack:* 10 Tablets, extract from pregnant mare's urine; 11 tablets, medrogestone (p.1557·1); extract from pregnant mare's urine.
*Menopausal disorders; menstrual disorders; osteoporosis.*

**Presoquim** *Kener, Mex.†.*
Diltiazem (p.901·3).

**Prespir** *Remexa, Mex.*
Aluminium chloride (p.1142·1).
*Hyperhidrosis.*

**Press-12** *Genepharm, Gr.*
Lisinopril (p.946·3).
*Heart failure; hypertension; myocardial infarction.*

**Pressalolo** *Locatelli, Ital.†.*
Labetalol hydrochloride (p.943·3).
*Hypertension.*

**Pressalolo Diuretico** *Locatelli, Ital.†.*
Labetalol hydrochloride (p.943·3); chlortalidone (p.882·3).
*Hypertension.*

**Pressamina** *Teofarma, Ital.*
Dimetofrine hydrochloride (p.902·3).
*Hypotension.*

**Pressat** *Biolab Sanus, Braz.*
Amlodipine besilate (p.862·1).
*Hypertension.*

**Pressel** *Legrand, Braz.†.*
Enalapril maleate (p.909·2).
*Hypertension.*

**Presselin All** *Presselin, Ger.*
Homoeopathic preparation.

**Presselin Arterien K 5 P** *Presselin, Ger.*
Crataegus (p.1677·1); hypericum (p.299·1); garlic (p.1691·1); barlauchkraut; java tea (p.1702·3); mistletoe (p.1715·3).
*Circulatory disorders.*

**Presselin Blahungs K 4 N** *Presselin, Ger.*
Peppermint leaf (p.1283·2); caraway (p.1667·2); fennel (p.1687·2); chamomile (p.1669·3); calamus (p.1664·1); absinthium (p.1645·1); sage (p.1741·2); melissa (p.1711·1).
*Digestive-system disorders.*

**Presselin BN Nieren-Blasen** *Presselin, Ger.†.*
Homoeopathic preparation.

**Presselin Cpl 87 N** *Presselin, Ger.†.*
Homoeopathic preparation.

**Presselin Dysmen Olin 3 N** *Presselin, Ger.†.*
Viburnum prunifolium; agnus castus (p.1649·1); anserina; shepherd's purse (p.1744·1); cimicifuga (p.1671·3).
*Menopausal disorders; menstrual disorders.*

**Presselin Dyspeptikum** *Presselin, Ger.*
Chamomile (p.1669·3); lavender (p.1705·1); sage (p.1741·2); caraway (p.1667·2); cardamom (p.1667·3); coriander (p.1676·1); fennel (p.1687·2); absinthium (p.1645·1); ginger (p.1267·1).
*Biliary disorders; dyspepsia; liver disorders.*

**Presselin Gold N** *Presselin, Ger.*
Homoeopathic preparation.

**Presselin Heilozon P** *Presselin, Ger.*
Magnesium citrate (p.1272·1).
*Magnesium deficiency.*

**Presselin Hepaticum P** *Presselin, Ger.*
Taraxacum (p.1751·3); greater celandine (p.1695·3); silybum marianum (p.1043·3).
*Liver and biliary-tract disorders.*

**Presselin HK Herz-Kreislauf** *Presselin, Ger.*
Homoeopathic preparation.

**Presselin MIG F** *Presselin, Ger.*
Homoeopathic preparation.

**Presselin MIG M** *Presselin, Ger.*
Homoeopathic preparation.

**Presselin 218 N** *Presselin, Ger.†.*
Homoeopathic preparation.

**Presselin Nerven K 1 N** *Presselin, Ger.*
Hypericum (p.299·1); valerian (p.1762·2); lupulus (p.1708·1); passion flower (p.1729·1).
*Depression; nervous disorders; sleep disorders.*

**Presselin Nervennahrung N** *Presselin, Ger.*
Homoeopathic preparation.

**Presselin Nieren-Blasen K 3** *Presselin, Ger.*
Birch leaf (p.1660·3); java tea (p.1702·3); equisetum (p.1684·1); urtica root (p.1762·1); solidago virgaurea (p.1748·3); lovage root (p.1708·1); ononis (p.1723·3); bearberry (p.1659·2).
*Urinary-tract disorders.*

**Presselin Olin 5** *Presselin, Ger.†.*
Homoeopathic preparation.

**Presselin Osteo** *Presselin, Ger.*
Homoeopathic preparation.

**Presselin Stoffwechsel-Tee Hapeka 225 N**
*Presselin, Ger.*
Chamomile (p.1669·3); stoechados; senna (p.1288·2); fennel (p.1687·2); juniper (p.1703·1); phaseolus (seed-free); equisetum (p.1684·1); couch-grass (p.1676·2).
*Constipation.*

**Presselin VE** *Presselin, Ger.†.*
Melilotus officinalis.
*Venous disorders.*

**Pressimed** *Wild, Switz.†.*
Dihydroergocristine mesilate (p.1680·1); bendroflumethiazide (p.867·3); reserpine (p.995·1).
*Hypertension.*

**Pressimedin** *Kwizda, Austria†.*
Dihydroergocristine mesilate (p.1680·1); bendroflumethiazide (p.867·3); reserpine (p.995·1).
*Hypertension.*

**Pressin**
*Alphapharm, Austral.; Utopian, Thai.*
Prazosin hydrochloride (p.985·1).
*Benign prostatic hyperplasia; heart failure; hypertension; Raynaud's syndrome.*

**Pressitan** *Iquinosa, Spain.*
Enalapril maleate (p.909·2).
*Heart failure; hypertension.*

**Pressitan Plus** *Iquinosa, Spain.*
Enalapril maleate (p.909·2); hydrochlorothiazide (p.933·2).
*Hypertension.*

**Pressodipin** *Genepharm, Gr.*
Nitrendipine (p.973·3).
*Hypertension.*

**Pressolat** *Agis, Israel.*
Nifedipine (p.966·2).
*Hypertension.*

**Pressomax** *Kinder, Braz.*
Captopril (p.879·2).
*Hypertension.*

**Pressotec** *Teuto, Braz.*
Enalapril maleate (p.909·2).
*Hypertension.*

**Pressunic Compositum** *Unipharm, Israel†.*
Reserpine (p.995·1); dihydralazine (p.900·1).
*Hypertension.*

**Pressural** *Polifarma, Ital.*
Indapamide (p.938·2).
*Hypertension.*

**Pressuril** *Phoinix Pharm (Φοινιξ Φαρμ), Gr.*
Lisinopril (p.946·3).
*Heart failure; hypertension; myocardial infarction.*

**Pressyn** *Ferring, Canad.*
Vasopressin (p.1342·2).
*Adjunct in abdominal radiography; diabetes insipidus; postoperative abdominal distension.*

**Prestim**
*Leo, Irl.†; ICN, UK.*
Timolol maleate (p.1012·2); bendroflumethiazide (p.867·3).
*Hypertension.*

**Prestodol** *Rayere, Mex.*
Clonixin lysine (p.26·3).
*Pain.*

**Prestole** *Pharmafarm, Fr.*
Triamterene (p.1016·2); hydrochlorothiazide (p.933·2).
*Hypertension.*

**Presun**
*Note. This name is used for preparations of different composition.*
*Westwood-Squibb, Canad.†; Westwood, USA.*
*Cream SPF 15:* Padimate O (p.1155·1); oxybenzone (p.1154·3).
*Sunscreen.*

*Westwood-Squibb, Canad.†; Westwood, USA.*
*Lotion SPF 15:* Aminobenzoic acid (p.1142·2); padimate O (p.1155·1); oxybenzone (p.1154·3).
*Sunscreen.*

*Westwood-Squibb, Canad.; Westwood, USA.*
*SPF 8; SPF 39:* Padimate O (p.1155·1); oxybenzone (p.1154·3).
*Sunscreen.*

*Westwood-Squibb, Canad.*
*SPF 15:* Octinoxate (p.1154·3); octisalate (p.1154·3); oxybenzone (p.1154·3).
*SPF 29:* Octinoxate (p.1154·3); octisalate (p.1154·3); oxybenzone (p.1154·3).
*SPF 15; SPF 27; SPF 30:* Octinoxate (p.1154·3); octisalate (p.1154·3); oxybenzone (p.1154·3); avobenzone (p.1142·3).
*SPF 21; SPF 28:* Titanium dioxide (p.1160·3).
*Sunscreen.*

**Presun Active** *Bristol-Myers Products, USA.*
*SPF 15; SPF 30:* Octinoxate (p.1154·3); oxybenzone (p.1154·3); octisalate (p.1154·3).
*Sunscreen.*

**Presun Facial** *Westwood, USA.*
*SPF 15:* Padimate O (p.1155·1); oxybenzone (p.1154·3).
*Sunscreen.*

**Presun for Kids** *Westwood, USA; Bristol-Myers Products, USA.*
Octinoxate (p.1154·3); oxybenzone (p.1154·3); octisalate (p.1154·3).
*Sunscreen.*

**Presun Lip Stick** *Westwood, USA.*
*SPF 15:* Padimate O (p.1155·1); oxybenzone (p.1154·3).
*Sunscreen.*

**Presun Moisturizing** *Bristol-Myers Products, USA.*
*SPF 46:* Padimate O (p.1155·1); oxybenzone (p.1154·3).
*Sunscreen.*

**Presun Moisturizing with Keri** *Bristol-Myers Products, USA.*
*SPF 15:* Padimate O (p.1155·1); oxybenzone (p.1154·3).
*SPF 25:* Octinoxate (p.1154·3); oxybenzone (p.1154·3); octisalate (p.1154·3).
*Sunscreen.*

**Presun Sensitive Skin** *Westwood, USA; Bristol-Myers Products, USA.*
*SPF 15; SPF 29:* Octinoxate (p.1154·3); oxybenzone (p.1154·3); octisalate (p.1154·3).
*Sunscreen.*

**Presun Spray Mist** *Bristol-Myers Products, USA.*
*SPF 23:* Octinoxate (p.1154·3); padimate O (p.1155·1); oxybenzone (p.1154·3); octisalate (p.1154·3).
*Sunscreen.*

**Presun Ultra** *Westwood-Squibb, USA.*
*SPF 30:* Avobenzone (p.1142·3); octinoxate (p.1154·3); octisalate (p.1154·3); oxybenzone (p.1154·3).
*Sunscreen.*

**Presyc** *Pasteur, Chile.*
Capsaicin (p.24·2).
*Diabetic neuropathy; musculoskeletal and joint pain; phantom-limb pain; postherpetic neuralgia; pruritus.*

**Preterax**
*Servier, Arg.; Servier, Austria; Servier, Braz.†; Therval, Fr.; Servier, Irl.; Servier, Ital.; Servier, Singapore.*
Perindopril erbumine (p.980·2); indapamide (p.938·2).
*Hypertension.*

**Pretts Diet Aid** *Milance, USA.*
Alginic acid (p.1576·3); carmellose sodium (p.1577·3); sodium bicarbonate (p.1223·2).

**Pretuval** *Roche, Switz.*
Dextromethorphan hydrobromide (p.1117·3); pseudoephedrine hydrochloride (p.1129·2); paracetamol (p.76·2).
*Cold symptoms.*

**Pretuval C** *Roche, Switz.*
Dextromethorphan hydrobromide (p.1117·3); pseudoephedrine hydrochloride (p.1129·2); paracetamol (p.76·2); ascorbic acid (p.1460·2).
*Cold symptoms.*

**Pretz**
*Note. This name is used for preparations of different composition.*
*Alcon, Hong Kong.*
Eriodictyon (p.1121·2).
*Nasal dryness.*

*Parnell, Irl.*
Moisturising nasal spray.
*Nasal dryness.*

*Parnell, USA.*
Sodium chloride (p.1233·3).
*Inflammation and dryness of nasal membranes.*

**Pretz-D** *Parnell, USA.*
Ephedrine sulfate (p.1120·1).
*Nasal congestion.*

**Prevacid**
*Abbott, Canad.; Takeda, Malaysia; Takeda, Singapore; Takeda, Thai.; TAP, USA.*
Lansoprazole (p.1269·3).
*Dyspepsia; gastro-oesophageal reflux; peptic ulcer; Zollinger-Ellison syndrome.*

**Prevacid NapraPAC** *TAP, USA.*
Naproxen (p.65·1).
Lansoprazole (p.1269·3) is included in this preparation in an attempt to limit adverse effects on the gastrointestinal mucosa.
*Musculoskeletal and joint disorders.*

**Prevagin-Premaril** *Dexxon, Israel.*
Conjugated oestrogens (p.1543·2).
*Menopausal vulvovaginal disorders.*

**Prevalin** *Chefaro, Neth.†.*
Sodium cromoglicate (p.795·3).
*Allergic conjunctivitis; allergic rhinitis.*

**Prevalina** *Silesia, Chile.*
Mianserin hydrochloride (p.306·3).
*Depression.*

**Prevalite** *Upsher-Smith, USA.*
Colestyramine (p.889·3).

**Prevalon** *Abello, Spain.*
Multivitamin and amino-acid preparation (p.1417·1).
*Tonic.*

**Prevax** *Biosintetica, Braz.*
Calcium folinate (p.1431·1).

**Prevecilina** *Grunenthal, Port.*
Clemizole penicillin (p.194·1); benzylpenicillin sodium (p.163·2).
Lidocaine hydrochloride (p.1377·3) is included in the intramuscular injection to alleviate the pain of injection.
*Bacterial infections.*

**Prevegyne** *Farmalight, Port.*
Ascorbic acid (p.1460·2).
*Vulvovaginal disorders.*

**Preven** *Gynetics, USA.*
Levonorgestrel (p.1563·2); ethinylestradiol (p.1553·2).
*Postcoital oral contraceptive.*

**Prevenar**
*Wyeth, Arg.; Wyeth, Austral.; Wyeth Lederle, Austria; Wyeth, Chile; Wyeth Lederle, Denm.; Wyeth Lederle, Fin.; Wyeth Lederle, Fr.; Wyeth, Ger.; Wyeth, Irl.; Wyeth Lederle, Ital.; Wyeth Lederle, Norw.; Wyeth Lederle, Port.; Wyeth, Spain; Wyeth Lederle, Swed.; Lederle, Switz.; Wyeth, UK.*
A pneumococcal conjugate vaccine (7-valent) (p.1633·1).
*Active immunisation in infants and children.*

**Prevencal** *Lalco, Canad.†.*
Calcium carbonate (p.1254·2).

**Prevencal & D** *Lalco, Canad.†.*
Calcium carbonate (p.1254·2); vitamin D (p.1461·2).

**Prevencal & D & Fer** *Lalco, Canad.†.*
Calcium carbonate (p.1254·2); vitamin D (p.1461·2); ferrous fumarate (p.1427·3).

**Prevencal & D & Magnesium** *Lalco, Canad.†.*
Calcium carbonate (p.1254·2); vitamin D (p.1461·2); magnesium oxide (p.1272·3).

**Prevencor** *Almirall, Spain.*
Atorvastatin calcium (p.866·1).
*Hyperlipidaemias.*

**Prevent** *Agropharm, UK.*
Pyrethrins (p.1509·3); piperonyl butoxide (p.1509·2).
*Insectic repellent.*

**Preventan** *Grunenthal, Chile.*
Prednisolone (p.1108·1).
*Corticosteroid.*

**Prevepen** *Grunenthal, Chile.*
Clemizole penicillin (p.194·1).
*Bacterial infections.*

**Prevepen Forte** *Grunenthal, Chile.*
Benzylpenicillin sodium (p.163·2); clemizole penicillin (p.194·1); lidocaine hydrochloride (p.1377·3).
Lidocaine hydrochloride (p.1377·3) is included in this preparation to alleviate the pain of injection.
*Bacterial infections.*

**Prevex**
*Note. This name is used for preparations of different composition.*
*Trans Canaderm, Canad.*
*Cream:* Cyclomethicone (p.1482·1); yellow soft paraffin (p.1479·3).
*Barrier cream for hands.*
*Lotion:* Moisturiser.

*Simesa, Ital.*
Felodipine (p.914·3).
*Angina pectoris; hypertension.*

*Stiefel, Thai.*
Barrier gel.

**Prevex B**
*Trans Canaderm, Canad.; Stiefel, Thai.*
Betamethasone valerate (p.1093·2).
*Skin disorders.*

**Prevex Diaper Rash Cream** *Trans Canaderm, Canad.†.*
Zinc oxide (p.1163·2).
*Barrier cream.*

**Prevex HC**
*Trans Canaderm, Canad.; Stiefel, Thai.*
Hydrocortisone (p.1103·3).
*Skin disorders.*

**Prevident** *Colgate Oral, USA.*
Sodium fluoride (p.1444·3).
*Dental caries prophylaxis.*

**Previfem** *Andrx, USA.*
Norgestimate (p.1563·2); ethinylestradiol (p.1553·2).
*Combined oral contraceptive.*

**Previgrip** *Socopharm, Fr.*
Inactivated influenza vaccine (p.1620·2).
*Active immunisation.*

**Previnfec** *Lacefa, Arg.*
Chloroxylenol (p.1177·2).
*Disinfection.*

**Previscan**
*Note. This name is used for preparations of different composition.*
*Hexal, Arg.*
Pentoxifylline (p.979·3).
*Intermittent claudication.*

*Procter & Gamble, Fr.*
Fluindione (p.918·2).
*Thromboembolic disorders.*

**Previum** *Chefaro, Neth.†.*
Aciclovir (p.626·1).
*Herpes simplex infections.*

**Prevnar**
*Wyeth-Ayerst, Canad.; Wyeth-Ayerst, USA.*
A pneumococcal conjugate vaccine (7-valent) (p.1633·1).
*Active immunisation.*

**Prevolac** *Cosmopharm, Gr.*
Azelaic acid (p.1142·3).
*Acne.*

**Prevpac** *TAP, USA.*
Capsules, lansoprazole (Prevacid) (p.1269·3); capsules, amoxicillin trihydrate (Trimox) (p.155·3); tablets, clarithromycin (Biaxin) (p.192·2).
*Duodenal ulcer associated with Helicobacter pylori infection.*

**Prewash** *Pharmacia Upjohn, Hong Kong†.*
Triclosan (p.1195·2).
*Acne.*

**Prexan** *Lafare, Ital.*
Naproxen (p.65·1).
*Musculoskeletal, joint, peri-articular, and soft-tissue disorders; neuralgias.*

**Prexene** *Herbaline, Ital.†.*
Garlic (p.1691·1); crataegus (p.1677·1); olive oil (p.1723·2); silver birch (p.1660·3).
*Hypertension; tachycardia.*

**Prexidine** *Pharmascience, Fr.*
Chlorhexidine gluconate (p.1173·2).
*Mouth infections.*

**Prezal** *Aventis, Neth.*
Lansoprazole (p.1269·3).
*Gastro-oesophageal reflux; peptic ulcer; Zollinger-Ellison syndrome.*

**Prezatim** *Merck, Braz.*
Prezatide copper acetate (p.1156·1).
*Cicatrisation.*

**Prezolon** *Nycomed, Gr.*
Prednisolone (p.1108·1).
*Corticosteroid.*

**Priadel**
*Sanofi Synthelabo, Belg.; Sanofi Synthelabo, Irl.; Sanofi Synthelabo, Malaysia; Sanofi Synthelabo, Neth.; Bamford, NZ; Sanofi Synthelabo, Port.; Sanofi Synthelabo, Singapore; Synthelabo, Switz.; Sanofi Synthelabo, UK.*
Lithium carbonate (p.301·1) or lithium citrate (p.301·1).
*Aggressive or self-harming behaviour; bipolar disorder; depression; mania.*

**Priamide** *Janssen-Cilag, Belg.†.*
Isopropamide iodide (p.485·2).
*Diarrhoea; gastrointestinal spasm.*

**Priaxim** *Ravizza, Ital.†.*
Flunoxaprofen (p.43·3).
*Gynaecological inflammation; musculoskeletal, joint, peri-articular, and soft-tissue disorders; venous disorders.*

**Pricam** *Mintlab, Chile.*
Piroxicam (p.84·2).
*Inflammation; pain.*

**Priciasol** *Labima, Belg.*
Naphazoline nitrate (p.1124·3).
*Nasal congestion.*

**Pricillin** *Malayan, Singapore.*
Ampicillin trihydrate (p.157·2).
*Bacterial infections.*

**Prickly Heat Powder** *Carter-Wallace, Austral.†.*
Zinc oxide (p.1163·2).
*Chafed skin; eczema; heat rash; prickly heat.*

**Pridam** *Pisa, Mex.*
Noradrenaline (p.974·3).

**Pridana** *Novartis, Port.*
Pirisudanol maleate (p.1732·3).
*Mental function disorders.*

**Pridecil** *Farmalab, Braz.*
Bromopride (p.1254·1).
*Nausea and vomiting.*

**Pri-De-Sid** *Polipharm, Thai.†.*
Cisapride (p.1259·2).
*Dyspepsia; gastro-oesophageal reflux; gastrointestinal motility disorders; gastroparesis.*

**Pridinol** *Millet Roux, Braz.†.*
Terfenadine (p.441·1).
*Hypersensitivity reactions.*

**Pridio** *Quimifar, Spain.*
Caffeine (p.782·1); chlorphenamine maleate (p.427·3); paracetamol (p.76·2); salicylamide (p.87·3).
*Fever; nasal congestion; pain.*

**Priftin**
*Hoechst Marion Roussel, Braz.†; Hoechst Marion Roussel, USA.*
Rifapentine (p.253·3).
*Leprosy; tuberculosis.*

**Prigost** *Rider, Chile.*
Bromocriptine mesilate (p.1200·3).
*Hyperprolactinaemia; parkinsonism.*

**Prilace** *Aventis, Ital.*
Ramipril (p.994·1); piretanide (p.983·3).
*Hypertension.*

**Prilagin** *Gambar, Ital.†.*
Miconazole (p.405·2) or miconazole nitrate (p.405·3).
*Candidiasis; Gram-positive bacterial infections.*

**Prilan** *Sofex, Port.*
Enalapril maleate (p.909·2).
*Heart failure; hypertension.*

**Prilosec** *AstraZeneca, USA.*
Omeprazole (p.1278·2) or omeprazole magnesium (p.1278·2).
*Gastro-oesophageal reflux; heartburn; peptic ulcer; Zollinger-Ellison syndrome.*

**Prilovase** *CPH, Port.*
Captopril (p.879·2).
*Heart failure; hypertension.*

**Prilpressin** *Legrand, Braz.*
Amlodipine besilate (p.862·1).
*Hypertension.*

**Priltam** *Atache, Spain†.*
Capsaicin (p.24·2).
*Muscle and joint pain.*

**Priltenk** *Biotenk, Arg.*
Enalapril maleate (p.909·2).
*Heart failure; hypertension; myocardial infarction.*

**Primacaine** *IMS, Ital.*
Articaine hydrochloride (p.1370·3).
Adrenaline hydrochloride (p.852·3) is included in this preparation as a vasoconstrictor to diminish absorption and localise the effect of the local anaesthetic.
*Local anaesthesia.*

**Prima-Cal** *Prima, Thai.*
Calcium carbonate (p.1254·2).
*Calcium supplement.*

**Prima-Cal Plus Vit D** *Prima, Thai.*
Calcium carbonate (p.1254·2); vitamin D (p.1461·2).
*Calcium and vitamin D supplement.*

**Primacard** *Matara, Fr.†.*
Pregnancy test (p.1734·3).

**Primacin** *Boucher & Muir, Austral.*
Primaquine phosphate (p.456·2).
*Malaria.*

**Primacine** *Pinewood, Irl.*
Erythromycin ethyl succinate (p.208·1) or erythromycin stearate (p.208·2).
*Bacterial infections.*

**Primacor**
*Sanofi Synthelabo, Austral.; Sanofi Synthelabo, Braz.; Sanofi Synthelabo, Canad.; Sanofi Synthelabo, Hong Kong; Sanofi Winthrop, Israel; Sanofi Synthelabo, Malaysia; Sanofi Synthelabo, Mex.; Sanofi Synthelabo, NZ; Sanofi Synthelabo, Singapore; Sanofi Synthelabo, Thai.; Sanofi Synthelabo, UK; Sanofi Winthrop, USA.*
Milrinone lactate (p.959·2).
*Heart failure.*

**Primacton** *Streuli, Switz.*
Spironolactone (p.1003·1).
*Cirrhosis; hyperaldosteronism; hypertension; nephrotic syndrome; oedema.*

**Primacy C+AHA** *Dispolab, Chile.*
Ascorbic acid (p.1460·2); glycolic acid (p.1147·3); lactic acid (p.1704·1); zinc sulfate (p.1469·3).
*Acne; skin pigmentation disorders.*

**Primacy Phyto +** *Dispolab, Chile.*
Kojic acid (p.1151·2); bearberry (p.1659·2); thyme (p.1755·2); pepino; citrus bioflavonoids (p.1688·2).
*Skin pigmentation disorders.*

**Primaderm** *Aventis, Arg.*
Prednicarbate (p.1107·3).
*Skin disorders.*

**Primafen** *Aventis, Spain†.*
Cefotaxime sodium (p.175·3).
Lidocaine (p.1377·3) is included in the intramuscular injection to alleviate the pain of injection.
*Bacterial infections.*

**Primafluor** *Prima, Braz.*
Sodium fluoride (p.1444·3).
*Dental caries prophylaxis.*

**Primahex** *Convatec, UK†.*
Chlorhexidine (p.1173·2); alcohol (p.1166·1).
*Skin disinfection.*

**Primakinder** *Kinder, Braz.*
Primaquine phosphate (p.456·2).
*Malaria.*

**Primalan**
*Pierre Fabre, Arg.; Inava, Fr.; Pierre Fabre, Ital.; Pierre Fabre, Port.; Rhone-Poulenc Sante, Thai.†; May & Baker, UK†.*
Mequitazine (p.437·2).
*Hypersensitivity reactions.*

**Primamed** *Sanofi Synthelabo, Ger.†.*
Aluminium chlorohydrate (p.1142·1).
*Burns; skin disorders; wounds.*

**Primanol** *Jamieson, Canad.*
Evening primrose oil (p.1686·3).

**Primanol-Borage** *Jamieson, Canad.*
Evening primrose oil (p.1686·3); borage oil (p.1661·3).

**Primaquin** *Osteolab, Chile.*
Estradiol (p.1550·1).
*Menopausal disorders.*

**Primaquin MP** *Osteolab, Chile.*
18 Tablets, estradiol (p.1550·1); 12 tablets, estradiol; medroxyprogesterone acetate (p.1557·2).
*Menopausal disorders.*

**Primaquin MP Continuo** *Osteolab, Chile.*
Estradiol (p.1550·1); medroxyprogesterone acetate (p.1557·2).
*Menopausal disorders.*

**Primasept Med** *Schulke & Mayr, Ger.*
Propyl alcohol (p.1191·2); isopropyl alcohol (p.1184·3); orthophenylphenol (p.1187·2).
*Hand disinfection.*

**Primasone** *Aventis, Braz.†.*
Mequitazine (p.437·2).
*Hypersensitivity reactions.*

**Primaspan** *Orion, Fin.*
Aspirin (p.15·1).
*Musculoskeletal, joint and peri-articular disorders; pain; thromboembolism prophylaxis.*

**Primastick** *Matara, Fr.*
Pregnancy test (p.1734·3).

**Primatene** *Whitehall-Robins, USA.*
Ephedrine hydrochloride (p.1120·1); guaifenesin (p.1122·1).
Formerly contained ephedrine hydrochloride and theophylline.
*Bronchial asthma.*

**Primatene Dual Action** *Whitehall, USA†.*
Theophylline (p.798·3); ephedrine hydrochloride (p.1120·1); guaifenesin (p.1122·1).
*Asthma.*

**Primatene Mist** *Whitehall, USA.*
Adrenaline (p.852·2).
*Bronchial asthma.*

**Primatene Mist Suspension** *Whitehall, USA.*
Adrenaline acid tartrate (p.852·2).
*Bronchial asthma.*

**Primatenol** *Streuli, Switz.*
Atenolol (p.865·2).
*Angina; arrhythmias; hypertension; myocardial infarction.*

**Primatenol Plus** *Streuli, Switz.*
Atenolol (p.865·2); chlortalidone (p.882·3).
*Hypertension.*

**Primatime** *Matara, Fr.*
Fertility test (p.1734·3).

**Primatour** *Viatris, Neth.*
Chlorcyclizine hydrochloride (p.427·2); cinnarizine (p.428·3).
*Motion sickness.*

**Primatuss Cough Mixture 4** *Rugby, USA.*
Chlorphenamine maleate (p.427·3); dextromethorphan hydrobromide (p.1117·3).
*Coughs and cold symptoms.*

**Primatuss Cough Mixture 4D** *Rugby, USA.*
Pseudoephedrine hydrochloride (p.1129·2); dextromethorphan hydrobromide (p.1117·3); guaifenesin (p.1122·1).
*Coughs.*

**Primavax** *Pasteur Merieux, Ital.†.*
A diphtheria, tetanus, and hepatitis B vaccine.
*Active immunisation.*

**Primavera-N** *Fabra, Arg.*
Metoclopramide hydrochloride (p.1274·3).
*Dyspepsia; nausea and vomiting.*

**Primaxin**
*Merck Sharp & Dohme, Austral.; Merck Frosst, Canad.; Vianex (Βιανεξ), Gr.; Merck Sharp & Dohme, NZ; Merck Sharp & Dohme, UK; Merck, USA.*
Imipenem (p.221·1); cilastatin sodium (p.188·1).
*Bacterial infections.*

**Primbactam** *Menarini, Ital.*
Aztreonam (p.160·3).
*Gram-negative bacterial infections.*

**Primcillin** *AstraZeneca, Denm.*
Phenoxymethylpenicillin potassium (p.242·1).
*Bacterial infections.*

**Prime Time** *Quest, Canad.†.*
Multivitamin and mineral preparation (p.1417·1).

**Primene**
*Baxter Immuno, Arg.; Baxter, Austral.; Baxter, Austria; Baxter, Canad.; Baxter, Fr.; Baxter, Ger.; Baxter, Irl.; Baxter, Mex.; Baxter, Spain; Baxter, UK.*
Amino-acid infusion (p.1417·1).
*Parenteral nutrition in infants.*

**Primera** *Eurofarma, Braz.*
Desogestrel (p.1547·2); ethinylestradiol (p.1553·2).
*Combined oral contraceptive.*

**Primeral**
*Note. This name is used for preparations of different composition.*
*Sanofi Synthelabo, Braz.*
Bromopride (p.1254·1); dimethicone (p.1289·2); pepsin (p.1729·3); α-amylase (p.1654·2); lipase.
*Digestive disorders; nausea and vomiting.*

*Master Pharma, Ital.†.*
Naproxen sodium (p.65·1).
*Musculoskeletal and joint disorders; pain.*

**Primeran** *Sanofi Synthelabo, Gr.*
Metoclopramide (p.1274·3) or metoclopramide hydrochloride (p.1274·3).
*Acid aspiration; aid in diagnostic procedures; delayed gastric emptying; gastro-oesophageal reflux disease; nausea and vomiting.*

**Primesin** *Schwarz, Ital.*
Fluvastatin sodium (p.918·2).
*Hypercholesterolaemia.*

**Primil** *Francia, Ital.*
Magnesium; potassium; vitamins (p.1417·1).
*Nutritional supplement.*

**Primiprost** *AstraZeneca, India.*
Dinoprostone (p.1515·1).
*Labour induction.*

**Primobolan**
*Schering, Austral.; Schering, Austria†; Schering, Ger.; Schering, Mex.; Schering, Norw.†; Schering, S.Afr.*
Metenolone acetate (p.1559·2) or metenolone enantate (p.1559·3).
*Anabolic; aplastic anaemia; breast cancer; liver disorders; osteoporosis.*

**Primobolan Depot**
*Shepa, Gr.; Schering, Ital.†; Schering, Spain.*
Metenolone enantate (p.1559·3).
*Anabolic; anaemia in chronic renal failure; aplastic anaemia; breast cancer; osteoporosis.*

**Primobolan S** *Schering, Neth.*
Metenolone acetate (p.1559·2).
*Aplastic anaemia.*

**Primocef** *Julphar, UAE.*
Cefotaxime sodium (p.175·3).
*Bacterial infections.*

**Primodian Depot**
*Schering, S.Afr.; Schering, Thai.*
Estradiol valerate (p.1550·2); testosterone enantate (p.1570·1).
*Menopausal disorders; osteoporosis.*

**Primodium** *Janssen-Cilag, Swed.*
Loperamide oxide (p.1271·1).
*Diarrhoea.*

**Primofenac** *Streuli, Switz.*
Diclofenac sodium (p.32·1).
*Gout; inflammation; musculoskeletal, joint, and peri-articular disorders; pain.*

**Primofol Depot** *Schering, Chile.*
Estradiol valerate (p.1550·2).
*Amenorrhoea; oestrogen deficiency.*

**Primogonyl** *Schering, Ger.*
Chorionic gonadotrophin (p.1320·3).
*Cryptorchidism, hypogonadism, and delayed puberty in males; infertility in females.*

**Primogyn** *Schering, Mex.*
Estradiol valerate (p.1550·2).
*Amenorrhoea; menorrhagia; oestrogen deficiency; uterine hypoplasia.*

**Primogyn Depot**
*Schering, Austral.; Schering, S.Afr.*
Estradiol valerate (p.1550·2).
*Amenorrhoea; dysfunctional uterine bleeding; uterine hypoplasia.*

**Primogyna**
*Schering, Braz.; Schering, Chile.*
Estradiol valerate (p.1550·2).
*Menopausal disorders; osteoporosis.*

**Primolut Depot**
*Schering, Chile; Schering, Mex.; Schering, S.Afr.†.*
Hydroxyprogesterone caproate (p.1556·3).
*Amenorrhoea; female infertility; threatened or recurrent miscarriage; uterine hypoplasia.*

**Primolut N**
*Schering, Austral.; Schering, Fin.; Schering, Hong Kong; German Remedies, India; Schering, Irl.; Schering, Malaysia; Schering, Neth.; Schering, Norw.; Schering, NZ; Schering, S.Afr.; Schering, Singapore; Schering, Switz.; Schering, Thai.; Schering, UK.*
Norethisterone (p.1562·2).
*Dysfunctional uterine bleeding; endometriosis; mastopathy; menstrual disorders.*

**Primolut-Nor**
*Schering, Arg.; Schering, Austria; Schering, Belg.; Schering, Braz.; Schering, Chile; Schering, Fin.; Schering, Fr.; Schering, Ger.; Shepa, Gr.; Schering, Israel; Schering, Ital.; Schering, Mex.; Schering, Port.; Schering, Spain; Schering, Swed.; Schering, Switz.†.*
Norethisterone acetate (p.1562·2).
*Breast cancer; dysfunctional uterine bleeding; endometriosis; mastopathy; menstrual disorders; uterine hypoplasia.*

**Primoniat Depot** *Schering, Chile.*
Testosterone propionate (p.1570·1); testosterone enantate (p.1570·1).
Some injections contain only testosterone enantate.
*Aplastic anaemia; breast cancer; male hypogonadism.*

**Primonil** *Teva, Israel.*
Imipramine hydrochloride (p.300·1).
*Depression; nocturnal enuresis.*

**Primoris** *Herbarium, Braz.*
Linoleic acid (p.1690·2); oleic acid (p.1481·3); gamolenic acid (p.1690·2).

**Primosiston**
*Note. This name is used for preparations of different composition.*
*Schering, Arg.; Schering, Mex.; Schering, Switz.*
*Injection:* Hydroxyprogesterone caproate (p.1556·3); estradiol benzoate (p.1550·1).
*Metrorrhagia.*

*Schering, Austria; Schering, Braz.; Schering, Chile; Schering, Ger.; Schering, Spain†; Schering, Switz.*
*Tablets:* Norethisterone acetate (p.1562·2); ethinylestradiol (p.1553·2).
*Dysfunctional uterine bleeding; menstrual disorders.*

**Primostat** *Schering, Mex.*
Gestonorone caproate (p.1556·2).
*Benign prostatic hyperplasia; endometrial cancer.*

**Primoteston Depot**
*Note. This name is used for preparations of different composition.*
*Schering, Austral.; Schering, Mex.; Schering, NZ; Schering, UK†.*
Testosterone enantate (p.1570·1).
*Aplastic anaemia; breast cancer; endometrial cancer; male androgen deficiency; male hypogonadism.*

*Schering, Norw.*
Testosterone enantate (p.1570·1); testosterone propionate (p.1570·1).
Some injections contain only testosterone enantate.
*Androgenic; genital cancer in females; hypogonadism in males.*

**Primotussan** *Galenika, Ger.†.*
Cowslip rhizome (p.1735·1); thyme (p.1755·2).
*Cold symptoms.*

**Primover** *Alcon Cusi, Spain.*
Sodium cromoglicate (p.795·3).
*Allergic conjunctivitis.*

**Primovist** *Schering, Swed.*
Gadoxetate disodium (p.1063·1).
*Contrast medium for magnetic resonance imaging of the liver.*

**Primovlar** *Schering, Braz.†.*
Norgestrel (p.1563·2); ethinylestradiol (p.1553·2).
*Combined oral contraceptive.*

**Primoxil** *Bayer, Ital.†.*
Moexipril hydrochloride (p.961·2).
*Hypertension.*

**Primperan**
*Sanofi Synthelabo, Belg.; Sanofi Winthrop, Denm.; Sanofi Synthelabo, Fin.; Sanofi Synthelabo, Fr.; Sanofi Synthelabo, Hong Kong; Fujisawa, Jpn; Sanofi Synthelabo, Malaysia; Sanofi Synthelabo, Mex.; Lorex Synthelabo, Neth.†; Sanofi Synthelabo, Norw.; Sanofi Synthelabo, Port.; Sanofi Synthelabo, Singapore; Sanofi Synthelabo, Spain; Sanofi Synthelabo, Swed.; Synthelabo, Switz.; Berk, UK.*
Metoclopramide (p.1274·3) or metoclopramide hydrochloride (p.1274·3).
*Adjunct in gastrointestinal examination; gastro-oesophageal reflux; gastrointestinal motility disorders; nausea and vomiting.*

**Primperan Complex** *Synthelabo, Spain†.*
Dimethicone (p.1289·2); metoclopramide (p.1274·3); sorbitol (p.1446·3).
*Aerophagia; dyspepsia; hiatus hernia; meteorism; vomiting.*

**Primperil** *Lacefa, Arg.*
Metoclopramide (p.1274·3).
*Nausea and vomiting.*

**Primperoxane** *Synthelabo, Fr.†.*
Metoclopramide (p.1274·3); dimethicone (p.1289·2).
*Dyspepsia.*

**Primpesasy** *Sanofi Synthelabo, Mex.*
Metoclopramide hydrochloride (p.1274·3); dimeticone (p.1289·2).
*Aid to gastrointestinal examination; gastritis; hiatus hernia; nausea and vomiting; oesophagitis; peptic ulcer.*

**Primsol** *Ascent, USA.*
Trimethoprim hydrochloride (p.273·2).
*Otitis media; urinary-tract infections.*

**Primum** *Labinca, Arg.*
Flunitrazepam (p.698·2).
*Hypnotic.*

**Primyxine** *Alpharma, Fr.*
Oxytetracycline hydrochloride (p.241·1); polymyxin B sulfate (p.245·1).
*Skin and wound infections.*

**Prinachol** *Zurita, Braz.*
Cynara (p.1678·3); boldo (p.1661·2).
*Liver disorders.*

**Prinactizide** *Irex, Fr.†.*
Altizide (p.858·1); spironolactone (p.1003·1).
*Hypertension; oedema.*

**Princi B1 + B6** *Sanofi Synthelabo, Neth.*
Thiamine hydrochloride (p.1455·1); pyridoxine hydrochloride (p.1456·3).
*Vitamin B deficiency associated with alcoholism.*

**Princi-B**
*Bournonville, Belg.†.*
Vitamin B substances (p.1417·1).
*Alcoholism; cardiovascular disorders; drug intoxication; neurogenic pain; rheumatic pain.*

*SERP, Mon.*
Pyridoxine hydrochloride; thiamine nitrate (p.1417·1).
*Asthenia.*

*Sanofi Synthelabo, Thai.*
Vitamin $B_1$ (p.1455·2); vitamin $B_6$ (p.1457·2); vitamin $B_{12}$ (p.1458·2).
*Beri-beri; neuritis.*

**Princi-B Fort**
*Sanofi Synthelabo, Hong Kong; Sanofi Synthelabo, Malaysia; Sanofi Synthelabo, Singapore.*
Vitamin $B_1$ (p.1455·2); vitamin $B_6$ (p.1457·2); vitamin $B_{12}$ (p.1458·2).
*Neuralgias; neuritis; tonic; vitamin B deficiency.*

**Principen** *Apothecon, USA.*
Ampicillin trihydrate (p.157·2).
*Bacterial infections.*

**Princol** *Provit, Mex.*
Lincomycin hydrochloride (p.226·2).
*Bacterial infections.*

**Prindex** *Abbott, Mex.*
Pseudoephedrine hydrochloride (p.1129·2); carbinoxamine maleate (p.426·3).
*Upper respiratory-tract congestion.*

**Prinil** *Merck Sharp & Dohme, Switz.*
Lisinopril (p.946·3).
*Heart failure; hypertension.*

**Prinivil**
*Amrad, Austral.; Merck Sharp & Dohme, Austria; Prodome, Braz.; Merck Frosst, Canad.; Bristol-Myers Squibb, Fr.; Vianex (Βιανεξ), Gr.; Merck Sharp & Dohme, Hong Kong; Bristol-Myers Squibb, Ital.; Merck Sharp & Dohme, Malaysia; Merck Sharp & Dohme, Mex.; Merck Sharp & Dohme, NZ; Merck Sharp & Dohme, Port.; Merck Sharp & Dohme, S.Afr.; Merck Sharp & Dohme, Singapore; Bristol-Myers Squibb, Spain; Merck, USA.*
Lisinopril (p.946·3).
*Diabetic nephropathy; heart failure; hypertension; myocardial infarction.*

**Prinivil Plus** *Bristol-Myers Squibb, Spain.*
Lisinopril (p.946·3); hydrochlorothiazide (p.933·2).
*Hypertension.*

**Prinol Plus** *Rivero, Arg.*
Preparation for enteral nutrition (p.1417·1).

**Prinox** *Andromaco, Arg.*
Alprazolam (p.668·3).
*Anxiety; panic attacks; phobias.*

**Prinsyl** *Coventry, UK†.*
Chloroxylenol (p.1177·2).

**Printan** *Raffo, Chile.*
Sodium chloride (p.1233·3).
*Nasal congestion; nasal hygiene.*

**Printania** *Clintec, Fr.†.*
High protein nutritional supplement (p.1417·1).

**Printol** *Coventry, UK†.*
Tar acids (p.1193·3).

**Prinzide**
*Prodome, Braz.; Merck Frosst, Canad.; Bristol-Myers Squibb, Fr.; Bristol-Myers Squibb, Ital.; Merck Sharp & Dohme, Mex.; Merck Sharp & Dohme, NZ†; Merck Sharp & Dohme, Port.; Merck Sharp & Dohme, Switz.; Merck, USA.*
Lisinopril (p.946·3); hydrochlorothiazide (p.933·2).
*Hypertension.*

**Prioderm**
*Viatris, Belg.; Norpharma, Denm.; Mundipharma, Fin.; Sarget, Fr.; SSL, Irl.; Rafa, Israel; Viatris, Neth.; Mundipharma, Norw.; SSL, NZ; Mundipharma, Swed.; Mundipharma, Switz.; SSL, UK.*
Malathion (p.1507·1).
*Pediculosis; scabies.*

**Priorin**
*Roche, Austria; Roche Nicholas, Ger.*
Millet; calcium pantothenate; cystine (p.1417·1).
*Hair and nail disorders.*

*Roche, Ital.†.*
Millet; calcium pantothenate; cystine; wheat-germ oil (p.1417·1).
*Skin disorders.*

**Priorin Biotin** *Roche Nicholas, Ger.†.*
Biotin (p.1423·2).
*Biotin deficiency.*

**Priorin N** *Roche, Switz.*
Millet; calcium pantothenate; cystine; wheat-germ oil (p.1417·1).
*Hair and nail disorders.*

**Priorix**
*GlaxoSmithKline, Austral.; GlaxoSmithKline, Austria; GlaxoSmithKline, Belg.; GlaxoSmithKline, Braz.; GlaxoSmithKline, Canad.; GlaxoSmithKline, Fin.; GlaxoSmithKline, Fr.; GlaxoSmithKline, Ger.; SmithKline Beecham, Gr.; GlaxoSmithKline, Hong Kong; GlaxoSmithKline, Irl.; SmithKline Beecham, Israel; GlaxoSmithKline, Ital.; GlaxoSmithKline, Malaysia; SmithKline Beecham, Mex.; Smith Kline & French, Port.†; GlaxoSmithKline, S.Afr.; GlaxoSmithKline, Singapore; GlaxoSmithKline, Spain; GlaxoSmithKline, Swed.; SmithKline Beecham, Switz.; GlaxoSmithKline, Thai.; GlaxoSmithKline, UK.*
A measles, mumps, and rubella vaccine (attenuated Schwarz, Jeryl Lynn, and Wistar RA 27/3 strains respectively) (p.1625·1).
*Active immunisation.*

**Priovit 12** *SIT, Ital.*
Multivitamin preparation (p.1417·1).

**Priper** *Armstrong, Arg.*
Pipemidic acid (p.243·1).
*Genito-urinary tract infections; infected wounds, burns, and ulcers.*

**Priper Plus** *Armstrong, Arg.*
Pipemidic acid (p.243·1); phenazopyridine (p.83·2).
*Genito-urinary tract infections.*

**Pripsen**
*Note. This name is used for preparations of different composition.*
*Thornton & Ross, Irl.*
Piperazine phosphate (p.111·2); sennosides (p.1288·2).
*Ascariasis; enterobiasis.*

Thornton & Ross, UK.
*Elixir:* Piperazine citrate (p.111·2).
*Ascariasis; enterobiasis.*
*Oral powder:* Piperazine phosphate (p.111·2); senna (p.1288·2).
*Ascariasis; enterobiasis.*
*Tablets:* Mebendazole (p.108·2).
*Enterobiasis.*

**Priscol** *Ciba Vision, Ger.†.*
Tolazoline hydrochloride (p.1015·1).
*Vascular eye disorders.*

**Priscoline**
*Novartis, Austral.†; Novartis, NZ†; Ciba, USA†.*
Tolazoline hydrochloride (p.1015·1).
*Persistent pulmonary hypertension of the newborn.*

**Prisdal** *Almirall, Spain.*
Citalopram hydrobromide (p.289·1).
*Anxiety; depression; obsessive-compulsive disorder.*

**Prisma**
*Note. This name is used for preparations of different composition.*
*Pasteur, Chile.*
Citalopram (p.289·1).
*Depression.*
*Thiemann, Ger.*
Mianserin hydrochloride (p.306·3).
*Depression.*
*Mediolanum, Ital.; Medinfar, Port.*
Mesoglycan sodium (p.1714·1).
*Cerebral and peripheral vascular disorders; hyperlipidaemias; thromboembolic disorders.*

**Prisoventril** *Simoes, Braz.*
Phenolphthalein (p.1284·1); cascara (p.1255·1).
*Constipation.*

**Pristine**
*Xepa-Soul Pattinson, Hong Kong; Xepa-Soul Pattinson, Malaysia; Xepa-Soul Pattinson, Singapore.*
Ketoconazole (p.403·3).
*Dandruff; pityriasis versicolor; seborrhoeic dermatitis.*

**Pristinex**
*Xepa-Soul Pattinson, Hong Kong; Xepa-Soul Pattinson, Malaysia; Xepa-Soul Pattinson, Singapore.*
Ketoconazole (p.403·3).
*Fungal infections.*

**Pritor**
*GlaxoSmithKline, Arg.; GlaxoSmithKline, Austral.; GlaxoSmithKline, Braz.; GlaxoSmithKline, Fr.; Glaxo Wellcome, Gr.; GlaxoSmithKline, Ital.; Glaxo Wellcome, Port.; Glaxo Wellcome, Spain.*
Telmisartan (p.1010·1).
*Hypertension.*

**Pritor Plus** *GlaxoSmithKline, Spain.*
Telmisartan (p.1010·1); hydrochlorothiazide (p.933·2).
*Hypertension.*

**Pritoral** *GlaxoSmithKline, Chile.*
Telmisartan (p.1010·1).
*Hypertension.*

**PritorPlus** *GlaxoSmithKline, Fr.*
Telmisartan (p.1010·1); hydrochlorothiazide (p.933·2).
*Hypertension.*

**Privacom** *Typharm, UK.*
Clotrimazole (p.396·2).
*Vaginal candidiasis.*

**Privin**
*Novartis, Austria; Novartis Consumer, Ger.*
Naphazoline nitrate (p.1124·3).
*Aid to cystoscopy and rhinoscopy; nasal congestion.*

**Privina**
*Novartis, Arg.; Novartis, Braz.*
Naphazoline nitrate (p.1124·3).
*Nasal congestion.*

**Privine** *Ciba, USA.*
Naphazoline hydrochloride (p.1124·3).
*Nasal congestion.*

**Privituss** *Mitim, Ital.*
Cloperastine fendizoate (p.1117·2).
*Coughs.*

**Prixar** *Lepetit, Ital.*
Levofloxacin (p.225·3).
*Bacterial infections.*

**Prixin** *Richmond, Arg.*
Ampicillin (p.157·1); sulbactam (p.257·2).
*Bacterial infections.*

**Prizem** *Solfran, Mex.*
Diazepam (p.690·1).

**Prizma** *Unipharm, Israel.*
Fluoxetine hydrochloride (p.292·1).
*Bulimia nervosa; depression; obsessive-compulsive disorder.*

**Pro Dorm** *Synthelabo, Ger.†.*
Lorazepam (p.704·1).
*Anxiety; sleep disorders.*

**Pro Lertus** *Tecnofarma, Chile.*
Diclofenac colestyramine (p.33·1).
*Inflammation; musculoskeletal and joint disorders; pain.*

**Pro Ulco** *Solvay, Spain.*
Lansoprazole (p.1269·3).
*Gastro-oesophageal reflux; peptic ulcer.*

**Pro-Actidil**
*Glaxo Wellcome, Austria†; Wellcome, Israel; Wellcome, Spain.*
Triprolidine hydrochloride (p.442·3).
*Hypersensitivity reactions; skin disorders.*

**Proaf** *Abic, Israel.*
Isoflupredone acetate (p.1105·3); ephedrine hydrochloride (p.1120·1); naphazoline nitrate (p.1124·3).
*Rhinitis; sinusitis.*

**Proagil** *Marien, Austria.*
Homoeopathic preparation.

**Proaller** *Pekana, Ger.*
Homoeopathic preparation.

**ProAmatine** *Shire Richwood, USA.*
Midodrine hydrochloride (p.959·2).
*Orthostatic hypotension.*

**Proampi** *GlaxoSmithKline Sante, Fr.*
Pivampicillin (p.244·1).
*Bacterial infections.*

**Proartinal** *Provit, Mex.*
Ibuprofen (p.45·3).
*Inflammation; pain.*

**Proasma-T** *Progress, Thai.*
Terbutaline sulfate (p.797·2).
*Obstructive airways disease; premature labour.*

**Pro-Banthine**
*Sigma, Austral.; Searle, Belg.†; Roberts, Canad.†; Searle, Denm.†; RPG, India; Baker Norton, Irl.†; Searle, Israel†; Sigma, NZ; Searle, S.Afr.; Searle, Switz.†; Hansam, UK; Schiapparelli Searle, USA.*
Propantheline bromide (p.489·1).
*Adjunct in gastrointestinal diagnostic procedures; gastrointestinal disorders; hyperhidrosis; nocturnal enuresis; peptic ulcer; renal colic.*

**Probase 3** *Schering-Plough, UK.*
Emollient.
*Dry skin.*

**Probax** *Fischer, USA.*
Propolis (p.1735·2).
*Skin disorders.*

**Probec** *Farmoquimica, Braz.*
Ambroxol hydrochloride (p.1114·3).
*Respiratory-tract congestion.*

**Probecid**
*AstraZeneca, Fin.; AstraZeneca, Norw.; Astra, Swed.*
Probenecid (p.416·3).
*Adjunct to beta-lactam antibacterials; gout.*

**Probecilin** *Eurofarma, Braz.†.*
Procaine benzylpenicillin (p.246·1).
Probenecid (p.416·3) is included in this preparation to reduce renal tubular excretion of the antibiotic.
*Bacterial infections.*

**Probec-T** *J&J-Merck, USA.*
Vitamin B substances with vitamin C (p.1417·1).

**Probeks** *Hebron, Braz.*
Aloe vera (p.1141·3).
*Skin disorders.*

**Proben** *Quatromed, S.Afr.*
Probenecid (p.416·3).
*Gout.*

**Probenxil** *Cimed, Braz.*
Diclofenac potassium (p.32·1).
*Inflammation.*

**Probenzima** *Farmoquimica, Braz.†.*
Ampicillin sodium (p.157·1).
*Bacterial infections.*

**Probenzima Ampicilina** *Farmoquimica, Braz.†.*
Ampicillin (p.157·1); trypsin (p.1758·3); chymotrypsin (p.1671·2).
*Bacterial infections; inflammation.*

**Probenzima Analgesico** *Farmoquimica, Braz.†.*
Paracetamol (p.76·2); trypsin (p.1758·3); chymotrypsin (p.1671·2).
*Inflammation; pain.*

**Probeta** *Allergan, Canad.*
Levobunolol hydrochloride (p.946·2); dipivefrine hydrochloride (p.1681·2).
*Glaucoma; ocular hypertension.*

**Probi-Albumin** *Probifasa, Mex.*
Albumin (p.740·3).
*Acute barbiturate overdosage; burns; hypoproteinaemia; nephrotic syndrome; pancreatitis; plasma volume expansion; shock.*

**Probigol** *Biohorma, Ital.*
Propolis (p.1735·2); echinacea (p.1683·2).
*Oral hygiene.*

**Pro-Bionate** *Natren, USA.*
*Lactobacillus acidophilus* (p.1704·2).
*Dietary supplement.*

**Probiophyt V** *OTW, Ger.†.*
Silybum marianum (p.1043·3).
*Liver disorders.*

**Probiox** *Baif, Ital.†.*
Vitamin B substances (p.1417·1); lactic-acid-producing organisms (p.1704·2).
*Gastrointestinal disorders.*

**Probi-Rho D** *Probifasa, Mex.*
An anti-D immunoglobulin (p.1608·1).
*Prevention of rhesus sensitisation.*

**Probi-Tet** *Probifasa, Mex.*
Tetanus immunoglobulin (p.1640·3).
*Passive immunisation.*

**Probitor**
*Biochemie, Austral.; Tyrol, Austria; Novartis, Gr.; Biochemie, Thai.; Novartis, Thai.*
Omeprazole (p.1278·2).
*Gastro-oesophageal reflux; peptic ulcer; Zollinger-Ellison syndrome.*

**Probofex** *Wockhardt, India.*
Ferrous fumarate (p.1427·3); folic acid (p.1429·1); vitamin $B_1$; vitamin $B_6$; vitamin $B_{12}$; nicotinamide (p.1417·1).
Vitamin C (p.1460·2) is included in this preparation to increase the absorption and availability of iron.
*Iron-deficiency anaemia.*

**Probufen** *Nakornpatana, Thai.*
Ibuprofen (p.45·3).
*Musculoskeletal and joint disorders.*

**Pro-C** *Procare, Austral.†.*
Ascorbic acid (p.1460·2).
*Vitamin C supplement.*

**Pro-30C** *Capo Sole, Ital.*
Propolis (p.1735·2).

**Procadax** *Fulford, India.*
Ceftibuten (p.182·1).
*Bacterial infections.*

**Procadil** *Recordati, Ital.*
Procaterol hydrochloride (p.791·1).
*Obstructive airways disease.*

**Procal**
*Note. A similar name is used for preparations of different composition (see below).*
*Christiaens, Belg.*
Sodium fluoride (p.1444·3).
*Osteoporosis.*

**Pro-Cal**
*Note. A similar name is used for preparations of different composition (see above).*
*Vitaflo, Irl.; Vitaflo, UK.*
Preparation for enteral nutrition (p.1417·1).

**ProcalAmine**
*Braun McGaw, Hong Kong†.*
Amino-acid infusion (p.1417·1).
*Parenteral nutrition.*
*Pisa, Mex.*
Amino-acid, glycerol, and electrolyte preparation (p.1417·1).
*Parenteral nutrition.*
*McGaw, NZ†.*
Amino-acid, carbohydrate, and electrolyte infusion (p.1417·1).
*Parenteral nutrition.*
*McGaw, USA.*
Amino-acid and electrolyte infusion (p.1417·1).
*Parenteral nutrition.*

**Procal-D** *Kato, Singapore†.*
Calcium (p.1225·1); vitamin D (p.1461·2).
*Calcium and vitamin D deficiency.*

**Pro-Cal-Sof** *Vangard, USA†.*
Docusate calcium (p.1262·1).
*Constipation.*

**Procamide**
*Zambon, Braz.; Zambon, Ital.†.*
Procainamide hydrochloride (p.987·1).
*Arrhythmias.*

**Procan** *Pfizer, Canad.*
Procainamide hydrochloride (p.987·1).
*Arrhythmias.*

**Procanbid** *Monarch, USA.*
Procainamide hydrochloride (p.987·1).
Formerly called Procan SR.
*Ventricular arrhythmias.*

**Procanest** *Gray, Arg.*
Procaine hydrochloride (p.1383·2).
*Local anaesthesia.*

**Procaneural** *RAN, Ger.*
Procaine hydrochloride (p.1383·2); caffeine (p.782·1).
*Nervous system disorders.*

**Procaptan** *Stroder, Ital.*
Perindopril erbumine (p.980·2).
*Heart failure; hypertension.*

**Procardia** *Pfizer, USA.*
Nifedipine (p.966·2).
*Angina pectoris; hypertension.*

**Procardin** *Medochemie, Singapore†.*
Dipyridamole (p.903·1).
*Thromboembolic disorders.*

**Procardol** *Adelco, Gr.*
Isosorbide mononitrate (p.942·1).
*Angina; heart failure.*

**Pro-Cas** *Milk Industries, Israel.*
Protein supplement (p.1417·1).

**Procavit** *EMS, Braz.*
Multivitamin, mineral, and amino-acid preparation (p.1417·1).

**Proceane Hypertonique** *Proceane, Fr.*
Mineral preparation (p.1417·1).
*Nutritional supplement.*

**Proceane Isotonique** *Proceane, Fr.*
*Nasal spray:* Sea water (p.1233·3).
*Nasal cleansing; nasal dryness.*
*Oral solution:* Mineral preparation (p.1417·1).
*Nutritional supplement.*

**Procef**
*Bristol-Myers Squibb, Austria; Bristol-Myers Squibb, Chile; Bristol-Myers Squibb, Fin.†; Bristol-Myers Squibb, Gr.; Bristol-Myers Squibb, Hong Kong; Dompe, Ital.; Bristol-Myers Squibb, Malaysia; Bristol-Myers Squibb, Mex.; Bristol-Myers Squibb, Port.; Bristol-Myers Squibb, Singapore; Bristol-Myers Squibb, Switz.; Bristol-Myers Squibb, Thai.*
Cefprozil (p.179·2).
*Bacterial infections.*

**Procelac** *Armstrong, Arg.*
Omeprazole (p.1278·2).
*Gastritis; gastro-oesophageal reflux; peptic ulcer; Zollinger-Ellison syndrome.*

**Procephal** *Provit, Mex.*
Erythromycin estolate (p.208·1).
*Bacterial infections.*

**Proceptin** *Beximco, Singapore.*
Omeprazole (p.1278·2).
*Acid aspiration; gastro-oesophageal reflux; gastrointestinal haemorrhage; gastrointestinal hyperacidity; peptic ulcer; Zollinger-Ellison syndrome.*

**Procetoken** *Microsules Bernabo, Arg.*
Fenofibrate (p.915·2).
*Hyperlipidaemias.*

**Prochieve** *Columbia, USA.*
Progesterone (p.1566·2).
*Amenorrhoea; female infertility.*

**Prochlor**
*Upha, Malaysia.*
Prochlorperazine (p.716·2).
*Nausea and vomiting; psychoses.*
*Beacons, Singapore.*
Prochlorperazine maleate (p.716·3).
*Anxiety; nausea and vomiting.*

**Prochol** *Procare, Austral.†.*
Nicotinic acid (p.1441·1); oat bran (p.1253·2).
*Hyperlipidaemias.*

**Prochor** *Protein, Mex.†.*
Propranolol (p.990·1).

**Prociclide** *Crinos, Ital.*
Defibrotide (p.892·1).
*Thrombosis prophylaxis.*

**Pro-Cid** *Pharmalab, Austral.*
Probenecid (p.416·3).
*Adjunct to beta-lactam antibacterials; gout; reduction of cidofovir-associated nephrotoxicity.*

**Procilin** *IQFA, Mex.*
Benzylpenicillin sodium (p.163·2); procaine benzylpenicillin (p.246·1).
*Bacterial infections.*

**Procillin** *Caps, S.Afr.*
Procaine benzylpenicillin (p.246·1).
*Bacterial infections.*

**Procimeti** *Provit, Mex.*
Cimetidine (p.1255·3).
*Peptic ulcer.*

**Procin** *Schering-Plough, Braz.*
Ciprofloxacin (p.188·2) or ciprofloxacin hydrochloride (p.188·2).
*Bacterial infections.*

**Procion** *Medipharm, Chile.*
Prednisone (p.1109·3).
*Corticosteroid.*

**Procirex** *KG, Ital.*
Bromopride hydrochloride (p.1254·1).
*Digestive disorders.*

**Proclim** *Fournier, Canad.†.*
Medroxyprogesterone acetate (p.1557·2).
*Menstrual disorders.*

**Proclimine** *Progress, Thai.*
Oxyphencyclimine hydrochloride (p.487·2).
*Gastrointestinal disorders; genito-urinary disorders.*

**Proclor** *Pentafarma, Port.*
Omeprazole (p.1278·2).

**Procloril** *Provit, Mex.*
Chloramphenicol (p.185·1).
*Bacterial infections.*

**Proclozine** *Pharmasant, Thai.*
Prochlorperazine maleate (p.716·3).
*Alcoholism; anxiety; mania; schizophrenia.*

**Procodin** *DHA, Singapore.*
Codeine phosphate (p.27·1); promethazine hydrochloride (p.439·1).
*Coughs.*

**Procodine** *Medipharma, Hong Kong.*
Promethazine hydrochloride (p.439·1); codeine phosphate (p.27·1); ephedrine hydrochloride (p.1120·1).
*Cold and influenza symptoms.*

**Procof** *Aspen, S.Afr.*
Diphenhydramine hydrochloride (p.431·3); pholcodine (p.1128·3); guaifenesin (p.1122·1).
*Coughs.*

**Procofen** *Alcon, Braz.†.*
Suprofen (p.93·1).
*Inflammatory eye disorders.*

**Procold** *Procare, Austral.†.*
Ascorbic acid (p.1460·2); horseradish (p.1697·3); verbascum thapsus (p.1764·1); euphorbia hirta (p.1686·3); garlic (p.1691·1).
*Respiratory-tract disorders.*

**Pro-Coll** *DMG, Ital.†.*
Amino acids, vitamin C, yeast, and minerals (p.1417·1).
*Nutritional supplement.*

**Procomfrin** *Planta, Canad.†.*
Comfrey (p.1675·2).
*Bruises; sprains; wounds.*

**Procomvax**
*Chiron Behring, Ger.; Vianex (Βιανέξ), Gr.; Aventis Pasteur, Ital.*
A haemophilus influenzae and hepatitis B vaccine (p.1616·3).
*Active immunisation.*

**Proconfial** *Schwabe, Arg.*
Drotaverine hydrochloride (p.1683·1).
*Smooth muscle spasm.*

**Procor**
*Note. This name is used for preparations of different composition.*
*Boehringer de Angeli, Braz.†.*
Dipyridamole (p.903·1).
*Ischaemic heart disease; thromboembolism prophylaxis.*

*Unipharm, Israel.*
Amiodarone hydrochloride (p.859·2).
*Angina pectoris; arrhythmias; heart failure; myocardial infarction.*

**Procor S** *Boehringer de Angeli, Braz.†.*
Dipyridamole (p.903·1); salicylic acid (p.1157·1).
*Thromboembolism prophylaxis.*

**Procordal**
*Muller Goppingen, Ger.; Staufen, Ger.*
Homoeopathic preparation.

**Procordal Gold** *Staufen, Ger.*
Homoeopathic preparation.

**Procort** *Roberts, USA.*
Hydrocortisone (p.1103·3).
*Corticosteroid.*

**Procorum**
*Ebewe, Austria; Abbott, Ger.; Abbott, Ital.; Knoll, Mex.; Knoll, Thai.*
Gallopamil hydrochloride (p.922·3).
*Angina pectoris; arrhythmias; hypertension; ischaemic heart disease; myocardial infarction.*

**Procosamine** *Usana, Hong Kong.*
Glucosamine sulfate (p.1694·1); calcium ascorbate (p.1460·2); manganese; silicon.
*Osteoarthritis.*

**Procoutol** *Spirig, Switz.*
Triclosan (p.1195·2).
*Skin disorders.*

**Procren**
*Abbott, Denm.; Abbott, Fin.; Abbott, Norw.; Abbott, Swed.*
Leuprorelin acetate (p.1331·1).
Formerly known as Lupron in *Swed.*
*Breast cancer; endometriosis; prostatic cancer; uterine fibroma.*

**Procrin** *Abbott, Spain.*
Leuprorelin acetate (p.1331·1).
*Endometriosis; female infertility; precocious puberty; prostatic cancer; uterine fibroma.*

**Procrit** *Ortho Biotech, USA.*
Epoetin alfa (p.747·2).
*Anaemia in cancer patients on chemotherapy; anaemia in zidovudine-treated HIV-infected patients; anaemia of chronic renal failure; pre-operative anaemias.*

**Proctalgen** *BC Lutz, Switz.*
Hamamelis (p.1696·3); diethylamine salicylate (p.34·1).
*Anorectal disorders.*

**Proctase-P** *Meiji, Thai.*
Proctase; pancreatin (p.1725·3).
*Haematoma; inflammation; oedema; respiratory-tract congestion.*

**Proctena** *Infosint, Ital.*
Hamamelis; aesculus; paeonia officinalis; cardiospermum halicacabum.

**Proctidol** *Novartis Consumer, Ital.*
Hydrocortisone acetate (p.1103·3); benzocaine (p.1370·3).
*Haemorrhoids.*

**Proctil** *Byk, Braz.†.*
Policresulen (p.1190·1); cinchocaine hydrochloride (p.1373·2).
*Haemorrhoids.*

**Proctium**
*Allergan-Frumtost, Braz.†; Esteve, Spain.*
Calcium dobesilate (p.1664·2); lidocaine hydrochloride (p.1377·3); prednisolone (p.1108·1).
*Anorectal disorders.*

**Procto** *Cophar, Switz.†.*
Fluocinolone acetonide (p.1101·2); lidocaine hydrochloride (p.1377·3).
*Anorectal disorders.*

**Procto Synalar** *Minerva (Μινερβα), Gr.*
Fluocinolone acetonide (p.1101·2); lidocaine hydrochloride (p.1377·3).
*Haemorrhoids.*

**Proctoacid** *Byk Gulden, Mex.*
Policresulen (p.1190·1); cinchocaine hydrochloride (p.1373·2).
*Anorectal disorders.*

**Proctocort**
*Boehringer Ingelheim, Fr.; Monarch, USA.*
Hydrocortisone (p.1103·3) or hydrocortisone acetate (p.1103·3).
*Anorectal disorders; Crohn's disease; haemorrhagic colitis.*

**Proctocream HC** *Stafford-Miller, UK†.*
Hydrocortisone acetate (p.1103·3); pramocaine hydrochloride (p.1382·2).
*Anorectal disorders.*

**Proctocream HC 2.5%** *Schwarz, USA.*
Hydrocortisone acetate (p.1103·3).
Proctocream HC formerly contained hydrocortisone acetate and pramocaine hydrochloride.
*Skin disorders.*

**Proctodan-HC** *Odan, Canad.*
Pramocaine hydrochloride (p.1382·2); hydrocortisone acetate (p.1103·3); zinc sulfate (p.1469·3).
*Anorectal disorders.*

**Proctofoam**
*Note. This name is used for preparations of different composition.*
*Omnimed, S.Afr.*
Hydrocortisone acetate (p.1103·3); pramocaine hydrochloride (p.1382·2).
*Anorectal disorders.*

*Schwarz, USA.*
Pramocaine hydrochloride (p.1382·2).
*Anorectal disorders.*

**Proctofoam-HC**
*Reed & Carnrick, Canad.; Stafford-Miller, Irl.; Medis, Israel; Stafford-Miller, Ital.; Meda, UK; Schwarz, USA.*
Hydrocortisone acetate (p.1103·3); pramocaine hydrochloride (p.1382·2).
*Anorectal disorders.*

**Proctogel** *Maver, Chile.*
Tribenoside (p.1757·3); lidocaine hydrochloride (p.1377·3).
*Haemorrhoids.*

**Procto-Glyvenol**
*Novartis, Austria†; Novartis, Braz.; Novartis, Chile; Novartis, Israel; Novartis, Mex.; Novartis Consumer, Port.; Novartis Consumer, Switz.*
Tribenoside (p.1757·3); lidocaine (p.1377·3) or lidocaine hydrochloride (p.1377·3).
*Haemorrhoids.*

**Procto-Ikatral** *Baliarda, Arg.*
OPC; lidocaine hydrochloride (p.1377·3); hydrocortisone acetate (p.1103·3).
*Haemorrhoids.*

**Procto-Jellin** *Grunenthal, Ger.*
Fluocinolone acetonide (p.1101·2); lidocaine hydrochloride (p.1377·3).
*Anorectal disorders.*

**Procto-Kaban** *Asche, Ger.*
Clocortolone pivalate (p.1096·1); clocortolone caproate (p.1096·1); cinchocaine hydrochloride (p.1373·2).
*Anorectal disorders.*

**Proctolog**
*Pfizer, Fr.; Menarini, Port.; Parke, Davis, Singapore; Juste, Spain.*
Ruscogenin (p.1741·1); trimebutine (p.1758·1).
*Anorectal disorders.*

**Proctolyn** *Recordati, Ital.*
Fluocinolone acetonide (p.1101·2); ketocaine hydrochloride (p.1377·1).
*Anorectal disorders.*

**Proctomyxin** *Sabex, Canad.*
Hydrocortisone (p.1103·3); framycetin sulfate (p.215·1); cinchocaine hydrochloride (p.1373·2); esculoside (p.1648·2).
*Anorectal disorders.*

**Proctonet** *Uniderm, Ital.*
Mallow (p.1709·3); aesculus (p.1648·2); almond oil (p.1651·1); hamamelis (p.1696·3).
*Anorectal disorders; personal hygiene.*

**Proctonostrum** *Nostrum, Port.*
Aluminium acetate (p.1652·3); hydrocortisone acetate (p.1103·3); lidocaine (p.1377·3); zinc oxide (p.1163·2).
*Anorectal disorders.*

**Proctoparf** *Whitehall-Much, Ger.†.*
Bufexamac (p.21·3); bismuth subgallate (p.1252·2); lidocaine hydrochloride (p.1377·3); titanium dioxide (p.1160·3).
*Anorectal disorders.*

**Proctoplex** *Knop, Chile.*
Hamamelis (p.1696·3); aesculus (p.1648·2); lidocaine hydrochloride (p.1377·3).
*Anorectal disorders.*

**Proctopure** *Dermofarma, Ital.*
Aescin (p.1648·2); aesculus (p.1648·2); hamamelis (p.1696·3); calendula (p.1665·2); liquorice (p.1270·2); melaleuca (p.1710·2).
*Anorectal disorders.*

**Proctor's Pinelyptus** *Ernest Jackson, UK.*
Eucalyptus oil (p.1686·2); menthol (p.1711·3); oleum pini sylvestris; siberian fir oil.
*Coughs; throat irritation.*

**Proctosan** *Hertz, Braz.†.*
Azulene (p.1658·3); hamamelis (p.1696·3); lidocaine (p.1377·3); menthol (p.1711·3); aesculus (p.1648·2).
*Haemorrhoids.*

**Proctosedyl**
*Note. This name is used for preparations of different composition.*
*Aventis, Austral.; Hoechst Marion Roussel, Israel†; Aventis, NZ; Aventis, UK.*
Cinchocaine hydrochloride (p.1373·2); hydrocortisone (p.1103·3).
*Anorectal disorders.*

*Aventis, Canad.; Aventis, Denm.; Aventis, Fin.; Aventis, Hong Kong; Aventis, Irl.; Aventis, Malaysia; Aventis, Norw.; Aventis, S.Afr.; Aventis, Singapore; Aventis, Swed.; Aventis, Thai.*
Cinchocaine hydrochloride (p.1373·2); hydrocortisone (p.1103·3); framycetin sulfate (p.215·1); esculoside (p.1648·2).
*Anorectal disorders.*

*Aventis, India.*
Hydrocortisone acetate (p.1103·3); heparin (p.927·3); framycetin sulfate (p.215·1); esculoside (p.1648·2); benzocaine (p.1370·3); butyl aminobenzoate (p.1373·1).
*Haemorrhoids.*

*Roche, Ital.*
*Ointment:* Amylocaine (p.1370·3); benzocaine (p.1370·3); hydrocortisone acetate (p.1103·3); esculoside (p.1648·2).
*Suppositories:* Benzocaine (p.1370·3); hydrocortisone acetate (p.1103·3); esculoside (p.1648·2).
*Anal pruritus; haemorrhoids.*

*Aventis, Neth.*
Cinchocaine hydrochloride (p.1373·2); hydrocortisone (p.1103·3); framycetin sulfate (p.215·1).
*Haemorrhoids.*

**Proctosoll** *Wassermann, Ital.*
Benzocaine (p.1370·3); hydrocortisone acetate (p.1103·3); heparin sodium (p.928·1).
*Haemorrhoids.*

**Proctosone**
*Note. This name is used for preparations of different composition.*
*Technilab, Canad.*
Cinchocaine hydrochloride (p.1373·2); hydrocortisone acetate (p.1103·3); framycetin sulfate (p.215·1); esculoside (p.1648·2).
Formerly contained cinchocaine hydrochloride, hydrocortisone acetate, neomycin sulfate, and esculoside.
*Anorectal disorders.*

*Technilab, Hong Kong.*
Cinchocaine hydrochloride (p.1373·2); hydrocortisone (p.1103·3); neomycin sulfate (p.235·1); esculoside (p.1648·2).
*Haemorrhoids.*

**Proctosor** *Soria Natural, Spain.*
Shepherd's purse (p.1744·1); hydrastis canadensis (p.1698·3); cupressus sempervirens.
*Haemorrhoids; menstrual disorders; uterine fibroids; varices.*

**Proctospre**
*Hennig, Ger.; Sanofi, Switz.†.*
Cinchocaine (p.1373·2); chlorquinaldol (p.187·3); diphenylpyraline (p.432·3).
*Anogenital disorders; anorectal disorders.*

**Proctosteroid** *Aldo, Spain.*
Triamcinolone diacetate (p.1110·2).
*Proctitis; proctosigmoiditis; ulcerative colitis.*

**Procto-Synalar**
*Note. This name is used for preparations of different composition.*
*Grunenthal, Austria.*
Fluocinolone acetonide (p.1101·2); lidocaine hydrochloride (p.1377·3).
*Anorectal disorders.*

*Yamanouchi, Belg.*
Fluocinolone acetonide (p.1101·2); lidocaine hydrochloride (p.1377·3); bismuth subgallate (p.1252·2); menthol (p.1711·3).
*Anorectal disorders.*

**Procto-Synalar N** *Grunenthal, Switz.*
Fluocinolone acetonide (p.1101·2); lidocaine hydrochloride (p.1377·3).
Procto-Synalar formerly contained fluocinolone acetonide, lidocaine hydrochloride, menthol, and bismuth subgallate.
*Anorectal disorders.*

**Proctozorin-N** *Teva, Israel.*
Hydrocortisone (p.1103·3); allantoin (p.1141·3); benzocaine (p.1370·3); aluminium acetotartrate (p.1652·3); menthol (p.1711·3); zinc oxide (p.1163·2).
*Anorectal disorders.*

**Proctyl**
*Byk, Arg.; Altana, Braz.*
Policresulen (p.1190·1); cinchocaine hydrochloride (p.1373·2).
*Anorectal disorders.*

**Proculin** *Chauvin ankerpharm, Ger.*
Naphazoline hydrochloride (p.1124·3).
*Conjunctivitis.*

**Procur** *Douglas, Austral.*
Cyproterone acetate (p.1544·1).
*Androgenisation in females; prostatic cancer; sexual deviation in males.*

**Pro-Cure** *Merck Sharp & Dohme, Israel.*
Finasteride (p.1554·2).
*Benign prostatic hyperplasia.*

**Procuta** *Pharmascience, Fr.*
Isotretinoin (p.1148·3).
*Acne.*

**Procutan**
*Note. This name is used for preparations of different composition.*
*Sankyo, Braz.*
Chloramphenicol (p.185·1); fibrinolysin (p.916·2); dornase alfa (p.1119·1).
*Skin infections.*

*Schering-Plough, S.Afr.*
Hydrocortisone (p.1103·3).
*Skin disorders.*

**Pro-Cute** *Ferndale, USA.*
Emollient and moisturiser.

**Procyclid** *ICN, Canad.*
Procyclidine hydrochloride (p.488·2).
*Parkinsonism.*

**Procyclo** *Organon, Ger.*
11 Tablets, estradiol valerate (p.1550·2); 10 tablets, estradiol valerate; medroxyprogesterone acetate (p.1557·2).
*Menopausal disorders.*

**Procythol** *Sanofi Synthelabo, Gr.*
Selegiline hydrochloride (p.1214·1).
*Parkinsonism.*

**Procytox** *Asta Medica, Canad.*
Cyclophosphamide (p.540·2).
*Malignant neoplasms.*

**Pro-Dafalgan**
*Bristol-Myers Squibb, Belg.; Bristol-Myers Squibb, Denm.; Bristol-Myers Squibb, Fin.; UPSA, Fr.†; Bristol-Myers Squibb, Norw.; Bristol-Myers Squibb, Port.; Bristol-Myers Squibb, Swed.; Upsamedica, Switz.*
Propacetamol hydrochloride (p.85·3).
*Fever; pain.*

**Prodafem**
*Pharmacia, Austria; Pharmacia, Switz.*
Medroxyprogesterone acetate (p.1557·2).
*Amenorrhoea; endometriosis; menopausal disorders; menorrhagia.*

**Prodamox** *Rubio, Spain.*
Proglumetacin maleate (p.85·2).
*Musculoskeletal, joint, and peri-articular disorders.*

**Prodasone**
*Pharmacia, Chile; Pharmacia Upjohn, Fr.†.*
Medroxyprogesterone acetate (p.1557·2).
*Amenorrhoea; breast and endometrial cancers; dysfunctional uterine bleeding; endometrial hyperplasia.*

**Prodazol** *Protein, Mex.†.*
Mebendazole (p.108·2).

**Prodeine** *Sanofi Synthelabo, Austral.*
Paracetamol (p.76·2); codeine phosphate (p.27·1).
*Fever; pain.*

**Prodel** *Pasteur, Chile.*
Chlorphenamine maleate (p.427·3).
*Hypersensitivity reactions.*

**Prodel B** *Pasteur, Chile.*
Betamethasone (p.1093·1); chlorphenamine maleate (p.427·3).
*Hypersensitivity reactions.*

**Prodep**
*Sun, Singapore†; Sun, Thai.*
Fluoxetine hydrochloride (p.292·1).
*Mixed anxiety depressive states; obsessive-compulsive disorder.*

**Proderm**
*Note. This name is used for preparations of different composition.*
*Galderma, Braz.*
Triclosan (p.1195·2).
*Skin disinfection.*

*Intra Pharma, Irl.*
Barrier preparation.

*Dow, USA.*
Castor oil (p.1668·2); peru balsam (p.1730·2).
*Decubitus ulcers.*

**Proderma** *Cantabria, Spain.*
Doxycycline hyclate (p.206·2).
*Bacterial infections.*

**Prodessal** *Almirall, Spain†.*
Cyanocobalamin (p.1458·2); cyclobutyrol (p.1678·2); cytidine; electrolytes (p.1217·1); uridine (p.1760·3).
*Liver disorders; oral hygiene.*

**Pro-Diaban**
*Schering, Austria; Bayer, Ger.†.*
Glisoxepide (p.333·1).
*Diabetes mellitus.*

**Prodicard** *AstraZeneca, Neth.†.*
Isosorbide dinitrate (p.941·1).
*Angina pectoris.*

**Prodiem Plain** *Novartis Consumer, Canad.*
Psyllium hydrophilic mucilloid (p.1268·1).
*Constipation; fibre supplement.*

**Prodiem Plus** *Novartis Consumer, Canad.*
Psyllium hydrophilic mucilloid (p.1268·1); senna pod (p.1288·2).
*Constipation.*

**Prodifer** *Provit, Mex.*
Ampicillin (p.157·1).
*Bacterial infections.*

**Prodigrip** *Aventis Pasteur, Spain.*
An influenza vaccine (p.1620·2).
*Active immunisation.*

**Prodil** *Farmasa, Braz.*
Doxazosin (p.909·1).
*Benign prostatic hyperplasia.*

**Prodilantin** *Pfizer, Fr.*
Fosphenytoin sodium (p.361·3).
*Epilepsy.*

**Prodis** *Procare, Austral.†.*
Multivitamins, amino acids, ginseng, and minerals (p.1417·1).
*Dietary supplement.*

**Prodium**
*Note. This name is used for preparations of different composition.*
*Propan, S.Afr.*
Loperamide hydrochloride (p.1271·1).
*Diarrhoea; ostomy management.*

*Breckenridge, USA.*
Phenazopyridine hydrochloride (p.83·1).
*Irritation of the lower urinary tract.*

**Prodiuret** *Sabona, Ger.*
Equisetum (p.1684·1).
*Oedema; urinary-tract disorders.*

**Prodolina** *Promeco, Mex.*
Dipyrone (p.35·3).
*Fever; pain.*

**Prodon** *Tika, Swed.*
Ketoprofen (p.51·2).
*Musculoskeletal and joint disorders.*

**Prodop** *Protein, Mex.†.*
Methyldopa (p.953·2).

**Prodopa** *Pacific, NZ.*
Methyldopa (p.953·2).
*Hypertension.*

**Prodorol** *Be-Tabs, S.Afr.*
Propranolol hydrochloride (p.989·3).
*Angina pectoris; anxiety; arrhythmias; hypertension; hyperthyroidism; phaeochromocytoma.*

**Prodoxidil** *Prodotti, Braz.*
Piroxicam (p.84·2).

**Prodoxil** *Prodotti, Braz.*
Amoxicillin trihydrate (p.155·3).
*Bacterial infections.*

**Prodoxin** *Prodotti, Braz.*
Ceftriaxone sodium (p.182·3).
*Bacterial infections.*

**Prodren** *Alcon, Israel.*
Dipivefrine hydrochloride (p.1681·2).
*Glaucoma.*

**Product Code 889** *Scientific Hospital Supplies, Austral.*
Preparation for enteral nutrition (p.1417·1).
*Methylmalonic acidaemia; propionic acidaemia.*

**Produvir** *Prodotti, Braz.*
Zidovudine (p.658·2).
*HIV infection.*

**Pro-Efferalgan**
*Upsa, Ital.; Upsamedica, Spain.*
Propacetamol hydrochloride (p.85·3).
*Pain.*

**Proendotel** *Fidia, Ital.*
Cloricromen hydrochloride (p.889·1).
*Thrombotic disorders.*

**Proepa** *Prodome, Braz.*
Polyunsaturated fatty acids (p.1417·1).
*Thrombosis prophylaxis.*

**Pro-Epanutin**
*Pfizer, Austral.†; Pfizer, Austria; Pfizer, Denm.; Pfizer, Fin.; Pfizer, Gr.; Parke, Davis, Irl.; Parke, Davis, Neth.; Pfizer, Norw.; Parke, Davis, Port.†; Pfizer, Swed.; Pfizer, UK.*
Fosphenytoin sodium (p.361·3).
*Epilepsy; seizures associated with neurosurgery and head trauma.*

**Proesten** *Procare, Austral.†.*
Vitamins; minerals (p.1417·1); garlic (p.1691·1); cimicifuga (p.1671·3); viburnum opulus; passion flower (p.1729·1); sarsaparilla (p.1742·1).
*Dietary supplement; menopausal disorders.*

**Proetzonide** *Dallas, Arg.*
Budesonide (p.1094·2).
*Asthma.*

**Proetztotal** *Dallas, Arg.*
*Nasal spray:* Phenylephrine hydrochloride (p.1126·3); neomycin sulfate (p.235·1); chlorphenamine maleate (p.427·3); gramicidin (p.220·2).
*Nebuliser solution:* Phenylephrine hydrochloride (p.1126·3); neomycin sulfate (p.235·1); dexamethasone sodium phosphate (p.1097·2); chlorphenamine maleate (p.427·3).

**Prof** *Elvetium, Arg.*
Galactosaminoglucuronoglycan sulfate.
*Degenerative joint disorders.*

**Profact** *Aventis, Ger.*
Buserelin acetate (p.1319·2).
*Prostatic cancer.*

**Profamid**
*Orion, Denm.; Orion, Fin.*
Flutamide (p.556·2).
*Prostatic cancer.*

**Profar** *Infar, India.*
Allylestrenol (p.1541·3).
*Benign prostatic hyperplasia.*

**Profargil** *Profarb, Braz.†.*
Metronidazole (p.607·2); vitamin $B_1$; vitamin $B_2$; vitamin $B_6$ (p.1417·1).
*Alcoholism; protozoal infections.*

**Profasi**
*Serono, Arg.; Serono, Austral.; Serono, Austria; Novartis, Chile; Serono, Denm.; Serono, Fin.; Serono, Gr.; Serono, Hong Kong; Serum Institute, India; Serono, Irl.; Serono, Malaysia; Serono, Mex.; Serono, Neth.; Serono, Norw.; Serono, NZ; Serono, S.Afr.; Serono, Singapore; Serono, Swed.; Serono, Switz.; Serono, Thai.; Serono, UK†; Serono, USA.*
Chorionic gonadotrophin (p.1320·3).
*Cryptorchidism; delayed puberty; hypogonadotrophic hypogonadism; male and female infertility; threatened or recurrent miscarriage.*

**Profasi HP**
*Serono, Braz.; Serono, Canad.; Serono, Ital.; Serono, Port.; Serono, Spain.*
Chorionic gonadotrophin (p.1320·3).
*Cryptorchidism; delayed puberty; hypogonadotrophic hypogonadism; male and female infertility; threatened or recurrent miscarriage.*

**Profed** *Progress, Thai.*
Triprolidine hydrochloride (p.442·3); pseudoephedrine hydrochloride (p.1129·2).
*Allergic rhinitis; cold symptoms; hay fever; nasal congestion.*

**Profelina** *Farcoral, Mex.†.*
Dipyrone (p.35·3).

**Profelixir** *Farcoral, Mex.*
Vitamin preparation (p.1417·1).
*Tonic.*

**Profemina** *Laboratorios Chile, Chile.*
Conjugated oestrogens (p.1543·2).
*Menopausal disorders; osteoporosis.*

**Profemina CC** *Laboratorios Chile, Chile.*
Conjugated oestrogens (p.1543·2); medroxyprogesterone (p.1557·3).
*Menopausal disorders; osteoporosis.*

**Profemina MP** *Laboratorios Chile, Chile.*
18 Tablets, conjugated oestrogens (p.1543·2); 12 tablets, conjugated oestrogens; medroxyprogesterone acetate (p.1557·2).
*Menopausal disorders; osteoporosis.*

**Profen** *Wakefield, USA†.*
Phenylpropanolamine hydrochloride (p.1127·3); guaifenesin (p.1122·1).
*Upper respiratory-tract symptoms.*

**Profen II** *Ivax, USA.*
Pseudoephedrine hydrochloride (p.1129·2); guaifenesin (p.1122·1).
Formerly contained phenylpropanolamine hydrochloride and guaifenesin.
*Coughs.*

**Profen II DM** *Ivax, USA.*
Pseudoephedrine hydrochloride (p.1129·2); guaifenesin (p.1122·1); dextromethorphan hydrobromide (p.1117·3).
Formerly contained phenylpropanolamine hydrochloride, guaifenesin, and dextromethorphan hydrobromide.
*Coughs.*

**Profen Forte DM** *Ivax, USA.*
Pseudoephedrine hydrochloride (p.1129·2); dextromethorphan hydrobromide (p.1117·3); guaifenesin (p.1122·1).
Formerly contained phenylpropanolamine hydrochloride, dextromethorphan hydrobromide, and guaifenesin.
*Coughs.*

**Profena** *Pond's, Thai.*
Ibuprofen (p.45·3).
*Musculoskeletal and joint disorders.*

**Profenal** *Alcon, USA.*
Suprofen (p.93·1).
*Inhibition of intra-operative miosis.*

**Profenda** *Jamieson, Canad.†.*
Betacarotene, vitamin C, and vitamin E (p.1417·1).

**Profenid**
*Aventis, Arg.; Aventis, Austria; Aventis, Braz.; Aventis, Chile; Aventis, Fr.; Aventis, Israel; Aventis, Mex.; Vitoria, Port.; Aventis, Thai.*
Ketoprofen (p.51·2).
*Gout; inflammation; musculoskeletal, joint, peri-articular, and soft-tissue disorders; pain.*

**Profenil** *Pascual, Hong Kong.*
Alverine citrate (p.1250·2).
*Gastrointestinal spasm.*

**Profeno** *Milano, Thai.*
Ibuprofen (p.45·3).
*Pain.*

**Profenzol** *Farcoral, Mex.*
Mebendazole (p.108·2).
*Worm infections.*

**Profer**
*Aesculapius, Ital.†; Tedec Meiji, Spain.*
Ferritin (p.1427·2).
*Iron deficiency; iron-deficiency anaemias.*

**Profergan** *Teuto, Braz.*
Promethazine hydrochloride (p.439·1).
*Nausea and vomiting; sedative; vertigo.*

**Profex** *Dragenopharm, Israel.*
Propafenone hydrochloride (p.988·3).
*Arrhythmias.*

**Profiber** *Sherwood, USA.*
Lactose-free preparation for enteral nutrition (p.1417·1).

**Profibra** *Support, Braz.*
Dietary fibre supplement (soya polysaccharides) (p.1417·1).

**Profil** *Atral, Port.*
Amantadine (p.1198·2).

**Profilasmim-Ped** *Stiefel, Braz.*
Ketotifen fumarate (p.788·1).
*Allergic conjunctivitis; allergic rhinitis; asthma; urticaria.*

**Profilate**
*Grifols, Ger.; Alpha, Israel.*
A factor VIII preparation (p.751·1).
*Haemorrhagic disorders.*

**Profilnine**
*Alpha, Hong Kong; Alpha, Israel; Alpha Therapeutic, Malaysia; Alpha Therapeutic, Singapore; Alpha Therapeutic, Thai.; Alpha Therapeutic, USA.*
A factor IX complex (p.752·2).
*Haemorrhagic disorders.*

**Profinal** *Julphar, UAE.*
Ibuprofen (p.45·3).
*Fever; inflammation; musculoskeletal, joint, peri-articular and soft-tissue disorders; pain.*

**Profisin** *Instituto Sanitas, Chile.*
Dicycloverine hydrochloride (p.481·2); chlordiazepoxide hydrochloride (p.674·2).
*Smooth muscle spasm.*

**Profiten** *Pharma Clal, Israel.*
Ketotifen fumarate (p.788·1).
*Hypersensitivity reactions.*

**Profium** *De Mayo, Braz.*
Mebendazole (p.108·2); tiabendazole (p.114·2).
*Worm infections.*

**Proflag** *Salus, Mex.†.*
Metronidazole (p.607·2).

**Proflam** *Eurofarma, Braz.*
Aceclofenac (p.11·2).
*Inflammation; pain.*

**Proflavanol**
*Usana, Hong Kong.*
Vitamin C (p.1460·2) grape seed; ascorbyl palmitate (p.1168·2).
*Antioxidant; vitamin C supplement.*

*USANA, USA.*
Vitamin C (p.1460·2); flavonoids from grape seed (p.1688·2).
*Nutritional supplement.*

**Proflavanol C** *Usana, Canad.*
Calcium ascorbate (p.1460·2); potassium ascorbate (p.1233·1); magnesium ascorbate (p.1227·3); zinc ascorbate (p.1461·1).
*Vitamin C supplement.*

**Proflax** *Sidus, Arg.*
Timolol maleate (p.1012·2).
*Angina pectoris; glaucoma; hypertension; migraine; myocardial infarction; ocular hypertension.*

**Proflex**
*Novartis Consumer, Irl.; Novartis Consumer, UK.*
Ibuprofen (p.45·3).
*Musculoskeletal, joint, peri-articular, and soft-tissue disorders.*

**Proflo** *Procare, Austral.†.*
Vitamins; minerals (p.1417·1); bioflavonoids (p.1688·2); ruscus aculeatus; aesculus (p.1648·2); hamamelis (p.1696·3); pulsatilla (p.1737·1).
*Dietary supplement; peripheral vascular disorders.*

**Proflox**
*Note. This name is used for preparations of different composition.*
*Therabel, Belg.*
Moxifloxacin (p.233·1).
*Bacterial infections.*

*Sigma, Braz.; Pharmasant, Thai.*
Ciprofloxacin (p.188·2).
*Bacterial infections.*

*Cipla, India.*
Pefloxacin mesilate (p.241·3).
*Bacterial eye infections.*

*Bialfar, Port.; Esteve, Spain.*
Moxifloxacin hydrochloride (p.233·1).
*Bacterial infections.*

**Profloxin** *Hexal, Austral.*
Ciprofloxacin hydrochloride (p.188·2).
*Bacterial infections.*

**Profluid** *Procare, Austral.†.*
Taraxacum (p.1751·3); parsley piert (p.1729·1); bearberry (p.1659·2); juniper (p.1703·1).
*Bladder disorders; cystitis; fluid retention.*

**Profol** *Medley, Braz.*
Buclizine hydrochloride (p.426·3); lysine; tryptophan; vitamin $B_6$; vitamin $B_{12}$ (p.1417·1).
*Tonic.*

**Profolen** *Blausiegel, Braz.*
Propofol (p.1305·3).
*General anaesthesia.*

**Profort** *Abbott, Braz.*
Preparation for enteral nutrition (p.1417·1).

**ProFree** *Allergan, USA.*
Papain (p.1727·3) (p.1164·2).
*Cleansing solution for contact lenses.*

**Profrin-A** *Allergan, Port.*
Mepyramine maleate (p.437·1); phenylephrine hydrochloride (p.1126·3); phenazone (p.82·3).
*Eye irritation.*

**Profungal** *Dankos, Singapore.*
Ketoconazole (p.403·3).
*Fungal infections.*

**Profylac** *ALK, Fin.*
Infant feed (p.1417·1).
*Lactose intolerance; milk allergy; soya protein intolerance.*

**Progandol** *Almirall, Spain.*
Doxazosin mesilate (p.908·3).
*Benign prostatic hyperplasia; hypertension.*

**Progastrit** *Hexal, Ger.*
*Chewable tablets:* Aluminium hydroxide (p.1249·2); magnesium hydroxide (p.1272·2); magnesium trisilicate (p.1272·3).
*Oral suspension:* Aluminium hydroxide (p.1249·2); magnesium hydroxide (p.1272·2).
*Gastrointestinal disorders.*

**Progediol** *Diba, Mex.*
Progesterone (p.1566·2); estradiol benzoate (p.1550·1).
*Menstrual disorders.*

**Progeffik**
*Effik, Ital.; Effik, Spain.*
Progesterone (p.1566·2).
*Female infertility; menopausal disorders; menstrual disorders; threatened or habitual miscarriage.*

**Progemox** *Proge, Ital.*
Amoxicillin trihydrate (p.155·3).
*Bacterial infections.*

**Progenar** *Menarini, Port.*
Progesterone (p.1566·2).
*Benign breast disorders.*

**Progendo** *Gynopharm, Chile.*
Progesterone (p.1566·2).

**Proger-F** *Streger, Mex.*
Progesterone (p.1566·2); estradiol benzoate (p.1550·1).
*Menstrual disorders.*

**Progeril**
*Sanofi Winthrop, Mex.†; Sanofi Synthelabo, Switz.†.*
Co-dergocrine mesilate (p.1674·1).
*Headache; peripheral and cerebral vascular disorders.*

**Progesic** *Xepa-Soul Pattinson, Hong Kong.*
Paracetamol (p.76·2).
*Pain.*

**Progest**
*Note. This name is used for preparations of different composition.*
*Elea, Arg.; Samarth, India.*
Progesterone (p.1566·2).
*Benign breast disorders; dysfunctional uterine bleeding; female infertility; menopausal disorders; menstrual disorders; recurrent and threatened miscarriage.*

*Heralds, Braz.†.*
Estradiol benzoate (p.1550·1); progesterone (p.1566·2); hydroxyprogesterone (p.1556·3); ethinylestradiol (p.1553·2).
*Menopausal disorders; menstrual disorders.*

**Progestan** *Nourypharma, Neth.*
Progesterone (p.1566·2).
*Hormone replacement therapy; menstrual disorders.*

**Progestasert**
*Theraplix, Fr.†; Alza, USA.*
Progesterone (p.1566·2).
*Progestogen-only intra-uterine contraceptive device.*

**Progesteron-Depot** *Jenapharm, Ger.*
Hydroxyprogesterone caproate (p.1556·3).
*Female infertility; menstrual disorders; threatened or recurrent miscarriage.*

**Progesterone-retard Pharlon** *Schering, Fr.*
Hydroxyprogesterone caproate (p.1556·3).
*Female infertility; premature labour; progestogen; threatened or recurrent miscarriage.*

**Progestogel**
*Besins, Belg.; Besins, Fr.; Kade, Ger.; Besins, Ger.; Besins, Hong Kong; Lusofarmaco, Ital.; Quimedical, Port.; Seid, Spain; Golaz, Switz.; Piette, Thai.*
Progesterone (p.1566·2).
*Benign breast disorders.*

**Progestol** *Sanofi Synthelabo, Ital.*
Progesterone (p.1566·2).
*Acne; seborrhoea; seborrhoeic alopecia.*

**Progestosol** *Besins, Fr.†.*
Progesterone (p.1566·2).
*Hyperseborrhoea.*

**Progestrol** *IBSA, Hong Kong†.*
Algestone acetophenide (p.1541·3); estradiol enantate (p.1550·1).
*Endometriosis; injectable contraceptive; menstrual disorders.*

**Progevera**
*IFET (ΙΦΕΤ), Gr.; Pharmacia, Spain.*
Medroxyprogesterone acetate (p.1557·2).
*Cancer of breast, kidney, and endometrium; contraception; endometriosis; female infertility; menometrorrhagia; menopausal disorders; menstrual disorders.*

**Progevera 250** *Pharmacia, Spain.*
Medroxyprogesterone acetate (p.1557·2).
*Breast cancer; endometrial cancer.*

**Progezzard** *Pizzard, Mex.†.*
Medroxyprogesterone (p.1557·3).

**Proginkgo** *Procare, Austral.†.*
Ginkgo biloba (p.1692·3).
*Cerebral and peripheral vascular disorders; tonic.*

**Proglan** *Procare, Austral.†.*
Black currant seed oil (p.1661·1).
*Dietary supplement; source of polyunsaturated fatty acids.*

**Proglicem**
*Key, Arg.; Schering-Plough, Fr.; Essex, Ger.; Schering-Plough, Ital.; Schering-Plough, Neth.; Essex, Switz.*
Diazoxide (p.893·2).
*Hypertension; hypoglycaemia.*

**Proglycem**
*Schering, Canad.; IFET (ΙΦΕΤ), Gr.; Baker Norton, USA.*
Diazoxide (p.893·2).
*Hypertensive episodes in nephropathy; hypoglycaemia.*

**Pro-Gola** *Cabassi, Ital.*
Propolis (p.1735·2).

**Progona** *MIP, Ger.†.*
Glucosamine sulfate (p.1694·1).
*Gonarthroses.*

**Progor** *SMB, Belg.*
Diltiazem hydrochloride (p.900·1).
*Hypertension.*

**Progout**
*Alphapharm, Austral.; Pacific, Hong Kong; Pacific, NZ; Alphapharm, Singapore; Merck, Singapore; CP Pharmaceuticals, UK†.*
Allopurinol (p.412·2).
*Gout; hyperuricaemia; renal calculi.*

**Prograf**
*Gador, Arg.; Janssen-Cilag, Austral.; Fujisawa, Austria; Janssen-Cilag, Braz.; Fujisawa, Canad.; Pharma Investi, Chile; Fujisawa, Denm.; Fujisawa, Fin.; Fujisawa, Fr.; Fujisawa, Ger.; Vianex (Βιανέξ), Gr.; Fujisawa, Hong Kong; Fujisawa, Irl.; Fujisawa, Israel; Fujisawa, Ital.; Fujisawa, Jpn; Janssen-Cilag, Malaysia; Cilag, Mex.; Fujisawa, Norw.; Janssen-Cilag, NZ; Fujisawa, Port.; Adcock Ingram Critical Care, S.Afr.; Janssen-Cilag, Singapore; Fujisawa, Spain; Fujisawa, Swed.; Vifor, Switz.; Janssen-Cilag, Thai.; Fujisawa, UK; Fujisawa, USA.*
Tacrolimus (p.1363·3).
*Graft-versus-host disease; liver, kidney, and heart, transplant rejection; myasthenia gravis.*

**Prograft** *Fujisawa, Belg.*
Tacrolimus (p.1363·3).
*Transplant rejection.*

**PRO'gram** *Montebello, Fr.*
High protein food for special diets (p.1417·1).

**Progras** *Temis, Arg.*
Sorbitol (p.1446·3).

**Progray** *Gray, Arg.*
Propanidid (p.1305·3).
*General anaesthesia.*

**Progress**
*Note. A similar name is used for preparations of different composition (see below).*
*Procare, Austral.†.*
Ginseng; garlic; multivitamins; minerals; bladderwrack; cramp bark (p.1417·1).
*Dietary supplement.*

**Progresse**
*Note. A similar name is used for preparations of different composition (see above).*
*Biosintetica, Braz.*
Gabapentin (p.362·2).
*Epilepsy.*

**Proguval** *Eberth, Ger.*
Plantago lanceolata (p.1738·2).
*Catarrh; mouth and throat inflammation.*

**Progyluton**
*Schering, Chile; Schering, Israel; Schering, Malaysia; Schering, Mex.; Schering, Port.; Schering, Singapore; Schering, Spain.*
11 Tablets, estradiol valerate (p.1550·2); 10 tablets, estradiol valerate; norgestrel (p.1563·2).
*Menopausal disorders; menstrual disorders; osteoporosis.*

**Progynon**
*Schering, Arg.; Schering, Austria; Schering, Denm.; Schering, Swed.; Schering, Thai.*
Estradiol valerate (p.1550·2).
*Dysfunctional uterine bleeding; menopausal disorders; menstrual disorders; oestrogen deficiency; osteoporosis.*

**Progynon C**
*Schering, Austria; Schering, Ger.; Schering, Israel.*
Ethinylestradiol (p.1553·2).
*Dysfunctional uterine bleeding; endometrial hyperplasia; oestrogen deficiency.*

**Progynon Depot**
*Schering, Ital.†; Schering, Spain†.*
Estradiol valerate (p.1550·2).
*Menstrual disorders; oestrogen deficiency.*

**Progynon Depot 10**
*Schering, Ger.; Schering, Neth.; Schering, Switz.†.*
Estradiol valerate (p.1550·2).
*Endometrial hyperplasia; menstrual disorders; oestrogen deficiency.*

**Progynova**
*Schering, Austral.; Schering, Austria; Schering, Belg.; Schering, Fin.; Schering, Fr.; Schering, Ger.; Schering, Hong Kong; Schering, Israel; Schering, Ital.; Schering, Malaysia; Schering, Neth.; Schering, Norw.; Schering, NZ; Schering, S.Afr.; Schering, Singapore; Schering, Spain; CIC, Spain; Schering, Switz.; Schering, Thai.; Schering, UK.*
Estradiol (p.1550·1) or estradiol valerate (p.1550·2).
*Menopausal disorders; osteoporosis.*

**Prohair**
*Uniao Quimica, Braz.; Merck Sharp & Dohme, Chile.*
Finasteride (p.1554·2).
*Alopecia androgenetica; benign prostatic hyperplasia.*

**Prohance**
*Regional Health, Austral.; Gerot, Austria; Byk, Belg.; Squibb Diagnostics, Canad.†; Bracco, Denm.; Astra Tech, Fin.; Byk, Fr.; Byk Gulden, Ger.; Merck, Irl.; Bracco, Ital.; Eisai, Jpn; Byk, Neth.; Bracco, Norw.; Rovi, Spain; Astra Tech, Swed.; Bracco, Switz.; Bracco, UK; Bracco, USA.*
Gadoteridol (p.1062·3).
*Contrast medium for magnetic resonance imaging.*

**Pro-HDL** *Wockhardt, India.*
Lovastatin (p.949·1).
*Hypercholesterolaemia.*

**Prohelmin** *Hebron, Braz.*
Mebendazole (p.108·2); tiabendazole (p.114·2).
*Worm infections.*

**Prohep** *Aventis, S.Afr.*
Liver hydrolysate; vitamin $B_{12}$ (p.1458·2); choline bitartrate (p.1424·3); cysteine (p.1426·3); inositol (p.1701·2).
*Liver disorders.*

**Proheparum** *Knoll, Thai.†.*
Cysteine (p.1426·3); choline bitartrate (p.1424·3); inositol (p.1701·2); liver hydrolysate.
*Liver disorders.*

**Prohexal** *Hexal, S.Afr.*
Fluoxetine hydrochloride (p.292·1).
*Bulimia; depression; obsessive-compulsive disorder.*

**ProHIBiT**
*Aventis Pasteur, Austria; Pasteur Merieux, USA.*
A haemophilus influenzae conjugate vaccine (diphtheria toxoid conjugate) (p.1616·1).
*Active immunisation.*

**Prohist** *Be-Tabs, S.Afr.*
Promethazine hydrochloride (p.439·1).
*Hypersensitivity reactions; premedication; sedative.*

**Projuvex** *Merck, Port.†.*
Co-dergocrine mesilate (p.1674·1); deanol acetamidobenzoate (p.1585·3); rutoside (p.1688·2); pyridoxine; vitamin E; potassium gluconate (p.1417·1).
*Cerebral and peripheral vascular disorders; mental function disorders.*

**Proken M** *Kendrick, Mex.*
Metoprolol tartrate (p.957·1).
*Angina pectoris; hypertension; myocardial infarction.*

**Prokids** *Procare, Austral.†.*
Multivitamin and mineral preparation (p.1417·1).

**Prokinate** *Julphar, UAE†.*
Cisapride (p.1259·2).
*Gastrointestinal motility disorders.*

**Prokinyl** *Techni-Pharma, Mon.*
Metoclopramide hydrochloride (p.1274·3).
*Aid to gastrointestinal examination; dyspepsia; nausea and vomiting.*

**Prol** *Procare, Austral.†.*
Silybum marianum (p.1043·3).
*Liver disorders.*

**Prolacam** *Schering, Austria.*
Lisuride maleate (p.1210·3).
*Acromegaly; amenorrhoea; female infertility; galactorrhoea; lactation inhibition; mastitis.*

**Proladone**
*Abbott, Austral.; Abbott, NZ†.*
Oxycodone pectinate (p.75·3).
*Pain.*

**Prolair** *3M, Fr.*
Beclometasone dipropionate (p.1091·1).
*Asthma.*

**Prolaken** *Fustery, Mex.*
Metoprolol tartrate (p.957·1).
*Angina pectoris; arrhythmias; hypertension.*

**Prolan** *Procare, Austral.†.*
Multivitamin and mineral preparation (p.1417·1).
*Anxiety; dietary supplement.*

**Prolastin**
*Bayer, Canad.; Bayer, Ger.; Bayer Biological, Hong Kong†; Bayer, USA.*
Alpha$_1$-proteinase inhibitor (p.1651·2).
*Congenital alpha$_1$ antitrypsin deficiency.*

**Prolastina**
*Bayer, Ital.; Bayer, Spain.*
Alpha$_1$-proteinase inhibitor (p.1651·2).
*Congenital alpha$_1$ antitrypsin deficiency.*

**Prolax**
*Note. A similar name is used for preparations of different composition (see below).*
*Procare, Austral.†.*
Senna (p.1288·2); prune (p.1285·1).
*Constipation.*

**Pro-Lax**
*Note. A similar name is used for preparations of different composition (see above).*
*Rivex, Canad.†.*
Polyethylene glycol (p.1708·2); electrolytes (p.1217·1).
*Constipation.*

**Prolert** *Pensa, Spain†.*
Caffeine (p.782·1).
*Fatigue.*

**Proleukin**
*Raffo, Arg.; CSL, Austral.; Caleo, Austria; Chiron, Belg.; Zodiac, Braz.; Chiron, Canad.; Chiron, Denm.; Chiron, Fr.; Chiron, Ger.; Roche, Gr.; Chiron, Hong Kong; Chiron, Israel; Chiron, Ital.; Asofarma, Mex.; Chiron, Neth.; CSL, NZ; Roche, Port.†; Chiron, Singapore; Chiron, Spain; Roche, Switz.; Chiron, UK; Chiron, USA.*
Aldesleukin (p.562·3).
*Metastatic melanoma; metastatic renal-cell carcinoma.*

**Prolidon** *Carnot, Mex.†.*
Progesterone (p.1566·2).
*Amenorrhoea; functional uterine haemorrhage; recurrent miscarriage.*

**Prolief** *Propan, S.Afr.*
Paracetamol (p.76·2).
*Fever; pain.*

**Prolifen** *Chiesi, Ital.*
Clomifene citrate (p.1542·2).
*Anovulatory infertility.*

**Prolift**
*Pharmacia, Arg.; Pharmacia, Braz.; Pharmacia, Chile.*
Reboxetine mesilate (p.316·3).
*Depression.*

**Prolipase**
*Janssen-Cilag, Arg.; Janssen-Cilag, Austria†; Janssen-Cilag, Switz.*
Pancrelipase (p.1725·3).
*Pancreatic insufficiency.*

**Prolisina E2** *Pharmacia, Arg.*
Dinoprostone (p.1515·1).
*Labour induction.*

**Prolisina VR** *Pharmacia, Arg.*
Alprostadil (p.1512·3).
*Maintenance of patent ductus arteriosus.*

**Prolitrol** *Millet Roux, Braz.†.*
Pygeum africanum (p.1568·2).
*Benign prostatic hyperplasia.*

**Prolixan**
*Jacoby, Austria; Unipharma, Gr.; Viatris, Neth.; Neves, Port.; Siegfried, Switz.†.*
Azapropazone (p.20·1).
*Gout; inflammation; musculoskeletal, joint, and periarticular disorders.*

**Prolixana** *Siegfried, Swed.†.*
Azapropazone (p.20·1).
*Musculoskeletal and joint disorders.*

**Prolixin** *Apothecon, USA; Princeton, USA.*
Fluphenazine decanoate (p.699·3).
*Psychoses.*

**Prolmon** *Tokyo Tanabe, Hong Kong†.*
Protoporphyrin IX disodium (p.1735·3).
*Cholecystitis; cholelithiasis.*

**Proloid S** *Parke, Davis, Mex.*
Levothyroxine sodium (p.1600·1); liothyronine sodium (p.1602·2).
*Adjunct in hyperthyroidism; hypothyroidism.*

**Prolol**
*Merck, Hong Kong; Dexxon, Israel; Atlantic, Thai.*
Propranolol hydrochloride (p.989·3).
*Angina pectoris; arrhythmias; hypertension; hypertrophic obstructive cardiomyopathy; migraine; myocardial infarction; phaeochromocytoma; tremor.*

**Prolong** *Maver, Chile.*
Lidocaine (p.1377·3).
*Erectile dysfunction.*

**Prolopa**
*Roche, Belg.; Roche, Braz.; Roche, Canad.; Roche, Chile.*
Levodopa (p.1205·2); benserazide hydrochloride (p.1200·2).
*Parkinsonism.*

**Proloprim**
*GlaxoSmithKline, Canad.; Glaxo Wellcome, USA.*
Trimethoprim (p.272·2).
*Bacterial infections of the urinary tract.*

**Proluton**
*Schering, Arg.; Schering, Austral.; Schering, Thai.†.*
Progesterone (p.1566·2).
*Progesterone test in secondary amenorrhoea.*

**Proluton Depot**
*Schering, Arg.; Schering, Austria; Schering, Ger.; Shepa, Gr.; Schering, Hong Kong†; German Remedies, India; Schering, Israel; Schering, Ital.; Schering, Malaysia; Schering, Neth.; Schering, Singapore; Schering, Switz.†; Schering, Thai.; Schering, UK†.*
Hydroxyprogesterone caproate (p.1556·3).
Formerly known as Primolut Depot in the *UK*.
*Amenorrhoea; cancer of breast, uterus, or kidney; endometriosis; female infertility; metrorrhagia; progestogen deficiency; threatened or recurrent miscarriage; uterine hypoplasia.*

**Promac** *Provit, Mex.†.*
Nitrofurantoin (p.237·2).

**Promacet** *MCR, USA.*
Paracetamol (p.76·2); butalbital (p.673·3).
*Pain.*

**Promal** *Allen, Austria.*
Atovaquone (p.601·3); proguanil hydrochloride (p.457·1).
*Malaria.*

**Promani** *SmithKline Beecham, Canad.†.*
Triclosan (p.1195·2).
*Dry or irritated skin.*

**Promanum N**
*Braun, Ger.; Braun, Switz.*
Alcohol (p.1166·1); isopropyl alcohol (p.1184·3).
*Hand disinfection.*

**Promatussin DM** *Lioh, Canad.*
Promethazine hydrochloride (p.439·1); dextromethorphan hydrobromide (p.1117·3); pseudoephedrine (p.1129·2).
*Coughs.*

**Promaxol** *Otsuka, Spain†.*
Procaterol hydrochloride (p.791·1).
*Obstructive airways disease.*

**Promeal** *Volchem, Ital.*
Preparation for enteral nutrition (p.1417·1).

**Promecilina** *Promeco, Mex.†.*
Ampicillin (p.157·1).
*Bacterial infections.*

**Promedyl**
*Note. This name is used for preparations of different composition.*
*Upha, Malaysia.*
Codeine phosphate (p.27·1); promethazine (p.439·1).
*Coughs.*

*Beacons, Singapore.*
Codeine phosphate (p.27·1); promethazine hydrochloride (p.439·1); ephedrine hydrochloride (p.1120·1).
*Coughs.*

**Promega** *Parke, Davis, USA.*
Omega-3 marine triglycerides with vitamin E (p.976·2).
*Dietary supplement.*

**Promelatonin** *Laborest, Ital.*
Tryptophan; niacin; magnesium (p.1417·1).
*Nutritional supplement; sleep disorders.*

**Promensil** *Novogen, Austral.*
Red clover (p.1737·3).
*Menopausal disorders.*

**Prometax**
*Biosintetica, Braz.; Sigma-Tau, Ital.; Medibial, Port.; Esteve, Spain.*
Rivastigmine hydrogen tartrate (p.1497·1).
*Alzheimer's disease.*

**Prometh with Dextromethorphan** *Barre-National, USA.*
Promethazine hydrochloride (p.439·1); dextromethorphan hydrobromide (p.1117·3).
*Coughs and cold symptoms.*

**Prometh VC Plain** *Warner Chilcott, USA; Goldline, USA; Barre-National, USA.*
Promethazine hydrochloride (p.439·1); phenylephrine hydrochloride (p.1126·3).
*Allergic rhinitis; nasal congestion.*

**Promethawern** *Wernigerode, Ger.*
Promethazine teoclate (p.439·2).
*Anxiety; hypersensitivity reactions; nausea and vomiting; premedication; sleep disorders.*

**Promethazine Compound Linctus** *Medipharma, Hong Kong.*
Promethazine hydrochloride (p.439·1); dextromethorphan hydrobromide (p.1117·3); ephedrine hydrochloride (p.1120·1).
*Cold and influenza symptoms.*

**Promethazine Expectorants** *Vitamed, Israel.*
Promethazine hydrochloride (p.439·1); ipecacuanha (p.1122·3); sulfogaiacol (p.1131·1).
*Coughs.*

**Promethazine VC with Codeine** *Warner Chilcott, USA.*
Promethazine hydrochloride (p.439·1); phenylephrine hydrochloride (p.1126·3); codeine phosphate (p.27·1).

**Prometidine** *Cazi, Braz.*
Cimetidine (p.1255·3).
*Peptic ulcer.*

**Prometrium**
*Schering, Canad.; Rottapharm, Ital.; Solvay, USA.*
Progesterone (p.1566·2).
*Female infertility; menopausal disorders; menstrual disorders; threatened or habitual miscarriage.*

**Promibasol** *Rayere, Mex.*
Metronidazole (p.607·2).
*Amoebiasis; giardiasis; trichomoniasis.*

**Promibasol-Plus** *Rayere, Mex.*
Fluocinolone acetonide (p.1101·2); metronidazole (p.607·2); nystatin (p.406·3).
*Vulvovaginal infections.*

**Promiced** *IQFA, Mex.*
Metoprolol (p.956·3).
*Angina pectoris; arrhythmias; hypertension.*

**Promictuline** *Ashbourne, UK†.*
Oxybutynin hydrochloride (p.486·3).
*Neurogenic bladder; unstable bladder.*

**Promidan** *Mintlab, Chile.*
Chlormezanone (p.675·1); diazepam (p.690·1).
*Skeletal muscle spasm.*

**Promifen** *Wiener, Mex.†.*
Prednisone (p.1109·3).
*Corticosteroid.*

**Prominal**
*Sanofi Synthelabo, Austral.†; Merck, Spain†; Sanofi Synthelabo, UK†.*
Methylphenobarbital (p.366·3).
*Epilepsy.*

**Promincil** *Chefaro Ardeval, Fr.*
*Capsules:* Bladderwrack (p.1742·3); paullinia (p.1765·3); java tea (p.1702·3).
Formerly contained fucus, meadowsweet, and equisetum.
*Topical gel:* Hedera helix leaf; guarana (p.1765·3).
*Herbal slimming preparation.*

**Prominol** *MCR, USA.*
Butalbital (p.673·3); paracetamol (p.76·2).
*Pain.*

**Promise**
*Wyeth, Mex.; Wyeth, Singapore.*
Nutritional supplement for children (p.1417·1).

**Promit**
*Medical Specialties, Austral.; Torrex, Austria; Pharmacia Upjohn, Fr.†; Pharmalink, Ger.; Alliance, S.Afr.; Braun, Switz.; Pharmacia, USA.*
Dextran 1 (p.745·2).
*Prevention of anaphylactic reactions to infusions of dextrans.*

**Promiten**
*Pharmalink, Denm.; Pharmalink, Norw.; Pharmalink, Swed.*
Dextran 1 (p.745·2).
*Prevention of anaphylactic reactions to infusions of dextrans.*

**Promix** *Capo Sole, Ital.*
Propolis (p.1735·2); agrumi; echinacea (p.1683·2); clove (p.1673·2).

**Promix 3** *Capo Sole, Ital.*
Propolis (p.1735·2); myrtillus (p.1718·3); echinacea (p.1683·2); agrumi oil.

**Promixin** *Profile, UK.*
Colistimethate sodium (p.199·1).
*Gram-negative bacterial infections.*

**Promocard**
*AstraZeneca, Belg.; AstraZeneca, Neth.*
Isosorbide mononitrate (p.942·1).
*Angina pectoris.*

**ProMod**
*Abbott, Austral.; Abbott, Braz.; Abbott, Canad.; Abbott, Ital.; Abbott, NZ; Abbott, Singapore; Abbott Nutrition, UK; Ross, USA.*
Dietary protein supplement (p.1417·1).

**Promogran**
*Note. This name is used for preparations of different composition.*
*Johnson & Johnson, Fr.*
Oxidised cellulose (p.757·1); collagen (p.1674·3).
*Ulcers; wounds.*

*Johnson & Johnson, Ger.*
Collagen (p.1674·3).
*Wounds.*

**Promolan** *Sarabhai Piramal, India.*
High-protein dietary supplement (p.1417·1).

**Promote** *Abbott, Ital.*
Preparation for enteral nutrition (p.1417·1).

**Promoxil** *Medpro, S.Afr.*
Amoxicillin (p.155·3).
*Bacterial infections.*

**Prompt**
*Temis, Arg.*
Ispaghula (p.1268·1); sennosides (p.1288·2).
*Constipation.*

*Procter & Gamble, Braz.†.*
Ispaghula (p.1268·1); senna (p.1288·2).
*Constipation.*

**Promune** *Procare, Austral.†.*
Multivitamin, amino-acid, and mineral preparation with thymus extract (p.1417·1).
*Dietary supplement.*

**Promyrtil** *Organon, Chile.*
Mirtazapine (p.307·3).
*Depression.*

**Pronaestin** *Rekah, Israel.*
Benzocaine (p.1370·3); methylthioninium chloride (p.1042·2); thymol (p.1194·2).
*Gingivitis; mouth hygiene; stomatitis.*

**Pronasteron** *Sanval, Braz.*
Finasteride (p.1554·2).
*Benign prostatic hyperplasia.*

**Pro-Nat**
*Note. A similar name is used for preparations of different composition (see below).*
*Pro-Nat, Fr.†.*
A range of organ extracts (bovine) (p.1709·3).

**Pronat**
*Note. A similar name is used for preparations of different composition (see above).*
*Solfran, Mex.*
Naproxen (p.65·1).
*Inflammation.*

**Pronaxen**
*Orion, Fin.; Orion, Swed.*
Naproxen (p.65·1).
*Fever; gout; inflammation; musculoskeletal and joint disorders; pain.*

**Pronaxil** *Streger, Mex.*
Naproxen (p.65·1).
*Gout; musculoskeletal, joint, and peri-articular disorders.*

**Pronax-P** *Kener, Mex.†.*
Naproxen sodium (p.65·1).

**Pronazol** *Diffucap, Braz.*
Fluconazole (p.398·1).
*Fungal infections.*

**Pronemia Hematinic** *Lederle, USA.*
Ferrous fumarate (p.1427·3); intrinsic factor concentrate; vitamin $B_{12}$ substances (p.1458·2); folic acid (p.1429·1).
Vitamin C (p.1460·2) is included in this preparation to increase the absorption and availability of iron.
*Anaemias.*

**Pronerv** *Gerot, Austria.*
Thiamine hydrochloride (p.1455·1) or thiamine nitrate (p.1455·1); pyridoxine hydrochloride (p.1456·3); cyanocobalamin (p.1458·2).
*Neuralgia; neuritis; neuropathies.*

**Pronervon Phyto** *Scheffler, Ger.*
Valerian (p.1762·2); passion flower (p.1729·1); melissa (p.1711·1).
*Agitation; sleep disorders.*

**Pronervon T** *Scheffler, Ger.*
Temazepam (p.723·2).
*Sleep disorders.*

**Pronest** *BPL-Meizler, Braz.*
Propofol (p.1305·3).
*General anaesthesia.*

**Pronestyl**
*Bristol-Myers Squibb, Austral.; Squibb, Canad.; IFET (ΙΦΕΤ), Gr.; Bristol-Myers Squibb, Hong Kong; Sarabhai Piramal, India; Bristol-Myers Squibb, Irl.; Bristol-Myers Squibb, Israel; Bristol-Myers Squibb, Neth.; Bristol-Myers Squibb, NZ; Bristol-Myers Squibb, S.Afr.†; Bristol-Myers Squibb, Switz.†; Bristol-Myers Squibb, Thai.†; Bristol-Myers Squibb, UK; Apothecon, USA†.*
Procainamide hydrochloride (p.987·1).
*Arrhythmias.*

**Proneurin** *Hexal, Ger.*
Promethazine hydrochloride (p.439·1).
*Anxiety; hypersensitivity reactions; sleep disorders; vomiting.*

**Proneurit** *Demo, Gr.*
Lorazepam (p.704·1).
*Anxiety disorders; insomnia; status epilepticus.*

**Pronicol** *Bioresearch, Mex.*
Chloramphenicol (p.185·1).
*Gastrointestinal infections.*

**Pronitol** *Fournier SA, Spain.*
Pygeum africanum (p.1568·2).
*Benign prostatic hyperplasia.*

**Pronivel** *Elea, Arg.*
Epoetin (p.747·1).
*Anaemias.*

**Pronoctan** *Schering, Denm.*
Lormetazepam (p.705·2).
*Insomnia; premedication.*

**Pronose** *Lusofarmaco, Ital.*
Cetirizine hydrochloride (p.427·1); pseudoephedrine hydrochloride (p.1129·2).
*Rhinitis.*

**Pronosil** *Silom, Thai.†.*
Propranolol hydrochloride (p.989·3).
*Angina pectoris; arrhythmias; hypertension.*

**Pronovan** *AFI, Norw.†.*
Propranolol hydrochloride (p.989·3).
*Angina pectoris; arrhythmias; hypertension; hyperthyroidism; migraine; myocardial infarction; tremor.*

**Pronoxen** *Farcoral, Mex.*
Naproxen (p.65·1).
*Inflammation.*

**Prontalgin** *GiEnne, Ital.*
Tramadol hydrochloride (p.94·3).
*Pain.*

**Prontalgine** *Boehringer Ingelheim, Fr.*
Paracetamol (p.76·2); codeine phosphate (p.27·1); caffeine (p.782·1).
*Pain.*

**Prontamid** *SIT, Ital.†.*
Sulfacetamide sodium (p.257·3).
*Eye infections.*

**Prontinal** *Dompe, Ital.*
Beclometasone dipropionate (p.1091·1).
*Obstructive airways disease; rhinitis.*

**Pronto**
*Note. This name is used for preparations of different composition.*
*Del, Canad.*
Pyrethrin (p.1509·3); piperonyl butoxide (p.1509·2).

*Del, USA.*
*Shampoo:* Pyrethrins (p.1509·3); piperonyl butoxide (p.1509·2).
*Pediculosis.*

*Surface spray:* Phenothrin (p.1509·1).
*Lice infestation.*

**Pronto Emoform** *Byk Gulden, Ital.†.*
Sodium monofluorophosphate (p.1446·2); sodium fluoride (p.1444·3).
*Oral hygiene.*

**Pronto Platamine** *Pharmacia Upjohn, Ital.*
Cisplatin (p.538·1).
*Malignant neoplasms.*

**Prontoalivio** *Laborsil, Braz.†.*
Methyl salicylate (p.59·3); turpentine oil (p.1760·1); camphor (p.1665·3).
*Musculoskeletal and joint disorders.*

**Prontobario**
*Gerot, Austria; Bracco, Ital.; Bracco, Port.†.*
Barium sulfate (p.1061·1).
Simeticone (p.1289·2) is included in some preparations to eliminate gas from the gastrointestinal tract before radiography.
*Contrast medium for gastrointestinal radiography.*

**Prontocid N** *Braun, Ger.*
Formaldehyde (p.1179·3); glutaral (p.1180·3).
*Instrument disinfection.*

**Prontodex** *Procter & Gamble, Austria.*
Dextromethorphan (p.1117·3).
*Coughs.*

**Prontoferro** *Amsa, Ital.*
Ferrous gluconate (p.1428·1).
Ascorbic acid (p.1460·2) is included in this preparation to increase the absorption and availability of iron.
*Iron-deficiency anaemia.*

**Prontofort** *Medix, Mex.*
Tramadol hydrochloride (p.94·3).
*Pain.*

**Prontogest** *Amsa, Ital.*
Progesterone (p.1566·2).
*Adjunct in gynaecological surgery; menstrual disorders; postnatal depression; threatened or recurrent miscarriage.*

**Prontokef** *Master Pharma, Ital.†.*
Cefoperazone sodium (p.174·3).
Lidocaine hydrochloride (p.1377·3) is included in this preparation to alleviate the pain of injection.
*Bacterial infections.*

**Prontoket** *CSC, Austria.*
Ketoprofen (p.51·2).
*Musculoskeletal, joint, peri-articular, and soft-tissue disorders.*

**Prontol** *Novag, Mex.*
Metoprolol (p.956·3).

**Prontolax** *Streuli, Switz.*
Bisacodyl (p.1251·3).
*Bowel evacuation; constipation.*

**Prontomixin** *Farmila, Ital.†.*
Lactic-acid-producing organisms (p.1704·2); vitamin B substances; passion flower; pineapple; carrot (p.1417·1).
*Maintenance of normal gastrointestinal flora.*

**Prontomucil** *Francia, Ital.*
Guacetisal (p.1121·3).
*Respiratory-tract congestion.*

**Prontopyrin plus** *Mack, Illert., Ger.*
Paracetamol (p.76·2); caffeine (p.782·1).
*Pain.*

**Prontovent** *Salus, Ital.*
Clenbuterol hydrochloride (p.784·2).
*Obstructive airways disease.*

**Propa** *Jean-Marie, Hong Kong.*
Propranolol (p.990·1).
*Angina pectoris; anxiety; arrhythmias; essential tremor; hypertension; migraine; myocardial infarction.*

**Propa PH** *Del, Canad.*
Salicylic acid (p.1157·1).
*Acne.*

**Propabloc** *Azupharma, Ger.*
Propranolol hydrochloride (p.989·3).
*Angina pectoris; anxiety; arrhythmias; essential tremor; hypertension; hyperthyroidism; migraine.*

**Propac** *Sherwood, USA.*
Dietary protein supplement (p.1417·1).

**Propace** *Protein, Mex.†.*
Metoclopramide (p.1274·3).

**Propacet** *Lemmon, USA.*
Dextropropoxyphene napsilate (p.28·3); paracetamol (p.76·2).
*Pain.*

**Propacil** *Halewood, Thai.†.*
Propylthiouracil (p.1603·1).
*Hyperthyroidism.*

**Propacor** *Bunker, Braz.*
Propranolol hydrochloride (p.989·3).

**Propaderm**
*Shire, Canad.; GlaxoSmithKline, UK.*
Beclometasone dipropionate (p.1091·1).
*Skin disorders.*

**Propafen** *BASF, Ger.†.*
Propafenone hydrochloride (p.988·3).
*Arrhythmias.*

**Propagest** *Carnrick, USA†.*
Phenylpropanolamine hydrochloride (p.1127·3).
*Nasal congestion.*

**Propain**
*Note. This name is used for preparations of different composition.*
*Restan, S.Afr.*
*Syrup:* Promethazine hydrochloride (p.439·1); paracetamol (p.76·2).
*Tablets:* Paracetamol (p.76·2); codeine phosphate (p.27·1); diphenhydramine hydrochloride (p.431·3); caffeine (p.782·1).
*Pain and associated tension.*

*Sankyo, UK.*
Paracetamol (p.76·2); codeine phosphate (p.27·1); diphenhydramine hydrochloride (p.431·3); caffeine (p.782·1).
*Cold and influenza symptoms; fever; pain.*

**Propain Forte** *Mer-National, S.Afr.*
Paracetamol (p.76·2); codeine phosphate (p.27·1); diphenhydramine hydrochloride (p.431·3); caffeine (p.782·1); phenobarbital (p.367·3).
*Pain and associated tension.*

**Propain Plus** *Sankyo, UK.*
Paracetamol (p.76·2); doxylamine succinate (p.432·3); caffeine (p.782·1); codeine phosphate (p.27·1).
*Pain.*

**Propal** *Durascan, Denm.*
Propranolol hydrochloride (p.989·3).
*Angina pectoris; arrhythmias; hypertension; hyperthyroidism; migraine; myocardial infarction; tremor; variceal haemorrhage.*

**Propalem** *Lemery, Mex.*
Propranolol hydrochloride (p.989·3).
*Hypertension.*

**Propalen** *Zerboni, Mex.†.*
Propranolol (p.990·1).

**Propalgin** *Kener, Mex.†.*
Propranolol (p.990·1).

**Propalgina Plus** *Roche, Spain.*
Ascorbic acid (p.1460·2); chlorphenamine maleate (p.427·3); dextromethorphan hydrobromide (p.1117·3); phenylephrine hydrochloride (p.1126·3); paracetamol (p.76·2).
*Upper respiratory-tract disorders.*

**Propalgina PS Hot Lemon** *Roche, Spain†.*
Dextromethorphan hydrobromide (p.1117·3); paracetamol (p.76·2); pseudoephedrine hydrochloride (p.1129·2).
*Upper-respiratory-tract disorders.*

**Propalong** *TRB, Arg.*
Propranolol hydrochloride (p.989·3).

**Propam** *Pacific, NZ.*
Diazepam (p.690·1).
*Alcohol withdrawal syndrome; anxiety; epilepsy; premedication; skeletal muscle spasm; sleep disorders; spasticity.*

**Propamerck** *Merck dura, Ger.*
Propafenone hydrochloride (p.988·3).
*Arrhythmias.*

**Propamide**
*Atlantic, Malaysia; Atlantic, Singapore; Atlantic, Thai.*
Chlorpropamide (p.330·3).
*Diabetes mellitus.*

**Propan**
*Note. This name is used for preparations of different composition.*
*UCI, Braz.*
Buclizine hydrochloride (p.426·3); vitamin B substances; lysine hydrochloride (p.1417·1).
*Reduced appetite; tonic.*

*Rhone-Poulenc Rorer, Hong Kong†.*
Buclizine (p.426·3); vitamin B substances (p.1417·1).
*Tonic.*

**Propan Gel-S** *Propan, S.Afr.*
Aluminium hydroxide (p.1249·2); magnesium oxide (p.1272·3); dicycloverine hydrochloride (p.481·2); dimethicone (p.1289·2).
*Gastrointestinal disorders associated with hyperacidity.*

**Propanol** *Upha, Malaysia.*
Propranolol hydrochloride (p.989·3).
*Angina pectoris; anxiety; arrhythmias; essential tremor; hypertension; hyperthyroidism; hypertrophic obstructive cardiomyopathy; migraine; myocardial infarction; phaeochromocytoma.*

**Propantel** *Gastroenterologicos, Mex.†.*
Propantheline bromide (p.489·1).

**Propanthel** *ICN, Canad.*
Propantheline bromide (p.489·1).
*Anticholinergic.*

**PropapH** *Del, USA.*
Salicylic acid (p.1157·1).
*Acne.*

**Propaphenin** *Rodleben, Ger.*
Chlorpromazine hydrochloride (p.675·2).
*Anxiety; hiccups; nausea; pain; premedication; pruritus; psychoses; sleep disorders; vomiting.*

**Proparakain-POS** *Ursapharm, Ger.*
Proxymetacaine hydrochloride (p.1384·1).
*Local anaesthesia.*

**Propargile** *Holistica, Fr.*
Propolis (p.1735·2); pollen; clay.
*Digestive disorders.*

**Proparin** *Galen, Mex.*
Heparin sodium (p.928·1).
*Anticoagulation in blood transfusion, extracorporeal circulation, and dialysis; thromboembolic disorders.*

**Propass**
*Hormel, Hong Kong; Hormel, Singapore.*
Dietary protein supplement (p.1417·1).
*Preparation for enteral nutrition.*

**Propast** *CaDiGroup, Ital.*
Zinc oxide (p.1163·2); propolis (p.1735·2); undecenoic acid (p.410·3).
*Skin disorders.*

**Propastad** *Stada, Ger.†.*
Propafenone hydrochloride (p.988·3).
*Arrhythmias.*

**Propavan** *Sanofi Synthelabo, Swed.*
Propiomazine maleate (p.440·3).
*Sleep disorders.*

**Propavent** *GlaxoSmithKline, Arg.*
Beclometasone dipropionate (p.1091·1).
*Asthma.*

**Propavente** *Glaxo Wellcome, Port.*
Guaifenesin (p.1122·1); salbutamol (p.791·3).
*Coughs.*

**Propayerst** *Wyeth, Arg.*
Propranolol hydrochloride (p.989·3).
*Angina pectoris; arrhythmias; hypertension; hypertrophic subaortic stenosis; migraine; myocardial infarction; phaeochromocytoma; tremor.*

**Propayerst Plus** *Wyeth, Arg.*
Propranolol hydrochloride (p.989·3); hydrochlorothiazide (p.933·2).
*Hypertension.*

**Propecia**
*Merck Sharp & Dohme, Arg.; Merck Sharp & Dohme, Austral.; Merck Sharp & Dohme, Braz.; Merck Frosst, Canad.; Merck Sharp & Dohme, Denm.; Merck Sharp & Dohme, Fin.; Merck Sharp & Dohme-Chibret, Fr.; Merck Sharp & Dohme, Ger.; Merck Sharp & Dohme, Hong Kong; Merck Sharp & Dohme, Israel; Merck Sharp & Dohme, Ital.; Merck Sharp & Dohme, Malaysia; Merck Sharp & Dohme, NZ; Merck Sharp & Dohme, Port.; Merck Sharp & Dohme, S.Afr.; Merck Sharp & Dohme, Singapore; Merck Sharp & Dohme, Spain; Merck Sharp & Dohme, Swed.; Merck Sharp & Dohme, Switz.; Merck Sharp & Dohme, Thai.; Merck Sharp & Dohme, UK; Merck, USA.*
Finasteride (p.1554·2).
*Alopecia androgenetica.*

**Propedil** *Yauquimia, Mex.†.*
Pipenzolate (p.487·3).

**Properil** *Royal, Chile.*
Captopril (p.879·2).
*Heart failure; hypertension.*

**Propeshia** *Merck Sharp & Dohme, Mex.*
Finasteride (p.1554·2).
*Alopecia androgenetica.*

**Propess**
*Ferring, Austria; Ferring, Denm.†; Ferring, Fin.; Ferring, Fr.; Ferring, Ger.; Chemipharma, Gr.; Zeneca, Hong Kong†; Ferring, Israel; Ferring, Ital.; Zeneca, Mex.†; Ferring, Neth.; Ferring, Port.; Ferring, S.Afr.; Ferring, Spain; Ferring, Swed.; Ferring, Switz.; Ferring, UK.*
Dinoprostone (p.1515·1).
*Labour induction; termination of pregnancy.*

**Prophage** *Progress, Thai.*
Metformin hydrochloride (p.342·3).
*Diabetes mellitus.*

**Prophedin** *Siam Bheasach, Thai.*
Triprolidine hydrochloride (p.442·3); pseudoephedrine hydrochloride (p.1129·2).
*Cold symptoms; hay fever; rhinitis; upper respiratory-tract congestion.*

**Pro-Phree**
*Abbott, Austral.; Ross, USA.*
Protein-free infant feed supplement (p.1417·1).

**Prophthal** *Procare, Austral.†.*
Myrtillus (p.1718·3); ginkgo biloba (p.1692·3).
*Herbal supplement.*

**Prophyllin** *Rystan, USA.*
Sodium propionate (p.408·1); chlorophyllin copper complex (p.1057·1).
*Contact dermatoses; dermatophytosis; eczemas; minor burns.*

**Prophylux** *Hennig, Ger.*
Propranolol hydrochloride (p.989·3).
*Angina pectoris; anxiety; arrhythmias; essential tremor; migraine; myocardial infarction.*

**Propibay** *Bayer, Mex.†.*
Propicillin potassium (p.246·3).
*Bacterial infections.*

**Propiden** *Durascan, Denm.*
Loperamide hydrochloride (p.1271·1).
*Diarrhoea.*

**Propil** *Pharmacia, Braz.*
Propylthiouracil (p.1603·1).
*Hyperthyroidism.*

**Propilracil** *Biolab Sanus, Braz.*
Propylthiouracil (p.1603·1).
*Hyperthyroidism.*

**Propimex** *Ross, USA.*
A range of methionine- and valine-free preparations for enteral nutrition including an infant feed (p.1417·1).
*Methylmalonic acidaemia; propionic acidaemia.*

**Propine**
*Allergan, Arg.; Allergan, Austral.; Allergan, Belg.; Allergan, Braz.; Allergan, Canad.; Allergan, Denm.; Allergan, Fin.; Allergan, Fr.; Allergan, Hong Kong; Allergan, Irl.; Allergan, Israel; Allergan, Ital.; Allergan, Malaysia; Allergan, Norw.; Allergan, NZ†; Allergan, Port.; Allergan, S.Afr.; Allergan, Singapore; Allergan, Swed.; Allergan, Thai.; Allergan, UK; Allergan, USA.*
Dipivefrine hydrochloride (p.1681·2).
*Ocular hypertension; open-angle glaucoma.*

**Propiochrone** *Schering-Plough, Gr.*
Betamethasone sodium phosphate (p.1093·1); betamethasone dipropionate (p.1093·1).
*Corticosteroid.*

**Propiocine** *Aventis, Fr.†.*
Erythromycin propionate (p.208·2).
*Bacterial infections.*

**Propioform** *Schering-Plough, Gr.*
Betamethasone dipropionate (p.1093·1).
*Topical corticosteroid.*

**Propionat** *Farmigea, Ital.*
Sodium propionate (p.408·1).
*Eye disorders.*

**Propiosalic** *Schering-Plough, Gr.*
Salicylic acid (p.1157·1); betamethasone dipropionate (p.1093·1).
*Skin disorders.*

**Propiosol** *Neo Quimica, Braz.*
Clobetasol propionate (p.1095·2).
*Skin disorders.*

**Propiral** *Yauquimia, Mex.†.*
Dipyrone (p.35·3).

**Proplax** *Hebron, Braz.†.*
Propolis (p.1735·2); sodium fluoride (p.1444·3); cetylpyridinium chloride (p.1173·1).

**Proplex**
*Baxter, Israel; Baxter, UK†.*
A factor IX preparation (p.752·2).
*Haemorrhagic disorders.*

**Proplex T**
*Baxter-Hyland, Hong Kong; Baxter, Malaysia; Baxter, Singapore†; Baxter, Spain†; Baxter, USA.*
A factor IX preparation (p.752·2).
*Haemorrhagic disorders.*

**Pro-Plus** *Roche Consumer, UK.*
Caffeine (p.782·1).
*Fatigue.*

**Propoabbott** *Abbott, Braz.*
Propofol (p.1305·3).
*General anaesthesia.*

**Propocam** *Abbott, Mex.*
Propofol (p.1305·3).
*General anaesthesia; sedative.*

**Propofan** *Aventis, Fr.*
Dextropropoxyphene (p.28·3); paracetamol (p.76·2); caffeine (p.782·1).
*Pain.*

**Propol** *Sydenham, Mex.†.*
Propranolol (p.990·1).

**Propolcream** *Bucaneve, Ital.*
Propolis (p.1735·2).

**Propoleos** *Natufarma, Arg.*
Propolis (p.1735·2).
*Dietary supplement.*

**Propolisept Urtinktur** *Johanser, Ger.*
Homoeopathic preparation.

**Propolisept-Salbe** *Johanser, Ger.*
Propolis (p.1735·2).
*Skin disorders.*

**Propomill** *CaDiGroup, Ital.*
Propolis (p.1735·2); chamomile (p.1669·3).
*Skin irritation.*

**Proponol** *Help, Gr.*
Piroxicam (p.84·2).
*Dysmenorrhoea; gout; inflammation; musculoskeletal and joint disorders; pain.*

**Propoten** *Biochimico, Braz.*
Cefoxitin sodium (p.177·2).
*Bacterial infections.*

**Propovan** *Cristalia, Braz.*
Propofol (p.1305·3).
*General anaesthesia.*

**propra** *CT, Ger.*
Propranolol hydrochloride (p.989·3).
*Angina pectoris; arrhythmias; hypertension; hyperthyroidism; tremor.*

**Propra comp** *Ratiopharm, Ger.*
Propranolol hydrochloride (p.989·3); triamterene (p.1016·2); hydrochlorothiazide (p.933·2).
*Hypertension.*

**Proprahexal** *Hexal, Austria.*
Propranolol hydrochloride (p.989·3).
*Angina pectoris; anxiety disorders; arrhythmias; hypertension; hyperthyroidism; migraine; phaeochromocytoma; tremor.*

**Propral** *Orion, Fin.*
Propranolol hydrochloride (p.989·3).
*Angina pectoris; arrhythmias; digitalis toxicity; essential tremor; hypertension; hyperthyroidism; migraine and cluster headache; myocardial infarction; phaeochromocytoma.*

**Propranet** *Nettopharma, Denm.†.*
Propranolol hydrochloride (p.989·3).
*Angina pectoris; arrhythmias; hypertension; hyperthyroidism; migraine; myocardial infarction; tremor; variceal haemorrhage.*

**Propranur** *Stegropharm, Ger.*
Propranolol hydrochloride (p.989·3).
*Angina pectoris; arrhythmias; hypertension; hyperthyroidism.*

**Propra-ratiopharm** *Ratiopharm, Ger.*
Propranolol (p.990·1) or propranolol hydrochloride (p.989·3).
*Angina pectoris; arrhythmias; hypertension; hyperthyroidism; tremor.*

**Pro-PS** *Procare, Austral.†.*
*Cream:* Disodium fumarate (p.1147·3); cetrimide (p.1172·1); chlorhexidine gluconate (p.1173·2).
*Tablets:* Disodium fumarate (p.1147·3); fumaric acid (p.1147·3); vitamins; minerals (p.1417·1).
*Psoriasis.*

**Propulm** *SIT, Ital.*
Procaterol hydrochloride (p.791·1).
*Obstructive airways disease.*

**Propulsid** *Janssen, USA†.*
Cisapride (p.1259·2).
*Gastro-oesophageal reflux.*

**Propulsin** *Janssen-Cilag, Ger.†.*
Cisapride (p.1259·2).
*Gastrointestinal disorders.*

**Propycil**
*Solvay, Ger.; Solvay, Port.*
Propylthiouracil (p.1603·1).
*Hyperthyroidism.*

**Propyderm** *ACO Hud, Swed.*
Emollient.
*Dry skin.*

**Propyl** *Sriprasit, Thai.*
Propylthiouracil (p.1603·1).
*Hyperthyroidism.*

**Propy-Lacticare** *Stiefel, Fr.*
Lactic acid (p.1704·1); propylene glycol (p.1735·2).
*Dry skin disorders.*

**Propyless** *Schering-Plough, Swed.*
Emollient.
*Dry skin.*

**Propylthiocil** *Teva, Israel.*
Propylthiouracil (p.1603·1).
*Hyperthyroidism.*

**Propyl-Thyracil** *Merck Frosst, Canad.*
Propylthiouracil (p.1603·1).
*Hyperthyroidism.*

**Propyre T** *Salvat, Spain†.*
Aspirin (p.15·1); caffeine (p.782·1); theobromine (p.798·2).
*Fever; inflammation; pain.*

**Pro-Q** *CollaGenex, USA.*
Dimeticone (p.1482·1).
*Barrier preparation.*

**Proquin** *Douglas, Austral.*
Ciprofloxacin hydrochloride (p.188·2).
*Bacterial infections.*

**P-Roquine** *PP Lab, Thai.*
Chloroquine phosphate (p.448·2).
*Malaria.*

**Prorhinel**
*Novartis Sante, Fr.*
Benzododecinium bromide (p.1170·2); polysorbate 80 (p.1415·2).
*Rhinopharyngeal infections.*

*Interdelta, Switz.*
Benzododecinium bromide (p.1170·2); sodium chloride (p.1233·3); polysorbate 80 (p.1415·2).
*Nasal disorders.*

**Prorynorm** *Hexal, Ger.†.*
Propafenone hydrochloride (p.988·3).
*Arrhythmias.*

**Pro-Sabona Uno** *Sabona, Ger.*
Urtica (p.1762·1).
*Benign prostatic hyperplasia.*

**Prosatietil** *Equilibre Attitude, Fr.*
Lactoserum glycomacropeptides; red cherry; magnesium oxide; griffonia simplicifolia (p.1696·1) (p.1417·1).
*Obesity.*

**Proscar**
*Merck Sharp & Dohme, Arg.; Merck Sharp & Dohme, Austral.; Merck Sharp & Dohme, Austria; Merck Sharp & Dohme, Belg.; Merck Sharp & Dohme, Braz.; Merck Frosst, Canad.; Merck Sharp & Dohme, Chile; Merck Sharp & Dohme, Denm.; Merck Sharp & Dohme, Fin.; MSD Chibropharm, Ger.; Vianex (Βιανεξ), Gr.; Merck Sharp & Dohme, Hong Kong; Merck Sharp & Dohme, Irl.; Merck Sharp & Dohme, Ital.; Merck Sharp & Dohme, Malaysia; Merck Sharp & Dohme, Mex.; Merck Sharp & Dohme, Neth.; Merck Sharp & Dohme, Norw.; Merck Sharp & Dohme, NZ; Merck Sharp & Dohme, Port.; Merck Sharp & Dohme, S.Afr.; Merck Sharp & Dohme, Singapore; Merck Sharp & Dohme, Spain; Merck Sharp & Dohme, Swed.; Merck Sharp & Dohme, Switz.; Merck Sharp & Dohme, Thai.; Merck Sharp & Dohme, UK; Merck, USA.*
Finasteride (p.1554·2).
*Benign prostatic hyperplasia.*

**Proscope** *Tanabe, Jpn.*
Iopromide (p.1065·2).
*Radiographic contrast medium.*

**Prosedar** *Schering-Plough, Port.*
Quazepam (p.718·2).

**Prosed/DS** *Star, USA.*
Methenamine (p.230·1); salol (p.88·1); methylthioninium chloride (p.1042·2); benzoic acid (p.1169·3); atropine sulfate (p.477·1); hyoscyamine sulfate (p.485·1).
*Pain and discomfort of the urinary tract.*

**Prosed-X** *Procare, Austral.†.*
Valerian (p.1762·2); lupulus (p.1708·1); passion flower (p.1729·1).
*Anxiety; insomnia.*

**Proser** *Ibirn, Ital.†.*
Saw palmetto (p.1569·1).
*Prostatic hyperplasia.*

**Prosgutt** *Farmasa, Mex.*
Saw palmetto (p.1569·1); urtica (p.1762·1).
*Benign prostatic hyperplasia; urinary-tract disorders.*

**Pro-Shape** *Procare, Austral.†.*
Garcinia quaesita; chromium trichloride (p.1425·1); pectin (p.1580·3); methylcellulose (p.1580·2); magnesium amino acid chelate (p.1229·1).
*Dietary fibre supplement; obesity.*

**Prosicca** *Agepha, Austria.*
Hypromellose (p.1579·3).
*Eye irritation.*

**ProSight Lutein** *Major, USA.*
Vitamin and mineral preparation (p.1417·1).

**Prosiston** *Schering, Ger.*
Norethisterone acetate (p.1562·2); ethinylestradiol (p.1553·2).
*Menstrual disorders.*

**Proskin**
*Note. This name is used for preparations of different composition.*
*Teofarma, Spain.*
Dimethicone (p.1482·1); thiomersal (p.1194·1); zinc oxide (p.1163·2).
*Skin disorders.*

*Julphar, UAE.*
Zinc oxide (p.1163·2).
*Nappy rash; skin irritation.*

**Proslender** *Procare, Austral.†.*
Gymnema silvestre; dietary fibre (p.1253·2).
*Obesity.*

**Proslim-Lipid** *Procare, Austral.†.*
Purified bile extract (p.1660·3).
*Obesity.*

**Prosmin** *Biotenk, Arg.*
Finasteride (p.1554·2).
*Benign prostatic hyperplasia.*

**Prosobee**
*Bristol-Myers Squibb, Arg.; Mead Johnson, Austral.†; Mead Johnson, Braz.; Mead Johnson Nutritionals, Canad.†; Mead Johnson Nutritionals, Fin.; Mead Johnson, Fr.; Mead Johnson, Hong Kong; Mead Johnson, Irl.; Mead Johnson, Israel†; Mead Johnson, Ital.; Mead Johnson, Malaysia; Mead Johnson, NZ†; Mead Johnson, Port.; Mead Johnson, Singapore; Mead Johnson Nutritionals, Thai.; Mead Johnson Nutritionals, UK; Mead Johnson Nutritionals, USA.*
Infant feed (p.1417·1).
*Cow's milk intolerance; galactokinase deficiency; galactosaemia; gluten sensitivity; lactose or sucrose intolerance.*

**Prosom** *Abbott, USA.*
Estazolam (p.697·3).
*Insomnia.*

**Pro-Sope** *Rougier, Canad.†.*
Sodium lauril ether sulfate (p.1574·3).
*Instrument disinfection.*

**Prosoyal** *FDC, India.*
Infant feed (p.1417·1).
*Intolerance to animal milk; lactose intolerance.*

**Prospan**
*Sanova, Austria; Madaus, Fr.; Engelhard, Ger.; Engelhard, Malaysia; Engelhard, Switz.†.*
Hedera helix.
*Coughs; respiratory-tract disorders associated with excess viscous mucus.*

**Prospec** *Protein, Mex.†.*
Ambroxol (p.1114·3).

**Prost-I** *Procare, Austral.†.*
Vitamins; amino acids; minerals (p.1417·1); devil's claw root (p.28·2); yucca (p.1766·2); salix (p.87·3); green-lipped mussel (p.1696·1); bromelains (p.1662·2); papain (p.1727·3).
*Dietary supplement; musculoskeletal and joint disorders.*

**Prosta** *Procare, Austral.†.*
Saw palmetto (p.1569·1).
*Benign prostatic hyperplasia.*

**Prosta Fink forte** *GlaxoSmithKline Consumer, Ger.*
Cucurbita (p.1677·3).
*Prostatic disorders.*

**Prosta Fink N** *SmithKline Beecham OTC, Ger.†.*
Saw palmetto (p.1569·1); cucurbita (p.1677·3).
*Prostatic disorders.*

**Prosta Urgenin Uno** *Hoyer, Ger.*
Saw palmetto (p.1569·1).
*Benign prostatic hyperplasia.*

**Prostabiol** *Yves Ponroy, Fr.*
Cucurbita; acerola; zinc gluconate; pollen (p.1417·1).
*Urinary-tract disorders in men.*

**Prosta-Caps Chassot N** *Mavena, Switz.*
Cucurbita (p.1677·3); cucurbita oil (p.1677·3); saw palmetto (p.1569·1); echinacea angustifolia (p.1683·2); java tea (p.1702·3); ononis (p.1723·3).
Formerly contained cucurbita, cucurbita oil, saw palmetto, echinacea angustifolia, rubia tinctorum, java tea, and ononis.
*Benign prostatic hyperplasia.*

**Prosta-Caps Fink** *SmithKline Beecham Consumer, Switz.†.*
Cucurbita (p.1677·3); cucurbita oil (p.1677·3); saw palmetto (p.1569·1).
*Benign prostatic hyperplasia.*

**Prostacur**
*Note. This name is used for preparations of different composition.*
*Finadiet, Arg.*
Sitosterol (p.982·3).
*Benign prostatic hyperplasia.*

*Prasfarma, Spain.*
Flutamide (p.556·2).
*Prostatic cancer.*

**Prostadilat** *Pfizer, Austria.*
Doxazosin mesilate (p.908·3).
*Benign prostatic hyperplasia; hypertension.*

**Prostadirex** *Irex, Fr.*
Flutamide (p.556·2).
*Prostatic cancer.*

**Prostaflor**
*Sanova, Austria; Roche, Switz.*
Pollen extracts.
*Benign prostatic hyperplasia.*

**Prostafort** *Knop, Chile.*
Saw palmetto (p.1569·1).
*Benign prostatic hyperplasia.*

**Prostaforton** *Biocur, Ger.*
Urtica root (p.1762·1).
*Benign prostatic hyperplasia.*

**Prostagalen** *Galenika, Ger.*
Urtica root (p.1762·1).
*Prostatic disorders.*

**Prostagutt** *Austroplant, Austria.*
Saw palmetto (p.1569·1); populi trem. (p.1733·3); urtica dioica (p.1762·1).
*Bladder disorders; prostatic disorders.*

**Prostagutt forte** *Schwabe, Ger.*
Saw palmetto (p.1569·1); urtica root (p.1762·1).
*Prostatic disorders.*

**Prostagutt mono** *Schwabe, Ger.*
Saw palmetto (p.1569·1).
*Benign prostatic hyperplasia.*

**Prostagutt uno** *Schwabe, Ger.*
Saw palmetto (p.1569·1).
*Benign prostatic hyperplasia.*

**Prostagutt-F** *Schwabe, Switz.*
Saw palmetto (p.1569·1); urtica (p.1762·1).
*Benign prostatic hyperplasia.*

**Prostaherb N** *Cesra, Ger.*
Urtica root (p.1762·1).
*Benign prostatic hyperplasia.*

**Prostakan** *Schwabe, Malaysia; Bio-Pharmaceuticals, Malaysia.*
Saw palmetto (p.1569·1); urtica (p.1762·1).
*Benign prostatic hyperplasia.*

**Prostal**
*Note. This name is used for preparations of different composition.*
*Motima, Fr.*
Pollen.
*Tonic.*

*Teikoku, Jpn.*
Chlormadinone acetate (p.1542·1).
*Prostatic cancer; prostatic hyperplasia.*

**Prostalium** *Teuto, Braz.*
Saw palmetto (p.1569·1).
*Benign prostatic hyperplasia.*

**Prostall** *Recalcine, Chile.*
Tamsulosin hydrochloride (p.1009·2).
*Prostatic disorders.*

**Prostalog** *Byk Tosse, Ger.†; Byk Gulden, Ger.†.*
Cucurbita (p.1677·3).
*Prostatic disorders.*

**Prostamal** *Almirall, Spain†.*
Pygeum africanum (p.1568·2).
*Benign prostatic hyperplasia.*

**Prostamed**
*Klein, Ger.; Distrifarma, Port.*
Cucurbita (p.1677·3); solidago virgaurea (p.1748·3); poplar leaf (p.1733·3).
*Prostatic and urinary-tract disorders.*

**Prostamed Urtica** *Klein, Ger.*
Urtica (p.1762·1).
*Micturition disorders associated with prostatic cancer.*

**Prostamid** *BDH, India.*
Flutamide (p.556·2).
*Prostatic cancer.*

**Prostamustin** *Azupharma, Ger.*
Estramustine meglumine phosphate (p.551·2) or estramustine sodium phosphate (p.551·1).
*Prostatic cancer.*

**Prostan** *Progress, Thai.*
Mefenamic acid (p.55·2).
*Pain.*

**Prostandin** *Ono, Jpn.*
Alprostadil alfadex (p.1512·3).
*Controlled hypotension in surgery; peripheral vascular disorders.*

**Prostaneurin** *Sanofi Synthelabo, Ger.*
Urtica root (p.1762·1).
*Benign prostatic hyperplasia.*

**Prostanovag** *Gobbi, Arg.*
Finasteride (p.1554·2).
*Benign prostatic hyperplasia.*

**Prostap**
*Wyeth, Irl.; Wyeth, UK.*
Leuprorelin acetate (p.1331·1).
*Endometriosis; prostatic cancer; uterine fibroids.*

**Prostaphlin-A** *Bristol-Myers Squibb, Israel†.*
Cloxacillin sodium (p.198·2).
*Staphylococcal infections.*

**Prostarell** *Sanorell, Ger.*
Homoeopathic preparation.

**Prostasal** *TAD, Ger.*
Sitosterol (p.982·3).
*Prostatic disorders.*

**Prostasan** *Bioforce, Switz.*
Saw palmetto (p.1569·1).
*Benign prostatic hyperplasia.*

**Prostascint Kit** *Cytogen, Israel.*
Indium-111 capromab pendetide (p.1523·3).
*Diagnosis of prostatic cancer.*

**Prostaselect** Dreluso, Ger.†.
Homoeopathic preparation.

**Prostaserene** Therabel, Belg.
Saw palmetto (p.1569·1).
*Micturition disorders due to benign prostatic hyperplasia.*

**Prostasyx** Syxyl, Ger.†.
Homoeopathic preparation.

**Prostata** Stada, Ger.
Urtica root (p.1762·1).
*Prostatic disorders.*

**Prostata-Gastreu N R25** Reckeweg, Ger.
Homoeopathic preparation.

**Prostata-Komplex N Ho-Fu-Complex** Liebermann, Ger.
Homoeopathic preparation.

**Prostata-Kurbis S** Twardy, Ger.†.
Cucurbita (p.1677·3); cucurbita oil (p.1677·3); sago palm.
*Prostatic disorders; urinary-tract disorders.*

**Prostatal** Herbarium, Braz.
Saw palmetto (p.1569·1).
*Benign prostatic hyperplasia.*

**Prostate Support** Reese, USA.
Sitosterol (p.982·3); zinc citrate.

**Prostatin F** Abbott, Ger.
Bearberry (p.1659·2); urtica root (p.1762·1).
*Prostatitis.*

**Prostatonin**
Madaus, Austria; Pharmaton, Switz.
Pygeum africanum (p.1568·2); urtica (p.1762·1).
*Benign prostatic hyperplasia.*

**Prosta-Urgenin**
Madaus, Austria; Madaus, Belg.; Madaus, Ger.†.
Saw palmetto (p.1569·1).
*Benign prostatic hyperplasia.*

**Prosta-Urgenine** Biomed, Switz.
Saw palmetto (p.1569·1).
*Benign prostatic hyperplasia.*

**Prostavasin**
Sidus, Arg.; Gebro, Austria; Biosintetica, Braz.; Schwarz, Ger.; Schwarz, Hong Kong; Schwarz, Ital.
Alprostadil alfadex (p.1512·3).
*Peripheral arterial occlusion.*

**Prostawern** Wernigerode, Ger.
Urtica root (p.1762·1).
*Prostatic disorders.*

**Prostazosina** Kampel Martian, Arg.
Doxazosin (p.909·1).
*Benign prostatic hyperplasia.*

**Prostease** Jamieson, Canad.
Cranberry (p.1676·3); cucurbita seed oil (p.1677·3); pygeum bark (p.1568·2); saw palmetto berry (p.1569·1).

**Prostec** CSC, Austria.
Mepartricin (p.405·2).
*Benign prostatic hyperplasia.*

**Prostem** Baldacci, Braz.
Pygeum africanum (p.1568·2).
*Benign prostatic hyperplasia.*

**Prostem Plus** Baldacci, Braz.
Pygeum africanum (p.1568·2); urtica (p.1762·1).
*Benign prostatic hyperplasia.*

**Prostene** Armstrong, Arg.
Finasteride (p.1554·2).
*Benign prostatic hyperplasia.*

**Prosteo** Procare, Austral.†.
Calcium gluconate (p.1225·2); calcium carbonate (p.1254·2); colecalciferol (p.1461·3); dolomite.
*Calcium supplement.*

**Prostep**
Elan, Canad.; Lederle, USA.
Nicotine (p.1720·1).
*Aid to smoking withdrawal.*

**Prosteren** Crinos, Ital.
Saw palmetto (p.1569·1).
*Benign prostatic hyperplasia.*

**Prostess** TAD, Ger.
Saw palmetto (p.1569·1).
*Benign prostatic hyperplasia.*

**Prostetin** Takeda, Jpn†.
Oxendolone (p.1565·2).
*Prostatic hyperplasia.*

**Prostex** Medix, Mex.
Saw palmetto (p.1569·1).
*Benign prostatic hyperplasia.*

**ProstGard** Holista, Canad.
Cucurbita seed oil (p.1677·3); saw palmetto berry (p.1569·1); vitamin $B_6$ (p.1457·2); zinc gluconate (p.1469·2).

**Prostica** TAD, Ger.
Flutamide (p.556·2).
*Prostatic cancer.*

**Prostide**
Libbs, Braz.; Sigma-Tau, Ital.
Finasteride (p.1554·2).
*Benign prostatic hyperplasia.*

**Prostigmin**
ICN, Arg.; Dermatech, Austral.; ICN, Austria; ICN, Canad.; ICN, Hong Kong; Roche, Irl.†; ICN, Malaysia; ICN, Neth.; Medilink, Norw.†; ICN, Thai.; ICN, USA.
Neostigmine (p.1492·2), neostigmine bromide (p.1492·2), or neostigmine metilsulfate (p.1492·2).
*Intestinal atony; myasthenia gravis; postoperative distension and urinary retention; reversal of competitive neuromuscular blockade.*

**Prostigmina** ICN, Ital.
Neostigmine metilsulfate (p.1492·2).
*Gastrointestinal atony; myasthenia gravis; reversal of competitive neuromuscular blockade.*

**Prostigmine**
Sanico, Belg.†; ICN, Braz.; Roche, Chile; CSP, Fr.; IFET (ΙΦΕΤ), Gr.; Roche, Israel†; ICN, Mex.; ICN, Port.; ICN, Spain; ICN, Switz.
Neostigmine bromide (p.1492·2) or neostigmine metilsulfate (p.1492·2).
*Ileus; meteorism; myasthenia gravis; postoperative intestinal atony; postoperative urinary retention; reversal of competitive neuromuscular blockade.*

**Prostin** Pharmacia, Singapore.
Dinoprostone (p.1515·1).
*Labour induction.*

**Prostin E2**
Pharmacia, Austral.; Pharmacia, Austria; Pharmacia, Belg.; Pharmacia, Canad.; Pharmacia-Upjohn, Gr.; Pharmacia, Hong Kong; Pharmacia, Irl.; Pharmacia Upjohn, Israel; Pharmacia Upjohn, Ital.; Pharmacia, Malaysia; Pharmacia, Neth.; Pharmacia, NZ; Pharmacia, Port.; Pharmacia, S.Afr.; Pharmacia, Switz.; Pharmacia, Thai.; Pharmacia, UK; Pharmacia Upjohn, USA.
Dinoprostone (p.1515·1).
*Hydatidiform mole; labour induction; termination of pregnancy.*

**Prostin F2** Pharmacia, Irl.
Dinoprost trometamol (p.1514·3).
*Labour induction.*

**Prostin F2 Alpha**
Pharmacia, Austral.; Pharmacia, Hong Kong; Pharmacia Upjohn, Israel; Pharmacia, NZ; Pharmacia, S.Afr.
Dinoprost trometamol (p.1514·3).
*Hydatidiform mole; labour induction; termination of pregnancy.*

**Prostin Pediatrico** Pharmacia, Chile.
Alprostadil (p.1512·3).
*Maintenance of patent ductus arteriosus.*

**Prostin VR**
Pharmacia, Austral.; Pharmacia, Belg.; Pharmacia, Canad.; Pharmacare, Gr.; Pharmacia, Hong Kong; Pharmacia Upjohn, India; Pharmacia Upjohn, Israel; Pharmacia Upjohn, Ital.; Pharmacia, Malaysia; Pharmacia, Neth.; Pharmacia, NZ; Pharmacia, Port.; Pharmacia, S.Afr.; Pharmacia, Switz.; Pharmacia, Thai.; Pharmacia, UK; Upjohn, USA.
Alprostadil (p.1512·3).
*Maintenance of patent ductus arteriosus.*

**Prostine $E_2$** Pharmacia, Fr.
Dinoprostone (p.1515·1).
*Hydatidiform mole; labour induction; termination of pregnancy.*

**Prostine $F_2$ Alpha** Pharmacia Upjohn, Fr.†.
Dinoprost trometamol (p.1514·3).
*Labour induction.*

**Prostine VR** Pharmacia, Fr.
Alprostadil (p.1512·3).
*Maintenance of patent ductus arteriosus.*

**Prostinfenem**
Pharmacia, Denm.; Pharmacia, Swed.
Carboprost trometamol (p.1514·2).
*Intra-uterine death; postpartum haemorrhage; termination of pregnancy.*

**Prostin/15M**
Pharmacia, Belg.; Pharmacia, Neth.; Pharmacia, NZ.
Carboprost trometamol (p.1514·2).
*Intra-uterine death; postpartum haemorrhage; termination of pregnancy.*

**Prostivas**
Pharmacia, Denm.; Pharmacia, Fin.; Pharmacia, Norw.; Pharmacia, Swed.
Alprostadil (p.1512·3).
*Maintenance of patent ductus arteriosus.*

**Prostodin** AstraZeneca, India.
Carboprost trometamol (p.1514·2).
*Postpartum haemorrhage; termination of pregnancy.*

**Prostogenat** Azupharma, Ger.
Flutamide (p.556·2).
*Prostatic cancer.*

**Prosturol** Farmasierra, Spain.
Benzydamine hydrochloride (p.21·1); pygeum africanum (p.1568·2).
*Prostatic adenoma.*

**Prost-X** Homeocan, Canad.
Homoeopathic preparation.

**Prosulf**
CP Pharmaceuticals, Hong Kong; CP, Israel; CP Pharmaceuticals, UK.
Protamine sulfate (p.1050·3).
*Neutralisation of heparin activity.*

**Prosure**
Abbott, Irl.; Abbott Nutrition, UK.
Preparation for enteral nutrition (p.1417·1).

**Prosymbioflor** Peithner, Austria.
Autolysate of *Escherichia coli*; *Enterococcus faecalis* (p.1704·2).
*Immunotherapy.*

**Pro-Symbioflor** Symbiopharm, Ger.
Autolysates of: *Escherichia coli*; *Enterococcus faecalis* (p.1704·2).
*Gastrointestinal disorders.*

**Prota** Samarth, India.
Protamine sulfate (p.1050·3).
*Antidote to heparin.*

**Protact** Coloplast, Fr.
Barrier cream.

**Protactyl** Hexal, Ger.
Promazine hydrochloride (p.717·3).
*Anxiety; neurogenic pain; premedication; pruritus; psychoses; sleep disorders; vomiting.*

**Protagent**
Alcon, Austria; Bournonville, Belg.†; Alcon, Ger.; Alkon (Αλκον), Gr.; Alcon, Hong Kong; Alcon, Ital.; Alcon, Switz.
Povidone (p.1581·2).
*Dry eyes; eye irritation.*

**Protalgia** Reig Jofre, Spain†.
Fosfosal (p.44·2).
*Fever; musculoskeletal, joint, and soft-tissue disorders; pain.*

**Protamide**
Note. This name is used for preparations of different composition.
Therabel, Belg.†.
Stomach extract.
*Postherpetic neuralgia.*

Ferraz, Lynce, Port.†.
Amino-acids, peptones, and polypeptides (p.1417·1).

**Protan** Protein, Mex.†.
Dextromethorphan (p.1117·3).

**Protangix** Expanpharm, Fr.†.
Dipyridamole (p.903·1).
*Coronary disorders; thromboembolic disorders.*

**Protanol** Teuto, Braz.
Amitriptyline hydrochloride (p.280·3).
*Depression.*

**Protaphan**
Novo Nordisk, Fin.; Novo Nordisk, Ger.
Neutral isophane insulin injection (human) (p.333·3).
*Diabetes mellitus.*

**Protaphane**
Novo Nordisk, Austral.; Novo Nordisk, NZ.
Isophane insulin injection (human, monocomponent) (p.333·3).
*Diabetes mellitus.*

**Protaphane HM**
Novo Nordisk, Gr.; Novo Nordisk, Hong Kong; Novo Nordisk, Ital.; Novo Nordisk, S.Afr.
Isophane insulin injection (human, monocomponent) (p.333·3).
*Diabetes mellitus.*

**Protaphane MC**
Novo Nordisk, Braz.; Novo Nordisk, Hong Kong†.
Neutral isophane insulin injection (porcine, monocomponent) (p.333·3).
*Diabetes mellitus.*

**Protarin** Wayne, Mex.†.
Medroxyprogesterone (p.1557·3).

**Protasol** Alcon, Austria†.
Comfort drops for hard contact lenses (p.1164·2).

**Protat** Potter's, UK.
Corn silk (p.1676·1).
Formerly contained corn silk and kava.
*Bladder discomfort.*

**Protaxil**
Delta, Port.; Rottapharm, Spain†.
Proglumetacin maleate (p.85·2).
*Inflammation; musculoskeletal, joint, peri-articular, and soft-tissue disorders.*

**Protaxol** Provit, Mex.
Co-trimoxazole (p.199·3).
*Bacterial infections.*

**Protaxon**
Sanofi Synthelabo, Austria; Opfermann, Ger.
Proglumetacin maleate (p.85·2).
*Gout; musculoskeletal joint, peri-articular, and soft-tissue disorders.*

**Protease** Richmond, Arg.
Nevirapine (p.650·2).
*HIV infection.*

**Proteazone** IMS, Ital.
Adazone.
*Instrument disinfection.*

**Protec** Protec, UK.
Dioctyl adipate (p.1504·2).
*Insect repellent.*

**Pro-Tec Sport** Allergan, Canad.
*SPF 20:* Octinoxate (p.1154·3); octisalate (p.1154·3); oxybenzone (p.1154·3).
*Sunscreen.*

**Protec T** Implementos Plasticos, Mex.†.
Copper-wound plastic (p.1425·3).
*Intra-uterine contraceptive device.*

**Proteccion Ultra** Rider, Chile.
*SPF 30:* Octinoxate (p.1154·3); oxybenzone (p.1154·3); octisalate (p.1154·3); meradimate (p.1151·3); homosalate (p.1148·1).
*Sunscreen.*

**ProTech** Triton, USA.
Povidone-iodine (p.1190·3); lidocaine hydrochloride (p.1377·3).
*Burns; cuts.*

**Protecor** Duopharm, Ger.
Crataegus (p.1677·1); magnesium complex with acid hydrolysate of corn starch; alpha tocoferil acetate (p.1465·1).
*Cardiovascular disorders.*

**Protectaid**
Axcan, Canad.; Axcan, Hong Kong; Sinclair, UK.
Nonoxinol 9 (p.1413·3); sodium cholate; benzalkonium chloride (p.1168·3).
*Contraceptive.*

**Protecteur Levres** Lancome, Canad.†.
*SPF 15:* Octinoxate (p.1154·3); titanium dioxide (p.1160·3).
*Sunscreen.*

**Protectina** Gross, Braz.
Doxycycline hyclate (p.206·2).
*Bacterial infections.*

**Protecto** National Care, Canad.
Benzethonium chloride (p.1169·2); zinc oxide (p.1163·2).
*Barrier cream.*

**Protecto-Derm** Ingram & Bell, Canad.†.
Silicone (p.1482·1).
*Barrier cream.*

**Protectol** Daniels, USA.
Calcium undecenoate (p.410·3).
*Bromhidrosis; fungal skin infections; hyperhidrosis; minor skin irritation; nappy rash.*

**Protector** Quimifar, Spain.
Loperamide (p.1271·2).
Formerly contained diphenoxylate hydrochloride.
*Diarrhoea.*

**Protegra Antioxid** Wyeth-Whitehall, Arg.
Vitamin and mineral preparation (p.1417·1).

**Proteigeno** Poen, Arg.
β-Aminoethanol phosphoric acid; amino acids; pyridoxine (p.1417·1).
*Tonic.*

**Proteika** Leman, Fr.†.
Nutritional supplement (p.1417·1).

**Protein Free Diet (Product 80056)** Mead Johnson, Austral.
Preparation for infant enteral nutrition (p.1417·1).
*Disorders of amino acid metabolism.*

**Protein Plus** Nutricia, Austral.†.
High protein enteral feed (p.1417·1).

**Protein-Free**
Mead Johnson, Hong Kong; Mead Johnson, Ital.
Food for low-protein diets (p.1417·1).

**Proteinsteril Hepa** Fresenius, Belg.†.
Amino-acid infusion (p.1417·1).
*Parenteral nutrition in liver failure.*

**Proteinsteril KE** Fresenius, Belg.†.
Amino-acid infusion with electrolytes (p.1417·1).
*Parenteral nutrition.*

**Proteita** Janssen-Cilag, Arg.
Collagen (p.1674·3).
*Ulcers; wounds.*

**Protemp** Procare, Austral.†.
Vitamins; minerals (p.1417·1); bearberry (p.1659·2); parsley piert (p.1729·1); juniper (p.1703·1); viburnum opulus.
*Dietary supplement; dysmenorrhoea; premenstrual syndrome.*

**Proten Plus** Fresenius Kabi, Port.†.
Preparation for enteral nutrition (p.1417·1).

**Protenac** Enila, Braz.
Preparation for enteral nutrition (p.1417·1).

**Protenate**
Baxter-Hyland, Hong Kong†; Hyland, USA.
Plasma protein fraction (p.758·2).
*Burns; hypoalbuminaemia; hypovolaemia.*

**Protensin-M** Bristol-Myers Squibb, S.Afr.
Hydroflumethiazide (p.937·2); reserpine (p.995·1).
*Hypertension.*

**Proteoferrina** Bayer, Ital.
Iron succinyl-protein complex (p.1438·1).
*Iron deficiency; iron-deficiency anaemia.*

**Proteozym** Wiedemann, Ger.
Bromelains (p.1662·2).
*Inflammation; oedema.*

**Proterenal** Phoenix, Arg.
Isoprenaline hydrochloride (p.940·2).
*Heart block; shock.*

**Proteval** Protein, Mex.†.
Valproic acid (p.380·1).

**Protevis** Allergan, Arg.
Timolol maleate (p.1012·2).
*Glaucoma; ocular hypertension.*

**Protexel** Lab Francais du Fractionnement, Fr.
Protein C (p.759·2).
*Thromboembolic disorders.*

**Prothanon** Riemser, Ger.
Dioxopromethazine hydrochloride (p.440·1).
*Skin disorders.*

**Prothanon cromo** Chauvin ankerpharm, Ger.†.
Sodium cromoglicate (p.795·3).
*Allergic conjunctivitis; allergic rhinitis.*

**Prothazin** Rodleben, Ger.; Wernigerode, Ger.
Promethazine hydrochloride (p.439·1).
*Allergic disorders; anxiety; insomnia; premedication; psychoses; vomiting.*

**Prothazine** Strand, Malaysia.
Promethazine hydrochloride (p.439·1).
*Hypersensitivity reactions; motion sickness; nausea and vomiting.*

**Prothiaden**
Abbott, Austral.; Knoll, Belg.; Abbott, Denm.; Teofarma, Fr.; Abbott, Hong Kong; Knoll, India; Abbott, Irl.; Abbott, Malaysia; Knoll, Neth.; Abbott, NZ; Knoll, S.Afr.; Abbott, Singapore; Alter, Spain; Boots, Thai.; Abbott, UK.
Dosulepin hydrochloride (p.291·1).
*Depression; mixed anxiety depressive states.*

**Prothiazide** *Pacific, NZ†.*
Cyclopenthiazide (p.890·3).
*Heart failure; hypertension; oedema.*

**Prothiazine** *CTI, Israel.*
Promethazine hydrochloride (p.439·1).
*Anxiety; coughs; hypersensitivity reactions; insomnia; nausea; pain; parkinsonism; premedication.*

**Prothiazine Expectorant** *CTI, Israel.*
Promethazine hydrochloride (p.439·1); guaifenesin (p.1122·1); ipecacuanha (p.1122·3).
*Coughs.*

**Prothicid** *Themis Chemicals, India.*
Protionamide (p.246·3).
*Tuberculosis.*

**Prothil** *Solvay, Ger.*
Medrogestone (p.1557·1).
*Menopausal disorders; progestagenic.*

**Prothiucil** *Sanova, Austria.*
Propylthiouracil (p.1603·1).
*Hyperthyroidism; ulcerative colitis.*

**Prothrombinex** *CSL, NZ.*
A factor IX preparation (p.752·2).
*Haemorrhagic disorders.*

**Prothrombinkomplex BaWu** *Intersero, Ger.*
A factor IX preparation (p.752·2).
*Haemorrhagic disorders.*

**Prothromplex**
*Baxter, Spain; Immuno, UK†.*
A factor IX preparation (p.752·2).
*Haemorrhagic disorders.*

**Prothromplex S-TIM 4**
*Immuno, Austria; Immuno, Ger.†.*
A factor IX preparation (p.752·2).
*Haemorrhagic disorders.*

**Prothromplex Total S-TIM 4** *Baxter, Switz.*
A factor IX preparation (p.752·2).
*Haemorrhagic disorders.*

**Prothromplex-T** *Immuno, Braz.†.*
A factor IX preparation (p.752·2).
*Haemorrhagic disorders.*

**Prothromplex-T TIM 4** *Adcock Ingram Critical Care, S.Afr.*
A factor IX preparation (p.752·2).
*Haemorrhagic disorders.*

**Prothuril** *Unipharma, Gr.*
Propylthiouracil (p.1603·1).
*Hyperthyroidism.*

**Prothyrid**
*Sanofi Synthelabo, Austria; Henning, Ger.*
Levothyroxine sodium (p.1600·1); liothyronine hydrochloride (p.1602·2).
*Hypothyroidism; thyroiditis.*

**Prothyrysat** *Ysatfabrik, Ger.*
Lycopus europaeus.
*Hyperthyroidism.*

**Proti 5** *Pharmygiene, Fr.*
Nutritional supplement (p.1417·1).

**Protiaden**
*Teofarma, Ital.; Knoll, Switz.*
Dosulepin hydrochloride (p.291·1).
*Depression; mixed anxiety depressive states.*

**Protiadene** *Abbott, Port.*
Dosulepin hydrochloride (p.291·1).
*Depression.*

**Protical** *Pharmygiene, Fr.*
High protein foods for special diets (p.1417·1).

**Protid** *Lunsco, USA.*
Paracetamol (p.76·2); chlorphenamine maleate (p.427·3); phenylephrine hydrochloride (p.1126·3).

**Protideal** *Protiforme, Fr.*
High protein foods for special diets (p.1417·1).

**Protiderm** *Panalab, Arg.*
Miconazole nitrate (p.405·3); zinc oxide (p.1163·2).
*Fungal nappy rash.*

**Protidiet** *Protidiet, Fr.*
Nutritional protein supplement (p.1417·1).

**Protifar**
*Nutricia, Austral.; Nutricia, Fin.; Nutricia, Fr.; Nutricia, Irl.; Nutricia, Ital.; Baxter, NZ; Nutricia, NZ; Nutricia, Thai.; Nutricia Clinical, UK.*
Dietary protein supplement (p.1417·1).

**Protifar Plus** *Nutricia, Port.*
High protein nutritional supplement (p.1417·1).

**Protifortf** *Pharmygiene, Fr.†.*
Preparation for enteral nutrition (p.1417·1).

**Protifortifiant** *Pharmygiene, Fr.*
Protein enriched nutritional supplement (p.1417·1).

**Protil** *Diepal, Fr.†.*
High protein nutritional supplement (p.1417·1).

**Protilase** *Rugby, USA†.*
Pancrelipase (p.1725·3).
*Pancreatic enzyme deficiency.*

**Protina G** *Fresenius Kabi, Ital.*
Preparation for enteral nutrition (p.1417·1).

**Protina Torre MP** *Fresenius Kabi, Ital.*
Preparation for enteral nutrition (p.1417·1).

**Protinex** *Pfizer, India.*
High-protein dietary supplement (p.1417·1).

**Protinin** *Probifasa, Mex.*
Aprotinin (p.742·3).
*Cardiopulmonary bypass; extracorporeal circulation; haemorrhage.*

**Protinules** *Alembic, India.*
High-protein dietary supplement (p.1417·1).

**Protinutril** *Pharmacia Upjohn, Fr.†.*
Amino-acid, vitamin, and mineral infusion (p.1417·1).
*Parenteral nutrition.*

**Protipharm** *DHN, Fr.†.*
A range of nutritional supplements (p.1417·1).

**Protireal** *Novartis Nutrition, Fr.†.*
Preparation for enteral nutrition (p.1417·1).

**Protium**
*Abbott, Irl.; Altana, UK.*
Pantoprazole sodium (p.1283·1).
*Gastro-oesophageal reflux; peptic ulcer; Zollinger-Ellison syndrome.*

**Protobex** *Centaur, India.*
Nutritional supplement (p.1417·1).

**Proto-Boric** *Bell, India.*
Boric acid (p.1662·1); borax (p.1661·3); naphazoline hydrochloride (p.1124·3); camphor (p.1665·3); menthol (p.1711·3).
*Corneal ulcer; inflammatory eye infections.*

**Protocide** *Unipharm, Israel.*
Tinidazole (p.617·1).
*Anaerobic bacterial infections; protozoal infections.*

**Protogyl**
*Xepa-Soul Pattinson, Hong Kong†; Xepa-Soul Pattinson, Malaysia; Xepa-Soul Pattinson, Singapore†.*
Metronidazole (p.607·2).
*Amoebiasis; genito-urinary-tract infections; trichomoniasis.*

**Protol** *Procare, Austral.†.*
Vitamins; minerals (p.1417·1); garlic (p.1691·1).
*Dietary supplement; viral infections.*

**Proton**
*Note. This name is used for preparations of different composition.*
*Heralds, Braz.†.*
Vitamin $B_1$ (p.1455·2).
*Vitamin $B_1$ deficiency; vitamin $B_1$ supplement.*

*Medinfar, Port.*
Omeprazole (p.1278·2).
*Gastro-oesophageal reflux; peptic ulcer; Zollinger-Ellison syndrome.*

**Protonix** *Wyeth-Ayerst, USA.*
Pantoprazole sodium (p.1283·1).
*Gastro-oesophageal reflux; Zollinger-Ellison syndrome.*

**Protopam**
*Wyeth-Ayerst, Canad.; Wyeth-Ayerst, USA.*
Pralidoxime chloride (p.1050·1).
*Anticholinesterase antagonist; organophosphorus insecticide poisoning.*

**Protopic**
*Fujisawa, Irl.; Fujisawa, Jpn; Fujisawa, Port.; Fujisawa, Spain; Fujisawa, UK; Fujisawa, USA.*
Tacrolimus (p.1363·3).
*Atopic eczema.*

**Protosin** *Streger, Mex.*
Quinfamide (p.615·2).
*Intestinal amoebiasis.*

**Protosol** *Kamada, Israel.*
Aprotinin (p.742·3).
*Hyperfibrinolytic haemorrhage; reduction of blood loss in cardiopulmonary bypass.*

**Protostat** *Ortho Pharmaceutical, USA.*
Metronidazole (p.607·2).
*Amoebiasis; anaerobic bacterial infections; trichomoniasis.*

**Protovit**
*Roche, Belg.; Roche, Braz.; Roche, Ital.; Roche, Spain.*
Multivitamin preparation (p.1417·1).

*Roche Nicholas, Fr.*
Vitamin and mineral preparation (p.1417·1).

**Protovit N** *Roche, Port.*
Multivitamin preparation (p.1417·1).

**Protozone** *Techniiab, Hong Kong†.*
Hydrocortisone acetate (p.1103·3); cinchocaine hydrochloride (p.1373·2); neomycin sulfate (p.235·1); esculoside (p.1648·2).
*Haemorrhoids.*

**Protromplex** *Baxter Immuno, Arg.*
A factor IX preparation (p.752·2).
*Haemorrhagic disorders.*

**Protromplex TIM 3** *Baxter, Ital.*
Factor IX (p.752·2).
*Deficiency of factors II, IX, and X.*

**Protropin**
*Roche, Canad.; Genentech, USA.*
Somatrem (p.1327·2).
*Growth hormone deficiency.*

**Protuss** *Horizon, USA.*
Hydrocodone tartrate (p.45·1); sulfogaiacol (p.1131·1).
*Coughs.*

**Protussa** *Knoll, India.*
Dextromethorphan hydrobromide (p.1117·3); chlorphenamine maleate (p.427·3).
*Coughs.*

**Protuss-D** *Horizon, USA.*
Hydrocodone tartrate (p.45·1); pseudoephedrine hydrochloride (p.1129·2); sulfogaiacol (p.1131·1).
*Coughs.*

**Protuss-DM** *Horizon, USA.*
Guaifenesin (p.1122·1); pseudoephedrine hydrochloride (p.1129·2); dextromethorphan hydrobromide (p.1117·3).
*Coughs.*

**Pro-Uro** *Ghimas, Ital.†.*
Pipemidic acid (p.243·1).
*Urinary-tract infections.*

**Provacsin Nasal** *Inmunolab, Arg.*
Neomycin (p.235·1); naphazoline (p.1124·3).
*Nasal congestion.*

**Provail**
*CCM, Malaysia; CCM, Singapore.*
Ketoprofen (p.51·2).
*Inflammation; musculoskeletal, joint, and peri-articular disorders; pain.*

**Provames** *Aventis, Fr.*
Estradiol (p.1550·1).
*Menopausal disorders; osteoporosis.*

**Provamicina** *Aventis, Mex.*
Spiramycin (p.255·3).
*Bacterial infections; toxoplasmosis.*

**Provas** *Schwarz, Ger.; Sanol, Ger.*
Valsartan (p.1018·3).
*Hypertension.*

**Provas comp** *Schwarz, Ger.; Sanol, Ger.*
Valsartan (p.1018·3); hydrochlorothiazide (p.933·2).
*Hypertension.*

**Provascul** *Gerot, Austria.*
Bamethan succinate (p.866·3).
*Peripheral vascular disorders.*

**Provatine** *Duopharma, Hong Kong.*
Fluoxetine hydrochloride (p.292·1).
*Depression.*

**Provax** *Probios, Port.*
Lysates of *Staphylococcus aureus*; *Streptococcus pyogenes*; *Streptococcus viridans*; *Klebsiella pneumoniae*; *Klebsiella ozaenae*; *Streptococcus pneumoniae*; *Haemophilus influenzae*; *Moraxella cattarhalis*.
*Respiratory-tract infections.*

**Provegol** *SVR, Fr.*
Pyrithione zinc (p.1156·2).
*Scalp disorders.*

**Provelle** *Pharmacia, Austral.*
Maroon tablets, conjugated oestrogens (Premarin) (p.1543·2); blue tablets, medroxyprogesterone acetate (Provera) (p.1557·2).
*Menopausal disorders; osteoporosis.*

**Provenal** *Pulitzer, Ital.*
A heparinoid (p.931·1).
*Vascular disorders with a risk of thrombosis.*

**Provenen**
*Austroplant, Austria; Schwabe, Spain.*
Aesculus (p.1648·2).
*Venous insufficiency.*

**Proveno N** *Madaus, Ger.*
Aescin (p.1648·2).
*Vascular disorders.*

**Pro-Vent** *Wellcome, Irl.†.*
Theophylline (p.798·3).
*Bronchospasm.*

**Proventil** *Schering, USA.*
Salbutamol (p.791·3) or salbutamol sulfate (p.791·3).
*Bronchospasm.*

**Provera**
*Pharmacia, Austral.; Pharmacia, Austria; Pharmacia, Belg.; Pharmacia, Braz.; Pharmacia, Canad.; Pharmacia, Chile; Pharmacia, Denm.; Pharmacia, Fin.; Pharmacia-Upjohn, Gr.; Pharmacia, Hong Kong; Pharmacia, Irl.; Pharmacia Upjohn, Israel; Pharmacia Upjohn, Ital.; Pharmacia, Malaysia; Pharmacia Upjohn, Mex.; Pharmacia, Neth.; Pharmacia, Norw.; Pharmacia, NZ; Pharmacia, Port.; Pharmacia, S.Afr.; Pharmacia, Singapore; Pharmacia, Swed.; Pharmacia, Thai.; Pharmacia, UK; Pharmacia Upjohn, USA.*
Medroxyprogesterone acetate (p.1557·2).
*Dysfunctional uterine bleeding; endometriosis; malignant neoplasms; menopausal disorders; menstrual disorders; threatened or recurrent miscarriage.*

**Provertin-UM TIM 3** *Baxter, Ital.*
Factor VII (p.750·3).
*Factor VII deficiency.*

**Provetal** *Protein, Mex.†.*
Valproic acid (p.380·1).

**Provette Continuous** *Pharmacia Upjohn, NZ†.*
28 Tablets, conjugated oestrogens (p.1543·2); 28 tablets, medroxyprogesterone acetate (p.1557·2).
*Menopausal disorders; osteoporosis.*

**Provette Sequential** *Pharmacia Upjohn, NZ†.*
28 Tablets, conjugated oestrogens (p.1543·2); 14 tablets, medroxyprogesterone acetate (p.1557·2).
*Menopausal disorders; osteoporosis.*

**Provical** *Stevia, Braz.†.*
Vitamin D; vitamin $B_{12}$; calcium chloride; calcium phosphate; fluoride; sorbitol (p.1417·1).
*Nutritional supplement.*

**Provictol** *SVR, Fr.*
Ichthammol (p.1148·2); salicylic acid (p.1157·1); urea (p.1162·2); tridecyl salicylate; allantoin (p.1141·3).
*Dandruff.*

**Provide** *Fresenius Kabi, Irl.*
Gluten-, lactose-, and milk-free food for special diets (p.1417·1).
*Bowel disorders; nutritional supplement.*

**Providex** *Baldassari, Braz.†.*
Neomycin (p.235·1); benzocaine (p.1370·3); chlorobutanol (p.1176·3).
*Ear infections.*

**ProvideXtra**
*Fresenius Kabi, Fin.; Fresenius Kabi, UK.*
Preparation for enteral nutrition (p.1417·1).

**Provigil**
*Organon, Belg.; Cephalon, Irl.; Lafon, Israel; Dompe Biotec, Ital.; Cephalon, UK; Cephalon, USA.*
Modafinil (p.1591·1).
*Narcoleptic syndrome; shift-work sleep disorders; sleep apnoea.*

**Provimin** *Ross, USA.*
A protein, vitamin, and mineral preparation for enteral nutrition (p.1417·1).

**Proviodine**
*Rougier, Canad.; Rougier, Hong Kong.*
Povidone-iodine (p.1190·3).
*Burns; skin and mucous membrane disinfection; vaginal infections; wounds.*

**Proviron**
*Schering, Austral.; Schering, Austria; Schering, Belg.; Schering, Braz.; Schering, Chile; Schering, Fin.; Schering, Fr.†; Schering, Ger.; Shepa, Gr.; Schering, Hong Kong; Schering, Israel; Schering, Ital.; Schering, Mex.; Schering, Neth.; Schering, Port.; Schering, S.Afr.; Schering, Spain; Schering, Switz.†; Schering, UK.*
Mesterolone (p.1559·1).
*Androgen deficiency; aplastic anaemia; erectile dysfunction; male hypogonadism; male infertility.*

**Provironum**
*German Remedies, India; Schering, Malaysia; Schering, Singapore; Schering, Thai.*
Mesterolone (p.1559·1).
*Androgen deficiency; erectile dysfunction; hypogonadism; male infertility.*

**Provisc**
*Alcon, Arg.; Alcon, Austral.; Alcon, Belg.†; Alcon, Fr.; Alcon, Ger.; Alcon, Hong Kong; Alcon, Irl.; Alcon, Ital.; Alcon, Malaysia; Alcon, NZ; Alcon, S.Afr.; Alcon, Singapore; Alcon, Swed.†; Alcon, Thai.; Alcon, UK†.*
Sodium hyaluronate (p.1697·3).
*Adjunct in eye surgery.*

**Provisual** *Poen, Arg.*
Gentamicin sulfate (p.217·1).
*Bacterial eye infections.*

**Provisual Compuesto** *Poen, Arg.*
Gentamicin sulfate (p.217·1); dexamethasone (p.1097·1); tetryzoline hydrochloride (p.1131·2).
*Infected eye disorders.*

**Provita** *Scherer, Thai.*
Multivitamin and mineral preparation (p.1417·1).

**Provitamin A + D + E** *Klein, Ger.*
Multivitamin preparation (p.1417·1).

**Provitamin A-E** *Cielle, Ital.*
Vitamin A (p.1451·2); vitamin E (p.1464·3); royal jelly (p.1740·3).
*Nutritional supplement.*

**Proviton** *Upha, Malaysia.*
Multivitamin and mineral preparation with ginseng, lecithin, and lysine (p.1417·1).

**Provive** *Zeus, Braz.*
Propofol (p.1305·3).
*General anaesthesia.*

**Provixen-N** *Zekides, Gr.*
Ambroxol hydrochloride (p.1114·3).
*Respiratory disorders associated with viscous mucus.*

**Provocholine**
*Methapharm, Canad.; Methapharm, USA.*
Methacholine chloride (p.1492·1).
*Diagnosis of bronchial hyperreactivity.*

**Provokit** *Lindopharm, Ger.*
Methacholine chloride (p.1492·1).
*Diagnosis of bronchial hyperreactivity.*

**Provotest** *Hoechst, Ger.†.*
Dichlorodifluoromethane (p.1236·1).
*Diagnostic agent.*

**Prowess** *Harley Street Supplies, UK†.*
Yohimbine hydrochloride (p.1766·2); pemoline (p.1591·2); methyltestosterone (p.1559·3).
*Erectile dysfunction.*

**Prowess Plain** *Harley Street Supplies, UK.*
Yohimbine hydrochloride (p.1766·2).
*Erectile dysfunction.*

**Pro-Whey** *Milk Industries, Israel.*
Protein supplement (p.1417·1).

**ProWohl** *Eurim, Ger.†.*
Magaldrate (p.1271·3).
*Gastrointestinal disorders.*

**Proxacin** *Neo Quimica, Braz.*
Ciprofloxacin hydrochloride (p.188·2).
*Bacterial infections.*

**Proxalin** *Degorts, Mex.*
Naproxen (p.65·1).
*Gout; inflammation; musculoskeletal, joint, and periarticular disorders; pain.*

**Proxalin-Plus** *Degorts, Mex.*
Naproxen (p.65·1); paracetamol (p.76·2).
*Fever; pain.*

**Proxalyoc** *Lafon, Fr.*
Piroxicam (p.84·2).
*Musculoskeletal and joint disorders.*

**Proxen**
*Roche, Austral.; Grunenthal, Austria; Syntex, Ger.; Roche, Ger.; Medochemie, Hong Kong; Grunenthal, Switz.; Pharmaland, Thai.*
Naproxen (p.65·1).
*Gout; inflammation; musculoskeletal, joint, peri-articular, and soft-tissue disorders.*

*Almirall, Spain†.*
Naproxen lysine (p.65·3).

Lidocaine (p.1377·3) is included in the injection to alleviate the pain of injection.
*Fever; gout; musculoskeletal, joint, peri-articular, and soft-tissue disorders; pain.*

**Proxidin** Procare, Austral.†.
Vitamins; minerals; garlic; eleutherococcus senticosis (p.1417·1).
*Dietary supplement.*

**Proxigel** Reed & Carnrick, USA†.
Urea hydrogen peroxide (p.1195·3).
*Oral inflammation.*

**Proxil** Rottapharm, Ital.
Proglumetacin maleate (p.85·2).
*Inflammation; pain.*

**Proxin** Strand, Malaysia.
Cloxacillin sodium (p.198·2).
*Bacterial infections.*

**Proxine** Del Saz & Filippini, Ital.†.
Naproxen (p.65·1).
*Musculoskeletal and joint disorders; pain.*

**Proxinor** Progress, Thai.
Norfloxacin (p.238·3).
*Bacterial infections.*

**Proxitec** Tecnofarma, Mex.
Ciprofloxacin (p.188·2).
*Bacterial infections.*

**Proxol** Sam-On, Israel.
Dextropropoxyphene hydrochloride (p.28·3); paracetamol (p.76·2).
*Fever; pain.*

**Proxytab** Wockhardt, India.
Dextropropoxyphene hydrochloride (p.28·3); paracetamol (p.76·2).
*Pain.*

**Proxyvon** Wockhardt, India.
Dextropropoxyphene hydrochloride (p.28·3); paracetamol (p.76·2).
*Pain.*

**Proyeast** Procare, Austral.†.
Garlic (p.1691·1); echinacea (p.1683·2); ascorbic acid (p.1460·2); chaparral (p.1670·1); zinc gluconate (p.1469·2); vitamin A (p.1451·2); pau d'arco.
*Candidiasis.*

**Prozac**
Lilly, Arg.; Lilly, Austral.; Lilly, Belg.; Lilly, Braz.; Lilly, Canad.; Lilly, Chile; Lilly, Fr.; Lilly, Hong Kong; Lilly, Irl.; Lilly, Israel; Lilly, Ital.; Lilly, Malaysia; Lilly, Mex.; Lilly, Neth.; Lilly, NZ; Lilly, Port.; Lilly, S.Afr.; Lilly, Singapore; Dista, Spain; Lilly, Thai.; Lilly, UK; Lilly, USA.
Fluoxetine hydrochloride (p.292·1).
*Bulimia; depression; obsessive-compulsive disorder; panic disorder; premenstrual dysphoric disorder.*

**Prozamel** Clonmel, Irl.
Fluoxetine hydrochloride (p.292·1).
*Bulimia; depression; obsessive-compulsive disorder.*

**Prozatan** UCB, Irl.
Fluoxetine hydrochloride (p.292·1).
*Bulimia; depression; obsessive-compulsive disorder.*

**Prozef** Bristol-Myers Squibb, S.Afr.
Cefprozil (p.179·2).
*Bacterial infections.*

**Prozen** Teuto, Braz.
Fluoxetine hydrochloride (p.292·1).
*Depression.*

**Proziere** Ashbourne, UK.
Prochlorperazine maleate (p.716·3).

**Prozin** Lusofarmaco, Ital.
Chlorpromazine hydrochloride (p.675·2).
*Hiccups; pain; premedication; psychiatric disorders; vomiting.*

**Prozina** Apsen, Braz.†.
Oxaprozin (p.75·1).

**Prozine**
Note. This name is used for preparations of different composition.
Utopian, Thai.
Chlorpromazine hydrochloride (p.675·2).
*Psychoses.*

Hauck, USA.
Promazine hydrochloride (p.717·3).
*Psychoses.*

**Prozit**
Pinewood, Irl.; Pinewood, UK.
Fluoxetine hydrochloride (p.292·1).
*Bulimia; depression; obsessive-compulsive disorder.*

**Prozitel** Farcoral, Mex.
Praziquantel (p.112·2).
*Neurocysticercosis.*

**Prozolin** Liferpal, Mex.
Metronidazole benzoate (p.607·2).

**ProZone** Darier, Mex.
*SPF 30:* Melanin; octinoxate (p.1154·3); octisalate (p.1154·3); oxybenzone (p.1154·3); butyl methoxycinnamate; homosalate (p.1148·1).
*Sunscreen.*

**ProZone Body** Darier, Mex.
*SPF 25:* Melanin; octinoxate (p.1154·3); oxybenzone (p.1154·3); avobenzone (p.1142·3); titanium dioxide (p.1160·3).
*Sunscreen.*

**ProZone Face** Darier, Mex.
*SPF 25:* Melanin; octinoxate (p.1154·3); oxybenzone (p.1154·3); octisalate (p.1154·3).
*Sunscreen.*

**ProZone Ultra** Darier, Mex.
*SPF 80:* Melanin; octocrilene (p.1154·3); octinoxate (p.1154·3); octisalate (p.1154·3); oxybenzone (p.1154·3); avobenzone (p.1142·3); titanium dioxide (p.1160·3).
*Sunscreen.*

**Prozyme** Procare, Austral.†.
Outer layer, pepsin (p.1729·3); bromelains (p.1662·2); glutamic acid hydrochloride (p.1433·2); inner layer, pancreatin (p.1725·3); papain (p.1727·3); bromelains.
*Dyspepsia.*

**Prozyn** Adcock Ingram, S.Afr.†.
Fluoxetine hydrochloride (p.292·1).
*Bulimia nervosa; mixed anxiety depressive states; obsessive-compulsive disorder.*

**Prudencial** Northia, Arg.
Nifedipine (p.966·2).
*Angina pectoris; hypertension.*

**Pruderm** Euroderm, Arg.
Camphor (p.1665·3); menthol (p.1711·3).
*Pruritus.*

**Prueboi** Temis, Arg.
Egg yolk; soya lecithin; sunflower oil.

**Pruina** Faes, Spain.
Senna (p.1288·2); cassia fistula (p.1255·2); coriander (p.1676·1); tamarind (p.1293·2).
*Constipation.*

**Prulit** Vinas, Spain.
Menthol (p.1711·3).
Formerly known as Nopika.
*Insect stings; muscle sprains and strains; pruritus.*

**Prunasine** Christiaens, Belg.
Senna fruit (p.1288·2).
*Constipation.*

**Prunodiet** DHN, Fr.
Dietary fibre supplement (p.1417·1).
*Constipation.*

**Prunogil** Novartis Nutrition, Fr.†.
Dietary fibre supplement (p.1417·1).
*Constipation.*

**Prunus-Bad** Weleda, Austria.
Prunus spinosa.
*Tonic.*

**Prurex** Agepha, Austria.
Diphenhydramine hydrochloride (p.431·3).
*Allergic skin disorders; burns; insect bites; pruritus; sunburn.*

**Pruriced** Uriage, Fr.
*Cream:* Calamine (p.1144·1); borage oil (p.1661·3); Uriage thermal water.
*Topical gel:* Calamine (p.1144·1); glycine (p.1433·3); Uriage thermal water.
*Skin irritation.*

**Pruridermase** Sofex, Port.
Calamine (p.1144·1); diphenhydramine (p.431·3); menthol (p.1711·3).
Formerly contained calamine, diphenhydramine, menthol, and hamamelis.
*Pruritus; skin irritation.*

**Pruridol** Cazi, Braz.
Benzyl benzoate (p.1500·2).
*Pediculosis; scabies.*

**Prurigel** Fortbenton, Arg.
Triclosan (p.1195·2); mallow (p.1709·3); chamomile (p.1669·3).
*Scalp disorders.*

**Pruri-med** Permamed, Switz.
Sodium sulfosuccinated undecenoic acid monoethanolamide (p.411·1); lauromacrogol 400 (p.1412·3).
*Skin disorders.*

**Prurimix** Metochem, Austria.
Talc (p.1159·1); zinc oxide (p.1163·2); lauromacrogol 400 (p.1412·3); menthol (p.1711·3); diphenylpyraline hydrochloride (p.432·3).
*Skin disorders.*

**Pruripelen** ICN, Arg.
Calamine (p.1144·1); benzocaine (p.1370·3); diphenhydramine hydrochloride (p.431·3); camphor (p.1665·3); menthol (p.1711·3).
*Pruritus; skin irritation.*

**Prurisedan** Andromaco, Arg.
*Lotion:* Phenol (p.1188·1); camphor (p.1665·3); zinc oxide (p.1163·2); diphenhydramine hydrochloride (p.431·3); neocalamine (p.1144·1).
*Topical powder:* Phenol (p.1188·1); camphor (p.1665·3); boric acid (p.1662·1); zinc stearate (p.1575·3); zinc oxide (p.1163·2).
*Allergic skin disorders; insect bites; pruritus; sunburn; urticaria.*

**Prurisedan Antimicotico** Andromaco, Arg.
Bifonazole (p.395·1); diphenhydramine hydrochloride (p.431·3).
*Fungal skin and nail infections.*

**Prurisedan Biotic** Andromaco, Arg.
Gentamicin sulfate (p.217·1); ketoconazole (p.403·3); hydrocortisone acetate (p.1103·3).
*Infected skin disorders.*

**Pruritrat** Newlab, Braz.†.
Lindane (p.1506·3).
*Pediculosis; scabies.*

**Prurix**
Stiefel, Arg.; Stiefel, Braz.†; Stiefel, Chile; Stiefel, Mex.
Camphor (p.1665·3); menthol (p.1711·3).
*Pruritus.*

**Prurizin** Darrow, Braz.
Hydroxyzine hydrochloride (p.434·3).
*Hypersensitivity reactions.*

**Pryleugan** Temmler, Ger.
Imipramine hydrochloride (p.300·1).
*Depression; nocturnal enuresis; pain.*

**Pryndette** Aventis, NZ.
Paracetamol (p.76·2); doxylamine succinate (p.432·3).
*Fever; pain; sedative.*

**Prysma** UCB, Spain.
Omeprazole (p.1278·2).
*Gastro-oesophageal reflux; peptic ulcer; Zollinger-Ellison syndrome.*

**Prysoline** Rekah, Israel.
Primidone (p.376·3).
*Epilepsy.*

**PSE CPM** Boca, USA.
Pseudoephedrine hydrochloride (p.1129·2); chlorphenamine maleate (p.427·3).
*Upper respiratory-tract disorders.*

**PSE MSC** Cypress, USA.
Pseudoephedrine hydrochloride (p.1129·2); hyoscine methonitrate (p.483·3).
*Cold symptoms; rhinitis; sinusitis.*

**Pselac** Fresenius Kabi, Austria.
Lactitol (p.1269·1).
*Constipation; hepatic encephalopathy.*

**Pserhofer's** Agepha, Austria.
Aloes (p.1248·2); frangula (p.1266·3).
*Constipation.*

**Pseudo** Major, USA.
Pseudoephedrine hydrochloride (p.1129·2).
*Nasal congestion.*

**Pseudo-Car DM** Geneva, USA.
Pseudoephedrine hydrochloride (p.1129·2); carbinoxamine maleate (p.426·3); dextromethorphan hydrobromide (p.1117·3).
*Coughs and cold symptoms.*

**Pseudocef**
Grunenthal, Austria†; Takeda, Ger.†.
Cefsulodin sodium (p.180·2).
Lidocaine hydrochloride (p.1377·3) may be included in the intramuscular injection to alleviate the pain of injection.
*Bacterial infections.*

**Pseudo-Chlor** Geneva, USA; Major, USA.
Pseudoephedrine hydrochloride (p.1129·2); chlorphenamine maleate (p.427·3).
*Upper respiratory-tract symptoms.*

**Pseudofrin** Trianon, Canad.
Pseudoephedrine hydrochloride (p.1129·2).
*Congestion.*

**Pseudo-Gest** Major, USA.
Pseudoephedrine hydrochloride (p.1129·2).
*Nasal congestion.*

**Pseudo-Gest Plus** Major, USA.
Pseudoephedrine hydrochloride (p.1129·2); chlorphenamine maleate (p.427·3).
*Upper respiratory-tract symptoms.*

**Pseudono** Milano, Thai.†.
Pseudoephedrine hydrochloride (p.1129·2).
*Rhinitis; upper respiratory-tract congestion.*

**Pseudophage** Servier, Fr.
Sodium alginate (p.1577·1); agar (p.1576·3).
*Obesity.*

**Psico Blocan** Estedi, Spain.
Chlordiazepoxide hydrochloride (p.674·2); hyoscine methobromide (p.483·3).
*Gastrointestinal spasm.*

**Psicoasten** Beta, Arg.
Paroxetine hydrochloride (p.311·2).
*Depression; obsessive-compulsive disorder; panic attacks; social phobia.*

**Psicocen** Centrum, Spain.
Sulpiride (p.722·2).
*Anxiety disorders; psychoses; vertigo.*

**Psicofar** Sifarma, Ital.†.
Chlordiazepoxide hydrochloride (p.674·2).
*Anxiety disorders; behaviour disorders in children.*

**Psicoglut** Sanofi Winthrop, Braz.†.
Piracetam (p.1732·1); cyanocobalamin; glutamine; DL-serine; iosine (p.1417·1).
*Impaired mental function.*

**Psicosedin** Farmasa, Braz.
Chlordiazepoxide (p.674·2).
*Adjuvant in general anaesthesia; alcohol withdrawal syndrome; anxiety; panic attacks; tension headache; tremor.*

**Psicosoma Solucion** Ferrer, Spain.
Magnesium glutamate hydrobromide (p.1709·2); promethazine hydrochloride (p.439·1).
*Insomnia; night terrors; sedative.*

**Psilo-Balsam N** Stada, Ger.†.
Diphenhydramine hydrochloride (p.431·3); cetylpyridinium chloride (p.1173·1).
Formerly contained diphenhydramine hydrochloride, cetylpyridinium chloride, and butoxycaine hydrochloride.
*First-degree burns; insect stings; nettle rash; skin irritation; sunburn; wind burns.*

**Psilumax** Columbia, Mex.
Psyllium seed (p.1268·1); wheat fibre (p.1253·2).
*Bowel evacuation; constipation.*

**Psipax** Merck, Port.
Fluoxetine hydrochloride (p.292·1).
*Depression.*

**Psiquial** Merck, Braz.
Fluoxetine hydrochloride (p.292·1).
*Depression.*

**Psiu** Teuto, Braz.
Cetylpyridinium chloride (p.1173·1); ammonium chloride (p.1115·2).
Formerly contained cetylpyridinium chloride, ammonium chloride, sodium citrate, and sodium benzoate.
*Respiratory-tract congestion.*

**Psocortene** Medifa, Fr.†.
Flumetasone pivalate (p.1101·1); salicylic acid (p.1157·1); coal tar (p.1159·2).
*Skin disorders.*

**Psodermil** Edol, Port.
Betamethasone dipropionate (p.1093·1); salicylic acid (p.1157·1).
*Skin and scalp disorders.*

**Pso-Rad** Pentamedical, Ital.
Mallow oil; lappa; aloe; bladderwrack; calendula; lavender; tormentil; helichrysum.
*Skin disorders.*

**Psoraderm 5**
Pharmascience, Fr.; Democal, Switz.†.
5-Methoxypsoralen (p.1154·1).
*Psoriasis.*

**Psoradexan**
Hermal, Ger.; Procter & Gamble, Switz.†.
Dithranol (p.1146·1); urea (p.1162·2).
*Psoriasis.*

**Psoradrate** Procter & Gamble, Irl.†.
Dithranol (p.1146·1); urea (p.1162·2).
*Psoriasis.*

**Psoralon MT** Hermal, Ger.
Dithranol (p.1146·1); salicylic acid (p.1157·1).
*Psoriasis.*

**Psorantral** Isdin, Spain†.
Dithranol (p.1146·1); salicylic acid (p.1157·1).
*Psoriasis.*

**Psor-a-set** Hogil, USA.
Salicylic acid (p.1157·1).

**Psor-Asist** Sunspot, Austral.
*Cream:* Sulfur (p.1158·2); salicylic acid (p.1157·1); coal tar (p.1159·2).
*Psoriasis.*
*Lotion:* Sulfur (p.1158·2); salicylic acid (p.1157·1); aloe vera (p.1141·3); urea (p.1162·2).
*Psoriasis of the scalp.*

**Psorasolv** Potter's, UK.
Starch (p.1449·1); sublimed sulfur (p.1158·2); zinc oxide (p.1163·2); pokeroot (p.1733·1); clivers (p.1673·2).
*Psoriasis.*

**Psorcon** Dermik, USA.
Diflorasone diacetate (p.1099·3).
*Skin disorders.*

**Psorcutan**
Schering, Austria; Schering, Ger.; Asche, Ger.; Schering, Ital.
Calcipotriol (p.1144·1).
*Psoriasis.*

**Psorex** GlaxoSmithKline, Braz.
Clobetasol propionate (p.1095·2).
*Skin disorders.*

**Psoriacen** Sanitas, Port.
Calaguala.
*Dermatitis; psoriasis.*

**Psoriacreme** Bradleys, NZ†.
Coal tar (p.1159·2).
*Eczema; psoriasis.*

**Psoriasdin** Isdin, Spain.
Coal tar (p.1159·2).
*Keratinisation disorders; psoriasis.*

**Psoriasis-Bad** Balneopharm, Ger.
Fumaric acid (p.1147·3); disodium fumarate (p.1147·3).
*Bath additive; psoriasis.*

**Psoriasis-Salbe M** Balneopharm, Ger.†.
Fumaric acid (p.1147·3); coal tar (p.1159·2); allantoin (p.1141·3); methyl salicylate (p.59·3); salicylic acid (p.1157·1).
*Psoriasis.*

**Psoriasis-Salbe S** Balneopharm, Ger.
Fumaric acid (p.1147·3); allantoin (p.1141·3); methyl salicylate (p.59·3); salicylic acid (p.1157·1).
*Psoriasis.*

**Psoriasis-Solution** Balneopharm, Ger.
Sodium fumarate (p.1147·3).
*Psoriasis.*

**Psoriasis-Sulfur L12** Homeocan, Canad.
Homoeopathic preparation.

**Psoriasis-Tabletten** Balneopharm, Ger.
Sodium fumarate (p.1147·3).
*Psoriasis.*

**Psoriasol** Lalco, Canad.†.
Tar (p.1159·3).
*Psoriasis.*

**Psoriatec** Sirius, USA.
Dithranol (p.1146·1).
Formerly known as Micanol.
*Psoriasis.*

**Psoricreme** Schering-Plough, Neth.
Dithranol (p.1146·1).
*Psoriasis.*

**Psoriderm**
Note. This name is used for preparations of different composition.
Dermal Laboratories, Irl.; Dermal Laboratories, UK.
Coal tar (p.1159·2).
*Psoriasis.*

Mipharm, Ital.
Dithranol (p.1146·1).
*Psoriasis.*

**Psorigel**
Galderma, Austral.; Galderma, Canad.†; Galderma, Chile; Galderma, Hong Kong†; Galderma, Irl.†; Galderma, NZ; Galderma, S.Afr.†; Healthpoint, USA.
Coal tar (p.1159·2).
*Eczema; psoriasis.*

**Psorigerb N** Cesra, Ger.
Salicylic acid (p.1157·1); coal tar (p.1159·2); urea (p.1162·2).
*Eczema; psoriasis.*

**Psorimed**
Wolff, Ger.; Leo, Ger.; Leo, Irl.; Leo, Port.
Salicylic acid (p.1157·1).
*Psoriasis of the scalp.*

**Psorin**
Note. This name is used for preparations of different composition.
Kinder, Braz.
Clobetasol propionate (p.1095·2).
*Skin disorders.*

LPC, UK.
*Ointment:* Dithranol (p.1146·1); salicylic acid (p.1157·1); coal tar (p.1159·2).
*Scalp gel:* Dithranol (p.1146·1); salicylic acid (p.1157·1); methyl salicylate (p.59·3).
*Psoriasis.*

**Psorinase** IDI, Ital.
Salicylic acid (p.1157·1); tretinoin (p.1161·1); betamethasone valero-acetate (p.1093·2).
*Psoriasis.*

**Psychobald** Sigmapharm, Austria.
Valerian (p.1762·2); bitter orange (p.1723·3).
*Anxiety disorders; sleep disorders.*

**Psychoneuroticum (Rowo-578)** Pharmakon, Ger.
Homoeopathic preparation.

**Psychopax**
Sigmapharm, Austria; Sigmapharm, Switz.
Diazepam (p.690·1).
*Anxiety disorders; epilepsy; febrile convulsions; premedication; skeletal muscle spasm; sleep disorders.*

**Psychotonin**
Madaus, Austria; Steigerwald, Ger.
Hypericum (p.299·1).
*Anxiety; depression.*

**Psychotonin M** Steigerwald, Ger.
Hypericum (p.299·1).
*Anxiety; depression.*

**Psychotonin-sed** Steigerwald, Ger.†.
Hypericum (p.299·1); valerian (p.1762·2).
*Anxiety; depression; sleep disorders.*

**Psycoton** Esseti, Ital.
Piracetam (p.1732·1).
*Mental function impairment.*

**Psylia** Techni-Pharma, Mon.
Ispaghula (p.1268·1).
*Constipation.*

**Psymion** Declimed, Ger.†.
Maprotiline hydrochloride (p.306·1).
*Depression.*

**Psyquil**
Sanofi Synthelabo, Austria; Sanofi Synthelabo, Ger.
Triflupromazine (p.727·1) or triflupromazine hydrochloride (p.727·1).
*Agitation; nausea and vomiting; neuroleptanalgesia; premedication; schizophrenia; sedative.*

**Psyrazine** Condrugs, Thai.
Trifluoperazine (p.726·3).
*Anxiety; nausea and vomiting; psychoses.*

**PSY-stabil** Pekana, Ger.
Homoeopathic preparation.

**PTA** Neuropharma, Arg.
Alprazolam (p.668·3).
*Anxiety; depression.*

**P-Tanna** Prasco, USA.
Phenylephrine tannate (p.1127·2); mepyramine tannate (p.437·1).
*Upper respiratory-tract disorders.*

**PTE** American Pharmaceutical, USA.
A range of trace element preparations (p.1417·1).
*Parenteral nutrition.*

**Ptinolin** Help, Gr.
Ranitidine hydrochloride (p.1285·2).
*Conditions where gastric acid reduction is beneficial; gastric hypersecretion including Zollinger-Ellison syndrome; peptic ulcer.*

**Puamin** Schwarzhaupt, Ger.†.
Lign. muira puama; yohimbe; nicametate citrate monohydrate; alpha tocoferil acetate.
*Erectile dysfunction; tonic.*

**Pubergen** Uni-Sankyo, India.
Chorionic gonadotrophin (p.1320·3).
*Cryptorchidism; delayed puberty; female infertility; habitual miscarriage; hypogonadotrophic hypogonadism; oligospermia; pituitary dwarfism.*

**Pudan-Lebertran-Zinksalbe** Bano, Austria.
Zinc oxide (p.1163·2); peru balsam (p.1730·2); cod-liver oil (p.1425·2).
*Burns; decubitus ulcer; nappy rash; wounds.*

**Puernol** Formenti, Ital.
Paracetamol (p.76·2).
*Fever; pain.*

**Puersan** Heralds, Braz.†.
Cichorium intybus; rhubarb (p.1287·3); fennel (p.1687·2).
*Gastrointestinal spasm.*

**Puerzym** FIRMA, Ital.†.
Pepsinogen.
*Digestive system disorders.*

**Pulbil** Fujisawa, Ger.
Sodium cromoglicate (p.795·3).
*Asthma.*

**Pulbronc** Recalcine, Chile.
Clobutinol hydrochloride (p.1117·1); orciprenaline sulfate (p.790·2); ammonium chloride (p.1115·2).
*Coughs.*

**Pulbronc Simple** Recalcine, Chile.
Clobutinol hydrochloride (p.1117·1).
*Coughs.*

**Pulibex** Medinova (Μεντινοβα), Gr.
Aciclovir (p.626·1).
*Labial and genital herpes simplex infections.*

**Pulin**
YSP, Malaysia; Yung Shin, Singapore.
Metoclopramide hydrochloride (p.1274·3).
*Nausea and vomiting.*

**Pulkrin** Kinder, Braz.
Co-trimoxazole (p.199·3).
*Bacterial infections.*

**Pulmadil**
3M, Denm.†; 3M, Neth.†.
Rimiterol hydrobromide (p.791·3).
*Bronchospasm.*

**Pulmagol** Pasteur, Chile.
Codeine phosphate (p.27·1); ephedrine hydrochloride (p.1120·1); sodium benzoate (p.1169·3); drosera (p.1683·1); lobelia (p.1589·1).
*Respiratory-tract disorders.*

**Pulmarin** NCSN, Ital.
Sulfogaiacol (p.1131·1); cineole (p.1672·1); pine oil; menthol (p.1711·3).
*Catarrh.*

**Pulmax** Zyma, Fr.†.
Peru balsam (p.1730·2); camphor (p.1665·3); eucalyptus oil (p.1686·2); rosemary oil (p.1740·2).
*Respiratory-tract congestion.*

**Pulmaxan** AstraZeneca, Ital.
Budesonide (p.1094·2).
*Asthma.*

**Pulmeno** Novartis, Spain.
Theophylline (p.798·3).
*Heart failure; obstructive airways disease; paroxysmal dyspnoea.*

**Pulmex**
Note. This name is used for preparations of different composition.
Novartis Consumer, Austria; Novartis, Chile; Novartis Consumer, Switz.
Peru balsam (p.1730·2); camphor (p.1665·3); eucalyptus oil (p.1686·2); rosemary oil (p.1740·2).
*Cold symptoms; coughs.*

Novartis Consumer, Belg.
Benzyl benzoate (p.1500·2); benzyl cinnamate; peru balsam (p.1730·2); camphor (p.1665·3); rosemary oil (p.1740·2); eucalyptus oil (p.1686·2).
*Cold symptoms.*

Novartis, Israel.
Peru balsam (p.1730·2); camphor (p.1665·3).
*Bronchitis; catarrh; cold symptoms; coughs.*

Novartis Consumer, Switz.
*Bath additive:* Thyme oil (p.1755·3); pine needle oil; eucalyptus oil (p.1686·2); rosemary oil (p.1740·2); lavender oil (p.1705·2); niaouli oil (p.1719·3).
*Cough and cold symptoms.*

**Pulmex Baby**
Note. This name is used for preparations of different composition.
Novartis Consumer, Belg.
Benzyl benzoate (p.1500·2); benzyl cinnamate; peru balsam (p.1730·2); rosemary oil (p.1740·2); eucalyptus oil (p.1686·2).
*Cold symptoms.*

Novartis Consumer, Switz.
Peru balsam (p.1730·2); eucalyptus oil (p.1686·2); rosemary oil (p.1740·2).
*Cold symptoms; coughs.*

**Pulmiben** ITF, Port.
Carbocisteine (p.1116·2).
*Respiratory-tract disorders associated with increased or viscous mucus.*

**Pulmicort**
AstraZeneca, Austral.; AstraZeneca, Austria; AstraZeneca, Belg.; AstraZeneca, Braz.; AstraZeneca, Canad.; AstraZeneca, Chile; AstraZeneca, Fin.; AstraZeneca, Fr.; AstraZeneca, Ger.; Stern, Ger.; AstraZeneca, Gr.; AstraZeneca, Hong Kong; AstraZeneca, India; AstraZeneca, Irl.; AstraZeneca, Malaysia; Astra, Mex.; AstraZeneca, Neth.; AstraZeneca, Norw.; AstraZeneca, NZ; AstraZeneca, Port.; Astra, S.Afr.; AstraZeneca, Singapore; AstraZeneca, Spain; Draco, Swed.; AstraZeneca, Switz.; AstraZeneca, Thai.; AstraZeneca, UK; Astra, USA.
Budesonide (p.1094·2).
*Asthma; croup; nasal polyps; rhinitis.*

**Pulmicret** AstraZeneca, Ger.; Stern, Ger.
Acetylcysteine (p.1112·3).
*Respiratory-tract disorders associated with increased or viscous mucus.*

**Pulmictan** Antibioticos, Spain.
Budesonide (p.1094·2).
*Asthma.*

**Pulmidur**
AstraZeneca, Austria; AstraZeneca, Ger.; Stern, Ger.
Theophylline (p.798·3).
*Obstructive airways disease.*

**Pulmilide** Boehringer Ingelheim, Austria.
Flunisolide (p.1101·1).
*Asthma.*

**Pulminflamatoria** Ern, Spain.
Ampicillin sodium (p.157·1); ampicillin benzathine (p.158·1); bromhexine hydrochloride (p.1115·3).
*Respiratory-tract infections.*

**Pulmison** Boehringer Ingelheim, S.Afr.
Prednisone (p.1109·3).
*Obstructive airways disease.*

**Pulmist** Promedica, Ital.
Flunisolide (p.1101·1).
*Asthma; bronchitis; rhinitis.*

**Pulmo Bailly**
Bailly, Fr.; DDD, UK.
Codeine (p.27·1); guaiacol (p.1122·1).
*Coughs.*

Bengue, Irl.†.
Codeine phosphate (p.27·1); guaiacol (p.1122·1).
*Coughs.*

**Pulmo Borbalan** Spyfarma, Spain.
Amoxicillin trihydrate (p.155·3); bromhexine hydrochloride (p.1115·3).
*Respiratory-tract infections.*

**Pulmo Diet** Support, Braz.
Preparation for enteral nutrition (p.1417·1).

**Pulmo Grey Balsam** Orravan, Spain†.
Camphor (p.1665·3); allyl sulfide; cineole (p.1672·1); niaouli oil (p.1719·3); guaiacol (p.1122·1).
*Respiratory-tract disorders.*

**Pulmo Lisoflam** Pharmacia, Arg.
Budesonide (p.1094·2).
*Allergic rhinitis; asthma; nasal polyps.*

**Pulmo Menal** Alacan, Spain.
Bromhexine hydrochloride (p.1115·3); guaifenesin (p.1122·1); sodium benzoate (p.1169·3); co-trimoxazole (p.199·3).
*Respiratory-tract infections.*

**Pulmocare**
Abbott, Arg.; Abbott, Austral.; Abbott, Braz.; Abbott, Canad.; Ross, Hong Kong; Abbott, Irl.; Ross, Israel; Abbott, Ital.; Abbott, Mex.; Abbott, NZ; Abbott, Singapore; Abbott, Thai.; Abbott Nutrition, UK; Ross, USA.
Preparation for enteral nutrition (p.1417·1).
*Respiratory system disorders.*

**Pulmocilin** Eurofarma, Braz.†.
Benzylpenicillin potassium (p.163·2); procaine benzylpenicillin (p.246·1).
*Bacterial infections.*

**Pulmocis** Schering, UK.
Technetium-99m human albumin macroaggregates (p.1525·2).
*Scintigraphic imaging of the lung.*

**Pulmoclase**
Bios, Belg.†; UCB, Fin.†; UCB, Gr.; UCB, Irl.; UCB, Neth.†; UCB, Port.
Carbocisteine (p.1116·2).
*Respiratory-tract disorders associated with viscous mucus.*

**Pulmocler** Monserrat, Arg.
Bromhexine hydrochloride (p.1115·3); butetamate citrate (p.1116·2).
*Respiratory-tract disorders.*

**Pulmocod**
Note. A similar name is used for preparations of different composition (see below).
Warner-Lambert, Fr.†.
Codeine (p.27·1); sodium benzoate (p.1169·3); cineole (p.1672·1).
*Coughs.*

**Pulmo-Cod**
Note. A similar name is used for preparations of different composition (see above and below).
Stadmed, India.
Multivitamin and calcium preparation (p.1417·1).

**Pulmo-Cod (C & G)**
Note. A similar name is used for preparations of different composition (see above).
Stadmed, India.
Vitamins and calcium (p.1417·1); creosote (p.1117·2); sulfogaiacol (p.1131·1).
*Bronchitis.*

**Pulmocordio forte** Hevert, Ger.†.
Ammi visnaga; belladonna; ipecacuanha; kalium jodat.; thyme (p.1755·2); castanae; ephedrine hydrochloride (p.1120·1); sulfogaiacol (p.1131·1).
*Coughs and associated respiratory-tract disorders.*

**Pulmocordio mite SL** Hevert, Ger.
Anise oil (p.1655·2); fennel oil (p.1687·3); liquorice (p.1270·2); thyme (p.1755·2).
*Respiratory-tract disorders.*

**Pulmo-cyl Ho-Len-Complex** Liebermann, Ger.
Homoeopathic preparation.

**Pulmodexane** Bailly, Fr.
Dextromethorphan hydrobromide (p.1117·3).
*Coughs.*

**Pulmodex-C** Baldassari, Braz.†.
Dipyrone (p.35·3); vitamin C (p.1460·2); cineole (p.1672·1); guaifenesin (p.1122·1).
*Cold and influenza symptoms.*

**Pulmofasa** Generfarma, Spain.
Ammonium camphocarbonate diaminopyridine carboxylate (p.1585·1); calcium pantothenate (p.1442·3); cineole (p.1672·1); senega (p.1130·2); sodium benzoate (p.1169·3); sulfogaiacol (p.1131·1); tolu balsam (p.1131·3); pinus sylvestris; anethole (p.1654·3).
*Respiratory-tract disorders.*

**Pulmofasa Antihist** Sabater, Spain†.
Ammonium camphocarbonate (p.1585·1); calcium pantothenate (p.1442·3); cineole (p.1672·1); diphenhydramine hydrochloride (p.431·3); sodium benzoate (p.1169·3); sulfogaiacol (p.1131·1); senega (p.1130·2); tolu balsam (p.1131·3); pinus sylvestris; anethole (p.1654·3).
*Upper respiratory-tract disorders.*

**Pulmofluide Simple** Pfizer Sante, Fr.
Terpin (p.1131·1); cineole (p.1672·1); sodium benzoate (p.1169·3); guaifenesin (p.1122·1).
*Respiratory-tract congestion.*

**Pulmoflux** Neo Quimica, Braz.
Salbutamol sulfate (p.791·3).
*Obstructive airways disease.*

**Pulmofor** Vifor, Switz.
Dextromethorphan hydrobromide (p.1117·3).
*Coughs.*

**Pulmoformil** Uniao Quimica, Braz.†.
Guaifenesin (p.1122·1); ephedrine hydrochloride (p.1120·1); homatropine methylbromide (p.483·2); lobelia (p.1589·1); grindelia (p.1696·1); tolu balsam (p.1131·3).
*Respiratory-tract congestion.*

**Pulmoforte** Osorio de Moraes, Braz.†.
Sodium benzoate (p.1169·3); guaifenesin (p.1122·1); lobelia (p.1589·1); potassium iodide (p.1598·1).
*Coughs.*

**Pulmogripe** Breves, Braz.†.
Sulfureto de alila; niaouli oil (p.1719·3); cineole (p.1672·1); benzyl cinnamate; camphor (p.1665·3).
*Cold and influenza symptoms.*

**Pulmoiodo** Bunker, Braz.†.
Belladonna (p.479·1); jaborandi; eucalyptus (p.1686·1); ginger (p.1267·1); siparuna guyanensis; lantana camara; mikania.
*Respiratory-tract congestion.*

**Pulmolite** REM, Braz.†.
Albumin (p.740·3).
*Diagnostic agent.*

**Pulmoll** GlaxoSmithKline Sante, Fr.
Terpin (p.1131·1); menthol (p.1711·3); amylocaine hydrochloride (p.1370·2).
*Throat disorders.*

**Pulmoll au menthol et a l'eucalyptus** SmithKline Beecham Sante, Fr.
Menthol (p.1711·3); peppermint oil (p.1283·2); eucalyptus oil (p.1686·2).
*Throat disorders.*

**Pulmonar**
Rudefsa, Mex.
Lysate of *Streptococcus pneumoniae*; *Klebsiella pneumoniae*; *Streptococcus haemolyticus*; *Staphylococcus aureus*; *Moraxella catarrhalis*; *Haemophilus influenzae*.
*Respiratory-tract infections.*

OM, Port.
Lysates of *Haemophilus influenzae*; *Streptococcus pneumoniae*; *Klebsiella pneumoniae*; *Staphylococcus aureus*; *Streptococcus pyogenes*; *Moraxella catarrhalis*.
*Respiratory-tract infections.*

**Pulmonase** Monin, Fr.†.
Codeine (p.27·1); sodium benzoate (p.1169·3); cherry-laurel; aconite root (p.1646·3); drosera (p.1683·1); tolu balsam (p.1131·3).
*Coughs.*

**Pulmonilo Synergium** Aristegui, Spain†.
Oxytetracycline (p.241·1); calcium guaiacolate; niaouli oil (p.1719·3); cineole (p.1672·1).
*Respiratory-tract infections.*

**Pulmonium N** Wala, Ger.†.
Plantago lanceolata (p.1738·2); Norway spruce; petasites officinalis (p.1663·3).
*Respiratory-tract disorders.*

**Pulmonix** Luper, Braz.
Potassium iodide (p.1598·1); sulfogaiacol (p.1131·1); tolu balsam (p.1131·3).
*Respiratory-tract congestion.*

**Pulmophyllin** Propan, S.Afr.
Theophylline (p.798·3).
*Obstructive airways disease.*

**Pulmophylline** Riva, Canad.†.
Theophylline (p.798·3).
*Bronchoconstriction.*

**Pulmoquin** Labomed, Chile.
Codeine phosphate (p.27·1); ammonium chloride (p.1115·2).
*Coughs.*

**Pulmorell** Sanorell, Ger.
Homoeopathic preparation.

**Pulmo-Rest** Stadmed, India.
Bromhexine hydrochloride (p.1115·3); salbutamol (p.791·3); guaifenesin (p.1122·1).
*Coughs.*

**Pulmo-Rest Expectorant** Stadmed, India.
Bromhexine hydrochloride (p.1115·3); salbutamol (p.791·3); guaifenesin (p.1122·1); menthol (p.1711·3).
*Coughs.*

**Pulmorex DM** Prodemdis, Canad.
Diphenhydramine hydrochloride (p.431·3); dextromethorphan hydrobromide (p.1117·3); ammonium chloride (p.1115·2).

**Pulmorien** Sinteropico, Braz.†.
Sodium camsilate; dipyrone (p.35·3); ascorbic acid (p.1460·2).
*Cold and influenza symptoms.*

**Pulmorphan** Riva, Canad.
Dextromethorphan hydrobromide (p.1117·3); guaifenesin (p.1122·1); pheniramine maleate (p.438·3); phenylephrine hydrochloride (p.1126·3).
*Coughs.*

**Pulmorphan Pediatrique** Riva, Canad.
Dextromethorphan hydrobromide (p.1117·3); pheniramine maleate (p.438·3); phenylephrine hydrochloride (p.1126·3).
*Coughs.*

**Pulmosan**
Note. A similar name is used for preparations of different composition (see below).
Gezzi, Arg.
Bromhexine hydrochloride (p.1115·3).
*Coughs.*

**Pulmo-San**
Note. A similar name is used for preparations of different composition (see above).
Zimaia, Port.
Brovanexine hydrochloride (p.1116·1).
*Coughs.*

**Pulmoserum** Bailly, Fr.
Codeine (p.27·1); guaiacol (p.1122·1).
Formerly contained codeine, guaiacol, and phosphoric acid.
*Coughs.*

**Pulmosin** Fresenius Kabi, Austria†.
Sodium cromoglicate (p.795·3).
*Asthma.*

**Pulmosina** Labomed, Chile.
Eucalyptus (p.1686·1); avocado; pectoral flowers; tolu balsam (p.1131·3); honey (p.1434·2).
*Coughs.*

**Pulmosodyl** Bridoux, Fr.†.
Pholcodine (p.1128·3); sodium benzoate (p.1169·3); tolu balsam (p.1131·3).
*Coughs.*

**Pulmospin** Spyfarma, Spain†.
Guaifenesin (p.1122·1); ampicillin trihydrate (p.157·2).
*Respiratory-tract infections.*

**Pulmosterin Duo** Normon, Spain.
Bromhexine (p.1115·3); guaifenesin (p.1122·1); co-trimoxazole (p.199·3).
*Respiratory-tract infections.*

**Pulmosterin Retard** Normon, Spain.
Ampicillin sodium (p.157·1); ampicillin benzathine (p.158·1); guaifenesin (p.1122·1).
*Respiratory-tract infections.*

**Pulmotide** Taro, Israel.
Budesonide (p.1094·2).
*Asthma.*

**Pulmo-Timelets**
Temmler, Denm.; Temmler, Ger.
Theophylline (p.798·3).
*Obstructive airways disease.*

**Pulmotin** Serum-Werk Bernburg, Ger.
*Ointment:* Anise oil (p.1655·2); camphor (p.1665·3); eucalyptus oil (p.1686·2); thyme oil (p.1755·3); conifer oil; thymol (p.1194·2).
*Respiratory-tract disorders.*
*Oral liquid:* Thyme (p.1755·2); guaifenesin (p.1122·1).
*Bronchitis; catarrh; coughs.*

**Pulmotosse** Delta, Braz.
Diphenhydramine hydrochloride (p.431·3); ammonium chloride (p.1115·2).
*Coughs.*

**Pulmotropic** Robert, Spain.
Doxycycline guaiacolsulfonate (p.206·3); muramidase hydrochloride (p.1717·2).
*Respiratory-tract infections.*

**Pulmovax** Merck Sharp & Dohme, Mex.
A pneumococcal vaccine (23-valent) (p.1633·1).
*Active immunisation.*

**Pulmovent** Boehringer Ingelheim, Austria.
Acetylcysteine (p.1112·3).
*Respiratory-tract disorders.*

**Pulmoverina** Prima, Braz.
Sodium dibunate (p.1130·2); sulfogaiacol (p.1131·1); sodium benzoate (p.1169·3).
*Coughs.*

**Pulmovital** Ifusa, Mex.
Sulfogaiacol (p.1131·1); sodium benzoate (p.1169·3).
*Coughs.*

**Pulmozyme**
Roche, Arg.; Roche, Austral.; Roche, Austria; Roche, Belg.; Roche, Braz.; Roche, Canad.; Roche, Denm.; Roche, Fin.; Roche, Fr.; Roche, Ger.; Roche, Gr.; Roche, Irl.; Roche, Israel; Roche, Ital.; Roche, Mex.; Roche, Neth.; Roche, Norw.; Roche, NZ; Roche, Port.; Roche, S.Afr.; Roche, Spain; Roche, Swed.; Roche, Switz.; Roche, UK; Genentech, USA.
Dornase alfa (p.1119·1).
*Cystic fibrosis.*

**Pulpomixine** Septodont, Switz.†.
Dexamethasone acetate (p.1097·1); framycetin sulfate (p.215·1); polymyxin B sulfate (p.245·1).
*Dental disorders.*

**Pulsalux** Ciba Vision, Ital.
Soya oil (p.1447·2); ginkgo biloba (p.1692·3); melilotus; rutoside (p.1688·2).
*Circulatory disorders.*

**Pulsar**
Note. This name is used for preparations of different composition.
Phoenix, Arg.
Cisapride (p.1259·2).
*Gastro-oesophageal reflux.*
Medosan, Ital.
Colextran hydrochloride (p.890·3).
*Glucose metabolic disorders; hyperlipidaemia; obesity.*

**Pulsar Enzimatico** Phoenix, Arg.
Cisapride (p.1259·2); pancreatin (p.1725·3); simeticone (p.1289·2).
*Digestive disorders; gastro-oesophageal reflux; meteorism.*

**Pulsar Plus** Phoenix, Arg.
Cisapride (p.1259·2); simeticone (p.1289·2).
*Gastro-oesophageal reflux; meteorism.*

**Pulsatilla Med Complex** Dynamit, Austria.
Homoeopathic preparation.

**Pulsit** Precimex, Mex.†.
Haloperidol (p.701·2).

**Pulsitil** Janssen-Cilag, Austria†.
Cisapride (p.1259·2).
*Constipation; dyspepsia; gastro-oesophageal reflux; intestinal pseudo-obstruction.*

**Pulsol** Galen, Mex.
Enalapril maleate (p.909·2).
*Heart failure; hypertension.*

**Pulsor** Tecnimede, Port.
Calcium pangamate (p.1727·2).

**Pulsoton** Chinoin, Mex.†.
Methyldopa (p.953·2).

**Pulverizador Nasal** Collado, Spain†.
Phenylephrine hydrochloride (p.1126·3).
*Nasal congestion.*

**Pulvhydrops Mono** Lomapharm, Ger.
Equisetum (p.1684·1).
*Oedema; urinary-tract disorders.*

**Pulvicin** Biolab, Thai.
Co-trimoxazole (p.199·3).
*Bacterial infections.*

**Pulvinal Beclometasone Dipropionate** Trinity, UK.
Beclometasone dipropionate (p.1091·1).
*Asthma.*

**Pulvinal Salbutamol** Trinity, UK.
Salbutamol (p.791·3).
*Obstructive airways disease.*

**Pulvis-3** Bayer, Ital.†.
Propoxur (p.1509·2).
*Pediculosis.*

**Pulvispray** Peters, Fr.†.
Mixed aldehydes; alcohol (p.1166·1); isopropyl alcohol (p.1184·3).
*Disinfection.*

**Pulvo** Urgo, Ger.
Catalase (p.1668·3); hexamidine isetionate (p.1181·3).
*Ulcers; wounds.*

**Pulvo 47**
Fournier, Belg.†; Fournier, Fr.; Fournier, Thai.
Catalase (p.1668·3); hexamidine isetionate (p.1181·3).
*Burns; skin irritation; ulcers; wounds.*

**Pulvo Neomycin** Urgo, Ger.
Catalase (p.1668·3); neomycin sulfate (p.235·1).
*Burns; infected skin disorders; ulcers; wounds.*

**Pulvo Neomycine** Fournier, Belg.†.
Catalase (p.1668·3); neomycin sulfate (p.235·1).
*Burns; skin irritation; wounds.*

**Pulvo 47 Neomycine** Fournier, Fr.
Catalase (p.1668·3); neomycin sulfate (p.235·1).
*Ulcers; wounds.*

**Pumilene Vapo** Montefarmaco, Ital.
Pumilio pine oil (p.1737·1); cineole (p.1672·1); peppermint oil (p.1283·2).

**Pumilen-N** Tosse, Ger.†.
Eucalyptus oil (p.1686·2); pumilio pine oil (p.1737·1); oleum pini sylvestris; peppermint oil (p.1283·2); thymol (p.1194·2).
*Colds; nasal congestion.*

**Pumilsan** Montefarmaco, Ital.
Dequalinium chloride (p.1178·1).
*Mouth and throat disinfection.*

**Pumonal eco natura** Ecosol, Switz.
Hedera helix.
*Coughs.*

**Pumpan** Bittner, Austria.
Homoeopathic preparation.

**Pump-Hep**
IFET (ΙΦΕΤ), Gr.; Leo, UK†.
Heparin sodium (p.928·1).
Now known as Heparin Sodium ampoules in the *UK*.
*Thromboembolic disorders.*

**Puncto E** Viatris, Ger.
*d*-Alpha tocopherol (p.1464·3).
*Vitamin E deficiency.*

**Pungino** Whitehall, Ital.†.
Vitamin $B_1$ (p.1455·2); citronella oil (p.1673·2).
*Insect repellent.*

**Punktyl** Krewel, Ger.†.
Lorazepam (p.704·1).
*Anxiety; sleep disorders.*

**Puntol** Velka, Gr.
Ambroxol hydrochloride (p.1114·3).
*Respiratory disorders associated with viscous mucus.*

**Puntual** Lainco, Spain.
Calcium sennoside A (p.1288·3); calcium sennoside B (p.1288·3).
*Constipation.*

**Puntualex** Lainco, Spain.
Calcium sennoside A (p.1288·3); calcium sennoside B (p.1288·3).
*Bowel evacuation.*

**Pupiletto** Bell, India.
Phenylephrine hydrochloride (p.1126·3).
*Glaucoma; production of mydriasis.*

**Pupilla** Wassermann, Ital.
Naphazoline nitrate (p.1124·3).
*Inflammatory and allergic eye disorders.*

**Pupilla Antistaminico** Wassermann, Ital.
Naphazoline nitrate (p.1124·3); thonzylamine hydrochloride (p.442·2).
*Inflammatory and allergic eye disorders.*

**Pupilla Light** Wassermann, Ital.
Benzalkonium chloride (p.1168·3); hypromellose; chamomile water; hyssop water; rose water; plantaginis water; mallow water; myrtillus water.
*Eye disinfection; eye irritation.*

**Puraloe** Neo Dermos, Arg.
Aloe vera (p.1141·3); tretinoin (p.1161·1).
*Keratinisation disorders.*

**Puralube**
Note. This name is used for preparations of different composition.
Metapharma, Canad.
Liquid paraffin (p.1479·1); soft paraffin (p.1479·3).
Fougera, USA.
*Eye drops:* Polyvinyl alcohol (p.1581·1).
*Eye ointment:* White soft paraffin (p.1479·3); light liquid paraffin (p.1479·1).
*Dry eyes.*

**Puran T4** Sanofi Synthelabo, Braz.
Levothyroxine sodium (p.1600·1).
*Hypothyroidism.*

**Purata** Aspen, S.Afr.
Oxazepam (p.712·2).
*Alcohol withdrawal syndrome; anxiety.*

**Purbac** Aspen, S.Afr.
Co-trimoxazole (p.199·3).
*Bacterial infections.*

**Pur-Bloka** Aspen, S.Afr.
Propranolol hydrochloride (p.989·3).
*Angina pectoris; arrhythmias; hypertension; hyperthyroidism; migraine; phaeochromocytoma.*

**Pure Health** Lexon, UK.
Aspirin (p.15·1).
*Thrombosis prophylaxis.*

**Pure Omega** BritHealth, UK.
Fish oil concentrate (p.976·1).

**Pure Plan** Cedar Health, UK.
Birch; meadowsweet; cynara; taraxacum; lappa; wild pansy; fennel; bladderwrack; tamarind; prune; green tea (p.1417·1).

**Pureduct** Rosen, Ger.
Allopurinol (p.412·2).
*Gout; hyperuricaemia; renal calculi.*

**Puregon**
Organon, Arg.; Organon, Austral.; Organon, Austria; Organon, Belg.; Organon, Braz.; Organon, Canad.; Organon, Chile; Organon, Denm.; Organon, Fin.; Organon, Fr.; Organon, Ger.; Organon (Οργκανον), Gr.; Organon, Hong Kong; Organon, Irl.; Organon, Israel; Organon, Ital.; Organon, Malaysia; Organon, Mex.; Organon, Neth.; Organon, Norw.; Organon, NZ; Organon, Port.; Donmed, S.Afr.; Organon, Singapore; Organon, Spain; Organon, Swed.; Organon, Switz.; Organon, Thai.; Organon, UK.
Follitropin beta (p.1324·2).
*Male and female infertility.*

**Pureness Blemish Control** Shiseido, Canad.†.
Sulfur (p.1158·2).
*Acne.*

**Puresis** Aspen, S.Afr.
Furosemide (p.919·3).
*Hypertension; oedema.*

**Puretam** Biotrends, Gr.
Tamoxifen citrate (p.584·1).
*Breast cancer.*

**Purethal**
Hal, Ger.
Modified allergen extracts of grass, tree and weed pollen(p.1650·1).
*Allergen immunotherapy.*
Hal, Neth.
Aluminium hydroxide adsorbed grass or tree pollen and house dust mite (p.1650·2) allergen extracts(p.1650·1).
*Allergen immunotherapy.*

**Purfalox** Kleva, Gr.
Tolfenamic acid (p.94·2).
*Dysmenorrhoea; inflammation; musculoskeletal and joint disorders; pain.*

**Purfilx** Filaxis, Arg.
Cyproterone acetate (p.1544·1).

**Purganol** Saunier-Daguin, Fr.†.
Phenolphthalein (p.1284·1).
*Constipation.*

**Purgante** Orravan, Spain†.
Phenolphthalein (p.1284·1).
*Constipation.*

**Purgazen** Agepha, Austria.
Bisacodyl (p.1251·3); dimeticone (p.1289·2).
*Bowel evacuation; constipation.*

**Purge** Fleming, USA.
Castor oil (p.1668·2).
*Constipation.*

**Purgoleite** Virtus, Braz.†.
Phenolphthalein (p.1284·1); cascara (p.1255·1); calcium phosphate (p.1225·3).
*Constipation.*

**Purgo-Pil** Qualiphar, Belg.
Bisacodyl (p.1251·3).
*Bowel evacuation; constipation.*

**Purgoxin** Aspen, S.Afr.
Digoxin (p.895·2).
*Cardiac disorders.*

**Puricin** Shiwa, Thai.
Allopurinol (p.412·2).
*Gout; hyperuricaemia.*

**Puricos** Aspen, S.Afr.
Allopurinol (p.412·2).
*Gout; hyperuricaemia.*

**Purid** Aventis, Chile.
Pipemidic acid (p.243·1).
*Urinary-tract infections.*

**Puride** Polipharm, Thai.
Allopurinol (p.412·2).
*Gout; hyperuricaemia.*

**Purigoa** Wyeth Lederle, Austria.
Bisacodyl (p.1251·3); docusate sodium (p.1262·2).
*Constipation.*

**Purilon** Coloplast, Fr.
Carmellose sodium (p.1577·3); calcium alginate (p.745·1).
*Ulcers; wounds.*

**Puri-Nethol**
GlaxoSmithKline, Arg.; GlaxoSmithKline, Austral.; GlaxoSmithKline, Austria; GlaxoSmithKline, Belg.; GlaxoSmithKline, Braz.; GlaxoSmithKline, Canad.; GlaxoSmithKline, Chile; GlaxoSmithKline, Fr.; GlaxoSmithKline, Ger.; GlaxoSmithKline, Hong Kong; GlaxoSmithKline, India; Wellcome, Irl.; Wellcome, Israel; GlaxoSmithKline, Ital.; Glaxo Wellcome, Mex.; GlaxoSmithKline, Neth.; GlaxoSmithKline, Norw.; GlaxoSmithKline, NZ; GlaxoSmithKline, S.Afr.; GlaxoSmithKline, Singapore; GlaxoSmithKline, Swed.; GlaxoSmithKline, Switz.; GlaxoSmithKline, Thai.; GlaxoSmithKline, UK; Gate, USA.
Mercaptopurine (p.567·2).
*Leukaemias.*

**Purinol**
Ratiopharm, Austria; Pinewood, Irl.
Allopurinol (p.412·2).
*Gout; hyperuricaemia; prophylaxis of uric acid and calcium oxalate stones.*

**Puriphyl** Adam, Mon.
Caprylylcollagenic acid.
*Acne.*

**Purisole**
Fresenius Kabi, Port.; Fresenius Kabi, Switz.†.
Sorbitol (p.1446·3); mannitol (p.950·2).
*Bladder irrigation.*

**Puritabs**
Dermatech, Austral.†; Balmar, NZ.
Sodium dichloroisocyanurate (p.1191·3).
*Water disinfection.*

**Puritenk** Biotenk, Arg.
Allopurinol (p.412·2).
*Gout; hyperuricaemia; renal calculi.*

**Purmolax** Hua, Thai.
Phenolphthalein (p.1284·1).
*Constipation.*

**Purmycin** Aspen, S.Afr.
Erythromycin estolate (p.208·1).
*Bacterial infections.*

**Purochin** Nuovo ISM, Ital.†.
Urokinase (p.1018·2).
*Thromboembolic disorders.*

**Purofilina** Rhein, Mex.†.
Proxyphylline (p.791·2).

**Purol** Bravir, Braz.†.
Liquid paraffin (p.1479·1).
*Constipation.*

**Puromylon** Aspen, S.Afr.
Nalidixic acid (p.234·1).
*Gram-negative bacterial urinary-tract infections.*

**Purporent** Rowa, Malaysia.
Nicotinaldehyde; cineole (p.1672·1); camphor (p.1665·3); ammonii anisatus; pumilio pine oil (p.1737·1); rosemary oil (p.1740·2); aroma oils.
*Respiratory-tract congestion.*

**Purpose** Johnson & Johnson, USA; Merck, USA.
A range of emollient, cleansing, and moisturising preparations.

**Purpose Alpha Hydroxy** Johnson & Johnson, Canad.†.
*SPF 15:* Octinoxate (p.1154·3); octisalate (p.1154·3); oxybenzone (p.1154·3).
*Sunscreen.*

**Purpose Dual** Johnson & Johnson, Canad.†.
*SPF 15:* Meradimate (p.1151·3); octinoxate (p.1154·3); titanium dioxide (p.1160·3).
*Sunscreen.*

**Purpuralin**
Alcon, Braz.; Alcon, Hong Kong.
Anthocyanosides; betacarotene (p.1422·3).
*Eye disorders.*

**Pur-Rutin** Andreabal, Switz.
Troxerutin (p.1688·3).
*Peripheral vascular disorders.*

**Pursana** Zeller, Switz.
Sorbitol (p.1446·3); fig (p.1266·3).
*Constipation.*

**Pursenid** *Novartis Consumer, Spain.*
Calcium sennoside A (p.1288·3); calcium sennoside B (p.1288·3).
*Constipation.*

**Pursennid**
*Novartis Consumer, Austria; Novartis, Denm.; Novartis, Israel†; Novartis Consumer, Ital.; Novartis, Norw.*
Calcium sennoside A (p.1288·3); calcium sennoside B (p.1288·3).
*Bowel evacuation; constipation.*

*Novartis, Fin.; Novartis, Gr.; Novartis, Swed.*
Senna (p.1288·2).
*Bowel evacuation; constipation.*

**Pursennid Complex** *Novartis, Ital.†.*
Senna (p.1288·2); polycarbophil calcium (p.1284·2).
*Constipation.*

**Pursennid Fibra** *Novartis, Ital.†.*
Polycarbophil calcium (p.1284·2).
*Constipation; diarrhoea.*

**Pursennide**
*Novartis Sante, Fr.; Novartis Consumer, Port.; Novartis Consumer, Switz.*
Calcium sennosides (p.1288·3) (p.1288·3).
*Constipation.*

**Pursennid-In** *Novartis, India.*
Sennosides (p.1288·2); docusate sodium (p.1262·2).
*Bowel evacuation; constipation.*

**Pursept A** *Merz, Ger.†.*
Alcohol (p.1166·1); glyoxal (p.1181·1); quaternary ammonium compounds.
*Surface and instrument disinfection.*

**Puru-C** *Vitabalans, Fin.*
Ascorbic acid (p.1460·2); sodium ascorbate (p.1460·2).
*Vitamin C deficiency.*

**Pusiran**
*Atlantic, Hong Kong; Atlantic, Malaysia; Atlantic, Singapore; Vana, Thai.*
Dextromethorphan hydrobromide (p.1117·3).
*Coughs.*

**Putaren** *PD, Thai.*
Diclofenac sodium (p.32·1).
*Musculoskeletal and joint disorders.*

**Putatone** *Silom, Thai.†.*
Indometacin (p.47·3).
*Gout; musculoskeletal and joint disorders.*

**Puvadin**
*Medochemie, Hong Kong; Medochemie, Malaysia.*
Trioxysalen (p.1162·2).
*Vitiligo.*

**Puvasoralen** *Crawford, UK.*
Methoxsalen (p.1152·1).
Available on a named-patient basis only.
*Mycosis fungoides; psoriasis; vitiligo.*

**PV Carpine**
*Allergan, Austral.; Allergan, NZ†.*
Pilocarpine hydrochloride (p.1495·1).
*Glaucoma; reversal of mydriasis.*

**PVA** *Allergan, Austral.*
Polyvinyl alcohol (p.1581·1).
*Dry eyes.*

**P-vate** *Osoth, Thai.*
Clobetasol propionate (p.1095·2).
*Skin disorders.*

**PVF** *Frosst, Canad.†.*
Benzathine phenoxymethylpenicillin (p.163·2).
*Bacterial infections.*

**PVFK** *Lioh, Canad.*
Phenoxymethylpenicillin potassium (p.242·1).
*Bacterial infections.*

**P-Vidine** *PP Lab, Thai.*
Povidone-iodine (p.1190·3).
*Skin, mucous membrane, and wound disinfection.*

**PVK** *Lilly, Austral.†.*
Phenoxymethylpenicillin potassium (p.242·1).
*Bacterial infections.*

**PVPI** *Geyer, Braz.*
Povidone-iodine (p.1190·3).
*Skin disinfection.*

**P-V-Tussin** *Numark, USA.*
*Syrup:* Hydrocodone tartrate (p.45·1); pseudoephedrine hydrochloride (p.1129·2); chlorphenamine maleate (p.427·3).
*Coughs and cold symptoms.*
*Tablets:* Hydrocodone tartrate (p.45·1); phenindamine tartrate (p.438·2); guaifenesin (p.1122·1).
*Coughs.*

**Pyal** *Sanico, Belg.†.*
Sulfanilamide (p.263·2); sulfathiazole (p.264·1); cod-liver oil (p.1425·2); colecalciferol (p.1461·3).
*Burns; wounds.*

**Pycnogenol Plus** *Reese, USA.*
Bioflavonoids (p.1688·2); grape seed; pycnogenol (p.1688·2).

**Pyelodion** *Neo Quimica, Braz.†.*
Sulfacetamide (p.257·3); methenamine (p.230·1); belladonna (p.479·1).
*Urinary-tract infections.*

**Pygmal** *URPAC, Fr.*
2,4,5-Trichlorophenol complex with tri-isobutyl phosphate; zinc oxide (p.1163·2); zinc carbonate (p.1163·2).
*Acne.*

**Pygosal** *Salus, Mex.†.*
Ispaghula (p.1268·1).

**Pykaryl T** *Rodleben, Ger.*
Benzyl nicotinate (p.21·2).
*Peripheral vascular disorders; rheumatic disorders; soft-tissue injuries.*

**Pykno** *Procare, Austral.†.*
Vitis vinifera; myrtillus (p.1718·3).
*Peripheral vascular disorders; tonic.*

**Pylobactel** *Galenica, Gr.*
Carbon-13 (p.1667·3) labelled urea.
*Diagnosis of Helicobacter pylori infection.*

**Pylobactell**
*Italchimici, Ital.; Torbet Laboratories, UK.*
Carbon-13 (p.1667·3) labelled urea.
*Diagnosis of Helicobacter pylori infection.*

**Pylori 13** *Medical Instruments, Switz.*
Carbon-13 labelled urea (p.1667·3).
*Test for Helicobacter pylori infection.*

**Pylori Chek** *Sorin, Spain.*
Carbon-13 labelled urea (p.1667·3).
*Test for Helicobacter pylori infection.*

**Pylorid**
*GlaxoSmithKline, Arg.; GlaxoSmithKline, Belg.; GlaxoSmithKline, Braz.; Glaxo Wellcome, Canad.†; GlaxoSmithKline, Denm.; GlaxoSmithKline, Fin.; Glaxo Wellcome, Gr.; GlaxoSmithKline, Hong Kong; Glaxo Wellcome, Irl.; GlaxoSmithKline, Ital.; GlaxoSmithKline, Neth.; GlaxoSmithKline, Norw.; Glaxo Wellcome, Port.; Glaxo Wellcome, Singapore†; Glaxo Wellcome, Spain; GlaxoSmithKline, Switz.; GlaxoSmithKline, Thai.; GlaxoSmithKline, UK.*
Ranitidine bismuth citrate (p.1287·2).
*Peptic ulcer.*

**Pylorid-KA** *GlaxoSmithKline, Austral.*
*Combination pack:* Tablets, ranitidine bismuth citrate (Pylorid) (p.1287·2); tablets, clarithromycin (p.192·2); capsules, amoxicillin trihydrate (p.155·3).
*Helicobacter pylori-associated peptic ulcer.*

**Pyloripac** *Medley, Braz.*
Capsules, amoxicillin (p.155·3); tablets, clarithromycin (p.192·2); capsules, lansoprazole (p.1269·3).
*Helicobacter pylori-associated peptic ulcer.*

**Pyloriset** *Orion, USA.*
Test for gastrointestinal disorders.

**Pylorisin** *GlaxoSmithKline, Austria.*
Ranitidine bismuth citrate (p.1287·2).
*Peptic ulcer.*

**Pynamic** *Condrugs, Thai.*
Mefenamic acid (p.55·2).
*Pain.*

**Pynclear** *Libra, S.Afr.*
Paracetamol (p.76·2); doxylamine succinate (p.432·3); caffeine (p.782·1); codeine phosphate (p.27·1).
*Pain and tension.*

**Pynmed** *Medpro, S.Afr.*
*Syrup:* Paracetamol (p.76·2); codeine phosphate (p.27·1); promethazine hydrochloride (p.439·1).
*Pain with tension.*
*Tablets:* Paracetamol (p.76·2); codeine phosphate (p.27·1); caffeine (p.782·1); meprobamate (p.706·2).
*Pain and associated tension.*

**Pynstop** *Covan, S.Afr.*
Paracetamol (p.76·2); codeine phosphate (p.27·1); caffeine (p.782·1); doxylamine succinate (p.432·3).
*Fever; pain and associated tension.*

**Pyocefal** *Takeda, Fr.†.*
Cefsulodin sodium (p.180·2).
Lidocaine (p.1377·3) is included in the intramuscular injection to alleviate the pain of injection.
*Bacterial infections.*

**Pyocoline** *Millet Roux, Braz.†.*
Ammonium chloride (p.1115·2); hydroxyquinoline hydrochloride; terpin hydrate (p.1131·1).
*Urinary-tract infections.*

**Pyodontyl** *Sanofi Synthelabo, Hong Kong.*
Metesculetol sodium (p.1714·1); allantoin (p.1141·3).
*Gum disorders.*

**Pyolysin** *Serum-Werk Bernburg, Ger.*
Extract of staphylococci, streptococci, escherichia coli, pseudomonas aeruginosa, micrococcus-ovis-Buillon; zinc oxide (p.1163·2); salicylic acid (p.1157·1).
*Burns; infected skin disorders; skin ulcers; wounds.*

**Pyoralene** *Expanpharm, Fr.†.*
Maize (p.1449·1).
*Mouth disorders.*

**Pyoredol** *Roussel, Fr.†.*
Phenytoin sodium (p.370·2).
*Gum disorders.*

**Pyorex** *Bailly, Fr.*
Ethacridine lactate (p.1165·3); sodium ricinoleate (p.1575·3).
*Oral hygiene.*

**Pyostacine**
*Aventis, Belg.†; Aventis, Fr.; Aventis, Israel.*
Pristinamycin (p.246·1).
*Bacterial infections.*

**Pyracon** *Hua, Thai.*
Paracetamol (p.76·2).
*Fever; pain.*

**Pyradol** *Xixia, S.Afr.*
Paracetamol (p.76·2).
*Fever; pain.*

**Pyrafat**
*Kolassa, Austria; Fatol, Ger.; Fatol, Hong Kong.*
Pyrazinamide (p.246·3).
*Mycobacterial infections.*

**Pyralfin** *Lupin, India.*
Pyrimethamine (p.458·1); sulfadoxine (p.259·3).
*Malaria.*

**Pyralin** *Pharmacia, Austral.*
Sulfasalazine (p.1291·1).
*Crohn's disease; rheumatoid arthritis; ulcerative colitis.*

**Pyralvex**
*Lazar, Arg.; Norgine, Hong Kong; Norgine, Thai.*
Anthraquinone glycosides; salicylic acid (p.1157·1).
*Mouth and throat disorders.*

*Norgine, Austral.; Norgine, Austria; Norgine, Belg.; Norgine, Fr.; Norgine, Ger.; Norgine, Irl.; Norgine, Ital.; Norgine, Neth.; Helsinn, Port.; Norgine, S.Afr.; Norgine, Singapore; Norgine, Spain; Norgine, Switz.; Norgine, UK.*
Rhubarb (p.1287·3); salicylic acid (p.1157·1).
*Mouth and throat disorders.*

**Pyranol** *Solfran, Mex.*
Dipyrone (p.35·3).
*Pain.*

**Pyrantin** *Biopharm, Hong Kong.*
Pyrantel embonate (p.113·2).
*Worm infections.*

**Pyrantrin** *Biopharm, Hong Kong.*
Pyrantel embonate (p.113·2).
*Worm infections.*

**Pyrapam** *General Drugs, Thai.*
Pyrantel embonate (p.113·2).
*Worm infections.*

**Pyratab** *Shiwa, Thai.*
Pyrazinamide (p.246·3).
*Tuberculosis.*

**Pyrazide** *Aventis, S.Afr.*
Pyrazinamide (p.246·3).
*Tuberculosis.*

**Pyrcon** *Krewel, Ger.*
Pyrvinium embonate (p.113·3).
*Enterobiasis.*

**Pyreazid** *Salvat, Spain†.*
Isoniazid (p.222·2).
*Tuberculosis.*

**Pyrecol** *Polipharm, Thai.*
Paracetamol (p.76·2); chlorphenamine maleate (p.427·3); phenylephrine hydrochloride (p.1126·3).
*Cold symptoms; hay fever.*

**Pyreflor** *Clement-Thekan, Fr.*
*Lotion:* Permethrin (p.1508·3); piperonyl butoxide (p.1509·2); enoxolone (p.36·2).
*Shampoo:* Permethrin (p.1508·3); piperonyl butoxide (p.1509·2).
*Pediculosis.*

**Pyretal** *Shiwa, Thai.*
Paracetamol (p.76·2).
*Fever; pain.*

**Pyrethrum Spray** *Nelson, UK.*
Homoeopathic preparation.

**Pyrexon** *Wockhardt, India.*
Paracetamol (p.76·2).
*Fever; pain.*

**Pyribenzamine** *Novartis Consumer, Canad.†.*
Tripelennamine hydrochloride (p.442·3).
*Hypersensitivity reactions.*

**Pyricontin** *Modi-Mundipharma, India.*
Vitamin $B_6$ (p.1457·2).
*Vitamin $B_6$ deficiency.*

**Pyridiate** *Rugby, USA.*
Phenazopyridine hydrochloride (p.83·1).
*Irritation of the lower urinary tract.*

**Pyridium**
*Pfizer, Braz.; Pfizer, Canad.; Parke, Davis, Chile; Pfizer, Hong Kong; Parke, Davis, India; Pfizer Consumer, S.Afr.; Warner Chilcott, USA.*
Phenazopyridine hydrochloride (p.83·1).
*Pain and irritation of the urinary tract.*

**Pyridium Plus** *Warner Chilcott, USA.*
Phenazopyridine hydrochloride (p.83·1); hyoscyamine hydrobromide (p.485·1); butalbital (p.673·3).
*Urinary-tract pain and spasm, with apprehension.*

**Pyrifin** *Hoechst Marion Roussel, S.Afr.†.*
Rifampicin (p.250·2); isoniazid (p.222·2); pyrazinamide (p.246·3).
*Tuberculosis.*

**Pyrifoam**
*Dermatech, Austral.; Balmar, NZ.*
Permethrin (p.1508·3).
*Pediculosis.*

**Pyrigesic** *East India Pharma, India.*
Paracetamol (p.76·2).
*Fever; pain.*

**Pyril** *Vitae, Mex.†.*
Dipyrone (p.35·3).
*Fever; pain.*

**Pyrilax** *Berlin-Chemie, Ger.*
Bisacodyl (p.1251·3).
*Bowel evacuation; constipation.*

**Pyrimel** *Catarinense, Braz.*
Paracetamol (p.76·2).
*Fever; pain.*

**Pyrimon** *FDC, India.*
Dexamethasone (p.1097·1); chloramphenicol (p.185·1).
*Allergic eye disorders; eye infections; eye trauma.*

**Pyrinex** *Ambix, USA†.*
Pyrethrins (p.1509·3); piperonyl butoxide (p.1509·2).
*Pediculosis.*

**Pyrinyl II** *Barre-National, USA.*
Pyrethrins (p.1509·3); piperonyl butoxide technical (p.1509·2).
*Pediculosis.*

**Pyrinyl Plus** *Rugby, USA.*
Pyrethrins (p.1509·3); piperonyl butoxide (p.1509·2).
*Pediculosis.*

**Pyriped** *Mintlab, Chile.*
Ibuprofen (p.45·3).
*Fever; inflammation; pain.*

**Pyrisept** *Weifa, Norw.*
Cetylpyridinium chloride (p.1173·1).
*Disinfection of hands and skin; minor skin infections.*

**Pyritil**
*Biolab, Malaysia; Biolab, Thai.*
Pyritinol hydrochloride (p.1737·2).
*Organic brain disorders.*

**Pyrocaps** *Be-Tabs, S.Afr.*
Piroxicam (p.84·2).
*Gout; musculoskeletal and joint disorders.*

**Pyrogallic** *Gordon, USA.*
Pyrogallol (p.1156·2).
*Calluses; verrucas.*

**Pyrogastrone**
*Note. This name is used for preparations of different composition.*
*Sanofi Synthelabo, Irl.*
Carbenoxolone sodium (p.1254·3); alginic acid (p.1576·3); aluminium hydroxide (p.1249·2); magnesium trisilicate (p.1272·3); sodium bicarbonate (p.1223·2).
*Flatulence; gastro-oesophageal reflux; heartburn; hiatus hernia; peptic ulcer.*

*Sanofi Synthelabo, UK.*
*Oral suspension†:* Carbenoxolone sodium (p.1254·3); aluminium hydroxide (p.1249·2); sodium alginate (p.1577·1); potassium bicarbonate (p.1223·1).
*Tablets:* Carbenoxolone sodium (p.1254·3); alginic acid (p.1576·3); aluminium hydroxide (p.1249·2); magnesium trisilicate (p.1272·3); sodium bicarbonate (p.1223·2).
*Gastro-oesophageal reflux.*

**Pyrogenium** *Hanosan, Ger.*
Homoeopathic preparation.

**Pyromed** *Sanofi Synthelabo, Ger.*
Paracetamol (p.76·2).
*Fever; pain.*

**Pyron** *Reuffer, Mex.†.*
Dipyrone (p.35·3).
*Fever; pain.*

**Pyroxin** *Aventis, Austral.*
Pyridoxine hydrochloride (p.1456·3).
*Alcoholism; anaemias; homocystinuria; nausea and vomiting in pregnancy; premenstrual syndrome; radiation sickness.*

**Pyroxy** *Shiwa, Thai.*
Piroxicam (p.84·2).
*Gout; musculoskeletal, joint, peri-articular, and soft-tissue disorders.*

**Pyr-Pam** *UCI, Braz.*
Pyrvinium embonate (p.113·3).
*Enterobiasis.*

**Pyrvin** *Orion, Fin.*
Pyrvinium embonate (p.113·3).
*Worm infections.*

**Pytazen** *Douglas, NZ.*
Dipyridamole (p.903·1).
*Thromboembolic disorders.*

**Pytest** *Tri-Med, USA.*
Carbon-14 (p.1523·1) labelled urea.
*Diagnosis of Helicobacter pylori infection.*

**Pyverm** *Cifarma, Braz.†.*
Pyrvinium embonate (p.113·3).
*Worm infections.*

**Pyzin** *Lupin, India.*
Pyrazinamide (p.246·3).
*Tuberculosis.*

**PZA**
*Hefa, Ger.; Biochemie, Malaysia; Novartis, Malaysia; Biochemie, Singapore†; Biochemie, Thai.; Novartis, Thai.*
Pyrazinamide (p.246·3).
*Tuberculosis.*

**PZA-Ciba** *Novartis, India.*
Pyrazinamide (p.246·3).
*Tuberculosis.*

**P-Zide** *Cadila Pharma, India.*
Pyrazinamide (p.246·3).
*Tuberculosis.*

**Q200** *Pacific, NZ.*
Quinine sulfate (p.460·2).
*Malaria; myotonia; nocturnal cramps.*

**Q300** *Pacific, NZ.*
Quinine sulfate (p.460·2).
*Malaria; myotonia; nocturnal cramps.*

**Q 10** *Sidefarma, Port.*
Ubidecarenone (p.1760·2).
*Drug-induced cardiotoxicity; heart failure.*

**Q-Age** *Bracco, Ital.†.*
Vitamins; ubidecarenone (p.1417·1).

**Qari** *Mediolanum, Ital.*
Rufloxacin hydrochloride (p.254·3).
*Bacterial infections.*

**QDALL** *Atley, USA.*
Pseudoephedrine hydrochloride (p.1129·2); chlorphenamine maleate (p.427·3).
*Upper respiratory-tract disorders.*

**QED** *Omega, Irl.*
Test for alcohol in saliva.

**QED A-150** *Prieto, Arg.*
Test for alcohol in blood.

**Qiftrin** *Hexal, Braz.*
Co-trimoxazole (p.199·3).
*Bacterial infections; Pneumocystis carinii pneumonia; protozoal infections.*

**Qinolon** *Great Eastern, Thai.; Therapharma, Thai.*
Ofloxacin (p.239·3).
*Bacterial infections.*

**QM Integratore** *Mavi, Ital.†.*
Trace-element preparation with vitamin B substances and vitamin C (p.1417·1).
*Nutritional supplement.*

**QT** *Schering-Plough, USA.*
*SPF 2:* Octinoxate (p.1154·3); dihydroxyacetone (p.1145·2).
*Sunscreen.*

**Q-Tech** *Lifetech, Hong Kong†.*
Phentolamine mesilate (p.982·1).
*Peripheral vascular disorders.*

**QTest** *Quidel, USA.*
Pregnancy test (p.1734·3).

**QTest Ovulation** *Quidel, USA.*
Fertility test (p.1734·3).

**Quadblock** *Hamilton, Austral.†.*
*Cream SPF 30+; topical milk SPF 30+:* Octinoxate (p.1154·3); titanium dioxide (p.1160·3); enzacamene (p.1147·1).
*Stick SPF 30+:* Oxybenzone (p.1154·3); octinoxate (p.1154·3); avobenzone (p.1142·3); titanium dioxide (p.1160·3).
*Sunscreen.*

**Quadezyme** *Pascual, Hong Kong.*
Muramidase hydrochloride (p.1717·2); dequalinium chloride (p.1178·1).
*Allergic rhinitis; mouth and throat disorders; sinusitis.*

**Quadion** *Fortbenton, Arg.*
Ketoconazole (p.403·3).
*Dandruff.*

**Quadracel** *Aventis Pasteur, Canad.*
A diphtheria, tetanus, pertussis and inactivated poliomyelitis vaccine (p.1615·1).
*Active immunisation.*

**Quadra-Hist D** *Ethex, USA†.*
Phenylpropanolamine hydrochloride (p.1127·3); phenyltoloxamine citrate (p.439·1); mepyramine maleate (p.437·1); pheniramine maleate (p.438·3).
*Coughs and cold symptoms.*

**Quadramet**
*ARI, Austral.; CIS, Fr.; Schering, Ital.; Schering, Port.; Schering, Spain; Schering, UK; Du Pont, USA.*
Samarium-153 lexidronam (p.1525·2).
*Metastatic bone pain.*

**Quadrasa**
*Norgine, Fr.; Norgine, Ital.*
Sodium aminosalicylate (p.155·1).
*Ulcerative colitis.*

**Quadrax** *Boehringer Ingelheim Promeco, Mex.*
Ibuprofen (p.45·3).
*Inflammation; pain.*

**Quadriderm**
*Key, Arg.; Schering-Plough, Braz.; Schering-Plough, Hong Kong; Schering-Plough, S.Afr.; Schering-Plough, Singapore; Essex, Switz.; Schering-Plough, Thai.†.*
Betamethasone valerate (p.1093·2); gentamicin sulfate (p.217·1); tolnaftate (p.410·1); clioquinol (p.196·3).
*Infected skin disorders.*

**Quadriderm CD** *Key, Arg.*
Betamethasone dipropionate (p.1093·1); clotrimazole (p.396·2); gentamicin sulfate (p.217·1).
*Infected skin disorders.*

**Quadriderm NF** *Schering-Plough, Mex.*
Betamethasone dipropionate (p.1093·1); clotrimazole (p.396·2); gentamicin sulfate (p.217·1).
*Infected skin disorders.*

**Quadriderme** *Schering-Plough, Port.*
Betamethasone dipropionate (p.1093·1); clotrimazole (p.396·2); gentamicin sulfate (p.217·1).
*Infected skin disorders.*

**Quadrikin** *Kinder, Braz.*
Betamethasone valerate (p.1093·2); gentamicin sulfate (p.217·1); tolnaftate (p.410·1); clioquinol (p.196·3).
*Infected skin disorders.*

**Quadrilon** *Neo Quimica, Braz.*
Betamethasone valerate (p.1093·2); gentamicin sulfate (p.217·1); tolnaftate (p.410·1); clioquinol (p.196·3).
*Infected skin disorders.*

**Quadrinal** *Knoll, USA.*
Ephedrine hydrochloride (p.1120·1); phenobarbital (p.367·3); theophylline calcium salicylate (p.804·3); potassium iodide (p.1598·1).
*Chronic respiratory disease.*

**Quadriplus** *Delta, Braz.*
Betamethasone valerate (p.1093·2); gentamicin sulfate (p.217·1); tolnaftate (p.410·1); clioquinol (p.196·3).
*Infected skin disorders.*

**Quadronal ASS comp** *AWD, Ger.*
Aspirin (p.15·1); caffeine (p.782·1).
*Pain.*

**Quadronal comp** *AWD, Ger.*
Paracetamol (p.76·2); caffeine (p.782·1).
*Pain.*

**Quadropril**
*Asta Medica, Austria; AWD, Ger.*
Spirapril hydrochloride (p.1003·1).
*Hypertension.*

**Quagu-Test** *Fada, Arg.*
Aprotinin (p.742·3).

**Quait** *SIT, Ital.†.*
Lorazepam (p.704·1).
*Anxiety disorders; premedication.*

**Qual** *Silanes, Mex.*
Paracetamol (p.76·2); dextropropoxyphene hydrochloride (p.28·3); diazepam (p.690·1).
*Pain; painful muscle spasm.*

**Qualecon** *Duncan, Arg.*
Fenofibrate (p.915·2).
*Hyperlipidaemias.*

**Qualiton** *TO-Chemicals, Thai.*
Guaifenesin (p.1122·1); theophylline (p.798·3).
*Coughs; obstructive airways disease.*

**Quam** *Stada, Ger.†.*
Garlic (p.1691·1).
*Lipid disorders; vascular disorders.*

**Quamatel** *Gedeon Richter, Hong Kong.*
Famotidine (p.1265·2).
*Gastro-oesophageal reflux; peptic ulcer; Zollinger-Ellison syndrome.*

**Quanil** *Teofarma, Ital.*
Meprobamate (p.706·2).
*Anxiety disorders.*

**Quantaffirm** *Organon Teknika, USA.*
Test for infectious mononucleosis.

**Quantalan**
*Bristol-Myers Squibb, Austria; Bristol-Myers Squibb, Ger.; Bristol-Myers Squibb, Port.; Bristol-Myers Squibb, Switz.*
Colestyramine (p.889·3).
*Biliary-tract disorders; hypercholesterolaemia; poisoning with phenprocoumon; pruritus associated with biliary obstruction.*

**Quantor** *Almirall, Spain.*
Ranitidine hydrochloride (p.1285·2).
*Acid aspiration; gastro-oesophageal reflux; gastrointestinal haemorrhage; gastrointestinal hyperacidity; peptic ulcer; Zollinger-Ellison syndrome.*

**Quardin** *Mepha, Port.*
Ranitidine hydrochloride (p.1285·2).
*Acid aspiration; gastro-oesophageal reflux; gastrointestinal haemorrhage; peptic ulcer; Zollinger-Ellison syndrome.*

**Quarelin** *Chinoin, Hung.*
Dipyrone (p.35·3); caffeine (p.782·1); drotaverine hydrochloride (p.1683·1).
*Migraine.*

**Quark** *Poliframa, Ital.*
Ramipril (p.994·1).
*Heart failure; hypertension; myocardial infarction; renal insufficiency.*

**Quartamon Med** *Schulke & Mayr, Ger.†.*
Benzalkonium chloride (p.1168·3).
*Surface disinfection.*

**Quarzan** *Roche, USA†.*
Clidinium bromide (p.480·2).
*Peptic ulcer (adjunct).*

**Quasar** *Ravizza, Ital.†.*
Verapamil hydrochloride (p.1019·1).
*Hypertension.*

**Quatohex** *Braun, Ger.*
Didecyldimethylammonium chloride (p.1178·3); benzalkonium chloride (p.1168·3); biguanidinium acetate; polymeric biguanides.
*Surface disinfection.*

**Quatro-Soda** *Aspen, S.Afr.*
Sodium citrate (p.1223·2); sodium bicarbonate (p.1223·2); tartaric acid (p.1752·1); citric acid (p.1673·1).
*Gastrointestinal hyperacidity; urinary alkalisation.*

**Quatro-Virelon** *Chiron Behring, Ger.*
A diphtheria, tetanus, pertussis, and poliomyelitis vaccine (p.1615·1).
*Active immunisation.*

**Quazium** *Schering-Plough, Ital.*
Quazepam (p.718·2).
*Insomnia.*

**Quefeno** *Helfarma, Port.*
Ketotifen fumarate (p.788·1).
*Allergic rhinitis; asthma; urticaria.*

**Quelacid** *Enila, Braz.*
Aluminium and calcium chelate.
*Gastrointestinal hyperacidity.*

**Quelicin**
*Abbott, Braz.; Abbott, Canad.; Abbott, USA.*
Suxamethonium chloride (p.1406·2).
*Depolarising neuromuscular blocker.*

**Quelidrine** *Abbott, USA.*
Dextromethorphan hydrobromide (p.1117·3); chlorphenamine maleate (p.427·3); ephedrine hydrochloride (p.1120·1); phenylephrine hydrochloride (p.1126·3); ammonium chloride (p.1115·2); ipecac fluidextract (p.1122·3).
*Coughs.*

**Quellada**
*Note. This name is used for preparations of different composition.*
*GlaxoSmithKline Consumer, Austral.; Stafford-Miller, Hong Kong.*
Permethrin (p.1508·3).
*Pediculosis; scabies.*

*GlaxoSmithKline Consumer, Belg.†; Stafford-Miller, Irl.; Searle, S.Afr.†.*
Lindane (p.1506·3).
*Pediculosis; scabies.*

**Quellada H** *Block, Ger.†.*
Lindane (p.1506·3).
*Pediculosis.*

**Quellada M** *GlaxoSmithKline Consumer, UK.*
Malathion (p.1507·1).
*Pediculosis; scabies.*

**Quellada P**
*Note. This name is used for preparations of different composition.*
*Block, Ger.†.*
Pyrethrum flower (p.1509·3); piperonyl butoxide (p.1509·2).
*Pediculosis.*

*Stafford-Miller, NZ†.*
Permethrin (p.1508·3).
*Pediculosis; scabies.*

**Quelodin** *Ariston, Braz.*
Menthol (p.1711·3); menthone; α-pinene; cineole (p.1672·1); camphene; greater celandine (p.1695·3); phenylpropanol (p.1731·1); olive oil (p.1723·2).
*Gallstones.*

**Quelodin F** *Ariston, Arg.*
Chelidonium (p.1695·3); taraxacum (p.1751·3); silybum marianum (p.1043·3); linoleic acid (p.1690·2) or magnesium linoleate.
*Biliary-tract disorders.*

**Quem Plus** *Prodava, Arg.*
Allantoin (p.1141·3); wool fat (p.1483·1).
*Barrier cream.*

**Quemicetina**
*Rontag, Arg.; Pharmacia, Braz.; Pharmacia, Chile; Pharmacia Upjohn, Mex.*
Chloramphenicol (p.185·1), chloramphenicol palmitate (p.185·1), or chloramphenicol sodium succinate (p.185·1).
*Bacterial infections.*

**Quemicetina con Hidrocortisona** *Rontag, Arg.*
Chloramphenicol (p.185·1); hydrocortisone acetate (p.1103·3).
*Infected skin disorders.*

**Quemox** *YSP, Malaysia.*
Mebendazole (p.108·2).
*Worm infections.*

**Quenobilan** *Estedi, Spain.*
Chenodeoxycholic acid (p.1670·1).
*Gallstones.*

**Quenocol** *Zambon, Spain.*
Chenodeoxycholic acid (p.1670·1).
*Gallstones.*

**Quensyl** *Sanofi Synthelabo, Ger.*
Hydroxychloroquine sulfate (p.452·3).
*Chronic polyarthritis; lupus erythematosus; malaria.*

**Quentakehl** *Sanum-Kehlbeck, Ger.*
Homoeopathic preparation.

**Queratil** *Reig Jofre, Spain†.*
Cineole (p.1672·1); ichthammol (p.1148·2); trinitrophenol (p.1758·1); ergocalciferol (p.1462·1); tannic acid (p.1751·2); zinc oxide (p.1163·2); vitamin A (p.1451·2).
*Burns.*

**Quercetol Hemostatico** *Ferrer, Spain†.*
Carbazochrome (p.745·1); quercetin (p.1688·2); creatinine sulfate.
*Haemorrhage.*

**Quercetol K** *Ferrer, Spain†.*
Ascorbic acid (p.1460·2); calcium gluconate (p.1225·2); carbazochrome (p.745·1); menadione sodium bisulfite (p.1466·3); quercetin (p.1688·2).
*Capillary fragility; haemorrhage.*

**Querto** *Byk Gulden, Ger.*
Carvedilol (p.881·1).
*Angina pectoris; heart failure; hypertension.*

**Quest Gamma Oil** *Quest, Malaysia.*
Evening primrose oil (p.1686·3).
*Dietary supplement.*

**Questran**
*Bristol-Myers Squibb, Arg.; Bristol-Myers Squibb, Austral.; Bristol-Myers Squibb, Belg.; Bristol-Myers Squibb, Braz.; Bristol, Canad.; Bristol-Myers Squibb, Denm.; Bristol-Myers Squibb, Fin.; Bristol-Myers Squibb, Fr.; IFET (ΙΦΕΤ), Gr.; Bristol-Myers Squibb, Hong Kong; Bristol-Myers Squibb, Irl.; Bristol-Myers Squibb, Israel†; Bristol-Myers Squibb, Ital.; Bristol-Myers Squibb, Malaysia; Mead Johnson, Mex.†; Bristol-Myers Squibb, Neth.; Bristol-Myers Squibb, Norw.; Bristol-Myers Squibb, NZ; Bristol-Myers Squibb, S.Afr.; Bristol-Myers Squibb, Singapore; Bristol-Myers, Spain; Bristol-Myers Squibb, Swed.; Bristol-Myers Squibb, Thai.; Bristol-Myers Squibb, UK; Par, USA.*
Colestyramine (p.889·3).
*Adjunct in organophosphorus pesticide poisoning; diarrhoea; hypercholesterolaemia; pruritus associated with biliary obstruction.*

**Quetidin** *Drugtech, Chile.*
Quetiapine (p.719·1).
*Schizophrenia.*

**Quetzal** *Smaller, Spain.*
Hypericum (p.299·1).
*Tonic.*

**Qugyl** *RPG, India.*
Diloxanide furoate (p.604·1); metronidazole (p.607·2).
*Amoebiasis; giardiasis.*

**Quiacort** *Euroderm, Arg.*
Betamethasone (p.1093·1).
*Skin disorders.*

**Quiacort G** *Euroderm, Arg.*
Betamethasone (p.1093·1); gentamicin (p.219·1).
*Infected skin disorders.*

**Quiacort G Plus** *Euroderm, Arg.*
Betamethasone (p.1093·1); gentamicin (p.219·1); clotrimazole (p.396·2).
*Infected skin disorders.*

**Quibron**
*Note. This name is used for preparations of different composition.*
*Bristol-Myers Squibb, Thai.†.*
Theophylline (p.798·3).
*Obstructive airways disease.*

*Apothecon, USA.*
Theophylline (p.798·3); guaifenesin (p.1122·1).
*Bronchospasm.*

**Quibron-T**
*Bristol, Canad.; Roberts, USA.*
Theophylline (p.798·3).
*Obstructive airways disease.*

**Quick N Easy** *KK, UK.*
Pregnancy test (p.1734·3).

**Quick Pep** *Thompson, USA†.*
Caffeine (p.782·1).
*Fatigue.*

**Quickcal** *Vitaflo, Irl.*
Preparation for enteral nutrition (p.1417·1).

**QuickCal** *Vitaflo, UK.*
High energy food fortifier (p.1417·1).

**QuickCare** *Ciba Vision, Canad.*
Range of cleaning, disinfecting, rinsing, and storage solutions for soft contact lenses (p.1164·2).

**QuickVue** *Quidel, USA.*
Pregnancy test (p.1734·3).

**Quiedorm** *Menarini, Spain.*
Quazepam (p.718·2).
*Insomnia.*

**Quiens** *Antonetto, Ital.*
Hypericum (p.299·1).
*Depression.*

**Quies** *Quies, Fr.†.*
Eschscholtzia californica.
*Nervous disorders.*

**Quiet Days** *Cantassium Co., UK.*
Skullcap (p.1746·3); lupulus (p.1708·1); valerian (p.1762·2).

**Quiet Life** *Lane, UK.*
Motherwort (p.1717·1); wild lettuce (p.1765·2); lupulus (p.1708·1); passion flower (p.1729·1); valerian (p.1762·2); thiamine hydrochloride (p.1455·1); riboflavin (p.1456·1); nicotinamide (p.1441·2).
*Insomnia; stresses and strains.*

**Quiet Nite** *Cantassium Co., UK.*
Valerian (p.1762·2); lupulus (p.1708·1); lettuce (p.1765·2); passion flower (p.1729·1).
*Insomnia.*

**Quiet Tyme** *Cantassium Co., UK.*
Skullcap (p.1746·3); lupulus (p.1708·1); passion flower (p.1729·1); valerian (p.1762·2); gentian (p.1692·2); vitamin B substances (p.1417·1).

**Quietan** *Roche, Ital.†.*
Valerian (p.1762·2); passion flower (p.1729·1); crataegus (p.1677·1).
*Insomnia.*

**Quietiline** *Sciencex, Fr.*
Bromazepam (p.671·3).
*Anxiety.*

**Quietude** *Boiron, Fr.*
Homoeopathic preparation.

**Quiflox** *Teuto, Braz.*
Ciprofloxacin hydrochloride (p.188·2).
*Bacterial infections.*

**Quifloxona** *Farmaco, Mex.*
Ciprofloxacin (p.188·2).
*Bacterial infections.*

**Quik** *Valeas, Ital.*
Cloperastine fendizoate (p.1117·2).
*Coughs.*

**Quilagen** *Randall, Mex.†.*
Gentamicin (p.219·1).
*Bacterial infections.*

**Qui-Lea** *Elea, Arg.*
Quinestrol (p.1568·2).
*Menopausal disorders.*

**Quilla simplex** *Pharmacia, Swed.*
Ammonium chloride (p.1115·2); quillaia (p.1416·1).
*Respiratory-tract disorders.*

**Quilonorm**
*GlaxoSmithKline, Austria; Doetsch, Grether, Switz.*
Lithium acetate (p.305·1) or lithium carbonate (p.301·1).
*Bipolar disorder; depression; mania.*

**Quilonum**
*GlaxoSmithKline, Austral.; GlaxoSmithKline, Ger.; GlaxoSmithKline, S.Afr.*
Lithium acetate (p.305·1) or lithium carbonate (p.301·1).
*Bipolar disorder; cluster headache; depression; mania.*

**Quimalan** *Quimica y Farmacia, Mex.*
Enalapril maleate (p.909·2).
*Heart failure; hypertension.*

**Quimefuran** *IQFA, Mex.*
Kaolin (p.1268·3); pectin (p.1580·3).
Formerly contained furazolidone.
*Diarrhoea.*

**Quimio-Ped** *Stiefel, Braz.*
Co-trimoxazole (p.199·3).
*Bacterial infections; Pneumocystis carinii pneumonia; protozoal infections.*

**Quimio-Ped Balsamico** *Stiefel, Braz.†.*
Co-trimoxazole (p.199·3); guaifenesin (p.1122·1); ammonium chloride (p.1115·2).
*Bacterial infections.*

**Quimobrom** *Maver, Mex.*
Erythromycin (p.208·1); bromhexine (p.1115·3).
*Bacterial infections.*

**Quimocyclar** *Grossman, Mex.*
Tetracycline hydrochloride (p.266·2).
*Bacterial infections.*

**Quimodril** *Italfarmaco, Spain.*
Trypsin (p.1758·3); chymotrypsin (p.1671·2); teclothiazide potassium (p.1010·1).
*Oedema.*

**Quimolactona** *Quimica y Farmacia, Mex.*
Spironolactone (p.1003·1).
*Hypertension.*

**Quimolauril** *Maver, Mex.*
Erythromycin (p.208·1).
*Bacterial infections.*

**Quimosporina** *Quimica y Farmacia, Mex.*
Cefalexin (p.168·1).
*Bacterial infections.*

**Quimotrase** *Alcon Cusi, Spain†.*
Chymotrypsin (p.1671·2).
*Aid in cataract surgery.*

**Quimotrip** *Collins, Mex.*
Tetracycline (p.266·2); enzymes.
*Bacterial infections.*

**Quimpe Amida** *Quimpe, Spain†.*
Sulfanilamide (p.263·2); zinc oxide (p.1163·2).
*Bacterial skin infections.*

**Quimpe Antibiotico** *Quimpe, Spain.*
Tetracycline hydrochloride (p.266·2).
*Bacterial infections.*

**Quimpe Vitamin** *Quimpe, Spain†.*
Vitamin B substances and amino-acid preparation (p.1417·1).

**Quimpedor** *Quimpe, Spain.*
Caffeine (p.782·1); phenazone (p.82·3); pyridoxine hydrochloride (p.1456·3); propyphenazone (p.85·3); thiamine hydrochloride (p.1455·1).
*Fever; pain.*

**Quinaband**
*SSL, Austral.; SSL, UK.*
Calamine (p.1144·1); clioquinol (p.196·3); zinc oxide (p.1163·2).
*Leg ulcers; medicated bandage.*

**Quinaglute**
*Schering, S.Afr.†; Berlex, USA†.*
Quinidine gluconate (p.991·3).
*Arrhythmias.*

**Quinalan** *Lannett, USA†.*
Quinidine gluconate (p.991·3).
*Arrhythmias.*

**Quinate**
*Note. This name is used for preparations of different composition.*
*Aventis, Austral.*
Quinine sulfate (p.460·2).
*Diagnosis of myasthenia gravis; malaria; muscle cramps; myotonia congenita.*

*Rougier, Canad.†.*
Quinidine gluconate (p.991·3).
*Arrhythmias.*

**Quinax**
*Alcon, Hong Kong; Alcon, Singapore; Alcon, Thai.*
Azapentacene polysulfonate sodium.
*Cataract.*

**Quinazide** *Malesci, Ital.*
Quinapril hydrochloride (p.991·1); hydrochlorothiazide (p.933·2).
*Hypertension.*

**Quinazil** *Malesci, Ital.*
Quinapril hydrochloride (p.991·1) or quinaprilat (p.991·2).
*Heart failure; hypertension.*

**Quinbisul** *Alphapharm, Austral.*
Quinine bisulfate (p.460·1).
*Malaria; nocturnal leg cramps.*

**Quindoleina** *Gastroenterologicos, Mex.†.*
Clioquinol (p.196·3).

**Quineuron** *Euromex, Mex.†.*
Quinidine (p.991·3).

**Quinfamex** *Ofimex, Mex.†.*
Quinfamide (p.615·2).

**Quini** *Astra, Mex.*
Quinidine bisulfate (p.991·3).
*Arrhythmias.*

**Quinicardina** *Berenguer Infale, Spain†.*
Quinidine sulfate (p.991·3).
*Arrhythmias.*

**Quinicardine** *Barrenne, Braz.*
Quinidine sulfate (p.991·3).
*Arrhythmias.*

**Quinidex**
*Wyeth-Ayerst, Canad.†; Robins, USA.*
Quinidine sulfate (p.991·3).
*Arrhythmias.*

**Quiniduran** *Teva, Israel.*
Quinidine bisulfate (p.991·3).
*Arrhythmias.*

**Quinidurule** *AstraZeneca, Fr.†.*
Quinidine bisulfate (p.991·3).
*Arrhythmias.*

**Quinimax** *Sanofi Synthelabo, Fr.*
Quinine gluconate (p.462·1) or quinine hydrochloride (p.460·2); quinidine gluconate (p.991·3) or quinidine hydrochloride (p.993·2); cinchonine hydrochloride (p.1672·1); cinchonidine hydrochloride (p.1672·1).
Formerly contained quinine-resorcinol dihydrochloride, quinidine-resorcinol dihydrochloride, cinchonine-resorcinol dihydrochloride, and cinchonidine-resorcinol dihydrochloride.
*Malaria.*

**Quininga** *Inga, India.*
Quinine dihydrochloride (p.460·1) or quinine sulfate (p.460·2).
*Malaria; muscle cramps.*

**Quinisedine** *Sodia, Fr.*
Quinine benzoate (p.462·1); crataegus (p.1677·1).
*Cramps.*

**Quinivax-in** *Valda, Ital.*
A diphtheria, tetanus, pertussis, poliomyelitis, and Haemophilus influenzae vaccine (p.1615·1).
*Active immunisation.*

**Quinobact** *Nicholas Piramal, India.*
Ciprofloxacin (p.188·2) or ciprofloxacin lactate (p.188·3).
*Bacterial infections.*

**Quinobarb** *Rougier, Canad.†.*
Quinidine phenylethylbarbiturate (p.993·2).
*Arrhythmias; sedative.*

**Quinobiot** *Andromaco, Chile.*
Levofloxacin (p.225·3).
*Bacterial infections.*

**Quinoc** *Douglas, NZ†.*
Quinine sulfate (p.460·2).
*Malaria; myotonia; nocturnal cramps.*

**Quinocarbine** *GNR, Fr.†.*
Aluminium orthoxyquinoleate; activated charcoal (p.1030·2).
*Diarrhoea; meteorism.*

**Quinocort**
*Quinoderm, Irl.; Adams, UK†.*
Potassium hydroxyquinoline sulfate (p.1734·2); hydrocortisone (p.1103·3).
*Infected skin disorders.*

**Quinoctal** *Fawns & McAllan, Austral.*
Quinine sulfate (p.460·2).
*Malaria; nocturnal cramps.*

**Quinoderm**
*Quinoderm, Irl.; Aventis, S.Afr.; Quinoderm, Switz.†; Ferndale, UK.*
Benzoyl peroxide (p.1143·2); potassium hydroxyquinoline sulfate (p.1734·2).
*Acne; folliculitis.*

**Quinoderm Antibacterial Face Wash** *Ferndale, UK.*
Chlorhexidine gluconate (p.1173·2); cetrimide (p.1172·1); detergents.
*Skin cleanser; soap substitute.*

**Quinoderm-H** *Hoechst Marion Roussel, S.Afr.†.*
Benzoyl peroxide (p.1143·2); potassium hydroxyquinoline sulfate (p.1734·2); hydrocortisone (p.1103·3).
*Skin disorders.*

**Quinodermil** *Oftalder, Port.*
Clioquinol (p.196·3).

**Quinodermil-AS** *Edol, Port.*
Salicylic acid (p.1157·1); clioquinol (p.196·3).
*Infected skin disorders.*

**Quinodis**
*Grunenthal, Austria; Roche, Belg.†; Roche, Denm.†; Grunenthal, Ger.; Grunenthal, Switz.†.*
Fleroxacin (p.213·2).
*Bacterial infections.*

**Quinoflex** *Mepha, Port.*
Norfloxacin (p.238·3).
*Bacterial infections.*

**Quinoflox**
*Note. This name is used for preparations of different composition.*
*Biolab Sanus, Braz.*
Ciprofloxacin hydrochloride (p.188·2) or ciprofloxacin lactate (p.188·3).
*Bacterial infections.*

*Diba, Mex.*
Ciprofloxacin hydrochloride (p.188·2); lidocaine hydrochloride (p.1377·3).
*Bacterial ear infections.*

**Quinoform** *EMS, Braz.*
Norfloxacin (p.238·3).
*Bacterial infections.*

**Quinoforme** *Sanofi Synthelabo, Fr.*
Basic quinine formate (p.462·1).
*Malaria.*

**Quinomed** *Biocumed, Arg.*
Ofloxacin (p.239·3).
*Bacterial eye infections.*

**Quinoped** *Adams, UK†.*
Benzoyl peroxide (p.1143·2); potassium hydroxyquinoline sulfate (p.1734·2).
*Fungal skin infections.*

**Quinora** *Key, USA†.*
Quinidine sulfate (p.991·3).
*Arrhythmias.*

**Quinoret** *Darier, Mex.*
Hydroquinone (p.1148·1); vitamin A (p.1451·2).
*Skin pigmentation disorders; sun-induced skin damage.*

**Quinortar** *Iquinosa, Spain.*
Coal tar (p.1159·2); chlorquinaldol (p.187·3); titanium dioxide (p.1160·3).
*Skin disorders.*

**Quinox** *Labesfal, Port.*
Ciprofloxacin (p.188·2).
*Bacterial infections.*

**Quinoxan** *Teuto, Braz.*
Ofloxacin (p.239·3).
*Bacterial infections.*

**Quinradon** *Hua, Thai.†.*
Diiodohydroxyquinoline (p.603·3); boric acid (p.1662·1); phosphoric acid (p.1731·2).
*Vaginal infections.*

**Quinradon-N** *Hua, Thai.*
Diiodohydroxyquinoline (p.603·3); nystatin (p.406·3); boric acid (p.1662·1); phosphoric acid (p.1731·2).
*Vaginal infections.*

**Quinsana Plus** *Mennen, USA.*
Tolnaftate (p.410·1).
*Fungal skin infections.*

**Quinsul** *Alphapharm, Austral.*
Quinine sulfate (p.460·2).
*Malaria; nocturnal leg cramps.*

**Quintabs** *Freeda, USA.*
A range of vitamin preparations (p.1417·1).

**Quintasa**
*Ferring, Canad.†; Ferring, Spain†.*
Mesalazine (p.1273·2).
*Inflammatory bowel disease.*

**Quintelmin** *EMS, Braz.*
Mebendazole (p.108·2).
*Worm infections.*

**Quintex** *Therabel, Belg.*
Butamirate citrate (p.1116·2).
Formerly contained dioxethedrin hydrochloride, promethazine hydrochloride, and codeine phosphate.
*Coughs.*

**Quintex Pediatrique** *Therabel, Belg.*
Butamirate citrate (p.1116·2).
Formerly contained dioxethedrin hydrochloride, promethazine hydrochloride pholcodine, and sulfogaiacol.
*Coughs.*

**Quintonine** *GlaxoSmithKline Sante, Fr.*
Cinnamon (p.1672·2); kola (p.1765·3); dried bitter-orange peel (p.1723·3); cinchona bark (p.1671·3); quassia (p.1737·2); gentian (p.1692·2).
*Asthenia.*

**Quintopan** *GlaxoSmithKline Sante, Fr.*
Chlorphenamine maleate (p.427·3); dextromethorphan hydrobromide (p.1117·3); sodium benzoate (p.1169·3).
*Coughs.*

**Quintopan Enfant** *SmithKline Beecham Sante, Fr.†.*
Promethazine hydrochloride (p.439·1); pholcodine (p.1128·3); sulfogaiacol (p.1131·1); dioxethedrin hydrochloride (p.1119·1).
*Coughs.*

**Quipro** *Ciclum, Spain.*
Ciprofloxacin hydrochloride (p.188·2).
*Bacterial infections.*

**Quiralam** *Guidotti, Spain.*
Dexketoprofen trometamol (p.51·2).
*Pain.*

**Quirgel** *Retrain, Spain.*
Dexketoprofen trometamol (p.51·2).
*Inflammation; pain.*

**Quiss** *Jagson, India.*
Betamethasone valerate (p.1093·2); gentamicin sulfate (p.217·1); tolnaftate (p.410·1); clioquinol (p.196·3).
*Infected skin disorders.*

**Quit** *Aspen, S.Afr.*
Nicotine (p.1720·1).
*Aid to smoking withdrawal.*

**Quitadrill** *Pierre Fabre Sante, Fr.*
Mequitazine (p.437·2).
*Hypersensitivity.*

**Quitaxon**
*Roche, Belg.†; Ercopharm, Denm.†; Nepalm, Fr.*
Doxepin hydrochloride (p.291·2).
*Depression.*

**Quitoso**
*Elisium, Arg.; Lepori, Port.*
Pyrethrins (p.1509·3); piperonyl butoxide (p.1509·2).
*Pediculosis.*

**QuitX** *Alphapharm, Austral.*
Nicotine (p.1720·1).
*Aid to smoking withdrawal.*

**Quixil** *Omrix, Israel.*
Human clottable proteins; human alpha thrombin (p.760·1); calcium chloride (p.1225·1).
*Haemorrhage.*

**Quixin** *Santen, USA.*
Levofloxacin (p.225·3).
*Bacterial conjunctivitis.*

**Quocel** *Rayere, Mex.*
Quinfamide (p.615·2).
*Amoebiasis.*

**Quocin** *Isdin, Spain.*
Acetic acid (p.1645·2); salicylic acid (p.1157·1).
*Callosities.*

**Quoderm** *Isdin, Spain†.*
Meclocycline sulfosalicylate (p.229·1).
*Acne.*

**Quomem**
*Allen, Austria; Glaxo Allen, Ital.; Esteve, Spain; GlaxoSmithKline, Thai.*
Bupropion hydrochloride (p.287·2).
*Aid to smoking withdrawal.*

**Quool** *Allmi-Care, UK.*
Menthol (p.1711·3).
*Musculoskeletal pain.*

**Quosten** *Ibi, Ital.†.*
Calcitonin (salmon) (p.768·2).
*Hypercalcaemia; osteoporosis; Paget's disease of bone; reflex sympathetic dystrophy.*

**Quotal NF** *Bristol-Myers Squibb, Arg.*
Chloramphenicol sodium succinate (p.185·1).
*Bacterial infections.*

**Quotane** *Zambon, Fr.*
Quinisocaine hydrochloride (p.1384·2).
*Pruritus.*

**Quotivit O.E.** *Mayoly-Spindler, Fr.*
Multivitamin and mineral preparation (p.1417·1).

**Qura** *Microsules Bernabo, Arg.*
Astemizole (p.424·2); bromhexine hydrochloride (p.1115·3); pseudoephedrine sulfate (p.1129·2); paracetamol (p.76·2).
*Influenza symptoms.*

**QV**
*Ego, Austral.; Ego, Hong Kong; Ego, Malaysia; Ego, NZ; Ego, Singapore.*
A range of emollients and soap substitutes.
*Skin disorders.*

**QV Flare Up** *Ego, Singapore.*
Benzalkonium chloride (p.1168·3); triclosan (p.1195·2); light liquid paraffin (p.1479·1).
*Eczema.*

**QV Lip Balm**
*Ego, Austral.†; Ego, Hong Kong; Ego, Malaysia; Ego, NZ; Ego, Singapore.*
Avobenzone (p.1142·3); octinoxate (p.1154·3).
*Dry, cracked, or chapped lips; sunscreen.*

**Qvar**
*3M, Arg.; 3M, Austral.; UCB, Belg.; 3M, Canad.; 3M, Fr.; 3M, Hong Kong; 3M, Irl.; 3M, Malaysia; 3M, Neth.; Aventis, NZ; 3M, S.Afr.; 3M, Singapore; UCB, Spain; Ivax, UK; Ivax, USA.*
Beclometasone dipropionate (p.1091·1).
*Asthma.*

**Q-Vax** *CSL, Austral.*
An inactivated Q fever vaccine (p.1635·3).
*Active immunisation.*

**R & C**
*Reed & Carnrick, Canad.; Reed & Carnrick, USA†.*
Pyrethrins (p.1509·3); piperonyl butoxide (p.1509·2).
*Pediculosis; surface and textile insecticide.*

**R Calm** *Labima, Belg.*
Diphenhydramine hydrochloride (p.431·3).
*Allergic conjunctivitis; allergic rhinitis; pruritus; urticaria.*

**R Calm + B6** *Labima, Belg.†.*
Dimenhydrinate (p.431·1); pyridoxine (p.1457·2).
*Motion sickness; urticaria.*

**RA Lotion** *Medco, USA.*
Resorcinol (p.1156·3); calamine (p.1144·1); borax (p.1661·3).
*Acne.*

**RA Morph** *Pharmacia, NZ.*
Morphine hydrochloride (p.60·1).
*Pain.*

**Rabarbaroni** *Max Farma, Ital.†.*
Rhubarb (p.1287·3); cinchona (p.1671·3); bitter orange (p.1723·3); liquorice (p.1270·2).
*Constipation.*

**RabAvert** *Chiron, USA.*
A rabies vaccine (p.1635·3).
*Active immunisation.*

**Rabec** *Phoenix, Arg.*
Rabeprazole sodium (p.1285·1).
*Gastro-oesophageal reflux; peptic ulcer.*

**Rabeloc** *Cadila Pharma, India.*
Rabeprazole (p.1285·1).
*Gastro-oesophageal reflux; peptic ulcer.*

**Rabies Gamma** *Biagini, Ital.†.*
A rabies immunoglobulin (p.1635·3).
*Passive immunisation.*

**Rabies-Imovax**
*Aventis Pasteur, Denm.; Aventis Pasteur, Fin.; Aventis Pasteur, Norw.; Aventis Pasteur, Swed.*
A rabies vaccine (Wistar PM/WI 38-1503-3M) (p.1635·3).
*Active immunisation.*

**Rabigam** *NBI, S.Afr.*
A rabies immunoglobulin (p.1635·3).
*Passive immunisation.*

**Rabipor** *Biovac, S.Afr.*
A rabies vaccine (p.1635·3).
*Active immunisation.*

**Rabipur**
*Grunenthal, Austria; Chiron Behring, Ger.; Aventis, India; Chiron, Thai.; Masta, UK.*
A rabies vaccine (Flury strain grown on chicken fibroblast cultures) (p.1635·3).
*Active immunisation.*

**Rabivac** *Chiron Behring, Ger.*
A rabies vaccine (Pitman-Moore strain grown on human diploid cell cultures) (p.1635·3).
*Active immunisation.*

**Rablas** *Medichrom, Gr.*
Enalapril maleate (p.909·2).
*Heart failure; hypertension.*

**Raboldo** *IMO, Ital.†.*
Cascara (p.1255·1); boldo (p.1661·2); rhubarb (p.1287·3).
*Constipation.*

**Rabro** *Vitafarma, Spain†.*
Calcium carbonate (p.1254·2); frangula bark (p.1266·3); liquorice (p.1270·2); magnesium oxide (p.1272·3); dimethicone (p.1289·2).
*Flatulence; gastritis; hyperchlorhydria; peptic ulcer.*

**Rabro N** *Teofarma, Ger.*
Calcium carbonate (p.1254·2); liquorice (p.1270·2); magnesium oxide (p.1272·3).
*Gastrointestinal hyperacidity; heartburn.*

**Rabugen** *Unison, Hong Kong.*
Domperidone (p.1263·2).
*Gastrointestinal disorders; nausea and vomiting.*

**Rabuman**
*Berna, Hong Kong; Berna, Ital.†; Berna, Switz.; Berna, Thai.†.*
A rabies immunoglobulin (p.1635·3).
*Passive immunisation.*

**Racestyptin** *Austrodent, Austria†.*
Aluminium chloride (p.1142·1); hydroxyquinoline sulfate (p.1700·1).
*Adjunct in dental procedures.*

**Racestyptine** *Septodont, Switz.*
*Solution:* Aluminium chloride (p.1142·1).
*Thread†:* Aluminium chloride (p.1142·1); lidocaine (p.1377·3); hydroxyquinoline (p.1700·1).
*Dental and gum disorders.*

**Racetam** *Samjin, Singapore.*
Piracetam (p.1732·1).
*Cerebral trauma; cerebrovascular disorders.*

**Ra-Cliss** *Fresenius Kabi, Ital.†.*
Monobasic sodium phosphate (p.1230·3); dibasic sodium phosphate (p.1231·1).
*Bowel evacuation; constipation.*

**Racovel** *Cryopharma, Mex.*
Levodopa (p.1205·2); carbidopa (p.1204·3).
*Parkinsonism.*

**Radacef** *Bristol-Myers Squibb, Gr.*
Ceforanide (p.175·2).
*Bacterial infections.*

**Radalgin** *Streuli, Switz.*
Nonivamide (p.67·2); methyl nicotinate (p.59·2); glycol salicylate (p.44·3); histamine hydrochloride (p.1697·1).
*Musculoskeletal pain; sports injuries.*

**Radan** *Marjan, Braz.*
Ranitidine hydrochloride (p.1285·2).
*Gastro-oesophageal reflux; gastrointestinal haemorrhage; peptic ulcer; Zollinger-Ellison syndrome.*

**Radanil** *Roche, Arg.*
Benznidazole (p.602·3).
*Protozoal infections.*

**Radecol** *Asta Medica, Ger.†.*
Nicotinyl alcohol tartrate (p.966·2).
*Hyperlipidaemias; vascular disorders.*

**Radedorm** *AWD, Ger.*
Nitrazepam (p.710·1).
*Sleep disorders.*

**Radenarcon** *Asta Medica, Ger.†.*
Etomidate (p.1299·1).
*General anaesthesia.*

**Radepur** *AWD, Ger.*
Chlordiazepoxide (p.674·2).
*Anxiety disorders; insomnia.*

**RadiaGel** *Carrington, USA.*
Acemannan (p.1645·2).
*Radiation wounds.*

**Radialar 280** *Juste, Spain.*
Meglumine amidotrizoate (p.1060·2).
*Radiographic contrast medium.*

**Radian** *Roche, S.Afr.†.*
*Cream:* Menthol (p.1711·3); camphor (p.1665·3); methyl salicylate (p.59·3); capsicum oleoresin (p.1667·1); camphor oil.
*Liniment:* Menthol (p.1711·3); aspirin (p.15·1); camphor (p.1665·3); methyl salicylate (p.59·3).
*Pain.*

**Radian-B**
*Note. This name is used for preparations of different composition.*
*Roche Consumer, Austral.*
*Liniment:* Menthol (p.1711·3); camphor (p.1665·3); ammonium salicylate (p.14·2); methyl salicylate (p.59·3); ethyl salicylate (p.37·3).
*Musculoskeletal and joint disorders; soft-tissue disorders.*
*Roche Consumer, Austral.; Radiol, Israel; Ransom, UK.*
*Topical rub:* Menthol (p.1711·3); camphor (p.1665·3); methyl salicylate (p.59·3); capsicum oleoresin (p.1667·1).
*Musculoskeletal, joint, and soft-tissue disorders.*
*Roche Consumer, Irl.*
*Topical rub:* Menthol (p.1711·3); camphor (p.1665·3); methyl salicylate (p.59·3); camphor oil; capsaicin (p.24·2).
*Musculoskeletal and soft-tissue disorders.*
*Roche Consumer, Irl.; Ransom, UK.*
*Liniment; topical spray:* Menthol (p.1711·3); camphor (p.1665·3); ammonium salicylate (p.14·2); salicylic acid (p.1157·1).
*Musculoskeletal and joint disorders.*
*Radiol, Israel.*
*Liniment; topical spray:* Aspirin (p.15·1); menthol (p.1711·3); camphor (p.1665·3); methyl salicylate (p.59·3).
*Musculoskeletal, joint, and soft-tissue disorders.*

**Radian-B Ibuprofen** *Ransom, UK.*
Ibuprofen (p.45·3).
*Musculoskeletal pain; sports injuries.*

**Radian-B Red Oils** *Roche Consumer, UK.*
Methyl nicotinate (p.59·2); expressed mustard oil (p.1718·2).
*Musculoskeletal and joint pain.*

**Radicura** *Walker, Arg.*
Boldo (p.1661·2); carqueja; canchalagua.
*Digestive disorders.*

**Radicut** *Mitsubishi, Jpn.*
Edaravone (p.909·2).
*Cerebral infarction.*

**Radigen** *Medipharm, Chile.*
Risperidone (p.719·2).
*Psychoses.*

**Radikal**
*Note. This name is used for preparations of different composition.*
*Sandipro, Belg.*
Malathion (p.1507·1).
*Pediculosis.*
*Maurer, Ger.†.*
Clotrimazole (p.396·2).
*Fungal skin infections.*

**Radilem** *Lemery, Mex.*
Methylprednisolone acetate (p.1106·1).
*Corticosteroid.*

**Radin** *Dexa, Hong Kong.*
Ranitidine hydrochloride (p.1285·2).
*Peptic ulcer; Zollinger-Ellison syndrome.*

**Radina** *Amhof, Arg.*
Tobramycin (p.271·2).
*Bacterial eye infections.*

**Radina Dex** *Amhof, Arg.*
Tobramycin (p.271·2); dexamethasone (p.1097·1).
*Infected eye disorders.*

**Radine** *Pond's, Thai.*
Ranitidine hydrochloride (p.1285·2).
*Gastro-oesophageal reflux; peptic ulcer; Zollinger-Ellison syndrome.*

**Radio Salil** *Vinas, Spain.*
*Cream:* Camphor (p.1665·3); methyl nicotinate (p.59·2); methyl salicylate (p.59·3); salicylic acid (p.1157·1); menthol (p.1711·3).
*Spray:* Camphor (p.1665·3); diethylamine salicylate (p.34·1); menthol (p.1711·3).
*Musculoskeletal, joint, peri-articular, and soft-tissue disorders.*

**Radioced** *Interfarma, Ital.†.*
Dimethicone (p.1482·1).
*Barrier preparation.*

**Radiogardase** *Heyl, USA.*
Prussian blue (p.1051·2).
*Exposure to caesium-137 or thallium.*

**Radiogardase-Cs** *Heyl, Ger.*
Prussian blue (p.1051·2).
*Reduction in body-half-life of radiocaesium.*

**Radiomiron** *Schering, Chile.*
Iopamidol (p.1064·3).
*Radiographic contrast medium.*

**Radiopaque** *Dabur, India.*
Iohexol (p.1064·2).
*Radiographic contrast medium.*

**Radioselectan** *Schering, Fr.*
Sodium amidotrizoate (p.1060·2); meglumine amidotrizoate (p.1060·2).
*Radiographic contrast medium.*

**Radol** *Julphar, UAE.*
Dichloroxylenol (p.1178·3); clorophene (p.1177·3).
*Disinfectant.*

**Rado-Salil** *Will-Pharma, Belg.*
Ethyl salicylate (p.37·3); methyl salicylate (p.59·3); glycol salicylate (p.44·3); salicylic acid (p.1157·1); camphor (p.1665·3); menthol (p.1711·3); capsicum oleoresin (p.1667·1).
*Lumbago; muscle and joint pain.*

**Rado-Spray** *Will-Pharma, Belg.*
Lidocaine hydrochloride (p.1377·3); glycol salicylate (p.44·3); methyl nicotinate (p.59·2).
*Musculoskeletal pain; sports injuries.*

**Raductil**
*Abbott, Arg.; Knoll, Mex.*
Sibutramine hydrochloride (p.1593·1).
*Obesity.*

**Radyn** *Arlex, Mex.†.*
Ranitidine (p.1285·2).

**Rafacalcin** *Rafarm, Gr.*
Calcitonin (p.768·2).
*Osteoporosis.*

**Rafapen V-K** *Rafa, Israel.*
Phenoxymethylpenicillin (p.242·1).
*Bacterial infections.*

**Rafapen Mega** *Rafa, Israel.*
Phenoxymethylpenicillin (p.242·1).
*Bacterial endocarditis prophylaxis.*

**Rafassal** *Rafa, Israel.*
Mesalazine (p.1273·2).
*Inflammatory bowel disease.*

**Rafathricin** *Rafa, Israel†.*
Tyrothricin (p.275·1).
*Mouth and throat infections.*

**Rafathricin with Benzocaine** *Rafa, Israel.*
Tyrothricin (p.275·1); benzocaine (p.1370·3).
*Mouth and throat disorders.*

**Rafazocine** *Rafa, Israel.*
Pentazocine (p.79·3).
*Pain.*

**Rafazocine X** *Rafa, Israel†.*
Pentazocine hydrochloride (p.79·3); naloxone hydrochloride (p.1044·3).
*Pain.*

**Rafen** *Alphapharm, Austral.*
Ibuprofen (p.45·3).
*Fever; inflammation; musculoskeletal and joint disorders; pain.*

**Raffo-Ca** *Raffo, Arg.*
Calcium citrate (p.1225·1).
*Osteoporosis.*

**Raffolutil** *Raffo, Arg.*
Bicalutamide (p.530·1).

**Raffonin** *Raffo, Chile.*
Fluticasone propionate (p.1102·3).
*Allergic rhinitis.*

**Raffreddoremed** *Iodosan, Ital.*
Paracetamol (p.76·2); isopropamide iodide (p.485·2); dimetofrine hydrochloride (p.902·3); caffeine (p.782·1); chlorphenamine maleate (p.427·3); ascorbic acid (p.1460·2).
*Cold and influenza symptoms.*

**Rafocilina** *Raffo, Arg.*
Ofloxacin (p.239·3).
*Bacterial ear infections.*

**Raftace** *Wockhardt, India.*
*Oral liquid:* Sodium alginate (p.1577·1); magnesium trisilicate (p.1272·3); aluminium hydroxide (p.1249·2).
*Tablets:* Alginic acid (p.1576·3); magnesium trisilicate (p.1272·3); aluminium hydroxide (p.1249·2); sodium bicarbonate (p.1223·2).
*Dyspepsia; gastro-oesophageal reflux; hiatus hernia.*

**Raft-Eze** *Pinewood, UK.*
Sodium bicarbonate (p.1223·2); sodium alginate (p.1577·1); calcium carbonate (p.1254·2).
*Gastro-oesophageal reflux.*

**Rafton** *Ferring, Canad.*
Alginic acid (p.1576·3) or sodium alginate (p.1577·1); aluminium hydroxide (p.1249·2).
*Heartburn.*

**Rafuzone** *Rafa, Israel†.*
Nitrofurazone (p.238·2).
*Infected burns.*

**Ragaden** *Ganassini, Ital.*
Cetylpyridinium chloride (p.1173·1).
*Nipple disinfection.*

**Ragonil** *Roche, Ecuad.*
Benznidazole (p.602·3).
*Protozoal infections.*

**Raikocef** *Mediolanum, Ital.*
Cefonicid sodium (p.174·2).
Lidocaine hydrochloride (p.1377·3) is included in the intramuscular injection to alleviate the pain of injection.
*Gram-negative bacterial infections.*

**Ralcidin** *Amadeus, India.*
Chlorphenamine maleate (p.427·3); paracetamol (p.76·2); phenylephrine hydrochloride (p.1126·3); caffeine (p.782·1).
*Cold symptoms; hypersensitivity reactions.*

**Ralgex** *SSL, UK.*
*Cream:* Glycol salicylate (p.44·3); methyl nicotinate (p.59·2); capsicum oleoresin (p.1667·1).
*Topical stick:* Glycol salicylate (p.44·3); ethyl salicylate (p.37·3); methyl salicylate (p.59·3); capsicum oleoresin (p.1667·1); menthol (p.1711·3).
*Musculoskeletal and joint disorders.*

**Ralgex Freeze Spray** *SSL, UK.*
Isopentane; dimethyl ether (p.1236·1); glycol monosalicylate (p.44·3).
*Musculoskeletal and joint disorders.*

**Ralgex Heat Spray (low-odour)** *SSL, UK.*
Glycol monosalicylate (p.44·3); methyl nicotinate (p.59·2).
*Musculoskeletal and joint disorders.*

**Ralicid** *Sanochemia, Austria.*
Indometacin (p.47·3).
*Gout; inflammation; musculoskeletal, joint, and periarticular disorders; oedema; pain.*

**Ralinet** *Coup, Gr.*
Loratadine (p.436·1).
*Allergic rhinitis; pruritus.*

**Ralodantin** *Pharmacia, Austral.*
Nitrofurantoin (p.237·2).
*Urinary-tract infections.*

**Ralofekt** *Temmler, Ger.*
Pentoxifylline (p.979·3).
*Peripheral vascular disorders; vascular disorders of the eye or ear.*

**Ralogaine** *Kenral, Austral.†.*
Minoxidil (p.960·1).
*Alopecia androgenetica.*

**Ralopar** *Aventis, Port.*
Cefotaxime sodium (p.175·3).
*Bacterial infections.*

**Ralovera** *Pharmacia, Austral.*
Medroxyprogesterone acetate (p.1557·2).
*Abnormal uterine bleeding; adjunct to oestrogen therapy; amenorrhoea; endometriosis; malignant neoplasms.*

**Ralozam** *Pharmacia, Austral.†.*
Alprazolam (p.668·3).
*Anxiety; panic disorders.*

**Ralsifen-X** *Serral, Mex.*
Tamoxifen (p.585·3).
*Breast cancer.*

**Ralur** *Drossapharm, Switz.*
Heparin sodium (p.928·1); indometacin (p.47·3); lauromacrogol 400 (p.1412·3).
*Musculoskeletal, joint, peri-articular, and soft-tissue disorders.*

**Ramace**
*Aventis, Austral.; AstraZeneca, Belg.; AstraZeneca, Denm.; AstraZeneca, Fin.; Astra, Mex.; AstraZeneca, S.Afr.*
Ramipril (p.994·1).
*Diabetic nephropathy; heart failure; hypertension; myocardial infarction.*

**Ramavit** *Leiras, Fin.†.*
Vitamin B substances with iron (p.1417·1).
*Vitamin B and iron deficiency.*

**Ramend** *Queisser, Ger.*
Senna (p.1288·2).
*Constipation.*

**Ramend Krauter** *Queisser, Ger.*
Senna (p.1288·2); maté (p.1765·3); coriander (p.1676·1); fennel (p.1687·2); aniseed (p.1655·2).
*Constipation.*

**Ramet Cade** *CS, Fr.†.*
Cade oil (p.1159·2).
*Skin disorders.*

**Ramet Dalibour** *CS, Fr.†.*
Copper sulfate (p.1426·1); zinc sulfate (p.1469·3).
*Skin cleaning and disinfection.*

**Ramet Pain** *CS, Fr.†.*
Copper sulfate (p.1426·1); zinc sulfate (p.1469·3).
*Skin cleansing and disinfection.*

**Ramfin**
*Biolab, Malaysia; Biolab, Thai.*
Rifampicin (p.250·2).
*Gonorrhoea; leprosy; tuberculosis.*

**Rami Slijmoplossende** *Warner-Lambert, Neth.*
Carbocisteine (p.1116·2).
*Coughs.*

**Rami-Dextromethorphan** *Warner-Lambert, Neth.*
Dextromethorphan hydrobromide (p.1117·3).
Formerly contained codeine and antimony potassium tartrate.
*Coughs.*

**Ramidox** *Errekappa, Ital.*
Loperamide oxide (p.1271·1).
*Diarrhoea.*

**Ramipres** *Pasteur, Chile.*
Ramipril (p.994·1).
*Heart failure; hypertension.*

**Ramistos** *Pasteur, Chile.*
Codeine (p.27·1); bromoform (p.1663·1); belladonna (p.479·1); lobelia (p.1589·1); drosera (p.1683·1); grindelia (p.1696·1).
*Respiratory-tract disorders.*

**Ramivan** *Medipharm, Chile.*
Roxithromycin (p.254·2).
*Bacterial infections.*

**Ramno Fix** *Piam, Ital.*
*Lactobacillus rhamnosus*; *Lactobacillus casei casei*; *Lactobacillus acidophilus* (p.1704·2).
*Digestive disorders.*

**Ramno-Flor** *Piam, Ital.*
Lactic-acid-producing organisms (p.1704·2).
*Nutritional supplement.*

**Ramol** *Nakornpatana, Thai.*
Paracetamol (p.76·2).
*Pain.*

**Ramp** *MediMar, UK†.*
Pregnancy test (p.1734·3).

**Rampicin** *Shiwa, Thai.*
Rifampicin (p.250·2).
*Gonorrhoea; leprosy; tuberculosis.*

**Ramses**
*Durex, Canad.; Schmid, USA†.*
Nonoxinol 9 (p.1413·3).
*Contraceptive.*

**Ramysis** *Isis, UK†.*
Doxycycline hyclate (p.206·2).
*Bacterial infections.*

**Ran** *Helsinn, Port.*
Ranitidine hydrochloride (p.1285·2).
*Gastro-oesophageal reflux; peptic ulcer; Zollinger-Ellison syndrome.*

**Ran H2** *Seid, Spain.*
Ranitidine hydrochloride (p.1285·2).
*Acid aspiration; gastro-oesophageal reflux; peptic ulcer; Zollinger-Ellison syndrome.*

**Ran Lich** *Lichtenstein, Ger.*
Ranitidine hydrochloride (p.1285·2).
*Acid aspiration; gastro-oesophageal reflux; gastrointestinal haemorrhage; peptic ulcer; Zollinger-Ellison syndrome.*

**Ranacid** *Nycomed, Norw.†.*
Ranitidine hydrochloride (p.1285·2).
*Acid aspiration syndrome; gastro-oesophageal reflux; peptic ulcer; Zollinger-Ellison syndrome.*

**Ranamp** *Ranbaxy, S.Afr.*
Ampicillin sodium (p.157·1).
*Bacterial infections.*

**Ranceph** *Ranbaxy, S.Afr.*
Cefalexin (p.168·1).
*Bacterial infections.*

**Rancil** *Ranbaxy, Thai.*
Amoxicillin trihydrate (p.155·3).
*Bacterial infections.*

**Ranclav**
*Ranbaxy, S.Afr.*
Amoxicillin (p.155·3); clavulanic acid (p.193·3).
*Bacterial infections.*

*Ranbaxy, Thai.*
Potassium clavulanate (p.193·3); amoxicillin (p.155·3).
*Bacterial infections.*

**Ranclosil** *Ranbaxy, S.Afr.*
Ampicillin (p.157·1); cloxacillin (p.198·2).
*Bacterial infections.*

**Randex** *Randall, Mex.*
Ambroxol hydrochloride (p.1114·3).
*Respiratory-tract disorders associated with viscous mucus.*

**Randoclin** *Ranbaxy, S.Afr.*
Doxycycline (p.206·2).
*Bacterial infections; malaria.*

**Randum** *Teofarma, Ital.*
Metoclopramide hydrochloride (p.1274·3).
*Gastrointestinal disorders.*

**Ranepal** *Liferpal, Mex.*
Ranitidine (p.1285·2).
*Peptic ulcer.*

**Ranfen** *Ranbaxy, S.Afr.*
Ibuprofen (p.45·3).
*Fever; inflammation; musculoskeletal, joint, and soft-tissue disorders; pain.*

**Ranfradin** *Ranbaxy, S.Afr.*
Cefradine (p.179·3).
*Bacterial infections.*

**Rani**
*ABZ, Ger.; Alpharma-Isis, Ger.; Denk, Singapore.*
Ranitidine hydrochloride (p.1285·2).
*Acid aspiration; gastro-oesophageal reflux; gastrointestinal haemorrhage; peptic ulcer; Zollinger-Ellison syndrome.*

**Rani 2** *Alphapharm, Austral.*
Ranitidine hydrochloride (p.1285·2).
*Gastro-oesophageal reflux; peptic ulcer; Zollinger-Ellison syndrome.*

**Raniben** *FIRMA, Ital.*
Ranitidine hydrochloride (p.1285·2).
*Gastro-oesophageal reflux; gastrointestinal hyperacidity; peptic ulcer; Zollinger-Ellison syndrome.*

**Raniberl** *Berlin-Chemie, Ger.*
Ranitidine hydrochloride (p.1285·2).
*Acid aspiration; gastro-oesophageal reflux; gastrointestinal haemorrhage; peptic ulcer; Zollinger-Ellison syndrome.*

**Ranibeta** *Betapharm, Ger.*
Ranitidine hydrochloride (p.1285·2).
*Acid aspiration; gastro-oesophageal reflux; gastrointestinal haemorrhage; peptic ulcer; Zollinger-Ellison syndrome.*

**Ranibloc**
*Wolff, Ger.; Glaxo Allen, Ital.*
Ranitidine hydrochloride (p.1285·2).
*Acid aspiration; gastro-oesophageal reflux; gastrointestinal haemorrhage; peptic ulcer; Zollinger-Ellison syndrome.*

**Ranic**
*Hexal, Austria; Glaxo Wellcome, Belg.†.*
Ranitidine hydrochloride (p.1285·2).
*Gastro-oesophageal haemorrhage; gastro-oesophageal reflux; peptic ulcer; Zollinger-Ellison syndrome.*

**Ranicel** *Laboratorios Chile, Chile.*
Ranitidine hydrochloride (p.1285·2).
*Dyspepsia; gastric hyperacidity.*

**Ranicid** *M & H, Thai.*
Ranitidine hydrochloride (p.1285·2).
*Gastro-oesophageal reflux; peptic ulcer; Zollinger-Ellison syndrome.*

**Raniclon** *Novartis, Gr.*
Ranitidine hydrochloride (p.1285·2).
*Conditions where gastric acid reduction is beneficial; gastric hypersecretion including Zollinger-Ellison syndrome; peptic ulcer.*

**Ranicodan** *Pharmacodane, Denm.*
Ranitidine (p.1285·2).
*Acid aspiration; gastro-oesophageal reflux; peptic ulcer; Zollinger-Ellison syndrome.*

**Ranicur** *Pharmacia, Fin.*
Ranitidine hydrochloride (p.1285·2).
*Acid aspiration; gastro-oesophageal reflux; peptic ulcer; Zollinger-Ellison syndrome.*

**Ranicux** *TAD, Ger.*
Ranitidine hydrochloride (p.1285·2).
*Acid aspiration; gastro-oesophageal reflux; gastrointestinal haemorrhage; peptic ulcer; Zollinger-Ellison syndrome.*

**Ranidil** *Menarini, Ital.*
Ranitidine hydrochloride (p.1285·2).
*Gastrointestinal hyperacidity; peptic ulcer gastro-oesophageal reflux; Zollinger-Ellison syndrome.*

**Ranidin**
*Uniao Quimica, Braz.; Faes, Spain.*
Ranitidine hydrochloride (p.1285·2).
*Acid aspiration; gastro-oesophageal reflux; gastrointestinal hyperacidity; peptic ulcer; short-bowel syndrome; Zollinger-Ellison syndrome.*

**Ranidina** *Bunker, Braz.*
Ranitidine hydrochloride (p.1285·2).
*Peptic ulcer.*

**Ranidine**
*Biolab, Singapore; Biolab, Thai.*
Ranitidine (p.1285·2).
*Gastro-oesophageal reflux; peptic ulcer; Zollinger-Ellison syndrome.*

**Ranidura T** *Merck dura, Ger.*
Ranitidine hydrochloride (p.1285·2).
*Acid aspiration; gastro-oesophageal reflux; gastrointestinal haemorrhage; peptic ulcer; Zollinger-Ellison syndrome.*

**Ranifarma** *Continentales, Mex.†.*
Ranitidine (p.1285·2).

**Raniflex** *Royton, Braz.*
Ranitidine hydrochloride (p.1285·2).
*Peptic ulcer.*

**Ranifur** *Fustery, Mex.*
Ranitidine (p.1285·2) or ranitidine hydrochloride (p.1285·2).
*Acid aspiration; gastro-oesophageal reflux; gastrointestinal haemorrhage; peptic ulcer; Zollinger-Ellison syndrome.*

**Ranigyl** *Raza, Malaysia; Pharmaniaga, Malaysia.*
Metronidazole (p.607·2).
*Amoebiasis; anaerobic bacterial infections; giardiasis; trichomoniasis.*

**Ranihexal**
*Hexal, Austral.; Hexal, S.Afr.*
Ranitidine hydrochloride (p.1285·2).
*Acid aspiration; gastro-oesophageal reflux; peptic ulcer; Zollinger-Ellison syndrome.*

**Ranikur** *Opco, Denm.*
Ranitidine (p.1285·2).
*Acid aspiration; gastro-oesophageal reflux; peptic ulcer; Zollinger-Ellison syndrome.*

**Ranil** *Gea, Fin.*
Ranitidine hydrochloride (p.1285·2).
*Acid aspiration; dyspepsia; gastro-oesophageal reflux; peptic ulcer; Zollinger-Ellison syndrome.*

**Ranilonga** *Sanofi Synthelabo, Spain†.*
Ranitidine hydrochloride (p.1285·2).
*Acid aspiration; gastro-oesophageal reflux; peptic ulcer; short-bowel syndrome; Zollinger-Ellison syndrome.*

**Ranimed** *Ecosol, Switz.*
Ranitidine hydrochloride (p.1285·2).
*Gastro-oesophageal reflux; peptic ulcer; Zollinger-Ellison syndrome.*

**Ranimerck** *Merck dura, Ger.*
Ranitidine hydrochloride (p.1285·2).
*Acid aspiration; gastro-oesophageal reflux; gastrointestinal haemorrhage; peptic ulcer; Zollinger-Ellison syndrome.*

**Ranimex** *Orion, Fin.*
Ranitidine hydrochloride (p.1285·2).
*Acid aspiration; dyspepsia; gastro-oesophageal reflux; peptic ulcer; Zollinger-Ellison syndrome.*

**Rani-nerton** *Dolorgiet, Ger.*
Ranitidine hydrochloride (p.1285·2).
*Acid aspiration; gastro-oesophageal reflux; gastrointestinal haemorrhage; peptic ulcer; Zollinger-Ellison syndrome.*

**Raniplex** *Fournier, Fr.*
Ranitidine hydrochloride (p.1285·2).
*Gastro-oesophageal reflux; gastrointestinal haemorrhage; peptic ulcer; Zollinger-Ellison syndrome.*

**Raniprotect** *Riemser, Ger.*
Ranitidine hydrochloride (p.1285·2).
*Acid aspiration; gastro-oesophageal reflux; gastrointestinal haemorrhage; peptic ulcer; Zollinger-Ellison syndrome.*

**Rani-Q** *Scand Pharm, Swed.*
Ranitidine hydrochloride (p.1285·2).
*Gastro-oesophageal reflux; heartburn.*

**Ranisen** *Senosiain, Mex.*
Ranitidine hydrochloride (p.1285·2).
*Acid aspiration; gastro-oesophageal reflux; gastrointestinal haemorrhage; peptic ulcer; Zollinger-Ellison syndrome.*

**Ranisifar** *Siphar, Switz.*
Ranitidine hydrochloride (p.1285·2).
*Gastro-oesophageal reflux; gastrointestinal haemorrhage; peptic ulcer; Zollinger-Ellison syndrome.*

**Ranitak** *Luper, Braz.*
Ranitidine hydrochloride (p.1285·2).
*Peptic ulcer.*

**Ranitax** *Saval, Chile.*
Ranitidine (p.1285·2).
*Gastritis; gastro-oesophageal reflux; peptic ulcer; Zollinger-Ellison syndrome.*

**Ranitic**
*Hexal, Arg.; Hexal, Austral.; Hexal, Ger.; Rowex, Irl.; Tillomed, UK.*
Ranitidine hydrochloride (p.1285·2).
*Acid aspiration; chronic dyspepsia; gastro-oesophageal reflux; gastrointestinal haemorrhage; peptic ulcer; Zollinger-Ellison syndrome.*

**Ranitidi GNO** *Arion, Arg.*
Ranitidine (p.1285·2).
*Peptic ulcer.*

**Ranitidoc** *Docpharm, Ger.*
Ranitidine hydrochloride (p.1285·2).
*Acid aspiration; gastro-oesophageal reflux; peptic ulcer; Zollinger-Ellison syndrome.*

**Ranitil** *EMS, Braz.*
Ranitidine hydrochloride (p.1285·2).
*Acid aspiration; gastro-oesophageal reflux; gastrointestinal haemorrhage; peptic ulcer; Zollinger-Ellison syndrome.*

**Ranitine** *Azevedos, Port.*
Ranitidine hydrochloride (p.1285·2).
*Gastro-oesophageal reflux; peptic ulcer; Zollinger-Ellison syndrome.*

**Ranitinol** *Ducto, Braz.*
Ranitidine hydrochloride (p.1285·2).
*Peptic ulcer.*

**Ranition** *Sanval, Braz.*
Ranitidine hydrochloride (p.1285·2).
*Peptic ulcer.*

**Ranitral** *Sanitas, Arg.*
Ranitidine hydrochloride (p.1285·2).
*Gastritis; gastro-oesophageal reflux; peptic ulcer; Zollinger-Ellison syndrome.*

**Ranitrat** *Cazi, Braz.*
Ranitidine hydrochloride (p.1285·2).
*Peptic ulcer.*

**Ranitul** *Oriental, Arg.*
Ranitidine (p.1285·2).
*Peptic ulcer.*

**Ranityrol** *Tyrol, Austria.*
Ranitidine hydrochloride (p.1285·2).
*Acid aspiration; gastro-oesophageal haemorrhage; gastro-oesophageal reflux; peptic ulcer; Zollinger-Ellison syndrome.*

**Ranivel** *Duncan, Spain†.*
Ranitidine hydrochloride (p.1285·2).
*Gastrointestinal hyperacidity.*

**Ranix** *Abbott, Spain.*
Ranitidine hydrochloride (p.1285·2).
*Acid aspiration; gastro-oesophageal reflux; gastrointestinal hyperacidity; peptic ulcer; short-bowel syndrome; Zollinger-Ellison syndrome.*

**Ranixal** *Ratiopharm, Fin.*
Ranitidine hydrochloride (p.1285·2).
*Acid aspiration; gastro-oesophageal reflux; peptic ulcer; Zollinger-Ellison syndrome.*

**Ranmoxy** *Ranbaxy, S.Afr.*
Amoxicillin trihydrate (p.155·3).
*Bacterial infections.*

**Ranolta** *Jean-Marie, Hong Kong.*
Ranitidine hydrochloride (p.1285·2).
*Gastro-oesophageal reflux; peptic ulcer; Zollinger-Ellison syndrome.*

**Ranopine** *Pinewood, Irl.*
Ranitidine hydrochloride (p.1285·2).
*Gastric hyperacidity; gastro-oesophageal reflux; peptic ulcer; Zollinger-Ellison syndrome.*

**Ranoprin** *Ratiopharm, Fin.*
Propranolol hydrochloride (p.989·3).
*Angina pectoris; arrhythmias; essential tremor; glaucoma; hypertension; hyperthyroidism; hypertrophic obstructive cardiomyopathy; migraine; myocardial infarction.*

**Ranoxyl**
*Note. This name is used for preparations of different composition.*
*Douglas, Austral.*
Ranitidine hydrochloride (p.1285·2).
*Gastro-oesophageal reflux; peptic ulcer; Zollinger-Ellison syndrome.*

*Ranbaxy, Singapore†.*
Amoxicillin trihydrate (p.155·3).
*Bacterial infections.*

**Ranozol** *ST, Thai.*
Miconazole nitrate (p.405·3).
*Fungal skin infections.*

**Ranpuric** *Triomed, S.Afr.†.*
Allopurinol (p.412·2).
*Gout; hyperuricaemia.*

**Rantac** *Unique, India.*
Ranitidine hydrochloride (p.1285·2).
*Dyspepsia; gastro-oesophageal reflux; gastrointestinal hyperacidity; peptic ulcer; Zollinger-Ellison syndrome.*

**Rantag** *Julphar, UAE.*
Ranitidine hydrochloride (p.1285·2).
*Acid aspiration; dyspepsia; gastro-oesophageal reflux; gastrointestinal haemorrhage; peptic ulcer; Zollinger-Ellison syndrome.*

**Rantec** *Berk, UK.*
Ranitidine hydrochloride (p.1285·2).
*Acid aspiration; dyspepsia; gastro-oesophageal reflux; gastrointestinal haemorrhage; peptic ulcer; Zollinger-Ellison syndrome.*

**Ranteen** *Aspen, S.Afr.*
Ranitidine hydrochloride (p.1285·2).
*Acid aspiration; gastro-oesophageal reflux; peptic ulcer; Zollinger-Ellison syndrome.*

**Ranthrocin** *Ranbaxy, Singapore.*
Erythromycin ethyl succinate (p.208·1).
*Bacterial infections.*

**Rantudal** *Menarini, Gr.*
Acemetacin (p.11·3).
*Dysmenorrhoea; gout; inflammation; musculoskeletal disorders; pain; spondyloarthritis.*

**Rantudil**
*Tropon, Ger.; Bayer, Mex.; Bial, Port.; Bayer, Singapore†.*
Acemetacin (p.11·3).
*Gout; inflammation; musculoskeletal, joint, peri-articular, and soft-tissue disorders; pain; thrombophlebitis; vasculitis.*

**Ranuber** *ICN, Spain.*
Ranitidine hydrochloride (p.1285·2).
*Acid aspiration; gastro-oesophageal reflux; gastrointestinal haemorrhage; gastrointestinal hyperacidity; peptic ulcer; short-bowel syndrome; Zollinger-Ellison syndrome.*

**Ranulin** *Pisa, Mex.*
Ranitidine (p.1285·2).

**Ranvil** *Gentili, Ital.*
Nicardipine hydrochloride (p.965·1).
*Angina pectoris; heart failure; hypertension.*

**Ranvir** *Ranbaxy, Thai.*
Aciclovir (p.626·1).
*Herpesvirus infections.*

**Ranxas** *Labinca, Arg.*
Doxorubicin hydrochloride (p.547·3).
*Malignant neoplasms.*

**Ranzac** *Eastern Pharmaceuticals, UK.*
Ranitidine hydrochloride (p.1285·2).
*Dyspepsia; gastric hyperacidity; heartburn.*

**Ranzil** *Tocogino, Mex.†.*
Ranitidine (p.1285·2).

**Ranzol** *Ranbaxy, S.Afr.*
Cefazolin sodium (p.170·3).
*Bacterial infections.*

**Rapaid Antiseptic** *Rye, Austral.*
Melaleuca oil (p.1710·2).
*Minor wounds; skin infections.*

**Rapaid First Aid** *Rye, Austral.†.*
Melaleuca oil (p.1710·2).
*Bites; minor wounds; skin infections; skin irritation; stings.*

**Rapaid Medicated** *Rye, Austral.†.*
Melaleuca oil (p.1710·2); zinc oxide (p.1163·2).
*Skin disorders.*

**Rapaid Rash-Relief** *Rye, Austral.*
*Cream:* Melaleuca oil (p.1710·2); aloe vera (p.1141·3).
*Skin disorders.*

**Rapako comp** *Truw, Ger.*
Homoeopathic preparation.

**Rapako xylo** *Truw, Ger.*
Xylometazoline hydrochloride (p.1132·2).
*Rhinitis.*

**Rapamic** *Cipan, Port.*
Ketoconazole (p.403·3).
*Fungal infections.*

**Rapamune**
*Wyeth, Arg.; Wyeth, Austral.; Wyeth, Belg.; Wyeth, Braz.; Wyeth-Ayerst, Canad.; Wyeth, Chile; Wyeth, Denm.; Wyeth Lederle, Fin.; Wyeth Lederle, Fr.; Wyeth, Ger.; Wyeth, Gr.; Wyeth, Irl.; Ayerst, Israel; Wyeth Lederle, Ital.; Wyeth, Mex.; Wyeth Lederle, Norw.; Wyeth, NZ; Wyeth, Spain; Wyeth Lederle, Swed.; Wyeth, Switz.; Wyeth, UK; Wyeth-Ayerst, USA.*
Sirolimus (p.1363·1).
*Renal transplant rejection.*

**Rap-eze** *Roche Consumer, UK.*
Calcium carbonate (p.1254·2).
*Dyspepsia; heartburn.*

**Raphanus S Potier** *Pharmethic, Belg.†.*
Raphanus sativus niger.
*Dyspepsia associated with biliary dyskinesia.*

**Rapicort** *Malesci, Ital.†.*
Hydrocortisone sodium succinate (p.1104·1).
*Shock.*

**Rapid Gel** *Biokosma, Braz.†.*
Trolamine (p.1758·2).
*Pain.*

**Rapid Strand** *Amersham, Austral.*
Iodine-125 (p.1524·2) titanium capsules welded into a silver rod.
*Prostatic cancer.*

**Rapidal** *Bial, Spain.*
Terfenadine (p.441·1).
*Hypersensitivity reactions.*

**Rapidica** *Sarabhai Piramal, India.*
Neutral insulin injection (porcine, highly purified) (p.333·3).
*Diabetes mellitus.*

**Rapidocaine** *Sintetica, Switz.*
Lidocaine hydrochloride (p.1377·3).
Adrenaline hydrochloride (p.852·3) is included in some injections as a vasoconstrictor to diminish absorption and localise the effect of the local anaesthetic.
*Arrhythmias; local anaesthesia.*

**Rapidol**
*Note. This name is used for preparations of different composition.*
*Pharmonta, Austria.*
Paracetamol (p.76·2); propyphenazone (p.85·3); caffeine (p.782·1).
*Fever; pain.*

*Pfizer, Chile; Ranbaxy, Malaysia; Ranbaxy, Singapore.*
Paracetamol (p.76·2).
*Fever; pain.*

**RapidVue** *Quidel, USA.*
Pregnancy test (p.1734·3).

**Rapifen**
*AstraZeneca, Austral.; Janssen-Cilag, Austria; Janssen-Cilag, Belg.; Janssen-Cilag, Braz.; Janssen-Cilag, Chile; Janssen-Cilag, Denm.; Orion, Fin.; Janssen-Cilag, Fr.; Janssen-Cilag, Ger.; IFET (ΙΦΕΤ), Gr.; Janssen, Hong Kong; Janssen-Cilag, Irl.; Janssen-Cilag, Israel; Janssen-Cilag, Malaysia; Janssen, Mex.; Janssen-Cilag, Neth.; Janssen-Cilag, Norw.; Janssen-Cilag, NZ; Janssen-Cilag, S.Afr.; Janssen-Cilag, Swed.; Janssen-Cilag, Switz.; Janssen-Cilag, UK.*
Alfentanil hydrochloride (p.12·2).
*Induction of general anaesthesia; pain during surgical procedures.*

**Rapignost Basic Screen Plus** *Advance Diagnostic, Irl.*
Test for ascorbic acid, glucose, protein, blood, pH, and nitrites in urine.

**Rapignost Diabetes Profile** *Advance Diagnostic, Irl.*
Test for ketones, ascorbic acid, and glucose in urine.

**Rapignost Total Screen LSG** *Advance Diagnostic, Irl.*
Test for bilirubin, urobilinogen, pH, glucose, protein, ketones, blood, nitrite, ascorbic acid, and leucocytes in urine.

**Rapilax**
*Merck, Arg.; Hertz, Braz.†.*
Sodium picosulfate (p.1289·3).
*Constipation.*

**Rapilax Fibras** *Merck, Arg.*
Ispaghula (p.1268·1); senna (p.1288·2).
*Constipation.*

**Rapilin** *Sun, India.*
Repaglinide (p.344·3).
*Diabetes mellitus.*

**Rapilysin**
*Roche, Austral.; Roche, Austria; Roche, Belg.; Roche, Denm.; Roche, Fin.; Roche, Fr.; Roche, Ger.; Roche, Irl.; Roche, Ital.; Roche, Neth.; Roche, Norw.; Roche, NZ; Roche, Port.; Roche, Spain; Roche, Swed.; Roche, Switz.; Roche, UK.*
Reteplase (p.995·2).
*Myocardial infarction.*

**Rapimix** *Sarabhai Piramal, India.*
A mixture of insulin injection (porcine, highly purified) 30% and isophane insulin (porcine, highly purified) 70% (p.333·3).
*Diabetes mellitus.*

**Rapi-snooze** *Medinaturals, UK†.*
Melatonin (p.1710·2); pyridoxine (p.1457·2); valerian (p.1762·2).

**Rapitard MC** *Novo Nordisk, Switz.†.*
Biphasic insulin injection (bovine crystalline 75%, porcine soluble 25%, monocomponent) (p.333·3).
*Diabetes mellitus.*

**Rapitil** *Aventis, UK.*
Nedocromil sodium (p.789·3).
*Allergic conjunctivitis; keratoconjunctivitis.*

**Rapitux** *Sigma-Tau, Ital.*
Levodropropizine (p.1119·3).
*Coughs.*

**Rapivir** *Glaxo Wellcome, Mex.*
Valaciclovir hydrochloride (p.656·1).
*Herpes simplex infections; varicella-zoster infections.*

**Raplon** *Organon, USA†.*
Rapacuronium bromide (p.1405·2).
*Competitive neuromuscular blocker.*

**Rapolyte**
*Ergha, Irl.; Provalis, UK.*
Sodium chloride; potassium chloride; sodium citrate; glucose (p.1222·2).
*Diarrhoea; oral rehydration therapy.*

**Rappell** *Pfizer Consumer, UK.*
Piperonal (p.1509·1).
*Head lice repellent.*

**Raptiva** *Genentech, USA.*
Efalizumab (p.1146·3).
*Psoriasis.*

**Rapura** *Globopharm, Switz.*
Peru balsam (p.1730·2); camphor (p.1665·3); thymol (p.1194·2); zinc oxide (p.1163·2).
*Minor skin lesions.*

**Raquiferol** *Spedrog, Arg.*
Vitamin D (p.1461·2).
*Hypoparathyroidism; osteomalacia; renal osteodystrophy; vitamin D deficiency.*

**Rarical** *Janssen-Cilag, Braz.*
Multivitamin and mineral preparation (p.1417·1).

**Raricap** *Ethnor, India.*
Calcium ferrous citrate (p.1436·1); folic acid (p.1429·1); vitamin $B_2$; vitamin $B_6$; vitamin $B_{12}$ (p.1417·1).
Vitamin C (p.1460·2) is included in this preparation to increase the absorption and availability of iron.
*Iron-deficiency anaemia.*

**Raricap L** *Ethnor, India.*
Calcium ferrous citrate (p.1436·1); vitamin A palmitate; colecalciferol; vitamin $B_1$; vitamin $B_2$; nicotinamide; lysine hydrochloride (p.1417·1).
*Iron-deficiency anaemia.*

**Rariplex** *Uniao Quimica, Braz.†.*
Multivitamin and mineral preparation (p.1417·1).

**RAS** *Wiedemann, Ger.†.*
Antireticular serum (rabbit).
*Tonic.*

**Rasal** *Ipsen, Spain.*
Olsalazine sodium (p.1278·1).
*Ulcerative colitis.*

**Raset** *Unison, Thai.*
Bezafibrate (p.873·2).
*Hyperlipidaemias.*

**Rashfree** *Abbott, India.*
Benzalkonium chloride (p.1168·3); zinc oxide (p.1163·2).
*Nappy rash; skin disinfection.*

**Rasilvax** *Chiron Vaccines, Ital.*
A rabies vaccine (human diploid cell) (p.1635·3).
*Active immunisation.*

**Rastinon**
*Aspen, Austral.; Hoechst Marion Roussel, Austria†; Hoechst, Ger.†; Hoechst Marion Roussel, Hong Kong†; Hoechst Marion Roussel, Ital.†; Aventis, Mex.; Hoechst Marion Roussel, Neth.†; Hoechst Marion Roussel, S.Afr.†; Aventis, Spain†.*
Tolbutamide (p.348·1).
*Diabetes mellitus.*

**Ratacand** *AstraZeneca, Ital.*
Candesartan cilexetil (p.878·3).
*Hypertension.*

**Ratacand Plus** *AstraZeneca, Ital.*
Candesartan cilexetil (p.878·3); hydrochlorothiazide (p.933·2).
*Hypertension.*

**Rati Salil Crema** *Gramon, Arg.*
Amyl salicylate (p.14·3); camphor (p.1665·3); turpentine oil (p.1760·1); salicylic acid (p.1157·1); capsaicin (p.24·2).
*Musculoskeletal and joint disorders.*

**Rati Salil E** *Gramon, Arg.*
Magnesium salicylate (p.55·1).
*Musculoskeletal, joint, and soft-tissue disorders.*

**Rati Salil Flex** *Gramon, Arg.*
Salicylic acid (p.1157·1); diethylamine salicylate (p.34·1).
*Musculoskeletal, joint, peri-articular, and soft-tissue disorders; neuralgia.*

**Rati Salil Gel** *Gramon, Arg.*
Methyl salicylate (p.59·3).
*Musculoskeletal, joint, peri-articular, and soft-tissue disorders; neuralgia.*

**Rati Salil Ice** *Gramon, Arg.*
Menthol (p.1711·3).
*Musculoskeletal, joint, peri-articular, and soft-tissue disorders.*

**Rati Salil Pro** *Gramon, Arg.*
Methyl salicylate (p.59·3); menthol (p.1711·3).
*Musculoskeletal, joint, peri-articular, and soft-tissue disorders.*

**Ratic** *Atlantic, Thai.*
Ranitidine (p.1285·2).
*Peptic ulcer; Zollinger-Ellison syndrome.*

**Ratica** *LBS, Thai.*
Ranitidine (p.1285·2).
*Gastro-oesophageal reflux; peptic ulcer.*

**Raticina** *Microsules Bernabo, Arg.*
Ranitidine hydrochloride (p.1285·2).
*Peptic ulcer.*

**ratioAllerg** *Ratiopharm, Ger.*
*Cream:* Hydrocortisone (p.1103·3).
*Skin disorders.*
*Nasal spray:* Beclometasone dipropionate (p.1091·1).
*Hay fever.*
*Topical gel:* Diphenhydramine hydrochloride (p.431·3).
*Hypersensitivity reactions.*

**ratioDolor**
*Ratiopharm, Austria; Ratiopharm, Ger.*
Ibuprofen lysine (p.46·3).
*Fever; pain.*

**ratioGast** *Ratiopharm, Ger.*
*Capsules:* Tormentil (p.1757·2).
*Diarrhoea.*
*Oral drops:* Anise oil (p.1655·2); fennel oil (p.1687·3); caraway oil (p.1667·3).
*Dyspepsia.*

**ratioGrippal + C** *Ratiopharm, Ger.†.*
Aspirin (p.15·1); paracetamol (p.76·2); ascorbic acid (p.1460·2).
*Cold symptoms.*

**ratioHepar** *Ratiopharm, Ger.*
Cynara (p.1678·3).
*Biliary disorders.*

**ratioMobil** *Ratiopharm, Ger.*
Piroxicam (p.84·2).
*Musculoskeletal, joint, peri-articular, and soft-tissue disorders.*

**Rationale** *Manetti Roberts, Ital.*
Colextran hydrochloride (p.890·3).
*Hyperlipidaemias.*

**Rationasal** *Ratiopharm, Spain†.*
Xylometazoline hydrochloride (p.1132·2).
*Nasal congestion; sinusitis.*

**Ratiopyrin**
*Ratiopharm, Austria; Ratiopharm, Ger.*
Aspirin (p.15·1); paracetamol (p.76·2); caffeine (p.782·1).
*Pain.*

**ratioSept**
*Ratiopharm, Austria; Ratiopharm, Ger.*
Rhatany root (p.1738·1).
*Mouth inflammation.*

**Raudil** *Novag, Mex.*
Ranitidine (p.1285·2).
*Acid aspiration; gastro-oesophageal reflux; gastrointestinal haemorrhage; peptic ulcer; Zollinger-Ellison syndrome.*

**Raudopen** *Farmabion, Spain†.*
Amoxicillin trihydrate (p.155·3).
*Bacterial infections.*

**Raufuncton N** *Knoll, Ger.†.*
Rauwolfiae vomitoria (p.994·3); squill (p.1130·3); convallaria (p.1675·3); adonis vernalis (p.1648·1).
*Arrhythmias; hypertension.*

**Rauserpin** *Breves, Braz.†.*
Reserpine (p.995·1).
*Hypertension; Raynaud's syndrome.*

**RauwolfiaViscomp** *Schuck, Ger.*
Homoeopathic preparation.

**Rauwolsan H** *Pfluger, Ger.*
Homoeopathic preparation.

**Rauwoplant** *Schwabe, Ger.†.*
Rauwolfia (p.994·3); crataegus (p.1677·1).
*Hypertension.*

**Rauzide** *Apothecon, USA.*
Rauwolfia serpentina (p.994·3); bendroflumethiazide (p.867·3).
*Hypertension.*

**Ravalgen** *GlaxoSmithKline Consumer, Ger.*
Garlic oil (p.1691·2).
*Age-related vascular changes.*

**Ravalton** *Rafarm, Gr.*
Ciprofloxacin hydrochloride (p.188·2).
*Bacterial infections.*

**Ravamil** *Merck, S.Afr.*
Verapamil hydrochloride (p.1019·1).
*Angina pectoris; arrhythmias; hypertension.*

**Ravenol** *Caber, Ital.*
A heparinoid (p.931·1).
*Vascular disorders with a risk of thrombosis.*

**Raveron**
*Germania, Austria†; Asta Medica, Braz.†.*
Prostate extract.
*Benign prostatic hyperplasia.*

**Ravigona** *Roche Nicholas, Spain†.*
Vitamin A palmitate (p.1453·1); tocoferil acetate (p.1465·1).
*Eye disorders; male infertility.*

**Ravocaine and Novocain** *Cook-Waite, USA†.*
Propoxycaine hydrochloride (p.1384·1); procaine (p.1383·2).
Noradrenaline (p.974·3) is included as a vasoconstrictor to diminish absorption and localise the effect of the local anaesthetic.
*Local anaesthesia.*

**Ravotril** *Roche, Chile.*
Clonazepam (p.359·1).
*Anxiety; epilepsy; panic attacks; social phobia.*

**Raw Prostate** *Natural Life, Arg.*
Prostate extract.
*Dietary supplement.*

**Raxamida** *Arlex, Mex.†.*
Loperamide (p.1271·2).

**Raxedin** *Quimica y Farmacia, Mex.†.*
Loperamide (p.1271·2).

**Raxeto** *Dosa, Arg.*
Raloxifene (p.1568·3).
*Osteoporosis.*

**Ray Block** *Del-Ray, USA.*
*SPF 15:* Padimate O (p.1155·1); oxybenzone (p.1154·3).
*Sunscreen.*

**Raycept** *Zambon, Port.*
Calcium levofolinate (p.1431·1).
*Anaemias; methotrexate toxicity.*

**Rayepen** *Rayere, Mex.†.*
Ampicillin (p.157·1).
*Bacterial infections.*

**Rayetetra** *Rayere, Mex.†.*
Tetracycline (p.266·2).
*Bacterial infections.*

**Rayne** *Fustery, Mex.†.*
Diazepam (p.690·1).

**Rayvist** *Schering, Switz.†.*
Meglumine ioglicate (p.1064·1) or meglumine ioglicate and sodium ioglicate (p.1064·2).
*Radiographic contrast medium.*

**Rayvist 180** *Schering, Austria†.*
Meglumine ioglicate (p.1064·1).
*Radiographic contrast medium.*

**Razagleda Plus** *Dallas, Arg.*
Benzocaine (p.1370·3); carmellose (p.1577·3).
*Obesity.*

**Razene** *Pacific, NZ.*
Cetirizine hydrochloride (p.427·1).
*Allergic conjunctivitis; allergic rhinitis; insect bites; urticaria.*

**RBC**
*Note. This name is used for preparations of different composition.*
*Rybar, Irl.*
Antazoline hydrochloride (p.424·2); calamine (p.1144·1); cetrimide (p.1172·1).
*Pruritus; skin irritation.*
*Co-Pharma, UK.*
Calamine (p.1144·1); dibrompropamidine isetionate (p.1178·2).
Formerly contained antazoline hydrochloride, calamine, and cetrimide.
*Insect bites and stings.*

**R-Cetate** *GHP, Thai.*
Electrolyte infusion with or without glucose (p.1217·1).
*Carbohydrate source; fluid and electrolyte disorders.*

**RCF** *Ross, USA.*
Carbohydrate-free soy protein feed (p.1417·1).
*Carbohydrate intolerance; ketogenic diet.*

**R-Cin** *Lupin, India.*
Rifampicin (p.250·2).
*Tuberculosis.*

**R-Cinex** *Lupin, India.*
Rifampicin (p.250·2); isoniazid (p.222·2).
*Tuberculosis.*

**R-Cinex Z** *Lupin, India.*
Rifampicin (p.250·2); isoniazid (p.222·2); pyrazinamide (p.246·3).
*Tuberculosis.*

**R-Den** *Nakorn, Thai.*
21 Tablets, levonorgestrel (p.1563·2); ethinylestradiol (p.1553·2); 7 tablets, inert.
*Combined oral contraceptive.*

**Reabilan**
*Nestle, Fr.; Clintec, Irl.†; Galagen, USA.*
A range of preparations for enteral nutrition (p.1417·1).

**Reacel-A** *Offenbach, Mex.*
Tretinoin (p.1161·1).
*Acne; keratinisation disorders.*

**Reach Junior Fluoride** *Johnson & Johnson, Irl.†.*
Sodium fluoride (p.1444·3).
*Dental care.*

**Reactine**
*Pfizer Consumer, Canad.; Pfizer, Norw.*
Cetirizine hydrochloride (p.427·1).
*Allergic conjunctivitis; allergic rhinitis; allergic skin disorders.*

**Reactine Plus** *Pfizer Consumer, Canad.†.*
Tablets, cetirizine hydrochloride (p.427·1); extended-release capsules, pseudoephedrine hydrochloride (p.1129·2).
*Allergic rhinitis; urticaria.*

**Reactivan** *Merck, S.Afr.*
Fencamfamin hydrochloride (p.1588·2); vitamins (p.1417·1).
*Tonic.*

**Reafix** *Gemballa, Braz.*
Oral rehydration solution (p.1222·2).
*Oral rehydration therapy.*

**Reagin** *Baliarda, Arg.*
Citicoline (p.1672·3).

**Reagin Vascular** *Baliarda, Arg.*
Citicoline (p.1672·3); co-dergocrine mesilate (p.1674·1).
*Cerebrovascular disorders.*

**Real Lemon Cold Powders** *Sterwin, UK†.*
Paracetamol (p.76·2); phenylephrine (p.1126·3); ascorbic acid (p.1460·2).
*Cold symptoms.*

**Realderm** *Reall, Switz.*
Zinc oxide (p.1163·2); glycerol (p.1694·3); aluminium acetotartrate (p.1652·3).
*Nappy rash; skin irritation.*

**Realdiet** *Celia, Fr.*
A range of preparations for enteral nutrition (p.1417·1).

**Realdrax** *Liferpal, Mex.*
Ibuprofen (p.45·3).
*Inflammation; pain.*

**Real-Vit** *Solfran, Mex.*
Multivitamin preparation (p.1417·1).

**Reanima** *Benitol, Arg.*
Caffeine (p.782·1); paracetamol (p.76·2).
*Fever; pain.*

**Reapam** *Parke, Davis, Neth.*
Prazepam (p.716·2).
*Anxiety.*

**Reasec**
*Janssen-Cilag, Belg.†; Janssen-Cilag, Ger.†; Janssen-Cilag, Ital.†; Janssen-Cilag, Switz.†.*
Diphenoxylate hydrochloride (p.1261·3).
Atropine sulfate (p.477·1) is included in this preparation to discourage abuse.
*Diarrhoea.*

**Re-Azo** *Reese, USA.*
Phenazopyridine hydrochloride (p.83·1).

**Rebacil** *Lisapharma, Ital.*
Bacampicillin hydrochloride (p.161·2).
*Bacterial infections.*

**ReBalance** *Zeller, Switz.*
Hypericum (p.299·1).
*Anxiety disorders; insomnia.*

**Rebaten** *Sigma, Braz.*
Propranolol hydrochloride (p.989·3).
*Hypertension.*

**Rebetol**
*Schering-Plough, Austria; Schering-Plough, Belg.; Schering-Plough, Braz.; Schering-Plough, Chile; Schering-Plough, Denm.; Schering-Plough, Fin.; Schering-Plough, Fr.; Essex, Ger.; Schering-Plough, Gr.; Schering-Plough, Hong Kong; Schering-Plough, Irl.; Schering-Plough, Israel; Schering-Plough, Ital.; Schering-Plough, Malaysia; Schering-Plough, Neth.; Schering-Plough, Norw.; Schering-Plough, Port.; Schering-Plough, Singapore; Schering-Plough, Spain; Schering-Plough, Swed.; Schering-Plough, Thai.; Schering-Plough, UK.*
Ribavirin (p.652·1).
For use in combination with interferon alfa-2b.
*Hepatitis C.*

**Rebetron**
*Essex, Arg.; Schering-Plough, Austral.; Schering, Canad.; Schering-Plough, S.Afr.; Schering, USA.*
Injection, interferon alfa-2b (Intron A) (p.640·3); capsules, ribavirin (Rebetol) (p.652·1).
*Chronic hepatitis C.*

**Rebif**
*Serono, Arg.; Serono, Austral.; Serono, Austria; Serono, Braz.; Serono, Canad.; Serono, Denm.; Serono, Fin.; Serono, Fr.; Serono, Ger.; Serono, Gr.; Serono, Hong Kong; Serono, Irl.; Serono, Israel; Serono, Ital.; Serono, Malaysia; Serono, Mex.; Serono, Neth.; Serono, Norw.; Serono, Port.; Serono, S.Afr.; Serono, Singapore; Serono, Spain; Serono, Swed.; Serono, Switz. Serono, Thai.; Serono, UK; Serono, USA.*
Interferon beta-1a (p.645·3).
*Multiple sclerosis.*

**Rebladerm** *Dermoteca, Port.*
Urea (p.1162·2).
*Dry skin disorders.*

**Rebone**
*Note. A similar name is used for preparations of different composition (see below).*
*Ache, Braz.*
Ipriflavone (p.773·2).
*Osteoporosis.*

**Re-BONE**
*Note. A similar name is used for preparations of different composition (see above).*
*Mallinckrodt, Switz.*
Rhenium-186 disodium etidronate (p.1525·1).
*Painful bone metastases in prostatic cancer.*

**Reca** *Cantabria, Spain.*
Enalapril maleate (p.909·2).
*Heart failure; hypertension.*

**Recaflex** *Recalcine, Chile.*
Tenoxicam (p.93·1).
*Gout; inflammation; musculoskeletal, joint, and soft-tissue disorders.*

**Recal** *New Farma, Ital.*
Calcium carbonate (p.1254·2).
*Calcium deficiency.*

**Recalfe** *Hebron, Braz.*
Alendronic acid (p.765·3).
*Osteoporosis.*

**Recalplex** *Cazi, Braz.*
Vitamin B substances (p.1417·1).
*Nutritional supplement.*

**Recamicina** *Lafi, Chile.*
Levofloxacin (p.225·3).
*Bacterial infections.*

**Recarcin** *Sanum-Kehlbeck, Ger.*
*Bacillus firmus.*
*Immunotherapy; joint disorders; rheumatism; sciatica.*

**Recatol Algin** *Riemser, Ger.*
Alginic acid (p.1576·3); carmellose sodium (p.1577·3).
*Obesity.*

**Recatol mono** *Riemser, Ger.*
Phenylpropanolamine hydrochloride (p.1127·3).
*Obesity.*

**Recatol N** *Riemser, Ger.†.*
Phenylpropanolamine hydrochloride (p.1127·3); thiamine hydrochloride (p.1455·1); pyridoxine hydrochloride (p.1456·3); ascorbic acid (p.1460·2).
*Obesity.*

**Receant** *Remedina, Gr.*
Cefuroxime sodium (p.184·1).
*Bacterial infections.*

**Recef** *Uno, Ital.*
Cefazolin sodium (p.170·3).
*Bacterial infections.*

**Receptozine** *Be-Tabs, S.Afr.*
Promethazine hydrochloride (p.439·1).
*Hypersensitivity.*

**Recessan** *Kreussler, Ger.*
Lauromacrogol 400 (p.1412·3).
*Mouth and throat inflammation.*

**Recilugo** *Ariston, Braz.†.*
Ethenzamide (p.37·2); nicotinylpyrazolone; orphenadrine (p.486·2).
*Skeletal muscle spasm.*

**Recipect** *Orion, Fin.*
Codeine phosphate (p.27·1); guaifenesin (p.1122·1).
*Coughs.*

**Recital** *Unipharm, Israel.*
Citalopram hydrobromide (p.289·1).
*Depression; panic attacks.*

**Reclomide** *Major, USA.*
Metoclopramide hydrochloride (p.1274·3).
*Nausea and vomiting.*

**Reclor** *Sarabhai Piramal, India.*
Chloramphenicol (p.185·1).
*Bacterial infections.*

**Rececef** *Julphar, UAE.*
Cefaclor (p.167·1).
*Bacterial infections.*

**Recofen** *Reese, USA.*
Guaifenesin (p.1122·1); dextromethorphan hydrobromide (p.1117·3).

**Recofen-D** *Reese, USA.*
Guaifenesin (p.1122·1); dextromethorphan hydrobromide (p.1117·3).

**Recofol**
*Gobbi, Arg.; Alphapharm, Austral.; Leiras, Denm.†; Leiras, Fin.; Leiras, Israel; Schering, Israel; Pisa, Mex.; Schering, Norw.; Pacific, NZ; Organon, Port.; Leiras, Singapore; Schering, Spain; Schering, Swed.; Narco-Med, Switz.; Leiras, Thai.*
Propofol (p.1305·3).
*General anaesthesia; sedative.*

**Recombinant H-B Vax II** *Merck Sharp & Dohme, Israel.*
A hepatitis B vaccine (p.1618·1).
*Active immunisation.*

**Recombinate**
*Baxter, Arg.; Baxter, Austral.; Baxter, Austria; Baxter, Belg.†; Baxter, Canad.; Baxter, Denm.; Baxter, Fin.; Baxter, Fr.; Baxter, Ger.; Baxter, Gr.; Hyland, Hong Kong; Baxter, Ital.; Baxtor, Jpn; Baxter, NZ; Baxter, Port.†; Baxter, Spain; Baxter, Swed.; Baxter, Switz.; Baxter Bio-Science, UK; Baxter, USA.*
A factor VIII preparation (recombinant) (p.751·1).
*Haemorrhagic disorders.*

**Recombivax HB**
*Merck Sharp & Dohme, Braz.; Merck Frosst, Canad.; Pasteur Merieux, Ital.; Aventis, Port.; Aventis Pasteur, Spain; Merck, USA.*
A hepatitis B vaccine (recombinant DNA) (p.1618·1).
*Active immunisation.*

**Recomvax B** *Aventis Pasteur, Chile.*
A hepatitis B vaccine (p.1618·1).
*Active immunisation.*

**Reconvan**
*Fresenius Kabi, Ger.; Fresenius Kabi, Port.; Fresenius Kabi, Switz.; Fresenius Kabi, UK.*
Preparation for enteral nutrition (p.1417·1).

**Recormon**
*Roche, Arg.; Roche, Austria; Boehringer Mannheim, Belg.†; Asta Medica, Braz.; Roche, Braz.; Roche, Chile; Ercopharm, Denm.†; Boehringer Mannheim, Fr.†; Boehringer Mannheim, Ger.†; Roche, Hong Kong; Boehringer Mannheim, Irl.†; Roche Diagnostics, Israel; Roche, Mex.; Boehringer Mannheim, Norw.†; Roche, NZ; Boehringer Mannheim, Port.; Roche, S.Afr.; Roche, Singapore; Roche, Switz.; Roche, Thai.*
Epoetin beta (p.747·2).
*Anaemias; autologous blood transfusions.*

**Recort Plus** *Reese, USA.*
Hydrocortisone (p.1103·3).
*Skin disorders.*

**Recoveron** *Armstrong, Mex.*
Sodium acexamate (p.1646·2).
*Burns; ulcers; wounds.*

**Recoveron N** *Armstrong, Mex.*
Sodium acexamate (p.1646·2); neomycin sulfate (p.235·1).
*Infected wounds; skin infections.*

**Recoveron NC** *Armstrong, Mex.*
Sodium acexamate (p.1646·2) neomycin sulfate (p.235·1).
*Wounds.*

**Recovery Food** *Milupa, Irl.†.*
Food for special diet (p.1417·1).

**Recozil** *Recon, Singapore.*
Gemfibrozil (p.923·1).
*Hyperlipidaemias.*

**Recrea** *Antula, Swed.*
Minoxidil (p.960·1).
*Alopecia androgenetica.*

**Rectacaine** *Reese, USA.*
*Ointment:* Phenylephrine hydrochloride (p.1126·3); shark-liver oil.
*Suppositories:* Phenylephrine hydrochloride (p.1126·3).

**Rectagene Medicated Balm** *Pfeiffer, USA.*
Yeast (p.1469·1); shark-liver oil.
*Haemorrhoids.*

**Rectagene Medicated Rectal Balm** *Pfeiffer, USA.*
Benzocaine (p.1370·3); phenylephrine hydrochloride (p.1126·3); bismuth subgallate (p.1252·2); zinc oxide (p.1163·2); mepyramine maleate (p.437·1).
*Anorectal disorders.*

**Rectalad** *Carter-Wallace, Austral.*
Docusate sodium (p.1262·2).
*Bowel evacuation; constipation.*

**Rectamigdol** *Diviser Aquilea, Spain.*
Bismuth camphocarbonate (p.1253·1).
*Sore throat.*

**Rectanus** *Heralds, Braz.†.*
Tribenoside (p.1757·3); lidocaine (p.1377·3).
*Haemorrhoids.*

**Rectinol** *Pfizer Consumer, Austral.*
Adrenaline (p.852·2); benzocaine (p.1370·3); zinc oxide (p.1163·2).
*Anorectal disorders.*

**Rectinol HC** *Pfizer Consumer, Austral.*
Cinchocaine hydrochloride (p.1373·2); hydrocortisone (p.1103·3).
*Anorectal disorders.*

**Rectiole** *Caldeira & Metelo, Port.†.*
Glycerol (p.1694·3).
*Bowel evacuation; constipation.*

**Recto Bronco Tosse** *Labocor, Port.†.*
Quinine sulfate (p.460·2); camphor (p.1665·3); niaouli oil (p.1719·3); terpin hydrate (p.1131·1).
*Coughs.*

**Recto Menaderm** *Menarini, Spain†.*
Beclometasone dipropionate (p.1091·1); clioquinol (p.196·3); heparin (p.927·3); cod-liver oil (p.1425·2); lidocaine hydrochloride (p.1377·3).
*Anorectal disorders.*

**Recto Menaderm NF** *Menarini, Spain.*
Beclometasone dipropionate (p.1091·1).
*Anorectal disorders.*

**Rectocort**
*Welcker-Lyster, Canad.†; Rougier, Hong Kong†.*
Hydrocortisone acetate (p.1103·3).
*Haemorrhoids.*

**Rectodelt** *Trommsdorff, Ger.*
Prednisone (p.1109·3).
*Rectal corticosteroid.*

**Rectogel** *Riva, Canad.*
Benzocaine (p.1370·3); zinc sulfate (p.1469·3).
*Anorectal disorders.*

**Rectogel HC** *Riva, Canad.*
Benzocaine (p.1370·3); zinc sulfate (p.1469·3); hydrocortisone acetate (p.1103·3).
*Anorectal disorders.*

**Rectogesic** *Cellegy, Austral.*
Glyceryl trinitrate (p.923·2).
*Anal fissure.*

**Rectopanbiline** *Sarget, Fr.*
Bile extract (p.1660·3); gelatin (p.754·3); glycerol (p.1694·3).
*Bowel evacuation; constipation.*

**Rectophedrol** *Martin, Fr.†.*
Cineole (p.1672·1); guaiacol carbonate (p.1122·1); wild thyme oil; camphor (p.1665·3); ephedrine (p.1120·1); procaine hydrochloride (p.1383·2).
*Respiratory-tract disorders.*

**Rectoplexil**
*Note. This name is used for preparations of different composition.*
*Rhone-Poulenc Rorer, Belg.†.*
Oxomemazine (p.438·2); guaifenesin (p.1122·1); sodium benzoate (p.1169·3); paracetamol (p.76·2).
*Coughs.*

*Theraplix, Fr.†.*
Oxomemazine (p.438·2).
Formerly contained oxomemazine, guaifenesin, sodium benzoate, and paracetamol.
*Coughs.*

**Rectopred** *Jacoby, Austria.*
Prednisolone sodium phosphate (p.1108·1).
*Croup.*

**Rectopulmo Adultos** *Salusif, Port.*
Camphor (p.1665·3); cineole (p.1672·1); niaouli oil (p.1719·3); quinine sulfate (p.460·2).
*Respiratory-tract disorders.*

**Rectopulmo Infantil** *Salusif, Port.*
Camphor (p.1665·3); cineole (p.1672·1); niaouli oil (p.1719·3).
*Respiratory-tract disorders.*

**Rectoquintyl** *Sodip, Switz.†.*
Ethyl orthoformate (p.1121·2); wild thyme oil; cineole (p.1672·1).
*Coughs.*

**Rectoquintyl-Promethazine** *Sanofi, Switz.†.*
Ethyl orthoformate (p.1121·2); promethazine (p.439·1); wild thyme oil; cineole (p.1672·1).
*Coughs.*

**Rectoquotane** *Zambon, Fr.*
Quinisocaine hydrochloride (p.1384·2); cetrimide (p.1172·1).
*Anorectal disorders.*

**Recto-Reparil** *Madaus, Ital.*
Aescin (p.1648·2); tetracaine hydrochloride (p.1385·1).
*Anorectal disorders.*

**Rectosan** *Terramin, Austria†.*
Naphazoline hydrochloride (p.1124·3); menthol (p.1711·3); benzocaine (p.1370·3).
*Anorectal disorders.*

**Rectosellan** *Mann, Ger.†.*
Aesculus (p.1648·2); melilotus officinalis.
*Haemorrhoids.*

**Rectosellan H** *Mann, Ger.†.*
*Ointment:* Lauromacrogol 400 (p.1412·3); zinc oxide (p.1163·2).
*Anorectal disorders.*
*Suppositories:* Zinc oxide (p.1163·2); benzocaine (p.1370·3).
*Haemorrhoids.*

**Rectoseptal-Neo bismuthe** *Actipharm, Switz.*
Bismuth succinate (p.1253·1); cineole (p.1672·1); terpin hydrate (p.1131·1); potassium hydroxyquinoline sulfate hydrate (p.1734·2).
*Pharyngeal disorders.*

**Rectoseptal-Neo Pholcodine** *Actipharm, Switz.†.*
Guaiacol (p.1122·1); cineole (p.1672·1); terpin hydrate (p.1131·1); pholcodine (p.1128·3).
*Respiratory-tract disorders.*

**Rectoseptal-Neo simple** *Actipharm, Switz.*
Cineole (p.1672·1); terpin hydrate (p.1131·1); potassium hydroxyquinoline sulfate (p.1734·2).
Formerly contained guaiacol, cineole, terpin hydrate, and potassium hydroxyquinoline sulfate.
*Respiratory-tract disorders.*

**Rectovalone**
*Jouveinal, Canad.†; Parke, Davis, Fr.†; Byk, Neth.†; Juste, Spain†.*
Tixocortol pivalate (p.1110·1).
*Haemorrhagic rectocolitis; ulcerative colitis.*

**Rectovasol** *Qualiphar, Belg.*
Bismuth subgallate (p.1252·2); bismuth oxyiodogallate (p.1253·1); zinc oxide (p.1163·2); aesculus (p.1648·2); hamamelis (p.1696·3); amylocaine (p.1370·3); peru balsam (p.1730·2).
*Haemorrhoids.*

**Rectozorin** *Teva, Israel.*
*Ointment:* Bismuth oxychloride (p.1253·1); thymol iodide (p.1194·3); zinc oxide (p.1163·2); benzocaine (p.1370·3); menthol (p.1711·3).
*Suppositories:* Bismuth subgallate (p.1252·2); thymol iodide (p.1194·3); zinc oxide (p.1163·2); benzocaine (p.1370·3); menthol (p.1711·3); tannic acid (p.1751·2).
*Haemorrhoids.*

**Recugel** *Bausch & Lomb, Arg.*
Dexpanthenol (p.1727·2).
*Corneal lesions.*

**Recupex** *Wockhardt, India.*
Nutritional supplement (p.1417·1).

**Recvalysat** *Ysatfabrik, Ger.*
Valerian (p.1762·2).
*Agitation; sleep disorders.*

**Recycline** *Rekah, Israel.*
Tetracycline hydrochloride (p.266·2).
*Bacterial eye and skin infections.*

**Red Away** *Rivex Ophthalmics, Canad.*
Naphazoline hydrochloride (p.1124·3).

**Red Cross Toothache** *Mentholatum, USA.*
Eugenol (p.1686·2).
*Toothache.*

**Red Kooga** *Peter Black, UK.*
Ginseng (p.1693·1).
*Tonic.*

**Red Kooga Betalife** *Peter Black, UK†.*
Multivitamin preparation with ginseng, selenium, and fish oil (p.1417·1).

**Red Kooga Co-Q-10 and Ginseng** *Peter Black, UK.*
Ginseng (p.1693·1); ubidecarenone (p.1760·2).
*Tonic.*

**Red Kooga Sport** *English Grains, UK†.*
Multivitamin preparation with ginseng, iron, and glucose (p.1417·1).
*Tonic.*

**Red Off** *Laboratorios Chile, Chile.*
Naphazoline (p.1124·3).
*Eye irritation.*

**Red Off Plus** *Laboratorios Chile, Chile.*
Antazoline (p.424·2); naphazoline (p.1124·3).
*Eye irritation.*

**Red Oil** *Nella, UK.*
Methyl nicotinate (p.59·2); volatile mustard oil (p.1718·2); clove oil (p.1673·3); arachis oil (p.1656·1).
*Muscle pain.*

**Red Seal Liquid Calcium** *Ancient, Austral.†.*
Calcium carbonate (p.1254·2); ergocalciferol (p.1462·1).
*Osteoporosis.*

**Redac** *Gerolimatos (Γερολυματος), Gr.*
Tenoxicam (p.93·1).
*Dysmenorrhoea; gout; inflammation; osteoarthritis; pain; rheumatoid arthritis; spondyloarthropathies.*

**Redacid** *Maver, Mex.*
Ranitidine (p.1285·2).
*Peptic ulcer.*

**Redactiv**
*Wassermann, Ital.†; Glaxo Wellcome, Mex.*
Rifaximin (p.254·1).
*Bacterial skin infections; gastrointestinal infections.*

**Redaflam** *Maver, Mex.*
Nimesulide (p.67·1).
*Fever; inflammation; pain.*

**Redalip** *Maver, Mex.*
Bezafibrate (p.873·2).
*Hypercholesterolaemia.*

**Redap** *Galderma, Denm.*
Adapalene (p.1141·1).
*Acne.*

**Redaxa fit** *Riemser, Ger.*
Equisetum (p.1684·1).
*Water retention.*

**Redaxa Lax** *Palmicol, Ger.†.*
Rhubarb (p.1287·3); aloes (p.1248·2).
*Constipation.*

**Redentil** *Ibefar, Braz.†.*
Aspirin (p.15·1); caffeine (p.782·1); paracetamol (p.76·2).
Aluminium hydroxide (p.1249·2) is included in this preparation in an attempt to limit adverse effects on the gastrointestinal mucosa.
*Fever; pain.*

**Redeptin** *Janssen-Cilag, Irl.*
Fluspirilene (p.701·1).
*Schizophrenia.*

**Redergin** *Lek, Thai.*
Co-dergocrine mesilate (p.1674·1).
*Cerebrovascular disorders; hypertension; migraine and other vascular headache; peripheral vascular disorders.*

**Redergot** *OM, Port.*
Co-dergocrine mesilate (p.1674·1).
*Cerebral and peripheral vascular disorders.*

**Rediarin** *Maver, Mex.*
Loperamide (p.1271·2).
*Diarrhoea.*

**Redicres Rapido** *Deutsche, Chile.*
Glucomannan (p.1693·3).
*Hypercholesterolaemia; obesity.*

**Redimune** *ZLB, Switz.*
A normal immunoglobulin (p.1627·2).
*Auto-immune disorders; bone marrow transplantation; idiopathic thrombocytopenic purpura; immunodeficiency; Kawasaki disease.*

**Redipred**
*Aspen, Austral.; Aventis, NZ.*
Prednisolone sodium phosphate (p.1108·1).
*Corticosteroid.*

**Redisol** *Merck Sharp & Dohme, Thai.*
Cyanocobalamin (p.1458·2).
*Schilling test; vitamin $B_{12}$ deficiency.*

**Redken Solve Acid Balance** *Redken, Canad.†.*
Pyrithione zinc (p.1156·2).
*Dandruff.*

**Redol** *Elvetium, Arg.*
Capsicum oleoresin (p.1667·1).
*Neuralgia; osteoarthritis; rheumatoid arthritis.*

**Redol Comp** *Orion, Fin.*
Dextromethorphan hydrobromide (p.1117·3); salbutamol sulfate (p.791·3).
*Respiratory-tract disorders.*

**Redolet** *Solfran, Mex.*
Oxyphenbutazone (p.76·1).
*Inflammation.*

**Redomex** *Lundbeck, Belg.*
Amitriptyline hydrochloride (p.280·3).
*Depression.*

**ReDormin**
*Note. This name is used for preparations of different composition.*
*Flordis, Austral.*
Valerian (p.1762·2); lupulus (p.1708·1).
*Sleep disorders.*

*Zeller, Switz.*
*Syrup:* Valerian (p.1762·2).
*Tablets:* Valerian (p.1762·2); lupulus (p.1708·1).
*Sleep disorders.*

**Redotex NF** *Medix, Mex.*
Pseudoephedrine hydrochloride (p.1129·2); atropine sulfate (p.477·1); aloin (p.1248·3).
*Obesity.*

**Redotrin** *Coup, Gr.*
Roxithromycin (p.254·2).
*Bacterial infections.*

**Redox-Injektopas** *Pascoe, Ger.†.*
Multivitamin preparation (p.1417·1).
Procaine hydrochloride (p.1383·2) is included in this preparation to alleviate the pain of injection.

**Redoxon**
*Roche, Arg.; Roche Consumer, Austral.†; Roche, Austria; Roche, Belg.; Roche, Braz.; Roche, Canad.; Roche, Chile; Roche, Hong Kong; Roche Consumer, Irl.; Roche, Israel; Roche, Ital.; Roche, Mex.; Roche Consumer, Neth.; Roche, NZ†; Roche, Port.; Roche, S.Afr.†; Roche Consumer, Singapore†; Roche, Spain; Roche, Switz.; Roche, Thai.†; Roche Consumer, UK.*
Ascorbic acid (p.1460·2), calcium ascorbate (p.1460·2), or sodium ascorbate (p.1460·2).
*Malabsorption syndromes; methaemoglobinaemia; vitamin C deficiency; vitamin C supplement.*

**Redoxon A** *Roche, Arg.*
Ascorbic acid (p.1460·2); vitamin A palmitate (p.1453·1).
*Vitamin supplement.*

**Redoxon Calciovit** *Roche, Spain.*
Ascorbic acid (p.1460·2); calcium carbonate (p.1254·2); colecalciferol (p.1461·3); pyridoxine hydrochloride.
*Bone and dental disorders; calcium deficiency; osteomalacia; rickets.*

**Redoxon Complex** *Roche, Spain.*
Multivitamin and mineral preparation (p.1417·1).

**Redoxon Double Action**
*Roche, NZ; Roche Consumer, Singapore; Roche Consumer, UK.*
Vitamin C (p.1460·2); zinc (p.1469·2).
*Dietary supplement.*

**Redoxon Protector** *Roche Consumer, UK†.*
Multivitamin and mineral preparation (p.1417·1).

**Redoxon-B** *Roche, Canad.*
Ascorbic acid; vitamin B substances; magnesium salts (p.1417·1).
*Nutritional supplement.*

**Redoxon-Cal** *Roche, Canad.*
Ascorbic acid; ergocalciferol; pyridoxine hydrochloride; calcium carbonate (p.1417·1).
*Bone and dental disorders; delayed wound and fracture healing; nutritional supplement; osteomalacia; osteoporosis.*

**Redrate** *Sanofi Synthelabo, Port.*
Glucose; sodium chloride; sodium bicarbonate; potassium chloride (p.1222·2).
*Diarrhoea; oral rehydration therapy.*

**Redrocin** *Unison, Thai.*
Erythromycin ethyl succinate (p.208·1).
*Bacterial infections.*

**Reducap** *Casmar, Mex.†.*
Phentermine (p.1592·2).

**Reducealin** *Propan, S.Afr.*
Propylhexedrine (p.1592·3); vitamin B substances (p.1417·1).
*Obesity.*

**Reducelle** *Alsitan, Ger.†.*
Aloes (p.1248·2); birch leaf (p.1660·3); cascara (p.1255·1); ononis (p.1723·3); phaseolus vulgaris.
*Bowel evacuation; constipation.*

**Reducin** *Finadiet, Arg.*
Soya lecithin (p.1706·1).
*Dietary supplement.*

**Reducin-A** *Unique, India.*
Ibuprofen (p.45·3); paracetamol (p.76·2).
*Fever; inflammation; pain.*

**Reducol**
*Note. This name is used for preparations of different composition.*
*Prodome, Braz.*
Lovastatin (p.949·1).
*Hyperlipidaemias.*

*Saninter, Port.*
Oxidised glycerol triester.
*Cicatrisation; wounds.*

**Reductel** *Degorts, Mex.*
Captopril (p.879·2).
*Heart failure; hypertension; myocardial infarction.*

**Reducterol** *Elfor, Spain.*
Bezafibrate (p.873·2).
*Hyperlipidaemias.*

**Reductil**
*Abbott, Austral.; Ebewe, Austria; Knoll, Belg.; Abbott, Braz.; Abbott, Chile; Abbott, Denm.; Abbott, Fin.; Abbott, Ger.; Abbott, Hong Kong; Abbott, Irl.; Teva, Israel; Abbott, Ital.; Knoll, Neth.; Abbott, NZ; Abbott, Port.; Knoll, S.Afr.; Abbott, Singapore; Abbott, Spain; Abbott, Swed.; Knoll, Switz.; Abbott, Thai.; Abbott, UK.*
Sibutramine hydrochloride (p.1593·1).
*Obesity.*

**Reducto** *Sanova, Austria.*
Monobasic potassium phosphate (p.1230·3); dibasic sodium phosphate (p.1231·1).
*Calcium oxalate stones; hypercalcaemia.*

**Reducto-special** *Asta Medica, Switz.†.*
Monobasic potassium phosphate (p.1230·3); dibasic sodium phosphate dihydrate (p.1231·1).
*Calcium oxalate stones; hypercalcaemia; phosphate supplement.*

**Reducto-spezial** *Temmler, Ger.*
Monobasic potassium phosphate (p.1230·3); dibasic sodium phosphate dihydrate (p.1231·1).
*Calcium oxalate stones; hypercalcaemia; phosphate supplement.*

**Redudiet** *AM, Arg.*
Garcinia cambogia; centella (p.1144·3); alginic acid (p.1576·3); vitamin E (p.1464·3).
*Obesity.*

**Redufen** *Zollweiden, Switz.†.*
Ibuprofen (p.45·3).
*Fever; pain.*

**Redulip** *Hexal, Braz.*
Tiratricol (p.1604·3).
*Obesity.*

**Redupon** *Aventis, S.Afr.*
Ephedrine hydrochloride (p.1120·1); caffeine (p.782·1); phenolphthalein (p.1284·1).
*Obesity.*

**Redupres**
*Note. A similar name is used for preparations of different composition (see below).*
*Leti, Spain†.*
Verapamil hydrochloride (p.1019·1).
*Angina pectoris; arrhythmias; hypertension.*

**Redupress**
*Note. A similar name is used for preparations of different composition (see above).*
*Ache, Braz.*
Losartan potassium (p.947·2).
*Hypertension.*

**Reduprost** *Raffo, Arg.*
Tamsulosin (p.1009·3).
*Benign prostatic hyperplasia.*

**Redurate** *Alliance, S.Afr.*
Allopurinol (p.412·2).
*Gout; hyperuricaemia.*

**Redusa** *Jean-Marie, Hong Kong.*
Phentermine hydrochloride (p.1592·2).
*Obesity.*

**Redusan** *Farmalight, Port.†.*
Poliglusam; vitamin C.
*Slimming aid.*

**Redusan Plus** *Farmalight, Port.*
Poliglusam; vitamin C; nicotinic acid; chromium (p.1417·1).
*Slimming aid.*

**Reduscar** *UCI, Braz.*
Finasteride (p.1554·2).
*Benign prostatic hyperplasia.*

**Redusterol** *Raffo, Arg.*
Simvastatin (p.997·1).
*Hypercholesterolaemia.*

**Redutemp** *International Ethical, USA.*
Paracetamol (p.76·2).

**Reduten** *Instituto Sanitas, Chile.*
Sibutramine hydrochloride (p.1593·1).
*Obesity.*

**Redutensil** *Beta, Arg.*
Valsartan (p.1018·3).
*Hypertension.*

**Reduterm** *SFD, Port.†.*
Oxidised glycerol triester.
*Burns; cicatrisation.*

**Redutona** *Faes, Spain.*
Phenytoin (p.370·2); phenobarbital (p.367·3); aminohydroxybutyric acid (p.353·2); pyridoxine hydrochloride (p.1456·3).
*Epilepsy.*

**Reduvit** *Technikon, S.Afr.*
Multivitamin and mineral preparation (p.1417·1).

**Re-Dux** *Microsules Bernabo, Arg.*
Bismuth citrate (p.1252·1).
*Peptic ulcer.*

**Reduxade** *Abbott, Ital.*
Sibutramine hydrochloride (p.1593·1).
*Obesity.*

**Reduxpain** *Kenyaku, Thai.*
Methyl salicylate (p.59·3); menthol (p.1711·3); eugenol (p.1686·2).
*Musculoskeletal, joint, and soft-tissue disorders.*

**Redvit** *Bunker, Braz.*
Multivitamin, mineral, and amino-acid preparation (p.1417·1).

**Reedvit** *Lafedar, Arg.*
Cyanocobalamin (p.1458·2).
*Anaemia; neuralgia; neuritis.*

**Reef Deep Sun Tan Oil** *Boots Healthcare, Austral.*
*SPF6:* Octinoxate (p.1154·3); oxybenzone (p.1154·3).
*Sunscreen.*

**Reef Sun Tan Oil** *Boots Healthcare, Austral.*
*SPF15:* Octinoxate (p.1154·3); octocrilene (p.1154·3).
*Sunscreen.*

**Reef Sun'n Surf** *Boots Healthcare, Austral.*
*SPF 15:* Octinoxate (p.1154·3); oxybenzone (p.1154·3); titanium dioxide (p.1160·3).
*Sunscreen.*

**Reef Tanning Lotion** *Boots, Austral.†.*
*SPF 6:* Octinoxate (p.1154·3).
*SPF 15+:* Octinoxate (p.1154·3); oxybenzone (p.1154·3).
*Sunscreen.*

**Reemplazante Gastri Mein** *Fresenius Kabi, Spain†.*
Ammonium chloride; potassium chloride; sodium chloride (p.1217·1).
*Fluid and electrolyte depletion.*

**Reemplazante Intesti** *Mein, Spain†.*
Glucose; potassium chloride; sodium chloride; sodium lactate (p.1222·2).
*Fluid depletion.*

**Reese's Pinworm** *Reese, USA.*
Pyrantel embonate (p.113·2).
*Worm infections.*

**ReFacto**
*Wyeth, Arg.; Wyeth, Austral.; Genetics Institute, Austria; Wyeth Lederle, Belg.; Genetics Institute, Denm.; Wyeth Lederle, Fin.; Wyeth Lederle, Fr.; Wyeth, Ger.; Genetics, Gr.; Wyeth, Irl.; Wyeth Lederle, Ital.; Wyeth Lederle, Port.; Wyeth, Spain; Wyeth Lederle, Swed.; Pharmacia, Swed.; Genetics Institute, Switz.; Wyeth, UK; Genetics Institute, USA.*
Moroctocog alfa (p.751·2).
*Haemorrhagic disorders.*

**Refenax Caramelos Expectorantes** *Monserrat, Arg.*
Tolu balsam (p.1131·3); niaouli oil (p.1719·3); lidocaine (p.1377·3); hexylresorcinol (p.1182·1); cineole (p.1672·1); menthol (p.1711·3).
*Coughs; sore throat.*

**Refenax Colirio** *Monserrat, Arg.*
Naphazoline hydrochloride (p.1124·3); pheniramine maleate (p.438·3).
*Eye disorders.*

**Refenax Gotas Nasales** *Monserrat, Arg.*
Naphazoline hydrochloride (p.1124·3); diphenhydramine hydrochloride (p.431·3).
*Nasal congestion.*

**Refenax Jarabe** *Monserrat, Arg.*
Butetamate citrate (p.1116·2); ammonium chloride (p.1115·2); guaifenesin (p.1122·1); pseudoephedrine (p.1129·2); sodium benzoate (p.1169·3); sodium citrate (p.1223·2).
*Coughs.*

**Refenesen** *Reese, USA.*
Guaifenesin (p.1122·1).

**Refenesen Plus** *Reese, USA.*
Guaifenesin (p.1122·1); pseudoephedrine hydrochloride (p.1129·2).

**Refesan T** *Hanosan, Ger.*
Homoeopathic preparation.

**Refex** *Raza, Malaysia; Pharmaniaga, Malaysia.*
Cefalexin (p.168·1).
*Bacterial infections.*

**Reflax** *Merck, Braz.*
Cefaclor (p.167·1).
*Bacterial infections.*

**Reflex**
*Note. This name is used for preparations of different composition.*
*Boots Healthcare, Fr.†.*
Picolamine salicylate (p.84·1).
*Musculoskeletal and joint pain.*

*Boots Healthcare, Spain.*
Camphor (p.1665·3); methyl salicylate (p.59·3); turpentine oil (p.1760·1); menthol (p.1711·3).
*Rheumatic and muscle pain.*

**Reflexan** *Pharma Investi, Chile.*
Cyclobenzaprine hydrochloride (p.1393·1).
*Skeletal muscle spasm.*

**Reflexgel** *Boots Healthcare, Belg.*
Methyl salicylate (p.59·3); camphor (p.1665·3); menthol (p.1711·3).
*Musculoskeletal, joint, peri-articular, and soft-tissue pain and inflammation.*

**Reflexspray** *Boots Healthcare, Belg.*
Methyl salicylate (p.59·3); turpentine oil (p.1760·1); camphor (p.1665·3); menthol (p.1711·3).
*Musculoskeletal, joint, peri-articular, and soft-tissue pain and inflammation.*

**Reflin** *Ranbaxy, India.*
Cefazolin sodium (p.170·3).
*Bacterial infections.*

**Reflocheck** *Roche Diagnostics, Ital.†.*
Test for glucose in blood (p.1694·2).

**Reflor** *Sanova, Austria.*
*Enterococcus faecium* (p.1704·2).
*Gastrointestinal disorders.*

**Reflotron** *Roche Diagnostics, Irl.*
Test for a range of cardiac risk factors in blood, serum, or plasma.

**Refludan**
*Aventis, Austral.†; Hoechst Marion Roussel, Austria; Aventis, Belg.†; Hoechst Marion Roussel, Braz.†; Aventis, Canad.; Schering, Denm.; Aventis, Fin.; Aventis, Fr.; Aventis, Ger.; Hoechst Marion Roussel, Gr.; Pharmion, Irl.; Aventis, Ital.; Aventis, Neth.; Schering, Norw.; Aventis, Port.†; Aventis, Swed.; Aventis, Switz.; Pharmion, UK; Hoechst Marion Roussel, USA.*
Lepirudin (p.945·2).
*Thromboembolic disorders in patients with heparin-associated thrombocytopenia.*

**Refludin**
*Aventis, S.Afr.†; Aventis, Spain.*
Lepirudin (p.945·2).
*Thromboembolic disorders.*

**Reflux** *IPS, Neth.†.*
Methenamine mandelate (p.230·2).
*Urinary-tract infections.*

**Refluxin** *Orion, Fin.†.*
Sodium alginate (p.1577·1); sodium bicarbonate (p.1223·2); calcium carbonate (p.1254·2).
*Gastro-oesophageal reflux; hiatus hernia.*

**Refluxine** *Spirig, Switz.*
Alginic acid (p.1576·3); sodium bicarbonate (p.1223·2); aluminium hydroxide-magnesium carbonate co-dried gel (p.1250·1).
*Gastro-oesophageal reflux.*

**Refobacin**
*Merck, Austria; Hermal, Ger.; Merck, Ger.*
Gentamicin sulfate (p.217·1).
*Bacterial infections.*

**Refobacin-Palacos R**
*Merck, Austria†; Biomet Merck, Ger.; Merck, Singapore; Merck, Thai.*
Gentamicin sulfate (p.217·1); methylmethacrylate/methylacrylate copolymer (p.1714·3).
*Bone cement for orthopaedic surgery.*

**Refolinon**
*Pharmacia Upjohn, S.Afr.†.*
Folinic acid (p.1431·1).
*Antidote to folic acid antagonists; megaloblastic anaemias.*

*Pharmacia, UK.*
Calcium folinate (p.1431·1).
*Antidote to folic acid antagonists; megaloblastic anaemia.*

**Reforce** *Atral, Port.*
Fluconazole (p.398·1).
*Fungal infections.*

**Reforgan** *Nikkho, Braz.*
Arginine aspartate (p.1421·1).
*Nutritional supplement.*

**Refortrix** *GlaxoSmithKline, Braz.*
A diphtheria and tetanus vaccine (p.1613·1).
*Active immunisation.*

**Refotax** *Uno, Ital.*
Cefotaxime sodium (p.175·3).
Lidocaine (p.1377·3) is included in the intramuscular injection to alleviate the pain of injection.
*Gram-negative bacterial infections.*

**Refrane Bronce** *Neo Dermos, Arg.*
Benzophenone (p.1143·1); octinoxate (p.1154·3); tyrosine (p.1451·1).
*Sunscreen; tanning agent.*

**Refrane Gel** *Neo Dermos, Arg.*
*SPF 20:* Titanium dioxide (p.1160·3).
*Sunscreen.*

**Refresh**
*Allergan, Austral.; Allergan, Braz.; Allergan, Canad.; Allergan, Fr.; Alvia (Αλβια), Gr.; Allergan, Israel; Allergan, Malaysia; Allergan, Mex.; Allergan, NZ; Allergan, S.Afr.; Allergan, Singapore; Allergan, Thai.; Allergan, USA.*
Polyvinyl alcohol (p.1581·1); povidone (p.1581·2).
*Dry eyes.*

*Allergan, UK.*
Polyvinyl alcohol (p.1581·1).
Formerly contained polyvinyl alcohol and povidone.
*Dry eyes.*

**Refresh Free** *Allergan, Arg.*
Polyvinyl alcohol (p.1581·1); povidone (p.1581·2).
*Dry eyes.*

**Refresh Gel** *Allergan, Arg.*
Carbomer (p.1577·2).
*Dry eyes.*

**Refresh Liquigel** *Allergan, Austral.*
Carmellose sodium (p.1577·3).
*Dry eyes.*

**Refresh Plus**
*Allergan, Canad.; Allergan, Hong Kong; Allergan, Singapore; Allergan, USA.*
Carmellose sodium (p.1577·3).
*Dry eyes.*

**Refresh PM** *Allergan, USA.*
White soft paraffin (p.1479·3); liquid paraffin (p.1479·1); wool alcohols (p.1482·3).
*Dry eyes.*

**Refresh Tears**
*Allergan, Arg.; Allergan, Canad.; Allergan, Chile; Allergan, Hong Kong; Allergan, Mex.; Allergan, USA.*
Carmellose sodium (p.1577·3).
*Dry eyes.*

**Refresh Tears Plus**
*Allergan, Austral.; Allergan, NZ.*
Carmellose sodium (p.1577·3).
*Dry eyes.*

**Refrianex** *Montpellier, Arg.*
Paracetamol (p.76·2); pseudoephedrine sulfate (p.1129·2); bromhexine hydrochloride (p.1115·3).
*Respiratory-tract disorders.*

**Refrianex Compuesto** *Montpellier, Arg.*
Paracetamol (p.76·2); pseudoephedrine sulfate (p.1129·2); bromhexine hydrochloride (p.1115·3); chlorphenamine maleate (p.427·3).
*Respiratory-tract disorders.*

**Reftax** *Ranbaxy, S.Afr.*
Cefotaxime sodium (p.175·3).
*Bacterial infections.*

**Refulgin** *Spyfarma, Spain†.*
Adenosine triphosphate (p.1648·1); hydroxocobalamin acetate (p.1458·2); pyritinol hydrochloride (p.1737·2); prosultiamine (p.1455·1).
*Mental function disorders.*

**Refusal** *Artu, Neth.*
Disulfiram (p.1681·3).
*Chronic alcoholism.*

**Regadrin B** *Berlin-Chemie, Ger.*
Bezafibrate (p.873·2).
*Hyperlipidaemias.*

**Regain** *R&D, USA.*
Nutritional supplement in renal failure (p.1417·1).

**Regaine**
*Pharmacia, Austria; Pharmacia, Belg.; Pharmacia, Braz.; Pharmacia, Chile; Pharmacia, Denm.; Pharmacia, Fin.; Pharmacia, Fr.; Pharmacia, Ger.; Pharmacia, Hong Kong; Pharmacia, Irl.; Pharmacia Upjohn, Israel; Pharmacia Upjohn, Ital.; Pharmacia, Malaysia; Pharmacia Upjohn, Mex.; Pharmacia, Neth.; Pharmacia, Norw.; Pharmacia, Port.; Pharmacia, S.Afr.; Pharmacia, Singapore; Pharmacia, Spain; Pharmacia, Swed.; Pharmacia, Switz.; Pharmacia, Thai.; Pfizer Consumer, UK.*
Minoxidil (p.960·1).
*Alopecia androgenetica.*

**Regal** *Andromaco, Chile.*
Docusate sodium (p.1262·2).
*Constipation.*

**Regalil** *Farmoquimica, Braz.†.*
Ranitidine (p.1285·2).
*Gastro-oesophageal reflux; gastrointestinal haemorrhage; peptic ulcer; Zollinger-Ellison syndrome.*

**Regalisa** *Microsules, Arg.*
Cisapride (p.1259·2).

**Regamint** *Soria Natural, Spain.*
Peppermint leaf (p.1283·2); pimpinella; liquorice (p.1270·2).
*Gastrointestinal disorders.*

**Regard** *Smith & Nephew, S.Afr.*
Glycerol (p.1694·3).
*Lubrication.*

**Regasinum antallergicum** *Rowa, Ger.*
Homoeopathic preparation.

**Regasinum antiinfectiosum N** *Rowa, Ger.*
Homoeopathic preparation.

**Regasinum cardiale N** *Rowa, Ger.*
Homoeopathic preparation.

**Regasinum hepaticum N** *Rowa, Ger.*
Homoeopathic preparation.

**Regavasal N** *Rowa, Ger.*
Homoeopathic preparation.

**Regelan**
*Zeneca, Austria†; Zeneca, Switz.†.*
Clofibrate (p.884·3).
*Hyperlipidaemias.*

**Regelan N** *Zeneca, Ger.†.*
Clofibrate (p.884·3).
*Hyperlipidaemias.*

**Regena-Haut G** *Regenaplex, Ger.*
Homoeopathic preparation.

**Regena-Haut W** *Regenaplex, Ger.*
Homoeopathic preparation.

**Regenaplex** *Regenaplex, Ger.*
A range of homoeopathic preparations.

**Regender**
*IPI, Port.; Alacan, Spain.*
Polypodium leucotomos.
*Skin disorders.*

**Regeneresen** *Dyckerhoff, Ger.*
Ribonucleic acid (p.1738·2).
*Tonic.*

**Regenerin** *Sanova, Austria.*
Procaine hydrochloride (p.1383·2); vitamin A (p.1451·2); vitamin E (p.1464·3).
*Reduced mental and physical capacity in the elderly.*

**Regenesis** *Elea, Arg.*
Alendronate sodium (p.765·3).
*Osteoporosis; Paget's disease of bone.*

**Regenom** *Genom, Braz.*
Vitamin A acetate (p.1453·1); chloramphenicol (p.185·1); methionine (p.1042·1).
*Infected eye disorders.*

**Regenon**
*Sanova, Austria†; Trenker, Belg.†; Temmler, Denm.†; Temmler, Ger.†; Asta Medica, Switz.; Temmler, Thai.; TTN, Thai.*
Diethylpropion hydrochloride (p.1587·1).
*Obesity.*

**Regental** *Tecnofarma, Chile.*
Nimodipine (p.972·3).
*Alzheimer's disease; cerebrovascular insufficiency; mental function impairment; neurological deficit following subarachnoid haemorrhage.*

**Regepar**
*Sanofi Synthelabo, Austria; Sanofi, Switz.†.*
Selegiline hydrochloride (p.1214·1).
*Parkinsonism.*

**Regepithel**
*Alcon, Ger.*
Vitamin A palmitate (p.1453·1); thiamine hydrochloride (p.1455·1); calcium pantothenate (p.1442·3).
*Corneal defects.*

*Alcon, Hong Kong.*
Vitamin A (p.1451·2); thiamine (p.1455·2); calcium pantothenate (p.1442·3).
*Eye disorders.*

**Regibloc** *Intramed, S.Afr.†.*
Bupivacaine hydrochloride (p.1371·1).
*Local anaesthesia.*

**Regina Royal Concorde** *Regina, UK.*
Royal jelly (p.1740·3); ginseng (p.1693·1); damiana aphrodisiaca (p.1679·1); saw palmetto (p.1569·1).

**Regina Royal Five** *Regina, UK.*
Royal jelly (p.1740·3); bee pollen; pure honey (p.1434·2).

**Regina Royal One Hundred** *Regina, UK.*
Royal jelly (p.1740·3).

**Regiocaina** *Richmond, Arg.*
Lidocaine (p.1377·3).
*Local anaesthesia.*

**Regitin** *Novartis, Denm.*
Phentolamine mesilate (p.982·1).
*Adrenaline or noradrenaline overdose; erectile dysfunction; phaeochromocytoma.*

**Regitina**
*Novartis, Arg.; Novartis, Braz.*
Phentolamine mesilate (p.982·1).
*Erectile dysfunction.*

**Regitine**
*Novartis, Austral.; Novartis, Belg.; Novartis, Israel; Novartis, Neth.; Novartis, NZ; Novartis, S.Afr.; Novartis, Switz.; Novartis, USA†.*
Phentolamine mesilate (p.982·1).
*Noradrenaline extravasation; phaeochromocytoma.*

*IFET (ΙΦΕΤ), Gr.*
Phentolamine hydrochloride (p.982·2).
*Phaeochromocytoma.*

**Regla pH**
*UCB, Belg.*
Algeldrate (p.1249·2); light magnesium oxide (p.1272·3).
*Gastrointestinal disorders associated with hyperacidity.*

*UCB, Gr.*
Aluminium hydroxide (p.1249·2); magnesium oxide (p.1272·3).
*Antacid.*

*UCB, Neth.*
*Chewable tablets:* Aluminium hydroxide-magnesium carbonate co-dried gel (p.1250·1) magnesium hydroxide (p.1272·2).
*Oral suspension:* Aluminium hydroxide (p.1249·2); magnesium hydroxide (p.1272·2).
*Gastritis; gastro-oesophageal reflux; heartburn; peptic ulcer.*

**Regla pH Forte** *UCB, Belg.*
Algeldrate (p.1249·2); light magnesium oxide (p.1272·3); aluminium hydroxide-magnesium carbonate co-dried gel(p.1250·1).
*Gastric hyperacidity; peptic ulcer.*

**Reglan**
*Wyeth-Ayerst, Canad.†; CFL, India; Sanofi Synthelabo, Port.; Schwarz, USA.*
Metoclopramide hydrochloride (p.1274·3).
*Adjunct in gastrointestinal procedures; gastrointestinal motility disorders; nausea and vomiting.*

**ReglaPh** *UCB, Gr.*
Aluminium hydroxide-magnesium carbonate co-dried gel (p.1250·1).
*Antacid.*

**Reglosedyl** *Medifarma, Mex.*
Paregoric (camphorated opium tincture) (p.74·2); viburnum.
*Gastrointestinal spasm.*

**Reglovar** *Quimioterapica, Braz.†.*
Estradiol benzoate (p.1550·1).
*Breast cancer; menopausal disorders; oestrogen deficiency; osteoporosis; prostatic cancer.*

**Reglumax** *Max Farma, Ital.*
Reduced glutathione sodium (p.1040·3).
*Drug and alcohol poisoning.*

**Reglusan** *Novag, Mex.*
Glibenclamide (p.331·2).
*Diabetes mellitus.*

**Regolact Plus** *Naturmed, Ital.*
Lactic-acid-producing organisms (p.1704·2).
*Maintenance of normal gastrointestinal flora.*

**Regolpause** *Provita, Ital.†.*
Multivitamin and mineral preparation (p.1417·1).

**Regomed** *Interpharm, Austria†.*
Enalapril maleate (p.909·2).
*Heart failure; hypertension.*

**Regonol**
*Organon, Canad.†; Organon, USA†.*
Pyridostigmine bromide (p.1496·1).
*Myasthenia gravis; reversal of competitive neuromuscular blockade.*

**Regran** *Delta, Braz.†.*
Papaverine (p.1728·1); belladonna (p.479·1); viburnum prunifolium; Jamaica dogwood (p.1702·3); valerian (p.1762·2).
*Dysmenorrhoea.*

**Regranex**
*Janssen-Ortho, Canad.; Janssen-Cilag, Fr.; Janssen-Cilag, Ger.; Janssen-Cilag, Israel; Cilag, Mex.; Janssen-Cilag, Neth.; Janssen-Cilag, Singapore†; Janssen-Cilag, Swed.†; Janssen-Cilag, Switz.; Janssen-Cilag, UK; Johnson & Johnson, USA.*
Becaplermin (p.1143·1).
*Diabetic neuropathic ulcers.*

**Regro**
*DHA, Malaysia; DHA, Singapore.*
Minoxidil (p.960·1).
*Alopecia androgenetica; alopecia areata.*

**Regroton** *Rhone-Poulenc Rorer, USA.*
Chlortalidone (p.882·3); reserpine (p.995·1).
*Hypertension.*

**Regrowth** *Progress, Thai.*
Minoxidil (p.960·1).
*Alopecia androgenetica.*

**Regubil** *Riva, Canad.†.*
Biliary salts (p.1660·3); dehydrocholic acid (p.1679·2); deoxycholic acid (p.1660·3).
*Biliary-tract disorders.*

**Regucal** *Baliarda, Arg.*
Calcium pidolate (p.1226·1).
*Calcium supplement.*

**Regucal D** *Baliarda, Arg.*
Calcium citrate (p.1225·1); colecalciferol (p.1461·3).
*Calcium and vitamin D supplement.*

**Regucel** *Terapia, Mex.†.*
Ferrous sulfate (p.1428·2).

**Regudig** *Beta, Arg.*
Guar gum (p.333·2).
*Diabetes mellitus; obesity.*

**Regufer** *Terapia, Mex.†.*
Ferrous fumarate (p.1427·3).

**Regulacid** *Lazar, Arg.*
Omeprazole (p.1278·2).
*Gastro-oesophageal reflux; peptic ulcer; Zollinger-Ellison syndrome.*

**Regulacor-POS** *Ursapharm, Ger.*
Crataegus (p.1677·1).
*Cardiac disorders.*

**Regulact** *ICN, Mex.*
Lactulose (p.1269·1).
*Constipation; hepatic encephalopathy.*

**Regulador Blumen** *Luper, Braz.†.*
Cotton root bark; plumeria lancifolia; berberis laurina.
*Dysmenorrhoea.*

**Regulador Gesteira** *CIF, Braz.†.*
Paracetamol (p.76·2); viburnum prunifolium.
*Dysmenorrhoea.*

**Regulador Xavier n-1** *Hepacholan, Braz.†.*
Viburnum; gossypium; belladonna (p.479·1); calcium chloride (p.1225·1).
*Menstrual disorders.*

**Regulador Xavier n-2** *Hepacholan, Braz.†.*
Rhubarb (p.1287·3); savin; belladonna (p.479·1); ferric ammonium citrate (p.1427·2); citric acid (p.1673·1).
*Menstrual disorders.*

**Regulan**
*Procter & Gamble, Irl.; Procter & Gamble, UK.*
Ispaghula (p.1268·1).
*Constipation; diverticular disease; irritable bowel syndrome.*

**Regulane** *Finadiet, Arg.*
Loperamide hydrochloride (p.1271·1).
*Diarrhoea.*

**Regulane AF** *Finadiet, Arg.*
Loperamide hydrochloride (p.1271·1); simeticone (p.1289·2).
*Diarrhoea; flatulence.*

**Regular Iletin I** *Lilly, USA†.*
Insulin injection (bovine and porcine) (p.333·3).
*Diabetes mellitus.*

**Regular Iletin II** *Lilly, USA.*
Insulin injection (porcine) (p.333·3).
*Diabetes mellitus.*

**Regular Strength Bayer** *Sterling Health, USA.*
Aspirin (p.15·1).
Formerly known as Therapy Bayer.
*Fever; inflammation; myocardial infarction; pain; transient ischaemic attacks.*

**Regular Strength Cold Daytime Relief** *West-Can, Canad.*
Pseudoephedrine hydrochloride (p.1129·2); dextromethorphan hydrobromide (p.1117·3); paracetamol (p.76·2).

**Regular Strength Cold Nighttime Relief** *West-Can, Canad.*
Pseudoephedrine hydrochloride (p.1129·2); dextromethorphan hydrobromide (p.1117·3); paracetamol (p.76·2); chlorphenamine maleate (p.427·3).

**Regular Strength Sinus** *Stanley, Canad.*
Pseudoephedrine hydrochloride (p.1129·2); paracetamol (p.76·2).

**Regulaten** *Juste, Spain.*
Eprosartan mesilate (p.912·1).
*Hypertension.*

**Regulax** *Hexal, Braz.*
Cotton root bark; plumeria lancifolia; berberis laurina.
*Dysmenorrhoea.*

**Regulax N** *Krewel, Ger.*
Senna (p.1288·2).
*Constipation.*

**Regulax Picosulfat** *Krewel, Ger.*
Sodium picosulfate (p.1289·3).
*Constipation.*

**Regulax SS** *Republic, USA.*
Docusate sodium (p.1262·2).
*Constipation.*

**Reguletts** *Husler, Switz.*
Phenolphthalein (p.1284·1).
*Constipation.*

**Regulex** *Whitehall-Robins, Canad.*
Docusate sodium (p.1262·2).
*Constipation.*

**Regulex-D** *Whitehall-Robins, Canad.†.*
Dantron (p.1261·1); docusate sodium (p.1262·2).
*Constipation.*

**Regulim**
*Atlantic, Hong Kong†; Atlantic, Singapore; Atlantic, Thai.*
Phenolphthalein (p.1284·1).
*Bowel evacuation; constipation.*

**Regulin**
*Note. This name is used for preparations of different composition.*
*Vitasan, Austria.*
Cynara (p.1678·3).
*Digestive disorders.*

*Gea, Denm.*
Glibenclamide (p.331·2).
*Diabetes mellitus.*

**Regulip** *Raffo, Arg.*
Salmon oil (p.976·1).
*Hyperlipidaemias.*

**Reguloid** *Rugby, USA.*
Psyllium hydrophilic mucilloid (p.1268·1).
*Constipation.*

**Regulose** *Novartis Consumer, UK.*
Lactulose (p.1269·1).
*Constipation.*

**Regulton**
*Knoll, Belg.*
Amezinium metilsulfate (p.858·2).
*Hypotension.*

*Teofarma, Ger.*
Amezinium metilsulfate (p.858·2).
*Hypotension.*

**Regunon** *Schering, Swed.†.*
Levonorgestrel (p.1563·2); ethinylestradiol (p.1553·2).
*Combined oral contraceptive.*

**Regurin**
*Galen, Irl.; Galen, UK.*
Trospium chloride (p.491·2).
*Bladder instability.*

**Rehalyt** *SAD, Denm.*
Electrolyte infusion with glucose (p.1217·1).
*Carbohydrate source; fluid and electrolyte disorders.*

**Rehidrat**
*Eurofarma, Braz.*
Potassium chloride; sodium citrate dihydrate; sodium chloride; glucose (p.1222·2).
*Diarrhoea; oral rehydration therapy.*

*Pharmacia, Irl.; Pharmacia, UK†.*
Sodium chloride; potassium chloride; sodium bicarbonate; citric acid; glucose; sucrose; fructose (p.1222·2).
*Diarrhoea; oral rehydration therapy.*

*Searle, Israel†.*
Sodium chloride; potassium chloride; sodium bicarbonate; citric acid; glucose (p.1222·2).
*Diarrhoea; oral rehydration therapy.*

*Pharmacia, S.Afr.*
Sodium chloride; potassium chloride; sodium bicarbonate; glucose; sucrose (p.1222·2).
*Diarrhoea; oral rehydration therapy.*

**Rehsal** *Laboratorios Chile, Chile.*
Electrolytes; glucose (p.1222·2).
*Oral rehydration therapy.*

**Rehydralyte**
*Abbott, Canad.; Abbott, Thai.; Ross, USA.*
Oral rehydration solution (p.1222·2).
*Diarrhoea; oral rehydration therapy.*

**Rehydrex med glucos**
*Fresenius Kabi, Norw.; Fresenius Kabi, Swed.*
Electrolyte infusion with glucose (p.1217·1).
*Fluid and electrolyte disorders.*

**Rehydrex med Glucose** *Fresenius Kabi, Denm.*
Electrolyte infusion with glucose (p.1217·1).
*Carbohydrate source; fluid and electrolyte disorders.*

**Reidramax** *Cazi, Braz.*
Glucose; sodium citrate; potassium chloride; sodium chloride (p.1222·2).
*Oral rehydration therapy.*

**Reidrax** *Bonomelli, Ital.†.*
Electrolytes; glucose (p.1222·2).
*Oral rehydration therapy.*

**Reise Superpep-K** *Pharmacal, Switz.†.*
Dimenhydrinate (p.431·1).
*Motion sickness; nausea; vertigo; vomiting.*

**Reisedragee Eu Rho** *Eu Rho, Ger.*
Diphenhydramine hydrochloride (p.431·3); 8-chlorotheophylline.
*Nausea; vomiting.*

**Reisegold** *Whitehall-Much, Ger.*
*Sugar-coated tablets:* Diphenhydramine hydrochloride (p.431·3); caffeine (p.782·1); 8-chlorotheophylline; pyridoxine hydrochloride (p.1456·3).
*Tablets:* Dimenhydrinate (p.431·1).
*Motion sickness.*

**Reisetabletten** *Ratiopharm, Ger.; Stada, Ger.*
Dimenhydrinate (p.431·1).
*Motion sickness; nausea; vertigo; vomiting.*

**Reisevit** *Agepha, Austria.*
Pyridoxine hydrochloride (p.1456·3).
*Motion sickness; nausea and vomiting; vitamin $B_6$ deficiency.*

**Rejuva** *Stiefel, Canad.†.*
*SPF 15:* Avobenzone (p.1142·3); octinoxate (p.1154·3).
*Sunscreen.*

**Rejuva-A** Stiefel, Canad.
Tretinoin (p.1161·1).
*Photodamaged skin.*

**Rejuvesol** Cytosol, Israel.
Sodium pyruvate; inosine; adenine; dibasic sodium phosphate; monobasic sodium phosphate.
*Extracorporeal rejuvenation.*

**Rekamide** Rekah, Israel.
Loperamide hydrochloride (p.1271·1).
*Diarrhoea.*

**Rekasitin** Rekah, Israel.
Zinc oxide (p.1163·2); cod-liver oil (p.1425·2); allantoin (p.1141·3).
*Barrier preparation; burns; nappy rash; skin disorders.*

**Rekawan**
Solvay, Austria†; Rekawan, Ger.
Potassium chloride (p.1232·2).
*Potassium deficiency.*

**Rekiv** Rekah, Israel.
Magnesium carbonate (p.1272·1); bismuth subnitrate (p.1252·2); sodium bicarbonate (p.1223·2); frangula bark (p.1266·3); calamus (p.1664·1).
*Gastritis; gastrointestinal hyperacidity; peptic ulcer.*

**Rekod** Rekah, Israel.
Codeine phosphate (p.27·1).
*Coughs; pain.*

**Rekont** Madaus, Austria.
Trospium chloride (p.491·2).
*Bladder function disorders.*

**Rekord B12** Sigma-Tau, Ital.
Amino-acid and vitamin B substances (p.1417·1).
*Tonic.*

**Rekord Ferro** Sigma-Tau, Ital.
Iron succinyl-protein complex (p.1438·1).
*Iron deficiency; iron-deficiency anaemia.*

**Relacon-DM** Cypress, USA.
Dextromethorphan hydrobromide (p.1117·3); guaifenesin (p.1122·1); pseudoephedrine hydrochloride (p.1129·2).
*Coughs; nasal congestion.*

**Relacon-HC** Cypress, USA.
Hydrocodone tartrate (p.45·1); chlorphenamine maleate (p.427·3); phenylephrine hydrochloride (p.1126·3).
*Coughs; upper respiratory-tract congestion.*

**Relact** Kora, Irl.
Lactic acid (p.1704·1).
*Vaginal discharge.*

**Relafen**
GlaxoSmithKline, Canad.; SmithKline Beecham, USA.
Nabumetone (p.63·3).
*Osteoarthritis; rheumatoid arthritis.*

**Relaflex** Galenogal, Braz.†.
Dipyrone (p.35·3); orphenadrine citrate (p.486·1); caffeine (p.782·1).
*Pain; smooth muscle spasm.*

**Relampago** Ibefar, Braz.†.
Thymol (p.1194·2); menthol (p.1711·3); neotutocaina; eugenol (p.1686·2).

**Relapamil** Orion, Fin.
Quinine hydrochloride (p.460·2); diazepam (p.690·1).
*Muscle spasm.*

**Relar** Pharmaland, Thai.
Orphenadrine citrate (p.486·1); paracetamol (p.76·2).
*Muscle pain; tension headache.*

**Relasan** Bioquimico, Mex.†.
Diazepam (p.690·1).

**Relaten** Herbaline, Ital.†.
Chamomile (p.1669·3); crataegus (p.1677·1); eschscholtzia californica; red-poppy (p.1058·1).
*Agitation; anxiety; insomnia.*

**Relatene** Mintlab, Chile.
Ketoprofen (p.51·2).
*Inflammation; pain.*

**Relatrac** Pisa, Mex.
Atracurium besilate (p.1399·1).
*Competitive neuromuscular blocker.*

**Relavit Fosforo** Seber, Port.
Glutamine (p.1433·2); thiamine; calcium magnesium fytate.
*Adjunct in epilepsy; depression; mental function disorders.*

**Relax** Zeller, Switz.
Petasites (p.1663·3); valerian (p.1762·2); passion flower (p.1729·1); melissa (p.1711·1).
*Anxiety; sleep disorders.*

**Relax B$^+$** Vitalia, UK.
Valerian (p.1762·2); lupulus (p.1708·1); passion flower (p.1729·1); vitamin B substances (p.1417·1).

**Relax and Sleep** Jamieson, Canad.
Cataria; lupulus (p.1708·1); passion flower (p.1729·1); valerian (p.1762·2).
*Sleep disorders.*

**Relaxan** Gea, Denm.†.
Gallamine triethiodide (p.1403·2).
*Competitive neuromuscular blocker.*

**Relaxaplex** Vitaplex, Austral.†.
Valerian (p.1762·2); skullcap (p.1746·3); passion flower (p.1729·1); lupulus (p.1708·1); gentian (p.1692·2).
*Herbal sedative.*

**Relaxar** Bouty, Ital.
Mephenesin (p.1394·3); methyl nicotinate (p.59·2).
*Neuromuscular pain; soft-tissue disorders.*

**Relaxa-Tabs** Woods, Austral.
Mepyramine maleate (p.437·1).
*Insomnia; nervous tension.*

**Relaxedans** Salvat, Spain†.
Chlordiazepoxide (p.674·2); pyridoxine (p.1457·2).
*Anxiety.*

**Relaxibys** Belmac, Spain.
Carisoprodol (p.1392·1); paracetamol (p.76·2).
*Musculoskeletal spasticity.*

**Relaxil** Dansk-Flama, Braz.
Bromazepam (p.671·3).
*Anxiety.*

**Relaxine**
Trenker, Belg.; Warner-Lambert, Fr.†.
Valerian (p.1762·2).
*Insomnia; nervous disorders.*

**Relaxin-P** Jean-Marie, Hong Kong.
Chlorzoxazone (p.1392·3); paracetamol (p.76·2).
*Painful skeletal muscle spasm.*

**Relaxit**
Note. This name is used for preparations of different composition.
Abigo, Swed.
Sodium bicarbonate (p.1223·2); potassium acid tartrate (p.1284·3); calcium silicate (p.1226·1).
*Constipation; faecal incontinence.*

Crawford, UK.
Sodium citrate (p.1223·2); sodium laurilsulfate (p.1574·2); sorbic acid (p.1192·3); glycerol (p.1694·3); sorbitol (p.1446·3).
*Constipation.*

**Relaxoddi** Leurquin, Fr.†.
Butacaine (p.1372·3); oleic acid (p.1481·3).
*Dyspepsia.*

**Relaxophen** Tanta, Canad.
Paracetamol (p.76·2); methocarbamol (p.1395·1).

**Relaxyl**
Note. This name is used for preparations of different composition.
Nycomed, Austria.
Dibasic sodium phosphate (p.1231·1); monobasic sodium phosphate (p.1230·3).
*Bowel evacuation; constipation.*

Franco-Indian, India.
*Ointment:* Mephenesin (p.1394·3); methyl nicotinate (p.59·2); capsicum oleoresin (p.1667·1).
*Musculoskeletal, joint, and soft-tissue disorders.*
*Slow-release tablets; tablets:* Diclofenac sodium (p.32·1).
*Gout; musculoskeletal and joint disorders.*
*Topical gel:* Diclofenac diethylamine (p.32·1).
*Soft-tissue disorders.*

Thornton & Ross, UK.
Alverine citrate (p.1250·2).
*Irritable bowel syndrome.*

**Relaxyl Plus** Franco-Indian, India.
Diclofenac sodium (p.32·1); paracetamol (p.76·2).
*Gout; musculoskeletal and joint disorders.*

**Relazepam** Pisa, Mex.
Diazepam (p.690·1).

**Relcofen** Alpharma, UK.
Ibuprofen (p.45·3).
*Pain.*

**Releaf for PMS** Lake, USA.
Pyridoxine hydrochloride (p.1456·3) in a base of natural herbs.
*Premenstrual syndrome.*

**Release** New Vision, Canad.
Vitamin C; manganese (p.1417·1).

**Relefact** Hoechst Marion Roussel, Gr.
Protirelin (p.1337·3).
*Thyroid function test.*

**Relefact LH-RH**
Aventis, Austria; Aventis, Ger.; Hoechst Marion Roussel, Gr.; Aventis, Israel; Aventis, Neth.
Gonadorelin (p.1325·1).
*Diagnosis of hypothalamic-pituitary-gonadal dysfunction.*

**Relefact TRH**
Aventis, Austria; Aventis, Canad.; Aventis, Ger.; Aventis, Israel; Aventis, Neth.; Aventis, Switz.
Protirelin (p.1337·3).
*Diagnosis of thyroid and pituitary dysfunction.*

**Relenza**
GlaxoSmithKline, Arg.; GlaxoSmithKline, Austral.; GlaxoSmithKline, Austria; GlaxoSmithKline, Belg.; Glaxo Wellcome, Braz.†; GlaxoSmithKline, Canad.; GlaxoSmithKline, Chile; GlaxoSmithKline, Denm.; GlaxoSmithKline, Fin.; GlaxoSmithKline, Fr.; GlaxoSmithKline, Ger.; Glaxo Wellcome, Gr.; GlaxoSmithKline, Hong Kong; Glaxo Wellcome, Irl.; GlaxoSmithKline, Israel; GlaxoSmithKline, Ital.; Glaxo Wellcome, Mex.; GlaxoSmithKline, Neth.; GlaxoSmithKline, Norw.; GlaxoSmithKline, NZ; Glaxo Wellcome, Port.; GlaxoSmithKline, S.Afr.; Glaxo Wellcome, Singapore†; GlaxoSmithKline, Spain; GlaxoSmithKline, Swed.; GlaxoSmithKline, Switz.; GlaxoSmithKline, UK; Glaxo Wellcome, USA.
Zanamivir (p.658·1).
*Influenza.*

**Relepax** Pfizer, Fr.
Eletriptan hydrobromide (p.467·1).
*Migraine.*

**Relert**
Pfizer, Fin.; Mack, Israel; Pfizer, Spain.
Eletriptan hydrobromide (p.467·1).
*Migraine.*

**Reless** Alk-Scherax, Ger.
Bee venom extract (p.1650·2) or wasp venom extract (p.1650·2).
*Allergen immunotherapy.*

**Relestat** Allergan, UK.
Epinastine hydrochloride (p.433·3).
*Allergic conjunctivitis.*

**Relexic** Sunward, Singapore†.
Chlormezanone (p.675·1); paracetamol (p.76·2).
*Pain; skeletal muscle spasm.*

**Relexil** Laboratorios Chile, Chile.
Cyclobenzaprine hydrochloride (p.1393·1).
*Skeletal muscle spasm.*

**Reliberan** Geymonat, Ital.
Chlordiazepoxide hydrochloride (p.674·2).
*Anxiety disorders.*

**Relief** Allergan, USA.
Phenylephrine hydrochloride (p.1126·3).
*Minor eye irritation.*

**Relief Rub** Greenridge, Austral.†.
Echinacea purpurea (p.1683·2); melaleuca oil (p.1710·2); eucalyptus oil (p.1686·2); thyme oil (p.1755·3); turpentine oil (p.1760·1); cajuput oil (p.1664·1); peppermint oil (p.1283·2).
*Cold and influenza symptoms; musculoskeletal and joint pain.*

**Relief-Coff** PD Pharm, S.Afr.
Diphenhydramine hydrochloride (p.431·3); ammonium chloride (p.1115·2); sodium citrate (p.1223·2).
*Coughs.*

**Reliev**
Justesa Imagem, Braz.†; Schering, Chile.
Meglumine amidotrizoate (p.1060·2).
*Radiographic contrast medium.*

**Reliev 76%** Schering, Chile.
Sodium amidotrizoate (p.1060·2); meglumine amidotrizoate (p.1060·2).
*Radiographic contrast medium.*

**Relievol Allergy Sinus** Tanta, Canad.
Pseudoephedrine hydrochloride (p.1129·2); chlorphenamine maleate (p.427·3); paracetamol (p.76·2).

**Relievol PMS** Tanta, Canad.
Paracetamol (p.76·2); pamabrom (p.978·2); mepyramine maleate (p.437·1).

**Relievol Sinus** Tanta, Canad.
Pseudoephedrine hydrochloride (p.1129·2); paracetamol (p.76·2).

**Relif** SmithKline, Spain.
Nabumetone (p.63·3).
*Osteoarthritis; rheumatoid arthritis.*

**Relifen**
Sanwa, Jpn; GlaxoSmithKline, S.Afr.
Nabumetone (p.63·3).
*Musculoskeletal, joint, peri-articular, and soft-tissue disorders.*

**Relifex**
GlaxoSmithKline, Braz.; Meda, Denm.; GlaxoSmithKline, Fin.; SmithKline Beecham, Gr.; GlaxoSmithKline, Hong Kong; Meda, Irl.; SmithKline Beecham, Israel; SmithKline Beecham, Mex.; Meda, Norw.; SmithKline Beecham, Singapore†; Meda, Swed.; GlaxoSmithKline, Thai.; Meda, UK.
Nabumetone (p.63·3).
*Gout; inflammation; musculoskeletal and joint disorders.*

**Relisan** Xixia, S.Afr.
Nabumetone (p.63·3).
*Musculoskeletal and joint disorders.*

**Reliser**
Serono, Arg.; Serono, Braz.; Serono, Mex.
Leuprorelin acetate (p.1331·1).
*Endometriosis; female infertility; prostatic cancer; uterine fibroids.*

**Relisorm** Serono, Canad.†.
Gonadorelin acetate (p.1325·2).
*Diagnosis of hypothalamic-pituitary-gonadal dysfunction.*

**Relisorm L**
Serono, Braz.†; Serono, Hong Kong; Serono, Mex.†; Serono, Switz.
Gonadorelin acetate (p.1325·2).
*Test of hypothalamic-pituitary-gonadal function.*

**Relitone** Garec, S.Afr.
Nabumetone (p.63·3).
*Musculoskeletal and joint disorders.*

**Reliv** Recip, Swed.
Paracetamol (p.76·2).
*Fever; pain.*

**Reliveran** Novartis, Arg.
Metoclopramide (p.1274·3).
*Nausea and vomiting.*

**Relivora Komplex** Sanum-Kehlbeck, Ger.
Homoeopathic preparation.

**Relmus** Sanofi Synthelabo, Port.
Thiocolchicoside (p.1395·2).
*Neuromuscular pain; parkinsonism; skeletal muscle spasticity.*

**Relmus Compositum** Sanofi Synthelabo, Port.
Thiocolchicoside (p.1395·2); aescin (p.1648·2).
*Inflammation; musculoskeletal, joint, and soft-tissue injury; oedema; phlebitis; thrombophlebitis.*

**Reloxyl**
Note. This name is used for preparations of different composition.
RDC, Ital.
Benzoyl peroxide (p.1143·2).
*Acne; skin disinfection.*

Cheminova, Spain.
Amoxicillin trihydrate (p.155·3).
*Bacterial infections.*

**Reloxyl Mucolitico** Cheminova, Spain.
Amoxicillin trihydrate (p.155·3); guaifenesin (p.1122·1).
*Respiratory-tract infections.*

**Relpax**
EMS, Braz.†; Pfizer, Braz.†; Pfizer, Denm.; Pfizer, Fr.; Pfizer, Ital.; Pfizer, Mex.; Pfizer, Norw.; Pfizer, Spain; Pfizer, Swed.; Pfizer, Switz.; Pfizer, UK; Pfizer, USA.
Eletriptan hydrobromide (p.467·1).
*Migraine.*

**Relvene** Pharmascience, Fr.
Oxerutins (p.1688·2).
*Chronic venous insufficiency.*

**Relyomycin** Relyo, Gr.
Doxycycline hyclate (p.206·2).
*Bacterial infections.*

**Relyovix** Relyo, Gr.
Propylene glycol cefatrizine (p.170·3).
*Bacterial infections.*

**Rem** Chobet, Arg.
Midazolam (p.707·1).
*General anaesthesia; premedication; sedative.*

**Remafen**
Xepa-Soul Pattinson, Hong Kong; Xepa-Soul Pattinson, Malaysia; Xepa-Soul Pattinson, Singapore.
Diclofenac sodium (p.32·1).
*Gout; musculoskeletal and joint disorders.*

**Remdue** Biomedica, Ital.
Flurazepam dihydrochloride (p.700·3).
*Insomnia.*

**Remedacen** Aventis, Ger.
Dihydrocodeine polistirex (p.35·2).
*Coughs.*

**Remedeine** Napp, UK.
Paracetamol (p.76·2); dihydrocodeine tartrate (p.34·3).
*Pain.*

**Remederm** Widmer, Ger.
Urea (p.1162·2); vitamin A palmitate (p.1453·1); alpha tocoferil acetate (p.1465·1); dexpanthenol (p.1727·2).
*Skin disorders.*

**Remederm HC** Widmer, Ger.
Hydrocortisone (p.1103·3).
*Skin disorders.*

**Remedium Nervinum N EKF** Biomedica, Ger.†.
Homoeopathic preparation.

**Remedium Sinutale N EKF** Biomedica, Ger.†.
Homoeopathic preparation.

**Remedol** Remedica, Singapore.
Paracetamol (p.76·2).
*Fever; pain.*

**Remeflin** Recordati, Ital.
Dimefline hydrochloride (p.1587·2).
*Respiratory and circulatory disorders.*

**Remegel**
Warner-Lambert, Irl.†; Warner-Lambert, Ital.†; SSL, UK.
Calcium carbonate (p.1254·2).
*Gastric hyperacidity.*

**Remegel Wind Relief** SSL, UK.
Calcium carbonate (p.1254·2); simeticone (p.1289·2).
*Dyspepsia; flatulence; heartburn.*

**Remen** Parke, Davis, Ital.†.
Pramiracetam sulfate (p.1734·3).
*Mental function impairment.*

**Remena** Remedina, Gr.
Ciprofloxacin hydrochloride (p.188·2).
*Bacterial infections.*

**Remens** Bittner, Austria.
Homoeopathic preparation.

**Remergil** Organon, Ger.; Thiemann, Ger.
Mirtazapine (p.307·3).
*Depression.*

**Remergon** Organon, Belg.
Mirtazapine (p.307·3).
*Depression.*

**Remeron**
Organon, Arg.; Organon, Austral.; Organon, Austria; Organon, Braz.; Organon, Canad.; Organon, Denm.; Organon, Fin.; Organon Teknika (Οργκανον Τεχνικα), Gr.; Organon, Hong Kong; Organon, Israel; Organon, Ital.; Organon, Malaysia; Organon, Mex.; Nourypharma, Neth.; Organon, Norw.; Organon, Port.; Donmed, S.Afr.; Organon, Singapore; Organon, Swed.; Organon, Switz.; Organon, Thai.; Organon, USA.
Mirtazapine (p.307·3).
*Depression.*

**Remestan**
Wyeth Lederle, Austria; ICN, Ger.
Temazepam (p.723·2).
*Sleep disorders.*

**Remethan**
Remedica, Hong Kong; Remedica, Malaysia; Remedica, Singapore; Remedica, Thai.
Diclofenac diethylamine (p.32·1) or diclofenac sodium (p.32·1).
*Gout; inflammation; musculoskeletal, joint, peri-articular, and soft-tissue disorders; pain.*

**Remexal** Permamed, Switz.
Lauromacrogol 600 (p.1412·3); dimethyl sulfoxide (p.1473·2); glycol salicylate (p.44·3); dexpanthenol (p.1727·2); menthol (p.1711·3); camphor (p.1665·3).
*Musculoskeletal, joint, and peri-articular disorders.*

**Remicade**
White, Arg.; Schering-Plough, Austral.; Schering-Plough, Belg.; Schering-Plough, Braz.†; Schering, Canad.; Schering-Plough, Chile; Centocor, Denm.; Schering-Plough, Fin.; Schering-Plough, Fr.; Essex, Ger.; Centocor, Gr.; Schering-Plough, Irl.; Schering-Plough, Israel; Schering-

*Plough, Ital.; Schering-Plough, Mex.; Schering-Plough, Neth.; Schering-Plough, Norw.; Schering-Plough, NZ; Schering-Plough, Port.†; Schering-Plough, Spain; Schering-Plough, Swed.; Essex, Switz.; Schering-Plough, UK; Centocor, USA.*
Infliximab (p.50·1).
*Ankylosing spondylitis; Crohn's disease; rheumatoid arthritis.*

**Remicaine** *Adcock Ingram Generics, S.Afr.*
Lidocaine hydrochloride (p.1377·3).
*Arrhythmias; local anaesthesia.*

**Remicard** *Adcock Ingram Generics, S.Afr.*
Lidocaine hydrochloride (p.1377·3).
*Arrhythmias.*

**Remid** *TAD, Ger.*
Allopurinol (p.412·2).
*Gout; hyperuricaemia; renal calculi.*

**Remiderm** *Elvetium, Arg.*
Centella (p.1144·3).

**Remidol** *Farmasierra, Spain.*
Ibuprofen (p.45·3).
*Musculoskeletal, joint, peri-articular, and soft-tissue disorders.*

**Remifemin**
*Schaper & Brummer, Ger.; Schaper & Brummer, Malaysia; Bionax, Malaysia; Schaper & Brummer, Singapore; Farmasierra, Spain; Asta Medica, Switz.†; Schaper & Brummer, Thai.*
Cimicifuga (p.1671·3).
*Menopausal disorders; menstrual disorders.*

**Remifemin plus** *Schaper & Brummer, Ger.*
Hypericum (p.299·1); cimicifuga (p.1671·3).
*Menopausal disorders; menstrual disorders.*

**Remikin** *Remedina, Gr.*
Amikacin sulfate (p.154·1).
*Bacterial infections.*

**Reminyl**
*Janssen-Cilag, Arg.; Janssen-Cilag, Austral.; Janssen-Cilag, Austria; Janssen-Cilag, Belg.; Janssen-Cilag, Braz.; Janssen-Ortho, Canad.; Janssen-Cilag, Denm.; Janssen-Cilag, Fin.; Janssen-Cilag, Fr.; Janssen-Cilag, Ger.; Janssen-Cilag, Gr.; Shire, Irl.; Janssen-Cilag, Ital.; Janssen-Cilag, Norw.; Janssen-Cilag, NZ; Janssen-Cilag, S.Afr.; Janssen-Cilag, Singapore; Janssen-Cilag, Spain; Janssen-Cilag, Swed.; Janssen-Cilag, Switz.; Janssen-Cilag, Thai.; Shire, UK; Janssen, USA.*
Galantamine hydrobromide (p.1491·2).
*Alzheimer's disease.*

**Remiprostan uno** *Schaper & Brummer, Ger.*
Saw palmetto (p.1569·1).
*Benign prostatic hyperplasia.*

**Remisan** *Vir, Spain.*
Amoxicillin trihydrate (p.155·3).
*Bacterial infections.*

**Remisan Mucolitico** *Vir, Spain.*
Amoxicillin trihydrate (p.155·3); bromhexine hydrochloride (p.1115·3).
*Respiratory-tract infections.*

**Remisol** *Degorts, Mex.*
Methocarbamol (p.1395·1).
*Skeletal muscle spasm.*

**Remisol-PLS** *Degorts, Mex.*
Methocarbamol (p.1395·1); aspirin (p.15·1).
*Musculoskeletal pain.*

**Remitex** *Bago, Chile.*
Cetirizine hydrochloride (p.427·1).
*Hypersensitivity reactions.*

**Remitex D** *Bago, Chile.*
Cetirizine hydrochloride (p.427·1); pseudoephedrine sulfate (p.1129·2).
*Allergic rhinitis.*

**Remnos** *DDSA Pharmaceuticals, UK.*
Nitrazepam (p.710·1).
*Insomnia.*

**Remodil** *Remedica, Singapore.*
Diphenoxylate hydrochloride (p.1261·3).
Atropine sulfate (p.477·1) is included in this preparation to discourage abuse.
*Diarrhoea.*

**Remodulin**
*United Therapeutics, Israel; United Therapeutics, USA.*
Treprostinil sodium (p.1521·2).
*Pulmonary hypertension.*

**Remontal** *Vita, Spain.*
Nimodipine (p.972·3).
*Cognitive impairment in the elderly; neurological deficit following subarachnoid haemorrhage.*

**Remoplexe** *Lehning, Fr.†.*
Copper gluconate (p.1425·3).
*Musculoskeletal and joint disorders; viral infections.*

**Remotil** *Azevedos, Port.*
Domperidone (p.1263·2).
*Aid in gastrointestinal examination; dyspepsia; nausea; vomiting.*

**Remotiv**
*Bayer, Arg.; Flordis, Austral.; Bayer, Austria; Bayer, Chile; Bayer, Ger.†; Knoll, Mex.; Knoll, S.Afr.; Zeller, Switz.*
Hypericum (p.299·1).
*Anxiety; depression; sleep disorders.*

**Remotive** *Biofutura, Ital.*
Hypericum (p.299·1).
*Depression.*

**Remotrox** *Pharmaceutical Enterprises, S.Afr.*
Dicycloverine hydrochloride (p.481·2); dried aluminium hydroxide gel (p.1249·2); light magnesium oxide (p.1272·3).
*Gastrointestinal disorders.*

**Remov** *Piam, Ital.*
Nimesulide (p.67·1).
*Fever; inflammation; pain.*

**Remove** *Smith & Nephew, Austral.*
Dipropylene glycol methyl ether.
*Adhesive remover.*

**Remular-S** *International Ethical, USA.*
Chlorzoxazone (p.1392·3).
*Musculoskeletal pain.*

**Remy** *Sella, Ital.*
Camphor (p.1665·3); ethyl salicylate (p.37·3); menthol (p.1711·3); capsicum oleoresin (p.1667·1).
*Rheumatism.*

**Remycin**
*Remedica, Hong Kong.*
Doxycycline hyclate (p.206·2).
*Bacterial infections.*

*Remedica, Singapore.*
Doxycycline (p.206·2).
*Bacterial infections.*

**Remydrial** *Winzer, Ger.†.*
Dapiprazole hydrochloride (p.1679·1).
*Reversal of mydriasis.*

**Ren Hematocis** *REM, Braz.†.*
Sodium pyrophosphate.
*Diagnostic agent.*

**Rena** *Pharmaland, Thai.*
Orphenadrine citrate (p.486·1); paracetamol (p.76·2).
*Muscle pain; skeletal muscle spasm.*

**Renacalcio** *Biocontrol, Arg.*
Calcium carbonate (p.1254·2).
*Calcium supplement; hypocalcaemia; osteoporosis.*

**Renacidin**
*Note. This name is used for preparations of different composition.*
*Ingens, Arg.*
Finasteride (p.1554·2).
*Alopecia androgenetica.*

*Guardian, USA.*
Anhydrous citric acid (p.1673·1); gluconic acid; magnesium carbonate (p.1272·1).
*Renal calculi.*

**Renacor** *Dieckmann, Ger.*
Enalapril maleate (p.909·2); hydrochlorothiazide (p.933·2).
*Hypertension.*

**Renagel**
*Genzyme, Canad.; Genzyme, Denm.; Genzyme, Fr.; Genzyme, Ger.; Genzyme, Gr.; Genzyme, Irl.; Genzyme, Israel; Dompe Biotec, Ital.; Genzyme, Neth.; Enzifarma, Port.; Genzyme, Spain; Genzyme, Swed.; Genzyme, UK; Genzyme, USA.*
Sevelamer hydrochloride (p.1051·2).
*Hyperphosphataemia.*

**Renal Caps** *Cypress, USA.*
Multivitamin preparation (p.1417·1).

**Renal Care** *Abbott, Ital.*
Preparation for enteral nutrition in renal failure (p.1417·1).

**Renalapril** *Neo Quimica, Braz.*
Enalapril maleate (p.909·2).
*Hypertension.*

**Renal-Vit** *Nutrovit, Braz.†.*
Vitamin and mineral preparation (p.1417·1).

**Renamel** *Clonmel, Irl.*
Oxybutynin hydrochloride (p.486·3).
*Neurogenic bladder; nocturnal enuresis; unstable bladder.*

**RenAmin** *Clintec, USA.*
Amino-acid infusion (p.1417·1).
*Parenteral nutrition in renal impairment.*

**Renapur** *Schering-Plough, Swed.*
Anhydrous potassium citrate (p.1223·1); anhydrous sodium citrate (p.1223·2); anhydrous citric acid (p.1673·1).
*Renal calculi.*

**Renase** *Pharmaland, Thai.*
Amiloride hydrochloride (p.858·2); hydrochlorothiazide (p.933·2).
*Hepatic cirrhosis with ascites and oedema; hypertension; oedema.*

**Renaton** *Korea United, Singapore.*
Enalapril maleate (p.909·2).
*Heart failure; hypertension.*

**Rena-Vite** *Cypress, USA.*
Vitamin B substances; vitamin C (p.1417·1).

**Renax** *Everett, USA.*
Multivitamin and mineral preparation in renal failure (p.1417·1).

**Renbiocid** *Ist. Chim. Inter., Ital.*
Cefonicid sodium (p.174·2).
Lidocaine hydrochloride (p.1377·3) is included in this preparation to alleviate the pain of injection.
*Gram-negative bacterial infections.*

**Rencef** *EciFarma, Chile.*
Lactulose (p.1269·1).
*Bowel evacuation; constipation; hepatic encephalopathy.*

**Rendells** *Prisfar, Port.*
Nonoxinol 9 (p.1413·3).
*Contraceptive.*

**Rendells Plus** *Rendell, NZ.*
Nonoxinol 9 (p.1413·3).
*Contraceptive.*

**Renedil**
*Aventis, Belg.; Aventis, Canad.; Aventis, Neth.*
Felodipine (p.914·3).
*Angina pectoris; hypertension.*

**Re/Neph** *Pisa, Mex.*
Nutritional supplement in renal failure (p.1417·1).

**Renese**
*Pfizer, Belg.; Pfizer, USA†.*
Polythiazide (p.984·2).
*Hypertension; oedema.*

**Renese R** *Pfizer, USA.*
Polythiazide (p.984·2); reserpine (p.995·1).
*Hypertension.*

**Reneuron** *Juste, Spain.*
Fluoxetine hydrochloride (p.292·1).
*Bulimia; depression; obsessive-compulsive disorder.*

**Reneuu Invisible Glove** *Hoe, Malaysia.*
Barrier cream.

**Renezide** *Aspen, S.Afr.*
Triamterene (p.1016·2); hydrochlorothiazide (p.933·2).
*Hypertension; oedema.*

**Renidur** *Merck Sharp & Dohme, Port.*
Enalapril maleate (p.909·2); hydrochlorothiazide (p.933·2).
*Hypertension.*

**Renilon** *Nutricia, Port.*
Preparation for enteral nutrition (p.1417·1).
*Renal failure.*

**Renipress** *Cazi, Braz.*
Enalapril maleate (p.909·2).
*Hypertension.*

**Renipril** *APS, Port.*
Enalapril maleate (p.909·2).
*Heart failure; hypertension.*

**Renipril Plus** *APS, Port.*
Enalapril maleate (p.909·2); hydrochlorothiazide (p.933·2).
*Hypertension.*

**Renistad** *Stada, Austria.*
Enalapril maleate (p.909·2).
*Heart failure; hypertension.*

**Renitec**
*Merck Sharp & Dohme, Arg.; Merck Sharp & Dohme, Austral.; Merck Sharp & Dohme, Austria; Merck Sharp & Dohme, Belg.; Merck Sharp & Dohme, Braz.; Merck Sharp & Dohme, Denm.; Merck Sharp & Dohme, Fin.; Merck Sharp & Dohme-Chibret, Fr.; Vianex (Βιανεξ), Gr.; Merck Sharp & Dohme, Hong Kong; Merck Sharp & Dohme, Malaysia; Merck Sharp & Dohme, Mex.; Merck Sharp & Dohme, Neth.; Merck Sharp & Dohme, Norw.; Merck Sharp & Dohme, NZ; Merck Sharp & Dohme, Port.; Merck Sharp & Dohme, S.Afr.; Merck Sharp & Dohme, Singapore; Merck Sharp & Dohme, Spain; Merck Sharp & Dohme, Swed.; Merck Sharp & Dohme, Thai.*
Enalapril (p.909·2), enalapril maleate (p.909·2), or enalaprilat (p.909·3).
*Angina pectoris; heart failure; hypertension; myocardial infarction.*

**Renitec Comp**
*Merck Sharp & Dohme, Fin.; Merck Sharp & Dohme, Norw.; Merck Sharp & Dohme, Swed.*
Enalapril maleate (p.909·2); hydrochlorothiazide (p.933·2).
*Hypertension.*

**Renitec Plus**
*Merck Sharp & Dohme, Austral.; Merck Sharp & Dohme, Austria; Merck Sharp & Dohme, Fin.; Merck Sharp & Dohme, Neth.*
Enalapril maleate (p.909·2); hydrochlorothiazide (p.933·2).
*Hypertension.*

**Renitecmax** *Merck Sharp & Dohme, Spain.*
Enalapril maleate (p.909·2); hydrochlorothiazide (p.933·2).
*Hypertension.*

**Reniten** *Merck Sharp & Dohme, Switz.*
Enalapril maleate (p.909·2) or enalaprilat (p.909·3).
*Heart failure; hypertension; left ventricular dysfunction.*

**Reniten Plus** *Merck Sharp & Dohme, Switz.*
Enalapril maleate (p.909·2); hydrochlorothiazide (p.933·2).
*Hypertension.*

**Rennie**
*Roche, Arg.; Roche, Belg.; Roche, Braz.; Roche, Fin.; Roche Nicholas, Fr.; Roche Nicholas, Ger.; Roche, Hong Kong†; Roche Nicholas, Israel; Roche, Ital.; Roche Consumer, Neth.; Roche Consumer, Singapore; Roche, Spain; Roche, Swed.; Roche, Switz.; Roche Consumer, UK.*
Calcium carbonate (p.1254·2); magnesium carbonate (p.1272·1).
*Dyspepsia; flatulence; heartburn.*

**Rennie Defarin** *Roche Nicholas, Ger.*
Calcium carbonate (p.1254·2); heavy magnesium carbonate (p.1272·1); simeticone (p.1289·2).
*Gastrointestinal disorders with meteorism.*

**Rennie Deflatine**
*Roche Nicholas, Fr.; Roche Consumer, Irl.; Roche Consumer, Neth.; Roche, Switz.; Roche Consumer, UK.*
Calcium carbonate (p.1254·2); magnesium carbonate (p.1272·1); simeticone (p.1289·2).
*Dyspepsia; flatulence; heartburn.*

**Rennie Digestif**
*Roche Consumer, Austral.; Roche, Port.*
Calcium carbonate (p.1254·2); magnesium carbonate (p.1272·1).
*Dyspepsia; gastric hyperacidity.*

**Rennie Duo**
*Roche, Austria; Roche Consumer, Irl.; Roche Consumer, UK.*
Calcium carbonate (p.1254·2); magnesium carbonate (p.1272·1); alginic acid (p.1576·3) or sodium alginate (p.1577·1).
*Dyspepsia; gastro-oesophageal reflux.*

**Rennie Gold** *Roche Consumer, UK†.*
Calcium carbonate (p.1254·2).
*Dyspepsia; flatulence.*

**Rennie Peppermint** *Roche Consumer, Irl.*
Calcium carbonate (p.1254·2); magnesium carbonate (p.1272·1).
*Gastric hyperacidity; heartburn.*

**Rennie Rap-Eze** *Roche Consumer, Irl.*
Calcium carbonate (p.1254·2).
*Gastric hyperacidity; heartburn.*

**Rennie Refluxine** *Roche Nicholas, Fr.†.*
Calcium carbonate (p.1254·2); light magnesium carbonate (p.1272·1); sodium alginate (p.1577·1).
*Gastric hyperacidity; gastro-oesophageal reflux.*

**Rennie Soft Chews** *Roche Consumer, UK.*
Calcium carbonate (p.1254·2).
*Dyspepsia; flatulence; heartburn.*

**Renob Blasen- und Nierentee** *Pfleger, Ger.*
Birch leaf (p.1660·3); couch-grass rhizome (p.1676·2); solidago virgaurea (p.1748·3); ononis (p.1723·3); liquorice root (p.1270·2).
*Urinary-tract disorders.*

**Renocil** *Farma Lepori, Spain.*
Sodium cromoglicate (p.795·3).
*Rhinitis.*

**Renocis** *Schering, UK.*
Technetium-99m succimer (p.1525·2).
*Radionuclide imaging of the kidney.*

**Renoclear** *Transphyto, Fr.†.*
Cleansing, disinfection and soaking of soft contact lenses (p.1164·2).

**Renofundina** *Braun, Port.†.*
Glucose; calcium chloride; magnesium chloride; potassium chloride; sodium acetate; sodium chloride (p.1221·1).
*Haemodialysis.*

**Renografin**
*Squibb Diagnostics, Canad.†; Squibb Diagnostics, USA.*
Meglumine amidotrizoate (p.1060·2); sodium amidotrizoate (p.1060·2).
*Radiographic contrast medium.*

**Renolip** *Remedina, Gr.*
Gemfibrozil (p.923·1).
*Hyperlipidaemias.*

**Reno-M**
*Squibb Diagnostics, Canad.†; Squibb Diagnostics, USA.*
Meglumine amidotrizoate (p.1060·2).
*Radiographic contrast medium.*

**Renopen** *Ativus, Braz.*
Saw palmetto (p.1569·1).
*Benign prostatic hyperplasia.*

**Renorell** *Sanorell, Ger.*
Homoeopathic preparation.

**Renormax**
*Schering-Plough, Ital.; Italfarmaco, Spain.*
Spirapril hydrochloride (p.1003·1).
*Hypertension.*

**Renotol** *Raza, Malaysia; Pharmaniaga, Malaysia.*
Atenolol (p.865·2).
*Angina pectoris; hypertension.*

**Renova**
*Ortho Dermatological, Canad.; Janssen-Cilag, S.Afr.; Janssen-Cilag, Thai.; Ortho Dermatological, USA.*
Tretinoin (p.1161·1).
*Photoageing of the skin.*

**Renovator** *Hertz, Braz.†.*
Yohimbine (p.1766·2); tocoferol (p.1464·3).
*Erectile dysfunction.*

**Renpress** *ICN, Spain.*
Spirapril hydrochloride (p.1003·1).
*Hypertension.*

**Rentamine Pediatric** *Major, USA.*
Phenylephrine tannate (p.1127·2); ephedrine tannate (p.1120·3); chlorphenamine tannate (p.428·1); pentoxyverine tannate (p.1126·3).
*Coughs and cold symptoms.*

**Rentibloc** *Shire, Ger.*
Sotalol hydrochloride (p.1001·3).
*Arrhythmias.*

**Rentylin** *Shire, Ger.*
Pentoxifylline (p.979·3).
*Peripheral and ocular vascular disorders.*

**Renu**
*Bausch & Lomb, Braz.; Bausch & Lomb, Canad.; Bausch & Lomb, Fr.†; Bausch & Lomb, NZ; Bausch & Lomb, USA.*
Range of solutions for soft contact lenses (p.1164·2).

**Renu Enzymatic Cleaner** *Bausch & Lomb, USA.*
Subtilisin-A (p.1164·2).
*Cleansing solution for soft contact lenses.*

**Renu Multiplus** *Bausch & Lomb, UK.*
Solution for cleansing, disinfecting, and removal of protein from contact lenses (p.1164·2).

**Renu Plus** *Bausch & Lomb, Braz.*
Cleaning solution for contact lenses (p.1164·2).

**Ren-Ur** *Lafedar, Arg.*
Hydrochlorothiazide (p.933·2); amiloride hydrochloride (p.858·2).
*Hypertension.*

**Renusor** *Soria Natural, Spain.*
Corn silk (p.1676·1); couch-grass (p.1676·2); betula alba (p.1660·3); solidago (p.1748·3).
*Fluid retention.*

**Renutrin** *Heralds, Braz.†.*
Ferrous fumarate (p.1427·3); vitamins (p.1417·1).
*Iron deficiency; iron-deficiency anaemias.*

**Renutryl** *Germania, Austria.*
Preparation for enteral nutrition (p.1417·1).

**Renutryl 500** *Nestle, Fr.*
Nutritional supplement (p.1417·1).

**Reocol** *Also, Ital.*
Tartaric acid; sodium bicarbonate (p.1223·2); anhydrous citric acid; magnesium sulfate (p.1228·2).
*Constipation; dyspepsia.*

**Reodyn** *Orion, Fin.*
Carbocisteine (p.1116·2).
*Respiratory-tract disorders.*

**Reoferol** *Zimaia, Port.*
Tocoferil nicotinate (p.1015·1).

**Reoflus** *Pulitzer, Ital.*
Heparin calcium (p.927·3).
*Thromboembolic disorders.*

**Reolase** *Pulitzer, Ital.*
Telmesteine (p.1131·1).
*Respiratory-tract disorders.*

**Reomax** *Pfizer, Ital.*
Etacrynic acid (p.913·2) or sodium etacrynate (p.913·3).
*Oedema.*

**Reomucil** *DOC, Ital.*
Carbocisteine (p.1116·2).
*Respiratory-tract congestion.*

**ReoPro**
*Lilly, Arg.; Lilly, Austral.; Centocor, Austria; Lilly, Belg.; Lilly, Braz.; Lilly, Canad.; Lilly, Chile; Centocor, Denm.; Lilly, Fin.; Lilly, Fr.; Lilly, Ger.; Pharmaserve Lilly (Φαρμασερβ Λιλλυ), Gr.; Lilly, Hong Kong; Lilly, India; Lilly, Irl.; Centocor, Israel; Lilly, Ital.; Lilly, Malaysia; Lilly, Mex.; Centocor, Neth.; Centocor, Norw.; Lilly, NZ; Lilly, S.Afr.; Lilly, Singapore; Lilly, Spain; Lilly, Swed.; Lilly, Switz.; Lilly, Thai.; Lilly, UK; Centocor, USA; Lilly, USA.*
Abciximab (p.841·3).
*Prevention of ischaemic cardiac complications during angioplasty, atherectomy or stent placement; unstable angina pectoris.*

**Reotan** *Medicus, Gr.*
Calcium folinate (p.1431·1).
*Antidote to folic acid antagonists; megaloblastic anaemia.*

**Repalyte**
*Aventis, Austral.; DHA, Singapore.*
Glucose and electrolytes (p.1222·2).
*Diarrhoea; oral rehydration therapy.*

**Repan** *Everett, USA.*
Butalbital (p.673·3); caffeine (p.782·1); paracetamol (p.76·2).
*Pain.*

**Repan CF** *Everett, USA.*
Paracetamol (p.76·2); butalbital (p.673·3).
*Pain.*

**Reparcillin** *New Research, Ital.*
Piperacillin sodium (p.243·1).
Lidocaine hydrochloride (p.1377·3) is included in this preparation to alleviate the pain of injection.
*Bacterial infections.*

**Reparex** *Drugtech, Chile.*
Vitamin E; selenium (p.1417·1).
*Antioxidant preparation.*

**Reparil**
*Note. This name is used for preparations of different composition.*
*Madaus, Austria; Altana, Braz.; Madaus, Ger.†; Madaus, Thai.*
*Injection:* Sodium aescinate (p.1648·2).
*Back pain; inflammation; oedema; vascular disorders.*
*Madaus, Austria; Madaus, Belg.; Altana, Braz.; Madaus, Ger.; Madaus, Hong Kong; Madaus, Ital.; Biomed, Switz.; Madaus, Thai.*
*Tablets:* Aescin (p.1648·2).
*Inflammation; oedema; thrombophlebitis; venous insufficiency.*
*Madaus, Austria; Byk Madaus, S.Afr.*
*Topical gel:* Aescin (p.1648·2); diethylamine salicylate (p.34·1).
*Muscle and joint pain; soft-tissue injury; vascular disorders.*
*Madaus, Belg.; Altana, Braz.; Madaus, Fr.; Madaus, Hong Kong; Biomed, Switz.; Madaus, Thai.*
*Topical gel:* Aescin (p.1648·2); sodium aescin polysulfate (p.1648·2); diethylamine salicylate (p.34·1).
*Haematomas; inflammation; soft-tissue disorders; tenosynovitis; thrombophlebitis; varicose veins; venous insufficiency.*
*Madaus, Ital.*
*Topical gel:* Aescin (p.1648·2); heparin sodium (p.928·1); diethylamine salicylate (p.34·1).
*Soft-tissue disorders.*

**Reparil N** *Biomed, Switz.†.*
Aescin (p.1648·2); diethylamine salicylate (p.34·1).
*Soft-tissue injury.*

**Reparil-Gel N** *Madaus, Ger.*
Aescin (p.1648·2); diethylamine salicylate (p.34·1).
*Soft-tissue disorders.*

**Repariven** *Roche, Chile.*
Aescin (p.1648·2); a heparinoid (p.931·1); diethylamine salicylate (p.34·1).
*Phlebitis; soft-tissue injury; varices.*

**Repasma** *Pharmador, S.Afr.†.*
Amobarbital (p.670·1); aminophylline (p.780·2); ephedrine hydrochloride (p.1120·1).
*Asthma.*

**RepaVen** *Madaus, Ital.*
Aesculus (p.1648·2); melilotus; rutoside (p.1688·2).
*Oedema; venous insufficiency.*

**Rep-Cartil** *Farmoterapia, Arg.*
Collagen (p.1674·3); cartilage.
*Dietary supplement.*

**Repelente Rep** *Aulo Gelio, Arg.*
*Cream; lotion:* Citronella oil (p.1673·2).
*Topical spray:* Citronella oil (p.1673·2); jojoba oil.
*Insect repellent.*

**Repelex** *Instituto Sanitas, Chile.*
Compound 5734.
*Insect repellent.*

**Repeltin** *Pierre Fabre, Ger.*
Alimemazine (p.424·1).
*Bronchial asthma or asthma-like complaints; pruritus.*

**Repentil** *Raffo, Arg.*
Melatonin (p.1710·2).
*Regulation of circadian rhythm.*

**Repervit** *Scherer, Ital.*
Vitamin A palmitate (p.1453·1).
*Vitamin A deficiency.*

**Repevax**
*Aventis Pasteur, Ger.; Aventis Pasteur, UK.*
A diphtheria, tetanus, pertussis (acellular), and poliomyelitis (inactivated) vaccine (p.1615·1).
*Active immunisation.*

**Repha Orphon** *Repha, Ger.*
Java tea (p.1702·3).
*Gout; rheumatism; urinary-tract disorders.*

**Rephacimin** *Repha, Ger.†.*
Homoeopathic preparation.

**Rephacratin** *Repha, Ger.†.*
Crataegus (p.1677·1).
*Cardiac disorders.*

**Rephahyval** *Repha, Ger.†.*
Hypericum (p.299·1).
*Anxiety disorders; depression.*

**Rephalgin** *Repha, Ger.*
Homoeopathic preparation.

**Rephalysin C** *Repha, Ger.*
*Escherichia coli.*
*Gastrointestinal disorders.*

**Repha-Os** *Repha, Ger.*
Tormentil root (p.1757·2); rhatany root (p.1738·1); myrrh (p.1718·3); anise oil (p.1655·2); eucalyptus oil (p.1686·2); peppermint oil (p.1283·2); clove oil (p.1673·3); menthol (p.1711·3).
*Mouth and throat disorders.*

**Rephaprossan** *Repha, Ger.†.*
Homoeopathic preparation.

**Rephastasan** *Repha, Ger.*
Homoeopathic preparation.

**Rephenyl** *Reese, USA†.*
Guaifenesin (p.1122·1); phenylpropanolamine hydrochloride (p.1127·3).

**Repilysin** *Roche, Gr.*
Reteplase (p.995·2).
*Myocardial infarction.*

**Repisan** *Bittner, Austria.*
Homoeopathic preparation.

**Repivate** *Xeragen, S.Afr.*
Betamethasone valerate (p.1093·2).
*Skin disorders.*

**Replagal**
*TKT, Denm.; TKT, Fr.; TKT, Ger.; TKT, Israel; TKT, Spain.*
Agalsidase alfa (p.1651·1).
*Fabry disease.*

**Replasyn** *TRB, Arg.*
Estradiol (p.1550·1).
*Menopausal disorders; osteoporosis.*

**Replavit** *Stanley, Canad.*
Multivitamin preparation (p.1417·1).

**Replavite** *Sussex, UK†.*
Oral rehydration solution (p.1222·2).
*Diarrhoea.*

**Replena** *Abbott, Braz.*
Preparation for enteral nutrition (p.1417·1).

**Replenate** *BPL, UK.*
A factor VIII preparation (p.751·1).
Formerly known as 8SM.
*Haemophilia A.*

**Replenine**
*BPL-Meizler, Braz.; BPL, Israel; BPL, Singapore; BPL, UK.*
A factor IX preparation (p.752·2).
*Haemophilia B.*

**Replenine VF** *Bio Products, Malaysia.*
A factor IX preparation (p.752·2).
*Haemophilia B.*

**Replens**
*Sanofi Synthelabo, Austral.; Wolfs, Belg.; Wellspring, Canad.; Mipharm, Ital.; Sanofi Winthrop, Port.†; Ipsen, Spain; Meda, Swed.; Warner-Lambert, USA.*
Polycarbophil (p.1284·2).
*Vaginal dryness.*
*Columbia, Fr.; Ethical Research, Irl.†; Teva, Israel; Adcock Ingram, S.Afr.; Vifor, Switz.; Anglian, UK.*
Vaginal lubricant.
*Vaginal dryness; vaginal irritation.*

**Replete** *Clintec, USA.*
Lactose-free, gluten-free preparation for enteral nutrition (p.1417·1).

**Replicare** *Smith & Nephew Healthcare, UK.*
Hydrocolloid dressing.
*Burns; ulcers; wounds.*

**Repligen** *Panalab, Arg.*
Metronidazole (p.607·2).
*Rosacea.*

**Repogen** *Libbs, Braz.*
Conjugated oestrogens (p.1543·2).
*Menopausal disorders.*

**Repogen Ciclo** *Libbs, Braz.*
14 Tablets, conjugated oestrogens (p.1543·2); 14 tablets, conjugated oestrogens; medroxyprogesterone acetate (p.1557·2).
*Menopausal disorders; oestrogen deficiency; osteoporosis.*

**Repogen Conti** *Libbs, Braz.*
Conjugated oestrogens (p.1543·2); medroxyprogesterone acetate (p.1557·2).
*Menopausal disorders.*

**Reposans** *Wesley, USA†.*
Chlordiazepoxide hydrochloride (p.674·2).
*Alcohol withdrawal syndrome; anxiety.*

**Reposo-Mono** *Medgenix, Belg.*
Meprobamate (p.706·2).
*Insomnia.*

**Reposton** *Provit, Mex.*
Liver extract.
*Anaemias.*

**Repotin** *Bioclones, S.Afr.*
Epoetin (p.747·1).
*Anaemias; autologous blood transfusions.*

**Repovit** *Sigma, Braz.*
Vitamin and mineral preparation (p.1417·1).

**Repowine mono** *Truw, Ger.*
Scoparium (p.1742·2).
*Cardiac disorders.*

**Repowinon** *Truw, Ger.†.*
Homoeopathic preparation.

**Repriadol** *Nycomed, Denm.†.*
Morphine sulfate (p.60·2).
*Pain.*

**Repronex** *Ferring, USA.*
Menotrophin (p.1330·1).
*Infertility.*

**Reprost** *Andromaco, Chile.*
Naproxen (p.65·1).
*Gout; musculoskeletal, joint, and peri-articular disorders; pain.*

**Reproven N** *Hanosan, Ger.*
Homoeopathic preparation.

**Reptilase**
*Disperga, Austria; Pharmadeveloppement, Fr.; Troikaa, India; Difa, Ital.†; Neves, Port.; Llorente, Spain†.*
Haemocoagulase (p.743·3).
*Haemorrhage.*

**Repursan** *Biokanol, Ger.*
Muira puama; kola; vitamins (p.1417·1).
*Tonic.*

**Repursan M** *Boots, Ger.†.*
Cort. yohimbe.; nuces colae; lign. muir. puam.; testes; vitamins; minerals (p.1417·1).
*Tonic.*

**Repursan ST** *Biokanol, Ger.†.*
Pausinystalia yohimbe; kola (p.1765·3); ephedra (p.1119·3); vitamins; minerals (p.1417·1).
*Sexual fatigue.*

**Requiesan** *Klein, Ger.*
Eschscholtzia californica; avena (p.1658·2).
*Sleep disorders.*

**Requip**
*GlaxoSmithKline, Arg.; GlaxoSmithKline, Austria; GlaxoSmithKline, Belg.; GlaxoSmithKline, Canad.; GlaxoSmithKline, Chile; GlaxoSmithKline, Denm.; GlaxoSmithKline, Fr.; GlaxoSmithKline, Ger.; SmithKline Beecham, Gr.; GlaxoSmithKline, Hong Kong; GlaxoSmithKline, Irl.; SmithKline Beecham, Israel; GlaxoSmithKline, Ital.; SmithKline Beecham, Neth.; GlaxoSmithKline, Norw.; Beecham, Port.; GlaxoSmithKline, S.Afr.; GlaxoSmithKline, Singapore; GlaxoSmithKline, Spain; GlaxoSmithKline, Swed.; SmithKline Beecham, Switz.; GlaxoSmithKline, UK; SmithKline Beecham, USA.*
Ropinirole hydrochloride (p.1213·3).
*Parkinsonism.*

**Res Vin** *Geymonat, Ital.*
Vitamins; mineral; rutoside; proanthyocyanidins; resveratrol (p.1417·1).
*Circulatory disorders; nutritional supplement.*

**Resaid** *Geneva, USA†.*
Phenylpropanolamine hydrochloride (p.1127·3); chlorphenamine maleate (p.427·3).
*Upper respiratory-tract symptoms.*

**Resakal** *Puerto Galiano, Spain.*
Paracetamol (p.76·2).
*Fever; pain.*

**Resalt** *Aspen, S.Afr.*
Sodium chloride; potassium chloride; glucose; sodium bicarbonate (p.1222·2).
*Diarrhoea; oral rehydration therapy.*

**Resaltex**
*Procter & Gamble, Austria†; Procter & Gamble, Ger.†.*
Hydrochlorothiazide (p.933·2); reserpine (p.995·1); triamterene (p.1016·2).
*Hypertension.*

**Resan Mucolitico** *Alacan, Spain†.*
Ampicillin sodium (p.157·1); bromhexine (p.1115·3).
Lidocaine (p.1377·3) is included in this preparation to alleviate the pain of injection.
*Respiratory-tract infections.*

**Resan Retard** *Alacan, Spain†.*
Ampicillin sodium (p.157·1); ampicillin benzathine (p.158·1); bromhexine hydrochloride (p.1115·3).
Lidocaine hydrochloride (p.1377·3) is included in this preparation to alleviate the pain of injection.
*Respiratory-tract infections.*

**Resata** *Rafarm, Gr.*
Budesonide (p.1094·2).
*Allergic rhinitis; topical corticosteroid.*

**Rescaps-D SR** *Geneva, USA†.*
Phenylpropanolamine hydrochloride (p.1127·3); caramiphen edisilate (p.1116·2).
*Coughs.*

**Rescold** *Klinger, Braz.*
Phenylephrine hydrochloride (p.1126·3); chlorphenamine maleate (p.427·3); paracetamol (p.76·2).
*Cold and influenza symptoms.*

**Rescon** *Capellon, USA†.*
*Capsules:* Pseudoephedrine hydrochloride (p.1129·2); chlorphenamine maleate (p.427·3).
*Liquid:* Phenylpropanolamine hydrochloride (p.1127·3); chlorphenamine maleate (p.427·3).
*Upper respiratory-tract symptoms.*

**Rescon-DM** *Capellon, USA.*
Dextromethorphan hydrobromide (p.1117·3); pseudoephedrine hydrochloride (p.1129·2); chlorphenamine maleate (p.427·3).
*Coughs and cold symptoms.*

**Rescon-ED** *Capellon, USA†.*
Pseudoephedrine hydrochloride (p.1129·2); chlorphenamine maleate (p.427·3).
*Upper respiratory-tract symptoms.*

**Rescon-GG** *Capellon, USA.*
Phenylephrine hydrochloride (p.1126·3); guaifenesin (p.1122·1).
*Coughs.*

**Rescon-Jr** *Capellon, USA.*
Phenylephrine hydrochloride (p.1126·3); chlorphenamine maleate (p.427·3).
*Upper respiratory-tract disorders.*

**Rescon-MX** *Capellon, USA.*
Phenylephrine hydrochloride (p.1126·3); chlorphenamine maleate (p.427·3); hyoscine methonitrate (p.483·3).
Formerly contained pseudoephedrine hydrochloride, chlorphenamine maleate, and hyoscine methonitrate.
*Upper respiratory-tract disorders.*

**Rescriptor**
*Pfizer, Austral.; Pharmacia, Braz.†; Agouron, Canad.; Pharmacia Upjohn, Mex.; Pharmacia Upjohn, USA.*
Delavirdine mesilate (p.630·2).
*HIV infection.*

**RescueFlow**
*Biophausia, Denm.; Biophausia, Ger.; Bioquest, Ger.; Biophausia, Norw.; Biophausia, Swed.; Vitaline, UK.*
Dextran 70 (p.746·2) in sodium chloride.
*Plasma volume expansion.*

**Rescuesol** *Pisa, Mex.*
Dextran 60 (p.746·1) in sodium chloride.

**Rescula**
*Novartis Ophthalmics, Arg.; Novartis Ophthalmics, Braz.; Novartis, Chile; Ueno, Jpn; Novartis, Mex.; Novartis Ophthalmics, Singapore; Novartis Ophthalmics, Switz.; Novartis, Thai.; Novartis Ophthalmics, USA.*
Unoprostone isopropyl (p.1521·3).
*Glaucoma; ocular hypertension.*

**Rescuvolin**
*Nycomed, Austria; Asta Oncologia, Braz.; Nettopharma, Denm.; Nycomed, Fin.; Medac, Ger.; Chemipharma, Gr.; Pharmachemie, Israel†; Pharmachemie, Malaysia; Nycomed, Norw.; Asta Medica, NZ; Pharmachemie, S.Afr.; Pharmachemie, Singapore; Nycomed, Swed.; Pharmachemie, Thai.; Teva, Thai.*
Calcium folinate (p.1431·1).
*Adjunct to fluorouracil in colorectal cancer; antidote to folic acid antagonists; folic acid deficiency; megaloblastic anaemia; reduction of methotrexate toxicity.*

**Resdan** *Whitehall-Robins, Canad.†.*
Cetrimide (p.1172·1).
*Dandruff.*

**Resectal** *Fresenius Kabi, Austria.*
Sorbitol (p.1446·3); mannitol (p.950·2).
*Bladder and prostate surgery.*

**Resectisol**
*McGaw, NZ†; Kendall McGaw, USA.*
Mannitol (p.950·2).
*Irrigation solution.*

**Reser** *TO-Chemicals, Thai.*
Reserpine (p.995·1); hydralazine hydrochloride (p.931·2); hydrochlorothiazide (p.933·2).
*Hypertension.*

**Reseril** *Bristol-Myers Squibb, Ital.†.*
Nefazodone hydrochloride (p.309·2).
*Depression.*

**Reserpina** *British Dispensary, Thai.†.*
Reserpine (p.995·1).
*Hypertension; sedative.*

**Reset** *Biomedica, Ital.†.*
Aniracetam (p.1655·1).
*Mental function impairment.*

**Resfenol** *Galenogal, Braz.†.*
Paracetamol (p.76·2); chlorphenamine maleate (p.427·3); phenylephrine hydrochloride (p.1126·3).
*Cold and influenza symptoms.*

**Resfin** *Jofrain, Mex.†.*
Paracetamol (p.76·2).
*Fever; pain.*

**Resfolin** *Piam, Ital.*
Calcium folinate (p.1431·1).
*Anaemias; antidote to folic acid antagonists; folate deficiency; reduction of aminopterin and methotrexate toxicity.*

**Resfrialgina** *Farmedica, Braz.†.*
Dipyrone (p.35·3); vitamin C (p.1460·2).
*Cold and influenza symptoms.*

**Resfry** *Neo Quimica, Braz.*
*Syrup:* Paracetamol (p.76·2); dexchlorpheniramine maleate (p.427·3); caffeine (p.782·1); ascorbic acid (p.1460·2).
*Tablets:* Green tablets, paracetamol (p.76·2); dexchlorpheniramine maleate (p.427·3); caffeine (p.782·1); yellow tablets, ascorbic acid (p.1460·2).
*Cold and influenza symptoms.*

**Resfry Infantil** *Neo Quimica, Braz.†.*
Salicylamide (p.87·3); chlorphenamine maleate (p.427·3); caffeine (p.782·1); ascorbic acid (p.1460·2).
*Cold and influenza symptoms.*

**Resical** *Fresenius Medical, Port.*
Calcium polystyrene sulfonate (p.1032·3).

**Residex P55** *Agropharm, UK.*
Permethrin (p.1508·3).
*Mosquito repellent for nets and clothing.*

**Resilar** *Orion, Fin.*
Dextromethorphan hydrobromide (p.1117·3).
*Coughs.*

**Resimatil** *Sanofi Synthelabo, Ger.*
Primidone (p.376·3).
*Epilepsy.*

**Resina Carbolica Dentilin** *Ghimas, Ital.†.*
Guaiacol (p.1122·1); lidocaine hydrochloride (p.1377·3); alcohol (p.1166·1); camphor (p.1665·3); thymol (p.1194·2).
*Dental disinfection; dental pain.*

**Resincalcio**
*Omedir, Arg.; Rubio, Spain.*
Calcium polystyrene sulfonate (p.1032·3).
*Hyperkalaemia.*

**Resincolestiramina**
*Rubio, Singapore; Rubio, Spain; Rubio, Thai.; TTN, Thai.*
Colestyramine (p.889·3).
*Diarrhoea; hyperlipidaemias; pruritus associated with biliary obstruction.*

**Resinol** *Mentholatum, USA†.*
Calamine (p.1144·1); zinc oxide (p.1163·2); resorcinol (p.1156·3).
*Minor skin irritation.*

**Resinsodio**
*Rubio, Singapore; Rubio, Spain; Rubio, Thai.†; TTN, Thai.†.*
Sodium polystyrene sulfonate (p.1053·1).
*Hyperkalaemia.*

**Resistan** *Truw, Ger.*
Homoeopathic preparation.

**Resisten Retard** *Smaller, Spain†.*
Ampicillin sodium (p.157·1); ampicillin benzathine (p.158·1); bromhexine hydrochloride (p.1115·3).
Lidocaine hydrochloride (p.1377·3) is included in this preparation to alleviate the pain of injection.
*Respiratory-tract infections.*

**Resivit** *Rhone-Poulenc Rorer, Spain†.*
Multivitamin preparation (p.1417·1).

**Resma** *UCB, Belg.*
Zafirlukast (p.807·1).
*Asthma.*

**Resnedal** *Byk Leo, Spain†.*
Chlortalidone (p.882·3); spironolactone (p.1003·1); reserpine (p.995·1).
*Hypertension.*

**Resochin**
*Bayer, Austria; Bayer, Ger.; Bayer, India; Bayer, Spain.*
Chloroquine phosphate (p.448·2).
*Amoebiasis; lupus erythematosus; malaria; rheumatoid arthritis.*

**Resochina** *Bayer, Port.*
Chloroquine phosphate (p.448·2).
*Amoebiasis; lupus erythematosus; malaria; rheumatoid arthritis.*

**Resochine** *Bayer, Switz.†.*
Chloroquine phosphate (p.448·2).
*Amoebiasis; lupus erythematosus; malaria; rheumatoid arthritis.*

**Resodermil** *Edol, Port.*
Sulfur (p.1158·2); resorcinol (p.1156·3).
*Acne.*

**Resoferon**
*Ciba-Geigy, Belg.†; Novartis, Gr.; Novartis, Switz.*
Ferrous sulfate (p.1428·2).
Succinic acid may be included to increase the absorption and availability of iron.
*Iron deficiency; iron-deficiency anaemia.*

**Resol**
*Note. This name is used for preparations of different composition.*
*Terramin, Austria†.*
Camphor (p.1665·3); terpineol (p.1752·2); eucalyptus oil (p.1686·2); pumilio pine oil (p.1737·1); menthol (p.1711·3); thymol (p.1194·2).
*Catarrh; rheumatism.*

*Wyeth-Ayerst, USA.*
Glucose; sodium chloride; potassium citrate; citric acid; sodium phosphate; magnesium chloride; calcium chloride; sodium citrate (p.1222·2).
*Diarrhoea; oral rehydration therapy.*

**Resolution** *Phoenix Health, UK†.*
Nicotine (p.1720·1); vitamins (p.1417·1).
*Aid to smoking withdrawal.*

**Resolutivo Regium** *Miquel Garriga, Spain.*
Boldo (p.1661·2); chumbera; equisetum (p.1684·1); sideritide; rosemary (p.1740·2); cynodon; arenaria; melissa (p.1711·1).
*Diuresis.*

**Resolve**
*Note. This name is used for preparations of different composition.*
*Ego, Austral.*
*Balm:* Miconazole nitrate (p.405·3); bufexamac (p.21·3).
Formerly known as Fungo.
*Fungal skin infections.*
*Cream; powder; topical solution:* Miconazole (p.405·2) or miconazole nitrate (p.405·3).
Formerly known as Fungo.
*Fungal skin and nail infections.*

*SSL, UK.*
Paracetamol (p.76·2); anhydrous citric acid (p.1673·1); sodium bicarbonate (p.1223·2); potassium bicarbonate (p.1223·1); anhydrous sodium carbonate (p.1747·1); ascorbic acid (p.1460·2).
*Dyspepsia; headache.*

**Resolve Extra** *SSL, UK.*
Paracetamol (p.76·2); sodium bicarbonate (p.1223·2); caffeine (p.782·1).
*Dyspepsia; headache.*

**Resolve Plus** *Ego, Austral.*
Miconazole nitrate (p.405·3); hydrocortisone (p.1103·3).
Formerly known as Fungocort.
*Fungal skin infections with inflammation.*

**Resolve Thrush** *Ego, Austral.*
Miconazole nitrate (p.405·3).
Formerly known as Fungo.
*Vulvovaginal candidiasis.*

**Resolve/GP** *Allergan, USA.*
Cleansing solution for hard and gas permeable contact lenses (p.1164·2).

**Resonium**
*Sanofi Winthrop, Denm.; Sanofi Synthelabo, Fin.; Irex, Port.; Sanofi Synthelabo, Swed.*
Sodium polystyrene sulfonate (p.1053·1).
*Hyperkalaemia.*

**Resonium A**
*Sanofi Synthelabo, Austral.; Sanofi Synthelabo, Austria; Sanofi Synthelabo, Ger.; Sanofi Synthelabo, Hong Kong; Sanofi Synthelabo, Irl.; Sanofi Synthelabo, Malaysia; Sanofi Synthelabo, Neth.; Sanofi Synthelabo, NZ; Sanofi Synthelabo, Switz.; Sanofi Synthelabo, Thai.; Sanofi Synthelabo, UK.*
Sodium polystyrene sulfonate (p.1053·1).
*Hyperkalaemia.*

**Resonium Calcium**
*Sanofi Synthelabo, Canad.; Sanofi Winthrop, Denm.; Sanofi Synthelabo, Norw.; Sanofi Synthelabo, Swed.*
Calcium polystyrene sulfonate (p.1032·3).
*Hyperkalaemia.*

**Resorbane** *Spirig, Switz.*
Cineole (p.1672·1); camphor (p.1665·3); niaouli oil (p.1719·3).
*Respiratory-tract disorders.*

**Resorborina** *Belmac, Spain.*
*Mouthwash:* Benzalkonium chloride (p.1168·3); dexamethasone (p.1097·1); resorcinol (p.1156·3); tetracaine hydrochloride (p.1385·1).
*Throat spray:* Benzalkonium chloride (p.1168·3); betamethasone valerate (p.1093·2); tetracaine hydrochloride (p.1385·1).
*Mouth and throat inflammation.*

**Resostyl** *Medinova (Μεντινοβα), Gr.*
Selegiline hydrochloride (p.1214·1).
*Parkinsonism.*

**Resource**
*Novartis, Arg.; Novartis Consumer, Austral.; Novartis, Braz.; Novartis Nutrition, Canad.; Novartis, Fin.; Novartis Nutrition, Fr.; Novartis Nutrition, Hong Kong; Novartis Consumer, Port.; Novartis Nutrition, Singapore; Novartis, UK; Novartis Nutrition, USA.*
A range of preparations for enteral nutrition (p.1417·1).

**Resource Benefiber**
*Novartis Consumer, Ital.*
Dietary fibre supplement (p.1253·2).

*Novartis, UK.*
Guar gum (p.333·2).
*Nutritional supplement.*

**Resource Energy** *Novartis Consumer, Ital.*
Preparation for enteral nutrition (p.1417·1).

**Resource Fruit** *Novartis Consumer, Ital.*
Preparation for enteral nutrition (p.1417·1).

**Resource Gelificata** *Novartis Consumer, Ital.*
Carrageenan (p.1578·2); xanthan gum (p.1582·3); guar gum (p.333·2).
*Dysphagia.*

**Resource Meritene** *Novartis Consumer, Ital.*
A range of preparations for enteral nutrition (p.1417·1).

**Resource ThickenUp**
*Novartis, Irl.; Novartis Consumer, Ital.; Novartis, NZ; Novartis, UK.*
Nutritional supplement for thickening foods (p.1417·1).
*Dysphagia.*

**Resovist**
*Schering, Austral.; Schering, Fin.; Schering, Ger.; Schering, Port.; Schering, Swed.; Schering, Switz.*
Ferucarbotran (p.1061·3).
*Contrast medium for magnetic resonance imaging.*

**Respa-ARM** *Respa, USA†.*
Phenylephrine hydrochloride (p.1126·3); phenylpropanolamine hydrochloride (p.1127·3); chlorphenamine maleate (p.427·3); belladonna alkaloids (p.479·1).

**Respacal**
*UCB, Belg.; UCB, UK†.*
Tulobuterol hydrochloride (p.806·3).
*Bronchospasm.*

**Respa-DM** *Respa, USA.*
Dextromethorphan hydrobromide (p.1117·3); guaifenesin (p.1122·1).
*Coughs; respiratory-tract congestion.*

**Respa-GF** *Respa, USA†.*
Guaifenesin (p.1122·1).

**Respahist** *Respa, USA.*
Pseudoephedrine hydrochloride (p.1129·2); brompheniramine maleate (p.426·1).

**Respaire** *Laser, USA.*
Pseudoephedrine hydrochloride (p.1129·2); guaifenesin (p.1122·1).
*Coughs and cold symptoms; nasal congestion.*

**Respalis** *Nestle, Fr.*
Preparation for enteral nutrition (p.1417·1).
*Respiratory insufficiency.*

**Respalor**
*Mead Johnson, Hong Kong†; Mead Johnson Nutritionals, Thai.†; Mead Johnson Nutritionals, USA.*
Preparation for enteral nutrition (p.1417·1).
*Respiratory system disorders.*

**Respa-1st** *Respa, USA.*
Pseudoephedrine hydrochloride (p.1129·2); guaifenesin (p.1122·1).
*Respiratory-tract disorders associated with increased or viscous mucus.*

**Respatona Decongestant Formula** *Brauer, Austral.†.*
Anise oil (p.1655·2); althaea (p.1651·3); bryonia (p.1663·1); iceland moss; chamomile (p.1669·3); thyme (p.1755·2); urtica (p.1762·1); ammonium causticum; aconitum napellus; coccus cacti; corallium rubrum; drosera rotundifolia; ipecacuanha; kali bich.; kreosotum; spongia tosta; sticta pulmonaria.
*Coughs and cold symptoms.*

**Respatona Plus Bronchial Cough Relief** *Brauer, Austral.†.*
Anise oil (p.1655·2); althaea (p.1651·3); bryonia (p.1663·1); iceland moss; echinacea angustifolia (p.1683·2); chamomile (p.1669·3); thyme (p.1755·2); urtica (p.1762·1); aconitum napellus; coccus cacti; corallium rubrum; drosera rotundifolia; ipecacuanha; kali bich.; kreosotum; spongia tosta; sticta pulmonaria.
*Coughs.*

**Respax**
*Pharmacia Upjohn, Austral.; Pharmacia Upjohn, Hong Kong†; Pharmacia Upjohn, NZ†.*
Salbutamol (p.791·3) or salbutamol sulfate (p.791·3).
*Obstructive airways disease.*

**Respbid** *Boehringer Ingelheim, USA.*
Theophylline (p.798·3).
*Obstructive airways disease.*

**Respexil** *Prodome, Braz.*
Norfloxacin (p.238·3).
*Bacterial infections.*

**Respibien** *Cinfa, Spain.*
Oxymetazoline hydrochloride (p.1126·1).
*Nasal congestion.*

**Respibron** *Andromaco, Chile.*
Oxolamine citrate (p.1126·1) or oxolamine phosphate (p.1126·1).
*Coughs.*

**Respicilin** *Haller, Braz.*
Amoxicillin trihydrate (p.155·3).
*Bacterial infections.*

**Respicort** *Mundipharma, Ger.*
Budesonide (p.1094·2).
*Obstructive airways disease.*

**Respicur**
*Byk, Austria; Byk Gulden, Ital.*
Theophylline (p.798·3).
*Obstructive airways disease.*

**RespiGam** *Medimmune, USA.*
Respiratory syncytial virus immunoglobulins (p.1637·2).
*Passive immunisation.*

**Respilene**
*Note. This name is used for preparations of different composition.*
*Sanofi Synthelabo OTC, Fr.*
Pholcodine (p.1128·3).
*Coughs.*

*Columbia, Mex.*
Zipeprol (p.1132·3).
*Bronchitis; coughs.*

**Respimex** *Pharmacia, Arg.*
Ketotifen fumarate (p.788·1).
*Asthma; hypersensitivity reactions.*

**Respimox** *Wockhardt, India.*
Amoxicillin trihydrate (p.155·3); bromhexine hydrochloride (p.1115·3).
*Respiratory-tract infections.*

**Respinol** *Pharmaceutical Enterprises, S.Afr.*
Phenylephrine hydrochloride (p.1126·3); chlorphenamine maleate (p.427·3); hyoscine methonitrate (p.483·3).
*Cold symptoms; sinusitis; vasomotor rhinitis.*

**Respinol Compound** *Pharmaceutical Enterprises, S.Afr.*
Pholcodine (p.1128·3); pseudoephedrine hydrochloride (p.1129·2); chlorphenamine maleate (p.427·3); hyoscine methonitrate (p.483·3).
*Cold symptoms; coughs; rhinitis; sinusitis.*

**Respir** *Schering-Plough, Spain.*
Oxymetazoline hydrochloride (p.1126·1).
*Nasal congestion.*

**Respir Balsamico** *Schering-Plough, Spain†.*
Camphor (p.1665·3); cineole (p.1672·1); oxymetazoline hydrochloride (p.1126·1); menthol (p.1711·3).
*Nasal congestion.*

**Respiral** *Sanofi Synthelabo, Port.†.*
Zipeprol hydrochloride (p.1132·3).
*Coughs.*

**Respiret** *Klonal, Arg.*
Salbutamol (p.791·3).
*Obstructive airways disease.*

**Respiro** *Byk Gulden, Ital.*
Xylometazoline hydrochloride (p.1132·2).
*Nasal congestion.*

**Respirol** *Remedina, Gr.*
Ambroxol hydrochloride (p.1114·3).
*Respiratory disorders associated with viscous mucus.*

**Respiroma** *Fournier SA, Spain.*
Salbutamol sulfate (p.791·3).
Formerly contained iodinated glycerol and salbutamol sulfate.
*Obstructive airways disease.*

**Respisniffers** *Aspen Consumer, S.Afr.†.*
Cineole (p.1672·1); pine oil; chloroxylenol (p.1177·2); turpentine oil (p.1760·1); menthol (p.1711·3).
*Bronchitis; cold symptoms; nasal congestion.*

**Respitol** *Cinfa, Spain†.*
Sodium chloride (p.1233·3).
*Nasal congestion.*

**Resplant** *Spitzner, Ger.*
Echinacea purpurea (p.1683·2).
*Respiratory- and urinary-tract infections.*

**Respocort**
*3M, Austral.†; Lavipharm, Gr.; 3M, NZ.*
Beclometasone dipropionate (p.1091·1).
*Obstructive airways disease.*

**Respolin**
*3M, Austral.†; 3M, Chile; 3M, Hong Kong; 3M, Malaysia; 3M, NZ; 3M, Singapore; 3M, Thai.*
Salbutamol sulfate (p.791·3).
*Obstructive airways disease.*

**Responsar** *Bayer, Ital.*
Cyfluthrin (p.1502·3).
*Insecticide.*

**Respontin**
*GlaxoSmithKline, Norw.; Allen & Hanburys, UK.*
Ipratropium bromide (p.787·1).
*Obstructive airways disease.*

**Resprax** *Prodotti, Braz.*
Green tablets, salicylamide (p.87·3); caffeine (p.782·1); chlorphenamine maleate (p.427·3); yellow tablets, vitamin C (p.1460·2).
Aluminium hydroxide (p.1249·2) is included in the green tablets in an attempt to limit adverse effects on the gastrointestinal mucosa.
*Cold and influenza symptoms.*

**Respreve** *Pharmacia, Hong Kong.*
Salbutamol (p.791·3).
*Bronchospasm.*

**Resprim**
*Alphapharm, Austral.; Teva, Israel; Alphapharm, Malaysia; Merck, Malaysia.*
Co-trimoxazole (p.199·3).
*Bacterial infections; Pneumocystis carinii pneumonia.*

**Resprin**
*Note. This name is used for preparations of different composition.*
*Johnson & Johnson, Braz.*
Paracetamol (p.76·2); carbinoxamine maleate (p.426·3); pentoxyverine citrate (p.1126·2); phenylephrine hydrochloride (p.1126·3).
*Cold and influenza symptoms.*

*Rice Steele, Irl.*
Aspirin (p.15·1).
*Fever; inflammation; pain.*

**Restal** *SFD, Port.*
Oxidised glycerol triester.
*Cicatrisation; cracked lips; dry skin.*

**Restameth-SR** *Restan, S.Afr.*
Indometacin (p.47·3).
*Gout; musculoskeletal and joint disorders.*

**Restandol**
*Organon, Denm.; Organon (Οργκανον), Gr.; Organon, Irl.; Organon, UK.*
Testosterone undecylate (p.1570·1).
*Male hypogonadism; osteoporosis.*

**Restasis** *Allergan, USA.*
Ciclosporin (p.1351·2).
*Dry eyes.*

**Restaslim** *Restan, S.Afr.*
Phenylpropanolamine hydrochloride (p.1127·3).
*Obesity.*

**Restaurene** *Armstrong, Arg.*
Chlorhexidine gluconate (p.1173·2); sodium acexamate (p.1646·2).
*Cracked nipples; ulcers; wounds.*

**Restavit** *Woods, Austral.*
Doxylamine succinate (p.432·3).
*Insomnia.*

**Resteclin** *Sarabhai Piramal, India.*
Tetracycline hydrochloride (p.266·2).
*Bacterial infections.*

**Restenil** *Recip, Swed.†.*
Meprobamate (p.706·2).
*Anxiety; headache; skeletal muscle spasm; sleep disorders.*

**Restex** *Roche, Ger.*
Levodopa (p.1205·2); benserazide hydrochloride (p.1200·2).
*Restless-leg syndrome.*

**Restful** *Bros, Gr.*
Sulpiride (p.722·2).
*Psychoses.*

**Restin** *Restan, S.Afr.*
Valerian (p.1762·2); vitamin B substances (p.1417·1); ascorbic acid.
*Nonpsychotic mental disorders.*

**Restol** *Laboratorios Chile, Chile.*
Domperidone (p.1263·2).
*Aid in gastrointestinal investigation; nausea and vomiting; regurgitation in infants.*

**Restopon** *Bros, Gr.*
Ranitidine hydrochloride (p.1285·2).
*Conditions where gastric acid reduction is beneficial; gastric hypersecretion including Zollinger-Ellison syndrome; peptic ulcer.*

**Restorativ Glucosamine Muscle and Joint** *Holista, Canad.*
Borage oil; boswellia; frankincense; camphor oil; devil's claw; evening primrose oil; glucosamine sulfate; grape seed oil; peppermint oil; rosemary oil (p.1417·1).

**Restore** *InAgra, USA†.*
Psyllium hydrophilic mucilloid (p.1268·1).

**Restoril**
*Note. This name is used for preparations of different composition.*
*Novartis, Canad.; Novartis, USA.*
Temazepam (p.723·2).
*Insomnia.*

*Silesia, Chile.*
Chlormezanone (p.675·1).
*Skeletal muscle spasm.*

**Restovar** *Organon, Swed.*
Lynestrenol (p.1557·1); ethinylestradiol (p.1553·2).
*Combined oral contraceptive.*

**Restrical** *Merck Medication Familiale, Fr.*
Liquid paraffin (p.1479·1).
*Constipation.*

**Restructa forte ST** *Fides, Ger.*
Homoeopathic preparation.

**Restwel** *Covan, S.Afr.*
Doxylamine succinate (p.432·3).
*Insomnia.*

**Restylane** *Q-Med, Singapore.*
Hyaluronic acid (p.1697·3).
*Lip enhancement; skin contour defects.*

**Resulax** *Tika, Swed.*
Sorbitol (p.1446·3).
*Bowel evacuation; constipation.*

**Resulin** *Ist. Chim. Inter., Ital.*
Nimesulide (p.67·1).
*Fever; inflammation; pain.*

**Resurmide** *Ibi, Ital.*
Somatostatin acetate (p.1339·3).
*Gastrointestinal haemorrhage.*

**Resvelife** *Nuovo ICT, Ital.*
Resveratrol.
*Skin irritation.*

**Resyl**
*Novartis Consumer, Austria; Novartis, Israel; Novartis Consumer, Ital.; Novartis, Swed.; Novartis Consumer, Switz.*
Guaifenesin (p.1122·1).
*Coughs; respiratory-tract congestion.*

**Resyl DM** *Novartis Consumer, Ital.*
Guaifenesin (p.1122·1); dextromethorphan hydrobromide (p.1117·3).
*Coughs.*

**Resyl mit Codein** *Novartis Consumer, Austria.*
Guaifenesin (p.1122·1); codeine phosphate (p.27·1).
*Coughs.*

**Resyl Plus** *Novartis Consumer, Switz.*
Guaifenesin (p.1122·1); codeine phosphate (p.27·1).
*Coughs.*

**Retabolin forte** *Medika, Switz.*
Vitamin B substances (p.1417·1).
*Neuralgia; neuritis.*

**Retacillin compositum** *Jenapharm, Ger.*
Benzylpenicillin sodium (p.163·2); procaine benzylpenicillin (p.246·1); benzathine benzylpenicillin (p.162·3).
*Bacterial infections.*

**Retacnyl**
*Galderma, Arg.; Galderma, Braz.; Galderma, Chile; Galderma, Fr.; Galderma, Hong Kong; Galderma, Malaysia; Galderma, Mex.; Galderma, S.Afr.; Galderma, Singapore; Galderma, Thai.*
Tretinoin (p.1161·1).
*Acne; keratinisation disorders; photoageing of the skin.*

**Retafer**
*Orion, Fin.; Orion, Singapore†.*
Ferrous sulfate (p.1428·2).
*Iron deficiency; iron-deficiency anaemia.*

**Retafyllin**
*Orion, Fin.; Orion, Malaysia; Orion, Singapore; Orion, Thai.*
Theophylline (p.798·3).
*Obstructive airways disease.*

**Retalzem** *Menarini, Hong Kong.*
Diltiazem hydrochloride (p.900·1).
*Heart failure; hypertension; ischaemic heart disease.*

**Retan** *Microsules, Arg.*
Alprazolam (p.668·3).
*Anxiety.*

**Ret-A-Pres** *Precimex, Mex.†.*
Tretinoin (p.1161·1).

**Retardent** *Periproducts, UK†.*
Stabilised chlorine dioxide (CloSYS II) (p.1176·2).
*Halitosis.*

**Retardex** *Periproducts, UK.*
Stabilised chlorine dioxide (CloSYS II) (p.1176·2).
*Halitosis.*

**Retardin** *Janssen-Cilag, Denm.†.*
Diphenoxylate hydrochloride (p.1261·3).
Atropine sulfate (p.477·1) is included in this preparation to discourage abuse.
*Diarrhoea.*

**Retarpen**
*Biochemie, Austria; Biochemie, Malaysia; Biochemie, Singapore.*
Benzathine benzylpenicillin (p.162·3).
*Bacterial infections.*

*Septa, Spain.*
Ampicillin sodium (p.157·1); ampicillin benzathine (p.158·1).
Lidocaine (p.1377·3) is included in this preparation to alleviate the pain of injection.
*Bacterial infections.*

**Retarpen Balsamico** *Reig Jofre, Spain.*
Ampicillin sodium (p.157·1); ampicillin benzathine (p.158·1); cineole (p.1672·1); guaifenesin (p.1122·1).
Lidocaine hydrochloride (p.1377·3) is included in this preparation to alleviate the pain of injection.
*Respiratory-tract infections.*

**Retarpen compositum** *Biochemie, Austria.*
Benzylpenicillin sodium (p.163·2); procaine benzylpenicillin (p.246·1); benzathine benzylpenicillin (p.162·3).
*Bacterial infections.*

**Retarpen Mucolitico** *Reig Jofre, Spain.*
Ampicillin sodium (p.157·1); ampicillin benzathine (p.158·1); bromhexine hydrochloride (p.1115·3).
Lidocaine hydrochloride (p.1377·3) is included in this preparation to alleviate the pain of injection.
*Respiratory-tract infections.*

**Retavase**
*Biovail, Canad.; Boehringer Mannheim, USA.*
Reteplase (p.995·2).
*Myocardial infarction.*

**Retavit** *CTI, Israel.*
Tretinoin (p.1161·1).
*Acne.*

**Retcin** *DDSA Pharmaceuticals, UK†.*
Erythromycin (p.208·1).

**Retebem** *Pharmacia, Arg.*
Oxybutynin (p.487·1).
*Bladder instability.*

**Retef**
*AB-Consult, Austria; Galderma, Ger.†.*
Hydrocortisone aceponate (p.1104·2).
*Skin disorders.*

**Retemic** *Apsen, Braz.*
Oxybutynin hydrochloride (p.486·3).
*Neurogenic bladder; urinary incontinence.*

**Retens** *Chiesi, Spain.*
Doxycycline hyclate (p.206·2).
*Bacterial infections; malaria.*

**Reticulogen** *Lilly, Ital.†.*
Cyanocobalamin (p.1458·2).
*Megaloblastic anaemia; vitamin $B_{12}$ deficiency.*

**Reticulogen Fortificado** *Lilly, Spain.*
Cyanocobalamin (p.1458·2).
*Vitamin $B_{12}$ deficiency.*

**Reticus** *Euroderm, Ital.*
Desonide (p.1096·3).
*Skin disorders.*

**Retimax** *Alcon Cusi, Spain.*
Pentoxifylline (p.979·3).
*Cerebral and peripheral vascular disorders.*

**Retin-A**
*Janssen-Cilag, Arg.; Janssen-Cilag, Austral.; Janssen-Cilag, Austria; Janssen-Cilag, Braz.; Ortho Dermatological, Canad.; Janssen-Cilag, Chile; Janssen-Cilag, Fr.; Cilag, Hong Kong; Janssen-Cilag, Irl.; Janssen-Cilag, Israel; Janssen-Cilag, Ital.; Janssen-Cilag, Malaysia; Cilag, Mex.; Janssen-Cilag, NZ; Janssen-Cilag, Port.; Janssen-Cilag, S.Afr.; Janssen-Cilag, Singapore; Janssen-Cilag, Switz.; Janssen-Cilag, Thai.; Janssen-Cilag, UK; Ortho Dermatological, USA.*
Tretinoin (p.1161·1).
*Acne; keratinisation disorders; photoageing of the skin.*

**Retinar** *Bunker, Braz.*
Vitamin A (p.1451·2).

**Retinol** *INTES, Ital.*
Myrtillus (p.1718·3).
*Eye disorders.*

**Retinol-A** *Young Again Nutrients, USA.*
Vitamin A palmitate (p.1453·1).
*Minor skin disorders.*

**Retinova**
*RoC, Belg.†; Janssen-Cilag, Braz.; RoC, Fr.; Janssen-Cilag, NZ; Janssen-Cilag, Singapore; Johnson & Johnson, Spain; Janssen-Cilag, Swed.; Johnson & Johnson, UK.*
Tretinoin (p.1161·1).
*UV-induced skin damage.*

**Retinovit** *INTES, Ital.*
Myrtillus (p.1718·3); vitamin A (p.1451·2); vitamin E (p.1464·3).
*Circulatory disorders of the eye.*

**Retirides** *OTC, Spain.*
Tretinoin (p.1161·1).
*Acne; sunlight-induced skin damage.*

**Retisdin** *Isdin, Port.*
Vitamin A betadex; various sunscreens.
*UV-induced skin damage.*

**Retisol-A** *Stiefel, Canad.*
Tretinoin (p.1161·1).
*Acne.*

**Retitop** *Roche-Posay, Fr.†.*
Tretinoin (p.1161·1).
*Acne; keratinisation disorders.*

**Retodol Compositum** *Rimsa, Mex.*
Hyoscine butylbromide (p.483·3); dipyrone (p.35·3).
*Pain; smooth muscle spasm.*

**Retofar** *Searle, Mex.†.*
Metronidazole (p.607·2).
*Amoebiasis; anaerobic bacterial infections.*

**Retolen** *Altana, Spain†.*
Astemizole (p.424·2).
*Hypersensitivity reactions.*

**Retoxil** *Alcon, Arg.*
Vitamin, mineral, and trace element preparation (p.1417·1).

**ReTrieve** *Dermatech, Austral.*
Tretinoin (p.1161·1).
*Acne.*

**Retrovir**
*GlaxoSmithKline, Arg.; GlaxoSmithKline, Austral.; GlaxoSmithKline, Austria; GlaxoSmithKline, Belg.; GlaxoSmithKline, Braz.; GlaxoSmithKline, Canad.; GlaxoSmithKline, Chile; GlaxoSmithKline, Denm.; GlaxoSmithKline, Fin.; GlaxoSmithKline, Fr.; GlaxoSmithKline, Ger.; Glaxo Wellcome, Gr.; GlaxoSmithKline, Hong Kong; GlaxoSmithKline, India; Wellcome, Irl.; Wellcome, Israel; GlaxoSmithKline, Ital.; GlaxoSmithKline, Malaysia; Glaxo Wellcome, Mex.; GlaxoSmithKline, Neth.; GlaxoSmithKline, Norw.; GlaxoSmithKline, NZ; Wellcome, Port.; GlaxoSmithKline, S.Afr.; GlaxoSmithKline, Singapore; GlaxoSmithKline, Spain; GlaxoSmithKline, Swed.; GlaxoSmithKline, Switz.; GlaxoSmithKline, Thai.; GlaxoSmithKline, UK; Glaxo Wellcome, USA.*
Zidovudine (p.658·2).
*HIV infection.*

**Retrovir/3TC Post-HIV Exposure** *GlaxoSmithKline, S.Afr.*
Capsules, zidovudine (Retrovir) (p.658·2); tablets, lamivudine (3TC) (p.648·2).
*Prophylaxis of HIV infection.*

**Rettavate** *Allen, Gr.*
Clobetasone butyrate (p.1095·3).
*Topical corticosteroid.*

**Retterspitz Aerosol** *Retterspitz, Ger.†.*
Ephedrine hydrochloride (p.1120·1); pumilio pine oil (p.1737·1); siberian fir oil; thyme oil (p.1755·3); eucalyptus oil (p.1686·2); menthol (p.1711·3).
*Respiratory-tract infections.*

**Retterspitz Ausserlich** *Retterspitz, Ger.†.*
Rosemary oil (p.1740·2); citric acid (p.1673·1); tartaric acid (p.1752·1); alum (p.1652·1); thymol (p.1194·2).
*Inflammatory disorders.*

**Retterspitz Gelee** *Retterspitz, Ger.†.*
Thymol (p.1194·2); allantoin (p.1141·3); rosemary oil (p.1740·2); tartaric acid (p.1752·1); alum (p.1652·1); citric acid (p.1673·1).
*Skin disorders.*

**Retterspitz Heilsalbe** *Retterspitz, Ger.†.*
Pumilio pine oil (p.1737·1); siberian fir oil; thymol (p.1194·2); allantoin (p.1141·3).
*Haemorrhoids; skin disorders.*

**Retterspitz Innerlich** *Retterspitz, Ger.†.*
Citric acid (p.1673·1); tartaric acid (p.1752·1); alum (p.1652·1); thyme oil (p.1755·3).
*Gastrointestinal disorders.*

**Retterspitz Quick** *Retterspitz, Ger.†.*
Rosemary oil (p.1740·2); camphor (p.1665·3); menthol (p.1711·3); thymol (p.1194·2).
*Chest disorders; joint disorders; myalgia.*

**Reucam**
*CT, Ital.; Maver, Mex.*
Piroxicam (p.84·2).
*Inflammation; musculoskeletal, joint, and peri-articular disorders; pain.*

**Reudene** *ABC, Ital.*
Piroxicam (p.84·2).
*Musculoskeletal, joint, and peri-articular disorders.*

**Reufel** *Ehlinger, Mex.†.*
Piroxicam (p.84·2).

**Reufirron** *Reuffer, Mex.†.*
Ferrous fumarate (p.1427·3).

**Reuflodol** *Nattermann, Spain†.*
Pinazone (p.43·2).
*Musculoskeletal, joint, and peri-articular disorders; pain.*

**Reugast** *Basi, Port.*
Fenbufen (p.39·1).

**Reugot** *Igefarma, Braz.†.*
Colchicine (p.415·1).
*Gout.*

**Reukamicin** *Reuffer, Mex.†.*
Kanamycin (p.225·2).

**Reumacid** *Remek, Gr.*
Indometacin (p.47·3).
*Gout; inflammation; musculoskeletal and joint disorders; pain.*

**Reumacort** *Teofarma, Ital.*
Hydrocortisone acetate (p.1103·3); methyl gentisate (p.59·2).
*Muscle and joint pain.*

**Reumadil** *Heralds, Braz.†.*
Diclofenac (p.32·1).
*Gout; inflammation; musculoskeletal, joint, and peri-articular disorders; pain.*

**Reumagel** *Sanofi Winthrop, Mex.†.*
Etofenamate (p.38·1).

**Reumagil** *KBR, Ital.*
Piroxicam (p.84·2).
*Musculoskeletal, joint, and peri-articular disorders.*

**Reumaless** *Pharmaton, Ger.†.*
*Balsam:* Methyl salicylate (p.59·3); benzyl nicotinate (p.21·2).
*Musculoskeletal, joint, and soft-tissue disorders; neuralgia.*
*Capsules:* Urtica (p.1762·1).
*Rheumatism.*

**Reumaren** *QIF, Braz.†.*
Diclofenac sodium (p.32·1).
*Gout; inflammation; musculoskeletal, joint, and peri-articular disorders; pain.*

**Reumat** *Sinteropico, Braz.†.*
Bromelains (p.1662·2); phenylbutazone (p.83·2).

**Reumatosil** *Saba, Ital.†.*
Nifenazone (p.66·3).
*Neuralgias; neuritis; rheumatic disorders.*

**Reumazine** *Luper, Braz.†.*
Prednisolone (p.1108·1); oxyphenbutazone (p.76·1).
*Inflammation.*

**Reumilase Plus** *MDM, Ital.*
Glucosamine hydrochloride; chondroitin sodium sulfate; collagen; devil's claw root; vitamins (p.1417·1).
*Joint disorders.*

**Reumin** *Willmar, Mex.†.*
Indometacin (p.47·3).

**Reumine** *Poen, Arg.*
Amino-acid, vitamin A, and mineral preparation (p.1417·1).
Lidocaine (p.1377·3) is included in the injection to alleviate the pain of injection.
*Musculoskeletal and joint disorders.*

**Reumix** *Makros, Braz.†.*
Betamethasone (p.1093·1); phenylbutazone (p.83·2).
Aluminium glycinate (p.1249·1) is included in this preparation in an attempt to limit adverse effects on the gastrointestinal mucosa.
*Inflammation.*

**Reumo** *UCB, Spain.*
Indometacin (p.47·3).
*Gout; inflammation; musculoskeletal, joint, and peri-articular disorders; pain.*

**Reumol** *Cabuchi, Arg.*
Camphor (p.1665·3); menthol (p.1711·3); salicylic acid (p.1157·1).

**Reumon** *Bial, Port.*
Etofenamate (p.38·1).
*Gout; inflammation; musculoskeletal, joint, peri-articular, and soft-tissue disorders; neuralgia; pain.*

**Reumophan** *Grisi, Mex.*
Ketoprofen (p.51·2); chlorzoxazone (p.1392·3).
*Gout; musculoskeletal, joint, and peri-articular disorders.*

**Reumoquin** *Nattermann, Spain†.*
Ketoprofen (p.51·2).
*Gout; musculoskeletal, joint, and peri-articular disorders; pain.*

**Reumoxican** *Medinfar, Port.*
Piroxicam (p.84·2).
*Inflammation; pain.*

**Reupax** *CPH, Port.*
Flurbiprofen (p.43·3).
*Musculoskeletal, joint, and peri-articular disorders.*

**Reuplex** *Farmasa, Braz.*
Ibuprofen (p.45·3); paracetamol (p.76·2).
*Fever; inflammation; pain.*

**Reuprofen** *Terapeutico, Ital.*
Ketoprofen (p.51·2).
*Musculoskeletal, joint, peri-articular, and soft-tissue disorders.*

**Reusan** *Reuffer, Mex.†.*
Dexamethasone (p.1097·1).
*Corticosteroid.*

**Reusin** *Sankyo, Spain.*
Indometacin (p.47·3).
*Gout; inflammation; musculoskeletal, joint, peri-articular, and soft-tissue disorders; pain.*

**Reutaren** *Miller, Braz.†.*
Diclofenac potassium (p.32·1).

**Reutenox** *Solvay, Spain.*
Tenoxicam (p.93·1).
*Calcium stones; musculoskeletal, joint, and peri-articular disorders.*

**Reutricam** *Liferpal, Mex.*
Piroxicam (p.84·2).
*Fever; musculoskeletal and joint disorders; pain.*

**Reuxen** *Tecnifar, Port.*
Naproxen (p.65·1).
*Fever; gout; inflammation; musculoskeletal, joint, peri-articular, and soft-tissue disorders; pain.*

**Revalid**
*Geymonat, Ital.†.*
Amino acids; millet; wheat-germ; dried yeast; soya protein; minerals; vitamins (p.1417·1).
*Skin, hair, and nail disorders.*

Vifor, Switz.
Multivitamins and minerals (p.1417·1); amino-acids; aminobenzoic acid; milii flavi; tritici embryonis; faex medicinal.
*Hair and nail disorders.*

**Revange** Biosintetica, Braz.
Isosorbide mononitrate (p.942·1).
*Angina pectoris.*

**Revanil** Cambridge, UK†.
Lisuride maleate (p.1210·3).
Now known as Lisuride Tablets.
*Parkinsonism.*

**Revapol** AF, Mex.
Mebendazole (p.108·2).
*Worm infections.*

**Revasc**
Aventis, Austral.; Aventis, Braz.†; Rhone-Poulenc Rorer, Fin.†; Aventis, Fr.; Aventis, Ger.; Novartis, Ger.; Rhone-Poulenc Rorer, Irl.†; Aventis, Norw.; Aventis, NZ†; Aventis, Spain; Rhone-Poulenc Rorer, Swed.†; Aventis, Switz.; Aventis, UK†.
Desirudin (p.892·3).
*Venous thrombosis prophylaxis.*

**Revastin** Neo Quimica, Braz.
Simvastatin (p.997·1).
*Hypercholesterolaemia.*

**Revaton** Pharmco, S.Afr.†.
Haematoporphyrin (p.1696·2); vitamin $B_{12}$ (p.1458·2); ascorbic acid (p.1460·2); yeast extract (p.1469·1).
*Tonic.*

**Revaxis**
Aventis Pasteur, Belg.; Aventis Pasteur, Fr.; Aventis Pasteur, Ger.; Vianex (Βιανεξ), Gr.; Aventis Pasteur, Irl.; Aventis Pasteur, Ital.; Pro Vaccine, Switz.; Aventis Pasteur, UK.
A diphtheria, tetanus, and poliomyelitis vaccine (p.1615·2).
*Active immunisation.*

**Reve** IMO, Ital.
Valerian (p.1762·2); passion flower (p.1729·1).
*Insomnia.*

**Reveal** BR Pharmaceuticals, UK.
Pregnancy test (p.1734·3).

**Revectina** Sintofarma, Braz.
Ivermectin (p.105·3).
*Filariasis.*

**Revelatest** Pierre Fabre Sante, Fr.
Pregnancy test (p.1734·3).

**Revellex**
Essex, Arg.; Schering-Plough, S.Afr.
Infliximab (p.50·1).
*Crohn's disease; rheumatoid arthritis.*

**Revelplac** Naf, Arg.
Erythrosine (p.1057·2).
*Plaque disclosing agent.*

**Revelplac 2001** Naf, Arg.
Erythrosine (p.1057·2); fluoride.
*Plaque disclosing agent.*

**Revenil** Aventis, Braz.
Bufylline (p.781·3); doxylamine succinate (p.432·3); etafedrine hydrochloride (p.1121·2).
*Bronchospastic disorders.*

**Revenil Dospan** Aventis, Braz.
Bufylline (p.781·3); doxylamine succinate (p.432·3); etafedrine hydrochloride (p.1121·2); phenylephrine hydrochloride (p.1126·3).
*Brochospastic disorders.*

**Revenil Expectorante** Hoechst Marion Roussel, Braz.†.
Bufylline (p.781·3); doxylamine succinate (p.432·3); etafedrine hydrochloride (p.1121·2); guaifenesin (p.1122·1).
*Bronchospastic disorders.*

**Revenox** Collins, Mex.
Melatonin (p.1710·2).
*Sleep disorders.*

**Reverin** Hoechst Marion Roussel, Canad.†.
Rolitetracycline (p.254·1).
*Bacterial infections.*

**Reversa** Dermtek, Canad.
Glycolic acid (p.1147·3).
*Skin disorders requiring exfoliation.*

**Reversa AHA HQ** Dermtek, Canad.†.
Glycolic acid (p.1147·3); hydroquinone (p.1148·1).
*Skin disorders requiring exfoliation.*

**Reversa UV** Dermtek, Canad.
Glycolic acid (p.1147·3); strontium chloride (p.1749·3).
*Skin disorders.*

**Reversol** Organon, USA.
Edrophonium chloride (p.1490·3).
*Diagnosis of myasthenia gravis; evaluation of emergency treatment of myasthenic crises; reversal of competitive neuromuscular blockade.*

**Revex** Baxter, USA.
Nalmefene hydrochloride (p.1044·1).
*Opioid poisoning.*

**Rev-Eyes** Bausch & Lomb, USA.
Dapiprazole hydrochloride (p.1679·1).
*Reversal of mydriasis.*

**Revez** Chobet, Arg.
Naltrexone hydrochloride (p.1046·1).
*Alcohol withdrawal syndrome; opioid withdrawal syndrome.*

**Revia**
Orphan, Austral.; Torrex, Austria; Cristalia, Braz.; Du Pont, Canad.; Bristol-Myers Squibb, Denm.; Meda, Fin.; Bristol-Myers Squibb, Fr.; Du Pont, Hong Kong; Boots, Hong Kong; Du Pont, Irl.; Du Pont, Israel; Armstrong, Mex.; Du Pont, Norw.; Baxter, NZ; Sanofi Synthelabo, S.Afr.; Bristol-Myers Squibb, Spain; Bristol-Myers Squibb, Swed.; Boots, Thai.; Bristol-Myers Squibb, Thai.; Barr, USA.
Naltrexone hydrochloride (p.1046·1).
*Alcohol withdrawal syndrome; opioid withdrawal syndrome.*

**Revic** Alcon Cusi, Spain†.
Carbomer (p.1577·2).
*Dry eyes; eye irritation.*

**Revicain** Wiedemann, Ger.
Procaine hydrochloride (p.1383·2); vitamins (p.1417·1).
*Tonic.*

**Revicain comp** Wiedemann, Ger.
Procaine hydrochloride (p.1383·2); aescin (p.1648·2); minerals (p.1417·1).
*Tonic.*

**Revicain comp plus** Wiedemann, Ger.
Procaine hydrochloride (p.1383·2); aescin (p.1648·2); haematoporphyrin (p.1696·2); vitamins; minerals (p.1417·1).
*Tonic.*

**Revicon**
United American, Hong Kong; United American, Malaysia; United American, Singapore; Great Eastern, Thai.; United American, Thai.
Multivitamin and mineral preparation with yeast and methionine (p.1417·1).

**Revil** Tecnofarma, Chile.
Cyproheptadine hydrochloride (p.430·1); vitamins.
*Reduced appetite.*

**Revimine** Uniao Quimica, Braz.
Dopamine hydrochloride (p.907·1).
*Heart failure; hypotension.*

**Revion** Norma (Νορμα), Gr.
Ciprofloxacin hydrochloride (p.188·2).
*Bacterial infections.*

**Revirax** Blausiegel, Braz.
Zidovudine (p.658·2).
*HIV infection.*

**Revit** ICN, Canad.†.
Multivitamin preparation (p.1417·1).

**Revital**
Ranbaxy, Malaysia.
Multivitamin and mineral preparation with ginseng, choline, and methionine (p.1417·1).

Basi, Port.
Multivitamin preparation (p.1417·1).

**Revitaleyes** Allergan, Canad.†.
Polyvinyl alcohol (p.1581·1).
*Dry eyes.*

**Revitalizing** Crinos, Ital.
Glycolic acid (p.1147·3).
*Skin disorders.*

**Revitalose** UCB, Fr.
Ampoule A, magnesium aspartate (p.1227·3); L-leucine (p.1439·1); L-lysine hydrochloride (p.1439·2); L-phenylalanine (p.1443·1); L-valine (p.1451·2); ampoule B, sodium ascorbate (p.1460·2).
*Asthenia.*

**Revitalose C**
Note. This name is used for preparations of different composition.
UCB, Belg.
Amino acids and sodium ascorbate (p.1417·1).
*Tonic.*

Rivex, Canad.
Ascorbic acid (p.1460·2).
*Vitamin C supplement.*

UCB, Switz.
Amino acids; vitamin C (p.1417·1).
*Tonic.*

**Revitam** Biolab Sanus, Braz.
A range of multivitamin preparations with or without minerals (p.1417·1).

**Revitan** Ranbaxy, Thai.
Ginseng (p.1693·1); multivitamins and minerals (p.1417·1).
*Tonic.*

**Revitex** Gerbex, Canad.
Multivitamin preparation preparation with calcium and iron (p.1417·1).

**Revitonil** Lichtwer, UK.
Echinacea (p.1683·2); peppermint (p.1283·2); clove (p.1673·2); aniseed (p.1655·2); liquorice (p.1270·2); fennel (p.1687·2); eucalyptus (p.1686·1).
*Cold symptoms.*

**Revitonus C** Sabex, Canad.
Ascorbic acid (p.1460·2); suprarenal cortex extract (p.1110·1); testicular extract (p.1569·3); brain extract (p.1709·3).
*Vitamin C supplement.*

**Revivan**
Zambon, Braz.; AstraZeneca, Ital.
Dopamine hydrochloride (p.907·1).
*Heart failure; hypotension; shock.*

**Revive**
Note. This name is used for preparations of different composition.
Pfizer, NZ†.
Tetryzoline hydrochloride (p.1131·2); macrogol 400 (p.1709·1).
*Eye irritation.*

Allergan, UK†.
Carmellose (p.1577·3) (p.1164·2).
*Comfort drops for use with soft contact lenses.*

**Revivona** Nycomed, Austria.
Multivitamin preparation (p.1417·1).

**Revixil** Gador, Arg.
Stavudine (p.654·2).
*HIV infection.*

**Revocon** Sun, India.
Tetrabenazine (p.1752·2).
*Ballism; chorea; dyskinesias; dystonias.*

**Revolyt** Gunnar Kjems, Denm.
Glucose; potassium chloride; magnesium sulfate; sodium citrate; sodium chloride (p.1222·2).
*Diarrhoea; oral rehydration therapy.*

**Revulsan** Faria, Braz.
Papaverine diethylbarbiturate (p.1728·2); belladonna (p.479·1); pentetrazol (p.1592·1).
*Smooth muscle spasm.*

**Rewodina** AWD, Ger.
Diclofenac sodium (p.32·1).
*Gout; inflammation; musculoskeletal, joint, and soft-tissue disorders; pain.*

**Rex** MDM, Ital.
Calcium lactate gluconate (p.1225·3); calcium carbonate (p.1254·2).
*Bone disorders; hypocalcaemia.*

**Rexachlor** Be-Tabs, S.Afr.†.
Paracetamol (p.76·2); chlormezanone (p.675·1).
*Pain and associated tension.*

**Rexacin**
Unison, Hong Kong; Unison, Thai.
Norfloxacin (p.238·3).
*Bacterial infections.*

**Rexalgan** Dompe, Ital.
Tenoxicam (p.93·1).
*Musculoskeletal and joint disorders.*

**Rexall Daily Sunblock** Tanning Research, Canad.
*SPF 15:* Octinoxate (p.1154·3); oxybenzone (p.1154·3).
*Sunscreen.*

**Rexall Kids Daily Sunblock** Tanning Research, Canad.
*SPF 30:* Homosalate (p.1148·1); octinoxate (p.1154·3); octisalate (p.1154·3); oxybenzone (p.1154·3).
*Sunscreen.*

**Rexall Oil-Free Daily Sunblock** Tanning Research, Canad.
*SPF 30:* Octinoxate (p.1154·3); octisalate (p.1154·3); oxybenzone (p.1154·3).
*Sunscreen.*

**Rexall Sport Sunblock** Tanning Research, Canad.
*SPF 30:* Octinoxate (p.1154·3); octisalate (p.1154·3); oxybenzone (p.1154·3).
*Sunscreen.*

**Rexall Sunblock** Tanning Research, Canad.
*SPF 30:* Homosalate (p.1148·1); octinoxate (p.1154·3); octisalate (p.1154·3); oxybenzone (p.1154·3).
*Sunscreen.*

**Rexamat** Pharmacia, Arg.
Calcitriol (p.1461·2).
*Hypoparathyroidism; osteoporosis renal osteodystrophy; rickets.*

**Rexan** Ist. Chim. Inter., Ital.
Aciclovir (p.626·1).
*Herpesvirus infections.*

**Rexer** Organon, Spain.
Mirtazapine (p.307·3).
*Depression.*

**Rexgenta** Areu, Spain.
Gentamicin sulfate (p.217·1).
*Bacterial infections.*

**Rexichlor** Esoform, Ital.
Chlorhexidine gluconate (p.1173·2); benzalkonium chloride (p.1168·3).
*Skin disinfection.*

**Rexigen Forte** Ion, USA†.
Phendimetrazine tartrate (p.1592·1).

**Rexilen** Serra Pamies, Spain.
Doxycycline hyclate (p.206·2).
*Bacterial infections; malaria.*

**Rexiluven S** Novartis Consumer, Ger.
Aesculus (p.1648·2).
*Venous insufficiency.*

**Reximide** Duopharma, Hong Kong.
Loperamide hydrochloride (p.1271·1).
*Diarrhoea; ostomy management.*

**Rexitene** Roche, Austria†.
Guanabenz acetate (p.926·2).
*Hypertension.*

**Rexitol** Rekah, Israel.
Chloroxylenol (p.1177·2); terpineol (p.1752·2).
*Disinfection.*

**Rexivin** Collins, Mex.
Methocarbamol (p.1395·1).
*Inflammation.*

**Rexolate** Hyrex, USA.
Sodium thiosalicylate (p.90·2).
*Gout; pain; rheumatic fever.*

**Rexophtal N** Bausch & Lomb, Switz.
Phenylephrine hydrochloride (p.1126·3).
Formerly contained chlorhexidine gluconate and phenylephrine hydrochloride.
*Conjunctivitis.*

**Rexort** Takeda, Fr.
Citicoline (p.1672·3).
*Cerebrovascular disorders.*

**Rexorubia**
Homeocan, Canad.; Lehning, Fr.
Homoeopathic preparation.

**Reyataz**
Bristol-Myers Squibb, UK; Bristol-Myers Squibb, USA.
Atazanavir sulfate (p.629·1).
*HIV infection.*

**Rezamid**
Note. This name is used for preparations of different composition.
ICN, Arg.
Triamcinolone acetonide (p.1110·2); neomycin sulfate (p.235·1).
*Infected skin disorders.*

Summers, USA.
Resorcinol (p.1156·3); sulfur (p.1158·2).
*Acne.*

**Rezamid D, Rezamid F, Rezamid M** ICN, Arg.
Triamcinolone acetonide (p.1110·2).
*Skin disorders.*

**Rezulin**
Parke, Davis, Austral.†; Parke, Davis, Mex.†; Parke, Davis, USA†.
Troglitazone (p.348·2).
*Diabetes mellitus.*

**Rezult** Sun, India.
Rosiglitazone maleate (p.345·2).
*Diabetes mellitus.*

**RFG-Kit** Poen, Arg.
Fluorescein sodium (p.1689·1).
*Aid to eye examination.*

**R-Gel** Healthline, USA.
Capsaicin (p.24·2).

**R-Gen** Goldline, USA.
Iodinated glycerol (p.1122·3).
*Coughs.*

**R-Gene** Kabivitrum, USA.
Arginine hydrochloride (p.1421·1).
*Test to assess pituitary reserve for growth hormone.*

**Rhabarex B** Palmicol, Ger.†.
Bisacodyl (p.1251·3).
*Constipation; stool softener.*

**Rheaban Maximum Strength** Pfizer, USA.
Activated attapulgite (p.1251·1).
*Diarrhoea.*

**Rhefluin**
Kytta, Ger.†; Medika, Switz.
Amiloride hydrochloride (p.858·2); hydrochlorothiazide (p.933·2).
*Ascites; hypertension; oedema.*

**Rheila Medicated Cough Drops** Hilarys, Canad.†.
Liquorice (p.1270·2); menthol (p.1711·3).

**Rheila Stringiet N** Diedenhofen, Ger.†.
Benzalkonium chloride (p.1168·3).
*Mouth and throat infections.*

**Rhem** Andromaco, Chile.
Zaleplon (p.727·3).
*Insomnia.*

**Rhemofenax** Duopharma, Hong Kong.
Diclofenac sodium (p.32·1).
*Musculoskeletal and joint disorders.*

**Rhenus med** APS, Ger.
Ruscus aculeatus.
*Venous insufficiency.*

**Rheobral** Niverpharm, Fr.
Troxerutin (p.1688·3); vincamine (p.1764·2).
*Mental function impairment in the elderly.*

**Rheoflux** Niverpharm, Fr.
Troxerutin (p.1688·3).
*Haemorrhoids; venous insufficiency.*

**Rheofusin** Fresenius Kabi, Austria.
Dextran 40 (p.745·3) with electrolytes.
*Microcirculatory disorders; thrombosis prophylaxis.*

**Rheogen**
Note. This name is used for preparations of different composition.
Robugen, Ger.
Aloes (p.1248·2).
Formerly known as Rheogen N and contained rhubarb and aloes.
*Constipation.*

Robugen, Hong Kong†.
Rhubarb (p.1287·3); aloes (p.1248·2); belladonna (p.479·1).
*Constipation.*

**Rheohes** Braun, Ger.
Pentastarch (p.750·1).
*Circulatory disorders; plasma volume expansion.*

**Rheomacrodex**
Medical Specialties, Austral.†; Torrex, Austria; Braun, Braz.†; Medisan, Canad.†; Pharmalink, Denm.; Pharmacia Upjohn, Fr.†; Pharmalink, Ger.; IFET (ΙΦΕΤ), Gr.; Pharmacia Upjohn, Israel; Pisa, Mex.; Pharmalink, Norw.; Alliance, S.Afr.; Fresenius Kabi, Spain; Pharmalink, Swed.; Braun, Switz.; Cambridge, UK†; Pharmacia, USA.
Dextran 40 (p.745·3) in glucose or sodium chloride.
*Plasma volume expansion; thrombosis prophylaxis.*

**rheotromb** Curasan, Ger.
Urokinase (p.1018·2).
*Thromboembolic disorders.*

**Rhesogam**
Aventis Behring, Austria; Aventis Behring, Ger.
An anti-D immunoglobulin (p.1608·1).
*Prevention of rhesus sensitisation.*

**Rhesogamma**
Centeon, Mex.†; Aventis Behring, Norw.; Aventis Behring, Spain; Aventis Behring, Swed.
An anti-D immunoglobulin (p.1608·1).
*Prevention of rhesus sensitisation.*

**Rhesogamma P**
Aventis Pasteur, Chile; Statens Serum Institut, Denm.; Gerolimatos (Γερολυματος), Gr.
An anti-D immunoglobulin (p.1608·1).
*Prevention of rhesus sensitisation.*

**Rhesonativ**
Darrow, Braz.†; Pharmacia, Irl.; Pharmacia, Malaysia; Pharmacia Upjohn, Norw.†; Biovitrum, Swed.
An anti-D immunoglobulin (p.1608·1).
*Prevention of rhesus sensitisation.*

**Rhesugam** NBI, S.Afr.
An anti-D immunoglobulin (p.1608·1).
*Prevention of rhesus sensitisation.*

**Rhesuman**
Berna, Belg.†; Berna, Hong Kong†; Berna, Ital.†; Berna, Port.; Berna, Spain†; Berna, Switz.†; Berna, Thai.†.
An anti-D immunoglobulin (p.1608·1).
*Prevention of rhesus sensitisation.*

**Rheu** Vitasan, Austria.
Homoeopathic preparation.

**Rheubalmin** Hoernecke, Ger.†.
Diethylamine salicylate (p.34·1); benzyl nicotinate (p.21·2).
*Musculoskeletal and joint disorders; neuralgia.*

**Rheubalmin Bad** Hoernecke, Ger.
Methyl salicylate (p.59·3); isobornyl acetate; camphor (p.1665·3).
*Bath additive; circulatory disorders; musculoskeletal, joint, and soft-tissue disorders; neuralgia; respiratory-tract disorders.*

**Rheubalmin Bad Nico** Hoernecke, Ger.†.
Benzyl nicotinate (p.21·2).
*Bath additive; circulatory disorders; musculoskeletal and joint disorders; neuralgia.*

**Rheubalmin Indo** Hoernecke, Ger.
Indometacin (p.47·3).
*Musculoskeletal, joint, peri-articular, and soft-tissue disorders.*

**Rheubalmin N** Hoernecke, Ger.
Glycol salicylate (p.44·3).
*Musculoskeletal and joint disorders; neuralgia.*

**Rheubalmin Thermo** Hoernecke, Ger.
*Ointment:* Glycol salicylate (p.44·3); benzyl nicotinate (p.21·2).
*Topical solution*†*:* Glycol salicylate (p.44·3); benzyl nicotinate (p.21·2); camphor (p.1665·3).
*Musculoskeletal and joint disorders; neuralgia; peripheral vascular disorders.*

**Rheucastin** Pfluger, Ger.
Homoeopathic preparation.

**Rheucostan M** Hanosan, Ger.†.
Homoeopathic preparation.

**Rheufenac** Helvepharm, Switz.†.
Diclofenac sodium (p.32·1).
Now known as Diclofenac Helvepharm.
*Gout; inflammation; musculoskeletal, joint, and peri-articular disorders; oedema; pain; renal and biliary colic.*

**Rheuferm Phyto** Wiedemann, Ger.
Devil's claw root (p.28·2).
*Degenerative joint disorders.*

**Rheugesal** Mucos, Austria.
Diethylamine salicylate (p.34·1); flufenamic acid (p.43·2); myrtecaine (p.1381·3).
*Musculoskeletal, joint, peri-articular, and soft-tissue disorders.*

**Rheugesic** Medpro, S.Afr.
Piroxicam (p.84·2).
*Gout; musculoskeletal, joint, and soft-tissue disorders; pain.*

**Rheuma**
Note. This name is used for preparations of different composition.
Peithner, Austria.
Homoeopathic preparation.

Weleda, Austria.
Aconitum napellus (p.1646·3); arnica (p.1656·3); betula folium (p.1660·3); mandragora radix; formica; rosemary oil (p.1740·2).
*Musculoskeletal and joint disorders.*

**Rheuma Lindofluid** Lindopharm, Ger.†.
Flufenamic acid (p.43·2).
*Musculoskeletal, joint, peri-articular, and soft-tissue disorders.*

**Rheuma V + T Bad N** Spitzner, Ger.†.
Glycol salicylate (p.44·3); diethylamine salicylate (p.34·1); oleum pini sylvestris.
*Bath additive; cold symptoms; musculoskeletal, joint, peri-articular, and soft-tissue disorders; neuralgia.*

**RheumaASS** Ratiopharm, Austria.
Aspirin (p.15·1).
*Fever; pain; rheumatism.*

**Rheuma-Bad** Eu Rho, Ger.†.
Glycol salicylate (p.44·3); benzyl nicotinate (p.21·2); camphor (p.1665·3); diethylamine salicylate (p.34·1).
*Cold symptoms; musculoskeletal and joint disorders; neuralgia; peripheral vascular disorders.*

**Rheumabene** Merckle, Ger.
Dimethyl sulfoxide (p.1473·2).
*Musculoskeletal, joint, and peri-articular disorders.*

**Rheumacin**
Pacific, NZ; Hillcross, UK.
Indometacin (p.47·3).
*Fever; gout; inflammation; musculoskeletal, joint, and peri-articular disorders; pain.*

**Rheumadoron**
Weleda, Austria; Weleda, Fr.; Weleda, UK.
Homoeopathic preparation.

**Rheumadyn PMD** Plantamed, Ger.
Homoeopathic preparation.

**Rheuma-Gastreu R46** Reckeweg, Ger.
Homoeopathic preparation.

**Rheuma-Gel** Ratiopharm, Ger.
Etofenamate (p.38·1).
*Musculoskeletal, joint, and soft-tissue disorders.*

**Rheuma-Hek** Strathmann, Ger.
Urtica (p.1762·1).
*Musculoskeletal and joint disorders.*

**Rheuma-Hevert** Hevert, Ger.
Homoeopathic preparation.

**Rheumajecta** Enzypharm, Neth.†.
Sulfate adenyltransferase; chondroitin sulfotransferase; catalase (p.1668·3).
*Rheumatic disorders.*

**Rheumakaps** Steigerwald, Ger.
Salix (p.87·3).
*Fever; headache; musculoskeletal and joint disorders.*

**Rheumalan** Hilarys, Canad.
Methyl salicylate (p.59·3); camphor (p.1665·3); menthol (p.1711·3); belladonna (p.479·1); capsicum oleoresin (p.1667·1); croton oil (p.28·2); eucalyptus oil (p.1686·2); expressed mustard oil (p.1718·2); salicylic acid (p.1157·1).

**Rheumaliment N** Galenika, Ger.†.
Camphor (p.1665·3); eucalyptus oil (p.1686·2); turpentine oil (p.1760·1).
*Musculoskeletal and joint pain.*

**Rheuma-Liquidum** Eu Rho, Ger.†.
Glycol salicylate (p.44·3); benzyl nicotinate (p.21·2); nonivamide (p.67·2).
*Musculoskeletal, joint, peri-articular, and soft-tissue disorders; neuralgia; peripheral vascular disorders.*

**rheuma-loges** Loges, Ger.
Homoeopathic preparation.

**Rheumanox** Charoen, Thai.
Ibuprofen (p.45·3).
*Gout; musculoskeletal, joint, and peri-articular disorders.*

**Rheuma-Pasc** Pascoe, Ger.
Homoeopathic preparation.

**Rheuma-Pasc N** Pascoe, Ger.†.
Rosemary oil (p.1740·2); methyl salicylate (p.59·3); hamamelis (p.1696·3).
*Neuralgia; neuritis.*

**Rheuma-Plantina** Plantina, Ger.†.
Homoeopathic preparation.

**Rheumaplast N** Beiersdorf, Ger.†.
Cayenne pepper (p.1667·1).
*Musculoskeletal and joint disorders.*

**Rheumasalbe** CT, Ger.
Nonivamide (p.67·2); benzyl nicotinate (p.21·2); eucalyptus oil (p.1686·2).
*Musculoskeletal, joint, and soft-tissue disorders; neuralgia.*

**Rheuma-Salbe**
Note. This name is used for preparations of different composition.
Stada, Ger.
Glycol salicylate (p.44·3); benzyl nicotinate (p.21·2).
*Musculoskeletal, joint, and soft-tissue disorders; peripheral vascular disorders.*

Twardy, Ger.†.
Camphor (p.1665·3); menthol (p.1711·3); clove oil (p.1673·3).
*Rheumatic disorders; sports injuries.*

**Rheuma-Salbe N** Lichtenstein, Ger.
Glycol salicylate (p.44·3); benzyl nicotinate (p.21·2).
*Musculoskeletal, joint, and soft-tissue disorders; peripheral vascular disorders.*

**Rheumasan** Kwizda, Austria.
Salicylic acid (p.1157·1); sodium humate; norway spruce oil; camphor (p.1665·3); eucalyptus oil (p.1686·2); menthol (p.1711·3).
*Bath additive; cold symptoms; musculoskeletal and joint disorders.*

**Rheumasan Moor-Bad S** Sanofi Synthelabo, Ger.
Sodium humate.
Rheumasan Moor-Bad formerly contained diethylamine salicylate and sodium humate.
*Bath additive; musculoskeletal and joint disorders.*

**Rheumasan N** Sanofi Synthelabo, Ger.
*Ointment*†*:* Salicylic acid (p.1157·1); methyl nicotinate (p.59·2).
*Bruising; muscle, joint, and nerve disorders.*
*Topical rub:* Salicylic acid (p.1157·1); benzyl nicotinate (p.21·2).
*Musculoskeletal, joint, and soft-tissue disorders; neuralgia.*

**Rheumaselect** Dreluso, Ger.
Homoeopathic preparation.

**Rheuma-Sern** Truw, Ger.
Devil's claw root (p.28·2).
*Musculoskeletal and joint disorders.*

**Rheumasit** Medice, Ger.
Dexamethasone (p.1097·1); benzyl nicotinate (p.21·2).
*Musculoskeletal, joint, peri-articular, and soft-tissue disorders; neuralgia.*

**Rheumasol** Peter Black, UK†.
Guaiacum resin (p.1696·2); prickly ash bark (p.1766·3).
*Rheumatic and muscular pain and stiffness.*

**Rheumatab Salicis** Schuck, Ger.
Salix (p.87·3).
*Headache; rheumatic disorders.*

**Rheumatabletten N** Cosmochema, Ger.
Homoeopathic preparation.

**Rheumatac** Sovereign, UK.
Diclofenac sodium (p.32·1).
*Gout; inflammation; musculoskeletal, joint, and peri-articular disorders; pain.*

**Rheuma-Teufelskralle HarpagoMega** Twardy, Ger.†.
Devil's claw root (p.28·2).
*Appetite loss; dyspepsia; musculoskeletal and joint disorders.*

**Rheumatex** Wampole, USA.
Test for rheumatoid factor in serum.

**Rheumatic Pain** Cantassium Co., UK.
Guaiacum resin (p.1696·2); taraxacum (p.1751·3); celery (p.1669·1); menyanthes (p.1712·1).
*Muscle and joint pain.*

**Rheumatic Pain Relief** Herbal Concepts, UK.
Menyanthes (p.1712·1); guaiacum resin (p.1696·2); capsicum (p.1667·1); capsicum oleoresin (p.1667·1); celery oil (p.1669·1).
*Musculoskeletal and joint pain.*

**Rheumatic Pain Remedy** Potter's, UK.
Menyanthes (p.1712·1); lappa root (p.1704·3); achillea (p.1646·2); guaiacum resin (p.1696·2).
*Musculoskeletal and joint disorders.*

**Rheumatic Pain Tablets** Healthcrafts, UK†.
Guaiacum resin (p.1696·2); menyanthes (p.1712·1); celery seed (p.1669·1).
*Rheumatic pain.*

**Rheumatica** Nelson, UK.
Homoeopathic preparation.

**Rheumatism Rhus Tox** Homeocan, Canad.
Homoeopathic preparation.

**Rheumaton**
Carter-Wallace, Switz.†; Wampole, USA.
Test for rheumatoid factor in serum or synovial fluid.

**Rheumatrex**
Wyeth-Ayerst, Canad.†; Stada, USA.
Methotrexate (p.568·2) or methotrexate sodium (p.568·3).
*Psoriasis; rheumatoid arthritis.*

**Rheumatropfen N** Cosmochema, Ger.
Homoeopathic preparation.

**Rheumavek** Faran, Gr.
Diclofenac sodium (p.32·1).
*Dysmenorrhoea; inflammation; musculoskeletal and joint disorders; pain.*

**Rheumax** Hoernecke, Ger.†.
Methyl salicylate (p.59·3).
*Musculoskeletal and joint disorders.*

**Rheumed** Phytomed, Switz.
Homoeopathic preparation.

**Rheumeda** Madaus, Ger.
Homoeopathic preparation.

**Rheumesser** Gerot, Austria.
Kebuzone (p.51·1); salamidacetic acid (p.87·3); dexamethasone (p.1097·1); cyanocobalamin (p.1458·2) or hydroxocobalamin acetate (p.1458·2).
Lidocaine (p.1377·3) is included in this preparation to alleviate the pain of injection.
*Musculoskeletal and joint disorders.*

**Rheumex** Gebro, Austria.
Glycol salicylate (p.44·3); benzyl nicotinate (p.21·2); allantoin (p.1141·3).
*Musculoskeletal and joint disorders; sports injuries.*

**Rheumichthol Bad** Ichthyol, Ger.†.
Light ammonium bituminosulphonate (p.1148·2); glycol salicylate (p.44·3); diethylamine salicylate (p.34·1).
*Bath additive; musculoskeletal and joint disorders.*

**Rheumitin** Krewel, Ger.
Piroxicam (p.84·2).
*Gout; musculoskeletal, joint, and soft-tissue disorders.*

**Rheumodoron 1** Weleda, Ger.
Homoeopathic preparation.

**Rheumodoron 2** Weleda, Ger.
Homoeopathic preparation.

**Rheumodoron 102 A** Weleda, Ger.
Homoeopathic preparation.

**Rheumon**
Kolassa, Austria; Tropon, Ger.; Drossapharm, Switz.
Etofenamate (p.38·1).
*Inflammation; musculoskeletal, joint, peri-articular, and soft-tissue disorders; pain.*

**Rheumox**
Goldshield, Irl.; Goldshield, UK.
Azapropazone (p.20·1).
*Acute gout; ankylosing spondylitis; rheumatoid arthritis.*

**Rheunervol N** Riemser, Ger.
Camphor (p.1665·3).
*Musculoskeletal and joint disorders.*

**Rheutrop** Kolassa, Austria.
Acemetacin (p.11·3).
*Gout; inflammation; musculoskeletal and joint disorders; thrombophlebitis; vasculitis.*

**Rhewlin**
Upha, Malaysia; Beacons, Singapore.
Diclofenac diethylamine (p.32·1) or diclofenac sodium (p.32·1).
*Inflammation; musculoskeletal, joint, and soft-tissue disorders; pain.*

**Rhinaaxia**
Agepha, Austria; Thea, Fr.; Proel, Gr.; Inpharzam, Switz.
Magnesium isospaglumate (p.1702·2).
*Allergic rhinitis.*

Allergan-Frumtost, Braz.†; Zambon, Ital.
Sodium spaglumate.
*Allergic rhinitis.*

**Rhinadine** Farmaline, Thai.
Brompheniramine maleate (p.426·1); pseudoephedrine hydrochloride (p.1129·2).
*Nasal congestion.*

**Rhinadvil** Whitehall, Fr.
Ibuprofen (p.45·3); pseudoephedrine hydrochloride (p.1129·2).
*Fever; headache; rhinitis with nasal congestion.*

**Rhinal** Ahimsa, Arg.
Naphazoline (p.1124·3).
*Nasal congestion.*

**Rhinalar**
Roche, Canad.; Roche, Hong Kong†.
Flunisolide (p.1101·1).
*Allergic rhinitis.*

**Rhinall** Scherer, USA.
Phenylephrine hydrochloride (p.1126·3).
*Nasal congestion.*

**Rhinallergy** Boiron, Fr.
Homoeopathic preparation.

**Rhinamide**
Note. This name is used for preparations of different composition.
Vitalpharma, Belg.†.
Diphenylpyraline hydrochloride (p.432·3); sulfanilamide (p.263·2); ephedrine hydrochloride (p.1120·1).
*Nasal congestion.*

Bailly, Fr.
Ephedrine hydrochloride (p.1120·1); benzoic acid (p.1169·3).
*Congestion of the nose and throat.*

**Rhinar** TP, Thai.
Carbinoxamine maleate (p.426·3); pseudoephedrine hydrochloride (p.1129·2).
*Cold symptoms; rhinitis; upper respiratory-tract congestion.*

**Rhinaris** Pharmascience, Canad.
Macrogol (p.1708·2); propylene glycol (p.1735·2).
*Rhinitis.*

**Rhinaris Saline** Pharmascience, Canad.
Sodium chloride (p.1233·3).
*Nasal disorders.*

**Rhinatate** Major, USA.
Phenylephrine tannate (p.1127·2); chlorphenamine tannate (p.428·1); mepyramine tannate (p.437·1).
*Upper respiratory-tract symptoms.*

**Rhinatate-NF** Major, USA.
Phenylephrine tannate (p.1127·2); chlorphenamine tannate (p.428·1).
*Upper respiratory-tract disorders.*

**Rhinathiol**
Note. This name is used for preparations of different composition.
Sanofi Synthelabo, Fr.
Biclotymol (p.1171·1).
*Mouth and throat infections.*

Sanofi Synthelabo OTC, Fr.; Sanofi Synthelabo, Hong Kong; Sanofi Synthelabo, Malaysia; Lorex Synthelabo, Neth.†; Sanofi Synthelabo, Singapore; Synthelabo, Switz.; Sanofi Synthelabo, Thai.
Carbocisteine (p.1116·2).
*Otitis media; respiratory-tract disorders associated with increased or viscous mucus; sinusitis.*

**Rhinathiol Antirhinitis** Sanofi Synthelabo, Belg.
Phenylephrine hydrochloride (p.1126·3); chlorphenamine maleate (p.427·3).
*Rhinitis; sinusitis.*

**Rhinathiol Promethazine**
Sanofi Synthelabo OTC, Fr.; Sanofi Synthelabo, Hong Kong; Sanofi Synthelabo, Malaysia; Sanofi Synthelabo, Singapore†; Synthelabo, Switz.
Carbocisteine (p.1116·2); promethazine hydrochloride (p.439·1).
*Coughs.*

**Rhinathiol Tosse Seca** Sanofi Synthelabo, Port.†.
Dextromethorphan hydrobromide (p.1117·3).
*Coughs.*

**Rhinathiol Toux Seche** Sanofi Synthelabo OTC, Fr.†.
Dextromethorphan hydrobromide (p.1117·3).
*Coughs.*

**Rhinathiol Toux Seche Pholcodine** Sanofi Synthelabo OTC, Fr.
Pholcodine (p.1128·3).
*Coughs.*

**RhinATP** Aerocid, Fr.†.
Adenosine triphosphate, disodium salt (p.1648·1); sulfasuccinamide (p.264·1).
*Infections of the nose and throat.*

**Rhinedrine** Cooperation Pharmaceutique, Fr.
Benzododecinium bromide (p.1170·2).
*Nose and throat infections.*

**Rhinedrine Lubricant** Jamieson, Canad.†.
Carbowax; propylene glycol (p.1735·2).

**Rhinedrine Moisturizing** Jamieson, Canad.
Glycerol (p.1694·3); propylene glycol (p.1735·2).

**Rhinex**
Note. This name is used for preparations of different composition.
Wernigerode, Ger.
Naphazoline hydrochloride (p.1124·3).
*Nasal congestion; rhinitis; sinusitis.*

Prima, Thai.
Carbocisteine (p.1116·2).
*Coughs associated with increased or viscous mucus.*

**Rhinidine** Pfizer Consumer, Belg.
Xylometazoline hydrochloride (p.1132·2).
*Nasal congestion and irritation.*

**Rhinipan** Pharmacal, Switz.†.
Phenylephrine hydrochloride (p.1126·3); dequalinium diacetate (p.1178·1); chlorhexidine gluconate (p.1173·2).
*Catarrh; rhinitis; sinusitis.*

**Rhiniramine** DHA, Singapore.
Dexchlorpheniramine maleate (p.427·3).
*Hypersensitivity reactions.*

**Rhinirex** Irex, Fr.†.
Beclometasone dipropionate (p.1091·1).
*Rhinitis.*

**Rhinisan** Alcon, Ger.
Triamcinolone acetonide (p.1110·2).
*Allergic rhinitis.*

**Rhinitisan** Bioforce, Switz.
Homoeopathic preparation.

**Rhinivict** Fujisawa, Ger.
Beclometasone dipropionate (p.1091·1).
*Rhinitis.*

**Rhinobeta** Betapharm, Ger.
Electrolyte solution (p.1217·1).
*Nasal disorders.*

**Rhinobiotal** Martin, Fr.†.
Framycetin sulfate (p.215·1).
*Nose and throat infections.*

**Rhinocap**
Note. This name is used for preparations of different composition.
Grossmann, Hong Kong; Grossmann, Switz.
Phenylephrine hydrochloride (p.1126·3); dimenhydrinate (p.431·1); caffeine (p.782·1).
*Allergic rhinitis; cold symptoms; nasal congestion; sinus congestion.*

Inibsa, Spain.
Phenylephrine hydrochloride (p.1126·3); carbinoxamine maleate (p.426·3).
*Nasal congestion.*

**Rhinocaps**
Note. This name is used for preparations of different composition.
Vemedia, Neth.†.
Camphor (p.1665·3); chlorothymol (p.1177·2); cineole (p.1672·1); menthol (p.1711·3); terpineol (p.1752·2).
*Cold symptoms.*

Ferndale, USA†.
Phenylpropanolamine hydrochloride (p.1127·3); aspirin (p.15·1); paracetamol (p.76·2).
*Upper respiratory-tract symptoms.*

**Rhinocillin B** Medicopharm, Austria†.
Bacitracin (p.161·3).

**Rhinoclir**
Note. This name is used for preparations of different composition.
Febena, Ger.
Dexpanthenol (p.1727·2).
*Nasal disorders.*

Agis, Israel.
Oxymetazoline hydrochloride (p.1126·1).
*Nasal congestion.*

**Rhinocort**
Note. This name is used for preparations of different composition.
AstraZeneca, Austral.; AstraZeneca, Austria; AstraZeneca, Belg.; AstraZeneca, Canad.; AstraZeneca, Denm.; AstraZeneca, Fin.; AstraZeneca, Fr.; AstraZeneca, Hong Kong; AstraZeneca, India; AstraZeneca, Irl.; AstraZeneca, Ital.; AstraZeneca, Malaysia; Astra, Mex.; AstraZeneca, Neth.; AstraZeneca, Norw.; AstraZeneca, NZ†; Astra, S.Afr.; AstraZeneca, Singapore; AstraZeneca, Spain; Draco, Swed.; AstraZeneca, Switz.; AstraZeneca, Thai.; AstraZeneca, UK; Astra, USA.
Budesonide (p.1094·2).
*Nasal polyps; rhinitis.*

Agis, Israel; Teijin, Jpn.
Beclometasone dipropionate (p.1091·1).
*Rhinitis.*

**Rhinocortol** AstraZeneca, Austria.
Budesonide (p.1094·2).
*Nasal polyps; rhinitis.*

**Rhinocure** Medibel, Switz.†.
Polysorbate 80 (p.1415·2); sodium chloride (p.1233·3); matricaria (p.1669·3); benzethonium chloride (p.1169·2).
*Rhinopharyngeal disorders.*

**Rhinocure Simplex** Medibel, Switz.†.
Polysorbate 80 (p.1415·2); sodium chloride (p.1233·3); benzethonium chloride (p.1169·2).
*Rhinopharyngeal disorders.*

**Rhinodex** INQ, Braz.†.
Naphazoline (p.1124·3); benzalkonium chloride (p.1168·3).
*Nasal congestion.*

**Rhinodoron** Weleda, Fr.
Sodium chloride (p.1233·3); potassium chloride (p.1232·2); aloe vera (p.1141·3).
*Nasal cleansing; nasal dryness.*

**Rhinodrin** Montavit, Austria.
Diphenhydramine hydrochloride (p.431·3); naphazoline hydrochloride (p.1124·3).
*Rhinitis.*

**Rhinofeb** Martin, Fr.†.
Paracetamol (p.76·2); chlorphenamine maleate (p.427·3); phenylpropanolamine hydrochloride (p.1127·3).
*Cold symptoms.*

**Rhinofebral**
Martin, Fr.; Martin, Switz.
Paracetamol (p.76·2); chlorphenamine maleate (p.427·3); ascorbic acid (p.1460·2).
*Rhinopharyngeal disorders.*

**Rhinofebryl** Aventis, Belg.
Chlorphenamine maleate (p.427·3); paracetamol (p.76·2).
*Rhinitis with fever and/or headache.*

**Rhinofluimucil** Zambon, Fr.
Acetylcysteine (p.1112·3); tuaminoheptane sulfate (p.1132·1); benzalkonium chloride (p.1168·3).
*Rhinopharyngeal congestion.*

**Rhino-Gastreu N R49** Reckeweg, Ger.
Homoeopathic preparation.

**Rhinogen** IBSA, Switz.
Sodium hyaluronate (p.1697·3).
*Nasal dryness.*

**Rhinoguttae Argenti diacetylotannici proteinici** Leyh, Ger.
Silver protein acetyl tannate (p.1746·2).
*Cold symptoms.*

**Rhinoguttae Dexamethasoni cum Naphazolino** Leyh, Ger.
Dexamethasone (p.1097·1); naphazoline hydrochloride (p.1124·3).
*Cold symptoms; rhinitis.*

**Rhinoguttae pro Infantibus N** Leyh, Ger.
Silver protein acetyl tannate (p.1746·2).
Rhinoguttae pro Infantibus formerly contained ephedrine hydrochloride and silver protein acetyl tannate.
*Bacterial nose infections.*

**Rhinohist** Seng, Thai.
Carbinoxamine maleate (p.426·3); pseudoephedrine hydrochloride (p.1129·2).
*Allergic rhinitis; hay fever; upper respiratory-tract congestion.*

**Rhino-Lacteol** Lacteol, Fr.†.
*Lactobacillus acidophilus* (p.1704·2).
*Infections of the nose and throat.*

**Rhinolar-EX** McGregor, USA†.
Phenylpropanolamine hydrochloride (p.1127·3); chlorphenamine maleate (p.427·3).
*Upper respiratory-tract symptoms.*

**Rhinolast**
Astra, Ger.†; Stern, Ger.†; Orion, Irl.; Asta Medica, Israel; 3M, NZ†; Mer-National, S.Afr.; Viatris, UK.
Azelastine hydrochloride (p.425·2).
*Allergic rhinitis.*

**Rhinolex** Remek, Gr.
Ephedrine hydrochloride (p.1120·1).
*Nasal congestion.*

**Rhinomer**
Novartis Consumer, Ger.; Novartis Consumer, Port.; Novartis Consumer, Switz.; Novartis Consumer, UK†.
Isotonic sea water (p.1233·3).
*Nasal disorders.*

**Rhino-Mex** Charton, Canad.†.
Naphazoline hydrochloride (p.1124·3); amylocaine hydrochloride (p.1370·2).
*Nasal congestion.*

**Rhino-Mex-N** Charton, Canad.†.
Naphazoline hydrochloride (p.1124·3).
*Nasal congestion.*

**Rhinon** Petrasch, Austria.
*Nasal ointment:* Naphazoline hydrochloride (p.1124·3); sulfadiazine (p.258·2).
*Rhinitis; sinusitis.*

*Nose drops:* Naphazoline hydrochloride (p.1124·3).
*Rhinitis.*

**Rhinoperd** Agepha, Austria.
Naphazoline hydrochloride (p.1124·3).
*Aid in rhinoscopy; rhinitis; sinusitis.*

**Rhinoperd comp** Agepha, Austria.
Naphazoline hydrochloride (p.1124·3); diphenhydramine hydrochloride (p.431·3).
*Cold symptoms; rhinitis.*

**Rhinophen-C** Maxi, Thai.
Brompheniramine maleate (p.426·1); vitamin C (p.1460·2).
*Hypersensitivity reactions.*

**Rhinopront**
Note. This name is used for preparations of different composition.
Pfizer, Austria; Mack, Belg.; Grunenthal, Chile; Mack, Illert., Ger.; Mack, Hong Kong; Mack, Malaysia; Mack, Singapore; Mack, Switz.; Mack, Thai.
*Capsules:* Carbinoxamine maleate (p.426·3); phenylephrine hydrochloride (p.1126·3).
*Cold symptoms; hay fever; rhinitis; sinusitis.*

Pfizer, Austria; Mack, Illert., Ger.; Mack, Hong Kong; Mack, Singapore†; Mack, Switz.; Mack, Thai.†.
*Syrup:* Phenylpropanolamine polistirex (p.1128·2); carbinoxamine polistirex (p.426·3).
*Cold symptoms; hay fever; rhinitis; sinusitis.*

Grunenthal, Chile.
*Oral suspension:* Carbinoxamine maleate (p.426·3); phenylpropanolamine (p.1127·3).
*Cold and influenza symptoms; rhinitis; sinusitis.*

Mack, Illert., Ger.
*Nasal spray:* Tetryzoline hydrochloride (p.1131·2).
*Catarrh; colds; hay fever.*

**Rhinopront Top** Mack, Switz.
Tetryzoline hydrochloride (p.1131·2).
*Rhinopharyngeal disorders.*

**Rhinopten** Debat, Fr.†.
Antigens of: *Staphylococcus aureus* 634, 636; *Streptococcus* 147, 155 *Streptococcus pneumoniae* 209; *Moraxella catarrhalis* 987.
*Disorders of the ear, nose, and throat.*

**Rhinosept** Delta, Braz.
Naphazoline hydrochloride (p.1124·3); diphenhydramine hydrochloride (p.431·3); neomycin sulfate (p.235·1).
*Nasal congestion.*

**Rhinoside** Biomedica-Chemica, Gr.
Budesonide (p.1094·2).
*Allergic rhinitis.*

**Rhinosol** AstraZeneca, Denm.
Budesonide (p.1094·2).
*Hay fever.*

**Rhinosovil** Eu Rho, Ger.
Naphazoline nitrate (p.1124·3); pheniramine maleate (p.438·3).
*Nasal congestion; rhinitis.*

**Rhinospray**
Boehringer Ingelheim, Belg.; Boehringer Ingelheim, Ger.; Boehringer Ingelheim, Port.; Fher, Spain.
Tramazoline hydrochloride (p.1131·3).
*Nasal congestion; otitis media; sinusitis.*

**Rhinospray Antialergico** Fher, Spain.
Tramazoline hydrochloride (p.1131·3); chlorphenamine maleate (p.427·3).
*Nasal congestion.*

**Rhinospray Atlantik** Boehringer Ingelheim, Ger.
Sea water (p.1233·3).
*Nasal disorders.*

**Rhinospray Plus**
Boehringer Ingelheim, Austria; Boehringer Ingelheim, Ger.
Tramazoline hydrochloride (p.1131·3); cineole (p.1672·1); menthol (p.1711·3); camphor (p.1665·3).
*Nasal congestion.*

**Rhino-stas** Stada, Ger.†.
Xylometazoline hydrochloride (p.1132·2).
*Rhinitis; sinusitis.*

**Rhinostop** IBSA, Switz.
Xylometazoline hydrochloride (p.1132·2).
*Otitis media; rhinitis; sinusitis.*

**Rhino-Sulfuryl** Richelet, Fr.
Sodium thiosulfate (p.1053·3); ephedrine hydrochloride (p.1120·1).
*Rhinopharyngeal congestion.*

**Rhinosyn** Great Southern, USA.
Pseudoephedrine hydrochloride (p.1129·2); chlorphenamine maleate (p.427·3).
*Upper respiratory-tract symptoms.*

**Rhinosyn-DM** Great Southern, USA.
Pseudoephedrine hydrochloride (p.1129·2); chlorphenamine maleate (p.427·3); dextromethorphan hydrobromide (p.1117·3).
*Coughs and cold symptoms.*

**Rhinosyn-DMX** Great Southern, USA.
Dextromethorphan hydrobromide (p.1117·3); guaifenesin (p.1122·1).
*Coughs.*

**Rhinosyn-X** Great Southern, USA.
Pseudoephedrine hydrochloride (p.1129·2); dextromethorphan hydrobromide (p.1117·3); guaifenesin (p.1122·1).
*Coughs.*

**Rhinothricinol** Plan, Switz.
Tyrothricin (p.275·1); eucalyptus oil (p.1686·2).
*Rhinopharyngeal infections.*

**Rhinoton plus** Krewel, Ger.
Sea salt (p.1233·3).
*Nasal dryness.*

**Rhinotrophyl** Jolly-Jatel, Fr.
Thenoate monoethanolamine (p.269·2).
Formerly contained thenoate monoethanolamine and framycetin sulfate.
*Infections of the nose and throat.*

**Rhinotussal**
Note. This name is used for preparations of different composition.
Mack, Illert., Ger.; Mack, Switz.
*Capsules:* Phenylephrine hydrochloride (p.1126·3); carbinoxamine maleate (p.426·3); dextromethorphan hydrobromide (p.1117·3).
*Coughs and associated respiratory-tract disorders.*

Mack, Illert., Ger.; Mack, Switz.
*Syrup:* Phenylpropanolamine resin (p.1128·2); carbinoxamine resin (p.426·3); dextromethorphan resin (p.1118·1).
*Coughs and associated respiratory-tract disorders.*

Mack, Thai.†.
Phenylpropanolamine polistirex (p.1128·2); carbinoxamine polistirex (p.426·3); dextromethorphan polistirex (p.1118·1).
*Coughs; rhinitis.*

**Rhinovac** Darrow, Braz.
Antigen extracts (p.1650·1).
*Allergen immunotherapy.*

**Rhinovalon** Almirall, Belg.
Tixocortol pivalate (p.1110·1).
*Rhinitis.*

**Rhinovalon Neomycine** Almirall, Belg.
Tixocortol pivalate (p.1110·1); neomycin sulfate (p.235·1).
*Infective rhinitis.*

**Rhinovent** Boehringer Ingelheim, Switz.
Ipratropium bromide (p.787·1).
*Rhinitis.*

**Rhinovis** CTI, Israel.
Carbinoxamine maleate (p.426·3); phenylephrine hydrochloride (p.1126·3).
*Rhinitis; sinusitis.*

**Rhinox** Nycomed, Norw.
Oxymetazoline hydrochloride (p.1126·1).
*Nasal congestion.*

**Rhinureflex** Boots Healthcare, Fr.
Ibuprofen (p.45·3); pseudoephedrine hydrochloride (p.1129·2).
*Fever; headache; nasal congestion; rhinitis.*

**Rhinyl** Pierre Fabre Sante, Fr.†.
Framycetin sulfate (p.215·1); sodium propionate (p.408·1).
*Colds.*

**Rhodacine** Rhoxalpharma, Canad.
Indometacin (p.47·3).
*Gout; musculoskeletal and joint disorders.*

**Rhodamer** Rhone-Poulenc Rorer, Mex.†.
Methotrexate (p.568·2).

**Rhodiaprox** Rhodiapharm, Canad.†.
Naproxen (p.65·1).
*Fever; inflammation; pain.*

**Rhodine** Rhone-Poulenc Rorer, Belg.†.
Aspirin (p.15·1).
*Dental pain; fever; headache; rheumatic pain.*

**Rhodis** Rhodiapharm, Canad.
Ketoprofen (p.51·2).
*Musculoskeletal and joint disorders.*

**Rhodogil** Aventis, Spain.
Spiramycin (p.255·3); metronidazole (p.607·2).
*Bacterial infections.*

**RhoGAM**
Ortho, Hong Kong; Ortho Diagnostic, USA.
An anti-D immunoglobulin (p.1608·1).
*Prevention of rhesus sensitisation.*

**Rhoival** Byk Tosse, Ger.; Byk Gulden, Ger.
Agrimony (p.1649·1); solidago virgaurea (p.1748·3); hypericum (p.299·1); shepherd's purse (p.1744·1); arnica (p.1656·3); valerian (p.1762·2).
*Urinary-tract disorders.*

**Rhonal**
Rhone-Poulenc Rorer, Belg.†; Rhone-Poulenc Rorer, Israel†; Rhone-Poulenc Rorer, Mex.†; Aventis, Spain.
Aspirin (p.15·1).
*Fever; musculoskeletal, joint and peri-articular disorders; pain; thromboembolism prophylaxis.*

**Rhonuracil** Rhone-Poulenc Rorer, Mex.†.
Fluorouracil (p.554·2).

**Rhophylac**
ZLB, Switz.; ZLB, UK.
An anti-D immunoglobulin (p.1608·1).
*Prevention of rhesus sensitisation.*

**Rhotral** Rhodiapharm, Canad.
Acebutolol hydrochloride (p.848·1).
*Angina pectoris; hypertension.*

**Rhotrimine** Rhodiapharm, Canad.
Trimipramine maleate (p.320·2).
*Depression.*

**Rhovail** Rhodiapharm, Canad.
Ketoprofen (p.51·2).
*Musculoskeletal and joint disorders.*

**Rhovane** Rhodiapharm, Canad.
Zopiclone (p.729·3).
*Insomnia.*

**Rhuaka** Anglian, UK†.
Cascara (p.1255·1); rhubarb (p.1287·3); senna (p.1288·2).
*Constipation.*

**Rhuli Gel** Rydelle, USA†.
Benzyl alcohol (p.1170·2); menthol (p.1711·3); camphor (p.1665·3).
*Minor skin irritation.*

**Rhuli Spray** Rydelle, USA†.
Calamine (p.1144·1); camphor (p.1665·3); benzocaine (p.1370·3).
*Minor skin irritation.*

**Rhum Creosotado** Dansk-Flama, Braz.
Creosote (p.1117·2); sodium hypophosphite; calcium hypophosphite (p.1226·3); benzoic acid (p.1169·3).
*Respiratory-tract congestion.*

**Rhumagrip** Cooperation Pharmaceutique, Fr.
Paracetamol (p.76·2); pseudoephedrine hydrochloride (p.1129·2).
*Cold symptoms.*

**Rhumalgan** Sandoz, UK.
Diclofenac sodium (p.32·1).
*Gout; inflammation; musculoskeletal, joint, and periarticular disorders; pain.*

**Rhumanol** TO-Chemicals, Thai.
Diclofenac diethylamine (p.32·1).
*Musculoskeletal, joint, and peri-articular disorders.*

**Rhumantin** Gea, Denm.†.
Penicillamine (p.1046·3).
*Cystinuria; heavy metal poisoning; rheumatoid arthritis; Wilson's disease.*

**Rhumatisme** Gerbex, Canad.
Methyl salicylate (p.59·3); camphor (p.1665·3); capsicum oleoresin (p.1667·1); trimethylcyclohexanol.
Formerly known as Rheumatisme.

**Rhume** Pharmacard, Switz.
Xylometazoline hydrochloride (p.1132·2).
*Nasal congestion.*

**Rhus Med Complex** Dynamit, Austria.
Homoeopathic preparation.

**Rhus Opodeldoc** *Knop, Chile.*
Camphor (p.1665·3); rosemary (p.1740·2); thyme (p.1755·2); rhus toxicodendron (p.1738·1); ammonia (p.1653·3).
*Musculoskeletal, joint, and soft-tissue disorders.*

**Rhus toxicodendron Oligoplex** *Madaus, Ger.*
Homoeopathic preparation.

**Rhus-Rheuma-Gel N** *DHU, Ger.*
Rhus toxicodendron (p.1738·1); ledum; comfrey (p.1675·2).
*Muscle and joint disorders.*

**Rhythmocor** *Lannacher, Austria.*
Propafenone hydrochloride (p.988·3).
*Arrhythmias.*

**Rhythmy** *Shionogi, Jpn.*
Rilmazafone hydrochloride.
*Insomnia; premedication.*

**Riabal**
*Chiesi, Fr.; Ibi, Ital.; Fujisawa, Thai.*
Prifinium bromide (p.488·2).
*Smooth muscle spasm.*

**Riacen** *Promedica, Ital.*
Piroxicam (p.84·2).
*Musculoskeletal, joint, and peri-articular disorders.*

**Riamet**
*Novartis, Austral.; Novartis, Austria; Novartis, Ger.; Novartis, Hong Kong; Novartis, Norw.; Novartis, Switz.; Novartis, UK.*
Artemether (p.447·2); lumefantrine (p.453·3).
*Malaria.*

**Ribastamin** *Beta, Arg.*
Risedronate sodium (p.774·3).
*Osteoporosis.*

**Ribatra** *Panalab, Arg.*
Clobetasol (p.1095·3).
*Eczema.*

**Ribatran** *Ferlux, Fr.*
Trypsin (p.1758·3); ribonuclease (p.1738·1); chymotrypsinogen.
*Oedema following trauma or surgery.*

**Ribav** *Biosintetica, Braz.*
Ribavirin (p.652·1).
*Viral infections.*

**Ribavin** *Lupin, India.*
Ribavirin (p.652·1).
*Hepatitis; herpesvirus infections; respiratory syncytial virus infection.*

**Ribaviron C** *Pizarro, Braz.*
Ribavirin (p.652·1).
*Viral infections.*

**Ribelfan** *Pharmacia Upjohn, Ital.†.*
Propyphenazone (p.85·3); noscapine (p.1125·3).
*Cold and influenza symptoms.*

**Ribex** *Merck, Arg.*
Vincamine (p.1764·2); cinnarizine (p.428·3).
*Cerebral and peripheral vascular disorders.*

**Ribex Flu** *Pfizer Consumer, Ital.*
Diclofenac sodium (p.32·1).
*Fever; influenza symptoms; pain.*

**Ribex Nasale** *Pfizer Consumer, Ital.*
Phenylephrine hydrochloride (p.1126·3).
*Nasal congestion.*

**Ribex Tosse** *Pfizer Consumer, Ital.*
Dropropizine (p.1119·3).
*Coughs.*

**Ribexen con Espettorante** *Pfizer Consumer, Ital.*
Dropropizine (p.1119·3); guaifenesin (p.1122·1).
*Coughs.*

**Ribocarbo** *Ribosepharm, Ger.*
Carboplatin (p.533·3).
*Malignant neoplasms.*

**Ribociclina** *Formenti, Ital.†.*
Doxycycline hyclate (p.206·2).
*Bacterial infections.*

**Ribodoxo-L** *Ribosepharm, Ger.*
Doxorubicin hydrochloride (p.547·3).
*Malignant neoplasms.*

**Ribofluor** *Ribosepharm, Ger.*
Fluorouracil (p.554·2).
*Malignant neoplasms.*

**Ribofolin**
*Klinge, Austria; Ribosepharm, Ger.*
Calcium folinate (p.1431·1).
*Adjunct to fluorouracil therapy; antidote to folic acid antagonists; methotrexate toxicity.*

**Ribolac** *Gebro, Switz.†.*
*Lactobacillus acidophilus* (p.1704·2); vitamins (p.1417·1).
*Diarrhoea.*

**Ribomicin** *Farmigea, Ital.*
Gentamicin sulfate (p.217·1).
*Bacterial eye infections.*

**Ribomunyl**
*Germania, Austria; Silesia, Chile; Inava, Fr.; Pierre Fabre, Ger.; Pierre Fabre, Port.; Pierre Fabre, Spain†; Robapharm, Switz.*
Ribosomal fractions of *Klebsiella pneumoniae*; *Streptococcus pneumoniae*; *Streptococcus pyogenes*; *Haemophilus influenzae*; membrane fraction of *Klebsiella pneumoniae*.
*Respiratory-tract infections.*

**Ribomustin** *Ribosepharm, Ger.*
Bendamustine hydrochloride (p.529·3).
*Malignant neoplasms.*

**Ribon** *Therabel, Belg.*
Riboflavin (p.1456·1).
*Muscle cramps; vitamin $B_2$ deficiency.*

**Riboposid** *Ribosepharm, Ger.*
Etoposide (p.551·3).
*Malignant neoplasms.*

**Ribostat** *Valeas, Ital.†.*
Ribostamycin sulfate.
*Gastrointestinal infections.*

**Ribotrex** *Pierre Fabre, Ital.*
Azithromycin (p.159·1).
*Bacterial infections.*

**Ribotripsin** *Grin, Mex.*
Trypsin (p.1758·3); chymotrypsin (p.1671·2).

**Ribovac**
*Pierre Fabre, Arg.; Schering-Plough, Mex.*
Ribosomal fractions of *Klebsiella pneumoniae*; *Streptococcus pneumoniae*; *Streptococcus pyogenes*; *Haemophilus influenzae*; membrane fraction of *Klebsiella pneumoniae*.
*Respiratory-tract infections.*

**Ribovir** *Plants, Ital.*
Royal jelly (p.1740·3); echinacea (p.1683·2); black currant (p.1661·1).
*Nutritional supplement.*

**Ribo-Wied** *Wiedemann, Ger.*
Spleen; liver; heart; placenta (p.1709·3).
*Tonic.*

**Ribozym** *Sofex, Port.*
Ribonucleic acids; glycerophosphates; kola; nicotinamide; thiamine; calcium; sodium (p.1417·1).
*Tonic.*

**Ribrain**
*Yamanouchi, Ger.†; Galenica, Gr.*
Betahistine mesilate (p.1660·1).
*Meniere's disease; vertigo.*

**Ribufen** *Jofrain, Mex.†.*
Ibuprofen (p.45·3).

**Ribujet** *Chiesi, Spain.*
Budesonide (p.1094·2).
*Asthma.*

**Ribusol** *Wasserman, Spain†.*
Budesonide (p.1094·2).
*Asthma; nasal polyps; rhinitis; skin disorders.*

**RIC Calcio** *Dominguez, Arg.*
Calcium polystyrene sulfonate (p.1032·3).
*Hyperkalaemia.*

**Rical** *Rigers, Mex.†.*
Calcium gluconate (p.1225·2).

**Riccomycine** *Kropf, Switz.†.*
Neomycin sulfate (p.235·1); ichthammol (p.1148·2); matricaria (p.1669·3); vitamin A palmitate (p.1453·1); ergocalciferol (p.1462·1); hamamelis (p.1696·3).
*Burns; superficial infected wounds.*

**Riccovitan** *Kropf, Switz.*
Vitamin A palmitate (p.1453·1); ergocalciferol (p.1462·1); ichthammol (p.1148·2); hamamelis (p.1696·3); chamomile (p.1669·3); zinc oxide (p.1163·2).
*Burns; skin inflammation; superficial wounds.*

**Ricelyt** *MM, India.*
Sodium chloride; potassium chloride; sodium citrate; rice (p.1222·2).
*Oral rehydration therapy.*

**Ricerca System** *Johnson & Johnson, Ital.*
Multivitamin, mineral, and amino-acid preparation (p.1417·1).
*Skin, hair, and nail disorders.*

**Ricerca System Anagen** *Dermoteca, Port.†.*
Vitamin, mineral, amino-acid, and lipid preparation (p.1417·1).
*Hair and nail disorders.*

**Ricerca System Elios** *Dermoteca, Port.†.*
Vitamin, mineral, amino-acid, and lipid preparation (p.1417·1).
*Sunlight-induced skin disorders.*

**Ricerca System Hidra** *Dermoteca, Port.†.*
Vitamins, minerals, amino-acids, and borage oil (p.1417·1).
*Emollient.*

**Ricerca System Iposeb** *Dermoteca, Port.†.*
Vitamins, minerals, amino-acids, and cucurbita oil (p.1417·1).
*Acne; seborrhoeic dermatitis.*

**Richmond Antiseptic Cream** *Eastern Pharmaceuticals, UK.*
Cetrimide (p.1172·1).
*Burns; skin irritation; wounds.*

**Ricilin** *Galen, Mex.†.*
Rifampicin (p.250·2).

**Ricilina** *Recalcine, Chile.*
Azithromycin hydrochloride (p.159·3).
*Bacterial infections.*

**Ricin**
*Atlantic, Hong Kong; Atlantic, Thai.*
Rifampicin (p.250·2).
*Bacterial infections including tuberculosis and gonorrhoea.*

**Ricinis**
*Atlantic, Hong Kong†; Atlantic, Thai.†.*
Rifampicin (p.250·2); isoniazid (p.222·2).
*Tuberculosis.*

**Ricino Koki** *Calmante Vitaminado, Spain†.*
Castor oil (p.1668·2).
*Bowel evacuation.*

**Ricola** *Cedar Health, UK.*
Menthol (p.1711·3); peppermint oil (p.1283·2).
*Coughs; nasal congestion; sore throat.*

**Riconazol** *Bunker, Braz.*
Fluconazole (p.398·1).
*Fungal infections.*

**Ricridene** *Lipha Sante, Fr.*
Nifurzide (p.237·2).
*Diarrhoea.*

**Ricura** *Pekana, Ger.*
Homoeopathic preparation.

**RID** *Pfizer, USA.*
Pyrethrins (p.1509·3); piperonyl butoxide (p.1509·2).
*Pediculosis.*

**Ridamin**
*Unison, Singapore; Unison, Thai.*
Loratadine (p.436·1).
*Allergic rhinitis; allergic skin reactions.*

**Rid-a-Pain** *Pfeiffer, USA.*
Benzocaine (p.1370·3); menthol (p.1711·3); cineole (p.1672·1).
*Oral lesions.*

**Rid-a-Pain HP** *Pfeiffer, USA.*
Capsaicin (p.24·2).
*Pain.*

**Ridaq** *Aspen, S.Afr.*
Hydrochlorothiazide (p.933·2).
*Hypertension; oedema.*

**Ridasa** *Manuell, Mex.*
Ribonuclease (p.1738·1); dornase alfa (p.1119·1).
*Viral infections.*

**Ridaura**
*Link, Austral.; SmithKline Beecham, Austria; Yamanouchi, Belg.; GlaxoSmithKline, Braz.; Paladin, Canad.; Goldshield, Denm.; Goldshield, Fin.; Yamanouchi, Ger.; Vianex (Βιανεξ), Gr.; IFET (ΙΦΕΤ), Gr.; Goldshield, Hong Kong; Goldshield, Irl.; Goldshield, Israel; Yamanouchi, Ital.; SmithKline Beecham, Mex.†; Yamanouchi, Neth.; Goldshield, Norw.; Link, NZ; Yamanouchi, Port.; Pharmafrica, S.Afr.; SmithKline Beecham, Singapore†; Recordati, Spain; Goldshield, Swed.; Doetsch, Grether, Switz.; SmithKline Beecham, Thai.†; Yamanouchi, UK; SmithKline Beecham, USA.*
Auranofin (p.19·1).
*Juvenile idiopathic arthritis; psoriatic arthritis; rheumatoid arthritis.*

**Ridauran** *Robapharm, Fr.*
Auranofin (p.19·1).
*Rheumatoid arthritis.*

**Ridazin** *Taro, Israel.*
Thioridazine hydrochloride (p.724·2).
*Aggression; agitation; anxiety.*

**Ridazine** *Atlantic, Thai.*
Thioridazine hydrochloride (p.724·2).
*Anxiety; depression; mania; schizophrenia.*

**Ridene** *Syntex, Mex.†.*
Nicardipine hydrochloride (p.965·1).
*Angina pectoris; cerebrovascular ischaemia; hypertension.*

**Ridenol** *RID, USA.*
Paracetamol (p.76·2).

**Rideril** *DDSA Pharmaceuticals, UK.*
Thioridazine (p.724·2).
*Schizophrenia.*

**Ridersweet** *Rider, Chile.*
Aspartame (p.1422·1).
*Sugar substitute.*

**Ridinox** *Bell, India.*
Idoxuridine (p.637·3).
*Herpetic keratitis.*

**Ridiodent** *Ogna, Ital.*
Sodium fluoride (p.1444·3); cetylpyridinium chloride (p.1173·1).
*Dental caries prophylaxis.*

**Ri-Donna** *DermoDuemila, Ital.*
Vitamins; selenium; betaine; soya; rhodiola; bacopa moniera; dioscorea; borage (p.1417·1).
*Nutritional supplement for women.*

**Riduton Ergo** *Francia, Ital.*
Carnitine; betacarotene; glutathione; vitamin C; vitamin E (p.1417·1).
*Nutritional supplement.*

**Ridutox** *SoSe, Ital.*
Glutathione (p.1040·3).
*Alcohol and drug poisoning; radiation sickness.*

**Riduvir** *Francia, Ital.*
Aciclovir (p.626·1).
*Herpesvirus infections.*

**Rielex** *Sanval, Braz.*
Dipyrone (p.35·3); orphenadrine citrate (p.486·1); caffeine (p.782·1).
*Skeletal muscle spasm.*

**Rifa**
*Note. This name is used for preparations of different composition.*
*Grunenthal, Ger.*
Rifampicin (p.250·2) or rifampicin sodium (p.252·3).
*Tuberculosis.*

*Concept, India.*
Rifampicin (p.250·2); isoniazid (p.222·2); vitamin $B_6$ (p.1457·2).
*Tuberculosis.*

**Rifa E** *Concept, India.*
Rifampicin (p.250·2); isoniazid (p.222·2); ethambutol (p.212·2); vitamin $B_6$ (p.1457·2).
*Tuberculosis.*

**Rifacilin** *Pharmaceutical Co, India.*
Rifampicin (p.250·2).
*Tuberculosis.*

**Rifacol** *Formenti, Ital.*
Rifaximin (p.254·1).
*Adjuvant in hyperammonaemia; gastrointestinal infections.*

**Rifacom E-Z** *Indoco, India.*
1 Tablet, rifampicin (p.250·2); isoniazid (p.222·2); 2 tablets, pyrazinamide (p.246·3); 1 tablet, ethambutol (p.212·2).
*Tuberculosis.*

**Rifadecina** *Klonal, Arg.*
Rifampicin (p.250·2).
*Bacterial infections including tuberculosis.*

**Rifadin**
*Aventis, Arg.; Aventis, Austral.; Aventis, Canad.; Hoechst Marion Roussel, Gr.; IFET (ΙΦΕΤ), Gr.; Aventis, Hong Kong; Aventis, Irl.; Lepetit, Ital.; Aventis, Mex.; Aventis, Neth.; Pharmacia Upjohn, Norw.†; Aventis, NZ; Aventis, Port.; Aventis, S.Afr.; Aventis, Swed.; Aventis, Thai.; Aventis, UK; Hoechst Marion Roussel, USA.*
Rifampicin (p.250·2) or rifampicin sodium (p.252·3).
*Bacterial infections including tuberculosis and leprosy; bacterial meningitis prophylaxis.*

**Rifadine**
*Aventis, Belg.; Aventis, Fr.*
Rifampicin (p.250·2) or rifampicin sodium (p.252·3).
*Bacterial infections including tuberculosis and leprosy; prophylaxis of meningococcal meningitis.*

**Rifafour** *Aventis, S.Afr.*
Rifampicin (p.250·2); isoniazid (p.222·2); pyrazinamide (p.246·3); ethambutol (p.212·2).
*Tuberculosis.*

**Rifagen**
*Note. This name is used for preparations of different composition.*
*Genepharm, Gr.*
Fluconazole (p.398·1).
*Fungal infections.*

*Llorente, Spain; General Drugs, Thai.*
Rifampicin (p.250·2).
*Mycobacterial infections.*

**Rifaldin**
*Aventis, Braz.; Aventis, Spain.*
Rifampicin (p.250·2) or rifampicin sodium (p.252·3).
*Mycobacterial infections; staphylococcal infections.*

**Rifam** *Siam Bheasach, Thai.*
Rifampicin (p.250·2).
*Bacterial infections.*

**Rifamate** *Hoechst Marion Roussel, USA.*
Rifampicin (p.250·2); isoniazid (p.222·2).
*Tuberculosis.*

**Rifamcilin** *Galen, Mex.†.*
Rifampicin (p.250·2).

**Rifamcin** *Pond's, Thai.*
Rifampicin (p.250·2).
*Tuberculosis.*

**Rifamiso** *Siam Bheasach, Thai.†.*
Rifampicin (p.250·2); isoniazid (p.222·2).
*Tuberculosis.*

**Rifamp** *Neo Quimica, Braz.*
Rifampicin (p.250·2).

**Rifam-P** *PP Lab, Thai.*
Rifampicin (p.250·2).
*Gonorrhoea; leprosy; tuberculosis.*

**Rifampyzid** *Pond's, Thai.*
Rifampicin (p.250·2); isoniazid (p.222·2); pyrazinamide (p.246·3).
*Tuberculosis.*

**Rifamycin** *Biochem, India.*
Rifampicin (p.250·2).
*Tuberculosis.*

**Rifan** *Neo Quimica, Braz.*
Rifamycin sodium (p.253·2).

**Rifanicozid** *Piam, Ital.†.*
Rifampicin (p.250·2); isoniazid (p.222·2).
*Tuberculosis.*

**Rifano** *Milano, Thai.†.*
Rifampicin (p.250·2).
*Gonorrhoea; leprosy; tuberculosis.*

**Rifapiam** *Piam, Ital.*
Rifampicin (p.250·2).
*Bacterial infections including tuberculosis.*

**Rifaprim**
*Aventis, Arg.; Aventis, Mex.*
Rifampicin (p.250·2); trimethoprim (p.272·2).
*Bacterial infections.*

**Rifasynt**
*Medochemie, Hong Kong; Medochemie, Malaysia; Medochemie, Thai.*
Rifampicin (p.250·2).
*Bacterial infections including tuberculosis and leprosy.*

**Rifater**
*Aventis, Austria; Aventis, Canad.; Aventis, Fr.; Grunenthal, Ger.; Aventis, Hong Kong; Aventis, Irl.; Lepetit, Ital.; Aventis, Mex.; Aventis, Port.; Aventis, S.Afr.†; Hoechst Marion Roussel, Singapore†; Aventis, Spain; Aventis, Switz.; Aventis, Thai.; Aventis, UK; Hoechst Marion Roussel, USA.*
Rifampicin (p.250·2); isoniazid (p.222·2); pyrazinamide (p.246·3).
*Tuberculosis.*

**Rifazida** *Pharmacia, Spain.*
Isoniazid (p.222·2); rifampicin (p.250·2).
*Tuberculosis.*

**Rifedot** *Alacan, Spain.*
Astemizole (p.424·2).
*Hypersensitivity reactions.*

**Rifex** *Sanofi Synthelabo, Port.*
Rifampicin (p.250·2).
*Gram-positive bacterial infections; tuberculosis.*

**Rifinah** Aventis, Arg.; Aventis, Fr.; Grunenthal, Ger.; Hoechst Marion Roussel, Gr.; Aventis, Hong Kong; Aventis, Irl.; Lepetit, Ital.; Aventis, Mex.; Aventis, Neth.; Aventis, NZ; Aventis, Port.; Aventis, S.Afr.; Hoechst Marion Roussel, Singapore†; Aventis, Spain; Aventis, Switz.; Aventis, Thai.; Aventis, UK.
Rifampicin (p.250·2); isoniazid (p.222·2).
*Tuberculosis.*

**Rifocin** Aventis, Austria; Lepetit, Ital.
Rifamycin sodium (p.253·2).
Lidocaine hydrochloride (p.1377·3) may be included in the intramuscular injection to alleviate the pain of injection.
*Bacterial infections.*

**Rifocina**
Note. This name is used for preparations of different composition.
Aventis, Arg.; Aventis, Port.
Rifamycin (p.253·3).
*Bacterial infections including tuberculosis.*

Aventis, Braz.
Rifamycin sodium (p.253·2).
*Staphylococcal infections.*

Aventis, Spain†.
Rifamycin sodium (p.252·3).
*Asymptomatic carriers of Neisseria meningitidis; bacterial infections; tuberculosis.*

**Rifocine** Aventis, Belg.; Marion Merrell, Fr.†.
Rifamycin (p.253·3).
*Bacterial infections.*

**Rifocort** Medley, Braz.
Rifamycin sodium (p.253·2); prednisolone acetate (p.1108·1).
*Skin disorders.*

**Rifocyna** Aventis, Mex.
Rifamycin sodium (p.253·2).
*Impetigo; infected burns and wounds.*

**Rifoldin** Aventis, Austria.
Rifampicin (p.250·2).
*Asymptomatic Haemophilus influenzae carriers; asymptomatic meningococcal carriers; brucellosis; leprosy; staphylococcal infections; tuberculosis.*

**Rifoldin INH** Aventis, Austria.
Rifampicin (p.250·2); isoniazid (p.222·2).
*Tuberculosis.*

**Rifun** Schwarz, Ger.; Sanol, Ger.
Pantoprazole sodium (p.1283·1).
*Gastro-oesophageal reflux; peptic ulcer.*

**Riganpil** Rigers, Mex.†.
Ampicillin (p.157·1).
*Bacterial infections.*

**Rigentex** Bracco, Ital.
*d*-Alpha tocopherol (p.1464·3).
*Vitamin E deficiency.*

**Riget** Biolab, Thai.
21 Tablets, levonorgestrel (p.1563·2); ethinylestradiol (p.1553·2); 7 tablets, inert.
*Combined oral contraceptive.*

**Rigevidon** Gedeon Richter, Hong Kong; Gedeon Richter, Malaysia; Gedeon Richter, Thai.
Levonorgestrel (p.1563·2); ethinylestradiol (p.1553·2).
28-Day packs also contain 7 inert tablets.
*Combined oral contraceptive; menstrual disorders.*

**Rigidur** Ferring, Denm.†; Ferring, Fin.†.
Alprostadil alfadex (p.1512·3).
*Erectile dysfunction.*

**Rigidur Duo** Ferring, Swed.†.
Alprostadil alfadex (p.1512·3).
*Erectile dysfunction.*

**Rigix** UCB, Austria.
Cetirizine hydrochloride (p.427·1).
*Hypersensitivity reactions.*

**Rigmoz** Elvetium, Arg.
Granisetron hydrochloride (p.1267·1).
*Nausea and vomiting.*

**Rigoletten** Tendem, Neth.
Aluminium hydroxide-magnesium carbonate co-dried gel (p.1250·1); magnesium hydroxide (p.1272·2).
*Gastrointestinal disorders associated with hyperacidity.*

**Rigoran** Vita, Spain.
Ciprofloxacin hydrochloride (p.188·2) or ciprofloxacin lactate (p.188·3).
*Bacterial infections.*

**Rigotax** Prater, Chile.
Cetirizine (p.427·2).
*Hypersensitivity reactions.*

**Riklinak** Rivero, Arg.
Amikacin sulfate (p.154·1).
*Bacterial infections.*

**Rikodeine** 3M, Austral.
Dihydrocodeine tartrate (p.34·3).
*Coughs.*

**Rikoderm** 3M, Austral.
Light liquid paraffin (p.1479·1); dewaxed wool fat (p.1483·1).
*Dry skin disorders.*

**Rikospray** 3M, Ital.
Aldioxa (p.1141·2); cetylpyridinium chloride (p.1173·1); terpineol (p.1752·2); dimethicone (p.1482·1).
*Barrier preparation; skin disinfection.*

**Rilamir** Gea, Denm.
Triazolam (p.725·3).
*Insomnia.*

**Rilan** UCI, Braz.
Sodium cromoglicate (p.795·3).
*Allergic rhinitis.*

**Rilaprost** Guidotti, Ital.
Saw palmetto (p.1569·1).
*Benign prostatic hyperplasia.*

**Rilaquin** Microsules, Arg.
Metoclopramide hydrochloride (p.1274·3).
*Gastrointestinal motility disorders; nausea and vomiting.*

**Rilastil** Dermoteca, Port.
*SPF 10:* Octinoxate (p.1154·3); avobenzone (p.1142·3); zinc oxide (p.1163·2).
*Sunscreen.*

**Rilastil Anti-Oxidante** Dermoteca, Port.
Fish oil; borage; zinc-enriched yeast; lecithin; glyceryl stearate; selenium-enriched yeast; betacarotene; tocoferil acetate (p.1417·1).
*Antioxidant; nutritional supplement.*

**Rilastil Dermo Solar** Dermoteca, Port.
Tyrosine (p.1451·1); borage oil (p.1661·3); wheat; betacarotene (p.1422·3); bearberry (p.1659·2); alpha tocopherol (p.1464·3); selenium (p.1444·1).

**Rilaten** Guidotti, Ital.
Rociverine (p.1740·1).
*Smooth muscle spasm.*

**Rilatine** Novartis, Belg.
Methylphenidate hydrochloride (p.1590·2).
*Attention deficit hyperactivity disorder; narcoleptic syndrome.*

**Rilcapton** Medochemie, Hong Kong; Medochemie, Singapore†.
Captopril (p.879·2).
*Heart failure; hypertension.*

**Rilex** Gry, Ger.
Tetrazepam (p.724·1).
*Skeletal muscle spasticity; skeletal muscle tension.*

**Rilfit** Apomedica, Austria.
Aspirin (p.15·1); paracetamol (p.76·2); salicylamide (p.87·3); caffeine (p.782·1).
*Fever; pain.*

**Rilutek** Aventis, Arg.; Aventis, Austral.; Rhone-Poulenc Rorer, Austria; Aventis, Belg.; Aventis, Braz.; Aventis, Canad.; Aventis, Denm.; Aventis, Fin.; Aventis, Fr.; Aventis, Ger.; Rhone-Poulenc Rorer, Gr.; Aventis, Hong Kong; Aventis, Irl.; Aventis, Israel; Lepetit, Ital.; Rhone-Poulenc Rorer, Jpn; Aventis, Mex.; Aventis, Neth.; Aventis, Norw.; Aventis, Port.; Aventis, S.Afr.; Aventis, Singapore; Aventis, Spain; Aventis, Swed.; Aventis, Switz.; Aventis, Thai.; Aventis, UK; Rhone-Poulenc Rorer, USA.
Riluzole (p.1738·3).
*Amyotrophic lateral sclerosis.*

**Rimacid** Ranbaxy, UK.
Indometacin (p.47·3).

**Rimacillin** Ranbaxy, UK.
Ampicillin (p.157·1).
*Bacterial infections.*

**Rimactan** Biochemie, Austria; Ciba-Geigy, Belg.†; Biochemie, Denm.; Novartis, Fr.; Ciba, Ger.†; Biochemie, Israel; Novartis, Mex.; Novartis, Neth.; Biochemie, Norw.; Geminis, Spain; Swedish Orphan, Swed.; Medika, Switz.
Rifampicin (p.250·2) or rifampicin sodium (p.252·3).
*Bacterial infections including tuberculosis and leprosy; prophylaxis of meningococcal meningitis.*

**Rimactan + INH** Biochemie, Austria.
Rifampicin (p.250·2); isoniazid (p.222·2).
*Tuberculosis.*

**Rimactane** Novartis, Hong Kong; Novartis, India; Swedish Orphan, Irl.; Novartis, Malaysia; Biochemie, Malaysia; Rolab, S.Afr.; Biochemie, Singapore; Novartis, Thai.; Biochemie, Thai.; Orphan, UK; Geneva, USA.
Rifampicin (p.250·2) or rifampicin sodium (p.252·3).
*Bacterial infections including leprosy and tuberculosis; prophylaxis of meningococcal meningitis.*

**Rimactazid** Novartis, Gr.; Swedish Orphan, Irl.; Novartis, Malaysia; Biochemie, Malaysia; Rolab, S.Afr.; Biochemie, Singapore; Geminis, Spain; Biochemie, Thai.; Novartis, Thai.; Orphan, UK.
Rifampicin (p.250·2); isoniazid (p.222·2).
*Tuberculosis.*

**Rimactazid + Z** Novartis, India.
1 Tablet, rifampicin (p.250·2); isoniazid (p.222·2); 2 tablets, pyrazinamide (p.246·3).
*Tuberculosis.*

**Rimactazide** Novartis, Switz.†.
Rifampicin (p.250·2); isoniazid (p.222·2).
*Tuberculosis.*

**Rimactazide + Z** Ciba, Switz.†.
Tablets, rifampicin (p.250·2); isoniazid (p.222·2); tablets, pyrazinamide (p.246·3).
*Tuberculosis.*

**Rimafen** Ranbaxy, UK.
Ibuprofen (p.45·3).

**Rimafungol** Belmac, Spain.
Ciclopirox olamine (p.396·1).
*Fungal infections.*

**Rimagrip** Belmac, Spain.
Aspirin (p.15·1); ascorbic acid (p.1460·2); chlorphenamine maleate (p.427·3); kola (p.1765·3).
*Coughs; fever; nasal congestion; pain.*

**Rimapam** Ranbaxy, UK.
Diazepam (p.690·1).

**Rimapen**
Note. This name is used for preparations of different composition.
Orion, Fin.
Rifampicin (p.250·2).
*Tuberculosis.*

Rima, UK†.
Phenoxymethylpenicillin potassium (p.242·1).

**Rimapurinol** Ranbaxy, UK.
Allopurinol (p.412·2).

**Rimarex** Sun, India.
Moclobemide (p.308·2).
*Depression; phobias.*

**Rimarin** Rima, UK†.
Chlorphenamine (p.428·1).

**Rimasal** Rima, UK†.
Salbutamol (p.791·3).

**Rimastine** Armstrong, Mex.
Sulpiride (p.722·2).
*Depression; nausea and vomiting; obsessive-compulsive disorder; schizophrenia; vertigo.*

**Rimbol** Esteve, Spain†.
Astemizole (p.424·2).
*Hypersensitivity reactions.*

**Rimcure** Rolab, S.Afr.
Rifampicin (p.250·2); isoniazid (p.222·2); pyrazinamide (p.246·3).
*Tuberculosis.*

**Rimcure 3-FDC** Biochemie, Thai.; Novartis, Thai.
Rifampicin (p.250·2); isoniazid (p.222·2); pyrazinamide (p.246·3).
*Tuberculosis.*

**Rimevax** SmithKline Beecham, Austral.; SmithKline Beecham, Belg.†; SmithKline Beecham, Israel; SmithKline Beecham, Ital.†; GlaxoSmithKline, Malaysia; SmithKline Beecham, Mex.; GlaxoSmithKline, NZ†; GlaxoSmithKline, S.Afr.; GlaxoSmithKline, Spain; SmithKline Beecham, Switz.; SmithKline Beecham, Thai.†.
A measles vaccine (Schwarz strain) (p.1623·1).
*Active immunisation.*

**Rimexel** Thiemann, Ger.
Rimexolone (p.1110·1).
*Musculoskeletal and joint disorders.*

**Rimidol** UCB, Swed.
Naphazoline hydrochloride (p.1124·3).
*Eye irritation.*

**Rimifon** Laphal, Fr.; Roche, Spain†; Labatec, Switz.
Isoniazid (p.222·2).
*Tuberculosis and other mycobacterial infections.*

**Rimodar** Anglo-French Drugs, India.
Sulfadoxine (p.259·3); pyrimethamine (p.458·1).
*Malaria.*

**Rimoxallin** Ranbaxy, UK.
Amoxicillin trihydrate (p.155·3).
*Bacterial infections.*

**Rimoxol** Rimsa, Mex.
Ambroxol (p.1114·3).
*Coughs.*

**Rimoxyn** Rima, UK†.
Naproxen (p.65·1).

**Rimpazid** Cadila, India.
Rifampicin (p.250·2); isoniazid (p.222·2).
*Tuberculosis.*

**Rimsalin** Rimsa, Mex.
Lincomycin hydrochloride (p.226·2).
*Bacterial infections.*

**Rimso** Shire, Canad.; Britannia Pharmaceuticals, UK; Research Industries Corp., USA.
Dimethyl sulfoxide (p.1473·2).
*Interstitial cystitis.*

**Rimycin** Alphapharm, Austral.
Rifampicin (p.250·2).
*Leprosy; prophylaxis of Haemophilus influenzae type B infection; prophylaxis of meningococcal infection; tuberculosis.*

**Rin Up** Farma Lepori, Spain.
Phenylephrine hydrochloride (p.1126·3).
*Upper respiratory-tract congestion.*

**Rinade BID** Econo Med, USA.
Pseudoephedrine hydrochloride (p.1129·2); chlorphenamine maleate (p.427·3).
*Upper respiratory-tract symptoms.*

**Rinadine** Pharmaland, Thai.
Cimetidine (p.1255·3).
*Peptic ulcer; Zollinger-Ellison syndrome.*

**Rinafed** Raza, Malaysia; Pharmaniaga, Malaysia.
Pseudoephedrine hydrochloride (p.1129·2); triprolidine hydrochloride (p.442·3).
*Nasal congestion.*

**Rinafort** Schering-Plough, Belg.†; Schering-Plough, Malaysia; Schering-Plough, Singapore.
Dexbrompheniramine maleate (p.426·1); pseudoephedrine sulfate (p.1129·2).
*Upper respiratory-tract congestion.*

**Rinalix** Xepa-Soul Pattinson, Malaysia; Xepa-Soul Pattinson, Singapore.
Indapamide (p.938·2).
*Hypertension.*

**Rinantipiol** Ottolenghi, Ital.
Silver protein (p.1746·2); resorcinol (p.1156·3); niaouli oil (p.1719·3); adrenaline hydrochloride (p.852·3); procaine hydrochloride (p.1383·2).
*Nasal congestion.*

**Rinatec** Boehringer Ingelheim, Irl.; Boehringer Ingelheim, UK.
Ipratropium bromide (p.787·1).
*Rhinitis.*

**Rinatrol** Windson, Braz.†.
Naphazoline (p.1124·3); panthenol (p.1727·2).
*Nasal congestion.*

**Rinaze** Boehringer Ingelheim, S.Afr.†.
Beclometasone dipropionate (p.1091·1).
*Allergic rhinitis.*

**Rinazina** GlaxoSmithKline Consumer, Ital.
Naphazoline nitrate (p.1124·3).
*Nasal congestion.*

**Rince Bouche Antiseptique** Atlas, Canad.
Cetylpyridinium chloride (p.1173·1).

**Rinedrone** Deca, Ital.†.
Dexamethasone (p.1097·1); tonzonium bromide (p.1757·2).
*Rhinitis; rhinosinusitis.*

**Rinelon** Malesci, Ital.; Schering-Plough, Mex.; Schering-Plough, S.Afr.; Menarini, Spain; Schering-Plough, Thai.
Mometasone furoate (p.1107·2).
*Rhinitis; sinusitis.*

**Rinerge** Atral, Port.
Oxymetazoline hydrochloride (p.1126·1).
*Nasal congestion.*

**Rinex** Triomed, S.Afr.
Chlorphenamine maleate (p.427·3); phenylpropanolamine hydrochloride (p.1127·3); phenylephrine hydrochloride (p.1126·3).
*Allergic rhinitis; cold and influenza symptoms.*

**Rinexin** Recip, Fin.; Recip, Norw.; Recip, Swed.
Phenylpropanolamine hydrochloride (p.1127·3).
*Rhinitis; sinusitis; urinary incontinence.*

**Ring N** Mack, Illert., Ger.
Aspirin (p.15·1); caffeine (p.782·1); ascorbic acid (p.1460·2).
*Cold symptoms; fever; pain.*

**Ringersteril** Baxter, Fin.
Electrolyte infusion with or without glucose (p.1217·1).
*Fluid and electrolyte disorders.*

**Ringworm Ointment** Douglas, Austral.
Tolnaftate (p.410·1).
*Ringworm.*

**Rinil** Recip, Swed.
Sodium cromoglicate (p.795·3).
*Allergic conjunctivitis; allergic rhinitis.*

**Rinilyn** Chefaro, Spain.
Sodium cromoglicate (p.795·3).
*Hay fever; rhinitis.*

**Rinisone** Medley, Braz.
Prednisolone sodium phosphate (p.1108·1); ephedrine hydrochloride (p.1120·1); naphazoline nitrate (p.1124·3).
Formerly contained fluprednisolone, ephedrine, and naphazoline.
*Nasal disorders.*

**Rinnova** Sefarma, Ital.
Calcium glycerophosphate; colecalciferol; soya isoflavones (p.1417·1).
*Menopausal disorders.*

**Rino Calyptol** Aventis, Ital.
Oxymetazoline hydrochloride (p.1126·1).
*Nasal congestion.*

**Rino Clenil** Chiesi, Hong Kong†; Chiesi, Ital.; Chiesi, Singapore.
Beclometasone dipropionate (p.1091·1).
*Rhinitis; sinusitis.*

**Rino Dexa** Sanofi Synthelabo, Spain.
Chlorphenamine maleate (p.427·3); dexamethasone sodium phosphate (p.1097·2); muramidase hydrochloride (p.1717·2); neomycin sulfate (p.235·1).
*Rhinitis; rhinopharyngeal infection; sinusitis.*

**Rino Ebastel** Almirall, Spain.
Pseudoephedrine hydrochloride (p.1129·2); ebastine (p.433·1).
*Allergic rhinitis.*

**Rino Naftazolina** Bruschettini, Ital.
Naphazoline hydrochloride (p.1124·3).
*Nasal congestion.*

**Rino Resfenol** Galenogal, Braz.†.
Naphazoline (p.1124·3).
*Nasal congestion.*

**Rino Spray** Heralds, Braz.†.
Oxymetazoline (p.1126·2).
*Nasal congestion.*

**Rino-Azetin** UCI, Braz.
Azelastine hydrochloride (p.425·2).
*Hypersensitivity reactions.*

**Rino-B** Cassara, Arg.
Budesonide (p.1094·2).
*Laryngitis; pharyngitis; rhinitis.*

**Rinobactil** CEPA, Spain.
Ebastine (p.433·1); pseudoephedrine hydrochloride (p.1129·2).
*Allergic rhinitis.*

**Rinobalsamiche** Farmatre, Ital.; Ramini, Ital.; Sella, Ital.
Menthol (p.1711·3); niaouli oil (p.1719·3).
*Nasal congestion.*

**Rinobanedif**
*Note. This name is used for preparations of different composition.*
*Bago, Chile.*
Bacitracin zinc (p.161·3); neomycin sulfate (p.235·1); xylometazoline hydrochloride (p.1132·2); antazoline phosphate (p.424·2).
*Rhinitis; sinusitis.*
*Roche, Spain.*
Bacitracin zinc (p.161·3); phenylephrine hydrochloride (p.1126·3); neomycin sulfate (p.235·1); prednisolone (p.1108·1); cineole (p.1672·1); niaouli oil (p.1719·3).
*Upper respiratory-tract disorders.*

**Rinoben** *Cazi, Braz.*
Sodium chloride (p.1233·3).
*Nasal congestion.*

**Rinoblanco** *Alcon Cusi, Spain.*
Xylometazoline hydrochloride (p.1132·2).
*Nasal congestion.*

**Rinoblanco Dexa Antibio** *Alcon Cusi, Spain†.*
Dexamethasone sodium phosphate (p.1097·2); neomycin sulfate (p.235·1); xylometazoline hydrochloride (p.1132·2).
*Upper respiratory-tract disorders.*

**Rinocidina** *Valeas, Ital.*
Tyrothricin (p.275·1); naphazoline nitrate (p.1124·3).
*Rhinitis; sinusitis.*

**Rinocorin** *Sanofi Synthelabo, Spain†.*
Oxymetazoline hydrochloride (p.1126·1).
*Nasal congestion.*

**Rinocron** *Neo Quimica, Braz.†.*
Naphazoline (p.1124·3); tyrothricin (p.275·1); thiomersal (p.1194·1); nitrofurazone (p.238·2).
*Nasal congestion.*

**Rinocusi Vitaminico** *Sanofi Synthelabo, Spain.*
Vitamin A (p.1451·2).
*Nasal congestion; nasal irritation.*

**Rinodan** *Medipharm, Chile.*
Sodium chloride (p.1233·3).
*Nasal congestion; nasal hygiene; rhinitis.*

**Rinodif** *Roche, Spain†.*
Oxymetazoline hydrochloride (p.1126·1).
*Nasal congestion.*

**Rinofen** *Delta, Braz.†.*
Diosfenol; cineole (p.1672·1); menthol (p.1711·3); sumatra benzoin (p.1751·1); lavender (p.1705·1).
*Nasal congestion.*

**Rinofilax AG M** *Raffo, Arg.*
Naphazoline (p.1124·3); neomycin (p.235·1).
*Nasal congestion.*

**Rinofluimucil**
*Note. This name is used for preparations of different composition.*
*Zambon, Braz.*
Acetylcysteine (p.1112·3); tuaminoheptane sulfate (p.1132·1); fludrocortisone acetate (p.1100·1).
*Rhinitis.*
*Zambon, Hong Kong; Zambon, Ital.; Zambon, Spain†; Inpharzam, Switz.; Zambon, Thai.*
Acetylcysteine (p.1112·3); tuaminoheptane sulfate (p.1132·1).
*Rhinitis; sinusitis.*

**Rinofluimucil-S** *Zambon, Ger.*
Acetylcysteine (p.1112·3); tuaminoheptane sulfate (p.1132·1).
*Rhinitis; sinusitis.*

**Rinoflumil** *Zambon, Spain.*
Acetylcysteine (p.1112·3); tuaminoheptane sulfate (p.1132·1).
*Rhinitis.*

**Rinoflux** *IMA, Braz.*
Sodium chloride (p.1233·3).
*Nasal congestion.*

**Rinofomentil** *SIT, Ital.*
Silver protein (p.1746·2); naphazoline nitrate (p.1124·3); niaouli oil (p.1719·3).
*Nasal disorders.*

**Rinofren** *Carnot, Mex.*
Chlorphenamine maleate (p.427·3); pseudoephedrine hydrochloride (p.1129·2); paracetamol (p.76·2).
Formerly contained chlorphenamine maleate, phenylpropanolamine hydrochloride, paracetamol, and caffeine.
*Allergic rhinitis; hay fever; rhinopharyngitis; sinusitis.*

**Rinofren Pediatrico** *Carnot, Mex.*
Chlorphenamine maleate (p.427·3); paracetamol (p.76·2).
*Cold and influenza symptoms.*

**Rinofrenal**
*Note. This name is used for preparations of different composition.*
*Monsanto, Ital.*
Sodium cromoglicate (p.795·3); chlorphenamine maleate (p.427·3).
*Rhinitis.*
*Sigma-Tau, Spain.*
Sodium cromoglicate (p.795·3).
*Hay fever; rhinitis.*

**Rinofrenal Plus** *Sigma-Tau, Spain.*
Chlorphenamine maleate (p.427·3); sodium cromoglicate (p.795·3).
*Hay fever; rhinitis.*

**Rinofrim** *Laboratorios Chile, Chile.*
Phenylephrine hydrochloride (p.1126·3); phenylpropanolamine hydrochloride (p.1127·3); phenyltoloxamine citrate (p.439·1); carbinoxamine maleate (p.426·3).
*Cold and influenza symptoms; otitis media; rhinitis; sinusitis.*

**Rinogan** *Confar, Port.*
Chlorphenamine (p.428·1); phenylpropanolamine (p.1127·3); ascorbic acid (p.1460·2).

**Rinogel** *Cassara, Arg.*
Sodium cromoglicate (p.795·3); naphazoline hydrochloride (p.1124·3).
*Allergic rhinitis; epistaxis; nasal surgery.*

**Rinogerol** *Brasmedica, Braz.†.*
Neomycin sulfate (p.235·1); bacitracin (p.161·3).

**Rinoglin** *Seber, Port.*
Chlorphenamine maleate (p.427·3); sodium cromoglicate (p.795·3).
*Conjunctivitis; eye irritation; rhinitis.*

**Rinogutt Antiallergico Spray** *Boehringer Ingelheim, Ital.*
Tramazoline hydrochloride (p.1131·3); chlorphenamine maleate (p.427·3).
*Allergic rhinitis.*

**Rinogutt Eucalipto-Fher** *Boehringer Ingelheim, Ital.*
Tramazoline hydrochloride (p.1131·3); cineole (p.1672·1); menthol (p.1711·3); camphor (p.1665·3).
*Nasal congestion.*

**Rinogutt Spray-Fher** *Boehringer Ingelheim, Ital.*
Tramazoline hydrochloride (p.1131·3).
*Nasal congestion.*

**Rinojet** *Valeas, Ital.*
Betamethasone (p.1093·1); phenylephrine hydrochloride (p.1126·3).
*Rhinitis; rhinopharyngitis; sinusitis.*

**Rinojet SF** *Valeas, Ital.*
Neomycin sulfate (p.235·1); polymyxin B sulfate (p.245·1).
*Infections of the upper respiratory tract.*

**Rinoklin** *Klinger, Braz.†.*
Naphazoline (p.1124·3).
*Nasal congestion.*

**Rinolan** *Berman, Mex.*
Phenylephrine (p.1126·3).

**Rino-Lastin** *Asta Medica, Braz.*
Azelastine hydrochloride (p.425·2).
*Nasal congestion.*

**Rinolergan** *Grunenthal, Chile.*
Phenylephrine tannate (p.1127·2); chlorphenamine tannate (p.428·1); mepyramine tannate (p.437·1).
*Cold symptoms; rhinitis; sinusitis.*

**Rinomar**
*Note. This name is used for preparations of different composition.*
*Janssen-Cilag, Belg.*
Pseudoephedrine hydrochloride (p.1129·2).
Formerly contained cinnarizine, phenylpropanolamine hydrochloride, and isopropamide iodide.
*Rhinitis.*
*Recip, Fin.; Pharmacia Upjohn, Norw.†; Recip, Swed.*
Cinnarizine (p.428·3); phenylpropanolamine hydrochloride (p.1127·3).
*Nasal congestion; rhinitis.*

**Rinomax** *Ern, Spain.*
Carbinoxamine maleate (p.426·3); pseudoephedrine (p.1129·2).
*Nasal congestion.*

**Rinomex** *Recalcine, Chile.*
Loratadine (p.436·1); pseudoephedrine (p.1129·2).
*Cold symptoms; otitis media; rhinitis; sinusitis.*

**Rinomicine** *Fardi, Spain.*
*Oral sachets:* Ascorbic acid (p.1460·2); caffeine (p.782·1); chlorphenamine maleate (p.427·3); phenylephrine hydrochloride (p.1126·3); paracetamol (p.76·2); salicylamide (p.87·3).
*Tablets:* Caffeine (p.782·1); chlorphenamine maleate (p.427·3); phenylephrine hydrochloride (p.1126·3); paracetamol (p.76·2); salicylamide (p.87·3).
*Influenza and cold symptoms; nasal congestion.*

**Rinomicine Activada** *Fardi, Spain.*
Caffeine (p.782·1); chlorphenamine maleate (p.427·3); phenylephrine hydrochloride (p.1126·3); paracetamol (p.76·2); salicylamide (p.87·3).
*Influenza and cold symptoms; nasal congestion.*

**Rinopaidolo** *Deca, Ital.*
Niaouli oil (p.1719·3); eucalyptus oil (p.1686·2).
*Nasal congestion.*

**Rinopanteina** *DMG, Ital.*
Dexpanthenol (p.1727·2); vitamin A (p.1451·2).
*Nasal hygiene.*

**Rinoparin** *Pasteur, Chile.*
Pseudoephedrine hydrochloride (p.1129·2); chlorphenamine maleate (p.427·3).
*Cold symptoms.*

**Rino-Ped** *Stiefel, Braz.*
Sodium chloride (p.1233·3).
*Nasal congestion.*

**Rinoretard** *Warner-Lambert, Spain†.*
Carbinoxamine (p.426·3); phenylpropanolamine (p.1127·3).
*Nasal congestion.*

**Rinorix** *Boehringer Ingelheim, Austria.*
Tramazoline hydrochloride (p.1131·3).
*Rhinitis.*

**Rinos** *Molteni, Ital.†.*
Xylometazoline hydrochloride (p.1132·2); thymol (p.1194·2); cineole (p.1672·1).
*Nasal congestion.*

**Rinos-A** *Farmasa, Braz.*
Naphazoline hydrochloride (p.1124·3).
*Nasal congestion.*

**Rinosbon** *Eversil, Braz.*
Dexamethasone (p.1097·1); phenylephrine hydrochloride (p.1126·3); chlorphenamine maleate (p.427·3).
*Nasal disorders.*

**Rinosedin** *Streuli, Switz.*
Xylometazoline hydrochloride (p.1132·2).
*Adjunct in rhinoscopy; cold symptoms; otitis; sinus disorders.*

**Rinosil** *Zeta, Ital.†.*
Cetylpyridinium chloride (p.1173·1); chlorobutanol; menthol; cineole; camphor.
*Nasal disinfection.*

**Rinosite** *Sanval, Braz.*
Naphazoline hydrochloride (p.1124·3); diphenhydramine hydrochloride (p.431·3); neomycin sulfate (p.235·1).
*Nasal congestion.*

**Rinosol**
*Cassara, Arg.; Zekides, Gr.*
Beclometasone dipropionate (p.1091·1).
*Allergic rhinitis; asthma.*

**Rinosone** *Faes, Spain.*
Fluticasone propionate (p.1102·3).
*Nasal polyps; rhinitis.*

**Rinosoro** *Farmasa, Braz.*
Sodium chloride (p.1233·3); benzalkonium chloride (p.1168·3).
*Nasal congestion.*

**Rinospray** *Recordati, Ital.†.*
Dequalinium chloride (p.1178·1); naphazoline hydrochloride (p.1124·3).
*Disinfection and decongestion of the upper respiratory tract.*

**Rinostat** *RPG, India.*
Paracetamol (p.76·2); chlorphenamine (p.427·3); pseudoephedrine hydrochloride (p.1129·2).
*Cold symptoms.*

**Rinostil** *Deca, Ital.*
Eucalyptus oil (p.1686·2); camphor (p.1665·3); thymol (p.1194·2); menthol (p.1711·3).
*Rhinopharyngeal congestion.*

**Rinotil** *Brasmedica, Braz.†.*
Sodium chloride (p.1233·3); benzalkonium chloride (p.1168·3).
*Nasal congestion.*

**Rinotricina** *SIT, Ital.*
Tyrothricin (p.275·1).
*Rhinitis; sinusitis.*

**Rinovagos** *Valeas, Ital.*
Ipratropium bromide (p.787·1).
*Rhinitis.*

**Rinoval** *Saval, Chile.*
Mometasone furoate (p.1107·2).
*Rhinitis.*

**Rinovel** *Ern, Spain.*
Naphazoline nitrate (p.1124·3); neomycin sulfate (p.235·1); prednisolone (p.1108·1).
*Congestion and infection of the nose and ear.*

**Rinoven** *Medipharm, Chile.*
Pseudoephedrine hydrochloride (p.1129·2); chlorphenamine maleate (p.427·3).
*Allergic rhinitis; upper respiratory-tract congestion.*

**Rinoven Compuesto** *Medipharm, Chile.*
Paracetamol (p.76·2); pseudoephedrine hydrochloride (p.1129·2); chlorphenamine maleate (p.427·3).
*Bronchitis; cold and influenza symptoms; otitis; rhinitis; sinusitis.*

**Rinovit** *SIT, Ital.*
Ephedrine (p.1120·1); cineole (p.1672·1); niaouli oil (p.1719·3).
*Nasal congestion.*

**Rinovit Nube** *SIT, Ital.†.*
Silver protein (p.1746·2); naphazoline nitrate (p.1124·3); niaouli oil (p.1719·3).
*Congestion of the upper respiratory tract.*

**Rinowash** *Markos-Mefar, Ital.*
Sodium chloride (p.1233·3).
*Nasal cleansing.*

**Rinox Adulto** *Cibran, Braz.†.*
Naphazoline (p.1124·3).
*Nasal congestion.*

**Rinox Pediatrico** *Cibran, Braz.†.*
Sodium chloride (p.1233·3).
*Nasal congestion.*

**Rinozin** *QIF, Braz.†.*
Naphazoline hydrochloride (p.1124·3); dexpanthenol (p.1727·2).
*Nasal congestion.*

**Rinsoderm** *Nycomed, Norw.†.*
Pyrethrum extract (p.1509·3); piperonyl butoxide (p.1509·2).
*Pediculosis.*

**Rinstead** *Schering-Plough, UK.*
*Contact pastille†:* Lidocaine hydrochloride (p.1377·3).
*Mouth irritation; mouth ulcers.*
*Pastilles:* Menthol (p.1711·3); cetylpyridinium chloride (p.1173·1).
*Denture irritation; mouth ulcers.*
*Topical gel:* Benzocaine (p.1370·3); chloroxylenol (p.1177·2).
*Mouth pain; mouth ulcers.*

**Rinstead Teething Gel** *Schering-Plough, UK†.*
Lidocaine (p.1377·3); cetylpyridinium chloride (p.1173·1).
*Mouth ulcers; teething pain.*

**Rintac** *Raza, Malaysia; Pharmaniaga, Malaysia.*
Ranitidine hydrochloride (p.1285·2).
*Gastro-oesophageal reflux; peptic ulcer; Zollinger-Ellison syndrome.*

**Rinurel** *Warner-Lambert, Fr.†.*
Phenylpropanolamine hydrochloride (p.1127·3); phenyltoloxamine citrate (p.439·1); paracetamol (p.76·2).
*Disorders of the ear, nose, and throat.*

**Rinutan** *Pfizer Sante, Fr.†.*
Paracetamol (p.76·2); phenylpropanolamine hydrochloride (p.1127·3); phenyltoloxamine citrate (p.439·1).
*Cold symptoms.*

**Riodine** *Orion, NZ.*
Povidone-iodine (p.1190·3).
*Skin and wound disinfection; skin infections.*

**Rio-Josipyrin N** *CPF, Ger.†.*
Aspirin (p.15·1); paracetamol (p.76·2); caffeine (p.782·1).
*Headache; influenza; neuralgia.*

**Riomet** *Ranbaxy, USA.*
Metformin (p.342·3).
*Diabetes mellitus.*

**Riopan**
*Note. This name is used for preparations of different composition.*
*Byk, Arg.; Byk, Austria; Byk, Belg.; Altana, Braz.; Whitehall-Robins, Canad.; Byk, Fr.; Byk Gulden, Ger.; Roland, Ger.; Nycomed, Gr.; Byk Gulden, Ital.; Byk, Neth.; Byk, Port.; Altana, Switz.; Whitehall, USA.*
Magaldrate (p.1271·3).
*Gastrointestinal disorders associated with hyperacidity.*
*Byk Gulden, Mex.*
Magaldrate (p.1271·3); dimeticone (p.1289·2).
*Gastrointestinal disorders associated with hyperacidity.*

**Riopan Plus**
*Altana, Braz.; Whitehall-Robins, Canad.; Whitehall, USA.*
Magaldrate (p.1271·3); simeticone (p.1289·2).
*Gastrointestinal disorders associated with hyperacidity.*

**Riopone** *Akromed, S.Afr.†.*
Magaldrate (p.1271·3).
*Gastrointestinal hyperacidity.*

**Riostatin** *Mer-National, S.Afr.*
Tetracycline hydrochloride (p.266·2); nystatin (p.406·3); vitamin B substances (p.1417·1); ascorbic acid.
*Bacterial infections.*

**Riotane** *Orion, NZ.*
Chlorhexidine gluconate (p.1173·2).
*Skin, wound, and instrument disinfection.*

**Riotapen** *Fermentaciones y Sintesis, Spain†.*
Amoxicillin sodium (p.155·3) or amoxicillin trihydrate (p.155·3).
*Bacterial infections.*

**Rioven** *Willmar, Mex.†.*
Vitamin B substances (p.1417·1).

**Ripason** *Knoll, Mex.†.*
Liver extract.

**Riphenidate** *Technilab, Canad.*
Methylphenidate hydrochloride (p.1590·2).

**Ripix**
*Ciba Vision, Ital.; Novartis Ophthalmics, Switz.*
Metipranolol (p.955·3); pilocarpine hydrochloride (p.1495·1).
*Glaucoma; ocular hypertension.*

**Ripol** *Laboratorios Chile, Chile.*
Sildenafil (p.1744·2).
*Erectile dysfunction.*

**Riposon** *Vianex (Βιανέξ), Gr.*
Tibezonium iodide (p.1756·2).
*Mouth infections.*

**Risatarun** *Ravensberg, Ger.*
Deanol aceglumate (p.1585·3).
*Nervous system disorders.*

**Riscalon** *Boehringer Mannheim, Spain†.*
*Cream:* Fentiazac (p.43·1).
*Musculoskeletal, joint, peri-articular, and soft-tissue disorders.*

**Rischiaril** *Piam, Ital.*
Deanol hemisuccinate (p.1585·3).
*Mental function impairment.*

**Risek** *Julphar, UAE.*
Omeprazole (p.1278·2).
*Acid aspiration; gastro-oesophageal reflux; peptic ulcer; Zollinger-Ellison syndrome.*

**Riselle** *Organon, Braz.*
Estradiol (p.1550·1).
*Oestrogen deficiency.*

**Risicordin** *Heumann, Ger.*
Spironolactone (p.1003·1); hydrochlorothiazide (p.933·2).
*Ascites; hyperaldosteronism; hypertension; liver cirrhosis; oedema.*

**Risidon** *Merck, Port.*
Metformin hydrochloride (p.342·3).
*Diabetes mellitus.*

**Risinetten** *Hexal, Austria.*
Althaea (p.1651·3).
*Coughs.*

**Risocalm** *Medifive, Thai.*
Tolperisone hydrochloride (p.1396·3).
*Skeletal muscle spasm.*

**Risolid**
*Alpharma, Denm.; Alpharma, Fin.*
Chlordiazepoxide (p.674·2).
*Alcohol withdrawal syndrome; anxiety disorders; insomnia.*

**Risoltuss** Magis, Ital.†.
Cloperastine fendizoate (p.1117·2).
*Coughs.*

**Risoniac** Klonal, Arg.
Isoniazid (p.222·2); rifampicin (p.250·2).
*Tuberculosis.*

**Risordan**
Note. This name is used for preparations of different composition.
Elvetium, Arg.
Vitamin E acetate (p.1465·1).
*Vitamin E deficiency.*

Aventis, Fr.
Isosorbide dinitrate (p.941·1).
*Angina pectoris; heart failure; pulmonary oedema.*

**Risperdal**
Janssen-Cilag, Arg.; Janssen-Cilag, Austral.; Janssen-Cilag, Austria; Janssen-Cilag, Belg.; Janssen-Cilag, Braz.; Janssen-Ortho, Canad.; Janssen-Cilag, Chile; Janssen-Cilag, Denm.; Janssen-Cilag, Fin.; Janssen-Cilag, Fr.; Organon, Fr.; Janssen-Cilag, Ger.; Organon, Ger.; Janssen-Cilag, Gr.; Janssen, Hong Kong; Janssen-Cilag, Irl.; Janssen-Cilag, Israel; Janssen-Cilag, Ital.; Janssen-Kyowa, Jpn; Janssen-Cilag, Malaysia; Janssen, Mex.; Janssen-Cilag, Neth.; Janssen-Cilag, Norw.; Janssen-Cilag, NZ; Janssen-Cilag, Port.; Janssen-Cilag, S.Afr.; Janssen-Cilag, Singapore; Janssen-Cilag, Spain; Janssen-Cilag, Swed.; Organon, Swed.; Janssen-Cilag, Switz.; Janssen-Cilag, Thai.; Janssen-Cilag, UK; Janssen, USA.
Risperidone (p.719·2) or risperidone tartrate.
*Psychoses.*

**Risperin** Gador, Arg.
Risperidone (p.719·2).
*Schizophrenia.*

**Rispid** Panacea, India.
Risperidone (p.719·2).
*Psychoses.*

**Ristalen** Tedec Meiji, Spain†.
Enalapril maleate (p.909·2).
*Heart failure; hypertension.*

**Risthal** Pasteur, Chile.
Aluminium hydroxide (p.1249·2).
*Antacid.*

**Risto** Progress, Thai.
Triamcinolone acetonide (p.1110·2).
*Skin disorders.*

**Ristolzit** Leovan, Gr.
Nimesulide (p.67·1).
*Inflammation; musculoskeletal disorders; pain.*

**Ritalin**
Novartis, Austral.; Novartis, Austria; Novartis, Canad.; Novartis, Chile; Novartis, Denm.; Novartis, Ger.; Novartis, Hong Kong; Novartis, Irl.; Novartis, Israel; Novartis, Malaysia; Novartis, Mex.; Novartis, Neth.; Novartis, Norw.; Novartis, NZ; Novartis, S.Afr.; Novartis, Singapore; Novartis, UK; Novartis, USA.
Methylphenidate hydrochloride (p.1590·2).
*Attention deficit hyperactivity disorder; narcoleptic syndrome.*

**Ritalina**
Novartis, Arg.; Novartis, Braz.
Methylphenidate hydrochloride (p.1590·2).
*Attention-deficit hyperactivity disorder; narcoleptic syndrome.*

**Ritaline**
Novartis, Fr.; Novartis, Switz.
Methylphenidate hydrochloride (p.1590·2).
*Attention-deficit hyperactivity disorder; narcoleptic syndrome.*

**Ritalmex** Alkaloida, Thai.†.
Mexiletine (p.958·3).
*Arrhythmias.*

**Ritamine** Demo, Gr.
Nimesulide (p.67·1).
*Inflammation; musculoskeletal disorders; pain.*

**Ritaphen** Triomed, S.Afr.
Methylphenidate hydrochloride (p.1590·2).
*Attention-deficit hyperactivity disorder; narcoleptic syndrome.*

**Riteban** Centrum, Spain.
Minoxidil (p.960·1).
*Alopecia androgenetica.*

**Rite-Diet**
SHS, Fr.; Nutricia, Irl.†; Nutricia Dietary, UK.
Gluten-free food for special diets (p.1417·1).

**Rition** Piam, Ital.
Glutathione sodium (p.1040·3).
*Alcohol and drug poisoning; radiation trauma.*

**Ritmocardyl**
Sanofi Synthelabo, Arg.
Amiodarone (p.859·2).
*Arrhythmias.*

Bago, Chile.
Amiodarone hydrochloride (p.859·2).
*Angina pectoris; arrhythmias.*

**Ritmocit** Asofarma, Arg.
Diltiazem (p.901·3).
*Angina pectoris; hypertension.*

**Ritmocor**
Note. This name is used for preparations of different composition.
Drugtech, Chile.
Propafenone hydrochloride (p.988·3).
*Arrhythmias.*

Malesci, Ital.
Quinidine polygalacturonate (p.991·3).
*Arrhythmias.*

**Ritmodan**
Aventis, Ital.; Aventis, Port.
Disopyramide (p.903·3) or disopyramide phosphate (p.903·3).
*Arrhythmias.*

**Ritmoforine** Aventis, Neth.
Disopyramide phosphate (p.903·3).
*Arrhythmias.*

**Ritmogel** Terapeutico, Ital.
Royal jelly (p.1740·3).
*Nutritional supplement.*

**Ritmolol** Cryopharma, Mex.
Metoprolol tartrate (p.957·1).
*Angina pectoris; arrhythmias; heart failure; hypertension; hyperthyroidism; migraine; myocardial infarction.*

**Ritmoneuran** Hertz, Braz.†.
Adonis vernalis (p.1648·1); erythrina mulungu (p.1717·2); passion flower (p.1729·1).

**Ritmonorm** Abbott, Braz.
Propafenone hydrochloride (p.988·3).
*Arrhythmias.*

**Ritopar**
Elea, Arg.; Agis, Israel.
Ritodrine hydrochloride (p.1739·2).
*Fetal distress during labour; premature labour.*

**Ritro** Benedetti, Ital.
Flurithromycin ethyl succinate (p.214·2).
*Bacterial infections.*

**Ritrocel** Silesia, Chile.
Methylphenidate hydrochloride (p.1590·2).
*Attention-deficit hyperactivity disorder; narcoleptic syndrome.*

**Ritromine** Hexa-Medinova, Arg.
Norfloxacin (p.238·3).
*Bacterial infections.*

**Ritroprim** Klonal, Arg.
Rifampicin (p.250·2); trimethoprim (p.272·2).
*Bacterial infections.*

**Rituxan**
Roche, Canad.; IDEC, USA; Genentech, USA.
Rituximab (p.582·3).
*Non-Hodgkin's lymphoma.*

**Ritvir** Rontag, Arg.
Nevirapine (p.650·2).
*HIV infection.*

**Rityne** Osoth, Thai.
Loratadine (p.436·1).
*Allergic rhinitis; allergic skin disorders.*

**Rivacefin** Rivero, Arg.
Ceftriaxone (p.183·3).
*Bacterial infections.*

**Rivanase** Riva, Canad.
Beclometasone dipropionate (p.1091·1).
*Corticosteroid.*

**Rivanol** Chinosolfabrik, Ger.
Ethacridine lactate (p.1165·3).
*Antiseptic.*

**Rivasa** Riva, Canad.
Aspirin (p.15·1).

**Rivasol** Riva, Canad.
Zinc sulfate (p.1469·3).
*Anorectal disorders.*

**Rivasol HC** Riva, Canad.
Zinc sulfate (p.1469·3); hydrocortisone acetate (p.1103·3).
*Anorectal disorders.*

**Rivasone** Riva, Canad.†.
Betamethasone valerate (p.1093·2).
*Skin disorders.*

**Rivatril** Roche, Fin.
Clonazepam (p.359·1).
*Epilepsy.*

**Rivecrum** Rivero, Arg.
Vecuronium bromide (p.1409·3).
*Competitive neuromuscular blocker.*

**Rivela** Beiersdorf, Ital.†.
Pregnancy test (p.1734·3).

**Riveparin** Rivero, Arg.
Heparin (p.927·3).
*Anticoagulant.*

**Rivervan** Rivero, Arg.
Vancomycin hydrochloride (p.275·2).
*Bacterial infections.*

**Rivescal Tar** Pergam, Ital.
Coal tar (p.1159·2); salicylic acid (p.1157·1).
*Seborrhoeic dermatitis.*

**Rivescal ZPT** Pergam, Ital.
Pyrithione zinc (p.1156·2).
*Seborrhoeic dermatitis.*

**Rivial** Rivero, Arg.
Multivitamin preparation for infusion (p.1417·1).

**Rividose** Rigers, Mex.†.
Vitamin B substances (p.1417·1).

**Rivistel** Delagrange, Port.
Alpiropride (p.465·3).
*Migraine.*

**Rivitin BC** Lannacher, Austria.
Vitamin B substances and vitamin C (p.1417·1).

**Rivodarone** Rivopharm, Switz.
Amiodarone hydrochloride (p.859·2).
*Arrhythmias.*

**Rivodol** Rivopharm, Switz.
Paracetamol (p.76·2).
*Fever; pain.*

**Rivoltan** Lichtwer, Ger.
Devil's claw root (p.28·2).
*Degenerative joint disorders.*

**Rivopen-V** Rivopharm, Switz.†.
Phenoxymethylpenicillin potassium (p.242·1).
*Bacterial infections.*

**Rivostatin** Rivopharm, Switz.†.
Nystatin (p.406·3).
*Fungal infections.*

**Rivotril**
Roche, Arg.; Roche, Austral.; Roche, Austria; Roche, Belg.; Roche, Braz.; Roche, Canad.; Roche, Denm.; Roche, Fr.; Roche, Ger.; Roche, Gr.; IFET (ΙΦΕΤ), Gr.; Roche, Hong Kong; Roche, Irl.; Roche, Israel; Roche, Ital.; Roche, Mex.; Roche, Neth.; Roche, Norw.; Roche, NZ; Roche, Port.; Roche, S.Afr.; Roche, Singapore†; Roche, Spain; Roche, Switz.; Roche, Thai.; Roche, UK.
Clonazepam (p.359·1).
*Epilepsy; status epilepticus.*

**Rivovit** Rivopharm, Switz.†.
Multivitamin preparation (p.1417·1).

**Rivoxicillin** Rivopharm, Switz.†.
Amoxicillin (p.155·3).
*Bacterial infections.*

**Rivozol** Rivopharm, Switz.
Metronidazole (p.607·2) or metronidazole benzoate (p.607·2).
*Anaerobic bacterial infections; protozoal infections.*

**Riwa Franzbranntwein** Gerlach, Ger.
Camphor (p.1665·3); alcohol (p.1166·1).
*Musculoskeletal, joint, and soft-tissue disorders; poor circulation.*

**α-Rix** GlaxoSmithKline, Belg.
An influenza vaccine (p.1620·2).
*Active immunisation.*

**Rixapen** Menarini, Belg.
Clometocillin potassium (p.198·1).
*Bacterial infections.*

**Rizaben** Kissei, Jpn.
Tranilast (p.806·3).
*Allergic conjunctivitis; allergic rhinitis; asthma; atopic dermatitis; keloids.*

**Rizalief** Merck Sharp & Dohme, Austria.
Rizatriptan benzoate (p.471·1).
*Migraine.*

**Rizaliv** Neopharmed, Ital.
Rizatriptan benzoate (p.471·1).
*Migraine.*

**Rizalt** Merck Sharp & Dohme, Israel.
Rizatriptan (p.471·2).
*Migraine.*

**Rize** Yoshitomi, Jpn.
Clotiazepam (p.685·2).
*Anxiety states; autonomic disorders; premedication; sleep disorders.*

**Rizen** Formenti, Ital.
Clotiazepam (p.685·2).
*Anxiety disorders; sleep disorders.*

**R-Loc** Cadila, India.
Ranitidine hydrochloride (p.1285·2).
*Dyspepsia; gastric hyperacidity; gastro-oesophageal reflux; peptic ulcer; Zollinger-Ellison syndrome.*

**RMS**
Note. This name is used for preparations of different composition.
Reith & Petrasch, Ger.
Lactic acid (p.1704·1) or calcium lactate (p.1225·3).
*Skin disorders.*

Baxter, NZ†; Upsher-Smith, USA.
Morphine sulfate (p.60·2).
*Pain.*

**RN13 Regeneresen** Dyckerhoff, Ger.
Ribonucleic acid (p.1738·2).
*Tonic.*

**Roaccutan**
Roche, Arg.; Roche, Austria; Roche, Denm.; Roche, Fin.; Roche, Ger.; Roche, Gr.; Roche, Ital.; Roche, Mex.; Roche, Port.
Isotretinoin (p.1148·3).
*Acne.*

**Roaccutane**
Roche, Austral.; Roche, Belg.; Roche, Fr.; Roche, Hong Kong; Roche, Irl.; Roche, Israel; Roche, Neth.; Roche, NZ; Roche, S.Afr.; Roche, Singapore; Roche, Switz.; Roche, Thai.; Roche, UK.
Isotretinoin (p.1148·3).
*Acne.*

**Roacnetan** Roche, Chile.
Isotretinoin (p.1148·3).
*Acne.*

**Roacutan**
Roche, Braz.; Roche, Spain.
Isotretinoin (p.1148·3).
*Acne.*

**Ro-A-Vit** Roche, NZ†.
Vitamin A palmitate (p.1453·1).
*Vitamin A deficiency.*

**Robafen AC Cough** Major, USA.
Guaifenesin (p.1122·1); codeine phosphate (p.27·1).
*Coughs.*

**Robafen CF** Major, USA†.
Phenylpropanolamine hydrochloride (p.1127·3); dextromethorphan hydrobromide (p.1117·3); guaifenesin (p.1122·1).
*Coughs.*

**Robafen DAC** Major, USA.
Pseudoephedrine hydrochloride (p.1129·2); codeine phosphate (p.27·1); guaifenesin (p.1122·1).
*Coughs.*

**Robafen DM** Major, USA.
Dextromethorphan hydrobromide (p.1117·3); guaifenesin (p.1122·1).
*Coughs.*

**Robanul** Richmond, Arg.
Epirubicin (p.550·3).
*Malignant neoplasms.*

**Robatar** Rougier, Canad.†.
Tar (p.1159·3).
*Skin disorders of the scalp.*

**RoBathol** Pharmaceutical Specialties, USA.
Emollient.

**Robaxacet** Whitehall-Robins, Canad.
Methocarbamol (p.1395·1); paracetamol (p.76·2).
*Musculoskeletal, peri-articular, and soft-tissue pain.*

**Robaxacet-8** Whitehall-Robins, Canad.
Methocarbamol (p.1395·1); paracetamol (p.76·2); codeine phosphate (p.27·1).
*Musculoskeletal, peri-articular and soft-tissue pain.*

**Robaxifen** Wyeth, Mex.
Methocarbamol (p.1395·1); paracetamol (p.76·2).
*Musculoskeletal pain.*

**Robaxin**
Whitehall-Robins, Canad.; Wyeth Lederle, Fin.†; Robins, Hong Kong; Wyeth, Mex.†; Aspen, S.Afr.; Ipsen, Spain; Wyeth Lederle, Swed.†; Whitehall, Thai.; Shire, UK; Wyeth-Ayerst, USA; Schwarz, USA.
Methocarbamol (p.1395·1).
*Skeletal muscle spasm.*

**Robaxisal**
Whitehall-Robins, Canad.; Shire, Irl.†; Wyeth, Mex.; Aspen, S.Afr.; Ipsen, Spain; Robins, USA†.
Methocarbamol (p.1395·1); aspirin (p.15·1).
*Musculoskeletal pain.*

**Robaxisal Compuesto** Ipsen, Spain.
Methocarbamol (p.1395·1); paracetamol (p.76·2).
*Musculoskeletal pain.*

**Robaxisal Forte** Wyeth Lederle, Swed.†.
Methocarbamol (p.1395·1); aspirin (p.15·1).
*Skeletal muscle spasm.*

**Robaxisal-C** Whitehall-Robins, Canad.
Methocarbamol (p.1395·1); aspirin (p.15·1); codeine phosphate (p.27·1).
*Musculoskeletal, peri-articular and soft-tissue pain.*

**Robaz** Lavipharm, Gr.
Metronidazole (p.607·2).
*Acne rosacea.*

**Roberfarin** Robert, Spain.
Dequalinium chloride (p.1178·1); enoxolone (p.36·2); hydrocortisone acetate (p.1103·3); oxetacaine (p.1382·1); tyrothricin (p.275·1).
*Mouth and throat inflammation.*

**Robervital** Robert, Spain.
Oxaceprol (p.1725·1); tocoferil sodium succinate.
*Dermatomyositis; musculoskeletal and joint disorders.*

**Robidone** Wyeth-Ayerst, Canad.†.
Hydrocodone tartrate (p.45·1).
*Coughs.*

**Robidrine** Whitehall-Robins, Canad.†.
Pseudoephedrine hydrochloride (p.1129·2).
*Nasal congestion.*

**Robiflam** Khandelwal, India.
Methocarbamol (p.1395·1); ibuprofen (p.45·3).
*Skeletal muscle spasm.*

**Robi-Flu** Wyeth Consumer, Chile.
Paracetamol (p.76·2); pseudoephedrine hydrochloride (p.1129·2); chlorphenamine maleate (p.427·3).
*Cold and influenza symptoms.*

**Robigesic** Whitehall-Robins, Canad.
Paracetamol (p.76·2).
*Fever; pain.*

**Robimycin Robitabs** Robins, USA.
Erythromycin (p.208·1).
*Bacterial infections.*

**Robinax** Khandelwal, India.
Methocarbamol (p.1395·1).
*Skeletal muscle spasm.*

**Robinaxol** Khandelwal, India.
Methocarbamol (p.1395·1); paracetamol (p.76·2).
*Skeletal muscle spasm.*

**Robinaz** Whitehall, Port.†.
Oxymetazoline hydrochloride (p.1126·1).
*Nasal congestion.*

**Robinia Med Complex** Dynamit, Austria.
Homoeopathic preparation.

**Robinia Ro-Plex (Rowo-99)** Pharmakon, Ger.†.
Homoeopathic preparation.

**Robinul**
Wyeth, Austral.; Wyeth Lederle, Austria; Wyeth Lederle, Belg.; Wyeth-Ayerst, Canad.†; Meda, Denm.; Wyeth Lederle, Fin.; Riemser, Ger.; Robins, Hong Kong; Antigen, Irl.†; Wyeth, Neth.†; Wyeth Lederle, Norw.; Wyeth, NZ; Aspen, S.Afr.; Meda, Swed.; Wyeth, Switz.†; Anpharm, UK; Horizon, USA.
Glycopyrronium bromide (p.482·3).
*Adjunct in peptic ulcer; hyperhidrosis; intra-operative management of cardiac vagal reflexes; premedication; protection against muscarinic effects of anticholinesterases used to reverse neuromuscular blockade.*

**Robinul-Neostigmin**
Meda, Denm.; Wyeth Lederle, Fin.; Wyeth Lederle, Norw.; Wyeth Lederle, Swed.
Neostigmine metilsulfate (p.1492·2).

Glycopyrronium bromide (p.482·3) is included in this preparation to protect against the muscarinic actions.
*Reversal of competitive neuromuscular blockade.*

**Robinul-Neostigmine** Wyeth Lederle, Belg.; Antigen, Irl.†; Wyeth, Switz.; Anpharm, UK.
Neostigmine metilsulfate (p.1492·2).
Glycopyrronium bromide (p.482·3) is included in this preparation to protect against the muscarinic actions.
*Reversal of competitive neuromuscular blockade.*

**Robitussin** Wyeth-Whitehall, Arg.; Whitehall-Robins, Canad.; Robins, Israel; Wyeth, Mex.; Wyeth Consumer, Singapore; Wyeth, Spain; Whitehall, Thai.; Robins, USA.
Guaifenesin (p.1122·1).
*Coughs.*

**Robitussin AC**
Note. This name is used for preparations of different composition.
Whitehall-Robins, Canad.
Guaifenesin (p.1122·1); pheniramine maleate (p.438·3); codeine phosphate (p.27·1).
*Coughs.*

Robins, USA.
Guaifenesin (p.1122·1); codeine phosphate (p.27·1).
*Coughs.*

**Robitussin Caramelos** Wyeth-Whitehall, Arg.
Menthol (p.1711·3).
*Coughs.*

**Robitussin CF** Robins, Hong Kong†; Robins, USA†.
Guaifenesin (p.1122·1); phenylpropanolamine hydrochloride (p.1127·3); dextromethorphan hydrobromide (p.1117·3).
*Coughs.*

**Robitussin Chesty Cough** Wyeth Consumer, Irl.
Guaifenesin (p.1122·1).
Formerly known as Robitussin Expectorant.
*Coughs.*

**Robitussin for Chesty Coughs** Wyeth Consumer, UK.
Guaifenesin (p.1122·1).
*Coughs.*

**Robitussin for Chesty Coughs with Congestion** Wyeth Consumer, UK.
Guaifenesin (p.1122·1); pseudoephedrine hydrochloride (p.1129·2).
Formerly known as Robitussin Plus.
*Coughs; nasal congestion.*

**Robitussin Childrens Cough & Cold** Whitehall-Robins, Canad.
Dextromethorphan hydrobromide (p.1117·3); pseudoephedrine hydrochloride (p.1129·2).
Formerly known as Robitussin Pediatric Cough & Cold.
*Coughs and cold symptoms.*

**Robitussin Childrens Cough DM** Whitehall-Robins, Canad.
Dextromethorphan hydrobromide (p.1117·3).
*Coughs.*

**Robitussin Children's Night Relief** Whitehall, NZ.
Chlorphenamine maleate (p.427·3); dextromethorphan hydrobromide (p.1117·3); pseudoephedrine hydrochloride (p.1129·2).
*Coughs and cold symptoms.*

**Robitussin with Codeine** Whitehall-Robins, Canad.
Guaifenesin (p.1122·1); pheniramine maleate (p.438·3); codeine phosphate (p.27·1).
*Coughs.*

**Robitussin Cold** Wyeth Consumer, Singapore.
Guaifenesin (p.1122·1); pseudoephedrine hydrochloride (p.1129·2).
*Coughs; nasal congestion.*

**Robitussin Cold & Cough** Wyeth Consumer, Singapore; Robins, USA.
Guaifenesin (p.1122·1); dextromethorphan hydrobromide (p.1117·3); pseudoephedrine hydrochloride (p.1129·2).
*Coughs; nasal congestion.*

**Robitussin Cold, Cough & Flu** Wyeth Consumer, Singapore.
Paracetamol (p.76·2); guaifenesin (p.1122·1); dextromethorphan hydrobromide (p.1117·3); pseudoephedrine hydrochloride (p.1129·2).
*Cold and flu symptoms; coughs; nasal congestion.*

**Robitussin Cough Calmers** Robins, USA†.
Dextromethorphan hydrobromide (p.1117·3).
*Coughs.*

**Robitussin Cough & Cold** Whitehall-Robins, Canad.
Guaifenesin (p.1122·1); dextromethorphan hydrobromide (p.1117·3); pseudoephedrine hydrochloride (p.1129·2).
*Coughs and cold symptoms.*

**Robitussin Cough, Cold & Flu** Whitehall-Robins, Canad.
Guaifenesin (p.1122·1); dextromethorphan hydrobromide (p.1117·3); pseudoephedrine hydrochloride (p.1129·2); paracetamol (p.76·2).
*Cold and flu symptoms; coughs.*

**Robitussin Cough Drops** Robins, USA.
Menthol (p.1711·3); eucalyptus oil (p.1686·2).

**Robitussin D** Wyeth-Whitehall, Arg.
Guaifenesin (p.1122·1); pseudoephedrine hydrochloride (p.1129·2).
*Coughs; nasal congestion.*

**Robitussin DAC** Robins, USA.
Guaifenesin (p.1122·1); pseudoephedrine hydrochloride (p.1129·2); codeine phosphate (p.27·1).
*Coughs.*

**Robitussin DM** Whitehall Consumer, Austral.; Whitehall-Robins, Canad.; Robins, Hong Kong; Robins, Israel; Wyeth, Mex.; Whitehall, NZ; Wyeth Consumer, Singapore; Whitehall, Thai.; Robins, USA.
Guaifenesin (p.1122·1); dextromethorphan hydrobromide (p.1117·3).
*Coughs.*

**Robitussin DM Antitusivo** Wyeth, Spain.
Dextromethorphan hydrobromide (p.1117·3).
*Coughs.*

**Robitussin DM-P** Whitehall Consumer, Austral.; Whitehall, NZ.
Dextromethorphan hydrobromide (p.1117·3); pseudoephedrine hydrochloride (p.1129·2).
*Coughs; nasal and sinus congestion.*

**Robitussin Dry Cough** Wyeth Consumer, Irl.
Dextromethorphan hydrobromide (p.1117·3).
Formerly known as Robitussin Cough Soother.
*Coughs.*

**Robitussin for Dry Coughs** Wyeth Consumer, UK.
Dextromethorphan hydrobromide (p.1117·3).
*Coughs.*

**Robitussin DX** Whitehall Consumer, Austral.; Whitehall, NZ.
Dextromethorphan hydrobromide (p.1117·3).
*Coughs.*

**Robitussin EX** Whitehall Consumer, Austral.; Whitehall, NZ.
Guaifenesin (p.1122·1).
*Coughs.*

**Robitussin Expectorant**
Note. This name is used for preparations of different composition.
Robins, Hong Kong.
Guaifenesin (p.1122·1).
*Coughs.*

Whitehall-Robins, Switz.
Acetylcysteine (p.1112·3).
*Coughs with viscous mucus.*

**Robitussin Honey Cough** Whitehall, NZ.
Dextromethorphan hydrobromide (p.1117·3); honey (p.1434·2).
*Coughs.*

**Robitussin Honey Cough DM** Whitehall-Robins, Canad.
Dextromethorphan hydrobromide (p.1117·3).
*Coughs.*

**Robitussin Honey Cough Syrup** Whitehall Consumer, Austral.
Dextromethorphan hydrobromide (p.1117·3).
*Coughs.*

**Robitussin Junior** Whitehall, UK†.
Dextromethorphan hydrobromide (p.1117·3).
*Coughs.*

**Robitussin Maximum Strength Cough** Robins, Hong Kong.
Dextromethorphan hydrobromide (p.1117·3).
*Coughs.*

**Robitussin Maximum Strength Cough & Cold** Robins, USA.
Dextromethorphan hydrobromide (p.1117·3); pseudoephedrine hydrochloride (p.1129·2).
*Coughs and cold symptoms.*

**Robitussin ME** Whitehall Consumer, Austral.; Whitehall, NZ.
Guaifenesin (p.1122·1); bromhexine hydrochloride (p.1115·3).
*Coughs; respiratory-tract congestion.*

**Robitussin Night Relief** Robins, USA.
Pseudoephedrine hydrochloride (p.1129·2); dextromethorphan hydrobromide (p.1117·3); mepyramine maleate (p.437·1); paracetamol (p.76·2).
*Coughs and cold symptoms.*

**Robitussin Night-Time** Whitehall, UK†.
Brompheniramine maleate (p.426·1); codeine phosphate (p.27·1); pseudoephedrine hydrochloride (p.1129·2).
*Coughs.*

**Robitussin Paediatric Cough** Robins, Hong Kong.
Dextromethorphan hydrobromide (p.1117·3).
*Coughs.*

**Robitussin PE** Robins, Hong Kong; Wyeth Consumer, Singapore; Whitehall, Thai.; Robins, USA.
Guaifenesin (p.1122·1); pseudoephedrine hydrochloride (p.1129·2).
*Coughs; nasal congestion.*

**Robitussin Pediatric** Robins, USA.
Dextromethorphan hydrobromide (p.1117·3).
*Coughs.*

**Robitussin Pediatric Cough & Cold Formula** Robins, USA.
Dextromethorphan hydrobromide (p.1117·3); pseudoephedrine hydrochloride (p.1129·2).
*Coughs and cold symptoms.*

**Robitussin Plus** Wyeth Consumer, Irl.
Guaifenesin (p.1122·1); pseudoephedrine hydrochloride (p.1129·2).
Formerly known as Robitussin Expectorant Plus.
*Coughs; nasal congestion.*

**Robitussin PM Cough & Cold** Wyeth Consumer, USA.
Dextromethorphan hydrobromide (p.1117·3); chlorphenamine maleate (p.427·3); pseudoephedrine hydrochloride (p.1129·2).
*Upper respiratory-tract disorders.*

**Robitussin PS** Whitehall Consumer, Austral.; Whitehall, NZ.
Guaifenesin (p.1122·1); pseudoephedrine hydrochloride (p.1129·2).
*Coughs; nasal congestion.*

**Robitussin Severe Congestion** Robins, USA.
Guaifenesin (p.1122·1); pseudoephedrine hydrochloride (p.1129·2).

**Robovites** Vita Health, Singapore.
Multivitamin preparation with or without iron or zinc (p.1417·1).

**Robovites Multivitamin** Vita Health, Singapore.
Multivitamins; cod-liver oil; evening primrose oil; echinacea; ginkgo biloba (p.1417·1).

**Roburis** Ripari-Gero, Ital.†.
Ubidecarenone (p.1760·2).
*Cardiac disorders; coenzyme Q10 deficiency.*

**Roburvit** Echo, Ital.
Royal jelly (p.1740·3).

**Robuvalen** Robugen, Ger.
Zinc oxide (p.1163·2).
*Eczema; skin lesions.*

**RoC Sunscreen Stick** RoC, UK.
Dibenzoylmethane (p.1145·2); a cinnamic ester.
*Sunscreen.*

**RoC Total Sunblock** RoC, UK.
*SPF 25:* Octinoxate (p.1154·3); avobenzone (p.1142·3); titanium dioxide (p.1160·3).
*Sunscreen.*

**Rocal** ANB, Thai.
Dextromethorphan hydrobromide (p.1117·3); guaifenesin (p.1122·1); terpin hydrate (p.1131·1).
*Coughs.*

**Rocaltrol** Roche, Austral.; Roche, Austria; Roche, Belg.; Roche, Braz.; Roche, Canad.; Roche, Chile; Roche, Denm.; Roche, Fr.; Roche, Ger.; Roche, Hong Kong; Roche, Irl.; Roche, Ital.; Roche, Jpn; Roche, Mex.; Roche, Neth.; Roche, Norw.; Roche, NZ; Roche, Port.; Roche, S.Afr.; Roche, Singapore; Roche, Spain; Roche, Swed.; Roche, Switz.; Roche, Thai.; Roche, UK; Roche, USA.
Calcitriol (p.1461·2).
*Hypoparathyroidism; osteomalacia; renal osteodystrophy; rickets; vitamin D deficiency.*

**Rocanal Imediat** Medirel, Switz.†.
Povidone-iodine (p.1190·3).
*Dental disinfection.*

**Rocanal Permanent Gangrene** Medirel, Switz.†.
Powder, hydrocortisone acetate (p.1103·3); paraformaldehyde (p.1187·3); zinc oxide (p.1163·2); zinc stearate (p.1575·3); zinc acetate (p.1469·2); liquid, eugenol (p.1686·2).
*Dental infections.*

**Rocanal Permanent Vital** Medirel, Switz.†.
Powder, paraformaldehyde (p.1187·3); zinc oxide (p.1163·2); zinc stearate (p.1575·3); zinc acetate (p.1469·2); liquid, eugenol (p.1686·2).
*Dental disorders.*

**Roccal** Sanofi Winthrop, Irl.†.
Benzalkonium chloride (p.1168·3).
*Skin disinfection.*

**Roccaxin** Nakorn, Thai.
Piroxicam (p.84·2).
*Musculoskeletal, joint, peri-articular, and soft-tissue disorders.*

**Rocefalin** Roche, Spain.
Ceftriaxone sodium (p.182·3).
Lidocaine (p.1377·3) is included in the intramuscular injection to alleviate the pain of injection.
*Bacterial infections.*

**Rocefin** Roche, Braz.; Roche, Ital.
Ceftriaxone sodium (p.182·3).
Lidocaine hydrochloride (p.1377·3) may be included in the intramuscular injection to alleviate the pain of injection.
*Gram-negative bacterial infections.*

**Rocephalin** Roche, Denm.; Roche, Fin.; Roche, Norw.; Roche, Swed.
Ceftriaxone sodium (p.182·3).
Lidocaine hydrochloride (p.1377·3) may be included in some injections to alleviate the pain of injection.
*Bacterial infections.*

**Rocephin** Roche, Austral.; Roche, Austria; Roche, Canad.; Roche, Ger.; Roche, Gr.; Roche, Hong Kong; Roche, Irl.; Roche, Israel; Roche, Jpn; Roche, Mex.; Roche, Neth.; Roche, NZ; Roche, Port.; Roche, S.Afr.; Roche, Singapore; Roche, Thai.; Roche, UK; Roche, USA.
Ceftriaxone sodium (p.182·3).
Lidocaine hydrochloride (p.1377·3) may be included in the intramuscular injection to alleviate the pain of injection.
*Bacterial infections.*

**Rocephine** Roche, Belg.; Roche, Fr.; Roche, Switz.
Ceftriaxone sodium (p.182·3).
Lidocaine hydrochloride (p.1377·3) is included in the intramuscular preparation to alleviate the pain of injection.
*Bacterial infections.*

**Roceron** Roche, Norw.
Interferon alfa-2a (p.640·3).
*Chronic active hepatitis B; chronic hepatitis C; malignant neoplasms.*

**Roceron-A** Roche, Denm.
Interferon alfa-2a (p.640·3).
*Chronic hepatitis B or C; malignant neoplasms.*

**Rocgel** Chiesi, Fr.
Boehmite.
*Gastrointestinal disorders.*

**Rochagan** Roche, Braz.
Benznidazole (p.602·3).
*American trypanosomiasis.*

**Roche** Syntex, Canad.†.
Naproxen sodium (p.65·1).
*Inflammation; pain.*

**Rochevit** Roche, Spain.
Multivitamin and mineral preparation (p.1417·1).

**Rociclyn** Zambon, Neth.
Tolfenamic acid (p.94·2).
*Osteoarthritis; rheumatoid arthritis.*

**Rocid** Max Farma, Ital.
Cefonicid sodium (p.174·2).
Lidocaine hydrochloride (p.1377·3) is included in this preparation to alleviate the pain of injection.
*Gram-negative bacterial infections.*

**Rocilin** Rosco, Denm.; Rosco, Norw.
Phenoxymethylpenicillin potassium (p.242·1).
*Bacterial infections.*

**Rocmaline** Calea, Austria; Chiesi, Fr.
Arginine (p.1421·1); malic acid (p.1709·2).
*Liver disorders.*

**Rocodin** Brunel, S.Afr.†.
Paracetamol (p.76·2); codeine phosphate (p.27·1).
*Fever; pain.*

**Rocof** Roche, Thai.†.
Dextromethorphan hydrobromide (p.1117·3); chlorphenamine maleate (p.427·3); pseudoephedrine hydrochloride (p.1129·2).
*Coughs.*

**Rocornal** UCB, Austria; UCB, Ger.
Trapidil (p.1016·2).
*Ischaemic heart disease; prevention of restenosis following percutaneous transluminal coronary angioplasty.*

**Roctylan** Pharmedia (Φαρμεντια), Gr.
Butamirate citrate (p.1116·2).
*Cough.*

**Rodakin** Kener, Mex.†.
Loratadine (p.436·1).

**Rodase** Pond's, Thai.
Serrapeptase (p.1743·2).
*Inflammation; respiratory-tract congestion; wounds.*

**Rodavan** Asta Medica, Ger.†.
Chlorphenoxamine hydrochloride (p.428·3); caffeine (p.782·1); 8-chlorotheophylline.
*Motion sickness; nausea; vertigo; vomiting.*

**Rodazol** Novartis, Ger.†.
Aminoglutethimide (p.526·3).
*Breast cancer; Cushing's syndrome.*

**Rodenal** Rekah, Israel.
Trihexyphenidyl hydrochloride (p.490·2).
*Parkinsonism.*

**Rodepan** Pharma Investi, Chile.
Cyproheptadine hydrochloride (p.430·1); thiamine hydrochloride; pyridoxine hydrochloride; riboflavine sodium phosphate; nicotinamide; ascorbic acid (p.1417·1).
*Reduced appetite; tonic.*

**Rodermil** Edol, Port.
Metronidazole (p.607·2).
*Rosacea.*

**Rodinac** Geminis, Arg.
Diclofenac (p.32·1).
*Inflammation; pain.*

**Rodinac Biotic** Geminis, Arg.
Amoxicillin (p.155·3); diclofenac (p.32·1).
*Bacterial infections.*

**Rodinac Flex** Geminis, Arg.
Pridinol (p.1395·2); diclofenac (p.32·1).
*Inflammation; muscle spasm; pain.*

**Rodinac Gesic** Geminis, Arg.
Paracetamol (p.76·2); diclofenac (p.32·1).
*Inflammation; pain.*

**Rodogyl** Aventis, Fr.; Aventis, Mex.
Spiramycin (p.255·3); metronidazole (p.607·2).
*Mouth infections.*

**Rodopsin Plus** Baldacci, Ital.
Vitamin E; copper; zinc; red vine (p.1417·1).

**Rodovit** Allen, Mex.
Vitamin preparation with or without minerals (p.1417·1).

**RO-Dry Eyes** Richmond Ophthalmics, Canad.†.
Polyvinyl alcohol (p.1581·1).
*Dry eyes.*

**RO-Eye Drops** Richmond Ophthalmics, Canad.†.
Tetryzoline hydrochloride (p.1131·2).

**RO-Eyewash** Richmond Ophthalmics, Canad.†.
Boric acid (p.1662·1).

**Rofact** ICN, Canad.
Rifampicin (p.250·2).
*Tuberculosis.*

**Rofatuss** MIP, Ger.
Clobutinol hydrochloride (p.1117·1).
*Coughs.*

**Rofenid** *Aventis, Belg.*
Ketoprofen (p.51·2).
*Inflammation; musculoskeletal, joint, and peri-articular disorders; oedema; pain.*

**Rofepain** *LBS, Thai.*
Ketoprofen (p.51·2).
*Gout; musculoskeletal, joint, peri-articular, and soft-tissue disorders; pain.*

**Roferon-A**
*Roche, Arg.; Roche, Austral.; Roche, Austria; Roche, Belg.; Roche, Braz.; Roche, Canad.; Roche, Chile; Roche, Fin.; Roche, Fr.; Roche, Ger.; Roche, Gr.; Roche, Hong Kong; Nicholas Piramal, India; Roche, Irl.; Roche, Israel; Roche, Ital.; Roche, Jpn; Roche, Mex.; Roche, Neth.; Roche, NZ; Roche, Port.; Roche, S.Afr.; Roche, Singapore; Roche, Spain; Roche, Swed.; Roche, Switz.; Roche, Thai.; Roche, UK; Roche, USA.*
Interferon alfa-2a (rbe) (p.640·3).
*Hepatitis B; hepatitis C; malignant neoplasms.*

**Rofetab** *Centaur, India.*
Rofecoxib (p.86·3).
*Musculoskeletal and joint disorders; pain.*

**Rofex** *Nicholas Piramal, India.*
Cefalexin (p.168·1).
*Bacterial infections.*

**Rofiz** *Wockhardt, India.*
Rofecoxib (p.86·3).
*Musculoskeletal, joint, and soft-tissue disorders; pain.*

**Roflatol Phyto (Rowo-146)** *Pharmakon, Ger.†.*
Chamomile (p.1669·3); caraway oil (p.1667·3); fennel oil (p.1687·3); peppermint oil (p.1283·2).
*Gastrointestinal disorders.*

**Rofoxin** *Royton, Braz.*
Ceftriaxone sodium (p.182·3).
Lidocaine (p.1377·3) is included in the intramuscular injection to alleviate the pain of injection.
*Bacterial infections.*

**Rogaan** *Abic, Israel.*
Dextropropoxyphene hydrochloride (p.28·3); aspirin (p.15·1); paracetamol (p.76·2); caffeine (p.782·1).
*Cold symptoms; pain.*

**Rogadermis** *Lacefa, Arg.*
Vitamin A (p.1451·2).
*Burns.*

**Rogaine**
*Pharmacia, Austral.; Pharmacia, Austria; McNeil Consumer, Canad.; Pharmacia, NZ; Pharmacia, USA.*
Minoxidil (p.960·1).
Formerly known as Regaine in *Austral.* and *NZ.*
*Alopecia androgenetica.*

**Rogal** *Galen, Mex.†.*
Piroxicam (p.84·2).
*Gout; musculoskeletal, joint, peri-articular, and soft-tissue disorders; pain.*

**Rogasti** *Pacific, Israel.*
Famotidine (p.1265·2).
*Duodenal ulcer; gastro-oesophageal reflux; Zollinger-Ellison syndrome.*

**Rogastril** *Roemmers, Arg.*
Cinitapride acid tartrate (p.1259·2).
*Gastro-oesophageal reflux; gastrointestinal motility disorders.*

**Roge** *Pastor Farina, Ital.†.*
Anhydrous citric acid (p.1673·1); magnesium carbonate (p.1272·1).
*Constipation.*

**Rogelina** *Geminis, Arg.*
Sodium picosulfate (p.1289·3).
*Constipation.*

**Rogitine**
*Novartis, Canad.; Alliance, UK.*
Phentolamine mesilate (p.982·1).
*Dermal necrosis and sloughing following intravenous administration of noradrenaline; phaeochromocytoma.*

**roha-Fenchel-Tee** *Roha, Ger.†.*
Fennel (p.1687·2).
*Gastrointestinal disorders.*

**rohasal** *Roha, Ger.*
Absinthium (p.1645·1); aniseed (p.1655·2); kaolin (p.1268·3); calcium phosphate (p.1225·3); dried magnesium sulfate (p.1229·1); calcium carbonate (p.1254·2); heavy magnesium carbonate (p.1272·1); sodium bicarbonate (p.1223·2).
*Gastrointestinal disorders.*

**rohasal N** *Roha, Ger.*
Sodium bicarbonate (p.1223·2); calcium carbonate (p.1254·2); heavy magnesium carbonate (p.1272·1).
*Gastrointestinal disorders.*

**Rohipnol** *Roche, Spain.*
Flunitrazepam (p.698·2).
*Anxiety; general anaesthesia; insomnia.*

**Rohto Zi** *Mentholatum, UK.*
Camphor (p.1665·3).
*Eye irritation.*

**Rohto Zi Contact** *Mentholatum, Austral.*
Hyetellose (p.1579·2).
*Dry eyes.*

**Rohto Zi Fresh** *Mentholatum, Austral.*
Povidone (p.1581·2).
*Dry eyes.*

**Rohypnol**
*Roche, Arg.; Roche, Austral.†; Roche, Austria; Roche, Belg.; Roche, Braz.; Roche, Chile; Roche, Denm.; Roche, Fr.; Roche, Ger.; Roche, Hong Kong; Roche, Irl.; Roche, Israel†; Roche, Mex.; Roche, Neth.; Roche, Norw.; Roche, Port.; Roche, S.Afr.; Roche, Swed.; Roche, Switz.; Roche, Thai.; Roche, UK†.*
Flunitrazepam (p.698·2).
*Insomnia.*

**Roical** *Shin Poong, Singapore.*
Calcitriol (p.1461·2).
*Hypoparathyroidism; osteomalacia; osteoporosis; renal osteodystrophy; rickets.*

**Roidhemo**
*Cusi, Hong Kong†; Pan Quimica, Spain.*
Aesculus (p.1648·2); benzyl phenol; benzyl salicylate; ephedrine hydrochloride (p.1120·1); hamamelis (p.1696·3); lactic acid (p.1704·1).
*Anorectal disorders.*

**Roiplon** *Menarini, Gr.*
Etofenamate (p.38·1).
*Inflammation; musculoskeletal and joint disorders; pain.*

**Roipnol** *Roche, Ital.*
Flunitrazepam (p.698·2).
*Insomnia.*

**Rojema** *Self-Care Products, UK.*
Royal jelly (p.1740·3).

**Rojobacter** *Ferro, Arg.*
Dibromo hydroxymercuric fluorescein sodium.
*Bacterial infections.*

**Rokacet** *Taro, Israel.*
Paracetamol (p.76·2); caffeine (p.782·1); codeine phosphate (p.27·1).
*Coughs fever; pain.*

**Rokacet Plus** *Taro, Israel.*
Paracetamol (p.76·2); caffeine (p.782·1); codeine phosphate (p.27·1).
*Coughs; fever; pain.*

**Rokadin** *Kener, Mex.*
Loratadine (p.436·1).
*Hypersensitivity.*

**Rokal** *Taro, Israel.*
Aspirin (p.15·1); caffeine (p.782·1); codeine phosphate (p.27·1).
*Coughs; fever; pain; rheumatism.*

**Rokal Plus** *Taro, Israel.*
Aspirin (p.15·1); caffeine (p.782·1); codeine phosphate (p.27·1).
*Coughs; fever; pain; rheumatism.*

**Rokamol** *Taro, Israel.*
Paracetamol (p.76·2).
*Fever; pain.*

**Rokamol Plus Codeine** *Taro, Israel.*
Paracetamol (p.76·2); codeine phosphate (p.27·1).
*Coughs; fever; pain.*

**Rokan**
*Andromaco, Chile; Spitzner, Ger.*
Ginkgo biloba leaf (p.1692·3).
*Mental function disorders; peripheral circulatory disorders.*

**Rokanite** *Taro, Israel.*
Aspirin (p.15·1); codeine phosphate (p.27·1).
*Coughs; fever; pain; rheumatism.*

**Rokital** *Formenti, Ital.*
Rokitamycin (p.254·1).
*Bacterial infections.*

**Rolac Plus** *Wyeth, India.*
Magaldrate (p.1271·3); simeticone (p.1289·2).
*Flatulence; gastric hyperacidity; gastritis; peptic ulcer.*

**Rolaids** *Pfizer Consumer, Canad.*
Calcium carbonate (p.1254·2); magnesium hydroxide (p.1272·2).
*Dyspepsia.*

**Rolaket** *Elpen (Ελπεν), Gr.*
Nimesulide (p.67·1).
*Inflammation; musculoskeletal disorders; pain.*

**Rolap** *Teva Tuteur, Arg.*
Tamoxifen (p.585·3).

**Rolar** *Pharmaland, Thai.*
Codeine phosphate (p.27·1); guaifenesin (p.1122·1).
Formerly contained codeine phosphate, guaifenesin, and phenylpropanolamine hydrochloride.
*Cold symptoms; coughs; nasal congestion.*

**Rolatuss Expectorant** *Huckaby, USA.*
Phenylephrine hydrochloride (p.1126·3); codeine phosphate (p.27·1); chlorphenamine maleate (p.427·3); ammonium chloride (p.1115·2).
*Coughs.*

**Rolatuss with Hydrocodone** *Major, USA†.*
Phenylpropanolamine hydrochloride (p.1127·3); phenylephrine hydrochloride (p.1126·3); mepyramine maleate (p.437·1); pheniramine maleate (p.438·3); hydrocodone tartrate (p.45·1).
*Coughs and cold symptoms.*

**Rolatuss Plain** *Major, USA.*
Phenylephrine hydrochloride (p.1126·3); chlorphenamine maleate (p.427·3).
*Upper respiratory-tract symptoms.*

**Roleca Wacholder** *Riemser, Ger.*
Juniper oil (p.1703·1).
*Diuretic.*

**Roleca-S** *Medichemie Bioline, Switz.†.*
Juniper oil (p.1703·1).
*Gastrointestinal disorders.*

**Rolene** *Riva, Canad.†.*
Betamethasone dipropionate (p.1093·1).
*Skin disorders.*

**Rolip** *LED, Fr.*
*alpha*-Acetyl mandelic acid (p.228·3).
*Dry lips.*

**Roliwol** *Stada, Switz.†.*
Methyl salicylate (p.59·3); camphor (p.1665·3); methyl nicotinate (p.59·2); menthol (p.1711·3); turpentine oil (p.1760·1); eucalyptus oil (p.1686·2); mint oil (p.1715·2); thymol (p.1194·2); nutmeg oil (p.1722·3).
*Musculoskeletal and joint pain; sports injuries.*

**Roliwol B** *Stada, Switz.†.*
Glycol salicylate (p.44·3); camphor (p.1665·3); diethylamine salicylate (p.34·1); pine oil.
*Musculoskeletal, joint, and peri-articular pain.*

**Roliwol S** *Stada, Switz.†.*
Glycol salicylate (p.44·3); benzyl nicotinate (p.21·2); nonivamide (p.67·2).
*Musculoskeletal, joint, and peri-articular disorders.*

**Roll-bene** *Mepha, Switz.†.*
Heparin sodium (p.928·1); dimethyl sulfoxide (p.1473·2); dexpanthenol (p.1727·2).
*Inflammation; musculoskeletal, joint, peri-articular, and soft-tissue disorders; pain; peripheral vascular disorders.*

**Roll-On** *Shaklee, Canad.*
Aluminium chlorohydrate (p.1142·1).
*Hyperhidrosis.*

**Roloken** *Kendrick, Mex.†.*
Biperiden (p.479·3).

**Rolsical** *Sun, India.*
Calcitriol (p.1461·2).
*Hypocalcaemia; hypoparathyroidism; osteoporosis; rickets.*

**Romadin** *Grunenthal, Spain†.*
Astemizole (p.424·2).
*Hypersensitivity reactions.*

**Romarene** *Beaufour, Fr.*
Rosemary (p.1740·2); taraxacum (p.1751·3); kinkeliba (p.1703·3); potassium sodium tartrate (p.1284·3); sodium citrate (p.1223·2).
*Gastrointestinal disorders.*

**Romarinex** *Aerocid, Fr.*
Rosemary (p.1740·2); kinkeliba (p.1703·3).
*Biliary-tract disorders.*

**Romarinex-Choline** *Aerocid, Fr.†.*
Rosemary (p.1740·2); cynara (p.1678·3); boldo (p.1661·2); taraxacum (p.1751·3); kinkeliba (p.1703·3); choline citrate (p.1424·3).
*Gastrointestinal disorders.*

**Romazicon** *Roche, USA.*
Flumazenil (p.1038·3).
Formerly known as Mazicon.
*Benzodiazepine overdosage; reversal of benzodiazepine-induced sedation.*

**Rombay** *Apotheke Heiligen Dreifaltigkeit, Austria.*
Talc (p.1159·1); zinc oxide (p.1163·2); peru balsam (p.1730·2).
*Skin irritation.*

**Rombellin**
*Simons, Ger.; Adroka, Switz.*
Biotin (p.1423·2).
*Biotin deficiency.*

**Rombox** *Glaxo Wellcome, Mex.*
Cefalexin (p.168·1); ambroxol hydrochloride (p.1114·3).
*Respiratory-tract infections.*

**Romesa** *Rhone-Poulenc Rorer, Mex.†.*
Warfarin sodium (p.1022·2).

**Romesec**
*Ranbaxy, Malaysia; Ranbaxy, Singapore.*
Omeprazole (p.1278·2).
*Dyspepsia; gastro-oesophageal reflux; peptic ulcer; Zollinger-Ellison syndrome.*

**Romet** *Mitsubishi, Jpn.*
Repirinast (p.791·2).
*Asthma.*

**Romicin** *Pacific, NZ.*
Roxithromycin (p.254·2).
*Bacterial infections.*

**Romidon** *Relyo, Gr.*
Dextropropoxyphene hydrochloride (p.28·3).
*Pain.*

**Romigal** *Romigal, Ger.†.*
Aspirin (p.15·1).
*Fever; inflammation; musculoskeletal, joint, and soft-tissue disorders; pain; thromboembolic disorders.*

**Romilar**
*Note. This name is used for preparations of different composition.*
*Roche, Arg.; Roche, Mex.†; Roche, Spain; Roche, Thai.*
Dextromethorphan hydrobromide (p.1117·3).
*Coughs.*

*Roche, Ital.†.*
Dextromethorphan hydrobromide (p.1117·3); ammonium chloride (p.1115·2).
*Coughs.*

*Roche, Thai.*
*Syrup:* Dextromethorphan hydrobromide (p.1117·3); ammonium chloride (p.1115·2); dexpanthenol (p.1727·2).
*Coughs.*

**Romilar AC** *Scot-Tussin, USA.*
Codeine phosphate (p.27·1); guaifenesin (p.1122·1).
*Coughs.*

**Romilar Antitussivum** *Roche, Belg.*
Dextromethorphan hydrobromide (p.1117·3).
*Coughs.*

**Romilar Mucolyticum** *Roche, Belg.*
Carbocisteine (p.1116·2).
*Respiratory-tract disorders associated with accumulation of mucus.*

**Rominafort** *Garden House, Arg.*
Betacarotene; collagen; alpha tocopherol (p.1417·1).
*Dietary supplement.*

**Romir** *Diba, Mex.*
Captopril (p.879·2).
*Heart failure; hypertension; myocardial infarction.*

**Romiver** *Rafarm, Gr.*
Terbinafine (p.408·2).
*Fungal skin infections.*

**Rommix** *Ashbourne, UK.*
Erythromycin (p.208·1).

**Romulin** *Chew, Thai.*
Bromhexine hydrochloride (p.1115·3).
*Respiratory-tract disorders associated with increased or viscous mucus.*

**Ronabin** *Unimed, Israel.*
Dronabinol (p.1264·2).
*Nausea and vomiting induced by cytotoxic therapy.*

**Ronal**
*Note. This name is used for preparations of different composition.*
*Aventis, Braz.†.*
Aspirin (p.15·1).
*Fever; inflammation; pain; thromboembolism prophylaxis.*

*Durascan, Denm.*
Flunitrazepam (p.698·2).
*Insomnia.*

**Roname** *Lacer, Spain.*
Glimepiride (p.332·2).
*Diabetes mellitus.*

**RO-Naphz** *Richmond Ophthalmics, Canad.†.*
Naphazoline hydrochloride (p.1124·3).
*Eye congestion.*

**Rondamine-DM** *Major, USA.*
Pseudoephedrine hydrochloride (p.1129·2); dextromethorphan hydrobromide (p.1117·3); brompheniramine maleate (p.426·1).
Formerly contained pseudoephedrine hydrochloride, dextromethorphan hydrobromide, and carbinoxamine maleate.
*Coughs and cold symptoms.*

**Rondec**
*Note. This name is used for preparations of different composition.*
*Abbott, Arg.; Abbott, Ital.†; Abbott, Spain†; Biovail, USA.*
Carbinoxamine maleate (p.426·3); pseudoephedrine hydrochloride (p.1129·2).
*Allergic and vasomotor rhinitis; nasal congestion.*

*Biovail, USA.*
*Syrup:* Brompheniramine maleate (p.426·1); pseudoephedrine hydrochloride (p.1129·2).
*Upper respiratory-tract disorders.*

**Rondec Compositum** *Abbott, Arg.*
Carbinoxamine maleate (p.426·3); pseudoephedrine hydrochloride (p.1129·2); bromhexine hydrochloride (p.1115·3); paracetamol (p.76·2).
*Respiratory-tract disorders.*

**Rondec-DM**
*Abbott, Thai.; Dura, USA.*
Carbinoxamine maleate (p.426·3); pseudoephedrine hydrochloride (p.1129·2); dextromethorphan hydrobromide (p.1117·3).
*Coughs and cold symptoms; respiratory symptoms of allergy.*

**Rondimen** *Asta Medica, Ger.†.*
Mefenorex hydrochloride (p.1589·2).
*Obesity.*

**Ronemox** *Nicholas Piramal, India.*
Amoxicillin trihydrate (p.155·3).
*Bacterial infections.*

**Ronexine** *Rekah, Israel.*
Levomepromazine maleate (p.703·2).
*Anxiety; behaviour disorders; tension.*

**Ronfase** *Pharmacia, Arg.*
Estradiol (p.1550·1).
*Menopausal disorders.*

**Ronfnyl**
*Note. This name is used for preparations of different composition.*
*Anben, Fr.*
Natural polysaccharides.
*Snoring.*

*Veron, Ger.; Anben, Malaysia.*
Xanthan gum (p.1582·3).
*Snoring.*

**Ronic** *Edol, Port.*
Dexamethasone (p.1097·1).
*Inflammatory eye disorders.*

**Ronmix** *Ashbourne, UK†.*
Erythromycin (p.208·1).

**Ronpirin APCQ** *Mitchell, UK†.*
Paracetamol (p.76·2); aspirin (p.15·1); caffeine (p.782·1); quinine hydrochloride (p.460·2).

**Ronpirin Cold Remedy** *Mitchell, UK†.*
Promethazine hydrochloride (p.439·1); dextromethorphan hydrochloride; paracetamol (p.76·2).
*Cold symptoms.*

**Rontafor** *Pharmacia, Arg.*
Calcium folinate (p.1431·1).
*Antidote to folic acid antagonists; colorectal cancer; megaloblastic anaemia; reduction of methotrexate toxicity.*

**Rontagel** *Pharmacia, Arg.*
Estradiol (p.1550·1).
*Menopausal disorders; osteoporosis.*

**Rontilona**
*Alodial, Port.; Alter, Spain.*
Fluticasone propionate (p.1102·3).
*Nasal polyps; rhinitis.*

**Ronvan** *Asta Oncologia, Braz.*
Fosfestrol sodium (p.1555·3).
*Breast cancer; prostatic cancer.*

**Ronvir** *Pharmacia, Arg.*
Didanosine (p.630·3).
*HIV infection.*

**Ropect** *Scherer, Thai.*
Codeine phosphate (p.27·1); guaifenesin (p.1122·1).
Formerly contained codeine phosphate, guaifenesin, and phenylpropanolamine hydrochloride.
*Coughs.*

**Rophelin** *Rolmex, Canad.*
Ammonium chloride (p.1115·2); tolu balsam (p.1131·3); white pine compound; wild cherry bark (p.1765·2).

**Ropion** *Kaken, Jpn.*
Flurbiprofen axetil (p.44·2).
*Pain.*

**Ropril** *Aegis, Hong Kong.*
Captopril (p.879·2).
*Heart failure; hypertension.*

**R.O.R.** *Aventis Pasteur, Fr.*
A measles, mumps, and rubella vaccine (Edmonston 749D, Jeryl Lynn, and Wistar RA 27/3 strains respectively) (p.1625·1).
*Active immunisation.*

**Rosac** *Stiefel, USA.*
Sulfacetamide sodium (p.257·3); sulfur (p.1158·2).
*Acne.*

**Rosagenus** *Leovan, Gr.*
Famotidine (p.1265·2).
*Conditions where gastric acid reduction is beneficial; gastric hypersecretion including Zollinger-Ellison syndrome; peptic ulcer.*

**Rosalgin**
*Lepori, Port.; Farma Lepori, Spain.*
Benzydamine hydrochloride (p.21·1).
*Cervicitis; vulvovaginitis.*

**Rosalox** *Drossapharm, Switz.*
Metronidazole (p.607·2).
*Rosacea.*

**Rosanil** *Galderma, USA.*
Sulfur (p.1158·2); sulfacetamide sodium (p.257·3).
*Acne.*

**Rosarthron** *Steierl, Ger.*
Rosemary oil (p.1740·2); pumilio pine oil (p.1737·1).
*Circulatory disorders; gout; musculoskeletal and joint disorders; neuritis; respiratory-tract disorders.*

**Rosarthron forte** *Steierl, Ger.†.*
Rosemary oil (p.1740·2); methyl salicylate (p.59·3); benzyl nicotinate (p.21·2).
*Circulatory disorders; gout; musculoskeletal and joint disorders; neuritis; respiratory-tract disorders.*

**Rosased** *Pierre Fabre, Ital.*
Metronidazole (p.607·2).
*Rosacea.*

**Rosatil BB** *Novag, Mex.*
Zinc oxide (p.1163·2).
*Nappy rash; skin irritation.*

**Roscillin** *Ranbaxy, India.*
Ampicillin sodium (p.157·1) or ampicillin trihydrate (p.157·2).
*Bacterial infections.*

**Roseliane Creme** *Saninter, Port.†.*
Moisturiser.

**Roseliane Lait** *Saninter, Port.†.*
Soap substitute.

**Rosets** *Akorn, USA.*
Rose bengal sodium (p.1740·1).
*Ophthalmic diagnostic agent.*

**Rosiced** *Pierre Fabre, Fr.*
Metronidazole (p.607·2).
*Rosacea.*

**Rosiden** *Shin Poong, Singapore.*
Piroxicam (p.84·2).
*Gout; inflammation; musculoskeletal, joint, and periarticular disorders; pain.*

**Rosig** *Sigma, Austral.*
Piroxicam (p.84·2).
*Ankylosing spondylitis; osteoarthritis; rheumatoid arthritis.*

**Rosilan** *Vitoria, Port.*
Deflazacort (p.1096·2).
*Corticosteroid.*

**Rosils** *Boots Healthcare, Belg.*
Noscapine (p.1125·3); phenylephrine hydrochloride (p.1126·3).
*Coughs; upper respiratory-tract congestion.*

**Rosital** *Faran, Gr.*
Nimodipine (p.972·3).
*Neurological deficit following subarachnoid haemorrhage.*

**Rosken Skin Repair**
*Note. This name is used for preparations of different composition.*
*Pfizer Consumer, Austral.*
Dimethicone (p.1482·1).
*Dermatitis; dry skin.*

*Pfizer, NZ.*
Dimethicone (p.1482·1); glycerol (p.1694·3).
*Barrier cream; bedsores; dry skin.*

**Rosol-Gamma** *Biagini, Ital.†.*
A rubella immunoglobulin (p.1637·3).
*Passive immunisation.*

**Rosone** *Riva, Canad.†.*
Betamethasone dipropionate (p.1093·1).
*Skin disorders.*

**Rosovax** *Nuovo ISM, Ital.†.*
A rubella vaccine (Wistar RA 27/3 strain) (p.1637·3).
*Active immunisation.*

**Rossepar** *KBR, Ital.*
Sodium ferric gluconate complex (p.1444·3).
*Iron deficiency; iron-deficiency anaemias.*

**Rossitrol** *Polifarma, Ital.*
Roxithromycin (p.254·2).
*Bacterial infections.*

**Rossofolin** *Errekappa, Ital.*
Multivitamin and mineral preparation (p.1417·1).

**Ro-Strumal NEU (Rowo-221)** *Pharmakon, Ger.*
Spongia tosta; ovi putamen tosta; magnesium hydrogen phosphate; anhydrous sodium phosphate; terra silicea purificata.
*Iodine deficiency.*

**Rosula** *Doak, USA.*
Sulfacetamide sodium (p.257·3); sulfur (p.1158·2); urea (p.1162·2).
*Acne.*

**Rotane** *Aventis, India.*
Roxatidine acetate hydrochloride (p.1288·1).
*Gastro-oesophageal reflux; peptic ulcer.*

**Roter** *Roter, Thai.†.*
Bismuth subnitrate (p.1252·2); magnesium carbonate (p.1272·1); sodium bicarbonate (p.1223·2); frangula bark (p.1266·3).
*Dyspepsia; gastric hyperacidity; gastritis; gastrointestinal spasm; heartburn; peptic ulcer.*

**Roter Complex** *Farma Lepori, Spain†.*
Bismuth subnitrate (p.1252·2); magnesium carbonate (p.1272·1); sodium bicarbonate (p.1223·2); frangula bark (p.1266·3); calamus root (p.1664·1); sulpiride (p.722·2).
*Duodenitis; gastritis; hyperchlorhydria; peptic ulcer.*

**Rotersept** *Roterpharma, Irl.†.*
Chlorhexidine gluconate (p.1173·2).
*Cracked nipples; mastitis.*

**Rotesan** *Abbott, Spain†.*
Roxithromycin (p.254·2).
*Bacterial infections.*

**Rothacin** *Julphar, UAE.*
Indometacin (p.47·3).
*Dysmenorrhoea; musculoskeletal, joint, and peri-articular disorders.*

**Rothonal** *Vilco, Gr.*
Ranitidine hydrochloride (p.1285·2).
*Conditions where gastric acid reduction is beneficial; gastric hypersecretion including Zollinger-Ellison syndrome; peptic ulcer.*

**Rothricin** *Siam Bheasach, Thai.*
Roxithromycin (p.254·2).
*Bacterial infections.*

**Roth's RKT Tropfen** *Infirmarius-Rovit, Ger.*
Homoeopathic preparation.

**Roth's Ropulmin N** *Infirmarius-Rovit, Ger.*
Homoeopathic preparation.

**Roth's Rotacard** *Infirmarius-Rovit, Ger.*
Homoeopathic preparation.

**Rotilen** *Terapeutico, Ital.*
Methacycline hydrochloride (p.230·1).
*Bacterial infections.*

**Rotol** *Jukunda, Ger.†.*
Hypericum (p.299·1).
*Joint pain; nervous disorders; wounds.*

**Rotram** *Ranbaxy, Braz.*
Roxithromycin (p.254·2).
*Bacterial infections.*

**Rotramin** *Celltech, Spain.*
Roxithromycin (p.254·2).
*Bacterial infections.*

**Rotuss** *Scherer, Thai.*
Codeine phosphate (p.27·1); guaifenesin (p.1122·1).
Formerly contained codeine phosphate, guaifenesin, and phenylpropanolamine.
*Coughs.*

**Roubac** *Rougier, Canad.†.*
Co-trimoxazole (p.199·3).
*Bacterial infections.*

**Roug-mycin** *Pharmanik (Φαρμανικ), Gr.*
Erythromycin stearate (p.208·2).
*Bacterial infections.*

**Rouhex-G** *Rougier, Canad.†.*
Chlorhexidine gluconate (p.1173·2).
*Acne; skin disinfection; surface and instrument disinfection.*

**Rounox** *Rougier, Canad.†.*
Paracetamol (p.76·2).
*Fever; pain.*

**Rouphylline**
*Rougier, Canad.†; Rougier, Hong Kong†.*
Choline theophyllinate (p.784·2).
*Bronchospasm.*

**Rouvax**
*Aventis Pasteur, Braz.; Aventis Pasteur, Fr.; Pasteur Merieux, Hong Kong†; Pasteur Merieux, Israel; Aventis Pasteur, Ital.; Aventis, S.Afr.; Aventis Pasteur, Thai.*
A measles vaccine (Schwarz strain) (p.1623·1).
*Active immunisation.*

**Rouvax Merieux** *Vianex (Βιανεξ), Gr.*
A measles vaccine (p.1623·1).
*Active immunisation.*

**Rovacor**
*Stancare, India; Ranbaxy, Singapore.*
Lovastatin (p.949·1).
*Atherosclerosis; hyperlipidaemias.*

**Rovalcyte** *Roche, Fr.*
Valganciclovir (p.656·3).
*Cytomegalovirus retinitis.*

**Rovamicina**
*Aventis, Braz.; Aventis, Ital.*
Spiramycin (p.255·3).
*Bacterial infections.*

**Rovamycin**
*Gerot, Austria; Aventis, Denm.†; Nicholas Piramal, India; Aventis, Norw.; Aventis, Thai.*
Spiramycin (p.255·3).
*Bacterial infections; toxoplasmosis.*

**Rovamycine**
*Aventis, Arg.; Aventis, Belg.; Aventis, Canad.; Aventis, Fr.; Teofarma, Ger.; Aventis, Gr.; Aventis, Hong Kong; Aventis, Israel; Aventis, Malaysia; Rhone-Poulenc Rorer, Neth.; Aventis, Port.; Aventis, Singapore; Aventis, Spain; Aventis, Switz.*
Spiramycin (p.255·3) or spiramycin adipate (p.256·1).
*Bacterial infections; cryptosporidiosis; toxoplasmosis.*

**Rovericlin** *Chrispa (Χρισπα), Gr.*
Amikacin sulfate (p.154·1).
*Bacterial infections.*

**Roveril** *Roux-Ocefa, Arg.*
Ibuprofen (p.45·3); pseudoephedrine hydrochloride (p.1129·2).
*Fever; nasal congestion; pain.*

**Rovigon**
*Roche, Austria; Roche, Belg.; Roche, Chile; Roche Nicholas, Fr.; Piramal, India; Roche, Ital.; Roche, Port.; Roche, Switz.; Roche, Thai.†.*
Vitamin A (p.1451·2); vitamin E (p.1464·3).
*Vitamin A and E deficiency.*

**Rovigon G** *Roche Nicholas, Ger.*
Vitamin A palmitate (p.1453·1); alpha tocoferil acetate (p.1465·1).
*Vitamin A and E deficiency.*

**Rovit** *Rolab, S.Afr.*
Multivitamin preparation (p.1417·1).

**Rovit C** *Rolab, S.Afr.*
Vitamin C (p.1460·2).
*Vitamin C supplement.*

**Rowachol**
*Note. This name is used for preparations of different composition.*
*Rosch & Handel, Austria; Rowa, Ger.; Rowa, Irl.*
Menthol (p.1711·3); menthone; α-pinene; β-pinene; borneol; camphene; cineole (p.1672·1).
*Hepatobiliary disorders.*

*Raffo, Chile.*
Natural terpenes.
*Biliary-tract disorders; liver disorders.*

*Rowa, Hong Kong; Rowa, Israel; Rowa, Malaysia; Rowa, Thai.; Meadow, UK.*
Menthol (p.1711·3); menthone; pinene; borneol; camphene; cineole (p.1672·1).
*Hepatobiliary disorders.*

*Nexis, Spain.*
Menthol (p.1711·3); pinenes; borneol; camphene; cineole (p.1672·1); emodin; oxidised terpenes.
*Anorexia; hepatobiliary disorders.*

**Rowachol comp** *Rowa, Ger.*
Menthol (p.1711·3); menthone; α-pinene; β-pinene; borneol; camphene; cineole (p.1672·1); deanol benzilate hydrochloride (p.1585·3).
*Biliary-tract disorders.*

**Rowachol-Digestiv** *Rowa, Ger.*
Menthol (p.1711·3); menthone; α-pinene; β-pinene; borneol; camphene; cineole (p.1672·1).
*Digestive system disorders; hepatobiliary disorders.*

**Rowaclimax** *Rowa, Ger.†.*
Agnus castus; alchemilla; aletris farinosa; capsella bursa pastoris; chamomile; valerian.
*Gynaecological disorders.*

**Rowadermat** *Rosch & Handel, Austria.*
Carbenoxolone sodium (p.1254·3).
*Aphthous ulcers; herpes labialis.*

**Rowalind**
*Rosch & Handel, Austria; Rowa, Irl.†.*
Nicotinaldehyde; ammonium chloride (p.1115·2); ammonia solution (p.1653·3); camphor (p.1665·3); menthol (p.1711·3); rosemary oil (p.1740·2); lavender oil (p.1705·2).
*Musculoskeletal, joint, and soft-tissue disorders; neuralgia; neuritis.*

**Rowanefrin** *Nexis, Spain.*
Anethole (p.1654·3); borneol; camphene; rubia tinctorum; oxidised terpenes; pinenes; fenchone; cineole (p.1672·1).
*Renal calculi; urinary-tract disorders.*

**Rowapraxin**
*Rowa, Ger.*
Pipoxolan (p.1732·1).
*Smooth muscle spasms.*

*Rowa, Hong Kong; Rowa, Irl.†; Rowa, Malaysia.*
Pipoxolan hydrochloride (p.1732·1).
*Smooth muscle spasm.*

**Rowarolan**
*Note. This name is used for preparations of different composition.*
*Rowa, Irl.*
Calcium carbonate (p.1254·2).
*Adsorbent in ulcers and sores.*

*Rowa, Malaysia.*
Mineral and trace element preparation (p.1417·1).
*Minor wounds; ulcers.*

**Rowasa**
*Solvay, Fr.; Solvay, USA.*
Mesalazine (p.1273·2).
*Inflammatory bowel disease.*

**Rowatanal**
*Note. This name is used for preparations of different composition.*
*Rowa, Hong Kong; Rowa, Malaysia; Rowa, Singapore.*
Bismuth subgallate (p.1252·2); menthol (p.1711·3); zinc oxide (p.1163·2); calcium carbonate (p.1254·2).
*Anorectal disorders.*

*Rowa, Irl.*
Bismuth subgallate (p.1252·2); menthol (p.1711·3); zinc oxide (p.1163·2).
*Anal irritation; haemorrhoids.*

**Rowatinex**
*Note. This name is used for preparations of different composition.*
*Rosch & Handel, Austria; Rowa, Ger.; Rowa, Irl.*
α-Pinene; β-pinene; camphene; borneol; anethole (p.1654·3); fenchone; cineole (p.1672·1).
*Urinary-tract disorders.*

*Raffo, Chile; Rowa, Hong Kong; Rowa, Israel; Rowa, Malaysia; Rowa, Thai.; Monmouth, UK†.*
Pinene; camphene; borneol; anethole (p.1654·3); fenchone; cineole (p.1672·1).
*Urinary-tract disorders.*

**Rowo-52** *Pharmakon, Ger.†.*
Homoeopathic preparation.
Lidocaine hydrochloride (p.1377·3) is included in this preparation to alleviate the pain of injection.

**Rowo-216** *Pharmakon, Ger.†.*
Homoeopathic preparation.
Lidocaine hydrochloride (p.1377·3) is included in this preparation to alleviate the pain of injection.

**Rowo-298** *Pharmakon, Ger.*
Homoeopathic preparation.
Lidocaine hydrochloride (p.1377·3) is included in this preparation to alleviate the pain of injection.

**Rowo-629** *Pharmakon, Ger.*
Lidocaine hydrochloride (p.1377·3).
*Local anaesthesia.*

**Rowo-849 Echinacea Ro-Plex (Rowo-849)** *Pharmakon, Ger.†.*
Homoeopathic preparation.

**Rowo Rytesthin Ro-Plex (Rowo-318)** *Pharmakon, Ger.†.*
Homoeopathic preparation.

**Rowo-778 Symphytum Ro-Plex T (Rowo-778)** *Pharmakon, Ger.*
Homoeopathic preparation.

**Rowo-Rytesthin (Rowo-576)** *Pharmakon, Ger.†.*
Homoeopathic preparation.

**Rowo-Sedaphin 138 (Rowo-138)** *Pharmakon, Ger.*
Homoeopathic preparation.

**Roxacilin** *Royton, Braz.*
Oxacillin (p.240·3).
*Bacterial infections.*

**Roxalia** *Boiron, Canad.*
Homoeopathic preparation.

**Roxane**
*Hoechst Marion Roussel, Austria†; Hoechst Marion Roussel, Singapore†.*
Roxatidine acetate hydrochloride (p.1288·1).
*Gastro-oesophageal reflux; peptic ulcer.*

*Lavipharm, Gr.*
Roxatidine (p.1288·1).
*Peptic ulcer.*

**Roxanol** *aai, USA.*
Morphine sulfate (p.60·2).
*Pain.*

**Roxatine** *Hexal, Austral.†.*
Paroxetine hydrochloride (p.311·2).
*Depression; obsessive-compulsive disorder; panic attacks; social phobia.*

**Roxazin** *Basi, Port.*
Piroxicam (p.84·2).

**Roxcin**
*Biolab, Malaysia; Biolab, Thai.*
Roxithromycin (p.254·2).
*Bacterial infections.*

**Roxen** *Hua, Thai.*
Naproxen (p.65·1).
*Gout; musculoskeletal and joint disorders.*

**Roxene** *Benedetti, Ital.*
Piroxicam (p.84·2).
*Inflammation; musculoskeletal, joint, peri-articular, and soft-tissue disorders; pain.*

**Roxenil** *Caber, Ital.*
Piroxicam (p.84·2).
*Musculoskeletal, joint, and peri-articular disorders.*

**Roxeptin** *Ipca, India.*
Roxithromycin (p.254·2).
*Bacterial infections.*

**Roxflan** *Merck, Braz.*
Amlodipine besilate (p.862·1).
*Hypertension.*

**Roxi** TAD, Ger.
Roxithromycin (p.254·2).
*Bacterial infections.*

**Roxibion** Leiras, Fin.
Roxithromycin (p.254·2).
*Bacterial infections.*

**Roxicam** Sanofi Synthelabo, Arg.
Piroxicam (p.84·2).
*Musculoskeletal and joint disorders; pain.*

**Roxicet**
Boehringer Ingelheim, Canad.†; Roxane, USA.
Oxycodone hydrochloride (p.75·2); paracetamol (p.76·2).
*Pain.*

**Roxicilline** Medichrom, Gr.
Roxithromycin (p.254·2).
*Bacterial infections.*

**Roxicin**
Atlantic, Hong Kong; Atlantic, Thai.
Roxithromycin (p.254·2).
*Bacterial infections.*

**Roxicodone** aai, USA.
Oxycodone hydrochloride (p.75·2).
*Pain.*

**Roxid**
Teuto, Braz.; Alembic, India.
Roxithromycin (p.254·2).
*Bacterial infections.*

**Roxiden** Pulitzer, Ital.
Piroxicam (p.84·2).
*Musculoskeletal, joint, and peri-articular disorders.*

**Roxidura** Merck dura, Ger.
Roxithromycin (p.254·2).
*Bacterial infections.*

**Roxifen** TO-Chemicals, Thai.
Piroxicam (p.84·2).
*Musculoskeletal, joint, and peri-articular disorders.*

**Roxigrun** Grunenthal, Ger.
Roxithromycin (p.254·2).
*Bacterial infections.*

**Roxiklinge** Fujisawa, Ger.
Roxithromycin (p.254·2).
*Bacterial infections.*

**Roxilan** Olan-Kemed, Thai.
Roxithromycin (p.254·2).
*Bacterial infections.*

**Roxillin** Rowex, Irl.†.
Amoxicillin trihydrate (p.155·3).
*Bacterial infections.*

**Roxilox** Roxane, USA.
Oxycodone hydrochloride (p.75·2); paracetamol (p.76·2).
*Pain.*

**Roximin** Pharmaland, Thai.
Roxithromycin (p.254·2).
*Bacterial infections.*

**Roximin-Galenica** Iasis, Gr.
Roxithromycin (p.254·2).
*Bacterial infections.*

**Roxin** Arrow, Austral.
Norfloxacin (p.238·3).
*Bacterial infections.*

**Roxina** Cazi, Braz.
Roxithromycin (p.254·2).
*Bacterial infections.*

**Roxine** Duopharma, Hong Kong.
Dequalinium chloride (p.1178·1).
*Mouth and throat disorders.*

**Roxinox** Charoen Bhaesaj, Malaysia.
Roxithromycin (p.254·2).
*Bacterial infections.*

**Roxiprin** Roxane, USA.
Oxycodone hydrochloride (p.75·2); oxycodone terephthalate (p.75·2); aspirin (p.15·1).
*Pain.*

**Roxi-Puren** Alpharma-Isis, Ger.
Roxithromycin (p.254·2).
*Bacterial infections.*

**Roxit**
Aventis, Ger.; Aventis, Ital.; Knoll, Neth.; Hoechst Marion Roussel, S.Afr.†.
Roxatidine acetate hydrochloride (p.1288·1).
*Gastro-oesophageal reflux; peptic ulcer.*

**Roxitan** Remedica, Malaysia.
Piroxicam (p.84·2).
*Gout; musculoskeletal and joint disorders.*

**Roxithro-Lich** Lichtenstein, Ger.
Roxithromycin (p.254·2).
*Bacterial infections.*

**Roxithrostad** Stada, Austria.
Roxithromycin (p.254·2).
*Bacterial infections.*

**Roxithroxyl** Bangkok Lab & Cosmetic, Thai.
Roxithromycin (p.254·2).
*Bacterial infections.*

**Roxitin** TP, Thai.
Roxithromycin (p.254·2).
*Bacterial infections.*

**Roxitran** Neo Quimica, Braz.
Roxithromycin (p.254·2).
*Bacterial infections.*

**Roxitricina** Hexal, Braz.
Roxithromycin (p.254·2).
*Bacterial infections.*

**Roxitrol** Ofimex, Mex.†.
Roxithromycin (p.254·2).

**Roxitrom** Biolab Sanus, Braz.
Roxithromycin (p.254·2).
*Bacterial infections.*

**Roxitromin** Sanval, Braz.
Roxithromycin (p.254·2).
*Bacterial infections.*

**Roxium** M & H, Thai.
Piroxicam (p.84·2).
*Musculoskeletal, joint, peri-articular, and soft-tissue disorders.*

**Roxiwas** Chiesi, Spain.
Roxatidine acetate (p.1288·1).
*Gastro-oesophageal reflux; peptic ulcer.*

**Roxlecon** Pond's, Thai.
Roxithromycin (p.254·2).
*Bacterial infections.*

**Roxo** Unipharm, Israel.
Roxithromycin (p.254·2).
*Bacterial infections.*

**Roxomycin** Silom, Thai.
Roxithromycin (p.254·2).
*Bacterial infections.*

**Roxorin** Richmond, Arg.
Doxorubicin (p.547·3).
*Malignant neoplasms.*

**Roxthomed** Progress, Thai.
Roxithromycin (p.254·2).
*Bacterial infections.*

**Roxthrin** TO-Chemicals, Thai.
Roxithromycin (p.254·2).
*Bacterial infections.*

**Roxto** M & H, Thai.
Roxithromycin (p.254·2).
*Bacterial infections.*

**Roxtrocin** Greater Pharma, Thai.
Roxithromycin (p.254·2).
*Bacterial infections.*

**Roxy**
Note. This name is used for preparations of different composition.
Mer-National, S.Afr.
Oxytetracycline hydrochloride (p.241·1).
*Bacterial infections.*

Sriprasit, Thai.
Roxithromycin (p.254·2).
*Bacterial infections.*

**Roxycam** Greater Pharma, Thai.
Piroxicam (p.84·2).
*Gout; musculoskeletal and joint disorders.*

**Roxyn** Raza, Malaysia; Pharmaniaga, Malaysia.
Naproxen (p.65·1).
*Gout; musculoskeletal and joint disorders; pain.*

**Roxyrol** Concept, India.
Roxithromycin (p.254·2).
*Bacterial infections.*

**Roxyspes** Specifar (Σπεσιφαρ), Gr.
Roxithromycin (p.254·2).
*Bacterial infections.*

**Royal E** Cielle, Ital.
Royal jelly (p.1740·3); vitamin E (p.1464·3).
*Nutritional supplement.*

**Royal Galanol** Lifeplan, UK†.
Evening primrose oil (p.1686·3); royal jelly (p.1740·3).
*Nutritional supplement.*

**Royal Life** Bioceuticals, UK.
Multivitamin, mineral, and amino-acid preparation (p.1417·1).

**Royalin** TO-Chemicals, Thai.
Salbutamol sulfate (p.791·3); guaifenesin (p.1122·1).
*Coughs; obstructive airways disease.*

**Roycefax** Royton, Braz.
Ceftazidime (p.180·2).
*Bacterial infections.*

**Roychlor** Waymar, Canad.
Potassium chloride (p.1232·2).
*Potassium deficiency.*

**Royen**
Omedir, Arg.; Rubio, Spain.
Calcium acetate (p.1225·1).
*Calcium supplement; hyperphosphataemia.*

**Royflex** Waymar, Canad.†.
Trolamine salicylate (p.95·3).
*Musculoskeletal and joint disorders.*

**Royl 6** Mer-National, S.Afr.
Vitamin B substances with vitamin C (p.1417·1).

**Roytrin** Royton, Braz.
Co-trimoxazole (p.199·3).
*Bacterial infections; Pneumocystis carinii pneumonia; protozoal infections.*

**Royvac Kit** Waymar, Canad.
Oral solution, magnesium citrate (p.1272·1); 3 tablets, bisacodyl (p.1251·3); 1 suppository, bisacodyl.
*Bowel evacuation.*

**Rozacreme** Biorga, Fr.
Metronidazole (p.607·2).
*Rosacea.*

**Rozagel** Biorga, Fr.
Metronidazole (p.607·2).
*Rosacea.*

**Rozex**
Galderma, Arg.; Galderma, Austral.; AB-Consult, Austria; Galderma, Belg.; Galderma, Braz.; Galderma, Denm.; Galderma, Fin.; Galderma, Fr.; Galderma, Hong Kong; Galderma, Irl.; Galderma, Israel; Galderma, Ital.; Galderma, Malaysia; Galderma, Neth.; Galderma, Norw.; Galderma, NZ; Galderma, S.Afr.; Galderma, Singapore; Galderma, Spain; Galderma, Swed.; Galderma, Switz.; Galderma, UK.
Metronidazole (p.607·2).
*Rosacea.*

**Rozicel** Bristol-Myers Squibb, Ital.
Cefprozil (p.179·2).
*Bacterial infections.*

**Rozovin** Pharmanik (Φαρμανικ), Gr.
Ibuprofen (p.45·3).
*Dysmenorrhoea; inflammation; musculoskeletal and joint disorders; pain.*

**RP-Pose** Pose, Thai.†.
Rifampicin (p.250·2).
*Bacterial infections including tuberculosis, leprosy, and gonorrhoea.*

**R-Rax** Progress, Thai.
Hydroxyzine hydrochloride (p.434·3).
*Pruritus.*

**R-Tanna**
Note. This name is used for preparations of different composition.
Duramed, USA.
*Suspension:* Phenylephrine tannate (p.1127·2); mepyramine tannate (p.437·1).
*Upper respiratory-tract disorders.*

Prasco, USA.
*Tablets:* Phenylephrine tannate (p.1127·2); chlorphenamine tannate (p.428·1).
*Upper respiratory-tract disorders.*

**R-Tanna S Pediatric** Prasco, USA.
Phenylephrine tannate (p.1127·2); chlorphenamine tannate (p.428·1).
*Upper respiratory-tract disorders.*

**R-Tannamine** Qualitest, USA.
Phenylephrine tannate (p.1127·2); chlorphenamine tannate (p.428·1); mepyramine tannate (p.437·1).
*Upper respiratory-tract symptoms.*

**R-Tannate** Warner Chilcott, USA; Copley, USA; Schein, USA.
Phenylephrine tannate (p.1127·2); chlorphenamine tannate (p.428·1); mepyramine tannate (p.437·1).
*Allergic rhinitis; nasal congestion.*

**R-Tannic-S** Cypress, USA.
Phenylephrine tannate (p.1127·2); mepyramine tannate (p.437·1).
*Allergic rhinitis; cold symptoms; sinusitis.*

**RTH** Ferring, Braz.†.
Protirelin (p.1337·3).
*Diagnostic agent.*

**R-Tyflam** Rayere, Mex.
Piroxicam (p.84·2).
*Inflammation; pain.*

**Rubacina** Rubio, Spain.
Famotidine (p.1265·2).
*Gastro-oesophageal reflux; peptic ulcer; Zollinger-Ellison syndrome.*

**Rubeaten**
Kwizda, Austria; Berna, Hong Kong†; Berna, Ital.†; Berna, Port.; Byk Madaus, S.Afr.†; Berna, Singapore†; Berna, Spain†; Berna, Switz.; Berna, Thai.†.
A rubella vaccine (attenuated Wistar RA 27/3 strain) (p.1637·3).
*Active immunisation.*

**Rubellovac** Chiron Behring, Ger.
A rubella vaccine (Wistar RA 27/3 strain) (p.1637·3).
*Active immunisation.*

**Rubesal**
Hamilton, Austral.; Hamilton, Hong Kong.
Diethylamine salicylate (p.34·1); camphor (p.1665·3); menthol (p.1711·3).
*Muscular pain; soft-tissue disorders.*

**Rubeuman** Berna, Ital.†.
A rubella immunoglobulin (p.1637·3).
*Passive immunisation.*

**Rubex**
Note. This name is used for preparations of different composition.
Bristol-Myers Squibb, Braz.; Bristol-Myers Squibb Oncology, USA.
Doxorubicin hydrochloride (p.547·3).
*Malignant neoplasms.*

Rice Steele, Irl.
Ascorbic acid (p.1460·2).
*Vitamin C deficiency.*

**Rubia Paver** Medical, Spain†.
Atropine sulfate (p.477·1); papaverine hydrochloride (p.1728·1); rubia tinctorum.
*Renal calculi.*

**Rubicalm** Julphar, UAE.
Diethylamine salicylate (p.34·1); menthol (p.1711·3).
*Musculoskeletal pain.*

**Rubicolan F** Syxyl, Ger.
Homoeopathic preparation.

**Rubi-Dex** Cazi, Braz.
Menthol (p.1711·3); methyl salicylate (p.59·3).
Formerly contained methacholine chloride, menthol, and methyl salicylate.
*Musculoskeletal and joint disorders.*

**Rubidiosin Composto** SIT, Ital.†.
Rubidium iodide (p.1741·1); potassium iodide (p.1598·1); testosterone hemisuccinate (p.1571·2); lidocaine (p.1377·3); heparin sodium (p.928·1).
*Cataracts.*

**Rubidox** Pharmacia, Arg.
Cyproterone acetate (p.1544·1).
*Androgenisation in females; prostatic cancer; sexual deviation in males.*

**RubieDorm** Rubiepharm, Ger.†.
Valerian oil.
*Agitation; sleep disorders.*

**RubieFol** Rubiepharm, Ger.
Folic acid (p.1429·1).
*Folic acid deficiency.*

**RubieMag + E** Rubiepharm, Ger.
*d*-Alpha-Tocoferil acetate (p.1465·1); magnesium oxide (p.1272·3).
*Vitamin E and magnesium deficiency.*

**RubieMen** Rubiepharm, Ger.
Dimenhydrinate (p.431·1).
*Motion sickness; nausea and vomiting; vertigo.*

**RubieMol** Rubiepharm, Ger.
Paracetamol (p.76·2).
*Fever; pain.*

**RubieNex mono** Rubiepharm, Ger.†.
Ergotamine tartrate (p.467·2).
*Headache; migraine.*

**RubieNex spezial** Rubiepharm, Ger.
Ergotamine tartrate (p.467·2); propyphenazone (p.85·3).
*Menstrual disorders; migraine.*

**RubieSed** Rubiepharm, Ger.
Valerian (p.1762·2); melissa (p.1711·1); passion flower (p.1729·1).
*Agitation; sleep disorders.*

**Rubifarm** Pharmacia, Arg.
Epirubicin hydrochloride (p.550·2).
*Malignant neoplasms.*

**Rubifen**
Omedir, Arg.; AFT, NZ; Rubio, Singapore; Rubio, Spain; Rubio, Thai.; TTN, Thai.
Methylphenidate hydrochloride (p.1590·2).
*Attention deficit hyperactivity disorder; mood disorders; narcoleptic syndrome.*

**Rubifort** Kinder, Braz.
Vitamin A palmitate; colecalciferol (p.1417·1).
*Vitamin A and D supplement.*

**Rubilax** Pharmachoice, S.Afr.
Charcoal (p.1030·2); rhubarb (p.1287·3); senna (p.1288·2).
*Constipation.*

**Rubilem** Lemery, Mex.
Daunorubicin hydrochloride (p.545·3).
*Malignant neoplasms.*

**Rubilin** Medeva, UK†.
A rubella vaccine (live attenuated Wistar RA 27/3) (p.1637·3).
*Active immunisation.*

**Rubina** Euroforma, Braz.
Epirubicin hydrochloride (p.550·2).
*Malignant neoplasms.*

**Rubio N** Worwag, Ger.†.
Urea (p.1162·2).
*Dry skin disorders.*

**Rubion** Desbergers, Canad.†.
Cyanocobalamin (p.1458·2).
*Anaemias.*

**Rubiron** Sidus, Arg.
Ferrous sulfate (p.1428·2); folic acid (p.1429·1); cyanocobalamin (p.1458·2).
Ascorbic acid (p.1460·2) is included in this preparation to increase the absorption and availability of iron.
*Iron-deficiency anaemia; nutritional supplement.*

**Rubiron B12** Klinger, Braz.†.
Ferrous sulfate (p.1428·2); vitamin B substances (p.1417·1).
Ascorbic acid (p.1460·2) is included in this preparation to increase the absorption and availability or iron.
*Anaemias.*

**Rubisan**
Peithner, Austria; DHU, Ger.; Omida, Switz.
Homoeopathic preparation.

**Rubistenol** Fermenti, Ital.†.
Rubidium iodide (p.1741·1); sodium iodide (p.1598·1); potassium iodide (p.1598·1); sodium formate (p.1689·3); strychnine glycerophosphate.
*Eye disorders.*

**Rubiten** Rafarm, Gr.
Diltiazem (p.901·3).
*Angina; hypertension.*

**Rubiulcer** Rubio, Spain.
Ranitidine hydrochloride (p.1285·2).
*Acid aspiration; gastro-oesophageal reflux; gastrointestinal hyperacidity; peptic ulcer; short-bowel syndrome; Zollinger-Ellison syndrome.*

**Rubizon-Rheumagel** Makara, Austria.
Glycol salicylate (p.44·3); camphor (p.1665·3); benzyl nicotinate (p.21·2); capsaicin (p.24·2).
*Chilblains; musculoskeletal and joint disorders; neuralgia.*

**Rubizuel** Sedabel, Braz.†.
Hydroxocobalamin (p.1458·2); thiamine (p.1455·2).
*Vitamin supplement.*

**Rubjovit** SIFI, Ital.
Rubidium iodide (p.1741·1); sodium iodide (p.1598·1); calcium formate (p.1689·3); sodium ascorbate (p.1460·2); thiamine hydrochloride (p.1455·1).
*Cataracts.*

**Rublex D** Don, Israel.
Menthol (p.1711·3); camphor (p.1665·3); methyl salicylate (p.59·3); salicylic acid (p.1157·1).
*Musculoskeletal and joint disorders.*

**Rublex Massage Cream** Don, Israel.
Menthol (p.1711·3); camphor (p.1665·3); methyl salicylate (p.59·3); capsicum oleoresin (p.1667·1).
*Musculoskeletal and joint disorders.*

**Rubocord** Rafarm, Gr.
Clobetasol propionate (p.1095·2).
*Topical corticosteroid.*

**Ruboderm** Labcatal, Fr.†.
Zinc gluconate (p.1469·2); copper gluconate (p.1425·3).
*Skin and hair disorders.*

**Ruboril** Darier, Mex.
Barrier cream.

**Rubozinc** Labcatal, Fr.
Zinc gluconate (p.1469·2).
*Acne; acrodermatitis enteropathica.*

**Rubracobal** Medquimica, Braz.†.
Vitamin B substances with amino acids and gastric mucosa extract (p.1417·1).

**Rubralong** Dovalle, Braz.
Ferrous fumarate (p.1427·3); vitamin B substances (p.1417·1).
Vitamin C (p.1460·2) is included in this preparation to increase the absorption and availability of iron.
*Iron deficiency; iron-deficiency anaemias.*

**Rubramin** Squibb, Canad.†.
Vitamin $B_{12}$ (p.1458·2).
*Schilling test; vitamin $B_{12}$ deficiency.*

**Rubranova** Mead Johnson, Braz.
Hydroxocobalamin (p.1458·2).
*Megaloblastic anaemia; vitamin $B_{12}$ deficiency.*

**Rubraplex** Sarabhai Piramal, India.
Ferric ammonium citrate (p.1427·2); folic acid (p.1429·1).
*Anaemia.*

**Rubrargil** IQB, Braz.
Ferrous sulfate (p.1428·2); vitamin $B_1$; vitamin $B_{12}$; copper sulfate (p.1417·1).
Vitamin C (p.1460·2) is included in this preparation to increase the absorption and availability of iron.
*Iron deficiency; iron-deficiency anaemias.*

**Rubriment**
Note. This name is used for preparations of different composition.
Nycomed, Austria.
Benzyl nicotinate (p.21·2); nonivamide (p.67·2); glycol salicylate (p.44·3); salicylamide (p.87·3); camphor (p.1665·3); turpentine oil (p.1760·1).
*Frostbite; joint, muscle, and nerve disorders; peripheral vascular disorders; sport massage.*

Riemser, Ger.
*Bath additive:* Benzyl nicotinate (p.21·2).
*Bath additive; peripheral vascular disorders; rheumatism.*

*Ointment:* Benzyl nicotinate (p.21·2); nonivamide (p.67·2).
*Frostbite; inflammation; musculoskeletal and joint disorders; peripheral vascular disorders.*

**Rubriment-N** Riemser, Ger.
Benzyl nicotinate (p.21·2); glycol salicylate (p.44·3); camphor (p.1665·3).
*Frostbite; musculoskeletal, joint, and peri-articular disorders; peripheral vascular disorders.*

**Rubrina** Solfran, Mex.
Hydroxocobalamin (p.1458·2).

**Rubrobion** Sintofarma, Braz.
Ferric ammonium citrate (p.1427·2); vitamin B substances; inositol; liver extract (p.1417·1).
*Iron deficiency; iron-deficiency anaemias.*

**Rubrocalcium** Caber, Ital.†.
Calcium levulinate (p.1225·3).
*Calcium deficiency.*

**Rubrociclina** DMG, Ital.
Demeclocycline hydrochloride (p.204·3); erythromycin estolate (p.208·1).
*Bacterial infections.*

**Rubrocortin** Farma Lepori, Spain.
Cyanocobalamin (p.1458·2); suprarenal cortex extract (p.1110·1); liver extract; inosine (p.1701·2).
*Anaemias; tonic.*

**Rubroferrina** NCSN, Ital.
Sodium ferric gluconate complex (p.1444·3).
*Anaemias.*

**Rubus Complex** Blackmores, Austral.†.
Raspberry leaf (p.1737·3); spirulina (p.1749·2); ascorbic acid; mitchella repens; hesperidin (p.1688·2); rutoside (p.1688·2); *d*-alpha tocoferil acid succinate; vitamin B substances (p.1417·1); choline bitartrate; inositol.
*Obstetric and gynaecological disorders.*

**Rucaina** Rudefsa, Mex.†.
Lidocaine (p.1377·3).

**Rucaten Forte** Armstrong, Arg.
Acemetacin (p.11·3); chlorzoxazone (p.1392·3).
*Musculoskeletal, joint, and peri-articular disorders.*

**Rucaten Prednisolona** Armstrong, Arg.
Acemetacin (p.11·3); prednisolone (p.1108·1); thiamine hydrochloride; cyanocobalamin (p.1417·1).
*Gout; musculoskeletal and joint disorders; neuralgia.*

**Rucin** General Drugs, Thai.
Roxithromycin (p.254·2).
*Bacterial infections.*

**Rudd-U** Frankin, Hong Kong.
Oxyphencyclimine hydrochloride (p.487·2); methiosulfonium chloride (p.1714·1).
Formerly contained oxyphencyclimine hydrochloride, methiosulfonium chloride, aluminium hydroxide, magnesium trisilicate, and simeticone.
*Stomach discomfort.*

**Rudesol** Pharmacos, Mex.†.
Phenylbutazone (p.83·2).
*Musculoskeletal and joint disorders.*

**Rudi-Rouvax**
Aventis Pasteur, Braz.; Aventis Pasteur, Thai.
A measles and rubella vaccine (Schwarz and Wistar RA 27/3 strains respectively) (p.1624·3).
*Active immunisation.*

**Rudistrol** Boiron, Canad.
Homoeopathic preparation.

**Rudivax**
Aventis Pasteur, Braz.; Aventis Pasteur, Fr.; Aventis Pasteur, Hong Kong; Pasteur Merieux, Israel; Aventis Pasteur, Ital.; Aventis, S.Afr.; Pasteur Merieux, Singapore†; Aventis Pasteur, Thai.
A live attenuated rubella vaccine (Wistar RA 27/3M strain) (p.1637·3).
*Active immunisation.*

**Rudocaine** Streuli, Switz.
Articaine hydrochloride (p.1370·3).
Adrenaline hydrochloride (p.852·3) is included in this preparation as a vasoconstrictor to diminish absorption and localise the effect of the local anaesthetic.
*Local anaesthesia.*

**Rudocycline** Streuli, Switz.
Doxycycline hyclate (p.206·2).
*Bacterial infections.*

**Rudolac** Streuli, Switz.
Lactulose (p.1269·1).
*Constipation; hepatic encephalopathy.*

**Rudotel** AWD, Ger.
Medazepam (p.706·1).
*Anxiety disorders.*

**Ru-Ef-Tb** Rudefsa, Mex.†.
Isomicotin hydrazide.

**Ruflox** Eurofarma, Braz.†.
Rufloxacin hydrochloride (p.254·3).
*Bacterial infections.*

**Rufol** Fournier, Fr.
Sulfamethizole (p.260·3).
*Cystitis.*

**Ru-lets** Rugby, USA.
A range of vitamin preparations (p.1417·1).

**Rulicalcin** Aventis, Ital.
Calcitonin (salmon) (p.768·2).
*Hypercalcaemia; osteoporosis; Paget's disease of bone; reflex sympathetic dystrophy.*

**Rulid**
Aventis, Arg.; Aventis, Belg.; Aventis, Braz.; Aventis, Fr.; Aventis, Ger.; Hoechst Marion Roussel, Gr.; Aventis, Hong Kong; Aventis, Israel; Lepetit, Ital.; Aventis, Malaysia; Aventis, Mex.; Aventis, Singapore; Aventis, Switz.; Aventis, Thai.
Roxithromycin (p.254·2).
*Bacterial infections.*

**Rulide**
Aventis, Austral.; Aventis, Austria; Aventis, Neth.; Aventis, NZ†; Aventis, Port.; Aventis, S.Afr.; Aventis, Spain.
Roxithromycin (p.254·2).
*Bacterial infections.*

**Rulivan** Europharma, Spain†.
Nefazodone hydrochloride (p.309·2).
*Depression.*

**Rulofer G** Lomapharm, Ger.
Ferrous gluconate (p.1428·1).
*Iron deficiency.*

**Rulofer N** Lomapharm, Ger.
Ferrous fumarate (p.1427·3).
*Iron deficiency.*

**RuLox** Rugby, USA.
Aluminium hydroxide (p.1249·2); magnesium hydroxide (p.1272·2).
*Hyperacidity.*

**RuLox Plus** Rugby, USA.
Aluminium hydroxide (p.1249·2); magnesium hydroxide (p.1272·2); simeticone (p.1289·2).
*Hyperacidity.*

**Rulun** Lacer, Spain.
Hydrochlorothiazide (p.933·2); rauwolfia (p.994·3); trichlormethiazide (p.1017·2); xantinol nicotinate (p.1029·1).
Formerly contained hydrochlorothiazide, rauwolfia, trichlormethiazide, xantinol nicotinate, and pentosan polysulfate.
*Hypertension.*

**Rumadene** Chew, Thai.
Piroxicam (p.84·2).
*Gout; musculoskeletal, joint, and peri-articular disorders.*

**Rumalon**
Asta Medica, Braz.; Recalcine, Chile.
Cartilage; bone-marrow extract.
*Osteoarthritis.*

**Rumasian** Asian Pharm, Thai.
Ibuprofen (p.45·3).
*Musculoskeletal and joint disorders.*

**Rumatab** Pharmaland, Thai.
Diclofenac sodium (p.32·1).
*Gout; inflammation; musculoskeletal and joint disorders.*

**Rumatifen** Chew, Thai.
Ibuprofen (p.45·3).
*Dysmenorrhoea; gout; musculoskeletal and joint disorders.*

**Rumatifen-Plus** Chew, Thai.
Ibuprofen (p.45·3); paracetamol (p.76·2).
*Fever; pain.*

**Rumicine** Schering-Plough, Fr.†.
Aspirin (p.15·1); chlorphenamine maleate (p.427·3); caffeine (p.782·1).
*Cold symptoms.*

**Rumisedan** Lafage, Arg.
Piroxicam (p.84·2); ascorbic acid (p.1460·2).
*Inflammation; pain.*

**Rumisedan Fuerte** Lafage, Arg.
Piroxicam (p.84·2); carisoprodol (p.1392·1); ascorbic acid; vitamin B substances (p.1417·1).
*Inflammation; pain.*

**Rumitex** Beckerath, Ger.†.
Homoeopathic preparation.

**Rum-K** Fleming, USA.
Potassium chloride (p.1232·2).
*Hypokalaemia.*

**Runde** Rafarm, Gr.
Tetramethrin (p.1510·2); piperonyl butoxide (p.1509·2).
*Head, body, and crab lice.*

**Rupan**
Medochemie, Hong Kong; Medochemie, Malaysia; Medochemie, Thai.
Ibuprofen (p.45·3).
*Musculoskeletal, joint, and soft-tissue disorders; pain.*

**Rupecef** Duncan, Arg.
Cefalotin (p.168·3).
*Bacterial infections.*

**Rupediz** Duncan, Arg.
Diazepam (p.690·1).
*Anxiety.*

**Rupegen** Duncan, Arg.
Gentamicin (p.219·1).
*Bacterial infections.*

**Rupe-N** Duncan, Arg.
Hyoscine (p.483·3).
*Muscle spasm.*

**Rupe-N Compuesto** Duncan, Arg.
Hyoscine (p.483·3); dipyrone (p.35·3).
*Muscle spasm.*

**Rupton** Dexo, Thai.†.
Brompheniramine maleate (p.426·1); phenylpropanolamine hydrochloride (p.1127·3).
*Cold and flu symptoms; hay fever; sinusitis.*

**Rupton Chronules**
Dexo, Fr.†; Dexo, Switz.
Brompheniramine maleate (p.426·1); phenylpropanolamine hydrochloride (p.1127·3).
*Upper respiratory-tract disorders.*

**Ruscimel** Soria Natural, Spain.
Hamamelis (p.1696·3); aesculus (p.1648·2); cupressus sempervirens; ruscus aculeatus.
*Haemorrhoids; venous disorders.*

**Ruscorectal**
Heumann, Ger.†; Juste, Spain.
Ruscogenin (p.1741·1).
*Anorectal disorders.*

**Ruscoroid** Inverni della Beffa, Ital.
Ruscogenin (p.1741·1); tetracaine hydrochloride (p.1385·1).
*Anorectal disorders.*

**Ruscovarin** Alpinamed, Switz.†.
Heparin (p.927·3).
*Peripheral vascular disorders.*

**Ruscus** Llorens, Spain.
Cinchocaine hydrochloride (p.1373·2); prednisolone (p.1108·1); ruscogenin (p.1741·1); zinc oxide (p.1163·2); menthol (p.1711·3).
*Anorectal disorders.*

**Rusedal** OPW, Ger.
Medazepam (p.706·1).
*Anxiety disorders.*

**Russedyl** Strand, Malaysia.
Promethazine hydrochloride (p.439·1); codeine phosphate (p.27·1).
*Allergic rhinitis; coughs; sinusitis.*

**Rusyde** CP Pharmaceuticals, UK.
Furosemide (p.919·3).
*Oedema.*

**Ruta-Gastreu N R55** Reckeweg, Ger.
Homoeopathic preparation.

**Ruticalzon** Brady, Austria.
Colecalciferol (p.1461·3); rutoside (p.1688·2); vitamin C (p.1460·2); calcium citrate (p.1225·1).
*Capillary haemorrhage; infections.*

**Ruticalzon VC** Stegropharm, Ger.
Rutoside (p.1688·2); ascorbic acid (p.1460·2).
*Haemorrhagic disorders.*

**Rutice Fuerte** Teofarma, Spain†.
Ascorbic acid (p.1460·2); rutoside (p.1688·2).
*Vascular disorders.*

**Rutinice Fortissimo** Menarini, Port.
Rutoside (p.1688·2); ascorbic acid (p.1460·2).
*Haemorrhage.*

**Rutinion** Biomo, Ger.
Rutoside (p.1688·2).
*Venous insufficiency.*

**Rutisan CE** Carlo Erba OTC, Ital.
Rutoside (p.1688·2); vitamin C (p.1460·2); vitamin E (p.1464·3).
*Vascular disorders.*

**Rutiscorbin** Calea, Austria.
Rutoside (p.1688·2); ascorbic acid (p.1460·2).
*Haemorrhage; infections.*

**Rutisept extra** Henkel, Ger.
Isopropyl alcohol (p.1184·3); triclosan (p.1195·2).
*Hand disinfection.*

**Rutiviscal** Sanidom, Austria.
Garlic (p.1691·1); crataegus (p.1677·1); mistletoe (p.1715·3); rutoside (p.1688·2).
*Atherosclerosis.*

**Ru-Tuss** Boots, USA†.
*Oral liquid:* Phenylephrine hydrochloride (p.1126·3); chlorphenamine maleate (p.427·3).
*Tablets:* Phenylephrine hydrochloride (p.1126·3); phenylpropanolamine hydrochloride (p.1127·3); chlorphenamine maleate (p.427·3); hyoscyamine sulfate (p.485·1); atropine sulfate (p.477·1); hyoscine hydrobromide (p.483·3).
*Upper respiratory-tract symptoms.*

**Ru-Tuss DE** Boots, USA†.
Pseudoephedrine hydrochloride (p.1129·2); guaifenesin (p.1122·1).
*Coughs.*

**Ru-Tuss Expectorant** Boots, USA†.
Pseudoephedrine hydrochloride (p.1129·2); dextromethorphan hydrobromide (p.1117·3); guaifenesin (p.1122·1).
*Coughs.*

**Ru-Tuss with Hydrocodone** Boots, USA†.
Hydrocodone tartrate (p.45·1); phenylephrine hydrochloride (p.1126·3); phenylpropanolamine hydrochloride (p.1127·3); pheniramine maleate (p.438·3); mepyramine maleate (p.437·1).
*Cough, cold, and hay fever symptoms.*

**Ruvamed** Coup, Gr.
Piroxicam (p.84·2).
*Dysmenorrhoea; gout; inflammation; musculoskeletal and joint disorders; pain.*

**Ruvominox** Rafarm, Gr.
Diclofenac sodium (p.32·1).
*Dysmenorrhoea; inflammation; musculoskeletal and joint disorders; pain; prevention of miosis in ophthalmic surgery.*

**Ruxicolan** Rafarm, Gr.
Ticlopidine (p.1012·1).
*Thromboembolic disorders.*

**RV Paque**
Note. This name is used for preparations of different composition.
ICN, Canad.; ICN, NZ.
Zinc oxide (p.1163·2); octinoxate (p.1154·3).
Formerly contained zinc oxide and cinoxate in *Canad.*
*Sunscreen.*

ICN, Hong Kong†; ICN, Malaysia; ICN, Singapore; ICN, USA.
Zinc oxide (p.1163·2); cinoxate (p.1145·1).
*Sunscreen.*

**R-Vac** Serum Institute, India.
A rubella vaccine (Wistar RA 27/3 strain) (p.1637·3).
*Active immunisation.*

**RVHB Maxamaid** Scientific Hospital Supplies, Austral.†.
Food for special diets (p.1417·1).
*Homocystinuria; hypermethioninaemia.*

**Ryccard** Propan, S.Afr.†.
Cyclizine hydrochloride (p.429·3).
*Nausea; vestibular disorders; vomiting.*

**Rydene** Yamanouchi, Belg.
Nicardipine hydrochloride (p.965·1).
*Angina pectoris; hypertension.*

**Rye** Rafarm, Gr.
Bifonazole (p.395·1).
*Fungal skin infections.*

**Rylosol** ICN, Canad.†.
Sotalol hydrochloride (p.1001·3).
*Arrhythmias.*

**Rymed** Edwards, USA.
Pseudoephedrine hydrochloride (p.1129·2); guaifenesin (p.1122·1).
*Coughs.*

**Rymed-TR** Edwards, USA†.
Phenylpropanolamine hydrochloride (p.1127·3); guaifenesin (p.1122·1).
*Coughs.*

**Ryna** Wallace, USA.
Pseudoephedrine hydrochloride (p.1129·2); chlorphenamine maleate (p.427·3).
*Upper respiratory-tract symptoms.*

**Ryna-12** Wallace, USA.
Mepyramine tannate (p.437·1); phenylephrine tannate (p.1127·2).
*Nasal congestion; rhinitis.*

**Ryna-C** Wallace, USA.
Pseudoephedrine hydrochloride (p.1129·2); chlorphenamine maleate (p.427·3); codeine phosphate (p.27·1).
*Coughs and cold symptoms.*

**Rynacrom**
Aventis, Austral.; Rhone-Poulenc Rorer, Canad.†; Fisons, Irl.; Aventis, Mex.; Aventis, NZ; Aventis, Port.; Aventis, S.Afr.†; Aventis, Singapore; Aventis, Thai.; Pantheon, UK.
Sodium cromoglicate (p.795·3).
*Allergic rhinitis.*

**Rynacrom Allergy** Pantheon, UK†.
Sodium cromoglicate (p.795·3); xylometazoline hydrochloride (p.1132·2).
*Allergic rhinitis with associated nasal congestion.*

**Rynacrom Composto** Aventis, Port.†.
Sodium cromoglicate (p.795·3); xylometazoline hydrochloride (p.1132·2).
*Allergic rhinitis; nasal congestion.*

**Rynacrom Compound**
Rhone-Poulenc Rorer, Hong Kong†; Rhone-Poulenc Rorer, Irl.†; Avent-

*is, Malaysia; Fisons, Singapore†; Rhone-Poulenc Rorer, Singapore†; Aventis, Thai.; Pantheon, UK.*
Sodium cromoglicate (p.795·3); xylometazoline hydrochloride (p.1132·2).
*Allergic rhinitis with associated nasal congestion.*

**Rynacrom M** *Rhone-Poulenc Rorer, Hong Kong†.*
Sodium cromoglicate (p.795·3).
*Allergic rhinitis.*

**Ryna-CX** *Wallace, USA.*
Pseudoephedrine hydrochloride (p.1129·2); guaifenesin (p.1122·1); codeine phosphate (p.27·1).
*Coughs.*

**Rynatan** *Wallace, USA.*
Azatadine maleate (p.425·1); pseudoephedrine sulfate (p.1129·2).
Formerly contained phenylephrine tannate, chlorphenamine tannate, and mepyramine tannate.
*Cold symptoms.*

**Rynatanic** *Novartis, Arg.*
Phenylephrine tannate (p.1127·2); chlorphenamine tannate (p.428·1); mepyramine tannate (p.437·1).

**Rynatus** *Novartis, Arg.*
Pentoxyverine tannate (p.1126·3); phenylephrine tannate (p.1127·2) ephedrine tannate (p.1120·3); chlorphenamine tannate (p.428·1).

**Rynatuss** *Wallace, USA.*
Pentoxyverine tannate (p.1126·3); chlorphenamine tannate (p.428·1); ephedrine tannate (p.1120·3); phenylephrine tannate (p.1127·2).
*Coughs.*

**Ryol** *Hoyer, Ger.*
Oxybutynin hydrochloride (p.486·3).
*Bladder instability.*

**Ryped** *Propan, S.Afr.†.*
Erythromycin estolate (p.208·1).
*Bacterial infections.*

**Rythmex** *Teva, Israel.*
Propafenone hydrochloride (p.988·3).
*Arrhythmias.*

**Rythmical** *Unipharm, Israel.*
Disopyramide phosphate (p.903·3).
*Arrhythmias.*

**Rythmodan**
*Aventis, Austral.; Aventis, Austria; Aventis, Belg.; Aventis, Canad.; Aventis, Fr.; Hoechst Marion Roussel, Gr.; Aventis, Irl.; Aventis, Neth.; Aventis, NZ; Aventis, S.Afr.; Borg, UK.*
Disopyramide (p.903·3) or disopyramide phosphate (p.903·3).
*Arrhythmias.*

**Rythmodul** *Aventis, Ger.*
Disopyramide phosphate (p.903·3).
*Arrhythmias.*

**Rythmogastryl** *Rafarm, Gr.*
Omeprazole (p.1278·2).
*Acid aspiration; eradication of Helicobacter pylori in combination with antimicrobials; peptic ulcer; reflux oesophagitis; Zollinger-Ellison syndrome.*

**Rythmol**
*Abbott, Canad.; Knoll, Fr.; Knoll, S.Afr.; Abbott, USA.*
Propafenone hydrochloride (p.988·3).
*Arrhythmias.*

**Rythmonopm** *Vianex (Βιανεξ), Gr.*
Propafenone hydrochloride (p.988·3).
*Arrythmias.*

**Rythocin** *Masa, Thai.†.*
Erythromycin stearate (p.208·2).
*Bacterial infections.*

**Rytmobeta** *Abbott, Ital.*
Sotalol hydrochloride (p.1001·3).
*Arrhythmias.*

**Rytmogenat** *Azupharma, Ger.*
Propafenone hydrochloride (p.988·3).
*Arrhythmias.*

**Rytmonorm**
*Knoll, Belg.; Abbott, Chile; Abbott, Denm.; Abbott, Fin.; Abbott, Ger.; Abbott, Hong Kong; Abbott, Ital.; Abbott, Malaysia; Knoll, Neth.; Abbott, NZ; Abbott, Port.; Abbott, Singapore; Abbott, Spain; Abbott, Swed.; Knoll, Switz.; Abbott, Thai.*
Propafenone hydrochloride (p.988·3).
*Arrhythmias.*

**Rytmonorma** *Ebewe, Austria.*
Propafenone hydrochloride (p.988·3).
*Arrhythmias.*

**Rytmopasc** *Pascoe, Ger.*
Homoeopathic preparation.

**Rytmo-Puren** *Alpharma-Isis, Ger.*
Propafenone hydrochloride (p.988·3).
*Arrhythmias.*

**Ry-Tuss** *Cypress, USA.*
Pentoxyverine tannate (p.1126·3); chlorphenamine tannate (p.428·1); ephedrine tannate (p.1120·3); phenylephrine tannate (p.1127·2).
*Coughs.*

**S-2** *Nephron, USA.*
Racepinefrine hydrochloride (p.854·1).
*Bronchospasm.*

**S.8** *Chefaro, Ger.*
Diphenhydramine hydrochloride (p.431·3).
*Sleep disorders.*

**S Amet** *Europharma, Spain.*
Ademetionine (p.1647·2).
*Depression; liver disorders.*

**S-26 AR**
*Wyeth Health, Austral.; Wyeth, Chile; Wyeth, Hong Kong; Wyeth, NZ; Wyeth Lederle, Port.; Wyeth, Singapore.*
Infant feed (p.1417·1).
*Regurgitation.*

**S-26 HA** *Wyeth, Hong Kong.*
Infant feed (p.1417·1).
*Cow's milk protein allergy.*

**S-26 LF**
*Wyeth Health, Austral.; Wyeth, Hong Kong; Wyeth, NZ; Wyeth, Singapore.*
Infant feed (p.1417·1).
*Lactose intolerance.*

**S-26 sem Lactose** *Wyeth Lederle, Port.*
Infant feed (p.1417·1).
*Lactose intolerance.*

**Saak** *Yungjin, Singapore.*
Methyl salicylate (p.59·3); glycol salicylate (p.44·3) menthol (p.1711·3); benzyl alcohol (p.1170·2).
*Musculoskeletal and joint pain.*

**SAB** *Parke, Davis, Austria†.*
Simeticone (p.1289·2); magnesium hydroxide (p.1272·2); aluminium hydroxide (p.1249·2).
*Flatulence, dyspepsia; peptic ulcer.*

**SAB Simplex**
*Pfizer, Austria; Parke, Davis, Ger.*
Simeticone (p.1289·2).
*Detergent poisoning; meteorism; reduction of intestinal gas before gastrointestinal procedures.*

**Saba** *Lampugnani, Ital.*
Saw palmetto (p.1569·1).
*Prostatic hyperplasia.*

**Sabacur uno** *Biocur, Ger.*
Saw palmetto (p.1569·1).
*Benign prostatic hyperplasia.*

**Sabadilla Med Complex** *Dynamit, Austria.*
Homoeopathic preparation.

**Sabal**
*Note. This name is used for preparations of different composition.*
*Pierre Fabre, Arg.; Ducray, Fr.*
*Shampoo:* Saw palmetto (p.1569·1); zinc salicylate (p.1157·2).
*Seborrhoeic dermatitis.*

*Pierre Fabre, Arg.*
*Topical emulsion:* Saw palmetto (p.1569·1); zinc pidolate.
*Seborrhoea.*

*Ducray, Fr.†.*
*Topical gel; topical emulsion:* Saw palmetto (p.1569·1); zinc pidolate; keluamid (p.1151·2).
*Seborrhoea.*

*Duopharm, Ger.; Stada, Ger.*
Saw palmetto (p.1569·1).
*Benign prostatic hyperplasia.*

**Sabal uno** *Apogepha, Ger.*
Saw palmetto (p.1569·1).
*Benign prostatic hyperplasia.*

**Sabalia** *Boiron, Canad.*
Homoeopathic preparation.

**Sabalin** *Lichtwer, UK.*
Saw palmetto (p.1569·1).
*Male urinary discomfort.*

**Sabalvit** *Bional, Ger.*
Saw palmetto (p.1569·1).
*Benign prostatic hyperplasia.*

**Sabanotropico** *Perez Gimenez, Spain.*
Bismuth subgallate (p.1252·2); dexamethasone sodium phosphate (p.1097·2); phenol (p.1188·1); sulfathiazole (p.264·1); tannic acid (p.1751·2); menthol (p.1711·3).
*Chilblains; cold-induced skin damage.*

**Sabatif** *Apomedica, Austria.*
Simeticone (p.1289·2); activated charcoal (p.1030·2); sulfur (p.1158·2); rhubarb (p.1287·3); senna leaf (p.1288·2); caraway oil (p.1667·3); fennel oil (p.1687·3).
*Dyspepsia; flatulence; laxative.*

**Sabax Fosenema** *Adcock Ingram, S.Afr.*
Monobasic sodium phosphate (p.1230·3); dibasic sodium phosphate (p.1231·1).
*Bowel evacuation.*

**Sabax Gentamix** *Adcock Ingram, S.Afr.*
Gentamicin sulfate (p.217·1).
*Bacterial infections.*

**SabCaps** *Medichemie Bioline, Switz.*
Saw palmetto (p.1569·1).
*Benign prostatic hyperplasia.*

**Sabima** *Atlantis, Mex.*
Secnidazole (p.615·3).
*Amoebiasis; giardiasis; trichomoniasis.*

**Sabin**
*Aventis Pasteur, Arg.; GlaxoSmithKline, Belg.*
An oral poliomyelitis vaccine (p.1633·3).
*Active immunisation.*

**Sabofen** *Geyer, Braz.*
Povidone-iodine (p.1190·3).
*Skin disinfection.*

**Sabonal Uno** *Sabona, Ger.*
Saw palmetto (p.1569·1).
*Benign prostatic hyperplasia.*

**Sabonete Sulfuroso** *Simoes, Braz.*
Sublimed sulfur (p.1158·2).
*Seborrhoea.*

**Sabril**
*Aventis, Arg.; Aventis, Austral.; Aventis, Austria; Aventis, Belg.; Aventis, Braz.; Aventis, Canad.; Aventis, Chile; Aventis, Fr.; Aventis, Ger.; Aventis, Hong Kong; Aventis, Irl.; Rhone-Poulenc Aventis, Ital.; Aventis, Mex.; Yamanouchi, Neth.; Aventis, NZ; Aventis, Port.; Aventis, S.Afr.; Aventis, Singapore; Aventis, Switz.; Aventis, UK.*
Vigabatrin (p.383·2).
*Epilepsy.*

**Sabrilan** *Agis, Israel.*
Vigabatrin (p.383·2).
*Epilepsy.*

**Sabrilex**
*Aventis, Denm.; Aventis, Fin.; Aventis, Norw.; Aventis, Spain; Aventis, Swed.*
Vigabatrin (p.383·2).
*Epilepsy.*

**Sabro** *Senosiain, Mex.*
Aloglutamol (p.1248·3).
*Gastritis; gastro-oesophageal reflux; gastrointestinal hyperacidity; hiatus hernia; peptic ulcer.*

**Saburgen-N** *Weber & Weber, Ger.*
Homoeopathic preparation.

**Sabutol** *Malaysia Chemist, Singapore.*
Salbutamol sulfate (p.791·3).
*Obstructive airways disease.*

**Sacietyl** *Finadiet, Arg.*
Sibutramine (p.1593·2).
*Obesity.*

**Sacin** *Labomed, Chile.*
Diethylpropion (p.1587·1).
*Obesity.*

**Sacnel** *Teofarma, Ital.*
Colloidal sulfur (p.1158·2); zinc oxide (p.1163·2); titanium dioxide (p.1160·3); dithiosalicylic acid (p.1146·1); hamamelis leaves (p.1696·3).
*Acne; seborrhoeic dermatitis.*

**Sacolene** *EG, Fr.*
Methylenated milk proteins.
*Diarrhoea.*

**Sacsol** *Eagle, Austral.†.*
Hexane (p.1475·1); camphor (p.1665·3).
*Surgical cement solvent for stoma patients.*

**Sacsol NF** *Eagle, Austral.†.*
Trichloroethane (p.1477·3); camphor (p.1665·3).
*Non-flammable surgical cement solvent for stoma patients.*

**Sactabs** *PSM, NZ.*
Saccharin (p.1443·2).
*Artificial sweetener.*

**Sadefen** *Roche Nicholas, Spain†.*
Ibuprofen (p.45·3).
*Fever; pain.*

**Sadeltan F** *Hautel, Arg.*
Aloe vera (p.1141·3); urea (p.1162·2).
*Emollient.*

**Sadol** *Catarinense, Braz.*
Iron (p.1434·3); pyridoxine; nicotinamide; caffeine; citric acid (p.1417·1).
*Iron deficiency; iron-deficiency anaemias.*

**SAE** *Pasteur, Chile.*
Propyphenazone (p.85·3); adiphenine hydrochloride (p.1648·1); trasentine.
*Smooth muscle spasm.*

**Saetil** *Robapharm, Spain.*
Ibuprofen arginine (p.46·3).
*Fever; musculoskeletal, joint, and peri-articular disorders; pain.*

**Safarol** *Medichrom, Gr.*
Butamirate citrate (p.1116·2).
*Cough.*

**Saf-Clens** *Calgon Vestal, USA.*
Wound cleanser.

**Safe Tussin 30** *Kramer, USA.*
Guaifenesin (p.1122·1); dextromethorphan hydrobromide (p.1117·3).
*Coughs.*

**Safeway Cough Lozenges** *Sutton, Canad.†.*
Menthol (p.1711·3).

**Safeway Nasal** *Prodemdis, Canad.*
Sodium chloride (p.1233·3).

**Saforelle** *Biosaude, Port.*
Lappa (p.1704·3).
*Soap substitute.*

**Safyr Bleu Antihistamine** *MDI, S.Afr.*
Antazoline hydrochloride (p.424·2); tetryzoline hydrochloride (p.1131·2).
*Allergic conjunctivitis; hay fever.*

**Sagadreps** *Diepharmex, Fr.*
Biclotymol (p.1171·1).
Formerly known as Hexadreps.
*Mouth and throat infections.*

**Sagamicin**
*Kyowa, Jpn; Kyowa, Singapore.*
Micronomicin sulfate (p.231·3).
*Bacterial infections.*

**Sagamicina** *Tubilux, Ital.†.*
Micronomicin sulfate (p.231·3).
*Bacterial eye infections.*

**Sagitta Kamillbad** *BASF, Ger.†.*
Chamomile oil (p.1669·3).
*Bath additive; skin and mucous-membrane disorders.*

**Sagittacin N** *BASF, Ger.†.*
Tetracycline hydrochloride (p.266·2).
*Respiratory-tract infections.*

**Sagittacortin** *BASF, Ger.†.*
Hydrocortisone (p.1103·3) or hydrocortisone acetate (p.1103·3).
*Skin disorders.*

**Sagittamuc** *BASF, Ger.†.*
Ambroxol hydrochloride (p.1114·3); doxycycline hyclate (p.206·2).
*Respiratory-tract infections.*

**Sagittaproct** *BASF, Ger.†.*
*Injection:* Quinine dihydrochloride (p.460·1).
*Haemorrhoids.*

*Suppositories; ointment:* Hamamelis (p.1696·3); bismuth subgallate (p.1252·2).
*Haemorrhoids.*

*Topical gel:* Lidocaine hydrochloride (p.1377·3).
*Local anaesthesia.*

**Sagittaproct S** *BASF, Ger.†.*
Lauromacrogol 400 (p.1412·3); zinc oxide (p.1163·2); bismuth subnitrate (p.1252·2).
*Haemorrhoids.*

**Sagrada-Lax** *Falqui, Ital.†.*
Cascara sagrada (p.1255·1).
*Constipation.*

**Sagrosept** *Schulke & Mayr, Ger.*
*Lotion:* Isopropyl alcohol (p.1184·3); propyl alcohol (p.1191·2); lactic acid (p.1704·1).
*Hand disinfection.*

*Medicated wipes:* Isopropyl alcohol (p.1184·3); propyl alcohol (p.1191·2); benzoic acid (p.1169·3); lactic acid (p.1704·1).
*Skin disinfection; surface disinfection; wounds.*

**Saintbois** *Vifor, Switz.*
Ethylmorphine hydrochloride (p.37·3); sulfogaiacol (p.1131·1); sodium benzoate (p.1169·3); belladonna (p.479·1); hyssopus officinalis; tolu balsam (p.1131·3).
*Coughs; respiratory-tract disorders.*

**Sais Andrews** *Sterling, Port.†.*
Citric acid (p.1673·1); magnesium sulfate (p.1228·2); sodium bicarbonate (p.1223·2).

**Sais de Frutos** *Confar, Port.†.*
Tartaric acid (p.1752·1); sodium carbonate (p.1747·1).

**Sais Zitos** *Zimaia, Port.†.*
Tartaric acid (p.1752·1); sodium carbonate (p.1747·1); sodium tartrate (p.1290·1).

**Saizen**
*Serono, Arg.; Serono, Austral.; Serono, Austria; Serono, Braz.; Serono, Canad.; Serono, Fin.; Serono, Fr.; Serono, Ger.; Serono, Gr.; Serono, Hong Kong; Serum Institute, India; Serono, Irl.; Serono, Israel†; Serono, Ital.; Serono, Malaysia; Serono, Mex.; Serono, Norw.; Serono, NZ; Serono, Port.; Serono, S.Afr.; Serono, Singapore; Serono, Spain; Serono, Swed.; Serono, Switz.; Serono, UK; Serono, USA.*
Somatropin (p.1327·2).
*Growth disorders in renal failure; growth hormone deficiency; Turner's syndrome.*

**Sal de Andrews** *GlaxoSmithKline, Braz.*
Magnesium sulfate (p.1228·2); sodium bicarbonate (p.1223·2).
*Gastrointestinal hyperacidity.*

**Sal de Fruta Eno**
*Note. This name is used for preparations of different composition.*
*GlaxoSmithKline, Arg.*
Sodium bicarbonate (p.1223·2); sodium carbonate (p.1747·1); tartaric acid (p.1752·1).
*Gastric hyperacidity.*

*GlaxoSmithKline, Braz.*
Sodium bicarbonate (p.1223·2); sodium carbonate (p.1747·1).
*Gastrointestinal hyperacidity.*

*GlaxoSmithKline, Chile.*
Sodium bicarbonate (p.1223·2); citric acid (p.1673·1).
*Gastrointestinal disorders.*

*SmithKline Beecham, Spain.*
Citric acid (p.1673·1); sodium bicarbonate (p.1223·2); sodium carbonate (p.1747·1).
*Gastrointestinal hyperacidity.*

**Sal De Yasta** *Bayer, Chile.*
Sodium bicarbonate (p.1223·2).
*Antacid.*

**Sal Dietetica** *Reccius, Chile.*
Potassium chloride (p.1232·2).
*Dietary salt substitute.*

**Sal Lite** *Rider, Chile.*
Sodium chloride (p.1233·3); potassium chloride (p.1232·2).
*Dietary salt substitute.*

**Sal Liviana En Sodio** *Reccius, Chile.*
Sodium chloride (p.1233·3); potassium chloride (p.1232·2).
*Dietary salt substitute.*

**Salac**
*Note. This name is used for preparations of different composition.*
*Andromaco, Arg.*
Clobetasol propionate (p.1095·2).
*Skin disorders.*

*Medicis, Canad.†; GenDerm, USA.*
Salicylic acid (p.1157·1).
*Acne.*

**Sal-Acid** *Pedinol, USA.*
Salicylic acid (p.1157·1).
*Warts.*

**Salact** *Knoll, Austral.†.*
Salicylic acid (p.1157·1).
*Acne.*

**Salactic Film** *Pedinol, USA.*
Salicylic acid (p.1157·1).
*Warts.*

**Salactol**
*Dermal Laboratories, Irl.; Dermal Laboratories, UK.*
Salicylic acid (p.1157·1); lactic acid (p.1704·1); flexible collodion.
*Calluses; corns; verrucas; warts.*

**Salagen**
Novartis, Austria; Pharmacia, Canad.; Novartis, Fin.; Novartis Ophthalmics, Fr.; Novartis Ophthalmics, Ger.; Biotrends, Gr.; Novartis, Irl.; MGI, Israel; Novartis, Ital.; Chiron, Neth.; Novartis Ophthalmics, Port.; Novartis Ophthalmics, Swed.; Novartis, UK; MGI, USA.
Pilocarpine hydrochloride (p.1495·1).
*Radiation-induced xerostomia; Sjögren's syndrome.*

**Salagesic** Blackmores, Austral.†.
Salix (p.87·3); wood betony; cimicifuga (p.1671·3); phenylalanine; magnesium phosphate; glycine; iron phosphate.
*Pain.*

**Salamol**
Ivax, Hong Kong; Ivax, Irl.; Ivax, Singapore; Norton Healthcare, Singapore; Ivax, UK.
Salbutamol (p.791·3) or salbutamol sulfate (p.791·3).
*Asthma; bronchospasm.*

**Salapin** Pinewood, UK.
Salbutamol sulfate (p.791·3).
*Asthma.*

**Salatac**
Dermal Laboratories, Irl.; Dermal, Israel.
Salicylic acid (p.1157·1); lactic acid (p.1704·1).
*Calluses; corns; verrucas; warts.*

**Salatac Gel** Dermal Laboratories, UK.
Salicylic acid (p.1157·1); lactic acid (p.1704·1).
*Calluses; corns; verrucas; warts.*

**Salazine** CTI, Israel†.
Sulfasalazine (p.1291·1).
*Ulcerative colitis.*

**Salazopirina** Jaba, Port.
Sulfasalazine (p.1291·1).
*Inflammatory bowel disease; rheumatoid arthritis.*

**Salazoprin** Cazi, Braz.
Sulfasalazine (p.1291·1).
*Inflammatory bowel disease.*

**Salazopyrin**
Pharmacia, Austral.; Pharmacia, Austria; Pharmacia, Canad.; Pharmacia, Denm.; Pharmacia, Fin.; Pharmacia, Hong Kong; Pharmacia, Irl.; Pharmacia Upjohn, Israel; Pharmacia Upjohn, Ital.; Pharmacia, Malaysia; Pharmacia, Norw.; Pharmacia, NZ; Pharmacia, S.Afr.; Pharmacia, Singapore; Pharmacia, Swed.; Pharmacia, Switz.; Pharmacia, Thai.; Pharmacia, UK.
Sulfasalazine (p.1291·1).
*Inflammatory bowel disease; pyoderma gangrenosum; rheumatoid arthritis.*

**Salazopyrina** Pharmacia, Spain.
Sulfasalazine (p.1291·1).
*Proctitis; ulcerative colitis.*

**Salazopyrine**
Pharmacia, Belg.; Pharmacia, Fr.; Pharmacia, Neth.
Sulfasalazine (p.1291·1).
*Inflammatory bowel disease; rheumatoid arthritis.*

**Salbei Curarina** Harras-Curarina, Ger.
Sage (p.1741·2).
*Mouth and throat inflammation.*

**Salbei-Halspastillen** Bioflora, Austria.
Sage oil (p.1741·2); calcium pantothenate (p.1442·3); chlorhexidine hydrochloride (p.1173·3).
*Mouth and throat disorders.*

**Salbetol** FDC, India.
Salbutamol sulfate (p.791·3).
*Obstructive airways disease.*

**Salbu** Orion, Ger.; Fatol, Ger.
Salbutamol sulfate (p.791·3).
*Obstructive airways disease.*

**Salbudan** Norton, Denm.
Salbutamol (p.791·3).
*Obstructive airways disease.*

**Salbufax** Master Pharma, Ital.
Salbutamol sulfate (p.791·3).
*Asthma; bronchospastic disorders.*

**Salbuhexal** Hexal, Ger.
Salbutamol sulfate (p.791·3).
*Obstructive airways disease.*

**Salbulair** 3M, Ger.
Salbutamol sulfate (p.791·3).
*Obstructive airways disease.*

**Salbulin**
3M, Denm.†; Riker, Mex.†; 3M, S.Afr.; 3M, UK.
Salbutamol (p.791·3) or salbutamol sulfate (p.791·3).
*Obstructive airways disease.*

**Salbulind** Lindopharm, Ger.
Salbutamol sulfate (p.791·3).
*Obstructive airways disease.*

**Salbumol** GlaxoSmithKline, Fr.
Salbutamol sulfate (p.791·3).
*Asthma; premature labour.*

**Salbunova** Lavipharm, Gr.
Salbutamol sulfate (p.791·3).
*Asthma; chronic respiratory failure.*

**Salbupp** Dermapharm, Ger.
Salbutamol sulfate (p.791·3).
*Obstructive airways disease.*

**Salburin** Luper, Braz.
Salbutamol sulfate (p.791·3).
*Obstructive airways disease.*

**Salbusian** Asian Pharm, Thai.
Salbutamol sulfate (p.791·3).
*Obstructive airways disease.*

**Salbutac** Polipharm, Thai.
Salbutamol sulfate (p.791·3).
*Obstructive airways disease.*

**Salbutalan** Quimica y Farmacia, Mex.
Salbutamol (p.791·3).

**Salbutalin** Hebron, Braz.
Salbutamol (p.791·3).
*Obstructive airways disease.*

**Salbutam** Bunker, Braz.
Salbutamol sulfate (p.791·3).
*Obstructive airways disease.*

**Salbutamax** Uniao Quimica, Braz.
Salbutamol sulfate (p.791·3).
*Obstructive airways disease.*

**Salbutard**
United Nordic, Denm.†; Lusofarmaco, Ital.
Salbutamol sulfate (p.791·3).
*Asthma; bronchospastic disorders.*

**Salbuterol** IG, Malaysia; Medidata, Malaysia.
Salbutamol (p.791·3).
*Asthma.*

**Salbutib** Ibfarma, Braz.†.
Salbutamol (p.791·3).
*Obstructive airways disease.*

**Salbutol** Danes, Arg.
Salbutamol (p.791·3) or salbutamol sulfate (p.791·3).
*Obstructive airways disease.*

**Salbutol Beclo** Danes, Arg.
Salbutamol (p.791·3); beclometasone dipropionate (p.1091·1).
*Obstructive airways disease.*

**Salbuvent**
Nycomed, Denm.; Leiras, Fin.; Nycomed, Norw.†; Douglas, NZ†.
Salbutamol (p.791·3) or salbutamol sulfate (p.791·3).
*Obstructive airways disease.*

**Salcacam** Salvat, Spain†.
Piroxicam (p.84·2).
*Gout; musculoskeletal, joint, and peri-articular disorders; pain.*

**Salcal** Saval, Chile.
Fenproporex hydrochloride (p.1588·3).
*Obesity.*

**Salcat** Pharmacia, Port.
Calcitonin (salmon) (p.768·2).
*Hypercalcaemia; osteolysis of malignancy; osteoporosis; Paget's disease of bone.*

**Salcedogen** Fardi, Spain†.
Citric acid (p.1673·1); magnesium chloride (p.1228·1); sodium bicarbonate (p.1223·2); sodium citrate (p.1223·2); mannitol (p.950·2).
*Constipation; hepatobiliary disorders; hypomagnesaemia; lithiasis; uric acidaemia.*

**Salcedol** Fardi, Spain.
Potassium sulfate (p.1232·2); sodium bicarbonate (p.1223·2); sodium sulfate (p.1290·1); tartaric acid (p.1752·1).
*Constipation; digestive disorders; hepatobiliary disorders.*

**Salcemetic** Fardi, Spain.
Cyclobutyrol (p.1678·2); metoclopramide hydrochloride (p.1274·3); mannitol (p.950·2).
*Gastrointestinal disorders.*

**Salceryl** Ranbaxy, Thai.†.
Salbutamol sulfate (p.791·3); guaifenesin (p.1122·1).
*Coughs; obstructive airways disease.*

**Salco** Lisapharm, Israel.
Calcitonin (salmon) (p.768·2).
*Hypercalcaemia; osteoporosis; Paget's disease of bone.*

**Salcoat** Teijin, Jpn.
Beclometasone dipropionate (p.1091·1).
*Stomatitis.*

**Salcotan** Scherer, Hong Kong†.
Ubidecarenone (p.1760·2).
*Cardiac disorders; cerebral metabolic disorders; muscular disorders.*

**Saldac**
Douglas, Austral.†; Douglas, NZ†.
Sulindac (p.91·2).
*Musculoskeletal, joint, and peri-articular disorders.*

**Salder S** Medley, Braz.
Salicylic acid (p.1157·1); sulfur (p.1158·2).
*Acne; pityriasis versicolor.*

**Saldeva**
Note. This name is used for preparations of different composition.
Montpellier, Arg.
Benzoic acid sulfonamide; atropine methobromide (p.476·3); metamizole magnesium (p.36·1).
*Dysmenorrhoea; premenstrual syndrome.*

Roche, Spain.
Caffeine (p.782·1); dimenhydrinate (p.431·1); paracetamol (p.76·2).
*Dysmenorrhoea.*

**Salena** Novartis, Arg.
Flumetasone pivalate (p.1101·1); salicylic acid (p.1157·1).
*Skin disorders.*

**Sales de Frutas P G** Perez Gimenez, Spain.
Citric acid (p.1673·1); sodium bicarbonate (p.1223·2); tartaric acid (p.1752·1).
*Constipation; gastrointestinal hyperacidity.*

**Sales Fruta Mag Viviar** Viviar, Spain.
Magnesium carbonate (p.1272·1); sodium bicarbonate (p.1223·2); tartaric acid (p.1752·1).
*Constipation; gastrointestinal hyperacidity.*

**Saleto** Roberts, USA.
Paracetamol (p.76·2); aspirin (p.15·1); salicylamide (p.87·3); caffeine (p.782·1).
The name Saleto is also used for a preparation containing ibuprofen.
*Pain.*

**Saleto-200** Roberts, USA.
Ibuprofen (p.45·3).
The name Saleto is also used for a preparation containing paracetamol, aspirin, salicylamide, and caffeine.
*Fever; osteoarthritis; pain; rheumatoid arthritis.*

**Saleto-D** Roberts, USA†.
Phenylpropanolamine hydrochloride (p.1127·3); paracetamol (p.76·2); caffeine (p.782·1); salicylamide (p.87·3).
*Upper respiratory-tract symptoms.*

**Salflex** Carnrick, USA.
Salsalate (p.88·1).
*Musculoskeletal and joint disorders.*

**Salf-Pas** Salf, Ital.
Sodium aminosalicylate (p.155·1).
*Tuberculosis.*

**Salguer** Fada, Arg.
Povidone-iodine (p.1190·3).
*Disinfection.*

**Salgydal a la noramidopyrine** Bouchara-Recordati, Fr.
Dipyrone (p.35·3); paracetamol (p.76·2); codeine phosphate (p.27·1).
*Pain.*

**Salhumin** Sanova, Austria.
*Bath additive:* Sodium humate; salicylic acid (p.1157·1).
*Rheumatic disorders.*

*Liniment:* Sodium humate; capsicum (p.1667·1); salicylic acid (p.1157·1); eucalyptus oil (p.1686·2); rosemary oil (p.1740·2); turpentine oil (p.1760·1); camphor (p.1665·3).
*Circulatory disorders; muscle, joint, and nerve pain.*

**Salhumin Gel** Bastian, Ger.
Glycol salicylate (p.44·3).
*Soft-tissue injury.*

**Salhumin Gel N** Bastian, Ger.†.
Glycol salicylate (p.44·3); benzyl nicotinate (p.21·2); camphor (p.1665·3).
*Neuralgia; peripheral vascular disorders; rheumatism; sports injuries.*

**Salhumin Rheuma-Bad** Bastian, Ger.
Salicylic acid (p.1157·1); sodium humate.
*Bath additive; musculoskeletal and joint disorders.*

**Salhumin Sitzbad N** Bastian, Ger.
Salicylic acid (p.1157·1); sodium humate.
*Bath additive; gynaecological disorders.*

**Salhumin Teilbad N** Bastian, Ger.
Salicylic acid (p.1157·1); sodium humate; esculoside (p.1648·2).
*Bath additive; circulatory disorders.*

**Sali D'Achille** Terme di Salsomaggiore, Ital.
Mineral salt preparation.
*Sore feet.*

**Sali di Salsomaggiore** Terme di Salsomaggiore, Ital.
Mineral salt preparation.
*Gynaecological disorders; nose and throat disorders.*

**Sali Iodati di Montecatini** Terme di Montecatini, Ital.†.
Mineral salt preparation.
*Constipation.*

**Sali Lassativi di Chianciano** Terme di Chianciano, Ital.†.
Mineral salt preparation.
*Constipation; digestive-system disorders.*

**Sali Tamerici di Montecatini** Terme di Montecatini, Ital.†.
Mineral salt preparation.
*Constipation.*

**Sali-Adalat** Bayer, Ger.
Nifedipine (p.966·2); mefruside (p.951·3).
*Hypertension.*

**Sali-Aldopur**
Kwizda, Austria; Hormosan, Ger.
Spironolactone (p.1003·1); bendroflumethiazide (p.867·3).
*Hyperaldosteronism; hypertension; hypokalaemia; liver cirrhosis and ascites; oedema.*

**Salibra** Brothier, Fr.†.
Monobasic calcium phosphate; monobasic magnesium phosphate; monobasic sodium phosphate; monobasic manganese phosphate; monobasic potassium phosphate; monobasic lithium phosphate (p.1417·1).
*Tonic.*

**Salic** Darrow, Braz.
Lactic acid (p.1704·1); salicylic acid (p.1157·1).
*Keratinisation disorders.*

**Salicairine** Richelet, Fr.
Salicaria.
*Diarrhoea.*

**Salicalcium** CT, Ital.
Calcium carbonate (p.1254·2).
*Calcium deficiency; calcium supplement.*

**SaliCept** Carrington, USA.
Acemannan (p.1645·2).
*Wounds, injuries, and ulcers of the oral mucosa.*

**Salicil**
Note. This name is used for preparations of different composition.
Ducto, Braz.
Aspirin (p.15·1).
*Fever; pain.*

Bersan, Ital.
Salicylic acid (p.1157·1).
*Scalp disorders.*

**Salicilato de Bismuto Composto** Simoes, Braz.
Bismuth salicylate (p.1252·1); sodium bicarbonate (p.1223·2); magnesium oxide (p.1272·3); calcium carbonate (p.1254·2); belladonna (p.479·1).
*Diarrhoea; gastrointestinal hyperacidity.*

**Salicina** Ratiopharm, Ital.
Aspirin (p.15·1); ascorbic acid (p.1460·2).
*Cold and influenza symptoms; pain.*

**Salicin-C** Amnol, Ital.
Salix; echinacea; minerals; vitamin C (p.1417·1).
*Nutritional supplement.*

**Salicort** Cassara, Arg.
Triamcinolone acetonide (p.1110·2); salicylic acid (p.1157·1).
*Skin disorders.*

**Salicort-R** Kattwiga, Ger.
Homoeopathic preparation.

**Salicrem** Gezzi, Arg.
Diethylamine salicylate (p.34·1); benzocaine (p.1370·3).
*Musculoskeletal and joint disorders.*

**Salicrem K** Gezzi, Arg.
Ketoprofen (p.51·2).
*Musculoskeletal and joint disorders.*

**Salicrem Miconazol** Gezzi, Arg.
Miconazole nitrate (p.405·3).
*Fungal skin infections.*

**Salicyl** Galderma, Denm.
Salicylic acid (p.1157·1).
*Keratinisation disorders.*

**Salicylcafeina** Menarini, Port.
Aspirin (p.15·1); caffeine (p.782·1).
*Fever; pain.*

**Sali-Decoderm**
Merck, Austria†; Hermal, Ger.
Fluprednidene acetate (p.1102·2); salicylic acid (p.1157·1).
*Scalp disorders (tincture); skin disorders.*

**Salidex** Braun, Norw.
Anhydrous glucose (p.1432·2); sodium chloride (p.1233·3).
*Carbohydrate source; fluid and electrolyte disorders.*

**Salidur** Omega, Spain.
Furosemide (p.919·3); triamterene (p.1016·2).
*Hypertension; oedema.*

**Saliject** Omega, Canad.
Sodium salicylate (p.90·1).
*Sclerotherapy.*

**Salikaren** Rekah, Israel.
Salicylic acid (p.1157·1).
*Keratinisation disorders.*

**Saliker**
Note. This name is used for preparations of different composition.
Roche-Posay, Arg.
Salicylic acid (p.1157·1); piroctone olamine (p.1155·2); iodopropynyl butyl carbamate (Glicacil).
*Scalp disorders.*

Roche-Posay, Braz.; Roche-Posay, Fr.
Salicylic acid (p.1157·1); piroctone olamine (p.1155·2); iodopropynyl butyl carbamate (Glicacil); capryloyl salicylate; capryloyl glycine.
*Dandruff; seborrhoeic dermatitis.*

Roche-Posay, Irl.
Salicylic acid (p.1157·1); piroctone olamine (p.1155·2).
*Dandruff; seborrhoeic dermatitis.*

**Salilax**
Orion, Denm.; Orion, Swed.
Magnesium oxide (p.1272·3).
*Bowel evacuation.*

**Salimar-Bad L** Li-il, Ger.†.
Sodium salicylate (p.90·1); salicylic acid (p.1157·1).
*Bath additive; musculoskeletal and joint disorders.*

**Saliment** Vida, Hong Kong.
Methyl salicylate (p.59·3); eucalyptus oil (p.1686·2); menthol (p.1711·3).
*Musculoskeletal and joint pain.*

**Salimetin** Luper, Braz.
Methyl salicylate (p.59·3); turpentine oil (p.1760·1); menthol (p.1711·3); camphor (p.1665·3); chlorophyllin copper complex sodium (p.1057·1); lavender oil (p.1705·2).
Formerly contained methyl salicylate, turpentine oil, and camphor.
*Musculoskeletal and joint disorders.*

**Salimidin** Kampel Martian, Arg.
Itraconazole (p.401·3).
*Fungal infections.*

**Salimont** Pharmonta, Austria.
Aspirin (p.15·1).
*Fever; pain.*

**Salinal** Julphar, UAE.
Simeticone (p.1289·2).
*Adjunct in gastroscopy and bowel radiography; flatulence.*

**Salinex**
Sabex, Canad.; Muro, USA.
Sodium chloride (p.1233·3).
*Nasal hygiene; nasal irritation.*

**Salinol** Sabex, Canad.
Macrogol (p.1708·2); propylene glycol (p.1735·2).
*Nasal lubricant.*

**Salipads** Galderma, Braz.
Salicylic acid (p.1157·1).
*Keratinisation disorders; seborrhoea.*

**Salipax** *Mepha, Port.*
Fluoxetine hydrochloride (p.292·1).
*Depression.*

**Salipran** *Celltech, Fr.*
Benorilate (p.20·3).
*Pain.*

**Sali-Prent** *Bayer, Ger.*
Acebutolol hydrochloride (p.848·1); mefruside (p.951·3).
*Hypertension.*

**Sali-Puren** *Alpharma-Isis, Ger.*
Triamterene (p.1016·2); hydrochlorothiazide (p.933·2).
*Heart failure; hypertension; oedema.*

**Salisoap** *Darrow, Braz.*
Salicylic acid (p.1157·1); sulfur (p.1158·2).
*Seborrhoeic dermatitis.*

**Salisol** *Rekah, Israel.*
Salicylic acid (p.1157·1); alcohol (p.1166·1).
*Keratinisation disorders; skin disinfection.*

**Sali-Spiroctan** *Roche, Switz.†.*
Spironolactone (p.1003·1); butizide (p.878·2).
*Hyperaldosteronism.*

**Salisteril** *Fresenius Kabi, Switz.*
Electrolyte infusion (p.1217·1).
*Fluid and electrolyte disorders.*

**Salistoperm** *Ursapharm, Ger.*
Salicylamide (p.87·3); benzocaine (p.1370·3).
*Musculoskeletal, joint, peri-articular, and soft-tissue disorders; neuralgia.*

**Salitanol Estreptomicina** *Quimpe, Spain.*
Albumin tannate (p.1248·1); dihydrostreptomycin sulfate (p.205·3); sulfathiazole (p.264·1).
*Gastrointestinal infections.*

**Saliton** *Planta, Canad.†.*
Salix (p.87·3).
*Fever; pain.*

**Saliva medac** *Medac, Ger.*
Mucin (porcine) (p.1579·1).
*Saliva substitute.*

**Saliva Orthana** *A.S., UK.*
*Lozenges:* Mucin (p.1579·1); xylitol (p.1469·1).
*Oral spray:* Mucin (p.1579·1); xylitol (p.1469·1); sodium fluoride (p.1444·3).
*Saliva substitute.*

**Salivace** *Penn, UK†.*
Carmellose sodium (p.1577·3); xylitol (p.1469·1); electrolytes (p.1217·1).
*Dry mouth.*

**Salivan** *Apsen, Braz.†.*
Carmellose sodium (p.1577·3).
*Dry mouth.*

**Salivart**
*Gebauer, Canad.; Master, Chile; Gebauer, Hong Kong; Gebauer, USA.*
Carmellose sodium (p.1577·3); sorbitol (p.1446·3); electrolytes (p.1217·1).
*Dry mouth.*

**Saliveze** *Wyvern, UK.*
Electrolytes (p.1217·1).
*Dry mouth.*

**Salivix** *Provalis, UK.*
Malic acid (p.1709·2); calcium lactate (p.1225·3); sodium phosphate (p.1231·1).
*Dry mouth.*

**Salix** *Scandinavian Natural Health & Beauty, USA.*
Artificial saliva.

**Salmagne** *Fardi, Spain.*
Magnesium citrate (p.1272·1); magnesium sulfate (p.1228·2); sodium bicarbonate (p.1223·2); tartaric acid (p.1752·1); mannitol (p.950·2).
*Constipation; digestive disorders.*

**Salmaplon** *Khandelwal, India.*
Salbutamol (p.791·3).
*Obstructive airways disease.*

**Salmax** *CCM, Malaysia.*
Salbutamol sulfate (p.791·3).
*Obstructive airways disease.*

**Salmetedur** *Menarini, Ital.*
Salmeterol xinafoate (p.795·1).
*Bronchospastic disorders.*

**Salmeter** *Reddy's, India.*
Salmeterol (p.795·2).
*Asthma.*

**Salmiak** *Soldan, Ger.*
Ammonium chloride (p.1115·2); liquorice (p.1270·2); anise oil (p.1655·2).
*Respiratory-tract disorders.*

**Salmocalcin**
*Sanofi Synthelabo, Arg.; Ripari-Gero, Ital.†.*
Calcitonin (salmon) (p.768·2).
*Hypercalcaemia; osteoporosis; Paget's disease of bone; reflex sympathetic dystrophy.*

**Salmocide** *Atlantis, Mex.*
Furazolidone (p.605·2).
*Gastrointestinal infections.*

**Salmofar** *Lafare, Ital.*
Calcitonin (salmon) (p.768·2).
*Hypercalcaemia; osteoporosis; Paget's disease of bone; reflex sympathetic dystrophy.*

**Salmol**
*Atlantic, Hong Kong; Biolab, Malaysia; Atlantic, Singapore; Atlantic, Thai.; Biolab, Thai.*
Salbutamol sulfate (p.791·3).
*Obstructive airways disease; premature labour.*

**Salmol Expectorant** *Biolab, Thai.*
Salbutamol sulfate (p.791·3); guaifenesin (p.1122·1).
*Obstructive airways disease.*

**Salmoten** *Adipharm (Αδηφαρμ), Gr.*
Calcitonin (salmon) (p.768·2).
*Hypercalcaemia; osteoporosis; Paget's disease of bone.*

**Salmundin** *Mundipharma, Ger.*
Salbutamol sulfate (p.791·3).
*Obstructive airways disease.*

**Salodiur** *Gerot, Austria.*
Triamterene (p.1016·2); hydrochlorothiazide (p.933·2).
*Hypertension; oedema.*

**Salofalk**
*Orphan, Austral.; Merck, Austria; Axcan, Canad.; EciFarma, Chile; Falk, Ger.; Galenica, Gr.; Falk, Hong Kong; Antigen, Irl.; Abbott, Ital.; Falk, Malaysia; Farmasa, Mex.; Tramedico, Neth.; Falk, Port.; Falk, Singapore; Medichemie, Switz.; Falk, Thai.; Provalis, UK.*
Mesalazine (p.1273·2).
*Inflammatory bowel disease.*

**Sal-Oil-T** *Syosset, USA.*
Coal tar (p.1159·2); salicylic acid (p.1157·1).
*Seborrhoea.*

**Salomethyl** *Mitsubishi-Tokyo, Hong Kong.*
Methyl salicylate (p.59·3); glycol salicylate (p.44·3); menthol (p.1711·3); camphor (p.1665·3); eucalyptus oil (p.1686·2); thymol (p.1194·2); capsaicin (p.24·2); benzyl nicotinate (p.21·2).
*Headache; insect bites; musculoskeletal and soft-tissue disorders; neuralgia.*

**Salomol** *Clonmel, Irl.†.*
Salbutamol (p.791·3) or salbutamol sulfate (p.791·3).
*Obstructive airways disease.*

**Salonair** *Salonpas, UK.*
Methyl salicylate (p.59·3); menthol (p.1711·3); camphor (p.1665·3); benzyl nicotinate (p.21·2); glycol salicylate (p.44·3).
*Muscle and joint pain.*

**Salongo** *Madaus, Spain.*
Oxiconazole nitrate (p.407·3).
*Fungal infections.*

**Salonpas**
*Note. This name is used for preparations of different composition.*
*Hisamitsu, Braz.†.*
Methyl salicylate (p.59·3); menthol (p.1711·3); camphor (p.1665·3); thymol (p.1194·2); glycol salicylate (p.44·3).
*Musculoskeletal and joint disorders.*

*Silesia, Chile.*
Methyl salicylate (p.59·3); menthol (p.1711·3); camphor (p.1665·3); tocoferol acetate (p.1465·1).
*Musculoskeletal and joint pain; neuralgia.*

*Farmila, Ital.*
*Medicated bandage:* Menthol (p.1711·3); methyl salicylate (p.59·3); camphor (p.1665·3); glycol salicylate (p.44·3); thymol (p.1194·2).
*Topical spray:* Methyl salicylate (p.59·3); menthol (p.1711·3); camphor (p.1665·3); benzyl nicotinate (p.21·2); glycol salicylate (p.44·3).
*Musculoskeletal, joint, and soft-tissue pain.*

*Hisamitsu, Malaysia.*
Methyl salicylate (p.59·3); glycol salicylate (p.44·3); menthol (p.1711·3); thymol (p.1194·2); camphor (p.1665·3); tocoferil acetate (p.1465·1).
*Musculoskeletal, joint, and soft-tissue pain and inflammation.*

*Hisamitsu, NZ; Pharmaco, NZ.*
Camphor (p.1665·3); methyl salicylate (p.59·3); menthol (p.1711·3).
*Inflammation; pain.*

*Salonpas, UK.*
Methyl salicylate (p.59·3); glycol salicylate (p.44·3).
*Musculoskeletal and joint pain.*

**Salopyrine** *Adelco, Gr.*
Sulfasalazine (p.1291·1).
*Inflammatory bowel disease.*

**Salospir** *Unipharma, Gr.*
Aspirin (p.15·1).
*Fever; inflammation; pain; thrombosis prophylaxis.*

**Salpad** *Pharmatrix, Arg.*
Salicylic acid (p.1157·1).
*Acne; keratinisation disorders.*

**Sal-Plant** *Pedinol, USA.*
Salicylic acid (p.1157·1).
*Warts.*

**Salseb** *Draxis, Canad.*
Salicylic acid (p.1157·1).

**Salsitab** *Upsher-Smith, USA.*
Salsalate (p.88·1).
*Fever; inflammation; pain.*

**Salsol** *Kee, India.*
Salbutamol sulfate (p.791·3).
*Bronchospasm.*

**Salsyvase** *Ipex, Swed.*
Salicylic acid (p.1157·1).
Formerly known as Salicylsyrevaselin.
*Skin disorders.*

**Saltadol** *Lindopharm, Ger.*
Potassium chloride; sodium chloride; sodium bicarbonate; glucose (p.1222·2).
*Diarrhoea; oral rehydration therapy.*

**Saltamol**
*Zambon, Braz.†; Ranbaxy, Thai.†.*
Salbutamol (p.791·3).
*Obstructive airways disease.*

Salbutamol sulfate (p.791·3).
*Obstructive airways disease.*

**Saltermox** *Propan, S.Afr.†.*
Amoxicillin (p.155·3).
*Bacterial infections.*

**Salterpyn** *Propan, S.Afr.*
*Syrup:* Paracetamol (p.76·2); codeine phosphate (p.27·1); promethazine hydrochloride (p.439·1).
*Fever; pain.*
*Tablets:* Paracetamol (p.76·2); codeine phosphate (p.27·1); caffeine (p.782·1); meprobamate (p.706·2).
*Pain with tension.*

**Saltos** *Roux-Ocefa, Arg.*
Noscapine ascorbate (p.1125·3); papaverine hydrochloride (p.1728·1); ephedrine hydrochloride (p.1120·1); guaifenesin (p.1122·1); hydroxyfylline.
*Coughs.*

**Saltrates** *Uhlmann-Eyraud, Switz.*
*Cream:* Triclosan (p.1195·2); methylchloroisothiazolinone (p.1185·1); menthol (p.1711·3); chamomile oil (p.1669·3); hypericum oil (p.299·2); citronella oil (p.1673·2); lavender oil (p.1705·2).
*Dry or painful feet.*
*Topical gel:* Sodium hydroxide (p.1747·3); trometamol (p.1758·2).
*Calluses; corns.*

**Saltrates Rodell** *Uhlmann-Eyraud, Switz.*
Chamomile (p.1669·3); hypericum (p.299·1); sodium bicarbonate (p.1223·2); anhydrous sodium carbonate (p.1747·1); sodium sesquicarbonate; sodium perborate (p.1192·2).
*Foot disorders.*

**Sal-Tropine** *Hope, USA.*
Atropine sulfate (p.477·1).

**Saltucin**
*Roche, Austria†; Boehringer Mannheim, Ger.†.*
Butizide (p.878·2).
*Diabetes insipidus; heart failure; hypertension; oedema; renal calculi.*

**Salubion** *Merck, Chile.*
Vitamins; minerals; rutin (p.1417·1).
*Tonic.*

**Salucur** *Salus, Fr.†.*
Urtica (p.1762·1); saw palmetto (p.1569·1); cucurbita (p.1677·3); vitamin B substances; vitamin C (p.1417·1).
*Prostatic disorders; urinary-tract disorders.*

**Saludopin** *SIT, Ital.*
Methyldopa (p.953·2); butizide (p.878·2).
*Hypertension.*

**Salugliben** *Salus, Mex.†.*
Glibenclamide (p.331·2).
*Diabetes mellitus.*

**Saluket-H I** *Salus, Mex.*
Ketotifen (p.788·2).
*Asthma.*

**Salures** *Pharmacia, Swed.*
Bendroflumethiazide (p.867·3).
*Hypertension; oedema; renal calculi.*

**Salures-K** *Pharmacia, Swed.*
Bendroflumethiazide (p.867·3); potassium chloride (p.1232·2).
*Hypertension; oedema; renal calculi.*

**Saluretin** *Zeneca, Switz.†.*
Spironolactone (p.1003·1); bendroflumethiazide (p.867·3).
*Hyperaldosteronism; hypertension; oedema.*

**Saluric** *Merck Sharp & Dohme, Irl.†.*
Chlorothiazide (p.882·1).
*Hypertension; oedema.*

**Salurin** *Julphar, UAE.*
Furosemide (p.919·3).
*Oedema.*

**Saluron** *Apothecon, USA.*
Hydroflumethiazide (p.937·2).
*Hypertension; oedema.*

**Salus** *Salushaus, Ger.†.*
Devil's claw root (p.28·2).
*Tonic.*

**Salus Abfuhr-Tee Nr. 2** *Salushaus, Ger.†.*
Rose fruit (p.1740·1); chamomile (p.1669·3); calendula (p.1665·2); buckthorn (p.1254·1); senna (p.1288·2); fennel (p.1687·2).
*Constipation.*

**Salus Augenschutz-Kapseln NA** *Salushaus, Ger.*
Myrtillus (p.1718·3); vitamin A palmitate (p.1453·1).
*Hypersensitivity to light; night blindness.*

**Salus Bronchial-Tee Nr.8** *Salushaus, Ger.†.*
Fennel (p.1687·2); calendula (p.1665·2); Iceland moss; verbascum (p.1764·1); tilia (p.1756·2); cowslip flower (p.1735·1); lamium album; thyme (p.1755·2); knotgrass; raspberry leaf (p.1737·3).
*Coughs and associated respiratory-tract disorders.*

**Salus Herz-Schutz-Kapseln** *Salushaus, Ger.*
Crataegus (p.1677·1); alpha tocoferil acetate (p.1465·1); magnesium complex with acid hydrolysate of maize starch.
*Cardiovascular disorders.*

**Salus Leber-Galle-Tee Nr.18** *Salushaus, Ger.†.*
Cynara (p.1678·3); fennel (p.1687·2); chamomile (p.1669·3); taraxacum (p.1751·3); stoechados; calendula (p.1665·2); achillea (p.1646·2); peppermint leaf (p.1283·2).
*Liver and biliary disorders.*

**Salus Mistel-Tropfen** *Salushaus, Ger.*
Mistletoe (p.1715·3).
*Atherosclerosis.*

**Salus Multi-Vitamin-Energetikum** *Salushaus, Ger.*
Multivitamin preparation with plant extracts (p.1417·1).
*Tonic; vitamin deficiency.*

**Salus Nerven-Schlaf-Tee Nr.22** *Salushaus, Ger.†.*
Chamomile (p.1669·3); bellis perennis; paeonia officinalis; stoechados; fennel (p.1687·2); lupulus (p.1708·1); hypericum (p.299·1); lavender (p.1705·1); melissa (p.1711·1); sweet orange (p.1724·1).
*Nervous disorders.*

**Salus Rheuma-Tee Krautertee Nr. 12** *Salushaus, Ger.†.*
Birch leaf (p.1660·3); urtica (p.1762·1); fennel (p.1687·2); taraxacum (p.1751·3); calendula (p.1665·2); equisetum (p.1684·1); achillea (p.1646·2); juniper (p.1703·1).
*Rheumatic disorders.*

**Salus Venen Krauter Dragees N** *Salushaus, Ger.*
Aesculus (p.1648·2); melilotus.
*Venous insufficiency.*

**Salus Zinnkraut** *Salushaus, Ger.†.*
Equisetum (p.1684·1).
*Oedema.*

**Salusa** *Novartis Consumer, S.Afr.*
Procaine hydrochloride (p.1383·2); vitamins; haematoporphyrin (p.1417·1).

**Salusan** *Salushaus, Ger.†.*
Crataegus (p.1677·1); mistletoe (p.1715·3); ammi visnaga fruit (p.1653·3); equisetum (p.1684·1); dried bitter-orange peel (p.1723·3); lemon peel (p.1706·2); passion flower (p.1729·1); melissa (p.1711·1); valerian (p.1762·2); hypericum (p.299·1); lupulus (p.1708·1); rosemary (p.1740·2); cymbopogon citratus; bearberry (p.1659·2); wheat germ; tinct. germen. hordeoli.
*Cardiovascular disorders.*

**Salutaris** *Incaico, Arg.*
Ispaghula (p.1268·1); coriander (p.1676·1); soluble fibre (p.1253·2).
*Hypercholesterolaemia; obesity.*

**Salutensin** *Shire Richwood, USA.*
Hydroflumethiazide (p.937·2); reserpine (p.995·1).
*Hypertension.*

**Salutina** *Bergamo, Braz.†.*
Kola (p.1765·3); carqueja; iodine (p.1598·1); potassium iodide (p.1598·1); calcium dihydrogen phosphate (p.1664·2); glycerol; alcohol.

**Salva Infantes** *Camps, Spain†.*
Magnesium carbonate (p.1272·1); magnesium sulfate (p.1228·2); betanaphthyl benzoate (p.103·2).
*Gastrointestinal disorders.*

**Salvacam** *Biomed, Spain.*
Piroxicam (p.84·2).
*Gout; musculoskeletal, joint, peri-articular, and soft-tissue disorders; pain.*

**Salvacolina NF** *Salvat, Spain.*
Loperamide hydrochloride (p.1271·1).
Salvacolina formerly contained albumin tannate and opium.
*Diarrhoea.*

**Salvacolon** *Salvat, Spain.*
*Bacillus subtilis*; vitamins and amino acids (p.1417·1).
*Cystitis; gastrointestinal disorders; restoration of the gastrointestinal flora.*

**Salvalerg** *GlaxoSmithKline, Arg.*
Cetirizine (p.427·2).
*Hypersensitivity reactions.*

**Salvalion** *Normon, Spain†.*
Raubasine (p.994·3); almitrine (p.1584·2).
*Cerebrovascular disorders; vestibular disorders.*

**Salvapen** *Salvat, Spain.*
Amoxicillin trihydrate (p.155·3).
*Bacterial infections.*

**Salvapen Mucolitico** *Salvat, Spain.*
Amoxicillin trihydrate (p.155·3); bromhexine hydrochloride (p.1115·3).
*Respiratory-tract infections.*

**Salvara** *Bittner, Austria.*
Homoeopathic preparation.

**Salvarina** *Salvat, Spain.*
Caffeine (p.782·1); dimenhydrinate (p.431·1); ibuprofen (p.45·3).
*Dysmenorrhoea.*

**Salvatrim** *Salvat, Spain†.*
Co-trimoxazole (p.199·3).
*Bacterial infections; Pneumocystis carinii pneumonia.*

**Salvaxil** *Fada, Arg.*
Loperamide (p.1271·2).
*Diarrhoea.*

**Salvent** *Wolff, Ger.*
Salbutamol (p.791·3).
*Obstructive airways disease.*

**Salvesept** *Cederroth, Spain†.*
Alcohol (p.1166·1); chlorhexidine hydrochloride (p.1173·3).
*Wound disinfection.*

**salvi CAL E-G** *Baxter, Ger.†.*
Glucose and electrolyte infusion (p.1417·1).
*Parenteral nutrition.*

**salvi CAL GX** *Baxter, Ger.†.*
Glucose monohydrate (p.1432·2); xylitol (p.1469·1) (p.1417·1).
*Parenteral nutrition.*

**salviamin X-E** Baxter, Ger.†.
Amino-acid, xylitol, and electrolyte infusion (p.1417·1).
*Parenteral nutrition.*

**salviamin G-E** Baxter, Ger.
Amino-acid, glucose, and electrolyte infusion (p.1417·1).
*Parenteral nutrition.*

**salviamin GX-E** Baxter, Ger.†.
Amino-acid, glucose, xylitol, and electrolyte infusion (p.1417·1).
*Parenteral nutrition.*

**salviamin hepar** Baxter, Ger.
Amino-acid and electrolyte infusion (p.1417·1).
*Parenteral nutrition in liver disease.*

**Salviathymol N** Galenika, Ger.
Sage oil (p.1741·2); eucalyptus oil (p.1686·2); peppermint oil (p.1283·2); cinnamon oil (p.1672·2); clove oil (p.1673·3); fennel oil (p.1687·3); anise oil (p.1655·2); menthol (p.1711·3); thymol (p.1194·2).
*Mouth and throat disorders.*

**Salvibest** CT, Ger.†.
Rhatany root (p.1738·1).
*Mouth and gum disorders.*

**Salvicutan** Lazar, Arg.
Protoporphyrin; vitamin A palmitate (p.1453·1); dequalinium; cetrimonium bromide (p.1173·1).
*Burns; skin infections; skin irritation; ulcers; wounds.*

**Salviette H** Whitehall, Ital.
Hamamelis water (p.1696·3); glycerol (p.1694·3).
*Anal cleansing; haemorrhoids.*

**salvilipid** Baxter, Ger.
Soya oil (p.1447·2).
Contains egg lecithin.
*Lipid infusion for parenteral nutrition.*

**Salvit M** Belfar, Braz.†.
Vitamin and mineral preparation (p.1417·1).

**Salvital** Reckitt & Colman, Austral.†.
Magnesium sulfate (p.1228·2); sodium bicarbonate (p.1223·2); tartaric acid (p.1752·1).
*Dyspepsia; nausea.*

**Salvituss** FIRMA, Ital.
Levodropropizine (p.1119·3).
*Coughs.*

**Salvyl** Petrasch, Austria.
Undecenoic acid (p.410·3) sulfur (p.1158·2) complex; betanaphthol (p.103·2); salicylic acid (p.1157·1).
*Acne; erythrasma; fungal skin infections.*

**Salvysat**
Mayrhofer, Austria; Ysatfabrik, Ger.
Sage leaves (p.1741·2).
*Hyperhidrosis; mouth and throat inflammation.*

**Salycilina** Upsifarma, Port.
Aspirin (p.15·1).
*Fever; pain.*

**Salzone** Wallace Mfg Chem., UK.
Paracetamol (p.76·2).
*Fever; pain.*

**Samarin** Berlin Pharm, Thai.
Silymarin (p.1043·3).
*Liver disorders.*

**Sambil** Lacer, Spain†.
Boldine (p.1661·2); hydroxymethylnicotinamide (p.1700·1).
*Digestive-system disorders.*

**Sambuco (Specie Composta)** Dynacren, Ital.
Tilia (p.1756·2); sambucus (p.1741·3); spiraea (p.1710·1); rose fruit (p.1740·1).
*Cold symptoms.*

**Sambucol** Biopura, Port.†.
Sambucus (p.1741·3).
*Cold and influenza symptoms.*

**Sambucus Complex** Blackmores, Austral.†.
Sambucus (p.1741·3); euphrasia (p.1686·3); echinacea angustifolia (p.1683·2); hydrastis (p.1698·3); euphorbia hirta (p.1686·3); *d*-alpha tocoferil acid succinate (p.1465·1); vitamin A acetate (p.1453·1).
*Conjunctivitis; otorrhoea; upper respiratory-tract disorders.*

**Same Plast** Savoma, Ital.
Emollient.

**Samertan** Bago, Chile.
Telmisartan (p.1010·1).
*Hypertension.*

**Same-Seb** Savoma, Ital.
Colloidal sulfur (p.1158·2); salicylic acid (p.1157·1).
*Acne; seborrhoea.*

**Same-Seb Beta** Savoma, Ital.
Salicylic acid (p.1157·1); glycolic acid (p.1147·3).
*Acne.*

**Samilstin** LPB, Ital.
Octreotide (p.1333·3).
*Acromegaly; diarrhoea associated with immunodeficiency; endocrinal tumours of the gastrointestinal tract; pancreatic fistula; postoperative complications of pancreatic surgery; variceal haemorrhage.*

**Samonil** IQFA, Mex.
Metronidazole (p.607·2).
*Amoebiasis; giardiasis; trichomoniasis.*

**Samonter** Sanitas, Arg.
Mazindol (p.1589·1).
*Obesity.*

**Samox** Seven Stars, Thai.
Amoxicillin (p.155·3).
*Bacterial infections.*

**Samoxin** Sriprasit, Thai.
Amoxicillin (p.155·3).
*Bacterial infections.*

**Samyr**
Abbott, Ital.; Knoll, Mex.
Ademetionine sulfate tosilate (p.1647·2).
*Depression; liver disorders.*

**Sanabronchiol** Falqui, Ital.
Dextromethorphan hydrobromide (p.1117·3).
*Coughs.*

**Sanaco** PD, Thai.
Chlorophyll (p.1057·1); benzalkonium chloride (p.1168·3).
*Personal hygiene; vaginal douche.*

**Sanacol** Sydney Ross, Braz.†.
Aspirin (p.15·1); cinnamedrine hydrochloride (p.1672·2); caffeine (p.782·1).
*Smooth muscle spasm.*

**Sanacorte** Labortecne, Braz.†.
Schinus terebenthifolius; piptadenia columbriana; cereus hildfmanianus; salis angulata.
*Cicatrisation.*

**Sanaden Reforzado** Calmante Vitaminado, Spain†.
Creosote (p.1117·2); benzocaine (p.1370·3); niaouli oil (p.1719·3).
*Toothache.*

**Sanaderm**
Note. This name is used for preparations of different composition.
Febena, Ger.
Hamamelis (p.1696·3); zinc oxide (p.1163·2).
*Burns; skin disorders; wounds.*

Herbaline, Ital.†.
Echinacea (p.1683·2); calendula (p.1665·2); viola tricolor; helichrysum italicum; bergamot oil (p.1659·3); lavender oil (p.1705·2); thyme oil (p.1755·3); geranium oil (p.1692·2).
*Burns; skin irritation; wounds.*

**Sanadermil** Vifor, Switz.
Hydrocortisone acetate (p.1103·3).
*Skin disorders.*

**Sanadiar** Ibefar, Braz.†.
Phthalylsulfathiazole (p.242·3); sulfaguanidine (p.260·3); pectin (p.1580·3); aluminium hydroxide (p.1249·2).
*Diarrhoea.*

**Sanador** Virtus, Braz.†.
Methyl salicylate (p.59·3); turpentine oil (p.1760·1); camphor (p.1665·3); menthol (p.1711·3); chlorophyll (p.1057·1).
*Musculoskeletal and joint disorders.*

**Sanadorn** Jacoby, Austria.
Crataegus (p.1677·1).
*Heart disorders.*

**Sanafen** SmithKline Beecham, Braz.†.
Ibuprofen (p.45·3).

**Sanaform** Esoform, Ital.
Benzalkonium chloride (p.1168·3).
*Surface disinfection.*

**Sanagas** Ducto, Braz.
Dimethicone (p.1289·2).
*Flatulence.*

**Sanalepsi N** Roche, Switz.
Doxylamine succinate (p.432·3).
*Hypersensitivity reactions; nervous disorders.*

**Sanaler** Instituto Sanitas, Chile.
Cetirizine hydrochloride (p.427·1).
*Allergic conjunctivitis; allergic rhinitis; allergic skin disorders.*

**Sanaler-D** Instituto Sanitas, Chile.
Cetirizine (p.427·2); pseudoephedrine sulfate (p.1129·2).
*Allergic rhinitis.*

**Sanalgin** Interlogim, Neth.
Paracetamol (p.76·2); propyphenazone (p.85·3); caffeine (p.782·1).
*Fever; pain.*

**Sanalgin N** Gebro, Switz.
Paracetamol (p.76·2); caffeine (p.782·1).
Sanalgin formerly contained paracetamol, propyphenazone, and caffeine.
*Pain.*

**Sanamidol** Inkeysa, Spain.
Omeprazole (p.1278·2).
*Gastro-oesophageal reflux; peptic ulcer; Zollinger-Ellison syndrome.*

**Sanaprav**
Sankyo, Austria; Sankyo, Ital.; Sankyo, Port.
Pravastatin sodium (p.984·3).
*Atherosclerosis; hypercholesterolaemia.*

**Sana-Scrub** Forder, Arg.
Carica papaya; polyethylene granules.
*Skin cleansing.*

**Sanasepton** Ritsert, Ger.
Erythromycin (p.208·1) or erythromycin ethyl succinate (p.208·1).
*Bacterial infections.*

**Sana-Sol** Nycomed, Fin.
Multivitamin preparation (p.1417·1).

**Sanasthmax** Cascan, Ger.; GlaxoSmithKline, Ger.
Beclometasone dipropionate (p.1091·1).
*Asthma; bronchitis.*

**Sanasthmyl** Cascan, Ger.; GlaxoSmithKline, Ger.
Beclometasone dipropionate (p.1091·1).
*Asthma; bronchitis; tracheitis.*

**Sanatison Mono** Taurus, Ger.
Hydrocortisone (p.1103·3).
*Burns; skin disorders.*

**Sanatogen**
Key, Austral.†; Roche, Hong Kong†; German Remedies, India; Roche Consumer, Irl.; Roche, S.Afr.†; Roche Consumer, Singapore†; Roche Consumer, UK.
A range of vitamin, mineral, and nutritional preparations (p.1417·1).

**Sanato-Rhev** Hotz, Ger.†.
Camphor (p.1665·3); isopropyl alcohol (p.1184·3).
*Muscle and joint pain; soft-tissue disorders; superficial circulatory disorders.*

**Sanaven** Sankyo, Ger.
A heparinoid (p.931·1); phenylephrine hydrochloride (p.1126·3).
*Venous disorders.*

**Sanaven Venentabletten** Sankyo, Ger.†.
Aesculus (p.1648·2).
*Venous disorders.*

**Sanavir** Biologici Italia, Ital.
Aciclovir (p.626·1).
*Herpesvirus infections.*

**Sanavitan S** Bottger, Ger.
*dl*-Alpha tocoferil acetate (p.1465·1).
*Vitamin E deficiency.*

**Sanaxin** Tyrol, Austria.
Cefalexin (p.168·1).
*Bacterial infections.*

**Sanblex** Medipharm, Chile.
Sulpiride (p.722·2).
*Behaviour disorders; depression; irritability.*

**Sancago**
Chinta, Thai.†.
Indometacin (p.47·3); methocarbamol (p.1395·1).
*Gout; musculoskeletal and joint disorders.*

Chinta, Thai.
*Cream:* Methyl salicylate (p.59·3); menthol (p.1711·3); eugenol (p.1686·2).
*Insect bites; musculoskeletal, joint and soft-tissue disorders.*

**Sancap** Novartis, Gr.
Captopril (p.879·2).
*Heart failure; hypertension; myocardial infarction.*

**Sancipro** United Nordic, Denm.
Ciprofloxacin hydrochloride (p.188·2).
*Bacterial infections.*

**Sancor Biosalud** Sancor, Arg.
A range of preparations for enteral nutrition (p.1417·1).

**Sanctura** Indevus, USA; Odyssey, USA.
Trospium chloride (p.491·2).
*Bladder instability.*

**Sanderson's Throat Specific** Sandersons, UK.
*Mixture:* Acetic acid (p.1645·2); quassia (p.1737·2); squill (p.1130·3); capsicum (p.1667·1).
*Pastilles:* Honey (p.1434·2); squill vinegar (p.1130·3); capsicum (p.1667·1); tolu (p.1131·3); menthol (p.1711·3); cinnamic acid (p.1177·3); benzoic acid (p.1169·3); eucalyptus oil (p.1686·2).
*Catarrh; sore throat.*

**Sandimmun**
Novartis, Arg.; Novartis, Austral.; Novartis, Austria; Novartis, Belg.; Novartis, Braz.; Novartis, Chile; Novartis, Denm.; Novartis, Fin.; Novartis, Fr.; Novartis, Ger.; Novartis, Gr.; Novartis, Hong Kong; Novartis, Irl.; Novartis, Israel; Novartis, Ital.; Novartis, Malaysia; Novartis, Mex.; Novartis, Norw.; Novartis, NZ; Novartis, Port.; Novartis, S.Afr.; Novartis, Spain; Novartis, Swed.; Novartis, Switz.; Novartis, Thai.; Novartis, UK.
Ciclosporin (p.1351·2).
*Atopic dermatitis; graft-versus-host disease; nephrotic syndrome; psoriasis; rheumatoid arthritis; transplant rejection; uveitis.*

**Sandimmun Neoral**
Novartis, Gr.; Novartis, India; Novartis, Singapore†.
Ciclosporin (p.1351·2).
*Atopic dermatitis; graft-versus-host disease; nephrotic syndrome; psoriasis; rheumatoid arthritis; transplant rejection; uveitis.*

**Sandimmune**
Novartis, Canad.; Novartis, Neth.; Novartis, USA.
Ciclosporin (p.1351·2).
*Graft-versus-host disease; transplant rejection.*

**Sandival** Bouzen, Arg.
Paracetamol (p.76·2); pseudoephedrine hydrochloride (p.1129·2); chlorphenamine maleate (p.427·3).
*Influenza symptoms.*

**Sandival Desleible** Bouzen, Arg.
Benzydamine (p.21·1).
*Inflammation; pain.*

**Sandival NF** Bouzen, Arg.
Paracetamol (p.76·2); pseudoephedrine (p.1129·2).
*Influenza symptoms.*

**Sandocal**
Note. This name is used for preparations of different composition.
Novartis Consumer, Austral.†; Novartis, Fr.†; Novartis Consumer, Irl.; Novartis Consumer, Port.; Novartis Consumer, UK.
Calcium lactate gluconate (p.1225·3); calcium carbonate (p.1254·2).
*Calcium deficiencies; osteomalacia; osteoporosis; rickets.*

Novartis, India.
Calcium carbonate (p.1254·2).
*Calcium deficiency; calcium supplement.*

**Sandocal-D** Azupharma, Ger.
Calcium carbonate (p.1254·2); colecalciferol (p.1461·3).
*Calcium and vitamin D deficiency; osteoporosis.*

**Sandoglobulin**
CSL, Austral.; Novartis, Austria; Novartis, Fin.†; Novartis, Ger.; Novartis, Gr.; Novartis, Irl.†; Novartis, Israel; CSL, NZ; Novartis, Swed.†; ZLB, UK; Novartis, USA†.
A normal immunoglobulin (p.1627·2).
*Guillain-Barré syndrome; idiopathic thrombocytopenic purpura; immunodeficiency; Kawasaki disease; passive immunisation.*

**Sandoglobulina**
Novartis, Arg.; Novartis, Braz.; Novartis, Chile; Novartis, Ital.; Novartis, Mex.; Novartis, Port.
A normal immunoglobulin (p.1627·2).
*Guillain-Barré syndrome; hypogammaglobulinaemia; idiopathic thrombocytopenic purpura; Kawasaki disease; passive immunisation.*

**Sandoglobuline**
Novartis, Belg.; Novartis, Fr.†; Novartis, Switz.†.
A normal immunoglobulin (p.1627·2).
*Guillain-Barré syndrome; hypogammaglobulinaemia; idiopathic thrombocytopenic purpura; Kawasaki disease; passive immunisation.*

**Sando-K** HK Pharma, UK.
Potassium bicarbonate (p.1223·1); potassium chloride (p.1232·2).
*Hypokalaemia.*

**Sandolanid** Novartis, Austria†.
Acetyldigoxin (p.851·1).
*Arrhythmias.*

**Sandomigran**
Novartis, Arg.; Novartis, Austral.; Novartis, Austria†; Novartis, Belg.; Novartis, Braz.; Novartis, Canad.; Novartis, Ger.†; Novartis, Hong Kong; Novartis, Israel†; Novartis, Ital.; Novartis, Malaysia; Novartis, Neth.; Novartis, NZ; Novartis, S.Afr.; Novartis, Spain.
Pizotifen malate (p.470·3).
*Cluster headache; migraine; vasomotor headache.*

**Sandomigrin**
Novartis, Denm.; Novartis, Swed.
Pizotifen malate (p.470·3).
*Cluster headache; migraine.*

**Sandonorm**
Novartis, Austria; Novartis, Switz.
Bopindolol malonate (p.875·3).
*Angina pectoris; hypertension.*

**Sandoparin** Novartis, Austria.
Certoparin sodium (p.882·1).
*Thromboembolic disorders.*

**Sandoparine** Novartis, Switz.
Certoparin sodium (p.882·1).
*Thrombosis prophylaxis.*

**Sandopart** Sandoz, Ital.†.
Demoxytocin (p.1322·3).
*Induction of labour; post-partum uterine involution; prevention of breast engorgement and mastitis; stimulation of lactation.*

**Sandoretic** Novartis, Switz.
Bopindolol malonate (p.875·3); chlortalidone (p.882·3).
*Hypertension.*

**Sandosource**
Novartis Consumer, Austral.; Novartis, Braz.; Novartis, Irl.; Novartis Consumer, Ital.†; Novartis, UK.
Preparation for enteral nutrition (p.1417·1).

**Sandosource Peptide**
Novartis, Arg.; Novartis Nutrition, Canad.†.
Preparation for enteral nutrition (p.1417·1).

**Sandostatin**
Novartis, Arg.; Novartis, Austral.; Novartis, Austria; Novartis, Braz.; Novartis, Canad.; Novartis, Chile; Novartis, Denm.; Novartis, Fin.; Novartis, Ger.; Novartis, Gr.; Novartis, Hong Kong; Novartis, India; Novartis, Irl.; Novartis, Israel; Novartis, Malaysia; Novartis, Norw.; Novartis, NZ; Novartis, S.Afr.; Novartis, Singapore; Novartis, Spain; Novartis, Swed.; Novartis, Thai.; Novartis, UK; Novartis, USA.
Octreotide (p.1333·3) or octreotide acetate (p.1333·1).
*Acromegaly; AIDS-associated refractory diarrhoea; gastrointestinal endocrine tumours; prevention of complications following pancreatic surgery; variceal haemorrhage.*

**Sandostatina**
Novartis, Ital.; Novartis, Mex.; Novartis, Port.
Octreotide (p.1333·3).
*Acromegaly; AIDS-associated refractory diarrhoea; gastrointestinal endocrine tumours; pancreatic and gastrointestinal fistulas; prevention of complications following pancreatic surgery; variceal haemorrhage.*

**Sandostatine**
Novartis, Belg.; Novartis, Fr.; Novartis, Neth.; Novartis, Switz.
Octreotide (p.1333·3) or octreotide acetate (p.1333·1).
*Acromegaly; AIDS-associated refractory diarrhoea; gastrointestinal endocrine tumours; prevention of complications following pancreatic surgery; variceal haemorrhage.*

**Sandovac** Novartis, Austria.
An inactivated influenza vaccine (p.1620·2).
*Active immunisation.*

**Sandoven** Novartis, Austria†.
Dihydroergocristine mesilate (p.1680·1); esculoside (p.1648·2); rutoside (p.1688·2).
*Thrombophlebotic disorders; venous insufficiency.*

**Sandoz Ca-D** Novartis Consumer, Belg.
Calcium carbonate (p.1254·2); colecalciferol (p.1461·3).
*Osteoporosis.*

**Sandoz Calcium** Novartis Consumer, Belg.
*Effervescent tablets; oral powder:* Calcium lactate gluconate (p.1225·3); calcium carbonate (p.1254·2).
Formerly known as Calcium-Sandoz.
*Bone demineralisation; calcium supplement; osteoporosis; tetany.*
*Injection:* Calcium glubionate (p.1225·1).

Formerly known as Calcium-Sandoz.
*Hypocalcaemia; potassium poisoning; rickets; tetany.*

**Sandoz Calcium + Vitamine C** Novartis Consumer, Belg.
Ascorbic acid (p.1460·2); calcium carbonate (p.1254·2); calcium lactate gluconate (p.1225·3).
Formerly known as Ca-C.
*Calcium and vitamin C deficiency.*

**Sandoz Calcium-C** Novartis Consumer, S.Afr.
Calcium lactate gluconate (p.1225·3); calcium carbonate (p.1254·2); vitamin C (p.1460·2).
*Vitamin C and calcium supplement.*

**Sandrena**
Organon, Austral.; Organon, Austria; Organon, Braz.; Organon, Chile; Organon, Denm.; Organon, Ger.; Organon, Ital.; Organon, Mex.; Organon, Neth.; Organon, NZ; Organon, Switz.; Organon, UK.
Estradiol (p.1550·1).
*Menopausal disorders; osteoporosis.*

**Sanein** Almirall, Spain.
Aceclofenac (p.11·2).
*Musculoskeletal, joint, and peri-articular disorders; pain.*

**Sanelor**
Note. This name is used for preparations of different composition.
Chefaro, Belg.
Loratadine (p.436·1).
*Allergic rhinitis; urticaria.*

Instituto Sanitas, Chile.
Lovastatin (p.949·1).
*Hypercholesterolaemia.*

**Sanepa Forte** Maver, Chile.
Omega-3 marine triglycerides (p.976·2).

**Sanerva** Royal, Chile.
Alprazolam (p.668·3).
*Anxiety; panic attacks.*

**Sangcya**
Lilly, Israel; Sangstat, UK†.
Ciclosporin (p.1351·2).
*Atopic dermatitis; graft-versus-host disease; nephrotic syndrome; psoriasis; rheumatoid arthritis; transplant rejection; uveitis.*

**Sangen** Marco Viti, Ital.
Benzalkonium chloride (p.1168·3).
*Disinfection of wounds and burns.*

**Sangen Casa** Marco Viti, Ital.
*Liquid:* Benzethonium chloride (p.1169·2); benzalkonium chloride (p.1168·3).
*Spray:* Orthophenylphenol (p.1187·2); benzalkonium chloride (p.1168·3).
*Surface disinfection.*

**Sangen Sapone Disinfettante** Marco Viti, Ital.
Triclocarban (p.1195·1).
*Skin disinfection.*

**Sangenor** Mundipharma, Austria.
Arginine aspartate (p.1421·1).
*Tonic.*

**Sangerol** Novartis Consumer, Switz.
Lidocaine hydrochloride (p.1377·3); muramidase hydrochloride (p.1717·2); tyrothricin (p.275·1).
*Mouth and throat disorders.*

**Sangobion**
Merck, Malaysia; Merck, Singapore; Merck, Thai.†.
Ferrous gluconate (p.1428·1); folic acid (p.1429·1); vitamin $B_{12}$ (p.1458·2); minerals (p.1417·1).
Vitamin C (p.1460·2) is included in this preparation to increase the absorption and availability of iron.
*Anaemias.*

**Sangotone** Gemballa, Braz.
Ferrous citrate (p.1436·1); choline citrate; copper gluconate; vitamin B substances (p.1417·1).
*Iron deficiency; iron-deficiency anaemias.*

**Sanguisan N** Coradol, Ger.
Homoeopathic preparation.

**Sanguisorbis N** Sabona, Ger.
Homoeopathic preparation.

**Sangur-Test** Roche Diagnostics, Austral.
Test for blood in urine.

**Sanhelios 333** Pharmacia Upjohn, Switz.†.
Garlic (p.1691·1).
*Atherosclerosis.*

**Sanhelios Capsules a la vitamine A** Ars Vitae, Switz.
Vitamin A palmitate (p.1453·1); wheat-germ oil.
*Vitamin A deficiency.*

**Sanhelios Einschlaf** Bregenzer, Austria.
Valerian root (p.1762·2); lupulus (p.1708·1).
*Sleep disorders.*

**Sanhelios Leber-Galle** Bregenzer, Austria.
Silybum marianum (p.1043·3); turmeric (p.1058·3).
*Digestive disorders; hepatobiliary disorders.*

**Sanhelios Venen** Pharmacia Upjohn, Switz.†.
Aesculus (p.1648·2).
*Venous insufficiency.*

**Sanhelios-Entwasserungsdragees** Bregenzer, Austria.
Birch leaf (p.1660·3).
*Urinary-tract disorders.*

**Sanicel** Squibb, Spain.
Amphotericin B (p.391·2); tetracycline hydrochloride (p.266·2).
*Vulvovaginal infections.*

**Sanicolax** Sanico, Belg.†.
Phenolphthalein (p.1284·1); podophyllum (p.1155·2); aloin (p.1248·3); belladonna (p.479·1); hyoscyamus (p.485·2); nux vomica (p.1722·3).
*Constipation.*

**Sanicopyrine** Sanico, Belg.†.
Paracetamol (p.76·2).
*Fever; pain.*

**SaniDrox** Sanitas, Ital.
Peracetic acid (p.1187·3).
*Instrument disinfection.*

**Sanieb** Puerto Galiano, Spain.
Glycine (p.1433·3); arginine (p.1421·1); brassica oleracea.
*Gastritis; gastrointestinal hyperacidity; peptic ulcer.*

**Sanifer** Esseti, Ital.
Sodium ferric gluconate complex (p.1444·3).
*Anaemias; oligohaemia in infants.*

**Saniflor Collutorio** Esseti, Ital.
Benzydamine hydrochloride (p.21·1).
*Gingivitis.*

**Saniflor Vena** Esseti, Ital.†.
Benzydamine hydrochloride (p.21·1).
*Peripheral vascular disorders.*

**Sanifolin** Fargim, Ital.
Calcium folinate (p.1431·1).
*Anaemias; antidote to folic acid antagonists; folate deficiency; reduction of aminopterin and methotrexate toxicity.*

**Sanifug** Wolff, Ger.†.
Loperamide hydrochloride (p.1271·1).
*Diarrhoea.*

**Sanigermin** Instituto Sanitas, Chile.
Triclosan (p.1195·2).
*Hand disinfection; skin infections.*

**Sanil Menta Bucal** Hertz, Braz.†.
Menthol (p.1711·3); cetylpyridinium chloride (p.1173·1).
*Oral hygiene.*

**Sanilin** Hertz, Braz.†.
Benzocaine (p.1370·3); cetylpyridinium chloride (p.1173·1); menthol (p.1711·3).

**Sanipresin** Instituto Sanitas, Chile.
Losartan potassium (p.947·2).
*Hypertension.*

**Sanipresin-D** Instituto Sanitas, Chile.
Losartan potassium (p.947·2); hydrochlorothiazide (p.933·2).
*Hypertension.*

**Saniprostol** Instituto Sanitas, Chile.
Finasteride (p.1554·2).
*Benign prostatic hyperplasia.*

**Saniquiet** Sanitalia, Ital.
Passion flower; tilia; birch; magnesium; lithium; manganese (p.1417·1).

**SaniSteril Deterferri** Sanitas, Ital.
Benzalkonium chloride (p.1168·3).
*Instrument disinfection.*

**SaniSteril Sterilferri** Sanitas, Ital.
Glutaral (p.1180·3).
*Instrument disinfection.*

**SaniSteril Strumenti Alcolico** Sanitas, Ital.
Benzalkonium chloride (p.1168·3); isopropyl alcohol (p.1184·3).
*Instrument disinfection.*

**Sani-Supp** G & W, USA.
Glycerol (p.1694·3).
*Constipation.*

**Saniter Compuesto** Instituto Sanitas, Chile.
Levodopa (p.1205·2); carbidopa (p.1204·3).
*Parkinsonism.*

**Sanitos** DB, Fr.
Salicylic acid (p.1157·1).
*Calluses; corns; warts.*

**Sanivit** Scherer, Thai.
Multivitamin and mineral preparation with procaine hydrochloride, royal jelly, and lecithin (p.1417·1).

**Sanjin Royal Jelly** Super Mayoreo Naturista, Mex.
Ginseng (p.1693·1).
*Tonic.*

**Sankombi** Sanum-Kehlbeck, Ger.
Homoeopathic preparation.

**Sanmigran** Novartis, Fr.
Pizotifen malate (p.470·3).
*Migraine.*

**Sano Tuss** Welti, Switz.
Emetine hydrochloride (p.604·3); ethylmorphine hydrochloride (p.37·3); ephedrine hydrochloride (p.1120·1); codeine phosphate (p.27·1); guaifenesin (p.1122·1); cherry-laurel; tolu balsam (p.1131·3).
*Catarrh; coughs.*

**Sanobamat** Sanico, Belg.†.
Meprobamate (p.706·2).
*Anxiety disorders; sleep disorders.*

**Sanoclorofila** Veafarm, Braz.†.
Iodine (p.1598·1); salicylic acid (p.1157·1); menthol (p.1711·3); chlorophyll (p.1057·1).
*Fungal skin infections.*

**Sanoderm** Reccius, Chile.
Allantoin (p.1141·3); zinc oxide (p.1163·2); vitamin A (p.1451·2); vitamin D (p.1461·2).
*Skin disorders.*

**Sanodin** Altana, Spain.
Carbenoxolone sodium (p.1254·3).
*Gingivitis; mouth ulcers.*

**Sanoformine** Mayoly-Spindler, Fr.†.
Anhydrous copper sulfate (p.1426·1); sodium fluoride (p.1444·3).
*Disinfection of mucous membranes.*

**Sanogyl** Tonipharm, Fr.
*Pink toothpaste:* Sodium monofluorophosphate (p.1446·2); sodium fluoride (p.1444·3).
*White toothpaste:* Sodium fluoride (p.1444·3).
*Oral hygiene.*

**Sanogyl Bianco** Berna, Ital.†.
Sodium monofluorophosphate (p.1446·2); acetarsol sodium (p.600·2).
*Gingivitis; oral hygiene.*

**Sanogyl Fluo** Tonipharm, Fr.
Sodium monofluorophosphate (p.1446·2); sodium fluoride (p.1444·3).
*Dental caries prophylaxis.*

**Sanogyl Junior** Tonipharm, Fr.
Sodium monofluorophosphate (p.1446·2); sodium fluoride (p.1444·3).
*Dental caries prophylaxis.*

**Sanoma** Heilit, Ger.†.
Carisoprodol (p.1392·1).
*Skeletal muscle spasm.*

**Sanomigran**
Novartis, Irl.; Novartis, UK.
Pizotifen malate (p.470·3).
*Migraine and other vascular headaches.*

**Sanopinwern** Wernigerode, Ger.
*Inhalation:* Eucalyptus oil (p.1686·2); oleum pini sylvestris.
*Cold symptoms.*
*Oral drops:* Thyme (p.1755·2).
*Bronchitis; catarrh; coughs.*

**Sanopinwern T** Wernigerode, Ger.
Tetryzoline hydrochloride (p.1131·2).
*Nasal congestion.*

**Sanor**
Biolab, Malaysia; Biolab, Thai.
Dipotassium clorazepate (p.685·1).
*Anxiety.*

**Sanoral**
Note. This name is used for preparations of different composition.
Novartis, Austria.
Tyrothricin (p.275·1); muramidase hydrochloride (p.1717·2); lidocaine hydrochloride (p.1377·3).
*Mouth and throat inflammation.*

Bioprogress, Ital.†.
Chlorhexidine gluconate (p.1173·2).
*Mouth disinfection.*

**Sanorex**
Novartis, Canad.; Novartis, Mex.; Novartis, USA†.
Mazindol (p.1589·1).
*Obesity.*

**Sanorvil** Pharmaten (Φαρματεν), Gr.
Betamethasone valerate (p.1093·2).
*Topical corticosteroid.*

**Sanostol** Schmidgall, Austria.
Multivitamin preparation (p.1417·1).

**Sanovit** Byk Gulden, Mex.
Cobamamide (p.1459·1).

**Sanoxit** Galderma, Ger.
Benzoyl peroxide (p.1143·2).
*Acne.*

**Sanoyodo** Cinfa, Spain.
Povidone-iodine (p.1190·3).
*Skin and wound disinfection.*

**Sanpronol** Sanval, Braz.
Propranolol hydrochloride (p.989·3).
*Angina pectoris; arrhythmias; hypertension.*

**Sans Soleil Skin Ceuticals** Dispolab, Chile.
Dihydroxyacetone (p.1145·2).
*Suntanning agent.*

**Sans-Acne** Galderma, Canad.
Erythromycin (p.208·1); alcohol (p.1166·1).
*Acne.*

**Sansacne** Galderma, Mex.
Erythromycin (p.208·1).
*Acne.*

**Sansanal** Rottapharm, Ger.†.
Captopril (p.879·2).
*Heart failure; hypertension.*

**Sansert**
Novartis, Canad.; Novartis, USA†.
Methysergide maleate (p.469·3).
*Vascular headache.*

**Sansudor** Boehringer Ingelheim, Switz.
Aluminium chlorohydrex (p.1142·1).
*Hyperhidrosis; intertrigo.*

**Santa Flora S** Madaus, Ger.
Homoeopathic preparation.

**Santaherba**
Homeocan, Canad.; Lehning, Fr.
Homoeopathic preparation.

**Santalyt** Asche, Ger.
Sodium chloride; glucose; potassium chloride; sodium bicarbonate (p.1222·2).
*Diarrhoea; oral rehydration therapy.*

**Santamex-Expectorant** Santa, Gr.
Carbocisteine (p.1116·2).
*Respiratory disorders associated with viscous mucus.*

**Santane $A_4$** Iphym, Fr.†.
Meadowsweet flowers (p.1710·1); black currant leaf (p.1661·1); salix leaf (p.87·3); heather flowers; orange leaf (p.1723·3); juniper berry (p.1703·1); chamomile flowers (p.1669·3); matricaria flowers; vervain leaf (p.1764·1).
*Musculoskeletal disorders.*

**Santane $C_6$** Iphym, Fr.†.
Frangula bark (p.1266·3); senna leaf (p.1288·2); boldo leaf (p.1661·2); vervain leaf (p.1764·1); peppermint leaf (p.1283·2); mallow flowers (p.1709·3); centaurea cyanus flowers; pale rose flowers; caraway seed (p.1667·2).
*Constipation.*

**Santane $D_5$** Iphym, Fr.†.
Melissa leaf (p.1711·1); origanum flowers; peppermint leaf (p.1283·2); fennel seed (p.1687·2); aniseed (p.1655·2); lupulus flowers (p.1708·1); matricaria flowers (p.1669·3); thyme flowers (p.1755·2); rosemary leaf (p.1740·2); caraway seed (p.1667·2); cinnamon bark (p.1672·2).
*Gastrointestinal disorders.*

**Santane $F_{10}$** Iphym, Fr.†.
Boldo leaf (p.1661·2); box leaf; peppermint leaf (p.1283·2); tetragonum leaf; calendula flower (p.1665·2); rosemary leaf (p.1740·2); chamomile flower (p.1669·3); caraway seed (p.1667·2); cinnamon bark (p.1672·2).
*Hepato-biliary insufficiency.*

**Santane $H_7$** Iphym, Fr.†.
Mistletoe leaf (p.1715·3); olive leaf; crataegus flower and leaf (p.1677·1); melilot flower; calendula flower (p.1665·2); myrtillus berry (p.1718·3); peppermint leaf (p.1283·2); vervain leaf (p.1764·1); broom flower (p.1742·2); fennel seed (p.1687·2); sweet orange peel (p.1724·1).
*Hypertension.*

**Santane $N_9$** Iphym, Fr.†.
Tilia flowers (p.1756·2); crataegus flowers and leaves (p.1677·1); pale rose flowers; peppermint leaf (p.1283·2); melissa leaf (p.1711·1); bitter-orange leaves and buds (p.1723·3); origanum flowers; lupulus flowers (p.1708·1); lavender flowers (p.1705·1).
*Nervous disorders.*

**Santane $O_1$** Iphym, Fr.†.
Heather flowers; bearberry leaf (p.1659·2); peppermint leaf (p.1283·2); pulegium (p.1736·1); meadowsweet flowers (p.1710·1); rosemary leaf (p.1740·2); mallow flowers (p.1709·3); tilia flowers (p.1756·2); eucalyptus leaf (p.1686·1); laurel leaf; caraway seed (p.1667·2); bitter orange leaves (p.1723·3).
*Nutritional disorders.*

**Santane $R_8$** Iphym, Fr.†.
Bearberry leaf (p.1659·2); heather flowers; black currant leaf (p.1661·1); rosemary leaf (p.1740·2); peppermint leaf (p.1283·2); broom flowers (p.1742·2); lavender flowers (p.1705·1); juniper berry (p.1703·1); thyme flowers (p.1755·2); meadowsweet flowers (p.1710·1); cinnamon bark (p.1672·2).
*Kidney disorders.*

**Santane $V_3$** Iphym, Fr.†.
Artemisia leaf; peppermint leaf (p.1283·2); sage leaf (p.1741·2); crataegus flowers and leaf (p.1677·1); broom flowers (p.1742·2); green tea flowers (p.1765·3); cupressus sempervirens leaf; melilotus officinalis flower and leaf; sweet orange peel (p.1724·1); bitter orange leaf (p.1723·3).
*Vascular disorders.*

**Santasal N** Merckle, Ger.
Aspirin (p.15·1).
*Fever; pain.*

**Santasapina V** Bioforce, Ger.
Pine needle.
*Catarrh.*

**Santasapina Nouvelle formule** Bioforce, Switz.
Pine buds.
*Upper respiratory-tract disorders.*

**Santax S** Asche, Ger.
*Saccharomyces boulardii* (p.1704·2).
*Diarrhoea.*

**Santenol** Coop. Farm., Ital.†.
Lefetamine hydrochloride (p.53·1).
Lidocaine hydrochloride (p.1377·3) is included in this preparation to alleviate the pain of injection.
*Pain.*

**Santevini** Novartis, India.
Vitamin B substances; peptone; calcium gluconate (p.1417·1).
*Tonic.*

**Santin** ISA, Arg.
Magnesium; vitamin C; vitamin $B_6$; passion flower; tilia (p.1417·1).
*Dietary supplement.*

**Santus** Bittner, Austria.
Homoeopathic preparation.

**Santussal** Novartis, Braz.
Pimethixene (p.439·1); proxyphylline (p.791·2); ammonium chloride (p.1115·2).
*Coughs.*

**Santyl**
Smith & Nephew, Canad.; Knoll, USA.
Collagenase (p.1675·1).
*Debridement of dermal ulcers and severe burns.*

**Sanukehl** Sanum-Kehlbeck, Ger.
Homoeopathic preparation.

**Sanutri Osseo** Novartis Nutrition, Port.†.
Calcium-enriched nutritional supplement (p.1417·1).
*Osteoporosis.*

**Sanuvis** Sanum-Kehlbeck, Ger.
Homoeopathic preparation.

**Sanvapress** Sanval, Braz.
Enalapril maleate (p.909·2).
*Hypertension.*

**Sanvita Bronchial** Sanomed, Austria.
Eucalyptus oil (p.1686·2); peppermint oil (p.1283·2); thyme oil (p.1755·3).
*Catarrh; coughs.*

**Sanvita Enerlecit** *Sanamed, Austria.*
Lecithin; vitamins (p.1417·1).
*Tonic.*

**Sanvita Leber-Galle** *Sanamed, Austria.*
Cynara (p.1678·3); turmeric (p.1058·3); taraxacum (p.1751·3).
*Hepatobiliary disorders.*

**Sanvita Magen** *Sanamed, Austria.*
Ginger (p.1267·1); caraway oil (p.1667·3); gentian root (p.1692·2).
*Dyspepsia; motion sickness; nausea; vomiting.*

**Sanxon** *Mayo, Mex.†.*
A multivitamin preparation (p.1417·1).

**Sanyrene** *Urgo, Fr.*
Barrier preparation.

**Sanytol** *Ideal, Fr.*
Permethrin (p.1508·3); phenothrin (p.1509·1); benzyl benzoate (p.1500·2); didecyldimethylammonium chloride (p.1178·3); triclosan (p.1195·2).
*House dust mite acaricide.*

**Sanzur** *Garec, S.Afr.*
Fluoxetine hydrochloride (p.292·1).
*Bulimia nervosa; depression; obsessive-compulsive disorder.*

**Sanzyme-DS** *Uni-Sankyo, India.*
Amylase (p.1654·2); aluminium hydroxide (p.1249·2); magnesium hydroxide (p.1272·2); sodium bicarbonate (p.1223·2); simeticone (p.1289·2).
*Dyspepsia; flatulence.*

**Sanzyme-S** *Sankyo, Thai.*
Cellulase (p.1669·1); lipase; pancreatin (p.1725·3); sanzyme-N.
*Digestive disorders.*

**Sapec** *Riemser, Ger.*
Garlic (p.1691·1).
*Hyperlipidaemias.*

**Sapoderm**
*Note. This name is used for preparations of different composition.*
*Reckitt Benckiser, Austral.*
Triclosan (p.1195·2).
*Skin cleansing.*

*Ingram & Bell, Canad.†.*
Hexachlorophene (p.1181·2).
*Antisepsis.*

**Sapresta** *Taiho, Jpn.*
Aranidipine (p.864·2).
*Hypertension.*

**Sapriken** *Kener, Mex.*
Cisapride (p.1259·2).

**Sapucai** *Geminis, Arg.*
*Cream:* Permethrin (p.1508·3).
*Pediculosis.*
*Shampoo:* Benzyl benzoate (p.1500·2); benzocaine (p.1370·3); permethrin (p.1508·3).
*Pediculosis; scabies.*

**Saquat** *Ramini, Ital.*
Benzalkonium chloride (p.1168·3).
*Disinfection of wounds and burns.*

**Sara** *Nakorn, Thai.*
Paracetamol (p.76·2).
*Fever; pain.*

**Sarafem** *Warner Chilcott, USA.*
Fluoxetine hydrochloride (p.292·1).
*Premenstrual dysphoric disorder.*

**Sarapin** *High Chemical, USA.*
Sarracenia purpurea distillate (p.88·2).
*Neuromuscular or neuralgic pain.*

**Saratoga** *Blair, USA.*
Zinc oxide (p.1163·2); boric acid (p.1662·1); cineole (p.1672·1); peru balsam (p.1730·2).
*Minor skin irritation.*

**Sarcoderma** *Confar, Port.*
Lindane (p.1506·3).
*Pediculosis; scabies.*

**Sarcop** *Unipharma, Spain.*
Permethrin (p.1508·3).
*Scabies.*

**Sarcoton** *Medley, Braz.*
Disulfiram (p.1681·3).
Formerly contained disulfiram and metronidazole.
*Alcoholism.*

**Sarf** *Julphar, UAE.*
Ciprofloxacin hydrochloride (p.188·2).
*Bacterial infections.*

**Sargenor**
*Sarget, Fr.; Asta Medica, Ital.; Viatris, Port.; Viatris, Spain.*
Arginine aspartate (p.1421·1).
*Tonic.*

**Sargenor a la Vitamine C** *Viatris, Fr.*
Arginine aspartate (p.1421·1); vitamin C (p.1460·2).
*Tonic.*

**Sargepirine** *Asta Medica, Fr.†.*
Aspirin (p.15·1).
Glycine (p.1433·3) is included in this preparation in an attempt to limit adverse effects on the gastrointestinal mucosa.
*Fever; pain.*

**Saridine** *Atlantic, Thai.*
Sulfasalazine (p.1291·1).
*Ulcerative colitis.*

**Saridon**
*Note. This name is used for preparations of different composition.*
*Roche, Arg.; Roche, Austria; Roche, Belg.; Roche, Braz.; Roche Nicholas, Ger.; Roche, Hong Kong; Roche, Ital.; Roche Consumer, Neth.; Roche, Spain; Roche, Switz.*
Paracetamol (p.76·2); propyphenazone (p.85·3); caffeine (p.782·1).
*Fever; pain.*

*Roche, Chile; Roche, Mex.†.*
Paracetamol (p.76·2); caffeine (p.782·1).
*Fever; pain.*

*Roche, Thai.†.*
Paracetamol (p.76·2).
*Fever; pain.*

**Saridon N** *Roche, Port.*
Paracetamol (p.76·2); propyphenazone (p.85·3); caffeine (p.782·1).
*Pain.*

**Sarilen** *Normon, Spain†.*
Roxatidine acetate (p.1288·1).
*Gastro-oesophageal reflux; peptic ulcer.*

**Sarna**
*Stiefel, Austral.; Stiefel, Malaysia; Stiefel, Singapore; Stiefel, Thai.*
Camphor (p.1665·3); menthol (p.1711·3); phenol (p.1188·1).
*Dry skin; pruritus.*

**Sarna Anti-Itch** *Stiefel, USA.*
Camphor (p.1665·3); menthol (p.1711·3).
*Poison ivy; poison oak; pruritus; sunburn.*

**Sarna HC** *Stiefel, Canad.*
Hydrocortisone (p.1103·3).
*Skin disorders.*

**Sarna-P** *Stiefel, Canad.*
Pramocaine hydrochloride (p.1382·2); camphor (p.1665·3); menthol (p.1711·3).
*Skin irritation.*

**Sarnapen** *Dovalle, Braz.*
Bioallethrin (p.1500·3); piperonyl butoxide (p.1509·2).
*Pediculosis; scabies.*

**Sarnaton** *Royton, Braz.*
Benzyl benzoate (p.1500·2).
*Scabies.*

**Sarnigal** *QIF, Braz.†.*
Benzyl benzoate (p.1500·2).
*Pediculosis; scabies.*

**Sarnisan** *Eurofarma, Braz.†.*
Benzyl benzoate (p.1500·2).
*Pediculosis; scabies.*

**Sarnodex** *Bunker, Braz.*
Benzyl benzoate (p.1500·2).
*Pediculosis; scabies.*

**Sarnol** *Stiefel, Fr.*
Camphor (p.1665·3); menthol (p.1711·3).
*Skin disorders.*

**Sarolin** *Sobral, Braz.†.*
Salbutamol (p.791·3).
*Obstructive airways disease.*

**Saromet** *Pharmacia, Arg.*
Diazepam (p.690·1).
*Alcohol withdrawal syndrome; anxiety; convulsions; skeletal muscle spasm.*

**Saroten**
*Lundbeck, Austria; Lundbeck, Denm.; Lundbeck, Fin.; Bayer, Ger.; Lundbeck, Gr.; Lundbeck, S.Afr.†; Lundbeck, Swed.; Lundbeck, Switz.*
Amitriptyline hydrochloride (p.280·3).
*Depression; insomnia; nocturnal enuresis; pain.*

**Sarotena** *Lundbeck, India.*
Amitriptyline hydrochloride (p.280·3).
*Depression; nocturnal enuresis.*

**Sarotex**
*Lundbeck, Neth.; Lundbeck, Norw.*
Amitriptyline hydrochloride (p.280·3).
*Depression; nocturnal enuresis; pain.*

**Sarpiol** *INQ, Braz.†.*
Lindane (p.1506·3).
*Pediculosis; scabies.*

**Sarpul** *Toyama, Jpn.*
Aniracetam (p.1655·1).
*Cerebral infarction.*

**Sarsaparol Uro** *Sabona, Ger.*
Homoeopathic preparation.

**Sarsapsor** *Ysatfabrik, Ger.*
Homoeopathic preparation.

**Sartol** *Stiefel, Spain.*
Menthol (p.1711·3); camphor (p.1665·3).
*Insect bites; pruritus; urticaria.*

**Sartuzin** *Help, Gr.*
Fluoxetine hydrochloride (p.292·1).
*Depression; obsessive-compulsive disorder; panic disorder.*

**SAS** *ICN, Canad.*
Sulfasalazine (p.1291·1).
*Ulcerative colitis.*

**Saspryl** *Inibsa, Spain.*
Aspirin (p.15·1).
*Fever; musculoskeletal, joint and peri-articular disorders; pain; thromboembolism prophylaxis.*

**Sastid**
*Note. This name is used for preparations of different composition.*
*Stiefel, Arg.; Stiefel, Braz.; Stiefel, Canad.†; Stiefel, Hong Kong; Stiefel, Malaysia; Stiefel, Mex.; Stiefel, S.Afr.; Stiefel, Singapore; Stiefel, Spain; Stiefel, Thai.*
Precipitated sulfur (p.1158·2); salicylic acid (p.1157·1).
*Acne; pityriasis versicolor; seborrhoea.*

*Stiefel, USA.*
Precipitated sulfur (p.1158·2).
Formerly contained precipitated sulfur and salicylic acid.

**Sastid Anti-Fungal** *Stiefel, Singapore.*
Clotrimazole (p.396·2).
*Fungal skin and vaginal infections.*

**Sastid Jabon** *Stiefel, Chile.*
Salicylic acid (p.1157·1); sulfur (p.1158·2).
*Acne; pityriasis versicolor; seborrhoea.*

**Sasulen** *Faes, Spain.*
Piroxicam (p.84·2).
*Gout; musculoskeletal, joint, peri-articular, and soft-tissue disorders; pain.*

**Satedon** *Protein, Mex.†.*
Azathioprine (p.1349·1).

**Satigene** *Microsules, Arg.*
Irinotecan (p.564·3).
*Malignant neoplasms.*

**Satinique Anti-Dandruff** *Amway, Canad.*
Pyrithione zinc (p.1156·2).

**Sativol** *Boiron, Canad.†.*
Homoeopathic preparation.

**Saton** *Saval, Chile.*
Sibutramine (p.1593·2).
*Obesity.*

**Saturnil** *Adelco, Gr.*
Alprazolam (p.668·3).
*Anxiety disorders; mixed anxiety-depressive states.*

**Saugella** *Rottapharm, Fr.*
Thyme (p.1755·2); sage (p.1741·2); milk serum; lactic acid (p.1704·1).
*Skin cleansing.*

**Saugella Gel** *Rottapharm, Ital.*
Vaginal lubricant.

**Saugella Idrocrema** *Rottapharm, Ital.*
Vaginal lubricant.

**Saugella Intilac** *Rottapharm, Ital.*
Lactic acid (p.1704·1).
*Maintenance of vaginal pH.*

**Saugella Salviettine** *Rottapharm, Ital.*
Sage (p.1741·2); lactic acid (p.1704·1).
*Personal hygiene.*

**Saugella Uomo** *Rottapharm, Ital.*
Helichrysum italicum; clove (p.1673·2).
*Male personal hygiene.*

**Sauran** *Abello, Spain†.*
Citicoline (p.1672·3) or citicoline sodium (p.1672·3).
*Cerebrovascular disorders.*

**Saurat** *Armstrong, Arg.*
Fluoxetine hydrochloride (p.292·1).
*Depression.*

**Savacol Mouth and Throat Rinse** *Colgate Oral Care, Austral.†.*
Chlorhexidine gluconate (p.1173·2).
*Minor oral infections; mouth ulcers.*

**Savarine** *AstraZeneca, Fr.*
Proguanil hydrochloride (p.457·1); chloroquine phosphate (p.448·2).
*Malaria.*

**Savecal** *Ibirn, Ital.*
Calcium carbonate (p.1254·2).
*Calcium deficiency; calcium supplement.*

**Saventrine**
*IFET (ΙΦΕΤ), Gr.; Pharmax, Hong Kong†; Pharmax, Irl.; Pharmax, Singapore; Forest Laboratories, UK†.*
Isoprenaline hydrochloride (p.940·2).
*Bradycardia; cardiogenic or endotoxic shock; evaluation of congenital heart defects; heart block; Stokes-Adams attacks.*

**Savex** *Sabex, Canad.*
Camphor (p.1665·3); menthol (p.1711·3).

**Savex 15** *Sabex, Canad.*
*SPF 15:* Octinoxate (p.1154·3); oxybenzone (p.1154·3); camphor (p.1665·3).
*Sunscreen.*

**Savex with PABA** *Sabex, Canad.*
Padimate O (p.1155·1); camphor (p.1665·3); menthol (p.1711·3); salicylic acid (p.1157·1).
*Sunscreen.*

**Savex Sunblock** *Sabex, Canad.*
*SPF 15:* Padimate O (p.1155·1); oxybenzone (p.1154·3).
*Sunscreen.*

**Savex with Sunscreen** *Sabex, Canad.*
Camphor (p.1665·3); menthol (p.1711·3); salicylic acid (p.1157·1).

**Savilen** *Sanofi Synthelabo, Gr.*
Ciprofibrate (p.884·2).
*Hyperlipidaemias.*

**Savior** *Abic, Israel; Teva, Israel.*
Chlorhexidine gluconate (p.1173·2); cetrimide (p.1172·1).
*Burns; skin disinfection; wounds.*

**Savlodil** *AstraZeneca, Canad.*
Cetrimide (p.1172·1); chlorhexidine gluconate (p.1173·2).
*Wound disinfection.*

**Savlon**
*Note. This name is used for preparations of different composition.*
*AstraZeneca, Canad.†; Novartis Consumer, Irl.; Boots Healthcare, NZ; Zeneca, Port.†; Pharmedica, S.Afr.†; Johnson & Johnson, Singapore.*
Cetrimide (p.1172·1); chlorhexidine gluconate (p.1173·2).
*Burns; disinfection; wounds.*

*Whitehall-Robins, Canad.†.*
Cetrimide (p.1172·1).
*Skin disorders.*

**Savlon Antiseptic**
*Boots, Austral.†.*
*Topical powder; liquid treatment:* Povidone-iodine (p.1190·3).
*Burns; fungal skin infections; skin abrasions; wounds.*

*Boots Healthcare, Austral.*
*Cream; topical liquid:* Cetrimide (p.1172·1); chlorhexidine (p.1173·2).
*Skin abrasions; wounds.*

**Savlon Antiseptic Cream** *Novartis Consumer, UK.*
Cetrimide (p.1172·1); chlorhexidine gluconate (p.1173·2).
*Skin disinfection.*

**Savlon Antiseptic Liquid** *Novartis Consumer, UK.*
Cetrimide (p.1172·1); chlorhexidine gluconate (p.1173·2).
Formerly known as Savlon Concentrated Antiseptic.
*Skin disinfection.*

**Savlon Antiseptic Wound Wash** *Novartis Consumer, UK.*
Chlorhexidine gluconate (p.1173·2).
*Skin disinfection.*

**Savlon Dry** *Novartis Consumer, UK.*
Povidone-iodine (p.1190·3).
*Skin disinfection.*

**Savlon Natural Antiseptic** *Novartis Consumer, UK.*
Melaleuca oil (p.1710·2).
*Skin irritation.*

**Savlon Natural First Aid for Bruises** *Novartis Consumer, UK.*
Arnica (p.1656·3).
*Bruises.*

**Savlon Natural First Aid for Burns** *Novartis Consumer, UK.*
Calendula (p.1665·2); echinacea (p.1683·2); hypericum (p.299·1); urtica (p.1762·1).
*Burns.*

**Savlon Natural First Aid for Cuts & Sores** *Novartis Consumer, UK.*
Calendula (p.1665·2); hypericum (p.299·1).
*Minor wounds.*

**Savlon Natural First Aid for Insect Bites & Stings** *Novartis Consumer, UK.*
Hypericum (p.299·1); yellow dock (p.1766·1); echinacea angustifolia (p.1683·2); ledum palustre; calendula (p.1665·2); arnica (p.1656·3); pyrethrum (p.1509·3).
*Insect bites and stings.*

**Savoral** *Novartis Nutrition, Fr.†.*
Preparation for enteral nutrition (p.1417·1).

**Savorix T** *Cesam, Port.†.*
Piroctone olamine (p.1155·2); sulfur (p.1158·2).
*Dandruff; seborrhoeic dermatitis.*

**Saw Palmetto Formula** *Quest, Canad.*
Buchu leaf; cayenne; corn silk; kelp; parsley leaf; pumpkin seed; saw palmetto berry (p.1417·1).

**Sawmetto Vivo-Livo** *Panpharma, Hong Kong.*
Saw palmetto (p.1569·1); cucurbita oil (p.1677·3); soya oil (p.1447·2).
*Benign prostatic hyperplasia.*

**Sayomol** *Cinfa, Spain†.*
Promethazine hydrochloride (p.439·1).
*Cutaneous hypersensitivity reactions.*

**Sazo** *Wallace, India.*
Sulfasalazine (p.1291·1).
*Crohn's disease; rheumatoid arthritis; ulcerative colitis.*

**SBOB** *Nakorn, Thai.*
Loperamide hydrochloride (p.1271·1).
*Diarrhoea.*

**SBPA Analgesic/Calmative** *SBPA, Austral.†.*
Paracetamol (p.76·2); codeine phosphate (p.27·1); doxylamine succinate (p.432·3).
*Fever; pain.*

**SC-300** *Hamilton, Austral.†.*
Coconut oil derivatives.
*Barrier cream; skin cleansing.*

**Scabecid** *Stiefel, Fr.*
Lindane (p.1506·3).
*Pediculosis; scabies.*

**Scabene**
*Note. This name is used for preparations of different composition.*
*Medican, Canad.*
Esdepallethrine (p.1505·1); piperonyl butoxide (p.1509·2).
*Scabies.*

*Stiefel, Mex.†.*
Lindane (p.1506·3).

**Scabenzil** *Delta, Braz.*
Benzyl benzoate (p.1500·2).
*Pediculosis; scabies.*

**Scabexyl** *Stiefel, Chile.*
Lindane (p.1506·3).
*Pediculosis; scabies.*

**Scabicin**
*Fischer, Israel; Cosmofarma, Port.*
Crotamiton (p.1145·1).
*Pruritus; scabies.*

**Scabiex** *Rekah, Israel.*
Benzyl benzoate (p.1500·2).
*Scabies.*

**Scabine** *Stadmed, India.*
Lindane (p.1506·3); cetrimide (p.1172·1).
*Pediculosis; scabies.*

**Scabioderm** *Bajer, Arg.*
Bioallethrin (p.1500·3); piperonyl butoxide (p.1509·2); benzyl benzoate (p.1500·2).
*Pediculosis; scabies.*

**Scabioid** *Legrand, Braz.*
Benzyl benzoate (p.1500·2).
*Scabies.*

**Scabisan** *Chinoin, Mex.*
Lindane (p.1506·3).
*Pediculosis; scabies.*

**Scabisan Plus** *Chinoin, Mex.*
Lindane (p.1506·3); benzyl benzoate (p.1500·2).
*Scabies.*

**Scadan**
*Note. This name is used for preparations of different composition.*
*Medipharm, Chile.*
Chlorphenamine maleate (p.427·3).
*Hypersensitivity reactions.*

*Miles, USA.*
Trimethyltetradecylammonium bromide (p.1172·3); stearyl dimethyl benzyl ammonium chloride.
*Seborrhoea.*

**Scaflam**
*Schering-Plough, Braz.; Lavipharm, Gr.*
Nimesulide (p.67·1).
*Fever; inflammation; musculoskeletal disorders; pain.*

**Scalid** *Uniao Quimica, Braz.*
Nimesulide (p.67·1).
*Fever; inflammation; pain.*

**Scalpicin**
*Note. This name is used for preparations of different composition.*
*Combe, Ital.*
Hydrocortisone (p.1103·3); menthol (p.1711·3).
*Skin irritation.*

*Combe, USA.*
Salicylic acid (p.1157·1); menthol (p.1711·3).
Formerly contained hydrocortisone, and menthol.

**Scalpicin Anti-Dandruff Anti-Itch** *Combe, Canad.*
Menthol (p.1711·3); salicylic acid (p.1157·1).

**Scalpicin Capilar** *Combe, Spain.*
Hydrocortisone (p.1103·3).
*Scalp disorders.*

**Scalpin** *Specifar (Σπεσιφαρ), Gr.*
Ketoconazole (p.403·3).
*Fungal scalp infections.*

**Scalpvit** *Kemiprogress, Ital.*†.
Vitamins, selenium, yeast, and amino acids (p.1417·1).
*Nutritional supplement.*

**Scandicain**
*AstraZeneca, Austria; AstraZeneca, Ger.; Dentsply, Ger.; AstraZeneca, Switz.*
Mepivacaine hydrochloride (p.1381·2).
*Local anaesthesia.*

**Scandicaine**
*AstraZeneca, Belg.; DFL, Braz.*†*; AstraZeneca, Neth.*
Mepivacaine hydrochloride (p.1381·2).
Adrenaline (p.852·2) or adrenaline acid tartrate (p.852·2) is included in some injections as a vasoconstrictor to diminish absorption and localise the effect of the local anaesthetic.
*Local anaesthesia.*

**Scandine**
*Zambon, Belg.; Zambon, Ital.; Zambon, Port.*
Ibopamine hydrochloride (p.937·3).
*Heart failure.*

**Scandinibsa**
*Inibsa, Port.; Inibsa, Spain.*
Mepivacaine hydrochloride (p.1381·2).
Adrenaline (p.852·2) or adrenaline acid tartrate (p.852·2) is included in some injections as a vasoconstrictor to diminish absorption and localise the effect of the local anaesthetic.
*Local anaesthesia.*

**Scandinor** *DFL, Braz.*†.
Mepivacaine hydrochloride (p.1381·2).
Noradrenaline acid tartrate (p.974·3) is included in this preparation as a vasoconstrictor to diminish absorption and localise the effect of the local anaesthetic.
*Local anaesthesia.*

**Scandishake**
*Nutricia, Austral.; Nutricia, Fin.; Scientific Hospital Supplies, Irl.; Scandipharm, Israel; Nutricia, Ital.; Baxter, NZ; Nutricia, NZ; Scientific Hospital Supplies, UK.*
Preparation for enteral nutrition (p.1417·1).

**Scandonest**
*Septodont, Austral.; Austrodent, Austria; Septodont, Denm.; Ogna, Ital.; Septodont, Norw.; Dental Warehouse, S.Afr.; Septodont, Switz.*
Mepivacaine hydrochloride (p.1381·2).
Adrenaline (p.852·2) or noradrenaline acid tartrate (p.974·3) is included in some injections as a vasoconstrictor to diminish absorption and localise the effect of the local anaesthetic.
*Local anaesthesia.*

**Scanlux**
*Sanochemia, Austria; Sanochemia, UK.*
Iopamidol (p.1064·3).
*Radiographic contrast medium.*

**Scannotrast** *Gerot, Austria.*
Barium sulfate (p.1061·1).
*Radiographic contrast medium for CT scanning.*

**Scarfade** *GAR, Singapore.*
Dimeticone (p.1482·1); cyclomethicone; polysiloxane.
*Scars.*

**Scavenger** *Aesculapius, Ital.*
Glutathione (p.1040·3).
*Alcohol or drug poisoning; ionising radiation trauma.*

**Schamill** *Ritsert, Ger.*†.
Achillea (p.1646·2).
*Dyspepsia.*

**Scheinpharm Artificial Tears** *Schein, Canad.*
Polyvinyl alcohol (p.1581·1).

**Scheinpharm Artificial Tears Plus** *Schein, Canad.*
Polyvinyl alcohol (p.1581·1); povidone (p.1581·2).

**Scheinpharm Testone-Cyp** *Schein, Canad.*†.
Testosterone cipionate (p.1569·3).
*Androgen.*

**Scheinpharm Triamcine-A** *Schein, Canad.*†.
Triamcinolone acetonide (p.1110·2).
*Corticosteroid.*

**Scheribar** *Schering, Arg.*
Barium sulfate (p.1061·1).
*Contrast medium for gastrointestinal radiography.*

**Scheribase** *Schering, Port.*†.
Emollient.
*Pharmaceutical diluent; skin disorders.*

**Schericur**
*Schering, Arg.; Schering, Austria*†*; Schering, Spain.*
Hydrocortisone (p.1103·3).
*Skin disorders.*

**Scheriderm**
*Schering, Arg.; Schering, Mex.*
Diflucortolone valerate (p.1099·3); isoconazole nitrate (p.401·3); neomycin sulfate (p.235·1).
*Infected skin disorders.*

**Schering Base** *Schering, Canad.*
Emollient.
*Dry skin; topical diluent.*

**Schering PC4** *Schering, UK*†.
Norgestrel (p.1563·2); ethinylestradiol (p.1553·2).
*Postcoital oral contraceptive.*

**Scheriproct**
*Note. This name is used for preparations of different composition.*
*Schering, Arg.; Schering, Austral.; Schering, Austria; Schering, Belg.; Schering, Chile; Schering, Fin.; Schering, Ger.; Asche, Ger.; Schering, Irl.; Schering, Mex.; Schering, Norw.; Schering, Port.; Schering, S.Afr.; Schering, Spain; Schering, Switz.; Schering, UK.*
Prednisolone caproate (p.1108·1); cinchocaine hydrochloride (p.1373·2).
*Anorectal disorders.*

*Schering, Thai.*
Prednisolone caproate (p.1108·1); cinchocaine hydrochloride (p.1373·2); clemizole undecylate (p.429·2).
*Anorectal disorders.*

**Scheriproct N** *Schering, Swed.*
Prednisolone caproate (p.1108·1); cinchocaine hydrochloride (p.1373·2).
*Anorectal disorders.*

**Scheriproct Neo** *Shepa, Gr.*
Cinchocaine hydrochloride (p.1373·2); prednisolone caproate (p.1108·1).
*Haemorrhoids.*

**Scherogel**
*Schering, Austria; Schering, Belg.*†*; Asche, Ger.; Schering, Ital.*†.
Benzoyl peroxide (p.1143·2).
*Acne.*

**Schias-Amaro Medicinale** *AFOM, Ital.*
Rhubarb (p.1287·3); boldo (p.1661·2); cascara (p.1255·1).
*Constipation; digestive disorders.*

**Schiwalys Hemofiltration** *Baxter, Swed.*
Electrolyte solution for haemofiltration (p.1221·1).
Some solutions also contain glucose.

**Schizopol** *Polipharm, Thai.*
Haloperidol (p.701·2).

**Schlaf- und Nerventee** *Bad Heilbrunner, Ger.*
Valerian (p.1762·2); melissa (p.1711·1); lupulus (p.1708·1).
*Nervous disorders.*

**SchlafTabs** *Ratiopharm, Ger.*
Doxylamine succinate (p.432·3).
*Sleep disorders.*

**Schlehepar N** *Hanosan, Ger.*
Homoeopathic preparation.

**Schleimhaut-Komplex Ho-Fu-Complex** *Liebermann, Ger.*
Homoeopathic preparation.

**Schmerz-Dolgit** *Dolorgiet, Ger.*
Ibuprofen (p.45·3).
*Fever; pain; rheumatism.*

**Schneckensaft N** *Hotz, Ger.*†.
Thyme (p.1755·2); castanea vulgaris; limacin.
*Bronchitis; coughs.*

**Schneckensirup** *Alsitan, Ger.*†.
Alfalfa (p.1649·1); thyme (p.1755·2).
*Cold symptoms.*

**schnupfen endrine** *Asche, Ger.*
Xylometazoline hydrochloride (p.1132·2).
*Nasal congestion.*

**Scholl Athlete's Foot**
*Note. This name is used for preparations of different composition.*
*Schering-Plough, Canad.*
Butenafine hydrochloride (p.395·2).
*Tinea pedis.*

*SSL, UK.*
Tolnaftate (p.410·1).
*Tinea pedis.*

**Scholl Athlete's Foot Preparations** *Schering-Plough, Canad.*
*Gel; powder; spray powder:* Tolnaftate (p.410·1).
*Tinea pedis.*

**Scholl Callus Removal** *SSL, UK.*
Salicylic acid (p.1157·1).
*Calluses.*

**Scholl Callus Remover** *Schering-Plough, Canad.*
Salicylic acid (p.1157·1).
*Calluses; corns.*

**Scholl Clear Away** *Schering-Plough, Canad.*
Salicylic acid (p.1157·1).
*Warts.*

**Scholl Corn, Callus Plaster Preparation** *Schering-Plough, Canad.*†.
Salicylic acid (p.1157·1).
*Calluses; corns.*

**Scholl Corn & Callus Removal Liquid** *SSL, UK.*
Salicylic acid (p.1157·1); camphor (p.1665·3).
*Calluses; corns.*

**Scholl Corn Removal** *SSL, UK.*
Salicylic acid (p.1157·1).
*Corns.*

**Scholl Corn Remover** *Schering-Plough, Canad.*
Salicylic acid (p.1157·1).
*Calluses; corns.*

**Scholl Corn Salve** *Schering-Plough, Canad.*†.
Salicylic acid (p.1157·1).
*Calluses; corns.*

**Scholl Corn/Callous Removers** *Scholl, Israel.*
Salicylic acid (p.1157·1).
*Corns.*

**Scholl 2-Drop Corn Remedy** *Schering-Plough, Canad.*
Salicylic acid (p.1157·1).
*Calluses; corns.*

**Scholl Dry Antiperspirant Foot Spray** *Schering-Plough, Canad.*
Aluminium chlorohydrate (p.1142·1).
*Foot odour; foot perspiration.*

**Scholl One Step** *Schering-Plough, Canad.*
Salicylic acid (p.1157·1).
*Calluses; corns; warts.*

**Scholl Seal & Heal** *SSL, UK.*
Salicylic acid (p.1157·1); camphor (p.1665·3).
*Calluses; corns; verrucas; warts.*

**Scholl Verucca Removal** *SSL, UK.*
Salicylic acid (p.1157·1).
*Verrucas; warts.*

**Scholl Wart Remover** *Schering-Plough, Canad.*†.
Salicylic acid (p.1157·1).
*Warts.*

**Scholl Zino** *Schering-Plough, Canad.*
Salicylic acid (p.1157·1).
*Corns.*

**Schoolife** *Lifeplan, UK*†.
Multinutrient preparation (p.1417·1).

**Schoum** *Pharmygiene, Fr.*
Fumitory (p.1690·1); ononis (p.1723·3); Jamaica dogwood (p.1702·3); sorbitol (p.1446·3); alverine citrate (p.1250·2).
*Gastrointestinal and kidney disorders.*

**Schrundensalbe Dermi-cyl** *Liebermann, Ger.*
Salicylic acid (p.1157·1).
*Skin disorders.*

**Schufen** *Kenyaku, Thai.*
Ibuprofen (p.45·3).
*Fever; inflammation; pain.*

**Schupps Baldrian Sedativbad** *Schupp, Ger.*†.
Valerian (p.1762·2); valerian oil; citronella oil (p.1673·2); lupulus (p.1708·1).
*Bath additive; nervous disorders; sleep disorders.*

**Schupps Fichte-Menthol Olbad** *Schupp, Ger.*†.
Norway spruce oil; eucalyptus oil (p.1686·2); menthol (p.1711·3).
*Bath additive; catarrh.*

**Schupps Heilkrauter Erkaltungsbad** *Schupp, Ger.*†.
Eucalyptus oil (p.1686·2); thyme oil (p.1755·3); peppermint oil (p.1283·2).
*Bath additive; cold symptoms.*

**Schupps Heilkrauter Rheumabad** *Schupp, Ger.*†.
Methyl salicylate (p.59·3); camphor (p.1665·3); rosemary oil (p.1740·2); Norway spruce oil; sage oil (p.1741·2); juniper oil (p.1703·1).
*Bath additive; musculoskeletal and joint disorders.*

**Schupps Kohlensaurebad** *Schupp, Ger.*†.
Sodium bicarbonate (p.1223·2); aluminium sulfate (p.1653·1).
*Bath additive; circulatory disorders; hypertension.*

**Schupps Latschenkiefer Olbad** *Schupp, Ger.*†.
Pumilio pine oil (p.1737·1); pine-needle oil; Norway spruce oil; turpentine oil (p.1760·1); juniper oil (p.1703·1).
*Bath additive; musculoskeletal and joint disorders; nervous disorders.*

**Schupps Melissen Olbad** *Schupp, Ger.*
Citronella oil (p.1673·2).
*Bath additive; nervous disorders.*

**Schwarze-Salbe** *Lichtenstein, Ger.*†.
Ichthammol (p.1148·2).
*Skin disorders.*

**Schwarzwalder Heublumen-Extrakt** *Schupp, Ger.*†.
Hay flowers.
*Rheumatism.*

**Schweden-Mixtur H nouvelle formulation**
*Hanseler, Switz.*
Aloes (p.1248·2); senna (p.1288·2); rhubarb (p.1287·3).
*Constipation.*

**Schwedentrunk** *Infirmarius-Rovit, Ger.*†.
Aloes (p.1248·2); senna (p.1288·2); manna (p.1273·1); myrrh (p.1718·3); angelica (p.1655·1); carlina; gentian (p.1692·2); zedoary; camphor (p.1665·3); saffron (p.1058·2); theriacale; vitamin C (p.1460·2).
*Gastrointestinal disorders.*

**Schwedentrunk Elixier** *Infirmarius-Rovit, Ger.*
Angelica (p.1655·1); gentian (p.1692·2); cardamom fruit (p.1667·3); cinnamon (p.1672·2); valerian (p.1762·2).
*Digestive-system disorders.*

**Schwedentrunk mit Ginseng** *Infirmarius-Rovit, Ger.*†.
Aloes (p.1248·2); senna (p.1288·2); manna (p.1273·1); myrrh (p.1718·3); angelica (p.1655·1); carlina; gentian (p.1692·2); zedoary; camphor (p.1665·3); saffron (p.1058·2); theriacale; vitamin C (p.1460·2); ginseng (p.1693·1).
*Gastrointestinal disorders.*

**Schwefelbad Dr Klopfer**
*Note. This name is used for preparations of different composition.*
*Austroplant, Austria; Protina, Ger.*
Sulfur (p.1158·2); sodium thiosulfate (p.1053·3).
*Bath additive; musculoskeletal and joint disorders; skin disorders.*

*Protina, Switz.*†.
Zinc sulfide; sodium sulfite (p.1193·1); sodium bisulfite (p.1193·1); colloidal sulfur (p.1158·2); pine oil; turpentine oil (p.1760·1).
Formerly known as Bain Soufre du Dr Klopfer.
*Circulatory disorders; hyperhidrosis; musculoskeletal and joint disorders; skin disorders.*

**Schwefelbad-Saar** *CPF, Ger.*†.
Sulfurated potash (p.1158·3).
*Bath additive; rheumatic disorders; skin disorders.*

**Schwefel-Diasporal** *Protina, Ger.*†.
*Cream:* Sulfur (p.1158·2).
*Topical solution:* Sulfur (p.1158·2); camphor (p.1665·3).
*Skin disorders.*

**Schwohepan S** *Schworer, Ger.*
Silybum marianum (p.1043·3); greater celandine (p.1695·3).
*Biliary and gastrointestinal spasm; liver disorders.*

**Schwoneural** *Schworer, Ger.*
Homoeopathic preparation.

**Schworalgan** *Schworer, Ger.*
Paracetamol (p.76·2); propyphenazone (p.85·3).
*Fever; pain.*

**Schworocard** *Schworer, Ger.*
Homoeopathic preparation.

**Schworocor** *Schworer, Ger.*
Homoeopathic preparation.

**Schworosin** *Schworer, Ger.*
Homoeopathic preparation.

**Schworotox** *Schworer, Ger.*
Homoeopathic preparation.

**Schworotox N** *Schworer, Ger.*
Homoeopathic preparation.

**Sciargo** *Potter's, UK.*
Shepherd's purse (p.1744·1); wild carrot (p.1765·1); clivers (p.1673·2); bearberry (p.1659·2); juniper berry oil (p.1703·1).
*Lumbago; sciatica.*

**Scillacor** *Steigerwald, Ger.*
Homoeopathic preparation.

**Scillase N** *Ziethen, Ger.*
Squill (p.1130·3).
*Heart failure; kidney disorders.*

**Scintadren** *Nycomed Amersham, UK.*
Selenium-75 (p.1525·2) in the form of 6β-(methyl($^{75}$Se)seleno)methyl-19-norcholest-5(10)-en-3β-ol.
*Adrenal gland imaging.*

**Sciomir** *CT, Ital.*
Thiocolchicoside (p.1395·2).
*Neuromuscular pain; parkinsonism; spasticity.*

**Sciroppo Berta** *Berta, Ital.*
Liquorice (p.1270·2); sulfogaiacol (p.1131·1).
*Catarrh; coughs.*

**Sciroppo Fenoglio** *AFOM, Ital.*
Ferric ammonium citrate (p.1427·2).
*Anaemias.*

**Sciroppo Merck all'Efetonina** *Bracco, Ital.*†.
Racephedrine hydrochloride (Efetonina) (p.1120·3); thyme (p.1755·2).
*Coughs; respiratory-tract disorders.*

**Scitropin**
*Scigen, Austral.; Scigen, Hong Kong; Scigen, Singapore.*
Somatropin (p.1327·2).
*Growth disorders in renal failure; growth hormone deficiency; Turner's syndrome.*

**Sclane** *Llorente, Spain*†.
Betamethasone acetate (p.1093·1); betamethasone sodium phosphate (p.1093·1).
*Corticosteroid.*

**Scleramin** *Ibirn, Ital.*†.
Vinburnine phosphate (p.1764·2).
*Cerebrovascular disorders.*

**Scleremo** *Bailleul, Fr.*
Chrome alum (p.1670·2); glycerol (p.1694·3).
*Varicose veins.*

**Scleril** *AGIPS, Ital.*
Fenofibrate (p.915·2).
*Exudative diabetic retinopathy; hyperlipidaemias; xanthoma.*

**Sclerobion** *Merck, India.*
Vitamin A (p.1451·2); vitamin $B_6$ (p.1457·2); vitamin E (p.1464·3).
*Corneal and conjunctival xerosis; senile macular degeneration; vitamin A and E deficiency.*

**Sclerocalcine** *Lehning, Fr.*
Homoeopathic preparation.

**Sclerodex** *Omega, Canad.*
Glucose (p.1432·2); sodium chloride (p.1233·3); phenethyl alcohol (p.1188·1).
*Sclerotherapy.*

**Sclerodine** *Omega, Canad.*
Iodine (p.1598·1); sodium iodide (p.1598·1).
*Sclerotherapy.*

**Sclerofin** *Armstrong, Arg.*
Fenofibrate (p.915·2).
*Hyperlipidaemias.*

**Scleromate** *Palisades, USA.*
Sodium morrhuate (p.1748·1).
*Varicose veins.*

**Sclerosol** *Bryan, USA.*
Sterile talc (p.1159·1).
*Malignant pleural effusion.*

**Sclerovein** *Resinag, Switz.*
Lauromacrogol 600 (p.1412·3); alcohol (p.1166·1).
*Variceal sclerosis.*

**SCMC**
*Upha, Malaysia; Beacons, Singapore.*
Carbocisteine (p.1116·2).
*Respiratory-tract disorders associated with increased or viscous mucus.*

**SCMC Promethazine** *Upha, Malaysia.*
Carbocisteine (p.1116·2); promethazine hydrochloride (p.439·1).
*Coughs.*

**S-Coaltar** *Ducray, Fr.†.*
Coal tar (p.1159·2); salicylic acid (p.1157·1).
*Dandruff.*

**Scoburen** *Renaudin, Fr.*
Hyoscine butylbromide (p.483·3).
*Biliary-tract disorders; gynaecological pain; smooth muscle spasm Gastrointestinal disorders.*

**Scoline**
*Mayne, Austral.; GlaxoSmithKline, S.Afr.*
Suxamethonium chloride (p.1406·2).
*Depolarising neuromuscular blocker.*

**Scolybil** *Windson, Braz.†.*
Acetylmethionine; choline citrate (p.1424·3); sorbitol (p.1446·3).
*Liver disorders.*

**Scopace** *Hope, USA.*
Hyoscine hydrobromide (p.483·3).
*Parkinsonism.*

**Scopanil** *Recalcine, Chile.*
Pargeverine (p.487·3); metamizole magnesium (p.36·1).
*Smooth muscle spasm and pain.*

**Scopas** *Asian Pharm, Thai.*
Hyoscine butylbromide (p.483·3).
*Gastro-duodenitis; nausea and vomiting; peptic ulcer; smooth muscle spasm.*

**Scope**
*Note. This name is used for preparations of different composition.*
*Procter & Gamble, Canad.†.*
Cetylpyridinium chloride (p.1173·1); domiphen bromide (p.1179·1).
Formerly known as Scope with Oraseptate.
*Oral hygiene.*
*Procter & Gamble, USA.*
Cetylpyridinium chloride (p.1173·1).
*Minor mouth or throat irritation.*

**Scopex** *Propan, S.Afr.; Restan, S.Afr.*
Hyoscine butylbromide (p.483·3).
*Gastrointestinal spasm.*

**Scopex Co** *Propan, S.Afr.*
Hyoscine butylbromide (p.483·3); dipyrone (p.35·3).
*Gastrointestinal spasm; urinary-tract spasm.*

**Scopinal** *Julphar, UAE.*
Hyoscine butylbromide (p.483·3).
*Smooth muscle spasm.*

**Scopoderm**
*Novartis, Austria; Novartis, Denm.; Novartis, Fin.; Novartis, Norw.; Novartis, Swed.*
Hyoscine (p.483·3).
*Motion sickness.*

**Scopoderm TTS**
*Novartis Sante, Fr.; Novartis Consumer, Ger.; Novartis, Hong Kong; Novartis Consumer, Neth.; Enzpharma, NZ; Novartis Nutrition, Singapore†; Novartis, Switz.†; Novartis Consumer, UK.*
Hyoscine (p.483·3).
*Intractable cough in terminal illness; motion sickness.*

**Scorbex** *Aspen, S.Afr.*
Vitamin C (p.1460·2).
*Vitamin C deficiency.*

**Scordal** *Kattwiga, Ger.*
*Capsules:* Herba teucrii.
*Oral drops:* Herba teucrii; magnesium chloride (p.1228·1).
*Cardiovascular disorders; gastrointestinal disorders.*

**Scorotox** *Kattwiga, Ger.*
Homoeopathic preparation.

**Scott Dandruff Shampoo** *Scott, Canad.*
Pyrithione zinc (p.1156·2).
*Scalp disorders.*

**Scottopect** *Nycomed, Austria.*
*Gel:* Turpentine oil (p.1760·1); eucalyptus oil (p.1686·2); thyme oil (p.1755·3); menthol (p.1711·3); camphor (p.1665·3).
*Oral drops:* Thyme (p.1755·2).
*Oral liquid:* Thyme (p.1755·2); wild thyme; plantago lanceolata (p.1738·2).
*Bronchitis; catarrh.*

**Scott's Cod Liver** *GlaxoSmithKline, Thai.*
Vitamins A and D (p.1417·1).

**Scott's Emulsion**
*Note. This name is used for preparations of different composition.*
*GlaxoSmithKline, Hong Kong.*
Cod-liver oil (p.1425·2).
*Dietary supplement.*
*SmithKline Beecham Consumer, UK†.*
Cod-liver oil (p.1425·2); calcium hypophosphite (p.1226·3); sodium hypophosphite.
*SmithKline Beecham, USA.*
Vitamins A and D (p.1417·1).

**Scott's Emulsion Orange** *SmithKline Beecham, Hong Kong.*
Cod-liver oil (p.1425·2); calcium hypophosphite (p.1226·3).
*Dietary supplement.*

**Scott's Emulsion Original** *SmithKline Beecham, Hong Kong.*
Cod-liver oil; capelin oil; calcium hypophosphite; sodium hypophosphite (p.1417·1).
*Dietary supplement.*

**Scot-Tussin Allergy** *Scot-Tussin, USA.*
Diphenhydramine hydrochloride (p.431·3).

**Scot-Tussin DM** *Scot-Tussin, USA.*
Chlorphenamine maleate (p.427·3); dextromethorphan hydrobromide (p.1117·3).
*Coughs and cold symptoms.*

**Scot-Tussin DM Cough Chasers** *Scot-Tussin, USA.*
Dextromethorphan hydrobromide (p.1117·3).
*Coughs.*

**Scot-Tussin Expectorant** *Scot-Tussin, USA.*
Guaifenesin (p.1122·1).
*Coughs.*

**Scot-Tussin Original 5-Action** *Scot-Tussin, USA.*
Phenylephrine hydrochloride (p.1126·3); pheniramine maleate (p.438·3); sodium citrate (p.1223·2); sodium salicylate (p.90·1); caffeine citrate (p.782·1).
*Upper respiratory-tract symptoms.*

**Scot-Tussin Senior Clear** *Scot-Tussin, USA.*
Guaifenesin (p.1122·1); dextromethorphan hydrobromide (p.1117·3).
*Coughs.*

**SCR** *Pickles, UK.*
Salicylic acid (p.1157·1).
*Cradle cap.*

**Scriptolyte** *Propan, S.Afr.*
Potassium chloride; sodium chloride; sodium citrate; glucose (p.1222·2).
*Diarrhoea; oral rehydration therapy.*

**Scripto-Metic** *Propan, S.Afr.*
Prochlorperazine maleate (p.716·3).
*Anxiety disorders; migraine; nausea and vomiting; vestibular disorders.*

**Scullcap & Gentian Tablets** *Dorwest, UK.*
Skullcap (p.1746·3); valerian (p.1762·2); vervain (p.1764·1); gentian (p.1692·2).
*Anxiety; insomnia; irritability.*

**SD-Hermal** *Hermal, Ger.*
Clotrimazole (p.396·2).
*Pityriasis versicolor; seborrhoeic dermatitis.*

**SDL** *Bencard, Ger.†.*
Allergen extracts (p.1650·1).
*Allergen immunotherapy.*

**SDV** *Teomed, Switz.†.*
Pollen allergen extracts (p.1650·1).
*Allergen immunotherapy.*

**Sea Breeze** *Bristol-Myers Squibb, Canad.†.*
Alcohol (p.1166·1); camphor (p.1665·3); benzoic acid (p.1169·3).
*Skin cleansing.*

**Seabell** *Pond's, Thai.*
Flunarizine hydrochloride (p.434·1).
*Cerebral and peripheral vascular disorders; memory disorders; vestibular disorders.*

**Sea-Cal** *Bioceuticals, UK.*
Calcium carbonate (p.1254·2).

**Seacor** *SPA, Ital.*
Omega-3 triglycerides (p.976·1).
*Hypertriglyceridaemia.*

**Seal On** *Alltracel, Hong Kong.*
Calcium oxidised cellulose (p.757·2); sodium oxidised cellulose (p.757·2).
*Haemorrhage.*

**Sealdin** *Lacer, Spain.*
Sertraline hydrochloride (p.317·2).
*Depression; obsessive-compulsive disorder; panic disorder.*

**Sea-Legs**
*Boots Healthcare, NZ; SSL, UK.*
Meclozine hydrochloride (p.436·3).
*Motion sickness.*

**Seale's Lotion** *C & M, USA.*
Sulfur (p.1158·2); borax (p.1661·3); zinc oxide (p.1163·2).
*Acne.*

**Seal-On**
*Alltracel, Irl.; Beta Healthcare, UK.*
Calcium oxidised cellulose (p.757·2); sodium oxidised cellulose (p.757·2).
*Capillary haemorrhage.*

**SeaMist** *Schein, USA.*
Sodium chloride (p.1233·3).
*Inflammation and dryness of nasal membranes.*

**Sea-Omega** *Rugby, USA.*
Omega-3 marine triglycerides with vitamin E (p.976·2).
*Dietary supplement.*

**Seasonale** *Duramed, USA.*
84 Tablets, levonorgestrel (p.1563·2); ethinylestradiol (p.1553·2); 7 tablets, inert.
*Combined oral contraceptive.*

**Seasorb Soft** *Coloplast, UK.*
Calcium alginate (p.745·1); carmellose (p.1577·3).
*Exudating wounds.*

**Seatone** *Peter Black, UK.*
Green-lipped mussel (p.1696·1).

**Sebacnol** *Boots Healthcare, Ital.*
*Lotion:* Mimosa tenuiflora; glycolic acid (p.1147·3).
*Topical gel:* Mimosa tenuiflora; urtica (p.1762·1); thyme (p.1755·2); tilia (p.1756·2).
*Acne.*

**Sebaklen** *Fumouze, Fr.†.*
Xenysalate hydrochloride (p.1163·1).
*Seborrhoeic dermatitis.*

**Sebamed**
*Sebapharma, Hong Kong; Sebapharma, Thai.*
A range of skin cleansers and emollients.

**Sebamed Suncream 20** *Sebapharma, Thai.*
Octinoxate (p.1154·3); avobenzone (p.1142·3); enzacamene (p.1147·1).
*Sunscreen.*

**Sebamed Suncream 28** *Sebapharma, Thai.*
Octinoxate (p.1154·3); titanium dioxide (p.1160·3).
*Sunscreen.*

**Sebamed Sunlotion** *Sebapharma, Thai.*
*SPF 20:* Octinoxate (p.1154·3); avobenzone (p.1142·3); enzacamene (p.1147·1).
*Sunscreen.*

**Seba-Nil** *Healthpoint, USA.*
Skin cleanser.
*Acne.*

**Sebaquin** *Summers, USA.*
Diiodohydroxyquinoline (p.603·3).
*Scalp disorders.*

**Sebasorb** *Summers, USA.*
Sulfur (p.1158·2); salicylic acid (p.1157·1).
*Acne.*

**Sebaveen**
*Rydelle, Ital.†; Dermoteca, Port.†.*
Avena (p.1658·2); salicylic acid (p.1157·1); carbocisteine (p.1116·2).
*Seborrhoeic dermatitis.*

**Sebcur** *Dermtek, Canad.*
Salicylic acid (p.1157·1).
*Seborrhoea of the scalp.*

**Sebcur/T** *Dermtek, Canad.*
Salicylic acid (p.1157·1); coal tar (p.1159·2).
*Psoriasis of the scalp.*

**Sebercim** *GlaxoSmithKline, Ital.*
Norfloxacin (p.238·3).
*Urinary-tract infections.*

**Sebex** *Rugby, USA.*
Salicylic acid (p.1157·1); sulfur (p.1158·2).
*Seborrhoea.*

**Sebexol** *Devesa, Ger.*
Emollient.
*Skin disorders.*

**Sebexol cum urea** *Devesa, Ger.*
Urea (p.1162·2).
*Skin disorders.*

**Sebex-T** *Rugby, USA.*
Coal tar (p.1159·2); sulfur (p.1158·2); salicylic acid (p.1157·1).
*Seborrhoea.*

**Sebiprox**
*Stiefel, Ger.; Stiefel, Spain.*
Ciclopirox olamine (p.396·1).
*Seborrhoeic dermatitis.*

**Sebirinse**
*Ego, Austral.†; Ego, NZ.*
Diacetyldimonium chloride; dexpanthenol (p.1727·2); phenethyl alcohol (p.1188·1).
*Dry scalp and hair disorders.*

**Sebitar**
*Ego, Austral.; Ego, Hong Kong; Ego, NZ; Ego, Singapore.*
Tar (p.1159·3); coal tar (p.1159·2); salicylic acid (p.1157·1); undecylenamide (p.411·1).
*Skin and scalp disorders.*
*Ego, Malaysia.*
Pine tar (p.1159·3); coal tar (p.1159·2); salicylic acid (p.1157·1); undecenoic acid diethanolamide.
*Skin and scalp disorders.*

**Sebium K2** *Polaris, Ital.†.*
Salicylic acid (p.1157·1).
*Acne.*

**Sebizole**
*Douglas, Austral.; Douglas, Hong Kong; Douglas, NZ; Douglas, Singapore.*
Ketoconazole (p.403·3).
*Dandruff; seborrhoeic dermatitis.*

**Sebizon** *Schering, USA†.*
Sulfacetamide sodium (p.257·3).
*Bacterial skin infections; seborrhoeic dermatitis of the scalp.*

**Sebo** *Chew, Thai.*
Betamethasone valerate (p.1093·2).
*Scalp disorders.*

**Sebo Concept D/A** *Marcel, Canad.†.*
Resorcinol (p.1156·3); salicylic acid (p.1157·1); sulfur (p.1158·2).

**Sebo Creme** *Widmer, Switz.*
Vitamins (p.1417·1); urea (p.1162·2); triclosan (p.1195·2).
*Acne; seborrhoea.*

**Sebo Shampooing** *Widmer, Switz.*
Pyrithione zinc (p.1156·2); sodium sulfosuccinated undecenoic acid monoethanolamide (p.411·1); triclosan (p.1195·2).
*Scalp disorders.*

**Sebolic** *Finn Vita, Chile.*
Melaleuca oil (p.1710·2).
*Skin and scalp disorders.*

**Sebolith** *Widmer, Switz.*
Econazole (p.397·1).
*Pityriasis versicolor.*

**Sebomin** *Alpharma, UK.*
Minocycline hydrochloride (p.231·3).
*Acne.*

**Sebophane** *Saninter, Port.†.*
Abietic acid; copper pidolate; zinc pidolate.
*Seborrhoeic dermatitis.*

**Sebo-Psor** *Widmer, Switz.*
Dexamethasone (p.1097·1); tretinoin (p.1161·1); urea (p.1162·2).
*Scalp disorders.*

**Seborrol**
*Ego, Austral.†; Ego, Hong Kong†; Ego, NZ.*
Salicylic acid (p.1157·1); resorcinol (p.1156·3); undecylenamide (p.411·1).
*Scalp disorders.*

**Sebosel**
*Taro, Israel; Taro, Thai.*
Selenium sulfide (p.1157·3).
*Dandruff; pityriasis versicolor; seborrhoeic dermatitis.*

**Sebo-Soufrol** *Gebro, Switz.*
Pyrithione zinc (p.1156·2); sulfur (p.1158·2).
*Scalp disorders.*

**Sebosquam** *Paraphar, Fr.†.*
Ictasol (p.1148·3); cade oil (p.1159·2); climbazole (p.396·2).
*Seborrhoeic dermatitis.*

**Sebrane** *Menarini, Fr.†.*
Dextromethorphan hydrobromide (p.1117·3).
*Coughs.*

**Sebrane Rhume** *Menarini, Fr.†.*
Phenylpropanolamine hydrochloride (p.1127·3); brompheniramine maleate (p.426·1).
*Cold symptoms.*

**Sebryl** *Bioclon, Mex.*
Allantoin (p.1141·3); clioquinol (p.196·3); coal tar (p.1159·2).
*Dandruff; seborrhoeic dermatitis.*

**Sebryl Plus** *Bioclon, Mex.*
Allantoin (p.1141·3); clioquinol (p.196·3); coal tar (p.1159·2); triclosan (p.1195·2).
*Dandruff; seborrhoeic dermatitis.*

**Sebucare** *Westwood-Squibb, USA.*
Salicylic acid (p.1157·1).
*Seborrhoea.*

**Sebulex**
*Note. This name is used for preparations of different composition.*
*Panalab, Arg.*
Panthenol (p.1727·2); salicylic acid (p.1157·1).
*Seborrhoea.*
*Westwood-Squibb, Canad.; Westwood-Squibb, USA.*
Sulfur (p.1158·2); salicylic acid (p.1157·1).
*Scalp disorders.*

**Sebulon** *Westwood-Squibb, Canad.*
Pyrithione zinc (p.1156·2).
*Scalp disorders.*

**Sebumselen** *Juventus, Spain.*
Benzalkonium chloride (p.1168·3); selenium sulfide (p.1157·3).
*Skin and scalp disorders.*

**Sebutone**
*Westwood-Squibb, Canad.; Westwood, Singapore†.*
Coal tar (p.1159·2); salicylic acid (p.1157·1); sulfur (p.1158·2).
*Scalp disorders.*

**Secabiol** *Normon, Spain.*
Carnitine (p.1423·3).
*Cardiac disorders; carnitine deficiency.*

**Secadine** *Xixia, S.Afr.*
Cimetidine (p.1255·3).
*Gastrointestinal disorders.*

**Secadrex**
*Rhone-Poulenc Rorer, Hong Kong†; Aventis, Neth.; Aventis, S.Afr.†; Italfarmaco, Spain; Aventis, UK.*
Acebutolol hydrochloride (p.848·1); hydrochlorothiazide (p.933·2).
*Hypertension.*

**Secalan** *Max Ritter, Switz.†.*
Chlorhexidine gluconate (p.1173·2); isopropyl alcohol (p.1184·3).
*Minor skin lesions; skin disinfection.*

**Secalbum** *Nutricia-Bago, Arg.*
Calcium caseinate.
*Dietary protein supplement.*

**Secale (Hevertoplex 147)** *Hevert, Ger.†.*
Homoeopathic preparation.

**Secale Med Complex** *Dynamit, Austria.*
Homoeopathic preparation.

**Secalip**
*Fournier, Fr.; Fournier SA, Spain.*
Fenofibrate (p.915·2).
*Hyperlipidaemias.*

**Secalosan N** *Hanosan, Ger.*
Homoeopathic preparation.

**Secalysat** *Ysatfabrik, Ger.*
Homoeopathic preparation.

**Secalysat EM** *Ysatfabrik, Ger.†.*
Ergometrine maleate (p.1684·1).
*Gynaecological bleeding.*

**Secamin** *Lab, Port.*
Co-dergocrine mesilate (p.1674·1).
*Cerebral and peripheral vascular disorders; mental function disorders.*

**Secand** *Royal, Chile.*
Sorbitol (p.1446·3); malic acid (p.1709·2); electrolytes (p.1217·1).
*Saliva substitute.*

**Secaris** *Pharmascience, Canad.*
Macrogol (p.1708·2); propylene glycol (p.1735·2).
*Rhinitis.*

**Seclodin** *Much, Ger.†.*
Ibuprofen (p.45·3).
*Fever; pain.*

**Secnid** *Cifarma, Braz.†.*
Secnidazole (p.615·3).
*Bacterial infections; protozoal infections.*

**Secnidal**
*Aventis, Braz.; Aventis, Mex.*
Secnidazole (p.615·3).
*Amoebiasis; giardiasis; trichomoniasis.*

**Secnidalin** *Ducto, Braz.*
Secnidazole (p.615·3).
*Amoebiasis; trichomoniasis.*

**Secnil** *Nicholas Piramal, India.*
Secnidazole (p.615·3).
*Amoebiasis; bacterial vaginosis; giardiasis; trichomonal vaginitis.*

**Secni-Plus** *Farmoquimica, Braz.*
Secnidazole (p.615·3).
*Amoebiasis; giardiasis.*

**Secnizol** *UCI, Braz.*
Secnidazole (p.615·3).
*Bacterial infections; protozoal infections.*

**Secnol** *IPRAD, Fr.*
Secnidazole (p.615·3).
*Amoebiasis; giardiasis; trichomoniasis.*

**Seco** *Sriprasit, Thai.*
Codeine phosphate (p.27·1); guaifenesin (p.1122·1); terpin hydrate (p.1131·1).
*Coughs.*

**Secokapton** *Strallhofer, Austria.*
Ergotamine tartrate (p.467·2); caffeine (p.782·1).
*Migraine.*

**Seconal**
*Lilly, Canad.†; Lilly, Irl.†; Lilly, S.Afr.†; Flynn, UK; Lilly, USA.*
Secobarbital sodium (p.721·2).
*Insomnia; sedative.*

**Secotex**
*Boehringer Ingelheim, Arg.; Boehringer de Angeli, Braz.; Boehringer Ingelheim, Chile; Promeco, Mex.*
Tamsulosin hydrochloride (p.1009·2).
*Benign prostatic hyperplasia.*

**Secpel** *Medinfar, Port.*
Lactic acid (p.1704·1); lecithin (p.1706·1).
*Seborrhoeic dermatitis of the scalp.*

**Secpel Composto** *Medinfar, Port.*
Ichthammol (p.1148·2); lactic acid (p.1704·1); lecithin (p.1706·1).
*Psoriasis; scalp disorders.*

**Secran** *Scherer, USA.*
Multivitamin preparation (p.1417·1).

**SecreFlo** *RepliGen, USA.*
Secretin (synthetic) (p.1742·3).
*Assessment of pancreatic function.*

**Secrelux** *Goldham, Ger.*
Secretin hydrochloride (p.1743·1).
*Diagnosis of Zollinger-Ellison syndrome; test of pancreatic function.*

**Secrepat** *Abbott, Spain.*
Aluminium hydroxide (p.1249·2); calcium carbonate (p.1254·2); magnesium trisilicate (p.1272·3); aluminium glycinate (p.1249·1).
*Gastrointestinal hyperacidity.*

**Secrepina** *AstraZeneca, Spain†.*
Omeprazole (p.1278·2) or omeprazole sodium (p.1278·2).
*Gastro-oesophageal reflux; peptic ulcer; Zollinger-Ellison syndrome.*

**Secresol** *Permamed, Switz.†.*
Acetylcysteine (p.1112·3).
*Respiratory-tract disorders associated with increased or viscous mucus.*

**Secret 28** *Elea, Arg.*
24 Tablets, gestodene (p.1556·1); ethinylestradiol (p.1553·2); 4 tablets, inert.
*Combined oral contraceptive.*

**Secretil** *Caber, Ital.*
Ambroxol hydrochloride (p.1114·3).
*Respiratory-tract congestion.*

**Sectam** *Locatelli, Ital.†.*
Latamoxef disodium (p.225·3).
*Bacterial infections.*

**Sectral**
*Rhone-Poulenc Rorer, Austria†; Aventis, Belg.; Aventis, Canad.; Aventis, Fr.; Aventis, Hong Kong; Aventis, Irl.; Aventis, Israel; Aventis, Ital.; Aventis, Malaysia; Aventis, Neth.; Aventis, S.Afr.; Aventis, Singapore; Italfarmaco, Spain; Aventis, Switz.; Aventis, UK; ESP, USA.*
Acebutolol hydrochloride (p.848·1).
*Angina pectoris; arrhythmias; hypertension.*

**Sectrazide** *Aventis, Belg.*
Acebutolol hydrochloride (p.848·1); hydrochlorothiazide (p.933·2).
*Hypertension.*

**Secubar** *Elan, Spain.*
Lisinopril (p.946·3).
*Diabetic nephropathy; heart failure; hypertension; myocardial infarction.*

**Secubar Diu** *Elan, Spain.*
Lisinopril (p.946·3); hydrochlorothiazide (p.933·2).
*Hypertension.*

**Secuentex-21** *Searle, Mex.*
15 Tablets, mestranol (p.1559·2); 6 tablets, chlormadinone acetate (p.1542·1); mestranol.
*Sequential oral contraceptive.*

**Se-Cure** *Everett, USA.*
Shark cartilage; vitamin E; vitamin C; zinc oxide; selenium (p.1417·1).
*Nutritional supplement.*

**Securgin** *Menarini, Ital.*
Desogestrel (p.1547·2); ethinylestradiol (p.1553·2).
*Combined oral contraceptive.*

**Securo** *ICN, Arg.*
Ivermectin (p.105·3).
*Onchocerciasis; scabies.*

**Securon** *Abbott, UK.*
Verapamil hydrochloride (p.1019·1).
*Angina pectoris; arrhythmias; hypertension; myocardial infarction.*

**Securopen**
*Bayer, Austria†; Bayer, Ger.†; Bayer, Irl.†; Bayer, Ital.†; Bayer, Norw.†.*
Azlocillin sodium (p.160·2).
*Pseudomonal infections.*

**Securpres** *Monsanto, Ital.*
Indenolol hydrochloride (p.939·1).
*Angina pectoris; arrhythmias; hypertension.*

**Seczol** *Medley, Braz.*
Tioconazole (p.409·3); tinidazole (p.617·1).
*Vaginal infections.*

**Seda Kneipp N** *Kneipp, Ger.†.*
Valerian (p.1762·2); lupulus (p.1708·1).
*Nervous disorders; sleep disorders.*

**Sedabarb** *Be-Tabs, S.Afr.†.*
Phenobarbital (p.367·3).

**Sedabel** *Sedabel, Braz.*
Hyoscine (p.483·3); dipyrone (p.35·3); atropine sulfate (p.477·1).
*Pain; smooth muscle spasm.*

**Sedaben** *Labima, Belg.*
Lormetazepam (p.705·2).
*Insomnia.*

**Sedacalman** *Schwarzwalder, Ger.*
Homoeopathic preparation.

**Sedacollyre** *Cooperation Pharmaceutique, Fr.*
Oxedrine tartrate (p.977·3); berberine hydrochloride (p.1659·3); benzododecinium bromide (p.1170·2).
*Eye congestion.*

**Sedacoron**
*Ebewe, Austria; Ebewe, Hong Kong.*
Amiodarone hydrochloride (p.859·2).
*Arrhythmias.*

**Sedacris** *Elea, Arg.*
Theophylline (p.798·3); guaifenesin (p.1122·1).
*Coughs; obstructive airways disease.*

**Sedactrim** *Sedar, Braz.†.*
Co-trimoxazole (p.199·3).
*Bacterial infections; Pneumocystis carinii pneumonia; protozoal infections.*

**Sedactrim Balsamico** *Sedar, Braz.†.*
Co-trimoxazole (p.199·3); guaifenesin (p.1122·1); ammonium chloride (p.1115·2).
*Bacterial infections.*

**Sedacur** *Schaper & Brummer, Ger.*
Valerian (p.1762·2); lupulus (p.1708·1); melissa (p.1711·1).
*Nervous disorders; sleep disorders.*

**Seda-Do** *Grasler, Ger.*
Homoeopathic preparation.

**Sedadom** *Sanidom, Austria.*
Valerian (p.1762·2); lupulus (p.1708·1).
*Anxiety disorders; sleep disorders.*

**Seda-Gel** *Key, Austral.*
*Lotion:* Cetylpyridinium chloride (p.1173·1); chlorhexidine acetate (p.1173·2); lidocaine (p.1377·3).
*Mouth ulcers; teething and denture pain.*
*Oral gel:* Choline salicylate (p.26·2); menthol (p.1711·3).
*Painful mouth disorders.*

**Sedagin** *Biocontrolfarm, Ital.†.*
Eschscholtzia californica.

**Seda-Grandelat** *Synpharma, Austria.*
Lupulus (p.1708·1); melissa leaf (p.1711·1); orange flower (p.1723·3).
*Anxiety disorders.*

**Sedagripe** *Novaquimica, Braz.†.*
Chlorphenamine maleate (p.427·3); aspirin (p.15·1); methoxyphenamine (p.1124·2); caffeine (p.782·1).
*Cold and influenza symptoms.*

**Sedagul** *Wild, Switz.*
Lidocaine hydrochloride (p.1377·3).
*Local anaesthesia.*

**Sedakatt** *Kattwiga, Ger.*
Homoeopathic preparation.

**Sedalen Cort** *Montefarmaco, Ital.*
Hydrocortisone acetate (p.1103·3); benzocaine (p.1370·3); hamamelis (p.1696·3); aesculus (p.1648·2).
*Anorectal disorders.*

**Sedalene** *Cristalia, Braz.; Gunther, Braz.*
Dipyrone (p.35·3); homatropine methylbromide (p.483·2); papaverine hydrochloride (p.1728·1); adiphenine (p.1648·1).
*Smooth muscle spasm.*

**Sedalex** *Teuto, Braz.*
Orphenadrine citrate (p.486·1); dipyrone (p.35·3); caffeine (p.782·1).
*Pain; smooth muscle spasm.*

**Sedalgina** *Teuto, Braz.*
Isometheptene mucate (p.1702·1); dipyrone (p.35·3); caffeine (p.782·1).
*Pain.*

**Sedalin**
*Note. This name is used for preparations of different composition.*
*Dinafarma, Braz.†.*
Passion flower (p.1729·1); erythrina mulungu (p.1717·2); crataegus (p.1677·1).
*Chi Sheng, Thai.*
Ceftriaxone sodium (p.182·3).
*Bacterial infections.*

**Sedalint Baldrian** *Madaus, Ger.†.*
Valerian root (p.1762·2).
*Nervous disorders; sleep disorders.*

**Sedalint Kava** *Madaus, Ger.†.*
Kava (p.1703·2).
*Anxiety disorders.*

**Sedalipid** *Steigerwald, Ger.*
Magnesium-pyridoxal-5′-phosphate-glutaminate.
*Hyperlipidaemias.*

**Sedalito** *Merck, Mex.*
Paracetamol (p.76·2).
*Fever; pain.*

**Sedalmerck**
*Note. This name is used for preparations of different composition.*
*Merck, Braz.*
Paracetamol (p.76·2); caffeine (p.782·1).
*Fever; pain.*
*Merck, Chile; Merck, Mex.*
Paracetamol (p.76·2); caffeine (p.782·1); pseudoephedrine hydrochloride (p.1129·2).
*Fever; nasal congestion; pain; rhinitis; sinusitis.*
*Merck, Spain.*
Caffeine (p.782·1); ephedrine hydrochloride (p.1120·1); ethylmorphine hydrochloride (p.37·3); propyphenazone (p.85·3).
*Pain.*

**Sedalmerck TH** *Merck, Mex.*
Paracetamol (p.76·2); pseudoephedrine hydrochloride (p.1129·2); dextromethorphan hydrobromide (p.1117·3).
*Allergic rhinitis; coughs; fever; nasal congestion; pain; sinusitis.*

**Sedalozia** *Iphym, Fr.†.*
Crataegus (p.1677·1); eschscholtzia californica; valerian (p.1762·2).
*Insomnia; nervous disorders.*

**Sedalpan** *Teofarma, Ital.*
Methyl nicotinate (p.59·2); diethylamine salicylate (p.34·1).
*Musculoskeletal, joint, and soft-tissue disorders.*

**Sedanium-R** *Coup, Gr.*
Famotidine (p.1265·2).
*Conditions where gastric acid reduction is beneficial; gastric hypersecretion including Zollinger-Ellison syndrome; peptic ulcer.*

**Sedans** *Ganassini, Ital.*
Amitriptyline hydrochloride (p.280·3); chlordiazepoxide hydrochloride (p.674·2).
*Nervous disorders.*

**Sedante Arceli** *Gezzi, Arg.*
Passion flower (p.1729·1); melissa (p.1711·1); valerian (p.1762·2); sage (p.1741·2); tilia (p.1756·2).
*Sedative.*

**Sedante Dia** *Serranita, Arg.*
Passion flower (p.1729·1); valerian (p.1762·2); tilia (p.1756·2).
*Sedative.*

**Sedante Nativa** *Argenfarma, Arg.*
Valerian (p.1762·2).
*Sedative.*

**Sedante Noche** *Serranita, Arg.*
Passion flower (p.1729·1).
*Insomnia.*

**Sedantol**
*Note. This name is used for preparations of different composition.*
*Dovalle, Braz.†.*
Valerian (p.1762·2); melissa (p.1711·1); passion flower (p.1729·1).
*Sedative.*
*Recalcine, Chile.*
Diazepam (p.690·1); chlormezanone (p.675·1).
*Anxiety; insomnia; skeletal muscle spasm.*

**Sedapain** *Garec, S.Afr.*
Paracetamol (p.76·2); doxylamine succinate (p.432·3); caffeine (p.782·1); codeine phosphate (p.27·1).
*Pain with tension.*

**Sedapap** *Merz, USA.*
Paracetamol (p.76·2); butalbital (p.673·3).
*Tension headache.*

**Sedaplaie** *Medeva, Fr.†.*
Dodeclonium bromide (p.1178·3); amylocaine hydrochloride (p.1370·2).
*Burns; wounds.*

**Seda-Plantina** *Plantina, Ger.*
Valerian (p.1762·2); lupulus (p.1708·1); melissa (p.1711·1); passion flower (p.1729·1); rosemary (p.1740·2).
*Agitation; sleep disorders.*

**Sedaplus** *Chephasaar, Ger.; Rosen, Ger.*
Doxylamine succinate (p.432·3).
*Hypersensitivity reactions; nocturnal enuresis; premedication; sleep disorders.*

**Seda-Rash** *Key, Austral.†.*
Zinc oxide (p.1163·2); castor oil (p.1668·2).
*Eczema; heat rash; intertrigo; nappy rash.*

**Sedarene** *Theratech, Fr.*
Paracetamol (p.76·2); codeine phosphate (p.27·1).
*Fever; pain.*

**Sedariston** *Steiner, Ger.*
Valerian root (p.1762·2); hypericum (p.299·1); melissa leaf (p.1711·1).
*Nervous disorders.*

**Sedariston Konzentrat** *Steiner, Ger.*
Hypericum (p.299·1); valerian root (p.1762·2).
*Anxiety disorders; sleep disorders.*

**Sedartryl** *Oberlin, Fr.*
Methyl nicotinate (p.59·2); amyl salicylate (p.14·3); menthol (p.1711·3).
Formerly contained methyl nicotinate, amyl salicylate, salicylic acid, menthol, camphor, turpentine oil, and volatile mustard oil.
*Musculoskeletal and joint pain.*

**Sedaselect** *Dreluso, Ger.*
Homoeopathic preparation.

**Sedaselect D** *Dreluso, Ger.*
Lupulus (p.1708·1); valerian (p.1762·2).
Sedaselect N formerly contained lupulus, valerian, passion flower, and melissa.
*Nervous disorders; sleep disorders.*

**Sedasept**
*Note. This name is used for preparations of different composition.*
*Michaux, Belg.†.*
Chlorhexidine gluconate (p.1173·2); lidocaine hydrochloride (p.1377·3).
Formerly contained acetarsol sodium, sulfanilamide, and thymol.
*Mouth and throat disorders.*
*Sanico, Switz.*
Cineole (p.1672·1); peppermint oil (p.1283·2); thyme oil (p.1755·3); menthol (p.1711·3); thymol (p.1194·2); methyl salicylate (p.59·3).
*Dental inflammation; oral hygiene.*

**Sedasol eco natura** *Ecosol, Switz.*
Valerian (p.1762·2).
*Nervous disorders; sleep disorders.*

**Sedasor** *Soria Natural, Spain.*
Valerian (p.1762·2); crataegus (p.1677·1); passion flower (p.1729·1); spike lavender (p.1749·2).
*Anxiety; insomnia; nervous disorders.*

**Sedaspir** *Bride, Fr.*
Codeine phosphate (p.27·1); caffeine (p.782·1); aspirin (p.15·1).
*Pain.*

**Sedastip** *Milte, Ital.*
Fibre (p.1253·2); vitamins (p.1417·1).
*Constipation.*

**Sedasyx** *Syxyl, Ger.*
Valerian (p.1762·2); lupulus (p.1708·1); melissa (p.1711·1).
*Nervous disorders; sleep disorders.*

**Sedatif PC**
*Boiron, Canad.; Boiron, Fr.; Boiron, Port.; Boiron, Switz.*
Homoeopathic preparation.

**Sedatif Tiber** *Phytoprevent, Fr.*
Crataegus (p.1677·1); passion flower (p.1729·1); potassium bromide (p.1663·1); sodium bromide (p.1663·1).
*Anxiety; insomnia.*

**Sedatival**
*Note. This name is used for preparations of different composition.*
*Raffo, Arg.*
Lorazepam (p.704·1).
*Anxiety.*

Recalcine, Chile.
Ketazolam (p.703·1).
*Anxiety; skeletal muscle spasm.*

**Sedativum-Hevert** Hevert, Ger.
Diphenhydramine hydrochloride (p.431·3).
*Anxiety; hypersensitivity reactions; motion sickness; nausea; sleep disorders; vomiting.*

**Sedatol** EG, Ital.
*Capsules:* Passion flower (p.1729·1); valerian (p.1762·2); crataegus (p.1677·1); chamomile (p.1669·3); piscidia (p.1702·3).
*Syrup:* Passion flower (p.1729·1); chamomile (p.1669·3); crataegus (p.1677·1); piscidia (p.1702·3); melissa (p.1711·1).
*Insomnia.*

**Sedatonyl** Lipha Sante, Fr.†.
Phenobarbital (p.367·3); crataegus (p.1677·1).
*Anxiety; insomnia.*

**Sedatoss** Janssen-Cilag, Braz.†.
Fedrilate (p.1121·2).
*Coughs.*

**Sedatruw S** Truw, Ger.†.
Valerian (p.1762·2); lupulus (p.1708·1); melissa (p.1711·1).
*Nervous disorders; sleep disorders.*

**Sedatus** Elvetium, Arg.
Bromazepam (p.671·3).
*Anxiety.*

**Sedatuss** Trianon, Canad.†.
Dextromethorphan hydrobromide (p.1117·3); chlorphenamine maleate (p.427·3); guaiacol (p.1122·1); pseudoephedrine hydrochloride (p.1129·2).
*Coughs.*

**Sedatuss DM** Trianon, Canad.
Dextromethorphan hydrobromide (p.1117·3).

**Sedatux** EMS, Braz.
Potassium iodide (p.1598·1); lobelia (p.1589·1); hyoscyamus (p.485·2).
*Respiratory-tract congestion.*

**Sedauric** Laborsil, Braz.†.
Tyrothricin (p.275·1); urea (p.1162·2).
*Ear infections.*

**Sedazin** Lagap, Switz.
Lorazepam (p.704·1).
*Anxiety; premedication; sleep disorders.*

**Sedergine**
Bristol-Myers Squibb, Belg.; Bristol-Myers Squibb, Port.†; Uriach, Spain.
Aspirin (p.15·1).
*Fever; musculoskeletal, joint and peri-articular disorders; pain; thromboembolism prophylaxis.*

**Sedergine C**
Bristol-Myers Squibb, Belg.; Uriach, Spain.
Aspirin (p.15·1); ascorbic acid (p.1460·2).
*Fever; pain.*

**Sedermyl** Cooperation Pharmaceutique, Fr.
Isothipendyl hydrochloride (p.435·2).
*Insect stings; pruritus.*

**Sedesterol** Poen, Arg.
Dexamethasone (p.1097·1).
*Inflammatory eye disorders.*

**Sedevil** Collins, Mex.
Pseudoephedrine (p.1129·2); chlorphenamine (p.428·1).
*Cold and influenza symptoms.*

**Sedex** Janssen-Cilag, Port.
Flunitrazepam (p.698·2).

**Sediat** Pfleger, Ger.
Diphenhydramine hydrochloride (p.431·3).
*Sleep disorders.*

**Sedibaine** Marion Merrell, Fr.†.
Phenobarbital (p.367·3); crataegus (p.1677·1); ballota; valerian (p.1762·2).
Formerly contained strophanthus, phenobarbital, hyoscyamus, crataegus, ballota, valerian, and belladonna.
*Nervous disorders.*

**Sedicepan** Serra Pamies, Spain.
Lorazepam (p.704·1).
*Alcohol withdrawal syndrome; anxiety; insomnia; nausea; premedication; vomiting.*

**Sediclon** Degorts, Mex.
Dicycloverine (p.481·2).

**Sediel** Sumitomo, Jpn.
Tandospirone citrate (p.723·2).
*Anxiety; depression; phobias; sleep disorders.*

**Sedilax** Teuto, Braz.
Carisoprodol (p.1392·1); diclofenac sodium (p.32·1); paracetamol (p.76·2); caffeine (p.782·1).
*Pain; smooth muscle spasm.*

**Sedilene Procto** Montefarmaco, Ital.
Benzocaine (p.1370·3); aesculus (p.1648·2); hamamelis (p.1696·3).
*Anorectal disorders.*

**Sedilit** Instituto Sanitas, Chile.
Diazepam (p.690·1); chlormezanone (p.675·1).
*Anxiety; insomnia; skeletal muscle spasm.*

**Sedilix**
Note. This name is used for preparations of different composition.
Xepa-Soul Pattinson, Malaysia.
Promethazine hydrochloride (p.439·1); codeine phosphate (p.27·1).
*Coughs.*

Xepa-Soul Pattinson, Singapore.
Codeine phosphate (p.27·1); promethazine hydrochloride (p.439·1); ephedrine hydrochloride (p.1120·1).
*Coughs.*

**Sedilix DM**
Xepa-Soul Pattinson, Hong Kong†; Xepa-Soul Pattinson, Malaysia; Xepa-Soul Pattinson, Singapore.
Dextromethorphan hydrobromide (p.1117·3); pseudoephedrine hydrochloride (p.1129·2); promethazine hydrochloride (p.439·1).
*Coughs; nasal congestion.*

**Sedilor** Dolisos, Canad.
Homoeopathic preparation.

**Sedinal** Melisana, Belg.
Crataegus (p.1677·1); ballota; passion flower (p.1729·1).
*Nervous disorders.*

**Sedinfant N** Biocur, Ger.
Valerian (p.1762·2); melissa (p.1711·1); passion flower (p.1729·1).
*Agitation; excitability; sleep disorders.*

**Sedinol** Aspen, S.Afr.
Doxylamine succinate (p.432·3); paracetamol (p.76·2); codeine phosphate (p.27·1); caffeine (p.782·1).
*Pain and associated tension.*

**Sedioton** Wyeth Lederle, Port.
Ambutonium bromide (p.1653·2); oxazepam (p.712·2).

**Sedisan** Bioquimico, Mex.†.
Trifluoperazine (p.726·3).

**Sediten** Taro, Israel†.
Fluphenazine hydrochloride (p.699·3).
*Anxiety.*

**Sediver** Maver, Mex.†.
Diazepam (p.690·1).
*Anxiety; muscle spasm; sedative.*

**Sedizepan** Septa, Spain†.
Lorazepam (p.704·1).
*Alcohol withdrawal syndrome; anxiety; epilepsy; insomnia; nausea; vomiting.*

**Sedo** Rapide, Spain†.
Methadone (p.58·3).
*Diamorphine detoxification; opioid withdrawal; pain.*

**Sedobex** Ecobi, Ital.†.
Sodium dibunate (p.1130·2); grindelia (p.1696·1); cardamom (p.1667·3); lattuca sativa; sodium benzoate (p.1169·3).
*Bronchial disorders; coughs.*

**Sedobion** Sintofarma, Braz.†.
Dipyrone (p.35·3); hyoscine methobromide (p.483·3).
*Smooth muscle spasm.*

**Sedobrina** Vinas, Spain†.
Lormetazepam (p.705·2).
*Insomnia.*

**Sedocalcio** Deca, Ital.
Calcium lactate (p.1225·3); sodium benzoate (p.1169·3).
*Mouth and throat disorders.*

**Sedocardin** Pfluger, Ger.
Homoeopathic preparation.

**Sedodermil** Vifor, Switz.†.
Methyl anthranilate (p.1154·1); pentyl valerate; bornyl salicylate (p.21·2); laurus nobilis oil; menthol (p.1711·3).
*Musculoskeletal and joint pain.*

**Sedofan** Julphar, UAE.
Triprolidine hydrochloride (p.442·3); pseudoephedrine hydrochloride (p.1129·2).
*Cold symptoms; upper respiratory-tract congestion.*

**Sedofan II** Julphar, UAE.
Pseudoephedrine hydrochloride (p.1129·2).
*Nasal congestion; otitis media; sinusitis.*

**Sedofan DM** Julphar, UAE.
Triprolidine hydrochloride (p.442·3); pseudoephedrine hydrochloride (p.1129·2); dextromethorphan hydrobromide (p.1117·3).
*Upper respiratory-tract disorders.*

**Sedofan P** Julphar, UAE.
Dextromethorphan hydrobromide (p.1117·3).
*Coughs.*

**Sedofan T** Julphar, UAE.
Triprolidine hydrochloride (p.442·3).
*Allergic rhinitis; hypersensitivity reactions.*

**Sedofantil** Pharmafina, Chile.
Calcium bromolactobionate (p.674·1).
*Hyperactivity in children.*

**Sedofarin** Pensa, Spain.
Dequalinium chloride (p.1178·1); dexamethasone (p.1097·1); benzocaine (p.1370·3); tyrothricin (p.275·1).
*Mouth and throat disorders.*

**Sedofit** Body Spring, Ital.
Magnesium (p.1227·3); crataegus (p.1677·1); eschscholtzia; passion flower (p.1729·1); tilia (p.1756·2); pyridoxine (p.1457·2).
*Anxiety; insomnia.*

**Sedogastrol** Recalcine, Chile.
Chlordiazepoxide hydrochloride (p.674·2); clidinium bromide (p.480·2).
*Gastrointestinal motility disorders; smooth muscle spasm.*

**Sedogelat** Metochem, Austria.
Valerian root (p.1762·2); melissa (p.1711·1); passion flower (p.1729·1).
*Anxiety disorders; sleep disorders.*

**Sedogelat forte** Metochem, Austria.
Valerian (p.1762·2); melissa (p.1711·1).
*Anxiety disorders; sleep disorders.*

**Sedol**
Note. This name is used for preparations of different composition.
Cazi, Braz.
Isometheptene hydrochloride (p.1702·1) or isometheptene mucate (p.1702·1); dipyrone (p.35·3); caffeine (p.782·1).

OFF, Ital.
Propyphenazone (p.85·3); caffeine (p.782·1).
*Fever; influenza symptoms; neuralgia.*

**Sedonat** Soria Natural, Spain.
Passion flower (p.1729·1); crataegus (p.1677·1); valerian (p.1762·2); bitter orange oil (p.1723·3).
*Insomnia; sedative; stress.*

**Sedonium**
Lichtwer, Ger.; Medichemie Bioline, Switz.; Lichtwer, UK.
Valerian (p.1762·2).
*Agitation; insomnia.*

**Sedopal** Lehning, Fr.
Crataegus (p.1677·1); eschscholtzia californica; melilotus officinalis.
*Insomnia; nervous disorders.*

**Sedopect** Silesia, Chile.
Pseudoephedrine hydrochloride (p.1129·2); chlorphenamine maleate (p.427·3); codeine phosphate (p.27·1).
*Cold and influenza symptoms; coughs.*

**Sedophon** Mayoly-Spindler, Fr.†.
Ethylmorphine hydrochloride (p.37·3); aconite (p.1646·3); guaifenesin (p.1122·1).
*Coughs.*

**Sedopretten** Schoning-Berlin, Ger.
Diphenhydramine hydrochloride (p.431·3).
*Insomnia.*

**Sedopuer F** SIT, Ital.
Passion flower (p.1729·1); valerian (p.1762·2); crataegus (p.1677·1); calcium glycerophosphate (p.1225·2).
*Insomnia; nervous disorders.*

**Sedoran** Raffo, Chile.
Sertraline (p.317·3).
*Depression; obsessive-compulsive disorder.*

**Sedorrhoide** Cooperation Pharmaceutique, Fr.†.
Dodeclonium (p.1178·3); benzocaine (p.1370·3); esculoside (p.1648·2); enoxolone (p.36·2).
*Anorectal disorders.*

**Sedosan N** Grossmann, Switz.
Crataegus (p.1677·1).
Sedosan formerly contained crataegus and passion flower.
*Nervous disorders.*

**Sedosil** Vifor, Switz.†.
Pimethixene (p.439·1).
*Nervous disorders.*

**Sedosolvin** Ipca, India.
Dextromethorphan hydrobromide (p.1117·3); chlorphenamine maleate (p.427·3); bromhexine (p.1115·3).
*Coughs.*

**Sedotensil** Sanofi Synthelabo, Arg.
Lisinopril (p.946·3).
*Heart failure; hypertension.*

**Sedotime** Iquinosa, Spain.
Ketazolam (p.703·1).
*Anxiety; insomnia; skeletal muscle spasm.*

**Sedotus** Andromaco, Chile.
Tolu (p.1131·3); pectoral; drosera (p.1683·1); quillaia (p.1416·1).
*Coughs.*

**Sedotusse** Helsinn, Port.
Codeine phosphate (p.27·1); ephedrine hydrochloride (p.1120·1).
*Coughs.*

**Sedotussin**
Note. This name is used for preparations of different composition.
UCB, Austria; UCB, Ger.
Pentoxyverine (p.1126·2), pentoxyverine citrate (p.1126·2), or pentoxyverine hydrochloride (p.1126·3).
*Coughs.*

UCB, Switz.
*Oral drops:* Pentoxyverine citrate (p.1126·2); terpin hydrate (p.1131·1); cineole (p.1672·1); menthol (p.1711·3); thymol (p.1194·2); guaifenesin (p.1122·1).
*Suppositories:* Pentoxyverine (p.1126·2); terpin hydrate (p.1131·1); terpineol (p.1752·2); cineole (p.1672·1); guaifenesin (p.1122·1).
*Syrup†:* Pentoxyverine citrate (p.1126·2); terpin hydrate (p.1131·1); cineole (p.1672·1); menthol (p.1711·3); thyme (p.1755·2).
*Coughs and associated respiratory-tract disorders.*

**Sedotussin Efeu** UCB, Ger.
Hedera helix.
*Bronchitis; catarrh.*

**Sedotussin Expectorans** UCB, Ger.†.
*Oral drops:* Pentoxyverine citrate (p.1126·2); terpin (p.1131·1); cineole (p.1672·1); menthol (p.1711·3); thymol (p.1194·2); guaifenesin (p.1122·1).
*Syrup:* Pentoxyverine citrate (p.1126·2); terpin (p.1131·1); cineole (p.1672·1); menthol (p.1711·3); thyme (p.1755·2).
*Coughs and associated respiratory-tract disorders.*

**Sedotussin muco** UCB, Ger.
Carbocisteine (p.1116·2).
*Respiratory-tract disorders with excess or viscous mucus.*

**Sedotussin plus** UCB, Ger.
Pentoxyverine citrate (p.1126·2); chlorphenamine maleate (p.427·3).
*Coughs.*

**Sedovegan** Wolff, Ger.
Hypericum (p.299·1).
*Depression.*

**Sedovegan Novo** Wolff, Ger.†.
Diphenhydramine hydrochloride (p.431·3).
*Insomnia.*

**Sedovent** Schworer, Ger.
Cinnamon (p.1672·2); dried bitter-orange peel (p.1723·3); achillea (p.1646·2); gentian (p.1692·2).
*Gastrointestinal disorders.*

**Sedoxil** Medibial, Port.
Mexazolam (p.707·1).
*Anxiety disorders.*

**Sedural** Rekah, Israel.
Phenazopyridine hydrochloride (p.83·1).
*Urinary-tract pain and irritation.*

**Seduspar** QIF, Braz.†.
Buspirone hydrochloride (p.672·2).
*Anxiety.*

**Sefal** Sepi, Ital.
Alfacalcidol (p.1461·2).
*Hypoparathyroidism; osteomalacia; osteoporosis; renal osteodystrophy; rickets.*

**Sefaretic**
Unison, Hong Kong; Unison, Thai.
Amiloride hydrochloride (p.858·2); hydrochlorothiazide (p.933·2).
*Heart failure; hepatic cirrhosis with ascites; hypertension.*

**Sefasin** Macrophar, Thai.
Cefalexin (p.168·1).
*Bacterial infections.*

**Sefdene** Unison, Hong Kong.
Piroxicam (p.84·2).
*Gout; musculoskeletal and joint disorders.*

**Sefdin** Unichem, India.
Cefdinir (p.171·3).
*Bacterial infections.*

**Seferin** General Drugs, Thai.
Aspirin (p.15·1).
*Inflammation; musculoskeletal and joint disorders; pain.*

**Sefloc** Unison, Hong Kong.
Metoprolol tartrate (p.957·1).
*Angina pectoris; arrhythmias; hypertension.*

**Sefmal**
Unison, Hong Kong; Unison, Singapore; Unison, Thai.
Tramadol hydrochloride (p.94·3).
*Pain.*

**Sefmex**
Unison, Hong Kong; Unison, Thai.
Selegiline hydrochloride (p.1214·1).
*Alzheimer's disease; parkinsonism.*

**Sefmic**
Unison, Hong Kong; Unison, Thai.
Mefenamic acid (p.55·2).
*Pain.*

**Sefnor** Unison, Singapore.
Norfloxacin (p.238·3).
*Bacterial infections.*

**Seforman** Valdecasas, Mex.†.
Furazolidone (p.605·2).

**Seftem** Shionogi, Jpn.
Ceftibuten (p.182·1).
*Bacterial infections.*

**Seftil**
Unison, Hong Kong; Unison, Malaysia; Unison, Thai.
Tenoxicam (p.93·1).
*Gout; inflammation; musculoskeletal, joint, and periarticular disorders.*

**Sefulken** Kendrick, Mex.
Diazoxide (p.893·2).
*Hypertension.*

**Segel** Diba, Mex.
Aluminium hydroxide (p.1249·2); glycine (p.1433·3); calcium carbonate (p.1254·2); dimeticone (p.1289·2).
*Gastrointestinal hyperacidity.*

**Seglor**
Schwarz, Fr.; Pharmafar, Ital.; Sanofi Synthelabo, Port.
Dihydroergotamine mesilate (p.465·3).
*Headache; migraine; orthostatic hypotension; peripheral vascular disorders; vertigo.*

**Segurex** Gador, Arg.
Sildenafil (p.1744·2).
*Erectile dysfunction.*

**Seguril** Aventis, Spain.
Furosemide (p.919·3).
*Forced diuresis; heart failure; hypertension; nephrotic syndrome; oedema; oliguria; renal failure.*

**Seide** Rafarm, Gr.
Roxithromycin (p.254·2).
*Bacterial infections.*

**Seikivita** Ortoquimica, Braz.†.
Cyanocobalamin; pyridoxine hydrochloride; linolenic acid (p.1417·1).

**Seis-B** Apsen, Braz.
Pyridoxine hydrochloride (p.1456·3).
*Vitamin $B_6$ deficiency.*

**Sejungin B** Bock, Ger.†.
Homoeopathic preparation.

**Sekalax** Kener, Mex.
Sennosides A and B (p.1288·2).
*Constipation.*

**Seki**
Zambon, Braz.; Zambon, Ital.
Cloperastine fendizoate (p.1117·2) or cloperastine hydrochloride (p.1117·2).
*Coughs.*

**Sekin** Almirall, Belg.
Cloperastine fendizoate (p.1117·2) or cloperastine hydrochloride (p.1117·2).
*Coughs.*

**Sekisan** Almirall, Spain.
Cloperastine fendizoate (p.1117·2) or cloperastine hydrochloride (p.1117·2).
*Coughs.*

**Sekitol** Sinteropico, Braz.†.
Diphenhydramine (p.431·3); ammonium chloride (p.1115·2).
*Coughs.*

**Sekretolin** Hoechst, Ger.†.
Secretin hydrochloride (p.1743·1).
*Diagnosis of pancreatic disorders and Zollinger-Ellison syndrome.*

**Sekretovit**
Boehringer Ingelheim, Austria; Boehringer Ingelheim, Mex.
Ambroxol hydrochloride (p.1114·3).
*Respiratory-tract congestion.*

**Sekretovit Amoxi** Boehringer Ingelheim, Mex.
Ambroxol hydrochloride (p.1114·3); amoxicillin trihydrate (p.155·3).
*Respiratory-tract infections.*

**Sekretovit Ex** Boehringer Ingelheim, Mex.
Ambroxol hydrochloride (p.1114·3); clenbuterol hydrochloride (p.784·2).
*Respiratory-tract congestion.*

**Sekucid**
Note. This name is used for preparations of different composition.
Paragerm, Fr.
Glutaral (p.1180·3).
*Instrument disinfection.*

Henkel, Ital.
Glutaral (p.1180·3); isopropyl alcohol (p.1184·3).
*Instrument disinfection.*

**Sekucid konz** Henkel, Ger.
Glutaral (p.1180·3); isopropyl alcohol (p.1184·3); ethylhexanal.
*Instrument disinfection.*

**Sekudrill**
Henkel, Ger.; Henkel, Ital.
Potassium hydroxide (p.1734·2); propylene glycol (p.1735·2).
*Instrument disinfection.*

**Sekugerm** Henkel, Ital.†.
Glutaral (p.1180·3); glyoxal (p.1181·1).
*Disinfection of fibre-optic equipment; endoscope disinfection.*

**Sekumatic** Henkel, Ital.
Glutaral (p.1180·3); alcohol (p.1166·1); chloroform; acetone.
*Instrument disinfection.*

**Sekumatic FD** Henkel, Ger.
Glutaral (p.1180·3).
*Instrument disinfection.*

**Sekumatic FDR** Henkel, Ger.
Glucoprotamine (p.1180·3); didecylmethylpoly(oxyethyl) ammonium propionate; tributyltetradecylphosphonium chloride.
*Surface and instrument disinfection.*

**Sekusept** Henkel, Ger.
Peracetic acid (p.1187·3).
*Instrument and surface disinfection.*

**Sekusept Extra N**
Henkel, Ger.; Henkel, Ital.
Benzalkonium chloride (p.1168·3); glutaral (p.1180·3).
*Instrument disinfection.*

**Sekusept forte** Henkel, Ger.
Formaldehyde (p.1179·3); glyoxal (p.1181·1); glutaral (p.1180·3); benzalkonium chloride (p.1168·3).
*Instrument disinfection.*

**Sekusept forte S** Henkel, Ger.
Formaldehyde (p.1179·3); glutaral (p.1180·3).
*Instrument disinfection.*

**Sekusept N** Henkel, Ital.
Peracetic acid (p.1187·3).
*Instrument disinfection.*

**Sekusept Plus** Henkel, Ger.
Glucoprotamine (p.1180·3).
*Instrument disinfection.*

**Sel D** Pharmadeveloppement, Fr.
Sodium chloride; sodium phosphate; sodium sulfate; sodium iodide; sodium bromide (p.1417·1).
*Dietary salt substitute.*

**Sel d'Ems** Siemens, Switz.
Natural sels d'Ems.
*Upper respiratory-tract disorders.*

**Seladin**
YSP, Malaysia; Yung Shin, Singapore.
Naproxen (p.65·1).
*Gout; musculoskeletal and joint disorders.*

**Selan** Iquinosa, Spain.
Cefuroxime axetil (p.184·1).
*Bacterial infections.*

**Selanac** Whitehall, Braz.†.
Magaldrate (p.1271·3).
*Gastrointestinal hyperacidity.*

**Selanir** Selvi, Ital.
Cefaclor (p.167·1).
*Bacterial infections.*

**Selax** Odan, Canad.
Docusate sodium (p.1262·2).
*Constipation.*

**Selaxa** Proel, Gr.
Amikacin sulfate (p.154·1).
*Bacterial infections.*

**Selbex**
Eisai, Jpn; Eisai, Thai.
Teprenone (p.1293·3).
*Gastric ulcer; gastritis.*

**Sel'bis** Expanpharm, Fr.†.
Potassium chloride (p.1417·1); ammonium chloride; calcium formate; glutamic acid.
*Dietary salt substitute.*

**Seldane** Hoechst Marion Roussel, Canad.†.
Terfenadine (p.441·1).
*Hypersensitivity reactions.*

**Selebound** Slopak, Arg.
Selenium (p.1444·1).
*Dietary supplement.*

**Selecid** Leo, Port.
Pivmecillinam hydrochloride (p.244·2).
*Salmonella enteritis; urinary-tract infections.*

**Selecim** Cimex, Switz.
Selegiline hydrochloride (p.1214·1).
*Parkinsonism.*

**Selecom** Fulton, Ital.
Selegiline hydrochloride (p.1214·1).
*Parkinsonism.*

**Select 1/35** Dispensapharm, Canad.
Norethisterone (p.1562·2); ethinylestradiol (p.1553·2).
*Combined oral contraceptive.*

**Selectadoce** Diba, Mex.
Thiamine (p.1455·2); pyridoxine (p.1457·2); hydroxocobalamin (p.1458·2).
*Anaemias; neuritis.*

**Selectadril** Diba, Mex.
Metoprolol tartrate (p.957·1).
*Hypertension; myocardial infarction.*

**Selectafer N** Dreluso, Ger.
Iron sucrose (p.1438·2); cyanocobalamin (p.1458·2); folic acid (p.1429·1).
*Primary and secondary anaemias; tonic.*

**Selectan** Schering, Arg.
Norethisterone acetate (p.1562·2).
*Adjunct in hormone replacement therapy.*

**Selecten** Unipharm, Israel†.
Fluphenazine hydrochloride (p.699·3).
*Anxiety; psychoses.*

**Selectin** Bristol-Myers Squibb, Ital.
Pravastatin sodium (p.984·3).
*Atherosclerosis; hypercholesterolaemia.*

**Selecto** Diba, Mex.
Pancreatin (p.1725·3).
*Pancreatic insufficiency.*

**Selectocalcio** Asta Medica, Braz.
Calcium lactate; ergocalciferol; calcium phosphate; cyanocobalamin; sodium fluoride (p.1417·1).
*Nutritional supplement.*

**Selecto-D** Diba, Mex.
Pancreatin (p.1725·3); dimeticone (p.1289·2).
*Gastrointestinal disorders.*

**Selectofen** Diba, Mex.
Diclofenac sodium (p.32·1).
*And soft-tissue disorders; gout; inflammation; musculoskeletal, joint; pain.*

**Selectofur** Diba, Mex.
Furosemide (p.919·3).
*Hypertension; oedema.*

**Selectografin** Schering, Ital.†.
Sodium amidotrizoate (p.1060·2); meglumine amidotrizoate (p.1060·2).
*Contrast medium for urography and angiography.*

**Selectol**
Gerot, Austria; Pharmacia, Belg.; Aventis, Chile; Leiras, Fin.; Pharmacia, Ger.; Aventis, Gr.; Aventis, Hong Kong; Aventis, Irl.; Shinyaku, Jpn; Aventis, NZ†; Aventis, Switz.
Celiprolol hydrochloride (p.881·3).
*Angina pectoris; arrhythmias; hypertension.*

**Selectomycin** Grunenthal, Ger.
Spiramycin (p.255·3).
*Bacterial infections; toxoplasmosis.*

**Selectovit** Diba, Mex.
Vitamin B substances (p.1417·1).

**Selectrim** Ciforma, Braz.†.
Co-trimoxazole (p.199·3).
*Bacterial infections.*

**Selecturon** Gerot, Austria.
Celiprolol hydrochloride (p.881·3); chlortalidone (p.882·3).
*Hypertension.*

**Selectus**
Note. This name is used for preparations of different composition.
Purissimus, Arg.
Dextromethorphan hydrobromide (p.1117·3); bromhexine hydrochloride (p.1115·3).
*Coughs.*

BA Farma, Port.
Fluoxetine hydrochloride (p.292·1).
*Bulimia nervosa; depression; mixed anxiety depressive disorders; obsessive-compulsive disorder.*

BA Farma, Port.
Fluoxetine (p.296·3).

**Selectus FN** Purissimus, Arg.
Clofedanol hydrochloride (p.1117·1); bromhexine hydrochloride (p.1115·3).
*Coughs.*

**Seledat** Master Pharma, Ital.
Selegiline hydrochloride (p.1214·1).
*Psychiatric disorders.*

**Seledie** Inverni della Beffa, Ital.
Nadroparin calcium (p.963·3).
*Venous thrombosis.*

**Selefusin** Pisa, Mex.
Selenium (p.1444·1).

**Selegam** Hexal, Ger.
Selegiline hydrochloride (p.1214·1).
*Parkinsonism.*

**Selegel**
Pierre Fabre, Arg.; Ducray, Fr.
Selenium sulfide (p.1157·3).
*Seborrhoeic dermatitis.*

**Selegil** Diba, Mex.
Metronidazole (p.607·2) or metronidazole benzoate (p.607·2).
*Amoebiasis; giardiasis; trichomoniasis.*

**Selegos**
Medochemie, Hong Kong; Medochemie, Malaysia; Medochemie, Singapore.
Selegiline hydrochloride (p.1214·1).
*Parkinsonism.*

**Selektine** Bristol-Myers Squibb, Neth.
Pravastatin sodium (p.984·3).
*Hypercholesterolaemia.*

**Selemax** Novartis Consumer, Ital.†.
Selenium; betacarotene; vitamin E; vitamin C; zinc; copper (p.1417·1).
*Antoxidant nutritional supplement.*

**Selemerck** Merck dura, Ger.
Selegiline hydrochloride (p.1214·1).
*Parkinsonism.*

**Selemite-B** Blackmores, Austral.†.
Selenomethionine.
*Selenium deficiency.*

**Selemix** Provita, Ital.†.
Vitamins; minerals; ubidecarenone (p.1417·1).

**Selemun** Biosyn, Ger.
Sodium selenite (p.1444·1).
*Selenium deficiency.*

**Selemycin**
Medochemie, Hong Kong; Medochemie, Malaysia; Medochemie, Singapore†.
Amikacin sulfate (p.154·1).
*Bacterial infections.*

**Selen** Fresenius Kabi, Austria.
Sodium selenite (p.1444·1).
*Dietary supplement.*

**Selenarell** Sanorell, Ger.
Homoeopathic preparation.

**Selenase**
Richter, Austria; Biosyn, Ger.; Biosyn, Switz.
Sodium selenite (p.1444·1).
*Selenium deficiency.*

**Selene** Eurofarma, Braz.
Ethinylestradiol (p.1553·2); cyproterone acetate (p.1544·1).
*Androgenic symptoms in women; polycystic ovary syndrome.*

**Selenio Composto** Catarinense, Braz.
Vitamin and mineral preparation (p.1417·1).

**Selenion** Labcatal, Fr.
Selenium (p.1444·1).
*Muscular disorders; skin disorders.*

**Selenium Bonus** Lifeplan, UK.
Selenium; chromium; zinc; vitamins (p.1417·1).
*Antoxidant preparation.*

**Selenium E** Biomedica, Austral.†.
Selenomethionine; *d*-alpha tocoferil acid succinate (p.1465·1).
*Dietary supplement.*

**Selenium Med Complex** Dynamit, Austria.
Homoeopathic preparation.

**Selenium Plus** Sisu, Canad.
Selenium (p.1444·1); methionine (p.1042·1).

**Selenium-ACE**
Richelet, Fr.; Helsinn, Port.; Wassen, UK†.
Selenium yeast (p.1444·1); vitamins A, C, and E (p.1417·1).

Wassen, Ital.
Selenium (p.1444·1); vitamins A, C, and E; betacarotene (p.1417·1).

**Selenix** Novartis Consumer, Port.
Selenium sulfide (p.1157·3).
*Dandruff; pityriasis versicolor.*

**Seleno-6** Solgar, UK†.
Selenomethionine.
*Dietary supplement.*

**Selenokehl** Sanum-Kehlbeck, Ger.
Homoeopathic preparation.

**Selenol** Propharma, Denm.
Selenium sulfide (p.1157·3).
*Pityriasis versicolor; seborrhoeic dermatitis.*

**Selen-Wied** Wiedemann, Ger.
Homoeopathic preparation.

**Sele-Pak** Smith & Nephew SoloPak, USA.
Selenious acid (p.1444·1).
*Parenteral nutrition.*

**Seleparina** Italfarmaco, Ital.
Nadroparin calcium (p.963·3).
*Thrombosis prophylaxis.*

**Selepark** Betapharm, Ger.
Selegiline hydrochloride (p.1214·1).
*Parkinsonism.*

**Selepen**
Fujisawa, Hong Kong; American Pharmaceutical, USA.
Selenious acid (p.1444·1).
*Parenteral nutrition.*

**Seleplus** Chemedica, Switz.†.
Selenium yeast; vitamins A, C, and E (p.1417·1).
*Selenium deficiency.*

**Seler** Pasteur, Chile.
Sildenafil citrate (p.1744·2).
*Erectile dysfunction.*

**Seles Beta** Schwarz, Ital.
Atenolol (p.865·2).
*Angina pectoris; hypertension.*

**Selexid**
Leo, Austria; Leo, Belg.; Leo, Canad.; Leo, Denm.; Leo, Fin.; Leo, Fr.; Leo, Norw.; CSL, NZ; Leo, NZ; Leo, Swed.; Leo, UK.
Mecillinam (p.228·3), pivmecillinam (p.244·2), or pivmecillinam hydrochloride (p.244·2).
*Bacterial infections of the urinary tract.*

**Selexid N** Leo (Λεο), Gr.
Mecillinam (p.228·3).
*Bacterial infections.*

**Selezen** Teofarma, Ital.
Imidazole salicylate (p.47·2).
*Fever; inflammation; pain.*

**Selg** Promefarm, Ital.
Macrogol 4000 (p.1709·1); electrolytes (p.1217·1).
*Bowel evacuation; constipation.*

**Selgene**
Alphapharm, Austral.; Pacific, NZ; Merck, Thai.†.
Selegiline hydrochloride (p.1214·1).
*Parkinsonism.*

**Selg-Esse** Promefarm, Ital.
Macrogol 4000 (p.1709·1); simeticone (p.1289·2); electrolytes (p.1217·1).
*Bowel evacuation.*

**Selgimed** Hennig, Ger.
Selegiline hydrochloride (p.1214·1).
*Parkinsonism.*

**Selgin** Intas, India.
Selegiline hydrochloride (p.1214·1).
*Parkinsonism.*

**Selgina** Andromaco, Chile.
Selegiline hydrochloride (p.1214·1).
*Parkinsonism.*

**Selgine** Teofarma, Fr.
Sodium chloride (p.1233·3); sea salt.
*Mouth disorders.*

**Selimax** Libbs, Braz.
Azithromycin (p.159·1).
*Bacterial infections.*

**Seline** Berlin Pharm, Thai.
Selegiline hydrochloride (p.1214·1).
*Parkinsonism.*

**Selinol** Orion, Swed.
Atenolol (p.865·2).
*Angina pectoris; arrhythmias; hypertension.*

**Selipran**
Bristol-Myers Squibb, Austria; Bristol-Myers Squibb, Switz.
Pravastatin sodium (p.984·3).
*Coronary atherosclerosis; hypercholesterolaemia.*

**Selit** Biosyn, Ger.†.
Sodium selenite (p.1444·1).
*Selenium deficiency.*

**Selm** Precimex, Mex.†.
Methyldopa (p.953·2).

**Selobloc** Lagap, Switz.†.
Atenolol (p.865·2).
*Angina pectoris; arrhythmias; hypertension.*

**Selocomp ZOC** Pharmacia, Fin.
Metoprolol succinate (p.957·1); hydrochlorothiazide (p.933·2).
*Hypertension.*

**Selokeen** AstraZeneca, Neth.
Metoprolol succinate (p.957·1) or metoprolol tartrate (p.957·1).
*Angina pectoris; arrhythmias; hypertension; hyperthyroidism; migraine; myocardial infarction.*

**Seloken**
AstraZeneca, Austria; AstraZeneca, Belg.; AstraZeneca, Braz.; AstraZeneca, Denm.; AstraZeneca, Fin.; AstraZeneca, Fr.; AstraZeneca, Ital.; Astra, Jpn; AstraZeneca, Mex.; AstraZeneca, Norw.; AstraZeneca, Spain†; Hassle, Swed.
Metoprolol succinate (p.957·1) or metoprolol tartrate (p.957·1).
*Angina pectoris; arrhythmias; cardiomyopathy; hypertension; hyperthyroidism; migraine; myocardial infarction.*

**Seloken retard Plus** Sanova, Austria.
Metoprolol succinate (p.957·1); hydrochlorothiazide (p.933·2).
*Hypertension.*

**Seloken ZOC**
AstraZeneca, Fin.; Hassle, Swed.
Metoprolol succinate (p.957·1).
*Angina pectoris; arrhythmias; hypertension; migraine; myocardial infarction.*

**Seloken ZOC/ASA** AstraZeneca, Fin.; Hassle, Swed.
Tablet I, metoprolol succinate (p.957·1); tablet II, aspirin (p.15·1).
*Angina pectoris; myocardial infarction.*

**Selokomb** AstraZeneca, Neth.†.
Metoprolol succinate (p.957·1) or metoprolol tartrate (p.957·1); hydrochlorothiazide (p.933·2).
*Hypertension.*

**Selon** Truw, Ger.
Valerian (p.1762·2); lupulus (p.1708·1).
*Agitation; sleep disorders.*

**Selopral** Orion, Fin.
Metoprolol tartrate (p.957·1).
*Angina pectoris; arrhythmias; hypertension; hyperthyroidism; migraine; myocardial infarction.*

**Selopres**
AstraZeneca, India.
Metoprolol tartrate (p.957·1); hydrochlorothiazide (p.933·2).
*Hypertension.*

AstraZeneca, Mex.
Metoprolol succinate (p.957·1); hydrochlorothiazide (p.933·2).
*Hypertension.*

**Selopresin** Pharmacia, Spain.
Metoprolol tartrate (p.957·1); hydrochlorothiazide (p.933·2).
*Hypertension.*

**Selopress** AstraZeneca, Braz.
Metoprolol succinate (p.957·1) or metoprolol tartrate (p.957·1); hydrochlorothiazide (p.933·2).
*Hypertension.*

**Selozide**
Pharmacia, Belg.; Monsanto, Ital.
Metoprolol tartrate (p.957·1); hydrochlorothiazide (p.933·2).
*Hypertension.*

**Selo-Zok**
AstraZeneca, Belg.; AstraZeneca, Braz.; AstraZeneca, Denm.; AstraZeneca, Norw.
Metoprolol succinate (p.957·1).
*Angina pectoris; arrhythmias; hypertension; hyperthyroidism; migraine; myocardial infarction; tremor.*

**Selpar** Therabel, Ital.†.
Selegiline hydrochloride (p.1214·1).
*Parkinsonism.*

**Selpiran** Diba, Mex.
Hyoscine butylbromide (p.483·3); dipyrone (p.35·3).
*Smooth muscle spasm and pain.*

**Selpiran-S** Diba, Mex.
Hyoscine butylbromide (p.483·3).
*Smooth muscle spasm.*

**Sels Calcaires Nutritifs** Weleda, Fr.
*Combination pack:* Homoeopathic preparation.

**Selso** Luchon, Fr.
Sodium chloride (p.1233·3); sulfur (p.1158·2).
*Nasal irrigation.*

**Selsun**
Abbott, Arg.; Carter-Wallace, Austral.; Abbott, Austria; Abbott, Belg.; Abbott, Braz.†; Abbott, Canad.; Abbott, Chile; Abbott, Denm.; Abbott, Fin.; Abbott, Fr.; Abbott, Ger.; Abbott, Gr.; Abbott, Hong Kong; Abbott, Irl.; Abbott, Israel; Abbott, Malaysia; Abbott, Norw.; Carter, NZ; Wilson, NZ; Abbott, Port.†; Abbott, S.Afr.; Abbott, Swed.; Abbott, Switz.; Abbott, Thai.; Abbott, UK; Chattem, USA.
Selenium sulfide (p.1157·3).
*Dandruff; pityriasis versicolor; seborrhoeic dermatitis of the scalp.*

**Selsun Blu** Abbott, Ital.
Selenium sulfide (p.1157·3).
*Dandruff.*

**Selsun Plus** Abbott, Ital.
Selenium sulfide (p.1157·3); menthol (p.1711·3).
*Dandruff.*

**Selsun with Provitamin $B_5$** Abbott, Canad.
Selenium sulfide (p.1157·3); panthenol (p.1727·2).

**Selsun-R** Abbott, Neth.
Selenium sulfide (p.1157·3).
*Pityriasis versicolor.*

**Seltoc** Apomedica, Austria.
Ethenzamide (p.37·2); diphenhydramine hydrochloride (p.431·3); quinine hydrochloride (p.460·2); ascorbic acid (p.1460·2).
*Cold symptoms.*

**Seltomylon** Diba, Mex.
Nalidixic acid (p.234·1).
*Urinary-tract infections.*

**Seltouch** Teikoku Seiyaku, Jpn.
Felbinac (p.39·1).
*Inflammation; musculoskeletal, joint, and peri-articular disorders; pain.*

**Seltrans** Niddapharm, Ger.
Sodium selenite (p.1444·1).
*Selenium deficiency.*

**Selukos**
Ipex, Austria†; Ipex, Fin.; Ipex, Ger.; Ipex, Norw.; Ipex, Swed.
Selenium sulfide (p.1157·3).
*Pityriasis versicolor; seborrhoeic dermatitis of the scalp.*

**Selva N** Unipharma, Gr.
Sodium chloride (p.1233·3).
*Nasal congestion.*

**Selvigon**
Asta Medica, Austria†; Asta Medica, Braz.; Sanfer, Mex.
Pipazetate hydrochloride (p.1129·1).
*Coughs.*

**Selvigon Hustensaft** Asta Medica, Ger.†.
Pipazetate hydrochloride (p.1129·1).
*Coughs.*

**Selvjgon** Aventis, Ital.
Pipazetate hydrochloride (p.1129·1).
*Coughs.*

**Semap**
Janssen-Cilag, Austria; Janssen-Cilag, Belg.; Janssen-Cilag, Braz.; Janssen-Cilag, Denm.; Janssen-Cilag, Fr.; Janssen-Cilag, Israel; Janssen, Mex.; Janssen-Cilag, Neth.; Janssen-Cilag, Switz.
Penfluridol (p.713·2).
*Psychoses.*

**Semax** Andromaco, Chile.
Citalopram (p.289·1).
*Depression.*

**Semble** Merisant, Arg.
Saccharin sodium (p.1443·3); cyclamate; sucrose (p.1450·1).
*Sugar substitute.*

**Sembrina**
Boehringer Mannheim, Ger.†; Boehringer Mannheim, Neth.†.
Methyldopa (p.953·2).
*Hypertension.*

**Semeth** Greater Pharma, Thai.
Simeticone (p.1289·2).
*Flatulence; meteorism; preparation of gastrointestinal tract for radiological examination or gastroscopy.*

**Semibiocin** Orion, Ger.†.
Erythromycin ethyl succinate (p.208·1).
*Bacterial infections.*

**Semicid** Whitehall, USA.
Nonoxinol 9 (p.1413·3).
*Contraceptive.*

**Semi-Daonil**
Aventis, Austral.; Aventis, Hong Kong; Aventis, India; Aventis, Irl.; Aventis, NZ†; Aventis, Port.; Aventis, Switz.; Aventis, UK.
Glibenclamide (p.331·2).
*Diabetes mellitus.*

**Semi-Euglucon**
Roche, Austria; Roche, Fin.; Roche, Hong Kong; Nicholas Piramal, India; Boehringer Mannheim, Neth.†; Roche, Port.; Roche, Switz.; Roche, Thai.
Glibenclamide (p.331·2).
*Diabetes mellitus.*

**Semi-Euglucon N** Aventis, Ger.
Glibenclamide (p.331·2).
*Diabetes mellitus.*

**Semiglen** Biochemie, Austria.
Omeprazole (p.1278·2).
*Gastro-oesophageal reflux; peptic ulcer; Zollinger-Ellison syndrome.*

**Semi-Gliben-Puren N** Isis Puren, Ger.†.
Glibenclamide (p.331·2).
*Diabetes mellitus.*

**Semilente** Novo Nordisk, Ger.
Insulin zinc suspension (porcine, monocomponent) (p.333·3).
*Diabetes mellitus.*

**Semilente MC** Novo Nordisk, Switz.
Insulin zinc suspension (amorphous) (porcine, monocomponent) (p.333·3).
*Diabetes mellitus.*

**Semipenil** Magis, Ital.
Piperacillin sodium (p.243·1).
Lidocaine hydrochloride (p.1377·3) is included in this preparation to alleviate the pain of injection.
*Bacterial infections.*

**Semper** Semper, Fin.
Range of nutritional preparations (p.1417·1).

**Sempera** Janssen-Cilag, Ger.; GlaxoSmithKline, Ger.
Itraconazole (p.401·3).
*Fungal infections.*

**Semprex**
GlaxoSmithKline, Austria; Warner-Lambert, Denm.†; Pfizer, Fin.; GlaxoSmithKline, Fin.; GlaxoSmithKline, Hong Kong; GlaxoSmithKline, Ital.; GlaxoSmithKline, Malaysia; GlaxoSmithKline, Neth.; GlaxoSmithKline, S.Afr.; GlaxoSmithKline, Singapore; GlaxoSmithKline, Swed.; GlaxoSmithKline, Switz.; GlaxoSmithKline, Thai.; GlaxoSmithKline, UK†.
Acrivastine (p.423·3).
*Allergic conjunctivitis; allergic rhinitis; allergic skin disorders.*

**Semprex-D** Celltech, USA.
Acrivastine (p.423·3); pseudoephedrine hydrochloride (p.1129·2).
*Allergic rhinitis.*

**Semuele** Doctum, Gr.
Ranitidine hydrochloride (p.1285·2).
*Conditions where gastric acid reduction is beneficial; gastric hypersecretion including Zollinger-Ellison syndrome; peptic ulcer.*

**Senagar** Sigma, Austral.
Senega (p.1130·2); ammonium bicarbonate (p.1115·1); camphor (p.1665·3).
*Coughs.*

**Senalsor** Soria Natural, Spain.
Senna (p.1288·2); althaea (p.1651·3); fennel (p.1687·2).
*Constipation.*

**Sendoxan**
Baxter, Denm.; Asta Medica, Fin.; Asta Medica, Norw.; Asta Medica, Swed.
Cyclophosphamide (p.540·2).
*Immune system disorders; malignant neoplasms.*

**Sene Composta** Infabra, Braz.†.
Senna (p.1288·2); cassia (p.1255·2); coriander (p.1676·1); liquorice (p.1270·2).
*Constipation.*

**Senecion** Klein, Ger.†.
Senecio (p.1743·1); ascorbic acid (p.1460·2).
*Haemorrhagic disorders.*

**Senefor** Pierre Fabre, Ital.†.
Phosphatidyl serine (p.1731·2).
*Mental function impairment.*

**Senega and Ammonia** McGloin, Austral.†.
Ammonium bicarbonate (p.1115·1); camphor (p.1665·3); liquorice (p.1270·2); senega root (p.1130·2); ammonia solution (p.1653·3).
*Cold symptoms.*

**Seneuval** Qualiphar, Belg.†.
Valerian (p.1762·2); passion flower (p.1729·1); crataegus (p.1677·1).
Formerly contained valerian and melissa.
*Insomnia; nervousness.*

**Senexon**
Note. This name is used for preparations of different composition.
Gador, Arg.
Betacarotene; vitamin E; vitamin C (p.1417·1).
*Dietary supplement in vascular disease.*

Rugby, USA.
Senna (p.1288·2).
*Constipation.*

**Senexon E** Gador, Arg.
*d*-Alpha tocoferil acetate (p.1465·1).
*Cardiovascular and neurological disorders; vitamin E deficiency.*

**Senexon Plus** Gador, Arg.
Betacarotene; vitamin E; vitamin C; selenium; zinc; manganese; copper (p.1417·1).
*Antioxidant preparation.*

**Senicor** Duopharm, Ger.
Crataegus (p.1677·1).
*Heart failure.*

**Senikolp** Leiras, Fin.
Sodium estrone sulfate (p.1553·1); estradiol (p.1550·1); broxyquinoline (p.165·3).
*Menopausal disorders; oestrogen deficiency.*

**Senilezol** Edwards, USA.
Vitamin B substances with iron (p.1417·1).

**Senior** Strathmann, Ger.†.
Pemoline (p.1591·2).
*Mental function disorders.*

**Senior Formula** Pharmavite, Canad.†.
Multivitamin and mineral preparation (p.1417·1).

**Senior Multi-One** Swiss Herbal, Canad.
Multivitamin and mineral preparation (p.1417·1).

**Senioral** Belmac, Spain†.
Clocinizine hydrochloride (p.429·2); phenylpropanolamine hydrochloride (p.1127·3).
Formerly contained buzepide metiodide, clocinizine hydrochloride, and pholcodine.
*Upper respiratory-tract congestion.*

**Seniospray** Belmac, Spain.
Oxymetazoline hydrochloride (p.1126·1); chlorphenamine maleate (p.427·3).
*Nasal congestion.*

**Seniovita aktiv** Cesra, Ger.
Homoeopathic preparation.

**Senlax** Intercare, UK†.
Senna (p.1288·2).
*Constipation.*

**Senna-Gen** Goldline, USA.
Senna (p.1288·2).
*Constipation.*

**SennaPlus** Fleet, Austral.
Senna (p.1288·2).
*Constipation.*

**Sennapur** Pharmia, Fin.
Senna (p.1288·2).
*Constipation.*

**Senna-Specie Composta** Dynacren, Ital.
Senna (p.1288·2); peppermint leaf (p.1283·2); chamomile (p.1669·3); fennel (p.1687·2).
*Constipation.*

**Sennesoft** Herron, Austral.
Docusate sodium (p.1262·2); sennosides (p.1288·2).
*Constipation.*

**Sennetabs** Herron, Austral.†.
Sennosides (p.1288·2).
*Constipation.*

**Sennocol** Viatris, Neth.
Senna (p.1288·2).
*Constipation.*

**Senociclin** Senosiain, Mex.†.
Tetracycline (p.266·2).
*Bacterial infections.*

**Senodin-AN** Bristol-Myers Squibb, Ital.
Pheniramine maleate (p.438·3); codeine phosphate (p.27·1).
*Coughs.*

**Senokot**
Reckitt Benckiser, Austral.; Reckitt Benckiser, Irl.; Columbia, Mex.; Reckitt Benckiser, NZ; Reckitt Benckiser, S.Afr.; Reckitt Benckiser, Thai.
Sennosides (p.1288·2).
*Constipation.*

Reckitt & Colman, Belg.†; Purdue, Canad.; Sarget, Fr.; Reckitt Benckiser, Hong Kong; Reckitt Benckiser, Malaysia; Mundipharma, Norw.; Reckitt Benckiser, Singapore; Reckitt Benckiser, UK; Purdue Frederick, USA.
Senna (p.1288·2).
*Constipation.*

**Senokot Direct Relief** Reckitt Benckiser, UK.
Glycerol (p.1694·3).
*Constipation.*

**Senokot-S**
Purdue, Canad.; Purdue Frederick, USA.
Senna (p.1288·2); docusate sodium (p.1262·2).
*Constipation.*

**Senokotxtra** Purdue Frederick, USA.
Senna (p.1288·2).
*Constipation.*

**Senol**
Note. This name is used for preparations of different composition.
Gemballa, Braz.
Allantoin (p.1141·3); aminoacridine (p.1165·3); cinchocaine hydrochloride (p.1373·2); benzocaine (p.1370·3); hydroxyquinoline sulfate (p.1700·1).
*Skin disorders.*

Bier, Ital.
Cetrimonium bromide (p.1173·1).
*Nipple disinfection.*

**Senolax**
Neolab, Canad.†; Codilab, Port.
Sennosides A and B (p.1288·2).
*Constipation.*

**Senophile**
Note. This name is used for preparations of different composition.
Prima, Braz.
*Ointment:* Bismuth subnitrate (p.1252·2).
*Topical powder:* Bismuth subnitrate (p.1252·2); bismuth subgallate (p.1252·2); boric acid (p.1662·1); zinc oxide (p.1163·2).
*Skin disorders.*

Braun, Fr.
Zinc oxide (p.1163·2); cholesteryl benzoate.
*Skin irritation.*

**Senorm** Sun, Thai.†.
Haloperidol decanoate (p.701·3).
*Schizophrenia.*

**Senosan** Cos Farma, Ital.
Emollient.

**Senro** Biosarto, Spain.
Norfloxacin (p.238·3).
*Genito-urinary tract infections.*

**Sensaid con Fluor** Dentaid, Chile.
Potassium nitrate (p.1190·1); sodium fluoride (p.1444·3).
*Dental hypersensitivity.*

**Sensaval** Lundbeck, Swed.
Nortriptyline hydrochloride (p.310·2).
*Depression.*

**Sensibit** Liomont, Mex.
Loratadine (p.436·1).
*Hypersensitivity.*

**Sensibit D** Liomont, Mex.
Loratadine (p.436·1); pseudoephedrine sulfate (p.1129·2).
*Allergic rhinitis; nasal congestion.*

**Sensicutan** Harras-Curarina, Ger.
Levomenol (p.1707·1); heparin sodium (p.928·1).
*Skin disorders.*

**Sensiderme** Neo Quimica, Braz.
Nitrofurazone (p.238·2).

**Sensifluid**
Ducray, Fr.; Pierre Fabre, Hong Kong†.
Avena (p.1658·2).
*Soap substitute.*

**Sensigard** Copernico, Ital.
Ranitidine hydrochloride (p.1285·2).
*Gastric hyperacidity; gastro-oesophageal reflux; peptic ulcer; Zollinger-Ellison syndrome.*

**Sensigel**
Note. This name is used for preparations of different composition.
Sidus, Arg.; Pierre Fabre Sante, Fr.; Pierre Fabre, Singapore.
Nicomethanol hydrofluoride; potassium nitrate (p.1190·1).
*Hypersensitive teeth.*

Pergam, Ital.
Allantoin (p.1141·3); vitamin A; vitamin E; lactic acid (p.1704·1).
*Vaginal lubricant.*

**Sensilacer** Andromaco, Chile.
Potassium nitrate (p.1190·1); sodium monofluorophosphate (p.1446·2).
*Caries prophylaxis; dental hypersensitivity.*

**Sensilube** CCD, Fr.
Polyacrylamide; phenoxyethanol; nipastat; citric acid.
*Instrument lubricant; vaginal lubricant.*

**Sensinerv forte** Cesra, Ger.
Valerian root (p.1762·2); lupulus (p.1708·1).
*Nervous disorders; sleep disorders.*

**Sensiotin** Steigerwald, Ger.
Homoeopathic preparation.

**Sensipar** Amgen, USA.
Cinacalcet hydrochloride (p.770·2).
*Hypercalcaemia in parathyroid carcinoma; hyperparathyroidism in chronic renal dialysis.*

**Sensiquell** Pergam, Ital.
Milk protein; allantoin (p.1141·3); lactic acid (p.1704·1).
*Maintenance of vaginal pH.*

**Sensit** *Organon, Austria; Thiemann, Ger.; Organon Teknika (Οργανον Τεχνικα), Gr.*
Fendiline hydrochloride (p.915·1).
*Ischaemic heart disease.*

**Sensitex** *Kinder, Braz.*
Betamethasone valerate (p.1093·2).
*Skin disorders.*

**Sensit-F** *Organon, Ital.†.*
Fendiline hydrochloride (p.915·1).
*Ischaemic heart disease; myocardial infarction.*

**Sensitiner** *Statens Serum Institut, Denm.*
Antigens from *Mycobacterium* spp. (p.1650·1).
*Diagnosis of mycobacterial infections.*

**Sensitive Care** *Asta Medica, Port.†.*
Potassium citrate (p.1223·1); sodium monofluorophosphate (p.1446·2).
*Dental caries prophylaxis; dental hypersensitivity.*

**Sensitive Eyes** *Bausch & Lomb, Canad.; Bausch & Lomb, NZ; Bausch & Lomb, USA.*
Range of solutions for contact lenses (p.1164·2).

**Sensitivity Protection Crest** *Procter & Gamble, USA.*
Potassium nitrate (p.1190·1); sodium fluoride (p.1444·3).
*Sensitive teeth.*

**Sensitram** *Libbs, Braz.*
Tramadol hydrochloride (p.94·3).
*Pain.*

**Sensival** *Wallace, India.*
Nortriptyline hydrochloride (p.310·2).
*Bipolar disorder; depression.*

**Sensivision au plantain** *Chauvin, Fr.*
Plantain (p.1733·1).
*Eye disorders.*

**Sensodent** *Stafford-Miller, Switz.*
Strontium chloride (p.1749·3).
*Hypersensitive teeth.*

**Sensodyne** *Block, Canad.*
Strontium chloride (p.1749·3).
*Hypersensitive teeth.*

**Sensodyne Antitartaro** *GlaxoSmithKline, Braz.*
Potassium nitrate (p.1190·1); sodium fluoride (p.1444·3).
*Hypersensitive teeth.*

**Sensodyne C/Bicarbonato de Sodio** *GlaxoSmithKline, Braz.*
Potassium nitrate (p.1190·1); sodium fluoride (p.1444·3).
*Hypersensitive teeth.*

**Sensodyne Formula Original** *GlaxoSmithKline, Braz.*
Strontium chloride (p.1749·3).
*Hypersensitive teeth.*

**Sensodyne Fresh Mint** *GlaxoSmithKline, Braz.*
Potassium nitrate (p.1190·1); sodium fluoride (p.1444·3).
*Hypersensitive teeth.*

**Sensodyne med** *Block, Austria.*
Strontium chloride (p.1749·3).
*Hypersensitive teeth.*

**Sensodyne Mint** *GlaxoSmithKline, UK.*
Sodium fluoride (p.1444·3); strontium acetate.
*Hypersensitive teeth.*

**Sensodyne Original** *GlaxoSmithKline, UK.*
Strontium chloride (p.1749·3).
*Hypersensitive teeth.*

**Sensodyne Protecao Total** *GlaxoSmithKline, Braz.*
Potassium nitrate (p.1190·1); sodium fluoride (p.1444·3).
*Hypersensitive teeth.*

**Sensodyne-F**
*Note. This name is used for preparations of different composition.*
*Block, Canad.; Block, USA.*
Potassium nitrate (p.1190·1); sodium fluoride (p.1444·3) or sodium monofluorophosphate (p.1446·2).
*Hypersensitive teeth.*

*Stafford-Miller, UK.*
Potassium chloride (p.1232·2); sodium fluoride (p.1444·3); triclosan (p.1195·2).
*Dental caries prophylaxis; hypersensitive teeth.*

**Sensodyne-SC** *Block, USA.*
Strontium chloride (p.1749·3).
*Hypersensitive teeth.*

**SensoGARD** *Block, USA.*
Benzocaine (p.1370·3).
*Mouth and throat disorders.*

**Sensorcaine**
*AstraZeneca, Canad.; Astra, USA.*
Bupivacaine hydrochloride (p.1371·1).
Adrenaline (p.852·2) or adrenaline acid tartrate (p.852·2) is included in some injections as a vasoconstrictor to diminish absorption and localise the effect of the local anaesthetic.
*Local anaesthesia.*

**Sensoricaine** *AstraZeneca, India.*
Bupivacaine hydrochloride (p.1371·1).
*Local anaesthesia.*

**Sens-Out** *Careiatrics, Arg.*
Sodium fluoride (p.1444·3); potassium nitrate (p.1190·1).
*Hypersensitive teeth.*

**Sentidol** *Medipharm, Chile.*
Venlafaxine (p.322·3).
*Anxiety; depression.*

**Sentril** *Biomedis, Thai.; Great Eastern, Thai.*
Dequalinium chloride (p.1178·1); cetylpyridinium chloride (p.1173·1); ascorbic acid (p.1460·2).
*Mouth and throat infections.*

**Sepan** *Janssen-Cilag, Denm.*
Cinnarizine (p.428·3).
*Allergic rhinitis; hay fever; motion sickness; urticaria.*

**Sepatren** *Sumitomo, Jpn.*
Cefpiramide sodium (p.178·2).
*Bacterial infections.*

**Sepazon** *Sankyo, Hong Kong†.*
Cloxazolam (p.685·3).
*Anxiety disorders.*

**Sepcen** *Centrum, Spain.*
Ciprofloxacin hydrochloride (p.188·2).
*Bacterial infections.*

**Sepdine** *PD, Thai.*
Chlorhexidine gluconate (p.1173·2); cetrimide (p.1172·1).
*Skin, instrument, and wound disinfection.*

**Sepex** *Key, Arg.*
Ceftibuten (p.182·1).
*Bacterial infections.*

**Sepexin**
*Note. This name is used for preparations of different composition.*
*Lyka, India.*
Cefalexin (p.168·1).
*Bacterial infections.*

*Schering-Plough, S.Afr.*
Ceftibuten (p.182·1).
*Bacterial infections.*

**Sepfadine** *Nakorn, Thai.*
Povidone-iodine (p.1190·3).
*Burns; skin and soft-tissue disinfection; wounds.*

**Sephros** *YSP, Malaysia.*
Cefradine (p.179·3).
*Bacterial infections.*

**Sepmax** *GlaxoSmithKline, India.*
Co-trimoxazole (p.199·3).
*Bacterial infections; Pneumocystis carinii pneumonia; toxoplasmosis.*

**Se-Power** *Cantassium Co., UK.*
Selenium yeast (p.1444·1); myrtillus (p.1718·3); euphrasia (p.1686·3); vitamin E (p.1464·3); zinc gluconate (p.1469·2); vitamin A (p.1451·2); riboflavin (p.1456·1).

**Seprafilm**
*Genzyme, UK; Genzyme, USA.*
Sodium hyaluronate (p.1697·3); carmellose (p.1577·3).
*Prevention of surgical adhesions.*

**Sepram**
*Lundbeck, Austria; Bayer, Ger.*
Citalopram hydrobromide (p.289·1) or citalopram hydrochloride (p.289·1).
*Depression; obsessive-compulsive disorder; panic attacks.*

**Sepsilem** *Lemery, Mex.*
Cefotaxime sodium (p.175·3).
*Bacterial infections.*

**Sepso J** *Hofmann & Sommer, Ger.*
Povidone-iodine (p.1190·3).
*Burns; infected skin disorders; skin, hand, and mucous membrane disinfection; wounds.*

**Sepsol** *Upha, Malaysia.*
Chlorhexidine gluconate (p.1173·2).
*Skin disinfection.*

**Septa** *Circle, USA†.*
Polymyxin B sulfate (p.245·1); neomycin sulfate (p.235·1); bacitracin (p.161·3).
*Bacterial skin infections.*

**Septacare** *Teva, Israel.*
Chlorhexidine acetate (p.1173·2); cetrimide (p.1172·1).
*Burns; genito-urinary disinfection; skin disinfection; wounds.*

**Septacef** *Reig Jofre, Spain; Septa, Spain.*
Cefradine (p.179·3).
*Bacterial infections.*

**Septacin** *Chinoin, Mex.*
Ambroxol hydrochloride (p.1114·3).
*Respiratory-tract congestion.*

**Septacin Amoxi** *Chinoin, Mex.*
Ambroxol hydrochloride (p.1114·3); amoxicillin trihydrate (p.155·3).
*Respiratory-tract infections.*

**Septacin Ex** *Chinoin, Mex.*
Ambroxol hydrochloride (p.1114·3); clenbuterol hydrochloride (p.784·2).
*Respiratory-tract disorders.*

**Septacord** *Muller Goppingen, Ger.*
Potassium aspartate (p.1233·1); magnesium aspartate (p.1227·3); crataegus (p.1677·1).
*Cardiac disorders.*

**Septadine**
*Note. This name is used for preparations of different composition.*
*Floris, Israel.*
Alcohol (p.1166·1); chlorhexidine (p.1173·2).
*Skin disinfection.*

*Be-Tabs, S.Afr.*
Povidone-iodine (p.1190·3).
*Minor throat infections; skin infections; wound and burn disinfection.*

**Septadine Scrub** *Floris, Israel.*
Chlorhexidine gluconate (p.1173·2).
*Skin disinfection; wound disinfection.*

**Septal** *Teva, Israel.*
Chlorhexidine gluconate (p.1173·2).
*Skin disinfection; wounds.*

**Septalibour** *Ducray, Fr.*
Avena (p.1658·2); copper sulfate (p.1426·1); zinc sulfate (p.1469·3).
*Cleansing of atopic skin.*

**Septalone** *Teva, Israel.*
Chlorhexidine gluconate (p.1173·2).
*Burns; disinfection in obstetrics; skin and instrument disinfection; wounds.*

**Septanest**
*Austrodent, Austria; DFL, Braz.†; Septodont, Denm.; Ogna, Ital.; Septodont, Switz.; Deproco, UK.*
Articaine hydrochloride (p.1370·3).
Adrenaline (p.852·2) or adrenaline acid tartrate (p.852·2) is included in this preparation as a vasoconstrictor to diminish absorption and localise the effect of the local anaesthetic.
*Local anaesthesia.*

**Septeal** *Sinbio, Fr.*
Chlorhexidine gluconate (p.1173·2).
*Skin and wound disinfection.*

**Septi-Aid** *Raza, Malaysia; Pharmaniaga, Malaysia.*
Povidone-iodine (p.1190·3).
*Skin and wound disinfection.*

**Septicide** *Bago, Arg.*
Ciprofloxacin hydrochloride (p.188·2).
*Bacterial infections.*

**Septicol**
*Note. This name is used for preparations of different composition.*
*Willmar, Mex.†.*
Thiomersal (p.1194·1).

*Streuli, Switz.*
Chloramphenicol (p.185·1).
*Bacterial eye infections.*

**Septicon** *Ciba Vision, Austria†.*
*Combination pack:* Lensept, hydrogen peroxide (p.1182·2); Lensrins NT, storage and rinsing solution (p.1164·2).
*Care of soft contact lenses.*

**Septicortin** *Streuli, Switz.†.*
Cortisone acetate (p.1096·1); chloramphenicol (p.185·1).
*Inflammatory eye infections.*

**Septidiaryl** *Martin-Johnson & Johnson, Fr.*
Nifuroxazide (p.237·2).

**Septidine** *Osoth, Thai.*
Povidone-iodine (p.1190·3).
*Burns; skin disinfection; wounds.*

**Septidron** *Aventis, S.Afr.*
Pipemidic acid (p.243·1).
*Urinary-tract infections.*

**Septil** *Azevedos, Port.*
Povidone-iodine (p.1190·3).
*Burns; skin disinfection; skin infections; ulcers; wounds.*

**Septilisin**
*Note. This name is used for preparations of different composition.*
*Bago, Arg.*
Cefalexin (p.168·1).
*Bacterial infections.*

*Grin, Mex.*
Polymyxin B sulfate (p.245·1); neomycin sulfate (p.235·1); gramicidin (p.220·2).
*Bacterial eye infections.*

**Septiolan** *Climax, Braz.*
Co-trimoxazole (p.199·3).
*Bacterial infections; Pneumocystis carinii pneumonia; protozoal infections.*

**Septiolan Balsamico** *Climax, Braz.†.*
Co-trimoxazole (p.199·3); guaifenesin (p.1122·1); ammonium chloride (p.1115·2).
*Bacterial infections.*

**Septirose** *Sudo, Singapore†.*
Serrapeptase (p.1743·2).
*Inflammation; respiratory-tract congestion.*

**Septisan** *Cederroth, Spain.*
Chlorhexidine gluconate (p.1173·2).
*Disinfection of skin, burns, and wounds.*

**Septisept** *Chefaro Ardeval, Fr.†.*
Cetrimide (p.1172·1).
Formerly known as Asepto 7.
*Burns; wounds.*

**Septi-Soft** *Calgon Vestal, USA.*
Triclosan (p.1195·2).
*Skin cleanser.*

**Septisol**
*Note. This name is used for preparations of different composition.*
*Monot, Fr.†.*
Salicylic acid (p.1157·1).
*Chronic conjunctivitis.*

*Calgon Vestal, USA.*
*Foam:* Hexachlorophene (p.1181·2).
*Skin disinfection.*

*Solution:* Triclosan (p.1195·2).
*Skin cleanser; skin disinfection.*

**Septison** *Orion, Fin.*
Prednisolone (p.1108·1); dequalinium chloride (p.1178·1).
*Skin disorders.*

**Septisooth** *Pharmachoice, S.Afr.*
Povidone-iodine (p.1190·3).
*Burns; skin infections; ulcers; wounds.*

**Septivon** *Chefaro Ardeval, Fr.*
Triclocarban (p.1195·1); detergents.
*Skin and mucous membrane disinfection.*

**Septivon N** *SSL, Switz.*
Triclocarban (p.1195·1); cetrimonium chloride (p.1173·1).
*Hand disinfection; minor skin lesions.*

**Septobore** *Cooper (Κοπερ), Gr.*
Naphazoline nitrate (p.1124·3); boric acid (p.1662·1).
*Ocular irritation.*

**Septocaine**
*Septodont, Denm.; Septodont, Norw.; Septodont, USA.*
Articaine hydrochloride (p.1370·3).
Adrenaline (p.852·2) is included in this preparation as a vasoconstrictor to reduce absorption and localise the effect of the local anaesthetic.
*Local anaesthesia.*

**Septocipro** *Lesvi, Spain.*
Ciprofloxacin hydrochloride (p.188·2) or ciprofloxacin lactate (p.188·3).
*Bacterial infections.*

**Septocoll** *Biomet Merck, Ger.*
Collagen (bovine) (p.1674·3); gentamicin sulfate (p.217·1).
*Wounds.*

**Septol** *Teva, Israel.*
Chlorhexidine gluconate (p.1173·2).
*Skin disinfection.*

**Septolit** *Henkel, Ger.*
Benzalkonium chloride (p.1168·3); oligo(di(iminoimidocarbonyl)iminohexamethylene).
*Surface disinfection.*

**Septomandolo** *IPA, Ital.*
Cefamandole nafate (p.169·3).
Lidocaine hydrochloride (p.1377·3) is included in the intramuscular injection to alleviate the pain of injection.
*Gram-negative bacterial infections.*

**Septomixine** *Septodont, Switz.*
Hydrocortisone acetate (p.1103·3); framycetin sulfate (p.215·1).
Formerly contained dexamethasone, polymyxin B sulfate, tyrothricin, and neomycin sulfate.
*Dental infections.*

**Septone** *Shiwa, Thai.*
Chlorhexidine gluconate (p.1173·2); cetrimide (p.1172·1).
*Burns; skin and instrument disinfection; wounds.*

**Septonsil** *Pekana, Ger.*
Homoeopathic preparation.

**Septopal**
*Merck, Arg.; Biomet, Austral.; Merck, Austria; Mediplant, Belg.†; Merck, Braz.; Merck, Denm.; Merck, Fin.; Biomet Merck, Ger.; Galenica, Gr.; Merck, Hong Kong; Merck, India; Merck, Irl.†; Merck, Malaysia; Ortomed, Neth.; Merck, Norw.; Merck, S.Afr.; Merck, Singapore; Scandimed, Swed.; Merck, Switz.; Merck, Thai.; Biomet Merck, UK.*
Gentamicin sulfate (p.217·1); polymethylmethacrylate-methylmethacrylate copolymer (p.1714·3).
*Bacterial infections of bone and soft tissues.*

**Septoprin** *Medley, Braz.†.*
Co-trimoxazole (p.199·3).
*Bacterial infections; Pneumocystis carinii pneumonia; protozoal infections.*

**Septoral** *Merck, Port.†.*
Cetylpyridinium chloride (p.1173·1).

**Septosan**
*Note. This name is used for preparations of different composition.*
*Stiefel, Fr.*
Triclocarban (p.1195·1); triclosan (p.1195·2).
*Disinfection.*

*Stiefel, Mex.*
*Soap:* Triclocarban (p.1195·1); triclosan (p.1195·2).
*Skin cleansing.*

*Topical lotion:* Triclosan (p.1195·2).
*Soap substitute.*

**Septosol** *Xerogen, S.Afr.*
Phenol (p.1188·1).
*Sore throat.*

**Septra**
*GlaxoSmithKline, Canad.; Monarch, USA.*
Co-trimoxazole (p.199·3).
*Bacterial infections; Pneumocystis carinii pneumonia.*

**Septran**
*GlaxoSmithKline, India; GlaxoSmithKline, S.Afr.*
Co-trimoxazole (p.199·3).
*Bacterial infections; Pneumocystis carinii pneumonia; toxoplasmosis.*

**Septrin**
*Sigma, Austral.; GlaxoSmithKline, Chile; Glaxo Wellcome, Gr.; Sigma, Hong Kong; Glaxo Wellcome, Irl.; Wellcome, Israel; Glaxo Wellcome, Mex.; Wellcome, Port.; GlaxoSmithKline, Singapore; Celltech, Spain; GlaxoSmithKline, Thai.; GlaxoSmithKline, UK.*
Co-trimoxazole (p.199·3).
*Bacterial infections; nocardiosis; Pneumocystis carinii pneumonia; toxoplasmosis.*

**Sepurin** *Gross, Braz.*
Methenamine (p.230·1); methylthioninium chloride (p.1042·2).
*Vulvovaginal infections.*

**Sequals G** *Lagos, Arg.*
Rosemary (p.1740·2); enebro (p.1159·2); crataegus (p.1677·1); birch (p.1660·3).
*Scalp disorders.*

**Sequax** *Elvetium, Arg.*
Clozapine (p.685·3).
*Schizophrenia.*

**Sequennia** Wyeth Lederle, Austria.
14 Tablets, conjugated oestrogens (p.1543·2); 14 tablets, conjugated oestrogens; medroxyprogesterone acetate (p.1557·2).
*Menopausal disorders; osteoporosis.*

**Sequilar**
Schering, Austria; Schering, Ger.; Schering, Switz.†.
Levonorgestrel (p.1563·2); ethinylestradiol (p.1553·2).
28-Day packs also contain 7 inert tablets.
*Biphasic oral contraceptive.*

**Sequilar ED** Schering, Austral.
21 Tablets, levonorgestrel (p.1563·2); ethinylestradiol (p.1553·2); 7 tablets, inert.
*Biphasic oral contraceptive.*

**Sequinan** Pharmacia, Arg.
Risperidone (p.719·2).
*Psychoses.*

**Sequostat** Jenapharm, Ger.
6 Tablets, ethinylestradiol (p.1553·2); 15 tablets, ethinylestradiol; norethisterone acetate (p.1562·2).
*Sequential oral contraceptive.*

**Seracalm** Demopharm, Switz.†.
Valerian (p.1762·2); melissa (p.1711·1); neroli oil (p.1719·2); lavender oil (p.1705·2).
*Sleep disorders.*

**Seraccel** Serum Institute, India.
Gelatin (p.754·3).
*Priming of heart-lung machine and artificial kidney; shock.*

**Seracin** Pharmaland, Thai.
Ofloxacin (p.239·3).
*Bacterial infections.*

**Seractil**
Gebro, Austria; Byk, Neth.; Gebro, Spain; Gebro, Switz.
Dexibuprofen (p.46·1).
*Fever; gout; inflammation; musculoskeletal, joint, and peri-articular disorders; pain.*

**Seractiv** Nordic Drugs, Denm.
Dexibuprofen (p.46·1).
*Dysmenorrhoea; osteoarthritis.*

**Serad** Pfizer Consumer, Ital.†.
Sertraline hydrochloride (p.317·2).
*Depression.*

**Serag-HAES** Serag-Wiessner, Ger.
Pentastarch (p.750·1) in sodium chloride.
*Hypovolaemia; plasma volume expansion.*

**Seraim** Anglo-French Drugs, India.
Serrapeptase (p.1743·2).
*Breast engorgement; inflammation; pain.*

**Seralbuman** ISI, Ital.†.
Albumin (p.740·3).
*Hypoalbuminaemia.*

**Seralbumin** Probifasa, Mex.
Albumin (p.740·3).
*Hypoalbuminaemia; plasma volume expansion; shock.*

**Seramed** Medifive, Thai.
Serrapeptase (p.1743·2).
*Inflammation; respiratory-tract congestion.*

**Seranex sans codeine** Democal, Switz.
Phenazone (p.82·3); propyphenazone (p.85·3); ethenzamide (p.37·2); benzyl mandelate; caffeine (p.782·1).
*Pain.*

**Ser-Ap-Es**
Novartis, Canad.†; Novartis, Thai.; Ciba, USA.
Reserpine (p.995·1); hydralazine hydrochloride (p.931·2); hydrochlorothiazide (p.933·2).
*Hypertension.*

**Serasa** Serono, Mex.†.
Asparaginase (p.528·3).

**Seravit**
SHS, Fr.; Scientific Hospital Supplies, Irl.; Scientific Hospital Supplies, UK.
A range of multivitamin and mineral preparations (p.1417·1).

**Serax**
Wyeth-Ayerst, Canad.†; Alpharma, USA.
Oxazepam (p.712·2).
*Alcohol withdrawal syndrome; anxiety.*

**Serc**
Solvay, Austral.; Solvay, Canad.; Solvay, Fr.; Solvay, Irl.; Byk Gulden, Mex.; Solvay, NZ; Solvay, S.Afr.; Solvay, Spain; Solvay, Thai.; Solvay, UK.
Betahistine hydrochloride (p.1660·1).
*Ménière's disease.*

**Sercerin** Farmasa, Braz.
Sertraline hydrochloride (p.317·2).
*Depression.*

**Sercim** IQFA, Mex.
Cimetidine (p.1255·3).

**Serdolect**
Lundbeck, Austria†; Lundbeck, Denm.†; Lundbeck, Ger.†; Lundbeck, Norw.†; Lundbeck, Switz.; Lundbeck, UK.
Sertindole (p.721·3).
*Schizophrenia.*

**Serebon** Sankyo, Hong Kong†.
Oxazolam (p.712·3).
*Anxiety; depression; premedication; sleep disorders.*

**Serecid** Douglas, NZ.
Hydroxyzine hydrochloride (p.434·3).
*Anxiety; asthma; pruritus; urticaria.*

**Serecor** Sanofi Synthelabo, Fr.
Hydroquinidine hydrochloride (p.937·3).
*Arrhythmias.*

**Seredyn** Degorts, Mex.†.
Diazepam (p.690·1).

**Serefrex** Janssen-Cilag, Arg.
Ketanserin (p.943·1).
*Hypertension.*

**Sereine** Optikem, USA.
Range of solutions for hard contact lenses (p.1164·2).

**Sere-Mit** Mitim, Ital.†.
Saw palmetto (p.1569·1).
*Prostatic hyperplasia.*

**Serenace**
Sigma, Austral.; Pharmacia, Hong Kong; RPG, India; Ivax, Irl.; Pharmacia, Malaysia; Sigma, NZ; Pharmacia, S.Afr.; Pharmacia, Singapore; Searle, Thai.†; Ivax, UK.
Haloperidol (p.701·2).
*Agitation; alcoholism; anxiety; childhood behaviour disorders; motor tics; nausea and vomiting; psychoses; Tourette syndrome.*

**Serenade** Alter, Spain†.
Nitrazepam (p.710·1).
*Insomnia.*

**Serenal** Wyeth Lederle, Port.
Oxazepam (p.712·2).

**Serenase**
Note. This name is used for preparations of different composition.
Almirall, Belg.
Lorazepam (p.704·1).
*Anxiety; insomnia; premedication.*

QIF, Braz.†.
Passion flower (p.1729·1); chamomile (p.1669·3); erythrina mulungu (p.1717·2).
*Sedative.*

Janssen-Cilag, Denm.; Orion, Fin.; Lusofarmaco, Ital.
Haloperidol (p.701·2) or haloperidol decanoate (p.701·3).
*Alcohol withdrawal syndrome; hiccups; movement disorders; pain; psychoses; vomiting.*

**Serene** Pharmaland, Thai.
Dipotassium clorazepate (p.685·1).
*Anxiety.*

**Serenelfi** Lusofarmaco, Port.
Haloperidol (p.701·2).

**Serenex** Sintofarma, Braz.†.
Zopiclone (p.729·3).
*Insomnia.*

**Serengrav** Baldacci, Ital.
Folic acid (p.1429·1).
*Prevention of neural tube defects during pregnancy.*

**Serenight** Montefarmaco, Ital.†.
Vitamin $B_6$; magnesium; kava; lupulus; eschscholtzia (p.1417·1).

**Serenil** Natufarma, Arg.
Passion flower (p.1729·1); valerian (p.1762·2); tilia (p.1756·2).
*Sedative.*

**Serenoa Complex** Blackmores, Austral.†.
Equisetum (p.1684·1); saw palmetto (p.1569·1); buchu (p.1663·1); *d*-alpha tocoferil acid succinate (p.1465·1); zinc amino acid chelate (p.1469·3).
*Prostate disorders; urinary-tract disorders.*

**Serenoa-C** Wassen, UK†.
Saw palmetto (p.1569·1); vitamins; minerals (p.1417·1).

**Serenol** Dolisos, Canad.
Homoeopathic preparation.

**Serentil**
Novartis, Canad.†; Boehringer Ingelheim, USA.
Mesoridazine besilate (p.706·3).
*Alcohol withdrawal syndrome; psychoses.*

**Serenus** Biolab Sanus, Braz.
Passion flower (p.1729·1); crataegus (p.1677·1); adonis vernalis (p.1648·1).
*Sedative.*

**Serepax**
Sigma, Austral.; Wyeth, Chile; Wyeth Lederle, Denm.; Wyeth, India; Wyeth Lederle, Norw.†; Wyeth, NZ†; Akromed, S.Afr.
Oxazepam (p.712·2).
*Alcohol withdrawal syndrome; anxiety disorders.*

**Serepress** Formenti, Ital.
Ketanserin tartrate (p.943·1).
*Hypertension.*

**Sereprid** Labomed, Chile.
Tiapride hydrochloride (p.725·1).
*Alcohol withdrawal syndrome; behaviour disorders; headache; movement disorders.*

**Sereprile** Sanofi Synthelabo, Ital.
Tiapride hydrochloride (p.725·1).
*Gastrointestinal dyskinesia; movement and behaviour disorders.*

**Sereprostat**
Pierre Fabre, Arg.; Robapharm, Spain.
Saw palmetto (p.1569·1).
*Prostatic disorders.*

**Seresis**
Boehringer Ingelheim, Chile.
Ascorbic acid; grape; tomato; selenium; vitamin E; betacaroteno (p.1417·1).
*Dietary supplement.*

Pharmaton, Switz.†.
Vitamins; lycopene; proanthocyanidines; selenium (p.1417·1).

**Seresta**
Wyeth Lederle, Belg.; Wyeth Lederle, Fr.; Eurocept, Neth.; Wyeth, Switz.
Oxazepam (p.712·2).
*Alcohol withdrawal syndrome; anxiety; sleep disorders.*

**Seretaide** Glaxo Wellcome, Port.
Salmeterol xinafoate (p.795·1); fluticasone propionate (p.1102·3).
*Asthma.*

**Seretide**
GlaxoSmithKline, Arg.; Allen & Hanburys, Austral.; GlaxoSmithKline, Austria; GlaxoSmithKline, Belg.; GlaxoSmithKline, Braz.; GlaxoSmithKline, Chile; GlaxoSmithKline, Denm.; GlaxoSmithKline, Fin.; GlaxoSmithKline, Fr.; Allen, Gr.; GlaxoSmithKline, Hong Kong; Allen & Hanburys, Irl.; GlaxoSmithKline, Israel; GlaxoSmithKline, Ital.; GlaxoSmithKline, Malaysia; Glaxo Wellcome, Mex.; GlaxoSmithKline, Neth.; GlaxoSmithKline, Norw.; GlaxoSmithKline, S.Afr.; GlaxoSmithKline, Singapore; GlaxoSmithKline, Spain; GlaxoSmithKline, Swed.; GlaxoSmithKline, Switz.; GlaxoSmithKline, Thai.; Allen & Hanburys, UK.
Salmeterol xinafoate (p.795·1); fluticasone propionate (p.1102·3).
*Obstructive airways disease.*

**Seretran** Drugtech, Chile.
Paroxetine hydrochloride (p.311·2).
*Depression.*

**Sereupin** Abbott, Ital.
Paroxetine hydrochloride (p.311·2).
*Anxiety; depression; obsessive-compulsive disorder; panic disorders.*

**Serevent**
GlaxoSmithKline, Arg.; Allen & Hanburys, Austral.; GlaxoSmithKline, Austria; GlaxoSmithKline, Belg.; GlaxoSmithKline, Braz.; GlaxoSmithKline, Canad.; GlaxoSmithKline, Chile; GlaxoSmithKline, Denm.; GlaxoSmithKline, Fin.; GlaxoSmithKline, Fr.; GlaxoSmithKline, Ger.; Cascan, Ger.; Glaxo Wellcome, Gr.; GlaxoSmithKline, Hong Kong; Allen & Hanburys, Irl.; GlaxoSmithKline, Israel; GlaxoSmithKline, Ital.; GlaxoSmithKline, Malaysia; Glaxo Wellcome, Mex.; GlaxoSmithKline, Neth.; GlaxoSmithKline, Norw.; GlaxoSmithKline, NZ; Glaxo Wellcome, Port.; GlaxoSmithKline, S.Afr.; GlaxoSmithKline, Singapore; GlaxoSmithKline, Spain; GlaxoSmithKline, Swed.; GlaxoSmithKline, Switz.; GlaxoSmithKline, Thai.; Allen & Hanburys, UK; Glaxo Wellcome, USA.
Salmeterol xinafoate (p.795·1).
*Obstructive airways disease.*

**Serezac** Pulitzer, Ital.
Fluoxetine hydrochloride (p.292·1).
*Bulimia nervosa; depression; obsessive-compulsive disorder.*

**Serfabiotic** Serra Pamies, Spain†.
Metampicillin sodium (p.229·3).
*Bacterial infections.*

**Serfinato** Basi, Port.
Reserpine (p.995·1).
*Hypertension.*

**Serformin** Biochemie, Thai.; Novartis, Thai.
Metformin hydrochloride (p.342·3).
*Diabetes mellitus.*

**Serfoxide** Beecham, Spain†.
Pyridoxine phosphoserinate (p.1457·2).
*Chronic alcoholism; vitamin $B_6$ deficiency.*

**Sergast** Truw, Ger.
Turmeric (p.1058·3).
*Digestive system disorders.*

**Serianon** Fada, Arg.
Heparin (p.927·3).
*Thromboembolic disorders.*

**Seriglutan B12** Serpero, Ital.†.
Amino-acid and vitamin $B_{12}$ preparation (p.1417·1).
*Tonic.*

**Serimol** Raza, Malaysia; Pharmaniaga, Malaysia.
Paracetamol (p.76·2).
*Fever; pain.*

**Serivo** Pasteur, Chile.
Sertraline hydrochloride (p.317·2).
*Depression; obsessive-compulsive disorder; panic attacks; post-traumatic stress disorder.*

**Serlain** Pfizer, Belg.
Sertraline hydrochloride (p.317·2).
*Depression; obsessive-compulsive disorder; panic disorders.*

**Serless** Truw, Ger.
Urtica root (p.1762·1).
*Benign prostatic hyperplasia.*

**Sermaka** Lilly, Ger.†.
Fludroxycortide (p.1100·3).
*Skin disorders.*

**Sermetrol** Serral, Mex.
Metoprolol (p.956·3).

**Sermion**
Pharmacia, Arg.; Pharmacia, Austria; Pharmacia, Braz.; Pharmacia, Chile; Aventis, Fr.; Pharmacia, Ger.; Pharmacia, Hong Kong; Pharmacia Upjohn, Ital.; Pharmacia Upjohn, Mex.; Pharmacia, Port.; Kenfarma, Spain; Pharmacia, Switz.; Pharmacia, Thai.
Nicergoline (p.1719·3) or nicergoline tartrate (p.1720·1).
*Cerebral, eye, and ear vascular disorders; hypertension; mental function impairment.*

**Sermonil** Pharmaland, Thai.
Imipramine hydrochloride (p.300·1).
*Depression; nocturnal enuresis.*

**Serobid** Cipla, India.
Salmeterol xinafoate (p.795·1).
*Asthma.*

**Serobif** Serono, Ital.
Interferon beta (p.645·3).
*Malignant neoplasms; viral infections.*

**Serocalcin**
Serono, Braz.
Calcitonin (salmon) (p.768·2).
*Osteoporosis.*

Serono, Mex.†.
Calcitonin (p.768·2).

**Serocryptin**
Serono, Arg.; Serono, Hong Kong; Serono, Mex.; Serono, Singapore†; Serono, Switz.†; Serono, Thai.†.
Bromocriptine mesilate (p.1200·3).
*Acromegaly; benign breast disorders; female infertility; galactorrhoea; lactation inhibition; male hypogonadism; menstrual disorders; parkinsonism; pituitary adenoma.*

**Serocytol** Serolab, Switz.
A range of equine antisera raised against body tissues and organs.

**Serodox** Serono, Mex.†.
Doxorubicin.

**Serofene**
Serono, Arg.; Serono, Braz.; Novartis, Chile; Serono, Ital.
Clomifene citrate (p.1542·2).
*Anovulatory infertility; functional uterine haemorrhage; polycystic ovary syndrome.*

**Seroflo** Cipla, India.
Salmeterol (p.795·2); fluticasone propionate (p.1102·3).
*Asthma.*

**Serofusine** Braun, Switz.
Electrolyte infusion with or without glucose (p.1217·1).
*Fluid and electrolyte disorders.*

**Seroglubin**
Gador, Arg.; Probifasa, Mex.
A normal immunoglobulin (p.1627·2).
*Passive immunisation.*

**Seromex** Ratiopharm, Fin.
Fluoxetine hydrochloride (p.292·1).
*Bulimia nervosa; depression; obsessive-compulsive disorder.*

**Seromida** Serono, Mex.†.
Ifosfamide (p.561·1).

**Seromycin**
Lilly, Canad.†; Lilly, Hong Kong; Dura, USA.
Cycloserine (p.202·1).
*Tuberculosis; urinary-tract infections.*

**Seronex** Medix, Mex.
Domperidone (p.1263·2).
*Gastrointestinal motility disorders; nausea and vomiting.*

**Seronil** Orion, Fin.
Fluoxetine hydrochloride (p.292·1).
*Bulimia nervosa; depression; obsessive-compulsive disorder.*

**Serophene**
Serono, Austral.; Serono, Austria; Serono, Canad.; Serono, Hong Kong; Serono, Irl.†; Serono, Malaysia; Serono, Mex.; Serono, Neth.; Serono, S.Afr.; Serono, Singapore; Serono, Switz.; Serono, Thai.; Serono, UK†; Serono, USA.
Clomifene citrate (p.1542·2).
*Anovulatory infertility; male infertility.*

**Serophy**
Monal, Fr.†; Interdelta, Switz.
Sodium chloride (p.1233·3).
*Nasal disorders.*

**Seroplatin** Serono, Mex.†.
Cisplatin (p.538·1).

**Seroposide** Serono, Mex.†.
Etoposide (p.551·3).

**Seropram**
Lundbeck, Austria; Lundbeck, Fr.; Lundbeck, Gr.; Lundbeck, Ital.; Organon, Mex.; Lundbeck, Spain; Lundbeck, Switz.
Citalopram hydrobromide (p.289·1) or citalopram hydrochloride (p.289·1).
*Depression; obsessive-compulsive disorder; panic disorder.*

**Seroquel**
Bago, Arg.; AstraZeneca, Austral.; AstraZeneca, Austria; AstraZeneca, Belg.; AstraZeneca, Braz.; AstraZeneca, Canad.; AstraZeneca, Chile; AstraZeneca, Denm.; AstraZeneca, Fin.; AstraZeneca, Ger.; Astra-Zeneca, Gr.; AstraZeneca, Hong Kong; AstraZeneca, Irl.; Zeneca, Israel; AstraZeneca, Ital.; AstraZeneca, Malaysia; Zeneca, Mex.; AstraZeneca, Neth.; AstraZeneca, Norw.; AstraZeneca, NZ; Astra-Zeneca, Port.; Zeneca, S.Afr.; AstraZeneca, Singapore; AstraZeneca, Spain; AstraZeneca, Switz.; AstraZeneca, Thai.; AstraZeneca, UK; Zeneca, USA.
Quetiapine fumarate (p.718·2).
*Psychoses.*

**Seroscand** Scand Pharm, Swed.
Fluoxetine hydrochloride (p.292·1).
*Bulimia; depression; obsessive-compulsive disorder.*

**Serostim**
Serono, Arg.; Serono, Canad.; Serono, Hong Kong; Serono, Mex.; Serono, Singapore†; Serono, USA.
Somatropin (p.1327·2).
*AIDS-related cachexia.*

**Serotabir** Serono, Mex.†.
Cytarabine (p.543·1).

**Sero-Tet** Green Cross, Malaysia.
A tetanus immunoglobulin (p.1640·3).
*Passive immunisation.*

**Serotone**
Temis, Arg.; Japan Tobacco, Jpn.
Azasetron hydrochloride (p.1251·1).
*Nausea and vomiting associated with antineoplastic therapy.*

**Serotron** Serono, Mex.†.
Mitoxantrone.

**Serotulle** *SSL, UK.*
Chlorhexidine acetate (p.1173·2).
*Wounds.*

**Serovidina** *Serono, Mex.†.*
Zidovudine (p.658·2).

**Serovin** *Serono, Mex.†.*
Vinblastine (p.592·1).

**Seroxat**
*GlaxoSmithKline, Austria; GlaxoSmithKline, Belg.; GlaxoSmithKline, Denm.; GlaxoSmithKline, Fin.; GlaxoSmithKline, Ger.; SmithKline Beecham, Gr.; GlaxoSmithKline, Hong Kong; GlaxoSmithKline, Irl.; SmithKline Beecham, Israel; GlaxoSmithKline, Ital.; GlaxoSmithKline, Malaysia; GlaxoSmithKline, Neth.; GlaxoSmithKline, Norw.; Beecham, Port.; GlaxoSmithKline, Singapore; GlaxoSmithKline, Spain; GlaxoSmithKline, Swed.; GlaxoSmithKline, Thai.; GlaxoSmithKline, UK.*
Paroxetine hydrochloride (p.311·2).
*Depression; obsessive-compulsive disorder; panic disorders; post-traumatic stress disorder; social anxiety disorder.*

**Serozinc** *Roche-Posay, Fr.*
Sodium chloride (p.1233·3); zinc sulfate (p.1469·3).
*Skin disorders; wound and ulcer cleansing.*

**Serpafar** *Faran, Gr.*
Clomifene citrate (p.1542·2).
*Anovulatory infertility; diagnosis of hormonal disorders.*

**Serpax** *Wyeth Lederle, Ital.*
Oxazepam (p.712·2).
*Alcohol withdrawal syndrome; anxiety; depression; insomnia.*

**Serpens** *Lisapharma, Ital.*
Saw palmetto (p.1569·1).
*Prostatic hyperplasia.*

**Serradase** *Siam Bheasach, Thai.*
Serrapeptase (p.1743·2).
*Inflammation; respiratory-tract congestion; wounds.*

**Serranit** *Serral, Mex.*
Ranitidine (p.1285·2).
*Peptic ulcer.*

**Serrano** *M & H, Thai.*
Serrapeptase (p.1743·2).
*Breast engorgement; cystitis; epididymitis; inflammation; oedema; sinusitis.*

**Serrao** *Masa, Thai.*
Serrapeptase (p.1743·2).
*Inflammation; respiratory-tract congestion; wounds.*

**Serrapep** *Asian Pharm, Thai.*
Serrapeptase (p.1743·2).
*Inflammation; respiratory-tract congestion; wounds.*

**Serrason** *Unison, Thai.*
Serrapeptase (p.1743·2).
*Breast engorgement; cystitis; epididymitis; inflammation; sinusitis; wisdom tooth pericoronitis; wounds.*

**Serratol** *Serral, Mex.*
Difenidol (p.1261·1).
*Nausea and vomiting; vertigo.*

**Serrazyme** *Shin Poong, Singapore.*
Serrapeptase (p.1743·2).
*Inflammation; respiratory-tract congestion.*

**Serrin** *Macrophar, Thai.*
Serrapeptase (p.1743·2).
*Inflammation; respiratory-tract congestion.*

**Serta** *Unichem, India.*
Sertraline hydrochloride (p.317·2).
*Depression; obsessive-compulsive disorder; panic disorder; post-traumatic stress disorder.*

**Sertacream** *Geymonat, Ital.*
Sertaconazole nitrate (p.408·1).
*Fungal skin infections.*

**Sertadie** *Geymonat, Ital.*
Sertaconazole nitrate (p.408·1).
*Vaginal candidiasis.*

**Sertagyn** *Shire, Ital.*
Sertaconazole nitrate (p.408·1).
*Vaginal candidiasis.*

**Sertal** *Roemmers, Arg.*
Pargeverine (p.487·3).
*Smooth muscle spasm.*

**Sertal Compuesto** *Roemmers, Arg.*
Pargeverine (p.487·3); clonixin lysine (p.26·3).
*Smooth muscle spasm.*

**Sertalia** *Theramex, Mon.*
Copper-wound polyethylene (p.1425·3).
*Intra-uterine contraceptive device; postcoital contraceptive.*

**Serterol** *Serral, Mex.*
Probucol (p.986·3).
*Hypercholesterolaemia.*

**Sertidine** *Serral, Mex.*
Famotidine (p.1265·2).
*Peptic ulcer.*

**Sertinal** *Bouzen, Arg.*
Phenylpropanolamine (p.1127·3); caffeine (p.782·1).
*Obesity.*

**Sertopic** *CPH, Port.*
Sertaconazole nitrate (p.408·1).
*Fungal skin infections; vulvovaginal candidiasis.*

**Sertrixen** *Serral, Mex.*
Naproxen (p.65·1).
*Inflammation; pain.*

**Serutan** *Menley & James, USA.*
Psyllium seed (p.1268·1).
*Constipation.*

**Servambutol** *Biochemie, Thai.; Novartis, Thai.*
Ethambutol hydrochloride (p.211·3).
*Tuberculosis.*

**Servamox**
*Novartis, Mex.; Servipharm, Switz.†.*
Amoxicillin trihydrate (p.155·3).
*Bacterial infections.*

*Biochemie, Thai.; Novartis, Thai.*
Amoxicillin (p.155·3).
*Bacterial infections.*

**Servamox CLV** *Novartis, Mex.*
Amoxicillin trihydrate (p.155·3); potassium clavulanate (p.193·3).
*Bacterial infections.*

**Servamox-F** *Novartis, Mex.*
Amoxicillin trihydrate (p.155·3).
*Bacterial infections.*

**Servanolol** *Novartis, Thai.†; Servipharm, Thai.†.*
Propranolol hydrochloride (p.989·3).
*Angina pectoris; hypertension; myocardial infarction.*

**Servatrin** *Aspen, S.Afr.*
Timolol maleate (p.1012·2); amiloride hydrochloride (p.858·2); hydrochlorothiazide (p.933·2).
*Hypertension.*

**Servazolin** *Biochemie, Austria.*
Cefazolin sodium (p.170·3).
*Bacterial infections.*

**Servetinal** *Salusif, Port.*
Bismuth salicylate (p.1252·1); belladonna (p.479·1); calcium carbonate (p.1254·2); magnesium hydroxide (p.1272·2); peppermint oil (p.1283·2); sodium bicarbonate (p.1223·2).
*Gastric hyperacidity.*

**Servicef**
*Note. This name is used for preparations of different composition.*
*Novartis, Mex.*
Cefalexin (p.168·1).
*Bacterial infections.*

*Servipharm, Switz.†.*
Cefazolin sodium (p.170·3).
*Bacterial infections.*

**Servicillin** *Novartis, Thai.†; Servipharm, Thai.†.*
Ampicillin trihydrate (p.157·2).
*Bacterial infections.*

**Servicimet** *Novartis, Thai.†; Servipharm, Thai.†.*
Cimetidine (p.1255·3).
*Gastro-oesophageal reflux; peptic ulcer; Zollinger-Ellison syndrome.*

**Serviclazide** *Biochemie, Thai.; Novartis, Thai.*
Gliclazide (p.332·1).
*Diabetes mellitus.*

**Serviclor** *Novartis, Mex.*
Cefaclor (p.167·1).
*Bacterial infections.*

**Serviclox** *Biochemie, Thai.; Novartis, Thai.*
Cloxacillin sodium (p.198·2).
*Bacterial infections.*

**Servicol** *Novartis, Thai.†; Servipharm, Thai.†.*
Chloramphenicol (p.185·1) or chloramphenicol palmitate (p.185·1).
*Bacterial infections.*

**Servicyclin** *Novartis, Thai.†; Servipharm, Thai.†.*
Oxytetracycline hydrochloride (p.241·1).
*Bacterial infections.*

**Servidapsone** *Biochemie, Thai.; Novartis, Thai.*
Dapsone (p.202·2).
*Dermatitis herpetiformis; leprosy.*

**Servidiclox** *Biochemie, Thai.; Novartis, Thai.*
Dicloxacillin sodium (p.205·2).
*Bacterial infections.*

**Servidipine** *Novartis, Thai.†; Servipharm, Thai.†.*
Nifedipine (p.966·2).
*Hypertension; ischaemic heart disease.*

**Servidopa** *Biochemie, Thai.; Novartis, Thai.*
Methyldopa (p.953·2).
*Hypertension.*

**Servidoxyne**
*Servipharm, Hong Kong†; Servipharm, Singapore†; Biochemie, Thai.; Novartis, Thai.*
Doxycycline hyclate (p.206·2).
*Bacterial infections.*

**Servidrat**
*Biochemie, Singapore; Novartis, Thai.†; Servipharm, Thai.†.*
Glucose; electrolytes (p.1222·2).
*Diarrhoea; oral rehydration therapy.*

**Servidrat Low Sodium** *Servipharm, Malaysia.*
Glucose; sodium chloride; potassium chloride; citric acid; sodium bicarbonate (p.1222·2).
*Diarrhoea; oral rehydration therapy.*

**Serviflox** *Novartis, Thai.*
Ciprofloxacin (p.188·2).
*Bacterial infections.*

**Servigenta**
*Novartis, Mex.; Servipharm, Switz.†; Novartis, Thai.†; Servipharm, Thai.†.*
Gentamicin sulfate (p.217·1).
*Bacterial infections.*

**Servin** *Condrugs, Thai.*
Mianserin hydrochloride (p.306·3).
*Depression.*

**Servinadine** *Novartis, Thai.†; Servipharm, Thai.†.*
Terfenadine (p.441·1).
*Allergic conjunctivitis; allergic rhinitis.*

**Servinaprox** *Servipharm, Switz.†.*
Naproxen (p.65·1).
*Inflammation; pain.*

**Servindomet** *Novartis, Thai.†; Servipharm, Thai.†.*
Indometacin (p.47·3).
*Gout; musculoskeletal and joint disorders; pain.*

**Servipen-V** *Biochemie, Thai.; Novartis, Thai.*
Phenoxymethylpenicillin potassium (p.242·1).
*Bacterial infections.*

**Servipep**
*Servipharm, Hong Kong; Servipharm, Singapore†; Novartis, Thai.†; Servipharm, Thai.†.*
Famotidine (p.1265·2).
*Gastro-oesophageal reflux; peptic ulcer; Zollinger-Ellison syndrome.*

**Serviprofen**
*Servipharm, Switz.†; Novartis, Thai.†; Servipharm, Thai.†.*
Ibuprofen (p.45·3).
*Fever; gout; inflammation; musculoskeletal and joint disorders; pain.*

**Serviproxan** *Biochemie, Thai.; Novartis, Thai.*
Naproxen sodium (p.65·1).
*Gout; musculoskeletal and joint disorders; pain.*

**Serviradine** *Novartis, Mex.*
Ranitidine hydrochloride (p.1285·2).
*Acid aspiration; gastro-oesophageal reflux; gastrointestinal haemorrhage; peptic ulcer; Zollinger-Ellison syndrome.*

**Servispor**
*Servipharm, Switz.†; Novartis, Thai.†; Servipharm, Thai.†.*
Cefalexin (p.168·1).
*Bacterial infections.*

**Servitamol**
*Servipharm, Switz.†; Novartis, Thai.†; Servipharm, Thai.†.*
Salbutamol (p.791·3).
*Obstructive airways disease.*

**Servitenol** *Servipharm, Switz.†.*
Atenolol (p.865·2).
*Angina pectoris; hypertension; myocardial infarction.*

**Servitet** *Novartis, Thai.†; Servipharm, Thai.†.*
Tetracycline hydrochloride (p.266·2).
*Bacterial infections.*

**Servithiazid** *Novartis, Thai.†; Servipharm, Thai.†.*
Hydrochlorothiazide (p.933·2).
*Hypertension; oedema.*

**Servitifen** *Novartis, Thai.†; Servipharm, Thai.†.*
Ketotifen (p.788·2).
*Allergic bronchitis; asthma; hay fever.*

**Servitrim**
*Novartis, Mex.; Novartis, Thai.†; Servipharm, Thai.†.*
Co-trimoxazole (p.199·3).
*Bacterial infections; Pneumocystis carinii pneumonia.*

**Servitrocin**
*Servipharm, Hong Kong†; Servipharm, Singapore†; Servipharm, Switz.†; Biochemie, Thai.; Novartis, Thai.*
Erythromycin ethyl succinate (p.208·1) or erythromycin stearate (p.208·2).
*Bacterial infections.*

**Servium** *Teva, Israel†.*
Chlordiazepoxide (p.674·2).
*Anxiety; insomnia; premedication; sedative.*

**Servizol**
*Novartis, Mex.; Servipharm, Singapore†; Servipharm, Switz.†; Novartis, Thai.†; Servipharm, Thai.†.*
Metronidazole (p.607·2) or metronidazole benzoate (p.607·2).
*Anaerobic infections; protozoal infections.*

**Serzone**
*Bristol-Myers Squibb, Austral.†; Bristol-Myers Squibb, Braz.†; Bristol-Myers Squibb, Canad.†; Bristol-Myers Squibb, Hong Kong†; Bristol-Myers Squibb, Mex.†; Bristol-Myers Squibb, NZ†; Bristol-Myers Squibb, S.Afr.†; Bristol-Myers Squibb, Singapore†; Bristol-Myers Squibb, Thai.†; Bristol-Myers Squibb, USA†.*
Nefazodone hydrochloride (p.309·2).
*Depression.*

**Serzonil** *Bristol-Myers Squibb, Israel†.*
Nefazodone hydrochloride (p.309·2).
*Depression.*

**Sesal** *Ophtha, Denm.*
Antazoline hydrochloride (p.424·2); naphazoline hydrochloride (p.1124·3).
*Allergic conjunctivitis.*

**Sesalgin** *Willmar, Mex.†.*
Dipyrone (p.35·3).

**Sesame Street** *McNeil Consumer, USA.*
A range of vitamin preparations (p.1417·1).

**Sesden**
*Tanabe, Jpn; Tanabe, Singapore.*
Timepidium bromide (p.489·3).
*Premedication for examination of the gastrointestinal or urinary tract; smooth muscle spasm.*

**Sessoforte** *Denk, Hong Kong.*
Vitamins; methyltestosterone; kola; damiana; yohimbine; strychnos; ephedra; testis extract (p.1417·1).
*Tonic.*

**Sestrine** *Beta, Arg.*
Repaglinide (p.344·3).
*Diabetes mellitus.*

**Setacol** *Hamilton, Austral.*
Hyoscine butylbromide (p.483·3).

**Setamol**
*Reckitt Benckiser, Austral.; Hovid, Hong Kong; Hovid, Singapore†.*
Paracetamol (p.76·2).
*Fever; pain.*

**Setarin** *Strand, Malaysia.*
Miconazole nitrate (p.405·3).
*Fungal skin infections.*

**Setarin H** *Strand, Malaysia.*
Miconazole (p.405·2); hydrocortisone acetate (p.1103·3).
*Infected skin disorders.*

**Setcillin** *Strand, Malaysia.*
Ampicillin trihydrate (p.157·2).
*Bacterial infections.*

**Sethro** *Strand, Malaysia.*
Erythromycin ethyl succinate (p.208·1) or erythromycin stearate (p.208·2).
*Bacterial infections.*

**Setin** *Alliance, S.Afr.*
Metoclopramide hydrochloride (p.1274·3).
*Gastrointestinal disorders.*

**Setlers**
*Note. This name is used for preparations of different composition.*
*Block, Austria.*
Simeticone (p.1289·2).
*Flatulence.*

*Thornton & Ross, UK.*
Calcium carbonate (p.1254·2).
*Dyspepsia; flatulence; heartburn; nausea.*

**Setlers Heartburn & Indigestion Liquid** *Stafford-Miller, UK.*
Calcium carbonate (p.1254·2); sodium bicarbonate (p.1223·2); sodium alginate (p.1577·1).
*Dyspepsia; gastro-oesophageal reflux; heartburn.*

**Setlers Tums** *SmithKline Beecham Consumer, Irl.†.*
Calcium carbonate (p.1254·2).
*Dyspepsia; flatulence; heartburn; nausea.*

**Setlinctus** *Strand, Malaysia.*
Codeine phosphate (p.27·1).
*Coughs.*

**Setmenate** *Strand, Malaysia.*
Dimenhydrinate (p.431·1).
*Ménière's disease; migraine; nausea and vomiting; vertigo.*

**Setmotil** *Strand, Malaysia.*
Diphenoxylate hydrochloride (p.1261·3).
Atropine sulfate (p.477·1) is included in this preparation to discourage abuse.
*Diarrhoea; ostomy management.*

**Setmoxil** *Strand, Malaysia.*
Amoxicillin trihydrate (p.155·3).
*Bacterial infections.*

**Setprodine** *Raza, Hong Kong.*
Pseudoephedrine hydrochloride (p.1129·2); triprolidine hydrochloride (p.442·3).
*Allergic rhinitis; coughs; sinusitis; upper respiratory-tract congestion.*

**Setrilan** *Essex, Ital.*
Spirapril hydrochloride (p.1003·1).
*Hypertension.*

**Setromol** *Strand, Malaysia.*
Paracetamol (p.76·2).
*Fever; pain.*

**Setron** *Agis, Israel.*
Granisetron (p.1267·2).
*Nausea and vomiting induced by cytotoxic therapy.*

**Setronges**
*Raza, Hong Kong; Strand, Malaysia.*
Cetylpyridinium chloride (p.1173·1); benzocaine (p.1370·3).
*Mouth and throat disorders.*

**Setronil** *Chemopharma, Chile.*
Citalopram hydrobromide (p.289·1).
*Depression; panic attacks.*

**Setrosone** *Strand, Malaysia.*
Betamethasone valerate (p.1093·2).
*Skin disorders.*

**Setrozole** *Strand, Malaysia.*
Metronidazole (p.607·2).
*Amoebiasis; trichomoniasis.*

**Setsolone** *Strand, Malaysia.*
Prednisolone (p.1108·1).
*Corticosteroid.*

**Setux** *Aventis, Braz.*
Codeine resinate (p.27·3); phenyltoloxamine resinate (p.439·1).
*Coughs.*

**Setux Expectorante** *Aventis, Braz.*
Codeine resinate (p.27·3); guaifenesin (p.1122·1); phenyltoloxamine resinate (p.439·1).
*Coughs.*

**Seudotabs** *Parmed, USA.*
Pseudoephedrine hydrochloride (p.1129·2).
*Nasal congestion.*

**Seven Seas**
*British Cod Liver Oils, Hong Kong; Seven Seas, Singapore; Merck, Thai.; Seven Seas, UK.*
A range of vitamin, mineral, and nutritional preparations (p.1417·1).

**Sevenal** *Chinoin, Mex.†.*
Phenobarbital sodium (p.367·3).

**Sevenaleta** *Chinoin, Mex.†.*
Phenobarbital sodium (p.367·3).

**Severin** *Chinoin, Mex.*
Nimesulide (p.67·1).
*Fever; inflammation; pain.*

**Severon** *Profarma, Thai.*
Omeprazole (p.1278·2).
*Gastro-oesophageal reflux; peptic ulcer; Zollinger-Ellison syndrome.*

**Sevinol** *Schering-Plough, Belg.*
Fluphenazine hydrochloride (p.699·3).
*Psychoses.*

**Sevium** *Ni-The, Gr.*
Haloperidol (p.701·2).
*Huntington's chorea; psychoses; tics.*

**Sevocris** *Cristalia, Braz.*
Sevoflurane (p.1307·3).
*General anaesthesia.*

**Sevorane**
*Abbott, Arg.; Abbott, Austral.; Abbott, Austria; Abbott, Belg.; Abbott, Braz.; Abbott, Canad.; Abbott, Denm.; Abbott, Fin.; Abbott, Fr.; Abbott, Ger.; Abbott, Gr.; Abbott, Hong Kong; Abbott, Irl.; Abbott, Israel; Abbott, Ital.; Abbott, Malaysia; Abbott, Mex.; Abbott, Neth.; Abbott, Norw.; Abbott, NZ; Abbott, Singapore; Abbott, Spain; Abbott, Swed.; Abbott, Switz.; Abbott, Thai.*
Sevoflurane (p.1307·3).
*General anaesthesia.*

**Sevorex** *Tika, Swed.*
Precipitated sulfur (p.1158·2); salicylic acid (p.1157·1).
*Scalp disorders.*

**Sevredol**
*Viatris, Fr.; Mundipharma, Ger.; Napp, Irl.; Viatris, Neth.; Douglas, NZ; Viatris, Port.; Viatris, Spain; Mundipharma, Switz.; Napp, UK.*
Morphine sulfate (p.60·2).
*Pain.*

**Sevre-Long** *Mundipharma, Switz.*
Morphine sulfate (p.60·2).
*Pain.*

**Sevrium** *Vinas, Spain†.*
Tetrabamate, a complex of febarbamate (p.698·2), difebarbamate (p.697·2), and phenobarbital (p.367·3).
*Alcohol withdrawal syndrome.*

**Sexadien** *Leo, Denm.*
Dienestrol (p.1547·3).
*Vulvovaginal disorders.*

**Sexormom** *INQ, Braz.†.*
Methyltestosterone (p.1559·3); yohimbine (p.1766·2); caffeine (p.782·1); tocopherol (p.1464·3); ephedrine (p.1120·1).
*Erectile dysfunction.*

**SF Gel** *Cypress, USA.*
Sodium fluoride (p.1444·3).
*Dental caries prophylaxis.*

**SFC Lotion** *Stiefel, USA.*
Stearyl alcohol (p.1482·3).
*Skin cleanser.*

**S/Gel** *Neutrogena, Fr.†.*
Salicylic acid (p.1157·1).
*Scalp disorders.*

**Sguardi** *Farmigea, Ital.*
Benzalkonium chloride (p.1168·3).
*Eye disinfection.*

**SH-206** *Pharmascience, Canad.*
Acetic acid (p.1645·2); camphor (p.1665·3).
*Pediculosis.*

**Shade**
*Note. This name is used for preparations of different composition.*
*Schering-Plough, Canad.†.*
*SPF 15:* Octinoxate (p.1154·3); oxybenzone (p.1154·3).
*SPF 25:* Oxybenzone (p.1154·3); octinoxate (p.1154·3); octisalate (p.1154·3).
*SPF 30:* Oxybenzone (p.1154·3); octinoxate (p.1154·3); homosalate (p.1148·1); octisalate (p.1154·3).
*SPF 45:* Octinoxate (p.1154·3); octocrilene (p.1154·3); octisalate (p.1154·3); oxybenzone (p.1154·3).
*Sunscreen.*
*Essex, Chile.*
*SPF 30; SPF 45:* Homosalate (p.1148·1); octinoxate (p.1154·3); oxybenzone (p.1154·3); octisalate (p.1154·3); imidazolidinyl urea.
*Sunscreen.*
*Schering-Plough, USA.*
*Gel SPF 30:* Octinoxate (p.1154·3); oxybenzone (p.1154·3); homosalate (p.1148·1).
*Lotion SPF 30; stick SPF 30:* Octinoxate (p.1154·3); oxybenzone (p.1154·3); homosalate (p.1148·1); octisalate (p.1154·3).
*SPF 15:* Octinoxate (p.1154·3); oxybenzone (p.1154·3).
*SPF 45:* Octinoxate (p.1154·3); oxybenzone (p.1154·3); octocrilene (p.1154·3); octisalate (p.1154·3).
*Sunscreen.*

**Shade UVAGuard** *Schering-Plough, USA.*
Octinoxate (p.1154·3); avobenzone (p.1142·3); oxybenzone (p.1154·3).
*Sunscreen.*

**Shak Iso** *Clintec, Fr.†.*
Preparation for enteral nutrition (p.1417·1).

**Shaklee Dandruff Control** *Shaklee, Canad.*
Pyrithione zinc (p.1156·2).

**Shaklee Lip Protection Stick** *Shaklee, Canad.*
*SPF 15:* Padimate O (p.1155·1); oxybenzone (p.1154·3).
*Sunscreen.*

**Shaklee Sunscreen** *Shaklee, Canad.†.*
*SPF 30:* Octinoxate (p.1154·3); octisalate (p.1154·3); oxybenzone (p.1154·3).
*Sunscreen.*

**Shamday Antiforfora** *Euroderm, Ital.*
Piroctone olamine (p.1155·2); urtica (p.1762·1).
*Seborrhoeic dermatitis.*

**Shampoo SDE Tar** *Essex, Ital.*
Coal tar (p.1159·2).
*Scalp disorders.*

**Shampoo SDE Zinc** *Essex, Ital.*
Pyrithione zinc (p.1156·2).
*Seborrhoeic dermatitis.*

**Shampoo Tersa-Tar** *Dermaclin, Mex.*
Coal tar (p.1159·2).
*Scalp disorders.*

**Shampooing Anti-Pelliculaire** *Atlas, Canad.*
Pyrithione zinc (p.1156·2).

**Shampooing extra-doux** *Widmer, Switz.*
Triclosan (p.1195·2).
*Scalp disorders.*

**Shampooing Traitant Antipelliculaire** *Ducray, Fr.*
Pyrithione zinc (p.1156·2).
*Dandruff.*

**Shampoux** *Qualiphar, Belg.†.*
Permethrin (p.1508·3); piperonyl butoxide (p.1509·2).
*Pediculosis.*

**Shampoux Repel** *Qualiphar, Belg.†.*
(N-Butyl-N-acetyl)-3-ethylaminopropionate.
*Pediculosis.*

**Shanvac-B** *Shanta, India.*
A hepatitis B vaccine (p.1618·1).
*Active immunisation.*

**Sharkoferrol** *Alembic, India.*
Ferric ammonium citrate; malt extract; vitamins (p.1417·1).
*Nutritional supplement.*

**Sharkomalt** *Haffkine, India.*
Vitamin A (p.1451·2); vitamin D (p.1461·2); malt extract.
*Vitamin A and D deficiency.*

**Sharkovit** *Haffkine, India.*
Vitamin A (p.1451·2); vitamin D (p.1461·2).
*Vitamin A and D deficiency.*

**Sheik** *Durex, Canad.*
Nonoxinol 9 (p.1413·3).
*Contraceptive.*

**Sheik Elite** *Schmid, USA.*
Nonoxinol 9 (p.1413·3).
*Contraceptive.*

**Sheko** *Medipharma, Hong Kong.*
Zinc oxide (p.1163·2); methyl salicylate (p.59·3).
*Skin disorders.*

**Shellgel** *Cytosol, USA.*
Sodium hyaluronate (p.1697·3).
*Aid in ophthalmic surgery.*

**Shemol** *Grin, Mex.*
Timolol maleate (p.1012·2).
*Glaucoma; ocular hypertension.*

**Shepard's** *Dermik, USA.*
Emollient and moisturiser.

**Shield** *GlaxoSmithKline, India.*
Lidocaine (p.1377·3); hydrocortisone acetate (p.1103·3); zinc oxide (p.1163·2); allantoin (p.1141·3).
*Anorectal disorders.*

**Shields** *Ansell, Canad.*
Nonoxinol 9 (p.1413·3).
*Contraceptive.*

**Shii-ta-ker** *Holistica, Fr.*
Lentinus edodes.
*Immunostimulant.*

**Shin-Biofermin S** *Takeda, Hong Kong.*
*Bifidobacterium bifidum* (p.1704·2); *Lactobacillus acidophilus* (p.1704·2); *Enterococcus faecalis* (p.1704·2).
*Constipation; diarrhoea; meteorism.*

**Shinbit** *Schering, Jpn.*
Nifekalant hydrochloride (p.972·2).
*Arrhythmias.*

**Shincef** *Shin Poong, Singapore.*
Cefuroxime sodium (p.184·1).
*Bacterial infections.*

**Shincort**
*YSP, Malaysia; Yung Shin, Singapore; Yung Shin, Thai.*
Triamcinolone acetonide (p.1110·2).
*Corticosteroid.*

**Shinfomycin** *YSP, Malaysia.*
Cefoperazone sodium (p.174·3).
*Bacterial infections.*

**Shingles Pain Relief** *Procare, Austral.†.*
Capsicum (p.1667·1).
*Arthritic and rheumatic pain; postherpetic neuralgia.*

**Shinoxol**
*YSP, Malaysia; Yung Shin, Singapore.*
Ambroxol hydrochloride (p.1114·3).
*Respiratory-tract disorders associated with viscous mucus.*

**Shintamet**
*YSP, Malaysia; Yung Shin, Singapore.*
Cimetidine (p.1255·3).
*Dyspepsia; gastro-oesophageal reflux; gastrointestinal hypersecretion; peptic ulcer.*

**Shiomarin** *Shionogi, Jpn.*
Latamoxef sodium (p.225·3).
Lidocaine (p.1377·3) is included in the intramuscular injection to alleviate the pain of injection.
*Bacterial infections.*

**Shiseido Benefiance Daytime** *Shiseido, Canad.*
*Cream:* Octinoxate (p.1154·3); oxybenzone (p.1154·3).
*Emulsion:* Octinoxate (p.1154·3).
*Sunscreen.*

**Shiseido Skincare Day Essential** *Shiseido, Canad.*
*SPF 10:* Avobenzone (p.1142·3); octinoxate (p.1154·3).
*Sunscreen.*

**Shiseido Skincare Day Protective** *Shiseido, Canad.*
*SPF 15:* Titanium dioxide (p.1160·3).
*Sunscreen.*

**Shiseido Skincare Protective** *Shiseido, Canad.*
Avobenzone (p.1142·3); octinoxate (p.1154·3); oxybenzone (p.1154·3).
*Sunscreen.*

**Shiseido Sun Block Stick** *Shiseido, Canad.*
Octinoxate (p.1154·3); titanium dioxide (p.1160·3).
*Sunscreen.*

**Shiseido Sun Protection** *Shiseido, Canad.*
*SPF 8:* Octinoxate (p.1154·3).
*Sunscreen.*

**Shiseido Sunblock** *Shiseido, Canad.*
*SPF 19:* Octinoxate (p.1154·3); oxybenzone (p.1154·3).
*Sunscreen.*

**Shiseido Sunblock Face Cream** *Shiseido, Canad.*
Octinoxate (p.1154·3); oxybenzone (p.1154·3); ensulizole (p.1147·1); titanium dioxide (p.1160·3).
*Sunscreen.*

**Shiseido Sunblock Lip Treatment** *Shiseido, Canad.*
Octinoxate (p.1154·3).
*Sunscreen.*

**Shiseido Tanning** *Shiseido, Canad.†.*
*SPF 4:* Octinoxate (p.1154·3).
*Sunscreen.*

**Shiseido Translucent Sun Block** *Shiseido, Canad.*
Octinoxate (p.1154·3); oxybenzone (p.1154·3); titanium dioxide (p.1160·3).
*Sunscreen.*

**Shiseido Vital-Perfection** *Shiseido, Canad.*
*Cream:* Octinoxate (p.1154·3); oxybenzone (p.1154·3); titanium dioxide (p.1160·3).
*Stick:* Octinoxate (p.1154·3).
*Sunscreen.*

**Shiwalax** *Shiwa, Thai.*
Tolperisone hydrochloride (p.1396·3).
*Musculoskeletal pain; parkinsonism.*

**Shur-Seal** *Milex, USA.*
Nonoxinol 9 (p.1413·3).
*Contraceptive.*

**Si o No** *Fresh Ones, Arg.*
Pregnancy test (p.1734·3).

**Siadocin** *Siam Bheasach, Thai.*
Doxycycline hyclate (p.206·2).
*Bacterial infections.*

**Sialexin** *Siam Bheasach, Thai.*
Cefalexin (p.168·1).
*Bacterial infections.*

**Sialin** *Sigmapharm, Austria.*
Carmellose sodium (p.1577·3); electrolytes (p.1217·1).
*Saliva substitute.*

**Sialor** *Paladin, Canad.*
Anethole trithione (p.1655·1).
*Dry mouth.*

**Siamdopa** *Siam Bheasach, Thai.*
Methyldopa (p.953·2).
*Hypertension.*

**Siamformet** *Siam Bheasach, Thai.*
Metformin hydrochloride (p.342·3).
*Diabetes mellitus.*

**Siamidine** *Siam Bheasach, Thai.*
Cimetidine (p.1255·3).
*Gastric hyperacidity; gastro-oesophageal reflux; peptic ulcer.*

**Siamik** *Siam Bheasach, Thai.*
Amikacin sulfate (p.154·1).
*Bacterial infections.*

**Sia-Mox** *Siam Bheasach, Thai.*
Amoxicillin trihydrate (p.155·3).
*Bacterial infections.*

**Siampicil** *Siam Bheasach, Thai.*
Ampicillin trihydrate (p.157·2).
*Bacterial infections.*

**Siampraxol** *Siam Bheasach, Thai.*
Alprazolam (p.668·3).
*Anxiety; mixed anxiety depressive states.*

**Siarizine** *Siam Bheasach, Thai.*
Cinnarizine (p.428·3).
*Cerebrovascular disorders; migraine; motion sickness; peripheral vascular disorders; vestibular disorders.*

**Siaten** *Italfarmaco, Spain.*
Zopiclone (p.729·3).
*Insomnia.*

**Sibelium**
*Janssen-Cilag, Arg.; Janssen-Cilag, Austria; Janssen-Cilag, Belg.; Janssen-Cilag, Braz.; Pharmascience, Canad.; Janssen-Cilag, Chile; Janssen-Cilag, Denm.; Janssen-Cilag, Fr.; Janssen-Cilag, Ger.; Janssen, Hong Kong; Janssen-Cilag, Irl.; Janssen-Cilag, Ital.; Janssen-Cilag, Malaysia; Janssen, Mex.; Janssen-Cilag, Neth.; Janssen-Cilag, Port.; Janssen-Cilag, S.Afr.; Janssen-Cilag, Singapore; Esteve, Spain; Janssen-Cilag, Switz.; Janssen-Cilag, Thai.*
Flunarizine hydrochloride (p.434·1).
*Migraine; vestibular disorders.*

**Sibelium Plus** *Janssen-Cilag, Arg.*
Flunarizine hydrochloride (p.434·1); nicergoline (p.1719·3).
*Migraine; vertigo.*

**Sibicort** *Orion, Fin.*
Hydrocortisone (p.1103·3); chlorhexidine gluconate (p.1173·2).
*Infected skin disorders.*

**Sibudan** *Teva Tuteur, Arg.*
Irinotecan (p.564·3).
*Malignant neoplasms.*

**Sibu-Estirol** *Bouzen, Arg.*
Sibutramine (p.1593·2).
*Obesity.*

**Sibutral** *Knoll, Fr.*
Sibutramine hydrochloride (p.1593·1).
*Obesity.*

**Sicadentol Plus** *Geminis, Arg.*
*Tablets:* Naproxen (p.65·1).
*Inflammation; pain.*
*Topical liquid:* Procaine (p.1383·2); eugenol (p.1686·2).

**Sicadol** *Rider, Chile.*
Mefenamic acid (p.55·2).
*Pain.*

**Sical**
*Rottapharm, Ital.†; Rottapharm, Spain.*
Calcitonin (salmon) (p.768·2).
*Hypercalcaemia; metastatic bone pain; osteoporosis; Paget's disease of bone.*

**Sicaril** *Sanofi Synthelabo, Gr.*
Malathion (p.1507·1).
*Head and crab lice; scabies.*

**Sicatem** *Richmond, Arg.*
Cisplatin (p.538·1).
*Malignant neoplasms.*

**Sicazine**
*Smith & Nephew, Fr.; Inibsa, Port.†.*
Sulfadiazine silver (p.259·1).
*Burns; wounds.*

**Siccafluid**
*Sidus, Arg.; Thea, Fr.; Thea, Ital.; Thea, Spain.*
Carbomer (p.1577·2).
*Dry eyes; eye irritation.*

**Siccagent** *Alcon, Belg.*
Povidone (p.1581·2).
*Dry eyes.*

**Siccalix** *Drossapharm, Switz.*
Sea salt (p.1233·3); dexpanthenol (p.1727·2).
*Nasal dryness.*

**Siccapos** *Ursapharm, Ger.*
Carbomer 980 (p.1577·2).
*Dry eyes.*

**Siccaprotect**
*Croma, Austria; Ursapharm, Ger.*
Dexpanthenol (p.1727·2); polyvinyl alcohol (p.1581·1).
*Dry eyes.*

**Sicca-Stulln** *Stulln, Ger.*
Hypromellose (p.1579·3).
*Dry eyes.*

**Sicco** *AWD, Ger.*
Indapamide (p.938·2).
*Hypertension.*

**Siccoral** *Sanova, Austria.*
Acetylcysteine (p.1112·3).
*Respiratory-tract disorders associated with viscous mucus.*

**Sicef** *Infosint, Ital.*
Cefazolin sodium (p.170·3).
Lidocaine hydrochloride (p.1377·3) is included in this preparation to alleviate the pain of injection.
*Bacterial infections.*

**Si-Cliss** *SIFRA, Ital.†.*
Sorbitol (p.1446·3); sodium citrate (p.1223·2); sodium lauril sulfoacetate (p.1574·3).
*Constipation.*

**Sico Relax** *Rottapharm, Spain.*
Diazepam (p.690·1).
*Alcohol withdrawal syndrome; anxiety; epilepsy; premedication; skeletal muscle spasticity; sleep disorders.*

**Sicobal** *Siam Bheasach, Thai.*
Mecobalamin (p.1459·1).
*Peripheral neuropathies.*

**Sicombyl** *Christiaens, Belg.*
Salicylic acid (p.1157·1).
*Hygiene of the umbilicus in neonates.*

**Sic-Ophtal** *Winzer, Ger.*
Hypromellose (p.1579·3).
*Dry eyes.*

**Sicoplus** *Disprovent, Arg.*
Idebenone (p.1700·3).
*Cerebrovascular disorders.*

**Sicorten**
*Novartis Consumer, Austria; Novartis Consumer, Belg.†; Bioglan, Ger.; Novartis, Hong Kong; Novartis, Israel†; Novartis, Neth.; Novartis Consumer, Port.; Geminis, Spain; Novartis, Switz.*
Halometasone (p.1103·3).
*Skin disorders.*

**Sicorten Plus**
*Bioglan, Ger.; Novartis, Hong Kong; Novartis, Israel; Novartis Consumer, Port.; Geminis, Spain; Novartis, Switz.*
Halometasone (p.1103·3); triclosan (p.1195·2).
*Infected skin disorders.*

**Sicriptin** *Serum Institute, India.*
Bromocriptine mesilate (p.1200·3).
*Acromegaly; amenorrhoea; female infertility; galactorrhoea; lactation inhibition; parkinsonism.*

**Sicrit** *Wyeth, Chile.*
Medroxyprogesterone acetate (p.1557·2).

**Sidenar** *Armstrong, Arg.*
Lorazepam (p.704·1).
*Anxiety; behaviour disorders; neuroses.*

**Sideralce** *Lafedar, Arg.*
Ferrous sulfate (p.1428·2); folic acid (p.1429·1).
Ascorbic acid (p.1460·2) is included in this preparation to increase the absorption and availability of iron.

**Siderblut** *Disprovent, Arg.*
Ferrous sulfate (p.1428·2).
*Iron-deficiency anaemia.*

**Siderfol** *Raptakos, India.*
Ferrous fumarate (p.1427·3); folic acid; vitamin B$_{12}$; vitamin B$_6$; copper sulfate (p.1417·1).
Vitamin C (p.1460·2) is included in this preparation to increase the absorption and availability of iron.
*Anaemias.*

**Sideril** *Senosiain, Mex.†.*
Trazodone (p.320·1).

**Sideroglobina** *Pharmacia Upjohn, Ital.*
Ferritransferrin.
*Iron-deficiency anaemia.*

**Sidervim** *Lafare, Ital.*
Ferrous gluconate (p.1428·1).
Ascorbic acid (p.1460·2) is included in this preparation to increase the absorption and availability of iron.
*Iron-deficiency anaemia.*

**Sidroga Brust-Husten-Tee** *Jacoby, Austria.*
Althaea (p.1651·3); plantago lanceolata (p.1738·2); thyme leaf (p.1755·2); aniseed (p.1655·2); orange flower (p.1723·3).
*Catarrh; coughs.*

**Sidroga Erkaltungstee** *Jacoby, Austria.*
Rose fruit (p.1740·1); wild thyme; chamomile flower (p.1669·3); sambucus (p.1741·3); tilia (p.1756·2).
*Respiratory-tract disorders.*

**Sidroga Herz-Kreislauf-Tee** *Jacoby, Austria.*
Crataegus (p.1677·1); melissa leaf (p.1711·1); rosemary leaf (p.1740·2); orange flower (p.1723·3); spearmint (p.1749·1).
*Anxiety disorders; cardiac disorders.*

**Sidroga Kindertee** *Jacoby, Austria.*
Fennel (p.1687·2); chamomile flower (p.1669·3); melissa leaf (p.1711·1); peppermint leaf (p.1283·2); tilia (p.1756·2).
*Gastrointestinal disorders; sleep disorders.*

**Sidroga Leber-Galle-Tee** *Jacoby, Austria.*
Taraxacum (p.1751·3); silybum marianum fruit (p.1043·3); achillea (p.1646·2); peppermint leaf (p.1283·2); caraway (p.1667·2).
*Gastrointestinal and biliary disorders.*

**Sidroga Magen-Darm-Tee** *Jacoby, Austria.*
Calamus root (p.1664·1); centaury (p.1669·2); chamomile flower (p.1669·3); achillea (p.1646·2); melissa leaf (p.1711·1); spearmint (p.1749·1).
*Gastrointestinal disorders.*

**Sidroga Nerven- und Schlaftee** *Jacoby, Austria.*
Lupulus (p.1708·1); melissa leaf (p.1711·1); valerian root (p.1762·2); spearmint (p.1749·1); orange flower (p.1723·3).
*Anxiety disorders; sleep disorders.*

**Sidroga Nieren- und Blasentee** *Jacoby, Austria.*
Bearberry leaf (p.1659·2); silver birch leaf (p.1660·3); solidago virgaurea (p.1748·3); java tea (p.1702·3); couch-grass (p.1676·2); peppermint leaf (p.1283·2).
*Urinary-tract disorders.*

**Sidroga Stoffwechseltee** *Jacoby, Austria.*
Spearmint (p.1749·1); taraxacum (p.1751·3); urtica (p.1762·1); prunus spinosa.
*Digestive disorders; renal disorders.*

**Siduol** *Eisai, Thai.*
Alpha tocoferil calcium succinate (p.1465·3); phytomenadione (p.1467·1); rutoside (p.1688·2); muramidase hydrochloride (p.1717·2); pluronic F-68.
*Haemorrhoids.*

**Siduro** *Ipex, Swed.*
Ketoprofen (p.51·2).
*Musculoskeletal pain.*

**Siepex** *Aventis, Spain†.*
Dextromethorphan hydrobromide (p.1117·3).
*Cough.*

**Sieral** *Vilco, Gr.*
Omeprazole (p.1278·2).
*Acid aspiration; eradication of Helicobacter pylori in combination with antimicrobials; peptic ulcer; reflux oesophagitis; Zollinger-Ellison syndrome.*

**Siero Antiofidico** *Sclavo, Ital.†.*
European viper venom antiserum (p.1639·1).
*European viper bite.*

**Sies** *Senosiain, Mex.*
Hidrosmin (p.1688·3).
*Capillary fragility; haemorrhoids; oedema; venous insufficiency.*

**Siesta-1** *Welti, Switz.*
Anhydrous citric acid (p.1673·1); tartaric acid (p.1752·1); magnesium sulfate (p.1228·2); sodium bicarbonate (p.1223·2).
*Constipation.*

The symbol † denotes a preparation no longer actively marketed

**Siete Mares Higado Bacal** *Grifols, Spain†.*
Cod-liver oil (p.1425·2); tocopherol.
*Vitamin A and D deficiencies.*

**Sifaclor** *Siam Bheasach, Thai.*
Cefaclor (p.167·1).
*Bacterial infections.*

**Sifamic** *SIFI, Ital.†.*
Amikacin sulfate (p.154·1).
*Eye infections.*

**Sificetina** *SIFI, Ital.*
Chloramphenicol (p.185·1).
*Eye infections.*

**Sificrom**
*Craveri, Arg.; SIFI, Ital.; SIFI, Singapore.*
Sodium cromoglicate (p.795·3).
*Conjunctivitis; keratoconjunctivitis.*

**Sifiviral** *SIFI, Ital.*
Aciclovir (p.626·1).
*Herpes simplex keratitis.*

**Siframin** *Fresenius Kabi, Ital.*
Amino-acid infusion (p.1417·1).
*Parenteral nutrition.*

**Sifrol**
*Boehringer Ingelheim, Arg.; Boehringer de Angeli, Braz.; Boehringer Ingelheim, Chile; Boehringer Ingelheim, Denm.; Boehringer Ingelheim, Fin.; Boehringer Ingelheim, Ger.; Boehringer Ingelheim, Neth.; Boehringer Ingelheim, Norw.; Boehringer Ingelheim, Swed.; Boehringer Ingelheim, Switz.*
Pramipexole hydrochloride (p.1212·2).
*Parkinsonism.*

**Sigabloc** *Alpharma-Isis, Ger.*
Atenolol (p.865·2); chlortalidone (p.882·3).
*Hypertension.*

**Sigabroxol** *Alpharma-Isis, Ger.*
Ambroxol hydrochloride (p.1114·3).
*Respiratory-tract disorders with increased or viscous mucus.*

**Sigacalm** *Alpharma-Isis, Ger.*
Oxazepam (p.712·2).
*Anxiety; sleep disorders.*

**Sigacap Cor** *Alpharma-Isis, Ger.*
Captopril (p.879·2).
*Heart failure; hypertension.*

**Sigacefal** *Alpharma-Isis, Ger.*
Cefaclor (p.167·1).
*Bacterial infections.*

**Sigacimet** *Alpharma-Isis, Ger.*
Cimetidine (p.1255·3).
*Gastro-oesophageal reflux; peptic ulcer; Zollinger-Ellison syndrome.*

**Sigacora** *Alpharma-Isis, Ger.*
Isosorbide mononitrate (p.942·1).
*Angina pectoris; heart failure; pulmonary hypertension.*

**Sigadoc** *Alpharma-Isis, Ger.*
Indometacin (p.47·3).
*Musculoskeletal, joint, and soft-tissue disorders; sports injuries.*

**Sigadoxin**
*Jacoby, Austria†; Maver, Chile; Alpharma-Isis, Ger.; Neves, Port.; Medika, Switz.*
Doxycycline (p.206·2) or doxycycline hyclate (p.206·2).
*Bacterial infections.*

**Sigafam** *Rhein, Mex.*
Famotidine (p.1265·2).
*Gastro-oesophageal reflux; peptic ulcer; Zollinger-Ellison syndrome.*

**Sigafenac** *Alpharma-Isis, Ger.*
Diclofenac sodium (p.32·1).
*Gout; inflammation; musculoskeletal, joint, and soft-tissue disorders; pain.*

**Sigamopen** *Alpharma-Isis, Ger.*
Amoxicillin trihydrate (p.155·3).
*Bacterial infections.*

**Sigamuc** *Alpharma-Isis, Ger.*
Doxycycline hyclate (p.206·2); ambroxol hydrochloride (p.1114·3).
*Bacterial infections of the respiratory tract.*

**Sigamucil** *Dumex, Ger.†.*
Acetylcysteine (p.1112·3).
*Respiratory-tract disorders associated with increased or viscous mucus.*

**Sigaperidol**
*Alpharma-Isis, Ger.; Medika, Switz.*
Haloperidol (p.701·2).
*Anxiety; pain; psychoses; vomiting.*

**Sigaprim**
*Alpharma-Isis, Ger.; Medika, Switz.*
Co-trimoxazole (p.199·3).
*Bacterial infections; Pneumocystis carinii pneumonia.*

**Sigaprolol** *Alpharma-Isis, Ger.*
Metoprolol tartrate (p.957·1).
*Arrhythmias; hypertension; ischaemic heart disease; migraine; myocardial infarction.*

**Sigapurol**
*Medika, Switz.; Siegfried, Thai.†.*
Allopurinol (p.412·2).
*Gout; hyperuricaemia; renal calculi.*

**Sigas** *Polipharm, Thai.*
Simeticone (p.1289·2).
*Flatulence.*

**Sigasalur** *Dumex, Ger.†.*
Furosemide (p.919·3).
*Hypertension; oedema.*

**Sigatricin** *Trahan, Thai.*
Tyrothricin (p.275·1); benzocaine (p.1370·3); benzethonium chloride (p.1169·2).
*Mouth and throat disorders.*

**Sigma Liquid Antacid** *Sigma, Austral.*
Aluminium hydroxide (p.1249·2); magnesium hydroxide (p.1272·2); simeticone (p.1289·2).
*Dyspepsia; flatulence; heartburn.*

**Sigma Relief**
*Note. This name is used for preparations of different composition.*
*Sigma, Austral.*
Dextromethorphan hydrobromide (p.1117·3); pseudoephedrine hydrochloride (p.1129·2); guaifenesin (p.1122·1); sodium citrate (p.1223·2).
*Cold and influenza symptoms; coughs.*

*Sigma, Hong Kong.*
Dextromethorphan hydrobromide (p.1117·3); pseudoephedrine hydrochloride (p.1129·2); guaifenesin (p.1122·1).
*Coughs; respiratory-tract congestion.*

**Sigma Relief Chest Rub** *Sigma, Austral.*
Camphor (p.1665·3); menthol (p.1711·3).

**Sigma Relief Junior**
*Sigma, Austral.*
Dextromethorphan hydrobromide (p.1117·3); pseudoephedrine hydrochloride (p.1129·2); sodium citrate.
*Cold and influenza symptoms; coughs.*

*Sigma, Hong Kong.*
Dextromethorphan hydrobromide (p.1117·3); pseudoephedrine hydrochloride (p.1129·2).
*Coughs; respiratory-tract congestion.*

**Sigmacort** *Sigma, Austral.*
Hydrocortisone acetate (p.1103·3).
*Skin disorders.*

**Sigmafon** *Lafare, Ital.†.*
Mebutamate (p.951·2).
*Hypertension.*

**Sigmalin B$_6$** *Sigmapharm, Austria.*
Salicylamide (p.87·3); paracetamol (p.76·2); caffeine (p.782·1); pyridoxine hydrochloride (p.1456·3).
*Fever; pain.*

**Sigmalin B$_6$ forte** *Sigmapharm, Austria.*
Salicylamide (p.87·3); paracetamol (p.76·2); dextropropoxyphene hydrochloride (p.28·3); caffeine (p.782·1); pyridoxine hydrochloride (p.1456·3).
*Fever; pain.*

**Sigmalin B$_6$ ohne Coffein** *Sigmapharm, Austria.*
Salicylamide (p.87·3); paracetamol (p.76·2); pyridoxine hydrochloride (p.1456·3).
*Fever; pain.*

**Sigman-Haustropfen** *Sigmapharm, Austria.*
Peppermint oil (p.1283·2); caraway oil (p.1667·3); dexpanthenol (p.1727·2); chamomile flower (p.1669·3); condurango bark (p.1675·3); liquorice root (p.1270·2); absinthium (p.1645·1); gentian root (p.1692·2); bitter orange peel (p.1723·3).
Formerly contained peppermint oil, caraway oil, dexpanthenol, chamomile flower, condurango bark, liquorice root, absinthium, gentian root, bitter orange peel, senna, and frangula bark.
*Gastrointestinal and biliary-tract disorders.*

**Sigmart** *Chugai, Jpn.*
Nicorandil (p.965·3).
*Angina pectoris.*

**Sigmasporin**
*Sigma, Braz.†; Julphar, UAE.*
Ciclosporin (p.1351·2).
*Atopic eczema; nephrotic syndrome; psoriasis; rheumatoid arthritis; transplant rejection.*

**Sigmatriol** *Sigma, Braz.†.*
Calcitriol (p.1461·2).
*Vitamin D supplement.*

**Sigmaxin** *Fawns & McAllan, Austral.*
Digoxin (p.895·2).

**Sigmetadine** *Sigma, Austral.*
Cimetidine (p.1255·3).
*Gastro-oesophageal reflux; peptic ulcer; Zollinger-Ellison syndrome.*

**Signal** *Green Turtle Bay Vitamin Co., USA.*
Omega triglycerides (p.1417·1).
*Tonic.*

**Sigtab-M** *Roberts, USA.*
Multivitamin and mineral preparation (p.1417·1).

**Siguent Hycor** *Sigma, Austral.*
Hydrocortisone acetate (p.1103·3).
*Inflammatory eye disorders.*

**Siguent Neomycin** *Sigma, Austral.*
Neomycin sulfate (p.235·1).
*Skin infections.*

**SIL-1000, -5000** *DORC, Neth.*
Silicone oil (p.1482·1).
*Ophthalmic tamponade.*

**Silace**
*Tanta, Canad.; Silarx, USA.*
Docusate sodium (p.1262·2).
*Constipation.*

**Silace-C** *Silarx, USA†.*
Casanthranol (p.1255·1); docusate sodium (p.1262·2).
*Constipation.*

**Silact** *Sofar, Ital.*
Tilactase (p.1756·2).
*Lactose intolerance.*

**Siladryl** *Silarx, USA.*
Diphenhydramine hydrochloride (p.431·3).
*Hypersensitivity reactions.*

**Silafed** *Silarx, USA.*
Pseudoephedrine hydrochloride (p.1129·2); triprolidine hydrochloride (p.442·3).
*Upper respiratory-tract symptoms.*

**Silain** *Teva, Israel.*
Simeticone (p.1289·2); aluminium hydroxide-magnesium carbonate co-dried gel (p.1250·1).
*Flatulence; gastrointestinal hyperacidity.*

**Silaminic Cold** *Silarx, USA†.*
Phenylpropanolamine hydrochloride (p.1127·3); chlorphenamine maleate (p.427·3).
*Cold symptoms.*

**Silaminic Expectorant** *Silarx, USA†.*
Phenylpropanolamine hydrochloride (p.1127·3); guaifenesin (p.1122·1).
*Coughs.*

**Sil-A-Mox** *Silom, Thai.*
Amoxicillin trihydrate (p.155·3).
*Bacterial infections.*

**Silan** *Smith & Nephew, Denm.*
Dimeticone (p.1482·1); zinc oxide (p.1163·2).
*Dry skin; skin irritation.*

**Silapap** *Silarx, USA.*
Paracetamol (p.76·2).
*Fever; pain.*

**Silarine** *Vir, Spain.*
Silymarin (p.1043·3).
*Toxic hepatitis.*

**Silartrin** *Silesia, Chile.*
Ibuprofen (p.45·3); dipyrone (p.35·3).
Aluminium hydroxide (p.1249·2) is included in this preparation in an attempt to limit adverse effects on the gastrointestinal mucosa.
*Inflammation; musculoskeletal and joint disorders; pain.*

**Silastic** *Dow Corning, UK†.*
Liquid silicone (p.1482·1); stannous octoate.
*Open granulating wounds.*

**Silaxa** *Temis, Arg.*
Monobasic sodium phosphate (p.1230·3); dibasic sodium phosphate (p.1231·1).
*Bowel evacuation.*

**Silaxon** *Restan, S.Afr.†.*
Sennosides A and B (p.1288·2).
*Constipation.*

**Silbecor** *Biotech, S.Afr.*
Sulfadiazine silver (p.259·1).
*Burns.*

**Silbephylline** *Minerva (Μινερβα), Gr.*
Diprophylline (p.784·3).
*Asthma; chronic obstructive pulmonary disease.*

**Silberne** *Brady, Austria.*
Cascara (p.1255·1); rhubarb (p.1287·3); ox bile (p.1660·3).
*Constipation.*

**Silcon** *Faulding Consumer, Austral.*
Dimethicone (p.1482·1); wool fat (p.1483·1).
*Barrier preparation.*

**Silcor** *Galderma, Arg.*
Calcitriol (p.1461·2).
*Psoriasis.*

**Sildec-DM** *Silarx, USA.*
*Oral drops:* Carbinoxamine maleate (p.426·3); pseudoephedrine hydrochloride (p.1129·2); dextromethorphan hydrobromide (p.1117·3).
*Syrup:* Brompheniramine maleate (p.426·1); pseudoephedrine hydrochloride (p.1129·2); dextromethorphan hydrobromide (p.1117·3).
*Coughs.*

**Sildefil** *Pfizer, Arg.*
Sildenafil citrate (p.1744·2).
*Erectile dysfunction.*

**Sildicon-E** *Silarx, USA†.*
Phenylpropanolamine hydrochloride (p.1127·3); guaifenesin (p.1122·1).
*Coughs.*

**Silencium** *Aventis, Braz.*
*Pastilles:* Dextromethorphan (p.1117·3); benzocaine (p.1370·3).
*Syrup:* Dextromethorphan hydrobromide (p.1117·3); doxylamine succinate (p.432·3); sodium citrate (p.1223·2).
*Coughs.*

**Silentan** *Krewel, Ger.*
Nefopam hydrochloride (p.66·2).
Formerly contained diazepam and aspirin.
*Pain.*

**Silepar** *Ibirn, Ital.†.*
Silymarin (p.1043·3).
*Liver disorders.*

**Sileton** *Silesia, Chile.*
Vitamin and mineral preparation (p.1417·1).
*Tonic.*

**Silettum** *Jaldes, Fr.*
Equisetum; hydrolysed sesame protein; vitamin B substances (p.1417·1).
*Hair disorders.*

**Silfedrine** *Silarx, USA.*
Pseudoephedrine hydrochloride (p.1129·2).
*Nasal congestion.*

**Silflam** *Silom, Thai.*
Diclofenac diethylamine (p.32·1).
*Musculoskeletal, joint, and peri-articular disorders.*

**Silfox** *Armstrong, Arg.*
Rofecoxib (p.86·3).
*Osteoarthritis; pain.*

**Silgel** *Nagor, UK.*
Silicone (p.1482·1).
*Hypertrophic and keloid scars.*

**Silibene** *Merckle, Ger.*
Silybum marianum (p.1043·3).
*Liver disorders.*

**Silic** *Ego, NZ.*
Dimethicone (p.1482·1); glycerol (p.1694·3).
*Barrier preparation; bed sores; eczema.*

**Silic 15**
*Ego, Austral.; Ego, Hong Kong; Ego, Malaysia; Ego, Singapore.*
Dimeticone (p.1482·1).
*Barrier preparation.*

**Silica L11** *Homeocan, Canad.*
Homoeopathic preparation.

**Silica-OK** *Wassen, UK.*
Silica; selenium; vitamins (p.1417·1).

**Silicare** *Orion, NZ.*
Dimethicone (p.1482·1).
*Barrier agent.*

**Silicic Complex** *Procare, Austral.†.*
Equisetum (p.1684·1); silica (p.1581·3); calcium (p.1225·1); potassium (p.1232·1).
*Brittle nails and hair; tissue repair.*

**Silicin** *Greater Pharma, Thai.*
Cinnarizine (p.428·3).
*Cerebrovascular disorders; migraine; motion sickness; peripheral vascular disorders; vestibular disorders.*

**Silicol** *Szama, Arg.*
Barrier cream.
*Dermatitis; nappy rash; skin irritation.*

**Silicur** *Biocur, Ger.*
Silybum marianum (p.1043·3).
*Liver disorders.*

**Silidermil** *Fides Ecopharma, Spain.*
*Ointment:* Dimethicone (p.1482·1); zinc oxide (p.1163·2).
*Topical powder:* Cetylpyridinium chloride (p.1173·1); dimethicone (p.1482·1); zinc oxide (p.1163·2).
*Skin disorders.*

**Silidral** *Spedrog, Arg.*
Alendronate sodium (p.765·3).
*Osteoporosis.*

**Silidron** *GlaxoSmithKline, Braz.*
Dimeticone (p.1289·2).
*Flatulence.*

**Siligaz**
*Bio-Sante, Canad.; Arkomedika, Fr.*
Simeticone (p.1289·2).
*Meteorism.*

**Siligel** *Stafford-Miller, Braz.†.*
Aluminium hydroxide (p.1249·2); magnesium trisilicate (p.1272·3); dimethicone (p.1289·2).
*Flatulence; gastrointestinal hyperacidity.*

**Silimag** *Faes, Spain†.*
Magnesium trisilicate (p.1272·3).
*Dyspepsia; peptic ulcer.*

**Silimalon** *Nikkho, Braz.*
Methionine (p.1042·1); silymarin (p.1043·3).
*Liver disorders.*

**Silimarin** *Benedetti, Ital.*
Silymarin (p.1043·3).
*Liver disorders.*

**Silimarit** *Bionorica, Ger.*
Silybum marianum (p.1043·3).
*Liver disorders.*

**Silimazu** *Farmasur, Spain.*
Silymarin (p.1043·3).
*Toxic hepatitis.*

**Sili-Met-San**
*Note. This name is used for preparations of different composition.*
*Therabel, Belg.*
Dimethicone (p.1289·2).
Formerly contained dimethicone, and calcium pantothenate.
*Aid to gastrointestinal radiographic examination; trapped gastrointestinal gas.*

*UCB, Switz.*
*Oral suspension†:* Dimethicone (p.1289·2).
*Tablets:* Dimethicone (p.1289·2); calcium pantothenate (p.1442·3).
*Aid to radiologic examination; flatulence.*

**Siliprele** *Herbaxt, Fr.*
Equisetum (p.1684·1).
*Gastrointestinal and renal disorders.*

**Silirex** *Lampugnani, Ital.*
Silymarin (p.1043·3).
*Liver disorders.*

**Silisan** *Merck, Ital.*
Simeticone (p.1289·2); calcium pantothenate (p.1442·3).
*Gastrointestinal disorders associated with excess gas; preparation of the stomach for endoscopy and surgery.*

**Siliver** *Farmasa, Braz.*
Silymarin (p.1043·3).
*Liver disorders.*

**Silkis**
*AB-Consult, Austria; Galderma, Belg.; Galderma, Braz.; Galderma, Fin.; Galderma, Fr.; Galderma, Ger.; Galderma, Neth.; Galderma, Switz.; Galderma, UK.*
Calcitriol (p.1461·2).
*Psoriasis.*

**Silliver** *Abbott, Ital.*
Silymarin (p.1043·3).
*Liver disorders.*

**Sillix** *Giuliani, Ital.*
Dried yeast (p.1469·1); vitamin B substances (p.1417·1).

**Sillix C** *Giuliani, Ital.*
Dried yeast (p.1469·1); vitamin B substances; vitamin C (p.1417·1).
*Nutritional supplement.*

**Sillix Donna** *Giuliani, Ital.†.*
Minerals; dried yeast; vitamin E; vitamin $B_6$; folic acid (p.1417·1).
*Nutritional supplement.*

**Silmar** *Hennig, Ger.*
Silybum marianum (p.1043·3).
*Liver disorders.*

**Silmycetin** *Silom, Thai.*
Chloramphenicol (p.185·1).
*Bacterial eye or ear infections.*

**Sil-Norboral** *Silanes, Mex.*
Glibenclamide (p.331·2); metformin (p.342·3).
*Diabetes mellitus.*

**Siloderm** *Suyog, India.*
Dimethicone (p.1482·1); zinc oxide (p.1163·2); calamine (p.1144·1); cetrimide (p.1172·1).
*Dermatitis.*

**Silomat**
*Note. This name is used for preparations of different composition.*
*Boehringer Ingelheim, Arg.; Boehringer Ingelheim, Austria; Boehringer Ingelheim, Belg.; Boehringer de Angeli, Braz.; Boehringer Ingelheim, Chile; Boehringer Ingelheim, Fin.; Boehringer Ingelheim, Fr.; Boehringer Ingelheim, Ger.; Boehringer Ingelheim, Gr.; Boehringer Ingelheim, Malaysia; Boehringer Ingelheim, Port.; Boehringer Ingelheim, Singapore; Boehringer Ingelheim, Thai.*
Clobutinol hydrochloride (p.1117·1).
*Coughs.*

*Boehringer Ingelheim, Fr.*
*Syrup:* Clobutinol hydrochloride (p.1117·1); sodium benzoate (p.1169·3).
*Coughs.*

**Silomat Compositum** *Boehringer Ingelheim, Thai.†.*
Clobutinol hydrochloride (p.1117·1); orciprenaline sulfate (p.790·2).
*Coughs.*

**Silomat DA** *Boehringer Ingelheim, S.Afr.*
Clobutinol hydrochloride (p.1117·1); orciprenaline sulfate (p.790·2).
*Coughs.*

**Silomat Plus** *Boehringer de Angeli, Braz.*
Clobutinol hydrochloride (p.1117·1); doxylamine succinate (p.432·3).
*Coughs.*

**Silomat-Fher** *Boehringer Ingelheim, Ital.*
Clobutinol hydrochloride (p.1117·1).
*Coughs.*

**Silon** *Smith & Nephew, Swed.*
Dimethicone (p.1482·1); zinc oxide (p.1163·2).
*Barrier cream.*

**Silostar** *Uriach, Spain.*
Nebivolol hydrochloride (p.964·3).
*Hypertension.*

**Silox-50** *Jean-Marie, Hong Kong.*
Aluminium hydroxide (p.1249·2); magnesium trisilicate (p.1272·3); simeticone (p.1289·2).
*Flatulence; gastritis; gastrointestinal hyperacidity; heartburn.*

**Siloxan** *Nycomed, Norw.*
Simeticone (p.1289·2).
*Flatulence; postoperative intestinal gas retention.*

**Siloxogene** *RPG, India.*
Aluminium hydroxide (p.1249·2); magnesium hydroxide (p.1272·2); simeticone (p.1289·2).
*Gastrointestinal hyperacidity.*

**Silphen** *Silarx, USA.*
Diphenhydramine hydrochloride (p.431·3).

**Silphen DM** *Silarx, USA.*
Dextromethorphan hydrobromide (p.1117·3).
*Coughs.*

**Silpin** *Laborsil, Braz.†.*
Co-trimoxazole (p.199·3).
*Bacterial infections; Pneumocystis carinii pneumonia; protozoal infections.*

**Silrelax** *Silesia, Chile.*
Chlormezanone (p.675·1); dipyrone (p.35·3).
*Musculoskeletal and joint disorders; pain.*

**Siltapp** *Silarx, USA†.*
Brompheniramine maleate (p.426·1); phenylpropanolamine hydrochloride (p.1127·3); dextromethorphan hydrobromide (p.1117·3).
*Upper respiratory-tract symptoms.*

**Sil-Tex** *Silarx, USA†.*
Phenylephrine hydrochloride (p.1126·3); phenylpropanolamine hydrochloride (p.1127·3); guaifenesin (p.1122·1).
*Coughs.*

**Siltussin**
*Note. This name is used for preparations of different composition.*
*Silom, Thai.*
Guaifenesin (p.1122·1); ammonium chloride (p.1115·2); menthol (p.1711·3).
*Coughs.*

*Silarx, USA.*
Guaifenesin (p.1122·1).
*Coughs.*

**Siltussin DM** *Silarx, USA.*
Guaifenesin (p.1122·1); dextromethorphan hydrobromide (p.1117·3).
*Coughs.*

**Siltussin-CF** *Silarx, USA†.*
Guaifenesin (p.1122·1); phenylpropanolamine hydrochloride (p.1127·3); dextromethorphan hydrobromide (p.1117·3).
*Coughs.*

**Silubin**
*Andromaco, Spain.*
Buformin (p.330·3).
*Diabetes mellitus.*

*Grunenthal, Switz.*
Buformin hydrochloride (p.330·3).
*Diabetes mellitus.*

**Siludrox** *Eurofarma, Braz.*
Dimeticone (p.1289·2); aluminium hydroxide (p.1249·2); magnesium hydroxide (p.1272·2).
*Flatulence; gastrointestinal hyperacidity.*

**Silvadene**
*Aventis, Mex.; Hoechst Marion Roussel, USA.*
Sulfadiazine silver (p.259·1).
*Infected burns.*

**Silvadiazin** *Julphar, UAE.*
Sulfadiazine silver (p.259·1).
*Burns; ulcers; wounds.*

**Silvana** *Molteni, Ital.†.*
Benzalkonium chloride (p.1168·3); glacial acetic acid (p.1645·2).
*Skin disinfection.*

**Silvaysan** *Sanum-Kehlbeck, Ger.*
Silybum marianum (p.1043·3).
*Liver disorders.*

**Silvazine**
*Smith & Nephew, Austral.; Smith & Nephew, NZ; Smith & Nephew, Singapore.*
Sulfadiazine silver (p.259·1); chlorhexidine gluconate (p.1173·2).
*Prevention of infection in burns, ulcers, and wounds.*

**Silvederma**
*Asmopul, Arg.*
Sulfadiazine (p.258·2).
*Bacterial infections.*

*Aldo, Spain.*
Sulfadiazine silver (p.259·1).
*Burns; skin ulcers; wounds.*

**Silvedine** *Silvestre, Braz.†.*
Povidone-iodine (p.1190·3).
*Disinfection of skin, mucous membranes, wounds, and instruments.*

**Silver Clove Medicated Balm** *Sportbalm, Austral.†.*
Clove bud oil (p.1673·3); menthol (p.1711·3); cajuput oil (p.1664·1); peppermint oil (p.1283·2); camphor (p.1665·3).
*Musculoskeletal and joint pain.*

**Silvercef** *Uno, Ital.*
Cefonicid sodium (p.174·2).
Lidocaine hydrochloride (p.1377·3) is included in this preparation to alleviate the pain of injection.
*Gram-negative bacterial infections.*

**Silverex** *Crosslands, India.*
Sulfadiazine silver (p.259·1); chlorhexidine gluconate (p.1173·2).
*Burns; leg ulcers; pressure sores.*

**Silverol**
*Abic, Hong Kong†; Abic, Israel; Abic-Teva, Thai.*
Sulfadiazine silver (p.259·1).
*Infected burns; infected skin ulcers; infected wounds.*

**Silvertone** *Resinag, Switz.*
Sulfadiazine silver (p.259·1).
*Infected burns; infected wounds.*

**Silybon** *Micro, India.*
Silymarin (p.1043·3).
*Liver disorders.*

**Silybum Complex** *Blackmores, Austral.†.*
Silybum marianum (p.1043·3); garlic (p.1691·1); taraxacum (p.1751·3); nicotinic acid (p.1441·1); sodium sulfate (p.1290·1).
*Hypercholesterolaemia; liver and biliary-tract disorders.*

**Silyhexal** *Hexal, Austria.*
Silybum marianum (p.1043·3).
*Liver disorders.*

**Silymarin Phytosome** *Eagle, Austral.†.*
Silybum marianum (p.1043·3).
*Digestive disorders.*

**Sily-Sabona** *Sabona, Ger.*
Silybum marianum (p.1043·3).
*Liver disorders.*

**Silzolin** *Savio, Ital.*
Cefazolin sodium (p.170·3).
Lidocaine hydrochloride (p.1377·3) is included in this preparation to alleviate the pain of injection.
*Bacterial infections.*

**Simaal Gel 2** *Schein, USA.*
Aluminium hydroxide (p.1249·2); magnesium hydroxide (p.1272·2); simeticone (p.1289·2).
*Hyperacidity.*

**Simacort** *Siam Bheasach, Thai.*
Triamcinolone (p.1110·2) or triamcinolone acetonide (p.1110·2).
*Musculoskeletal, joint, and peri-articular disorders; skin disorders.*

**Simagel**
*Note. This name is used for preparations of different composition.*
*Philopharm, Ger.*
Almasilate (p.1248·2).
*Gastrointestinal disorders.*

*Atlantic, Malaysia; Atlantic, Thai.†.*
Dried aluminium hydroxide gel (p.1249·2); magnesium hydroxide (p.1272·2); simeticone (p.1289·2).
*Flatulence; gastric hyperacidity; gastritis; heartburn; peptic ulcer.*

**Simaglen**
*Unison, Hong Kong; Unison, Thai.*
Cimetidine (p.1255·3).
*Gastro-oesophageal reflux; peptic ulcer; Zollinger-Ellison syndrome.*

**Simaphil** *Philopharm, Ger.*
Magaldrate (p.1271·3).
*Gastrointestinal disorders.*

**Simar** *Ofimex, Mex.†.*
Rifampicin (p.250·2).

**Simatin** *Chemomedica, Austria†.*
Ethosuximide (p.360·1).
*Absence seizures.*

**Simbion** *Merck, Chile.*
Vitamin and mineral preparation (p.1417·1).
*Dietary supplement.*

**Simcone** *TO-Chemicals, Thai.*
Simeticone (p.1289·2).
*Flatulence.*

**Simdax**
*Orion, Fin.; Orion, Norw.; Abbott, Spain; Orion, Swed.*
Levosimendan (p.946·2).
*Heart failure.*

**Simeco**
*Note. This name is used for preparations of different composition.*
*Wyeth, Gr.; Wyeth, India; Whitehall, Singapore†; Whitehall, Thai.; Wyeth, UK†.*
*Oral suspension:* Aluminium hydroxide (p.1249·2); magnesium hydroxide (p.1272·2); simeticone (p.1289·2).
*Dyspepsia; flatulence.*

*Wyeth, Gr.; Wyeth, Hong Kong; Whitehall, Singapore†; Whitehall, Thai.; Wyeth, UK.*
*Tablets:* Aluminium hydroxide-magnesium carbonate co-dried gel (p.1250·1); magnesium hydroxide (p.1272·2); simeticone (p.1289·2).
*Dyspepsia; flatulence.*

**Simeco Plus**
*Eurofarma, Braz.; Wyeth Consumer, Chile.*
Aluminium hydroxide (p.1249·2); magnesium hydroxide (p.1272·2); simeticone (p.1289·2).
*Gastrointestinal hyperacidity; meteorism.*

**Simecon**
*Sanitas, Arg.; Chinta, Thai.*
Simeticone (p.1289·2).
*Gastrointestinal disorders with excess gas; infant flatulence.*

**Simecon Antiacido** *Sanitas, Arg.*
Aluminium hydroxide (p.1249·2); magnesium hydroxide (p.1272·2); simeticone (p.1289·2).
*Flatulence; gastrointestinal hyperacidity.*

**Simegel** *Medipharma, Hong Kong.*
Aluminium hydroxide (p.1249·2); magnesium trisilicate (p.1272·3); simeticone (p.1289·2).
*Dyspepsia; flatulence; gastrointestinal hyperacidity; peptic ulcer.*

**Simepar**
*Mepha, Hong Kong; Mepha, Malaysia; Mepha, Singapore; Mepha, Switz.*
Silymarin (p.1043·3); vitamin B substances (p.1417·1).
*Liver disorders.*

**Simetac** *Vida, Hong Kong.*
Ranitidine hydrochloride (p.1285·2).
*Gastro-oesophageal reflux; peptic ulcer.*

**Simet-AF** *Soma, Switz.*
Simeticone (p.1289·2).
*Aid in gastrointestinal procedures; detergent intoxication; flatulence.*

**Simetyl** *M & H, Thai.*
Simeticone (p.1289·2).
*Flatulence.*

**Simex** *Hua, Thai.*
Cimetidine (p.1255·3).
*Peptic ulcer; Zollinger-Ellison syndrome.*

**Simic** *Zyma, Switz.†.*
Urtica root (p.1762·1).
*Benign prostatic hyperplasia.*

**Simicol** *CTI, Israel.*
Simeticone (p.1289·2).
*Colic; flatulence; griping pain.*

**Similac Advance HA** *Abbott, Port.*
Infant feed (p.1417·1).
*Milk protein allergy.*

**Similac Advance LF** *Abbott, Mex.*
Lactose-free infant feed (p.1417·1).
*Lactose intolerance.*

**Similac Advance Sin Lactosa** *Abbott, Chile.*
Infant feed (p.1417·1).
*Lactose intolerance.*

**Similac Isomil** *Abbott, Israel.*
Infant feed (p.1417·1).
*Cows milk protein sensitivity.*

**Similac Lactose Free** *Ross, USA.*
Lactose-free infant feed (p.1417·1).
*Lactose intolerance.*

**Similac LF**
Abbott, Canad.; Abbott, Hong Kong; Abbott, Ital.; Abbott, Malaysia; Abbott, Thai.
Lactose-free infant feed (p.1417·1).
*Lactose intolerance.*

**Similac PM 60/40** Ross, USA.
Low-mineral infant feed (p.1417·1).
*Hypocalcaemia; renal impairment.*

**Similac RA** Abbott, Ital.
Infant feed (p.1417·1).
*Hypersensitivity.*

**Similasan I** Ocusoft, USA.
Artificial tears.

**Similia** Hochstetter, Chile.
Hamamelis (p.1696·3).
*Haemorrhoids.*

**Similibus** Knop, Chile.
Homoeopathic preparation.

**Simoph Tears** Siam Bheasach, Thai.
Hypromellose (p.1579·3) (p.1164·2).
*Dry eye; wetting solution for hard contact lenses.*

**Simovil** Merck Sharp & Dohme, Israel.
Simvastatin (p.997·1).
*Hyperlipidaemias.*

**Simoxil** Infosint, Ital.
Amoxicillin trihydrate (p.155·3).
*Bacterial infections.*

**Simoyiam** Siam Bheasach, Thai.
Flunarizine hydrochloride (p.434·1).
*Cerebrovascular disorders; migraine.*

**Simp** Esoform, Ital.
Chlorhexidine gluconate (p.1173·2); benzalkonium chloride (p.1168·3).
*Skin and wound disinfection.*

**Simperten** Laboratorios Chile, Chile.
Losartan potassium (p.947·2).
*Hypertension.*

**Simperten-D** Laboratorios Chile, Chile.
Losartan potassium (p.947·2); hydrochlorothiazide (p.933·2).
*Hypertension.*

**Simplamox** ISF, Ital.
Amoxicillin trihydrate (p.155·3).
*Bacterial infections.*

**Simple** Agepha, Austria.
Disinfection and storage solution for contact lenses (p.1164·2).

**Simple Cleaner** Agepha, Austria.
Cleaning solution for contact lenses (p.1164·2).

**Simplene**
Chauvin, Irl.†; Smith & Nephew, S.Afr.†; Chauvin, UK†.
Adrenaline (p.852·2).
*Open-angle glaucoma.*

**Simplet** Major, USA.
Pseudoephedrine hydrochloride (p.1129·2); chlorphenamine maleate (p.427·3); paracetamol (p.76·2).
*Upper respiratory-tract symptoms.*

**Simplex** Ophtha, Norw.
Liquid paraffin (p.1479·1); white soft paraffin (p.1479·3).
*Sore and dry skin in the eyelid area.*

**Simplex-Fieberblasen** Nycomed, Austria.
Aciclovir (p.626·1).
*Herpes labialis.*

**Simplicity** Stanley, Canad.
Pregnancy test and fertility test (p.1734·3).

**Simplotan**
Pfizer, Austral.; Pfizer, Ger.; Pierre Fabre, Ger.
Tinidazole (p.617·1).
*Anaerobic bacterial infections; protozoal infections.*

**Simply Cough** McNeil Pharmaceutical, USA.
Dextromethorphan hydrobromide (p.1117·3).
*Coughs.*

**Simply Sleep**
McNeil Consumer, Canad.; McNeil, USA.
Diphenhydramine hydrochloride (p.431·3).
*Insomnia.*

**Simply Stuffy** McNeil Pharmaceutical, USA.
Pseudoephedrine hydrochloride (p.1129·2).
*Nasal congestion.*

**Simpottantacinque** Esoform, Ital.
Benzalkonium chloride (p.1168·3); chlorhexidine gluconate (p.1173·2); alcohol (p.1166·1).
*Disinfection of skin, hands, and wounds.*

**Simprox** Areu, Spain.
Astemizole (p.424·2).
*Hypersensitivity reactions.*

**Simpsons** Medico-Biological Laboratories, UK.
Zinc stearate (p.1575·3); zinc oxide (p.1163·2); sublimed sulfur (p.1158·2); salicylic acid (p.1157·1).
*Skin disorders.*

**Simron Plus** SmithKline Beecham, USA.
Vitamin B substances with vitamin C, iron, and folic acid (p.1417·1).

**Simrose** Serum Institute, India.
Evening primrose oil (p.1686·3).
*Premenstrual syndrome.*

**Simtec** CCM, Malaysia.
Cetirizine hydrochloride (p.427·1).
*Allergic rhinitis; urticaria.*

**Simulcium G3**
Note. This name is used for preparations of different composition.
Gandhour, Fr.†.
Monomethyltrisilanol mannuronate.
*Skin disorders.*

Dermoteca, Port.
Emollient and moisturiser.
*Skin disorders.*

**Simulect**
Novartis, Arg.; Novartis, Austral.; Novartis, Belg.; Novartis, Braz.; Novartis, Canad.; Novartis, Chile; Novartis, Denm.; Novartis, Fin.; Novartis, Fr.; Novartis, Ger.; Novartis, Gr.; Novartis, Hong Kong; Novartis, Irl.; Novartis, Israel; Novartis, Ital.; Novartis, Malaysia; Novartis, Mex.; Novartis, Neth.; Novartis, Norw.; Novartis, NZ; Novartis, Port.; Novartis, S.Afr.; Novartis, Singapore†; Novartis, Spain; Novartis, Swed.; Novartis, Switz.; Novartis, Thai.; Novartis, UK; Novartis, USA.
Basiliximab (p.1351·1).
*Renal transplant rejection.*

**Simultan** Silesia, Chile.
Thioridazine hydrochloride (p.724·2).
*Childhood behaviour disorders; depression; psychoses.*

**Simusol** Siam Bheasach, Thai.
Ambroxol hydrochloride (p.1114·3).
*Respiratory-tract disorders associated with increased or viscous mucus.*

**Simvacol** APS, Port.
Simvastatin (p.997·1).
*Hyperlipidaemias.*

**Simvacor** Unipharm, Israel.
Simvastatin (p.997·1).
*Hypercholesterolaemia.*

**Simvador** Discovery, UK.
Simvastatin (p.997·1).
*Hypercholesterolaemia; secondary prevention of coronary heart disease.*

**Simvast** Julphar, UAE.
Simvastatin sodium (p.999·2).
*Atherosclerosis; hypercholesterolaemia.*

**Simvasten** Spyfarma, Spain.
Simvastatin hydrochloride (p.997·1).
*Hyperlipidaemias.*

**Simvor** Ranbaxy, Thai.
Simvastatin (p.997·1).
*Hypercholesterolaemia.*

**Simvotin** Stancare, India.
Simvastatin (p.997·1).
*Hypercholesterolaemia.*

**Sin Mareo x 4** Perez Gimenez, Spain.
Dimenhydrinate (p.431·1); belladonna (p.479·1).
*Nausea; vertigo; vomiting.*

**Sin-A Crud** Quimica y Farmacia, Mex.
Paracetamol (p.76·2); caffeine (p.782·1); aluminium hydroxide (p.1249·2); magnesium hydroxide (p.1272·2); calcium carbonate (p.1254·2).
*Symptoms of overindulgence with food or alcohol.*

**Sinacarb** Amrad, Austral.†.
Levodopa (p.1205·2); carbidopa (p.1204·3).
*Parkinsonism.*

**Sinacid** Rider, Chile.
Myrtecaine laurilsulfate (p.1381·3); galactane sulfate; aluminium glycinate (p.1249·1).
*Gastrointestinal disorders.*

**Si-Nade** GlaxoSmithKline, S.Afr.
Paracetamol (p.76·2); phenylpropanolamine hydrochloride (p.1127·3).
*Cold and influenza symptoms; sinusitis.*

**Sinadrin Plus** Reese, USA.
Paracetamol (p.76·2); pseudoephedrine hydrochloride (p.1129·2); dexbrompheniramine maleate (p.426·1).

**Sinaf** Taro, Israel.
Oxymetazoline hydrochloride (p.1126·1); phenylephrine hydrochloride (p.1126·3).
*Nasal congestion.*

**Sin-A-Gen** Byk Gulden, Mex.
Polysaccharide polysulfuric acid ester.
*Vaginal contraceptive.*

**Sinaler** Cassara, Arg.
Loratadine (p.436·1).
*Allergic rhinitis; allergic skin disorders; laryngitis; sinusitis.*

**Sinaler B** Cassara, Arg.
Loratadine (p.436·1); betamethasone (p.1093·1).
*Allergic rhinitis; allergic skin disorders; laryngitis; sinusitis.*

**Sinalfa**
Abbott, Denm.; Abbott, Norw.; Abbott, Swed.
Terazosin hydrochloride (p.1010·3).
*Benign prostatic hyperplasia; hypertension.*

**Sinalgia** Silesia, Chile.
Fepradinol hydrochloride (p.43·1).
*Musculoskeletal, joint, peri-articular, and soft-tissue disorders.*

**Sinalgico** Microsules Bernabo, Arg.
Ketorolac (p.52·3) or ketorolac trometamol (p.52·1).
*Pain.*

**Sin-Algin** Instituto Sanitas, Chile.
Paracetamol (p.76·2); chlormezanone (p.675·1).
*Musculoskeletal and joint disorders; pain.*

**Sinamida Cicatrizante** Gezzi, Arg.
Ergocalciferol (p.1462·1); zinc oxide (p.1163·2).
*Wounds.*

**Sinamida Econazol** Gezzi, Arg.
Econazole nitrate (p.397·2).
*Fungal skin and vaginal infections.*

**Sinamida Pies** Gezzi, Arg.
Undecenoic acid (p.410·3); zinc undecenoate (p.411·1).
*Fungal skin infections.*

**Sinamida-D** Gezzi, Arg.
Zinc oxide (p.1163·2).
*Skin disorders.*

**Sinapause**
Organon, Chile; Organon, Mex.
Estriol succinate (p.1552·3).
*Genito-urinary tract disorders associated with oestrogen deficiency.*

**Sinapet** Silesia, Chile.
Fenproporex hydrochloride (p.1588·3).
*Obesity.*

**Sinapils** Pfeiffer, USA†.
Phenylpropanolamine hydrochloride (p.1127·3); chlorphenamine maleate (p.427·3); paracetamol (p.76·2); caffeine (p.782·1).
*Upper respiratory-tract symptoms.*

**Sinapisme Rigollot** Chefaro Ardeval, Fr.
Defatted black mustard paper (p.1718·2).
*Respiratory-tract congestion.*

**Sinaplin** Rimsa, Mex.
Ampicillin sodium (p.157·1) or ampicillin trihydrate (p.157·2).
*Bacterial infections.*

**Sinapsan** Rodleben, Ger.; Vedim, Ger.
Piracetam (p.1732·1).
*Organic brain disorders.*

**Sinaqua** Sofex, Port.
Barrier preparation.

**Sinarest**
Note. This name is used for preparations of different composition.
Centaur, India.
*Nasal drops:* Oxymetazoline hydrochloride (p.1126·1).
*Nasal congestion.*

*Oral drops:* Paracetamol (p.76·2); pseudoephedrine hydrochloride (p.1129·2); chlorphenamine maleate (p.427·3).

*Syrup:* Paracetamol (p.76·2); pseudoephedrine hydrochloride (p.1129·2); chlorphenamine maleate (p.427·3); sodium citrate (p.1223·2); menthol (p.1711·3).

*Tablets:* Paracetamol (p.76·2); pseudoephedrine hydrochloride (p.1129·2); chlorphenamine maleate (p.427·3); caffeine (p.782·1).

*Allergic rhinitis; cold and influenza symptoms; otitis media; sinusitis.*

Ciba, USA.
Pseudoephedrine hydrochloride (p.1129·2); chlorphenamine maleate (p.427·3); paracetamol (p.76·2).
*Upper respiratory-tract symptoms.*

**Sinarest Linctus** Centaur, India.
Dextromethorphan hydrobromide (p.1117·3); chlorphenamine maleate (p.427·3); menthol (p.1711·3).
*Coughs.*

**Sinarest Vapocaps** Centaur, India.
Camphor (p.1665·3); chlorothymol (p.1177·2); cineole (p.1672·1); menthol (p.1711·3); terpineol (p.1752·2).
*Cold symptoms; pharyngitis; sinusitis; upper respiratory-tract congestion.*

**Sinarest-PD** Centaur, India.
Oxymetazoline hydrochloride (p.1126·1).
*Nasal congestion.*

**Sinarona** Kener, Mex.†.
Amiodarone hydrochloride (p.859·2).

**Sinartrol**
Silesia, Chile; Pharmanel, Gr.; SPA, Ital.
Piroxicam cinnamate (p.85·1).
*Gout; inflammation; musculoskeletal and joint disorders; pain.*

**Sinaryl** Homberger, Switz.†.
Homoeopathic preparation.

**Sinase** Douglas, NZ†.
Beclometasone dipropionate (p.1091·1).
*Allergic rhinitis.*

**Sinasmal** Laboratorios Chile, Chile.
Salbutamol (p.791·3).
*Obstructive airways disease.*

**Sinaspril-Paracetamol** Roche Consumer, Neth.
Paracetamol (p.76·2).
*Fever; pain.*

**Sinaxial**
TRB, Arg.
Sialogangliosides (porcine).
*Cerebral trauma; peripheral neuropathy.*

TRB, Braz.
Polysiagoside (p.1691·1).
*Cerebrovascular disorders.*

**Sincerck** Salus, Mex.†.
Praziquantel (p.112·2).

**Sincerum** Dallas, Arg.
Sodium carbonate (p.1747·1); phenazone (p.82·3); neomycin sulfate (p.235·1); cetrimide (p.1172·1).
*Ear disorders.*

**Sincerum Biotic** Dallas, Arg.
Neomycin sulfate (p.235·1); dexamethasone (p.1097·1).
*Infected ear disorders.*

**Sincerum Biotic L** Dallas, Arg.
Neomycin sulfate (p.235·1); dexamethasone (p.1097·1); polymyxin B sulfate (p.245·1); lidocaine hydrochloride (p.1377·3).
*Infected ear disorders.*

**Sincon** Tika, Swed.
Polyvinyl alcohol (p.1581·1).
*Dry eyes.*

**Sincosan** Omisan, Ital.†.
Benzalkonium chloride (p.1168·3).
*Surface disinfection.*

**Sincrivit** AGIPS, Ital.
Multivitamin preparation (p.1417·1).

**Sindol** Ahimsa, Arg.
Ibuprofen (p.45·3).
*Inflammation; pain.*

**Sindopa** Pacific, NZ.
Carbidopa (p.1204·3); levodopa (p.1205·2).
*Parkinsonism.*

**Sindrat** Windson, Braz.†.
Oral rehydration solution (p.1222·2).
*Diarrhoea; oral rehydration therapy.*

**Sindrolen** Temis, Arg.
*Injection:* Piroxicam (p.84·2); dexamethasone sodium phosphate (p.1097·2); pyridoxine hydrochloride (p.1456·3); hydroxocobalamin (p.1458·2).
*Inflammation; muscle spasm; neuritis.*

*Topical gel:* Piroxicam (p.84·2).
*Inflammation.*

**Sindrolen Vitaminado** Temis, Arg.
Piroxicam (p.84·2); paracetamol (p.76·2); vitamin $B_1$; vitamin $B_6$.
*Inflammation; pain.*

**Sine-Aid IB** McNeil Consumer, USA.
Pseudoephedrine (p.1129·2); ibuprofen (p.45·3).

**Sine-Aid Maximum Strength** McNeil Consumer, USA.
Paracetamol (p.76·2); pseudoephedrine hydrochloride (p.1129·2).
*Sinus headache.*

**Sinease** Schering-Plough, Austral.
Loratadine (p.436·1); pseudoephedrine sulfate (p.1129·2).
*Allergic rhinitis.*

**Sinecod**
Novartis Consumer, Belg.; Novartis, Gr.; Novartis Consumer, Port.; Novartis Consumer, Switz.; Novartis, Thai.
Butamirate citrate (p.1116·2).
*Coughs.*

**Sinecod Bocca** Novartis Consumer, Ital.†.
Benzoxonium chloride (p.1170·2).
*Oral antiseptic.*

**Sinecod Tosse Fluidificante** Novartis Consumer, Ital.
Carbocisteine (p.1116·2).
*Catarrh; coughs.*

**Sinecod Tosse Sedativo** Novartis Consumer, Ital.
Butamirate citrate (p.1116·2).
*Coughs.*

**Sinedal** Synpharma, Switz.
Propyphenazone (p.85·3); paracetamol (p.76·2); caffeine (p.782·1).
*Fever; pain.*

**Sinedol** Italmex, Mex.
Paracetamol (p.76·2).
*Fever; pain.*

**Sinedopa** Duopharma, Hong Kong.
Carbidopa (p.1204·3); levodopa (p.1205·2).
*Parkinsonism.*

**Sinedyston** Steiner, Ger.†.
Co-dergocrine mesilate (p.1674·1); hypericum (p.299·1).
*Mental function disorders.*

**Sinefricol** Sanofi Synthelabo, Spain†.
Caffeine (p.782·1); phenylephrine hydrochloride (p.1126·3); paracetamol (p.76·2); thenyldiamine hydrochloride (p.442·1).
*Catarrh; influenza symptoms.*

**Sinegastrin**
Note. This name is used for preparations of different composition.
Novag, Mex.
Cimetidine (p.1255·3).
*Peptic ulcer.*

Ferrer, Spain†.
Almasilate (p.1248·2).
*Dyspepsia; gastritis; gastro-oesophageal reflux; peptic ulcer.*

**Sinemet**
Sidus, Arg.; Merck Sharp & Dohme, Austral.; Merck Sharp & Dohme, Austria; Merck Sharp & Dohme, Belg.; Prodome, Braz.; Du Pont, Canad.; Merck Sharp & Dohme, Chile; Merck Sharp & Dohme, Denm.; Merck Sharp & Dohme, Fin.; Bristol-Myers Squibb, Fr.; Vianex (Βιανεξ), Gr.; Merck Sharp & Dohme, Hong Kong; Du Pont, Irl.; Merck Sharp & Dohme, Israel; Bristol-Myers Squibb, Ital.; Merck Sharp & Dohme, Malaysia; Merck Sharp & Dohme, Mex.; Merck Sharp & Dohme, Neth.; Merck Sharp & Dohme, Norw.; Merck Sharp & Dohme, NZ; Merck Sharp & Dohme, Port.; Merck Sharp & Dohme, S.Afr.; Merck Sharp & Dohme, Singapore; Bristol-Myers Squibb, Spain; Merck Sharp & Dohme, Swed.; Merck Sharp & Dohme, Switz.; Merck Sharp & Dohme, Thai.; Bristol-Myers Squibb, UK; Bristol-Myers Squibb, USA.
Carbidopa (p.1204·3); levodopa (p.1205·2).
These ingredients can be described by the British Approved Name Co-careldopa.
*Parkinsonism.*

**Sine-Off Allergy** SmithKline Beecham Consumer, Canad.†.
Paracetamol (p.76·2); chlorphenamine maleate (p.427·3); phenylpropanolamine hydrochloride (p.1127·3).

**Sine-Off Maximum Strength Allergy/Sinus** *SmithKline Beecham, USA.*
Paracetamol (p.76·2); chlorphenamine maleate (p.427·3); pseudoephedrine hydrochloride (p.1129·2).
*Upper respiratory-tract symptoms.*

**Sine-Off Maximum Strength No Drowsiness Formula** *SmithKline Beecham Consumer, USA.*
Paracetamol (p.76·2); pseudoephedrine hydrochloride (p.1129·2).
*Upper respiratory-tract symptoms.*

**Sine-Off ND** *SmithKline Beecham Consumer, Canad.†.*
Paracetamol (p.76·2); phenylpropanolamine hydrochloride (p.1127·3).

**Sine-Off Sinus Medicine** *SmithKline Beecham Consumer, USA†.*
Aspirin (p.15·1); chlorphenamine maleate (p.427·3); phenylpropanolamine hydrochloride (p.1127·3).
*Upper respiratory-tract symptoms.*

**Sinequan**
*Pfizer, Austral.; Pfizer, Austria; Pfizer, Belg.; Pfizer, Canad.; Pfizer, Denm.; Pfizer, Gr.; Pfizer, Hong Kong; Pfizer, Irl.; Pfizer, Mex.; Pfizer, Neth.; Pfizer, Norw.; Farmasierra, Spain; Pfizer, Thai.; Pfizer, UK; Pfizer, USA.*
Doxepin hydrochloride (p.291·2).
*Anxiety disorders; depression.*

**Sinerbe** *Plough, Port.*
Dexchlorpheniramine maleate (p.427·3); pseudoephedrine sulfate (p.1129·2); guaifenesin (p.1122·1).
*Coughs and associated respiratory-tract disorders.*

**Sinergen** *Biosintetica, Braz.*
Amlodipine besilate (p.862·1); enalapril maleate (p.909·2).
*Hypertension.*

**Sinergina** *Faes, Spain.*
Phenytoin (p.370·2).
*Epilepsy.*

**Sinertec** *Merck Sharp & Dohme, Ital.*
Enalapril maleate (p.909·2); hydrochlorothiazide (p.933·2).
*Hypertension.*

**Sinesalin** *Zeneca, Switz.†.*
Bendroflumethiazide (p.867·3).
*Hypertension; oedema.*

**Sinestic** *Biofutura, Ital.*
Budesonide (p.1094·2); formoterol fumarate (p.786·1).
*Asthma.*

**Sinestron** *Medix, Mex.*
Lorazepam (p.704·1).
*Anxiety; mixed anxiety depressive states.*

**Sinevrile** *Serpero, Ital.†.*
Hydroxocobalamin (p.1458·2); monophosphothiamine chloride (p.1455·2).
Lidocaine hydrochloride (p.1377·3) is included in this preparation to alleviate the pain of injection.
*Alcoholic neuritis; diabetic neuritis; neuritis; polyneuritis; sciatica; trigeminal neuralgia.*

**Sinex**
*Note. This name is used for preparations of different composition.*
*Procter & Gamble, Mex.*
Oxymetazoline hydrochloride (p.1126·1).
*Nasal congestion.*
*Richardson-Vicks, USA.*
Phenylephrine hydrochloride (p.1126·3).
*Nasal congestion.*

**Sinezan** *Esoform, Ital.*
Pyrethrum flower (p.1509·3); piperonyl butoxide (p.1509·2); diethyltoluamide (p.1503·3).
Formerly contained diethyltoluamide.
*Insect repellent.*

**Sinfrontal** *Muller Goppingen, Ger.*
Homoeopathic preparation.

**Singastril** *Andromaco, Chile.*
Pantoprazole sodium (p.1283·1).
*Gastro-oesophageal reflux; peptic ulcer.*

**Singlauc** *Biocumed, Arg.*
Carteolol hydrochloride (p.880·3).
*Glaucoma; ocular hypertension.*

**Singlet** *SmithKline Beecham Consumer, USA.*
Pseudoephedrine hydrochloride (p.1129·2); chlorphenamine maleate (p.427·3); paracetamol (p.76·2).
*Upper respiratory-tract symptoms.*

**Singril** *Offenbach, Mex.*
Moroxydine hydrochloride (p.649·3); chlorphenamine (p.428·1); dipyrone (p.35·3).
*Cold and influenza symptoms.*

**Singrilen** *Offenbach, Mex.*
Moroxydine hydrochloride (p.649·3); paracetamol (p.76·2); phenylephrine (p.1126·3); chlorphenamine (p.428·1).
*Cold and influenza symptoms.*

**Singulair**
*Merck Sharp & Dohme, Arg.; Merck Sharp & Dohme, Austral.; Merck Sharp & Dohme, Austria; Merck Sharp & Dohme, Belg.; Merck Sharp & Dohme, Braz.; Merck Frosst, Canad.; Merck Sharp & Dohme, Chile; Merck Sharp & Dohme, Denm.; Merck Sharp & Dohme, Fin.; Merck Sharp & Dohme-Chibret, Fr.; Dieckmann, Ger.; Vianex (Βιανεξ), Gr.; Merck Sharp & Dohme, Hong Kong; Merck Sharp & Dohme, Irl.; Merck Sharp & Dohme, Israel; Merck Sharp & Dohme, Ital.; Merck Sharp & Dohme, Malaysia; Merck Sharp & Dohme, Mex.; Merck Sharp & Dohme, Neth.; Merck Sharp & Dohme, Norw.; Merck Sharp & Dohme, NZ; Merck Sharp & Dohme, Port.; Merck Sharp & Dohme, S.Afr.; Merck Sharp & Dohme, Singapore; Merck Sharp & Dohme, Spain; Merck Sharp & Dohme, Swed.; Merck Sharp & Dohme, Switz.; Merck Sharp & Dohme, Thai.; Merck Sharp & Dohme, UK; Merck, USA.*
Montelukast sodium (p.788·3).
*Allergic rhinitis; asthma.*

**Sinhcloran** *Vitae, Mex.†.*
Ranitidine (p.1285·2).
*Peptic ulcer.*

**Siniphen** *Singer, Switz.†.*
*Suppositories:* Salicylamide (p.87·3); propyphenazone (p.85·3); caffeine (p.782·1); lidocaine hydrochloride (p.1377·3).
*Tablets:* Salicylamide (p.87·3); propyphenazone (p.85·3); caffeine (p.782·1).
*Fever; pain.*

**Sinketol** *Locatelli, Ital.†.*
Ketoprofen (p.51·2).
*Gout; musculoskeletal, joint, and peri-articular disorders.*

**Sinkron** *Ripari-Gero, Ital.*
Citicoline sodium (p.1672·3).
*Cerebrovascular disorders; mental function disorders.*

**Sinlergia** *Sanitas, Arg.*
Pseudoephedrine hydrochloride (p.1129·2); terfenadine (p.441·1).
*Respiratory-tract disorders.*

**Sinmaren** *Schering, Spain.*
Tamoxifen citrate (p.584·1).
*Breast cancer.*

**Sinmol** *Maxfarma, Spain.*
Paracetamol (p.76·2).
*Fever; pain.*

**Sinobid** *Biospray, Gr.*
Norfloxacin (p.238·3).
*Urinary tract infections.*

**Sinogan**
*Aventis, Chile.*
Levomepromazine (p.703·2).
*Anxiety; depression; pain; psychoses; sleep disorders.*
*Aventis, Mex.*
Levomepromazine hydrochloride (p.703·2) or levomepromazine maleate (p.703·2).
*Psychoses.*
*Aventis, Spain.*
Levomepromazine hydrochloride (p.703·2).
*Anxiety; depression; pain; psychoses; sleep disorders.*

**Sinografin**
*Squibb Diagnostics, Canad.†; Squibb Diagnostics, USA.*
Meglumine amidotrizoate (p.1060·2); meglumine adipiodone (p.1060·1).
*Contrast medium for hysterosalpingography.*

**Sinolax-Milder** *Synpharma, Austria.*
Fig (p.1266·3); fennel (p.1687·2); manna (p.1273·1).
*Constipation; stool softener.*

**Sinomarin** *Belolab, Fr.*
Sea water.
*Nasal cleansing; nasal congestion.*

**Sinop** *Craveri, Arg.*
Amlodipine (p.862·2).
*Angina pectoris; hypertension.*

**Sinophenin** *Rodleben, Ger.*
Promazine hydrochloride (p.717·3).
*Anxiety disorders; pain; pre- and postoperative sedative; pruritus; psychoses; sleep disorders; vomiting; withdrawal symptoms.*

**Sinopil** *GlaxoSmithKline, India.*
Lacidipine (p.944·2).
*Hypertension.*

**Sinoral**
*Biolab, Malaysia; Biolab, Thai.*
Tenoxicam (p.93·1).
*Gout; musculoskeletal, joint, and peri-articular disorders.*

**Sinotar** *Lane, UK.*
Althaea (p.1651·3); echinacea (p.1683·2); sambucus (p.1741·3).
*Blocked sinuses; catarrh.*

**Sinovula** *Asche, Ger.*
Norethisterone (p.1562·2); ethinylestradiol (p.1553·2).
*Combined oral contraceptive; menstrual disorders.*

**Sinoxis** *Hosbon, Spain.*
Buflomedil hydrochloride (p.877·2).
*Vascular disorders.*

**Sinozol** *Best, Mex.*
Itraconazole (p.401·3).
*Fungal infections.*

**Sinozzard** *Cryopharma, Mex.*
Prazosin hydrochloride (p.985·1).
*Hypertension.*

**Sinpasmon** *Instituto Sanitas, Chile.*
Pipenzolate bromide (p.487·3); phenobarbital (p.367·3).
*Gastrointestinal disorders.*

**Sinpet** *Pharmacos Abug, Mex.*
Phentermine hydrochloride (p.1592·2).
*Obesity.*

**Sinpor** *Neves, Port.*
Simvastatin (p.997·1).
*Hypercholesterolaemia.*

**Sinpro N** *Worwag, Ger.*
Paracetamol (p.76·2).
*Fever; pain.*

**Sinquan** *Pfizer, Ger.*
Doxepin hydrochloride (p.291·2).
*Anxiety; depression; sleep disorders; withdrawal syndromes.*

**Sinquane** *Pfizer, Switz.*
Doxepin hydrochloride (p.291·2).
*Anxiety disorders; depression.*

**Sinsia** *Seoul Pharma, Singapore.*
Serrapeptase (p.1743·2).
*Inflammation; respiratory-tract congestion.*

**Sinsurrene** *Parke, Davis, Ital.†.*
Hydrocortisone sodium hemisuccinate (p.1104·1); desoxycortone sodium hemisuccinate (corticosterone) (p.1097·1); aldosterone sodium hemisuccinate (p.1091·1); prasterone sodium sulfate (p.1566·1).
*Adrenal insufficiency.*

**Sintalgin** *Sintofarma, Braz.*
Nimesulide (p.67·1).
*Fever; inflammation; pain.*

**Sintamin** *Fresenius Kabi, Ital.*
Amino-acid infusion (p.1417·1).
*Parenteral nutrition.*

**Sintebron** *Sintesina, Arg.*
Ephedrine (p.1120·1); guaifenesin (p.1122·1).
*Coughs.*

**Sintegran** *Sintesina, Arg.*
Metoclopramide (p.1274·3).
*Nausea and vomiting.*

**Sintemicina** *Sintesina, Arg.*
Mitomycin (p.573·3).
*Malignant neoplasms.*

**Sintenyl** *Sintetica, Switz.*
Fentanyl citrate (p.40·1).
*Pain.*

**Sintepul** *Sintesina, Arg.*
Gentamicin (p.219·1).
*Bacterial infections.*

**Sinteroid** *Breves, Braz.†.*
A heparinoid (p.931·1); clofibrate (p.884·3).
*Hyperlipidaemias.*

**Sinthrome** *Alliance, UK.*
Acenocoumarol (p.848·3).
*Thromboembolic disorders.*

**Sintisone**
*Pharmacia Upjohn, Hong Kong†; Pharmacia, Port.*
Prednisolone steaglate (p.1108·2).
*Corticosteroid.*

**Sintobil** *Molteni, Ital.†.*
Fencibutirol (p.1687·1); boldo (p.1661·2); cascara (p.1255·1); frangula (p.1266·3).
*Constipation.*

**Sintocalcin** *Biagini, Ital.†.*
Elcatonin (p.768·3).
*Hypercalcaemia; osteoporosis; Paget's disease of bone; reflex sympathetic dystrophy.*

**Sintocef** *Pulitzer, Ital.*
Cefonicid sodium (p.174·2).
Lidocaine hydrochloride (p.1377·3) is included in the intramuscular injection to alleviate the pain of injection.
*Gram-negative bacterial infections.*

**Sintoclar** *Pulitzer, Ital.*
Citicoline (p.1672·3).
*Cerebrovascular disorders; mental function disorders.*

**Sintodian** *Pharmacia Upjohn, Ital.*
Droperidol (p.697·2).
*Anaesthesia; psychoses.*

**Sintofenac** *Sintofarma, Braz.*
Diclofenac sodium (p.32·1).

**Sintoftona** *SMB, Chile.*
Chloramphenicol (p.185·1); prednisolone acetate (p.1108·1).
*Infected eye disorders.*

**Sintolatt** *Lampugnani, Ital.*
Lactulose (p.1269·1).
*Constipation; disturbances in intestinal flora.*

**Sintomicetina** *Medley, Braz.*
Chloramphenicol (p.185·1) or chloramphenicol sodium succinate (p.185·1).
*Bacterial infections.*

**Sintomodulina** *Italfarmaco, Ital.*
Thymopentin (p.1756·1).
*Immunodeficiency.*

**Sintonal** *Europharma, Spain.*
Brotizolam (p.672·1).
*Insomnia.*

**Sintopen** *Magis, Ital.*
Amoxicillin trihydrate (p.155·3).
*Bacterial infections.*

**Sintoplus** *PH&T, Ital.*
Piperacillin sodium (p.243·1).
Lidocaine hydrochloride (p.1377·3) is included in this preparation to alleviate the pain of injection.
*Bacterial infections.*

**Sintotrat** *Bracco, Ital.*
Hydrocortisone acetate (p.1103·3).
*Skin irritation.*

**Sintozima** *Sintofarma, Braz.*
Pancreatin (p.1725·3); metoclopramide hydrochloride (p.1274·3); bromelains (p.1662·2); dehydrocholic acid (p.1679·2); cellulase (p.1669·1); dimethicone (p.1289·2).
*Digestive disorders.*

**Sintrocid** *Collins, Mex.*
Levothyroxine (p.1601·3).
*Hypothyroidism.*

**Sintrogel** *Roche Nicholas, Spain†.*
Aluminium hydroxide (p.1249·2); magnesium carbonate (p.1272·1); magnesium oxide (p.1272·3).
*Gastrointestinal hyperacidity.*

**Sintrom**
*Novartis, Arg.; Novartis, Austria; Novartis, Belg.; Novartis, Canad.; Novartis, Fr.; Novartis, Gr.; Novartis, Israel; Novartis, Ital.; Novartis, Mex.; Novartis, Port.; Novartis, Spain; Novartis, Switz.*
Acenocoumarol (p.848·3).
*Thromboembolic disorders.*

**Sintrom Mitis** *Novartis, Neth.*
Acenocoumarol (p.848·3).
*Thromboembolic disorders.*

**Sinuberase** *Rudefsa, Mex.*
Lactic-acid-producing organisms (p.1704·2).
*Diarrhoea; restoration of normal intestinal flora.*

**Sinuc** *Biocur, Ger.*
Hedera helix.
*Bronchitis; catarrh.*

**Sinuclear** *Garec, S.Afr.*
Paracetamol (p.76·2); phenylpropanolamine hydrochloride (p.1127·3).
*Upper respiratory-tract congestion.*

**Sinuclear P** *Garec, S.Afr.*
Paracetamol (p.76·2); triprolidine hydrochloride (p.442·3); pseudoephedrine hydrochloride (p.1129·2).
*Cold and influenza symptoms; nasal congestion.*

**Sinucon** *Salters, S.Afr.*
Paracetamol (p.76·2); ephedrine hydrochloride (p.1120·1); caffeine (p.782·1); chlorphenamine maleate (p.427·3).
*Cold and influenza symptoms; hay fever; sinus congestion.*

**Sinufed** *Trima, Israel.*
Pseudoephedrine hydrochloride (p.1129·2).
*Nasal congestion; sinus congestion.*

**Sinufed Kid Day** *Trima, Israel.*
Pseudoephedrine hydrochloride (p.1129·2).
*Nasal and sinus congestion.*

**Sinufed Kid Night** *Trima, Israel.*
Triprolidine hydrochloride (p.442·3); pseudoephedrine hydrochloride (p.1129·2).
*Allergic disorders; nasal and sinus congestion.*

**Sinufed Timecelles** *Roberts, USA.*
Pseudoephedrine hydrochloride (p.1129·2); guaifenesin (p.1122·1).
*Coughs and cold symptoms; nasal congestion.*

**Sinuforce** *Bioforce, Switz.*
Homoeopathic preparation.

**Sinuforton** *Sanofi Synthelabo, Ger.*
*Capsules:* Anise oil (p.1655·2); cowslip rhizome (p.1735·1); thyme (p.1755·2).
*Upper respiratory-tract congestion.*
*Oral drops:* Anise oil (p.1655·2); eucalyptus oil (p.1686·2); thyme (p.1755·2).
*Upper respiratory-tract congestion.*
*Oral liquid:* Cowslip rhizome (p.1735·1); thyme (p.1755·2).
*Cold symptoms.*

**Sinugesic** *Triomed, S.Afr.*
Paracetamol (p.76·2); pseudoephedrine hydrochloride (p.1129·2).
*Fever; pain; upper respiratory-tract congestion.*

**Sinugex** *Frega, Canad.†.*
Diphenylpyraline hydrochloride (p.432·3); paracetamol (p.76·2); caffeine (p.782·1).

**Sinulen** *Medibrands, Israel.*
Oxymetazoline hydrochloride (p.1126·1).
*Nasal congestion.*

**Sinulin**
*Note. This name is used for preparations of different composition.*
*Flordis, Austral.*
Gentian (p.1692·2); primrose.
*Respiratory-tract infections; sinusitis.*
*Carnrick, USA†.*
Paracetamol (p.76·2); chlorphenamine maleate (p.427·3); phenylpropanolamine hydrochloride (p.1127·3).
*Cold symptoms; nasal congestion.*

**Sinumax** *Janssen-Cilag, S.Afr.*
Paracetamol (p.76·2); pseudoephedrine hydrochloride (p.1129·2).
*Cold symptoms.*

**Sinumax Allergy Sinus** *Janssen-Cilag, S.Afr.*
Paracetamol (p.76·2); pseudoephedrine hydrochloride (p.1129·2); chlorphenamine maleate (p.427·3).
*Cold symptoms; nasal congestion.*

**Sinumax Co** *Janssen-Cilag, S.Afr.*
Paracetamol (p.76·2); pseudoephedrine hydrochloride (p.1129·2); codeine phosphate (p.27·1).
*Fever; pain; upper respiratory-tract congestion.*

**Sinumax Cold & Flu Plus Cough** *Janssen-Cilag, S.Afr.*
Paracetamol (p.76·2); pseudoephedrine hydrochloride (p.1129·2); dextromethorphan hydrobromide (p.1117·3); chlorphenamine maleate (p.427·3).
*Cold and influenza symptoms.*

**Sinumax IB** *Janssen-Cilag, S.Afr.*
Pseudoephedrine hydrochloride (p.1129·2); ibuprofen (p.45·3).
*Cold and influenza symptoms; sinusitis.*

**Sinumed** *Triomed, S.Afr.*
Pseudoephedrine hydrochloride (p.1129·2).
*Upper respiratory-tract congestion.*

**Sinumine** *Maxi, Thai.*
Carbinoxamine maleate (p.426·3).
*Hypersensitivity reactions.*

**Sinumist-SR** *Hauck, USA†.*
Guaifenesin (p.1122·1).
*Coughs.*

**Sinupan** Ion, USA.
Guaifenesin (p.1122·1); phenylephrine hydrochloride (p.1126·3).
*Coughs and cold symptoms; nasal congestion.*

**Sinupas N** Pascoe, Ger.
Homoeopathic preparation.

**Sinupret**
Austroplant, Austria; Bionorica, Ger.; Bionorica, Hong Kong; Bionorica, Singapore; Biomed, Switz.; Bionorica, Thai.
Gentian root (p.1692·2); cowslip flower (p.1735·1); sorrel (p.1749·1); sambucus flower (p.1741·3); vervain (p.1764·1).
*Respiratory-tract inflammation.*

**Sinurit** Microsules, Arg.
Roxithromycin (p.254·2).
*Bacterial infections.*

**Sinus**
Note. This name is used for preparations of different composition.
Hearst, Braz.†.
Naphazoline hydrochloride (p.1124·3); diphenhydramine hydrochloride (p.431·3); neomycin sulfate (p.235·1).
*Nasal congestion.*

Homeocan, Canad.
Homoeopathic preparation.

**Sinus & Congestion Relief** WestCan, Canad.†.
Pseudoephedrine hydrochloride (p.1129·2); paracetamol (p.76·2).

**Sinus Excedrin** Bristol-Myers Squibb, USA.
Paracetamol (p.76·2); pseudoephedrine hydrochloride (p.1129·2).
*Nasal congestion.*

**Sinus and Hayfever** Vitaglow, Austral.†.
Horseradish (p.1697·3); fenugreek (p.1688·1); ascorbic acid (p.1460·2); betacarotene (p.1422·3); zinc amino acid chelate (p.1469·3).
*Hay fever; sinusitis; upper respiratory-tract congestion.*

**Sinus Inhalaciones** Boots Healthcare, Spain.
Camphor (p.1665·3); cineole (p.1672·1); peppermint oil (p.1283·2); oleum pini sylvestris; menthol (p.1711·3); eucalyptus oil (p.1686·2).
*Nasal congestion.*

**Sinus Medication** Stanley, Canad.†.
Pseudoephedrine hydrochloride (p.1129·2); paracetamol (p.76·2).

**Sinus Pain & Nasal Congestion Relief** WestCan, Canad.
Pseudoephedrine hydrochloride (p.1129·2); paracetamol (p.76·2).

**Sinus Relief** Brauer, Austral.†.
Homoeopathic preparation.

**Sinusaid** Sriprasit, Thai.
Triprolidine hydrochloride (p.442·3); pseudoephedrine hydrochloride (p.1129·2).
*Nasal congestion.*

**Sinusal** Sam-On, Israel†.
Paracetamol (p.76·2); phenylpropanolamine hydrochloride (p.1127·3).
*Cold symptoms; nasal congestion; rhinitis; sinus congestion; sinusitis.*

**Sinusalia** Boiron, Canad.
Homoeopathic preparation.

**Sinuselect** Dreluso, Ger.
Homoeopathic preparation.

**Sinusitis Hevert N** Hevert, Ger.
Homoeopathic preparation.

**Sinusitis PMD** Plantamed, Ger.†.
Homoeopathic preparation.

**Sinusitis-Komplex N** Staufen, Ger.†.
Homoeopathic preparation.

**Sinusitis-Weliplex** Weber & Weber, Ger.
Homoeopathic preparation.

**Sinusol** Richter, Austria.
Gentian root (p.1692·2); cowslip flower (p.1735·1); vervain (p.1764·1).
*Catarrh.*

**Sinusol-Schleimlosender Tee** Richter, Austria.
Cowslip flower (p.1735·1); sambucus flower (p.1741·3); vervain (p.1764·1).
*Catarrh.*

**Sinuspax**
Homeocan, Canad.; Lehning, Fr.
Homoeopathic preparation.

**Sinus-Relief** Major, USA.
Pseudoephedrine hydrochloride (p.1129·2); paracetamol (p.76·2).
*Upper respiratory-tract symptoms.*

**Sinustat** Xixia, S.Afr.
Paracetamol (p.76·2); phenylpropanolamine hydrochloride (p.1127·3).
*Cold and influenza symptoms.*

**Sinustop Pro** Murdock, USA.
Pseudoephedrine hydrochloride (p.1129·2).
*Nasal congestion.*

**Sinustrat** Zurita, Braz.
Lufta operculata; sodium chloride (p.1233·3).
*Nasal congestion.*

**Sinustrat Solucao Natural** Zurita, Braz.
Sodium chloride (p.1233·3).
*Nasal congestion.*

**Sinustrat Vasoconstritor** Zurita, Braz.
Sodium chloride (p.1233·3); naphazoline hydrochloride (p.1124·3).
*Nasal congestion.*

**Sinusyx** Syxyl, Ger.
Homoeopathic preparation.

**Sinutab**
Note. This name is used for preparations of different composition.
Parke, Davis, Arg.; Pfizer Consumer, Belg.; Ache, Braz.†; Parke, Davis, Chile; Warner-Lambert, Hong Kong†; Pfizer Consumer, S.Afr.
Paracetamol (p.76·2); phenylpropanolamine hydrochloride (p.1127·3); phenyltoloxamine citrate (p.439·1).
*Cold and influenza symptoms; rhinitis; sinusitis.*

Pfizer Consumer, Irl.
Paracetamol (p.76·2); phenylpropanolamine hydrochloride (p.1127·3).
*Allergic rhinitis; cold and influenza symptoms; sinusitis.*

Parke, Davis, S.Afr.†.
*Nasal spray:* Xylometazoline hydrochloride (p.1132·2).
*Nasal congestion.*

Warner-Lambert, Spain†.
Chlorphenamine maleate (p.427·3); paracetamol (p.76·2); pseudoephedrine hydrochloride (p.1129·2).
*Fever; influenza and cold symptoms; pain.*

**Sinutab II** Pfizer Consumer, Port.
Paracetamol (p.76·2); pseudoephedrine hydrochloride (p.1129·2).
*Nasal congestion; sinusitis.*

**Sinutab with Codeine**
Note. This name is used for preparations of different composition.
Pfizer Consumer, Canad.
Paracetamol (p.76·2); pseudoephedrine hydrochloride (p.1129·2); chlorphenamine maleate (p.427·3); codeine phosphate (p.27·1).
*Cold symptoms; nasal congestion.*

Pfizer Consumer, S.Afr.
Paracetamol (p.76·2); phenylpropanolamine hydrochloride (p.1127·3); phenyltoloxamine citrate (p.439·1); codeine phosphate (p.27·1).
*Cold and influenza symptoms; sinus headache.*

**Sinutab Extra Strength** Warner-Lambert, Canad.†.
Paracetamol (p.76·2); pseudoephedrine hydrochloride (p.1129·2); chlorphenamine maleate (p.427·3).
*Cold symptoms; nasal congestion.*

**Sinutab Extra Strength Daytime/Nightime**
Pfizer Consumer, Canad.
Tablets (Daytime), pseudoephedrine hydrochloride (p.1129·2); paracetamol (p.76·2); tablets (Nighttime), pseudoephedrine hydrochloride; paracetamol; diphenhydramine hydrochloride (p.431·3).
*Cold symptoms; rhinitis; sinusitis.*

**Sinutab Maximum Strength Sinus Allergy**
Warner-Lambert, USA.
Pseudoephedrine hydrochloride (p.1129·2); chlorphenamine maleate (p.427·3); paracetamol (p.76·2).
*Upper respiratory-tract symptoms.*

**Sinutab ND** Pfizer Consumer, S.Afr.
Paracetamol (p.76·2); phenylpropanolamine hydrochloride (p.1127·3).
*Cold and influenza symptoms.*

**Sinutab Nightime**
Note. This name is used for preparations of different composition.
Pfizer Consumer, Canad.
Paracetamol (p.76·2); diphenhydramine hydrochloride (p.431·3); pseudoephedrine hydrochloride (p.1129·2).
Formerly contained paracetamol, chlorphenamine, and pseudoephedrine.
*Cold symptoms; nasal congestion.*

Warner-Lambert, UK†.
Paracetamol (p.76·2); phenylpropanolamine hydrochloride (p.1127·3); phenyltoloxamine citrate (p.439·1).
*Congestion.*

**Sinutab Non-Drying** Warner-Lambert, USA.
Pseudoephedrine hydrochloride (p.1129·2); guaifenesin (p.1122·1).
*Coughs.*

**Sinutab Sinus & Allergy** Pfizer Consumer, Canad.
Paracetamol (p.76·2); pseudoephedrine hydrochloride (p.1129·2); chlorphenamine maleate (p.427·3).
Formerly known as Sinutab Regular.
*Cold symptoms; nasal congestion.*

**Sinutab Sinus & Allergy 12 Hour** Warner-Lambert, Canad.†.
Paracetamol (p.76·2); phenylpropanolamine hydrochloride (p.1127·3); phenyltoloxamine citrate (p.439·1).
Formerly known as Sinutab SA.
*Cold symptoms; nasal congestion.*

**Sinutab Sinus Allergy & Pain Relief**
Pfizer Consumer, Austral.; Pfizer, NZ.
Paracetamol (p.76·2); pseudoephedrine hydrochloride (p.1129·2); chlorphenamine maleate (p.427·3).
*Allergic rhinitis; cold symptoms; sinus headache.*

**Sinutab Sinus (Daytime) Non Drowsy** Pfizer Consumer, Canad.
Paracetamol (p.76·2); pseudoephedrine hydrochloride (p.1129·2).
Formerly known as Sinutab ND Daytime Formula.
*Cold symptoms; nasal congestion.*

**Sinutab Sinus Non Drowsy** Pfizer Consumer, Canad.
Paracetamol (p.76·2); pseudoephedrine hydrochloride (p.1129·2).
Formerly known as Sinutab No Drowsiness.
*Cold symptoms; nasal congestion.*

**Sinutab Sinus & Pain Relief**
Pfizer Consumer, Austral.; Pfizer, NZ.
Paracetamol (p.76·2); pseudoephedrine hydrochloride (p.1129·2).
*Cold symptoms; sinus headache.*

**Sinutab Without Drowsiness** Warner-Lambert, USA.
Pseudoephedrine hydrochloride (p.1129·2); paracetamol (p.76·2).
*Upper respiratory-tract symptoms.*

**SINUtuss DM** WE, USA.
Dextromethorphan hydrobromide (p.1117·3); guaifenesin (p.1122·1); phenylephrine hydrochloride (p.1126·3).
*Coughs.*

**SINUvent** WE, USA†.
Phenylpropanolamine hydrochloride (p.1127·3); guaifenesin (p.1122·1).
*Coughs and cold symptoms; nasal congestion.*

**Sinuvent PE** WE, USA.
Phenylephrine hydrochloride (p.1126·3); guaifenesin (p.1122·1).
*Upper respiratory-tract disorders.*

**Sinuzin** Biolab, Malaysia.
Chlorphenamine maleate (p.427·3); paracetamol (p.76·2).
*Allergic rhinitis; cold and influenza symptoms; hay fever; respiratory-tract congestion.*

**Sinuzin-D**
Biolab, Singapore†; Biolab, Thai.†.
Chlorphenamine maleate (p.427·3); paracetamol (p.76·2); phenylpropanolamine hydrochloride (p.1127·3).
*Cold symptoms; rhinitis; upper respiratory-tract disorders.*

**Sinvacor** Merck Sharp & Dohme, Ital.
Simvastatin (p.997·1).
*Coronary atherosclerosis; hypercholesterolaemia.*

**Sinvascor** Baldacci, Braz.
Simvastatin (p.997·1).
*Atherosclerosis; hypercholesterolaemia.*

**Sinvastacor** Hexal, Braz.
Simvastatin (p.997·1).
*Hypercholesterolaemia.*

**Sinvastil** Neo-Farmaceutica, Port.
Simvastatin (p.997·1).
*Hyperlipidaemias.*

**Sinvatrox** Legrand, Braz.
Simvastatin (p.997·1).
*Hypercholesterolaemia.*

**Siochrome** David, India.
*Injection:* Carbazochrome (p.745·1).
*Tablets:* Carbazochrome (p.745·1); menadione sodium bisulfite (p.1466·3); vitamin C (p.1460·2); calcium hydrogen phosphate (p.1225·2).
*Epistaxis; haemoptysis; menstrual disorders; retinal haemorrhage.*

**Siofor** Berlin-Chemie, Ger.
Metformin hydrochloride (p.342·3).
*Diabetes mellitus.*

**Siokof-P** David, India.
Dextromethorphan hydrobromide (p.1117·3); pseudoephedrine hydrochloride (p.1129·2); bromhexine hydrochloride (p.1115·3); ammonium chloride (p.1115·2); menthol (p.1711·3).
*Respiratory-tract congestion.*

**Sioneuron** David, India.
Vitamin $B_1$ (p.1455·2); vitamin $B_6$ (p.1457·2); vitamin $B_{12}$ (p.1458·2); nicotinamide (p.1441·2); calcium pantothenate (p.1442·3) or dexpanthenol (p.1727·2).
*Peripheral neuropathy.*

**Siopel**
Bioglan, Irl.; Genop, S.Afr.†; Centrapharm, UK.
Cetrimide (p.1172·1); dimeticone 1000 (p.1482·1).
*Barrier cream; napkin rash.*

**Sioplex** David, India.
Vitamin B substances; vitamin C (p.1417·1).
*Vitamin B and C deficiency.*

**Sioplex Lysine** David, India.
Vitamin B substances with lysine hydrochloride (p.1417·1).
*Vitamin B deficiency.*

**Sioplex-Z** David, India.
Multivitamin preparation with zinc (p.1417·1).
*Vitamin B and C deficiency.*

**Sioril** David, India.
Oxyphenbutazone (p.76·1).
*Ankylosing spondylitis.*

**Siosol** Febena, Ger.†.
Greater celandine (p.1695·3).
*Biliary and gastrointestinal spasm.*

**Siozwo** Febena, Ger.
*Nasal ointment:* Naphazoline hydrochloride (p.1124·3); peppermint oil (p.1283·2).
*Catarrh; nasal congestion; rhinitis.*
*Nasal solution:* Isotonic electrolyte solution (p.1217·1).
*Nasal irrigation.*

**Siozwo N** Febena, Ger.†.
Bismuth subgallate (p.1252·2); hamamelis (p.1696·3); zinc oxide (p.1163·2).
*Burns; skin disorders; wounds.*

**Sipam** Siam Bheasach, Thai.
Diazepam (p.690·1).
*Anxiety; insomnia.*

**Sipcar** Microsules Bernabo, Arg.
Bromazepam (p.671·3).
*Anxiety.*

**Sipental** Siam Bheasach, Thai.
Pentoxifylline (p.979·3).
*Cerebral, ocular, and peripheral vascular disorders.*

**Siphene** Serum Institute, India.
Clomifene citrate (p.1542·2).
*Female infertility.*

**Sipirac** Chemopharma, Chile.
Diclofenac diethylamine (p.32·1) or diclofenac sodium (p.32·1).
*Gout; inflammation; musculoskeletal, joint, peri-articular, and soft-tissue disorders; pain.*

**Siprofen** Labima, Belg.
Ibuprofen (p.45·3).
*Fever; pain.*

**Siqualine** Bristol-Myers Squibb, Mex.†.
Fluphenazine (p.699·3).

**Siqualone**
Bristol-Myers Squibb, Denm.; Bristol-Myers Squibb, Fin.; Bristol-Myers Squibb, Norw.; Bristol-Myers Squibb, Swed.
Fluphenazine decanoate (p.699·3) or fluphenazine hydrochloride (p.699·3).
*Psychoses.*

**Siquial** Merck, Mex.
Fluoxetine hydrochloride (p.292·1).
*Bulimia nervosa; depression; obsessive-compulsive disorder.*

**Siquil**
Sarabhai Piramal, India; Bristol-Myers Squibb, Neth.†.
Triflupromazine hydrochloride (p.727·1).
*Anxiety; bipolar disorder; nausea and vomiting; psychoses.*

**Siran**
Temmler, Ger.; Temmler, Israel.
Acetylcysteine (p.1112·3).
*Respiratory-tract disorders associated with viscous mucus.*

**Sirani** Ofimex, Mex.†.
Ranitidine (p.1285·2).

**Sirben** Uniao Quimica, Braz.
Mebendazole (p.108·2).
*Worm infections.*

**Sirdalud**
Novartis, Arg.; Novartis, Austria; Novartis, Belg.; Novartis, Braz.; Novartis, Chile; Novartis, Denm.; Novartis, Fin.; Sanofi Synthelabo, Ger.; Novartis, Gr.; Novartis, India; Novartis, Ital.; Novartis, Mex.; Novartis, Neth.; Novartis, Port.; Novartis, Spain; Novartis, Switz.; Novartis, Thai.
Tizanidine hydrochloride (p.1395·3).
*Skeletal muscle spasm; spasticity.*

**Sirepar** Gedeon Richter, Thai.
Liver extract.
*Liver disorders.*

**Siridone** Chemopharma, Chile.
Cinnarizine (p.428·3).
*Cerebral and peripheral vascular disorders; migraine; vestibular disorders.*

**Sirigen** Adivar, Ital.
Benzalkonium chloride (p.1168·3).
*Disinfection of wounds and burns.*

**Sirmia Abfuhrkapseln** Niedermaier, Ger.†.
Senna (p.1288·2); peppermint oil (p.1283·2); caraway oil (p.1667·3).
*Constipation.*

**Sirmia Artischockenelixier N** Niedermaier, Ger.†.
Cynara (p.1678·3); taraxacum (p.1751·3).
*Hepatobiliary disorders.*

**Sirmia Knoblauchsaft N** Niedermaier, Ger.†.
Garlic (p.1691·1).
*Hyperlipidaemia.*

**Sirmiosta Nervenelixier N** Niedermaier, Ger.†.
Melissa (p.1711·1); passion flower (p.1729·1); valerian (p.1762·2).
*Agitation; insomnia.*

**Sirodina** Clariana, Spain.
Pyridoxine (p.1457·2); sulpiride (p.722·2).
*Nervous disorders; vertigo.*

**Sirolax** Pharbita, Israel†.
Lactulose (p.1269·1).
*Constipation; hepatic coma.*

**Sirop antitussif Wyss a base de codeine** Wyss, Switz.†.
Codeine phosphate (p.27·1); cherry-laurel; ipecacuanha (p.1122·3); senega root (p.1130·2); althaea (p.1651·3).
*Coughs.*

**Sirop Boin** Picot, Fr.†.
Codeine (p.27·1); menthol (p.1711·3); adrenaline (p.852·2); guaiacol (p.1122·1); aconite (p.1646·3); cherry laurel.
*Respiratory disorders.*

**Sirop Cocillana Codeine** Atlas, Canad.
Codeine phosphate (p.27·1); cocillana (p.1117·2); euphorbia (p.1686·3); senega (p.1130·2); squill (p.1130·3); wild lettuce (p.1765·2).

**Sirop contre la toux nouvelle formule** Zeller, Switz.†.
Hedera helix.
*Bronchial disorders with viscous mucus.*

**Sirop Dentition** Sabex, Canad.†.
Benzocaine (p.1370·3).

**Sirop des Vosges Expectorant** GlaxoSmithKline Sante, Fr.
Carbocisteine (p.1116·2).
*Respiratory-tract congestion.*

**Sirop Des Vosges Toux Seche** GlaxoSmithKline Sante, Fr.
Pholcodine (p.1128·3).
*Coughs.*

**Sirop DM** *Marc-O, Canad.†.*
Dextromethorphan hydrobromide (p.1117·3).

**Sirop Expectorant** *Technilab, Canad.*
Guaifenesin (p.1122·1).

**Sirop Passi-Par** *Parsenn, Switz.*
Passion flower (p.1729·1); crataegus (p.1677·1).
*Anxiety; insomnia.*

**Sirop Pectoral adulte** *Oberlin, Fr.†.*
Ethylmorphine hydrochloride (p.37·3); aconite (p.1646·3); bromoform (p.1663·1); sodium benzoate (p.1169·3); sulfogaiacol (p.1131·1); cherry laurel; belladonna (p.479·1); drosera (p.1683·1); eucalyptus oil (p.1686·2); senega (p.1130·2); ipecacuanha (p.1122·3) tolu balsam (p.1131·3).
*Coughs.*

**Sirop pectoral DP1** *DP-Medica, Switz.†.*
Guaifenesin (p.1122·1); codeine phosphate (p.27·1); ephedrine hydrochloride (p.1120·1); sodium benzoate (p.1169·3); althaea (p.1651·3); tolu balsam (p.1131·3); plantain (p.1733·1); thyme (p.1755·2); pine buds; pectoral syrup.
*Bronchitis; catarrh; coughs.*

**Sirop pectoral DP2, DP3** *DP-Medica, Switz.†.*
Guaifenesin (p.1122·1); codeine phosphate (p.27·1); ephedrine hydrochloride (p.1120·1); sodium benzoate (p.1169·3); belladonna (p.479·1); althaea (p.1651·3); tolu balsam (p.1131·3); plantain (p.1733·1); thyme (p.1755·2); pine buds; pectoral syrup.
*Bronchitis; catarrh; coughs.*

**Sirop Pectoral enfant** *Oberlin, Fr.†.*
Sodium benzoate (p.1169·3); sulfogaiacol (p.1131·1); sodium bromide (p.1663·1); drosera (p.1683·1); eucalyptus oil (p.1686·2); frangula (p.1266·3); ethylmorphine hydrochloride (p.37·3); tolu balsam (p.1131·3).
*Coughs.*

**Sirop Pectoral Vicks** *Lachartre, Fr.†.*
Pentoxyverine citrate (p.1126·2).
Formerly contained pentoxyverine citrate, guaifenesin, and sodium citrate.
*Coughs.*

**Sirop pour le sommeil** *Zeller, Switz.*
Valerian (p.1762·2).
*Sleep disorders.*

**Sirop S contre la toux et la bronchite** *Sympharma, Switz.*
Codeine phosphate (p.27·1); drosera (p.1683·1); hyoscyamus (p.485·2); liquorice (p.1270·2) primula root (p.1735·1).
*Coughs.*

**Sirop Teyssedre** *Therica, Fr.†.*
Calcium bromide (p.1663·1); cloral hydrate (p.684·1); calamint.
*Sleep disorders in children.*

**Sirop Toux du Larynx** *Qualiphar, Belg.†.*
Codeine phosphate (p.27·1); belladonna (p.479·1); aconite (p.1646·3); lobelia (p.1589·1); cherry-laurel water; drosera (p.1683·1); erysimin.
*Coughs.*

**Sirop Wyss contre la toux** *Wyss, Switz.†.*
Cherry-laurel; ipecacuanha (p.1122·3); senega root (p.1130·2); althaea (p.1651·3).
*Coughs.*

**Siros** *Janssen-Cilag, Ger.*
Itraconazole (p.401·3).
*Vulvovaginal candidiasis.*

**Sirotamicin BG** *Maigal, Arg.*
Betamethasone (p.1093·1); gentamicin (p.219·1).

**Sirotamicin HC** *Maigal, Arg.*
Hydrocortisone (p.1103·3).
*Skin disorders.*

**Siroxyl** *Aventis, Belg.*
Carbocisteine (p.1116·2).
*Respiratory-tract disorders associated with retention of bronchial secretions.*

**Sirtal**
*Sanofi Synthelabo, Austria; Merck dura, Ger.*
Carbamazepine (p.353·3).
*Alcohol withdrawal syndrome; bipolar disorder; diabetes insipidus; diabetic neuropathy; epilepsy; multiple sclerosis; neuralgia.*

**Sisare** *Nourypharma, Ger.*
11 Tablets, estradiol valerate (p.1550·2); 10 tablets, estradiol valerate; medroxyprogesterone acetate (p.1557·2).
*Menopausal disorders.*

**Sisare mono** *Nourypharma, Ger.*
Estradiol (p.1550·1).
*Menopausal disorders.*

**Sisomina** *Schering-Plough, Spain†.*
Sisomicin sulfate (p.254·3).
*Bacterial infections.*

**Sisoptin** *Themis Chemicals, India.*
Sisomicin sulfate (p.254·3).
*Bacterial infections.*

**Sistalgina** *Merck, Chile.*
Pramiverine (p.1734·3); dipyrone (p.35·3).
*Smooth muscle spasm and pain.*

**Sita** *Hoyer, Ger.*
Saw palmetto (p.1569·1).
*Benign prostatic hyperplasia.*

**Sitem** *Inpa, Gr.*
Phenothrin (p.1509·1).
*Head, body, and crab lice.*

**Siterone** *Rex, NZ.*
Cyproterone acetate (p.1544·1).
*Androgen-dependent alopecia and hirsutism in females; hypersexuality in males; prostatic cancer.*

**Siticox** *Sarabhai Piramal, India.*
Rifampicin (p.250·2).
*Tuberculosis.*

**Siticox-INH** *Sarabhai Piramal, India.*
Rifampicin (p.250·2); isoniazid (p.222·2).
*Tuberculosis.*

**Sito-Lande** *Sanofi Synthelabo, Ger.*
Sitosterol (p.982·3).
*Hyperlipidaemias.*

**Sitrac** *BPL-Meizler, Braz.*
Atracurium besilate (p.1399·1).
*Competitive neuromuscular blocker.*

**Sitriol** *Alphapharm, Austral.*
Calcitriol (p.1461·2).
*Hypocalcaemia; osteoporosis.*

**Sitzmarks**
*Note. This name is used for preparations of different composition.*
*Dominguez, Arg.*
Radio-opaque markers.
*Investigation of gastrointestinal motility.*

*Konsyl, USA.*
Radio-opaque polyvinyl chloride.
*Contrast medium for gastrointestinal radiography.*

**Sivastin** *Sigma-Tau, Ital.*
Simvastatin (p.997·1).
*Atherosclerosis; hypercholesterolaemia; ischaemic heart disease.*

**Sivlor** *Sidus, Arg.*
Lovastatin (p.949·1).
*Hypercholesterolaemia.*

**Sizopin** *Sun, India.*
Clozapine (p.685·3).
*Schizophrenia.*

**SJ Liniment** *International Dermatologicals, Canad.*
Methyl salicylate (p.59·3); menthol (p.1711·3); ammonia (p.1653·3); coal tar (p.1159·2).

**Skaelud** *Propharma, Denm.*
Pyrithione zinc (p.1156·2).
*Pityriasis versicolor; seborrhoeic dermatitis.*

**Skeeter Stik** *Triton, USA.*
Lidocaine (p.1377·3); phenol (p.1188·1).
*Skin disorders.*

**Skelan** *Great Eastern, Thai.; Therapharma, Thai.*
Ibuprofen (p.45·3); paracetamol (p.76·2).
*Pain.*

**Skelan IB** *Biomedis, Thai.; Great Eastern, Thai.*
Ibuprofen (p.45·3).
*Gout; musculoskeletal, joint, and peri-articular disorders; pain.*

**Skelaxin** *King, USA.*
Metaxalone (p.1395·1).
*Painful musculoskeletal conditions.*

**Skelid**
*Mayne, Austral.; Sanofi Synthelabo, Austria; Sanofi Synthelabo, Belg.; Sanofi Synthelabo, Braz.†; Sanofi Synthelabo, Fin.; Sanofi Synthelabo, Fr.; Sanofi Synthelabo, Ger.; Sanofi Synthelabo, Neth.; Sanofi Synthelabo, Spain; Sanofi Synthelabo, Swed.; Sanofi Synthelabo, Switz.; Sanofi Synthelabo, UK; Sanofi Winthrop, USA.*
Tiludronate sodium (p.776·1).
*Paget's disease of bone.*

**Skema** *Pentamedical, Ital.*
*Cream:* Zinc oxide (p.1163·2); titanium dioxide (p.1160·3).
*Lotion:* Octinoxate (p.1154·3); avobenzone (p.1142·3).
*Sunscreen.*

**Skenan**
*Upsamedica, Belg.†; UPSA, Fr.; Upsa, Ital.; Bristol-Myers Squibb, Port.; Upsamedica, Spain.*
Morphine sulfate (p.60·2).
*Pain.*

**Skezide** *Masa, Thai.†.*
Hydrochlorothiazide (p.933·2); triamterene (p.1016·2).
*Hypertension; oedema.*

**SK-F, BIC-F** *Fresenius Medical, Switz.†.*
Acidic and basic haemodialysis concentrates (p.1221·1).

**Skiacol** *Alcon, Fr.*
Cyclopentolate hydrochloride (p.480·3).
*Production of cycloplegia and mydriasis.*

**Skiatropine** *Bausch & Lomb, Switz.*
Atropine sulfate (p.477·1).
*Eye disorders; production of mydriasis and cycloplegia.*

**Skid** *Lichtenstein, Ger.*
Minocycline hydrochloride (p.231·3).

**Skid E** *Lichtenstein, Ger.†.*
Erythromycin (p.208·1).
*Acne.*

**Skilax** *Almirall, Spain.*
Sodium picosulfate (p.1289·3).
*Constipation.*

**Skin Bond Cement** *Smith & Nephew, Austral.†.*
Appliance adhesive.

**Skin C** *Dispolab, Chile.*
Emollient containing vitamin C (p.1460·2).

**Skin Cap**
*Volta, Chile; Medix, Mex.†.*
Pyrithione zinc (p.1156·2).
*Dandruff; seborrhoeic dermatitis.*

**Skin Care Nutrients** *Lifeplan, UK.*
Vitamins; minerals; bioflavonoids; cysteine; lecithin; choline; inositol (p.1417·1).
*Dietary supplement.*

**Skin Cleanser & Deodorizer** *National Care, Canad.*
Benzethonium chloride (p.1169·2).
*Skin hygiene in incontinent patients.*

**Skin Cleansing** *Cantassium Co., UK.*
Lappa (p.1704·3); senna (p.1288·2); fumitory (p.1690·1); clivers (p.1673·2).

**Skin Clear** *Potter's, UK.*
*Ointment:* Starch (p.1449·1); sublimed sulfur (p.1158·2); zinc oxide (p.1163·2); melaleuca oil (p.1710·2).
*Tablets:* Echinacea root (p.1683·2).
*Skin disorders.*

**Skin Conditioner & Bath Oil** *Arjo, Canad.†.*
Light liquid paraffin (p.1479·1).
*Dry skin; pruritus.*

**Skin Cure** *Young Again Nutrients, USA.*
Pyrithione zinc (p.1156·2).
*Skin disorders.*

**Skin Dry** *Darier, Mex.*
Aluminium tetrachlorohydrate (p.1142·1).
*Dry skin.*

**Skin Eruptions Mixture** *Potter's, UK.*
Blue flag (p.1702·1); lappa root (p.1704·3); yellow dock (p.1766·1); sarsaparilla (p.1742·1); buchu (p.1663·1); cascara (p.1255·1).
*Skin disorders.*

**Skin Hair & Nails** *Natural Life, Arg.*
Vitamins; calcium; iron (p.1417·1).
*Dietary supplement.*

**Skin Healing Cream** *Brauer, Austral.†.*
Calendula (p.1665·2); hypericum (p.299·1).
*Bruised fingers and toes; cuts and abrasions; insect bites; skin irritation.*

**Skin Prep** *Smith & Nephew, Austral.†.*
Film dressing.

**Skin Repair**
*Rosken, Hong Kong; Pfizer Consumer, Singapore.*
Dimeticone (p.1482·1).
*Cracked and dry skin; eczema.*

**Skin Repair Daily Care** *Rosken, Singapore†.*
Emollient and barrier preparation.

**Skin Shield**
*Del, Canad.†; Del, USA.*
Dyclonine hydrochloride (p.1376·2); benzethonium chloride (p.1169·2).
*Liquid bandage.*

**Skin So Soft Antibacterial** *Avon, Canad.*
*Lotion:* Triclosan (p.1195·2).
*Topical gel:* Alcohol (p.1166·1).

**Skin Sol P** *Maigal, Arg.*
Titanium dioxide (p.1160·3).
*Sunscreen.*

**Skin Sol T** *Maigal, Arg.*
Octinoxate (p.1154·3) titanium dioxide (p.1160·3); octisalate (p.1154·3).
*Sunscreen.*

**Skinat** *Teofarma, Ital.*
Collagen (p.1674·3).
*Prevention of scarring.*

**Skincalm** *Boots Healthcare, NZ.*
Hydrocortisone acetate (p.1103·3).
*Skin disorders.*

**Skin-Cap** *Catalysis, Arg.*
Pyrithione zinc (p.1156·2).
*Dandruff; seborrhoea.*

**Skinderm A** *Maigal, Arg.*
Vitamin A (p.1451·2).
*Skin disorders.*

**Skindure** *March, Thai.*
Miconazole nitrate (p.405·3).
*Fungal skin and nail infections.*

**Skinfect** *Bangkok Lab & Cosmetic, Thai.*
Gentamicin sulfate (p.217·1).
*Bacterial skin infections.*

**Skinicles** *Skinicles, Canad.†.*
Hydroquinone (p.1148·1); padimate O (p.1155·1).

**Skinman Intensiv** *Henkel, Ger.†.*
Alcohol (p.1166·1); chlorhexidine gluconate (p.1173·2).
*Skin disinfection.*

**Skinman Soft** *Henkel, Ger.*
Isopropyl alcohol (p.1184·3); benzalkonium chloride (p.1168·3); undecenoic acid (p.410·3).
*Skin disinfection.*

**Skinocyclin** *Asche, Ger.*
Minocycline hydrochloride (p.231·3).
*Acne.*

**Skinoderm** *Pharma Clal, Israel.*
Azelaic acid (p.1142·3).
*Acne.*

**Skinola-Fett** *Medika, Switz.*
Bath additive.
*Dry skin disorders.*

**Skinoren**
*Schering, Austral.; Schering, Austria; Schering, Belg.; Schering, Denm.; Schering, Fin.; Schering, Fr.†; Schering, Ger.; Asche, Ger.; Shepa, Gr.; Schering, Hong Kong; Schering, Ital.; Schering, Malaysia; Schering, Norw.; Schering, NZ; Schering, Port.; Schering, S.Afr.; Schering, Singapore; Schering, Spain; Schering, Swed.; Schering, Switz.; Schering, Thai.; Schering, UK.*
Azelaic acid (p.1142·3).
*Acne.*

**Skinsept** *Henkel, Austria.*
Alcohol (p.1166·1); isopropyl alcohol (p.1184·3).
*Skin disinfection.*

**Skinsept F** *Henkel, Ger.*
Isopropyl alcohol (p.1184·3); chlorhexidine gluconate (p.1173·2); hydrogen peroxide (p.1182·2).
*Skin disinfection.*

**Skinsept G** *Henkel, Ger.*
Alcohol (p.1166·1); isopropyl alcohol (p.1184·3).
*Skin disinfection.*

**Skinsept mucosa**
*Henkel, Austria; Henkel, Ger.*
Alcohol (p.1166·1); hydrogen peroxide 30% (p.1182·3); chlorhexidine gluconate (p.1173·2).
*Mucous membrane disinfection.*

**Skintex** *Lloyd, Aimee, UK.*
Chloroxylenol (p.1177·2); camphor (p.1665·3).
*Skin disorders.*

**SkinVit** *Pharmadass, UK.*
Multivitamin, mineral, and amino-acid preparation (p.1417·1).

**Skleremo** *Elvetium, Arg.*
Chrome alum (p.1670·2); glycerol (p.1694·3).
*Varices.*

**Sklerofibrat** *Merckle, Ger.*
Bezafibrate (p.873·2).
*Hyperlipidaemias.*

**Sklerosol N** *Febena, Ger.*
Colloidal silicon dioxide (p.1581·3).
*Hair and nail disorders.*

**Sklerovenol N** *Febena, Ger.*
Aesculus (p.1648·2).
Formerly contained aesculus and rutoside sodium sulfate.
*Soft-tissue inflammation; venous insufficiency.*

**Sklerovitol** *Lannacher, Austria.*
Nicotinoylprocaine hydrochloride; vitamin B substances (p.1417·1); rutoside (p.1688·2).
*Peripheral vascular disorders; reduced mental and physical capacity in the elderly; tonic.*

**Skudal** *White, Arg.*
Meloxicam (p.56·1).
*Musculoskeletal and joint disorders.*

**Slap** *Temis, Arg.*
Aspartame (p.1422·1).
*Sugar substitute.*

**Sleep Aid**
*Tanta, Canad.; Stanley, Canad.; Technilab, Canad.; Galpharm, UK.*
Diphenhydramine hydrochloride (p.431·3).
*Insomnia.*

**Sleepeaze** *Galpharm, UK.*
Diphenhydramine hydrochloride (p.431·3).
*Insomnia.*

**Sleep-Ettes D** *Reese, USA.*
Diphenhydramine hydrochloride (p.431·3).
*Insomnia.*

**Sleep-eze 3** *Whitehall, USA†.*
Diphenhydramine hydrochloride (p.431·3).
*Insomnia.*

**Sleep-Eze D** *Medtech, Canad.*
Diphenhydramine hydrochloride (p.431·3).
*Insomnia.*

**Sleep-Eze V Natural** *Medtech, Canad.*
Valerian (p.1762·2).
*Sleep disorders.*

**Sleepeze PM** *Aspen, S.Afr.*
Diphenhydramine hydrochloride (p.431·3).
*Insomnia.*

**Sleepia**
*Pfizer, Austria; Pfizer, Ger.; Pfizer, Switz.*
Diphenhydramine hydrochloride (p.431·3).
*Insomnia.*

**Sleeplessness & Insomnia Relief** *Brauer, Austral.†.*
Homoeopathic preparation.

**Sleepwell 2-nite** *Rugby, USA.*
Diphenhydramine hydrochloride (p.431·3).
*Insomnia.*

**Slepan** *Staufen, Ger.*
Homoeopathic preparation.

**Slim Caps** *Amino, Switz.*
Phenylpropanolamine hydrochloride (p.1127·3).
*Obesity.*

**Slim Mint**
*Note. This name is used for preparations of different composition.*
*Stella, Canad.†.*
Benzocaine (p.1370·3); methylcellulose (p.1580·2).
*Obesity.*

*Thompson, USA†.*
Benzocaine (p.1370·3).
*Obesity.*

**Slim 'n Trim** *Covan, S.Afr.*
Cathine (p.1585·2).
*Obesity.*

**Slimase** *Sessa, Ital.†.*
Ananas.
*Inflammation.*

**SlimLinea** *Bifarma, Ital.†.*
Bladderwrack (p.1742·3); betula (p.1660·3).

**Slimmer** *Baif, Ital.*
Piscidia erythrina; fucus vesiculosus; ananas sativa; equisetum arvense; betula alba; ononis spinosa; centella asiatica; orthosiphon stamineus; ruscus aculeatus; lespedeza capitata (p.1417·1).
*Nutritional supplement.*

**Slimomin** Eurodrug, Hong Kong†.
Phenylpropanolamine hydrochloride (p.1127·3).
*Obesity.*

**Slimum** Ferrier, Fr.
Homoeopathic preparation.

**Slippery Elm Stomach Tablets** Potter's, UK.
Slippery elm bark (p.1747·1); cinnamon oil (p.1672·2); anise oil (p.1655·2); peppermint oil (p.1283·2).
*Dyspepsia; flatulence.*

**Sloan** Warner-Lambert, Ital.
Capsicum oleoresin (p.1667·1); glycol monosalicylate (p.44·3); white camphor oil; pine oil; menthol (p.1711·3); eucalyptus oil (p.1686·2); benzyl nicotinate (p.21·2).
*Musculoskeletal, joint, and soft-tissue pain.*

**Sloan Baume** Soma, Switz.†.
Ethyl nicotinate (p.37·2); menthol (p.1711·3); camphor (p.1665·3); methyl salicylate (p.59·3); capsicum oleoresin (p.1667·1); eucalyptus oil (p.1686·2); pine oil; turpentine oil (p.1760·1).
*Musculoskeletal and joint disorders.*

**Sloan Liniment** Soma, Switz.†.
Camphor (p.1665·3); methyl salicylate (p.59·3); capsicum oleoresin (p.1667·1); pine oil; turpentine oil (p.1760·1).
*Musculoskeletal and joint disorders.*

**Sloan's balsem** Warner-Lambert, Neth.
Capsicum (p.1667·1); camphor (p.1665·3); benzyl nicotinate (p.21·2); glycol salicylate (p.44·3).
*Muscle and joint pain.*

**Slo-Bid**
Rhone-Poulenc Rorer, Canad.†; Rhone-Poulenc Rorer, Hong Kong†; Aventis, Mex.; Rhone-Poulenc Rorer, USA.
Theophylline (p.798·3).
*Obstructive airways disease.*

**Slofedipine** Sterwin, UK.
Nifedipine (p.966·2).
*Angina pectoris; hypertension.*

**Slofenac** Sterwin, UK.
Diclofenac sodium (p.32·1).

**Slo-Indo** Generics, UK.
Indometacin (p.47·3).
*Inflammation; pain.*

**Slo-Morph** Helsinn Birex, Irl.
Morphine sulfate (p.60·2).
*Pain.*

**Slo-Niacin** Upsher-Smith, USA.
Nicotinic acid (p.1441·1).
*Hyperlipidaemia (adjunct); nicotinic acid deficiency; pellagra.*

**Slo-Phyllin**
Aventis, Irl.; Merck, UK; Rhone-Poulenc Rorer, USA.
Theophylline (p.798·3).
*Obstructive airways disease.*

**Slo-Phyllin GG** Rhone-Poulenc Rorer, USA.
Theophylline (p.798·3); guaifenesin (p.1122·1).
*Asthma; bronchospasm.*

**Slo-Salt-K** Mission Pharmacal, USA.
Sodium chloride (p.1233·3); potassium chloride (p.1232·2).
*Dehydration; heat prostration; sodium depletion; volume depletion.*

**Slo-Theo** Ethypharm, Hong Kong.
Theophylline (p.798·3).
*Obstructive airways disease.*

**Slow Deralin** Abic, Israel.
Propranolol hydrochloride (p.989·3).
*Angina pectoris; hypertension; hyperthyroidism; migraine; tremor.*

**Slow Fe with Folic Acid** Novartis Consumer, USA.
Dried ferrous sulfate (p.1428·3); folic acid (p.1429·1).
*Iron and folic acid deficiency.*

**Slow K** Novartis, Chile.
Potassium chloride (p.1232·2).
*Hypokalaemia.*

**Slow Release Mega C** Vitaglow, Austral.†.
Calcium ascorbate (p.1460·2); ascorbic acid (p.1460·2).
*Bruising; cold and influenza symptoms; maintenance of oral health; vitamin supplement; wounds.*

**Slow Release Mega Multi** Vitaglow, Austral.†.
Multivitamin and mineral preparation (p.1417·1).

**Slow-Fe**
Novartis Consumer, Canad.; Novartis, Israel; Novartis Consumer, UK; Novartis Consumer, USA.
Dried ferrous sulfate (p.1428·3).
*Iron deficiency; iron-deficiency anaemia.*

**Slow-Fe Folic**
Novartis Consumer, Canad.; Novartis, Israel; Novartis Consumer, UK.
Dried ferrous sulfate (p.1428·3); folic acid (p.1429·1).
*Iron and folic acid deficiency in pregnancy.*

**Slow-K**
Novartis, Austral.; Allergan-Frumtost, Braz.†; Novartis, Canad.; Novartis, Hong Kong; Novartis, Irl.; Novartis, Israel; Novartis, Malaysia; Novartis, Neth.; Novartis, NZ; Novartis, S.Afr.; Alliance, UK; Summit, USA.
Potassium chloride (p.1232·2).
*Hypokalaemia.*

**Slow-Lopresor**
Novartis, Belg.; Novartis, NZ.
Metoprolol tartrate (p.957·1).
*Angina pectoris; arrhythmias; hypertension; hyperthyroidism; migraine; myocardial infarction.*

**Slow-Mag**
Wellspring, Canad.; Merck, S.Afr.; Purdue, USA.
Magnesium chloride (p.1228·1).
*Magnesium deficiency.*

The symbol † denotes a preparation no longer actively marketed

**Slow-Sodium**
Novartis, Austral.; Novartis, Irl.†; HK Pharma, UK.
Sodium chloride (p.1233·3).
*Hyponatraemia.*

**Slow-Trasicor**
Novartis, Canad.; Novartis, Irl.†; Novartis, NZ; Novartis, Switz.; Novartis, UK.
Oxprenolol hydrochloride (p.978·1).
*Angina pectoris; anxiety; arrhythmias; hypertension; myocardial infarction.*

**Slow-Trasitensine** Novartis, Switz.
Oxprenolol hydrochloride (p.978·1); chlortalidone (p.882·3).
*Hypertension.*

**Slozem** Merck, UK.
Diltiazem hydrochloride (p.900·1).
*Angina pectoris; hypertension.*

**SLT** C & M, USA.
Coal tar (p.1159·2); salicylic acid (p.1157·1); lactic acid (p.1704·1).
*Seborrhoea.*

**Slumber** Seven Seas, UK.
Lupulus (p.1708·1); piscidia (p.1702·3); passion flower (p.1729·1); wild lettuce (p.1765·2).
*Insomnia.*

**SM-33** Roche Consumer, Austral.
Salicylic acid (p.1157·1); lidocaine (p.1377·3); tannic acid (p.1751·2); menthol (p.1711·3); thymol (p.1194·2); glycerol (p.1694·3); alcohol.
*Mouth ulcers; oral abrasions; teething and denture pain.*

**SM-33 Adult Formula** Roche Consumer, Austral.
Lidocaine (p.1377·3); salicylic acid (p.1157·1); tannins; alcohol; rhubarb (p.1287·3).
*Mouth ulcers; oral abrasions.*

**SMA AR** Wyeth, Mex.
Infant feed (p.1417·1).
*Gastro-oesophageal reflux.*

**SMA High Energy** SMA Nutrition, Irl.
Infant feed (p.1417·1).
*Growth failure; malabsorption; malnutrition.*

**SMA LF** SMA Nutrition, Irl.
Infant feed (p.1417·1).
*Lactose intolerance.*

**SMA Sin Lactosa** Wyeth, Mex.
Infant feed (p.1417·1).
*Lactose intolerance.*

**Smaril** Coup, Gr.
Ranitidine hydrochloride (p.1285·2).
*Conditions where gastric acid reduction is beneficial; gastric hypersecretion including Zollinger-Ellison syndrome; peptic ulcer.*

**Smart Fizz** Thompson, Austral.†.
A range of multivitamin and mineral preparations (p.1417·1).

**Smecta**
Beaufour, Fr.; Beaufour-Ipsen, Hong Kong; Beaufour-Ipsen, Malaysia; Emerging Pharma, Malaysia; Beaufour-Ipsen, Singapore; Beaufour-Ipsen, Thai.
Dioctahedral smectite.
*Diarrhoea.*

**Smilitene** Rafarm, Gr.
Doxycycline hyclate (p.206·2).
*Bacterial infections.*

**Smok Quits** Eagle, Austral.†.
Homoeopathic preparation.

**Smoke-Eze** Brauer, Austral.†.
Homoeopathic preparation.

**Smokeless** Inibsa, Spain.
Lobeline sulfate (p.1589·1).
*Aid to smoking withdrawal.*

**Smokerette** Medinex, Canad.†.
Silver acetate (p.1746·1).
*Aid to smoking withdrawal.*

**Smoking Withdrawal Support** Homeocan, Canad.
Homoeopathic preparation.

**SMZ-TMP** Apothecon, USA.
Co-trimoxazole (p.199·3).

**Snake Bite** CSL, Austral.†.
A range of monovalent and polyvalent snake antisera (brown snake, tiger snake, death adder, taipan, black snake) (p.1639·1).
*Passive immunisation.*

**Snap Skin Cleanser Normal** Stella, Canad.†.
Isopropyl alcohol (p.1184·3); hamamelis (p.1696·3).

**Snap Skin Cleanser Sensitive** Stella, Canad.†.
Hamamelis (p.1696·3).

**Snaplets-DM** Baker Cummins, USA†.
Phenylpropanolamine hydrochloride (p.1127·3); dextromethorphan hydrobromide (p.1117·3).
*Coughs and cold symptoms.*

**Snaplets-EX** Baker Cummins, USA†.
Phenylpropanolamine hydrochloride (p.1127·3); guaifenesin (p.1122·1).
*Coughs.*

**Snaplets-Multi** Baker Cummins, USA†.
Phenylpropanolamine hydrochloride (p.1127·3); dextromethorphan hydrobromide (p.1117·3); chlorphenamine maleate (p.427·3).
*Coughs and cold symptoms.*

**Snell Cell** Wassen, Ital.
Kola; guarana; maté; garcinia cambogia; coleus; aesculus (p.1417·1).
*Cellulitis.*

**Snell'it** Wassen, Ital.
Apple vinegar; inulin (p.1702·1).

**Snif** Eurofarma, Braz.
Sodium chloride (p.1233·3).
*Nasal congestion.*

**Snip** Medochemie, Hong Kong.
Paracetamol (p.76·2); chlorphenamine maleate (p.427·3); pseudoephedrine hydrochloride (p.1129·2).
*Cold symptoms.*

**Sno Phenicol** Chauvin, UK†.
Chloramphenicol (p.185·1).
*Bacterial eye infections.*

**Sno Pro** Scientific Hospital Supplies, Irl.
Low-protein, low-phenylalanine food for special diets (p.1417·1).
*Disorders of amino-acid metabolism; milk substitute.*

**Sno Strips**
Smith & Nephew, Irl.†; Akorn, USA.
Test for tear production.

**Sno Tears**
Chauvin, Irl.; Bausch & Lomb, UK.
Polyvinyl alcohol (p.1581·1).
*Dry eyes.*

**Snoffocin** Seven Stars, Thai.
Norfloxacin (p.238·3).
*Bacterial infections.*

**Snooze Fast** BDI, USA.
Diphenhydramine hydrochloride (p.431·3).
*Insomnia.*

**Sno-Pro** Nutricia, Ital.
Food for special diets (p.1417·1).
*Phenylketonuria; renal failure.*

**Snor-Away** Munro, UK.
Almond oil (p.1651·1); olive oil (p.1723·2); peppermint oil (p.1283·2); sesame oil (p.1743·3); sunflower oil (p.1451·1); vitamins.
*Snoring.*

**Snore Calm** BSSAA, UK.
Euphrasia officinalis (p.1686·3).
*Snoring.*

**Snore Eze**
Note. A similar name is used for preparations of different composition (see below).
Brauer, Austral.†.
Homoeopathic preparation.

**Snoreeze**
Note. A similar name is used for preparations of different composition (see above).
Passion for Life, Singapore.
Glycerol; olive oil; peppermint oil; soya lecithin; sunflower oil; sweet almond oil; sesame oil; vitamin E; vitamin $B_6$ (p.1417·1).
*Snoring.*

**Snore No More**
Note. A similar name is used for preparations of different composition (see below).
Homeocan, Canad.
Homoeopathic preparation.

**Snore-No-More**
Note. A similar name is used for preparations of different composition (see above).
Anben, Israel.
Polysaccharides; phosphate; sodium chloride (p.1233·3).
*Nasal dryness; snoring.*

**Snore Stop** Nutravite, Canad.
Homoeopathic preparation.

**Snorenz**
Enzpharma, NZ; Passion for Life, UK†.
Peppermint oil (p.1283·2); olive oil (p.1723·2); sunflower oil (p.1451·1); sesame oil (p.1743·3); almond oil (p.1651·1); vitamins E, C, and $B_6$ (p.1417·1).
*Snoring.*

**Snowfire** Pickles, UK.
Benzoin (p.1751·1); citronella (p.1673·2); thyme oil (p.1755·3); lemon thyme (p.1755·2); clove oil (p.1673·3); cade oil (p.1159·2).
*Chapped hands; chilblains.*

**SNP** Quatromed, S.Afr.
Sodium nitroprusside hydrochloride.
*Hypertension; production of controlled hypotension during surgery.*

**Snufflebabe** Pickles, UK.
Menthol (p.1711·3); thyme oil (p.1755·3); eucalyptus oil (p.1686·2).
*Congestion.*

**Snufflebabe Cradle Cap** Pickles, UK.
Salicylic acid (p.1157·1).
*Cradle cap.*

**Snup** Stada, Ger.
Xylometazoline hydrochloride (p.1132·2).
*Catarrh; rhinitis.*

**Soaclens**
Alcon, Austral.; Alcon, Braz.†; Alcon, Canad.; Alcon, Fr.†; Alcon, NZ; Alcon, USA.
Wetting, soaking, and storage solution for contact lenses (p.1164·2).

**Soam** Edol, Port.
Emollient.

**Soapex** Galderma, Braz.
Triclosan (p.1195·2).
*Skin disinfection.*

**Sobelin**
Note. This name is used for preparations of different composition.
Pharmacia, Ger.
Clindamycin hydrochloride (p.194·2), clindamycin palmitate hydrochloride (p.194·2) or clindamycin phosphate (p.194·2).
*Bacterial infections.*

TO-Chemicals, Thai.
Flunarizine (p.434·2).
*Cerebrovascular disorders; migraine; motion sickness; peripheral vascular disorders; vestibular disorders.*

**Sobrepin**
Farmasa, Braz.; Roche, Ital.; Tedec Meiji, Spain.
Sobrerol (p.1130·2).
*Respiratory-tract congestion.*

**Sobrepina** Baldacci, Port.
Nimodipine (p.972·3).
*Cerebral ischaemia; cerebral vasospasm following subarachnoid haemorrhage.*

**Sobrial** Merck, S.Afr.
Acamprosate calcium (p.668·1).
*Alcoholism.*

**Sobril**
Pharmacia, Norw.; Pharmacia, Swed.
Oxazepam (p.712·2).
*Alcohol withdrawal syndrome; anxiety disorders; premedication; sleep disorders.*

**Sobrius** Fada, Arg.
Heparin (p.927·3).
*Thromboembolic disorders.*

**Socian**
Sanofi Synthelabo, Braz.; Sanofi Synthelabo, Chile; Sanofi Synthelabo, Port.
Amisulpride (p.669·3).
*Depression; psychoses.*

**Socloxin** Olan-Kemed, Thai.
Cloxacillin sodium (p.198·2).
*Bacterial infections.*

**Socosep** Cetus, Arg.
Ketoconazole (p.403·3).
*Fungal infections.*

**Sodemethin** Vilco, Gr.
Glyceryl trinitrate (p.923·2).
*Angina; heart failure.*

**Soden** DHA, Singapore.
Naproxen sodium (p.65·1).
*Gout; musculoskeletal and joint disorders; pain.*

**Soderm** Dermapharm, Ger.
Betamethasone valerate (p.1093·2).
*Skin disorders.*

**Soderm Plus** Dermapharm, Ger.
Betamethasone valerate (p.1093·2); salicylic acid (p.1157·1).
*Skin disorders.*

**Sodexx** Kwizda, Austria.
Cimetidine (p.1255·3).
*Gastro-oesophageal reflux.*

**Sodibic** Aspen, Austral.
Sodium bicarbonate (p.1223·2).
*Bicarbonate replacement in renal failure.*

**Sodiclo** Brissenco, S.Afr.†.
Diclofenac sodium (p.32·1).
*Inflammation; rheumatic disorders.*

**Sodilen** Motima, Fr.
Pollen.
*Antoxidant.*

**Sodilin** Collins, Mex.
Procaine benzylpenicillin (p.246·1).
*Bacterial infections.*

**Sodiofolin** Medac, UK.
Sodium folinate (p.1431·2).
*Adjunct to fluorouracil in colorectal cancer; methotrexate toxicity.*

**Sodiopen** Reig Jofre, Spain.
Benzylpenicillin sodium (p.163·2).
*Bacterial infections.*

**Sodioral con Inulina** CaDiGroup, Ital.
Oral rehydration solution with inulin (p.1222·2).
*Diarrhoea.*

**Sodiparin** Baxter Immuno, Arg.
Heparin sodium (p.928·1).
*Thromboembolic disorders.*

**Sodipen** Antibioticos, Mex.
Benzylpenicillin sodium (p.163·2).
*Bacterial infections.*

**Sodipental** Pisa, Mex.
Thiopental sodium (p.1309·1).
*Convulsions; general anaesthesia; increased intracranial pressure in neurosurgery.*

**Sodip-phylline** Sanofi, Switz.
Theophylline (p.798·3).
*Obstructive airways disease.*

**Sodipryl retard** Sanofi, Switz.
Naftidrofuryl oxalate (p.964·1).
*Peripheral and cerebral vascular disorders.*

**Sodium Sulamyd**
Schering, Canad.; Schering, USA.
Sulfacetamide sodium (p.257·3).
*Eye infections.*

**Sodixen** Rayere, Mex.
Naproxen sodium (p.65·1).
*Fever; musculoskeletal and joint disorders; pain.*

**Sodol Compound** *Major, USA.*
Aspirin (p.15·1); carisoprodol (p.1392·1).
*Musculoskeletal pain.*

**Sodolac** *Sofex, Port.*
Etodolac (p.37·3).
*Gout; musculoskeletal, joint, and peri-articular disorders; pain.*

**Sodorant** *Stiefel, Arg.*
*Cream:* Guaiazulene (p.1696·2); aluminium chlorohydrate (p.1142·1); triclocarban (p.1195·1).
*Deodorant bar:* Triclocarban (p.1195·1).
*Deodorant roll-on:* Aluminium chlorohydrate (p.1142·1).
*Hyperhidrosis.*

**Sofarcid** *Sofar, Ital.*
Cefonicid sodium (p.174·2).
Lidocaine hydrochloride (p.1377·3) is included in this preparation to alleviate the pain of injection.
*Gram-negative bacterial infections.*

**Sofargen** *Sofar, Ital.*
Sulfadiazine silver (p.259·1).
*Bacterial skin infections; burns; wounds.*

**Sofasin** *Faran, Gr.*
Norfloxacin (p.238·3).
*Urinary tract infections.*

**Sofenol** *C & M, USA.*
Emollient and moisturiser.

**Soffodex** *Dexxon, Israel.*
Dibasic sodium phosphate (p.1231·1); monobasic sodium phosphate (p.1230·3).
*Bowel evacuation; constipation.*

**Soficlor**
*Xepa-Soul Pattinson, Hong Kong; Xepa-Soul Pattinson, Malaysia; Xepa-Soul Pattinson, Singapore.*
Cefaclor (p.167·1).
*Bacterial infections.*

**Sofidrox**
*Xepa-Soul Pattinson, Hong Kong; Xepa-Soul Pattinson, Malaysia; Xepa-Soul Pattinson, Singapore.*
Cefadroxil (p.167·2).
*Bacterial infections.*

**Sofilex**
*Xepa-Soul Pattinson, Hong Kong; Xepa-Soul Pattinson, Malaysia; Xepa-Soul Pattinson, Singapore.*
Cefalexin (p.168·1).
*Bacterial infections.*

**Soflax**
*Note. This name is used for preparations of different composition.*
*Pharmascience, Canad.*
Docusate sodium (p.1262·2).
*Constipation.*
*Cipla-Medpro, S.Afr.*
Senna (p.1288·2).
*Constipation.*
*Julphar, UAE.*
Lactulose (p.1269·1).
*Constipation; hepatic encephalopathy.*

**Soflax EX** *Pharmascience, Canad.*
Bisacodyl (p.1251·3).
*Constipation.*

**Sofloran** *Pisa, Mex.*
Isoflurane (p.1301·1).
*General anaesthesia.*

**Sof/Pro Clean** *Sherman, Israel†.*
Cleansing solution for soft contact lenses (p.1164·2).

**Sofracort**
*Aventis, Canad.*
Framycetin sulfate (p.215·1); gramicidin (p.220·2); dexamethasone (p.1097·1).
*Ear disorders; eye disorders.*
*Aventis, India.*
Framycetin sulfate (p.215·1); dexamethasone sodium metasulfobenzoate (p.1097·2); gramicidin (p.220·2).
*Infected eye disorders.*

**Sofradex**
*Aventis, Austral.; Aventis, Denm.; Aventis, Fin.; Aventis, Hong Kong; Aventis, India; Aventis, Irl.; Aventis, Malaysia; Aventis, Neth.; Hoechst Marion Roussel, Norw.; Aventis, NZ; Aventis, S.Afr.; Aventis, Singapore; Hoechst Marion Roussel, Swed.†; Aventis, Switz.; Aventis, Thai.; Florizel, UK.*
Dexamethasone (p.1097·1) or dexamethasone sodium metasulfobenzoate (p.1097·2); framycetin sulfate (p.215·1); gramicidin (p.220·2).
*Infected eye and ear disorders.*

**Sofradex-F** *Aventis, India.*
Dexamethasone acetate (p.1097·1); framycetin sulfate (p.215·1); clotrimazole (p.396·2).
*Skin disorders.*

**Sofraline** *Aventis, Belg.*
Framycetin sulfate (p.215·1); naphazoline nitrate (p.1124·3).
*Respiratory-tract disorders.*

**Soframycin**
*Note. This name is used for preparations of different composition.*
*Aventis, Austral.; Erfa, Canad.; Aventis, India; Aventis, Irl.; Hoechst Marion Roussel, Neth.†; Aventis, NZ; Hoechst Marion Roussel, S.Afr.†; Hoechst Marion Roussel, Singapore†; Aventis, Switz.; Florizel, UK.*
*Eye/ear drops; eye/ear ointment:* Framycetin sulfate (p.215·1).
*Bacterial eye and ear infections.*
*Aventis, Austral.; Erfa, Canad.; Aventis, Irl.; Aventis, NZ.*
*Ointment:* Framycetin sulfate (p.215·1); gramicidin (p.220·2).
*Bacterial skin infections.*
*Erfa, Canad.*
*Nasal spray:* Framycetin sulfate (p.215·1); gramicidin (p.220·2); phenylephrine hydrochloride (p.1126·3).
*Bacterial nasal infections; nasal congestion.*

**Soframycine**
*Aventis, Belg.; Theraplix, Fr.†.*
Framycetin sulfate (p.215·1).
*Bacterial nose and throat infections.*

**Soframycine Hydrocortisone** *Theraplix, Fr.†.*
Framycetin sulfate (p.215·1); hydrocortisone (p.1103·3).
*Bacterial nose and throat infections with inflammation.*

**Soframycine Naphazoline** *Theraplix, Fr.†.*
Framycetin sulfate (p.215·1); naphazoline nitrate (p.1124·3).
*Congestion and bacterial infection of the nose and throat.*

**Sofrasolone** *Aventis, Belg.*
Prednisolone acetate (p.1108·1); framycetin sulfate (p.215·1); naphazoline nitrate (p.1124·3).
*Allergy or infections of the upper respiratory-tract.*

**Sofra-Tull**
*Aventis, Austria; Aventis, Ger.*
Framycetin sulfate (p.215·1).
*Burns; skin infections; ulcers; wounds.*

**Sofra-Tulle**
*Aventis, Austral.; Aventis, Canad.; Hoechst Marion Roussel, Denm.†; Aventis, Fin.; Aventis, Hong Kong; Aventis, India; Hoechst Marion Roussel, Irl.†; Aventis, Israel; Aventis, Malaysia; Aventis, Neth.; Aventis, Norw.; Aventis, NZ†; Aventis, S.Afr.; Aventis, Singapore; Hoechst Marion Roussel, Swed.†; Aventis, Switz.; Aventis, Thai.; Aventis, UK.*
Framycetin sulfate (p.215·1).
*Burns; infected skin disorders; ulcer; wounds.*

**Sof-Sof** *CTS, Israel.*
Phenothrin (p.1509·1).
*Pediculosis.*

**Sof-T**
*Gynetics, Singapore; Doetsch, Grether, Switz.†.*
Copper-wound plastic (p.1425·3).
*Intra-uterine contraceptive device.*

**Soft Kilnits** *Andromaco, Chile.*
Acetic acid (p.1645·2).
*Pediculosis.*

**Soft Lips** *Mentholatum, Canad.*
*SPF 17:* Octinoxate (p.1154·3); oxybenzone (p.1154·3); padimate O (p.1155·1); dimethicone (p.1482·1).
*Sunscreen.*

**Soft Lips Crystal Ice** *Mentholatum, Canad.*
Octinoxate (p.1154·3); octisalate (p.1154·3); oxybenzone (p.1154·3).
*Sunscreen.*

**Soft Lips French Vanilla** *Mentholatum, Canad.*
*SPF 20:* Octinoxate (p.1154·3); octisalate (p.1154·3); oxybenzone (p.1154·3).
*Sunscreen.*

**Soft Lips Sparkle** *Mentholatum, Canad.*
*SPF 10:* Octinoxate (p.1154·3).
*Sunscreen.*

**Soft Lips Ultra** *Mentholatum, Canad.*
*SPF 30:* Avobenzone (p.1142·3); octinoxate (p.1154·3); octisalate (p.1154·3).
*Sunscreen.*

**Soft Mate**
*Barnes Hind, NZ; Pilkington Barnes-Hind, USA.*
Range of solutions for soft contact lenses (p.1164·2).

**Soft Mate Consept** *Pilkington Barnes-Hind, USA.*
Hydrogen peroxide (p.1182·2) (p.1164·2).
*Disinfecting solution for soft contact lenses.*

**Soft Mate Consept I** *Willvonseder, Austria†.*
Hydrogen peroxide (p.1182·2) (p.1164·2).
*Cleansing and disinfecting solution for soft contact lenses.*

**Soft Mate Consept 2** *Willvonseder, Austria†.*
Rinsing and neutralising solution for soft contact lenses (p.1164·2).

**Soft Mate Enzyme Plus Cleaner** *Pilkington Barnes-Hind, USA.*
Subtilisin-A (p.1164·2).
*Cleansing solution for soft contact lenses.*

**Softa Man**
*Braun, Ger.; Braun, Ital.*
Alcohol (p.1166·1); propyl alcohol (p.1191·2).
*Hand disinfection.*

**Softab** *Alcon, NZ†.*
Sodium dichloroisocyanurate (p.1191·3) (p.1164·2).
*Disinfection of soft contact lenses.*

**Softasept N**
*Braun, Ger.; Braun, Switz.*
Alcohol (p.1166·1); isopropyl alcohol (p.1184·3).
*Skin disinfection.*

**Softene** *Melisana, Belg.*
Docusate sodium (p.1262·2); bisacodyl (p.1251·3).
*Constipation.*

**Softin** *Dexcel, Israel†.*
Vaginal lubricant.

**Softixol** *Schering-Plough, Mex.*
Ambroxol hydrochloride (p.1114·3).
*Respiratory-tract disorders associated with viscous mucus.*

**Softon** *Banner, Hong Kong†.*
Docusate sodium (p.1262·2).
*Constipation.*

**Softon Plus** *Banner, Hong Kong†.*
Docusate sodium (p.1262·2); casanthranol (p.1255·1).
*Constipation.*

**Softwash** *Palmolive Skincare, Austral.†.*
Triclosan (p.1195·2).
*Hand disinfection.*

**Softwear**
*Ciba Vision, Austral.†; Ciba Vision, Canad.*
Sodium chloride (p.1233·3) (p.1164·2).
*Rinsing and storage solution for soft contact lenses.*
*Ciba Vision, NZ.*
Rinsing solution for contact lenses (p.1164·2).

**Sogilen** *Pharmacia, Spain.*
Cabergoline (p.1203·3).
*Parkinsonism.*

**Sogoon** *Steiner, Ger.*
Devil's claw root (p.28·2).
*Joint disorders.*

**Soijatutteli** *Valio, Fin.*
Infant feed (p.1417·1).
*Cow's milk allergy; lactose intolerance.*

**Soin Autobronzant** *Clarins, Canad.*
*SPF 15:* Avobenzone (p.1142·3); octinoxate (p.1154·3); octisalate (p.1154·3); oxybenzone (p.1154·3).
*Sunscreen.*

**Sojar Men** *Sojar, Arg.*
Soya isoflavones (p.1447·2).
*Dietary supplement.*

**Sojar Plus-Calcio** *Sojar, Arg.*
Soya protein; calcium; soya isoflavones (p.1417·1).
*Dietary supplement.*

**Sojar Pro** *Sojar, Arg.*
Soya protein (p.1447·2).
*Dietary supplement.*

**Sojarlech** *Sojar, Arg.*
Soya protein; vitamins; minerals (p.1417·1).
*Dietary supplement.*

**Soklinal** *Allergan, Ger.†.*
Phenylmercuric nitrate (p.1189·2) (p.1164·2).
*Storage and rinsing solution for contact lenses.*

**Sol Bronce Vital** *AM, Arg.*
Betacarotene (p.1422·3); canthaxanthin (p.1056·3).
*Tanning aid.*

**Solacap** *SAT, Spain.*
Fluconazole (p.398·1).
*Fungal infections.*

**Solacid** *Dey's, India.*
Aluminium hydroxide (p.1249·2); magnesium hydroxide (p.1272·2); magnesium trisilicate (p.1272·3); simeticone (p.1289·2).
*Flatulence; gastrointestinal hyperacidity.*

**Solacy** *Grimberg, Fr.*
Cystine (p.1426·3); sulfur (p.1158·2); vitamin A acetate (p.1453·1); yeast (p.1469·1).
*Upper respiratory-tract disorders.*

**Solage** *Galderma, USA.*
Mequinol (p.1151·3); tretinoin (p.1161·1).
*Sun-induced skin hyperpigmentation.*

**Solamin** *Fresenius Kabi, Ital.*
Amino-acid infusion (p.1417·1).
*Parenteral nutrition.*

**Solan-M** *Winzer, Ger.*
Vitamin A palmitate (p.1453·1).
*Eye disorders.*

**Solantal** *Fujisawa, Jpn.*
Tiaramide hydrochloride (p.94·1).
*Inflammation; pain.*

**Solapsor** *Ysatfabrik, Ger.*
Dulcamara (p.1683·1).
*Eczema.*

**Solaquin**
*Note. This name is used for preparations of different composition.*
*ICN, Braz.; ICN, Mex.*
Hydroquinone (p.1148·1); padimate O (p.1155·1); octinoxate (p.1154·3); oxybenzone (p.1154·3).
*Skin hyperpigmentation.*
*ICN, Hong Kong; ICN, Singapore; ICN, USA.*
Hydroquinone (p.1148·1).
*Skin hyperpigmentation.*
*Crawford, UK.*
Hydroquinone (p.1148·1) with sunscreens.
*Skin hyperpigmentation.*

**Solaquin Forte**
*Note. This name is used for preparations of different composition.*
*ICN, Arg.*
Hydroquinone (p.1148·1); padimate O (p.1155·1); dioxybenzone (p.1145·3).
*Skin hyperpigmentation.*
*ICN, Canad.*
Hydroquinone (p.1148·1); padimate (p.1155·1); dioxybenzone (p.1145·3); oxybenzone (p.1154·3).
Formerly contained hydroquinone, roxadimate, dioxybenzone, and oxybenzone.
*Skin hyperpigmentation.*
*ICN, Malaysia.*
*SPF 17:* Hydroquinone (p.1148·1) with sunscreens.
*Skin hyperpigmentation.*
*ICN, USA.*
*Cream:* Hydroquinone (p.1148·1); padimate O (p.1155·1); dioxybenzone (p.1145·3); oxybenzone (p.1154·3).
*Topical gel:* Hydroquinone (p.1148·1); padimate O (p.1155·1); dioxybenzone (p.1145·3).
*Skin hyperpigmentation.*

**Solar Block** *Mentholatum, Austral.*
Octinoxate (p.1154·3); avobenzone (p.1142·3); enzacamene (p.1147·1); octocrilene (p.1154·3).
*Sunscreen.*

**Solar Block Baby** *Mentholatum, Austral.*
Octinoxate (p.1154·3); enzacamene (p.1147·1); zinc oxide (p.1163·2).
*Sunscreen.*

**Solar Block Surf/Sport** *Mentholatum, Austral.*
Octinoxate (p.1154·3); avobenzone (p.1142·3); enzacamene (p.1147·1); octocrilene (p.1154·3); octil triazone (p.1154·3).
*Sunscreen.*

**Solaraze**
*Bioglan, Ger.; Bioglan, Swed.; Shire, UK; Skye, USA.*
Diclofenac sodium (p.32·1).
*Actinic keratoses.*

**Solarcaine**
*Note. This name is used for preparations of different composition.*
*Schering-Plough, Braz.; Balmar, NZ.*
*Topical spray:* Benzocaine (p.1370·3).
*Local anaesthesia; skin irritation.*
*Schering-Plough, Canad.; Schering-Plough, Hong Kong†; Schering-Plough, UK; Schering-Plough, USA.*
Benzocaine (p.1370·3); triclosan (p.1195·2).
*Minor skin lesions and burns; skin irritation.*
*Balmar, NZ.*
*Lotion:* Benzocaine (p.1370·3); camphor (p.1665·3); menthol (p.1711·3); triclosan (p.1195·2).
*Sunburn.*
*Schering-Plough, Spain†.*
Benzocaine (p.1370·3); hexachlorophene (p.1181·2).
*Burns; insect stings; skin disorders.*
*Democal, Switz.*
Lidocaine (p.1377·3).
*Minor skin lesions and burns.*
*Schering-Plough, UK†.*
*Topical gel:* Aloe vera (p.1141·3); lidocaine (p.1377·3).
*Cuts; insect bites; sunburn.*

**Solarcaine Aloe Extra Burn Relief** *Schering-Plough, USA.*
Lidocaine (p.1377·3); aloe vera (p.1141·3).
*Local anaesthesia.*

**Solarcaine Aloe Vera** *Balmar, NZ.*
Aloe vera (p.1141·3).
*Minor burns; skin irritation; sunburn.*

**Solarcaine Aloe Vera Gel** *Essex, Chile.*
Lidocaine hydrochloride (p.1377·3); aloe vera (p.1141·3).
*Sunburn.*

**Solarcaine Lidocaine** *Schering-Plough, Canad.*
Lidocaine (p.1377·3) or lidocaine hydrochloride (p.1377·3).
*Sunburn; wounds.*

**Solarcaine Spray Aerosol** *Essex, Chile.*
Isopropyl alcohol (p.1184·3); triclosan (p.1195·2); benzocaine (p.1370·3).
*Skin irritation.*

**Solarcaine Stop Itch** *Schering-Plough, Canad.†.*
Papain (p.1727·3).
*Skin pain and irritation.*

**Solardril Composto** *Bunker, Braz.*
Calamine (p.1144·1); diphenhydramine hydrochloride (p.431·3); camphor (p.1665·3).

**Solart** *Pfizer, Ital.*
Acemetacin (p.11·3).
*Musculoskeletal and joint disorders.*

**Solatran**
*GlaxoSmithKline, Belg.; GlaxoSmithKline, S.Afr.; Doetsch, Grether, Switz.*
Ketazolam (p.703·1).
*Anxiety disorders; nervous disorders; sedative; skeletal muscle spasm.*

**Solaurit** *Polcopharma, Austral.†.*
Homoeopathic preparation.

**Solavert** *Arrow, Austral.*
Sotalol hydrochloride (p.1001·3).
*Arrhythmias.*

**Solaxin** *Eisai, Hong Kong.*
Chlorzoxazone (p.1392·3).
*Painful skeletal muscle spasm.*

**SolBar**
*Note. This name is used for preparations of different composition.*
*Person & Covey, Canad.; Dispolab, Chile; Person & Covey, USA.*
*SPF 30; SPF 50:* Octocrilene (p.1154·3); octinoxate (p.1154·3); oxybenzone (p.1154·3).
*Sunscreen.*
*Person & Covey, USA.*
*SPF 15:* Octinoxate (p.1154·3); oxybenzone (p.1154·3).
*Sunscreen.*

**SolBar Plus** *Person & Covey, Canad.†.*
*SPF 15:* Oxybenzone (p.1154·3); roxadimate (p.1157·1).
*Sunscreen.*

**Solblastin** *Faulding, Port.*
Vinblastine sulfate (p.591·2).

**Solciclina** *Solfran, Mex.*
Amoxicillin trihydrate (p.155·3).
*Bacterial infections.*

**Solclin** *Solfran, Mex.*
Tetracycline (p.266·2).
*Bacterial infections.*

**Solcode** *Reckitt Benckiser, Austral.*
Aspirin (p.15·1); codeine phosphate (p.27·1).
*Fever; pain.*

**Solcoderm**
*Solco, Hong Kong; Solco, Malaysia; Solco, Switz.*
Nitric acid (p.1722·1); glacial acetic acid (p.1645·2); oxalic acid dihydrate (p.1725·1); lactic acid (p.1704·1); copper nitrate trihydrate.
*Benign skin growths.*

**Solco-Derman** *ICN, Ger.*
Glacial acetic acid (p.1645·2); oxalic acid (p.1725·1); nitric acid (p.1722·1); lactic acid (p.1704·1); copper nitrate.
*Skin disorders.*

**Solcogyn** *Solco, Switz.*
Nitric acid (p.1722·1); glacial acetic acid (p.1645·2); oxalic acid dihydrate (p.1725·1); zinc nitrate hexahydrate.
*Benign cervical lesions.*

**Solcoseryl**
*Poen, Arg.; Solco, Austria; Solco, Hong Kong; Asta Medica, Ital.†; Solco, Malaysia; ICN, Neth.; Diafarm, Spain; Solco, Switz.; Merck, Thai.; Solco, Thai.*
Protein-free calf blood extract.
*Burns; cerebral and peripheral vascular disorders; eye disorders; peptic ulcer; skin disorders; soft-tissue disorders; wounds.*

**Solcoseryl Dental**
*Kamp, Arg.; Solco, Austria; Solco, Ger.; Solco, Hong Kong; Solco, Malaysia; Solco, Switz.; Merck, Thai.; Solco, Thai.*
Protein-free calf blood extract; lauromacrogol 400 (p.1412·3).
*Mouth disorders.*

**Solcosplen** *Strathmann, Ger.*
Calf spleen extract.
*Menopausal disorders.*

**Solco-Trichovac**
*Solco, Hong Kong†.*
Lactobacilli (p.1704·2).
*Bacterial vaginitis; trichomoniasis.*

*Solco, Switz.*
*Lactobacillus acidophilus* (p.1704·2).
*Vaginal infections.*

**Soldactone**
*Continental Pharma, Belg.; Searle, Denm.†; Searle, Fin.†; Searle, Neth.; Pharmacia, Norw.; Searle, Swed.†; Pharmacia, Switz.*
Potassium canrenoate (p.984·2).
*Ascites; hyperaldosteronism; hypokalaemia; oedema.*

**Soldermil Ecran Total** *Edol, Port.*
*SPF 24:* Zinc oxide (p.1163·2); titanium dioxide (p.1160·3).
*Sunscreen.*

**Soldermil Protector solar** *Edol, Port.*
*SPF 15:* Sunscreen.

**Soldesam** *Farmacologico Milanese, Ital.*
Dexamethasone sodium phosphate (p.1097·2).
*Corticosteroid.*

**Soldesanil** *Diapit, Gr.*
Dexamethasone sodium phosphate (p.1097·2).
*Corticosteroid.*

**Soldrin**
*Note. This name is used for preparations of different composition.*
*Andromaco, Chile.*
Tiabendazole (p.114·2).
*Worm infections.*

*Columbia, Mex.*
*Ear drops:* Hydrocortisone (p.1103·3); chloramphenicol (p.185·1); benzocaine (p.1370·3).
*Otitis externa.*
*Eye drops:* Dexamethasone sodium phosphate (p.1097·2); neomycin sulfate (p.235·1).
*Infected eye disorders.*

**Solecin** *Echo, Ital.*
Soya lecithin (p.1706·1); wheat germ; gelatin (p.754·3); glycerol (p.1694·3); betacarotene (p.1422·3).
*Nutritional supplement.*

**Soledum** *Cassella-med, Ger.*
Cineole (p.1672·1).
*Bronchitis; sinusitis.*

**Soledum Balsam** *Cassella-med, Ger.*
Cineole (p.1672·1).
*Respiratory-tract disorders.*

**Soledum Hustensaft** *Cassella-med, Ger.*
Thyme (p.1755·2).
*Bronchitis; catarrh; coughs.*

**Soledum Hustentropfen** *Cassella-med, Ger.*
Thyme (p.1755·2).
*Bronchitis; catarrh; coughs.*

**Soledum med** *Cassella-med, Ger.*
Chamomile oil (p.1669·3).
*Nasal congestion; rhinitis.*

**Soleil Ecran** *Osler, Fr.*
*SPF 20; SPF 30:* Octinoxate (p.1154·3); titanium dioxide (p.1160·3); avobenzone (p.1142·3).
*Sunscreen.*

**Solemar** *Delta, Braz.†.*
Salicylic acid (p.1157·1); sulfur (p.1158·2).
*Seborrhoea.*

**Solemil** *Neckerman, Braz.†.*
Neomycin sulfate (p.235·1); benzethonium chloride (p.1169·2); vitamin A (p.1451·2); vitamin D (p.1461·2).
*Skin infections.*

**Solevita** *Permamed, Switz.*
Hypericum (p.299·1).
*Agitation; depression; sleep disorders.*

**Solex A15** *Dermol, USA.*
Padimate O (p.1155·1); oxybenzone (p.1154·3).
*Sunscreen.*

**Solexa**
*Pharmacia, Austria; Pfizer, Ital.; Pharmacia, Neth.; Medinfar, Port.*
Celecoxib (p.25·2).
*Osteoarthritis; rheumatoid arthritis.*

**Soleze** *Pickles, UK†.*
Dibrompropamidine isetionate (p.1178·2); hydroviton.
*Burns; sunburn.*

**Solfa** *Takeda, Jpn.*
Amlexanox (p.781·1).
*Allergic rhinitis; asthma.*

**Solfac** *Bayer, Ital.*
Cyfluthrin (p.1502·3).
*Insecticide.*

**Solfen** *Antigen, Irl.*
Ibuprofen (p.45·3).
*Fever; pain.*

**Solfidin** *Pharmacia, Arg.*
Clonazepam (p.359·1).
*Epilepsy; panic attacks.*

**Solfomucil** *Locatelli, Ital.†.*
Carbocisteine (p.1116·2).
*Otorhinolaryngeal disorders; respiratory-tract congestion.*

**Solfoton** *ECR, USA†.*
Phenobarbital (p.367·3).
*Epilepsy; insomnia; sedative.*

**Solfranicol** *Solfran, Mex.*
Chloramphenicol (p.185·1); tetracycline (p.266·2).
*Bacterial infections.*

**Solfurol** *Solfran, Mex.*
Furazolidone (p.605·2); clioquinol (p.196·3).
*Diarrhoea.*

**Solganal**
*Schering, Canad.; Schering-Plough, Israel†; Schering, USA.*
Aurothioglucose (p.19·3).
*Rheumatoid arthritis.*

**Solgeretik** *Bristol-Myers Squibb, Austria†.*
Nadolol (p.963·1); bendroflumethiazide (p.867·3).
*Hypertension.*

**Solgol**
*Bristol-Myers Squibb, Austria†; Bristol-Myers Squibb, Ger.; Sanofi Synthelabo, Spain.*
Nadolol (p.963·1).
*Angina pectoris; arrhythmias; hypertension; migraine.*

**Solian**
*Sanofi Synthelabo, Austral.; Sanofi Synthelabo, Austria; Sanofi Synthelabo, Belg.; Sanofi Synthelabo, Fr.; Sanofi Synthelabo, Ger.; Sanofi Synthelabo, Hong Kong; Sanofi Synthelabo, Irl.; Synthelabo, Israel; Sanofi Synthelabo, Ital.; Sanofi Synthelabo, Norw.; Sanofi Synthelabo, S.Afr.; Sanofi Synthelabo, Singapore; Sanofi Synthelabo, Spain; Synthelabo, Switz.; Sanofi Synthelabo, UK.*
Amisulpride (p.669·3).
*Schizophrenia.*

**Solibay** *Bayer, Mex.*
Bezafibrate (p.873·2).
*Hyperlipidaemias.*

**Solicam** *SMB, Belg.*
Piroxicam (p.84·2).
*Gout; musculoskeletal and joint disorders; pain.*

**Solidago M** *Pilsensee, Ger.†.*
Solidago virgaurea (p.1748·3).
*Urinary-tract disorders.*

**Solidagoren N** *Klein, Ger.*
Solidago virgaurea (p.1748·3); potentilla anserina; equisetum (p.1684·1).
*Renal disorders.*

**Solidagosan N** *Hanosan, Ger.*
Homoeopathic preparation.

**Solidon** *Adelco, Gr.*
Chlorpromazine hydrochloride (p.675·2).
*Agitation; psychoses.*

**Solin** *Saval, Chile.*
Lidocaine hydrochloride (p.1377·3).
*Pain during injection.*

**Solinase** *Yamanouchi, Jpn.*
Pamiteplase (p.978·3).

**Solinitrina** *Almirall, Spain.*
Glyceryl trinitrate (p.923·2).
*Angina pectoris; heart failure; induction of hypotension in surgery; myocardial infarction.*

**Solipid** *Laevosan, Austria†.*
Soya oil (p.1447·2).
Some preparations contain egg lecithin.
*Lipid infusion for parenteral nutrition.*

**Solisan** *Synpharma, Austria.*
Ononis root (p.1723·3); taraxacum (p.1751·3); centaury (p.1669·2).
Formerly contained ononis root, bearberry, and centaury.
*Urinary-tract disorders.*

**Solitab** *Hermes, Ger.†.*
Magnesium trisilicate (p.1272·3).
*Gastrointestinal disorders associated with hyperacidity.*

**Solivito N**
*Pharmacia, Irl.; Fresenius Kabi, UK.*
Water-soluble vitamin preparation (p.1417·1).
*Parenteral nutrition.*

**Sol-Jod** *Ecobi, Ital.*
Iodine (p.1598·1).
*Oral antisepsis.*

**Solkan** *Solfran, Mex.*
Kanamycin (p.225·2).
*Bacterial infections.*

**Sollival** *Sirval, Ital.*
Emollient.

**Solmag** *Ecosol, Switz.*
Magnesium aspartate (p.1227·3).
*Arrhythmias; magnesium deficiency; magnesium supplement.*

**Solmucaine** *IBSA, Switz.*
Acetylcysteine (p.1112·3); tyrothricin (p.275·1); lidocaine hydrochloride (p.1377·3).
*Upper respiratory-tract disorders with viscous mucus.*

**Solmucalm** *IBSA, Switz.*
Acetylcysteine (p.1112·3); chlorphenamine maleate (p.427·3).
*Coughs.*

**Solmucol**
*Genevrier, Fr.; IBSA, Hong Kong; Fidia, Ital.; Aspen, S.Afr.; Genevrier, Singapore; Bioiberica, Spain; IBSA, Switz.*
Acetylcysteine (p.1112·3).
*Eye disorders; paracetamol overdosage; respiratory-tract congestion.*

**Solmux**
*Westmont, Hong Kong; Great Eastern, Thai.; Pediatrica, Thai.; Westmont, Thai.*
Carbocisteine (p.1116·2).
*Respiratory-tract disorders associated with increased or viscous mucus.*

**Soloc** *Goldshield, UK.*
Bisoprolol fumarate (p.875·1).
*Angina pectoris; hypertension.*

**Solocalm** *Microsules Bernabo, Arg.*
Piroxicam (p.84·2) or piroxicam betadex (p.84·2).
*Gout; musculoskeletal, joint, peri-articular, and soft-tissue disorders; pain.*

**Solocalm Plus** *Microsules Bernabo, Arg.*
Piroxicam (p.84·2); carisoprodol (p.1392·1); dexamethasone (p.1097·1); pyridoxine hydrochloride; hydroxocobalamin.
*Musculoskeletal, joint, and peri-articular disorders.*

**Solocalm-B** *Microsules Bernabo, Arg.*
Piroxicam (p.84·2); thiamine hydrochloride; pyridoxine hydrochloride; cyanocobalamin.
*Inflammation; neuritis.*

**Solocalm-Flex** *Microsules Bernabo, Arg.*
Piroxicam (p.84·2); carisoprodol (p.1392·1).
*Musculoskeletal and joint disorders.*

**Solo-care**
*Ciba Vision, Austral.†; Ciba Vision, Braz.; Ciba Vision, Canad.*
Cleansing, rinsing, disinfecting, and storage solution for contact lenses (p.1164·2).

**Solocare** *Ciba Vision, NZ.*
Cleaning, disinfecting, rinsing, and storage solution for soft contact lenses (p.1164·2).

**Solo-care Hard**
*Ciba Vision, Austria†; Ciba Vision, Canad.*
Cleansing, rinsing, conditioning, storage, and wetting solution for hard and gas permeable contact lenses (p.1164·2).

**Solo-care Soft** *Ciba Vision, Austria†.*
Rinsing, storage, and disinfecting solution for soft contact lenses (p.1164·2).

**Solomet** *Orion, Fin.*
Methylprednisolone (p.1106·1), methylprednisolone acetate (p.1106·1), or methylprednisolone sodium succinate (p.1106·2).
*Corticosteroid.*

**Solomet c bupivacain hydrochlorid** *Orion, Fin.*
Methylprednisolone acetate (p.1106·1); bupivacaine hydrochloride (p.1371·1).
*Musculoskeletal, joint, and peri-articular disorders.*

**Solone** *Fawns & McAllan, Austral.*
Prednisolone (p.1108·1).
*Corticosteroid.*

**Solosa**
*Hoechst Marion Roussel, Gr.; Rhone-Poulenc Aventis, Ital.*
Glimepiride (p.332·2).
*Diabetes mellitus.*

**Solosin** *Aventis, Ger.*
Theophylline (p.798·3).
*Obstructive airways disease.*

**SoloSite** *Smith & Nephew, Austral.*
Carmellose sodium (p.1577·3); allantoin (p.1141·3).
*Wounds.*

**Solosprin** *Zydus, India.*
Isosorbide mononitrate (p.942·1); aspirin (p.15·1).
*Angina pectoris; myocardial infarction.*

**Solotrim** *Fresenius Kabi, Austria.*
Trimethoprim (p.272·2).
*Bacterial infections.*

**Solotron** *General Nutrition, Canad.*
Multivitamin and mineral preparation (p.1417·1).

**Solovite** *Solgar, UK.*
Multivitamin and mineral preparation (p.1417·1).

**Solpadeine** *GlaxoSmithKline, Irl.*
Paracetamol (p.76·2); codeine phosphate (p.27·1); caffeine (p.782·1).
*Cold and influenza symptoms; pain.*

**Solpadeine Max** *GlaxoSmithKline Consumer, UK.*
Paracetamol (p.76·2); codeine phosphate (p.27·1).
These ingredients can be described by the British Approved Name Co-codamol.
*Fever; pain.*

**Solpadeine Plus** *GlaxoSmithKline Consumer, UK.*
Paracetamol (p.76·2); codeine phosphate (p.27·1); caffeine (p.782·1).
*Fever; pain.*

**Solpadol**
*Sanofi Synthelabo, Irl.; Sanofi Synthelabo, UK.*
Paracetamol (p.76·2); codeine phosphate (p.27·1).
These ingredients can be described by the British Approved Name Co-codamol 30/500.
*Pain.*

**Solpaflex**
*Note. This name is used for preparations of different composition.*
*SmithKline Beecham, Denm.*
Ibuprofen (p.45·3).
*Inflammation; musculoskeletal and joint disorders; pain.*

*GlaxoSmithKline Consumer, UK.*
*Tablets:* Ibuprofen (p.45·3); codeine phosphate (p.27·1).
*Fever; pain.*

*SmithKline Beecham Consumer, UK†.*
*Topical gel:* Ketoprofen (p.51·2).
*Oedema; pain; peri-articular and soft-tissue disorders.*

**Solpat** *Parggon, Mex.*
Ambroxol hydrochloride (p.1114·3).
*Respiratory-tract congestion.*

**Solphyllex** *Adcock Ingram, S.Afr.*
Theophylline (p.798·3); etofylline (p.785·1); diphenylpyraline hydrochloride (p.432·3); ammonium chloride (p.1115·2); sodium citrate (p.1223·2).
*Coughs.*

**Solphyllin** *Adcock Ingram, S.Afr.*
Theophylline (p.798·3); etofylline (p.785·1).
*Obstructive airways disease.*

**Solpic** *Medical, Port.*
Mepyramine maleate (p.437·1); calamine (p.1144·1); benzocaine (p.1370·3).
*Skin irritation.*

**Solplex 40** *Fresenius Kabi, Ital.*
Dextran 40 (p.745·3) in sodium chloride.
*Peripheral arteriopathy; plasma volume expansion.*

**Solplex 70** *Fresenius Kabi, Ital.*
Dextran 70 (p.746·2) in sodium chloride.
*Plasma volume expansion; thrombosis prophylaxis.*

**Solprene** *Farmigea, Ital.*
Prednisolone sodium phosphate (p.1108·1); neomycin sulfate (p.235·1).
*Infected eye disorders.*

**Solprin**
*Reckitt Benckiser, Austral.*
Aspirin (p.15·1).
*Fever; inhibition of platelet aggregation; pain.*

*Reckitt Benckiser, NZ.*
Calcium aspirin (p.17·3).
*Inflammation; pain.*

**Solsavit** *Solfran, Mex.*
Vitamin $B_{12}$; vitamin $B_6$ (p.1417·1).

**Solsolona** *Cryopharma, Mex.†.*
Methylprednisolone acetate (p.1106·1).
*Corticosteroid.*

**Soltamox** *Rosemont, UK.*
Tamoxifen citrate (p.584·1).
*Anovulatory infertility; breast cancer.*

**Soltice** *Chattem, USA.*
Methyl salicylate (p.59·3); camphor (p.1665·3); menthol (p.1711·3).
*Muscle, joint, and soft-tissue pain; neuralgia.*

**Soltric** *ICN, Mex.*
Mebendazole (p.108·2).
*Worm infections.*

**Soltrictor con Lagrifilm** *Allergan, Mex.*
Naphazoline hydrochloride (p.1124·3); polyvinyl alcohol (p.1581·1).
*Eye irritation.*

**Soltrim** *Almirall, Spain.*
Sulfamethoxazole lysine (p.262·3); trimethoprim (p.272·2).
*Bacterial infections; Pneumocystis carinii pneumonia.*

**Soltrimox** *Richmond, Arg.*
Ceftriaxone (p.183·3).
*Bacterial infections.*

**Solubacter**
*Boots Healthcare, Fr.; Innotech, Port.†.*
Triclocarban (p.1195·1).
*Disinfection of skin and mucous membranes.*

**Solubeol**
*Note. This name is used for preparations of different composition.*
*Piette, Belg.†.*
Guaifenesin (p.1122·1); phenoxyethanol (p.1189·1).
*Solvent for painful intramuscular injections.*

*Azevedos, Port.*
Cypress oil; eucalyptus oil (p.1686·2); hyssop oil; lavender oil (p.1705·2); oleum pini sylvestris.
*Respiratory-tract disorders.*

**Solu-Biloptin** *Schering, UK.*
Calcium iopodate (p.1065·2).
*Contrast medium for biliary-tract radiography.*

**Solubitrat** *Sanova, Austria.*
Birch leaf (p.1660·3); solidago virgaurea (p.1748·3); java tea (p.1702·3); fennel oil (p.1687·3).
*Urinary-tract disorders.*

**Solucalcine** *Prima, Braz.†.*
Calcium chloride (p.1225·1).
*Hypocalcaemia.*

**Solucamphre**
*Note. This name is used for preparations of different composition.*
*Synthelabo, Belg.†.*
Codeine (p.27·1); ethylmorphine (p.37·3); ephedrine (p.1120·1); piperazine hydrate (p.111·2); camsylic acid; aconite (p.1646·3); belladonna (p.479·1); ipecacuanha (p.1122·3); senna (p.1288·2).
*Coughs.*

*Synthelabo, Fr.†.*
Piperazine camsilate (p.112·1).
*Hypotension.*

**Solucao ABC** *Hertz, Braz.†.*
Benzoic acid (p.1169·3); iodine (p.1598·1); potassium iodide (p.1598·1).
*Fungal skin infections.*

**Solucao Aminon** *Fresenius, Braz.*
Amino-acid infusion (p.1417·1).
*Parenteral nutrition.*

**Solucao Aminorin** *Fresenius, Braz.*
Amino-acid infusion (p.1417·1).
*Parenteral nutrition.*

**Solucao Anticoagulante** *Hypofarma, Braz.†.*
Citric acid (p.1673·1); glucose (p.1432·2); sodium citrate (p.1223·2).
*Anticoagulant for blood transfusions.*

**Solucao Nasal de Nafazolina** *Bergamo, Braz.†.*
Naphazoline (p.1124·3); nitrofurazone (p.238·2); panthenol (p.1727·2).
*Nasal congestion.*

**Solucao Stago** *Merck, Port.†.*
Boldo (p.1661·2); comfrey (p.1675·2); chamomile (p.1669·3); cinchona bark (p.1671·3); sarsaparilla (p.1742·1); black pine; euonymus (p.1265·2); buchu (p.1663·1); junco.
*Dyspepsia.*

**Solucaps** *Medix, Mex.*
Mazindol (p.1589·1).
*Obesity.*

**Solucel** *Stiefel, Spain.*
Benzoyl peroxide (p.1143·2).
*Acne.*

**Solu-Celestan** *Aesca, Austria.*
Betamethasone disodium phosphate (p.1093·1).
*Corticosteroid.*

**Solucer** *Fortbenton, Arg.*
Trolamine polypeptide oleate-condensate (p.1758·2).
*Ear wax removal.*

**Soluchrom** *Cooperation Pharmaceutique, Fr.*
Merbromin sodium (p.1185·3).
*Skin, burn and wound disinfection.*

**Solucion De Lugol** *Volta, Chile.*
Iodine (p.1598·1); sodium iodide (p.1598·1).
*Disinfection.*

**Solucion Detergente** *Reccius, Chile.*
Sodium lauril ether sulfate (p.1574·3).

**Solucion DP** *Pisa, Mex.*
Glucose; sodium chloride; calcium chloride; magnesium chloride; sodium lactate (p.1221·1).
*Peritoneal dialysis.*

**Solucion Fisio** *Cinfa, Spain.*
Sodium chloride (p.1233·3).
*Nasal congestion.*

**Solucion Schoum** *Pharmascience, Spain.*
Boldo (p.1661·2); fumitory (p.1690·1); hamamelis (p.1696·3); melissa (p.1711·1); rhubarb (p.1287·3); piscidia (p.1702·3); peppermint oil (p.1283·2); hydrastis canadensis (p.1698·3); ethyl alcohol; glycerol.
*Hepatobiliary disorders.*

**Solucionic** *Diviser Aquilea, Spain†.*
Povidone-iodine (p.1190·3).
*Bacterial vaginosis.*

**Solucis** *Aesculapius, Ital.*
Carbocisteine (p.1116·2).
*Respiratory-tract congestion.*

**Solucol** *PSM, NZ†.*
Sodium bicarbonate (p.1223·2); tartaric acid (p.1752·1); thymol (p.1194·2).
*Oral hygiene.*

**Solucort** *Merck Sharp & Dohme-Chibret, Fr.†.*
Prednisolone sodium phosphate (p.1108·1).
*Corticosteroid.*

**Solu-Cortef**
*Pharmacia, Austral.; Pharmacia, Belg.; Pharmacia, Braz.; Pharmacia, Canad.; Pharmacia, Chile; Pharmacia, Denm.; Pharmacia, Fin.; Pharmacia-Upjohn, Gr.; Pharmacia, Hong Kong; Pharmacia, Irl.; Pharmacia Upjohn, Israel; Pharmacia Upjohn, Ital.; Pharmacia, Malaysia; Pharmacia, Neth.; Pharmacia, Norw.; Pharmacia, NZ; Pharmacia, Port.; Pharmacia, S.Afr.; Pharmacia, Singapore; Pharmacia, Swed.; Pharmacia, Switz.; Pharmacia, Thai.; Pharmacia, UK; Upjohn, USA.*
Hydrocortisone sodium succinate (p.1104·1).
*Corticosteroid.*

**Solu-Crom** *Sabex, Canad.*
Sodium cromoglicate (p.795·3).
*Allergic conjunctivitis.*

**Solu-Dacortin** *Merck, Austria.*
Prednisolone sodium succinate (p.1108·2).
*Corticosteroid.*

**Soludacortin** *Bracco, Ital.*
Prednisolone sodium succinate (p.1108·2).
*Corticosteroid.*

**Solu-Dacortin H** *Merck, Spain†.*
Prednisolone sodium succinate (p.1108·2).
*Corticosteroid.*

**Solu-Dacortina** *Merck, Port.*
Prednisolone sodium succinate (p.1108·2).
*Corticosteroid.*

**Solu-Dacortine**
*Merck, Belg.; Merck, Switz.*
Prednisolone sodium succinate (p.1108·2).
*Corticosteroid.*

**Soludactone** *Pharmacia, Fr.*
Potassium canrenoate (p.984·2).
*Ascites; hyperaldosteronism; hypokalaemia; oedema.*

**Soludecadron** *Merck Sharp & Dohme-Chibret, Fr.†.*
Dexamethasone sodium phosphate (p.1097·2).
*Corticosteroid.*

**Solu-Decortin-H** *Merck, Ger.*
Prednisolone sodium succinate (p.1108·2).
*Parenteral corticosteroid.*

**Soluderme** *Schering-Plough, Port.*
Betamethasone dipropionate (p.1093·1).
*Skin disorders.*

**Soludial** *Soludia, Fr.†.*
Sodium bicarbonate (p.1223·2).
*Haemodialysis.*

**Soludor** *Lehning, Fr.*
Homoeopathic preparation.

**Solufen**
*Note. This name is used for preparations of different composition.*
*Irex, Fr.; Whitehall-Robins, Switz.†.*
Ibuprofen (p.45·3).
*Fever; pain.*

*Rigers, Mex.†.*
Chloramphenicol (p.185·1).
*Bacterial infections.*

**Solufena** *UCB, Spain†.*
Ibuprofen (p.45·3).
*Fever; pain.*

**Solufilina** *BOI, Spain.*
Etamiphylline hydrochloride (p.785·1).
*Angina pectoris; heart failure; myocardial infarction; obstructive airways disease.*

**Solufilina Sedante** *BOI, Spain†.*
Etamiphylline hydrochloride (p.785·1); phenobarbital (p.367·3).
*Obstructive airways disease; precordial pain.*

**Solufilina Simple** *BOI, Spain†.*
Etamiphylline hydrochloride (p.785·1).
*Angina pectoris; heart failure; myocardial infarction; obstructive airways disease.*

**Solu-Flur** *Germiphene, Canad.†.*
Sodium fluoride (p.1444·3).
*Dental caries prophylaxis.*

**Solufos** *Busto, Spain.*
Fosfomycin calcium (p.214·2) or fosfomycin sodium (p.214·3).
Lidocaine (p.1377·3) is included in the intramuscular injection to alleviate the pain of injection.
*Bacterial infections.*

**Solugastril**
*Sanova, Austria; Pharmacia, Ger.*
Aluminium hydroxide (p.1249·2); calcium carbonate (p.1254·2).
*Duodenitis; dyspepsia; gastritis; gastro-oesophageal reflux; peptic ulcer.*

**Solugel**
*Note. This name is used for preparations of different composition.*
*Stiefel, Arg.; Stiefel, Braz.; Stiefel, Canad.; Stiefel, Chile; Stiefel, Mex.*
Benzoyl peroxide (p.1143·2).
*Acne.*

*Johnson & Johnson, Austral.*
Hydrogel dressing.
*Burns; wounds.*

**Solukapton** *Strallhofer, Austria.*
Aspirin (p.15·1); caffeine (p.782·1).
*Fever; pain.*

**Solulexin** *Duopharma, Hong Kong.*
Cefalexin (p.168·1).
*Bacterial infections.*

**Solulip** *Pharmanik (Φαρμανικ), Gr.*
Gemfibrozil (p.923·1).
*Hyperlipidaemias.*

**Solumag**
*Note. This name is used for preparations of different composition.*
*Kolassa, Austria; Boehringer Ingelheim, Fr.; Geymonat, Ital.*
Magnesium pidolate (p.1228·2).
*Anxiety related hyperventilation; dysmenorrhoea; eclampsia; magnesium deficiency; premature labour.*

*Hexal, S.Afr.*
Magnesium oxide (p.1272·3).
*Magnesium deficiency.*

**Solu-Medrol**
*Pharmacia, Arg.; Pharmacia, Austral.; Pharmacia, Austria; Pharmacia, Belg.; Pharmacia, Braz.; Pharmacia, Canad.; Pharmacia, Chile; Pharmacia, Denm.; Pharmacia, Fin.; Pharmacia, Fr.; Pharmacia, Hong Kong; Pharmacia Upjohn, India; Pharmacia Upjohn, Israel; Pharmacia Upjohn, Ital.; Pharmacia, Malaysia; Pharmacia Upjohn, Mex.; Pharmacia, Neth.; Pharmacia, Norw.; Pharmacia, NZ ;Pharmacia, Port.; Pharmacia, S.Afr.; Pharmacia, Singapore; Pharmacia, Swed.; Pharmacia, Switz.; Pharmacia, Thai.; Pharmacia Upjohn, USA.*
Methylprednisolone sodium succinate (p.1106·2).
*Corticosteroid.*

*Pharmacia-Upjohn, Gr.*
Methylprednisolone hydrogen succinate (p.1106·1) or methylprednisolone sodium succinate (p.1106·2).
*Corticosteroid.*

**Solu-Medrone**
*Pharmacia, Irl.; Pharmacia, UK.*
Methylprednisolone sodium succinate (p.1106·2).
*Corticosteroid.*

**Solumerin** *Ariston, Arg.*
Benzethonium chloride (p.1169·2); tyrothricin (p.275·1); cetylpyridinium chloride (p.1173·1); butimerin.
*Burns; mouth disorders; skin infections; ulcers; wounds.*

**Solumidazol** *Diba, Mex.*
Metronidazole (p.607·2).
*Amoebiasis; trichomoniasis.*

**Solu-Moderin** *Pharmacia, Spain.*
Methylprednisolone sodium succinate (p.1106·2).
*Corticosteroid.*

**Solumol** *C & M, USA.*
Vehicle for topical preparations.

**Soluna** *Elea, Arg.*
Quinestrol (p.1568·2); etynodiol diacetate (p.1554·2).
*Combined oral contraceptive; dysmenorrhoea.*

**Solunac** *Systopic, India.*
Diclofenac (p.32·1).
*Gout; musculoskeletal and joint disorders.*

**Solupen** *Bial, Spain†.*
Doxycycline hyclate (p.206·2).
*Bacterial infections; malaria.*

**Solupen Enzimatico** *Bial, Spain†.*
Doxycycline hyclate (p.206·2); chymotrypsin (p.1671·2); trypsin (p.1758·3).
*Bacterial infections.*

**Solupen N** *Winzer, Ger.*
Dexamethasone sodium phosphate (p.1097·2).
*Rhinitis; sinusitis.*

**Solupen-D** *Winzer, Ger.†.*
Oxedrine tartrate (p.977·3); naphazoline hydrochloride (p.1124·3); dexamethasone sodium phosphate (p.1097·2).
*Rhinitis; sinusitis.*

**Solupred** *Aventis, Fr.*
Prednisolone metasulfobenzoate sodium (p.1108·1).
*Corticosteroid.*

**Soluprick SQ**
*ALK, Denm.; ALK, Fin.; ALK, Swed.*
Allergen extracts (p.1650·1).
*Diagnosis of hypersensitivity.*

**Solupsa** *Upsamedica, Belg.†.*
Carbasalate calcium (p.25·1).
*Cardiovascular disorders.*

**Solupsan** *UPSA, Fr.†.*
Carbasalate calcium (p.25·1).
*Fever; pain; rheumatic disorders.*

**Solurex** *Hyrex, USA.*
Dexamethasone acetate (p.1097·1) or dexamethasone sodium phosphate (p.1097·2).
*Corticosteroid.*

**Soluric** *Unipharma, Gr.*
Allopurinol (p.412·2).
*Gout; hyperuricaemia associated with cancer chemotherapy; kidney stones.*

**Solurin** *Farmarin, Braz.*
Electrolytes (p.1221·1).
*Haemodialysis solution.*

**Solurrinol** *Teofarma, Spain.*
Potassium chlorate (p.1734·2); sodium bicarbonate (p.1223·2); sodium chloride (p.1233·3).
*Upper-respiratory-tract disorders.*

**Solurutine Papaverine F. Retard** *Synthelabo, Fr.†.*
Ethoxazorutoside (p.1688·2); ascorbic acid (p.1460·2); papaverine hydrochloride (p.1728·1).
*Cerebral and peripheral vascular disorders.*

**Solus** *Lifeplan, UK.*
Multivitamin, mineral, and nutritional preparation (p.1417·1).

**Solusprin** *Bioresearch, Spain.*
Lysine aspirin (p.54·3).
*Fever; musculoskeletal, joint and peri-articular disorders; pain; thromboembolism prophylaxis.*

**Solusteril** *Urgo, Fr.†.*
Sodium dichloroisocyanurate (p.1191·3).
*Infant feeding equipment disinfection.*

**Soluston** *Rafa, Israel.*
Chenodeoxycholic acid (p.1670·1).
*Cholesterol gallstones.*

**Solustrep** *Caps, S.Afr.*
Streptomycin sulfate (p.256·2).
*Tuberculosis.*

**Solustres** *Finadiet, Arg.*
Tetracycline hydrochloride (p.266·2); papain (p.1727·3).
*Bacterial infections.*

**Solutina** *Alcon, Mex.*
Pheniramine maleate (p.438·3); naphazoline hydrochloride (p.1124·3).
*Conjunctivitis.*

**Solutio Cordes**
*Ichthyol, Austria†; Ichthyol, Ger.*
Ictasol (p.1148·3).
*Scalp disorders.*

**Solutio Cordes Dexa N** *Ichthyol, Ger.*
Dexamethasone (p.1097·1).
*Scalp disorders.*

**Solution Antiseptique** *Stella, Belg.*
Alcohol (p.1166·1); ether (p.1474·2).
*Skin and instrument disinfection.*

**Solution ChKM du Prof Dr Walkhoff** *Haupt, Switz.†.*
Parachlorophenol (p.1187·3); camphor (p.1665·3); menthol (p.1711·3).
*Dental inflammation.*

**Solution Stago Diluee** *Pharmadeveloppement, Fr.*
Boldo (p.1661·2); chamomile (p.1669·3); kinkeliba (p.1703·3); golden rod (p.1748·3).
*Digestive disorders.*

**Solutrast** *Byk Gulden, Ger.*
Iopamidol (p.1064·3).
*Radiographic contrast medium.*

**Solutrat** *Labinca, Arg.*
Ursodeoxycholic acid (p.1760·3).
*Gallstones.*

**Solutricine** *Schieffer, Switz.†.*
Tyrothricin (p.275·1); ascorbic acid (p.1460·2).
*Mouth and throat disorders.*

**Solutricine Expectorant** *Theraplix, Fr.*
Carbocisteine (p.1116·2).
*Respiratory-tract congestion.*

**Solutricine Maux de Gorge** *Theraplix, Fr.*
Tetracaine hydrochloride (p.1385·1); hexamidine isetionate (p.1181·3).
*Mouth and throat disorders.*

**Solutricine Tetracaine** *Theraplix, Fr.*
Tyrothricin (p.275·1); tetracaine hydrochloride (p.1385·1).
*Mouth and throat disorders.*

**Solutricine Vitamine C** *Theraplix, Fr.*
Tyrothricin (p.275·1); ascorbic acid (p.1460·2).
*Mouth and throat infections.*

**Soluver** *Dermtek, Canad.*
Salicylic acid (p.1157·1).
*Verrucas.*

**Soluver Plus** *Dermtek, Canad.*
Salicylic acid (p.1157·1).
*Warts.*

**Soluvit**
*Pharmacia Upjohn, Belg.†; Fresenius Kabi, Denm.; Fresenius Kabi, Fin.; Fresenius Kabi, Fr.; Fresenius Kabi, Gr.; Fresenius Kabi, Ital.; Fresenius Kabi, Norw.; Fresenius Kabi, S.Afr.; Fresenius Kabi, Spain; Fresenius Kabi, Swed.; Fresenius Kabi, Switz.*
Multivitamin preparation (p.1417·1).
*Parenteral nutrition.*

**Soluvit N**
*Hamilton, Austral.†; Baxter, Ger.; Fresenius Kabi, Hong Kong; Pharmacia Upjohn, Israel; Fresenius Kabi, Malaysia; Fresenius Kabi, Neth.; Baxter, NZ; Fresenius Kabi, NZ; Fresenius Kabi, Port.; Fresenius Kabi, Singapore; Fresenius Kabi, Thai.*
Multivitamin preparation (p.1417·1).
*Parenteral nutrition.*

**Soluvit Neu** *Fresenius Kabi, Austria.*
Multivitamin preparation (p.1417·1).
*Parenteral nutrition.*

**Soluvite** *Pharmics, USA.*
Multivitamin preparation with fluoride (p.1444·3)(p.1417·1).
*Dental caries prophylaxis; dietary supplement.*

**Solu-Volon A** *Bristol-Myers Squibb, Austria.*
Triamcinolone acetonide dipotassium phosphate (p.1110·3).
*Corticosteroid.*

**Soluzione Composta Alcoolica Saponosa di Coaltar** *Bruni, Ital.†.*
Coal tar (p.1159·2); quillaia (p.1416·1); methyl salicylate (p.59·3); alcohol (p.1166·1).
*Eczema.*

**Soluzione Darrow** *Diaco, Ital.*
Electrolyte infusion (p.1217·1).
*Infantile diarrhoea.*

**Soluzione Schoum** *Aventis, Ital.*
Fumitory (p.1690·1); ononis (p.1723·3); piscidia (p.1702·3).
*Painful spasm of the urinary and biliary tracts.*

**Soluzyme** *Lupin, India.*
Trypsin (p.1758·3); chymotrypsin (p.1671·2).
*Inflammation; oedema.*

**Solvanol** *Medipharm, Chile.*
Clobutinol hydrochloride (p.1117·1); orciprenaline sulfate (p.790·2); ammonium chloride (p.1115·2).
*Coughs.*

**Solvazinc** *Provalis, UK.*
Zinc sulfate (p.1469·3).
*Zinc deficiency.*

**Solve Dandruff** *Redken, Canad.*
Pyrithione zinc (p.1156·2).
*Scalp disorders.*

**Solvente Indoloro** *Apolo, Arg.; Duncan, Arg.; Fada, Arg.; Monserrat, Arg.; Northia, Arg.; Pharmacia, Arg.; Veinfar, Arg.*
Lidocaine (p.1377·3) or lidocaine hydrochloride (p.1377·3).
*Pain during injection.*

**Solvetan** *Glaxo Wellcome, Gr.*
Ceftazidime (p.180·2).
*Bacterial infections.*

**Solvex**
*Note. This name is used for preparations of different composition.*
*Merz, Ger.*
Reboxetine mesilate (p.316·3).
*Depression.*

*Teva, Israel.*
Bromhexine hydrochloride (p.1115·3).
*Respiratory-tract congestion.*

**Solvex Liquido Fungicida** *Schering, Arg.*
Benzoic acid (p.1169·3); salicylic acid (p.1157·1); chlorothymol (p.1177·2).
*Fungal skin infections.*

**Solvezink**
AstraZeneca, Austria; AstraZeneca, Denm.†; AstraZeneca, Fin.†; AstraZeneca, Ger.; Stern, Ger.; AstraZeneca, Norw.; Tika, Swed.
Zinc sulfate (p.1469·3).
*Acne; acrodermatitis enteropathica; leg ulcer.*

**Solviflu** Boots Healthcare, Ital.
Ibuprofen (p.45·3); pseudoephedrine hydrochloride (p.1129·2).
*Cold and influenza symptoms.*

**Solvin**
Note. This name is used for preparations of different composition.
Mexin, India.
Bromhexine hydrochloride (p.1115·3); pseudoephedrine hydrochloride (p.1129·2).
*Respiratory-tract congestion.*

Loren, Mex.
Povidone-iodine (p.1190·3).
*Oral hygiene; skin disinfection.*

**Solving** MDM, Ital.
Nimesulide (p.67·1).
*Fever; inflammation; pain.*

**Solvipect** Nycomed, Norw.
Guaifenesin (p.1122·1); liquorice (p.1270·2).
*Coughs.*

**Solvipect comp** Nycomed, Norw.
Guaifenesin (p.1122·1); liquorice (p.1270·2); ethylmorphine hydrochloride (p.37·3).
*Coughs.*

**Solvisol** Solfran, Mex.
Multivitamin preparation (p.1417·1).

**Solvium** Chefaro, Spain.
Ibuprofen (p.45·3).
*Musculoskeletal, joint, peri-articular, and soft-tissue disorders.*

**Solvobil**
Note. This name is used for preparations of different composition.
Farmasa, Braz.
Cynara (p.1678·3); boldo (p.1661·2); cascara (p.1255·1); belladonna (p.479·1); peppermint leaf (p.1283·2); juniper oil (p.1703·1).
*Liver disorders.*

Master, Chile.
Ursodeoxycholic acid (p.1760·3).
*Gallstones.*

Recordati, Ital.
Sodium cholate; nicotinamide (p.1441·2); boldo (p.1661·2); cascara (p.1255·1).
*Constipation.*

**Solvolin** Genera, Switz.†.
Bromhexine hydrochloride (p.1115·3).
*Respiratory-tract disorders with viscous mucus.*

**Solvomed** Kwizda, Austria†.
Acetylcysteine (p.1112·3).
*Bronchitis.*

**Solvopret** Bionorica, Thai.
Thyme (p.1755·2); hedera helix.
*Bronchitis.*

**Solvopret TP** Bionorica, Thai.
Thyme (p.1755·2); cowslip rhizome (p.1735·1).
*Bronchitis.*

**Solyptol** Faulding, Austral.
*Cream:* Benzalkonium chloride (p.1168·3); allantoin (p.1141·3).
*Abrasions; burns; cuts; insect bites.*
*Soap:* Triclosan (Irgasan) (p.1195·2).
*Topical liquid:* Pine oil; chloroxylenol (p.1177·2).
*Abrasions; cuts; insect bites.*

**Som** Satori, Fr.
A range of nutritional supplements (p.1417·1).

**Soma**
Note. This name is used for preparations of different composition.
Novaquimica, Braz.†.
Ampicillin benzathine (p.158·1); ampicillin sodium (p.157·1).
*Bacterial infections.*

Carter Horner, Canad.; Wallace, USA.
Carisoprodol (p.1392·1).
*Musculoskeletal disorders.*

**Soma Balsamico** Novaquimica, Braz.†.
Ampicillin benzathine (p.158·1); ampicillin sodium (p.157·1); guaifenesin (p.1122·1); cineole (p.1672·1); niaouli oil (p.1719·3).
Lidocaine (p.1377·3) is included in this preparation to alleviate the pain of injection.
*Bacterial infections.*

**Soma Complex** Teofarma, Ital.
Carisoprodol (p.1392·1); dipyrone (p.35·3).
*Musculoskeletal and joint pain and spasm.*

**Soma Compound** Wallace, USA.
Carisoprodol (p.1392·1); aspirin (p.15·1).
*Musculoskeletal disorders.*

**Soma Compound with Codeine** Wallace, USA.
Carisoprodol (p.1392·1); aspirin (p.15·1); codeine phosphate (p.27·1).
*Musculoskeletal disorders.*

**Somabion** Medicus, Gr.
Somatostatin acetate (p.1339·3).
*Upper gastrointestinal tract haemorrhage.*

**Somac**
Pharmacia, Austral.; Pharmacia, Fin.; Byk Gulden, Norw.; Pharmacia, NZ.
Pantoprazole sodium (p.1283·1).
*Gastro-oesophageal reflux; peptic ulcer; Zollinger-Ellison syndrome.*

**Somacid** Collins, Mex.
Carisoprodol (p.1392·1).
*Skeletal muscle spasm.*

**Somac-MA** Pharmacia, Austral.†.
Tablets, pantoprazole sodium (Somac) (p.1283·1); capsules, amoxicillin trihydrate (Amoxil) (p.155·3); tablets, metronidazole (Flagyl) (p.607·2).
*Peptic ulcer.*

**Somadril**
Alpharma, Denm.; Alpharma, Norw.; Alpharma, Swed.
Carisoprodol (p.1392·1).
*Pain; skeletal muscle spasm.*

**Somadril Comp**
Alpharma, Fin.; Alpharma, Swed.
Carisoprodol (p.1392·1); paracetamol (p.76·2); caffeine (p.782·1).
*Musculoskeletal and joint disorders; pain.*

**Somaflam** Wallace, India.
Carisoprodol (p.1392·1); ibuprofen (p.45·3).
*Inflammation; pain; skeletal muscle spasm.*

**Somaflex**
Note. This name is used for preparations of different composition.
Sigma, Braz.†.
Carisoprodol (p.1392·1); dipyrone (p.35·3).
*Skeletal muscle spasm.*

Cosmopharm, Gr.
Disodium etidronate (p.771·2).
*Osteoporosis; Paget's disease of bone.*

**Somagerol** Riemser, Ger.
Lorazepam (p.704·1).
*Anxiety disorders; premedication; sleep disorders.*

**Somalgen** Bago, Arg.
Talniflumate.
*Inflammation.*

**Somalgesic** Carter-Wallace, Mex.
Naproxen (p.65·1); carisoprodol (p.1392·1).
*Musculoskeletal, joint, and peri-articular disorders.*

**Somalgin** Sigma, Braz.
Aspirin (p.15·1).
Aluminium glycinate (p.1249·1) and magnesium carbonate (p.1272·1) are included in this preparation in an attempt to limit adverse effects on the gastrointestinal mucosa.
*Fever; inflammation; pain; thrombosis prophylaxis.*

**Somalium** Ache, Braz.
Bromazepam (p.671·3).
*Anxiety; insomnia.*

**Somanol** Braun, Swed.†.
Sorbitol (p.1446·3); mannitol (p.950·2).
*Urological irrigation.*

**Somanol + Ethanol** Braun, Fin.
Sorbitol (p.1446·3); mannitol (p.950·2); alcohol (p.1166·1).
*Urological irrigation.*

**Somapam** Pacific, NZ.
Temazepam (p.723·2).
*Insomnia; premedication.*

**Somaplus** Cazi, Braz.
Diazepam (p.690·1).
*Alcohol withdrawal syndrome; anxiety; epilepsy; insomnia; premedication; sedative; skeletal muscle spasm.*

**Somarexin** Lalco, Canad.
Vitamin B substances and iron (p.1417·1).

**Somarexin & C** Lalco, Canad.
Vitamin B substances, vitamin C, calcium, and iron (p.1417·1).

**Somasedin** Heralds, Braz.†.
Papaverine hydrochloride (p.1728·1); homatropine methylbromide (p.483·2); adiphenine hydrochloride (p.1648·1).
*Smooth muscle spasm.*

**Somastin** Faran, Gr.
Somatostatin (p.1339·3).
*Upper gastrointestinal tract haemorrhage.*

**Somatarax** Vedim, Spain†.
Brallobarbital calcium (p.671·3); hydroxyzine dihydrochloride (p.434·3); secobarbital sodium (p.721·2).
*Insomnia.*

**Somatin** Torrex, Austria.
Somatostatin acetate (p.1339·3).
*Gastrointestinal haemorrhage; prevention of complications following pancreatic surgery.*

**Somatofalk** Falk, Neth.†.
Somatostatin acetate (p.1339·3).
*Gastrointestinal haemorrhage.*

**Somatolan** Lannacher, Austria.
Somatostatin acetate (p.1339·3).
*Gastrointestinal haemorrhage; prevention of complications following pancreatic surgery.*

**Somatoline** Manetti Roberts, Ital.
Levothyroxine (p.1601·3); aescin (p.1648·2).
*Adipose states with cellulite.*

**Somatosan** Curamed, Thai.†.
Somatostatin acetate (p.1339·3).
*Gastrointestinal haemorrhage; pancreatic and duodenal fistulae; prevention of complications following pancreatic surgery.*

**Somatran** Andromaco, Chile.
Sumatriptan (p.473·1).
*Migraine.*

**Somatrel** Ferring, Denm.
Somatorelin acetate (p.1339·2).
*Test for growth hormone deficiency.*

**Somatron** Volchem, Ital.
L-Arginine (p.1421·1); L-ornithine (p.1442·3).
*Nutritional supplement.*

**Somatrop** Biosintetica, Braz.
Somatropin (p.1327·2).
*Growth hormone deficiency.*

**Somatropil** Klinger, Braz.†.
Somatropin (p.1327·2).
*Growth hormone deficiency.*

**Somatulin** Ipsen, Switz.
Lanreotide acetate (p.1330·3).
*Acromegaly.*

**Somatulina**
Ipsen, Port.; Ipsen, Spain.
Lanreotide acetate (p.1330·3).
*Acromegaly; neuroendocrine tumours.*

**Somatuline**
Sidus, Arg.; Ipsen, Austral.; Ipsen, Austria†; Ipsen, Belg.; Ipsen, Fin.; Beaufour, Fr.; Ipsen, Gr.; Beaufour-Ipsen, Hong Kong; Ipsen, Irl.; Pharma Biotech, Israel; Beaufour-Ipsen, Singapore; Ipsen, Swed.; Ipsen, UK.
Lanreotide acetate (p.1330·3).
*Acromegaly; neuroendocrine tumours; thyrotrophic adenoma.*

**Somatyl** Teofarma, Ital.
Betaine sodium aspartate (p.1660·2).
*Digestive disorders.*

**Somavert**
Pfizer, UK; Pharmacia, USA.
Pegvisomant (p.1337·2).
*Acromegaly.*

**Somazina**
Temis, Arg.; Sintofarma, Braz.; Andromaco, Chile; Novag, Mex.†; CPH, Port.; Ferrer, Spain.
Citicoline (p.1672·3) or citicoline sodium (p.1672·3).
*Cerebral oedema; cerebral trauma; cerebrovascular disorders; dyskinesia; mental function impairment; parkinsonism.*

**Somese**
Pharmacia, Chile; Pharmacia, Malaysia; Pharmacia Upjohn, Singapore†.
Triazolam (p.725·3).
*Insomnia.*

**Somiaton** Serono, Spain.
Somatostatin acetate (p.1339·3).
*Pancreatic fistulae; variceal haemorrhage.*

**Somin**
YSP, Malaysia; Yung Shin, Singapore.
Dexchlorpheniramine maleate (p.427·3).
*Hypersensitivity reactions.*

**Sominex**
Note. This name is used for preparations of different composition.
EMS, Braz.
Passion flower (p.1729·1); crataegus (p.1677·1); valerian (p.1762·2).
*Sedative.*

GlaxoSmithKline Consumer, Canad.; SmithKline Beecham Consumer, USA.
Diphenhydramine hydrochloride (p.431·3).
*Insomnia.*

Prater, Chile.
Valerian (p.1762·2).
*Sleep disorders.*

Thornton & Ross, UK.
Promethazine hydrochloride (p.439·1).
*Insomnia.*

**Sominex Pain Relief** SmithKline Beecham Consumer, USA.
Diphenhydramine hydrochloride (p.431·3); paracetamol (p.76·2).
*Insomnia.*

**Somit** Gador, Arg.
Zolpidem (p.729·2).
*Insomnia.*

**Somnal** Stada, Austria.
Zopiclone (p.729·3).
*Insomnia.*

**Somnatrol** Abbott, Arg.
Estazolam (p.697·3).
*Insomnia.*

**Somnil**
Note. This name is used for preparations of different composition.
Tecnofarma, Chile.
Zolpidem (p.729·2).
*Insomnia.*

Aspen, S.Afr.
Doxylamine succinate (p.432·3).
*Insomnia.*

**Somnipax** Bago, Chile.
Zaleplon (p.727·3).
*Sleep disorders.*

**Somnipron** Instituto Sanitas, Chile.
Zolpidem (p.729·2).
*Insomnia.*

**Somnite**
Norgine, Irl.; Norgine, UK.
Nitrazepam (p.710·1).
*Insomnia.*

**Somnium**
Fresenius Kabi, Austria; Medichemie, Switz.
Lorazepam (p.704·1); diphenhydramine hydrochloride (p.431·3).
*Sleep disorders.*

**Somno** Saval, Chile.
Zolpidem (p.729·2).
*Insomnia.*

**Somnol** Carter Horner, Canad.†.
Flurazepam monohydrochloride (p.700·3).
*Insomnia.*

**Somnosan** Hormosan, Ger.
Zopiclone (p.729·3).
*Sleep disorders.*

**Somnovit** Aventis, Spain.
Loprazolam (p.704·1).
*Insomnia.*

**Somnubene** Ratiopharm, Austria.
Flunitrazepam (p.698·2).
*Sleep disorders.*

**Somnuvis S** Truw, Ger.
Valerian (p.1762·2); lupulus (p.1708·1); passion flower (p.1729·1); kava (p.1703·2).
*Nervous disorders; sleep disorders.*

**Somoblon** Vannier, Arg.
Co-dergocrine mesilate (p.1674·1).
*Cerebrovascular disorders.*

**Somol** Maver, Chile.
Diphenhydramine hydrochloride (p.431·3).
*Insomnia.*

**Somonal** Juste, Spain.
Somatostatin acetate (p.1339·3).
*Bleeding oesophageal varices; pancreatic fistulas.*

**Sompraz** Sun, India.
Esomeprazole (p.1265·1).
*Gastro-oesophageal reflux; peptic ulcer.*

**Somsanit** Kohler, Ger.
Sodium oxybate (p.1308·3).
*General anaesthesia.*

**Sonacide** Wyeth-Ayerst, Canad.†.
Glutaral (p.1180·3).
*Instrument disinfection.*

**Sonadryl** Allergan, Arg.
Pilocarpine nitrate (p.1495·1).
*Glaucoma; ocular hypertension.*

**Sonalent** Medinova (Μεντνοβα), Gr.
Azelaic acid (p.1142·3).
*Acne.*

**Sonata**
Wyeth Lederle, Belg.; Wyeth, Braz.; Wyeth Lederle, Denm.; Wyeth Lederle, Fin.; Wyeth, Ger.; Wyeth, Gr.; Wyeth, Irl.; Wyeth Lederle, Ital.; Wyeth, Mex.; Biohorm, Spain; Wyeth Lederle, Swed.; Wyeth, Switz.; Wyeth, UK; King, USA.
Zaleplon (p.727·3).
*Insomnia.*

**Sondalis**
Nestle, Fr.; Nestle Clinical, Irl.; Nestle, Ital.; Nestle, UK.
A range of preparations for enteral nutrition (p.1417·1).

**Sone** Fawns & McAllan, Austral.
Prednisone (p.1109·3).
*Corticosteroid.*

**Sonebon** Sigma, Braz.
Nitrazepam (p.710·1).
*Epilepsy; insomnia.*

**Soneriper** Pharmasant, Thai.
Tolperisone hydrochloride (p.1396·3).
*Skeletal muscle spasm.*

**Soneryl** Hansam, UK.
Butobarbital (p.673·3).
*Insomnia.*

**Songar** Valeas, Ital.
Triazolam (p.725·3).
*Insomnia.*

**Songha**
Bender, Austria; Boehringer Ingelheim, Belg.; Boehringer Ingelheim, Port.
Valerian (p.1762·2); melissa (p.1711·1).
*Anxiety disorders; sleep disorders.*

**Songha Day** Pharmaton, Switz.†.
Kava (p.1703·2).
*Anxiety.*

**Songha Night**
Pharmaton, Israel; Pharmaton, Switz.†.
Valerian (p.1762·2); melissa (p.1711·1).
*Insomnia; nervous disorders.*

**Sonhare** Boehringer de Angeli, Braz.†.
Valerian (p.1762·2); melissa (p.1711·1).
*Sedative.*

**Sonicur** Solvay, Spain.
Anethole trithione (p.1655·1).
*Dry mouth.*

**Sonidal** Specifar (Σπεσιφαρ), Gr.
Budesonide (p.1094·2).
*Topical corticosteroid.*

**Sonidar** Julphar, UAE.
Budesonide (p.1094·2).
*Asthma.*

**Sonide** Gufic, India.
Sodium nitroprusside (p.1000·2).
*Hypertension; mitral regurgitation.*

**Sonifilan** Kaken, Jpn.
Sizofiran (p.583·3).
*Radiotherapy enhancement for uterine cervical cancer.*

**Sonin**
Note. This name is used for preparations of different composition.
Asta Medica, Braz.
Pimethixene maleate.
*Respiratory-tract disorders in children.*

Merck, Ger.
Loprazolam (p.704·1).
*Sleep disorders.*

**Soni-Slo** *Helsinn Birex, Irl.†; Lipha, Irl.†.*
Isosorbide dinitrate (p.941·1).
*Angina pectoris.*

**Sonnenbrandspray** *Jacoby, Austria.*
Homoeopathic preparation.

**Sonnenbraun** *Twardy, Ger.†.*
Betacarotene (p.1422·3); biotin (p.1423·2); calcium pantothenate (p.1442·3).
*Sunburn.*

**Sonodor** *Vitafarma, Spain.*
Diphenhydramine hydrochloride (p.431·3).
*Hypersensitivity reactions; insomnia.*

**Sonofit** *Arkochim, Spain†.*
Crataegus (p.1677·1); eschscholtzia californica; passion flower (p.1729·1).
*Insomnia; nervous disorders.*

**Sonoripan** *Marjan, Braz.*
Valerian (p.1762·2).
*Sedative.*

**SonoRx** *Bracco, USA.*
Simeticone coated cellulose (p.1289·2).
*Adjunct in ultrasound imaging.*

**Sonotabs** *Galenogal, Braz.†.*
Passion flower (p.1729·1); crataegus (p.1677·1).
*Sedative.*

**Sonotrat** *Medley, Braz.†.*
Nitrazepam (p.710·1).
*Epilepsy; insomnia.*

**Sonotryl** *Singer, Switz.†.*
Propyphenazone (p.85·3); paracetamol (p.76·2); caffeine (p.782·1); drofenine hydrochloride (p.482·1).
*Painful smooth muscle spasm.*

**SonoVue**
*Byk, Belg.; Bracco, Denm.; Bracco, Ital.; Byk, Neth.; Astra Tech, Norw.; Bracco, Port.; Astra Tech, Swed.*
Sulfur hexafluoride (p.1067·3).
*Ultrasound contrast medium.*

**Sonrisal** *GlaxoSmithKline, Braz.*
Aspirin (p.15·1); sodium carbonate anhydrous (p.1747·1); sodium bicarbonate (p.1223·2); citric acid (p.1673·1).
*Dyspepsia; pain.*

**Sons Piral** *Sons, Mex.*
Paracetamol (p.76·2).
*Fever; pain.*

**Sontedril** *Willmar, Mex.†.*
Diphenhydramine (p.431·3).

**Soolan** *Julphar, UAE.*
Chlorphenamine maleate (p.427·3); phenylephrine hydrochloride (p.1126·3); guaifenesin (p.1122·1).
*Coughs and cold symptoms.*

**Soor-Gel** *Engelhard, Ger.†.*
Dequalinium salicylate (p.1178·1).
*Fungal and bacterial mouth and throat infections.*

**Soorphenesin** *Kade, Ger.*
Chlorphenesin (p.396·1).
*Fungal and bacterial infections of the vagina.*

**Sootha** *Nelson, UK.*
Homoeopathic preparation.

**Soothaderm** *Pharmakon, USA.*
Mepyramine maleate (p.437·1); benzocaine (p.1370·3); zinc oxide (p.1163·2).
*Pruritus.*

**Soothake Toothache Gel** *Pickles, UK.*
Clove oil (p.1673·3).
Formerly contained benzocaine and clove oil.
*Toothache.*

**Soothake Toothache Tincture** *Pickles, UK.*
Clove oil (p.1673·3); lidocaine (p.1377·3).

**Soothe Aid** *Zee, Canad.*
Hexylresorcinol (p.1182·1).

**Soothelip**
*Bayer, Irl.; Bayer Consumer, UK.*
Aciclovir (p.626·1).
*Herpes labialis.*

**Soothe'n Heal** *Mentholatum, Austral.†.*
Hydrous wool fat (p.1483·2); glycerol (p.1694·3); benzyl alcohol (p.1170·2).
*Dry skin.*

**Soothex** *Jamieson, Canad.*
Allantoin (p.1141·3).

**Soothing Ice Rub** *Stanley, Canad.*
Menthol (p.1711·3).

**Soothol** *Ayrton, UK.*
Cajuput oil (p.1664·1); rosemary oil (p.1740·2); arachis oil (p.1656·1).
*Ear wax removal.*

**Soov Bite**
*Ego, Austral.; Ego, Hong Kong; Ego, Malaysia; Ego, NZ; Ego, Singapore.*
Lidocaine hydrochloride (p.1377·3); cetrimide (p.1172·1); menthol (p.1711·3).
*Insect bites; pruritus; stings.*

**Soov Burn**
*Ego, Austral.; Ego, NZ.*
Lidocaine hydrochloride (p.1377·3); cetrimide (p.1172·1).
*Minor burns; sunburn.*

**Soov Cream**
*Ego, Austral.; Ego, NZ; Ego, Singapore.*
Lidocaine hydrochloride (p.1377·3); cetrimide (p.1172·1); chlorhexidine gluconate (p.1173·2).
*Haemorrhoids; minor cuts, abrasions, and burns; sunburn.*

**Soov Prickly Heat**
*Ego, Austral.; Ego, Hong Kong; Ego, Malaysia; Ego, Singapore.*
Salicylic acid (p.1157·1); zinc oxide (p.1163·2); light liquid paraffin (p.1479·1) or liquid paraffin (p.1479·1).
*Heat rash.*

**Sopa-K** *Pharmanik (Φαρμανικ), Gr.*
Potassium gluconate (p.1232·2).
*Hypokalaemia; potassium depletion.*

**Sopalamin 3B** *Melisana, Belg.*
Vitamin B substances (p.1417·1).
*Alcoholism; neurogenic pain; vitamin B deficiency.*

**Sopalamine 3B** *Technilab, Canad.*
Vitamin B substances (p.1417·1).
*Vitamin B deficiency.*

**Sopalamine 3B Plus** *Charton, Canad.†.*
Multivitamin preparation (p.1417·1).

**Sopalamine 3B Plus C** *Technilab, Canad.*
Multivitamin preparation (p.1417·1).

**Sopax** *Zimaia, Port.*
Nordazepam (p.710·3).
*Anxiety.*

**Sophidone** *UPSA, Fr.*
Hydromorphone hydrochloride (p.45·2).
*Pain.*

**Sophipren** *Sophia, Mex.*
Prednisolone acetate (p.1108·1).
*Eye disorders.*

**Sophixin** *Sophia, Mex.*
Ciprofloxacin hydrochloride (p.188·2).
*Bacterial eye infections.*

**Sophtal** *Alcon, Fr.*
*Eye drops:* Salicylic acid (p.1157·1); chlorhexidine gluconate (p.1173·2).
*Eye lotion:* Salicylic acid (p.1157·1); borax (p.1661·3); rose water.
*Eye disorders.*

**Sophtal-POS N** *Ursapharm, Ger.*
Salicylic acid (p.1157·1).
*Eye irritation; inflammatory eye disorders.*

**Soporin** *Herbamed, Switz.*
Valerian (p.1762·2); passion flower (p.1729·1); lupulus (p.1708·1); melissa (p.1711·1).
*Sleep disorders.*

**Soprol**
*Wyeth Lederle, Fr.; Helsinn Birex, Irl.*
Bisoprolol fumarate (p.875·1).
*Angina pectoris; hypertension.*

**Soproxen**
*Berlin Pharm, Singapore; Berlin Pharm, Thai.*
Naproxen sodium (p.65·1).
*Gout; musculoskeletal, joint, and soft-tissue inflammation; pain.*

**Sopulmin** *Scharper, Ital.*
Sobrerol (p.1130·2).
*Respiratory-tract disorders.*

**Soquette** *Barnes Hind, Arg.*
Polyvinyl alcohol (p.1581·1); benzalkonium chloride (p.1168·3) (p.1164·2).
*Wetting and storage solution for contact lenses.*

**Soraderm** *Stafford-Miller, Norw.*
Coal tar (p.1159·2).
*Psoriasis; seborrhoeic dermatitis.*

**Soral** *Help, Gr.*
Tenoxicam (p.93·1).
*Dysmenorrhoea; gout; inflammation; osteoarthritis; pain; rheumatoid arthritis; spondyloarthropathies.*

**Soramin** *Darrow, Braz.*
Amino-acid infusion (p.1417·1).
*Parenteral nutrition.*

**Sorbalgon** *Hartmann, Fr.*
Calcium alginate (p.745·1).
*Ulcers; wounds.*

**Sorbangil**
*Pharmacia, Norw.; Pharmacia, Swed.*
Isosorbide dinitrate (p.941·1).
*Angina pectoris; heart failure.*

**Sorbecal** *QIF, Braz.†.*
Calcium phosphate; calcium pantothenate; ergocalciferol; vitamin $B_{12}$ (p.1417·1).
*Nutritional supplement.*

**Sorbenor** *Casen Fleet, Spain.*
Arginine aspartate (p.1421·1).
*Tonic.*

**Sorbicet** *Bouzen, Arg.*
Cetrimide (p.1172·1).
*Disinfection.*

**Sorbichew** *AstraZeneca, UK†.*
Isosorbide dinitrate (p.941·1).
*Angina pectoris.*

**Sorbiclis** *SIT, Ital.*
Sorbitol (p.1446·3); docusate sodium (p.1262·2).
*Constipation.*

**Sorbid** *AstraZeneca, UK†.*
Isosorbide dinitrate (p.941·1).
*Angina pectoris.*

**Sorbidilat**
*Astra, Austria†; AstraZeneca, Switz.*
Isosorbide dinitrate (p.941·1).
*Angina pectoris; heart failure; hypertension; myocardial infarction.*

**Sorbidin**
*Alphapharm, Austral.; Alphapharm, Malaysia; Merck, Malaysia; Merck, Thai.*
Isosorbide dinitrate (p.941·1).
*Angina pectoris; heart failure; ischaemic heart disease.*

**Sorbidon Hydrate** *Gordon, USA.*
Emollient.
*Dry skin; hyperkeratosis.*

**Sorbifer** *Astra, Hong Kong†.*
Ferrous sulfate (p.1428·2).
*Iron deficiency; iron-deficiency anaemia.*

**Sorbilax** *Pharmacia, Austral.*
Sorbitol (p.1446·3).
*Constipation.*

**Sorbiline** *Franco-Indian, India.*
Tricholine citrate (p.1424·3); sorbitol (p.1446·3).
*Biliary and liver disorders.*

**Sorbimon** *Ratiopharm, Austria†.*
Isosorbide mononitrate (p.942·1).
*Angina pectoris; heart failure; myocardial infarction; pulmonary hypertension.*

**Sorbisal** *Allergan, NZ†.*
Irrigation and rinsing solution for contact lenses (p.1164·2).

**Sorbisterit**
*Fresenius Medical, Austria; Fresenius Medical, Ger.; Fresenius Medical, Switz.*
Calcium polystyrene sulfonate (p.1032·3).
*Hyperkalaemia.*

**Sorbitrate**
*Zeneca, Belg.†; Nicholas Piramal, India; AstraZeneca, Thai.†; Astra-Zeneca, UK†; Zeneca, USA.*
Isosorbide dinitrate (p.941·1).
*Angina pectoris; heart failure.*

**Sorbitur** *Baxter, Swed.†.*
Sorbitol (p.1446·3).
*Bladder irrigation.*

**Sorbon** *Unipharm, Israel.*
Buspirone hydrochloride (p.672·2).
*Anxiety disorders.*

**Sorbsan**
*Maersk, Austral.; Braun, Fr.†; Braun, Ital.; Maersk, UK.*
Calcium alginate (p.745·1).
*Burns; skin ulceration; wounds.*

**Sorcal**
*Note. This name is used for preparations of different composition.*
*Wyeth, Braz.*
Calcium polystyrene sulfonate (p.1032·3).
*Hypercalcaemia.*
*Polipharm, Thai.*
Calcium carbonate (p.1254·2).
*Calcium supplement.*

**Sorciclina** *Inexfa, Spain†.*
Doxycycline hyclate (p.206·2); prolase.
*Bacterial infections.*

**Sore Mouth Gel** *Boots, Thai.*
Lidocaine (p.1377·3); cetylpyridinium chloride (p.1173·1); menthol (p.1711·3); cineole (p.1672·1).
*Oral pain.*

**Sore Throat Chewing Gum** *Or-Dov, Austral.†.*
Dichlorobenzyl alcohol (p.1178·3); amylmetacresol (p.1168·2); vitamin C (p.1460·2).
*Sore throat.*

**Sore Throat L39** *Homeocan, Canad.*
Homoeopathic preparation.

**Sore Throat Lozenges** *Sutton, Canad.*
Benzocaine (p.1370·3); menthol (p.1711·3).

**Sore Throat Relief** *Brauer, Austral.†.*
Homoeopathic preparation.

**Sorebral** *Condrugs, Thai.*
Cinnarizine (p.428·3).
*Cerebrovascular disorders; migraine; peripheral vascular disorders; vestibular disorders.*

**Soredine** *Cooper (Κοπερ), Gr.*
Ranitidine hydrochloride (p.1285·2).
*Conditions where gastric acid reduction is beneficial; gastric hypersecretion including Zollinger-Ellison syndrome; peptic ulcer.*

**Soren** *Daewon, Hong Kong.*
Naproxen sodium (p.65·1).
*Gout; musculoskeletal, joint, and peri-articular disorders; pain.*

**Sorgoa** *Scheurich, Ger.†.*
Tolnaftate (p.410·1).
*Fungal skin infections.*

**Sorgoran** *Sanova, Austria†.*
Tolnaftate (p.410·1).
*Fungal skin and nail infections.*

**Soriacur** *Medica, Arg.*
Coal tar (p.1159·2).
*Psoriasis.*

**Sorial** *Fortbenton, Arg.*
Coal tar (p.1159·2).
*Psoriasis.*

**Soriatane**
*Roche, Canad.; Roche, Fr.; Roche, USA.*
Acitretin (p.1140·2).
*Keratinisation disorders; psoriasis.*

**Soridermal** *Mintlab, Chile.*
Ketoconazole (p.403·3).
*Fungal skin infections.*

**Sorine Adulto** *Ache, Braz.*
Benzalkonium chloride (p.1168·3); sodium chloride (p.1233·3); naphazoline (p.1124·3).
*Nasal congestion.*

**Sorine Infantil** *Ache, Braz.*
Benzalkonium chloride (p.1168·3); sodium chloride (p.1233·3).
*Nasal congestion.*

**Sormodren**
*Ebewe, Austria; Abbott, Ger.; Teofarma, Ital.; Knoll, Mex.†.*
Bornaprine hydrochloride (p.480·1).
*Drug-induced extrapyramidal disorders; hyperhidrosis; parkinsonism.*

**Sormon** *Gerard, Irl.*
Isosorbide mononitrate (p.942·1).
*Angina pectoris.*

**Sornil** *Utopian, Thai.*
Isosorbide dinitrate (p.941·1).
*Angina pectoris.*

**Soro de Manutencao H** *Labesfal, Port.*
Electrolyte infusion with glucose (p.1217·1).
*Carbohydrate source; fluid and electrolyte disorders.*

**Soro Nasal** *Osorio de Moraes, Braz.*
Sodium chloride (p.1233·3); benzalkonium chloride (p.1168·3).
*Nasal congestion.*

**Soroliv** *Teuto, Braz.*
Sodium chloride (p.1233·3).
*Nasal congestion.*

**Soronal** *Cimed, Braz.†.*
Sodium chloride (p.1233·3); benzalkonium chloride (p.1168·3).
*Nasal congestion.*

**Soroneo** *Neo Quimica, Braz.*
Sodium chloride (p.1233·3).
*Nasal congestion; nasal hygiene.*

**Soropon** *Purdue, Canad.*
Tyrothricin (p.275·1); trolamine polypeptide cocoate condensate (p.1758·2).
*Scalp disorders.*

**Sorot**
*Petrasch, Austria; Ravensberg, Ger.*
Dequalinium chloride (p.1178·1).
*Mouth and throat infections.*

**Sorquetan** *Basotherm, Ger.†.*
Tinidazole (p.617·1).
*Bacterial or protozoal infections.*

**Sorsis** *Fortbenton, Arg.*
*Cream:* Allantoin (p.1141·3); coal tar (p.1159·2); triamcinolone (p.1110·2).
*Skin disorders.*
*Shampoo:* Salicylic acid (p.1157·1); coal tar (p.1159·2).
*Dandruff; seborrhoea.*

**Sorsis Beta** *Fortbenton, Arg.*
Salicylic acid (p.1157·1); betamethasone (p.1093·1); coal tar (p.1159·2).
*Skin disorders.*

**Sortis**
*Pfizer, Austria; Godecke, Ger.; Mack, Illert., Ger.; Parke, Davis, Ger.; Pfizer, Ger.; Pfizer, Switz.*
Atorvastatin calcium (p.866·1).
*Hyperlipidaemias.*

**Sosegon**
*Yamanouchi, Jpn; Sanofi Synthelabo, Port.; Sanofi Synthelabo, Spain; Sanofi Synthelabo, Thai.*
Pentazocine (p.79·3), pentazocine hydrochloride (p.79·3), or pentazocine lactate (p.79·3).
*Pain.*

**Sosenol** *Adcock Ingram, S.Afr.*
Pentazocine (p.79·3).
*Pain.*

**Sostac** *Laboratorios Chile, Chile.*
Fluoxetine (p.296·3).
*Depression.*

**Sostatin** *Faran, Gr.*
Ketoconazole (p.403·3).
*Fungal infections.*

**Sostenon** *Organon, Mex.*
Testosterone propionate (p.1570·1); testosterone phenylpropionate (p.1570·1); testosterone isocaproate (p.1570·1); testosterone decanoate (p.1570·1).
*Androgen deficiency.*

**Sostilar** *Pharmacia, Belg.*
Cabergoline (p.1203·3).
*Hyperprolactinaemia.*

**Sostril** *GlaxoSmithKline, Ger.*
Ranitidine hydrochloride (p.1285·2).
*Acid aspiration; gastro-oesophageal reflux; gastrointestinal haemorrhage; gastrointestinal hyperacidity; peptic ulcer; Zollinger-Ellison syndrome.*

**Sota** *1A, Ger.; ABZ, Ger.*
Sotalol hydrochloride (p.1001·3).
*Arrhythmias.*

**Sota Lich** *Lichtenstein, Ger.*
Sotalol hydrochloride (p.1001·3).
*Arrhythmias.*

**Sotab** *Douglas, Austral.*
Sotalol hydrochloride (p.1001·3).
*Arrhythmias.*

**Sotabet**
*Gea, Denm.; Gea, Swed.*
Sotalol hydrochloride (p.1001·3).
*Arrhythmias.*

**Sotabeta** *Betapharm, Ger.*
Sotalol hydrochloride (p.1001·3).
*Arrhythmias.*

**Sotacor**
*Hexal, Arg.; Bristol-Myers Squibb, Austral.; Bristol-Myers Squibb, Austria; Bristol-Myers Squibb, Braz.; Bristol, Canad.; Bristol-Myers Squibb, Denm.; Bristol-Myers Squibb, Fin.; Bristol-Myers Squibb, Hong Kong; Bristol-Myers Squibb, Irl.; Bristol-Myers Squibb, Israel; Bristol-Myers Squibb, Jpn; Bristol-Myers Squibb, Malaysia; Bristol-Myers Squibb, Neth.; Bristol-Myers Squibb, Norw.; Bristol-Myers Squibb, NZ; Bristol-Myers Squibb, S.Afr.; Bristol-Myers Squibb, Singapore; Bristol-Myers Squibb, Swed.; Bristol-Myers Squibb, Thai.†; Bristol-Myers Squibb, UK.*
Sotalol hydrochloride (p.1001·3).
*Angina pectoris; arrhythmias; hypertension; hyperthyroidism; myocardial infarction.*

**Sotagamma** *Worwag, Ger.*
Sotalol hydrochloride (p.1001·3).
*Arrhythmias.*

**Sota-Gry** *Teva, Ger.†.*
Sotalol hydrochloride (p.1001·3).
*Arrhythmias.*

**Sotahexal**
*Hexal, Austral.; Hexal, Austria; Hexal, Ger.; Hexal, S.Afr.*
Sotalol hydrochloride (p.1001·3).
*Angina pectoris; arrhythmias; hypertension; hyperthyroidism; myocardial infarction.*

**Sotalex**
*Bristol-Myers Squibb, Belg.; Bristol-Myers Squibb, Fr.; Bristol-Myers Squibb, Ger.; Bristol-Myers Squibb, Ital.; Bristol-Myers Squibb, Switz.*
Sotalol hydrochloride (p.1001·3).
*Arrhythmias; hypertension; myocardial infarction.*

**Sotalin** *Ratiopharm, Fin.*
Sotalol hydrochloride (p.1001·3).
*Arrhythmias.*

**Sotalodoc** *Docpharm, Ger.*
Sotalol hydrochloride (p.1001·3).
*Arrhythmias.*

**Sotamed** *S Med, Austria.*
Sotalol hydrochloride (p.1001·3).
*Arrhythmias.*

**Sotamol** *Technilab, Canad.†.*
Sotalol hydrochloride (p.1001·3).
*Arrhythmias.*

**Sotanorm** *Medicopharm, Austria.*
Sotalol hydrochloride (p.1001·3).
*Arrhythmias.*

**Sotaper** *Bristol-Myers Squibb, Mex.*
Sotalol (p.1002·2).
*Arrhythmias; hypertension.*

**Sotapor** *Bristol-Myers, Spain.*
Sotalol hydrochloride (p.1001·3).
*Arrhythmias.*

**Sota-Puren** *Alpharma-Isis, Ger.*
Sotalol hydrochloride (p.1001·3).
*Arrhythmias.*

**Sotaryt** *Azupharma, Ger.*
Sotalol hydrochloride (p.1001·3).
*Arrhythmias.*

**Sota-saar** *Rosen, Ger.*
Sotalol hydrochloride (p.1001·3).
*Arrhythmias.*

**Sotastad**
*Stada, Austria; Stada, Ger.*
Sotalol hydrochloride (p.1001·3).
*Arrhythmias.*

**Sotatyrol** *Tyrol, Austria.*
Sotalol hydrochloride (p.1001·3).
*Arrhythmias.*

**Sotaziden N** *Bristol-Myers Squibb, Ger.*
Nadolol (p.963·1); bendroflumethiazide (p.867·3).
*Hypertension.*

**Sotilen**
*Medochemie, Hong Kong; Medochemie, Singapore†; Medochemie, Thai.*
Piroxicam (p.84·2).
*Gout; musculoskeletal and joint disorders.*

**Sotoger** *Gerard, Irl.*
Sotalol hydrochloride (p.1001·3).
*Arrhythmias.*

**Sotomycin** *Bros, Gr.*
Clindamycin phosphate (p.194·2).
*Acne.*

**Sotradecol** *Elkins-Sinn, USA.*
Sodium tetradecyl sulfate (p.1575·1).
*Varicose veins.*

**Sotret** *Ranbaxy, USA.*
Isotretinoin (p.1148·3).
*Acne.*

**Soufrane** *Sanofi Synthelabo OTC, Fr.*
Thenoate sodium (p.269·2).
*Nasopharyngeal infections.*

**Soufrol** *Gebro, Switz.*
Mesulphen (p.1152·1).
*Bath additive; musculoskeletal and joint disorders; skin disorders.*

**Soufrol TP** *Gebro, Switz.*
Medicinal mud; sulfur (p.1158·2).
*Musculoskeletal and joint disorders.*

**Soufrol ZNP** *Gebro, Switz.†.*
Sulfur (p.1158·2); pyrithione zinc (p.1156·2).
*Scalp disorders.*

**Sovel** *Novartis, Ger.*
Norethisterone acetate (p.1562·2).
*Menstrual disorders.*

**Soventol**
*Note. This name is used for preparations of different composition.*
*Ebewe, Austria; Rentschler, Ger.*
Bamipine lactate (p.425·3).
*Burns; frostbite; insect and jellyfish stings; pruritus; sunburn; urticaria.*

*Nicholas Piramal, India.*
Bamipine lactate (p.425·3); ammonium chloride (p.1115·2); sodium citrate (p.1223·2); menthol (p.1711·3).
*Bronchitis; coughs.*

*Knoll, Mex.†.*
Bamipine (p.425·3).

**Soventol HC** *Rentschler, Ger.*
Hydrocortisone acetate (p.1103·3).
*Skin disorders.*

**Soviclor** *Collins, Mex.*
Aciclovir (p.626·1).
*Herpesvirus infections.*

**Sovipan** *Sanofi Synthelabo, Gr.*
Aceclofenac (p.11·2).
*Ankylosing spondylitis; inflammation; osteoarthritis; pain; rheumatoid arthritis.*

**Soy Forte with Block Cohosh** *Cenovis, Austral.†.*
Soya (p.1447·2); cimicifuga (p.1671·3); calcium hydrogen phosphate (p.1225·2); colecalciferol (p.1461·3); magnesium oxide (p.1272·3).
*Menopausal disorders; osteoporosis.*

**Soya Diet** *Support, Braz.*
A range of soya-based preparations for enteral nutrition (p.1417·1).

**Soyac** *Support, Braz.*
Soy protein preparation for enteral nutrition (p.1417·1).

**Soyacal**
*Grifols, Arg.; Grifols, Ital.; Grifols, Spain.*
Soya oil (p.1447·2).
Contains egg phospholipids.
*Lipid infusion for parenteral nutrition.*

**Soyal** *FDC, India.*
Food for special diets (p.1417·1).
*Lactose intolerance; milk intolerance.*

**Soyalac** *Nutricia-Loma Lindar, USA.*
Lactose-free soy protein infant feed (p.1417·1).

**Soyaloid** *Serral, Mex.*
Soya flour (p.1447·2); povidone (p.1581·2).
*Bath additive; skin disorders.*

**Soyaven** *Delicias, Mex.*
Food for special diets (p.1417·1).
*Food allergies; lactose and cow's milk intolerance.*

**Soydex** *Darier, Mex.*
Soya flour (p.1447·2); povidone (p.1581·2).
*Bath additive; skin disorders.*

**Soymen** *Irmed, Ital.*
Soya (p.1447·2); vitamins (p.1417·1).
*Menopausal disorders.*

**SoyPlus** *Lifeplan, UK.*
Soya isoflavones; folic acid (p.1417·1).
*Dietary supplement.*

**SP** *Sussex, UK†.*
Paracetamol (p.76·2); caffeine (p.782·1); phenylephrine hydrochloride (p.1126·3).

**SP54** *Bene-Chemie, Hong Kong.*
Pentosan polysulfate sodium (p.979·2).
*Thromboembolic disorders.*

**SP95** *DHN, Fr.*
Protein and vitamin preparation (p.1417·1).
*Nutritional supplement.*

**SP Betaisodona** *Mundipharma, Ger.†.*
Povidone-iodine (p.1190·3).
*Hand disinfection; skin and mucous membrane disinfection.*

**SP Cream** *Curacel, Austral.*
Melaleuca oil (p.1710·2); salicylic acid (p.1157·1); solanum lycopersicum leaf; urea (p.1162·2).
*Keratoses; sunspots; warts.*

**SP Troches**
*Meiji, Malaysia; Meiji, Singapore.*
Dequalinium chloride (p.1178·1).
*Mouth and throat disorders.*

**Spablock** *Masa, Thai.*
Drotaverine hydrochloride (p.1683·1).
*Smooth muscle spasm.*

**Spaciclina** *SPA, Ital.†.*
Tetracycline hydrochloride (p.266·2).
*Bacterial and protozoal infections.*

**Spagall** *Sanova, Austria.*
*p*,α-Dimethylbenzyl alcohol nicotinate (p.1680·3); naphthylacetic acid (p.1719·1); caroverine (p.1668·1).
*Hepatobiliary disorders.*

**Spagulax** *Pharmafarm, Fr.*
Ispaghula (p.1268·1).
*Constipation.*

**Spagulax au Citrate de Potassium** *Pharmafarm, Fr.*
Ispaghula (p.1268·1); potassium citrate (p.1223·1).
*Constipation.*

**Spagulax au Sorbitol** *Pharmafarm, Fr.*
Ispaghula (p.1268·1); sorbitol (p.1446·3).
*Constipation.*

**Spagulax Mucilage** *Pharmafarm, Fr.*
Ispaghula (p.1268·1).
*Constipation.*

**Spagymun** *Spagyros, Switz.*
Echinacea angustifolia flowers and roots; echinacea purpura flowers and roots (p.1683·2); eupatorium perfoliatum.
*Immune stimulant.*

**Spagyrom** *Spagyros, Switz.*
Echinacea angustifolia flowers and roots; echinacea purpura flowers and roots (p.1683·2); clove oil (p.1673·3); cinnamon oil (p.1672·2); juniper oil (p.1703·1); lavender oil (p.1705·2); chamomile oil (p.1669·3); peppermint oil (p.1283·2); rosemary oil (p.1740·2); savory oil; thyme oil (p.1755·3).
*Common cold; mouth and throat disorders.*

**Spai** *INTES, Ital.†.*
Sodium chloride; potassium chloride; calcium chloride; magnesium chloride; sodium acetate; sodium citrate (p.1217·1).
*Adjunct in otorhinolaryngeal procedures; cleaning solution for contact lens; ocular irrigation.*

**Spalgin** *SPA, Ital.†.*
Pipethanate ethobromide (p.487·3).
*Premedication; smooth muscle spasticity.*

**Spalt**
*Note. This name is used for preparations of different composition.*
*Sanova, Austria.*
Phenazone salicylate (p.82·3); salicylamide (p.87·3); caffeine (p.782·1).
*Pain.*

*Much, Ger.†.*
Aspirin (p.15·1).
*Cold symptoms; fever; pain.*

*Whitehall-Much, Ger.*
Ibuprofen (p.45·3).
*Fever; pain.*

**Spalt N**
*Note. This name is used for preparations of different composition.*
*Whitehall, Swed.†.*
Phenazone (p.82·3).
*Fever; pain.*

*Whitehall-Robins, Switz.†.*
Paracetamol (p.76·2).
*Fever; pain.*

**Spalt Schmerz-Gel** *Whitehall-Much, Ger.*
Diisopropanolamine felbinac (p.39·1).
*Musculoskeletal, joint, and soft-tissue disorders.*

**Spalt Schmerztabletten** *Whitehall-Much, Ger.*
Aspirin (p.15·1); paracetamol (p.76·2).
*Pain.*

**Spamus** *T Man, Thai.*
Tolperisone hydrochloride (p.1396·3).
*Parkinsonism; skeletal muscle spasm.*

**Span C** *Freeda, USA.*
Citrus bioflavonoids complex (p.1688·2); ascorbic acid (p.1460·2).
*Capillary bleeding.*

**Spanidin** *Kayaku, Jpn.*
Gusperimus hydrochloride (p.1360·2).
*Renal transplant rejection.*

**Spanish Tummy Mixture** *Potter's, UK.*
Blackberry root bark; catechu (p.1668·3).
*Diarrhoea.*

**Span-K**
*Aspen, Austral.; Aspen, Hong Kong; Aventis, NZ†.*
Potassium chloride (p.1232·2).
*Potassium deficiency.*

**Spanor** *Bailleul, Fr.*
Doxycycline hyclate (p.206·2).
*Bacterial infections.*

**Spanplex** *Collins, Mex.*
Vitamin preparation (p.1417·1).

**Spara** *Dainippon, Jpn.*
Sparfloxacin (p.255·1).
*Bacterial infections.*

**Sparaplaie** *Urgo, Fr.*
Benzalkonium chloride (p.1168·3).
*Wounds.*

**Spardac** *Cadila, India.*
Sparfloxacin (p.255·1).
*Bacterial infections.*

**Sparine**
*Wyeth, Austral.†; Wyeth Lederle, Denm.; Wyeth Lederle, Fin.; Wyeth, Gr.; Wyeth, Irl.†; Akromed, S.Afr.†; Genus, UK†; Wyeth-Ayerst, USA†.*
Promazine embonate (p.717·3) or promazine hydrochloride (p.717·3).
*Agitation; alcohol withdrawal syndrome; anxiety; hiccup; nausea; premedication; psychoses; sedative; vomiting.*

**Sparkal**
*Gea, Denm.; Gea, Fin.; Gea, Swed.*
Amiloride hydrochloride (p.858·2); hydrochlorothiazide (p.933·2).
*Hypertension; liver cirrhosis with ascites; oedema.*

**Sparkles** *Lafayette, USA.*
Sodium bicarbonate (p.1223·2); citric acid (p.1673·1); simeticone (p.1289·2).
*Adjunct in endoscopy; flatulence.*

**Sparkling White Eye Drops** *Propan, S.Afr.*
Oxymetazoline hydrochloride (p.1126·1).
*Allergic eye inflammation.*

**Sparksol** *Asta Medica, Ital.*
Amino-acid preparation with vitamin $B_6$ (p.1417·1).

**Spartiol** *Klein, Ger.*
Sarothamnus scoparius (p.1742·2).
*Arrhythmias.*

**Spartocine**
*UCB, Belg.; UCB, Fin.*
Ferrous aspartate (p.1427·3).
*Iron deficiency; iron-deficiency anaemias.*

**Spartocine N** *UCB, Ger.*
Ferrous aspartate (p.1427·3).
*Iron-deficiency anaemia.*

**Sparx** *Wockhardt, India.*
Sparfloxacin (p.255·1).
*Bacterial infections.*

**Spascopan** *Bangkok Lab & Cosmetic, Thai.*
Hyoscine butylbromide (p.483·3).
*Smooth muscle spasm.*

**Spasdic** *Progress, Thai.*
Flavoxate hydrochloride (p.482·2).
*Urinary-tract disorders.*

**Spasen** *FIRMA, Ital.*
*Suppositories†:* Otilonium bromide (p.1725·1); lidocaine hydrochloride (p.1377·3).
*Gastrointestinal spasm.*

*Tablets:* Otilonium bromide (p.1725·1).
*Gastrointestinal pain and spasm.*

**Spasen Somatico** *FIRMA, Ital.*
Otilonium bromide (p.1725·1); diazepam (p.690·1).
*Gastrointestinal pain and spasm.*

**Spasfon**
*Therabel, Belg.; Lafon, Fr.; Demo, Gr.*
Phloroglucinol (p.1731·1); trimethylphloroglucinol (p.1731·1).
*Smooth muscle spasm.*

**Spasfon-Lyoc** *Lafon, Fr.*
Phloroglucinol (p.1731·1).
*Smooth muscle spasm.*

**Spasgone** *Chew, Thai.*
Paracetamol (p.76·2); hyoscine butylbromide (p.483·3).
*Smooth muscle spasm.*

**Spasgone-H** *Chew, Thai.*
Hyoscine butylbromide (p.483·3).
*Smooth muscle spasm.*

**Spasma** *Stella, Belg.*
Morphine hydrochloride (p.60·1); hyoscine hydrobromide (p.483·3).
*Biliary and renal colic; pain; premedication.*

**Spasmag** *Grimberg, Fr.*
*Capsules; oral solution:* Magnesium sulfate (p.1228·2); dried yeast (p.1469·1).
*Magnesium deficiency.*

*Injection:* Magnesium sulfate (p.1228·2).
*Eclampsia; magnesium deficiency.*

**Spasmalgan** *Apogepha, Ger.*
Denaverine hydrochloride.
*Smooth muscle spasm.*

**Spasmalgin** *Sam-On, Israel.*
Atropine sulfate (p.477·1); papaverine hydrochloride (p.1728·1); paracetamol (p.76·2); codeine phosphate (p.27·1).
*Smooth muscle spasm.*

**Spasman** *Merckle, Ger.*
Demelverine hydrochloride; trihexyphenidyl hydrochloride (p.490·2).
*Smooth muscle spasm.*

**Spasman scop** *Merckle, Ger.*
Hyoscine butylbromide (p.483·3).
*Smooth muscle spasm.*

**Spasmaverine** *Aventis, Fr.†.*
*Suppositories:* Alverine (p.1250·2); benzocaine (p.1370·3).
*Tablets:* Alverine citrate (p.1250·2).
*Smooth muscle spasm.*

**Spasmend** *Restan, S.Afr.*
Paracetamol (p.76·2); mephenesin (p.1394·3).
*Pain; skeletal muscle spasm.*

**Spasmeridan** *UCB, Ital.*
Diazepam (p.690·1); hyoscine methobromide (p.483·3).
*Gastrointestinal pain and spasm.*

**Spasmex**
*Note. This name is used for preparations of different composition.*
*Biol, Arg.; Rider, Chile; Pfleger, Ger.*
Trospium chloride (p.491·2).
*Smooth muscle spasms; urinary incontinence.*

*Scharper, Ital.*
*Injection:* Phloroglucinol (p.1731·1).
*Tablets; suppositories:* Phloroglucinol (p.1731·1); trimethylphloroglucinol (p.1731·1).
*Painful spasm of the biliary and urinary tracts.*

**Spasmhalt** *Stanley, Canad.*
Paracetamol (p.76·2); codeine phosphate (p.27·1); methocarbamol (p.1395·1).

**Spasmhalt-ASA** *Stanley, Canad.*
Aspirin (p.15·1); codeine phosphate (p.27·1); methocarbamol (p.1395·1).

**Spasmidenal** *Jolly-Jatel, Fr.†.*
Crataegus (p.1677·1); valerian (p.1762·2); phenobarbital (p.367·3).
*Insomnia; nervous disorders.*

**Spasmine**
*Note. This name is used for preparations of different composition.*
*Norgine, Belg.*
Alverine citrate (p.1250·2).
*Irritable bowel syndrome.*

*Jolly-Jatel, Fr.*
Valerian (p.1762·2); crataegus (p.1677·1).
*Insomnia; nervous disorders.*

**Spasmium** *Sanova, Austria.*
Caroverine (p.1668·1) or caroverine hydrochloride (p.1668·1).
*Smooth muscle spasm; tinnitus.*

**Spasmium comp** *Sanova, Austria.*
Caroverine (p.1668·1); metamizole calcium (p.36·1).
*Painful smooth muscle spasm.*

**Spasmo Claim** *Apomedica, Austria.*
Turmeric (p.1058·3); benzyl mandelate; *p*,α-dimethylbenzyl alcohol (p.1680·3); peppermint oil (p.1283·2); caraway oil (p.1667·3); fennel oil (p.1687·3); lemon oil (p.1706·2); camphor (p.1665·3); thymol (p.1194·2); guaiazulene (p.1696·2).
*Gastrointestinal disorders.*

**spasmo gallo sanol** *Sanol, Ger.*
Greater celandine (p.1695·3); turmeric (p.1058·3).
*Biliary and gastrointestinal spasm.*

**spasmo gallo sanol mint** *Sanol, Ger.; Schwarz, Ger.*
Peppermint oil (p.1283·2).
*Biliary-tract spasm.*

**Spasmo Inalgon Neu** *Calea, Austria.*
Dipyrone (p.35·3).
*Painful smooth muscle spasm.*

**Spasmo Nil** *Duchesnay, Canad.†.*
Aluminium hydroxide (p.1249·2); magnesium trisilicate (p.1272·3); dicycloverine hydrochloride (p.481·2); simeticone (p.1289·2).

**Spasmo-Barbamin** *Streuli, Switz.*
Propyphenazone (p.85·3); adiphenine hydrochloride (p.1648·1); diphenhydramine hydrochloride (p.431·3).
*Painful smooth muscle spasm.*

**Spasmo-Barbamine compositum** *Streuli, Switz.*
Propyphenazone (p.85·3); adiphenine hydrochloride (p.1648·1); diphenhydramine hydrochloride (p.431·3); codeine phosphate (p.27·1).
*Painful smooth muscle spasm.*

**Spasmo-Bomaleb** *Hevert, Ger.†.*
Homoeopathic preparation.

**Spasmo-Canulase**
*Novartis Consumer, S.Afr.; Novartis Consumer, Switz.*
Metixene hydrochloride (p.485·3); dimethicone (p.1289·2); pancreatin (p.1725·3); cellulase (p.1669·1); pepsin (p.1729·3); glutamic acid hydrochloride (p.1433·2); sodium dehydrocholate (p.1679·2).
*Gastrointestinal disorders.*

**Spasmo-Cibalgin** *Novartis Consumer, Switz.*
Propyphenazone (p.85·3); drofenine hydrochloride (p.482·1).
*Painful smooth muscle spasm.*

**Spasmo-Cibalgin comp** *Novartis Consumer, Switz.*
Propyphenazone (p.85·3); drofenine hydrochloride (p.482·1); codeine phosphate (p.27·1).
*Painful smooth muscle spasm.*

**Spasmo-Cibalgin compositum S** *Novartis, Ger.†.*
Propyphenazone (p.85·3); drofenine hydrochloride (p.482·1); codeine phosphate (p.27·1).
*Smooth muscle spasm.*

**Spasmo-Cibalgin S** *Novartis, Ger.*
Propyphenazone (p.85·3); drofenine hydrochloride (p.482·1).
*Smooth muscle spasm.*

**Spasmo-Cibalgina** *Novartis, Ital.*
Propyphenazone (p.85·3); drofenine hydrochloride (p.482·1).
*Painful smooth muscle spasm.*

**Spasmo-Cibalgine** *Ciba-Geigy, Belg.†.*
Propyphenazone (p.85·3); drofenine hydrochloride (p.482·1).
*Dysmenorrhoea; smooth muscle spasm.*

**Spasmocor** *Asta Medica, Austria.*
Glyceryl trinitrate (p.923·2); pentaerithrityl tetranitrate (p.979·1); nicotinic acid (p.1441·1); benzyl mandelate.
*Angina pectoris; heart failure; peripheral vascular spasm.*

**Spasmoctyl**
*Menarini, Arg.; Guidotti, Spain.*
Otilonium bromide (p.1725·1).
*Gastrointestinal spasm; irritable bowel syndrome.*

**Spasmocyclon** *3M, Ger.*
Cyclandelate (p.890·3).
*Cerebrovascular disorders; migraine; vestibular disorders.*

**Spasmodene** *Edochim, Ital.†.*
Pipethanate ethobromide (p.487·3).
*Biliary and urinary-tract spasm and dyskinesia; gastrointestinal spasm; premedication for endoscopy and radiography.*

**Spasmodex** *Crinex, Fr.*
Dihexyverine hydrochloride (p.481·3).
*Gastrointestinal disorders.*

**Spasmodil** *ABC, Ital.*
Pipethanate ethobromide (p.487·3).
*Gastrointestinal spasm and hypermotility; premedication for endoscopy and radiography; urinary and biliary spasm and dyskinesia.*

**Spasmofen** *Abigo, Swed.*
Hyoscine methonitrate (p.483·3); papaverine hydrochloride (p.1728·1); morphine hydrochloride (p.60·1); noscapine hydrochloride (p.1125·3); codeine hydrochloride (p.27·1).
*Pain; smooth muscle spasm.*

**Spasmofides S** *Fides, Ger.*
Homoeopathic preparation.

**Spasmogel** *Alliance, S.Afr.*
Dicycloverine hydrochloride (p.481·2); light magnesium oxide (p.1272·3); aluminium hydroxide (p.1249·2).
*Dyspepsia; flatulence; gastritis; gastro-oesophageal reflux; heartburn; peptic ulcer.*

**Spasmo-Granobil-Krampf- und Reizhusten**
*Synpharma, Austria.*
Aniseed (p.1655·2); helianthus annuus; thyme (p.1755·2).
*Coughs.*

**Spasmoliv**
*Xepa-Soul Pattinson, Malaysia; Xepa-Soul Pattinson, Singapore.*
Hyoscine butylbromide (p.483·3).
*Smooth muscle spasm.*

**Spasmolyt**
*Madaus, Austria; Hoyer, Ger.*
Trospium chloride (p.491·2).
*Bladder function disorders; smooth muscle spasm.*

**Spasmo-Lyt**
*Madaus, Denm.; Madaus, Thai.*
Trospium chloride (p.491·2).
*Bladder function disorders.*

**Spasmomen**
*Menarini, Belg.; Menarini, Hong Kong; Menarini, Ital.*
Otilonium bromide (p.1725·1).
*Gastrointestinal spasm; premedication for gastrointestinal procedures.*

**Spasmomen Somatico** *Menarini, Ital.*
Otilonium bromide (p.1725·1); diazepam (p.690·1).
*Gastrointestinal spasm.*

**Spasmo-Mucosolvan** *Boehringer Ingelheim, Ger.*
Clenbuterol hydrochloride (p.784·2); ambroxol hydrochloride (p.1114·3).
*Respiratory-tract disorders.*

**Spasmonal**
*Note. This name is used for preparations of different composition.*
*Trenker, Belg.*
Mebeverine hydrochloride (p.1273·1).
*Irritable bowel syndrome.*

*Norgine, Hong Kong; Norgine, Irl.; Norgine, Malaysia; Norgine, Singapore; Norgine, Thai.; Norgine, UK.*
Alverine citrate (p.1250·2).
*Smooth muscle spasm.*

**Spasmonal Fibre** *Norgine, UK†.*
Sterculia (p.1290·2); alverine citrate (p.1250·2).
*Hypertonic colon; irritable bowel syndrome.*

**Spasmo-Nervogastrol** *Sanofi Synthelabo, Ger.*
Butinoline phosphate (p.1663·3); calcium carbonate (p.1254·2); bismuth subnitrate (p.1252·2).
*Gastrointestinal disorders.*

**Spasmo-Oxepam** *Wyeth Lederle, Fin.†.*
Oxazepam (p.712·2); ambutonium bromide (p.1653·2).
*Anxiety disorders; gastrointestinal motility disorders.*

**Spasmoplex** *Neo-Farmaceutica, Port.*
Trospium chloride (p.491·2).
*Urinary incontinence.*

**Spasmoplus**
*Note. This name is used for preparations of different composition.*
*Novartis, Austria; Novartis, Belg.*
Propyphenazone (p.85·3); drofenine hydrochloride (p.482·1); codeine phosphate (p.27·1).
*Painful smooth muscle spasm.*

*Novartis, Ital.*
Propyphenazone (p.85·3); codeine phosphate (p.27·1).
*Pain.*

**Spasmopriv**
*Note. This name is used for preparations of different composition.*
*Irex, Fr.*
Mebeverine hydrochloride (p.1273·1).
*Gastrointestinal and biliary-tract spasm.*

*Senosiain, Mex.; Eurodrug, Singapore; Eurodrug, Thai.*
Fenoverine (p.1687·3).
*Smooth muscle spasm.*

**Spasmo-Proxyvon** *Wockhardt, India.*
*Capsules:* Dicycloverine hydrochloride (p.481·2); dextropropoxyphene hydrochloride (p.28·3); paracetamol (p.76·2).
*Injection:* Dicycloverine (p.481·2).
*Smooth muscle spasm.*

**Spasmo-Proxyvon Forte** *Wockhardt, India.*
Dicycloverine (p.481·2); diclofenac sodium (p.32·1).
*Smooth muscle spasm.*

**Spasmo-Rhoival TC** *Byk Gulden, Ger.; Byk Tosse, Ger.*
Trospium chloride (p.491·2).
*Bladder function disorders.*

**Spasmosarto** *Biosarto, Spain†.*
Trospium chloride (p.491·2).
*Urinary incontinence.*

**Spasmosedine**
*Note. This name is used for preparations of different composition.*
*Pharmethic, Belg.†.*
Crataegus (p.1677·1); phenobarbital (p.367·3); quinine hydrobromide (p.460·2); meprobamate (p.706·2).
*Arrhythmias; vascular spasm.*

*DB, Fr.*
Crataegus (p.1677·1).
Formerly contained crataegus and phenobarbital.
*Cardiac disorders; nervous disorders.*

**Spasmosol** *Streuli, Switz.*
Morphine hydrochloride (p.60·1); codeine hydrochloride (p.27·1); noscapine hydrochloride (p.1125·3); atropine sulfate (p.477·1); papaverine hydrochloride (p.1728·1).
*Pain.*

**Spasmo-Solugastril**
*Sanova, Austria; Pharmacia, Ger.*
Aluminium hydroxide (p.1249·2); butinoline phosphate (p.1663·3); calcium carbonate (p.1254·2).
*Gastrointestinal disorders.*

**Spasmosyx F** *Syxyl, Ger.*
Homoeopathic preparation.

**Spasmotropin** *Legrand, Braz.*
Dipyrone (p.35·3); papaverine hydrochloride (p.1728·1); homatropine methylbromide (p.483·2).
*Smooth muscle spasm.*

**Spasmo-Urgenin**
*Madaus, Austria; Neo-Farmaceutica, Port.; Byk Madaus, S.Afr.; Madaus, Spain; Madaus, Thai.*
Trospium chloride (p.491·2); echinacea (p.1683·2); saw palmetto (p.1569·1).
*Prostatic and urinary-tract spasm and pain.*

**Spasmo-Urgenin TC** *Hoyer, Ger.*
Trospium chloride (p.491·2).
*Bladder function disorders.*

**Spasmo-Urgenine Neo** *Biomed, Switz.*
Trospium chloride (p.491·2).
Spasmo-Urgenine formerly contained trospium chloride, echinacea angustifolia, and saw palmetto.
*Urinary-tract disorders.*

**Spasmowern** *Wernigerode, Ger.*
Hyoscine butylbromide (p.483·3).
*Smooth muscle spasm.*

**Spasmoxyl** *Berner, Fin.*
Oxybutynin hydrochloride (p.486·3).
*Bladder function disorders.*

**Spassirex** *Irex, Fr.*
Phloroglucinol (p.1731·1).
*Smooth muscle pain and spasm.*

**Spastrex** *Propan, S.Afr.*
Oxyphenonium bromide (p.487·2).
*Gastrointestinal and urinary-tract spasm.*

**Spasuret** *Pierre Fabre, Ger.*
Flavoxate hydrochloride (p.482·2).
*Urinary-tract disorders.*

**Spasuri** *Pharmasant, Thai.*
Flavoxate hydrochloride (p.482·2).
*Urinary-tract disorders.*

**Spasyt** *TAD, Ger.*
Oxybutynin hydrochloride (p.486·3).
*Bladder instability; urinary incontinence.*

**Spatab** *Sriprasit, Thai.*
Hyoscine butylbromide (p.483·3).
*Gastrointestinal and urinary-tract disorders; smooth muscle spasm.*

**Spatix** *Bioprogress, Ital.*
Suleparoid (p.1009·1).
*Vascular disorders with a risk of thrombosis.*

**Spaziron** *Vilco, Gr.*
Sodium cromoglicate (p.795·3).
*Allergic conjunctivitis.*

**Spazol** *Siam Bheasach, Thai.*
Itraconazole (p.401·3).
*Fungal infections.*

**Speciafoldine** *Theraplix, Fr.*
Folic acid (p.1429·1).
*Nutritional deficiency; prevention of neural tube disorders.*

**Special Defense Sun Block** *Clinique, Canad.†.*
*SPF 25:* Titanium dioxide (p.1160·3).
*Sunscreen.*

**Specicef-N** *Specifar (Σπεσιφαρ), Gr.*
Propylene glycol cefatrizine (p.170·3).
*Bacterial infections.*

**Speci-Chol** *Pekana, Ger.*
Homoeopathic preparation.

**Species Carvi comp** *Weleda, Austria.*
Aniseed (p.1655·2); urtica (p.1762·1); fennel (p.1687·2); caraway (p.1667·2).
*Flatulence; gastrointestinal cramp.*

**Species nervinae** *Kwizda, Austria.*
Hypericum (p.299·1); valerian (p.1762·2); melissa leaf (p.1711·1); peppermint leaf (p.1283·2).
*Anxiety disorders; sleep disorders.*

**Specifthir** *Specifar (Σπεσιφαρ), Gr.*
Malathion (p.1507·1).
*Head and crab lice; scabies.*

**Specilid** *Specifar (Σπεσιφαρ), Gr.*
Nimesulide (p.67·1).
*Inflammation; musculoskeletal disorders; pain.*

**Specinor** *Specifar (Σπεσιφαρ), Gr.*
Ranitidine hydrochloride (p.1285·2).
*Conditions where gastric acid reduction is beneficial; gastric hypersecretion including Zollinger-Ellison syndrome; gastro-intesinal ulcer.*

**Spec-T**
*Note. This name is used for preparations of different composition.*
*Apothecon, USA†.*
Dextromethorphan hydrobromide (p.1117·3); benzocaine (p.1370·3).
*Coughs.*

*Squibb, USA†.*
Benzocaine (p.1370·3).
*Sore throat.*

**Spec-T Sore Throat/Decongestant** *Apothecon, USA†.*
Phenylpropanolamine hydrochloride (p.1127·3); phenylephrine hydrochloride (p.1126·3); benzocaine (p.1370·3).
*Upper respiratory-tract symptoms.*

**Spectazole** *Ortho Dermatological, USA.*
Econazole nitrate (p.397·2).
*Fungal skin infections.*

**Spectra** *Solus, India.*
Doxepin (p.291·2).
*Depression.*

**Spectraban**
*Note. This name is used for preparations of different composition.*
*Stiefel, Arg.; Stiefel, Mex.*
*SPF 20:* Oxybenzone (p.1154·3); homosalate (p.1148·1); octinoxate (p.1154·3).
*Sunscreen.*

*Stiefel, Braz.*
Aminobenzoic acid (p.1142·2).
*Sunscreen.*

*Stiefel, Chile.*
Oxybenzone (p.1154·3); octinoxate (p.1154·3); homosalate (p.1148·1).
*Sunscreen.*

*Stiefel, S.Afr.†.*
*SPF 4:* Padimate O (p.1155·1).
*Sunscreen.*

*Stiefel, Thai.*
*SPF 19:* Zinc oxide (p.1163·2).
*Sunscreen.*

*Stiefel, UK.*
*SPF 25:* Padimate O (p.1155·1); aminobenzoic acid (p.1142·2).
*Sunscreen.*

**Spectraban 55**
*Stiefel, Chile; Stiefel, Mex.*
*SPF 55:* Octinoxate (p.1154·3); oxybenzone (p.1154·3); sulisobenzone (p.1158·3); titanium dioxide (p.1160·3).
*Sunscreen.*

**Spectraban T** *Stiefel, Braz.*
Padimate O (p.1155·1); avobenzone (p.1142·3); titanium dioxide (p.1160·3).
*Sunscreen.*

**Spectraban Ultra**
*Note. This name is used for preparations of different composition.*
*Stiefel, Chile.*
Padimate O (p.1155·1); avobenzone (p.1142·3); oxybenzone (p.1154·3).
*Sunscreen.*

*Stiefel, Mex.*
*SPF 30 (UVB); SPF 6 (UVA):* Padimate O (p.1155·1); oxybenzone (p.1154·3); avobenzone (p.1142·3); titanium dioxide (p.1160·3).
*Sunscreen.*

*Stiefel, Thai.; Stiefel, UK.*
*SPF 28:* Padimate O (p.1155·1); avobenzone (p.1142·3); oxybenzone (p.1154·3); titanium dioxide (p.1160·3).
*Sunscreen.*

**Spectracef** *Purdue, USA.*
Cefditoren pivoxil (p.172·1).
*Bacterial infections.*

**Spectracil** *Alliance, S.Afr.*
Ampicillin trihydrate (p.157·2).
*Bacterial infections.*

**Spectramedryn** *Allergan, Ger.†.*
Medrysone (p.1106·1).
*Allergic and inflammatory disorders of the eye.*

**Spectramox** *Alliance, S.Afr.*
Amoxicillin trihydrate (p.155·3).
*Bacterial infections.*

**Spectrapain** *Alliance, S.Afr.*
Paracetamol (p.76·2); codeine phosphate (p.27·1).
*Pain.*

**Spectrapain Forte** *Alliance, S.Afr.*
Paracetamol (p.76·2); codeine phosphate (p.27·1); caffeine (p.782·1); meprobamate (p.706·2).
*Pain and associated tension.*

**Spectrasone** *Alliance, S.Afr.*
Erythromycin estolate (p.208·1).
*Bacterial infections.*

**Spectratet** *Alliance, S.Afr.†.*
Oxytetracycline (p.241·1).
*Bacterial infections.*

**Spectrim** *Alliance, S.Afr.*
Co-trimoxazole (p.199·3).
*Bacterial infections.*

**Spectro Derm** *Block, Canad.*
Skin cleanser.
*Cleansing of abraded and irritated skin.*

**Spectro Gluvs** *Block, Canad.*
Barrier cream.

**Spectro Gram** *Block, Canad.*
Chlorhexidine gluconate (p.1173·2).
*Disinfection of skin and hands.*

**Spectro Jel** *Block, Canad.*
Skin cleanser.

**Spectro Tar** *Spectropharm, Canad.*
*Shampoo:* Chlorhexidine gluconate (p.1173·2); coal tar (p.1159·2).
*Scalp disorders.*
*Skin wash:* Coal tar (p.1159·2).
*Eczema; psoriasis.*

**Spectrobid** *Pfizer, USA†.*
Bacampicillin hydrochloride (p.161·2).
*Bacterial infections.*

**Spectrocef** *Epifarma, Ital.*
Cefotaxime sodium (p.175·3).
Lidocaine hydrochloride (p.1377·3) is included in this preparation to alleviate the pain of injection.
*Gram-negative bacterial infections.*

**Spectrocin** *Iquinosa, Spain.*
Gramicidin (p.220·2); neomycin sulfate (p.235·1).
*Infected burns; infected wounds; skin infections; superficial eye infections.*

**Spectrocin Plus** *Numark, USA.*
Neomycin sulfate (p.235·1); polymyxin B sulfate (p.245·1); bacitracin (p.161·3); lidocaine (p.1377·3).
*Bacterial skin infections.*

**Spectro-Jel** *Recsei, USA.*
Soap-free skin cleanser.

**Spectroxyl** *Ecosol, Switz.*
Amoxicillin (p.155·3).
*Bacterial infections.*

**Spectrum**
*Note. This name is used for preparations of different composition.*
*KSL, Canad.†.*
Multivitamin and mineral preparation (p.1417·1).

*Sigma-Tau, Ital.*
Ceftazidime (p.180·2).
*Bacterial infections.*

*Johnson & Johnson Medical, UK.*
Alcohol (p.1166·1); quaternary ammonium compounds.
Formerly contained alcohol, chlorhexidine gluconate, and quaternary ammonium compounds.
*Surface disinfection.*

**Specyton cartilage-parathyroide** *Menarini, Fr.†.*
Cartilage and parathyroid antisera.
*Arthritis.*

**Spedifen** *Inpharzam, Switz.*
Ibuprofen arginine (p.46·3).
*Fever; inflammation; pain.*

**Spedralgin sans codeine** *Democal, Switz.*
Paracetamol (p.76·2); phenazone (p.82·3); propyphenazone (p.85·3); caffeine (p.782·1).
*Fever; pain.*

**Spedro** *Demopharm, Switz.†.*
Codeine phosphate (p.27·1); ephedrine hydrochloride (p.1120·1); belladonna (p.479·1); ipecacuanha (p.1122·3); guaifenesin (p.1122·1); sodium benzoate (p.1169·3); terpin hydrate (p.1131·1).
*Coughs and associated respiratory-tract disorders.*

**Spektramox**
*AstraZeneca, Denm.; AstraZeneca, Fin.; Astra, Swed.*
Amoxicillin trihydrate (p.155·3); potassium clavulanate (p.193·3).
*Bacterial infections.*

**Spel** *Silesia, Chile.*
Betamethasone valerate (p.1093·2).
*Skin disorders.*

**Spencer's Bronchitis** *McGloin, Austral.†.*
Ammonium chloride (p.1115·2); codeine phosphate (p.27·1); phenylpropanolamine hydrochloride (p.1127·3).
*Cold symptoms; throat irritation.*

**Spenglersan** *Apotheke Roten Krebs, Austria.*
A range of homoeopathic bacterial antigens.

**Spenglersan Kolloid** *Meckel, Ger.*
Homoeopathic preparation.

**Spersacarbachol** *Ciba Vision, Switz.†.*
Carbachol (p.1488·1).
*Glaucoma; ocular hypertension.*

**Spersacarpin** *Novartis Ophthalmics, Ger.*
Pilocarpine hydrochloride (p.1495·1).
*Glaucoma; reversal of mydriasis.*

**Spersacarpine**
*Novartis Ophthalmics, Hong Kong; Novartis Ophthalmics, Malaysia; Novartis Ophthalmics, Switz.*
Pilocarpine hydrochloride (p.1495·1).
*Glaucoma; ocular hypertension.*

*Ciba Vision, Singapore†.*
Pilocarpine nitrate (p.1495·1).
*Glaucoma.*

**Spersacet**
*Novartis Ophthalmics, Hong Kong; Novartis Ophthalmics, Switz.*
Sulfacetamide sodium (p.257·3).
*Bacterial eye infections; dacryocystitis.*

**Spersacet C**
*Ciba Vision, Hong Kong†; Restan, S.Afr.; Novartis Ophthalmics, Switz.; Ciba Vision, Thai.†.*
Sulfacetamide sodium (p.257·3); chloramphenicol (p.185·1).
*Bacterial eye infections.*

**Spersadex**
*Novartis Ophthalmics, Ger.; Novartis Ophthalmics, Hong Kong; Novartis, Norw.; Restan, S.Afr.; Novartis Ophthalmics, Switz.*
Dexamethasone sodium phosphate (p.1097·2).
*Inflammatory eye disorders.*

**Spersadex Comp**
*Novartis, Chile; Novartis, Denm.; Novartis Ophthalmics, Ger.; Novartis Ophthalmics, Hong Kong; Novartis Ophthalmics, Malaysia; Restan, S.Afr.; Novartis Ophthalmics, Singapore; Novartis Ophthalmics, Switz.*
Dexamethasone sodium phosphate (p.1097·2); chloramphenicol (p.185·1).
*Inflammatory eye infections.*

**Spersadex med kloramfenikol** *Novartis, Norw.*
Dexamethasone sodium phosphate (p.1097·2); chloramphenicol (p.185·1).
*Inflammatory eye infections.*

**Spersadexolin** *Novartis Ophthalmics, Ger.*
Dexamethasone sodium phosphate (p.1097·2); chloramphenicol (p.185·1); tetryzoline hydrochloride (p.1131·2).
*Eye disorders.*

**Spersadexoline**
*Novartis Ophthalmics, Hong Kong; Novartis Ophthalmics, Malaysia; Restan, S.Afr.; Novartis Ophthalmics, Singapore; Novartis Ophthalmics, Switz.; Novartis, Thai.*
Dexamethasone (p.1097·1) or dexamethasone sodium phosphate (p.1097·2); chloramphenicol (p.185·1); tetryzoline hydrochloride (p.1131·2).
*Inflammatory eye infections.*

**Spersallerg**
*Novartis, Chile; Novartis Ophthalmics, Ger.; Novartis Ophthalmics, Hong Kong; Novartis Ophthalmics, Malaysia; Novartis, Norw.; Restan, S.Afr.; Novartis Ophthalmics, Singapore; Novartis Ophthalmics, Switz.; Novartis, Thai.*
Antazoline hydrochloride (p.424·2); tetryzoline hydrochloride (p.1131·2).
*Allergic conjunctivitis.*

**Spersamide** *Restan, S.Afr.*
Sulfacetamide sodium (p.257·3).
*Eye infections.*

**Spersanicol**
*Novartis Ophthalmics, Hong Kong; Novartis Ophthalmics, Malaysia; Novartis, Mex.†; Restan, S.Afr.; Novartis Ophthalmics, Singapore; Novartis Ophthalmics, Switz.*
Chloramphenicol (p.185·1).
*Eye infections; lachrymo-nasal irrigation.*

**Spersapolymyxin**
*Ciba Vision, Hong Kong†; Novartis Ophthalmics, Switz.; Novartis, Thai.*
Polymyxin B sulfate (p.245·1); neomycin sulfate (p.235·1).
*Bacterial eye infections.*

**Spersatear** *Restan, S.Afr.*
Hypromellose (p.1579·3).
*Dry eyes.*

**Sperti Plus Preparacion H** *Wyeth-Whitehall, Arg.*
Shark-liver oil; phenylephrine hydrochloride (p.1126·3).
*Haemorrhoids.*

**Sperti Praparation H**
*Note. This name is used for preparations of different composition.*
*Wyeth Lederle, Austria.*
*Rectal gel:* Hamamelis (p.1696·3).
*Rectal ointment; suppositories:* Yeast (p.1469·1); shark-liver oil.
*Haemorrhoids.*

*Whitehall-Much, Ger.*
Yeast (p.1469·1); shark-liver oil.
*Haemorrhoids.*

**Sperti Preparacao H** *Wyeth Consumer, Port.*
Yeast (p.1469·1); shark-liver oil.
*Anorectal disorders.*

**Sperti Preparacion H** *Wyeth-Whitehall, Arg.*
Shark-liver oil.
*Haemorrhoids.*

**Sperti (Preparacion H) Clear Gel** *Wyeth Consumer, Chile.*
Hamamelis (p.1696·3).
*Haemorrhoids.*

**Sperti Preparation H**
*Wyeth Consumer, Neth.; Whitehall-Robins, Switz.*
Yeast (p.1469·1); shark-liver oil.
*Haemorrhoids.*

**Sperti (Preparation H)** *Wyeth Consumer, Chile.*
Yeast (p.1469·1); shark-liver oil.
*Anorectal disorders.*

**Spesicor** *Leiras, Fin.*
Metoprolol succinate (p.957·1) or metoprolol tartrate (p.957·1).
*Angina pectoris; arrhythmias; hypertension; hyperthyroidism; migraine; myocardial infarction.*

**Speton** *Temmler, Port.*
Halazone (p.1181·2).

**Spevin** *Expanpharm, Fr.†.*
Cascara sagrada (p.1255·1); quassia amara (p.1737·2).
*Constipation.*

**SPF 15 For Body** *Shaklee, Canad.*
*SPF 15:* Octinoxate (p.1154·3); oxybenzone (p.1154·3).
*Sunscreen.*

**Spherex** *Pharmacia, Ger.*
Amilomer 25-45 (p.1653·2).
*Adjuvant to antineoplastics in liver cancer.*

**Spherulin** *ALK, USA.*
Coccidioidin (p.1674·1).
*Skin test for coccidioidomycosis.*

**Sphingogel** *LED, Fr.*
Phytosphingosine; mandelic acid (p.228·3); malic acid (p.1709·2); citric acid (p.1673·1); salicylic acid (p.1157·1).
*Acne.*

**S.P.H.P.** *Cantassium Co., UK.*
Prostate gland; spinal cord (p.1709·3); calcium hypophosphite (p.1226·3); nicotinamide (p.1441·2); lecithin (p.1706·1); wheat germ; kola (p.1765·3); vitamin A (p.1451·2); vitamin D (p.1461·2).

**Spicline** *Socopharm, Fr.†.*
Minocycline hydrochloride (p.231·3).
*Bacterial infections.*

**Spidifen**
*Zambon, Belg.*
Ibuprofen (p.45·3).
*Fever; musculoskeletal and joint disorders; pain.*

*Zambon, Port.*
Ibuprofen arginine (p.46·3).
*Inflammation; pain.*

**Spidox** *Phoinix Pharm (Φοινιξ Φαρμ), Gr.*
Nitrendipine (p.973·3).
*Hypertension.*

**Spidufen** *Zambon, Braz.*
Ibuprofen arginine (p.46·3).
*Inflammation; pain.*

**Spigelon** *Peithner, Austria.*
Homoeopathic preparation.

**Spilacnet** *Nettopharma, Denm.†.*
Spironolactone (p.1003·1).
*Hyperaldosteronism; hypertension; oedema.*

**Spilan** *Kanoldt, Ger.†.*
Hypericum (p.299·1).
*Anxiety disorders; depression.*

**Spir** *Inava, Fr.*
Beclometasone dipropionate (p.1091·1).
*Asthma.*

**Spiracin** *TO-Chemicals, Thai.*
Spiramycin (p.255·3).
*Bacterial infections.*

**Spiractin**
*Alphapharm, Austral.; Aspen, S.Afr.*
Spironolactone (p.1003·1).
*Heart failure; hepatic cirrhosis with ascites or oedema; hirsutism in females; hyperaldosteronism; hypertension; nephrotic syndrome; oedema.*

**Spiralgin** *Spirig, Switz.*
Mefenamic acid (p.55·2).
*Fever; inflammation; pain.*

**Spiraphan** *Kattwiga, Ger.*
Homoeopathic preparation.

**Spiravet** *Merial, Denm.†.*
Spiramycin (p.255·3).
*Bacterial infections.*

**Spirbon** *Calea, Austria.*
Chlorphenoxamine hydrochloride (p.428·3); ephedrine hydrochloride (p.1120·1); emetine hydrochloride (p.604·3).
*Respiratory-tract disorders.*

**Spiresis** *Orion, Fin.*
Spironolactone (p.1003·1).
*Hyperaldosteronism; hypertension; liver cirrhosis with ascites; oedema.*

**Spiretic** *DDSA Pharmaceuticals, UK†.*
Spironolactone (p.1003·1).

**Spirial**
*SVR, Fr.; SVR, Ital.*
Aluminium chlorohydrate (p.1142·1).
*Hyperhidrosis.*

**Spiricort** *Spirig, Switz.*
Prednisolone (p.1108·1).
*Corticosteroid.*

**Spiridazide** *SIT, Ital.*
Spironolactone (p.1003·1); hydrochlorothiazide (p.933·2).
*Hyperaldosteronism.*

**Spiridon** *Orion, Singapore†.*
Spironolactone (p.1003·1).
*Heart failure; hyperaldosteronism; hypertension; liver cirrhosis; nephrotic syndrome; oedema.*

**Spirillon** *Worwag, Ger.*
Mineral (p.1217·1) and trace element (p.1417·1) preparation.

**Spirit Salicyl** *Floris, Israel.*
Salicylic acid (p.1157·1); alcohol (p.1166·1).
*Keratinisation disorders; skin disinfection.*

**Spirit Whitfield** *Floris, Israel.*
Salicylic acid (p.1157·1); benzoic acid (p.1169·3).
*Fungal skin infections.*

**Spiriva**
*Boehringer Ingelheim, Austral.; Boehringer Ingelheim, Chile; Boehringer Ingelheim, Irl.; Boehringer Ingelheim, Port.; Boehringer Ingelheim, UK; Boehringer Ingelheim, USA; Pfizer, USA.*
Tiotropium bromide (p.806·2).
*Obstructive airways disease.*

**Spirix**
*Nycomed, Denm.; Nycomed, Fin.; Nycomed, Norw.; Nycomed, Swed.*
Spironolactone (p.1003·1).
*Hyperaldosteronism; hypertension; liver cirrhosis with ascites; oedema.*

**spiro** *CT, Ger.*
Spironolactone (p.1003·1).
*Ascites; hyperaldosteronism; oedema.*

**Spiro comp** *Ratiopharm, Ger.*
Spironolactone (p.1003·1); furosemide (p.919·3).
*Ascites; hyperaldosteronism; liver cirrhosis; nephrotic syndrome; oedema.*

**Spirobene** *Ratiopharm, Austria.*
Spironolactone (p.1003·1).
*Hyperaldosteronism; hypertension; oedema.*

**Spirobeta** *Betapharm, Ger.*
Spironolactone (p.1003·1).
*Ascites; hyperaldosteronism; oedema.*

**Spiro-Co** *Norton, UK†.*
Spironolactone (p.1003·1); hydroflumethiazide (p.937·2).
These ingredients are present in such proportions that together they can be described by the British Approved Name Co-flumactone.
*Heart failure.*

**Spirocort**
*AstraZeneca, Arg.; AstraZeneca, Denm.; Simesa, Ital.*
Budesonide (p.1094·2).
*Asthma; nasal polyps; rhinitis.*

**Spiroctan**
*Ferlux, Fr.; Roche, Switz.†.*
Potassium canrenoate (p.984·2) or spironolactone (p.1003·1).
*Adjuvant in myasthenia; hyperaldosteronism; hypertension; oedema.*

**Spiroctazine** *Ferlux, Fr.*
Spironolactone (p.1003·1); altizide (p.858·1).
*Hypertension; oedema.*

**Spiro-D** *Lichtenstein, Ger.*
Spironolactone (p.1003·1); furosemide (p.919·3).
*Ascites; hyperaldosteronism; oedema.*

**Spiroderm** *Monsanto, Ital.*
Spironolactone (p.1003·1).
*Acne.*

**Spirofur** *Bruno, Ital.*
Spironolactone (p.1003·1); furosemide (p.919·3).
*Hypertension; oedema.*

**Spirogamma** *Worwag, Ger.*
Spironolactone (p.1003·1).
*Ascites; hyperaldosteronism; oedema.*

**Spirogel** *Worndli, Switz.†.*
Camphor (p.1665·3); phenol (p.1188·1); cinnamic acid (p.1177·3); cinnamaldehyde; guaiacol (p.1122·1); phenazone (p.82·3); chlorobutanol (p.1176·3); thymol iodide (p.1194·3); thymol (p.1194·2); anethole (p.1654·3); safrole (p.1742·1); eugenol (p.1686·2).
*Dental disorders.*

**Spirohexal** *Hexal, Austria.*
Spironolactone (p.1003·1).
*Hyperaldosteronism; hypertension; oedema.*

**Spirolair** *3M, Belg.†.*
Pirbuterol acetate (p.790·3).
*Asthma; bronchitis; emphysema.*

**Spirolang** *SIT, Ital.*
Spironolactone (p.1003·1).
*Hyperaldosteronism; hypertension.*

**Spirolept** *Thea, Fr.*
An inactivated leptospirosis vaccine (p.1622·2).
*Active immunisation.*

**Spirometon** *Belmac, Spain.*
Bendroflumethiazide (p.867·3); spironolactone (p.1003·1).
*Hypertension; oedema.*

**Spiromide** *RPG, India.*
Furosemide (p.919·3); spironolactone (p.1003·1).
*Hypertension; oedema.*

**Spiromix** *Pulitzer, Ital.*
Spiramycin (p.255·3).
*Bacterial infections.*

**Spiron**
*Note. This name is used for preparations of different composition.*
*Andromaco, Chile.*
Risperidone (p.719·2).
*Schizophrenia.*

*Orion, Denm.*
Spironolactone (p.1003·1).
*Ascites; hyperaldosteronism; oedema.*

**Spironex** *PP Lab, Thai.*
Spironolactone (p.1003·1).
*Ascites; hypertension; oedema; primary aldosteronism.*

**Spirono**
*Genericon, Austria; Alpharma-Isis, Ger.*
Spironolactone (p.1003·1).
*Hyperaldosteronism; hypertension; liver cirrhosis with ascites and oedema; oedema.*

**Spirono comp** *Genericon, Austria.*
Spironolactone (p.1003·1); furosemide (p.919·3).
*Hyperaldosteronism; oedema.*

**Spironol** *Pharbita, Israel.*
Spironolactone (p.1003·1).
*Heart failure; hepatic cirrhosis; hypertension; hypokalaemia; oedema; primary hyperaldosteronism.*

**Spironolacton Plus** *Heumann, Ger.*
Spironolactone (p.1003·1) furosemide (p.919·3).
*Ascites; oedema.*

**Spironone** *Dexo, Fr.*
Spironolactone (p.1003·1).
*Adjuvant in myasthenia; hyperaldosteronism; hypertension; oedema.*

**Spironothiazid**
*Desma, Ger.; Synthelabo, Switz.†.*
Spironolactone (p.1003·1); hydrochlorothiazide (p.933·2).
*Ascites; hyperaldosteronism; hypertension; oedema.*

**Spiropal** *Nycomed, Norw.†.*
Spironolactone (p.1003·1).
*Hyperaldosteronism; hypertension; oedema.*

**Spiropent**
*Boehringer Ingelheim, Austria; Boehringer Ingelheim, Ger.; Boehringer Ingelheim, Gr.; Boehringer Ingelheim, Ital.; Teijin, Jpn; Promeco, Mex.; Boehringer Ingelheim, Spain.*
Clenbuterol hydrochloride (p.784·2).
*Obstructive airways disease.*

**Spiroscand** *Enapharm, Swed.*
Spironolactone (p.1003·1).
*Hyperaldosteronism; hypertension; liver cirrhosis with ascites; oedema.*

**Spirosine** *Faran, Gr.*
Cefotaxime sodium (p.175·3).
*Bacterial infections.*

**Spirospare** *Ashbourne, UK.*
Spironolactone (p.1003·1).
*Ascites; heart failure; nephrotic syndrome; oedema; primary hyperaldosteronism.*

**Spirostada comp** *Stada, Ger.*
Spironolactone (p.1003·1); bendroflumethiazide (p.867·3).
*Ascites; hyperaldosteronism; hypertension; oedema.*

**Spiro-Tablinen** *Sanorania, Ger.†.*
Spironolactone (p.1003·1).
*Ascites; hyperaldosteronism; oedema.*

**Spirotone** *Pacific, NZ.*
Spironolactone (p.1003·1).
*Aldosteronism; heart failure; hepatic cirrhosis with ascites; hirsutism; hypertension; hypokalaemia; nephrotic syndrome; oedema.*

**Spirox** *Agepha, Austria†.*
Spironolactone (p.1003·1).
*Hyperaldosteronism; hypertension; nephrotic syndrome; oedema.*

**Spirsa** *Alter, Spain.*
Chlorphenamine maleate (p.427·3); phenylephrine hydrochloride (p.1126·3); paracetamol (p.76·2).
*Cold and influenza symptoms.*

**Spitacid** *Henkel, Ger.*
Alcohol (p.1166·1); isopropyl alcohol (p.1184·3); benzyl alcohol (p.1170·2).
*Hand disinfection.*

**Spitaderm**
*Paragerm, Fr.; Henkel, Ital.*
Isopropyl alcohol (p.1184·3); chlorhexidine gluconate (p.1173·2); hydrogen peroxide (p.1182·2).
*Skin disinfection.*

**Spitalen** *Erfa, Belg.*
Virginiamycin (p.277·3); neomycin sulfate (p.235·1).
*Bacterial infections.*

**Spizef**
*Grunenthal, Austria; Takeda, Austria; Grunenthal, Ger.*
Cefotiam hydrochloride (p.177·2).
Lidocaine hydrochloride (p.1377·3) may be included in the intramuscular injection to alleviate the pain of injection.
*Bacterial infections.*

**SPL** *Delmont, USA.*
Two strains of lysed *Staphylococcus aureus* in solution (p.1640·2).
*Staphylococcal infection.*

**Splendil**
*AstraZeneca, Braz.; AstraZeneca, Chile; Astra, Jpn.*
Felodipine (p.914·3).
*Angina pectoris; hypertension.*

**Splenocarbine** *Lesourd, Fr.*
Activated charcoal (p.1030·2).
*Gastrointestinal disorders.*

**Splenofigon** *Hertz, Braz.†.*
Vitamin B substances; lysine; sodium glutamate (p.1417·1).
*Digestive disorders.*

**Splen-Uvocal** *Stroschein, Ger.†.*
Spleen extract.
*Immunotherapy.*

**Spm-OK** *Wassen, Ital.*
Vitamins; magnesium; zinc; borage oil; griffonia simplicifolia; agnus castus (p.1417·1).
*Nutritional supplement.*

**Spolera** *OTW, Ger.*
Acmella ciliata.
*Insect stings; soft-tissue injuries.*

**Spondylon** *Riemser, Ger.*
*Capsules:* Ketoprofen (p.51·2).
*Gout; inflammation; musculoskeletal, joint, and soft-tissue disorders; pain.*
*Embrocation:* Methyl nicotinate (p.59·2); camphor (p.1665·3).
*Muscular and neuromuscular disorders.*

**Spondylonal** *ICN, Ger.*
Multivitamin preparation (p.1417·1).

**Spondyvit** *ICN, Ger.*
*d*-Alpha tocoferil acetate (p.1465·1).
*Vitamin E deficiency.*

**Spongostan** *Ethicon, Ital.†.*
Absorbable gelatin sponge (p.754·3).
*Haemorrhage.*

**Sponsin** *Farmasan, Ger.*
Co-dergocrine mesilate (p.1674·1).
*Adjuvant for mental function disorders; cervical disc syndrome; hypertension.*

**Sponwiga** *Kattwiga, Ger.*
Homoeopathic preparation.

**Sporacid** *IMS, Ital.*
Glutaral (p.1180·3).
*Instrument disinfection.*

**Sporahexal** *Hexal, Austral.*
Cefalexin (p.168·1).
*Bacterial infections.*

**Sporal** *Janssen-Cilag, Thai.*
Itraconazole (p.401·3).
*Fungal infections.*

**Sporanox**
*Janssen-Cilag, Arg.; Janssen-Cilag, Austral.; Janssen-Cilag, Austria; Janssen-Cilag, Belg.; Janssen-Cilag, Braz.; Janssen-Ortho, Canad.; Janssen-Cilag, Chile; Janssen-Cilag, Denm.; Janssen-Cilag, Fin.; Janssen-Cilag, Fr.; Janssen-Cilag, Gr.; Janssen, Hong Kong; Janssen-Cilag, Irl.; Janssen-Cilag, Israel; Janssen-Cilag, Ital.; Janssen-Cilag, Malaysia; Janssen, Mex.; Janssen-Cilag, Norw.; Janssen-Cilag, NZ; Janssen-Cilag, Port.; Janssen-Cilag, S.Afr.; Janssen-Cilag, Singapore; Janssen-Cilag, Spain; Janssen-Cilag, Swed.; Janssen-Cilag, Switz.; Janssen-Cilag, UK; Janssen, USA.*
Itraconazole (p.401·3).
*Fungal infections.*

**Sporasec** *Janssen, Mex.*
Itraconazole (p.401·3); secnidazole (p.615·3).
*Bacterial and fungal vaginosis.*

**Sporcid** *Fresenius Kabi, Ger.*
Glutaral (p.1180·3); formaldehyde (p.1179·3).
Formerly contained 2-alkoxi-3,4-dihydro-2-H-pyran aldehyde adduct, formaldehyde, glyoxal, ricinoleic acid propylamidotrimethylammonium methosulfate, and oleylaminooxyethylate.
*Instrument disinfection.*

**Sporex**
*Note. This name is used for preparations of different composition.*
*Rougier, Canad.†.*
Formaldehyde (p.1179·3); benzalkonium chloride (p.1168·3); sodium nitrite (p.1052·3).
*Instrument sterilisation.*

*IMS, Ital.*
Glutaral (p.1180·3).
*Instrument disinfection.*

**Sporicef** *Ranbaxy, Thai.*
Cefalexin (p.168·1).
*Bacterial infections.*

**Sporicidin** *IMS, Ital.*
Glutaral-phenate complex (p.1181·1).
*Instrument and surface disinfection.*

**Sporidex**
*Ranbaxy, India; Ranbaxy, Malaysia; Ranbaxy, Singapore; Ranbaxy, Thai.*
Cefalexin (p.168·1).
*Bacterial infections.*

**Sporidox Plus** *IMS, Ital.*
Peracetic acid (p.1187·3).
*Instrument disinfection.*

**Sporiline** *Schering-Plough, Fr.*
Tolnaftate (p.410·1).
*Fungal skin infections.*

**Sporinex** *Medochemie, Thai.*
Tinidazole (p.617·1).
*Amoebiasis; giardiasis; trichomoniasis.*

**Sporlab** *Biolab, Thai.*
Itraconazole (p.401·3).
*Fungal infections.*

**Sporlac** *Uni-Sankyo, India.*
*Lactobacillus sporogenes* (p.1704·2).
*Antibiotic-associated diarrhoea; moniliasis.*

**Spornar** *Charoen Bhaesaj, Thai.*
Itraconazole (p.401·3).
*Fungal infections.*

**Sporostatin** *Schering-Plough, Braz.*
Griseofulvin (p.400·3).
*Fungal infections.*

**Sporoxyl** *Bangkok Lab & Cosmetic, Thai.*
Ketoconazole (p.403·3).
*Fungal infections.*

**Sport Sunblock** *Avon, Canad.†.*
*SPF 30:* Octinoxate (p.1154·3); octisalate (p.1154·3); oxybenzone (p.1154·3).
*Sunscreen.*

**Sportenine**
*Boiron, Canad.; Boiron, Port.†.*
Homoeopathic preparation.

**Sportino** *Harras-Curarina, Ger.*
Heparin sodium (p.928·1).
*Soft-tissue injury; superficial vascular disorders.*

**Sportino Akut**
*Kwizda, Austria; Harras-Curarina, Ger.*
Glycol salicylate (p.44·3); arnica (p.1656·3).
*Musculoskeletal, joint, and soft-tissue disorders.*

**Sportium** *Lyron, Switz.*
Heparin sodium (p.928·1); allantoin (p.1141·3); dexpanthenol (p.1727·2).
*Soft-tissue injuries; venous insufficiency.*

**Sports Eze Bruising Relief** *Brauer, Austral.†.*
*Oral spray:* Homoeopathic preparation.
*Topical gel:* Arnica (p.1656·3).
*Soft-tissue injuries.*

**Sports Eze Joint & Muscle** *Brauer, Austral.†.*
Homoeopathic preparation.

**Sports Multi** *Cenovis, Austral.†.*
Multivitamin and mineral preparation (p.1417·1).

**Sportscreme** *Thompson, USA.*
Trolamine salicylate (p.95·3).
*Muscle, joint, and soft-tissue pain; neuralgia.*

**Sportscreme Ice** *Thompson, USA.*
Menthol (p.1711·3).
*Muscle, joint, and soft-tissue pain; neuralgia.*

**Sportsman Rub** *Salters, S.Afr.†.*
Capsicum oleoresin (p.1667·1); methyl nicotinate (p.59·2); methyl salicylate (p.59·3).
*Musculoskeletal pain.*

**Sportsmega** *Cantassium Co., UK.*
Multivitamin and mineral preparation (p.1417·1).

**Sportupac M** *Terra-Bio, Ger.*
Aesculus (p.1648·2); aescin (p.1648·2).
Sportupac N formerly contained aesculus, aescin, and heparin sodium.
*Bruising.*

**Sportusal** *Permamed, Switz.*
Lauromacrogol 400 (p.1412·3); dimethyl sulfoxide (p.1473·2); heparin sodium (p.928·1); glycol salicylate (p.44·3); dexpanthenol (p.1727·2).
*Soft-tissue trauma; superficial thrombophlebitis; varices.*

**Sportusal Spray sine heparino** *Permamed, Switz.*
Lauromacrogol 400 (p.1412·3); dimethyl sulfoxide (p.1473·2); glycol salicylate (p.44·3); dexpanthenol (p.1727·2); menthol (p.1711·3); camphor (p.1665·3).
*Soft-tissue disorders.*

**Sportz Sunscreen** *Scott, Canad.†.*
*SPF 15:* Octinoxate (p.1154·3); octisalate (p.1154·3); oxybenzone (p.1154·3).
*Sunscreen.*

**Spotof** *CCD, Fr.*
Tranexamic acid (p.760·3).
*Haemorrhage.*

**Spotoway** *Health & Diet Food Co., UK.*
Chlorhexidine (p.1173·2).
*Skin irritation and spots.*

**Spozal** *Chong Kun Dang, Singapore†.*
Ketoconazole (p.403·3).
*Dandruff; fungal scalp infections.*

**Spozol** *Delta, Braz.*
Itraconazole (p.401·3).
*Fungal infections.*

**Spray Anti-Septico** *Johnson & Johnson, Braz.*
Lidocaine hydrochloride (p.1377·3); benzethonium chloride (p.1169·2).

**Spray Auto-Bronzant** *Clarins, Canad.*
*SPF 15:* Avobenzone (p.1142·3); octinoxate (p.1154·3); octisalate (p.1154·3); oxybenzone (p.1154·3).
Formerly contained avobenzone, octocrilene, octinoxate, octisalate, and oxybenzone.
*Sunscreen.*

**Spray de Proteccion Total** *Pierre Fabre Dermo-Cosmetique, Arg.*
Titanium dioxide (p.1160·3); cinnamate.
*Sunscreen.*

**Spray Solaire Bronzage Rapide** *Clarins, Canad.*
*SPF 6:* Avobenzone (p.1142·3); octinoxate (p.1154·3).
*Sunscreen.*

**Spray Solaire Bronzage Securite** *Clarins, Canad.*
*SPF 15:* Octocrilene (p.1154·3); octinoxate (p.1154·3); octisalate (p.1154·3); oxybenzone (p.1154·3).
*Sunscreen.*

**Spraychrome** *Beige, S.Afr.†.*
Merbromin (p.1185·3).
*Minor wound disinfection.*

**Spray-on Bande** *Eagle, Austral.†.*
Povidone and vinyl acetate copolymer.
*Plastic skin preparation for colostomies and ileostomies.*

**Spray-Pax** *Pharmygiene, Fr.*
Pyrethrum (p.1509·3); piperonyl butoxide (p.1509·2).
*Pediculosis.*

**Spray-Tish** *Boehringer Ingelheim, Austral.*
Tramazoline hydrochloride (p.1131·3).
*Nasal congestion.*

**Spray-U-Thin** *Caprice Greystoke, USA†.*
Phenylpropanolamine hydrochloride (p.1127·3).

**Sprediol** *Stroder, Ital.*
Estradiol (p.1550·1).
*Menopausal disorders.*

**Spregal**
*Note. This name is used for preparations of different composition.*
*Pharmygiene, Fr.; Medpro, S.Afr.*
Esdepallethrine (p.1505·1); piperonyl butoxide (p.1509·2).
*Scabies.*

*Wolff, Ger.*
Bioallethrin (p.1500·3); piperonyl butoxide (p.1509·2).
*Scabies.*

**Spren** *Sigma, Austral.*
Aspirin (p.15·1).
*Fever; inhibition of platelet aggregation; pain.*

**Spreor** *Inava, Fr.*
Salbutamol (p.791·3).
*Obstructive airways disease.*

**Sprilon**
*Smith & Nephew, Irl.; Smith & Nephew Healthcare, UK.*
Dimethicone (p.1482·1); zinc oxide (p.1163·2).
*Barrier preparation; eczema; pressure sores; skin fissures; skin ulcers.*

**Sprinsol** *Fortune, Hong Kong.*
Chlorphenamine maleate (p.427·3).
*Hypersensitivity reactions.*

**Sprintec** *Barr, USA.*
21 Tablets, ethinylestradiol (p.1553·2); norgestimate (p.1563·2); 7 tablets, inert.
*Combined oral contraceptive.*

**SPS** *Carolina, USA.*
Sodium polystyrene sulfonate (p.1053·1).
*Hyperkalaemia.*

**SPZ** *Douglas, NZ†.*
Sulfinpyrazone (p.417·3).
*Gout; thromboembolic disorders.*

**Squad** *Irex, Fr.†.*
Flavodate sodium (p.1688·2).
*Menorrhagia; peripheral vascular disorders.*

**Squam** *Gador, Arg.*
*Dental gel:* Disodium etidronate (p.771·2); sodium fluoride (p.1444·3); sodium monofluorophosphate (p.1446·2).
*Toothpaste:* Disodium etidronate (p.771·2); calcium pyrophosphate; sodium fluoride (p.1444·3).
*Dental caries prevention.*

**Squamasol**
*Ichthyol, Austria†; Ichthyol, Ger.*
Salicylic acid (p.1157·1).
*Scalp disorders.*

**Squa-med** *Permamed, Switz.*
Pyrithione zinc (p.1156·2); sodium undecylamide MEA-sulfosuccinate; urea (p.1162·2).
*Scalp disorders.*

**Squaphane**
*Uriage, Fr.; Saninter, Port.†.*
*Shampoo:* Malic acid (p.1709·2); resorcinol (p.1156·3); piroctone olamine (p.1155·2); cade oil (p.1159·2).
*Scalp disorders.*

*Uriage, Fr.; Saninter, Port.†.*
*Lotion:* Malic acid (p.1709·2); piroctone olamine (p.1155·2); cade oil (p.1159·2).
*Scalp disorders.*

**Squibb-HC** *Bristol-Myers Squibb, Austral.†.*
Hydrocortisone acetate (p.1103·3).
*Skin disorders.*

**SRC Expectorant** *Edwards, USA.*
Pseudoephedrine hydrochloride (p.1129·2); guaifenesin (p.1122·1); hydrocodone tartrate (p.45·1).
*Coughs.*

**Srilane**
*Merck, Belg.; Lipha Sante, Fr.; Merck-Lipha, Hong Kong.*
Idrocilamide (p.1394·3).
*Pain in peri-articular and soft-tissue disorders; skeletal muscle spasm; superficial phlebitis.*

**SRM-Rhotard**
*Alliance, S.Afr.; Ethical, Singapore.*
Morphine sulfate (p.60·2).
*Pain.*

**SRO** *Rivero, Arg.*
Sodium chloride; potassium chloride; sodium citrate; glucose (p.1222·2).
*Oral rehydration.*

**SSD**
*Abbott, Canad.; Par, USA.*
Sulfadiazine silver (p.259·1).
*Burns; wounds.*

**SSKI** *Upsher-Smith, USA.*
Potassium iodide (p.1598·1).
*Respiratory-tract disorders.*

**SST**
*Lafon, Fr.; Sinclair, UK.*
Sorbitol (p.1446·3); macrogol (p.1708·2); malic acid (p.1709·2); sodium citrate (p.1223·2).
*Dry mouth.*

**SSZ** *Gufic, India.*
Sulfadiazine silver (p.259·1).
*Fungal corneal infections.*

**ST-52** *Baxter Oncology, Fr.*
Fosfestrol sodium (p.1555·3).
*Prostatic cancer.*

**ST 37** *Menley & James, USA.*
Hexylresorcinol (p.1182·1).
*Antiseptic.*

**St Bonifatius-Tee** *Kolassa, Austria.*
Equisetum (p.1684·1); frangula bark (p.1266·3); senna leaf (p.1288·2); valerian root (p.1762·2); bitter orange (p.1723·3); tilia flower (p.1756·2); boldo leaf (p.1661·2); juniper wood (p.1703·1); rhubarb (p.1287·3).
*Diuretic; gastrointestinal motility disorders.*

**S-T Cort** *Scot-Tussin, USA†.*
Hydrocortisone (p.1103·3).
*Skin disorders.*

**S-T Forte** *Scot-Tussin, USA†.*
Hydrocodone tartrate (p.45·1); phenylephrine hydrochloride (p.1126·3); phenylpropanolamine hydrochloride (p.1127·3); pheniramine maleate (p.438·3); guaifenesin (p.1122·1).
*Coughs and cold symptoms; nasal congestion.*

**S-T Forte 2** *Scot-Tussin, USA.*
Chlorphenamine maleate (p.427·3); hydrocodone tartrate (p.45·1).
*Coughs and cold symptoms.*

**St. Jakobs-Balsam Mono** *Riemser, Ger.*
Zinc oxide (p.1163·2).
*Burns; skin disorders; wounds.*

**St James Balm** *Medico-Biological Laboratories, UK.*
Zinc oxide (p.1163·2); ichthammol (p.1148·2); salicylic acid (p.1157·1); urea (p.1162·2).
*Skin disorders.*

**St Johnswort Compound** *Potter's, UK.*
Juniper oil (p.1703·1); hypericum (p.299·1); salix (p.87·3); cimicifuga (p.1671·3); skullcap (p.1746·3).
*Sciatica.*

**St. Joseph Adult Chewable** *Schering-Plough, USA.*
Aspirin (p.15·1).

**St. Joseph Cold Tablets For Children** *Schering-Plough, USA†.*
Phenylpropanolamine hydrochloride (p.1127·3); paracetamol (p.76·2).
*Upper respiratory-tract symptoms.*

**St. Joseph Cough Suppressant** *Schering-Plough, USA†.*
Dextromethorphan hydrobromide (p.1117·3).
*Coughs.*

**St Luke's Oil** *British Dispensary, Thai.*
Methyl salicylate (p.59·3); menthol (p.1711·3); camphor (p.1665·3); thyme oil (p.1755·3).
*Muscle pain; soft-tissue injury.*

**St Luke's Sports Oil** British Dispensary, Thai.
Methyl salicylate (p.59·3); menthol (p.1711·3); camphor (p.1665·3); eucalyptus oil (p.1686·2).
*Muscle pain; soft-tissue injury.*

**St Mary's Thistle Plus** Eagle, Austral.†.
Silybum marianum (p.1043·3); myrtillus (p.1718·3); taraxacum (p.1751·3).
*Liver tonic; peripheral vascular disorders; psoriasis.*

**St Radegunder Abfuhrtee mild** Synpharma, Austria.
Prunus spinosa; cichorium intybus; fennel (p.1687·2); mallow flower (p.1709·3).
*Constipation.*

**St Radegunder Beruhigungs- und Einschlaftee** Synpharma, Austria.
Valerian root (p.1762·2); lupulus (p.1708·1); orange flower (p.1723·3); melissa leaf (p.1711·1).
*Anxiety disorders; sleep disorders.*

**St Radegunder Blahungstreibender Tee** Synpharma, Austria.
Fennel (p.1687·2); caraway (p.1667·2); peppermint leaf (p.1283·2); chamomile flower (p.1669·3).
*Dyspepsia; flatulence.*

**St Radegunder Bronchialtee** Synpharma, Austria.
Fennel (p.1687·2); thyme (p.1755·2); eucalyptus leaf (p.1686·1); veronica officinalis; verbascum flower (p.1764·1).
*Catarrh.*

**St Radegunder Entschlackungs-Elixier** Synpharma, Austria.
Taraxacum (p.1751·3); pansy; manna (p.1273·1); bitter orange peel (p.1723·3); rose fruit (p.1740·1).
*Diuretic.*

**St Radegunder Entwasserungs-Elixier** Synpharma, Austria.
Birch leaf (p.1660·3); equisetum (p.1684·1); urtica (p.1762·1).
*Urinary-tract disorders.*

**St Radegunder Entwasserungstee** Synpharma, Austria.
Ononis root (p.1723·3); birch leaf (p.1660·3); equisetum (p.1684·1); urtica (p.1762·1).
*Urinary-tract disorders.*

**St Radegunder Fiebertee** Synpharma, Austria.
Tilia flower (p.1756·2); sambucus flower (p.1741·3); chamomile flower (p.1669·3); melissa leaf (p.1711·1).
*Cold symptoms.*

**St Radegunder Herz-Kreislauf-Tonikum** Synpharma, Austria.
Crataegus (p.1677·1); melissa leaf (p.1711·1); rosemary leaf (p.1740·2); bitter orange peel (p.1723·3).
*Cardiac disorders.*

**St Radegunder Herz-Kreislauf-unterstutzender Tee** Synpharma, Austria.
Crataegus (p.1677·1); rosemary leaf (p.1740·2); melissa leaf (p.1711·1); lavender flower (p.1705·1).
*Cardiac disorders.*

**St Radegunder Hustentee** Synpharma, Austria.
Wild thyme; plantago lanceolata (p.1738·2); althaea (p.1651·3); galeopsis ochroleuca; mallow flower (p.1709·3).
*Coughs.*

**St Radegunder Leber-Galle-Tee** Synpharma, Austria.
Cichorium intybus root; taraxacum (p.1751·3); marrubium vulgare root (p.1124·1); peppermint leaf (p.1283·2).
*Gastrointestinal and biliary-tract disorders.*

**St Radegunder Magenberuhigungstee** Synpharma, Austria.
Melissa leaf (p.1711·1); peppermint leaf (p.1283·2); fennel fruit (p.1687·2); mallow flower (p.1709·3).
*Gastrointestinal disorders.*

**St Radegunder Nerventee** Synpharma, Austria.
Melissa leaf (p.1711·1); valerian root (p.1762·2); lupulus (p.1708·1); delphinium consolida flower.
*Nervous disorders; sleep disorders.*

**St Radegunder Nerven-Tonikum** Synpharma, Austria.
Valerian root (p.1762·2); lupulus (p.1708·1); melissa leaf (p.1711·1).
*Nervous disorders; sleep disorders.*

**St Radegunder Nierentee** Synpharma, Austria.
Bearberry (p.1659·2); equisetum (p.1684·1); herniaria (p.1697·1); ononis (p.1723·3).
*Urinary-tract disorders.*

**St Radegunder Reizmildernder Magentee** Synpharma, Austria.
Chamomile flower (p.1669·3); mallow flower and leaf (p.1709·3)(p.1709·3); fennel (p.1687·2); melissa leaf (p.1711·1).
*Gastrointestinal disorders.*

**St Radegunder Rosmarin-Wein** Synpharma, Austria.
Rosemary leaf (p.1740·2); melissa leaf (p.1711·1).
*Circulatory disorders.*

**St Radegunder Tee gegen Durchfall** Synpharma, Austria.
Hamamelis leaf (p.1696·3); strawberry; chamomile flower (p.1669·3); juglans regia; fennel (p.1687·2).
*Diarrhoea.*

**St Radegunder Thorasan-Krauterhustensaft** Synpharma, Austria.
Cowslip (p.1735·1); thyme (p.1755·2); plantago lanceolata (p.1738·2).
*Catarrh; coughs.*

**St Radegunder Verdauungstee** Synpharma, Austria.
Absinthium (p.1645·1); centaury (p.1669·2); bitter orange peel (p.1723·3); caraway (p.1667·2); gentian root (p.1692·2).
*Gastrointestinal disorders.*

**Stabicilline** Vifor, Switz.
Phenoxymethylpenicillin potassium (p.242·1).
*Bacterial infections.*

**Stabilanol** Pharmaten (Φαρματεν), Gr.
Fluconazole (p.398·1).
*Fungal infections.*

**Stablon**
Servier, Arg.; Servier, Austria; Servier, Braz.; Ardix, Fr.; Serdia, India; Servier, Malaysia; Sanfer, Mex.†; Servier, Port.; Servier, Singapore; Servier, Thai.
Tianeptine (p.318·2) or tianeptine sodium (p.318·2).
*Depression; mixed anxiety depressive states.*

**Stacer** Atral, Port.
Ranitidine hydrochloride (p.1285·2).
*Gastro-oesophageal reflux; peptic ulcer; Zollinger-Ellison syndrome.*

**Stacho-Zym N** Kattwiga, Ger.†.
Pancreatin (p.1725·3); enzymes from Aspergillus.
*Digestive system disorders.*

**Stacin** Macrophar, Thai.
Erythromycin (p.208·1).
*Bacterial infections.*

**Stacort-A** Standard, Hong Kong†.
Triamcinolone acetonide (p.1110·2).
*Corticosteroid.*

**Stadaglicin**
Stada, Hong Kong; Stada, Malaysia; Stada, Singapore†; Stada, Thai.†.
Sodium cromoglicate (p.795·3).
*Allergic rhinitis; conjunctivitis.*

**Stadalax** Stada, Ger.
Bisacodyl (p.1251·3).
*Constipation.*

**Stadelant** Chrispa (Χρισπα), Gr.
Enalapril maleate (p.909·2).
*Heart failure; hypertension.*

**Stadol**
Bristol-Myers Squibb, Canad.; Bristol-Myers Squibb, Chile; Bristol-Myers Squibb, Israel†; Bristol-Myers Squibb, Mex.; Bristol-Myers Squibb, USA; Cephalon, USA.
Butorphanol tartrate (p.23·3).
*Pain.*

**Stadovir** Stada, Austria.
Aciclovir (p.626·1).
*Herpes labialis.*

**Stadyl** Medipharma, Hong Kong.
Codeine phosphate (p.27·1); ephedrine hydrochloride (p.1120·1); chlorphenamine maleate (p.427·3); ammonium chloride (p.1115·2).
*Cold and influenza symptoms.*

**Staficilin N** Bristol-Myers Squibb, Braz.
Oxacillin sodium (p.240·2).
*Bacterial infections.*

**Staficyn** FIRMA, Ital.†.
Meticillin sodium (p.230·3).
*Staphylococcal infections.*

**Stafilon** AGIPS, Ital.
Methacycline hydrochloride (p.230·1).
*Bacterial infections.*

**Staflocil** Orion, Fin.
Cloxacillin sodium (p.198·2).
*Bacterial infections.*

**Stafoxil**
Yamanouchi, Irl.†; Yamanouchi, Neth.
Flucloxacillin sodium (p.213·3).
*Bacterial infections.*

**Stagesic** Huckaby, USA.
Hydrocodone tartrate (p.45·1); paracetamol (p.76·2).
*Pain.*

**Stagid**
Lipha Sante, Fr.; Merck, Port.
Metformin embonate (p.342·3).
*Diabetes mellitus.*

**Stago** Synthelabo, Switz.†.
Greater celandine (p.1695·3); turmeric (p.1058·3); cynara scolymus (p.1678·3); boldo (p.1661·2).
*Biliary-tract disorders; constipation; nausea.*

**Stahist** Huckaby, USA.
Pseudoephedrine hydrochloride (p.1129·2); phenylephrine hydrochloride (p.1126·3); chlorphenamine maleate (p.427·3); hyoscyamine sulfate (p.485·1); hyoscine hydrobromide (p.483·3); atropine sulfate (p.477·1).
Formerly contained phenylpropanolamine hydrochloride, phenylephrine hydrochloride, chlorphenamine maleate, hyoscyamine sulfate, hyoscine hydrobromide, and atropine sulfate.
*Upper respiratory-tract symptoms.*

**Stalcin** Locatelli, Ital.†.
Calcitonin (salmon) (p.768·2).
*Hypercalcaemia; osteoporosis; Paget's disease.*

**Stalene** Unison, Thai.
Fluconazole (p.398·1).
*Fungal infections.*

**Stalevo** Orion, UK.
Levodopa (p.1205·2); carbidopa (p.1204·3); entacapone (p.1205·1).
*Parkinsonism.*

**Stallergenes MRV** Stallergenes, Fr.†.
*Staphylococcus aureus*; *Staphylococcus albus*; Streptococcus spp.; *Streptococcus pneumoniae*; *Haemophilus influenzae*; *Klebsiella pneumoniae*; *Moraxella catarrhalis*.
*Respiratory-tract infections.*

**Staloral**
Stallergenes, Ital.
An allergen extract (p.1650·1).
*Allergen immunotherapy.*

Stallergenes, Switz.
Pollen allergen extracts(p.1650·1).
*Allergen immunotherapy.*

**Staltor** Bayer, Fr.†.
Cerivastatin (p.881·3).
*Hypercholesterolaemia.*

**Stamar** Kampel Martian, Arg.
Stavudine (p.654·2).
*HIV infection.*

**Stamaril**
Aventis Pasteur, Arg.; Aventis Pasteur, Austral.; Aventis Pasteur, Belg.; Aventis Pasteur, Chile; Aventis Pasteur, Denm.; Aventis Pasteur, Fin.; Pasteur Vaccins, Fr.; Aventis Pasteur, Ger.; Aventis Pasteur, Irl.; Aventis Pasteur, Ital.; Aventis Pasteur, Malaysia; Aventis Pasteur, Neth.; Aventis Pasteur, Norw.; Aventis, S.Afr.; Aventis Pasteur, Singapore; Aventis Pasteur, Swed.; Pro Vaccine, Switz.; Aventis, UK.
A yellow fever vaccine (17D strain) (p.1644·2).
*Active immunisation.*

**Stamina** Chi Sheng, Thai.
Vitamin B substances with glucose (p.1417·1).

**Stamoist E** Huckaby, USA.
Pseudoephedrine hydrochloride (p.1129·2); guaifenesin (p.1122·1).
*Coughs.*

**Stamoist LA** Huckaby, USA†.
Phenylpropanolamine hydrochloride (p.1127·3); guaifenesin (p.1122·1).
*Coughs and cold symptoms; nasal congestion.*

**Stamoneyrol** Biostam (Βιοσταμ), Gr.
Sulpiride (p.722·2).
*Psychoses.*

**Stancare** Stanley, Canad.†.
Wool fat (p.1483·1); liquid paraffin (p.1479·1).

**Standacillin**
Biochemie, Austria; Biochemie, Malaysia; Biochemie, Singapore.
Ampicillin sodium (p.157·1) or ampicillin trihydrate (p.157·2).
*Bacterial infections.*

**Standard III** Aguettant, Fr.
Electrolyte preparation (p.1217·1).
*Parenteral nutrition.*

**Stangyl**
Rhone-Poulenc Rorer, Austria†; Aventis, Ger.
Trimipramine maleate (p.320·2) or trimipramine mesilate (p.320·3).
*Depression; pain.*

**Stanhexidine** Omega, Canad.
Chlorhexidine gluconate (p.1173·2).

**Stanilo** Pharmacia, Ger.
Spectinomycin hydrochloride (p.255·2).
*Gonorrhoea.*

**Stanno-Bardane** Pharmacobel, Belg.†.
Tin (p.1756·3); lappa (p.1704·3).
*Staphylococcal infections.*

**Stanol** Body Research, Thai.
Stanozolol (p.1569·2).
*Anabolic; hereditary angioedema.*

**Stapenor**
Bayer, Austria; Bayer, Ger.†.
Oxacillin sodium (p.240·2).
*Benzylpenicillin-resistant staphylococcal infections.*

**Staphlex**
Alphapharm, Malaysia; Merck, Malaysia; Pacific, NZ.
Flucloxacillin sodium (p.213·3).
*Gram-positive bacterial infections.*

Merck, Singapore; Pacific, Singapore.
Flucloxacillin (p.213·3).
*Bacterial infections.*

**Staphycid** Trenker, Belg.
Flucloxacillin magnesium (p.213·3) or flucloxacillin sodium (p.213·3).
*Bacterial infections.*

**Staphyclox** Norma (Νορμα), Gr.
Cloxacillin sodium (p.198·2).
*Bacterial infections.*

**Staphylase** Prima, Braz.†.
Dried yeast (p.1469·1); white wine; glycerol.
*Digestive disorders.*

**Staphylex**
Alphapharm, Austral.; GlaxoSmithKline, Ger.
Flucloxacillin magnesium (p.213·3) or flucloxacillin sodium (p.213·3).
*Bacterial infections.*

**Staphypan** Berna, Switz.
Staphylococci.
*Staphylococcal infections.*

**Staporos** Hoechst Marion Roussel, Braz.†.
Calcitonin (pork) (p.768·2).
*Hypercalcaemia; osteoporosis; Paget's disease of bone.*

**Starcef** FIRMA, Ital.
Ceftazidime (p.180·2).
*Gram-negative bacterial infections.*

**Starem** Hoechst, Fr.†.
Dextropropoxyphene hydrochloride (p.28·3); paracetamol (p.76·2).
*Pain.*

**Staril** Bristol-Myers Squibb, UK.
Fosinopril sodium (p.919·1).
*Heart failure; hypertension.*

**Starlep** Farma Lepori, Spain†.
Metoclopramide glycyrrhizinate (p.1276·1); sodium bicarbonate (p.1223·2); tartaric acid (p.1752·1).
*Gastritis, nausea; gastrointestinal hyperacidity; hepatobiliary disorders; vomiting.*

**Starlix**
Novartis, Arg.; Novartis, Braz.; Novartis, Chile; Novartis, Denm.; Novartis, Fin.; Novartis, Ger.; Novartis, Gr.; Novartis, Hong Kong; Novartis, Irl.; Novartis, Malaysia; Novartis, Norw.; Novartis, NZ; Novartis, S.Afr.; Novartis, Singapore; Novartis, Spain; Novartis, Swed.; Novartis, Switz.; Novartis, UK; Novartis, USA.
Nateglinide (p.343·3).
*Diabetes mellitus.*

**Starnoc** Servier, Canad.
Zaleplon (p.727·3).
*Insomnia.*

**Starogyn** Leiras, Fin.
Broxyquinoline (p.165·3).
*Vaginal infections.*

**Star-Otic** Stellar, USA.
Glacial acetic acid (p.1645·2); aluminium acetate (p.1652·3); boric acid (p.1662·1).
*Ear infection.*

**Starox** Grunenthal, Chile.
Gatifloxacin (p.216·2).
*Bacterial infections.*

**Star-Pen** Tyrol, Austria.
Benzathine phenoxymethylpenicillin (p.163·2) or phenoxymethylpenicillin potassium (p.242·1).
*Bacterial infections.*

**Start NP** ICN, Arg.
Gentamicin sulfate (p.217·1); hydrocortisone acetate (p.1103·3); ketoconazole (p.403·3).
*Infected skin disorders.*

**Startonyl**
Wyeth Lederle, Austria; Seber, Port.
Citicoline (p.1672·3).
*Cerebrovascular disorders; head injury.*

**Stas Akut** Stada, Ger.†.
Acetylcysteine (p.1112·3).
*Respiratory-tract disorders with excess mucus.*

**stas Erkaltungssalbe** Stada, Ger.
Camphor (p.1665·3); eucalyptus oil (p.1686·2); pine needle oil.
*Cold symptoms.*

**stas Erkaltungssalbe mild** Stada, Ger.
Eucalyptus oil (p.1686·2); pine needle oil.
*Cold symptoms.*

**Stas Gurgellosung** Stada, Ger.†.
Hexetidine (p.1182·1).
*Inflammatory disorders and infections of the oropharynx.*

**stas Halsschmerz-Tabletten** Stada, Ger.†.
Cetylpyridinium chloride(p.1173·1); dequalinium chloride (p.1178·1).
*Bacterial infections of the mouth and throat.*

**stas Nasentropfen, Nasenspray** Stada, Ger.
Xylometazoline hydrochloride (p.1132·2).
*Nasal congestion; rhinitis.*

**stas-Hustenloser** Stada, Ger.
Ambroxol hydrochloride (p.1114·3).
*Respiratory-tract disorders associated with increased or viscous mucus.*

**stas-Hustenstiller N** Stada, Ger.
Clobutinol hydrochloride (p.1117·1).
*Coughs.*

**Stat-Crit** Wampole, USA.
Test for haematocrit/haemoglobin measurement.

**Statex**
Pharmascience, Canad.; Pharmascience, Singapore.
Morphine sulfate (p.60·2).
*Pain.*

**Staticin**
Westwood-Squibb, Canad.; Westwood, USA.
Erythromycin (p.208·1).
*Acne.*

**Staticine** Bristol-Myers Squibb, Switz.†.
Erythromycin (p.208·1).
*Acne.*

**Staticum** Uriach, Spain.
Glisentide (p.333·1).
*Diabetes mellitus.*

**Statiflex G** Braun, Switz.
Electrolyte infusion with glucose (p.1217·1).
*Carbohydrate source; fluid and electrolyte disorders.*

**Statinclyne** Cazi, Braz.
Tetracycline hydrochloride (p.266·2).
*Bacterial infections.*

**Stativa** Chiesi, Ital.†.
Cerivastatin sodium (p.881·3).
*Hypercholesterolaemia.*

**Statrol**
Note. This name is used for preparations of different composition.
Alcon, Belg.; Alkon (Αλκον), Gr.; Alcon, Thai.†.
Neomycin sulfate (p.235·1); polymyxin B sulfate (p.245·1).
*Bacterial eye infections.*

Alcon Cusi, Spain†.
Neomycin sulfate (p.235·1); polymyxin B sulfate (p.245·1); phenylephrine hydrochloride (p.1126·3).
*Eye infections.*

**Statuss Expectorant** *Huckaby, USA†.*
Phenylpropanolamine hydrochloride (p.1127·3); codeine phosphate (p.27·1); guaifenesin (p.1122·1).
*Coughs.*

**Statuss Green** *Huckaby, USA†.*
Pheniramine maleate (p.438·3); mepyramine maleate (p.437·1); phenylephrine hydrochloride (p.1126·3); phenylpropanolamine hydrochloride (p.1127·3); hydrocodone tartrate (p.45·1).
*Coughs and cold symptoms.*

**Staurodorm**
*Sanova, Austria; Madaus, Belg.*
Flurazepam (p.700·3).
*Insomnia.*

**Staurodorm Neu** *Dolorgiet, Ger.*
Flurazepam (p.700·3).
*Sleep disorders.*

**Stavacin** *Biol, Arg.*
*Staphylococcus aureus.*
*Staphylococcal infections.*

**Stavir** *Cipla, India.*
Stavudine (p.654·2).
*HIV infection.*

**Stay Alert** *Apothecary, USA.*
Caffeine (p.782·1).
*Fatigue.*

**Stay-Wet 3** *Sherman, USA.*
Cleansing, wetting, and soaking solution for gas permeable contact lenses (p.1164·2).

**Stay-Wet 4** *Sherman, USA.*
Wetting solutions for hard contact lenses (p.1164·2).

**STD** *Intramed, S.Afr.†.*
Sodium tetradecyl sulfate (p.1575·1).
*Varicose veins.*

**Stecort-NM** *Stancare, India.*
Beclometasone dipropionate (p.1091·1); neomycin sulfate (p.235·1); miconazole nitrate (p.405·3).
*Infected skin lesions.*

**Stediril**
*Wyeth Lederle, Fr.; Wyeth, Ger.*
Norgestrel (p.1563·2); ethinylestradiol (p.1553·2).
*Combined oral contraceptive; endometriosis; menstrual disorders.*

**Stediril 30**
*Wyeth Lederle, Belg.; Wyeth, Ger.; Wyeth, Switz.*
Levonorgestrel (p.1563·2); ethinylestradiol (p.1553·2).
28-Day packs also contain 7 inert tablets.
*Combined oral contraceptive.*

**Stediril D**
*Wyeth Lederle, Austria; Wyeth Lederle, Belg.; Wyeth, Ger.; Wyeth, Switz.*
Levonorgestrel (p.1563·2); ethinylestradiol (p.1553·2).
*Combined oral contraceptive; endometriosis; menstrual disorders.*

**Stediril 30, Stediril D** *Wyeth, Neth.*
Levonorgestrel (p.1563·2); ethinylestradiol (p.1553·2).
*Combined oral contraceptive.*

**Stedon** *Adelco, Gr.*
Diazepam (p.690·1).
*Alcohol withdrawal syndrome; anxiety disorders; premedication; skeletal muscle spasm; sleep disorders; status epilepticus; tetanus.*

**Stefolant** *Chrispa (Χρισπα), Gr.*
Ambroxol hydrochloride (p.1114·3).
*Respiratory disorders associated with viscous mucus.*

**Steicardin N** *Steigerwald, Ger.*
Homoeopathic preparation.

**Steicorton** *Steigerwald, Ger.*
Crataegus (p.1677·1).
*Heart failure.*

**Steigal** *Steigerwald, Ger.†.*
Turmeric (p.1058·3); greater celandine (p.1695·3).
*Biliary colic.*

**Steinaclox** *Medichrom, Gr.*
Norfloxacin (p.238·3).
*Urinary tract infections.*

**Steiprostat** *Steigerwald, Ger.*
Saw palmetto (p.1569·1).
*Benign prostatic hyperplasia.*

**Steirocall N** *Steierl, Ger.*
Homoeopathic preparation.

**Steiroplex** *Steierl, Ger.*
Homoeopathic preparation.

**Steitonit** *Lopes, Braz.†.*
Podophyllum (p.1155·2); rhubarb (p.1287·3); senna (p.1288·2); olive oil (p.1723·2); peppermint leaf (p.1283·2); castor oil (p.1668·2).
*Calculi.*

**Stelabid**
*GlaxoSmithKline, Canad.; SmithKline Beecham, Irl.†; Armstrong, Mex.*
Isopropamide iodide (p.485·2); trifluoperazine hydrochloride (p.726·3).
*Gastrointestinal disorders.*

**Stelapar**
*Kirby, Arg.; GlaxoSmithKline, Braz.*
Trifluoperazine hydrochloride (p.726·3); tranylcypromine sulfate (p.318·3).
*Mixed anxiety depressive states; psychoses.*

**Stelazine**
*Kirby, Arg.; Link, Austral.; GlaxoSmithKline, Braz.; SmithKline Beecham, Canad.†; Vianex (Βιανεξ), Gr.; Goldshield, Irl.; SmithKline Beecham, Mex.; Link, NZ; Pharmafrica, S.Afr.; Goldshield, UK GlaxoSmithKline, USA†.*
Trifluoperazine hydrochloride (p.726·3).
*Agitation; anxiety; nausea and vomiting; psychoses.*

**Stelea** *Elea, Arg.*
Stavudine (p.654·2).
*HIV infection.*

**Stelium** *Ni-The, Gr.*
Trifluoperazine hydrochloride (p.726·3).
*Psychoses.*

**Stella**
*Note. This name is used for preparations of different composition.*
*Alpharma, Fin.*
Zolpidem tartrate (p.728·3).
*Insomnia.*

*Jean-Marie, Hong Kong†.*
Prochlorperazine mesilate (p.716·3).
*Anxiety; nausea.*

**Stellamicina** *Pierrel, Ital.†.*
Erythromycin estolate (p.208·1).
*Bacterial infections.*

**Stellatropine** *Stella, Belg.*
Atropine sulfate (p.477·1).
*Arrhythmias; cholinesterase inhibitor intoxication; premedication.*

**Stellisept** *Beiersdorf, Switz.†.*
Orthophenylphenol (p.1187·2); sodium laurilsulfate (p.1574·2).
*Skin and hand disinfection.*

**Stellorphinad** *Stella, Belg.*
Morphine hydrochloride (p.60·1).
*Pain.*

**Stellorphine** *Stella, Belg.*
Morphine hydrochloride (p.60·1).
*Acute pulmonary oedema; pain; premedication; severe trauma.*

**Stemetil**
*Aventis, Austral.; Aventis, Canad.; Aventis, Denm.; Aventis, Fin.; Aventis, Hong Kong; Nicholas Piramal, India; Aventis, Irl.; Aventis, Ital.; Aventis, Malaysia; Aventis, Neth.; Aventis, Norw.; Aventis, NZ; Aventis, S.Afr.; Aventis, Singapore; Aventis, Swed.; Aventis, Thai.; Castlemead, UK.*
Prochlorperazine (p.716·2), prochlorperazine maleate (p.716·3), or prochlorperazine mesilate (p.716·3).
*Alcohol and opioid withdrawal syndromes; anxiety; migraine; nausea and vomiting; psychoses; vestibular disorders.*

**Stemgen**
*Amgen, Austral.; Amgen, Canad.*
Ancestim (p.742·2).
*Mobilisation of autologous peripheral blood progenitor cells.*

**Stemiz** *Cadila, India.*
Astemizole (p.424·2).
*Allergic conjunctivitis; allergic rhinitis; allergic skin disorders.*

**Stemzine** *Aventis, Austral.*
Prochlorperazine maleate (p.716·3).
*Nausea and vomiting; psychoses; vertigo.*

**Sten** *Atlantis, Mex.*
Prasterone (p.1565·3); testosterone propionate (p.1570·1); testosterone cipionate (p.1569·3).
*Androgenic; breast cancer; erectile dysfunction; hypogonadism; loss of libido in females.*

**Stenobronchial** *Giovanardi, Ital.*
Sulfogaiacol (p.1131·1); wild thyme; tolu balsam (p.1131·3).
*Coughs, catarrh.*

**Stenocrat** *Schwabe, Ger.*
Ammi visnaga fruit (p.1653·3); crataegus leaves, flowers, and fruit (p.1677·1).
*Angina pectoris.*

**steno-loges N** *Loges, Ger.†.*
Ammi visnaga (p.1653·3).
*Cardiac disorders; obstructive airways disease.*

**Stenoptin** *Teofarma, Ger.*
Verapamil hydrochloride (p.1019·1); isosorbide dinitrate (p.941·1).
*Angina pectoris; myocardial infarction.*

**Stenosara** *Ibefar, Braz.†.*
Vitamin B substances; minerals (p.1417·1).

**Stenox** *Atlantis, Mex.*
Fluoxymesterone (p.1555·3).
*Androgenic; erectile dysfunction; hypogonadism.*

**Steocalcin** *Christiaens, Belg.*
Calcitonin (salmon) (p.768·2).
*Hypercalcaemia; osteolysis; osteoporosis; Paget's disease of bone; reflex sympathetic dystrophy.*

**Steocar** *Christiaens, Belg.*
Calcium carbonate (p.1254·2).
*Calcium deficiency; calcium supplement; osteoporosis.*

**Steocin** *SoSe, Ital.*
Calcitonin (salmon) (p.768·2).
*Hypercalcaemia; osteoporosis; Paget's disease of bone.*

**Steovit D3** *Christiaens, Belg.*
Calcium carbonate (p.1254·2); colecalciferol (p.1461·3).
*Calcium and vitamin D deficiency; osteoporosis.*

**Step 2** *Candioli, Ital.*
Extract of *Triticum sativum*.
*Aid to removal of lice eggs.*

**Stephadilat-S** *Bros, Gr.*
Fluoxetine hydrochloride (p.292·1).
*Depression; obsessive-compulsive disorder; panic disorder.*

**Sterac**
*Note. This name is used for preparations of different composition.*
*Galen, UK†.*
Sterile water (p.1765·1).
*Diluent for antiseptic solutions; wounds.*

*Galen, UK†.*
Sodium chloride (p.1233·3).
*Irrigation solution.*

**Steradent** *Reckitt Benckiser, India.*
Sodium perborate (p.1192·2).
*Denture cleanser.*

**Sterades** *Galderma, Ital.*
Desonide (p.1096·3).
*Skin disorders.*

**Steramin** *Formenti, Ital.*
Benzalkonium chloride (p.1168·3).
*Disinfection of wounds, burns, and mucous membranes.*

**Steramina G** *Formenti, Ital.*
Benzalkonium chloride (p.1168·3).
*Disinfection of wounds, burns, vagina, hands, instruments, surfaces, and skin.*

**Steranabol Ritardo** *Pharmacia Upjohn, Ital.†.*
Oxabolone cipionate (p.1565·1).
*Osteoporosis.*

**Steranios** *Anios, Fr.*
Glutaral (p.1180·3).
*Instrument disinfection.*

**Sterapred** *Merz, USA.*
Prednisone (p.1109·3).
*Corticosteroid.*

**Sterax**
*Galderma, Belg.; Galderma, Chile; Galderma, Ger.†; Galderma, Switz.*
Desonide (p.1096·3).
*Skin disorders.*

**Ster-Dex** *Novartis Ophthalmics, Fr.*
Oxytetracycline (p.241·1); dexamethasone (p.1097·1).
*Eye disorders.*

**Sterets** *SSL, UK.*
Isopropyl alcohol (p.1184·3).
*Skin disinfection.*

**Sterets H**
*Seton, Israel.*
Isopropyl alcohol (p.1184·3); chlorhexidine gluconate (p.1173·2).
*Skin disinfection.*

*SSL, UK.*
Isopropyl alcohol (p.1184·3); chlorhexidine acetate (p.1173·2).
*Skin disinfection.*

**Sterets Unisept** *SSL, UK†.*
Chlorhexidine gluconate (p.1173·2).
*Skin disinfection.*

**Sterex** *International Dermatologicals, Canad.*
Coal tar (p.1159·2); salicylic acid (p.1157·1); sulfur (p.1158·2).

**Sterexidine** *Galen, UK†.*
Chlorhexidine gluconate (p.1173·2).
*Antiseptic irrigation solution.*

**Stericlens** *CD Medical, UK.*
Sodium chloride (p.1233·3).
*Wound irrigation.*

**Steridine** *Xeragen, S.Afr.*
Povidone-iodine (p.1190·3).
*Burns; mouth and throat infections; skin infections; wounds.*

**Steridol** *Biocure, Ital.*
Chlorhexidine gluconate (p.1173·2); cetrimide (p.1172·1).
*Disinfection.*

**Steridrolo** *Molteni, Ital.*
Tosylchloramide sodium (p.1194·3).
*Disinfection of wounds, burns, and external genitals.*

**Steridrolo a rapida idrolisi** *Molteni, Ital.*
Halazone (p.1181·2).
*Water purification.*

**Sterigel** *SSL, UK.*
Hemicellulose (p.1578·3).
*Ulcers; wounds.*

**Sterigin** *Merck, Austria.*
Estradiol (p.1550·1).
*Menopausal disorders; osteoporosis.*

**Sterigynon** *Arcana, Austria.*
Cyproterone acetate (p.1544·1); ethinylestradiol (p.1553·2).
*Acne and hirsutism in women; oral contraceptive in women with androgen-associated symptoms.*

**Steril Zeta** *Zeta, Ital.*
*Cream:* Triclosan (p.1195·2); usnic acid (p.1762·1); hamamelis (p.1696·3); cod-liver oil (p.1425·2).
*Topical powder:* Triclosan (p.1195·2); usnic acid (p.1762·1); zinc oxide (p.1163·2); zinc stearate (p.1575·3).
*Disinfection of burns and wounds.*

**Sterilene** *Amsa, Ital.*
Cetrimonium tosilate (p.1173·1).
*Vaginal disinfection.*

**Sterilent** *SIFI, Ital.†.*
Sterilising solution for hard contact lenses (p.1164·2).

**Sterilite** *Coventry, UK†.*
Tar acids (p.1193·3).

**Sterillium**
*Bode, Austria; Rivadis, Fr.; Bode, Ger.*
Mecetronium etilsulfate (p.1185·2); isopropyl alcohol (p.1184·3); propyl alcohol (p.1191·2).
*Skin disinfection.*

**Sterillium Virugard** *Bode, Ger.*
Alcohol (p.1166·1).
*Hand disinfection.*

**Sterilon**
*Boots Healthcare, Belg.; Boots Healthcare, Neth.; Boots, Spain†.*
Chlorhexidine gluconate (p.1173·2) or chlorhexidine hydrochloride (p.1173·3).
*Skin and wound disinfection.*

**Sterimar**
*Merck, Austria; Fumouze, Fr.; Veron, Ger.; Intra Pharma, Irl.; Fumouze, Israel; Baldacci, Ital.; Viatris, Port.; Doetsch, Grether, Switz.; Carter-Wallace, UK.*
Isotonic sea water (p.1233·3).
*Nasal dryness; nasal hygiene.*

**Sterimar Cu** *Baldacci, Ital.*
Sea water (p.1233·3); copper (p.1425·3).
*Nasal cleansing.*

**Sterimycine** *Novartis Ophthalmics, Fr.*
Kanamycin sulfate (p.225·1); polymyxin B sulfate (p.245·1).
*Eye infections.*

**Steri-Neb Cromogen** *Norton Waterford, Irl.†.*
Sodium cromoglicate (p.795·3).
*Asthma.*

**Steri-Neb Salamol** *Ivax, Irl.*
Salbutamol sulfate (p.791·3).
*Obstructive airways disease.*

**Sterinet** *Consol, Ital.†.*
Cetylpyridinium chloride (p.1173·1).
*Skin and hand disinfection.*

**Sterinor**
*Heumann, Ger.; ABC, Ital.†.*
Co-tetroxazine (p.199·3).
*Bacterial infections.*

**Sterinova** *Medentech, Irl.†.*
Sodium dichloroisocyanurate (p.1191·3).
*Sterilisation of infant feeding equipment.*

**Steripaste** *SSL, UK.*
Zinc oxide (p.1163·2).
*Ulcers.*

**Steripod** *SSL, UK.*
Sodium chloride (p.1233·3).
Formerly known as Steripod Blue.
*Irrigation solution.*

**Steripod Chlorhexidine Gluconate** *SSL, UK.*
Chlorhexidine gluconate (p.1173·2).
Formerly known as Steripod Pink.
*Skin disinfection.*

**Steripod Chlorhexidine Gluconate with Cetrimide** *SSL, UK.*
Chlorhexidine gluconate (p.1173·2); cetrimide (p.1172·1).
Formerly known as Steripod Yellow.
*Skin disinfection.*

**Sterisol** *Warner-Lambert, NZ†.*
Hexetidine (p.1182·1).
*Mouth and throat infections.*

**Steri/Sol** *Pfizer Consumer, Canad.*
Hexetidine (p.1182·1).
*Mouth and throat disorders.*

**Steriwipe** *Helapet, UK.*
Isopropyl alcohol (p.1184·3).
*Surface disinfection.*

**Sterk hostesirup** *Nycomed, Norw.†.*
Ethylmorphine hydrochloride (p.37·3); codeine phosphate (p.27·1).
*Coughs.*

**Sterlane**
*Note. This name is used for preparations of different composition.*
*Hoechst Marion Roussel, Braz.†.*
Lauryloxypropyl-β-aminobutyric acid; dodecylaminopropyl-β-aminobutyric acid.
*Skin disinfection.*

*Pharmadeveloppement, Fr.*
Lauryloxypropyl-β-aminobutyric acid; dodecylaminopropyl-β-aminobutyric acid; miristalkonium chloride (p.1186·3).
*Skin cleansing; skin infections.*

**Stern Biene Fenchelhonig**
*Makara, Austria†; Roland, Ger.†.*
Fennel oil (p.1687·3).
*Upper respiratory-tract disorders associated with viscous mucus.*

**Stern Biene Fenchelsirup** *Altana, Ger.*
Fennel oil (p.1687·3).
*Upper respiratory-tract disorders associated with viscous mucus.*

**Sterocort** *Taro, Israel.*
Triamcinolone (p.1110·2).
*Corticosteroid.*

**Sterodelta** *Metapharma, Ital.†.*
Diflorasone diacetate (p.1099·3).
*Skin disorders.*

**Sterodex** *Fischer, Israel.*
Dexamethasone sodium phosphate (p.1097·2).
*Eye inflammation.*

**Sterofrin** *Alcon, Austral.*
Prednisolone acetate (p.1108·1).
*Inflammatory and allergic eye disorders.*

**Sterofundin** *Braun, Ger.*
Electrolyte infusion (p.1217·1).
*Fluid and electrolyte disorders.*

**Sterofundin A** *Braun, Austria.*
Potassium-free electrolyte infusion with glucose (p.1217·1).
*Carbohydrate source; fluid and electrolyte disorders.*

**Sterofundin B, Sterofundin G, Sterofundin HG** *Braun, Austria.*
Electrolyte infusion with glucose (p.1217·1).
*Carbohydrate source; fluid and electrolyte disorders.*

**Sterofundin BG** *Braun, Ger.*
Electrolyte infusion with glucose (p.1217·1).
*Carbohydrate source; fluid and electrolyte disorders.*

**Sterofundin BX** *Braun, Ger.†.*
Electrolyte infusion with xylitol (p.1217·1).
*Carbohydrate source; fluid and electrolyte disorders.*

**Sterofundin HEG** *Braun, Ger.*
Electrolyte infusion with glucose (p.1217·1).
*Carbohydrate source; fluid and electrolyte disorders.*

**Sterofundin R** *Braun, Austria†.*
Electrolyte infusion (p.1217·1) with rutoside sodium sulfate (p.1688·3).
*Fluid and electrolyte disorders.*

**Sterofundin, Sterofundin K** *Braun, Austria.*
Electrolyte infusion (p.1217·1).
*Fluid and electrolyte disorders.*

**Sterofundin VG** *Braun, Ger.*
Electrolyte infusion with glucose (p.1217·1).
*Carbohydrate source; fluid and electrolyte disorders.*

**Sterogyl**
*Aventis, Fr.; IFET (ΙΦΕΤ), Gr.*
Ergocalciferol (p.1462·1).
*Vitamin D deficiency.*

**Sterolone** *Francia, Ital.*
Fluocinolone acetonide (p.1101·2).
*Skin disorders.*

**Steromien** *Aspen, S.Afr.*
Betamethasone (p.1093·1).
*Corticosteroid.*

**Steron** *West-Coast, Thai.*
Norethisterone (p.1562·2).
*Endometriosis; menstrual disorders.*

**Steronase Aq** *Aventis, Israel.*
Triamcinolone acetonide (p.1110·2).
*Allergic rhinitis.*

**Steronide** *Galderma, Braz.*
Desonide (p.1096·3).
*Skin disorders.*

**Steropotassium** *Sterop, Belg.*
Potassium chloride (p.1232·2).
*Hypokalaemia.*

**Steroprim** *Sterop, Belg.*
Co-trimoxazole (p.199·3).
*Bacterial infections.*

**Sterosan** *Lachifarma, Ital.*
Benzalkonium chloride (p.1168·3); orthophenylphenol (p.1187·2).
*Skin, wound, and burn disinfection.*

**Steros-Anal**
*Bristol-Myers Squibb, Austria; Bristol-Myers Squibb, Ger.*
Triamcinolone acetonide (p.1110·2); lidocaine hydrochloride (p.1377·3).
*Anorectal disorders.*

**Sterosone** *Raza, Malaysia; Pharmaniaga, Malaysia.*
Prednisolone (p.1108·1).
*Corticosteroid.*

**Sterostatine** *Sterop, Belg.*
Nystatin (p.406·3).
*Fungal infections.*

**Ster-Zac** *SSL, UK.*
*Bath additive:* Triclosan (p.1195·2).
*Skin cleanser:* Hexachlorophene (p.1181·2).
*Skin disinfection.*

**Stesiron**
*Alpharma, Denm.; Alpharma, Fin.; Alpharma, Norw.*
Buspirone hydrochloride (p.672·2).
*Alcoholism; anxiety disorders.*

**Stesolid**
*Chemomedica, Austria; Alpharma, Denm.; Alpharma, Fin.; Alpharma-Isis, Ger.; Remek, Gr.; Alpharma, Hong Kong; Dumex, Irl.; CTI, Israel; Alpharma, Norw.; CSL, NZ; Dumex, NZ; Alpharma, Port.; Alpharma, Singapore; Ipsen, Spain; Alpharma, Swed.; Alpharma, Switz.; Dumex-Alpharma, Thai.; Alpharma, UK.*
Diazepam (p.690·1).
*Alcohol withdrawal syndrome; anxiety; eclampsia; epilepsy; febrile convulsions; neuroses; premedication; skeletal muscle spasm; sleep disorders; status epilepticus; tetanus.*

**Stetic** *Abbott, Braz.†.*
Aspartame (p.1422·1).
*Sugar substitute.*

**Stevencillin** *Rafarm, Gr.*
Amoxicillin (p.155·3).
*Bacterial infections.*

**Stevia Dulri** *Tanki, Arg.*
Stevia rebaudiana.
*Sugar substitute for diabetics.*

**Sthenorex** *Pharmygiene, Fr.*
Fenugreek (p.1688·1); pollen.
*Anorexia.*

**Stick Ecran Solaire** *Clarins, Canad.†.*
*SPF 19:* Octinoxate (p.1154·3); oxybenzone (p.1154·3); titanium dioxide (p.1160·3).
*Sunscreen.*

**Stick Ecran Total** *Vichy, Canad.*
*SPF 25:* Octinoxate (p.1154·3); titanium dioxide (p.1160·3).
*Sunscreen.*

**Stick Labial de Proteccion Total** *Pierre Fabre Dermo-Cosmetique, Arg.*
Titanium dioxide (p.1160·3); cinnamate.
*Sunscreen.*

**Stick Solaire Haute Protection** *Clarins, Canad.*
*SPF 30:* Octinoxate (p.1154·3); oxybenzone (p.1154·3).
*Sunscreen.*

**Stiebenyl** *Pharmanel, Gr.*
Ramipril (p.994·1).
*Hypertension.*

**Stiedex** *Stiefel, UK.*
Desoximetasone (p.1096·3); salicylic acid (p.1157·1).
*Skin and scalp disorders.*

**Stiedex LP** *Stiefel, UK.*
Desoximetasone (p.1096·3).
*Skin disorders.*

**Stiefcortil**
*Stiefel, Arg.; Stiefel, Braz.*
Hydrocortisone (p.1103·3).
*Skin disorders.*

**Stiefderm** *Stiefel, Braz.†.*
Triclocarban (p.1195·1).
*Skin disinfection.*

**Stiefotrex** *Stiefel, Gr.*
Isotretinoin (p.1148·3).
*Acne.*

**Stiemycin**
*Stiefel, Arg.; Stiefel, Braz.; Stiefel, Hong Kong; Stiefel, Irl.; Stiefel, Malaysia; Stiefel, Mex.; Stiefel, Neth.; Stiefel, NZ; Stiefel, S.Afr.; Stiefel, Singapore; Stiefel, Thai.; Stiefel, UK.*
Erythromycin (p.208·1).
*Acne.*

**Stiemycine**
*Sanova, Austria; Stiefel, Ger.; Stiefel, Switz.*
Erythromycin (p.208·1).
*Acne.*

**Stieprox**
*Stiefel, Irl.; Stiefel, Singapore; Stiefel, Thai.*
Ciclopirox olamine (p.396·1).
*Scalp disorders.*

**Stieva-A**
*Stiefel, Austral.; Stiefel, Canad.; Stiefel, Chile; Stiefel, Hong Kong; Stiefel, Malaysia; Stiefel, Mex.; Stiefel, Singapore; Stiefel, Thai.*
Tretinoin (p.1161·1).
*Acne.*

**Stievamycin**
*Stiefel, Canad.; Stiefel, Chile; Stiefel, Mex.*
Tretinoin (p.1161·1); erythromycin (p.208·1).
*Acne.*

**Stigmicarpin** *Bros, Gr.*
Nimodipine (p.972·3).
*Neurological deficit following subarachnoid haemorrhage.*

**Stilamin**
*Serono, Arg.; Serono, Austria; Serono, Braz.; Serono, Canad.; Vianex (Βιανεξ), Gr.; Serono, Hong Kong; Serum Institute, India; Serono, Ital.; Serono, Mex.; Serono, Port.; Serono, S.Afr.; Serono, Singapore†; Serono, Switz.; Serono, Thai.*
Somatostatin acetate (p.1339·3).
*Diabetic ketoacidosis; gastrointestinal haemorrhage; pancreatic, biliary, and intestinal fistulae; postoperative complications following pancreatic surgery.*

**Stilaze** *Sandipro, Belg.*
Lormetazepam (p.705·2).
*Insomnia.*

**Stilene** *Pfizer Consumer, Belg.*
Dipropylene glycol salicylate (p.44·3); capsicum oleoresin (p.1667·1).
*Musculoskeletal, joint, nerve, and soft-tissue pain.*

**Stilex**
*Note. This name is used for preparations of different composition.*
*Pharmanik (Φαρμανικ), Gr.*
Butamirate citrate (p.1116·2).
*Cough.*

*Vifor, Switz.*
*Cream:* Mepyramine maleate (p.437·1); lidocaine hydrochloride (p.1377·3); calcium levulinate (p.1225·3); menthol (p.1711·3).
*Topical gel; fluigel; topical spray:* Mepyramine maleate (p.437·1); lidocaine hydrochloride (p.1377·3); dexpanthenol (p.1727·2).
*Skin disorders.*

**Stilgrip** *Hertz, Braz.†.*
Chlorphenamine (p.428·1); phenylephrine (p.1126·3); paracetamol (p.76·2).
*Cold and influenza symptoms.*

**Still** *Allergan, Braz.*
Diclofenac sodium (p.32·1).
*Inflammatory eye disorders.*

**Stilla**
*Note. This name is used for preparations of different composition.*
*Warner-Lambert, Fr.†.*
Phenylephrine hydrochloride (p.1126·3); methylthioninium chloride (p.1042·2).
*Eye disorders.*

*Abic, Israel.*
Tetryzoline hydrochloride (p.1131·2).
*Eye irritation.*

**Stilla Decongestionante** *Angelini, Ital.*
Tetryzoline hydrochloride (p.1131·2).
*Eye irritation.*

**Stilla Delicato** *Angelini, Ital.*
Benzalkonium chloride (p.1168·3).
*Eye disinfection; eye irritation.*

**Stillacor** *Wolff, Ger.*
β-Acetyldigoxin (p.851·1).
*Arrhythmias; heart failure.*

**Stillargol** *Mayoly-Spindler, Fr.*
Silver protein (p.1746·2).
*Infections of the eye and nose.*

**Stilnoct**
*Sanofi Synthelabo, Belg.; Sanofi Winthrop, Denm.; Sanofi Synthelabo, Fin.; Sanofi Synthelabo, Irl.; Sanofi Synthelabo, Neth.; Sanofi Synthelabo, Norw.; Sanofi Synthelabo, Swed.; Sanofi Synthelabo, UK.*
Zolpidem tartrate (p.728·3).
*Insomnia.*

**Stilnox**
*Sanofi Synthelabo, Austral.; Sanofi Synthelabo, Braz.; Sanofi Synthelabo, Fr.; Sanofi Synthelabo, Ger.; Sanofi Synthelabo, Gr.; Sanofi Synthelabo, Hong Kong; Synthelabo, Israel; Sanofi Synthelabo, Ital.; Sanofi Synthelabo, Malaysia; Sanofi Synthelabo, Mex.; Sanofi Synthelabo, Port.; Sanofi Synthelabo, S.Afr.; Sanofi Synthelabo, Singapore; Sanofi Synthelabo, Spain; Synthelabo, Switz.; Sanofi Synthelabo, Thai.*
Zolpidem tartrate (p.728·3).
*Insomnia.*

**Stilomagic** *Antipiol, Ital.*
Ammonia (p.1653·3); hamamelis (p.1696·3); almond oil (p.1651·1).
*Insect repellent.*

**Stilpane** *Aspen, S.Afr.*
*Capsules:* Paracetamol (p.76·2); codeine phosphate (p.27·1); meprobamate (p.706·2).
*Pain and associated tension.*
*Syrup:* Paracetamol (p.76·2); codeine phosphate (p.27·1); promethazine hydrochloride (p.439·1); camphorated opium tincture (p.74·2).
*Fever; pain.*
*Tablets:* Paracetamol (p.76·2); codeine phosphate (p.27·1); caffeine (p.782·1); meprobamate (p.706·2).
*Pain and associated tension.*

**Stilphostrol** *Miles, USA†.*
Fosfestrol (p.1555·3) or fosfestrol sodium (p.1555·3).
*Prostatic cancer.*

**Stimate** *Centeon, USA.*
Desmopressin acetate (p.1322·3).
*Haemophilia A; von Willebrand's disease.*

**Stimilfar** *Lusofarmaco, Port.*
Piracetam (p.1732·1); vincamine (p.1764·2).

**Stimlor** *Berk, UK†.*
Naftidrofuryl oxalate (p.964·1).
*Cerebral and peripheral vascular disorders.*

**Stimol** *Biocodex, Fr.*
Citrulline malate (p.1425·2).
*Asthenia.*

**Stimolfit** *Body Spring, Ital.*
Senna (p.1288·2); rhubarb (p.1287·3); cascara (p.1255·1); peppermint leaf (p.1283·2); threonine (p.1451·1); inositol (p.1701·2).
*Gastrointestinal disorders.*

**Stimtes** *Lilly, Ital.*
Collagen (bovine) (p.1674·3).
*Skin ulcers; wounds.*

**Stimu-ACTH** *Ferring, Fr.*
Corticorelin triflutate (p.1321·3).
*Diagnosis of adrenocortical dysfunction.*

**Stimubral** *Lusofarmaco, Port.*
Piracetam (p.1732·1).

**Stimu-GH** *Ferring, Fr.*
Somatorelin acetate (p.1339·2).
*Diagnosis of hypothalamic-pituitary dysfunction.*

**Stimul** *Celltech, Belg.†.*
Pemoline (p.1591·2).
*Attention deficit hyperactivity disorder; narcoleptic syndrome.*

**Stimulance**
*Baxter, NZ; Nutricia, NZ; Nutricia, Port.*
Dietary fibre supplement (p.1253·2).

**Stimulex** *Cipan, Port.*
Vitamin B substances (p.1417·1).
*Tonic; vitamin B deficiency.*

**Stimu-LH** *Ferring, Fr.*
Gonadorelin (p.1325·1).
*Diagnosis of hypothalamic-pituitary-gonadal dysfunction.*

**Stimulnerv** *Disprovent, Arg.*
Ginseng; glucuronolactone; phosphorylcolamine; potassium aspartate; magnesium aspartate; vitamin $_{12}$ (p.1417·1).
*Tonic.*

**Stimunal** *Poirier, Fr.*
*Capsules; syrup:* Vitamin and mineral preparation (p.1417·1).
*Spray:* Zinc pidolate; copper pidolate; manganese pidolate; ascorbic acid; pyridoxine hydrochloride; calendula officinalis.
*Cleansing of nose, mouth, and throat.*

**Stimuplexe** *Lehning, Fr.*
Cobalt gluconate; manganese glycerophosphate; zinc gluconate; copper gluconate; lysine hydrochloride; phosphoric acid (p.1417·1).
*Asthenia.*

**Stimu-TSH** *Ferring, Fr.*
Protirelin (p.1337·3).
*Diagnosis of hypothalamic-pituitary-thyroid dysfunction.*

**Stimuzim** *Biotekfarma, Ital.†.*
Inosine pranobex (p.640·2).
*Immunodeficiency; viral infections.*

**Stimycine** *Stiefel, Fr.*
Erythromycin (p.208·1).
*Acne.*

**Stin** *Medquimica, Braz.†.*
Buclizine (p.426·3); lysine; thiamine; pyridoxine; cyanocobalamin (p.1417·1).
*Tonic.*

**Sting-Eze** *Wisconsin Pharmacal, USA.*
Diphenhydramine hydrochloride (p.431·3); camphor (p.1665·3); phenol (p.1188·1); benzocaine (p.1370·3); cineole (p.1672·1).
*Pruritus.*

**Sting-Kill** *Randob, USA.*
Benzocaine (p.1370·3); menthol (p.1711·3).
*Insect bites and stings; minor skin irritation.*

**Stingose**
*Pfizer Consumer, Austral.; Hamilton, Hong Kong; Hamilton, Israel†; Pfizer, NZ; Eden, S.Afr.; Ayrton, UK.*
Aluminium sulfate (p.1653·1).
*Bites and stings.*

**Stioxyl** *Sylak, Swed.*
Benzoyl peroxide (p.1143·2).
*Acne.*

**Stipo** *Repha, Ger.*
Thuja; lycopodium; lemna min.; pulsatilla; mezereum; kal. bichrom.; hydrastis; benzocaine (p.1370·3); ephedrine hydrochloride (p.1120·1); naphazoline hydrochloride (p.1124·3).
*Nasal disorders.*

**Stiprox**
*Stiefel, Braz.; Stiefel, Chile; Stiefel, Fr.; Stiefel, Ital.; Stiefel, Mex.*
Ciclopirox olamine (p.396·1).
*Dandruff; fungal skin infections; seborrhoeic dermatitis.*

**Stiproxal** *Stiefel, Fr.*
Ciclopirox olamine (p.396·1); salicylic acid (p.1157·1).
*Dandruff.*

**Stivane** *Beaufour, Fr.†.*
Pirisudanol maleate (p.1732·3).
*Tonic.*

**Stivate** *Stiefel, Thai.*
Clobetasol propionate (p.1095·2).
*Skin disorders.*

**Stobcon** *Chew, Thai.†.*
Brompheniramine maleate (p.426·1); phenylpropanolamine hydrochloride (p.1127·3).
*Cold symptoms; hypersensitivity reactions; nasal congestion.*

**Stocof** *Chew, Thai.*
Guaifenesin (p.1122·1); chlorphenamine maleate (p.427·3); terpin hydrate (p.1131·1).
*Coughs; nasal congestion.*

**Stocrin**
*Merck Sharp & Dohme, Arg.; Merck Sharp & Dohme, Austral.; Merck Sharp & Dohme, Belg.; Merck Sharp & Dohme, Braz.; Merck Sharp & Dohme, Chile; Merck Sharp & Dohme, Denm.; Merck Sharp & Dohme, Fin.; Merck, Gr.; Merck Sharp & Dohme, Hong Kong; Merck Sharp & Dohme, Israel; Merck Sharp & Dohme, Malaysia; Merck Sharp & Dohme, Mex.; Merck Sharp & Dohme, Neth.; Merck Sharp & Dohme, Norw.; Merck Sharp & Dohme, NZ; Merck Sharp & Dohme, Port.; Merck Sharp & Dohme, S.Afr.; Merck Sharp & Dohme, Singapore; Merck Sharp & Dohme, Swed.; Merck Sharp & Dohme, Switz.; Merck Sharp & Dohme, Thai.*
Efavirenz (p.632·2).
*HIV infection.*

**Stodal**
*Note. This name is used for preparations of different composition.*
*Boiron, Canad.; Boiron, Fr.*
Homoeopathic preparation.

*Boiron, Port.*
Pulsatilla; rumex crispus; bryonia dioica; ipeca; spongia tosta; sticta pulmonaria; antimonium tartaricum; myocarde; coccus cacti; drosera; tolu balsam (p.1131·3); senega (p.1130·2).
*Coughs.*

**Stodal for Children** *Boiron, Canad.*
Homoeopathic preparation.

**Stofilan**
*Christiaens, Belg.; Lek, Hong Kong†.*
Co-dergocrine mesilate (p.1674·1).
*Mental function impairment; vascular disorders.*

**Stogar** *Fujirebio, Jpn.*
Lafutidine (p.1269·3).
*Peptic ulcer.*

**STOI-X** *Apomedica, Austria.*
Selenium disulfide (p.1157·3).
*Dandruff.*

**Stolina** *Almirall, Spain.*
Cyproheptadine cyclamate (p.430·2); amino acids and cyanocobalamin (p.1417·1).
*Anorexia; tonic; weight loss.*

**Stoma Anestesia Dental** *Bucca, Spain†.*
Lidocaine hydrochloride (p.1377·3); potassium hydroxyquinoline sulfate (p.1734·2).
Adrenaline (p.852·2) and noradrenaline acid tartrate (p.974·3) are included in this preparation as vasoconstrictors to diminish absorption and localise the effect of the local anaesthetic.
*Local anaesthesia.*

**Stomaax** *Theralab, Canad.*
Aluminium hydroxide (p.1249·2); magnesium hydroxide (p.1272·2).

**Stomaax Plus** *Therapex, Canad.*
Aluminium hydroxide (p.1249·2); magnesium hydroxide (p.1272·2); simeticone (p.1289·2).

**Stomac** *Greater Pharma, Thai.*
*Oral liquid:* Aluminium hydroxide (p.1249·2); magnesium hydroxide (p.1272·2); simeticone (p.1289·2).
*Tablets:* Aluminium hydroxide (p.1249·2); magnesium trisilicate (p.1272·3); atropine sulfate (p.477·1); peppermint oil (p.1283·2).
*Gastric hyperacidity; gastritis; peptic ulcer.*

**Stomach Calm** *Brauer, Austral.†.*
Homoeopathic preparation.

**Stomach Mixture** *Potter's, UK.*
Bismuth and ammonium citrate (p.1253·1); taraxacum (p.1751·3); gentian root (p.1692·2); compound rhubarb tincture (p.1287·3).
*Dyspepsia.*

**Stomachicon N** *Syxyl, Ger.†.*
Chamomile (p.1669·3); peppermint leaf (p.1283·2); caraway (p.1667·2); dried bitter-orange peel (p.1723·3).
*Appetite loss; dyspepsia.*

**Stomachysat N** *Ysatfabrik, Ger.*
Absinthium (p.1645·1); achillea (p.1646·2); gnaphalium dioicum; peppermint leaf (p.1283·2).
*Gastrointestinal disorders.*

**Stomacine** *Plan, Switz.*
Pepsin (p.1729·3); condurango (p.1675·3); cardamom (p.1667·3); quassia (p.1737·2).
*Gastrointestinal disorders.*

**Stoma-Gastreu S R5** *Reckeweg, Ger.*
Homoeopathic preparation.

**Stomagel N** *CPF, Ger.†.*
Aluminium hydroxide gel (p.1249·2); magnesium oxide (p.1272·3).
*Gastritis; gastrointestinal hyperacidity; peptic ulcer.*

**Stomahesive**
*Note. This name is used for preparations of different composition.*
*Convatec, Austral.*
*Topical paste:* Butyl monoester polymer with ethanol.
*Colostomies and ileostomies.*

*Convatec, Austral.; Bristol-Myers Squibb, NZ; Convatec, UK.*
*Topical wafer:* Carmellose sodium (p.1577·3); gelatin (p.754·3); pectin (p.1580·3); polyisobutylene.
*Stoma care.*

*Convatec, Fr.*
Barrier paste.
*Fistulae; stoma care.*

*Bristol-Myers Squibb, NZ.*
*Topical paste; topical powder:* Carmellose sodium (p.1577·3); gelatin (p.754·3); pectin (p.1580·3).
*Stoma care.*

**Stomakon** *Biolab Sanus, Braz.*
Cimetidine (p.1255·3).
*Acid aspiration; gastro-oesophageal reflux; gastrointestinal haemorrhage; peptic ulcer; Zollinger-Ellison syndrome.*

**Stomasal Med** *Mauermann, Ger.*
Aluminium hydroxide (p.1249·2); magnesium oxide (p.1272·3); lupulus (p.1708·1); peppermint leaf (p.1283·2); agrimony (p.1649·1); calamus (p.1664·1); chlorophyllin (p.1057·1).
*Gastrointestinal disorders.*

**Stomec** *Progress, Thai.*
Omeprazole (p.1278·2).
*Gastro-oesophageal reflux; peptic ulcer; Zollinger-Ellison syndrome.*

**Stomedine** *GlaxoSmithKline Sante, Fr.*
Cimetidine (p.1255·3).
*Gastro-oesophageal reflux; gastrointestinal hyperacidity.*

**Stomet**
*Farmoquimica, Braz.†; Valda, Ital.*
Cimetidine (p.1255·3).
*Gastro-oesophageal reflux; gastrointestinal haemorrhage; peptic ulcer; Zollinger-Ellison syndrome.*

**Stomidros** *Stomygen, Ital.†.*
Calcium hydroxide (p.1664·3).
*Dental capping; infection of the dental canal.*

**Stomigen** *Steiner, Ger.*
Magnesium hydroxide (p.1272·2); calcium carbonate (p.1254·2).
*Gastrointestinal hyperacidity; peptic ulcer.*

**Stomosan** *Vicente, Spain†.*
Bismuth subnitrate (p.1252·2); marrubium vulgare (p.1124·1); sodium bromide (p.1663·1); sodium citrate (p.1223·2).
*Gastritis; gastrointestinal hyperacidity; peptic ulcer.*

**Stomygen** *Stomygen, Ital.*
Sodium monofluorophosphate (p.1446·2); cetylpyridinium chloride (p.1173·1).
*Oral hygiene.*

**Stongel** *Cazi, Braz.*
Aluminium hydroxide (p.1249·2); magnesium hydroxide (p.1272·2).
*Gastrointestinal hyperacidity.*

**Stop**
*Oral-B, UK†; Oral-B, USA.*
Stannous fluoride (p.1448·3).
*Dental caries prophylaxis.*

**Stop Espinilla Normaderm** *Capilares, Spain.*
Benzoyl peroxide (p.1143·2).
*Acne.*

**Stop Hemo**
*Brothier, Fr.; Brothier, Switz.†.*
Calcium alginate (p.745·1).
*Superficial haemorrhage.*

**Stop Itch**
*Note. A similar name is used for preparations of different composition (see Stopitch, below).*
*Dermatech, Austral.†; Schering-Plough, Canad.; Balmar, NZ.*
Papain (p.1727·3).
*Skin irritation.*

**Stopain**
*Note. This name is used for preparations of different composition.*
*Britisfarma, Spain†.*
Paracetamol (p.76·2).
*Fever; pain.*

*Chew, Thai.*
*Cream:* Methyl salicylate (p.59·3); menthol (p.1711·3); eugenol (p.1686·2); thymol (p.1194·2); eucalyptus oil (p.1686·2); turpentine oil (p.1760·1).
*Topical gel:* Menthol (p.1711·3).
*Musculoskeletal pain.*

**Stopaler** *Kampel Martian, Arg.*
Cetirizine (p.427·2).

**Stop-Allerg** *Genop, S.Afr.*
Sodium cromoglicate (p.795·3).
Formerly known as Vistacrom.
*Allergic conjunctivitis.*

**Stoparen** *Anpharm (Ανφαρμ), Gr.*
Cefotaxime sodium (p.175·3).
*Bacterial infections.*

**Stopayne** *Adcock Ingram, S.Afr.*
*Syrup:* Paracetamol (p.76·2); codeine phosphate (p.27·1); promethazine hydrochloride (p.439·1).
*Tablets; capsules:* Paracetamol (p.76·2); codeine phosphate (p.27·1); caffeine (p.782·1); meprobamate (p.706·2).
*Fever; pain.*

**Stopcold** *UCB, Spain.*
Cetirizine hydrochloride (p.427·1); pseudoephedrine hydrochloride (p.1129·2).
*Allergic rhinitis.*

**Stopen** *Berman, Mex.*
Di-iodo-kaolin-pectin-sulfa.
*Diarrhoea; gastrointestinal infections.*

**Stopex** *Medical, Port.*
Sulfathiazole (p.264·1).
*Vaginal infections.*

**Stopit** *Rafa, Israel.*
Loperamide hydrochloride (p.1271·1).
*Diarrhoea.*

**Stopitch**
*Note. A similar name is used for preparations of different composition (see Stop Itch, above).*
*Restan, S.Afr.*
Hydrocortisone acetate (p.1103·3).
*Skin disorders.*

**Stoppers** *Charwell Pharmaceuticals, UK†.*
Nicotine (p.1720·1).
*Aid to smoking withdrawal.*

**Stoptoss** *Delta, Braz.*
Ammonium chloride (p.1115·2); diphenhydramine hydrochloride (p.431·3).
*Coughs.*

**Stovalid N** *Cesra, Ger.*
Peppermint leaf (p.1283·2); absinthium (p.1645·1); fennel (p.1687·2); chamomile (p.1669·3); aniseed (p.1655·2); caraway (p.1667·2); angelica root (p.1655·1); calamus root (p.1664·1); gentian root (p.1692·2).
*Appetite loss; dyspepsia.*

**Stoxil**
*Dermatech, Austral.; ICN, Hong Kong†; ICN, Singapore†.*
Idoxuridine (p.637·3).
*Herpes simplex skin infections.*

**Strafortin** *Strathmann, Ger.*
Calcium carbonate (p.1254·2); colecalciferol (p.1461·3).
*Osteoporosis.*

**Strains Cream** *Nelson, UK.*
Homoeopathic preparation.

**Stranoval** *Teofarma, Ital.*
Betamethasone valerate (p.1093·2); dextran sulfate (p.1679·2).
*Peripheral vascular disorders; soft-tissue disorders.*

**Stratene** *Gerda, Fr.†.*
Cetiedil citrate (p.882·1).
*Intermittent claudication.*

**Strattera**
*Lilly, Austral.; Lilly, UK; Lilly, USA.*
Atomoxetine hydrochloride (p.1585·1).
*Attention-deficit hyperactivity disorder.*

**Strefen** *Crookes Healthcare, UK.*
Flurbiprofen (p.43·3).
*Sore throat.*

**Streflam** *Crookes Healthcare, UK†.*
Flurbiprofen (p.43·3).
*Sore throat.*

**Strength** *Potter's, UK.*
Damiana (p.1679·1); kola (p.1765·3); saw palmetto (p.1569·1).
*Tonic.*

**Strepfen**
*Boots Healthcare, Austral.; Boots Healthcare, NZ; Boots Healthcare, Port.*
Flurbiprofen (p.43·3).
*Sore throat.*

**Strepsils**
*Boots Healthcare, Austral.; Boots Healthcare, Belg.; Schering-Plough, Canad.; Boots, Denm.; Boots, Fin.; Boots Healthcare, Fr.; Boots, Hong Kong; Boots Healthcare, Irl.; Boots, Israel; Boots Healthcare, Malaysia; Boots Healthcare, Neth.; Boots Healthcare, NZ; Boots Healthcare, S.Afr.; Boots, Singapore; Boots Healthcare, Spain; Astra, Swed.†; Crookes Healthcare, UK.*
Dichlorobenzyl alcohol (p.1178·3); amylmetacresol (p.1168·2).
*Sore throat.*

**Strepsils I** *Schering-Plough, Canad.†.*
Amylmetacresol (p.1168·2).
*Sore throat.*

**Strepsils con Anestesico** *Boots Healthcare, Spain.*
Dichlorobenzyl alcohol (p.1178·3); amylmetacresol (p.1168·2); lidocaine (p.1377·3).
*Mouth and throat disorders.*

**Strepsils con Vitamina C** *Boots Healthcare, Spain.*
Sodium ascorbate (p.1460·2); ascorbic acid (p.1460·2); dichlorobenzyl alcohol (p.1178·3); amylmetacresol (p.1168·2).
*Sore throat.*

**Strepsils Cough**
*Boots Healthcare, NZ; Crookes Healthcare, UK†.*
Dextromethorphan hydrobromide (p.1117·3).
*Coughs.*

**Strepsils Cough Relief** *Boots Healthcare, Austral.*
Dextromethorphan hydrobromide (p.1117·3).
*Coughs.*

**Strepsils Dry Cough** *Boots Healthcare, NZ.*
Dextromethorphan hydrobromide (p.1117·3).
*Coughs.*

**Strepsils Dual Action**
*Boots, Hong Kong; Boots Healthcare, Irl.; Boots Healthcare, Malaysia; Boots, Singapore.*
Amylmetacresol (p.1168·2); dichlorobenzyl alcohol (p.1178·3); lidocaine (p.1377·3) or lidocaine hydrochloride (p.1377·3).
*Sore throat.*

**Strepsils Echinacea Defence** *Boots Healthcare, NZ.*
Ascorbic acid (p.1460·2); echinacea (p.1683·2).
*Cold symptoms.*

**Strepsils Eucalyptus Menthol** *Boots Healthcare, S.Afr.*
Dichlorobenzyl alcohol (p.1178·3); amylmetacresol (p.1168·2); menthol (p.1711·3).
*Sore throat.*

**Strepsils Extra**
*Boots Healthcare, Austral.; Crookes Healthcare, UK.*
Hexylresorcinol (p.1182·1).
*Sore throat.*

**Strepsils Lidocaine** *Boots, Fr.*
Amylmetacresol (p.1168·2); dichlorobenzyl alcohol (p.1178·3); lidocaine hydrochloride (p.1377·3).
*Mouth disorders; sore throat.*

**Strepsils + Lidocaine** *Boots Healthcare, Belg.*
Dichlorobenzyl alcohol (p.1178·3); amylmetacresol (p.1168·2); lidocaine (p.1377·3).
*Sore throat.*

**Strepsils Menthol**
*Boots Healthcare, Belg.; Boots, Fin.*
Dichlorobenzyl alcohol (p.1178·3); amylmetacresol (p.1168·2); menthol (p.1711·3).
*Mouth and throat disorders.*

**Strepsils Menthol en Eucalyptus** *Boots Healthcare, Neth.*
Amylmetacresol (p.1168·2); dichlorobenzyl alcohol (p.1178·3); menthol (p.1711·3); eucalyptus oil (p.1686·2).
*Sore throat.*

**Strepsils Miel-Citron** *Boots Healthcare, Fr.*
Amylmetacresol (p.1168·2); dichlorobenzyl alcohol (p.1178·3).
*Sore throat.*

**Strepsils Orange-C** *Boots Healthcare, S.Afr.*
Dichlorobenzyl alcohol (p.1178·3); amylmetacresol (p.1168·2); ascorbic acid (p.1460·2); menthol (p.1711·3).
*Sore throat.*

**Strepsils Pain Relief Plus** *Crookes Healthcare, UK†.*
Lidocaine (p.1377·3); dichlorobenzyl alcohol (p.1178·3); amylmetacresol (p.1168·2).
Formerly known as Strepsils Dual Action.
*Sore throat.*

**Strepsils Plus**
*Boots Healthcare, Austral.; Boots, Israel; Boots Healthcare, S.Afr.*
Dichlorobenzyl alcohol (p.1178·3); amylmetacresol (p.1168·2); lidocaine hydrochloride (p.1377·3).
*Sore throat.*

**Strepsils Plus Anaesthetic**
*Boots Healthcare, NZ; Boots, Thai.*
Dichlorobenzyl alcohol (p.1178·3); amylmetacresol (p.1168·2); lidocaine hydrochloride (p.1377·3).
*Sore throat.*

**Strepsils Plus Vit C** *Boots, Thai.*
Dichlorobenzyl alcohol (p.1178·3); amylmetacresol (p.1168·2); vitamin C (p.1460·2).
*Sore throat.*

**Strepsils Sinaasappel en Vitamine C** *Boots Healthcare, Neth.*
Dichlorobenzyl alcohol (p.1178·3); amylmetacresol (p.1168·2); ascorbic acid (p.1460·2).
*Sore throat.*

**Strepsils Soothing Honey & Lemon** *Boots Healthcare, S.Afr.†.*
Dichlorobenzyl alcohol (p.1178·3); amylmetacresol (p.1168·2).
*Sore throat.*

**Strepsils Sugar Free** *Boots, Thai.*
Amylmetacresol (p.1168·2); dichlorobenzyl alcohol (p.1178·3).
*Sore throat.*

**Strepsils Vit C** *Boots Healthcare, Belg.*
Dichlorobenzyl alcohol (p.1178·3); amylmetacresol (p.1168·2); ascorbic acid (p.1460·2); sodium ascorbate (p.1460·2).
*Sore throat.*

**Strepsils Vitamin C** *Boots Healthcare, Irl.*
Dichlorobenzyl alcohol (p.1178·3); amylmetacresol (p.1168·2); vitamin C (p.1460·2).
*Sore throat.*

**Strepsils with Vitamin C**
*Boots, Israel; Boots Healthcare, NZ; Crookes Healthcare, UK.*
Dichlorobenzyl alcohol (p.1178·3); amylmetacresol (p.1168·2); vitamin C (p.1460·2).
*Sore throat.*

**Strepsils Vitamine C** *Boots Healthcare, Fr.*
Amylmetacresol (p.1168·2); dichlorobenzyl alcohol (p.1178·3); ascorbic acid (p.1460·2); sodium ascorbate (p.1460·2).
*Sore throat.*

**Strepsils Zinc Cold Relief** *Boots, Austral.†.*
Zinc gluconate (p.1469·2); sodium ascorbate (p.1460·2); ascorbic acid (p.1460·2).
*Cold symptoms.*

**Strepsils Zinc Defence** *Crookes Healthcare, UK.*
Zinc gluconate (p.1469·2); ascorbic acid (p.1460·2).

**Strepsilspray Lidocaine** *Boots Healthcare, Fr.*
Amylmetacresol (p.1168·2); dichlorobenzyl alcohol (p.1178·3); lidocaine (p.1377·3).
*Mouth disorders; sore throat.*

**Streptase**
*Aventis, Austral.; Aventis, Austria; Aventis, Belg.†; Aventis Behring, Braz.; Aventis, Canad.; Aventis, Chile; Aventis Behring, Denm.; Aventis Behring, Fin.; Aventis Behring, Fr.; Aventis Behring, Ger.; Hoechst Marion Roussel, Gr.; Aventis, Hong Kong; Aventis, India; Aventis, Irl.; Behring, Israel; Aventis, Ital.; Aventis, Malaysia; Aventis, Mex.; Aventis Behring, Neth.; Aventis Behring, Norw.; Zuellig, NZ; Aventis, Port.; Aventis, S.Afr.; Hoechst Marion Roussel, Singapore†; Aventis Behring, Spain; Aventis Behring, Swed.; Aventis, Switz.; Aventis, Thai.; Aventis Behring, UK; Aventis, USA.*
Streptokinase (p.1005·2).
*Thromboembolic disorders.*

**Strepto** *General Drugs, Thai.*
Streptomycin sulfate (p.256·2).
*Bacterial infections including tuberculosis.*

**Streptocol** *Molteni, Ital.†.*
Streptomycin sulfate (p.256·2).
*Bacterial infections of the gastrointestinal tract.*

**Strepto-Erbazide** *Mac, India.*
Streptomycin sulfate (p.256·2); methaniazide sodium.
*Tuberculosis.*

**Strepto-Fatol** *Fatol, Ger.*
Streptomycin sulfate (p.256·2).
*Bacterial infections including tuberculosis.*

**Strepto-Hefa** *Hefa, Ger.*
Streptomycin sulfate (p.256·2).
*Bacterial infections including tuberculosis.*

**Streptomagma** *Wyeth Lederle, Ital.*
*Oral suspension:* Dried aluminium hydroxide (p.1249·2); heavy kaolin (p.1268·3); pectin (p.1580·3).
*Tablets:* Activated attapulgite (p.1251·1); pectin (p.1580·3); dried aluminium hydroxide (p.1249·2).
*Diarrhoea.*

**Streptonase** *Blausiegel, Braz.*
Streptokinase (p.1005·2).
*Thromboembolic disorders.*

**Strepto-Plus** *Molteni, Ital.†.*
Co-trimoxazole (p.199·3).
*Bacterial infections.*

**Streptosil con Neomicina-Fher** *Boehringer Ingelheim, Ital.*
Neomycin sulfate (p.235·1); sulfathiazole (p.264·1).
*Bacterial skin infections.*

**Streptosil L PMC** *Fher, Ital.*
Benzalkonium chloride (p.1168·3).
*Skin disinfection.*

**Streptozyme**
*Carter-Wallace, Switz.†; Wampole, USA.*
Test for streptococcal extracellular antigens in blood, plasma, and serum.

**Streptuss** *Boots Healthcare, Spain.*
Dextromethorphan hydrobromide (p.1117·3).
*Coughs.*

**Stresam** *Biocodex, Fr.*
Etifoxine hydrochloride (p.698·1).
*Anxiety.*

**Stress** *Homeocan, Canad.*
Homoeopathic preparation.

**Stress 600** *Nion, USA.*
Multivitamin and mineral preparation (p.1417·1).

**Stress B Complex**
*Pharmavite, Canad.; Moore, USA.*
A range of vitamin preparations with or without minerals (p.1417·1).

**Stress Formula**
*Wampole, Canad.; Nature's Bounty, USA.*
A range of vitamin preparations with or without minerals (p.1417·1).

**Stress Formula B Compound plus Vitamin C** *Quest, Canad.*
Vitamin B substances and vitamin C (p.1417·1).

**Stress Formula c/Zinc** *Natural Life, Arg.*
Vitamins; copper; zinc (p.1417·1).

**Stress Plex C** *Jamieson, Canad.*
Vitamin B substances, vitamin C, and zinc (p.1417·1).

**Stress Relief** *Brauer, Austral.†.*
Homoeopathic preparation.

**Stress Tab** *Shoppers Drug Mart, Canad.*
Vitamin B substances and vitamin C (p.1417·1).

**Stress Tab with Iron** *Shoppers Drug Mart, Canad.*
Multivitamin preparation with iron (p.1417·1).

**Stress Tab with Zinc** *Shoppers Drug Mart, Canad.*
Multivitamin preparation with zinc (p.1417·1).

**Stress Tablets** *DC Labs, Canad.*
Vitamin B substances and vitamin C (p.1417·1).

**Stressan** *Teuto, Braz.*
Vitamin and mineral preparation (p.1417·1).

**Stresscaps**
*Gilton, Braz.†.*
Vitamin B substances (p.1417·1).
*Nutritional supplement.*

*Wyeth Lederle, India.*
Vitamin B substances with vitamin C (p.1417·1).

**Stressease** *Jamieson, Canad.*
Multivitamin and mineral preparation (p.1417·1).

**Stressen** *Medosan, Ital.*
Amino-acid and vitamin preparation (p.1417·1).
*Tonic.*

**StressForm "605" with Iron** *Nature's Bounty, USA†.*
Multivitamin preparation with iron (p.1417·1).

**Stressigal** *Anpharm (Ανφαρμ), Gr.*
Buspirone hydrochloride (p.672·2).
*Generalised anxiety.*

**Stressless** *Dendron, UK.*
Lupulus (p.1708·1); skullcap (p.1746·3); valerian (p.1762·2); vervain (p.1764·1).
*Stress.*

**Stresson**
*Nutricia, Austral.; Support, Braz.; Nutricia, Fin.; Nutricia, Irl.; Nutricia, Ital.; Baxter, NZ; Nutricia, NZ.*
Preparations for enteral nutrition (p.1417·1).

**Stresson Multifibra** *Nutricia, Port.*
Preparation for enteral nutrition (p.1417·1).

**Stresstabs**
*Wyeth-Whitehall, Arg.; Whitehall, Braz.; Whitehall-Robins, Canad.; Wyeth, Hong Kong; Wyeth, Mex.; Wyeth Consumer, Port.; Whitehall, Thai.; Lederle, USA.*
A range of vitamin preparations with or without minerals (p.1417·1).

**Stresstabs with Zinc** *Lederle, Israel.*
Multivitamin and mineral preparation (p.1417·1).

**Stresstein** *Sandoz Nutrition, USA.*
Preparation for enteral nutrition (p.1417·1).
*Stress.*

**Strialisin** *MDM, Ital.*
Thiocolchicoside (p.1395·2).
*Neuromuscular pain; parkinsonism; spasticity.*

**Striant**
*Ardana, UK; Columbia, USA.*
Testosterone (p.1569·3).
*Male hypogonadism; testosterone deficiency.*

**Striaton** *Abbott, Ger.*
Levodopa (p.1205·2); carbidopa (p.1204·3).
*Parkinsonism.*

**Striatridin** *Opfermann, Ger.†.*
Cetostearyl octanoate; amino acids; ethyl nicotinate (p.37·2).
*Skin disorders.*

**Strictus** *Fada, Arg.*
Chlorhexidine (p.1173·2).
*Disinfection.*

**Stri-Dex Antibacterial Cleansing** *Sterling, USA.*
Triclosan (p.1195·2).

**Stri-Dex Clear** *Sterling, USA.*
Salicylic acid (p.1157·1).

**Stri-Dex Face Wash** *Sterling Health, USA.*
Triclosan (p.1195·2).
*Skin cleanser.*

**Stri-Dex Pads** *Glenbrook, USA.*
Salicylic acid (p.1157·1); alcohol (p.1166·1).
*Acne.*

**Stringan** *Strallhofer, Austria.*
Polyphloretin phosphate; phenylephrine (p.1126·3).
*Nasal congestion.*

**Strocain**
*Eisai, Hong Kong; Eisai, Jpn; Eisai, Singapore; Eisai, Thai.*
Oxetacaine (p.1382·1).
*Gastrointestinal disorders.*

**Strodival** *Herbert, Ger.*
Ouabain (p.977·3).
*Arrhythmias; heart failure.*

**Strogen** *Strathmann, Ger.*
Saw palmetto (p.1569·1).
*Benign prostatic hyperplasia.*

**Stromba**
*Sanofi Synthelabo, Belg.†; Sanofi Synthelabo, Irl.; Sanofi Synthelabo, Neth.†; Sanofi Synthelabo, UK†.*
Stanozolol (p.1569·2).
*Angioedema; cutaneous vasculitis; osteoporosis; Raynaud's syndrome; scleroderma; thromboembolic disorders.*

**Strombaject** *Sanofi Synthelabo, Belg.†.*
Stanozolol (p.1569·2).
*Anabolic.*

**Stromectol**
*Merck Sharp & Dohme, Austral.; Merck Sharp & Dohme-Chibret, Fr.; Merck, USA.*
Ivermectin (p.105·3).
*Lymphatic filariasis; onchocerciasis; scabies; strongyloidiasis.*

**Stromic** *Strathmann, Ger.*
Solidago virgaurea (p.1748·3).
*Urinary-tract disorders.*

**217 Strong** *Frosst, Canad.†.*
Aspirin (p.15·1); caffeine citrate (p.782·1).
*Fever; inflammation; pain.*

**StrongStart** *Savage, USA.*
Multivitamin and mineral preparation (p.1417·1).

**Strongus** *Franconpharm, Ger.*
Garlic (p.1691·1).
*Hyperlipidaemia.*

**Strophantab** *Fides, Ger.*
Homoeopathic preparation.

**Strophanthin-Herztabletten compositum**
*Cosmochema, Ger.*
Homoeopathic preparation.

**Strophanthus** *Phytomed, Switz.*
Homoeopathic preparation.

**Stropheupas-forte** *Pascoe, Ger.†.*
Homoeopathic preparation.

**Strotan** *Strathmann, Ger.*
Agnus castus (p.1649·1).
*Mastalgia; menstrual disorders.*

**Strovite** *Everett, USA.*
A range of vitamin and mineral preparations (p.1417·1).

**Strox** *Dabur, India.*
Ciprofloxacin hydrochloride (p.188·2).
*Bacterial infections.*

**Strubelin** *Phoinix Pharm (Φοινιξ Φαρμ), Gr.*
Ambroxol hydrochloride (p.1114·3).
*Respiratory disorders associated with viscous mucus.*

**Structolipid**
*Fresenius Kabi, Austria; Fresenius Kabi, Denm.; Fresenius Kabi, Fin.; Fresenius Kabi, Gr.; Fresenius Kabi, Norw.; Baxter, NZ; Fresenius Kabi, NZ; Fresenius Kabi, Port.; Fresenius Kabi, Spain; Fresenius Kabi, Swed.; Fresenius Kabi, Switz.; Fresenius Kabi, UK.*
Soya oil (p.1447·2); triglycerides from coconut oil or palm kernel oil (p.1440·3).
Contains egg phospholipids.
*Lipid infusion for parenteral nutrition.*

**Structolipide** *Fresenius Kabi, Fr.*
Triglycerides from coconut oil (p.1440·3) and soya oil (p.1447·2).
Contains egg lecithin.
*Lipid infusion for parenteral nutrition.*

**Structum**
*Sidus, Arg.; Pierre Fabre, Fr.; Robapharm, Switz.*
Chondroitin sulfate sodium (p.1670·2).
*Osteoarthritis.*

**Strumazol**
*Christiaens, Belg.; Nourypharma, Neth.*
Thiamazole (p.1603·3).
*Hyperthyroidism.*

**Strumedical 400** *Henning, Ger.†.*
Diiodotyrosine (p.1597·3).
*Iodine-deficiency disorders.*

**Strumex** *Robugen, Ger.*
Sodium iodide (p.1598·1).
*Iodine-deficiency disorders.*

**Stryphnasal** *Truw, Ger.*
Adrenalone hydrochloride (p.1648·2).
Formerly known as Stryphonasal.
*Epistaxis.*

**Stryphnon** *Sanova, Denm.*
Adrenalone hydrochloride (p.1648·2).
*Haemorrhage.*

**St-Tissues** *Bode, Ger.*
Isopropyl alcohol (p.1184·3); propyl alcohol (p.1191·2); mecetronium etilsulfate (p.1185·2).
*Surface disinfection.*

**Stuart Formula** *J&J-Merck, USA.*
Multivitamin and mineral preparation with iron and folic acid (p.1417·1).

**Stuart Prenatal** *Integrity, USA.*
Multivitamin and mineral preparation with folic acid and iron (p.1417·1).
*Dietary supplement in pregnancy.*

**Stuartnatal 1+1** *Wyeth-Ayerst, USA.*
Multivitamin and mineral preparation with iron and folic acid (p.1417·1).
*Dietary supplement in pregnancy.*

**Stuartnatal Plus** *Integrity, USA.*
Multivitamin and mineral preparation (p.1417·1).

**Stud** *Pound International, UK.*
Lidocaine (p.1377·3).
*Premature ejaculation.*

**Stud 100**
*Key, Austral.†; Trupharm, Israel.*
Lidocaine (p.1377·3).
*Premature ejaculation.*

**Stugerina** *Hexal, Braz.*
Cinnarizine (p.428·3).
*Vertigo.*

**Stugeron**
*Janssen-Cilag, Arg.; Janssen-Cilag, Belg.; Janssen-Cilag, Braz.; Janssen-Cilag, Chile; Janssen-Cilag, Gr.; Janssen, Hong Kong; Ethnor, India; Janssen-Cilag, Irl.; Janssen-Cilag, Ital.; Janssen-Cilag, Malaysia; Janssen, Mex.; Janssen-Cilag, Port.; Janssen-Cilag, S.Afr.; Janssen-Cilag, Singapore; Esteve, Spain; Janssen-Cilag, Switz.; Janssen-Cilag, Thai.; Janssen-Cilag, UK; Johnson & Johnson MSD Consumer, UK.*
Cinnarizine (p.428·3).
*Cerebrovascular disorders; migraine; motion sickness; peripheral vascular disorders; vestibular disorders.*

**Stullmaton** *Stulln, Ger.*
Centaury (p.1669·2); arnica (p.1656·3); melissa (p.1711·1); chamomile (p.1669·3); absinthium (p.1645·1); spruce tips; trace elements.
*Gastrointestinal disorders.*

**Stunarone** *Janssen-Cilag, Israel.*
Cinnarizine (p.428·3).
*Vestibular disorders.*

**Stuno** *Milano, Thai.*
Cinnarizine (p.428·3).
*Cerebral and peripheral vascular disorders; motion sickness; vestibular disorders.*

**Stutgeron**
*Janssen-Cilag, Austria; Janssen-Cilag, Ger.†.*
Cinnarizine (p.428·3).
*Cerebral and peripheral vascular disorders; vestibular disorders.*

**STV** *Elvetium, Arg.*
Stavudine (p.654·2).
*HIV infection.*

**Stye** *Del, USA.*
Yellow mercuric oxide (p.1712·3).
*Minor eye infections.*

**Stylo Sport** *Lancome, Canad.†.*
*SPF 15:* Octinoxate (p.1154·3); titanium dioxide (p.1160·3).
*Sunscreen.*

**stypro** *Curasan, Ger.*
Gelatin (p.754·3).
*Haemostatic.*

**Styptanon**
*Organon, Austria.*
Estriol sodium succinate (p.1552·3).
*Capillary haemorrhage.*

*Organon, Braz.*
Estriol succinate (p.1552·3).
*Haemorrhage; thrombocytopenia.*

**Styptin** *German Remedies, India.*
Norethisterone acetate (p.1562·2).
*Endometriosis; mastalgia; menstrual disorders.*

**Stypto-Caine** *Pedinol, USA.*
Aluminium chloride (p.1142·1); tetracaine (p.1385·1); hydroxyquinoline sulfate (p.1700·1).
*Bleeding in minor wounds.*

**Styptocid** *Stadmed, India.*
*Injection:* Carbazochrome (p.745·1).
*Tablets:* Carbazochrome (p.745·1); menadione sodium bisulfite (p.1466·3); rutoside (p.1688·2); vitamin C (p.1460·2); vitamin D (p.1461·2); calcium hydrogen phosphate (p.1225·2).
*Epistaxis; haemoptysis; menstrual disorders; retinal haemorrhage.*

**Styptysat** *Ysatfabrik, Ger.*
Shepherd's purse (p.1744·1).
*Haemorrhagic disorders.*

**Suadian** *Schering, Ital.*
Naftifine hydrochloride (p.406·2).
*Fungal skin and nail infections.*

**Sual** *Del Bel, Arg.*
Bladderwrack (p.1742·3).
*Dietary supplement.*

**Sualim** *Fouchard, Chile.*
Soap substitute.

**Sualyn** *Vita, Spain†.*
Bismuth subnitrate (p.1252·2); magnesium carbonate (p.1272·1); metoclopramide hydrochloride (p.1274·3); sorbitol (p.1446·3).
*Gastric spasms; gastritis; nausea; peptic ulcer; vomiting.*

**Suamoxil** *Cantabria, Spain†.*
Amoxicillin trihydrate (p.155·3).
*Bacterial infections.*

**Suavene** *Remexa, Mex.*
Avena (p.1658·2).

**Suavigel** *Fouchard, Chile.*
Levomenol (p.1707·1); enoxolone (p.36·2).
*Emollient.*

**Suavisan** *Medical, Arg.*
Hexylresorcinol (p.1182·1); benzocaine (p.1370·3); tyrothricin (p.275·1).
*Mouth and throat disorders.*

**Suavisan N** *Medical, Arg.*
Hexylresorcinol (p.1182·1); neomycin (p.235·1); benzocaine (p.1370·3).
*Mouth and throat disorders.*

**Suavisol** *Barnes Hind, Arg.*
Cleansing solution for soft contact lenses (p.1164·2).

**Suavit Calcio** *Dinafarma, Braz.†.*
Vitamin $B_{12}$; ergocalciferol; calcium chloride (p.1417·1).
*Nutritional supplement.*

**Suaviter** *Ico, Ital.*
Aspartame (p.1422·1).
*Sugar substitute.*

**Suavithiol** *Lersan, Arg.*
Naphazoline hydrochloride (p.1124·3); chlorphenamine maleate (p.427·3).
*Eye disorders.*

**Suavuret** *Organon, Spain.*
Ethinylestradiol (p.1553·2); desogestrel (p.1547·2).
*Combined oral contraceptive; menstrual disorders.*

**Sub Tensin** *Altana, Spain.*
Nitrendipine (p.973·3).
*Hypertension.*

**Subamycin** *Dey's, India.*
Tetracycline hydrochloride (p.266·2).
*Bacterial infections.*

**Subcutin N** *Ritsert, Ger.*
Benzocaine (p.1370·3).
*Mouth and throat disorders.*

**Subcuvia** *Baxter, UK.*
A normal immunoglobulin (p.1627·2).
*Immunodeficiency.*

**Subdue**
*Mead Johnson Nutritionals, Canad.; Mead Johnson, NZ.*
Preparation for enteral nutrition (p.1417·1).
*Inflammatory bowel disease; malabsorption disorders.*

**Subitan** *Eurofarma, Braz.†.*
Potassium iodide (p.1598·1); ammonium chloride (p.1115·2); mepyramine maleate (p.437·1); ephedrine hydrochloride (p.1120·1); lobelia (p.1589·1); hyoscyamus (p.485·2).
*Respiratory-tract congestion.*

**Sublimaze**
*Janssen-Cilag, Arg.; Janssen-Cilag, Austral.; Janssen-Ortho, Canad.†; Janssen-Cilag, Irl.; Janssen-Cilag, NZ; Janssen-Cilag, S.Afr.; Janssen-Cilag, UK; Janssen, USA.*
Fentanyl citrate (p.40·1).
*Adjunct to anaesthesia; neuroleptanalgesia; pain.*

**Sublivac** *Hal, Ger.*
Allergen extracts of pollen, house dust mites (p.1650·2), and skin (p.1650·2) (p.1650·1).
*Allergen immunotherapy.*

**Sublivac B.E.S.T.** *Hal, Neth.*
Allergen extracts (glycerolinated) (p.1650·1).
*Allergen immunotherapy.*

**Suboffen** *Offenbach, Mex.*
Pseudoephedrine (p.1129·2).
*Nasal congestion.*

**Suboxone** *Reckitt Benckiser, USA.*
Buprenorphine hydrochloride (p.21·3); naloxone hydrochloride (p.1044·3).
*Opioid withdrawal syndrome.*

**Subreum**
*Byk, Austria; Byk Tosse, Ger.; Byk Gulden, Ger.; OM, Port.*
*Escherichia coli* extract.
*Chronic polyarthritis.*

**Substi** *Abbott, Fr.†.*
Preparation for enteral nutrition (p.1417·1).

**Substitol** *Mundipharma, Austria.*
Morphine sulfate (p.60·2).
*Substitution therapy in opiate dependence.*

**Subsyde** *Raptakos, Thai.*
Diclofenac sodium (p.32·1).
*Gout; musculoskeletal and joint disorders; pain.*

**Subutex**
*Reckitt Benckiser, Austral.; Aesca, Austria; Schering-Plough, Belg.; Schering-Plough, Denm.; Schering-Plough, Fin.; Schering-Plough, Fr.; Essex, Ger.; Schering-Plough, Gr.; Schering-Plough, Hong Kong; Schering-Plough, Israel; Essex, Ital.; Schering-Plough, Malaysia; Schering-Plough, Norw.; Schering-Plough, Port.; Schering-Plough, Singapore; Schering-Plough, Spain; Schering-Plough, Swed.; Essex, Switz.; Schering-Plough, UK; Reckitt Benckiser, USA.*
Buprenorphine hydrochloride (p.21·3).
*Opioid withdrawal syndrome.*

**Sucadermil** *Edol, Port.*
Salicylic acid (p.1157·1); sulfur (p.1158·2); cade oil (p.1159·2).

**Sucari** *Jean-Marie, Hong Kong.*
Sucralfate (p.1290·2).
*Gastritis; peptic ulcer.*

**Sucaryl**
*Note. This name is used for preparations of different composition.*
*Merisant, Arg.; Abbott, Austral.†; Rider, Chile; Abbott, Fr.; Abbott, NZ.*
Calcium cyclamate (p.1426·2) or sodium cyclamate (p.1426·2); saccharin sodium (p.1443·3).
*Sugar substitute.*

*Abbott, Braz.†.*
Sodium cyclamate (p.1426·2).
*Sugar substitute.*

*Abbott, Canad.*
Sodium cyclamate (p.1426·2) with or without glucose.
*Sugar substitute.*

**Successia** *Wyeth Lederle, Fr.*
16 Tablets, estradiol (p.1550·1); 12 tablets, estradiol; gestodene (p.1556·1).
*Menopausal disorders; osteoporosis.*

**Succi** *Scott-Cassara, Arg.*
Suxamethonium (p.1408·3).
*Depolarising neuromuscular blocker.*

**Succi Pharmacetin** *Olan-Kemed, Thai.†.*
Chloramphenicol sodium succinate (p.185·1).
*Bacterial infections.*

**Succicaptal** *SERB, Fr.*
Succimer (p.1054·2).
*Mercury and lead poisoning.*

**Succicuran** *Rodleben, Ger.†.*
Suxamethonium chloride (p.1406·2).
*Depolarising neuromuscular blocker.*

**Succilate** *Aspen, S.Afr.†.*
Erythromycin estolate (p.208·1).
*Bacterial infections.*

**Succin** Abbott, S.Afr.†.
Erythromycin ethyl succinate (p.208·1).
*Bacterial infections.*

**Succinolin** Amino, Switz.
Suxamethonium chloride (p.1406·2).
*Depolarising neuromuscular blocker.*

**Succinyl**
Taro, Israel; Asta Medica, Malaysia; Asta Medica, Thai.
Suxamethonium chloride (p.1406·2).
*Depolarising neuromuscular blocker.*

**Succosa** Tika, Swed.†.
Sucralfate (p.1290·2).
*Peptic ulcer.*

**Succus Cineraria Maritima** Walker Pharmacal, USA.
Senecio (p.1743·1); hamamelis (p.1696·3); boric acid (p.1662·1).
*Cataract opacity.*

**Sucedal** Pharma Investi, Chile.
Zolpidem (p.729·2).
*Sleep disorders.*

**Sucee** Biolab, Thai.
Cyproterone acetate (p.1544·1); ethinylestradiol (p.1553·2).
*Androgen-dependent acne, alopecia, and hirsutism in females; oral contraceptive in women with androgenic symptoms.*

**Sucontral** Harras-Curarina, Ger.
Coutarea latiflora (p.1676·3).
*Diabetes mellitus.*

**Sucrabest** Combustin, Ger.
Sucralfate (p.1290·2).
*Peptic ulcer.*

**Sucrafen** LSP, Thai.
Sucralfate (p.1290·2).
*Gastritis; gastro-oesophageal reflux; peptic ulcer.*

**Sucrafilm** Sigma, Braz.
Sucralfate (p.1290·2).
*Peptic ulcer.*

**Sucrager** Nutrifar, Ital.
Sucralfate (p.1290·2).
*Gastritis; gastro-oesophageal reflux; peptic ulcer.*

**Sucraid** Orphan Medical, USA.
Sacrosidase (p.1741·2).
*Sucrase deficiency.*

**Sucral**
Bioprogress, Ital.; Ranbaxy, Thai.
Sucralfate (p.1290·2).
*Gastritis; gastro-oesophageal reflux; peptic ulcer.*

**Sucralan** Lannacher, Austria.
Sucralfate (p.1290·2).
*Gastro-oesophageal reflux; peptic ulcer.*

**Sucralbene** Ratiopharm, Austria.
Sucralfate (p.1290·2).
*Gastro-oesophageal reflux; peptic ulcer.*

**Sucralfin** Inverni della Beffa, Ital.
Sucralfate (p.1290·2).
*Gastritis; gastro-oesophageal reflux; peptic ulcer.*

**Sucralmax** Quesada, Arg.
Sucralfate (p.1290·2).
*Peptic ulcer.*

**Sucralose** Julphar, UAE.
Sucralfate (p.1290·2).
*Gastro-oesophageal reflux; peptic ulcer.*

**Sucralstad** Stada, Austria.
Sucralfate (p.1290·2).
*Peptic ulcer.*

**Sucralum** Inibsa, Port.
Sucralfate (p.1290·2).
*Gastritis; gastro-oesophageal reflux; peptic ulcer.*

**Sucramal** Sanofi Synthelabo, Ital.
Sucralfate (p.1290·2).
*Gastritis; gastro-oesophageal reflux; peptic ulcer.*

**Sucramed** S Med, Austria.
Sucralfate (p.1290·2).
*Peptic ulcer.*

**Sucraphil** Philopharm, Ger.
Sucralfate (p.1290·2).
*Gastro-oesophageal reflux; peptic ulcer.*

**Sucrate**
Lisapharma, Ital.; Lisapharma, Thai.
Sucralfate (p.1290·2).
*Gastritis; gastro-oesophageal reflux; peptic ulcer.*

**Sucrato** Armstrong, Mex.
Tripotassium dicitratobismuthate (p.1252·2).
*Peptic ulcer.*

**Sucratyrol** Tyrol, Austria.
Sucralfate (p.1290·2).
*Gastro-oesophageal reflux; peptic ulcer.*

**Sucredulcor** Pierre Fabre Sante, Fr.
Saccharin (p.1443·2).
*Sugar substitute.*

**Sucret** Sintofarma, Braz.†.
Aspartame (p.1422·1).
*Sugar substitute.*

**Sucrets**
Note. This name is used for preparations of different composition.
GlaxoSmithKline Consumer, Canad.; SmithKline Beecham Consumer, USA.
Dyclonine hydrochloride (p.1376·2).
*Sore throat.*

SmithKline Beecham, Israel.
Hexylresorcinol (p.1182·1).
*Sore throat.*

**Sucrets Children's Formula** SmithKline Beecham, Israel.
Dyclonine hydrochloride (p.1376·2).
*Sore throat.*

**Sucrets Cough Control**
GlaxoSmithKline Consumer, Canad.
Dextromethorphan (p.1117·3).
*Sore throat.*

SmithKline Beecham, USA†.
Dextromethorphan hydrobromide (p.1117·3).
*Coughs.*

**Sucrets Extra Strength** GlaxoSmithKline Consumer, Canad.
Hexylresorcinol (p.1182·1).
*Sore throat.*

**Sucrets 4-Hour Cough** SmithKline Beecham Consumer, USA†.
Dextromethorphan (p.1117·3).
*Coughs.*

**Sucrets for Kids** GlaxoSmithKline Consumer, Canad.
Dyclonine hydrochloride (p.1376·2).

**Sucrets Maximum Strength** SmithKline Beecham, Israel.
Dyclonine hydrochloride (p.1376·2).
*Sore throat.*

**Sucrets Sore Throat** SmithKline Beecham Consumer, USA.
Hexylresorcinol (p.1182·1).
*Sore throat.*

**Sucrin** Rafa, Israel.
Sodium cyclamate (p.1426·2); saccharin sodium (p.1443·3).
*Sugar substitute.*

**Sucroril** Sofar, Ital.
Sucralfate (p.1290·2).
*Gastritis; gastro-oesophageal reflux; peptic ulcer.*

**Suczulen mono** Abbott, Ger.
Liquorice (p.1270·2).
*Peptic ulcer.*

**Sudafed**
Pfizer Consumer, Austral.; GlaxoSmithKline, Fr.; Glaxo Wellcome, Hong Kong†; GlaxoSmithKline, India; Calmic, Irl.; Glaxo Wellcome, Mex.; Pfizer Consumer, Port.; GlaxoSmithKline, S.Afr.; GlaxoSmithKline, Singapore; Warner-Lambert, USA.
Pseudoephedrine hydrochloride (p.1129·2).
*Nasal and sinus congestion.*

**Sudafed for Children** Pfizer, NZ.
Pseudoephedrine hydrochloride (p.1129·2).
*Nasal congestion.*

**Sudafed Cold & Allergy** Warner-Lambert, USA.
Pseudoephedrine hydrochloride (p.1129·2); chlorphenamine maleate (p.427·3).

**Sudafed Cold & Cough**
Note. This name is used for preparations of different composition.
Pfizer Consumer, Canad.
Pseudoephedrine hydrochloride (p.1129·2); dextromethorphan hydrobromide (p.1117·3); paracetamol (p.76·2).
*Coughs and cold symptoms.*

Warner-Lambert, USA.
Pseudoephedrine hydrochloride (p.1129·2); dextromethorphan hydrobromide (p.1117·3); paracetamol (p.76·2); guaifenesin (p.1122·1).
*Coughs and cold symptoms.*

**Sudafed Cold & Flu** Pfizer Consumer, Canad.
Paracetamol (p.76·2); dextromethorphan hydrobromide(p.1117·3); guaifenesin (p.1122·1); pseudoephedrine hydrochloride (p.1129·2).
*Coughs and cold symptoms.*

**Sudafed Cold & Sinus** Warner-Lambert, USA.
Pseudoephedrine hydrochloride (p.1129·2); paracetamol (p.76·2).
*Nasal congestion.*

**Sudafed Congestion & Sinus Pain Relief** Pfizer Consumer, Austral.
Pseudoephedrine hydrochloride (p.1129·2); ibuprofen (p.45·3).

**Sudafed Day/Nightime Relief** Pfizer, NZ.
Day tablets, pseudoephedrine hydrochloride (p.1129·2); paracetamol (p.76·2); night tablets, pseudoephedrine hydrochloride; paracetamol; triprolidine hydrochloride (p.442·3).
*Cold and influenza symptoms.*

**Sudafed Daytime/Nightime Relief** Pfizer Consumer, Austral.
Day tablets, pseudoephedrine hydrochloride (p.1129·2); paracetamol (p.76·2); night tablets, pseudoephedrine hydrochloride; paracetamol; triprolidine hydrochloride (p.442·3).

**Sudafed Decongestant** Pfizer Consumer, Canad.
Pseudoephedrine hydrochloride (p.1129·2).
*Nasal congestion.*

**Sudafed DM** Warner-Lambert, Canad.†.
Pseudoephedrine hydrochloride (p.1129·2); dextromethorphan hydrobromide (p.1117·3).
*Cold symptoms; nasal congestion.*

**Sudafed Expectorant**
GlaxoSmithKline, Hong Kong; Calmic, Irl.†; GlaxoSmithKline, S.Afr.; GlaxoSmithKline, Singapore.
Pseudoephedrine hydrochloride (p.1129·2); guaifenesin (p.1122·1).
*Coughs; upper respiratory-tract congestion.*

**Sudafed Head Cold & Sinus** Pfizer Consumer, Canad.
Pseudoephedrine hydrochloride (p.1129·2); paracetamol (p.76·2).
*Cold symptoms; sinus pain.*

**Sudafed 12 Hour Relief** Pfizer, NZ.
Pseudoephedrine hydrochloride (p.1129·2).
*Nasal congestion.*

**Sudafed Non-Drying Sinus** Warner-Lambert, USA.
Pseudoephedrine hydrochloride (p.1129·2); guaifenesin (p.1122·1).
*Coughs and cold symptoms.*

**Sudafed Plus**
Note. This name is used for preparations of different composition.
Pfizer Consumer, UK.
Pseudoephedrine hydrochloride (p.1129·2); triprolidine hydrochloride (p.442·3).
*Allergic rhinitis.*

Wellcome, USA.
Pseudoephedrine hydrochloride (p.1129·2); chlorphenamine maleate (p.427·3).
*Upper respiratory-tract symptoms.*

**Sudafed Severe Cold** Warner-Lambert, USA.
Pseudoephedrine hydrochloride (p.1129·2); dextromethorphan hydrobromide (p.1117·3); paracetamol (p.76·2).
*Coughs and cold symptoms.*

**Sudafed Sinus** Warner-Lambert, USA.
Pseudoephedrine hydrochloride (p.1129·2); paracetamol (p.76·2).
*Nasal congestion.*

**Sudafed Sinus Advance** Pfizer Consumer, Canad.
Pseudoephedrine hydrochloride (p.1129·2); ibuprofen (p.45·3).
*Cold symptoms; sinusitis.*

**Sudafed Sinus & Nasal Decongestant**
Warner-Lambert, Austral.†; Pfizer, NZ.
Pseudoephedrine hydrochloride (p.1129·2).
*Nasal and sinus congestion.*

**Sudafed Sinus Pain & Allergy Relief**
Pfizer Consumer, Austral.; Pfizer, NZ.
Pseudoephedrine hydrochloride (p.1129·2); paracetamol (p.76·2); triprolidine hydrochloride (p.442·3).
*Allergic rhinitis; hay fever; nasal congestion; sinus pain.*

**Sudafed Sinus Pain Relief**
Pfizer Consumer, Austral.; Pfizer, NZ.
Pseudoephedrine hydrochloride (p.1129·2); paracetamol (p.76·2).
*Nasal congestion; sinus pain.*

**Sudagesic** GlaxoSmithKline, S.Afr.
Pseudoephedrine hydrochloride (p.1129·2); paracetamol (p.76·2).
*Cold and influenza symptoms.*

**Sudal** Atley, USA.
Pseudoephedrine hydrochloride (p.1129·2); guaifenesin (p.1122·1).
*Coughs.*

**Suda-Tussin** Reese, USA†.
Phenylpropanolamine hydrochloride (p.1127·3); guaifenesin (p.1122·1); dextromethorphan hydrobromide (p.1117·3).

**Sudevil Vita** Byk, Arg.
Cyproheptadine hydrochloride (p.430·1); vitamins.
*Reduced appetite.*

**Sudhinol** Ranbaxy, India.
Dextropropoxyphene (p.28·3); paracetamol (p.76·2).
*Pain.*

**Sudis** Andromaco, Mex.
Paracetamol (p.76·2).
*Fever; inflammation; pain.*

**Sudocrem**
Tosara, Irl.†; Tosara, UK.
Zinc oxide (p.1163·2); benzyl benzoate (p.1500·2); benzyl cinnamate; benzyl alcohol (p.1170·2).
*Acne; chilblains; eczema; minor burns; napkin rash; pressure sores; sunburn; wounds.*

**Sudodrin** ICN, Canad.†.
Pseudoephedrine hydrochloride (p.1129·2).

**Sudol** Coventry, UK†.
Tar acids (p.1193·3).

**Sudomyl** PSM, NZ.
Pseudoephedrine hydrochloride (p.1129·2).
*Nasal congestion.*

**Sudonol** Hearst, Braz.†.
Benzoic acid (p.1169·3); salicylic acid (p.1157·1); iodine (p.1598·1).
*Fungal skin infections.*

**Sudosian** Asian Pharm, Thai.
Pseudoephedrine hydrochloride (p.1129·2).
*Nasal congestion; obstructive airways disease; rhinitis.*

**Sudosin** Medea, Spain†.
Formaldehyde (p.1179·3); lindane (p.1506·3); aminobenzoic acid (p.1142·2); salicylic acid (p.1157·1); talc; thymol (p.1194·2); lavender essence.
*Skin disorders.*

**Suero Antiofidico Polivalente** Biol, Arg.
Viper venom antiserum (*Crotalus durissus, Bothrops alternatus, Bothrops neuwiedii*) (p.1639·1).
*Passive immunisation.*

**Suero Fisiologico**
Rider, Chile; Cinfa, Spain.
Sodium chloride (p.1233·3).
*Fluid and electrolyte disorders; nasal congestion.*

**Suero Fisiologico Vitulia** Ern, Spain.
Sodium chloride (p.1233·3).
*Fluid and electrolyte depletion; hypovolaemia.*

**Suero Glucosado Vitulia** Ern, Spain.
Glucose (p.1432·2).
*Carbohydrate source; fluid depletion.*

**Suero Glucosalino Vitulia** Ern, Spain.
Sodium chloride (p.1233·3); glucose (p.1432·2).
*Carbohydrate source; fluid and electrolyte depletion.*

**Suero Levulosado Vitulia** Ern, Spain†.
Fructose (p.1431·3).
*Carbohydrate source; fluid depletion.*

**Suero Potassico Bieffe ME** Bieffe, Spain.
Potassium chloride (p.1232·2); sodium chloride (p.1233·3).
*Diabetic ketoacidosis; hypokalaemia.*

**Suero Ringer Braun** Braun, Spain.
Electrolyte infusion (p.1217·1).
*Fluid and electrolyte depletion.*

**Suero Ringer Lactato Vitulia** Ern, Spain.
Electrolyte infusion (p.1217·1).
*Fluid and electrolyte depletion.*

**Sueroral** Casen Fleet, Spain.
Glucose; potassium chloride; sodium citrate; sodium chloride (p.1222·2).
*Diarrhoea; oral rehydration therapy; vomiting.*

**Suevitine** Augot, Fr.†.
Vitamin, mineral, and trace element preparation (p.1417·1).

**Sufenta**
Janssen-Cilag, Arg.; Janssen-Cilag, Austria; Janssen-Cilag, Belg.; Janssen-Cilag, Braz.; Janssen-Ortho, Canad.; Janssen-Cilag, Chile; Janssen-Cilag, Denm.; Janssen-Cilag, Fin.; Janssen-Cilag, Fr.; Janssen-Cilag, Ger.; Janssen-Cilag, Malaysia; Janssen-Cilag, Neth.; Janssen-Cilag, Norw.; Janssen-Cilag, S.Afr.; Janssen-Cilag, Swed.; Janssen-Cilag, Switz.; Taylor, USA.
Sufentanil citrate (p.90·2).
*Analgesia in anaesthesia; general anaesthesia; pain.*

**Suffisance** Plumbland, Arg.
Sulfur (p.1158·2).
*Acne.*

**Sufil** Elfar, Spain.
Mebendazole (p.108·2).
*Worm infections.*

**Sufisal** Silanes, Mex.
Pentoxifylline (p.979·3).
*Vascular disorders.*

**Sufortan** Sanfer, Mex.
Penicillamine (p.1046·3).
*Cystinuria; heavy-metal poisoning; rheumatoid arthritis; Wilson's disease.*

**Sufortanon** Asta Medica, Spain†.
Penicillamine (p.1046·3).
*Cystinuria; heavy-metal poisoning; rheumatoid arthritis; Wilson's disease.*

**Sufralem** Solvay, Port.
Anethole trithione (p.1655·1).
*Dry eyes; dry mouth.*

**Sufrexal**
Janssen-Cilag, Belg.; Janssen-Cilag, Ital.†; Janssen-Cilag, Port.; Janssen-Cilag, Thai.
Ketanserin tartrate (p.943·1).
*Hypertension.*

Janssen, Mex.
Ketanserin (p.943·1).
*Burns; cervical ulcers; skin ulcers; wounds.*

**Suganril** Sarabhai Piramal, India.
Piroxicam (p.84·2).
*Gout; musculoskeletal and joint disorders.*

**Sugar** Uno, Ital.
Sucralfate (p.1290·2).
*Gastritis; gastro-oesophageal reflux; peptic ulcer.*

**Sugar Bloc** Cantassium Co., UK.
Gymnema silvestre; chromium orotate (p.1724·3).
*Diet aid.*

**Sugarbil** Novag, Spain.
Cyclobutyrol sodium (p.1678·2); magnesium sulfate (p.1228·2); sorbitol (p.1446·3).
*Constipation; hepatobiliary disorders.*

**Sugarceton** Novag, Spain†.
Calcium fructose diphosphate; hydroxocobalamin hydrochloride (p.1459·1); promethazine hydrochloride (p.439·1); thiamine phosphate (p.1455·2); trometamol acefyllinate (p.1758·3); trometamol thioctate (p.1754·3); sorbitol (p.1446·3); glucose (p.1432·2).
*Acetonaemia; acidosis.*

**Sugarless C** Cenovis, Austral.†; Vitelle, Austral.†.
Ascorbic acid (p.1460·2); sodium ascorbate (p.1460·2).
*Vitamin C supplement.*

**Sugast** Selvi, Ital.
Sucralfate (p.1290·2).
*Gastritis; gastro-oesophageal reflux; peptic ulcer.*

**Sugiran** Pensa, Spain.
Alprostadil alfadex (p.1512·3).
*Peripheral vascular disease.*

**Sugril** Siam Bheasach, Thai.
Glibenclamide (p.331·2).
*Diabetes mellitus.*

**Suguan** Hoechst, Ital.
Glibenclamide (p.331·2); phenformin hydrochloride (p.344·1).
*Diabetes mellitus.*

**Suguan M** Hoechst, Ital.
Glibenclamide (p.331·2); metformin hydrochloride (p.342·3).
*Diabetes mellitus.*

**Suifac** Novartis, Mex.
Omeprazole (p.1278·2).
*Gastro-oesophageal reflux; peptic ulcer; Zollinger-Ellison syndrome.*

**Suiflox** *Novartis, Mex.*
Ciprofloxacin hydrochloride (p.188·2).
*Bacterial infections.*

**Suimel** *Oriental, Arg.*
Saccharin sodium (p.1443·3); glucose (p.1432·2); cyclamate.
*Sugar substitute.*

**Suipen** *Novartis, Mex.*
Procaine benzylpenicillin (p.246·1); benzylpenicillin sodium (p.163·2).
*Bacterial infections.*

**Sukar-Sin** *Laboratorios Chile, Chile.*
*Liquid:* Sodium cyclamate (p.1426·2); saccharin sodium (p.1443·3).
*Tablets:* Saccharin sodium (p.1443·3).
*Sugar substitute.*

**Sukcee** *Indian Drugs, India.*
Ascorbic acid (p.1460·2); sodium ascorbate (p.1460·2).
*Infections; scurvy; wounds.*

**Sukepar** *Biochimico, Braz.*
Liver extract.
*Liver disorders.*

**Sukir** *Brasifa, Braz.*†.
Saccharin sodium (p.1443·3).
*Sugar substitute.*

**Sukolin** *Orion, Fin.*
Suxamethonium chloride (p.1406·2).
*Depolarising neuromuscular blocker.*

**Sul 10** *Grin, Mex.*
Sulfacetamide sodium (p.257·3).
*Bacterial eye infections.*

**Sulamid** *Baldacci, Ital.*
Amisulpride (p.669·3).
*Depression.*

**Sular**
*AstraZeneca, Belg.; Zeneca, Mex.†; AstraZeneca, Neth.†; AstraZeneca, Spain; Horizon, USA.*
Nisoldipine (p.973·2).
*Angina pectoris; hypertension.*

**Sulartrene** *NCSN, Ital.*†.
Sulindac (p.91·2).
*Gout; musculoskeletal, joint, peri-articular, and soft-tissue disorders.*

**Sulazine** *Chatfield Laboratories, UK.*
Sulfasalazine (p.1291·1).
*Inflammatory bowel disease; rheumatoid arthritis.*

**Sulbacin** *Unichem, India.*
*Injection:* Sulbactam (p.257·2); ampicillin (p.157·1).
*Tablets:* Sultamicillin tosilate (p.264·2).
*Bacterial infections.*

**Sulbacta** *Olan-Kemed, Thai.*
Co-trimoxazole (p.199·3).
*Bacterial infections.*

**Sulbamox** *Bago, Chile.*
Amoxicillin sodium (p.155·3) or amoxicillin trihydrate (p.155·3); pivsulbactam (p.257·2) or sulbactam sodium (p.257·2).
*Bacterial infections.*

**Sulcain**
*Shinyaku, Hong Kong; Shinyaku, Singapore; Shinyaku, Thai.*
Ethyl *p*-piperidinoacetylaminobenzoate (p.1376·3); magcerin (magnesia alumina hydrate).
*Gastric pain; gastritis; nausea; pyrosis.*

*Shinyaku, Jpn.*
Ethyl *p*-piperidinoacetylaminobenzoate (p.1376·3).
*Gastritis.*

**Sulcoline** *Teva Tuteur, Arg.*
Vinorelbine (p.594·2).
*Malignant neoplasms.*

**Sulcran** *Silesia, Chile.*
Sucralfate (p.1290·2).
*Peptic ulcer.*

**Sulcrate** *Aventis, Canad.*
Sucralfate (p.1290·2).
*Gastrointestinal haemorrhage; peptic ulcer.*

**Suldiamin** *Fortbenton, Arg.*
Sulfur (p.1158·2).
*Seborrhoea.*

**Sulen** *Farmacologico Milanese, Ital.*
Sulindac (p.91·2).
*Gout; musculoskeletal, joint, and peri-articular disorders.*

**Suleo-M** *SSL, UK.*
Malathion (p.1507·1).
*Pediculosis.*

**Sulf-10** *Novartis Ophthalmics, USA.*
Sulfacetamide sodium (p.257·3).
*Eye infections.*

**Sulfa 10** *Viatris, Belg.*
Sulfacetamide sodium (p.257·3).
*Bacterial eye infections.*

**Sulfa Cloran** *Grin, Mex.*
Chloramphenicol (p.185·1); sulfacetamide sodium (p.257·3).
*Bacterial eye infections.*

**Sulfa Hidro** *Grin, Mex.*
Hydrocortisone acetate (p.1103·3); sulfacetamide sodium (p.257·3).
*Infected eye disorders.*

**Sulfac** *Ocusoft, USA.*
Sulfacetamide sodium (p.257·3).
*Bacterial eye infections.*

**Sulfacet** *Llorens, Spain*†.
Sulfacetamide sodium (p.257·3).
*Bacterial eye infections.*

**Sulfacetam** *Medical, Spain.*
Sulfacetamide sodium (p.257·3).
*Eye infections.*

**Sulfacet-R**
*Dermik, Canad.; Dermik, USA.*
Sulfacetamide sodium (p.257·3); sulfur (p.1158·2).
*Acne; rosacea; seborrhoeic dermatitis.*

**Sulfachloramphenicol** *Novartis, Gr.*
Chloramphenicol (p.185·1); sulfacetamide sodium (p.257·3).
*Eye infections.*

**Sulfacid** *Fischer, Israel.*
Sulfacetamide sodium (p.257·3).
*Eye infections.*

**Sulfacollyre** *Sterop, Belg.*
Sulfacetamide sodium (p.257·3).
*Bacterial eye infections.*

**Sulfaderm** *Kinder, Braz.*
Sulfadiazine silver (p.259·1).

**Sulfadiazina de Plata** *Denver, Arg.*
Sulfadiazine silver (p.259·1); vitamin A (p.1451·2); lidocaine (p.1377·3).

**Sulfadiazinac** *Catarinense, Braz.*
Sulfadiazine (p.258·2).
*Bacterial infections.*

**Sulfafer** *Protein, Mex.*†.
Ferrous sulfate (p.1428·2).

**Sulfagine** *Tocogino, Mex.*†.
Sulfathiazole (p.264·1).

**Sulfagrand** *Ahimsa, Arg.*
Co-trimoxazole (p.199·3).
*Bacterial infections.*

**Sulfamide** *Medical Ophthalmics, USA.*
Prednisolone acetate (p.1108·1); sulfacetamide sodium (p.257·3).
*Infected eye disorders.*

**Sulfamylon** *Bertek, USA.*
Mafenide acetate (p.228·2).
*Burns.*

**Sulfanicole** *Cooper (Κοπερ), Gr.*
Chloramphenicol (p.185·1); sulfacetamide sodium (p.257·3).
*Eye infections.*

**Sulfanil** *Allergan-Frumtost, Braz.*†.
Sulfacetamide (p.257·3).
*Bacterial eye infections.*

**Sulfanoral T** *Sidus, Arg.*
Tyrothricin (p.275·1); cresol (p.1177·3); benzocaine (p.1370·3).
*Mouth and throat disorders.*

**Sulfaplat** *Lafedar, Arg.*
Sulfadiazine silver (p.259·1); vitamin A palmitate (p.1453·1); lidocaine (p.1377·3).

**Sulfarlem**
*Solvay, Belg.†; Solvay, Canad.†; Solvay, Fr.; Solvay, Hong Kong†; Hoechst Marion Roussel, S.Afr.†; Solvay, Switz.*
Anethole trithione (p.1655·1).
*Biliary-tract disorders; dry eye; dry mouth; hypersensitivity reactions; liver disorders.*

**Sulfarlem Choline** *Solvay, Belg.*†.
Anethole trithione (p.1655·1); choline bitartrate (p.1424·3).
*Liver disorders; steatosis.*

**Sulfarlem S 25** *Solvay, Belg.*
Anethole trithione (p.1655·1).
*Dry mouth.*

**Sulfaryl** *Zeneca, Belg.*†.
Acetarsol (p.600·2); sulfanilamide (p.263·2); sodium perborate (p.1192·2).
*Mouth disorders.*

**Sulfatina** *Geyer, Braz.*
Atropine sulfate (p.477·1).

**Sulfato Ferroso Composto** *Legrand, Braz.*
Ferrous sulfate (p.1428·2); thiamine nitrate (p.1455·1); copper sulfate (p.1426·1).
Ascorbic acid (p.1460·2) is included in this preparation to increase the absorption and availability of iron.
*Anaemias.*

**Sulfatofer** *Neo Quimica, Braz.*
*Oral drops; oral liquid:* Ferrous sulfate (p.1428·2).
*Iron-deficiency anaemia.*
*Tablets:* Ferrous sulfate (p.1428·2); copper sulfate (p.1426·1); thiamine hydrochloride (p.1455·1); riboflavin (p.1456·1).
*Anaemias.*

**Sulfatral** *LA, Arg.*
Sulfadiazine (p.258·2).
*Bacterial skin infections.*

**Sulfatral-Cerio** *LA, Arg.*
Sulfadiazine (p.258·2); cerous nitrate (p.1144·3).
*Bacterial skin infections.*

**Sulfatrex** *QIF, Braz.*†.
Co-trimoxazole (p.199·3); guaifenesin (p.1122·1); ammonium chloride (p.1115·2).
*Bacterial infections.*

**Sulfatril** *Hua, Thai.*
Sulfadiazine (p.258·2); sulfadimidine (p.259·2); sulfamerazine (p.260·3).
*Bacterial infections.*

**Sulfatrim**
*Vitamed, Israel; Schein, USA.*
Co-trimoxazole (p.199·3).
*Bacterial infections; Pneumocystis carinii pneumonia.*

**Sulfa+Trim** *Braskap, Braz.*†.
Co-trimoxazole (p.199·3).
*Bacterial infections.*

**Sulfawal** *Novag, Mex.*
Co-trimoxazole (p.199·3).
*Bacterial infections.*

**Sulfer Plus** *Delta, Braz.*
Ferrous sulfate (p.1428·2).
*Iron-deficiency anaemia.*

**Sulferro** *Fontovit, Braz.*
Ferrous sulfate (p.1428·2).
*Iron-deficiency anaemia.*

**Sulferrol** *Bunker, Braz.*
Ferrous sulfate (p.1428·2).
*Iron deficiency; iron-deficiency anaemia.*

**Sulfestrep** *Pisa, Mex.*
Streptomycin (p.256·1).
*Bacterial infections.*

**Sulfex**
*Charton, Canad.†; Xepa-Soul Pattinson, Hong Kong.*
Sulfacetamide sodium (p.257·3).
*Bacterial eye infections.*

**Sulfile**
*Monsanto, Ital.*
Arginine timonacicate (p.1421·2).
*Liver disorders.*

*Lepori, Port.*
Arginine tidiacicate (p.1421·2).
*Liver disorders.*

**Sulfinona** *Basi, Port.*
Sulfinpyrazone (p.417·3).

**Sulfintestin Neom** *Hosbon, Spain*†.
Formosulfathiazole (p.214·2); neomycin sulfate (p.235·1).
*Gastrointestinal infections.*

**Sulfintestin Neomicina** *Normon, Spain.*
Dihydrostreptomycin sulfate (p.205·3); formosulfathiazole (p.214·2); neomycin sulfate (p.235·1).
*Gastrointestinal infections.*

**Sulfiselen** *Diviser Aquilea, Spain*†.
Selenium sulfide (p.1157·3); thiram disulfide (p.1755·1).
*Dandruff.*

**Sulfitrat** *Teuto, Braz.*
Sulfiram (p.1510·1).

**Sulfix** *Allo Pro, Austria*†.
Methylmethacrylate/polymethylmethacrylate (p.1714·3).
*Bone cement.*

**Sulfizax** *Remir, Mex.*†.
Sulfafurazole (p.260·1).
*Bacterial infections.*

**Sulfoam** *Doak, USA.*
Sulfur (p.1158·2).
Formerly contained salicylic acid.
*Dandruff; seborrhoea.*

**Sulfoid Trimetho** *Valdecasas, Mex.*
Co-trimoxazole (p.199·3).
*Bacterial infections.*

**Sulfoil** *C & M, USA.*
Soap-free skin cleanser.

**Sulfometh** *Hua, Thai.*
Co-trimoxazole (p.199·3).
*Bacterial infections.*

**Sulfona**
*Zimaia, Port.; Orsade, Spain.*
Dapsone (p.202·2).
*Leprosy.*

**Sulfo-Olbad Cordes** *Ichthyol, Ger.*
Shale oil; soya oil (p.1447·2).
*Bath additive; skin disorders.*

**Sulfopino** *Schoning-Berlin, Ger.*
Colloidal sulfur (p.1158·2).
*Bath additive; joint disorders; neuralgia; skin disorders.*

**Sulforcin** *Healthpoint, USA.*
Sulfur (p.1158·2); resorcinol (p.1156·3).
*Acne.*

**Sulfort** *Alpha, Mex.*†.
Co-trimoxazole (p.199·3).
*Bacterial infections.*

**Sulfo-Salicyl** *Life, Israel.*
Salicylic acid (p.1157·1); sulfur (p.1158·2); Dead Sea minerals.
*Psoriasis; seborrhoea.*

**Sulfo-Schwefelbad** *Strallhofer, Austria.*
Sulfur (p.1158·2); sodium hydroxide (p.1747·3).
*Musculoskeletal and joint disorders; skin disorders.*

**Sulfo-Selenium** *Asta Medica, Belg.*†.
Hydrocortisone (p.1103·3); selenium disulfide (p.1157·3).
*Squamous blepharitis.*

**Sulfotrim** *Gea, Denm.*
Co-trimoxazole (p.199·3).
*Bacterial infections; Pneumocystis carinii pneumonia.*

**Sulfoxyl**
*Stiefel, Canad.†; Stiefel, USA.*
Benzoyl peroxide (p.1143·2); sulfur (p.1158·2).
*Acne.*

**Sulfredox** *Rubiepharm, Ger.*
*Oral granules*†*:* Aluminium sodium silicate (p.1250·2); sulfur (p.1158·2); calcium carbonate (p.1254·2); magnesium oxide (p.1272·3); sodium ascorbate; trace elements.
*Tablets:* Aluminium sodium silicate (p.1250·2); sulfur (p.1158·2); calcium carbonate (p.1254·2); sodium ascorbate; trace elements.
*Digestive system disorders.*

**Sulf+Trim** *Sinterapico, Braz.*†.
Co-trimoxazole (p.199·3).
*Bacterial infections.*

**Sulfur Med Complex** *Dynamit, Austria.*
Homoeopathic preparation.

**Sulfurell** *Sanorell, Ger.*
Homoeopathic preparation.

**Sulfuretten** *Stulln, Ger.*
Sulfur (p.1158·2); sodium thiosulfate (p.1053·3).
*Dermatoses; lead, arsenic, or mercury poisoning; metabolic disorders.*

**Sulfuryl** *Richelet, Fr.*
*Bath additive:* Sulfurated aluminium sodium silicate (p.1250·2); precipitated sulfur (p.1158·2).
*Arthroses; skin disorders.*
*Chewable tablets; inhalation tablets:* Sulfurated aluminium sodium silicate (p.1250·2).
*Respiratory-tract congestion.*
*Soap:* Sulfurated aluminium sodium silicate (p.1250·2); precipitated sulfur (p.1158·2).
*Skin disorders.*

**Sulgan 99** *Klosterfrau, Austria.*
*Ointment; suppositories:* Ethyl linoleate; ethyl linolenate; benzocaine (p.1370·3); dichlorobenzyl alcohol (p.1178·3); aluminium chlorohydrate (p.1142·1); hamamelis (p.1696·3); camphor (p.1665·3); menthol (p.1711·3); zinc oxide (p.1163·2).
*Rectal wipes:* Benzocaine (p.1370·3); dichlorobenzyl alcohol (p.1178·3); hamamelis (p.1696·3); chamomile water (p.1669·3); camphor (p.1665·3); menthol (p.1711·3).
*Anorectal disorders.*

**Sulgan N** *Doetsch, Grether, Switz.*
*Ointment; suppositories:* Ethyl linoleate; ethyl linolenate; lidocaine (p.1377·3) or lidocaine hydrochloride (p.1377·3); dichlorobenzyl alcohol (p.1178·3); camphor (p.1665·3); menthol (p.1711·3); triclosan (p.1195·2).
*Wipes:* Dichlorobenzyl alcohol (p.1178·3); lidocaine hydrochloride (p.1377·3); camphor (p.1665·3); menthol (p.1711·3).
*Anorectal disorders.*

**Sulidamor** *Damor, Ital.*
Nimesulide (p.67·1).
*Fever; inflammation; pain.*

**Sulide** *Infosint, Ital.*
Nimesulide (p.67·1).
*Fever; inflammation; pain.*

**Sulimed** *Inibsa, Port.*
Nimesulide (p.67·1).
*Inflammation; musculoskeletal, joint, and peri-articular disorders; pain.*

**Sulindal** *Chibret, Spain.*
Sulindac (p.91·2).
*Gout; inflammation; musculoskeletal, joint, and peri-articular disorders; pain.*

**Sulindor** *Millet Roux, Braz.*†.
Dipyrone (p.35·3); isometheptene (p.1702·2); caffeine (p.782·1).
*Smooth muscle spasm.*

**Sulinol** *ICT, Ital.*†.
Sulindac (p.91·2).
*Gout; musculoskeletal, joint, and peri-articular disorders; neuritis; sciatica.*

**Sulkine** *Zambon, Spain.*
Levosulpiride (p.722·2).
*Dyspepsia.*

**Sulmasque** *C & M, USA.*
Sulfur (p.1158·2).
*Acne.*

**Sulmetin** *Sanofi Synthelabo, Spain.*
Magnesium sulfate (p.1228·2).
Procaine hydrochloride (p.1383·2) is included in the intramuscular injection to alleviate the pain of injection.
*Convulsions; tachycardia; vertigo.*

**Sulmetin Papaver** *Sanofi Synthelabo, Spain.*
Atropine methobromide (p.476·3); magnesium sulfate (p.1228·2); papaverine hydrochloride (p.1728·1); propyphenazone (p.85·3).
*Pain due to smooth muscle spasm.*

**Sulmetin Papaverina** *Sanofi Synthelabo, Spain.*
*Injection:* Magnesium sulfate (p.1228·2); papaverine hydrochloride (p.1728·1).
Procaine hydrochloride (p.1383·2) is included in the intramuscular injection to alleviate the pain of injection.
*Convulsions; hypertension; smooth muscle spasm; tachycardia.*
*Tablets:* Atropine methobromide (p.476·3); magnesium gluconate (p.1228·1); papaverine hydrochloride (p.1728·1); propyphenazone (p.85·3).
*Pain due to smooth muscle spasm.*

**Sulmycin**
*Aesca, Austria; Essex, Ger.; Nycomed, Ger.*
Gentamicin sulfate (p.217·1).
*Bacterial infections.*

**Sulmycin mit Celestan-V** *Essex, Ger.*
Gentamicin sulfate (p.217·1); betamethasone valerate (p.1093·2).
*Infected skin disorders.*

**Sulmyn** *Sons, Mex.*
Kanamycin (p.225·2).
*Bacterial infections.*

**Sulnil** *Allergan, Braz.*
Chloramphenicol (p.185·1); sulfacetamide sodium (p.257·3).
*Bacterial eye infections.*

**Sulobil** *Atlantis, Mex.*
Chenodeoxycholic acid (p.1670·1).
*Cholesterol gallstones.*

**Sulocten** *Microsules, Arg.*
Enalapril maleate (p.909·2).
*Hypertension.*

**Sulorane** *Zeneca, Israel.*
Desflurane (p.1297·2).
*General anaesthesia.*

**Sulotil** *Lafi, Chile.*
Nifedipine (p.966·2).
*Angina pectoris; hypertension.*

**Suloves** *Lampugnani, Ital.†.*
A heparinoid (p.931·1).
*Thrombosis prophylaxis.*

**Sulp** *Hexal, Ger.*
Sulpiride (p.722·2).
*Depression; schizophrenia; vestibular disorders.*

**Sulpan** *Sanofi Synthelabo, Braz.*
Sulpiride (p.722·2); bromazepam (p.671·3).
*Depression.*

**Sulparex** *Bristol-Myers Squibb, UK†.*
Sulpiride (p.722·2).
*Schizophrenia.*

**Sulperazon**
*Note. This name is used for preparations of different composition.*
*Pfizer, Arg.; Pfizer, Hong Kong; Pfizer, Thai.*
Sulbactam sodium (p.257·2); cefoperazone sodium (p.174·3).
*Bacterial infections.*

*Pfizer, Chile; Pfizer, Malaysia.*
Sulbactam (p.257·2); cefoperazone (p.175·1).
*Bacterial infections.*

*Pfizer, Jpn.*
Ampicillin sodium (p.157·1); sulbactam sodium (p.257·2).
*Bacterial infections.*

**Sulphamide** *Vitamed, Israel†.*
Sulfacetamide sodium (p.257·3).
*Bacterial eye infections.*

**Sulpho-Lac** *Doak, USA.*
Sulfur (p.1158·2); zinc sulfate (p.1469·3).
*Acne.*

**Sulpilan** *Labomed, Chile.*
Sulpiride (p.722·2).
*Depression; psychoses.*

**Sulpiren** *Medochemie, Hong Kong†.*
Sulpiride (p.722·2).
*Gastrointestinal disorders.*

**Sulpitil** *Pharmacia, UK.*
Sulpiride (p.722·2).
*Schizophrenia.*

**Sulpivert** *Hennig, Ger.*
Sulpiride (p.722·2).
*Depression; schizophrenia; vestibular disorders.*

**Sulpor** *Rosemont, UK.*
Sulpiride (p.722·2).
*Schizophrenia.*

**Sulpril** *AstraZeneca, Denm.†.*
Sulpiride (p.722·2).
*Schizophrenia.*

**Sulprim** *Berman, Mex.*
Co-trimoxazole (p.199·3).
*Bacterial infections.*

**Sulpyrin** *CCPC, Hong Kong†.*
Dipyrone (p.35·3).
*Fever.*

**Sulquibron** *Bohm, Spain†.*
Ampicillin (p.157·1); citiolone (p.1672·3).
*Respiratory-tract infections.*

**Sulquipen** *Bohm, Spain.*
Cefalexin (p.168·1).
*Bacterial infections.*

**Sultanol**
*GlaxoSmithKline, Austria; GlaxoSmithKline, Ger.; Schwarz, Ger.*
Salbutamol sulfate (p.791·3).
*Obstructive airways disease.*

**Sulterline** *TP, Thai.*
Terbutaline sulfate (p.797·2).
*Obstructive airways disease.*

**Sultiprim** *Columbia, Mex.*
Co-trimoxazole (p.199·3).
*Bacterial infections.*

**Sulton** *Geymonat, Ital.*
Calcium folinate (p.1431·1).
*Anaemias; antidote to folic acid antagonists; reduction of aminopterin and methotrexate toxicity.*

**Sultrin**
*Janssen-Cilag, Austral.†; Janssen-Cilag, Belg.; Janssen-Ortho, Canad.†; Janssen-Cilag, Irl.; Janssen-Cilag, Port.; Janssen-Cilag, S.Afr.; Janssen-Cilag, UK; Ortho McNeil, USA.*
Sulfabenzamide (p.257·3); sulfacetamide (p.257·3); sulfathiazole (p.264·1).
*Cervicitis; vaginitis.*

**Sultrona** *Cryopharma, Mex.*
Conjugated oestrogens (p.1543·2).
*Menopausal disorders; osteoporosis.*

**Sultroquin** *Farcoral, Mex.*
Clioquinol (p.196·3); homatropine (p.483·2); phthalylsulfathiazole (p.242·3).
*Gastrointestinal disorders.*

**Sumacal** *Sherwood, USA.*
Glucose polymers (p.1417·1).
*Carbohydrate source.*

**Sumaclina** *Alodial, Port.*
Simvastatin (p.997·1).
*Hypercholesterolaemia.*

**Sumal** *Purissimus, Arg.*
Bendroflumethiazide (p.867·3); homatropine methylbromide (p.483·2); dipyrone (p.35·3).
*Premenstrual syndrome.*

**Sumapen** *Great Eastern, Thai.; Westmont, Thai.*
Ampicillin trihydrate (p.157·2).
*Bacterial infections.*

**Sumax** *Libbs, Braz.*
Sumatriptan succinate (p.471·2).
*Migraine.*

**Sumedium** *Milano, Thai.*
Phenazopyridine hydrochloride (p.83·1).
*Urinary-tract pain.*

**Sumenan** *Spedrog, Arg.*
Zolpidem tartrate (p.728·3).
*Insomnia.*

**Sumial** *Icaro, Spain.*
Propranolol hydrochloride (p.989·3).
*Angina pectoris; arrhythmias; gastrointestinal haemorrhage; hypertension; hyperthyroidism; migraine; myocardial infarction; obstructive cardiomyopathy; phaeochromocytoma; tremor.*

**Sumidin** *Pharmaland, Thai.*
Serrapeptase (p.1743·2).
*Inflammation; oedema; respiratory-tract congestion.*

**Sumiferon** *Sumitomo, Jpn.*
Interferon alfa (p.640·3).
*Hepatitis B and C; malignant neoplasms; myelopathy; subacute sclerosing panencephalitis.*

**Sumigrene** *Sigma-Tau, Ital.*
Sumatriptan succinate (p.471·2).
*Cluster headache; migraine.*

**Suminat** *Sun, India.*
Sumatriptan succinate (p.471·2).
*Migraine.*

**Sumir** *Craveri, Arg.*
Azithromycin (p.159·1).
*Bacterial infections.*

**Summavac** *Cassara, Arg.*
A range of bacterial and fungal allergen extracts (p.1650·1).
*Hypersensitivity reactions.*

**Summavit** *Bioprogress, Ital.*
Multivitamin preparation (p.1417·1).

**Summavit ME** *Armstrong, Arg.*
Vitamin and mineral preparation (p.1417·1).

**Summers Eve**
*Fleet, Singapore; De Witt, UK; Fleet, USA.*
A range of feminine hygiene preparations.

**Summers Eve Disposable**
*Note. This name is used for preparations of different composition.*
*Fleet, Austral.†.*
*Fresh Scent:* Phenol (p.1188·1).
*Herbal Scented; White Flowers; Hint of Musk:* Octoxinol 9 (p.1414·1).
*Vinegar and Water:* Vinegar (p.1645·2).
*Vaginal cleanser.*

*Fleet, USA.*
*Regular solution:* Sodium citrate (p.1223·2); citric acid (p.1673·1); sodium benzoate (p.1169·3).
*Scented solution:* Sodium citrate (p.1223·2); citric acid (p.1673·1); sodium benzoate (p.1169·3); octoxinol 9 (p.1414·1).
*Solution:* Vinegar (p.1645·2).
*Vaginal disorders.*

**Summers Eve Feminine** *Fleet, Austral.†.*
*Bath additive; topical liquid; topical spray:* Soap substitute.
*Vaginal hygiene.*
*Topical powder:* Octoxinol 9 (p.1414·1); benzethonium chloride (p.1169·2).
*Intertrigo; vaginal irritation.*
*Towelettes:* Octoxinol 9 (p.1414·1).
*Vaginal hygiene.*

**Summer's Eve Hierbas** *Rider, Chile.*
Citric acid (p.1673·1); sodium benzoate (p.1169·3); sodium citrate (p.1223·2); octoxinol 9 (p.1414·1).
*Vaginal hygiene.*

**Summers Eve Medicated**
*Fleet, Malaysia; Dewitt, Malaysia; Fleet, Singapore†; Fleet, USA.*
Povidone-iodine (p.1190·3).
*Vaginal disorders.*

**Summers Eve Post-Menstrual** *Fleet, USA.*
Sodium laurilsulfate (p.1574·2); monobasic sodium phosphate (p.1230·3); dibasic sodium phosphate (p.1231·1); sodium chloride (p.1233·3); edetic acid (p.1038·2).
*Vaginal disorders.*

**Summer's Eve Vinagre y Agua** *Rider, Chile.*
Vinegar (p.1645·2); benzoic acid (p.1169·3).
*Vaginal hygiene.*

**Sumo** *Interbelle, Arg.*
Phenothrin (p.1509·1).
*Pediculosis.*

**Sumycin** *Apothecon, USA.*
Tetracycline hydrochloride (p.266·2).
*Bacterial infections.*

**Sun Buffer** *Clinique, Canad.†.*
*SPF 15:* Octinoxate (p.1154·3).
*Sunscreen.*

**Sun Defense Lip Block** *Norman, Canad.*
*SPF 15:* Octinoxate (p.1154·3); oxybenzone (p.1154·3).
*Sunscreen.*

**Sun Defense Sunblock** *Norman, Canad.*
*SPF 25:* Octinoxate (p.1154·3); homosalate (p.1148·1); octisalate (p.1154·3); oxybenzone (p.1154·3).
*Sunscreen.*

**Sun Defense Sunscreen** *Norman, Canad.*
*SPF 8:* Octinoxate (p.1154·3); oxybenzone (p.1154·3).
*Sunscreen.*

**Sun High Protection Kids Sunblock** *Avon, Canad.*
*SPF 40:* Avobenzone (p.1142·3); homosalate (p.1148·1); octinoxate (p.1154·3); octisalate (p.1154·3); oxybenzone (p.1154·3).
*Sunscreen.*

**Sun Lip Balm** *Avon, Canad.*
*SPF 15:* Octinoxate (p.1154·3); oxybenzone (p.1154·3).
*Sunscreen.*

**Sun Management Extensive Protection** *Kay, Canad.*
Octinoxate (p.1154·3); octisalate (p.1154·3); oxybenzone (p.1154·3).
*Sunscreen.*

**Sun Management Intensive Protection** *Kay, Canad.†.*
*SPF 20:* Octinoxate (p.1154·3); octisalate (p.1154·3); oxybenzone (p.1154·3).
*Sunscreen.*

**Sun Management Lip Protection** *Kay, Canad.*
*SPF 15:* Octinoxate (p.1154·3); oxybenzone (p.1154·3).
*Sunscreen.*

**Sun Management Sensible Protection** *Kay, Canad.*
Octinoxate (p.1154·3); oxybenzone (p.1154·3).
*Sunscreen.*

**Sun Pacer** *Amway, Canad.*
*SPF 30:* Octocrilene (p.1154·3); octinoxate (p.1154·3); octisalate (p.1154·3); oxybenzone (p.1154·3).
*SPF 8; SPF 15:* Octinoxate (p.1154·3); oxybenzone (p.1154·3).
*Sunscreen.*

**Sun Pacer Protective** *Amway, Canad.†.*
*SPF 8:* Oxybenzone (p.1154·3); padimate O (p.1155·1).
*SPF 15:* Octinoxate (p.1154·3); oxybenzone (p.1154·3); padimate O (p.1155·1).
*SPF 30:* Octinoxate (p.1154·3); oxybenzone (p.1154·3); padimate O (p.1155·1); titanium dioxide (p.1160·3).
*Sunscreen.*

**Sun Pacer Sunless Tanning** *Amway, Canad.†.*
*SPF 15:* Octinoxate (p.1154·3); octisalate (p.1154·3); oxybenzone (p.1154·3).
*Sunscreen.*

**Sun Tanning** *Solar, Canad.†.*
*SPF 4:* Octinoxate (p.1154·3).
*Sunscreen.*

**Sun-Benz** *Sun, Canad.*
Benzydamine hydrochloride (p.21·1).
*Oropharyngeal mucositis; sore throat.*

**Sunblock** *Estee Lauder, Canad.†.*
*SPF 15; SPF 25:* Titanium dioxide (p.1160·3).
*Sunscreen.*

**Sunblock for Face** *Estee Lauder, Canad.*
*SPF 30:* Octinoxate (p.1154·3); oxybenzone (p.1154·3); titanium dioxide (p.1160·3); zinc oxide (p.1163·2).
*Sunscreen.*

**Sunblock Lotion** *Tanning Research, Canad.*
*SPF 15:* Octinoxate (p.1154·3); oxybenzone (p.1154·3).
*SPF 30:* Homosalate (p.1148·1); octinoxate (p.1154·3); octisalate (p.1154·3); oxybenzone (p.1154·3).
*Sunscreen.*

**Suncodin** *Aventis, S.Afr.*
Paracetamol (p.76·2); codeine phosphate (p.27·1); phenyltoloxamine citrate (p.439·1); caffeine (p.782·1).
*Fever; pain; sinus congestion.*

**Sundays Maximum Protection** *Nutri-Metics, Canad.†.*
*SPF 15:* Avobenzone (p.1142·3); octinoxate (p.1154·3).
*Sunscreen.*

**Sundown**
*Note. This name is used for preparations of different composition.*
*Johnson & Johnson, Austral.†; Johnson & Johnson, Braz.; Johnson & Johnson, USA.*
*SPF 8; SPF 15; SPF 20; SPF 30:* Octinoxate (p.1154·3); octisalate (p.1154·3); oxybenzone (p.1154·3); titanium dioxide (p.1160·3).
*Sunscreen.*

*Johnson & Johnson, Braz.*
*SPF 50:* Octinoxate (p.1154·3); meradimate (p.1151·3); oxybenzone (p.1154·3); octocrilene (p.1154·3); titanium dioxide (p.1160·3).
*Sunscreen.*

**Sundown Active** *Johnson & Johnson, Austral.†.*
*SPF 15:* Titanium dioxide (p.1160·3); zinc oxide (p.1163·2).
*Sunscreen.*

**Sundown Baby** *Johnson & Johnson, Braz.*
*SPF 30:* Titanium dioxide (p.1160·3); zinc oxide (p.1163·2).
*Sunscreen.*

**Sundown Cabelos** *Johnson & Johnson, Braz.*
*SPF 15:* Octinoxate (p.1154·3); oxybenzone (p.1154·3); octisalate (p.1154·3).
*Sunscreen.*

**Sundown Clear Gel** *Johnson & Johnson, Braz.*
*SPF 15:* Octinoxate (p.1154·3); homosalate (p.1148·1); oxybenzone (p.1154·3).
*Sunscreen.*

**Sundown C/Repelente** *Johnson & Johnson, Braz.*
*SPF 15:* Octinoxate (p.1154·3); oxybenzone (p.1154·3); octisalate (p.1154·3); titanium dioxide (p.1160·3).
*Sunscreen.*

**Sundown with Insect Repellent** *Johnson & Johnson, Austral.†.*
*SPF 15+:* Octinoxate (p.1154·3); avobenzone (p.1142·3); titanium dioxide (p.1160·3); di-*N*-propyl isocinchomeronate; piperonyl butoxide (p.1509·2); *N*-octylbicycloheptene dicarboximide; pyrethrins (p.1509·3).
*Sunscreen and insect repellent.*

**Sundown Kids** *Johnson & Johnson, Braz.*
*SPF 30:* Octinoxate (p.1154·3); octocrilene (p.1154·3); oxybenzone (p.1154·3); titanium dioxide (p.1160·3).
*Sunscreen.*

**Sundown Kids Colour** *Johnson & Johnson, Braz.*
*SPF 30:* Octocrilene (p.1154·3); octinoxate (p.1154·3); oxybenzone (p.1154·3); octisalate (p.1154·3); titanium dioxide (p.1160·3).
*Sunscreen.*

**Sundown Sport**
*Note. This name is used for preparations of different composition.*
*Johnson & Johnson, Braz.*
*SPF 15:* Octinoxate (p.1154·3); oxybenzone (p.1154·3); octisalate (p.1154·3); titanium dioxide (p.1160·3).
*Sunscreen.*

*Johnson & Johnson, USA.*
*SPF 15:* Zinc oxide (p.1163·2); titanium dioxide (p.1160·3).
*Sunscreen.*

**Sundown Spray** *Johnson & Johnson, Braz.*
*SPF 15:* Octinoxate (p.1154·3); octocrilene (p.1154·3); oxybenzone (p.1154·3).
*Sunscreen.*

**Sundown Toddler** *Johnson & Johnson, Austral.†.*
*SPF 15+:* Octinoxate (p.1154·3); oxybenzone (p.1154·3); octisalate (p.1154·3); avobenzone (p.1142·3).
*Sunscreen.*

**SuNerven** *Lane, UK.*
Motherwort (p.1717·1); vervain (p.1764·1); valerian (p.1762·2); passion flower (p.1729·1).
*Stresses and strains.*

**Sunfilter** *Estee Lauder, Canad.†.*
*SPF 15:* Avobenzone (p.1142·3); octinoxate (p.1154·3); titanium dioxide (p.1160·3).
*Sunscreen.*

**Sun-Glizide**
*Sunward, Malaysia; Sunward, Singapore†.*
Gliclazide (p.332·1).
*Diabetes mellitus.*

**Suniderma** *Galderma, Spain.*
Hydrocortisone aceponate (p.1104·2).
*Skin disorders.*

**Sunkist** *Ciba, USA.*
Ascorbic acid (p.1460·2).

**Sunmax 30** *Stiefel, Braz.*
Oxybenzone (p.1154·3); homosalate (p.1148·1); OMC; eusolex 6300 (p.1147·1).
*Sunscreen.*

**Sunmax 60** *Stiefel, Braz.*
Avobenzone (p.1142·3); titanium dioxide (p.1160·3); octil triazone (p.1154·3); homosalate (p.1148·1).
*Sunscreen.*

**Sunnie** *Green Turtle Bay Vitamin Co., USA.*
Vitamins; minerals; glutamine; hypericum; betaine; ginkgo biloba (p.1417·1).
*Tonic.*

**Sunolut** *Sunward, Malaysia.*
Norethisterone (p.1562·2).
*Dysfunctional uterine bleeding; endometriosis; menopausal disorders; menstrual disorders.*

**Sunprox**
*Sunward, Malaysia; Sunward, Singapore†.*
Naproxen sodium (p.65·1).
*Gout; musculoskeletal, joint, and peri-articular disorders; pain.*

**Sunrythm** *Suntory, Jpn.*
Pilsicainide hydrochloride (p.983·1).
*Arrhythmias.*

**Sunsan-Heillotion** *Richter, Austria.*
Diphenhydramine hydrochloride (p.431·3); dexpanthenol (p.1727·2); allantoin (p.1141·3).
*Inflammatory skin disorders; skin irritation.*

**Sunscreen Lotion**
*Note. This name is used for preparations of different composition.*
*Norwood, Canad.*
*SPF 30:* Octinoxate (p.1154·3); octisalate (p.1154·3); oxybenzone (p.1154·3); titanium dioxide (p.1160·3).
*SPF 45:* Octinoxate (p.1154·3); octocrilene (p.1154·3); octisalate (p.1154·3); oxybenzone (p.1154·3).
*SPF 8; SPF 15:* Octinoxate (p.1154·3); oxybenzone (p.1154·3); titanium dioxide (p.1160·3).
*Sunscreen.*

*Scott, Canad.*
*SPF 15:* Oxybenzone (p.1154·3); octinoxate (p.1154·3); octisalate (p.1154·3).
*Sunscreen.*

*Therapex, Canad.*
*SPF 15:* Avobenzone (p.1142·3); octinoxate (p.1154·3); oxybenzone (p.1154·3).
*SPF 30:* Avobenzone (p.1142·3); octinoxate (p.1154·3); oxybenzone (p.1154·3); titanium dioxide (p.1160·3).
*Sunscreen.*

**Sunscreen Lotion Ecran** *Prodemdis, Canad.*
*SPF 15:* Avobenzone (p.1142·3); octinoxate (p.1154·3); oxybenzone (p.1154·3).
*SPF 30:* Avobenzone (p.1142·3); enzacamene (p.1147·1); octinoxate (p.1154·3); ensulizole (p.1147·1).
*Sunscreen.*

**Sunseekers** *Avon, Canad.*
*SPF 15:* Octinoxate (p.1154·3); oxybenzone (p.1154·3).
*SPF 6; SPF 30:* Octinoxate (p.1154·3); octisalate (p.1154·3); oxybenzone (p.1154·3).
*Sunscreen.*

**Sunsense**
*Note. This name is used for preparations of different composition.*
*Ego, Hong Kong; Ego, Malaysia.*
*Cream SPF 30+:* Octinoxate (p.1154·3); oxybenzone (p.1154·3); titanium dioxide (p.1160·3); avobenzone (p.1142·3).
*Sunscreen.*

*Ego, Hong Kong; Ego, Malaysia.*
*Topical gel:* Amiloxate (p.1142·2); octinoxate (p.1154·3); enzacamene (p.1147·1); avobenzone (p.1142·3); oxybenzone (p.1154·3).
*Sunscreen.*

*Ego, Hong Kong; Ego, Malaysia.*
*Ultra SPF 30+; Face Milk SPF 30+:* Octinoxate (p.1154·3); oxybenzone (p.1154·3); titanium dioxide (p.1160·3).
*Sunscreen.*

*Ego, NZ.*
*SPF 15+:* Titanium dioxide (p.1160·3); oxybenzone (p.1154·3); avobenzone (p.1142·3); ethylhexyl cinnamate.
*Sunscreen.*

*Ego, Singapore.*
*Cream SPF 30+; Ultra SPF 30+; Face Milk SPF 30+:* Octinoxate (p.1154·3); oxybenzone (p.1154·3); titanium dioxide (p.1160·3).
*Sunscreen.*

**Sunsense Aftersun** *Ego, Austral.†.*
Emollient.
*Dry skin.*

**Sunsense Clear** *Ego, Singapore.*
Amiloxate (p.1142·2); octinoxate (p.1154·3); enzacamene (p.1147·1); avobenzone (p.1142·3); oxybenzone (p.1154·3).
*Sunscreen.*

**Sunsense Daily Face**
*Ego, Austral.†; Ego, Hong Kong; Ego, Malaysia; Ego, Singapore.*
*SPF 30+:* Octinoxate (p.1154·3); titanium dioxide (p.1160·3); enzacamene (p.1147·1).
*Sunscreen.*

**Sunsense Lip Balm**
*Ego, Austral.†; Ego, Hong Kong; Ego, Malaysia; Ego, Singapore.*
*SPF 30+:* Octinoxate (p.1154·3); oxybenzone (p.1154·3); titanium dioxide (p.1160·3); avobenzone (p.1142·3).
*Sunscreen.*

**Sunsense Low Irritant**
*Ego, Austral.†; Ego, Hong Kong; Ego, Malaysia; Ego, Singapore.*
*SPF 20:* Titanium dioxide (p.1160·3).
*Sunscreen.*

**Sunsense Sport**
*Note. This name is used for preparations of different composition.*
*Ego, Austral.†; Ego, Hong Kong; Ego, Malaysia.*
*Cream SPF 30+:* Octinoxate (p.1154·3); oxybenzone (p.1154·3); titanium dioxide (p.1160·3); enzacamene (p.1147·1).
*Sunscreen.*

*Ego, Hong Kong; Ego, Malaysia.*
*Milk SPF 30+:* Titanium dioxide (p.1160·3); octinoxate (p.1154·3); enzacamene (p.1147·1); oxybenzone (p.1154·3); avobenzone (p.1142·3); ensulizole (p.1147·1).
*Sunscreen.*

**Sunsense Sport Cream** *Ego, Singapore.*
*SPF 30+:* Octinoxate (p.1154·3); oxybenzone (p.1154·3); titanium dioxide (p.1160·3); enzacamene (p.1147·1).
*Sunscreen.*

**Sunsense Sport Milk** *Ego, Singapore.*
*SPF 30+:* Octinoxate (p.1154·3); oxybenzone (p.1154·3); titanium dioxide (p.1160·3); enzacamene (p.1147·1); avobenzone (p.1142·3); ensulizole (p.1147·1).
*Sunscreen.*

**Sunsense and Sunsense Ultra** *Ego, Austral.†.*
*SPF 30+:* Octinoxate (p.1154·3); oxybenzone (p.1154·3); titanium dioxide (p.1160·3).
*Sunscreen.*

**Sunsense Toddler Milk**
*Ego, Austral.†; Ego, Hong Kong; Ego, Malaysia; Ego, Singapore.*
*SPF 30+:* Octinoxate (p.1154·3); oxybenzone (p.1154·3); titanium dioxide (p.1160·3); amiloxate (p.1142·2).
*Sunscreen.*

**Sunsense Ultra**
*Ego, Malaysia; Sandoz, UK.*
Octinoxate (p.1154·3); oxybenzone (p.1154·3); titanium dioxide (p.1160·3).
*Sunscreen.*

**Sunsmackers** *Bonne Bell, Canad.†.*
*SPF 6; SPF 30:* Octinoxate (p.1154·3); oxybenzone (p.1154·3); padimate O (p.1155·1).
*Sunscreen.*

**Sunspot**
*Note. This name is used for preparations of different composition.*
*Sunspot, Austral.*
Salicylic acid (p.1157·1).
*Hard skin; solar keratoses.*

*Surf Ski International, UK†.*
Camphor (p.1665·3); benzoin (p.1751·1); ethyl glycol.; benzalkonium chloride (p.1168·3); allantoin (p.1141·3); isopropyl alcohol (p.1184·3).
*Herpes labialis.*

**Supa C** *Vitaplex, Austral.†.*
Calcium ascorbate (p.1460·2).
*Vitamin C deficiency.*

**Supa-Boost** *Vitaplex, Austral.†.*
Multivitamin and mineral preparation with rutoside (p.1417·1).

**Supac** *Mission Pharmacal, USA†.*
Paracetamol (p.76·2); aspirin (p.15·1); caffeine (p.782·1).
*Pain.*

**Supacef** *GlaxoSmithKline, India.*
Cefuroxime (p.184·1) or cefuroxime sodium (p.184·1).
*Bacterial infections.*

**Supadol** *Whitehall, Fr.*
Paracetamol (p.76·2); codeine phosphate (p.27·1).
*Pain.*

**Supartz**
*Smith & Nephew, UK; Smith & Nephew, USA.*
Sodium hyaluronate (p.1697·3).
*Osteoarthritis of the knee; synovial fluid replacement.*

**Super Active Multi** *Quest, Canad.†.*
Multivitamin and mineral preparation (p.1417·1).

**Super Antioxidant Plus** *Lifeplan, UK.*
Vitamins; minerals; fish oil; starflower oil; garlic oil (p.1417·1).
*Antoxidant preparation.*

**Super Anti-Oxydant Formula** *Equilibre Attitude, Fr.*
Nutritional supplement (p.1417·1).

**Super AO Formula** *Seroyal, Canad.†.*
Betacarotene, selenium, vitamin C, vitamin D, and zinc (p.1417·1).

**Super B** *Vitaglow, Austral.†.*
Vitamin B substances with ascorbic acid (p.1417·1).
*Dietary supplement.*

**Super B Complex** *Sisu, Canad.*
Vitamin B substances (p.1417·1).
*Nutritional supplement.*

**Super B Plus** *Vitaglow, Austral.†.*
Vitamin B substances; vitamin C; lysine hydrochloride; magnesium oxide; potassium sulfate; zinc amino acid chelate (p.1417·1).
*Dietary supplement; tonic.*

**Super B Plus Liver Tonic** *Vitaglow, Austral.†.*
Silybum marianum (p.1043·3); vitamins; minerals (p.1417·1).
*Dietary supplement; digestive system disorders.*

**Super B Stress** *Roche Consumer, Austral.†.*
Vitamin B substances; vitamin C; minerals; passion flower (p.1417·1).
*Dietary supplement.*

**Super Banish** *Smith & Nephew, Austral.*
Silver nitrate (p.1746·1); ethylene thiourea.
*Ostomy deodorant.*

**Super C** *Quest, Canad.*
Ascorbic acid (p.1460·2).

**Super Cal-C Bio** *Eagle, Austral.†.*
Calcium ascorbate (p.1460·2); bioflavonoids (p.1688·2).
*Vitamin C deficiency.*

**Super Cal-Mag** *Seroyal, Canad.†.*
Mineral preparation with vitamin D (p.1417·1).

**Super Cold Tabs** *Reese, USA†.*
Paracetamol (p.76·2); phenylpropanolamine hydrochloride (p.1127·3); chlorphenamine (p.428·1).
*Cold symptoms.*

**Super Cough** *Medipharma, Hong Kong.*
Ephedrine hydrochloride (p.1120·1); codeine phosphate (p.27·1); promethazine hydrochloride (p.439·1).
*Cold and influenza symptoms.*

**Super Cromer Orto** *Normon, Spain.*
Merbromin (p.1185·3).
*Wound disinfection.*

**Super D Perles** *Roberts, USA.*
Vitamins A and D (p.1417·1).

**Super Daily** *Lee-Adams, Canad.*
Multivitamin and mineral preparation (p.1417·1).

**Super Energex Plus** *Sante Naturelle, Canad.*
Vitamin B substances, minerals, kola, and liver extract (p.1417·1).

**Super 28 Formula** *Reese, USA.*
Multivitamin, mineral, and herbal preparation (p.1417·1).

**Super Galanol** *Lifeplan, UK†.*
Borage oil (p.1661·3).
*Nutritional supplement.*

**Super Gamma Oil with Vitamin E** *Quest, Canad.†.*
Evening primrose oil (p.1686·3); vitamin E (p.1464·3).

**Super GammaOil Marine** *Quest, UK†.*
Evening primrose oil (p.1686·3); borage oil (p.1661·3); concentrated fish oil (p.976·2).

**Super GLA** *Cantassium Co., UK.*
Gamma linolenic acid (from vegetable oils) (p.1690·2).

**Super Hi Potency** *Nion, USA.*
Multivitamin and mineral preparation (p.1417·1).

**Super Ivy Dry** *Ivy Corp, USA.*
Zinc acetate (p.1469·2); benzyl alcohol (p.1170·2).
*Minor skin irritation.*

**Super Kids** *Swiss Herbal, Canad.*
Multivitamin and mineral preparation (p.1417·1).

**Super Mega B+C** *Quest, UK.*
Vitamin B and C substances (p.1417·1); valerian (p.1762·2); passion flower (p.1729·1); peppermint oil (p.1283·2); wood betony; cimicifuga root (p.1671·3); skullcap (p.1746·3); lupulus (p.1708·1); ginger root (p.1267·1).

**Super Once A Day**
*Quest, Canad.; Quest, UK.*
Multivitamin and mineral preparation (p.1417·1).

**Super Orti-Vite** *Seroyal, Canad.†.*
Multivitamin and mineral preparation (p.1417·1).

**Super Plenamins**
*3M, Irl.†; 3M, UK†.*
Multivitamin and mineral preparation (p.1417·1).

**Super Quints** *Freeda, USA.*
Vitamin B substances (p.1417·1).

**Super Soluble Maxipro HBV** *Scientific Hospital Supplies, Austral.*
Preparation for enteral nutrition (p.1417·1).
*Hypoproteinaemia.*

**Super Strength Sinadrin** *Reese, USA†.*
Paracetamol (p.76·2); phenylpropanolamine hydrochloride (p.1127·3); chlorphenamine (p.428·1).

**Super Stress Mega B plus Vitamin C** *Quest, Canad.*
Vitamin B substances and vitamin C (p.1417·1).

**Super Vikaps** *Reese, USA.*
Multivitamin and mineral preparation (p.1417·1).

**Super Vita Vim**
*Jamieson, Canad.†; Jamieson, Hong Kong.*
Multivitamin and mineral preparation (p.1417·1).

**Super Vitalex** *Carmaran, Canad.†.*
Vitamin B substances and iron (p.1417·1).

**Super Wate-On** *DDD, UK†.*
Nutritional supplement with vitamins (p.1417·1).

**Superan** *Sanofi Synthelabo, Braz.*
Alizapride hydrochloride (p.1248·1).
*Nausea and vomiting.*

**Superantioxidante** *Natural Life, Arg.*
Betacarotene; vitamin C; vitamin E; selenium (p.1417·1).
*Antoxidant preparation.*

**Superdophilus** *Natren, USA.*
*Lactobacillus acidophilus* (p.1704·2).
*Dietary supplement.*

**SuperEPA** *Advanced Nutritional Technology, USA.*
Omega-3 marine triglycerides (p.976·2).
*Dietary supplement.*

**Superfade** *Sunspot, Austral.†.*
Hydroquinone (p.1148·1); salicylic acid (p.1157·1); dexpanthenol (p.1727·2); padimate O (p.1155·1); vitamin E.
*Skin hyperpigmentation.*

**Supergan** *Sanochemia, Austria†.*
Dihydroergocristine mesilate (p.1680·1); reserpine (p.995·1); hydrochlorothiazide (p.933·2).
*Hypertension.*

**Superhist** *Eurofarma, Braz.*
Chlorphenamine maleate (p.427·3); ascorbic acid (p.1460·2); aspirin (p.15·1); caffeine (p.782·1).
Aluminium hydroxide (p.1249·2) is included in this preparation in an attempt to limit adverse effects on the gastrointestinal mucosa.
Formerly contained phenindamine, ascorbic acid, aspirin, and caffeine.
*Cold and influenza symptoms.*

**Superlipid** *Almirall, Spain.*
Probucol (p.986·3).
*Hyperlipidaemias.*

**Supermin** *Vitaglow, Austral.†.*
Mineral and trace element preparation with vitamin D and lecithin (p.1417·1).

**Supero** *Lifepharma, Ital.*
Cefuroxime sodium (p.184·1).
Lidocaine hydrochloride (p.1377·3) is included in this preparation to alleviate the pain of injection.
*Gram-negative bacterial infections.*

**Superol** *Tendem, Neth.*
Hydroxyquinoline sulfate (p.1700·1).
*Sore throat.*

**Superpeni** *Aventis, Spain†.*
Amoxicillin trihydrate (p.155·3).
*Bacterial infections.*

**Superpep**
*Hermes, Ger.; Democal, Switz.†.*
Dimenhydrinate (p.431·1).
*Motion sickness; nausea; vertigo; vomiting.*

**Superplex-T** *Major, USA.*
Vitamin B substances with vitamin C (p.1417·1).

**Supersan** *Merck, Port.†.*
Cyproheptadine hydrochloride (p.430·1).
*Appetite stimulant.*

**SuperSkin** *CliniMed, UK.*
Enbucrilate (p.1678·1).
*Barrier preparation.*

**Supertar** *ICN, Arg.*
Coal tar (p.1159·2).
*Scalp disorders.*

**Supertendin 2000 N** *Thiemann, Ger.*
Dexamethasone (p.1097·1); lidocaine hydrochloride (p.1377·3).
*Neuralgia; neuritis; painful inflammatory musculoskeletal and joint disorders.*

**Supertendin-Depot** *Thiemann, Ger.*
Dexamethasone acetate (p.1097·1); lidocaine hydrochloride (p.1377·3).
*Musculoskeletal, joint, and peri-articular disorders; neuritis.*

**Superthiol** *Francia, Ital.†.*
Carbocisteine (p.1116·2) or carbocisteine sodium (p.1116·3).
*Respiratory-tract congestion.*

**Supertonic** *Diafarm, Spain.*
Amino-acid preparation with cyanocobalamin (p.1417·1).
*Tonic.*

**Supervit** *QIF, Braz.†.*
Vitamin B substances (p.1417·1).
*Nutritional supplement.*

**Supeudol** *Sabex, Canad.*
Oxycodone hydrochloride (p.75·2).
*Pain.*

**Suplac**
*Biolab, Singapore; Biolab, Thai.*
Bromocriptine mesilate (p.1200·3).
*Amenorrhoea; female and male infertility; galactorrhoea; lactation inhibition.*

**Suplan** *Hebron, Braz.*
Glucose; vitamins; minerals (p.1417·1).
*Nutritional supplement.*

**Suplasyn**
*Paladin, Canad.†; Merckle, Ger.; Pliva, UK.*
Sodium hyaluronate (p.1697·3).
*Osteoarthritis; synovial fluid replacement.*

**Supledin** *Luper, Braz.*
Multivitamin preparation with or without minerals (p.1417·1).

**Suplena**
*Abbott, Arg.; Abbott, Austral.; Abbott, Canad.†; Abbott, Hong Kong; Abbott, Irl.; Ross, Israel; Abbott, Mex.; Abbott, NZ; Abbott Nutrition, UK; Ross, USA.*
Preparation for enteral nutrition (p.1417·1).
Formerly known as Replena in the *USA*.
*Renal failure.*

**Suplevit**
*EMS, Braz.; Riva, Canad.*
Multivitamin and mineral preparation (p.1417·1).

**Supligol** *Lazar, Arg.*
Estradiol cipionate (p.1550·1); testosterone enantate (p.1570·1).
*Menopausal disorders; osteoporosis.*

**Supo Gliz** *Perez Gimenez, Spain.*
Glycerol (p.1694·3).
*Constipation; laxative dependence.*

**Supo Kristal** *CEPA, Spain†.*
Glycerol (p.1694·3).
*Constipation; laxative dependence.*

**Supofen** *Basi, Port.*
Paracetamol (p.76·2).
*Fever; pain.*

**Supositorio Hamamelis Composto** *Simoes, Braz.*
Hamamelis (p.1696·3); aesculus (p.1648·2); lidocaine hydrochloride (p.1377·3).
*Haemorrhoids.*

**Supositorios Senosiain** *Senosiain, Mex.*
Glycerol (p.1694·3).
*Constipation.*

**Supotron** *Remedina, Gr.*
Enalapril maleate (p.909·2).
*Heart failure; hypertension.*

**Supoviol** *Master, Chile.*
Nonoxinol 9 (p.1413·3).
*Vaginal contraceptive.*

**Supplamins F** *3M, Israel†.*
Multivitamin and mineral preparation (p.1417·1).

**Supplemaman** *Yves Ponroy, Fr.†.*
Vitamin B substances, fatty acids, magnesium, and iron (p.1417·1).
*Nutritional supplement during pregnancy.*

**Suppletive** *Dermoteca, Port.*
Moisturiser.
*Dry skin.*

**Supplex** *Cedar Health, UK.*
Green-lipped mussel (p.1696·1).
*Joint disorders.*

**Suppomaline** *Solvay, Fr.*
Belladonna (p.479·1); codeine phosphate (p.27·1); caffeine (p.782·1); paracetamol (p.76·2).
*Fever; pain.*

**Supportan**
*Fresenius Kabi, Fin.†; Fresenius Kabi, Ital.; Fresenius Kabi, Port.; Fresenius Kabi, Switz.*
Preparation for enteral nutrition (p.1417·1).

**Supprelin** *Roberts, USA.*
Histrelin acetate (p.1329·3).
*Precocious puberty.*

**Suppress**
*Note. This name is used for preparations of different composition.*
*Stanley, Canad.*
Diphenhydramine hydrochloride (p.431·3); codeine phosphate (p.27·1); ammonium chloride (p.1115·2).

*Ferndale, USA†.*
Dextromethorphan hydrobromide (p.1117·3).
*Coughs.*

**Supra** *ICN, Mex.*
Lidamidine hydrochloride (p.1270·2).
*Gastrointestinal disorders.*

**Supraalox** *Aventis, Spain.*
Aluminium hydroxide (p.1249·2); magnesium hydroxide (p.1272·2).
*Dyspepsia; peptic ulcer.*

**Supracaine** *Hoechst Marion Roussel, Canad.†.*
Tetracaine (p.1385·1).
*Oral soft-tissue pain; reduction of gag reflex.*

**Supracam** *Asofarma, Arg.*
Pantoprazole sodium (p.1283·1).
*Gastro-oesophageal reflux; peptic ulcer.*

**Supracef** *Orion, Fin.†.*
Cefixime (p.172·3).
*Bacterial infections.*

**Supracid** *Asta Medica, Austria.*
Spironolactone (p.1003·1); hydrochlorothiazide (p.933·2).
*Hyperaldosteronism; hypertension; oedema.*

**Supracombin**
*Grunenthal, Austria; Grunenthal, Ger.; Grunenthal, Switz.*
Co-trimoxazole (p.199·3).
*Bacterial infections; Pneumocystis carinii pneumonia.*

**Supracortin 3** *Hermal, Thai.; Boots, Thai.*
Fluprednidene acetate (p.1102·2); neomycin sulfate (p.235·1); clioxquine (p.220·3).
*Infected skin disorders.*

**Supracream** *Boots, Thai.; Hermal, Thai.*
Emollient barrier cream.
*Dry skin; nappy rash.*

**Supracyclin**
*Grunenthal, Austria; Grunenthal, Ger.*
Doxycycline (p.206·2).
*Bacterial infections.*

**Supracycline** *Grunenthal, Switz.*
Doxycycline (p.206·2).
*Bacterial infections.*

**Supradol** *Liomont, Mex.*
Ketorolac trometamol (p.52·1).
*Pain.*

**Supradyn**
*Roche, Arg.; Roche Consumer, Austral.; Roche, Austria; Roche, Belg.†; Roche, Braz.; Roche, Chile; Roche Nicholas, Ger.†; Roche, Hong Kong; Piramal, India; Roche, Ital.; Roche, Mex.; Roche Consumer, Neth.; Roche, NZ; Roche, Port.; Roche Consumer, Singapore; Roche, Switz.; Roche, Thai.; Roche Consumer, UK.*
A range of multivitamin and multivitamin and mineral preparations (p.1417·1).

**Supradyn Ginseng** *Roche, Chile.*
Vitamins; minerals; ginseng; rutoside (p.1417·1).
*Dietary supplement.*

**Supradyn N** *Roche, Israel.*
Multivitamin and mineral preparation (p.1417·1).

**Supradyn Vital 50+** *Roche, Switz.*
Multivitamin and mineral preparation with ginseng (p.1417·1)(p.1693·1).

**Supradyne** *Roche Nicholas, Fr.*
Multivitamin and mineral preparation (p.1417·1).

**Supradynvital** *Roche Nicholas, Fr.*
Multivitamin and mineral preparation with ginseng (p.1417·1).

**Supragesic**
*Note. This name is used for preparations of different composition.*
*Beta, Arg.*
Dextropropoxyphene hydrochloride (p.28·3) or dextropropoxyphene napsilate (p.28·3) ibuprofen (p.45·3) or ibuprofen lysine (p.46·3).
*Pain.*

*Pharmaceutical Enterprises, S.Afr.*
*Capsules:* Paracetamol (p.76·2); codeine phosphate (p.27·1); caffeine (p.782·1); meprobamate (p.706·2).
*Pain.*

*Syrup:* Paracetamol (p.76·2); codeine phosphate (p.27·1).
*Fever; pain.*

**Supralan** *Siam Bheasach, Thai.*
Fluocinolone acetonide (p.1101·2).
*Skin disorders.*

**Supralan-N** *Siam Bheasach, Thai.*
Fluocinolone acetonide (p.1101·2); neomycin sulfate (p.235·1).
*Infected skin disorders.*

**Supralef** *Martin, Spain†.*
Hydrocortisone acetate (p.1103·3).
*Skin disorders.*

**Supralip** *Fournier, UK.*
Fenofibrate (p.915·2).
*Hyperlipidaemias.*

**Supralox**
*Aventis, Fr.†; Rhone-Poulenc Rorer, Ger.†.*
Aluminium hydroxide (p.1249·2); magnesium hydroxide (p.1272·2).
*Gastrointestinal disorders.*

**Supramol** *Sam-On, Israel.*
Paracetamol (p.76·2).
*Fever; pain.*

**Supramox**
*Grunenthal, Austria.*
Amoxicillin trihydrate (p.155·3).
*Bacterial infections.*

*Grunenthal, Switz.*
Amoxicillin (p.155·3).
*Bacterial infections.*

**Supramycin** *Grunenthal, Ger.*
Tetracycline hydrochloride (p.266·2).
*Bacterial infections.*

**Supran** *Teva, Israel.*
Cefixime (p.172·3).
*Bacterial infections.*

**Suprane**
*Baxter Immuno, Arg.; Zeneca, Austral.†; Baxter, Austria; Pharmacia Upjohn, Belg.†; Baxter, Braz.†; Baxter, Canad.; Baxter, Denm.; Baxter, Fin.; Baxter, Ger.; Baxter, Gr.; Pharmacia Upjohn, Irl.†; Baxter, Ital.; Zeneca, Mex.†; Baxter, Neth.; Pharmacia Upjohn, Norw.†; Baxter, NZ; Zeneca, S.Afr.; AstraZeneca, Singapore†; Baxter, Spain; Baxter, Swed.; Baxter, Switz.; Baxter Anaesthesia, UK; Ohmeda, USA.*
Desflurane (p.1297·2).
*General anaesthesia.*

**Supranitrin** *Gap, Gr.*
Glyceryl trinitrate (p.923·2).
*Angina; heart failure.*

**Suprapen** *GlaxoSmithKline, S.Afr.*
Amoxicillin (p.155·3); flucloxacillin (p.213·3).
*Bacterial infections.*

**Supraproct-S** *Julphar, UAE.*
Betamethasone valerate (p.1093·2); cinchocaine hydrochloride (p.1373·2).
*Anorectal disorders.*

**Suprarenin**
*Aventis, Austria; Aventis, Ger.*
Adrenaline hydrochloride (p.852·3).
*Adjunct to local anaesthesia; circulatory collapse; hypersensitivity reactions; shock.*

**Suprasec** *Janssen-Cilag, Arg.*
Loperamide (p.1271·2).
*Diarrhoea.*

**Suprasten** *Gross, Braz.*
Suprarenal cortex (p.1110·1); ascorbic acid (p.1460·2); pentetrazol (p.1592·1).
*Impaired mental function.*

**Suprastin** *EGIS, Hung.*
Chloropyramine hydrochloride (p.427·3).
*Hypersensitivity reactions.*

**Supratonin** *Grunenthal, Ger.*
Amezinium metilsulfate (p.858·2).
*Hypotension.*

**Supra-Vir** *Trima, Israel.*
Aciclovir (p.626·1).
*Herpesvirus infections.*

**Supraviran** *Grunenthal, Ger.*
Aciclovir (p.626·1) or aciclovir sodium (p.626·1).
*Herpesvirus infections.*

**Supravite**
*Nobel, Canad.*
Vitamin B substances and iron (p.1417·1).

*Pharmavite, Canad.†.*
A range of vitamin preparations with or without minerals (p.1417·1).

**Supravite C** *Nobel, Canad.*
Vitamin B substances, vitamin C, and iron (p.1417·1).

**Suprax**
*Aventis, Canad.; Fujisawa, Ger.; Aventis, Irl.; Wyeth Lederle, Ital.; Aventis, UK; Lupin, USA.*
Cefixime (p.172·3).
*Bacterial infections.*

**Suprecur**
*Aventis, Austria; Aventis, Denm.; Aventis, Fin.; Aventis, Ger.; Aventis, Hong Kong; Aventis, Irl.; Aventis, Neth.; Aventis, Norw.; Hoechst Marion Roussel, Singapore†; Aventis, Swed.; Aventis, UK.*
Buserelin acetate (p.1319·2).
*Endometriosis; ovulation induction.*

**Suprefact**
*Aventis, Arg.; Aventis, Austria; Aventis, Belg.; Aventis, Braz.; Aventis, Canad.; Aventis, Denm.; Aventis, Fin.; Aventis, Fr.; Hoechst Marion Roussel, Gr.; Hoechst Marion Roussel, Hong Kong†; Aventis, Irl.; Aventis, Ital.; Aventis, Malaysia; Aventis, Mex.; Aventis, Neth.; Aventis, Norw.; Aventis, NZ; Aventis, Port.; Aventis, S.Afr.; Aventis, Singapore; Aventis, Spain; Aventis, Swed.; Aventis, Switz.; Aventis, Thai.; Aventis, UK.*
Buserelin acetate (p.1319·2).
*Endometriosis; ovulation induction; prostatic cancer; uterine fibroids.*

*Aventis, Israel.*
Buserelin (p.1319·2) or buserelin acetate (p.1319·2).
*Endometriosis; ovulation induction; prostatic cancer; uterine fibroids.*

**Suprema** *Biolab Sanus, Braz.*
Norethisterone acetate (p.1562·2); estradiol (p.1550·1).
*Menopausal disorders.*

**Supremase** *Tecnimede, Port.*
Fluconazole (p.398·1).
*Fungal infections.*

**Suprenoat** *Roche, Austria†.*
Spironolactone (p.1003·1); butizide (p.878·2); reserpine (p.995·1).
*Hypertension.*

**Supres** *Merck Frosst, Canad.*
Methyldopa (p.953·2); chlorothiazide (p.882·1).
*Hypertension.*

**Supresol** *Biologici Italia, Ital.*
Methylprednisolone sodium succinate (p.1106·2).
*Parenteral corticosteroid.*

**Supressin** *Pfizer, Austria.*
Doxazosin mesilate (p.908·3).
*Benign prostatic hyperplasia; hypertension.*

**Suprexon**
*Ciba Vision, Denm.†; Ciba Vision, Ger.†; Ciba Vision, Neth.†; Ciba Vision, Switz.†.*
Guanethidine monosulfate (p.926·3); adrenaline (p.852·2).
*Glaucoma.*

**Sup-Rhinite** *SmithKline Beecham Sante, Fr.†.*
Chlorphenamine maleate (p.427·3); phenylephrine hydrochloride (p.1126·3).
*Rhinopharyngeal congestion.*

**Suprim**
*Note. This name is used for preparations of different composition.*
*Degorts, Mex.*
Dipyrone (p.35·3).
*Fever; pain.*

*Hovid, Singapore.*
Co-trimoxazole (p.199·3).
*Bacterial infections; protozoal infections.*

**Suprimal** *IPS, Neth.†.*
Meclozine hydrochloride (p.436·3).
*Motion sickness.*

**Suprimox** *Rexcel, India.*
Amoxicillin (p.155·3); cloxacillin (p.198·2).
*Bacterial infections.*

**Supristol** *Knoll, Mex.†.*
Co-trimoxazole (p.199·3).
*Bacterial infections.*

**Suprium** *Sanofi Synthelabo, Fin.*
Sulpiride (p.722·2).
*Depression; psychoses.*

**Suprotide** *Fresenius Kabi, Ital.*
Nutritional supplement (p.1417·1).

**Suracton** *Actipharm, Switz.*
Minerals; pyridoxine hydrochloride (p.1456·3).
*Tonic.*

**Suralgan** *Monsanto, Ital.*
Tiaprofenic acid (p.93·3).
*Inflammation; pain.*

**Surazem** *Pharmacia, Neth.*
Diltiazem hydrochloride (p.900·1).
*Hypertension.*

**Surbex**
*Abbott, Canad.*
Vitamin B substances with ascorbic acid (p.1417·1).
*Nutritional supplement.*

*Abbott, USA.*
A range of vitamin preparations (p.1417·1).

**Surbex with C** *Abbott, Hong Kong.*
Vitamin B substances with vitamin C (p.1417·1).
*Vitamin B and C deficiencies.*

**Surbex C** *Abbott, Malaysia.*
Vitamin B substances; vitamin C (p.1417·1).

**Surbex with C** *Abbott, Singapore.*
Vitamin B substances with vitamin C (p.1417·1).

**Surbex plus Iron** *Abbott, Canad.*
Vitamin B substances with ascorbic acid and ferrous sulfate (p.1417·1).
*Nutritional supplement.*

**Surbex plus Zinc** *Abbott, Canad.*
Vitamin B substances with ascorbic acid and zinc sulfate (p.1417·1).
*Nutritional supplement.*

**Surbex T**
*Abbott, Hong Kong; Abbott, Singapore; Abbott, Thai.*
Vitamin B substances with vitamin C (p.1417·1).
*Vitamin B and C deficiencies.*

*Abbott, India.*
Vitamin B substances with vitamin C and liver (p.1417·1).

**Surbex with Zinc**
*Abbott, Hong Kong; Abbott, Malaysia; Abbott, Singapore.*
Vitamin B substances; vitamin C; vitamin E; zinc (p.1417·1).

**Surbronc**
*Boehringer Ingelheim, Belg.; Boehringer Ingelheim, Fr.*
Ambroxol hydrochloride (p.1114·3).
*Respiratory-tract congestion.*

**Surbu-Gen-T** *Goldline, USA.*
Vitamin B substances with vitamin C (p.1417·1).

**Surdolin** *Ofimex, Mex.†.*
Tiaprofenic acid (p.93·3).

**SureLac** *Caraco, USA.*
Tilactase (p.1756·2).
*Lactose intolerance.*

**Sure-Lax**
*Note. This name is used for preparations of different composition.*
*Islacan, Spain†; English Grains, UK†.*
Phenolphthalein (p.1284·1).
*Constipation.*

*Chefaro, UK.*
Senna (p.1288·2).
*Constipation.*

**Sure-Lax (Herbal)** *Chefaro, UK.*
Aloes (p.1248·2); fennel (p.1687·2); valerian (p.1762·2); cnicus benedictus (p.1673·3).
*Constipation.*

**Surelen** *Roche Nicholas, Fr.*
Nutritional supplement (p.1417·1).
*Tonic.*

**Surem** *Roche, Spain†.*
Butalamine hydrochloride (p.878·2).
*Vascular disorders.*

**Sureptil**
*Sanofi Synthelabo, Braz.; Sanofi Synthelabo, Fr.†.*
Cinnarizine (p.428·3); heptaminol acefyllinate (p.786·3).
*Mental function impairment; vascular disorders.*

**Sureskin** *Euromedex, Fr.*
Carmellose sodium (p.1577·3).
*Burns; ulcers; wounds.*

**Suretin** *Recordati, Ital.†.*
Tazarotene (p.1160·2).
*Psoriasis.*

**Surfa-Base** *Rougier, Canad.†.*
Emollient and vehicle.

**Surfactal** *Boehringer Ingelheim, Ital.*
Ambroxol hydrochloride (p.1114·3).
*Neonatal surfactant deficiency; prevention of bronchopulmonary complications following surgery.*

**Surfactante B** *Richet, Arg.*
Bovine pulmonary surfactant (p.1736·2).

**Surfacten** *Mitsubishi, Jpn.*
Bovine pulmonary extract (p.1736·1).
*Respiratory distress syndrome.*

**Surfactil** *Farmion, Braz.*
Ambroxol hydrochloride (p.1114·3).
*Respiratory-tract congestion.*

**Surfak**
*Aventis, Canad.*
Docusate sodium (p.1262·2).
*Constipation.*

*Upjohn, USA.*
Docusate calcium (p.1262·1).
*Constipation.*

**Surfaz** *Franco-Indian, India.*
*Ear drops:* Clotrimazole (p.396·2); lidocaine (p.1377·3).
*Fungal ear infections.*

*Topical solution; cream; vaginal tablets:* Clotrimazole (p.396·2).
*Fungal skin and vaginal infections.*

**Surfaz-SN** *Franco-Indian, India.*
Clotrimazole (p.396·2); betamethasone dipropionate (p.1093·1); neomycin sulfate (p.235·1).
*Infected skin disorders.*

**Surfexo Neonatal** *GlaxoSmithKline, Fr.†.*
Colfosceril palmitate (p.1736·2).
*Respiratory distress syndrome in premature infants.*

**Surfol** *Stiefel, USA.*
Emollient.

**Surfolase**
*Monsanto, Ital.; Lepori, Port.*
Ambroxol acefyllinate (p.1114·3).
*Obstructive airways disease.*

**Surfont** *Ardeypharm, Ger.*
Mebendazole (p.108·2).
*Worm infections.*

**Surfortan** *Diepharmex, Fr.*
Lysine; potassium phosphate; pyridoxine hydrochloride (p.1417·1).
*Tonic.*

**Surgam**
*Aventis, Austral.; Tramedico, Belg.†; Aventis, Canad.; Aventis, Fr.; Aventis, Ger.; Aventis, Irl.; Aventis, Neth.; Aventis, NZ; Aventis, Port.; Aventis, S.Afr.; Aventis, Thai.; Aventis, UK.*
Tiaprofenic acid (p.93·3).
*Gout; inflammation; musculoskeletal, joint, peri-articular and soft-tissue disorders; pain.*

*Aventis, Mex.*
Tiaprofenic acid (p.93·3) or tiaprofenic acid, trometamol salt (p.94·1).
*Gout; inflammation; musculoskeletal, joint, and peri-articular disorders; pain.*

**Surgamic** *Aventis, Spain†.*
Tiaprofenic acid (p.93·3).
*Inflammation; musculoskeletal, joint, and peri-articular disorders; pain.*

**Surgamyl**
*Aventis, Denm.; Aventis, Fin.; Scharper, Ital.*
Tiaprofenic acid (p.93·3).
Lidocaine (p.1377·3) may be included in the intramuscular injection to alleviate the pain of injection.
*Inflammation; musculoskeletal and joint disorders; pain.*

**Surgel** *Ulmer, USA.*
Carmellose sodium (p.1577·3); propylene glycol (p.1735·2); glycerol (p.1694·3).
*Vaginal lubricant.*

**Surgestone**
Aventis, Fr.; Aventis, Port.
Promegestone (p.1568·1).
*Fibroids; mastalgia; menopausal disorders; menstrual disorders.*

**Surgicel**
Ethicon, Fr.; Johnson & Johnson Medical, UK†; Johnson & Johnson Medical, USA.
Oxidised regenerated cellulose (p.757·1).
*Haemorrhage.*

**Surgicoll** MBP, Ger.
Collagen (p.1674·3).
*Haemorrhage.*

**Surgident** Mini, Switz.†.
Adrenaline hydrochloride (p.852·3).
*Gingival haemorrhage.*

**Surgi-Gel** Orion, NZ.
Lubricating gel.

**Surgras Physiologique** Roche-Posay, Arg.
Soap substitute.

**Surifarm** Reig Jofre, Spain†.
Aluminium hydroxide (p.1249·2); dimethicone (p.1289·2); magnesium trisilicate (p.1272·3); metoclopramide (p.1274·3).
*Aerophagia; digestive disorders; meteorism.*

**Suril** Ibirn, Ital.
Sucralfate (p.1290·2).
*Gastritis; gastro-oesophageal reflux; peptic ulcer.*

**Sur-Lax**
Jean-Marie, Hong Kong; Jean-Marie, Singapore†.
Sodium picosulfate (p.1289·3).
*Constipation; stool softener.*

**Surlid**
Aventis, Denm.; Aventis, Fin.; Hoechst Marion Roussel, Mex.†; Aventis, Swed.
Roxithromycin (p.254·2).
*Bacterial infections.*

**Surmenalit** Faes, Spain.
Sulbutiamine (p.1455·1).
*Vitamin B1 deficiency.*

**Surmontil**
Aventis, Austral.; Aventis, Belg.†; Aventis, Canad.; Aventis, Denm.; Aventis, Fin.; Aventis, Fr.; Aventis, Hong Kong; Nicholas Piramal, India; Aventis, Irl.; Aventis, Israel; Aventis, Ital.; Aventis, Neth.; Aventis, Norw.; Aventis, NZ; Vitoria, Port.; Aventis, S.Afr.; Aventis, Spain; Aventis, Swed.; Aventis, Switz.; Aventis, UK; Wyeth-Ayerst, USA.
Trimipramine (p.320·2), trimipramine maleate (p.320·2), or trimipramine mesilate (p.320·3).
*Anxiety; depression; insomnia; pain.*

**Surmoruine** Bournonville, Belg.†.
Cod-liver oil (p.1425·2).
*Osteomalacia; osteoporosis; rickets; vitamin A and D deficiency.*

**Surnox** Aventis, Spain.
Ofloxacin (p.239·3) or ofloxacin hydrochloride (p.240·1).
*Bacterial infections.*

**Suronit**
Note. This name is used for preparations of different composition.
Degorts, Mex.
Nitrofurantoin (p.237·2).
*Urinary-tract infections.*

Ehlinger, Mex.†.
Ranitidine (p.1285·2).

**Surpass** Wrigley, USA.
Calcium carbonate (p.1254·2).
*Dyspepsia; heartburn.*

**Surplex** Seng, Thai.
Vitamin B substances; ascorbic acid (p.1417·1).
*Intravenous vitamin supplement.*

**Surquina** Innotech, Fr.
Quinine hydrochloride (p.460·2).
*Malaria.*

**Sursum** Abiogen, Ital.
Alpha tocopherol (p.1464·3).
*Vitamin E deficiency.*

**Survanta**
Abbott, Arg.; Abbott, Austral.; Abbott, Austria; Abbott, Belg.; Abbott, Braz.; Abbott, Canad.; Abbott, Fr.; Abbott, Ger.; Ross, Hong Kong; Abbott, Mex.; Abbott, Neth.; Abbott, NZ; Abbott, S.Afr.; Abbott, Singapore; Abbott, Spain; Abbott, Switz.; Abbott, Thai.; Abbott, UK; Ross, USA.
Beractant (p.1736·2).
*Neonatal respiratory distress syndrome.*

**Survanta-Vent**
Abbott, Norw.; Abbott, Swed.
Beractant (p.1736·2).
*Neonatal respiratory distress syndrome.*

**Survector**
Servier, Braz.; Teravix, Port.
Amineptine hydrochloride (p.280·3).
*Depression.*

**Survimed**
Fresenius Kabi, Irl.; Fresenius Kabi, Ital.; Fresenius Kabi, Port.; Fresenius Kabi, Switz.; Fresenius Kabi, UK.
Range of preparations for enteral nutrition (p.1417·1).

**Survitine** Roche Nicholas, Fr.†.
Multivitamin and mineral preparation (p.1417·1).
*Nutritional disorders.*

**Susano** Halsey, USA.
Atropine sulfate (p.477·1); hyoscine hydrobromide (p.483·3); hyoscyamine hydrobromide (p.485·1) or hyoscyamine sulfate (p.485·1); phenobarbital (p.367·3).
*Gastrointestinal disorders.*

**Suscard**
Pharmax, Irl.; AstraZeneca, Norw.†; Hassle, Swed.; Forest Laboratories, UK.
Glyceryl trinitrate (p.923·2).
*Angina pectoris; heart failure.*

**Suspectim** Delta, Braz.†.
Furazolidone (p.605·2); homatropine (p.483·2); pectin (p.1580·3).
*Diarrhoea.*

**Sus-Phrine** Forest Pharmaceuticals, USA†.
Adrenaline (p.852·2).
*Asthma; bronchospasm.*

**Suss** Hoechst Marion Roussel, Braz.†.
Co-trimoxazole (p.199·3).
*Bacterial infections; Pneumocystis carinii pneumonia; protozoal infections.*

**Suss Balsamico** Hoechst Marion Roussel, Braz.†.
Co-trimoxazole (p.199·3); guaifenesin (p.1122·1); ammonium chloride (p.1115·2).
*Bacterial infections.*

**Sustac**
Note. This name is used for preparations of different composition.
Pharmacia, Arg.
Ranitidine hydrochloride (p.1285·2).
*Gastritis; gastro-oesophageal reflux; peptic ulcer; Zollinger-Ellison syndrome.*

Pharmax, Irl.; Forest Laboratories, UK.
Glyceryl trinitrate (p.923·2).
*Angina pectoris.*

**Sustacal**
Mead Johnson, Austral.†; Mead Johnson, Braz.; Mead Johnson Nutritionals, Canad.†; Mead Johnson, Hong Kong†; Mead Johnson, Israel; Mead Johnson Nutritionals, Thai.†; Mead Johnson Nutritionals, USA.
A range of preparations for enteral nutrition (p.1417·1).

**Sustagen**
Bristol-Myers Squibb, Arg.; Novartis Consumer, Austral.; Mead Johnson, Braz.; Mead Johnson, Chile; Mead Johnson, Hong Kong; Mead Johnson, NZ; Mead Johnson Nutritionals, Thai.; Mead Johnson Nutritionals, USA.
A range of preparations for enteral nutrition (p.1417·1).

**Sustain**
Note. This name is used for preparations of different composition.
Support, Braz.
Preparation for enteral nutrition (p.1417·1).

Zee, USA.
Sodium chloride; calcium carbonate; potassium chloride (p.1217·1).

**Sustained Release Buffered C** Blackmores, Austral.†.
Vitamin C (p.1460·2); bioflavonoids (p.1688·2); hesperidin (p.1688·2); rose fruit (p.1740·1); rutoside (p.1688·2).
*Vitamin C supplement.*

**Sustained Release Executive B Plus Herbs**
Blackmores, Austral.†.
Vitamins; minerals; passion flower; avena (p.1417·1).
*Nutritional supplement; stress.*

**Sustaire** Pfizer, USA.
Theophylline (p.798·3).
*Asthma; bronchospastic disorders.*

**Sustanon**
Organon, Belg.; Organon, Hong Kong; Organon, Ital.; Organon, NZ.
Testosterone propionate (p.1570·1); testosterone phenylpropionate (p.1570·1); testosterone isocaproate (p.1570·1); testosterone decanoate (p.1570·1).
*Male hypogonadism; masculinisation in gender reassignment of females.*

**Sustanon 100**
Organon, Austral.; Infar, India; Organon, Irl.; Organon, Neth.; Organon, UK.
Testosterone propionate (p.1570·1); testosterone phenylpropionate (p.1570·1); testosterone isocaproate (p.1570·1).
*Androgen deficiency; breast cancer; delayed puberty; male hypogonadism; osteoporosis.*

**Sustanon 250**
Organon, Arg.; Organon, Austral.; Organon, Fin.; Infar, India; Organon, Irl.; Organon, Israel; Organon, Malaysia; Organon, Neth.; Donmed, S.Afr.; Organon, Singapore; Organon, UK.
Testosterone propionate (p.1570·1); testosterone phenylpropionate (p.1570·1); testosterone isocaproate (p.1570·1); testosterone decanoate (p.1570·1).
*Androgen deficiency; breast cancer; delayed puberty; male hypogonadism; osteoporosis.*

**Sustemial** Malesci, Ital.
Ferrous gluconate (p.1428·1).
*Anaemias; iron deficiency.*

**Sustenan** Organon, Chile.
Testosterone undecylate (p.1570·1).
*Male hypogonadism; osteoporosis.*

**Sustenan 250** Organon, Chile.
Testosterone propionate (p.1570·1); testosterone phenylpropionate (p.1570·1); testosterone isocaproate (p.1570·1); testosterone decanoate (p.1570·1).
*Male hypogonadism; osteoporosis.*

**Sustenium** Menarini, Ital.
Fosfocreatinine disodium (p.1689·3).
*Muscle disorders.*

**Sustenon 250** Organon, Port.
Testosterone propionate (p.1570·1); testosterone phenylpropionate (p.1570·1); testosterone isocaproate (p.1570·1); testosterone decanoate (p.1570·1).
*Male hypogonadism; osteoporosis.*

**Sustiva**
Du Pont, Canad.; Bristol-Myers Squibb, Fr.; Bristol-Myers Squibb, Ger.; Du Pont, Irl.; Bristol-Myers Squibb, Ital.; Bristol-Myers Squibb, Spain; Bristol-Myers Squibb, UK; Bristol-Myers Squibb, USA.
Efavirenz (p.632·2).
*HIV infection.*

**Sustrate** Bristol-Myers Squibb, Braz.
Propatylnitrate (p.989·3).
*Angina pectoris.*

**Sustress Plus** Sankyo, Braz.
Vitamin and mineral preparation (p.1417·1).

**Sutac** Sripasit, Thai.
Cetirizine hydrochloride (p.427·1).
*Allergic conjunctivitis; allergic rhinitis; allergic skin disorders.*

**Sutif** Farma Lepori, Spain.
Terazosin hydrochloride (p.1010·3).
*Benign prostatic hyperplasia; hypertension.*

**Sutin** Loren, Mex.
Vitamin A (p.1451·2); colecalciferol (p.1461·3); cod-liver oil (p.1425·2); benzalkonium chloride (p.1168·3); zinc oxide (p.1163·2).
*Keratinisation disorders.*

**Sutrico** Kampel Martian, Arg.
Finasteride (p.1554·2).
*Alopecia.*

**Sutrico Tar** Kampel Martian, Arg.
Coal tar (p.1159·2).
*Scalp disorders.*

**Sutril** Novag, Spain.
Torasemide (p.1015·3) or torasemide sodium (p.1015·3).
*Hypertension; oedema.*

**Su-Tuss DM** Cypress, USA.
Dextromethorphan hydrobromide (p.1117·3); guaifenesin (p.1122·1).
*Coughs.*

**Su-Tuss HD** Cypress, USA.
Hydrocodone tartrate (p.45·1); pseudoephedrine hydrochloride (p.1129·2); guaifenesin (p.1122·1).

**Suvalan** Arrow, Austral.
Sumatriptan succinate (p.471·2).
*Migraine.*

**Suvipen** Thera, Fr.†.
Metampicillin sodium (p.229·3).
*Bacterial infections.*

**Suxar** Biolab Sanus, Braz.†.
Salbutamol (p.791·3).
*Obstructive airways disease.*

**Suxidina** Seid, Spain.
*Aspergillus oryzae*; dimethicone (p.1289·2); metoclopramide hydrochloride (p.1274·3); oxazepam hemisuccinate (p.712·3).
*Aerophagia; digestive disorders; meteorism.*

**Suxilep** Jenapharm, Ger.
Ethosuximide (p.360·1).
*Absence seizures.*

**Suxinutin**
Pfizer, Austria; Pfizer, Fin.; Parke, Davis, Ger.; Pfizer, Swed.; Pfizer, Switz.
Ethosuximide (p.360·1).
*Absence seizures.*

**Svedocain Sin Vasoconstr** Inibsa, Spain.
Bupivacaine hydrochloride (p.1371·1).
*Local anaesthesia.*

**Sviroxit** Rafarm, Gr.
Disodium etidronate (p.771·2).
*Osteoporosis; Paget's disease of bone.*

**Svitalark** Leovan, Gr.
Buspirone hydrochloride (p.672·2).
*Generalised anxiety.*

**SVR 50B** SVR, Fr.
*SPF 50:* Titanium dioxide (p.1160·3); zinc oxide (p.1163·2).
*Sunscreen.*

**SVR Creme Antimoustique** SVR, Fr.
Dimethyl phthalate (p.1504·1); metatoluamide.
*Insect repellent.*

**Swarm** Pickles, UK.
Hamamelis (p.1696·3); dibrompropamidine isetionate (p.1178·2); calamine (p.1144·1).
*Insect bites and stings.*

**Sweatosan N** Novartis Consumer, Ger.
Sage (p.1741·2).
*Hyperhidrosis.*

**Swecon** YSP, Malaysia.
Hydrotalcite (p.1267·3).
*Gastric hyperacidity; gastritis; peptic ulcer.*

**Sween Cream** Coloplast, USA.
Barrier cream.

**Sweet Touch** Farmacologico Milanese, Ital.†.
Aspartame (p.1422·1).
*Sugar substitute.*

**Sweetabb** Pose, Thai.†.
Aspartame (p.1422·1).
*Sugar substitute.*

**Sweetex** Boots Healthcare, NZ†.
Saccharin sodium (p.1443·3).
*Sweetening agent.*

**Swiff** Berlin Pharm, Thai.
Monobasic sodium phosphate (p.1230·3); dibasic sodium phosphate (p.1231·1).
*Bowel evacuation; constipation.*

**Swim-Ear**
Metapharma, Canad.; Co-Pharma, UK; Fougera, USA.
Isopropyl alcohol (p.1184·3); glycerol (p.1694·3).
*Removal of trapped ear water.*

**Swiss Herb Cough Drops** Ricola, Canad.
Althaea (p.1651·3); burnet (p.1663·2); horehound (p.1124·1); mallow (p.1709·3); menthol (p.1711·3); parsley piert (p.1729·1); peppermint oil (p.1283·2); plantago cordata; thyme (p.1755·2); veronica officinalis with or without ascorbic acid (p.1460·2).

**Swiss One** Swiss Herbal, Canad.
Multivitamin and mineral preparation (p.1417·1).

**Swiss-Kal Eff** Byk Madaus, S.Afr.†.
Potassium citrate (p.1223·1); potassium bicarbonate (p.1223·1).
*Hypokalaemia in hyperchloraemic acidosis.*

**Swiss-Kal SR** Byk Madaus, S.Afr.
Potassium chloride (p.1232·2).

**SX Carduus** Schwabe Extracta, Ger.†.
Silybum marianum (p.1043·3).
*Liver disorders.*

**SX Mentha** Schwabe Extracta, Ger.†.
Peppermint oil (p.1283·2).
*Irritable bowel syndrome.*

**SX Sabal** Schwabe Extracta, Ger.†.
Saw palmetto (p.1569·1).
*Benign prostatic hyperplasia.*

**SX Valeriana comp** Schwabe Extracta, Ger.†.
Valerian (p.1762·2); melissa (p.1711·1).
*Agitation; sleep disorders.*

**Sycold** Siam Bheasach, Thai.†.
Phenylpropanolamine hydrochloride (p.1127·3); paracetamol (p.76·2); chlorphenamine maleate (p.427·3).
*Cold and influenza symptoms; hay fever; sinusitis; upper respiratory-tract disorders.*

**Sycot** Stadmed, India.
Trifluoperazine hydrochloride (p.726·3); trihexyphenidyl hydrochloride (p.490·2).
*Schizophrenia.*

**Sydolil** Columbia, Mex.
Ergotamine tartrate (p.467·2); caffeine (p.782·1); aspirin (p.15·1).
*Headache including migraine.*

**Sygen** TRB, Braz.
Monosialoganglioside sodium (p.1691·1); electrolytes.
*Cerebrovascular disorders.*

**Sykofen** Silom, Thai.
Ketotifen fumarate (p.788·1).
*Asthma; bronchitis; hypersensitivity reactions.*

**Sylador** Sanofi Synthelabo, Braz.
Tramadol hydrochloride (p.94·3).
*Pain.*

**Syllact** Wallace, USA.
Ispaghula (p.1268·1).
*Constipation.*

**Syllamalt** Wallace, USA†.
Malt extract (p.1439·2); ispaghula (p.1268·1).
*Constipation.*

**Symadal M** Chauvin ankerpharm, Ger.
Dimethicone 200 (p.1482·1).
*Barrier preparation.*

**Symax** Capellon, USA.
Hyoscyamine sulfate (p.485·1).
*Control of gastrointestinal secretions; cystitis; gastrointestinal spasm; heart block; parkinsonism; renal colic; rhinitis.*

**Symbial** Galderma, Neth.
Urea (p.1162·2); sodium chloride (p.1233·3).
*Skin disorders.*

**Symbicort**
AstraZeneca, Arg.; AstraZeneca, Austral.; AstraZeneca, Austria; AstraZeneca, Belg.; AstraZeneca, Braz.; AstraZeneca, Chile; AstraZeneca, Denm.; AstraZeneca, Fin.; AstraZeneca, Fr.; AstraZeneca, Ger.; Promed, Ger.; Stern, Ger.; AstraZeneca, Hong Kong; AstraZeneca, Irl.; AstraZeneca, Israel; AstraZeneca, Neth.; AstraZeneca, Norw.; AstraZeneca, NZ; AstraZeneca, Port.; AstraZeneca, Singapore; AstraZeneca, Spain; Draco, Swed.; AstraZeneca, Switz.; AstraZeneca, Thai.; AstraZeneca, UK.
Budesonide (p.1094·2); formoterol fumarate (p.786·1).
*Asthma.*

**Symbiocort** AstraZeneca, Ital.
Budesonide (p.1094·2); formoterol fumarate (p.786·1).
*Asthma.*

**Symbioflor I** Peithner, Austria.
Live cells and autolysate of *Enterococcus faecalis* (p.1704·2).
*Gastrointestinal disorders; infections.*

**Symbioflor I** Symbiopharm, Ger.
Cells and autolysate of *Enterococcus faecalis* (p.1704·2).
*Immunotherapy.*

**Symbioflor II** Peithner, Austria.
Live cells and autolysate of *Escherichia coli.*
*Gastrointestinal disorders; infections.*

**Symbioflor 2** Symbiopharm, Ger.
Cells and autolysate of *Escherichia coli.*
*Gastrointestinal disorders.*

**Symbioflor-Antigen** Symbiopharm, Ger.
*Escherichia coli.*
*Immunotherapy.*

**Symbyax** Lilly, USA.
Olanzapine (p.710·3); fluoxetine hydrochloride (p.292·1).
*Bipolar disorder.*

**Symfona N** Medichemie, Switz.
Ginkgo biloba (p.1692·3).
*Cerebrovascular disorders.*

**Symmetrel**
Novartis, Austral.; Du Pont, Canad.; Novartis, Gr.; Novartis, Hong Kong; Novartis, Irl.; Novartis, Israel†; Novartis, Neth.; Novartis, NZ;

*Novartis, S.Afr.; Novartis, Singapore; Novartis, Switz.; Alliance, UK; Endo, USA.*
Amantadine hydrochloride (p.1197·2).
*Drug-induced extrapyramidal disorders; herpes zoster; influenza A; parkinsonism.*

**Symoron** *Yamanouchi, Neth.*
Methadone hydrochloride (p.57·2).
*Opioid addiction; pain.*

**Symoxyl** *Sarabhai Piramal, India.*
Amoxicillin (p.155·3) or amoxicillin trihydrate (p.155·3).
*Bacterial infections.*

**Sympal** *Berlin-Chemie, Ger.*
Dexketoprofen trometamol (p.51·2).
*Pain.*

**Sympalept** *Streuli, Switz.*
Oxedrine tartrate (p.977·3).
*Circulatory disorders; hypotension.*

**Sympaneurol** *DB, Fr.*
Crataegus (p.1677·1); passion flower (p.1729·1); valerian (p.1762·2).
Formerly contained phenobarbital, crataegus, passion flower, and valerian.
*Nervous disorders; sleep disorders.*

**Sympathyl** *Innotech, Fr.*
Crataegus (p.1677·1); eschscholtzia californica; magnesium oxide (p.1272·3).
Formerly contained phenobarbital and crataegus.
*Nervous disorders; sleep disorders.*

**Sympatol**
*Boehringer Ingelheim, Austria; Boehringer Ingelheim, Ger.†; Boehringer Ingelheim, Ital.*
Oxedrine tartrate (p.977·3).
*Hypotension.*

**Sympavagol** *Novartis Sante, Fr.*
Passion flower (p.1729·1); crataegus (p.1677·1).
*Nervous disorders; sleep disorders.*

**Symphocal** *Abic, Israel.*
Oxolamine citrate (p.1126·1).
*Coughs.*

**Symphytum Ro-Plex (Rowo-776)** *Pharmakon, Ger.*
Homoeopathic preparation.

**Symphytum-Komplex** *Woelm, Ger.*
Homoeopathic preparation.

**Symptofed** *Propan, S.Afr.*
Pseudoephedrine hydrochloride (p.1129·2).
*Upper respiratory-tract congestion.*

**Syn MD**
*Synthelabo, Belg.†; Kramer, Switz.†.*
Sorbitol (p.1446·3).
*Bowel evacuation; constipation; dyspepsia.*

**Synacol CF** *Roberts, USA.*
Dextromethorphan hydrobromide (p.1117·3); guaifenesin (p.1122·1).
*Coughs.*

**Synacort** *Syntex, USA.*
Hydrocortisone (p.1103·3).
*Skin disorders.*

**Synacthen**
*Novartis, Austral.; Novartis, Austria; Novartis, Belg.; Novartis, Chile; Novartis, Denm.; Novartis, Ger.; Novartis, Irl.; Novartis, Israel; Novartis, Ital.; Novartis, Neth.; Novartis, NZ; Novartis, Port.; Novartis, Swed.; Novartis, Switz.; Alliance, UK.*
Tetracosactide (p.1340·2), tetracosactide hexa-acetate (p.1340·3), or tetracosactide hexa-acetate zinc phosphate complex (p.1340·3).
*Adrenocorticotrophic hormone; diagnosis of adrenocortical insufficiency; infantile spasms; multiple sclerosis.*

**Synacthen Depot**
*Novartis, Canad.; Novartis, Ger.; Novartis, S.Afr.; Alliance, UK.*
Tetracosactide acetate zinc phosphate complex (p.1340·3), tetracosactide hexa-acetate (p.1340·3), or tetracosactide zinc hydroxide complex (p.1340·2).
*Adrenocorticotrophic hormone; diagnosis of adrenocortical insufficiency.*

**Synacthen Retard** *Novartis, Switz.*
Tetracosactide hexaacetate zinc complex (p.1340·3).
*Adrenocorticotrophic hormone.*

**Synacthene**
*Novartis, Fr.; IFET (ΙΦΕΤ), Gr.*
Tetracosactide (p.1340·2).
*Adrenocorticotrophic hormone; diagnosis of adrenocortical insufficiency; infantile spasm; multiple sclerosis.*

**Syn-A-Gen** *Democal, Switz.*
Nonoxinol 9 (p.1413·3).
*Contraceptive.*

**Synagis**
*Abbott, Arg.; Abbott, Austral.; Abbott, Belg.; Abbott, Braz.; Abbott, Denm.; Abbott, Fin.; Abbott, Fr.; Abbott, Ger.; Abbott, Gr.; Med Immune, Hong Kong; Abbott, Irl.; Abbott, Ital.; Abbott, Mex.; Abbott, Neth.; Abbott, Norw.; Abbott, NZ; Abbott, S.Afr.; Abbott, Singapore; Abbott, Spain; Abbott, Swed.; Abbott, Switz.; Abbott, UK; Medimmune, USA.*
Palivizumab (p.1637·2).
*Respiratory syncytial virus infections.*

**Synalar**
*Grunenthal, Austria; Yamanouchi, Belg.; Aventis, Braz.†; Medicis, Canad.; Bioglan, Denm.; Aventis, Fr.; Bioglan, Hong Kong; Bioglan, Irl.; Bioglan, Malaysia; Syntex, Mex.; Bioglan, Norw.; AFT, NZ; Janssen-Cilag, Port.; Genop, S.Afr.†; Bioglan, Singapore†; Yamanouchi, Spain; Bioglan, Swed.; Grunenthal, Switz.; Sanofi Synthelabo, Thai.; GP, UK; Medicis, USA.*
Fluocinolone acetonide (p.1101·2).
*Skin disorders.*

**Synalar Bi-Otic**
*Yamanouchi, Belg.; Yamanouchi, Neth.*
Fluocinolone acetonide (p.1101·2); neomycin sulfate (p.235·1); polymyxin B sulfate (p.245·1).
*Inflammatory ear infections.*

**Synalar C**
*Bioglan, Irl.; Syntex, Mex.; Genop, S.Afr.†; Bioglan, Singapore†; GP, UK.*
Fluocinolone acetonide (p.1101·2); clioquinol (p.196·3).
*Infected skin disorders.*

**Synalar med Chinoform**
*Bioglan, Denm.; Bioglan, Norw.*
Fluocinolone acetonide (p.1101·2); clioquinol (p.196·3).
*Infected skin disorders.*

**Synalar N**
*Note. This name is used for preparations of different composition.*
*Grunenthal, Austria; Bioglan, Hong Kong; Bioglan, Irl.; Bioglan, Malaysia; Genop, S.Afr.†; Bioglan, Singapore†; Grunenthal, Switz.; Sanofi Synthelabo, Thai.; GP, UK.*
Fluocinolone acetonide (p.1101·2); neomycin sulfate (p.235·1).
*Infected skin disorders.*

*Syntex, Mex.*
Fluocinolone acetonide (p.1101·2); polymyxin B sulfate (p.245·1); neomycin sulfate (p.235·1); phenylephrine hydrochloride (p.1126·3).
*Nasal and sinus disorders.*

**Synalar Nasal** *Yamanouchi, Spain.*
Phenylephrine hydrochloride (p.1126·3); fluocinolone acetonide (p.1101·2); neomycin sulfate (p.235·1); polymyxin B sulfate (p.245·1).
*Nasal congestion and infection.*

**Synalar Neo** *Syntex, Mex.*
Fluocinolone acetonide (p.1101·2); neomycin sulfate (p.235·1).
*Infected skin disorders.*

**Synalar Neomicina** *Yamanouchi, Spain.*
Fluocinolone acetonide (p.1101·2); neomycin sulfate (p.235·1).
*Infected skin disorders.*

**Synalar Neomycine** *Cassenne, Fr.†.*
Fluocinolone acetonide (p.1101·2); neomycin sulfate (p.235·1).
*Infected skin disorders.*

**Synalar O** *Syntex, Mex.*
Fluocinolone acetonide (p.1101·2); polymyxin B sulfate (p.245·1); neomycin sulfate (p.235·1); lidocaine hydrochloride (p.1377·3).
*Otitis externa.*

**Synalar Oftalmico** *Syntex, Mex.*
Fluocinolone acetonide (p.1101·2); polymyxin B sulfate (p.245·1); neomycin sulfate (p.235·1).
*Infected eye disorders.*

**Synalar Otico** *Yamanouchi, Spain.*
Fluocinolone acetonide (p.1101·2); neomycin sulfate (p.235·1); polymyxin B sulfate (p.245·1).
*Ear disorders.*

**Synalar Rectal**
*Janssen-Cilag, Port.; Yamanouchi, Spain.*
Bismuth subgallate (p.1252·2); fluocinolone acetonide (p.1101·2); lidocaine hydrochloride (p.1377·3); menthol (p.1711·3).
*Anorectal disorders.*

**Synalar Rectal Simple** *Yamanouchi, Spain.*
Fluocinolone acetonide (p.1101·2).
*Anorectal disorders.*

**Synalar Simple** *Minerva (Μινερβα), Gr.*
Fluocinolone acetonide (p.1101·2).
*Topical corticosteroid.*

**Synaleve** *Mer-National, S.Afr.*
*Capsules:* Paracetamol (p.76·2); codeine phosphate (p.27·1); meprobamate (p.706·2).
*Pain and associated tension.*
*Syrup†:* Paracetamol (p.76·2); codeine phosphate (p.27·1); promethazine hydrochloride (p.439·1).
*Fever; pain.*
*Tablets†:* Paracetamol (p.76·2); codeine phosphate (p.27·1); caffeine (p.782·1); meprobamate (p.706·2).
*Pain and associated tension.*

**Synalgo** *Geymonat, Ital.*
Naproxen aminobutanol (p.65·3).
*Gout; musculoskeletal and joint disorders; neuralgia; sciatica.*

**Synalgos-DC** *Wyeth-Ayerst, USA.*
Dihydrocodeine tartrate (p.34·3); aspirin (p.15·1); caffeine (p.782·1).
*Pain.*

**Synap** *Restan, S.Afr.*
Paracetamol (p.76·2); dextropropoxyphene napsilate (p.28·3); diphenhydramine hydrochloride (p.431·3); caffeine (p.782·1).
*Pain.*

**Synapausa** *Organon, Port.*
Estriol succinate (p.1552·3).
*Oestrogen deficiency.*

**Synapause**
*Donmed, S.Afr.; Organon, Spain†.*
Estriol succinate (p.1552·3).
*Oestrogen deficiency.*

**Synapause E** *Nourypharma, Ger.*
Estriol (p.1552·3).
*Menopausal disorders.*

**Synapause-E$_3$** *Organon, Neth.*
Estriol (p.1552·3).
*Adjunct in cervical smear tests; menopausal disorders; oestrogen deficiency.*

**Synarel**
*Pharmacia, Austral.; Searle, Belg.†; Pharmacia, Braz.; Pharmacia, Canad.; Pharmacia, Fr.; Pharmacia, Hong Kong; Pharmacia, Irl.; Searle, Israel; Searle, Mex.; Pharmacia, Neth.; Pharmacia, NZ; Pharmacia, S.Afr.; Seid, Spain; Pharmacia, UK; Searle, USA.*
Nafarelin acetate (p.1332·3).
*Endometriosis; ovarian stimulation in in-vitro fertilisation; precocious puberty; uterine fibroids.*

**Synarela**
*Pharmacia, Denm.; Pharmacia, Fin.; Pharmacia, Ger.; Pharmacia, Norw.; Pharmacia, Swed.*
Nafarelin acetate (p.1332·3).
*Endometriosis; ovarian stimulation for in-vitro fertilisation; uterine fibroids.*

**Synarome** *Faran, Gr.*
Atenolol (p.865·2).
*Angina; arrythmias; hypertension.*

**Synastone** *Auden McKenzie, UK.*
Methadone hydrochloride (p.57·2).
*Opioid withdrawal syndrome.*

**Synbetamine** *Synco, Hong Kong.*
Betamethasone (p.1093·1); dexchlorpheniramine maleate (p.427·3).
*Hypersensitivity reactions; inflammatory eye disorders.*

**Synbrozil** *Synco, Hong Kong.*
Gemfibrozil (p.923·1).
*Hyperlipidaemias.*

**Syncarpin-N** *Winzer, Ger.*
Pilocarpine hydrochloride (p.1495·1); neostigmine bromide (p.1492·2).
Syncarpin formerly contained pilocarpine borate, neostigmine bromide, and naphazoline hydrochloride.
*Glaucoma; reversal of mydriasis.*

**Synchlolim** *Atlantic, Thai.*
Chloramphenicol sodium succinate (p.185·1).
*Bacterial infections.*

**Synchrocell** *Dermoteca, Port.*
Acediosmin; aescin (p.1648·2); acetyl glucosamine; glucuronic acid.
*Cellulite.*

**Synchro-Levels** *Alphrema, Ital.*
Vitamin, amno-acid, mineral, and fatty acid preparation (p.1417·1).

**Synchrorose** *Dermoteca, Port.*
Silymarin (p.1043·3); acetyl glucosamine; *dl*-alpha tocoferil acetate (p.1465·1); hyaluronic acid (p.1697·3).
*High skin coloration.*

**Synchrovit** *Dermoteca, Port.*
Vitamin A palmitate (p.1453·1); alpha tocoferil acetate (p.1465·1); acetyl glucosamine; glucuronic acid; hyaluronic acid (p.1697·3).
*High skin coloration.*

**Syncillin** *Infectopharm, Ger.†.*
Azidocillin sodium (p.159·1).
*Bacterial infections.*

**Synclovir** *Synco, Hong Kong.*
Aciclovir (p.626·1).
*Herpes simplex infections.*

**Synco-CFN** *Synco, Hong Kong.*
Clotrimazole (p.396·2); fluocinolone acetonide (p.1101·2); neomycin sulfate (p.235·1).
*Infected skin disorders.*

**Syncoforte** *Synco, Hong Kong.*
Vitamin B substances (p.1417·1).
*Vitamin B deficiencies.*

**Syncomet** *Synco, Hong Kong.*
Cimetidine (p.1255·3).
*Gastritis; gastro-oesophageal reflux; peptic ulcer.*

**Syncoquin** *Synco, Hong Kong.*
Chloroquine phosphate (p.448·2).
*Amoebic hepatitis; lupus erythematosus; malaria; rheumatoid arthritis.*

**Syncortyl** *Aventis, Fr.*
Desoxycortone acetate (p.1097·1).
*Mineralocorticoid deficiency.*

**Syncro** *Fontovit, Braz.*
Vitamin and mineral preparation (p.1417·1).

**Syndette** *Adcock Ingram, S.Afr.†.*
Paracetamol (p.76·2); doxylamine succinate (p.432·3).
*Fever; pain; sedative.*

**Syndol**
*Note. This name is used for preparations of different composition.*
*Roche, Chile.*
Ketorolac trometamol (p.52·1).
*Pain.*

*SSL, Irl.; Adcock Ingram, S.Afr.; SSL, UK.*
Paracetamol (p.76·2); codeine phosphate (p.27·1); doxylamine succinate (p.432·3); caffeine (p.782·1).
*Pain.*

*Mer-National, S.Afr.†.*
*Syrup:* Paracetamol (p.76·2); doxylamine succinate (p.432·3); codeine phosphate (p.27·1).
*Fever; pain with tension.*

**Syndopa**
*Sun, India; Sun, Thai.*
Carbidopa (p.1204·3); levodopa (p.1205·2).
*Parkinsonism.*

**Synedil** *Yamanouchi, Fr.*
Sulpiride (p.722·2).
*Nervous disorders; psychoses.*

**Synemol** *Medicis, USA.*
Fluocinolone acetonide (p.1101·2).
*Skin disorders.*

**Synerbiol** *Nutergia, Fr.*
Marine fish oil (p.976·2).
*Nutritional supplement.*

**Synercid**
*Aventis, Arg.; Aventis, Austral.; Aventis, Austria; Aventis, Braz.; Aventis, Canad.; Aventis, Fin.; Aventis, Fr.; Aventis, Ger.; Aventis, Irl.; Aventis, Israel; Aventis, Ital.; Aventis, Mex.; Aventis, Neth.; Aventis, S.Afr.; Aventis, Spain; Aventis, Swed.; Aventis, Switz.; Aventis, UK; Monarch, USA.*
Quinupristin (p.248·3) or quinupristin mesilate (p.248·2); dalfopristin (p.248·3) or dalfopristin mesilate (p.248·1).
*Bacterial infections.*

**Synerga** *Laves, Ger.*
Cell-free lysate of *Escherichia coli*.
*Allergies.*

**Synergistic Manganese** *Quest, Canad.†.*
Manganese, vitamin A, and vitamin C (p.1417·1).

**Synergistic Selenium** *Quest, Canad.*
Selenium, vitamin C, and vitamin E (p.1417·1).

**Synergomycin** *Abbott, Ger.*
Erythromycin ethyl succinate (p.208·1); bromhexine hydrochloride (p.1115·3).
*Bacterial infections of the respiratory tract.*

**Synergon** *Lipha Sante, Fr.*
Progesterone (p.1566·2); estrone (p.1553·1).
*Amenorrhoea.*

**Synergyl** *Monsanto, Fr.†.*
Multivitamin and mineral preparation (p.1417·1).

**Synermox** *Douglas, NZ.*
Amoxicillin trihydrate (p.155·3); potassium clavulanate (p.193·3).
*Bacterial infections.*

**Synerpril**
*Merck Sharp & Dohme, Austria; Merck Sharp & Dohme, Denm.; Merck Sharp & Dohme, Swed.*
Enalapril maleate (p.909·2); hydrochlorothiazide (p.933·2).
*Hypertension.*

**Syneudon** *Krewel, Ger.*
Amitriptyline hydrochloride (p.280·3).
*Depression.*

**Synfase**
*Pharmacia, Norw.; Pharmacia, Swed.*
Norethisterone (p.1562·2); ethinylestradiol (p.1553·2).
28-Day packs also contains 7 inert tablets.
*Triphasic oral contraceptive.*

**Synflex**
*Altimed, Canad.; Roche, Hong Kong; Roche, Irl.; Recordati, Ital.; Roche, NZ; Roche, S.Afr.; Roche, Singapore†; Roche, Thai.; Roche, UK.*
Naproxen sodium (p.65·1).
*Gout; inflammation; musculoskeletal, joint and periarticular disorders; pain.*

**Syngel** *Will-Pharma, Belg.*
Aluminium hydroxide-magnesium carbonate co-dried gel (p.1250·1); magnesium hydroxide (p.1272·2); magnesium trisilicate (p.1272·3); lidocaine hydrochloride (p.1377·3).
*Gastritis; gastro-oesophageal reflux.*

**Syngynon** *Jenapharm, Ger.*
Hydroxyprogesterone caproate (p.1556·3); estradiol benzoate (p.1550·1).
*Menstrual disorders.*

**Synitidine** *Synco, Hong Kong.*
Ranitidine hydrochloride (p.1285·2).
*Dyspepsia; gastro-oesophageal reflux; oesophagitis; peptic ulcer; Zollinger-Ellison syndrome.*

**Synizoral** *Synco, Hong Kong.*
Ketoconazole (p.403·3).
*Fungal infections.*

**Synkapton** *Strallhofer, Austria.*
Ergotamine tartrate (p.467·2); dimenhydrinate (p.431·1); caffeine (p.782·1).
*Migraine and other vascular headaches.*

**Synkavit** *Cambridge, UK†.*
Menadiol sodium phosphate (p.1466·3).
Now known as Menadiol Diphosphate Tablets.
*Factor VII deficiency; hypoprothrombinaemia.*

**Synobel** *Yamanouchi, Spain.*
Clioquinol (p.196·3); fluocinolone acetonide (p.1101·2).
*Infected skin disorders.*

**Synogin** *Chinta, Thai.†.*
Naproxen (p.65·1).
*Gout; musculoskeletal and joint disorders.*

**Synoxicam** *Synco, Hong Kong.*
Piroxicam (p.84·2).
*Gout; inflammation; musculoskeletal and joint disorders; pain.*

**Synpharma Aromatische Tinktur** *Synpharma, Austria.*
Cinnamon (p.1672·2); clove (p.1673·2); ginger (p.1267·1).
*Dyspepsia; flatulence.*

**Synpharma Bronchial** *Synpharma, Austria.*
Anise oil (p.1655·2); eucalyptus oil (p.1686·2); thyme oil (p.1755·3).
*Catarrh; coughs.*

**Synpharma Instant-Blasen- und Nierentee**
*Synpharma, Austria.*
Birch leaf (p.1660·3); equisetum (p.1684·1); urtica (p.1762·1).
*Urinary-tract disorders.*

**Synpharma Instant-Brust- und Hustentee** *Synpharma, Austria.*
Althaea (p.1651·3); cowslip (p.1735·1); thyme (p.1755·2).
*Respiratory-tract disorders.*

**Synpharma Instant-Nerventee** *Synpharma, Austria.*
Valerian (p.1762·2); melissa leaf (p.1711·1); orange (p.1723·3).
*Nervous disorders; sleep disorders.*

**Synphase**
*Pharmacia, Hong Kong; Pharmacia, UK.*
Ethinylestradiol (p.1553·2); norethisterone (p.1562·2).
*Triphasic oral contraceptive.*

**Synphasec** *Grunenthal, Ger.*
Ethinylestradiol (p.1553·2); norethisterone (p.1562·2).
*Triphasic oral contraceptive.*

**Synphasic**
*Pharmacia, Austral.; Pharmacia, Canad.; Pharmacia, NZ.*
Ethinylestradiol (p.1553·2); norethisterone (p.1562·2).
28-Day packs also contain 7 inert tablets.
*Triphasic oral contraceptive.*

**Synrelin** *Pharmacia, Arg.*
Nafarelin acetate (p.1332·3).
*Endometriosis; female infertility; precocious puberty.*

**Synrelina** *Pharmacia, Switz.*
Nafarelin acetate (p.1332·3).
*Endometriosis.*

**Syn-Rx** *Medeva, USA†.*
Dark blue tablets, pseudoephedrine hydrochloride (p.1129·2); guaifenesin (p.1122·1); light green tablets, guaifenesin.
*Respiratory-tract congestion.*

**Syn-Rx DM** *Medeva, USA†.*
Light blue tablets, pseudoephedrine hydrochloride (p.1129·2); guaifenesin (p.1122·1); yellow tablets, dextromethorphan hydrobromide (p.1117·3); guaifenesin.
*Coughs; nasal congestion.*

**Syntaris**
*Roche, Austria†; Roche, Belg.; Dermapharm, Ger.; Roche, Irl.; Recordati, Ital.; Roche, Neth.; Roche, S.Afr.†; Roche, Switz.; Ivax, UK.*
Flunisolide (p.1101·1).
*Allergic rhinitis.*

**Syntestan** *Syntex, Ger.; Roche, Ger.*
Cloprednol (p.1096·1).
*Asthma; polyarthritis.*

**Synthamin**
*Baxter, Austral.; Baxter, Ger.; Baxter, Irl.; Baxter, NZ; Fresenius Kabi, S.Afr.†; Baxter, Spain; Baxter, Switz.; Baxter, UK.*
Amino-acid infusion with or without electrolytes (p.1417·1).
*Parenteral nutrition.*

**Synthocilin** *Pharmaceutical Co, India.*
Ampicillin sodium (p.157·1) or ampicillin trihydrate (p.157·2).
*Bacterial infections.*

**Synthol**
*Note. This name is used for preparations of different composition.*
*Bournonville, Belg.†.*
Cloral hydrate (p.684·1); menthol (p.1711·3); resorcinol (p.1156·3); salicylic acid (p.1157·1); veratrol.
*Skin and mucous membrane disorders.*

*GlaxoSmithKline Sante, Fr.*
Menthol (p.1711·3); resorcinol (p.1156·3); salicylic acid (p.1157·1); veratrol.
Formerly contained cloral hydrate, menthol, resorcinol, salicylic acid, and veratrol.
*Mouth and throat disorders; soft-tissue trauma.*

**Synthomanet** *Remedina, Gr.*
Ranitidine hydrochloride (p.1285·2).
*Conditions where gastric acid reduction is beneficial; gastric hypersecretion including Zollinger-Ellison syndrome; peptic ulcer.*

**Synthomycine** *Abic, Israel; Biogal, Israel; Rekah, Israel.*
Chloramphenicol (p.185·1) or chloramphenicol sodium succinate (p.185·1).
*Bacterial infections.*

**Synthroid**
*Abbott, Braz.; Abbott, Canad.; Abbott, USA.*
Levothyroxine sodium (p.1600·1).
*Hypothyroidism; thyroid-stimulating hormone suppression.*

**Synti** *Medochemie, Malaysia.*
Dequalinium chloride (p.1178·1).
*Mouth and throat disorders.*

**Syntocinon**
*Novartis, Arg.; Novartis, Austral.; Novartis, Austria; Novartis, Belg.; Novartis, Braz.; Novartis, Chile; Novartis, Denm.; Novartis, Fin.; Novartis, Fr.; Novartis, Ger.; Novartis, Hong Kong; Novartis, India; Novartis, Irl.; Novartis, Israel†; Novartis, Ital.; Novartis, Malaysia; Novartis, Mex.; Novartis, Neth.; Novartis, Norw.; Novartis, NZ; Novartis, Port.; Novartis, S.Afr.; Novartis, Singapore; Novartis, Spain; Novartis, Swed.; Novartis, Switz.; Novartis, Thai.†; Alliance, UK.*
Oxytocin (p.1336·1).
*Caesarean section; incomplete abortion; induction and maintenance of labour; lactation disorders; postpartum haemorrhage; postpartum uterine atony.*

**Syntoclox** *Codal Synto, Thai.*
Cloxacillin sodium (p.198·2).
*Bacterial infections.*

**Syntofene** *GlaxoSmithKline Sante, Fr.†.*
Ibuprofen (p.45·3).
*Soft-tissue disorders.*

**Syntometrin** *Novartis, Ger.*
Methylergometrine maleate (p.1714·2); oxytocin (p.1336·1).
*Delivery of the placenta; postpartum haemorrhage.*

**Syntometrine**
*Novartis, Austral.; Novartis, Hong Kong; Novartis, Irl.; Novartis, Israel†; Novartis, Malaysia; Novartis, NZ; Novartis, S.Afr.; Alliance, UK.*
Ergometrine maleate (p.1684·1); oxytocin (p.1336·1).
*Management of third-stage labour; postpartum haemorrhage.*

**Syntonol** *Codal Synto, Thai.*
Propranolol hydrochloride (p.989·3).
*Angina pectoris; anxiety; arrhythmias; hypertension; phaeochromocytoma; tremor.*

**Syntopressin** *Novartis, Irl.†.*
Lypressin (p.1342·3).
*Diabetes insipidus.*

**Synum C** *Biosyn, Ger.*
Ascorbic acid (p.1460·2).
*Methaemoglobinaemia; vitamin C deficiency.*

**Synuretic** *DDSA Pharmaceuticals, UK†.*
Hydrochlorothiazide (p.933·2); amiloride hydrochloride (p.858·2).
These ingredients can be described by the British Approved Name Co-amilozide.
*Ascites; heart failure; hypertension.*

**Synureticum** *Medisa, Switz.†.*
Spironolactone (p.1003·1); hydrochlorothiazide (p.933·2).
*Heart failure; hypertension; nephrotic syndrome; oedema.*

**Synvisc**
*Novartis, Arg.; Bayer, Austral.; Novartis, Braz.; Genzyme, Canad.; Novartis, Chile; Boehringer Ingelheim, Fr.; Wyeth, Ger.; Biomatrix, Hong Kong†; Biomatrix, Israel; Bayer, Malaysia; Novartis, Mex.; Bayer, NZ; Roche, S.Afr.†; Bayer, Singapore; Biomatrix, Swed.; Biomatrix, Switz.; Bayer, Thai.; Biomatrix, UK; Wyeth-Ayerst, USA.*
Hylan G-F 20 (p.1697·3).
*Osteoarthritis of the knee.*

**Synvomin** *Synco, Hong Kong.*
Promethazine teoclate (p.439·2).
*Nausea and vomiting.*

**Syprine** *Merck, USA.*
Trientine dihydrochloride (p.1055·2).
Formerly known as Cuprid.
*Wilson's disease.*

**Syprol** *Rosemont, UK.*
Propranolol hydrochloride (p.989·3).

**Syracol CF** *Roberts, USA.*
Guaifenesin (p.1122·1); dextromethorphan hydrobromide (p.1117·3).
*Coughs.*

**Syraprim** *Galen, Mex.*
Co-trimoxazole (p.199·3).
*Bacterial infections.*

**Syrea** *Medac, Ger.*
Hydroxycarbamide (p.559·1).
*Chronic myeloid leukaemia; essential thrombocythaemia; polycythaemia vera.*

**Syrup DM** *Therapex, Canad.*
Dextromethorphan hydrobromide (p.1117·3).

**Syrup DM-D** *Therapex, Canad.*
Dextromethorphan hydrobromide (p.1117·3); pseudoephedrine hydrochloride (p.1129·2).

**Syrup DM-D-E** *Therapex, Canad.*
Dextromethorphan hydrobromide (p.1117·3); pseudoephedrine hydrochloride (p.1129·2); guaifenesin (p.1122·1).

**Syrup DM-E** *Therapex, Canad.*
Dextromethorphan hydrobromide (p.1117·3); guaifenesin (p.1122·1).

**Syrvite** *Barre-National, USA; Major, USA; Moore, USA.*
Multivitamin preparation (p.1417·1).

**Syscan** *Torrent, India.*
Fluconazole (p.398·1).
*Fungal infections.*

**Syscor**
*Bayer, Austria; Bayer, Belg.; AstraZeneca, Braz.; Bayer, Fin.; Bayer, Gr.; Bayer, Ital.; Zeneca, Mex.†; AstraZeneca, Neth.†; Zeneca, S.Afr.; AstraZeneca, Spain; Bayer, Swed.†; AstraZeneca, Switz.; Forest Laboratories, UK.*
Nisoldipine (p.973·2).
*Angina pectoris; heart failure; hypertension.*

**Systaflam** *Systopic, India.*
Chlorzoxazone (p.1392·3); diclofenac sodium (p.32·1); paracetamol (p.76·2).
*Painful skeletal muscle spasm.*

**Systen**
*Janssen-Cilag, Austria; Janssen-Cilag, Belg.; Janssen-Cilag, Braz.; Janssen-Cilag, Fr.; Janssen-Cilag, Ital.; Cilag, Mex.; Janssen-Cilag, Neth.; Janssen-Cilag, Switz.*
Estradiol (p.1550·1).
*Menopausal disorders; osteoporosis.*

**Systen Conti** *Janssen-Cilag, Switz.*
Estradiol (p.1550·1); norethisterone acetate (p.1562·2).
*Menopausal disorders.*

**Systen Sequi** *Janssen-Cilag, Switz.*
4 Patches, estradiol (p.1550·1) (Systen); 4 patches, estradiol; norethisterone acetate (p.1562·2) (Systen Conti).
*Menopausal disorders.*

**Systepin** *Klinge, Irl.*
Nifedipine (p.966·2).
*Hypertension; ischaemic heart disease.*

**Systodin** *Nycomed, Norw.†.*
Quinidine sulfate (p.991·3).
*Arrhythmias.*

**Systral**
*Fresenius Kabi, Austria†; Viatris, Ger.; Asta Medica, Hong Kong; Sideforma, Port.; Asta Medica, Thai.*
Chlorphenoxamine hydrochloride (p.428·3).
*Allergic skin reactions; skin irritation.*

**Systral C**
*Asta Medica, Austria†; Viatris, Ger.*
Chlorphenoxamine hydrochloride (p.428·3); caffeine (p.782·1).
*Hypersensitivity reactions.*

**Systral Hydrocort** *Viatris, Ger.*
Hydrocortisone (p.1103·3).
*Skin disorders.*

**Systrason** *Asta Medica, Austria†.*
Chlorphenoxamine (p.428·3); hydrocortisone acetate (p.1103·3).
*Skin disorders.*

**Sytron** *Link, UK.*
Sodium feredetate (p.1444·3).
*Iron-deficiency anaemia.*

**Syu** *Anglo-French Drugs, India.*
Nutritional supplement (p.1417·1).

**Syviman N** *Muller Goppingen, Ger.*
Comfrey (p.1675·2); mistletoe (p.1715·3).
*Joint disorders.*

**Syxal** *Syxyl, Ger.*
Hypericum (p.299·1).
*Depression.*

**Syxyl-Vitamin-Comb** *Syxyl, Ger.†.*
Vitamin B substances (p.1417·1).
*Vitamin B deficiency.*

**Szillosan forte** *Henk, Ger.†.*
Squill (p.1130·3); crataegus (p.1677·1).
*Heart failure.*

**T3** *Unipharma, Gr.*
Liothyronine sodium (p.1602·2).
*Hypothyroidism.*

**T4**
*Montpellier, Arg.; Unipharma, Gr.*
Levothyroxine sodium (p.1600·1).
*Hypothyroidism; thyroid cancer; thyroiditis.*

**T5** *MC, Ital.*
Glutaral (p.1180·3).
*Instrument disinfection.*

**T. Polio** *Aventis Pasteur, Fr.*
A tetanus and poliomyelitis (inactivated) vaccine (p.1641·3).
*Active immunisation.*

**T & T Antioxidant** *Procare, Austral.†.*
Silybum marianum (p.1043·3); camellia sinensis (p.1765·3).
*Adjunct in detoxification regimens; exposure to chemical and environmental toxins and tobacco smoke; inflammation.*

**TA Baume** *Bencard, Ger.*
Allergen extracts of tree pollen(p.1650·1).
Formerly known as TA Baumpollen.
*Allergen immunotherapy.*

**TA Graser** *Bencard, Ger.*
Allergen extracts of grass pollen(p.1650·1).
Formerly known as TA Graserpollen.
*Allergen immunotherapy.*

**TA MIX** *Bencard, Ger.*
Allergen extracts of mixed pollens(p.1650·1).
*Allergen immunotherapy.*

**Tab Vaccine** *Berna, Singapore†.*
*Salmonella typhi.*
*Active immunisation.*

**Tabalon**
*Teofarma, Ger.; Aventis, Mex.*
Ibuprofen (p.45·3).
*Fever; gout; inflammation; musculoskeletal and joint disorders; pain.*

**Tabarell** *Sanorell, Ger.*
Homoeopathic preparation.

**Tab-A-Vite** *Major, USA.*
A range of vitamin preparations (p.1417·1).

**Tabcin** *Bayer, Austria.*
Ibuprofen (p.45·3).
*Pain.*

**Tabcin Antigripal** *Bayer, Arg.*
Paracetamol (p.76·2); butetamate citrate (p.1116·2); caffeine (p.782·1); phenylephrine hydrochloride (p.1126·3).
*Cold and influenza symptoms.*

**Tabcin Compuesto** *Bayer, Arg.*
Chlorphenamine maleate (p.427·3); pseudoephedrine hydrochloride (p.1129·2); paracetamol (p.76·2).
*Cold and influenza symptoms.*

**Tabcin Expectorante** *Bayer, Arg.*
Ambroxol hydrochloride (p.1114·3).
*Coughs.*

**Taben 450** *Wassen, Ital.*
Magnesium; potassium; sodium; taurine (p.1417·1).
*Nutritional supplement.*

**Tabine** *BPL-Meizler, Braz.*
Cytarabine (p.543·1).
*Malignant neoplasms.*

**Tabletas Antiacidas** *Pasteur, Chile.*
Magnesium hydroxide (p.1272·2).
*Gastric hyperacidity.*

**Tabletas Phillips** *GlaxoSmithKline, Chile.*
Calcium carbonate (p.1254·2); aluminium hydroxide-sorbitol complex (p.1249·2) (p.1446·3); magnesium hydroxide (p.1272·2).
*Gastric hyperacidity.*

**Tabletas Quimpe** *Quimpe, Spain.*
Atropine methonitrate (p.477·1); codeine phosphate (p.27·1); diphenhydramine hydrochloride (p.431·3); ephedrine hydrochloride (p.1120·1); phenazone (p.82·3); propyphenazone (p.85·3).
*Upper respiratory-tract disorders.*

**Tabletes Valda** *Canonne, Braz.†.*
Menthol (p.1711·3); cineole (p.1672·1); terpineol (p.1752·2); thymol (p.1194·2).
*Mouth and throat disorders.*

**Tabloid** *GlaxoSmithKline, USA.*
Tioguanine (p.588·2).
*Acute myeloid leukaemia.*

**Taborcil** *Lacer, Spain†.*
Gemfibrozil (p.923·1).
*Hyperlipidaemias.*

**Tabotamp**
*Johnson & Johnson, Ger.†; Ethicon, Ital.†.*
Oxidised cellulose (p.757·1).
*Surgical haemorrhage.*

**Tabrin** *Hoechst Marion Roussel, Gr.*
Ofloxacin (p.239·3) or oflaxacin hydrochloride (p.240·1).
*Bacterial infections.*

**Tabritis** *Potter's, UK.*
Sambucus (p.1741·3); achillea (p.1646·2); prickly ash bark (p.1766·3); lappa (p.1704·3); clivers (p.1673·2); poplar bark (p.1733·3); bearberry (p.1659·2); senna (p.1288·2).
*Musculoskeletal and joint disorders.*

**Tac** *Parnell, USA.*
Triamcinolone acetonide (p.1110·2).
*Corticosteroid.*

**TAC Esofago** *Bracco, Ital.*
Barium sulfate (p.1061·1).
*Contrast medium for computerised tomography of the oesophagus.*

**Tacardia** *Richmond, Arg.*
Losartan (p.948·2).
*Hypertension.*

**Tacef**
*Grunenthal, Austria; Takeda, Ger.†.*
Cefmenoxime hydrochloride (p.173·2).
*Bacterial infections.*

**Tacex** *Galen, Mex.*
Ceftriaxone sodium (p.182·3).
*Bacterial infections.*

**Tachidol** *Angelini, Ital.*
Paracetamol (p.76·2); codeine phosphate (p.27·1).
*Fever; pain.*

**Tachiflu** *Angelini, Ital.*
Paracetamol (p.76·2); ascorbic acid (p.1460·2).
*Fever; influenza symptoms; pain.*

**Tachifludec** *Angelini, Ital.*
Paracetamol (p.76·2); ascorbic acid (p.1460·2); phenylephrine hydrochloride (p.1126·3).
*Fever; influenza symptoms; pain.*

**Tachipirina** *Angelini, Ital.*
Paracetamol (p.76·2).
*Fever; pain.*

**Tachmalcor** *AWD, Ger.*
Detajmium bitartrate (p.893·1).
*Arrhythmias.*

**Tachmalin** *Dresden, Ger.†.*
Ajmaline (p.856·1).
*Arrhythmias.*

**TachoComb**
*Nycomed, Austria; Nycomed, Ger.; Nycomed, Hong Kong; Nycomed, Thai.*
Equine collagen (p.1674·3); human fibrinogen (p.753·2); bovine thrombin (p.760·1); bovine aprotinin (p.742·3).
*Haemorrhage.*

**Tacholiquin**
*Sigmapharm, Austria; Bene, Ger.*
Tyloxapol (p.1416·3).
*Respiratory-tract disorders associated with increased or viscous mucus.*

**Tachotop N** *Nycomed, Ger.*
Collagen (p.1674·3).
*Haemorrhage.*

**Tachydaron** *AWD, Ger.*
Amiodarone hydrochloride (p.859·2).
*Arrhythmias.*

**Tachyfenon** *Dresden, Ger.†.*
Propafenone hydrochloride (p.988·3).
*Arrhythmias.*

**Tachynerg Campher Herzsalbe** *Eberth, Ger.*
Benzyl nicotinate (p.21·2); camphor (p.1665·3).
*Cardiac disorders.*

**Tachynerg N** *Eberth, Ger.†.*
Testosterone propionate (p.1570·1); benzyl nicotinate (p.21·2); camphor (p.1665·3); menthol (p.1711·3); lemon oil (p.1706·2).
*Cardiac disorders.*

**Tachystin** *Chauvin ankerpharm, Ger.*
Dihydrotachysterol (p.1461·3).
*Hypoparathyroidism; pseudohypoparathyroidism.*

**Tachytalol** *Asta Medica, Ger.†.*
Sotalol hydrochloride (p.1001·3).
*Arrhythmias.*

**Tacid-4** *Roche, S.Afr.†.*
Aluminium hydroxide-magnesium carbonate co-dried gel (p.1250·1); calcium carbonate (p.1254·2); magnesium hydroxide (p.1272·2); sodium bicarbonate (p.1223·2).
*Hyperchlorhydria.*

**Tacidina** *Sedar, Braz.†.*
Aspirin (p.15·1); caffeine (p.782·1).
*Fever; pain.*

**Tacinol** *Polipharm, Thai.*
Triamcinolone acetonide (p.1110·2).
*Skin disorders.*

**Taclipaxol** *Biochimico, Braz.*
Paclitaxel (p.577·3).
*Malignant neoplasms.*

**Tacrinal** *Biosintetica, Braz.*
Tacrine hydrochloride (p.1497·2).
*Alzheimer's disease.*

**Tacron**
*Note. This name is used for preparations of different composition.*
*Korea United, Singapore.*
Ticlopidine hydrochloride (p.1011·2).
*Atherosclerosis; peripheral vascular disease.*

*Farmasierra, Spain.*
Naproxen (p.65·1).
*Fever; gout; musculoskeletal and joint disorders; pain.*

**Tacryl** *Abigo, Denm.*
Methdilazine (p.437·2).
*Hay fever; rhinitis; urticaria.*

**tactu-nerval** *Feldhoff, Ger.*
Bovine testicular extract (p.1569·3); bovine placental extract.
*Musculoskeletal disorders; nervous disorders.*

**TAD**
*Note. A similar name is used for preparations of different composition (see below).*
*Biomedica, Hong Kong.*
Glutathione (p.1040·3).
*Alcohol or drug poisoning; liver disorders; radiation injury.*

*Biomedica, Ital.*
Glutathione sodium (p.1040·3).
*Alcohol or drug poisoning; ionising radiation damage.*

**TAD+**
*Note. A similar name is used for preparations of different composition (see above).*
*Seroyal, Canad.†.*
Multivitamins with zinc (p.1417·1).

**Tadenan**
*Roche, Austria; Fournier, Fr.; Debat, Hong Kong†; Fournier, Ital.; Fournier, Port.; Fournier, Switz.; Debat, Thai.*
Pygeum africanum (p.1568·2).
*Benign prostatic hyperplasia.*

**Tadenom** *Aventis, Mex.*
Pygeum africanum (p.1568·2).
*Benign prostatic hyperplasia.*

**Tadex** *Orion, Fin.*
Tamoxifen citrate (p.584·1).
*Breast cancer.*

**Tafenil** *Asofarma, Mex.*
Flutamide (p.556·2).
*Prostatic cancer.*

**Tafil**
*Pharmacia, Denm.; Pharmacia, Ger.; Pharmacia Upjohn, Mex.*
Alprazolam (p.668·3).
*Alcohol withdrawal syndrome; anxiety; panic disorders.*

**Tafirol** *Sidus, Arg.*
Paracetamol (p.76·2).
*Fever; pain.*

**Tafloc** *Aspen, S.Afr.*
Ofloxacin (p.239·3).
*Bacterial infections.*

**Taflox** *Faribérica, Port.*
Norfloxacin (p.238·3).
*Bacterial infections.*

**Tagadine** *Duopharma, Hong Kong.*
Cimetidine (p.1255·3).
*Gastro-oesophageal reflux; gastrointestinal haemorrhage; peptic ulcer; Zollinger-Ellison syndrome.*

**Tagagel** *SmithKline Beecham, Ger.†.*
Cimetidine (p.1255·3).
*Gastro-oesophageal reflux; peptic ulcer; Zollinger-Ellison syndrome.*

**Tagal** *Galen, Mex.*
Ceftazidime (p.180·2).
*Bacterial infections.*

**Tagaliv** *Teuto, Braz.*
Cimetidine (p.1255·3).
*Peptic ulcer.*

**Tagamet**
*Key, Arg.; GlaxoSmithKline, Austral.; GlaxoSmithKline, Belg.; GlaxoSmithKline, Braz.; GlaxoSmithKline, Canad.; SmithKline Beecham, Denm.†; Enteris, Fr.; GlaxoSmithKline, Ger.; Vianex (Βιανεξ), Gr.; GlaxoSmithKline, Hong Kong; GlaxoSmithKline, Irl.; SmithKline Beecham, Israel; GlaxoSmithKline, Ital.; GlaxoSmithKline, Malaysia; SmithKline Beecham, Mex.; GlaxoSmithKline, Neth.; GlaxoSmithKline, Norw.; SmithKline Beecham, NZ†; Smith Kline & French, Port.; GlaxoSmithKline, S.Afr.; GlaxoSmithKline, Singapore; GlaxoSmithKline, Spain; GlaxoSmithKline, Swed.; SmithKline Beecham, Switz.; GlaxoSmithKline, Thai.; Chemidex, UK; GlaxoSmithKline, UK; SmithKline Beecham, USA.*
Cimetidine (p.1255·3) or cimetidine hydrochloride (p.1255·3).
*Acid aspiration; dyspepsia; gastro-oesophageal reflux; gastrointestinal haemorrhage; pancreatic insufficiency; peptic ulcer; short bowel syndrome; Zollinger-Ellison syndrome.*

**TAGG** *Eagle, Austral.†.*
Benzalkonium chloride (p.1168·3); lauromacrogol 400 (p.1412·3).
Formerly contained benzododecinium chloride.
*Deodorant detergent for ostomies.*

**Tagonis** *GlaxoSmithKline, Ger.; Janssen-Cilag, Ger.*
Paroxetine hydrochloride (p.311·2).
*Anxiety; depression; obsessive-compulsive disorder; panic attacks; post-traumatic stress disorder.*

**Tagozzard** *Pizzard, Mex.†.*
Psyllium seed (p.1268·1).

**Taguinol** *Spyfarma, Spain.*
Loperamide hydrochloride (p.1271·1).
*Diarrhoea.*

**Taharmayim** *Medentech, Israel.*
Sodium dichloroisocyanurate (p.1191·3).
*Water purification.*

**Taharsept** *Medentech, Israel.*
Sodium dichloroisocyanurate (p.1191·3).
*Instrument, surface, and equipment disinfection.*

**Tahartaf** *Medentech, Israel.*
Sodium dichloroisocyanurate (p.1191·3).
*Equipment disinfection.*

**Tahor** *Pfizer, Fr.*
Atorvastatin calcium (p.866·1).
*Hypercholesterolaemia.*

**Tai Ginseng N**
*Note. This name is used for preparations of different composition.*
*Poehlmann, Ger.*
Ginseng; crataegus; vitamins (p.1417·1).
*Tonic.*

*Poehlmann, Switz.†.*
Ginseng (p.1693·1); crataegus (p.1677·1); hypericum (p.299·1); vitamins (p.1417·1).
*Tonic.*

**Taido** *Cetem, Fr.*
Glycerol (p.1694·3); honey (p.1434·2); collagen (p.1674·3).
*Vaginal lubricant.*

**Taigalor** *Formenti, Ital.*
Lornoxicam (p.54·2).
*Inflammation; pain.*

**Taingel** *Ghimas, Ital.*
Royal jelly; pollen; ginseng; eleutherococcus (p.1417·1).
*Nutritional supplement.*

**Tairal** *Rottapharm, Spain.*
Famotidine (p.1265·2).
*Gastro-oesophageal reflux; peptic ulcer; Zollinger-Ellison syndrome.*

**Takadol** *Pharmascience, Fr.*
Tramadol hydrochloride (p.94·3).
*Pain.*

**Takata** *Madariaga, Spain.*
Senna (p.1288·2).
Formerly contained aloin, belladonna, and phenolphthalein.
*Constipation.*

**Takecef** *Sofar, Ital.*
Cefaclor (p.167·1).
*Bacterial infections.*

**Takepron**
*Takeda, Hong Kong; Takeda, Jpn.*
Lansoprazole (p.1269·3).
*Dyspepsia; gastro-oesophageal reflux; peptic ulcer; Zollinger-Ellison syndrome.*

**Takesulin** *Takeda, Jpn.*
Cefsulodin sodium (p.180·2).
Mepivacaine hydrochloride (p.1381·2) is included in the intramuscular injection to alleviate the pain of injection.
*Pseudomonal infections.*

**Taketiam** *Takeda, Fr.*
Cefotiam hexetil hydrochloride (p.177·2).
*Bacterial infections.*

**Takil** *Marjan, Braz.*
Tinidazole (p.617·1); tioconazole (p.409·3).
*Vaginal infections.*

**Taks**
*Codal Synto, Malaysia; Codal Synto, Thai.*
Diclofenac sodium (p.32·1).
*Inflammation; musculoskeletal and joint disorders.*

**Takus** *Pharmacia, Ger.*
Ceruletide tris(diethylamine) (p.1669·2).
*Diagnostic agent; paralytic ileus; postoperative atony.*

**Talacen** *Sanofi Winthrop, USA.*
Pentazocine hydrochloride (p.79·3); paracetamol (p.76·2).
*Pain.*

**Talam** *Arrow, Austral.*
Citalopram hydrobromide (p.289·1).
*Depression.*

**Talasa NF** *Andromaco, Arg.*
Butamirate citrate (p.1116·2).
*Coughs.*

**Talavir** *Sigma-Tau, Ital.*
Valaciclovir hydrochloride (p.656·1).
*Herpes zoster infections.*

**Talcid**
*Bayer, Austria; Bayer, Ger.; Bayer, Gr.; Bayer, Israel; Bayer, Mex.; Bayer, Spain.*
Hydrotalcite (p.1267·3).
*Gastrointestinal hyperacidity.*

**Talco Alivio** *Simoes, Braz.*
Purified talc (p.1159·1); starch (p.1449·1); zinc oxide (p.1163·2); salol (p.88·1); boric acid (p.1662·1); sulfur (p.1158·2); menthol (p.1711·3); camphor (p.1665·3); salicylic acid (p.1157·1).
*Pruritus.*

**Talco Antihistam Calber** *Pentafarm, Spain†.*
Calamine (p.1144·1); zinc oxide (p.1163·2); bismuth subnitrate (p.1252·2); kaolin; diphenhydramine hydrochloride (p.431·3); menthol (p.1711·3); talc (p.1159·1).
*Cutaneous hypersensitivity reactions.*

**Talerc** *Boehringer de Angeli, Braz.*
Epinastine hydrochloride (p.433·3).
*Hypersensitivity reactions.*

**Talflex** *Bago, Chile.*
Ketoprofen (p.51·2).
*Gout; inflammation; musculoskeletal, joint peri-articular, and soft-tissue disorders; pain.*

**Talidat**
*Merck, Austria; Merck, Ger.; Merck, Spain†.*
Hydrotalcite (p.1267·3).
*Gastrointestinal disorders associated with hyperacidity.*

**Talion** *Tanabe, Jpn.*
Bepotastine (p.425·3).
*Allergic rhinitis; allergic skin disorders.*

**Talizer** *Serral, Mex.*
Talomida.
*Adjunct in HIV infection; leprosy.*

**Talkosona** *Vita, Spain†.*
Benzalkonium chloride (p.1168·3); bismuth subnitrate (p.1252·2); dexamethasone (p.1097·1); talc; tannic acid (p.1751·2); zinc oxide (p.1163·2).
*Skin infections with inflammation.*

**Talofen** *Fournier, Ital.*
Promazine hydrochloride (p.717·3).
*Anxiety; pain; psychoses; vomiting.*

**Talofilina** *Novartis, Braz.*
Theophylline (p.798·3).
*Obstructive airways disease.*

**Talohexal** *Hexal, Austral.*
Citalopram hydrobromide (p.289·1).
*Depression.*

**Taloken** *Kendrick, Mex.*
Ceftazidime (p.180·2).
*Bacterial infections.*

**Talol** *Saval, Chile.*
Allopurinol (p.412·2).
*Gout; hyperuricaemia; renal calculi.*

**Talowin** *Costec, Arg.*
*Cream:* Aloe vera (p.1141·3); dexpanthenol (p.1727·2).
*Emollient.*

*Shampoo:* Chloroxylenol (p.1177·2).
*Dandruff; seborrhoea.*

**Taloxa**
*Aesca, Austria; Schering-Plough, Belg.; Schering-Plough, Fr.; Essex, Ger.; Schering-Plough, Ital.; Schering-Plough, Neth.; Schering-Plough, Norw.; Schering-Plough, Port.; Schering-Plough, Spain†; Schering-Plough, Swed.; Essex, Switz.*
Felbamate (p.361·1).
Formerly known as Taloxoral in *Norw.*
*Lennox-Gastaut syndrome.*

**Talpramin** *Psicofarma, Mex.*
Imipramine hydrochloride (p.300·1).
*Depression; nocturnal enuresis; parasomnias.*

**Talquis Cusi** *Synthelabo, Spain†.*
Diphenhydramine hydrochloride (p.431·3); zinc oxide (p.1163·2); talc (p.1159·1).
*Allergic skin disorders.*

**Talquissar** *Vita, Spain†.*
Bismuth subnitrate (p.1252·2); boric acid (p.1662·1); calamine (p.1144·1); talc (p.1159·1); tannic acid (p.1751·2).
*Skin disorders.*

**Talquistina** *Vita, Spain.*
Calamine (p.1144·1).
Formerly contained calamine and diphenhydramine hydrochloride.
*Insect bites; pruritus.*

**Talseclin** *Bristol-Myers Squibb, Chile.*
Tetracycline (p.266·2); amphotericin b (p.391·2).
*Fungal vulvovaginal infections; trichomoniasis.*

**Talso** *Sanofi Synthelabo, Ger.*
Saw palmetto (p.1569·1).
*Benign prostatic hyperplasia.*

**Talsutin**
*Bristol-Myers Squibb, Braz.; Bristol-Myers Squibb, Hong Kong; Bristol-Myers Squibb, Malaysia.*
Tetracycline hydrochloride (p.266·2); amphotericin B (p.391·2).
*Bacterial and fungal vaginal infections.*

**Taludon** *Sigma, Braz.*
Phenytoin (p.370·2); glutamic acid (p.1433·2).
*Epilepsy.*

**Talusin**
*Knoll, Austral.†; Knoll, Fin.†; Abbott, Ger.; Knoll, Switz.†.*
Proscillaridin (p.990·3).
*Heart failure.*

**Taluvian**
*Abbott, Ital.; Esteve, Spain.*
Apomorphine hydrochloride (p.1199·1).
*Erectile dysfunction.*

**Talval** *Lipha, Switz.*
Idrocilamide (p.1394·3).
*Musculoskeletal and joint disorders.*

**Talvosilen**
*Sigmapharm, Austria; Bene, Ger.; Milupa, Switz.*
Codeine phosphate (p.27·1); paracetamol (p.76·2).
*Pain.*

**Talwin**
*Abbott, Canad.; Sanofi Synthelabo, Canad.; Sanofi Winthrop, Israel; Abbott, Ital.; Abbott, Singapore†; Sanofi Synthelabo, Singapore†; Sanofi Winthrop, USA.*
Pentazocine hydrochloride (p.79·3) or pentazocine lactate (p.79·3).
*Adjunct to general anaesthesia; pain; premedication.*

**Talwin Compound** *Sanofi Winthrop, USA.*
Pentazocine hydrochloride (p.79·3); aspirin (p.15·1).
*Pain.*

**Talwin NX**
*Sanofi Winthrop, Israel; Sanofi Winthrop, USA.*
Pentazocine hydrochloride (p.79·3).
Naloxone hydrochloride (p.1044·3) is included in this preparation to discourage abuse.
*Pain.*

**Tam** *Alacan, Spain.*
Ciprofloxacin hydrochloride (p.188·2).
*Bacterial infections.*

**Tamagon**
*Medochemie, Hong Kong; Medochemie, Malaysia; Medochemie, Thai.†.*
Terfenadine (p.441·1).
*Hypersensitivity reactions.*

**Tamanybonsan** *Salushaus, Ger.†.*
Salix (p.87·3).
*Fever; headache; rheumatic disorders.*

**Tamaril** *Marjan, Braz.*
Senna (p.1288·2); tamarind (p.1293·2); cassia pulp (p.1255·2); liquorice (p.1270·2); coriander (p.1676·1).
*Constipation.*

**Tamarine**
*Note. This name is used for preparations of different composition.*
*GlaxoSmithKline, Arg.*
Tamarind (p.1293·2); anthraquinone glycosides.
*Constipation.*

*SmithKline Beecham, Belg.†; Barrenne, Braz.; Whitehall, Ital.; Whitehall-Robins, Switz.†.*
Tamarind (p.1293·2); cassia (p.1255·2); senna (p.1288·2); coriander (p.1676·1); liquorice (p.1270·2).
*Constipation.*

*Barrenne, Braz.*
*Capsules:* Tamarind (p.1293·2); cassia (p.1255·2); senna (p.1288·2); coriander (p.1676·1).
*Constipation.*

*GlaxoSmithKline, Chile.*
Senna (p.1288·2); tamarind (p.1293·2); prune (p.1285·1); apple.
*Constipation.*

*GlaxoSmithKline Sante, Fr.*
Tamarind (p.1293·2); senna (p.1288·2).
*Constipation.*

**Tamarix** *Hebron, Braz.*
Tamarind (p.1293·2); cassia pulp (p.1255·2); senna (p.1288·2); coriander (p.1676·1); liquorice (p.1270·2).
*Constipation.*

**Tamax** *Fresenius Kabi, Austria.*
Tamoxifen citrate (p.584·1).
*Breast cancer; endometrial cancer.*

**Tamaxin** *Orion, Swed.†.*
Tamoxifen citrate (p.584·1).
*Breast cancer.*

**Tambocor**
*3M, Austral.; 3M, Belg.; 3M, Canad.; 3M, Chile; 3M, Denm.; 3M, Fin.; 3M, Ger.; 3M, Hong Kong; 3M, Irl.; 3M, Israel; 3M, Malaysia; 3M, Mex.; 3M, Neth.; 3M, Norw.; 3M, NZ; 3M, S.Afr.; 3M, Singapore; 3M, Swed.; 3M, Switz.; 3M, Thai.; 3M, UK; 3M, USA.*
Flecainide acetate (p.916·2).
*Arrhythmias.*

**Tambocur** *3M, Arg.*
Flecainide acetate (p.916·2).
*Arrhythmias.*

**Tambutec** *Tecnofarma, Mex.*
Ethambutol (p.212·2).

**Tamec** *Ecosol, Switz.*
Tamoxifen citrate (p.584·1).
*Breast cancer.*

**Tameran** *Semar, Spain†.*
Famotidine (p.1265·2).
*Gastro-oesophageal reflux; peptic ulcer; Zollinger-Ellison syndrome.*

**Tametin** *Caber, Ital.†.*
Cimetidine (p.1255·3).
*Gastric hyperacidity; peptic ulcer; Zollinger-Ellison syndrome.*

**Tamexin** *Ratiopharm, Fin.*
Tamoxifen citrate (p.584·1).
*Breast cancer.*

**Tamifen** *Medochemie, Hong Kong.*
Tamoxifen citrate (p.584·1).
*Anovulatory infertility; breast cancer.*

**Tamiflu**
*Roche, Arg.; Roche, Austral.; Roche, Braz.; Roche, Canad.; Roche, Chile; Roche, Fr.; Roche, Hong Kong; Roche, Irl.; Roche, Israel; Chugai, Jpn; Roche, NZ; Roche, Port.; Roche, Singapore; Roche, Switz.; Roche, UK; Roche, USA.*
Oseltamivir phosphate (p.651·1).
*Influenza.*

**Tamigen** *Solfran, Mex.*
Gentamicin (p.219·1).
*Bacterial infections.*

**Tamik**
IPRAD, Fr.; Marcofina, Hong Kong.
Dihydroergotamine mesilate (p.465·3).
*Migraine; orthostatic hypotension; venous insufficiency.*

**Tamilan** Gador, Arg.
Magnesium pemoline (p.1591·3).
*Fatigue; mental function impairment.*

**Tamin** Merck Sharp & Dohme, Spain.
Famotidine (p.1265·2).
*Gastro-oesophageal reflux; peptic ulcer; Zollinger-Ellison syndrome.*

**Tamine SR** Geneva, USA†.
Phenylpropanolamine hydrochloride (p.1127·3); phenylephrine hydrochloride (p.1126·3); brompheniramine maleate (p.426·1).
*Upper respiratory-tract symptoms.*

**Tamisa** Eurofarma, Braz.
Ethinylestradiol (p.1553·2); gestodene (p.1556·1).
*Combined oral contraceptive.*

**Tamizam** Zambon, Belg.
Tamoxifen citrate (p.584·1).
*Breast cancer; endometrial cancer.*

**Tamobeta** Betapharm, Ger.†.
Tamoxifen citrate (p.584·1).
*Breast cancer.*

**Tamofen**
Hexal, Arg.; Schering, Austria; Aventis, Braz.†; Aventis, Canad.; Aventis, Denm.; Leiras, Fin.; Rhone-Poulenc Rorer, Ger.†; Douglas, Hong Kong†; Pharmacia, Irl.; Rhodia, Israel; Rhone-Poulenc Rorer, Mex.†; Leiras, Norw.†; Douglas, NZ; Leiras, Singapore; Douglas, Thai.; TTN, Thai.; Pharmacia, UK†.
Tamoxifen citrate (p.584·1).
*Anovulatory infertility; breast cancer; endometrial cancer.*

**Tamofene** Aventis, Fr.
Tamoxifen citrate (p.584·1).
*Breast cancer.*

**Tamokadin** Kade, Ger.
Tamoxifen citrate (p.584·1).
*Breast cancer.*

**Tamolan** Olan-Kemed, Thai.
Tramadol hydrochloride (p.94·3).
*Pain.*

**Tamolem** Laboratorios Chile, Chile.
Tamoxifen citrate (p.584·1).
*Breast cancer; endometrial cancer.*

**Tamone** Pharmacia Upjohn, Canad.†.
Tamoxifen citrate (p.584·1).
*Breast cancer.*

**Tamooex** BPL-Meizler, Braz.
Tamoxifen citrate (p.584·1).
*Breast cancer.*

**Tamopham** Phamos, Ger.
Tamoxifen citrate (p.584·1).
*Breast cancer.*

**Tamophar** Julphar, UAE.
Tamoxifen citrate (p.584·1).
*Anovulatory infertility; breast cancer.*

**Tamoplex**
Nycomed, Austria; Asta Oncologia, Braz.; Chemipharma, Gr.; Pharmachemie, Israel†; Pharmachemie, Malaysia; Pharmachemie, S.Afr.; Pharmachemie, Singapore†; Pharmachemie, Thai.; Teva, Thai.
Tamoxifen citrate (p.584·1).
*Breast cancer; endometrial cancer.*

**Tamosin** Sigma, Austral.
Tamoxifen citrate (p.584·1).
*Breast cancer.*

**Tamox**
Cristalia, Braz.; 1A, Ger.; ABZ, Ger.; Gry, Ger.; Alpharma-Isis, Ger.; Teva, Ger.; Rowex, Irl.
Tamoxifen citrate (p.584·1).
*Breast cancer; endometrial cancer.*

**Tamoxan**
Kener, Mex.†; Tecnimede, Port.
Tamoxifen citrate (p.584·1).

**Tamoxasta** Baxter Oncology, Ger.
Tamoxifen citrate (p.584·1).
*Breast cancer.*

**Tamoxen**
Douglas, Austral.; CTI, Israel.
Tamoxifen citrate (p.584·1).
*Breast cancer.*

**Tamoxene** Lisapharma, Ital.
Tamoxifen citrate (p.584·1).
*Breast cancer.*

**Tamoxi** Generics, Israel.
Tamoxifen citrate (p.584·1).
*Breast cancer.*

**Tamoxigenat** Azupharma, Ger.†.
Tamoxifen citrate (p.584·1).
*Breast cancer.*

**Tamoximerck** Merck dura, Ger.
Tamoxifen citrate (p.584·1).
*Breast cancer.*

**Tamoxin** Eurofarma, Braz.
Tamoxifen citrate (p.584·1).
*Breast cancer.*

**Tamoxis** Gautier, Arg.
Tamoxifen (p.585·3).
*Breast cancer; melanoma; ovarian cancer.*

**Tamoxistad** Stada, Ger.
Tamoxifen citrate (p.584·1).
*Breast cancer.*

**Tamper** Gap, Gr.
Cimetidine (p.1255·3).
*Conditions where gastric acid reduction is beneficial; gastric hypersecretion including Zollinger-Ellison syndrome; peptic ulcer.*

**Tampo** Nakorn, Thai.
Co-trimoxazole (p.199·3).
*Bacterial infections.*

**Tamposit N** Scheffler, Ger.
Lauromacrogol 400 (p.1412·3) zinc oxide (p.1163·2); bismuth subnitrate (p.1252·2).
*Anorectal disorders.*

**Tampositorien H** Scheffler, Ger.
Hamamelis (p.1696·3).
*Anorectal disorders.*

**Tampositorien mit Belladonna** Provita, Austria.
Belladonna (p.479·1); guaiazulene (p.1696·2); hamamelis (p.1696·3).
*Anorectal disorders.*

**Tampovagan** Co-Pharma, UK†.
Diethylstilbestrol (p.1548·1); lactic acid (p.1704·1).
*Postmenopausal vaginitis.*

**Tampovagan c Acid lact** Sanofi Synthelabo, Ger.†.
Lactic acid (p.1704·1).
*Vaginitis.*

**Tamyl** Ci & Di, Ital.
Propylene glycol cefatrizine (p.170·3).
*Bacterial infections.*

**Tan Express** Banana Boat, Canad.†.
*SPF 4:* Octinoxate (p.1154·3); octisalate (p.1154·3); oxybenzone (p.1154·3).
*Sunscreen.*

**Tanac**
Note. This name is used for preparations of different composition.
Del, Canad.; Del, USA.
*Topical gel:* Allantoin (p.1141·3); dyclonine hydrochloride (p.1376·2).
*Herpes labialis.*

Del, Canad.
*Topical liquid:* Benzocaine (p.1370·3); benzalkonium chloride (p.1168·3); tannic acid (p.1751·2).

Del, USA.
*Lipstick:* Benzocaine (p.1370·3); benzalkonium chloride (p.1168·3); tannic acid (p.1751·2).
*Sore lips.*
*Topical liquid:* Benzocaine (p.1370·3); benzalkonium chloride (p.1168·3).
*Mouth ulcers; sore gums.*

**Tanac Dual Core** Del, USA.
Benzocaine (p.1370·3); tannic acid (p.1751·2); allantoin (p.1141·3); benzalkonium chloride (p.1168·3); padimate O (p.1155·1).
*Oral lesions.*

**Tanacet**
Ashbury, Canad.; Herbal Laboratories, UK.
Feverfew (p.469·1).
*Migraine.*

**Tanadopa** Tanabe, Jpn.
Docarpamine (p.906·3).
*Heart failure.*

**Tanafed** Horizon, USA†.
Chlorphenamine tannate (p.428·1); pseudoephedrine tannate (p.1130·1).
*Upper respiratory-tract symptoms.*

**Tanafed DM** First Horizon, USA†.
Dextromethorphan tannate; chlorphenamine tannate (p.428·1); pseudoephedrine tannate (p.1130·1).
*Upper respiratory-tract disorders.*

**Tanafed DMX** First Horizon, USA.
Dextromethorphan tannate (p.1118·1); dexchlorpheniramine tannate (p.428·1); pseudoephedrine tannate (p.1130·1).
*Upper respiratory-tract disorders.*

**Tanafed DP** First Horizon, USA.
Pseudoephedrine tannate (p.1130·1); dexchlorpheniramine tannate (p.428·1).
*Upper respiratory-tract disorders.*

**Tanagel** Durban, Spain.
Belladonna (p.479·1); gelatin tannate (p.1751·3); opium (p.74·2).
*Colitis; diarrhoea; gastroenteritis.*

**Tanagel Papeles** Durban, Spain.
Gelatin tannate (p.1751·3).
*Diarrhoea.*

**Tanakan**
Phoenix, Arg.; Abbott, Braz.; Beaufour, Fr.; Beaufour-Ipsen, Hong Kong; Beaufour-Ipsen, Malaysia; Emerging Pharma, Malaysia; Knoll, Mex.; Beaufour-Ipsen, Singapore; Beaufour-Ipsen, Thai.
Ginkgo biloba (p.1692·3).
*Cerebral and peripheral vascular disorders; dizziness; tinnitus; vertigo.*

**Tanakene**
Ipsen, Spain; Intersan, Switz.
Ginkgo biloba (p.1692·3).
*Vascular disorders.*

**Tanalbina** Knoll, Port.†.
Albumin tannate (p.1248·1).
*Diarrhoea.*

**Tanalone** Labima, Belg.
Albumin tannate (p.1248·1); pectin (p.1580·3).
*Diarrhoea.*

**Tanasid** Pfizer Lambert, Spain.
Aluminium hydroxide (p.1249·2); sodium carbonate (p.1747·2).
*Gastrointestinal hyperacidity.*

**Tanatril**
Craveri, Arg.; Gerot, Austria; Algol, Fin.; Beaufour, Fr.; Hormosan, Ger.; Gerolimatos (Γερολυματος), Gr.; Tanabe, Hong Kong; Rottapharm, Ital.†; Tanabe, Jpn; Delta, Port.; Tanabe, Singapore; Tanabe, Thai.; Trinity, UK.
Imidapril hydrochloride (p.938·2).
*Hypertension.*

**Tanavat** Microsules, Arg.
Simvastatin (p.997·1).
*Hypercholesterolaemia.*

**Tancilina** Raymos, Arg.
Tetracycline (p.266·2).
*Bacterial infections.*

**Tandax** Novartis, Mex.
Naproxen sodium (p.65·1).
*Inflammation; pain.*

**Tandem Icon** Britpharm, UK†.
Pregnancy test (p.1734·3).

**Tandene** Bunker, Braz.
Carisoprodol (p.1392·1); diclofenac sodium (p.32·1); paracetamol (p.76·2); caffeine (p.782·1).
Formerly contained carisoprodol.
*Smooth muscle spasm.*

**Tanderalgin** Delta, Braz.
Carisoprodol (p.1392·1); caffeine (p.782·1); diclofenac sodium (p.32·1); paracetamol (p.76·2).

**Tanderil** Ciba Vision, Austria.
Oxyphenbutazone (p.76·1).
*Eye disorders.*

**Tanderon** Pharmaland, Thai.
Tolperisone hydrochloride (p.1396·3).
*Skeletal muscle spasm.*

**Tandial** Solfran, Mex.
Diazepam (p.690·1).

**Tandiur** Raymos, Arg.
Hydrochlorothiazide (p.933·2).

**Tandix** Azevedos, Port.
Indapamide (p.938·2).
*Hypertension.*

**Tandorene** Vitae, Mex.†.
Oxyphenbutazone (p.76·1).
*Inflammation; musculoskeletal and joint disorders.*

**Tandrex** Sintofarma, Braz.†.
Oxyphenbutazone (p.76·1).
Aluminium hydroxide (p.1249·2) and magnesium trisilicate (p.1272·3) are included in this preparation in an attempt to limit adverse effects on the gastrointestinal mucosa.
*Musculoskeletal and joint disorders.*

**Tandrex A** Sintofarma, Braz.†.
Oxyphenbutazone (p.76·1); paracetamol (p.76·2).
Aluminium hydroxide (p.1249·2) and magnesium trisilicate (p.1272·3) are included in this preparation in an attempt to limit adverse effects on the gastrointestinal mucosa.
*Musculoskeletal and joint disorders.*

**Tandrexin** Sintofarma, Braz.
Ampicillin (p.157·1).
*Bacterial infections.*

**Tandriflan** Uniao Quimica, Braz.
Paracetamol (p.76·2); carisoprodol (p.1392·1); diclofenac sodium (p.32·1); caffeine (p.782·1).

**Tandrilax** Ache, Braz.
Paracetamol (p.76·2); carisoprodol (p.1392·1); diclofenac sodium (p.32·1); caffeine (p.782·1).
*Skeletal muscle spasm.*

**Tanezox** Microsules, Arg.
Azithromycin (p.159·1).
*Bacterial infections.*

**Tanganil** Pierre Fabre, Fr.
Acetylleucine (p.1646·1).
*Vertigo.*

**Tangenol** Bucca, Spain.
Eugenol (p.1686·2); procaine hydrochloride (p.1383·2); tannic acid (p.1751·2).
*Dental disorders.*

**Tanidina** Robert, Spain.
Ranitidine hydrochloride (p.1285·2).
*Acid aspiration; gastro-oesophageal reflux; gastrointestinal hyperacidity; peptic ulcer; short-bowel syndrome; Zollinger-Ellison syndrome.*

**Tanizona** Offenbach, Mex.
Naproxen (p.65·1).
*Inflammation.*

**Tannacomp** Rentschler, Ger.
Albumin tannate (p.1248·1); ethacridine lactate (p.1165·3).
*Diarrhoea.*

**Tannalbin**
Medicopharm, Austria; Rentschler, Ger.; Knoll, Neth.
Albumin tannate (p.1248·1).
*Diarrhoea.*

**Tannic-12** Cypress, USA.
Pentoxyverine tannate (p.1126·3); chlorphenamine tannate (p.428·1).
*Coughs.*

**Tannidin Plus** GD, Ital.
Betacarotene (p.1422·3); selenium (p.1444·1); vitamin E (p.1464·3).
*Antoxidant.*

**Tannisol** GD, Ital.
Betacarotene (p.1422·3).
*Sunscreen.*

**Tannolact** Galderma, Ger.
Condensation product of urea-sodium cresolsulfonic acid.
*Hyperhidrosis; skin disorders.*

**Tannolil** Li-il, Ger.
Tannic acid (p.1751·2); aluminium sulfate (p.1653·1).
*Haemorrhoids; hyperhidrosis; skin irritation.*

**Tannopon** Orion, Fin.
Opium (p.74·2); belladonna (p.479·1); bismuth salicylate (p.1252·1); albumin tannate (p.1248·1).
*Diarrhoea.*

**Tannosynt**
Note. This name is used for preparations of different composition.
Hermal, Austria.
2,6-Bis-N' (2-hydroxy-3-sulfo (5-methyl-)benzyl)-ureidomethyl-phenol(ev. p-cresol) disodium.
*Skin disorders.*

Hermal, Ger.
Tannic acid (p.1751·2).
*Burns; hyperhidrosis; skin disorders.*

Hermal, Port.†.
Dimethyl urea; phenol (p.1188·1); sodium phenolsulfonate.
*Skin disorders.*

Boots Healthcare, Switz.
Phenol cresol sulfonic acid-formaldehyde condensation product.
Formerly contained tannic acid or sodium tannate.
*Skin disorders.*

**Tanoral** Parmed, USA.
Phenylephrine tannate (p.1127·2); chlorphenamine tannate (p.428·1); mepyramine tannate (p.437·1).
*Upper respiratory-tract symptoms.*

**Tanrix** GlaxoSmithKline, Ital.
An adsorbed tetanus vaccine (p.1640·3).
*Active immunisation.*

**Tanser** Ciclum, Spain.
Atenolol (p.865·2).
*Angina pectoris; arrhythmias; hypertension; myocardial infarction.*

**Tanston** Parke, Davis, Chile.
Mefenamic acid (p.55·2).
*Inflammation; pain.*

**Tantacol DM** Tanta, Canad.†.
Phenylpropanolamine hydrochloride (p.1127·3); pheniramine maleate (p.438·3); mepyramine maleate (p.437·1); dextromethorphan hydrobromide (p.1117·3).
*Cold symptoms; coughs.*

**Tantafed** Tanta, Canad.
Pseudoephedrine hydrochloride (p.1129·2).

**Tantaphen** Tanta, Canad.
Paracetamol (p.76·2).
*Fever; pain.*

**Tantapp** Tanta, Canad.†.
Phenylephrine hydrochloride (p.1126·3); phenylpropanolamine hydrochloride (p.1127·3); brompheniramine maleate (p.426·1).

**Tantol Skin Cleanser** Quatromed, S.Afr.†.
Triclosan (p.1195·2); phenonip; phenoxyethanol (p.1189·1).
*Skin disinfection.*

**Tantol Skin Lotion** Quatromed, S.Afr.†.
Soap substitute.

**Tantum**
Note. This name is used for preparations of different composition.
CSC, Austria; 3M, Canad.; Angelini, Ital.; Chefaro, Neth.†; Lepori, Port.; Farma Lepori, Spain.
Benzydamine hydrochloride (p.21·1).
*Gynaecological disorders; inflammation; mouth and throat disorders; pain; peri-articular and soft-tissue disorders; phlebitis; venous insufficiency.*

Farma Lepori, Spain.
*Throat spray:* Benzydamine hydrochloride (p.21·1); hexamidine di-isetionate (p.1181·3).
*Mouth and throat disorders.*

**Tantum Ciclina** Farma Lepori, Spain†.
Benzydamine hydrochloride (p.21·1); tetracycline hydrochloride (p.266·2).
*Acne; bacterial infections.*

**Tantum Rosa** Lepori, Port.
Benzydamine hydrochloride (p.21·1); trimethylcetylammonium toluenesulfonate.
*Vulvovaginal infections.*

**Tantum Verde**
Note. This name is used for preparations of different composition.
Solvay, Ger.; Lepori, Port.; Farma Lepori, Spain.
Benzydamine hydrochloride (p.21·1).
*Mouth and throat pain and inflammation.*

Lepori, Port.
*Pastilles:* Benzydamine hydrochloride (p.21·1); benzocaine (p.1370·3).
*Mouth and throat pain and inflammation.*

**Tantumar** CSC, Austria.
Benzydamine hydrochloride (p.21·1).
*Mouth and throat disorders; soft-tissue injury.*

**Tanvimil** Raymos, Arg.
A range of vitamin preparations with or without minerals (p.1417·1).

**Tanyl**
Taro, Israel; Intramed, S.Afr.†.
Fentanyl citrate (p.40·1).
*Adjunct to general anaesthesia; pain.*

**Tanzal** Iquinosa, Spain†.
Oxatomide (p.438·1).
*Hypersensitivity reactions.*

**TAO** Pfizer, USA.
Troleandomycin (p.274·1).
*Bacterial infections.*

**Tapal-2** *GlaxoSmithKline, Chile.*
Aspirin (p.15·1); caffeine (p.782·1); cinnamedrine hydrochloride (p.1672·2).
*Menstrual disorders.*

**Tapanol** *Republic, USA.*
Paracetamol (p.76·2).
*Fever; pain.*

**Tapazol**
*Lilly, Braz.; Lilly, Mex.*
Thiamazole (p.1603·3).
*Hyperthyroidism.*

**Tapazole**
*Paladin, Canad.; Lilly, Hong Kong†; Lilly, Israel; Lilly, Ital.; Disto, Switz.; Lilly, Thai.; Lilly, USA.*
Thiamazole (p.1603·3).
*Hyperthyroidism.*

**Taponoto** *Teofarma, Spain.*
Potassium carbonate.
*Removal of ear wax.*

**Taporin** *Galen, Mex.*
Cefotaxime sodium (p.175·3).
*Bacterial infections.*

**Taprodex** *Provit, Mex.*
Dexamethasone (p.1097·1).
*Corticosteroid.*

**Tapsin 2 Analgesico** *Maver, Chile.*
Paracetamol (p.76·2); caffeine (p.782·1).
*Fever; pain.*

**Tapsin Analgesico** *Maver, Chile.*
Paracetamol (p.76·2); caffeine (p.782·1).
*Fever; pain.*

**Tapsin Compuesto** *Maver, Chile.*
Paracetamol (p.76·2); noscapine hydrochloride (p.1125·3); caffeine (p.782·1); sodium ascorbate (p.1460·2).
*Cold and influenza symptoms.*

**Tapsin Compuesto con Clorfenamina** *Maver, Chile.*
Paracetamol (p.76·2); noscapine hydrochloride (p.1125·3); caffeine (p.782·1); sodium ascorbate (p.1460·2); chlorphenamine maleate (p.427·3).
*Cold and influenza symptoms.*

**Tapsin Compuesto Dia/Noche Plus** *Maver, Chile.*
Day sachet, paracetamol (p.76·2); noscapine hydrochloride (p.1125·3); caffeine (p.782·1); sodium ascorbate (p.1460·2); night sachet, paracetamol (p.76·2); noscapine hydrochloride (p.1125·3); caffeine (p.782·1); sodium ascorbate (p.1460·2); chlorphenamine maleate (p.427·3).
*Cold and influenza symptoms.*

**Tapsin Periodo Menstrual** *Maver, Chile.*
Paracetamol (p.76·2); pamabrom (p.978·2); mepyramine maleate (p.437·1).
*Menstrual disorders.*

**Tapsin sin Cafeina** *Maver, Chile.*
Paracetamol (p.76·2).
*Fever; pain.*

**Tapzol** *Rayere, Mex.†.*
Kaolin (p.1268·3); pectin (p.1580·3).
*Diarrhoea.*

**Tapzol con Neomicina** *Rayere, Mex.*
Kaolin (p.1268·3); pectin (p.1580·3); neomycin (p.235·1).
*Diarrhoea.*

**Taquicord** *Knoll, Braz.†.*
Amiodarone (p.859·2).
*Arrhythmias.*

**Tar Doak** *Trans Canaderm, Canad.†.*
Coal tar (p.1159·2).
*Skin disorders.*

**Tar Isdin Champu** *Isdin, Spain.*
Coal tar (p.1159·2).
*Scalp disorders.*

**Tar Isdin Plus** *Isdin, Spain.*
Coal tar (p.1159·2); salicylic acid (p.1157·1).
*Scalp disorders.*

**Tara** *Polipharm, Thai.*
Miconazole nitrate (p.405·3).
*Fungal skin, hair, and nail infections.*

**Tara Abfuhrsirup** *Disperga, Austria†.*
Senna (p.1288·2).
*Bowel evacuation; constipation; stool softener.*

**Taradyl** *Roche, Belg.*
Ketorolac trometamol (p.52·1).
*Pain.*

**Taraleon** *Zilly, Ger.*
Taraxacum (p.1751·3).
*Biliary-tract disorders; diuretic; dyspepsia; loss of appetite.*

**Taraphilic** *Medco, USA.*
Coal tar (p.1159·2).
*Skin disorders.*

**Tara-Plus** *Polipharm, Thai.*
Miconazole nitrate (p.405·3); triamcinolone acetonide (p.1110·2).
*Fungal skin and nail infections.*

**Tarassaco (Specie Composta)** *Dynacren, Ital.*
Taraxacum (p.1751·3); silymarin (p.1043·3); zedoary; peppermint leaf (p.1283·2); caraway (p.1667·2).
*Biliary disorders; herbal tea.*

**Taraten** *Polipharm, Thai.*
Clotrimazole (p.396·2).
*Fungal skin infections.*

**Taraxacum Compuesto** *Hochstetter, Chile.*
Homoeopathic preparation.

**Taraxacum Med Complex** *Dynamit, Austria.*
Homoeopathic preparation.

**Taraxin** *TO-Chemicals, Thai.*
Hydroxyzine hydrochloride (p.434·3).
*Allergic skin disorders; pruritus; sedative.*

**Tarband**
*Seton Scholl, Austral.; SSL, UK†.*
Coal tar (p.1159·2); zinc oxide (p.1163·2).
*Leg ulcers; medicated bandage; skin disorders.*

**Tardan** *Odan, Canad.*
Salicylic acid (p.1157·1); coal tar (p.1159·2).
*Seborrhoea.*

**Tardigal** *Lilly, Ger.*
Digitoxin (p.894·3).
*Heart failure.*

**Tardocillin** *Infectopharm, Ger.*
Benzathine benzylpenicillin (p.162·3).
Tolycaine hydrochloride (p.1385·3) is included in this preparation to alleviate the pain of injection.
*Long-term treatment of rheumatic fever.*

**Tardotol** *Orion, Denm.†.*
Carbamazepine (p.353·3).
*Alcohol withdrawal syndrome; diabetes insipidus; epilepsy; trigeminal neuralgia.*

**Tardyferon**
*Germania, Austria; Robapharm, Fr.; Robapharm, Switz.*
Ferrous sulfate (p.1428·2); mucoproteose.
Ascorbic acid (p.1460·2) may be included in this preparation to increase the absorption and availability of iron.
*Iron deficiency; iron-deficiency anaemia.*

*Pierre Fabre, Ger.; Pharmafabre (Φαρμαφαμπρ), Gr.; Knoll, Mex.†; Pierre Fabre, Port.; Pierre Fabre, Spain.*
Ferrous sulfate (p.1428·2).
Ascorbic acid (p.1460·2) may be included in this preparation to increase the absorption and availability of iron.
*Iron deficiency; iron-deficiency anaemia.*

**Tardyferon $B_9$**
*Robapharm, Fr.*
Ferrous sulfate (p.1428·2); folic acid (p.1429·1); mucoproteose.
Ascorbic acid (p.1460·2) is included in this preparation to increase the absorption and availability of iron.
*Iron and folic acid deficiency.*

*Pierre Fabre, Singapore.*
Ferrous sulfate (p.1428·2); folic acid (p.1429·1).
*Iron and folic acid deficiency.*

**Tardyferon-Fol**
*Germania, Austria.*
Ferrous sulfate (p.1428·2); folic acid (p.1429·1); mucoproteose.
*Folic acid deficiency; iron-deficiency anaemias.*

*Pierre Fabre, Ger.*
Ferrous sulfate (p.1428·2); folic acid (p.1429·1).
Ascorbic acid (p.1460·2) is included in this preparation to increase the absorption and availability of iron.
*Iron and folic acid deficiency; iron-deficiency anaemias.*

*Pierre Fabre, Port.*
Ferrous sulfate (p.1428·2); folic acid (p.1429·1).
*Iron and folic acid deficiency.*

**Tareg**
*Biosintetica, Braz.; Novartis, Chile; Novartis, Fr.; Novartis, Ital.; Helsinn, Port.*
Valsartan (p.1018·3).
*Hypertension.*

**Tareg-D** *Novartis, Chile.*
Valsartan (p.1018·3); hydrochlorothiazide (p.933·2).
*Hypertension.*

**Tarflex** *Stiefel, Braz.*
Coal tar (p.1159·2).
*Skin disorders.*

**Targel**
*Logos, Arg.; Odan, Canad.*
Coal tar (p.1159·2).
*Psoriasis; scalp disorders.*

**Targel SA** *Odan, Canad.*
Coal tar solution (p.1159·2); salicylic acid (p.1157·1).
*Psoriasis.*

**Target**
*Note. This name is used for preparations of different composition.*
*Wyeth Lederle, Austria; Lederle, Switz.†.*
Felbinac (p.39·1).
*Musculoskeletal, joint, peri-articular, and soft-tissue disorders.*

*Whitehall-Much, Ger.†.*
Felbinac iminobispropanol salt (p.39·1).
*Musculoskeletal, joint, and soft-tissue disorders.*

*Lisapharma, Hong Kong; Lisapharma, Ital.*
Atenolol (p.865·2); chlortalidone (p.882·3).
*Hypertension.*

**Targifor** *Aventis, Braz.*
Arginine aspartate (p.1421·1).
*Nutritional supplement.*

**Targifor C** *Aventis, Braz.*
Arginine aspartate (p.1421·1); ascorbic acid (p.1460·2).
*Nutritional supplement.*

**Targocid**
*Aventis, Arg.; Aventis, Austral.; Wyeth Lederle, Austria; Aventis, Belg.; Aventis, Braz.; Aventis, Denm.; Aventis, Fin.; Aventis, Fr.; Aventis, Ger.; Vianex (Βιανέξ), Gr.; Aventis, Hong Kong; Aventis, India; Aventis, Irl.; Aventis, Israel; Hoechst Marion Roussel, Jpn; Aventis, Malaysia; Aventis, Mex.; Aventis, Neth.; Aventis, Norw.; Aventis, NZ; Aventis, S.Afr.; Aventis, Singapore; Aventis, Spain; Aventis, Swed.; Aventis, Switz.; Aventis, Thai.; Aventis, UK.*
Teicoplanin (p.264·3).
*Gram-positive bacterial infections.*

**Targosid**
*Lepetit, Ital.; Aventis, Port.*
Teicoplanin (p.264·3).
*Gram-positive bacterial infections.*

**Targretin**
*Elan, Irl.; Ferrer, Spain; Elan, UK; Ligand, USA.*
Bexarotene (p.529·3).
*Cutaneous T-cell lymphoma.*

**Targus** *Abbott, Braz.*
Flurbiprofen (p.43·3).

**Tarisdin** *Isdin, Spain†.*
Coal tar (p.1159·2); salicylic acid (p.1157·1).
*Skin disorders.*

**Taritux** *Monot, Fr.†.*
Dextromethorphan hydrobromide (p.1117·3).
*Coughs.*

**Tarivid**
*Aventis, Austria; Aventis, Belg.; Aventis, Denm.; Aventis, Fin.; Aventis, Ger.; Daiichi, Hong Kong; Santen, Hong Kong; Aventis, India; Aventis, Irl.; Aventis, Israel Daiichi, Jpn; Santen, Jpn; Daiichi, Malaysia; Aventis, Neth.; Aventis, Norw.; Aventis, Port.; Aventis, S.Afr.; Daiichi, Singapore; Hoechst Marion Roussel, Spain†; Aventis, Swed.; Aventis, Switz.; Daiichi, Thai.; Aventis, UK.*
Ofloxacin (p.239·3) or ofloxacin hydrochloride (p.240·1).
*Bacterial infections.*

**Tarjen** *Samakeephaesaj, Thai.*
Diclofenac sodium (p.32·1).
*Musculoskeletal, joint, peri-articular, and soft-tissue disorders.*

**Tarjena** *Samakeephaesaj, Thai.*
Diclofenac sodium (p.32·1).
*Gout; musculoskeletal and joint disorders.*

**Tarka**
*Ebewe, Austria; Roche, Braz.†; Abbott, Denm.; Abbott, Fin.; Knoll, Fr.; Abbott, Ger.; Abbott, Ital.; Knoll, Mex.; Knoll, Neth.; Knoll, S.Afr.; Abbott, Spain; Abbott, Swed.; Knoll, Switz.; Abbott, UK; Abbott, USA.*
Trandolapril (p.1016·1); verapamil hydrochloride (p.1019·1).
*Hypertension.*

**Tarlene** *Medco, USA.*
Coal tar (p.1159·2); salicylic acid (p.1157·1).
*Seborrhoea.*

**Tarmed**
*Stiefel, Chile; Stiefel, Ger.; Stiefel, Gr.; Stiefel, Ital.†; Stiefel, Mex.; Stiefel, Port.; Stiefel, Spain.*
Coal tar (p.1159·2).
*Scalp disorders.*

**Taro Gel**
*Taro, Canad.*
Sterile lubricating jelly.

*Taro, Israel.*
Propylene glycol (p.1735·2); glycerol (p.1694·3).
*Lubricating gel.*

*AFT, NZ.*
Lubricating gel.

**Tarocidin** *Taro, Israel.*
Chloramphenicol (p.185·1); polymyxin B sulfate (p.245·1).
*Blepharitis; conjunctivitis.*

**Tarocidin D** *Taro, Israel.*
Chloramphenicol (p.185·1); polymyxin B sulfate (p.245·1); dexamethasone sodium phosphate (p.1097·2).
*Blepharitis; conjunctivitis.*

**Taroctyl** *Taro, Israel.*
Chlorpromazine hydrochloride (p.675·2).
*Psychiatric disorders; vomiting.*

**Tarocyn** *Taro, Israel†.*
Oxytetracycline hydrochloride (p.241·1); polymyxin B sulfate (p.245·1).
*Bacterial infections.*

**Tarodent** *Taro, Israel.*
Chlorhexidine gluconate (p.1173·2).
*Mouth disorders.*

**Tarodex** *Taro, Israel.*
Dextromethorphan hydrobromide (p.1117·3).
*Coughs.*

**Tarophed** *Taro, Israel.*
Pseudoephedrine hydrochloride (p.1129·2).
*Aural and nasal congestion.*

**Tarophenicol** *Taro, Israel†.*
Chloramphenicol (p.185·1).
*Blepharitis; conjunctivitis.*

**Taro-Sone** *Taro, Canad.*
Betamethasone dipropionate (p.1093·1).
*Skin disorders.*

**Tarseb** *Draxis, Canad.*
Tar (p.1159·3).

**Tarsum** *Summers, USA.*
Coal tar (p.1159·2); salicylic acid (p.1157·1).
*Seborrhoea.*

**Tartar Control Listerine** *Pfizer Consumer, UK.*
Zinc chloride (p.1469·2).
*Tooth tartar.*

**Tartephedreel** *Peithner, Austria.*
Homoeopathic preparation.

**Tartrina** *Mead Johnson, Mex.†.*
Dextromethorphan (p.1117·3).

**Tarvexol** *Labinca, Arg.*
Paclitaxel (p.577·3).
*Malignant neoplasms.*

**Tarytar** *Stiefel, Chile.*
Cade oil (p.1159·2); tar (p.1159·3); arachis oil (p.1656·1); coal tar (p.1159·2).
*Scalp disorders.*

**Tasakal** *Offenbach, Mex.*
Sodium dibunate (p.1130·2); guaifenesin (p.1122·1); homatropine methylbromide (p.483·2).
*Coughs.*

**Tasedan** *Hormona, Mex.*
Estazolam (p.697·3).
*Insomnia; premedication.*

**Tasep** *IPS, Spain.*
Cefazolin sodium (p.170·3).
*Bacterial infections.*

**Tasmaderm** *Gebro, Switz.*
Motretinide (p.1154·2).
*Acne.*

**Tasmar**
*Roche, Arg.; Roche, Austria; Roche, Braz.; Roche, Chile; Roche, Hong Kong; Roche, Mex.†; Roche, Norw.†; Roche, NZ; Roche, S.Afr.; Roche, Singapore†; Roche, Switz.; Roche, Thai.†; Roche, USA.*
Tolcapone (p.1216·1).
*Parkinsonism.*

**Tasty C** *Nutrition Care, Austral.†.*
Vitamin C (p.1460·2); vitamin E; betacarotene; rutoside; zinc amino-acid chelate (p.1417·1).
*Vitamin C deficiency.*

**Tatig** *Bioindustria, Ital.*
Sertraline hydrochloride (p.317·2).
*Depression; obsessive-compulsive disorder; panic disorder.*

**Tationil** *Roche, Ital.*
Glutathione sodium (p.1040·3).
*Alcohol or drug poisoning; ionising radiation trauma.*

**Tau Kit** *Isomed, Spain.*
Carbon-13 labelled urea (p.1667·3).
*Test for gastrointestinal Helicobacter pylori infection.*

**Taucor** *Sigma-Tau, Spain.*
Lovastatin (p.949·1).
*Atherosclerosis; hypercholesterolaemia.*

**Tauglicolo**
*SIT, Ital.*
Bromhexine hydrochloride (p.1115·3); sulfogaiacol (p.1131·1).
*Respiratory-tract congestion.*

*IBI, Thai.*
Bromhexine hydrochloride (p.1115·3); guaifenesin (p.1122·1).
*Respiratory-tract disorders associated with increased or viscous mucus.*

**Tauliz** *Aventis, Ital.*
Piretanide (p.983·3).
*Hypertension; oedema.*

**Tauma** *IMO, Ital.†.*
Salix (p.87·3); passion flower (p.1729·1); crataegus (p.1677·1).
*Insomnia.*

**Taural** *Roemmers, Arg.*
Ranitidine (p.1285·2) or ranitidine hydrochloride (p.1285·2).
*Gastritis; gastro-oesophageal reflux; peptic ulcer.*

**Taurargin** *Baldacci, Braz.*
Arginine; taurine; ditetraethylammonium phosphate (p.1417·1).
*Nutritional supplement.*

**Tauredon**
*Byk, Austria; Byk Tosse, Ger.; Byk Gulden, Ger.; Byk, Port.; Altana, Switz.*
Sodium aurothiomalate (p.88·2).
*Juvenile idiopathic arthritis; psoriatic arthritis; rheumatoid arthritis.*

**Tauro** *Teofarma, Ital.*
Tauroursodeoxycholic acid (p.1761·1).
*Gallstones.*

**Taurobetina** *Zambon, Spain.*
Adenosine phosphate dipotassium (p.1647·3); cyanocobalamin (p.1458·2); pyridoxine hydrochloride (p.1456·3); uridine phosphate (p.1760·3); taurine (p.1752·1).
*Neuromuscular metabolic disorders.*

**Taurolin**
*Chemomedica, Austria; Boehringer Ingelheim, Ger.; Geistlich, Switz.*
Taurolidine (p.264·2).
*Bacterial infections.*

**Taurovit** *Bruschettini, Ital.†.*
Mineral and vitamin preparation with taurine (p.1417·1).
*Nutritional supplement.*

**Tautoss** *Sigma-Tau, Spain.*
Levodropropizine (p.1119·3).
*Coughs.*

**Tauval** *Sigma-Tau, Spain†.*
Valerian (p.1762·2).
*Anxiety; insomnia.*

**Tauxolo** *SIT, Ital.*
Ambroxol hydrochloride (p.1114·3).
*Respiratory-tract congestion.*

**Tavanic**
*Aventis, Arg.; Hoechst Marion Roussel, Austria; Aventis, Belg.; Aventis, Braz.; Aventis, Chile; Aventis, Fin.; Aventis, Fr.; Aventis, Ger.; Hoechst Marion Roussel, Gr.; Aventis, India; Aventis, Irl.; Aventis, Isra-*

el; Aventis, Ital.; Aventis, Mex.; Aventis, Neth.; Aventis, Port.; Aventis, S.Afr.; Aventis, Spain; Aventis, Swed.; Aventis, Switz.; Aventis, UK.
Levofloxacin (p.225·3).
*Bacterial infections.*

**Tavan-SP 54** *Aventis, S.Afr.*
Pentosan polysulfate sodium (p.979·2).
*Hyperlipidaemias; thromboembolic disorders.*

**Tavegil**
*Novartis Consumer, Ger.; Novartis, Irl.†; Novartis Consumer, Ital.; Novartis Consumer, Neth.; Novartis Consumer, Spain; Novartis Consumer, UK.*
Clemastine fumarate (p.429·1).
*Hypersensitivity reactions; insect bites; pruritus; sunburn.*

**Tavegyl**
*Novartis, Austria; Novartis, Denm.; Novartis Consumer, Port.; Novartis Consumer, S.Afr.; Novartis, Swed.; Novartis Consumer, Switz.*
Clemastine fumarate (p.429·1).
*Hypersensitivity reactions; skin disorders.*

**Taver**
*Medochemie, Malaysia; Medochemie, Thai.*
Carbamazepine (p.353·3).
*Epilepsy; glossopharyngeal neuralgia; trigeminal neuralgia.*

**Tavidan** *Baldacci, Ital.*
Suleparoid (p.1009·1).
*Thrombosis prophylaxis.*

**Tavinex** *Hexa-Medinova, Arg.*
Tyrothricin (p.275·1); benzocaine (p.1370·3).
*Mouth and throat disorders.*

**Tavinex Expectorante** *Hexa-Medinova, Arg.*
Ambroxol hydrochloride (p.1114·3).
*Respiratory-tract disorders with viscous mucus.*

**Tavinex Expectotabs** *Hexa-Medinova, Arg.*
Ambroxol hydrochloride (p.1114·3).
*Respiratory-tract disorders with viscous mucus.*

**Tavipec**
*Montavit, Austria; Montavit, Thai.*
Spike lavender oil (p.1749·2).
*Respiratory-tract disorders.*

**Tavist**
*Novartis Consumer, Canad.†; Novartis, Mex.; Novartis Consumer, Port.; Novartis, USA†.*
Clemastine fumarate (p.429·1).
*Hypersensitivity reactions; pruritus.*

**Tavist Allergy** *Novartis, USA.*
Clemastine fumarate (p.429·1).
Formerly known as Tavist-1.
*Allergic rhinitis.*

**Tavist ND** *Novartis, USA.*
Loratadine (p.436·1).
*Allergic rhinitis; urticaria.*

**Tavist-D**
*Novartis Consumer, Canad.†; Novartis, Mex.; Novartis, USA†.*
Clemastine fumarate (p.429·1); phenylpropanolamine hydrochloride (p.1127·3).
*Allergic rhinitis; nasal congestion.*

**Tavolax** *Singer, Switz.†.*
Aloes (p.1248·2); belladonna (p.479·1); matricaria (p.1669·3); cascara (p.1255·1); senna (p.1288·2); bisacodyl (p.1251·3); docusate sodium (p.1262·2).
*Bowel evacuation; constipation.*

**Tavolax nouvelle formule** *Singer, Switz.*
Bisacodyl (p.1251·3).
*Bowel evacuation; constipation.*

**Tavonin**
*Flordis, Austral.; VSM, Neth.*
Ginkgo biloba (p.1692·3).
*Age-related mental function disorders; peripheral vascular disorders.*

**Tavor**
*Note. This name is used for preparations of different composition.*
*Tecnofarma, Chile.*
Fluconazole (p.398·1).
*Fungal infections.*

*Wyeth, Ger.; Wyeth, Gr.; Wyeth Lederle, Ital.*
Lorazepam (p.704·1).
*Anxiety disorders; premedication; psychoses; sleep disorders; status epilepticus.*

*Asofarma, Mex.*
Oxybutynin chloride (p.486·3).
*Neurogenic bladder.*

**Taxagon** *Elvetium, Arg.*
Trazodone hydrochloride (p.319·1).
*Depression.*

**Taxfeno** *Raffo, Arg.*
Tamoxifen (p.585·3).

**Taxifur** *Fustery, Mex.*
Ceftazidime (p.180·2).
*Bacterial infections.*

**Taxilan**
*Lundbeck, Ger.; Byk, Neth.†.*
Perazine dimalonate (p.713·3).
*Agitation; depression; mania; psychoses.*

**Taxocris** *Kampel Martian, Arg.*
Paclitaxel (p.577·3).
*Malignant neoplasms.*

**Taxodiol** *Tecnofarma, Chile.*
Paclitaxel (p.577·3).
*Ovarian cancer.*

**Taxofen** *Blausiegel, Braz.*
Tamoxifen (p.585·3).
*Breast cancer.*

**Taxol**
*Bristol-Myers Squibb, Arg.; Bristol-Myers Squibb, Austral.; Bristol-Myers Squibb, Austria; Bristol-Myers Squibb, Belg.; Bristol-Myers Squibb, Braz.; Bristol-Myers Squibb, Canad.; Bristol-Myers Squibb, Denm.; Bristol-Myers Squibb, Fin.; Bristol-Myers Squibb, Fr.; Bristol-Myers Squibb, Ger.; Bristol-Myers Squibb, Gr.; Bristol-Myers Squibb, Hong Kong; Bristol-Myers Squibb, Irl.; Bristol-Myers Squibb, Israel; Bristol-Myers Squibb, Ital.; Bristol-Myers Squibb, Jpn; Bristol-Myers Squibb, Malaysia; Bristol-Myers Squibb, Neth.; Bristol-Myers Squibb, Norw.; Bristol-Myers Squibb, NZ; Bristol-Myers Squibb, Port.; Bristol-Myers Squibb, S.Afr.; Bristol-Myers Squibb, Singapore; Bristol-Myers, Spain; Bristol-Myers Squibb, Swed.; Bristol-Myers Squibb, Switz.; Bristol-Myers Squibb, Thai.; Bristol-Myers Squibb, UK; Bristol-Myers Squibb Oncology, USA.*
Paclitaxel (p.577·3).
*AIDS-related Kaposi's sarcoma; breast cancer; non-small cell lung cancer; ovarian cancer.*

**Taxotere**
*Aventis, Arg.; Aventis, Austral.; Sanova, Austria; Aventis, Belg.; Aventis, Braz.; Aventis, Canad.; Aventis, Denm.; Aventis, Fin.; Aventis, Fr.; Aventis, Ger.; Rhone-Poulenc Rorer, Gr.; Aventis, Hong Kong; Aventis, Irl.; Aventis, Israel; Aventis, Ital.; Rhone-Poulenc Rorer, Jpn; Aventis, Malaysia; Aventis, Mex.; Aventis, Neth.; Aventis, Norw.; Aventis, NZ; Aventis, Port.; Aventis, S.Afr.; Aventis, Singapore; Aventis, Spain; Aventis, Swed.; Aventis, Switz.; Aventis, Thai.; Aventis, UK; Aventis, USA.*
Docetaxel (p.547·1).
*Breast cancer; non small-cell lung cancer; ovarian cancer.*

**Taxus**
*Note. This name is used for preparations of different composition.*
*Beta, Arg.*
Calcium carbonate (p.1254·2); colecalciferol (p.1461·3).
*Calcium and vitamin D deficiency; osteoporosis.*

*Tecnofarma, Chile; Asofarma, Mex.*
Tamoxifen citrate (p.584·1).
*Breast cancer; endometrial cancer; prostatic cancer.*

**Taxyl** *Solfran, Mex.*
Dexamethasone (p.1097·1).
*Corticosteroid.*

**Taycovit** *Elvetium, Arg.*
Paclitaxel (p.577·3).
*Breast cancer; ovarian cancer.*

**Tazac** *Lilly, Austral.*
Nizatidine (p.1277·2).
*Gastro-oesophageal reflux; peptic ulcer.*

**Tazepin** *Climax, Braz.*
Ranitidine hydrochloride (p.1285·2).
*Peptic ulcer.*

**Tazicef** *SmithKline Beecham, USA; Bristol-Myers Squibb, USA.*
Ceftazidime (p.180·2).
*Bacterial infections.*

**Tazidem** *Eurofarma, Braz.†.*
Ceftazidime (p.180·2).
*Bacterial infections.*

**Tazidime**
*Lilly, Canad.; Lilly, USA.*
Ceftazidime (p.180·2).
*Bacterial infections.*

**Taziken** *Kendrick, Mex.*
Terbutaline sulfate (p.797·2).
*Obstructive airways disease; premature labour.*

**Tazobac**
*Wyeth, Ger.; IRBI, Ital.†; Wyeth Lederle, Port.; Lederle, Switz.*
Piperacillin sodium (p.243·1); tazobactam sodium (p.264·3).
*Bacterial infections.*

**Tazocel** *Wyeth, Spain.*
Piperacillin sodium (p.243·1); tazobactam sodium (p.264·3).
*Bacterial infections.*

**Tazocilline** *Wyeth Lederle, Fr.*
Piperacillin sodium (p.243·1); tazobactam sodium (p.264·3).
*Bacterial infections.*

**Tazocin**
*Wyeth, Austral.; Wyeth Lederle, Belg.; Wyeth, Braz.; Wyeth-Ayerst, Canad.; Wyeth Lederle, Denm.; Wyeth Lederle, Fin.; Wyeth, Gr.; Wyeth, Hong Kong; Wyeth, Irl.; Lederle, Israel; Wyeth Lederle, Ital.; Wyeth, Malaysia; Wyeth, Mex.; Wyeth, Neth.; Wyeth Lederle, Norw.; Lederle, NZ; Wyeth, S.Afr.; Wyeth, Singapore; Wyeth Lederle, Swed.; Wyeth-Ayerst, Thai.; Wyeth, UK.*
Piperacillin sodium (p.243·1); tazobactam sodium (p.264·3).
Lidocaine hydrochloride (p.1377·3) is included in the intramuscular injection to alleviate the pain of injection.
*Bacterial infections.*

**Tazonam**
*Wyeth, Arg.; Wyeth Lederle, Austria; Wyeth, Chile.*
Piperacillin sodium (p.243·1); tazobactam sodium (p.264·3).
*Bacterial infections.*

**Tazorac**
*Allergan, Canad.; Allergan, USA.*
Tazarotene (p.1160·2).
*Acne; psoriasis.*

**Taztia** *Andrx, USA.*
Diltiazem hydrochloride (p.900·1).
*Hypertension.*

**Tazusin** *Efarmes, Spain.*
Terazosin hydrochloride (p.1010·3).
*Benign prostatic hyperplasia; hypertension.*

**T-BMP** *Seroyal, Canad.†.*
Vitamin $B_1$ and choline tartrate (p.1417·1).

**TBV** *Seroyal, Canad.†.*
Vitamin $B_1$, vitamin $B_3$, and magnesium (p.1417·1).

**3TC**
*GlaxoSmithKline, Arg.; GlaxoSmithKline, Austral.; GlaxoSmithKline, Canad.; GlaxoSmithKline, Hong Kong; GlaxoSmithKline, Malaysia; Glaxo Wellcome, Mex.; GlaxoSmithKline, NZ; GlaxoSmithKline, S.Afr.; GlaxoSmithKline, Switz.*
Lamivudine (p.648·2).
*HIV infection.*

**3TC Complex** *GlaxoSmithKline, Arg.*
Lamivudine (p.648·2); zidovudine (p.658·2).
*HIV infection.*

**3TC/Epivir** *GlaxoSmithKline, Chile.*
Lamivudine (p.648·2).
*HIV infection.*

**3TC/AZT** *Elea, Arg.*
Lamivudine (p.648·2); zidovudine (p.658·2).
*HIV infection.*

**TCK-21** *REM, Braz.†.*
Technetium-99m sodium oxidronate (p.1525·2).
*Diagnostic agent.*

**TCK 6** *REM, Braz.†.*
Pentetic acid (p.1050·1).
*Diagnostic agent.*

**TCK 18** *REM, Braz.†.*
Sodium fytate (p.1052·3).
*Diagnostic agent.*

**TCK 7 Angiocis** *REM, Braz.†.*
Sodium pyrophosphate.
*Diagnostic agent.*

**TCK-1 Hematocis** *REM, Braz.†.*
Potassium perrenate; sodium thiosulfate (p.1053·3).
*Diagnostic agent.*

**TCK-17 Nanocis** *REM, Braz.†.*
Renio sulfate.
*Diagnostic agent.*

**TCO** *Seroyal, Canad.†.*
Vitamin and mineral preparation (p.1417·1).

**TCP** *Pfizer Consumer, UK.*
*Cream:* Chloroxylenol (p.1177·2); triclosan (p.1195·2); halogenated phenols; phenol (p.1188·1); sodium salicylate (p.90·1).
*Minor skin disorders; skin disinfection.*

*Liquid:* Halogenated phenols; phenol (p.1188·1).
Formerly contained halogenated phenols, phenol, and sodium salicylate.
*Minor skin disorders; mouth ulcers; sore throat.*

*Lozenges:* Hexylresorcinol (p.1182·1).
*Sore throat.*

*Ointment:* Iodine (p.1598·1); phenol (p.1188·1); sodium salicylate (p.90·1); methyl salicylate (p.59·3); precipitated sulfur (p.1158·2); tannic acid (p.1751·2); camphor (p.1665·3); salicylic acid (p.1157·1).
*Haemorrhoids; minor skin disorders; pruritus.*

**TD** *GlaxoSmithKline, Spain.*
A diphtheria and tetanus vaccine (p.1613·1).
*Active immunisation.*

**TD Spray Iso Mack** *Mack, Illert., Ger.*
Isosorbide dinitrate (p.941·1).
*Ischaemic heart disease.*

**Td-Impfstoff** *Aventis Pasteur, Ger.*
An adsorbed diphtheria and tetanus vaccine (p.1613·1).
*Active immunisation of older children and adults.*

**Td-Polio** *Aventis Pasteur, Canad.*
An adsorbed diphtheria, tetanus, and inactivated poliomyelitis vaccine (p.1615·2).
*Active immunisation.*

**Td-pur**
*Grunenthal, Austria; Chiron Behring, Ger.*
An adsorbed diphtheria and tetanus vaccine (p.1613·1).
*Active immunisation of older children and adults.*

**Td-Rix** *GlaxoSmithKline, Ger.*
An adsorbed diphtheria and tetanus vaccine (p.1613·1).
*Active immunisation of older children and adults.*

**Td-Vaccinol** *Procter & Gamble, Ger.†.*
An adsorbed diphtheria and tetanus vaccine (p.1613·1).
*Active immunisation of older children and adults.*

**Td-Virelon** *Chiron Behring, Ger.*
A diphtheria, tetanus, and poliomyelitis vaccine (p.1615·2).
*Active immunisation.*

**Te Anatoxal**
*Kwizda, Austria; Berna, Hong Kong; Berna, Malaysia; Swiss Serum, Malaysia; Berna, NZ; Berna, Singapore; Berna, Thai.; Swiss Serum, Thai.; Berna, USA.*
An adsorbed tetanus vaccine (p.1640·3).
*Active immunisation.*

**Tea Test** *Asofarma, Arg.*
Pregnancy test (p.1734·3).

**Tea Tree & Witch Hazel Cream** *Lane, UK.*
Hamamelis (p.1696·3); eucalyptus oil (p.1686·2); methyl salicylate (p.59·3); camphor (p.1665·3); melaleuca oil (p.1710·2); zinc oxide (p.1163·2).
*Skin disorders.*

**Tealep** *Raffo, Arg.*
Finasteride (p.1554·2).
*Benign prostatic hyperplasia.*

**Tealine** *Arkopharma, Fr.*
Java tea (p.1702·3); green tea (p.1765·3).
*Slimming aid.*

**Teardrops**
*Novartis Ophthalmics, Austral.†; Novartis Ophthalmics, Canad.; Ciba Vision, NZ†.*
Polyvinyl alcohol (p.1581·1); povidone (p.1581·2).
*Dry eyes.*

**TearGard** *Lee, USA.*
Hyetellose (p.1579·2).
*Artificial tears.*

**Teargel**
*Novartis Ophthalmics, Arg.; Restan, S.Afr.*
Carbomer (p.1577·2).
*Dry eyes.*

**Tear-Gel** *Novartis Ophthalmics, Canad.*
Carbomer 940 (p.1577·2).
*Dry eyes.*

**Teargen** *Goldline, USA.*
Artificial tear solution.
*Dry eyes.*

**Tearisol** *Novartis Ophthalmics, USA.*
Hypromellose (p.1579·3).
*Dry eyes.*

**Tears Again** *Ocusoft, USA.*
*Eye drops:* Carmellose sodium (p.1577·3).
*Eye drops:* Polyvinyl alcohol (p.1581·1).
*Eye ointment:* White soft paraffin (p.1479·3); liquid paraffin (p.1479·1).
*Dry eyes.*

**Tears Again MC** *Ocusoft, USA.*
Hypromellose (p.1579·3).
*Dry eyes.*

**Tears Encore** *Dioptic, Canad.*
Polysorbate 80 (p.1415·2).
*Dry eyes.*

**Tears Humectante** *Alcon Cusi, Spain.*
Dextran 70 (p.746·2); hypromellose (p.1579·3).
*Dry eyes.*

**Tears Lubricante** *Alcon Cusi, Spain.*
Wool fat (p.1483·1); white soft paraffin (p.1479·3).
Formerly known as Tears Gel.
*Dry eyes.*

**Tears Natural** *Alkon (Αλκον), Gr.*
Dextran 70 (p.746·2); hypromellose (p.1579·3).
*Dry eyes.*

**Tears Naturale**
*Note. This name is used for preparations of different composition.*
*Alcon, Austral.; Alcon, Belg.; Alcon, Canad.; Alcon, Chile; Alcon, Irl.; Alcon, Israel; Alcon, Malaysia; Alcon, Norw.; Alcon, NZ; Alcon, Port.; Alcon, S.Afr.; Alcon, Singapore; Alcon, Swed.†; Alcon, Switz.; Alcon, Thai.; Alcon, UK; Alcon, USA.*
Dextran 70 (p.746·2); hypromellose (p.1579·3).
*Dry eyes.*

*Alcon, Austria.*
Carbomer 974P (p.1577·2).
*Dry eyes.*

*Alcon, Hong Kong.*
Duasorb water-soluble polymeric system.
*Dry eyes.*

**Tears Night & Day** *Ocusoft, USA†.*
Carmellose sodium (p.1577·3); povidone (p.1581·2).
*Dry eyes.*

**Tears Plus**
*Allergan, Austral.; Allergan, Canad.; Allergan, NZ; Allergan, S.Afr.; Allergan, Switz.; Allergan, USA.*
Polyvinyl alcohol (p.1581·1); povidone (p.1581·2).
*Dry eyes.*

**Tears Renewed** *Akorn, USA.*
*Eye drops:* Dextran 70 (p.746·2); hypromellose (p.1579·3).
*Eye ointment:* White soft paraffin (p.1479·3); light liquid paraffin (p.1479·1).
*Dry eyes.*

**Teatrois** *DB, Fr.*
Tiratricol (p.1604·3).
*Thyroid disorders.*

**Tebamide** *G & W, USA.*
Trimethobenzamide hydrochloride (p.442·2).
*Nausea and vomiting.*

**Tebasedan** *Windson, Braz.†.*
Dipyrone (p.35·3); homatropine methylbromide (p.483·2); papaverine hydrochloride (p.1728·1).
*Smooth muscle spasm.*

**Tebege-Tannin** *Fresenius Kabi, Austria†.*
Tannic acid (p.1751·2); acriflavinium chloride (p.1165·3).
*Anal fissures; burns; frostbite; infected skin disorders; sunburn; ulcers.*

**Tebertin** *Berenguer Infale, Spain†.*
Inosine (p.1701·2).
*Digitalis intoxication; heart failure; hepatitis; radiation toxicity.*

**tebesium** *Hefa, Ger.*
Isoniazid (p.222·2).
Pyridoxine hydrochloride (p.1456·3) is included in this preparation for the prophylaxis of peripheral neuropathy.
*Tuberculosis.*

**tebesium-s** *Hefa, Ger.*
Isoniazid (p.222·2).
*Tuberculosis.*

**Tebetane Composto** *Ferraz, Lynce, Port.†.*
Alanine (p.1421·1); glycine (p.1433·3); glutamic acid (p.1433·2); prunus arborea.

**Tebetane Compuesto** *Elfar, Spain.*
Alanine (p.1421·1); glycine (p.1433·3); glutamic acid (p.1433·2); pygeum africanum (p.1568·2).
*Prostatic disorders.*

**Tebezide** *Be-Tabs, S.Afr.†.*
Pyrazinamide (p.246·3).
*Tuberculosis.*

**Tebloc** *Lafare, Ital.*
Loperamide hydrochloride (p.1271·1).
*Diarrhoea.*

**Tebofortan** *Austroplant, Austria.*
Ginkgo biloba (p.1692·3).
*Cerebral and peripheral vascular disorders.*

**Tebofortin** *Schwabe, Switz.*
Ginkgo biloba (p.1692·3).
*Tonic.*

**Tebokan**
*Grunenthal, Chile; Beaufour-Ipsen, Singapore†; Emerging Pharma, Singapore†; Schwabe, Switz.*
Ginkgo biloba (p.1692·3).
*Cerebal and peripheral vascular disorders; intermittent claudication; mental function impairment.*

**Tebonin**
*Austroplant, Austria; Altana, Braz.; Schwabe, Ger.; Farmasa, Mex.*
Ginkgo biloba (p.1692·3).
*Cerebral and peripheral vascular disorders; intermittent claudication; mental function disorders; vestibular disorders.*

**Teboven** *Farmasa, Mex.*
Troxerutin (p.1688·3).
*Venous insufficiency.*

**Te-Br** *Provit, Mex.*
Tetracycline hydrochloride (p.266·2).
*Bacterial infections.*

**Tebraxin** *Bracco, Ital.*
Rufloxacin hydrochloride (p.254·3).
*Bacterial infections.*

**Tebrazid**
*Continental Pharma, Belg.; ICN, Canad.*
Pyrazinamide (p.246·3).
*Tuberculosis.*

**Teceeme** *Nutricia-Bago, Arg.*
Medium-chain triglycerides (p.1440·3).
*Nutritional supplement.*

**Tecelac** *Biotest, Ger.*
Antithymocyte globulin (p.1348·3).
*Cardiac transplant rejection.*

**Tecfazolina** *Bohm, Spain.*
Cefazolin sodium (p.170·3).
Lidocaine (p.1377·3) is included in this preparation to alleviate the pain of injection.
*Bacterial infections.*

**Tecfoline** *Tecnofarma, Mex.†.*
Folinic acid (p.1431·1).

**TechneScan DMSA** *Mallinckrodt, Braz.†.*
Technetium-99m dimercaptosuccinic acid (p.1525·2).
*Diagnostic agent.*

**TechneScan DTPA** *Mallinckrodt, Braz.†.*
Technetium-99m trisodium calcium pentetate (p.1525·2).
*Diagnostic agent.*

**TechneScan Enxofre** *Mallinckrodt, Braz.†.*
Technetium-99m sodium thiosulfate (p.1525·2).
*Diagnostic agent.*

**TechneScan HDP**
*Mallinckrodt, Braz.†; Tyco, Spain; Mallinckrodt, USA.*
Technetium-99m disodium oxidronate (p.1525·2).
*Bone scanning agent.*

**TechneScan MAA** *Mallinckrodt, Braz.†.*
Technetium-99m albumin (p.1525·2).
*Diagnostic agent.*

**TechneScan MAG3**
*BSM, Austria; Mallinckrodt, Braz.†; Byk Gulden, Ital.; Tyco, Spain.*
Technetium-99m betiatide (p.1525·2).
*Contrast medium for renal imaging.*

**TechneScan MDB** *Mallinckrodt, Braz.†.*
Technetium-99m medronate (p.1525·2).
*Diagnostic agent.*

**TechneScan PYP** *Mallinckrodt, Braz.†.*
Technetium-99m pyrophosphate (p.1525·2).
*Diagnostic agent.*

**TechneScan Q12** *Mallinckrodt, Braz.†.*
Technetium-99m furomine/trifosmin (p.1525·2).
*Diagnostic agent.*

**Techniques Anti-Dandruff** *Avon, Canad.*
Pyrithione zinc (p.1156·2).
*Scalp disorders.*

**Teclind** *Eurofarma, Braz.†.*
Lincomycin hydrochloride (p.226·2).
*Bacterial infections.*

**Tecnal** *Technilab, Canad.*
Butalbital (p.673·3); caffeine (p.782·1); aspirin (p.15·1).
*Pain; tension.*

**Tecnal C** *Technilab, Canad.*
Butalbital (p.673·3); caffeine (p.782·1); aspirin (p.15·1); codeine phosphate (p.27·1).
*Pain; tension.*

**Tecnemab K1** *Amersham, Spain†.*
Antimelanoma antibody.
*Diagnosis of melanoma.*

**Tecnid** *Ativus, Braz.*
Secnidazole (p.615·3).
*Bacterial infections; protozoal infections.*

**Tecnocarb** *Zodiac, Braz.*
Carboplatin (p.533·3).
*Malignant neoplasms.*

**Tecnocris** *Zodiac, Braz.*
Vincristine sulfate (p.592·2).
*Malignant neoplasms.*

**Tecnofen** *Columbia, Mex.†.*
Tamoxifen citrate (p.584·1).
*Breast cancer.*

**Tecnoflut** *Zodiac, Braz.*
Flutamide (p.556·2).
*Prostatic cancer.*

**Tecnolip** *Tecnifar, Port.*
Lovastatin (p.949·1).
*Atherosclerosis; hypercholesterolaemia.*

**Tecnomicina** *Zodiac, Braz.*
Bleomycin sulfate (p.530·2).
*Malignant neoplasms.*

**Tecnoplatin**
*Zodiac, Braz.; Columbia, Mex.†.*
Cisplatin (p.538·1).
*Malignant neoplasms.*

**Tecnosal** *Tecnifar, Port.*
Triflusal (p.1017·3).
*Thromboembolic disorders.*

**Tecnotax** *Zodiac, Braz.*
Tamoxifen citrate (p.584·1).
*Breast cancer.*

**Tecnotecan** *Zodiac, Braz.*
Irinotecan hydrochloride (p.564·1).
*Malignant neoplasms.*

**Tecnovorin** *Zodiac, Braz.*
Calcium folinate (p.1431·1).
*Adjunct to fluorouracil in colorectal cancer; antidote to folic acid antagonists; megaloblastic anaemias.*

**Teconam** *Asian Pharm, Thai.*
Tenoxicam (p.93·1).
*Gout; musculoskeletal and joint disorders.*

**Tecyn** *Jofrain, Mex.†.*
Tetracycline (p.266·2).
*Bacterial infections.*

**Teczem** *Hoechst Marion Roussel, USA.*
Enalapril maleate (p.909·2); diltiazem malate (p.901·3).
*Hypertension.*

**Teczol** *Hexal, Braz.†.*
Fluconazole (p.398·1).
*Fungal infections.*

**Teddy-C** *Community Pharmacy, Thai.*
Ascorbic acid (p.1460·2).
*Vitamin C deficiency.*

**Tedec Profer** *Tedec Meiji, Spain†.*
Ferritin (p.1427·2).
*Iron-deficiency anaemia.*

**Tedicumar** *Estedi, Spain.*
Warfarin sodium (p.1022·2).
*Thromboembolic disorders.*

**Tediprima** *Estedi, Spain.*
Trimethoprim (p.272·2).
*Genito-urinary infections.*

**Tedipulmo** *Estedi, Spain.*
Terbutaline sulfate (p.797·2).
*Obstructive airways disease.*

**Tedivax** *GlaxoSmithKline, Belg.*
An adsorbed diphtheria and tetanus vaccine (p.1613·1).
*Active immunisation.*

**Tedol** *Edol, Port.*
Ketoconazole (p.403·3).
*Fungal infections.*

**Tedral** *Parke, Davis, Canad.†.*
Theophylline (p.798·3); ephedrine hydrochloride (p.1120·1); phenobarbital (p.367·3).
*Bronchospasm.*

**Tedralan** *SERP, Mon.*
Theophylline (p.798·3).
*Obstructive airways disease.*

**Tedrigen** *Goldline, USA.*
Theophylline (p.798·3); ephedrine hydrochloride (p.1120·1); phenobarbital (p.367·3).
*Bronchospasm.*

**Teedex** *Rice Steele, Irl.*
Paracetamol (p.76·2); diphenhydramine hydrochloride (p.431·3).
*Fever; pain.*

**Teejel**
*Viatris, Belg.; Purdue, Canad.; SSL, Irl.; Rafa, Israel.*
Choline salicylate (p.26·2).
*Gum and mouth pain.*

**Teekanne Blasen- und Nierentee** *Teekanne, Austria.*
Equisetum (p.1684·1); birch leaf (p.1660·3); solidago virgaurea (p.1748·3); ononis (p.1723·3); peppermint leaf (p.1283·2).
*Urinary-tract disorders.*

**Teekanne Erkaltungstee** *Teekanne, Austria.*
Sambucus (p.1741·3); tilia (p.1756·2); thyme (p.1755·2).
*Cold symptoms.*

**Teekanne Herz- und Kreislauftee** *Teekanne, Austria.*
Crataegus (p.1677·1); rosemary (p.1740·2); fennel (p.1687·2); spearmint (p.1749·1).
*Cardiac disorders.*

**Teekanne Husten- und Brusttee** *Teekanne, Austria.*
Fennel (p.1687·2); aniseed (p.1655·2); wild thyme; sage leaf (p.1741·2); thyme (p.1755·2).
*Coughs.*

**Teekanne Leber- und Galletee** *Teekanne, Austria.*
Fennel (p.1687·2); Javanese turmeric (p.1759·3); chamomile (p.1669·3); taraxacum (p.1751·3).
*Liver and biliary disorders.*

**Teekanne Magen- und Darmtee** *Teekanne, Austria.*
Chamomile (p.1669·3); peppermint leaf (p.1283·2); cinnamon (p.1672·2); melissa (p.1711·1).
*Gastrointestinal disorders.*

**Teekanne Schlaf- und Nerventee** *Teekanne, Austria.*
Lavender (p.1705·1); peppermint leaf (p.1283·2); melissa (p.1711·1); valerian (p.1762·2).
*Sleep disorders.*

**Teen Derm** *Fouchard, Chile.*
Glycolic acid (p.1147·3).

**Teen Formula** *Avon, Canad.*
Multivitamin and mineral preparation (p.1417·1).

**Teen Vitamins** *Adams, Canad.†.*
Multivitamin and mineral preparation (p.1417·1).

**Teenstick** *Arkopharma, UK.*
Clove oil (p.1673·3); geranium oil (p.1692·2); palmarosa oil; melaleuca oil (p.1710·2); ylang ylang oil; Dixeol.
*Acne.*

**Teer-Linola-Fett** *Wolff, Ger.*
Coal tar (p.1159·2).
*Skin disorders.*

**Teerol** *Max Ritter, Switz.†.*
Coal tar (p.1159·2).
*Skin disorders.*

**Teerol-H** *Max Ritter, Switz.†.*
Coal tar (p.1159·2); allantoin (p.1141·3); triclosan (p.1195·2).
*Scalp disorders.*

**Teeth Tough** *Vitamed, Israel.*
Sodium fluoride (p.1444·3).
*Dental caries.*

**Teetha** *Nelson, UK.*
Homoeopathic preparation.
Formerly known as Teething Granules.

**Teething** *Hylands, Canad.*
Homoeopathic preparation.

**Teething Relief** *Brauer, Austral.†.*
Homoeopathic preparation.

**Tefaclor** *TO-Chemicals, Thai.*
Cefaclor (p.167·1).
*Bacterial infections.*

**Tefamin** *Recordati, Ital.*
Aminophylline (p.780·2) or theophylline (p.798·3).
*Asthma; bronchospasm.*

**Tefavinca** *Bohm, Spain.*
Vincamine (p.1764·2).
*Cerebral trauma; cerebrovascular disorders; circulatory disorders of the eye, ear, nose, and throat; vestibular disorders.*

**Tefilin** *Hermal, Ger.*
Tetracycline hydrochloride (p.266·2).
*Bacterial skin infections.*

**Tefizox** *Teva, Israel†.*
Ceftizoxime sodium (p.182·2).
*Bacterial infections.*

**Teflan** *Uniao Quimica, Braz.*
Tenoxicam (p.93·1).

**Tegagen** *3M, Arg.*
Calcium alginate (p.745·1).
*Ulcers; wounds.*

**Tegasorb**
*Note. This name is used for preparations of different composition.*
*Novartis, Arg.*
Hydrocolloid dressing.
*Burns; ulcers; wounds.*

*3M, Fr.†.*
Carmellose (p.1577·3).
*Burns; ulcers.*

**Tegeline** *Lab Francais du Fractionnement, Fr.*
A normal immunoglobulin (p.1627·2).
*Hypogammaglobulinaemia; idiopathic thrombocytopenic purpura; Kawasaki disease; passive immunisation; retinochoroiditis.*

**Tegens** *Inverni della Beffa, Ital.*
Myrtillus (p.1718·3).
*Capillary disorders.*

**Tegisec**
*Roussel, Port.†.*
Fenproporex (p.1588·3).

*Roussel, Spain†.*
Fenproporex hydrochloride (p.1588·3).
*Obesity.*

**Tegison** *Roche, USA†.*
Etretinate (p.1147·1).
*Psoriasis.*

**Tegopen** *Bristol, Canad.†.*
Cloxacillin sodium (p.198·2).
*Bacterial infections.*

**Tegra** *Hermes, Ger.†; Sanapharm, Ger.†.*
Garlic oil (p.1691·2).
*Hyperlipidaemias.*

**Tegreen** *Pharmanex, USA.*
Green tea (p.1765·3).
*Dietary supplement.*

**Tegretal**
*Novartis, Chile; Novartis, Ger.*
Carbamazepine (p.353·3).
*Alcohol withdrawal syndrome; bipolar disorder; diabetic neuropathy; epilepsy; multiple sclerosis; neuralgias.*

**Tegretard** *Cristalia, Braz.*
Carbamazepine (p.353·3).
*Alcohol withdrawal syndrome; epilepsy; neuralgias.*

**Tegretol**
*Novartis, Arg.; Novartis, Austral.; Novartis, Austria; Novartis, Belg.; Novartis, Braz.; Novartis, Canad.; Novartis, Denm.; Novartis, Fin.; Novartis, Fr.; Novartis, Gr.; Novartis, Hong Kong; Novartis, Irl.; Novartis, Israel; Novartis, Ital.; Novartis, Malaysia; Novartis, Mex.; Novartis, Neth.; Novartis, Norw.; Novartis, NZ; Novartis, Port.; Novartis, S.Afr.; Novartis, Singapore; Novartis, Spain; Novartis, Swed.; Novartis, Switz.; Novartis, Thai.; Novartis, UK; Novartis, USA.*
Carbamazepine (p.353·3).
*Alcohol withdrawal syndrome; bipolar disorder; diabetes insipidus; diabetic neuropathy; epilepsy; glossopharyngeal neuralgia; mania; trigeminal neuralgia.*

**Tegrex** *Neo Quimica, Braz.*
Carbamazepine (p.353·3).
*Epilepsy.*

**Tegrezin** *Cazi, Braz.*
Carbamazepine (p.353·3).
*Epilepsy.*

**Tegrin**
*Note. This name is used for preparations of different composition.*
*Block, Canad.†; Reedco, USA.*
Coal tar (p.1159·2).
*Skin and scalp disorders.*

*GlaxoSmithKline, Port.†.*
Allantoin (p.1141·3); coal tar (p.1159·2).
*Psoriasis.*

**Tegrin Medicated** *Block, USA†.*
Coal tar (p.1159·2).
*Skin disorders.*

**Tegrin-HC** *Block, USA.*
Hydrocortisone (p.1103·3).
*Skin disorders.*

**Tegrin-LT** *Block, USA†.*
Pyrethrins (p.1509·3); piperonyl butoxide (p.1509·2).

**Tegrital** *Novartis, India.*
Carbamazepine (p.353·3).
*Bipolar disorder; epilepsy; trigeminal neuralgia.*

**Tegunal** *CEPA, Spain†.*
Dimethicone (p.1482·1); benzethonium chloride (p.1169·2); talc (p.1159·1); zinc oxide (p.1163·2).
*Skin disorders.*

**Teguphen** *Lupin, India.*
Terfenadine (p.441·1); guaifenesin (p.1122·1); phenylephrine hydrochloride (p.1126·3).
*Coughs.*

**Teguran** *Tegur, Mex.†.*
Nitrofurantoin (p.237·2).

**Teicomid** *Hoechst Marion Roussel, Ital.†.*
Teicoplanin (p.264·3).
*Gram-positive bacterial infections.*

**Teicox** *Richmond, Arg.*
Teicoplanin (p.264·3).
*Bacterial infections.*

**Teiklonal** *Klonal, Arg.*
Teicoplanin (p.264·3).
*Bacterial infections.*

**Tejel** *Johnson & Johnson, Spain.*
Coal tar (p.1159·2).
*Scalp disorders.*

**Tejuntivo** *Iquinosa, Spain.*
Oxaceprol (p.1725·1).
*Musculoskeletal, joint, and peri-articular disorders; osteoporosis; soft-tissue injury.*

**Tekaval** *Asofarma, Arg.*
Valproate semisodium (p.380·1).
*Epilepsy.*

**Tekfema** *Rivero, Arg.*
Monobasic sodium phosphate (p.1230·3); dibasic sodium phosphate (p.1231·1).
*Bowel evacuation.*

**Teladar** *Dermol, USA.*
Betamethasone dipropionate (p.1093·1).
*Skin disorders.*

**Telament** *Restan, S.Afr.*
Simeticone (p.1289·2).
*Gripe; infant colic.*

**Telarix** *Help, Gr.*
Cetirizine hydrochloride (p.427·1).
*Allergic conjunctivitis; allergic rhinitis; pruritus.*

**Telaroid** *Cetus, Arg.*
Meloxicam (p.56·1).
*Inflammation.*

**Telbibur N** *Fatol, Ger.*
Cyanocobalamin (p.1458·2); nicotinamide (p.1441·2); pyridoxine hydrochloride (p.1456·3).
Lidocaine hydrochloride (p.1377·3) is included in this preparation to alleviate the pain of injection.
*Liver disorders.*

**Telbon** *Novartis, Braz.†.*
Sulfogaiacol (p.1131·1); chlorphenamine maleate (p.427·3).
*Respiratory-tract congestion.*

**Teldafen** *Hoechst Marion Roussel, Braz.†.*
Terfenadine (p.441·1); pseudoephedrine hydrochloride (p.1129·2).
*Allergic rhinitis.*

**Teldane**
*Aventis, Austral.†; Hoechst Marion Roussel, Braz.†; Marion Merrell, Fr.†; Hoechst Marion Roussel, Ger.†; Hoechst Marion Roussel, Hong Kong†; Aventis, Mex.*
Terfenadine (p.441·1).
*Hypersensitivity reactions; pruritic skin disorders.*

**Teldane D** *Aventis, Mex.*
Terfenadine (p.441·1); pseudoephedrine (p.1129·2).
*Allergic rhinitis.*

**Teldanex**
*Aventis, Denm.; Hoechst Marion Roussel, Fin.†; Aventis, Norw.; Aventis, Swed.*
Terfenadine (p.441·1).
*Allergic conjunctivitis; allergic rhinitis; allergic skin disorders.*

**Teldrin** *SmithKline Beecham Consumer, USA.*
Chlorphenamine maleate (p.427·3).
*Hypersensitivity reactions.*

**Telebar** *Guerbet, Braz.†.*
Barium sulfate (p.1061·1).
Dimeticone (p.1289·2) is included in this preparation to eliminate gas from the gastrointestinal tract before radiography.
*Contrast medium for gastrointestinal radiography.*

**Telebrix**
*Codali, Belg.; Mallinckrodt, Canad.; Guerbet, Denm.†; Guerbet, Israel.*
Meglumine ioxitalamate (p.1066·3) and/or sodium ioxitalamate (p.1066·3).
*Radiographic contrast medium.*

**Telebrix 12**
*Guerbet, Fr.; Guerbet, Neth.†; Guerbet, Port.; Guerbet, Switz.*
Sodium ioxitalamate (p.1066·3).
*Radiographic contrast medium.*

**Telebrix 30**
*Guerbet, Braz.†; Rider, Chile; Guerbet, Fr.; Guerbet, Ital.†; Guerbet, Neth.†; Guerbet, Port.; Guerbet, Switz.*
Meglumine ioxitalamate (p.1066·3).
*Radiographic contrast medium.*

**Telebrix 35**
*Guerbet, Braz.; Rider, Chile; Guerbet, Fr.; Guerbet, Port.; Guerbet, Switz.*
Meglumine ioxitalamate (p.1066·3); sodium ioxitalamate (p.1066·3).
*Radiographic contrast medium.*

**Telebrix 38**
*Temis, Arg.; Guerbet, Braz.†; Guerbet, Ital.†.*
Meglumine ioxitalamate (p.1066·3); sodium ioxitalamate (p.1066·3).
*Radiographic contrast medium.*

**Telebrix 350**
*Guerbet, Neth.†; Guerbet, Port.†.*
Meglumine ioxitalamate (p.1066·3); sodium ioxitalamate (p.1066·3).
*Radiographic contrast medium.*

**Telebrix Coronar** *Guerbet, Braz.†.*
Meglumine ioxitalamate (p.1066·3); sodium ioxitalamate (p.1066·3).
*Radiographic contrast medium.*

**Telebrix Coronario** *Temis, Arg.*
Meglumine ioxitalamate (p.1066·3); sodium ioxitalamate (p.1066·3).
*Radiographic contrast medium.*

**Telebrix Gastro**
*Codali, Belg.; Guerbet, Fr.; Guerbet, Ger.; R+N, Gr.; Guerbet, Israel; Guerbet, Neth.†; Guerbet, Port.; Guerbet, Switz.*
Meglumine ioxitalamate (p.1066·3).
*Contrast medium for gastrointestinal radiography.*

**Telebrix Hystero**
*Temis, Arg.; Codali, Belg.; Guerbet, Braz.; Guerbet, Fr.; R+N, Gr.; Guerbet, Port.*
Meglumine ioxitalamate (p.1066·3).
*Contrast medium for hysterosalpingography.*

**Telebrix N 180 and 300** *Guerbet, Ger.*
Meglumine ioxitalamate (p.1066·3).
*Contrast medium for urinary-tract radiography.*

**Telebrix Polyvidone** *Guerbet, Neth.†.*
Meglumine ioxitalamate (p.1066·3); povidone.
Formerly known as Vasurix-Polyvidone.
*Contrast medium for hysterosalpingography and urinary-tract radiography.*

**Telebrix TC** *Guerbet, Braz.†.*
Meglumine ioxitalamate (p.1066·3).
*Radiographic contrast medium.*

**Telen** *Yamanouchi, Ger.*
Tripotassium dicitratobismuthate (p.1252·2).
*Duodenal ulcer.*

**Telepaque**
*Nycomed, Austral.†; Sanofi Synthelabo, Braz.†; Sanofi Winthrop, Canad.†; Nycomed, USA.*
Iopanoic acid (p.1065·1).
*Contrast medium for cholecystography.*

**Telergon II** *Medicafarm, Ital.*
Royal jelly (p.1740·3).
*Nutritional supplement.*

**Telesol** *Ipsen, Spain†.*
Oxitriptan (p.311·1).
*Depression; epilepsy.*

**Tele-Stulln** *Stulln, Ger.*
Naphazoline hydrochloride (p.1124·3) or naphazoline nitrate (p.1124·3).
Formerly contained actinoquinol sodium and naphazoline nitrate.
*Blepharitis; conjunctivitis.*

**Telfast**
*Aventis, Austral.; Hoechst Marion Roussel, Austria; Aventis, Belg.; Aventis, Denm.; Aventis, Fin.; Aventis, Fr.; Aventis, Ger.; Procter & Gamble, Ger.; Aventis, Hong Kong; Aventis, Irl.; Aventis, Israel; Lepetit, Ital.; Hoechst Marion Roussel, Neth.; Aventis, Norw.; Aventis, NZ; Aventis, Port.; Aventis, S.Afr.; Aventis, Singapore; Aventis, Spain; Aventis, Swed.; Orion, Swed.; Aventis, Switz.; Aventis, Thai.; Aventis, UK.*
Fexofenadine hydrochloride (p.433·3).
*Allergic rhinitis; urticaria.*

**Telfast Decongestant**
*Aventis, Austral.; Aventis, NZ.*
Fexofenadine hydrochloride (p.433·3); pseudoephedrine hydrochloride (p.1129·2).
*Allergic rhinitis; nasal congestion.*

**Telfast-D** *Aventis, Hong Kong.*
Fexofenadine hydrochloride (p.433·3); pseudoephedrine hydrochloride (p.1129·2).
*Allergic rhinitis.*

**Telmitin** *Nakornpatana, Thai.*
Niclosamide (p.110·1).
*Cestode infections.*

**Telo Cypro** *Relax, Ital.*
Copper wire (p.1425·3).
*Headache; insomnia; muscle spasm; musculoskeletal and joint disorders; pain.*

**Telos** *Merckle, Ger.*
Lornoxicam (p.54·2).
*Musculoskeletal and joint disorders.*

**Telset** *Medipharm, Chile.*
Tioconazole (p.409·3).
*Fungal and Gram-positive bacterial skin infections.*

**Teltonal** *Biocur, Ger.*
Devil's claw root (p.28·2).
*Joint disorders.*

**Telugren** *Alpes Chemie, Chile.*
Clotrimazole (p.396·2).
*Fungal skin infections.*

**Telugren Plus** *Alpes Chemie, Chile.*
Clotrimazole (p.396·2); dexamethasone acetate (p.1097·1).
*Fungal and Gram-positive bacterial skin infections with inflammation.*

**Teluron** *Schering, Jpn.*
Terguride (p.1216·1).
*Galactorrhoea; hyperprolactinaemia; suppression of lactation.*

**Telus** *Elvetium, Arg.*
Ranitidine (p.1285·2).
*Peptic ulcer.*

**Telvodin** *Armstrong, Arg.*
Atenolol (p.865·2).
*Angina pectoris; arrhythmias; hypertension.*

**Temaco** *Nakornpatana, Thai.*
Theophylline (p.798·3).
*Obstructive airways disease.*

**Temador** *Sanico, Belg.†.*
Temazepam (p.723·2).
*Anxiety disorders; premedication; sleep disorders.*

**Temaze** *Alphapharm, Austral.*
Temazepam (p.723·2).
*Insomnia.*

**temazep** *CT, Ger.*
Temazepam (p.723·2).
*Sleep disorders.*

**Temazin Cold** *Trenier, USA†.*
Phenylpropanolamine hydrochloride (p.1127·3); chlorphenamine maleate (p.427·3).
*Upper respiratory-tract symptoms.*

**Temazine** *Pinewood, Irl.†.*
Temazepam (p.723·2).
*Insomnia.*

**Temesta**
*Wyeth Lederle, Austria; Wyeth Lederle, Belg.; Wyeth Lederle, Denm.; Wyeth Lederle, Fin.; Wyeth Lederle, Fr.; Wyeth, Neth.; Wyeth Lederle, Swed.; Wyeth, Switz.*
Lorazepam (p.704·1).
*Alcohol withdrawal syndrome; anxiety; insomnia; nausea and vomiting; premedication; status epilepticus.*

**Temetex** *Roche, Ital.*
Diflucortolone valerate (p.1099·3).
*Skin disorders.*

**Temgesic**
*Kirby, Arg.; Reckitt Benckiser, Austral.; Aesca, Austria; Schering-Plough, Belg.; Schering-Plough, Denm.; Schering-Plough, Fin.; Schering-Plough, Fr.; Essex, Ger.; Grunenthal, Ger.; Reckitt Benckiser, Hong Kong; Schering-Plough, Hong Kong; Reckitt Benckiser, Irl.; Schering-Plough, Ital.; Schering-Plough, Malaysia; Schering-Plough, Mex.; Schering-Plough, Neth.; Schering-Plough, Norw.; Reckitt Benckiser, NZ; Schering-Plough, S.Afr.; Schering-Plough, Singapore; Schering-Plough, Swed.; Essex, Switz.; Schering-Plough, Thai.; Schering-Plough, UK.*
Buprenorphine hydrochloride (p.21·3).
*Pain.*

*Schering-Plough, Braz.*
Buprenorphine (p.21·3) or buprenorphine hydrochloride (p.21·3).
*Pain.*

**Temgesic-nX** *Reckitt Benckiser, NZ†.*
Buprenorphine hydrochloride (p.21·3).
Naloxone hydrochloride (p.1044·3) is included in this preparation to discourage abuse.
*Pain.*

**Temic** *Uno, Ital.*
Cimetidine (p.1255·3).
*Gastric hyperacidity; gastro-oesophageal reflux; gastrointestinal haemorrhage; peptic ulcer; Zollinger-Ellison syndrome.*

**Temigran** *Teva, Israel.*
Ergotamine tartrate (p.467·2); chlorcyclizine (p.427·3); caffeine (p.782·1); codeine phosphate (p.27·1).
*Vascular headache.*

**Temodal**
*Essex, Arg.; Schering-Plough, Austral.; Schering-Plough, Austria; Schering-Plough, Belg.; Schering-Plough, Braz.; Schering, Canad.; Schering-Plough, Chile; Schering-Plough, Denm.; Schering-Plough, Fin.; Schering-Plough, Fr.; Essex, Ger.; Schering-Plough, Gr.; Schering-Plough, Hong Kong; Schering-Plough, Irl.; Schering-Plough, Israel; Schering-Plough, Ital.; Schering-Plough, Mex.; Schering-Plough, Neth.; Schering-Plough, Norw.; Schering-Plough, NZ; Schering-Plough, Port.†; Schering-Plough, Singapore; Schering-Plough, Spain; Schering-Plough, Swed.; Essex, Switz.; Schering-Plough, Thai.; Schering-Plough, UK.*
Temozolomide (p.587·1).
*Astrocytoma; glioblastoma multiforme; malignant glioma.*

**Temodar** *Schering, USA.*
Temozolomide (p.587·1).
*Anaplastic astrocytoma.*

**Temolan** *Olan-Kemed, Thai.†.*
Paracetamol (p.76·2).
Lidocaine hydrochloride (p.1377·3) is included in this preparation to alleviate the pain of injection.
*Fever; pain.*

**Temovate** *Glaxo Wellcome, USA.*
Clobetasol propionate (p.1095·2).
*Skin disorders.*

**Temoxol** *Schering-Plough, S.Afr.*
Temozolomide (p.587·1).
*Malignant glioma.*

**Temperal**
*Allen, Mex.; Diviser Aquilea, Spain.*
Paracetamol (p.76·2).
*Fever; pain.*

**Temperax** *Bago, Chile.*
Citalopram hydrobromide (p.289·1).
*Depression.*

**Tempil** *Temmler, Ger.*
Ibuprofen (p.45·3).
*Fever; pain.*

**Tempil N** *Temmler, Ger.*
Diphenylpyraline hydrochloride (p.432·3); metamfepramone hydrochloride (p.1714·1); aspirin (p.15·1).
*Cold symptoms.*

**Tempire** *Collins, Mex.*
Paracetamol (p.76·2).
*Fever; pain.*

**Templadol** *Master, Chile.*
Mefenamic acid (p.55·2).
*Pain.*

**Tempo** *Thompson, USA.*
Aluminium hydroxide (p.1249·2); magnesium hydroxide (p.1272·2); simeticone (p.1289·2); calcium carbonate (p.1254·2).
*Hyperacidity.*

**Tempofin** *Collins, Mex.*
Paracetamol (p.76·2).
*Pain.*

**Tempolax** *Hommel, Ger.*
Bisacodyl (p.1251·3).
*Bowel evacuation; constipation.*

**Tempo-Rinolo** *Aventis, Ital.*
Phenylpropanolamine hydrochloride (p.1127·3); chlorphenamine maleate (p.427·3).
*Nasal congestion.*

**Temporol** *Orion, Irl.*
Carbamazepine (p.353·3).
*Alcohol withdrawal syndrome; deafferentation pain; epilepsy; trigeminal neuralgia.*

**Temposil** *Wyeth-Ayerst, Canad.†.*
Calcium carbimide (p.1664·2).
*Alcoholism.*

**Tempra**
*Note. This name is used for preparations of different composition. Mead Johnson, Austral.†; Bristol-Myers Squibb, Belg.†; Mead Johnson Nutritionals, Canad.; Bristol-Myers Squibb, Mex.; Mead Johnson, Singapore†; Upsamedica, Spain†; Mead Johnson Nutritionals, Thai.; Mead Johnson Nutritionals, USA.*
Paracetamol (p.76·2).
*Fever; pain.*

*Bristol-Myers Squibb, Mex.*
*Injection:* Propacetamol hydrochloride (p.85·3).
*Fever; pain.*

**Tempra CD** *Bristol-Myers Squibb, Mex.*
Paracetamol (p.76·2); codeine phosphate (p.27·1).
*Pain.*

**Tempra MF** *Bristol-Myers Squibb, Mex.*
Paracetamol (p.76·2); caffeine (p.782·1).
*Fever; pain.*

**Temprin** *Continentales, Mex.†.*
Paracetamol (p.76·2).
*Fever; pain.*

**Temserin** *Vianex (Βιανεξ), Gr.*
Timolol maleate (p.1012·2).
*Glaucoma.*

**Temtabs** *Sigma, Austral.*
Temazepam (p.723·2).
*Insomnia.*

**Temzzard** *Pizzard, Mex.*
Paracetamol (p.76·2).
*Fever; pain.*

**Tenacid** *Sigma-Tau, Ital.*
Imipenem (p.221·1); cilastatin sodium (p.188·1).
Lidocaine hydrochloride (p.1377·3) is included in the intramuscular injection to alleviate the pain of injection.
*Bacterial infections.*

**Tenadin** *Opco, Denm.*
Terfenadine (p.441·1).
*Allergic conjunctivitis; allergic rhinitis; hay fever; urticaria.*

**Tenadren** *Wyeth, Braz.*
Propranolol hydrochloride (p.989·3); hydrochlorothiazide (p.933·2).
*Hypertension.*

**Tenadrin** *Hua, Thai.*
Diphenhydramine hydrochloride (p.431·3); ammonium chloride (p.1115·2); sodium citrate (p.1223·2); menthol (p.1711·3).
*Coughs; nasal congestion.*

**Tenag** *Marjan, Braz.*
Agnus castus (p.1649·1).

**Tenalgin** *Vida, Port.*
Tenoxicam (p.93·1).
*Gout; musculoskeletal, joint, and peri-articular disorders.*

**Tenalif** *Columbia, Mex.*
Oxeladin citrate (p.1126·1); ambroxol hydrochloride (p.1114·3).
*Respiratory-tract disorders with increased or viscous mucus.*

**Tenaron**
*Labinca, Arg.; Pharma Investi, Chile.*
Meloxicam (p.56·1).
*Inflammation; musculoskeletal, joint, peri-articular, and soft-tissue disorders; pain.*

**Tenat** *Helvepharm, Switz.†.*
Atenolol (p.865·2).
Now known as Atenolol Helvepharm.
*Angina pectoris; arrhythmias; hypertension; myocardial infarction.*

**Tenax** *Siam Bheasach, Thai.*
Tenoxicam (p.93·1).
*Gout; musculoskeletal, joint, and peri-articular disorders.*

**Tenben** *Galen, UK†.*
Atenolol (p.865·2); bendroflumethiazide (p.867·3).
*Hypertension.*

**Ten-Bloka** *Aspen, S.Afr.*
Atenolol (p.865·2).
*Angina pectoris; hypertension.*

**Tencef** *Tedec Meiji, Spain.*
Cefminox sodium (p.174·1).
*Bacterial infections.*

**Tencet** *Hauck, USA.*
Paracetamol (p.76·2); butalbital (p.673·3); caffeine (p.782·1).
Formerly known as G-1.
*Pain.*

**Tenchlor**
*Aspen, S.Afr.; Berk, UK.*
Atenolol (p.865·2); chlortalidone (p.882·3).
These ingredients can be described by the British Approved Name Co-tenidone.
*Hypertension.*

**Tencilan** *Finadiet, Arg.*
Dipotassium clorazepate (p.685·1).
*Anxiety.*

**Tencon** *International Ethical, USA.*
Paracetamol (p.76·2); butalbital (p.673·3).

**Tender Age** *Jamieson, Canad.†.*
Multivitamin preparation (p.1417·1).

**TenderWet** *IVF, Switz.*
Xanthan gum (p.1582·3).
*Wounds.*

**Tendolon** *Elpen (Ελπεν), Gr.*
Calcitonin (p.768·2).
*Hypercalcaemia; osteoporosis; Paget's disease of bone.*

**Tendrin** *Pisa, Mex.*
Ephedrine (p.1120·1).

**Tenelid** *Allergan-Frumtost, Braz.†.*
Guanabenz acetate (p.926·2).
*Hypertension.*

**Teneretic** *AstraZeneca, Ger.*
Atenolol (p.865·2); chlortalidone (p.882·3).
*Hypertension.*

**Tenex** *ESP, USA.*
Guanfacine hydrochloride (p.927·2).
*Hypertension.*

**Tenibex** *Lemery, Mex.*
Albendazole (p.101·2).

**Tenidon** *Gerard, Denm.*
Atenolol (p.865·2); chlortalidone (p.882·3).
*Hypertension.*

**Tenif**
*AstraZeneca, Belg.; AstraZeneca, UK.*
Atenolol (p.865·2); nifedipine (p.966·2).
*Angina pectoris; hypertension.*

**Teniken** *Kener, Mex.†.*
Praziquantel (p.112·2).

**Tenitran** *Pfizer, Ital.*
Tenitramine (p.1010·3).
*Angina pectoris; heart failure.*

**Teniverme** *Basi, Port.*
Flubendazole (p.105·2).

**Ten-K** *Summit, USA.*
Potassium chloride (p.1232·2).
*Hypokalaemia; potassium depletion.*

**Tenkafruse** *CP Pharmaceuticals, UK†.*
Furosemide (p.919·3).
*Hypercalcaemia; hypertension; oedema; oliguria.*

**Tenkdol** *Biotenk, Arg.*
Ketorolac trometamol (p.52·1).
*Pain.*

**Tenliv** *Ativus, Braz.*
Feverfew (p.469·1).
*Migraine.*

**Tenlol** *Amrad, Austral.†.*
Atenolol (p.865·2).
*Angina pectoris; arrhythmias; hypertension; myocardial infarction.*

**Teno** *BASF, Ger.†.*
Atenolol (p.865·2).
*Arrhythmias; hypertension; ischaemic heart disease.*

**Tenoblock** *Leiras, Fin.*
Atenolol (p.865·2).
*Angina pectoris; arrhythmias; hypertension; hyperthyroidism; myocardial infarction.*

**Tenocam**
*Eurofarma, Braz.; M & H, Thai.*
Tenoxicam (p.93·1).
*Gout; musculoskeletal and joint disorders.*

**Tenocard** *Klonal, Arg.*
Nimodipine (p.972·3).

**Tenoclor** *ICI, India.*
Atenolol (p.865·2); chlortalidone (p.882·3).
*Hypertension.*

**Tenocor** *Merck, Thai.*
Atenolol (p.865·2).
*Angina pectoris; arrhythmias; hypertension; myocardial infarction.*

**Tenofed** *Ipca, India.*
Atenolol (p.865·2); nifedipine (p.966·2).
*Angina pectoris; hypertension.*

**Tenolin** *Technilab, Canad.*
Atenolol (p.865·2).
*Angina pectoris; hypertension.*

**Tenolol**
*Ipca, India; IPCA, Singapore; Siam Bheasach, Thai.*
Atenolol (p.865·2).
*Angina pectoris; arrhythmias; hypertension; myocardial infarction.*

**Tenolone** *Lusofarmaco, Ital.*
Atenolol (p.865·2); chlortalidone (p.882·3).
*Hypertension.*

**Tenomax** *Boniscontro & Gazzone, Ital.*
Atenolol (p.865·2).
*Angina pectoris; arrhythmias; hypertension; myocardial infarction.*

**Tenon** *Biolab, Thai.†.*
Astemizole (p.424·2).
*Allergic conjunctivitis; allergic rhinitis; hypersensitivity reactions; pruritus; urticaria.*

**Tenopres** *Sidus, Arg.*
Losartan potassium (p.947·2).
*Hypertension.*

**Tenopres D** *Sidus, Arg.*
Losartan potassium (p.947·2); hydrochlorothiazide (p.933·2).
*Hypertension.*

**Tenoprin** *Ratiopharm, Fin.*
Atenolol (p.865·2).
*Angina pectoris; arrhythmias; hypertension; hyperthyroidism; myocardial infarction.*

**Tenopt** *Sigma, Austral.*
Timolol maleate (p.1012·2).
*Glaucoma; ocular hypertension.*

**Tenordate** *AstraZeneca, Fr.*
Nifedipine (p.966·2); atenolol (p.865·2).
*Hypertension.*

**Tenoret**
*AstraZeneca, Hong Kong; AstraZeneca, Irl.; AstraZeneca, Malaysia; AstraZeneca, NZ†; AstraZeneca, Singapore; AstraZeneca, Thai.; AstraZeneca, UK.*
Atenolol (p.865·2); chlortalidone (p.882·3).
These ingredients can be described by the British Approved Name Co-tenidone.
*Hypertension.*

**Tenoretic**
*AstraZeneca, Austria; AstraZeneca, Belg.; AstraZeneca, Braz.; AstraZeneca, Canad.; AstraZeneca, Chile; Pharmacia, Denm.; AstraZeneca, Fr.; AstraZeneca, Hong Kong; AstraZeneca, Irl.; AstraZeneca, Ital.; AstraZeneca, Malaysia; Zeneca, Mex.; Zeneca, Neth.; AstraZeneca, NZ†; AstraZeneca, Port.; Zeneca, S.Afr.; AstraZeneca, Singapore; AstraZeneca, Spain; AstraZeneca, Switz.; AstraZeneca, Thai.; AstraZeneca, UK; Zeneca, USA.*
Atenolol (p.865·2); chlortalidone (p.882·3).
These ingredients can be described by the British Approved Name Co-tenidone.
*Hypertension.*

**Tenoric** *Ipca, India.*
Atenolol (p.865·2); chlortalidone (p.882·3).
*Hypertension.*

**Tenormin**
*AstraZeneca, Austral.; AstraZeneca, Austria; AstraZeneca, Belg.; AstraZeneca, Canad.; AstraZeneca, Chile; Pharmacia, Denm.; AstraZeneca, Ger.; Cana, Gr.; AstraZeneca, Hong Kong; ICI, India; AstraZeneca, Irl.; AstraZeneca, Ital.; AstraZeneca, Malaysia; Zeneca, Mex.; Zeneca, Neth.; Pharmacia, Norw.; AstraZeneca, NZ†; AstraZeneca, Port.; AstraZeneca, S.Afr.; AstraZeneca, Singapore; AstraZeneca, Spain; Pharmacia, Swed.; AstraZeneca, Switz.; AstraZeneca, Thai.; AstraZeneca, UK; Zeneca, USA.*
Atenolol (p.865·2).
*Angina pectoris; arrhythmias; hypertension; hyperthyroidism; migraine; myocardial infarction.*

**Tenormine** *AstraZeneca, Fr.*
Atenolol (p.865·2).
*Angina pectoris; arrhythmias; hypertension; myocardial infarction.*

**Ten-O-Six** *Bonne Bell, Canad.†.*
Salicylic acid (p.1157·1).
*Acne.*

**Tenotec** *Ache, Braz.*
Tenoxicam (p.93·1).

**Tenovate** *GlaxoSmithKline, India.*
Clobetasol propionate (p.1095·2).
*Skin disorders.*

**Tenovate G** *GlaxoSmithKline, India.*
Clobetasol propionate (p.1095·2); gentamicin sulfate (p.217·1).
*Infected skin disorders.*

**Tenovate M** *GlaxoSmithKline, India.*
Clobetasol propionate (p.1095·2); miconazole nitrate (p.405·3).
*Infected skin disorders.*

**Tenox**
*Note. This name is used for preparations of different composition.*
*Orion, Fin.; Orion, Irl.*
Temazepam (p.723·2).
*Anxiety; insomnia; premedication.*

*Charoen, Thai.*
Tenoxicam (p.93·1).
*Gout; musculoskeletal, joint, and peri-articular disorders.*

**Tenoxen** *Biosintetica, Braz.*
Tenoxicam (p.93·1).
*Musculoskeletal, joint, and peri-articular disorders.*

**Tenoxil** *Olan-Kemed, Thai.*
Tenoxicam (p.93·1).
*Musculoskeletal, joint, and peri-articular disorders.*

**Tenoxol** *Pulitzer, Ital.*
Neltenexine (p.1125·2).
*Respiratory-tract disorders.*

**Tenpril** *Lisapharma, Ital.*
Captopril (p.879·2).
*Heart failure; hypertension; myocardial infarction.*

**Ten-Quat** *Esoform, Ital.*
Benzalkonium chloride (p.1168·3).
*Surface disinfection.*

**Tens** *Boehringer Ingelheim, Port.*
Lacidipine (p.944·2).
*Hypertension.*

**Tensadiur** *Savio, Ital.*
Benazepril hydrochloride (p.867·2); hydrochlorothiazide (p.933·2).
*Hypertension.*

**Tensaldin** *Delta, Braz.*
Caffeine (p.782·1); isometheptene hydrochloride (p.1702·1) or isometheptene mucate (p.1702·1); dipyrone (p.35·3).
*Migraine.*

**Tensaliv** *Neo Quimica, Braz.*
Amlodipine besilate (p.862·1).
*Hypertension.*

**Tensamon** *Instituto Sanitas, Chile.*
Cyclobenzaprine hydrochloride (p.1393·1).
*Musculoskeletal disorders.*

**Tensan** *Klinge, Austria.*
Nilvadipine (p.972·2).
*Hypertension.*

**Tensanil** *Savio, Ital.*
Benazepril hydrochloride (p.867·2).
*Heart failure; hypertension.*

**Tensazol** *Tecnifar, Port.*
Enalapril maleate (p.909·2).
*Heart failure; hypertension; ischaemic heart disease; myocardial infarction; unstable angina pectoris.*

**Tensiben** *Soria Natural, Spain.*
Olive oil (p.1723·2); crataegus (p.1677·1); betula alba (p.1660·3).
*Arrhythmias; hypertension.*

**Tensidol** *Kenyaku, Thai.*
Haloperidol (p.701·2).
*Anxiety; psychiatric disorders.*

**Tensig** *Sigma, Austral.*
Atenolol (p.865·2).
*Angina pectoris; arrhythmias; hypertension; myocardial infarction.*

**Tensikey** *Inkeysa, Spain.*
Lisinopril (p.946·3).
*Diabetic nephropathy; heart failure; hypertension; myocardial infarction.*

**Tensikey Complex** *Inkeysa, Spain.*
Lisinopril (p.946·3); hydrochlorothiazide (p.933·2).
*Hypertension.*

**Tensil** *Sintofarma, Braz.†.*
Chlordiazepoxide (p.674·2).
*Alcohol withdrawal syndrome; anxiety; tension headache; tremor.*

**Tensilon**
*ICN, Canad.†; Roche, S.Afr.†; ICN, USA.*
Edrophonium chloride (p.1490·3).
*Diagnosis of myasthenia gravis; reversal of competitive neuromuscular blockade.*

**Tensimin** *Unique, India.*
Atenolol (p.865·2).
*Hypertension.*

**Tensiocap** *Giscard, Arg.*
Pilocarpine (p.1494·3).

**Tensiocomplet** *Medea, Spain.*
Hydralazine hydrochloride (p.931·2); hydrochlorothiazide (p.933·2); reserpine (p.995·1).
*Hypertension.*

**Tensiomax** *Bago, Chile.*
Cyclobenzaprine hydrochloride (p.1393·1).
*Skeletal muscle spasm.*

**Tensiomin**
*Thiemann, Ger.; Egis, Hong Kong; Egis, Thai.*
Captopril (p.879·2).
*Heart failure; hypertension.*

**Tensiomin-Cor** *Thiemann, Ger.*
Captopril (p.879·2).
*Heart failure; hypertension.*

**Tensionorme** *Lisapharm, Fr.*
Bendroflumethiazide (p.867·3); reserpine (p.995·1).
*Hypertension.*

**Tensioval** *Sanval, Braz.*
Methyldopa (p.953·2).
*Hypertension.*

**Tensipine** *Genus, UK.*
Nifedipine (p.966·2).
*Angina pectoris; hypertension.*

**Tensiplex** *Francia, Ital.*
Vinburnine phosphate (p.1764·2).
*Cerebrovascular disorders; mental function impairment.*

**Tensispes** *Specifar (Σπεσιφαρ), Gr.*
Buspirone hydrochloride (p.672·2).
*Generalised anxiety.*

**Tensitruw** *Truw, Ger.†.*
Crataegus (p.1677·1).
*Cardiac disorders.*

**Tensium**
*Note. This name is used for preparations of different composition.*
*Baliarda, Arg.*
Alprazolam (p.668·3).
*Alcohol withdrawal syndrome; anxiety; mixed anxiety depressive states; panic attacks.*

*DDSA Pharmaceuticals, UK.*
Diazepam (p.690·1).
*Alcohol withdrawal syndrome; anxiety; epilepsy; insomnia; premedication; skeletal muscle spasm.*

**Tenso Stop** *Esteve, Spain.*
Fosinopril sodium (p.919·1).
*Heart failure; hypertension.*

**Tenso Stop Plus** *Esteve, Spain.*
Fosinopril sodium (p.919·1); hydrochlorothiazide (p.933·2).
*Hypertension.*

**Tensobon**
*Schwarz, Ger.; Upsamedica, Switz.†.*
Captopril (p.879·2).
*Diabetic nephropathy; heart failure; hypertension.*

**Tensobon comp**
*Schwarz, Ger.; Upsamedica, Switz.*
Captopril (p.879·2); hydrochlorothiazide (p.933·2).
*Heart failure; hypertension.*

**Tensocardil** *Esteve, Spain.*
Fosinopril sodium (p.919·1).
*Heart failure; hypertension.*

**Tensoderm** *Ferraz, Lynce, Port.†.*
Zinc oxide (p.1163·2); sulfur (p.1158·2); camphor (p.1665·3).
*Acne; seborrhoea.*

**Tensodin** *Ativus, Braz.*
Amlodipine besilate (p.862·1).
*Hypertension.*

**Tensodox** *Lafi, Chile.*
Cyclobenzaprine (p.1393·2).
*Skeletal muscle spasm.*

**Tensofar** *Pharma Investi, Chile.*
Nitrendipine (p.973·3).
*Hypertension.*

**Tensoflux** *Hennig, Ger.*
Bendroflumethiazide (p.867·3); amiloride hydrochloride (p.858·2).
*Ascites; hypertension; oedema; renal calculi.*

**Tensogard** *Bristol-Myers Squibb, Ital.*
Fosinopril sodium (p.919·1).
*Heart failure; hypertension.*

**Tensogradal** *Almirall, Spain.*
Nitrendipine (p.973·3).
*Hypertension.*

**Tensoliv** *Laboratorios Chile, Chile.*
Chlordiazepoxide (p.674·2); clidinium bromide (p.480·2).
*Irritable colon.*

**Tensolve** *Aspen, S.Afr.*
Paracetamol (p.76·2); diphenhydramine hydrochloride (p.431·3); codeine phosphate (p.27·1); caffeine (p.782·1).
*Pain.*

**Tensoprel**
*Rubio, Singapore; Rubio, Spain.*
Captopril (p.879·2).
*Diabetic nephropathy; heart failure; hypertension; myocardial infarction.*

**Tensopril**
*Note. This name is used for preparations of different composition.*
*Armstrong, Arg.; Merck Sharp & Dohme, Israel.*
Lisinopril (p.946·3).
*Heart failure; hypertension.*

*Ivax, Irl.; Irex, Port.; Ivax, UK.*
Captopril (p.879·2).
*Heart failure; hypertension.*

**Tensopril D** *Armstrong, Arg.*
Lisinopril (p.946·3); hydrochlorothiazide (p.933·2).
*Hypertension.*

**Tensopyn** *Parke-Med, S.Afr.†.*
Paracetamol (p.76·2); codeine phosphate (p.27·1); doxylamine succinate (p.432·3); caffeine (p.782·1).
*Pain and associated tension.*

**Tensostad** *Stada, Ger.*
Captopril (p.879·2).
*Heart failure; hypertension.*

**Tensotin** *Julphar, UAE.*
Atenolol (p.865·2).
*Angina pectoris; arrhythmias; hypertension.*

**Tensozide** *Bristol-Myers Squibb, Ital.*
Fosinopril sodium (p.919·1); hydrochlorothiazide (p.933·2).
*Hypertension.*

**Tenstaten** *Beaufour, Fr.*
Cicletanine hydrochloride (p.883·2).
*Hypertension.*

**Tenston** *Covan, S.Afr.*
*Sustained-release capsules; sustained-release tablets:* Paracetamol (p.76·2); caffeine (p.782·1); codeine phosphate (p.27·1); meprobamate (p.706·2).
*Fever; pain.*
*Syrup:* Promethazine hydrochloride (p.439·1); paracetamol (p.76·2); codeine phosphate (p.27·1).
*Fever; pain.*
*Tablets:* Aspirin (p.15·1); paracetamol (p.76·2); caffeine (p.782·1); codeine phosphate (p.27·1); meprobamate (p.706·2).
*Pain.*

**Tensulan** *Marjan, Braz.*
Vitamin preparation (p.1417·1).

**Tensuril** *Cristalia, Braz.*
Diazoxide (p.893·2).
*Hypertension; hypoglycaemia.*

**Tentrini**
*Nutricia, Austral.; Nutricia, Fr.; Nutricia, Irl.; Nutricia Clinical, UK.*
A range of preparations for enteral nutrition (p.1417·1).

**Tenualax** *Bago, Arg.*
Lactulose (p.1269·1).
*Constipation; gastrointestinal enteropathy; hepatic encephalopathy.*

**Tenuate**
*Aventis, Austral.; Aventis, Canad.; Aventis, USA.*
Diethylpropion hydrochloride (p.1587·1).
*Obesity.*

**Tenuate Dospan**
*Hoechst Marion Roussel, Belg.†; Bruno, Ital.†; Hoechst Marion Roussel, Mex.†; Aventis, NZ; Mer-National, S.Afr.*
Diethylpropion hydrochloride (p.1587·1).
*Obesity.*

**Tenuate Retard**
*Artegodan, Ger.†; Hoechst Marion Roussel, Switz.†.*
Diethylpropion hydrochloride (p.1587·1).
*Obesity.*

**Tenuatina** *Rottapharm, Spain†.*
Dihydroergotamine mesilate (p.465·3).
*Circulatory disorders; migraine; orthostatic hypotension.*

**Tenutex** *Recip, Swed.*
Disulfiram (p.1681·3); benzyl benzoate (p.1500·2).
*Pediculosis; scabies.*

**Tenvatil** *Drugtech, Chile.*
Trihexyphenidyl hydrochloride (p.490·2).
*Parkinsonism.*

**Tenzone** *Tocogino, Mex.†.*
Methyldopa (p.953·2).

**Teobid** *Vita, Ital.†.*
Theophylline (p.798·3).
*Asthma; bronchospasm.*

**Teoden** *Biosintetica, Braz.*
Salbutamol (p.791·3).
*Obstructive airways disease.*

**Teodosis** *Welt, Arg.*
Theophylline (p.798·3).
*Obstructive airways disease.*

**Teodrin** *Prodotti, Braz.†.*
Aminophylline (p.780·2); ephedrine (p.1120·1).
*Obstructive airways disease.*

**Teofylamin** *Medic, Denm.*
Aminophylline (p.780·2).
*Obstructive airways disease.*

**Teogrand** *Ahimsa, Arg.*
Ranitidine (p.1285·2).
*Peptic ulcer.*

**Teolixir** *Biogalenica, Spain.*
Theophylline (p.798·3).
*Heart failure; obstructive airways disease; paroxysmal dyspnoea.*

**Teolixir Compositum** *Biogalenica, Spain.*
Guaifenesin (p.1122·1); prednisolone (p.1108·1); theophylline (p.798·3).
*Obstructive airways disease.*

**Teolong**
*Abbott, Braz.; Knoll, Mex.*
Theophylline (p.798·3).
*Obstructive airways disease.*

**Teonibsa** *Inibsa, Port.*
Theophylline (p.798·3).
*Heart failure; obstructive airways disease; pulmonary oedema.*

**Teonim** *Mipharm, Ital.†.*
Nimesulide (p.67·1).
*Fever; inflammation; pain.*

**Teonova** *Corvi, Ital.†.*
Theophylline (p.798·3).
*Obstructive airways disease.*

**Teophyl** *IQB, Braz.*
Theophylline (p.798·3).
*Obstructive airways disease.*

**Teoptic**
*Ciba Vision, Irl.; Novartis, Neth.; Restan, S.Afr.; Novartis, UK.*
Carteolol hydrochloride (p.880·3).
*Glaucoma; ocular hypertension.*

**Teoremac** *Sanfer, Mex.*
Glucametacin (p.44·3).
*Inflammation; pain.*

**Teoremin** *Asta Medica, Braz.*
Glucametacin (p.44·3).
*Musculoskeletal and joint disorders.*

**Teosona** *Phoenix, Arg.*
Theophylline (p.798·3).
*Obstructive airways disease.*

**Teosona Sol** *Phoenix, Arg.*
Theophylline (p.798·3); theophylline monoethanolamine (p.804·3).
*Obstructive airways disease.*

**Teoston** *Ariston, Braz.*
Theophylline (p.798·3).
*Asthma; bronchodilator.*

**Teovent**
*Note. This name is used for preparations of different composition.*
*Pharmacia Upjohn, Norw.†; Recip, Swed.*
Choline theophyllinate (p.784·2).
*Obstructive airways disease.*

*Schering-Plough, Port.*
Theophylline (p.798·3).
*Asthma.*

**Teovit** *Inexfa, Spain†.*
Aceglutamide (p.1645·2); hydroxocobalamin acetate (p.1458·2); pyridoxine hydrochloride (p.1456·3); thiamine phosphate (p.1455·2).
*Vitamin B deficiency.*

**Tepam** *BASF, Ger.†.*
Tetrazepam (p.724·1).
*Skeletal muscle tension and spasticity.*

**Tepanil** *Norma (Νορμα), Gr.*
Nitrendipine (p.973·3).
*Hypertension.*

**Tepavil** *Almirall, Spain.*
Sulpiride (p.722·2).
*Anxiety; psychoses; vertigo.*

**Tepazepan** *Almirall, Spain.*
Diazepam (p.690·1); pyridoxine (p.1457·2); sulpiride (p.722·2).
*Anxiety; neurosis; psychoses; psychosomatic disorders.*

**Tepilta**
*Note. This name is used for preparations of different composition.*
*Wyeth Lederle, Austria; Wyeth, Spain†.*
Aluminium hydroxide (p.1249·2); magnesium hydroxide (p.1272·2); oxetacaine (p.1382·1).
*Dyspepsia; gastritis; gastro-oesophageal reflux; heartburn; hiatus hernia; peptic ulcer.*

*ICN, Ger.*
Aluminium hydroxide (p.1249·2); light magnesium carbonate (p.1272·1) or magnesium hydroxide (p.1272·2); oxetacaine (p.1382·1).
*Gastrointestinal disorders.*

**Tepox Cal** *Ciclum, Spain.*
Calcium pidolate (p.1226·1).
*Calcium deficiency.*

**Tequin**
*Bristol-Myers Squibb, Arg.; Bristol-Myers Squibb, Austral.; Bristol-Myers Squibb, Braz.; Bristol-Myers Squibb, Canad.; Bristol-Myers Squibb, Malaysia; Bristol-Myers Squibb, Mex.; Bristol-Myers Squibb, S.Afr.; Bristol-Myers Squibb, Singapore; Bristol-Myers Squibb, Thai.; Bristol-Myers Squibb, USA.*
Gatifloxacin (p.216·2).
*Bacterial infections.*

**Teraciton** *Ariston, Braz.*
Tetracycline (p.266·2).
*Bacterial infections.*

**Teraclox** *Fustery, Mex.*
Cefaclor (p.167·1).
*Bacterial infections.*

**Teradyl** *Hua, Thai.*
Codeine phosphate (p.27·1); promethazine hydrochloride (p.439·1).
*Coughs.*

**Terafluss** *Epiforma, Ital.*
Terazosin hydrochloride (p.1010·3).
*Benign prostatic hyperplasia; hypertension.*

**Teragran**
*Bristol-Myers Squibb, Chile.*
Multivitamin and iron preparation (p.1417·1).
*Dietary supplement in children.*

*Bristol-Myers Squibb, Mex.*
Vitamin and mineral preparation (p.1417·1).

**Teragran Junior** *Bristol-Myers Squibb, Braz.†.*
Multivitamin preparation (p.1417·1).

**Teragran M** *Bristol-Myers Squibb, Braz.*
Multivitamin and mineral preparation (p.1417·1).

**Terak** *Akorn, USA.*
Oxytetracycline hydrochloride (p.241·1); polymyxin B sulfate (p.245·1).
*Bacterial eye infections.*

**Teralithe** *Aventis, Fr.*
Lithium carbonate (p.301·1).
*Bipolar disorder; psychoses.*

**Teramic** *Andromaco, Chile.*
Itraconazole (p.401·3).
*Fungal infections.*

**Teranic** *Biolab, Thai.†.*
Terfenadine (p.441·1).
*Allergic conjunctivitis; allergic rhinitis; urticaria.*

**Terapova** *Fustery, Mex.*
Conjugated oestrogens (p.1543·2).
*Menopausal disorders; osteoporosis.*

**Teraprost** *Malesci, Ital.*
Terazosin hydrochloride (p.1010·3).
*Benign prostatic hyperplasia.*

**Terasep** *Fada, Arg.*
Cefotaxime (p.176·3).
*Bacterial infections.*

**Teraumon** *Smaller, Spain.*
Terazosin hydrochloride (p.1010·3).
*Benign prostatic hyperplasia; hypertension.*

**Terazol**
*Janssen-Ortho, Canad.; Janssen-Cilag, Denm.†; Janssen-Cilag, S.Afr.†; Janssen-Cilag, Swed.†; Ortho McNeil, USA.*
Terconazole (p.409·3).
*Vulvovaginal candidiasis.*

**Terbac** *Syntex, Mex.*
Ceftriaxone sodium (p.182·3).
Lidocaine (p.1377·3) is included in the intramuscular injection to alleviate the pain of injection.
*Bacterial infections.*

**Terbasmin** *Ern, Spain.*
Terbutaline sulfate (p.797·2).
*Obstructive airways disease.*

**Terbasmin Expectorante** *Ern, Spain.*
Guaifenesin (p.1122·1); terbutaline sulfate (p.797·2).
*Obstructive airways disease.*

**Terbolan** *Hoechst Marion Roussel, Braz.†.*
Furosemide (p.919·3); reserpine (p.995·1).
*Hypertension.*

**Terbosil** *Silom, Thai.*
Terbutaline sulfate (p.797·2); guaifenesin (p.1122·1).
*Coughs; obstructive airways disease.*

**Terbron**
*Biolab, Hong Kong; Biopharm, Hong Kong; Biolab, Malaysia; Biolab, Thai.*
Terbutaline sulfate (p.797·2).
*Obstructive airways disease.*

**Terbron Expectorant** *Biolab, Thai.*
Terbutaline sulfate (p.797·2); guaifenesin (p.1122·1).
*Obstructive airways disease.*

**Terbuken** *Kener, Mex.†.*
Terbutaline sulfate (p.797·2).

**Terbul** *Teofarma, Ger.*
Terbutaline sulfate (p.797·2).
*Obstructive airways disease.*

**Terbulin**
*Vitamed, Israel; IG, Malaysia; Medidata, Malaysia; Great Eastern, Thai.; Westmont, Thai.*
Terbutaline sulfate (p.797·2).
*Obstructive airways disease; premature labour.*

**Terbulin Expectorant** *Chinta, Thai.†.*
Terbutaline sulfate (p.797·2); guaifenesin (p.1122·1).
*Obstructive airways disease.*

**Terbuno** *Milano, Thai.*
Terbutaline sulfate (p.797·2).
*Obstructive airways disease.*

**Terbutastad** *Stada, Austria.*
Terbutaline sulfate (p.797·2).
*Obstructive airways disease.*

**Terbuturmant** *Dermapharm, Ger.*
Terbutaline sulfate (p.797·2).
*Obstructive airways disease.*

**Tercian**
*Aventis, Fr.; Vitoria, Port.*
Cyamemazine (p.689·2) or cyamemazine tartrate (p.689·2).
*Anxiety; depression; psychoses; withdrawal syndromes.*

**Terco-C** *Hua, Thai.*
Codeine phosphate (p.27·1); guaifenesin (p.1122·1); terpin hydrate (p.1131·1).
*Coughs.*

**Terco-D** *Hua, Thai.*
Dextromethorphan hydrobromide (p.1117·3); guaifenesin (p.1122·1); terpin hydrate (p.1131·1).
*Coughs.*

**Terden** *Shiwa, Thai.†.*
Terfenadine (p.441·1).
*Allergic skin disorders; hay fever; rhinitis; rhinoconjunctivitis.*

**Terdine** *Silom, Thai.†.*
Terfenadine (p.441·1).
*Allergic conjunctivitis; allergic rhinitis; allergic skin disorders; hay fever; urticaria.*

**Terekol** *Panalab, Arg.*
Terbinafine hydrochloride (p.408·2).
*Fungal skin, hair, and nail infections.*

**Terelit** *Farmasan, Ger.*
Doxycycline hyclate (p.206·2); ambroxol hydrochloride (p.1114·3).
*Respiratory-tract infections associated with increased or viscous mucus.*

**Terfadine** *Samakeephaesaj, Thai.†.*
Terfenadine (p.441·1).
*Allergic conjunctivitis; allergic rhinitis; allergic skin disorders.*

**Terfedura** *Merck dura, Ger.*
Terfenadine (p.441·1).
*Allergic conjunctivitis; allergic rhinitis; allergic skin disorders.*

**Terfegen** *General Drugs, Thai.†.*
Terfenadine (p.441·1).
*Allergic rhinitis; allergic skin disorders.*

**Terfemax** *Temis, Arg.*
Terfenadine (p.441·1).
*Hypersensitivity reactions.*

**Terfemundin** *Mundipharma, Ger.*
Terfenadine (p.441·1).
*Allergic conjunctivitis; allergic rhinitis; allergic skin disorders.*

**Terfen** *Siam Bheasach, Thai.†.*
Terfenadine (p.441·1).
*Allergic conjunctivitis; allergic rhinitis; urticaria.*

**Terfenadina DG** *Phoenix, Arg.*
Terfenadine (p.441·1); pseudoephedrine hydrochloride (p.1129·2).
*Allergic rhinitis; otitis media; sinusitis.*

**Terfenor** *Norton, S.Afr.†.*
Terfenadine (p.441·1).
*Allergic rhinitis; allergic skin disorders.*

**Terfenor Antihistamine** *Norton, UK†.*
Terfenadine (p.441·1).
*Allergic rhinitis; allergic skin disorders.*

**Terfex** *Gynopharm, Chile.*
Terbinafine hydrochloride (p.408·2).
*Fungal infections.*

**Terfin** *Pharmacodane, Denm.*
Terfenadine (p.441·1).
*Allergic conjunctivitis; allergic rhinitis; hay fever; urticaria.*

**Terfium** *Hexal, Ger.†.*
Terfenadine (p.441·1).
*Hypersensitivity reactions.*

**Terfluzine**
*ICN, Canad.†; Aventis, Fr.†; Rhone-Poulenc Rorer, Israel†; Rhone-Poulenc Rorer, Neth.†.*
Trifluoperazine hydrochloride (p.726·3).
*Agitation; psychoses.*

**Tergil** *MM, India.*
Terbutaline sulfate (p.797·2); guaifenesin (p.1122·1).
*Obstructive airways disease.*

**Tergil-T** *MM, India.*
Terbutaline sulfate (p.797·2); theophylline (p.798·3).
*Obstructive airways disease.*

**Tergynan** *Bouchara, Fr.†.*
Ternidazole (p.616·3); neomycin sulfate (p.235·1); nystatin (p.406·3); prednisolone metasulfobenzoate sodium (p.1108·1).
*Vaginitis.*

**Tericin AT** *Ativus, Braz.*
Tetracycline hydrochloride (p.266·2); amphotericin B (p.391·2).
*Bacterial and fungal vulvovaginal infections.*

**Teril**
*Alphapharm, Austral.; Alphapharm, Hong Kong; Taro, Israel; Pacific, NZ; Taro, UK; Taro, USA.*
Carbamazepine (p.353·3).
*Bipolar disorder; diabetes insipidus; epilepsy; trigeminal neuralgia.*

**Terivalidin** *Gerot, Austria.*
Terizidone (p.266·2).
*Bacterial infections.*

**Terlane** *Mundipharma, Austria†.*
Terfenadine (p.441·1).
*Hypersensitivity reactions.*

**Terloc**
*Armstrong, Arg.*
Amlodipine besilate (p.862·1).
*Angina pectoris; hypertension.*

*Laboratorios Chile, Chile.*
Amlodipine (p.862·2).
*Angina pectoris; hypertension.*

**Terloc Duo** *Armstrong, Arg.*
Amlodipine besilate (p.862·1); benazepril (p.867·2).
*Hypertension.*

**Terlomexin** *Effik, Fr.*
Fenticonazole nitrate (p.397·3).
*Candidiasis.*

**Termalgin**
*Novartis, Spain; Novartis Consumer, Switz.†.*
Paracetamol (p.76·2).
*Fever; pain.*

**Termalgin Codeina** *Novartis, Spain.*
Codeine phosphate (p.27·1); paracetamol (p.76·2).
*Pain.*

**Termizol** *Fustery, Mex.*
Ketoconazole (p.403·3).
*Fungal infections.*

**Termofren** *Roemmers, Arg.*
Paracetamol (p.76·2).
*Fever; pain.*

**Termogripe C** *Luper, Braz.*
*Syrup:* Chlorphenamine maleate (p.427·3); caffeine (p.782·1); salicylamide (p.87·3); ascorbic acid (p.1460·2).
*Tablets:* Green tablets, chlorphenamine maleate (p.427·3); caffeine (p.782·1); salicylamide (p.87·3); yellow tablets, ascorbic acid (p.1460·2).
*Cold and influenza symptoms.*

**Termol** *Uniao Quimica, Braz.*
Paracetamol (p.76·2).
*Fever; pain.*

**Termonal** *Sanval, Braz.*
Dipyrone (p.35·3).
*Fever; pain.*

**Termonil** *Liferpal, Mex.*
Dipyrone (p.35·3).
*Fever; pain.*

**Termo-Ped** *Stiefel, Braz.*
Paracetamol (p.76·2).
*Fever; pain.*

**Termoprin** *Cazi, Braz.*
Dipyrone (p.35·3).
*Fever; pain.*

**Termopriona** *Neo Quimica, Braz.*
Dipyrone (p.35·3).
*Fever; pain.*

**Termosan** *Dom, Spain.*
Camphor (p.1665·3); methyl salicylate (p.59·3); salicylic acid (p.1157·1); turpentine oil (p.1760·1); menthol (p.1711·3); lavender oil (p.1705·2); thyme oil (p.1755·3); eucalyptus oil (p.1686·2).
Formerly contained camphor, capsicum oleoresin, methyl salicylate, salicylic acid, turpentine oil, menthol, lavender oil, thyme oil, and eucalyptus oil.
*Muscle pain; soft-tissue disorders; upper respiratory-tract disorders.*

**Termotrin** *Loren, Mex.*
Paracetamol (p.76·2).
*Fever; pain.*

**Ternadin** *Cantabria, Spain.*
Terfenadine (p.441·1).
*Hypersensitivity reactions.*

**Ternalin** *Agis, Israel†.*
Terfenadine (p.441·1).
*Allergic rhinitis; allergic skin disorders.*

**Ternalin-D** *Agis, Israel†.*
Terfenadine (p.441·1); pseudoephedrine (p.1129·2).
*Allergic rhinitis.*

**Ternel** *Chrispa (Χρισπα), Gr.*
Diltiazem (p.901·3).
*Angina; hypertension.*

**Terneurine** *Bristol-Myers Squibb, Fr.†.*
Vitamin B substances (p.1417·1).
*Asthenia.*

**Ternolol**
*Hovid, Malaysia; Hovid, Singapore.*
Atenolol (p.865·2).
*Angina pectoris; arrhythmias; hypertension; myocardial infarction.*

**Terocaps** *Medix, Mex.*
Garcinia cambogia.
*Hypercholesterolaemia; obesity.*

**Terodul** *Degorts, Mex.*
Ranitidine hydrochloride (p.1285·2).
*Gastro-oesophageal reflux; peptic ulcer; Zollinger-Ellison syndrome.*

**Terol** *Mavi, Mex.†.*
Paracetamol (p.76·2).
*Fever; pain.*

**Terolut** *Solvay, Fin.*
Dydrogesterone (p.1549·2).
*Endometriosis; menopausal disorders; menstrual disorders.*

**Teromol** *Aldo, Spain.*
Theophylline (p.798·3).
*Heart failure; obstructive airways disease.*

**Teronac**
*Novartis, Israel; Novartis, Neth.†; Novartis, Singapore; Novartis, Switz.*
Mazindol (p.1589·1).
*Obesity.*

**Terost** *Ativus, Braz.*
Alendronic acid (p.765·3).
*Osteoporosis.*

**Terostrant** *Chrispa (Χρισπα), Gr.*
Gemfibrozil (p.923·1).
*Hyperlipidaemias.*

**Terpalate** *Ferrer, Spain†.*
Aluminium hydroxide (p.1249·2); attapulgite (p.1251·1); enoxolone aluminium (p.1264·3); magnesium oxide (p.1272·3); sodium citrate (p.1223·2).
*Gastritis; gastrointestinal hyperacidity; peptic ulcer.*

**Terpect** *Themis Chemicals, India.*
Terbutaline sulfate (p.797·2); bromhexine hydrochloride (p.1115·3); guaifenesin (p.1122·1); menthol (p.1711·3).
*Obstructive airways disease.*

**Terpestrol H** *Medopharm, Ger.†.*
Turpentine oil (p.1760·1).
*Respiratory-tract disorders.*

**Terphylin** *Themis Chemicals, India.*
Terbutaline sulfate (p.797·2); etofylline (p.785·1).
*Obstructive airways disease.*

**Terpine des Monts-Dore** *Centrapharm, Fr.†.*
Terpin (p.1131·1).
*Respiratory-tract congestion.*

**Terpine Gonnon**
*Note. This name is used for preparations of different composition.*
*Monot, Fr.†.*
*Tablets:* Terpin (p.1131·1); codeine (p.27·1).
*Respiratory-tract disorders.*

*Pharminter, Fr.†.*
*Oral liquid:* Terpin (p.1131·1); tolu balsam (p.1131·3).
*Respiratory-tract disorders.*

**Terpoin** *Houghs Healthcare, UK†.*
Codeine phosphate (p.27·1); menthol; cineole.
*Coughs.*

**Terpone** *Rosa-Phytopharma, Fr.*
Terpin (p.1131·1); Siberian fir oil; niaouli oil (p.1719·3); eucalyptus oil (p.1686·2).
*Respiratory-tract disorders.*

**Terponil** *Vitafarma, Spain.*
Oxidised terpenes; terpin (p.1131·1).
*Respiratory-tract disorders.*

**Terposen** *Vir, Spain.*
Ranitidine hydrochloride (p.1285·2).
*Acid aspiration; gastro-oesophageal reflux; gastrointestinal hyperacidity; peptic ulcer; short-bowel syndrome; Zollinger-Ellison syndrome.*

**Terra-Cortil** *Pfizer, Gr.*
Hydrocortisone (p.1103·3); oxytetracycline hydrochloride (p.241·1).
*Infected and inflamed skin conditions.*

**Terra-Cortril**
*Note. This name is used for preparations of different composition.*
*Pfizer, Arg.; Pfizer, Belg.; Pfizer, Braz.; Pfizer, Fin.; Pfizer, Irl.†; Pfizer, Norw.; Pfizer, UK.*
*Ointment:* Oxytetracycline (p.241·1) or oxytetracycline hydrochloride (p.241·1); hydrocortisone (p.1103·3).
*Infected skin disorders.*

*Pfizer, Belg.; Pfizer, S.Afr.; Farmasierra, Spain.*
*Eye/ear drops; eye/ear ointment:* Oxytetracycline hydrochloride (p.241·1); hydrocortisone acetate (p.1103·3); polymyxin B sulfate (p.245·1).
*Ear infections; eye infections.*

*Pfizer, S.Afr.; Farmasierra, Spain; Pfizer, USA.*
*Ointment:* Oxytetracycline hydrochloride (p.241·1); hydrocortisone acetate (p.1103·3).
*Eye inflammation with bacterial infection; infected skin disorders.*

**Terracortril**
*Note. This name is used for preparations of different composition.*
*Mann, Ger.; Pfizer, Switz.*
*Cream; ointment; topical spray:* Oxytetracycline hydrochloride (p.241·1); hydrocortisone (p.1103·3); polymyxin B sulfate (p.245·1).
*Burns; infected skin disorders; wounds.*

*Mann, Ger.; Pfizer, Switz.*
*Eye/ear drops; eye ointment:* Oxytetracycline hydrochloride (p.241·1); hydrocortisone acetate (p.1103·3); polymyxin B sulfate (p.245·1).
*Ear infections; inflammatory disorders of the eye.*

*Pfizer, Swed.*
Oxytetracycline hydrochloride (p.241·1); hydrocortisone (p.1103·3).
*Infected skin disorders; otitis externa.*

**Terra-Cortril com Polimixina B** *Pfizer, Braz.†.*
Oxytetracycline hydrochloride (p.241·1); hydrocortisone (p.1103·3); polymyxin B sulfate (p.245·1).
*Infected skin disorders.*

**Terra-Cortril Gel Steraject met polymyxine-B** *Pfizer, Neth.*
Oxytetracycline calcium (p.241·1); hydrocortisone (p.1103·3); polymyxin B sulfate (p.245·1).
*Sinusitis.*

**Terracortril med polymyxin B** *Pfizer, Swed.*
Oxytetracycline hydrochloride (p.241·1); hydrocortisone acetate (p.1103·3); polymyxin B sulfate (p.245·1).
*Infected ear and eye disorders; otitis externa.*

**Terra-Cortril met polymyxine-B** *Pfizer, Neth.*
Oxytetracycline hydrochloride (p.241·1); hydrocortisone acetate (p.1103·3); polymyxin B sulfate (p.245·1).
*Blepharitis squamosa; inflammatory ear infections.*

**Terracortril N** *Mann, Ger.*
Betamethasone sodium phosphate (p.1093·1); gentamicin sulfate (p.217·1).
*Infected and inflammatory eye disorders.*

**Terra-Cortril Nistatina** *Pfizer, Arg.*
Oxytetracycline calcium (p.241·1) or oxytetracycline hydrochloride (p.241·1); hydrocortisone (p.1103·3); nystatin (p.406·3).
*Infected skin disorders.*

**Terra-Cortril Nystatin**
*Pfizer, Irl.†; Pfizer, UK†.*
Oxytetracycline calcium (p.241·1); hydrocortisone (p.1103·3); nystatin (p.406·3).
*Infected skin disorders.*

**Terra-Cortril P** *Pfizer, Fin.*
Oxytetracycline hydrochloride (p.241·1); hydrocortisone acetate (p.1103·3); polymyxin B sulfate (p.245·1).
*Infected ear disorders; infected eye disorders.*

**Terra-Cortril Polymyxin B** *Pfizer, Norw.*
Oxytetracycline hydrochloride (p.241·1); hydrocortisone acetate (p.1103·3); polymyxin B sulfate (p.245·1).
*Ear disorders.*

**Terradermina** *Flopen, Braz.†.*
Salicylic acid (p.1157·1); sulfur (p.1158·2).
*Acne.*

**Terrados** *Pfizer, Mex.*
Oxytetracycline (p.241·1).
*Bacterial infections.*

**Terrafor** *Terrafor, Fr.*
Octalite.
*Digestive disorders.*

**Terrakal** *Offenbach, Mex.*
Tetracycline (p.266·2).
*Bacterial infections.*

**Terralin** *Schulke & Mayr, Ger.†.*
Benzalkonium chloride (p.1168·3); phenoxypropanol (p.1189·1).
*Surface disinfection.*

**Terramicina**
*Note. This name is used for preparations of different composition.*
*Pfizer, Arg.; Pfizer, Braz.; Pfizer, Mex.; Farmasierra, Spain.*
*Capsules; eye ointment; injection; tablets:* Oxytetracycline (p.241·1) or oxytetracycline hydrochloride (p.241·1).
Lidocaine (p.1377·3) may be included in the intramuscular injection to alleviate the pain of injection.
*Bacterial infections.*

*Pfizer, Mex.*
*Eye ointment; ointment:* Oxytetracycline (p.241·1); polymyxin B sulfate (p.245·1).
*Bacterial infections.*

*Farmasierra, Spain.*
*Ointment:* Oxytetracycline hydrochloride (p.241·1); polymyxin B sulfate (p.245·1).
*Skin infections.*

**Terramicina con Polimixina B** *Pfizer, Arg.*
Oxytetracycline hydrochloride (p.241·1); polymyxin B sulfate (p.245·1).
*Bacterial skin infections.*

**Terramicina Pomada** *Pfizer, Braz.*
Oxytetracycline hydrochloride (p.241·1); polymyxin B sulfate (p.245·1).
*Bacterial eye infections; bacterial skin infections.*

**Terramycin**
*Note. This name is used for preparations of different composition.*
*Mann, Ger.; Pfizer, Israel; Pfizer, Malaysia; Pfizer, S.Afr.; Pfizer, Singapore; Pfizer, Thai.*
*Eye ointment; ointment:* Oxytetracycline (p.241·1) or oxytetracycline hydrochloride (p.241·1); polymyxin B (p.245·2) or polymyxin B sulfate (p.245·1).
*Eye infections; infected skin disorders.*

*Pfizer, Gr.; Pfizer, Hong Kong†; Pfizer, India; Pfizer, Singapore; Pfizer, Thai.†; Pfizer, UK†; Pfizer, USA.*
Oxytetracycline (p.241·1) or oxytetracycline hydrochloride (p.241·1).
Lidocaine hydrochloride (p.1377·3) may be included in the injection to alleviate the pain of injection.
*Bacterial infections.*

**Terramycin met polymyxine-B** *Pfizer, Neth.†.*
Oxytetracycline hydrochloride (p.241·1); polymyxin B sulfate (p.245·1).
*Bacterial infections.*

**Terramycin N** *Mann, Ger.*
Gentamicin sulfate (p.217·1).
*Bacterial eye infections.*

**Terramycin with Polymyxin** *Pfizer, Gr.*
Oxytetracycline hydrochloride (p.241·1); polymyxin B sulfate (p.245·1).
*Skin infections.*

**Terramycin Polymyxin B**
*Pfizer, Denm.; Pfizer, Norw.; Pfizer, Swed.*
Oxytetracycline hydrochloride (p.241·1); polymyxin B sulfate (p.245·1).
*Bacterial skin and eye infections.*

**Terramycin with Polymyxin B**
*Pfizer, Hong Kong; Pfizer, USA.*
Oxytetracycline hydrochloride (p.241·1); polymyxin B sulfate (p.245·1).
*Bacterial eye and skin infections.*

**Terramycin SF** *Pfizer, India.*
Oxytetracycline hydrochloride (p.241·1); vitamin B substances (p.1454·3).
*Bacterial infections.*

**Terramycine**
*Pfizer, Belg.; Pfizer, Switz.†.*
Oxytetracycline hydrochloride (p.241·1); polymyxin B sulfate (p.245·1).
*Eye infections; skin infections.*

**Terramycine Solu-Retard** *Pfizer, Fr.†.*
Oxytetracycline (p.241·1).
Lidocaine (p.1377·3) is included in this preparation to alleviate the pain of injection.
*Bacterial infections.*

**Terranilo** *Biol, Spain†.*
Chymotrypsin (p.1671·2); tetracycline hydrochloride (p.266·2).
*Bacterial infections.*

**Terranumonyl** *Sanofi Winthrop, Mex.†.*
Tetracycline (p.266·2).
*Bacterial infections.*

**Terrasil** *Silom, Thai.*
Oxytetracycline (p.241·1); polymyxin B sulfate (p.245·1).
*Eye infections.*

**Terricil** *Edol, Port.*
Oxytetracycline hydrochloride (p.241·1).
*Bacterial eye infections.*

**Tersac** *Trans Canaderm, Canad.†.*
Salicylic acid (p.1157·1); triclosan (p.1195·2).
*Acne.*

**Tersaseptic**
*Note. This name is used for preparations of different composition.*
*Trans Canaderm, Canad.*
Triclosan (p.1195·2).
*Skin cleanser; skin disorders.*

*Dermaclin, Mex.; Doak, USA.*
Soap substitute.
*Acne.*

**Tersa-Tar** *Trans Canaderm, Canad.*
Coal tar (p.1159·2).
*Psoriasis; seborrhoea.*

**Tersatar** *Doak, Hong Kong†.*
Tar (p.1159·3).
*Feminine hygiene; skin and scalp disorders.*

**Tersif** *Baliarda, Arg.*
Lisinopril (p.946·3).
*Hypertension.*

**Tersigat** *3M, Fr.*
Oxitropium bromide (p.790·3).
*Obstructive airways disease.*

**Tersoderm Anticaspa** *Defuen, Arg.*
Biotin (p.1423·2); undecenoic acid diethanolamide; piroctone olamine (p.1155·2); jojoba oil.
*Scalp disorders.*

**Tersoderm Cabellos Grasos** *Defuen, Arg.*
Biotin sulfur (p.1158·2); undecenoic acid amide; triclosan (p.1195·2); coconut oil (p.1481·1).
*Scalp disorders.*

**Tersoderm Plus** *Defuen, Arg.*
Ketoconazole (p.403·3).
*Dandruff; seborrhoeic dermatitis.*

**Tertensif** *Servier, Spain.*
Indapamide (p.938·2).
*Hypertension; oedema.*

**Tertroxin**
*Boots Healthcare, Austral.; GlaxoSmithKline, NZ; GlaxoSmithKline, S.Afr.; GlaxoSmithKline, Thai.; Goldshield, UK.*
Liothyronine sodium (p.1602·2).
*Hyperthyroidism; hypothyroidism; myxoedema coma.*

**Tervalon** *Lazar, Arg.*
Amlodipine besilate (p.862·1).
*Angina pectoris; hypertension.*

**Terveson** *Doctum, Gr.*
Lovastatin (p.949·1).
*Primary hypercholesterolaemia.*

**Terzine** *Seven Stars, Thai.*
Cetirizine hydrochloride (p.427·1).
*Allergic rhinitis; allergic skin disorders.*

**Terzolin**
*Janssen-Cilag, Ger.; Janssen-Cilag, Switz.*
Ketoconazole (p.403·3).
*Pityriasis versicolor; seborrhoeic dermatitis.*

**Tesacof** *Novartis, Mex.*
Bromhexine hydrochloride (p.1115·3).
*Respiratory-tract congestion.*

**Tesalon** *Novartis, Mex.*
Benzonatate (p.1115·3).
*Coughs.*

**Tesamone** *Dunhall, USA†.*
Testosterone (p.1569·3).
*Androgen replacement therapy; delayed puberty.*

**Tesical** *Sintesina, Arg.*
Mebendazole (p.108·2).
*Worm infections.*

**Teslac**
*Bristol-Myers Squibb, Chile; Bristol-Myers Squibb Oncology, USA.*
Testolactone (p.587·3).
*Breast cancer.*

**Teslascan**
*Nycomed, Austria; Nycomed, Belg.†; Amersham, Denm.; Amersham, Fin.; Amersham, Fr.; Amersham, Ger.; Nycomed, Gr.; Nycomed, Ital.; Nycomed Imaging, Norw.; Amersham, NZ; Amersham, Spain; Amersham, Swed.; Nycomed Amersham, Switz.; Nycomed Amersham, UK; Nycomed, USA.*
Mangafodipir trisodium (p.1067·1).
*Contrast medium for magnetic resonance imaging of the liver.*

**Tesopalmed Forte cum Yohimbine** *Trima, Israel.*
Yohimbine hydrochloride (p.1766·2); strychnine nitrate (p.1750·1).
*Erectile dysfunction.*

**Tesopen** *Collins, Mex.*
Benzonatate (p.1115·3).
*Coughs.*

**Tesoprel** *Thiemann, Ger.*
Bromperidol (p.672·1) or bromperidol lactate (p.672·1).
*Schizophrenia.*

**Tesor-C** *Segix, Ital.†.*
16 Tablets, estradiol (p.1550·1); 12 tablets, estradiol; norethisterone acetate (p.1562·2).
*Menopausal disorders; osteoporosis.*

**Tesos** *Altana, Spain†.*
Tetridamine maleate (p.93·2).
*Vaginitis.*

**Tess** *Troikaa, India.*
Triamcinolone acetonide (p.1110·2).
*Oral lesions and inflammation.*

**Tessalon** *Forest Pharmaceuticals, USA.*
Benzonatate (p.1115·3).
*Coughs.*

**Tessifol** *Esfar, Port.*
Atenolol (p.865·2).
*Angina pectoris; arrhythmias; hypertension; myocardial infarction.*

**Tessofort** *Bustillos, Mex.†.*
Multivitamin preparation (p.1417·1).

**Test Pack Plus**
*Abbott, Chile; Abbott, UK.*
Pregnancy test (p.1734·3).

**Testac** *Medac, Ger.†.*
Flutamide (p.556·2).
*Prostatic cancer.*

**Testanon 25** *Infar, India.*
Testosterone propionate (p.1570·1).
*Androgen deficiency; osteoporosis.*

**Testanon 50** *Infar, India.*
Testosterone phenylpropionate (p.1570·1).
*Androgen deficiency; osteoporosis.*

**Tes-Tape**
*Lilly, Austral.; Lilly, Canad.; Lilly, Irl.†; Lilly, Ital.†; Lilly, NZ†; Lilly, S.Afr.†; Lilly, Switz.†.*
Test for glucose in urine (p.1694·2).

**testasa e** *Chefaro, Ger.*
Yohimbe extract.
*Male sexual exhaustion.*

**Testerell** *Sanorell, Ger.*
Homoeopathic preparation.

**Test-Estro** *Rugby, USA†.*
Estradiol cipionate (p.1550·1); testosterone cipionate (p.1569·3).
*Menopausal vasomotor symptoms; prevention of postpartum breast engorgement.*

**Testex** *Altana, Spain.*
Testosterone cipionate (p.1569·3) or testosterone propionate (p.1570·1).
*Aplastic anaemia; endometriosis; female breast cancer; lactation inhibition; male hypogonadism and androgen deficiency; menopausal disorders; osteoporosis.*

**Testiculi** *Disperga, Austria†.*
Testis extract (p.1569·3).
*Androgen deficiency; hypogonadism.*

**Testim** *Auxilium, USA.*
Testosterone (p.1569·3).
*Hypogonadism.*

**Testinfex** *Flopen, Braz.†.*
Neomycin (p.235·1); sulfamethoxypyridazine (p.263·1); sulfadiazine (p.258·2); sulfaguanidine (p.260·3).
*Diarrhoea.*

**Testiormina** *Sanval, Braz.†.*
Testosterone cipionate (p.1569·3).
*Androgen; breast cancer in females; delayed puberty; male hypogonadism.*

**Testisan** *Mintlab, Chile.*
Phthalylsulfathiazole (p.242·3); nifuroxazide (p.237·2).

**Testo** *Baldassari, Braz.†.*
Guarana; erythroxylon catuaba; ginseng; arginine; lysine; ptychopetalum uncinatum; gelatin; testis extract; wheat germ; kola (p.1417·1).

**Testoderm**
*Ferring, Austria; Ferring, Belg.†; Ferring, Ger.†; Ferring, Neth.; Ferring, Switz.; Ferring, UK†; Alza, USA.*
Testosterone (p.1569·3).
*Testosterone deficiency.*

**Testo-Enant** *Geymonat, Ital.*
Testosterone enantate (p.1570·1).
*Androgenic; breast cancer; fibroids.*

**Testofran** *Faria, Braz.†.*
Yohimbine (p.1766·2); vitamin $B_1$; vitamin E; calcium inositohexaphosphate; magnesium inositohexaphosphate; magnesium stearate.
*Erectile dysfunction.*

**Testogel** *Schering, UK.*
Testosterone (p.1569·3).
*Hypogonadism.*

**Testonus** *Profarb, Braz.†.*
Methyltestosterone (p.1559·3); vitamin $B_1$; vitamin E.
*Breast cancer in females; cryptorchidism; delayed puberty in males; erectile dysfunction; hypogonadism in males.*

**Testopel** *Bartor Pharmacal, USA.*
Testosterone (p.1569·3).
*Androgen deficiency; delayed puberty.*

**Testosterone Implants** *Organon, UK.*
Testosterone (p.1569·3).
*Male hypogonadism.*

**Testotard** *Chephasaar, Ger.*
Flutamide (p.556·2).
*Prostatic cancer.*

**Testotonic B** *Sam-On, Israel†.*
Methyltestosterone (p.1559·3).
*Erectile dysfunction.*

**Testoviron** *Shepa, Gr.*
Testosterone enantate (p.1570·1).
*Androgen deficiency; aplastic anaemia; breast cancer; male hypogonadism.*

**Testoviron 100**
*Schering, Austria†; Schering, Thai.*
Testosterone propionate (p.1570·1); testosterone enantate (p.1570·1).
*Aplastic anaemia in men; erectile dysfunction; female breast cancer; male hypogonadism.*

**Testoviron 250**
*Schering, Austria; Schering, Thai.*
Testosterone enantate (p.1570·1).
*Aplastic anaemia in men; erectile dysfunction; female breast cancer; male hypogonadism.*

**Testoviron Depot**
*Note. This name is used for preparations of different composition.*
*Schering, Belg.†; Schering, Hong Kong; Schering, Neth.; Schering, Port.; Schering, Singapore†; Schering, Swed.; Schering, Switz.*
Testosterone enantate (p.1570·1).
*Breast cancer; male hypogonadism.*

*German Remedies, India; Schering, Israel; Schering, Ital.*
Testosterone enantate (p.1570·1); testosterone propionate (p.1570·1).
*Aplastic anaemia; breast cancer; endometrial cancer; erectile dysfunction; male hypogonadism.*

**Testoviron Depot 50** *Schering, Ger.*
Testosterone enantate (p.1570·1); testosterone propionate (p.1570·1).
*Hypogonadism in men.*

**Testoviron Depot 100** Schering, Arg.; Schering, Ger.; Schering, Spain.
Testosterone enantate (p.1570·1); testosterone propionate (p.1570·1).
*Female breast cancer; haematopoietic disorders; hepatic cirrhosis; male hypogonadism and androgen deficiency; male infertility; osteoporosis.*

**Testoviron Depot 135** Schering, Denm.
Testosterone enantate (p.1570·1); testosterone propionate (p.1570·1).
*Breast cancer; male hypogonadism.*

**Testoviron Depot 250** Schering, Arg.; Schering, Denm.; Schering, Ger.; Schering, Spain.
Testosterone enantate (p.1570·1).
*Female breast cancer; haematopoietic disorders; hepatic cirrhosis; male hypogonadism and androgen deficiency; male infertility; osteoporosis.*

**Testovis** SIT, Ital.
Testosterone propionate (p.1570·1).
*Androgenic; breast disorders; fibroids; menstrual disorders.*

**Testozzard** Pizzard, Mex.†.
Testosterone (p.1569·3).

**Testpack hCG-Urine** Abbott, Irl.
Pregnancy test (p.1734·3).

**TestPack Plus hCG-Urine** Abbott, USA.
Pregnancy test (p.1734·3).

**Testred** ICN, USA.
Methyltestosterone (p.1559·3).
*Androgen replacement therapy; breast cancer.*

**Tesurene** A Natureza, Braz.†.
Testosterone propionate (p.1570·1); vitamin E (p.1464·3).
*Androgenic; breast cancer in females; lichen sclerosus.*

**Teta Extra** Fresenius Kabi, Ger.
Didecyldimethylammonium chloride (p.1178·3); polihexanide (p.1190·1).
*Surface disinfection.*

**Tetabulin** Baxter Immuno, Arg.; Immuno, Austria; Immuno, Hong Kong; Immuno, Irl.; Baxter, Ital.; Baxter BioScience, UK.
A tetanus immunoglobulin (p.1640·3).
Formerly known as Humotet in the *UK*.
*Passive immunisation.*

**Tetabuline** Baxter, Belg.†; Immuno, Switz.†.
A tetanus immunoglobulin (p.1640·3).
*Passive immunisation.*

**Tetacid** Interpharm, Austria.
Famotidine (p.1265·2).
*Gastric hyperacidity; gastro-oesophageal reflux; heartburn.*

**Tetagam** Aventis Behring, Austria; NBI, S.Afr.
A tetanus immunoglobulin (p.1640·3).
*Passive immunisation.*

**Tetagam N** Aventis Behring, Ger.
A tetanus immunoglobulin (p.1640·3).
*Passive immunisation.*

**Tetagamma** Nuovo ISM, Ital.
A tetanus immunoglobulin (p.1640·3).
*Passive immunisation.*

**Tetagamma P** Aventis Behring, Spain.
An tetanus immunoglobulin (p.1640·3).
*Passive immunisation.*

**Tetagam-P** Gerolimatos (Γερολυματος), Gr.; Zydus, India.
A tetanus immunoglobulin (p.1640·3).
*Passive immunisation.*

**Tetaglobulina** Pasteur Merieux, Braz.†.
A tetanus immunoglobulin (p.1640·3).
*Passive immunisation.*

**Tetaglobuline** Pasteur Merieux, Israel.
A tetanus immunoglobulin (p.1640·3).
*Passive immunisation.*

**Tetagrip** Aventis Pasteur, Fr.
A tetanus and influenza vaccine (p.1641·3).
*Active immunisation.*

**Tetamer** Pasteur Merieux, Belg.†.
An adsorbed tetanus vaccine (p.1640·3).
*Active immunisation.*

**Tetamun SSW** SmithKline Beecham, Ger.
A tetanus vaccine (p.1640·3).
*Active immunisation.*

**Tetamyn** Bioclon, Mex.
A tetanus vaccine (p.1640·3).
*Active immunisation.*

**Tetanobulin** Immuno, Braz.†; Baxter, Ger.
A tetanus immunoglobulin (p.1640·3).
*Passive immunisation.*

**Tetanogamma** Aventis Behring, Braz.; Centeon, Mex.†.
A tetanus immunoglobulin (p.1640·3).
*Passive immunisation.*

**Tetanol** Elea, Arg.; Grunenthal, Austria; Chiron Behring, Ger.; Aventis, Mex.
A tetanus vaccine (p.1640·3).
*Active immunisation.*

**Tetanosimultan** Immuno, Austria†.
A tetanus immunoglobulin (p.1640·3).
*Passive immunisation.*

**Tetanus-Gamma** Kedrion, Ital.
A tetanus immunoglobulin (p.1640·3).
*Passive immunisation.*

**Teta-S** Fresenius Kabi, Ger.
Didecylmethylalkoxiammonium propionate; cocospropylenediamineguanidinium diacetate; polihexanide (p.1190·1).
*Surface disinfection.*

**Tetasorbat SSW** SmithKline Beecham, Ger.†.
An adsorbed tetanus vaccine (p.1640·3).
*Active immunisation.*

**Tetatox** Berna, Ital.
An adsorbed tetanus vaccine (p.1640·3).
*Active immunisation.*

**Tetavax** Aventis Pasteur, Arg.; Aventis Pasteur, Braz.; Aventis Pasteur, Chile; Pasteur Merieux, Ger.†; Aventis Pasteur, Hong Kong; Aventis Pasteur, Malaysia; Pasteur Merieux, Neth.; Aventis Pasteur, Norw.; Aventis, S.Afr.; Aventis Pasteur, Thai.; Pasteur Merieux, UK†.
An adsorbed tetanus vaccine (p.1640·3).
*Active immunisation.*

**Tetaven** Baxter, Ital.
A tetanus immunoglobulin (p.1640·3).
*Passive immunisation.*

**Tetavenin** Immuno, Austria.
A tetanus immunoglobulin (p.1640·3).
*Passive immunisation.*

**Tetefit Vitamin E** Medra, Austria.
Alpha tocopherol (p.1464·3).
*Tonic.*

**Tetesept**
Note. This name is used for preparations of different composition.
Kolassa, Austria†.
*Balsam:* Camphor (p.1665·3); menthol (p.1711·3); eucalyptus oil (p.1686·2); pumilio pine oil (p.1737·1); turpentine oil (p.1760·1); rosemary oil (p.1740·2); sage oil (p.1741·2).
*Coughs and cold symptoms.*
Kolassa, Austria.
*Pastilles:* Dequalinium chloride (p.1178·1); cetylpyridinium chloride (p.1173·1); hesperidin methyl chalcone (p.1688·3); ascorbic acid (p.1460·2).
*Bacterial infections of the mouth and throat.*
Medra, Austria.
*Oral liquid:* Plantago lanceolata (p.1738·2).
*Catarrh; coughs.*

**Tetesept Calcium** Medra, Austria.
Calcium carbonate (p.1254·2).
*Calcium supplement.*

**Tetesept Magnesium** Medra, Austria.
Magnesium carbonate (p.1272·1).
*Magnesium deficiency.*

**Tetesept Vitamin C** Medra, Austria.
Ascorbic acid (p.1460·2).
*Vitamin C deficiency.*

**Tethexal** Hexal, Ger.
Tetrazepam (p.724·1).
*Skeletal muscle tension and spasticity.*

**Tetinox** Silanes, Mex.
A tetanus vaccine (p.1640·3).
*Active immunisation.*

**Tetmosol** AstraZeneca, Braz.; ICI, India; AstraZeneca, Mex.; Zeneca, S.Afr.; AstraZeneca, Singapore.
Sulfiram (p.1510·1).
*Scabies.*

**Tetra** Atlantis, Mex.
Tetracycline (p.266·2).
*Bacterial infections.*

**Tetra Caplets** Reese, USA†.
Paracetamol (p.76·2); phenylpropanolamine hydrochloride (p.1127·3).

**Tetra Central** Pharmasant, Thai.
Tetracycline hydrochloride (p.266·2).
*Bacterial infections.*

**Tetra Hubber** ICN, Spain.
Tetracycline hydrochloride (p.266·2).
*Bacterial infections.*

**Tetra Tripsin** Torlan, Spain†.
Novobiocin (p.239·2); protease; tetracycline phosphate (p.266·2).
*Bacterial infections.*

**Tetrabioptal** Farmila, Ital.†.
Tetracycline (p.266·2) or tetracycline hydrochloride (p.266·2).
*Bacterial infections of the eye.*

**Tetrabronco** Flopen, Braz.†.
Potassium iodide (p.1598·1); guaifenesin (p.1122·1); oxeladin (p.1126·1).
*Respiratory-tract congestion.*

**Tetracap** Circle, USA†.
Tetracycline hydrochloride (p.266·2).
*Bacterial infections.*

**Tetracem** Crown, S.Afr.
Oxytetracycline (p.241·1).
*Bacterial infections.*

**Tetracina** Bunker, Braz.
Tetracycline hydrochloride (p.266·2).
*Bacterial infections.*

**Tetraclin** Teuto, Braz.
Tetracycline hydrochloride (p.266·2).
*Bacterial infections.*

**Tetracoq** Aventis Pasteur, Belg.; Aventis Pasteur, Braz.; Aventis Pasteur, Fr.†; Pasteur Merieux, Hong Kong†; Pasteur Merieux, Israel; Aventis Pasteur, Malaysia; Aventis Pasteur, Thai.
An adsorbed diphtheria, tetanus, pertussis, and poliomyelitis (inactivated) vaccine (p.1615·1).
*Active immunisation.*

**Tetract-HIB** Pasteur Merieux, Belg.†; Aventis Pasteur, Braz.; Aventis Pasteur, Chile; Pasteur Merieux, Israel; Pasteur Merieux, Ital.†; Aventis Pasteur, Malaysia; Aventis Pasteur, Singapore; Aventis Pasteur, Spain; Aventis Pasteur, Thai.
A diphtheria, tetanus, pertussis, and haemophilus influenzae vaccine (p.1614·2).
*Active immunisation.*

**Tetracyn** Pfizer, Canad.†.
Tetracycline hydrochloride (p.266·2).
*Bacterial infections.*

**Tetraderm** Teuto, Braz.
Betamethasone valerate (p.1093·2); gentamicin sulfate (p.217·1); tolnaftate (p.410·1); clioquinol (p.196·3).
Formerly contained betamethasone valerate, neomycin sulfate, tolnaftate, and clioquinol.
*Infected skin disorders.*

**Tetradin** Caldeira & Metelo, Port.
Disulfiram (p.1681·3).
*Chronic alcoholism; nickel dermatitis.*

**Tetradox** Ranbaxy, Singapore; Ranbaxy, Thai.
Doxycycline hyclate (p.206·2).
*Bacterial infections.*

**Tetrafluor** Stomygen, Ital.†.
Ammonium fluoride (p.1445·3); potassium fluoride (p.1445·3); sodium fluoride (p.1444·3); sodium monofluorophosphate (p.1446·2).
*Oral hygiene.*

**Tetrafosammina** FIRMA, Ital.†.
Tetracycline phosphate complex (p.266·2).
*Bacterial infections.*

**Tetra-Gelomyrtol** Sanova, Austria; Pohl, Ger.
Oxytetracycline hydrochloride (p.241·1); myrtol.
*Bronchitis; sinusitis.*

**Tetragynon** Schering, Denm.; Schering, Fr.; Schering, Ger.; Schering, Norw.; Schering, Port.†; Schering, Switz.
Levonorgestrel (p.1563·2); ethinylestradiol (p.1553·2).
*Postcoital oral contraceptive.*

**Tetrahelmin** Luper, Braz.
Mebendazole (p.108·2).
*Worm infections.*

**Tetralgin** Craveri, Arg.
Ergotamine (p.468·3); caffeine (p.782·1); chlorphenamine (p.428·1); dipyrone (p.35·3); metoclopramide (p.1274·3).
*Migraine.*

**Tetralgin Novo** Craveri, Arg.
Ergotamine (p.468·3); caffeine (p.782·1); chlorphenamine (p.428·1); dipyrone (p.35·3); domperidone (p.1263·2).
*Migraine.*

**Tetralim** Vana, Thai.
Tetracycline phosphate complex (p.266·2).
*Bacterial infections.*

**Tetralisal** Galderma, Mex.
Lymecycline (p.228·2).
*Acne.*

**Tetralution** Merckle, Ger.
Tetracycline hydrochloride (p.266·2).
*Bacterial infections.*

**Tetralysal** Galderma, Arg.; AB-Consult, Austria; Galderma, Belg.; Galderma, Braz.; Galderma, Denm.; Galderma, Fin.; Galderma, Fr.; Galderma, Irl.; Galderma, Ital.; Galderma, Norw.; Galderma, S.Afr.; Galderma, Swed.; Galderma, UK.
Lymecycline (p.228·2).
*Bacterial infections.*

**Tetram** Nycomed, Norw.†.
Piroxicam (p.84·2).
*Dysmenorrhoea; musculoskeletal and joint disorders.*

**Tetra-Mag** Cypress, USA.
Magnesium salicylate (p.55·1); phenyltoloxamine citrate (p.439·1).

**Tetramax** Luper, Braz.
Tetracycline hydrochloride (p.266·2).
*Bacterial infections.*

**Tetramdura** Merck dura, Ger.
Tetrazepam (p.724·1).
*Skeletal muscle spasm.*

**Tetramel** Aspen, S.Afr.
Oxytetracycline hydrochloride (p.241·1).
*Bacterial infections.*

**Tetramicin** EMS, Braz.
Tetracycline hydrochloride (p.266·2) or tetracycline phosphate complex (p.266·2).
*Bacterial infections.*

**Tetramil** Farmigea, Ital.
Tetryzoline hydrochloride (p.1131·2); pheniramine maleate (p.438·3).
*Conjunctivitis; eye irritation and congestion.*

**Tetramizol Composto** Iodo Suma, Braz.†.
Tetramisole (p.114·1); tiabendazole (p.114·2).
*Nematode infections.*

**Tetramizotil** Osorio de Moraes, Braz.
Tetramisole (p.114·1).
*Nematode infections.*

**Tetramune** Wyeth-Ayerst, Canad.†; Wyeth-Ayerst, Hong Kong†; Wyeth, Mex.†; Lederle, NZ†; Wyeth, Singapore†; Lederle, Switz.†; Lederle, USA†.
A diphtheria, tetanus, pertussis, and haemophilus influenzae vaccine (p.1614·2).
*Active immunisation.*

**Tetrana** Vana, Thai.
Tetracycline (p.266·2).
*Bacterial infections.*

**Tetranase** Rottapharm, Fr.†.
Oxytetracycline hydrochloride (p.241·1).
Formerly contained oxytetracycline hydrochloride and bromelains.
*Bacterial infections.*

**Tetrano** Milano, Thai.
Tetracycline hydrochloride (p.266·2).
*Bacterial infections.*

**Tetranovax** Pisa, Mex.†.
Tetracycline (p.266·2).
*Bacterial infections.*

**Tetrapres** Precimex, Mex.†.
Tetracycline (p.266·2).
*Bacterial infections.*

**Tetraprocyn** Protein, Mex.†.
Tetracycline (p.266·2).
*Bacterial infections.*

**Tetrapulmo** Eversil, Braz.
*Capsules; syrup:* Sodium camsilate; chlorphenamine maleate (p.427·3); dipyrone (p.35·3); guaifenesin (p.1122·1); terpin hydrate (p.1131·1).
*Injection:* Dipyrone (p.35·3); chlorphenamine maleate (p.427·3); guaifenesin (p.1122·1); cineole (p.1672·1); niaouli oil (p.1719·3); sodium camsilate.
*Cold and influenza symptoms.*

**Tetra-saar** Chephasaar, Ger.
Tetrazepam (p.724·1).
*Skeletal muscle tension and spasticity.*

**Tetrasan** CEPA, Spain†.
Doxycycline hyclate (p.206·2).
*Bacterial infections.*

**Tetrasine** Optopics, USA.
Tetryzoline hydrochloride (p.1131·2).
*Minor eye irritation.*

**Tetrasine Extra** Optopics, USA.
Tetryzoline hydrochloride (p.1131·2); macrogol 400 (p.1708·2).
*Minor eye irritation.*

**Tetra-Tablinen** Sanorania, Ger.†.
Oxytetracycline hydrochloride (p.241·1).
*Bacterial infections.*

**TetraTITER** Wyeth, S.Afr.†.
A diphtheria, tetanus, pertussis, and haemophilus influenzae vaccine (p.1614·2).
*Active immunisation.*

**Tetratoss** Heralds, Braz.†.
Sodium camsilate; cineole (p.1672·1); menthol (p.1711·3); guaifenesin (p.1122·1); oxeladin citrate (p.1126·1).
*Respiratory-tract congestion.*

**Tetravac** Aventis Pasteur, Belg.; Aventis Pasteur, Fr.; Aventis Pasteur, Ger.; Vianex (Βιανεξ), Gr.; Aventis Pasteur, Irl.; Aventis Pasteur, Ital.; Pro Vaccine, Switz.
A diphtheria, tetanus, pertussis, and poliomyelitis vaccine (p.1615·1).
*Active immunisation.*

**Tetraxil** Delta, Braz.
Tetracycline hydrochloride (p.266·2).
*Bacterial infections.*

**Tetrazep** 1A, Ger.; ABZ, Ger.; CT, Ger.
Tetrazepam (p.724·1).
*Skeletal muscle tension and spasticity.*

**Tetrazil** Arlex, Mex.†.
Tetracycline (p.266·2).
*Bacterial infections.*

**Tetrerba** Pharmacia Upjohn, Mex.†.
Tetracycline (p.266·2).
*Bacterial infections.*

**Tetrex** Bristol-Myers Squibb, Austral.; Bristol-Myers Squibb, Mex.; Bristol-Myers Squibb, S.Afr.†.
Tetracycline hydrochloride (p.266·2).
*Adjunct in intestinal amoebiasis; bacterial infections; malaria.*
Bristol-Myers Squibb, Braz.
Tetracycline phosphate complex (p.266·2).
*Bacterial infections.*

**Tetrex-F** Bristol-Myers Squibb, S.Afr.†.
Tetracycline hydrochloride (p.266·2); nystatin (p.406·3).
*Bacterial infections; candidiasis.*

**Tetrib** Ibfarma, Braz.†.
Tetracycline (p.266·2).
*Bacterial infections.*

**Tetrilin** MIP, Ger.
Tetryzoline hydrochloride (p.1131·2).
*Nasal congestion.*

**Tetrim** IQFA, Mex.
Tetracycline (p.266·2).
*Bacterial infections.*

**Tetrisal** MIP, Ger.
Sodium chloride (p.1233·3).
*Dry nose; nasal congestion.*

**Tetroid** Ache, Braz.
Levothyroxine sodium (p.1600·1).
*Hypothyroidism.*

**Tet-Tox** CSL, Austral.; CSL, NZ.
An adsorbed tetanus vaccine (p.1640·3).
*Active immunisation.*

**Tetuman**
*Berna, Belg.†; Berna, Hong Kong; Berna, Ital.†; Berna, Malaysia; Swiss Serum, Malaysia; Berna, Port.; Byk Madaus, S.Afr.†; Berna, Spain; Berna, Switz.; Berna, Thai.†.*
A tetanus immunoglobulin (p.1640·3).
*Passive immunisation.*

**Teufelskralle** *Merck dura, Ger.*
Devil's claw root (p.28·2).
*Joint disorders.*

**Teutocilin** *Teuto, Braz.*
Oxacillin sodium (p.240·2).
*Bacterial infections.*

**Teutoformin** *Teuto, Braz.*
Metformin hydrochloride (p.342·3).
*Diabetes mellitus.*

**Teutolax** *Teuto, Braz.†.*
Phenolphthalein (p.1284·1).
*Constipation.*

**Teutomicina** *Teuto, Braz.*
Neomycin sulfate (p.235·1); bacitracin zinc (p.161·3).

**Teutonico** *Teuto, Braz.†.*
Ferrous sulfate (p.1428·2); phosphoric acid (p.1731·2).
*Iron deficiency; iron-deficiency anaemias.*

**Teutoss** *Teuto, Braz.*
Potassium iodide (p.1598·1); ephedrine hydrochloride (p.1120·1); belladonna (p.479·1); stramonium (p.489·2).
*Respiratory-tract congestion.*

**Teutrin** *Teuto, Braz.*
Co-trimoxazole (p.199·3).
*Bacterial infections; Pneumocystis carinii pneumonia; protozoal infections.*

**Teutrin Balsamico** *Teuto, Braz.†.*
Co-trimoxazole (p.199·3); guaifenesin (p.1122·1); ammonium chloride (p.1115·2).
*Bacterial infections.*

**Tevacaine** *Teva, Israel.*
Mepivacaine hydrochloride (p.1381·2).
*Local anaesthesia.*

**Tevacor** *Teva, Israel.*
Oxprenolol hydrochloride (p.978·1).
*Angina pectoris; arrhythmias; hypertension.*

**Tevacutan** *Teva, Israel.*
Clotrimazole (p.396·2); dexamethasone (p.1097·1); neomycin sulfate (p.235·1).
*Fungal skin infections.*

**Tevacycline** *Teva, Israel.*
Tetracycline hydrochloride (p.266·2).
*Bacterial infections.*

**Tevapirin** *Teva, Israel.*
Aspirin (p.15·1).
*Thromboembolism prophylaxis.*

**Tevax** *GlaxoSmithKline, Belg.*
An adsorbed tetanus vaccine (p.1640·3).
*Active immunisation.*

**Teveten**
*Solvay, Austral.; Solvay, Austria; Solvay, Belg.; SmithKline Beecham, Braz.†; Solvay, Canad.; Solvay, Denm.; Orion, Fin.; Solvay, Fr.; Aventis, Ger.; Solvay, Ger.; Solvay, Gr.; Solvay, Irl.; Solvay, Neth.; Solvay, Norw.; Solvay, Port.; Solvay, Swed.; Solvay, Switz.; Solvay, UK; SmithKline Beecham, USA.*
Eprosartan mesilate (p.912·1).
*Hypertension.*

**Teveten HCT** *Biovail, USA.*
Eprosartan mesilate (p.912·1); hydrochlorothiazide (p.933·2).
*Hypertension.*

**Teveten Plus** *Solvay, Austral.*
Eprosartan mesilate (p.912·1); hydrochlorothiazide (p.933·2).
*Hypertension.*

**Tevetens** *Solvay, Spain.*
Eprosartan mesilate (p.912·1).
*Hypertension.*

**Tevetenz** *Solvay, Ital.*
Eprosartan mesilate (p.912·1).
*Hypertension.*

**Tevoril** *Proel, Gr.*
Ambroxol hydrochloride (p.1114·3).
*Respiratory disorders associated with viscous mucus.*

**Tev-Tropin** *Gate, USA.*
Somatropin (p.1327·2).
*Growth hormone deficiency.*

**Texacort**
*GenDerm, Canad.†; GenDerm, USA.*
Hydrocortisone (p.1103·3).
*Skin disorders.*

**Texate** *Columbia, Mex.†.*
Methotrexate (p.568·2).
*Malignant neoplasms.*

**Texicam** *Deutsche, Chile.*
Tenoxicam (p.93·1).
*Inflammation; musculoskeletal and joint disorders.*

**Texodil** *Aventis, Fr.*
Cefotiam hexetil hydrochloride (p.177·2).
*Bacterial infections of the respiratory-tract.*

**Texot** *Filaxis, Arg.*
Docetaxel (p.547·1).
*Malignant neoplasms.*

**Texoven** *Tecnofarma, Mex.*
Benzonatate (p.1115·3).
*Coughs.*

**Texx** *Krewel, Ger.*
Hypericum (p.299·1).
*Anxiety; depression.*

**Teylor** *Dom, Spain.*
Simvastatin (p.997·1).
*Hyperlipidaemias; secondary prophylaxis of ischaemic heart disease.*

**TFE** *Seroyal, Canad.†.*
Vitamin A, vitamin E, and zinc (p.1417·1).

**TFT**
*Alcon, Ger.†; Bausch & Lomb, S.Afr.*
Trifluridine (p.655·3).
*Herpes simplex keratitis.*

**TFT Ophtiole**
*Tramedico, Belg.†; Tramedico, Neth.*
Trifluridine (p.655·3).
*Viral eye infections.*

**T/Gel**
*Note. This name is used for preparations of different composition.*
*Neutrogena, Fr.†.*
Salicylic acid (p.1157·1); piroctone olamine (p.1155·2).
*Scalp and hair disorders.*

*Neutrogena, Israel; Johnson & Johnson, UK.*
Coal tar (Neutar) (p.1159·2).
*Scalp disorders.*

**T-Gen** *Goldline, USA.*
Trimethobenzamide hydrochloride (p.442·2).
*Nausea and vomiting.*

**T-Gesic** *Williams, USA.*
Paracetamol (p.76·2); hydrocodone tartrate (p.45·1).
*Pain.*

**THA** *Woods, Austral.*
Tacrine hydrochloride (p.1497·2).
*Postoperative respiratory stimulant; reversal of competitive neuromuscular blockade.*

**Thacapzol** *Recip, Swed.*
Thiamazole (p.1603·3).
*Hyperthyroidism.*

**Thaden**
*Aspen, S.Afr.; Trinity, UK†.*
Dosulepin hydrochloride (p.291·1).
*Depression; mixed anxiety depressive states.*

**Thais** *Besins, Fr.*
Estradiol (p.1550·1).
*Menopausal disorders.*

**Thalamonal**
*Janssen-Cilag, Austria†; Janssen-Cilag, Belg.†; Janssen-Cilag, Ger.†; Janssen-Cilag, Neth.†.*
Droperidol (p.697·2); fentanyl citrate (p.40·1).
*General anaesthesia; neuroleptanalgesia; premedication.*

**Thalaris** *Technilab, Canad.†.*
Sodium chloride (p.1233·3).
*Oral hygiene.*

**Thalitone** *Monarch, USA.*
Chlortalidone (p.882·3).
*Hypertension; oedema.*

**Thalomid** *Celgene, USA.*
Thalidomide (p.1752·3).
*Erythema nodosum leprosum.*

**Tham**
*Abbott, Austral.; Kohler, Ger.*
Trometamol (p.1758·2) with or without electrolytes.
*Metabolic acidosis.*

**Thamacetat** *Bellon, Fr.†.*
Trometamol (p.1758·2).
*Metabolic acidosis.*

**Thamesol** *Diaco, Ital.*
Trometamol (p.1758·2).
*Metabolic acidosis.*

**t/h-basan** *Schonenberger, Switz.*
Triamterene (p.1016·2); hydrochlorothiazide (p.933·2).
*Hypertension; oedema.*

**The Brioni** *Husler, Switz.†.*
Sambucus (p.1741·3); melissa (p.1711·1); peppermint leaf (p.1283·2); senna (p.1288·2); fennel (p.1687·2); agrimony (p.1649·1).
*Constipation.*

**The Chambard-Tee** *Brady, Austria.*
Senna leaf (p.1288·2); althaea leaf (p.1651·3); peppermint leaf (p.1283·2); melissa leaf (p.1711·1); hyssopus officinalis; anthyllidis flower; calendula (p.1665·2); cyanae flower.
*Constipation.*

**The Franklin** *Noveal, Switz.†.*
Senna (p.1288·2); couch-grass (p.1676·2); fennel (p.1687·2); melissa (p.1711·1); boldo (p.1661·2); hyssopus officinalis; cuminum cyminum; peppermint leaf (p.1283·2); aniseed (p.1655·2).
*Constipation.*

**The Ginseng King** *Medicafarm, Ital.*
Fish milk; fish brain extract; cod-liver extract; myrtillus; acacia honey; fructose; ginseng (p.1417·1).
*Nutritional supplement.*

**The laxatif Solubilax** *Heumann, Switz.†.*
Senna (p.1288·2); frangula bark (p.1266·3).
*Bowel evacuation; constipation.*

**Thedox** *Mer-National, S.Afr.†.*
Doxycycline polyphosphate sodium complex (p.206·2).
*Bacterial infections.*

**Theinol** *Bailly, Fr.*
Paracetamol (p.76·2); caffeine (p.782·1).
Formerly contained sodium salicylate, phenazone, and caffeine.
*Fever; pain.*

**Thelban** *Biolab, Malaysia.*
Albendazole (p.101·2).
*Worm infections.*

**Thelmox** *Remedica, Malaysia.*
Mebendazole (p.108·2).
*Worm infections.*

**Themibutol** *Themis Chemicals, India.*
Ethambutol hydrochloride (p.211·3).
*Tuberculosis.*

**theo** *CT, Ger.*
Theophylline (p.798·3) or theophylline sodium glycinate (p.804·3).
*Obstructive airways disease.*

**Theo-24**
*Monsanto, Ital.; UCB, USA.*
Theophylline (p.798·3).
*Obstructive airways disease.*

**Theo Max** *Desarrollo, Spain.*
Theophylline (p.798·3).
*Heart failure; obstructive airways disease; paroxysmal dyspnoea.*

**Theo PA** *GlaxoSmithKline, India.*
Theophylline (p.798·3).
*Bronchospasm.*

**Theo-Asthalin** *Cipla, India.*
Salbutamol sulfate (p.791·3); theophylline (p.798·3).
*Obstructive airways disease.*

**Theobid Duracaps** *Russ, USA.*
Theophylline (p.798·3).
*Asthma; chronic bronchitis; emphysema.*

**Theobric** *Remidex, India.*
Terbutaline sulfate (p.797·2); theophylline (p.798·3).
*Asthma; bronchitis.*

**Theo-Bronc** *Rougier, Canad.*
Guaifenesin (p.1122·1); potassium iodide (p.1598·1); theophylline (p.798·3); mepyramine maleate (p.437·1).
*Obstructive airways disease.*

**Theo-Bros** *Bros, Gr.*
Theophylline (p.798·3).
*Asthma; chronic obstructive pulmonary disease; neonatal apnoea and bradycardia.*

**Theochron**
*Riva, Canad.†; Forest Pharmaceuticals, USA.*
Theophylline (p.798·3).
*Obstructive airways disease.*

**Theocol** *Beige, S.Afr.†.*
Diphenhydramine hydrochloride (p.431·3); ammonium chloride (p.1115·2); sodium citrate (p.1223·2); menthol (p.1711·3).
*Coughs.*

**Theodrine** *Rugby, USA.*
Theophylline (p.798·3); ephedrine hydrochloride (p.1120·1); phenobarbital (p.367·3).
*Bronchospasm.*

**Theo-Dur**
*AstraZeneca, Arg.; AstraZeneca, Austral.†; Astra, Belg.†; AstraZeneca, Canad.; AstraZeneca, Denm.; AstraZeneca, Fin.; Lavipharm, Gr.; AstraZeneca, Hong Kong; Astra, Irl.†; Recordati, Ital.; AstraZeneca, Norw.; AstraZeneca, NZ†; Astra, S.Afr.†; AstraZeneca, Singapore†; Pharmacia, Spain; Draco, Swed.; AstraZeneca, Thai.†; AstraZeneca, UK†; Key, USA†.*
Theophylline (p.798·3).
*Obstructive airways disease; paroxysmal dyspnoea.*

**Theofol** *Leiras, Fin.*
Theophylline (p.798·3).
*Obstructive airways disease.*

**Theofol Comp** *Leiras, Fin.*
Theophylline (p.798·3); guaifenesin (p.1122·1).
*Obstructive airways disease.*

**Theogel** *SAN, Ital.†.*
Royal jelly (p.1740·3).

**Theohexal** *Hexal, Austria†.*
Theophylline (p.798·3).
*Obstructive airways disease.*

**Theolair**
*3M, Belg.; 3M, Canad.; 3M, Fr.†; 3M, Ger.; 3M, Ital.; 3M, Neth.; 3M, Spain; 3M, Switz.; 3M, USA.*
Theophylline (p.798·3).
*Obstructive airways disease; paroxysmal dyspnoea.*

**Theolan** *Elan, Irl.†.*
Theophylline (p.798·3).
*Bronchospasm.*

**Theolin**
*Upha, Malaysia; AstraZeneca, Neth.†; Beacons, Singapore.*
Theophylline (p.798·3).
*Obstructive airways disease.*

**Theolong** *Eisai, Jpn.*
Theophylline (p.798·3).
*Obstructive airways disease.*

**Theomax DF** *Barre-National, USA; Schein, USA.*
Theophylline (p.798·3); ephedrine sulfate (p.1120·1); hydroxyzine hydrochloride (p.434·3).
*Bronchospasm.*

**Theophar** *Julphar, UAE.*
Theophylline (p.798·3).
*Obstructive airways disease.*

**Theophen** *Aspen, S.Afr.*
Theophylline (p.798·3); etofylline (p.785·1).
*Obstructive airways disease.*

**Theophen Comp** *Aspen, S.Afr.*
Theophylline (p.798·3); etofylline (p.785·1); diphenylpyraline hydrochloride (p.432·3); ammonium chloride (p.1115·2).
*Coughs.*

**Theophyllaminum** *Leiras, Fin.†.*
Aminophylline hydrate (p.780·2).
*Obstructive airways disease.*

**Theophyllard**
*Byk, Belg.†; OPW, Ger.†.*
Theophylline (p.798·3).
*Obstructive airways disease.*

**Theopirina** *Dovalle, Braz.*
Orphenadrine (p.486·2); dipyrone (p.35·3); caffeine (p.782·1).
*Skeletal muscle spasm.*

**Theoplus**
*Germania, Austria; Pharmafabre (Φαρμαφαμπρ), Gr.; Byk Madaus, S.Afr.; Pierre Fabre, Singapore; Pierre Fabre, Spain.*
Theophylline (p.798·3).
*Heart failure; obstructive airways disease; paroxysmal dyspnoea.*

**Theosal** *Ranbaxy, Thai.†.*
Theophylline (p.798·3); salbutamol (p.791·3).
*Obstructive airways disease.*

**Theospan-SR** *Laser, USA†.*
Theophylline (p.798·3).

**Theospirex** *Gebro, Austria.*
Theophylline (p.798·3) or theophylline sodium glycinate (p.804·3).
*Obstructive airways disease.*

**Theo-SR** *Rhone-Poulenc Rorer, Canad.†.*
Theophylline (p.798·3).
*Obstructive airways disease.*

**Theostat**
*Note. This name is used for preparations of different composition.*
*Inava, Fr.*
Theophylline hydrate (p.798·3).
*Asthma; obstructive airways disease.*

*Lagamed, S.Afr.†.*
Etofylline (p.785·1).
*Obstructive airways disease.*

**Theo-Talusin** *Knoll, Switz.†.*
Proscillaridin (p.990·3); etofylline (p.785·1).
*Cardiac disorders.*

**Theotard** *CTI, Israel.*
Theophylline (p.798·3).
*Obstructive airways disease.*

**Theotex** *Terapeutico, Ital.*
Metalkonium chloride (p.1185·3).
*Personal hygiene; skin disinfection.*

**Theotrim**
*Trima, Israel; Trima, Thai.*
Theophylline (p.798·3).
*Obstructive airways disease.*

**Theovent**
*Schering-Plough, Hong Kong†; Schering, USA.*
Theophylline (p.798·3).
*Asthma; reversible bronchospasm.*

**Theo-X** *Carnrick, USA.*
Theophylline (p.798·3).
*Obstructive airways disease.*

**Thephorin** *Sinclair, Irl.†.*
Phenindamine tartrate (p.438·2).
*Hypersensitivity reactions.*

**Theprubicine** *Aventis, Fr.*
Pirarubicin (p.580·1).
*Breast cancer.*

**Thera Hematinic** *Major, USA.*
Ferrous fumarate (p.1427·3); folic acid (p.1429·1); multivitamins and minerals (p.1417·1).
*Iron-deficiency anaemias.*

**Thera Tears** *Novartis, Mex.*
Carmellose (p.1577·3).
*Dry eyes; eye irritation.*

**Therabid** *Mission Pharmacal, USA.*
Multivitamin preparation (p.1417·1).

**Therac** *C & M, USA.*
Sulfur (p.1158·2); salicylic acid (p.1157·1).
*Acne.*

**Theracap** *Nycomed Amersham, UK.*
Iodine-131 (p.1524·2) as sodium iodide.
*Hyperthyroidism; thyroid cancer.*

**Theracaps** *Reese, USA†.*
Paracetamol (p.76·2); phenylpropanolamine hydrochloride (p.1127·3); mepyramine maleate (p.437·1); dextromethorphan hydrobromide (p.1117·3).

**Theraclox** *Great Eastern, Thai.; Therapharma, Thai.*
Cloxacillin (p.198·2).
*Bacterial infections.*

**Theracne** *Igefarma, Braz.†.*
Triclosan (p.1195·2).
*Acne.*

**Theracof Plus** *Reese, USA.*
Paracetamol (p.76·2); phenylephrine hydrochloride (p.1126·3); guaifenesin (p.1122·1); diphenhydramine hydrochloride (p.431·3).

**Theracort** *Igefarma, Braz.†.*
Triamcinolone acetonide (p.1110·2).
*Skin disorders.*

**TheraCys** *Pasteur Merieux, USA.*
A BCG vaccine (p.1609·2).
*Bladder cancer.*

**Theradol** *Therabel, Neth.*
Tramadol hydrochloride (p.94·3).
*Pain.*

**TheraFlu** *Novartis, Mex.*
Paracetamol (p.76·2); pseudoephedrine hydrochloride (p.1129·2); chlorphenamine maleate (p.427·3).
*Cold and influenza symptoms.*

**TheraFlu Flu and Cold** *Novartis, USA.*
Chlorphenamine maleate (p.427·3); pseudoephedrine hydrochloride (p.1129·2); paracetamol (p.76·2).
*Cold and flu symptoms.*

**TheraFlu Flu, Cold & Cough**
*Sandoz, Canad.†; Novartis, USA.*
Chlorphenamine maleate (p.427·3); pseudoephedrine hydrochloride (p.1129·2); paracetamol (p.76·2); dextromethorphan hydrobromide (p.1117·3).
*Coughs and cold symptoms.*

**TheraFlu Vapor Stick** *Novartis, USA.*
Camphor (p.1665·3); menthol (p.1711·3).
*Musculoskeletal pain; upper respiratory-tract congestion.*

**Thera-Flur** *Colgate-Hoyt, USA.*
Sodium fluoride (p.1444·3).
*Dental caries prophylaxis.*

**Theragen** *Reese, USA.*
Capsaicin (p.24·2).

**Theragenerix** *Goldline, USA.*
A range of vitamin preparations (p.1417·1).

**Theragenerix-H** *Goldline, USA.*
Ferrous fumarate (p.1427·3); folic acid (p.1429·1); multivitamins and minerals (p.1417·1).
*Iron-deficiency anaemias.*

**Thera-gesic** *Mission Pharmacal, USA.*
Methyl salicylate (p.59·3); menthol (p.1711·3).
*Musculoskeletal and joint pain.*

**Theragran** *Mead Johnson Nutritionals, USA.*
A range of vitamin preparations (p.1417·1).

**Theragran AntiOxidant** *Bristol-Myers Squibb, USA.*
Vitamins A, C, and E with minerals (p.1417·1).

**Theragran Hematinic** *Apothecon, USA†.*
Multivitamin and mineral preparation with iron and folic acid (p.1417·1).
*Iron-deficiency anaemias.*

**Theragran-M**
*Sarabhai Piramal, India; Bristol-Myers Squibb, S.Afr.†; Bristol-Myers Squibb, Thai.*
Multivitamin and mineral preparation (p.1417·1).

**Thera-Hist** *Major, USA†.*
Phenylpropanolamine hydrochloride (p.1127·3); chlorphenamine maleate (p.427·3).
*Upper respiratory-tract symptoms.*

**Theralen** *Aventis, Swed.*
Alimemazine tartrate (p.423·3).
*Anxiety; behaviour disorders; hypersensitivity reactions; premedication; sleep disorders; vomiting.*

**Theralene**
*Aventis, Belg.*
Alimemazine (p.424·1).
*Coughs; cramps; dystonias; hypersensitivity reactions; insomnia; psychiatric disorders; tics.*

*Celltech, Fr.*
Alimemazine tartrate (p.423·3).
*Cough; hypersensitivity reactions; insomnia; premedication; pruritus.*

**Theralene Pectoral** *Rhone-Poulenc Rorer, Belg.†.*
Alimemazine tartrate (p.423·3); ethylmorphine hydrochloride (p.37·3); ephedrine hydrochloride (p.1120·1); ammonium acetate (p.1115·1).
*Coughs.*

**Theralene Pectoral Nourrisson** *Celltech, Fr.*
Alimemazine tartrate (p.423·3); ammonium acetate (p.1115·1); tolu balsam (p.1131·3).
*Coughs.*

**Thera-M** *Major, USA.*
Multivitamin preparation with minerals and folic acid (p.1417·1).

**Theramycin Z** *Medicis, USA†.*
Erythromycin (p.208·1).
*Acne.*

**Theranal** *Roche Consumer, Neth.*
Bismuth subnitrate (p.1252·2); zinc oxide (p.1163·2); lidocaine (p.1377·3).
*Haemorrhoids.*

**Theranyl** *Abigo, Swed.*
Nicotinic acid (p.1441·1); salicylic acid (p.1157·1).
*Musculoskeletal and joint disorders.*

**TheraPatch Cold Sore** *Lectec, USA.*
Lidocaine (p.1377·3); camphor (p.1665·3).
*Herpes labialis.*

**Therapeutic Bath** *Goldline, USA.*
Emollient and moisturiser.

**Therapeutic Bath Oil**
*Note. This name is used for preparations of different composition.*
*Avant Garde, Canad.†.*
Liquid paraffin (p.1479·1).

*Scott, Canad.*
Liquid paraffin (p.1479·1); wool fat (p.1483·1).

**Therapeutic Mineral Ice** *Bristol-Myers Products, USA.*
Menthol (p.1711·3).
*Muscle, joint, and soft-tissue pain; neuralgia.*

**Therapeutic Skin Lotion** *Scott, Canad.*
Lanolin oil (p.1483·1); liquid paraffin (p.1479·1).

**Therapeutic Soothing Ice** *Jamieson, Canad.*
Methyl salicylate (p.59·3); camphor (p.1665·3); menthol (p.1711·3); eucalyptus oil (p.1686·2).

**Theraplex T** *Medicis, USA†.*
Coal tar (p.1159·2).
*Scalp disorders.*

**Theraplex Z** *Medicis, USA†.*
Pyrithione zinc (p.1156·2).
*Dandruff; seborrhoeic dermatitis.*

**Therapsor** *Igefarma, Braz.†.*
Clobetasol propionate (p.1095·2).
*Skin disorders.*

**Therasa** *Pharmachemie, Belg.*
Aspirin (p.15·1).
*Thromboembolic disorders.*

**Therasona** *Igefarma, Braz.†.*
Hydrocortisone (p.1103·3).
*Skin disorders.*

**Theratar** *Igefarma, Braz.†.*
Coal tar (p.1159·2).
*Skin disorders.*

**Theravee** *Vangard, USA.*
A range of vitamin preparations (p.1417·1).

**Theravee Hematinic** *Vangard, USA.*
Iron (p.1434·3); folic acid (p.1429·1); multivitamins and minerals (p.1417·1).
*Iron-deficiency anaemias.*

**Theravim** *Nature's Bounty, USA.*
A range of vitamin preparations (p.1417·1).

**Theravite** *Barre-National, USA.*
Multivitamin preparation (p.1417·1).

**Therems** *Rugby, USA.*
A range of vitamin preparations (p.1417·1).

**Therevac Plus** *Jones, USA.*
Docusate sodium (p.1262·2); glycerol (p.1694·3); benzocaine (p.1370·3); soft soap (p.1575·2).
*Constipation.*

**Therevac SB** *Jones, USA.*
Docusate sodium (p.1262·2); glycerol (p.1694·3); soft soap (p.1575·2).
*Constipation.*

**Therma Ayoral** *Rayere, Mex.†.*
Dipyrone (p.35·3).
*Fever; pain.*

**Thermal**
*Provita, Austria; Alpharma, Norw.*
Ethyl nicotinate (p.37·2); diethylamine salicylate (p.34·1).
*Musculoskeletal and joint disorders; neuralgia.*

**Thermalife** *Thermalife, Austral.†.*
Protein and trace metal complex (Peptophen).
*Arthritic pain; bath additive; bed sores; emollient; muscular pain.*

**Thermalife C** *Thermalife, Austral.†.*
Protein/trace metal complex (Peptophen); capsicum oleoresin (p.1667·1).
*Arthritic pain; muscular pain.*

**Thermazene** *Sherwood, USA.*
Sulfadiazine silver (p.259·1).
*Infected burns.*

**Thermo Burger** *Ysatfabrik, Ger.*
Capsicum (p.1667·1).
*Musculoskeletal, joint, and soft-tissue disorders; neuralgia.*

**Thermo Mobilisin** *Sankyo, Ger.†.*
Flufenamic acid (p.43·2); a heparinoid (p.931·1); benzyl nicotinate (p.21·2).
*Musculoskeletal and joint disorders; neuralgia.*

**Thermo Rub** *Rolmex, Canad.*
Methyl salicylate (p.59·3); menthol (p.1711·3); cineole (p.1672·1).

**Thermocream** *Pharmacobel, Belg.*
Methyl salicylate (p.59·3); menthol (p.1711·3); capsicum (p.1667·1).
*Musculoskeletal disorders.*

**Thermocutan** *Streuli, Switz.*
Nonivamide (p.67·2); ethyl nicotinate (p.37·2); benzyl nicotinate (p.21·2); aminophenazone salicylate (p.14·2).
*Chilblains; musculoskeletal, joint, peri-articular, and soft-tissue disorders.*

**Thermodent** *Mentholatum, Austral.†.*
Potassium nitrate (p.1190·1); sodium monofluorophosphate (p.1446·2).
*Desensitising toothpaste.*

**Thermo-Gel** *Prodemdis, Canad.*
Camphor (p.1665·3); menthol (p.1711·3); benzocaine (p.1370·3); thymol (p.1194·2).

**Thermogene** *Montefarmaco, Ital.*
Capsicum oleoresin (p.1667·1).
*Musculoskeletal and joint pain.*

**thermo-loges** *Loges, Ger.†.*
Benzyl nicotinate (p.21·2); pine needle oil; rosemary oil (p.1740·2).
*Circulatory disorders; musculoskeletal, joint, and soft-tissue disorders.*

**Thermo-Menthoneurin** *Byk Gulden, Ger.; Roland, Ger.*
Glycol salicylate (p.44·3); benzyl nicotinate (p.21·2).
*Musculoskeletal, joint, peri-articular, and soft-tissue disorders; neuralgia.*

**Thermo-Menthoneurin Bad** *Tosse, Ger.†.*
Glycol salicylate (p.44·3); benzyl nicotinate (p.21·2); methyl nicotinate (p.59·2).
*Bath additive; musculoskeletal and joint disorders; peripheral circulatory disorders.*

**Thermo-Rheumon**
*Kolassa, Austria; Tropon, Ger.*
Etofenamate (p.38·1); benzyl nicotinate (p.21·2).
*Musculoskeletal, joint, peri-articular, and soft-tissue disorders.*

**Thermorub**
*Note. A similar name is used for preparations of different composition (see below).*
*Raza, Malaysia; Pharmaniaga, Malaysia.*
Methyl salicylate (p.59·3); eucalyptus oil (p.1686·2); turpentine oil (p.1760·1).
*Musculoskeletal pain.*

**Thermo-Rub**
*Note. A similar name is used for preparations of different composition (see above).*
*Propan, S.Afr.*
Methyl salicylate (p.59·3).
*Muscular pain; rheumatism.*

**Thermosenex** *Riemser, Ger.*
Camphor (p.1665·3); glycol salicylate (p.44·3); benzyl nicotinate (p.21·2).
*Musculoskeletal and joint disorders; neuralgia; sprains.*

**Thesit** *Gepepharm, Ger.*
Lauromacrogol 400 (p.1412·3); mepivacaine hydrochloride (p.1381·2).
*Burns; insect stings; skin disorders.*

**Thesit P** *Gepepharm, Ger.†.*
Lauromacrogol 400 (p.1412·3); promethazine hydrochloride (p.439·1); prednisolone acetate (p.1108·1).
*Skin disorders.*

**Thevier** *GlaxoSmithKline, Ger.*
Levothyroxine sodium (p.1600·1).
*Hypothyroidism.*

**Thex Forte** *Lee, USA.*
Vitamin B and C preparation (p.1417·1).

**Thiaben** *UCI, Braz.*
Tiabendazole (p.114·2).
*Nematode infections.*

**Thiabena** *UCI, Braz.*
Tiabendazole (p.114·2); neomycin sulfate (p.235·1).
*Skin infections.*

**Thiabet** *Wolff, Ger.*
Metformin hydrochloride (p.342·3).
*Diabetes mellitus.*

**Thiacomin** *Medichrom, Gr.*
Thiocolchicoside (p.1395·2).
*Muscle spasm.*

**Thiamcin** *General Drugs, Thai.*
Thiamphenicol (p.269·2).
*Bacterial infections.*

**Thiaminose** *Climax, Braz.*
Ascorbic acid (p.1460·2); thiamine hydrochloride (p.1455·1).
*Nutritional supplement.*

**Thianax** *Cazi, Braz.*
Tiabendazole (p.114·2).
*Worm infections.*

**Thiavit** *Julphar, UAE.*
Thiamine hydrochloride (p.1455·1).
*Vitamin $B_1$ deficiency.*

**Thiazid-comp** *Wolff, Ger.*
Triamterene (p.1016·2); hydrochlorothiazide (p.933·2).
*Hypertension; oedema.*

**Thick & Easy**
*Hormel, Hong Kong; Hormel, Singapore.*
Food thickener (p.1417·1).
*Dysphagia.*

**Thickened Juice** *Baxter, NZ; Nutricia, NZ.*
Nutritional supplement (p.1417·1).
*Dysphagia.*

**Thierry** *Makara, Austria†.*
Fennel oil (p.1687·3); purified honey (p.1434·2).
*Catarrh; colds; coughs.*

**Thilo Tears** *Bournonville, Belg.†.*
Carbomer (p.1577·2).
*Dry eyes.*

**Thilo Wet** *Alcon, Austria†.*
A wetting solution for contact lenses (p.1164·2).

**Thiloadren** *Alcon, Austria.*
Dipivefrine hydrochloride (p.1681·2); pilocarpine hydrochloride (p.1495·1).
*Glaucoma.*

**Thiloadren N** *Alcon, Ger.*
Dipivefrine hydrochloride (p.1681·2); pilocarpine hydrochloride (p.1495·1).
*Glaucoma.*

**Thilocanfol** *Alcon, Ger.*
Azidamfenicol (p.159·1).
*Bacterial eye infections.*

**Thilocanfol C** *Alcon, Ger.*
Chloramphenicol (p.185·1).
*Bacterial eye infections.*

**Thilocof** *Alkon (Αλκον), Gr.*
Chloramphenicol (p.185·1).
*Eye infections.*

**Thilocombin**
*Note. This name is used for preparations of different composition.*
*Alcon, Austria†.*
Theophylline (p.798·3); heptaminol (p.1697·1) or heptaminol hydrochloride (p.1697·1); nicotinyl alcohol (p.966·1) or nicotinyl alcohol tartrate (p.966·2).
*Angina pectoris; migraine; peripheral, coronary, and cerebral vascular disorders; thromboembolic disorders.*

*Alkon (Αλκον), Gr.*
Dipivefrine hydrochloride (p.1681·2); pilocarpine (p.1494·3).
*Glaucoma.*

**Thilodexine** *Pharmex (Φαρμεξ), Gr.*
Dexamethasone sodium metasulfobenzoate (p.1097·2).
*Inflammatory eye disorders.*

**Thilodigon**
*Alcon, Austria; Alcon, Ger.*
Guanethidine monosulfate (p.926·3); dipivefrine hydrochloride (p.1681·2).
*Glaucoma.*

**Thilodrin** *Alkon (Αλκον), Gr.*
Dipivefrine hydrochloride (p.1681·2).
*Glaucoma.*

**Thilogel** *Alkon (Αλκον), Gr.*
Carbomer (p.1577·2).
*Dry eyes.*

**Thilol** *Pharmex (Φαρμεξ), Gr.*
Trifluridine (p.655·3).
*Herpes simplex infections in the eye.*

**Thilo-micine** *Alkon (Αλκον), Gr.*
Tobramycin (p.271·2).
*Eye infections.*

**Thilomide** *Alkon (Αλκον), Gr.*
Lodoxamide trometamol (p.1707·3).
*Allergic conjunctivitis.*

**Thilorbin** *Alcon, Ger.*
Oxybuprocaine hydrochloride (p.1382·1); fluorescein sodium (p.1689·1).
*Ophthalmic procedures.*

**Thilo-Tears**
*Alcon, Ger.; Alcon, Switz.†.*
Carbomer (p.1577·2).
*Dry eyes.*

**Thilotim** *Alkon (Αλκον), Gr.*
Timolol maleate (p.1012·2).
*Glaucoma.*

**Thiloxedine** *Pharmex (Φαρμεξ), Gr.*
Dexamethasone (p.1097·1).
*Topical corticosteroid.*

**Thinz** *Aspen, S.Afr.*
Cathine hydrochloride (p.1585·2).
*Obesity.*

**Thiobitum** *Riemser, Ger.*
Ichthammol (p.1148·2).
*Skin disorders.*

**Thioctacid**
*Asta Medica, Austria; Viatris, Ger.*
Thioctic acid (p.1754·3) or trometamol thioctate (p.1754·3).
*Diabetic neuropathy.*

**Thiodantol** *Rekah, Israel.*
Isothipendyl hydrochloride (p.435·2).
*Skin irritation.*

**Thiodeol** *Breves, Braz.†.*
Sulfogaiacol (p.1131·1); iodine (p.1598·1); adrenal extract; calcium glycerophosphate (p.1225·2); neroli oil (p.1719·2).
*Respiratory-tract disorders.*

**Thioderon** *Shionogi, Jpn.*
Mepitiostane (p.1559·1).
*Breast cancer; renal anaemia.*

**Thiogamma** *Worwag, Ger.*
Meglumine thioctate or thioctic acid (p.1754·3).
*Diabetic neuropathy.*

**Thiola**
*Sigma, Austral.; Santen, Hong Kong; Coop. Farm., Ital.; Mission Pharmacal, USA.*
Tiopronin (p.1054·3).
*Cataract; liver disorders; mercury poisoning; prevention of cystine renal calculi.*

**Thiomed** *Medifive, Thai.*
Thioridazine hydrochloride (p.724·2).
*Anxiety; mania; schizophrenia.*

**Thiomucase** *Farmasa, Braz.*
Mucopolysaccharidase (p.1755·1); amylase (p.1654·2); chymotrypsin (p.1671·2).
*Oedema.*

**Thionembutal** *Abbott, Braz.*
Thiopental sodium (p.1309·1).
*General anaesthesia.*

**Thiopentax** *Cristalia, Braz.*
Thiopental sodium (p.1309·1).
*General anaesthesia.*

**Thiophenicol** *Sanofi Synthelabo, Fr.*
Thiamphenicol (p.269·2) or thiamphenicol glycinate hydrochloride (p.269·2).
*Bacterial infections.*

**Thioplex**
*Wyeth Lederle, Ital.; Amgen, USA.*
Thiotepa (p.588·1).
*Malignant neoplasms.*

**Thiopon** *Amido, Fr.†.*
Thiophenic oil.
*Respiratory-tract inflammation.*

**Thiopon Balsamique** *Amido, Fr.†.*
Thiophenic oil; eucalyptus oil (p.1686·2); pine oil; niaouli oil (p.1719·3).
*Upper respiratory-tract infections.*

**Thiopon Pantothenique** *Amido, Fr.†.*
Thiophenic oil; calcium pantothenate (p.1442·3).
*Respiratory-tract inflammation.*

**Thioprine**
*Alphapharm, Austral.; Pacific, NZ.*
Azathioprine (p.1349·1).
*Auto-immune disorders; transplant rejection.*

**Thioril** *Torrent, India.*
Thioridazine hydrochloride (p.724·2).
*Schizophrenia.*

**Thiorubrol** *Adroka, Switz.*
*Bath additive*†: Sodium thioricinol sulfonate; sodium thiosulfate (p.1053·3); sodium sulfate (p.1290·1).
*Musculoskeletal and joint disorders; skin disorders.*
*Bath oil:* Trolamine thioricinol sulfate.
*Muscle and joint pain; skin disorders.*

**Thiosan** *Azevedos, Port.*
Sulfiram (p.1510·1).
*Pediculosis; scabies.*

**Thiosedal** *Zyma, Fr.*†.
Ethylmorphine hydrochloride (p.37·3); hyoscyamus (p.485·2); sulfogaiacol (p.1131·1).
*Coughs.*

**Thiosept** *Terrapharm, Austria.*
Shale oil.
*Hyperhidrosis; inflammation; musculoskeletal and joint disorders; peripheral vascular disorders; skin disorders.*

**Thiosia** *Asian Pharm, Thai.*
Thioridazine hydrochloride (p.724·2).
*Anxiety; depression.*

**Thiosol** *Coop. Farm., Ital.*
Tiopronin (p.1054·3).
*Respiratory-tract congestion.*

**Thiospot** *Dermoteca, Port.*
Thiolin; ascorbyl palmitate (p.1168·2); tartaric acid (p.1752·1); salicylic acid (p.1157·1).
*Hyperpigmentation disorders.*

**Thiosulfil Forte** *Wyeth-Ayerst, USA*†.
Sulfamethizole (p.260·3).
*Urinary-tract infections.*

**Thiovalone** *Pfizer, Fr.*
Tixocortol pivalate (p.1110·1); chlorhexidine gluconate (p.1173·2).
*Inflammation of the mouth and throat.*

**Thioxene** *Esseti, Ital.*
Glutathione sodium (p.1040·3).
*Alcohol or drug poisoning; ionising radiation damage.*

**Thiozine** *Pinewood, Irl.*
Thioridazine hydrochloride (p.724·2).
*Anxiety; behaviour disorders; psychoses; senile confusion; tension.*

**Thiprasolan** *Bajer, Arg.*
Alprazolam (p.668·3).
*Anxiety; depression.*

**Thirial** *Dolisos, Fr.*†.
Garlic (p.1691·1).
*Circulatory disorders.*

**Thixit** *Douglas, NZ.*
Tiotixene hydrochloride (p.725·2).
*Psychoses.*

**Thohelur I** *Truw, Ger.*†.
Mineral preparation (p.1417·1).

**Thohelur II** *Truw, Ger.*†.
Mineral preparation with colecalciferol (p.1417·1).

**Thomaeamin X E** *DeltaSelect, Ger.*
Amino-acid, electrolyte, and xylitol infusion (p.1417·1).
*Parenteral nutrition.*

**Thomaeamin hepar** *DeltaSelect, Ger.*
Amino-acid infusion (p.1417·1).
*Parenteral nutrition in liver failure.*

**Thomaeamin n** *DeltaSelect, Ger.*
Amino-acid infusion with or without electrolytes (p.1417·1).
*Parenteral nutrition.*

**Thomaedex 40** *Delta, Ger.*†.
Dextran 40 (p.745·3) in sodium chloride.
*Plasma volume expansion; thrombosis prophylaxis; vascular disorders.*

**Thomaedex 60** *Delta, Ger.*†.
Dextran 60 (p.746·1) in sodium chloride.
*Plasma volume expansion; thrombosis prophylaxis.*

**Thomaegelin** *DeltaSelect, Ger.*
Gelatin polysuccinate (p.754·3) in Ringer acetate.
*Hypovolaemia.*

**Thomaejonin** *DeltaSelect, Ger.*
A range of electrolyte infusions with or without carbohydrate (p.1217·1).
*Fluid and electrolyte disorders.*

**Thomaemannit** *DeltaSelect, Ger.*
Mannitol (p.950·2).
*Fluid retention; renal failure.*

**Thomapyrin**
*Boehringer Ingelheim, Austria; Boehringer Ingelheim, Ger.*
Aspirin (p.15·1); paracetamol (p.76·2); caffeine (p.782·1).
*Fever; pain.*

**Thomapyrin akut** *Boehringer Ingelheim, Ger.*
Aspirin (p.15·1).
*Fever; pain.*

**Thomapyrin C** *Boehringer Ingelheim, Ger.*
Aspirin (p.15·1); paracetamol (p.76·2); ascorbic acid (p.1460·2).
*Pain.*

**Thomapyrin mit Vitamin C** *Boehringer Ingelheim, Austria.*
Aspirin (p.15·1); paracetamol (p.76·2); ascorbic acid (p.1460·2).
*Cold symptoms.*

**Thomapyrine** *Boehringer Ingelheim, Switz.*
Aspirin (p.15·1); paracetamol (p.76·2); caffeine (p.782·1).
*Fever; pain.*

**Thomasin** *Apogepha, Ger.*
Etilefrine hydrochloride (p.914·1).
*Hypotension.*

**Thombran** *Boehringer Ingelheim, Ger.*
Trazodone hydrochloride (p.319·1).
*Depression.*

**Thorazine** *SmithKline Beecham, USA.*
Chlorpromazine (p.675·1) or chlorpromazine hydrochloride (p.675·2).
*Acute intermittent porphyria; adjunct in tetanus; bipolar disorder; hiccups; nausea and vomiting; premedication; psychoses; severe behavioural disorders in children.*

**THR** *Seroyal, Canad.*†.
Vitamin E, magnesium, and potassium (p.1417·1).

**Threamine DM** *Barre-National, USA*†.
Phenylpropanolamine hydrochloride (p.1127·3); chlorphenamine maleate (p.427·3); dextromethorphan hydrobromide (p.1117·3).
*Coughs and cold symptoms.*

**Threchop** *Collins, Mex.*
Diiodohydroxyquinoline (p.603·3); furazolidone (p.605·2); homatropine (p.483·2).
*Amoebic dysentery.*

**Threolone** *Abic, Israel.*
Prednisolone (p.1108·1); chloramphenicol (p.185·1).
*Infected skin disorders.*

**Threptin Micromix** *Raptakos, India.*
Nutritional supplement (p.1417·1).

**Thriazol** *Alpharma, Mex.*
Co-trimoxazole (p.199·3).
*Bacterial infections.*

**Thrioniren** *Antor, Gr.*
Nimodipine (p.972·3).
*Neurological deficit following subarachnoid haemorrhage.*

**Thriostaxil** *Medinova (Μεντνοβα), Gr.*
Roxithromycin (p.254·2).
*Bacterial infections.*

**Thriusedon** *Zekides, Gr.*
Lisinopril (p.946·3).
*Heart failure; hypertension; myocardial infarction.*

**Throat** *Dumex-Alpharma, Denm.*†.
Benzoic acid (p.1169·3); lidocaine (p.1377·3); menthol (p.1711·3).
*Stomatitis.*

**Throat Discs** *SmithKline Beecham, USA.*
Capsicum (p.1667·1); peppermint oil (p.1283·2); liquid paraffin (p.1479·1).
*Sore throat.*

**Throat Lozenges**
*Note. This name is used for preparations of different composition.*
*Novopharm, Canad.*
Benzocaine (p.1370·3); cetylpyridinium chloride (p.1173·1).
*Novopharm, Canad.*
Cetylpyridinium chloride (p.1173·1).
*Stanley, Canad.*†.
Hexylresorcinol (p.1182·1).

**Throaties Anti-Bacterial Pastilles** *Ernest Jackson, UK.*
Amylmetacresol (p.1168·2).
*Sore throat.*

**Throaties Pastilles** *Ernest Jackson, UK.*
*Blackcurrant flavour:* Honey (p.1434·2); menthol (p.1711·3).
*Original flavour:* Benzoin tincture (p.1751·1); menthol (p.1711·3).
*Coughs; sore throat.*

**Thrombace** *Drossapharm, Switz.*†.
Aloxiprin (p.14·1).
*Thromboembolic disorders.*

**Thrombace Neo** *Drossapharm, Switz.*
Aspirin (p.15·1).
*Thromboembolism prophylaxis.*

**Thrombareduct** *Azupharma, Ger.*
Heparin sodium (p.928·1).
*Soft-tissue disorders; soft-tissue injury.*

**Thrombate**
*Bayer, Canad.; Bayer Biological, Hong Kong*†.
Antithrombin III (p.742·2).
*Antithrombin III deficiency.*

**Thrombate III** *Bayer, USA.*
Antithrombin III (p.742·2).
*Antithrombin III deficiency.*

**Thrombhibin** *Immuno, Austria.*
Antithrombin III (p.742·2).
*Antithrombin III deficiency.*

**Thrombinar** *Jones, USA.*
Thrombin (p.760·1).
*Minor haemorrhage.*

**Thrombo AS** *Merck, Chile.*
Aspirin (p.15·1).
*Thromboembolism prophylaxis.*

**Thrombo ASS** *Lannacher, Austria.*
Aspirin (p.15·1).
*Thrombosis prophylaxis.*

**Thrombocid**
*Note. This name is used for preparations of different composition.*
*Sigmapharm, Austria; Bene, Ger.; Neo-Farmaceutica, Port.; Milupa, Switz.*
*Ointment:* Pentosan polysulfate sodium (p.979·2); guaiazulene (p.1696·2); thymol (p.1194·2).
*Burns; insect bites; soft-tissue disorders; superficial vascular disorders.*
*Bene, Ger.; Bene-Chemie, Hong Kong; Neo-Farmaceutica, Port.*
*Suppositories:* Pentosan polysulfate sodium (p.979·2); guaiazulene (p.1696·2).
*Anorectal disorders.*
*Bene, Ger.; Neo-Farmaceutica, Port.; Milupa, Switz.*
*Topical gel:* Pentosan polysulfate sodium (p.979·2); rosemary oil (p.1740·2); pumilio pine oil (p.1737·1); melissa oil (p.1711·2).
*Soft-tissue disorders; superficial vascular disorders.*
*Lacer, Spain.*
Pentosan polysulfate sodium (p.979·2).
Formerly contained pentosan polysulfate sodium and thymol.
*Burns; haemorrhoids; peripheral vascular disorders; soft-tissue disorders.*

**Thrombocoll** *Johnson & Johnson, Ger.*†.
Thrombin (p.760·1).
*Haemorrhage.*

**Thrombodine** *Lannacher, Austria.*
Ticlopidine hydrochloride (p.1011·2).
*Thrombosis prophylaxis.*

**Thrombogen** *Johnson & Johnson Medical, USA.*
Thrombin (p.760·1).
*Bleeding from small blood vessels.*

**Thrombohexal** *Hexal, Austria.*
Dipyridamole (p.903·1); aspirin (p.15·1).
*Glomerulonephritis; peripheral arterial disorders.*

**Thrombophob**
*Note. This name is used for preparations of different composition.*
*Ebewe, Austria; German Remedies, India; Hoechst Marion Roussel, S.Afr.*†.
*Ointment:* Heparin (p.927·3) or heparin sodium (p.928·1); benzyl nicotinate (p.21·2).
*Soft-tissue injuries; superficial vascular disorders.*
*Ebewe, Austria; Abbott, Ger.; German Remedies, India; Aventis, S.Afr.*
*Topical gel:* Heparin (p.927·3) or heparin sodium (p.928·1).
*Soft-tissue injuries; superficial vascular disorders.*

**Thrombophob-S** *Ebewe, Austria.*
Heparin sodium (p.928·1).
*Soft-tissue injury; superficial vascular disorders.*

**Thrombosantin** *Boehringer Ingelheim, Austria.*
Dipyridamole (p.903·1); aspirin (p.15·1).
*Glomerulonephritis; peripheral vascular disorders.*

**Thrombostat**
*Pfizer, Austral.; Pfizer, Canad.; Pfizer, NZ; Parke, Davis, Singapore*†*; Parke, Davis, USA.*
Thrombin (p.760·1).
*Minor haemorrhage.*

**Thrombotrol** *CSL, NZ.*
Antithrombin III (p.742·2).
*Antithrombin III deficiency.*

**Thrombotrol-VF** *CSL, Austral.*
Antithrombin III (p.742·2).
*Antithrombin III deficiency.*

**Thuja Med Complex** *Dynamit, Austria.*
Homoeopathic preparation.

**Thuja Oligoplex** *Madaus, Ger.*
Homoeopathic preparation.

**Thujaderm** *Knop, Chile.*
Thuja (p.1755·1).
*Warts.*

**Thunas Bilettes** *Thuna, Canad.*†.
Aloin (p.1248·3); cascara (p.1255·1); phenolphthalein (p.1284·1).

**Thunas Eye Drops** *Thuna, Canad.*
Boric acid (p.1662·1); borax (p.1661·3).

**Thunas Hyperacidity Tablets** *Thuna, Canad.*
Magnesium hydroxide (p.1272·2); aluminium hydroxide-magnesium carbonate co-dried gel (p.1250·1); simeticone (p.1289·2).

**Thunas Laxative** *Thuna, Canad.*
Cascara (p.1255·1); senna (p.1288·2); bryony; fennel (p.1687·2); liquorice (p.1270·2); juglans; leptandra.

**Thunas Pile** *Thuna, Canad.*
Benzocaine (p.1370·3); bismuth subcarbonate (p.1252·1); ephedrine sulfate (p.1120·1); zinc oxide (p.1163·2).
*Haemorrhoids.*

**Thunas Salve for Rheumatic Pains** *Thuna, Canad.*
Methyl salicylate (p.59·3); camphor (p.1665·3); menthol (p.1711·3).

**Thunas Tab for Menstrual Pain** *Thuna, Canad.*
Motherwort (p.1717·1); senecio (p.1743·1); sodium salicylate (p.90·1); teucrium scorodonia; viburnum.

**Thybon** *Henning, Ger.*
Liothyronine hydrochloride (p.1602·2).
*Hypothyroidism.*

**Thycapzol** *Gea, Denm.*
Thiamazole (p.1603·3).
*Hyperthyroidism.*

**Thymi Syrup** *Vitamed, Israel.*
Thyme (p.1755·2).
*Coughs.*

**Thymian Erkaltungs-Bad** *Li-il, Ger.*
Thyme oil (p.1755·3).
*Bath additive; respiratory-tract disorders; skin disorders.*

**Thymi-Fips** *Lichtenstein, Ger.*†.
Thyme (p.1755·2).
*Respiratory-tract disorders.*

**Thymipin N** *Novartis Consumer, Ger.*
*Cream:* Thyme (p.1755·2); camphor (p.1665·3); eucalyptus oil (p.1686·2).
*Syrup; oral drops; suppositories:* Thyme (p.1755·2).
*Bronchitis; catarrh; coughs.*

**Thymiverlan** *Verla, Ger.*
Thyme (p.1755·2).
*Respiratory-tract disorders.*

**Thymodrosin** *Gubler, Switz.*†.
Guaifenesin (p.1122·1); codeine phosphate (p.27·1); thyme (p.1755·2); drosera (p.1683·1); plantaginis (p.1738·2); castanea vulgaris; ipecacuanha (p.1122·3); belladonna (p.479·1); liquorice (p.1270·2).
*Coughs.*

**Thymodrosin N** *Gubler, Switz.*
Guaifenesin (p.1122·1); thyme (p.1755·2); drosera (p.1683·1); plantaginis (p.1738·2); liquorice (p.1270·2).
*Respiratory-tract disorders.*

**Thymo-Glanduretten** *Biosyn, Ger.*
Bovine thymus extract (p.1756·1).
*Immunotherapy.*

**Thymoglobulin**
*Imtix, Ger.; IFET (ΙΦΕΤ), Gr.*
An antithymocyte immunoglobulin (p.1348·3).
*Aplastic anaemia; graft-versus-host disease; transplant rejection.*

**Thymoglobuline**
*Imtix, Belg.*†*; Aventis Pasteur, Braz.; Imtix, Denm.; Imtix, Fr.; Pasteur Merieux, Hong Kong*†*; Imtix Sangstat, Israel; Imtix, Ital.; Sangstat, Neth.; Aventis, S.Afr.; Sangstat, Singapore; Pacific Biosciences, Singapore; Imtix, Switz.; Aventis Pasteur, Thai.*
An antithymocyte immunoglobulin (rabbit) (p.1348·3).
*Aplastic anaemia; graft-versus-host disease; transplant rejection.*

**Thymoject** *Biosyn, Ger.*
Bovine thymus extract (p.1756·1).
*Immunological disorders.*

**Thymol Mouthwash Red**
*Pharmacia Upjohn, Austral.*†*; Orion, NZ.*
Thymol (p.1194·2); menthol (p.1711·3).
*Halitosis; mouth and throat infections.*

**Thymophysin** *CytoChemia, Ger.*
Thymus extract (p.1756·1).
*Immunotherapy.*

**Thymorell** *Sanorell, Ger.*
Homoeopathic preparation.

**Thymoseptine** *Tilman, Belg.*
Thyme (p.1755·2); wild thyme.
*Respiratory-tract disorders; sore throat.*

**Thymoval** *Smetana, Austria.*
Cowslip (p.1735·1); valerian (p.1762·2); thyme (p.1755·2).
*Coughs.*

**Thymowied** *Wiedemann, Ger.*
Calf thymus extract (p.1756·1).
*Immunotherapy.*

**Thymunes** *Eagle, Austral.*†.
Thymus (p.1756·1).

**Thym-Uvocal** *Strathmann, Ger.*
Calf thymus extract (p.1756·1).
*Immunotherapy.*

**Thypinone** *Abbott, USA*†.
Protirelin (p.1337·3).
*Diagnostic assessment of thyroid function.*

**Thyradin-S** *Teikoku, Jpn.*
Levothyroxine sodium (p.1600·1).
*Goitre; hypothyroidism.*

**Thyrar** *Rhone-Poulenc Rorer, USA*†.
Thyroid (bovine) (p.1604·2).
*Hypothyroidism; thyroid cancer.*

**Thyrax**
*Organon, Belg.; Nourypharma, Neth.; Organon, Port.; Organon, Spain*†.
Levothyroxine sodium (p.1600·1).
*Diagnostic suppression of thyroid activity; hypothyroidism; thyroid cancer.*

**Thyrefact**
*Aventis, Denm.*†*; Hoechst Marion Roussel, Swed.*†.
Protirelin (p.1337·3).
*Test of thyroid or pituitary-hypothalamic function; thyroid disorders.*

**Thyrel-TRH** *Ferring, USA*†.
Protirelin (p.1337·3).
Formerly called Relefact TRH.
*Diagnosis of thyroid dysfunction.*

**Thyreocomb N** *Berlin-Chemie, Ger.*
Levothyroxine (p.1601·3); potassium iodide (p.1598·1).
*Iodine-deficiency disorders.*

**Thyreogutt** *Austroplant, Austria.*
Motherwort (p.1717·1); lycopus europaeus.
*Hyperthyroidism; mastalgia; tachycardia.*

**Thyreogutt mono** *Schwabe, Ger.*
Motherwort (p.1717·1).
*Mastalgia; mild hyperthyroidism.*

**thyreo-loges comp** *Loges, Ger.*
Homoeopathic preparation.

**thyreo-loges N** *Loges, Ger.*
Lycopus europaeus.
*Hyperthyroidism; mastalgia.*

**Thyreo-Pasc N** *Pascoe, Ger.*
Homoeopathic preparation.

**Thyreostat II** *Herbrand, Ger.; Berlin-Chemie, Ger.*
Propylthiouracil (p.1603·1).
*Hyperthyroidism.*

**Thyreotom** *Berlin-Chemie, Ger.*
Liothyronine (p.1602·2); levothyroxine (p.1601·3).
*Hypothyroidism.*

**Thyrex** *Biochemie, Austria.*
Levothyroxine sodium (p.1600·1).
*Hypothyroidism.*

**Thyro-4** *Faran, Gr.*
Levothyroxine sodium (p.1600·1).
*Hypothyroidism.*

**Thyro-Block**
*Carter Horner, Canad.; Wallace, USA.*
Potassium iodide (p.1598·1).
*Blockade of thyroid uptake of radioiodine.*

**Thyrogen**
*Biobras, Braz.; Genzyme, Denm.; Genzyme, Ger.; Genzyme, Israel; Genzyme, Ital.; Genzyme, Norw.; Genzyme, Spain; Nycomed, Swed.; Genzyme, UK; Genzyme, USA.*
Thyrotropin alfa (p.1341·1).
*Detection of thyroid remnants and thyroid cancer in post-thyroidectomy patients; measurement of serum thyroglobulin.*

**Thyrohormone** *Ni-The, Gr.*
Levothyroxine sodium (p.1600·1).
*Hypothyroidism.*

**Thyrolar** *Forest Pharmaceuticals, USA.*
Liothyronine sodium (p.1602·2); levothyroxine sodium (p.1600·1).
*Evaluation of thyroid function; hypothyroidism; TSH suppression.*

**Thyroliberin** *Merck, Ger.*
Protirelin (p.1337·3).
*Assessment of pituitary and thyroid function.*

**Thyroliberin TRH** *Merck, Austria.*
Protirelin (p.1337·3).
*Test for thyroid-pituitary function.*

**Thyronajod** *Henning, Ger.*
Levothyroxine sodium (p.1600·1); potassium iodide (p.1598·1).
*Hypothyroidism.*

**Thyrosit** *Sriprasit, Thai.*
Levothyroxine sodium (p.1600·1).
*Hypothyroidism.*

**Thyrostat** *Ni-The, Gr.*
Carbimazole (p.1596·2).
*Hyperthyroidism.*

**Thyrotardin N** *Henning, Ger.*
Liothyronine hydrochloride (p.1602·2).
*Hypothyroidism.*

**Thyrozol**
*Merck, Ger.; Merck, Singapore.*
Thiamazole (p.1603·3).
*Hyperthyroidism.*

**Thytropar**
*USV, Israel; Armour, USA†.*
Thyrotrophin (p.1341·1).
*Diagnosis of thyroid disorders.*

**TI Baby Natural** *Fischer, USA.*
*SPF 16:* Titanium dioxide (p.1160·3).
*Sunscreen.*

**TI Lite** *Fischer, USA.*
*SPF 15:* Octinoxate (p.1154·3); titanium dioxide (p.1160·3).
*Sunscreen.*

**TI Screen** *Pedinol, USA.*
*SPF 30:* Octinoxate (p.1154·3); oxybenzone (p.1154·3); octisalate (p.1154·3); octocrilene (p.1154·3).
*SPF 8; SPF 15:* Octinoxate (p.1154·3); oxybenzone (p.1154·3).
*Sunscreen.*

**TI Screen Natural** *Pedinol, USA.*
*SPF 16:* Titanium dioxide (p.1160·3).
*Sunscreen.*

**TI Screen Sunless** *Pedinol, USA.*
*SPF 17; SPF 23:* Octinoxate (p.1154·3); oxybenzone (p.1154·3).
*Sunscreen.*

**Tiabenzol** *Teuto, Braz.*
Tiabendazole (p.114·2).
*Worm infections.*

**Tiabexol** *Offenbach, Mex.*
Cyanocobalamin (p.1458·2); thiamine (p.1455·2).
*Vitamin supplement.*

**Tiabiose** *UCI, Braz.†.*
Tiabendazole (p.114·2).
*Nematode infections.*

**Tiabrenolo** *NCSN, Ital.†.*
Tiadenol (p.1011·2).
*Hyperlipidaemias.*

**Tiacid** *Draxis, Canad.*
Salicylic acid (p.1157·1); lactic acid (p.1704·1).

**Tiaden**
*Note. This name is used for preparations of different composition.*
*Gap, Gr.*
Amiloride hydrochloride (p.858·2); hydrochlorothiazide (p.933·2).
*Heart failure; hypertension; oedema.*

*Malesci, Ital.†.*
Tiadenol (p.1011·2).
*Hyperlipidaemias.*

**Tiadil**
*Zambon, Neth.; Basi, Port.*
Diltiazem hydrochloride (p.900·1).
*Hypertension.*

**Tiadilon** *Crinex, Fr.†.*
Arginine tidiacicate (p.1421·2).
*Liver disorders.*

**Tiadipona** *Abbott, Spain.*
Bentazepam (p.671·3).
*Anxiety; insomnia.*

**Tiadyl** *Abbott, Arg.*
Candesartan cilexetil (p.878·3).
*Hypertension.*

**Tiadyl Plus** *Abbott, Arg.*
Candesartan cilexetil (p.878·3); hydrochlorothiazide (p.933·2).
*Hypertension.*

**Tiakem** *Vita, Ital.†.*
Diltiazem hydrochloride (p.900·1).
*Hypertension; ischaemic heart disease.*

**Tial** *Lindopharm, Ger.*
Tramadol hydrochloride (p.94·3).
*Pain.*

**Tiamate** *Hoechst Marion Roussel, USA†.*
Diltiazem malate (p.901·3).
*Angina pectoris; hypertension.*

**Tiamidexal** *Silanes, Mex.*
1 Ampoule, cyanocobalamin (p.1458·2); thiamine hydrochloride (p.1455·1); 1 ampoule, dexamethasone sodium phosphate (p.1097·2).
*Gout; musculoskeletal, joint, and peri-articular disorders; neuritis.*

**Tiamin** *Ducto, Braz.*
Vitamin B substances (p.1417·1).

**Tiaminal $B_{12}$** *Silanes, Mex.*
Cyanocobalamin (p.1458·2); thiamine hydrochloride (p.1455·1).
Lidocaine hydrochloride (p.1377·3) is included in this preparation to alleviate the pain of injection.
*Neuralgia; neuritis; vitamin B deficiencies.*

**Tiaminal $B_{12}$ Trivalente** *Silanes, Mex.*
Cyanocobalamin (p.1458·2) or hydroxocobalamin (p.1458·2); thiamine hydrochloride (p.1455·1); pyridoxine hydrochloride (p.1456·3).
*Neuralgia; neuritis; pernicious anaemia; vitamin B deficiencies.*

**Tiamol** *Optimapharma, Canad.*
Fluocinonide (p.1101·3).
*Skin disorders.*

**Tiamon Mono** *Temmler, Ger.*
Dihydrocodeine tartrate (p.34·3).
*Coughs.*

**Tiaplex** *Delta, Braz.*
Tiabendazole (p.114·2).
*Worm infections.*

**Tiapridal**
*Sanofi Synthelabo, Belg.; Sanofi Synthelabo, Braz.; Sanofi Synthelabo, Fr.; Sanofi Synthelabo, Hong Kong; Sanofi Synthelabo, Neth.; Sanofi Synthelabo, Port.; Sanofi Synthelabo, Singapore†; Synthelabo, Switz.*
Tiapride hydrochloride (p.725·1).
*Aggression; alcohol withdrawal syndrome; anxiety; behaviour disorders; movement disorders; pain.*

**Tiapridex** *Sanofi Synthelabo, Ger.*
Tiapride hydrochloride (p.725·1).
*Parkinsonism and other hyperkinetic disorders.*

**Tiaprizal** *Sanofi Synthelabo, Spain.*
Tiapride hydrochloride (p.725·1).
*Anxiety; attention-deficit hyperactivity disorder; movement disorders; nausea and vomiting.*

**Tiaprofen** *Bioprogress, Ital.*
Tiaprofenic acid (p.93·3).
*Inflammation; pain.*

**Tiaprorex** *Lampugnani, Ital.†.*
Tiaprofenic acid (p.93·3).
*Inflammation; pain.*

**Tiatral 100 SR** *Novartis, Switz.*
Aspirin (p.15·1).
*Thromboembolic disorders.*

**Tiaven** *Loren, Mex.*
Vitamin B substances (p.1417·1).

**Tiazac**
*Biovail, Canad.; Forest Pharmaceuticals, USA.*
Diltiazem hydrochloride (p.900·1).
*Angina pectoris; hypertension.*

**Tiazen** *Bioprogress, Ital.†.*
Diltiazem hydrochloride (p.900·1).
*Hypertension; ischaemic heart disease.*

**Tiazolidin** *Solvay, Ital.†.*
Timonacic (p.1756·2).
*Liver disorders.*

**Tiba** *Pharmaland, Thai.*
Gemfibrozil (p.923·1).
*Hyperlipidaemias.*

**Tiberal**
*Roche, Belg.; Roche, Fr.; Roche, Israel†; Roche, Ital.†; Roche, Mex.†; Roche, NZ; Roche, Switz.*
Ornidazole (p.612·2).
*Anaerobic bacterial infections; protozoal infections.*

**Tibifor** *Lisapharma, Ital.*
Cefaclor (p.167·1).
*Bacterial infections.*

**Tibinide** *Recip, Swed.*
Isoniazid (p.222·2).
*Tuberculosis.*

**Tibirim** *Ranbaxy, Thai.†.*
Rifampicin (p.250·2).
*Tuberculosis.*

**Tibirim INH** *Stancare, India.*
Rifampicin (p.250·2); isoniazid (p.222·2).
*Tuberculosis.*

**Tibitol** *Pharmaceutical Co, India.*
Ethambutol (p.212·2).
*Tuberculosis.*

**Tibofem** *Organon, Arg.*
Tibolone (p.1572·3).
*Menopausal disorders.*

**Tiburon** *Monot, Fr.†.*
Ibuprofen (p.45·3).
*Fever; musculoskeletal and joint disorders; pain; soft-tissue disorders.*

**Ticalma** *Kelemata, Ital.*
Valerian root (p.1762·2).
*Sedative.*

**Ticar**
*SmithKline Beecham, Canad.†; GlaxoSmithKline, USA.*
Ticarcillin sodium (p.270·2).
*Bacterial infections.*

**Ticarpen**
*GlaxoSmithKline, Fr.; SmithKline Beecham, Neth.; SmithKline Beecham, Spain.*
Ticarcillin sodium (p.270·2).
*Bacterial infections.*

**Ticdine** *Fascino, Thai.*
Ticlopidine hydrochloride (p.1011·2).
*Intermittent claudication; stroke prophylaxis; thromboembolism prophylaxis; unstable angina pectoris.*

**Tice** *Organon, USA.*
A BCG vaccine (p.1609·2).
*Active immunisation; bladder cancer.*

**Tickly Cough & Sore Throat Relief** *Herbal Concepts, UK.*
Hyssop; senega (p.1130·2); liquorice (p.1270·2).
*Coughs and cold symptoms; sore throat.*

**Ticlid**
*Sanofi Synthelabo, Arg.; Roche, Austral.; Sanofi Synthelabo, Belg.; Sanofi Synthelabo, Braz.; Roche, Canad.; Sanofi Synthelabo, Chile; Sanofi Synthelabo, Fr.; Sanofi Synthelabo, Gr.; Sanofi Synthelabo, Hong Kong; Sanofi Synthelabo, Malaysia; Syntex, Mex.; Sanofi Synthelabo, Norw.; Roche, NZ†; Sanofi Synthelabo, S.Afr.; Sanofi Synthelabo, Singapore; Sanofi Synthelabo, Swed.; Sanofi Winthrop, Switz.†; Sanofi Synthelabo, Thai.; Sanofi Synthelabo, UK†; Roche, USA.*
Ticlopidine hydrochloride (p.1011·2).
*Intermittent claudication; maintenance of extracorporeal circulation; thromboembolism prophylaxis.*

**Ticlidil** *CTI, Israel.*
Ticlopidine hydrochloride (p.1011·2).
*Stroke prophylaxis.*

**Ticlobal** *Baldacci, Braz.*
Ticlopidine hydrochloride (p.1011·2).
*Thromboembolism prophylaxis.*

**Ticlodix** *Vitoria, Port.*
Ticlopidine hydrochloride (p.1011·2).
*Thromboembolism prophylaxis.*

**Ticlodone**
*Sanofi Synthelabo, Austria; Gerolimatos (Γερολυματος), Gr.; Sigma-Tau, Ital.; Almirall, Spain.*
Ticlopidine hydrochloride (p.1011·2).
*Thromboembolism prophylaxis.*

**Ticlogi** *Ibirn, Ital.*
Ticlopidine hydrochloride (p.1011·2).
*Thrombosis prophylaxis.*

**Ticlomed** *Leurquin, Fr.*
Ticlopidine hydrochloride (p.1011·2).
*Intermittent claudication; maintenance of extracorporeal circulation; thrombosis prophylaxis.*

**Ticlop** *Zydus, India.*
Ticlopidine hydrochloride (p.1011·2).
*Thrombosis.*

**Ticlopat** *Biosaude, Port.*
Ticlopidine hydrochloride (p.1011·2).
*Intermittent claudication; maintenance of extracorporeal circulation; stroke prophylaxis; thromboembolism prophylaxis.*

**Ticloproge** *Proge, Ital.*
Ticlopidine hydrochloride (p.1011·2).
*Thrombosis prophylaxis.*

**Ticoflex** *Uno, Ital.*
Naproxen aminobutanol (p.65·3).
*Gout; musculoskeletal, joint, peri-articular, and soft-tissue disorders; neuralgias.*

**Ticolcin** *Tecnofarma, Mex.*
Colchicine (p.415·1).
*Gout; liver cirrhosis.*

**Ticon** *Hauck, USA.*
Trimethobenzamide hydrochloride (p.442·2).
*Nausea and vomiting.*

**Ticovac** *Baxter, Fr.†.*
A tick-borne encephalitis vaccine (p.1642·1).
*Active immunisation.*

**Tidact**
*YSP, Malaysia; Yung Shin, Singapore.*
Clindamycin hydrochloride (p.194·2).
*Bacterial infections.*

**Tiddy** *Sriprasit, Thai.*
Multivitamin and mineral preparation with lysine (p.1417·1).

**Tidigesic** *Sun, India.*
Buprenorphine (p.21·3).
*Pain.*

**Tielle**
*Johnson & Johnson, Ger.; Ethicon, Ital.; Johnson & Johnson Medical, UK.*
Foamed hydrogel.
*Skin ulcers; wounds.*

**Tiempe** *DDSA Pharmaceuticals, UK†.*
Trimethoprim (p.272·2).

**Tienam**
*Merck Sharp & Dohme, Belg.; Merck Sharp & Dohme, Braz.; Merck Sharp & Dohme, Chile; Merck Sharp & Dohme, Denm.; Merck Sharp & Dohme, Fin.; Merck Sharp & Dohme-Chibret, Fr.; Merck Sharp & Dohme, Hong Kong; Merck Sharp & Dohme, Israel; Merck Sharp & Dohme, Ital.; Merck Sharp & Dohme, Malaysia; Merck Sharp & Dohme, Mex.; Merck Sharp & Dohme, Neth.; Merck Sharp & Dohme, Norw.; Merck Sharp & Dohme, Port.; Merck Sharp & Dohme, S.Afr.; Merck Sharp & Dohme, Singapore; Merck Sharp & Dohme, Spain; Merck Sharp & Dohme, Swed.; Merck Sharp & Dohme, Switz.; Merck Sharp & Dohme, Thai.*
Imipenem (p.221·1); cilastatin sodium (p.188·1).
Lidocaine hydrochloride (p.1377·3) may be included in the intramuscular injection to alleviate the pain of injection.
*Bacterial infections.*

**Tienor** *Farmaka, Ital.*
Clotiazepam (p.685·2).
*Anxiety; insomnia.*

**Tierlite** *Bros, Gr.*
Fluconazole (p.398·1).
*Fungal infections.*

**Tifell** *Bucca, Spain.*
Cineole (p.1672·1); cresol (p.1177·3); eugenol (p.1686·2); formaldehyde (p.1179·3).
*Mouth infections.*

**Tifen** *Andromaco, Chile.*
Ibuprofen (p.45·3).
*Fever; inflammation; pain.*

**Tifenso** *Clinced, Austria†.*
Benzyl nicotinate (p.21·2); choline salicylate (p.26·2).

**Tiffy**
*Note. This name is used for preparations of different composition.*
*Medochemie, Hong Kong.*
Paracetamol (p.76·2).
*Fever; pain.*

*Nakorn, Thai.*
*Syrup:* Paracetamol (p.76·2); chlorphenamine maleate (p.427·3); phenylephrine hydrochloride (p.1126·3).
Formerly contained paracetamol, phenylpropanolamine hydrochloride, chlorphenamine maleate, and phenylephrine hydrochloride.
*Tablets:* Paracetamol (p.76·2); chlorphenamine maleate (p.427·3); phenylpropanolamine hydrochloride (p.1127·3).
*Cold and influenza symptoms; hay fever.*

**Tiffy Fu** *Nakorn, Thai.*
Paracetamol (p.76·2); chlorphenamine maleate (p.427·3); pseudoephedrine hydrochloride (p.1129·2).
*Cold symptoms.*

**Tiffyrub** *Nakorn, Thai.*
Menthol (p.1711·3); camphor (p.1665·3); turpentine oil (p.1760·1); eucalyptus oil (p.1686·2); nutmeg oil (p.1722·3).
*Cold symptoms; coughs; nasal congestion.*

**Tifox** *Chong Kun Dang, Ital.*
Cefoxitin sodium (p.177·2).
Lidocaine hydrochloride (p.1377·3) is included in the intramuscular injection to alleviate the pain of injection.
*Gram-negative bacterial infections.*

**Tigan**
*Note. This name is used for preparations of different composition.*
*SmithKline Beecham, Mex.†.*
Trimethobenzamide (p.442·2).

*Roberts, USA.*
*Suppositories:* Trimethobenzamide hydrochloride (p.442·2); benzocaine (p.1370·3).
*Nausea and vomiting.*

*Roberts, USA; Monarch, USA.*
*Capsules; injection:* Trimethobenzamide hydrochloride (p.442·2).
*Nausea and vomiting.*

**Tigason**
*Roche, Braz.†; Roche, Ital.†; Chugai, Jpn.*
Etretinate (p.1147·1).
*Keratinisation disorders; oral lichen planus; psoriasis.*

**Tigel IRM** *Koni-Cofarm, Chile.*
Coal tar (p.1159·2).
*Scalp disorders.*

**Tiger Balm** *SSL, UK.*
Cajuput oil (p.1664·1); camphor (p.1665·3); clove oil (p.1673·3); menthol (p.1711·3).
*Musculoskeletal pain.*

**Tiger Balm Liquid** *LRC Products, UK†.*
Cajuput oil (p.1664·1); camphor (p.1665·3); cinnamon oil (p.1672·2); clove oil (p.1673·3); menthol (p.1711·3); peppermint oil (p.1283·2).
*Muscle ache.*

**Tiger Balm Red** *Haw Par, Canad.*
Camphor (p.1665·3); menthol (p.1711·3); cajuput oil (p.1664·1); cinnamon oil (p.1672·2); clove oil (p.1673·3); peppermint oil (p.1283·2).

**Tiger Balm White** *Haw Par, Canad.*
Camphor (p.1665·3); menthol (p.1711·3); cajuput oil (p.1664·1); clove oil (p.1673·3); peppermint oil (p.1283·2).

**Tiger Balsam Rot** *Klosterfrau, Austria.*
Camphor (p.1665·3); menthol (p.1711·3); cajuput oil (p.1664·1); peppermint oil (p.1283·2); clove oil (p.1673·3); cinnamon oil (p.1672·2).
*Muscle pain.*

**Tiger Liniment** *Haw Par, Canad.*
Methyl salicylate (p.59·3); menthol (p.1711·3); eucalyptus oil (p.1686·2).

**Tiger Snake** *Commonwealth Serum, Hong Kong.*
A tiger snake venom antisera (p.1639·1).
*Snake bite.*

**Tiglio (Specie Composta)** *Dynacren, Ital.*
Tilia (p.1756·2); sambucus (p.1741·3); meadowsweet (p.1710·1).
*Cold symptoms; herbal tea.*

**Tigridol** *Phytomedica, Fr.*
Camphor (p.1665·3); menthol (p.1711·3); clove oil (p.1673·3); eucalyptus oil (p.1686·2); peppermint oil (p.1283·2); cinnamon oil (p.1672·2).
*Pain.*

**Tikacillin** *Tika, Swed.*
Phenoxymethylpenicillin potassium (p.242·1).
*Bacterial infections.*

**Tikl** *Monserrat, Arg.*
Ketoconazole (p.403·3).
*Scalp disorders.*

**Tikleen** *Ipca, India.*
Ticlopidine hydrochloride (p.1011·2).
*Thrombosis.*

**Tiklid**
*Sanofi Synthelabo, Austria; Sanofi Synthelabo, Ital.; Sanofi Synthelabo, Spain.*
Ticlopidine hydrochloride (p.1011·2).
*Thromboembolism prophylaxis.*

**Tiklyd**
*Sanofi Synthelabo, Ger.; Sanofi Synthelabo, Port.*
Ticlopidine hydrochloride (p.1011·2).
*Thrombosis prophylaxis.*

**Tikosyn** *Pfizer, USA.*
Dofetilide (p.906·3).
*Arrhythmias.*

**Tilad** *Aventis, Spain.*
Nedocromil sodium (p.789·3).
*Asthma.*

**Tilade**
*Aventis, Austral.; Aventis, Austria; Aventis, Braz.; Aventis, Canad.; Aventis, Denm.; Aventis, Fin.; Aventis, Fr.†; Aventis, Ger.; Aventis, Gr.; Aventis, Hong Kong; Fisons, Irl.; Aventis, Israel; Aventis, Ital.; Aventis, Neth.; Aventis, NZ; Aventis, S.Afr.†; Aventis, Switz.; Pantheon, UK; Monarch, USA.*
Nedocromil sodium (p.789·3).
*Allergic conjunctivitis; allergic rhinitis; asthma.*

**Tilaire** *Rhone-Poulenc Rorer, Mex.†.*
Nedocromil sodium (p.789·3).
*Obstructive airways disease.*

**Tilarin**
*Aventis, Austria; Aventis, Fin.; Aventis, Ital.; Aventis, NZ†; Aventis, Switz.*
Nedocromil sodium (p.789·3).
*Allergic rhinitis.*

**Tilatil** *Roche, Braz.*
Tenoxicam (p.93·1).
*Musculoskeletal, joint, and peri-articular disorders.*

**Tilavist**
*Aventis, Austria; Aventis, Denm.; Aventis, Fin.; Aventis, Fr.; Fisons, Irl.; Aventis, Israel; Aventis, Ital.; Aventis, Neth.; Aventis, Norw.; Aventis, NZ†; Aventis, Port.; Fisons, Singapore†; Rhone-Poulenc Rorer, Singapore†; Aventis, Spain; Aventis, Swed.; Aventis, Switz.*
Nedocromil sodium (p.789·3).
*Conjunctivitis.*

**Tilazem**
*Parke, Davis, Arg.; Parke, Davis, Chile; Parke, Davis, Mex.; Pfizer, S.Afr.*
Diltiazem hydrochloride (p.900·1).
*Angina pectoris; hypertension.*

**Tilcitin** *Roche, Gr.*
Tenoxicam (p.93·1).
*Dysmenorrhoea; gout; inflammation; osteoarthritis; pain; rheumatoid arthritis; spondyloarthropathies.*

**Tilcotil**
*Roche, Austral.†; Roche, Austria; Roche, Belg.; Roche, Chile; Roche, Denm.; Roche, Fin.; Roche, Fr.; Roche, Ger.†; Roche, Hong Kong; Roche, Ital.; Chugai, Jpn; Roche, Mex.; Roche, Neth.; Roche, NZ; Roche, Port.; Roche, S.Afr.; Roche, Singapore†; Roche, Spain; Roche, Switz.; Roche, Thai.*
Tenoxicam (p.93·1).
*Gout; musculoskeletal, joint, peri-articular, and soft-tissue disorders.*

**Tildiem**
*Sanofi Synthelabo, Belg.; Chemopharma, Chile; Sanofi Synthelabo, Fr.; Sanofi Synthelabo, Gr.; Synthelabo, Hong Kong†; Sanofi Synthelabo, Irl.; Sanofi Synthelabo, Ital.; Sanofi Synthelabo, Neth.; Sanofi Synthelabo, Singapore†; Synthelabo, Switz.; Sanofi Synthelabo, Thai.†; Sanofi Synthelabo, UK.*
Diltiazem hydrochloride (p.900·1).
*Angina pectoris; arrhythmias; hypertension; myocardial ischaemia.*

**Tilekin** *Kinder, Braz.*
Paracetamol (p.76·2).
*Pain.*

**Tilene** *Francia, Ital.*
Fenofibrate (p.915·2).
*Hyperlipidaemias.*

**Tilexim** *Caber, Ital.*
Cefuroxime axetil (p.184·1).
*Bacterial infections.*

**Tilfilin** *Funk, Spain†.*
Carbocisteine (p.1116·2); chlorphenamine maleate (p.427·3); phenylephrine hydrochloride (p.1126·3); choline theophyllinate (p.784·2).
*Obstructive airways disease.*

**Tili** *ABZ, Ger.*
Tilidine hydrochloride (p.94·1).
Naloxone hydrochloride (p.1044·3) is included in this preparation to discourage abuse.
*Pain.*

**Tili Comp** *1A, Ger.*
Tilidine hydrochloride (p.94·1).
Naloxone hydrochloride (p.1044·3) is included in this preparation to discourage abuse.
*Pain.*

**Tilicomp** *Betapharm, Ger.*
Tilidine hydrochloride (p.94·1).
Naloxone hydrochloride (p.1044·3) is included in this preparation to discourage abuse.
*Pain.*

**Tilidalor** *Hexal, Ger.*
Tilidine hydrochloride (p.94·1).
Naloxone hydrochloride (p.1044·3) is included in this preparation to discourage abuse.
*Pain.*

**Tilidin comp** *Aliud, Ger.; Basics, Ger.; Heumann, Ger.; Stada, Ger.*
Tilidine hydrochloride (p.94·1).
Naloxone hydrochloride (p.1044·3) is included in this preparation to discourage abuse.
*Pain.*

**Tilidin N** *Lichtenstein, Ger.*
Tilidine hydrochloride (p.94·1).
Naloxone hydrochloride (p.1044·3) is included in this preparation to discourage abuse.
*Pain.*

**Tilidin plus** *Ratiopharm, Ger.*
Tilidine hydrochloride (p.94·1).
Naloxone hydrochloride (p.1044·3) is included in this preparation to discourage abuse.
*Pain.*

**Tilidin-saar** *Chephasaar, Ger.*
Tilidine hydrochloride (p.94·1).
Naloxone hydrochloride (p.1044·3) is included in this preparation to discourage abuse.
*Pain.*

**Tilidura** *Merck dura, Ger.*
Tilidine hydrochloride (p.94·1).
Naloxone hydrochloride (p.1044·3) is included in this preparation to discourage abuse.
*Pain.*

**Tiligetic** *Azupharma, Ger.*
Tilidine hydrochloride (p.94·1).
Naloxone hydrochloride (p.1044·3) is included in this preparation to discourage abuse.
*Pain.*

**Tilimerck** *Merck dura, Ger.*
Tilidine hydrochloride (p.94·1).
Naloxone hydrochloride (p.1044·3) is included in this preparation to discourage abuse.
*Pain.*

**Tili-Puren** *Alpharma-Isis, Ger.*
Tilidine hydrochloride (p.94·1).
Naloxone hydrochloride (p.1044·3) is included in this preparation to discourage abuse.
*Pain.*

**Tilitrate** *Parke, Davis, Spain†.*
Tilidine hydrochloride (p.94·1).
*Pain.*

**Tilker**
*Sanofi Winthrop, Denm.; Sanofi Synthelabo, Norw.; Sanofi Synthelabo, Spain.*
Diltiazem hydrochloride (p.900·1).
*Angina pectoris; hypertension.*

**Till** *Amnol, Ital.*
Triclosan (p.1195·2); alkylamidobetaine.
*Personal hygiene.*

**tilnalox** *CT, Ger.*
Tilidine hydrochloride (p.94·1).
Naloxone hydrochloride (p.1044·3) is included in this preparation to discourage abuse.
*Pain.*

**Tilodene** *Alphapharm, Austral.*
Ticlopidine hydrochloride (p.1011·2).
*Thromboembolism prophylaxis.*

**Tiloptic** *Merck Sharp & Dohme, Israel.*
Timolol maleate (p.1012·2).
*Glaucoma; ocular hypertension.*

**Tiloryth** *Tillomed, UK.*
Erythromycin (p.208·1).
*Bacterial infections.*

**Tilosin** *Wayne, Mex.†.*
Hyoscine butylbromide (p.483·3).

**Tiloxican** *Hexal, Braz.*
Tenoxicam (p.93·1).

**Tilstigmin** *Tablets, India.*
Neostigmine bromide (p.1492·2) or neostigmine metilsulfate (p.1492·2).
*Myasthenia gravis.*

**Tiltab** *SmithKline Beecham, Braz.†.*
Rosiglitazone maleate (p.345·2).
*Diabetes mellitus.*

**Tiltis** *Euroderm, Arg.*
Benzoyl peroxide (p.1143·2).
*Acne.*

**Ti-Lub** *Draxis, Canad.*
Liquid paraffin (p.1479·1) or light liquid paraffin (p.1479·1).

**Tilur** *Drossapharm, Switz.*
Acemetacin (p.11·3).
*Musculoskeletal and joint disorders; superficial thrombophlebitis.*

**TIM** *Seroyal, Canad.†.*
Vitamins A, C, and E, and zinc (p.1417·1).

**Timabak**
*Agepha, Austria; Allergan-Frumtost, Braz.†; Andromaco, Chile; Thea, Fr.; Thea, Hong Kong; Pharmacia, Singapore.*
Timolol maleate (p.1012·2).
*Glaucoma; ocular hypertension.*

**Timacar** *Merck Sharp & Dohme, Denm.*
Timolol maleate (p.1012·2).
*Angina pectoris; glaucoma; hypertension; migraine; myocardial infarction.*

**Timacor** *Merck Sharp & Dohme-Chibret, Fr.*
Timolol maleate (p.1012·2).
*Angina pectoris; hypertension; myocardial infarction.*

**Tim-Ak** *Dioptic, Canad.*
Timolol maleate (p.1012·2).
*Raised intra-ocular pressure.*

**Timarol** *Laboratorios Chile, Chile.*
Tramadol hydrochloride (p.94·3).
*Pain.*

**Timasen** *Asta Medica, Braz.*
Tramadol hydrochloride (p.94·3).
*Pain.*

**Timax** *Agepha, Austria.*
Timolol maleate (p.1012·2).
*Glaucoma; ocular hypertension.*

**Time Action B Complex with C** *Hall, Canad.*
Vitamins B and C (p.1417·1).

**Time Released Balanced B** *Lee-Adams, Canad.*
Vitamin B substances (p.1417·1).

**Timecef**
*Aventis, Austria; Aventis, Braz.†; Lepetit, Ital.*
Cefodizime sodium (p.174·1).
Lidocaine hydrochloride (p.1377·3) is included in some intramuscular injections to alleviate the pain of injection.
*Gram-negative bacterial infections.*

**Timed** *Biocumed, Arg.*
Timolol maleate (p.1012·2).
*Glaucoma; ocular hypertension.*

**Timed Action Balanced B** *Hall, Canad.*
Vitamin B substances (p.1417·1).

**Timed D** *Biocumed, Arg.*
Timolol maleate (p.1012·2); dorzolamide hydrochloride (p.908·3).
*Glaucoma; ocular hypertension.*

**Timed Release C** *Jamieson, Canad.*
Ascorbic acid (p.1460·2).

**Timed Release Ester C** *General Nutrition, Canad.*
Vitamin C substances (p.1460·2).

**Timed Release Mega Men** *General Nutrition, Canad.*
Multivitamin and mineral preparation (p.1417·1).

**Timed Release Swiss One** *Swiss Herbal, Canad.*
Range of multivitamin and mineral preparations (p.1417·1).

**Timed Release Ultra Mega** *General Nutrition, Canad.*
Range of multivitamin and mineral preparations (p.1417·1).

**Timed Release Vita-Vim** *Jamieson, Canad.†.*
Multivitamin and mineral preparation (p.1417·1).

**Timed Release Womens Ultra Mega** *General Nutrition, Canad.*
Multivitamin and mineral preparation (p.1417·1).

**Timelit** *Lundbeck, Ital.†.*
Lofepramine hydrochloride (p.305·3).
*Depression.*

**Timenten** *SmithKline Beecham, Switz.*
Ticarcillin sodium (p.270·2); potassium clavulanate (p.193·3).
*Bacterial infections.*

**Timentin**
*GlaxoSmithKline, Austral.; GlaxoSmithKline, Belg.; GlaxoSmithKline, Braz.; GlaxoSmithKline, Canad.; SmithKline Beecham, Gr.; GlaxoSmithKline, Hong Kong; GlaxoSmithKline, India; SmithKline Beecham, Irl.; SmithKline Beecham, Israel; GlaxoSmithKline, Ital.; SmithKline Beecham, Mex.; SmithKline Beecham, Neth.; GlaxoSmithKline, NZ; GlaxoSmithKline, UK; SmithKline Beecham, USA.*
Ticarcillin sodium (p.270·2); potassium clavulanate (p.193·3).
*Bacterial infections.*

**Timezol** *Richmond, Arg.*
Omeprazole (p.1278·2).
*Peptic ulcer.*

**Timi** *Sriprasit, Thai.*
Miconazole nitrate (p.405·3); triamcinolone acetonide (p.1110·2).
*Fungal skin and nail infections with inflammation.*

**Timicolid** *Pfizer Consumer, Ital.*
Dithranol (p.1146·1).
*Psoriasis.*

**Timicon** *Merck Sharp & Dohme, Ital.*
Timolol maleate (p.1012·2); pilocarpine hydrochloride (p.1495·1).
*Glaucoma; ocular hypertension.*

**Timisol** *Ecosol, Switz.*
Timolol maleate (p.1012·2).
*Glaucoma; ocular hypertension.*

**T-Immun**
*Immuno, Austria†; Immuno, Ger.†.*
A tetanus vaccine (p.1640·3).
*Active immunisation.*

**Timo (Specie Composta)** *Dynacren, Ital.*
Thyme (p.1755·2); fennel (p.1687·2); plantago lanceolata (p.1738·2); liquorice (p.1270·2).
*Coughs; herbal tea.*

**Timocomod** *Ioltech, Fr.*
Timolol maleate (p.1012·2).
*Glaucoma; ocular hypertension.*

**Timo-COMOD**
*Ursapharm, Ger.; Ursapharm, Neth.*
Timolol maleate (p.1012·2).
*Glaucoma; ocular hypertension.*

**Timodine**
*Reckitt Benckiser, Irl.; Reckitt Benckiser, UK.*
Nystatin (p.406·3); hydrocortisone (p.1103·3).
*Infected skin disorders.*

**Timodrop** *Biolab, Thai.*
Timolol maleate (p.1012·2).
*Glaucoma; ocular hypertension.*

**TimoEDO** *Mann, Ger.*
Timolol maleate (p.1012·2).
*Glaucoma; ocular hypertension.*

**Timoferol** *Elerte, Fr.*
Ferrous sulfate (p.1428·2).
Ascorbic acid (p.1460·2) is included in this preparation to increase the absorption and availability of iron.
*Anaemias.*

**Timoftal** *Agepha, Austria.*
Timolol maleate (p.1012·2).
*Glaucoma; ocular hypertension.*

**Timoftol** *Merck Sharp & Dohme, Spain.*
Timolol maleate (p.1012·2).
*Glaucoma; ocular hypertension.*

**Timogel** *Thea, Spain.*
Timolol maleate (p.1012·2).
*Glaucoma; ocular hypertension.*

**Timoglau** *Edol, Port.*
Timolol maleate (p.1012·2).
*Ocular hypertension.*

**Timoglau Plus** *Edol, Port.*
Timolol maleate (p.1012·2); pilocarpine hydrochloride (p.1495·1).
*Glaucoma.*

**Timoglobulina**
*Aventis Pasteur, Arg.; Aventis Pasteur, Chile; Imtix, Spain.*
Antithymocyte immunoglobulin (rabbit) (p.1348·3).
*Aplastic anaemia; graft-versus-host disease; transplant rejection.*

**Timohexal**
*Hexal, Austria; Hexal, Ger.*
Timolol maleate (p.1012·2).
*Cataracts; glaucoma; ocular hypertension.*

**Timolabak** *Thea, Ital.*
Timolol maleate (p.1012·2).
*Glaucoma; ocular hypertension.*

**Timolen** *Davi, Port.*
Timolol maleate (p.1012·2).
*Glaucoma; ocular hypertension.*

**Timoler** *Lersan, Arg.*
Timolol maleate (p.1012·2).
*Ocular hypertension.*

**Timolide**
*Merck Frosst, Canad.; Merck, USA.*
Timolol maleate (p.1012·2); hydrochlorothiazide (p.933·2).
*Hypertension.*

**Timolo** *Bell, India.*
Timolol maleate (p.1012·2).
*Glaucoma; ocular hypertension.*

**Timolux** *Tubilux, Ital.*
Timolol maleate (p.1012·2).
*Glaucoma; ocular hypertension.*

**Timomann** *Mann, Ger.*
Timolol maleate (p.1012·2).
*Glaucoma; ocular hypertension.*

**Timonil**
*Desitin, Ger.; Desitin, Hong Kong†; Desitin, Israel; Desitin, Switz.; CP Pharmaceuticals, UK.*
Carbamazepine (p.353·3).
*Alcohol withdrawal syndrome; bipolar disorder; diabetic neuropathy; epilepsy; neuralgias; nonepileptic seizures in multiple sclerosis.*

**Timo-Optal** *Olan-Kemed, Thai.*
Timolol maleate (p.1012·2).
*Glaucoma; ocular hypertension.*

**Timop** *Laboratorios Chile, Chile.*
Timolol maleate (p.1012·2).
*Glaucoma.*

**Tim-Ophtal**
*Agepha, Austria; Winzer, Ger.*
Timolol maleate (p.1012·2).
*Glaucoma; ocular hypertension.*

**Timoptic**
*Merck Sharp & Dohme, Arg.; Merck Sharp & Dohme, Austria; Merck Frosst, Canad.; Merck Sharp & Dohme, Switz.; Merck, USA.*
Timolol maleate (p.1012·2).
*Glaucoma; ocular hypertension.*

**Timoptol**
*Merck Sharp & Dohme, Austral.; Merck Sharp & Dohme, Belg.; Merck Sharp & Dohme, Braz.; Merck Sharp & Dohme-Chibret, Fr.; Merck Sharp & Dohme, Hong Kong; Merck Sharp & Dohme, Irl.; Merck Sharp & Dohme, Ital.; Merck Sharp & Dohme, Malaysia; Merck Sharp & Dohme, Mex.; Merck Sharp & Dohme, Neth.; Merck Sharp*

& Dohme, NZ; Chibret, Port.; Merck Sharp & Dohme, S.Afr.; Merck Sharp & Dohme, Singapore; Merck Sharp & Dohme, Thai.; Merck Sharp & Dohme, UK.
Timolol maleate (p.1012·2).
*Glaucoma; ocular hypertension.*

**Timoptol-XE** Merck Sharp & Dohme, Austral.; Merck Sharp & Dohme, Chile.
Timolol maleate (p.1012·2).
*Glaucoma; ocular hypertension.*

**Timosan**
Note. This name is used for preparations of different composition.
Fund a Paiva, Braz.†.
Thymus polypeptides (bovine) (p.1756·1).
*Immunotherapy.*
Santen, Denm.; Santen, Fin.; Santen, Norw.; Santen, Swed.
Timolol maleate (p.1012·2).
*Glaucoma; ocular hypertension.*

**Timosil** Silom, Thai.
Timolol maleate (p.1012·2).
*Glaucoma; ocular hypertension.*

**Timosin** Sclavo, Ital.†.
Thymalfasin (p.1755·2).
*Influenza in immunodeficient patients.*

**Timosine** Chibret, Ger.
Timolol maleate (p.1012·2).
*Glaucoma; ocular hypertension.*

**Timosoft** Scharper, Ital.
Timolol maleate (p.1012·2).
*Glaucoma; ocular hypertension.*

**Timo-Stulln** Stulln, Ger.
Timolol maleate (p.1012·2).
*Glaucoma; ocular hypertension.*

**Timox** Desitin, Ger.
Oxcarbazepine (p.366·3).
*Epilepsy.*

**Timozzard** Pizzard, Mex.
Timolol maleate (p.1012·2).
*Glaucoma; ocular hypertension.*

**Timpanol** Hexal, Braz.
Procaine hydrochloride (p.1383·2); phenol (p.1188·1).
*Ear infections; earache.*

**Timpilo**
Merck Sharp & Dohme, Arg.; Merck Sharp & Dohme, Austral.; Merck Sharp & Dohme, Austria; Merck Frosst, Canad.; Merck Sharp & Dohme, Denm.; Merck Sharp & Dohme, Fin.; Merck Sharp & Dohme-Chibret, Fr.; Chibret, Ger.; Merck Sharp & Dohme, Hong Kong; Merck Sharp & Dohme, Israel; Merck Sharp & Dohme, Malaysia; Merck Sharp & Dohme, Mex.†; Merck Sharp & Dohme, Neth.; Merck Sharp & Dohme, Norw.; Merck Sharp & Dohme, NZ; Merck Sharp & Dohme, Singapore; Merck Sharp & Dohme, Swed.; Merck Sharp & Dohme, Switz.
Timolol maleate (p.1012·2); pilocarpine hydrochloride (p.1495·1).
*Glaucoma; ocular hypertension.*

**Timpron** Berk, UK†.
Naproxen (p.65·1).
*Gout; musculoskeletal and joint disorders.*

**Timsopt** Merck Sharp & Dohme, Austria.
Dorzolamide hydrochloride (p.908·3); timolol maleate (p.1012·2).
*Glaucoma.*

**Timunox** Janssen-Cilag, Ital.†.
Thymopentin (p.1756·1).
*Immunodeficiency.*

**Tina** Biolab, Thai.†.
Cyproterone acetate (p.1544·1); ethinylestradiol (p.1553·2).
*Androgen-dependent acne, alopecia, and hirsutism in females; oral contraceptive in women with androgenic symptoms.*

**Tinacef** Richmond, Arg.
Ceftazidime (p.180·2).
*Bacterial infections.*

**Tinactin**
Schering-Plough, Canad.; Schering-Plough, USA.
Tolnaftate (p.410·1).
*Fungal skin infections.*

**Tinaderm**
Key, Arg.; Schering-Plough, Austral.; Schering-Plough, Chile; Fulford, India; Schering-Plough, Irl.; Schering-Plough, Ital.; Schering-Plough, Malaysia; Schering-Plough, Mex.; Schering-Plough, NZ; Schering-Plough, S.Afr.; Schering-Plough, Singapore; Schering-Plough, Spain†; Schering-Plough, UK.
Tolnaftate (p.410·1).
*Fungal skin and nail infections.*

**Tinaderm Extra** Schering-Plough, Austral.
Clotrimazole (p.396·2).
*Fungal skin infections.*

**Tinaderme** Plough, Port.
Tolnaftate (p.410·1).
*Fungal skin and nail infections.*

**Tinaderm-M**
Schering-Plough, Irl.; Schering-Plough, UK.
Tolnaftate (p.410·1); nystatin (p.406·3).
*Fungal skin and nail infections.*

**Tinagel** Schering-Plough, Belg.†.
Benzoyl peroxide (p.1143·2).
*Acne.*

**Tinaroc-Combi** Orion, Fin.†.
Tablets (morning), phenylpropanolamine hydrochloride (Tinaroc) (p.1127·3); tablets (evening), phenylpropanolamine hydrochloride; carbinoxamine maleate (Tinaroc-A) (p.426·3).
*Allergic rhinitis.*

**Tinasol** Fischer, Israel†.
Tolnaftate (p.410·1).
*Fungal skin infections.*

**Tinasolve** Rye, Singapore.
Melaleuca oil (p.1710·2); triclosan (p.1195·2).
*Fungal skin infections.*

**Tinatox** Riemser, Ger.
Tolnaftate (p.410·1).
*Fungal skin infections.*

**Tinax** Euroforma, Braz.
Epoetin (p.747·1).
*Anaemias.*

**Tinazol** Darrow, Braz.†.
Tioconazole (p.409·3).
*Fungal infections.*

**Tinazole** General Drugs, Thai.
Tinidazole (p.617·1).
*Amoebiasis; giardiasis; trichomoniasis.*

**TinBen** Ferndale, USA.
Barrier preparation.

**TinCoBen** Ferndale, USA.
Barrier preparation.

**Tinctura Justi** Pascoe, Ger.†.
Homoeopathic preparation.

**Tine Test PPD** Lederle, USA†.
Tuberculin purified protein derivative (p.1759·1).
*Diagnosis of tuberculosis.*

**Tineafax** Douglas, Austral.
Tolnaftate (p.410·1).
*Tinea pedis.*

**Tinerol** Roche, Spain.
Ornidazole (p.612·2).
*Amoebiasis; anaerobic bacterial infections; giardiasis.*

**Ting** Heritage Consumer, USA.
Miconazole nitrate (p.405·3).
Formerly contained tolnaftate.
*Fungal skin infections.*

**Tingosan** Bittner, Austria.
Homoeopathic preparation.

**Tini** Codal Synto, Thai.
Tinidazole (p.617·1).
*Amoebiasis; anaerobic bacterial infections; giardiasis; trichomoniasis.*

**Tiniazol** Liferpal, Mex.
Ketoconazole (p.403·3).
*Fungal skin, nail, and vaginal infections.*

**Tinidafyl** Jagson, India.
Tinidazole (p.617·1).
*Anaerobic bacterial infections; protozoal infections.*

**Tinidafyl Plus** Jagson, India.
Tinidazole (p.617·1); diloxanide furoate (p.604·1); methylpolysiloxane (p.1482·1).
*Amoebiasis.*

**Tinnitin** Sanova, Austria.
Caroverine hydrochloride (p.1668·1).
*Smooth muscle spasm; tinnitus.*

**Tinok AF** Rekah, Israel.
Sodium chloride (p.1233·3).
*Nasal congestion.*

**Tinoral** Uniao Quimica, Braz.
Tinidazole (p.617·1).
*Fungal infections.*

**Tinox** Osteolab, Chile.
Tibolone (p.1572·3).
*Menopausal disorders.*

**Tinsenol** Medipharm, Chile.
Thioridazine (p.724·2).
*Attention-deficit disorder; behaviour disorders; sleep disorders.*

**Tinset**
Janssen-Cilag, Arg.; Janssen-Cilag, Austria; Janssen-Cilag, Belg.; Janssen-Cilag, Chile; Janssen-Cilag, Fr.; Janssen-Cilag, Ger.†; Janssen-Cilag, Gr.; Cilag, Hong Kong; Formenti, Ital.; Janssen, Mex.; Janssen-Cilag, Neth.; Janssen-Cilag, Port.; Janssen-Cilag, S.Afr.; Janssen-Cilag, Thai.
Oxatomide (p.438·1).
*Hypersensitivity reactions.*

**Tintorine** Bipharma, Neth.†.
Salicylic acid (p.1157·1); lactic acid (p.1704·1).
*Warts.*

**Tintu. Mertiolato Asens** Asens, Spain†.
Thiomersal (p.1194·1); monoethanolamine.
*Skin disinfection.*

**Tintura Benjui** Orion, Fin.
Camphor (p.1665·3); menthol (p.1711·3).
*Respiratory-tract congestion.*

**Tintura de Salsa Caroba e Manaca** Dansk-Flama, Braz.†.
Parsley (p.1728·3); jacaranda caroba; brunfelsia hopeana; sassafras (p.1742·1); sarsaparilla (p.1742·1).

**Tintus** Orion, Fin.
Guaifenesin (p.1122·1).
*Coughs.*

**Tinver** Pilkington Barnes-Hind, USA.
Sodium thiosulfate (p.1053·3); salicylic acid (p.1157·1); isopropyl alcohol (p.1184·3).
*Pityriasis versicolor.*

**Tiobarbital** Braun, Spain.
Thiopental sodium (p.1309·1).
*Epilepsy; general anaesthesia.*

**Tiobec** Laborest, Ital.
Thioctic acid (p.1754·3); vitamins (p.1417·1).
*Neuropathies; nutritional supplement.*

**Tiocalmina** Ottolenghi, Ital.
Sulfogaiacol (p.1131·1); dropropizine (p.1119·3).
*Coughs.*

**Tioconax** Delta, Braz.
Tioconazole (p.409·3).
*Fungal infections.*

**Tiocosol** OFF, Ital.
Sulfogaiacol (p.1131·1); sodium benzoate (p.1169·3).
*Catarrh; coughs.*

**Tioctan**
Purissimus, Arg.; Rothpharma, Austria; Fujisawa, Jpn.
Thioctic acid (p.1754·3).
*Diabetic neuropathy; subacute necrotising encephalomyelopathy; thioctic acid supplement; vestibular deafness.*

**Tioctan-S** Leiras, Fin.
Vitamin B substances; ascorbic acid; dehydrocholic acid (p.1417·1).
*Vitamin B deficiency.*

**Tiof**
Saval, Chile; Columbia, Mex.
Timolol maleate (p.1012·2).
*Glaucoma; ocular hypertension.*

**Tiofeniclin** Sanofi Synthelabo, Mex.
Thiamphenicol (p.269·2).
*Bacterial infections.*

**Tioguaialina** Montefarmaco, Ital.
Sulfogaiacol (p.1131·1).
*Catarrh; coughs.*

**Tioguanina** IFET (ΙΦΕΤ), Gr.
Tioguanine (p.588·2).
*Acute leukaemias.*

**Tiomicol** Panalab, Arg.
Tioconazole (p.409·3).
*Fungal skin and nail infections.*

**Tionamil** Ideco, Ital.
Sulfogaiacol (p.1131·1); sodium benzoate (p.1169·3); terpin hydrate (p.1131·1).
*Coughs.*

**Tionazen** Cazi, Braz.
Tioconazole (p.409·3).
*Fungal infections.*

**Tioner** Andromaco, Spain.
Tramadol hydrochloride (p.94·3).
*Pain.*

**Tiorfan**
GlaxoSmithKline, Braz.; Bioprojet, Fr.; Ferrer, Spain.
Racecadotril (p.1285·2).
*Diarrhoea.*

**Tiorilene** Boniscontro & Gazzone, Ital.
Thiocolchicoside (p.1395·2).
*Neuromuscular pain; parkinsonism; spasticity.*

**Tiosalis** Teva Tuteur, Arg.
Ondansetron (p.1281·1).
*Nausea and vomiting.*

**Tiosalprin** Salus, Mex.†.
Azathioprine (p.1349·1).

**Tioscina** Inverni della Beffa, Ital.†.
Aescin (p.1648·2); thiocolchicoside (p.1395·2).
*Inflammation; musculoskeletal and soft-tissue disorders.*

**Tioside** Ibi, Ital.
Thiocolchicoside (p.1395·2).
*Neuromuscular pain; parkinsonism; spasticity.*

**Tiosol** Uniao Quimica, Braz.†.
Sulfiram (p.1510·1).
*Scabies.*

**Tiotau** Damor, Ital.
Taurosteine.
*Respiratory-tract congestion.*

**Tioten** Therabel, Ital.†.
Stepronin sodium (p.1130·3).
*Respiratory-tract congestion.*

**Tiotil** Abigo, Swed.
Propylthiouracil (p.1603·1).
*Hyperthyroidism.*

**Tiovalone** Juste, Spain.
Tixocortol pivalate (p.1110·1).
*Nasal polyps; rhinitis.*

**Tioxal** Solfran, Mex.
Vitamin $B_{12}$; vitamin $B_6$ (p.1417·1).

**TIP** Farmalider, Spain†.
Dextromethorphan hydrobromide (p.1117·3).
*Coughs.*

**Tipac** Mintlab, Chile.
Ranitidine hydrochloride (p.1285·2).
*Peptic ulcer.*

**Tiparol** Astra, Swed.
Tramadol hydrochloride (p.94·3).
*Pain.*

**Tiperal** Clonmel, Irl.
Propranolol hydrochloride (p.989·3).
*Angina pectoris; anxiety; arrhythmias; essential tremor; hypertension; migraine; myocardial infarction; obstructive cardiomyopathy; phaeochromocytoma.*

**Tipidin** DHA, Singapore.
Ticlopidine hydrochloride (p.1011·2).
*Intermittent claudication; stroke prophylaxis.*

**Tipidine** Seven Stars, Thai.
Ticlopidine hydrochloride (p.1011·2).
*Diabetic retinopathy; intermittent claudication; thromboembolism prophylaxis; unstable angina pectoris.*

**Tipkin** TP, Thai.
Amikacin sulfate (p.154·1).
*Gram-negative bacterial infections.*

**Tiplac** Euro-Labor, Port.; Grunenthal, Port.
Lysine aspirin (p.54·3).
*Thrombosis prophylaxis.*

**Tipodex** Ern, Spain.
Famotidine (p.1265·2).
*Gastro-oesophageal reflux; peptic ulcer; Zollinger-Ellison syndrome.*

**Tipotaf** Vitamed, Israel.
Sodium chloride (p.1233·3).
*Eye wash; nasal congestion.*

**Tiprocin** Clonmel, Irl.†.
Erythromycin ethyl succinate (p.208·1).
*Bacterial infections.*

**Tipuric** Clonmel, Irl.
Allopurinol (p.412·2).
*Gout; prophylaxis of uric acid and calcium oxalate stones.*

**Tiq'Aouta** Clement-Thekan, Fr.
Diethyltoluamide (p.1503·3); dimethyl phthalate (p.1504·1); enoxolone (p.36·2).
*Insect repellent.*

**Tirabicin** Kleva, Gr.
Roxithromycin (p.254·2).
*Bacterial infections.*

**Tiracaspa** Hexal, Braz.
Cetrimonium bromide (p.1173·1).
*Seborrhoeic dermatitis.*

**Tiracrin** Geymonat, Ital.
Levothyroxine sodium (p.1600·1).
*Hypothyroidism.*

**Tiradine** British Dispensary, Thai.
Loratadine (p.436·1).
*Allergic rhinitis; allergic skin disorders.*

**Tirakallos** Dakota, Braz.†.
Salicylic acid (p.1157·1); lactic acid (p.1704·1).
*Keratinisation disorders.*

**Tiralcol** Sidepal, Braz.
Homoeopathic preparation.

**Tiratosse** DM, Braz.†.
Guaifenesin (p.1122·1); oxomemazine (p.438·2); paracetamol (p.76·2); sodium benzoate (p.1169·3).
*Coughs.*

**Tirgon** Woelm, Ger.
Bisacodyl (p.1251·3).
*Constipation.*

**Tirlor** Biochemie, Thai.; Novartis, Thai.
Loratadine (p.436·1).
*Allergic skin disorders; asthma (adjunct); hay fever.*

**Tirocal** Cryopharma, Mex.
Calcitriol (p.1461·2).
*Hypocalcaemia; hypoparathyroidism; osteoporosis; renal osteodystrophy; rickets.*

**Tirocular**
Angelini, Ital.; Lepori, Port.
Acetylcysteine (p.1112·3).
*Corneal disorders; dry eyes.*

**Tirodril** Estedi, Spain.
Thiamazole (p.1603·3).
*Hyperthyroidism.*

**Tiroide Amsa** Amsa, Ital.
Levothyroxine sodium (p.1600·1); liothyronine sodium (p.1602·2).
*Hypothyroidism.*

**Tiroide Vister** Teofarma, Ital.
Thyroglobulin (p.1604·1).
*Hypothyroidism.*

**Tiroidine** Rudefsa, Mex.
Levothyroxine sodium (p.1600·1).
*Hypothyroidism.*

**Tirolaxo** Edigen, Spain†.
Docusate sodium (p.1262·2).
*Constipation.*

**Tiroler Adler Leber- und Gallentee** Apotheke Tiroler Adler, Austria.
Taraxacum (p.1751·3); peppermint leaf (p.1283·2); cynara (p.1678·3); silybum marianum (p.1043·3); chamomile (p.1669·3).
*Biliary-tract disorders.*

**Tiroler Adler Schwedenbitter** Apotheke Tiroler Adler, Austria.
Cynara (p.1678·3); fennel (p.1687·2); silybum marianum (p.1043·3); calamus; zedoary; juniper berry; absinthium; peppermint leaf; taraxacum; bitter orange peel; angelica; gentian; pimpinella saxifraga; myrrh; cnicus benedictus; camphor.
*Gastrointestinal disorders.*

**Tiroler Steinol** Tiroler, Austria.
Yellow soft paraffin (p.1479·3); yellow beeswax (p.1480·2); hydrous wool fat (p.1483·2); white soft paraffin (p.1479·3).
*Skin disorders.*

**Tirosint** Amsa, Ital.
Levothyroxine sodium (p.1600·1).
*Hypothyroidism.*

**Tirotax** Novartis, Mex.
Cefotaxime sodium (p.175·3).
*Bacterial infections.*

**Tirovel** Duncan, Arg.
Piroxicam (p.84·2).
*Inflammation; pain.*

**Tirozol 5/10** Merck, Chile.
Thiamazole (p.1603·3).
*Hyperthyroidism.*

**Tirs** *Difa, Ital.*
Benzalkonium chloride (p.1168·3); hypromellose (p.1579·3).
*Dry eyes; eye disinfection.*

**Tisamid** *Orion, Fin.*
Pyrazinamide (p.246·3).
*Tuberculosis.*

**Tisana Arnaldi** *Arnaldi-Uscio, Ital.†.*
Senna (p.1288·2); frangula bark (p.1266·3); liquorice (p.1270·2); boldo leaves (p.1661·2); chinese rhubarb (p.1287·3); greater celandine (p.1695·3); couch-grass root (p.1676·2); saponaria root; dulcamara (p.1683·1); melissa leaves (p.1711·1); angelica root (p.1655·1); viola tricolor flowers.
*Constipation.*

**Tisana Cisbey** *Geymonat, Ital.†.*
Rhubarb (p.1287·3); liquorice (p.1270·2); couch-grass (p.1676·2); peppermint leaf (p.1283·2); parietaria; melissa (p.1711·1); fennel (p.1687·2); coriander (p.1676·1); mallow (p.1709·3).
*Digestive disorders; sleep disorders.*

**Tisana Kelemata** *Kelemata, Ital.*
*Tablets; granules:* Senna (p.1288·2).
*Teabags; tea:* Senna (p.1288·2); couch-grass (p.1676·2); guaiacum; hyssop; parietaria; peppermint leaf (p.1283·2); sarsaparilla (p.1742·1); aniseed (p.1655·2); melissa (p.1711·1).
*Constipation.*

**Tisane Antibiliaire et Stomachique** *Denolin, Belg.†.*
Senna (p.1288·2); frangula bark (p.1266·3); althaea (p.1651·3); peppermint leaf (p.1283·2); cnicus benedictus (p.1673·3); rosemary (p.1740·2); melilotus officinalis; liquorice (p.1270·2); calendula flower (p.1665·2); mallow flower (p.1709·3); fennel (p.1687·2); aniseed (p.1655·2); tilia (p.1756·2).
*Biliary-tract congestion; digestive disorders.*

**Tisane antiflatulente pour nourissons et enfants** *Sidroga, Switz.*
Fennel (p.1687·2); chamomile (p.1669·3); tilia (p.1756·2); melissa (p.1711·1); peppermint leaf (p.1283·2); vervain (p.1764·1).
*Flatulence.*

**Tisane antirhumatismale** *Sidroga, Switz.*
Spearmint (p.1749·1); passion flower (p.1729·1); salix (p.87·3); stevia rebaudiana.
*Rheumatism.*

**Tisane calmante pour les enfants** *Sidroga, Switz.*
Valerian (p.1762·2); lupulus (p.1708·1); melissa (p.1711·1); orange flowers (p.1723·3); passion flower (p.1729·1).
*Nervous excitement; sleep disorders.*

**Tisane Clairo** *Weleda, Fr.†.*
Aniseed (p.1655·2); clove (p.1673·2); peppermint leaf (p.1283·2); senna leaflets (p.1288·2).
*Constipation.*

**Tisane Contre la Tension** *Denolin, Belg.†.*
Mistletoe (p.1715·3); frangula bark (p.1266·3); crataegus (p.1677·1); orthosiphonis stamineus (p.1702·3); bearberry (p.1659·2); Javanese turmeric (p.1759·3); passion flower (p.1729·1); olive leaf; star anise; peppermint leaf (p.1283·2).
*Hypertension.*

**Tisane contre les refroidissements** *Sidroga, Switz.*
Rose fruit (p.1740·1); sambucus (p.1741·3); chamomile (p.1669·3); tilia (p.1756·2); wild thyme.
*Cold symptoms.*

**Tisane Depurative "les 12 Plantes"** *Denolin, Belg.†.*
Sarsaparilla (p.1742·1); lappa (p.1704·3); fumitory (p.1690·1); parietaria; saponaria; senna (p.1288·2); frangula bark (p.1266·3); liquorice (p.1270·2); peppermint leaf (p.1283·2); mallow flower (p.1709·3); calendula flower (p.1665·2); fennel (p.1687·2); angelica (p.1655·1); star anise.
*Digestive disorders; kidney disorders; skin eruptions.*

**Tisane des Familles** *Monot, Fr.†.*
Equisetum (p.1684·1); tilia (p.1756·2); senna (p.1288·2); peppermint (p.1283·2); althaea (p.1651·3); liquorice (p.1270·2); parietaria; fennel (p.1687·2); melissa (p.1711·1); caraway (p.1667·2); sambucus (p.1741·3); ash; vervain (p.1764·1); cynara (p.1678·3); boldo (p.1661·2); aniseed (p.1655·2); frangula (p.1266·3); meadowsweet (p.1710·1).
*Constipation.*

**Tisane Digestive Weleda** *Weleda, Fr.†.*
Achillea (p.1646·2); aniseed (p.1655·2); caraway (p.1667·2); fennel (p.1687·2); chamomile (p.1669·3).
*Gastrointestinal disorders.*

**Tisane Diuretique**
*Note. This name is used for preparations of different composition.*
*Denolin, Belg.†.*
Bearberry (p.1659·2); juniper (p.1703·1); meadowsweet (p.1710·1); fraxinus excelsior; cynodontis root; liquorice (p.1270·2); calendula flower (p.1665·2); star anise; calluna; angelica (p.1655·1); fennel (p.1687·2); tritici root.
*Kidney and urinary disorders.*

*Sidroga, Switz.*
Birch (p.1660·3); bean pods; urtica (p.1762·1); equisetum (p.1684·1).
*Urinary-tract disorders.*

**Tisane favorisant l'allaitement** *Sidroga, Switz.*
Aniseed (p.1655·2); fennel (p.1687·2); caraway (p.1667·2); melissa (p.1711·1).
*Lactation stimulant.*

**Tisane Grande Chartreuse** *Aerocid, Fr.†.*
Marjoram; althaea (p.1651·3); liquorice (p.1270·2); senna (p.1288·2); frangula (p.1266·3); melissa (p.1711·1); peppermint (p.1283·2); ash; parietaria; coriander (p.1676·1).
*Constipation; skin disorders of digestive origin.*

**Tisane Hepatique de Hoerdt** *Wieger, Fr.*
Absinthium (p.1645·1); achillea (p.1646·2); agrimony (p.1649·1); boldo (p.1661·2); centaury (p.1669·2); couch-grass (p.1676·2); menyanthes (p.1712·1); sage (p.1741·2).
*Liver and biliary-tract disorders.*

**Tisane hepatique et biliaire** *Sidroga, Switz.*
Cynara (p.1678·3); boldo (p.1661·2); taraxacum (p.1751·3); silybum marianum (p.1043·3); peppermint leaf (p.1283·2); achillea (p.1646·2).
*Digestive system disorders.*

**Tisane laxative** *Sidroga, Switz.*
Fennel (p.1687·2); senna (p.1288·2); star anise; liquorice (p.1270·2).
Formerly contained frangula bark, fennel, senna, star anise, and liquorice.
*Constipation.*

**Tisane laxative H nouvelle formulation** *Hanseler, Switz.*
Senna (p.1288·2).
Formerly contained sambucus, senna, aniseed, fennel, and mint.
*Constipation.*

**Tisane laxative Natterman no 13** *Piraud, Switz.†.*
Senna (p.1288·2); aniseed (p.1655·2); caraway (p.1667·2); coriander (p.1676·1); fennel (p.1687·2); juniper (p.1703·1); liquorice (p.1270·2).
*Constipation.*

**Tisane laxative Natterman no 13 instant** *Piraud, Switz.†.*
Senna (p.1288·2); liquorice (p.1270·2).
*Constipation.*

**Tisane Mexicaine** *Medecine Vegetale, Fr.†.*
Red vine leaf; boldo leaf (p.1661·2); frangula bark (p.1266·3); hyssop; rosemary (p.1740·2); ash leaf; senna leaf (p.1288·2).
*Venous-lymphatic insufficiency.*

**Tisane Orientale Soker** *Medecine Vegetale, Fr.†.*
Arenaria; parietaria; couch-grass root (p.1676·2); bearberry leaves (p.1659·2); corn silk (p.1676·1).
*Urinary infections; water retention.*

**Tisane Pectorale** *Denolin, Belg.†.*
Poppy capsule (p.1129·1); star anise; liquorice (p.1270·2); carrageenan (p.1578·2); hedera terrestris (p.1696·1); hyssop; angelica (p.1655·1); althaea (p.1651·3); mallow flower (p.1709·3); calendula flower (p.1665·2); tilia (p.1756·2).
*Coughs.*

**Tisane pectorale et antitussive** *Sidroga, Switz.*
Sage (p.1741·2); althaea (p.1651·3); fennel (p.1687·2); iceland moss; red-poppy petal (p.1058·1); plantaginis (p.1738·2); star anise; liquorice (p.1270·2); thyme (p.1755·2).
*Coughs and congestion.*

**Tisane pectorale pour les enfants** *Sidroga, Switz.*
Althaea (p.1651·3); cowslip flower (p.1735·1); plantain (p.1733·1); liquorice (p.1270·2); thyme (p.1755·2).
*Cold symptoms.*

**Tisane pour Dormir** *Denolin, Belg.†.*
Poppy capsule (p.1129·1); bitter orange (p.1723·3); chamomile (p.1669·3); crataegus (p.1677·1); star anise; sage (p.1741·2); peppermint leaf (p.1283·2).
*Insomnia; nervous disorders.*

**Tisane pour le coeur et la circulation** *Sidroga, Switz.*
Birch (p.1660·3); motherwort (p.1717·1); spearmint (p.1749·1); melissa (p.1711·1); crataegus (p.1677·1).
*Cardiac and circulatory disorders.*

**Tisane pour le Foie** *Denolin, Belg.†.*
Javanese turmeric (p.1759·3); fabianae imbricatae; boldo (p.1661·2); cynara scolymus (p.1678·3); kinkeliba (p.1703·3); senna (p.1288·2); peppermint leaf (p.1283·2); melissa (p.1711·1); aniseed (p.1655·2); vervain (p.1764·1); liquorice (p.1270·2); tilia (p.1756·2); calendula flower (p.1665·2).
*Biliary-tract congestion; digestive disorders.*

**Tisane pour le sommeil et les nerfs** *Sidroga, Switz.*
Valerian (p.1762·2); lupulus (p.1708·1); spearmint (p.1749·1); melissa (p.1711·1); orange flower (p.1723·3).
*Nervousness; sleep disorders.*

**Tisane pour les enfants** *Sidroga, Switz.†.*
Fennel (p.1687·2); matricaria (p.1669·3); tilia (p.1756·2); melissa (p.1711·1); peppermint leaf (p.1283·2); vervain (p.1764·1).
*Agitation; muscular contractures; sleep disorders.*

**Tisane pour les reins et la vessie** *Sidroga, Switz.*
Bearberry (p.1659·2); birch (p.1660·3); Java tea (p.1702·3); lovage root (p.1708·1); peppermint leaf (p.1283·2); juniper (p.1703·1).
Formerly contained bearberry, birch, boldo, angelica, rose fruit, lovage, tilia, mallow flowers, orthosiphon, peppermint leaf, equisetum, juniper, and juglans regia.
*Urinary-tract disorders.*

**Tisane pour l'estomac** *Sidroga, Switz.*
Calamus (p.1664·1); matricaria (p.1669·3); spearmint (p.1749·1); melissa (p.1711·1); achillea (p.1646·2); centaury (p.1669·2).
*Gastrointestinal disorders.*

**Tisane Provencale No l** *Tisane Provencale, Switz.*
Senna (p.1288·2); althaea (p.1651·3).
*Constipation.*

**Tisane Purgative** *Denolin, Belg.†.*
Senna (p.1288·2); frangula bark (p.1266·3); peppermint leaf (p.1283·2); althaea (p.1651·3); fennel (p.1687·2); aniseed (p.1655·2); calendula flower (p.1665·2); mallow flower (p.1709·3); angelica (p.1655·1); liquorice (p.1270·2); melissa (p.1711·1).
*Constipation; digestive disorders.*

**Tisane relaxante N** *Sidroga, Switz.*
Valerian (p.1762·2); lavender flower (p.1705·1); melissa (p.1711·1); passion flower (p.1729·1).
*Nervous tension.*

**Tisane Sedative Weleda** *Weleda, Fr.†.*
Lavender (p.1705·1); valerian (p.1762·2); mallow flowers (p.1709·3).
*Insomnia; nervous disorders.*

**Tisane Touraine** *Pharmacie Principale, Fr.†.*
Ash; vervain (p.1764·1); asperule; parietaria; meadowsweet (p.1710·1); fragaria vesca; peppermint (p.1283·2); melissa (p.1711·1); frangula (p.1266·3); centaurea cyanus; senna (p.1288·2).
*Constipation.*

**Tisanes de l'Abbe Hamon no 3** *Aerocid, Fr.†.*
Frangula (p.1266·3); viola; convallaria (p.1675·3); equisetum (p.1684·1); ash; meadowsweet (p.1710·1); maize (p.1676·1); centaurea cyanus; hazel.
*Arthritis; gout; pain; sciatica.*

**Tisanes de l'Abbe Hamon no 6** *Aerocid, Fr.†.*
Asperule; oranger (p.1723·3); passion flower (p.1729·1); water-lily; sage (p.1741·2); calendula (p.1665·2); mistletoe (p.1715·3); tilia (p.1756·2); lyciet.
*Nervous disorders.*

**Tisanes de l'Abbe Hamon no 11** *Aerocid, Fr.†.*
Bladderwrack (p.1742·3); yellow dock (p.1766·1); couch-grass (p.1676·2); liquorice (p.1270·2); hazel.
*Obesity.*

**Tisanes de l'Abbe Hamon no 14** *Aerocid, Fr.†.*
Groundsel; achillea (p.1646·2); viburnum; shepherd's purse (p.1744·1); oak (p.1722·3); cupressus sempervirens; lemon verbena (p.1706·3); asperule; liquorice (p.1270·2); hazel; calendula (p.1665·2); centaurea cyanus; euphorbia (p.1686·3).
*Circulatory disorders.*

**Tisanes de l'Abbe Hamon no 15** *Aerocid, Fr.†.*
Elecampane (p.1119·3); comfrey (p.1675·2); erysimum; marrube (p.1124·1); borage (p.1661·3); bugloss; eucalyptus (p.1686·1); hazel; sticta pulmonaria.
*Respiratory-tract disorders.*

**Tisanes de l'Abbe Hamon no 16** *Aerocid, Fr.†.*
Lappa (p.1704·3); carrot; centaury (p.1669·2); thistle-roland; scoparium (p.1742·2); gratiola; convallaria (p.1675·3); hazel; liquorice (p.1270·2).
*Liver disorders.*

**Tisanes de l'Abbe Hamon no 17** *Aerocid, Fr.†.*
Globulaire; frangula (p.1266·3); mint (p.1749·1); mercurial; hazel; rhapontic rhubarb (p.1288·1).
*Constipation.*

**Tisatin** *Arlex, Mex.†.*
Phenylbutazone (p.83·2).

**Tisept**
*Seton, Israel; SSL, UK.*
Cetrimide (p.1172·1); chlorhexidine gluconate (p.1173·2).
*Disinfection of burns and wounds; skin disinfection.*

**Tisercin** *Thiemann, Ger.†.*
Levomepromazine (p.703·2) or levomepromazine maleate (p.703·2).
*Pain; psychoses.*

**Tisit** *Pfeiffer, USA.*
Pyrethrins (p.1509·3); piperonyl butoxide (p.1509·2).
*Pediculosis.*

**Tisobrif** *Alcala, Spain.*
Isoniazid (p.222·2); rifampicin (p.250·2).
Pyridoxine hydrochloride (p.1456·3) is included in this preparation for the prophylaxis of peripheral neuropathy.
*Tuberculosis.*

**Tisogen** *Gautier, Arg.*
Topotecan hydrochloride (p.589·1).
*Ovarian cancer; small-cell lung cancer.*

**Tisorek** *Microsules Bernabo, Arg.*
Celecoxib (p.25·2).
*Osteoarthritis; rheumatoid arthritis.*

**Tisplal** *Rhone-Poulenc Rorer, Mex.†.*
Cisplatin (p.538·1).

**Tispol Ibu-DD** *Woelm, Ger.*
Ibuprofen lysine (p.46·3).
*Fever; pain.*

**Tispol S** *Woelm, Ger.†.*
Propyphenazone (p.85·3); paracetamol (p.76·2).
*Toothache.*

**Tisseel**
*Baxter, Canad.; Immuno, Hong Kong; Immuno, Irl.†; Immuno, Israel; Adcock Ingram Critical Care, S.Afr.; Baxter BioScience, UK.*
1 Vial, fibrinogen (p.753·2); fibronectin (p.1688·1); factor XIII (p.753·1); plasminogen (p.984·1); 1 vial, aprotinin (p.742·3); 1 vial, calcium chloride (p.1225·1); 1 vial, thrombin (p.760·1).
On mixing this forms a fibrin glue (p.753·1).
*Dural sealing; haemorrhage; wounds.*

**Tisseel Duo** *Baxter, Austral.*
1 syringe, aprotinin (p.742·3); fibrinogen (p.753·2); fibronectin (p.1688·1); factor XIII (p.753·1); 1 syringe, calcium chloride (p.1225·1); thrombin (p.760·1).
On mixing this forms a fibrin glue (p.753·1).
*Adjunct in colostomy closure; haemostasis during surgery.*

**Tisseel Duo Quick**
*Baxter, Denm.; Baxter, Fin.; Baxter, Swed.*
1 Vial, fibrinogen (p.753·2); fibronectin (p.1688·1); factor XIII (p.753·1); plasminogen (p.984·1); aprotinin (p.742·3); albumin (p.740·3); 1 vial, thrombin (p.760·1); plasma protein (p.758·2); calcium chloride (p.1225·1).
On mixing this forms a fibrin glue (p.753·1).
*Haemorrhage; wounds.*

**Tissucol**
*Baxter Immuno, Arg.; Baxter, Austria; Baxter, Belg.†; Immuno, Braz.†; Baxter, Fr.; Baxter, Ital.; Baxter, Switz.*
1 Vial, fibrinogen (p.753·2); fibronectin (p.1688·1); factor XIII (p.753·1); plasminogen (p.984·1); 1 vial, aprotinin (p.742·3); 2 vials, thrombin (p.760·1); 1 vial, calcium chloride (p.1225·1).
On mixing this forms a fibrin glue (p.753·1).
*Haemorrhage; wounds.*

**Tissucol Duo** *Baxter, Spain.*
1 Vial, fibrinogen (p.753·2); fibronectin (p.1688·1); factor XIII (p.753·1); plasminogen (p.984·1); aprotinin (p.742·3); 1 vial, thrombin (p.760·1); calcium chloride (p.1225·1).
On mixing this forms a fibrin glue (p.753·1).
*Haemorrhage.*

**Tissucol Duo Quick**
*Baxter Immuno, Arg.; Baxter, Austria.*
1 Vial, fibrinogen (p.753·2); fibronectin (p.1688·1); factor XIII (p.753·1); plasminogen (p.984·1); aprotinin (p.742·3); 1 vial, thrombin (p.760·1); calcium chloride (p.1225·1).
On mixing this forms a fibrin glue (p.753·1).
*Wounds.*

**Tissucol Duo S**
*Baxter, Ger.; Baxter, Switz.*
1 Vial, plasma protein (p.758·2); fibrinogen (p.753·2); fibronectin (p.1688·1); aprotinin (p.742·3); factor XIII (p.753·1); plasminogen (p.984·1); 1 vial, thrombin (p.760·1); calcium chloride (p.1225·1).
On mixing this forms a fibrin glue (p.753·1).
*Haemorrhage; wounds.*

**Tissucol Fibrinkleber tiefgefroren** *Immuno, Ger.†.*
1 Ampoule: plasma protein fraction (p.758·2); fibrinogen (p.753·2); fibronectin (p.1688·1); factor XIII (p.753·1); plasminogen (p.984·1); 1 application set: aprotinin (p.742·3); calcium chloride (p.1225·1); lotion: calcium chloride; thrombin (p.760·1).
On mixing this forms a fibrin glue (p.753·1).
*Wounds.*

**Tissucol-Kit** *Baxter, Ger.*
1 Ampoule: plasma protein fraction (p.758·2); fibrinogen (p.753·2); fibronectin (p.1688·1); factor XIII (p.753·1); plasminogen (p.984·1); 1 ampoule: aprotinin (p.742·3); 2 ampoules: thrombin (p.760·1); 1 ampoule: calcium chloride (p.1225·1).
On mixing this forms a fibrin glue (p.753·1).
*Wounds.*

**TissuCone** *Baxter BioScience, Ger.*
Collagen (p.1674·3).
*Haemorrhage.*

**TissuFleece** *Baxter BioScience, Ger.*
Collagen (p.1674·3).
*Haemorrhage.*

**TissuFoil** *Baxter BioScience, Ger.*
Collagen (p.1674·3).
*Haemorrhage.*

**TissuVlies** *Immuno, Ger.†.*
Collagen (p.1674·3).
*Haemorrhage.*

**Tisuderma** *Cinfa, Spain.*
Hydrocortisone acetate (p.1103·3); neomycin sulfate (p.235·1).
*Skin infections with inflammation.*

**Tis-U-Sol** *Baxter, USA.*
Electrolytes (p.1217·1).
*Irrigation solution.*

**Titan**
*Note. This name is used for preparations of different composition.*
*Barnes Hind, Arg.; Pilkington Barnes-Hind, USA.*
Cleansing solution for hard contact lenses (p.1164·2).

*Durex, Canad.†.*
Nonoxinol 9 (p.1413·3).
*Contraceptive.*

**Titanorein** *Abello, Spain†.*
Carrageenan (p.1578·2); titanium dioxide (p.1160·3); lidocaine (p.1377·3).
*Haemorrhoids.*

**Titanoreine**
*Note. This name is used for preparations of different composition.*
*Martin, Fr.*
Carrageenan (p.1578·2); titanium dioxide (p.1160·3); zinc oxide (p.1163·2).
*Anorectal disorders.*

*Martin, Switz.*
*Ointment:* Carrageenan (p.1578·2); titanium dioxide (p.1160·3); zinc oxide (p.1163·2); lidocaine (p.1377·3).
*Suppositories:* Carrageenan (p.1578·2); titanium dioxide (p.1160·3); zinc oxide (p.1163·2).
*Anorectal disorders.*

**Titanoreine Lidocaine** *Martin, Fr.*
Carrageenan (p.1578·2); titanium dioxide (p.1160·3); zinc oxide (p.1163·2); lidocaine (p.1377·3).
*Anorectal disorders.*

**Titanox** *Demo, Gr.*
Promethazine hydrochloride (p.439·1).
*Hypersensitivity reactions.*

**Tition** *Pharmazam, Spain†.*
Reduced glutathione (p.1040·3).
*Hepatitis.*

**Titmus Losung I** *Ciba Vision, Austria†.*
Hydrogen peroxide (p.1182·2) (p.1164·2).
*Disinfection and storage of contact lenses.*

**Titmus Losung 2** *Ciba Vision, Austria†.*
Catalase (p.1668·3) (p.1164·2).
*Neutralisation and rinsing of contact lenses.*

**Titralac**
*Benitol, Arg.; 3M, Austral.; 3M, Canad.†; 3M, Hong Kong; Nycomed, Norw.; 3M, NZ; 3M, S.Afr.; 3M, UK†.*
Calcium carbonate (p.1254·2); glycine.
*Calcium supplement; gastrointestinal disorders; hyperphosphataemia.*

**Titralac Extra Strength** *3M, USA.*
Calcium carbonate (p.1254·2).
*Hyperacidity.*

**Titralac Plus** *3M, USA.*
Calcium carbonate (p.1254·2); simeticone (p.1289·2).
*Hyperacidity.*

**Titralac-Sil**
*3M, Austral.; 3M, Malaysia; 3M, NZ; 3M, Singapore.*
Calcium carbonate (p.1254·2); simeticone (p.1289·2); glycine.
*Dyspepsia; flatulence; gastric hyperacidity; gastritis; heartburn; peptic ulcer.*

**Titralgan** *Berlin-Chemie, Ger.*
Phenazone (p.82·3); paracetamol (p.76·2); caffeine (p.782·1).
*Fever; pain.*

**Titrane** *CEPA, Spain†.*
Isosorbide mononitrate (p.942·1).
*Angina pectoris; heart failure.*

**Ti-Tre** *Teofarma, Ital.*
Liothyronine sodium (p.1602·2).
*Hypothyroidism.*

**Titretta** *Berlin-Chemie, Ger.*
Propyphenazone (p.85·3); codeine phosphate (p.27·1).
*Pain.*

**Titus** *Help, Gr.*
Lorazepam (p.704·1).
*Anxiety disorders; insomnia; status epilepticus.*

**Ti-U-Lac** *Draxis, Canad.*
Urea (p.1162·2).

**Ti-U-Lac HC** *Spectropharm, Canad.†.*
Hydrocortisone (p.1103·3); urea (p.1162·2).
*Skin disorders.*

**Ti-UVA-B** *Draxis, Canad.*
*SPF 22:* Octinoxate (p.1154·3); oxybenzone (p.1154·3).
*Sunscreen.*

**Tivision** *Bell, India.*
Lidocaine hydrochloride (p.1377·3).
*Eye-strain.*

**Tivitis** *Llorens, Spain.*
Gramicidin (p.220·2); methylthioninium chloride (p.1042·2); neomycin sulfate (p.235·1); polymyxin B sulfate (p.245·1); tetryzoline hydrochloride (p.1131·2).
*Bacterial eye infections.*

**Tixair** *Byk, Fr.*
Acetylcysteine (p.1112·3).
*Respiratory-tract congestion.*

**Tixobar**
*Justesa Imagen, Arg.; AstraZeneca, Austral.†.*
Barium sulfate (p.1061·1).
*Radiography of gastrointestinal tract.*

**Tixycolds** *Novartis Consumer, UK.*
Diphenhydramine hydrochloride (p.431·3); pseudoephedrine hydrochloride (p.1129·2).
*Cold and influenza symptoms.*

**Tixycolds Cold and Allergy** *Novartis Consumer, UK.*
Xylometazoline hydrochloride (p.1132·2).
*Nasal congestion; rhinitis; sinusitis.*

**Tixycolds Cold and Hayfever** *Novartis Consumer, UK†.*
Camphor (p.1665·3); menthol (p.1711·3); turpentine oil (p.1760·1); eucalyptus oil (p.1686·2).
Formerly known as Tixylix Inhalant.
*Nasal congestion.*

**Tixylix**
*Note. This name is used for preparations of different composition.*
*Nicholas Piramal, India; Intercare, Irl.†.*
Promethazine hydrochloride (p.439·1); pholcodine citrate (p.1128·3); phenylpropanolamine hydrochloride (p.1127·3).
*Cold symptoms; coughs.*

*Aventis, Malaysia; Aventis, NZ; Alps, S.Afr.*
Promethazine hydrochloride (p.439·1); pholcodine (p.1128·3).
Formerly contained promethazine hydrochloride, pholcodine, and phenylpropanolamine hydrochloride.
*Coughs and cold symptoms.*

**Tixylix Baby Syrup** *Novartis Consumer, UK.*
Glycerol (p.1694·3).
*Coughs.*

**Tixylix Catarrh** *Novartis Consumer, UK†.*
Diphenhydramine hydrochloride (p.431·3); menthol (p.1711·3).
*Nasal congestion.*

**Tixylix Chest Rub**
*Aventis, Austral.; Aventis, NZ.*
Cineole (p.1672·1); pine oil; rosemary oil (p.1740·2); thyme oil (p.1755·3); terpineol (p.1752·2).
*Nasal congestion.*

**Tixylix Chesty Cough**
*Novartis Consumer, Irl.; Novartis Consumer, UK.*
Guaifenesin (p.1122·1).
*Coughs.*

**Tixylix Cough & Cold** *Novartis Consumer, UK.*
Pseudoephedrine hydrochloride (p.1129·2); chlorphenamine maleate (p.427·3); pholcodine (p.1128·3).
*Coughs and cold symptoms.*

**Tixylix Daytime** *Novartis Consumer, UK.*
Pholcodine (p.1128·3).
*Coughs.*

**Tixylix Flu** *Quatromed, S.Afr.*
Triprolidine hydrochloride (p.442·3); pseudoephedrine hydrochloride (p.1129·2).
*Nasal congestion.*

**Tixylix Nightime**
*Aventis, Austral.; Rhone-Poulenc Rorer, Hong Kong†.*
Promethazine hydrochloride (p.439·1); pholcodine (p.1128·3).
*Coughs.*

**Tixylix Night-Time** *Novartis Consumer, UK.*
Promethazine hydrochloride (p.439·1); pholcodine (p.1128·3).
*Coughs.*

**Tixymol** *Novartis Consumer, UK†.*
Paracetamol (p.76·2).
*Fever; pain.*

**Tixyplus** *Novartis Consumer, UK.*
Paracetamol (p.76·2); diphenhydramine hydrochloride (p.431·3).
*Cold and influenza symptoms.*

**Tizoxim** *Richmond, Arg.*
Cefotaxime (p.176·3).
*Bacterial infections.*

**TKC** *Grunenthal, Chile.*
Ketoconazole (p.403·3).
*Scalp disorders.*

**T-KI** *Seroyal, Canad.†.*
Vitamin A and vitamin C (p.1417·1).

**T-Koff** *Williams, USA†.*
Phenylpropanolamine hydrochloride (p.1127·3); phenylephrine hydrochloride (p.1126·3); chlorphenamine maleate (p.427·3); codeine phosphate (p.27·1).
*Coughs and cold symptoms.*

**T-LI** *Seroyal, Canad.†.*
Vitamin B substances, vitamin C, copper, and iron (p.1417·1).

**TLM** *Seroyal, Canad.†.*
Vitamin C and minerals (p.1417·1).

**T-LU** *Seroyal, Canad.†.*
Vitamins A, C, and E (p.1417·1).

**T-MA** *Seroyal, Canad.†.*
Vitamin A, vitamin E, and zinc (p.1417·1).

**T-Medevax** *Ribosepharm, Ger.†.*
An adsorbed tetanus vaccine (p.1640·3).
*Active immunisation.*

**TMG Folic** *Douglas, NZ.*
Betaine; folic acid; vitamin $B_{12}$ (p.1417·1).
*Nutritional supplement.*

**TMP**
*Ratiopharm, Ger.; Pacific, NZ.*
Trimethoprim (p.272·2).
*Bacterial infections of the urinary tract.*

**TMS** *TAD, Ger.*
Co-trimoxazole (p.199·3).
*Bacterial infections.*

**TNKase** *Genentech, USA.*
Tenecteplase (p.1010·2).
*Myocardial infarction.*

**Toa** *Wyeth, Mex.*
Dextromethorphan hydrobromide (p.1117·3); pseudoephedrine hydrochloride (p.1129·2).
*Coughs; nasal congestion.*

**Toallet Benzal** *Terrier, Mex.†.*
Benzalkonium.

**Tobacin** *Aristo, India.*
Tobramycin (p.271·2).
*Bacterial eye infections.*

**Tobazon** *Bell, India.*
Tobramycin sulfate (p.271·3); dexamethasone sodium phosphate (p.1097·2).
*Inflammation and infection following cataract surgery.*

**Tobe** *Laboratorios Chile, Chile.*
Tibolone (p.1572·3).
*Menopausal disorders; osteoporosis.*

**Tobedoce** *Jofrain, Mex.†.*
Vitamin B substances (p.1417·1).

**Tobi**
*Teva Tuteur, Arg.; Amrad, Austral.; Croma, Austria; Chiron, Canad.; Pathogenesis, Denm.; Orphan, Fin.; Chiron, Fr.; Dermapharm, Ger.; Pathogenesis, Gr.; Pathogenesis, Irl.; Chiron, Israel; Dompe, Ital.; Pathogenesis, Norw.; Baxter, NZ; Chiron, NZ; Chiron, Spain; Swedish Orphan, Swed.; Chiron, UK; Pathogenesis, USA.*
Tobramycin (p.271·2).
*Pseudomonal infections in cystic fibrosis.*

**Tobitil**
*Ranbaxy, India; Ranbaxy, S.Afr.*
Tenoxicam (p.93·1).
*Dysmenorrhoea; gout; musculoskeletal, joint, and peri-articular disorders.*

**Tobra** *Lilly, Mex.*
Tobramycin sulfate (p.271·3).
*Bacterial infections.*

**Tobra Gobens**
*APS, Port.; Normon, Spain.*
Tobramycin sulfate (p.271·3).
*Bacterial infections.*

**Tobrabact** *Novartis, Spain.*
Tobramycin (p.271·2).
*Bacterial eye infections.*

**Tobra-cell** *Cell Pharm, Ger.*
Tobramycin sulfate (p.271·3).
*Bacterial infections.*

**Tobracil** *Oftalder, Port.†.*
Tobramycin sulfate (p.271·3).
*Bacterial eye infections.*

**Tobracort** *Genom, Braz.*
Tobramycin (p.271·2); dexamethasone (p.1097·1).
*Infected eye disorders.*

**Tobradex**
*Alcon, Arg.; Alcon, Austria; Alcon, Belg.; Alcon, Braz.; Alcon, Canad.; Alcon, Chile; Alcon, Fr.; Alcon, Hong Kong; Alcon, Ital.; Alcon, Malaysia; Alcon, Mex.; Alcon, NZ; Alcon, S.Afr.; Alcon, Singapore; Alcon Cusi, Spain; Alcon, Switz.; Alcon, Thai.; Alcon, UK; Alcon, USA.*
Tobramycin (p.271·2); dexamethasone (p.1097·1).
*Infected eye disorders.*

**Tobradistin** *Dista, Spain.*
Tobramycin sulfate (p.271·3).
*Bacterial infections.*

**Tobrafen** *Alcon, Switz.*
Diclofenac sodium (p.32·1); tobramycin (p.271·2).
*Postoperative eye inflammation.*

**Tobragan**
*Allergan, Arg.; Allergan, Braz.; Allergan, Chile.*
Tobramycin (p.271·2).
*Bacterial eye infections.*

**Tobral** *Alcon, Ital.*
Tobramycin (p.271·2).
*Bacterial infections of the eye and external ear.*

**Tobralex** *Alcon, Irl.*
Tobramycin (p.271·2).
*Bacterial eye infections.*

**Tobra-M** *Bausch & Lomb, Braz.*
Tobramycin (p.271·2).
*Bacterial infections.*

**Tobramaxin** *Alcon, Ger.*
Tobramycin (p.271·2).
*Bacterial eye infections.*

**Tobramina** *Lilly, Braz.*
Tobramycin sulfate (p.271·3).
*Bacterial infections.*

**Tobraneg** *Lilly, India.*
Tobramycin sulfate (p.271·3).
*Bacterial infections.*

**Tobranom** *Genom, Braz.*
Tobramycin (p.271·2).
*Bacterial eye infections.*

**Tobrasix** *Lilly, Austria.*
Tobramycin sulfate (p.271·3).
*Bacterial infections.*

**Tobrasol** *Ocusoft, USA.*
Tobramycin (p.271·2).
*Bacterial eye infections.*

**Tobrasone** *Alcon, NZ†.*
Tobramycin (p.271·2); fluorometholone acetate (p.1102·2).
*Infected inflammatory eye disorders.*

**Tobrex**
*Alcon, Arg.; Alcon, Austral.; Alcon, Austria; Alcon, Belg.; Alcon, Braz.; Alcon, Canad.; Alcon, Chile; Alcon, Denm.; Alcon, Fin.; Alcon, Fr.; Alcon (Λλκον), Gr.; Alcon, Hong Kong; Alcon, Israel; Alcon, Malaysia; Alcon, Mex.; Alcon, Norw.; Alcon, NZ; Alcon, Port.; Alcon, S.Afr.; Alcon, Singapore; Alcon Cusi, Spain; Alcon, Swed.; Alcon, Switz.; Alcon, Thai.; Alcon, USA.*
Tobramycin (p.271·2).
*Bacterial eye infections.*

*FIRMA, Ital.†.*
Tobramycin sulfate (p.271·3).
*Bacterial infections.*

**Tobridavi** *Davi, Port.*
Tobramycin (p.271·2).
*Bacterial eye infections.*

**Tobrin** *Laboratorios Chile, Chile.*
Tobramycin (p.271·2).
*Bacterial eye infections.*

**Tobrin-D** *Laboratorios Chile, Chile.*
Tobramycin (p.271·2); dexamethasone (p.1097·1).
*Bacterial eye infections with inflammation.*

**Tobutol** *General Drugs, Thai.*
Ethambutol hydrochloride (p.211·3).
*Tuberculosis.*

**Tocalfa** *Marvecs, Ital.*
*dl*-Alpha tocoferil acetate (p.1465·1); vitamin A (p.1451·2).
*Vitamin A and E deficiency.*

**Tocalm** *Prater, Chile.*
Ambroxol (p.1114·3).
*Respiratory-tract congestion.*

**Tocid** *TO-Chemicals, Singapore†.*
Aluminium hydroxide-magnesium carbonate co-dried gel (p.1250·1); dicycloverine hydrochloride (p.481·2); simeticone (p.1289·2).
*Duodenitis; dyspepsia; flatulence; gastric hyperacidity; gastritis; gastro-oesophageal reflux; gastrointestinal motility disorders; heartburn; peptic ulcer; pylorospasm.*

**Toclapekt** *UCB, Fin.*
Carbocisteine (p.1116·2).
*Respiratory-tract congestion.*

**Toclase**
*UCB, Denm.; UCB, Fin.; UCB, Hong Kong; UCB, Norw.; Vedim, Port.†; UCB, Swed.; UCB, Thai.*
Pentoxyverine citrate (p.1126·2) or pentoxyverine hydrochloride (p.1126·3).
*Coughs.*

**Toclase Expectorant**
*Note. This name is used for preparations of different composition.*
*UCB, Fin.*
Pentoxyverine citrate (p.1126·2); terpin hydrate (p.1131·1).
*Coughs.*

*UCB, Fr.*
Carbocisteine (p.1116·2).
*Respiratory-tract disorders.*

**Toclase Toux Seche** *UCB, Fr.*
Pentoxyverine citrate (p.1126·2).
*Coughs.*

**Toco** *Pharma 2000, Fr.*
Alpha tocoferil acetate (p.1465·1).
*Hyperlipidaemia.*

**Tocodrine** *Medichemie, Switz.*
Buphenine hydrochloride (p.1663·2).
*Inhibition of uterine contraction.*

**Tocogen** *Abiogen, Ital.†.*
*d*-Alpha tocoferil acetate (p.1465·1).
*Cardiac stenosis; diabetes mellitus; disorders of the female reproductive system; muscular dystrophy; peripheral vascular disorders.*

**Tocogestan** *Theramex, Mon.†.*
Hydroxyprogesterone enantate (p.1556·3); progesterone (p.1566·2); *dl*-alpha tocoferil palmitate (p.1465·3).
*Premature labour; threatened miscarriage.*

**Tocolion** *Sciencex, Fr.*
Alpha tocoferil acetate (p.1465·1).
*Hyperlipidaemias.*

**Tocomine** *Pfizer, Fr.†.*
*dl*-Alpha tocoferil acetate (p.1465·1).
*Vitamin E deficiency.*

**Tocomizol** *Tocogino, Mex.†.*
Ketoconazole (p.403·3).
*Fungal infections.*

**Toconal** *Cryopharma, Mex.*
Ketoconazole (p.403·3).
*Fungal infections.*

**Tocopa** *Arkopharma, Fr.*
Alpha tocoferil acetate (p.1465·1).
Formerly known as Tocophan.
*Hyperlipidaemias.*

**Tocorell** *Sanorell, Ger.*
*d*-Alpha tocopherol (p.1464·3) or *d*-α-tocoferil acetate (p.1465·1).
*Vitamin E deficiency.*

**Tocovenos**
*Fresenius Kabi, Austria; Fresenius, Ger.†.*
*dl*-Alpha tocoferil acetate (p.1465·1).
*Vitamin E deficiency.*

**Tocovid** *Hovid, Singapore.*
Vitamin E; squalene; phytosterol complex; phyto-carotenoid complex (p.1417·1).
*Vitamin E supplement.*

**Tocovid Suprabio** *Hovid, Malaysia.*
Vitamin E; squalene; phytosterol complex; phytocarotenoid complex (p.1417·1).
*Dietary supplement.*

**Tocovital** *Steigerwald, Ger.*
*d*-Alpha tocoferol (p.1464·3).
*Vitamin E deficiency.*

**Tocrat** *Sanofi Synthelabo, Arg.*
Nitrendipine (p.973·3).
*Hypertension.*

**Todalgil** *Aldo, Spain†.*
Ibuprofen (p.45·3).
*Fever; musculoskeletal, joint, and peri-articular disorders; pain.*

**Today** *Wyeth, UK†.*
Nonoxinol 9 (p.1413·3).
*Contraceptive.*

**Today Ovulation Test** *Omega, Irl.*
Fertility test (p.1734·3).

**Todexona** *SMB, Chile.*
Tobramycin (p.271·2); dexamethasone (p.1097·1).
*Bacterial eye infections with inflammation.*

**Todolac** *Norpharma, Denm.*
Etodolac (p.37·3).
*Gout; inflammation; musculoskeletal and joint disorders.*

**Toepedo** *Dendron, UK.*
Benzoic acid (p.1169·3); salicylic acid (p.1157·1).
*Fungal skin infections.*

**Tofen**
*Note. This name is used for preparations of different composition.*
*Beximco, Singapore.*
Ketotifen (p.788·2).
*Asthma; hypersensitivity reactions.*

*Utopian, Thai.*
Ibuprofen (p.45·3).
*Inflammation; musculoskeletal and joint disorders; pain.*

**Toflamixina**
*Novartis Ophthalmics, Arg.; Novartis Ophthalmics, Braz.*
Tobramycin (p.271·2).
*Bacterial eye infections.*

**Toflamixina Plus** *Novartis Ophthalmics, Arg.*
Tobramycin (p.271·2); dexamethasone (p.1097·1).
*Infected eye disorders.*

**Toflex** *TO-Chemicals, Thai.*
Cefalexin (p.168·1).
*Bacterial infections.*

**Tofranil**
*Novartis, Arg.; Novartis, Austral.; Novartis, Austria; Novartis, Belg.;*

*Novartis, Braz.; Novartis, Canad.; Novartis, Fr.; Novartis, Ger.; Novartis, Hong Kong; Novartis, Irl.; Novartis, Israel; Novartis, Ital.; Novartis, Mex.; Novartis, Neth.; CSL, NZ; Novartis, Port.; Novartis, S.Afr.; Novartis, Spain; Novartis, Swed.; Novartis, Switz.; Novartis, Thai.†; Novartis, UK; Novartis, USA.*
Imipramine (p.300·1), imipramine embonate (p.300·1), or imipramine hydrochloride (p.300·1).
*Depression; nocturnal enuresis; pain; panic attacks.*

**Tofranil-PM** *Novartis, USA.*
Imipramine embonate (p.300·1).
*Depression.*

**Togal**
*Note. This name is used for preparations of different composition.*
*Sanova, Austria†.*
Aspirin (p.15·1); lithium citrate (p.301·1); quinine dihydrochloride (p.460·1).
*Cold symptoms; pain.*
*Togal, Ger.*
*Suppositories:* Paracetamol (p.76·2).
*Fever; pain.*
*Tablets:* Aspirin (p.15·1); lithium citrate (p.301·1); quinine dihydrochloride (p.460·1).
*Fever; inflammation; pain.*

**Togal ASS**
*Togal, Ger.; Togal, Switz.*
Aspirin (p.15·1).
*Fever; inflammation; pain.*

**Togal Ibuprofen** *Togal, Ger.*
Ibuprofen (p.45·3).
*Fever; pain.*

**Togal Kopfschmerzbrause + Vit C** *Togal, Ger.*
Aspirin (p.15·1); ascorbic acid (p.1460·2); caffeine (p.782·1).
*Pain.*

**Togal Mobil Rheuma-Bad** *Togal, Ger.†.*
Camphor (p.1665·3); benzyl nicotinate (p.21·2); Norway spruce oil; rosemary oil (p.1740·2).
*Bath additive; circulatory disorders; musculoskeletal, joint, peri-articular, and soft-tissue disorders.*

**Togal Mobil-Gel** *Togal, Ger.*
Glycol salicylate (p.44·3); benzyl nicotinate (p.21·2).
*Musculoskeletal and soft-tissue disorders.*

**Togal Mono** *Sanova, Austria.*
Aspirin (p.15·1).
*Fever; pain.*

**Togamycin**
*Pharmacia, Arg.; Pharmacia Upjohn, Israel.*
Spectinomycin hydrochloride (p.255·2).
*Gonorrhoea.*

**Togasan** *Togal, Ger.*
*d*-Alpha tocopherol (p.1464·3) or *d*-alpha tocoferil acetate (p.1465·1).
*Vitamin E deficiency.*

**Togine** *Utopian, Thai.*
Co-dergocrine mesilate (p.1674·1).
*Cerebral and peripheral vascular disorders.*

**Togrel** *Armstrong, Arg.*
Levomepromazine maleate (p.703·2).
*Pain; psychoses.*

**Togrisol** *Solfran, Mex.*
Aspirin (p.15·1); caffeine (p.782·1).
*Cold symptoms.*

**Toilax**
*Orion, Denm.; Orion, Fin.; Orion, Irl.; Orion, Norw.; Orion, Swed.*
Bisacodyl (p.1251·3).
*Bowel evacuation; constipation.*

**Tokovitan** *Orion, Fin.*
*d*-Alpha tocoferil acetate (p.1465·1).
*Vitamin E deficiency.*

**Tol** *Eco, S.Afr.*
Allergen extracts (p.1650·1).
*Hyposensitisation.*

**Tol 12** *Saval, Chile.*
Thiamine hydrochloride (p.1455·1); pyridoxine hydrochloride (p.1456·3); vitamin $B_{12}$ (p.1458·2).
*Neuralgia; neuritis; reduced appetite; tonic.*

**Tol Total** *Saval, Chile.*
Vitamin preparation with or without minerals (p.1417·1).
*Dietary supplement.*

**Tolan** *Solfran, Mex.*
Methyl salicylate (p.59·3).
*Soft-tissue injury.*

**Tolanase**
*Pharmacia Upjohn, Irl.†; Pharmacia Upjohn, UK†.*
Tolazamide (p.348·1).
*Diabetes mellitus.*

**Tolbetol** *Raza, Malaysia; Pharmaniaga, Malaysia.*
Labetalol hydrochloride (p.943·3).
*Angina pectoris; hypertension.*

**Tolbin**
*Unison, Hong Kong; Unison, Singapore.*
Terbutaline sulfate (p.797·2).
*Obstructive airways disease; premature labour.*

**Tolchicine** *TO-Chemicals, Thai.*
Colchicine (p.415·1).
*Gout.*

**Toldex** *Bial, Port.*
Aspirin (p.15·1).

**Tolecen** *Centrum, Spain†.*
Hypericum (p.299·1).
*Asthenia; sleep disorders.*

**Tolectin**
*Janssen-Cilag, Austria; Janssen-Cilag, Belg.†; Janssen-Ortho, Canad.; Janssen-Cilag, Denm.†; Janssen-Cilag, Irl.†; Janssen-Cilag, Ital.†; Cilag, Mex.; Janssen-Cilag, Neth.; Janssen-Cilag, S.Afr.†; Janssen-Cilag, Switz.; Ortho McNeil, USA.*
Tolmetin (p.94·3) or tolmetin sodium (p.94·2).
*Inflammation; musculoskeletal, joint, peri-articular, and soft-tissue disorders; pain.*

**Tolep** *Novartis, Ital.*
Oxcarbazepine (p.366·3).
*Epilepsy.*

**Tolerance Extreme** *Pierre Fabre Dermo-Cosmetique, Arg.*
Emollient; skin cleanser.
*Skin irritation.*

**Tolerane**
*Note. This name is used for preparations of different composition.*
*Alcon, Arg.*
Flurbiprofen (p.43·3).
*Inflammatory eye disorders.*
*Bago, Chile.*
Disulfiram (p.1681·3).
*Alcoholism.*

**Tolerex**
*Novartis Nutrition, Canad.†; Novartis, Israel†; Procter & Gamble, USA.*
Preparation for enteral nutrition (p.1417·1).

**Toleriane**
*Roche-Posay, Arg.; Roche-Posay, Braz.; Roche-Posay, Irl.*
A range of emollient preparations.

**Tolestan** *Roemmers, Arg.*
Cloxazolam (p.685·3).
*Anxiety.*

**Tolexine**
*Biorga, Fr.; Biorga, Hong Kong†.*
Doxycycline (p.206·2).
*Bacterial infections.*

**Tolfamic** *Faran, Gr.*
Tolfenamic acid (p.94·2).
*Dysmenorrhoea; inflammation; musculoskeletal and joint disorders; pain.*

**Tolfrinic** *Ascher, USA.*
Ferrous fumarate (p.1427·3); cyanocobalamin (p.1458·2).
Ascorbic acid (p.1460·2) is included in this preparation to increase the absorption and availability of iron.
*Iron-deficiency anaemias.*

**Tolgin** *Saval, Chile.*
Vitamins; minerals; ginseng (p.1417·1).
*Asthenia; tonic.*

**Tolid** *Dolorgiet, Ger.*
Lorazepam (p.704·1).
*Anxiety; premedication; sleep disorders.*

**Toliken** *Norma (Νορμα), Gr.*
Clindamycin (p.194·2).
*Acne.*

**Toliman** *Scharper, Ital.*
Cinnarizine (p.428·3).
*Cerebral and peripheral vascular disorders.*

**Tolimed** *Medifive, Thai.*
Mianserin hydrochloride (p.306·3).
*Depression.*

**Tolinase**
*Pharmacia Upjohn, Swed.†; Upjohn, USA.*
Tolazamide (p.348·1).
*Diabetes mellitus.*

**Tolindol** *Meuse, Belg.*
Proglumetacin maleate (p.85·2).
*Musculoskeletal, joint, and peri-articular disorders.*

**Tollwutglobulin** *Pasteur Merieux, Ger.†.*
A rabies immunoglobulin (p.1635·3).
*Passive immunisation.*

**Tollwut-Impfstoff (HDC)** *Aventis Pasteur, Ger.*
A rabies vaccine (human diploid cell) (p.1635·3).
*Active immunisation.*

**Tolmicen**
*Pharmacia Upjohn, Hong Kong†; Pharmacia Upjohn, Ital.; Pharmacia, NZ; Pharmacia Upjohn, Port.*
Tolciclate (p.410·1).
*Fungal skin infections.*

**Tolmicil** *Pharmacia-Upjohn, Gr.*
Tolciclate (p.410·1).
*Fungal skin infections.*

**Tolmicol** *Pharmacia, Braz.*
Tolciclate (p.410·1).
*Fungal skin infections.*

**Tolmin** *Durascan, Denm.*
Mianserin hydrochloride (p.306·3).
*Depression.*

**Tolnaderm**
*Sterfil, India; Quimica y Farmacia, Mex.†.*
Tolnaftate (p.410·1).
*Fungal skin infections.*

**Tolodina** *Estedi, Spain.*
Amoxicillin trihydrate (p.155·3).
*Bacterial infections.*

**Toloran** *Rayere, Mex.*
Ketorolac trometamol (p.52·1).
*Pain.*

**Toloxane** *Beta, Arg.*
Rofecoxib (p.86·3).
*Dysmenorrhoea; osteoarthritis.*

**Toloxim** *Merck, Port.*
Mebendazole (p.108·2).
*Worm infections.*

**Toloxin**
*Note. This name is used for preparations of different composition.*
*Biolab Sanus, Braz.*
Metamizole magnesium (p.36·1).
*Fever; pain.*
*TO-Chemicals, Thai.*
Digoxin (p.895·2).
*Arrhythmias; heart failure.*

**Tolrest** *Biosintetica, Braz.*
Sertraline hydrochloride (p.317·2).
*Depression.*

**Toltem** *Temis, Arg.*
Tolterodine tartrate (p.489·3).
*Bladder instability.*

**Toluidinblau** *Kohler, Ger.*
Tolonium chloride (p.1757·1).
*Methaemoglobinaemia.*

**Tolu-Sed DM** *Scherer, USA.*
Dextromethorphan hydrobromide (p.1117·3); guaifenesin (p.1122·1).
*Coughs.*

**Tolusil** *INQ, Braz.†.*
Potassium iodide (p.1598·1); sodium benzoate (p.1169·3); ephedrine hydrochloride (p.1120·1); erythrina mulungu (p.1717·2).
*Respiratory-tract congestion.*

**Tolvin** *Organon, Ger.*
Mianserin hydrochloride (p.306·3).
*Depression.*

**Tolvon**
*Organon, Austral.; Organon, Austria; Organon, Braz.; Organon, Denm.; Organon, Fin.; Organon, Hong Kong; Organon, Irl.; Organon, Mex.; Nourypharma, Neth.; Organon, Norw.; Organon, NZ; Organon, Port.; Organon, Singapore†; Organon, Swed.; Organon, Switz.; Organon, Thai.*
Mianserin hydrochloride (p.306·3).
*Depression.*

**Tolyprin** *Du Pont, Ger.†.*
Azapropazone (p.20·1).
*Gout; inflammation; musculoskeletal, joint, and soft-tissue disorders; pain.*

**Tomabef** *Salus, Ital.*
Cefoperazone sodium (p.174·3).
Lidocaine hydrochloride (p.1377·3) is included in this preparation to alleviate the pain of injection.
*Gram-negative bacterial infections.*

**Tomag** *Temis, Arg.*
Ranitidine hydrochloride (p.1285·2).
*Gastric hyperacidity.*

**Tomanil** *Byk, Arg.*
Diclofenac diethylamine (p.32·1) or diclofenac sodium (p.32·1).
*Gout; inflammation; musculoskeletal, joint, peri-articular, and soft-tissue disorders; neuritis; oedema.*

**Tomcin** *General Drugs, Thai.*
Erythromycin estolate (p.208·1) or erythromycin stearate (p.208·2).
*Bacterial infections.*

**Tomevis** *Brasifa, Braz.†.*
Multivitamin and mineral preparation (p.1417·1).

**Tomevit** *Spyfarma, Spain.*
Adenosine triphosphate; arginine aspartate; glutathione; hydroxocobalamin acetate; lysine hydrochloride; pyritinol hydrochloride (p.1417·1).
*Tonic.*

**Tomid** *Gufic, India.*
Metoclopramide hydrochloride (p.1274·3).
*Motion sickness; vomiting.*

**Tomiporan** *Toyama, Jpn.*
Cefbuperazone sodium (p.171·2).
*Bacterial infections.*

**Tomiron** *Toyama, Jpn.*
Cefteram pivoxil (p.181·3).
*Bacterial infections.*

**Tomocat** *Lafayette, USA.*
Barium sulfate (p.1061·1).
*Contrast medium for gastrointestinal radiography.*

**Tomoray** *Varifarma, Arg.*
Meglumine amidotrizoate (p.1060·2) with/without sodium amidotrizoate (p.1060·2).
*Radiographic contrast medium.*

**Tomudex**
*AstraZeneca, Arg.; AstraZeneca, Austral.; AstraZeneca, Austria; AstraZeneca, Belg.; AstraZeneca, Braz.; AstraZeneca, Canad.; AstraZeneca, Fin.; AstraZeneca, Fr.; AstraZeneca, Hong Kong; AstraZeneca, Irl.; AstraZeneca, Ital.; Zeneca, Mex.; AstraZeneca, Neth.; AstraZeneca, Norw.; AstraZeneca, Port.; Zeneca, S.Afr.; AstraZeneca, Singapore; AstraZeneca, Spain; AstraZeneca, Switz.; AstraZeneca, UK.*
Raltitrexed (p.582·1).
*Colorectal cancer.*

**Tomycin** *Orion, Fin.*
Tobramycin sulfate (p.271·3).
*Bacterial infections.*

**Tomycine** *Novartis Ophthalmics, Canad.*
Tobramycin (p.271·2).
*Bacterial eye infections.*

**Ton Was** *Chiesi, Spain.*
Vitamin B substances (p.1417·1); ginseng (p.1693·1).
*Tonic.*

**Tonactil** *Arkopharma, Fr.*
Kola (p.1765·3); ginseng (p.1693·1).
*Asthenia.*

**Tonactiv** *Herboline, Ital.†.*
Angelica (p.1655·1); fennel (p.1687·2); laurus nobilis; aniseed (p.1655·2).
*Depression; hypotension; tonic.*

**Tonalgen** *Andromaco, Chile.*
Cyclobenzaprine hydrochloride (p.1393·1).
*Musculoskeletal pain.*

**Tonamil** *Ecobi, Ital.*
Thonzylamine (p.442·2).
*Conjunctivitis; rhinitis; skin irritation.*

**Tonaril** *Laboratorios Chile, Chile.*
Trihexyphenidyl (p.490·3).
*Drug-induced exptrapyramidal disorders; parkinsonism.*

**Tonaton** *Sankyo, Braz.*
Yohimbine (p.1766·2); fevillea trilobata; labiadas; ephedrine hydrochloride (p.1120·1); atropine methonitrate (p.477·1).
*Erectile dysfunction.*

**Tonavir** *Richmond, Arg.*
Stavudine (p.654·2).
*HIV infection.*

**Tonavital** *Recalcine, Chile.*
Amino acids; vitamins; minerals (p.1417·1).
*Tonic.*

**Toncard-Do** *Grasler, Ger.*
Homoeopathic preparation.

**Toncils** *Vitabalans, Fin.*
Chlorhexidine hydrochloride (p.1173·3); benzocaine (p.1370·3).
*Mouth and throat disorders.*

**Tondex** *Hormona, Mex.*
Gentamicin sulfate (p.217·1).
*Bacterial infections.*

**Tondinel H** *Pfluger, Ger.*
Homoeopathic preparation.

**Tonekin** *Assistance, Arg.*
Chromium tripicolinate (p.1425·1).

**Tonekin Plus** *Assistance, Arg.*
Chromium tripicolinate (p.1425·1); levocarnitine (p.1423·3).
*Dietary supplement.*

**Toneon** *Raffo, Arg.*
Minoxidil (p.960·1).
*Alopecia.*

**Toness** *Angelini, Ital.*
Proxazole citrate (p.1735·3).
*Smooth muscle relaxant; vascular disorders.*

**Tonex** *Boehringer Ingelheim, Switz.†.*
Tetracaine hydrochloride (p.1385·1); chamomile (p.1669·3); sage (p.1741·2); aluminium formate; mint oil (p.1715·2); menthol (p.1711·3).
*Minor skin lesions; mouth disorders.*

**Tonexis**
*Clintec, Fr.†; Clintec, Irl.†; Clintec, Ital.†.*
A range of preparations for enteral nutrition (p.1417·1).

**Tonexis HP** *Clintec, Fr.†.*
High-protein nutritional supplement (p.1417·1).

**Tongill** *Novartis, Austria.*
Tyrothricin (p.275·1); muramidase hydrochloride (p.1717·2); lidocaine hydrochloride (p.1377·3).
*Mouth and throat disorders.*

**Tonginal** *Bittner, Austria.*
Homoeopathic preparation.

**Toniazol** *Nicholas Piramal, India.*
Vitamin B substances (p.1454·3); glucose (p.1432·2); bitter orange peel (p.1723·3); absinthium (p.1645·1).
*Tonic.*

**Tonible** *Novartis Consumer, Ital.†.*
Multivitamin and mineral preparation (p.1417·1).

**Tonibral** *GNR, Port.*
Deanol hemisuccinate (p.1585·3).
*Tonic.*

**Tonibral Adulte** *GNR, Fr.†.*
Deanol hemisuccinate (p.1585·3).
*Tonic.*

**Tonic Yeast** *Seven Seas, UK.*
Yeast (p.1469·1); vitamin B substances (p.1417·1).
Formerly known as Phillips P.T.Y. Yeast Tablets.

**Tonicalcium**
*Therabel, Belg.†; Bouchara-Recordati, Fr.*
DL-Lysine ascorbate (p.1461·1); calcium ascorbate (p.1460·2).
*Asthenia; vitamin C deficiency.*

**Tonice** *Confar, Port.*
*Oral liquid:* Deanol pyroglutamate (p.1585·3); magnesium aminobenzoate; ascorbic acid.
*Syrup:* Deanol pyroglutamate (p.1585·3); calcium gluceptate; lysine hydrochloride.
*Tonic.*

**Tonico Blumen** *Luper, Braz.*
Ferrous sulfate (p.1428·2); phosphoric acid; aloes; myrrh; mace; cinnamon.
*Anaemias.*

**Tonico Juventus** *Juventus, Spain.*
Cyproheptadine hydrochloride (p.430·1); cobamamide (p.1459·1).
*Tonic.*

**Tonico No I** *QIF, Braz.†.*
Ferrous sulfate (p.1428·2); phosphoric acid (p.1731·2).
*Iron deficiency; iron-deficiency anaemias.*

**Tonico Pasteur** *Pasteur, Chile.*
Vitamin and mineral preparation (p.1417·1).
*Tonic.*

**Tonico Prata** Uniao Quimica, Braz.†.
Manganese sulfate; sodium glycerophosphate; ferric ammonium citrate (p.1427·2).
*Iron deficiency; iron-deficiency anaemias.*

**Tonicol & ADC** Multi-Pro, Canad.†.
Multivitamin and iron preparation (p.1417·1).

**Tonicum**
Petrasch, Austria.
Vitamins (p.1417·1); caffeine; lactic acid.
*Tonic.*

SIT, Ital.
Amino-acid and vitamin preparation (p.1417·1).

**Tonid** Milano, Thai.
Tinidazole (p.617·1).
*Amoebiasis; anaerobic bacterial infections; giardiasis; trichomoniasis.*

**Tonilax** Monot, Fr.†.
Frangula bark (p.1266·3); aloes (p.1248·2).

**Tonimax** Soria Natural, Spain.
Eleutherococcus senticosis (p.1744·1); rosemary oil (p.1740·2); savory oil.
*Fatigue.*

**Tonimed** Interpharm, Austria.
Piroxicam (p.84·2).
*Musculoskeletal, joint, and soft-tissue disorders.*

**Tonimer** Dermoteca, Port.
Sea water (p.1233·3).
*Nasal cleansing; nasal disorders.*

**Tonimol** Herbes Universelles, Canad.
Multivitamin preparation (p.1417·1).

**Tonipan** Alpharma, Norw.
Vitamin B substances with manganese (p.1417·1).
*Vitamin B deficiency.*

**Tonique D nouvelle formule** Democal, Switz.
Multivitamin and minerals with plant extracts (p.1417·1).
*Tonic.*

**Tonique Vegetal** Lehning, Fr.
Homoeopathic preparation.

**Tonisan** Dolisos, Fr.†.
Ginseng (p.1693·1); black tea (p.1765·3).
*Tonic.*

**Tonizin** Betapharm, Ger.
Hypericum (p.299·1).
*Anxiety; depression; nervous disorders.*

**Tono** Milano, Thai.
Tolnaftate (p.410·1).
*Fungal skin infections.*

**Tonobexol** Novartis Ophthalmics, Arg.
Betaxolol hydrochloride (p.873·1).
*Glaucoma.*

**Tonocalcin**
Wassermann, Ital.; Merck, Mex.; Alfa Wassermann, Thai.
Calcitonin (salmon) (p.768·2).
*Hypercalcaemia; osteoporosis; Paget's disease of bone; reflex sympathetic dystrophy.*

**Tonocaltin**
Zambon, Port.; Zambon, Spain.
Calcitonin (salmon) (p.768·2).
*Hypercalcaemia; metastatic bone pain; Paget's disease of bone; postmenopausal osteoporosis.*

**Tonocard**
AstraZeneca, Canad.†; Astra, Hong Kong†; AstraZeneca, Neth.†; Hassle, Swed.†; AstraZeneca, Thai.†; AstraZeneca, UK†; Astra, USA†.
Tocainide hydrochloride (p.1014·1).
*Ventricular arrhythmias.*

**Tono-Cis** Laboratorios Chile, Chile.
Cisapride (p.1259·2).
*Gastro-oesophageal reflux; gastrointestinal motility disorders.*

**Tonoferon** East India Pharma, India.
*Oral drops:* Colloidal iron hydroxide; lysine hydrochloride (p.1439·2); vitamin $B_{12}$ (p.1458·2); folic acid (p.1429·1).
*Syrup; paediatric syrup:* Colloidal iron hydroxide; folic acid (p.1429·1); vitamin $B_{12}$ (p.1458·2).
*Iron-deficiency anaemias.*

**Tonofit** Body Spring, Ital.
Vitamins; magnesium; phenylalanine; ginkgo biloba; eleutherococcus (p.1417·1).
*Tonic.*

**Tonoflex** Instituto Sanitas, Chile.
Paracetamol (p.76·2); chlorzoxazone (p.1392·3).
*Skeletal muscle spasm and pain.*

**Tonofolin** Teofarma, Ital.
Calcium folinate (p.1431·1).
*Megaloblastic anaemias.*

**Tonoftal** Essex, Ger.
Tolnaftate (p.410·1).
*Fungal skin infections.*

**Tonogen** ABC, Ital.
Haematoporphyrin hydrochloride (p.1696·2); cyanocobalamin (p.1458·2).
*Tonic.*

**Tonogen S** ABC, Ital.
Vitamin and mineral preparation with ginkgo biloba (p.1417·1).

**Tonoglutal** Wild, Switz.
Glutamic acid; sodium hydroxybenzylphosphinate; ascorbic acid; magnesium glycerophosphate; thiamine nitrate (p.1417·1).
*Tonic.*

The symbol † denotes a preparation no longer actively marketed

**Tonoklen** Farmabraz, Braz.†.
Ptychopetalum uncinatum; erythroxylon catuaba.
*Tonic.*

**Tonopan**
Novartis, Austria; Novartis, Braz.; Novartis, Mex.; Novartis, Spain; Novartis Consumer, Switz.
Caffeine (p.782·1); dihydroergotamine mesilate (p.465·3); propyphenazone (p.85·3).
*Migraine and other vascular headaches.*

**Tonopaque** Lafayette, USA.
Barium sulfate (p.1061·1).
*Contrast medium for gastrointestinal radiography.*

**Tonoplantin Mono** Palmicol, Ger.†.
Crataegus (p.1677·1).
*Heart failure.*

**Tonoplus** ABC, Ital.
Arginine oxoglurate (p.1421·2); aceglutamide (p.1645·2).
*Tonic.*

**Tonopres** Boehringer Ingelheim, Ger.†.
Dihydroergotamine mesilate (p.465·3).
*Hypotension; migraine and other vascular headaches.*

**Tonopron ACD** Instituto Sanitas, Chile.
Vitamin and mineral preparation (p.1417·1).
*Tonic.*

**Tonopron Fuerte Con Vit. B12** Instituto Sanitas, Chile.
Vitamin B substances with or without liver extract (p.1417·1).
*Tonic.*

**Tonoprotect** Dumex, Ger.†.
Atenolol (p.865·2).
*Angina pectoris; arrhythmias; hypertension.*

**Tonosai** QIF, Braz.†.
Ferric ammonium citrate (p.1427·2); vitamins (p.1417·1); liver extract; calcium glycerophosphate.
*Iron deficiency; iron-deficiency anaemias.*

**Tonosol** Unifa, Port.
Multivitamin preparation (p.1417·1).

**Tonotensil** Laboratorios Chile, Chile.
Lisinopril (p.946·3).
*Heart failure; hypertension.*

**Tonotensil D** Laboratorios Chile, Chile.
Lisinopril (p.946·3); hydrochlorothiazide (p.933·2).
*Hypertension.*

**Tonovin** Windson, Braz.†.
Multivitamin and mineral preparation (p.1417·1).

**Tonovital Antioxidante** Bago, Arg.
Tocopherol acetate; vitamin C; betacarotene; zinc; selenium (p.1417·1).
*Antioxidant preparation.*

**Tonovital E** Bago, Arg.
Tocopherol acetate (p.1464·3).

**Tonovital Plus Antioxidante** Bago, Arg.
Tocopherol acetate; vitamin C; betacarotene; zinc; copper; selenium; manganese (p.1417·1).
*Antioxidant preparation.*

**Tonovix** Sedabel, Braz.†.
Vitamin B substances with lysine (p.1417·1).

**Tonox** Utopian, Thai.
Tenoxicam (p.93·1).
*Gout; musculoskeletal, joint, and peri-articular disorders.*

**Tonsan akut** Bittner, Austria.
Homoeopathic preparation.

**Tonsan chronisch** Bittner, Austria.
Homoeopathic preparation.

**Tonsan-K** Bittner, Austria.
Homoeopathic preparation.

**Tonsicur** Agepha, Austria†.
Tyrothricin (p.275·1); benzalkonium chloride (p.1168·3).
*Mouth and throat disorders.*

**Tonsildrops** Eversil, Braz.†.
Cetylpyridinium chloride (p.1173·1); benzocaine (p.1370·3).
*Mouth and throat disorders.*

**Tonsilgon** Bionorica, Ger.
Althaea (p.1651·3); chamomile (p.1669·3); equisetum (p.1684·1); juglans regia; achillea (p.1646·2); oak bark (p.1722·3); taraxacum (p.1751·3).
*Respiratory-tract infections.*

**Tonsillitis PMD** Bionorica, Ger.
Homoeopathic preparation.

**Tonsillol** Ratiopharm, Austria.
Dequalinium chloride (p.1178·1).
*Mouth and throat infections.*

**Tonsillopas** Pascoe, Ger.
Homoeopathic preparation.

**Tonsillosyx** Syxyl, Ger.
Homoeopathic preparation.

**Tonsiotren** Peithner, Austria.
Homoeopathic preparation.

**Tonsiotren H** DHU, Ger.
Homoeopathic preparation.

**Tonterin** Fortune, Hong Kong.
Caffeine (p.782·1); propyphenazone (p.85·3); thiamine (p.1455·2).
*Fever; pain.*

**Tonum** Almirall, Spain.
Ketorolac trometamol (p.52·1).
*Pain.*

**Tonus** Lab, Port.
Distigmine bromide (p.1489·2).

**Tonus-forte-Tablinen** Sanorania, Ger.†.
Etilefrine hydrochloride (p.914·1).
*Hypotension.*

**Tonval** Saval, Chile.
Vitamins; yeast; calcium gluconate; lysine (p.1417·1).
*Tonic.*

**Toose** Juventus, Spain†.
Co-trimoxazole (p.199·3).
*Bacterial infections.*

**Toothache Drops** ICN, NZ.
Phenol (p.1188·1); benzocaine (p.1370·3); camphor (p.1665·3); peppermint oil (p.1283·2); clove oil (p.1673·3).
*Toothache.*

**Toothache Gel** Roberts, USA.
Benzocaine (p.1370·3); clove oil (p.1673·3).
*Toothache.*

**Top C** Lane, UK.
Rose fruit (p.1740·1); acerola; ascorbic acid (p.1460·2).
*Vitamin C deficiency.*

**Top Calcium** Esseti, Ital.
Calcium carbonate (p.1254·2).
*Calcium depletion; calcium supplement.*

**Top dent fluor** Pharmalink, Swed.
Sodium fluoride (p.1444·3).
*Dental caries prophylaxis.*

**Top Flog** Uniao Quimica, Braz.†.
Benzydamine hydrochloride (p.21·1).
*Inflammation.*

**Top Life Diet** Sidus, Arg.
Garcinia cambogia; trichromium picolinate; soya lecithin (p.1417·1).
*Dietary supplement.*

**Top Life Energizante** Sidus, Arg.
Ginseng; guarana; *dl*-alpha tocoferil acetate; magnesium oxide; levocarnitine; wheatgerm oil (p.1417·1).
*Dietary supplement.*

**Top Life Memory** Sidus, Arg.
Ginseng (p.1693·1); ginkgo biloba (p.1692·3).
*Dietary supplement.*

**Top Life Relax** Sidus, Arg.
Valerian (p.1762·2); passion flower (p.1729·1); tilia (p.1756·2).
*Dietary supplement.*

**Top Life Superantioxidante** Sidus, Arg.
*dl*-Alpha tocoferil acetate; calcium ascorbate; betacarotene; selenium (p.1417·1).
*Dietary supplement.*

**Top Marks** Lifeplan, UK†.
Multinutrient preparation (p.1417·1).

**Topaal** Pierre Fabre, Fr.
Alginic acid (p.1576·3); colloidal aluminium hydroxide (p.1249·2); magnesium carbonate (p.1272·1); silicon dioxide (p.1581·3).
*Gastro-oesophageal reflux.*

**Topaben-N** British Dispensary, Thai.
Betamethasone valerate (p.1093·2); neomycin sulfate (p.235·1).
*Skin disorders.*

**Topace** Sigma, Austral.
Captopril (p.879·2).
*Hypertension.*

**Topadol** Teva, Israel.
Ketorolac trometamol (p.52·1).
*Pain.*

**Topal** Ceuta, UK.
Aluminium hydroxide (p.1249·2); light magnesium carbonate (p.1272·1); alginic acid (p.1576·3).
*Gastric hyperacidity; gastritis; gastro-oesophageal reflux.*

**Topalgic** Aventis, Fr.
Tramadol hydrochloride (p.94·3).
*Pain.*

**Topamac**
Janssen-Cilag, Arg.; Janssen-Cilag, Gr.; Janssen-Cilag, India.
Topiramate (p.378·3).
*Epilepsy.*

**Topamax**
Janssen-Cilag, Austral.; Janssen-Cilag, Austria; Janssen-Cilag, Belg.; Janssen-Cilag, Braz.; Janssen-Ortho, Canad.; Janssen-Cilag, Chile; Janssen-Cilag, Ger.; Janssen, Hong Kong; Janssen-Cilag, Irl.; Janssen-Cilag, Israel; Janssen-Cilag, Ital.; Janssen-Cilag, Malaysia; Cilag, Mex.; Janssen-Cilag, Neth.; Janssen-Cilag, NZ; Janssen-Cilag, Port.; Janssen-Cilag, S.Afr.; Janssen-Cilag, Singapore; Janssen-Cilag, Spain; Janssen-Cilag, Switz.; Janssen-Cilag, Thai.; Janssen-Cilag, UK; Ortho McNeil, USA.
Topiramate (p.378·3).
*Epilepsy.*

**Toparal** Novag, Mex.
Methyldopa (p.953·2).
*Hypertension.*

**Topase** Medica Korea, Hong Kong.
Pancreatin (p.1725·3); ox bile (p.1660·3); dimethicone (p.1289·2); hemicellulase (p.1669·1).
*Adjunct in radiological procedures; dyspepsia.*

**Topasel** Boehringer Ingelheim, Spain.
Algestone acetophenide (p.1541·3); estradiol enantate (p.1550·1).
*Combined injectable contraceptive.*

**Topcal D3** Grunenthal, Belg.
Calcium citrate (p.1225·1); colecalciferol (p.1461·3).

**Top-Cat** Varifarma, Arg.
Barium sulfate (p.1061·1).
*Radiographic contrast medium.*

**Top-Dal** Randall, Mex.
Loperamide hydrochloride (p.1271·1).
*Diarrhoea.*

**Toperit** Kampel Martian, Arg.
Erythromycin (p.208·1).
*Acne.*

**Topestin** Labinca, Arg.
Topotecan hydrochloride (p.589·1).
*Malignant neoplasms.*

**Topfans** OP, Ital.
Diclofenac sodium (p.32·1).
*Musculoskeletal, joint, and peri-articular disorders.*

**Topfena** Alpharma, Fr.
Ketoprofen (p.51·2).
*Musculoskeletal, joint, peri-articular, and soft-tissue disorders; pain.*

**Topher-E** Scherer, Hong Kong.
α-Tocopherol (p.1464·3).
*Vitamin E supplement.*

**Topialyse**
Note. This name is used for preparations of different composition.
SVR, Fr.
Borage oil (p.1661·3); vitamin E (p.1464·3).
*Skin disorders.*

SVR, Ital.
Gamolenic acid (p.1690·2); borage oil (p.1661·3).
*Nutritional supplement.*

**Topic** Syntex, USA.
Benzyl alcohol (p.1170·2); camphor (p.1665·3); menthol (p.1711·3).
*Pruritus.*

**Topicaina**
Note. This name is used for preparations of different composition.
Braun, Spain.
Butyl aminobenzoate hydrochloride (p.1373·1); benzocaine (p.1370·3); tetracaine hydrochloride (p.1385·1).
*Local anaesthesia.*

Organon Teknika, Spain†.
Benzalkonium chloride (p.1168·3); butacaine sulfate (p.1372·3); butyl aminobenzoate (p.1373·1); cetrimide (p.1173·1); benzocaine (p.1370·3); tetracaine hydrochloride (p.1385·1).
*Local anaesthesia.*

**Topicaine** Hoechst Marion Roussel, Canad.†.
Benzocaine (p.1370·3).
*Local anaesthesia.*

**Topical** Tecnimede, Port.†.
Bifonazole (p.395·1).
*Fungal infections.*

**Topicasone** Franco-Indian, India.
Betamethasone benzoate (p.1093·1).
*Skin disorders.*

**Topicasone with Neomycin** Franco-Indian, India.
Betamethasone benzoate (p.1093·1); neomycin sulfate (p.235·1).
*Infected skin disorders.*

**Topicil**
Douglas, Hong Kong; Douglas, Malaysia; Douglas, NZ.
Clindamycin phosphate (p.194·2).
*Acne.*

**Topico Denticion Vera** Labitec, Spain.
Sodium bromide (p.1663·1); borax (p.1661·3); ethylene glycol; musk; anemone pulsatilla; menthol.
*Toothache.*

**Topicort**
Dermik, Canad.; Taro, USA.
Desoximetasone (p.1096·3).
*Skin disorders.*

**Topicorte**
Roussel, Fr.†; Aventis, Neth.; Hoechst Marion Roussel, Singapore†; Aventis, Thai.
Desoximetasone (p.1096·3).
*Skin disorders.*

**Topicorten V** Trima, Israel.
Flumetasone pivalate (p.1101·1); clioquinol (p.196·3).
*Infected skin disorders.*

**Topicorten-Tar** Trima, Israel.
Flumetasone pivalate (p.1101·1); coal tar (p.1159·2); salicylic acid (p.1157·1).
*Skin disorders.*

**Topicrem**
Note. This name is used for preparations of different composition.
Nigy, Singapore.
Urea (p.1162·2); glycerol (p.1694·3).
*Dry skin disorders.*

Aventis, Spain†.
Trolamine salicylate (p.95·3).
*Peri-articular and soft-tissue disorders.*

**Topicycline**
Shire, Irl.; Monmouth, UK; Procter & Gamble, USA†.
Tetracycline hydrochloride (p.266·2).
*Acne.*

**Topidexa** Kinder, Braz.
Dexamethasone acetate (p.1097·1).
*Skin disorders.*

**Topifort** Franco-Indian, India.
Clobetasol propionate (p.1095·2).
*Skin disorders.*

**Topifram** *Roussel, Fr.†; Hoechst Marion Roussel, Singapore†; Aventis, Thai.*
Desoximetasone (p.1096·3); framycetin sulfate (p.215·1); gramicidin (p.220·2).
*Infected skin disorders.*

**Topiglos** *Kinder, Braz.*
Cod-liver oil (p.1425·2); zinc oxide (p.1163·2).
*Barrieri preparation.*

**Topilact 12** *Fouchard, Chile.*
Ammonium lactate (p.1142·3).
*Dry skin.*

**Topilene** *Technilab, Canad.; Technilab, Hong Kong†.*
Betamethasone dipropionate (p.1093·1).
*Skin disorders.*

**Topilone** *Chew, Thai.*
Triamcinolone acetonide (p.1110·2).
*Skin disorders.*

**Topimax** *Janssen-Cilag, Denm.; Janssen-Cilag, Fin.; Janssen-Cilag, Norw.; Janssen-Cilag, Swed.*
Topiramate (p.378·3).
*Epilepsy.*

**Topionic** *Almirall, Spain.*
Povidone-iodine (p.1190·3).
*Skin, burn, and wound disinfection.*

**Topisalen** *Trima, Israel.*
Flumetasone pivalate (p.1101·1); salicylic acid (p.1157·1).
*Skin disorders.*

**Topisolon**
*Note. This name is used for preparations of different composition.*
*Aventis, Austria; Aventis, Ger.; Aventis, Irl.; Knoll, Switz.*
Desoximetasone (p.1096·3).
*Burns; skin disorders.*

*Aventis, Ger.*
*Topical solution:* Desoximetasone (p.1096·3); salicylic acid (p.1157·1).
*Scalp disorders; skin disorders.*

**Topisolon mit Salicylsaure** *Aventis, Austria.*
Desoximetasone (p.1096·3); salicylic acid (p.1157·1).
*Skin disorders.*

**Topisone** *Technilab, Canad.*
Betamethasone dipropionate (p.1093·1).
*Skin disorders.*

**Topivate** *Qestmed, S.Afr.*
Betamethasone valerate (p.1093·2).
*Skin disorders.*

**Toplexil**
*Note. This name is used for preparations of different composition.*
*Aventis, Belg.; Aventis, Braz.*
Oxomemazine (p.438·2) or oxomemazine hydrochloride (p.438·2); guaifenesin (p.1122·1); paracetamol (p.76·2); sodium benzoate (p.1169·3).
*Coughs.*

*Theraplix, Fr.*
Oxomemazine (p.438·2).
Formerly contained oxomemazine and guaifenesin.
*Coughs.*

*Aventis, Israel; Aventis, Neth.; Aventis, Switz.*
Oxomemazine (p.438·2); guaifenesin (p.1122·1); sodium benzoate (p.1169·3).
*Coughs.*

**Top-Mag** *Medipha, Fr.*
Magnesium pidolate (p.1228·2).
*Magnesium deficiency.*

**Top-Nitro** *Schering-Plough, Ital.*
Glyceryl trinitrate (p.923·2).
*Angina pectoris.*

**Topo Worth** *Dermopen, Braz.†.*
Cod-liver oil (p.1425·2); zinc oxide (p.1163·2); boric acid (p.1662·1).
*Barrier preparation; skin disorders.*

**Topoderm N** *Gepepharm, Ger.†.*
Diphenylpyraline hydrochloride (p.432·3); hydrocortisone (p.1103·3); neomycin sulfate (p.235·1).
*Haemorrhoids; infected skin disorders; skin disorders.*

**Topokebir** *Aspen, Arg.*
Topotecan hydrochloride (p.589·1).
*Ovarian cancer.*

**Toposar** *Gensia, USA.*
Etoposide (p.551·3).
*Small-cell lung cancer; testicular cancer.*

**Topotag** *Pharmacia, Arg.*
Topotecan hydrochloride (p.589·1).
*Ovarian cancer; small cell lung cancer.*

**Topotel** *Dabur, India.*
Topotecan hydrochloride (p.589·1).
*Ovarian cancer; small-cell lung cancer.*

**Toppyc** *Johnson & Johnson, Braz.*
Permethrin (p.1508·3).

**Topramine** *Condrugs, Thai.*
Imipramine (p.300·1).
*Depression; nocturnal enuresis.*

**Toprec** *Theraplix, Fr.*
Ketoprofen (p.51·2).
*Fever; pain.*

**Toprek**
*Rhone-Poulenc Rorer, Austria†; Aventis, Belg.†; Aventis, Ital.*
Ketoprofen (p.51·2).
*Musculoskeletal, joint and peri-articular disorders; pain.*

**Toprel** *Drugtech, Chile.*
Topiramate (p.378·3).
*Epilepsy.*

**Toprilem** *Lemery, Mex.*
Captopril (p.879·2).
*Diabetic nephropathy; heart failure; hypertension; myocardial infarction.*

**Toprim** *Nakorn, Thai.*
Co-trimoxazole (p.199·3).
*Bacterial infections.*

**Toprol XL**
*AstraZeneca, Austral.; AstraZeneca, USA.*
Metoprolol succinate (p.957·1).
*Angina pectoris; heart failure; hypertension.*

**Topromel** *Clonmel, Irl.†.*
Metoprolol tartrate (p.957·1).
*Angina pectoris; arrhythmias; hyperthyroidism; migraine; myocardial infarction.*

**Topron** *Chinoin, Mex.*
Nifuroxazide (p.237·2).
*Gastro-enteritis.*

**Top-Sabona** *Sabona, Ger.*
Peppermint oil (p.1283·2); eucalyptus oil (p.1686·2); rosemary oil (p.1740·2).
*Musculoskeletal and joint disorders; neuralgia.*

**Topsiton** *Triomed, S.Afr.*
Vitamins; anhydrous caffeine; calcium gluconate; calcium citrate (p.1417·1).
*Tonic.*

**Topster** *Valeas, Ital.*
Beclometasone dipropionate (p.1091·1).
*Inflammatory bowel disease.*

**Topsym**
*Grunenthal, Austria; Grunenthal, Ger.; Grunenthal, Switz.*
Fluocinonide (p.1101·3).
*Skin disorders.*

**Topsym polyvalent**
*Note. This name is used for preparations of different composition.*
*Grunenthal, Austria; Grunenthal, Switz.*
Fluocinonide (p.1101·3); gramicidin (p.220·2); neomycin sulfate (p.235·1); nystatin (p.406·3).
*Infected skin disorders.*

*Grunenthal, Ger.*
Fluocinonide (p.1101·3); neomycin sulfate (p.235·1); nystatin (p.406·3).
*Infected skin disorders.*

**Topsymin** *Grunenthal, Switz.*
Fluocinonide (p.1101·3).
*Skin disorders.*

**Topsymin F** *Grunenthal, Austria.*
Fluocinonide (p.1101·3).
*Skin disorders.*

**Topsyn**
*Medicis, Canad.; Teofarma, Ital.; Syntex, Mex.*
Fluocinonide (p.1101·3).
*Skin disorders.*

**Topsyne**
*Cassenne, Fr.†; Yamanouchi, Neth.*
Fluocinonide (p.1101·3).
*Skin disorders.*

**Topsyne Neomycine** *Cassenne, Fr.†.*
Fluocinonide (p.1101·3); neomycin sulfate (p.235·1).
*Infected skin disorders.*

**Topsyn-Y** *Syntex, Mex.*
Fluocinonide (p.1101·3); clioquinol (p.196·3).
*Infected skin disorders.*

**Toptabs** *Sussex, UK†.*
Aspirin (p.15·1); caffeine (p.782·1).

**Toquilone compositum** *Medichemie, Switz.*
Methaqualone (p.707·1); diphenhydramine hydrochloride (p.431·3).
*Sleep disorders.*

**Toradiur** *Roche, Ital.*
Torasemide sodium (p.1015·3).
*Ascites; heart failure; oedema; renal failure.*

**Toradol**
*Roche, Austral.; Roche, Canad.; Roche, Denm.; Roche, Fin.; Roche, Hong Kong; Roche, Norw.; Roche, Port.; Roche, Singapore; Roche, Spain; Roche, Swed.; Roche, UK; Roche, USA.*
Ketorolac trometamol (p.52·1).
*Pain.*

**Tora-Dol**
*Recordati, Ital.; Roche, S.Afr.; Roche, Switz.*
Ketorolac trometamol (p.52·1).
*Pain.*

**Toral** *Fustery, Mex.*
Ketorolac trometamol (p.52·1).
*Pain.*

**Toraseptol** *Lesvi, Spain.*
Azithromycin (p.159·1).
*Bacterial infections.*

**Torbetol**
*Note. This name is used for preparations of different composition.*
*Torbet, Irl.*
Cetrimide (p.1172·1); benzalkonium chloride (p.1168·3); hexachlorophene (p.1181·2).
*Acne.*

*Torbet Laboratories, UK.*
Cetrimide (p.1172·1); chlorhexidine gluconate (p.1173·2).
*Acne.*

**Torecan**
*Novartis, Austria; Novartis, Chile; Novartis, Ger.†; Novartis, Ital.; Novartis, Mex.; Novartis, Spain; Novartis, Swed.; Novartis, Switz.; Roxane, USA.*
Thiethylperazine (p.442·1), thiethylperazine malate (p.442·1), or thiethylperazine maleate (p.442·1).
*Nausea; vertigo; vomiting.*

**Torem**
*Berlin-Chemie, Ger.; Roche, Swed.; Roche, Switz.; Roche, UK.*
Torasemide (p.1015·3) or torasemide sodium (p.1015·3).
*Heart failure; hypertension; oedema; renal failure.*

**Torental**
*Aventis, Belg.; Aventis, Fr.*
Pentoxifylline (p.979·3).
*Mental function impairment in the elderly; vascular disorders.*

**Torfan** *Abbott, Ital.†.*
Dextromethorphan hydrobromide (p.1117·3); guaifenesin (p.1122·1); carbinoxamine maleate (p.426·3).
*Coughs.*

**Torfan H** *Abbott, Arg.*
Pseudoephedrine hydrochloride (p.1129·2); dextromethorphan hydrobromide (p.1117·3); guaifenesin (p.1122·1); carbinoxamine maleate (p.426·3).
*Coughs.*

**Torgyn** *Raffo, Arg.*
Clindamycin (p.194·2).
*Vaginal bacterial infections.*

**Toriac** *Rhone-Poulenc Rorer, Belg.†.*
Loperamide hydrochloride (p.1271·1).
*Diarrhoea.*

**Toriol** *Vita, Spain.*
Ranitidine hydrochloride (p.1285·2).
*Acid aspiration; gastro-oesophageal reflux; gastrointestinal haemorrhage; gastrointestinal hyperacidity; peptic ulcer; short-bowel syndrome; Zollinger-Ellison syndrome.*

**Torlanbulina Antitetani** *Torlan, Spain†.*
A tetanus immunoglobulin (p.1640·3).
*Passive immunisation.*

**Torlasporin** *Torlan, Spain.*
Cefalexin (p.168·1).
*Bacterial infections.*

**Tornalate** *Dura, USA.*
Bitolterol mesilate (p.781·3).
*Asthma; bronchospasm.*

**Tornix** *Steierl, Ger.*
Crataegus (p.1677·1); valerian (p.1762·2); passion flower (p.1729·1); rutoside (p.1688·2).
*Cardiac disorders.*

**Torolac** *Lupin, India.*
Ketorolac trometamol (p.52·1).
*Pain.*

**Torrat**
*Roche, Austria†; Roche, Ger.; Roche, Hong Kong.*
Metipranolol (p.955·3); butizide (p.878·2).
*Hypertension.*

**Torrem** *Roche, Belg.*
Torasemide (p.1015·3).
*Hypertension; oedema.*

**Torsilax** *Neo Quimica, Braz.*
Caffeine (p.782·1); carisoprodol (p.1392·1); diclofenac sodium (p.32·1); paracetamol (p.76·2).

**Torvast** *Pfizer, Ital.*
Atorvastatin calcium (p.866·1).
*Hyperlipidaemias.*

**Torymycin** *Chinta, Thai.*
Doxycycline hyclate (p.206·2).
*Bacterial infections.*

**Toryxil** *Baer, Ger.†.*
Diclofenac sodium (p.32·1).
*Inflammation; rheumatism.*

**T-OS** *Seroyal, Canad.†.*
Calcium, molybdenum, phosphorus, and vitamin D (p.1417·1).

**Tos Mai** *Edigen, Spain.*
Dextromethorphan hydrobromide (p.1117·3); benzocaine (p.1370·3); guaiacol (p.1122·1); sodium benzoate (p.1169·3).
*Respiratory-tract disorders.*

**Toscacalm** *Genepharm, Gr.*
Tenoxicam (p.93·1).
*Dysmenorrhoea; gout; inflammation; osteoarthritis; pain; rheumatoid arthritis; spondyloarthropathies.*

**Toscal** *Abbott, Spain†.*
*Syrup:* Ammonium chloride (p.1115·2); tolu balsam (p.1131·3); dextromethorphan hydrobromide (p.1117·3); ephedrine hydrochloride (p.1120·1); ipecacuanha (p.1122·3).
*Tablets:* Carbinoxamine maleate (p.426·3); dextromethorphan hydrobromide (p.1117·3).
*Respiratory-tract disorders.*

**Toscal Compuesto** *Abbott, Spain†.*
Ammonium chloride (p.1115·2); tolu balsam (p.1131·3); carbinoxamine maleate (p.426·3); dextromethorphan hydrobromide (p.1117·3); ephedrine hydrochloride (p.1120·1); ipecacuanha (p.1122·3).
*Upper respiratory-tract disorders.*

**Toscalmin** *Benitol, Arg.*
Bromhexine (p.1115·3).
*Coughs.*

**Toscamycin-R** *Genepharm, Gr.*
Roxithromycin (p.254·2).
*Bacterial infections.*

**Tosdetan** *Martin, Spain†.*
Citiolone (p.1672·3); co-trimoxazole (p.199·3).
*Respiratory-tract infections.*

**Tosdiazina** *Clariana, Spain.*
Tolu balsam (p.1131·3); erythromycin stearate (p.208·2); guaifenesin (p.1122·1).
*Respiratory-tract infections.*

**Tosdrope** *Schering-Plough, Port.*
Dexchlorpheniramine maleate (p.427·3); pseudoephedrine sulfate (p.1129·2); guaifenesin (p.1122·1).
*Coughs.*

**Toseina NF** *Italfarmaco, Spain.*
Codeine phosphate (p.27·1).
*Coughs; diarrhoea; pain.*

**Tosfriol** *Sanofi Synthelabo, Spain†.*
Dextromethorphan hydrobromide (p.1117·3).
*Coughs.*

**Tosicalcin** *Pharmanel, Gr.*
Calcitonin (p.768·2).
*Hypercalcaemia; osteoporosis; Paget's disease of bone.*

**Tosidrin** *Fardi, Spain.*
Dihydrocodeine tartrate (p.34·3).
*Coughs.*

**Tosifar** *Bial, Spain.*
Fominoben hydrochloride (p.1121·3).
*Respiratory-tract disorders.*

**Tosilab** *Labomed, Chile.*
Codeine phosphate (p.27·1); pseudoephedrine hydrochloride (p.1129·2); chlorphenamine maleate (p.427·3).
*Coughs.*

**Tosrhimatiol** *Sanofi Synthelabo, Spain.*
Dextromethorphan hydrobromide (p.1117·3).
*Coughs.*

**Tossamine** *Novartis Consumer, Switz.*
Codeine phosphate (p.27·1); noscapine (p.1125·3).
*Coughs.*

**Tossamine plus** *Novartis Consumer, Switz.*
White capsules, codeine phosphate (p.27·1); noscapine (p.1125·3); methylephedrine hydrochloride (p.1124·2); blue capsules, codeine phosphate; noscapine; diphenhydramine hydrochloride (p.431·3).
*Coughs.*

**Tossanil** *Galenogal, Braz.†.*
Sodium benzoate (p.1169·3); tolu balsam (p.1131·3); guaifenesin (p.1122·1); menthol (p.1711·3).
*Coughs.*

**Tossarel** *Aerocid, Fr.†.*
Elecampane (p.1119·3); marrubium (p.1124·1); terpin (p.1131·1); sodium benzoate (p.1169·3).
*Coughs.*

**Tossbel** *Riedel-Zabinka, Braz.†.*
Diphenhydramine hydrochloride (p.431·3); dextromethorphan hydrobromide (p.1117·3); ammonium chloride (p.1115·2).
*Coughs.*

**Tossec** *Klonal, Arg.*
Butamirate (p.1116·2).
*Coughs.*

**Tossedrin** *Hearst, Braz.†.*
Ephedrine (p.1120·1); sodium dibunate (p.1130·2).
*Coughs.*

**Tossefedrin** *Leofarma, Braz.†.*
Ephedrine hydrochloride (p.1120·1); bromoform (p.1663·1); sodium dibunate (p.1130·2).
*Respiratory-tract congestion.*

**Tossefin** *IQB, Braz.†.*
Sodium dibunate (p.1130·2); sulfogaiacol (p.1131·1).
*Coughs.*

**Tossefluid** *Ribex, Ital.*
Carbocisteine (p.1116·2).
*Catarrh; coughs.*

**Tosseina** *Bergamo, Braz.†.*
Umbauba; sodium benzoate (p.1169·3); ipecacuanha (p.1122·3); mikania glomerata; carqueja; eucalyptus (p.1686·1); lobelia (p.1589·1).
*Coughs.*

**Tossemed** *Iodosan, Ital.*
Dextromethorphan hydrobromide (p.1117·3); guaifenesin (p.1122·1).
*Coughs.*

**Tosseque** *Nostrum, Port.*
Bromhexine hydrochloride (p.1115·3).
*Respiratory-tract congestion.*

**Tossestop** *IMA, Braz.†.*
Diphenhydramine (p.431·3); ammonium chloride (p.1115·2).
*Coughs.*

**Tossex** *Sarabhai Piramal, India.*
Codeine phosphate (p.27·1); chlorphenamine maleate (p.427·3); menthol (p.1711·3); sodium citrate (p.1223·2).
*Coughs.*

**Tossex-S** *Sarabhai Piramal, India.*
Chlorphenamine maleate (p.427·3); codeine phosphate (p.27·1).
*Coughs.*

**Tossilerg** *Bunker, Braz.*
Diphenhydramine hydrochloride (p.431·3); ammonium chloride (p.1115·2).
*Coughs.*

**Tossimel** *Igefarma, Braz.†.*
Carbocisteine (p.1116·2).
*Respiratory-tract congestion.*

**Tossin** *Grunenthal, Chile.*
Codeine (p.27·1); phenyltoloxamine (p.439·1).
*Coughs.*

**Tossivitan** *Sedabel, Braz.*
Guaifenesin (p.1122·1); potassium iodide (p.1598·1); oxeladin (p.1126·1).
*Coughs.*

**Tossoral** *Recordati, Ital.*
Dextromethorphan hydrobromide (p.1117·3).
*Coughs.*

**Tosuman** *Berna, Ital.†.*
A pertussis immunoglobulin (p.1631·2).
*Passive immunisation.*

**Totacef**
*Bristol-Myers Squibb, Israel; Bristol-Myers Squibb, Ital.*
Cefazolin sodium (p.170·3).
*Bacterial infections.*

**Totacide** *Adams, Thai.†.*
Glutaral (p.1180·3).
*Instrument disinfection.*

**Totacillin** *SmithKline Beecham, USA†.*
Ampicillin trihydrate (p.157·2).
*Bacterial infections.*

**Totaforte**
*Asta Medica, Belg.†; Viatris, Neth.; Sidefarma, Port.*
Multivitamin and mineral preparation (p.1417·1).

**Total**
*Note. This name is used for preparations of different composition.*
*Allergan, Canad.*
Polyvinyl alcohol (p.1581·1) (p.1164·2).
*Cleansing, wetting, and soaking solution for hard and gas permeable contact lenses.*

*Allergan, Israel†; Allergan, USA.*
Cleansing, soaking and wetting solution for hard contact lenses (p.1164·2).

*Allergan, Port.†.*
Solution for contact lens care (p.1164·2).

**Total Care** *Allergan, Austral.†.*
A range of preparations for care of hard and gas permeable contact lenses (p.1164·2).

**Total Cover Sunblock** *Clinique, Canad.*
*SPF 30:* Octinoxate (p.1154·3); homosalate (p.1148·1); octisalate (p.1154·3); oxybenzone (p.1154·3).
*Sunscreen.*

**Total Eclipse** *Triangle, USA.*
*SPF 15:* Padimate O (p.1155·1); oxybenzone (p.1154·3); lisadimate (p.1151·2).
*Sunscreen.*

**Total Eclipse Moisturizing** *Triangle, USA.*
*SPF 15:* Padimate O (p.1155·1); oxybenzone (p.1154·3); octisalate (p.1154·3).
*Sunscreen.*

**Total Formula** *Vitaline, USA.*
A range of vitamin preparations (p.1417·1).

**Total Magnesiano** *Temis, Arg.*
Magnesium (as halogen salts) (p.1417·1).
*Tonic.*

**Total Magnesiano Antioxidante** *Temis, Arg.*
Magnesium lactate; alpha-tocoferil acetate (p.1417·1).
*Magnesium and vitamin E deficiency.*

**Total Magnesiano con Vit C** *Temis, Arg.*
Vitamin C; magnesium carbonate or magnesium chloride; magnesium fluoride; magnesium sulfate; magnesium phosphate (p.1417·1).
*Tonic.*

**Total Magnesiano E** *Temis, Arg.*
Oral powder, magnesium chloride; magnesium sulfate; magnesium phosphate; magnesium carbonate; ginseng; caffeine; tablets, vitamin E (p.1417·1).
*Tonic.*

**Total Magnesiano Energizante** *Temis, Arg.*
Vitamin B substances; ascorbic acid; calcium carbonate; magnesium carbonate; magnesium sulfate (p.1417·1).
*Tonic.*

**Total Magnesiano Fem** *Temis, Arg.*
Vitamin B substances; vitamin C; calcium carbonate; magnesium carbonate; magnesium sulfate (p.1417·1).
*Dietary supplement.*

**Total Magnesiano Limon** *Temis, Arg.*
Magnesium chloride; magnesium fluoride; magnesium sulfate; magnesium phosphate (p.1417·1).
*Magnesium deficiency; renal calculi.*

**Total Magnesiano Sport** *Temis, Arg.*
Magnesium (as halogen salts); ginseng; arginine aspartate; citrulline; B vitamins; ascorbic acid; trimethylxanthine; zinc sulfate; cobalt chloride (p.1417·1).
*Dietary supplement.*

**Total Magnesiano Stress** *Temis, Arg.*
Magnesium pidolate; thiamine hydrochloride; pyridoxine hydrochloride (p.1417·1).
*Magnesium deficiency; renal calculi.*

**Total Vitamins** *Natural Life, Arg.*
Vitamin and mineral preparation (p.1417·1).

**Total Woman** *Vitaglow, Austral.†.*
A range of multivitamin and mineral preparations (p.1417·1).
*Dietary supplement.*

**Totalbloc Maximum Protection** *Creative Brands, Austral.†.*
*SPF 15+:* Escalol 507; oxybenzone (p.1154·3); avobenzone (p.1142·3).
*Sunscreen.*

**TotalCare** *Allergan, Ger.†.*
Disinfecting, storage, and moistening solution for contact lenses (p.1164·2).

**Totalens** *Allergan-Frumtost, Braz.*
Polyvinyl alcohol (p.1581·1) (p.1164·2).
*Cleaning solution for contact lenses.*

**Totalflora** *Roux-Ocefa, Arg.*
*Lactobacillus acidophilus* (p.1704·2); *Lactobacillus bifidus*; *Bacillus subtilis*; yeast; bacteriophages.
*Restoration of gastrointestinal flora.*

**Totalip** *Guidotti, Ital.*
Atorvastatin calcium (p.866·1).
*Hyperlipidaemias.*

**Totalos Plus** *Sidus, Arg.*
Collagen (p.1674·3); proteoglycans; amino acids; hydroxyapatite (p.1699·3).
*Mineral supplement; osteogenesis imperfecta; osteomalacia; osteoporosis.*

**Totam**
*Hikma, Port.*
Cefotaxime sodium (p.175·3).
*Bacterial infections.*

*Cipla-Medpro, S.Afr.*
Cefotaxime (p.176·3).
*Bacterial infections.*

**Totamine** *Baxter, Fr.*
Amino-acid, electrolyte, and vitamin infusion (p.1417·1).
*Parenteral nutrition.*

**Totapen**
*Riedel-Zabinka, Braz.†.*
Ampicillin (p.157·1).
*Bacterial infections.*

*Bristol-Myers Squibb, Fr.*
Ampicillin sodium (p.157·1) or ampicillin trihydrate (p.157·2).
*Bacterial infections.*

**Totaretic** *CP Pharmaceuticals, UK.*
Atenolol (p.865·2); chlortalidone (p.882·3).
These ingredients can be described by the British Approved Name Co-tenidone.
*Hypertension.*

**Totasedan** *Recalcine, Chile.*
Bromazepam (p.671·3).
*Anxiety.*

**Totasex** *Aclimacao, Braz.†.*
Vitamin and mineral preparation (p.1417·1).

**Totatrom** *Tocogino, Mex.†.*
Erythromycin (p.208·1).
*Bacterial infections.*

**Totelle**
*Wyeth Lederle, Belg.; Wyeth, Chile; Wyeth, Denm.; Wyeth Lederle, Ital.*
14 Tablets, estradiol (p.1550·1); 14 tablets, estradiol; trimegestone (p.1573·3).
*Menopausal disorders; osteoporosis.*

**Totelle cyclo** *Wyeth Lederle, Austria.*
14 Tablets, estradiol (p.1550·1); 14 tablets, estradiol; trimegestone (p.1573·3).
*Menopausal disorders; osteoporosis.*

**Totelle Sekvens**
*Wyeth Lederle, Fin.; Wyeth Lederle, Swed.*
14 Tablets, estradiol (p.1550·1); 14 tablets, estradiol; trimegestone (p.1573·3).
*Menopausal disorders; osteoporosis.*

**Totelmin** *Dovalle, Braz.*
Albendazole (p.101·2).
*Worm infections.*

**Totephan** *Pharmascience, Fr.*
*Cream:* Glycerol; cholesterol; oleic acid; urea (p.1417·1).
*Oral powder:* Plant proteins; vitamins; minerals (p.1417·1).
*Hair and nail tonic.*

**Tot'Hema**
*Innotech, Fr.*
Ferrous gluconate (p.1428·1); manganese gluconate; copper gluconate (p.1417·1).
*Anaemia; nutritional supplement.*

*Innotech, Port.*
Ferrous gluconate (p.1428·1); manganese gluconate; copper gluconate; cobalt glutamate; vitamin $B_{12}$ (p.1417·1).
*Anaemia.*

**Totipen** *Liferpal, Mex.†.*
Ampicillin (p.157·1).
*Bacterial infections.*

**Totocortin** *Winzer, Ger.*
Dexamethasone sodium phosphate (p.1097·2).
*Eye disorders.*

**Totonik** *Pharmaceutical Enterprises, S.Afr.*
Vitamins; potassium glycerophosphate; caffeine; ferrous sulfate (p.1417·1).
*Tonic.*

**Toularynx** *Qualiphar, Belg.*
Codeine phosphate (p.27·1).
*Coughs.*

**Toulumad** *Ceninter, Spain†.*
Magnesium polygalacturonate.
*Gastric hyperacidity; peptic ulcer.*

**Touristil** *Janssen-Cilag, Belg.*
Cinnarizine (p.428·3); domperidone maleate (p.1263·2).
*Dyspepsia; motion sickness; nausea; sleep disorders; vertigo; vomiting.*

**Touro A & H** *Dartmouth, USA.*
Pseudoephedrine hydrochloride (p.1129·2); brompheniramine maleate (p.426·1).
*Allergic rhinitis; nasal congestion.*

**Touro Allergy** *Dartmouth, USA.*
Pseudoephedrine hydrochloride (p.1129·2); brompheniramine maleate (p.426·1).
*Rhinitis; upper respiratory-tract congestion.*

**Touro CC** *Dartmouth, USA.*
Pseudoephedrine hydrochloride (p.1129·2); dextromethorphan hydrobromide (p.1117·3); guaifenesin (p.1122·1).
*Coughs; nasal congestion.*

**Touro DM** *Dartmouth, USA.*
Dextromethorphan hydrobromide (p.1117·3); guaifenesin (p.1122·1).
*Coughs.*

**Touro Ex** *Dartmouth, USA.*
Guaifenesin (p.1122·1).
*Coughs.*

**Touro LA** *Dartmouth, USA.*
Pseudoephedrine hydrochloride (p.1129·2); guaifenesin (p.1122·1).
*Coughs and cold symptoms.*

**Toux seche** *Pharmacard, Switz.*
Dextromethorphan hydrobromide (p.1117·3).
*Coughs.*

**Touxium** *SMB, Belg.†.*
Dextromethorphan hydrobromide (p.1117·3).
*Coughs.*

**Tovene** *Redino, Ger.*
Diosmin (p.1688·2).
*Venous insufficiency.*

**Toverine** *TO-Chemicals, Thai.*
Drotaverine hydrochloride (p.1683·1).
*Smooth muscle spasm.*

**T.O.Vir** *TO-Chemicals, Thai.*
Zidovudine (p.658·2).
*HIV infection.*

**Toxal** *Rayere, Mex.*
Oxolamine (p.1126·1).
*Coughs.*

**Toxanal** *Columbia, Mex.†.*
A tetanus vaccine (p.1640·3).
*Active immunisation.*

**Toxepasi** *Roche, Ital.*
Cogalactoisomerase sodium (p.1674·3).
*Hyperbilirubinaemia.*

**Toxex** *Pekana, Ger.*
Homoeopathic preparation.

**Toxicarb** *SERB, Fr.*
Activated charcoal (p.1030·2).
*Poisoning.*

**Toxicerna** *Fides, Ger.*
Homoeopathic preparation.

**Toxicol** *Eagle, Austral.†.*
Vitamin B substances with mineral, herbal, and nutritional agents (p.1417·1).

**toxi-L 90 N** *Loges, Ger.*
Homoeopathic preparation.

**toxi-loges** *Loges, Ger.*
Homoeopathic preparation.

**toxi-loges N** *Loges, Ger.*
Homoeopathic preparation.

**Toximer** *Ratiopharm, Austria.*
*Suppositories:* Paracetamol (p.76·2); codeine phosphate (p.27·1).
*Pain.*
*Tablets:* Propyphenazone (p.85·3); paracetamol (p.76·2); codeine phosphate (p.27·1).
*Fever; pain.*

**Toximer C** *Merckle, Ger.*
Paracetamol (p.76·2); caffeine (p.782·1).
*Pain.*

**Toxiselect** *Dreluso, Ger.*
Homoeopathic preparation.

**Toxogonin**
*Merck, Austria; Merck, Chile; Merck, Denm.†; Merck, Ger.; Merck, Neth.; Merck, S.Afr.; Merck, Swed.*
Obidoxime chloride (p.1046·3).
*Organophosphorus pesticide poisoning.*

**Toxogonine** *Merck, Switz.*
Obidoxime chloride (p.1046·3).
*Organophosphorus poisoning.*

**TP-1**
*Serono, Braz.†; Serono, Spain†.*
Thymostimulin (p.1756·1).
*Immunotherapy.*

**T-PA** *Seroyal, Canad.†.*
Vitamin D and minerals (p.1417·1).

**TPE 1800 GX** *Baxter, Ger.*
Amino-acid, carbohydrate, and electrolyte infusion (p.1417·1).
*Parenteral nutrition.*

**TPH** *Baxter, Ital.*
Amino-acid infusion (p.1417·1).
*Parenteral nutrition for neonates and infants.*

**T-Phyl** *Purdue Frederick, USA.*
Theophylline (p.798·3).
*Asthma; bronchospasm.*

**TPN Additive** *DBL, Austral.†.*
Electrolytes (p.1217·1).
*Parenteral nutrition.*

**TP-Ophtal** *Winzer, Ger.*
Pilocarpine hydrochloride (p.1495·1); timolol maleate (p.1012·2).
*Glaucoma; ocular hypertension.*

**TPT** *Elvetium, Arg.*
Topotecan (p.589·1).
*Malignant neoplasms.*

**Trabar** *Mepha, Israel.*
Tramadol hydrochloride (p.94·3).
*Pain.*

**Trabilin** *Mepha, Braz.*
Tramadol hydrochloride (p.94·3).

**Trabit**
*Note. This name is used for preparations of different composition.*
*Mepha, Hong Kong†.*
*Injection:* 1 Ampoule, phenylbutazone sodium (p.84·1); orthocarbamoylphenoxyacetate sodium; dexamethasone (p.1097·1); 1 ampoule, vitamin $B_{12}$ (p.1458·2).
Lidocaine hydrochloride (p.1377·3) is included in this preparation to alleviate the pain of injection.
*Tablets:* Phenylbutazone (p.83·2); dexamethasone (p.1097·1); vitamin $B_1$; vitamin B12 (p.1417·1).
Aluminium glycinate (p.1249·1) is included in this preparation in an attempt to limit adverse effects on the gastrointestinal mucosa.
*Rheumatism.*

*Mepha, Hong Kong†; Mepha, Thai.*
*Rectal capsules:* Phenylbutazone (p.83·2); dexamethasone (p.1097·1); vitamin $B_{12}$ (p.1458·2).
*Musculoskeletal and joint disorders.*

*Mepha, Thai.*
*Injection:* Ampoule A, phenylbutazone sodium (p.84·1); salamidacetic acid (p.87·3); dexamethasone (p.1097·1); ampoule B, vitamin $B_{12}$ (p.1458·2).
Lidocaine hydrochloride (p.1377·3) is included in each ampoule to alleviate the pain of injection.
*Musculoskeletal and joint disorders.*

**Trablok** *Lemery, Mex.*
Atracurium besilate (p.1399·1).
*Competitive neuromuscular blocker.*

**Trabona** *Leiras, Fin.*
Diclofenac potassium (p.32·1) or diclofenac sodium (p.32·1).
*Inflammation; musculoskeletal and joint disorders; pain.*

**Trac Tabs 2X** *Hyrex, USA.*
Methenamine (p.230·1); salol (p.88·1); atropine sulfate (p.477·1); hyoscyamine sulfate (p.485·1); benzoic acid (p.1169·3); methylthioninium chloride (p.1042·2).
*Urinary-tract infections.*

**Tracefusin** *Pisa, Mex.*
Trace-element preparation (p.1417·1).

**Tracel**
*Fresenius Kabi, Denm.; Fresenius Kabi, Fin.; Fresenius Kabi, Norw.; Fresenius Kabi, Swed.*
Trace element infusion (p.1417·1).
*Parenteral nutrition.*

**Tracelyte**
*Sanderson, Chile; American Pharmaceutical, USA†.*
A range of trace element and electrolyte preparations (p.1217·1).
*Parenteral nutrition.*

**Tracer Glucose** *Boehringer Mannheim, Fr.†.*
Test for glucose in blood (p.1694·2).

**Tracheo Fresh** *Rappai, Switz.*
Sea salt (p.1233·3); macrogol 300 (p.1709·1).
*Tracheal lubricant; tracheostomy care.*

**Trachiform** *Philopharm, Ger.*
Cetylpyridinium chloride (p.1173·1); benzocaine (p.1370·3); mint oil (p.1715·2); menthol (p.1711·3).
*Mouth and throat disorders.*

**Trachisan**
*Note. This name is used for preparations of different composition.*
*Engelhard, Ger.; Engelhard, Hong Kong; Engelhard, Malaysia; Engelhard, Switz.†.*
Chlorhexidine gluconate (p.1173·2); lidocaine hydrochloride (p.1377·3); tyrothricin (p.275·1).
*Mouth and throat disorders.*

*Engelhard, Singapore.*
*Gargle:* Chlorhexidine gluconate (p.1173·2); lidocaine hydrochloride (p.1377·3).
*Lozenges:* Chlorhexidine gluconate (p.1173·2); lidocaine (p.1377·3); tyrothricin (p.275·1).
*Mouth and throat disorders.*

**Trachisan N** *Engelhard, Ger.*
Chlorhexidine gluconate (p.1173·2).
Trachisan formerly contained chlorhexidine gluconate and lidocaine hydrochloride.
*Mouth and throat disorders.*

**Trachitol** *Engelhard, Ger.†.*
Lidocaine hydrochloride (p.1377·3); propyl hydroxybenzoate (p.1183·3); alum (p.1652·1).
*Infections of the upper respiratory tract; inflammatory disorders of the oropharynx.*

**Trachyl** *Monal, Fr.†.*
Ethylmorphine hydrochloride (p.37·3).
*Coughs.*

**Tracilarin** *Norma (Νορμα), Gr.*
Cefradine (p.179·3).
*Bacterial infections.*

**Tracin** *Berman, Mex.†.*
Oxytetracycline (p.241·1).
*Bacterial infections.*

**Tracine** *Progress, Thai.*
Tramadol hydrochloride (p.94·3).
*Pain.*

**Tracitrans Plus**
*Fresenius Kabi, Ger.*
Electrolyte (p.1217·1) and trace element preparation (p.1417·1).
*Parenteral nutrition.*
*Fresenius Kabi, Mex.*
Trace-element preparation (p.1417·1).
*Parenteral nutrition.*

**Tracleer**
*Actelion, Austral.; Actelion, Irl.; Actelion, UK; Actelion, USA.*
Bosentan (p.875·3).
*Pulmonary hypertension.*

**Traconal** *Ache, Braz.*
Itraconazole (p.401·3).
*Fungal infections.*

**Tracozon** *Ariston, Braz.*
Itraconazole (p.401·3).
*Fungal infections.*

**Tracrium**
*GlaxoSmithKline, Arg.; GlaxoSmithKline, Austral.; GlaxoSmithKline, Austria; GlaxoSmithKline, Belg.; GlaxoSmithKline, Braz.; Glaxo Wellcome, Canad.†; GlaxoSmithKline, Chile; GlaxoSmithKline, Denm.; Glaxo Wellcome, Fin.†; GlaxoSmithKline, Fr.; GlaxoSmithKline, Ger.; Glaxo Wellcome, Gr.; GlaxoSmithKline, Hong Kong; GlaxoSmithKline, India; Wellcome, Irl.; Wellcome, Israel; GlaxoSmithKline, Ital.; GlaxoSmithKline, Malaysia; Glaxo Wellcome, Mex.; GlaxoSmithKline, Neth.; Glaxo Wellcome, Norw.†; GlaxoSmithKline, NZ; Wellcome, Port.†; GlaxoSmithKline, S.Afr.; GlaxoSmithKline, Singapore; GlaxoSmithKline, Spain; GlaxoSmithKline, Swed.; GlaxoSmithKline, Switz.; GlaxoSmithKline, Thai.; GlaxoSmithKline, UK; Glaxo Wellcome, USA.*
Atracurium besilate (p.1399·1).
*Competitive neuromuscular blocker.*

**Tractocile**
*Ferring, Arg.; Ferring, Belg.; Ferring, Denm.; Ferring, Fin.; Ferring, Fr.; Ferring, Ger.; Ferring, Hong Kong; Ferring, Irl.; Ferring, Ital.; Ferring, Neth.; Ferring, Norw.; Pharmaco, NZ; Ferring, Port.; Ferring, Spain; Ferring, Swed.; Ferring, UK.*
Atosiban acetate (p.1319·1).
*Premature labour.*

**Tractoven** *Amnol, Ital.*
*Capsules:* Centella; melilot; rutoside; vitamin E (p.1417·1).
*Nutritional supplement.*
*Cream:* Hedera; birch; aesculus; equisetum; myrtillus; centella; vitamin E (p.1417·1).

**Tractur** *Damor, Ital.†.*
Pipemidic acid (p.243·1).
*Bacterial infections of the urinary tract.*

**Tracur** *Cristalia, Braz.*
Atracurium besilate (p.1399·1).
*Competitive neuromuscular blocker.*

**Tracurix** *Richmond, Arg.*
Atracurium (p.1402·2).
*Competitive neuromuscular blocker.*

**Tracuron** *Scott-Cassara, Arg.*
Atracurium (p.1402·2).
*Competitive neuromuscular blocker.*

**Tracutil**
*Braun, Arg.; Braun, Chile; Braun, Fr.; Braun, Ger.; Braun, Switz.*
Trace-element preparation (p.1417·1).
*Parenteral nutrition.*

**Tracyne** *Raza, Malaysia; Pharmaniaga, Malaysia.*
Tetracycline hydrochloride (p.266·2).
*Bacterial infections.*

**Tradelia** *Wolff, Ger.*
Estradiol (p.1550·1).
*Menopausal disorders.*

**Tradexol** *Columbia, Mex.*
Ambroxol hydrochloride (p.1114·3).
*Respiratory-tract congestion.*

**Tradil** *Nordic, Swed.*
Dexibuprofen (p.46·1).
*Inflammation; pain.*

**Tradol**
*Alpharma-Isis, Ger.; Rowex, Irl.; Grunenthal, Mex.; Shin Poong, Singapore.*
Tramadol hydrochloride (p.94·3).
*Pain.*

**Tradolan**
*Lannacher, Austria; Lannacher, Denm.; Lannacher, Norw.; Nordic, Swed.*
Tramadol hydrochloride (p.94·3).
*Pain.*

**Tradolgesic** *Bangkok Lab & Cosmetic, Thai.*
Tramadol hydrochloride (p.94·3).
*Pain.*

**Tradon** *Lilly, Ger.*
Pemoline (p.1591·2).
*Hyperactivity in older children.*

**Tradonal**
*Viatris, Belg.; Asta Medica, Hong Kong; Viatris, Ital.; Viatris, Spain; Asta Medica, Thai.*
Tramadol hydrochloride (p.94·3).
*Pain.*

**Tradox** *Andromaco, Chile.*
Lamotrigine (p.363·3).

**Trafloxal**
*Tramedico, Belg.; Tramedico, Neth.*
Ofloxacin (p.239·3).
*Bacterial eye infections.*

**Trafuril** *Faran, Gr.*
Buspirone hydrochloride (p.672·2).
*Generalised anxiety.*

**Tralen** *Pfizer, Braz.*
Tioconazole (p.409·3).
*Fungal skin infections.*

**Tralgiol** *Ciclum, Spain.*
Tramadol hydrochloride (p.94·3).
*Pain.*

**Trali** *Pharmacia, Arg.*
Sodium picosulfate (p.1289·3).
*Constipation.*

**Tralic** *Andromaco, Mex.*
Tramadol hydrochloride (p.94·3).
*Pain.*

**Trama** *1A, Ger.; ABZ, Ger.; Kade, Ger.*
Tramadol hydrochloride (p.94·3).
*Pain.*

**Tramabene** *Ratiopharm, Austria.*
Tramadol hydrochloride (p.94·3).
*Pain.*

**Tramabeta** *Betapharm, Ger.*
Tramadol hydrochloride (p.94·3).
*Pain.*

**Tramacet** *Janssen-Cilag, UK.*
Tramadol hydrochloride (p.94·3); paracetamol (p.76·2).
*Pain.*

**Tramadex** *Dexcel, Israel.*
Tramadol hydrochloride (p.94·3).
*Pain.*

**Tramadin** *Ratiopharm, Fin.*
Tramadol hydrochloride (p.94·3).
*Pain.*

**Tramadoc** *Docpharm, Ger.*
Tramadol hydrochloride (p.94·3).
*Pain.*

**Tramadol-Dolgit** *Dolorgiet, Ger.*
Tramadol hydrochloride (p.94·3).
*Pain.*

**Tramadolor**
*Hexal, Austria; Hexal, Ger.; Mepha, Switz.†.*
Tramadol hydrochloride (p.94·3).
*Pain.*

**Tramadon** *Cristalia, Braz.*
Tramadol hydrochloride (p.94·3).
*Pain.*

**Trama-Dorsch** *Pharmaselect, Ger.*
Tramadol hydrochloride (p.94·3).
*Pain.*

**Tramadura** *Merck dura, Ger.*
Tramadol hydrochloride (p.94·3).
*Pain.*

**Tramagetic**
*Nycomed, Fin.; Azupharma, Ger.; Christiaens, Neth.; Nycomed, Norw.*
Tramadol hydrochloride (p.94·3).
*Pain.*

**Tramagit** *Krewel, Ger.*
Tramadol hydrochloride (p.94·3).
*Pain.*

**Tramahexal** *Hexal, S.Afr.*
Tramadol hydrochloride (p.94·3).
*Pain.*

**Tramake**
*Galen, Irl.; Galen, UK.*
Tramadol hydrochloride (p.94·3).
*Pain.*

**Trama-Klosidol** *Bago, Arg.*
Tramadol hydrochloride (p.94·3).
*Pain.*

**Tramal**
*Grunenthal, Arg.; CSL, Austral.; Grunenthal, Austria; Pharmacia, Braz.; Grunenthal, Chile; Orion, Fin.; Grunenthal, Ger.; Grunenthal, Hong Kong; Sanofi Synthelabo, Malaysia; Byk, Neth.; CSL, NZ; Grunenthal, Port.; Janssen-Cilag, S.Afr.; Sanofi Synthelabo, Singapore; Grunenthal, Switz.; Sanofi Synthelabo, Thai.*
Tramadol hydrochloride (p.94·3).
*Pain.*

**Tramalan**
*Hexal, Arg.; Olan-Kemed, Thai.†.*
Tramadol hydrochloride (p.94·3).
*Pain.*

**Tramamed**
*S Med, Austria; Medifive, Thai.*
Tramadol hydrochloride (p.94·3).
*Pain.*

**Tramamerck** *Merck dura, Ger.†.*
Tramadol hydrochloride (p.94·3).
*Pain.*

**Tramapine** *Pinewood, Irl.*
Tramadol hydrochloride (p.94·3).
*Pain.*

**Tramastad** *Stada, Austria.*
Tramadol hydrochloride (p.94·3).
*Pain.*

**Tramatyrol** *Tyrol, Austria.*
Tramadol hydrochloride (p.94·3).
*Pain.*

**Tramax** *Pond's, Thai.*
Tramadol hydrochloride (p.94·3).
*Pain.*

**Tramazac** *Cadila, India.*
Tramadol hydrochloride (p.94·3).
*Pain.*

**Trambo** *Alpharma, Fin.*
Tramadol hydrochloride (p.94·3).
*Pain.*

**Tramedphano** *Medphano, Ger.†.*
Tramadol hydrochloride (p.94·3).
*Pain.*

**Tramex** *Antigen, Irl.*
Tramadol hydrochloride (p.94·3).
*Pain.*

**Tramic** *TO-Chemicals, Thai.*
Tranexamic acid (p.760·3).
*Haemorrhagic disorders.*

**Tramil** *Wyeth Consumer, Irl.*
Paracetamol (p.76·2); caffeine (p.782·1).
*Fever; pain.*

**Tramisal** *URPAC, Fr.*
Ginkgo biloba (p.1692·3).
*Mental function impairment in the elderly; peripheral vascular disorders.*

**Tramo** *Jean-Marie, Hong Kong.*
Tramadol hydrochloride (p.94·3).
*Pain.*

**Tramoda** *LBS, Thai.*
Tramadol hydrochloride (p.94·3).
*Pain.*

**Tramsilione** *Greater Pharma, Thai.*
Triamcinolone acetonide (p.1110·2).
*Skin disorders.*

**Tramundal** *Mundipharma, Austria.*
Tramadol hydrochloride (p.94·3).
*Pain.*

**Tramundin** *Mundipharma, Ger.*
Tramadol hydrochloride (p.94·3).
*Pain.*

**Tranavan** *Polipharm, Thai.*
Lorazepam (p.704·1).
*Anxiety.*

**Tranazol** *Farmasa, Braz.*
Itraconazole (p.401·3).
*Fungal infections.*

**Trancap** *TP, Thai.*
Dipotassium clorazepate (p.685·1).
*Anxiety; insomnia.*

**Tranclor** *Siam Bheasach, Thai.*
Dipotassium clorazepate (p.685·1).
*Anxiety.*

**Trancolon** *Fujisawa, Jpn.*
Mepenzolate bromide (p.485·3).
*Irritable bowel syndrome.*

**Trancolon P** *Fujisawa, Jpn.*
Mepenzolate bromide (p.485·3); phenobarbital (p.367·3).
*Irritable bowel syndrome.*

**Trancon** *Condrugs, Thai.*
Dipotassium clorazepate (p.685·1).
*Anxiety.*

**Trancopal Dolo** *Henning, Ger.; Sanofi Synthelabo, Ger.*
Flupirtine maleate (p.43·3).
*Pain.*

**Trandate**
*Sigma, Austral.; GlaxoSmithKline, Austria; GlaxoSmithKline, Belg.; Shire, Canad.; GlaxoSmithKline, Chile; GlaxoSmithKline, Denm.; GlaxoSmithKline, Fr.; Sigma, Hong Kong; Celltech, Irl.; GlaxoSmithKline, Israel; Teofarma, Ital.; GlaxoSmithKline, Malaysia; GlaxoSmithKline, Neth.; GlaxoSmithKline, Norw.; GlaxoSmithKline, NZ; Glaxo Wellcome, Port.; GlaxoSmithKline, S.Afr.; Glaxo Wellcome, Singapore†; Kern, Spain; GlaxoSmithKline, Swed.; GlaxoSmithKline, Switz.; Celltech, UK; Faro, USA.*
Labetalol hydrochloride (p.943·3).
*Angina pectoris; controlled hypotension during anaesthesia; hypertension.*

**Trandiur** *Teofarma, Ital.*
Labetalol hydrochloride (p.943·3); chlortalidone (p.882·3).
*Hypertension.*

**Trandor** *Biolab Sanus, Braz.*
Fenoprofen calcium (p.39·2).
*Gout; inflammation; musculoskeletal, joint, and periarticular disorders; pain.*

**Trandrozine** *Asian Pharm, Thai.*
Hydroxyzine hydrochloride (p.434·3).
*Anxiety; pruritus.*

**Trane** *Omega, Arg.*
Chlorpropamide (p.330·3).
*Diabetes mellitus.*

**Tranex** *Malesci, Ital.*
Tranexamic acid (p.760·3).
*Haemorrhage.*

**Trangina** *Alpharma, UK.*
Isosorbide mononitrate (p.942·1).
Formerly known as Monosorb.
*Angina pectoris.*

**Trangorex** *Sanofi Synthelabo, Spain.*
Amiodarone hydrochloride (p.859·2).
*Arrhythmias.*

**Tranimet** *Royton, Braz.*
Cimetidine (p.1255·3).
*Peptic ulcer.*

**Trankilium** *Ni-The, Gr.*
Lorazepam (p.704·1).
*Anxiety disorders; insomnia; status epilepticus.*

**Trankimazin** *Pharmacia, Spain.*
Alprazolam (p.668·3).
*Anxiety.*

**Tranqipam** *Aspen, S.Afr.*
Lorazepam (p.704·1).
*Alcohol withdrawal syndrome; anxiety; premedication; sedative.*

**Tranquase** *Azupharma, Ger.*
Diazepam (p.690·1).
*Anxiety; premedication; skeletal muscle spasm.*

**Tranquil** *Pharmadass, UK.*
Crataegus (p.1677·1); tilia flower (p.1756·2); viburnum; hawthorn oil (p.1677·1).

**Tranquilyn** *Link, UK†.*
Methylphenidate hydrochloride (p.1590·2).
*Attention-deficit hyperactivity disorder.*

**Tranquinal**
*Bago, Arg.; Merck Bago, Braz.*
Alprazolam (p.668·3).
*Anxiety; insomnia.*

**Tranquinal Soma** *Bago, Arg.*
Alprazolam (p.668·3); sulpiride (p.722·2).
*Psychosomatic disorders.*

**Tranquirit** *Aventis, Ital.*
Diazepam (p.690·1).
*Anxiety; epilepsy; insomnia; psychoses.*

**Tranquital** *Novartis Sante, Fr.*
Valerian (p.1762·2); crataegus (p.1677·1).
*Insomnia; nervous disorders.*

**Tranquo** *Boehringer Ingelheim, Belg.*
Oxazepam (p.712·2).
*Anxiety disorders.*

**Transacalm** *Norgine, Fr.*
Trimebutine maleate (p.1758·1).
*Gastrointestinal disorders.*

**Transact** *Boots Healthcare, S.Afr.*
Flurbiprofen (p.43·3).
Formerly known as Trans Act$_{LAT}$.
*Musculoskeletal and joint disorders.*

**Transact Lat**
*Abbott, Ital.; Abbott, Port.*
Flurbiprofen (p.43·3).
*Musculoskeletal, joint, peri-articular, and soft-tissue disorders.*

**Transamin**
*Nikkho, Braz.; Nikolakopoulos (Νικολακοπουλος), Gr.; Daiichi, Hong Kong; Daiichi, Jpn; Daiichi, Malaysia; Daiichi, Thai.*
Tranexamic acid (p.760·3).
*Haemorrhagic disorders.*

**Transannon**
*Pharmacia, Ger.; Pharmacia, Switz.*
Conjugated oestrogens (p.1543·2).
28-Day packs also contain 7 inert tablets.
*Menopausal disorders; osteoporosis.*

**Transbil** *Hearst, Braz.†.*
Boldo (p.1661·2); solanum paniculatum; pichy.
*Liver disorders.*

**Transbilix**
*Codali, Belg.†; Guerbet, Fr.†.*
Meglumine adipiodone (p.1060·1).
*Contrast medium for biliary-tract radiography.*

**Transbronchin** *Viatris, Ger.*
Carbocisteine (p.1116·2).
*Respiratory-tract disorders associated with increased or viscous mucus.*

**Transbronquina** *Lab, Port.†.*
Codeine (p.27·1); trolamine (p.1758·2).
*Coughs.*

**Transbronquina Rectal** *Lab, Port.†.*
Camphor (p.1665·3); quinine (p.460·1).

**Transcop** *Recordati, Ital.*
Hyoscine (p.483·3).
*Motion sickness.*

**TransCyte**
*Smith & Nephew, UK; Smith & Nephew, USA.*
Bioengineered human skin equivalent (p.1158·1).
*Burns.*

**Transderm Scop** *Novartis Consumer, USA.*
Hyoscine (p.483·3).
*Motion sickness.*

**Transderma B** *Szama, Arg.*
Betamethasone valerate (p.1093·2).
*Skin disorders.*

**Transderma H** *Szama, Arg.*
Hydrocortisone (p.1103·3).
*Skin disorders.*

**Transdermal-NTG** *Warner Chilcott, USA.*
Glyceryl trinitrate (p.923·2).
*Angina pectoris.*

**Transderm-Nitro**
*Novartis, Canad.; Novartis, USA.*
Glyceryl trinitrate (p.923·2).
*Angina pectoris.*

**Transderm-V** *Novartis, Canad.*
Hyoscine (p.483·3).
*Motion sickness.*

**Transdiol** *Hexal, Arg.*
Estradiol (p.1550·1).
*Menopausal disorders.*

**Transene** *Sanofi Synthelabo, Ital.*
Dipotassium clorazepate (p.685·1).
*Anxiety; insomnia; nervous disorders.*

**Transferal** *Ferrer, Spain†.*
Tocofibrate (p.1015·1).
*Hyperlipidaemias.*

**Transfert** *Piam, Ital.*
Carnitine (p.1423·3).
*Carnitine deficiency.*

**Transformal** *Schwabe, Arg.*
Ginseng (p.1693·1).
*Tonic.*

**Transiderm-Nitro** *Novartis, Austral.; Novartis, Denm.†; Novartis, Fin.; Novartis, Irl.; Novartis, Neth.; Novartis, Norw.; Novartis, Swed.; Novartis, UK.*
Glyceryl trinitrate (p.923·2).
*Angina pectoris; prophylaxis of phlebitis and extravasation.*

**Transilane** *Innotech, Fr.*
Ispaghula (p.1268·1).
*Constipation.*

**Transimune** *Troikaa, India.*
Azathioprine (p.1349·1).
*Auto-immune disorders; organ transplantation.*

**Transipeg** *Roche, Arg.; Roche, Austria; Roche, Belg.; Roche Nicholas, Fr.; Syntex, Mex.†; Roche, Switz.*
Macrogol 3350 (p.1709·1); electrolytes (p.1217·1).
*Constipation.*

**Transipen** *Demo, Gr.*
Indapamide (p.938·2).
*Hypertension.*

**Transitol** *Schwarz, Fr.†.*
White soft paraffin (p.1479·3); light liquid paraffin (p.1479·1).
*Constipation.*

**Transix** *Christiaens, Belg.*
Senna (p.1288·2).
*Bowel evacuation; constipation.*

**Translet** *Rusch, UK.*
Barrier cream.

**Translet Plus One** *Rusch, UK.*
A deodorant liquid for use with colostomies and ileostomies.

**Translet Plus Two** *Rusch, UK.*
A deodorant liquid for use with colostomies and ileostomies.

**Translight** *Merck Sharp & Dohme-Chibret, Fr.†.*
Tyloxapol (p.1416·3)(p.1164·2).
*Hard contact lens cleaner.*

**Transmer** *Tradiphar, Fr.*
Promethazine hydrochloride (p.439·1); ephedrine hydrochloride (p.1120·1).
*Motion sickness.*

**Transmetil** *Boehringer Ingelheim, Arg.*
Ademetionine (p.1647·2).

*Abbott, Ital.*
Ademetionine butanedisulfonate (p.1647·2).
*Liver disorders.*

**Transoak** *Pabisch, Austria†.*
A rinsing and storage solution for hard and gas permeable contact lenses (p.1164·2).

**Transoddi** *Lipha Sante, Fr.†.*
Cinametic acid (p.1671·3).
*Dyspepsia.*

**Transol** *Pabisch, Austria†.*
A wetting solution for hard and gas permeable contact lenses (p.1164·2).

**Transoxyl** *Ferraz, Lynce, Port.*
Almitrine dimesilate (p.1584·2); raubasine (p.994·3).

**Trans-Plantar** *Westwood-Squibb, Canad.; Prater, Chile.*
Salicylic acid (p.1157·1).
*Keratinisation disorders; plantar warts.*

**Transpulmin** *Note. This name is used for preparations of different composition.*
*Asta Medica, Braz.*
*Suppositories:* Camphor (p.1665·3); guaiacol (p.1122·1); cineole (p.1672·1); menthol (p.1711·3).
*Respiratory-tract congestion.*
*Syrup:* Sodium camsilate; oxeladin citrate (p.1126·1); guaifenesin (p.1122·1); cineole (p.1672·1); menthol (p.1711·3).
*Coughs.*

*Asta Medica, Thai.*
Pipazetate hydrochloride (p.1129·1).
*Coughs.*

**Transpulmin Baby** *Viatris, Ger.*
Eucalyptus oil (p.1686·2); pine needle oil.
*Cold symptoms.*

**Transpulmin Balsam** *Viatris, Ger.*
Cineole (p.1672·1); menthol (p.1711·3); camphor (p.1665·3).
*Bronchitis; catarrh.*

**Transpulmin Balsamo** *Asta Medica, Braz.*
Camphor (p.1665·3); guaiacol (p.1122·1); cineole (p.1672·1); menthol (p.1711·3).
*Respiratory-tract congestion.*

**Transpulmin Kinderbalsam S** *Viatris, Ger.*
Eucalyptus oil (p.1686·2); pine needle oil.
*Cold symptoms.*

**Transpulmin Xarope** *Asta Medica, Braz.*
Guaifenesin (p.1122·1); oxeladin (p.1126·1); cineole (p.1672·1); menthol (p.1711·3); sodium camsilate.
*Respiratory-tract congestion.*

**Transpulmina** *Dogra, Port.*
Camphor (p.1665·3); cineole (p.1672·1); menthol (p.1711·3).
*Respiratory-tract disorders.*

**Transpulmina Gola** *Bayer, Ital.*
Dequalinium chloride (p.1178·1); menthol (p.1711·3); cineole (p.1672·1).
*Mouth and throat infections.*

**Transpulmina Tosse** *Bayer, Ital.*
*Pastilles:* Guaifenesin (p.1122·1); menthol (p.1711·3); cineole (p.1672·1); camphor (p.1665·3).
*Syrup:* Guaifenesin (p.1122·1); menthol (p.1711·3); cineole (p.1672·1).
*Catarrh; coughs.*

**Transtec** *Grunenthal, Belg.; Essex, Ger.; Grunenthal, Ger.; Napp, Irl.; Grunenthal, Port.; Grunenthal, Spain; Grunenthal, Switz.; Napp, UK.*
Buprenorphine (p.21·3).
*Pain.*

**Transulose** *Enteris, Fr.*
Lactulose (p.1269·1); liquid paraffin (p.1479·1); white soft paraffin (p.1479·3).
*Constipation.*

**Transvane** *Promedis, Belg.†.*
Thurfyl salicylate (p.93·3); hexyl nicotinate (p.45·1); ethyl nicotinate (p.37·2); benzocaine (p.1370·3).
*Musculoskeletal, joint, and soft-tissue disorders.*

**Transvasin** *Thornton & Ross, Irl.; Seton, NZ†; Sparks, NZ†; Meda, Swed.†.*
Ethyl nicotinate (p.37·2); hexyl nicotinate (p.45·1); thurfyl salicylate (p.93·3).
*Rheumatic and muscular pain; sprains; strains.*

**Transvasin Heat Rub** *Thornton & Ross, UK.*
Ethyl nicotinate (p.37·2); hexyl nicotinate (p.45·1); thurfyl salicylate (p.93·3).
*Musculoskeletal and joint pain; sprains; strains.*

**Transvasin Heat Spray** *Thornton & Ross, UK.*
Glycol salicylate (p.44·3); diethylamine salicylate (p.34·1); methyl nicotinate (p.59·2).
*Musculoskeletal and joint pain.*

**Transvercid** *Pierre Fabre Sante, Fr.*
Salicylic acid (p.1157·1).
*Warts.*

**Trans-Ver-Sal** *Westwood-Squibb, Canad.; Prater, Chile; Difa, Ital.; Darier, Mex.*
Salicylic acid (p.1157·1).
*Calluses; verrucas; warts.*

**Trans-Ver-Sal AdultPatch** *Doak, USA.*
Salicylic acid (p.1157·1).
*Verrucas.*

**Trans-Ver-Sal PediaPatch** *Doak, USA.*
Salicylic acid (p.1157·1).
Formerly known as PediaPatch.
*Warts.*

**Trans-Ver-Sal PlantarPatch** *Doak, USA.*
Salicylic acid (p.1157·1).
Formerly known as Trans-Plantar.
*Warts.*

**Transvital** *Gynopharm, Chile.*
Estradiol (p.1550·1).
*Menopausal disorders.*

**Transzone** *Par, USA.*
Melatonin (p.1710·2).

**Trantalol** *Pinewood, Irl.*
Atenolol (p.865·2).
*Angina pectoris; arrhythmias; hypertension; myocardial infarction.*

**Trantil** *Rudefsa, Mex.†.*
Carbamazepine (p.353·3).

**Tranvagal** *Essex, Chile.*
Parapenzolate bromide (p.487·2); chlordiazepoxide (p.674·2).
*Gastrointestinal disorders.*

**Tranxal** *CTI, Israel.*
Dipotassium clorazepate (p.685·1).
*Alcohol withdrawal syndrome; anxiety.*

**Tranxen** *Searle, Denm.†.*
Dipotassium clorazepate (p.685·1).
*Alcohol withdrawal syndrome; anxiety.*

**Tranxene** *Glaxo Wellcome, Austral.†; Sanofi Synthelabo, Belg.; Abbott, Canad.; Sanofi Synthelabo, Fr.; Sanofi Synthelabo, Gr.; Sanofi Synthelabo, Hong Kong; Boehringer Ingelheim, Irl.; Sanofi Synthelabo, Mex.; Sanofi Synthelabo, Neth.; Sanofi Synthelabo, Port.; Sanofi Synthelabo, S.Afr.; Sanofi Synthelabo, Singapore†; Sanofi Synthelabo, Thai.; Boehringer Ingelheim, UK; Abbott, USA.*
Dipotassium clorazepate (p.685·1).
*Alcohol withdrawal syndrome; anxiety; disturbed behaviour; epilepsy; premedication; sleep disorders.*

**Tranxilene** *Sanofi Synthelabo, Braz.*
Dipotassium clorazepate (p.685·1).
*Alcohol withdrawal syndrome; anxiety; epilepsy.*

**Tranxilium** *Sanofi Synthelabo, Austria; Rider, Chile; Sanofi Synthelabo, Ger.; Sanofi Synthelabo, Spain; Sanofi Synthelabo, Switz.*
Dipotassium clorazepate (p.685·1).
*Alcohol withdrawal syndrome; anxiety; convulsions; premedication; sleep disorders.*

**Tranxilium N** *Sanofi Synthelabo, Ger.*
Nordazepam (p.710·3).
*Anxiety; sleep disorders.*

**Tranzicalm** *Vocate, Gr.*
Nimesulide (p.67·1).
*Inflammation; musculoskeletal disorders; pain.*

**Trapanal** *Byk Gulden, Ger.*
Thiopental sodium (p.1309·1).
*General anaesthesia.*

**Trapax** *Wyeth, Arg.*
Lorazepam (p.704·1).
*Anxiety; epilepsy; nausea and vomiting; premedication.*

**Traqueobron** *Medquimica, Braz.†.*
Cetylpyridinium; ammonium chloride (p.1115·2); sodium benzoate (p.1169·3).
*Respiratory-tract congestion.*

**Traquivan** *Llorente, Spain†.*
Dihydrocodeine tartrate (p.34·3); co-trimoxazole (p.199·3).
*Respiratory-tract infections.*

**Trasedal** *Elerte, Fr.*
Tramadol hydrochloride (p.94·3).
*Pain.*

**Trasicor** *Novartis, Austria; Novartis, Belg.†; Novartis, Canad.; Novartis, Denm.; Novartis, Fr.; Novartis, Ger.; Novartis, Gr.; Novartis, Irl.†; Novartis, Israel†; Novartis, Neth.; Novartis, NZ†; Novartis, S.Afr.†; Novartis, Spain; Novartis, Switz.; Novartis, UK.*
Oxprenolol hydrochloride (p.978·1).
*Angina pectoris; anxiety; arrhythmias; hypertension; hyperthyroidism; hypertrophic obstructive cardiomyopathy; myocardial infarction; phaeochromocytoma.*

**Trasidrex** *Novartis, Irl.†; Novartis, S.Afr.†; Novartis, UK.*
Oxprenolol hydrochloride (p.978·1); cyclopenthiazide (p.890·3).
These ingredients can be described by the British Approved Name Co-prenozide.
*Hypertension.*

**Trasitensin** *Novartis, Austria; Novartis, Ger.; Novartis, Ital.; Novartis, Spain.*
Oxprenolol hydrochloride (p.978·1); chlortalidone (p.882·3).
*Hypertension.*

**Trasitensine** *Novartis, Fr.; Novartis, Switz.†.*
Oxprenolol hydrochloride (p.978·1); chlortalidone (p.882·3).
*Hypertension.*

**Trastocir** *Armstrong, Arg.*
Cilostazol (p.884·1).
*Peripheral vascular disorders.*

**Trasylol** *Bayer, Austral.; Bayer, Austria; Bayer, Belg.; Bayer, Braz.; Bayer, Canad.; Bayer, Chile; Bayer, Denm.; Bayer, Fin.; Bayer, Fr.; Bayer, Ger.; Bayer, Hong Kong; Bayer, Ital.†; Bayer, Malaysia; Bayer, Mex.; Bayer, Neth.; Bayer, NZ; Bayer, S.Afr.; Bayer, Singapore; Bayer, Spain; Bayer, Swed.; Bayer, Switz.; Bayer, Thai.; Bayer, UK; Bayer, USA.*
Aprotinin (p.742·3).
*Adjunct in open heart surgery and gynaecological surgery; antidote to thrombolytic therapy; hyperfibrinolytic haemorrhage; pulmonary embolism; shock.*

**Tratacne** *ICN, Arg.*
Tretinoin (p.1161·1); erythromycin (p.208·1).
*Acne.*

**Tratenamin** *Duncan, Arg.*
Lorazepam (p.704·1).
*Anxiety.*

**Tratobes** *Disprovent, Arg.*
Diethylpropion (p.1587·1); fenproporex (p.1588·3); diazepam (p.690·1).
*Obesity.*

**Tratocoli** *IMA, Braz.†.*
Furazolidone (p.605·2); phthalylsulfathiazole (p.242·3); pectin (p.1580·3).
*Diarrhoea.*

**Tratoderm** *IMA, Braz.†.*
Triclosan (p.1195·2); allantoin (p.1141·3).
*Skin disorders.*

**Tratul** *Gerot, Austria.*
Diclofenac (p.32·1) or diclofenac diethylamine (p.32·1) or diclofenac sodium (p.32·1).
*Biliary and renal colic; fever; gout; inflammation; musculoskeletal, joint, and peri-articular disorders; pain.*

**Trauma Relief** *Brauer, Austral.†.*
Homoeopathic preparation.

**Traumac** *Catarinense, Braz.*
Benzocaine (p.1370·3); camphor (p.1665·3); lavender (p.1705·1); turpentine oil (p.1760·1); menthol (p.1711·3); methyl salicylate (p.59·3).
*Musculoskeletal and joint disorders.*

**TraumaCal** *Mead Johnson, Austral.; Mead Johnson Nutritionals, Canad.; Mead Johnson, NZ; Mead Johnson, Singapore†; Mead Johnson Nutritionals, Thai.†; Mead Johnson Nutritionals, USA.*
Preparation for enteral nutrition (p.1417·1).
*Stress.*

**Traumacel P** *Synapse, Irl.*
Calcium oxidised cellulose (p.757·2).
*Capillary bleeding.*

**Trauma-cyl** *Liebermann, Ger.*
Chamomile oil (p.1669·3); sage oil (p.1741·2); arnica (p.1656·3); aesculus (p.1648·2); hamamelis (p.1696·3).
*Soft-tissue injury; vascular disorders.*

**Trauma-cyl N Complex** *Liebermann, Ger.*
Homoeopathic preparation.

**Trauma-Dolgit** *Dolorgiet, Ger.*
Ibuprofen (p.45·3).
*Musculoskeletal and joint disorders; sports injuries.*

**Traumadyn** *Plantamed, Ger.†.*
Homoeopathic preparation.

**Traumafusin** *Fresenius Kabi, Austria†.*
Amino-acid and electrolyte infusion (p.1417·1).
*Parenteral nutrition.*

**Traumagel** *Sanval, Braz.*
Methyl salicylate (p.59·3); camphor (p.1665·3); turpentine oil (p.1760·1).
*Musculoskeletal and joint disorders.*

**Traumal** *Novartis Consumer, Ital.*
Oxerutins (p.1688·2); a heparinoid (p.931·1).
*Bruises; sprains.*

**Traumalgyl** *Pharmadeveloppement, Fr.*
Mephenesin (p.1394·3); diethylamine salicylate (p.34·1); lidocaine (p.1377·3).
*Muscular pain.*

**Traumalitan** *3M, Ger.*
Heparin sodium (p.928·1).
*Soft-tissue injury; superficial vascular disorders.*

**Traumalix** *Drossapharm, Switz.*
Etofenamate (p.38·1).
*Musculoskeletal, joint, peri-articular, and soft-tissue disorders.*

**Traumanase** *Nattermann, Ger.; Aventis, Switz.*
Bromelains (p.1662·2).
*Inflammation with oedema.*

**Traumaparil** *Madaus, Austria.*
Aescin (p.1648·2).
*Soft-tissue disorders.*

**Traumaplant** *Kwizda, Austria; Harras-Curarina, Ger.*
Comfrey (p.1675·2).
*Musculoskeletal and joint disorders; sports injuries; wounds.*

**Trauma-Puren** *Alpharma-Isis, Ger.*
Heparin sodium (p.928·1); menthol (p.1711·3); glycol salicylate (p.44·3).
*Haematoma; inflammation; phlebitis.*

**Traumasalbe** *Provita, Austria.*
Capsicum (p.1667·1); methyl salicylate (p.59·3); turpentine oil (p.1760·1).
*Musculoskeletal, joint, peri-articular, and soft-tissue disorders.*

**Trauma-Salbe kuhlend** *Mayrhofer, Austria.*
Methyl salicylate (p.59·3); camphor (p.1665·3); menthol (p.1711·3).
*Musculoskeletal, joint, and soft-tissue disorders.*

**Trauma-Salbe Rodler 301 N** *Woelm, Ger.*
Camphor (p.1665·3); menthol (p.1711·3); methyl salicylate (p.59·3).
*Cold symptoms; musculoskeletal, joint, and peri-articular disorders.*

**Trauma-Salbe Rodler 302 N** *Woelm, Ger.*
Camphor (p.1665·3); turpentine oil (p.1760·1); eucalyptus oil (p.1686·2).
*Muscle and joint injuries.*

**Trauma-Salbe warmend** *Mayrhofer, Austria.*
Methyl salicylate (p.59·3); capsicum (p.1667·1); turpentine oil (p.1760·1).
*Musculoskeletal, joint, and soft-tissue disorders.*

**Traumasenex** *Riemser, Ger.*
Glycol salicylate (p.44·3).
*Rheumatism; soft-tissue disorders.*

**Traumasept** *Wolff, Ger.*
Povidone-iodine (p.1190·3).
*Burns; skin and mucous membrane disinfection; skin infections; ulcers; vaginal infections; wounds.*

**Traumasive** *Hexal, Ger.*
Hydrocolloid dressing.
*Burns; wounds.*

**Traumasport** *IBSA, Switz.†.*
Diclofenac epolamine (p.33·1).
*Musculoskeletal, joint, peri-articular and soft-tissue injuries.*

**Traumasteril kohlenhydratfrei** *Fresenius, Ger.†.*
Amino-acid and electrolyte infusion (p.1417·1).
*Parenteral nutrition.*

**Traumatociclina** *Biomedica, Ital.†.*
Meclocycline sulfosalicylate (p.229·1).
*Bacterial skin infections.*

**Traumazol** *Chinoin, Mex.*
Ethyl chloride (p.1376·2).
*Local anaesthesia.*

**Traumed** *Herbarium, Braz.*
Arnica (p.1656·3); ginkgo biloba (p.1692·3); aesculus (p.1648·2); menthol (p.1711·3); camphor (p.1665·3).

**Traumeel** *Peithner, Austria; Heel, USA.*
Homoeopathic preparation.

**Traumeel S** *Heel, Ger.; Heel, S.Afr.*
Homoeopathic preparation.

**Traumicid** *Note. This name is used for preparations of different composition.*
*Aventis Pasteur, Chile.*
Clonixin lysine (p.26·3).
*Inflammation; pain.*

*Montefarmaco, Ital.*
Methylbenzethonium chloride (p.1186·1); chlorothymol (p.1177·2).
*Wound disinfection.*

**Traumon** *Kolassa, Austria; Bayer, Ger.*
Etofenamate (p.38·1).
*Musculoskeletal, joint, peri-articular, and soft-tissue disorders.*

**Traumox** *Medpro, S.Afr.†.*
Naproxen (p.65·1).
*Dysmenorrhoea; gout; musculoskeletal and joint disorders.*

**Trausan** *Vitoria, Port.*
Citicoline (p.1672·3).
*Anxiety and depression in the elderly; cerebrovascular disorders; movement disorders; speech disorders; vertigo.*

**Travtil** *CEPA, Spain†.*
Cisapride (p.1259·2).
*Gastro-oesophageal reflux; gastroparesis.*

**Travacalm** *Key, Austral.*
Dimenhydrinate (p.431·1); hyoscine hydrobromide (p.483·3); caffeine (p.782·1).
*Motion sickness.*

**Travacalm HO** *Key, Austral.*
Hyoscine hydrobromide (p.483·3).
*Motion sickness.*

**Travacalm Natural** *Hamilton, Austral.†.*
Ginger (p.1267·1).
*Motion sickness.*

**Travad**
*Note. This name is used for preparations of different composition.*
*Baxter, Austral.*
Monobasic sodium phosphate (p.1230·3); dibasic sodium phosphate (p.1231·1).
*Bowel evacuation.*

*Baxter, Mex.*
Sodium citrate (p.1223·2); sodium phosphate (p.1231·1).
*Bowel evacuation.*

**Travahex** *Baxter, Fin.*
Chlorhexidine acetate (p.1173·2).
*Skin, wound, and mucous membrane disinfection.*

**Travamin** *Rekah, Israel.*
Dimenhydrinate (p.431·1).
*Motion sickness; radiation sickness.*

**Travamine** *ICN, Canad.*
Dimenhydrinate (p.431·1).

**Travasept**
*Baxter, Israel; Baxter, UK.*
Cetrimide (p.1172·1); chlorhexidine acetate (p.1173·2).
*Disinfection of burns and wounds; skin disinfection.*

**Travasol**
*Baxter Immuno, Arg.; Baxter, Canad.; Baxter, Mex.; Clintec, USA.*
A range of amino-acid infusions with or without carbohydrate and electrolytes (p.1417·1).
*Parenteral nutrition.*

**Travasorb** *Clintec, USA.*
A range of preparations for enteral nutrition (p.1417·1).

**Travatan**
*Alcon, Arg.; Alcon, Austral.; Alcon, Braz. Alcon, Chile; Alcon, Denm.; Alcon, Fr.; Alcon, Ger.; Alcon, Hong Kong; Alcon, Irl.; Alcon, Ital.; Alcon, Norw.; Alcon, Port.; Alcon, Singapore; Alcon Cusi, Spain; Alcon, Thai.; Alcon, UK; Alcon, USA.*
Travoprost (p.1521·1).
*Glaucoma; ocular hypertension.*

**Travel Aid** *WestCan, Canad.*
Dimenhydrinate (p.431·1).
*Nausea; vomiting.*

**Travel Calm** *Boots, UK†; Unichem, UK†.*
Hyoscine hydrobromide (p.483·3).
*Motion sickness.*

**Travel Sickness** *Cantassium Co., UK.*
Ginger (p.1267·1).

**Travel Sickness Cocculus** *Homeocan, Canad.*
Homoeopathic preparation.

**Travel Tabs** *WestCan, Canad.†.*
Dimenhydrinate (p.431·1).
*Motion sickness.*

**Travel Well** *Farmalider, Spain.*
Dimenhydrinate (p.431·1).
*Motion sickness.*

**Travelaide** *Yauyip, Austral.†.*
Ginger (p.1267·1); cardamom (p.1667·3); slippery elm (p.1747·1).
*Motion sickness.*

**Travelbac** *Healthcare Innovations, UK.*
Bacterial extracts; vitamin B substances; yeast (p.1417·1).
*Dietary supplement for travellers.*

**Travel-Caps** *English Grains, UK†.*
Ginger (p.1267·1); calumba (p.1665·2); chamomile (p.1669·3).

**Traveleeze** *Ernest Jackson, UK.*
Meclozine hydrochloride (p.436·3); ginger (p.1267·1).
*Motion sickness.*

**Travel-Gum**
*Asta Medica, Austria; Asta Medica, Port.†.*
Dimenhydrinate (p.431·1).
*Motion sickness; vestibular disorders.*

**Travelgum**
*Health-Care, Gr.; Asta Medica, Hong Kong†; Asta Medica, Ital.*
Dimenhydrinate (p.431·1).
*Motion sickness.*

**Travella** *Nelson, UK.*
Homoeopathic preparation.

**Travellers** *Phillips Yeast, UK†.*
Ginger (p.1267·1).
*Motion sickness.*

**Travello**
*Pharmacia, Denm.; Pharmacia, Norw.; Pharmacia, Swed.*
Loperamide hydrochloride (p.1271·1).
*Diarrhoea.*

**Travelmate** *Shoppers Drug Mart, Canad.†.*
Dimenhydrinate (p.431·1).

**Traveltabs** *Stanley, Canad.*
Dimenhydrinate (p.431·1).
*Nausea; vomiting.*

**Travert**
*Pharmacia Upjohn, Norw.†; Baxter, USA.*
Invert sugar (p.1434·3); electrolytes (p.1217·1).
*Carbohydrate source; fluid and electrolyte disorders.*

**Travex** *Viatris, Port.*
Tramadol hydrochloride (p.94·3).
*Pain.*

**Traviata** *Andromaco, Chile.*
Paroxetine hydrochloride (p.311·2).
*Depression; obsessive-compulsive disorder; panic attacks; social phobia.*

**Travilan** *Anpharm (Ανφαρμ), Gr.*
Ceftriaxone sodium (p.182·3).
*Bacterial infections.*

**Travisco**
*Farmalab, Braz.; Master Pharma, Ital.*
Trapidil (p.1016·2).
*Ischaemic heart disease; prevention of restenosis following angioplasty; thromboembolism prophylaxis.*

**Travocort**
*Schering, Austria; Schering, Belg.; Schering, Ger.; Asche, Ger.; Shepa, Gr.; Schering, Hong Kong; Schering, Irl.; Schering, Ital.; Schering, Malaysia; Schering, Port.; Schering, S.Afr.; Schering, Singapore; Schering, Switz.; Schering, Thai.*
Isoconazole nitrate (p.401·3); diflucortolone valerate (p.1099·3).
*Inflamed fungal skin infections.*

**Travogen**
*Schering, Austria; Schering, Belg.; Schering, Ger.; Asche, Ger.; Shepa, Gr.; Schering, Hong Kong; Schering, Ital.; Schering, Malaysia; Schering, Singapore; Schering, Switz.; Schering, Thai.*
Isoconazole (p.401·3) or isoconazole nitrate (p.401·3).
*Erythrasma; fungal infections of the nails, skin, vulva, and vagina.*

**Travogyn** *Ativus, Braz.*
Tioconazole (p.409·3); tiabendazole (p.114·2).

**Trawell** *Asta Medica, Switz.*
Dimenhydrinate (p.431·1).
*Motion sickness.*

**Traxam**
*Goldshield, Irl.; Wyeth Lederle, Ital.; Goldshield, UK.*
Felbinac (p.39·1).
*Musculoskeletal, joint, peri-articular, and soft-tissue disorders.*

**Traxamic** *Systopic, India.*
Tranexamic acid (p.760·3).
*Fibrinolysis; menorrhagia.*

**Traxaton** *Steigerwald, Ger.*
Oak bark (p.1722·3).
*Diarrhoea.*

**Tray-Te** *Gray, Arg.*
Tetracaine hydrochloride (p.1385·1).
*Local anaesthesia.*

**Trazidex** *Sophia, Mex.*
Tobramycin sulfate (p.271·3); dexamethasone (p.1097·1).
*Infected eye disorders.*

**Trazil** *Sophia, Mex.*
Tobramycin sulfate (p.271·3).
*Bacterial eye infections.*

**Trazinac** *Sophia, Mex.†.*
Diclofenac sodium (p.32·1); tobramycin sulfate (p.271·3).
*Adjunct to eye surgery; bacterial eye infections.*

**Trazodil** *Unipharm, Israel.*
Trazodone hydrochloride (p.319·1).
*Depression.*

**Trazograf**
*Darrow, Braz.†; Juste, Spain.*
Meglumine amidotrizoate (p.1060·2); sodium amidotrizoate (p.1060·2).
*Radiographic contrast medium.*

**Trazolan**
*Continental Pharma, Belg.; Pharmacia, Neth.*
Trazodone hydrochloride (p.319·1).
*Depression.*

**Trazone** *Tecnifar, Port.*
Trazodone hydrochloride (p.319·1).
*Depression.*

**Trazorel** *ICN, Canad.*
Trazodone hydrochloride (p.319·1).
*Depression.*

**Trazoteva** *Teva Tuteur, Arg.*
Docetaxel (p.547·1).
*Malignant neoplasms.*

**Trazyl** *Angelini, Ital.*
Ibopamine hydrochloride (p.937·3).
*Diagnosis of glaucoma; postoperative ocular hypotension; production of mydriasis.*

**TRCS-Verorab** *Aventis Pasteur, Thai.*
A rabies vaccine (p.1635·3).
*Active immunisation.*

**TRD-Contin** *Modi-Mundipharma, India.*
Tramadol hydrochloride (p.94·3).
*Pain.*

**Trebon** *Unipharma, Gr.*
Acetylcysteine (p.1112·3).
*Paracetamol poisoning.*

**Trebon-N** *Unipharma, Gr.*
Acetylcysteine (p.1112·3).
*Respiratory disorders associated with viscous mucus.*

**Trecalmo** *Bayer, Ger.†.*
Clotiazepam (p.685·2).
*Anxiety; sleep disorders.*

**Trecator**
*IFET (ΙΦΕΤ), Gr.; Wyeth-Ayerst, USA.*
Ethionamide (p.212·3).
*Tuberculosis.*

**Trecloran** *Collins, Mex.*
Chloramphenicol (p.185·1); tetracycline (p.266·2).
*Bacterial infections.*

**Treda** *Sanfer, Mex.*
Neomycin sulfate (p.235·1); pectin (p.1580·3); kaolin (p.1268·3).
*Gastro-enteritis.*

**Tredalat** *Bayer, Ger.*
Nifedipine (p.966·2); acebutolol hydrochloride (p.848·1).
*Angina pectoris; hypertension.*

**Tredemine**
*Aventis, Fr.; IFET (ΙΦΕΤ), Gr.*
Niclosamide (p.110·1).
*Tapeworm infections.*

**Tredol**
*Note. This name is used for preparations of different composition.*
*Aegis, Hong Kong.*
Atenolol (p.865·2).
*Angina pectoris; arrhythmias; hypertension; myocardial infarction.*

*Quimica y Farmacia, Mex.†.*
Dipyrone (p.35·3).

**Trefovital** *Vaillant, Ital.†.*
Royal jelly (p.1740·3).
*Nutritional supplement.*

**tregor** *Hormosan, Ger.*
Amantadine sulfate (p.1197·2).
*Parkinsonism.*

**Trelibec** *Mintlab, Chile.*
Co-trimoxazole (p.199·3).
*Bacterial infections.*

**Treloc** *AstraZeneca, Ger.; Promed, Ger.*
Metoprolol tartrate (p.957·1); hydrochlorothiazide (p.933·2); hydralazine hydrochloride (p.931·2).
*Hypertension.*

**Trelstar** *Pharmacia, USA.*
Triptorelin embonate (p.1341·2).
*Prostatic cancer.*

**Tremafarm** *Raffo, Chile.*
Fluoxetine (p.296·3).
*Mixed anxiety depressive states.*

**Tremaril** *LPB, Ital.*
Metixene hydrochloride (p.485·3).
*Parkinsonism.*

**Tremarit** *AWD, Ger.*
Metixene hydrochloride (p.485·3).
*Parkinsonism and other hyperkinetic disorders.*

**Tremblex**
*Janssen-Cilag, Belg.; Janssen-Cilag, Neth.*
Dexetimide hydrochloride (p.481·1).
*Drug-induced extrapyramidal disorders.*

**Tremexal** *Cosmopharm, Gr.*
Flutamide (p.556·2).
*Prostatic cancer.*

**Tremix** *Korhispana, Spain.*
Miconazole nitrate (p.405·3).
*Fungal skin infections.*

**Tremoforat** *Klein, Ger.*
Belladonna (p.479·1).
*Parkinsonism.*

**Tremopar** *Acis, Ger.*
Levodopa (p.1205·2); carbidopa (p.1204·3).
*Parkinsonism.*

**Tremoquil** *Astra, Swed.*
Metixene hydrochloride (p.485·3).
*Parkinsonism.*

**Tremorex** *Durascan, Denm.†.*
Selegiline hydrochloride (p.1214·1).
*Parkinsonism.*

**Tren** *YSP, Malaysia.*
Tranexamic acid (p.760·3).
*Haemorrhagic disorders.*

**Trenantone**
*Takeda, Austria; Takeda, Ger.*
Leuprorelin acetate (p.1331·1).
*Prostatic cancer.*

**Trendar PMS** *Whitehall-Robins, Canad.*
Paracetamol (p.76·2); pamabrom (p.978·2); mepyramine maleate (p.437·1).
*Premenstrual syndrome.*

**Trendinol** *Elan, Spain.*
Nitrendipine (p.973·3).
*Hypertension.*

**Trenelone** *Schering-Plough, Port.*
Dexchlorpheniramine maleate (p.427·3).

**Trenlin**
*CCM, Malaysia; CCM, Singapore.*
Pentoxifylline (p.979·3).
*Cerebral and peripheral vascular disorders.*

**Trentadil**
*Christiaens, Belg.; Celltech, Fr.*
Bamifylline hydrochloride (p.781·3).
*Asthma; obstructive airways disease.*

**Trental**
*Aventis, Arg.; Aventis, Austral.; Aventis, Austria; Aventis, Braz.; Aventis, Canad.; Aventis, Chile; Aventis, Denm.; Aventis, Fin.; Aventis, Ger.; Aventis, Hong Kong; Aventis, India; Aventis, Irl.; Aventis, Israel; Aventis, Ital.; Aventis, Malaysia; Aventis, Mex.; Aventis, Neth.; Aventis, Norw.; Aventis, NZ; Aventis, Port.; Aventis, S.Afr.; Aventis, Singapore; Aventis, Switz.; Aventis, Thai.; Aventis, UK; Hoechst Marion Roussel, USA.*
Pentoxifylline (p.979·3).
*Cerebral, ocular, and peripheral vascular disorders.*

**Treo**
*Note. This name is used for preparations of different composition.*
*Lundbeck, Denm.; Pharmacia, Fin.; Pharmacia, Swed.*
Aspirin (p.15·1); caffeine (p.782·1).
*Fever; pain.*

*Biopharm, USA.*
*SPF 8; SPF 15; SPF 30:* Octocrilene (p.1154·3); octinoxate (p.1154·3); oxybenzone (p.1154·3); octisalate (p.1154·3); citronella oil (p.1673·2).
*Sunscreen.*

**Treo comp** *Pharmacia, Swed.*
Aspirin (p.15·1); codeine phosphate (p.27·1); caffeine (p.782·1).
*Pain.*

**Treomycin** *Chew, Thai.*
Thiamphenicol (p.269·2).
*Bacterial infections.*

**Treparin** *NCSN, Ital.*
A heparinoid (p.931·1).
*Thrombosis prophylaxis.*

**Trepidan** *Max Farma, Ital.*
Prazepam (p.716·2).
*Anxiety.*

**Trepiline** *Aspen, S.Afr.*
Amitriptyline hydrochloride (p.280·3).
*Mixed anxiety depressive states.*

**Trepol** *Lemery, Mex.*
Dipyridamole (p.903·1).
*Cardiovascular disorders.*

**Trepress**
*Novartis, Austria; Azupharma, Ger.; Ciba, Switz.†.*
Oxprenolol hydrochloride (p.978·1); hydralazine hydrochloride (p.931·2); chlortalidone (p.882·3).
*Hypertension.*

**Tres Orix Forte**
*Almirall, Hong Kong; Almirall, Spain.*
Cyproheptadine orotate (p.430·2); amino acids and vitamins (p.1417·1).
*Anorexia; tonic; weight loss.*

**Tresal** *Tremedic, Swed.†.*
Sodium chloride (p.1233·3).
*Irrigation solution.*

**Tresite F** *Temis, Arg.*
Liothyronine (p.1602·2); flumetasone pivalate (p.1101·1).
*Skin disorders.*

**Tresium** *Prodes, Spain†.*
Bromhexine hydrochloride (p.1115·3); co-trimoxazole (p.199·3).
*Respiratory-tract infections.*

**Tresivac** *Serum Institute, India.*
A measles, mumps, and rubella vaccine (p.1625·1).
*Active immunisation.*

**Tresleen** *Pfizer, Austria.*
Sertraline hydrochloride (p.317·2).
*Depression; obsessive-compulsive disorder; panic attacks; post-traumatic stress disorder.*

**Tresos B** *Eagle, Austral.†.*
Multivitamin, amino-acid, and mineral preparation (p.1417·1).
*Dietary supplement.*

**Tretin** *Genepharm, Gr.*
Isotretinoin (p.1148·3).
*Acne.*

**Tretinoderm** *Defuen, Arg.*
Tretinoin (p.1161·1).
*Acne; photodamaged skin.*

**Tretinoine** *Widmer, Switz.†.*
Tretinoin (p.1161·1); urea (p.1162·2); triclosan (p.1195·2).
*Acne.*

**Tretinoine Kefrane** *RoC, Fr.†.*
Tretinoin (p.1161·1).
*Acne.*

**Tretinon**
*YSP, Malaysia; Wayne, Mex.†.*
Tretinoin (p.1161·1).
*Acne.*

**Treupel comp** *Asta Medica, Ger.†.*
Codeine phosphate (p.27·1); paracetamol (p.76·2).
*Fever; pain.*

**Treupel mono** *Asta Medica, Ger.†.*
Paracetamol (p.76·2).
*Fever; pain.*

**Treupel N** *Asta Medica, Switz.†.*
Paracetamol (p.76·2).
*Fever; pain.*

**Treupel sans codeine** *Asta Medica, Switz.*
Aspirin (p.15·1); paracetamol (p.76·2).
*Fever; pain.*

**Treupel simplex** *Asta Medica, Switz.*
Aspirin (p.15·1); paracetamol (p.76·2); ascorbic acid (p.1460·2).
*Fever; pain.*

**Treuphadol** *Treupha, Switz.*
Paracetamol (p.76·2).
*Fever; pain.*

**Treuphadol Plus** *Treupha, Switz.*
Paracetamol (p.76·2); codeine phosphate (p.27·1).
*Fever; pain.*

**Trevilor** *Wyeth, Ger.*
Venlafaxine hydrochloride (p.321·3).
*Anxiety; depression.*

**Trevina** *Orion, Denm.*
70 Tablets, estradiol valerate (p.1550·2); 14 tablets, estradiol valerate; medroxyprogesterone acetate (p.1557·2); 7 tablets, inert.
*Menopausal disorders; osteoporosis.*

**Trevis** *Kolassa, Austria.*
*Lactobacillus acidophilus* (p.1704·2); *Bifidobacterium animalis*; *Lactobacillus bulgaricus* (p.1704·2); *Streptococcus thermophilus* (p.1704·2).
*Diarrhoea.*

**Trewilor** *Wyeth Lederle, Austria†.*
Venlafaxine hydrochloride (p.321·3).
*Depression.*

**Trex** *Saval, Chile.*
Azithromycin (p.159·1).
*Bacterial infections.*

**Trexall** *Barr, USA.*
Methotrexate (p.568·2).
*Malignant neoplasms; psoriasis; rheumatoid arthritis.*

**Trexan**
*Note. This name is used for preparations of different composition.*
*Orion, Fin.*
Methotrexate (p.568·2).
*Malignant neoplasms; psoriasis; rheumatoid arthritis.*

*Bristol-Myers Squibb, Malaysia; Bristol-Myers Squibb, Singapore; Du Pont, USA.*
Naltrexone hydrochloride (p.1046·1).
*Opioid dependence.*

**Trexen** *Asofarma, Mex.*
Clindamycin phosphate (p.194·2).
*Bacterial vaginitis.*

**Trexeron** *Serono, Mex.†.*
Methotrexate (p.568·2).

**Trexirol NF** *Armstrong, Arg.*
Amoxicillin trihydrate (p.155·3); ambroxol hydrochloride (p.1114·3).
*Respiratory-tract infections.*

**Trexofin** *Cheil, Singapore.*
Ceftriaxone sodium (p.182·3).
*Bacterial infections.*

**Trexol** *Atlantis, Mex.*
Tramadol hydrochloride (p.94·3).
*Pain.*

**Trexydin** *Ranbaxy, Malaysia.*
Terfenadine (p.441·1); pseudoephedrine hydrochloride (p.1129·2).
*Allergic rhinitis.*

**Trexyl**
*Ranbaxy, India; Ranbaxy, Thai.†.*
Terfenadine (p.441·1).
*Allergic eye disorders; allergic rhinitis; allergic skin disorders.*

**Trezor** *Biosintetica, Braz.†.*
Galantamine hydrobromide (p.1491·2).
*Myasthenia.*

**TRH**
*Ferring, Arg.; UCB, Belg.; Ferring, Braz.†; Berlin-Chemie, Ger.; Ferring, Ger.; Ferring, Israel; Roche, Israel.*
Protirelin (p.1337·3).
*Assessment of hypothalamic-pituitary-thyroid function.*

**TRH Prem** *Novartis Consumer, Spain.*
Protirelin (p.1337·3).
*Evaluation of thyroid function.*

**Trhelea** *Elea, Arg.*
Protirelin (p.1337·3).
*Diagnosis of hypothalamic-pituitary-thyroid dysfunction.*

**Tri Hachemina** *Medea, Spain.*
Inositol (p.1701·2); calcium pantothenate (p.1442·3); aminobenzoic acid (p.1142·2) or sodium aminobenzoate (p.1747·1).
*Infertility; skin disorders.*

**Tri Vit with Fluoride** *Barre-National, USA.*
Multivitamin preparation with fluoride (p.1444·3)(p.1417·1).
*Dental caries prophylaxis; dietary supplement.*

**Triac** *Ache, Braz.*
Tiratricol (p.1604·3).
*Thyroid disorders.*

**Triacana**
*Sidus, Arg.; Andromaco, Chile; Laphal, Fr.*
Tiratricol (p.1604·3).
*Thyroid disorders; treatment of cellulite.*

**Triacel** *Aventis Pasteur, Arg.*
A diphtheria, tetanus, and pertussis vaccine (p.1613·3).
*Active immunisation.*

**Triacelluvax** *Chiron Vaccines, Ital.†.*
A diphtheria, tetanus, and acellular pertussis vaccine (p.1613·3).
*Active immunisation.*

**Triacet** *Lemmon, USA.*
Triamcinolone acetonide (p.1110·2).
*Skin disorders.*

**Triacilline** *Beecham, Belg.†.*
Ticarcillin sodium (p.270·2).
*Bacterial infections.*

**Triacomb**
*Technilab, Canad.; Technilab, Hong Kong.*
Triamcinolone acetonide (p.1110·2); nystatin (p.406·3); neomycin sulfate (p.235·1); gramicidin (p.220·2).
*Anal and vulvar pruritus; infected skin disorders.*

**Triactin** *Prometic, USA†.*
Phenylpropanolamine hydrochloride (p.1127·3); chlorphenamine maleate (p.427·3).
*Upper respiratory-tract disorders.*

**Triad** *Forest Pharmaceuticals, USA.*
Butalbital (p.673·3); paracetamol (p.76·2); caffeine (p.782·1).
*Tension headache.*

**Triada** *Loren, Mex.*
Vitamin B substances (p.1417·1).
Lidocaine (p.1377·3) is included in this preparation to alleviate the pain of injection.

**Triadapin** *Novopharm, Canad.†.*
Doxepin hydrochloride (p.291·2).
*Depression.*

**Tri-Adcortyl** *Bristol-Myers Squibb, UK.*
Nystatin (p.406·3); triamcinolone acetonide (p.1110·2); neomycin sulfate (p.235·1); gramicidin (p.220·2).
*Bacterial and fungal skin infections; otitis externa.*

**Triadene** *Schering, UK.*
Ethinylestradiol (p.1553·2); gestodene (p.1556·1).
*Triphasic oral contraceptive.*

**Triaderm** *Taro, Canad.*
Triamcinolone acetonide (p.1110·2).
*Skin disorders.*

**Triafed with Codeine** *Schein, USA†.*
Pseudoephedrine hydrochloride (p.1129·2); triprolidine hydrochloride (p.442·3); codeine phosphate (p.27·1).
*Coughs.*

**Triaformo** *Cusi, Hong Kong†.*
Clioquinol (p.196·3); triamcinolone acetonide (p.1110·2).
*Infected skin disorders.*

**Triagin** *Hertz, Braz.†.*
Camphor (p.1665·3); menthol (p.1711·3); turpentine; methyl salicylate (p.59·3).
*Musculoskeletal and joint disorders.*

**Triagynon** *Schering, Spain.*
Levonorgestrel (p.1563·2); ethinylestradiol (p.1553·2).
*Triphasic oral contraceptive.*

**Triaken** *Kendrick, Mex.*
Ceftriaxone sodium (p.182·3).
Lidocaine hydrochloride (p.1377·3) is included in the intramuscular injection to alleviate the pain of injection.
*Bacterial infections.*

**Trial AG** *Zee, USA.*
Aluminium hydroxide (p.1249·2); magnesium hydroxide (p.1272·2); simeticone (p.1289·2).
*Antacid; flatulence.*

**Trial Antacid** *Zee, USA.*
Calcium carbonate (p.1254·2).
*Antacid.*

**Trial Combi** *Beta, Arg.*
2 Patches, estradiol (p.1550·1); 2 patches, estradiol; norethisterone acetate (p.1562·2).
*Menopausal disorders; osteoporosis.*

**Trial Gel** *Beta, Arg.*
Estradiol (p.1550·1).
*Oestrogen deficiency.*

**Trial Gest** *Beta, Arg.*
Estradiol (p.1550·1); norethisterone acetate (p.1562·2).
*Menopausal disorders; osteoporosis.*

**Trial Pack** *Beta, Arg.*
Patches, estradiol (p.1550·1); norethisterone acetate (p.1562·2).
*Menopausal disorders.*

**Trial Sat** *Beta, Arg.*
Estradiol (p.1550·1).
*Menopausal disorders.*

**Trialix**
*Aventis, Austria; Aventis, Irl.; Aventis, Switz.*
Ramipril (p.994·1); piretanide (p.983·3).
*Hypertension.*

**Trialmin** *Menarini, Spain.*
Gemfibrozil (p.923·1).
*Hyperlipidaemias.*

**Trialona** *Alter, Spain.*
Fluticasone propionate (p.1102·3).
*Asthma.*

**Trialone** *Janssen-Cilag, S.Afr.*
Miconazole nitrate (p.405·3); triamcinolone acetonide (p.1110·2); neomycin sulfate (p.235·1).
*Infected skin disorders.*

**Trialyn DM** *Trianon, Canad.*
Dextromethorphan hydrobromide (p.1117·3); diphenhydramine hydrobromide (p.431·3); ammonium chloride (p.1115·2).
*Coughs.*

**Triam**
*Lichtenstein, Ger.; Wolff, Ger.*
Triamcinolone (p.1110·2) or triamcinolone acetonide (p.1110·2).
*Corticosteroid.*

*Denk, Singapore.*
Triamcinolone acetonide (p.1110·2).
*Corticosteroid.*

*Hyrex, USA.*
Triamcinolone diacetate (p.1110·2).
*Corticosteroid.*

**Triama** *Samakeephaesaj, Thai.*
Triamcinolone acetonide (p.1110·2).
*Skin disorders.*

**Triam-A** *Hyrex, USA.*
Triamcinolone acetonide (p.1110·2).
*Corticosteroid.*

**Triamaxco** *Ashbourne, UK.*
Triamterene (p.1016·2); hydrochlorothiazide (p.933·2).
These ingredients can be described by the British Approved Name Co-triamterzide.
*Hypertension; oedema.*

**Triamciterap**
*Note. This name is used for preparations of different composition.*
*Frasca, Arg.*
Triamcinolone (p.1110·2).
*Skin disorders.*

*Medica, Arg.*
Emollient.

**Triam-Co** *Ivax, Hong Kong.*
Hydrochlorothiazide (p.933·2); triamterene (p.1016·2).
*Hypertension; oedema.*

**Triamco** *Ivax, UK.*
Hydrochlorothiazide (p.933·2); triamterene (p.1016·2).
These ingredients can be described by the British Approved Name Co-triamterzide.
*Hypertension; oedema.*

**Triamcort** *Helvepharm, Switz.*
Triamcinolone acetonide (p.1110·2).
*Corticosteroid.*

**TriamCreme** *Lichtenstein, Ger.*
Triamcinolone acetonide (p.1110·2).
*Skin disorders.*

**Triamer** *Aventis Pasteur, Belg.*
An adsorbed diphtheria, tetanus, and pertussis vaccine (p.1613·3).
*Active immunisation of infants and young children.*

**Triamgalen** *Galen, Ger.*
Triamcinolone acetonide (p.1110·2).
*Skin disorders.*

**Triamhexal** *Hexal, Ger.*
Triamcinolone acetonide (p.1110·2).
*Corticosteroid.*

**Triamid** *Beta, Arg.*
Azithromycin (p.159·1).
*Bacterial infections.*

**Triaminic**
*Note. This name is used for preparations of different composition.*
*Sandoz, Canad.†; Novartis Consumer, S.Afr.†.*
*Sustained-release tablets:* Phenylpropanolamine hydrochloride (p.1127·3); pheniramine maleate (p.438·3); mepyramine maleate (p.437·1).
*Nasal and sinus congestion.*

*Novartis Sante, Fr.†; Wander, India.*
*Tablets:* Phenylpropanolamine hydrochloride (p.1127·3); pheniramine maleate (p.438·3).
Formerly contained phenylpropanolamine hydrochloride, mepyramine maleate, and pheniramine maleate in *Fr.*
*Cold symptoms; otitis media; rhinitis.*

*Wander, India; Novartis Consumer, USA†.*
*Syrup; oral drops:* Phenylpropanolamine hydrochloride (p.1127·3); chlorphenamine maleate (p.427·3).
Formerly contained mepyramine maleate, pheniramine maleate, and phenylpropanolamine hydrochloride in the *USA*.
*Cold symptoms; otitis media; rhinitis.*

*Novartis Consumer, Ital.*
*Nasal spray:* Chlorphenamine maleate (p.427·3); oxymetazoline hydrochloride (p.1126·1).
*Nasal congestion.*
*Tablets:* Phenylpropanolamine hydrochloride (p.1127·3); pheniramine maleate (p.438·3); mepyramine maleate (p.437·1); caffeine (p.782·1).
*Cold symptoms.*

**Triaminic-12** *Novartis Consumer, USA†.*
Phenylpropanolamine hydrochloride (p.1127·3); chlorphenamine maleate (p.427·3).
*Cold symptoms.*

**Triaminic Allergy** *Novartis Consumer, USA†.*
Phenylpropanolamine hydrochloride (p.1127·3); chlorphenamine maleate (p.427·3).
*Upper respiratory-tract symptoms.*

**Triaminic Allergy Congestion** *Novartis Consumer, Canad.*
Pseudoephedrine hydrochloride (p.1129·2).
*Nasal and sinus congestion.*

**Triaminic AM Cough & Decongestant Formula** *Novartis Consumer, USA.*
Pseudoephedrine hydrochloride (p.1129·2); dextromethorphan hydrobromide (p.1117·3).

**Triaminic AM Decongestant Formula** *Novartis Consumer, USA.*
Pseudoephedrine hydrochloride (p.1129·2).

**Triaminic Chewable** *Novartis Consumer, USA†.*
Phenylpropanolamine hydrochloride (p.1127·3); chlorphenamine maleate (p.427·3).
*Upper respiratory-tract symptoms.*

**Triaminic Cold** *Novartis Consumer, USA†.*
Phenylpropanolamine hydrochloride (p.1127·3); chlorphenamine maleate (p.427·3).
*Cold symptoms.*

**Triaminic Cold & Allergy**
*Note. This name is used for preparations of different composition.*
*Novartis Consumer, Canad.*
Chlorphenamine maleate (p.427·3); pseudoephedrine hydrochloride (p.1129·2).
Formerly contained chlorphenamine maleate and phenylpropanolamine hydrochloride.
*Nasal and sinus congestion.*

*Novartis, USA†.*
Phenylpropanolamine hydrochloride (p.1127·3); chlorphenamine maleate (p.427·3).
*Cold and allergy symptoms.*

**Triaminic Cold & Cough**
*Novartis Consumer, Canad.; Novartis, USA.*
Pseudoephedrine hydrochloride (p.1129·2); dextromethorphan hydrobromide (p.1117·3); chlorphenamine maleate (p.427·3).
*Coughs and cold symptoms.*

**Triaminic Cold, Cough & Fever** *Novartis Consumer, Canad.*
Paracetamol (p.76·2); chlorphenamine maleate (p.427·3); pseudoephedrine hydrochloride (p.1129·2); dextromethorphan hydrobromide (p.1117·3).
*Cold and influenza symptoms; coughs.*

**Triaminic Cold & Fever** *Novartis Consumer, Canad.*
Pseudoephedrine hydrochloride (p.1129·2); dextromethorphan hydrobromide (p.1117·3); paracetamol (p.76·2).

**Triaminic Cold & Night Time Cough** *Novartis Consumer, Canad.*
Chlorphenamine maleate (p.427·3); pseudoephedrine hydrochloride (p.1129·2); dextromethorphan hydrobromide (p.1117·3).
*Coughs and cold symptoms.*

**Triaminic Cough**
*Note. This name is used for preparations of different composition.*
*Novartis Consumer, Canad.*
Dextromethorphan hydrobromide (p.1117·3).
*Coughs.*

*Novartis Consumer, Canad.*
Pseudoephedrine hydrochloride (p.1129·2); dextromethorphan hydrobromide (p.1117·3).
*Coughs; nasal and sinus congestion.*

**Triaminic Cough & Congestion** *Novartis Consumer, Canad.*
Pseudoephedrine hydrochloride (p.1129·2); dextromethorphan hydrobromide (p.1117·3).
*Coughs; nasal congestion.*

**Triaminic Cough & Sore Throat** *Novartis Consumer, Canad.*
Paracetamol (p.76·2); pseudoephedrine hydrochloride (p.1129·2); dextromethorphan hydrobromide (p.1117·3).
*Coughs and cold symptoms.*

**Triaminic CS** *Wander, India.*
Dextromethorphan hydrobromide (p.1117·3); phenylpropanolamine (p.1127·3).
*Cold symptoms; otitis media; rhinitis.*

**Triaminic Decongestant & Expectorant** *Sandoz, Canad.†.*
Pseudoephedrine hydrochloride (p.1129·2); guaifenesin (p.1122·1).

**Triaminic DM**
*Note. This name is used for preparations of different composition.*
*Novartis Consumer, Canad.*
Dextromethorphan hydrobromide (p.1117·3).
*Coughs.*

*Novartis Consumer, USA†.*
Phenylpropanolamine hydrochloride (p.1127·3); dextromethorphan hydrobromide (p.1117·3).
*Coughs and cold symptoms.*

**Triaminic DM Daytime** *Novartis Consumer, Canad.†.*
Dextromethorphan hydrobromide (p.1117·3); phenylpropanolamine hydrochloride (p.1127·3); guaifenesin (p.1122·1).
*Coughs and cold symptoms.*

**Triaminic DM Expectorant** *Novartis Consumer, Canad.*
Dextromethorphan hydrobromide (p.1117·3); pseudoephedrine hydrochloride (p.1129·2); chlorphenamine maleate (p.427·3); guaifenesin (p.1122·1).
Formerly contained dextromethorphan hydrobromide, phenylpropanolamine hydrochloride, pheniramine maleate, mepyramine maleate, and guaifenesin.
*Coughs; nasal congestion.*

**Triaminic DM Nighttime** *Novartis Consumer, Canad.*
Dextromethorphan hydrobromide (p.1117·3); chlorphenamine maleate (p.427·3); pseudoephedrine hydrochloride (p.1129·2).
*Coughs; nasal congestion.*

**Triaminic DM-D** *Sandoz, Canad.†.*
Dextromethorphan hydrobromide (p.1117·3); pseudoephedrine hydrochloride (p.1129·2).
*Coughs; nasal and sinus congestion.*

**Triaminic Expectorant**
*Note. This name is used for preparations of different composition.*
*Novartis Consumer, Canad.*
Pseudoephedrine hydrochloride (p.1129·2); chlorphenamine maleate (p.427·3); guaifenesin (p.1122·1).
Formerly contained phenylpropanolamine hydrochloride, pheniramine maleate, mepyramine maleate, and guaifenesin.
*Coughs; nasal congestion.*

*Novartis Consumer, USA†.*
Phenylpropanolamine hydrochloride (p.1127·3); guaifenesin (p.1122·1).
*Coughs.*

**Triaminic Expectorant with Codeine** *Novartis Consumer, USA†.*
Codeine phosphate (p.27·1); phenylpropanolamine hydrochloride (p.1127·3); guaifenesin (p.1122·1).
*Coughs.*

**Triaminic Expectorant DH** *Sandoz, Canad.†; Novartis Consumer, USA†.*
Hydrocodone tartrate (p.45·1); phenylpropanolamine hydrochloride (p.1127·3); pheniramine maleate (p.438·3); mepyramine maleate (p.437·1); guaifenesin (p.1122·1).
*Coughs.*

**Triaminic Infant Oral Decongestant** *Novartis, USA.*
Pseudoephedrine hydrochloride (p.1129·2).
*Nasal congestion.*

**Triaminic Night Time Rub** *Sandoz, Canad.†.*
Camphor (p.1665·3); eucalyptus oil (p.1686·2); menthol (p.1711·3).

**Triaminic Nighttime Flu** *Novartis Consumer, Canad.*
Paracetamol (p.76·2); chlorphenamine maleate (p.427·3); pseudoephedrine hydrochloride (p.1129·2); dextromethorphan hydrobromide (p.1117·3).

**Triaminic Nite Light** *Novartis Consumer, USA.*
Pseudoephedrine hydrochloride (p.1129·2); chlorphenamine maleate (p.427·3); dextromethorphan hydrobromide (p.1117·3).
*Coughs and cold symptoms.*

**Triaminic Oral Infant** *Novartis Consumer, USA†.*
Phenylpropanolamine hydrochloride (p.1127·3); mepyramine maleate (p.437·1); pheniramine maleate (p.438·3).
*Upper respiratory-tract symptoms.*

**Triaminic Pediatric Drops** *Novartis Consumer, Canad.*
Pseudoephedrine hydrochloride (p.1129·2).

**Triaminic Severe Cold & Fever** *Novartis, USA.*
Paracetamol (p.76·2); pseudoephedrine hydrochloride (p.1129·2); dextromethorphan hydrobromide (p.1117·3); chlorphenamine maleate (p.427·3).
*Coughs and cold symptoms.*

**Triaminic Softchews** *Novartis, USA.*
Pseudoephedrine hydrochloride (p.1129·2); chlorphenamine maleate (p.427·3).
*Upper respiratory-tract disorders.*

**Triaminic Sore Throat Formula** *Novartis Consumer, USA.*
Pseudoephedrine hydrochloride (p.1129·2); dextromethorphan hydrobromide (p.1117·3); paracetamol (p.76·2).
*Coughs and cold symptoms.*

**Triaminic Throat Pain & Cough** *Novartis Consumer, Canad.*
Paracetamol (p.76·2); pseudoephedrine hydrochloride (p.1129·2); dextromethorphan hydrobromide (p.1117·3).
*Coughs and cold symptoms.*

*Novartis, USA.*
Paracetamol (p.76·2); pseudoephedrine (p.1129·2); dextromethorphan hydrobromide (p.1117·3).
*Coughs; sore throat.*

**Triaminicflu** *Novartis Consumer, Ital.*
Paracetamol (p.76·2); pheniramine maleate (p.438·3); phenylephrine hydrochloride (p.1126·3).
*Cold and influenza symptoms.*

**Triaminicin** *Novartis Consumer, Canad.†.*
Phenylpropanolamine hydrochloride (p.1127·3); mepyramine maleate (p.437·1); pheniramine maleate (p.438·3); paracetamol (p.76·2); caffeine (p.782·1).
*Cold symptoms.*

**Triaminicin Cold, Allergy, Sinus** *Novartis Consumer, USA†.*
Phenylpropanolamine hydrochloride (p.1127·3); chlorphenamine maleate (p.427·3); paracetamol (p.76·2).
*Upper respiratory-tract symptoms.*

**Triaminicol DM** *Novartis Consumer, Canad.*
Pseudoephedrine hydrochloride (p.1129·2); chlorphenamine maleate (p.427·3); dextromethorphan hydrobromide (p.1117·3).
Formerly contained phenylpropanolamine hydrochloride, mepyramine maleate, pheniramine maleate, and dextromethorphan hydrobromide.
*Coughs; nasal congestion.*

**Triaminicol Multi-Symptom Cough and Cold** *Novartis Consumer, USA†.*
Phenylpropanolamine hydrochloride (p.1127·3); chlorphenamine maleate (p.427·3); dextromethorphan hydrobromide (p.1117·3).
*Coughs and cold symptoms.*

**Triaminicol Multi-Symptom Relief** *Novartis Consumer, USA†.*
Phenylpropanolamine hydrochloride (p.1127·3); chlorphenamine maleate (p.427·3); dextromethorphan hydrobromide (p.1117·3).
*Coughs and cold symptoms.*

**Triamizide** *Pacific, NZ.*
Hydrochlorothiazide (p.933·2); triamterene (p.1016·2).
*Hypertension; oedema.*

**Triamonide** *Forest Pharmaceuticals, USA.*
Triamcinolone acetonide (p.1110·2).
*Corticosteroid.*

**Triampoen** *Poen, Arg.*
Triamcinolone (p.1110·2).
*Eye disorders.*

**Triampur compositum** *AWD, Ger.*
Triamterene (p.1016·2); hydrochlorothiazide (p.933·2).
*Heart failure; hypertension; oedema.*

**TriamSalbe** *Lichtenstein, Ger.*
Triamcinolone acetonide (p.1110·2).
*Skin disorders.*

**Triamsicort** *Diba, Mex.*
Triamcinolone (p.1110·2).
*Corticosteroid.*

**Triamteren comp** *Genericon, Austria; Ratiopharm, Ger.*
Triamterene (p.1016·2); hydrochlorothiazide (p.933·2).
*Heart failure; hypertension; oedema.*

**Triamteren-H** *3M, Ger.*
Triamterene (p.1016·2); hydrochlorothiazide (p.933·2).
*Heart failure; hypertension; oedema.*

**Triamteren/HCT** *Tyrol, Austria; Aliud, Ger.*
Triamterene (p.1016·2); hydrochlorothiazide (p.933·2).
*Heart failure; hypertension; oedema.*

**Triam-Tiazida R** *Normal, Port.*
Triamterene (p.1016·2); hydrochlorothiazide (p.933·2).
*Hypertension.*

**Triamvirgi** *Infosint, Ital.*
Triamcinolone acetonide (p.1110·2).
*Parenteral corticosteroid.*

**Trianal**
*Note. This name is used for preparations of different composition.*
*Will-Pharma, Belg.; Will-Pharma, Neth.*
Triamcinolone acetonide (p.1110·2); lidocaine hydrochloride (p.1377·3).
*Haemorrhoids; pruritus ani.*

*Trianon, Canad.*
Aspirin (p.15·1); caffeine (p.782·1); butalbital (p.673·3).
*Pain; sedative.*

**Trianal C** *Trianon, Canad.*
Aspirin (p.15·1); caffeine (p.782·1); butalbital (p.673·3); codeine phosphate (p.27·1).
*Pain; sedative.*

**Triancil** *Apsen, Braz.*
Triamcinolone acetonide (p.1110·2).
*Corticosteroid.*

**Tri-Anemul** *Medopharm, Ger.†.*
Triamcinolone acetonide (p.1110·2).
*Skin disorders.*

**Triapin** *Hoechst Marion Roussel, Austria; Aventis, Neth.; Aventis, UK.*
Felodipine (p.914·3); ramipril (p.994·1).
*Hypertension.*

**Triapten** *Riemser, Ger.*
Foscarnet sodium (p.634·2).
*Herpes simplex infections of the skin and mucous membranes.*

**Triarese** *Hexal, Ger.*
Triamterene (p.1016·2); hydrochlorothiazide (p.933·2).
*Heart failure; hypertension; oedema.*

**Triasox** *Berna, Spain.*
Tiabendazole (p.114·2).
*Worm infections.*

**Triaspar** *Beta, Arg.*
Cabergoline (p.1203·3).
*Parkinsonism.*

**Triasporin** *Italfarmaco, Ital.*
Itraconazole (p.401·3).
*Fungal infections.*

**Triastad HCT** *Stada, Austria.*
Triamterene (p.1016·2); hydrochlorothiazide (p.933·2).
*Hypertension; oedema.*

**Triastonal** *Hoyer, Ger.*
Sitosterol (p.982·3).
*Benign prostatic hyperplasia.*

**Triatec** *Aventis, Braz.; Aventis, Chile; Aventis, Denm.; Aventis, Fr.; Hoechst Marion Roussel, Gr.; Aventis, Ital.; Aventis, Norw.; Aventis, Port.; Aventis, Swed.; Aventis, Switz.*
Ramipril (p.994·1).
*Atherosclerosis; diabetic nephropathy; heart failure; hypertension; myocardial infarction.*

**Triatec-8** *Trianon, Canad.*
Paracetamol (p.76·2); codeine phosphate (p.27·1); caffeine citrate (p.782·1).
*Coughs; fever; pain.*

**Triatec-30** *Trianon, Canad.*
Paracetamol (p.76·2); codeine phosphate (p.27·1).
*Coughs; fever; pain.*

**Triatec Comp** *Aventis, Denm.; Aventis, Swed.; Aventis, Switz.*
Ramipril (p.994·1); hydrochlorothiazide (p.933·2).
*Hypertension.*

**Triatec Composto** *Aventis, Port.*
Ramipril (p.994·1); hydrochlorothiazide (p.933·2).
*Hypertension.*

**Triatec D** *Aventis, Braz.*
Ramipril (p.994·1); hydrochlorothiazide (p.933·2).
*Hypertension.*

**Triatec HCT** *Aventis, Ital.*
Ramipril (p.994·1); hydrochlorothiazide (p.933·2).
*Hypertension.*

**Triativ** *Ativus, Braz.*
Hypericum (p.299·1).
*Agitation; depression; sleep disorders.*

**Triatop** *Janssen-Cilag, Arg.; Janssen-Cilag, Austria; Janssen-Cilag, Ital.; Janssen-Cilag, Thai.*
Ketoconazole (p.403·3).
*Scalp disorders.*

**Triaval** *Orion, Switz.*
70 Tablets, estradiol valerate (p.1550·2); 14 tablets, estradiol valerate; medroxyprogesterone acetate (p.1557·2); 7 tablets, inert.
*Menopausal disorders; osteoporosis.*

**Triavil** *Merck Frosst, Canad.; Lotus, USA.*
Perphenazine (p.714·2); amitriptyline hydrochloride (p.280·3).
*Mixed anxiety depressive states; schizophrenia.*

**Tri-A-Vite F** *Major, USA.*
Multivitamin preparation with fluoride (p.1417·1).

**Triaxin** *Eurofarma, Braz.†.*
Ceftriaxone (p.183·3).
*Bacterial infections.*

**Triaxone** *Julphar, UAE.*
Ceftriaxone sodium (p.182·3).
*Bacterial infections.*

**Triaxton** *Ariston, Braz.*
Ceftriaxone (p.183·3).
*Bacterial infections.*

**Triaz** *Medicis, USA.*
Benzoyl peroxide (p.1143·2).
*Acne.*

**triazid** *CT, Ger.*
Triamterene (p.1016·2); hydrochlorothiazide (p.933·2).
*Heart failure; hypertension; oedema.*

**Triazine** *Aspen Consumer, S.Afr.†.*
Cyclizine hydrochloride (p.429·3).
*Motion sickness; vertigo.*

**Triazol** *Biolab Sanus, Braz.*
Fluconazole (p.398·1).
*Fungal infections.*

**Tribakin** *Farcoral, Mex.*
Co-trimoxazole (p.199·3).
*Bacterial infections.*

**Triban**
*Note. This name is used for preparations of different composition.*
*Solfran, Mex.*
Vitamin B$_{12}$; vitamin B$_1$ (p.1417·1).

*Great Southern, USA.*
Trimethobenzamide hydrochloride (p.442·2); benzocaine (p.1370·3).

**Tribdoze** *Labortecne, Braz.†.*
Vitamin and mineral preparation (p.1417·1).

**Tribe 12** *Pharmacos, Mex.*
Vitamin B substances (p.1417·1).
Lidocaine hydrochloride (p.1377·3) is included in this preparation to alleviate the pain of injection.

**Tribedex** *Medifarma, Mex.†.*
Vitamin B substances (p.1417·1).

**Tribedoxyl** *Aventis, Mex.*
*Capsules:* Cyanocobalamin (p.1458·2); benfotiamine (p.1454·3); pyridoxine hydrochloride (p.1456·3).
*Injection:* Hydroxocobalamin acetate (p.1458·2); thiamine hydrochloride (p.1455·1); pyridoxine hydrochloride (p.1456·3).
Lidocaine hydrochloride (p.1377·3) is included in this preparation to alleviate the pain of injection.
*Anaemias; neuralgias; neuritis; neuropathies.*

**Tribemin** *Sam-On, Israel.*
Vitamin B$_1$ (p.1455·2); vitamin B$_6$ (p.1457·2); vitamin B$_{12}$ (p.1458·2).
*Megaloblastic anaemia; neuralgias.*

**Tribesian** *Asian Pharm, Thai.*
Vitamin B$_1$ (p.1455·2); vitamin B$_6$ (p.1457·2); vitamin B$_{12}$ (p.1458·2).
*Anaemias; migraine; neuralgia; neuritis.*

**Tribesona** *ITF, Chile.*
Clotrimazole (p.396·2); dexamethasone acetate (p.1097·1).
*Infected skin disorders.*

**Tribeton** *Chemedica, Switz.†.*
Cyanocobalamin (p.1458·2) or hydroxocobalamin (p.1458·2); thiamine hydrochloride (p.1455·1); pyridoxine hydrochloride (p.1456·3).
Lidocaine hydrochloride (p.1377·3) is included in the injections to alleviate the pain of injection.
*Alcoholism; nerve pain; neuritis; pain; vitamin B deficiency.*

**Tribiot** *Grin, Mex.*
Neomycin sulfate (p.235·1); polymyxin B sulfate (p.245·1); bacitracin zinc (p.161·3).
*Bacterial eye infections.*

**Tribiotic Plus** *Thompson, USA†.*
Polymyxin B sulfate (p.245·1); neomycin sulfate (p.235·1); bacitracin (p.161·3); lidocaine (p.1377·3).

**Tri-Biozene** *Reese, USA.*
Bacitracin (p.161·3); polymyxin B sulfate (p.245·1); neomycin sulfate (p.235·1); pramocaine hydrochloride (p.1382·2).

**Tribonat** *Fresenius Kabi, Norw.; Fresenius Kabi, Swed.*
Trometamol (p.1758·2); electrolytes (p.1217·1).
*Buffer; metabolic and respiratory acidosis.*

**Tri-Buffered ASA** *Zee, Canad.*
Aspirin (p.15·1).
Calcium carbonate (p.1254·2), magnesium carbonate (p.1272·1), and magnesium oxide (p.1272·3) are included in this preparation in attempt to limit adverse effects on the gastrointestinal mucosa.

**Tricaine-MPS** *RPG, India.*
Oxetacaine (p.1382·1); simeticone (p.1289·2); aluminium hydroxide (p.1249·2); magnesium hydroxide (p.1272·2).
*Gastric hyperacidity; gastritis; gastro-oesophageal reflux; peptic ulcer.*

**Tri-Cal** *Medical Research, Hong Kong†.*
Calcium hydrogen phosphate (p.1225·2); calcium carbonate (p.1254·2); calcium gluconate (p.1225·2); vitamin D (p.1461·2); zinc oxide (p.1163·2); magnesium oxide (p.1272·3).
*Calcium supplement; osteoporosis.*

**Tricalcio com Fluor** *Bergamo, Braz.†.*
Vitamin and mineral preparation (p.1417·1).

**Trical-D** *Sigma, India.*
Calcium carbonate (p.1254·2); colecalciferol (p.1461·3).
*Calcium deficiency.*

**Tricalma Retard** *Sanofi Synthelabo, Chile.*
Alprazolam (p.668·3).
*Anxiety; mixed anxiety depressive states; panic attacks.*

**Tricalvit** *Gemballa, Braz.*
Vitamin and mineral preparation (p.1417·1).

**Trican** *Pfizer, Israel.*
Fluconazole (p.398·1).
*Fungal infections.*

**Tricandil** *Grunenthal, Belg.; SPA, Ital.; Prospa, Port.*
Mepartricin (p.405·2).
*Fungal vaginal infections; trichomoniasis.*

**Tricangine** *Asta Medica, Braz.*
Mepartricin (p.405·2); tetracycline (p.266·2).
*Bacterial and fungal vulvovaginal infections.*

**Tricef** *Merck, Austria; Merck, Chile; Bial, Port.; Astra, Swed.*
Cefixime (p.172·3).
*Bacterial infections.*

*Eurofarmaco, Ital.*
Propylene glycol cefatrizine (p.170·3).
*Bacterial infections.*

**Tricefin** *Dexa, Singapore.*
Ceftriaxone sodium (p.182·3).
*Bacterial infections.*

**Tricen** *Alter, Spain.*
Verapamil hydrochloride (p.1019·1); trandolapril (p.1016·1).
*Hypertension.*

**Tricephin** *Atlantic, Thai.*
Ceftriaxone sodium (p.182·3).
*Bacterial infections.*

**Tricept** *Cuprocept, S.Afr.*
Copper-wound plastic (p.1425·3).
*Intra-uterine contraceptive device.*

**Tricerol** *Pharmacia, Braz.; Armstrong, Mex.*
Etofibrate (p.914·2).
*Atherosclerosis; hyperlipidaemias.*

**Trichazole** *Bodene, S.Afr.; Aspen, S.Afr.*
Metronidazole (p.607·2).
*Anaerobic bacterial infections; protozoal infections.*

**Trichex** *Gerot, Austria.*
Metronidazole (p.607·2).
*Gardnerella vaginalis infections; trichomoniasis.*

**Tri-Chlor** *Gordon, USA.*
Trichloroacetic acid (p.1162·1).
*Warts.*

**Trichlorol** *Lysoform, Ger.*
Tosylchloramide sodium (p.1194·3).
*Surface disinfection.*

**Trichobiol** *Therasophia, Fr.*
Amino-acid, mineral, vitamin, and herbal preparation (p.1417·1).
*Hair and nail disorders.*

**Trichonas** *Pharmasant, Thai.*
Tinidazole (p.617·1).
*Amoebiasis; anaerobic bacterial infections; giardiasis; trichomoniasis.*

**Trichotine** *Schwarz, USA.*
Sodium laurilsulfate (p.1574·2); sodium perborate (p.1192·2); sodium chloride (p.1233·3).
*Vaginal disorders.*

**Trichozole** *Pacific, NZ.*
Metronidazole (p.607·2).
*Anaerobic bacterial infections; protozoal infections.*

**Tri-Ciclomex** *Gynopharm, Chile.*
Gestodene (p.1556·1); ethinylestradiol (p.1553·2).
*Triphasic oral contraceptive.*

**Triciclor** *Wyeth, Spain.*
Levonorgestrel (p.1563·2); ethinylestradiol (p.1553·2).
*Triphasic oral contraceptive.*

**Triciderm** *Ni-The, Gr.*
Tyrothricin (p.275·1).
*Skin infections.*

**Tricidine** *Pfizer Consumer, Belg.*
Tyrothricin (p.275·1); lidocaine hydrochloride (p.1377·3).
*Mouth and throat disorders.*

**Tricidine Dequalinium** *Pfizer Consumer, Belg.*
Dequalinium chloride (p.1178·1); lidocaine hydrochloride (p.1377·3).
*Mouth and throat disorders.*

**Tricifa** *Richet, Arg.*
Piroxicam (p.84·2).
*Inflammation.*

**TriCilest**
*Janssen-Cilag, Austria; Janssen-Cilag, S.Afr.*
Norgestimate (p.1563·2); ethinylestradiol (p.1553·2). 28-Day packs also contain 7 inert tablets.
Formerly known as Ortrel in *Austria.*
*Triphasic oral contraceptive.*

**Tricilon** *Organon, Braz.*
Medroxyprogesterone (p.1557·3).
*Injectable contraceptive.*

**Tricin** *Catarinense, Braz.*
Diclofenac potassium (p.32·1).
*Inflammation; pain.*

**Tricivir**
*GlaxoSmithKline, Arg.; GlaxoSmithKline, Chile.*
Abacavir sulfate (p.625·2); lamivudine (p.648·2); zidovudine (p.658·2).
*HIV infection.*

**Triclin** *Solfran, Mex.*
Tetracycline (p.266·2).
*Bacterial infections.*

**Tricloderm** *Merck, Hong Kong.*
Clotrimazole (p.396·2).
*Fungal skin infections.*

**Triclonam** *CTI, Israel.*
Triclofos sodium (p.726·2).
*Insomnia; sedative.*

**Tricloryl**
*GlaxoSmithKline, India.*
Triclofos sodium (p.726·2).
*Insomnia; sedative.*

*Galen, Irl.*
Triclofos (p.726·3).
*Hypnotic; sedative.*

**Triclose** *Q-Med, Ital.*
Azanidazole (p.602·3).
*Vaginal trichomoniasis.*

**Tri-Co** *Garec, S.Afr.†.*
Co-trimoxazole (p.199·3).
*Bacterial infections.*

**Tricocel** *UCI, Braz.†.*
Oxypyrantel.
*Worm infections.*

**Tricocet** *Legrand, Braz.*
Nystatin (p.406·3).
*Fungal infections.*

**Tricodein**
*Solco, Austria; Solco, Ger.†; Solco, Switz.*
Codeine phosphate (p.27·1).
*Coughs.*

**Tricodene Cough & Cold** *Pfeiffer, USA.*
Mepyramine maleate (p.437·1); codeine phosphate (p.27·1).
*Coughs and cold symptoms.*

**Tricodene Forte** *Pfeiffer, USA†.*
Phenylpropanolamine hydrochloride (p.1127·3); chlorphenamine maleate (p.427·3); dextromethorphan hydrobromide (p.1117·3).
*Coughs and cold symptoms.*

**Tricodene NN** *Pfeiffer, USA†.*
Phenylpropanolamine hydrochloride (p.1127·3); chlorphenamine maleate (p.427·3); dextromethorphan hydrobromide (p.1117·3).
*Coughs and cold symptoms.*

**Tricodene Pediatric Cough & Cold** *Pfeiffer, USA†.*
Phenylpropanolamine hydrochloride (p.1127·3); dextromethorphan hydrobromide (p.1117·3).
*Coughs and cold symptoms.*

**Tricodene Sugar Free** *Pfeiffer, USA.*
Chlorphenamine maleate (p.427·3); dextromethorphan hydrobromide (p.1117·3).
*Coughs and cold symptoms.*

**Tricoderm F** *Farmachimici, Ital.*
Salicylic acid (p.1157·1); piroctone olamine (p.1155·2); ichthammol (p.1148·2).
*Scalp disorders.*

**Tricodex** *Ecofarm, Ital.*
Amino-acid, vitamin, and mineral preparation (p.1417·1).
*Hair and nail disorders.*

**Tricofarma** *ICN, Arg.*
Finasteride (p.1554·2).
*Alopecia androgenetica.*

**Tricofin** *Raymos, Arg.*
Metronidazole (p.607·2).
*Anaerobic bacterial infections; protozoal infections.*

**Tricogyn** *Pharmaland, Thai.*
Tinidazole (p.617·1).
*Amoebiasis; giardiasis.*

**Tricolam** *Farmasierra, Spain.*
Tinidazole (p.617·1).
*Anaerobic bacterial infections; protozoal infections.*

**Tri-Cold**
*Note. A similar name is used for preparations of different composition (see below).*
*Labima, Belg.†.*
Diphenylpyraline hydrochloride (p.432·3); phenylephrine hydrochloride (p.1126·3); terpin hydrate (p.1131·1).
*Cold symptoms; hay fever; hypersensitivity reactions; nasal congestion; sinusitis.*

**Tricold**
*Note. A similar name is used for preparations of different composition (see above).*
*Agis, Israel†.*
Paracetamol (p.76·2); phenylephrine hydrochloride (p.1126·3); dextromethorphan hydrobromide (p.1117·3).
*Coughs and cold symptoms.*

**Tricolocion** *ICN, Arg.*
Minoxidil (p.960·1).
*Alopecia.*

**Tricolpex** *Bunker, Braz.*
Metronidazole (p.607·2); nystatin (p.406·3); urea (p.1162·2).
*Vulvovaginal infections.*

**Tricomed** *Hua, Thai.*
Metronidazole (p.607·2).
*Trichomoniasis.*

**Tricomox** *Pinewood, Irl.†.*
Co-trimoxazole (p.199·3).
*Bacterial infections.*

**Triconal** *ICN, Arg.*
Vitamin A; ascorbic acid; calcium pantothenate; methionine; arginine; pyridoxine hydrochloride; lecithin (p.1417·1).
*Dietary supplement.*

**Triconidazol** *Andromaco, Chile.*
Tinidazole (p.617·1).
*Anaerobic bacterial infections; protozoal infections.*

**Tricoplus** *Defuen, Arg.*
Minoxidil (p.960·1).
*Alopecia.*

**Tricoplus Conef** *Defuen, Arg.*
Lotion, minoxidil (p.960·1); tablets, finasteride (p.1554·2).
*Alopecia androgenetica.*

**Tricor** *Abbott, USA.*
Fenofibrate (p.915·2).
*Hyperlipidaemias.*

**Tricorex** *Provita, Ital.†.*
Amino-acid, vitamin, and mineral preparation (p.1417·1).
*Nutritional supplement.*

**Tricortin**
*Note. This name is used for preparations of different composition.*
*Fidia, Ital.*
Phosphatides (p.1706·1); cyanocobalamin (p.1458·2). Lidocaine hydrochloride (p.1377·3) is included in this preparation to alleviate the pain of injection.
*Peripheral and central nervous system disorders.*

*Fidia, Thai.*
Phospholipids; pyridoxine hydrochloride (p.1456·3); cyanocobalamin (p.1458·2).
*Metabolic and circulatory disorders of the brain.*

**Tricosten** *Farmion, Braz.†.*
Clotrimazole (p.396·2).
*Fungal skin and vaginal infections.*

**Tricovivax** *Medinfar, Port.*
Minoxidil (p.960·1).
*Alopecia androgenetica.*

**Tricowas B** *Chiesi, Spain.*
Metronidazole (p.607·2).
*Anaerobic bacterial infections; protozoal infections.*

**Tricox** *Themis Chemicals, India.*
Rifampicin (p.250·2); isoniazid (p.222·2); pyrazinamide (p.246·3).
*Tuberculosis.*

**Tricoxane**
*ICN, Arg.; ITF, Chile.*
Minoxidil (p.960·1).
*Alopecia androgenetica.*

**Tricoxidil** *Pfizer Consumer, Ital.*
Minoxidil (p.960·1).
*Alopecia androgenetica.*

**Tricozone** *Hua, Thai.*
Tinidazole (p.617·1).
*Amoebiasis; giardiasis; trichomoniasis.*

**Tri-Cyclen** *Janssen-Ortho, Canad.*
Norgestimate (p.1563·2); ethinylestradiol (p.1553·2).
*Acne; triphasic oral contraceptive.*

**Tridelta** *Ceccarelli, Ital.*
Colecalciferol (p.1461·3).
*Vitamin D deficiency.*

**Trident** *Adams, Canad.*
Xylitol (p.1469·1).
*Dental caries prophylaxis.*

**Triderm**
*Note. This name is used for preparations of different composition.*
*Schering-Plough, Hong Kong; Schering-Plough, Israel; Undra, Mex.; Schering-Plough, Singapore; Essex, Switz.*
Betamethasone dipropionate (p.1093·1); clotrimazole (p.396·2); gentamicin sulfate (p.217·1).
*Infected skin disorders.*

*Del-Ray, USA.*
Triamcinolone acetonide (p.1110·2).
*Skin disorders.*

**Triderm 5** *ICIM, Ital.*
Barrier preparation.

**Triderm Zeta** *ICIM, Ital.*
Zinc oxide (p.1163·2).
*Skin disorders.*

**Tridermal** *Panalab, Arg.*
Ketoconazole (p.403·3); hydrocortisone acetate (p.1103·3); gentamicin sulfate (p.217·1).
*Infected skin disorders.*

**Triderm-C** *Schering-Plough, Malaysia.*
Betamethasone dipropionate (p.1093·1); clotrimazole (p.396·2).
*Fungal skin infections.*

**Tridesilon**
*Note. This name is used for preparations of different composition.*
*Bayer, Canad.†; Bayer, USA.*
*Cream; ointment:* Desonide (p.1096·3).
*Skin disorders.*

*Bayer, USA.*
*Ear drops:* Desonide (p.1096·3); acetic acid (p.1645·2).
*Superficial ear infections with inflammation.*

**Tridesonit** *CS, Fr.*
Desonide (p.1096·3).
*Skin disorders.*

**Tridestan N** *Gador, Arg.*
Levonorgestrel (p.1563·2); ethinylestradiol (p.1553·2).
*Triphasic oral contraceptive.*

**Tridestra**
*Orion, Irl.†; Orion, UK.*
70 Tablets, estradiol valerate (p.1550·2); 14 tablets, estradiol valerate; medroxyprogesterone acetate (p.1557·2); 7 tablets, inert.
*Menopausal disorders; osteoporosis.*

**Tridette** *Gador, Arg.*
Norgestimate (p.1563·2); ethinylestradiol (p.1553·2).
*Triphasic oral contraceptive.*

**Tridigestivo Soubeiran** *Chobet, Arg.*
Pancreatin (p.1725·3); takadiastase; pepsin (p.1729·3).
*Digestive disorders.*

**Tridil**
*Cristalia, Braz.; Du Pont, Canad.†; Du Pont, Hong Kong; Boots, Hong Kong; Du Pont, Irl.†; Sanofi Synthelabo, S.Afr.; Faulding, USA.*
Glyceryl trinitrate (p.923·2).
*Control of blood pressure during surgery; heart failure; ischaemic heart disease.*

**Tridin**
*Note. This name is used for preparations of different composition.*
*Byk, Braz.†; Rottapharm, Chile; Rotta, Hong Kong; Rottapharm, Ital.*
Glutamine monofluorophosphate; calcium gluconate (p.1225·2); calcium citrate (p.1225·1).
*Osteoporosis.*

*Opfermann, Ger.*
Sodium monofluorophosphate (p.1446·2); calcium gluconate (p.1225·2); calcium citrate (p.1225·1).
*Osteoporosis.*

**Tridin Forte** *Opfermann, Ger.*
Sodium monofluorophosphate (p.1446·2); calcium carbonate (p.1254·2).
*Osteoporosis.*

**Triditol-G** *Loyal Advance, Hong Kong.*
Triamcinolone acetonide (p.1110·2); gentamicin sulfate (p.217·1); diphenhydramine hydrochloride (p.431·3); tolnaftate (p.410·1).
*Inflamed bacterial and fungal skin infections.*

**Tridocemine** *Aventis, Port.*
*Injection:* Vitamin $B_{12}$ (p.1458·2).
*Anaemia; neuralgia; neuritis; tonic.*

*Tablets†:* Benfotiamine (p.1454·3); pyridoxine hydrochloride (p.1456·3); hydroxocobalamin (p.1458·2).
*Neuralgia; neuritis; tonic.*

**Tridomose** *Aventis, S.Afr.*
Gestrinone (p.1556·2).
*Endometriosis.*

**Tridyl** *Condrugs, Thai.*
Trihexyphenidyl hydrochloride (p.490·2).
*Drug-induced extrapyramidal disorders; parkinsonism.*

**Triefect** *Geminis, Arg.*
Ketoconazole (p.403·3); gentamicin sulfate (p.217·1); hydrocortisone acetate (p.1103·3).
*Infected skin disorders.*

**Triella** *Janssen-Cilag, Fr.*
Norethisterone (p.1562·2); ethinylestradiol (p.1553·2).
*Triphasic oral contraceptive.*

**Tri-Emcortina** *Merck, Arg.*
Fluprednidene acetate (p.1102·2); neomycin sulfate (p.235·1); chloroquine (p.448·2).
*Infected skin disorders.*

**Triene** *Wassermann, Ital.*
Polyenacid.
*Barrier preparation; burns; skin irritation; wounds.*

**Triette** *Wyeth, Ger.*
Levonorgestrel (p.1563·2); ethinylestradiol (p.1553·2).
*Triphasic oral contraceptive.*

**Triexidyl** *Cristalia, Braz.*
Trihexyphenidyl hydrochloride (p.490·2).
*Parkinsonism.*

**Trifacilina** *Bago, Arg.*
Ampicillin (p.157·1).
*Bacterial infections.*

**Trifacta** *Nikkho, Braz.†.*
*Injection:* Vitamin B substances (p.1417·1); anti-anaemic fraction G.
*Anaemias.*

*Tablets:* Vitamin B substances (p.1417·1); anti-anaemic fraction G; ferrous sulfate (p.1428·2); copper chloride; manganese chloride.
*Anaemias; dietary supplement.*

**Trifamox**
*Note. This name is used for preparations of different composition.*
*Bago, Arg.*
Amoxicillin (p.155·3).
*Bacterial infections.*

*Merck Bago, Braz.*
Amoxicillin sodium (p.155·3) or amoxicillin trihydrate (p.155·3); sulbactam pivoxil or sulbactam sodium (p.257·2).
*Bacterial infections.*

**Trifamox Bronquial** *Bago, Arg.*
Amoxicillin trihydrate (p.155·3); brovanexine hydrochloride (p.1116·1).
*Bacterial infections of the respiratory tract.*

**Trifamox Duo** *Bago, Arg.*
Amoxicillin trihydrate (p.155·3).
*Bacterial infections.*

**Trifamox IBL**
*Bago, Arg.; Armstrong, Mex.*
Amoxicillin sodium (p.155·3) or amoxicillin trihydrate (p.155·3); pivsulbactam (p.257·2) or sulbactam sodium (p.257·2).
*Bacterial infections.*

**Trifas** *Silesia, Chile.*
Norgestimate (p.1563·2); ethinylestradiol (p.1553·2).
*Triphasic oral contraceptive.*

**Trifed** *Nakornpatana, Thai.*
Pseudoephedrine hydrochloride (p.1129·2); triprolidine hydrochloride (p.442·3).
*Allergic rhinitis; cold symptoms; hay fever; nasal congestion.*

**Trifed-C Cough** *Geneva, USA.*
Pseudoephedrine hydrochloride (p.1129·2); codeine phosphate (p.27·1); triprolidine hydrochloride (p.442·3).
*Coughs and cold symptoms.*

**Trifedrin** *Zest, Braz.*
Pseudoephedrine hydrochloride (p.1129·2); triprolidine hydrochloride (p.442·3); sulfogaiacol (p.1131·1).
*Coughs.*

**Trifeme**
*Wyeth, Austral.; Wyeth, NZ.*
21 Tablets, ethinylestradiol (p.1553·2); levonorgestrel (p.1563·2); 7 tablets, inert.
*Triphasic oral contraceptive.*

**Tri-Femoden** *Schering, Fin.*
Gestodene (p.1556·1); ethinylestradiol (p.1553·2).
*Triphasic oral contraceptive.*

**Trifen**
*Note. This name is used for preparations of different composition.*
*Hertz, Braz.†.*
Paracetamol (p.76·2).
*Fever; pain.*

*Be-Tabs, S.Afr.*
Triprolidine hydrochloride (p.442·3); pseudoephedrine hydrochloride (p.1129·2); codeine phosphate (p.27·1); guaifenesin (p.1122·1).
*Coughs.*

**Trifene** *Medinfar, Port.*
Ibuprofen (p.45·3).
*Fever; pain.*

**Triferon** *Salus, Ital.†.*
Thiamine hydrochloride (p.1455·1); pyridoxine hydrochloride (p.1456·3); hydroxocobalamin (p.1458·2).
*Neuralgia; neuritis; post-infection paresis; vitamin B deficiency.*

**Trifibra Mix** *Sanofi Synthelabo, Braz.†.*
Bran (p.1253·2).
*Constipation; dietary supplement.*

**Tri-Filena** *Organon, Austria†.*
White tablets, estradiol valerate (p.1550·2); blue tablets, estradiol valerate; medroxyprogesterone acetate (p.1557·2); yellow tablets, inert.
*Menopausal disorders; osteoporosis.*

**Triflucan**
*Pfizer, Arg.; Pfizer, Fr.; Pfizer, Israel.*
Fluconazole (p.398·1).
*Fungal infections.*

**Trifluid** *Otsuka, Jpn.*
Carbohydrate and electrolyte infusion (p.1417·1).
*Parenteral nutrition.*

**Triflumann** *Mann, Ger.*
Trifluridine (p.655·3).
*Herpesvirus keratitis.*

**Triflumed** *Medifive, Thai.*
Trifluoperazine (p.726·3).
*Anxiety; nausea and vomiting; psychoses.*

**Triflux** *Scharper, Ital.*
Triflusal (p.1017·3).
*Thromboembolic disorders.*

**Trifolium Complex** *Blackmores, Austral.†.*
Yellow dock (p.1766·1); taraxacum (p.1751·3); red clover (p.1737·3); lappa (p.1704·3); zinc amino acid chelate (p.1469·3); vitamin A acetate (p.1453·1).
*Skin disorders.*

**Trifosfaneurina** *Lepori, Port.*
Cocarboxylase chloride (p.1455·2).
*Acidosis; cardiopathy; diabetes mellitus; eclampsia; headache; neuralgia; neuritis; neuromuscular disorders; tonic; vomiting of pregnancy.*

**Trifosfaneurina B6** *Farma Lepori, Spain†.*
Cyanocobalamin; pyridoxal phosphate; riboflavin; thiamine phosphate (p.1417·1).
Lidocaine hydrochloride (p.1377·3) is included in this preparation to alleviate the pain of injection.
*Vitamin B deficiency.*

**Trifosfaneurina B2 B12** *Farma Lepori, Spain.*
Cyanocobalamin; riboflavin phosphate sodium; thiamine phosphate (p.1417·1).
*Vitamin B deficiency.*

**Trifyba**
Sanofi Synthelabo, Irl.; Sanofi Synthelabo, UK†.
Wheat grain extract (p.1253·2).
*Bowel disorders; constipation; haemorrhoids; stoma management.*

**Trigastril**
Sanova, Austria; Pharmacia, Ger.
Aluminium hydroxide gel (p.1249·2); magnesium hydroxide (p.1272·2); calcium carbonate (p.1254·2).
*Gastric hyperacidity; heartburn; peptic ulcer.*

**Tri-Gel** Vida, Hong Kong.
Triamcinolone acetonide (p.1110·2); lidocaine (p.1377·3); cetrimide (p.1172·1).
*Mouth lesions.*

**Trigen** Rimsa, Mex.
Ciprofloxacin hydrochloride (p.188·2).
*Bacterial infections.*

**Trigesico** Bristol-Myers Squibb, Chile.
Paracetamol (p.76·2); aspirin (p.15·1); caffeine (p.782·1).
*Cold symptoms; pain.*

**Triglicen** Prospa, Ital.†.
Omega-3 triglycerides (p.976·1).
*Dietary supplement; hypertriglyceridaemia.*

**Trigliceril CM** Support, Braz.
Preparation for enteral nutrition (p.1417·1).

**Triglobe**
AstraZeneca, Austria; AstraZeneca, Braz.; Astra, Ger.†; AstraZeneca, Malaysia; AstraZeneca, Singapore†; Astra, Spain†.
Sulfadiazine (p.258·2); trimethoprim (p.272·2).
*Bacterial infections.*

**Trigoa** Wyeth, Ger.
Levonorgestrel (p.1563·2); ethinylestradiol (p.1553·2).
*Triphasic oral contraceptive.*

**Trigogine**
Atlantic, Hong Kong; Atlantic, Singapore; Atlantic, Thai.
Co-dergocrine mesilate (p.1674·1).
*Cerebral and peripheral vascular disorders; mental function impairment in the elderly.*

**Trigon Depot** Squibb, Spain.
Triamcinolone acetonide (p.1110·2).
*Corticosteroid.*

**Trigon Rectal** Squibb, Spain.
Lidocaine (p.1377·3); triamcinolone acetonide (p.1110·2).
*Anorectal disorders.*

**Trigon Topico** Squibb, Spain.
Amphotericin B (p.391·2); gramicidin (p.220·2); neomycin sulfate (p.235·1); triamcinolone acetonide (p.1110·2).
*Infected skin disorders.*

**Trigyn** Continental Pharma, Thai.
Tinidazole (p.617·1).
*Amoebiasis; anaerobic bacterial infections; giardiasis; trichomoniasis.*

**Trigynera** Shepa, Gr.
Ethinylestradiol (p.1553·2); gestodene (p.1556·1).
*Combined oral contraceptive.*

**Tri-Gynera** Schering, Port.
Gestodene (p.1556·1); ethinylestradiol (p.1553·2).
*Triphasic oral contraceptive.*

**Trigynon**
Schering, Austria; Schering, Belg.; Schering, Ital.; Schering, Neth.
Levonorgestrel (p.1563·2); ethinylestradiol (p.1553·2).
*Triphasic oral contraceptive.*

**Trigynovin** Schering, Spain.
Gestodene (p.1556·1); ethinylestradiol (p.1553·2).
*Triphasic oral contraceptive.*

**TriHEMIC** Lederle, USA.
Ferrous fumarate (p.1427·3); vitamin $B_{12}$ substances (p.1458·2); intrinsic factor concentrate; folic acid (p.1429·1); vitamin E.
Vitamin C (p.1460·2) is included in this preparation to increase the absorption and availability of ferrous fumarate; docusate sodium (p.1262·2) is included to reduce the constipating effects of ferrous fumarate.
*Anaemias.*

**Triherpine**
Novartis Ophthalmics, Fr.†; Novartis Ophthalmics, Hong Kong; Ciba Vision, Ital.; Novartis Ophthalmics, Switz.; Novartis, Thai.
Trifluridine (p.655·3).
*Herpes simplex infections of the eye.*

**Trihexy** Geneva, USA.
Trihexyphenidyl hydrochloride (p.490·2).
*Parkinsonism.*

**TriHIBit** Pasteur Merieux, USA.
A diphtheria, tetanus, acellular pertussis, and haemophilus influenzae vaccine (p.1614·2).
*Active immunisation.*

**Trihistalex** Wolfs, Belg.
Diphenhydramine hydrochloride (p.431·3); cinchocaine hydrochloride (p.1373·2); nicotinamide (p.1441·2).
*Cutaneous hypersensitivity reactions; pain.*

**Trihistan**
Gea, Denm.; Weifa, Norw.
Chlorcyclizine hydrochloride (p.427·2).
*Hypersensitivity reactions; motion sickness; nausea; urticaria; vertigo.*

**Trihist-CS** Cypress, USA†.
Codeine phosphate (p.27·1); phenylpropanolamine hydrochloride (p.1127·3); brompheniramine maleate (p.426·1).

**Trihist-D** Cypress, USA†.
Phenylpropanolamine hydrochloride (p.1127·3); phenyltoloxamine citrate (p.439·1); mepyramine maleate (p.437·1); pheniramine maleate (p.438·3).
*Allergic rhinitis; sinusitis.*

**Trihist-DM** Cypress, USA†.
Phenylpropanolamine hydrochloride (p.1127·3); brompheniramine maleate (p.426·1); dextromethorphan hydrobromide (p.1117·3).

**Tri-Hydroserpine** Rugby, USA.
Hydrochlorothiazide (p.933·2); reserpine (p.995·1); hydralazine hydrochloride (p.931·2).
*Hypertension.*

**Tri-Immunol**
Wyeth-Ayerst, Canad.†; Lederle-Praxis, USA†.
An adsorbed diphtheria, tetanus and pertussis vaccine (p.1613·3).
*Active immunisation of infants and young children.*

**Triiodothyronine Injection** Goldshield, UK.
Liothyronine sodium (p.1602·2).
*Myxoedema coma.*

**Tri-K** Century, USA.
Potassium acetate (p.1232·1); potassium bicarbonate (p.1223·1); potassium citrate (p.1223·1).
*Hypokalaemia; potassium depletion.*

**Trikacide** Pharmascience, Canad.†.
Metronidazole (p.607·2).
*Bacterial infections; protozoal infections.*

**Trikof-D** Respa, USA†.
Guaifenesin (p.1122·1); dextromethorphan hydrobromide (p.1117·3); phenylpropanolamine hydrochloride (p.1127·3).
*Coughs; nasal congestion.*

**Tri-Kort** Keene, USA.
Triamcinolone acetonide (p.1110·2).
*Corticosteroid.*

**Trikozol** Orion, Fin.
Metronidazole (p.607·2).
*Anaerobic bacterial infections; antibiotic-associated colitis; Crohn's disease; eradication of Helicobacter pylori in peptic ulcer; protozoal infections.*

**Trikvilar** Schering, Fin.
Levonorgestrel (p.1563·2); ethinylestradiol (p.1553·2).
*Triphasic oral contraceptive.*

**Trilafon**
Schering-Plough, Belg.; Schering, Canad.; Schering-Plough, Denm.; Schering-Plough, Ital.; Schering-Plough, Mex.; Schering-Plough, Neth.; Schering-Plough, Norw.; Schering-Plough, S.Afr.; Schering-Plough, Swed.; Essex, Switz.; Schering, USA.
Perphenazine (p.714·2), perphenazine decanoate (p.714·2), or perphenazine enantate (p.714·2).
*Alcohol or opioid withdrawal syndromes; anxiety; hiccup; nausea; pain; premedication; pruritus; psychoses; vomiting.*

**Trilam** Gerard, Irl.
Triazolam (p.725·3).
*Insomnia.*

**Trilax** Hexal, Braz.
Carisoprodol (p.1392·1); diclofenac sodium (p.32·1); paracetamol (p.76·2); caffeine (p.782·1).

**Trileptal**
Novartis, Arg.; Novartis, Austral.; Novartis, Austria; Novartis, Belg.; Novartis, Braz.; Novartis, Chile; Novartis, Denm.; Novartis, Fin.; Novartis, Fr.; Novartis, Ger.; Novartis, Gr.; Novartis, Hong Kong; Novartis, Irl.; Novartis, Ital.†; Novartis, Malaysia; Novartis, Mex.; Novartis, Neth.; Novartis, Norw.; Novartis, NZ; Novartis, S.Afr.; Novartis, Spain; Novartis, Swed.; Novartis, Switz.; Novartis, UK; Novartis, USA.
Oxcarbazepine (p.366·3).
*Epilepsy.*

**Trileptin** Novartis, Israel.
Oxcarbazepine (p.366·3).
*Epilepsy.*

**Tri-Levlen** Berlex, USA.
Levonorgestrel (p.1563·2); ethinylestradiol (p.1553·2).
28-Day packs also contain 7 inert tablets.
*Triphasic oral contraceptive.*

**Trilifan** Schering-Plough, Fr.
Perphenazine enantate (p.714·2).
*Psychoses.*

**Trilisate**
Purdue, Canad.; Purdue Frederick, USA†.
Choline magnesium trisalicylate (p.26·2).
*Musculoskeletal and joint disorders.*

**Trillium Complex** Blackmores, Austral.†.
Trillium erectum; geranium maculatum; hydrastis (p.1698·3); ginseng (p.1693·1); *d*-alpha tocoferil acid succinate (p.1465·1).
*Menorrhagia.*

**Triloc** AstraZeneca, Austria.
Metoprolol tartrate (p.957·1); hydrochlorothiazide (p.933·2); hydralazine hydrochloride (p.931·2).
*Hypertension.*

**Trilog** Hauck, USA.
Triamcinolone acetonide (p.1110·2).
*Corticosteroid.*

**Trilombrin** Farmasierra, Spain.
Pyrantel embonate (p.113·2).
*Worm infections.*

**Trilon** Agepha, Austria.
Triamcinolone acetonide (p.1110·2); neomycin sulfate (p.235·1); gramicidin (p.220·2).
*Infected eye disorders.*

**Trilone** Hauck, USA.
Triamcinolone diacetate (p.1110·2).
*Corticosteroid.*

**Trilor** Loren, Mex.
*Oral suspension:* Furazolidone (p.605·2); clioquinol (p.196·3); homatropine (p.483·2); kaolin (p.1268·3); pectin (p.1580·3).
*Tablets:* Furazolidone (p.605·2); clioquinol (p.196·3); homatropine (p.483·2).
*Diarrhoea.*

**Trilosil** Silom, Thai.
Triamcinolone acetonide (p.1110·2).
*Skin disorders.*

**Trilosil N** Silom, Thai.†.
Triamcinolone acetonide (p.1110·2) neomycin sulfate (p.235·1).
*Infected skin disorders.*

**Triloxane** Vickmans, Hong Kong.
Magnesium hydroxide (p.1272·2) or magnesium trisilicate (p.1272·3); aluminium hydroxide (p.1249·2); simeticone (p.1289·2).
*Gastrointestinal disorders.*

**Triludan**
Aventis, Austria; Aventis, Belg.†; Hoechst Marion Roussel, Irl.†; Aventis, Neth.; Aventis, Port.; Aventis, S.Afr.
Terfenadine (p.441·1).
*Hypersensitivity reactions.*

**Trilufen** Marion Merrell Dow, Port.†.
Terfenadine (p.441·1); pseudoephedrine hydrochloride (p.1129·2).
*Allergic rhinitis.*

**Tri-Luma** Galderma, USA.
Hydroquinone (p.1148·1); tretinoin (p.1161·1); fluocinolone (p.1101·2).
*Facial melasma.*

**Trim**
Note. This name is used for preparations of different composition.
Saval, Chile.
Trimebutine maleate (p.1758·1).
*Gastrointestinal disorders.*

M & H, Malaysia; M & H, Thai.
Triamcinolone acetonide (p.1110·2).
*Oral lesions.*

**Tri-Mactex** Osteolab, Chile.
Norgestimate (p.1563·2); ethinylestradiol (p.1553·2).
*Triphasic oral contraceptive.*

**Trimadiaz Antrima** Doms-Adrian, Fr.†.
Co-trimazine (p.199·3).
Formerly known as Antrima.
*Bacterial infections; Pneumocystis carinii pneumonia.*

**Trimag** Uniao Quimica, Braz.
Tiratricol (p.1604·3).
*Thyroid disorders.*

**Trimasone** Pharmaland, Thai.†.
Triamcinolone acetonide (p.1110·2).
*Skin disorders.*

**Trimate-Ace** Sankyo, Thai.
Vitamin B substances with vitamin E (p.1417·1).

**Trimaze** Garec, S.Afr.
Clotrimazole (p.396·2).
*Fungal skin infections.*

**Trimazide** Major, USA.
Trimethobenzamide hydrochloride (p.442·2).
*Nausea and vomiting.*

**Trimazol** Upha, Malaysia.
Clotrimazole (p.396·2).
*Fungal skin infections.*

**Trimedal** Novartis, Braz.
Dimetindene maleate (p.431·2); rutoside (p.1688·2); paracetamol (p.76·2); ascorbic acid (p.1460·2); phenylephrine hydrochloride (p.1126·3).
*Cold and influenza symptoms.*

**Trimedat** Italfarmaco, Ital.
Trimebutine maleate (p.1758·1).
*Gastrointestinal spasm; irritable bowel disease; oesophageal motility disorders.*

**Trimedil** Novartis Consumer, Austria.
Paracetamol (p.76·2); phenylephrine hydrochloride (p.1126·3); dimetindene maleate (p.431·2); ascorbic acid (p.1460·2); oxerutins (p.1688·2).
*Cold symptoms.*

**Trimel** Douglas, NZ†.
Co-trimoxazole (p.199·3).
*Bacterial infections; nocardiosis; Pneumocystis carinii pneumonia; toxoplasmosis.*

**Trim-Elim** Reese, USA.
Caffeine (p.782·1); potassium salicylate; salicylamide (p.87·3).

**Trimepaz** Master, Chile.
Doxylamine succinate (p.432·3).
*Insomnia.*

**Trimesul** Universales, Mex.†.
Co-trimoxazole (p.199·3).
*Bacterial infections.*

**Trimesuxol** Ofimex, Mex.†.
Co-trimoxazole (p.199·3).
*Bacterial infections.*

**Trimetabol**
Note. This name is used for preparations of different composition.
Dansk-Flama, Braz.
Cyproheptadine acefyllinate (p.430·2); lysine hydrochloride; carnitine hydrochloride; vitamin B substances (p.1417·1).
*Reduced appetite; tonic.*

Zimaia, Port.
Cyproheptadine acefyllinate (p.430·2).
*Appetite stimulant.*

Uriach, Spain.
Cyproheptadine acefyllinate (p.430·2); amino acids and vitamins (p.1417·1).
*Anorexia; tonic; weight loss.*

**Trimetho comp** Strallhofer, Austria.
Co-trimoxazole (p.199·3).
*Bacterial infections.*

**Trimethox** Caps, S.Afr.
Co-trimoxazole (p.199·3).
*Bacterial infections.*

**Trimetin** Vitabalans, Fin.
Trimethoprim (p.272·2).
*Urinary-tract infections.*

**Trimetin Duplo** Vitabalans, Fin.
Sulfadiazine (p.258·2); trimethoprim (p.272·2).
*Respiratory-tract and urinary-tract infections.*

**Trimetoger** Streger, Mex.
Co-trimoxazole (p.199·3).
*Bacterial infections.*

**Trimeton** Schering-Plough, Ital.
Chlorphenamine maleate (p.427·3).
*Hypersensitivity reactions; motion sickness; vomiting.*

**Trimetoprim Balsamico** Prodotti, Braz.†.
Co-trimoxazole (p.199·3); guaifenesin (p.1122·1); ammonium chloride (p.1115·2).
*Bacterial infections.*

**Trimetoprim-Sulfa** Gea, Norw.
Co-trimoxazole (p.199·3).
*Bacterial infections; Pneumocystis carinii pneumonia.*

**Trimetox** Rimsa, Mex.
Co-trimoxazole (p.199·3).
*Bacterial infections.*

**Trimetrox** Richmond, Arg.
Tamoxifen (p.585·3).

**Trimex** Ratiopharm, Fin.
Trimethoprim (p.272·2).
*Urinary-tract infections.*

**Trimexazol**
Sanofi Synthelabo, Braz.; ICN, Mex.
Co-trimoxazole (p.199·3).
*Bacterial infections; Pneumocystis carinii pneumonia; protozoal infections.*

**Trimexazol Balsamico** Sanofi Winthrop, Braz.†.
Co-trimoxazole (p.199·3); guaifenesin (p.1122·1); ammonium chloride (p.1115·2).
*Bacterial infections.*

**Trimexazole**
Upha, Malaysia; Pharmasant, Thai.
Co-trimoxazole (p.199·3).
*Bacterial infections.*

**Trimexine** ICN, Mex.
Ambroxol hydrochloride (p.1114·3).
*Respiratory-tract congestion.*

**Trimexole** Rayere, Mex.
Co-trimoxazole (p.199·3).
*Bacterial infections; Pneumocystis carinii pneumonia.*

**Trimexole Compositum** Rayere, Mex.
Co-trimoxazole (p.199·3); guaifenesin (p.1122·1).
*Respiratory-tract infections.*

**Trimezole** Malayan, Singapore.
Co-trimoxazole (p.199·3).
*Bacterial infections.*

**Trim-Fit** Quest, Canad.
Bitter orange; enzyme blend; green tea; kelp; lipoic acid; hypericum; tonalin (p.1417·1).

**Tri-Micon**
Note. A similar name is used for preparations of different composition (see below).
Beacons, Singapore.
Betamethasone valerate (p.1093·2); miconazole nitrate (p.405·3); gentamicin sulfate (p.217·1).
*Infected skin disorders.*

**Trimicon**
Note. A similar name is used for preparations of different composition (see above).
Unison, Thai.
Miconazole nitrate (p.405·3); triamcinolone acetonide (p.1110·2).
*Infected skin disorders.*

**Trimicro** Microsules, Arg.
Ampicillin sodium (p.157·1) or ampicillin trihydrate (p.157·2).
*Bacterial infections.*

**Trimidura** Merck dura, Ger.
Trimipramine maleate (p.320·2).
*Depression.*

**Trimin sulfa** Astra, Swed.
Sulfadiazine (p.258·2); trimethoprim (p.272·2).
*Urinary-tract infections.*

**Trimineurin** Hexal, Ger.
Trimipramine maleate (p.320·2).
*Depression.*

**Triminol Cough** Rugby, USA†.
Phenylpropanolamine hydrochloride (p.1127·3); chlorphenamine maleate (p.427·3); dextromethorphan hydrobromide (p.1117·3).
*Coughs and cold symptoms.*

**Tri-Minulet**
Wyeth, Austral.; Wyeth Lederle, Austria; Wyeth Lederle, Belg.; Wyeth Lederle, Denm.; Wyeth Lederle, Fin.; Wyeth Lederle, Fr.; Wyeth, Gr.; Wyeth, Irl.; Wyeth Lederle, Ital.; Wyeth, Neth.; Wyeth Lederle, Port.; Akromed, S.Afr.; Wyeth, Spain; Wyeth, Switz.; Wyeth, UK.
Gestodene (p.1556·1); ethinylestradiol (p.1553·2).
28-Day packs also contain 7 inert tablets.
*Triphasic oral contraceptive.*

**Trimipramim** *TAD, Ger.*
Trimipramine maleate (p.320·2).
*Depression.*

**Trimiron** *Organon, Swed.*
Desogestrel (p.1547·2); ethinylestradiol (p.1553·2).
28-Day packs also contain 7 inert tablets.
*Triphasic oral contraceptive.*

**TriMix** *Fresenius Kabi, Austria.*
Amino-acid, carbohydrate, and lipid (from soya oil (p.1447·2)) infusions (p.1417·1).
Contains egg lecithin.
*Parenteral nutrition.*

**Trimogal** *Lagap, UK†.*
Trimethoprim (p.272·2).
*Bronchitis; urinary-tract infections.*

**Trimoks** *Docmed, S.Afr.†.*
Co-trimoxazole (p.199·3).
*Bacterial infections.*

**Trimol** *Julphar, UAE.*
Co-trimoxazole (p.199·3).
*Bacterial infections; nocardiosis; Pneumocystis carinii pneumonia; toxoplasmosis.*

**Trimol-A** *Julphar, UAE.*
Trimethoprim (p.272·2).
*Bacterial infections.*

**Trimonase** *Mipharm, Ital.*
Tinidazole (p.617·1).
*Amoebiasis; giardiasis; trichomoniasis.*

**Trimonil**
*Desitin, Denm.; Desitin, Fin.†; Desitin, Norw.; Desitin, Swed.*
Carbamazepine (p.353·3).
*Alcohol withdrawal syndrome; bipolar disorder; diabetes insipidus; diabetic neuropathy; epilepsy; mania; trigeminal neuralgia.*

**Trimono** *Procter & Gamble, Ger.†.*
Trimethoprim (p.272·2).
*Bacterial infections of the urinary tract.*

**Trimopan**
*Orion, Denm.; Orion, Fin.; Berk, UK.*
Trimethoprim (p.272·2).
*Urinary- and respiratory-tract infections.*

**Trimo-San** *Milex, USA.*
Hydroxyquinoline sulfate (p.1700·1); boric acid (p.1662·1); borax (p.1661·3); sodium laurilsulfate (p.1574·2); glycerol (p.1694·3).
*Vaginal deodoriser.*

**Trimovate** *GlaxoSmithKline, UK.*
Clobetasone butyrate (p.1095·3); oxytetracycline calcium (p.241·1); nystatin (p.406·3).
*Skin disorders with bacterial or fungal infection.*

**Trimovax**
*Aventis Pasteur, Arg.; Aventis Pasteur, Braz.; Aventis Pasteur, Hong Kong; Pasteur Merieux, Ital.†; Aventis, S.Afr.; Aventis Pasteur, Thai.*
A measles, mumps, and rubella vaccine (Schwarz, Urabe AM9, and Wistar RA27/3M strains, respectively) (p.1625·1).
*Active immunisation.*

**Trimox**
*Note. This name is used for preparations of different composition.*
*Delta, Braz.*
Amoxicillin (p.155·3).
*Bacterial infections.*

*Pose, Thai.†.*
Co-trimoxazole (p.199·3).
*Bacterial infections.*

*Apothecon, USA.*
Amoxicillin trihydrate (p.155·3).
*Bacterial infections.*

**Trimoxazole** *Biochemie, Austral.*
Co-trimoxazole (p.199·3).
*Bacterial infections.*

**Trimoxol** *Yamanouchi, Neth.*
Co-trimoxazole (p.199·3).
*Bacterial infections; Pneumocystis carinii pneumonia.*

**Trimoxzol** *Olan-Kemed, Thai.†.*
Co-trimoxazole (p.199·3).
*Bacterial infections.*

**Trimpex** *Roche, USA.*
Trimethoprim (p.272·2).
*Urinary-tract infections.*

**Trimstat** *Fada, Arg.*
Metronidazole (p.607·2).
*Bacterial infections; protozoal infections.*

**Trim-Vit** *Vitae, Mex.†.*
Co-trimoxazole (p.199·3).
*Bacterial infections.*

**Trimzol**
*Randall, Mex.†; Schwulst, S.Afr.†.*
Co-trimoxazole (p.199·3).
*Bacterial infections.*

**Trinaderm** *Schering, Braz.†.*
Tolnaftate (p.410·1).
*Fungal skin infections.*

**Trinagesic** *Propan, S.Afr.*
Meprobamate (p.706·2); paracetamol (p.76·2); codeine phosphate (p.27·1).
*Pain and associated tension.*

**Trinalgen** *Eurofarma, Braz.†.*
Hydroxocobalamin (p.1458·2); thiamine hydrochloride (p.1455·1); pyridoxine hydrochloride (p.1456·3).
Lidocaine hydrochloride (p.1377·3) is included in this preparation to alleviate the pain of injection.
*Megaloblastic anaemia; vitamin B deficiency.*

**Trinalin**
*Schering, Canad.; Schering-Plough, Mex.; Key, USA.*
Azatadine maleate (p.425·1); pseudoephedrine sulfate (p.1129·2).
*Allergic rhinitis; Eustachian tube congestion; nasal congestion.*

**Trinalion** *Neo-Farmaceutica, Port.*
Nimodipine (p.972·3).
*Cerebral ischaemia; cerebral vasospasm following subarachnoid haemorrhage.*

**Tri-Nasal** *Muro, USA.*
Triamcinolone acetonide (p.1110·2).
*Allergic rhinitis.*

**Trinate** *Cypress, USA.*
Multivitamin and mineral preparation with iron and folic acid (p.1417·1).

**Trinavet** *Collins, Mex.*
Vitamin preparation (p.1417·1).
*Neuritis.*

**Tri-Nefrin Extra Strength** *Pfeiffer, USA†.*
Phenylpropanolamine hydrochloride (p.1127·3); chlorphenamine maleate (p.427·3).
*Upper respiratory-tract symptoms.*

**Trinelax** *Protein, Mex.†.*
Co-trimoxazole (p.199·3).
*Bacterial infections.*

**Trinergic** *Unichem, India.*
Vitamin preparation with ginseng and zinc (p.1417·1).
*Tonic.*

**Trinergot** *Atlantis, Mex.*
Caffeine (p.782·1); ergotamine tartrate (p.467·2).
*Migraine and other vascular headaches.*

**TriNessa** *Watson, USA.*
21 Tablets, norgestimate (p.1563·2); ethinylestradiol (p.1553·2); 7 tablets, inert.
*Triphasic oral contraceptive.*

**Trinestril** *Aventis, Braz.*
Estradiol hexahydrobenzoate (p.1550·1); testosterone hexahydrobenzoate (p.1571·2); hydroxyprogesterone (p.1556·3).

**Trineurin** *Orion, Fin.*
Vitamin B substances (p.1417·1).
*Vitamin B deficiency.*

**Trinevral** *Eurofarma, Braz.†.*
Hydroxocobalamin (p.1458·2); thiamine hydrochloride (p.1455·1); pyridoxine hydrochloride (p.1456·3).
*Megaloblastic anaemia; vitamin B deficiency.*

**Trinevrina B6** *Guidotti, Ital.*
Thiamine hydrochloride (p.1455·1); pyridoxine hydrochloride (p.1456·3); cyanocobalamin (p.1458·2).
Lidocaine hydrochloride (p.1377·3) is included in the intramuscular injection to alleviate the pain of injection.
*Neuralgias; neuritis; radiation sickness; toxicosis.*

**Triniagar** *Almirall, Spain†.*
Mebutizide (p.951·2); triamterene (p.1016·2).
*Hypertension; oedema.*

**Trinicalm** *Torrent, India.*
Trifluoperazine (p.726·3).
*Anxiety; mixed anxiety depressive states; schizophrenia.*

**Trinicalm Forte** *Torrent, India.*
Chlorpromazine hydrochloride (p.675·2); trifluoperazine hydrochloride (p.726·3); trihexyphenidyl hydrochloride (p.490·2).
*Schizophrenia.*

**Trinicalm Plus** *Torrent, India.*
Trifluoperazine hydrochloride (p.726·3); trihexyphenidyl hydrochloride (p.490·2).
*Schizophrenia.*

**Trinidex** *Diaco, Ital.*
Glucose, vitamin, and sodium chloride infusion (p.1417·1).
*Carbohydrate source; fluid and electrolyte disorders.*

**Triniol** *Syntex, Spain†.*
Paramethasone acetate (p.1107·3); paramethasone disodium phosphate (p.1107·3).
*Corticosteroid.*

**Trinipatch**
*Fournier, Belg.; Sanofi Synthelabo, Canad.†; Sanofi Synthelabo, Fr.; Sanofi Synthelabo, Gr.; Lavipharm, Israel; Sanofi Synthelabo, Neth.; Helsinn, Port.; Sanofi Synthelabo, Spain.*
Glyceryl trinitrate (p.923·2).
*Angina pectoris.*

**Triniplas** *Novartis, Ital.*
Glyceryl trinitrate (p.923·2).
*Angina pectoris.*

**Triniscon** *Lilly, Hong Kong†.*
Liver and stomach concentrate; cobalamin (p.1458·2); ferrous fumarate (p.1427·3); folic acid (p.1429·1).
Vitamin C (p.1460·2) is included in this preparation to increase the absorption and availability of iron.
*Anaemias; iron deficiency.*

**Trinispray** *Sanofi Synthelabo, Spain.*
Glyceryl trinitrate (p.923·2).
*Angina pectoris.*

**Triniton** *Apogepha, Ger.*
Dihydralazine sulfate (p.899·3); hydrochlorothiazide (p.933·2); reserpine (p.995·1).
*Hypertension.*

**Trinitrina** *Pharmafar, Ital.*
Glyceryl trinitrate (p.923·2).
*Angina pectoris.*

**Trinitrine** *Sanofi, Switz.*
Glyceryl trinitrate (p.923·2).
*Angina pectoris; heart failure; pulmonary oedema.*

**Trinitrine Simple Laleuf** *Santa, Gr.*
Glyceryl trinitrate (p.923·2).
*Angina; heart failure.*

**Trinitron** *Quesada, Arg.*
Glyceryl trinitrate (p.923·2); caffeine (p.782·1).
*Angina pectoris.*

**Trinitrosan** *Merck, Ger.*
Glyceryl trinitrate (p.923·2).
*Angina pectoris; controlled hypotension; heart failure; hypertensive crisis; myocardial infarction.*

**Trinizol** *UCI, Braz.*
Tinidazole (p.617·1).
*Anaerobic bacterial infections; protozoal infections.*

**Trinizol M** *UCI, Braz.*
Tinidazole (p.617·1); miconazole nitrate (p.405·3).
*Vulvovaginal infections.*

**Trinolone** *Nida, Singapore.*
Triamcinolone acetonide (p.1110·2).
*Oral lesions.*

**Trinordiol**
*Wyeth, Arg.; Wyeth Lederle, Austria; Wyeth Lederle, Belg.; Wyeth, Braz.; Wyeth, Chile; Wyeth Lederle, Denm.; Wyeth Lederle, Fin.; Wyeth Lederle, Fr.; Wyeth, Ger.; Wyeth, Gr.; Wyeth, Hong Kong; Wyeth, Irl.; Wyeth-Ayerst, Israel; Wyeth Lederle, Ital.; Wyeth, Malaysia; Wyeth, Mex.; Wyeth, Neth.; Wyeth Lederle, Norw.; Wyeth Lederle, Port.; Wyeth, Singapore; Wyeth Lederle, Swed.; Wyeth, Switz.; Wyeth-Ayerst, Thai.†; Wyeth, UK.*
Levonorgestrel (p.1563·2); ethinylestradiol (p.1553·2).
28-Day packs also contain 7 inert tablets.
*Triphasic oral contraceptive.*

**Tri-Norinyl** *Searle, USA.*
Norethisterone (p.1562·2); ethinylestradiol (p.1553·2).
28-Day packs also contain 7 inert tablets.
*Triphasic oral contraceptive.*

**Trinorm** *Nycomed, Denm.*
18 Tablets, estradiol (p.1550·1); 10 tablets, estradiol; norethisterone (p.1562·2).
*Menopausal disorders; osteoporosis.*

**TRI-Normin** *AstraZeneca, Ger.*
Atenolol (p.865·2); chlortalidone (p.882·3); hydralazine hydrochloride (p.931·2).
*Hypertension.*

**Trinotecan** *Filaxis, Arg.*
Irinotecan hydrochloride (p.564·1).
*Colorectal cancer.*

**Trinotrex** *Faria, Braz.*
Tetracycline (p.266·2); muramidase (p.1717·2).
*Bacterial infections.*

**Trinovum**
*Janssen-Cilag, Austria; Janssen-Cilag, Belg.; Janssen-Cilag, Braz.; Janssen-Cilag, Denm.; Janssen-Cilag, Ger.; Cilag, Hong Kong; Janssen-Cilag, Irl.†; Janssen-Cilag, Ital.†; Janssen-Cilag, Neth.; Janssen-Cilag, S.Afr.; Janssen-Cilag, Swed.; Janssen-Cilag, Switz.; Janssen-Cilag, UK.*
Norethisterone (p.1562·2); ethinylestradiol (p.1553·2).
28-Day packs also contain 7 inert tablets.
*Triphasic oral contraceptive.*

**Trinsicon**
*Lilly, S.Afr.†.*
Vitamin $B_{12}$ (p.1458·2); ferrous fumarate (p.1427·3); folic acid (p.1429·1); intrinsic factor.
Vitamin C (p.1460·2) is included in this preparation to increase the absorption and availability of iron.
*Anaemias.*

*Lilly, Thai.*
Cobalamin (p.1458·2); ferrous fumarate (p.1427·3); folic acid (p.1429·1) liver and stomach concentrate.
Vitamin C (p.1460·2) is included in this preparation to increase the absorption and availability of iron.
*Anaemias.*

*UCB, USA.*
Ferrous fumarate (p.1427·3); vitamin $B_{12}$ substances (p.1458·2); intrinsic factor (liver-stomach preparation); folic acid (p.1429·1).
Ascorbic acid (p.1460·2) is included in this preparation to increase the absorption and availability of iron.
*Anaemias.*

**Trintek** *Goldshield, UK.*
Glyceryl trinitrate (p.923·2).
*Angina pectoris.*

**Trio D** *LED, Fr.*
Liquorice (p.1270·2).
*Hyperpigmentation disorders.*

**Trio S** *LED, Fr.*
Ensulizole (p.1147·1); octocrilene (p.1154·3); octinoxate (p.1154·3); titanium dioxide (p.1160·3).
*Hyperpigmentation disorders; sunscreen.*

**Trio Val** *Saval, Chile.*
Paracetamol (p.76·2); pseudoephedrine hydrochloride (p.1129·2); chlorphenamine maleate (p.427·3).
*Cold and influenza symptoms.*

**Trio Val Dia y Noche** *Saval, Chile.*
Night tablets, paracetamol (p.76·2); pseudoephedrine (p.1129·2); chlorphenamine (p.428·1); day tablets, paracetamol; pseudoephedrine.
*Cold and influenza symptoms.*

**TrioBe**
*Recip, Norw.*
Folic acid; cyanocobalamin; pyridoxine hydrochloride (p.1417·1).
*Vitamin B deficiency.*

*Recip, Swed.*
Folic acid; cyanocobalamin; pyridoxine (p.1417·1).
*Vitamin B and folic acid deficiency.*

**Triocalcio** *Heralds, Braz.†.*
Calcium carbonate (p.1254·2); vitamins A, C, and D (p.1417·1).

**Triocaps** *Vifor, Switz.*
Chlorphenamine maleate (p.427·3); phenylephrine hydrochloride (p.1126·3).
*Upper respiratory-tract disorders.*

**Triocetin** *OFF, Ital.*
Troleandomycin (p.274·1).
*Bacterial infections.*

**Trio-D** *Fouchard, Chile.*
Hydroquinone (p.1148·1); alpha hydroxy acids; ascorbic acid (p.1460·2).
*Skin pigmentation disorders.*

**Triodanin** *Norma (Νορμα), Gr.*
Amoxycillin trihydrate (p.155·3).
*Bacterial infections.*

**Triodeen** *Schering, Neth.*
Gestodene (p.1556·1); ethinylestradiol (p.1553·2).
*Triphasic oral contraceptive.*

**Trioden** *Schering, Austral.*
Gestodene (p.1556·1); ethinylestradiol (p.1553·2).
28-Day packs also contain 7 inert tablets.
*Triphasic oral contraceptive.*

**Triodena** *Schering, Austria.*
Gestodene (p.1556·1); ethinylestradiol (p.1553·2).
*Triphasic oral contraceptive.*

**Triodene**
*Schering, Belg.; Schering, Irl.; Schering, S.Afr.*
Gestodene (p.1556·1); ethinylestradiol (p.1553·2).
28-Day packs also contain 7 inert tablets.
*Triphasic oral contraceptive.*

**Triofan** *Vifor, Switz.*
Xylometazoline hydrochloride (p.1132·2); carbocisteine (p.1116·2).
*Upper respiratory-tract disorders.*

**Triofed**
*Pharmasant, Thai.; Barre-National, USA.*
Triprolidine hydrochloride (p.442·3); pseudoephedrine hydrochloride (p.1129·2).
*Allergic rhinitis; cold symptoms; hay fever; nasal congestion.*

**Triogene** *Medecine Vegetale, Fr.†.*
Kola (p.1765·3); gentian (p.1692·2); magnesium chloride (p.1228·1); ferrous gluconate (p.1428·1).
*Tonic.*

**Triogesic**
*Novartis Consumer, Irl.†; Novartis Consumer, UK†.*
Phenylpropanolamine hydrochloride (p.1127·3); paracetamol (p.76·2).
*Nasal and sinus congestion.*

**Triogestena** *Schering, Austria†.*
Gestodene (p.1556·1); ethinylestradiol (p.1553·2).
*Triphasic oral contraceptive.*

**Triogestin** *Wyeth Lederle, Austria†.*
Gestodene (p.1556·1); ethinylestradiol (p.1553·2).
*Triphasic oral contraceptive.*

**Triolax** *Herbes Universelles, Canad.†.*
Aloin (p.1248·3); cascara (p.1255·1); phenolphthalein (p.1284·1); bile salts (p.1660·3).

**Triolip** *Sofar, Ital.*
Omega-3 triglycerides (p.976·1).
*Dietary supplement.*

**TRI-OM** *OM, Switz.†.*
Aluminium magnesium silicate (p.1577·1); aluminium calcium silicate (p.1250·2).
*Gastrointestinal disorders.*

**Triomar**
*Pharmagic, Ital.; Prism, UK†.*
Omega-3 marine triglycerides (p.976·2).
*Hyperlipidaemias; joint disorders; skin disorders.*

**Triomer** *Vifor, Switz.*
Sterile sea water (p.1233·3).
*Nasal disorders.*

**Triomin** *Triomed, S.Afr.*
Minocycline hydrochloride (p.231·3).
*Bacterial infections.*

**Triominic**
*Novartis Consumer, Irl.†; Novartis Consumer, UK†.*
Phenylpropanolamine hydrochloride (p.1127·3); pheniramine maleate (p.438·3).
*Allergic rhinitis; nasal congestion.*

**Trionetta**
*Schering, Norw.; Schering, Swed.*
Levonorgestrel (p.1563·2); ethinylestradiol (p.1553·2).
28-Day packs also contain 7 inert tablets.
*Triphasic oral contraceptive.*

**Trioral/HCT** *Aliud, Austria.*
Triamterene (p.1016·2); hydrochlorothiazide (p.933·2).
*Heart failure; hypertension; oedema.*

**Triospan** *Extractum, Hung.*
Isopropamide iodide (p.485·2); drotaverine hydrochloride (p.1683·1); phenobarbital (p.367·3).
*Smooth muscle spasm.*

**Triostat** *Jones, USA.*
Liothyronine sodium (p.1602·2).
*Evaluation of thyroid function; hypothyroidism.*

**Triotann** *Prasco, USA.*
Phenylephrine tannate (p.1127·2); mepyramine tannate (p.437·1); chlorphenamine tannate (p.428·1).
*Allergic rhinitis; nasal congestion.*

**Tri-Otic** *Pharmics, USA.*
Chloroxylenol (p.1177·2); pramocaine hydrochloride (p.1382·2); hydrocortisone (p.1103·3).
*Inflammatory ear infections.*

**Triotonico** *Heralds, Braz.†.*
Multivitamin and mineral preparation (p.1417·1).

**Triovit** *Lane, UK†.*
A vitamin A, C, and D preparation (p.1417·1).

**Triox NF** *Andromaco, Chile.*
Naproxen sodium (p.65·1).
*Fever; musculoskeletal, joint, and soft-tissue disorders; pain.*

**Trioxina** *Uniao Quimica, Braz.*
Ceftriaxone (p.183·3).
*Bacterial infections.*

**Tri-P** *Cypress, USA†.*
Phenylpropanolamine hydrochloride (p.1127·3); pheniramine maleate (p.438·3); mepyramine maleate (p.437·1).

**Tripac-Cyano** *Covan, S.Afr.*
4 Vials, sodium thiosulfate (p.1053·3); 2 vials, sodium nitrite (p.1052·3); 6 vials, amyl nitrite (p.1032·1).
*Cyanide poisoning.*

**Tripacel**
*Aventis Pasteur, Austral.; Connaught, Canad.†; Aventis Pasteur, Hong Kong; Aventis Pasteur, Malaysia; Connaught, NZ; CSL, NZ; Aventis Pasteur, Singapore; Aventis Pasteur, Thai.*
A diphtheria, tetanus, and acellular pertussis vaccine (p.1613·3).
*Active immunisation.*

**Triparen** *Otsuka, Jpn.*
Carbohydrate and electrolyte infusion (p.1417·1).
*Parenteral nutrition.*

**Triparsean** *Pantofarma, Spain.*
Piketoprofen (p.84·1) or piketoprofen hydrochloride (p.84·1).
*Peri-articular and soft-tissue disorders.*

**Tripe P** *Universal, Hong Kong.*
Promethazine hydrochloride (p.439·1); pholcodine (p.1128·3); phenylpropanolamine hydrochloride (p.1127·3).
*Coughs and cold symptoms.*

**Tripedia** *Pasteur Merieux, USA.*
A diphtheria, tetanus, and acellular pertussis vaccine (p.1613·3).
*Active immunisation of infants and young children.*

**Triperidol**
*Janssen-Cilag, Ger.†; Ethnor, India.*
Trifluperidol (p.727·1) or trifluperidol hydrochloride (p.727·1).
*Autism; psychoses.*

**Triphacycline** *Tripharma, Switz.†.*
Tetracycline hydrochloride (p.266·2).
*Bacterial infections.*

**Triphasil**
*Wyeth, Austral.; Wyeth-Ayerst, Canad.; Wyeth, NZ; Akromed, S.Afr.; Wyeth-Ayerst, USA.*
Levonorgestrel (p.1563·2); ethinylestradiol (p.1553·2).
28-Day packs also contain 7 inert tablets.
*Triphasic oral contraceptive.*

**Tri-Phen-Chlor TR** *Rugby, USA†.*
Phenylpropanolamine hydrochloride (p.1127·3); phenylephrine hydrochloride (p.1126·3); chlorphenamine maleate (p.427·3); phenyltoloxamine citrate (p.439·1).
*Upper respiratory-tract symptoms.*

**Triphenyl** *Rugby, USA†.*
Phenylpropanolamine hydrochloride (p.1127·3); chlorphenamine maleate (p.427·3).
*Upper respiratory-tract symptoms.*

**Triphenyl Expectorant** *Rugby, USA†.*
Phenylpropanolamine hydrochloride (p.1127·3); guaifenesin (p.1122·1).
*Coughs.*

**Triphidus** *Motima, Fr.*
Lactobacillus acidophilus; bifidobacterium; lactobacillus bulgaricus (p.1704·2).
*Maintenance of gastrointestinal flora.*

**Triphosmag** *Boehringer Ingelheim, Fr.†.*
Phosphoric acid; dibasic sodium phosphate; magnesium chloride; magnesium glycerophosphate (p.1417·1).
*Tonic.*

**Triple X** *Carter-Wallace, USA†.*
Pyrethrins (p.1509·3); piperonyl butoxide (p.1509·2).
*Pediculosis.*

**Triple Antibiotic** *Dixon-Shane, USA†; Geneva, USA†; Marsam, USA†; Goldline, USA†; Lannett, USA†; Moore, USA†; NMC, USA†; Parmed, USA†; Rugby, USA†.*
Polymyxin B sulfate (p.245·1); neomycin sulfate (p.235·1); bacitracin (p.161·3).
*Bacterial skin infections.*

**Triple Antigen**
*CSL, Austral.†; Commonwealth Serum, Hong Kong.*
A diphtheria, tetanus and pertussis vaccine (p.1613·3).
*Active immunisation.*

**Triple Care Cleanser**
*Smith & Nephew, Austral.; Smith & Nephew, Canad.*
Emollient and skin cleanser.
*Ostomy care; skin disorders associated with incontinence.*

**Triple Care Cream** *Smith & Nephew, Canad.*
Zinc oxide (p.1163·2).

**Triple Paste** *Summers, USA.*
Zinc oxide (p.1163·2).
*Nappy rash.*

**Triple Protection** *Beiersdorf, Canad.*
*SPF 15:* Octinoxate (p.1154·3); octisalate (p.1154·3); oxybenzone (p.1154·3).
*Sunscreen.*

**Triple Sulfa** *Fougera, USA†; Goldline, USA†; Major, USA†; NMC, USA†; Rugby, USA†.*
Sulfathiazole (p.264·1); sulfacetamide (p.257·3); sulfabenzamide (p.257·3).
*Vaginitis due to Gardnerella vaginalis.*

**Tri-Plen** *Aventis, S.Afr.*
Ramipril (p.994·1); felodipine (p.994·3).
*Hypertension.*

**Triplex**
*Note. This name is used for preparations of different composition.*
*Kampel Martian, Arg.*
Miconazole (p.405·2); betamethasone (p.1093·1); gentamicin (p.219·1).
*Infected skin disorders.*

*Sriprasit, Thai.*
Trifluoperazine hydrochloride (p.726·3).
*Anxiety; nausea and vomiting; psychoses.*

**Tripo** *Hua, Thai.*
Triprolidine hydrochloride (p.442·3); pseudoephedrine hydrochloride (p.1129·2).
*Cold symptoms; hay fever; rhinitis; upper respiratory-tract congestion.*

**Tripondil** *Alphrema, Ital.*
Day tablets, levocarnitine tartrate; fennel; faseolamina; chromium polynicotinate; calcium phosphate; pyridoxine hydrochloride; night tablets, pineapple; selenium-rich yeast; bioflavonoids; equisetum (p.1417·1).
*Obesity.*

**Triposed** *Halsey, USA.*
Pseudoephedrine hydrochloride (p.1129·2); triprolidine hydrochloride (p.442·3).
*Upper respiratory-tract symptoms.*

**Tripress** *Pacific, NZ.*
Trimipramine maleate (p.320·2).
*Depression.*

**Triprim**
*Note. This name is used for preparations of different composition.*
*Sigma, Austral.; Ratiopharm, Austria; GlaxoSmithKline, NZ; Roche, S.Afr.*
Trimethoprim (p.272·2).
*Bacterial infections of the urinary tract.*

*Pharmaland, Thai.*
Co-trimoxazole (p.199·3).
*Bacterial infections.*

**Triprodrine** *Asian Pharm, Thai.*
Triprolidine hydrochloride (p.442·3); pseudoephedrine hydrochloride (p.1129·2).
*Cold symptoms; hay fever; respiratory-tract congestion; rhinitis.*

**Triprofed** *ICN, Canad.†.*
Pseudoephedrine hydrochloride (p.1129·2); triprolidine hydrochloride (p.442·3).

**Tri-Profen** *3M, Austral.*
Ibuprofen (p.45·3).
*Fever; inflammation; musculoskeletal and joint disorders; pain.*

**Tri-Profen Cold & Flu** *3M, Austral.*
Ibuprofen (p.45·3); pseudoephedrine hydrochloride (p.1129·2).
*Cold and influenza symptoms.*

**Tripsol** *Cazi, Braz.*
Amitriptyline hydrochloride (p.280·3).
*Depression.*

**Tripsor** *Orion, Fin.*
Trioxysalen (p.1162·2).
*Lichen obtusus; lichen planus; psoriasis.*

**Tripsyline** *Polipharm, Thai.*
Amitriptyline (p.280·3).
*Depression.*

**Tripta**
*Atlantic, Malaysia; Atlantic, Singapore; Atlantic, Thai.*
Amitriptyline hydrochloride (p.280·3).
*Depression.*

**Triptafen**
*Goldshield, Irl.†; Forley, UK.*
Amitriptyline hydrochloride (p.280·3); perphenazine (p.714·2).
*Mixed anxiety depressive states.*

**Triptil** *Merck Frosst, Canad.†.*
Protriptyline hydrochloride (p.316·2).
*Depression.*

**Triptizol** *SIT, Ital.*
Amitriptyline hydrochloride (p.280·3).
*Depression.*

**Tript-OH**
*Sigma-Tau, Ital.; Sigma-Tau, Switz.*
Oxitriptan (p.311·1).
*Depression; Down's syndrome; epilepsy; headache; insomnia; migraine; movement disorders; pain; parkinsonism; phenylketonuria.*

**Triptone** *Del, USA.*
Dimenhydrinate (p.431·1).
*Motion sickness.*

**Triptyl** *Orion, Fin.*
Amitriptyline hydrochloride (p.280·3).
*Depression; insomnia.*

**Triptyline** *Medifive, Thai.*
Amitriptyline hydrochloride (p.280·3).
*Depression.*

**Tripulmin**
*Note. This name is used for preparations of different composition.*
*Hexal, Braz.*
*Syrup:* Sodium camsilate; oxeladin citrate (p.1126·1); guaifenesin (p.1122·1); menthol (p.1711·3); cineole (p.1672·1).
*Respiratory-tract congestion.*

*QIF, Braz.†.*
*Ointment:* Camphor (p.1665·3); cineole (p.1672·1); menthol (p.1711·3); guaiacol (p.1122·1).
*Respiratory-tract congestion.*

**Tripulmin Balsamico** *Hexal, Braz.*
Camphor (p.1665·3); cineole (p.1672·1); guaiacol (p.1122·1); menthol (p.1711·3).
Formerly contained sodium camsilate, camphor, cineole, guaiacol, menthol, and oxeladin.
*Coughs.*

**Tripvac** *Biological E, India.*
A diphtheria, tetanus, and pertussis vaccine (p.1613·3).
*Active immunisation.*

**Triquilar**
*Schering, Arg.; Schering, Austral.; Schering, Braz.; Berlex, Canad.; Schering, Chile; Schering, Denm.; Schering, Ger.; Shepa, Gr.; Schering, Hong Kong; German Remedies, India; Schering, Malaysia; Schering, Mex.; Schering, NZ; Schering, Port.; Schering, Singapore; Schering, Switz.; Schering, Thai.*
Levonorgestrel (p.1563·2); ethinylestradiol (p.1553·2).
28-Day packs also contain 7 inert tablets.
*Triphasic oral contraceptive.*

**Tri-Regol**
*Gedeon Richter, Hong Kong; Gedeon Richter, Malaysia.*
Levonorgestrel (p.1563·2); ethinylestradiol (p.1553·2).
*Triphasic oral contraceptive.*

**Tririnol** *Biomedica, Ital.†.*
Xylometazoline hydrochloride (p.1132·2); dequalinium chloride (p.1178·1).
*Cold symptoms; sinusitis.*

**Trirubin** *Uniao Quimica, Braz.*
Vitamin $B_{12}$ (p.1458·2); vitamin $B_1$ (p.1455·2); vitamin $B_6$ (p.1457·2).
*Megaloblastic anaemia; vitamin B deficiency.*

**Trirutin** *Strathmann, Ger.†.*
Heparin sodium (p.928·1).
*Skin trauma; vascular disorders.*

**Trirutin N** *Strathmann, Ger.†.*
Troxerutin (p.1688·3).
Formerly contained troxerutin and etofylline.
*Vascular disorders.*

**Tris**
*Fresenius Kabi, Austria; Braun, Ger.*
Trometamol (p.1758·2).
*Citrate intoxication following blood transfusion; metabolic acidosis; respiratory acidosis.*

**Trisalgina** *Molteni, Ital.†.*
Dipyrone (p.35·3).
*Fever; pain.*

**Trisan** *Dermtek, Canad.*
Triclosan (p.1195·2).
*Skin cleanser.*

**Trisdazol** *Riedel-Zabinka, Braz.†.*
Metronidazole (p.607·2); nystatin (p.406·3); muramidase (p.1717·2).
*Vulvovaginal infections.*

**Trisekvens**
*Novo Nordisk, Denm.; Novo Nordisk, Fin.; Novo Nordisk, Norw.; Novo Nordisk, Swed.*
18 Tablets, estradiol (p.1550·1); 10 tablets, estradiol; norethisterone acetate (p.1562·2).
*Menopausal disorders; osteoporosis.*

**Trisel** *Klonal, Arg.*
Vitamin $B_{12}$; pyridoxine; thiamine (p.1417·1).

**Trisenox**
*Cell Therapeutics, UK; Cell Therapeutics, USA.*
Arsenic trioxide (p.1657·1).
*Acute promyelocytic leukaemia.*

**Triseptil**
*Note. This name is used for preparations of different composition.*
*Gedis, Ital.*
Chlorhexidine gluconate (p.1173·2).
*Hand disinfection.*

*Degorts, Mex.*
Tinidazole (p.617·1).
*Amoebiasis; giardiasis; trichomoniasis.*

**Trisequens**
*Note. This name is used for preparations of different composition.*
*Elea, Arg.; Novo Nordisk, Austral.; Novo Nordisk, Austria; Novo Nordisk, Belg.; Medley, Braz.; Silesia, Chile; Novo Nordisk, Fr.; Novo Nordisk, Hong Kong; Novo Nordisk, Irl.; Novo Nordisk, Ital.; Novo Nordisk, Malaysia; Novo Nordisk, Neth.; Novo Nordisk, NZ; Isdin, Port.; Novo Nordisk, S.Afr.; Novo Nordisk, Singapore; Isdin, Spain; Novo Nordisk, Switz.; Novo Nordisk, Thai.†; Novo Nordisk, UK.*
18 Tablets, estradiol (p.1550·1); 10 tablets, estradiol; norethisterone acetate (p.1562·2).
Formerly contained estradiol and estriol, and estradiol, estriol, and norethisterone acetate.
*Menopausal disorders; osteoporosis.*

*Novo Nordisk, Ger.*
16 Tablets, estradiol (p.1550·1); 12 tablets, estradiol; norethisterone acetate (p.1562·2).
*Menopausal disorders; osteoporosis.*

*Novo Nordisk, Gr.*
Estradiol (p.1550·1); norethisterone (p.1562·2).
*Hormone replacement therapy.*

*Novo Nordisk, Israel.*
Blue or yellow tablets, estradiol (p.1550·1); white tablets, estradiol; norethisterone acetate (p.1562·2); red tablets, estradiol.
*Menopausal disorders; osteoporosis.*

**Tri-Sinerge** *Atral, Port.†.*
Neomycin sulfate (p.235·1); streptomycin sulfate (p.256·2); bacitracin (p.161·3).
*Bowel sterilisation; gastrointestinal infections.*

**Trisiston** *Jenapharm, Ger.*
Ethinylestradiol (p.1553·2); levonorgestrel (p.1563·2).
*Triphasic oral contraceptive.*

**Trisofort** *Westmont, Hong Kong†.*
Isoniazid (p.222·2).
Vitamin B substances (p.1417·1) are included in this preparation for the prophylaxis of peripheral neuropathy.
*Tuberculosis.*

**Trisolvit** *Chauvin, Fr.†.*
Tocofersolan (p.1465·3); sodium ascorbate (p.1460·2); ethoxazorutoside (p.1688·2).
*Vascular eye disorders.*

**Trisoralen**
*ICN, Arg.; ICN, Canad.†; ICN, Hong Kong†; Lifepharma, Ital.†; ICN, USA†.*
Trioxysalen (p.1162·2).
*Intolerance to sunlight; vitiligo.*

**Trisorcin** *Merckle, Ger.*
Penicillamine (p.1046·3).
*Cystinuria; heavy-metal poisoning; polyarthritis; scleroderma; Wilson's disease.*

**Trisporal** *Janssen-Cilag, Neth.*
Itraconazole (p.401·3).
*Fungal infections.*

**Tri-Sprintec** *Barr, USA.*
21 Tablets, norgestimate (p.1563·2); ethinylestradiol (p.1553·2); 7 tablets, inert.
*Triphasic oral contraceptive.*

**Trissil** *Piam, Ital.†.*
Silymarin (p.1043·3).
*Liver disorders.*

**Tri-Statin II** *Rugby, USA.*
Triamcinolone acetonide (p.1110·2); nystatin (p.406·3).
*Skin disorders.*

**TriStep** *Asche, Ger.*
Levonorgestrel (p.1563·2); ethinylestradiol (p.1553·2).
*Triphasic oral contraceptive.*

**Tristina** *Mac, India.*
Diphenhydramine hydrochloride (p.431·3); ammonium chloride (p.1115·2); sodium citrate (p.1223·2); menthol (p.1711·3).
*Coughs.*

**Tristoject** *Mayrand, USA†.*
Triamcinolone diacetate (p.1110·2).
*Corticosteroid.*

**Trisufin** *Loren, Mex.*
Co-trimoxazole (p.199·3).
*Bacterial infections.*

**Trisul** *Pacific, NZ.*
Co-trimoxazole (p.199·3).
*Bacterial infections; Pneumocystis carinii pneumonia.*

**Trisulfaminic** *Shepherd, Canad.†.*
Phenylpropanolamine hydrochloride (p.1127·3); pheniramine maleate (p.438·3); mepyramine maleate (p.437·1); sulfadiazine (p.258·2); sulfamerazine (p.260·3); sulfadimidine (p.259·2).
*Congestion and infections of the upper respiratory-tract.*

**Trisulfose** *John Wyeth, India.*
Co-trimoxazole (p.199·3).
*Bacterial infections; Pneumocystis carinii pneumonia; toxoplasmosis.*

**Trisulprim** *Raza, Malaysia; Pharmaniaga, Malaysia.*
Sulfadiazine (p.258·2); trimethoprim (p.272·2).
*Urinary-tract infections.*

**Trisyn** *Baker Cummins, Canad.†.*
Fluocinonide (p.1101·3); procinonide (p.1110·1); ciprocinonide (p.1095·2).
*Skin disorders.*

**Tritab** *Sidus, Arg.*
Azithromycin (p.159·1).
*Bacterial infections.*

**Tritace**
*Aventis, Arg.; Aventis, Austral.; Aventis, Austria; Aventis, Belg.; Aventis, Hong Kong; Aventis, Irl.; Aventis, Israel; Aventis, Malaysia; Aventis, Mex.; Aventis, Neth.; Aventis, S.Afr.; Aventis, Singapore; Aventis, Thai.; Aventis, UK.*
Ramipril (p.994·1).
*Diabetic nephropathy; heart failure; hypertension; myocardial infarction; primary prophylaxis of atherosclerotic complications.*

**Tritace Comp** *Aventis, Israel.*
Ramipril (p.994·1); hydrochlorothiazide (p.933·2).
*Hypertension.*

**Tritace-HCT** *Aventis, Arg.*
Ramipril (p.994·1); hydrochlorothiazide (p.933·2).
*Hypertension.*

**Tritan** *Eon, USA.*
Chlorphenamine tannate (p.428·1); mepyramine tannate (p.437·1); phenylephrine tannate (p.1127·2).
*Allergic rhinitis; nasal congestion.*

**Tri-Tannate** *Rugby, USA.*
Phenylephrine tannate (p.1127·2); chlorphenamine tannate (p.428·1); mepyramine tannate (p.437·1).
*Upper respiratory-tract symptoms.*

**Tri-Tannate Plus Pediatric** *Rugby, USA.*
Phenylephrine tannate (p.1127·2); ephedrine tannate (p.1120·3); chlorphenamine tannate (p.428·1); pentoxyverine tannate (p.1126·3).
*Coughs and cold symptoms.*

**Tritanrix** *SmithKline Beecham, Ital.†.*
A diphtheria, tetanus, and pertussis vaccine (p.1613·3).
*Active immunisation.*

**Tritanrix HB**
*GlaxoSmithKline, India; GlaxoSmithKline, Malaysia; SmithKline Beecham, Spain; GlaxoSmithKline, Thai.*
A diphtheria, tetanus, pertussis, and hepatitis B vaccine (p.1614·3).
*Active immunisation.*

**Tritanrix HB-HIB** GlaxoSmithKline, Arg.
A diphtheria, tetanus, pertussis, haemophilus influenzae, and hepatitis B vaccine.
*Active immunisation.*

**Tritanrix HB/Hiberix** SmithKline Beecham, Mex.
Tritanrix, a diphtheria, tetanus, pertussis, and hepatitis B vaccine; Hiberix, a haemophilus influenzae conjugate vaccine.
Available in a dual presentation pack.
*Active immunisation.*

**Tritazide**
Aventis, Austria; Aventis, Belg.; Aventis, Mex.; Aventis, Neth.
Ramipril (p.994·1); hydrochlorothiazide (p.933·2).
*Hypertension.*

**Tritec** Glaxo Wellcome, USA†.
Ranitidine bismuth citrate (p.1287·2).
*Peptic ulcer.*

**Tritenk** Biotenk, Arg.
Co-trimoxazole (p.199·3).
*Bacterial infections; Pneumocystis carinii pneumonia.*

**Tritet** Akromed, S.Afr.†.
Tetracycline hydrochloride (p.266·2); chlortetracycline hydrochloride (p.187·3); demeclocycline hydrochloride (p.204·3).
*Bacterial infections.*

**Tri-Thiazid** Stada, Ger.
Triamterene (p.1016·2); hydrochlorothiazide (p.933·2).
*Heart failure; hypertension; oedema.*

**Tri-Thiazid Reserpin** Stada, Ger.
Triamterene (p.1016·2); hydrochlorothiazide (p.933·2); reserpine (p.995·1).
*Hypertension.*

**Triticum** Lepori, Port.
Trazodone hydrochloride (p.319·1).
*Depression.*

**Tritopan** Klonal, Arg.
Bromazepam (p.671·3).
*Anxiety.*

**Tri-Torrat** Roche, Ger.
Metipranolol (p.955·3); butizide (p.878·2); dihydralazine sulfate (p.899·3).
*Hypertension.*

**Trittico**
CSC, Austria; Faran, Gr.; Angelini, Hong Kong; Angelini, Ital.; ACRAF, Switz.
Trazodone hydrochloride (p.319·1).
*Anxiety; depression.*

Laboratorios Chile, Chile.
Trazodone (p.320·1) or trazodone hydrochloride (p.319·1).
*Alcohol withdrawal syndrome; anxiety; depression; schizophrenia.*

**Triv** Boyle, USA.
Hydroxyquinoline sulfate (p.1700·1); alkyl aryl sulfonate; edetic acid (p.1038·2); sodium sulfate (p.1290·1).
*Vaginal disorders.*

**Trivacuna** Leti, Spain†.
A diphtheria, tetanus, and pertussis vaccine (p.1613·3).
*Active immunisation of infants and young children.*

**Trivagel N** Marjan, Braz.
Dexamethasone phosphate (p.1097·2); neomycin sulfate (p.235·1); nystatin (p.406·3); tyrothricin (p.275·1).
*Vulvovaginal disorders.*

**Trivanex** Pharmasant, Thai.
Griseofulvin (p.400·3).
*Fungal infections.*

**Trivastal**
Servier, Arg.; Servier, Braz.; Eutherapie, Fr.; Servier, Ger.; Serdia, India; Servier, Malaysia; Servier, Port.; Servier, Singapore; Servier, Thai.
Piribedil (p.1212·2) or piribedil mesilate (p.1212·2).
*Mental function impairment in the elderly; parkinsonism; peripheral vascular disorders; vascular eye disorders; vestibular disorders.*

**Trivastan** Stroder, Ital.
Piribedil (p.1212·2).
*Vascular disorders.*

**Trivax** Wellcome, Irl.†.
A diphtheria, tetanus, and pertussis vaccine (p.1613·3).
*Active immunisation.*

**Trivax-AD**
Wellcome, Irl.†; Chiron Vaccines, UK.
An adsorbed diphtheria, tetanus, and pertussis vaccine (p.1613·3).
*Active immunisation of infants and young children.*

**Trivax-Hib** SmithKline Beecham, UK†.
A diphtheria, tetanus, pertussis, and haemophilus influenzae vaccine (p.1614·2).
*Active immunisation.*

**Trive**
Baxter, Fr.†; Baxter, Spain†; Baxter, Thai.†; Clintec, Thai.†.
Amino-acid, carbohydrate, and lipid (from soya oil (p.1447·2)) infusion (p.1417·1).
*Parenteral nutrition.*

**Trivemil** Baxter, Ital.
An amino-acid, lipid (from soya oil (p.1447·2)), and carbohydrate preparation (p.1417·1).
*Parenteral nutrition.*

**Trivermon** Bergamo, Braz.†.
Piperazine (p.111·2).
*Ascariasis; enterobiasis.*

**Tri-Vi-Flor**
Mead Johnson Nutritionals, Canad.; Mead Johnson Nutritionals, USA.
A range of vitamin preparations with fluoride (p.1444·3)(p.1417·1).
*Dental caries prophylaxis; dietary supplement.*

**Tri-Vi-Fluor**
Bristol-Myers Squibb, Arg.; Mead Johnson, Braz.
Multivitamin preparation with fluoride (p.1417·1) (p.1444·3).
*Dental caries prophylaxis; dietary supplement.*

**Triviken** Kener, Mex.†.
Vitamin B substances (p.1417·1).

**Trivina**
Pharmacia, Belg.; Aspen, S.Afr.; Orion, Swed.
White tablets, estradiol valerate (p.1550·2); blue tablets estradiol valerate; medroxyprogesterone acetate (p.1557·2); yellow tablets, inert.
*Menopausal disorders; osteoporosis.*

**Triviraten**
Raffo, Arg.; Berna, Hong Kong; Berna, Ital.†; Berna, Malaysia; Swiss Serum, Malaysia; Berna, NZ; Berna, Port.†; Byk Madaus, S.Afr.†; Berna, Spain; Berna, Switz.; Berna, Thai.; Swiss Serum, Thai.
A measles, mumps, and rubella vaccine (Edmonston-Zagreb, Rubini, and Wistar RA 27/3 strains, respectively) (p.1625·1).
*Active immunisation.*

**Tri-Vi-Sol**
Bristol-Myers Squibb, Arg.; Mead Johnson, Braz.; Mead Johnson Nutritionals, Canad.; Mead Johnson, Hong Kong; Bristol-Myers Squibb, Mex.; Mead Johnson Nutritionals, USA.
Multivitamin preparation (p.1417·1).

**Trivisol** Mead Johnson, Chile.
Vitamin A; vitamin C; vitamin D (p.1417·1).
*Vitamin supplement.*

**Tri-Vi-Sol with Fluoride** Mead Johnson Nutritionals, Canad.
Multivitamin preparation (p.1417·1) with fluoride (p.1444·3).
*Dental caries prophylaxis; vitamin supplement.*

**Tri-Vi-Sol with Iron** Mead Johnson Nutritionals, USA.
Multivitamin preparation with iron (p.1417·1).

**Tri-Vitamin** Schein, USA.
Vitamins A, C, and D (p.1417·1).

**Trivitamin Fluoride Drops** Schein, USA.
Multivitamin preparation with fluoride (p.1444·3)(p.1417·1).

**Trivitan** Merck, Spain†.
Pyridoxine (p.1457·2); vitamin A (p.1451·2); tocopherol (p.1464·3).
*Hyperkeratosis; keratoconjunctivitis; rhinitis; tonic; xerophthalmia.*

**Trivitana DM** Merck, Chile.
Vitamin A; vitamin $B_6$; vitamin E (p.1417·1).
*Dietary supplement.*

**Trivitana Q10** Merck, Chile.
Vitamin A; vitamin B; vitamin E; ubidecarenone (p.1417·1).
*Dietary supplement.*

**Trivit-B** TP, Thai.
Vitamin $B_1$ (p.1455·2); vitamin $B_6$ (p.1457·2); vitamin $B_{12}$ (p.1458·2).
*Neuritis; vitamin B deficiency.*

**Trivitol** Agepha, Austria.
Vitamins (p.1417·1); caffeine; kola.
*Tonic.*

**Trivon** Great Eastern, Thai.; Therapharma, Thai.
Vitamin $B_1$; vitamin $B_6$; vitamin $B_{12}$ (p.1417·1).
*Tonic.*

**Trivora** Watson, USA.
Levonorgestrel (p.1563·2); ethinylestradiol (p.1553·2).
28-Day packs also contain 7 inert tablets.
*Triphasic oral contraceptive.*

**Tri-Wycillina** Pharmacia Upjohn, Ital.
Benzathine benzylpenicillin (p.162·3); benzylpenicillin potassium (p.163·2); procaine benzylpenicillin (p.246·1).
*Bacterial infections.*

**Trixidine** Asta Medica, Ital.†.
Propylene glycol cefatrizine (p.170·3).
*Bacterial infections.*

**Trixilan** Pulitzer, Ital.†.
Propylene glycol cefatrizine (p.170·3).
*Bacterial infections.*

**Trixilem**
Laboratorios Chile, Chile; Lemery, Mex.; Lemery, Thai.
Methotrexate (p.568·2).
*Malignant neoplasms; mycosis fungoides; rheumatoid arthritis.*

**Trixne** Pharmatrix, Arg.
Erythromycin (p.208·1).
*Acne.*

**Trixol** Ferro, Arg.
Hyoscyamus (p.485·2); belladonna (p.479·1); boldo (p.1661·2); valerian (p.1762·2); atropine sulfate (p.477·1); phenobarbital sodium (p.367·3); papaverine hydrochloride (p.1728·1).

**Trixone** LBS, Thai.
Ceftriaxone sodium (p.182·3).
*Bacterial infections.*

**Trixotene** Labinca, Arg.
Docetaxel (p.547·1).
*Malignant neoplasms.*

**Trixzol** Great Eastern, Thai.; Westmont, Thai.
Co-trimoxazole (p.199·3).
*Bacterial infections.*

**Triyodisan** Bioquimico, Mex.†.
Liothyronine (p.1602·2).

**Triyosom** Justesa Imagen, Arg.
Meglumine amidotrizoate (p.1060·2); and/or sodium amidotrizoate (p.1060·2).
*Radiographic contrast medium.*

**Triyotex** Medix, Mex.
Liothyronine sodium (p.1602·2).
*Hypothyroidism.*

**Triz** Indoco, Thai.
Cetirizine hydrochloride (p.427·1).
*Allergic conjunctivitis; allergic rhinitis; allergic skin disorders.*

**Trizele** Choongwae, Hong Kong†.
Metronidazole (p.607·2).
*Anaerobic bacterial infections.*

**Trizid**
Douglas, Hong Kong†; Douglas, NZ†.
Triamterene (p.1016·2); hydrochlorothiazide (p.933·2).
*Hypertension; oedema.*

**Trizina** Francia, Ital.
Propylene glycol cefatrizine (p.170·3).
*Bacterial infections.*

**Trizivir**
GlaxoSmithKline, Austral.; GlaxoSmithKline, Belg.; Glaxo Wellcome, Denm.; GlaxoSmithKline, Fin.; GlaxoSmithKline, Fr.; GlaxoSmithKline, Ger.; GlaxoSmithKline, Irl.; GlaxoSmithKline, Israel; GlaxoSmithKline, Ital.; GlaxoSmithKline, Norw.; Glaxo Wellcome, Port.; GlaxoSmithKline, Singapore; Glaxo Wellcome, Spain; GlaxoSmithKline, Swed.; GlaxoSmithKline, Switz.; GlaxoSmithKline, UK; Glaxo Wellcome, USA.
Abacavir sulfate (p.625·2); lamivudine (p.648·2); zidovudine (p.658·2).
*HIV infection.*

**Trizol Balsamico** Riedel-Zabinka, Braz.†.
Co-trimoxazole (p.199·3); guaifenesin (p.1122·1).
*Bacterial infections.*

**Trizolin**
Remedica, Malaysia; Remedica, Singapore; Remedica, Thai.
Norfloxacin (p.238·3).
*Bacterial infections.*

**Trobicin**
Pharmacia, Austral.; Pharmacia, Austria; Pharmacia, Belg.; Pharmacia, Braz.; Pharmacia Upjohn, Canad.†; Pharmacia, Hong Kong; Pharmacia Upjohn, India; Pharmacia Upjohn, Irl.†; Pharmacia Upjohn, Ital.; Pharmacia Upjohn, Mex.†; Pharmacia, Port.; Pharmacia, S.Afr.; Pharmacia, Singapore; Pharmacia Upjohn, Swed.†; Pharmacia, Switz.; Pharmacia, Thai.; Pharmacia, USA†.
Spectinomycin hydrochloride (p.255·2).
*Gonorrhoea.*

**Trobicine** Pharmacia, Fr.
Spectinomycin hydrochloride (p.255·2).
*Gonorrhoea.*

**Troca Cationi** Laborest, Ital.
Magnesium; potassium; zinc (p.1217·1).
*Mineral deficiencies; stress; viral infections.*

**Troca Flu** Laborest, Ital.
Zinc; magnesium; vitamin C; vitamin A (p.1417·1).
*Candidiasis; viral infections.*

**Troca Flu Spray Nasale** Laborest, Ital.
Sodium chloride (p.1233·3); sulfur (p.1158·2).
*Nasal cleansing.*

**Trocacin** Nakornpatana, Thai.
Tyrothricin (p.275·1); benzocaine (p.1370·3).
*Mouth and throat disorders.*

**Trocaine** Roberts, USA.
Benzocaine (p.1370·3).
*Obesity; sore throat.*

**Trocal** Roberts, USA.
Dextromethorphan hydrobromide (p.1117·3).
*Coughs.*

**Trochain** Propan, S.Afr.
Cetrimide (p.1172·1); benzocaine (p.1370·3).
*Mouth and throat disorders.*

**Trocium** Strand, Malaysia.
Calcium lactate (p.1225·3).
*Calcium deficiency.*

**Trodrine** Malayan, Singapore.
Triprolidine hydrochloride (p.442·3); pseudoephedrine hydrochloride (p.1129·2).
*Allergic rhinitis; cold symptoms.*

**Trofalgon** Madariaga, Spain.
Cyanocobalamin (p.1458·2); muramidase hydrochloride (p.1717·2).
*Anorexia; tonic; weight loss.*

**Trofen** TP, Thai.
Ibuprofen (p.45·3).
*Fever; musculoskeletal and joint disorders; pain.*

**Trofentyl** Troikaa, India.
Fentanyl citrate (p.40·1).
*Analgesia in anaesthesia; neuroleptanalgesia.*

**Troferit** Chinoin, Mex.
Dropropizine (p.1119·3).
*Coughs.*

**Trofesil** Solfran, Mex.
Multivitamin preparation (p.1417·1).

**Trofi Milina** Europharma, Spain†.
*Capsules:* Phospholipids; pyridoxine hydrochloride (p.1456·3).
*Injection:* Cyanocobalamin (p.1458·2); phospholipids. Lidocaine hydrochloride (p.1377·3) is included in this preparation to alleviate the pain of injection.
*Dystonia; tonic.*

**Troficardil** Sintofarma, Braz.†.
Inosine (p.1701·2).
*Cardiovascular disorders.*

**Trofinan** Biol, Arg.
Dexamethasone phosphate (p.1097·2).
*Corticosteroid.*

**Trofinerv** Fidia, Ital.
Omega-3 marine triglycerides (p.976·2); vitamins (p.1417·1).
*Nutritional supplement.*

**Trofinerv Antiox** Fidia, Ital.
Omega-3 triglycerides (p.976·1); gamolenic acid (p.1690·2); vitamins; minerals (p.1417·1).
*Nutritional supplement.*

**Trofo 5** Uniderm, Ital.
Zinc oxide (p.1163·2); cod-liver oil (p.1425·2); hyaluronic acid (p.1697·3); chamomile oil (p.1669·3).
*Skin disorders.*

**Trofocalcium** Fournier, Ital.
Vitamin D and calcium preparation (p.1417·1).
*Calcium depletion; metabolic bone disorders.*

**Trofocard** Unipharma, Gr.
Magnesium aspartate (p.1227·3); magnesium chloride (p.1417·1).
*Hypomagnesaemia.*

**Trofodermin**
Note. This name is used for preparations of different composition.
Pharmacia, Braz.; Carlo Erba OTC, Ital.; Pharmacia, Thai.
Clostebol acetate (p.1543·2); neomycin sulfate (p.235·1).
*Burns; skin infections; skin ulcers; wounds.*

Pharmacia, Chile.
Clostebol (p.1543·2).
*Skin disorders.*

**Trofodermin Neomicina** Pharmacia, Chile.
Clostebol acetate (p.1543·2); neomycin sulfate (p.235·1).
*Infected skin disorders.*

**Trofodermin-S** Pharmacia Upjohn, Mex.†.
Clostebol (p.1543·2).
*Skin disorders.*

**Trofogin** Farmigea, Ital.
Estriol (p.1552·3).
*Cervicitis; menopausal disorders; oestrogen deficiency.*

**Trofomed** Trofomed, Ital.†.
Royal jelly (p.1740·3).

**Troforex Pepsico** Reig Jofre, Spain.
Cyproheptadine hydrochloride (p.430·1); amino acids and hydroxocobalamin (p.1417·1); pepsin (p.1729·3).
*Anorexia; tonic; weight-loss.*

**Trofoseptine** Boehringer Ingelheim, Fr.
Sodium acexamate (p.1646·2); neomycin sulfate (p.235·1).
Formerly contained clostebol acetate and neomycin sulfate.
*Infected ulcers.*

**Trojan** Carter Horner, Canad.
Nonoxinol 9 (p.1413·3).
*Contraceptive.*

**Troliber** Randall, Mex.†.
Dextropropoxyphene (p.28·3).

**Trolip** Dexa, Hong Kong.
Fenofibrate (p.915·2).
*Hyperlipidaemias.*

**Trolit** Silesia, Chile.
Levonorgestrel (p.1563·2); ethinylestradiol (p.1553·2).
*Menstrual disorders; triphasic oral contraceptive.*

**Trolovol**
Dexo, Fr.; Asta Medica, Ger.†.
Penicillamine (p.1046·3).
*Chronic polyarthritis; cystinuria; heavy-metal poisoning; rheumatoid arthritis; scleroderma; Wilson's disease.*

**Tromadil** Biolab, Thai.
Bromhexine hydrochloride (p.1115·3).
*Respiratory-tract disorders associated with increased or viscous mucus.*

**Tromagesic** Themis Chemicals, India.
Diclofenac sodium (p.32·1).
*Gout; musculoskeletal and joint disorders.*

**Tromalyt** Madaus, Spain.
Aspirin (p.15·1).
*Thrombosis prophylaxis.*

**Tromasin** Parke, Davis, Arg.
Papain (p.1727·3).
*Inflammation.*

**Tromasin con Aspirina** Parke, Davis, Arg.
Papain (p.1727·3); aspirin (p.1157·1).
*Inflammation; pain.*

**Trombenal** Bago, Arg.
Ticlopidine hydrochloride (p.1011·2).
*Thromboembolic disorders.*

**Trombenox** Menarini, Ital.†.
Enoxaparin sodium (p.910·3).
*Thromboembolic disorders.*

**Trombofob** Abbott, Braz.
*Ointment:* Heparin sodium (p.928·1); benzyl nicotinate (p.21·2).
*Soft-tissue injury; superficial vascular disorders.*
*Topical gel:* Heparin sodium (p.928·1).
*Superficial vascular disorders.*

**Tromboject** Omega, Canad.
Sodium tetradecyl sulfate (p.1575·1).
*Varicose veins.*

**Trombolisin** Proge, Ital.
Heparin calcium (p.927·3).
*Thromboembolic disorders.*

**Trombolysin** Nordic Healthcare, Denm.†.
Urokinase (p.1018·2).
*Myocardial infarction.*

**Tromboparin** *Baxter Immuno, Arg.*
Parnaparin (p.978·3).
*Thromboembolic disorders.*

**Trombopat** *Pentafarma, Port.*
Ticlopidine hydrochloride (p.1011·2).

**Trombosol** *Orion, Fin.*
Heparin sodium (p.928·1); benzyl nicotinate (p.21·2).
*Soft-tissue injury; superficial vascular disorders.*

**Trombovar**
*E-Z-EM, Canad.; Innothera, Fr.; Bouty, Ital.; Promedica, Malaysia.*
Sodium tetradecyl sulfate (p.1575·1).
*Cysts; oesophageal varices; varicose veins.*

**Tromboxanil** *Farmion, Braz.†.*
Dipyridamole (p.903·1); aspirin (p.15·1).
*Thromboembolism prophylaxis.*

**Trombyl** *Pharmacia, Swed.*
Aspirin (p.15·1).
*Angina pectoris; myocardial infarction; prevention of cerebrovascular ischaemia.*

**Tromcardin** *Trommsdorff, Ger.*
Potassium aspartate (p.1233·1); magnesium aspartate (p.1227·3).
*Arrhythmias; heart failure; myocardial infarction; potassium and magnesium deficiency.*

**Tromderm** *Silesia, Chile.*
Sertaconazole nitrate (p.408·1).
*Fungal skin infections; seborrhoeic dermatitis.*

**Tromedal** *Farcoral, Mex.*
Ketorolac trometamol (p.52·1).
*Pain.*

**Tromicol** *Willmar, Mex.†.*
Tetracycline (p.266·2).
*Bacterial infections.*

**Tromigal** *Galen, Mex.†.*
Erythromycin (p.208·1).
*Bacterial infections.*

**Tromir** *Ibirn, Ital.†.*
Suleparoid (p.1009·1).
*Thrombosis prophylaxis.*

**Tromlipon** *Trommsdorff, Ger.*
Thioctic acid (p.1754·3) or trometamol thioctate (p.1754·3).
*Diabetic neuropathy.*

**Trommcardin** *Jacoby, Austria.*
Potassium aspartate (p.1233·1); magnesium aspartate (p.1227·3).
*Arrhythmias; digitalis intoxication; heart failure; myocardial infarction; potassium and magnesium deficiency.*

**Trommgallol** *Jacoby, Austria.*
Cyclobutyrol sodium (p.1678·2); cynarine (p.1678·3); sorbitol (p.1446·3); magnesium sulfate (p.1228·2).
*Hepatobiliary disorders.*

**Trompersantin** *Boehringer Ingelheim, Mex.*
Dipyridamole (p.903·1).
*Thromboembolic disorders.*

**Tromphyllin** *Trommsdorff, Ger.*
Theophylline (p.798·3).
*Obstructive airways disease.*

**Tronan** *Roche, Ital.†.*
Suleparoid (p.1009·1).
*Thrombosis prophylaxis.*

**Troneo** *Nakorn, Thai.*
Tyrothricin (p.275·1); benzocaine (p.1370·3).
*Mouth and throat infections.*

**Tronex** *Tocogino, Mex.†.*
Ampicillin (p.157·1).
*Bacterial infections.*

**Tronolane** *Ross, USA.*
*Cream:* Pramocaine hydrochloride (p.1382·2); zinc oxide (p.1163·2).
*Suppositories:* Zinc oxide (p.1163·2).
Formerly contained pramocaine hydrochloride, pramocaine, and zinc oxide.
*Haemorrhoids.*

**Tronotene** *Abbott, Ital.*
Pramocaine hydrochloride (p.1382·2).
*Burns; haemorrhoids; pruritus.*

**Tronothane**
*Abbott, Fr.; Abbott, USA.*
Pramocaine hydrochloride (p.1382·2).
*Anal pain and pruritus; local anaesthesia.*

**Tronoxal** *Prasfarma, Spain.*
Ifosfamide (p.561·1).
*Malignant neoplasms.*

**Tropargal** *Sanofi Synthelabo, Spain.*
Diazepam (p.690·1); nortriptyline hydrochloride (p.310·2).
*Depression with anxiety or agitation.*

**Troparin** *Biochemie, Austria.*
Certoparin sodium (p.882·1).
*Thromboembolism prophylaxis.*

**Troparin compositum** *Biochemie, Austria.*
Certoparin sodium (p.882·1); dihydroergotamine mesilate (p.465·3).
Lidocaine hydrochloride (p.1377·3) is included in this preparation to alleviate the pain of injection.
*Thromboembolism prophylaxis.*

**Tropergen** *Goldshield, UK†.*
Diphenoxylate hydrochloride (p.1261·3).
Atropine sulfate (p.477·1) is included in this preparation to discourage abuse.
These ingredients can be described by the British Approved Name Co-phenotrope.
*Diarrhoea.*

**Tropex**
*Note. This name is used for preparations of different composition.*
*Rowa, Irl.*
Phenazone (p.82·3).
*Ear wax removal; otitis media.*

*Rowa, Singapore.*
Phenazone (p.82·3); glycerol (p.1694·3).
*Ear wax removal; otitis media.*

**Tropfen gegen Venenbeschwerden** *Jacoby, Austria.*
Homoeopathic preparation.

**Trophamine**
*Braun McGaw, Hong Kong†; Pisa, Mex.; McGaw, NZ†; Braun, Spain; McGaw, USA.*
Amino-acid infusion (p.1417·1).
*Parenteral nutrition in children.*

**Trophicard** *Kohler-Pharma, Ger.; Kohler, Ger.*
Potassium aspartate (p.1233·1); magnesium aspartate (p.1227·3).
*Cardiac disorders; magnesium or potassium deficiency.*

**Trophicreme** *Grunenthal, Fr.*
Estriol (p.1552·3).
*Postmenopausal vulvovaginal disorders.*

**Trophiderm** *Brothier, Fr.†.*
Calcium alginate (p.745·1).
*Ulcers.*

**Trophigil** *Grunenthal, Fr.*
*Lactobacillus caseivar rhamnosus* (p.1704·2); estriol (p.1552·3); progesterone (p.1566·2).
*Atrophic vaginitis; pre- and postoperative gynaecological care.*

**Trophires**
*Note. This name is used for preparations of different composition.*
*Sanofi Synthelabo OTC, Fr.*
*Suppositories:* Eucalyptus oil (p.1686·2); thenoate sodium (p.269·2).
*Respiratory-tract disorders.*
*Syrup:* Pholcodine (p.1128·3); thenoate sodium (p.269·2); eucalyptus oil (p.1686·2).
*Coughs.*

*Sanofi Synthelabo, Spain.*
*Nasal drops:* Cineole (p.1672·1); cypress oil; myrtle oil; thenoate sodium (p.269·2).
*Nasal cleansing.*
*Suppositories; syrup:* Pholcodine (p.1128·3).
*Cough.*

**Trophires Compose** *Sanofi Synthelabo OTC, Fr.*
Paracetamol (p.76·2); eucalyptus oil (p.1686·2); thenoate sodium (p.269·2).
*Fever; respiratory-tract disorders.*

**Trophoseptine** *Sanofi Synthelabo, Port.†.*
Promestriene (p.1568·2); chlorquinaldol (p.187·3).
*Vaginal infections.*

**Trophox** *Raptakos, India.*
High-protein dietary supplement (p.1417·1).

**Trophysan** *Baxter, Fr.*
Amino-acid, carbohydrate, mineral, and vitamin infusion (p.1417·1).
*Parenteral nutrition.*

**Tropicacyl** *Akorn, USA.*
Tropicamide (p.491·1).
*Induction of mydriasis and cycloplegia.*

**Tropical Blend** *Schering-Plough, Canad.†.*
Oxybenzone (p.1154·3).
*Sunscreen.*

**Tropical Blend Dark Tanning** *Schering-Plough, USA.*
*Lotion SPF 4:* Octinoxate (p.1154·3); oxybenzone (p.1154·3).
*Oil SPF 4:* Padimate O (p.1155·1); oxybenzone (p.1154·3).
*SPF 2:* Homosalate (p.1148·1).
*Sunscreen.*

**Tropical Blend Dry Oil** *Schering-Plough, USA.*
*SPF 2:* Homosalate (p.1148·1).
*SPF 4:* Homosalate (p.1148·1); oxybenzone (p.1154·3).
*Sunscreen.*

**Tropical Blend Tan Magnifier** *Schering-Plough, USA.*
*SPF 2; SPF 4:* Trolamine salicylate (p.95·3).
*Sunscreen.*

**Tropical Gold Dark Tanning** *Goldline, USA.*
*SPF 2:* Octinoxate (p.1154·3); padimate O (p.1155·1).
*SPF 4:* Octinoxate (p.1154·3); oxybenzone (p.1154·3).
*Sunscreen.*

**Tropical Gold Sunblock** *Goldline, USA.*
*SPF 15:* Octinoxate (p.1154·3); oxybenzone (p.1154·3).
*SPF 30:* Octinoxate (p.1154·3); octisalate (p.1154·3); homosalate (p.1148·1); oxybenzone (p.1154·3).
*Sunscreen.*

**Tropical Gold Sunscreen** *Goldline, USA.*
*SPF 8:* Octinoxate (p.1154·3); oxybenzone (p.1154·3).
*Sunscreen.*

**Tropicil Top** *Edol, Port.*
Tropicamide (p.491·1).
*Production of mydriasis and cycloplegia.*

**Tropico**
*Note. This name is used for preparations of different composition.*
*Bell, India.*
Tropicamide (p.491·1).
*Production of mydriasis and cycloplegia.*

*Perez Gimenez, Spain.*
Menthol (p.1711·3); eucalyptus oil (p.1686·2).
*Nasal congestion.*

**Tropicol** *Bournonville, Belg.†.*
Tropicamide (p.491·1).
*Production of mydriasis.*

**Tropicur** *Roche, Arg.*
Mefloquine hydrochloride (p.453·3).
*Malaria.*

**Tropimil** *Farmigea, Ital.*
Tropicamide (p.491·1).
*Production of mydriasis and cycloplegia.*

**Tropinal** *Sigma, Braz.*
Dipyrone (p.35·3); homatropine methylbromide (p.483·2); hyoscine butylbromide (p.483·3); hyoscyamine hydrobromide (p.485·1).
*Smooth muscle spasm.*

**Tropinom** *Genom, Braz.*
Tropicamide (p.491·1).
*Production of mydriasis and cycloplegia.*

**Tropiovent** *Ashbourne, UK†.*
Ipratropium bromide (p.787·1).
*Obstructive airways disease.*

**Tropisol** *Protein, Mex.†.*
Captopril (p.879·2).

**Tropium** *DDSA Pharmaceuticals, UK.*
Chlordiazepoxide hydrochloride (p.674·2).
*Alcohol withdrawal syndrome; anxiety.*

**Tropivag** *Finadiet, Arg.*
*Lactobacillus rhamnosus* (p.1704·2).
*Restoration of vaginal flora.*

**Tropivag Plus** *Finadiet, Arg.*
*Lactobacillus rhamnosus* (p.1704·2); progesterone (p.1566·2); estriol (p.1552·3).
*Vaginal disorders.*

**Tropixal** *Demo, Gr.*
Tropicamide (p.491·1).
*Production of mydriasis.*

**Tropoderm** *Kolassa, Austria.*
Neomycin sulfate (p.235·1); diphenylpyraline hydrochloride (p.432·3); buphenine hydrochloride (p.1663·2); hydrocortisone (p.1103·3).

**Tropyn** *Zafiro, Mex.*
Atropine sulfate (p.477·1).
*Gastrointestinal disorders; organophosphorus pesticide poisoning; premedication.*

**Trorix** *Asta Médica, Chile; Baxter, Chile.*
Ondansetron (p.1281·1).
*Nausea and vomiting.*

**Trosderm** *Pfizer Lambert, Spain.*
Tioconazole (p.409·3).
*Fungal skin infections.*

**Trosic** *General Drugs, Thai.*
Tramadol hydrochloride (p.94·3).
*Pain.*

**Trosid** *Pfizer Lambert, Spain.*
Tioconazole (p.409·3).
*Fungal skin and nail infections; vulvovaginal candidiasis.*

**Trospi** *Medac, Ger.*
Trospium chloride (p.491·2).
*Urinary-tract disorders.*

**Trosycort** *Pfizer, Fin.*
Tioconazole (p.409·3); hydrocortisone acetate (p.1103·3).
*Inflammatory fungal skin infections with secondary bacterial infection.*

**Trosyd**
*Pfizer, Arg.; Pfizer, Austria; Pfizer Consumer, Canad.; Pfizer, Fin.; Teofarma, Fr.; Pfizer, Hong Kong; Pfizer Consumer, Ital.; Pfizer, Malaysia; Pfizer, NZ†; Farminova, Port.; Pfizer, S.Afr.; Pfizer, Singapore; Pfizer, Switz.; Pfizer, Thai.*
Tioconazole (p.409·3).
*Fungal and bacterial infections of the skin, nails, and vagina; vaginal trichomoniasis.*

**Trosyl**
*Pfizer, Irl.; Pfizer, UK.*
Tioconazole (p.409·3).
*Fungal and bacterial infections of the nails.*

**Trova** *Pfizer, Israel†.*
Alatrofloxacin mesilate (p.154·1).
*Bacterial infections.*

**Trovan**
*Pfizer, Austral.†; Pfizer, Canad.; Pfizer, USA.*
*Injection:* Alatrofloxacin mesilate (p.154·1).
*Bacterial infections.*

*Pfizer, Austral.†; Pfizer, Braz.†; Pfizer, Canad.; Pfizer, Hong Kong†; Pfizer, Mex.†; Pfizer, USA.*
*Tablets:* Trovafloxacin mesilate (p.274·3).
*Bacterial infections.*

**Troxeven**
*Note. This name is used for preparations of different composition.*
*Typen, Arg.*
Troxerutin (p.1688·3) aescin (p.1648·2).
*Oedema; venous disorders.*

*Kreussler, Ger.*
Troxerutin (p.1688·3).
*Venous disorders.*

**Troxxil** *Laboratorios Chile, Chile.*
Tinidazole (p.617·1).
*Anaerobic bacterial infections; protozoal infections.*

**Troxyderm** *Ecofarm, Ital.*
Multivitamin, amino-acid, and mineral preparation with myrtillus (p.1417·1).
*Nutritional supplement; skin disorders.*

**Trozocina** *Sigma-Tau, Ital.*
Azithromycin (p.159·1).
*Bacterial infections.*

**Trozolet** *Tecnofarma, Chile.*
Anastrozole (p.528·1).
*Breast cancer.*

**Trozolite** *Raffo, Arg.*
Anastrozole (p.528·1).
*Malignant neoplasms.*

**Trozyman** *IQB, Braz.*
Azithromycin (p.159·1).
*Bacterial infections.*

**Tru**
*Note. This name is used for preparations of different composition.*
*Elea, Arg.*
Pyrvinium embonate (p.113·3).
*Oxyuriasis.*

*Pasteur, Chile.*
Sulfathiazole sodium (p.264·1); lidocaine hydrochloride (p.1377·3).
*Otitis.*

**Tru Compuesto** *Elea, Arg.*
Mebendazole (p.108·2); tinidazole (p.617·1).
*Worm infections.*

**True Illusion** *Maybelline, Canad.†.*
*Cream SPF 10:* Titanium dioxide (p.1160·3).
*Liquid SPF 10:* Octinoxate (p.1154·3).
*Sunscreen.*

**True Test**
*ALK, Denm.; Abello, Ger.†; Glaxo Wellcome, Mex.; Alk-Abello, NZ; CSL, NZ; Glaxo Wellcome, USA.*
A range of allergen-impregnated patches (p.1650·1).
*Diagnosis of allergic contact dermatitis.*

**Trufree**
*Cantassium Co., UK.*
*Tablets:* Multivitamin and mineral preparation (p.1417·1).

*Nutricia Dietary, UK.*
Gluten-free, wheat-free flours and foods for special diets (p.1417·1).
*Gluten sensitivity.*

**Trumsal** *Centrum, Spain.*
Diltiazem hydrochloride (p.900·1).
*Angina pectoris; hypertension.*

**Truoxin** *Helsinn Birex, Irl.*
Ciprofloxacin (p.188·2).
*Bacterial infections.*

**Truphylline** *G & W, USA.*
Aminophylline (p.780·2).
*Asthma; bronchospasm.*

**Truquil** *Lundbeck, Israel†.*
Chlorprothixene hydrochloride (p.682·3).
*Psychoses.*

**Trusopt**
*Merck Sharp & Dohme, Arg.; Merck Sharp & Dohme, Austral.; Merck Sharp & Dohme, Austria; Merck Sharp & Dohme, Belg.; Merck Sharp & Dohme, Braz.; Merck Frosst, Canad.; Merck Sharp & Dohme, Chile; Merck Sharp & Dohme, Denm.; Merck Sharp & Dohme, Fin.; Merck Sharp & Dohme-Chibret, Fr.; Chibret, Ger.; Vianex (Βιανεξ), Gr.; Merck Sharp & Dohme, Hong Kong; Merck Sharp & Dohme, Irl.; Merck Sharp & Dohme, Israel; Merck Sharp & Dohme, Ital.; Merck Sharp & Dohme, Malaysia; Merck Sharp & Dohme, Mex.; Merck Sharp & Dohme, Neth.; Merck Sharp & Dohme, Norw.; Merck Sharp & Dohme, NZ; Chibret, Port.; Merck Sharp & Dohme, S.Afr.; Merck Sharp & Dohme, Singapore; Merck Sharp & Dohme, Spain; Merck Sharp & Dohme, Swed.; Merck Sharp & Dohme, Switz.; Merck Sharp & Dohme, Thai.; Merck Sharp & Dohme, UK; Merck, USA.*
Dorzolamide hydrochloride (p.908·3).
*Glaucoma; ocular hypertension.*

**Truxa** *Raffo, Arg.*
Piroxicam (p.84·2).
*Inflammation.*

**Truxa R** *Raffo, Arg.*
Piroxicam (p.84·2).
Aluminium hydroxide (p.1249·2) is included in this preparation in an attempt to limit adverse effects on the gastrointestinal mucosa.
*Inflammation.*

**Truxal**
*Lundbeck, Austria; Lundbeck, Denm.; Lundbeck, Fin.; Lundbeck, Ger.; Lundbeck, Neth.; Lundbeck, Norw.; Lundbeck, Swed.; Lundbeck, Switz.*
Chlorprothixene (p.682·3), chlorprothixene acetate (p.682·3), chlorprothixene citrate (p.682·3), or chlorprothixene hydrochloride (p.682·3).
*Alcohol and drug withdrawal syndromes; anxiety disorders; behaviour disorders in children; neuroses; pain; psychoses; sleep disorders; vomiting.*

**Truxaletten**
*Lundbeck, Austria; Lundbeck, Switz.*
Chlorprothixene hydrochloride (p.682·3).
*Alcohol and drug withdrawal syndromes; anxiety disorders; behaviour disorders in children; neuroses; pain; psychoses; sleep disorders; vomiting.*

**Try** *Roche Nicholas, Fr.*
Vaginal lubricant.

**Tryasol** *Wernigerode, Ger.*
Codeine phosphate (p.27·1).
*Coughs.*

**Trycam**
*Douglas, NZ†; Douglas, Thai.; TTN, Thai.*
Triazolam (p.725·3).
*Insomnia.*

**Trymo** *Raptakos, India.*
Tripotassium dicitratobismuthate (p.1252·2).
*Peptic ulcer.*

**Tryptal** *Unipharm, Israel.*
Amitriptyline hydrochloride (p.280·3).
*Depression; nocturnal enuresis.*

**Tryptan** *ICN, Canad.*
Tryptophan (p.320·3).
*Adjunct in treatment of depression and bipolar disorder.*

**Tryptanol**
*Sidus, Arg.; Merck Sharp & Dohme, Austral.; Prodome, Braz.; Merck Sharp & Dohme, Hong Kong; Merck Sharp & Dohme, Malaysia; Merck Sharp & Dohme, Mex.; Merck Sharp & Dohme, NZ†; Merck Sharp & Dohme, S.Afr.; Merck Sharp & Dohme, Thai.*
Amitriptyline hydrochloride (p.280·3).
*Depression; nocturnal enuresis.*

**Tryptil** *Cristalia, Braz.†.*
Amitriptyline (p.280·3).
*Depression; nocturnal enuresis.*

**Tryptine** *Amrad, Austral.†.*
Amitriptyline hydrochloride (p.280·3).
*Depression; nocturnal enuresis.*

**Tryptizol**
*Merck Sharp & Dohme, Austria; Merck Sharp & Dohme, Belg.; Merck Sharp & Dohme, Denm.; Morson, Irl.†; Merck Sharp & Dohme, Neth.; Merck Sharp & Dohme, Norw.; Merck Sharp & Dohme, Port.; Neurogard, Spain; Merck Sharp & Dohme, Swed.; Merck Sharp & Dohme, Switz.*
Amitriptyline embonate (p.280·3) or amitriptyline hydrochloride (p.280·3).
*Depression; nocturnal enuresis.*

**Tryptoferm** *Gaschler, Ger.*
Pancreatin (p.1725·3).
*Inflammatory disorders.*

**Tryptomer** *Merind, India.*
Amitriptyline hydrochloride (p.280·3).
*Depression; nocturnal enuresis.*

**Trysul** *Savage, USA†.*
Sulfathiazole (p.264·1); sulfacetamide (p.257·3); sulfabenzamide (p.257·3).
*Vaginitis due to Gardnerella vaginalis.*

**T-Stat**
*Westwood-Squibb, Canad.; Bristol-Myers Squibb, Mex.; Westwood, Singapore; Westwood-Squibb, USA.*
Erythromycin (p.208·1).
*Acne.*

**Tsumura Bakumondo-to** *Tsumura, Jpn.*
Ophiopogon tuber; pinellia tuber; jujube; liquorice; ginseng; brown rice.
*Coughs.*

**Tsumura Dai-kenchu-to** *Tsumura, Jpn.*
Ginseng; zanthoxylum fruit; ginger.
*Gastrointestinal disorders.*

**Tsumura Gosha-jinki-gan** *Tsumura, Jpn.*
Rehmannia root; achyranthes root; cornus fruit; dioscorea rhizome; plantago seed; alisma rhizome; poria sclerotium; moutan bark; cinnamon bark; aconite tuber.
*Cold extremities; tonic; urinary-tract disorders.*

**Tsumura Hachimi-jio-gan** *Tsumura, Jpn.*
Rehmannia root; cornus fruit; dioscorea rhizome; alisma rhizome; poria sclerotium; moutan bark; cinnamon bark; aconite tuber.
*Cold extremities; tonic; urinary-tract disorders.*

**Tsumura Hochu-ekki-to** *Tsumura, Jpn.*
Astragalus root; atractylodes lancea rhizome; ginseng; angelica acutiloba root; bupleurum root; jujube; citrus unshiu peel; liquorice; cimicifuga rhizome; ginger.
*Gastrointestinal disorders; tonic.*

**Tsumura Kakkon-to** *Tsumura, Jpn.*
Pueraria root; jujube; ephedra herb; liquorice; cinnamon bark; peony root; ginger.
*Fever; headache; muscular disorders.*

**Tsumura Kami-shoyo-san** *Tsumura, Jpn.*
Bupleurum root; peony root; atractylodes lancea rhizome; angelica acutiloba root; poria sclerotium; gardenia fruit; moutan bark; liquorice; ginger; mentha herb.
*Menopausal disorders; menstrual disorders; tonic.*

**Tsumura Keishi-bukuryo-gan** *Tsumura, Jpn.*
Cinnamon bark; peony root; peach kernel; poria sclerotium; moutan bark.
*Menstrual and menopausal disorders; orchitis; respiratory-tract disorders.*

**Tsumura Rokumi-gan** *Tsumura, Jpn.*
Rehmannia root; cornus fruit; dioscorea rhizome; alisma rhizome; poria sclerotium; moutan bark.
*Pruritus; tonic; urinary-tract disorders.*

**Tsumura Sairei-to** *Tsumura, Jpn.*
Bupleurum root; alisma rhizome; pinellia tuber; scutellaria root; atractylodes lancea rhizome; jujube; polyporus sclerotium; ginseng; poria sclerotium; liquorice; cinnamon bark; ginger.
*Gastrointestinal disorders; oedema.*

**Tsumura Shakuyaku-kanzo-to** *Tsumura, Jpn.*
Liquorice; peony root.
*Muscle spasm; pain.*

**Tsumura Sho-saiko-to** *Tsumura, Jpn.*
Bupleurum root; pinellia tuber; scutellaria root; jujube; ginseng; liquorice; ginger.
*Gastrointestinal disorders; hepatitis; respiratory-tract infections.*

**Tsumura Sho-seiryu-to** *Tsumura, Jpn.*
Pinellia tuber; liquorice; cinnamon bark; schisandra fruit; asiasarum root; peony root; ephedra herb; ginger.
*Respiratory-tract disorders.*

**Tsumura Toki-shakuyaku-san** *Tsumura, Jpn.*
Peony root; atractylodes lancea rhizome; alisma rhizome; poria sclerotium; cnidium rhizome; angelica acutiloba root.
*Menstrual and menopausal disorders; tonic.*

**Tsumura Unkei-to** *Tsumura, Jpn.*
Ophiopogon tuber; pinellia tuber; angelica acutiloba root; liquorice; cinnamon bark; peony root; cnidium rhizome; ginseng; moutan bark; evodia fruit; ginger; gelatin.
*Circulatory disorders; insomnia; menstrual and menopausal disorders.*

**TTC** *Investigaciones Filosoficas y Cientificas, Mex.†.*
Thiamine (p.1455·2).

**TTD-$B_3$-$B_4$** *Tradiphar, Fr.*
Disulfiram (p.1681·3); nicotinamide (p.1441·2); adenine (p.1647·3).
*Alcoholism.*

**Tuaplex** *Cetus, Arg.*
Pyridoxine; phosphoserine; glutamine (p.1417·1).
*Tonic.*

**Tubarine** *Wellcome, Israel.*
Tubocurarine chloride (p.1409·2).
*Competitive neuromuscular blocker.*

**Tuberen** *Upsifarma, Port.†.*
Rifampicin (p.250·2); isoniazid (p.222·2); pyrazinamide (p.246·3).
*Tuberculosis.*

**Tubergen-Test** *Chiron Behring, Ger.*
Tuberculin (p.1759·1).
*Sensitivity test.*

**Tubersol**
*Aventis Pasteur, Canad.; CSL, NZ; Connaught, NZ; Pasteur Merieux, USA.*
Tuberculin purified protein derivative (p.1759·1).
*Diagnosis of tuberculosis.*

**Tubersol PPD** *Parisis, Spain.*
Tuberculins (p.1759·1).
*Diagnostic agent.*

**Tubertest** *Aventis Pasteur, Fr.*
Tuberculin (p.1759·1).
*Test for tuberculin sensitivity.*

**Tubetam** *Bioquimico, Mex.†.*
Ethambutol (p.212·2).

**Tubial 50B** *SVR, Fr.*
*SPF 50:* Titanium dioxide (p.1160·3); zinc oxide (p.1163·2).
*Sunscreen.*

**Tubilux** *Transdermal, UK.*
Sodium chloride (p.1233·3).
*Nasal dryness; nasal hygiene.*

**Tubilysin** *Orion, Fin.*
Isoniazid (p.222·2).
*Tuberculosis.*

**Tucks**
*Pfizer Consumer, Canad.; Warner-Lambert, USA.*
Hamamelis (p.1696·3); glycerol (p.1694·3).
*Haemorrhoids; perianal cleansing; vaginal cleansing.*

**Tuclase**
*UCB, Belg.; UCB, Ital.; UCB, Neth.*
Pentoxyverine citrate (p.1126·2) or pentoxyverine hydrochloride (p.1126·3).
*Coughs.*

**Tudcabil** *Pharmacia Upjohn, Ital.*
Tauroursodeoxycholic acid (p.1761·1).
*Biliary disorders.*

**Tueor** *Sofar, Ital.*
Barrier cream.

**Tuinal**
*Lilly, Canad.†; Lilly, Irl.†; Flynn, UK; Lilly, USA.*
Secobarbital sodium (p.721·2); amobarbital sodium (p.670·1).
*Insomnia; sedative.*

**Tukol** *Atlantis, Mex.*
Guaifenesin (p.1122·1).
*Coughs.*

**Tukson** *Sons, Mex.†.*
Oxolamine (p.1126·1).
*Coughs.*

**Tulgrasum Antibiotico** *Abbott, Spain.*
Bacitracin zinc (p.161·3) neomycin sulfate (p.235·1); polymyxin B sulfate (p.245·1).
*Burns; skin disorders; skin ulcers; wounds.*

**Tulgrasum Cicatrizante** *Abbott, Spain.*
Glycine; benzyl benzoate (p.1500·2); benzalkonium chloride (p.1168·3); amino acids.
*Burns; skin disorders; skin ulcers; wounds.*

**Tulip** *Pharmacia, Spain†.*
Flurbiprofen (p.43·3).
*Musculoskeletal, joint, and peri-articular disorders; pain.*

**Tulipe-R** *Coup, Gr.*
Astemizole (p.424·2).
*Allergic conjunctivitis; allergic rhinitis; pruritus.*

**Tulle Gras Lumiere**
*Solvay, Belg.†; Solvay, Fr.; Hefa, Ger.†.*
Peru balsam (p.1730·2).
*Burns; wounds.*

**Tulle Vaseline** *Stella, Belg.*
Yellow soft paraffin (p.1479·3); liquid paraffin (p.1479·1).
*Burns; wounds.*

**Tulotract** *Ardeypharm, Ger.*
Lactulose (p.1269·1).
*Constipation; hepatic encephalopathy; salmonella enteritis.*

**Tulox** *Mintlab, Chile.*
Oxolamine (p.1126·1).
*Coughs.*

**Tumarol**
*Note. This name is used for preparations of different composition.*
*Robugen, Ger.*
Eucalyptus oil (p.1686·2); camphor (p.1665·3); menthol (p.1711·3).
*Cold symptoms.*

*Renapharm, Switz.†.*
Camphor (p.1665·3); menthol (p.1711·3); cedar atlant. oil; eucalyptus oil (p.1686·2); turpentine oil (p.1760·1); thymol (p.1194·2).
*Cold symptoms.*

**Tumarol Kinderbalsam** *Robugen, Ger.*
Eucalyptus oil (p.1686·2); oleum pini sylvestris.
*Cold symptoms.*

**Tumarol-N** *Robugen, Ger.*
Camphor (p.1665·3); menthol (p.1711·3); eucalyptus oil (p.1686·2).
*Cold symptoms.*

**Tumax** *Sriprasit, Thai.*
Chlordiazepoxide hydrochloride (p.674·2); clidinium bromide (p.480·2).
*Gastrointestinal disorders; peptic ulcer; smooth muscle spasm.*

**Tumdi** *Sriprasit, Thai.*
Paracetamol (p.76·2).
*Fever; pain.*

**Tums**
*GlaxoSmithKline, Arg.; SmithKline Beecham, Braz.†; GlaxoSmithKline Consumer, Canad.; SmithKline Beecham, Gr.; GlaxoSmithKline Consumer, Irl.; SmithKline Beecham, Israel; GlaxoSmithKline Consumer, Port.; GlaxoSmithKline Consumer, UK; GlaxoSmithKline, USA.*
Calcium carbonate (p.1254·2).
*Calcium supplement; gastric hyperacidity.*

**Tums Plus** *SmithKline Beecham, USA.*
Calcium carbonate (p.1254·2); simeticone (p.1289·2).

**Tundra** *Frasca, Arg.*
Naproxen (p.65·1).
*Inflammation.*

**Tundrax** *Tecnobio, Spain†.*
Pseudoephedrine hydrochloride (p.1129·2); ebastine (p.433·1).
*Allergic rhinitis.*

**Tuneluz** *Baldacci, Port.*
Fluoxetine hydrochloride (p.292·1).
*Bulimia; depression.*

**Tunik** *Baliarda, Arg.*
Ademetionine (p.1647·2).
Lidocaine hydrochloride (p.1377·3) is included in this preparation to alleviate the pain of injection.
*Osteoarthritis.*

**Tunik B12** *Baliarda, Arg.*
Ademetionine (p.1647·2); vitamin $B_{12}$ (p.1458·2).
Lidocaine hydrochloride (p.1377·3) is included in this preparation to alleviate the pain of injection.
*Osteoarthritis.*

**Tunitol-BX** *Streger, Mex.*
Ambroxol hydrochloride (p.1114·3).
*Respiratory-tract congestion.*

**Tuosomin** *Leiras, Thai.*
Tamoxifen citrate (p.584·1).
*Anovulatory infertility; breast cancer; endometrial cancer.*

**Tupast** *Kleva, Gr.*
Ranitidine hydrochloride (p.1285·2).
*Conditions where gastric acid reduction is beneficial; gastric hypersecretion including Zollinger-Ellison syndrome; peptic ulcer.*

**Turbatherm** *Torfwerk Einfeld, Ger.†.*
Peat.
*Gastrointestinal disorders; musculoskeletal and joint disorders.*

**Turbaund** *Rafarm, Gr.*
Tolfenamic acid (p.94·2).
*Dysmenorrhoea; inflammation; musculoskeletal and joint disorders; pain.*

**Turbinal** *Valeas, Ital.*
Beclometasone dipropionate (p.1091·1).
*Rhinitis.*

**Turbocalcin**
*SmithKline Beecham, Braz.†; GlaxoSmithKline, Ital.*
Elcatonin (p.768·3).
*Hypercalcaemia; osteoporosis; Paget's disease of bone; reflex sympathetic dystrophy.*

**Turbogesic** *Laboratorios Chile, Chile.*
Diclofenac diethylamine (p.32·1).
*Musculoskeletal, joint, peri-articular, and soft-tissue disorders.*

**Turbovit** *Medipharm, Chile.*
Multivitamin preparation with or without minerals (p.1417·1).
*Tonic.*

**Turexan Capilla** *Turimed, Switz.*
Cetrimonium bromide (p.1173·1); urea (p.1162·2); dexpanthenol (p.1727·2).
*Scalp disorders.*

**Turexan Creme** *Turimed, Switz.*
Undecenoic acid (p.410·3); zinc undecenoate (p.411·1).
*Barrier cream; skin disorders.*

**Turexan Douche** *Turimed, Switz.*
Undecenoic acid (p.410·3).
*Skin disorders; soap substitute.*

**Turexan Emulsion** *Turimed, Switz.*
Undecenoic acid (p.410·3); zinc undecenoate (p.411·1); triclosan (p.1195·2).
*Skin disorders; soap substitute.*

**Turexan Lotion** *Turimed, Switz.*
Urea (p.1162·2); dexpanthenol (p.1727·2).
*Skin disorders.*

**Turfa** *Worwag, Ger.*
Triamterene (p.1016·2); hydrochlorothiazide (p.933·2).
*Hypertension; oedema.*

**Turgoral** *Medley, Braz.†.*
Glucose; sodium citrate; potassium chloride; sodium chloride (p.1417·1)(p.1222·2).

**Turicard** *Jenapharm, Ger.†.*
Glyceryl trinitrate (p.923·2).
*Cardiac disorders.*

**Turifarm** *Reuffer, Mex.†.*
Rifampicin (p.250·2).

**Turimonit** *Jenapharm, Ger.*
Isosorbide mononitrate (p.942·1).
*Cardiac disorders.*

**Turimycin** *Jenapharm, Ger.*
Clindamycin hydrochloride (p.194·2) or clindamycin phosphate (p.194·2).
*Bacterial infections.*

**Turinal**
*Gedeon Richter, Hong Kong; Gedeon Richter, Malaysia; Gedeon Richter, Singapore.*
Allylestrenol (p.1541·3).
*Premature labour; threatened or recurrent miscarriage.*

**Turineurin** *Jenapharm, Ger.*
Hypericum (p.299·1).
*Depression.*

**Turiplex** *Jenapharm, Ger.†.*
Cucurbita (p.1677·3).
*Urinary-tract disorders.*

**Turisan** *Turimed, Switz.*
Cetrimonium bromide (p.1173·1).
*Skin disinfection; skin infections.*

**Turisteron** *Jenapharm, Ger.*
Ethinylestradiol propanesulphonate (p.1553·2).
*Prostatic cancer.*

**Turixin** *GlaxoSmithKline, Ger.*
Mupirocin calcium (p.233·2).
*Nasal carriage of staphylococci.*

**Turmerik** *Knop, Chile.*
Turmeric (p.1058·3).
*Liver disorders; musculoskeletal and joint disorders.*

**Turoptin**
*Ciba Vision, Ital.; Novartis Ophthalmics, Switz.*
Metipranolol (p.955·3).
*Glaucoma; ocular hypertension.*

**Turpentine White Liniment** *McGloin, Austral.†.*
Turpentine oil (p.1760·1); camphor (p.1665·3).
*Muscle pain.*

**Turresis** *Irex, Port.*
Ethambutol hydrochloride (p.211·3).
*Tuberculosis.*

**Tusabron** *Bago, Chile.*
Clobutinol hydrochloride (p.1117·1); orciprenaline sulfate (p.790·2); ammonium chloride (p.1115·2).
*Coughs.*

**Tusant** *Lupin, India.*
Terfenadine (p.441·1); dextromethorphan hydrobromide (p.1117·3).
*Coughs.*

**Tusben** *Benedetti, Ital.*
Dimemorfan phosphate (p.1118·3).
*Coughs.*

**Tuscalman**
*Note. This name is used for preparations of different composition.*
*Kwizda, Austria; Berna, Ital.†; Berna, Switz.*
*Oral drops; suppositories:* Noscapine hydrochloride (p.1125·3); guaifenesin (p.1122·1).
*Respiratory-tract disorders.*

*Kwizda, Austria.*
*Syrup:* Noscapine hydrochloride (p.1125·3); guaifenesin (p.1122·1); althaea (p.1651·3); sambucus (p.1741·3).
*Bronchitis; catarrh; coughs; laryngitis; sore throat.*

*Berna, Spain.*
*Syrup; suppositories:* Noscapine hydrochloride (p.1125·3).
*Coughs.*

*Berna, Switz.*
*Syrup:* Noscapine hydrochloride (p.1125·3); guaifenesin (p.1122·1); althaea (p.1651·3).
*Respiratory-tract disorders.*

**Tusco** *Hua, Thai.*
Dextromethorphan hydrobromide (p.1117·3).
*Coughs.*

**Tuscolgen** *Great Eastern, Thai.; Westmont, Thai.*
Dextromethorphan hydrobromide (p.1117·3); guaifenesin (p.1122·1); chlorphenamine maleate (p.427·3).
*Coughs.*

**Tusehli** *Ehlinger, Mex.†.*
Benzonatate (p.1115·3).

**Tuselin Descongestivo** *Reig Jofre, Spain.*
Dextromethorphan hydrobromide (p.1117·3); phenylephrine hydrochloride (p.1126·3).
*Coughs; nasal congestion.*

**Tuselin Expectorante** *Reig Jofre, Spain†.*
Alloclamide hydrochloride (p.1114·2); ammonium chloride (p.1115·2); carbocisteine (p.1116·2); phenylephrine hydrochloride (p.1126·3); ipecacuanha (p.1122·3).
*Respiratory-tract disorders.*

**Tuseran** *Medichem, Hong Kong.*
Dextromethorphan hydrobromide (p.1117·3); phenylpropanolamine hydrochloride (p.1127·3); paracetamol (p.76·2).
Formerly contained dextromethorphan hydrobromide, guaifenesin, phenylpropanolamine hydrochloride, chlorphenamine maleate, and paracetamol.
*Coughs and cold symptoms.*

**Tusibron**
*Note. This name is used for preparations of different composition.*
*Kener, Mex.†.*
Ambroxol (p.1114·3).
*Kenwood, USA.*
Guaifenesin (p.1122·1).
*Coughs.*

**Tusibron-DM** *Kenwood, USA.*
Guaifenesin (p.1122·1); dextromethorphan hydrobromide (p.1117·3).
*Coughs.*

**Tusical** *Andromaco, Mex.*
Benzonatate (p.1115·3).
*Coughs.*

**Tusigen**
*Note. This name is used for preparations of different composition.*
*Bago, Chile.*
Chlorphenamine maleate (p.427·3); pseudoephedrine hydrochloride (p.1129·2); codeine phosphate (p.27·1).
*Coughs.*
*Liomont, Mex.*
Zipeprol hydrochloride (p.1132·3).
*Coughs.*

**Tusilen** *Allen, Mex.*
Dextromethorphan hydrobromide (p.1117·3); guaifenesin (p.1122·1); phenylephrine hydrochloride (p.1126·3).
*Coughs; respiratory-tract congestion.*

**Tusilen Pediatrico** *Allen, Mex.*
Dextromethorphan hydrobromide (p.1117·3); guaifenesin (p.1122·1); paracetamol (p.76·2).
*Coughs; fever.*

**Tusitato** *Fustery, Mex.*
Benzonatate (p.1115·3).
*Coughs.*

**Tusitinas** *Pensa, Spain.*
Dextromethorphan hydrobromide (p.1117·3).
*Coughs.*

**Tusminal** *Medipharm, Chile.*
Dextromethorphan (p.1117·3).
*Coughs.*

**Tusno** *Milano, Thai.*
Dextromethorphan hydrobromide (p.1117·3); guaifenesin (p.1122·1); bromhexine hydrochloride (p.1115·3).
*Coughs.*

**Tusofren** *Almirall, Spain†.*
Dropropizine (p.1119·3).
*Coughs.*

**Tusol** *Rhone-Poulenc Rorer, Mex.†.*
Oxolamine citrate (p.1126·1).

**Tusolven** *Vedim, Port.*
Ambroxol acefyllinate (p.1114·3).
*Obstructive airways disease.*

**Tusorama** *Quimifar, Spain.*
Dextromethorphan hydrobromide (p.1117·3).
*Coughs.*

**Tuspel** *Indoco, India.*
Diphenhydramine hydrochloride (p.431·3); ammonium chloride (p.1115·2); sodium citrate (p.1223·2); menthol (p.1711·3).
*Coughs.*

**Tuspel Plus** *Indoco, India.*
Bromhexine hydrochloride (p.1115·3); terbutaline (p.797·3); ammonium chloride (p.1115·2); menthol (p.1711·3).
*Coughs.*

**Tuspress** *Indoco, India.*
Dextromethorphan hydrobromide (p.1117·3); phenylpropanolamine hydrochloride (p.1127·3); chlorphenamine maleate (p.427·3); menthol (p.1711·3).
*Cold symptoms; coughs; nasal congestion.*

**Tusquelin** *Circle, USA†.*
Phenylpropanolamine hydrochloride (p.1127·3); dextromethorphan hydrobromide (p.1117·3); phenylephrine hydrochloride (p.1126·3); chlorphenamine maleate (p.427·3); ipecacuanha (p.1122·3); sulfogaiacol (p.1131·1).
*Coughs and cold symptoms.*

**Tusquit** *Xixia, S.Afr.*
Diphenhydramine hydrochloride (p.431·3); ammonium chloride (p.1115·2).
*Coughs.*

**Tuss** *Disperga, Austria†.*
Wild thyme; castanea vulgaris.
*Coughs and viscous mucus.*

**Tuss Hustenstiller** *Rentschler, Ger.*
Dextromethorphan hydrobromide (p.1117·3).
*Coughs.*

**Tussa** *Silom, Thai.*
Guaifenesin (p.1122·1).
*Coughs.*

**Tussafed** *Everett, USA.*
Carbinoxamine maleate (p.426·3); pseudoephedrine hydrochloride (p.1129·2); dextromethorphan hydrobromide (p.1117·3).
*Coughs and cold symptoms.*

**Tussafed HC** *Everett, USA.*
Hydrocodone tartrate (p.45·1); phenylephrine hydrochloride (p.1126·3); guaifenesin (p.1122·1).
*Coughs.*

**Tussafed-LA** *Everett, USA.*
Guaifenesin (p.1122·1); pseudoephedrine hydrochloride (p.1129·2); dextromethorphan hydrobromide (p.1117·3).
*Coughs; respiratory-tract congestion.*

**Tussafin Expectorant** *Rugby, USA.*
Pseudoephedrine hydrochloride (p.1129·2); guaifenesin (p.1122·1); hydrocodone tartrate (p.45·1).
*Coughs.*

**Tussafug**
*Robugen, Ger.; Medipharm, Switz.†.*
Benproperine embonate (p.1115·2) or benproperine phosphate (p.1115·2).
*Coughs.*

**Tuss-Allergine Modified TD** *Rugby, USA†.*
Phenylpropanolamine hydrochloride (p.1127·3); caramiphen edisilate (p.1116·2).
*Coughs.*

**Tussamag**
*Note. This name is used for preparations of different composition.*
*Montavit, Austria.*
*Ointment:* Spike lavender oil (p.1749·2); eucalyptus oil (p.1686·2); turpentine oil (p.1760·1); camphor (p.1665·3).
*Oral liquid:* Thyme (p.1755·2); castanea vulgaris.
*Bronchitis; catarrh; coughs.*
*Teofarma, Ital.*
Wild thyme; castanea leaves.
*Respiratory-tract congestion.*

**Tussamag Codeintropfen** *CT, Ger.†.*
Codeine phosphate (p.27·1).
*Coughs.*

**Tussamag Complex** *Teofarma, Ital.*
Wild thyme; dropropizine (p.1119·3).
*Coughs.*

**Tussamag Erkaltungsbalsam N** *CT, Ger.*
Eucalyptus oil (p.1686·2); pine needle oil.
*Catarrh.*

**Tussamag Halstabletten** *CT, Ger.†.*
Benzocaine (p.1370·3); menthol (p.1711·3); peppermint oil (p.1283·2); eucalyptus oil (p.1686·2).
*Pain, inflammation, and infection of the mouth and throat.*

**Tussamag Hustensaft N** *CT, Ger.*
Thyme (p.1755·2).
*Bronchitis; catarrh; coughs.*

**Tussamag Hustentropfen N** *CT, Ger.*
Thyme (p.1755·2).
*Bronchitis; catarrh; coughs.*

**Tussamed** *Hexal, Ger.†.*
Clobutinol hydrochloride (p.1117·1).
*Coughs.*

**Tussaminic C** *Sandoz, Canad.†.*
Codeine phosphate (p.27·1); phenylpropanolamine hydrochloride (p.1127·3); mepyramine maleate (p.437·1); pheniramine maleate (p.438·3).
*Coughs.*

**Tussaminic DH** *Sandoz, Canad.†.*
Hydrocodone tartrate (p.45·1); phenylpropanolamine hydrochloride (p.1127·3); mepyramine maleate (p.437·1); pheniramine maleate (p.438·3).
*Coughs.*

**Tussanil Compositum** *Vifor, Switz.*
Noscapine (p.1125·3); drosera (p.1683·1); liquorice (p.1270·2); eucalyptus oil (p.1686·2); peppermint oil (p.1283·2).
*Coughs.*

**Tussanil DH** *Misemer, USA.*
*Syrup:* Phenylephrine hydrochloride (p.1126·3); chlorphenamine maleate (p.427·3); hydrocodone tartrate (p.45·1).
*Coughs and cold symptoms.*
*Tablets†:* Phenylpropanolamine hydrochloride (p.1127·3); hydrocodone tartrate (p.45·1); guaifenesin (p.1122·1).
*Coughs.*

**Tussanil N** *Vifor, Switz.*
Noscapine hydrochloride (p.1125·3).
*Coughs.*

**Tussanil Plain** *Misemer, USA.*
Phenylephrine hydrochloride (p.1126·3); chlorphenamine maleate (p.427·3).
*Upper respiratory-tract symptoms.*

**Tussantiol** *Medisa, Switz.*
Carbocisteine (p.1116·2).
*Respiratory-tract disorders with increased mucus.*

**Tussanyl** *Giovanardi, Ital.*
Sulfogaiacol (p.1131·1); grindelia (p.1696·1).
*Catarrh; coughs.*

**Tussar-2** *Rhone-Poulenc Rorer, USA.*
Codeine phosphate (p.27·1); guaifenesin (p.1122·1); pseudoephedrine hydrochloride (p.1129·2).
*Coughs.*

**Tussar DM** *Rhone-Poulenc Rorer, USA.*
Dextromethorphan hydrobromide (p.1117·3); chlorphenamine maleate (p.427·3); pseudoephedrine hydrochloride (p.1129·2).
*Coughs and cold symptoms.*

**Tussar SF** *Rhone-Poulenc Rorer, USA.*
Codeine phosphate (p.27·1); guaifenesin (p.1122·1); pseudoephedrine hydrochloride (p.1129·2).
*Coughs.*

**Tusscodin** *Lannacher, Austria.*
Nicocodine hydrochloride (p.1125·2).
*Coughs.*

**Tuss-DM** *Hyrex, USA.*
Dextromethorphan hydrobromide (p.1117·3); guaifenesin (p.1122·1).
*Coughs.*

**Tussed** *Hexal, Ger.*
Clobutinol hydrochloride (p.1117·1).
*Coughs.*

**Tussefar** *Faran, Gr.*
Ambroxol hydrochloride (p.1114·3).
*Respiratory disorders associated with viscous mucus.*

**Tussend** *Monarch, USA.*
Hydrocodone tartrate (p.45·1); pseudoephedrine hydrochloride (p.1129·2); chlorphenamine maleate (p.427·3).
*Coughs.*

**Tussi-12** *Wallace, USA.*
Pentoxyverine tannate (p.1126·3); chlorphenamine tannate (p.428·1); phenylephrine tannate (p.1127·2).
*Coughs.*

**Tussi-12 D** *Wallace, USA.*
Pentoxyverine tannate (p.1126·3); mepyramine tannate (p.437·1); phenylephrine tannate (p.1127·2).
*Coughs.*

**Tussibron** *Sella, Ital.*
Oxolamine citrate (p.1126·1).
*Coughs.*

**Tussicare** *ST, Thai.*
Guaifenesin (p.1122·1); dextromethorphan hydrobromide (p.1117·3).
*Coughs.*

**Tussicon** *The Forty-Two, Thai.†.*
*Syrup:* Dextromethorphan hydrobromide (p.1117·3); guaifenesin (p.1122·1); sodium citrate (p.1223·2).
*Tablets:* Dextromethorphan hydrobromide (p.1117·3); phenylpropanolamine hydrochloride (p.1127·3); chlorphenamine maleate (p.427·3).
*Bronchitis; coughs; respiratory-tract disorders.*

**Tussi-12D S** *Wallace, USA.*
Pentoxyverine tannate (p.1126·3); mepyramine tannate (p.437·1); phenylephrine tannate (p.1127·2).
*Upper respiratory-tract disorders.*

**Tussidane** *Elerte, Fr.*
Dextromethorphan hydrobromide (p.1117·3).
*Coughs.*

**Tussidermil N** *Li-il, Ger.*
Eucalyptus oil (p.1686·2).
*Catarrh; musculoskeletal and joint disorders.*

**Tussidex** *Xepa-Soul Pattinson, Singapore.*
Dextromethorphan hydrobromide (p.1117·3).
*Coughs.*

**Tussidoron** *Weleda, Fr.*
Thyme (p.1755·2); drosera (p.1683·1).
*Coughs.*

**Tussidrill** *Pierre Fabre, Spain.*
Dextromethorphan hydrobromide (p.1117·3).
*Coughs.*

**Tussidyl** *Tika, Swed.†.*
Dextromethorphan hydrobromide (p.1117·3).
*Coughs.*

**Tussifed** *Warner-Lambert, Fr.†.*
Triprolidine hydrochloride (p.442·3); dextromethorphan hydrobromide (p.1117·3).
Formerly contained triprolidine hydrochloride, pseudoephedrine hydrochloride, and dextromethorphan hydrobromide.
*Coughs.*

**Tussifen** *Hexal, Braz.*
Belladonna (p.479·1); jaborandi; eucalyptus (p.1686·1); ginger (p.1267·1); siparuna guyanensis; lantana camara; mikania glomerulata.
*Respiratory-tract congestion.*

**Tussiflex** *Kemyos, Ital.†.*
Oxeladin citrate (p.1126·1); terpin hydrate (p.1131·1).
*Coughs.*

**Tussiflex D** *Abbott, Braz.*
Dropropizine (p.1119·3).
*Coughs.*

**Tussiflorin forte** *Pascoe, Ger.*
Hedera helix; primula root (p.1735·1); thyme (p.1755·2).
*Asthma; bronchitis.*

**Tussiflorin Hustensaft** *Pascoe, Ger.*
Vogelknoterichkraut; sanikelkraut; hohlzahnkraut; primula root (p.1735·1).
*Asthma; bronchitis; coughs.*

**Tussiflorin Hustenstiller** *Pascoe, Ger.*
Thyme (p.1755·2); drosera (p.1683·1).
*Cold symptoms; coughs.*

**Tussiflorin Hustentropfen** *Pascoe, Ger.*
Vogelknoterichkraut; sanikelkraut; hohlzahnkraut; primula root (p.1735·1).
*Asthma; bronchitis; coughs.*

**Tussiflorin N** *Pascoe, Ger.†.*
Knotgrass; sanicula europaea; galeopsis ochroleuca; equisetum (p.1684·1); cowslip rhizome (p.1735·1).
*Coughs and associated respiratory-tract disorders.*

**Tussigon** *Daniels, USA.*
Hydrocodone tartrate (p.45·1); homatropine methylbromide (p.483·2).
*Coughs and cold symptoms.*

**Tussilene** *Alpharma, Fr.*
Carbocisteine (p.1116·2).
*Respiratory-tract disorders.*

**Tussilinct** *Restan, S.Afr.*
Diphenhydramine hydrochloride (p.431·3); codeine phosphate (p.27·1); ammonium chloride (p.1115·2); sodium citrate (p.1223·2).
*Coughs.*

**Tussiliv** *Delta, Braz.*
Salbutamol sulfate (p.791·3).
*Obstructive airways disease.*

**Tussils**
*Boots, Hong Kong; Boots Healthcare, Malaysia; Boots, Singapore; Boots, Thai.*
Dextromethorphan hydrobromide (p.1117·3).
Formerly contained dextromethorphan hydrobromide and phenylephrine hydrochloride in *Hong Kong.*
*Coughs.*

**Tussimag Codein** *Montavit, Austria.*
Codeine phosphate (p.27·1); castanea vulgaris.
Formerly known as Tussamag mit Codein und Ephedrin and contained codeine phosphate, aesculus, and ephedrine hydrochloride.
*Bronchitis; catarrh; coughs.*

**Tussimont** *Pharmonta, Austria.*
*Ointment:* Camphor (p.1665·3); menthol (p.1711·3); eucalyptus oil (p.1686·2).
*Coughs and cold symptoms.*
*Oral drops:* Ammonium chloride (p.1115·2); thyme (p.1755·2); plantago lanceolata (p.1738·2).
*Coughs.*
*Oral liquid:* Senega (p.1130·2); thyme (p.1755·2).
*Coughs.*
*Tea:* Thyme (p.1755·2); plantago lanceolata (p.1738·2); althaea (p.1651·3); aniseed (p.1655·2); orange flower (p.1724·1).
*Catarrh; coughs; mouth and throat inflammation.*

**Tussin Antitussive** *Stanley, Canad.*
Dextromethorphan hydrobromide (p.1117·3).

**Tussin Antitussive, Expectorant, Decongestant** *Stanley, Canad.*
Pseudoephedrine hydrochloride (p.1129·2); dextromethorphan hydrobromide (p.1117·3); guaifenesin (p.1122·1).

**Tussin Children's DM** *Stanley, Canad.*
Pseudoephedrine hydrochloride (p.1129·2); dextromethorphan hydrobromide (p.1117·3).

**Tussin Expectorant** *Stanley, Canad.*
Guaifenesin (p.1122·1).

**TUSSinfant N** *Rubiepharm, Ger.*
Primula root (p.1735·1); thyme (p.1755·2).
*Cold symptoms.*

**Tussinol** *Pfizer Consumer, Austral.*
Pholcodine (p.1128·3).
*Coughs.*

**Tussinol Cough & Cold** *Pfizer Consumer, Austral.†.*
Chlorphenamine maleate (p.427·3); dextromethorphan hydrobromide (p.1117·3); pseudoephedrine hydrochloride (p.1129·2).
*Coughs and cold symptoms.*

**Tussinol Day-Time Cough & Cold** *Pfizer Consumer, Austral.†.*
Dextromethorphan hydrobromide (p.1117·3); pseudoephedrine hydrochloride (p.1129·2).
*Coughs and cold symptoms.*

**Tussinol for Dry Coughs** *Pfizer Consumer, Austral.*
Dextromethorphan hydrobromide (p.1117·3).
*Coughs.*

**Tussinol Expectorant** *Pfizer Consumer, Austral.*
Bromhexine hydrochloride (p.1115·3); guaifenesin (p.1122·1).
*Coughs.*

**Tussin-Pinho** *Gilton, Braz.†.*
Potassium iodide (p.1598·1); guaifenesin (p.1122·1).
*Respiratory-tract congestion.*

**Tussionex** *Aventis, Canad.*
Hydrocodone resin complex (p.45·1); phenyltoloxamine resin complex (p.439·1).
*Coughs.*

**Tussionex Pennkinetic** *Celltech, USA.*
Hydrocodone polistirex (p.45·1); chlorphenamine polistirex (p.428·1).
*Coughs and cold symptoms.*

**Tussi-Organidin DM NR** *Wallace, USA.*
Guaifenesin (p.1122·1); dextromethorphan hydrobromide (p.1117·3).
Tussi-Organidin DM formerly contained iodinated glycerol and dextromethorphan hydrobromide.
*Coughs.*

**Tussi-Organidin NR** *Wallace, USA.*
Codeine phosphate (p.27·1); guaifenesin (p.1122·1).
Tussi-Organidin formerly contained codeine phosphate and iodinated glycerol.
*Coughs.*

**Tussipax** *Bailleul, Fr.*
*Oral solution; tablets:* Ethylmorphine hydrochloride (p.37·3); codeine (p.27·1).
*Syrup:* Ethylmorphine hydrochloride (p.37·3); codeine (p.27·1); tolu balsam (p.1131·3); pectoral concentrate.
*Coughs.*

**Tussipax a l'Euquinine** *Therica, Fr.†.*
Ethylmorphine hydrochloride (p.37·3); codeine (p.27·1); pine oil; eucalyptus oil (p.1686·2); quinine etabonate (p.460·1).
*Coughs.*

**Tussipect** *Qualiphar, Belg.*
Dextromethorphan hydrobromide (p.1117·3).
*Coughs.*

**Tussiphane** *Celltech, Belg.†.*
Dextromethorphan hydrobromide (p.1117·3).
*Coughs.*

**Tussiplex** *Vifor, Switz.*
Chlorphenamine maleate (p.427·3); phenylephrine hydrochloride (p.1126·3); pholcodine (p.1128·3); guaifenesin (p.1122·1).
*Coughs.*

**Tussirex** *Scot-Tussin, USA.*
Codeine phosphate (p.27·1); pheniramine maleate (p.438·3); phenylephrine hydrochloride (p.1126·3); sodium citrate (p.1223·2); sodium salicylate (p.90·1); caffeine citrate (p.782·1); menthol (p.1711·3).
*Coughs.*

**Tussis**
*Note. This name is used for preparations of different composition.*
*OM, Port.†.*
Bibenzonium bromide (p.1115·3).
*Coughs.*
*Berlin Pharm, Thai.†.*
Diphenhydramine hydrochloride (p.431·3); ammonium chloride (p.1115·2); sodium citrate (p.1223·2); glycerol (p.1694·3); menthol (p.1711·3).
*Coughs; nasal congestion.*

**Tussisana N** *Muller Goppingen, Ger.*
Homoeopathic preparation.

**Tussisedal** *Elerte, Fr.*
Noscapine (p.1125·3); promethazine (p.439·1); polysorbate 85 (Tween 85).
*Coughs.*

**Tussistin** *DHU, Ger.*
Homoeopathic preparation.

**Tussistin N** *DHU, Ger.*
Homoeopathic preparation.

**Tussitot** *Restan, S.Afr.*
Diphenhydramine hydrochloride (p.431·3); codeine phosphate (p.27·1); ammonium chloride (p.1115·2); sodium citrate (p.1223·2).
*Coughs.*

**Tussiverlan** *Verla, Ger.†.*
Acetylcysteine (p.1112·3).
*Respiratory-tract disorders with viscous mucus.*

**Tussivit** *Ducto, Braz.*
Potassium iodide (p.1598·1); guaifenesin (p.1122·1).
*Coughs.*

**Tussizone** *Mallinckrodt, USA.*
Pentoxyverine tannate (p.1126·3); chlorphenamine tannate (p.428·1).
*Upper respiratory-tract disorders.*

**Tuss-LA** *Hyrex, USA.*
Pseudoephedrine hydrochloride (p.1129·2); guaifenesin (p.1122·1).
*Coughs.*

**Tusso** *BASF, Ger.†.*
Ambroxol hydrochloride (p.1114·3).
*Respiratory-tract disorders with increased or viscous mucus.*

**Tusso Rhinathiol** *Sanofi Synthelabo, Belg.*
Dextromethorphan hydrobromide (p.1117·3).
Formerly known as Rhinathiol Antitussivum.
*Coughs.*

**Tussocal** *Agis, Israel.*
Dextromethorphan hydrobromide (p.1117·3); phenylephrine hydrochloride (p.1126·3).
*Coughs; nasal congestion.*

**Tussodan DM** *Odan, Canad.*
Dextromethorphan hydrobromide (p.1117·3); pseudoephedrine hydrochloride (p.1129·2).

**Tussodina** *Dovalle, Braz.*
Sodium dibunate (p.1130·2); sodium benzoate (p.1169·3); sulfogaiacol (p.1131·1).
*Coughs.*

**Tussogest Extended-Release** *Major, USA†.*
Phenylpropanolamine hydrochloride (p.1127·3); caramiphen edisilate (p.1116·2).
*Coughs.*

**Tussol**
*Note. This name is used for preparations of different composition.*
*Ibefar, Braz.†.*
Oxomemazine hydrochloride (p.438·2); sodium benzoate (p.1169·3); guaifenesin (p.1122·1); potassium iodide (p.1598·1); ipecacuanha (p.1122·3).
*Coughs.*
*Amnol, Ital.*
Myrtillus (p.1718·3); thyme (p.1755·2); tilia (p.1756·2); liquorice (p.1270·2).
*Respiratory-tract disorders.*
*Nycomed, Norw.†.*
Guaifenesin (p.1122·1); ammonium chloride (p.1115·2); liquorice (p.1270·2); ammonium glycyrrhizinate (p.1115·2).
*Coughs.*

**Tussolvina** *Pfizer, Ital.*
Nepinalone hydrochloride (p.1125·2).
*Coughs.*

**Tussophedrine** *Trima, Israel.*
Ephedrine hydrochloride (p.1120·1); codeine phosphate (p.27·1); sulfogaiacol (p.1131·1); sodium benzoate (p.1169·3).
*Coughs.*

**Tussoret** *Fujisawa, Ger.*
Codeine phosphate (p.27·1).
Formerly known as Tussoretard SN.
*Coughs.*

**Tussoretardin** *Klinge, Austria.*
White day capsules, pentoxyverine citrate (p.1126·2); methylephedrine hydrochloride (p.1124·2); blue night capsules, pentoxyverine citrate; diphenhydramine hydrochloride (p.431·3).
*Coughs.*

**Tussosedan** *Teva, Israel.*
Pheniramine maleate (p.438·3); ephedrine hydrochloride (p.1120·1); codeine phosphate (p.27·1); ammonium chloride (p.1115·2).
*Coughs.*

**Tuss-Tan** *Econolab, USA.*
Pentoxyverine tannate (p.1126·3); chlorphenamine tannate (p.428·1); ephedrine tannate (p.1120·3).
*Upper respiratory-tract symptoms.*

**Tusstat** *Century, USA.*
Diphenhydramine hydrochloride (p.431·3).
*Coughs.*

**Tussucalman** *Ibefar, Braz.†.*
Sulfogaiacol (p.1131·1); sodium benzoate (p.1169·3); ammonium chloride (p.1115·2); ipecacuanha (p.1122·3); liquorice (p.1270·2); belladonna (p.479·1).
*Coughs.*

**Tussycalm** *Aventis, Ital.*
Dextromethorphan hydrobromide (p.1117·3).
*Coughs.*

**Tutiverm** *Elofar, Braz.†.*
Tiabendazole (p.114·2).
*Nematode infections.*

**Tutofusin**
*Fresenius Kabi, Austria†.*
Electrolyte infusion with glucose (p.1217·1).
*Carbohydrate source; fluid and electrolyte disorders.*
*Baxter, Ger.*
Electrolyte infusion (p.1217·1).
*Fluid and electrolyte disorders; peritoneal irrigation.*

**Tutofusin BG** *Baxter, Ger.*
Electrolyte infusion with glucose (p.1217·1).
*Carbohydrate source; fluid and electrolyte disorders.*

**Tutofusin BX** *Baxter, Ger.*
Electrolyte infusion with xylitol (p.1217·1).
*Carbohydrate source; fluid and electrolyte disorders.*

**Tutofusin G5** *Baxter, Ger.*
Electrolyte infusion with glucose (p.1217·1).
*Carbohydrate source; fluid and electrolyte disorders.*

**Tutofusin H G5** *Baxter, Ger.*
Electrolyte infusion with glucose (p.1217·1).
*Carbohydrate source; fluid and electrolyte disorders.*

**Tutofusin K 10** *Baxter, Ger.*
Electrolyte infusion (p.1217·1).
*Fluid and electrolyte disorders.*

**Tutofusin K 80** *Baxter, Ger.*
Electrolyte infusion with xylitol and glucose (p.1217·1).
*Potassium deficiency in cardiac disorders.*

**Tutofusin NS X** *Baxter, Ger.*
Electrolyte infusion with xylitol (p.1217·1).
*Fluid and electrolyte disorders.*

**Tutofusin OP** *Baxter, Ger.*
Electrolyte infusion (p.1217·1).
*Fluid and electrolyte disorders.*

**Tutofusin OP X** *Baxter, Ger.*
Electrolyte infusion with xylitol (p.1217·1).
*Carbohydrate source; fluid and electrolyte disorders.*

**Tutofusin OP G** *Baxter, Ger.*
Electrolyte infusion with glucose (p.1217·1).
*Carbohydrate source; fluid and electrolyte disorders.*

**Tutofusin S** *Baxter, Ger.*
Sodium chloride (p.1233·3); sodium acetate (p.1223·1); sorbitol (p.1446·3).
*Fluid retention; renal failure.*

**Tutoplast Dura** *Tutogen, Ger.*
Absorbable collagen from dehydrated human dura mater (p.1674·3).
*Repair or closure of body tissue.*

**Tutoplast Fascia lata** *Tutogen, Ger.*
Dehydrated human fascia lata (p.1674·3).
*Repair of joints and tendons.*

**Tutoseral** *Streuli, Switz.*
Electrolyte infusion (p.1217·1).
*Fluid and electrolyte disorders.*

**Tuttozem N** *Strathmann, Ger.†.*
Dexamethasone (p.1097·1).
*Burns; skin disorders.*

**Tux** *Pfizer Consumer, Belg.*
Ethylmorphine hydrochloride (p.37·3); codeine phosphate (p.27·1); ephedrine hydrochloride (p.1120·1); guaifenesin (p.1122·1); sodium benzoate (p.1169·3); sodium camsilate; senega (p.1130·2); senna (p.1288·2); tolu balsam (p.1131·3).
*Colds; coughs; respiratory disorders.*

**Tuxi**
*Leiras, Fin.; Weifa, Norw.*
Pholcodine (p.1128·3).
*Coughs.*

**Tuxidrin** *Weifa, Norw.†.*
Pholcodine (p.1128·3); ephedrine (p.1120·1).
*Coughs.*

**Tuxium** *Galephar, Fr.*
Dextromethorphan hydrobromide (p.1117·3).
*Coughs.*

**Tuzanil** *Bohm, Spain.*
Pygeum africanum (p.1568·2).
*Benign prostatic hyperplasia.*

**Tuzo** *Brasifa, Braz.†.*
Sodium benzoate (p.1169·3); ammonium chloride (p.1115·2); potassium iodide (p.1598·1); ephedrine hydrochloride (p.1120·1).
*Respiratory-tract congestion.*

**Tuzzil** *IQFA, Mex.*
Benzonatate (p.1115·3).
*Coughs.*

**T-Vites** *Freeda, USA.*
Multivitamin preparation with minerals (p.1417·1).

**Twice-A-Day** *Major, USA.*
Oxymetazoline hydrochloride (p.1126·1).
*Nasal congestion.*

**Twilite** *Pfeiffer, USA.*
Diphenhydramine hydrochloride (p.431·3).
*Insomnia.*

**Twina** *T Man, Thai.*
Clotrimazole (p.396·2); betamethasone valerate (p.1093·2).
*Inflammatory skin disorders.*

**Twin-K** *Boots, USA.*
Potassium gluconate (p.1232·2); potassium citrate (p.1223·1).
*Hypokalaemia; potassium depletion.*

**Twinrix**
*GlaxoSmithKline, Arg.; GlaxoSmithKline, Austral.; SmithKline Beecham, Austria; GlaxoSmithKline, Belg.; GlaxoSmithKline, Braz.; GlaxoSmithKline, Canad.; GlaxoSmithKline, Chile; SmithKline Beecham, Denm.; GlaxoSmithKline, Fin.; GlaxoSmithKline, Fr.; GlaxoSmithKline, Ger.; GlaxoSmithKline, Hong Kong; GlaxoSmithKline, Irl.; SmithKline Beecham, Israel; SmithKline Beecham, Ital.; SmithKline, Malaysia; SmithKline Beecham, Mex.; GlaxoSmithKline, Neth.; GlaxoSmithKline, Norw.; GlaxoSmithKline, NZ; Smith Kline & French, Port.; GlaxoSmithKline, S.Afr.; GlaxoSmithKline, Singapore; SmithKline Beecham, Spain; GlaxoSmithKline, Swed.; SmithKline Beecham, Switz.; GlaxoSmithKline, UK; SmithKline Beecham, USA.*
An inactivated hepatitis A and recombinant hepatitis B vaccine (p.1620·1).
Separate preparations are available for infants and children and for adults.
*Active immunisation.*

**Two Cal HN**
*Abbott, Austral.; Abbott, Irl.; Abbott, Mex.; Abbott, NZ.*
High-nitrogen preparation for enteral nutrition (p.1417·1).

**TwoCal** *Abbott, Ital.*
Preparation for enteral nutrition (p.1417·1).

**TwoCal HN**
*Abbott, Hong Kong; Abbott Nutrition, UK; Ross, USA.*
High calorie, high nitrogen preparation for enteral nutrition (p.1417·1).

**Tybikin** *M & H, Thai.*
Amikacin sulfate (p.154·1).
*Gram-negative bacterial infections.*

**Tycoytycoy** *Bouzen, Arg.*
Povidone-iodine (p.1190·3).
*Disinfection.*

**Tydamine** *Aspen, S.Afr.*
Trimipramine (p.320·2).
*Depression; nocturnal enuresis; obsessive-compulsive disorder.*

**Tyklid** *Sanofi Torrent, India.*
Ticlopidine hydrochloride (p.1011·2).
*Thrombosis.*

**Tylenol**
*Johnson & Johnson, Arg.; Johnson & Johnson, Austral.; Johnson & Johnson, Austria†; Janssen-Cilag, Braz.; McNeil Consumer, Canad.; Johnson & Johnson, Hong Kong; Johnson & Johnson, Irl.; Cilag, Mex.; Johnson & Johnson, Port.; Janssen-Cilag, S.Afr.; Abello, Spain; Janssen-Cilag, Switz.; Janssen-Cilag, Thai.; McNeil Consumer, USA.*
Paracetamol (p.76·2).
*Fever; pain.*

**Tylenol Aches & Strains** *McNeil Consumer, Canad.*
Chlorzoxazone (p.1392·3); paracetamol (p.76·2).
*Muscular aches and strains.*

**Tylenol Allergy Sinus** *Johnson & Johnson, Austral.*
Paracetamol (p.76·2); chlorphenamine maleate (p.427·3); pseudoephedrine hydrochloride (p.1129·2).
*Upper respiratory-tract symptoms.*

**Tylenol Allergy Sinus Day & Night** *McNeil, USA.*
Day capsules, pseudoephedrine hydrochloride (p.1129·2); chlorphenamine maleate (p.427·3); paracetamol (p.76·2); night capsules, pseudoephedrine hydrochloride; diphenhydramine hydrochloride (p.431·3); paracetamol.
*Upper respiratory-tract disorders.*

**Tylenol Allergy Sinus (Multi-Symptom Relief)** *McNeil Consumer, Canad.*
Paracetamol (p.76·2); chlorphenamine maleate (p.427·3); pseudoephedrine hydrochloride (p.1129·2).
*Allergy symptoms; sinus pain and congestion.*

**Tylenol Allergy Sinus (Nighttime)** *McNeil Consumer, Canad.*
Paracetamol (p.76·2); diphenhydramine hydrochloride (p.431·3); pseudoephedrine hydrochloride (p.1129·2).
*Allergy symptoms; sinus pain and congestion.*

**Tylenol Allergy-D** *McNeil Consumer, Canad.*
Paracetamol (p.76·2); diphenhydramine hydrochloride (p.431·3); pseudoephedrine hydrochloride (p.1129·2).
*Allergy symptoms; sinus pain and congestion.*

**Tylenol with Codeine**
*McNeil Consumer, Canad.; Janssen-Ortho, Canad.; Janssen-Cilag, Thai.; Ortho McNeil, USA.*
Paracetamol (p.76·2); codeine phosphate (p.27·1).
*Pain.*

**Tylenol with Codeine No 4** *McNeil Consumer, Canad.; Janssen-Ortho, Canad.*
Paracetamol (p.76·2); codeine phosphate (p.27·1).
*Fever; pain.*

**Tylenol with Codeine No 2 or No 3** *McNeil Consumer, Canad.; Janssen-Ortho, Canad.*
Paracetamol (p.76·2); caffeine (p.782·1); codeine phosphate (p.27·1).
*Fever; pain.*

**Tylenol Cold** *McNeil, Hong Kong.*
Paracetamol (p.76·2); pseudoephedrine hydrochloride (p.1129·2); dextromethorphan hydrobromide (p.1117·3); chlorphenamine maleate (p.427·3).
*Allergic rhinitis; cold symptoms.*

**Tylenol Cold (Chest Congestion)** *McNeil Consumer, Canad.*
Paracetamol (p.76·2); pseudoephedrine hydrochloride (p.1129·2); guaifenesin (p.1122·1); dextromethorphan hydrobromide (p.1117·3).
*Upper respiratory-tract symptoms.*

**Tylenol Cold Children's** *McNeil Consumer, Canad.*
Paracetamol (p.76·2); chlorphenamine maleate (p.427·3); pseudoephedrine hydrochloride (p.1129·2).
*Allergy symptoms; cold symptoms.*

**Tylenol Cold (Daytime)** *McNeil Consumer, Canad.*
Paracetamol (p.76·2); pseudoephedrine hydrochloride (p.1129·2); dextromethorphan hydrobromide (p.1117·3).
*Cold symptoms.*

**Tylenol Cold DM** *McNeil Consumer, Canad.*
Paracetamol (p.76·2); chlorphenamine maleate (p.427·3); pseudoephedrine hydrochloride (p.1129·2); dextromethorphan hydrobromide (p.1117·3).
*Cold symptoms.*

**Tylenol Cold & Flu**
*Note. This name is used for preparations of different composition.*
*Johnson & Johnson, Austral.*
Paracetamol (p.76·2); chlorphenamine maleate (p.427·3); pseudoephedrine hydrochloride (p.1129·2); dextromethorphan hydrobromide (p.1117·3).
*Cold and influenza symptoms.*
*Janssen-Cilag, S.Afr.*
Paracetamol (p.76·2); chlorphenamine maleate (p.427·3); pseudoephedrine hydrochloride (p.1129·2).
*Allergic rhinitis; cold symptoms.*

**Tylenol Cold & Flu (Nighttime Relief)** *McNeil Consumer, Canad.*
Paracetamol (p.76·2); chlorphenamine maleate (p.427·3); pseudoephedrine hydrochloride (p.1129·2); dextromethorphan hydrobromide (p.1117·3).
*Influenza symptoms.*

**Tylenol Cold & Flu Non-Drowsy** *Johnson & Johnson, Austral.*
Paracetamol (p.76·2); pseudoephedrine hydrochloride (p.1129·2); dextromethorphan hydrobromide (p.1117·3).
*Cold and influenza symptoms.*

**Tylenol Cold and Flu Powder** *McNeil Consumer, Canad.*
Paracetamol (p.76·2); chlorphenamine maleate (p.427·3); pseudoephedrine hydrochloride (p.1129·2); dextromethorphan hydrobromide (p.1117·3).
*Cold symptoms.*

**Tylenol Cold Infant's** *McNeil Consumer, Canad.*
Paracetamol (p.76·2); chlorphenamine maleate (p.427·3); pseudoephedrine hydrochloride (p.1129·2).
*Allergy symptoms; cold symptoms.*

**Tylenol Cold Medication** *McNeil Consumer, Canad.*
Paracetamol (p.76·2); chlorphenamine maleate (p.427·3); pseudoephedrine hydrochloride (p.1129·2).
*Cold symptoms.*

**Tylenol Cold (Nighttime)** *McNeil Consumer, Canad.*
Paracetamol (p.76·2); chlorphenamine maleate (p.427·3); pseudoephedrine hydrochloride (p.1129·2); dextromethorphan hydrobromide (p.1117·3).
*Cold symptoms.*

**Tylenol Cold No Drowsiness** *McNeil Consumer, USA.*
Paracetamol (p.76·2); pseudoephedrine hydrochloride (p.1129·2); dextromethorphan hydrobromide (p.1117·3).
*Coughs and cold symptoms.*

**Tylenol Cold Severe Congestion** *McNeil Consumer, USA.*
Paracetamol (p.76·2); pseudoephedrine hydrochloride (p.1129·2); dextromethorphan hydrobromide (p.1117·3); guaifenesin (p.1122·1).
*Coughs and cold symptoms.*

**Tylenol Cough** *McNeil Consumer, Canad.*
Paracetamol (p.76·2); dextromethorphan hydrobromide (p.1117·3).
*Coughs; fever; pain; sore throat.*

**Tylenol Cough with Decongestant** *McNeil Consumer, Canad.*
Paracetamol (p.76·2); dextromethorphan hydrobromide (p.1117·3); pseudoephedrine hydrochloride (p.1129·2).
*Coughs; fever; nasal congestion; pain; sore throat.*

**Tylenol Decongestant** *McNeil Consumer, Canad.*
Paracetamol (p.76·2); pseudoephedrine hydrochloride (p.1129·2).
*Cold and influenza symptoms.*

**Tylenol Flu (Daytime Relief)** *McNeil Consumer, Canad.*
Paracetamol (p.76·2); pseudoephedrine hydrochloride (p.1129·2); dextromethorphan hydrobromide (p.1117·3).
*Influenza symptoms.*

**Tylenol Flu Maximum Strength** *McNeil, USA.*
Pseudoephedrine hydrochloride (p.1129·2); diphenhydramine hydrochloride (p.431·3); paracetamol (p.76·2).
*Upper respiratory-tract disorders.*

**Tylenol Flu Night Time** *McNeil Consumer, USA.*
Paracetamol (p.76·2); diphenhydramine hydrochloride (p.431·3); pseudoephedrine hydrochloride (p.1129·2).

**Tylenol Flu (Nighttime Relief)** *McNeil Consumer, Canad.*
Paracetamol (p.76·2); pseudoephedrine hydrochloride (p.1129·2); diphenhydramine hydrochloride (p.431·3).
*Influenza symptoms.*

**Tylenol Flu No Drowsiness** *McNeil Consumer, USA.*
Paracetamol (p.76·2); dextromethorphan hydrobromide (p.1117·3); pseudoephedrine hydrochloride (p.1129·2).

**Tylenol Menstrual** *McNeil Consumer, Canad.*
Paracetamol (p.76·2); pamabrom (p.978·2); mepyramine maleate (p.437·1).
*Premenstrual syndrome.*

**Tylenol Night Pain** *Janssen-Cilag, S.Afr.*
Paracetamol (p.76·2); diphenhydramine hydrochloride (p.431·3).
*Insomnia with pain.*

**Tylenol No 1** *Janssen-Ortho, Canad.; McNeil Consumer, Canad.*
Paracetamol (p.76·2); caffeine (p.782·1); codeine phosphate (p.27·1).
*Pain.*

**Tylenol Severe Allergy** *McNeil Consumer, USA.*
Paracetamol (p.76·2); diphenhydramine hydrochloride (p.431·3).
*Hypersensitivity symptoms.*

**Tylenol Sinus**
*Note. This name is used for preparations of different composition.*
*Johnson & Johnson, Austral.; McNeil Consumer, Canad.*
Paracetamol (p.76·2); pseudoephedrine hydrochloride (p.1129·2).
*Cold symptoms; sinus and nasal congestion; sinus pain.*

*Cilag, Mex.*
Paracetamol (p.76·2); pseudoephedrine hydrochloride (p.1129·2); chlorphenamine maleate (p.427·3).
*Respiratory-tract congestion; rhinitis; rhinopharyngitis.*

**Tylenol Sinus (Daytime Relief)** *McNeil Consumer, Canad.*
Paracetamol (p.76·2); pseudoephedrine hydrochloride (p.1129·2).
*Cold symptoms; sinusitis.*

**Tylenol Sinus (Nighttime Relief)** *McNeil Consumer, Canad.*
Paracetamol (p.76·2); pseudoephedrine hydrochloride (p.1129·2); doxylamine succinate (p.432·3).
*Cold symptoms; sinusitis.*

**Tylephen** *IQB, Braz.*
Paracetamol (p.76·2).
*Fever; pain.*

**Tylex**
*Note. This name is used for preparations of different composition.*
*Janssen-Cilag, Braz.; Schwarz, Irl.; Schwarz, UK.*
Paracetamol (p.76·2); codeine phosphate (p.27·1).
These ingredients can be described by the British Approved Name Co-codamol 30/500.
*Pain.*

*Cilag, Mex.*
Paracetamol (p.76·2).
*Fever; pain.*

**Tylex CD** *Cilag, Mex.*
Paracetamol (p.76·2); codeine phosphate (p.27·1).
*Pain.*

**Tylex Flu** *Cilag, Mex.*
Paracetamol (p.76·2); pseudoephedrine hydrochloride (p.1129·2); chlorphenamine maleate (p.427·3); dextromethorphan hydrobromide (p.1117·3).
*Cold and influenza symptoms; coughs.*

**Tylidol** *Teuto, Braz.*
Paracetamol (p.76·2).
*Fever; pain.*

**Tyll** *Gilton, Braz.†.*
Pokeroot (p.1733·1).

**Tylox** *Ortho McNeil, USA.*
Oxycodone hydrochloride (p.75·2); paracetamol (p.76·2).
*Pain.*

**Tymelyt**
*Lundbeck, Austria; Lundbeck, Belg.†; Lundbeck, Denm.; Lundbeck, Swed.*
Lofepramine hydrochloride (p.305·3).
*Depression.*

**Tymol** *Pharmaland, Thai.*
Paracetamol (p.76·2).
*Fever; pain.*

**Tympagesic** *Savage, USA.*
Phenylephrine hydrochloride (p.1126·3); phenazone (p.82·3); benzocaine (p.1370·3).
*Earache.*

**Tympalgine** *Therabel, Belg.*
Phenazone (p.82·3); lidocaine hydrochloride (p.1377·3).
Formerly contained phenazone and procaine hydrochloride.
*Otitis.*

**Typherix**
*GlaxoSmithKline, Austral.; GlaxoSmithKline, Austria; GlaxoSmithKline, Belg.; GlaxoSmithKline, Canad.; GlaxoSmithKline, Fin.; GlaxoSmithKline, Fr.; GlaxoSmithKline, Ger.; GlaxoSmithKline, Irl.; SmithKline Beecham, Israel; GlaxoSmithKline, Ital.; GlaxoSmithKline, Neth.; GlaxoSmithKline, Norw.; GlaxoSmithKline, NZ; GlaxoSmithKline, Singapore; GlaxoSmithKline, Swed.; GlaxoSmithKline, UK.*
A typhoid vaccine (Vi capsular polysaccharide) (p.1642·2).
*Active immunisation.*

**Typhim Vi**
*Aventis Pasteur, Arg.; Aventis Pasteur, Austral.; Aventis, Austria; Aventis Pasteur, Belg.; Aventis Pasteur, Canad.; Aventis Pasteur, Chile; Aventis Pasteur, Denm.; Aventis Pasteur, Fin.; Pasteur Vaccins, Fr.; Aventis Pasteur, Ger.; Aventis Pasteur, Hong Kong; Aventis Pasteur, Irl.; Pasteur Merieux, Israel; Aventis Pasteur, Ital.; Aventis Pasteur, Malaysia; Aventis Pasteur, Neth.; Aventis Pasteur, Norw.; CSL, NZ; Aventis, S.Afr.; Pasteur Merieux, Singapore; Aventis Pasteur, Spain; Aventis Pasteur, Swed.; Aventis Pasteur, Thai.; Aventis Pasteur, UK; Pasteur Merieux, USA.*
A typhoid vaccine (Vi capsular polysaccharide) (p.1642·2).
*Active immunisation.*

**Typhoral** *Aventis, India.*
An attenuated oral typhoid vaccine (p.1642·2).
*Active immunisation.*

**Typhoral L** *Chiron Behring, Ger.*
A live oral typhoid vaccine (p.1642·2).
*Active immunisation.*

**Typhovax** *Green Cross, Malaysia.*
A typhoid vaccine (Vi capsular polysaccharide) (p.1642·2).
*Active immunisation.*

**Typh-Vax**
*CSL, Austral.; CSL, NZ.*
An oral typhoid vaccine (attenuated Ty21a Berna strain) (p.1642·2).
*Active immunisation.*

**Tyrazol** *Yamanouchi, Fin.*
Carbimazole (p.1596·2).
*Hyperthyroidism.*

**Tyrcine** *Oberlin, Fr.†.*
Tyrothricin (p.275·1); tetracaine hydrochloride (p.1385·1).
*Mouth and throat disorders.*

**Tyrenol** *Remedina, Gr.*
Astemizole (p.424·2).
*Allergic conjunctivitis; allergic rhinitis; pruritus.*

**Tyrex** *Ross, USA.*
Phenylalanine- and tyrosine-free preparation for enteral nutrition (p.1417·1).
*Tyrosinaemia types I, II, and III.*

**Tyrocaine** *Synco, Hong Kong.*
Tyrothricin (p.275·1); benzocaine (p.1370·3).
*Mouth and throat infections.*

**Tyrocombine** *Synpharma, Switz.*
*Ointment:* Tyrothricin (p.275·1); neomycin sulfate (p.235·1); benzethonium chloride (p.1169·2).
*Infected skin disorders; infected wounds.*
*Topical powder:* Tyrothricin (p.275·1); neomycin sulfate (p.235·1); benzethonium chloride (p.1169·2).
Formerly contained tyrothricin, neomycin sulfate, benzethonium chloride, and sulfathiazole.
*Infected skin disorders.*

**Tyrodone** *Major, USA.*
Hydrocodone tartrate (p.45·1); pseudoephedrine hydrochloride (p.1129·2).

**Tyro-Drops** *Centrapharm, Belg.*
Tyrothricin (p.275·1); lidocaine hydrochloride (p.1377·3).
*Mouth and throat disorders.*

**Tyromex** *Ross, USA†.*
Methionine-, phenylalanine-, and tyrosine-free infant feed (p.1417·1).
*Tyrosinaemia type I.*

**Tyroneomicin** *Alcala, Spain†.*
Bacitracin zinc (p.161·3); benzocaine (p.1370·3); hydrocortisone acetate (p.1103·3); neomycin sulfate (p.235·1); potassium chlorate (p.1734·2).
*Mouth and throat disorders.*

**Tyroplus** *Enila, Braz.*
Liothyronine sodium (p.1602·2); levothyroxine (p.1601·3).
*Thyroid disorders.*

**Tyroqualine** *Spirig, Switz.*
Tyrothricin (p.275·1); dequalinium chloride (p.1178·1); lidocaine hydrochloride (p.1377·3).
*Mouth and throat disorders.*

**Tyroseng** *Eagle, Austral.†.*
Tyrosine (p.1451·1); eleutherococcus senticosis (p.1744·1); calcium glycerophosphate (p.1225·2); phosphatidyl choline (p.1731·1); vitamin B substances (p.1417·1).
*Dietary supplement.*

**Tyrosin TU** *Bencard, Ger.*
Mixed allergen extracts (p.1650·1).
*Allergen immunotherapy.*

**Tyrosolvetten** *Altana, Ger.; Byk Gulden, Ger.*
Cetylpyridinium chloride (p.1173·1); benzocaine (p.1370·3).
*Mouth and throat disorders.*

**Tyrosolvetten-C** *Altana, Ger.; Byk Gulden, Ger.*
Cetylpyridinium chloride (p.1173·1); ascorbic acid (p.1460·2).
*Mouth and throat infections.*

**Tyrosum** *Summers, USA.*
Skin cleanser.

**Tyrosur**
*Note. This name is used for preparations of different composition.*
*Engelhard, Ger.*
*Topical gel:* Tyrothricin (p.275·1); cetylpyridinium chloride (p.1173·1).
*Infected skin disorders; infected wounds and burns.*
*Topical powder:* Tyrothricin (p.275·1).
*Infected skin disorders; infected wounds and burns.*

*Engelhard, Hong Kong.*
Tyrothricin (p.275·1).
*Infected skin disorders; infected wounds.*

**Tyrothricin** *Streuli, Switz.*
Tyrothricin (p.275·1); ethacridine lactate (p.1165·3); lidocaine hydrochloride (p.1377·3); menthol (p.1711·3); mint oil (p.1715·2).
*Mouth and throat disorders.*

**Tyrothricin Co** *Jean-Marie, Hong Kong.*
Tyrothricin (p.275·1); codeine phosphate (p.27·1); benzocaine (p.1370·3).
*Throat disorders.*

**Tyrothricin comp** *Provita, Austria.*
Tyrothricin (p.275·1); neomycin sulfate (p.235·1); benzalkonium chloride (p.1168·3); benzocaine (p.1370·3).
*Mouth and throat disorders.*

**Tyrothricin compositum** *Provita, Austria.*
Tyrothricin (p.275·1); neomycin sulfate (p.235·1); benzocaine (p.1370·3); camphor (p.1665·3).
*Ear disorders.*

**Tyrothricine + Gramicidine** *Democal, Switz.*
Tyrothricin (p.275·1); gramicidin (p.220·2); tetracaine hydrochloride (p.1385·1); benzethonium chloride (p.1169·2).
*Mouth and throat disorders.*

**Tyrothricine Lafran** *Lafran, Fr.†.*
Tyrothricin (p.275·1); butyl aminobenzoate (p.1373·1).
*Mouth and throat disorders.*

**Tyrozets**
*Merck Sharp & Dohme, Irl.; Merck Sharp & Dohme, Port.†; Johnson & Johnson MSD Consumer, UK.*
Tyrothricin (p.275·1); benzocaine (p.1370·3).
*Mouth and throat disorders.*

**Tytin** *Merind, India.*
Tyrothricin (p.275·1); benzocaine (p.1370·3); phenazone (p.82·3); hexylresorcinol (p.1182·1).
*Ear infections.*

**Tyzine**
*Pfizer, Denm.; Pfizer, Ger.; Pfizer, Switz.†; Kenwood, USA.*
Tetryzoline hydrochloride (p.1131·2).
*Conjunctivitis; eye irritation; nasal congestion; rhinitis; sinusitis.*

**T-ZA** *Siam Bheasach, Thai.†.*
Zidovudine (p.658·2).
*HIV infection.*

**Tzoali** *Kendrick, Mex.*
Diphenhydramine hydrochloride (p.431·3).
*Insomnia.*

**U Lactin** *Cosmofarma, Port.*
Urea (p.1162·2); alpha hydroxy acids.
*Dry skin disorders.*

**UAA** *Econo Med, USA.*
Methenamine (p.230·1); salol (p.88·1); atropine sulfate (p.477·1); hyoscyamine sulfate (p.485·1); benzoic acid (p.1169·3); methylthioninium chloride (p.1042·2).
*Urinary-tract infections.*

**UAD-Otic** *UAD, USA.*
Hydrocortisone (p.1103·3); neomycin sulfate (p.235·1); polymyxin B sulfate (p.245·1).
*Bacterial ear infections.*

**Ubenzima** *Pentafarma, Port.*
Ubidecarenone (p.1760·2).
*Cardiac disorders.*

**Ubicarden** *Locatelli, Ital.†.*
Ubidecarenone (p.1760·2).
*Cardiac disorders; coenzyme Q10 deficiency.*

**Ubicardio** *Tosi, Ital.*
Ubidecarenone (p.1760·2).
*Cardiac disorders; coenzyme Q10 deficiency.*

**Ubicondrial** *Medicamed, Port.*
Ubidecarenone (p.1760·2).
*Cardiac disorders.*

**Ubicor** *Magis, Ital.*
Ubidecarenone (p.1760·2).
*Cardiac disorders; coenzyme Q10 deficiency.*

**Ubidenone** *Esseti, Ital.*
Ubidecarenone (p.1760·2).
*Cardiac disorders; coenzyme Q10 deficiency.*

**Ubidex** *OFF, Ital.*
Ubidecarenone (p.1760·2).
*Cardiac disorders; coenzyme Q10 deficiency.*

**Ubifactor** *San Carlo, Ital.†.*
Ubidecarenone (p.1760·2).
*Cardiac disorders; coenzyme Q10 deficiency.*

**Ubimaior** *Chiesi, Ital.*
Ubidecarenone (p.1760·2).
*Cardiac disorders; coenzyme Q10 deficiency.*

**Ubisint** *Francia, Ital.†.*
Ubidecarenone (p.1760·2).
*Coenzyme Q10 deficiency: cardiac disorders.*

**Ubistesin**
*Espe, Austria; Espe, Ger.; Espe, Ital.; Espe, Switz.*
Articaine hydrochloride (p.1370·3).
Adrenaline hydrochloride (p.852·3) is included in this preparation as a vasoconstrictor to diminish absorption and localise the effect of the local anaesthetic.
*Local anaesthesia.*

**Ubiten**
*Note. This name is used for preparations of different composition.*
*Laboratorios, Chile.*
Carnitine fumarate; ubidecarenone; potassium; magnesium; vitamin C (p.1417·1).
*Dietary supplement.*

*Lifepharma, Ital.*
Ubidecarenone (p.1760·2).
*Cardiac disorders; coenzyme Q10 deficiency.*

**Ubivis** *AGIPS, Ital.*
Ubidecarenone (p.1760·2).
*Cardiac disorders; coenzyme Q10 deficiency.*

**Ubizol** *Alter, Port.*
Fluticasone propionate (p.1102·3).
*Skin disorders.*

**Ublosid** *Costec, Arg.*
Triclosan (p.1195·2); aluminium chlorohydrate (p.1142·1).

**Ubretid**
*Nycomed, Austria; Nycomed, Fin.; Nycomed, Ger.; Nycomed, Gr.; Nycomed, Hong Kong; Christiaens, Neth.; Aventis, NZ†; Roche, S.Afr.†; Nycomed, Singapore; Nycomed, Switz.; Aventis, UK.*
Distigmine bromide (p.1489·2).
*Myasthenia gravis; neurogenic bladder; postoperative gastrointestinal motility disorders; urinary retention.*

**Ubtest** *Otsuka, Spain.*
Carbon-13-labelled urea (p.1667·3).
*Test for Helicobacter pylori infection.*

**Ucecal**
*Asta Medica, Austria; UCB, Spain.*
Calcitonin (salmon) (p.768·2).
*Hypercalcaemia; hyperparathyroidism; immobilisation; osteolysis of malignancy; osteoporosis; Paget's disease of bone; pancreatic disorders; reflex sympathetic dystrophy; vitamin D intoxication.*

**Ucee D** *Merck, Ger.*
Dexpanthenol (p.1727·2).
*Skin lesions.*

**Ucemine PP** *UCB, Belg.*
Nicotinamide (p.1441·2).
*Vitamin PP deficiency.*

**Ucephan** *Ucyclyd, USA.*
Sodium benzoate (p.1169·3); sodium phenylacetate (p.1748·2).
*Hyperammonaemia.*

**Ucerax** *UCB, UK.*
Hydroxyzine hydrochloride (p.434·3).
*Anxiety; pruritus.*

**UCG-Slide** *Wampole, USA.*
Pregnancy test (p.1734·3).

**Ucholine** *M & H, Thai.*
Bethanechol chloride (p.1487·3).
*Neurogenic bladder; urinary retention.*

**Ucine** *Ashbourne, UK†.*
Sulfasalazine (p.1291·1).
*Inflammatory bowel disease.*

**Ucort** *YSP, Malaysia.*
Urea (p.1162·2); hydrocortisone acetate (p.1103·3).
*Dry skin disorders.*

**UDC** *Hexal, Ger.*
Ursodeoxycholic acid (p.1760·3).
*Biliary disorders; dyspepsia; gallstones.*

**UDCA** *Ferring, Arg.*
Ursodeoxycholic acid (p.1760·3).
*Liver and biliary-tract disorders.*

**Udesospray** *Faran, Gr.*
Budesonide (p.1094·2).
*Allergic rhinitis.*

**Udicil** *Pharmacia, Ger.*
Cytarabine (p.543·1).
*Malignant neoplasms.*

**Udiliv** *Solvay, India.*
Ursodeoxycholic acid (p.1760·3).
*Cholestatic liver disease; cholesterol gallstones.*

**Udima** *Dermapharm, Ger.*
Minocycline hydrochloride (p.231·3).
*Bacterial infections.*

**Udima Ery** *Dermapharm, Ger.†.*
Erythromycin (p.208·1).
*Acne.*

**Udramil** *Aventis, Ger.*
Verapamil hydrochloride (p.1019·1); trandolapril (p.1016·1).
*Hypertension.*

**Udrik** *Aventis, Ger.*
Trandolapril (p.1016·1).
*Heart failure following myocardial infarction; hypertension.*

**Ufarin** *Schering, Chile.*
Isoconazole nitrate (p.401·3).
*Fungal and Gram-positive bacterial vaginal infections; fungal skin infections.*

**Ufexil** *Demo, Gr.*
Ciprofloxacin hydrochloride (p.188·2) or ciprofloxacin lactate (p.188·3).
*Bacterial infections.*

**Ufocard** *Proel, Gr.*
Nitrendipine (p.973·3).
*Hypertension.*

**Ufonitren** *Proel, Gr.*
Omeprazole (p.1278·2).
*Acid aspiration; eradication of Helicobacter pylori in combination with antimicrobials; peptic ulcer; reflux oesophagitis; Zollinger-Ellison syndrome.*

**Ufor** *Valdecasas, Mex.*
Aluminium hydroxide (p.1249·2); magnesium hydroxide (p.1272·2).
*Gastrointestinal hyperacidity.*

**UFT**
*Bristol-Myers Squibb, Arg.; Bristol-Myers Squibb, Austria; Bristol-Myers Squibb, Belg.; Bristol-Myers Squibb, Braz.; Bristol-Myers Squibb, Fr.;*

Bristol-Myers Squibb, Ger.; Bristol-Myers Squibb, Hong Kong; Bristol-Myers Squibb, Israel; Bristol-Myers Squibb, Ital.; Taiho, Jpn; Taiho, Malaysia; Bristol-Myers Squibb, Mex.; Bristol-Myers Squibb, Norw.; Bristol-Myers Squibb, Port. Bristol-Myers Squibb, S.Afr.; Taiho, Singapore; Bristol-Myers, Spain; Bristol-Myers Squibb, Swed.; Bristol-Myers Squibb, Thai.
Tegafur (p.586·2); uracil.
*Malignant neoplasms.*

**Uftoral** Bristol-Myers Squibb, Denm.; Bristol-Myers Squibb, UK.
Tegafur (p.586·2); uracil.
*Colorectal cancer.*

**Ugal** Diba, Mex.
Cimetoxine.
*Peptic ulcer.*

**Ugrilon** Farmatrading, Port.†.
Caffeine (p.782·1); mepyramine maleate (p.437·1); paracetamol (p.76·2).
*Fever; pain.*

**Ugurol** Bayer, Ger.†; Rottapharm, Ital.
Tranexamic acid (p.760·3).
*Haemorrhagic disorders.*

**Ujostabil** Felgentrager, Ger.
Ammonium polystyrene sulfonate (p.1053·2); potassium polystyrene sulfonate (p.1050·1); magnesium polystyrene sulfonate (p.1053·2); sodium polystyrene sulfonate (p.1053·1).
*Renal calculi.*

**Ukidan** Serono, Austral.†; Serono, Austria†; Serono, Hong Kong†; Serum Institute, India; Serono, Israel†; Serono, Ital.†; Serono, Port.; Research Labs, S.Afr.†; Serono, Swed.†; Serono, Switz.†.
Urokinase (p.1018·2).
*Thromboembolic disorders.*

**UL 250** Merck, Port.
*Saccharomyces boulardii* (p.1704·2).
*Restoration of normal gastrointestinal flora.*

**U-Lactin Foot Cream** Fischer, Israel.
Urea (p.1162·2); lactic acid (p.1704·1); salicylic acid (p.1157·1).
*Skin disorders of the foot.*

**U-Lactin Forte** Fischer, Israel.
Urea (p.1162·2); lactic acid (p.1704·1).
*Skin disorders.*

**Ulcaid** Ranbaxy, S.Afr.
Ranitidine hydrochloride (p.1285·2).
*Acid aspiration; gastro-oesophageal reflux; peptic ulcer; Zollinger-Ellison syndrome.*

**Ulcar** Aventis, Fr.
Sucralfate (p.1290·2).
*Peptic ulcer.*

**Ulcecur** Ferring, Port.
Ranitidine hydrochloride (p.1285·2).
*Gastro-oesophageal reflux; peptic ulcer; Zollinger-Ellison syndrome.*

**Ulcedin**
Note. This name is used for preparations of different composition.
AGIPS, Ital.
Cimetidine (p.1255·3).
*Gastric hyperacidity; gastro-oesophageal reflux; gastrointestinal haemorrhage; peptic ulcer; Zollinger-Ellison syndrome.*

Sons, Mex.
Ranitidine hydrochloride (p.1285·2).
*Acid aspiration; gastro-oesophageal reflux; gastrointestinal haemorrhage; peptic ulcer; Zollinger-Ellison syndrome.*

**Ulcedine** Sanofi Synthelabo, Braz.; Great Eastern, Thai.; Westmont, Thai.
Cimetidine (p.1255·3).
*Acid aspiration; gastro-oesophageal reflux; gastrointestinal haemorrhage; peptic ulcer; Zollinger-Ellison syndrome.*

**Ulcedor** Brasifa, Braz.†.
Cimetidine (p.1255·3).
*Gastro-oesophageal reflux; gastrointestinal haemorrhage; peptic ulcer; Zollinger-Ellison syndrome.*

**Ulcefate** Abbott, S.Afr.†; Siam Bheasach, Thai.
Sucralfate (p.1290·2).
*Gastritis; gastro-oesophageal reflux; peptic ulcer.*

**Ulcefor** Elofar, Braz.
Omeprazole (p.1278·2).
*Peptic ulcer.*

**Ulcegel** TO-Chemicals, Thai.
Dried aluminium hydroxide gel (p.1249·2); magnesium hydroxide (p.1272·2); simeticone (p.1289·2).
*Gastric hyperacidity; heartburn; peptic ulcer.*

**Ulcekon** FDC, India.
Sucralfate (p.1290·2).
*Gastritis; peptic ulcer.*

**Ulcelac**
Note. This name is used for preparations of different composition.
Bago, Arg.
Famotidine (p.1265·2).
*Gastritis; gastro-oesophageal reflux; peptic ulcer; Zollinger-Ellison syndrome.*

Bago, Chile.
Omeprazole (p.1278·2).
*Gastro-oesophageal reflux; peptic ulcer; Zollinger-Ellison syndrome.*

**Ulcemet** TO-Chemicals, Thai.
Cimetidine (p.1255·3).
*Gastro-oesophageal reflux; peptic ulcer; Zollinger-Ellison syndrome.*

**Ulcemex** Lafi, Chile.
Pantoprazole sodium (p.1283·1).
*Peptic ulcer.*

**Ulcenon** Legrand, Braz.
Cimetidine (p.1255·3).
*Gastro-oesophageal reflux; gastrointestinal haemorrhage; peptic ulcer; Zollinger-Ellison syndrome.*

**Ulcepin** Rafa, Israel†.
Pirenzepine hydrochloride (p.488·1).
*Dyspepsia; gastric irritation; gastritis; gastrointestinal hyperacidity; peptic ulcer.*

**Ulcerac** Delta, Braz.
Cimetidine (p.1255·3).
*Peptic ulcer.*

**Ulceracid** Luper, Braz.
Cimetidine (p.1255·3).
*Gastro-oesophageal reflux; gastrointestinal haemorrhage; peptic ulcer; Zollinger-Ellison syndrome.*

**Ulceral**
Note. This name is used for preparations of different composition.
Aliud, Austria.
Sucralfate (p.1290·2).
*Gastro-oesophageal reflux; peptic ulcer.*

Tedec Meiji, Spain.
Omeprazole (p.1278·2).
*Gastro-oesophageal reflux; peptic ulcer; Zollinger-Ellison syndrome.*

**Ulceran** Medochemie, Hong Kong; Medochemie, Malaysia; Medochemie, Singapore†; Medochemie, Thai.
Famotidine (p.1265·2).
*Gastrointestinal haemorrhage; peptic ulcer; Zollinger-Ellison syndrome.*

**Ulcerase**
Note. This name is used for preparations of different composition.
Heralds, Braz.†.
Cimetidine (p.1255·3).
*Gastro-oesophageal reflux; gastrointestinal haemorrhage; peptic ulcer; Zollinger-Ellison syndrome.*

Knoll, Port.†.
Collagenase (p.1675·1).

**Ulcerease** Med-Derm, USA.
Liquefied phenol (p.1188·1).
*Mouth and throat pain.*

**Ulcerfen** Finadiet, Arg.
Cimetidine (p.1255·3).
*Peptic ulcer.*

**Ulceridine** Normal, Port.
Cimetidine (p.1255·3).

**Ulcerim** Rimsa, Mex.†.
Cimetidine (p.1255·3).

**Ulcerit** Hexal, Braz.
Ranitidine hydrochloride (p.1285·2).
*Peptic ulcer.*

**Ulcerlmin** Chugai, Jpn.
Sucralfate (p.1290·2).
*Gastritis; peptic ulcer.*

**Ulcermin** Bonafarma, Port.
Sucralfate (p.1290·2).
*Gastritis; gastro-oesophageal reflux; gastrointestinal haemorrhage; peptic ulcer.*

**Ulcerocin** Cimed, Braz.
Ranitidine (p.1285·2).
*Peptic ulcer.*

**Ulcerol** APS, Port.
Ranitidine hydrochloride (p.1285·2).
*Gastrointestinal hyperacidity; peptic ulcer.*

**Ulcerone** Pharmaplan, S.Afr.†.
Bismuth oxide (p.1252·1).
Formerly contained tripotassium dicitratobismuthate.
*Peptic ulcer.*

**Ulcerosol** Rio Preto, Braz.†.
Bismuth subnitrate (p.1252·2).
*Diarrhoea; duodenal ulcer; gastritis; gastrointestinal hyperacidity.*

**Ulcertec**
Note. This name is used for preparations of different composition.
DHA, Malaysia; DHA, Singapore.
Sucralfate (p.1290·2).
*Peptic ulcer.*

Neves, Port.
Lansoprazole (p.1269·3).
*Gastro-oesophageal reflux; peptic ulcer; Zollinger-Ellison syndrome.*

**Ulcesep** Centrum, Spain.
Omeprazole (p.1278·2).
*Gastro-oesophageal reflux; peptic ulcer; Zollinger-Ellison syndrome.*

**Ulcesium** Rhone-Poulenc Rorer, Mex.†.
Fentonium bromide (p.482·2).

**Ulcestop** Metapharma, Ital.†.
Cimetidine hydrochloride (p.1255·3).
*Gastro-oesophageal reflux; peptic ulcer; Zollinger-Ellison syndrome.*

**Ulcetrax** Salvat, Spain.
Famotidine (p.1265·2).
*Gastro-oesophageal reflux; peptic ulcer; Zollinger-Ellison syndrome.*

**Ulcevarin** Bajer, Arg.
Oxerutin (p.1688·2); vitamin A palmitate (p.1453·1).
*Inflammation; phlebitis; skin disorders.*

**Ulcex** Guidotti, Ital.
Ranitidine hydrochloride (p.1285·2).
*Gastritis or duodenitis associated with acid hypersecretion; gastro-oesophageal reflux; peptic ulcer; Zollinger-Ellison syndrome.*

**Ulcidine**
Note. This name is used for preparations of different composition.
ICN, Canad.
Famotidine (p.1265·2).

Raza, Malaysia; Pharmaniaga, Malaysia.
Cimetidine (p.1255·3).
*Acid aspiration; gastro-oesophageal reflux; peptic ulcer; Zollinger-Ellison syndrome.*

Spirig, Switz.
Ranitidine hydrochloride (p.1285·2).
*Gastrointestinal disorders associated with hyperacidity.*

**Ulcim** Quatromed, S.Afr.†.
Cimetidine (p.1255·3).
*Gastrointestinal disorders.*

**Ulcimet** Farmasa, Braz.; Polipharm, Thai.
Cimetidine (p.1255·3).
*Acid aspiration; gastro-oesophageal reflux; gastrointestinal haemorrhage; peptic ulcer; Zollinger-Ellison syndrome.*

**Ulcin** Ibirn, Ital.†.
Pirenzepine hydrochloride (p.488·1).
*Gastroduodenitis; peptic ulcer.*

**Ulcinax** Neo Quimica, Braz.
Cimetidine (p.1255·3).
*Peptic ulcer.*

**Ulcirex** Irex, Fr.†.
Ranitidine hydrochloride (p.1285·2).
*Gastro-oesophageal reflux; peptic ulcer; Zollinger-Ellison syndrome.*

**Ulcitag** Sedabel, Braz.
Cimetidine (p.1255·3).
*Gastro-oesophageal reflux; gastrointestinal haemorrhage; peptic ulcer; Zollinger-Ellison syndrome.*

**Ulcitrat** Bunker, Braz.
Cimetidine (p.1255·3).
*Peptic ulcer.*

**Ulco-cyl Ho-Len-Complex** Liebermann, Ger.
Homoeopathic preparation.

**Ulcoderma** Knoll, Mex.
Collagenase (p.1675·1); chloramphenicol (p.185·1).
*Burns; skin ulcers; wounds.*

**Ulcodina** SoSe, Ital.
Cimetidine (p.1255·3).
*Gastritis and duodenitis associated with acid hypersecretion; gastro-oesophageal reflux; peptic ulcer; Zollinger-Ellison syndrome.*

**Ulcofam** Codal Synto, Thai.
Famotidine (p.1265·2).
*Peptic ulcer; Zollinger-Ellison syndrome.*

**Ulcogant** Merck, Austria; Merck, Belg.; Merck, Ger.; Merck, Neth.; Merck, Switz.
Sucralfate (p.1290·2).
*Gastro-oesophageal reflux; peptic ulcer; stress-related gastrointestinal haemorrhage.*

**Ulcoid** Valdecasas, Mex.
Diphenhydramine hydrochloride (p.431·3).
*Hypersensitivity; sleep disorders.*

**Ulcoid-Zol** Valdecasas, Mex.
Astemizole (p.424·2).
*Hypersensitivity.*

**Ulcolind Amoxi** Lindopharm, Ger.†.
Amoxicillin trihydrate (p.155·3).
*Bacterial infections.*

**Ulcolind $H_2$** Lindopharm, Ger.†.
Cimetidine (p.1255·3).
*Acid aspiration; gastro-oesophageal reflux; gastrointestinal haemorrhage; peptic ulcer; Zollinger-Ellison syndrome.*

**Ulcolind Metro** Lindopharm, Ger.†.
Metronidazole (p.607·2).
*Anaerobic bacterial infections; protozoal infections.*

**Ulcolind Rani** Lindopharm, Ger.†.
Ranitidine hydrochloride (p.1285·2).
*Acid aspiration; gastro-oesophageal reflux; gastrointestinal haemorrhage; peptic ulcer; Zollinger-Ellison syndrome.*

**Ulcolind Wismut** Lindopharm, Ger.†.
Bismuth salicylate (p.1252·1).
*Gastritis; peptic ulcer.*

**Ulcomedina** De Salute, Ital.
Cimetidine (p.1255·3).
*Gastritis and duodenitis associated with acid hypersecretion; gastro-oesophageal reflux; peptic ulcer; Zollinger-Ellison syndrome.*

**Ulcomet** Medochemie, Hong Kong.
Cimetidine (p.1255·3).
*Acid aspiration; adjunct in pancreatic insufficiency; gastro-oesophageal reflux; gastrointestinal haemorrhage; peptic ulcer.*

**Ulcometin** Ratiopharm, Austria.
Cimetidine (p.1255·3) or cimetidine hydrochloride (p.1255·3).
*Acid aspiration; gastro-oesophageal reflux; gastrointestinal haemorrhage; hypersensitivity reactions; peptic ulcer; Zollinger-Ellison syndrome.*

**Ulcometion** Antibioticos, Spain.
Omeprazole (p.1278·2).
*Gastro-oesophageal reflux; peptic ulcer; Zollinger-Ellison syndrome.*

**Ulconar** Allergan-Frumtost, Braz.†.
Omeprazole (p.1278·2).
*Gastro-oesophageal reflux; gastrointestinal hyperacidity; peptic ulcer.*

**Ulcopir** Aesculapius, Ital.†.
Pirenzepine hydrochloride (p.488·1).
*Gastrointestinal disorders.*

**Ulcoprotect** Azupharma, Ger.
Pirenzepine hydrochloride (p.488·1).
*Gastrointestinal disorders.*

**Ulcoren** Medley, Braz.
Ranitidine hydrochloride (p.1285·2).
*Gastro-oesophageal reflux; gastrointestinal haemorrhage; peptic ulcer; Zollinger-Ellison syndrome.*

**Ulcosafe** BASF, Ger.†.
Pirenzepine hydrochloride (p.488·1).
*Gastrointestinal disorders.*

**Ulcosal** Lilly, Spain†.
Nizatidine (p.1277·2).
*Gastro-oesophageal reflux; peptic ulcer.*

**Ulcostad** Stada, Austria.
Cimetidine (p.1255·3) or cimetidine hydrochloride (p.1255·3).
*Acid aspiration; gastro-oesophageal reflux disease; gastrointestinal haemorrhage; hypersensitivity reactions; peptic ulcer; Zollinger-Ellison syndrome.*

**Ulcotenal** Recordati, Spain.
Pantoprazole sodium (p.1283·1).
*Gastro-oesophageal reflex; peptic ulcer.*

**Ulcotenk** Biotenk, Arg.
Ranitidine hydrochloride (p.1285·2).
*Peptic ulcer.*

**Ulcotruw N** Truw, Ger.†.
Peppermint leaf (p.1283·2); liquorice (p.1270·2); chamomile (p.1669·3).
*Gastrointestinal disorders.*

**Ulcourona** Neuropharma, Arg.
Idebenone (p.1700·3).
*Cerebrovascular disorders.*

**Ulc-Out** Raffo, Chile.
Omeprazole (p.1278·2).
*Gastro-oesophageal reflux; peptic ulcer; Zollinger-Ellison syndrome.*

**Ulcozol** Bago, Arg.; Merck Bago, Braz.
Omeprazole (p.1278·2) or omeprazole sodium (p.1278·2).
*Acid aspiration; gastro-oesophageal reflux; peptic ulcer; Zollinger-Ellison syndrome.*

**Ulcrafate** Polipharm, Thai.
Sucralfate (p.1290·2).
*Gastro-oesophageal reflux; peptic ulcer.*

**Ulcrast** Boniscontro & Gazzone, Ital.
Sucralfate (p.1290·2).
*Gastritis; gastro-oesophageal reflux; peptic ulcer.*

**Ulcrux** Prater, Chile.
Omeprazole (p.1278·2).
*Peptic ulcer.*

**Ulcubloc** Wolff, Ger.†.
Cimetidine (p.1255·3).
*Acid aspiration; gastro-oesophageal reflux; peptic ulcer; Zollinger-Ellison syndrome.*

**Ulcufato** Berenguer Infale, Spain†.
Sucralfate (p.1290·2).
*Gastrointestinal haemorrhage; peptic ulcer.*

**Ulcu-Pasc** Pascoe, Ger.
Liquorice (p.1270·2); chamomile (p.1669·3).
*Gastrointestinal disorders.*

**Ulcurilen** Austroplant, Austria.
Allantoin (p.1141·3); neomycin sulfate (p.235·1); chlorocresol (p.1177·1); alpha tocoferil acetate (p.1465·1).
*Ulcers; wounds.*

**Ulcurilen N** Spitzner, Ger.
*Ointment:* Allantoin (p.1141·3); chlorocresol (p.1177·1); neomycin sulfate (p.235·1).
*Topical powder:* Allantoin (p.1141·3); neomycin sulfate (p.235·1); alpha tocoferil acetate (p.1465·1).
*Infected skin disorders; wounds.*

**Ulcusan** Kwizda, Austria.
Famotidine (p.1265·2).
*Acid aspiration; gastro-oesophageal reflux; gastrointestinal haemorrhage; peptic ulcer; stress-related ulcer; Zollinger-Ellison syndrome.*

**Ulcyte** Alphapharm, Austral.
Sucralfate (p.1290·2).
*Peptic ulcer.*

**Uldadin** Collins, Mex.
Nizatidine (p.1277·2).
*Peptic ulcer.*

**Uldapril** Collins, Mex.
Lansoprazole (p.1269·3).
*Peptic ulcer.*

**Ulfamet** TO-Chemicals, Thai.
Famotidine (p.1265·2).
*Gastro-oesophageal reflux; peptic ulcer; Zollinger-Ellison syndrome.*

**Ulfon** Cephalon, Fr.†.
Aldioxa (p.1141·2); alcloxa (p.1141·2); calcium carbonate (p.1254·2).
*Gastrointestinal disorders.*

**Ulgarine** Geminis, Spain.
Famotidine (p.1265·2).
*Gastro-oesophageal reflux; peptic ulcer; Zollinger-Ellison syndrome.*

**Ulgastrin**
Note. This name is used for preparations of different composition.
Cibran, Braz.†.
Cimetidine (p.1255·3).
*Gastro-oesophageal reflux; gastrointestinal haemorrhage; peptic ulcer; Zollinger-Ellison syndrome.*

*Diedenhofen, Thai.*
Liquorice (p.1270·2); bismuth subnitrate (p.1252·2); aluminium sodium silicate (p.1250·2); anhydrous sodium sulfate (p.1290·1).
*Gastritis; heartburn; peptic ulcer.*

**Ulgastrin Bis** *Dolorgiet, Ger.†.*
Bismuth subnitrate (p.1252·2).
Formerly contained liquorice, bismuth subnitrate, aluminium sodium silicate, anhydrous sodium sulfate, and belladonna.
*Gastritis; peptic ulcer.*

**Ulgastrin Neu** *Dolorgiet, Ger.†.*
Liquorice (p.1270·2).
*Peptic ulcer.*

**Ulgel** *Dabur, India.*
Magaldrate (p.1271·3); simeticone (p.1289·2).
*Flatulence; gastritis; gastrointestinal hyperacidity; peptic ulcer.*

**Ulgescum** *Dolorgiet, Ger.†.*
Pirenzepine hydrochloride (p.488·1).
*Gastrointestinal disorders.*

**Ulgut** *Shionogi, Jpn.*
Benexate hydrochloride betadex (p.1251·2).
*Gastritis; peptic ulcer.*

**Ulis** *Lafare, Ital.*
Cimetidine (p.1255·3).
*Gastritis and duodenitis associated with acid hypersecretion; gastro-oesophageal reflux; peptic ulcer; Zollinger-Ellison syndrome.*

**Ulkodin** *Precimex, Mex.*
Ranitidine (p.1285·2).
*Peptic ulcer.*

**Ulkowis** *Temmler, Ger.*
Bismuth subnitrate (p.1252·2).
*Dyspepsia; peptic ulcer.*

**Ullus Blasen-Nieren-Tee N** *Polypharm, Ger.†.*
Birch leaf (p.1660·3); solidago virgaurea (p.1748·3); ononis (p.1723·3).
*Urinary-tract disorders.*

**Ullus Galle-Tee N** *Polypharm, Ger.†.*
Taraxacum (p.1751·3); peppermint leaf (p.1283·2); cynara (p.1678·3).
*Gastrointestinal spasm.*

**Ullus Kapseln N** *Polypharm, Ger.*
Liquorice (p.1270·2); chamomile (p.1669·3).
*Gastrointestinal disorders.*

**Ullus Magen-Tee N** *Polypharm, Ger.†.*
Fennel (p.1687·2); peppermint leaf (p.1283·2).
*Dyspepsia.*

**Ulogen** *Fustery, Mex.†.*
Cimetidine (p.1255·3).

**Ulone** *3M, Canad.*
Clofedanol hydrochloride (p.1117·1).
*Coughs.*

**Ulpax** *Hormona, Mex.*
Lansoprazole (p.1269·3).
*Gastro-oesophageal reflux; peptic ulcer; Zollinger-Ellison syndrome.*

**Ulprazole** *Polipharm, Thai.*
Omeprazole (p.1278·2).
*Gastro-oesophageal reflux; peptic ulcer; Zollinger-Ellison syndrome.*

**ULR-LA** *Geneva, USA†.*
Phenylpropanolamine hydrochloride (p.1127·3); guaifenesin (p.1122·1).
*Coughs and cold symptoms; nasal congestion.*

**Ulsal** *Gebro, Austria.*
Ranitidine hydrochloride (p.1285·2).
*Acid aspiration; gastro-oesophageal reflux; gastrointestinal haemorrhage; peptic ulcer; stress-related ulcer; Zollinger-Ellison syndrome.*

**Ulsanic**
*Chugai, Hong Kong; Teva, Israel; Aspen, S.Afr.; Chugai, Thai.*
Sucralfate (p.1290·2).
*Gastritis; gastro-oesophageal reflux; peptic ulcer.*

**Ulsaven** *Collins, Mex.*
Ranitidine hydrochloride (p.1285·2).
*Gastro-oesophageal reflux; hyperchlorhydria; peptic ulcer; Zollinger-Ellison syndrome.*

**Ulsen** *Senosiain, Mex.*
Omeprazole (p.1278·2).
*Gastro-oesophageal reflux; peptic ulcer; Zollinger-Ellison syndrome.*

**Ulserch** *Serch, Arg.*
Pantoprazole (p.1283·1).

**Ulserral** *Serral, Mex.*
Cimetidine (p.1255·3).
*Peptic ulcer.*

**Ultacit** *Aventis, Neth.*
Hydrotalcite (p.1267·3).
*Gastrointestinal disorders associated with hyperacidity.*

**Ultacite** *Roche Nicholas, Fr.†.*
Hydrotalcite (p.1267·3).
*Gastrointestinal disorders.*

**Ultak** *Cipla-Medpro, S.Afr.*
Ranitidine hydrochloride (p.1285·2).
*Acid aspiration; gastro-oesophageal reflux; peptic ulcer; Zollinger-Ellison syndrome.*

**Ultane**
*Abbott, S.Afr.; Abbott, USA.*
Sevoflurane (p.1307·3).
*General anaesthesia.*

**Ultec**
*Teva, Hong Kong†; Berk, UK.*
Cimetidine (p.1255·3).
*Dyspepsia; heartburn; peptic ulcer.*

**Ultexiv** *Alcon, Ger.†.*
Triamcinolone acetonide (p.1110·2); neomycin sulfate (p.235·1); gramicidin (p.220·2).
*Eye disorders.*

**Ulticadex** *Rafarm, Gr.*
Enalapril maleate (p.909·2).
*Heart failure; hypertension.*

**Ultidin** *Pharmacaps, Mex.†.*
Famotidine (p.1265·2).

**Ultilac N** *Bittermedizin, Ger.*
Almasilate (p.1248·2); calcium carbonate (p.1254·2); skimmed milk powder.
*Gastrointestinal disorders.*

**Ultimag** *Mirren, S.Afr.*
Magnesium chloride (p.1228·1); zinc oxide (p.1163·2).
*Magnesium and zinc supplement.*

**Ultiva**
*GlaxoSmithKline, Arg.; GlaxoSmithKline, Austral.; GlaxoSmithKline, Austria; GlaxoSmithKline, Belg.; GlaxoSmithKline, Braz.; Abbott, Canad.; GlaxoSmithKline, Chile; GlaxoSmithKline, Denm.; GlaxoSmithKline, Fin.; GlaxoSmithKline, Fr.; GlaxoSmithKline, Ger.; Glaxo Wellcome, Gr.; GlaxoSmithKline, Hong Kong; Elan, Irl.; GlaxoSmithKline, Israel; GlaxoSmithKline, Ital.; Glaxo Wellcome, Mex.†; GlaxoSmithKline, Neth.; GlaxoSmithKline, Norw.; GlaxoSmithKline, NZ; Glaxo Wellcome, Port.; GlaxoSmithKline, S.Afr.; GlaxoSmithKline, Singapore; GlaxoSmithKline, Spain; GlaxoSmithKline, Swed.; GlaxoSmithKline, Switz.; GlaxoSmithKline, UK; Glaxo Wellcome, USA.*
Remifentanil hydrochloride (p.86·1).
*Analgesia in anaesthesia.*

**Ultra** *Medgenix, Belg.†.*
Sulfacetamide sodium (p.257·3).
*Infected skin lesions.*

**Ultra Adsorb** *Lainco, Spain.*
Activated charcoal (p.1030·2).
*Diarrhoea.*

**Ultra Augenschutz** *Provita, Austria.*
Actinoquinol sodium (p.1647·2).
*Protection of the eyes from ultraviolet radiation.*

**Ultra Chloraseptic** *Prestige, UK.*
*Gargle:* Phenol (p.1188·1).
*Throat spray:* Benzocaine (p.1370·3).
*Sore throat.*

**Ultra Derm** *Reese, USA.*
Emollient and moisturiser.

**Ultra Energizer** *Equilibre Attitude, Fr.*
Guarana; mate; kola; avena; ginseng; ginkgo biloba; minerals; vitamins; octacosanol; sodium molybdate (p.1417·1).
*Tonic.*

**Ultra Heartburn Relief** *Galpharm, UK.*
Famotidine (p.1265·2).
*Dyspepsia; heartburn.*

**Ultra Mide**
*Paladin, Canad.; Baker Cummins, USA.*
Urea (p.1162·2).
*Dry skin; hyperkeratosis.*

**Ultra Strength Megadophilus** *Bullivants, Austral.†.*
*Lactobacillus acidophilus* (p.1704·2); *Bifidobacterium bifidum* (p.1704·2).
*Maintenance of normal gastrointestinal flora.*

**Ultra Tears**
*Alcon, Switz.†; Alcon, USA.*
Hypromellose (p.1579·3).
*Dry eyes.*

**Ultra Vita Time** *Nature's Bounty, USA.*
Multivitamin and mineral preparation with iron and folic acid (p.1417·1).

**Ultra Vita-Min** *Equilibre Attitude, Fr.*
Nutritional supplement (p.1417·1).

**Ultrabas** *Schering, Ger.†.*
Emollient.
*Diluent for Ultralan ointment.*

**Ultrabase**
*Schering, S.Afr.; Schering, UK.*
Emollient.
*Dry skin; pharmaceutical diluent.*

**Ultrabeta** *Vitoria, Port.*
Salmeterol xinafoate (p.795·1).
*Asthma.*

**Ultrabion** *Generfarma, Spain†.*
Ampicillin sodium (p.157·1); ampicillin benzathine (p.158·1).
*Bacterial infections.*

**Ultrabion Balsamico** *Sabater, Spain†.*
Ampicillin sodium (p.157·1); ampicillin benzathine (p.158·1); niaouli oil (p.1719·3); guaifenesin (p.1122·1).
*Respiratory-tract infections.*

**Ultrabiotic** *Bago, Chile.*
Mupirocin (p.233·1).
*Bacterial skin infections; infected burns and wounds.*

**ULTRAbrom** *WE, USA.*
Pseudoephedrine hydrochloride (p.1129·2); brompheniramine maleate (p.426·1).
*Upper respiratory-tract symptoms.*

**Ultrac** *Tecnofarma, Chile.*
Vitamins; minerals; ginseng; rutoside; deanol tartrate (p.1417·1).
*Dietary supplement; tonic.*

**Ultrac E** *Tecnofarma, Chile.*
Vitamins; minerals; ginseng; rutoside; deanol tartrate (p.1417·1).
*Dietary supplement; tonic.*

**Ultrac Q10** *Tecnofarma, Chile.*
Vitamins; minerals; ginseng; rutoside; ubidecarenone (p.1417·1).
*Dietary supplement.*

**Ultracain**
*Aventis, Ger.; Normon, Spain.*
Articaine hydrochloride (p.1370·3).
Adrenaline (p.852·2) may be included in this preparation as a vasoconstrictor to diminish absorption and localise the effect of the local anaesthetic.
*Local anaesthesia.*

**Ultracain Dental** *Aventis, Austria.*
Articaine hydrochloride (p.1370·3).
Adrenaline hydrochloride (p.852·3) is included in this preparation as a vasoconstrictor to diminish absorption and localise the effect of the local anaesthetic.
*Local anaesthesia.*

**Ultracain D-S**
*Aventis, Ger.; Novaxa, Ital.†; Aventis, Neth.*
Articaine hydrochloride (p.1370·3).
Adrenaline hydrochloride (p.852·3) is included in this preparation as a vasoconstrictor to diminish absorption and localise the effect of the local anaesthetic.
*Local anaesthesia.*

**Ultracain D-Suprarenin** *Aventis, Fin.*
Articaine hydrochloride (p.1370·3).
Adrenaline hydrochloride (p.852·3) is included in this preparation as a vasoconstrictor to diminish absorption and localise the effect of the local anaesthetic.
*Local anaesthesia.*

**Ultracain Hyperbaar** *Hoechst Marion Roussel, Neth.†.*
Articaine hydrochloride (p.1370·3).
*Local anaesthesia.*

**Ultracain hyperbar** *Aventis, Ger.*
Articaine hydrochloride (p.1370·3).
*Local anaesthesia.*

**Ultracain Suprarenin** *Aventis, Ger.*
Articaine hydrochloride (p.1370·3).
Adrenaline hydrochloride (p.852·3) is included in this preparation as a vasoconstrictor to diminish absorption and localise the effect of the local anaesthetic.
*Local anaesthesia.*

**Ultracaine D-S**
*Hoechst Marion Roussel, Canad.†; Aventis, Switz.*
Articaine hydrochloride (p.1370·3).
Adrenaline hydrochloride (p.852·3) is included in this preparation as a vasoconstrictor to diminish absorption and localise the effect of the local anaesthetic.
*Local anaesthesia.*

**Ultracal**
*Note. This name is used for preparations of different composition.*
*Baliarda, Arg.*
Saw palmetto (p.1569·1); pygeum africanum (p.1568·2).
*Prostate disorders.*

*Mead Johnson, Austral.; Mead Johnson, Hong Kong; Mead Johnson, NZ; Mead Johnson Nutritionals, Thai.†; Mead Johnson Nutritionals, USA.*
Preparation for enteral nutrition (p.1417·1).

**Ultracalcium** *Temis, Arg.*
Calcium carbonate (p.1254·2).
*Calcium supplement.*

**Ultracarbon**
*Merck, Ger.; Merck Consumer, Singapore; Merck, Thai.*
Activated charcoal (p.1030·2).
*Diarrhoea; flatulence; poisoning.*

**UltraCare**
*Note. A similar name is used for preparations of different composition (see below).*
*Allergan, Canad.; Allergan, USA.*
Disinfecting solution, hydrogen peroxide 3% (p.1182·2); neutralising tablets, catalase (p.1668·3) (p.1164·2).
*Contact lens care.*

**Ultracare**
*Note. A similar name is used for preparations of different composition (see above).*
*Optident, UK.*
Benzocaine (p.1370·3).
*Local anaesthesia.*

**UltraCare Daily Cleaner** *Allergan, Canad.*
Cleaning solution for soft contact lenses (p.1164·2).

**Ultracef**
*Note. This name is used for preparations of different composition.*
*Bristol-Myers Squibb, Irl.*
Cefadroxil (p.167·2).
*Bacterial infections.*

*Promeco, Mex.†.*
Ceftizoxime (p.182·3).
*Bacterial infections.*

**Ultracet** *Ortho McNeil, USA.*
Tramadol hydrochloride (p.94·3); paracetamol (p.76·2).
*Pain.*

**Ultracillin** *Caps, S.Afr.*
Benzathine benzylpenicillin (p.162·3); benzylpenicillin sodium (p.163·2); procaine benzylpenicillin (p.246·1).
*Bacterial infections.*

**Ultra-Clear-A-Med** *Procter & Gamble, Austria†.*
Benzoyl peroxide (p.1143·2).
*Acne.*

**Ultracorten H** *Novartis, Israel†.*
Prednisolone sodium tetrahydrophthalate (p.1109·1).
*Hypersensitivity reactions; shock.*

**Ultracortene-H** *Novartis, Switz.*
Prednisolone sodium tetrahydrophthalate (p.1109·1).
*Corticosteroid.*

**Ultracortenol**
*Novartis, Austria; Novartis, Denm.; Novartis, Fin.; Novartis Ophthalmics, Ger.; Novartis Ophthalmics, Hong Kong; Ciba Vision, Israel; Novartis, Neth.; Novartis, Norw.; Novartis Ophthalmics, Swed.; Novartis Ophthalmics, Switz.*
Prednisolone acetate (p.1108·1) or prednisolone pivalate (p.1108·1).
*Inflammatory eye disorders.*

**Ultracortin** *Collins, Mex.*
Clioquinol (p.196·3); hydrocortisone (p.1103·3).
*Inflammation.*

**Ultracur S** *Schering, Arg.*
Fluocortolone (p.1102·1); fluocortolone caproate (p.1102·1).
*Skin disorders.*

**Ultra-Demoplas** *Godecke, Ger.*
Dexamethasone (p.1097·1); prednisolone (p.1108·1); lidocaine hydrochloride (p.1377·3).
*Musculoskeletal and joint disorders.*

**Ultraderm**
*Note. A similar name is used for preparations of different composition (see below).*
*Ecobi, Ital.*
Fluocinolone acetonide (p.1101·2).
*Skin disorders.*

**Ultraderme**
*Note. A similar name is used for preparations of different composition (see above).*
*Richelet, Fr.*
*Saccharomyces boulardii* (p.1704·2).
*Seborrhoea.*

**Ultradermis** *ICN, Arg.*
Gentamicin sulfate (p.217·1).
*Bacterial skin infections.*

**Ultradina** *Brasmedica, Braz.†.*
Silver (p.1746·1).
*Diarrhoea.*

**Ultradol** *Procter & Gamble, Canad.*
Etodolac (p.37·3).
*Osteoarthritis; pain; rheumatoid arthritis.*

**Ultrafen** *Beximco, Singapore.*
Diclofenac (p.32·1).
*Gout; musculoskeletal and joint disorders; pain.*

**Ultraflu** *Pliva, Ital.*
Acetylcysteine (p.1112·3).
*Respiratory-tract congestion.*

**Ultrafort** *Brasmedica, Braz.†.*
Multivitamin, amino-acid, and mineral preparation (p.1417·1).

**Ultra-Freeda** *Freeda, USA.*
Multivitamin and mineral preparation (p.1417·1).

**Ultragin** *Wyeth, India.*
Paracetamol (p.76·2).
*Fever; pain.*

**Ultra-K** *Melisana, Belg.*
Potassium gluconate (p.1232·2).
*Potassium depletion.*

**Ultralan**
*Note. This name is used for preparations of different composition.*
*Schering, Austria; Schering, Ger.; Asche, Ger.; Schering, Ital.; Schering, Mex.*
*Lotion; cream:* Fluocortolone pivalate (p.1102·1); fluocortolone caproate (p.1102·1).
*Skin disorders.*

*Schering, Austria; Schering, Fr.; Schering, Ger.; Asche, Ger.; Schering, Hong Kong; Schering, Israel; Schering, Ital.*
*Fatty ointment; ointment:* Fluocortolone (p.1102·1); fluocortolone caproate (p.1102·1).
*Skin disorders.*

*Schering, Austria; Schering, Ger.; Asche, Ger.; Schering, Israel†; Schering, Ital.*
*Tablets:* Fluocortolone (p.1102·1).
*Corticosteroid.*

*Schering, Chile; Schering, Neth.; Schering, Switz.†.*
Fluocortolone (p.1102·1) or fluocortolone pivalate (p.1102·1); fluocortolone caproate (p.1102·1).
*Skin disorders.*

*Schering, Mex.*
*Ointment:* Fluocortolone caproate (p.1102·1); fluocortolone (p.1102·1).
*Skin disorders.*

*Galagen, USA.*
Lactose-free, gluten-free preparation for enteral nutrition (p.1417·1).

**Ultralan M** *Schering, Spain.*
Fluocortolone (p.1102·1).
*Skin disorders.*

**Ultralan-crinale** *Schering, Ger.†.*
Fluocortolone pivalate (p.1102·1); salicylic acid (p.1157·1).
*Scalp disorders; skin disorders.*

**Ultralanum Plain** *Meadow, UK.*
Fluocortolone (p.1102·1) or fluocortolone pivalate (p.1102·1); fluocortolone caproate (p.1102·1).
*Skin disorders.*

**Ultralente** *Novo Nordisk, USA.*
Insulin zinc suspension (bovine) (p.333·3).
*Diabetes mellitus.*

**Ultralente MC**
Novo Nordisk, Austral.†; Novo Nordisk, Switz.†.
Insulin zinc suspension (crystalline) (bovine, monocomponent) (p.333·3).
*Diabetes mellitus.*

**Ultra-Levura** Upsamedica, Spain.
*Saccharomyces boulardii* (p.1704·2).
*Restoration of the gastrointestinal flora.*

**Ultra-Levure**
Biocodex, Fr.; Petsiavas (Πετσιαβας), Gr.; Biomed, Switz.
*Saccharomyces boulardii* (p.1704·2).
*Diarrhoea; restoration of gastrointestinal flora.*

**Ultram** Ortho McNeil, USA.
Tramadol hydrochloride (p.94·3).
*Pain.*

**Ultra-Mag** Germania, Austria.
Magnesium gluconate (p.1228·1).
*Magnesium deficiency.*

**Ultra-Mg** Melisana, Belg.
Magnesium gluconate (p.1228·1).
*Magnesium deficiency; neuromuscular hyperexcitability.*

**Ultramicina**
Note. This name is used for preparations of different composition.
Lisopharma, Ital.
Fosfomycin calcium (p.214·2) or fosfomycin disodium (p.214·3).
Lidocaine hydrochloride (p.1377·3) is included in the intramuscular injection to alleviate the pain of injection.
*Bacterial infections.*

Dom, Spain.
Ciprofloxacin hydrochloride (p.188·2).
*Bacterial infections.*

**Ultramicina Plus** Dom, Spain.
Ciprofloxacin (p.188·2); fluocinolone acetonide (p.1101·2).
*Otitis externa.*

**Ultramidol** Irex, Port.
Bromazepam (p.671·3).
*Anxiety.*

**Ultramol** Sterwin, UK.
Paracetamol (p.76·2); codeine phosphate (p.27·1); caffeine (p.782·1).
*Fever; pain.*

**Ultramop** Canderm, Canad.
Methoxsalen (p.1152·1).
*Psoriasis; vitiligo.*

**Ultramox**
Royton, Braz.
Amoxicillin (p.155·3).
*Bacterial infections.*

Restan, S.Afr.†.
Amoxicillin trihydrate (p.155·3).
*Bacterial infections.*

**Ultran** Randall, Mex.
Ranitidine (p.1285·2).
*Acid aspiration; gastric hypersecretion; gastro-oesophageal reflux; gastrointestinal haemorrhage; peptic ulcer; Zollinger-Ellison syndrome.*

**Ultra-Natal** Ethex, USA.
Multivitamin and mineral preparation with carbonyl iron (p.1434·3) (p.1417·1).
*Nutritional supplement in pregnancy and postnatal period.*

**Ultrapenil** Vir, Spain.
Ampicillin sodium (p.157·1); ampicillin benzathine (p.158·1).
*Bacterial infections.*

**Ultraplex 31** Presselin, Ger.†.
Homoeopathic preparation.

**Ultraproct**
Note. This name is used for preparations of different composition.
Schering, Arg.; Schering, Austral.; Schering, Austria; Schering, Belg.; Schering, Chile; Schering, Fr.; Schering, Ger.; Asche, Ger.; Schering, Irl.; Schering, Ital.; Schering, Mex.; Schering, NZ; Schering, Switz.†; Meadow, UK.
Fluocortolone pivalate (p.1102·1); fluocortolone caproate (p.1102·1); cinchocaine hydrochloride (p.1373·2).
Formerly contained fluocortolone pivalate, fluocortolone caproate, cinchocaine hydrochloride, and clemizole undecylate.
*Anorectal disorders.*

Schering, Braz.; Schering, Hong Kong.
Fluocortolone pivalate (p.1102·1); fluocortolone caproate (p.1102·1); cinchocaine hydrochloride (p.1373·2); clemizole undecylate (p.429·2).
*Anorectal disorders.*

Schering, Port.
Fluocortolone pivalate (p.1102·1); lidocaine hydrochloride (p.1377·3).
Ultraproct cream formerly contained fluocortolone pivalate, lidocaine hydrochloride, and chlorquinaldol.
*Anorectal disorders.*

**Ultraquin** Canderm, Canad.
Hydroquinone (p.1148·1); padimate O (p.1155·1); oxybenzone (p.1154·3).
*Skin hyperpigmentation; sunscreen.*

**Ultraquin Plain** Canderm, Canad.
Hydroquinone (p.1148·1).
*Skin hyperpigmentation.*

**Ultra-R** Therapex, Canad.†.
Barium sulfate (p.1061·1).
*Contrast medium for radiography of the small bowel.*

**Ultra-Rich** Pierre Fabre, Hong Kong†.
Avena (p.1658·2).
*Bath additive; skin irritation.*

**Ultrase**
United Medical, Braz.†; Axcan, Canad.; Axcan, USA.
Pancrelipase (p.1725·3).
*Pancreatic enzyme deficiency.*

**Ultrasep** Rivadis, Fr.†.
Glutaral (p.1180·3); didecyldimethylammonium chloride (p.1178·3).
*Surface disinfection.*

**Ultrasept** Genpharm, S.Afr.†.
Co-trimoxazole (p.199·3).
*Bacterial infections.*

**Ultrasine** Schering, Ger.†.
Emollient base.
*Diluent for Ultralan lotion.*

**Ultrasol-F** Fresenius Kabi, Ger.
Formaldehyde (p.1179·3); glyoxal (p.1181·1); glutaral (p.1180·3); benzalkonium chloride (p.1168·3).
*Surface disinfection.*

**Ultrasol-S** Fresenius, Ger.†.
Formaldehyde (p.1179·3); glyoxal (p.1181·1); glutaral (p.1180·3); benzalkonium chloride (p.1168·3).
*Surface disinfection.*

**Ultrassol** Cosmofarma, Port.
Octinoxate (p.1154·3); avobenzone (p.1142·3); octisalate (p.1154·3); oxybenzone (p.1154·3); octocrilene (p.1154·3); zinc oxide (p.1163·2); titanium dioxide (p.1160·3).
*Sunscreen.*

**Ultratard**
Novo Nordisk, Austral.; Novo Nordisk, Fin.; Novo Nordisk, Irl.; Novo Nordisk, Neth.; Novo Nordisk, Norw.; Novo Nordisk, NZ; Novo Nordisk, Port.; Novo Nordisk, Spain; Novo Nordisk, Swed.; Novo Nordisk, UK.
Insulin zinc suspension (crystalline) (human) (p.333·3).
Formerly known as Human Ultratard in the *UK*.
*Diabetes mellitus.*

**Ultratard HM**
Novo Nordisk, Austria; Novo Nordisk, Belg.; Novo Nordisk, Fr.; Novo Nordisk, Ger.; Novo Nordisk, Hong Kong; Novo Nordisk, Ital.; Novo Nordisk, Malaysia; Novo Nordisk, S.Afr.; Novo Nordisk, Singapore; Novo Nordisk, Switz.; Novo Nordisk, Thai.†.
Insulin zinc suspension (crystalline) (recombinant, human, monocomponent) (p.333·3).
*Diabetes mellitus.*

**Ultrathon** 3M, UK†.
Diethyltoluamide (p.1503·3).
*Insect repellent.*

**Ultravate**
Westwood-Squibb, Canad.; Westwood-Squibb, USA.
Ulobetasol propionate (p.1111·3).
*Skin disorders.*

**Ultra-Vinca** Tecnimede, Port.
Vinpocetine (p.1764·2).

**Ultraviral** Raffo, Arg.
Lamivudine (p.648·2).
*HIV infection.*

**Ultraviral Duo** Raffo, Arg.
Lamivudine (p.648·2); zidovudine (p.658·2).
*HIV infection.*

**Ultraviro C** Covan, S.Afr.†.
Aspirin (p.15·1); caffeine (p.782·1); ascorbic acid (p.1460·2); chlorphenamine maleate (p.427·3).
*Cold symptoms; fever; pain.*

**Ultravisin** Farmigea, Ital.
Myrtillus (p.1718·3); *dl*-alpha tocoferil acetate (p.1465·1).
*Vascular retinopathy; vision disorders.*

**Ultravist**
Schering, Austral.; Schering, Austria; Schering, Belg.; Berlex, Canad.; Schering, Denm.; Schering, Fin.; Schering, Fr.; Schering, Ger.; Shepa, Gr.; Schering, Israel; Schering, Ital.; Schering, Neth.; Schering, Norw.; Schering, NZ; Schering, Port.; Schering, S.Afr.; Schering, Spain; Schering, Swed.; Schering, Switz.; Schering, UK; Berlex, USA.
Iopromide (p.1065·2).
*Radiographic contrast medium.*

**Ultravite** Stanley, Canad.
Multivitamin and mineral preparation (p.1417·1).
Formerly known as Ultravite with Minerals.

**Ultrazon N** Douglas, NZ†.
Betamethasone acetate (p.1093·1); neomycin sulfate (p.235·1).
*Infected eye and ear disorders.*

**Ultrazyme**
Allergan, Austral.†; Allergan-Frumtost, Braz.†; Allergan, Canad.; Allergan, Israel†; Allergan, NZ; Allergan, Port.†; Allergan, USA.
Subtilisin-A (p.1164·2).
*Cleanser for soft contact lenses.*

**Ultren** Sanova, Austria.
Vitamin A acetate (p.1453·1); ascorbic acid (p.1460·2).
*Cold and influenza symptoms; vitamin deficiency.*

**Ultreon** Pfizer, Ger.
Azithromycin (p.159·1).
*Mycobacterial infections.*

**Ultrex** Carrington, USA.
Acemannan (p.1645·2).
*Wounds.*

**Ultrimin** Mintlab, Chile.
Ergotamine tartrate (p.467·2); dipyrone (p.35·3); chlorphenamine maleate (p.427·3); caffeine (p.782·1).
*Migraine.*

**Ulxit** Tyrol, Austria.
Nizatidine (p.1277·2).
*Gastro-oesophageal reflux; peptic ulcer.*

**Ulzec** Triomed, S.Afr.
Omeprazole (p.1278·2).
*Gastro-oesophageal reflux; peptic ulcer; Zollinger-Ellison syndrome.*

**Ulzol** Dabur, India.
Omeprazole (p.1278·2).
*Gastro-oesophageal reflux; peptic ulcer; Zollinger-Ellison syndrome.*

**UM Instante** Farmabraz, Braz.†.
Tetracaine (p.1385·1); eugenol (p.1686·2); phenol (p.1188·1); menthol (p.1711·3).
*Mouth disorders.*

**Um Minuto** Kopkins, Braz.†.
Tetracaine hydrochloride (p.1385·1); phenol (p.1188·1); menthol (p.1711·3); methyl salicylate (p.59·3).
*Mouth disorders.*

**Um Segundo** Cibran, Braz.†.
Eugenol (p.1686·2); phenol (p.1188·1); iodine (p.1598·1); lidocaine (p.1377·3); menthol (p.1711·3); methyl salicylate (p.59·3).
*Mouth disorders.*

**Uman-Big** Kedrion, Ital.
A hepatitis B immunoglobulin (p.1617·2).
*Passive immunisation.*

**Uman-Cig** Kedrion, Ital.
A cytomegalovirus immunoglobulin (p.1612·1).
*Passive immunisation.*

**Uman-Complex DI** Kedrion, Ital.
A factor IX preparation (p.752·2).
*Deficiency of factors II, IX or X.*

**Uman-Cry DI** Kedrion, Ital.
Factor VIII (p.751·1).
*Factor VIII deficiency.*

**Uman-Fibrin** Biagini, Ital.†.
Fibrinogen (p.753·2).
*Hypofibrinogenaemia.*

**Uman-Gal E** Biagini, Ital.†.
Antilymphocyte immunoglobulin (horse) (p.1348·3).
*Immunosuppressant therapy.*

**Uman-Gamma** Kedrion, Ital.
A normal immunoglobulin (p.1627·2).
*Hypogammaglobulinaemia; passive immunisation.*

**Uman-Serum** Kedrion, Ital.
Plasma protein fraction (p.758·2).
*Hypoproteinaemia; shock.*

**Uman-Vzig** Kedrion, Ital.
A varicella-zoster immunoglobulin (p.1643·1).
*Passive immunisation.*

**Umasam** Szama, Arg.
Undecenoic acid monoethanolamide (p.411·1).
*Fungal skin infections; seborrhoea.*

**Umatrope** Lilly, Fr.
Somatropin (p.1327·2).
*Growth disorders in renal failure; growth hormone deficiency; Turner's syndrome.*

**Umbradol** Salvat, Spain†.
Salsalate (p.88·1).
*Musculoskeletal, joint, and peri-articular disorders.*

**Umbrium** Kwizda, Austria.
Diazepam (p.690·1).
*Anxiety disorders; skeletal muscle spasm; sleep disorders.*

**Umckaloabo**
Iso, Ger.; Farmasa, Mex.
Pelargonium sidoides.
*Respiratory-tract infections.*

**Umine**
Douglas, NZ; Douglas, Singapore.
Phentermine hydrochloride (p.1592·2).
*Obesity.*

**Umizan** Zerboni, Mex.†.
Phenazopyridine (p.83·2).

**Umoder** Rafarm, Gr.
Atenolol (p.865·2).
*Angina; arrythmias; hypertension.*

**Umolit** Rafarm, Gr.
Buspirone hydrochloride (p.672·2).
*Generalised anxiety.*

**Umoril** Synthelabo, Ital.†.
Toloxatone (p.318·2).
*Depression.*

**Umprel** Novartis, Austria.
Bromocriptine mesilate (p.1200·3).
*Parkinsonism.*

**Umuline Profil 20and 30** Lilly, Fr.
Mixtures of neutral insulin injection (human, prb) 20% and 30% and isophane insulin injection (human, prb) 80% and 70% respectively (p.333·3).
*Diabetes mellitus.*

**Umuline Protamine Isophane (NPH)** Lilly, Fr.
Isophane insulin injection (human, prb) (p.333·3).
*Diabetes mellitus.*

**Umuline Rapide** Lilly, Fr.
Neutral insulin injection (human, prb) (p.333·3).
*Diabetes mellitus.*

**Umuline Zinc** Lilly, Fr.
Insulin zinc suspension (human, prb) (crystalline) (p.333·3).
*Diabetes mellitus.*

**Umuline Zinc Compose** Lilly, Fr.
Insulin zinc suspension (human, prb) (amorphous 30%, crystalline 70%) (p.333·3).
*Diabetes mellitus.*

**UnA De Gato** Hochstetter, Chile.
Uncaria tomentosa.
*Inflammation.*

**Unacid** Pfizer, Ger.
Sulbactam sodium (p.257·2); ampicillin sodium (p.157·1).
*Bacterial infections.*

**Unacid PD** Pfizer, Ger.
Sultamicillin (p.264·2) or sultamicillin tosilate (p.264·2).
*Bacterial infections.*

**Unacil** FIRMA, Ital.†.
Doxycycline hyclate (p.206·2).
*Bacterial infections.*

**Unacim**
Note. This name is used for preparations of different composition.
Jouveinal, Fr.†.
*Tablets:* Sultamicillin tosilate (p.264·2).
*Bacterial infections.*

Pfizer, Fr.
*Injection:* Sulbactam sodium (p.257·2); ampicillin sodium (p.157·1).
Lidocaine hydrochloride (p.1377·3) is included in the intramuscular injection to alleviate the pain of injection.
*Bacterial infections.*

**Unakalm**
Pharmacia Upjohn, Belg.†; Pharmacia, Neth.; Tecnifar, Port.
Ketazolam (p.703·1).
*Anxiety.*

**Un-Alfa** Leo, Fr.
Alfacalcidol (p.1461·2).
*Hypocalcaemia; hypoparathyroidism; renal osteodystrophy; rickets.*

**Unalmes** Silesia, Chile†.
Algestone acetophenide (p.1541·3); estradiol enantate (p.1550·1).
*Combined injectable contraceptive.*

**Unamine** Unison, Thai.
Hydroxyzine hydrochloride (p.434·3).
*Anxiety; hypersensitivity reactions; pruritus.*

**Unamol** Senosiain, Mex.
Cisapride (p.1259·2).
*Constipation; dyspepsia; gastro-oesophageal reflux; gastroparesis.*

**UN-Aspirin** Zee, USA.
Paracetamol (p.76·2).
*Fever; pain.*

**Unasyn**
Note. This name is used for preparations of different composition.
Pfizer, Austria; Pfizer, Chile; Pfizer, Hong Kong; Pfizer, Israel; Pfizer, Ital.; Pfizer, Malaysia; Pfizer, Singapore; Farmasierra, Spain; Pfizer, Thai.; Pfizer, USA.
*Injection:* Ampicillin sodium (p.157·1); sulbactam sodium (p.257·2).
Lidocaine hydrochloride (p.1377·3) may be included in the intramuscular injection to alleviate the pain of injection.
*Bacterial infections.*

Pfizer, Austria; Pfizer, Ital.; Farmasierra, Spain.
*Tablets; oral suspension:* Sultamicillin tosilate (p.264·2).
*Bacterial infections.*

Pfizer, Hong Kong; Pfizer, Ital.; Pfizer, Malaysia; Pfizer, Singapore; Pfizer, Thai.
*Oral suspension; tablets:* Sultamicillin (p.264·2).
*Bacterial infections.*

**Unasyna**
Note. This name is used for preparations of different composition.
Pfizer, Chile; Pfizer, Mex.
*Tablets; oral suspension:* Sultamicillin (p.264·2).
*Bacterial infections.*

Pfizer, Mex.
*Injection:* Sulbactam sodium (p.257·2); ampicillin sodium (p.157·1).
*Bacterial infections.*

**Unasyn-S** Pfizer, Jpn.
Ampicillin sodium (p.157·1); sulbactam sodium (p.257·2).
*Bacterial infections.*

**Unat**
Roche, Austria; Roche, Chile; Roche, Ger.; Roche, Hong Kong; Lakeside, Mex.†; Roche, S.Afr.
Torasemide (p.1015·3) or torasemide sodium (p.1015·3).
*Heart failure; hypertension; oedema; renal insufficiency.*

**Unathen** Streuli, Switz.
Dexpanthenol (p.1727·2).
*Nasal disorders.*

**Unatol** Streuli, Switz.
Vitamin A palmitate (p.1453·1); dexpanthenol (p.1727·2); allantoin (p.1141·3).
*Nasal disorders.*

**Unava** Labinca, Arg.
Gliclazide (p.332·1).
*Diabetes mellitus.*

**Uncadol** Knop, Chile.
Uncaria tomentosa.
*Inflammation; musculoskeletal, joint, and peri-articular disorders.*

**Undecyl** Rekah, Israel.
Zinc undecenoate (p.411·1); undecenoic acid (p.410·3).
*Fungal skin infections.*

**Undelenic** Gordon, USA.
Undecenoic acid (p.410·3).
*Fungal skin infections.*

**Underan** *Saval, Chile.*
Mupirocin (p.233·1).
*Bacterial skin infections.*

**Undestor**
*Organon, Arg.; Organon, Belg.; Organon, Swed.*
Testosterone undecylate (p.1570·1).
*Male hypogonadism; osteoporosis.*

**Undex** *Melisana, Switz.*
Clotrimazole (p.396·2).
*Fungal foot infections.*

**Unergol** *Poli, Ital.†.*
Dihydroergocristine mesilate (p.1680·1).
*Hyperprolactinaemia; inhibition of lactation.*

**Unex Amarum** *Repha, Ger.*
Gentian (p.1692·2); absinthium (p.1645·1); ginger (p.1267·1).
*Appetite loss; dyspepsia; meteorism.*

**Unexym MD S** *Repha, Ger.*
Pancreatin (p.1725·3); betaine hydrochloride (p.1660·2).
Unexym MD formerly contained pancreatin, papain, and betaine hydrochloride (ROTE.00).
*Digestive disorders.*

**Unexym mono** *Repha, Ger.*
Pancreatin (p.1725·3).
*Pancreatic disorders.*

**Ung Vernleigh** *Propan, S.Afr.*
Sulfanilamide (p.263·2); merbromin (p.1185·3); peru balsam (p.1730·2); cod-liver oil (p.1425·2).
*Burns; wounds.*

**Ungel** *Stiefel, Arg.*
Triclocarban (p.1195·1).
*Dandruff.*

**Unguentacid** *Mucos, Ger.*
Linoleic acid triglyceride (p.1690·2); vitamin A palmitate (p.1453·1); *dl*-alpha tocoferil acetate (p.1465·1).
*Skin disorders.*

**Unguentine** *Mentholatum, USA.*
Phenol (p.1188·1); zinc oxide (p.1163·2); eucalyptus oil (p.1686·2); thyme oil (p.1755·3).
*Pain in minor burns.*

**Unguentine Plus** *Mentholatum, USA.*
Lidocaine hydrochloride (p.1377·3); chloroxylenol (p.1177·2); phenol (p.1188·1).
*Skin disorders.*

**Unguento Callicida Naion** *Puerto Galiano, Spain.*
Lactic acid (p.1704·1); salicylic acid (p.1157·1).
*Callosities.*

**Unguento Dermico Antibiotico**
*Note. This name is used for preparations of different composition.*
*Drag, Chile.*
Neomycin (p.235·1); polymyxin b (p.245·2).
*Bacterial skin infections.*
*Laboratorios Chile, Chile.*
Neomycin (p.235·1); bacitracin (p.161·3).
*Bacterial skin infections.*

**Unguento Leon** *Beiersdorf, Chile.*
Methyl salicylate (p.59·3); camphor (p.1665·3).
*Musculoskeletal and joint disorders.*

**Unguento Morry** *Teofarma, Spain.*
Salicylic acid (p.1157·1).
*Calluses.*

**Unguentolan** *Heyl, Ger.*
Cod-liver oil (p.1425·2).
*Wounds.*

**Unguentum Bossi** *Doak, USA†.*
Ammoniated mercury (p.1152·1); methenamine sulfosalicylate; coal tar (p.1159·2).
*Skin disorders.*

**Unguentum Lactisol** *Galactopharm, Ger.†.*
Lactic acid (p.1704·1).
*Skin disorders; wounds.*

**Unguentum lymphaticum** *PGM, Ger.*
Hemlock; colchicum (p.416·3); digitalis (p.894·2); podophyllum (p.1155·2); hyoscyamus (p.485·2); calendula (p.1665·2).
*Lymphatic disorders.*

**Unguentum M**
*Boots Healthcare, Irl.; Crookes Healthcare, UK.*
Emollient.
*Dry skin disorders; nappy rash; pharmaceutical diluent.*

**Unguentum Truw** *Truw, Ger.†.*
Homoeopathic preparation.

**Ungvita**
*Note. This name is used for preparations of different composition.*
*Roche Consumer, Austral.*
*Cream:* Zinc oxide (p.1163·2).
*Minor cuts and abrasions; skin disorders.*
*Ointment:* Vitamin A palmitate (p.1453·1).
*Traumatic skin disorders.*
*Roche, NZ.*
*Cream†:* Vitamin A palmitate (p.1453·1); calamine (p.1144·1); dimethicone (p.1482·1).
*Nappy rash; skin abrasions; skin irritation.*
*Ointment:* Vitamin A palmitate (p.1453·1).
*Chafed skin; cracked heels; cracked nipples; dry skin; minor burns.*

**Uni Amox** *Uniao Quimica, Braz.*
Amoxicillin trihydrate (p.155·3).
*Bacterial infections.*

**Uni B Complex Poliv** *Uniao Quimica, Braz.*
Vitamin B substances (p.1417·1).

**Uni Bromazepax** *Uniao Quimica, Braz.*
Bromazepam (p.671·3).
*Anxiety.*

**Uni Carbamaz** *Uniao Quimica, Braz.*
Carbamazepine (p.353·3).
*Epilepsy; neuritis.*

**Uni Cetotifen** *Uniao Quimica, Braz.*
Ketotifen fumarate (p.788·1).

**Uni Dexametason** *Uniao Quimica, Braz.*
Dexamethasone acetate (p.1097·1) or dexamethasone phosphate (p.1097·2).
*Corticosteroid.*

**Uni Diazepax** *Uniao Quimica, Braz.*
Diazepam (p.690·1).
*Anxiety.*

**Uni Doxiciclin** *Uniao Quimica, Braz.*
Doxycycline hyclate (p.206·2).
*Bacterial infections.*

**Uni Gliben** *Uniao Quimica, Braz.*
Glibenclamide (p.331·2).
*Diabetes mellitus.*

**Uni Haloper** *Uniao Quimica, Braz.*
Haloperidol (p.701·2).
*Psychoses.*

**Uni Hioscin** *Uniao Quimica, Braz.*
Hyoscine butylbromide (p.483·3).
*Muscle spasm.*

**Uni Masdil** *Esteve, Spain.*
Diltiazem hydrochloride (p.900·1).
*Angina pectoris; hypertension.*

**Uni Mist** *Asta Medica, Spain†.*
Morphine sulfate (p.60·2).
*Pain.*

**Uni Propralol** *Uniao Quimica, Braz.*
Propranolol hydrochloride (p.989·3).
*Arrhythmias; hypertension.*

**Uni Salve** *Smith & Nephew, Austral.*
Soft paraffin (p.1479·3).
*Barrier cream; minor skin irritations.*

**Uni Vir** *Uniao Quimica, Braz.*
Aciclovir (p.626·1).
*Herpesvirus infections.*

**Uni-Ace** *URL, USA.*
Paracetamol (p.76·2).

**Unibac** *Lilly, Belg.*
Dirithromycin (p.206·1).
*Bacterial infections.*

**Unibar** *Therapex, Canad.†.*
Barium sulfate (p.1061·1).
*Radiographic contrast medium.*

**Unibaryt** *Goldham, Ger.†.*
Sodium bicarbonate (p.1223·2); anhydrous citric acid (p.1673·1); simeticone (p.1289·2).
*Adjuvant to double contrast radiography; diagnostic agent.*

**Unibaryt-R** *IFET (ΙΦΕΤ), Gr.*
Barium sulfate (p.1061·1).
*Radiographic contrast medium.*

**Unibase** *Warner Chilcott, USA.*
Vehicle for topical preparations.

**Uni-Bent Cough** *URL, USA†.*
Diphenhydramine hydrochloride (p.431·3).

**Unibios Simple** *Fabra, Arg.*
Dipyrone (p.35·3).
*Fever; inflammation; pain.*

**Unicaine** *Bournonville, Belg.†.*
Oxybuprocaine hydrochloride (p.1382·1).
*Local anaesthesia.*

**Unical** *Sooft, Ital.*
Calcium carbonate (p.1254·2).
*Calcium deficiency; calcium supplement.*

**Unicalm** *Asofarma, Arg.*
Rofecoxib (p.86·3).
*Osteoarthritis; pain.*

**Unicap**
*Pharmacia, Braz.; Pharmacia Upjohn, Hong Kong†; Upjohn, UK†; Upjohn, USA.*
A range of vitamin and mineral preparations (p.1417·1).

**Unicap M** *Pharmacia Upjohn, Hong Kong†.*
Multivitamin and mineral preparation (p.1417·1).

**Unicarbazan** *Unichem, India.*
Diethylcarbamazine citrate (p.104·1); chlorphenamine maleate (p.427·3).
*Filariasis; tropical eosinophilia.*

**Unicef** *Ripari-Gero, Ital.†.*
Cefonicid sodium (p.174·2).
Lidocaine hydrochloride (p.1377·3) is included in this preparation to alleviate the pain of injection.
*Bacterial infections.*

**Uni-Check** *Exxe, Ital.*
Test for glucose in blood (p.1694·2).

**Unichew** *Ranbaxy, Thai.†.*
Dried aluminium hydroxide gel (p.1249·2); magnesium hydroxide (p.1272·2).
*Gastric hyperacidity; peptic ulcer.*

**Unichol** *Merck, Austria.*
Hymecromone (p.1700·1).
*Biliary-tract disorders.*

**Unicid** *Prospa, Ital.*
Cefonicid sodium (p.174·2).
Lidocaine hydrochloride (p.1377·3) is included in the intramuscular injection to alleviate the pain of injection.
*Gram-negative bacterial infections.*

**Unicide** *Unison, Thai.*
Niclosamide (p.110·1).
*Cestode infections.*

**Unicilin** *Universales, Mex.†.*
Ampicillin (p.157·1).
*Bacterial infections.*

**Unicilina** *Antibioticos, Spain.*
Benzylpenicillin sodium (p.163·2).
*Bacterial infections.*

**Uniclar**
*White, Arg.; Essex, Chile; Essex, Ital.; Undra, Mex.*
Mometasone furoate (p.1107·2).
*Rhinitis; sinusitis.*

**Uniclor** *Solfran, Mex.*
Chloramphenicol (p.185·1).
*Bacterial infections.*

**Uni-Colex** *Universal, Hong Kong.*
Guaifenesin (p.1122·1).
*Coughs.*

**Unicomplex-T & M** *Rugby, USA.*
Multivitamin and mineral preparation with iron and folic acid (p.1417·1).

**Unicontin**
*Modi-Mundipharma, India; Viatris, Port.*
Theophylline (p.798·3).
*Obstructive airways disease.*

**Unicordium** *Organon, Fr.*
Bepridil hydrochloride (p.868·3).
*Angina pectoris.*

**Unidasa** *Roux-Ocefa, Arg.*
Hyaluronidase (p.1698·2).

**Uni-Decon** *URL, USA†.*
Phenylpropanolamine hydrochloride (p.1127·3); phenylephrine hydrochloride (p.1126·3); chlorphenamine maleate (p.427·3); phenyltoloxamine citrate (p.439·1).
*Upper respiratory-tract symptoms.*

**Uniderm**
*Note. This name is used for preparations of different composition.*
*Smith & Nephew, Austral.*
Moisturiser.
*Schering-Plough, Denm.; Schering-Plough, Fin.†; Schering-Plough, Swed.*
Hydrocortisone (p.1103·3).
*Skin disorders.*
*Unison, Hong Kong; Unison, Singapore.*
Clobetasol propionate (p.1095·2).
*Skin disorders.*
*Raza, Malaysia; Pharmaniaga, Malaysia.*
Miconazole nitrate (p.405·3).
*Fungal skin and nail infections.*

**Unidermo** *Uniderm, Ital.*
Lactic acid (p.1704·1); collagen (p.1674·3).
*Skin cleansing.*

**Unidie** *Fournier SA, Spain.*
Cefonicid sodium (p.174·2).
*Bacterial infections.*

**Unidixina** *Universales, Mex.†.*
Nalidixic acid (p.234·1).

**Unidor** *Sanofi Synthelabo, Spain.*
Aspirin (p.15·1); caffeine (p.782·1).
*Fever; pain.*

**Unidose** *Cifarma, Braz.†.*
Etynodiol diacetate (p.1554·2); ethinylestradiol (p.1553·2).
*Combined oral contraceptive.*

**Unidox**
*Yamanouchi, Belg.†; Yamanouchi, Neth.*
Doxycycline (p.206·2).
*Bacterial infections.*

**Unidrol** *Unichem, India.*
Methylprednisolone acetate (p.1106·1).
*Corticosteroid.*

**Uni-Dur**
*Recordati, Ital.†; Schering-Plough, Mex.; Schering-Plough, S.Afr.†; Key, USA†.*
Theophylline (p.798·3).
*Obstructive airways disease.*

**Unienzyme c MPS** *Unichem, India.*
Amylase (p.1654·2); papain (p.1727·3); simeticone (p.1289·2); nicotinamide (p.1441·2); activated charcoal (p.1030·2).
*Dyspepsia; flatulence.*

**Unif** *Tek, Thai.*
Triamcinolone acetonide (p.1110·2).
*Skin and scalp disorders.*

**Uni-Febrin** *Universal, Hong Kong.*
Paracetamol (p.76·2).
*Fever; pain.*

**Uni-Fedra Compound** *Universal, Hong Kong.*
Triprolidine hydrochloride (p.442·3); pseudoephedrine hydrochloride (p.1129·2); codeine phosphate (p.27·1).
*Coughs; nasal congestion.*

**Unifenobarb** *Uniao Quimica, Braz.*
Phenobarbital (p.367·3).
*Epilepsy.*

**Unifer**
*Note. This name is used for preparations of different composition.*
*Rider, Chile.*
Ferrous gluceptate (p.1428·1).
*Iron deficiency; iron-deficiency anaemia.*
*Tosi, Ital.*
Iron sucrose (p.1438·2).
*Iron-deficiency anaemia.*
*Grossman, Mex.*
Iron carbonyl (p.1436·1).
*Iron-deficiency anaemia.*

**Unifiber** *Niche, USA.*
Powdered cellulose (p.1578·3).
*Constipation.*

**Unifibre** *Niche, Singapore†.*
Dietary fibre supplement (p.1417·1).
*Constipation.*

**Unifilin** *Uniao Quimica, Braz.*
Aminophylline (p.780·2).
*Asthma.*

**Uniflex**
*Xepa-Soul Pattinson, Malaysia; Xepa-Soul Pattinson, Singapore.*
Betamethasone valerate (p.1093·2).
*Skin disorders.*

**Uniflex-N**
*Xepa-Soul Pattinson, Malaysia; Xepa-Soul Pattinson, Singapore†.*
Betamethasone valerate (p.1093·2); neomycin sulfate (p.235·1).
*Infected skin disorders.*

**Uniflox** *Bayer, Fr.*
Ciprofloxacin hydrochloride (p.188·2).
*Cystitis; gonococcal urethritis.*

**Uniflu & Gregovite C** *Unigreg, Irl.†.*
Uniflu tablets, paracetamol (p.76·2); codeine phosphate (p.27·1); caffeine (p.782·1); diphenhydramine hydrochloride (p.431·3); phenylephrine hydrochloride (p.1126·3); Gregovite C tablets, ascorbic acid (p.1460·2).
*Colds and influenza symptoms.*

**Uniflu with Gregovite C** *Unigreg, UK.*
Uniflu tablets, phenylephrine hydrochloride (p.1126·3); caffeine (p.782·1); codeine phosphate (p.27·1); diphenhydramine hydrochloride (p.431·3); paracetamol (p.76·2); Gregovite C tablets, ascorbic acid (p.1460·2).
*Cold and influenza symptoms; nasal congestion.*

**Unifluid** *Thea, Fr.*
Povidone (p.1581·2).
*Dry eyes.*

**Unifyl**
*Mundipharma, Austria; Mundipharma, Switz.*
Theophylline (p.798·3).
*Obstructive airways disease.*

**Unigamol** *Norgine, Ger.*
Evening primrose oil (p.1686·3).
*Atopic eczema.*

**Unigan**
*Unison, Hong Kong; Unison, Thai.*
Hyoscine butylbromide (p.483·3); paracetamol (p.76·2).
*Smooth muscle pain and spasm.*

**Unigo** *Unison, Hong Kong.*
Metronidazole (p.607·2).
*Anaerobic bacterial infections; protozoal infections.*

**Uni-Gold hCG** *Kora, Irl.*
Pregnancy test (p.1734·3).

**Unigrip** *Uniao Quimica, Braz.*
Paracetamol (p.76·2).
*Fever; pain.*

**Unigyn** *Uniderm, Ital.*
Lactic acid (p.1704·1).
*Personal hygiene; vaginal douche.*

**Unihep**
*Leo, Irl.; Leo, UK†.*
Heparin sodium (p.928·1).
*Thromboembolic disorders.*

**Uni-Kaotin** *Universal, Hong Kong.*
Kaolin (p.1268·3); pectin (p.1580·3).
*Diarrhoea.*

**Uniket** *Lacer, Spain.*
Isosorbide mononitrate (p.942·1).
*Angina pectoris.*

**Unik-Zoru** *Therapex, Canad.†.*
Tartaric acid (p.1752·1); sodium bicarbonate (p.1223·2).
*Diagnostic agent.*

**Unilair**
*3M, Ger.; 3M, Neth.†.*
Theophylline (p.798·3).
*Obstructive airways disease.*

**Unilan** *Merck, Port.*
Alprazolam (p.668·3).
*Anxiety.*

**Unilarm** *Novartis Ophthalmics, Fr.*
Sodium chloride (p.1233·3).
*Dry eye.*

**Uniloc**
*Nycomed, Denm.; Nycomed, Fin.†; Nycomed, Norw.; Nycomed, Swed.*
Atenolol (p.865·2).
*Angina pectoris; arrhythmias; hypertension; hyperthyroidism; migraine; myocardial infarction.*

**Unilong** *Altana, Spain.*
Theophylline (p.798·3).
*Heart failure; obstructive airways disease; paroxysmal dyspnoea.*

**Unilux** *Goldham, Ger.*
Iopamidol (p.1064·3).
*Radiographic contrast medium.*

**Uni-Ma**
*Unison, Hong Kong; Unison, Thai.*
Monobasic sodium phosphate (p.1230·3); dibasic sodium phosphate (p.1231·1).
*Bowel evacuation; constipation.*

**Unimaalox** *Aventis, Spain†.*
Aluminium hydroxide (p.1249·2); magnesium hydroxide (p.1272·2).
*Dyspepsia; gastrointestinal hyperacidity.*

**Unimax**
*AstraZeneca, Austria; AstraZeneca, Fin.; AstraZeneca, Ger.; Promed, Ger.; AstraZeneca, Neth.; AstraZeneca, Switz.*
Felodipine (p.914·3); ramipril (p.994·1).
*Hypertension.*

**Unimazole** *Unipharma, Gr.*
Thiamazole (p.1603·3).
*Hyperthyroidism.*

**Unimer** *Diepharmex, Fr.*
Sea water.
*Nasal cleansing.*

**Unimest** *Astra, Spain†.*
Felodipine (p.914·3); ramipril (p.994·1).
*Hypertension.*

**Unimezol**
*Unichem, India; Ranbaxy, Thai.†.*
Metronidazole (p.607·2).
*Anaerobic bacterial infections; protozoal infections; ulcerative gingivitis.*

**Unimicebrina** *Sanofi Synthelabo, Spain.*
Ascorbic acid (p.1460·2).
*Adjunct in iron therapy; vitamin C deficiency.*

**Unimol** *Unison, Thai.*
Paracetamol (p.76·2).
*Fever; pain.*

**Unimox**
*Unison, Hong Kong; Unison, Singapore; Unison, Thai.*
Amoxicillin trihydrate (p.155·3).
*Bacterial infections.*

**Uniparin**
*Aventis, Austral.; CP Pharmaceuticals, Irl.†; CP Pharmaceuticals, UK†.*
Heparin calcium (p.927·3) or heparin sodium (p.928·1).
*Thromboembolic disorders.*

**Unipen** *Wyeth-Ayerst, USA†.*
Nafcillin sodium (p.233·3).
*Bacterial infections.*

**Unipexil** *Gifrer Barbezat, Fr.†.*
Minoxidil (p.960·1).
*Alopecia androgenetica.*

**Uni-Phen** *Universal, Hong Kong.*
Ammonium chloride (p.1115·2); sodium citrate (p.1223·2); diphenhydramine hydrochloride (p.431·3); menthol (p.1711·3).
*Coughs; nasal congestion.*

**Uni-Pholco** *Universal, Hong Kong.*
Pholcodine (p.1128·3).
*Coughs.*

**Uniphyl**
*Purdue, Canad.; Mundipharma, Hong Kong†; Adcock Ingram, S.Afr.; Purdue Frederick, USA.*
Theophylline (p.798·3).
*Obstructive airways disease.*

**Uniphyllin**
*Mundipharma, Ger.; Unipharma, Gr.*
Theophylline (p.798·3) or theophylline sodium glycinate (p.804·3).
*Obstructive airways disease.*

**Uniphyllin Continus**
*Napp, Irl.; Napp, UK.*
Theophylline (p.798·3).
*Heart failure; obstructive airways disease.*

**Unipine XL** *Genus, UK†.*
Nifedipine (p.966·2).
*Hypertension.*

**Uniplex**
*Note. This name is used for preparations of different composition.*
*Cimed, Braz.*
Amino-acid, vitamin, and mineral preparation (p.1417·1).

*Unipharma, Gr.*
Aciclovir (p.626·1).
*Herpes simplex infections.*

**Uniplus** *Angelini, Ital.*
Oxolamine citrate (p.1126·1); propyphenazone (p.85·3).
*Influenza symptoms; oral inflammation; otorhinolaryngeal inflammation; tracheobronchitis.*

**Uniprazol** *Uniao Quimica, Braz.*
Omeprazole (p.1278·2).
*Peptic ulcer.*

**Unipred** *Osoth, Thai.*
Prednisolone (p.1108·1); neomycin sulfate (p.235·1).
*Infected skin disorders.*

**Unipril** *AstraZeneca, Ital.*
Ramipril (p.994·1).
*Heart failure; hypertension; renal insufficiency.*

**Uniprildiur** *AstraZeneca, Ital.*
Ramipril (p.994·1); hydrochlorothiazide (p.933·2).
*Hypertension.*

**Uniprofen** *Uniao Quimica, Braz.*
Ibuprofen (p.45·3).
*Inflammation; pain.*

**Unique PH** *Alcon, Braz.*
Cleansing and wetting solution for hard contact lenses (p.1164·2).

**Unique Plus** *Eurofarma, Braz.*
Sodium monofluorophosphate (p.1446·2).
*Dental caries prophylaxis.*

**Uniquin**
*Biochemie, Austria; Wassermann, Ital.; Medinfar, Port.; Searle, S.Afr.*
Lomefloxacin hydrochloride (p.227·2).
*Bacterial infections.*

**Uni-Ramine** *Universal, Hong Kong.*
Chlorphenamine maleate (p.427·3).
*Hypersensitivity reactions.*

**Uni-Ramine CE** *Universal, Hong Kong.*
Codeine phosphate (p.27·1); ephedrine hydrochloride (p.1120·1); ammonium chloride (p.1115·2); chlorphenamine maleate (p.427·3).
*Coughs.*

**Uni-Ramine Expectorant** *Universal, Hong Kong.*
Chlorphenamine maleate (p.427·3); ammonium chloride (p.1115·2); sodium citrate (p.1223·2).
*Coughs.*

**Uniren**
*Unison, Hong Kong; Unison, Singapore; Unison, Thai.*
Diclofenac diethylamine (p.32·1) or diclofenac sodium (p.32·1).
*Musculoskeletal, joint, peri-articular, and soft-tissue disorders.*

**Uniretic** *Schwarz, USA.*
Moexipril hydrochloride (p.961·2); hydrochlorothiazide (p.933·2).
*Hypertension.*

**Unirhinol** *Union, Singapore†.*
Chlorphenamine maleate (p.427·3); paracetamol (p.76·2); phenylpropanolamine hydrochloride (p.1127·3).
*Cold symptoms.*

**Uniroid-HC** *Chemidex, UK.*
Cinchocaine hydrochloride (p.1373·2); hydrocortisone (p.1103·3).
*Anorectal disorders.*

**Unisal** *Merck Sharp & Dohme, Switz.*
Diflunisal (p.34·1).
*Inflammation; pain.*

**Uniscrub**
*Seton, Israel; SSL, UK†.*
Chlorhexidine gluconate (p.1173·2).
*Skin disinfection.*

**Unisedil** *Merck, Port.*
Diazepam (p.690·1).
*Alcohol withdrawal syndrome; anxiety disorders; skeletal muscle spasm.*

**Unisedyl** *Union, Singapore.*
Codeine phosphate (p.27·1); promethazine hydrochloride (p.439·1); ephedrine hydrochloride (p.1120·1).
*Coughs.*

**Unisept** *Seton, Israel.*
Chlorhexidine gluconate (p.1173·2).
*Disinfection of burns, mucous membranes, skin, and wounds.*

**Unisoil** *Therapex, Canad.†.*
Castor oil (p.1668·2).
*Constipation.*

**Unisol**
*Agepha, Austria; Alcon, USA.*
Rinsing and storage solutions for soft contact lenses (p.1164·2).

**Unisolve** *Smith & Nephew, Austral.*
Dipropylene glycol methyl ether; isopropyl alcohol (p.1184·3); isoparaffin.
*Medical adhesive remover.*

**Unisom**
*Note. This name is used for preparations of different composition.*
*Pfizer Consumer, Austral.; Pfizer Consumer, Canad.; Pfizer, Hong Kong; Pfizer, Mex.; Pfizer, NZ.*
Diphenhydramine hydrochloride (p.431·3).
*Insomnia.*

*Pfizer, Israel; Warner-Lambert, Spain†.*
Doxylamine succinate (p.432·3).
*Insomnia.*

**Unisom-2** *Pfizer Consumer, Canad.*
Doxylamine succinate (p.432·3).
*Insomnia.*

**Unisom Natural Source** *Pfizer Consumer, Canad.*
Valerian (p.1762·2).
*Insomnia.*

**Unisom with Pain Relief** *Pfizer Consumer, USA.*
Paracetamol (p.76·2); diphenhydramine hydrochloride (p.431·3).
*Insomnia; pain.*

**Unisom SleepTabs** *Pfizer Consumer, USA.*
Doxylamine succinate (p.432·3).
*Insomnia.*

**Unisom-C** *Pfizer, Canad.†.*
Diphenhydramine hydrochloride (p.431·3).
*Insomnia.*

**Unison Enema**
*Note. This name is used for preparations of different composition.*
*Unison, Hong Kong.*
Sodium chloride (p.1233·3).
*Constipation.*

*Unison, Thai.*
Macrogol (p.1708·2); sodium chloride.
*Constipation.*

**Unison Ointment** *Unison, Thai.*
Chloramphenicol (p.185·1).
*Bacterial skin infections.*

**Unistep hCG** *Orion, USA.*
Pregnancy test (p.1734·3).

**Unistin** *BPL-Meizler, Braz.*
Cisplatin (p.538·1).
*Malignant neoplasms.*

**Unitable** *INQ, Braz.†.*
Multivitamin and mineral preparation (p.1417·1).

**Unithroid** *Lannett, USA.*
Levothyroxine sodium (p.1600·1).
*Hypothyroidism.*

**Unitifed** *Union, Singapore.*
*Linctus:* Codeine phosphate (p.27·1); triprolidine hydrochloride (p.442·3); pseudoephedrine hydrochloride (p.1129·2).
Formerly known as Unitifed Compound.
*Syrup:* Triprolidine hydrochloride (p.442·3); pseudoephedrine hydrochloride (p.1129·2).
*Allergic rhinitis; cold symptoms; coughs; nasal and upper respiratory-tract congestion; sinusitis.*

**Unitimoftol** *Merck Sharp & Dohme, Spain†.*
Timolol maleate (p.1012·2).
*Glaucoma; ocular hypertension.*

**Unitinase** *BPL-Meizler, Braz.*
Streptokinase (p.1005·2).
*Thromboembolic disorders.*

**Unitone**
*Note. This name is used for preparations of different composition.*
*Fouchard, Chile.*
Nanotalasferas; betacarotene (p.1422·3).
*Skin pigmentation disorders.*

*Darier, Mex.*
Betacarotene (p.1422·3); octinoxate (p.1154·3); avobenzone (p.1142·3).
*Skin hyperpigmentation.*

**Uni-Tranxene** *Sanofi Synthelabo, Belg.*
Dipotassium clorazepate (p.685·1).
*Anxiety; mixed anxiety depressive states.*

**Unitrexate** *BPL-Meizler, Braz.*
Methotrexate (p.568·2).
*Malignant neoplasms.*

**Unitril** *Kener, Mex.†.*
Dimenhydrinate (p.431·1).

**Unitrim** *Master Pharma, Ital.†.*
Brodimoprim (p.165·3).
*Otorhinolaryngeal infections; respiratory-tract infections.*

**Unitrol** *Republic, USA†.*
Phenylpropanolamine hydrochloride (p.1127·3).
*Obesity.*

**Unitul Complex** *Bama, Spain.*
Sodium acexamate (p.1646·2); sulfadiazine silver (p.259·1).
*Burns; ulcers; wounds.*

**Unitulle**
*Aventis, Austral.; Cassenne, Fr.†.*
White soft paraffin (p.1479·3).
*Burns; skin ulcers; wounds.*

**Unituss** *Unison, Thai.*
Diphenhydramine hydrochloride (p.431·3); ammonium chloride (p.1115·2); sodium citrate (p.1223·2); menthol (p.1711·3).
*Coughs; nasal congestion.*

**Unituss HC** *URL, USA.*
Hydrocodone tartrate (p.45·1); phenylephrine hydrochloride (p.1126·3); chlorphenamine maleate (p.427·3).
*Upper respiratory-tract symptoms.*

**Uni-tussin** *URL, USA†.*
Guaifenesin (p.1122·1).
*Coughs.*

**Uni-tussin DM** *URL, USA.*
Dextromethorphan hydrobromide (p.1117·3); guaifenesin (p.1122·1).
*Coughs.*

**Unival**
*Note. This name is used for preparations of different composition.*
*Pharmafina, Chile.*
Lansoprazole (p.1269·3).
*Peptic ulcer.*

*Senosiain, Mex.*
Sucralfate (p.1290·2).
*Gastritis; peptic ulcer.*

**Univasc** *Schwarz, USA.*
Moexipril hydrochloride (p.961·2).
*Hypertension.*

**Uni-Vasin** *Universal, Hong Kong.*
Chlorphenamine maleate (p.427·3); phenylephrine hydrochloride (p.1126·3); phenylpropanolamine hydrochloride (p.1127·3).
*Upper respiratory-tract disorders.*

**Univate**
*Xepa-Soul Pattinson, Malaysia; Xepa-Soul Pattinson, Singapore.*
Clobetasol propionate (p.1095·2).
*Skin disorders.*

**Univer** *Elan, UK.*
Verapamil hydrochloride (p.1019·1).
*Angina pectoris; hypertension.*

**Universal Concentration Tablets** *Universal, S.Afr.†.*
Caffeine (p.782·1).
*Fatigue.*

**Universal Earache Drops** *Propan, S.Afr.†.*
Phenazone (p.82·3); procaine hydrochloride (p.1383·2); potassium hydroxyquinoline sulfate (p.1734·2).
*Ear disorders.*

**Universal Eye Drops** *Propan, S.Afr.†.*
Phenylephrine hydrochloride (p.1126·3); boric acid (p.1662·1).
*Eye inflammation; eye irritation.*

**Universal Nasal Drops** *Propan, S.Afr.†.*
Phenylephrine hydrochloride (p.1126·3); naphazoline nitrate (p.1124·3).
*Allergic rhinitis; sinusitis.*

**Universal Throat Lollies** *Propan, S.Afr.†.*
Cetylpyridinium chloride (p.1173·1).
*Mouth and throat infections.*

**Univol** *Carter Horner, Canad.*
Aluminium hydroxide (p.1249·2); magnesium hydroxide (p.1272·2).
*Gastrointestinal disorders associated with hyperacidity.*

**Uniwarfin** *Unichem, India.*
Warfarin sodium (p.1022·2).
*Thromboembolic disorders.*

**Uniwash** *Smith & Nephew, Austral.*
Skin cleanser.

**UniXan** *Norpharma, Denm.*
Theophylline (p.798·3).
*Obstructive airways disease.*

**Unixime** *FIRMA, Ital.*
Cefixime (p.172·3).
*Bacterial infections.*

**Unizen**
*Unison, Hong Kong; Unison, Malaysia; Unison, Singapore; Unison, Thai.*
Serrapeptase (p.1743·2).
*Inflammation; respiratory-tract congestion.*

**Unizink** *Kohler, Ger.; Kohler-Pharma, Ger.*
Zinc aspartate (p.1469·3).
*Zinc deficiency.*

**Unizitro** *Helfarma, Port.*
Azithromycin (p.159·1).
*Bacterial infections.*

**Unizol** *Farmoquimica, Braz.*
Fluconazole (p.398·1).
*Fungal infections.*

**Unizuric** *Quimica y Farmacia, Mex.*
Allopurinol (p.412·2).
*Hyperuricaemia.*

**Unizyme** *Ciba Vision, Canad.*
Subtilisin (p.1164·2).
*Protein removal from contact lenses.*

**UnoCardil** *Orion, Denm.†.*
Diltiazem hydrochloride (p.900·1).
*Hypertension.*

**Uno-Ciclo** *Biochimico, Braz.*
Algestone acetophenide (p.1541·3); estradiol enantate (p.1550·1).
*Injectable contraceptive.*

**Uno-Enantone** *Takeda, Ger.*
Leuprorelin acetate (p.1331·1).
*Prostatic cancer.*

**Uno-Lin** *3M, Denm.*
Theophylline hydrate (p.798·3).
*Obstructive airways disease.*

**Unoplex** *Offenbach, Mex.*
Vitamin preparation (p.1417·1).

**Unoprost**
*Note. This name is used for preparations of different composition.*
*Apsen, Braz.*
Doxazosin mesilate (p.908·3).
*Benign prostatic hyperplasia.*

*Guidotti, Ital.*
Terazosin hydrochloride (p.1010·3).
*Benign prostatic hyperplasia.*

**Unorox** *Centaur, India.*
Roxithromycin (p.254·2).
*Bacterial infections.*

**Unotex N feminin** *Bilgast, Ger.†.*
Homoeopathic preparation.

**Unotex N masculin** *Bilgast, Ger.†.*
Homoeopathic preparation.

**Uno-Vit** *Wiedemann, Ger.*
*dl*-Alpha tocopherol (p.1464·3).
*Vitamin E deficiency.*

**Unprozy** *Condrugs, Thai.*
Fluoxetine hydrochloride (p.292·1).
*Mixed anxiety depressive states; obsessive-compulsive disorder.*

**Unsayna** *Pfizer, Arg.*
*Injection:* Sulbactam sodium (p.257·2); ampicillin sodium (p.157·1).
*Tablets:* Sultamicillin tosilate (p.264·2).
*Bacterial infections.*

**Untano** *Rafarm, Gr.*
Miconazole nitrate (p.405·3).
*Fungal skin infections.*

**Untigex** *Heralds, Braz.†.*
Menthol (p.1711·3); methyl salicylate (p.59·3).
*Musculoskeletal and joint disorders.*

**Unwind Herbal Nytol** *GlaxoSmithKline Consumer, UK.*
Valerian (p.1762·2); lupulus (p.1708·1); wild lettuce (p.1765·2).
*Insomnia; stress.*

**UO** *YSP, Malaysia.*
Urea (p.1162·2).
*Dry skin disorders.*

**Uonin**
*Unison, Malaysia; Unison, Thai.*
Roxithromycin (p.254·2).
*Bacterial infections; meningitis prophylaxis.*

**Up Mep** *Cimed, Braz.†.*
Cimetidine (p.1255·3).
*Gastro-oesophageal reflux; gastrointestinal haemorrhage; peptic ulcer; Zollinger-Ellison syndrome.*

**U-Pasta** *Kowa, Jpn.*
Sucrose (p.1450·1); povidone-iodine (p.1190·3).
*Skin ulcers.*

**Upderm** *Genepharm, Gr.*
Clindamycin phosphate (p.194·2).
*Acne.*

**Upelva** *Pekana, Ger.*
Homoeopathic preparation.

**Upfen** *UPSA Conseil, Fr.*
Ibuprofen (p.45·3).
*Fever; pain.*

**Upha C** *Upha, Malaysia.*
Vitamin C (p.1460·2).
*Vitamin C deficiency; vitamin C supplement.*

**Upha Dextrophan** *Upha, Malaysia.*
Dextromethorphan hydrobromide (p.1117·3).
*Coughs.*

**Upha Lozenges** *Upha, Malaysia.*
Dequalinium chloride (p.1178·1); tyrothricin (p.275·1).
*Mouth and throat infections.*

**Uphacol** *Upha, Malaysia.*
Dicycloverine hydrochloride (p.481·2); simeticone (p.1289·2).
*Flatulence; gastrointestinal spasm.*

**Uphadeq** *Upha, Malaysia.*
Dequalinium chloride (p.1178·1).
*Mouth and throat infections.*

**Uphadyl CD** *Upha, Malaysia.*
Diphenhydramine hydrochloride (p.431·3); ammonium chloride (p.1115·2); codeine phosphate (p.27·1).
*Coughs.*

**Uphadyl Forte** *Upha, Malaysia.*
Diphenhydramine hydrochloride (p.431·3); ammonium chloride (p.1115·2).
*Coughs.*

**Uphageron** *Upha, Malaysia.*
Cinnarizine (p.428·3).
*Cerebral and peripheral vascular disorders; migraine; nausea; vertigo.*

**Uphalexin** *Upha, Malaysia.*
Cefalexin (p.168·1).
*Bacterial infections.*

**Uphalyte** *Upha, Malaysia.*
Glucose; sodium chloride; sodium bicarbonate; potassium chloride (p.1222·2).
*Diarrhoea; oral rehydration therapy.*

**Uphamol** *Upha, Malaysia.*
Paracetamol (p.76·2).
*Fever; pain.*

**Uphanormin** *Upha, Malaysia.*
Atenolol (p.865·2).
*Angina pectoris; arrhythmias; hypertension; myocardial infarction.*

**Uphastatin** *Upha, Malaysia.*
Nystatin (p.406·3).
*Candidiasis.*

**Uphavit Plus** *Upha, Malaysia.*
Multivitamin and mineral preparation (p.1417·1).

**Uphaxicam** *Upha, Malaysia.*
Piroxicam (p.84·2).
*Gout; musculoskeletal and joint disorders.*

**Uphazhexol** *Upha, Malaysia.*
Trihexyphenidyl hydrochloride (p.490·2).
*Drug-induced extrapyramidal disorders; parkinsonism.*

**Uprima**
*Abbott, Arg.; Abbott, Belg.; Abbott, Braz.; Abbott, Chile; Abbott, Denm.; Abbott, Fin.; Abbott, Fr.; Abbott, Ger.; Abbott, Gr.; Abbott, Hong Kong; Abbott, Irl.; Abbott, Ital.; Abbott, Norw.; Abbott, NZ; Abbott, Port.; Abbott, S.Afr.; Abbott, Spain; Abbott, Swed.; Abbott, UK.*
Apomorphine hydrochloride (p.1199·1).
*Erectile dysfunction.*

**U-Proxyn** *Unison, Thai.*
Naproxen (p.65·1).
*Gout; musculoskeletal and joint disorders.*

**Upsa C**
*Bristol-Myers Squibb, Belg.; Upsamedica, Spain†.*
Ascorbic acid (p.1460·2).
*Adjunct in treatment of iron supplementation; methaemoglobinaemia; vitamin C deficiency.*

**Upsa Plus** *Upsamedica, Ital.†.*
Oxolamine citrate (p.1126·1); propyphenazone (p.85·3).
*Influenza symptoms; respiratory-tract inflammation.*

**Upsadex** *Upsamedica, Spain†.*
Doxylamine succinate (p.432·3); sodium bromide; dibasic sodium phosphate; sodium sulfate (p.1217·1).
*Anxiety disorders; insomnia.*

**Upsalgin C** *Upsamedica, Switz.†.*
Aspirin (p.15·1); ascorbic acid (p.1460·2).
*Fever; pain.*

**Upsalgina**
*Upsamedica, Ital.†; Upsamedica, Spain†.*
Aspirin (p.15·1).
*Fever; inflammation; pain; thrombosis prophylaxis.*

**Upsalgine** *Upsamedica, Belg.†.*
Carbasalate calcium (p.25·1).
*Fever; pain.*

**Upsalgin-N** *Bristol-Myers Squibb, Gr.*
Aspirin (p.15·1).
*Fever; inflammation; pain.*

**Upsavit C** *Bristol-Myers Squibb, Belg.*
Ascorbic acid (p.1460·2).
*Methaemoglobinaemia; vitamin C deficiency.*

**Upset Stomach** *Homeocan, Canad.*
Homoeopathic preparation.

**Uracid**
*Note. This name is used for preparations of different composition.*
*Hassle, Swed.†.*
Aluminium hydroxide (p.1249·2); calcium carbonate (p.1254·2).
*Heartburn; hyperphosphataemia; peptic ulcer.*

*Wesley, USA.*
Methionine (p.1042·1).
*Odour, dermatitis, and ulceration in incontinent adults.*

**Uracil** *Pharmasant, Thai.*
Propylthiouracil (p.1603·1).
*Hyperthyroidism.*

**Uractazide** *Doc Pharma, Belg.†.*
Hydrochlorothiazide (p.933·2); spironolactone (p.1003·1).
*Hypertension; oedema.*

**Uractone**
*Doc Pharma, Belg.†; SPA, Ital.*
Spironolactone (p.1003·1).
*Hyperaldosteronism; hypertension; oedema.*

**Uractonum** *Medochemie, Singapore†.*
Spironolactone (p.1003·1).
*Heart failure; hyperaldosteronism; hypertension; liver cirrhosis with oedema; nephrotic syndrome.*

**Uracyst-S** *Stellar, Canad.*
Chondroitin sulfate sodium (p.1670·2).
*Replacement of glycosaminoglycan layer in the bladder.*

**Uracyst-S Test Kit** *Stellar, Canad.*
Chondroitin sulfate sodium (p.1670·2); potassium chloride (p.1232·2).
*Test for and treatment of bladder-wall glycosaminoglycan deficiency.*

**Ural**
*Abbott, Austral.; Abbott, Malaysia; Abbott, NZ.*
Sodium bicarbonate (p.1223·2); anhydrous sodium citrate (p.1223·2); anhydrous citric acid (p.1673·1); tartaric acid (p.1752·1).
*Dyspepsia; urinary alkalinisation.*

**Uralgin** *Ceccarelli, Ital.†.*
Nalidixic acid (p.234·1).
*Gram-negative bacterial infections of the urinary tract.*

**Uralyt** *Madaus, Spain†.*
Arnica (p.1656·3); convallaria (p.1675·3); equisetum arvense (p.1684·1); rubia tinctorum; solidago virgaurea (p.1748·3); echinacea angustifolia (p.1683·2); magnesium phosphate (p.1228·1).
*Renal calculi.*

**Uralyt Urato** *Madaus, Spain.*
Citric acid (p.1673·1); potassium citrate (p.1223·1).
Formerly contained citric acid, aescin, potassium citrate, ruberitric acid, and sodium citrate.
*Hypocitraturia; renal calculi; renal tubular acidosis.*

**Uralyt-U**
*Madaus, Austria; Madaus, Belg.; Hoyer, Ger.; Madaus, Israel; Madaus, Ital.; Neo-Farmaceutica, Port.; Byk Madaus, S.Afr.; Biomed, Switz.; Madaus, Thai.*
Potassium sodium hydrogen citrate (p.1224·1).
*Renal calculi; urinary alkalinisation.*

**Uramilon** *Biomedica-Chemica, Gr.*
Roxithromycin (p.254·2).
*Bacterial infections.*

**Uramox** *Taro, Israel.*
Acetazolamide (p.849·1).
*Acute mountain sickness; glaucoma; oedema.*

**Urantin** *Xixia, S.Afr.†.*
Nitrofurantoin (p.237·2).
*Urinary-tract infections.*

**Urantoin**
*Rafa, Israel†; DDSA Pharmaceuticals, UK†.*
Nitrofurantoin (p.237·2).
*Genito-urinary-tract infections.*

**Uraplex**
*Wassermann, Ital.; Madaus, Spain.*
Trospium chloride (p.491·2).
*Bladder instability; urinary incontinence.*

**Urapro** *Eagle, Austral.†.*
Saw palmetto (p.1569·1); lycopersicon esculentum; hydrastis (p.1698·3); urtica (p.1762·1); zinc gluconate (p.1469·2); nickel; ferrous phosphate.
*Nutritional supplement.*

**Urarthone**
*Homeocan, Canad.; Lehning, Fr.*
Homoeopathic preparation.

**Urasal** *Carter Horner, Canad.*
Methenamine (p.230·1).
*Urinary-tract infections.*

**Urasin** *Nakorn, Thai.*
Furosemide (p.919·3).
*Forced diuresis; heart failure; oedema.*

**Urazol** *Tecnofarma, Chile.*
Oxybutynin hydrochloride (p.486·3).
*Bladder instability.*

**Urbadan** *Hoechst Marion Roussel, Mex.†.*
Clobazam (p.358·2).

**Urbal** *Merck, Spain.*
Sucralfate (p.1290·2).
*Gastrointestinal haemorrhage; peptic ulcer.*

**Urbanil**
*Aventis, Braz.; Aventis, Port.*
Clobazam (p.358·2).
*Anxiety disorders; epilepsy.*

**Urbanol** *Sanofi Synthelabo, S.Afr.*
Clobazam (p.358·2).
*Alcohol withdrawal syndrome; anxiety; premedication.*

**Urbanyl**
*Sanofi Synthelabo, Fr.; Aventis, Switz.*
Clobazam (p.358·2).
*Alcohol withdrawal syndrome; anxiety; epilepsy.*

**Urbason**
*Aventis, Austria; Aventis, Ger.; Aventis, Ital.; Aventis, Spain; Hoechst Marion Roussel, Switz.†.*
Methylprednisolone (p.1106·1) or methylprednisolone sodium succinate (p.1106·2).
*Corticosteroid.*

**Urdes** *Errekappa, Ital.*
Ursodeoxycholic acid (p.1760·3).
*Biliary disorders.*

**Urdox** *CP Pharmaceuticals, UK.*
Ursodeoxycholic acid (p.1760·3).
*Cholesterol gallstones.*

**Urdrim** *Urbion, Spain.*
Astemizole (p.424·2).
*Hypersensitivity reactions.*

**Ureacin** *Pedinol, USA.*
Urea (p.1162·2).
*Dry skin; hyperkeratosis.*

**Ureadin** *Ingens, Arg.*
Urea (p.1162·2).
*Dry skin; hyperkeratotic skin disorders.*

**Ureadin 10 and 20**
*Andromaco, Chile; Isdin, Port.*
Urea (p.1162·2).
*Dry skin; hyperkeratotic skin disorders.*

**Ureadin 30** *Isdin, Port.*
Urea (p.1162·2); glycolic acid (p.1147·3); salicylic acid (p.1157·1).
*Hyperkeratotic skin disorders.*

**Ureadin Facial** *Isdin, Port.*
*SPF 10:* Urea (p.1162·2); glycerol (p.1694·3); borage oil (p.1661·3); sunscreens.
*Dry skin.*

**Ureadin Forte**
*Andromaco, Chile; Isdin, Port.*
Urea (p.1162·2); glycolic acid (p.1147·3); salicylic acid (p.1157·1); nicotinamide (p.1441·2).
*Dry skin disorders; hyperkeratotic skin disorders.*

**Ureadin Maos** *Isdin, Port.*
Urea (p.1162·2); glycerol (p.1694·3); lactic acid (p.1704·1).
*Dry skin.*

**Ureadin Pediatrics** *Andromaco, Chile.*
Urea (p.1162·2); gamolenic acid (p.1690·2).
*Skin disorders.*

**Ureadin 10 Plus** *Isdin, Port.*
Urea (p.1162·2); dexpanthenol (p.1727·2).
*Dry skin disorders.*

**Ureaphil** *Abbott, USA.*
Urea (p.1162·2).
*Cerebral oedema; raised intra-ocular pressure.*

**Ureata S** *Fides, Ger.*
Urea (p.1162·2); alpha tocoferil acetate (p.1465·1).
*Skin disorders; ulcers.*

**Urecare**
*Orion, Austral.; Delta West, Malaysia; Pharmacia, Singapore.*
Urea (p.1162·2).
*Dry skin disorders.*

**Urecholine**
*Merck Sharp & Dohme, Austral.†; Merck Frosst, Canad.†; Merck Sharp & Dohme, Israel; Merck Sharp & Dohme, Ital.†; Merck Sharp & Dohme, S.Afr.†; Merck Sharp & Dohme, Thai.; Odyssey, USA.*
Bethanechol chloride (p.1487·3).
*Congenital megacolon; neurogenic bladder; postoperative abdominal distension; urinary retention.*

**Urecrem**
*Ethicus, Arg.; Stiefel, Fr.†.*
Urea (p.1162·2).
*Dry skin disorders.*

**Urecrem Hidro** *Ethicus, Arg.*
Urea (p.1162·2); ammonium lactate (p.1142·3).
*Dry skin disorders.*

**Urederm**
*Hamilton, Austral.; Hamilton, Hong Kong.*
Urea (p.1162·2).
*Dry skin; skin irritation.*

**Uree** *Riva, Canad.*
Urea (p.1162·2).

**Uregyt** *Medphano, Ger.†.*
Etacrynic acid (p.913·2).
*Refractory oedema.*

**Ureina** *Confar, Port.*
Parietaria officinalis.

**Urekolin** *Grunenthal, Chile.*
Norfloxacin (p.238·3).
*Bacterial urinary-tract infections.*

**Urelief Plus** *Cypress, USA.*
Phenazopyridine hydrochloride (p.83·1); hyoscyamine hydrobromide (p.485·1); secbutabarbital sodium (p.721·2).
*Lower urinary-tract disorders.*

**Urelium Neu** *Europharm, Austria.*
Ammi visnaga fruit (p.1653·3); solidago virgaurea (p.1748·3); taraxacum (p.1751·3); aescin (p.1648·2).
*Renal calculi.*

**Urelle** *Pharmelle, USA.*
Methenamine (p.230·1); monobasic sodium phosphate (p.1230·3); salol (p.88·1); methylthioninium chloride (p.1042·2); hyoscyamine sulfate (p.485·1).
*Urinary-tract infections.*

**Urem**
*Mayrhofer, Austria; Kade, Ger.*
Ibuprofen (p.45·3).
*Fever; musculoskeletal, joint, peri-articular, and soft-tissue disorders; pain.*

**Uremiase** *Nogues, Fr.†.*
Kinkeliba (p.1703·3); calcium carbonate (p.1254·2).
Formerly contained silica, cholesterol, tricalcium phosphate, dibasic sodium phosphate, sodium chloride, kidney extract, combretum micranthum, heavy chalk.
*Gastrointestinal disorders.*

**Uremide**
*Alphapharm, Austral.; Propan, S.Afr.†.*
Furosemide (p.919·3).
*Hypertension; oedema.*

**Uremol** *Trans Canaderm, Canad.*
Urea (p.1162·2).
*Skin disorders.*

**Uremol-HC** *Trans Canaderm, Canad.*
Hydrocortisone acetate (p.1103·3); urea (p.1162·2).
*Skin disorders.*

**Uren** *Laboratorios Chile, Chile.*
Hydrochlorothiazide (p.933·2); triamterene (p.1016·2).
*Hypertension; oedema.*

**Ureotop** *Dermapharm, Ger.*
Urea (p.1162·2).
*Skin disorders.*

**Ureotop + VAS** *Dermapharm, Ger.*
Urea (p.1162·2); tretinoin (p.1161·1).
*Keratinisation disorders.*

**Urequin** *Craveri, Arg.*
Oxybutynin (p.487·1).
*Bladder instability.*

**Uretil** *Uniao Quimica, Braz.†.*
Phenazopyridine hydrochloride (p.83·1); nitrohydroxyquinoline.
*Urinary-tract infections.*

**Uretren Comp** *Orion, Fin.*
Triamterene (p.1016·2); trichlormethiazide (p.1017·2).
*Hypertension; oedema.*

**Uretron** *Marin, USA.*
Methenamine (p.230·1); monobasic sodium phosphate (p.1230·3); salol (p.88·1); methylthioninium chloride (p.1042·2); hyoscyamine sulfate (p.485·1).
*Urinary-tract infections.*

**Urex**
*Note. This name is used for preparations of different composition.*
*Fawns & McAllan, Austral.; Fawns & McAllan, Hong Kong.*
Furosemide (p.919·3).
*Hypertension; oedema; oliguria.*

*3M, USA.*
Methenamine hippurate (p.230·2).
*Urinary-tract infections.*

**Urfadyn PL** *Zambon, Belg.*
Nifurtoinol (p.237·2).
*Urinary-tract infections.*

**Urfadyne** *Inpharzam, Switz.†.*
Nifurtoinol (p.237·2).
*Urinary-tract infections.*

**Urfamycin**
*Zambon, Hong Kong; Zambon, Spain; Sermmitr, Thai.; Zambon, Thai.*
Thiamphenicol (p.269·2) or thiamphenicol glycinate hydrochloride (p.269·2).
*Bacterial infections.*

**Urfamycine**
*Zambon, Belg.; Inpharzam, Switz.*
Thiamphenicol (p.269·2) or thiamphenicol glycinate hydrochloride (p.269·2).
*Bacterial infections.*

**Urgendol** *Win-Medicare, India.*
Tramadol hydrochloride (p.94·3).
*Pain.*

**Urgenin**
*Note. This name is used for preparations of different composition.*
*Polcopharma, Austral.†; Madaus, Austria; Madaus, Belg.; Madaus, Hong Kong; Madaus, Israel.*
Echinacea (p.1683·2); saw palmetto (p.1569·1).
*Prostatic and urinary-tract disorders.*

*Madaus, Spain.*
Echinacea angustifolia (p.1683·2); saw palmetto (p.1569·1); esculoside (p.1648·2).
*Prostatic and urinary-tract disorders.*

**Urgenin Cucurbitae oleum** *Hoyer, Ger.*
Cucurbita seed oil (p.1677·3).
*Benign prostatic hyperplasia; urinary-tract disorders.*

**Urgenine** *Biomed, Switz.†.*
Echinacea purpurea (p.1683·2); saw palmetto (p.1569·1).
*Bladder irritability; prostatitis.*

**Urginol** *Panalab, Arg.*
Tolterodine tartrate (p.489·3).
*Bladder instability.*

**Urgis** *Cetus, Arg.*
Ranitidine (p.1285·2).
*Peptic ulcer.*

**Urgo Activ Huhneraugenpflaster** *Urgo, Ger.*
Salicylic acid (p.1157·1).
*Calluses; corns.*

**Urgocall** *Fournier SA, Spain.*
Salicylic acid (p.1157·1).
*Calluses; corns.*

**Urgofroid** *Urgo, Fr.*
Butane isobutane propane; menthol (p.1711·3).
*Peri-articular and soft-tissue disorders.*

**Urgomed** *Urgo, Fr.*
Carmellose (p.1577·3).
*Burns; wounds.*

**Urgosorb**
*Note. This name is used for preparations of different composition.*
*Urgo, Fr.*
Calcium alginate (p.745·1); carmellose (p.1577·3).
*Ulcers; wounds.*

*Urgo, Ger.*
Calcium alginate (p.745·1).
*Wounds.*

**Urgotul**
*Urgo, Fr.*
Carmellose (p.1577·3).
*Burns; ulcers; wounds.*

*Urgo, Ger.*
Carmellose sodium (p.1577·3).
*Burns; wounds.*

**Uriage**
*Note. This name is used for preparations of different composition.*
*Biorga, Fr.†.*
*SPF 25:* Octinoxate (p.1154·3); titanium dioxide (p.1160·3); dibenzoylmethane (p.1145·2).
*Sunscreen.*

*Saninter, Port.†.*
A range of emollients, moisturisers, and soap substitutes.

**Uriage Ecran Mineral** *Saninter, Port.†.*
*SPF 60:* Titanium dioxide (p.1160·3); zinc oxide (p.1163·2).
*Sunscreen.*

**Uriage Ecran Total** *Saninter, Port.†.*
*SPF 20; SPF 25:* Dibenzoylmethane (p.1145·2); cinnamate; titanium dioxide (p.1160·3).
*Sunscreen.*

**Uriage Ecran Total Mineral** *Biorga, Fr.†.*
*SPF 28:* Titanium dioxide (p.1160·3).
*Sunscreen.*

**Uriage Extreme** *Saninter, Port.†.*
*SPF60:* Cinnamate; titanium dioxide (p.1160·3).
*Sunscreen.*

**Uriage IP 90**
*Uriage, Fr.*
*SPF 100:* Octinoxate (p.1154·3); titanium dioxide (p.1160·3); zinc oxide (p.1163·2).
*Sunscreen.*

*Saninter, Port.†.*
Octinoxate (p.1154·3); titanium dioxide (p.1160·3); zinc oxide (p.1163·2).
*Sunscreen.*

**Uriage IP 60 Mineral** *Uriage, Fr.*
*SPF 100:* Titanium dioxide (p.1160·3); zinc oxide (p.1163·2).

**Uriage Stick Levres** *Uriage, Fr.*
*SPF 35:* Octinoxate (p.1154·3); titanium dioxide (p.1160·3).
*Sunscreen.*

**Uriage Stick Solaire Extreme** *Uriage, Fr.*
*SPF 90:* Octinoxate (p.1154·3); titanium dioxide (p.1160·3).
*Sunscreen.*

**Uri-Alk** *Medchem, S.Afr.*
Sodium citrate (p.1223·2); sodium bicarbonate (p.1223·2); tartaric acid (p.1752·1); anhydrous citric acid (p.1673·1).
*Gastrointestinal hyperacidity; urinary alkalinisation.*

**Uribac** *Precimex, Mex.†.*
Pipemidic acid (p.243·1).

**Uriben** *Rosemont, UK.*
Nalidixic acid (p.234·1).
*Urinary-tract infections.*

**Uribenz** *RAN, Ger.*
Allopurinol (p.412·2).
*Gout; hyperuricaemia; renal calculi.*

**Uricad** *Great Eastern, Thai.; Westmont, Thai.*
Allopurinol (p.412·2).
*Gout; hyperuricaemia; renal calculi.*

**Uricalm** *Cipla, Austral.*
Sodium bicarbonate (p.1223·2); anhydrous sodium citrate (p.1223·2); anhydrous citric acid (p.1673·1); tartaric acid (p.1752·1).
*Urinary alkalinisation.*

**Uricemil**
*Cristalia, Braz.; Molteni, Ital.*
Allopurinol (p.412·2).
*Gout; hyperuricaemia; renal calculi.*

**Uricodue** *Benedetti, Ital.*
Allopurinol (p.412·2); benziodarone (p.415·1).
*Hyperuricaemia.*

**Uriconorme** *Streuli, Switz.*
Allopurinol (p.412·2).
*Gout; hyperuricaemia; renal calculi.*

**Uricont**
*Rider, Chile; Teva, Israel.*
Oxybutynin hydrochloride (p.486·3).
*Neurogenic bladder; urinary incontinence.*

**Uricosal** *Biotech, Austral.*
citric acid monohydrate (p.1673·1); potassium citrate (p.1223·1).
*Urinary alkalinisation.*

**Uricovac** *Sanofi Synthelabo, Austria.*
Benzbromarone (p.414·3).
*Gout; hyperuricaemia; psoriasis; psoriatic arthritis.*

**Uricozyme**
*Sanofi Synthelabo, Fr.†; Sanofi Synthelabo, Ital.*
Urate oxidase (p.418·3).
*Hyperuricaemia.*

**Uridactone** *Faran, Gr.*
Spironolactone (p.1003·1).
*Heart failure; liver cirrhosis; malignant ascites; nephrotic syndrome; oedema; primary hyperaldosteronism.*

**Urideal** *Dolisos, Fr.*
Pilosella.
*Gastrointestinal disorders; renal disorders.*

**Uridon Modified** *Rugby, USA.*
Methenamine (p.230·1); salol (p.88·1); atropine sulfate (p.477·1); hyoscyamine sulfate (p.485·1); benzoic acid (p.1169·3); methylthioninium chloride (p.1042·2).
*Urinary-tract infections.*

**Uridoz** *Therabel, Fr.*
Fosfomycin trometamol (p.214·3).
*Cystitis.*

**Uriduct** *TAD, Ger.*
Doxazosin mesilate (p.908·3).
*Benign prostatic hyperplasia.*

**Uriflex C** *SSL, UK.*
Chlorhexidine gluconate (p.1173·2).
*Urinary catheter care.*

**Uriflex G** *SSL, UK.*
Citric acid (p.1673·1); sodium bicarbonate (p.1223·2); light magnesium oxide (p.1272·3); disodium edetate (p.1037·3).
*Urinary catheter care.*

**Uriflex R** *SSL, UK.*
Citric acid (p.1673·1); light magnesium carbonate (p.1272·1); gluconolactone; disodium edetate (p.1037·3).
*Urinary catheter care.*

**Uriflex S** *SSL, UK.*
Sodium chloride (p.1233·3).
*Urinary catheter care.*

**Uriflex W** *SSL, UK.*
Sterile pyrogen free water (p.1765·1).
*Urinary catheter care.*

**Uri-Flor** *AGIPS, Ital.*
Nalidixic acid (p.234·1).
*Gram-negative bacterial infections of the urinary tract.*

**Urifron** *Probiomed, Mex.*
Interferon alfa-2b (p.640·3).
*Hepatitis B; hepatitis C; malignant neoplasms.*

**Uriginex Urtica** *Repha, Ger.†.*
Urtica (p.1762·1).
*Rheumatic disorders.*

**Urigon** *Demo, Gr.*
Diclofenac sodium (p.32·1).
*Dysmenorrhoea; inflammation; musculoskeletal and joint disorders; pain.*

**Urigram** *Trima, Israel†.*
Nalidixic acid (p.234·1).
*Gram-negative bacterial urinary-tract infections.*

**Urihesive** *Convatec, Austral.†.*
Medical adhesive.

**Urikal** *Rafa, Israel.*
Sodium citrate (p.1223·2); sodium bicarbonate (p.1223·2); citric acid (p.1673·1); sodium carbonate (p.1747·1).
*Urinary-tract infections.*

**Uriken** *Kener, Mex.†.*
Pipemidic acid (p.243·1).

**Urilin** *Faria, Braz.*
Oxolinic acid (p.240·3).
*Urinary-tract infections.*

**Urimar-T** *Marnel, USA.*
Methenamine (p.230·1); monobasic sodium phosphate (p.1230·3); salol (p.88·1); methylthioninium chloride (p.1042·2); hyoscyamine sulfate (p.485·1).
*Urinary-tract infections.*

**Urimax** *Integrity, USA.*
Methenamine (p.230·1); monobasic sodium phosphate (p.1230·3); salol (p.88·1); methylthioninium chloride (p.1042·2); hyoscyamine sulfate (p.485·1).
*Lower urinary-tract disorders.*

**Urinase** *Eagle, Austral.†.*
Saw palmetto (p.1569·1); echinacea (p.1683·2); maize (p.1676·1); buchu (p.1663·1); hydrastis (p.1698·3); sassafras (p.1742·1); bearberry (p.1659·2); minerals.
*Prostatitis; urinary bladder disorders.*

**Urinefrol** *Lafage, Arg.*
Sarsaparilla (p.1742·1); liquorice (p.1270·2).

**Urinex** *Kern, Switz.*
Birch (p.1660·3); buchu (p.1663·1); barbiflore; bearberry (p.1659·2); haricot bean; equisetum (p.1684·1); solidago virgaurea (p.1748·3); meadowsweet (p.1710·1); calamus (p.1664·1); calendula (p.1665·2).
*Urinary-tract disorders.*

**Urinorm** *Sanofi Synthelabo, Spain.*
Benzbromarone (p.414·3).
*Gout; hyperuricaemia.*

**Urinox** *Charoen, Thai.*
Norfloxacin (p.238·3).
*Bacterial infections.*

**Urion**
*Byk, Austria; Zambon, Fr.; Byk Gulden, Ger.*
Alfuzosin hydrochloride (p.856·2).
*Benign prostatic hyperplasia.*

**Uripiser** *Serral, Mex.*
Pipemidic acid (p.243·1).
*Urinary-tract infections.*

**Uri-Plus Rubia** *Homeocan, Canad.*
Homoeopathic preparation.

**Uriprim** *Bial, Port.*
Allopurinol (p.412·2).
*Gout; hyperuricaemia.*

**Uripurinol** *Azupharma, Ger.*
Allopurinol (p.412·2).
*Gout; hyperuricaemia; renal calculi.*

**Urirex-K** *Aspen, S.Afr.*
Hydrochlorothiazide (p.933·2); potassium chloride (p.1232·2).
*Hypertension; oedema.*

**Urisan** *Tedec Meiji, Spain.*
Pipemidic acid (p.243·1).
*Urinary-tract infections.*

**Uriscreen** *Medical Industries, Austral.*
Test for bacteriuria, haematuria, and pyuria.

**Urisec** *Odan, Canad.*
Urea (p.1162·2).
*Dry skin conditions.*

**Urised** *PolyMedica, USA.*
Methenamine (p.230·1); salol (p.88·1); methylthioninium chloride (p.1042·2); benzoic acid (p.1169·3); atropine sulfate (p.477·1); hyoscyamine sulfate (p.485·1).
*Lower urinary-tract infection or spasm.*

**Urisept NF** *White, Arg.*
Co-trimoxazole (p.199·3); phenazopyridine hydrochloride (p.83·1).
*Urinary-tract infections.*

**Uriseptic** *SDA, USA.*
Methenamine (p.230·1); salol (p.88·1); methylthioninium chloride (p.1042·2); benzoic acid (p.1169·3); atropine sulfate (p.477·1); hyoscyamine sulfate (p.485·1).
*Urinary-tract infections.*

**Urisor** *Soria Natural, Spain.*
Bearberry (p.1659·2); calluna vulgaris; java tea (p.1702·3).
*Urinary-tract infections.*

**Urispadol** *Abigo, Denm.*
Flavoxate hydrochloride (p.482·2).
*Neurogenic bladder.*

**Urispas**
*Byk, Austria; Byk, Belg.; Paladin, Canad.; Negma, Fr.; Shire, Hong Kong; Bushnell, India; Shire, Irl.; Shire, Malaysia; Byk, Neth.; Byk, Port.; Pharmacia, S.Afr.; Shire, Singapore; Robapharm, Switz.; Shire, UK; SmithKline Beecham, USA.*
Flavoxate hydrochloride (p.482·2).
*Urinary-tract disorders.*

**Uristix**
*Bayer, Austral.; Bayer, Canad.†; Bayer Diagnostics, Irl.; Bayer Diagnostics, UK; Bayer, USA.*
Test for glucose and protein in urine.

**Uristix 2** *Bayer Diagnostici, Ital.†.*
Test for leucocytes and nitrites in urine.

**Uristix 4**
*Bayer, Canad.†; Bayer, USA.*
Test for glucose, protein, nitrite, and leucocytes in urine.

**Uritab** *Raza, Malaysia; Pharmaniaga, Malaysia.*
Allopurinol (p.412·2).
*Hyperuricaemia.*

**Uritact** *Cypress, USA.*
Hyoscyamine sulfate (p.485·1); methenamine (p.230·1); salol (p.88·1); atropine sulfate (p.477·1); methylthioninium chloride (p.1042·2); benzoic acid (p.1169·3).
*Lower urinary-tract disorders.*

**Uritest** *Bayer Diagnostics, Fr.*
Test for glucose, protein, nitrite, and leucocytes in urine.

**Uritest 2** *Bayer Diagnostics, Fr.*
Test for leucocytes and nitrites in urine.

**Uritracin** *Great Eastern, Thai.; United American, Thai.*
Norfloxacin (p.238·3).
*Gonorrhoea; urinary-tract infections.*

**Uritrat** *Libbs, Braz.*
Norfloxacin (p.238·3).
*Bacterial infections.*

**Uritrate** *Parke, Davis, Belg.†.*
Oxolinic acid (p.240·3).
*Gram-negative bacterial infections of the urinary tract.*

**Urival** *Zerboni, Mex.†.*
Nitrohydroxyquinoletina.

**Urizal** *Sigma, Braz.†.*
Co-trimoxazole (p.199·3); phenazopyridine (p.83·2).
*Urinary-tract infections.*

**Urizine**
*Unison, Singapore; Unison, Thai.*
Cinnarizine (p.428·3).
*Cerebral and peripheral vascular disorders; migraine; motion sickness; vestibular disorders.*

**Urizone** *Mer-National, S.Afr.*
Fosfomycin trometamol (p.214·3).
*Urinary-tract Escherichia coli infections.*

**Urlix** *Precimex, Mex.†.*
Nalidixic acid (p.234·1).

**Urmidin** *Ofimex, Mex.†.*
Pipemidic acid (p.243·1).

**Uro 3000** *Aguettant, Fr.†.*
Sodium chloride (p.1233·3), water, or glycine (p.1433·3) for irrigation.

**Uro Angiografin** *Schering, Spain.*
Meglumine amidotrizoate (p.1060·2).
*Radiographic contrast medium.*

**Uro Bac Septin** *Gilton, Braz.†.*
Co-trimoxazole (p.199·3); phenazopyridine (p.83·2).
*Urinary-tract infections.*

**Uro Bactrim** *Roche, Braz.†.*
Co-trimoxazole (p.199·3); phenazopyridine (p.83·2).
*Urinary-tract infections.*

**Uro Batrox** *Bergamo, Braz.†.*
Co-trimoxazole (p.199·3); phenazopyridine (p.83·2).
*Urinary-tract infections.*

**Uro Blue** *McNeil, USA.*
Methenamine (p.230·1); monobasic sodium phosphate (p.1230·3); salol (p.88·1); methylthioninium chloride (p.1042·2); hyoscyamine sulfate (p.485·1).
*Urinary-tract infections.*

**Uro Duoctrim** *Haller, Braz.†.*
Co-trimoxazole (p.199·3); phenazopyridine (p.83·2).
*Urinary-tract infections.*

**Uro Fink** *Fink, Ger.†.*
Silver birch leaf (p.1660·3); solidago virgaurea (p.1748·3); java tea (p.1702·3); black currant leaf (p.1661·1); bearberry (p.1659·2).
*Urinary-tract disorders.*

**Uro Furan** *Bunker, Braz.†.*
Nitrofurantoin (p.237·2).
*Urinary-tract infections.*

**Uro Heractrim** *Heralds, Braz.†.*
Co-trimoxazole (p.199·3); phenazopyridine (p.83·2).
*Urinary-tract infections.*

**Uro Septoprin** *Medley, Braz.†.*
Co-trimoxazole (p.199·3); phenazopyridine (p.83·2).
*Urinary-tract infections.*

**Uroalquine** *Rider, Chile.*
Sodium citrate (p.1223·2); potassium citrate (p.1223·1); anhydrous citric acid (p.1673·1).
*Acidosis; gout; renal calculi.*

**Urobac** *Ofimex, Mex.†.*
Nitrofurantoin (p.237·2).

**Urobacid**
*Tyrol, Austria; Biochemie, Malaysia; Biochemie, Singapore.*
Norfloxacin (p.238·3).
*Bacterial infections.*

**Urobactam** *Bristol-Myers, Spain.*
Aztreonam (p.160·3).
*Bacterial infections.*

**Uro-Bacteracin** *Teuto, Braz.†.*
Co-trimoxazole (p.199·3); phenazopyridine (p.83·2).
*Urinary-tract infections.*

**Urobactrex** *Sintofarma, Braz.†.*
Co-trimoxazole (p.199·3); phenazopyridine (p.83·2).
*Urinary-tract infections.*

**Uro-Bactrim** *Roche, Arg.*
Co-trimoxazole (p.199·3); phenazopyridine (p.83·2).
*Urinary-tract infections.*

**Uro-Baxapril** *Brasmedica, Braz.*
Co-trimoxazole (p.199·3); phenazopyridine (p.83·2).
*Urinary-tract infections.*

**Urobine** *Eshcol, Singapore.*
Yohimbine hydrochloride (p.1766·2).
*Erectile dysfunction.*

**Urobioctrin** *Cazi, Braz.†.*
Co-trimoxazole (p.199·3); phenazopyridine (p.83·2).
*Urinary-tract infections.*

**Urobiotic** *Hexal, Braz.*
Phenazopyridine hydrochloride (p.83·1); ampicillin (p.157·1).
*Urinary-tract infections.*

**Urobiotic-250** *Pfizer, USA.*
Oxytetracycline hydrochloride (p.241·1); sulfamethizole (p.260·3); phenazopyridine hydrochloride (p.83·1).
*Genito-urinary infections.*

**Uroc** *Lampugnani, Ital.*
Cinoxacin (p.188·1).
*Urinary-tract infections.*

**Urocalun**
*Shinyaku, Hong Kong; Shinyaku, Singapore.*
Quercus stenophylla (p.1722·3).
*Renal calculi.*

**Urocarb** *Hamilton, Austral.*
Bethanechol chloride (p.1487·3).
*Neurogenic bladder; urinary retention.*

**Urocarf** *SPA, Ital.†.*
Carfecillin sodium (p.166·3).
*Urinary-tract infections.*

**Urocaudal** *Pan Quimica, Spain†.*
Triamterene (p.1016·2).
*Obesity; oedema.*

**Urocaudal Tiazida** *Pan Quimica, Spain†.*
Hydrochlorothiazide (p.933·2); triamterene (p.1016·2).
*Hypertension; oedema.*

**Uro-Cephoral** *Merck, Ger.*
Cefixime (p.172·3).
*Bacterial infections.*

**Urochinasi** *IFET (ΙΦΕΤ), Gr.*
Urokinase (p.1018·2).
*Thromboembolic disorders.*

**Urocit-K**
*Orphan, Austral.; Mission Pharmacal, Hong Kong; Mission Pharma-*

*cal, Malaysia; Mission Pharmacal, Singapore†; Mission Pharmacal, USA.*
Potassium citrate (p.1223·1).
*Renal calculi; urinary alkalinising agent.*

**Urocrasina** *Sanobia, Port.†.*
Methenamine (p.230·1); piperazine hydrate (p.111·2); lithium benzoate (p.1707·2).
*Urinary-tract disorders.*

**Urocridin** *Fresenius, Ger.†.*
Ethacridine lactate (p.1165·3).
*Bladder irrigation for urinary-tract infections.*

**Uroctal**
*Almirall, Hong Kong; Almirall, Spain.*
Norfloxacin (p.238·3).
*Urinary-tract infections.*

**Uroctrin** *Legrand, Braz.*
Co-trimoxazole (p.199·3); phenazopyridine hydrochloride (p.83·1).
*Urinary-tract infections.*

**Urodene** *OFF, Ital.*
Pipemidic acid (p.243·1).
*Urinary-tract infections.*

**Urodie** *Abbott, Ital.*
Terazosin hydrochloride (p.1010·3).
*Benign prostatic hyperplasia.*

**Urodil Blasen-Nieren Arzneitee** *Selz, Ger.†.*
Java tea (p.1702·3); ononis (p.1723·3); birch leaf (p.1660·3); solidago virgaurea (p.1748·3); fennel (p.1687·2); rose fruit (p.1740·1); peppermint leaf (p.1283·2); calendula (p.1665·2); liquorice (p.1270·2).
*Urinary-tract disorders.*

**Urodil phyto** *Selz, Ger.*
Birch leaf (p.1660·3); solidago virgaurea (p.1748·3); java tea (p.1702·3).
*Urinary-tract disorders.*

**Urodin** *Streuli, Switz.*
Nitrofurantoin (p.237·2).
*Urinary-tract infections.*

**Urodonal** *Farmabraz, Braz.†.*
Theobromine (p.798·2); methenamine (p.230·1).
*Hyperuricaemia.*

**Urodyn** *Bionorica, Ger.†.*
Solidago virgaurea (p.1748·3).
*Urinary-tract disorders.*

**Urofar** *Elofar, Braz.†.*
Co-trimoxazole (p.199·3); phenazopyridine (p.83·2).
*Urinary-tract infections.*

**Urofen** *Teuto, Braz.*
Sulfamethoxypyridazine (p.263·1); nitrofurantoin (p.237·2); phenazopyridine hydrochloride (p.83·1).
*Urinary-tract infections.*

**Uroflan** *Biocur, Ger.†.*
Birch leaf (p.1660·3).
*Urinary-tract disorders.*

**Uroflo** *Abbott, Austria.*
Terazosin hydrochloride (p.1010·3).
*Benign prostatic hyperplasia.*

**Uroflox**
*Note. This name is used for preparations of different composition.*
*Farmion, Braz.; Bialfar, Port.*
Norfloxacin (p.238·3).
*Bacterial infections.*

*Armstrong, Mex.*
Rufloxacin hydrochloride (p.254·3).
*Urinary-tract infections.*

**Urofos** *Panalab, Arg.*
Norfloxacin (p.238·3).
*Bacterial infections.*

**Urofossat** *Dreluso, Ger.*
Homoeopathic preparation.

**Urogal** *Galen, Mex.†.*
Pipemidic acid (p.243·1).
*Urinary-tract infections.*

**Urogem** *Prodotti, Braz.*
Nitrofurantoin (p.237·2).
*Urinary-tract infections.*

**Urogesic**
*Atlantic, Singapore; Edwards, USA.*
Phenazopyridine hydrochloride (p.83·1).
*Irritation of the lower urinary tract.*

**Urogesic Blue** *Edwards, USA.*
Methenamine (p.230·1); monobasic sodium phosphate (p.1230·3); salol (p.88·1); methylthioninium chloride (p.1042·2); hyoscyamine sulfate (p.485·1).
*Urinary-tract infections.*

**Urogliss** *Montavit, Neth.*
Chlorhexidine hydrochloride (p.1173·3); lidocaine hydrochloride (p.1377·3).
*Catheterisation.*

**Urogliss-S** *Montavit, Neth.*
Chlorhexidine hydrochloride (p.1173·3).
*Catheterisation.*

**Urogotan A** *Silesia, Chile.*
Allopurinol (p.412·2).
*Gout; hyperuricaemia.*

**Urografin**
*Schering, Austral.; Schering, Austria; Schering, Denm.; Schering, Ger.†; German Remedies, India; Schering, Israel; Schering, Neth.; Schering, NZ; Schering, S.Afr.; Schering, Spain; Schering, Swed.; Schering, Switz.*
Meglumine amidotrizoate (p.1060·2); sodium amidotrizoate (p.1060·2).
*Radiographic contrast medium.*

**Urografin 150, 325, and 370** *Schering, UK.*
Meglumine amidotrizoate (p.1060·2); sodium amidotrizoate (p.1060·2).
*Radiographic contrast medium.*

**Urografin Meglumin** *Schering, Denm.*
Meglumine amidotrizoate (p.1060·2).
*Radiographic contrast medium.*

**Urografina**
*Schering, Arg.; Schering, Braz.†; Schering, Port.†.*
Meglumine amidotrizoate (p.1060·2); sodium amidotrizoate (p.1060·2).
*Radiographic contrast medium.*

**Urografine** *Schering, Belg.*
Meglumine amidotrizoate (p.1060·2); sodium amidotrizoate (p.1060·2).
*Radiographic contrast medium.*

**Urogram** *FIRMA, Ital.†.*
Nalidixic acid (p.234·1).
*Gram-negative bacterial infections of the genito-urinary tract.*

**Urogutt**
*Farmasa, Mex.; TTN, Thai.†; Willmar, Thai.†.*
Saw palmetto (p.1569·1).
*Benign prostatic hyperplasia.*

**Urokit** *Casasco, Arg.*
Potassium citrate (p.1223·1).
*Renal calculi.*

**Uroknop** *Knop, Chile.*
Lithium carbonicum; colchicum; methenamine (p.230·1); tartaric acid (p.1752·1).
*Gout; hyperuricaemia.*

**Uro-KP-Neutral** *Star, USA.*
Mineral preparation (p.1417·1).
*Phosphorus supplement.*

**Urol mono** *Hoyer, Ger.*
Solidago virgaurea (p.1748·3).
*Urinary-tract disorders.*

**uro-L 90 N** *Loges, Ger.*
Homoeopathic preparation.

**Urolene Blue** *Star, USA.*
Methylthioninium chloride (p.1042·2).
*Cyanide poisoning; cystitis; urethritis; drug-induced methaemoglobinaemia.*

**Uro-Leotrim** *Leofarma, Braz.†.*
Co-trimoxazole (p.199·3); phenazopyridine (p.83·2).
*Urinary-tract infections.*

**Uro-Linfol** *Omega, Arg.*
Norfloxacin (p.238·3).
*Bacterial infections of the urinary tract.*

**Urolithico** *Dansk-Flama, Braz.†.*
Persea americana; juglans regia; samambaia; phyllanthus niruri.
*Urinary-tract disorders.*

**Urologicum PMD** *Plantamed, Ger.†.*
Homoeopathic preparation.

**Urologicum-Echtroplex** *Weber & Weber, Ger.*
Homoeopathic preparation.

**Urologin** *Delta, Braz.*
Phenazopyridine hydrochloride (p.83·1).
*Urinary-tract disorders.*

**Urolosin** *Boehringer Ingelheim, Spain.*
Tamsulosin hydrochloride (p.1009·2).
*Benign prostatic hyperplasia.*

**Urolux Retro** *Goldham, Ger.*
Meglumine amidotrizoate (p.1060·2); sodium amidotrizoate (p.1060·2).
*Contrast medium for urinary-tract radiography.*

**Uro-Mag** *Blaine, USA.*
Magnesium oxide (p.1272·3).
*Hyperacidity; magnesium deficiency.*

**Uromethin** *Apogepha, Ger.*
Methionine (p.1042·1).
*Phosphate calculi; urinary acidification.*

**Uro-Micinovo** *Bago, Chile.*
Co-trimoxazole (p.199·3); phenazopyridine (p.83·2).
*Urinary-tract infections.*

**Uromil** *IPRAD, Fr.*
Bearberry (p.1659·2); green tea (p.1765·3).
*Urinary-tract disorders.*

**Uromiro**
*Gerot, Austria; Bracco, Port.†; Bracco, Switz.*
Meglumine iodamide (p.1063·2).
*Radiographic contrast medium.*

**Uromiro 24%, 36%, and 300** *Bracco, Ital.*
Meglumine iodamide (p.1063·2).
*Radiographic contrast medium.*

**Uromiro 340 and 420** *Bracco, Ital.*
Meglumine iodamide (p.1063·2); sodium iodamide (p.1063·2).
*Radiographic contrast medium.*

**Uromiro 300 Sodico** *Bracco, Ital.*
Sodium iodamide (p.1063·2).
*Radiographic contrast medium.*

**Uromiron** *Schering, Braz.†.*
Meglumine iodamide (p.1063·2).
*Radiographic contrast medium.*

**Uromitexan**
*Labinca, Arg.; Baxter, Austral.; Asta Medica, Austria; Baxter, Belg.; Asta Medica, Canad.; Asta Médica, Chile; Baxter, Chile; Baxter, Denm.; Asta Medica, Fin.; Baxter Oncology, Fr.; Baxter Oncology, Ger.; Baxter, Hong Kong; German Remedies, India; Asta Medica, Irl.; Asta Medica, Ital.; Baxter Oncology, Malaysia; Sanfer, Mex.; Viatris, Neth.; Asta Medica, Norw.; Asta Medica, NZ; Asta Medica, Port.; Aventis, S.Afr.; Baxter Oncology, Singapore; Prasfarma, Spain; Asta Medica, Swed.; Asta Medica, Switz.; Asta Medica, Thai.; Baxter Oncology, UK.*
Mesna (p.1041·2).
*Prevention of urotoxicity due to oxazaphosphorine antineoplastics.*

**Uromix** *Breves, Braz.†.*
Sulfamethizole (p.260·3); phenazopyridine (p.83·2); sulfacetamide (p.257·3).
*Urinary-tract infections.*

**Uromont** *Montavit, Austria.*
Dexamethasone (p.1097·1); chlorhexidine hydrochloride (p.1173·3); lidocaine hydrochloride (p.1377·3).
*Stricture prevention following transurethral procedures.*

**Uro-Munal** *Medice, Ger.*
*Escherichia coli.*
*Urinary-tract infections.*

**Uromykol** *Hoyer, Ger.*
Clotrimazole (p.396·2).
*Fungal infections of skin and vagina.*

**Uronalin** *Vitae, Mex.†.*
Nalidixic acid (p.234·1).
*Urinary-tract infections.*

**Uro-Nebacetin N** *Byk Gulden, Ger.*
Neomycin sulfate (p.235·1).
*Urinary-tract infections.*

**Uronefrex**
*Therabel, Belg.†; Cassenne, Fr.†; Robert, Spain.*
Acetohydroxamic acid (p.1645·3).
*Adjunct in urinary-tract infections with urea-splitting organisms; renal calculi due to bacterial urease.*

**Uroneotrim** *Neo Quimica, Braz.†.*
Co-trimoxazole (p.199·3); phenazopyridine (p.83·2).
*Urinary-tract infections.*

**Uronid** *Recordati, Spain.*
Flavoxate hydrochloride (p.482·2).
*Urinary-tract disorders.*

**Uronor** *Abbott, Ger.*
Potassium citrate (p.1223·1); potassium bicarbonate (p.1223·1); anhydrous citric acid (p.1673·1).
*Renal calculi.*

**Uronorm** *Wassermann, Ital.*
Cinoxacin (p.188·1).
*Urinary-tract infections.*

**Uronovag**
*Note. This name is used for preparations of different composition.*
*Gobbi, Arg.*
Norfloxacin (p.238·3).
*Bacterial infections.*

*Novag, Mex.*
Pipemidic acid (p.243·1).
*Urinary-tract infections.*

**Uropac** *EMS, Braz.*
Sulfamethoxypyridazine (p.263·1); nitrofurantoin (p.237·2); phenazopyridine hydrochloride (p.83·1).
*Urinary-tract infections.*

**Uro-Pasc** *Pascoe, Ger.†.*
Solidago virgaurea (p.1748·3); taraxacum (p.1751·3).
*Urinary-tract disorders.*

**Uro-Phosphate** *ECR, USA†.*
Methenamine (p.230·1); monobasic sodium phosphate (p.1230·3).
*Urinary-tract infections.*

**Urophytum** *Arkomedika, Fr.*
Buchu (p.1663·1); bearberry (p.1659·2).
*Urinary-tract disorders.*

**Uropielon** *Legrand, Braz.*
Ampicillin (p.157·1); phenazopyridine hydrochloride (p.83·1).
*Urinary-tract infections.*

**Uropimid** *CT, Ital.*
Pipemidic acid (p.243·1).
*Urinary-tract infections.*

**Uropimide** *Rider, Chile.*
Pipemidic acid (p.243·1).
*Urinary-tract infections.*

**Uropipedil** *Viamedica, Spain.*
Pipemidic acid (p.243·1).
*Urinary-tract infections.*

**Uropipemid** *AF, Mex.*
Pipemidic acid (p.243·1).
*Urinary-tract infections.*

**Uropirite** *INQ, Braz.†.*
Phenazopyridine (p.83·2); methenamine (p.230·1).
*Urinary-tract infections.*

**Uroplant** *Biomo, Ger.*
Solidago virgaurea (p.1748·3).
*Urinary-tract disorders.*

**Uroplex** *Sintofarma, Braz.*
Norfloxacin (p.238·3).
*Bacterial infections.*

**Uropol** *IMA, Braz.*
Co-trimoxazole (p.199·3); phenazopyridine (p.83·2).
*Urinary-tract infections.*

**Uro-POS** *Ursapharm, Ger.*
Urtica (p.1762·1).
*Prostatic hyperplasia.*

**Uro-Pract** *Ebewe, Austria.*
Sodium chloride (p.1233·3).
*Bladder irrigation; maintenance of bladder catheters.*

**Uro-Pract N** *Fresenius, Ger.†.*
Sodium chloride (p.1233·3).
*Maintenance of bladder catheters.*

**Uroprot**
*Laboratorios Chile, Chile; Lemery, Mex.*
Mesna (p.1041·2).
*Prevention of urotoxicity due to oxazaphosphorine antineoplastics.*

**Uropurat** *Kwizda, Austria.*
Bearberry (p.1659·2); herniaria (p.1697·1); equisetum (p.1684·1); ononis (p.1723·3).
*Urinary-tract disorders.*

**Uropyrine** *Pharmacobel, Belg.†.*
Phenazopyridine hydrochloride (p.83·1).
*Urinary-tract disorders.*

**Uroqid-Acid** *Beach, USA†.*
Methenamine mandelate (p.230·2); monobasic sodium phosphate monohydrate (p.1230·3).
*Urinary-tract infections.*

**Uroquidan** *UCB, Spain.*
Urokinase (p.1018·2).
*Intra-ocular haemorrhage; thromboembolic disorders.*

**Uroquina** *Rhone-Poulenc Rorer, Mex.†.*
Pefloxacin (p.241·3).

**Urorenal** *Schwabe, Ger.*
Birch leaf (p.1660·3).
*Urinary-tract disorders.*

**Uro-Ripirin** *Pharmacia Upjohn, Ger.†.*
Emepronium carrageenate (p.482·1).
*Urinary-tract disorders.*

**Urosalin** *Heralds, Braz.†.*
Methenamine (p.230·1); methylthioninium chloride (p.1042·2).
*Urinary-tract infections.*

**Urosan** *AGIPS, Ital.*
Pipemidic acid (p.243·1).
*Urinary-tract infections.*

**Uroselect** *Dreluso, Ger.*
Homoeopathic preparation.

**Uroseptal**
*Bago, Arg.; Merck Bago, Braz.*
Norfloxacin (p.238·3).
*Bacterial infections.*

**Uroseptin** *Gilton, Braz.†.*
Phenazopyridine (p.83·2); methylthioninium chloride (p.1042·2); methenamine mandelate (p.230·2); papaverine (p.1728·1).
*Urinary-tract disorders.*

**Uro-Septiolan** *Climax, Braz.†.*
Co-trimoxazole (p.199·3); phenazopyridine (p.83·2).
*Urinary-tract infections.*

**Uroseptol** *Fresenius Kabi, Ger.*
Ethacridine lactate (p.1165·3).
*Urinary-tract infections.*

**Urosetic** *Finmedical, Ital.*
Pipemidic acid (p.243·1).
*Urinary-tract infections.*

**Urosin**
*Note. This name is used for preparations of different composition.*
*Roche, Austria; Boehringer Mannheim, Ger.†.*
Allopurinol (p.412·2).
*Gout; hyperuricaemia; renal calculi.*

*YSP, Malaysia.*
Atenolol (p.865·2).
*Angina pectoris; hypertension.*

**Urosiphon** *Pierre Fabre Sante, Fr.†.*
Java tea (p.1702·3).
*Diuretic; slimming aid.*

**Urospasmon** *Heumann, Ger.*
Nitrofurantoin (p.237·2); sulfadiazine (p.258·2); phenazopyridine hydrochloride (p.83·1).
*Urinary-tract infections.*

**Urospasmon sine** *Heumann, Ger.*
Nitrofurantoin (p.237·2); sulfadiazine (p.258·2).
*Urinary-tract infections.*

**Urostei** *Steigerwald, Ger.†.*
Birch leaf (p.1660·3); solidago virgaurea (p.1748·3); java tea (p.1702·3).
*Urinary-tract disorders.*

**Uro-Stilloson** *Farco, Ger.*
Dexamethasone (p.1097·1); lidocaine hydrochloride (p.1377·3); chlorhexidine gluconate (p.1173·2).
*Urinary-tract disorders.*

**Urostix** *Bayer, India.*
Test for glucose and protein in urine.

**Uro-Tablinen** *Lichtenstein, Ger.*
Nitrofurantoin (p.237·2).
*Urinary-tract infections.*

**Uro-Tainer**
*Note. This name is used for preparations of different composition.*
*Braun, Belg.*
Chlorhexidine acetate (p.1173·2).
*Urinary catheter cre; urinary-bladder lavage.*

*Isramedcom, Israel.*
Sodium chloride (p.1233·3).
*Maintenance of indwelling urinary catheters.*

**Uro-Tainer M** *Braun, UK.*
Sodium chloride (p.1233·3).
*Vehicle for intravesical administration of drugs.*

**Uro-Tainer Solutio R** *Vifor Medical, Switz.†.*
Citric acid monohydrate (p.1673·1); gluconolactone; light magnesium carbonate (p.1272·1).
*Urinary catheter care.*

**Uro-Tainer Solution R** *Braun, UK.*
Citric acid (p.1673·1); gluconolactone; light magnesium carbonate (p.1272·1).
*Urinary catheter care.*

**Uro-Tainer Suby G**
Vifor Medical, Switz.†; Braun, UK.
Citric acid (p.1673·1); light magnesium oxide (p.1272·3); sodium bicarbonate (p.1223·2).
*Urinary catheter care.*

**Urotal** Lemery, Mex.†.
Pipemidic acid (p.243·1).

**Uro-Tarivid**
Aventis, Ger.; Aventis, Israel.
Ofloxacin (p.239·3).
*Bacterial infections.*

**Urotem** Temis, Arg.
Norfloxacin (p.238·3).
*Bacterial infections of the urinary tract.*

**Uro-Teutrim** Teuto, Braz.†.
Co-trimoxazole (p.199·3); phenazopyridine (p.83·2).
*Urinary-tract infections.*

**Urotonine** VHB, India.
Bethanechol chloride (p.1487·3).
*Neurogenic bladder; urinary retention.*

**Urotractan** Fujisawa, Ger.
Methenamine hippurate (p.230·2).
*Urinary-tract infections.*

**Urotractin**
Eurodrug, Hong Kong; GlaxoSmithKline, Ital.; Eurodrug, Malaysia; Eurodrug, Singapore; Eurodrug, Thai.
Pipemidic acid (p.243·1).
*Urinary-tract infections.*

**Urotrate** Parke, Davis, Fr.†.
Oxolinic acid (p.240·3).
*Urinary-tract infections.*

**Urotricef** Merck, Chile.
Cefixime (p.172·3).
*Bacterial infections.*

**Urotril** Hexal, Braz.
Phenazopyridine hydrochloride (p.83·1).
Formerly contained nitroxoline and phenazopyridine hydrochloride.
*Urinary-tract infections.*

**Urotrol** Almirall, Spain.
Tolterodine tartrate (p.489·3).
*Bladder instability.*

**Urotruw S** Truw, Ger.†.
Homoeopathic preparation.

**Uroval** FIRMA, Ital.†.
Pipemidic acid (p.243·1).
*Genito-urinary-tract infections.*

**Uro-Vaxom**
Sanofi Synthelabo, Ger.; Knoll, Mex.; OM, Port.; OM, Switz.
*Escherichia coli.*
*Urinary-tract infections.*

**Urovec** Collins, Mex.
Phenazopyridine (p.83·2); sulfamethoxazole (p.261·1); tetracycline (p.266·2).
*Urinary-tract infections.*

**Urovison**
Schering, Austria†; Schering, Ger.; Schering, Neth.
Meglumine amidotrizoate (p.1060·2); sodium amidotrizoate (p.1060·2).
*Radiographic contrast medium.*

**Urovisona** Schering, Arg.
Meglumine amidotrizoate (p.1060·2); sodium amidotrizoate (p.1060·2).
*Contrast medium for urography.*

**Uroxacin**
Note. This name is used for preparations of different composition.
Lazar, Arg.
Norfloxacin (p.238·3).
*Bacterial infections of the genito-urinary tract.*

Malesci, Ital.
Cinoxacin (p.188·1).
*Urinary-tract infections.*

**Uroxate** General Drugs, Thai.
Flavoxate hydrochloride (p.482·2).
*Urinary-tract disorders.*

**UroXatral**
Sanofi Synthelabo, Arg.; Sanofi Synthelabo, Chile; Sanofi Synthelabo, Ger.; Sanofi Synthelabo, USA.
Alfuzosin hydrochloride (p.856·2).
*Benign prostatic hyperplasia.*

**Uroxazol** Bunker, Braz.†.
Co-trimoxazole (p.199·3); phenazopyridine (p.83·2).
*Urinary-tract infections.*

**Uroxazol-N** Bunker, Braz.
Norfloxacin (p.238·3).
*Bacterial infections.*

**Uroxin**
Note. This name is used for preparations of different composition.
Unison, Singapore.
Ciprofloxacin hydrochloride (p.188·2).
*Bacterial infections.*

Unison, Thai.
Ciprofloxacin (p.188·2).
*Bacterial infections.*

Julphar, UAE.
Norfloxacin (p.238·3).
*Bacterial infections.*

**Uroxina** Farmalab, Braz.
Pipemidic acid (p.243·1).
*Urinary-tract infections.*

**Urozyl-SR** Restan, S.Afr.†.
Allopurinol (p.412·2).
*Gout; hyperuricaemia.*

**Ursacol**
Zambon, Braz.; Zambon, Ital.
Ursodeoxycholic acid (p.1760·3).
*Biliary-tract disorders.*

**Ursilon** Ibi, Ital.
Ursodeoxycholic acid (p.1760·3).
*Biliary-tract disorders.*

**Ursinus Inlay-Tabs** Novartis, USA.
Pseudoephedrine hydrochloride (p.1129·2); aspirin (p.15·1).
*Upper respiratory-tract symptoms.*

**Urso**
Axcan, Canad.; Heumann, Ger.; Mitsubishi, Jpn; Axcan, USA.
Ursodeoxycholic acid (p.1760·3).
*Biliary-tract disorders; cholesterol gallstones; liver disorders.*

**Urso Mix** Niddapharm, Ger.
Chenodeoxycholic acid (p.1670·1); ursodeoxycholic acid (p.1760·3).
*Cholesterol gallstones.*

**Ursobil** ABC, Ital.
Ursodeoxycholic acid (p.1760·3).
*Biliary-tract disorders.*

**Ursobilane** Estedi, Spain.
Ursodeoxycholic acid (p.1760·3).
*Gallstones.*

**Ursochol**
Zambon, Belg.; Zambon, Ger.; Zambon, Neth.; Zambon, Spain; Inpharzam, Switz.
Ursodeoxycholic acid (p.1760·3).
*Cholesterol gallstones; primary biliary cirrhosis.*

**Ursodamor** Damor, Ital.
Sodium succinate ursodeoxycholate (p.1761·1).
*Biliary-tract disorders.*

**Ursodexil** EG, Ital.
Ursodeoxycholic acid (p.1760·3).
*Biliary-tract disorders.*

**Ursodiol** Bioprogress, Ital.
Ursodeoxycholic acid (p.1760·3).
*Biliary-tract disorders.*

**Ursofalk**
Orphan, Austral.; Merck, Austria; Codali, Belg.; Jouveinal, Canad.†; EciFarma, Chile; Falk, Ger.; Galenica, Gr.; Falk, Hong Kong; Antigen, Irl.; Rafa, Israel; Abbott, Ital.; Falk, Malaysia; Farmasa, Mex.; Tramedico, Neth.; Falk, Norw.; Falk, Port.; Falk, Singapore; Meda, Swed.; Medichemie, Switz.; Falk, Thai.; Provalis, UK.
Ursodeoxycholic acid (p.1760·3).
*Cholesterol gallstones; primary biliary cirrhosis.*

**Ursofalk + Chenofalk** Falk, Ger.†.
White capsules, ursodeoxycholic acid (Ursofalk) (p.1760·3); yellow-orange capsules, chenodeoxycholic acid (Chenofalk) (p.1670·1).
*Cholesterol gallstones.*

**Ursoflor** SoSe, Ital.
Ursodeoxycholic acid (p.1760·3).
*Biliary-tract disorders.*

**Ursogal** Galen, UK.
Ursodeoxycholic acid (p.1760·3).
*Cholesterol gallstones.*

**Ursolac** Biomedica, Ital.
Ursodeoxycholic acid (p.1760·3).
*Biliary-tract disorders.*

**Ursolin** Berlin Pharm, Thai.
Ursodeoxycholic acid (p.1760·3).
*Biliary-tract disorders; liver disorders.*

**Ursolisin** Magis, Ital.
Ursodeoxycholic acid (p.1760·3).
*Biliary-tract disorders.*

**Ursolit** CTI, Israel.
Ursodeoxycholic acid (p.1760·3).
*Gallstones; liver disorders.*

**Ursolite** Vita, Spain†.
Ursodeoxycholic acid (p.1760·3).
*Gallstones.*

**Ursolvan**
Sanofi Synthelabo, Fr.; Sanofi Synthelabo, Hong Kong†; Sanofi Synthelabo, Singapore†.
Ursodeoxycholic acid (p.1760·3).
*Cholesterol gallstones.*

**Urson** Ripari-Gero, Ital.†.
Sodium succinate ursodeoxycholate (p.1761·1).
*Biliary-tract disorders.*

**Ursoproge** Proge, Ital.
Ursodeoxycholic acid (p.1760·3).
*Biliary-tract disorders.*

**Ursosan**
Mitsubishi-Tokyo, Hong Kong; Mitsubishi, Jpn.
Ursodeoxycholic acid (p.1760·3).
*Biliary-tract disorders; cholesterol gallstones; liver disorders.*

**Ursotan** Aventis, S.Afr.
Ursodeoxycholic acid (p.1760·3).
*Cholesterol gallstones.*

**Urtias** BASF, Ger.†.
Allopurinol (p.412·2).
*Gout; hyperuricaemia.*

**Urtica Plus** Europharm, Austria.
Urtica (p.1762·1).
*Urinary-tract disorders.*

**Urtica Plus N** Hoyer, Ger.†.
Urtica (p.1762·1).
*Benign prostatic hyperplasia.*

**Urticalcin**
Bioforce, Ger.; Bioforce, Switz.
Homoeopathic preparation.

**Urticaprostat uno** Azupharma, Ger.
Urtica (p.1762·1).
*Benign prostatic hyperplasia.*

**Urticur** Biocur, Ger.†.
Urtica (p.1762·1).
*Benign prostatic hyperplasia.*

**Urtigen** Sons, Mex.
Astemizole (p.424·2).
*Hypersensitivity.*

**Urtikalma** Fecofar, Arg.
Camphor (p.1665·3); calamine (p.1144·1); diphenhydramine (p.431·3).
*Pruritus.*

**Urtipret**
Bionorica, Ger.; Bionorica, Thai.†.
Urtica (p.1762·1).
*Benign prostatic hyperplasia.*

**Urtivac** Darrow, Braz.
Allergen extracts (p.1650·1).
*Allergen immunotherapy.*

**Urtivit** Bional, Ger.
Urtica (p.1762·1).
*Benign prostatic hyperplasia.*

**Urupan** Merckle, Ger.
Dexpanthenol (p.1727·2).
*Wounds.*

**Urzac** Quesada, Arg.
Ursodeoxycholic acid (p.1760·3).
*Gallstones.*

**Usanimals** Usana, Hong Kong.
Multivitamin and mineral preparation with hesperidin (p.1417·1).

**Usar Fibras** Phoenix, Arg.
Liquid paraffin (p.1479·1); cellulose (p.1578·3); agar (p.1576·3).
*Constipation.*

**Usedent** Neckerman, Braz.†.
Procaine (p.1383·2); phenol (p.1188·1); menthol (p.1711·3).
*Local anaesthesia.*

**Useton** Farmedica, Braz.†.
Buclizine (p.426·3); carnitine; lysine; gamma-aminobutyric acid; vitamin B substances (p.1417·1).
*Reduced appetite; tonic.*

**Usix** Raza, Malaysia; Pharmaniaga, Malaysia.
Furosemide (p.919·3).
*Ascites; hypertension; oedema.*

**Uskan**
Desitin, Ger.; Cimex, Switz.†.
Oxazepam (p.712·2).
*Anxiety; sleep disorders.*

**Usneabasan** Sanum-Kehlbeck, Ger.
Homoeopathic preparation.

**Usnicon** Eczane, Arg.
Benzalkonium chloride (p.1168·3).
*Disinfection.*

**U-Spa** Sriprasit, Thai.
Flavoxate hydrochloride (p.482·2).
*Urinary-tract disorders.*

**Ustilakehl** Sanum-Kehlbeck, Ger.
Homoeopathic preparation.

**Ustimon**
Sigmapharm, Austria; Lacer, Spain†.
Hexobendine hydrochloride (p.931·2).
*Cardiac disorders.*

**Ustiosan** Kelemata, Ital.
Procaine hydrochloride (p.1383·2); lidocaine hydrochloride (p.1377·3); hydroxyquinoline sulfate (p.1700·1).
*Minor wounds and burns; skin irritation.*

**UT 380** CCD, Fr.
Copper-wound plastic (p.1425·3).
*Intra-uterine contraceptive device.*

**Utabon** Uriach, Spain.
Oxymetazoline hydrochloride (p.1126·1).
*Nasal congestion.*

**Utefos** Prasfarma, Spain.
Tegafur (p.586·2).
*Malignant neoplasms.*

**Uteplex** Wyeth Lederle, Fr.
Trisodium uridine triphosphate (p.1760·3).
*Musculoskeletal disorders.*

**Utergin** Sigma, India.
Methylergometrine maleate (p.1714·2).
*Postpartum haemorrhage; puerperal sepsis; uterine bleeding; uterine subinvolution.*

**Uterine** Omega, Arg.
Isoxsuprine hydrochloride (p.1702·2).
*Premature labour; threatened miscarriage.*

**Uterovarol** Simoes, Braz.†.
Viburnum prunifolium; hydrastis (p.1698·3); valerian (p.1762·2); potassium bromide (p.1663·1).
*Dysmenorrhoea.*

**Uticox** Squibb, Spain.
Meloxicam (p.56·1).
*Ankylosing spondylitis; osteoarthritis; rheumatoid arthritis.*

**Utidol** Diba, Mex.
Dipyrone (p.35·3).
*Fever; pain.*

**Utilin** Sanum-Kehlbeck, Ger.
*Bacillus subtilis.*
*Immunotherapy.*

**Utilin H** Sanum-Kehlbeck, Ger.
Homoeopathic preparation.

**Utilin N** Sanum-Kehlbeck, Ger.
*Bacillus subtilis.*
*Gout; musculoskeletal and joint disorders; skin disorders.*

**Utilin S** Sanum-Kehlbeck, Ger.
*Mycobacterium phlei.*
*Immunotherapy.*

**Utin** Cipla-Medpro, S.Afr.
Norfloxacin (p.238·3).
*Urinary-tract infections.*

**Utinor**
Neopharmed, Ital.; Merck Sharp & Dohme, UK.
Norfloxacin (p.238·3).
*Bacterial infections of the urinary tract.*

**Utira** Hawthorn, USA.
Hyoscyamine sulfate (p.485·1); methylthioninium chloride (p.1042·2); monobasic sodium phosphate (p.1230·3); methenamine (p.230·1); salol (p.88·1).
*Urinary-tract pain and irritation.*

**Utisept** ST, Thai.
Trimethoprim (p.272·2).
*Urinary-tract infections.*

**utk** TAD, Ger.
Urtica (p.1762·1).
*Benign prostatic hyperplasia.*

**Utolid** Utopian, Thai.
Roxithromycin (p.254·2).
*Bacterial infections.*

**Utolincomycin** Utopian, Thai.
Lincomycin hydrochloride (p.226·2).
*Gram-positive bacterial infections.*

**Utoral** BPL-Meizler, Braz.
Fluorouracil (p.554·2).
*Malignant neoplasms.*

**Utovlan** Pharmacia, UK.
Norethisterone (p.1562·2).
*Breast cancer; endometriosis; menstrual disorders.*

**Utrim** Sanofi Winthrop, Braz.†.
Co-trimoxazole (p.199·3); phenazopyridine (p.83·2).
*Urinary-tract infections.*

**Utrogest** Kade, Ger.; Besins, Ger.
Progesterone (p.1566·2).
*Menopausal disorders.*

**Utrogestan**
Pharmacia, Arg.; Asta Medica, Austria; Besins, Belg.; Enila, Braz.; Besins, Fr.; Besins, Hong Kong; Aventis, Irl.; Besins-Iscovesco, Israel; Besins-Iscovesco, Malaysia; Atlantis, Mex.; Jaba, Port.; Scientific, S.Afr.; Besins-Iscovesco, Singapore; Seid, Spain; Golaz, Switz.; Piette, Thai.
Progesterone (p.1566·2).
*Benign breast disorders; female infertility; menopausal disorders; menstrual disorders; premature labour; threatened or recurrent miscarriage.*

**UV Protectant** Norwood, Canad.
*SPF 15:* Avobenzone (p.1142·3); octinoxate (p.1154·3); oxybenzone (p.1154·3).
*Sunscreen.*

**UV Sport Gel** Boots, Austral.†.
*SPF 15+:* Octinoxate (p.1154·3); octisalate (p.1154·3); octocrilene (p.1154·3); avobenzone (p.1142·3).
*Sunscreen.*

**UV Triplegard** Boots Healthcare, Austral.
*SPF 15:* Octinoxate (p.1154·3); oxybenzone (p.1154·3); titanium dioxide (p.1160·3).
*SPF 30+:* Octinoxate (p.1154·3); enzacamene (p.1147·1); zinc oxide (p.1163·2).
*Sunscreen.*

**UV Triplegard Hydrating Face Lotion** Boots Healthcare, Austral.
*SPF 20:* Octinoxate (p.1154·3); zinc oxide (p.1163·2); enzacamene (p.1147·1).
*Sunscreen.*

**UV Triplegard Kids** Boots Healthcare, Austral.
*SPF 30+:* Octinoxate (p.1154·3); enzacamene (p.1147·1); zinc oxide (p.1163·2).
*Sunscreen.*

**UV Triplegard Low Allergenic** Boots, Austral.†.
*SPF 15+:* Titanium dioxide (p.1160·3).
*Sunscreen.*

**UV Triplegard Sensitive Skin** Boots Healthcare, Austral.
*SPF 20:* Titanium dioxide (p.1160·3).
*Sunscreen.*

**UV Triplegard Sunscreen Cream - Water Resistant** Boots, Austral.†.
*SPF 15+:* Octinoxate (p.1154·3); oxybenzone (p.1154·3); titanium dioxide (p.1160·3).
*Sunscreen.*

**UV Triplegard Sunstick & Lip Balm** Boots Healthcare, Austral.
*SPF 30+:* Octinoxate (p.1154·3); octocrilene (p.1154·3); zinc oxide (p.1163·2).
*Sunscreen.*

**UV Triplegard Toddler Block Broad Spectrum Lotion - Water Resistant** Boots, Austral.†.
*SPF 15+:* Octinoxate (p.1154·3); oxybenzone (p.1154·3); titanium dioxide (p.1160·3).
*Sunscreen.*

**UV Triplegard Watersports** Boots Healthcare, Austral.
*SPF 30 +:* Octinoxate (p.1154·3); titanium dioxide (p.1160·3).
*Sunscreen.*

**UV Ultrablock** Boots Healthcare, NZ.
*SPF 15; SPF 20; SPF 30+:* Padimate O (p.1155·1); oxybenzone (p.1154·3).
This range formerly contained SPF 50+ preparations.
*Sunscreen.*

**Uvacin** Lichtwer, UK.
Taraxacum (p.1751·3); bearberry (p.1659·2).
*Female bladder discomfort.*

**Uvadex** Therakos, USA.
Methoxsalen (p.1152·1).
*T-cell lymphoma.*

**Uvalysat** Ysatfabrik, Ger.
Bearberry leaf (p.1659·2).
*Urinary-tract infections.*

**Uvamin** Mepha, Israel.
Nitrofurantoin (p.237·2).
*Urinary-tract infections.*

**Uvamine retard** Mepha, Switz.
Nitrofurantoin (p.237·2).
*Urinary-tract infections.*

**Uvanox** Knop, Chile.
Vitis vinifera.
*Lymphoedema; sight disorders; venous insufficiency.*

**Uvasal** GlaxoSmithKline, Arg.
Tartaric acid (p.1752·1); sodium bicarbonate (p.1223·2); citric acid (p.1673·1); caffeine (p.782·1); magnesium sulfate (p.1228·2).
*Dyspepsia.*

**Uva-Ursi Complex** Blackmores, Austral.†.
Taraxacum (p.1751·3); galium aparine (p.1673·2); bearberry (p.1659·2); buchu (p.1663·1).
*Bloating; dysuria; fluid retention; prostatitis; renal calculi; urethritis.*

**Uva-Ursi Plus** Eagle, Austral.†.
Bearberry (p.1659·2); parsley (p.1728·3); taraxacum (p.1751·3); zanthoxylum (p.1766·3).
*Cystitis; fluid retention.*

**Uvavit** Kolassa, Austria.
Multivitamin and mineral preparation (p.1417·1).
*Nutritional supplement in pregnancy.*

**Uvedose** Crinex, Fr.
Colecalciferol (p.1461·3).
*Vitamin D deficiency.*

**Uvega** Hormona, Mex.
Lidocaine hydrochloride (p.1377·3).
*Otitis externa.*

**Uveline** Martin, Fr.†.
Methylhydroxyquinoline metilsulfate (p.1714·2).
*UV-induced eye irritation.*

**Uvestat** Bournonville, Belg.†.
Methylhydroxyquinoline metilsulfate (p.1714·2).
*Light-induced eye irritation.*

**Uvesterol** Crinex, Fr.
Multivitamin preparation (p.1417·1).

**Uvesterol D** Crinex, Fr.
Ergocalciferol (p.1462·1).
*Vitamin D deficiency.*

**Uvicin** Steigerwald, Ger.
Homoeopathic preparation.

**Uvicol** Monot, Fr.†.
Actinoquinol (p.1647·2); oxedrine hydrochloride (p.977·3).
*Eye disorders.*

**Uvimag $B_6$** Laphal, Fr.
Magnesium glycerophosphate (p.1228·1); pyridoxine hydrochloride (p.1456·3).
*Vitamin and mineral supplementation.*

**Uvirgan mono** Abbott, Ger.
Cucurbita (p.1677·3).
*Urinary-tract disorders.*

**Uvirgan N** Abbott, Ger.
Urtica (p.1762·1); cucurbita (p.1677·3); ononis (p.1723·3).
*Urinary-tract disorders.*

**Uvistat**
Note. This name is used for preparations of different composition.
Eastern Pharmaceuticals, UK.
*SPF 15:* Octinoxate (p.1154·3); avobenzone (p.1142·3).
*Sunscreen.*

Windsor, UK†.
*SPF 10:* Mexenone (p.1154·2); octinoxate (p.1154·3); avobenzone (p.1142·3); titanium dioxide (p.1160·3).
*SPF 6; SPF 8:* Mexenone (p.1154·2); octinoxate (p.1154·3).
*Sunscreen.*

**Uvistat Babysun Cream** Windsor, UK†.
*SPF 12:* Mexenone (p.1154·2); octinoxate (p.1154·3).
*Sunscreen.*

**Uvistat Lipscreen** Boehringer Ingelheim, Irl.
*SPF 25; SPF 30:* Avobenzone (p.1142·3); titanium dioxide (p.1160·3).
*Sunscreen.*

**Uvistat Lotion** Boehringer Ingelheim, Irl.
*SPF 15; SPF 20; SPF 30; SPF 50:* Octinoxate (p.1154·3); avobenzone (p.1142·3); titanium dioxide (p.1160·3).
*Sunscreen.*

**Uvistat UV Protectant** Windsor, Irl.†.
*SPF 6; SPF 8; SPF 15:* Mexenone (p.1154·2); octinoxate (p.1154·3); avobenzone (p.1142·3); titanium dioxide (p.1160·3).
*Sunscreen.*

**UV-Luar** Luar, Arg.
Hydroxymethylquinoleine.
*Sunscreen.*

**Uxalun** Labinca, Arg.
Oxaliplatin (p.577·1).
*Malignant neoplasms.*

**Uxen** Aventis, Arg.
Amitriptyline hydrochloride (p.280·3).
*Depression.*

**Uxicolin** Pisa, Mex.
Suxamethonium chloride (p.1406·2).
*Depolarising neuromuscular blocker.*

**Uzara** Hertz, Braz.†.
Dipyrone (p.35·3); hyoscine (p.483·3).
*Pain; smooth muscle spasm.*

**Uzix** Rafarm, Gr.
Amikacin sulfate (p.154·1).
*Bacterial infections.*

**3V** Julphar, UAE.
Thiamine nitrate (p.1455·1); pyridoxine hydrochloride (p.1456·3); cyanocobalamin (p.1458·2).
*Migraine; neuralgia; neuritis; neuropathy; rheumatic pain.*

**V Day 1612** PP Lab, Thai.
Prosultiamine; vitamin $B_6$; vitamin $B_{12}$ (p.1417·1).
*Vitamin B deficiency.*

**V Day Lozenges** PP Lab, Thai.
Dequalinium chloride (p.1178·1).
*Mouth and throat infections.*

**V Day Milk** PP Lab, Thai.
Aluminium hydroxide (p.1249·2); magnesium hydroxide (p.1272·2); simeticone (p.1289·2).
*Gastric hyperacidity.*

**V Day Zepam** PP Lab, Thai.
Diazepam (p.690·1).
*Anxiety; insomnia.*

**V Infusionslosung** Baxter, Ger.
Electrolyte infusion (p.1217·1).
*Fluid and electrolyte disorders.*

**Vaben** Rafa, Israel.
Oxazepam (p.712·2).
*Agitation; anxiety.*

**Vabeta** Oftalder, Port.
Betamethasone valerate (p.1093·2).
*Skin disorders.*

**Vabicin** Vana, Thai.
Spectinomycin hydrochloride (p.255·2).
*Gonorrhoea.*

**Vabon**
Biolab, Malaysia; Biolab, Thai.
Danazol (p.1545·2).
*Benign breast disorders; endometriosis; gynaecomastia; hereditary angioedema; menorrhagia; precocious puberty.*

**Vac Antigrip Frac** Berna, Spain; Leti, Spain.
An influenza vaccine (p.1620·2).
*Active immunisation.*

**Vac Antimeningococic A+C** Aventis Pasteur, Spain.
A meningococcal vaccine (groups A and C) (p.1626·1).
*Active immunisation.*

**Vac Antiparotiditis** Aventis Pasteur, Spain.
A mumps vaccine (p.1626·3).
*Active immunisation.*

**Vac Antipolio Or** Celltech, Spain.
An oral poliomyelitis vaccine (p.1633·3).
*Active immunisation.*

**Vac Antipolio Oral** Glaxo Wellcome, Spain†.
An oral poliomyelitis vaccine (p.1633·3).
*Active immunisation.*

**Vac Antirrabica** Aventis Pasteur, Spain.
A rabies vaccine (p.1635·3).
*Active immunisation.*

**Vac Antirrubeola** Aventis Pasteur, Spain; SmithKline Beecham, Spain.
A rubella vaccine (RA 27/3) (p.1637·3).
*Active immunisation.*

**Vac Antitetanica** Medeva, Spain†.
A tetanus vaccine (p.1640·3).
*Active immunisation.*

**Vac Antitifica Or** Medeva, Spain†.
An oral typhoid vaccine (inactivated strain Ty21a) (p.1642·2).
*Active immunisation.*

**Vac Polio Sabin** GlaxoSmithKline, Spain.
An oral poliomyelitis vaccine (p.1633·3).
*Active immunisation.*

**Vac Poliomielitica** Berna, Spain.
A poliomyelitis vaccine (p.1633·3).
*Active immunisation.*

**Vac Triple MSD** Aventis Pasteur, Spain.
A measles, mumps, and rubella vaccine (attenuated Enders, Jeryl Lynn, and Wistar RA 27/3 strains respectively) (p.1625·1).
*Active immunisation.*

**Vacanyl** Vana, Thai.
Terbutaline sulfate (p.797·2).
*Obstructive airways disease.*

**Vaccin DTCP** Aventis Pasteur, Fr.†.
An adsorbed diphtheria, tetanus, pertussis, and poliomyelitis (inactivated) vaccine (p.1615·1).
*Active immunisation.*

**Vaccin DTP** Pasteur Vaccins, Fr.
A diphtheria, tetanus, and poliomyelitis (inactivated) vaccine (p.1615·2).
*Active immunisation.*

**Vaccin Meningococcique Merieux** Vianex (Βιανέξ), Gr.
A meningococcal vaccine (groups A and C, or A, C, Y, and W135) (p.1626·1).
*Active immunisation.*

**Vaccin Rubeole Merieux** Vianex (Βιανέξ), Gr.
A rubella vaccine (p.1637·3).
*Active immunisation.*

**Vaccin Tab** Berna, Switz.†.
A typhoid vaccine (p.1642·2).
*Active immunisation.*

**Vaccin TP** Pasteur Vaccins, Fr.
A tetanus and poliomyelitis (inactivated) vaccine (p.1641·3).
*Active immunisation.*

**Vaccine Antipoliomyelitique/Merieux** Vianex (Βιανέξ), Gr.
An oral poliomyelitis vaccine (Sabin) (p.1633·3).
*Active immunisation.*

**Vaccino Antipiogeno** Bruschettini, Ital.
A vaccine prepared from *Staphylococcus aureus*, *Pseudomonas aeruginosa*, *Escherichia coli*, *Streptococcus pyogenes*, and *Streptococcus pneumoniae*.
*Active immunisation against pyogenic bacterial infections.*

**Vaccino Antipneumocatarrale** Bruschettini, Ital.
A vaccine prepared from *Streptococcus pneumoniae*, *Streptococcus pyogenes*, *Haemophilus influenzae*, and *Moraxella catarrhalis*.
*Bacterial infections of the respiratory tract.*

**Vaccino Difto Tetano** ISI, Ital.†.
An adsorbed diphtheria and tetanus vaccine (p.1613·1).
*Active immunisation.*

**Vaccino DPT** ISI, Ital.†.
An adsorbed diphtheria, tetanus, and pertussis vaccine (p.1613·3).
*Active immunisation.*

**Vaccino Tab Te** Nuovo ISM, Ital.†.
A typhoid, paratyphoid A and B, and tetanus vaccine.
*Active immunisation.*

**Vacillin** Vana, Thai.
Ampicillin trihydrate (p.157·2).
*Bacterial infections.*

**Vacina Antipiogenica** Biolab Sanus, Braz.†.
A vaccine prepared from: *Streptococcus pyogenes*; *Streptococcus pneumoniae*; *Staphylococcus aureus*; *Pseudomonas aeruginosa*; *Escherichia coli*.
*Active immunisation against pyogenic bacterial infections.*

**Vacina Antipneumocatarral** Biolab Sanus, Braz.†.
A vaccine prepared from: *Streptococcus pyogenes*; *Streptococcus pneumoniae*; *Haemophilus influenzae*; *Moraxella catarrhalis*.
*Bacterial infections of the respiratory tract.*

**Vacina Catarral** Berna, Port.
Pneumococci; *Staphylococcus aureus*; *Staphylococcus albus*; streptococci; *Klebsiella pneumoniae*; *Moraxella catarrhalis*; *Haemophilus influenzae*.

**Vacina Dupla DT** Butantan, Braz.†.
A diphtheria and tetanus vaccine (p.1613·1).
*Active immunisation.*

**Vacina Meningococica A+C** Aventis Pasteur, Braz.
A meningococcal vaccine (groups A and C) (p.1626·1).
*Active immunisation.*

**Vacina Meningococica Conjugada Grupo C** Wyeth, Braz.
A meningococcal C conjugate vaccine (diphtheria $CRM_{197}$ protein conjugate) (p.1626·1).
*Active immunisation.*

**Vacina Pneumococica Conjugada 7-valate** Wyeth, Braz.
A pneumococcal conjugate vaccine (7-valent, diphtheria $CRM_{197}$ protein conjugate) (p.1633·1).
*Active immunisation.*

**Vacina Poliomielitica** Aventis Pasteur, Braz.
An oral poliomyelitis vaccine (p.1633·3).
*Active immunisation.*

**Vacina Triplice DPT** Butantan, Braz.†.
A diphtheria, tetanus, and pertussis vaccine (p.1613·3).
*Active immunisation.*

**Vacinolone** Vana, Thai.
Triamcinolone acetonide (p.1110·2).
*Skin disorders.*

**Vaclox** Vana, Thai.
Cloxacillin (p.198·2).
*Bacterial infections.*

**Vacolax** Vana, Thai.
Bisacodyl (p.1251·3).
*Constipation.*

**Vacontil**
Medochemie, Hong Kong; Medochemie, Malaysia; Medochemie, Singapore†; Medochemie, Thai.†.
Loperamide hydrochloride (p.1271·1).
*Diarrhoea.*

**Vacopan**
Atlantic, Malaysia; Atlantic, Singapore; Vana, Thai.
Hyoscine butylbromide (p.483·3).
*Gastro-duodenitis; nausea and vomiting; peptic ulcer; smooth muscle spasm.*

**Vacrax** Samchully, Singapore.
Aciclovir (p.626·1).
*Herpesvirus infections.*

**Vacromil** Gunopharm, Chile.
Goserelin acetate (p.1326·3).

**Vactyph** Zydus, India.
A typhoid vaccine (Vi capsular polysaccharide) (p.1642·2).
*Active immunisation of adults and children over 5 years.*

**Vacudol** Xixia, S.Afr.
Paracetamol (p.76·2); codeine phosphate (p.27·1); promethazine hydrochloride (p.439·1).
*Fever; pain.*

**Vacudol Forte** Xixia, S.Afr.
Paracetamol (p.76·2); codeine phosphate (p.27·1); caffeine (p.782·1); meprobamate (p.706·2).
*Pain and associated tension.*

**Vaculin** Biolab, Thai.†.
Co-dergocrine mesilate (p.1674·1).
*Mental function disorders.*

**Vacuna Antigripal**
Aventis Pasteur, Spain.
An influenza vaccine (p.1620·2).
*Active immunisation.*

Leti, Spain.
Inactivated polyvalent influenza vaccines (whole virion or split virion) (p.1620·2).
*Active immunisation.*

**Vacuna Antipiogena** Biol, Arg.
A vaccine containing micro-organisms responsible for skin infections.
*Active immunisation.*

**Vacuna Doble** Biol, Arg.
A diphtheria and tetanus vaccine (p.1613·1).
*Active immunisation.*

**Vacuna Haptenica** Puebla, Arg.
Polysaccharides from *Pseudomonas aeruginosa*; proteins from *Klebsiella pneumoniae*.
*Immunotherapy.*

**Vacuna Triple** Biol, Arg.; Purissimus, Arg.
A diphtheria, tetanus, and pertussis vaccine (p.1613·3).
*Active immunisation.*

**Vacuobil** Armstrong, Arg.
Methylenedioxycinnamic acid or potassium methylenedioxycinnamate.
*Liver and biliary-tract disorders.*

**Vacuobil Plus** Armstrong, Arg.
Methylenedioxycinnamic acid; metoclopramide hydrochloride (p.1274·3); simeticone (p.1289·2).
*Gastrointestinal disorders.*

**Vadarex** Bell, UK.
Methyl salicylate (p.59·3); menthol (p.1711·3); sweet birch oil (p.60·1); cajuput oil (p.1664·1); eucalyptus oil (p.1686·2).
*Musculoskeletal pain.*

**Vademin-Z** Roberts, USA; Hauck, USA.
Multivitamin and mineral preparation (p.1417·1).

**Vadicate** Inkeysa, Spain.
Vincamine hydrochloride (p.1764·2).
*Cerebral trauma; cerebrovascular disorders; circulatory disorders of the eye, ear, nose, and throat; vestibular disorders.*

**Vadilex**
Sanofi Synthelabo, Fr.; Sanofi Synthelabo, Hong Kong†; Sanofi Synthelabo, Singapore†.
Ifenprodil tartrate (p.938·1).
*Cerebral and peripheral vascular disorders; premature labour; threatened miscarriage; vascular ear disorders.*

**Vadinar** Serral, Mex.
Dipyridamole (p.903·1).
*Thromboembolic disorders.*

**Vadiral** Gynopharm, Chile.
Valaciclovir (p.656·2).
*Viral infections.*

**Vaditon** Madaus, Spain.
Fluvastatin sodium (p.918·2).
*Atherosclerosis; hyperlipidaemias.*

**Vadol** Phyteia, Switz.†.
Aspirin (p.15·1); caffeine (p.782·1).
*Fever; pain.*

**Vadolax** Ogna, Ital.
Cascara (p.1255·1); cynara (p.1678·3).
*Constipation.*

**Vadosilan** Bristol-Myers Squibb, Mex.
Isoxsuprine (p.1702·3).
*Peripheral and cerebral vascular disorders; premature labour.*

**Vafluson** Kleva, Gr.
Ketoconazole (p.403·3).
*Fungal infections.*

**Vag Oral** IQB, Braz.
Allergen extracts (p.1650·1).
*Allergen immunotherapy.*

**Vagaka** Vana, Thai.
Mebendazole (p.108·2).
*Worm infections.*

**Vagantin** Riemser, Ger.
Methanthelinium bromide (p.485·3).
*Gastrointestinal disorders.*

**Vagarne** Organon, Arg.
*Pessaries:* Nimorazole (p.611·3); clotrimazole (p.396·2).
*Tablets:* Nimorazole (p.611·3).
*Fungal infections; protozoal infections.*

**Vagarsol** Aspen, S.Afr.
Diiodohydroxyquinoline (p.603·3); cetylpyridinium chloride (p.1173·1); aminoacridine hydrochloride (p.1165·3); boric acid (p.1662·1).
*Vaginal infections.*

**Vagi Biotic** Cimed, Braz.†.
Nystatin (p.406·3); metronidazole (p.607·2); benzalkonium chloride (p.1168·3); urea (p.1162·2).
*Vulvovaginal infections.*

**Vagi-C** Taurus, Ger.
Ascorbic acid (p.1460·2).
*Vaginal disorders.*

**Vagicillin** Schur, Ger.
Neomycin sulfate (p.235·1).
*Vaginal infections.*

**Vagicin** Charoen, Thai.
Diiodohydroxyquinoline (p.603·3); nystatin (p.406·3); chloramphenicol (p.185·1).
*Vaginal infections.*

**Vagicural** Raymos, Arg.
Hydrocortisone (p.1103·3); neomycin (p.235·1); nitrofurazone (p.238·2); vitamin A (p.1451·2); thymol (p.1194·2); tyrothricin (p.275·1).

**Vagicural Plus** Raymos, Arg.
Centella (p.1144·3); metronidazole (p.607·2); miconazole (p.405·2); neomycin (p.235·1); polymyxin B (p.245·2).
*Vaginal infections.*

**Vagifem**
Novo Nordisk, Austral.; Novo Nordisk, Austria; Novo Nordisk, Belg.; Novo Nordisk, Denm.; Novo Nordisk, Fin.; Novo Nordisk, Ger.; Novo Nordisk, Gr.; Novo Nordisk, Irl.; Novo Nordisk, Israel; Novo Nordisk, Ital.; Novo Nordisk, Neth.; Novo Nordisk, Norw.; Novo Nordisk, NZ; Isdin, Port.; Novo Nordisk, S.Afr.; Novo Nordisk, Singapore; Isdin, Spain; Novo Nordisk, Swed.; Novo Nordisk, Switz.; Novo Nordisk, Thai.; Novo Nordisk, UK; Novo Nordisk, USA.
Estradiol (p.1550·1).
*Atrophic vaginitis.*

**Vagiflor** Asche, Ger.
*Lactobacillus acidophilus* (p.1704·2).
*Disorders of the vaginal flora; vaginitis.*

**Vagi-Gard Medicated Cream** Lake, USA.
Benzocaine (p.1370·3); benzalkonium chloride (p.1168·3).
*Vaginal irritation.*

**Vagi-Gard Medicated Disposable Douche** Lake, USA.
Octoxinol 9 (p.1414·1).
*Vaginal irritation and discharge.*

**Vagi-Gard Personal Lubricating Gel** Lake, USA.
Vaginal lubricant.

**Vagi-Hex**
Pierre Fabre, Ger.; Drossapharm, Switz.
Hexetidine (p.1182·1).
*Vaginitis.*

**Vagiklin** Kinder, Braz.
Tetracycline hydrochloride (p.266·2); amphotericin B (p.391·2).

**Vagil** PP Lab, Thai.
Metronidazole (p.607·2).
*Anaerobic bacterial infections.*

**Vagilen** Farmigea, Ital.
Metronidazole (p.607·2).
*Trichomoniasis.*

**Vagimax** Prodotti, Braz.
Metronidazole (p.607·2); nystatin (p.406·3).
*Vulvovaginal infections.*

**Vagimid** Apogepha, Ger.
Metronidazole (p.607·2).
*Anaerobic bacterial infections; protozoal infections.*

**Vaginex**
Schmid, Canad.†; QHP, USA.
Tripelennamine hydrochloride (p.442·3).
*External vaginal irritation.*

**Vaginyl** DDSA Pharmaceuticals, UK.
Metronidazole (p.607·2).

**Vagisan**
Note. This name is used for preparations of different composition.
Sidus, Arg.
Dihydrostreptomycin sulfate (p.205·3); tyrothricin (p.275·1); nitrofurazone (p.238·2).
*Vaginal infections.*

Wolff, Ger.
Lactic acid (p.1704·1); sodium lactate (p.1223·2).
*Vaginitis.*

**Vagisan Compuesto** Sidus, Arg.
Dihydrostreptomycin sulfate (p.205·3); tyrothricin (p.275·1); nitrofurazone (p.238·2); clotrimazole (p.396·2).
*Vaginal infections.*

**Vagisil**
Note. This name is used for preparations of different composition.
Combe, Canad.; Combe, Israel†.
Benzocaine (p.1370·3); resorcinol (p.1156·3).
*Vaginal irritation.*

Combe, Ital.
Lidocaine (p.1377·3); chlorothymol (p.1177·2).
*Anal and vulvar pruritus.*

Combe, UK.
Lidocaine (p.1377·3).
*Vaginal and rectal pruritus.*

Combe, USA.
*Cream:* Benzocaine (p.1370·3); resorcinol (p.1156·3).
*Skin disorders.*
*Topical powder:* Aloes (p.1248·2); liquid paraffin (p.1479·1); benzethonium chloride (p.1169·2).
*Vaginal disorders.*

**Vagistat** Bristol-Myers Squibb, USA.
Tioconazole (p.409·3).
*Vulvovaginal candidiasis.*

**Vagi-Sulfa** Janssen-Cilag, Braz.
Sulfathiazole (p.264·1); sulfacetamide (p.257·3); sulfabenzamide (p.257·3); urea (p.1162·2).
*Vaginal infections.*

**Vagitrene** Eurofarma, Braz.
Wheat germ.
*Vulvovaginal disorders.*

**Vagitrin-N** Bunker, Braz.
Dexamethasone phosphate (p.1097·2); nystatin (p.406·3); neomycin sulfate (p.235·1); tyrothricin (p.275·1); sodium propionate (p.408·1); boric acid (p.1662·1).
*Vulvovaginal infections.*

**Vagitrol-V** Roche, Mex.
Fluocinolone acetonide (p.1101·2); metronidazole (p.607·2); nystatin (p.406·3).
*Cervicitis; vaginitis; vulvitis.*

**Vagmicor** Zerboni, Mex.†.
Ketoconazole (p.403·3).

**Vagmycin** Bristol-Myers Squibb, S.Afr.
Tetracycline (p.266·2); amphotericin B (p.391·2).
*Vaginal infections.*

**Vagoclyss** Grossmann, Switz.
Lactic acid (p.1704·1).
*Vaginal infections and irritation.*

**Vagolisal** Biotekfarma, Ital.†.
Cimetidine (p.1255·3).
*Gastritis and duodenitis associated with acid hypersecretion; peptic ulcer.*

**Vagomine** Qualiphar, Belg.
Dimenhydrinate (p.431·1).
*Motion sickness; nausea; vertigo; vomiting.*

**Vagopax** Jaba, Port.
Propinox (p.487·3).
*Smooth muscle spasm.*

**Vagoplex** Makros, Braz.†.
Reserpine (p.995·1); homatropine methylbromide (p.483·2); hyoscine hydrobromide (p.483·3).
*Smooth muscle spasm.*

**Vagostabyl** Leurquin, Fr.
Crataegus (p.1677·1); calcium lactate (p.1225·3); melissa (p.1711·1); magnesium thiosulfate (p.1054·1).
*Nervous disorders.*

**Vagostal** Cantabria, Spain.
Famotidine (p.1265·2).
*Gastro-oesophageal reflux; peptic ulcer; Zollinger-Ellison syndrome.*

**Vagostesyl** Gross, Braz.
Atropine sulfate (p.477·1); papaverine hydrochloride (p.1728·1); phenobarbital (p.367·3); leptolobium elegans; passion flower (p.1729·1).
*Smooth muscle spasm.*

**Vagotrope-S** Sanofi Synthelabo, Port.†.
Hyoscine butylbromide (p.483·3).

**Vagran** Finadiet, Arg.
Astemizole (p.424·2).

**Vagran Descongestivo** Finadiet, Arg.
Astemizole (p.424·2); pseudoephedrine sulfate (p.1129·2).
*Rhinitis; sinusitis.*

**Vagyl** Vana, Thai.
Metronidazole (p.607·2).
*Amoebiasis; giardiasis; trichomoniasis.*

**Valamin 12** Pisa, Mex.
Hydroxocobalamin (p.1458·2).

**Valatux** Farmacologico Milanese, Ital.†.
Dextromethorphan hydrobromide (p.1117·3).
*Coughs.*

**Valavir**
Orion, Fin.; Alodial, Port.
Valaciclovir hydrochloride (p.656·1).
*Herpesvirus infections.*

**Valaxona** United Nordic, Denm.
Diazepam (p.690·1).
*Alcohol withdrawal syndrome; anxiety; spasticity.*

**Valbet**
Note. This name is used for preparations of different composition.
Delta, Braz.; Lupin, India; Biolab, Thai.
Betamethasone valerate (p.1093·2).
*Scalp disorders; skin disorders.*

Lupin, India.
*Cream:* Betamethasone valerate (p.1093·2); miconazole nitrate (p.405·3); neomycin sulfate (p.235·1).
*Infected skin disorders.*

**Valbet-N** Biolab, Thai.
Betamethasone (p.1093·1); neomycin (p.235·1).
*Infected skin disorders.*

**Valbil**
CHR, Ger.; CPH, Port.
Febuprol (p.1687·1).
*Biliary-tract dyskinesia; dyspepsia.*

**Valcaps** Pharmacaps, Mex.†.
Valproic acid (p.380·1).

**Valcatil** Panalab, Arg.
Methionine; cystine; gelatin (p.1417·1).
*Hair and nail disorders.*

**Valclair** Durbin, UK.
Diazepam (p.690·1).
*Alcohol withdrawal syndrome; anxiety; epilepsy; premedication; skeletal muscle spasm.*

**Valcote**
Abbott, Arg.; Abbott, Chile.
Valproic acid (p.380·1) or valproate semisodium (p.380·1).
*Bipolar disorder; epilepsy; migraine.*

**Valcyte**
Roche, Austral.; Roche, Irl.; Roche, NZ; Roche, UK; Roche, USA.
Valganciclovir hydrochloride (p.656·3).
*Cytomegalovirus retinitis.*

**Valda**
Note. This name is used for preparations of different composition.
Canonne, Braz.†.
Menthol (p.1711·3); cineole (p.1672·1); terpineol (p.1752·2); thymol (p.1194·2).
*Mouth disorders.*

Bayer Consumer, Canad.
Menthol (p.1711·3); cineole (p.1672·1); thymol (p.1194·2); terpin hydrate (p.1131·1); guaiacol (p.1122·1).
*Coughs.*

GlaxoSmithKline Sante, Fr.; GlaxoSmithKline, Hong Kong; SmithKline Beecham Consumer, Irl.; Sterling, Port.
Menthol (p.1711·3); cineole (p.1672·1); thymol (p.1194·2); terpineol (p.1752·2); guaiacol (p.1122·1).
*Throat disorders.*

**Valda F3** Sterling Midy, Ital.†.
Potassium fluoride (p.1445·3); sodium fluoride (p.1444·3); cicliomenol (p.1177·3); enoxolone (p.36·2).
*Dental disorders.*

**Valda Septol** SmithKline Beecham Sante, Fr.†.
Menthol (p.1711·3); cineole (p.1672·1); enoxolone (p.36·2); cicliomenol (p.1177·3).
*Mouth and throat infections.*

**Valdatos** Sterling Health, Spain†.
Dextromethorphan hydrobromide (p.1117·3).
*Coughs.*

**Valdefer** Valdecasas, Mex.
Ferrous sulfate (p.1428·2).
*Iron-deficiency anaemia.*

**Valderma**
Roche Consumer, Irl.; Ransom, UK.
*Cream:* Potassium hydroxyquinoline sulfate (p.1734·2); chlorocresol (p.1177·1).
*Acne.*

Roche Consumer, Irl.†; Roche Consumer, UK.
*Soap:* Triclocarban (p.1195·1).
*Acne.*

**Valdig-N Burger** Ysatfabrik, Ger.
Convallaria (p.1675·3).
*Heart failure.*

**Valdispert**
Solvay, Belg.; Solvay, Ger.; Vemedia, Neth.; Solvay, Port.; Solvay, Spain; Solvay, Switz.†.
Valerian (p.1762·2).
*Insomnia; nervous disorders.*

**Valdispert comp** Solvay, Ger.
Valerian (p.1762·2); lupulus (p.1708·1).
*Anxiety; sleep disorders.*

**Valdispert Complex** Solvay, Spain.
Passion flower (p.1729·1); valerian (p.1762·2).
*Insomnia; nervous disorders.*

**Valdorm** Valeas, Ital.
Flurazepam monohydrochloride (p.700·3).
*Insomnia.*

**Valeans** Valeas, Ital.
Alprazolam (p.668·3).
*Anxiety.*

**Valecid** Depofarma, Ital.
Cefonicid sodium (p.174·2).
Lidocaine hydrochloride (p.1377·3) is included in this preparation to alleviate the pain of injection.
*Gram-negative bacterial infections.*

**Valederm** Stiefel, Arg.
Betamethasone valerate (p.1093·2).
*Skin disorders.*

**Valena N** Spreewald, Ger.†.
Hypericum (p.299·1); passion flower (p.1729·1); valerian (p.1762·2).
*Anxiety; depression.*

**Valenium** Kenyaku, Thai.
Diazepam (p.690·1).
*Anxiety.*

**Valerbe** Bride, Fr.†.
Valerian (p.1762·2); vitamins (p.1417·1).
*Aid to smoking withdrawal.*

**Valerbet** Polipharm, Thai.
Betamethasone valerate (p.1093·2).
*Skin disorders.*

**Valerecen** Abigo, Swed.
Valerian (p.1762·2).
*Sedative.*

**Valergen** Hyrex, USA.
Estradiol valerate (p.1550·2).
*Female castration; female hypogonadism; menopausal vasomotor symptoms; prevention of breast engorgement; primary ovarian failure; prostatic cancer; vulval and vaginal atrophy.*

**Valerial** Zambon, Belg.
Valerian (p.1762·2).
*Nervous disorders; sleep disorders.*

**Valerian** Vitaplex, Austral.†.
Motherwort (p.1717·1); valerian (p.1762·2); skullcap (p.1746·3); populus (p.1733·3); capsicum (p.1667·1).
*Herbal sedative.*

**Valerian Passiflora and Hops** Lifeplan, UK.
Vitamins; minerals; kava kava; passion flower; motherwort; wild lettuce; scullcap; lupulus; valerian (p.1417·1).
*Herbal supplement.*

**Valerian Plus Herbal Plus Formula 12** Vitelle, Austral.†.
Valerian (p.1762·2); passion flower (p.1729·1); dibasic potassium phosphate (p.1230·3); magnesium oxide (p.1272·3).
*Insomnia; smooth muscle spasm.*

**Valeriana comp novum** Hevert, Ger.
Diphenhydramine hydrochloride (p.431·3); valerian (p.1762·2).
Valeriana comp formerly contained diphenhydramine hydrochloride, bitter-orange peel, chamomile, lupulus, kava, valerian, and peppermint oil.
*Anxiety; nervous disorders.*

**Valeriana forte N** Hevert, Ger.
Diphenhydramine hydrochloride (p.431·3); valerian (p.1762·2).
Valeriana forte formerly contained diphenhydramine hydrochloride, valerian, and lupulus.
*Sedative.*

**Valeriana mild** Hevert, Ger.
Valerian (p.1762·2); passion flower (p.1729·1); lupulus (p.1708·1).
*Nervous disorders; sleep disorders.*

**Valeriana Oligoplex** Madaus, Arg.
Melissa (p.1711·1); valerian (p.1762·2); avena (p.1658·2).
*Sedative.*

**Valeriana Orto** Normon, Spain.
Valerian (p.1762·2).
*Insomnia; nervous disorders.*

**Valeriana (Specie Composta)** Dynacren, Ital.
Valerian (p.1762·2); lupulus (p.1708·1); melissa (p.1711·1); peppermint leaf (p.1283·2); bitter-orange peel (p.1723·3).
*Insomnia.*

**Valerianaheel** Peithner, Austria.
Homoeopathic preparation.

**Valeric**
Atlantic, Singapore; Vana, Thai.
Allopurinol (p.412·2).
*Gout; hyperuricaemia.*

**Valerin** Fontovit, Braz.
Valerian (p.1762·2).
*Anxiety.*

**Valerina Day Time** Lichtwer, UK.
Valerian (p.1762·2); melissa (p.1711·1).
*Strain; stress.*

**Valerina Night-Time** Lichtwer, UK.
Valerian (p.1762·2); lupulus (p.1708·1); melissa (p.1711·1).
*Insomnia.*

**Valerix** Ativus, Braz.
Valerian (p.1762·2).
*Anxiety; sleep disturbances.*

**Valerocalma** Piam, Ital.
Centranthus ruber.
*Insomnia; sedative.*

**Valertest** Hyrex, USA†.
Estradiol valerate (p.1550·2); testosterone enantate (p.1570·1).
*Menopausal vasomotor symptoms; prevention of postpartum breast engorgement.*

**Valesono** Neves, Port.
Valerian (p.1762·2); passion flower (p.1729·1).
*Alcohol withdrawal syndrome; anxiety disorders; insomnia; smoking cessation.*

**Valeton** Rekah, Israel.
Valerian (p.1762·2).
*Nervous disorders.*

**Valette** Jenapharm, Ger.
Ethinylestradiol (p.1553·2); dienogest (p.1548·1).
*Androgen-dependent acne, seborrhoea, hirsutism, and alopecia in females; combined oral contraceptive.*

**Valezen** Teuto, Braz.
Valerian (p.1762·2).
*Anxiety.*

**Valfam** Valdecasas, Mex.
Loperamide (p.1271·2).
*Diarrhoea.*

**Valfiran** Sanval, Braz.
Sulfiram (p.1510·1).
*Pediculosis; scabies.*

**Valflex** Sanval, Braz.
Cefalexin (p.168·1).
*Bacterial infections.*

**Valherpes** Pensa, Spain.
Valaciclovir hydrochloride (p.656·1).
*Herpesvirus infections.*

**Valifol** Valdecasas, Mex.
Isoniazid (p.222·2).
*Tuberculosis.*

**Valin Baldrian** Sanova, Austria.
Valerian (p.1762·2); citronella oil (p.1673·2).
*Nervous disorders; sleep disorders.*

**Valinor** Baxter, Fr.
Amino-acid infusion (p.1417·1).
*Parenteral nutrition.*

**Valiquid** Roche, Ger.
Diazepam (p.690·1).
*Anxiety disorders; premedication; skeletal muscle spasm; sleep disorders.*

**Valirem** Genepharm, Gr.
Sulpiride (p.722·2).
*Psychoses.*

**Valisone** *Schering, Canad.; Schering, USA.*
Betamethasone valerate (p.1093·2).
*Skin disorders.*

**Valisone-G** *Schering, Canad.*
Betamethasone valerate (p.1093·2); gentamicin sulfate (p.217·1).
*Infected skin disorders.*

**Valium**
*Roche, Arg.; Roche, Austral.; Roche, Austria; Roche, Belg.; Roche, Braz.; Roche, Canad.; Roche, Denm.; Roche, Fr.; Roche, Ger.; Piramal, India; Roche, Irl.; Roche, Israel†; Roche, Ital.; Roche, Mex.; Roche, Neth.; Roche, Norw.; Roche, Port.; Roche, S.Afr.; Roche, Singapore†; Roche, Spain; Roche, Swed.†; Roche, Switz.; Roche, Thai.; Roche, UK†; Roche, USA.*
Diazepam (p.690·1).
*Alcohol withdrawal syndrome; anxiety disorders; childhood nightmares and somnambulism; convulsions; premedication; skeletal muscle spasm; status epilepticus; tetanus.*

**Valix** *Sintofarma, Braz.*
Diazepam (p.690·1).
*Anxiety.*

**Valken** *Kener, Mex.†.*
Valproic acid (p.380·1).

**Vallergan**
*Aventis, Austral.; Rhone-Poulenc Rorer, Denm.†; Rhone-Poulenc Rorer, Hong Kong†; Aventis, Irl.; Aventis, Norw.; Aventis, NZ; Aventis, S.Afr. Castlemead, UK.*
Alimemazine tartrate (p.423·3).
*Premedication; pruritus; urticaria.*

**Valmane**
*Note. This name is used for preparations of different composition.*
*Medicopharm, Austria.*
Valepotriates (p.1762·2).
*Anxiety disorders.*
*Sintofarma, Braz.; Solvay, Ger.†.*
Valerian (p.1762·2).
*Anxiety disorders; nervous disorders; sleep disorders.*

**Valmarin Bad N** *Hoernecke, Ger.†.*
Citronella oil (p.1673·2).
*Bath additive; insomnia; nervous disorders.*

**Valmicin** *Sanval, Braz.*
Erythromycin estolate (p.208·1).
*Bacterial infections.*

**Valnar** *Elvetium, Arg.*
Valproate semisodium (p.380·1).
*Bipolar disorder; epilepsy; migraine.*

**Valocordin-Diazepam** *Krewel, Ger.*
Diazepam (p.690·1).
*Anxiety disorders; sleep disorders.*

**Valoid**
*GlaxoSmithKline, Hong Kong; Wellcome, Irl.†; GlaxoSmithKline, NZ; GlaxoSmithKline, S.Afr.; CeNeS, UK.*
Cyclizine (p.429·3), cyclizine hydrochloride (p.429·3), or cyclizine lactate (p.429·3).
*Nausea; vestibular disorders; vomiting.*

**Valonorm** *Zenith, UK.*
Atropine sulfate (p.477·1); peppermint oil (p.1283·2); magnesium carbonate (p.1272·1); magnesium trisilicate (p.1272·3); calcium carbonate (p.1254·2); sodium bicarbonate (p.1223·2); aluminium hydroxide (p.1249·2).
*Dyspepsia; gastrointestinal spasm.*

**Valontan** *Recordati, Ital.*
Dimenhydrinate (p.431·1).
*Motion sickness.*

**Valopin** *Julphar, UAE.*
Sodium valproate (p.380·1).
*Epilepsy.*

**Valopride** *Pharmafar, Ital.*
Bromopride (p.1254·1).
*Gastrointestinal disorders.*

**Valoran**
*Medochemie, Hong Kong; Medochemie, Thai.*
Cefotaxime sodium (p.175·3).
*Bacterial infections.*

**Valorel** *Alpes Chemie, Chile.*
Etofenamate (p.38·1).
*Peri-articular and soft-tissue disorders.*

**Valoron**
*Parke, Davis, Belg.; Pfizer, S.Afr.; Pfizer, Switz.*
Tilidine hydrochloride (p.94·1).
*Pain.*

**Valoron N** *Godecke, Ger.; Parke, Davis, Ger.*
Tilidine hydrochloride (p.94·1) or tilidine phosphate (p.94·2).
Naloxone hydrochloride (p.1044·3) is included in this preparation to discourage abuse.
*Pain.*

**Valpakine** *Sanofi Synthelabo, Braz.*
Sodium valproate (p.380·1).
*Bipolar disorder; epilepsy.*

**Valpam** *Arrow, Austral.*
Diazepam (p.690·1).
*Anxiety disorders; skeletal muscle spasm; spasticity.*

**Valpar** *Valdecasas, Mex.*
Metronidazole benzoate (p.607·2).
*Amoebiasis; giardiasis; trichomoniasis.*

**Valparin**
*Torrent, India; Torrent, Thai.*
Sodium valproate (p.380·1).
*Epilepsy.*

**Valpax** *Recalcine, Chile.*
Clonazepam (p.359·1).
*Anxiety.*

**Valpeda** *Ransom, UK.*
Halquinol (p.220·3).
*Skin infections.*

**Valpex** *Armstrong, Arg.*
Donepezil hydrochloride (p.1489·2).
*Alzheimer's disease.*

**Valpiform** *General Dietary, UK.*
A range of gluten-free foods (p.1417·1).

**Valpin** *Recalcine, Chile.*
Octatropine methylbromide (p.486·1); phenobarbital (p.367·3).
*Colic; vomiting in infants.*

**Valpinax** *Crinos, Ital.*
Octatropine methylbromide (p.486·1); diazepam (p.690·1).
*Gastrointestinal spasm.*

**Val-Plus** *Edmond Pharma, Ital.*
Valerian (p.1762·2); passion flower (p.1729·1).
*Insomnia; sedative.*

**Valporal** *Teva, Israel.*
Valproic acid (p.380·1) or sodium valproate (p.380·1).
*Epilepsy.*

**Valprene** *Teuto, Braz.*
Sodium valproate (p.380·1).
*Epilepsy.*

**Valpression** *Menarini, Ital.*
Valsartan (p.1018·3).
*Hypertension.*

**Valpridol** *Sanofi Synthelabo, Spain†.*
Valaciclovir hydrochloride (p.656·1).
*Herpesvirus infections.*

**Valpro**
*Alphapharm, Austral.; TAD, Ger.; Alphapharm, Hong Kong.*
Sodium valproate (p.380·1).
*Epilepsy; mania.*

**Valpro Beta** *Betapharm, Ger.*
Sodium valproate (p.380·1).
*Epilepsy.*

**Valprodura** *Merck dura, Ger.*
Sodium valproate (p.380·1).
*Epilepsy.*

**Valproflux** *Hennig, Ger.*
Sodium valproate (p.380·1).
*Epilepsy.*

**Valprolept** *Hexal, Ger.*
Sodium valproate (p.380·1).
*Epilepsy.*

**ValproNa** *Teva, Ger.*
Sodium valproate (p.380·1).
*Epilepsy.*

**Valprosid** *Armstrong, Mex.*
Valproic acid (p.380·1) or sodium valproate (p.380·1).
*Epilepsy.*

**Valrian** *Leiras, Fin.*
Valerian (p.1762·2).
*Nervous disorders; sleep disorders.*

**Vals** *Esteve, Spain.*
Valsartan (p.1018·3).
*Hypertension.*

**Valsartan/HCTZ** *Novartis, Austria.*
Valsartan (p.1018·3); hydrochlorothiazide (p.933·2).
*Hypertension.*

**Valsera** *Polifarma, Ital.*
Flunitrazepam (p.698·2).
*Insomnia.*

**Valstar**
*Anthra, Israel; Celltech, USA.*
Valrubicin (p.590·3).
*Bladder cancer.*

**Valsweet** *Valma, Chile.*
Aspartame (p.1422·1).
*Sugar substitute.*

**Valtaxin** *Paladin, Canad.*
Valrubicin (p.590·3).
*Bladder cancer.*

**Valtran** *Pfizer, Belg.*
Tilidine hydrochloride (p.94·1).
Naloxone hydrochloride (p.1044·3) is included in this preparation to discourage abuse.
*Pain.*

**Valtrax** *Valeas, Ital.*
Diazepam (p.690·1); isopropamide iodide (p.485·2).
*Gastrointestinal spasm.*

**Valtrex**
*GlaxoSmithKline, Arg.; GlaxoSmithKline, Austral.; GlaxoSmithKline, Austria; GlaxoSmithKline, Braz.; GlaxoSmithKline, Canad.; GlaxoSmithKline, Chile; GlaxoSmithKline, Fin.; Cascan, Ger.; GlaxoSmithKline, Ger.; Glaxo Wellcome, Gr.; GlaxoSmithKline, Hong Kong; Wellcome, Irl.; Wellcome, Israel; GlaxoSmithKline, Malaysia; GlaxoSmithKline, Norw.; Wellcome, Port.; GlaxoSmithKline, Singapore; GlaxoSmithKline, Spain; GlaxoSmithKline, Swed.; GlaxoSmithKline, Switz.; GlaxoSmithKline, Thai.; GlaxoSmithKline, UK; Glaxo Wellcome, USA.*
Valaciclovir hydrochloride (p.656·1).
*Herpesvirus infections.*

**Val-Uno** *Edmond Pharma, Ital.*
Valerian (p.1762·2).
*Insomnia; sedative.*

**Valupass** *Knop, Chile.*
Valerian (p.1762·2); lupulus (p.1708·1); passiflora coerulea.
*Depression; insomnia; nervous disorders.*

**Valus** *Glenmark, India.*
Valdecoxib (p.96·1).
*Dysmenorrhoea; osteoarthritis; rheumatoid arthritis.*

**Valverde boutons de fievre creme** *Novartis Consumer, Switz.*
Melissa (p.1711·1).
*Herpes simplex or labialis.*

**Valverde Dragees laxatives** *Novartis Consumer, Switz.*
Fig (p.1266·3); senna (p.1288·2); petasites root (p.1663·3).
*Constipation.*

**Valverde Dragees pour la detente** *Novartis Consumer, Switz.*
Petasites root (p.1663·3); passion flower (p.1729·1); valerian (p.1762·2); melissa (p.1711·1).
*Nervous disorders.*

**Valverde Dragees pour le coeur** *Novartis Consumer, Switz.*
Crataegus leaves and fruit (p.1677·1); passion flower (p.1729·1); lupulus (p.1708·1); valerian root (p.1762·2).
*Cardiac disorders.*

**Valverde Dragees pour le sommeil** *Novartis Consumer, Switz.*
Lupulus (p.1708·1); valerian root (p.1762·2).
*Sleep disorders.*

**Valverde Efeu** *Novartis Consumer, Ger.†.*
Hedera helix.
*Bronchitis; catarrh.*

**Valverde Gouttes pour le coeur** *Novartis Consumer, Switz.*
Crataegus leaves and fruit (p.1677·1); passion flower (p.1729·1).
*Cardiac disorders.*

**Valverde Hyperval** *Zyma, Switz.†.*
Hypericum (p.299·1).
*Anxiety; tension.*

**Valverde prostate capsules** *Novartis Consumer, Switz.*
Urtica (p.1762·1).
*Prostate disorders.*

**Valverde regulateur du transit intestinal granules** *Novartis Consumer, Switz.*
Ispaghula (p.1268·1).
*Constipation.*

**Valverde Sabal** *Novartis Consumer, Ger.†.*
Saw palmetto (p.1569·1).
*Benign prostatic hyperplasia.*

**Valverde Sirop contre la toux** *Novartis Consumer, Switz.†.*
Hedera helix.
*Respiratory-tract disorders associated with excess mucus.*

**Valverde Sirop laxatif** *Novartis Consumer, Switz.*
Fig (p.1266·3); senna (p.1288·2).
*Constipation.*

**Valverde Sirop pour le sommeil** *Novartis Consumer, Switz.*
Valerian (p.1762·2).
*Sleep disorders.*

**Valverde Tablettes contre la toux** *Novartis Consumer, Switz.†.*
Hedera helix.
*Respiratory-tract disorders associated with excess mucus.*

**Valverde Traubensilberkerze** *Novartis Consumer, Ger.*
Cimicifuga (p.1671·3).
*Menopausal disorders.*

**Valverde Vitalite** *Novartis Consumer, Switz.*
Ginkgo biloba (p.1692·3).
*Tonic.*

**Vamazole** *Nakornpatana, Thai.*
Clotrimazole (p.396·2).
*Fungal skin infections.*

**Va-Mengoc-BC**
*Elea, Arg.; Enila, Braz.*
A meningococcal vaccine (groups B and C) (p.1626·1).
*Active immunisation.*

**Vamin**
*Fresenius Medical, Austral.; Fresenius Kabi, Austria; Pharmacia Upjohn, Belg.†; Baxter, Canad.; Fresenius Kabi, Denm.; Fresenius Kabi, Gr.; Fresenius Kabi, Hong Kong; Pharmacia Upjohn, Irl.†; Pharmacia Upjohn, Israel; Fresenius Kabi, Malaysia; Fresenius Kabi, Neth.; Fresenius Kabi, Norw.; Baxter, NZ; Fresenius Kabi, NZ; Fresenius Kabi, Port.; Fresenius Kabi, S.Afr.†; Fresenius Kabi, Swed.; Fresenius Kabi, UK.*
Amino-acid infusion with or without electrolytes (p.1417·1).
*Parenteral nutrition.*

**Vamin con Glucosa** *Fresenius Kabi, Spain.*
Amino-acid infusion with glucose and electrolytes (p.1417·1).
*Parenteral nutrition.*

**Vamin EF** *Fresenius Kabi, Ital.*
Amino-acid infusion (p.1417·1).
*Parenteral nutrition.*

**Vamin 18EF** *Fresenius Kabi, Singapore†.*
Amino-acid infusion (p.1417·1).
*Parenteral nutrition.*

**Vamin Glucose**
*Fresenius Medical, Austral.; Pharmacia Upjohn, Belg.†; Fresenius Kabi, Gr.; Fresenius Kabi, Hong Kong; Fresenius Kabi, Irl.; Pharmacia Upjohn, Israel; Fresenius Kabi, Malaysia; Fresenius Kabi, Neth.; Fresenius Kabi, Port.; Fresenius Kabi, S.Afr.†; Fresenius Kabi, Singapore†; Fresenius Kabi, Thai.; Fresenius Kabi, UK.*
Amino-acid, glucose, and electrolyte infusion (p.1417·1).
*Parenteral nutrition.*

**Vamin Glukos**
*Fresenius Kabi, Denm.; Fresenius Kabi, Fin.; Fresenius Kabi, Norw.; Fresenius Kabi, Swed.*
Amino-acid, glucose, and electrolyte infusion (p.1417·1).
*Parenteral nutrition.*

**Vamin Glukos Combi** *Fresenius Kabi, Fin.*
1 infusion, amino-acid, glucose, and electrolyte infusion (Vamin Glukos) (p.1417·1); 1 infusion, soya oil (Intralipid) (p.1447·2).
*Parenteral nutrition.*

**Vamin mit Glukose** *Fresenius Kabi, Austria.*
Amino-acid, glucose, and electrolyte infusion (p.1417·1).
*Parenteral nutrition.*

**Vamin N** *Fresenius Medical, Austral.*
Amino-acid and electrolyte infusion (p.1417·1).
*Parenteral nutrition.*

**Vamin N/I** *Fresenius Kabi, Fin.*
Amino-acid infusion (p.1417·1).
*Parenteral nutrition.*

**Vamina** *Fresenius Kabi, Switz.*
Amino-acid infusion (p.1417·1).
*Parenteral nutrition.*

**Vamina Glucose** *Fresenius Kabi, Switz.*
Amino-acid, carbohydrate, and electrolyte infusion (p.1417·1).
*Parenteral nutrition.*

**Vamine Glucose** *Fresenius Kabi, Fr.*
Amino-acid, glucose, and electrolyte infusion (p.1417·1).
*Parenteral nutrition.*

**Vaminolac**
*Fresenius Kabi, Denm.; Fresenius Kabi, Fin.; Fresenius Kabi, Norw.; Fresenius Kabi, Swed.*
Amino-acid infusion (p.1417·1).
*Parenteral nutrition.*

**Vaminolact**
*Fresenius Kabi, Austria; Pharmacia Upjohn, Belg.†; Fresenius Kabi, Fr.; Fresenius Kabi, Hong Kong; Pharmacia, Irl.; Pharmacia Upjohn, Israel; Fresenius Kabi, Malaysia; Fresenius Kabi, Neth.; Baxter, NZ; Fresenius Kabi, NZ.; Fresenius Kabi, Port.; Fresenius Kabi, Singapore; Fresenius Kabi, Switz.; Fresenius Kabi, Thai.; Fresenius Kabi, UK.*
Amino-acid infusion (p.1417·1).
*Parenteral nutrition.*

**Vanadiol** *Simoes, Braz.*
Vitamin B substances with sodium and calcium glycerophosphates (p.1417·1).
*Vitamin B deficiency; vitamin B supplement.*

**Vanafen** *Vana, Thai.*
Chloramphenicol (p.185·1).
*Bacterial eye or ear infections.*

**Vanafen-S**
*Atlantic, Hong Kong†; Atlantic, Singapore†.*
Chloramphenicol (p.185·1).
*Eye infections.*

**Vanamide** *Dermik, USA.*
Urea (p.1162·2).
*Dry skin.*

**Vanaurus** *Pisa, Mex.*
Vancomycin hydrochloride (p.275·2).
*Antibiotic-associated colitis due to Clostridium difficile; bacterial infections.*

**Vancam** *Abbott, Mex.*
Vancomycin hydrochloride (p.275·2).
*Antibiotic-associated colitis due to Clostridium difficile; bacterial infections.*

**Vancenase**
*Schering, Canad.†; Schering, USA.*
Beclometasone dipropionate (p.1091·1).
*Nasal polyps; rhinitis.*

**Vanceril**
*Schering, Canad.; Schering, USA†.*
Beclometasone dipropionate (p.1091·1).
*Asthma.*

**Vanclomin** *Teuto, Braz.*
Vancomycin hydrochloride (p.275·2).
*Bacterial infections.*

**Vanco**
*Azupharma, Ger.; Cell Pharm, Ger.; Pulitzer, Ital.*
Vancomycin hydrochloride (p.275·2).
*Bacterial infections.*

**Vancoabbott** *Abbott, Braz.*
Vancomycin hydrochloride (p.275·2).
*Bacterial infections.*

**Vancocid** *Biochimico, Braz.*
Vancomycin (p.275·2).
*Bacterial infections.*

**Vancocin**
*Lilly, Arg.; Lilly, Austral.; Lilly, Belg.; Lilly, Canad.; Lilly, Denm.; Lilly, Fin.; Lilly, Hong Kong; Lilly, India; Lilly, Irl.; Lilly, Israel; Lilly, Malaysia; Lilly, Mex.; Lilly, Neth.; Lilly, Norw.; Lilly, NZ; Rolab, S.Afr.; Lilly, Swed.; Lilly, Switz.; Lilly, Thai.; Lilly, UK; Lilly, USA.*
Vancomycin hydrochloride (p.275·2).
*Antibiotic-associated colitis; bacterial infections.*

**Vancocina**
*Lilly, Braz.; Lilly, Chile; Bayer, Ital.; Lilly, Port.*
Vancomycin hydrochloride (p.275·2).
*Bacterial infections.*

**Vancocine** *Lilly, Fr.*
Vancomycin hydrochloride (p.275·2).
*Bacterial infections.*

**Vancolan** *Julphar, UAE.*
Vancomycin hydrochloride (p.275·2).
*Bacterial infections.*

**Vancoled** Wyeth, Austral.†; Lederle, Israel; Lederle, Switz.†; Lederle, USA.
Vancomycin hydrochloride (p.275·2).
*Bacterial infections.*

**Vancomax** Klonal, Arg.
Vancomycin (p.275·2).

**Vancoplus** Royton, Braz.
Vancomycin hydrochloride (p.275·2).
*Bacterial infections.*

**Vanco-saar** Chephasaar, Ger.
Vancomycin hydrochloride (p.275·2).
*Bacterial infections.*

**Vancoscand** Scand Pharm, Swed.
Vancomycin hydrochloride (p.275·2).
*Gram-positive bacterial infections.*

**Vancoson** Ariston, Braz.
Vancomycin (p.275·2).
*Bacterial infections.*

**Vancotenk** Biotenk, Arg.
Vancomycin (p.275·2).
*Bacterial infections.*

**Vanco-Teva** Abic, Hong Kong†; Teva, Israel.
Vancomycin hydrochloride (p.275·2).
*Antibiotic-associated colitis; bacterial infections.*

**Vancox** Lemery, Mex.
Vancomycin hydrochloride (p.275·2).
*Bacterial infections.*

**Vanderbumin** Grossman, Mex.†.
Albumin (p.740·3).
*Barbiturate overdosage; burns; cerebral oedema; hypoproteinaemia; hypovolaemia; shock.*

**Vanderm** Agis, Israel.
Methylprednisolone aceponate (p.1106·3).
*Eczema; neurodermatitis.*

**Vandisul** Vannier, Arg.
Disulfiram (p.1681·3).
*Alcoholism.*

**Vandol** Schering-Plough, S.Afr.
Vitamin A (p.1451·2); vitamin D (p.1461·2).
*Skin disorders.*

**Vandral** Wyeth, Spain.
Venlafaxine hydrochloride (p.321·3).
*Anxiety; depression.*

**Vanesten** Atlantic, Singapore; Vana, Thai.
Clotrimazole (p.396·2).
*Fungal skin infections.*

**Vanex Expectorant** Abana, USA.
Pseudoephedrine hydrochloride (p.1129·2); guaifenesin (p.1122·1); hydrocodone tartrate (p.45·1).
*Coughs.*

**Vanex Forte** Abana, USA†.
Phenylpropanolamine hydrochloride (p.1127·3); phenylephrine hydrochloride (p.1126·3); chlorphenamine maleate (p.427·3); mepyramine maleate (p.437·1).
*Upper respiratory-tract symptoms.*

**Vanex Forte-R** Jones, USA†.
Phenylpropanolamine hydrochloride (p.1127·3); chlorphenamine maleate (p.427·3).
*Upper respiratory-tract disorders.*

**Vanex-HD** Abana, USA.
Phenylephrine hydrochloride (p.1126·3); chlorphenamine maleate (p.427·3); hydrocodone tartrate (p.45·1).
*Coughs and cold symptoms.*

**Vanicream** Pharmaceutical Specialties, USA.
Vehicle for topical preparations.

**Vanidene** Asta Medica, Belg.†.
Cyclovalone (p.1678·2).
*Liver disorders; skin disorders; vomiting with ketonuria.*

**Vanilone** Tradiphar, Fr.†.
Cyclovalone (p.1678·2).
*Dyspepsia.*

**Vaniqa** Women First, USA.
Eflornithine hydrochloride (p.604·2).
*Reduction of unwanted facial hair in women.*

**Vanmicina** Pisa, Mex.†.
Vancomycin hydrochloride (p.275·2).
*Antibiotic-associated colitis due to Clostridium difficile; bacterial infections.*

**Vanmycetin** FDC, India.
Chloramphenicol (p.185·1).
*Bacterial eye infections; corneal ulcer; trachoma.*

**Vanocin** Stratus, USA.
Sulfacetamide sodium (p.257·3).
*Acne; rosacea; seborrhoeic dermatitis.*

**Vanoxide** Dermik, USA†.
Benzoyl peroxide (p.1143·2).
*Acne.*

**Vanoxide-HC** Dermik, USA.
Benzoyl peroxide (p.1143·2); hydrocortisone (p.1103·3).
*Acne; seborrhoea.*

**Vanquin** Pfizer Consumer, Canad.; Pfizer, Denm.; Pfizer, Norw.; Pfizer, Swed.
Pyrvinium embonate (p.113·3).
*Enterobiasis.*

**Vanquish** Glenbrook, USA.
Aspirin (p.15·1); paracetamol (p.76·2); caffeine (p.782·1).
Aluminium hydroxide (p.1249·2) and magnesium hydroxide (p.1272·2) are included in this preparation in an attempt to limit adverse effects on the gastrointestinal mucosa.
*Pain.*

**Vansil** IFET (ΙΦΕΤ), Gr.; Pfizer, USA†.
Oxamniquine (p.110·3).
*Schistosomiasis.*

**Vantaggio** Gazzoni, Ital.†.
Aspartame (p.1422·1).
*Sugar substitute.*

**Vantal** Grossman, Mex.
Benzydamine hydrochloride (p.21·1).
*Mouth and throat inflammation; peri-articular disorders; soft-tissue disorders; vulvovaginitis.*

**Vanticon** Phoenix, Arg.
Zafirlukast (p.807·1).
*Asthma.*

**Vantin** Pharmacia Upjohn, USA.
Cefpodoxime proxetil (p.178·3).
*Bacterial infections.*

**Vantux** Grunenthal, Chile.
Zinc sulfate; gelatin; amino acids (p.1417·1).
*Hair and nail disorders.*

**Vanzor** Tocogino, Mex.†.
Diazepam (p.690·1).

**Vaopin N** Riemser, Ger.
Camphor (p.1665·3).
*Skin disorders.*

**Vap Air** DC Labs, Canad.
Camphor (p.1665·3); eucalyptus oil (p.1686·2); menthol (p.1711·3); pumilio pine oil (p.1737·1); thymol (p.1194·2).

**Vapex**
Note. This name is used for preparations of different composition.
Roche, Hong Kong†.
Menthol (p.1711·3); linalyl acetate; eucalyptus oil (p.1686·2); bornyl acetate (p.1662·2); camphor oil.
*Nasal congestion.*
Roche Consumer, Singapore†.
Menthol (p.1711·3); linalyl acetate; eucalyptus oil (p.1686·2); bornyl acetate (p.1662·2); camphor oil; lavender oil (p.1705·2).
*Nasal congestion.*

**Vapin** Lacer, Spain†.
Octatropine methylbromide (p.486·1).
*Adjunct in peptic ulcer; gastrointestinal spasm; irritable bowel syndrome.*

**Vapin Complex** Lacer, Spain†.
Dipyrone (p.35·3); octatropine methylbromide (p.486·1).
*Gastrointestinal spasm; pain.*

**Vapio** Millet Roux, Braz.†.
Piperonyl butoxide (p.1509·2); esdepallethrine (p.1505·1).
Formerly contained bioallethrin and piperonyl butoxide.
*Pediculosis.*

**Vapoflu** Lafi, Chile.
Clobutinol (p.1117·1); orciprenaline (p.790·2); ammonium chloride (p.1115·2).
*Coughs.*

**Vapolatum Inhalador** Maver, Chile.
Camphor (p.1665·3); methyl salicylate (p.59·3); menthol (p.1711·3).

**Vapolatum Labial** Maver, Chile.
Camphor (p.1665·3); methyl salicylate (p.59·3).

**Vapolatum Unguento** Maver, Chile.
Methyl salicylate (p.59·3); camphor (p.1665·3).

**Vapo-Myrtol** Marion Merrell, Fr.†.
Borneol; menthol (p.1711·3); myrtle oil; niaouli oil (p.1719·3); thyme oil (p.1755·3); cineole (p.1672·1).
*Respiratory-tract congestion.*

**Vaponefrin** Aventis, Canad.
Racepinefrine hydrochloride (p.854·1).
*Bronchospasm.*

**Vapor Flay** Chimicor, Ital.†.
Cymbopogon nardus oil; geranium oil (p.1692·2); pinus pinaster oil; verbena citriodora oil; peppermint oil (p.1283·2).
*Insect repellent.*

**Vapores Pyt** Fardi, Spain.
Peru balsam (p.1730·2); cupressus sempervirens; eucalyptus (p.1686·1); niaouli oil (p.1719·3); diplotaxis tenuifolia; abies pectinata; pinus sylvestris; beech.
*Upper respiratory-tract congestion.*

**Vaporil** Medical, Port.
Belladonna (p.479·1); eucalyptus oil (p.1686·2); benzoin (p.1751·1); thyme oil (p.1755·3); lavender oil (p.1705·2); camphor (p.1665·3).
*Catarrh.*

**Vaporisateur Medicamente**
Note. This name is used for preparations of different composition.
Alsi, Canad.
Camphor (p.1665·3); cineole (p.1672·1); menthol (p.1711·3); thymol (p.1194·2).
Multi-Pro, Canad.
Camphor (p.1665·3); eucalyptus oil (p.1686·2); menthol (p.1711·3); thymol (p.1194·2).

**Vaporisateur Nasal Decongestionnant** Prodemdis, Canad.†.
Xylometazoline hydrochloride (p.1132·2).

**Vaporizing Chest Rub** Stanley, Canad.
Camphor (p.1665·3); eucalyptus oil (p.1686·2); menthol (p.1711·3).

**Vaporizing Colds Rub** Scott, Canad.
Camphor (p.1665·3); eucalyptus oil (p.1686·2); menthol (p.1711·3).

**Vaporizing Ointment** Prodemdis, Canad.
Camphor (p.1665·3); cedar; eucalyptus oil (p.1686·2); menthol (p.1711·3); nutmeg oil (p.1722·3); thymol (p.1194·2); turpentine.

**Vapour Rub** Numark, UK.
Eucalyptus oil (p.1686·2); camphor (p.1665·3); menthol (p.1711·3).

**Vapresan** Temis, Arg.
Enalapril maleate (p.909·2).
*Heart failure; hypertension.*

**Vapresan Diur** Temis, Arg.
Enalapril maleate (p.909·2); hydrochlorothiazide (p.933·2).
*Hypertension.*

**VAQTA** Merck Sharp & Dohme, Arg.; Merck Sharp & Dohme, Austral.; Aventis Pasteur, Belg.; Merck Sharp & Dohme, Braz.; Merck Frosst, Canad.; Aventis Pasteur, Fin.; Aventis Pasteur, Fr.; Aventis Pasteur, Ger.; Vianex (Βιανέξ), Gr.; Merck Sharp & Dohme, Hong Kong; Aventis Pasteur, Irl.; Merck Sharp & Dohme, Israel; Aventis Pasteur, Ital.; Merck Sharp & Dohme, Malaysia; Merck Sharp & Dohme, Mex.; Merck Sharp & Dohme, NZ; Merck Sharp & Dohme, Singapore; Aventis Pasteur, Spain; Aventis Pasteur, Swed.; Pro Vaccine, Switz.; Merck Sharp & Dohme, Thai.; Aventis Pasteur, UK; Merck, USA.
A hepatitis A vaccine (p.1617·1).
Separate preparations are available for children and adolescents and for adults.
*Active immunisation.*

**Varedet** Fada, Arg.
Vancomycin (p.275·2).

**Varemoid** Novartis Consumer, S.Afr.†; Zyma, Switz.†; Novartis, Thai.†.
Oxerutins (p.1688·2).
*Anorectal disorders.*

**Varfine** Teofarma, Port.
Warfarin sodium (p.1022·2).

**Variargil** Logogen, Spain.
Alimemazine tartrate (p.423·3).
*Hypersensitivity reactions.*

**Varibiotic** Wyeth, Spain†.
Demeclocycline hydrochloride (p.204·3); streptodornase (p.1749·3); streptokinase (p.1005·2).
*Bacterial infections.*

**Varicare** Andromaco, Chile.
Aesculus (p.1648·2); hamamelis (p.1696·3).
*Haemorrhoids; venous insufficiency.*

**Varicela Biken** Aventis Pasteur, Arg.; Aventis Pasteur, Chile.
A live attenuated varicella-zoster vaccine (OKA strain) (p.1643·2).
*Active immunisation.*

**Varicell** Eversil, Braz.
Partially hydrolysed keratin; senna (p.1288·2); sublimed sulfur (p.1158·2); potassium acid tartrate (p.1284·3).

**Varicella** SmithKline Beecham, Austria†.
A varicella-zoster vaccine (OKA strain) (p.1643·2).
*Active immunisation.*

**Varicellon** Aventis Behring, Ger.
A varicella-zoster immunoglobulin (p.1643·1).
*Passive immunisation.*

**Varicex** Lohmann, Ital.
Zinc oxide (p.1163·2).
*Medicated dressing.*

**Varicofit** Body Spring, Ital.
Ginkgo biloba (p.1692·3); myrtillus (p.1718·3); pungitopo; taraxacum (p.1751·3); centella (p.1144·3); bioflavonoids (p.1688·2); vitamin C (p.1460·2).
*Circulatory disorders.*

**Varicogel** Wassermann, Ital.
Aesculus (p.1648·2); hamamelis (p.1696·3).
*Peripheral vascular disorders.*

**Varicose Ointment** Potter's, UK.
Cade oil (p.1159·2); hamamelis (p.1696·3); zinc oxide (p.1163·2).
*Skin irritation due to varicosity.*

**Varicylum** Chemosan, Austria.
Hamamelis (p.1696·3); chamomile oil (p.1669·3); arnica (p.1656·3).
*Skin disorders; soft-tissue disorders.*

**Varicylum N** Liebermann, Ger.
Homoeopathic preparation.

**Varicylum-S** Liebermann, Ger.
Chamomile oil (p.1669·3); sage oil (p.1741·2); arnica (p.1656·3); aesculus (p.1648·2); hamamelis (p.1696·3).
*Haemorrhoids; soft-tissue injury; vascular disorders.*

**Varidasa** Wyeth, Arg.; Wyeth, Mex.; Wyeth Lederle, Port.; Wyeth, Spain.
Streptokinase (p.1005·2); streptodornase (p.1749·3).
*Inflammation; local removal of blood clots; oedema.*

**Varidase** Wyeth, Austral.; Wyeth Lederle, Austria; Wyeth Lederle, Belg.†; Meda, Denm.; Wyeth Lederle, Fin.; Lederle, Ger.; Wyeth, Irl.; Lederle, Israel†; Wyeth Lederle, Ital.; Lederle, Neth.†; Wyeth Lederle, Norw.†; Lederle, NZ†; Wyeth, S.Afr.†; Meda, Swed.; Wyeth, UK.
Streptokinase (p.1005·2); streptodornase (p.1749·3).
*Inflammation; local removal of blood clots, fibrin, and purulent matter; oedema.*

**Varidoid** General Drugs, Thai.
A heparinoid (p.931·1).
*Haematoma; oedema; phlebitis; scars; sunburn; thrombosis; varicose veins.*

**Varigerm** Heralds, Braz.†.
Tyrothricin (p.275·1); hydroxyquinoline sulfate (p.1700·1); menthol (p.1711·3); mallow (p.1709·3); lactic acid (p.1704·1).
*Skin disorders.*

**Varigestrol** Varifarma, Arg.
Megestrol (p.1558·3).

**Varigloban** Kreussler, Ger.
Sodium iodide (p.1598·1); iodine (p.1598·1).
*Haemorrhoids; varicose veins.*

**Variglobin** Globopharm, Switz.
Sodium iodide (p.1598·1); iodine (p.1598·1).
*Varicose veins.*

**Varihes** Laevosan, Austria; Fresenius Kabi, Switz.
Hetastarch (p.750·1).
*Hypovolaemia.*

**Varihesive** Convatec, Port.
Carmellose sodium (p.1577·3); gelatin (p.754·3); pectin (p.1580·3).
*Skin ulcers; wounds.*

**Varihesive Hydroactive** Convatec, Switz.†.
Carmellose sodium (p.1577·3); gelatin (p.754·3); pectin (p.1580·3).
*Burns; skin ulcers; wounds.*

**Varikromo** Geyer, Braz.
Glycerol (p.1694·3); chrome alum (p.1670·2).

**Varilise** Ativus, Braz.
Aesculus (p.1648·2).
*Haemorrhoids; varices.*

**Varilisin** Knoll, Belg.†.
Collagenase (p.1675·1).
*Debridement of necrotic ulcers.*

**Varilrix** GlaxoSmithKline, Arg.; GlaxoSmithKline, Austral.; GlaxoSmithKline, Austria; GlaxoSmithKline, Belg.; GlaxoSmithKline, Braz.; GlaxoSmithKline, Chile; SmithKline Beecham, Denm.; GlaxoSmithKline, Fin.; GlaxoSmithKline, Ger.; GlaxoSmithKline, Hong Kong; GlaxoSmithKline, India; GlaxoSmithKline, Ital.; GlaxoSmithKline, Malaysia; SmithKline Beecham, Mex.; GlaxoSmithKline, Norw.; GlaxoSmithKline, NZ; GlaxoSmithKline, S.Afr.; GlaxoSmithKline, Singapore; GlaxoSmithKline, Spain; GlaxoSmithKline, Swed.; SmithKline Beecham, Switz.; GlaxoSmithKline, Thai.; GlaxoSmithKline, UK.
A live attenuated varicella-zoster vaccine (OKA strain) (p.1643·2).
*Active immunisation.*

**Varimer** Varifarma, Arg.
Mercaptopurine (p.567·2).
*Malignant neoplasms.*

**Varimesna** Varifarma, Arg.
Mesna (p.1041·2).

**Varimine** Atral, Port.
Multivitamin and mineral preparation (p.1417·1).

**Variplant** Knop, Chile.
Homoeopathic preparation.

**Variplastic** Virtus, Braz.†.
Digitoxin (p.894·3).
*Arrhythmias; heart failure.*

**Variplex** Knop, Chile.
Homoeopathic preparation.

**Varison** Euro-Labor, Port.; Grunenthal, Port.
Myrtillus (p.1718·3).
*Haemorrhoids; metrorrhagia; venous insufficiency.*

**Varitan N** Godecke, Ger.†.
Bismuth subgallate (p.1252·2); zinc oxide (p.1163·2); lauromacrogol 400 (p.1412·3).
*Anorectal disorders.*

**Varitect** Biotest, Austria; Biotest, Ger.; IFET (ΙΦΕΤ), Gr.; Biotest, Hong Kong; Intra Pharma, Irl.; Biotest, Israel; Biotest, Ital.; Biotest, Port.; Biotest, Singapore; Biotest, Switz.; Biotest, Thai.
A varicella-zoster immunoglobulin (p.1643·1).
*Passive immunisation.*

**Variton** Hormona, Mex.
Diosmin (p.1688·2); hesperidin (p.1688·2).
*Haemorrhoids; venous insufficiency.*

**Varivax** Merck Sharp & Dohme, Austral.; Merck Sharp & Dohme, Braz.; Merck Frosst, Canad.; Merck Sharp & Dohme, Hong Kong; Aventis Pasteur, Irl.; Aventis Pasteur, Ital.; Merck Sharp & Dohme, Malaysia; Merck Sharp & Dohme, Mex.; Merck Sharp & Dohme, Singapore; Aventis Pasteur, UK; Merck, USA.
A live attenuated varicella-zoster vaccine (OKA/Merck strain) (p.1643·2).
*Active immunisation.*

**Varizin** Heralds, Braz.†.
Aesculus (p.1648·2); hamamelis (p.1696·3).

**Varizol** Simoes, Braz.
*Oral solution:* Rutoside (p.1688·2); calcium pantothenate (p.1442·3); hamamelis (p.1696·3).
*Topical gel:* Rutoside (p.1688·2); panthenol (p.1727·2); aesculus (p.1648·2); hamamelis (p.1696·3); lidocaine (p.1377·3).
*Haemorrhoids.*

**Varlane** Schering, Belg.
Fluocortin butyl (p.1102·1).
*Burns; skin disorders; stings.*

**Varnoline** Organon, Fr.
Desogestrel (p.1547·2); ethinylestradiol (p.1553·2).
28-Day packs also contain 7 inert tablets.
*Combined oral contraceptive.*

**Varson** Almirall, Spain.
Nicergoline (p.1719·3).
*Vascular disorders.*

**Vartalan** *Drugtech, Chile.*
Valsartan (p.1018·3).
*Hypertension.*

**Vartalan D** *Drugtech, Chile.*
Valsartan (p.1018·3); hydrochlorothiazide (p.933·2).
*Hypertension.*

**Vartalon**
*Note. This name is used for preparations of different composition.*
*Labinca, Arg.*
Low-molecular-weight polypeptides; amino acids (p.1417·1).
*Osteoarthritis.*

*Asofarma, Mex.*
Glucosamine sulfate (p.1694·1).
Lidocaine hydrochloride (p.1377·3) is included in the injection to alleviate the pain of injection.
*Musculoskeletal and joint disorders.*

**Vartalon Complemento** *Labinca, Arg.*
Glucosamine sulfate (p.1694·1).
*Osteoarthritis.*

**Var-Zeta** *Alfa Biotech, Ital.†.*
A varicella-zoster immunoglobulin (p.1643·1).
*Passive immunisation.*

**Vas**
*Note. A similar name is used for preparations of different composition (see below).*
*Geymonat, Ital.*
Suleparoid (p.1009·1).
*Thrombosis prophylaxis.*

**V-AS**
*Note. A similar name is used for preparations of different composition (see above).*
*Progress, Thai.*
Aspirin (p.15·1).
*Fever; pain.*

**Vasactife** *Ferring, Port.*
Ginkgo biloba (p.1692·3).
*Vascular disorders.*

**Vasactin** *Ebewe, Austria.*
Calcium dobesilate (p.1664·2).
*Capillary disorders; venous insufficiency.*

**Vasa-Gastreu N R63** *Reckeweg, Ger.*
Homoeopathic preparation.

**Vascace**
*Roche, Gr.; Roche, Irl.; Roche, Israel; Roche, UK.*
Cilazapril (p.883·3).
*Heart failure; hypertension.*

**Vascace Plus** *Roche, Israel.*
Cilazapril (p.883·3); hydrochlorothiazide (p.933·2).
*Hypertension.*

**Vascal** *Schwarz, Ger.*
Isradipine (p.942·2).
*Hypertension.*

**Vascalpha** *Alpharma, UK.*
Felodipine (p.914·3).
*Hypertension.*

**Vascard** *Parke-Med, S.Afr.*
Nifedipine (p.966·2).
*Angina pectoris; hypertension.*

**Vascase**
*Roche, Braz.; Roche, Neth.; Pharmacia, Port.*
Cilazapril (p.883·3).
*Heart failure; hypertension.*

**Vascase Plus**
*Roche, Braz.; Roche, Neth.†; Pharmacia, Port.*
Cilazapril (p.883·3); hydrochlorothiazide (p.933·2).
*Hypertension.*

**Vascer** *Uniao Quimica, Braz.*
Pentoxifylline (p.979·3).
*Hypertension.*

**Vasclin** *Libbs, Braz.*
Aspirin (p.15·1); isosorbide mononitrate (p.942·1).
*Angina pectoris; myocardial infarction; unstable angina.*

**Vascocitrol** *Alpharma, Fr.*
Citroflavonoids (p.1688·2); ascorbic acid (p.1460·2); light magnesium carbonate (p.1272·1).
*Venous insufficiency.*

**Vascoman** *Takeda, Ital.*
Manidipine hydrochloride (p.950·2).
*Hypertension.*

**Vascopan** *Strand, Malaysia.*
Hyoscine butylbromide (p.483·3).
*Smooth muscle spasm.*

**Vascor** *Ortho McNeil, USA†.*
Bepridil hydrochloride (p.868·3).
*Angina pectoris.*

**Vascoray**
*Mallinckrodt, Braz.†.*
Meglumine iotalamate (p.1065·3).
*Radiographic contrast medium.*

*Mallinckrodt, USA†.*
Meglumine iotalamate (p.1065·3); sodium iotalamate (p.1065·3).
*Radiographic contrast medium.*

**Vascoten**
*Medochemie, Hong Kong; Medochemie, Malaysia; Medochemie, Singapore; Medochemie, Thai.*
Atenolol (p.865·2).
*Angina pectoris; arrhythmias; hypertension; myocardial infarction.*

**Vasculat**
*Boehringer de Angeli, Braz.; Boehringer Ingelheim, Spain†.*
Bamethan sulfate (p.866·3).
*Cerebral and peripheral vascular disorders.*

**Vasculene** *Finmedical, Ital.*
Flunarizine hydrochloride (p.434·1).
*Migraine; vertigo.*

**Vasculin**
*Biolab, Malaysia; Biolab, Thai.*
Co-dergocrine mesilate (p.1674·1).
*Mental function disorders.*

**Vasculine** *Desbergers, Canad.†.*
Multivitamin and mineral preparation (p.1417·1).

**Vasculoflex** *Baliarda, Arg.*
Flunarizine (p.434·2).
*Migraine.*

**Vascunormyl** *Alcon, Fr.*
Cyclandelate (p.890·3).
*Intermittent claudication; vascular eye disorders.*

**Vasdalat** *Kalbe, Singapore.*
Nifedipine (p.966·2).
*Angina pectoris; hypertension.*

**Vasdilat** *MDM, Ital.*
Isosorbide mononitrate (p.942·1).
*Ischaemic heart disease.*

**Vaselastic** *Recalcine, Chile.*
Buflomedil hydrochloride (p.877·2).
*Cerebral and peripheral vascular disorders; vestibular disorders.*

**Vaselatum** *Stiefel, Spain.*
Paraffin (p.1479·1); benzalkonium chloride (p.1168·3); triclosan (p.1195·2).
*Eczema.*

**Vaselina** *Uniao Quimica, Braz.*
White soft paraffin (p.1479·3).

**Vaselina Boricada** *Orravan, Spain; Puerto Galiano, Spain.*
Boric acid (p.1662·1); white soft paraffin (p.1479·3).
*Skin disorders; urethral or rectal lubricant.*

**Vaselina Mentolada**
*Note. This name is used for preparations of different composition.*
*Brum, Spain†.*
White soft paraffin (p.1479·3); menthol (p.1711·3); peppermint oil (p.1283·2).
*Skin disorders; urethral or rectal lubricant.*

*Puerto Galiano, Spain.*
White soft paraffin (p.1479·3); menthol (p.1711·3).
*Skin disorders; urethral or rectal lubricant.*

**Vaseline**
*Unilever, Canad.; Lever, UK.*
White soft paraffin (p.1479·3).
*Barrier preparation; dry skin; minor skin disorders.*

**Vaseline Gomenolee** *Gomenol, Fr.*
Niaouli oil (p.1719·3); white soft paraffin.
*Nasal disoreders.*

**Vaseline Intensive Care** *Chesebrough-Pond's, USA.*
*SPF 25:* Octinoxate (p.1154·3); oxybenzone (p.1154·3); octisalate (p.1154·3).
*SPF 30:* Octinoxate (p.1154·3); oxybenzone (p.1154·3); octisalate (p.1154·3); titanium dioxide (p.1160·3).
*SPF4; SPF 8; SPF 15:* Octinoxate (p.1154·3); oxybenzone (p.1154·3).
*Sunscreen.*

**Vaseline Intensive Care Active Sport** *Chesebrough-Pond's, USA.*
*SPF 8; SPF 15:* Octinoxate (p.1154·3); oxybenzone (p.1154·3).
*Sunscreen.*

**Vaseline Intensive Care Baby** *Chesebrough-Pond's, USA.*
*SPF 15:* Titanium dioxide (p.1160·3); zinc oxide (p.1163·2).
*SPF 30+:* Octinoxate (p.1154·3); oxybenzone (p.1154·3); octisalate (p.1154·3); titanium dioxide (p.1160·3).
*Sunscreen.*

**Vaseline Intensive Care Blockout** *Chesebrough-Pond's, USA.*
*SPF 40:* Padimate (p.1155·1); octinoxate (p.1154·3); oxybenzone (p.1154·3); octisalate (p.1154·3); titanium dioxide (p.1160·3).
*Sunscreen.*

**Vaseline Intensive Care No Burn No Bite** *Chesebrough-Pond's, USA.*
*SPF 8; SPF 15:* Octinoxate (p.1154·3); oxybenzone (p.1154·3).
*Sunscreen.*

**Vaseline Intensive Care-Total Care** *Unilever, Canad.*
*SPF 15:* Octinoxate (p.1154·3); oxybenzone (p.1154·3).
*Sunscreen.*

**Vaseline Lip Therapy** *Unilever, Canad.*
*SPF 15:* Octinoxate (p.1154·3); oxybenzone (p.1154·3); white soft paraffin.
*Sunscreen.*

**Vaselitulle** *Solvay, Fr.*
White soft paraffin (p.1479·3).
*Burns; wounds.*

**Vaselpin** *Faran, Gr.*
Roxithromycin (p.254·2).
*Bacterial infections.*

**Vaseretic**
*Merck Frosst, Canad.; Biovail, USA.*
Enalapril maleate (p.909·2); hydrochlorothiazide (p.933·2).
*Hypertension.*

**Vasesana-Vasoregulans** *Hotz, Ger.†.*
Aesculus (p.1648·2); mistletoe (p.1715·3); crataegus (p.1677·1); hamamelis (p.1696·3); arnica (p.1656·3); silybum marianum (p.1043·3).
*Haemorrhoids; vascular disorders.*

**Vasian** *Asian Pharm, Thai.*
Co-dergocrine mesilate (p.1674·1).
*Mental function disorders.*

**Vasican**
*DHA, Hong Kong; DHA, Malaysia; DHA, Singapore.*
Bromhexine hydrochloride (p.1115·3).
*Respiratory-tract disorders associated with increased or viscous mucus.*

**Vasil** *Pharmasant, Thai.†.*
Metoclopramide hydrochloride (p.1274·3).
*Nausea and vomiting.*

**Vasilium** *Medinfar, Port.*
Flunarizine hydrochloride (p.434·1).
*Migraine; vertigo.*

**Vaslip**
*Note. This name is used for preparations of different composition.*
*Biolab Sanus, Braz.*
Simvastatin (p.997·1).
*Hyperlipidaemias.*

*Ferrer, Spain†.*
Cerivastatin sodium (p.881·3).
*Hypercholesterolaemia.*

**Vasobrain** *Errekappa, Ital.*
Phospholipids; vitamin E; ginkgo biloba (p.1692·3) (p.1417·1).
*Mental function disorders.*

**Vasobral**
*Chiesi, Fr.; Logeais, Hong Kong; Chiesi, Hong Kong; Geymonat, Ital.*
Dihydroergocryptine mesilate (p.1680·1); caffeine (p.782·1).
*Cerebral and peripheral vascular disorders; headache.*

**Vasobrix** *Guerbet, Braz.†.*
Monoethanolamine ioxitalamate (p.1066·3); meglumine ioxitalamate (p.1066·3).
*Radiographic contrast medium.*

**Vasocardol** *Aventis, Austral.*
Diltiazem hydrochloride (p.900·1).
*Angina pectoris; hypertension.*

**Vasocedine** *Qualiphar, Belg.*
Naphazoline nitrate (p.1124·3).
*Nasal congestion.*

**Vasocedine Pseudoephedrine** *Qualiphar, Belg.*
Pseudoephedrine hydrochloride (p.1129·2).
*Rhinitis.*

**Vasocidin**
*Novartis Ophthalmics, Canad.; Novartis, USA.*
Prednisolone acetate (p.1108·1) or prednisolone sodium phosphate (p.1108·1); sulfacetamide sodium (p.257·3).
Formerly contained prednisolone sodium phosphate, phenylephrine hydrochloride, and sulfacetamide sodium in *Canad.*
*Eye inflammation with bacterial infection.*

**Vasocine** *Novartis Ophthalmics, USA†.*
Prednisolone acetate (p.1108·1); sulfacetamide sodium (p.257·3).
*Infected eye disorders.*

**VasoClear** *Novartis Ophthalmics, USA.*
Naphazoline hydrochloride (p.1124·3); polyvinyl alcohol (p.1581·1).
*Minor eye irritation.*

**VasoClear A** *Novartis Ophthalmics, USA.*
Naphazoline hydrochloride (p.1124·3); zinc sulfate (p.1469·3).
*Eye irritation.*

**Vasocon**
*Novartis Ophthalmics, Canad.; Ciba Vision, USA.*
Naphazoline hydrochloride (p.1124·3).
*Eye irritation.*

**Vasocon Ant** *Ciba Vision, Spain†.*
Naphazoline nitrate (p.1124·3); neomycin sulfate (p.235·1); zinc sulfate (p.1469·3).
*Eye congestion; eye infections.*

**Vasocon-A**
*Novartis Ophthalmics, Canad.; Novartis Ophthalmics, USA.*
Naphazoline hydrochloride (p.1124·3); antazoline phosphate (p.424·2).
*Eye irritation.*

**Vasoconstr** *Novartis, Spain†.*
Naphazoline nitrate (p.1124·3); zinc sulfate (p.1469·3).
*Eye irritation.*

**Vasoconstrictor Pensa** *Pensa, Spain.*
Naphazoline hydrochloride (p.1124·3).
*Nasal congestion.*

**Vasocor**
*Note. This name is used for preparations of different composition.*
*Azevedos, Port.*
Quinapril hydrochloride (p.991·1).
*Heart failure; hypertension.*

*Medika, Switz.*
Enalapril maleate (p.909·2).
*Hypertension.*

**Vasodexa** *Llorens, Spain.*
Dexamethasone phosphate (p.1097·2); tetryzoline hydrochloride (p.1131·2).
*Inflammatory eye disorders.*

**Vasodil** *Byk Gulden, Mex.*
Ginkgo biloba (p.1692·3).
*Vascular disorders.*

**Vasodilan** *Apothecon, USA.*
Isoxsuprine hydrochloride (p.1702·2).
*Cerebrovascular disorders; peripheral vascular disorders.*

**Vaso-Dilatan** *Agepha, Austria.*
Tolazoline hydrochloride (p.1015·1).
*Vascular disorders.*

**Vasodin** *Teofarma, Ital.*
Nicardipine hydrochloride (p.965·1).
*Angina pectoris; heart failure; hypertension.*

**Vasodip** *Dexcel, Israel.*
Lercanidipine hydrochloride (p.946·1).
*Hypertension.*

**Vasodipina** *Neo Quimica, Braz.*
Nimodipine (p.972·3).

**Vasodual** *Janssen-Cilag, Arg.*
Calcium dobesilate (p.1664·2); cinnarizine (p.428·3).
*Vascular disorders.*

**Vaso-E-Bion** *Rodisma, Ger.*
Troxerutin (p.1688·3); *dl*-alpha tocoferil acetate (p.1465·1).
*Vascular disorders.*

**Vasofed**
*Antigen, Irl.; Garec, S.Afr.†.*
Nifedipine (p.966·2).
*Angina pectoris; hypertension.*

**Vasofen** *Tubilux, Ital.*
Chloramphenicol sodium hemisuccinate (p.185·1); phenylephrine (p.1126·3); mepyramine maleate (p.437·1).
*Eye disorders.*

**Vasoflex** *Bago, Chile.*
Nimodipine (p.972·3).
*Cerebral ischaemia.*

**Vasofluina** *Zambon, Braz.†.*
Raubasine hydrochloride (p.994·3); dihydroergocristine mesilate (p.1680·1); dihydroergotamine mesilate (p.465·3).
*Vascular disorders.*

**Vasoforte N** *Krugmann, Ger.*
Aesculus (p.1648·2).
*Venous insufficiency.*

**Vasofrinic** *Trianon, Canad.*
Chlorphenamine maleate (p.427·3); pseudoephedrine hydrochloride (p.1129·2).
*Respiratory congestion.*

**Vasofrinic Plus** *Trianon, Canad.*
Dextromethorphan hydrobromide (p.1117·3); guaifenesin (p.1122·1); chlorphenamine maleate (p.427·3); pseudoephedrine hydrochloride (p.1129·2).
*Coughs; respiratory congestion.*

**Vasofyl** *Fustery, Mex.*
Pentoxifylline (p.979·3).
*Cerebral, ocular, and peripheral vascular disorders.*

**Vasogen**
*Pharmax, Irl.; Forest Laboratories, UK.*
Dimeticone (p.1482·1); zinc oxide (p.1163·2); calamine (p.1144·1).
*Barrier cream; nappy rash.*

**Vasojet** *Uniao Quimica, Braz.*
Lisinopril (p.946·3).
*Hypertension.*

**Vasolan** *Dexxon, Israel.*
Isoxsuprine hydrochloride (p.1702·2).
*Intermittent claudication; thromboangitis obliterans.*

**Vasolastine** *Enzypharm, Neth.†.*
Triacylglycerol lipase; acyl-CoA-dehydrogenase; amine oxidase.
*Vascular disorders.*

**Vasolat** *Prater, Chile.*
Enalapril maleate (p.909·2).
*Hypertension.*

**Vasolipid**
*Braun, Denm.†.*
Soya oil (p.1447·2).
Contains egg phospholipid.
*Lipid infusion for parenteral nutrition.*

*Braun, Fin.; Braun, Norw.; Braun, Swed.*
Soya oil (p.1447·2); medium-chain triglycerides (p.1440·3).
Contains egg lecithin.
*Lipid infusion for parenteral nutrition.*

**Vasomax** *Schering-Plough, Braz.†.*
Phentolamine hydrochloride (p.982·2).
*Erectile dysfunction.*

**Vasomed** *Chemopharma, Chile.*
Simvastatin (p.997·1).
*Hypercholesterolaemia.*

**Vasomil** *Aspen, S.Afr.*
Verapamil hydrochloride (p.1019·1).
*Angina pectoris; arrhythmias.*

**Vasomine** *Teuto, Braz.*
Dopamine hydrochloride (p.907·1).

**Vasomotal** *Solvay, Ger.*
Betahistine hydrochloride (p.1660·1).
*Ménière's disease.*

**Vasonase** *Yamanouchi, Spain.*
Nicardipine hydrochloride (p.965·1).
*Angina pectoris; cerebrovascular disorders; hypertension.*

**Vasonett** *INTES, Ital.*
Vincamine (p.1764·2).
*Cerebrovascular insufficiency.*

**Vasonit** *Lannacher, Austria.*
Pentoxifylline (p.979·3).
*Peripheral vascular disorders.*

**Vasonorm** *NCSN, Ital.†.*
Nicardipine hydrochloride (p.965·1).
*Angina pectoris; heart failure; hypertension.*

**Vasopos N** *Ursapharm, Ger.*
Tetryzoline hydrochloride (p.1131·2).
*Eye disorders.*

**Vasopressin** *Sandoz, Ger.†.*
Lypressin (p.1342·3).
*Diabetes insipidus.*

**Vasopril**
*Note. This name is used for preparations of different composition.*
*Biolab Sanus, Braz.*
Enalapril maleate (p.909·2).
*Hypertension.*
*Bristol-Myers Squibb, Israel.*
Fosinopril sodium (p.919·1).
*Heart failure; hypertension.*

**Vasopril Plus**
*Note. This name is used for preparations of different composition.*
*Biolab Sanus, Braz.*
Enalapril maleate (p.909·2); hydrochlorothiazide (p.933·2).
*Hypertension.*
*Bristol-Myers Squibb, Israel.*
Fosinopril sodium (p.919·1); hydrochlorothiazide (p.933·2).
*Hypertension.*

**Vasoprost** *Esteve, Port.*
Alprostadil alfadex (p.1512·3).
*Peripheral vascular disease.*

**Vasopt** *Fidia, Ital.*
Ginkgo biloba (p.1692·3); vitamin E acetate (p.1465·1); minerals (p.1417·1).
*Vascular disorders of the eye.*

**Vasopten** *Torrent, Thai.†.*
Verapamil hydrochloride (p.1019·1).
*Angina pectoris; arrhythmias; myocardial infarction.*

**Vasorbate** *Arcana, Austria.*
Isosorbide dinitrate (p.941·1).
*Angina pectoris; heart failure; myocardial infarction.*

**Vasorema** *Inverni della Beffa, Ital.*
Suleparoid (p.1009·1).
*Thrombosis prophylaxis.*

**Vasoretic** *Merck Sharp & Dohme, Ital.*
Enalapril maleate (p.909·2); hydrochlorothiazide (p.933·2).
*Hypertension.*

**Vasorinil** *Farmila, Ital.*
Tetryzoline hydrochloride (p.1131·2).
*Nasal congestion.*

**Vasosan** *Felgentrager, Ger.*
Colestyramine (p.889·3).
*Chologenic diarrhoea; hyperlipidaemias; pruritus.*

**Vasosterone** *Angelini, Ital.*
Hydrocortisone (p.1103·3); tetryzoline hydrochloride (p.1131·2).
*Nasal congestion.*

**Vasosterone Antibiotico** *Angelini, Ital.*
Hydrocortisone acetate (p.1103·3); tetryzoline hydrochloride (p.1131·2); neomycin sulfate (p.235·1); gramicidin (p.220·2).
*Rhinitis.*

**Vasosterone Collirio** *Angelini, Ital.*
Hydrocortisone acetate (p.1103·3); tetryzoline hydrochloride (p.1131·2); neomycin sulfate (p.235·1).
*Eye disorders.*

**Vasosterone Oto** *Angelini, Ital.*
Flumetasone pivalate (p.1101·1); gentamicin sulfate (p.217·1).
*Otitis externa.*

**Vasosulf**
*Ciba Vision, Canad.†; Ciba Vision, USA.*
Sulfacetamide sodium (p.257·3); phenylephrine hydrochloride (p.1126·3).
*Bacterial eye infections.*

**Vasosuprina Ilfi** *Lusofarmaco, Ital.*
Isoxsuprine hydrochloride (p.1702·2).
*Premature labour; threatened miscarriage.*

**Vasotec**
*Merck Frosst, Canad.; Biovail, USA.*
Enalapril maleate (p.909·2) or enalaprilat (p.909·3).
*Heart failure; hypertension.*

**Vasotenal**
*Roemmers, Arg.; Pharma Investi, Chile.*
Simvastatin (p.997·1).
*Atherosclerosis; hypercholesterolaemia.*

**Vasoton** *NCSN, Ital.†.*
Dihydroergocristine mesilate (p.1680·1).
*Cerebral and peripheral vascular disorders; dopamine deficiency; headache; hypertension; migraine.*

**Vasotonal** *Amnol, Ital.*
Aescin; caffeine; ruscus; centella; arnica; hedera; capsicum; ginkgo biloba; menthol.
*Skin disorders.*

**Vasotonin** *Merz, Ger.*
*Capsules:* Aesculus (p.1648·2).
*Haemorrhoids; vascular disorders.*
*Topical gel:* Arnica (p.1656·3).
*Musculoskeletal, joint, and soft-tissue disorders; superficial thrombophlebitis.*

**Vasotonin forte** *Merz, Ger.†.*
Aesculus (p.1648·2); mofebutazone (p.60·1).
*Superficial thrombophlebitis.*

**Vasotop** *Cipla, India.*
Nimodipine (p.972·3).
*Prevention of neurological deficits following subarachnoid haemorrhage.*

**Vasovitol** *Lannacher, Austria.*
Vitamin A palmitate (p.1453·1); alpha tocoferil acetate (p.1465·1).
*Vitamin A and E deficiency.*

**Vasoxine**
*Wellcome, Irl.; GlaxoSmithKline, UK†.*
Methoxamine hydrochloride (p.953·1).
*Hypotension.*

**Vasoxyl**
*Glaxo Wellcome, Canad.†; Glaxo Wellcome, USA†.*
Methoxamine hydrochloride (p.953·1).
*Control of blood pressure during surgery; postoperative collapse; supraventricular tachycardia.*

**Vasperdil** *Lacer, Spain†.*
Etamivan (p.1588·1); etofylline (p.785·1); hexobendine hydrochloride (p.931·2).
*Cerebrovascular disorders; circulatory disorders.*

**Vaspit**
*Asche, Ger.; Schering, Ital.; Schering, Spain.*
Fluocortin butyl (p.1102·1).
*Burns; insect stings; skin disorders.*

**Vastarel**
*Servier, Arg.; Servier, Braz.; Servier, Denm.; Biopharma, Fr.; Servier, Gr.; Servier, Hong Kong; Servier, Irl.; Stroder, Ital.; Servier, Malaysia; Servier, Port.; Servier, Singapore; Servier, Thai.*
Trimetazidine hydrochloride (p.1018·1).
*Angina pectoris; vascular eye disorders; vestibular disorders.*

**Vasten** *Aventis, Fr.*
Pravastatin sodium (p.984·3).
*Hypercholesterolaemia.*

**Vastensium** *Salvat, Spain.*
Nitrendipine (p.973·3).
*Hypertension.*

**Vastin**
*AstraZeneca, Austral.; AstraZeneca, NZ†.*
Fluvastatin sodium (p.918·2).
*Atherosclerosis; hypercholesterolaemia.*

**Vastina** *Richmond, Arg.*
Atorvastatin (p.866·2).
*Hypercholesterolaemia.*

**Vastinol** *TO-Chemicals, Thai.*
Trimetazidine hydrochloride (p.1018·1).
*Ischaemic heart disease.*

**Vastribil** *Farmasan, Ger.*
Troxerutin (p.1688·3).
*Vascular disorders.*

**Vastrictol** *Allergan-Frumtost, Braz.†.*
Naphazoline nitrate (p.1124·3); zinc sulfate (p.1469·3).
*Ocular congestion.*

**Vastripine** *Relyo, Gr.*
Nimodipine (p.972·3).
*Neurological deficit following subarachnoid haemorrhage.*

**Vastus**
*Note. This name is used for preparations of different composition.*
*Labinca, Arg.*
Albendazole (p.101·2).
*Worm infections.*
*Tecnofarma, Chile.*
Finasteride (p.1554·2).
*Benign prostatic hyperplasia.*

**Vasurix Polividona** *Guerbet, Braz.†.*
Meglumine ioxitalamate (p.1066·3); povidone.
*Radiographic contrast medium.*

**Vasylox** *Douglas, Austral.*
Oxymetazoline hydrochloride (p.1126·1); cineole (p.1672·1); menthol (p.1711·3).
*Nasal congestion.*

**Vatran** *Valeas, Ital.*
Diazepam (p.690·1).
*Anxiety; eclampsia; epilepsy; premedication; psychosomatic disorders; skeletal muscle spasm.*

**Vatrasin** *Synthelabo, Spain†.*
Nicardipine hydrochloride (p.965·1).
*Angina pectoris; cerebrovascular disorders; hypertension.*

**Vatrem** *Kener, Mex.†.*
Piroxicam (p.84·2).

**Vatrix-S** *Bioclon, Mex.†.*
Metronidazole (p.607·2).

**Vavifor** *Medifarma, Mex.*
Vitamin B substances; minerals (p.1417·1).
*Dietary supplement.*

**Vaxem Hib**
*Chiron Vaccines, Ital.; Fustery, Mex.; Chiron, Thai.*
A haemophilus influenzae conjugate vaccine (diphtheria toxoid conjugate) (p.1616·1).
*Active immunisation.*

**Vaxicoq** *Pasteur Merieux, Fr.†.*
An adsorbed pertussis vaccine (p.1631·2).
*Active immunisation.*

**Vaxicum NA** *Worwag, Ger.*
Camphor oil; rosemary oil (p.1740·2).
*Musculoskeletal, joint, peri-articular, and soft-tissue disorders; neuralgia.*

**Vaxidina** *VAAS, Ital.†.*
Chlorhexidine gluconate (p.1173·2).
*Skin disinfection; wound disinfection.*

**Vaxigrip**
*Aventis Pasteur, Arg.; Aventis Pasteur, Austral.; Aventis Pasteur, Austria; Aventis Pasteur, Belg.; Aventis Pasteur, Braz.; Aventis Pasteur, Canad.; Aventis Pasteur, Chile; Aventis Pasteur, Denm.; Aventis Pasteur, Fin.; Aventis Pasteur, Fr.; Vianex (Βιανεξ), Gr.; Aventis Pasteur, Hong Kong; Pasteur Merieux, Israel; Aventis Pasteur, Ital.; Aventis Pasteur, Malaysia; Pasteur Merieux, Neth.; Aventis Pasteur, Norw.; Aventis, NZ; Aventis Pasteur, Port.; Aventis, S.Afr.; Aventis Pasteur, Singapore; Aventis Pasteur, Swed.; Aventis Pasteur, Thai.*
An inactivated influenza vaccine (split virion) (p.1620·2).
*Active immunisation.*

**Vaxim HIB** *Aventis, India.*
A haemophilus influenzae conjugate vaccine (p.1616·1).
*Active immunisation.*

**Vaxipar** *Chiron Vaccines, Ital.*
A mumps vaccine (Urabe strain) (p.1626·3).
*Active immunisation.*

**Vaxitiol** *Bouty, Ital.*
*Lactobacillus sporogenes* (p.1704·2); *Lactobacillus acidophilus* (p.1704·2); *Streptococcus thermophilus* (p.1704·2); *Bifidobacterium bifidum* (p.1704·2); vitamins; minerals (p.1417·1).
*Maintenance of normal gastrointestinal flora.*

**Vazigam** *NBI, S.Afr.*
A varicella-zoster immunoglobulin (p.1643·1).
*Passive immunisation.*

**Vazosin** *Biotenk, Arg.*
Doxazosin (p.909·1).

**Vcanalare** *Vebas, Ital.*
Orthophenylphenol (p.1187·2).
*Root canal disinfection.*

**VCF**
*Silesia, Chile; Apothecus, Hong Kong†; Apothecus, USA.*
Nonoxinol 9 (p.1413·3).
*Contraceptive.*

**V-Cil-K** *Lilly, S.Afr.†.*
Phenoxymethylpenicillin potassium (p.242·1).
*Bacterial infections.*

**V-Cillin K** *Lilly, Canad.†.*
Phenoxymethylpenicillin potassium (p.242·1).
*Bacterial infections.*

**V-Crima** *Vitamed, Israel.*
Povidone (p.1581·2); hypromellose (p.1579·3).
*Dry eyes.*

**V-Dec-M** *Seatrace, USA.*
Pseudoephedrine hydrochloride (p.1129·2); guaifenesin (p.1122·1).
*Coughs.*

**Ve** *Tecnifar, Port.*
Vitamin E (p.1464·3).
*Vitamin E supplement.*

**Veafer** *Veafarm, Braz.†.*
Ferric ammonium citrate (p.1427·2); vitamin B substances (p.1417·1).
*Iron deficiency; iron-deficiency anaemias.*

**Veclam** *Malesci, Ital.*
Clarithromycin (p.192·2).
*Bacterial infections.*

**Vecredil** *Jagson, India.*
Ethacridine lactate (p.1165·3).
*Termination of pregnancy.*

**Vectarion**
*Servier, Belg.; Servier, Braz.; Servier, Denm.; Eutherapie, Fr.; Servier, Ger.†; Servier, Irl.; Servier, Port.†; Servier, Spain.*
Almitrine dimesilate (p.1584·2).
*Respiratory depression.*

**Vectavir**
*Novartis Consumer, Austral.; Novartis, Austria; Novartis, Belg.; Novartis, Denm.; Novartis, Fin.; Novartis, Ger.; Novartis, Gr.; Novartis, Hong Kong; Novartis, Israel; Novartis, Ital.; Novartis, Norw.; Novartis, NZ; Novartis, Spain; Novartis, Swed.; Novartis Consumer, UK.*
Penciclovir (p.651·2).
*Herpes labialis.*

**Vectidan** *Bago, Chile.*
Nicotinic acid (p.1441·1).
*Peripheral vascular disorders; skin ulcers.*

**Vectrin** *Warner Chilcott, USA†.*
Minocycline hydrochloride (p.231·3).
*Bacterial infections.*

**Vectrine** *Pharma 2000, Fr.*
Erdosteine (p.1121·1).
*Respiratory-tract congestion.*

**Vecural** *Richmond, Arg.*
Vecuronium bromide (p.1409·3).
*Competitive neuromuscular blocker.*

**Vecuron** *Scott-Cassara, Arg.*
Vecuronium bromide (p.1409·3).
*Competitive neuromuscular blocker.*

**Vedrin** *Polifarma, Ital.*
Xantinol nicotinate (p.1029·1).
*Peripheral vascular disorders.*

**Veemycin** *Osoth, Thai.*
Doxycycline hyclate (p.206·2).
*Bacterial infections.*

**Veenac** *Progress, Thai.*
Diclofenac sodium (p.32·1).
*Gout; inflammation; musculoskeletal and joint disorders; pain.*

**Veetids** *Apothecon, USA.*
Phenoxymethylpenicillin potassium (p.242·1).
*Bacterial infections.*

**Vefed** *PP Lab, Thai.*
Triprolidine hydrochloride (p.442·3); pseudoephedrine hydrochloride (p.1129·2).
*Allergic rhinitis; cold symptoms; nasal congestion.*

**Vefluxan** *Sanofi Synthelabo, Arg.*
Troxerutin (p.1688·3); bamethan (p.866·3).
*Haemorrhoids; varices.*

**Vefren** *Baliarda, Arg.*
*Cream:* Piroxicam (p.84·2).
*Inflammation; pain.*
*Tablets:* Piroxicam (p.84·2); paracetamol (p.76·2).
*Fever; inflammation; pain.*

**Vegadeine** *Warner-Lambert, Fr.†.*
Aspirin (p.15·1); paracetamol (p.76·2); codeine phosphate (p.27·1).
*Fever; pain.*

**Vegal** *Jofrain, Mex.†.*
Dipyrone (p.35·3).

**Veganin**
*Note. This name is used for preparations of different composition.*
*Pfizer Consumer, Austral.*
Aspirin (p.15·1); codeine phosphate (p.27·1).
*Fever; pain.*
*Warner-Lambert, Hong Kong†; Pfizer Consumer, Irl.; Warner-Lambert, Spain†.*
Aspirin (p.15·1); paracetamol (p.76·2); codeine phosphate (p.27·1).
*Fever; pain.*
*Pfizer Consumer, UK.*
Paracetamol (p.76·2); codeine phosphate (p.27·1); caffeine (p.782·1).
Formerly contained aspirin, paracetamol, and codeine phosphate.
*Fever; pain.*

**Veganin 3** *Aspen, S.Afr.*
Aspirin (p.15·1); paracetamol (p.76·2); codeine phosphate (p.27·1).
*Fever; pain.*

**Veganine**
*Note. This name is used for preparations of different composition.*
*Pfizer Sante, Fr.*
Paracetamol (p.76·2); caffeine (p.782·1).
*Fever; pain.*
*Warner-Lambert Consumer, Port.†.*
Aspirin (p.15·1); paracetamol (p.76·2); codeine phosphate (p.27·1).
*Fever; pain.*

**Vege Swiss One** *Swiss Herbal, Canad.*
Multivitamin and mineral preparation (p.1417·1).

**Vegebaby** *Clintec, Fr.†.*
Infant feed (p.1417·1).
*Milk intolerance.*

**Vegebom** *Jessel, Fr.*
Cineole (p.1672·1); cajuput oil (p.1664·1); sassafras oil (p.1742·1); cedar oil; camphor (p.1665·3); menthol (p.1711·3); nutmeg oil (p.1722·3); bay-laurel oil.
*Musculoskeletal, joint, and peri-articular disorders.*

**Vegebyl** *Roche, Ital.†.*
Boldo (p.1661·2); cynara (p.1678·3); rhubarb (p.1287·3); cascara (p.1255·1); chamomile (p.1669·3).
*Constipation; digestive disorders.*

**Vegelact** *Diepal, Fr.†.*
Infant feed (p.1417·1).
*Milk intolerance.*

**Vegelax** *Biologiques de l'Ile-de-France, Fr.*
Senna (p.1288·2); boldo (p.1661·2); cynara (p.1678·3).
*Constipation.*

**Vegelose** *Clintec, Fr.†.*
Gluten-free, milk-free nutritional supplement (p.1417·1).

**Vegesan** *Mack, Switz.†.*
Nordazepam (p.710·3).
*Anxiety disorders.*

**Vegestabil** *Labinca, Arg.*
Sulpiride (p.722·2); dipotassium clorazepate (p.685·1).

**Vegestabil Digest** *Labinca, Arg.*
Domperidone (p.1263·2); bromazepam (p.671·3); simeticone (p.1289·2).

**Vegetable Cough Remover** *Potter's, UK.*
Capsicum (p.1667·1); cimicifuga (p.1671·3); ipecacuanha (p.1122·3); lobelia (p.1589·1); pleurisy root (p.1733·1); skullcap (p.1746·3); skunk cabbage (p.1746·3); valerian (p.1762·2); elecampane (p.1119·3); marrubium (p.1124·1); hyssop; anise oil (p.1655·2); liquorice (p.1270·2).
*Coughs.*

**Vegetal Tonic** *Homeocan, Canad.*
Homoeopathic preparation.

**Vegetalin** *Genove, Spain†.*
Bearberry (p.1659·2); senna (p.1288·2); coriander (p.1676·1); hyssop; sage (p.1741·2).
*Constipation.*

**Vegetallumina** *Recordati, Ital.*
Camphor (p.1665·3); aluminium subacetate (p.1652·3); methyl salicylate (p.59·3); thyme oil (p.1755·3).
*Soft-tissue and peri-articular disorders.*

**Vegetarian Protein Supplement** *GNLD, Austral.†.*
Nutritional supplement (p.1417·1).

**Vegetex** *Lane, UK.*
Celery (p.1669·1); menyanthes (p.1712·1); cimicifuga (p.1671·3).
*Muscular pain.*

**Vegetoserum** *Alpharma, Fr.*
*Adult syrup:* Ethylmorphine hydrochloride (p.37·3); grindelia (p.1696·1).
Formerly contained ethylmorphine hydrochloride, aconite, belladonna, grindelia, and cherry-laurel.

*Paediatric syrup:* Ethylmorphine hydrochloride (p.37·3); orange flowers (p.1723·3).
*Coughs.*

**Vegicap Vegetarian** *Solgar, UK†.*
Multivitamin and mineral preparation (p.1417·1).

**Vegital** *Steierl, Ger.*
Homoeopathic preparation.

**Vehem** *Sandoz, Fr.†.*
Teniposide (p.587·2).
*Malignant neoplasms.*

**Veil** *Blake, UK.*
A covering cream.
*Concealment of birth marks, scars, and disfiguring skin disease.*

**Veinamitol**
*Negma, Belg.; Negma, Fr.; SEDR, Israel.*
Troxerutin (p.1688·3).
*Capillary impairment; haemorrhoids; venous insufficiency.*

**Veineva** *CCD, Fr.*
Diosmin (p.1688·2).
*Capillary disorders; haemorrhoids; venous insufficiency.*

**Veinobiase**
*Fournier, Fr.; Quimifar, Spain†.*
Ascorbic acid (p.1460·2); ruscus aculeatus; black currant (p.1661·1).
*Haemorrhoids; venous insufficiency.*

**Veinoconfort** *Yves Ponroy, Fr.†.*
Vitamin C substances (p.1417·1).
*Circulatory disorders.*

**Veinoglobuline** *Aventis Pasteur, Braz.†.*
A normal immunoglobulin (p.1627·2).
*Hypogammaglobulinaemia; idiopathic thrombocytopenic purpura; passive immunisation.*

**Veino-Gouttes-N** *Phytomed, Switz.*
Aesculus (p.1648·2); melilot; ruscus aculeatus.
*Venous insufficiency.*

**Veinophytum** *Arkopharma, Fr.*
Aesculus (p.1648·2); red vine.
*Capillary disorders; haemorrhoids; venous insufficiency.*

**Veinopress A3 and A4** *Innothera, Fr.*
Zinc oxide (p.1163·2).
*Care after variceal surgery; lymphoedema; post-sclerotherapy care; ulcers; venous insufficiency.*

**Veinosane** *Dolisos, Fr.†.*
Melilotus officinalis; red vine leaf.
*Haemorrhoids; venous insufficiency.*

**Veinostase** *Richelet, Fr.*
Aesculus (p.1648·2); hamamelis (p.1696·3); cupressus sempervirens; ascorbic acid (p.1460·2).
*Haemorrhoids; vascular disorders.*

**Veinotonyl** *Lipha Sante, Fr.*
Aesculus (p.1648·2); metesculetol sodium (p.1714·1).
*Peripheral vascular disorders.*

**Vekfazolin** *Faran, Gr.*
Cefuroxime sodium (p.184·1).
*Bacterial infections.*

**Velamox**
*Sigma, Braz.*
Amoxicillin (p.155·3).
*Bacterial infections.*

*GlaxoSmithKline, Ital.*
Amoxicillin sodium (p.155·3) or amoxicillin trihydrate (p.155·3).
*Bacterial infections.*

**Velaned** *Fada, Arg.*
Piroxicam (p.84·2).
*Inflammation.*

**Velasulin** *Novo Nordisk, Ger.†.*
Neutral insulin injection (crystalline) (porcine, highly-purified) (p.333·3).
*Diabetes mellitus.*

**Velasulin Human** *Novo Nordisk, Ger.†.*
Insulin injection (human) (p.333·3).
*Diabetes mellitus.*

**Velasulin MC** *Novo Nordisk, Ger.†.*
Insulin injection (porcine, monocomponent) (p.333·3).
*Diabetes mellitus.*

**Velaten** *Hoechst Marion Roussel, Ital.†.*
Sulfamethoxypyridazine (p.263·1); trimethoprim (p.272·2).
*Bacterial infections; Pneumocystis carinii pneumonia.*

**Velbacil** *Farmasierra, Spain†.*
Bacampicillin hydrochloride (p.161·2).
*Bacterial infections.*

**Velban**
*Lilly, Braz.; Lilly, USA.*
Vinblastine sulfate (p.591·2).
*Malignant neoplasms.*

**Velbe**
*Lilly, Arg.; Lilly, Austral.; Lilly, Austria; Lilly, Belg.; Lilly, Canad.†; Lilly, Chile; Lilly, Denm.; Lilly, Fin.; Lilly, Fr.; Lilly, Ger.; Pharmaserve Lilly (Φαρμασερβ Λιλλυ), Gr.; Lilly, Hong Kong; Lilly, Israel†; Lilly, Ital.; Lilly, Mex.; Centrafarm, Neth.; Lilly, Norw.; Lilly, Port.; Lilly, Swed.; Lilly, Switz.; Clonmel, UK.*
Vinblastine sulfate (p.591·2).
*Malignant neoplasms.*

**Velcade** *Ortho Biotech, UK; Millenium, USA.*
Bortezomib (p.532·1).
*Multiple myeloma.*

**Veldrol** *Collins, Mex.*
Tramadol (p.95·2).
*Pain.*

**Velexina** *Klonal, Arg.*
Cefalexin (p.168·1).
*Bacterial infections.*

**Veliten** *Zambon, Fr.*
Vitamins (p.1417·1); rutoside (p.1688·2).
*Vascular disorders.*

**Vellutan** *Abiogen, Ital.*
Tacalcitol (p.1158·3).
*Psoriasis.*

**Velmonit** *Esteve, Spain.*
Ciprofloxacin hydrochloride (p.188·2) or ciprofloxacin lactate (p.188·3).
*Bacterial infections.*

**Velocef** *Squibb, Spain.*
Cefradine (p.179·3).
*Bacterial infections.*

**Velodan** *Vita, Spain.*
Loratadine (p.436·1).
*Hypersensitivity reactions.*

**Velonarcon** *Asta Medica, Ger.†.*
Ketamine hydrochloride (p.1302·1).
*General anaesthesia; pain; status asthmaticus.*

**velopural** *Optimed, Ger.*
Hydrocortisone acetate (p.1103·3).
*Skin disorders.*

**Velorin**
*Remedica, Hong Kong; Remedica, Singapore; Remedica, Thai.*
Atenolol (p.865·2).
*Angina pectoris; arrhythmias; hypertension; myocardial infarction.*

**Velosalic** *División White's (Ver SCHERING PLOUGH).*
Mometasone furoate (p.1107·2); salicylic acid (p.1157·1).
*Hyperkeratotic skin disorders; psoriasis.*

**Velosef**
*Bristol-Myers Squibb, Belg.; Bristol-Myers Squibb, Chile; Bristol-Myers Squibb, Hong Kong; Bristol-Myers Squibb, Irl.; Bristol-Myers Squibb, Israel†; Bristol-Myers Squibb, Neth.; Bristol-Myers Squibb, NZ; Bristol-Myers Squibb, Port.; Bristol-Myers Squibb, UK; Apothecon, USA.*
Cefradine (p.179·3).
*Bacterial infections.*

**Velosulin**
*Novo Nordisk, Denm.†; Novo Nordisk, Fin.; Novo Nordisk, Jpn; Novo Nordisk, Neth.; Novo Nordisk, Norw.; Novo Nordisk, Swed.†; Novo Nordisk, UK.*
Neutral insulin injection (human, highly purified) (p.333·3).
Formerly known as Human Velosulin in the *UK.*
*Diabetes mellitus.*

**Velosulin HM**
*Novo Nordisk, Austria†; Novo Nordisk, Switz.*
Insulin injection (human, monocomponent) (p.333·3).
*Diabetes mellitus.*

**Velosulin Human BR** *Novo Nordisk, USA.*
Insulin injection (human, emp) (p.333·3).
*Diabetes mellitus.*

**Velosulin MC** *Novo Nordisk, Switz.†.*
Insulin injection (porcine, monocomponent) (p.333·3).
*Diabetes mellitus.*

**Velosuline Humanum** *Novo Nordisk, Belg.*
Insulin injection (human, emp) (p.333·3).
*Diabetes mellitus.*

**Veloudiet** *DHN, Fr.*
Preparation for enteral nutrition (p.1417·1).

**Velpro** *Alpharma, Mex.*
Benzonatate (p.1115·3).
*Coughs.*

**Velsay** *Sons, Mex.*
Naproxen (p.65·1).
*Musculoskeletal and joint disorders.*

**Veltex** *Mer-National, S.Afr.*
Diclofenac sodium (p.32·1).
*Gout; inflammation; musculoskeletal and joint disorders; pain.*

**Velutrix** *Eversil, Braz.†.*
Tetracycline phosphate complex (p.266·2); muramidase hydrochloride (p.1717·2).
*Bacterial infections.*

**Velvachol** *Healthpoint, USA.*
Vehicle for topical preparations.

**Velvelan** *Merck Sharp & Dohme, Canad.†; Frosst, Canad.†.*
Urea (p.1162·2).
*Dry skin disorders.*

**Vemizol** *Upha, Malaysia.*
Albendazole (p.101·2).
*Worm infections.*

**Vemol** *PP Lab, Thai.*
Paracetamol (p.76·2).
*Fever; pain.*

**Venacol** *Llorens, Spain.*
Aescin (p.1648·2); esculoside (p.1648·2); heparin sodium (p.928·1); ruscogenin (p.1741·1).
*Oedema; peripheral vascular disorders.*

**Venactive**
*Note. This name is used for preparations of different composition.*
*Euroderm, Ital.*
Centella (p.1144·3); aesculus (p.1648·2); hamamelis (p.1696·3).
*Tired legs.*

*Farmila, Ital.*
Bioflavonoids (p.1688·2); omega-3 triglycerides (p.976·1); centella (p.1144·3).
*Vascular disorders.*

**Venacton** *Klein, Ger.*
Aesculus (p.1648·2); scoparium (p.1742·2); hypericum (p.299·1); silybum marianum (p.1043·3); hamamelis (p.1696·3).
*Venous insufficiency.*

**Venactone** *Benedetti, Ital.*
Potassium canrenoate (p.984·2).
*Hyperaldosteronism; hypertension.*

**Venalisin** *AGIPS, Ital.†.*
Tribenoside (p.1757·3).
*Haemorrhoids; thrombophlebitis; varicose veins.*

**Venalitan** *3M, Ger.*
Heparin sodium (p.928·1).
*Soft-tissue injury; superficial vascular disorders.*

**Venalot**
*Note. This name is used for preparations of different composition.*
*Altana, Braz.; Schaper & Brummer, Ger.; Byk Gulden, Mex.*
Coumarin (p.1676·2); troxerutin (p.1688·3).
*Haemorrhoids; soft-tissue injury; superficial vascular disorders; venous and lymphatic insufficiency.*

*Asta Medica, Switz.†.*
*Liniment:* Melilotus; heparin (p.927·3).
*Peripheral vascular disorders.*

*Sustained-release tablets:* Coumarin (p.1676·2).
Formerly contained coumarin and troxerutin.
*Lymphoedema.*

**Venalot H** *Altana, Braz.*
Coumarin (p.1676·2); heparin (p.927·3).
*Soft-tissue injury.*

**Venalot mono** *Schaper & Brummer, Ger.*
Coumarin (p.1676·2).
*Soft-tissue injury.*

**Venalot N** *Schaper & Brummer, Ger.*
Coumarin (p.1676·2); rutoside sodium sulfate (p.1688·3).
*Peripheral vascular disorders.*

**Venalot novo** *Schaper & Brummer, Ger.*
Aesculus (p.1648·2).
*Venous insufficiency.*

**Venartel** *Andromaco, Chile.*
Citrus bioflavonoids (p.1688·2); diosmin (p.1688·2).
*Haemorrhoids; venous insufficiency.*

**Venastat**
*Boehringer Ingelheim, Arg.; Boehringer Ingelheim, Chile; Boehringer Ingelheim Promeco, Mex.; Pharmaton, Switz.†.*
Aesculus (p.1648·2).
*Venous insufficiency.*

**Venbig** *Kedrion, Ital.*
A hepatitis B immunoglobulin (p.1617·2).
*Passive immunisation.*

**Vencipon N** *Artesan, Ger.*
Ephedrine hydrochloride (p.1120·1); phenolphthalein (p.1284·1).
*Obesity.*

**Vendal** *Lannacher, Austria.*
Morphine hydrochloride (p.60·1).
*Pain.*

**Venderol** *Beacons, Singapore.*
Salbutamol (p.791·3).
*Obstructive airways disease.*

**Ven-Detrex** *Therabel, Belg.*
Diosmin (p.1688·2).
*Peripheral vascular disorders.*

**Vendrex** *IQB, Braz.*
Diclofenac sodium (p.32·1).

**Venelbin** *Hoechst, Ger.†.*
Dihydroergotamine mesilate (p.465·3); troxerutin (p.1688·3).
*Vascular disorders.*

**Venelbin N** *Hoechst, Ger.†.*
Heparin sodium (p.928·1).
*Superficial vascular disorders.*

**Venelbin ruscus** *Biocur, Ger.*
Ruscus aculeatus.
*Chronic venous insufficiency; haemorrhoids.*

**Venen-Dragees** *CT, Ger.*
Aesculus (p.1648·2).
*Venous insufficiency.*

**Venen-Fluid** *CT, Ger.*
Aesculus (p.1648·2).
*Phlebitis; soft-tissue injury; varices.*

**Venengel** *Ratiopharm, Ger.*
Heparin sodium (p.928·1); arnica (p.1656·3); aesculus (p.1648·2).
*Soft-tissue injury; vascular disorders.*

**Venen-Salbe** *Eu Rho, Ger.†.*
Aesculus (p.1648·2); arnica (p.1656·3).
*Haemorrhoids; soft-tissue injury; venous insufficiency.*

**Venen-Salbe N** *CT, Ger.*
Aesculus (p.1648·2); esculoside (p.1648·2).
*Bruising; oedema; varices.*

**Venen-Tabletten** *Stada, Ger.*
Aesculus (p.1648·2).
*Venous insufficiency.*

**Venentabs** *Ratiopharm, Ger.*
Aesculus (p.1648·2).
*Venous insufficiency.*

**Venen-Tropfen** *Eu Rho, Ger.†.*
Aesculus (p.1648·2).
*Haemorrhoids; thrombosis prophylaxis; venous insufficiency.*

**Venen-Tropfen N** *Bioforce, Ger.*
Aesculus (p.1648·2).
*Venous insufficiency.*

**Venex** *Decomed, Port.*
Diosmin (p.1688·2).
*Capillary fragility; haemorrhoids; menstrual disorders; orthostatic hypotension; venous insufficiency.*

**Vengesic** *Collins, Mex.*
Methocarbamol (p.1395·1); phenylbutazone (p.83·2); dexamethasone (p.1097·1); aluminium hydroxide (p.1249·2).
*Inflammation; musculoskeletal and joint disorders.*

**Venimmun**
*Aventis Behring, Ger.; Centeon, Ital.*
A normal immunoglobulin (p.1627·2).
*Hypogammaglobulinaemia; idiopathic thrombocytopenic purpura; passive immunisation.*

**Venimmun N** *Aventis Behring, Austria.*
A normal immunoglobulin (p.1627·2).
*Idiopathic thrombocytopenic purpura; passive immunisation.*

**Venimmuna** *Aventis Behring, Braz.*
A normal immunoglobulin (p.1627·2).
*Passive immunisation.*

**Venirene** *Irex, Fr.*
Diosmin (p.1688·2).
*Capillary disorders; haemorrhoids; venous insufficiency.*

**Veniten** *Whitehall-Robins, Switz.†.*
Troxerutin (p.1688·3).
*Peripheral vascular disorders.*

**Venitrin** *AstraZeneca, Ital.*
Glyceryl trinitrate (p.923·2).
*Angina pectoris; hypertensive crises; left-ventricular failure; myocardial infarction.*

**Venium** *Lubapharm Phlebologie, Switz.†.*
Coumarin (p.1676·2).
*Lymphoedema.*

**Venlax** *Saval, Chile.*
Venlafaxine (p.322·3) or venlafaxine hydrochloride (p.321·3).
*Anxiety; attention-deficit hyperactivity disorder; depression.*

**Venlor** *Cipla, India.*
Venlafaxine hydrochloride (p.321·3).
*Anxiety disorders; depression.*

**Veno** *Sanochemia, Austria†.*
Troxerutin (p.1688·3); dihydroergotamine tartrate (p.466·1).
*Chronic venous insufficiency.*

**Veno SL** *Ursapharm, Ger.*
Troxerutin (p.1688·3).
*Vascular disorders.*

**Venobene** *Ratiopharm, Austria.*
Heparin sodium (p.928·1); dexpanthenol (p.1727·2).
*Anorectal disorders; soft-tissue injury; superficial vascular disorders.*

**Venobiase** *Fournier, Ger.*
Ruscus aculeatus rhizome; black currant (p.1661·1).
*Venous insufficiency.*

**Venobiase mono** *Fournier, Ger.*
Ruscus aculeatus rhizome.
*Haemorrhoids; venous insufficiency.*

**veno-biomo** *Biomo, Ger.*
Aesculus (p.1648·2).
*Soft-tissue injury; venous insufficiency.*

**Venocaina** *Braun, Spain†.*
Procaine hydrochloride (p.1383·2).
*Local anaesthesia.*

**Venocur Triplex** *Abbott, Braz.*
Rutoside (p.1688·2); aesculus (p.1648·2); miroton.
*Venous insufficiency.*

**Venodin** *Tosi, Ital.†.*
Tribenoside (p.1757·3).
*Haemorrhoids; thrombophlebitis; varicose veins.*

**Venodura** *Merck dura, Ger.*
Aesculus (p.1648·2).
*Venous insufficiency.*

**Venofer**
*Andromaco, Chile; Vifor, Denm.; Therabel, Fr.; Fresenius Medical, Ger.; Vifor, Gr.; Vifor, Hong Kong; Vifor, Israel; Renapharma, Norw.; Ferraz, Lynce, Port.; Byk Madaus, S.Afr.; Vifor, Singapore; Uriach, Spain; Renapharma, Swed.; Vifor International, Switz.; SPB, Thai.†; Vifor, Thai.†; Syner-Med, UK; American Regent, USA.*
Iron sucrose (p.1438·2).
*Iron deficiency; iron-deficiency anaemia.*

**Venoferrum** *Byk Gulden, Mex.*
Iron sucrose (p.1438·2).
*Iron-deficiency anaemia.*

**Venofit**
*Note. This name is used for preparations of different composition.*
*Hochstetter, Chile.*
Homoeopathic preparation.

*Arkochim, Spain.*
Ruscus aculeatus; melilotus officinalis; hamamelis (p.1696·3).
*Peripheral vascular disorders.*

**Venofortan** *Ariston, Braz.*
Aescin (p.1648·2); vitamin $B_1$ (p.1455·2).
*Venous insufficiency.*

**Venoful** *Garden House, Arg.*
Centella (p.1144·3); ginkgo biloba (p.1692·3); hamamelis (p.1696·3); aesculus (p.1648·2).
*Haemorrhoids; oedema; varices.*

**Venogal** *Chinosolfabrik, Ger.†.*
Aesculus (p.1648·2).
*Venous insufficiency.*

**Venogamma** *Veripalvelu, Fin.*
A normal immunoglobulin (p.1627·2).
*Hypogammaglobulinaemia; idiopathic thrombocytopenic purpura.*

**Venogamma Anti-Rho (D)** *Alfa Biotech, Ital.†.*
An anti-D immunoglobulin (p.1608·1).
*Prevention of rhesus sensitisation.*

**Venogamma Polivalente** *Wassermann, Ital.†.*
A normal immunoglobulin (p.1627·2).
*Hypogammaglobulinaemia; passive immunisation.*

**Venoglobulin**
*Alpha, Israel; Alpha Therapeutic, Singapore; Alpha Therapeutic, USA.*
A normal immunoglobulin (p.1627·2).
*Hypogammaglobulinaemia; idiopathic thrombocytopenic purpura; immunodeficiency; Kawasaki disease.*

**Venoglobulin-H** *Mitsubishi, Jpn.*
A normal immunoglobulin (p.1627·2).
*Agammaglobulinaemia; hypogammaglobulinaemia; idiopathic thrombocytopenic purpura; Kawasaki disease; passive immunisation.*

**Venoglobulin-S**
*Alpha, Hong Kong; Alpha Therapeutic, Malaysia; Alpha Therapeutic, Thai.*
A normal immunoglobulin (p.1627·2).
*Idiopathic thrombocytopenic purpura; immunodeficiency; Kawasaki disease.*

**Venogyl** *Teva, Israel.*
Metronidazole (p.607·2).
*Anaerobic bacterial infections.*

**Veno-Hexanicit** *Promed, Ger.†.*
Inositol nicotinate (p.939·3); heptaminol hydrochloride (p.1697·1); troxerutin (p.1688·3).
*Inflammation; oedema; vascular disorders; vascular headache.*

**Veno-Kattwiga N** *Kattwiga, Ger.*
Aescin (p.1648·2); procaine hydrochloride (p.1383·2).
*Vascular disorders.*

**veno-L 90 N** *Loges, Ger.*
Homoeopathic preparation.

**Venolen** *Pharma Line, Ital.*
Troxerutin (p.1688·3).
*Haemorrhoids; varicose veins.*

**Venolep** *Farma Lepori, Spain.*
Hidrosmin (p.1688·3).
*Venous insufficiency.*

**Venomenhal** *Hal, Ger.*
Allergen extracts of bee venom (p.1650·2) and wasp venom (p.1650·2) (p.1650·1).
*Allergen immunotherapy.*

**Venomhal** *Hal, Neth.*
Aqueous bee venom (p.1650·2) and wasp venom (p.1650·2)(p.1650·1).
*Allergen immunotherapy.*

**Venomil**
*Bencard, Ger.; Miles, USA.*
Venoms of bee (p.1650·2), wasp (p.1650·2), hornet, yellow jacket, and mixed vespids (p.1650·1).
*Allergen immunotherapy.*

**Venoparil** *Neo-Farmaceutica, Port.*
*Tablets:* Aescin (p.1648·2).
*Haemorrhoids; joint pain; oedema; venous insufficiency.*
*Topical gel:* Aescin (p.1648·2); diethylamine salicylate (p.34·1).
*Musculoskeletal, joint, and soft-tissue injury; thrombophlebitis; varices.*

**Venoplant**
*Note. This name is used for preparations of different composition.*
*Schwabe, Ger.*
*Delayed-release tablets:* Aesculus (p.1648·2).
*Venous insufficiency.*
*Schwabe, Neth.†; Sanofi Synthelabo, Spain†.*
*Tablets; oral drops:* Silybum marianum (p.1043·3); aesculus (p.1648·2); hamamelis (p.1696·3).
*Vascular disorders.*
*Schwabe, Spain†.*
*Ointment:* Aesculus (p.1648·2); hamamelis (p.1696·3); heparin (p.927·3).
*Peripheral vascular disorders.*

**Venoplant AHS** *Schwabe, Ger.*
Aescin (p.1648·2); heparin sodium (p.928·1); glycol salicylate (p.44·3).
*Soft-tissue injury; venous insufficiency.*

**Venoplant comp** *Schwabe, Switz.*
Aescin (p.1648·2); heparin sodium (p.928·1); glycol salicylate (p.44·3).
*Musculoskeletal, joint, and soft-tissue injuries; scars; venous insufficiency.*

**Venoplant N** *Schwabe, Switz.*
Aesculus (p.1648·2); heparin sodium (p.928·1).
*Scars; soft-tissue injuries; vascular disorders.*

**Venoplant top** *Schwabe, Ger.*
Hamamelis (p.1696·3).
*Skin inflammation; varices.*

**Venoplus** *Also, Ital.*
Aesculus (p.1648·2); hamamelis (p.1696·3); silybum marianum (p.1043·3).
*Alterations in capillary permeability; varicose veins; venous dilatation.*

**Venopril** *Luper, Braz.*
Captopril (p.879·2).
*Hypertension.*

**Venopyronum** *Abbott, Ger.*
Aesculus (p.1648·2).
*Venous insufficiency.*

**Venopyronum N** *Abbott, Ger.*
Aesculus (p.1648·2).
*Venous insufficiency.*

**Venorell** *Sanorell, Ger.*
Homoeopathic preparation.

**Venoruton**
*Note. This name is used for preparations of different composition.*
*Novartis, Arg.; Novartis Consumer, Austria; Novartis Consumer, Belg.; Novartis, Chile; Novartis, Denm.; Novartis Consumer, Ger.; Novartis, Hong Kong; Novartis, Israel; Novartis Consumer, Ital.; Novartis Consumer, Neth.; Novartis Consumer, Port.; Novartis Consumer, Spain; Novartis Consumer, Switz.*
Oxerutins (p.1688·2).
*Chronic venous insufficiency; haemorrhoids; retinopathy; soft-tissue injury; vascular reactions following radiotherapy.*
*Novartis, Braz.; Novartis, Thai.*
Troxerutin (p.1688·3).
*Chronic venous insufficiency; haemorrhoids.*

**Venoruton Emulgel** *Novartis Consumer, Ger.*
Heparin sodium (p.928·1).
Formerly known as Venoruton Heparin.
*Soft-tissue injury; superficial vascular disorders.*

**Venoruton Heparin** *Novartis Consumer, Austria.*
Heparin sodium (p.928·1).
*Soft-tissue injury; superficial venous disorders.*

**Venos Cough Mixture** *GlaxoSmithKline Consumer, UK.*
Glucose (p.1432·2); treacle.
*Coughs.*

**Venos Expectorant**
*SmithKline Beecham Consumer, Irl.; GlaxoSmithKline Consumer, UK.*
Guaifenesin (p.1122·1); glucose (p.1432·2); treacle.
*Coughs.*

**Venos Honey & Lemon**
*Note. This name is used for preparations of different composition.*
*SmithKline Beecham Consumer, Irl.*
Ammonium chloride (p.1115·2); ipecacuanha (p.1122·3); liquid glucose (p.1432·2); honey (p.1434·2); lemon juice.
*Coughs.*
*GlaxoSmithKline Consumer, UK.*
Purified honey (p.1434·2); glucose (p.1432·2).
*Coughs; sore throat.*

**Venos for Kids** *GlaxoSmithKline Consumer, UK.*
Guaifenesin (p.1122·1).
*Coughs.*

**Venosan**
*Binesa, Spain†; Mack, Switz.†.*
Inositol nicotinate (p.939·3); pholedrine sulfate (p.982·3); troxerutin (p.1688·3).
*Vascular disorders.*

**Venoselect N** *Dreluso, Ger.*
Homoeopathic preparation.

**Venoserin** *Labomed, Chile.*
Ruscus aculeatus.
*Venous insufficiency.*

**Venosin** *Klinge, Austria.*
*Capsules; ointment; oral drops:* Aesculus (p.1648·2).
*Chronic venous insufficiency; haemorrhoids; oedema; superficial vascular disorders; thrombosis prophylaxis.*
*Topical gel:* Aescin (p.1648·2); heparin sodium (p.928·1); glycol salicylate (p.44·3).
*Chronic venous insufficiency; oedema; soft-tissue disorders.*

**Venosmil**
*Sidus, Arg.; Vitoria, Port.; Faes, Spain.*
Hidrosmin (p.1688·3).
*Cerebral and ocular vascular disorders; haemorrhoids; inflammatory skin disorders; venous insufficiency; vestibular disorders.*

**Venosmine** *Geymonat, Ital.*
Diosmin (p.1688·2).
*Peripheral vascular disorders.*

**Venostasin**
*Note. This name is used for preparations of different composition.*
*Ariston, Arg.; Klinge, Austria; Ariston, Braz.; Fujisawa, Ger.*
*Controlled-release capsules; ointment:* Aesculus (p.1648·2).
*Inflammation; venous insufficiency.*
*Ariston, Arg.*
*Tablets:* Aescin (p.1648·2); vitamin $B_1$ (p.1455·2).
*Venous insufficiency.*
*Ariston, Arg.; Fujisawa, Ger.*
*Topical gel:* Aescin (p.1648·2); heparin sodium (p.928·1); glycol salicylate (p.44·3).
*Soft-tissue injury; venous insufficiency.*

**Venostasin Composto** *Ariston, Braz.†.*
Heparin sodium (p.928·1); aescin (p.1648·2); glycol salicylate (p.44·3).
*Oedema; venous insufficiency.*

**Veno-Tebonin N** *Schwabe, Ger.*
Ginkgo biloba (p.1692·3); heptaminol hydrochloride (p.1697·1); troxerutin (p.1688·3).
*Haemorrhoids; vascular disorders.*

**Venotop** *Novartis, Austria.*
Dihydroergotamine tartrate (p.466·1); troxerutin (p.1688·3).
*Chronic venous insufficiency.*

**Venotrauma** *Also, Ital.*
Aesculus (p.1648·2); hamamelis (p.1696·3); heparin sodium (p.928·1).
*Soft-tissue disorders.*

**Venotrulan** *Bilgast, Ger.†.*
Hamamelis (p.1696·3); collinsonia canad.; paeonia offic.
*Haemorrhoids; vascular disorders.*

**Venotrulan N** *Truw, Ger.†.*
Aesculus (p.1648·2).
*Venous insufficiency.*

**Veno-V** *Inibsa, Port.*
Diosmin (p.1688·2).
*Oedema; vascular disorders.*

**Venovit** *Vaillant, Ital.†.*
Ruscus; hamamelis (p.1696·3); aesculus (p.1648·2).
*Venous insufficiency.*

**Vensa** *Bittner, Austria.*
Homoeopathic preparation.

**Vent Retard** *BOI, Spain.*
Theophylline (p.798·3).
*Heart failure; obstructive airways disease; paroxysmal dyspnoea.*

**Ventadur** *Celltech, Spain.*
Salbutamol sulfate (p.791·3).
*Obstructive airways disease.*

**Ventamol**
*Pinewood, Irl.*
Salbutamol (p.791·3).
*Obstructive airways disease.*
*Hovid, Malaysia.*
Salbutamol sulfate (p.791·3).
*Bronchospasm.*

**Ventamol Expectorant** *Hovid, Malaysia.*
Salbutamol sulfate (p.791·3); guaifenesin (p.1122·1).
*Bronchospasm.*

**Ventavis** *Schering, UK.*
Iloprost trometamol (p.1518·2).
*Pulmonary hypertension.*

**Venter** *Vent-3, Arg.*
Paracetamol (p.76·2); salicylamide (p.87·3); ascorbic acid (p.1460·2); phenylephrine hydrochloride (p.1126·3).
*Influenza symptoms.*

**Venterol** *Greater Pharma, Thai.*
Salbutamol sulfate (p.791·3).
*Obstructive airways disease.*

**Ventexxair** *Schwarz, Fr.*
Salbutamol (p.791·3).
*Obstructive airways disease.*

**Venteze** *Aspen, S.Afr.*
Salbutamol (p.791·3) or salbutamol sulfate (p.791·3).
*Obstructive airways disease.*

**Ventide**
*GlaxoSmithKline, Arg.; GlaxoSmithKline, Austria; GlaxoSmithKline, Chile; GlaxoSmithKline, Hong Kong; Glaxo Wellcome, Mex.; GlaxoSmithKline, Singapore; GlaxoSmithKline, Thai.; Allen & Hanburys, UK†.*
Salbutamol (p.791·3) or salbutamol sulfate (p.791·3); beclometasone dipropionate (p.1091·1).
*Obstructive airways disease.*

**Ventilan**
*Note. This name is used for preparations of different composition.*
*Sintofarma, Braz.†.*
Clenbuterol hydrochloride (p.784·2).
*Obstructive airways disease.*
*Glaxo Wellcome, Port.*
Salbutamol (p.791·3) or salbutamol sulfate (p.791·3).
*Obstructive airways disease; premature labour.*

**Ventilastin** *Viatris, Ger.*
Salbutamol sulfate (p.791·3).
*Obstructive airways disease.*

**Ventilat** *Boehringer Ingelheim, Ger.*
Oxitropium bromide (p.790·3).
*Obstructive airways disease.*

**Ventimax** *Norton, S.Afr.†.*
Salbutamol (p.791·3).
*Obstructive airways disease.*

**Ventisol** *Fustery, Mex.*
Ketotifen fumarate (p.788·1).
*Asthma; hypersensitivity.*

**Ventmax**
*Chiesi, Ital.*
Salbutamol (p.791·3).
*Obstructive airways disease.*
*Trinity, UK.*
Salbutamol sulfate (p.791·3).
*Obstructive airways disease.*

**Ventnaze** *Aspen, S.Afr.*
Beclometasone dipropionate (p.1091·1).
*Hay fever; rhinitis.*

**Ventodisk**
*GlaxoSmithKline, Canad.; Glaxo Wellcome, NZ†; GlaxoSmithKline, S.Afr.; GlaxoSmithKline, Switz.; Glaxo Wellcome, Thai.†.*
Salbutamol sulfate (p.791·3).
*Obstructive airways disease.*

**Ventodisks**
*GlaxoSmithKline, Fr.; GlaxoSmithKline, Hong Kong; Allen & Hanburys, Irl.; Allen & Hanburys, UK.*
Salbutamol sulfate (p.791·3).
*Bronchospasm; obstructive airways disease.*

**Ventoflu** *Finmedical, Ital.*
Flunisolide (p.1101·1).
*Asthma; bronchitis; rhinitis.*

**Ventolair** *3M, Ger.*
Beclometasone dipropionate (p.1091·1).
*Asthma.*

**Ventolase** *Juste, Spain.*
Clenbuterol hydrochloride (p.784·2).
*Obstructive airways disease.*

**Ventoliber** *Tecnimede, Port.*
Ambroxol hydrochloride (p.1114·3); clenbuterol hydrochloride (p.784·2).

**Ventolin**
*GlaxoSmithKline, Arg.; Allen & Hanburys, Austral.; GlaxoSmithKline, Belg.; GlaxoSmithKline, Canad.; GlaxoSmithKline, Hong Kong; Allen & Hanburys, Irl.; GlaxoSmithKline, Israel; GlaxoSmithKline, Ital.; GlaxoSmithKline, Malaysia; Glaxo Wellcome, Mex.; GlaxoSmithKline, Neth.; GlaxoSmithKline, NZ; GlaxoSmithKline, S.Afr.; GlaxoSmithKline, Singapore; GlaxoSmithKline, Spain; GlaxoSmithKline, Switz.; GlaxoSmithKline, Thai.; Allen & Hanburys, UK; Glaxo Wellcome, USA.*
Salbutamol (p.791·3) or salbutamol sulfate (p.791·3).
*Obstructive airways disease; premature labour; status asthmaticus.*

**Ventolin Compuesto** *GlaxoSmithKline, Arg.*
Salbutamol (p.791·3); guaifenesin (p.1122·1).
*Respiratory-tract congestion.*

**Ventolin Espettorante** *GlaxoSmithKline, Ital.*
Salbutamol sulfate (p.791·3); guaifenesin (p.1122·1).
*Bronchial congestion; bronchospasm.*

**Ventolin Expectorant**
*GlaxoSmithKline, Hong Kong; GlaxoSmithKline, Malaysia; GlaxoSmithKline, Thai.*
Salbutamol sulfate (p.791·3); guaifenesin (p.1122·1).
*Bronchospasm; respiratory-tract disorders associated with increased, viscous mucus.*

**Ventolin Flogo** *GlaxoSmithKline, Ital.*
Beclometasone dipropionate (p.1091·1); salbutamol (p.791·3).
*Obstructive airways disease.*

**Ventoline**
*GlaxoSmithKline, Denm.; GlaxoSmithKline, Fin.; GlaxoSmithKline, Fr.; GlaxoSmithKline, Norw.; GlaxoSmithKline, Swed.*
Salbutamol (p.791·3) or salbutamol sulfate (p.791·3).
*Obstructive airways disease; premature labour.*

**Ventomol** *Merck, Hong Kong.*
Salbutamol sulfate (p.791·3).
*Obstructive airways disease.*

**Ventor** *Rafarm, Gr.*
Nimesulide (p.67·1).
*Inflammation; musculoskeletal disorders; pain.*

**Ventorlin** *GlaxoSmithKline, India.*
Salbutamol sulfate (p.791·3); guaifenesin (p.1122·1).
*Obstructive airways disease.*

**Ventox** *Leiras, Fin.*
Oxitropium bromide (p.790·3).
*Obstructive airways disease.*

**Ventracid N** *Repha, Ger.*
Sodium bicarbonate (p.1223·2); pancreatin (p.1725·3); curcuma (p.1058·3).
*Gastrointestinal disorders.*

**Ventre Livre** *CIF, Braz.*
Cascara (p.1255·1); docusate sodium (p.1262·2).
*Constipation.*

**Ventricon N** *Syxyl, Ger.*
Bismuth subnitrate (p.1252·2); calcium carbonate (p.1254·2); magnesium oxide (p.1272·3).
*Gastrointestinal disorders.*

**Ventricor** *Faromed, Austria.*
Sotalol hydrochloride (p.1001·3).
*Arrhythmias.*

**Ventrigutt N** *Hanosan, Ger.*
Homoeopathic preparation.

**ventri-loges N** *Loges, Ger.*
Absinthium (p.1645·1); calamus (p.1664·1); gentian (p.1692·2).
*Appetite loss; dyspepsia.*

**Ventrimarin novo** *Steigerwald, Ger.†.*
Absinthium (p.1645·1); gentian (p.1692·2); angelica (p.1655·1).
*Appetite loss; dyspepsia; meteorism.*

**Ventrux** *Cernelle, Switz.*
*Enterococcus faecium* (p.1704·2).
*Gastrointestinal disorders; restoration of intestinal flora.*

**Ventzone** *Aspen, S.Afr.†.*
Beclometasone dipropionate (p.1091·1).
*Asthma.*

**Venucreme** *Permamed, Switz.*
Heparin sodium (p.928·1); glycol salicylate (p.44·3); dimethyl sulfoxide (p.1473·2); lauromacrogol 600 (p.1412·3); dexpanthenol (p.1727·2).
*Phlebitis; soft-tissue disorders; venous insufficiency.*

**Venugel** *Permamed, Switz.*
Heparin sodium (p.928·1); glycol salicylate (p.44·3); dimethyl sulfoxide (p.1473·2); lauromacrogol 600 (p.1412·3); dexpanthenol (p.1727·2).
*Phlebitis; soft-tissue disorders; venous insufficiency.*

**Venusmin** *Martin & Harris, India.*
Diosmin (p.1688·2).
*Haemorrhoids; menorrhagia; metrorrhagia; varicose veins.*

**Venustas Antiforfora** *BPR, Ital.*
Cinchona succirubra (p.1671·3).
*Seborrhoeic dermatitis.*

**Venustas Lozione Caduta** *BPR, Ital.†.*
Arnica (p.1656·3).
*Alopecia.*

**Venustas Shampoo per Capelli con Forfora e/o Grassi** *BPR, Ital.†.*
Urtica (p.1762·1).
*Seborrhoeic dermatitis.*

**Venutabs** *Lubapharm, Switz.*
Troxerutin (p.1688·3).
*Haemorrhoids; venous insufficiency.*

**Venyl** *Dolisos, Fr.*
Ruscus aculeatus; hesperidin methyl chalcone (p.1688·3); ascorbic acid (p.1460·2).
*Haemorrhoids; peripheral vascular disorders.*

**Vepan** *Indoco, India.*
Cefadroxil (p.167·2).
*Bacterial infections.*

**Vepar** *Savio, Ital.†.*
Suleparoid (p.1009·1).
*Peripheral vascular disorders.*

**Vepen** *Lacefa, Arg.*
Vitamin A; vitamin C; vitamin D; minerals (p.1417·1).

**Vepesid**
*Bristol-Myers Squibb, Arg.; Bristol-Myers Squibb, Austral.; Bristol-Myers Squibb, Austria; Bristol-Myers Squibb, Belg.; Bristol-Myers Squibb, Braz.; Bristol, Canad.; Bristol-Myers Squibb, Denm.; Bristol-Myers Squibb, Fin.; Bristol-Myers Squibb, Ger.; Bristol-Myers Squibb, Gr.; Bristol-Myers Squibb, Hong Kong; Bristol-Myers Squibb, Irl.; Bristol-Myers Squibb, Israel; Bristol-Myers Squibb, Ital.; Bristol-Myers Squibb, Malaysia; Bristol-Myers Squibb, Mex.; Bristol-Myers Squibb, Neth.; Bristol-Myers Squibb, Norw.; Bristol-Myers Squibb, NZ; Bristol-Myers Squibb, Port.; Bristol-Myers Squibb, S.Afr.; Bristol-Myers Squibb, Singapore; Bristol-Myers, Spain; Bristol-Myers Squibb, Swed.; Bristol-Myers Squibb, Switz.; Bristol-Myers Squibb, Thai.; Bristol-Myers Squibb, UK; Bristol-Myers Squibb Oncology, USA.*
Etoposide (p.551·3).
*Malignant neoplasms.*

**Vepeside** *Novartis, Fr.*
Etoposide (p.551·3).
*Malignant neoplasms.*

**Vepicombin** *Nycomed, Denm.*
Phenoxymethylpenicillin potassium (p.242·1).
*Bacterial infections.*

**Vera** *1A, Ger.; ABZ, Ger.; CT, Ger.; Heumann, Ger.*
Verapamil hydrochloride (p.1019·1).
*Angina pectoris; arrhythmias; hypertension.*

**Verabeta** *Betapharm, Ger.*
Verapamil hydrochloride (p.1019·1).
*Angina pectoris; arrhythmias; hypertension.*

**Veracaps** *Sigma, Austral.*
Verapamil hydrochloride (p.1019·1).
*Angina pectoris; hypertension.*

**Veracapt** *Ebewe, Austria.*
Verapamil hydrochloride (p.1019·1); captopril (p.879·2).
*Hypertension.*

**Veracef** *Bristol-Myers Squibb, Mex.*
Cefradine (p.179·3).
*Bacterial infections.*

**Veracim** *Cimex, Switz.†.*
Verapamil hydrochloride (p.1019·1).
*Arrhythmias; ischaemic heart disease.*

**Veracol** *Demo, Gr.*
Ceftriaxone sodium (p.182·3).
*Bacterial infections.*

**Veracolate**
*Note. This name is used for preparations of different composition.*
*Parke, Davis, Arg.; Pfizer, Thai.*
Bile salt (p.1660·3); cascara (p.1255·1); phenolphthalein (p.1284·1); capsicum oleoresin (p.1667·1).
*Biliary-tract disorders; intestinal motility disorders.*

*Aspen, S.Afr.*
Cascara sagrada (p.1255·1); phenolphthalein (p.1284·1).
*Constipation.*

*Numark, USA†.*
Cascara (p.1255·1); phenolphthalein (p.1284·1); capsicum oleoresin (p.1667·1).

**Veracor** *Dexxon, Israel.*
Verapamil hydrochloride (p.1019·1).
*Angina pectoris; arrhythmias; hypertension.*

**Veracoron** *Cibran, Braz.†.*
Verapamil hydrochloride (p.1019·1).
*Angina pectoris; arrhythmias; hypertension.*

**Veracur**
*Typharm, Irl.†; Typharm, UK.*
Formaldehyde (p.1179·3).
*Verrucas; warts.*

**Veracuril** *Fada, Arg.*
Oxytocin (p.1336·1).

**Veraday** *Pharmacia, Austria.*
Verapamil hydrochloride (p.1019·1).
*Angina pectoris; hypertension.*

**Veradin** *Novartis, Chile.*
Paracetamol (p.76·2); aspirin (p.15·1); caffeine (p.782·1).
*Pain.*

**Veradol** *Serch, Arg.*
Naproxen (p.65·1).
*Inflammation; pain.*

**Veragamma** *Worwag, Ger.*
Verapamil hydrochloride (p.1019·1).
*Angina pectoris; arrhythmias; hypertension.*

**Veragel**
*United American, Hong Kong; Great Eastern, Thai.; United American, Thai.*
Aluminium hydroxide-magnesium carbonate co-dried gel (p.1250·1); dimethicone (p.1289·2); dicycloverine hydrochloride (p.481·2).
*Dyspepsia; gastric hyperacidity; gastritis; heartburn; peptic ulcer.*

**Veragel DMS** *United American, Singapore.*
Aluminium hydroxide-magnesium carbonate co-dried gel (p.1250·1); dimeticone (p.1289·2); dicycloverine hydrochloride (p.481·2).
*Duodenitis; dyspepsia; flatulence; gastric hyperacidity; gastritis; gastro-oesophageal reflux; gastrointestinal motility disorders; heartburn; peptic ulcer; pylorospasm.*

**Verahexal**
*Hexal, Austral.; Hexal, Ger.; Hexal, S.Afr.*
Verapamil hydrochloride (p.1019·1).
*Angina pectoris; arrhythmias; hypertension.*

**Verakard** *Nycomed, Norw.*
Verapamil hydrochloride (p.1019·1).
*Angina pectoris; arrhythmias; hypertension.*

**Veraken** *Kener, Mex.†.*
Verapamil (p.1021·1).

**Veral** *Hexal, Arg.*
Verapamil hydrochloride (p.1019·1).
*Angina pectoris; arrhythmias; hypertension; myocardial infarction.*

**Veralan** *Quimica y Farmacia, Mex.†.*
Verapamil hydrochloride (p.1019·1).

**Veraldid** *Chobet, Arg.*
Troxerutin (p.1688·3); magnesium ascorbate (p.1227·3).
*Varices.*

**Vera-Lich** *Lichtenstein, Ger.*
Verapamil hydrochloride (p.1019·1).
*Angina pectoris; arrhythmias; hypertension.*

**Veraligral** *Sanofi Synthelabo, Mex.*
Veralipride (p.727·2).
*Menopausal disorders.*

**Veralipral** *Finadiet, Arg.*
Veralipride (p.727·2).
*Menopausal disorders.*

**Veralipral T** *Finadiet, Arg.*
Veralipride (p.727·2); bromazepam (p.671·3).
*Menopausal disorders.*

**Veralipril** *Sanofi Synthelabo, Ital.*
Veralipride (p.727·2).
*Menopausal disorders.*

**Veraloc**
*Orion, Denm.; Orion, Swed.†.*
Verapamil hydrochloride (p.1019·1).
*Angina pectoris; arrhythmias; hypertension; myocardial infarction.*

**Veralox** *Demo, Gr.*
Omeprazole (p.1278·2).
*Acid aspiration; eradication of Helicobacter pylori in combination with antimicrobials; peptic ulcer; reflux oesophagitis; Zollinger-Ellison syndrome.*

**Veramex** *Sanofi Synthelabo, Ger.*
Verapamil hydrochloride (p.1019·1).
*Angina pectoris; arrhythmias; hypertension; myocardial infarction.*

**Veramil**
*Ducto, Braz.; Orion, Irl.*
Verapamil hydrochloride (p.1019·1).
*Angina pectoris; arrhythmias; hypertension.*

*Themis Chemicals, India.*
Verapamil (p.1021·1).
*Angina pectoris; arrhythmias; hypertension.*

**Veramina** *Roux-Ocefa, Arg.*
Fosfomycin calcium (p.214·2) or fosfomycin sodium (p.214·3).
*Bacterial infections.*

**Veramon**
*Note. This name is used for preparations of different composition.*
*Schering-Plough, Braz.†.*
Aspirin (p.15·1); paracetamol (p.76·2); caffeine (p.782·1).
*Fever; pain.*

*Sofar, Ital.*
Propyphenazone (p.85·3); paracetamol (p.76·2).
*Fever; pain.*

**Veranorm** *Alpharma-Isis, Ger.*
Verapamil hydrochloride (p.1019·1).
*Angina pectoris; arrhythmias; hypertension.*

**Veranzol** *Collins, Mex.*
Albendazole (p.101·2).
*Worm infections.*

**Verap** *Rowex, Irl.*
Verapamil hydrochloride (p.1019·1).
*Angina pectoris; hypertension.*

**Verapabene** *Ratiopharm, Austria.*
Verapamil hydrochloride (p.1019·1).
*Angina pectoris; arrhythmias; heart failure; hypertension; hypertrophic obstructive cardiomyopathy.*

**Verapal** *Lafedar, Arg.*
Verapamil hydrochloride (p.1019·1).
*Angina pectoris; arrhythmias.*

**Verapam** *Streuli, Switz.*
Verapamil hydrochloride (p.1019·1).
*Angina pectoris; arrhythmias; cardiomyopathy; coronary spasm; hypertension; myocardial infarction.*

**Verapin** *Berlin Pharm, Thai.*
Verapamil hydrochloride (p.1019·1).
*Angina pectoris; arrhythmias; hypertension.*

**Veraplex**
*Teva Tuteur, Arg.*
Medroxyprogesterone (p.1557·3).

*Pharmachemie, Malaysia.*
Medroxyprogesterone acetate (p.1557·2).
*Breast cancer; endometrial cancer.*

**Verapress**
*Dexcel, Israel; Dexcel, UK.*
Verapamil hydrochloride (p.1019·1).
*Angina pectoris; hypertension.*

**Veraptin** *Boniscontro & Gazzone, Ital.*
Verapamil hydrochloride (p.1019·1).
*Angina pectoris; arrhythmias; hypertension; myocardial infarction.*

**Verasal** *TAD, Ger.*
Verapamil hydrochloride (p.1019·1).
*Angina pectoris; arrhythmias; hypertension.*

**Verasifar** *Siphar, Switz.†.*
Verapamil hydrochloride (p.1019·1).
*Hypertension.*

**Veraskin** *Mazal, Fr.*
Aloe vera (p.1141·3).
*Skin disorders; superficial burns and wounds.*

**Veraspir** *Alodial, Port.*
Salmeterol xinafoate (p.795·1).
*Asthma.*

**Verastad** *Stada, Austria.*
Verapamil hydrochloride (p.1019·1).
*Angina pectoris; arrhythmias; hypertension; hypertrophic cardiomyopathy; myocardial infarction.*

**Veratensin** *Farma Lepori, Spain†.*
Verapamil hydrochloride (p.1019·1).
*Angina pectoris; arrhythmias; hypertension.*

**Veratide** *Procter & Gamble, Ger.*
Verapamil hydrochloride (p.1019·1); triamterene (p.1016·2); hydrochlorothiazide (p.933·2).
*Hypertension.*

**Veratran** *Shire, Fr.*
Clotiazepam (p.685·2).
*Alcohol withdrawal syndrome; anxiety.*

**Veratropan Composto** *IQB, Braz.*
Hyoscine (p.483·3); dipyrone (p.35·3).
*Muscle spasm; pain.*

**Veratrum Med Complex** *Dynamit, Austria.*
Homoeopathic preparation.

**Veratyrol** *Tyrol, Austria.*
Verapamil hydrochloride (p.1019·1).
*Angina pectoris; arrhythmias; hypertension; hypertrophic cardiomyopathy; myocardial infarction.*

**Veraval** *Sanval, Braz.*
Verapamil hydrochloride (p.1019·1).
*Angina pectoris; arrhythmias; hypertension.*

**Veravorin** *Rafarm, Gr.*
Calcium folinate (p.1431·1).
*Antidote to folic acid antagonists; megaloblastic anaemia.*

**Verax**
*Tosi, Hong Kong; Tosi, Ital.*
Benzydamine hydrochloride (p.21·1).
*Mouth and throat disorders; phlebitis; venous insufficiency; vulvovaginal disorders.*

**Verazinc** *Forest Pharmaceuticals, USA.*
Zinc sulfate (p.1469·3).
*Dietary supplement.*

**Verbalem** *Lemery, Mex.†.*
Paracetamol (p.76·2).
*Fever; pain.*

**Verbascum Complex** *Blackmores, Austral.†.*
Verbascum thapsus (p.1764·1); marrubium vulgare (p.1124·1); pleurisy root (p.1733·1); liquorice (p.1270·2); ascorbic acid (p.1460·2); vitamin A acetate (p.1453·1).
*Respiratory system disorders.*

**Verbesol** *ICT, Ital.†.*
L-Verbenone.
*Respiratory-tract disorders.*

**Verbex** *Istoria, Ital.†.*
L-verbenone.
*Respiratory-tract disorders.*

**Verbital** *Faran, Gr.*
Bezafibrate (p.873·2).
*Hyperlipidaemias.*

**Verboril**
*Note. This name is used for preparations of different composition.*
*TRB, Arg.*
Doxycycline hyclate (p.206·2).
*Bacterial infections.*

*Faran, Gr.*
Diacerein (p.30·1).
*Osteoarthritis.*

**Vercef**
*Faulding, Austral.†; Ranbaxy, Malaysia; Ranbaxy, S.Afr.; Ranbaxy, Singapore; Ranbaxy, Thai.*
Cefaclor (p.167·1).
*Bacterial infections.*

**Vercite** *Abbott, Ital.*
Pipobroman (p.580·1).
*Chronic myeloid leukaemia; polycythaemia vera.*

**Vercol** *Viofar, Gr.*
Lisinopril (p.946·3).
*Heart failure; hypertension; myocardial infarction.*

**Vercyte** *Abbott, Fr.*
Pipobroman (p.580·1).
*Polycythaemia vera.*

**Verdal**
*Note. This name is used for preparations of different composition.*
*Olvos, Gr.*
Fluprednidene (p.1102·2); miconazole (p.405·2).
*Fungal skin infections with inflammation.*

*Falqui, Ital.*
Aspirin (p.15·1); paracetamol (p.76·2); caffeine (p.782·1).
*Fever; influenza symptoms; pain.*

**Verecolene CM** *GlaxoSmithKline Consumer, Ital.*
Bisacodyl (p.1251·3).
*Constipation.*

**Verel** *Yamanouchi, Ital.*
Salicylic acid (p.1157·1); lactic acid (p.1704·1); copper acetate.
*Hard skin; verrucas; warts.*

**Verelait** *Bouty, Ital.*
Lactulose (p.1269·1).
*Constipation.*

**Verelan**
*Wyeth-Ayerst, Canad.†; Elan, Irl.†; Schwarz, USA.*
Verapamil hydrochloride (p.1019·1).
*Hypertension.*

**Verexamil** *Fresenius Kabi, Austria†.*
Verapamil hydrochloride (p.1019·1).
*Angina pectoris; arrhythmias; hypertension.*

**Verfid** *Continentales, Mex.†.*
Piperazine (p.111·2).

**Vergentan** *Sanofi Synthelabo, Ger.*
Alizapride hydrochloride (p.1248·1).
*Nausea and vomiting; radiation sickness.*

**Vergeturine** *Bailleul, Fr.*
Vitamins (p.1417·1).
*Skin disorders.*

**Vergo** *Pacific, NZ.*
Betahistine hydrochloride (p.1660·1).
*Ménière's disease.*

**Vergon** *Marnel, USA.*
Meclozine hydrochloride (p.436·3).

**Vericaps** *Ovelle, Irl.*
Salicylic acid (p.1157·1).
*Warts.*

**Vericardine** *Medix, Fr.†.*
Crataegus (p.1677·1); passion flower (p.1729·1); valerian (p.1762·2).
Formerly contained phenobarbital and crataegus.
*Anxiety; insomnia; nervous disorders.*

**Vericordin** *Lazar, Arg.*
Atenolol (p.865·2).
*Angina pectoris; hypertension.*

**Vericordin Compuesto** *Lazar, Arg.*
Atenolol (p.865·2); hydrochlorothiazide (p.933·2); amiloride hydrochloride (p.858·2).
*Hypertension.*

**Vericort** *Viofar, Gr.*
Budesonide (p.1094·2).
*Allergic rhinitis; topical corticosteroid.*

**Veriderm** *Lachifarma, Ital.†.*
Sulfur (p.1158·2).
*Seborrhoea.*

**Veriga** *Frega, Canad.†.*
Piperazine citrate (p.111·2).

**Verilax** *Microsules Bernabo, Arg.*
Sodium picosulfate (p.1289·3).
*Constipation.*

**Verimex** *Vachon, Canad.†.*
Piperazine citrate (p.111·2).

**Verintex** *Pekana, Ger.*
Homoeopathic preparation.

**Verintex N** *Pekana, Ger.*
Homoeopathic preparation.

**Verisan** *Knoll, Mex.*
Aesculus (p.1648·2).
*Venous insufficiency.*

**Veriscal D** *Faes, Spain.*
Calcium carbonate (p.1254·2); colecalciferol (p.1461·3).
*Calcium deficiency; osteoporosis.*

**Verisop** *Gerard, Irl.*
Verapamil hydrochloride (p.1019·1).
*Angina pectoris; hypertension; supraventricular tachycardia.*

**Verladyn** *Verla, Ger.*
Dihydroergotamine mesilate (p.465·3).
*Hypotension; migraine and related vascular headaches.*

**Verla-Lipon** *Verla, Ger.*
Thioctic acid (p.1754·3) or ethylenediamine thioctate (p.1754·3).
*Diabetic polyneuropathy.*

**Verlim 3** *Saninter, Port.†.*
Collodion.
*Verrucas.*

**Verlin** *Sanval, Braz.†.*
Procaine hydrochloride (p.1383·2); zinc sulfate (p.1469·3); boric acid (p.1662·1).
*Eye disorders.*

**Verlost** *Rafarm, Gr.*
Ranitidine hydrochloride (p.1285·2).
*Conditions where gastric acid reduction is beneficial; gastric hypersecretion including Zollinger-Ellison syndrome; peptic ulcer.*

**Vermepen** *Dinafarma, Braz.†.*
Mebendazole (p.108·2).
*Worm infections.*

**Vermex** *Hua, Thai.*
Piperazine citrate (p.111·2).
*Ascariasis; enterobiasis.*

**Vermi** *Quimpe, Spain.*
Piperazine adipate (p.111·2).
*Worm infections.*

**Vermiclase** *Cifarma, Braz.†.*
Albendazole (p.101·2).
*Worm infections.*

**Vermicol** *Degorts, Mex.*
Mebendazole (p.108·2).
*Worm infections.*

**Vermidil** *Diba, Mex.*
Mebendazole (p.108·2).
*Worm infections.*

**Vermifran** *Faria, Braz.*
Piperazine hydrate (p.111·2).
*Ascariasis; enterobiasis.*

**Vermifuge** *Sorin-Maxim, Fr.*
Piperazine hydrate (p.111·2).
Formerly contained piperazine hydrate and sodium bromide.
*Intestinal nematode infections.*

**Vermilan** *Quimica y Farmacia, Mex.*
Albendazole (p.101·2).
*Worm infections.*

**Vermilen** *Quimioterapica, Braz.*
Piperazine (p.111·2).
*Ascariasis; enterobiasis.*

**Vermilen Composto** *Quimioterapica, Braz.*
Piperazine (p.111·2); tiabendazole (p.114·2).
*Worm infections.*

**Vermin**
Note. This name is used for preparations of different composition.
*Ratiopharm, Fin.*
Verapamil hydrochloride (p.1019·1).
*Angina pectoris; arrhythmias; hypertension; myocardial infarction.*

*Streger, Mex.*
Piperazine (p.111·2).
*Worm infections.*

**Vermin-Dazol** *Streger, Mex.*
Mebendazole (p.108·2).
*Worm infections.*

**Vermine** *Pharmasant, Thai.*
Verapamil hydrochloride (p.1019·1).
*Angina pectoris; arrhythmias; hypertension.*

**Verminon** *Simoes, Braz.*
Mebendazole (p.108·2).
*Worm infections.*

**Vermin-Plus** *Streger, Mex.*
Albendazole (p.101·2).
*Intestinal nematode infections.*

**Vermirax** *Johnson & Johnson, Braz.*
Mebendazole (p.108·2).
*Worm infections.*

**Vermis** *Utopian, Thai.*
Aciclovir (p.626·1).
*Herpes simplex infections.*

**Vermisen** *Novag, Mex.*
Albendazole (p.101·2).
*Worm infections.*

**Vermisol** *Khandelwal, India.*
Levamisole (p.107·1).
*Worm infections.*

**Vermital** *Elofar, Braz.*
Albendazole (p.101·2).
*Worm infections.*

**Vermixide** *Polipharm, Thai.*
Albendazole (p.101·2).
*Worm infections.*

**Vermizol** *Kinder, Braz.†.*
Tetramisole (p.114·1); pyrvinium embonate (p.113·3).
*Nematode infections.*

**Vermizym** *Bittermedizin, Ger.*
Papain (p.1727·3).
*Worm infections.*

**Vermol** *Faria, Braz.*
Mebendazole (p.108·2); tiabendazole (p.114·2).
*Worm infections.*

**Vermonon** *Brasifa, Braz.†.*
Mebendazole (p.108·2).
*Worm infections.*

**Vermoplex** *Cimed, Braz.*
Mebendazole (p.108·2).
*Worm infections.*

**Vermoral** *Legrand, Braz.*
Mebendazole (p.108·2).
*Worm infections.*

**Vermox**
*Janssen-Cilag, Austral.; Janssen-Cilag, Belg.; Janssen-Ortho, Canad.; Janssen-Cilag, Denm.; Janssen-Cilag, Ger.; Janssen-Cilag, Gr.; Janssen, Hong Kong; Janssen-Cilag, Irl.; Janssen-Cilag, Israel; Janssen-Cilag, Ital.; Janssen-Cilag, Malaysia; Janssen, Mex.; Janssen-Cilag, Neth.; Janssen-Cilag, Norw.; Janssen-Cilag, NZ; Janssen-Cilag, S.Afr.; Janssen-Cilag, Swed.; Janssen-Cilag, Switz.; Janssen-Cilag, UK; Janssen, USA.*
Mebendazole (p.108·2).
*Worm infections.*

**Vernarin** *Nakornpatana, Thai.*
Cinnarizine (p.428·3).
*Cerebral and peripheral vascular disorders; migraine; motion sickness; vestibular disorders.*

**Vernausin** *Ofimex, Mex.†.*
Difenidol (p.1261·1).

**Vernelan** *Verla, Ger.†.*
Magnesium aspartate hydrobromide (p.706·1).
*Nervous disorders; sleep disorders.*

**Vernies** *Parke, Davis, Spain.*
Glyceryl trinitrate (p.923·2).
*Angina pectoris; heart failure; myocardial infarction.*

**Vernleigh Baby Cream** *Propan, S.Afr.; Covan, S.Afr.*
Zinc oxide (p.1163·2); starch.
*Skin disorders.*

**Verolax**
*Angelini, Ital.; Lepori, Port.; Farma Lepori, Spain.*
Glycerol (p.1694·3).
*Constipation.*

**Veroptinstada** *Stada, Ger.*
Verapamil hydrochloride (p.1019·1).
*Angina pectoris; arrhythmias; hypertension.*

**Verorab**
*Aventis Pasteur, Arg.; Aventis Pasteur, Braz.; Aventis Pasteur, Chile; Aventis, S.Afr.*
A rabies vaccine (Wistar PM/WI 38-1503-3M strain) (p.1635·3).
*Active immunisation.*

**verospiron** *Hormosan, Ger.*
Spironolactone (p.1003·1).
*Oedema.*

**Verotina** *Libbs, Braz.*
Fluoxetine hydrochloride (p.292·1).
*Bulimia nervosa; depression; obsessive-compulsive disorder.*

**Verotonil** *Bago, Chile.*
Vitamins; minerals; ginseng; rutoside; lecithin (p.1417·1).
*Dietary supplement; tonic.*

**Veroven** *Lepori, Port.*
Hidrosmin (p.1688·3).
*Cerebral and ocular vascular disorders; haemorrhoids; venous insufficiency; vestibular disorders.*

**Veroxil**
Note. This name is used for preparations of different composition.
*Anpharm (Ανφαρμ), Gr.*
Lisinopril (p.946·3).
*Heart failure; hypertension; myocardial infarction.*

*Baldacci, Ital.*
Indapamide (p.938·2).
*Hypertension.*

**Verpacor** *Pharmacia Upjohn, Fin.†.*
Verapamil hydrochloride (p.1019·1).
*Angina pectoris; arrhythmias; hypertension; myocardial infarction.*

**Verpamil**
*Orion, Fin.; Orion, Malaysia; Pacific, NZ; Orion, Singapore.*
Verapamil hydrochloride (p.1019·1).
*Angina pectoris; arrhythmias; hypertension; myocardial infarction.*

**Verpir** *Kleva, Gr.*
Aciclovir (p.626·1).
*Labial and genital herpes simplex infections.*

**Verra-med** *Permamed, Switz.*
Tretinoin (p.1161·1); salicylic acid (p.1157·1); dimethyl sulfoxide (p.1473·2).
*Warts.*

**Verrucare** *Medinfar, Port.*
Salicylic acid (p.1157·1); lactic acid (p.1704·1); fluorouracil (p.554·2).
*Warts.*

**Verrucid** *Galen, Ger.*
Salicylic acid (p.1157·1).
*Calluses; corns; warts.*

**Verruclean** *LDA, Arg.*
Lactic acid (p.1704·1); salicylic acid (p.1157·1).
*Warts.*

**Verrucosal** *Monal, Fr.†.*
Salicylic acid (p.1157·1).
*Warts.*

**Verrufilm**
Note. This name is used for preparations of different composition.
*Biorga, Fr.; Isopharm, Hong Kong†.*
Lactic acid (p.1704·1); salicylic acid (p.1157·1).
*Warts.*

*Medinfar, Port.; SSL, Switz.*
Salicylic acid (p.1157·1).
Formerly contained lactic acid and salicylic acid in *Port.*
*Corns; verrucas; warts.*

**Verrugon** *Pickles, UK.*
Salicylic acid (p.1157·1).
*Verrucas.*

**Verrulia** *Boiron, Fr.*
Homoeopathic preparation.

**Verrulyse-Methionine**
*Bournonville, Belg.†.*
Magnesium oxide (p.1272·3); methionine (p.1042·1); calcium glycerophosphate (p.1225·2); ferric glycerophosphate (p.1695·2); manganese glycerophosphate (p.1695·2); magnesium glycerophosphate (p.1228·1).
*Warts.*

*CS, Fr.*
Magnesium oxide (p.1272·3); methionine (p.1042·1); calcium glycerophosphate (p.1225·2); ferric glycerophosphate (p.1695·2); manganese glycerophosphate (p.1695·2).
*Warts.*

**Verrumal**
Note. This name is used for preparations of different composition.
*Hermal, Ger.; Hermal, Hong Kong; Hermal, Israel; Hermal, Malaysia; Hermal, Singapore; Boots Healthcare, Switz.; Boots, Thai.; Hermal, Thai.*
Fluorouracil (p.554·2); salicylic acid (p.1157·1); dimethyl sulfoxide (p.1473·2).
*Warts.*

*Boots Healthcare, Port.*
Fluorouracil (p.554·2); salicylic acid (p.1157·1).
*Solar keratoses; warts.*

**Verrupan** *Pharmadeveloppement, Fr.*
Thuja (p.1755·1); salicylic acid (p.1157·1); lactic acid (p.1704·1).
*Warts.*

**Verrupatch** *Vinas, Spain.*
Salicylic acid (p.1157·1).
*Warts.*

**Verruplan** *Vinas, Spain.*
Salicylic acid (p.1157·1).
*Warts.*

**Verrupor** *Sella, Ital.*
Trichloroacetic acid (p.1162·1).
*Hard skin; verrucas; warts.*

**Verrutopic** *Andromaco, Arg.*
Salicylic acid (p.1157·1); lactic acid (p.1704·1).
*Hyperkeratosis; warts.*

**Verrutopic AS** *Andromaco, Arg.*
Salicylic acid (p.1157·1).
*Warts.*

**Verrutrix** *Pharmatrix, Arg.*
Salicylic acid (p.1157·1).
*Warts.*

**Verrux** *Igefarma, Braz.†.*
Salicylic acid (p.1157·1).
Also contained lactic acid in GM.97.
*Hard skin; keratinisation disorders; warts.*

**Verruxane** *ICN, Arg.*
Salicylic acid (p.1157·1).
*Warts.*

**Versacaps** *Seatrace, USA.*
Pseudoephedrine hydrochloride (p.1129·2); guaifenesin (p.1122·1).
*Coughs.*

**Versal**
*Schering-Plough, Denm.; Schering-Plough, Norw.; Pro Medica, Swed.*
Loratadine (p.436·1).
*Allergic conjunctivitis; allergic rhinitis; urticaria.*

**Versamiv** *Novag, Mex.*
Diiodohydroxyquinoline (p.603·3).
*Amoebiasis.*

**Versan** *Sanfer, Mex.†.*
Dextromethorphan (p.1117·3).

**Versatic** *Duncan, Arg.*
Cefadroxil (p.167·2).
*Bacterial infections.*

**Versed**
*Roche, Canad.; Roche, USA.*
Midazolam hydrochloride (p.707·2).
*General anaesthesia; premedication; sedative.*

*Roche, Fr.*
Midazolam (p.707·1).
*Sedative.*

**Versel** *Trans Canaderm, Canad.*
Selenium sulfide (p.1157·3).
*Fungal skin infections.*

**Versiclear** *Hope, USA.*
Sodium thiosulfate (p.1053·3); salicylic acid (p.1157·1).
*Fungal infections.*

**Versigen** *Chew, Thai.*
Gentamicin (p.219·1).
*Bacterial skin infections.*

**Versiva**
*Convatec, Ital.*
Foamed hydrogel.
*Wounds.*

*Convatec, Port.*
Hydrocolloid and hydrofibre dressing.
*Burns; wounds.*

**Versol** *Aguettant, Fr.*
Sodium chloride (p.1233·3) or water for irrigation.

**Verstadol** *Bristol-Myers, Spain†.*
Butorphanol tartrate (p.23·3).
*Pain; premedication.*

**Versus**
*CSC, Austria; Angelini, Ital.*
Bendazac (p.20·3).
*Skin disorders.*

**Vertab** *Trinity, UK.*
Verapamil hydrochloride (p.1019·1).
*Angina pectoris; hypertension.*

**Vertebralon N** *Eberth, Ger.*
Glycol salicylate (p.44·3); nonivamide (p.67·2); salicylic acid (p.1157·1).
*Musculoskeletal, joint, and soft-tissue disorders.*

**Vertel** *Bial, Port.*
Pyrantel embonate (p.113·2).

**Vertex** *Carnot, Mex.*
Mebendazole (p.108·2).
*Worm infections.*

**Vertiginkgo** *Midax, Ital.*
Ginkgo biloba (p.1692·3); vitamin C; vitamin E; manganese (p.1417·1).
*Nutritional supplement.*

**Vertigirex** *Irex, Fr.†.*
Betahistine hydrochloride (p.1660·1).
*Vestibular disorders.*

**Vertigoheel**
*Peithner, Austria; Heel, Ger.; Heel, S.Afr.; Heel, USA.*
Homoeopathic preparation.

**Vertigo-Hevert** *Hevert, Ger.*
Homoeopathic preparation.

**Vertigo-Meresa** *Dolorgiet, Ger.*
Sulpiride (p.722·2).
*Ménière's disease.*

**Vertigon** *Gerard, Irl.*
Betahistine hydrochloride (p.1660·1).
*Ménière's disease.*

**vertigo-neogama** *Hormosan, Ger.*
Sulpiride (p.722·2).
*Vertigo.*

**Vertigopas** *Pascoe, Ger.*
Homoeopathic preparation.

**Vertigo-Vomex** *Yamanouchi, Ger.*
Dimenhydrinate (p.431·1).
*Vertigo; vestibular disorders.*

**Vertin** *Solvay, India.*
Betahistine hydrochloride (p.1660·1).
*Ménière's syndrome; vertigo.*

**Vertipam** *Orion, Fin.*
Diazepam (p.690·1); cyclizine hydrochloride (p.429·3); nicotinic acid (p.1441·1).
*Vestibular disorders.*

**Vertirosan** *Sigmapharm, Austria.*
Dimenhydrinate (p.431·1).
*Migraine; motion sickness; nausea and vomiting; vestibular disorders.*

**Vertirosan Vitamin $B_6$** *Sigmapharm, Austria.*
Dimenhydrinate (p.431·1); pyridoxine hydrochloride (p.1456·3).
*Migraine; motion sickness; nausea and vomiting; vestibular disorders.*

**Vertisal** *Silanes, Mex.*
Metronidazole (p.607·2) or metronidazole benzoate (p.607·2).
*Amoebiasis; anaerobic bacterial infections; giardiasis; trichomoniasis.*

**Vertiserc** *Solvay, Ital.*
Betahistine hydrochloride (p.1660·1).
*Vestibular disorders.*

**Vertix** *Ache, Braz.*
Flunarizine hydrochloride (p.434·1).
*Vertigo.*

**Vertizine D** *Ache, Braz.*
Dihydroergocristine mesilate (p.1680·1); flunarizine hydrochloride (p.434·1).
*Vertigo.*

**Vertizole** *Rayere, Mex.*
Mebendazole (p.108·2).
*Worm infections.*

**Verucasep** *Galen, Irl.†.*
Glutaral (p.1180·3).
*Warts.*

**Verucca Removal System** *SSL, UK†.*
Salicylic acid (p.1157·1).
*Verrucas.*

**Verucid**
Note. This name is used for preparations of different composition.
*Galderma, Denm.; Yamanouchi, Ital.†; Galderma, Norw.*
Salicylic acid (p.1157·1); lactic acid (p.1704·1).
*Hard skin; verrucas; warts.*

*Agis, Israel.*
Salicylic acid (p.1157·1); fluorouracil (p.554·2); dimethyl sulfoxide (p.1473·2).
*Warts.*

*Lepori, Port.*
Salicylic acid (p.1157·1).

**Verufil** *Stiefel, Spain.*
Lactic acid (p.1704·1); salicylic acid (p.1157·1).
*Warts.*

**Verunec** *Savoma, Ital.*
Salicylic acid (p.1157·1); lactic acid (p.1704·1); urea (p.1162·2).
*Hard skin; verrucas; warts.*

**Verutal** *Stiefel, Fr.†.*
Glutaral (p.1180·3).
*Warts.*

**Verutex** *Roche, Braz.*
Fusidic acid (p.215·2).
*Bacterial skin infections.*

**Very-Test** *Serch, Arg.*
Pregnancy test (p.1734·3).

**Verytracin** *Diba, Mex.*
Erythromycin (p.208·1).
*Bacterial infections.*

**Very-Vit** *Diba, Mex.*
Vitamin and mineral preparation (p.1417·1).

**Verzol** *Delta, Braz.*
Mebendazole (p.108·2).
*Worm infections.*

**Verzum** *Elofar, Braz.*
Cinnarizine (p.428·3).
*Vertigo.*

**Vesadol** *Janssen-Cilag, Fr.*
Haloperidol (p.701·2); buzepide metiodide (p.480·2).
*Gastrointestinal spasms associated with anxiety.*

**Vesagex**
*Rybar, Irl.; Co-Pharma, UK.*
Cetrimide (p.1172·1).
*Burns; minor wounds; skin disorders.*

**Vesagex Heelbalm** *Co-Pharma, UK.*
Allantoin (p.1141·3); peppermint oil (p.1283·2); urea (p.1162·2); moisturisers.
*Dry, cracked skin on the heels and soles of the feet.*

**Vesalion** *Bristol-Myers Squibb, Arg.*
Diclofenac diethylamine (p.32·1), diclofenac potassium (p.32·1), or diclofenac sodium (p.32·1).
*Inflammation; musculoskeletal, joint, and peri-articular disorders; pain.*

**Vesalion B12** *Bristol-Myers Squibb, Arg.*
Diclofenac potassium (p.32·1); betamethasone (p.1093·1) or betamethasone sodium phosphate (p.1093·1); cyanocobalamin (p.1458·2) or hydroxocobalamin (p.1458·2).
*Neuralgias.*

**Vesalion Flex** *Bristol-Myers Squibb, Arg.*
Diclofenac sodium (p.32·1); pridinol mesilate (p.1395·2).
*Inflammation; muscle spasm; pain.*

**Vesalion Gesic** *Bristol-Myers Squibb, Arg.*
Diclofenac potassium (p.32·1); paracetamol (p.76·2).
*Inflammation; pain.*

**Vesalium**
*Janssen-Cilag, Austria†; Janssen-Cilag, Belg.†.*
Haloperidol (p.701·2); isopropamide iodide (p.485·2).
*Anxiety; psychosomatic disorders.*

**Vesanoid**
*Roche, Arg.; Roche, Austral.; Roche, Austria; Roche, Belg.; Roche, Braz.; Roche, Canad.; Roche, Chile; Roche, Fin.; Roche, Fr.; Roche, Ger.; Roche, Gr.; Roche, Hong Kong; Roche, Israel; Roche, Ital.; Roche, Mex.; Roche, Neth.; Roche, Norw.†; Roche, NZ; Roche, Port.; Roche, S.Afr.; Roche, Singapore; Roche, Swed.†; Roche, Switz.; Roche, UK; Roche, USA.*
Tretinoin (p.1161·1).
*Acute promyelocytic leukaemia.*

**Vesdil**
*AstraZeneca, Ger.; Promed, Ger.; AstraZeneca, Switz.*
Ramipril (p.994·1).
*Heart failure; hypertension; myocardial infarction; nephropathy.*

**Vesdil plus** *AstraZeneca, Ger.; Promed, Ger.*
Ramipril (p.994·1); hydrochlorothiazide (p.933·2).
*Hypertension.*

**Vesibil** *Flopen, Braz.†.*
Choline (p.1424·3); vitamin B substances (p.1417·1).
*Liver disorders.*

**Vesiherb** *Cesra, Ger.*
Cucurbita (p.1677·3).
Formerly known as Prostaherb Cucurbitae.
*Prostatic disorders.*

**Vesilax** *Frega, Canad.†.*
Cascara (p.1255·1); phenolphthalein (p.1284·1); bile salts (p.1660·3); pancreatin (p.1725·3); papain (p.1727·3).

**Vesirig** *Aguettant, Fr.*
Sodium chloride (p.1233·3).
*Lavage and irrigation.*

**Vesix** *Nycomed, Fin.*
Furosemide (p.919·3).
*Hypertension; oedema.*

**Vesparax**
*UCB, Belg.†; UCB, Neth.†; UCB, Port.; UCB, S.Afr.†.*
Hydroxyzine (p.435·1); brallobarbital (p.671·3); secobarbital (p.721·2).
*Insomnia.*

**Vesprin** *Apothecon, USA†.*
Triflupromazine hydrochloride (p.727·1).
*Nausea; psychoses; vomiting.*

**Vessel** *Farmion, Braz.*
Cinnarizine (p.428·3).
*Peripheral vascular disorders; vertigo.*

**Vessel Due F**
*Wassermann, Ital.; Wassermann, Malaysia.*
Sulodexide (p.1009·2).
*Thrombosis prophylaxis.*

**Vesselvite** *Bajamar, USA.*
Folic acid; vitamin $B_6$; vitamin $B_{12}$; vitamin E (p.1417·1).

**Vessiflex** *Wassermann, Ital.*
Sulodexide (p.1009·2); aminopropylone (p.14·2).
*Inflammation; injuries associated with pain and swelling.*

**Vestaclav** *Xepa-Soul Pattinson, Malaysia.*
Amoxicillin (p.155·3); clavulanic acid (p.193·3).
*Bacterial infections.*

**Vesyca** *YSP, Malaysia.*
Ranitidine (p.1285·2).
*Acid aspiration; gastro-oesophageal reflux; gastrointestinal haemorrhage; peptic ulcer; Zollinger-Ellison syndrome.*

**Vetamol** *Viofar, Gr.*
Norfloxacin (p.238·3).
*Urinary tract infections.*

**Vetedol** *Robert, Spain†.*
Benorilate (p.20·3).
*Fever; musculoskeletal, joint, and peri-articular disorders; pain.*

**Vethisel** *Rafarm, Gr.*
Cefradine (p.179·3).
*Bacterial infections.*

**Vethoine** *Wolfs, Belg.*
Phenytoin (p.370·2); phenobarbital (p.367·3); cascara (p.1255·1).
*Epilepsy.*

**Vetio** *Elvetium, Arg.*
Mitomycin (p.573·3).
*Malignant neoplasms.*

**Vetiprost** *Elvetium, Arg.*
Finasteride (p.1554·2).
*Benign prostatic hyperplasia.*

**Vetren**
*Byk, Austria; Byk Gulden, Ger.; Roland, Ger.*
Heparin sodium (p.928·1).
*Soft-tissue injury; venous insufficiency.*

**Vetuss HC** *Cypress, USA†.*
Hydrocodone tartrate (p.45·1); phenylephrine hydrochloride (p.1126·3); phenylpropanolamine hydrochloride (p.1127·3); mepyramine maleate (p.437·1); pheniramine maleate (p.438·3).
*Coughs and related respiratory-tract disorders.*

**Vexol**
*Alcon, Austria; Alcon, Braz.; Alcon, Canad.; Alcon, Denm.; Alcon, Fin.; Alcon, Fr.; Alcon, Ger.; Alkon (Αλκον), Gr.; Alcon, Hong Kong; Alcon, Irl.; Alcon, Ital.; Alcon, Mex.; Alcon, Norw.; Alcon, Port.; Alcon Cusi, Spain†; Alcon, Swed.; Alcon, Switz.; Alcon, UK; Alcon, USA.*
Rimexolone (p.1110·1).
*Inflammatory eye disorders.*

**Vexolon** *Alcon, Belg.*
Rimexolone (p.1110·1).
*Inflammatory eye disorders.*

**Vexurat** *Medinova (Μεντινοβα), Gr.*
Famotidine (p.1265·2).
*Conditions where gastric acid reduction is beneficial; gastric hypersecretion including Zollinger-Ellison syndrome; peptic ulcer.*

**Veybirol-Tyrothyricine** *Veyron-Froment, Fr.*
Solution A: formaldehyde (p.1179·3); solution B: tyrothricin (p.275·1).
*Mouth infections.*

**Vfend**
*Pfizer, Austral.; Pfizer, Fr.; Pfizer, Irl.; Pfizer, Port.; Pfizer, Spain; Pfizer, UK; Roerig, USA.*
Voriconazole (p.411·2).
*Fungal infections.*

**Via Mal** *Byk Gulden, Ital.*
Aspirin (p.15·1); caffeine (p.782·1).
Aluminium hydroxide (p.1249·2) is included in this preparation in an attempt to limit the adverse effects of aspirin on the gastrointestinal mucosa.
*Fever; pain.*

**Via Mal Traumagel** *Byk Gulden, Ital.*
Diethylamine salicylate (p.34·1); heparin sodium (p.928·1); menthol (p.1711·3).
*Soft-tissue disorders.*

**Viabom** *CPH, Port.*
Dimenhydrinate (p.431·1).
*Motion sickness; vertigo.*

**Viacin** *Aspen, S.Afr.†.*
Doxycycline hyclate (p.206·2).
*Bacterial infections.*

**Viactiv** *Mead Johnson Nutritionals, Canad.*
Calcium carbonate (p.1254·2); colecalciferol (p.1461·3).
*Calcium and vitamin D supplement.*

**Viadent**
*Note. This name is used for preparations of different composition.*
*Carter Horner, Canad.†.*
*Mouthwash:* Sanguinaria (p.1741·3).

*Colgate-Palmolive, Canad.*
*Toothpaste:* Sanguinaria (p.1741·3); sodium monofluorophosphate (p.1446·2).
*Dental plaque; gingivitis.*

**Viaderm-KC** *Taro, Canad.*
Triamcinolone acetonide (p.1110·2); neomycin sulfate (p.235·1); nystatin (p.406·3); gramicidin (p.220·2).
*Infected skin disorders.*

**Viadetres** *Alacan, Spain.*
Hydroxocobalamin (p.1458·2); pyritinol hydrochloride (p.1737·2); prosultiamine (p.1455·1).
*Vitamin B deficiency.*

**Viadil** *Pharma Investi, Chile.*
Pargeverine hydrochloride (p.487·3).
*Smooth muscle spasm.*

**Viadil Compuesto** *Pharma Investi, Chile.*
Pargeverine hydrochloride (p.487·3); metamizole magnesium (p.36·1).
*Smooth muscle spasm and pain.*

**Viadur** *Alza, USA.*
Leuprorelin acetate (p.1331·1).
*Prostatic cancer.*

**Viafen** *Novartis Consumer, Ital.*
Bufexamac (p.21·3).
*Dermatitis; insect stings; pruritus.*

**Viafurox** *Fada, Arg.*
Furosemide (p.919·3).
*Diuresis.*

**Viaggio** *Vifor, Switz.†.*
Dimenhydrinate (p.431·1); atropine sulfate (p.477·1); hyoscyamine sulfate (p.485·1); hyoscine hydrobromide (p.483·3); caffeine (p.782·1).
*Motion sickness; nausea; vomiting.*

**Viagra**
*Pfizer, Austral.; Pfizer, Austria; Pfizer, Belg.; Pfizer, Braz.; Pfizer, Canad.; Pfizer, Chile; Pfizer, Denm.; Pfizer, Fin.; Pfizer, Fr.; Pfizer, Ger.; Pfizer, Gr.; Pfizer, Hong Kong; Pfizer, Irl.; Pfizer, Israel; Pfizer, Ital.; Pfizer, Jpn; Pfizer, Malaysia; Pfizer, Mex.; Pfizer, Norw.; Pfizer, NZ; Pfizer, Port.; Pfizer, S.Afr.; Pfizer, Singapore; Pfizer, Spain; Pfizer, Swed.; Pfizer, Switz.; Pfizer, Thai.; Pfizer, UK; Pfizer, USA.*
Sildenafil citrate (p.1744·2).
*Erectile dysfunction.*

**Vial's tonischer Wein** *Eberth, Ger.*
Calcium phospholactate; beef extract; cinchonine; wine.
*Tonic.*

**Viamon** *Nadeau, Canad.†.*
Multivitamin and mineral preparation (p.1417·1).

**Viani**
*Allen, Austria; Cascan, Ger.; GlaxoSmithKline, Ger.; Glaxo Wellcome, Gr.*
Salmeterol xinafoate (p.795·1); fluticasone propionate (p.1102·3).
*Asthma.*

**Viapres** *Zambon, Ital.*
Lacidipine (p.944·2).
*Hypertension.*

**Viarex** *Schering-Plough, Israel.*
Beclometasone dipropionate (p.1091·1).
*Asthma.*

**Viarox**
*Essex, Ger.; Schering-Plough, S.Afr.*
Beclometasone dipropionate (p.1091·1).
*Asthma; rhinitis.*

**Viartril**
*Note. This name is used for preparations of different composition.*
*Spedrog, Arg.*
Rofecoxib (p.86·3).
*Osteoarthritis; pain.*

*Rottapharm, Chile.*
Glucosamine sulfate (p.1694·1).
Lidocaine hydrochloride (p.1377·3) is included in the injection to alleviate the pain of injection.
*Degenerative joint disorders.*

*Rotta, Hong Kong†; Rotta, Thai.*
*Injection:* Glucosamine sulfate (p.1694·1); glucosamine hydriodide (p.1694·1).
Lidocaine hydrochloride (p.1377·3) is included in this preparation to alleviate the pain of injection.
*Musculoskeletal and joint disorders.*

*Bioresearch, Mex.; Rotta, Thai.*
Glucosamine sulfate (p.1694·1).
*Musculoskeletal and joint disorders.*

**Viartril S**
*Rotta, Hong Kong; Rottapharm, Ital.; Rotta, Malaysia; Delta, Port.; Rotta, Singapore.*
Glucosamine sulfate (p.1694·1).
Lidocaine hydrochloride (p.1377·3) may be included in the injection to alleviate the pain of injection.
*Joint and cartilage disorders.*

**Viaspan**
*Du Pont, Canad.†; Bristol-Myers Squibb, Malaysia; Bristol-Myers Squibb, Singapore.*
Solution for flushing and cold storage of donor organs.

**ViATIM** *Aventis, UK.*
An inactivated hepatitis A and typhoid (Vi polysaccharide) vaccine (p.1620·1).
*Active immunisation.*

**Viatine** *Essex, Spain†.*
Loratadine (p.436·1).
*Hypersensitivity reactions.*

**Viatol** *Lacteol, Fr.*
Anhydrous glucose; sodium chloride; potassium citrate (p.1222·2).
*Diarrhoea; oral rehydration therapy.*

**Viavent** *Byk Madaus, S.Afr.†.*
Salbutamol sulfate (p.791·3).
*Obstructive airways disease.*

**Viaxol** *Maver, Mex.*
Ambroxol (p.1114·3).
*Respiratory-tract disorders.*

**Viazem**
*Biovail, Denm.; Gea, Swed.; Genus, UK.*
Diltiazem hydrochloride (p.900·1).
*Angina pectoris; hypertension.*

**Vibalgan** *Doms-Adrian, Fr.†.*
Hydroxocobalamin acetate (p.1458·2); cobamamide (p.1459·1).
*Vitamin $B_{12}$ deficiency.*

**Vi-Balsabron** *Lacefa, Arg.*
Noscapine (p.1125·3); guaifenesin (p.1122·1); chlorphenamine (p.428·1).
*Coughs.*

**Vibazine** *Medibios, India.*
Doxycycline hyclate (p.206·2).
*Bacterial infections.*

**Vibeden** *Gea, Denm.*
Hydroxocobalamin (p.1458·2).
*Megaloblastic anaemia; vitamin $B_{12}$ deficiency.*

**Vibee**
*Biolab, Malaysia; Biolab, Singapore.*
Vitamin $B_1$; vitamin $B_6$; vitamin $B_{12}$ (p.1417·1).
*Neuritis; vitamin B deficiency.*

**Viberol Tirotricina** *Teofarma, Spain.*
Formaldehyde (p.1179·3); tyrothricin (p.275·1).
*Mouth and throat inflammation; oral hygiene.*

**Vibetrat** *Cimed, Braz.†.*
Vitamin $B_1$ (p.1455·2); vitamin $B_6$ (p.1457·2); vitamin $B_{12}$ (p.1458·2).
*Vitamin B deficiency.*

**Vibetrat Dexa** *Cimed, Braz.†.*
Dexamethasone acetate (p.1097·1); vitamin $B_1$ (p.1455·2); vitamin $B_6$ (p.1457·2); vitamin $B_{12}$ (p.1458·2).
*Neuritis.*

**Vibion** *Jean-Marie, Hong Kong.*
Vitamin B substances (p.1417·1).
*Neuralgias; neuritis; neuropathies; vitamin B deficiencies.*

**Vibolex E** *MIP, Ger.*
*d*-Alpha tocoferil acetate (p.1465·1) or *dl*-alpha tocoferil acetate (p.1465·1).
*Vitamin E deficiency.*

**Vibracina** *Pfizer, Spain.*
Doxycycline hyclate (p.206·2).
*Bacterial infections; malaria.*

**Vibradox** *Durascan, Denm.*
Doxycycline (p.206·2).
*Bacterial infections.*

**Vibragel** *Novartis, Arg.*
Dimetindene maleate (p.431·2); phenylephrine (p.1126·3).
*Nasal congestion.*

**Vibral** *Sintofarma, Braz.*
Dropropizine (p.1119·3).
*Coughs.*

**Vibramicina**
*Pfizer, Arg.; Pfizer, Braz.; Pfizer, Chile; Pfizer, Mex.; Pfizer, Port.*
Doxycycline (p.206·2), doxycycline carrageenate (p.206·3), or doxycycline hyclate (p.206·2).
*Amoebiasis; bacterial infections; malaria.*

**Vibramycin**
*Pfizer, Austral.; Pfizer, Austria; Pfizer, Canad.†; Pfizer, Denm.; Pfizer, Ger.; Pfizer, Gr.; Pfizer, Hong Kong; Invicta, Irl.; Pfizer, Israel; Pfizer, Malaysia; Pfizer, Neth.; Pfizer, Norw.; Pfizer, S.Afr.; Pfizer, Singapore; Pfizer, Swed.; Pfizer, Thai.; Pfizer, UK; Pfizer, USA.*
Doxycycline (p.206·2), doxycycline calcium (p.206·2), doxycycline carrageenate (p.206·3), or doxycycline hyclate (p.206·2).
*Bacterial infections; intestinal amoebiasis; malaria.*

**Vibramycine**
*Pfizer, Belg.*
Doxycycline hyclate (p.206·2).
*Bacterial infections; malaria.*

*Pfizer, Switz.*
Doxycycline (p.206·2).
*Bacterial infections.*

**Vibramycine N** *CS, Fr.*
Doxycycline (p.206·2).
*Bacterial infections.*

**Vibra-S** *Pfizer, Neth.*
Doxycycline (p.206·2).
*Bacterial infections.*

**Vibratab** *Pfizer, Belg.*
Doxycycline (p.206·2).
*Bacterial infections; malaria.*

**Vibra-Tabs**
*Pfizer, Austral.; Pfizer, Canad.; Pfizer, USA.*
Doxycycline hyclate (p.206·2).
*Bacterial infections; intestinal amoebiasis; malaria.*

**Vibraveineuse**
*Pfizer, Fr.†; Pfizer, Switz.*
Doxycycline hyclate (p.206·2).
*Bacterial infections.*

**Vibravenos**
*Pfizer, Austria; Pfizer, Ger.; Pfizer, Israel†.*
Doxycycline (p.206·2) or doxycycline hyclate (p.206·2).
*Bacterial infections.*

**Vibravenosa** *Pfizer, Spain.*
Doxycycline hyclate (p.206·2).
*Bacterial infections; malaria.*

**Vibrocil**
*Note. This name is used for preparations of different composition.*
*Novartis Consumer, Austria; Novartis Consumer, Belg.; Novartis Consumer, Ger.; Novartis, Hong Kong; Novartis Consumer, Ital.; Novartis Consumer, Port.; Novartis Consumer, Switz.*
Dimetindene maleate (p.431·2); phenylephrine (p.1126·3).
*Otitis media; rhinitis; sinusitis.*

*Novartis Consumer, Belg.*
*Capsules:* Dimetindene maleate (p.431·2); pseudoephedrine hydrochloride (p.1129·2).
*Allergic rhinitis; sinusitis; vasomotor rhinitis.*

*Novartis Consumer, S.Afr.*
Dimetindene maleate (p.431·2); phenylephrine (p.1126·3); neomycin sulfate (p.235·1).
*Nasal disorders; sinusitis.*

**Vibrocil NF** *Novartis, Israel.*
Dimetindene maleate (p.431·2); phenylephrine (p.1126·3).
*Nasal congestion; otitis media; rhinitis; sinusitis.*

**Vibrocil-S** *Novartis Consumer, S.Afr.*
Dimetindene maleate (p.431·2); phenylephrine (p.1126·3).
*Nasal and sinus congestion.*

**Vibrumin** *General Drugs, Thai.*
Vitamin B substances (p.1417·1).

**Vibtil**
*Therabel, Belg.; Lafon, Fr.*
Tilia (p.1756·2).
*Dyspepsia.*

**Viburcol** *Heel, S.Afr.*
Homoeopathic preparation.

**Viburcol N** *Heel, Ger.*
Homoeopathic preparation.

**Viburnum Complex** *Blackmores, Austral.†.*
Viburnum opulus; cimicifuga (p.1671·3); angelica sinensis (p.1655·1); pulsatilla (p.1737·1); *d*-alpha tocoferil acid succinate (p.1465·1).
*Gynaecological disorders; muscle cramp.*

**Vi-C** *Sam-On, Israel.*
Ascorbic acid (p.1460·2).
*Vitamin C deficiency.*

**Vicam** *Keene, USA.*
Vitamin B substances (p.1417·1).
*Parenteral nutrition.*

**Vicapan N** *Merckle, Ger.*
Cyanocobalamin (p.1458·2).
*Vitamin $B_{12}$ deficiency.*

**Vi-Caps**
*Grossmann, Hong Kong; Grossmann, Switz.*
Multivitamin and mineral preparation (p.1417·1).

**Vicard** *Abbott, Austria.*
Terazosin hydrochloride (p.1010·3).
*Hypertension.*

**Viccillin** *Meiji, Thai.*
Ampicillin sodium (p.157·1) or ampicillin trihydrate (p.157·2).
*Bacterial infections.*

**Viccillin-S** *Meiji, Thai.*
Ampicillin (p.157·1); cloxacillin (p.198·2).
*Bacterial infections.*

**Vi-Ce** *Novartis, Braz.*
Ascorbic acid (p.1460·2).
*Vitamin C deficiency; vitamin C supplement.*

**Vicedent** *Terramin, Austria*†.
Ascorbic acid (p.1460·2).
*Gum disorders.*

**Vicefeno** *Fabra, Arg.*
Dextropropoxyphene (p.28·3); dipyrone (p.35·3).
*Pain.*

**Vicemex**
*Cimex, Hong Kong; Cimex, Switz.*
Ascorbic acid (p.1460·2).
*Vitamin C deficiency; vitamin C supplement.*

**Vicenrik** *Fada, Arg.*
Ascorbic acid (p.1460·2).
*Vitamin C supplement.*

**ViCetamol** *Gebro, Austria.*
Paracetamol (p.76·2); ascorbic acid (p.1460·2).
*Cold symptoms.*

**Vichy-Autobronzant** *Vichy, Canad.*
*SPF 7:* Avobenzone (p.1142·3); enzacamene (p.1147·1); ecamsule (p.1146·3).
*Sunscreen.*

**Vichy-Creme Ecran Total** *Vichy, Canad.*
*SPF 25:* Avobenzone (p.1142·3); octocrilene (p.1154·3); ecamsule (p.1146·3); titanium dioxide (p.1160·3).
*Sunscreen.*

**Vichy-Lait Ecran Enfants** *Vichy, Canad.*
*SPF 35:* Avobenzone (p.1142·3); octocrilene (p.1154·3); ecamsule (p.1146·3); titanium dioxide (p.1160·3).
*Sunscreen.*

**Vichy-Lait Ecran Extreme** *Vichy, Canad.*
*SPF 60:* Avobenzone (p.1142·3); enzacamene (p.1147·1); ecamsule (p.1146·3); titanium dioxide (p.1160·3).
*Sunscreen.*

**Vichy-Lait Protecteur** *Vichy, Canad.*
*SPF 15:* Avobenzone (p.1142·3); octocrilene (p.1154·3); ecamsule (p.1146·3); titanium dioxide (p.1160·3).
*Sunscreen.*

**Vici** *Monico, Ital.*
Ascorbic acid (p.1460·2).
*Vitamin C deficiency.*

**Vicilan** *Zeneca, Ital.*†.
Viloxazine hydrochloride (p.323·3).
*Depression.*

**Vicitina** *CT, Ital.*†.
Ascorbic acid (p.1460·2).
*Gingivitis; stomatitis; vitamin C deficiency.*

**Vick 44 Exp** *Procter & Gamble, Arg.*
Guaifenesin (p.1122·1).
*Coughs.*

**Vick Inalador** *Procter & Gamble, Braz.*
Camphor (p.1665·3); menthol (p.1711·3); methyl salicylate (p.59·3); Siberian fir oil.
*Nasal congestion.*

**Vick Pastilhas** *Procter & Gamble, Braz.*†.
Cineole (p.1672·1); menthol (p.1711·3); camphor (p.1665·3); tolu balsam (p.1131·3).

**Vick Pyrena** *Procter & Gamble, Braz.*
Paracetamol (p.76·2); vitamin C (p.1460·2).
*Cold and influenza symptoms.*

**Vick Sinex** *Procter & Gamble, Arg.*
Oxymetazoline hydrochloride (p.1126·1).
*Nasal congestion.*

**Vick Vaporub**
*Note. This name is used for preparations of different composition.*
*Procter & Gamble, Arg.*
Menthol (p.1711·3); camphor (p.1665·3); methyl salicylate (p.59·3); siberian fir oil.
*Nasal congestion.*

*Procter & Gamble, Braz.*
Menthol (p.1711·3); camphor (p.1665·3); eucalyptus oil (p.1686·2); nutmeg oil (p.1722·3); cedar leaf oil; turpentine oil (p.1760·1); thymol (p.1194·2).
*Nasal congestion.*

*Procter & Gamble, Mex.*
Menthol (p.1711·3); camphor (p.1665·3).
*Cold symptoms; nasal congestion.*

**Vick Vaporub NF** *Procter & Gamble, Arg.*
Menthol (p.1711·3); camphor (p.1665·3); eucalyptus oil (p.1686·2).
*Nasal congestion.*

**Vick Vitapyrena** *Procter & Gamble, Arg.*
Paracetamol (p.76·2).
*Fever; pain.*

**Vick Xarope** *Procter & Gamble, Braz.*
Guaifenesin (p.1122·1).
*Coughs.*

**Vicks Action** *Procter & Gamble, UK*†.
Ibuprofen (p.45·3); pseudoephedrine (p.1129·2).
*Cold symptoms.*

**Vicks Blue Drops** *Procter & Gamble, Austral.*†.
Menthol (p.1711·3); peppermint oil (p.1283·2).
*Throat irritation.*

**Vicks Chest Congestion Relief** *Procter & Gamble, Canad.*
Guaifenesin (p.1122·1).

**Vicks Children's Chloraseptic** *Procter & Gamble, USA.*
*Lozenges:* Benzocaine (p.1370·3).
*Throat spray:* Phenol (p.1188·1).
*Sore throat.*

**Vicks Children's NyQuil Allergy/Head Cold** *Richardson-Vicks, USA.*
Pseudoephedrine hydrochloride (p.1129·2); chlorphenamine maleate (p.427·3).
*Upper respiratory-tract symptoms.*

**Vicks Children's NyQuil Night-time Cold/Cough Liquid** *Richardson-Vicks, USA.*
Chlorphenamine maleate (p.427·3); pseudoephedrine hydrochloride (p.1129·2); dextromethorphan hydrobromide (p.1117·3).
*Coughs and cold symptoms.*

**Vicks Chloraseptic**
*Note. This name is used for preparations of different composition.*
*Procter & Gamble, Irl.*†; *Procter & Gamble, USA.*
Phenol (p.1188·1).
*Oral hygiene; sore throat.*

*Procter & Gamble (H&B Care), UK*†.
Phenol (p.1188·1); sodium phenolate.
*Oral hygiene; sore throat.*

**Vicks Chloraseptic Sore Throat** *Procter & Gamble, USA.*
Benzocaine (p.1370·3); menthol (p.1711·3).
*Sore throat.*

**Vicks Cold Care** *Procter & Gamble (H&B Care), UK*†.
Paracetamol (p.76·2); dextromethorphan (p.1117·3); phenylpropanolamine (p.1127·3).
*Cold symptoms.*

**Vicks Cough Drops** *Procter & Gamble, USA.*
Menthol (p.1711·3).
*Sore throat.*

**Vicks 44 Cough Relief** *Procter & Gamble, USA.*
Dextromethorphan hydrobromide (p.1117·3).
*Coughs.*

**Vicks Cough Silencers** *Richardson-Vicks, USA*†.
Dextromethorphan hydrobromide (p.1117·3); benzocaine (p.1370·3).
*Coughs.*

**Vicks Cough Syrup**
*Note. This name is used for preparations of different composition.*
*Procter & Gamble, Austral.*†.
Pentoxyverine citrate (p.1126·2); menthol (p.1711·3).
*Coughs.*

*Procter & Gamble, Canad.*†.
Ephedrine (p.1120·1); guaifenesin (p.1122·1); pentoxyverine citrate (p.1126·2).

**Vicks Cough Syrup for Chesty Coughs** *Procter & Gamble, Austral.*
Guaifenesin (p.1122·1).
*Coughs.*

**Vicks 44D Cough & Head Congestion** *Procter & Gamble, USA.*
Dextromethorphan hydrobromide (p.1117·3); pseudoephedrine hydrochloride (p.1129·2).
*Coughs and cold symptoms.*

**Vicks DayQuil** *Richardson-Vicks, USA.*
Pseudoephedrine hydrochloride (p.1129·2); dextromethorphan hydrobromide (p.1117·3); guaifenesin (p.1122·1); paracetamol (p.76·2).
*Coughs.*

**Vicks DayQuil Allergy Relief** *Procter & Gamble, USA*†.
Phenylpropanolamine hydrochloride (p.1127·3); brompheniramine maleate (p.426·1).

**Vicks DayQuil Sinus Pressure & Pain Relief** *Procter & Gamble, USA.*
Pseudoephedrine hydrochloride (p.1129·2); paracetamol (p.76·2).

**Vicks Dry Hacking Cough** *Procter & Gamble, USA*†.
Dextromethorphan hydrobromide (p.1117·3).
Formerly known as Vicks Formula 44.
*Coughs.*

**Vicks 44E** *Procter & Gamble, USA.*
Dextromethorphan hydrobromide (p.1117·3); guaifenesin (p.1122·1).
*Coughs.*

**Vicks Expectorant**
*Note. This name is used for preparations of different composition.*
*Lachartre, Fr.*
Guaifenesin (p.1122·1).
Formerly known as Vicks Vaposyrup Expectorant.
*Respiratory-tract congestion.*

*Procter & Gamble (H&B Care), UK*†.
Guaifenesin (p.1122·1); cetylpyridinium chloride (p.1173·1); sodium citrate (p.1223·2).
*Coughs.*

**Vicks Formel 44** *Procter & Gamble, Switz.*†.
Dextromethorphan (p.1117·3); benzocaine (p.1370·3); cetylpyridinium chloride (p.1173·1); menthol (p.1711·3); peppermint oil (p.1283·2).
*Coughs; sore throat.*

**Vicks Formula 44**
*Note. This name is used for preparations of different composition.*
*Procter & Gamble, NZ.*
Dextromethorphan hydrobromide (p.1117·3); menthol (p.1711·3).
*Coughs.*

*Procter & Gamble, Spain.*
Anethole (p.1654·3); cetylpyridinium chloride (p.1173·1); dextromethorphan (p.1117·3); benzocaine (p.1370·3); peppermint oil (p.1283·2); menthol (p.1711·3).
*Coughs.*

**Vicks Formula 44 Cough Control Discs** *Richardson-Vicks, USA*†.
Dextromethorphan hydrobromide (p.1117·3); benzocaine (p.1370·3).
*Coughs.*

**Vicks Formule 44 Calmine** *Procter & Gamble, Switz.*
Dextromethorphan (p.1117·3) or dextromethorphan hydrobromide (p.1117·3).
*Coughs.*

**Vicks Formule 44 Expectine** *Procter & Gamble, Switz.*
Guaifenesin (p.1122·1).
*Respiratory-tract disorders with viscous mucus.*

**Vicks Inalante** *Procter & Gamble, Ital.*
Menthol (p.1711·3); camphor (p.1665·3); methyl salicylate (p.59·3); pine oil.
*Nasal congestion.*

**Vicks Inhalador** *Procter & Gamble, Spain.*
Camphor (p.1665·3); menthol (p.1711·3).
Formerly contained camphor, methyl salicylate, sassafras oil, menthol, and bornyl acetate.
*Nasal congestion.*

**Vicks Inhaler**
*Note. This name is used for preparations of different composition.*
*Procter & Gamble, Austral.*†; *Procter & Gamble, NZ.*
Menthol (p.1711·3); camphor (p.1665·3); methyl salicylate (p.59·3); pumilio pine oil (p.1737·1).
*Nasal congestion.*

*Procter & Gamble, Canad.*
Menthol (p.1711·3); camphor (p.1665·3).
*Nasal congestion.*

*Procter & Gamble, Irl.*†.
Menthol (p.1711·3); camphor (p.1665·3); pine needle oil.
*Nasal congestion.*

*Richardson-Vicks, Israel*†.
Menthol (p.1711·3); camphor (p.1665·3); pine-needle oil; methyl salicylate (p.59·3).
*Nasal congestion.*

*Procter & Gamble (H&B Care), UK.*
Menthol (p.1711·3); camphor (p.1665·3); siberian fir oil.
*Nasal congestion.*

**Vicks Inhaler N** *Procter & Gamble, Switz.*
Menthol (p.1711·3); camphor (p.1665·3); methyl salicylate (p.59·3); pine needle oil.
*Nasal congestion.*

**Vicks 44M Cold, Flu & Cough LiquiCaps** *Procter & Gamble, USA.*
Dextromethorphan hydrobromide (p.1117·3); pseudoephedrine hydrochloride (p.1129·2); chlorphenamine maleate (p.427·3); paracetamol (p.76·2).

**Vicks Medinait**
*Note. This name is used for preparations of different composition.*
*Procter & Gamble, Ital.*
Dextromethorphan hydrobromide (p.1117·3); doxylamine succinate (p.432·3); paracetamol (p.76·2).
Formerly contained dextromethorphan hydrobromide, doxylamine succinate, ephedrine sulfate, and paracetamol.
*Cold and influenza symptoms.*

*Procter & Gamble, Spain; Procter & Gamble, Switz.*
Dextromethorphan hydrobromide (p.1117·3); doxylamine succinate (p.432·3); ephedrine sulfate (p.1120·1); paracetamol (p.76·2).
*Influenza and cold symptoms.*

**Vicks Medinite** *Procter & Gamble (H&B Care), UK.*
Dextromethorphan hydrobromide (p.1117·3); doxylamine succinate (p.432·3); pseudoephedrine hydrochloride (p.1129·2); paracetamol (p.76·2).
*Cold symptoms.*

**Vicks Menthol Cough Drops** *Procter & Gamble, USA.*
Menthol (p.1711·3); thymol (p.1194·2); eucalyptus oil (p.1686·2); camphor (p.1665·3); tolu balsam (p.1131·3).
*Sore throat.*

**Vicks 44 Non-Drowsy Cold & Cough LiquiCaps** *Procter & Gamble, USA.*
Dextromethorphan hydrobromide (p.1117·3); pseudoephedrine hydrochloride (p.1129·2).

**Vicks NyQuil LiquiCaps** *Richardson-Vicks, USA.*
Dextromethorphan hydrobromide (p.1117·3); paracetamol (p.76·2); pseudoephedrine hydrochloride (p.1129·2); doxylamine succinate (p.432·3).
*Coughs and cold symptoms.*

**Vicks NyQuil Multi-Symptom Cold Flu Relief** *Procter & Gamble, USA.*
Pseudoephedrine hydrochloride (p.1129·2); doxylamine succinate (p.432·3); dextromethorphan hydrobromide (p.1117·3); paracetamol (p.76·2).
*Cold symptoms.*

**Vicks Original Cough Syrup for Chesty Coughs** *Procter & Gamble, Irl.*†.
Guaifenesin (p.1122·1); cetylpyridinium chloride (p.1173·1); sodium citrate (p.1223·2).
*Coughs.*

**Vicks Pediatric Formula 44D Dry Hacking Cough & Head Congestion** *Procter & Gamble, USA*†.
Pseudoephedrine hydrochloride (p.1129·2); dextromethorphan hydrobromide (p.1117·3).
Formerly known as Vicks Formula 44D Pediatric.
*Coughs and cold symptoms.*

**Vicks Pediatric Formula 44E** *Richardson-Vicks, USA.*
Dextromethorphan hydrobromide (p.1117·3); guaifenesin (p.1122·1).
*Coughs.*

**Vicks Pediatric Formula 44M Multi-Symptom Cough & Cold** *Richardson-Vicks, USA.*
Pseudoephedrine hydrochloride (p.1129·2); dextromethorphan hydrobromide (p.1117·3); chlorphenamine maleate (p.427·3).
*Coughs and cold symptoms.*

**Vicks Rhume** *Lachartre, Fr.*
Ibuprofen (p.45·3); pseudoephedrine hydrochloride (p.1129·2).
*Rhinitis.*

**Vicks Sinex**
*Note. This name is used for preparations of different composition.*
*Procter & Gamble, Austral.; Procter & Gamble, Ital.; Procter & Gamble, NZ; Procter & Gamble, Switz.*
Oxymetazoline hydrochloride (p.1126·1); menthol (p.1711·3); camphor (p.1665·3); cineole (p.1672·1).
*Nasal congestion.*

*Procter & Gamble, Belg.; Procter & Gamble, Canad.; Procter & Gamble, Fin.; Procter & Gamble, Irl.*†; *Procter & Gamble, Neth.; Procter & Gamble (H&B Care), UK.*
Oxymetazoline hydrochloride (p.1126·1).
*Nasal congestion.*

**Vicks Sinex 12-Hour** *Procter & Gamble, USA.*
Oxymetazoline hydrochloride (p.1126·1).
Formerly known as Sinex Long Acting.
*Nasal congestion.*

**Vicks Spray** *Procter & Gamble, Spain.*
Oxymetazoline hydrochloride (p.1126·1); menthol (p.1711·3).
*Nasal congestion.*

**Vicks Throat Drops**
*Procter & Gamble, Austral.*†; *Procter & Gamble, Canad.*
Menthol (p.1711·3).
*Coughs; throat irritation.*

**Vicks Tosse Fluidificante** *Procter & Gamble, Ital.*
Guaifenesin (p.1122·1).
*Respiratory-tract congestion.*

**Vicks Tosse Pastiglie** *Procter & Gamble, Ital.*
Dextromethorphan (p.1117·3).
*Coughs.*

**Vicks Tosse Sedativo** *Procter & Gamble, Ital.*
Dextromethorphan hydrobromide (p.1117·3).
*Coughs.*

**Vicks Toux Seche** *Lachartre, Fr.*
Dextromethorphan hydrobromide (p.1117·3).
*Coughs.*

**Vicks Vapodrops** *Procter & Gamble, Austral.*†.
Menthol (p.1711·3); eucalyptus oil (p.1686·2).
*Nasal congestion; sore throat.*

**Vicks Vapodrops with Butter and Menthol** *Procter & Gamble, Austral.*†.
Menthol (p.1711·3).
*Nasal congestion; sore throat.*

**Vicks Vapor Inhaler** *Procter & Gamble, USA.*
Levmetamfetamine (p.1124·1).
*Nasal congestion.*

**Vicks Vaporub**
*Note. This name is used for preparations of different composition.*
*Procter & Gamble, Austral.*†.
Menthol (p.1711·3); camphor (p.1665·3); eucalyptus oil (p.1686·2); turpentine oil (p.1760·1); nutmeg oil (p.1722·3); cedar leaf oil.
*Cold symptoms; muscle pain.*

*Procter & Gamble, Belg.; Lachartre, Fr.; Procter & Gamble, NZ; Procter & Gamble, Swed.*
Menthol (p.1711·3); camphor (p.1665·3); eucalyptus oil (p.1686·2); turpentine oil (p.1760·1); nutmeg oil (p.1722·3); cedar wood oil; thymol (p.1194·2).
*Cold and influenza symptoms.*

*Procter & Gamble, Canad.*
Menthol (p.1711·3); camphor (p.1665·3); eucalyptus oil (p.1686·2).
*Cold symptoms.*

*Procter & Gamble, Fin.; Procter & Gamble, Neth.*
Menthol (p.1711·3); camphor (p.1665·3); eucalyptus oil (p.1686·2); turpentine oil (p.1760·1); thymol (p.1194·2).
*Cold and influenza symptoms.*

*Procter & Gamble, Irl.*†; *Procter & Gamble, Ital.; Procter & Gamble (H&B Care), UK.*
Menthol (p.1711·3); camphor (p.1665·3); eucalyptus oil (p.1686·2); turpentine oil (p.1760·1).
*Respiratory-tract congestion.*

*Procter & Gamble, Spain.*
Menthol (p.1711·3); camphor (p.1665·3); eucalyptus oil (p.1686·2); turpentine; thymol (p.1194·2).
*Upper-respiratory-tract disorders.*

*Procter & Gamble, USA.*
Menthol (p.1711·3); camphor (p.1665·3); eucalyptus oil (p.1686·2); cedar leaf oil.

**Vicks Vaporub N** Procter & Gamble, Switz.
Menthol (p.1711·3); camphor (p.1665·3); eucalyptus oil (p.1686·2); turpentine oil (p.1760·1); nutmeg oil (p.1722·3); cedar leaf oil; thymol (p.1194·2).
*Upper respiratory-tract disorders.*

**Vicks Vaposiroop** Procter & Gamble, Neth.
Dextromethorphan hydrobromide (p.1117·3).
*Coughs.*

**Vicks Vaposyrup** Procter & Gamble, Canad.†.
Menthol (p.1711·3).

**Vicks Vaposyrup Antitussif** Procter & Gamble, Belg.
Dextromethorphan hydrobromide (p.1117·3).
*Coughs.*

**Vicks Vaposyrup for Chesty Coughs** Procter & Gamble (H&B Care), UK.
Guaifenesin (p.1122·1).
*Coughs.*

**Vicks Vaposyrup for Dry Coughs** Procter & Gamble (H&B Care), UK.
Dextromethorphan hydrobromide (p.1117·3).
*Coughs.*

**Vicks Vaposyrup Expectorant** Procter & Gamble, Belg.
Guaifenesin (p.1122·1).
*Coughs; respiratory-tract disorders associated with mucus accumulation.*

**Vicks Vaposyrup for Tickly Coughs** Procter & Gamble (H&B Care), UK.
Menthol (p.1711·3).
*Coughs.*

**Vicks Vapotab** Procter & Gamble, Neth.
Dextromethorphan (p.1117·3).
*Coughs.*

**Vicks Victors Dual Action Cough Drops** Richardson-Vicks, USA.
Menthol (p.1711·3); eucalyptus oil (p.1686·2).

**Vicks Vital** Procter & Gamble (H&B Care), UK.
Ascorbic acid (p.1460·2); zinc acetate (p.1469·2).

**Vi-Claro** Abbott, Chile.
Naphazoline hydrochloride (p.1124·3).
*Eye irritation.*

**Viclor** Richet, Arg.
Paracetamol (p.76·2).
*Fever; pain.*

**Viclor Grip** Richet, Arg.
Paracetamol (p.76·2); ascorbic acid (p.1460·2); levophenylephrine (p.1127·2).

**Vicmafen** Offenbach, Mex.
Diclofenac sodium (p.32·1).
*Dysmenorrhoea; musculoskeletal, joint, and peri-articular disorders.*

**Vicnas** Sanofi Synthelabo, Spain†.
Norfloxacin (p.238·3).
*Urinary-tract infections.*

**Vicodin** Abbott, USA.
Hydrocodone tartrate (p.45·1); paracetamol (p.76·2).
*Pain.*

**Vicodin Tuss** Abbott, USA.
Hydrocodone tartrate (p.45·1); guaifenesin (p.1122·1).
*Coughs.*

**Vicoferell** Sanorell, Ger.†.
Multivitamin and iron preparation (p.1417·1).

**Vicombil** Bial, Port.
Multivitamin preparation (p.1417·1).

**Vicomin A C** Pfizer Lambert, Spain.
Ascorbic acid (p.1460·2); vitamin A palmitate (p.1453·1).
*Deficiency of vitamins A and C.*

**Vicon** UCB, USA.
A range of vitamin preparations with or without minerals (p.1417·1).

**Vicoprofen** Abbott, USA.
Hydrocodone tartrate (p.45·1); ibuprofen (p.45·3).
*Pain.*

**Vicortin** Vitae, Mex.†.
Hydrocortisone (p.1103·3).
*Skin disorders.*

**Vicrom**
Aventis, Israel; Aventis, NZ.
Sodium cromoglicate (p.795·3).
*Asthma; bronchitis.*

**Victan**
Sanofi Synthelabo, Arg.; Sanofi Synthelabo, Belg.; Sanofi Synthelabo, Fr.; Sanofi Synthelabo, Mex.; CPH, Port.; Sanofi Synthelabo, Thai.
Ethyl loflazepate (p.698·1).
*Alcohol withdrawal syndrome; anxiety; sleep disorders.*

**Victoril** Unipharm, Israel.
Dibenzepin (p.290·3).
*Depression.*

**Victrix** Farmasa, Braz.
Omeprazole (p.1278·2) or omeprazole sodium (p.1278·2).
*Gastro-oesophageal reflux; gastrointestinal hyperacidity; peptic ulcer.*

**Vida Brown Mixture** Vida, Hong Kong.
Liquorice (p.1270·2); camphorated opium (p.74·2).
*Catarrh; coughs.*

**Vida Cough** Vida, Hong Kong.
Chlorphenamine maleate (p.427·3); bromhexine hydrochloride (p.1115·3); pentoxyverine citrate (p.1126·2); guaifenesin (p.1122·1).
*Cold and influenza symptoms; coughs.*

**Vida Famodine** Vida, Hong Kong.
Famotidine (p.1265·2).
*Gastro-oesophageal reflux; gastrointestinal haemorrhage; peptic ulcer; Zollinger-Ellison syndrome.*

**Vida Fenadine** Vida, Hong Kong.
Terfenadine (p.441·1).
*Hypersensitivity reactions.*

**Vida Flatugel** Vida, Hong Kong.
Aluminium hydroxide (p.1249·2); magnesium hydroxide (p.1272·2); simeticone (p.1289·2).
*Gastrointestinal disorders.*

**Vida Neurotab** Vida, Hong Kong.
Vitamin $B_1$ (p.1454·3); vitamin $B_6$ (p.1456·3); vitamin $B_{12}$ (p.1458·2).
*Muscle and joint pain; neuralgia; neuritis; vitamin B deficiency.*

**Vida Salirub** Vida, Hong Kong.
Methyl salicylate (p.59·3); menthol (p.1711·3); eucalyptus oil (p.1686·2); cajuput oil (p.1664·1).
*Insect bites; muscle pain; soft-tissue disorders.*

**Vida-Butaline** Vida, Hong Kong.
Terbutaline sulfate (p.797·2).
*Asthma; chronic bronchitis.*

**Vidaclofen-Plus** Vida, Hong Kong.
Diclofenac sodium (p.32·1); vitamin $B_1$ (p.1454·3); vitamin $B_6$ (p.1456·3); vitamin $B_{12}$ (p.1458·2).
*Musculoskeletal, joint, and soft-tissue disorders; neuralgias; neuritis.*

**Vidaclovir** Vida, Hong Kong.
Aciclovir (p.626·1).
*Herpesvirus infections.*

**Vi-Dailin** Abbott, Port.
Multivitamin preparation (p.1417·1).

**Vidalat** Vida, Hong Kong.
Nifedipine (p.966·2).
*Angina pectoris; hypertension.*

**Vidalidine** Vida, Hong Kong.
Triprolidine hydrochloride (p.442·3); pseudoephedrine hydrochloride (p.1129·2).
*Allergic rhinitis; cold and influenza symptoms; nasal congestion.*

**Vidan** Vianex (Βιανεξ), Gr.
Mefenamic acid (p.55·2).
*Dysmenorrhoea; inflammation; musculoskeletal and joint disorders; pain.*

**Vidaperamide** Vida, Hong Kong.
Loperamide hydrochloride (p.1271·1).
*Diarrhoea.*

**Vidapirocam** Vida, Hong Kong.
Piroxicam (p.84·2).
*Musculoskeletal and joint disorders.*

**Vidapril** Helfarma, Port.
Captopril (p.879·2).
*Heart failure; hypertension.*

**Vidaspan** Vida, Hong Kong.
Hyoscine butylbromide (p.483·3).
*Smooth muscle spasm.*

**Vidatapp** Vida, Hong Kong.
Brompheniramine maleate (p.426·1); phenylephrine hydrochloride (p.1126·3); bromhexine hydrochloride (p.1115·3); paracetamol (p.76·2).
*Cold and influenza symptoms; rhinitis.*

**Vidatifen** Vida, Hong Kong.
Ketotifen fumarate (p.788·1).
*Asthma; hypersensitivity reactions.*

**Vidavit** Allen, Mex.†.
Vitamin $B_{12}$ (p.1458·2).

**Vi-Daylin**
Abbott, Canad.; Abbott, Hong Kong; Abbott, Malaysia; Abbott, NZ; Abbott, S.Afr.; Abbott, UK†; Ross, USA.
A range of vitamin preparations with or without minerals (p.1417·1).

**Vidaylin**
Abbott, India; Abbott, Singapore; Abbott, Thai.
A range of vitamin preparations with or without minerals or lysine (p.1417·1).

**Vi-Daylin plus Iron**
Abbott, Israel; Abbott, S.Afr.
Multivitamin preparation with iron (p.1417·1).

**Vi-Daylin/F** Ross, USA.
A range of vitamin and fluoride (p.1444·3) preparations (p.1417·1).

**Vidaza** Pharmion, USA.
Azacitidine (p.529·2).
*Myelodysplastic syndromes.*

**Vidcalm** Catarinense, Braz.†.
Chamomile (p.1669·3); espinheiro alvar; erythrina mulungu (p.1717·2); passion flower (p.1729·1); valerian (p.1762·2).
*Sedative.*

**Vi-De$_3$**
Sanova, Austria; Novartis, Switz.
Colecalciferol (p.1461·3).
*Hypoparathyroidism; osteomalacia; rickets; tetany.*

**Videne**
Adams, Hong Kong; Adams, Thai.; Adams, UK.
Povidone-iodine (p.1190·3).
*Burns; skin disinfection; wounds.*

**Video** Monot, Fr.†.
Phenylephrine hydrochloride (p.1126·3); rutoside sodium sulfate (p.1688·3).
*Conjunctivitis.*

**Video Capsule con Mirtillo** Farmila, Ital.†.
Vitamin E; betacarotene; zinc; ginkgo biloba; myrtillus (p.1417·1).
Formerly contained vitamin E, magnesium, betacarotene, selenium, and myrtillus.
*Antioxidant nutritional supplement.*

**Video-Light** Farmila, Ital.
Benzalkonium chloride (p.1168·3).
*Eye disinfection.*

**Video-Mill** Farmila, Ital.
Naphazoline nitrate (p.1124·3).
*Conjunctivitis.*

**Video-Net** Interdelta, Switz.
Phenylephrine hydrochloride (p.1126·3); rutoside sodium sulfate (p.1688·3).
*Eye irritation.*

**Videorelax** SIFI, Ital.
Chlorhexidine gluconate (p.1173·2); tilia (p.1756·2); chamomile (p.1669·3).
*Eye disinfection; eye irritation.*

**Viderm** Ganassini, Ital.
Hydroxyquinoline sulfate (p.1700·1); enoxolone (p.36·2).
*Wound disinfection.*

**Vidermina** Ganassini, Ital.
Copper usnate (p.1762·1).
*Vaginal disinfection.*

**Videx**
Bristol-Myers Squibb, Arg.; Bristol-Myers Squibb, Austral.; Bristol-Myers Squibb, Austria; Bristol-Myers Squibb, Belg.; Bristol-Myers Squibb, Braz.; Bristol, Canad.; Bristol-Myers Squibb, Chile; Bristol-Myers Squibb, Denm.; Bristol-Myers Squibb, Fin.; Bristol-Myers Squibb, Fr.; Bristol-Myers Squibb, Ger.; Bristol-Myers Squibb, Gr.; Bristol-Myers Squibb, Hong Kong; Bristol-Myers Squibb, Irl.; Bristol-Myers Squibb, Israel; Bristol-Myers Squibb, Ital.; Bristol-Myers Squibb, Malaysia; Bristol-Myers Squibb, Mex.; Bristol-Myers Squibb, Neth.; Bristol-Myers Squibb, Norw.; Bristol-Myers Squibb, NZ; Bristol-Myers Squibb, Port.; Bristol-Myers Squibb, S.Afr.; Bristol-Myers Squibb, Singapore; Bristol-Myers, Spain; Bristol-Myers Squibb, Swed.; Bristol-Myers Squibb, Switz.; Bristol-Myers Squibb, Thai.; Bristol-Myers Squibb, UK; Bristol-Myers Squibb, USA.
Didanosine (p.630·3).
*HIV infection.*

**Vidilac** Kite (Κιτε), Gr.
Hypromellose (p.1579·3).
*Dry eyes.*

**Vidirakt S** Mann, Ger.
Povidone (p.1581·2).
*Dry eyes.*

**Vidisept** Mann, Ger.
Povidone (p.1581·2).
*Dry eyes; eye irritation.*

**Vidisept EDO** Mann, Ger.
Povidone (p.1581·2).
*Dry eyes.*

**Vidisept N**
Mann, Malaysia; Mann, Singapore.
Povidone (p.1581·2).
*Dry eyes; eye irritation.*

**Vidiseptal EDO Sine** Mann, Ger.†.
Tetryzoline hydrochloride (p.1131·2).
*Eye irritation and inflammation.*

**Vidisic**
Riel, Austria; Tramedico, Belg.; Bausch & Lomb, Braz.; Mann, Ger.; Mann, Irl.; Mann, Malaysia; Tramedico, Neth.; Lepori, Port.; Mann, Singapore; Bausch & Lomb, Thai.; Mann, Thai.
Carbomer (p.1577·2).
*Dry eyes.*

**Vidora** Ferlux, Fr.
Indoramin hydrochloride (p.939·2).
*Migraine.*

**Vidox** Epicaris, Arg.
Mupirocin (p.233·1).
*Bacterial skin infections.*

**Vidyn** Sigma, Braz.
Multivitamin and mineral preparation (p.1417·1).

**Vie Ca Rad** Multi-Pro, Canad.
Betacarotene, selenium, vitamin C, and vitamin E (p.1417·1).

**Vieta** Bunker, Braz.
*dl*-Alpha tocoferil acetate (p.1465·1).

**Viewgam** Bacon, Arg.
Meglumine gadopentetate (p.1062·2).
*Contrast medium for magnetic resonance imaging.*

**Vifarcap** Farcoral, Mex.
Multivitamin and mineral preparation (p.1417·1).

**Vifazolin** Vianex (Βιανεξ), Gr.
Cefazolin sodium (p.170·3).
*Bacterial infections.*

**Vifenac** Vifor, Switz.
Diclofenac epolamine (p.33·1).
*Musculoskeletal and joint disorders.*

**Vi-Ferrin** Elofar, Braz.
Iron chelate (p.1436·1); folic acid (p.1429·1); cyanocobalamin (p.1458·2).
*Iron deficiency; iron-deficiency anaemias.*

**Vifolyt** Rayere, Mex.
Multivitamin and mineral preparation (p.1417·1).

**Vifortol** Parke, Davis, Arg.
Vitamin and mineral preparation (p.1417·1).

**Vig** Key, Austral.†.
*Chewable tablets:* Guarana (p.1765·3); ginseng (p.1693·1); ginkgo biloba (p.1692·3); glucose (p.1432·2).
*Tablets:* Guarana (p.1765·3); ginseng (p.1693·1); ginkgo biloba (p.1692·3).
*Tonic.*

**Vig Recovery** Key, Austral.†.
Guarana (p.1765·3); vitamin B substances; vitamin C (p.1417·1).
*Hangover.*

**Vigam**
BPL-Meizler, Braz.; BPL, Israel; Bio Products, Malaysia; BPL, Singapore; BPL, UK.
A normal immunoglobulin (p.1627·2).
*Hypogammaglobulinaemia; idiopathic thrombocytopenic purpura; Kawasaki disease.*

**Vigamox** Alcon, USA.
Moxifloxacin hydrochloride (p.233·1).
*Bacterial eye infections.*

**Vigam-S** BPL, Thai.
A normal immunoglobulin (p.1627·2).
*Hypogammaglobulinaemia; idiopathic thrombocytopenic purpura; immunodeficiency; Kawasaki disease.*

**Vigantol**
Merck, Ger.; Merck, Port.
Colecalciferol (p.1461·3).
*Osteomalacia; osteopathy; osteoporosis; rickets; vitamin D deficiency.*

**Vigantoletten**
Merck, Austria.
Colecalciferol-cholesterin.
*Rickets prophylaxis.*

Merck, Ger.
Colecalciferol (p.1461·3).
*Osteoporosis; rickets; vitamin D deficiency.*

**Vigarol** Vickmans, Hong Kong.
Liquid paraffin (p.1479·1).
*Constipation.*

**Vigem** Pharmavite, Canad.†.
Vitamin B substances (p.1417·1).

**Vigencial** Estedi, Spain.
Methylrosanilinium chloride (p.1186·1).
*Skin infections.*

**Vigicer** Beta, Arg.
Modafinil (p.1591·1).
*Narcoleptic syndrome.*

**Vigil** Merckle, Ger.
Modafinil (p.1591·1).
*Narcoleptic syndrome.*

**Vigilia** Grands Espaces, Fr.
Tilia (p.1756·2); vervain (p.1764·1).
*Sedative.*

**Vigilon** SSL, UK†.
Polyethylene oxide (p.1581·1).
*Hydrogel dressing; wounds.*

**Vigiten** Wyeth Lederle, Belg.
Lorazepam (p.704·1).
*Anxiety disorders; depression; mixed anxiety depressive states; obsessive-compulsive disorder.*

**Vigodana** Loges, Hong Kong.
α-Tocoferil acetate; orotic acid; procaine hydrochloride; haematoporphyrin; magnesium aspartate; magnesium oxide; magnesium sulfate (p.1417·1).
*Tonic.*

**vigodana N** Loges, Ger.
Alpha tocoferil acetate; orotic acid; haematoporphyrin; magnesium aspartate; magnesium oxide; dried magnesium sulfate (p.1417·1).
*Tonic.*

**Vigofortal** Pasteur, Chile.
Strychnine sulfate (p.1750·1); sodium phosphate; potassium phosphate; phosphoric acid (p.1417·1).
*Asthenia; tonic.*

**Vigogel** Farmetrusca, Ital.†.
Royal jelly (p.1740·3); liver extract; dried yeast (p.1469·1).

**Vigomar Forte** Marlop, USA.
Multivitamin and mineral preparation with iron (p.1417·1).

**Vigonal** Aclimacao, Braz.†.
Folic acid; cyanocobalamin; calcium glycerophosphate; sodium glycerophosphate; ergocalciferol (p.1417·1).
*Anaemias.*

**Vigoplus** Gazzoni, Ital.†.
Maltodextrin; fructose; vitamins; minerals (p.1417·1).
*Nutritional supplement.*

**Vigor Plus** Andromaco, Chile.
Vitamin and mineral preparation (p.1417·1).
*Dietary supplement.*

**Vigor-Ace** United American, Singapore.
Vitamin A; vitamin C; vitamin E; selenium; zinc; lecithin (p.1417·1).
*Tonic.*

**Vigoran** Golaz, Switz.
Ginseng (p.1693·1); deanol hydrogen tartrate (p.1585·3); magnesium orotate (p.1724·3).
*Tonic.*

**Vigorsan** Hoechst Marion Roussel, Ger.†.
Colecalciferol (p.1461·3).
*Osteopathy; osteoporosis; rickets; vitamin D deficiency.*

**Vigortol** Rugby, USA.
Multivitamin and mineral preparation (p.1417·1).

**Vigortonic** Arkochim, Spain.
Cinnamon (p.1672·2); ginseng (p.1693·1); kola (p.1765·3).
*Fatigue.*

**Vigour S** Restan, S.Afr.
Haematoporphyrin; cyanocobalamin; caffeine; yeast extract (p.1417·1).
*Tonic.*

**Vigranon B** *Wallace Mfg Chem., UK.*
Vitamin B substances (p.1417·1).

**Vikaman** *Disperga, Austria†.*
Menadione sodium bisulfite (p.1466·3).
*Haemorrhage.*

**Vikatron** *Ariston, Braz.*
Phytomenadione (p.1467·1).

**Vikela**
*Gerot, Austria; HRA, Fr.*
Levonorgestrel (p.1563·2).
*Postcoital oral contraceptive.*

**Viken** *Kendrick, Mex.*
Cefotaxime sodium (p.175·3).
Lidocaine hydrochloride (p.1377·3) is included in the intramuscular injection to alleviate the pain of injection.
*Bacterial infections.*

**Vilam** *Reuffer, Mex.†.*
Multivitamin and mineral preparation (p.1417·1).

**Vilan**
*Lannacher, Austria; Lannacher, Denm.; Nourypharma, Neth.; Synmedic, Switz.*
Nicomorphine hydrochloride (p.66·3).
*Pain; premedication.*

**Vilbine** *Richmond, Arg.*
Vinorelbine (p.594·2).
*Malignant neoplasms.*

**Vilerm** *Siam Bheasach, Thai.*
Aciclovir (p.626·1).
*Herpesvirus infections.*

**Vilne** *Dosa, Arg.*
Vinorelbine (p.594·2).
*Malignant neoplasms.*

**Vilona** *ICN, Mex.*
Ribavirin (p.652·1).
*Viral infections.*

**Viltar** *Dallas, Arg.*
Loperamide (p.1271·2).
*Diarrhoea.*

**Vilterm** *Drag, Chile.*
Betamethasone (p.1093·1); gentamicin (p.219·1).
*Infected skin disorders.*

**Vi-Magna** *Wyeth Lederle, India.*
Multivitamin preparation (p.1417·1).

**Vimax**
*Note. This name is used for preparations of different composition.*
*Roemmers, Arg.*
Sildenafil citrate (p.1744·2).
*Erectile dysfunction.*

*Bio2, Fr.*
Fish oil; yeast cultured in selenium-rich medium; vitamins; minerals (p.1417·1).
*Nutritional supplement.*

**Vimepan** *Collins, Mex.*
Vitamin preparation (p.1417·1).

**Vimeral** *ICN, Canad.*
Multivitamin and mineral preparation (p.1417·1).

**Viminate** *Barre-National, USA.*
Multivitamin and mineral preparation (p.1417·1).

**Vimineral** *Offenbach, Mex.*
Vitamin and mineral preparation (p.1417·1).

**Viminfort** *Solfran, Mex.*
Multivitamin and mineral preparation (p.1417·1).

**Vimoli** *Vitamed, Israel.*
Paracetamol (p.76·2).
*Fever; pain.*

**Vimotadine** *Casasco, Arg.*
Co-dergocrine (p.1674·1).
*Cerebrovascular disorders.*

**Vimultisa** *Fabra, Arg.*
Diclofenac (p.32·1).
*Inflammation.*

**Vin Tonique de Vial** *Eberth, Switz.*
Cinchona alkaloids (p.1671·3); calcium phosphate (p.1225·3); lactic acid (p.1704·1); beef extract; sweet wine.
*Tonic.*

**Vinarine** *Kampel Martian, Arg.*
Vinorelbine (p.594·2).
*Malignant neoplasms.*

**Vinatal**
*Triomed, S.Afr.†; British Dispensary, Thai.*
Multivitamin and mineral preparation (p.1417·1).

**Vinate GT** *Breckenridge, USA.*
Vitamin and mineral preparation with iron and folic acid (p.1417·1).
Docusate sodium (p.1262·2) is included in this preparation to reduce the constipating effects of iron.

**Vinca** *Substipharm, Fr.*
Vincamine (p.1764·2).
*Mental function impairment in the elderly.*

**Vincacen** *Centrum, Spain.*
Vincamine hydrochloride (p.1764·2).
*Cerebral trauma; cerebrovascular disorders; circulatory disorders of the eye, ear, nose, and throat; vestibular disorders.*

**Vincadar** *Aventis, Ital.*
Vincamine (p.1764·2).
*Cerebrovascular disorders.*

**Vincafolina** *Lampugnani, Ital.†.*
Vincamine (p.1764·2).
*Cerebrovascular disorders.*

**Vincafor** *Pharmafarm, Fr.†.*
Vincamine (p.1764·2).
*Mental function impairment in the elderly.*

**Vincagil**
*Aventis, Braz.†; Roussel, Port.*
Vincamine (p.1764·2).
*Cerebrovascular disorders.*

**Vincaminol** *Alacan, Spain.*
Vincamine hydrochloride (p.1764·2).
*Cerebral trauma; cerebrovascular disorders; circulatory disorders of the eye, ear, nose, and throat; vestibular disorders.*

**Vincapan** *Aventis, Mex.*
Vincamine (p.1764·2).
*Cerebrovascular disorders.*

**Vincapront** *Mack, Illert., Ger.†.*
Vincamine (p.1764·2).
*Ménière's disease; metabolic and circulatory disorders of the brain, retina, and inner ear.*

**Vinca-Ri** *INTES, Ital.*
Vincamine hydrochloride (p.1764·2).
*Disorders of cerebral, ocular, and vestibular perfusion.*

**Vincarutine** *SERP, Mon.*
Vincamine (p.1764·2); rutoside (p.1688·2).
*Mental function impairment in the elderly.*

**Vincasar** *Pharmacia Upjohn, Mex.†.*
Vincristine sulfate (p.592·2).

**Vincasar PFS** *Gensia, USA.*
Vincristine sulfate (p.592·2).
*Malignant neoplasms.*

**Vinca-Tablinen** *Sanorania, Ger.†.*
Vincamine (p.1764·2).
*Circulatory disorders of the brain, retina, and inner ear; Ménière's disease.*

**Vinca-Treis** *Ecobi, Ital.*
Vincamine (p.1764·2).
*Cerebrovascular disorders.*

**Vincent's Powders** *Roche Consumer, Austral.*
Aspirin (p.15·1).
*Fever; pain.*

**Vinces** *Elvetium, Arg.*
Vincristine sulfate (p.592·2).
*Malignant neoplasms.*

**Vincetron** *Biosintetica, Braz.*
Piracetam (p.1732·1); co-dergocrine mesilate (p.1674·1).
*Mental function impairment.*

**Vincidol** *Salvat, Spain.*
Aspirin (p.15·1); caffeine (p.782·1).
*Fever; pain.*

**Vincigrip** *Salvat, Spain.*
Chlorphenamine maleate (p.427·3); pseudoephedrine hydrochloride (p.1129·2); paracetamol (p.76·2).
Formerly contained chlorphenamine maleate, phenylpropanolamine hydrochloride, and paracetamol.
*Cold and influenza symptoms; fever; pain.*

**Vincigrip Balsamico** *Salvat, Spain†.*
Guaifenesin (p.1122·1); paracetamol (p.76·2).
*Influenza and cold symptoms; sinusitis.*

**Vincimax** *Synthelabo, Fr.†.*
Vincamine (p.1764·2).
*Cerebrovascular disorders; mental function impairment in the elderly.*

**Vinciseptil Otico** *Salvat, Spain.*
Benzydamine hydrochloride (p.21·1); fluocinolone acetonide (p.1101·2); neomycin sulfate (p.235·1); polymyxin B sulfate (p.245·1); tetracaine hydrochloride (p.1385·1).
*Ear disorders.*

**Vincitos** *Salvat, Spain.*
Dextromethorphan hydrobromide (p.1117·3); pseudoephedrine hydrochloride (p.1129·2).
*Coughs.*

**Vincizina** *Pharmacia, Braz.*
Vincristine sulfate (p.592·2).
*Malignant neoplasms.*

**Vinco Forte** *OTW, Ger.†.*
Bisacodyl (p.1251·3).
*Constipation.*

**Vinco-Abfuhr-Perlen** *OTW, Ger.*
Bisacodyl (p.1251·3).
*Constipation.*

**Vincosedan** *Reig Jofre, Spain.*
Diazepam (p.690·1).
Contains pyridoxine.
*Alcohol withdrawal syndrome; anxiety; febrile convulsions; insomnia; skeletal muscle spasm.*

**Vincrin** *Orion, Fin.†.*
Vincristine sulfate (p.592·2).
*Malignant neoplasms.*

**Vincristex** *Cristalia, Braz.*
Vincristine sulfate (p.592·2).
*Malignant neoplasms.*

**Vincrisul** *Irisfarma, Spain.*
Vincristine sulfate (p.592·2).
*Idiopathic thrombocytopenic purpura; malignant neoplasms.*

**Vinecort** *Genepharm, Gr.*
Budesonide (p.1094·2).
*Allergic rhinitis; topical corticosteroid.*

**Vinelbine** *Dabur, India.*
Vinorelbine (p.594·2).
*Breast cancer; non-small-cell lung cancer.*

**Vingel** *Bristol-Myers Squibb, Port.*
Aluminium hydroxide (p.1249·2); magnesium hydroxide (p.1272·2); simeticone (p.1289·2).
*Dyspepsia; gastritis; heartburn; peptic ulcer.*

**Vingional** *Fabra, Arg.*
Ranitidine (p.1285·2).
*Peptic ulcer.*

**Vinho Ferruginoso** *Luper, Braz.; Phos-Kola, Braz.; Teuto, Braz.*
Ferric ammonium citrate (p.1427·2).
*Iron deficiency; iron-deficiency anaemias.*

**Vinho Reconstituinte** *Hoechst Marion Roussel, Braz.†.*
Calcium (p.1225·1); peptone; cinchona bark (p.1671·3).

**Vinho Tonificante** *Stevia, Braz.†.*
Ferric ammonium citrate (p.1427·2).
*Iron deficiency; iron-deficiency anaemias.*

**Vinkhum** *Frasca, Arg.*
Vincamine (p.1764·2).

**Vinocard Q10** *Marjan, Braz.*
Ubidecarenone (p.1760·2).
*Co-enzyme Q10 deficiency.*

**Vinone** *Hikma, Port.*
Enoxacin (p.207·2).
*Bacterial infections.*

**Vinopepsin** *Terrapharm, Austria.*
Pepsin (p.1729·3); absinthium (p.1645·1).
*Gastrointestinal disorders.*

**Vinorgen** *Gautier, Arg.*
Vinorelbine tartrate (p.594·1).
*Breast cancer; non-small cell lung cancer.*

**Vinracine**
*BPL-Meizler, Braz.*
Vincristine (p.593·2).
*Malignant neoplasms.*

*Korean United, Malaysia.*
Vincristine sulfate (p.592·2).
*Malignant neoplasms.*

**Vinsal** *Salus, Ital.†.*
Vincamine (p.1764·2).
*Cerebrovascular disorders.*

**Vinsen** *Chew, Thai.*
Naproxen (p.65·1).
*Dysmenorrhoea; gout; musculoskeletal and joint disorders.*

**Vintec** *Columbia, Mex.†.*
Vincristine sulfate (p.592·2).
*Malignant neoplasms.*

**Vintene** *Baxter, Fr.*
Amino-acid infusion (p.1417·1).
*Parenteral nutrition.*

**Vinzam** *Almirall, Spain.*
Azithromycin (p.159·1).
*Bacterial infections.*

**Viobeta** *IDI, Ital.†.*
Betamethasone valero-acetate (p.1093·2); clioquinol (p.196·3).
*Infected skin disorders.*

**Viocidina** *IDI, Ital.†.*
Clioquinol (p.196·3); cod-liver oil (p.1425·2).
*Infected skin disorders.*

**Viocort** *Aspen, S.Afr.*
Hydrocortisone acetate (p.1103·3); diiodohydroxyquinoline (p.603·3).
*Skin disorders.*

**Viodenum** *Iquinosa, Spain†.*
Hidrosmin (p.1688·3).
*Peripheral vascular disorders.*

**Viodine**
*Orion, Austral.; Orion, NZ.*
Povidone-iodine (p.1190·3).
*Minor burns; skin disinfection; skin infections; wounds.*

**Viodor** *Aspen, S.Afr.*
Diiodohydroxyquinoline (p.603·3); benzocaine (p.1370·3).
*Skin infections with pruritus.*

**Vioform**
*FLAWA, Switz.†; Ciba, USA†.*
Clioquinol (p.196·3).
*Infected skin disorders.*

**Vioform-Hydrocortisone**
*Novartis, Canad.; Novartis Consumer, Irl.; Novartis Consumer, UK.*
Clioquinol (p.196·3); hydrocortisone (p.1103·3).
*Infected skin disorders.*

**Vioformio-Hidrocortisona** *Novartis, Braz.*
Clioquinol (p.196·3); hydrocortisone (p.1103·3).
*Skin disorders.*

**Vioformo** *Novartis, Mex.*
Clioquinol (p.196·3).
*Skin infections.*

**Vioformo-Cort** *Novartis, Mex.*
Clioquinol (p.196·3); hydrocortisone (p.1103·3).
*Infected skin disorders.*

**Viogen-C** *Goldline, USA.*
Vitamin B substances with vitamin C and minerals (p.1417·1).

**Viokase**
*Note. This name is used for preparations of different composition.*
*Wyeth, Austral.†; Wyeth, NZ†; Aspen, S.Afr.*
Pancreatin (p.1725·3).
*Pancreatic insufficiency.*

*Wolfs, Belg.†; Axcan, Canad.; Axcan, USA.*
Pancrelipase (p.1725·3).
*Pancreatic insufficiency.*

**Viola** *Sanopharm, Switz.*
Viola tricolor; zinc oxide (p.1163·2); almond oil (p.1651·1).
*Skin disorders.*

**Violgen** *INTES, Ital.†.*
Methylrosanilinium chloride (p.1186·1); lactic acid (p.1704·1).
*Vulvovaginitis.*

**Violin** *TO-Chemicals, Thai.*
Salbutamol (p.791·3).
*Obstructive airways disease.*

**Vioneurin**
*Note. This name is used for preparations of different composition.*
*Continental Pharma, Belg.*
Cyanocobalamin (p.1458·2); thiamine hydrochloride (p.1455·1); pyridoxine hydrochloride (p.1456·3).
*Neuritis; neuropathy; vitamin B deficiency.*

*Continental Pharma, Thai.†.*
Vitamin $B_1$ (p.1455·2); vitamin $B_{12}$ (p.1458·2).
*Malnutrition; musculoskeletal pain; neuralgia; neuritis.*

**Vioridon** *Viofar, Gr.*
Baclofen (p.1386·3).
*Spasticity.*

**Viotisone** *Unison, Thai.*
Ofloxacin (p.239·3).
*Bacterial infections.*

**Vioxx**
*Merck Sharp & Dohme, Arg.; Merck Sharp & Dohme, Austral.; Merck Sharp & Dohme, Austria; Merck Sharp & Dohme, Belg.; Merck Sharp & Dohme, Braz.; Merck Frosst, Canad.; Merck Sharp & Dohme, Denm.; Merck Sharp & Dohme, Fin.; Merck Sharp & Dohme-Chibret, Fr.; Merck Sharp & Dohme, Ger.; Vianex (Βιανεξ), Gr.; Merck Sharp & Dohme, Hong Kong; Merck Sharp & Dohme, Irl.; Merck Sharp & Dohme, Israel; Merck Sharp & Dohme, Ital.; Merck Sharp & Dohme, Malaysia; Merck Sharp & Dohme, Mex.; Merck Sharp & Dohme, Neth.; Merck Sharp & Dohme, Norw.; Merck Sharp & Dohme, NZ; Merck Sharp & Dohme, Port.; Merck Sharp & Dohme, S.Afr.; Merck Sharp & Dohme, Singapore; Merck Sharp & Dohme, Spain; Merck Sharp & Dohme, Swed.; Merck Sharp & Dohme, Switz.; Merck Sharp & Dohme, Thai.; Merck Sharp & Dohme, UK; Merck, USA.*
Rofecoxib (p.86·3).
*Osteoarthritis; pain; rheumatoid arthritis.*

**Vioxxalt** *Merck Sharp & Dohme, Denm.*
Rofecoxib (p.86·3).
*Pain.*

**Viperfav** *Aventis Pasteur, Fr.*
European viper venom antiserum (p.1639·1).
*European viper bite.*

**Vipirim** *INQ, Braz.†.*
Vitamin $B_1$ (p.1455·2); vitamin $B_2$ (p.1456·1); vitamin $B_6$ (p.1457·2); vitamin $B_{12}$ (p.1458·2).
*Vitamin B deficiency.*

**Viplex** *Riva, Canad.*
Vitamin B substances and iron (p.1417·1).

**Viplura** *IQFA, Mex.*
Vitamin preparation (p.1417·1).

**Viplus** *Parggon, Mex.*
Naproxen sodium (p.65·1); paracetamol (p.76·2).
*Fever; pain.*

**Vipocem** *Alter, Port.*
Vinpocetine (p.1764·2).
*Cerebrovascular disorders; vascular disorders of the eye and ear.*

**Vipodo** *Novag, Mex.*
Podophyllum (p.1155·2).
*Keratolytic.*

**Vipral** *Armstrong, Arg.*
Sulpiride (p.722·2).
*Dyspepsia; vomiting.*

**Vipratox** *Serum-Werk Bernburg, Ger.*
Vipera ammodytes toxin; methyl salicylate (p.59·3); camphor (p.1665·3).
*Musculoskeletal, joint, and soft-tissue disorders; neuralgias.*

**Vipres** *Vita, Spain.*
Enalapril maleate (p.909·2); nitrendipine (p.973·3).
*Hypertension.*

**Viprinex** *Abbott, Canad.†.*
Ancrod (p.863·2).
*Peripheral vascular disorders; thromboembolic disorders.*

**Vipro** *Scientific Hospital Supplies, UK†.*
Preparation for enteral nutrition (p.1417·1).

**Viprofen** *Iqfasa, Mex.†.*
Multivitamin and mineral preparation (p.1417·1).

**Vipsogal** *Harley Street Supplies, UK†.*
Betamethasone dipropionate (p.1093·1); fluocinonide (p.1101·3); gentamicin sulfate (p.217·1); salicylic acid (p.1157·1); panthenol (p.1727·2).
Available on a named-patient basis only.
*Skin disorders.*

**Viquin Forte** *ICN, Canad.*
Hydroquinone (p.1148·1); glycolic acid (p.1147·3) in a sunscreen basis.
*Skin pigmentation disorders.*

**Vira-A**
*Parke, Davis, Austral.†; Parke, Davis, NZ†; Monarch, USA†.*
Vidarabine (p.657·1).
*Herpes simplex keratitis and keratoconjunctivitis.*

**Viraban** *AFT, NZ.*
Aciclovir (p.626·1).
*Herpes labialis.*

**Virac** *Crosara, Ital.†.*
Inosine pranobex (p.640·2).
*Immunodeficiency; viral infections.*

**Viracept** *Roche, Arg.; Roche, Austral.; Roche, Austria; Roche, Belg.; Roche, Braz.; Agouron, Canad.; Roche, Chile; Roche, Denm.; Roche, Fin.; Roche, Fr.; Roche, Ger.; Roche, Gr.; Roche, Irl.; Roche, Israel; Roche, Ital.; Japan Tobacco, Jpn; Roche, Mex.; Roche, Neth.; Roche, Norw.; Roche, NZ; Roche, Port.; Roche, S.Afr.; Roche, Singapore; Roche, Spain; Roche, Swed.; Roche, Switz.; Roche, Thai.; Roche, UK; Agouron, USA.*
Nelfinavir mesilate (p.650·1).
*HIV infection.*

**Viracillina** *Infosint, Ital.*
Piperacillin sodium (p.243·1).
Lidocaine hydrochloride (p.1377·3) is included in this preparation to alleviate the pain of injection.
*Bacterial infections.*

**Virafer** *Aventis, Ital.*
Multivitamin and mineral preparation (p.1417·1).

**Viraferon** *Schering-Plough, Fr.; Schering-Plough, Mex.; Schering-Plough, Spain†; Schering-Plough, UK.*
Interferon alfa-2b (rbe) (p.640·3).
*Anogenital warts; hepatitis B; hepatitis C; malignant neoplasms.*

**ViraferonPeg** *Schering-Plough, Fr.; Schering-Plough, Irl.; Schering-Plough, UK.*
Peginterferon alfa-2b (rbe) (p.643·1).
*Chronic hepatitis C.*

**Viralief** *Clonmel, Irl.*
Aciclovir (p.626·1).
*Herpes simplex skin infections.*

**Viralin** *Magis, Ital.†.*
Inosine pranobex (p.640·2).
*Viral infections.*

**Viramid** *ICN, Braz.*
Ribavirin (p.652·1).
*Viral infections.*

**Vira-MP** *Pierre Fabre, Fr.†.*
Vidarabine sodium phosphate (p.657·1).
*Recurrent genital herpes infection.*

**Viramune** *Boehringer Ingelheim, Arg.; Boehringer Ingelheim, Austral.; Boehringer Ingelheim, Austria; Boehringer Ingelheim, Belg.; Boehringer de Angeli, Braz.†; Boehringer Ingelheim, Canad.; Boehringer Ingelheim, Chile; Boehringer Ingelheim, Denm.; Boehringer Ingelheim, Fin.; Boehringer Ingelheim, Fr.; Boehringer Ingelheim, Ger.; Boehringer Ingelheim, Gr.; Boehringer Ingelheim, Hong Kong; Boehringer Ingelheim, Irl.; Boehringer Ingelheim, Israel; Boehringer Ingelheim, Ital.; Boehringer Ingelheim, Jpn; Boehringer Ingelheim, Malaysia; Boehringer Ingelheim, Mex.; Boehringer Ingelheim, Neth.; Boehringer Ingelheim, Norw.; Boehringer Ingelheim, NZ; Boehringer Ingelheim, Port.; Boehringer Ingelheim, S.Afr.; Boehringer Ingelheim, Singapore; Boehringer Ingelheim, Spain; Boehringer Ingelheim, Swed.; Boehringer Ingelheim, Switz.; Boehringer Ingelheim, Thai.; Boehringer Ingelheim, UK; Roxane, USA.*
Nevirapine (p.650·2).
*HIV infection.*

**Viranet** *Kampel Martian, Arg.*
Valaciclovir (p.656·2).

**Virasolve** *Pfizer Consumer, Austral.; Rosken, Hong Kong; Pfizer, NZ.*
Idoxuridine (p.637·3); lidocaine hydrochloride (p.1377·3); benzalkonium chloride (p.1168·3).
*Herpes simplex infections of the mouth and skin.*

**Virasorb** *Thornton & Ross, UK.*
Aciclovir (p.626·1).
*Herpes labialis.*

**Viratin** *Raza, Malaysia; Pharmaniaga, Malaysia.*
Verapamil hydrochloride (p.1019·1).
*Angina pectoris; arrhythmias; hypertension.*

**Viravan** *Pediamed, USA.*
Phenylephrine tannate (p.1127·2); mepyramine tannate (p.437·1).

**Viravan-DM** *Pediamed, USA.*
Dextromethorphan tannate (p.1118·1); mepyramine tannate (p.437·1); phenylephrine tannate (p.1127·2).
*Upper respiratory-tract disorders.*

**Virax** *Alpharma-Isis, Ger.*
Aciclovir (p.626·1).
*Herpesvirus infections.*

**Viraxy** *General Drugs, Thai.*
Aciclovir (p.626·1).
*Herpesvirus infections.*

**Virazid** *ICN, Spain†.*
Ribavirin (p.652·1).
*Respiratory syncytial virus infections.*

**Virazide** *ICN, Austral.; Grossman, Mex.*
Ribavirin (p.652·1).
*Respiratory syncytial virus infections.*

**Virazole** *Sanico, Belg.†; UCI, Braz.; ICN, Canad.; ICN, Ger.; ICN, Hong Kong; ICN, Neth.; ICN, Singapore; ICN, Spain; Swedish Orphan, Swed.; ICN, UK; ICN, USA.*
Ribavirin (p.652·1).
*Respiratory syncytial virus infections.*

**Virazone** *Rayere, Mex.†.*
Aciclovir (p.626·1).

**Virbelte** *Korhispana, Spain†.*
Aciclovir (p.626·1).
*Herpes simplex infections.*

**Virdex** *Fulton, Ital.*
Ergotamine tartrate (p.467·2); caffeine (p.782·1); aminophenazone (p.14·2).
*Migraine.*

**Viread** *Gilead, Austral.; Gilead, Canad.; Gilead, Fr.; Gilead, Irl.; Gilead, Spain; Gilead, UK; Gilead, USA.*
Tenofovir disoproxil fumarate (p.655·1).
*HIV infection.*

**Viregyt** *Thiemann, Ger.†.*
Amantadine hydrochloride (p.1197·2).
*Parkinsonism.*

**Virelon C** *Chiron Behring, Ger.†.*
An inactivated poliomyelitis vaccine (p.1633·3).
*Active immunisation.*

**Virest** *Hovid, Malaysia; Hovid, Singapore.*
Aciclovir (p.626·1).
*Herpesvirus infections.*

**Virexen** *Will-Pharma, Belg.; Ferraz, Lynce, Port.; Vinas, Spain; Vinas, Switz.†.*
Idoxuridine (p.637·3) in dimethyl sulfoxide.
*Herpesvirus infections of the skin and mucous membranes.*

**Virfen** *Specifar (Σπεσιφαρ), Gr.*
Enalapril maleate (p.909·2).
*Heart failure; hypertension.*

**Virflutam** *Infosint, Ital.*
Flutamide (p.556·2).
*Prostatic cancer.*

**Virgamelis** *Pascoe, Ger.†.*
Hamamelis (p.1696·3).
*Skin irritation; wounds.*

**Virgan** *Sidus, Arg.; Thea, Fr.; Chauvin, UK.*
Ganciclovir (p.635·3).
*Herpes eye infections.*

**Virgilocard** *Sanova, Austria.*
Crataegus (p.1677·1); absinthium (p.1645·1).
*Cardiac disorders in the elderly.*

**Virginiana Gocce Verdi** *Kelemata, Ital.*
Naphazoline nitrate (p.1124·3).
*Eye congestion.*

**Virherpes** *Pensa, Spain.*
Aciclovir (p.626·1) or aciclovir sodium (p.626·1).
*Herpesvirus infections.*

**Viridal** *Orion, Denm.†; Hoyer, Ger.; Schwarz, Irl.; Schwarz, Ital.; Schwarz, UK.*
Alprostadil alfadex (p.1512·3).
*Erectile dysfunction.*

**Viridin** *Davi, Port.*
Trifluridine (p.655·3).
*Viral eye infections.*

**Virigen** *United Nordic, Denm.*
Yohimbine hydrochloride (p.1766·2).
*Erectile dysfunction.*

**Virilis-Gastreu S R41** *Reckeweg, Ger.*
Homoeopathic preparation.

**Virilisterona** *Sinterapico, Braz.†.*
Testosterone (p.1569·3).
*Androgen.*

**Virilit** *Jenapharm, Ger.*
Cyproterone acetate (p.1544·1).
*Erectile dysfunction; prostatic cancer.*

**Virilon**
*Note. This name is used for preparations of different composition.*
*Luper, Braz.*
Ginseng; catuaba; marapuama; vitamins (p.1417·1).

*Star, USA.*
*Capsules:* Methyltestosterone (p.1559·3).
*Androgen replacement therapy; breast cancer; male hypogonadism; postpartum breast engorgement; prepubertal cryptorchidism.*
*Injection:* Testosterone cipionate (p.1569·3).

**Virin** *Strand, Malaysia.*
Co-trimoxazole (p.199·3).
*Bacterial infections.*

**Virivac** *SBL, Denm.†; SBL, Swed.†.*
A measles, mumps, and rubella vaccine (Enders Edmonston B, Jeryl Lynn B, and RA 27/3 strains respectively) (p.1625·1).
*Active immunisation.*

**Virless** *YSP, Malaysia; Yung Shin, Singapore.*
Aciclovir (p.626·1).
*Herpesvirus infections.*

**Virlix** *UCB, Austria; Sanofi Synthelabo, Fr.; Mediolanum, Ital.; Glaxo Wellcome, Mex.; UCB, Norw.; Vedim, Port.; Lacer, Spain.*
Cetirizine hydrochloride (p.427·1).
*Hypersensitivity reactions.*

**Virlix-D** *Glaxo Wellcome, Mex.*
Cetirizine hydrochloride (p.427·1); pseudoephedrine hydrochloride (p.1129·2).
*Allergic rhinitis; eye irritation; nasal congestion.*

**Virman Plus** *Corypharma, Ital.*
Vitamin E; nicotinic acid; zinc (p.1417·1).
*Nutritional supplement.*

**Virmax** *Bago, Chile.*
Valaciclovir hydrochloride (p.656·1).
*Herpesvirus infections.*

**Virmen** *Menarini, Spain.*
Aciclovir (p.626·1).
*Herpesvirus infections.*

**Virobin** *Bock, Ger.†.*
Homoeopathic preparation.

**Virobis** *Aventis, S.Afr.*
*Cream:* Moroxydine hydrochloride (p.649·3); cetrimide (p.1172·1); diphenhydramine hydrochloride (p.431·3).
*Viral infections of the skin.*
*Tablets:* Moroxydine hydrochloride (p.649·3); atropine methonitrate (p.477·1); hyoscine methonitrate (p.483·3).
*Viral infections.*

**Virobron** *Temis, Arg.*
Nimesulide (p.67·1).
*Inflammation.*

**Virobron B12 NF** *Temis, Arg.*
Betamethasone (p.1093·1); vitamin $B_{12}$ (p.1458·2); diclofenac potassium (p.32·1).
*Musculoskeletal, joint, and peri-articular disorders; neuritis.*

**Viro-Do** *Grasler, Ger.*
Homoeopathic preparation.

**Virofral** *Novo Nordisk, Denm.†; Ferrosan, Swed.†.*
Amantadine hydrochloride (p.1197·2).
*Influenza A; parkinsonism.*

**Virogon** *Silom, Thai.*
Aciclovir (p.626·1).
*Herpesvirus infections.*

**Virohep-A** *Raffo, Arg.*
A hepatitis A vaccine (p.1617·1).
*Active immunisation.*

**Virolan** *Olan-Kemed, Thai.*
Aciclovir (p.626·1).
*Herpes simplex infections of the skin and mucous membranes.*

**ViroMed** *S Med, Austria.*
Aciclovir (p.626·1).
*Herpesvirus infections.*

**Viromed** *Progress, Thai.*
Aciclovir (p.626·1).
*Herpesvirus infections.*

**Viromidin** *Alcon Cusi, Spain.*
Trifluridine (p.655·3).
*Herpes simplex infections of the eye.*

**Viron Wart Lotion** *Odan, Canad.*
Glacial acetic acid (p.1645·2); lactic acid (p.1704·1); salicylic acid (p.1157·1).
*Verrucae.*

**Vironida** *Laboratorios Chile, Chile.*
Aciclovir (p.626·1).
*Herpesvirus infections.*

**Vironox** *Iketon, Ital.†.*
Nonoxinol 9 (p.1413·3); chloroxylenol (p.1177·2).
*Disinfection.*

**Viropect** *DHU, Ger.*
Homoeopathic preparation.

**Virophta** *Allergan, Fr.*
Trifluridine (p.655·3).
*Viral infections of the eye.*

**Viropox** *LSP, Thai.*
Aciclovir (p.626·1).
*Herpesvirus infections.*

**Viroptic** *Glaxo Wellcome, Canad.†; Glaxo Wellcome, USA; Monarch, USA.*
Trifluridine (p.655·3).
*Herpes simplex keratitis and keratoconjunctivitis.*

**Virormone** *Ferring, Austria; Paines & Byrne, Thai.; Nordic, UK.*
Testosterone (p.1569·3) or testosterone propionate (p.1570·1).
*Breast cancer; cryptorchidism; delayed puberty; male hypogonadism.*

**Virosol** *Phoenix, Arg.*
Amantadine hydrochloride (p.1197·2).
*Parkinsonism; viral infections.*

**Virostat** *Janssen-Ortho, Canad.†.*
Edoxudine (p.632·1).
*Genital herpes simplex infections.*

**Virovir** *Opus, UK.*
Aciclovir (p.626·1).
*Herpesvirus infections.*

**Viroxy** *Orion, Israel.*
Aciclovir sodium (p.626·1).
*Herpesvirus infections.*

**Virozid** *Teuto, Braz.*
Zidovudine (p.658·2).
*HIV infection.*

**Virtamox** *Infosint, Ital.*
Tamoxifen citrate (p.584·1).
*Breast cancer.*

**Virubact** *Biosyn, Ger.*
Homoeopathic preparation.

**Virucalm** *Inpharzam, Switz.*
Aciclovir (p.626·1).
*Herpes labialis.*

**Virucid** *Hofmann, Austria.*
Amantadine hydrochloride (p.1197·2).
*Influenza A; parkinsonism.*

**Viruderm** *Cinfa, Spain.*
Aciclovir (p.626·1).
*Herpes simplex infection.*

**Virudermin** *Robugen, Ger.; Iromedica, Switz.*
Zinc sulfate (p.1469·3).
*Herpes labialis.*

**Virudin** *Bracco, Ital.†.*
Foscarnet sodium (p.634·2).
*Cytomegalovirus retinitis.*

**Virulex**
*Note. This name is used for preparations of different composition.*
*Drossapharm, Switz.*
Greater celandine (p.1695·3).
*Herpes labialis.*

*Pose, Thai.*
Monopersulfate compound; sodium chloride; sulfamic acid.
*Instrument disinfection.*

**Virulex Forte** *Pascual, Hong Kong.*
Moroxydine hydrochloride (p.649·3); paracetamol (p.76·2); atropine methonitrate (p.477·1); hyoscine methonitrate (p.483·3).
*Viral infections.*

**Viru-Merz** *Kolassa, Austria; Therabel, Belg.; Grunenthal, Chile; Merz, Denm.†; Merz, Ger.; Merz, Hong Kong; Merz, Israel; Merz, Malaysia; Merz, Neth.; Medinfar, Port.; Merz, Singapore.*
Tromantadine hydrochloride (p.656·1).
*Herpesvirus infections of the skin and mucous membranes.*

**Viru-Merz Serol** *Pharmacare, Gr.; Merz, Switz.*
Tromantadine hydrochloride (p.656·1).
*Herpes simplex infections of the skin and mucous membranes.*

**Virunguent** *Hermal, Ger.; Hermal, Malaysia; Hermal, Port.; Hermal, Singapore; Boots Healthcare, Switz.*
Idoxuridine (p.637·3) in dimethyl sulfoxide.
*Herpes simplex infections of the skin and mucous membranes.*

**Virunguent P** *Hermal, Ger.*
Idoxuridine (p.637·3); prednisolone (p.1108·1).
*Herpes simplex infections.*

**Virupos** *Ursapharm, Ger.*
Aciclovir (p.626·1).
*Herpes simplex eye infections.*

**Viru-Salvysat** *Ysatfabrik, Ger.*
Sage (p.1741·2).
*Mouth and throat infections.*

**Virusan** *Rekah, Israel.*
Idoxuridine (p.637·3).
*Herpes simplex eye infections.*

**Viruseen** *Hommel, Ger.*
Aciclovir (p.626·1).
*Herpesvirus infections.*

**Viruserol** *Novartis Consumer, Ital.*
Tromantadine hydrochloride (p.656·1).
*Herpesvirus infections of the skin.*

**Viru-Serol** *Armstrong, Mex.; Lacer, Spain.*
Tromantadine hydrochloride (p.656·1).
*Herpesvirus infections of the skin and mucous membranes.*

**Virustat**
*Note. This name is used for preparations of different composition.*
*Sanus, Braz.†.*
Zidovudine (p.658·2).
*HIV infection.*

*Synthelabo, Hong Kong†.*
Moroxydine hydrochloride (p.649·3).
*Viral infections.*

**Virusteril** *Biospray, Gr.*
Aciclovir (p.626·1).
*Labial and genital herpes simplex infections.*

**Virustop** *Pulitzer, Ital.*
Inosine pranobex (p.640·2).
*Immunodeficiency; viral infections.*

**Viruxan** *Sigma-Tau, Ital.*
Inosine pranobex (p.640·2).
*Immunodeficiency; viral infections.*

**Virval** *Novag, Spain.*
Valaciclovir hydrochloride (p.656·1).
*Herpesvirus infections.*

**Virzin** *Dermapharm, Ger.*
Aciclovir (p.626·1).
*Herpesvirus infections.*

**Visacare** *Boehringer Ingelheim, Austria.*
Hypromellose (p.1579·3).
*Dry eyes.*

**Visadron** *Boehringer Ingelheim, Austria; Boehringer Ingelheim, Belg.; Alcon, Ger.; Boehringer Ingelheim, Ital.; Boehringer Ingelheim, Neth.†; Boehringer Ingelheim, Port.; Fher, Spain.*
Phenylephrine hydrochloride (p.1126·3).
*Eye irritation.*

**Visaline** *Bausch & Lomb, Switz.*
Buphenine hydrochloride (p.1663·2); betacarotene (p.1422·3); alpha tocopherol (p.1464·3); ascorbic acid (p.1460·2).
*Eye disorders.*

**Visalmin** *Bunker, Braz.*
Chloramphenicol (p.185·1).
*Bacterial eye infections.*

**Visamin** *Bittner, Austria.*
Homoeopathic preparation.

**Visano N** *Kade, Ger.*
Meprobamate (p.706·2).
*Anxiety disorders; gastrointestinal disorders; insomnia.*

**VisanoCor N** *Kade, Ger.*
Pentaerithrityl tetranitrate (p.979·1); diphenhydramine hydrochloride (p.431·3).
VisanoCor formerly contained pentaerithrityl tetranitrate, meprobamate, diphenhydramine hydrochloride, and nicotinic acid.
*Cardiac disorders.*

**Visano-mini N** *Kade, Ger.*
Meprobamate (p.706·2).
*Anxiety disorders; sleep disorders.*

**Viscaplus** *Sifarma, Ital.*
Marine cartilage; amino acids; minerals; antioxidants (p.1417·1).
*Alopecia; nutritional supplement.*

**Viscard** *Norma (Νορμα), Gr.*
Nifedipine (p.966·2).
*Angina; hypertension.*

**Viscasan** *Bioforce, Ger.*
Homoeopathic preparation.

**Visceralgine**
*Exel, Belg.*
Tiemonium iodide (p.489·3).
*Smooth muscle spasm.*

*Organon, Fr.*
Tiemonium metilsulfate (p.489·3).
*Smooth muscle spasms.*

**Visceralgine Compositum** *Exel, Belg.†.*
Tiemonium iodide (p.489·3); dipyrone (p.35·3); codeine phosphate (p.27·1).
*Smooth muscle spasm.*

**Visceralgine Forte** *Organon, Fr.*
*Injection; tablets:* Tiemonium metilsulfate (p.489·3); dipyrone (p.35·3).
The tablets formerly contained tiemonium metilsulfate, dipyrone, and codeine phosphate.
*Suppositories†:* Tiemonium metilsulfate (p.489·3); dipyrone (p.35·3); codeine phosphate (p.27·1).
*Pain; smooth muscle spasms.*

**Visclair**
*Sinclair, Irl.; Sinclair, UK.*
Mecysteine hydrochloride (p.1124·1).
*Respiratory-tract disorders with viscous mucus.*

**Viscoat**
*Alcon, Arg.; Alcon, Austral.; Alcon, Belg.†; Alcon, Fr.; Alcon, Ger.; Alcon, Hong Kong; Alcon, Ital.; Alcon, Malaysia; Alcon, NZ; Alcon, S.Afr.; Alcon, Singapore; Alcon, Switz.†; Alcon, Thai.; Alcon, UK†; Alcon, USA.*
Chondroitin sulfate sodium (p.1670·2); sodium hyaluronate (p.1697·3).
*Adjunct in eye surgery.*

**Viscocort** *Bournonville, Belg.†.*
Prednisolone acetate (p.1108·1); chloramphenicol (p.185·1).
*Infected inflammatory ear disorders.*

**Viscofresh** *Allergan, Spain.*
Carmellose sodium (p.1577·3).
*Dry eyes.*

**Viscolex** *Pinewood, Irl.*
Carbocisteine (p.1116·2).
*Respiratory-tract disorders with excessive or viscous mucus.*

**Viscolyt** *Gea, Denm.*
Bromhexine hydrochloride (p.1115·3).
*Dry eyes; respiratory-tract congestion.*

**Viscomucil** *ABC, Ital.*
Ambroxol hydrochloride (p.1114·3).
*Respiratory-tract congestion.*

**Visconisan N** *Hanosan, Ger.*
Homoeopathic preparation.

**Viscopaste** *Smith & Nephew, Irl.*
Zinc oxide (p.1163·2).
*Dermatitis; leg ulcers; medicated bandage; varicose eczema.*

**Viscopaste PB7**
*Smith & Nephew, Ital.; Smith & Nephew, S.Afr.†; Smith & Nephew, UK.*
Zinc oxide (p.1163·2).
*Medicated bandage.*

**Visc-Ophtal** *Winzer, Ger.*
Carbomer (p.1577·2).
*Dry eyes.*

**Viscophyll** *Krewel, Ger.*
Mistletoe (p.1715·3); bladderwrack (p.1742·3).
*Circulatory disorders.*

**Viscorapas duo** *Pascoe, Ger.*
Convallaria (p.1675·3); crataegus (p.1677·1).
*Heart failure.*

**Viscoseal**
*Chemedica, Ger.; Chemedica, Switz.*
Sodium hyaluronate (p.1697·3).
*Adjuvant in arthroscopy.*

**Viscotears**
*Novartis Ophthalmics, Arg.; Novartis, Austral.; Novartis Ophthalmics, Braz.; Novartis, Chile; Novartis, Denm.; Novartis, Fin.; Novartis Ophthalmics, Hong Kong; Ciba Vision, Israel; Novartis, Mex.; Novartis, Norw.; Novartis, NZ; Novartis, Spain; Novartis Ophthalmics, Swed.; Novartis Ophthalmics, Switz.; Novartis, UK.*
Carbomer 980 (p.1577·2).
*Dry eyes.*

**Viscoteina** *Iquinosa, Spain.*
Carbocisteine (p.1116·2).
*Respiratory-tract congestion.*

**Viscoter** *Novartis, Gr.*
Carbomer (p.1577·2).
*Dry eyes.*

**Viscotiol**
*Celltech, Fr.†; Searle, Ital.†.*
Letosteine (p.1123·3).
*Respiratory-tract congestion.*

**Viscotirs** *Ciba Vision, Ital.*
Carbomer (p.1577·2).
*Dry eyes.*

**Viscotraan** *Covan, S.Afr.*
Hypromellose (p.1579·3).
*Dry eyes.*

**Viscozyme** *Roche, Chile.*
Dornase alfa (p.1119·1).
*Cystic fibrosis.*

**Viscum album H** *Pflüger, Ger.*
Homoeopathic preparation.

**Viscysat** *Ysatfabrik, Ger.*
Mistletoe (p.1715·3).
*Circulatory disorders.*

**Visderm**
*Wyeth, Mex.; Wyeth-Ayerst, Thai.*
Amcinonide (p.1091·1).
*Skin disorders.*

**Visergil**
*LPB, Ital.†; Novartis, Spain†.*
Co-dergocrine mesilate (p.1674·1); thioridazine (p.724·2) or thioridazine hydrochloride (p.724·2).
*Cerebrovascular disorders; mixed anxiety depressive states.*

**Vi-Siblin**
*Pfizer, Denm.; Pfizer, Fin.; Pfizer, Norw.; Pfizer, Swed.*
Ispaghula (p.1268·1).
*Constipation; irritable bowel syndrome.*

**Vi-Siblin S** *Pfizer, Swed.*
Ispaghula (p.1268·1); sorbitol (p.1446·3).
*Constipation; irritable bowel syndrome.*

**Visicol** *Inkine, USA.*
Monobasic sodium phosphate (p.1230·3); dibasic sodium phosphate (p.1231·1).
*Bowel evacuation.*

**Visidic** *Laboratorios Chile, Chile.*
Polyvinyl alcohol (p.1581·1).
*Dry eyes; eye irritation.*

**Visinal** *Stada, Ger.†.*
Valerian (p.1762·2); lupulus (p.1708·1); passion flower (p.1729·1).
*Nervous disorders; sleep disorders.*

**Visine**
*Mack, Belg.†; Pfizer Consumer, Canad.; Pfizer, Fin.; Pfizer, Gr.; Pfizer, India; Pfizer, Israel; Pfizer Consumer, Ital.; Pfizer, Malaysia; Pfizer, NZ; Pfizer, Port.; Pfizer, Singapore; Pfizer, Switz.; Pfizer, Thai.*
Tetryzoline hydrochloride (p.1131·2).
*Eye irritation.*

**Visine AC** *Pfizer, Israel.*
Tetryzoline hydrochloride (p.1131·2); zinc sulfate (p.1469·3).
*Eye irritation.*

**Visine AD** *Pfizer, Mex.*
Oxymetazoline hydrochloride (p.1126·1).
*Eye irritation.*

**Visine Advanced Relief**
*Pfizer Consumer, Austral.; Pfizer, NZ.*
Tetryzoline hydrochloride (p.1131·2); dextran 70 (p.746·2); macrogol 400 (p.1709·1); povidone (p.1581·2).
*Dry eyes; eye irritation.*

**Visine Allergy**
*Pfizer, Austral.†; Pfizer Consumer, Canad.*
Tetryzoline hydrochloride (p.1131·2); zinc sulfate (p.1469·3).
Formerly known as Visine Plus in *Austral.* and Visine AC in *Canad.*
*Eye irritation.*

**Visine Allergy with Antihistamine**
*Pfizer Consumer, Austral.; Pfizer, NZ.*
Naphazoline hydrochloride (p.1124·3); pheniramine maleate (p.438·3).

**Visine Allergy Relief**
*Pfizer, Hong Kong; Pfizer, USA.*
Tetryzoline hydrochloride (p.1131·2); zinc sulfate (p.1469·3).
Formerly called Visine AC in the *USA*.
*Eye irritation.*

**Visine Contact Lens** *Pfizer Consumer, Canad.*
Hypromellose (p.1579·3)(p.1164·2).
*Eye irritation during contact lens wear.*

**Visine for Contacts** *Pfizer, Hong Kong.*
Hypromellose (p.1579·3); glycerol (p.1694·3) (p.1164·2).
*Eye irritation during contact lens wear.*

**Visine Extra** *Pfizer, Mex.*
Tetryzoline hydrochloride (p.1131·2); macrogol 400 (p.1709·1).
*Eye irritation.*

**Visine LR** *Pfizer Consumer, USA.*
Oxymetazoline hydrochloride (p.1126·1).
*Eye irritation.*

**Visine Moisturizing**
*Pfizer Consumer, Canad.; Pfizer, Hong Kong; Pfizer, USA.*
Tetryzoline hydrochloride (p.1131·2); macrogol 400 (p.1709·1).
Formerly called Visine Extra.
*Dry eyes; eye irritation.*

**Visine Original**
*Pfizer Consumer, Austral.; Pfizer, Hong Kong; Pfizer Consumer, USA.*
Tetryzoline hydrochloride (p.1131·2).
*Eye irritation.*

**Visine Revive** *Pfizer Consumer, Austral.†.*
Tetryzoline hydrochloride (p.1131·2); macrogol 400 (p.1709·1).
*Dry eyes; eye irritation.*

**Visine True Tears**
*Note. This name is used for preparations of different composition.*
*Pfizer Consumer, Austral.*
Glycerol (p.1694·3); hypromellose (p.1579·3); macrogol 400 (p.1709·1).
*Dry eyes.*

*Pfizer Consumer, Canad.*
Macrogol 400 (p.1709·1).

**Visine Workplace** *Pfizer Consumer, Canad.*
Oxymetazoline hydrochloride (p.1126·1).
Formerly known as Visine LR.
*Eye irritation.*

**Visiodose** *Cooperation Pharmaceutique, Fr.†.*
Chlorhexidine gluconate (p.1173·2); phenylephrine hydrochloride (p.1126·3).
*Conjunctivitis.*

**Visiolyre** *Urgo, Fr.†.*
Cadmium sulfate (p.1663·3); zinc sulfate (p.1469·3); phenylephrine hydrochloride (p.1126·3).
*Eye disorders.*

**Visio-Max** *Wassen, UK.*
Selenium; vitamins; bilberry (p.1417·1).

**Vision Care Enzymatic Cleaner** *Alcon, USA.*
Pancreatin (p.1725·3) (p.1164·2).
*Cleansing solution for soft contact lenses.*

**Visionace** *Vitabiotics, UK.*
Vitamin, mineral, and nutrient preparation (p.1417·1).
*Eye disorders.*

**Visional Gotas** *Maver, Chile.*
Tetryzoline hydrochloride (p.1131·2).
*Eye congestion.*

**VisionBlue** *DORC, Neth.*
Trypan blue (p.1758·3).
*Ophthalmic stain.*

**Visionom** *Genom, Braz.*
Hamamelis (p.1696·3); chamomile (p.1669·3).
*Eye disorders.*

**Visipaque**
*Amersham, Austral.; Nycomed, Austria; Nycomed, Belg.†; Nycomed Imaging, Canad.; Sanofi Synthelabo, Chile; Amersham, Denm.; Amersham, Fin.; Amersham, Fr.; Amersham, Ger.; Nycomed, Gr.; Nycomed, Israel; Nycomed, Ital.; Nycomed, Neth.†; Nycomed Imaging, Norw.; Amersham, NZ; Amersham, Spain; Amersham, Swed.; Nycomed, Switz.; Nycomed Amersham, UK; Nycomed, USA.*
Iodixanol (p.1063·3).
*Radiographic contrast medium.*

**Visiplex** *Bunker, Braz.*
Naphazoline hydrochloride (p.1124·3); zinc sulfate (p.1469·3); boric acid (p.1662·1); borax (p.1661·3).
*Ocular congestion.*

**Viskaldix**
*Novartis, Austria; Novartis, Belg.; Novartis, Braz.; Novartis, Chile; Novartis, Fr.; Novartis, Ger.; Novartis, Irl.; Novartis, Malaysia; Novartis, Neth.; Novartis, NZ†; Novartis, Switz.; Novartis, Thai.; Novartis, UK.*
Pindolol (p.983·2); clopamide (p.888·2).
*Hypertension.*

**Viskazide** *Novartis, Canad.*
Pindolol (p.983·2); hydrochlorothiazide (p.933·2).
*Hypertension.*

**Viskeen** *Novartis, Neth.*
Pindolol (p.983·2).
*Cardiovascular disorders.*

**Visken**
*Novartis, Austral.; Novartis, Austria; Novartis, Belg.; Novartis, Braz.; Novartis, Canad.; Novartis, Denm.; Novartis, Fin.; Novartis, Fr.; Novartis, Ger.; Novartis, Gr.; Novartis, Hong Kong; Novartis, India; Novartis, Irl.; Novartis, Israel†; Novartis, Ital.; Novartis, Mex.; Novartis, NZ†; Novartis, S.Afr.†; Novartis, Swed.; Sovereign, UK; Novartis, USA.*
Pindolol (p.983·2).
*Angina pectoris; arrythmias; hypertension; hyperthyroidism; hypertrophic obstructive cardiomyopathy; myocardial infarction; phaeochromocytoma.*

**Viskene** *Novartis, Switz.*
Pindolol (p.983·2).
*Cardiac disorders; hypertension.*

**Viskenit** *Novartis, Austria.*
Pindolol (p.983·2); isosorbide dinitrate (p.941·1).
*Angina pectoris.*

**Viskoferm** *Nordic, Swed.*
Acetylcysteine (p.1112·3).
*Bronchitis.*

**Viskose ojendraber** *Ophtha, Denm.*
Sodium chloride (p.1233·3).
*Dry eyes.*

**Vislin** *Alcon, Braz.*
Tetryzoline hydrochloride (p.1131·2); methylthioninium chloride (p.1042·2).
*Ocular congestion.*

**Vislube**
*Chemedica, Ger.; Chemedica, Switz.*
Sodium hyaluronate (p.1697·3) (p.1164·2).
*Contact lens lubricant; dry eyes.*

**Vismed**
*Hamilton, Austral.; Thea, Fr.; Chemedica, Ger.; Chemedica, Hong Kong; Tubilux, Ital.; Chemedica, Switz.*
Sodium hyaluronate (p.1697·3).
Formerly known as Vislube in *Hong Kong*.
*Dry eyes; lubrication for contact lens.*

**Visodin** *Allergan, Braz.*
Tetryzoline hydrochloride (p.1131·2); methylthioninium chloride (p.1042·2).
*Ocular congestion.*

**Visogenol** *INQ, Braz.†.*
Chlorobutanol (p.1176·3); boric acid (p.1662·1).
*Eye disorders.*

**Visolon** *Igefarma, Braz.†.*
Naphazoline (p.1124·3); benzalkonium chloride (p.1168·3); zinc sulfate (p.1469·3); berberine sulfate (p.1659·3).
*Ocular congestion.*

**Visolux** *Brasmedica, Braz.†.*
Tetryzoline (p.1131·2); methylthioninium chloride (p.1042·2).
*Eye disorders.*

**Visonest** *Allergan, Braz.*
Proxymetacaine hydrochloride (p.1384·1).
*Local anaesthesia.*

**Visopt** *Sigma, Austral.*
Phenylephrine (p.1126·3).
*Eye irritation and congestion.*

**Visotone** *British Dispensary, Thai.*
*Eye drops:* Phenylephrine hydrochloride (p.1126·3); boric acid (p.1662·1); borax (p.1661·3); sodium chloride (p.1233·3).
*Eye solution:* Boric acid (p.1662·1); borax (p.1661·3); salicylic acid (p.1157·1); zinc sulfate (p.1469·3).
*Eye irritation.*

**Visoy** *Wyeth Lederle, Port.*
Soy protein infant feed (p.1417·1).
*Gastro-enteritis; intolerance to cow's milk, lactose, or sucrose.*

**Vispring** *Pfizer Lambert, Spain.*
Tetryzoline hydrochloride (p.1131·2).
*Conjunctival congestion; eye irritation.*

**Vistabel** *Allergan, Fr.*
Botulinum A toxin (p.1388·3).
*Wrinkles.*

**Vistacarpin** *Allergan, Ger.†.*
Pilocarpine hydrochloride (p.1495·1).
*Glaucoma; production of miosis.*

**Vista-Cetamide** *Martindale, Hong Kong.*
Sulfacetamide (p.257·3).
NOTE. There is no connection between Martindale, The Complete Drug Reference and Martindale, Hong Kong.
*Eye infections.*

**Vistacloran** *Allergan, Arg.*
Chloramphenicol succinate (p.186·3); naphazoline hydrochloride (p.1124·3).
*Bacterial eye infections.*

**Vistacrom** *Allergan, Canad.†.*
Sodium cromoglicate (p.795·3).
*Conjunctivitis.*

**Vistafrin** *Allergan, Spain.*
Phenylephrine hydrochloride (p.1126·3).
*Eye irritation.*

**Vistagan**
*Allergan, Austria; Allergan, Ger.; Alvia (Αλβια), Gr.; Allergan, Ital.; Allergan, Switz.*
Levobunolol hydrochloride (p.946·2).
*Glaucoma; ocular hypertension.*

**Vistalbalon** *Allergan, Ger.†.*
Naphazoline hydrochloride (p.1124·3).
*Eye disorders.*

**Vista-Methasone** *Martindale Pharmaceuticals, UK.*
Betamethasone sodium phosphate (p.1093·1).
NOTE. There is no connection between Martindale, The Complete Drug Reference and Martindale Pharmaceuticals.
*Inflammatory disorders of the ear, eye, or nose.*

**Vista-Methasone N**
*Daniels, Irl.†; Martindale Pharmaceuticals, UK.*
Betamethasone sodium phosphate (p.1093·1); neomycin sulfate (p.235·1).
NOTE. There is no connection between Martindale, The Complete Drug Reference and Martindale Pharmaceuticals.
*Inflammatory disorders of the ear, eye, or nose with bacterial infection.*

**Vista-Phenicol** *Martindale, Hong Kong.*
Chloramphenicol (p.185·1).
NOTE. There is no connection between Martindale, The Complete Drug Reference and Martindale, Hong Kong.
*Blepharitis; conjunctivitis.*

**Vistaril** *Pfizer, USA.*
Hydroxyzine embonate (p.434·3).
*Anxiety; premedication; pruritus; sedative.*

**Vistazine** *Keene, USA†.*
Hydroxyzine hydrochloride (p.434·3).
*Anxiety; hypersensitivity reactions.*

**Vistide**
*Pharmacia, Austral.; Pharmacia, Austria; Pharmacia, Belg.; Pharmacia, Braz.†; Pharmacia, Fr.; Pharmacia, Ger.; Pharmacia Upjohn, Ital.; Pharmacia, Port.; Pharmacia, Spain; Pharmacia, Switz.; Pharmacia, UK; Gilead, USA.*
Cidofovir (p.629·2).
*Cytomegalovirus retinitis.*

**Vistimon**
*Jenapharm, Ger.; Jenapharm, Malaysia.*
Mesterolone (p.1559·1).
*Androgen deficiency.*

**Vistofilm** *Allergan, Ger.†.*
Polyvinyl alcohol (p.1581·1) (p.1164·2).
*Wetting solution for contact lenses.*

**Vistosan** *Allergan, Ger.†.*
Phenylephrine hydrochloride (p.1126·3).
*Eye disorders.*

**Vistoxyn** *Allergan, Ger.; Allergan, Switz.*
Oxymetazoline hydrochloride (p.1126·1).
*Conjunctivitis; eye irritation.*

**Visu Q10** *Visufarma, Ital.*
Ubidecarenone (p.1760·2); vitamin E; lutein (p.1417·1).
*Antoxidant.*

**Visual** *Hexal, Braz.*
Zinc sulfate (p.1469·3); boric acid (p.1662·1); borax (p.1661·3); naphazoline hydrochloride (p.1124·3).
Formerly contained zinc sulfate, procaine, boric acid, borax, naphazoline, and sodium sulfate.
*Ocular congestion.*

**Visual-Eyes** *Optopics, USA.*
Electrolyte solution (p.1217·1).
*Eye irrigation.*

**Visublefarite** *Visufarma, Ital.; Merck Sharp & Dohme, Spain†.*
Betamethasone (p.1093·1); sulfacetamide sodium (p.257·3); tetryzoline phosphate (p.1131·2).
*Eye disorders.*

**Visubril** *Allergan, Arg.*
Tetryzoline hydrochloride (p.1131·2); methylthioninium chloride (p.1042·2).
*Eye inflammation.*

**Visucloben** *Visufarma, Ital.*
Clobetasone butyrate (p.1095·3).
*Eye disorders.*

**Visucloben Antibiotico** *Visufarma, Ital.*
Clobetasone butyrate (p.1095·3); bekanamycin sulfate (p.162·2).
*Infected eye disorders.*

**Visucloben Decongestionante** *Visufarma, Ital.*
Clobetasone butyrate (p.1095·3); tetryzoline hydrochloride (p.1131·2).
*Eye congestion, irritation, and inflammation.*

**Visudyne** *Novartis Ophthalmics, Arg.; Novartis, Austral.; Novartis Ophthalmics, Braz.; Novartis Ophthalmics, Canad.; Novartis, Chile; Novartis, Denm.; Novartis, Fin.; Novartis Ophthalmics, Fr.; Novartis Ophthalmics, Ger.; Ciba, Gr.; Parkedale, Hong Kong; Novartis Ophthalmics, Hong Kong; Ciba Vision, Israel; Ciba Vision, Ital.; Novartis, Norw.; Novartis, NZ; Novartis Ophthalmics, Singapore; Novartis, Spain; Novartis Ophthalmics, Swed.; Novartis Ophthalmics, Switz.; Novartis, Thai.; Novartis Ophthalmics, UK; Novartis Ophthalmics, USA.*
Verteporfin (p.591·1).
*Age-related macular degeneration; choroidal neovascularisation.*

**Visuglican** *Visufarma, Ital.*
Sodium cromoglicate (p.795·3); chlorphenamine maleate (p.427·3).
*Conjunctivitis.*

**Visumetazone** *Visufarma, Ital.*
Dexamethasone (p.1097·1).
*Inflammatory eye disorders.*

**Visumetazone Antibiotico** *Visufarma, Ital.*
Bekanamycin sulfate (p.162·2); tetryzoline hydrochloride (p.1131·2); betamethasone (p.1093·1).
*Eye infections associated with inflammation and congestion.*

**Visumetazone Antistaminico** *Visufarma, Ital.*
Dexamethasone (p.1097·1); chlorphenamine maleate (p.427·3).
*Conjunctivitis.*

**Visumetazone Decongestionante** *Visufarma, Ital.*
Dexamethasone (p.1097·1); tetryzoline hydrochloride (p.1131·2).
*Conjunctivitis; eye congestion and irritation; scleritis.*

**Visumicina** *Visufarma, Ital.†.*
Bekanamycin sulfate (p.162·2); tetryzoline hydrochloride (p.1131·2).
*Bacterial eye infections.*

**Visumidriatic** *Visufarma, Ital.*
Tropicamide (p.491·1).
*Production of mydriasis.*

**Visumidriatic Antiflogistico** *Merck Sharp & Dohme, Ital.†.*
Betamethasone (p.1093·1); tropicamide (p.491·1).
*Inflammatory eye disorders.*

**Visumidriatic Fenilefrina** *Visufarma, Ital.*
Tropicamide (p.491·1); phenylephrine hydrochloride (p.1126·3).
*Production of mydriasis.*

**Visustrin** *Centra, Ital.*
Tetryzoline hydrochloride (p.1131·2); methylthioninium chloride (p.1042·2).
*Conjunctival oedema; eye congestion and irritation.*

**Visutensil** *Visufarma, Ital.†.*
Guanethidine monosulfate (p.926·3).
*Glaucoma.*

**Vi-Syneral** *Aventis Pasteur, Chile; Grossman, Mex.*
Multivitamin and mineral preparation (p.1417·1).
*USV, India.*
Multivitamin preparation (p.1417·1).

**Vi-Syneral GE** *Beta, Arg.*
Vitamin preparation with or without minerals (p.1417·1).

**Vi-Syneral Plus** *Sanofi Winthrop, Braz.†.*
Multivitamin preparation (p.1417·1).

**Vit Eparin** *Teofarma, Ital.*
Heparin sodium (p.928·1); tocoferil acetate (p.1465·1).
*Ocular haemorrhage and its sequelae.*

**Vita** *Poen, Arg.*
Vitamin A acetate; vitamin E; vitamin P (p.1417·1).
*Vitamin supplement.*

**Vita 3** *Novartis, Fr.†; Ciba Vision, Switz.†.*
Phenylephrine hydrochloride (p.1126·3); rutoside sodium sulfate (p.1688·3).
*Conjunctivitis; eye irritation.*

**Vita 3B** *Riva, Canad.*
Vitamin B substances (p.1417·1).

**Vita B6** *Vitaglow, Austral.†.*
Pyridoxine hydrochloride (p.1456·3).
*Premenstrual syndrome; vitamin $B_6$ supplement.*

**Vita B Compound 100** *Vita Pharm, Canad.*
Vitamin B substances (p.1417·1).

**Vita B plus C** *Romilo, Canad.†.*
Vitamin B substances and vitamin C (p.1417·1).

**Vita 3B plus C** *Riva, Canad.*
Vitamin B substances with vitamin C (p.1417·1).

**Vita Bee** *Rugby, USA.*
Multivitamin preparation (p.1417·1).

**Vita Buer-G-plus** *Altana, Switz.*
*Capsules:* Multivitamin and mineral preparation with kola and ginseng (p.1417·1).
*Oral liquid:* Multivitamin and mineral preparation with ginseng (p.1417·1).
*Tonic.*

**Vita Buerlecithin** *Altana, Ger.*
Lecithin (p.1706·1); vitamins (p.1417·1).
*Tonic.*
*Altana, Switz.*
Vitamin B preparation with lecithin (p.1706·1) (p.1417·1).
*Tonic.*

**Vita C** *Vitaglow, Austral.†.*
Calcium ascorbate (p.1460·2).
*Cold and influenza symptoms; wounds.*
*Upha, Malaysia.*
Vitamin C (p.1460·2).
*Vitamin C deficiency; vitamin C supplement.*

**Vita Calmag Zn** *Vita Health, Singapore.*
Calcium (p.1225·1); magnesium (p.1227·3); zinc (p.1469·2).
*Calcium deficiency; osteoporosis.*

**Vita Cris** *Cris Flower, Ital.*
Multivitamin preparation (p.1417·1).
*Nutritional supplement.*

**Vita Day** *Jamieson, Canad.†.*
Multivitamin and mineral preparation (p.1417·1).

**Vita Dino Buddies** *Vita Pharm, Canad.*
Multivitamin and mineral preparation (p.1417·1).

**Vita E** *Vitaglow, Austral.†.*
*d*-Alpha tocopherol (p.1464·3).
*Antoxidant; dry skin disorders; wounds.*

**Vita Ferin C** *Geistlich, Switz.*
Multivitamin and mineral preparation (p.1417·1).

**Vita Gerine** *Melisana, Switz.*
Deanol orotate; vitamins; minerals (p.1417·1); rutoside; choline bitartrate.
*Tonic.*

**Vita Grip** *Sinterapico, Braz.†.*
Ascorbic acid (p.1460·2); caffeine (p.782·1); salicylamide (p.87·3); chlorphenamine maleate (p.427·3).
*Cold and influenza symptoms.*

**Vita Menal** *Alacan, Spain.*
Cyproheptadine hydrochloride (p.430·1); amino acids; cyanocobalamin (p.1417·1); fosforylethanolamine.
*Tonic.*

**Vita Multicap** *Sriprasit, Thai.*
Multivitamin and mineral preparation (p.1417·1).

**Vita Senior** *Uniao Quimica, Braz.*
Vitamins; minerals; ginseng (p.1417·1).

**Vita Stress** *Vita Pharm, Canad.*
Multivitamin preparation (p.1417·1).

**Vita Truw** *Truw, Ger.†.*
Multivitamin and mineral preparation (p.1417·1).

**Vita Vim** *Jamieson, Canad.†.*
Multivitamin and mineral preparation (p.1417·1).

**Vita-B** *Shiwa, Thai.*
Vitamin $B_1$ (p.1455·2); vitamin $B_6$ (p.1457·2); vitamin $B_{12}$ (p.1458·2).
*Vitamin B deficiency.*

**Vita-B1** *Vitabalans, Fin.*
Thiamine hydrochloride (p.1455·1).
*Vitamin $B_1$ deficiency.*

**Vita-B2** *Vitabalans, Fin.*
Riboflavin (p.1456·1).
*Vitamin $B_2$ deficiency.*

**Vita-B6** *Vitabalans, Fin.*
Pyridoxine hydrochloride (p.1456·3).
*Vitamin $B_6$ deficiency.*

**Vitabact** *Novartis Ophthalmics, Fr.; Novartis Ophthalmics, Switz.*
Picloxydine dihydrochloride (p.1190·1).
*Bacterial eye infections.*

**Vitabase** *Heralds, Braz.†.*
Vitamin E (p.1464·3).
*Vitamin E deficiency.*

**Vitabase Complexo Vitaminico C/Minerais** *Johnson & Johnson, Braz.*
A vitamin and mineral preparation (p.1417·1).

**Vitabase Vitamina C** *Johnson & Johnson, Braz.*
Vitamin C (p.1460·2).

**Vitabe** *Silesia, Chile.*
Pyridoxine hydrochloride (p.1456·3).
*Vitamin $B_6$ deficiency.*

**Vita-Bel** *Offenbach, Mex.*
Vitamin B substances; lysine; iron (p.1417·1).
*Appetite loss.*

**Vitaber A E** *Llorens, Spain.*
Di-isopropylammonium dichloroacetate (p.900·1); vitamin A acetate (p.1453·1); tocoferil acetate (p.1465·1).
*Deficiency of vitamins A and E; eye disorders; infertility; recurrent miscarriage; skin disorders.*

**Vitaber PP + E** *Llorens, Spain†.*
Tocoferil nicotinate (p.1015·1).
*Hyperlipidaemias.*

**Vitableu** *Ciba Vision, Fr.†.*
Methylthioninium chloride (p.1042·2).
*Eye infections.*

**Vita-Bob** *Scot-Tussin, USA.*
Multivitamin preparation (p.1417·1).

**Vita-Brachont** *Azupharma, Ger.†.*
Cyanocobalamin (p.1458·2).
Lidocaine hydrochloride (p.1377·3) is included in this preparation to alleviate the pain of injection.
*Arthritis; neuralgia; neuritis; vitamin $B_{12}$ deficiency.*

**Vita-C** *Shaklee, Canad.; Vitabalans, Fin.; Freeda, USA.*
Ascorbic acid (p.1460·2).
*Scurvy; vitamin C deficiency.*

**Vitac** *Aventis, Chile.*
Ascorbic acid (p.1460·2).
*Vitamin C supplement.*

**Vita-C R15** *Reckeweg, Ger.*
Homoeopathic preparation.

**Vitacal** *Vita Health, Singapore.*
Calcium and vitamin D (p.1417·1).
*Calcium deficiency; osteoporosis.*

**Vita-Cal Mag with Zinc and Vitamin D** *Vita Pharm, Canad.*
Calcium; magnesium; zinc; vitamin D (p.1417·1).

**Vita-Cal Plus** *Shaklee, Canad.*
Multivitamin and mineral preparation (p.1417·1).

**Vitacap** *Medicap, Thai.*
Multivitamin and mineral preparation (p.1417·1).

**VitaCarn** *Kendall McGaw, USA.*
Carnitine (p.1423·3).
*Carnitine deficiency.*

**Vitace**
*Note. This name is used for preparations of different composition.*
*Pascoe, Ger.†.*
Multivitamin preparation (p.1417·1).
*Prisfar, Port.*
Echinacea purpurea (p.1683·2); vitamin C; zinc (p.1417·1).
*Tonic.*

**Vita-Ce** *Chemedica, Switz.*
Ascorbic acid (p.1460·2).
*Vitamin C deficiency; vitamin C supplement.*

**Vitacelsia Plus** *Prisfar, Port.*
Multivitamin and mineral preparation (p.1417·1).

**Vitacic** *Novartis Ophthalmics, Fr.*
Adenosine (p.851·2); thymidine (p.1755·3); cytidine; uridine (p.1760·3); disodium guanylate (p.1681·3).
*Corneal damage.*

**Vitacid** *Yabrofarma, Port.*
Tretinoin (p.1161·1).
*Acne.*

**Vitacimin** *Takeda, Thai.*
Ascorbic acid (p.1460·2).
*Vitamin C deficiency.*

**Vitacimin Sweetlet** *Takeda, Hong Kong.*
Ascorbic acid (p.1460·2); sodium ascorbate (p.1460·2).
*Vitamin C deficiency.*

**Vitacitrus** *Viternat, Braz.*
Ascorbic acid (p.1460·2).

**Vitacolor** *Heralds, Braz.†.*
Cod-liver oil (p.1425·2); zinc oxide (p.1163·2); boric acid (p.1662·1).
*Barrier preparation; skin disorders.*

**Vitacortil** *Hexa-Medinova, Arg.*
Betamethasone dipropionate (p.1093·1); gentamicin sulfate (p.217·1); clotrimazole (p.396·2).
*Infected skin disorders.*

**Vitacrecil** *Ferraz, Lynce, Port.*
Cystine; gelatin; zinc sulfate; ferrous sulfate; calcium pantothenate; pyridoxine hydrochloride (p.1417·1).
*Hair, skin, and nail disorders.*

**Vitactiv E** *HWS OTC, Austria.*
Alpha tocopherol (p.1464·3).
*Vitamin E deficiency.*

**Vitadece** *Klonal, Arg.*
Ascorbic acid; vitamin A; vitamin D (p.1417·1).
*Vitamin supplement.*

**Vita-Dermacide** *CS, Fr.*
Nicotinamide (p.1441·2); glutamic acid (p.1433·2); tryptophan (p.320·3).
*Irritative dermatitis.*

**Vitaderme** *Drogasil, Braz.†.*
Vitamin A; colecalciferol; vitamin E (p.1417·1); allantoin (p.1141·3).
*Barrier preparation.*

**Vitadesan** *Sanval, Braz.*
Vitamin A palmitate (p.1451·2); ergocalciferol (p.1462·1).

**Vita-D-Grin** *Grin, Mex.†.*
Ergocalciferol (p.1462·1).

**Vita-Diem** *Seven Seas, UK†.*
Multivitamin preparation (p.1417·1).

**Vitadol-C** *Karicare, NZ.*
Vitamin A, C, and D (p.1417·1).
*Vitamin supplement.*

**Vitadral** *Wernigerode, Ger.*
Vitamin A palmitate (p.1453·1).
*Vitamin A deficiency.*

**Vitadye** *Dermatech, Austral.; ICN, Malaysia.*
Dihydroxyacetone (p.1145·2).
*Vitiligo.*

**Vita-E** *Ache, Braz.; Shaklee, Canad.†; Vitabalans, Fin.; Worwag, Ger.; Cambridge Healthcare, UK.*
Vitamin E (p.1464·3).
*Dietary supplement.*

**Vita-E Plus Selenium** *Shaklee, Canad.†.*
Vitamin E (p.1464·3); selenium (p.1444·1).
*Dietary supplement.*

**Vitaendil C K P** *Wasserman, Spain†.*
Ascorbic acid (p.1460·2); menadione (p.1466·3); rutoside (p.1688·2).
*Haemorrhage.*

**VitaEPA** *Vita Health, Singapore.*
Docosahexaenoic acid (p.976·1); eicosapentaenoic acid (p.976·2).
*Hyperlipidaemias.*

**VitaEPA Plus** *Vita Health, Singapore.*
Eicosapentaenoic acid (p.976·2); evening primrose oil (p.1686·3).
*Circulatory disorders; hyperlipidaemias; inflammation.*

**Vitafardi C B12** *Fardi, Spain.*
Ascorbic acid (p.1460·2); hydroxocobalamin (p.1458·2).
*Deficiency of vitamins $B_{12}$ and C.*

**Vitafem** *Vita Pharm, Canad.*
Multivitamin and mineral preparation (p.1417·1).

**Vitaferro** *Hexal, Arg.; Hexal, Ger.*
Ferrous chloride (p.1427·3), ferrous gluconate (p.1428·1), or ferrous sulfate (p.1428·2).
*Iron deficiency; iron-deficiency anaemia.*

**Vitafissan N** *Uhlmann-Eyraud, Switz.*
Caseine hydrolysate (Labiline); vitamins A and E (p.1417·1); linoleic acid (p.1690·2); linolenic acid.
*Skin disorders.*

**Vitafluid** *Mann, Ger.*
Vitamin A palmitate (p.1453·1).
*Eye disorders.*

**Vitaflur** *Maver, Chile.*
Sodium fluoride (p.1444·3).

**Vitafol** *Everett, USA.*
*Syrup:* Ferric pyrophosphate (p.1427·2); folic acid (p.1429·1); vitamin B substances (p.1417·1).
*Tablets:* Ferrous fumarate (p.1427·3); folic acid (p.1429·1); multivitamins and minerals (p.1417·1).
*Iron-deficiency anaemias.*

**Vitaforte** *Rimsa, Mex.*
Multivitamin and mineral preparation (p.1417·1).

**Vitafran** *Faria, Braz.†.*
Vitamin C (p.1460·2).
*Vitamin C deficiency; vitamin C supplement.*

**Vitagama Fluor** *Almirall, Spain.*
Sodium fluoride (p.1444·3); multivitamins and minerals (p.1417·1).
*Vitamin and fluoride deficiencies.*

**Vitagama Fluor Complex** *Almirall, Spain†.*
Multivitamin preparation (p.1417·1) with ferrous sulfate (p.1428·2).
*Vitamin and iron deficiency.*

**Vita-Gard** *GNLD, Austral.†.*
Multivitamin and mineral preparation (p.1417·1).

**Vitagel** *Mann, Ger.*
Vitamin A palmitate (p.1453·1).
*Eye disorders.*

**Vitagenol**
*Note. This name is used for preparations of different composition.*
*Boehringer Ingelheim, Arg.*
Ginseng (p.1693·1).
*Mental function impairment; tonic.*
*Sanofi Synthelabo, Chile.*
Betacarotene; vitamin C; vitamin E; selenium (p.1417·1).
*Dietary supplement.*

**Vitagenol Plus** *Boehringer Ingelheim, Arg.*
Ginseng; minerals; vitamins (p.1417·1).
*Tonic.*

**Vitageran** *Odontofarma, Braz.†.*
Multivitamin and mineral preparation (p.1417·1).

**Vita-Gerin** *Chemomedica, Austria.*
Deanol orotate; vitamins; minerals; adenosine; choline bitartrate (p.1417·1).
*Tonic.*

**Vita-Gerin N** *Cassella-med, Ger.*
Deanol orotate; magnesium orotate; vitamins; minerals; choline bitartrate (p.1417·1).
*Tonic.*

**Vitageyer B** *Geyer, Braz.*
Vitamin B substances (p.1417·1).

**Vitageyer C** *Geyer, Braz.*
Ascorbic acid (p.1460·2).

**Vitaglow Selemite B** *Vitaglow, Austral.†.*
Selenium (p.1444·1); dried yeast (p.1469·1).
*Selenium deficiency.*

**Vitaglumil** *Salusif, Port.*
Vitamin B substances; ascorbic acid (p.1417·1).
*Tonic.*

**Vitagripe** *Berna, Spain.*
An influenza vaccine (p.1620·2).
*Active immunisation.*

**Vitagutt Knoblauch** *Schwarzhaupt, Ger.*
Garlic oil (p.1691·2).
*Circulatory disorders.*

**Vitagutt Vitamin E** *Schwarzhaupt, Ger.*
*dl*-Alpha tocoferil acetate (p.1465·1).
*Vitamin E deficiency.*

**Vita-Hexin** *Streuli, Switz.*
Chlorhexidine gluconate (p.1173·2); vitamin A palmitate (p.1453·1); cod-liver oil (p.1425·2); zinc oxide (p.1163·2).
*Skin lesions.*

**Vitaject** *Syxyl, Ger.*
Thiamine hydrochloride (p.1455·1); pyridoxine hydrochloride (p.1456·3); cyanocobalamin (p.1458·2).
*Vitamin B deficiency.*

**Vitakid** *Pharmaland, Thai.*
Multivitamin preparation with lysine (p.1417·1).
*Tonic.*

**Vita-Kid**
*Solgar, UK.*
Multivitamin preparation with folic acid (p.1417·1).

*Solgar, USA.*
Multivitamin preparation (p.1417·1).

**Vital** *Yu Sheng, Singapore.*
Glucosamine sulfate (p.1694·1).
*Joint and cartilage disorders.*

**Vital Eyes** *Novartis Consumer, UK.*
Lavender (p.1705·1); orange flower (p.1723·3); hamamelis (p.1696·3); euphrasia (p.1686·3).
*Eye irritation.*

**Vital Floramin** *Bennett, UK†.*
Mineral preparation (p.1417·1).
*Immune stimulant.*

**Vital High Nitrogen**
*Abbott, Hong Kong; Abbott, NZ; Ross, USA.*
A preparation for enteral nutrition (p.1417·1).

**Vital HN**
*Abbott, Austral.; Abbott, Canad.*
Preparation for enteral nutrition (p.1417·1).

**Vitalaif** *Medix, Mex.*
Multivitamin and mineral preparation with ginseng (p.1417·1).

**Vitalax** *Vita-Health, Hong Kong†.*
Psyllium hydrophilic mucilloid (p.1268·1).
*Constipation.*

**Vita-Lea** *Shaklee, Canad.*
Multivitamin and mineral preparation (p.1417·1).
*Dietary supplement.*

**Vitalen C** *Dovalle, Braz.*
Paracetamol (p.76·2); chlorphenamine (p.428·1); phenylephrine (p.1126·3); caffeine (p.782·1).
*Cold and influenza symptoms.*

**Vitaleph** *Aleph, Ital.†.*
Nutritional supplement (p.1417·1).

**Vitaler** *EMS, Braz.*
*Oral solution:* Buclizine (p.426·3); lysine; tryptophan; cyanocobalamin; vitamin $B_6$ (p.1417·1).
*Tablets:* Vitamin B substances; sodium glycerophosphate; calcium glycerophosphate; manganese hypophosphite; lysine hydrochloride; iron choline citrate (p.1417·1).
*Reduced appetite; tonic.*

**Vitalets** *Freeda, USA.*
Multivitamin and mineral preparation with iron (p.1417·1).

**Vitaleyes** *Novartis Ophthalmics, Fr.*
Multivitamin and trace-element preparation (p.1417·1).
*Nutritional supplement for healthy eyes.*

**Vitalgine** *Medecine Vegetale, Fr.†.*
Hamamelis (p.1696·3); viburnum.
*Haemorrhoids; peripheral vascular disorders.*

**Vitalin**
*Vitasan, Austria; Loges, Ger.†.*
Crataegus (p.1677·1).
*Heart failure.*

**Vitaline** *Bioglan, Austral.†.*
Lysine (p.1439·1); zinc oxide (p.1163·2).
*Herpes simplex lesions.*

**Vitalipid**
*Pharmacia Upjohn, Belg.†; Fresenius Kabi, Denm.; Fresenius Kabi, Fin.; Baxter, Ger.; Fresenius Kabi, Gr.; Fresenius Kabi, Ital.; Fresenius Kabi, Norw.; Baxter, NZ; Fresenius Kabi, NZ; Fresenius Kabi, Port.; Fresenius Kabi, S.Afr.†; Fresenius Kabi, Spain; Fresenius Kabi, Swed.; Fresenius Kabi, Thai.*
Vitamins A, $D_2$, E, and $K_1$ for infusion (p.1417·1).
*Parenteral nutrition.*

**Vitalipid N**
*Baxter, Austral.†; Fresenius Kabi, Hong Kong; Pharmacia Upjohn, Israel; Fresenius Kabi, Malaysia; Fresenius Kabi, Singapore; Fresenius Kabi, Switz.*
Vitamins A, $D_2$, E, and $K_1$ for infusion (p.1417·1).
*Parenteral nutrition.*

**Vitalipid Neu** *Fresenius Kabi, Austria.*
Vitamins A, D, E, and K for infusion (p.1417·1).
Contains egg lipid.
*Parenteral nutrition.*

**Vitalipide** *Fresenius Kabi, Fr.*
Vitamins A, $D_2$, E, and $K_1$ for infusion (p.1417·1).
*Parenteral nutrition.*

**Vitalisin** *Brasifa, Braz.†.*
Buclizine (p.426·3); lysine; carnitine; vitamin B substances (p.1417·1).
*Reduced appetite; tonic.*

**Vitalitan** *Ducto, Braz.*
A multivitamin and mineral preparation (p.1417·1).

**Vitalium** *Farma Lepori, Spain.*
Hypericum (p.299·1).
*Sleep disorders; tonic.*

**Vitalize** *Scot-Tussin, USA.*
Ferric pyrophosphate (p.1427·2); vitamin B substances with L-lysine (p.1417·1).
*Iron-deficiency anaemias.*

**Vital-Kapseln** *Ratiopharm, Ger.*
Eleutherococcus senticosus (p.1744·1).
*Tonic.*

**Vitalle** *Allen, Mex.*
Alpha tocopherol (p.1464·3).
*Vitamin E deficiency.*

**Vitalmin Nutraenergy** *Recalcine, Chile.*
Preparation for enteral nutrition (p.1417·1).

**Vitalmix Complex** *Montefarmaco, Ital.*
Myrtillus; guarana; ginseng; royal jelly; bioflavonoids; vitamins (p.1417·1).
*Nutritional supplement.*

**Vitalmix Fos** *Montefarmaco, Ital.*
Phosphorylserine; eleutherococcus; arginine aspartate; ginkgo biloba; royal jelly (p.1417·1).
*Nutritional supplement.*

**Vitalmix Junior** *Montefarmaco, Ital.*
Vitamin $B_{12}$; iron; folic acid; amino acids; phosphorylserine (p.1417·1).
*Nutritional supplement.*

**Vita-Logos** *Sigma-Tau, Switz.*
Cyanocobalamin; amino acids (p.1417·1).
*Tonic.*

**Vitalorange** *Glaxo Wellcome, Mex.*
Vitamin A (p.1451·2); colecalciferol (p.1461·3).
*Nutritional supplement.*

**Vitalpen** *Labomed, Chile.*
Flucloxacillin (p.213·3).
*Gram-positive bacterial infections.*

**Vitalux**
*Novartis Ophthalmics, Arg.; Novartis Ophthalmics, Canad.; Novartis, Chile; Ciba Vision, Fr.†; Novartis Ophthalmics, Hong Kong.*
A multivitamin and mineral preparation (p.1417·1).
*Eye disorders.*

*Ciba Vision, Braz.†.*
Vitamins; minerals; amino acids (p.1417·1).

*Novartis, Ital.*
Betacarotene; vitamins; minerals; soya lecithin; beeswax; wheat-germ oil (p.1417·1).
*Nutritional supplement.*

**Vitalux Plus** *Novartis, Ital.*
Vitamins; lecithin; luteine; gelatin; monoglycerides; iron oxides (p.1417·1).
*Nutritional supplement.*

**Vitalyn** *Fontovit, Braz.*
A multivitamin and mineral preparation (p.1417·1).

**Vitam Doce** *Frasca, Arg.*
Cyanocobalamin (p.1458·2).

**Vitamag** *Aspen, S.Afr.*
Vitamin B substances; magnesium; zinc (p.1417·1).
*Vitamin and mineral supplement.*

**Vita-Max** *Herbarium, Braz.*
Betacarotene; vitamin C; vitamin E; selenium (p.1417·1).

**Vitamedin**
*Sankyo, Hong Kong.*
Vitamin B substances (p.1417·1).
*Anaemias; neuritis; rheumatic disorders; sciatica.*

*Sankyo, Thai.*
Benfotiamine (p.1454·3); vitamin $B_6$ (p.1457·2); vitamin $B_{12}$ (p.1458·2).
*Anaemias; neural disorders.*

**Vita-Mefren** *Novartis Consumer, Belg.*
Chlorhexidine gluconate (p.1173·2); vitamin A palmitate (p.1453·1).
*Burns; infected skin disorders; wounds.*

**Vitamen** *Beta, Ital.*
Protein and multivitamin preparation (p.1417·1).

**Vita-Merfen** *Novartis Consumer, Switz.*
Chlorhexidine gluconate (p.1173·2); benzoxonium chloride (p.1170·2); vitamin A (p.1451·2).
*Minor wounds and burns.*

**Vita-Merfen NF** *Novartis, Israel.*
Chlorhexidine gluconate (p.1173·2); benzoxonium chloride (p.1170·2); vitamin A (p.1451·2).
*Burns; wounds.*

**Vita-Merfen Soins dermatologiques** *Novartis Consumer, Switz.*
Urea (p.1162·2).
*Dry skin.*

**Vitamfenicolo** *Tubilux, Ital.*
Chloramphenicol (p.185·1) or chloramphenicol sodium succinate (p.185·1).
*Bacterial eye infections.*

**Vitamidyne A and D** *Fischer, Israel.*
Vitamin A (p.1451·2); vitamin D (p.1461·2).
*Vitamin A and D deficiency.*

**Vitamil** *Laborsil, Braz.†.*
Buclizine (p.426·3); gamma-aminobutyric acid; vitamin B substances (p.1417·1).
*Reduced appetite; tonic.*

**Vitamin A Acid** *Dermik, Hong Kong.*
Tretinoin (p.1161·1).
*Acne.*

**Vitamin B duo** *Jenapharm, Ger.*
Thiamine hydrochloride (p.1455·1); pyridoxine hydrochloride (p.1456·3).
*Neurological system disorders.*

**Vitamin C-Calcium** *Herbrand, Ger.*
Calcium carbonate (p.1254·2); ascorbic acid (p.1460·2).
*Calcium deficiency; cold symptoms.*

**Vitamin F** *Klosterfrau, Austria.*
Ethyl linoleate.
*Skin disorders; wounds.*

**Vitamin for the Hair** *Natural Life, Arg.*
Vitamin and mineral preparation (p.1417·1).

**Vitamina C-Complex** *Natural Life, Arg.*
Rose fruit (p.1740·1); citrus bioflavonoids (p.1688·2); rutoside (p.1688·2); hesperidin (p.1688·2) complex; red cherry (p.1058·1).
*Vitamin C supplement.*

**Vitamina F99 Topica** *Vitafarma, Spain.*
Peru balsam (p.1730·2); vitamin F.
*Skin disorders.*

**Vitaminas Lorenzini** *Maxfarma, Spain†.*
Multivitamin and mineral preparation with ginseng (p.1417·1).

**Vitamine 15** *Solco, Switz.*
Multivitamin and mineral preparation (p.1417·1).

**Vitamine F99** *Doetsch, Grether, Switz.*
Ethyl linoleate; ethyl linolenate.
*Burns; skin disorders; wounds.*

**Vitaminer S** *Aventis, Braz.†.*
Multivitamin and mineral preparation (p.1417·1).

**Vitamineral** *ACO, Swed.*
Multivitamin and mineral preparation (p.1417·1).

**Vitaminex** *Ferrer, Spain†.*
Nucleosides; vitamins (p.1417·1).
*Tonic.*

**Vitaminic A-D** *Asta Medica, Belg.†.*
Vitamin A (p.1451·2); ergocalciferol (p.1462·1).
*Conjunctivitis; corneal burns and wounds; dry eyes.*

**Vita-Minis Cold & Flu** *Herron, Austral.†.*
Ascorbic acid (p.1460·2); sodium ascorbate (p.1460·2); echinacea angustifolia (p.1683·2); zinc (p.1469·2).
*Cold and influenza symptoms.*

**Vita-Minis Vitamin C Plus** *Herron, Austral.†.*
Calcium ascorbate (p.1460·2); bioflavonoids (p.1688·2).
*Vitamin C supplement.*

**Vitaminoftalmina** *Davi, Port.*
Vitamin A (p.1451·2).
*Eye disorders.*

**Vitaminol** *Bio-Sante, Canad.*
Multivitamin and mineral preparation (p.1417·1).

**Vitaminorum** *Sigma, Austral.*
Multivitamin preparation (p.1417·1).

**Vitamins Only** *Solgar, UK.*
Multivitamin preparation (p.1417·1).

**Vitamischka** *Bittner, Austria.*
Vitamin B substances (p.1417·1).

**Vitamon K** *Chefaro, Belg.*
Phytomenadione (p.1467·1).
*Vitamin K deficiency bleeding.*

**Vitamorrhuine** *Medgenix, Belg.†.*
Cod-liver oil (p.1425·2); vitamin A acetate (p.1453·1); colecalciferol (p.1461·3).
*Burns; skin disorders; wounds.*

**Vitamult** *CTI, Israel.*
Multivitamin preparation (p.1417·1).
*Tonic.*

**Vitamuruine** *Medgenix, Belg.*
Vitamin A acetate (p.1453·1).
*Burns; skin disorders; wounds.*

**Vitamycetin** *Wyeth, India.*
Chloramphenicol (p.185·1) or chloramphenicol palmitate (p.185·1).
*Bacterial infections.*

**Vitan** *Antigen, Irl.*
Multivitamin or multivitamin and mineral preparation (p.1417·1).

**Vit-A-N** *Farmigea, Ital.*
Vitamin A acetate (p.1453·1).
*Blepharitis; corneal ulcer; keratitis; keratoconjunctivitis.*

**Vitana-EZ** *Kenyaku, Thai.*
Multivitamin and mineral preparation with iron (p.1417·1).

**Vita-Nat** *Laboratorios Chile, Chile.*
Vitamin A; colecalciferol; ascorbic acid (p.1417·1).
*Vitamin A, D, and E supplement.*

**Vitanatur** *A Natureza, Braz.†.*
Vitamin B substances with minerals (p.1417·1).

**Vitaneed** *Sherwood, USA.*
Lactose-free preparation for enteral nutrition (p.1417·1).

**Vitaneuron** *Luper, Braz.*
Vitamin $B_{12}$ (p.1458·2); vitamin $B_1$ (p.1455·2).
*Megaloblastic anaemias; vitamin B deficiency.*

**Vitanol** *Stiefel, Spain.*
Tretinoin (p.1161·1).
*Acne; photodamaged skin.*

**Vitanol-A**
*Stiefel, Arg.; Stiefel, Braz.*
Tretinoin (p.1161·1).
*Acne; keratinisation disorders; skin hyperpigmentation.*

**Vitanor** *Medical, Port.†.*
Multivitamin preparation (p.1417·1).

**Vitanovit** *Flopen, Braz.†.*
Multivitamin and mineral preparation (p.1417·1).

**Vitapan** *Provita, Austria.*
Cod-liver oil (p.1425·2).
*Vitamin A and D deficiency.*

**Vitapantol** *Davigo, Belg.†.*
Calcium pantothenate (p.1442·3); vitamin A acetate (p.1453·1); nicotinamide (p.1441·2).
*Nasal disorders.*

**Vita-Ped** *Stiefel, Braz.*
Retinol palmitate; ascorbic acid; colecalciferol (p.1417·1).

**Vitapelen** *ICN, Arg.*
Vitamin A (p.1451·2); vitamin D (p.1461·2); zinc oxide (p.1163·2).
*Skin disorders.*

**Vitapen** *Vitamed, Israel.*
Ampicillin (p.157·1).
*Bacterial infections.*

**Vitaphakol**
*Novartis Ophthalmics, Fr.†; Ciba Vision, Port.†; Alcon Cusi, Spain; Ciba Vision, Switz.†.*
Adenosine (p.851·2); cytochrome C (p.1678·3); nicotinamide (p.1441·2); sodium succinate (p.1748·3); sorbitol (p.1446·3).
*Cataracts.*

**Vitaplex** *Provita, Austria.*
Multivitamin preparation (p.1417·1).

**Vitaplex comp** *Pharmacia Upjohn, Swed.†.*
Multivitamin preparation with iron (p.1417·1).

**Vitaplex mineral** *Pharmacia, Swed.*
Multivitamin and mineral preparation (p.1417·1).

**Vita-Plus** *Scot-Tussin, USA.*
A range of vitamin and mineral preparations (p.1417·1).

**Vitaplus B** *Douglas, NZ.*
Vitamin B substances; vitamin C; calcium (p.1417·1).
*Vitamin and calcium supplement.*

**Vitaplus B Plus** *Restan, S.Afr.*
Vitamin B substances; vitamin C; calcium (p.1417·1).
*Vitamin and calcium supplement.*

**Vitaplus C Plus** *Restan, S.Afr.*
Ascorbic acid (p.1460·2); calcium (p.1225·1).
*Vitamin C and calcium deficiencies.*

**Vita-Plus E** *Scot-Tussin, USA.*
Vitamin E (p.1464·3).
*Vitamin E deficiency.*

**Vita-PMS** *Bajamar, USA.*
Multivitamin and mineral preparation (p.1417·1).

**Vitapore** *Sunspot, Austral.†.*
Sulfur (p.1158·2); vitamin B substances (p.1417·1).
*Acne.*

**Vita-Preg** *Vitelle, Austral.†.*
Omega-3 marine triglycerides (p.976·2); folic acid (p.1429·1).
*Fatty-acid supplement in pregnancy; prevention of neural tube defects.*

**Vitaquick** *Vitaflo, Irl.*
Thickening agent (p.1417·1).
*Dysphagia.*

**Vitaral** *Kenyaku, Thai.*
Vitamins; minerals; rutoside; dehydrocholic acid; liver concentrate (p.1417·1).
*Vitamin and mineral deficiency.*

**Vitarex** *Pasadena, USA.*
Multivitamin and mineral preparation with iron (p.1417·1).

**Vitargenol** *Ciba Vision, Fr.†.*
Silver protein (p.1746·2).
*Eye disorders.*

**Vitarical** *Heralds, Braz.†.*
Multivitamin and mineral preparation (p.1417·1).

**Vitarnin**
*Grossmann, Hong Kong; Grossmann, Switz.*
Multivitamin and mineral preparation (p.1417·1).

**Vitarubin** *Streuli, Switz.*
Cyanocobalamin (p.1458·2) or hydroxocobalamin acetate (p.1458·2).
*Anaemias; neurological disorders; vitamin $B_{12}$ deficiency.*

**Vitarutine** *Novartis Ophthalmics, Fr.*
Rutoside sodium sulfate (p.1688·3); nicotinamide (p.1441·2).
*Conjunctival capillary fragility.*

**Vitasana** Boehringer Ingelheim, Austria†.
Vitamins; minerals; lecithin; deanol; ginseng (p.1417·1).

**Vitasana-Lebenstropfen** Riemser, Ger.
Gentian; calamus; menyanthes; melissa; achillea; peppermint leaf; crataegus; rosemary; rue; lupulus; valerian; juniper; aniseed; fennel; caraway; herba marjoranae.
*Tonic.*

**Vitasavoury** Vitaflo, UK.
High energy sip feed (p.1417·1).

**Vitasay** DM, Braz.†.
Multivitamin and mineral preparation (p.1417·1).

**Vitascarbol** Rhone-Poulenc Rorer, Israel†.
Vitamin C (p.1460·2).
*Vitamin C supplement.*

**Vita-Schlanktropfen** Schuck, Ger.†.
Cathine hydrochloride (p.1585·2).
*Obesity.*

**Vitascorb** Leofarma, Braz.†.
Vitamin C (p.1460·2).
*Vitamin C deficiency; vitamin C supplement.*

**Vitascorbol** Cooperation Pharmaceutique, Fr.
Ascorbic acid (p.1460·2) with or without sodium ascorbate (p.1460·2).
*Vitamin C deficiency.*

**Vitasedine** Ciba Vision, Fr.†.
Phenylephrine hydrochloride (p.1126·3); zinc sulfate (p.1469·3).
*Eye disorders.*

**Vitaseptine** Ciba Vision, Fr.†.
Sulfacetamide sodium (p.257·3).
Formerly contained sulfacetamide sodium, zinc sulfate, sodium iodide, and nicotinamide.
*Eye infections.*

**Vitaseptol** Novartis Ophthalmics, Fr.
Thiomersal (p.1194·1).
*Ocular antiseptic.*

**Vitaseve** Rider, Chile.
Calcium ascorbate (p.1460·2).
*Vitamin C supplement.*

**Vitasic** Germania, Austria†.
Adenosine (p.851·2); thymidine (p.1755·3); cytidine; uridine (p.1760·3); disodium guanylate (p.1681·3).
*Eye disorders.*

**Vitasma** Basi, Port.
Ephedrine hydrochloride (p.1120·1); meprobamate (p.706·2); prednisolone (p.1108·1); choline theophyllinate (p.784·2).

**VitaSohn** Antonetto, Ital.
Multivitamin and mineral preparation (p.1417·1).

**Vitasprint** Monsanto, Ital.
DL-Phosphoserine; cyanocobalamin (p.1458·2); glutamine (p.1433·2).
*Tonic.*

**Vitasprint $B_{12}$** Wyeth, Ger.
DL-Phosphoserine; cyanocobalamin (p.1458·2); glutamine (p.1433·2).
*Vitamin B deficiency.*

**Vitasprint Complex**
Monsanto, Ital.; Poli, Switz.
L-Phosphoserine; arginine hydrochloride (p.1421·1); L-phosphothreonine; glutamine (p.1433·2); hydroxocobalamin (p.1458·2).
*Tonic.*

**Vita-Squares** GNLD, Austral.†.
Multivitamin and mineral preparation (p.1417·1).

**Vitasten** Basi, Port.†.
Thiamine; vitamin $B_{12}$ (p.1417·1).

**Vita-Suple** Laborsil, Braz.†.
Multivitamin and mineral preparation (p.1417·1).

**Vitathion**
Eutherapie, Belg.†.
Ascorbic acid; glutathione; adenosine triphosphate; thiamine; inositocalcium; haemoglobin (p.1417·1).
*Asthenia; vitamin deficiency.*

Servier, Fr.
Ascorbic acid; thiamine hydrochloride; inositocalcium (p.1417·1).
*Asthenia.*

**Vita-Thion** Servier, S.Afr.
Vitamins; glutathione; sodium adenosine triphosphate; calcium inositol hexaphosphate (p.1417·1).
*Tonic.*

**Vitathion-ATP** Servier, Canad.
Ascorbic acid; adenosine triphosphate; calcium inositohexaphosphate; glutathione; magnesium inositohexaphosphate; thiamine (p.1417·1).
*Stress conditions.*

**Vitaton**
Allen, Mex.
Vitamin B substances (p.1417·1).

Vita Health, Singapore.
Vitamins; minerals; bee pollen; cysteine; ginseng; kelp; lecithin; lysine; royal jelly; yeast (p.1417·1).

**Vitatona** Brauer, Austral.†.
Angelica (p.1655·1); ascorbic acid (p.1460·2); kola nitida (p.1765·3); vitamin B substances (p.1417·1); hypericum (p.299·1); ginseng (p.1693·1); urtica urens (p.1762·1); aurum muriaticum; calcarea phosphorica; ferrum metallicum; ferrum phosphoricum; kali phosphoricum; magnesia phosphorica; phosphoric acid.
*Tonic.*

**Vitatonin** Ipex, Swed.
Multivitamins (p.1417·1); caffeine (p.782·1); vin. vermuth.; alcohol.
*Tonic.*

**Vitatonus Dexa** Bunker, Braz.
Vitamin B substances (p.1417·1); dexamethasone (p.1097·1) or dexamethasone phosphate (p.1097·2).

**Vitatron** VAAS, Ital.
Amino-acid preparation with vitamins and minerals (p.1417·1).
*Nutritional supplement.*

**Vitaveran Folico** Hormona, Mex.
Vitamin and mineral preparation (p.1417·1).

**Vitavir** Infosint, Ital.
Vitamins; minerals; carnitine tartrate; ginseng; ginkgo biloba (p.1417·1).
*Nutritional supplement.*

**Vitavitin** Sriprasit, Thai.
Multivitamin and mineral preparation (p.1417·1).

**Vitavox Pastillas** Escaned, Spain.
Camphor (p.1665·3); cineole (p.1672·1); chlorophyll (p.1057·1); ephedrine hydrochloride (p.1120·1); niaouli oil (p.1719·3); menthol (p.1711·3); sulfanilamide sodium mesilate (p.263·3); peppermint (p.1283·2).
*Mouth and throat disorders.*

**Vita-Worth B Complex** General Nutrition, Canad.
Vitamin B substances (p.1417·1).

**Vitawund** Novartis Consumer, Austria.
*Ointment:* Chlorhexidine gluconate (p.1173·2); halibut-liver oil (p.1434·1).
*Burns; wounds.*

*Topical powder:* Chlorhexidine acetate (p.1173·2).
*Prevention of wound infection.*

**Vitawund Baby** Novartis Consumer, Austria.
Lactose (p.1438·3).
*Care of umbilicus.*

**Vitax** Heralds, Braz.†.
Vitamin C (p.1460·2).
*Vitamin C deficiency; vitamin C supplement.*

**Vitax Derm** Ativus, Braz.
A multivitamin and mineral preparation (p.1417·1).

**Vitaxicam**
Ferrer, Singapore†; Robert, Spain.
Piroxicam (p.84·2).
*Gout; musculoskeletal, joint, peri-articular, and soft-tissue disorders; pain.*

**Vitayde C** Saval, Chile.
Vitamin A; vitamin C; vitamin D (p.1417·1).
*Dietary supplement.*

**Vitazell E** Kohler-Pharma, Ger.
*dl*-Alpha tocopherol (p.1464·3).
*Vitamin E deficiency.*

**Vitazinc** Ciba Vision, Fr.†.
Zinc sulfate (p.1469·3).
Formerly contained zinc sulfate and thiamine hydrochloride.
*Ocular antiseptic.*

**Vitazyme** East India Pharma, India.
*Capsules:* Amylase (p.1654·2); lactic acid bacillus (p.1704·2).

*Oral liquid; oral drops:* Amylase (p.1654·2); cinnamon oil (p.1672·2); caraway oil (p.1667·3); cardamom oil (p.1668·1).
*Dyspepsia.*

**Vitcaroten** Viternat, Braz.
Betacarotene (p.1422·3).
*Nutritional supplement.*

**Vit-C-Lutsch** Sanochemia, Austria.
Ascorbic acid (p.1460·2); calcium ascorbate (p.1460·2); hesperidin phosphate (p.1688·3).
*Vitamin C deficiency.*

**Vitec** Pharmaceutical Specialties, USA.
*dl*-Alpha tocoferil acetate (p.1465·1).
*Skin disorders.*

**Vitecaf** SIFI, Ital.
*Eye drops:* Rolitetracycline (p.254·1); chloramphenicol (p.185·1).

*Eye ointment:* Tetracycline hydrochloride (p.266·2); chloramphenicol (p.185·1); calcium pantothenate (p.1442·3).
*Infected eye disorders.*

**Vitef** Teofarma, Ital.
Polyenacid.
*Skin disorders.*

**Vitelle Nesentials** Fielding, USA.
Multivitamin and mineral preparation (p.1417·1).

**Vitelle Nestabs** Fielding, USA.
Multivitamin and mineral preparation with iron and folic acid (p.1417·1).
*Prenatal supplement.*

**Vitelle Nestrex** Fielding, USA.
Pyridoxine hydrochloride (p.1456·3).
*Pyridoxine deficiency.*

**Vitelsix** Unison, Thai.
Vitamin $B_1$; vitamin $B_6$; vitamin $B_{12}$ (p.1417·1).
*Loss of appetite; vitamin B deficiency.*

**Vitenur** Orion, Ger.†.
Acetylcysteine (p.1112·3).
*Respiratory-tract disorders with viscous mucus.*

**Viteral** Be-Tabs, S.Afr.
Multivitamin and mineral preparation (p.1417·1).
Formerly known as Be-Vital.

**Vitergan Master** Marjan, Braz.
Ginseng; vitamins; minerals (p.1417·1).

**Vitergan Pre-natal** Marjan, Braz.
A multivitamin and mineral preparation (p.1417·1).

**Vitergan Zinco** Marjan, Braz.
A range of multivitamin and mineral preparations (p.1417·1).

**Viternum**
Labomed, Chile; Senosiain, Mex.; OM, Port.; Juste, Spain.
Cyproheptadine pyridoxal phosphate (p.430·2).
*Allergic rhinitis; anorexia; urticaria.*

**Viternum Vitaminado** Labomed, Chile.
Cyproheptadine pyridoxal phosphate (p.430·2); vitamins (p.1417·1).
*Reduced appetite; tonic.*

**Viterra**
Pfizer Consumer, Ital.; Pfizer, Mex.; Pfizer, Port.; Pfizer Consumer, Spain†; Pfizer, Thai.
Multivitamin and mineral preparation (p.1417·1).

**Vitestable** Alcor, Spain.
Royal jelly; ginseng; tocopherol (p.1417·1).
*Tonic.*

**Vitex** Herbarium, Braz.
Agnus castus (p.1649·1).
*Menstrual disorders.*

**Vitexid** Sigma, India.
Spirulina (p.1749·2); vitamin B substances (p.1454·3); vitamin E (p.1464·3).
*Vitamin B and E deficiency.*

**Vitialgin** Marco Viti, Ital.†.
Propyphenazone (p.85·3); paracetamol (p.76·2).
*Fever; pain.*

**Viticromin** Auad, Braz.
Vitamin B substances (p.1417·1); brosimum gaudichaudii.
*Vitiligo.*

**Vitinoin** Pharmascience, Canad.†.
Tretinoin (p.1161·1).
*Acne.*

**Vitintra** Pharmacia Upjohn, Neth.
Vitamins A, $D_2$, E, and $K_1$ for infusion (p.1417·1).
*Parenteral nutrition.*

**Vitiral** Scherer, Thai.
Multivitamin and mineral preparation (p.1417·1).

**Vitiron**
Heralds, Braz.†.
Multivitamin preparation with iron (p.1417·1).

Mepha, Hong Kong.
Multivitamin and mineral preparation (p.1417·1).

Mepha, Singapore†.
Multivitamin and mineral preparation with methionine (p.1417·1).

Mepha, Switz.
Vitamins; minerals; choline bitartrate; inositol; methionine (p.1417·1).

**Vitiveine** Arkopharma, Fr.†.
Red vine.
*Haemorrhoids; peripheral vascular disorders.*

**ViTiX** Isis, Fr.
Cucurbita (p.1677·3).
*Skin depigmentation disorders.*

**Vitlipid N**
Pharmacia, Irl.; Fresenius Kabi, UK.
Vitamins A, $D_2$, E, and $K_1$ for infusion (p.1417·1).
*Parenteral nutrition.*

**Vitneurin** GlaxoSmithKline, India.
Vitamin $B_1$ (p.1455·2); vitamin $B_6$ (p.1457·2); vitamin $B_{12}$ (p.1458·2); dexpanthenol (p.1727·2).
*Neuropathies.*

**Vito Bronches** Duchesnay, Canad.
Diphenylpyraline hydrochloride (p.432·3); dextromethorphan hydrobromide (p.1117·3); potassium iodide (p.1598·1); sodium citrate (p.1223·2).

**Vitobasan N** BASF, Ger.†.
Thiamine hydrochloride (p.1455·1); pyridoxine hydrochloride (p.1456·3).
*Nervous system disorders.*

**Vitobel** Vianex (Βιανεξ), Gr.
Enalapril maleate (p.909·2).
*Heart failure; hypertension.*

**Vitogen** Stanley, Canad.
A range of vitamin preparations with or without minerals (p.1417·1).

**Vitogen Spectrum** Shoppers Drug Mart, Canad.†.
Multivitamin and mineral preparation (p.1417·1).

**Vitol** Orion, Fin.
Vitamin A or vitamin A palmitate; colecalciferol or ergocalciferol (p.1417·1).
*Vitamins A and D deficiency.*

**Vit-o-Mar** Asta Medica, Ger.†.
Silybum marianum (p.1043·3).
*Liver disorders.*

**Vitonic** Cypress, USA.
Vitamin B substances; minerals (p.1417·1).
*Dietary supplement.*

**Vitonico** Legrand, Braz.
Ferrous sulfate; phosphoric acid; aloes; myrrh; nutmeg; clove (p.1417·1).
*Iron-deficiency anaemias; tonic.*

**Vitonil** Gemballa, Braz.
Orotic acid; vitamin B substances (p.1417·1).
*Nutritional supplement.*

**Vitoral** Medifarma, Mex.†.
Multivitamin preparation (p.1417·1).

**Vitosal** Ziethen, Ger.
Vitamins (p.1417·1); rutoside sodium sulfate (p.1688·3); arnica (p.1656·3); sage (p.1741·2); peppermint oil (p.1283·2).
*Gum disorders.*

**Vitotal** Tecnofarma, Chile.
Ascorbic acid; vitamin E; betacarotene; magnesium (p.1417·1).
*Dietary supplement.*

**Vit-Porphyrin** Teofarma, Ital.
Haematoporphyrin dihydrochloride (p.1696·2); nicotinamide (p.1441·2).
*Tonic.*

**Vitrace** Aspen, S.Afr.
Multivitamin and mineral preparation (p.1417·1).
*Tonic.*

**Vitraday** Lifeplan, UK†.
Multinutrient preparation (p.1417·1).

**Vitrafem** Lifeplan, UK†.
Multinutrient preparation (p.1417·1).

**Vitrasert**
Bausch & Lomb, Austral.; Bausch & Lomb, UK†; Bausch & Lomb, USA.
Ganciclovir (p.635·3).
*Cytomegalovirus retinitis.*

**Vitravene**
Ciba Vision, Braz.†; Novartis, Denm.†; Novartis, Fin.†; Ciba Vision, Fr.†; Novartis Ophthalmics, Ger.†; Novartis, Irl.†; Ciba Vision, Ital.†; Novartis Ophthalmics, Swed.†; Novartis Ophthalmics, Switz.; Novartis Ophthalmics, UK†; Novartis Ophthalmics, USA.
Fomivirsen sodium (p.634·1).
*Cytomegalovirus retinitis.*

**Vitrax** Allergan, Fr.†.
Sodium hyaluronate (p.1697·3).
*Adjunct in eye surgery.*

**Vitreoclar** SIFI, Ital.
Red vine; minerals; vitamin E; amino acids (p.1417·1).
*Connective tissue disorders; nutritional supplement.*

**Vitreolent**
Novartis Ophthalmics, Hong Kong; Novartis Ophthalmics, Malaysia; Novartis Ophthalmics, Singapore; Novartis Ophthalmics, Switz.
Potassium iodide (p.1598·1); sodium iodide (p.1598·1).
*Eye disorders.*

**Vitreolent plus** Ciba Vision, Ger.†.
Cytochrome C (p.1678·3); adenosine (p.851·2); nicotinamide (p.1441·2).
*Cataracts.*

**Vitreolux** Novartis, Ital.
Vitamins; bioflavonoids; betacarotene; glucosamine; zinc; methionine; myrtillus; yeast (p.1417·1).
*Nutritional supplement.*

**Vitreosan** DMG, Ital.
Potassium bicarbonate; magnesium chloride; vitamin C (p.1417·1).
*Nutritional supplement.*

**Vitrical** Prodotti, Braz.†.
Multivitamin and mineral preparation (p.1417·1).

**Vitrimix**
Fresenius Kabi, Denm.; Fresenius Kabi, Norw.; Fresenius Kabi, Port.; Fresenius Kabi, Swed.; Fresenius Kabi, Switz.†; Fresenius Kabi, Thai.
Amino-acid, glucose, and lipid (from soya oil (p.1447·2)) infusion with or without electrolytes (p.1417·1).
Contains egg phospholipids.
*Parenteral nutrition.*

**Vitrimix KV**
Fresenius Kabi, Fr.; Fresenius Kabi, Hong Kong; Pharmacia, Irl.; Fresenius Kabi, Malaysia; Fresenius Kabi, Neth.; Fresenius Kabi, Singapore†; Fresenius Kabi, UK.
Amino-acid, glucose, and lipid (from soya oil (p.1447·2)) infusion with or without electrolytes (p.1417·1).
Contains fractionated egg phospholipids.
*Parenteral nutrition.*

**Vitrite** Seven Seas, UK†.
Multivitamin preparation (p.1417·1).

**Vitron** Pharmaland, Thai.
Vitamin $B_1$ (p.1455·2); vitamin $B_6$ (p.1457·2); vitamin $B_{12}$ (p.1458·2).
*Anorexia; neurasthenia; neurological disorders; neuropathy; toxaemia of pregnancy.*

**Vitron-C** Heritage Consumer, USA.
Ferrous fumarate (p.1427·3).
Ascorbic acid (p.1460·2) is included in this preparation to increase the absorption and availability of iron.
*Iron-deficiency anaemias.*

**Vitrosups** Llorens, Spain.
Glycerol (p.1694·3).
*Constipation; laxative dependence.*

**Vits** Profarb, Braz.†.
Multivitamin and mineral preparation (p.1417·1).

**Vitulpas** Drag, Chile.
Hydrocortisone (p.1103·3).
*Skin disorders.*

**Vit-u-pept** Plantina, Ger.
Weisskohl; bismuth subcarbonate (p.1252·1); heavy magnesium carbonate (p.1272·1); sodium bicarbonate (p.1223·2).
*Gastrointestinal disorders.*

**Vitussin**
Note. This name is used for preparations of different composition.
Vitamed, Israel.
Guaifenesin (p.1122·1).
*Coughs.*

Cypress, USA.
Hydrocodone tartrate (p.45·1); guaifenesin (p.1122·1).
*Coughs.*

**Vivabec** Lexon, UK.
Beclometasone dipropionate (p.1091·1).
*Hypersensitivity reactions.*

**Vivacor** Lexon, UK.
Bisoprolol fumarate (p.875·1).
*Angina pectoris; hypertension.*

**Vivactil** Merck, USA.
Protriptyline hydrochloride (p.316·2).
*Depression.*

**Vivadone** Lexon, UK.
Domperidone maleate (p.1263·2).
*Dyspepsia.*

**Viva-Drops** Vision, USA.
Polysorbate 80 (p.1415·2).
Formerly known as Vit-A-drops.
*Dry eyes.*

**Vival** Alpharma, Norw.
Diazepam (p.690·1).
*Anxiety; skeletal muscle spasm; sleep disorders.*

**Vivalan**
AstraZeneca, Belg.; Menarini, Belg.; AstraZeneca, Fr.; AstraZeneca, Ger.; Zeneca, Port.; AstraZeneca, UK†.
Viloxazine hydrochloride (p.323·3).
*Depression.*

**Vivalessence** Motima, Fr.
A range of preparations containing essential oils and plant extracts (p.1417·1).
*Tonic.*

**Vivamag** Byk, Fr.
Magnesium lactate (p.1228·1).
*Magnesium deficiency.*

**Vivamyne** Whitehall, Fr.
A range of vitamin preparations with or without minerals (p.1417·1).

**Vivance** Vivance, Fr.
Nutritional supplement (p.1417·1).

**Vivapryl** Asta Medica, UK†.
Selegiline hydrochloride (p.1214·1).
*Parkinsonism.*

**Vivarin** SmithKline Beecham Consumer, USA.
Caffeine (p.782·1).
*Fatigue.*

**Vivarint** AstraZeneca, Spain†.
Viloxazine hydrochloride (p.323·3).
*Depression.*

**Vivatak** Lexon, UK.
Ranitidine (p.1285·2).
*Dyspepsia; gastric hyperacidity; heartburn.*

**Vivatec**
Merck Sharp & Dohme, Denm.; Merck Sharp & Dohme, Fin.; Merck Sharp & Dohme, Norw.; Merck Sharp & Dohme, Swed.
Lisinopril (p.946·3).
*Heart failure; hypertension; myocardial infarction.*

**Vivatec Comp**
Merck Sharp & Dohme, Fin.; Merck Sharp & Dohme, Norw.
Lisinopril (p.946·3); hydrochlorothiazide (p.933·2).
*Hypertension.*

**Vivaxim** Aventis Pasteur, Austral.
A typhoid vaccine (Vi capsular polysaccharide) (p.1642·2).
*Active immunisation.*

**Vivaxine** Nakorn, Thai.
Sulfadoxine (p.259·3); pyrimethamine (p.458·1).
*Malaria.*

**Vivazid** Merck Sharp & Dohme, Denm.
Lisinopril (p.946·3); hydrochlorothiazide (p.933·2).
*Hypertension.*

**Vivelle**
Note. This name is used for preparations of different composition.
Janssen-Cilag, Austria.
Norgestimate (p.1563·2); ethinylestradiol (p.1553·2).
*Acne; triphasic oral contraceptive.*

Novartis, Canad.; Novartis, USA.
Estradiol (p.1550·1).
*Menopausal disorders; oestrogen deficiency; osteoporosis.*

**Vivena AR** Dieterba, Ital.
Infant feed (p.1417·1).
*Gastro-oesophageal reflux.*

**Vivena HA** Dieterba, Ital.
Infant feed (p.1417·1).
*Cow's milk intolerance.*

**Vivene** Theratech, Fr.
Aesculus (p.1648·2); troxerutin (p.1688·3).
*Haemorrhoids; peripheral vascular disorders.*

**Viverdal** Uniao Quimica, Braz.
Risperidone (p.719·2).
*Psychoses.*

**Vivicrom** Nucare, UK.
Sodium cromoglicate (p.795·3).
*Allergic conjunctivitis.*

**Vividrin**
Riel, Austria; Tramedico, Belg.†; Mann, Ger.; Kite (Kite), Gr.; Mann, Irl.; Mann, Malaysia; Mann, Neth.;Bausch & Lomb, S.Afr.; Mann, Singapore; Farma Lepori, Spain†; Gebro, Switz.; Bausch & Lomb, Thai.; Mann, Thai.; Pharma-Global, UK.
Sodium cromoglicate (p.795·3).
*Allergic conjunctivitis; allergic rhinitis; keratoconjunctivitis.*

**Vividrin comp** Mann, Ger.†.
Sodium cromoglicate (p.795·3); xylometazoline hydrochloride (p.1132·2).
*Allergic rhinitis.*

**Vividrin Loratadin** Mann, Ger.
Loratadine (p.436·1).
*Allergic conjunctivitis; allergic rhinitis; urticaria.*

**Vividrin mit Terfenadin** Mann, Ger.†.
Terfenadine (p.441·1).
*Hypersensitivity reactions.*

**Vividyl** Lilly, Ital.†.
Nortriptyline hydrochloride (p.310·2).
*Depression.*

**Vivimed**
Note. This name is used for preparations of different composition.
Riel, Austria.
Propyphenazone (p.85·3); paracetamol (p.76·2); caffeine (p.782·1).
*Fever; pain.*

Mann, Ger.†.
Paracetamol (p.76·2).
*Fever; pain.*

Mann, Irl.†.
Paracetamol (p.76·2); caffeine (p.782·1).
*Pain.*

**Vivin C**
Note. This name is used for preparations of different composition.
Menarini, Ital.; Alter, Spain†.
Aspirin (p.15·1); ascorbic acid (p.1460·2).
*Fever; pain.*

Alter, Port.†.
Ascorbic acid (p.1460·2).
*Cold and influenza symptoms; tonic.*

**Vivinox** Riel, Austria.
Valerian (p.1762·2); lupulus (p.1708·1); mistletoe (p.1715·3).
*Anxiety disorders.*

**Vivinox N** Mann, Ger.
Valerian (p.1762·2); lupulus (p.1708·1); passion flower (p.1729·1).
*Nervous disorders; sleep disorders.*

**Vivinox Stark** Mann, Ger.†.
Diphenhydramine hydrochloride (p.431·3).
*Sleep disorders.*

**Vivinox-Schlafdragees** Mann, Ger.†.
Diphenhydramine hydrochloride (p.431·3); valerian (p.1762·2); lupulus (p.1708·1).
*Sleep disorders.*

**Vivioptal**
Mann, Irl.; Pharma-Global, UK.
Multivitamin and mineral preparation (p.1417·1).

**Viviplus** Mann, Ger.
Hypericum (p.299·1).
*Depression.*

**Vivir** Unison, Thai.
Aciclovir (p.626·1).
*Herpesvirus infections.*

**ViviRhin S** Mann, Ger.†.
Xylometazoline hydrochloride (p.1132·2).
*Nasal congestion.*

**Vivisun** Mann, Ger.†.
Diphenhydramine hydrochloride (p.431·3); lauromacrogol 400 (p.1412·3).
*Hypersensitivity reactions of the skin.*

**Vivol** Carter Horner, Canad.†.
Diazepam (p.690·1).
*Anxiety; sedative.*

**Vivolan** Orion, Fin.
Emollient.
*Skin disorders; vehicle for topical drugs.*

**Vivonex**
Novartis, Arg.; Novartis Consumer, Austral.; Novartis, Braz.; Novartis Nutrition, Canad.†; Novartis Nutrition, Hong Kong; Promeco, Mex.; Novartis Nutrition, Singapore; Procter & Gamble, USA.
A range of preparations for enteral nutrition (p.1417·1).

**Vivotif**
Raffo, Arg.; Kwizda, Austria; Berna, Belg.; Berna, Canad.; Berna, Denm.; Berna, Fin.; Niddapharm, Ger.; Berna, Hong Kong; Celltech, Irl.; Swiss Serum Institute, Israel; Berna, Ital.; Berna, Malaysia; Swiss Serum, Malaysia; Berna, Norw.; Berna, Port.; Byk Madaus, S.Afr.; Berna, Singapore; Berna, Spain; Cortec, Swed.; Berna, Switz.; Berna, Thai.; Swiss Serum, Thai.; Masta, UK†; Berna, USA.
A live oral typhoid vaccine (attenuated Ty 21a strain) (p.1642·2).
*Active immunisation.*

**Vivradoxil** Alpharma, Mex.
Doxycycline (p.206·2).
*Bacterial infections.*

**Vivural** Procter & Gamble, Ger.
Calcium carbonate (p.1254·2).
*Calcium deficiency.*

**Vix Plex** Laborsil, Braz.†.
Multivitamin and mineral preparation (p.1417·1).

**Vixcef** Bago, Arg.
Cefixime (p.172·3).
*Bacterial infections.*

**Vixiderm E** ICN, Arg.
Benzoyl peroxide (p.1143·2).
*Acne.*

**Vixidone** ICN, Arg.
Dexamethasone (p.1097·1); chlorphenamine maleate (p.427·3).

**Vixidone T** ICN, Arg.
Dexamethasone (p.1097·1); terfenadine (p.441·1).

**Vixin** Sons, Mex.
Chloramphenicol (p.185·1).
*Bacterial infections.*

**Vixmicina** Uniao Quimica, Braz.
Chloramphenicol sodium succinate (p.185·1).
*Bacterial infections.*

**Vixorfit** Gezzi, Arg.
Glycerol (p.1694·3).
*Eye irritation.*

**Vi-Zac** UCB, USA.
Multivitamin and mineral preparation (p.1417·1).

**Vizax** Essex, Ital.†.
Isepamicin (p.222·2).
*Bacterial infections.*

**Vizerul** Montpellier, Arg.
Ranitidine hydrochloride (p.1285·2).
*Gastro-oesophageal reflux; peptic ulcer; Zollinger-Ellison syndrome.*

**Vizole** MM, India.
Levamisole (p.107·1) or levamisole hydrochloride (p.107·2).
*Worm infections.*

**Viz-On** Opus, UK†.
Sodium cromoglicate (p.795·3).
*Allergic conjunctivitis.*

**Vizoptal** Medical, Port.
Chlorobutanol (p.1176·3).

**Vizylac** Unichem, India.
*Lactobacillus sporogenes* (p.1704·2); vitamin B substances (p.1417·1).
*Imbalance of intestinal flora.*

**VM-2000** Solgar, UK.
Multivitamin and mineral preparation (p.1417·1).

**VM 26** Bristol-Myers Squibb, Ger.
Teniposide (p.587·2).
*Malignant neoplasms.*

**VM Drosan** Liferpal, Mex.†.
Multivitamin and mineral preparation (p.1417·1).

**Vobaderm** Hermal, Ger.
Fluprednidene acetate (p.1102·2); miconazole nitrate (p.405·3).
Formerly contained fluprednidene acetate.
*Infected skin disorders.*

**Vobamyk** Hermal, Ger.
Miconazole nitrate (p.405·3).
*Fungal and Gram-positive bacterial skin infections.*

**Vocadys** Chemineau, Fr.
Enoxolone (p.36·2); lidocaine hydrochloride (p.1377·3); erysimum.
*Sore throat.*

**Vocalzone** Kestrel, UK.
Menthol (p.1711·3); peppermint oil (p.1283·2); myrrh (p.1718·3); liquorice (p.1270·2).
*Throat irritation.*

**Vocara** Bittner, Austria.
Homoeopathic preparation.

**Vodol** Uniao Quimica, Braz.
Miconazole nitrate (p.405·3).
*Fungal skin infections.*

**Vofenal** Alcon, Canad.†.
Diclofenac sodium (p.32·1).
*Inflammatory eye disorders.*

**Vogalene**
Rhone-Poulenc Rorer, Belg.†; Aventis, Denm.; Schwarz, Fr.; Rhone-Poulenc Rorer, Israel†.
Metopimazine (p.1276·3).
*Nausea and vomiting.*

**Vogalib** Schwarz, Fr.
Metopimazine (p.1276·3).
*Nausea and vomiting.*

**Voglisan** Abbott, Braz.†.
Voglibose (p.348·3).
*Diabetes mellitus.*

**Voir** Velka, Gr.
Tenoxicam (p.93·1).
*Dysmenorrhoea; gout; inflammation; osteoarthritis; pain; rheumatoid arthritis; spondyloarthropathies.*

**Voker** YSP, Malaysia.
Famotidine (p.1265·2).
*Gastro-oesophageal reflux; peptic ulcer; Zollinger-Ellison syndrome.*

**Volamin** Volchem, Ital.
Amino-acid preparation (p.1417·1).
*Fatigue; liver disorders.*

**Volcidol-S** Pharmasant, Thai.
Tramadol hydrochloride (p.94·3).
*Pain.*

**Volcolon** Parke, Davis, Neth.
Ispaghula (p.1268·1).
*Constipation.*

**Voldal** Novartis, Fr.
Diclofenac sodium (p.32·1).
*Dysmenorrhoea; musculoskeletal, joint, and peri-articular disorders; renal colic.*

**Volfenac**
Collins, Mex.; General Drugs, Thai.
Diclofenac diethylamine (p.32·1) or diclofenac sodium (p.32·1).
*Gout; musculoskeletal, joint, peri-articular, and soft-tissue disorders; pain.*

**Vollmers praparierter gruner N** Salushaus, Ger.
Avena (p.1658·2); urtica (p.1762·1); alchemilla.
Formerly contained avena, urtica, alchemilla, and hypericum.
*Urinary-tract disorders.*

**Volmac** GlaxoSmithKline, Ger.; Cascan, Ger.
Salbutamol sulfate (p.791·3).
*Obstructive airways disease.*

**Volmax**
GlaxoSmithKline, Denm.; GlaxoSmithKline, Hong Kong; GlaxoSmithKline, Israel; Glaxo Allen, Ital.; GlaxoSmithKline, Malaysia; Glaxo Wellcome, Mex.; GlaxoSmithKline, NZ; Glaxo Wellcome, S.Afr.†; GlaxoSmithKline, Singapore; GlaxoSmithKline, Switz.; GlaxoSmithKline, Thai.; Allen & Hanburys, UK; Muro, USA†.
Salbutamol sulfate (p.791·3).
*Obstructive airways disease.*

**Volnac** TO-Chemicals, Thai.
Diclofenac sodium (p.32·1).
*Fever; inflammation; pain.*

**Vologen** Antigen, Irl.
Diclofenac sodium (p.32·1).
*Gout; inflammation; musculoskeletal, joint, and peri-articular disorders; pain.*

**Volon**
Bristol-Myers Squibb, Austria; Bristol-Myers Squibb, Ger.
Triamcinolone (p.1110·2).
*Corticosteroid.*

**Volon A**
Bristol-Myers Squibb, Austria; Bristol-Myers Squibb, Ger.
Triamcinolone acetonide (p.1110·2).
*Corticosteroid.*

**Volon A antibiotikahaltig** Bristol-Myers Squibb, Austria.
Triamcinolone acetonide (p.1110·2); neomycin sulfate (p.235·1); gramicidin (p.220·2).
*Skin disorders.*

**Volon A antibiotikahaltig N** Bristol-Myers Squibb, Ger.
Triamcinolone acetonide (p.1110·2); neomycin sulfate (p.235·1).
*Skin disorders.*

**Volon A Tinktur** Bristol-Myers Squibb, Austria.
Triamcinolone acetonide (p.1110·2); salicylic acid (p.1157·1).
*Otitis externa; skin disorders.*

**Volon A Tinktur N** Bristol-Myers Squibb, Ger.
Triamcinolone acetonide (p.1110·2); salicylic acid (p.1157·1).
*Otitis externa; skin disorders.*

**Volon A-Rhin** Bristol-Myers Squibb, Ger.
Triamcinolone acetonide (p.1110·2); phenylephrine hydrochloride (p.1126·3).
*Rhinitis; sinusitis.*

**Volon A-Schuttelmix** Bristol-Myers Squibb, Ger.
Triamcinolone acetonide (p.1110·2); zinc oxide (p.1163·2).
*Skin disorders.*

**Volon A-Zinklotion** Bristol-Myers Squibb, Austria.
Triamcinolone acetonide (p.1110·2); zinc oxide (p.1163·2).
*Skin disorders.*

**Volonimat** Bristol-Myers Squibb, Ger.
Triamcinolone acetonide (p.1110·2).
*Skin disorders.*

**Volonimat N** Bristol-Myers Squibb, Ger.
Triamcinolone acetonide (p.1110·2).
*Skin disorders.*

**Volonimat Plus N** Bristol-Myers Squibb, Ger.
Triamcinolone acetonide (p.1110·2); nystatin (p.406·3).
*Eczema with secondary yeast infection.*

**Volonten** Viofar, Gr.
Nimesulide (p.67·1).
*Inflammation; musculoskeletal disorders; pain.*

**Volplex** Cambridge, UK.
Succinylated gelatin (p.754·3) in sodium chloride.
*Blood volume expansion.*

**Volraman** Eastern Pharmaceuticals, UK.
Diclofenac sodium (p.32·1).
*Gout; inflammation; musculoskeletal disorders; pain.*

**Volsaid** Trinity, UK.
Diclofenac sodium (p.32·1).
*Inflammation; musculoskeletal, joint, and peri-articular disorders; pain.*

**Volta** T Man, Thai.
Diclofenac sodium (p.32·1).
*Musculoskeletal, joint, and peri-articular disorders.*

**Voltaflan** Bunker, Braz.
Diclofenac (p.32·1) or diclofenac sodium (p.32·1).

**Voltaflex** EMS, Braz.
Diclofenac sodium (p.32·1).
*Gout; inflammation; musculoskeletal, joint, and peri-articular disorders; pain.*

**Voltamicin**
Novartis, Austria; Ciba Vision, Braz.†; Ciba Vision, Ital.; Novartis Ophthalmics, Singapore; Novartis Ophthalmics, Switz.
Diclofenac sodium (p.32·1); gentamicin sulfate (p.217·1).
*Bacterial eye infections and inflammation.*

**Voltamicine** Novartis Ophthalmics, Fr.†.
Diclofenac sodium (p.32·1); gentamicin sulfate (p.217·1).
*Bacterial eye infections and inflammation following cataract surgery.*

**Voltanac** Pharmasant, Thai.
Diclofenac sodium (p.32·1).
*Musculoskeletal and joint disorders.*

**Voltaren**
Novartis, Arg.; Novartis, Austral.; Novartis, Austria; Novartis, Belg.; Novartis, Braz.; Novartis, Canad.; Novartis, Chile; Novartis, Denm.; Novartis, Fin.; Novartis, Ger.; Novartis Consumer, Ger.; Novartis, Gr.; Novartis, Hong Kong; Novartis, Israel; Ciba Vision, Ital.; Novartis, Ital.; Novartis, Malaysia; Novartis, Mex.; Novartis, Neth.; Novartis, Norw.;

*Novartis, NZ; Novartis, Port.; Novartis, S.Afr.; Novartis, Singapore; Novartis, Spain; Novartis, Swed.; Novartis, Thai.; Novartis, USA.*
Diclofenac (p.32·1), diclofenac diethylamine (p.32·1), diclofenac potassium (p.32·1), diclofenac resinate (p.33·1), or diclofenac sodium (p.32·1).
*Cystoid macular oedema; gout; inflammation; musculoskeletal, joint, peri-articular, and soft-tissue disorders; pain; prevention of intraoperative miosis; renal and biliary colic.*

**Voltaren Colirio**
*Novartis Ophthalmics, Arg.; Novartis Ophthalmics, Braz.*
Diclofenac sodium (p.32·1).
*Inflammatory eye disorders.*

**Voltaren Emulgel**
*Novartis, Spain; Novartis, Switz.*
Diclofenac diethylamine (p.32·1).
*Musculoskeletal, joint, peri-articular and soft-tissue disorders.*

**Voltaren Flex** *Novartis, Arg.*
Diclofenac sodium (p.32·1); pridinol mesilate (p.1395·2).
*Musculoskeletal and joint disorders.*

**Voltaren Forte** *Novartis, Arg.*
Diclofenac sodium (p.32·1); codeine phosphate (p.27·1).
*Pain.*

**Voltaren Ophta** *Novartis Ophthalmics, Switz.*
Diclofenac sodium (p.32·1).
*Eye disorders.*

**Voltaren Ophtha**
*Novartis, Austral.; Novartis Ophthalmics, Canad.; Novartis Ophthalmics, Ger.; Novartis Ophthalmics, Hong Kong; Ciba Vision, Israel; Novartis, Norw.; Novartis, NZ; Restan, S.Afr.; Novartis Ophthalmics, Singapore; Novartis Ophthalmics, Swed.*
Diclofenac sodium (p.32·1).
*Cystoid macular oedema; inflammatory eye disorders; prevention of miosis during cataract surgery.*

**Voltaren T** *Novartis, Swed.*
Diclofenac potassium (p.32·1).
*Pain.*

**Voltarene**
*Novartis, Fr.; Novartis, Switz.*
Diclofenac (p.32·1), diclofenac diethylamine (p.32·1), diclofenac resinate (p.33·1), or diclofenac sodium (p.32·1).
*Inflammation; musculoskeletal, joint, and peri-articular disorders; oedema; pain; renal colic.*

*Novartis Ophthalmics, Fr.*
*Eye drops:* Diclofenac sodium (p.32·1).
*Eye pain; inflammation following eye surgery; inhibition of intraoperative miosis.*

**Voltarene Rapide** *Novartis, Switz.*
Diclofenac potassium (p.32·1).
*Inflammation; pain.*

**Voltarol**
*Novartis, Irl.; Novartis, UK.*
Diclofenac (p.32·1), diclofenac diethylamine (p.32·1), diclofenac potassium (p.32·1), or diclofenac sodium (p.32·1).
*Gout; inflammation; musculoskeletal, joint, peri-articular, and soft-tissue disorders; pain.*

**Voltarol Ophtha**
*Novartis, Irl.; Novartis, UK.*
Diclofenac sodium (p.32·1).
*Anterior eye inflammation; inhibition of peri-operative miosis; prevention of cystoid macular oedema.*

**Voltax** *Poehlmann, Ger.*
Phospholipids; muira-puama; adenosine; vitamins (p.1417·1).
*Tonic.*

**Voltfast** *Novartis, Ital.*
Diclofenac potassium (p.32·1).
*Inflammation; pain.*

**Voltil** *Ardeypharm, Ger.*
Protein-free extract of bovine spleen.
*Gastrointestinal disorders; peripheral and cerebral vascular disorders; skin disorders.*

**Voltric** *UCB, Spain.*
Cetirizine hydrochloride (p.427·1).
*Allergic conjunctivitis; allergic rhinitis; pruritus; urticaria.*

**Voltrix** *Bunker, Braz.*
Diclofenac diethylamine (p.32·1) or diclofenac potassium (p.32·1).
*Gout; inflammation; musculoskeletal, joint, and periarticular disorders; pain.*

**Volumax D 40** *Blausiegel, Braz.*
Dextran 40 (p.745·3) in sodium chloride or glucose.
*Plasma volume expansion.*

**Volumax D 70** *Blausiegel, Braz.*
Dextran 70 (p.746·2) in sodium chloride or glucose.
*Plasma volume expansion.*

**Volutine** *Geymonat, Ital.*
Fenofibrate (p.915·2).
*Hyperlipidaemias.*

**Volutol** *Lemery, Mex.*
Carbamazepine (p.353·3).
*Epilepsy.*

**Voluven**
*Fresenius Kabi, Austria; Fresenius Kabi, Denm.; Fresenius Kabi, Fin.; Fresenius Kabi, Ger.; Fresenius Kabi, Ital.; Fresenius Kabi, Norw.; Fresenius Kabi, Port.; Fresenius Kabi, Spain; Fresenius Kabi, Swed.; Fresenius Kabi, Switz.; Fresenius Kabi, UK.*
An etherified starch (p.750·1).
*Plasma volume expansion.*

**Volverac** *TP, Thai.*
Diclofenac sodium (p.32·1).
*Inflammation following cataract surgery; postoperative cystoid macular oedema; prevention or reduction of intraoperative miosis.*

**Vomacur** *Hexal, Ger.*
Dimenhydrinate (p.431·1).
*Motion sickness; nausea; vertigo; vomiting.*

**Vomex A**
*Yamanouchi, Ger.; Galenica, Gr.*
Dimenhydrinate (p.431·1).
*Motion sickness; nausea and vomiting; premedication; vertigo.*

**Vomidon** *Be-Tabs, S.Afr.*
Domperidone (p.1263·2).
*Adjunct in gastrointestinal radiology; gastrointestinal disorders.*

**Vomidrine** *Azevedos, Port.*
Dimenhydrinate (p.431·1).
*Motion sickness.*

**Vomifene** *Mer-National, S.Afr.*
Buclizine hydrochloride (p.426·3); pyridoxine (p.1457·2).
*Motion sickness; nausea; vertigo; vomiting.*

**Vominar** *Charoen, Thai.*
Dimenhydrinate (p.431·1).
*Motion sickness; vertigo, nausea and vomiting.*

**Vominil** *Sedabel, Braz.*
Metoclopramide (p.1274·3); vitamin $B_6$ (p.1457·2).
*Nausea and vomiting.*

**Vomisin** *Rayere, Mex.*
Dimenhydrinate (p.431·1).
*Motion sickness; vestibular disorders.*

**Vomistop** *Medquimica, Braz.†.*
Metoclopramide (p.1274·3); vitamin $B_6$ (p.1457·2).
*Nausea and vomiting.*

**Vomitron** *Berlin Pharm, Thai.*
Ondansetron hydrochloride (p.1281·1).
*Nausea and vomiting induced by cytotoxics or radiotherapy.*

**Vomitusheel** *Peithner, Austria.*
Homoeopathic preparation.

**Vomix** *Natus, Braz.†.*
Metoclopramide (p.1274·3).
*Gastrointestinal motility disorders; nausea and vomiting.*

**Voncon** *Pharmaserve Lilly (Φαρμασερβ Λιλλυ), Gr.*
Vancomycin (p.275·2).
*Bacterial infections.*

**Vonifin** *Rudefsa, Mex.†.*
Metoclopramide (p.1274·3).

**Vonil** *UCI, Braz.†.*
Metoclopramide hydrochloride (p.1274·3).
*Gastrointestinal motility disorders; nausea and vomiting.*

**Vonil Enzimatico** *UCI, Braz.†.*
Metoclopramide (p.1274·3); pancreatin (p.1725·3); dimethicone (p.1289·2); sodium dehydrocholate (p.1679·2); bromelains (p.1662·2).
*Digestive disorders.*

**Vontrol**
*Enila, Braz.; GlaxoSmithKline, Chile; SmithKline Beecham, Mex.*
Difenidol hydrochloride (p.1261·1).
*Nausea and vomiting; vestibular disorders.*

**Vonum** *Gerot, Austria.*
Indometacin (p.47·3); lauromacrogol 400 (p.1412·3).
*Musculoskeletal, joint, and soft-tissue disorders.*

**Vopar** *Unison, Thai.*
Levodopa (p.1205·2); benserazide hydrochloride (p.1200·2).
*Parkinsonism.*

**Vopax** *Haller, Braz.*
Metoclopramide hydrochloride (p.1274·3).
Formerly contained metoclopramide and vitamin $B_6$.
*Nausea and vomiting.*

**V-Optic** *Vitamed, Israel.*
Timolol maleate (p.1012·2).
*Glaucoma.*

**Voraclor** *Lafare, Ital.*
Aciclovir (p.626·1).
*Herpesvirus infections.*

**Vorange**
*DHA, Hong Kong; DHA, Singapore.*
Vitamin C (p.1460·2).
*Vitamin C deficiency.*

**Vo-Remi** *Offenbach, Mex.*
Meclozine (p.436·3); pyridoxine (p.1457·2).
*Nausea and vomiting.*

**Voren**
*YSP, Malaysia; Yung Shin, Singapore; Yung Shin, Thai.†.*
Diclofenac diethylamine (p.32·1) or diclofenac sodium (p.32·1).
*Gout; inflammation; musculoskeletal, joint, peri-articular, and soft-tissue disorders; pain.*

**Voren Plus** *YSP, Malaysia.*
Diclofenac sodium (p.32·1); menthol (p.1711·3).
*Musculoskeletal, joint, and soft-tissue disorders.*

**Vorigeno** *Inibsa, Spain.*
Hyoscine hydrobromide (p.483·3).
*Motion sickness.*

**VoriNa** *Onkoworks, Ger.*
Sodium folinate (p.1431·2).

**Vorst** *Microsules Bernabo, Arg.*
Sildenafil citrate (p.1744·2).
*Erectile dysfunction.*

**VoSoL**
*Note. This name is used for preparations of different composition.*
*Carter-Wallace, Austral.†.*
Propylene glycol diacetate (p.1415·3).
*Otitis externa.*

*Carter Horner, Canad.; Wilson, NZ; Wallace, USA.*
Propylene glycol diacetate (p.1415·3); acetic acid (p.1645·2); benzethonium chloride (p.1169·2).
*Otitis externa.*

**VoSoL HC**
*Carter Horner, Canad.; Wallace, USA.*
Propylene glycol diacetate (p.1415·3); acetic acid (p.1645·2); benzethonium chloride (p.1169·2); hydrocortisone (p.1103·3).
*Otitis externa.*

**VoSpire** *Odyssey, USA.*
Salbutamol sulfate (p.791·3).
*Obstructive airways disease.*

**Vostar** *Medis, Denm.*
Diclofenac sodium (p.32·1).
*Inflammation; musculoskeletal and joint disorders.*

**Votag** *Ativus, Braz.*
Marine polyunsaturated fatty acids (p.976·2).
*Dietary supplement.*

**Votamed** *Medifive, Thai.*
Diclofenac sodium (p.32·1).
*Musculoskeletal and joint disorders.*

**Voveran** *Novartis, India.*
Diclofenac (p.32·1), diclofenac diethylamine (p.32·1), or diclofenac sodium (p.32·1).
*Allergic conjunctivitis; eye inflammation and trauma; gout; musculoskeletal and joint disorders; prevention of miosis in cataract surgery.*

**Voxpax**
*Homeocan, Canad.; Lehning, Fr.*
Homoeopathic preparation.

**Voxsuprine** *Major, USA.*
Isoxsuprine hydrochloride (p.1702·2).
*Cerebrovascular and peripheral vascular disorders.*

**V-Pen**
*Orion, Fin.*
Phenoxymethylpenicillin potassium (p.242·1).
*Bacterial infections.*

*Biochemie, Israel.*
Phenoxymethylpenicillin (p.242·1).
*Bacterial infections.*

**VP-Gen** *Gautier, Arg.*
Etoposide (p.551·3).
*Malignant neoplasms.*

**VP-Tec** *Columbia, Mex.†.*
Etoposide (p.551·3).
*Small cell lung cancer; testicular cancer.*

**VR** *Curacel, Austral.*
Dextran sulfate (p.1679·2); allantoin (p.1141·3); zinc oxide (p.1163·2); melaleuca oil (p.1710·2); alpha tocoferil acetate; vitamin A palmitate.
*Herpes labialis; postherpetic neuralgia; tinea pruritus.*

**Vraap** *Inverni della Beffa, Ital.*
Vincamine (p.1764·2).
*Disorders of cerebral, ocular, and vestibular circulation.*

**Vridol** *Rafa, Israel.*
Troxerutin (p.1688·3).
*Haemorrhoids; venous insufficiency.*

**V-Tablopen** *Viatris, Ger.*
Phenoxymethylpenicillin potassium (p.242·1).
*Bacterial infections.*

**V-Talgin** *Vitamed, Israel.*
Dipyrone (p.35·3).
*Fever; pain.*

**V-Tears** *Vitamed, Israel.*
Hyetellose (p.1579·2).
*Dry eyes.*

**Vuclodir** *Richmond, Arg.*
Lamivudine (p.648·2).
*HIV infection.*

**Vudirax** *Blausiegel, Braz.*
Lamivudine (p.648·2).

**Vueffe**
*Baldacci, Braz.; Baldacci, Ital.*
Peptides derived from the hydrolysis of bovine factor VIII (p.751·1).
*Haemorrhage.*

**Vulbegal** *Coup, Gr.*
Flunitrazepam (p.698·2).
*Insomnia.*

**Vulcase** *Teofarma, Fr.*
Aloes (p.1248·2).
*Constipation.*

**Vulcasid** *Atlantis, Mex.*
Omeprazole (p.1278·2).
*Gastro-oesophageal reflux; peptic ulcer; Zollinger-Ellison syndrome.*

**Vulgix** *Cazi, Braz.†.*
Tyrothricin (p.275·1); lactic acid (p.1704·1); lavender oil (p.1705·2); methylrosanilinium chloride (p.1186·1).
*Vulvovaginal infections.*

**Vulnofilin Compuesto** *Lazar, Arg.*
Red blood cells (p.759·3); protoporphyrin; papain (p.1727·3); tyrothricin (p.275·1); dequalinium.
*Wounds.*

**Vulnopur** *Deverge, Ital.*
Decylglucoside; sodium chloride (p.1233·3); aloe vera (p.1141·3); silver chloride (p.1746·1).
*Burns; cleansing of skin and mucous membranes; wounds.*

**Vulnostimulin** *Dermapharm, Ger.*
Wheat germ.
*Burns; wounds.*

**Vulpuran** *Rosch & Handel, Austria.*
Lead plaster-mass (p.1706·1); chamomile oil (p.1669·3); hypericum oil (p.299·2); cod-liver oil (p.1425·2); elemi; colophony (p.1675·1); emplastrum minii; turpentine oil (p.1760·1); peru balsam (p.1730·2); oxycholesterin.
*Furuncles; ulcers; wounds.*

**Vumon**
*Bristol-Myers Squibb, Arg.; Bristol-Myers Squibb, Austral.; Bristol-Myers Squibb, Austria; Bristol-Myers Squibb, Belg.; Bristol-Myers Squibb, Braz.; Bristol, Canad.; Bristol-Myers Squibb, Chile; Bristol-Myers Squibb, Denm.†; IFET (ΙΦΕΤ), Gr.; Bristol-Myers Squibb, Hong Kong; Bristol-Myers Squibb, Israel; Bristol-Myers Squibb, Ital.; Bristol-Myers Squibb, Malaysia; Bristol-Myers Squibb, Mex.; Bristol-Myers Squibb, Neth.; Bristol-Myers Squibb, NZ; Bristol-Myers Squibb, Port.; Bristol-Myers Squibb, S.Afr.; Bristol-Myers Squibb, Singapore; Bristol-Myers, Spain; Bristol-Myers Squibb, Swed.†; Bristol-Myers Squibb Oncology, USA.*
Teniposide (p.587·2).
*Malignant neoplasms.*

**Vunsu** *Costec, Arg.*
Padimate O (p.1155·1).
*Sunscreen.*

**Vurdon** *Help, Gr.*
Diclofenac sodium (p.32·1).
*Dysmenorrhoea; inflammation; musculoskeletal and joint disorders; pain.*

**VVS** *Econo Med, USA†.*
Sulfathiazole (p.264·1); sulfacetamide (p.257·3); sulfabenzamide (p.257·3).
*Vaginitis due to Gardnerella vaginalis.*

**Vykmin**
*ICN, Hong Kong; Seven Seas, UK†.*
Multivitamin and mineral preparation (p.1417·1).

**Vypen** *Douglas, NZ†.*
Pindolol (p.983·2).
*Angina pectoris; hypertension.*

**Vysorel** *Novipharm, Ger.†.*
Mistletoe (p.1715·3) from fir trees, apple trees or pine trees.
*Malignant neoplasms.*

**Vytinal** *Legrand, Braz.*
Multivitamin, amino-acid, and mineral preparation (p.1417·1).

**Vytone** *Dermik, USA.*
Hydrocortisone (p.1103·3); diiodohydroxyquinoline (p.603·3).

**Vytral** *Alpharma, Mex.*
Vitamin and mineral preparation (p.1417·1).

**V-Zoline** *Vitamed, Israel.*
Tetryzoline hydrochloride (p.1131·2).
*Eye irritation.*

**W5** *Aquamaid, UK†.*
Multivitamin and mineral preparation (p.1417·1).

**Wakamoto** *Wakamoto, Hong Kong.*
Aspergillus; *Eremothecium ashbyii*; lactobacteriaceae; dried yeast; diastase; protease; lipase; vitamin B substances; amino acids (p.1417·1).
*Tonic.*

**Wake-Up Tablets** *Adrem, Canad.*
Caffeine (p.782·1).
*Stimulant.*

**Walacort** *Wallace, India.*
Betamethasone (p.1093·1).
*Corticosteroid.*

**Walagesic** *Wallace, India.*
Dextropropoxyphene hydrochloride (p.28·3); paracetamol (p.76·2).
*Pain.*

**Walamycin** *Wallace, India.*
Colistin sulfate (p.198·3).
*Gastroenteritis.*

**Walaphage** *Wallace, India.*
Metformin hydrochloride (p.342·3).
*Diabetes mellitus.*

**Walavin** *Wallace, India.*
Griseofulvin (p.400·3).
*Fungal infections of the skin, hair, and nails.*

**Walekof** *MBD, Singapore†.*
Alimemazine tartrate (p.423·3); guaifenesin (p.1122·1); phenylpropanolamine hydrochloride (p.1127·3).
*Cold symptoms; nasal and respiratory-tract congestion.*

**Walesolone** *MBD, Singapore.*
Prednisolone (p.1108·1).
*Corticosteroid.*

**Walix** *Fidia, Ital.*
Oxaprozin (p.75·1).
*Musculoskeletal, joint, and peri-articular disorders.*

**Wallerox** *Novartis, Austria.*
Dihydroergotamine tartrate (p.466·1); troxerutin (p.1688·3).
*Venous insufficiency.*

**Walsedyl** *MBD, Singapore†.*
Codeine phosphate (p.27·1); ephedrine hydrochloride (p.1120·1); promethazine hydrochloride (p.439·1).
*Coughs; hay fever; hypersensitivity reactions; rhinitis.*

**Walyte** *Wallace, India.*
Sodium chloride; potassium chloride; sodium citrate; glucose (p.1222·2).
*Oral rehydration therapy.*

**Wampole Bronchial Cough Syrup** *Wampole, Canad.*
Ammonium chloride (p.1115·2); aralia racemosa; poplar buds (p.1733·3); sanguinaria (p.1741·3); senega (p.1130·2); white pine; wild cherry (p.1765·2).

**Wampole Vitamin Syrup** *Wampole, Canad.*
Vitamin B substances with iron (p.1417·1).

**Wandonorm** *Novartis, Ger.*
Bopindolol malonate (p.875·3).
*Hypertension.*

**Wanmycin**
*DHA, Hong Kong; DHA, Malaysia; DHA, Singapore.*
Doxycycline hyclate (p.206·2).
*Bacterial infections.*

**Wanse** *Yu Sheng, Singapore.*
Ferrous fumarate (p.1427·3); cyanocobalamin (p.1458·2); folic acid (p.1429·1).
*Anaemias.*

**War Lin** *Grisi, Mex.†.*
Lindane (p.1506·3).

**Waran** *Nycomed, Swed.*
Warfarin sodium (p.1022·2).
*Thromboembolic disorders.*

**Warca** *Pharmasant, Thai.*
Mebendazole (p.108·2).
*Worm infections.*

**Warfant** *Antigen, Irl.*
Warfarin sodium clathrate (p.1022·2).
*Thromboembolic disorders.*

**Warfilone** *Merck Frosst, Canad.†.*
Warfarin sodium (p.1022·2).
*Thromboembolic disorders.*

**WariActiv**
*Ritter, Ger.; Ritter, Hong Kong.*
Ethyl chloride (p.1376·2).
*Local anaesthesia.*

**Wari-Diclowal** *Ritter, Malaysia.*
Diclofenac sodium (p.32·1).
*Gout; inflammation; musculoskeletal, joint, and periarticular disorders; pain.*

**Waridipin** *Ritter, Hong Kong.*
Nifedipine (p.966·2).
*Angina pectoris; heart failure; hypertension.*

**Warimazol** *Ritter, Hong Kong.*
Clotrimazole (p.396·2).
*Fungal skin infections; vulvovaginitis.*

**Wari-Procomil**
*Ritter, Hong Kong; Ritter, Thai.*
Yohimbine hydrochloride (p.1766·2); methyltestosterone (p.1559·3); testes extract (p.1569·3); kola (p.1765·3); lecithin (p.1706·1); muira puama.
*Erectile dysfunction.*

**Wariviron** *Ritter, Hong Kong.*
Aciclovir (p.626·1).
*Herpes simplex infections.*

**Warix** *Drossopharm, Switz.*
Podophyllotoxin (p.1155·3).
*Anogenital warts.*

**Warme-Gel** *Ratiopharm, Ger.*
Glycol salicylate (p.44·3); benzyl nicotinate (p.21·2).
*Musculoskeletal, joint, peri-articular and soft-tissue disorders; neuralgia; peripheral vascular disorders.*

**Warm-Up** *Pharmco, S.Afr.†.*
Methyl salicylate (p.59·3); menthol (p.1711·3); eucalyptus oil (p.1686·2); turpentine oil (p.1760·1).
*Muscular pain and stiffness.*

**Wart Remover**
*Cress, Canad.†; Stiefel, USA; Glades, USA; Rugby, USA.*
Salicylic acid (p.1157·1).

**Wartec**
*Stiefel, Austral.; Stiefel, Braz.; Paladin, Canad.; Stiefel, Chile; Stiefel, Denm.; Stiefel, Fin.; Stiefel, Fr.; Stiefel, Ger.; Organon Teknika (Οργανον Τεχνικα), Gr.; Stiefel, Hong Kong; Stiefel, Ital.; Stiefel, Norw.; Stiefel, NZ; Stiefel, S.Afr.; Stiefel, Singapore; Fides Ecopharma, Spain; Sylak, Swed.*
Podophyllotoxin (p.1155·3).
*Anogenital warts.*

**Wartex** *Pickles, UK.*
Salicylic acid (p.1157·1).
*Warts.*

**Warticon**
*Stiefel, Irl.; Stiefel, UK.*
Podophyllotoxin (p.1155·3).
*Genital warts.*

**Wartner**
*Shield, Irl.; PSM, NZ; Passion for Life, UK.*
Dimethyl ether (p.1236·1); propane (p.1238·2).
*Verrucas; warts.*

**Wart-Off** *Pfizer, USA.*
Salicylic acid (p.1157·1).
*Warts.*

**Waruzol**
*Note. This name is used for preparations of different composition.*
*Pharmanik (Φαρμανικ), Gr.*
Astemizole (p.424·2).
*Allergic conjunctivitis; allergic rhinitis; pruritus.*

*Schlatter, Switz.*
Acetic acid (p.1645·2); lactic acid (p.1704·1); salicylic acid (p.1157·1).
*Warts.*

**Warz-ab Extor** *Ohropax, Switz.*
Salicylic acid (p.1157·1); lactic acid (p.1704·1).
*Calluses; corns; warts.*

**Warzen-Alldahin** *Roha, Ger.*
Salicylic acid (p.1157·1); lactic acid (p.1704·1).
*Calluses; warts.*

**Warzenmittel** *Sanova, Austria.*
Monochloroacetic acid (p.1154·2).
*Warts.*

**Warzin** *Rosch & Handel, Austria.*
Lactic acid (p.1704·1).
*Warts.*

**Wash E45** *Crookes Healthcare, UK.*
Soap substitute.
*Dry skin.*

**Wasp-Eze** *SSL, UK.*
*Ointment†:* Antazoline hydrochloride (p.424·2).
*Topical spray:* Mepyramine maleate (p.437·1); benzocaine (p.1370·3).
*Insect bites; stings.*

**Wassertrat** *Biolab Sanus, Braz.†.*
Sodium chloride; potassium chloride; sodium phosphate; magnesium citrate; sodium citrate; citric acid; calcium lactate (p.1222·2).
*Diarrhoea; oral rehydration therapy.*

**Water Babies**
*Note. This name is used for preparations of different composition.*
*Schering-Plough, Canad.*
*SPF 30; SPF 45:* Homosalate (p.1148·1); octinoxate (p.1154·3); oxybenzone (p.1154·3); octisalate (p.1154·3).
*Sunscreen.*

*Schering-Plough, USA.*
*SPF 15:* Octinoxate (p.1154·3); oxybenzone (p.1154·3).
*SPF 30:* Octinoxate (p.1154·3); oxybenzone (p.1154·3); homosalate (p.1148·1); octisalate (p.1154·3).
*SPF 45:* Octinoxate (p.1154·3); oxybenzone (p.1154·3); octocrilene (p.1154·3); octisalate (p.1154·3).
*Sunscreen.*

**Water Babies Little Licks** *Schering-Plough, USA.*
*SPF 30:* Octinoxate (p.1154·3); oxybenzone (p.1154·3); octisalate (p.1154·3).
*Sunscreen.*

**Water Babies UVGuard** *Schering-Plough, Canad.†.*
*SPF 15:* Avobenzone (p.1142·3); octinoxate (p.1154·3); oxybenzone (p.1154·3).
*SPF 30:* Avobenzone (p.1142·3); octinoxate (p.1154·3); octisalate (p.1154·3); oxybenzone (p.1154·3).
*Sunscreen.*

**Water Naturtabs** *Larkhall Laboratories, UK.*
Bladderwrack (p.1742·3); lappa (p.1704·3); ground ivy (p.1696·1); clivers (p.1673·2).

**Water Pill c Potasio** *Natural Life, Arg.*
Buchu (p.1663·1); bearberry (p.1659·2); parsley (p.1728·3); juniper (p.1703·1); potassium gluconate (p.1232·2).
*Diuretic.*

**Watershed** *Potter's, UK.*
*Oral mixture:* Wild carrot (p.1765·1); pellitory; buchu (p.1663·1); juniper (p.1703·1); clivers (p.1673·2).
*Tablets:* Buchu (p.1663·1); parsley piert (p.1729·1); bearberry (p.1659·2); juniper oil (p.1703·1).
*Water retention.*

**Waucosin** *Proel, Gr.*
Timolol maleate (p.1012·2).
*Glaucoma.*

**Waxolve** *Bell, India.*
Paradichlorobenzene (p.1728·3); benzocaine (p.1370·3); chlorobutanol (p.1176·3); turpentine oil (p.1760·1).
*Ear wax removal.*

**Waxsol**
*Norgine, Austral.; Norgine, Hong Kong; Norgine, Irl.; Norgine, Malaysia; Norgine, NZ; Zuellig, NZ; Norgine, Singapore; Norgine, Thai.; Norgine, UK.*
Docusate sodium (p.1262·2).
*Ear wax removal.*

**Waxsol NF** *Norgine, S.Afr.*
Docusate sodium (p.1262·2).
*Ear wax removal.*

**Waxwane** *Thornton & Ross, UK.*
Turpentine oil (p.1760·1); terpineol (p.1752·2); chloroxylenol (p.1177·2).
*Ear wax removal.*

**4-Way Fast Acting** *Bristol-Myers Products, USA.*
Phenylephrine hydrochloride (p.1126·3); naphazoline hydrochloride (p.1124·3); mepyramine maleate (p.437·1).
*Nasal congestion.*

**4-Way Long Lasting** *Bristol-Myers Products, USA.*
Oxymetazoline hydrochloride (p.1126·1).
*Nasal congestion.*

**Waycital** *Wayne, Mex.†.*
Praziquantel (p.112·2).

**Wayfrato** *Wayne, Mex.†.*
Bezafibrate (p.873·2).

**Waynazol** *Wayne, Mex.†.*
Fluconazole (p.398·1).
*Fungal infections.*

**Waysen** *Wayne, Mex.†.*
Diltiazem (p.901·3).

**Waysul** *Wayne, Mex.†.*
Ceftriaxone (p.183·3).
*Bacterial infections.*

**Waytifeno** *Wayne, Mex.†.*
Ketotifen (p.788·2).

**Waytrax** *Wayne, Mex.†.*
Ceftazidime (p.180·2).
*Bacterial infections.*

**WCS Dusting Powder** *Weleda, UK.*
Homoeopathic preparation.

**Wechseltee EF-EM-ES** *Smetana, Austria.*
Passion flower (p.1729·1); valerian (p.1762·2); lupulus (p.1708·1); hypericum (p.299·1); melissa (p.1711·1); crataegus (p.1677·1); mistletoe (p.1715·3).
*Anxiety disorders; menopausal disorders; nervousness; sleep disorders.*

**Weiche Zinkpaste** *Lichtenstein, Ger.†.*
Zinc oxide (p.1163·2).
*Skin disorders; wounds.*

**Weifapenin** *Weifa, Norw.*
Phenoxymethylpenicillin potassium (p.242·1).
*Bacterial infections.*

**Weight Control** *Homeocan, Canad.*
Homoeopathic preparation.

**Weight Loss Aid** *Herbal Concepts, UK.*
Taraxacum (p.1751·3); bladderwrack (p.1742·3); boldo (p.1661·2).
*Slimming aid.*

**Weight Loss Kit** *Dolisos, Canad.*
Homoeopathic preparation.

**Weight Watchers Punto** *Dieterba, Ital.†.*
*Oral granules:* Fructose (p.1431·3); sorbitol (p.1446·3); aspartame (p.1422·1).
*Tablets:* Aspartame (p.1422·1).
*Sugar substitute.*

**Weimerquin** *Biokanol, Ger.*
Chloroquine phosphate (p.448·2).
*Malaria.*

**Weiscal** *Valdecasas, Mex.*
Ambroxol hydrochloride (p.1114·3).
*Respiratory-tract congestion.*

**Weiscalina** *Valdecasas, Mex.*
Phenylephrine hydrochloride (p.1126·3).
*Nasal congestion.*

**Weisen-U** *Shigaken, Singapore.*
Methiosulfonium chloride (p.1714·1); amylase (p.1654·2); aluminium hydroxide (p.1249·2).
*Dyspepsia; flatulence; gastrointestinal hyperacidity; heartburn.*

**Welchol** *Sankyo, USA.*
Colesevelam hydrochloride (p.889·2).
*Hypercholesterolaemia.*

**Weleda Hamorrhoidalzapfchen** *Weleda, Ger.*
Hamamelis (p.1696·3); aesculus (p.1648·2); stibium metall.
*Anorectal disorders.*

**Weleda-Rheumasalbe M** *Weleda, Ger.*
Basilicumkraut; camphor (p.1665·3); fluorit; castanospermum oil; venice turpentine; sea water (p.1233·3); murmeltierfett; rosemary oil (p.1740·2).
*Frostbite; gout; musculoskeletal, joint, and soft-tissue disorders.*

**Wellbutrin**
*GlaxoSmithKline, Arg.; GlaxoSmithKline, Braz.; GlaxoSmithKline, Canad.; GlaxoSmithKline, Chile; Glaxo Wellcome, Mex.; GlaxoSmithKline, USA.*
Bupropion hydrochloride (p.287·2).
*Aid to smoking withdrawal; depression.*

**Wellcid** *Klinger, Braz.*
Permethrin (p.1508·3).

**Wellconal**
*GlaxoSmithKline, Hong Kong; GlaxoSmithKline, S.Afr.*
Dipipanone hydrochloride (p.35·3); cyclizine hydrochloride (p.429·3).
*Pain; vomiting.*

**Wellcoprim**
*GlaxoSmithKline, Austria; GlaxoSmithKline, Belg.†; GlaxoSmithKline, Fr.; GlaxoSmithKline, Neth.*
Trimethoprim (p.272·2) or trimethoprim lactate (p.273·2).
*Bacterial infections of the urinary tract.*

**Wellcovorin** *Glaxo Wellcome, USA†.*
Calcium folinate (p.1431·1).
*Megaloblastic anaemias; overdosage of folic acid antagonists.*

**Welldorm** *Smith & Nephew Healthcare, UK.*
Cloral betaine (p.684·1) or cloral hydrate (p.684·1).
Formerly contained dichloralphenazone.
*Insomnia.*

**Wellferon**
*Glaxo Wellcome, Austria†; Glaxo Wellcome, Braz.†; Glaxo Wellcome, Canad.†; Glaxo Wellcome, Fin.†; Glaxo Wellcome, Hong Kong†; Glaxo Wellcome, Israel†; GlaxoSmithKline, Ital.; Glaxo Wellcome, Mex.†; GlaxoSmithKline, NZ†; Glaxo Wellcome, Singapore†; Wellcome, Spain†; Glaxo Wellcome, Swed.†; Wellcome, Switz.†; GlaxoSmithKline, Thai.; Glaxo Wellcome, USA†.*
Interferon alfa-n1 (p.640·3).
*Chronic myeloid leukaemia; hairy-cell leukaemia; hepatitis B; hepatitis C; renal cell cancer.*

**Wellman** *Vitabiotics, UK.*
Multivitamin and mineral preparation (p.1417·1).

**Wellvone**
*GlaxoSmithKline, Austral.; GlaxoSmithKline, Austria; GlaxoSmithKline, Belg.; Glaxo Wellcome, Denm.†; GlaxoSmithKline, Fr.; GlaxoSmithKline, Ger.; Glaxo Wellcome, Gr.; GlaxoSmithKline, Ital.; GlaxoSmithKline, Neth.; GlaxoSmithKline, S.Afr.; Glaxo Wellcome, Spain†; GlaxoSmithKline, Swed.; GlaxoSmithKline, Switz.; GlaxoSmithKline, UK.*
Atovaquone (p.601·3).
*Pneumocystis carinii pneumonia.*

**Wellwoman** *Potter's, UK.*
*Herbal tea†:* Tilia (p.1756·2); skullcap (p.1746·3); achillea (p.1646·2); bearberry (p.1659·2).
*Tonic.*
*Tablets:* Achillea (p.1646·2); motherwort (p.1717·1); tilia (p.1756·2); skullcap (p.1746·3); valerian (p.1762·2).
*Menopausal disorders.*

**Welticilina** *Welt, Arg.*
Ampicillin (p.157·1).
*Bacterial infections.*

**Welt-Sulfazol** *Welt, Arg.*
Sulfathiazole (p.264·1).
*Burns; skin infections; wounds.*

**Wemid** *Microsules Bernabo, Arg.*
Erythromycin ethyl succinate (p.208·1) or erythromycin stearate (p.208·2).
*Bacterial infections.*

**Wepox** *Wockhardt, India.*
Epoetin alfa (p.747·2).
*Anaemias; autologous blood transfusion.*

**Weraplex Plain** *Weimer, Hong Kong†.*
Vitamin B substances (p.1417·1).
*Vitamin B deficiency; vitamin B supplement.*

**Westcan Century plus MV & Mineral** *Vita-Health, Hong Kong†.*
Multivitamin and mineral preparation (p.1417·1).

**Westcort**
*Bristol-Myers Squibb, Braz.; Westwood-Squibb, Canad.; Bristol-Myers Squibb, Mex.; Westwood-Squibb, USA.*
Hydrocortisone valerate (p.1104·2).
*Skin disorders.*

**Wet** *Fidia, Ital.*
Electrolytes (p.1217·1).
*Nasal irrigation.*

**Wetol** *Beta, Arg.*
Pilocarpine hydrochloride (p.1495·1).
*Radiotherapy-induced xerostomia; Sjögren's syndrome.*

**White Cloverine** *Medtech, USA.*
Barrier preparation.

**Whitfield** *Malaysia Chemist, Singapore.*
Salicylic acid (p.1157·1); benzoic acid (p.1169·3).
*Parasitic skin infections.*

**Whitfield Plus** *Sam-On, Israel†.*
Benzoic acid (p.1169·3); salicylic acid (p.1157·1); lidocaine hydrochloride (p.1377·3).
*Fungal skin infections.*

**Whitfields (Benzoic Acid Compound) Ointment** *McGloin, Austral.†.*
Benzoic acid (p.1169·3); salicylic acid (p.1157·1).
*Fungal skin infections.*

**Wibi**
*Galderma, Canad.†; Healthpoint, USA.*
Moisturiser.

**Wibophorin** *Pfluger, Ger.†.*
Homoeopathic preparation.

**Wibotin H** *Pfluger, Ger.*
Homoeopathic preparation.

**Wicaran** *Widmer, Fin.*
Tretinoin (p.1161·1); dexpanthenol (p.1727·2); urea (p.1162·2).
*Keratinisation disorders.*

**Wicarba** *Widmer, Fin.*
Vitamin A palmitate (p.1453·1); dexpanthenol (p.1727·2); urea (p.1162·2).
*Skin disorders.*

**Wick Daymed Erkaltungs** *Wick, Ger.*
*Capsules:* Dextromethorphan hydrobromide (p.1117·3); paracetamol (p.76·2); phenylpropanolamine hydrochloride (p.1127·3).
*Oral liquid:* Paracetamol (p.76·2); guaifenesin (p.1122·1); phenylephrine hydrochloride (p.1126·3); ascorbic acid (p.1460·2).
*Cold symptoms.*

**Wick Erkaltungs-Saft fur die Nacht** *Procter & Gamble, Austria.*
Doxylamine succinate (p.432·3); ephedrine sulfate (p.1120·1); dextromethorphan hydrobromide (p.1117·3); paracetamol (p.76·2).
*Cold symptoms.*

**Wick Formel 44** *Procter & Gamble, Austria.*
Dextromethorphan (p.1117·3).
*Coughs.*

**Wick Formel 44 Husten-Loser** *Wick, Ger.*
Guaifenesin (p.1122·1).
*Coughs and associated respiratory-tract disorders.*

**Wick Formel 44 Husten-Stiller** *Wick, Ger.*
Dextromethorphan hydrobromide (p.1117·3).
*Coughs.*

**Wick Formel 44 Plus Hustenloser** *Procter & Gamble, Austria.*
Guaifenesin (p.1122·1).
*Catarrh; coughs.*

**Wick Formel 44 plus Husten-Pastillen S** *Wick, Ger.*
Dextromethorphan (p.1117·3).
*Catarrh; coughs.*

**Wick Formel 44 Plus Hustenstiller** Procter & Gamble, Austria.
Dextromethorphan hydrobromide (p.1117·3).
*Coughs.*

**Wick Hustensaft** Procter & Gamble, Austria.
Dextromethorphan hydrobromide (p.1117·3); doxylamine succinate (p.432·3); sodium citrate (p.1223·2).
*Coughs.*

**Wick Inhalierstift N** Wick, Ger.
Menthol (p.1711·3); camphor (p.1665·3).
*Nasal congestion.*

**Wick Kinder Formel 44 Husten-Loser** Wick, Ger.†.
Guaifenesin (p.1122·1).
*Catarrh; coughs.*

**Wick Kinder Formel 44 Husten-Stiller** Wick, Ger.†.
Dextromethorphan hydrobromide (p.1117·3).
*Coughs.*

**Wick Medinait** Wick, Ger.
Doxylamine succinate (p.432·3); ephedrine sulfate (p.1120·1); dextromethorphan hydrobromide (p.1117·3); paracetamol (p.76·2).
*Cold and influenza symptoms.*

**Wick Sinex**
Note. This name is used for preparations of different composition.
Procter & Gamble, Austria.
Oxymetazoline hydrochloride (p.1126·1); menthol (p.1711·3); camphor (p.1665·3); cineole (p.1672·1).
*Cold symptoms.*

Wick, Ger.
Oxymetazoline hydrochloride (p.1126·1).
*Catarrh; nasal congestion.*

**Wick Sulagil** Wick, Ger.
Lidocaine (p.1377·3); dequalinium chloride (p.1178·1); cetylpyridinium chloride (p.1173·1).
*Mouth and throat disorders.*

**Wick Vapo Syrup** Procter & Gamble, Austria.
Menthol (p.1711·3).
*Catarrh; coughs.*

**Wick Vaporub**
Note. This name is used for preparations of different composition.
Procter & Gamble, Austria.
Menthol (p.1711·3); camphor (p.1665·3); eucalyptus oil (p.1686·2); nutmeg oil (p.1722·3); cedar wood oil; turpentine oil (p.1760·1); thymol (p.1194·2).
*Catarrh; coughs and cold symptoms.*

Wick, Ger.†.
Menthol (p.1711·3); camphor (p.1665·3); cineole (p.1672·1); turpentine oil (p.1760·1).
*Catarrh; cold symptoms; coughs.*

Wick, Ger.
*Ointment:* Menthol (p.1711·3); camphor (p.1665·3); eucalyptus oil (p.1686·2); turpentine oil (p.1760·1).
*Catarrh; cold symptoms; coughs.*

**Wick Vaposyrup** Wick, Ger.†.
Menthol (p.1711·3).
*Bronchitis; coughs.*

**Wicne** Widmer, Fin.
Triclosan (p.1195·2); salicylic acid (p.1157·1); colloidal sulfur (p.1158·2); colloidal silica (p.1581·3).
*Acne.*

**Wicnecarb** Widmer, Fin.
Pyridoxine hydrochloride (p.1456·3); triclosan (p.1195·2); colloidal sulfur (p.1158·2); urea (p.1162·2).
*Acne.*

**Wicnelact** Widmer, Fin.
Triclosan (p.1195·2); zinc sulfate (p.1469·3); lactic acid (p.1704·1); magnesium sulfate (p.1228·2); salicylic acid (p.1157·1).
*Acne; seborrhoea.*

**Wicnevit** Widmer, Fin.
Vitamin A palmitate (p.1453·1); triclosan (p.1195·2); pyridoxine hydrochloride (p.1456·3); dexpanthenol (p.1727·2); urea (p.1162·2).
*Acne; seborrhoea.*

**Wiedimmun** Wiedemann, Ger.
*Injection:* Homoeopathic preparation.
*Oral drops:* Echinacea purpurea (p.1683·2).
*Respiratory-tract infections.*

**Wifibrin** Willmar, Mex.†.
Paracetamol (p.76·2).
*Fever; pain.*

**Wigraine**
Note. This name is used for preparations of different composition.
Organon, Canad.†.
Ergotamine tartrate (p.467·2); belladonna alkaloids (p.479·1); caffeine (p.782·1).
*Migraine and other vascular headaches.*

Organon, USA.
Ergotamine tartrate (p.467·2); caffeine (p.782·1).
*Vascular headache.*

**Willlong**
Will-Pharma, Belg.; Willpharma, Thai.†.
Glyceryl trinitrate (p.923·2).
*Angina pectoris; heart failure.*

**Willospon**
Will-Pharma, Belg.†; Will-Pharma, Neth.
Gelatin foam (p.754·3).
*Haemostatic dressing.*

**Willospon Forte** Will-Pharma, Neth.
Collagen (p.1674·3).
*Haemostatic dressing.*

**Willowbark Plus Herbal Formula 11** Vitelle, Austral.†.
Skullcap (p.1746·3); devil's claw root (p.28·2); salix (p.87·3).
*Headache.*

**Wilpan** Microsules Bernabo, Arg.
Phenylephrine hydrochloride (p.1126·3); vitamin C (p.1460·2); pentoxyverine citrate (p.1126·2); paracetamol (p.76·2).
*Influenza symptoms.*

**Wilpan C** Microsules Bernabo, Arg.
Phenylephrine hydrochloride (p.1126·3); pentoxyverine citrate (p.1126·2); astemizole (p.424·2); vitamin C (p.1460·2).
*Influenza symptoms.*

**Wilprafen** Yamanouchi, Ger.
Josamycin (p.224·3) or josamycin propionate (p.224·3).
*Bacterial infections.*

**Wilyfenicol** Tocogino, Mex.†.
Chloramphenicol (p.185·1), chloramphenicol palmitate (p.185·1), or chloramphenicol sodium succinate (p.185·1).
*Bacterial infections.*

**Winar** Apogepha, Ger.
Urtica root (p.1762·1).
*Benign prostatic hyperplasia.*

**Winasma** Sanofi Synthelabo, Spain†.
Ephedrine sulfate (p.1120·1); phenobarbital (p.367·3); theophylline (p.798·3).
*Obstructive airways disease.*

**Winasorb**
Recalcine, Chile; Sanofi Synthelabo, Mex.
Paracetamol (p.76·2).
*Fever; pain.*

**Winasorb Flex** Recalcine, Chile.
Chlorzoxazone (p.1392·3); paracetamol (p.76·2).
*Skeletal muscle spasm and pain.*

**Wincef** Fujisawa, Jpn.
Cefoselis sulfate (p.175·2).
*Bacterial infections.*

**Wincoram**
Sanofi Synthelabo, Ger.
Amrinone (p.862·3).
*Heart failure.*

Sanofi Synthelabo, Spain.
Amrinone lactate (p.862·3).
*Heart failure.*

**Wind & Dyspepsia Relief** Herbal Concepts, UK.
Ginger (p.1267·1); hydrastis (p.1698·3); myrrh (p.1718·3); rhubarb (p.1287·3); valerian (p.1762·2); taraxacum (p.1751·3).
*Dyspepsia; flatulence.*

**Wind-Eze** GlaxoSmithKline Consumer, UK.
Simeticone (p.1289·2).
Formerly known as Setlers Wind-Eze.
*Flatulence.*

**Windol** Dermapharm, Ger.
Bufexamac (p.21·3).
*Inflammatory skin disorders.*

**Windol Basisbad** Dermapharm, Ger.
Liquid paraffin (p.1479·1); soya oil (p.1447·2).
*Bath additive; skin disorders.*

**Wingel** Sanofi Synthelabo, Mex.
Aluminium (p.1652·2); magnesium (p.1227·3); dimeticone (p.1289·2).
*Peptic ulcer.*

**Wink** Pharmco, S.Afr.†.
Naphazoline nitrate (p.1124·3); phenylephrine hydrochloride (p.1126·3).
*Eye irritation.*

**40 Winks** Roberts, USA.
Diphenhydramine hydrochloride (p.431·3).
*Insomnia.*

**Winlomylon** Adcock Ingram, S.Afr.
Nalidixic acid (p.234·1).
*Urinary-tract infections.*

**Winobanin** Sanofi Synthelabo, Ger.†.
Danazol (p.1545·2).
*Angioedema; benign breast disorders; endometriosis.*

**Winofit** Wockhardt, India.
Vitamin E; vitamin C; vitamin A; eicosapentaenoic acid; docosahexaenoic acid; zinc sulphate; folic acid; manganese sulfate; chromium tripicolinate; selenium dioxide (p.1417·1).
*Tonic.*

**Winol** Raffo, Arg.
Irinotecan hydrochloride (p.564·1).
*Colorectal cancer.*

**Winpac** Sanofi Synthelabo, Chile.
Paracetamol (p.76·2); pseudoephedrine hydrochloride (p.1129·2).
*Nasal congestion; pain; sinusitis.*

**Winpain** Brunel, S.Afr.
Paracetamol (p.76·2).
*Fever; pain.*

**Winpred** ICN, Canad.
Prednisone (p.1109·3).
*Corticosteroid.*

**WinRho**
CSL, Austral.; Cangene, Canad.; Cangene, Israel; CSL, NZ; Baxter, UK; Nabi, USA.
An anti-D immunoglobulin (p.1608·1).
*Idiopathic thrombocytopenic purpura; prevention of rhesus sensitisation.*

**Winstrol**
Zambon, Spain; Ovation, USA.
Stanozolol (p.1569·2).
*Anabolic; anaemia associated with renal insufficiency; female breast cancer; osteoporosis.*

**Winter AP** Merck, Braz.
Dexbrompheniramine maleate (p.426·1); pseudoephedrine sulfate (p.1129·2).

**Wintogeno** Alpharma, Singapore; Cox, Singapore.
Methyl salicylate (p.59·3); menthol (p.1711·3).
*Musculoskeletal, joint, and soft-tissue pain.*

**Wintomilon** Sanofi Synthelabo, Port.
Nalidixic acid (p.234·1).
*Urinary-tract infections.*

**Wintomylon**
Sanofi Synthelabo, Arg.; Sanofi Synthelabo, Braz.; Sanofi Synthelabo, Chile; Sanofi Synthelabo, Hong Kong; Sanofi Synthelabo, Mex.
Nalidixic acid (p.234·1).
*Gram-negative bacterial intestinal infections; urinary-tract infections.*

**Winton** Sanofi Synthelabo, Spain.
Aluminium hydroxide (p.1249·2); magnesium hydroxide (p.1272·2).
*Dyspepsia; gastrointestinal hyperacidity.*

**Wintonin** Sanofi Winthrop, Ger.†.
Gepefrine tartrate (p.923·2).
*Orthostatic hypotension.*

**Wisamt** Procter & Gamble, Austria.
Resorcinol (p.1156·3); sulfur (p.1158·2).
*Acne.*

**Wisamt N** Procter & Gamble, Ger.
Sulfur (p.1158·2); resorcinol (p.1156·3).
*Acne.*

**Wismut comp** Ratiopharm, Ger.
Bismuth subcarbonate (p.1252·1); anhydrous aluminium hydroxide (p.1249·2); dimethicone (p.1289·2); magnesium trisilicate gel (p.1272·3).
*Gastrointestinal disorders.*

**Witch Doctor**
Fleet, Austral.†; De Witt, UK.
Hamamelis (p.1696·3).
*Skin disorders.*

**Witch Sunsore** De Witt, UK.
Hamamelis (p.1696·3).
*Sunburn.*

**Witromin** Pisa, Mex.
Erythromycin (p.208·1).
*Bacterial infections.*

**Witte Kruis** Viatris, Neth.
Paracetamol (p.76·2); caffeine (p.782·1).
*Fever; pain.*

**Witty** Natural Health, Arg.
Permethrin (p.1508·3).
*Pediculosis.*

**Wobe-Mugos**
Note. This name is used for preparations of different composition.
Mucos, Austria.
Pancreatic proteolytic enzymes; calf thymus (p.1756·1); pisum sativum; lens esculenta; papain (p.1727·3).
*Adjunct to treatment of malignant neoplasms.*

Romsa, Mex.
Papain (p.1727·3); trypsin (p.1758·3); chymotrypsin (p.1671·2).
*Inflammatory and degenerative disorders; varicella-zoster infections.*

**Wobe-Mugos E** Mucos, Ger.
Trypsin (p.1758·3); chymotrypsin (p.1671·2); papain (p.1727·3).
*Malignant neoplasms; viral infections.*

**Wobe-Mugos Th** Mucos, Ger.†.
Trypsin (p.1758·3); papain (p.1727·3); bovine thymus extract (p.1756·1).
*Malignant neoplasms; viral infections.*

**Wobenzimal** Vitafarma, Spain.
*Ointment:* Papaya enzymes; lens sculenta enzymes; pisum sativum enzymes; pancreatin (p.1725·3); vitamin A (p.1451·2); thyme (p.1755·2); tocopherol (p.1464·3); vitamin F.
*Inflammation; oedema.*
*Tablets:* Papaya; lens sculenta; pisum sativum; pancreatin (p.1725·3); thyme (p.1755·2).
*Inflammation; oedema; peripheral vascular disorders.*

**Wobenzym**
Mucos, Austria; Romsa, Mex.
Pancreatin (p.1725·3); bromelains (p.1662·2); papain (p.1727·3); lipase; amylase (p.1654·2); trypsin (p.1758·3); chymotrypsin (p.1671·2); rutoside (p.1688·2).
*Musculoskeletal and joint inflammation; oedema.*

**Wobenzym N** Mucos, Ger.
*Ointment:* Bromelains (p.1662·2); trypsin (p.1758·3).
*Inflammation; oedema.*
*Tablets:* Pancreatin (p.1725·3); bromelains (p.1662·2); papain (p.1727·3); rutoside (p.1688·2).
*Inflammation; thrombophlebitis.*

**Woerisetten S** Kneipp, Switz.
Senna (p.1288·2).
*Constipation.*

**Wokadine** Wockhardt, India.
Povidone-iodine (p.1190·3).
*Burns; disinfection of hands, skin and mucous membranes; mouth and throat disorders; skin infections; vaginal infections; wounds.*

**Wokex-2** Wockhardt, India.
Rifampicin (p.250·2); isoniazid (p.222·2); vitamin $B_6$ (p.1457·2).
*Tuberculosis.*

**Wokex-3** Wockhardt, India.
1 Tablet, rifampicin (p.250·2); isoniazid (p.222·2); vitamin $B_6$ (p.1457·2); 1 tablet, ethambutol (p.212·2).
*Tuberculosis.*

**Wokex-4** Wockhardt, India.
1 Tablet, rifampicin (p.250·2); isoniazid (p.222·2); vitamin $B_6$ (p.1457·2); 2 tablets, pyrazinamide (p.246·3); 1 or 2 tablets, ethambutol (p.212·2).
*Tuberculosis.*

**Wolff Basis** Wolff, Ger.†.
Emollient.
*Pharmaceutical diluent; skin disorders.*

**Woloderma**
Adroka, Switz.†.
Soap substitute.
*Skin disorders.*

Adroka, Switz.
*Topical lotion:* Sodium lactate (p.1223·2); almond oil (p.1651·1).
*Skin disorders.*

**Woman Formula** Avon, Canad.
Multivitamin and mineral preparation (p.1417·1).

**Woman Kind** Windsor, UK†.
Pyridoxine (p.1457·2).
*Premenstrual syndrome.*

**Womens Change Formula** General Nutrition, Canad.
Multivitamin and mineral preparation (p.1417·1).

**Womens Exclusive Formula** Natural Life, Arg.
Vitamin and mineral preparation (p.1417·1).

**Women's Formula Herbal Formula 3** Vitelle, Austral.†.
Angelica (p.1655·1); cimicifuga (p.1671·3); blue cohosh (p.1661·2); pulsatilla (p.1737·1); agnus castus (p.1649·1).
*Menstrual disorders.*

**Womens Support** General Nutrition, Canad.
Multivitamin and mineral preparation (p.1417·1).

**Women's Timed Release Ultra Mega without Iron** General Nutrition, Canad.
Multivitamin and mineral preparation (p.1417·1).

**Womens Tylenol Multi-Symptom Menstrual Relief** McNeil Consumer, USA.
Paracetamol (p.76·2); pamabrom (p.978·2).

**Womosol Solar** Costec, Arg.
*SPF 12:* Padimate O (p.1155·1).
*Sunscreen.*

**Wonder Ice** Pedinol, USA.
Menthol (p.1711·3).
*Muscle, joint, and soft-tissue pain; neuralgia.*

**Wondergel** Lake, USA.
Vaginal lubricant.

**Wondra** Richardson-Vicks, USA.
Emollient and moisturiser.

**Woodwards Baby Chest Rub** SSL, UK†.
Menthol (p.1711·3); eucalyptus oil (p.1686·2); turpentine oil (p.1760·1).
*Nasal congestion and catarrh.*

**Woodwards Colic Drops** SSL, UK†.
Simeticone (p.1289·2).
*Colic; wind pain.*

**Woodward's Diaper Rash** Pharmacare, Canad.
Zinc oxide (p.1163·2).
*Nappy rash.*

**Woodwards Gripe Water**
Pharmacare, Canad.; LRC, Israel; SSL, UK.
Terpeneless dill seed oil (p.1680·2); sodium bicarbonate (p.1223·2).
*Infant colic.*

**Woodwards Inhalant** Aspen, S.Afr.
Cineole (p.1672·1); chloroxylenol (p.1177·2); pine oil; turpentine oil (p.1760·1); menthol (p.1711·3).
*Respiratory-tract disorders.*

**Woodwards Nappy Rash Ointment** Seton, UK†.
Zinc oxide (p.1163·2); cod-liver oil (p.1425·2).
*Nappy rash.*

**Woodwards Teething Gel** SSL, UK.
Lidocaine hydrochloride (p.1377·3); cetylpyridinium chloride (p.1173·1).
*Denture irritation; mouth ulcers; teething pain.*

**Worm** De Witt, UK†.
Piperazine citrate (p.111·2).
*Worm infections.*

**Wormex** Sussex, UK†.
Piperazine citrate (p.111·2).

**Wormgo** Aspen, S.Afr.
Mebendazole (p.108·2).
*Worm infections.*

**Wormin** Cadila Pharma, India.
Mebendazole (p.108·2).
*Worm infections.*

**Wormstop** Be-Tabs, S.Afr.
Mebendazole (p.108·2).
*Worm infections.*

**Wotinex** Wockhardt, India.
Tinidazole (p.617·1); diloxanide furoate (p.604·1).
*Amoebiasis.*

**Wound-A-Sept** Beige, S.Afr.†.
Cetrimide (p.1172·1).
*Minor wounds and burns.*

**Wright's Vaporizing Fluid** LRC Products, UK†.
Chlorocresol (p.1177·1).
*Cold symptoms; coughs.*

**Wrinkle Defence** *Sunspot, Austral.†.*
*SPF 15+:* Oxybenzone (p.1154·3); octinoxate (p.1154·3) in a moisturising base.
*Emollient; sunscreen.*

**W-Tropfen** *Hofmann & Sommer, Ger.*
Salicylic acid (p.1157·1); lactic acid (p.1704·1).
*Calluses; corns.*

**Wund- und Brand-Gel Eu Rho** *Eu Rho, Ger.†.*
Lidocaine hydrochloride (p.1377·3); allantoin (p.1141·3); cetylpyridinium chloride (p.1173·1); dexpanthenol (p.1727·2).
*Burns; wounds.*

**Wund- und Heilsalbe N** *Riemser, Ger.*
Dexpanthenol (p.1727·2).
*Skin disorders.*

**Wundesin** *Gebro, Austria.*
Povidone-iodine (p.1190·3).
*Wounds.*

**Wyamine** *Wyeth-Ayerst, USA.*
Mephentermine sulfate (p.952·1).
*Hypotension; shock.*

**Wyanoids Relief Factor** *Wyeth-Ayerst, USA.*
Live yeast cell derivative (p.1469·1); shark-liver oil.
*Haemorrhoids.*

**Wycillin** *Monarch, USA†.*
Procaine benzylpenicillin (p.246·1).
*Bacterial infections.*

**Wycillin R** *Eurofarma, Braz.*
Procaine benzylpenicillin (p.246·1); benzylpenicillin potassium (p.163·2).
*Bacterial infections.*

**Wycillina** *Pharmacia Upjohn, Ital.*
Benzathine benzylpenicillin (p.162·3).
*Bacterial infections.*

**Wycort** *Wyeth, India.*
Hydrocortisone acetate (p.1103·3).
*Corticosteroid.*

**Wycort c Neomycin** *Wyeth, India.*
Hydrocortisone acetate (p.1103·3); neomycin sulfate (p.235·1).
*Anal or vulval pruritus; burns; infected skin disorders; skin ulcers; wounds.*

**Wydase**
*Wyeth-Ayerst, Canad.†; Wyeth, Chile; Wyeth-Ayerst, USA†.*
Hyaluronidase (p.1698·2).
*Adjunct in subcutaneous urography; adjuvant to increase the absorption and dispersion of drugs; hypodermoclysis.*

**Wydora** *Riemser, Ger.*
Indoramin hydrochloride (p.939·2).
*Hypertension.*

**Wygesic**
*Wyeth, India; Wyeth-Ayerst, USA.*
Dextropropoxyphene hydrochloride (p.28·3); paracetamol (p.76·2).
*Fever; pain.*

**Wylaxine** *Whitehall, Belg.†.*
Bisoxatin acetate (p.1253·2).
*Bowel evacuation; constipation.*

**Wymesone** *Wyeth, India.*
Dexamethasone (p.1097·1).
*Corticosteroid.*

**Wymox** *Wyeth-Ayerst, USA†.*
Amoxicillin trihydrate (p.155·3).
*Bacterial infections.*

**Wypresin** *Wyeth Lederle, Austria.*
Indoramin hydrochloride (p.939·2).
*Hypertension.*

**Wysolone** *Wyeth, India.*
Prednisolone (p.1108·1).
*Corticosteroid.*

**Wysoy**
*Wyeth, Irl.; Wyeth, UK.*
Lactose-free food for special diets (p.1417·1).
*Cows' milk or lactose intolerance; galactokinase deficiency; galactosaemia.*

**Wytens** *Wyeth Lederle, Fr.*
Bisoprolol fumarate (p.875·1); hydrochlorothiazide (p.933·2).
*Hypertension.*

**Wytensin**
*Wyeth Lederle, Austria†; Wyeth-Ayerst, USA.*
Guanabenz acetate (p.926·2).
*Hypertension.*

**X-2** *Investigaciones Filosoficas y Cientificas, Mex.*
Cocarboxylase (p.1455·2).
*Thiamine deficiency.*

**Xacin** *Pharmasant, Thai.*
Norfloxacin (p.238·3).
*Bacterial infections.*

**X-Adene** *GNR, Fr.†.*
Procaine hydrochloride (p.1383·2); vitamin B substances (p.1417·1); polymerised sodium deoxyribonucleate.
*Tonic.*

**Xagrid** *Opopharma, Switz.*
Anagrelide hydrochloride (p.1654·3).
*Essential thrombocythaemia.*

**Xaken** *Kener, Mex.†.*
Methotrexate (p.568·2).

**Xal**
*Wolfs, Belg.†; Pharmadeveloppement, Fr.*
Potassium chloride; ammonium chloride; calcium formate; glutamic acid (p.1217·1).
*Dietary salt substitute.*

**Xalacom**
*Pharmacia, Austral.; Pharmacia, Belg.; Pharmacia, Chile; Pharmacia, Fr.; Pharmacia, Ger.; Pharmacia, Irl.; Pharmacia, Ital.; Pharmacia, Neth.; Pharmacia, Port.; Pharmacia, Singapore; Pharmacia, Spain; Pharmacia, Switz.; Pharmacia, UK.*
Latanoprost (p.1519·1); timolol maleate (p.1012·2).
*Glaucoma; ocular hypertension.*

**Xalatan**
*Pharmacia, Arg.; Pharmacia, Austral.; Pharmacia, Austria; Pharmacia, Belg.; Pharmacia, Braz.; Pharmacia, Canad.; Pharmacia, Chile; Pharmacia, Denm.; Pharmacia, Fin.; Pharmacia, Fr.; Pharmacia, Ger.; Pharmacia-Upjohn, Gr.; Pharmacia, Hong Kong; Pharmacia, Irl.; Pharmacia Upjohn, Israel; Pharmacia Upjohn, Ital.; Pharmacia, Malaysia; Pharmacia Upjohn, Mex.; Pharmacia, Neth.; Pharmacia, Norw.; Pharmacia, NZ; Pharmacia, Port.; Pharmacia, S.Afr.; Pharmacia, Singapore; Pharmacia, Spain; Pharmacia, Swed.; Pharmacia, Switz.; Pharmacia, Thai.; Pharmacia, UK; Pharmacia Upjohn, USA.*
Latanoprost (p.1519·1).
*Glaucoma; ocular hypertension.*

**Xalazin** *Caber, Ital.*
Mesalazine (p.1273·2).
*Inflammatory bowel disease.*

**Xalcom**
*Pharmacia, Denm.; Pharmacia, Fin.; Pharmacia, Norw.; Pharmacia, Swed.*
Latanoprost (p.1519·1); timolol maleate (p.1012·2).
*Glaucoma; ocular hypertension.*

**Xaliplat** *Richmond, Arg.*
Oxaliplatin (p.577·1).
*Malignant neoplasms.*

**Xalyn-Or** *Atlantis, Mex.*
Amoxicillin trihydrate (p.155·3).
*Bacterial infections.*

**Xamamina** *Bracco, Ital.*
Dimenhydrinate (p.431·1).
*Motion sickness.*

**Xanacine** *Progress, Thai.*
Alprazolam (p.668·3).
*Anxiety.*

**Xanagis** *Agis, Israel.*
Alprazolam (p.668·3).
*Anxiety; mixed anxiety depressive states; panic disorders.*

**Xanalin** *Silom, Thai.*
Neomycin sulfate (p.235·1); polymyxin B (p.245·2); gramicidin (p.220·2).
*Bacterial eye infections.*

**Xanax**
*Pharmacia, Arg.; Pharmacia, Austral.; Pharmacia, Belg.; Pharmacia, Canad.; Pharmacia, Fr.; Pharmacia, Ger.; Pharmacia-Upjohn, Gr.; Pharmacia, Hong Kong; Pharmacia, Irl.; Pharmacia Upjohn, Israel; Pharmacia Upjohn, Ital.; Pharmacia, Malaysia; Pharmacia, Neth.; Pharmacia, NZ; Pharmacia, Port.; Pharmacia, Singapore; Pharmacia, Switz.; Pharmacia, Thai.; Pharmacia, UK; Pfizer, USA.*
Alprazolam (p.668·3).
*Anxiety; mixed anxiety depressive states; panic disorder.*

**Xanbon** *Kissei, Jpn.*
Ozagrel sodium (p.1725·2).
*Cerebral thrombosis; cerebral vasospasm.*

**Xanef** *Merck Sharp & Dohme, Ger.*
Enalapril maleate (p.909·2) or enalaprilat (p.909·3).
*Heart failure; hypertension.*

**Xanidine**
*Berlin Pharm, Singapore.*
Ranitidine (p.1285·2).
*Acid aspiration; dyspepsia; gastro-oesophageal reflux; peptic ulcer; Zollinger-Ellison syndrome.*

*Berlin Pharm, Thai.*
Ranitidine hydrochloride (p.1285·2).
*Gastro-oesophageal reflux; peptic ulcer; Zollinger-Ellison syndrome.*

**Xanol**
*Note. This name is used for preparations of different composition.*
*Phoenix, Arg.*
Formoterol fumarate (p.786·1).
*Obstructive airways disease.*

*Pharmasant, Thai.*
Allopurinol (p.412·2).
*Gout; hyperuricaemia; renal calculi.*

**Xanolam** *Aspen, S.Afr.†.*
Alprazolam (p.668·3).
*Anxiety disorders; mixed anxiety depressive states; panic attacks.*

**Xanomel** *Clonmel, Irl.*
Ranitidine hydrochloride (p.1285·2).
*Gastric hyperacidity; gastro-oesophageal reflux; peptic ulcer; Zollinger-Ellison syndrome.*

**Xanor**
*Pharmacia, Austria; Pharmacia, Fin.; Pharmacia, Norw.; Pharmacia, S.Afr.; Pharmacia, Swed.*
Alprazolam (p.668·3).
*Anxiety disorders; mixed anxiety depressive states; panic attacks.*

**Xantervit** *SIFI, Ital.*
Xanthopterin; multivitamins (p.1417·1).
*Ocular trauma and lesions.*

**Xantervit Antibiotico** *SIFI, Ital.*
Xanthopterin; chloramphenicol (p.185·1); multivitamins (p.1417·1).
*Ocular trauma and lesions.*

**Xantervit Eparina** *SIFI, Ital.*
Xanthopterin; heparin sodium (p.928·1); multivitamins (p.1417·1).
*Ocular burns.*

**Xanthium**
*SMB, Belg.; Galephar, Fr.; SMB, Thai.*
Theophylline (p.798·3).
*Obstructive airways disease.*

**Xanthomax** *Ashbourne, UK.*
Allopurinol (p.412·2).

**Xantina B12** *Prodotti, Braz.*
Methionine (p.1042·1); choline (p.1424·3); vitamin B substances (p.1454·3); liver extract; with or without manganese (p.1440·1) and gastric mucosa extract.
*Liver disorders.*

**Xantinon B12** *Altana, Braz.*
Methionine (p.1042·1); vitamin B substances (p.1454·3); choline chloride (p.1424·3); liver extract; with or without manganese (p.1440·1) and gastric mucosa extract.
*Liver disorders.*

**Xantinon Complex** *Altana, Braz.*
Acetylmethionine; inositol (p.1701·2); choline citrate (p.1424·3); betaine hydrochloride (p.1660·2); cyanocobalamin (p.1458·2); pyridoxine hydrochloride (p.1456·3).
*Liver disorders.*

**Xantium** *Wyeth Lederle, Ital.*
Protirelin tartrate (p.1338·2).
*Neurological deficit.*

**Xantivent** *Essex, Switz.†.*
Theophylline (p.798·3).
*Bronchospasm.*

**Xantox** *Sinterapico, Braz.†.*
Cyanocobalamin (p.1458·2).

**Xantromid** *Richmond, Arg.*
Methotrexate (p.568·2).
*Malignant neoplasms.*

**Xanturenasi** *Teofarma, Ital.*
Pyridoxine hydrochloride (p.1456·3).
*Age-related metabolic disorders; epilepsy; migraine; skin disorders; tremor; vomiting in pregnancy.*

**Xao Pil** *Giscard, Arg.*
Pilocarpine (p.1494·3).
*Glaucoma; production of miosis.*

**Xao T** *Giscard, Arg.*
Tobramycin (p.271·2).
*Bacterial eye infections.*

**Xao-Dex** *Giscard, Arg.*
Tobramycin (p.271·2); dexamethasone (p.1097·1).
*Infected eye disorders.*

**Xapro** *Jenapharm, Ger.*
Estriol (p.1552·3).
*Vulvovaginal disorders.*

**Xarator** *Parke, Davis, Ital.*
Atorvastatin calcium (p.866·1).
*Hyperlipidaemias.*

**Xarope Antigripal** *Basi, Port.*
Codeine (p.27·1); ethylmorphine (p.37·3); sulfogaiacol (p.1131·1).
*Coughs.*

**Xarope Comp Mel e Agriao** *Sinterapico, Braz.†.*
Rorippa nasturtium aquaticum; aconite (p.1646·3); ipecacuanha (p.1122·3); senega (p.1130·2); mikania glomerata.
*Coughs.*

**Xarope das Criancas** *Sinterapico, Braz.†.*
Sodium dibunate (p.1130·2); sodium benzoate (p.1169·3); diphenhydramine hydrochloride (p.431·3).
*Coughs.*

**Xarope de Caraguata** *Sanval, Braz.*
Annona muricata; bromoform (p.1663·1); sodium benzoate (p.1169·3); aconite (p.1646·3); belladonna (p.479·1); tolu balsam (p.1131·3); grindelia (p.1696·1).
*Coughs.*

**Xarope de Eucalipto** *Teuto, Braz.†.*
Lobelia (p.1589·1); erysimum officinale; stramonium (p.489·2); eucalyptus (p.1686·1).
*Coughs.*

**Xarope de Iodeto de Potassio** *Uniao Quimica, Braz.†.*
Potassium iodide (p.1598·1); sulfogaiacol (p.1131·1).
*Coughs.*

**Xarope de Iodeto de Potassio Composto**
*Note. This name is used for preparations of different composition.*
*Kopkins, Braz.†.*
Potassium iodide (p.1598·1); lobelia (p.1589·1).
*Respiratory-tract congestion.*

*Laborsil, Braz.†.*
Potassium iodide (p.1598·1); sodium citrate (p.1223·2); carbinoxamine maleate (p.426·3).
*Respiratory-tract congestion.*

**Xarope de Limao Bravo**
*Note. This name is used for preparations of different composition.*
*Teuto, Braz.†.*
Sulfogaiacol (p.1131·1); sodium benzoate (p.1169·3); grindelia (p.1696·1); siparuna guyanensis.
*Respiratory-tract congestion.*

*Veafarm, Braz.†.*
Siparuna guyanensis; guaifenesin (p.1122·1); sodium benzoate (p.1169·3).
*Respiratory-tract congestion.*

**Xarope de Lobelia Composto** *Drogasil, Braz.†.*
Sulfogaiacol (p.1131·1); guaifenesin (p.1122·1); lobelia (p.1589·1).
*Respiratory-tract congestion.*

**Xarope de Macas Rainetas** *Medical, Port.*
Senna (p.1288·2); mannitol (p.950·2); apple pulp.
*Constipation.*

**Xarope 44E** *Procter & Gamble, Braz.*
Dextromethorphan hydrobromide (p.1117·3); guaifenesin (p.1122·1).
*Coughs.*

**Xarope Grindelia de Oliveira Junior** *Vitex, Braz.†.*
Ipecacuanha (p.1122·3); grindelia (p.1696·1).
*Respiratory-tract congestion.*

**Xarope Iodo-Suma** *Iodo Suma, Braz.*
Potassium iodide (p.1598·1); anchietea salutaris; bowdichia virgilloides; echinodorus macrophyllus; gentian (p.1692·2).
*Coughs.*

**Xarope Neo** *Neo Quimica, Braz.*
Potassium iodide (p.1598·1).
*Coughs.*

**Xarope Peitoral de Ameixa Composto** *Simoes, Braz.*
Sodium benzoate (p.1169·3); bromoform (p.1663·1); lobelia (p.1589·1); grindelia (p.1696·1); aconite (p.1646·3); eucalyptus oil (p.1686·2).
*Coughs.*

**Xarope Sao Joao** *Uniao Quimica, Braz.*
Bromoform (p.1663·1); sodium benzoate (p.1169·3); sulfogaiacol (p.1131·1); belladonna (p.479·1); aconite (p.1646·3); mulungu (p.1717·2); tar (p.1159·3); tolu balsam (p.1131·3).
Formerly contained bromoform and sodium benzoate.
*Coughs.*

**Xarope Valda** *Canonne, Braz.†.*
Cetylpyridinium chloride (p.1173·1); ammonium chloride (p.1115·2); sodium citrate (p.1223·2); sodium benzoate (p.1169·3).
*Respiratory-tract congestion.*

**Xarope Vick** *Procter & Gamble, Braz.†.*
Cetylpyridinium chloride (p.1173·1); sodium citrate (p.1223·2).
*Respiratory-tract congestion.*

**Xasmun** *Ciclum, Spain.*
Norfloxacin (p.238·3).
*Genito-urinary tract infections.*

**Xaten** *Biotherapie, Fr.†.*
Atenolol (p.865·2).
*Angina pectoris; hypertension.*

**Xatral**
*Sanofi Synthelabo, Austria; Sanofi Synthelabo, Belg.; Sanofi Synthelabo, Braz.†; Sanofi Winthrop, Denm.; Sanofi Synthelabo, Fin.; Sanofi Synthelabo, Fr.; Sanofi Synthelabo, Gr.; Sanofi Synthelabo, Hong Kong; Sanofi Synthelabo, Irl.; Synthelabo, Israel; Sanofi Synthelabo, Ital.; Sanofi Synthelabo, Malaysia; Sanofi Synthelabo, Neth.; Sanofi Synthelabo, Norw.; Sanofi Synthelabo, S.Afr.; Sanofi Synthelabo, Singapore; Sanofi Synthelabo, Swed.; Synthelabo, Switz.; Sanofi Synthelabo, Thai.; Sanofi Synthelabo, UK.*
Alfuzosin hydrochloride (p.856·2).
*Benign prostatic hyperplasia.*

**Xebramol** *Progress, Thai.*
Paracetamol (p.76·2).
*Fever; pain.*

**Xedenol** *Baliarda, Arg.*
Diclofenac sodium (p.32·1).
*Inflammation; musculoskeletal and joint disorders; pain.*

**Xedenol B12** *Baliarda, Arg.*
Diclofenac sodium (p.32·1); betamethasone (p.1093·1) or betamethasone phosphate (p.1093·2); cyanocobalamin (p.1458·2) or hydroxocobalamin (p.1458·2).
*Peri-articular disorders.*

**Xedenol Flex** *Baliarda, Arg.*
Diclofenac sodium (p.32·1); pridinol mesilate (p.1395·2).
*Musculoskeletal and joint disorders.*

**Xefo**
*Nycomed, Austria; Nycomed, Denm.; Nycomed, Fin.†; Nycomed, Gr.; Pharmacia, S.Afr.; Nycomed, Swed.; Nycomed, Thai.; CeNeS, UK†.*
Lornoxicam (p.54·2).
*Inflammation; musculoskeletal, joint, and peri-articular disorders; pain.*

**Xeloda**
*Roche, Arg.; Roche, Austral.; Roche, Belg.; Roche, Braz.; Roche, Canad.; Roche, Chile; Roche, Denm.; Roche, Fin.; Roche, Fr.; Roche, Ger.; Roche, Gr.; Roche, Hong Kong; Roche, Irl.; Roche, Israel; Roche, Ital.; Roche, Mex.; Roche, Norw.; Roche, NZ; Roche, Port.; Roche, S.Afr.; Roche, Singapore; Roche, Spain; Roche, Swed.; Roche, Switz.; Roche, Thai.; Roche, UK; Roche, USA.*
Capecitabine (p.533·2).
*Breast cancer; colorectal cancer.*

**Xeltic** *Unison, Hong Kong.*
Glibenclamide (p.331·2).
*Diabetes mellitus.*

**Xemos** *Recalcine, Chile.*
Salmeterol (p.795·2).
*Asthma.*

**Xenalon** *Mepha, Switz.*
Spironolactone (p.1003·1).
*Hyperaldosteronism; hypertension; nephrotic syndrome; oedema.*

**Xenar** *Wassermann, Ital.*
Naproxen (p.65·1).
*Musculoskeletal, joint, peri-articular, and soft-tissue disorders; neuralgia.*

**Xenazine**
*AFT, NZ; Cambridge, UK.*
Tetrabenazine (p.1752·2).
*Movement disorders.*

**Xenetix**
*Temis, Arg.; Guerbet, Austria; Codali, Belg.; Rider, Chile; Guerbet, Denm.; Guerbet, Fin.; Guerbet, Fr.; Guerbet, Ger.; R+N, Gr.; Guerbet,*

Israel; Guerbet, Ital.; Guerbet, Neth.†; Guerbet, Norw.; Guerbet, Port.; Guerbert, Spain; Gothia, Swed.; Guerbet, Switz.
Iobitridol (p.1063·1).
*Radiographic contrast medium.*

**Xenical**
Roche, Arg.; Roche, Austral.; Roche, Austria; Roche, Belg.; Roche, Braz.; Roche, Canad.; Roche, Chile; Roche, Denm.; Roche, Fin.; Roche, Fr.; Roche, Ger.; Roche, Gr.; Roche, Hong Kong; Roche, Irl.; Roche, Israel ;Roche, Ital.; Roche, Mex.; Roche, Neth.; Roche, Norw.; Roche, NZ; Roche, Port.; Roche, S.Afr.; Roche, Singapore; Roche, Spain; Roche, Swed.; Roche, Switz.; Roche, Thai.; Roche, UK; Roche, USA.
Orlistat (p.1724·2).
*Obesity.*

**Xenid** Aventis, Fr.
Diclofenac epolamine (p.33·1) or diclofenac sodium (p.32·1).
*Dysmenorrhoea; musculoskeletal, joint, and peri-articular disorders; renal colic.*

**Xenobid** Amadeus, India.
Naproxen (p.65·1) or naproxen sodium (p.65·1).
*Gout; musculoskeletal, joint, and soft-tissue disorders; pain.*

**Xenovate** Aspen, S.Afr.
Clobetasol propionate (p.1095·2).
*Skin disorders.*

**Xepagan** Xepa-Soul Pattinson, Singapore†.
Promethazine hydrochloride (p.439·1).
*Hypersensitivity reactions; sedative.*

**Xepamet**
Xepa-Soul Pattinson, Malaysia; Xepa-Soul Pattinson, Singapore.
Cimetidine (p.1255·3).
*Acid aspiration; adjunct in pancreatic insufficiency; dyspepsia; gastro-oesophageal reflux; peptic ulcer; Zollinger-Ellison syndrome.*

**Xepanicol**
Xepa-Soul Pattinson, Hong Kong; Xepa-Soul Pattinson, Malaysia; Xepa-Soul Pattinson, Singapore†.
Chloramphenicol (p.185·1).
*Bacterial eye infections.*

**Xepasone** Xepa-Soul Pattinson, Singapore.
Prednisolone (p.1108·1).
*Corticosteroid.*

**Xepin**
Bioglan, Irl.; Cambridge Healthcare, UK.
Doxepin hydrochloride (p.291·2).
*Pruritus.*

**Xerac AC**
Dispolab, Chile; Person & Covey, USA.
Aluminium chloride (p.1142·1); alcohol (p.1166·1).
*Hyperhidrosis.*

**Xeracil** Xerogen, S.Afr.†.
Amoxicillin (p.155·3).
*Bacterial infections.*

**Xeragel** Dispolab, Chile.
Silica (p.1581·3); dimeticone (p.1482·1).
*Barrier ointment; wounds.*

**Xeramax** Xerogen, S.Afr.
*Syrup:* Paracetamol (p.76·2); codeine phosphate (p.27·1); promethazine hydrochloride (p.439·1).
*Fever; pain.*
*Tablets:* Paracetamol (p.76·2); codeine phosphate (p.27·1); caffeine (p.782·1); meprobamate (p.706·2).
*Pain with tension.*

**Xeramel** Qestmed, S.Afr.
Erythromycin estolate (p.208·1).
*Bacterial infections.*

**Xerand**
Roche-Posay, Arg.; Roche-Posay, Irl.
Emollient.
*Dry skin; skin irritation.*

**Xeraspor** Qestmed, S.Afr.
Clotrimazole (p.396·2).
*Fungal skin infections; vulvovaginal candidiasis.*

**Xerazole** Qestmed, S.Afr.
Co-trimoxazole (p.199·3).
*Bacterial infections.*

**Xerenal** Kwizda, Austria.
Dosulepin hydrochloride (p.291·1).
*Depression.*

**Xerial** SVR, Ital.
Urea (p.1162·2); allantoin (p.1141·3); emollients.
*Dry skin.*

**Xerodent**
Alpharma, Fin.; Alpharma, Swed.
Sodium fluoride (p.1444·3); malic acid (p.1709·2).
*Dental caries prophylaxis; dry mouth.*

**Xeroderm**
Roche-Posay, Arg.; Dermol, USA.
Emollient.
*Dry skin disorders.*

**Xerogesic** Crown, S.Afr.
Paracetamol (p.76·2); codeine phosphate (p.27·1); caffeine (p.782·1); meprobamate (p.706·2).
*Pain and associated tension.*

**Xeroil** Roche-Posay, Irl.†.
Emollient.
*Dry skin.*

**Xeroprim** Crown, S.Afr.
Co-trimoxazole (p.199·3).
*Bacterial infections.*

**Xerotens** Covan, S.Afr.
Doxylamine succinate (p.432·3); paracetamol (p.76·2); codeine phosphate (p.27·1); caffeine (p.782·1).
*Pain and associated tension.*

**Xerumenex**
Viatris, Belg.; Viatris, Neth.
Trolamine polypeptide oleate-condensate (p.1758·2).
*Cleansing of external ear before otoscopy; removal of impacted ear wax.*

**Xet** Zydus, India.
Paroxetine (p.311·2).
*Anxiety disorders; depression; obsessive-compulsive disorder; panic disorder; post-traumatic stress disorder; social phobia.*

**Xflu**
SmithKline Beecham, Austral.†; GlaxoSmithKline, S.Afr.
An inactivated influenza vaccine (split virion) (p.1620·2).
*Active immunisation.*

**Xibornol Prodes** Almirall, Spain†.
*Oral suspension:* Bromhexine hydrochloride (p.1115·3); clofedanol hydrochloride (p.1117·1); xibornol (p.277·3).
*Suppositories:* Camphor (p.1665·3); niaouli oil (p.1719·3); xibornol (p.277·3).
*Respiratory-tract disorders.*

**Xicam** Pharmasant, Thai.
Piroxicam (p.84·2).
*Gout; musculoskeletal and joint disorders.*

**Xicane** Sanofi Synthelabo, Arg.
Naproxen (p.65·1).
*Gout: inflammation; musculoskeletal, joint, and periarticular disorders; pain.*

**Xicil** Rottapharm, Spain.
Glucosamine sulfate (p.1694·1).
*Rheumatic disorders.*

**Xiclav** Lannacher, Austria.
Amoxicillin trihydrate (p.155·3); potassium clavulanate (p.193·3).
*Bacterial infections.*

**Xiclovir** Lazar, Arg.
Aciclovir (p.626·1).
*Herpesvirus infections.*

**Xidanef**
Codal Synto, Malaysia; Codal Synto, Thai.
Ketotifen fumarate (p.788·1).
*Asthma; hypersensitivity reactions.*

**Xiemed** Medifive, Thai.
Alprazolam (p.668·3).
*Anxiety; mixed anxiety depressive states.*

**Xigris**
Lilly, Austral.; Lilly, Fr.; Lilly, Irl.; Lilly, NZ; Lilly, UK; Lilly, USA.
Drotrecogin alfa (activated) (p.759·2).
*Sepsis.*

**Xilinum** Farmila, Ital.
*Acinetobacter xilinum*; vitamins (p.1417·1).
*Diarrhoea; disturbances of the intestinal flora.*

**Xilodase** Apsen, Braz.
Neomycin sulfate (p.235·1); lidocaine (p.1377·3); hyaluronidase (p.1698·2).
*Infected skin disorders.*

**Xilo-Mynol** Molteni, Ital.†.
Lidocaine hydrochloride (p.1377·3).
Adrenaline acid tartrate (p.852·2) is included in some injections as a vasoconstrictor to diminish absorption and localise the effect of the local anaesthetic.
*Local anaesthesia.*

**Xilonibsa**
Note. This name is used for preparations of different composition.
Inibsa, Port.
*Injection; topical spray:* Lidocaine hydrochloride (p.1377·3).
Adrenaline (p.852·2) or noradrenaline (p.974·3) is included in the injection as a vasoconstrictor to diminish absorption and localise the effect of the local anaesthetic.
*Topical paste:* Lidocaine (p.1377·3); tetracaine (p.1385·1).
*Local anaesthesia.*
Inibsa, Spain.
Lidocaine (p.1377·3) or lidocaine hydrochloride (p.1377·3).
Adrenaline acid tartrate (p.852·2) is included in the injection as a vasoconstrictor to diminish absorption and localise the effect of the local anaesthetic.
*Local anaesthesia.*

**Xilopar**
Cephalon, Ger.; Segix, Ital.; Esteve, Port.
Selegiline hydrochloride (p.1214·1).
*Parkinsonism.*

**Ximaken** Kendrick, Mex.
Cefuroxime sodium (p.184·1).
*Bacterial infections.*

**Ximovan** Aventis, Ger.
Zopiclone (p.729·3).
*Insomnia.*

**Xinder** Fouchard, Chile.
Clobetasol (p.1095·3).
*Skin disorders.*

**Xinia** Finadiet, Arg.
Diclofenac sodium (p.32·1).
*Inflammation; musculoskeletal and joint disorders; pain.*

**Xintoprost** Richmond, Arg.
Vinblastine (p.592·1).
*Malignant neoplasms.*

**Xipamid** German Remedies, India.
Xipamide (p.1029·2).
*Hypertension; oedema.*

**Xipral** Silanes, Mex.
Pravastatin sodium (p.984·3).
*Hypercholesterolaemia.*

**Xiprine** Finn Vita, Chile.
Glipizide (p.332·2).
*Diabetes mellitus.*

**Xiprocan** Protein, Mex.†.
Amoxicillin (p.155·3).
*Bacterial infections.*

**Xiral** Hawthorn, USA.
Chlorphenamine maleate (p.427·3); pseudoephedrine hydrochloride (p.1129·2); hyoscine methonitrate (p.483·3).
*Allergic rhinitis; cold symptoms; sinusitis.*

**Xiratuss** Hawthorn, USA.
Pentoxyverine tannate (p.1126·3); chlorphenamine tannate (p.428·1); phenylephrine tannate (p.1127·2).
*Coughs; nasal congestion.*

**Xismox** Genus, UK.
Isosorbide mononitrate (p.942·1).

**Xiten** Grunenthal, Chile.
Beclometasone dipropionate (p.1091·1).
*Asthma; nasal polyps; rhinitis.*

**xitix** Woelm, Ger.†.
Ascorbic acid (p.1460·2); sodium ascorbate (p.1460·2).
*Vitamin C deficiency.*

**Xitocin** Cryopharma, Mex.
Oxytocin (p.1336·1).
*Labour induction; postpartum haemorrhage; uterine atony.*

**XLys Low Try Maxamaid** Scientific Hospital Supplies, UK.
Lysine- and tryptophan-free food (p.1417·1).
*Glutaric aciduria.*

**XMET Analog**
Scientific Hospital Supplies, Austral.; Scientific Hospital Supplies, Irl.
Food for special diets (p.1417·1).
*Homocystinuria; hypermethioninaemia.*

**XMET Maxamaid**
Scientific Hospital Supplies, Austral.; Scientific Hospital Supplies, Irl.; Scientific Hospital Supplies, UK.
Food for special diets (p.1417·1).
Formerly known as Maxamaid RVHB in the *UK*.
*Homocystinuria; hypermethioninaemia.*

**XMET Maxamum**
Scientific Hospital Supplies, Austral.; Support, Braz.; Scientific Hospital Supplies, Irl.
Food for special diets (p.1417·1).
*Homocystinuria.*

**XMET Maximum** Nutricia, NZ; Scientific Hospital Supplies, NZ.
Food for special diets (p.1417·1).
*Homocystinuria; hypermethioninaemia.*

**XMTVI Analog**
Scientific Hospital Supplies, Austral.; Support, Braz.
Infant feed (p.1417·1).
*Methylmalonic acidaemia; propionic acidaemia.*

**XMTVI Asadon** Scientific Hospital Supplies, Austral.
Food for special diets (p.1417·1).
*Methylmalonic acidaemia; propionic acidaemia.*

**XMTVI Maxamaid**
Scientific Hospital Supplies, Austral.; Support, Braz.; Scientific Hospital Supplies, UK.
Food for special diets (p.1417·1).
Formerly known as Maxamaid XMET, THRE, VAL, ISOLEU in the *UK*.
*Methylmalonic acidaemia; propionic acidaemia.*

**XMTVI Maxamum** Scientific Hospital Supplies, Austral.
Food for special diets (p.1417·1).
Formerly known as XMet, Thre, Val, Isoleu Maxamum.
*Methylmalonic acidaemia; propionic acidaemia.*

**Xolaam** Aventis, Fr.
Aluminium hydroxide (p.1249·2); magnesium hydroxide (p.1272·2).
*Gastrointestinal disorders.*

**Xolair** Genentech, USA.
Omalizumab (p.790·1).
*Asthma.*

**Xolof** Saval, Chile.
Tobramycin (p.271·2).
*Bacterial eye infections.*

**Xolof D** Saval, Chile.
Tobramycin (p.271·2); dexamethasone (p.1097·1).
*Infected eye disorders.*

**Xonatil** Precimex, Mex.†.
Ceftriaxone (p.183·3).
*Bacterial infections.*

**Xopenex** Sepracor, USA.
Levosalbutamol hydrochloride (p.788·2).
*Obstructive airways disease.*

**Xorox**
Kwizda, Austria; Kite (Κιτε), Gr.
Aciclovir (p.626·1) or aciclovir sodium (p.626·1).
*Cytomegalovirus infections; herpes simplex infections; varicella-zoster infections.*

**Xorpic** Andromaco, Port.; Grunenthal, Port.
Ciprofloxacin hydrochloride (p.188·2).
*Bacterial infections.*

**Xozacil** Columbia, Mex.
Benzylpenicillin sodium (p.163·2).
*Bacterial infections.*

**XP Analog**
Scientific Hospital Supplies, Austral.; Support, Braz.; Nutricia, Ital.; Nutricia, NZ; Scientific Hospital Supplies, NZ.
Food for special diets (p.1417·1).
*Phenylketonuria.*

**XP Analog LCP** SHS, Fr.
Food for special diets (p.1417·1).
Formerly known as Analog XP.
*Phenylketonuria.*

**XP Maxamaid**
Scientific Hospital Supplies, Austral.; Support, Braz.; SHS, Fr.; Scientific Hospital Supplies, Irl.; Nutricia, NZ; Scientific Hospital Supplies, NZ; Scientific Hospital Supplies, UK.
Food for special diets (p.1417·1).
*Phenylketonuria.*

**XP Maxamum**
Scientific Hospital Supplies, Austral.; Support, Braz.; SHS, Fr.; Scientific Hospital Supplies, Irl.; Nutricia, NZ; Scientific Hospital Supplies, NZ; Scientific Hospital Supplies, UK.
Food for special diets (p.1417·1).
*Phenylketonuria.*

**Xpe SPC** Faria, Braz.
Sulfogaiacol (p.1131·1); sodium benzoate (p.1169·3); bromoform (p.1663·1); grindelia (p.1696·1).
*Coughs.*

**XPhen, Tyr Analog** Scientific Hospital Supplies, Austral.
Food for special diets (p.1417·1).
*Tyrosinaemia.*

**XPhen, Tyr Maxamaid**
Scientific Hospital Supplies, Austral.; Scientific Hospital Supplies, UK.
Food for special diets (p.1417·1).
*Tyrosinaemia.*

**XPhen, Tyr Maxamum** Scientific Hospital Supplies, Austral.
Food for special diets (p.1417·1).
*Tyrosinaemia.*

**X-Praep** Viatris, Neth.
Sennosides (p.1288·2).
*Bowel evacuation; constipation.*

**X-Prep**
Mundipharma, Austria; Purdue, Canad.; Mundipharma, Ger.; Lavipharm, Gr.; Asta Medica, Ital.; Mundipharma, Norw.; Viatris, Port.; Mundipharma, Switz.; Gray, USA.
Senna (p.1288·2).
*Bowel evacuation.*
Viatris, Fr.; Rafa, Israel†; Adcock Ingram, S.Afr.; Viatris, Spain.
Sennosides A and B (p.1288·2).
*Bowel evacuation.*

**X-Prep Bowel Evacuant Kit-1** Gray, USA.
*Combination pack:* 2 tablets, standardised senna concentrate (p.1288·2); docusate sodium (p.1262·2) (Senokot-S); oral liquid, senna (X-Prep); 1 suppository, bisacodyl (Rectolax) (p.1251·3).
*Bowel evacuation.*

**X-Prep Bowel Evacuant Kit-2** Gray, USA†.
*Combination pack:* 1 dose oral granules, effervescent citrate/magnesium sulfate (Citralax) (p.1223·2) (p.1228·2); oral liquid, senna (X-Prep) (p.1288·2); 1 suppository, bisacodyl (Rectolax) (p.1251·3).
*Bowel evacuation.*

**XPT Tyrosidon** Scientific Hospital Supplies, UK.
Tyrosine- and phenylalanine-free amino-acid preparation (p.1417·1).
*Tyrosinaemia.*

**XPTM Tyrosidon**
Scientific Hospital Supplies, Austral.; Scientific Hospital Supplies, UK.
Food for special diets (p.1417·1).
*Tyrosinaemia.*

**X-Seb**
Paladin, Canad.; Baker Cummins, USA.
Salicylic acid (p.1157·1).
*Skin and scalp disorders.*

**X-Seb Plus**
Paladin, Canad.; Baker Cummins, USA.
Pyrithione zinc (p.1156·2); salicylic acid (p.1157·1).
*Scalp disorders.*

**X-Seb T**
Paladin, Canad.; Baker Cummins, USA.
Salicylic acid (p.1157·1); coal tar (p.1159·2).
*Scalp disorders.*

**X-Seb T Plus**
Paladin, Canad.; Baker Cummins, USA.
Salicylic acid (p.1157·1); coal tar (p.1159·2); menthol (p.1711·3).
*Scalp disorders.*

**XSP-Bena** Xepa-Soul Pattinson, Singapore†.
Diphenhydramine hydrochloride (p.431·3); sodium citrate (p.1223·2); ammonium chloride (p.1115·2).
*Coughs; nasal and bronchial congestion.*

**X'tac** Upha, Malaysia.
Ranitidine hydrochloride (p.1285·2).
*Gastric hyperacidity; gastro-oesophageal reflux; peptic ulcer; Zollinger-Ellison syndrome.*

**X-Tar** Dormer, Canad.
Salicylic acid (p.1157·1); coal tar (p.1159·2); menthol (p.1711·3).
*Scalp disorders.*

**Xuprin** Solvay, Austria.
Isoxsuprine resinate (p.1702·3).
*Peripheral vascular disorders.*

**Xusal** UCB, Ger.
Levocetirizine hydrochloride (p.435·3).
*Hypersensitivity reactions.*

**Xycam** Aspen, S.Afr.
Piroxicam (p.84·2).
*Gout; musculoskeletal and joint disorders.*

**Xylanaest** Gebro, Austria.
Lidocaine hydrochloride (p.1377·3).
Adrenaline (p.852·2) is included in some injections as a vasoconstrictor to diminish absorption and localise the effect of the local anaesthetic.
*Local anaesthesia.*

**Xylesine** Amino, Switz.
Lidocaine hydrochloride (p.1377·3).
*Local anaesthesia.*

**Xylestesin**
Note. This name is used for preparations of different composition.
Espe, Austria; Espe, Switz.
Lidocaine (p.1377·3); cetrimonium bromide (p.1173·1).
*Local anaesthesia.*

Cristalia, Braz.
Lidocaine (p.1377·3) or lidocaine hydrochloride (p.1377·3).
Adrenaline acid tartrate (p.852·2) or noradrenaline acid tartrate (p.974·3) is included in some injections as a vasoconstrictor to diminish absorption and localise the effect of the local anaesthetic.
*Local anaesthesia.*

**Xylestesin Pumpspray** 3M Espe, Ger.
Lidocaine (p.1377·3); cetrimonium bromide (p.1173·1).
*Local anaesthesia.*

**Xylestesin, Xylestesin-F** 3M Espe, Ger.
Lidocaine hydrochloride (p.1377·3).
Noradrenaline hydrochloride (p.975·1) is included in this preparation as a vasoconstrictor to diminish absorption and localise the effect of the local anaesthetic.
*Local anaesthesia.*

**Xylestesin-A, Xylestesin centro** 3M Espe, Ger.
Lidocaine hydrochloride (p.1377·3).
Adrenaline hydrochloride (p.852·3) is included in this preparation as a vasoconstrictor to diminish absorption and localise the effect of the local anaesthetic.
*Local anaesthesia.*

**Xylestesin-F** Espe, Switz.
Lidocaine hydrochloride (p.1377·3).
Noradrenaline hydrochloride (p.975·1) is included in this preparation as a vasoconstrictor to diminish absorption and localise the effect of the local anaesthetic.
*Local anaesthesia.*

**Xylestesin-S** 3M Espe, Ger.
Lidocaine hydrochloride (p.1377·3).
Noradrenaline hydrochloride (p.975·1) and adrenaline hydrochloride (p.852·3) are included in this preparation as vasoconstrictors to diminish absorption and localise the effect of the local anaesthetic.
*Local anaesthesia.*

**Xylestesin-S "special"** Espe, Switz.
Lidocaine hydrochloride (p.1377·3).
Adrenaline hydrochloride (p.852·3) and noradrenaline hydrochloride (p.975·1) are included in this preparation as vasoconstrictors to diminish absorption and localise the effect of the local anaesthetic.
*Local anaesthesia.*

**Xylestin-A** 3M, Hong Kong.
Lidocaine hydrochloride (p.1377·3).
Adrenaline hydrochloride (p.852·3) is included in this preparation as a vasoconstrictor to diminish absorption and localise the effect of the local anaesthetic.
*Local anaesthesia.*

**Xylit** Baxter, Ger.; Braun, Ger.; DeltaSelect, Ger.
Xylitol (p.1469·1).
*Carbohydrate source; fluid disorders.*

**Xylo** CT, Ger.
Xylometazoline hydrochloride (p.1132·2).
*Nasal congestion.*

**Xylo Siozwo** Febena, Ger.
Xylometazoline hydrochloride (p.1132·2).
*Nasal congestion.*

**Xylocain**
AstraZeneca, Austria; AstraZeneca, Denm.; AstraZeneca, Fin.; Dentsply, Fin.; AstraZeneca, Ger.; Dentsply, Ger.; AstraZeneca, Norw.; AstraZeneca, Swed.; AstraZeneca, Switz.
Lidocaine (p.1377·3) or lidocaine hydrochloride (p.1377·3).
Adrenaline (p.852·2) or adrenaline acid tartrate (p.852·2) is included in some injections as a vasoconstrictor to diminish absorption and localise the effect of the local anaesthetic.
*Local anaesthesia.*

**Xylocain $CO_2$** AstraZeneca, Switz.
Lidocaine (p.1377·3); carbon dioxide.
*Local anaesthesia.*

**Xylocain Comp** AstraZeneca, Denm.†.
Lidocaine (p.1377·3); bismuth subgallate (p.1252·2); zinc oxide (p.1163·2).
*Anorectal disorders.*

**Xylocain f.d. Kardiologie** AstraZeneca, Ger.
Lidocaine hydrochloride (p.1377·3).
*Arrhythmias; status epilepticus.*

**Xylocain Klorhexidin** AstraZeneca, Denm.†.
Lidocaine hydrochloride (p.1377·3); chlorhexidine gluconate (p.1173·2).
*Catheterisation; cystoscopy; local anaesthesia.*

**Xylocaina**
AstraZeneca, Arg.; AstraZeneca, Braz.; AstraZeneca, Ital.; Dentsply, Ital.; Astra, Mex.; AstraZeneca, Port.; Inibsa, Spain.
Lidocaine (p.1377·3) or lidocaine hydrochloride (p.1377·3).
Adrenaline (p.852·2), adrenaline acid tartrate (p.852·2), or noradrenaline (p.974·3) is included in some injections as a vasoconstrictor to diminish absorption and localise the effect of the local anaesthetic.
*Local anaesthesia.*

**Xylocaina 2%** AstraZeneca, Chile.
Lidocaine (p.1377·3) or lidocaine hydrochloride (p.1377·3).
*Local anaesthesia.*

**Xylocaine**
AstraZeneca, Austral.; Dentsply, Austral.; AstraZeneca, Belg.; AstraZeneca, Canad.; AstraZeneca, Fr.; Cana, Gr.; Astra-Zeneca, Gr.; AstraZeneca, Hong Kong; AstraZeneca, India; AstraZeneca, Irl.; Astra, Israel; AstraZeneca, Malaysia; AstraZeneca, Neth.; AstraZeneca, NZ; Astra, S.Afr.; AstraZeneca, Singapore AstraZeneca, Thai.; AstraZeneca, UK; Dentsply, UK; Astra, USA.
Lidocaine (p.1377·3) or lidocaine hydrochloride (p.1377·3).
Adrenaline (p.852·2) or adrenaline tartrate (p.852·2) is included in some injections as a vasoconstrictor to diminish absorption and localise the effect of the local anaesthetic.
*Local anaesthesia; ventricular arrhythmias.*

**Xylocaine Antiseptic** AstraZeneca, UK†.
Lidocaine hydrochloride (p.1377·3); chlorhexidine gluconate (p.1173·2).
*Local anaesthesia.*

**Xylocaine with Chlorhexidine** AstraZeneca, NZ.
Lidocaine hydrochloride (p.1377·3); chlorhexidine gluconate (p.1173·2).
*Local anaesthesia.*

**Xylocaine Jelly with Chlorhexidine** AstraZeneca, Austral.
Lidocaine hydrochloride (p.1377·3); chlorhexidine gluconate (p.1173·2).
*Catheterisation; endoscopy; local anaesthesia.*

**Xylocaine 2% Plain** AstraZeneca, UK†.
Lidocaine hydrochloride (p.1377·3).
Formerly known as Lignostab.
*Local anaesthesia.*

**Xylocaine Special Adhesive** AstraZeneca, Austral.
Lidocaine hydrochloride (p.1377·3).
*Topical anaesthesia in dentistry.*

**Xylocaine Visqueuse** AstraZeneca, Belg.
Lidocaine hydrochloride (p.1377·3).
*Adjunct in radiology and endoscopy; painful oral and oesophageal conditions.*

**Xylocard**
AstraZeneca, Austral.; AstraZeneca, Austria; AstraZeneca, Belg.; AstraZeneca, Canad.; AstraZeneca, Fr.; AstraZeneca, Hong Kong; AstraZeneca, India; Astra, Irl.†; AstraZeneca, Malaysia; AstraZeneca, Neth.†; Astra, Norw.†; AstraZeneca, NZ; AstraZeneca, Port.; AstraZeneca, Singapore†; Hassle, Swed.; AstraZeneca, Switz.; AstraZeneca, Thai.; AstraZeneca, UK†.
Lidocaine hydrochloride (p.1377·3).
*Ventricular arrhythmias.*

**Xylocitin** Jenapharm, Ger.
Lidocaine hydrochloride (p.1377·3).
Adrenaline acid tartrate (p.852·2) is included in some injections as a vasoconstrictor to diminish absorption and localise the effect of the local anaesthetic.
*Local anaesthesia.*

**Xylocitin cor** Jenapharm, Ger.
Lidocaine hydrochloride (p.1377·3).
*Ventricular arrhythmias.*

**Xylo-COMOD** Ursapharm, Ger.
Xylometazoline hydrochloride (p.1132·2).
*Nasal congestion.*

**Xylolin** Julphar, UAE.
Xylometazoline hydrochloride (p.1132·2).
*Nasal and sinus congestion.*

**Xyloma** Jean-Marie, Hong Kong.
Xylometazoline hydrochloride (p.1132·2).
*Nasal congestion; otitis media.*

**Xylonest**
AstraZeneca, Ger.; AstraZeneca, Switz.
Prilocaine hydrochloride (p.1382·3).
Adrenaline acid tartrate (p.852·2) or felypressin (p.1324·2) is included in some injections as a vasoconstrictor to diminish absorption and localise the effect of the local anaesthetic.
*Local anaesthesia.*

**Xylonest-Octapressin** Astra, Switz.†.
Prilocaine hydrochloride (p.1382·3).
Felypressin (p.1324·2) is included in this preparation as a vasoconstrictor to diminish absorption and localise the effect of the local anaesthetic.
*Local anaesthesia.*

**Xyloneural**
Gebro, Austria; Strathmann, Ger.; Gebro, Switz.
Lidocaine hydrochloride (p.1377·3).
*Headache; local anaesthesia; migraine; tinnitus; vertigo.*

**Xylonibsa** Inibsa, Spain†.
Cetylpyridinium chloride (p.1173·1); lidocaine hydrochloride (p.1377·3).
*Local anaesthesia.*

**Xylonor**
Note. This name is used for preparations of different composition.
Austrodent, Austria.
Lidocaine (p.1377·3); cetrimide (p.1172·1).
*Local anaesthesia.*

Ogna, Ital.
*Injection:* Lidocaine hydrochloride (p.1377·3).
Noradrenaline acid tartrate (p.974·3) or adrenaline acid tartrate (p.852·2) is included in some injections as a vasoconstrictor to diminish absorption and localise the effect of the local anaesthetic.
*Local anaesthesia.*

Ogna, Ital.; Prats, Spain; Septodont, Switz.
*Topical spray:* Lidocaine (p.1377·3); cetrimonium bromide (p.1173·1).
*Local anaesthesia.*

Septodont, Switz.†.
*Injection:* Lidocaine hydrochloride (p.1377·3).
Noradrenaline acid tartrate (p.974·3) or noradrenaline acid tartrate and adrenaline (p.852·2) are included in some injections as vasoconstrictors to diminish absorption and localise the effect of the local anaesthetic.
*Local anaesthesia.*

**Xylonor Especial** Prats, Spain.
Lidocaine hydrochloride (p.1377·3).
Adrenaline (p.852·2) and noradrenaline acid tartrate (p.974·3) are included in this preparation as vasoconstrictors to diminish absorption and localise the effect of the local anaesthetic.
*Local anaesthesia.*

**Xylonor 2% Sin Vasoconst** Prats, Spain.
Lidocaine hydrochloride (p.1377·3).
*Local anaesthesia.*

**Xylo-Pfan**
Pharmacia Upjohn, Canad.†; Adria, USA†.
Xylose (p.1766·1).
*Diagnosis of malabsorption.*

**Xyloproct**
Note. This name is used for preparations of different composition.
AstraZeneca, Austral.; Astra, Belg.†; AstraZeneca, Braz.; AstraZeneca, Fin.; AstraZeneca, Irl.; AstraZeneca, Ital.†; AstraZeneca, Malaysia; Astra, Mex.; AstraZeneca, Neth.†; AstraZeneca, Norw.; AstraZeneca, NZ; AstraZeneca, Singapore†; Tika, Swed.; AstraZeneca, Thai.†; AstraZeneca, UK.
Lidocaine (p.1377·3) or lidocaine hydrochloride (p.1377·3); hydrocortisone acetate (p.1103·3); aluminium acetate (p.1652·3) or aluminium subacetate (p.1652·3); zinc oxide (p.1163·2).
*Anorectal disorders.*

AstraZeneca, Hong Kong; Astra, Israel.
Lidocaine (p.1377·3); hydrocortisone acetate (p.1103·3).
Formerly contained lidocaine, hydrocortisone acetate, aluminium acetate, and zinc oxide.
*Anorectal disorders.*

**Xyloprocto** AstraZeneca, Arg.
Lidocaine (p.1377·3); hydrocortisone acetate (p.1103·3).

**Xylose-BMS** Bio-Medical, UK†.
Xylose (p.1766·1).
Formerly known as Xylomed.
*Diagnosis of malabsorption.*

**Xylotocan** AstraZeneca, Ger.
Tocainide hydrochloride (p.1014·1).
*Ventricular arrhythmias.*

**Xylotox**
Adcock Ingram, S.Afr.
Lidocaine hydrochloride(p.1377·3).
Adrenaline (p.852·2) or noradrenaline (p.974·3) is included in some preparations as a vasoconstrictor to diminish absorption and localise the effect of the local anaesthetic.
*Local anaesthesia.*

Dentsply, UK.
Lidocaine hydrochloride (p.1377·3).
Adrenaline acid tartrate (p.852·2) is included in this preparation as a vasoconstrictor to diminish absorption and localise the effect of the local anaesthetic.
*Local anaesthesia.*

**Xylovit** Vitamed, Israel.
Xylometazoline hydrochloride (p.1132·2).
*Nasal congestion.*

**Xymel** Clonmel, Irl.
Tramadol hydrochloride (p.94·3).
*Pain.*

**Xyrem** Orphan Medical, USA.
Sodium oxybate (p.1308·3).
*Cataplexy in patients with narcoleptic syndrome.*

**Xyzal**
UCB, Denm.; UCB, Fin.; UCB, Hong Kong; UCB, Irl.; UCB, Port.; UCB, UK.
Levocetirizine hydrochloride (p.435·3).
*Allergic conjunctivitis; allergic rhinitis; urticaria.*

**Xyzall** UCB, Fr.
Levocetirizine hydrochloride (p.435·3).
*Allergic rhinitis; urticaria.*

**Yacutin** Boots Healthcare, Spain.
Benzyl benzoate (p.1500·2); lindane (p.1506·3).
*Pediculosis; scabies.*

**Yadalan** Llorente, Spain†.
A nonoxinol (p.1413·2).
*Contraceptive.*

**Yadegal Compuesto** Rayere, Mex.
Dextromethorphan (p.1117·3); guaiacol (p.1122·1); chlorphenamine (p.428·1).
*Coughs.*

**Yakona N** Tentan, Switz.†.
Hypericum (p.299·1); kava (p.1703·2).
*Anxiety; nervous tension.*

**Yal**
Jacoby, Austria; Trommsdorff, Ger.; Gebro, Switz.
Docusate sodium (p.1262·2); sorbitol (p.1446·3).
*Bowel evacuation; constipation.*

**Yamalen** Aventis, Belg.†.
Dextropropoxyphene hydrochloride (p.28·3); paracetamol (p.76·2).
*Pain.*

**Yamatetan** Yamanouchi, Jpn.
Cefotetan disodium (p.177·1).
*Bacterial infections.*

**Yamcon** Sidus, Arg.
Wild yam.
*Menopausal disorders.*

**Yanal** Benitol, Arg.
Atropine (p.476·3); adrenaline (p.852·2).
*Asthma.*

**Yanurax** Fada, Arg.
Norfloxacin (p.238·3).
*Bacterial infections.*

**Yapamicin** Novag, Mex.
Ampicillin (p.157·1).
*Bacterial infections.*

**Yariba** Dendron, UK.
Kola (p.1765·3).
*Fatigue.*

**Yasmin**
Schering, Austral.; Schering, Austria; Schering, Belg.; Schering, Denm.; Schering, Ger.; Schering, Irl.; Schering, Israel; Schering, Norw.; Schering, Port.; Schering, Swed.; Schering, UK; Berlex, USA.
Drospirenone (p.1549·1); ethinylestradiol (p.1553·2).
28-Day packs also contain 7 inert tablets.
*Combined oral contraceptive.*

**Yasta**
Note. This name is used for preparations of different composition.
Bayer, Arg.
Sodium bicarbonate (p.1223·2); sodium carbonate (p.1747·1); caffeine (p.782·1); tartaric acid; sodium citrate.
*Dyspepsia; gastric hyperacidity.*

Bayer, Chile.
Aspirin (p.15·1); sodium bicarbonate (p.1223·2); citric acid (p.1673·1).
*Dyspepsia; pain.*

**Yatropan** Aventis, Braz.†.
Ephedrine (p.1120·1); menthol (p.1711·3); cineole (p.1672·1); tolu balsam (p.1131·3); lavender oil (p.1705·2); sumatra benzoin (p.1751·1); sulfanilamide (p.263·2); guaiacol (p.1122·1).
*Respiratory-tract congestion.*

**Yatrox** Vita, Spain.
Ondansetron hydrochloride (p.1281·1).
*Nausea and vomiting.*

**Yatushan Plus** Trima, Israel.
Diphenhydramine hydrochloride (p.431·3); diethyltoluamide (p.1503·3); dimethyl phthalate (p.1504·1).
*Insect bites.*

**Yavit** Ederka, Mex.†.
Multivitamin and mineral preparation (p.1417·1).

**Ydroquinidine Cooper** Cooper (Κοπερ), Gr.
Quinidine (p.991·3).
*Arrythmias.*

**Yeast Clear** Dolisos, Canad.
Homoeopathic preparation.

**Yeast Vite** Thornton & Ross, UK.
Caffeine (p.782·1); vitamin B substances (p.1417·1); dried yeast (p.1469·1).
*Tonic.*

**Yeast-Gard** Lake, USA.
Homoeopathic preparation.

**Yeast-X** Fleet, USA.
*Powder:* Corn starch (p.1449·1); zinc oxide (p.1163·2).
*Suppositories:* Pulsatilla (p.1737·1).

**Yectafer** AstraZeneca, Arg.
Iron sorbitol (p.1438·1).
*Iron-deficiency anaemia.*

**Yectafer Complex** AstraZeneca, Arg.
Iron sorbitol (p.1438·1); folic acid (p.1429·1); hydroxocobalamin (p.1458·2).
*Anaemias.*

**Yectames** Grossman, Mex.
Algestone acetophenide (p.1541·3); estradiol enantate (p.1550·1).
*Injectable contraceptive.*

**Yectamicina** Grossman, Mex.
Gentamicin sulfate (p.217·1).
*Bacterial infections.*

**Yectamid** Collins, Mex.
Amikacin sulfate (p.154·1).
*Gram-negative bacterial infections.*

**Yectofer** AstraZeneca, Spain†.
Iron sorbitol (p.1438·1).
*Anaemias.*

**Yedoc** Ciba Vision, Switz.†.
Gentamicin sulfate (p.217·1).
*Bacterial eye infections.*

**Yeiamin-2** YF Chem, Thai.†.
Amino-acid and carbohydrate infusion (p.1417·1).
*Parenteral nutrition.*

**Yelets** Freeda, USA.
Ferrous fumarate (p.1427·3); folic acid (p.1429·1); multivitamins and minerals (p.1417·1).
*Iron-deficiency anaemias.*

**Yelnac** BGA, Fr.
Minocycline hydrochloride (p.231·3).
*Bacterial infections.*

**Yendol** Faes, Spain.
Caffeine (p.782·1); chlorphenamine maleate (p.427·3); paracetamol (p.76·2); salicylamide (p.87·3).
*Cold and influenza symptoms; coughs.*

**Yermonil**
Novartis, Austria; Novartis, Ger.†; Ciba, Switz.†.
Ethinylestradiol (p.1553·2); lynestrenol (p.1557·1).
*Combined oral contraceptive.*

**Yesan** Rafarm, Gr.
Timolol maleate (p.1012·2).
*Glaucoma.*

**Yestamin** Peter Black, UK.
Vitamin B substances; ascorbic acid; iron (p.1417·1).

**Yewtaxan** *Pharmachemie, S.Afr.†.*
Paclitaxel (p.577·3).
*Breast cancer; ovarian cancer.*

**YF-Vax**
*Aventis Pasteur, Canad.; Pasteur Merieux, USA.*
A yellow fever vaccine (17D strain) (p.1644·2).
*Active immunisation.*

**Yirala** *Schering, Austria.*
Drospirenone (p.1549·1); ethinylestradiol (p.1553·2).
*Combined oral contraceptive.*

**Ylox** *Fortbenton, Arg.*
Minoxidil (p.960·1).
*Alopecia.*

**Yocon**
*Croma, Austria; Glenwood, Canad.; Laboratorios Chile, Chile; Glenwood, Ger.; Glenwood, Hong Kong†; Glenwood, USA.*
Yohimbine hydrochloride (p.1766·2).
*Erectile dysfunction.*

**Yocoral** *Intsel, Fr.*
Yohimbine hydrochloride (p.1766·2).
*Erectile dysfunction.*

**Yodacua** *Manuell, Mex.*
Povidone-iodine (p.1190·3).
*Water purification.*

**Yodine** *Manuell, Mex.*
Povidone-iodine (p.1190·3).
*Infected burns, ulcers, or wounds; mouth and throat infections; seborrhoeic dermatitis; skin infections; skin, mucous membrane, and instrument disinfection; vaginal infections.*

**Yodo Tio Calci** *Alcon Cusi, Spain†.*
Calcium chloride (p.1225·1); potassium iodide (p.1598·1); sodium thiosulfate (p.1053·3); sodium iodide (p.1598·1).
*Aspergillus eye infections; cataracts.*

**Yodofrixon Salicilado** *Purissimus, Arg.*
Methyl salicylate (p.59·3); iodine (p.1598·1).

**Yodolactina** *Manuell, Mex.*
Iodocasein (p.1598·3).
*Goitre; immunostimulant; obesity; obstructive airways disease; rheumatoid disorders; sclerosis; tuberculosis.*

**Yodolin** *Hexa-Medinova, Arg.*
Sodium picosulfate (p.1289·3).
*Constipation.*

**Yodon** *Sam-On, Israel.*
Povidone-iodine (p.1190·3).
*Burns; skin disorders; wounds.*

**Yodoxin** *Glenwood, USA.*
Diiodohydroxyquinoline (p.603·3).
*Intestinal amoebiasis.*

**Yodozona** *Offenbach, Mex.*
Furazolidone (p.605·2); clioquinol (p.196·3); pectin (p.1580·3); kaolin (p.1268·3); homatropine methylbromide (p.483·2).
*Diarrhoea.*

**Yohimex**
*Fortbenton, Arg.*
Yohimbine (p.1766·2).
*Kramer, USA†.*
Yohimbine hydrochloride (p.1766·2).
*Erectile dysfunction.*

**Yohydrol** *Riedel-Zabinka, Braz.†.*
Yohimbine (p.1766·2).
*Erectile dysfunction.*

**Yokel** *Bros, Gr.*
Cefuroxime sodium (p.184·1).
*Bacterial infections.*

**Yomax** *Apsen, Braz.*
Yohimbine hydrochloride (p.1766·2).
*Erectile dysfunction; orthostatic hypotension.*

**Yomesan**
*Bayer, Belg.; Bayer, Denm.; Bayer, Ger.; Bayer, Israel; Bayer, Ital.; Bayer, Neth.; Bayer, S.Afr.; Bayer, Swed.; Bayer, Thai.; IDIS, UK.*
Niclosamide (p.110·1).
Available on a named patient basis in the *UK*.
*Diphyllobothriasis; hymenolepiasis; taeniasis.*

**Yonka** *Silesia, Chile.*
Potassium gluconate (p.1232·2).
*Hypokalaemia.*

**Yopin** *Sydenham, Mex.†.*
Diiodohydroxyquinoline (p.603·3).

**Yoquin** *Arlex, Mex.†.*
Clioquinol (p.196·3).

**Youngflex Massage 168** *Youngflex, Canad.*
Menthol (p.1711·3); cajuput oil (p.1664·1); eucalyptus oil (p.1686·2).
*Musculoskeletal, joint, peri-articular, and soft-tissue disorders.*

**Your Choice** *Amcon, USA.*
Saline rinsing and storage solutions for soft contact lenses (p.1164·2) (p.1233·3).

**Yovis** *Fermenti, Ital.*
*Streptococcus salivarius* subsp. *thermophilus*; *Bifidobacterium breve*; *B. infantis*; *B. longum*; *Lactobacillus acidophilus*; *L. plantarum*; *L. casei*; *L. delbrueckii* subsp. *bulgaricus*; *Enterococcus faecium* (p.1704·2).
*Disturbance of gastrointestinal flora.*

**Yovita** *Pharma Italia, Ital.*
Lactic-acid-producing organisms (p.1704·2); vitamins; minerals; inulin (p.1417·1).
*Disturbances of the intestinal flora; nutritional supplement.*

**Ypsiloheel N** *Heel, Ger.*
Homoeopathic preparation.

**Yrelan** *Farmasa, Braz.†.*
Enalapril maleate (p.909·2); felodipine (p.914·3).
*Hypertension.*

**YSE** *Chatelut, Fr.*
Zinc gluconate (p.1469·2); kola (p.1765·3).
*Asthenia.*

**YSE Glutamique** *Chatelut, Fr.*
Zinc gluconate (p.1469·2); glutamic acid (p.1433·2).
*Asthenia.*

**Ysol 206** *Rabi & Solabo, Fr.*
Acetic acid (p.1645·2); camphor (p.1665·3); Java citronella oil (p.1673·2); sodium laurilsulfate (p.1574·2).
*Pediculosis.*

**Ystheal**
*Pierre Fabre Dermo-Cosmetique, Arg.; Silesia, Chile.*
Retinal.
*Photodamaged skin; pigmentation disorders.*

**Ytracis** *Schering, UK.*
Yttrium-90 (p.1526·3).

**Yucomy**
*YSP, Malaysia; Yung Shin, Singapore.*
Ketoconazole (p.403·3).
*Fungal infections.*

**Yurelax** *ICN, Spain.*
Cyclobenzaprine hydrochloride (p.1393·1).
*Skeletal muscle spasm.*

**Yuremetil D** *Willmar, Mex.†.*
Methyldopa (p.953·2).

**Yuremid** *Willmar, Mex.†.*
Furosemide (p.919·3).

**Yusin** *Maigal, Arg.*
Oxymetazoline (p.1126·2).
*Eye disorders; nasal congestion.*

**Yutopar**
*Solvay, Austral.†; Bristol, Canad.†; Solvay, Gr.; Solvay, Hong Kong; Solvay, India; Solvay, Irl.†; Solvay, Singapore†; Solvay, Thai.†; Durbin, UK; Astra, USA†.*
Ritodrine hydrochloride (p.1739·2).
*Fetal distress; premature labour.*

**Yuyo** *Incaico, Arg.*
Aloe vera (p.1141·3); cascara (p.1255·1).
*Constipation.*

**Yxin** *Pfizer, Ger.*
Tetryzoline hydrochloride (p.1131·2).
*Eye disorders.*

**Yxin Tears** *Pfizer, Ger.*
Povidone (p.1581·2).
*Dry eyes.*

**Z 300** *GlaxoSmithKline, NZ†.*
Allopurinol (p.412·2).
*Gout; hyperuricaemia.*

**Z Frin** *Grin, Mex.*
Zinc sulfate (p.1469·3); phenylephrine hydrochloride (p.1126·3).
*Eye disorders.*

**Z Span** *Goldshield, UK†.*
Zinc sulfate (p.1469·3).
*Zinc deficiency.*

**Zaart-H** *Cipla, India.*
Losartan potassium (p.947·2); hydrochlorothiazide (p.933·2).
*Hypertension.*

**Zaba** *Wyeth Lederle, Austria.*
Multivitamin and mineral preparation (p.1417·1).

**Zabysept** *Rafarm, Gr.*
Naphazoline nitrate (p.1124·3); zinc sulfate (p.1417·1).
*Ocular irritation.*

**Zacam** *Fournier, Ital.†.*
Piroxicam (p.84·2).
*Musculoskeletal, joint, and peri-articular disorders.*

**Zacetin** *Medica Korea, Singapore.*
Alprazolam (p.668·3).
*Anxiety; mixed anxiety depressive states.*

**Zacin**
*Elan, Irl.; Elan, UK.*
Capsaicin (p.24·2).
*Osteoarthritis.*

**Zacnan** *Lipha Sante, Fr.*
Minocycline hydrochloride (p.231·3).
*Bacterial infections.*

**Z-Acne** *Vitaglow, Austral.†.*
*Tablets:* Zinc amino acid chelate (p.1469·3); vitamins and minerals (p.1417·1); bioflavonoids (p.1688·2).
*Acne.*

**ZacPac** *Abbott, Ger.; Byk Gulden, Ger.*
Tablets, pantoprazole sodium (p.1283·1); tablets, amoxicillin trihydrate (p.155·3); tablets, clarithromycin (p.192·2).
*Peptic ulcer.*

**Zactin**
*Alphapharm, Austral.; Alphapharm, Singapore; Merck, Singapore.*
Fluoxetine hydrochloride (p.292·1).
*Depression; obsessive-compulsive disorder.*

**Zactos** *Lilly, Mex.*
Pioglitazone hydrochloride (p.344·1).
*Diabetes mellitus.*

**Zadaxin**
*Elvetium, Arg.; Sciclone, Ital.; Sciclone, Malaysia; Columbia, Mex.; Sciclone, Singapore; Sciclone, Thai.*
Thymalfasin (p.1755·2).
*Chronic hepatitis B; chronic hepatitis C; influenza vaccination in immunodeficient patients.*

**Zaden** *Raza, Malaysia; Pharmaniaga, Malaysia.*
Ketotifen fumarate (p.788·1).
*Asthma; hypersensitivity reactions.*

**Zad-G** *Gufic, India.*
Zinc sulfate (p.1469·3); sulfadiazine sodium (p.258·2).
*Bacterial skin infections.*

**Zadine**
*Note. This name is used for preparations of different composition.*
*Schering-Plough, Austral.; Schering-Plough, Hong Kong; Schering-Plough, Malaysia; Schering-Plough, NZ; Schering-Plough, Singapore.*
Azatadine maleate (p.425·1).
*Hypersensitivity reactions.*
*UCI, Braz.*
Ranitidine hydrochloride (p.1285·2).
*Gastro-oesophageal reflux; gastrointestinal haemorrhage; peptic ulcer; Zollinger-Ellison syndrome.*

**Zadino** *Milano, Thai.*
Ketotifen fumarate (p.788·1).
*Asthma; hypersensitivity reactions.*

**Zadipina** *Bayer, Ital.†.*
Nisoldipine (p.973·2).
*Angina pectoris; hypertension.*

**Zaditen**
*Novartis, Arg.; Novartis, Austria; Novartis, Belg.; Novartis, Braz.; Novartis Ophthalmics, Braz.; Novartis, Canad.; Novartis, Chile; Novartis, Denm.; Novartis, Fin.; Novartis, Fr.; Novartis, Ger.; Novartis, Gr.; Novartis, Hong Kong; Novartis, Irl.; Novartis, Israel; Novartis, Ital.; Novartis, Malaysia; Novartis, Mex.; Novartis, Neth.; Novartis, Norw.; Novartis, Port.; Novartis, S.Afr.; Novartis, Singapore; Novartis, Spain; Novartis Ophthalmics, Swed.; Novartis, Switz.; Novartis, Thai.; Novartis, UK.*
Ketotifen fumarate (p.788·1).
*Bronchial asthma; hypersensitivity reactions.*

**Zaditor**
*Novartis Ophthalmics, Canad.; Novartis Ophthalmics, USA.*
Ketotifen fumarate (p.788·1).
*Allergic conjunctivitis.*

**Zadolina** *Salus, Mex.*
Ceftazidime (p.180·2).
*Bacterial infections.*

**Zadorin**
*Mepha, Hong Kong; Mepha, Malaysia; Mepha, Switz.*
Doxycycline hyclate (p.206·2).
*Bacterial infections.*

**Zadstat**
*FL, Israel†; Lederle, UK†.*
Metronidazole (p.607·2).
*Anaerobic bacterial infections; protozoal infections.*

**Zadyl** *Thera, Fr.†.*
Cefradine (p.179·3).
*Bacterial infections.*

**Zaedoc** *Ashbourne, UK.*
Ranitidine hydrochloride (p.1285·2).
*Acid aspiration; dyspepsia; gastro-oesophageal reflux; gastrointestinal haemorrhage; peptic ulcer; Zollinger-Ellison syndrome.*

**Zafarismal** *Klonal, Arg.*
Zafirlukast (p.807·1).
*Asthma.*

**Zafen**
*Zambon, Ital.*
Ibuprofen arginine (p.46·3).
*Musculoskeletal, joint, and peri-articular disorders; pain.*
*Zambon, Neth.*
Ibuprofen (p.45·3).
*Fever; inflammation; musculoskeletal, joint, and peri-articular disorders; pain.*

**Zafibral**
*Medochemie, Hong Kong; Medochemie, Singapore†.*
Bezafibrate (p.873·2).
*Hyperlipidaemias.*

**Zafimida** *Zafiro, Mex.*
Furosemide (p.919·3).
*Forced diuresis; hypertension; oedema.*

**Zafirst** *Chiesi, Ital.*
Zafirlukast (p.807·1).
*Asthma.*

**Zafluox** *Infosint, Ital.*
Fluoxetine hydrochloride (p.292·1).
*Bulimia nervosa; depression; obsessive-compulsive disorder.*

**Zafor** *Mepha, Switz.†.*
Chlorzoxazone (p.1392·3); paracetamol (p.76·2).
*Painful skeletal muscle spasm.*

**Zagam**
*Aventis, Austria; Aventis, Fr.† ;Rhone-Poulenc Rorer, Ger.†; Rhone-Poulenc Rorer, Hong Kong†; Aventis, NZ† ;Rhone-Poulenc Rorer, S.Afr.†; Rhone-Poulenc Rorer, Switz.†; Rhone-Poulenc Rorer, Thai.†; Rhone-Poulenc Rorer, USA.*
Sparfloxacin (p.255·1).
*Bacterial infections of the respiratory-tract.*

**Zagastrol** *Riedel-Zabinka, Braz.†.*
Cimetidine (p.1255·3).
*Gastro-oesophageal reflux; gastrointestinal haemorrhage; peptic ulcer; Zollinger-Ellison syndrome.*

**Zagyl** *Xixia, S.Afr.†.*
Metronidazole (p.607·2).
*Anaerobic bacterial infections; protozoal infections.*

**Zahnerol N** *Dr Janssen, Ger.*
Benzocaine (p.1370·3).
*Dental disorders.*

**Zahnungstropfen Escatitona** *Madaus, Ger.*
Homoeopathic preparation.

**Zainexpect** *Strand, Malaysia.*
Diphenhydramine hydrochloride (p.431·3); ammonium chloride (p.1115·2).
*Coughs.*

**Zainexpect C & F** *Strand, Malaysia.*
Paracetamol (p.76·2); pseudoephedrine hydrochloride (p.1129·2); dextromethorphan (p.1117·3).
*Coughs and cold symptoms.*

**Zainexpect CD** *Strand, Malaysia.*
Codeine phosphate (p.27·1); diphenhydramine hydrochloride (p.431·3); ammonium chloride (p.1115·2).
*Coughs.*

**Zalain**
*Temis, Arg.; Pharmacia, Braz.; Andromaco, Chile; Trommsdorff, Ger.; Geymonat, Ital.; Ferrer, Malaysia; Ferrer, Singapore†; Cantabria, Spain.*
Sertaconazole nitrate (p.408·1).
*Fungal skin and nail infections.*

**Zaldiar**
*Grunenthal, Chile; Grunenthal, Fr.; Grunenthal, Switz.*
Tramadol hydrochloride (p.94·3); paracetamol (p.76·2).
*Pain.*

**Zalig** *Fournier, Ital.†.*
Propionyl erythromycin mercaptosuccinate (p.210·3).
*Bacterial infections.*

**Zalvor** *GlaxoSmithKline, Belg.*
Permethrin (p.1508·3).
*Pediculosis.*

**Zamacort** *Aventis, Mex.*
Triamcinolone acetonide (p.1110·2).
*Asthma.*

**Zamadol** *Viatris, UK.*
Tramadol hydrochloride (p.94·3).
*Pain.*

**Zamanon** *Aventis, S.Afr.*
Dolasetron mesilate (p.1262·3).
*Nausea and vomiting associated with cytotoxic therapy; postoperative nausea and vomiting.*

**Zambesil** *Gentili, Ital.†.*
Chlortalidone (p.882·3).
*Hypertension; oedema.*

**Zam-Buk**
*Note. This name is used for preparations of different composition.*
*Key, Austral.†.*
Eucalyptus oil (p.1686·2); camphor (p.1665·3); thyme oil (p.1755·3); colophony (p.1675·1); sassafras oil (p.1742·1).
*Minor skin disorders.*
*Roche, Hong Kong†; Roche Consumer, Singapore†.*
Eucalyptus oil (p.1686·2); camphor (p.1665·3); thyme oil (p.1755·3); colophony (p.1675·1).
*Bites and stings; chapped hands; cold sores; joint pain; minor wounds.*
*Roche, S.Afr.*
Eucalyptus oil (p.1686·2); camphor (p.1665·3); thyme oil (p.1755·3); sassafras oil (p.1742·1).
*Burns; chapped hands; insect bites; muscular pain; pruritus; wounds.*

**Zamene** *Menarini, Spain.*
Deflazacort (p.1096·2).
*Corticosteroid.*

**Zamocilline** *Zambon, Fr.†.*
Amoxicillin (p.155·3).
*Bacterial infections.*

**Zamudol** *Viatris, Fr.*
Tramadol hydrochloride (p.94·3).
*Pain.*

**Zanaflex**
*Draxis, Canad.; Elan, Irl.; Elan, UK; Athena Neurosciences, USA.*
Tizanidine hydrochloride (p.1395·3).
*Skeletal muscle spasticity.*

**Zanamet** *TO-Chemicals, Thai.*
Ranitidine (p.1285·2).
*Peptic ulcer; Zollinger-Ellison syndrome.*

**Zandine** *Duncan, Flockhart, Irl.*
Ranitidine hydrochloride (p.1285·2).
*Gastric hyperacidity; gastro-oesophageal reflux; peptic ulcer; Zollinger-Ellison syndrome.*

**Zanedip** *Recordati, Ital.*
Lercanidipine hydrochloride (p.946·1).
*Hypertension.*

**Zanfel** *Zanfel, USA.*
Polyethylene granules (p.1140·1) in a surfactant base.
*Urushiol-induced contact dermatitis.*

**Zanicor** *Delta, Port.*
Lercanidipine hydrochloride (p.946·1).
*Hypertension.*

**Zanidex** *Dexcel, Israel.*
Ranitidine hydrochloride (p.1285·2).
*Gastro-oesophageal reflux; gastrointestinal haemorrhage; peptic ulcer.*

**Zanidin** *Pacific, NZ†.*
Ranitidine hydrochloride (p.1285·2).
*Acid aspiration; dyspepsia; gastro-oesophageal reflux; gastrointestinal haemorrhage; peptic ulcer; Zollinger-Ellison syndrome.*

**Zanidip**
*Solvay, Austral.; Kwizda, Austria; Zambon, Belg.; Asta Medica, Braz.; Andromaco, Chile; UCB, Denm.; Leiras, Fin.; Bouchara-Recordati, Fr.; Galenica, Gr.; Schwarz, Hong Kong; UCB, Norw.; Recordati, Singapore; Recordati, Spain; Meda, Swed.; Napp, UK.*
Lercanidipine hydrochloride (p.946·1).
*Hypertension.*

**Zanizal** *Bruno, Ital.*
Nizatidine (p.1277·2).
*Gastro-oesophageal reflux; peptic ulcer.*

**Zanoc** *Delta, Braz.*
Ketoconazole (p.403·3).
*Fungal infections; seborrhoeic dermatitis.*

**Zanocin**
*Stancare, India; Ranbaxy, Malaysia.*
Ofloxacin (p.239·3).
*Bacterial infections.*

**Zanosar**
*Pharmacia, Canad.; Pharmacia, Fr.; IFET (ΙΦΕΤ), Gr.; Pharmacia Upjohn, Israel; Gensia, USA.*
Streptozocin (p.584·1).
*Pancreatic cancer.*

**Zanprol** *GlaxoSmithKline, UK.*
Omeprazole (p.1278·2).
*Gastro-oesophageal reflux.*

**Zantab** *Teva, Israel.*
Ranitidine hydrochloride (p.1285·2).
*Gastro-oesophageal reflux; gastrointestinal hyperacidity; peptic ulcer; Zollinger-Ellison syndrome.*

**Zantac**
*GlaxoSmithKline, Arg.; GlaxoSmithKline, Austral.; GlaxoSmithKline, Austria; GlaxoSmithKline, Belg.; GlaxoSmithKline, Canad.; Pfizer Consumer, Canad.; GlaxoSmithKline, Chile; GlaxoSmithKline, Denm.; GlaxoSmithKline, Fin.; Glaxo Wellcome, Gr.; GlaxoSmithKline, Hong Kong; GlaxoSmithKline, Irl.; GlaxoSmithKline, Israel; GlaxoSmithKline, Ital.; GlaxoSmithKline, Malaysia; GlaxoSmithKline, Neth.; GlaxoSmithKline, Norw.; GlaxoSmithKline, NZ; Glaxo Wellcome, Port.; GlaxoSmithKline, S.Afr.; GlaxoSmithKline, Singapore; GlaxoSmithKline, Spain; GlaxoSmithKline, Swed.; GlaxoSmithKline, Thai.; GlaxoSmithKline, UK; Glaxo Wellcome, USA.*
Ranitidine hydrochloride (p.1285·2).
*Acid aspiration; gastric hyperacidity; gastro-oesophageal reflux; gastrointestinal haemorrhage; peptic ulcer; Zollinger-Ellison syndrome.*

**Zantarac** *GlaxoSmithKline, Austria.*
Ranitidine hydrochloride (p.1285·2).
*Dyspepsia; heartburn.*

**Zantic**
*Boehringer Ingelheim, Ger.; GlaxoSmithKline, Ger.; GlaxoSmithKline, Switz.*
Ranitidine hydrochloride (p.1285·2).
*Acid aspiration; gastro-oesophageal reflux; gastrointestinal haemorrhage; gastrointestinal hyperacidity; peptic ulcer; Zollinger-Ellison syndrome.*

**Zantidon** *Siam Bheasach, Thai.*
Ranitidine (p.1285·2).
*Gastro-oesophageal reflux; peptic ulcer; Zollinger-Ellison syndrome.*

**Zantipres** *FIRMA, Ital.*
Zofenopril calcium (p.1029·3).
*Hypertension; myocardial infarction.*

**Zantril** *Abbott, Arg.*
Isoprenaline sulfate (p.940·2); calcium iodide (p.1116·2).
*Asthma.*

**Zantryl** *Ion, USA†.*
Phentermine hydrochloride (p.1592·2).

**Zanzipik** *Tipomark, Ital.*
Insect repellent.

**Zapain** *Goldshield, UK.*
Paracetamol (p.76·2); codeine phosphate (p.27·1).
These ingredients can be described by the British Approved Name Co-codamol.
*Pain.*

**Zaperin** *Sanabo, Austria†.*
Salbutamol (p.791·3).
*Asthma; bronchoconstriction.*

**Zaplon** *Torrent, India.*
Zaleplon (p.727·3).
*Insomnia.*

**Zappelin** *Iso, Ger.*
Homoeopathic preparation.

**Zaprin** *Willmar, Mex.†.*
Co-trimoxazole (p.199·3).
*Bacterial infections.*

**Zapto** *Aspen, S.Afr.*
Captopril (p.879·2).
*Heart failure; hypertension.*

**Zapto Co** *Aspen, S.Afr.*
Captopril (p.879·2); hydrochlorothiazide (p.933·2).
*Hypertension.*

**Zaramol** *Esfar, Port.*
Paracetamol (p.76·2).
*Fever; pain.*

**Zarator**
*Phoenix, Arg.; Pfizer, Chile; Pfizer, Denm.; Pfizer, Gr.; Pfizer, Port. Pfizer, Spain.*
Atorvastatin calcium (p.866·1).
*Hypercholesterolaemia.*

**Zarcop** *Mintlab, Chile.*
Doxylamine succinate (p.432·3).

**Zarent** *Aventis, Ital.*
Nedocromil sodium (p.789·3); salbutamol sulfate (p.791·3).
*Obstructive airways disease.*

**Zarex** *Dexcel, Israel.*
Famotidine (p.1265·2).
*Gastrointestinal hyperacidity; heartburn.*

**Zargus** *Biosintetica, Braz.*
Risperidone (p.719·2).
*Psychoses.*

**Zaricort**
*Xepa-Soul Pattinson, Malaysia; Xepa-Soul Pattinson, Singapore.*
Miconazole nitrate (p.405·3); hydrocortisone (p.1103·3).
*Fungal skin infections with inflammation.*

**Zarin**
*Xepa-Soul Pattinson, Malaysia; Xepa-Soul Pattinson, Singapore.*
Miconazole nitrate (p.405·3).
*Fungal infections of the skin, nails, and mucous membranes.*

**Zariviz** *Aventis, Ital.*
Cefotaxime sodium (p.175·3).
Lidocaine hydrochloride (p.1377·3) is included in the intramuscular injection to alleviate the pain of injection.
*Gram-negative bacterial infections.*

**Zarocs** *Pharmazam, Spain.*
Roxatidine acetate hydrochloride (p.1288·1).
*Gastro-oesophageal reflux; peptic ulcer.*

**Zarondan**
*Pfizer, Denm.; Warner-Lambert, Norw.†.*
Ethosuximide (p.360·1).
*Absence seizures.*

**Zarontin**
*Parke, Davis, Arg.; Pfizer, Austral.; Pfizer, Belg.; Pfizer, Canad.; Pfizer, Fr.; Pfizer, Gr.; Parke, Davis, Irl.; Parke, Davis, Israel; Parke, Davis, Ital.; Warner-Lambert, Mex.† Parke, Davis, Neth.; Pfizer, NZ; Pfizer, S.Afr.; Pfizer, Spain; Pfizer, UK; Parke, Davis, USA.*
Ethosuximide (p.360·1).
*Absence seizures.*

**Zaroxolyn**
*Aventis, Canad.; Heumann, Ger.; Celltech, Hong Kong; Medeva, Israel; Teofarma, Ital.; Rhone-Poulenc Rorer, Mex.†; Novartis, S.Afr.; Sanofi Winthrop, Swed.†; Celltech, USA.*
Metolazone (p.956·2).
*Hypertension; oedema.*

**Zaroxolyne** *Novartis, Switz.*
Metolazone (p.956·2).
*Hypertension; oedema.*

**Zasten** *Novartis, Spain.*
Ketotifen (p.788·2).
*Allergic rhinitis; asthma.*

**Zatinol** *Efarmes, Spain†.*
Paracetamol (p.76·2).
*Fever; pain.*

**Zatofug** *Wolff, Ger.*
Ketotifen fumarate (p.788·1).
*Asthma; hypersensitivity reactions.*

**Zatrol** *Andromaco, Chile.*
Omeprazole (p.1278·2).
*Gastro-oesophageal reflux; peptic ulcer; Zollinger-Ellison syndrome.*

**Zatur** *CCD, Fr.*
Oxybutynin hydrochloride (p.486·3).
*Neurogenic bladder disorders.*

**Zavedos**
*Pharmacia, Arg.; Pharmacia, Austral.; Pharmacia, Austria; Pharmacia, Belg.; Pharmacia, Braz.; Pharmacia, Chile; Pharmacia, Denm.; Pharmacia, Fin.; Pharmacia, Fr.; Pharmacia, Ger.; Pharmacia-Upjohn, Gr.; Pharmacia, Hong Kong; Pharmacia, Irl.; Pharmacia Upjohn, Israel; Pharmacia Upjohn, Ital.; Pharmacia, Malaysia; Pharmacia, Neth.; Pharmacia, Norw.; Pharmacia, NZ; Pharmacia, Port.; Pharmacia, S.Afr.; Pharmacia, Singapore; Kenfarma, Spain; Pharmacia, Swed.; Pharmacia, Switz.; Pharmacia, Thai.; Pharmacia, UK.*
Idarubicin hydrochloride (p.560·2).
*Malignant neoplasms.*

**Zavesca**
*Actelion, UK; Actelion, USA.*
Miglustat (p.1715·2).
*Gaucher disease.*

**Zayasel** *Salvat, Spain.*
Terazosin hydrochloride (p.1010·3).
*Benign prostatic hyperplasia; hypertension.*

**Z-Bec**
*Note. This name is used for preparations of different composition.*
*Whitehall-Robins, Canad.†; Whitehall, Thai.*
Multivitamin preparation with zinc (p.1417·1).

*Gap, Gr.*
Lisinopril (p.946·3).
*Heart failure; hypertension; myocardial infarction.*

*Robins, USA.*
Multivitamin and mineral preparation (p.1417·1).

**ZBM** *Blackmores, Austral.†.*
Zinc amino acid chelate (p.1469·3); vitamins and minerals (p.1417·1).
*Zinc deficiency.*

**ZBT** *Glenwood, USA†.*
Talc (p.1159·1); liquid paraffin (p.1479·1).
*Nappy rash.*

**Z-Cof** *Zyber, USA.*
Dextromethorphan hydrobromide (p.1117·3); guaifenesin (p.1122·1).
*Coughs.*

**Z-Cof HC** *Zyber, USA.*
Hydrocodone tartrate (p.45·1); chlorphenamine maleate (p.427·3); phenylephrine hydrochloride (p.1126·3).
*Upper respiratory-tract disorders.*

**Z-Dorm** *Rolab, S.Afr.*
Zopiclone (p.729·3).
*Insomnia.*

**Ze Caps** *Everett, USA.*
Zinc gluconate (p.1469·2); vitamin E (p.1464·3).
*Dietary supplement.*

**Zeadema** *Farmila, Ital.*
Multivitamin and mineral preparation with zeaxantina and red vine (p.1417·1).
*Antioxidant nutritional supplement.*

**ZeaSorb**
*Note. This name is used for preparations of different composition.*
*Stiefel, Arg.; Stiefel, Austral.; Stiefel, Canad.; Stiefel, Chile; Stiefel, Ger.†; Stiefel, Irl.; Stiefel, Thai.; Stiefel, UK.*
Aldioxa (p.1141·2); chloroxylenol (p.1177·2); cellulose (p.1578·3).
*Bromhidrosis; hyperhidrosis; intertrigo; prophylaxis of fungal skin infections.*

*Stiefel, Fr.*
Aldioxa (p.1141·2); cellulose (p.1578·3); magnesium silicate (p.1580·2).
*Hyperhidrosis.*

*Stiefel, Malaysia; Stiefel, Singapore.*
Aldioxa (p.1141·2); chloroxylenol (p.1177·2).
*Bromhidrosis; hyperhidrosis; intertrigo; tinea pedis.*

**ZeaSorb AF**
*Note. This name is used for preparations of different composition.*
*Stiefel, Canad.*
Tolnaftate (p.410·1).
*Fungal skin infections.*

*Stiefel, Chile; Stiefel, USA.*
Miconazole nitrate (p.405·3).
*Fungal skin infections.*

**Zeben** *Siam Bheasach, Thai.*
Albendazole (p.101·2).
*Worm infections.*

**Zebeta** *Barr, USA.*
Bisoprolol fumarate (p.875·1).
*Hypertension.*

**Zebrak** *Royal, Chile.*
Citalopram (p.289·1).
*Depression.*

**Zebu** *Pond's, Thai.*
Salbutamol (p.791·3).
*Bronchospasm.*

**Zeclar**
*Orion, Fin.; Abbott, Fr.*
Clarithromycin (p.192·2).
*Bacterial infections.*

**Zeclaren OD** *Abbott, Gr.*
Clarithromycin (p.192·2).
*Adjunct in Helicobacter pylori eradication; bacterial infections.*

**Zecnil** *Ferring, Ital.*
Somatostatin acetate (p.1339·3).
*Diabetic ketoacidosis; gastrointestinal haemorrhage; prevention of complications following pancreatic surgery.*

**Zedax** *Andromaco, Chile.*
Zopiclone (p.729·3).
*Insomnia.*

**Zedex** *Wockhardt, India.*
Bromhexine hydrochloride (p.1115·3); dextromethorphan hydrobromide (p.1117·3); ammonium chloride (p.1115·2); menthol (p.1711·3).
*Respiratory-tract congestion.*

**Zedex-P** *Wockhardt, India.*
Bromhexine hydrochloride (p.1115·3); dextromethorphan hydrobromide (p.1117·3); ammonium chloride (p.1115·2); menthol (p.1711·3); ephedrine hydrochloride (p.1120·1).
*Respiratory-tract congestion.*

**Zeefra**
*Bouchara-Recordati, Fr.; Bouchara-Recordati, Hong Kong.*
Cefradine (p.179·3).
*Bacterial infections.*

**Zeel**
*Heel, Ger.*
Homoeopathic preparation.

*Heel, S.Afr.*
*Injection:* Cartilago suis; funiculus umbilicalis suis; embryo suis; placenta suis; rhus toxicodendron; flor arnicae; dulcamara; symphytum; sanguinaria; sulfur; nadid; coenzyme A; thioctic acid; natrium oxalaceticum.
*Ointment; tablets:* Cartilago suis; funiculus umbilicalis suis; embryo suis; placenta suis; rhus toxicodendron; flor arnicae; dulcamara; symphytum; sanguinaria; sulfur; acidum silicicum colloidale; nadid; coenzyme A; thioctic acid; natrium oxalaceticum.
*Musculoskeletal and joint disorders.*

**Zeel comp** *Heel, Ger.*
Homoeopathic preparation.

**Zeel P** *Heel, Ger.*
Homoeopathic preparation.

**Zeel Plus** *Peithner, Austria.*
Homoeopathic preparation.

**Zeel T** *Heel, Ger.*
Homoeopathic preparation.

**Zee-Seltzer** *Zee, USA.*
Aspirin (p.15·1); citric acid (p.1673·1); sodium bicarbonate (p.1223·2).

**Zeet Expectorant** *Alembic, India.*
*Syrup:* Diphenhydramine hydrochloride (p.431·3); ammonium chloride (p.1115·2); guaifenesin (p.1122·1); bromhexine hydrochloride (p.1115·3); menthol (p.1711·3).
*Tablets:* Bromhexine hydrochloride (p.1115·3); phenylpropanolamine hydrochloride (p.1127·3).
*Coughs.*

**Zeet Linctus** *Alembic, India.*
Dextromethorphan hydrobromide (p.1117·3); guaifenesin (p.1122·1); phenylpropanolamine hydrochloride (p.1127·3).
*Coughs.*

**Zefa** *M & H, Thai.*
Cefazolin sodium (p.170·3).
*Bacterial infections.*

**Zefaxone** *M & H, Thai.*
Ceftriaxone sodium (p.182·3).
*Bacterial infections.*

**Zefazone** *Upjohn, USA.*
Cefmetazole sodium (p.173·3).
*Bacterial infections.*

**Zeffix**
*GlaxoSmithKline, Arg.; GlaxoSmithKline, Austral.; GlaxoSmithKline, Belg.; GlaxoSmithKline, Braz.; Glaxo Wellcome, Denm.; GlaxoSmithKline, Fin.; GlaxoSmithKline, Fr.; GlaxoSmithKline, Ger.; Glaxo Wellcome, Gr.; GlaxoSmithKline, Hong Kong; Glaxo Wellcome, Irl.; GlaxoSmithKline, Israel; GlaxoSmithKline, Ital.; GlaxoSmithKline, Malaysia; GlaxoSmithKline, NZ; Glaxo Wellcome, Port.; GlaxoSmithKline, Singapore; Glaxo Wellcome, Spain; GlaxoSmithKline, Swed.; GlaxoSmithKline, Switz.; GlaxoSmithKline, Thai.; GlaxoSmithKline, UK.*
Lamivudine (p.648·2).
*Hepatitis B.*

**Zefirol** *Bayer, Ital.†.*
Benzalkonium chloride (p.1168·3).
*Disinfection of skin, mucous membranes, and wounds; surface disinfection.*

**Zeftam** *M & H, Thai.*
Ceftazidime (p.180·2).
*Bacterial infections.*

**Zefxon** *Biolab, Thai.*
Omeprazole (p.1278·2).
*Gastro-oesophageal reflux; peptic ulcer; Zollinger-Ellison syndrome.*

**Zehu-Ze** *Biogal, Israel.*
Permethrin (p.1508·3).
*Pediculosis.*

**Zeisin** *3M, Ger.†.*
Pirbuterol acetate (p.790·3).
*Obstructive airways disease.*

**Zelapar** *Elan, UK.*
Selegiline hydrochloride (p.1214·1).
*Parkinsonism.*

**Zelderme** *Zeller, Port.†.*
Methylbenzethonium; zinc oxide (p.1163·2); vitamin A (p.1451·2); vitamin D (p.1461·2).
*Nappy rash.*

**Zeldox**
*Pfizer, Arg.; Pfizer, Braz.†; Pfizer, Chile; Pfizer, Denm.; Pfizer, Norw.; Pfizer, Swed.*
Ziprasidone hydrochloride (p.728·1) or ziprasidone mesilate (p.728·1).
*Psychoses.*

**Zelfin** *Randall, Mex.†.*
Albendazole (p.101·2).
*Worm infections.*

**Zelicrema** *Biomedica-Chemica, Gr.*
Azelaic acid (p.1142·3).
*Acne.*

**Zeliderm** *Vinas, Spain.*
Azelaic acid (p.1142·3).
*Acne.*

**Zelis** *Prospa, Ital.*
Piroxicam cinnamate (p.85·1).
*Musculoskeletal and joint disorders.*

**Zelitrex**
*GlaxoSmithKline, Belg.; GlaxoSmithKline, Denm.; GlaxoSmithKline, Fr.; GlaxoSmithKline, Ital.; GlaxoSmithKline, Neth.; GlaxoSmithKline, S.Afr.*
Valaciclovir hydrochloride (p.656·1).
*Herpesvirus infections.*

**Zelium** *Masa, Thai.*
Flunarizine (p.434·2).
*Cerebrovascular disorders; migraine.*

**Zelix** *Ativus, Braz.*
Fluconazole (p.398·1).
*Fungal infections.*

**Zellaforte** *Zellaforte, Switz.*
Multivitamin and mineral preparation (p.1417·1).

**Zellaforte N Plus** *Eurim, Ger.*
Nikethamide calcium thiocyanate (p.1591·2); inositol nicotinate (p.939·3); pholedrine sulfate (p.982·3).
*Tonic.*

**Zellaforte plus** *Solco, Austria.*
Procaine hydrochloride; haematoporphyrin; ferrous sulfate; vitamins (p.1417·1).
*Tonic.*

**Zeller-Augenwasser** *Herchemie, Austria.*
Saffron (p.1058·2); fennel oil (p.1687·3); zinc sulfate (p.1469·3).
*Eye inflammation and irritation.*

**Zellox-II**
*Hoe, Malaysia; Hoe, Singapore.*
Aluminium hydroxide (p.1249·2); magnesium hydroxide (p.1272·2); simeticone (p.1289·2).
*Dyspepsia; flatulence; gastric hyperacidity; gastritis; gastro-oesophageal reflux; heartburn.*

**Zelmac**
*Novartis, Austral.; Novartis, Braz.; Novartis, Singapore; Novartis, Switz.; Novartis, Thai.*
Tegaserod maleate (p.1293·2).
*Irritable bowel syndrome in females.*

**Zelmar** *Biomedica-Chemica, Gr.*
Loratadine (p.436·1).
*Allergic rhinitis; pruritus.*

**Zelnorm** *Novartis, USA.*
Tegaserod maleate (p.1293·2).
*Irritable bowel syndrome in women.*

**Zemaira** *Aventis Behring, USA.*
Alpha$_1$-proteinase inhibitor (p.1651·2).
*Alpha$_1$-proteinase inhibitor deficiency.*

**Zemalex** *ITF, Port.*
Piketoprofen (p.84·1) or piketoprofen hydrochloride (p.84·1).
*Musculoskeletal, joint, and peri-articular disorders.*

**Zemide** *Alpharma-Isis, Ger.*
Tamoxifen citrate (p.584·1).
*Breast cancer.*

**Zemplar** *Abbott, USA.*
Paricalcitol (p.1462·1).
*Hyperparathyroidism.*

**Zemtard** *Galen, UK.*
Diltiazem hydrochloride (p.900·1).
*Angina pectoris; hypertension.*

**Zemuron**
*Organon, Arg.; Organon, Canad.; Organon, USA.*
Rocuronium bromide (p.1405·2).
*Competitive neuromuscular blocker.*

**Zen** *Select, Ital.†.*
Piroxicam cinnamate (p.85·1).
*Musculoskeletal and joint disorders.*

**Zenalb**
*BPL-Meizler, Braz.; BPL, Hong Kong†; Bio Products, Malaysia; BPL, Singapore; BPL, Thai.; BPL, UK.*
Albumin (p.740·3).
*Burns; hypoalbuminaemia; hypovolaemic shock.*

**Zenapax**
*Roche, Arg.; Roche, Austral.; Roche, Austria; Roche, Belg.; Roche, Braz.; Roche, Canad.; Roche, Chile; Roche, Denm.; Roche, Fin.; Roche, Fr.; Roche, Ger.; Roche, Gr.; Roche, Hong Kong; Roche, Irl.; Roche, Israel; Roche, Ital.; Roche, Mex.; Roche, Neth.; Roche, NZ; Roche, Port.; Roche, S.Afr.; Roche, Singapore; Roche, Spain; Roche, Swed.; Roche, Switz.; Roche, Thai.; Roche, UK; Roche, USA.*
Daclizumab (p.1359·3).
*Renal transplant rejection.*

**Zenas**
*Fournier, Ger.†; Fournier SA, Spain†.*
Cerivastatin sodium (p.881·3).
*Hyperlipidaemias.*

**Zenavan** *Bial, Spain.*
Etofenamate (p.38·1).
*Pain; peri-articular disorders.*

**Zenaxin** *Maver, Mex.*
Albendazole (p.101·2).
*Worm infections.*

**Zenda** *Nakorn, Thai.*
Niclosamide (p.110·1); phenolphthalein (p.1284·1).
*Worm infections.*

**Zendhin** *DHA, Singapore.*
Ranitidine hydrochloride (p.1285·2).
*Dyspepsia; gastro-oesophageal reflux; peptic ulcer; Zollinger-Ellison syndrome.*

**Zendol** *Serum Institute, India.*
Danazol (p.1545·2).
*Benign breast disease; endometriosis; female infertility; menorrhagia; precocious puberty.*

**Zengac** *Fisiopharma, Ital.*
Vancomycin hydrochloride (p.275·2).
*Bacterial infections.*

**Zeniac** *LED, Fr.*
*Lotion:* Mandelic acid (p.228·3); salicylic acid (p.1157·1); ammonium lactate (p.1142·3).
*Acne.*
*Roll-on:* Mandelic acid (p.228·3); salicylic acid (p.1157·1); sulfur (p.1158·2).
*Acne.*
*Topical gel:* Lappa-biotin-zinc complex (p.1704·3) (p.1423·2) (p.1469·2).
*Skin cleansing.*

**Zeniac LP** *LED, Fr.*
Mandelic acid (p.228·3); salicylic acid (p.1157·1); ammonium lactate (p.1142·3); lappa-biotin-zinc complex (p.1704·3) (p.1423·2) (p.1469·2).
*Acne.*

**Zeniac LP Fort** *LED, Fr.*
Mandelic acid (p.228·3); tartaric acid (p.1752·1); salicylic acid (p.1157·1); ammonium lactate (p.1142·3).
*Acne.*

**Zenicide** *Douglas, NZ†.*
Glutaral (p.1180·3).
*Disinfection.*

**Zenium** *Alpharma, Fr.†.*
Co-dergocrine mesilate (p.1674·1).
*Mental function impairment.*

**Zenmolin** *DHA, Hong Kong.*
Salbutamol sulfate (p.791·3).
*Bronchospasm.*

**Zenodian** *CT, Ital.*
Sucralfate (p.1290·2).
*Gastritis; gastro-oesophageal reflux; peptic ulcer.*

**Zenoxone** *Biorex, UK.*
Hydrocortisone (p.1103·3).
*Skin disorders.*

**Zenpro** *Xepa-Soul Pattinson, Malaysia.*
Omeprazole (p.1278·2).
*Gastro-oesophageal reflux; peptic ulcer; Zollinger-Ellison syndrome.*

**Zensil** *Silom, Thai.*
Cetirizine hydrochloride (p.427·1).
*Allergic conjunctivitis; allergic rhinitis; allergic skin disorders.*

**Zentavion** *Vita, Spain.*
Azithromycin (p.159·1).
*Bacterial infections.*

**Zentel**
*GlaxoSmithKline, Austral.; GlaxoSmithKline, Braz.; GlaxoSmithKline, Chile; GlaxoSmithKline, Fr.; IFET (ΙΦΕΤ), Gr.; GlaxoSmithKline, India; GlaxoSmithKline, Ital.; GlaxoSmithKline Consumer, Malaysia; SmithKline Beecham, Mex.; GlaxoSmithKline Consumer, Port.; GlaxoSmithKline, S.Afr.; GlaxoSmithKline, Singapore; SmithKline Beecham, Switz.; GlaxoSmithKline, Thai.*
Albendazole (p.101·2).
*Giardiasis; worm infections.*

**Zentius**
*Roemmers, Arg.; Pharma Investi, Chile.*
Citalopram hydrobromide (p.289·1).
*Depression.*

**Zentralin** *Pasteur, Chile.*
Flunarizine hydrochloride (p.434·1).
*Cerebral and peripheral vascular disorders; vestibular disorders.*

**Zentramin Bastian N** *Bastian, Ger.*
Electrolyte preparation (p.1217·1).
*Hypersensitivity disorders; psychosomatic disorders; tetanus.*

**Zentropil** *BASF, Ger.†.*
Phenytoin (p.370·2) or phenytoin sodium (p.370·2).
*Epilepsy; trigeminal neuralgia.*

**Zenusin**
*Mepha, Port.; Mepha, Thai.†.*
Nifedipine (p.966·2).
*Angina pectoris; heart failure; hypertension; myocardial infarction; Raynaud's syndrome.*

**Zenzera** *Bangkok Lab & Cosmetic, Thai.*
Albendazole (p.101·2).
*Worm infections.*

**Zepac** *Ist. Chim. Inter., Ital.*
Heparin calcium (p.927·3).
*Thromboembolic disorders.*

**Zepan** *Jofrain, Mex.†.*
Diazepam (p.690·1).

**Zepelan** *Boehringer de Angeli, Braz.†.*
Feprazone (p.43·1).
*Musculoskeletal and joint disorders.*

**Zepelin**
*Boehringer Ingelheim, Austria†; Boehringer Ingelheim, Ital.*
Feprazone (p.43·1).
*Inflammation; musculoskeletal and joint disorders; pain.*

**Zepelindue** *Boehringer Ingelheim, Ital.*
Ketoprofen lysine (p.51·3).
*Inflammation; musculoskeletal, joint, peri-articular, and soft-tissue disorders; pain.*

**Zephiran**
*Sanofi Synthelabo, Canad.†; Sanofi Winthrop, USA.*
Benzalkonium chloride (p.1168·3).
*Eye, bladder, urethra, and body cavity irrigation; skin, mucous membrane, and wound disinfection; vaginal douching.*

**Zephirol** *Bayer, Thai.†.*
Benzalkonium chloride (p.1168·3).
*Instrument disinfection; skin and hand disinfection; vaginal and bladder irrigation.*

**Zepholin**
*Note. This name is used for preparations of different composition.*
*Genepharm, Gr.*
Cetirizine hydrochloride (p.427·1).
*Allergic conjunctivitis; allergic rhinitis; pruritus.*
*Klinge, Irl.*
Theophylline (p.798·3).
*Bronchospasm.*

**Zephrex** *Sanofi Synthelabo, USA.*
Pseudoephedrine hydrochloride (p.1129·2); guaifenesin (p.1122·1).
*Coughs.*

**Zepiken** *Kener, Mex.†.*
Carbamazepine (p.353·3).

**Zepilen** *Medochemie, Thai.*
Cefazolin sodium (p.170·3).
*Bacterial infections.*

**Zeplex** *M & H, Thai.*
Cefalexin (p.168·1).
*Bacterial infections.*

**Zepobrax** *Farmaline, Thai.*
Chlordiazepoxide (p.674·2); clidinium bromide (p.480·2).
*Smooth muscle spasm.*

**Zeprat** *Solfran, Mex.*
Diazepam (p.690·1).

**Zera** *Pentafarma, Port.*
Simvastatin (p.997·1).

**Zerandin** *Zerboni, Mex.†.*
Ranitidine (p.1285·2).

**Zerella**
*Schering, Austria; Theramex, Ital.*
Estradiol (p.1550·1).
*Menopausal disorders.*

**Zerene** *Biofutura, Ital.*
Zaleplon (p.727·3).
*Insomnia.*

**Zerfenazin** *Zerboni, Mex.†.*
Perphenazine (p.714·2).

**Zerinetta** *Boehringer Ingelheim, Ital.*
Paracetamol (p.76·2); chlorphenamine maleate (p.427·3).
*Cold and influenza symptoms.*

**Zerinetta-Fher** *Boehringer Ingelheim, Ital.†.*
Paracetamol (p.76·2); phenylpropanolamine hydrochloride (p.1127·3); chlorphenamine maleate (p.427·3).
*Cold and influenza symptoms.*

**Zerinoflu** *Boehringer Ingelheim, Ital.*
Paracetamol (p.76·2); chlorphenamine maleate (p.427·3); sodium ascorbate (p.1460·2).
*Cold and influenza symptoms.*

**Zerinol-Fher** *Boehringer Ingelheim, Ital.*
Paracetamol (p.76·2); chlorphenamine maleate (p.427·3).
Formerly contained paracetamol, phenylpropanolamine hydrochloride, and chlorphenamine maleate.
*Cold and influenza symptoms.*

**Zerit**
*Bristol-Myers Squibb, Arg.; Bristol-Myers Squibb, Austral.; Bristol-Myers Squibb, Austria; Bristol-Myers Squibb, Belg.; Bristol-Myers Squibb, Canad.; Bristol-Myers Squibb, Chile; Bristol-Myers Squibb, Denm.; Bristol-Myers Squibb, Fin.; Bristol-Myers Squibb, Fr.; Bristol-Myers Squibb, Ger.; Bristol-Myers Squibb, Gr.; Bristol-Myers Squibb, Hong Kong; Bristol-Myers Squibb, Irl.; Bristol-Myers Squibb, Israel; Bristol-Myers Squibb, Ital.; Bristol-Myers Squibb, Jpn; Bristol-Myers Squibb, Malaysia; Bristol-Myers Squibb, Mex.; Bristol-Myers Squibb, Neth.; Bristol-Myers Squibb, Norw.; Bristol-Myers Squibb, NZ; Bristol-Myers Squibb, Port.; Bristol-Myers Squibb, S.Afr.; Bristol-Myers Squibb, Singapore; Bristol-Myers, Spain; Bristol-Myers Squibb, Swed.; Bristol-Myers Squibb, Switz.; Bristol-Myers Squibb, Thai.; Bristol-Myers Squibb, UK; Bristol-Myers Squibb Oncology, USA.*
Stavudine (p.654·2).
*HIV infection.*

**Zeritavir** *Bristol-Myers Squibb, Braz.*
Stavudine (p.654·2).
*HIV infection.*

**Zermed** *Progress, Thai.*
Cetirizine hydrochloride (p.427·1).
*Allergic rhinitis; hypersensitivity reactions.*

**Zeroac** *Mavi, Ital.*
Azelaic acid (p.1142·3); phosphatidyl choline (p.1731·1).
*Acne.*

**Zerobase** *Zeroderma, UK.*
Liquid paraffin (p.1479·1).
*Diluent for topical steroids; dry skin; emollient.*

**Zeroflog** *Valeas, Ital.*
Diclofenac (p.32·1).
*Mouth and throat disorders.*

**Zeropenem** *Aventis, Arg.*
Meropenem (p.229·1).
*Bacterial infections.*

**Zeropyn** *Pharmco, S.Afr.†.*
Paracetamol (p.76·2); codeine phosphate (p.27·1).
*Fever; pain.*

**Zerosorin SN** *Schuck, Ger.*
Homoeopathic preparation.

**Zerospam** *Proel, Gr.*
Piroxicam (p.84·2).
*Dysmenorrhoea; gout; inflammation; musculoskeletal and joint disorders; pain.*

**Zertine** *Farmaline, Thai.*
Cetirizine hydrochloride (p.427·1).
*Allergic skin disorders.*

**Zesger** *Gerard, Irl.*
Lisinopril (p.946·3).
*Heart failure; hypertension; myocardial infarction.*

**Zestan** *Clonmel, Irl.*
Lisinopril (p.946·3).
*Heart failure; hypertension; myocardial infarction.*

**Zestomax** *Parke-Med, S.Afr.†.*
Lisinopril (p.946·3).
*Heart failure; hypertension; myocardial infarction.*

**Zestoretic**
*AstraZeneca, Arg.; AstraZeneca, Austria; AstraZeneca, Belg.; AstraZeneca, Braz.; AstraZeneca, Canad.; AstraZeneca, Chile; AstraZeneca, Denm.; AstraZeneca, Fr.; AstraZeneca, Hong Kong; AstraZeneca, Irl.; AstraZeneca, Ital.; Zeneca, Mex.; AstraZeneca, Neth.; AstraZeneca, Norw.; AstraZeneca, NZ†; AstraZeneca, Port.; AstraZeneca, S.Afr.; AstraZeneca, Spain; Hassle, Swed.; AstraZeneca, Switz.; AstraZeneca, UK; Zeneca, USA.*
Lisinopril (p.946·3); hydrochlorothiazide (p.933·2).
*Hypertension.*

**Zestril**
*AstraZeneca, Arg.; AstraZeneca, Austral.; AstraZeneca, Belg.; AstraZeneca, Braz.; AstraZeneca, Canad.; AstraZeneca, Chile; AstraZeneca, Denm.; AstraZeneca, Fin.; AstraZeneca, Fr.; Cana, Gr.; AstraZeneca, Hong Kong; AstraZeneca, Irl.; AstraZeneca, Ital.; AstraZeneca, Malaysia; Zeneca, Mex.; AstraZeneca, Neth.; AstraZeneca, Norw.; AstraZeneca, NZ; AstraZeneca, Port.; AstraZeneca, S.Afr.; AstraZeneca, Singapore; AstraZeneca, Spain; Hassle, Swed.; AstraZeneca, Switz.; AstraZeneca, Thai.; AstraZeneca, UK; AstraZeneca, USA.*
Lisinopril (p.946·3).
*Diabetic nephropathy; diabetic retinopathy; heart failure; hypertension; myocardial infarction.*

**Zeta N** *Bergamon, Ital.*
Usnic acid (p.1762·1).
*Vaginal disinfection.*

**Zetacet** *Stiefel, USA.*
Sulfur (p.1158·2); sulfacetamide sodium (p.257·3).
*Acne.*

**Zetagal** *Elpen (Ελπεν), Gr.*
Cefuroxime sodium (p.184·1).
*Bacterial infections.*

**Zetalax** *Zeta, Ital.*
Glycerol (p.1694·3).
*Constipation.*

**Zetalerg** *UCI, Braz.*
Cetirizine hydrochloride (p.427·1).
*Hypersensitivity reactions.*

**Zetamicin** *Menarini, Ital.*
Netilmicin sulfate (p.236·3).
*Bacterial infections.*

**Zetar**
*Dermik, Canad.; Dermik, Hong Kong; Dermik, USA.*
Coal tar (p.1159·2).
*Scalp disorders; skin disorders.*

**Zetarina** *Zafiro, Mex.*
Dopamine hydrochloride (p.907·1).
*Hypotension; shock.*

**Zetavir** *Liferpal, Mex.*
Aciclovir (p.626·1).
*Herpes simplex infections.*

**Zetavit** *Zeta, Ital.*
Multivitamin and mineral preparation (p.1417·1).

**Zetavudin** *Richmond, Arg.*
Zidovudine (p.658·2); lamivudine (p.648·2).

**Zetaxim** *Wockhardt, India.*
Cefotaxime sodium (p.175·3).
*Bacterial infections.*

**Zetia** *Merck, USA; Schering-Plough, USA.*
Ezetimibe (p.914·2).
*Hypercholesterolaemia.*

**Zetir**
*Abbott, Braz.; Rodleben, Ger.*
Cetirizine hydrochloride (p.427·1).
*Hypersensitivity reactions.*

**Zetir-D** *Abbott, Braz.†.*
Cetirizine hydrochloride (p.427·1); pseudoephedrine hydrochloride (p.1129·2).
*Nasal congestion.*

**Zetitec** *UCI, Braz.*
Ketotifen fumarate (p.788·1).
*Hypersensitivity reactions.*

**Zetix** *Pharmafina, Chile.*
Zopiclone (p.729·3).
*Insomnia.*

**Zeto** *Unipharm, Israel.*
Azithromycin (p.159·1).
*Bacterial infections.*

**Zetofen** *Parke-Med, S.Afr.*
Ketotifen fumarate (p.788·1).
*Allergic rhinitis; allergic skin disorders; asthma.*

**Zetomax** *Parke-Med, S.Afr.*
Lisinopril (p.946·3).
*Heart failure; hypertension; myocardial infarction.*

**Zetoridal** *Duncan, Arg.*
Haloperidol (p.701·2).

**Zetran** *Masa, Thai.*
Dipotassium clorazepate (p.685·1).
*Anxiety; insomnia.*

**Zetron** *Biolab, Thai.*
Ondansetron hydrochloride (p.1281·1).
*Nausea and vomiting induced by cytotoxics or radiotherapy; postoperative nausea and vomiting.*

**Zetrotax** *Richmond, Arg.*
Zidovudine (p.658·2).
*HIV infection.*

**Zevalin**
*Schering, UK; IDEC, USA.*
Ibritumomab tiuxetan (p.560·1).
For radiolabelling with indium-111 or yttrium-90.
*Non-Hodgkins lymphoma.*

**Zevin**
*Biolab, Hong Kong; Biolab, Malaysia; Biolab, Thai.*
Aciclovir (p.626·1).
*Herpes simplex infections of the skin and mucous membranes.*

**Z-gen** *Goldline, USA.*
Multivitamin and mineral preparation (p.1417·1).

**Ziac**
*Merck, Arg.; Merck, Chile; Barr, USA.*
Bisoprolol fumarate (p.875·1); hydrochlorothiazide (p.933·2).
*Hypertension.*

**Ziagen**
*GlaxoSmithKline, Austral.; GlaxoSmithKline, Belg.; GlaxoSmithKline, Canad.; GlaxoSmithKline, Chile; Glaxo Wellcome, Denm.; GlaxoSmithKline, Fin.; GlaxoSmithKline, Fr.; GlaxoSmithKline, Ger.; Glaxo Wellcome, Gr.; GlaxoSmithKline, Hong Kong; GlaxoSmithKline, Irl.; GlaxoSmithKline, Israel; GlaxoSmithKline, Ital.; GlaxoSmithKline, Norw.; GlaxoSmithKline, NZ; Glaxo Wellcome, Port.; GlaxoSmithKline, S.Afr.; GlaxoSmithKline, Singapore; Glaxo Wellcome, Spain; GlaxoSmithKline, Swed.; GlaxoSmithKline, Switz.; GlaxoSmithKline, UK; Glaxo Wellcome, USA.*
Abacavir sulfate (p.625·2).
*HIV infection.*

**Ziagenavir**
*GlaxoSmithKline, Arg.; GlaxoSmithKline, Braz.; Glaxo Wellcome, Mex.; GlaxoSmithKline, Thai.*
Abacavir sulfate (p.625·2).
*HIV infection.*

**Ziak** *Merck, S.Afr.*
Bisoprolol fumarate (p.875·1); hydrochlorothiazide (p.933·2).
*Hypertension.*

**Zibelant** *Chrispa (Χρισπα), Gr.*
Tenoxicam (p.93·1).
*Dysmenorrhoea; gout; inflammation; osteoarthritis; pain; rheumatoid arthritis; spondyloarthropathies.*

**Zibil** *Novartis, Mex.*
Salbutamol (p.791·3) or salbutamol sulfate (p.791·3).
*Obstructive airways disease.*

**Zibor** *Amdipharm, UK.*
Bemiparin sodium (p.867·1).

**Zibren** *Sigma-Tau, Ital.*
Acetylcarnitine or acetylcarnitine hydrochloride (p.1646·1).
*Cerebrovascular disorders; peripheral neuropathy.*

**Ziclin** *Knoll, S.Afr.*
Gliclazide (p.332·1).
*Diabetes mellitus.*

**Ziconal** *Raza, Malaysia; Pharmaniaga, Malaysia.*
Ketoconazole (p.403·3).
*Fungal infections.*

**Zidac** *Biotherapie, Fr.†.*
Ranitidine hydrochloride (p.1285·2).
*Gastro-oesophageal reflux; peptic ulcer; Zollinger-Ellison syndrome.*

**Zideron** *Norma (Νορμα), Gr.*
Dextropropoxyphene hydrochloride (p.28·3).
*Pain.*

**Zidicef** *Precimex, Mex.†.*
Ceftazidime (p.180·2).
*Bacterial infections.*

**Zidis** *Pond's, Thai.*
Zidovudine (p.658·2).
*HIV infection.*

**Zidix** *Euroforma, Braz.†.*
Zidovudine (p.658·2).
*HIV infection.*

**Zidolam** *Euroforma, Braz.*
Lamivudine (p.648·2); zidovudine (p.658·2).
*HIV infection.*

**Zidonil** *Rafarm, Gr.*
Fluconazole (p.398·1).
*Fungal infections.*

**Zidoval**
*3M, Denm.; 3M, Israel; 3M, Norw.; 3M, Swed.; 3M, UK.*
Metronidazole (p.607·2).
*Bacterial vaginosis.*

**Zidovimm** *Anpharm (Ανφαρμ), Gr.*
Aciclovir (p.626·1).
*Labial and genital herpes simplex infections.*

**Zidovir**
*Cristalia, Braz.; Cipla, India; Protein, Mex.†.*
Zidovudine (p.658·2).
*HIV infection.*

**Zidovusan** *Sanval, Braz.*
Zidovudine (p.658·2).
*HIV infectin.*

**Zienam**
*Merck Sharp & Dohme, Arg.; Merck Sharp & Dohme, Austria; Merck Sharp & Dohme, Ger.*
Imipenem (p.221·1); cilastatin sodium (p.188·1).
Lidocaine hydrochloride (p.1377·3) may be included in the intramuscular injection to alleviate the pain of injection.
*Bacterial infections.*

**Zifartel** *Continentales, Mex.†.*
Praziquantel (p.112·2).

**Zig C** *Falqui, Ital.†.*
Ascorbic acid (p.1460·2).

**Ziga-Gel** *Bangkok Lab & Cosmetic, Thai.*
Aluminium hydroxide (p.1249·2); magnesium hydroxide (p.1272·2); simeticone (p.1289·2).
*Flatulence; gastrointestinal hyperacidity; peptic ulcer.*

**Ziken** *Kendrick, Mex.*
Mesna (p.1041·2).
*Prevention of urotoxicity due to oxazaphosphorine antineoplastics.*

**Ziks** *Nnodum, USA.*
Methyl salicylate (p.59·3); menthol (p.1711·3); capsaicin (p.24·2).
*Musculoskeletal, joint, and soft-tissue disorders; neuralgia.*

**Zil** *Sarabhai Piramal, India.*
Tinidazole (p.617·1).
*Amoebiasis; anaerobic bacterial infections; giardiasis; trichomoniasis.*

**Zilaben** *Cristalia, Braz.*
Benzyl benzoate (p.1500·2).
*Pediculosis; scabies.*

**Zilactin**
*Zila, Canad.; Zila, USA.*
Benzyl alcohol (p.1170·2).
Formerly contained tannic acid in the *USA*.
*Lip lesions; mouth ulcers.*

**Zilactin Baby** *Zila, Canad.*
Benzocaine (p.1370·3).
*Teething.*

**Zilactin-B** *Zila, Canad.*
Benzocaine (p.1370·3).
*Mouth disorders.*

**Zilactin-B Medicated** *Zila, USA.*
Benzocaine (p.1370·3).
*Canker sores.*

**Zilactin-E** *Hexa-Medinova, Arg.*
Ergotamine tartrate (p.467·2); caffeine (p.782·1); aspirin (p.15·1).
*Migraine.*

**Zilactin-L**
*Zila, Canad.; Zila, USA.*
Lidocaine (p.1377·3).
*Herpes labialis.*

**Zilactin-Lip** *Zila, Canad.*
*SPF 24:* Octinoxate (p.1154·3); homosalate (p.1148·1); oxybenzone (p.1154·3); dimethicone (p.1482·1); menthol (p.1711·3).
*Herpes labialis.*

**Zilak** *Farmion, Braz.†.*
Ranitidine hydrochloride (p.1285·2).
*Peptic ulcer.*

**Zildem** *Parke-Med, S.Afr.*
Diltiazem hydrochloride (p.900·1).
*Angina pectoris; hypertension.*

**Zilden**
*Genepharm, Gr.; Dorom, Ital.†.*
Diltiazem hydrochloride (p.900·1).
*Angina pectoris; heart failure; myocardial infarction.*

**Zileze**
*Pinewood, Irl.; Opus, UK.*
Zopiclone (p.729·3).
*Insomnia.*

**Zilisten** *Demo, Gr.*
Cefuroxime sodium (p.184·1).
*Bacterial infections.*

**Zilium** *Wolfs, Belg.*
Domperidone maleate (p.1263·2).
*Delayed gastric emptying; nausea and vomiting.*

**Ziloxican** *Zimaia, Port.*
Meloxicam (p.56·1).

**Zilutrol** *Abbott, Switz.*
Meloxicam (p.56·1).
*Arthroses.*

**Zimadoce** *Rubio, Spain.*
Cobamamide (p.1459·1).
*Tonic.*

**Zimaina** *Zimaia, Port.*
Aspirin (p.15·1); caffeine (p.782·1).
*Fever; pain.*

**Zimalgin** *Amadeus, India.*
Paracetamol (p.76·2); caffeine (p.782·1); codeine phosphate (p.27·1).
*Pain.*

**Zimanel** *Proge, Ital.*
Cefotaxime sodium (p.175·3).
Lidocaine hydrochloride (p.1377·3) is included in this preparation to alleviate the pain of injection.
*Bacterial infections.*

**Zimaquin** *Gynopharm, Chile.*
Clomifene citrate (p.1542·2).
*Female infertility.*

**Zimbacol** *Link, UK.*
Bezafibrate (p.873·2).
*Hyperlipidaemias.*

**Zimerol** *Sons, Mex.†.*
Cimetidine (p.1255·3).
*Peptic ulcer.*

**Zimicina** *Hexal, Braz.*
Azithromycin (p.159·1).
*Bacterial infections.*

**Zimmex** *Silom, Thai.*
Simvastatin (p.997·1).
*Hypercholesterolaemia.*

**Zimocel** *SIT, Ital.*
Dried yeast (p.1469·1).

**Zimoclone** *Gerard, Irl.*
Zopiclone (p.729·3).
*Insomnia.*

**Zimor**
*Rubio, Singapore; Rubio, Spain.*
Omeprazole (p.1278·2).
*Gastro-oesophageal reflux; peptic ulcer; Zollinger-Ellison syndrome.*

**Zimovane**
*Aventis, Irl.; Aventis, UK.*
Zopiclone (p.729·3).
*Insomnia.*

**Zimox**
*Note. This name is used for preparations of different composition.*
*Faran, Gr.*
Levodopa (p.1205·2); carbidopa (p.1204·3).
*Parkinsonism.*

*Pharmacia Upjohn, Ital.*
Amoxicillin trihydrate (p.155·3).
*Bacterial infections.*

**Zinabol** *Makros, Braz.†.*
Cobamamide (p.1459·1).
*Reduced appetite; tonic.*

**Zinacef**
*GlaxoSmithKline, Belg.; GlaxoSmithKline, Braz.; GlaxoSmithKline, Canad.; GlaxoSmithKline, Denm.; GlaxoSmithKline, Fin.; GlaxoSmithKline, Ger.; Glaxo Wellcome, Gr.; GlaxoSmithKline, Hong Kong; GlaxoSmithKline, Irl.; GlaxoSmithKline, Israel; GlaxoSmithKline, Malaysia; GlaxoSmithKline, Neth.; GlaxoSmithKline, Norw.; GlaxoSmithKline, NZ; GlaxoSmithKline, S.Afr.; GlaxoSmithKline, Singapore; GlaxoSmithKline, Swed.; GlaxoSmithKline, Switz.; GlaxoSmithKline, Thai.; GlaxoSmithKline, UK; Glaxo Wellcome, USA.*
Cefuroxime sodium (p.184·1).
*Bacterial infections.*

**Zinaderm** *Technilab, Canad.*
Zinc oxide (p.1163·2).
*Skin disorders.*

**Zinadiur** *Errekappa, Ital.*
Benazepril hydrochloride (p.867·2); hydrochlorothiazide (p.933·2).
*Hypertension.*

**Zinadol** *Glaxo Wellcome, Gr.*
Cefuroxime axetil (p.184·1).
*Bacterial infections.*

**Zinadril** *Errekappa, Ital.*
Benazepril hydrochloride (p.867·2).
*Heart failure; hypertension.*

**Zinaf** *SoSe, Ital.†.*
Propylene glycol cefatrizine (p.170·3).
*Bacterial infections.*

**Zinalerg** *Darrow, Braz.†.*
Hydroxyzine hydrochloride (p.434·3).
*Hypersensitivity reactions.*

**Zinamide**
*Merck Sharp & Dohme, Austral.; Merck Sharp & Dohme, Irl.; Merck Sharp & Dohme, NZ; Merck Sharp & Dohme, UK†.*
Pyrazinamide (p.246·3).
*Tuberculosis.*

**Zinasen** *Atral, Port.*
Flunarizine hydrochloride (p.434·1).
*Migraine; vertigo.*

**Zinat** *GlaxoSmithKline, Switz.*
Cefuroxime axetil (p.184·1).
*Bacterial infections.*

**Zinaxin**
*Bionax, Hong Kong†; Bionax, Singapore†; Bionax, Thai.; Eurovita, Thai.; Vita Healthcare, UK.*
Ginger (p.1267·1).
*Musculoskeletal and joint disorders.*

**Zinaxin Plus** *Eurovita, Malaysia; Bionax, Malaysia.*
Ginger (p.1267·1); galanga.
*Musculoskeletal and joint disorders.*

**Zinc for Acne** *Natural Life, Arg.*
Zinc; vitamin C; Vitamin $B_6$; vitamin A; vitamin E (p.1417·1).

**Zinc B, E & C** *Puritan Quartz, Thai.*
Multivitamin preparation with zinc (p.1417·1).

**Zinc + C250** *Vitaplex, Austral.†.*
Zinc amino acid chelate (p.1469·3); ascorbic acid (p.1460·2).
*Zinc deficiency.*

**Zinc C Plus** *Vitaglow, Austral.†.*
Zinc amino acid chelate (p.1469·3); ascorbic acid (p.1460·2); vitamin B substances (p.1417·1).
*Inflammation; skin disorders; wounds.*

**Zinc Cream White** *McGloin, Austral.†.*
*SPF 15+:* Zinc oxide (p.1163·2).
*Burns; nappy rash; skin abrasions; skin irritation; sunscreen.*

**Zinc Defence** *Boots Healthcare, NZ.*
Ascorbic acid (p.1460·2); zinc (p.1469·2).
*Cold symptoms.*

**Zinc Lotion** *Vitamed, Israel.*
Zinc oxide (p.1163·2).
*Skin irritation.*

**Zinc Menthol** *Vitamed, Israel.*
Zinc oxide (p.1163·2); menthol (p.1711·3).
*Skin irritation.*

**Zinc Plus**
*Note. This name is used for preparations of different composition.*
*Cenovis, Austral.†; Vitelle, Austral.†.*
Zinc amino acid chelate (p.1469·3); vitamins and minerals (p.1417·1).
*Zinc deficiency.*

*Swiss Herbal, Canad.*
Zinc gluconate (p.1469·2); vitamin C (p.1460·2).

*Bio-Health, UK†.*
Zinc gluconate; vitamin $B_6$; magnesium (p.1417·1).

**Zinc Supplement** *Vitaplex, Austral.†.*
Zinc gluconate (p.1469·2); vitamins and minerals (p.1417·1).
*Zinc deficiency.*

**Zinc Zenith** *Eagle, Austral.†.*
Zinc gluconate (p.1469·2); zinc amino acid chelate (p.1469·3); alfalfa (p.1649·1); ascorbic acid (p.1460·2); maltase (p.1646·2); pyridoxine hydrochloride (p.1456·3); minerals (p.1417·1).
*Zinc, vitamin C and vitamin $B_6$ supplement.*

**Zincaband**
*SSL, Austral.; Smith & Nephew, Swed.†; SSL, UK.*
Zinc oxide (p.1163·2).
*Eczema; leg ulcers; medicated bandage.*

**Zinc-ACE** *Wassen, UK.*
Zinc; vitamins (p.1417·1).

**Zinca-Pak** *Smith & Nephew SoloPak, USA.*
Zinc sulfate (p.1469·3).
*Additive for intravenous total parenteral nutrition solutions.*

**Zincaps**
*Aspen, Austral.; Aspen, Hong Kong; Aventis, NZ; ST, Thai.*
Zinc sulfate (p.1469·3).
*Zinc supplement.*

**Zincate** *Paddock, USA.*
Zinc sulfate (p.1469·3).
*Dietary supplement.*

**Zincation** *Isdin, Spain.*
Pyrithione zinc (p.1156·2).
*Scalp disorders.*

**Zincation Plus** *Isdin, Spain.*
Pyrithione zinc (p.1156·2); coal tar (p.1159·2).
*Scalp disorders.*

**Zincfrin**
*Alcon, Austral.; Alcon, Belg.; Alcon, Canad.; Alcon, Denm.; Alcon, Fin.; Alcon, Ger.; Alcon, Malaysia; Alcon, NZ; Alcon Cusi, Spain; Alcon, Swed.; Alcon, Switz.†; Alcon, Thai.†; Alcon, USA.*
Phenylephrine hydrochloride (p.1126·3); zinc sulfate (p.1469·3).
*Eye irritation.*

**Zincfrin Antihistaminicum** *Alcon, Belg.*
Antazoline phosphate (p.424·2); naphazoline hydrochloride (p.1124·3); zinc sulfate (p.1469·3).
Formerly known as Zincfrin-A.
*Conjunctival congestion; eye irritation.*

**Zincfrin-A**
*Alcon, Canad.; Alcon, Fin.*
Antazoline phosphate (p.424·2); naphazoline hydrochloride (p.1124·3); zinc sulfate (p.1469·3).
*Allergic conjunctivitis.*

**Zinc-Ichtyol** *Viatris, Belg.†.*
Zinc oxide (p.1163·2); ichthammol (p.1148·2).
*Blepharitis; eczema and pruritus of the eye.*

**Zinc-Imizol** *Farmigea, Ital.*
Zinc sulfate (p.1469·3); naphazoline nitrate (p.1124·3).
*Conjunctivitis, alone or associated with blepharitis.*

**Zinco All' Acqua** *Sella, Ital.; Sella, Ital.*
Zinc oxide (p.1163·2).
*Skin disorders.*

**Zinco Sulpha** *Bell, India.*
Sulfacetamide sodium (p.257·3); zinc sulfate (p.1469·3).
*Eye infections.*

**Zincod** *Vitamed, Israel.*
Zinc oxide (p.1163·2); cod-liver oil (p.1425·2); kaolin (p.1268·3).
*Nappy rash; skin irritation.*

**Zincoderm**
*Taro, Canad.; Bersan, Ital.*
Zinc oxide (p.1163·2).
*Skin disorders.*

**Zincoderma** *Confar, Port.*
Zinc oxide (p.1163·2).

**Zincofax** *Pfizer Consumer, Canad.*
Zinc oxide (p.1163·2).
*Nappy rash.*

**Zincol** *Sam-On, Israel.*
Zinc sulfate (p.1469·3).
*Skin ulcers; wounds; zinc deficiency.*

**Zincolok** *Allergan, Braz.*
Zinc sulfate (p.1469·3); naphazoline hydrochloride (p.1124·3).
*Ocular congestion.*

**Zincometil** *Farmila, Ital.*
Benzalkonium chloride (p.1168·3); zinc sulfate (p.1469·3).
*Eye disinfection.*

**Zincon** *Lederle, USA.*
Pyrithione zinc (p.1156·2).
*Scalp disorders.*

**Zincopan** *Gunther, Braz.*
Zinc sulfate (p.1469·3).
*Zinc deficiency.*

**Zincoral** *Mavi, Ital.*
Zinc and copper supplement (p.1417·1).

**Zincosol** *Bioceuticals, UK.*
Zinc sulfate (p.1469·3).

**Zincotape** *Lohmann, Ital.†.*
Zinc oxide (p.1163·2).
*Medicated dressing.*

**Zincotex** *Lohmann, Ital.†.*
Zinc oxide (p.1163·2).
*Medicated dressing.*

**Zincovit** *Labomed, Chile.*
Vitamin A; vitamin C; vitamin E; zinc (p.1417·1).
*Dietary supplement.*

**Zincoxid** *Slapak, Arg.*
Zinc oxide (p.1163·2).
*Dietary supplement.*

**Zincream** *Medinova, Switz.*
Zinc oxide (p.1163·2).
*Nappy rash; wounds.*

**Zincstic** *Ideal Health, UK.*
Zinc oxide (p.1163·2); titanium dioxide (p.1160·3).
*Sunscreen.*

**Zinctab** *Pharmasant, Thai.*
Zinc (p.1469·2).
*Zinc supplement.*

**Zincum valerianicum-Hevert** *Hevert, Ger.*
Homoeopathic preparation.

**Zincvit** *Kenwood, USA.*
Multivitamin and mineral preparation (p.1417·1).

**Zindaclin** *Strakan, UK.*
Clindamycin phosphate (p.194·2).
*Acne.*

**Zindacline** *Fujisawa, Fr.*
Clindamycin (p.194·2).
*Acne.*

**Zinecard**
*Pharmacia, Canad.*
Dexrazoxane (p.1036·1).
*Prevention of doxorubicin cardiotoxicity.*

*Pharmacia Upjohn, USA.*
Dexrazoxane hydrochloride (p.1036·2).
*Prevention of doxorubicin cardiotoxicity.*

**Zineli** *Rafarm, Gr.*
Sodium cromoglicate (p.795·3).
*Allergic conjunctivitis; allergic rhinitis.*

**Zineryt**
*Yamanouchi, Belg.; Hermal, Ger.; Yamanouchi, Irl.; Yamanouchi, Ital.; Yamanouchi, Neth.; Yamanouchi, Port.; Yamanouchi, Spain; Yamanouchi, UK.*
Erythromycin (p.208·1); zinc acetate (p.1469·2).
*Acne.*

**Zinetac** *GlaxoSmithKline, India.*
Ranitidine hydrochloride (p.1285·2).
*Dyspepsia; gastro-oesophageal reflux; gastrointestinal hyperacidity; peptic ulcer; Zollinger-Ellison syndrome.*

**Zinetrin** *Stiefel, Braz.*
Cetirizine (p.427·2).
*Hypersensitivity reactions.*

**Zinga** *Ashbourne, UK†.*
Nizatidine (p.1277·2).
*Gastro-oesophageal reflux; peptic ulcer.*

**Zink beta** *Betapharm, Ger.*
Zinc sulfate (p.1469·3).
*Zinc deficiency.*

**Zink Verla** *Verla, Ger.*
Zinc gluconate (p.1469·2).
*Zinc deficiency.*

**Zinkamin**
*Merck, Austria; Falk, Ger.*
Bis(L-histadinato) zinc (p.1469·3).
*Zinc deficiency.*

**Zinkbrause** *Verla, Ger.*
Zinc sulfate (p.1469·3).
*Zinc deficiency.*

**Zink-Calmitol** *OBA, Denm.*
Camphor (p.1665·3); hyoscyamus oil (p.485·2); menthol (p.1711·3); zinc oxide (p.1163·2).
*Pruritus.*

**Zink-D Longoral** *Artesan, Ger.; Cassella-med, Ger.*
Zinc gluconate (p.1469·2).
*Zinc deficiency.*

**Zinkit** *Worwag, Ger.*
Zinc sulfate (p.1469·3).
*Zinc deficiency.*

**Zink'N'Swim** *Or-Dov, Austral.†.*
*SPF 15+:* Zinc oxide (p.1163·2).
*Sunscreen.*

**Zinkokehl** *Sanum-Kehlbeck, Ger.*
Homoeopathic preparation.

**Zinkolie** *Boots Healthcare, Neth.*
Zinc oxide (p.1163·2).
*Skin disorders.*

**Zinkorell** *Sanorell, Ger.*
*Injection:* Homoeopathic preparation.
*Tablets†:* Zinc oxide (p.1163·2).
*Zinc deficiency.*

**Zinkorot** *Worwag, Ger.*
Zinc orotate (p.1724·3).
*Zinc deficiency.*

**Zinkosalb** *Hilarys, Canad.†.*
Salicylic acid (p.1157·1); zinc oxide (p.1163·2).

**zinkotase** *Biosyn, Ger.*
Zinc aspartate (p.1469·3).
*Zinc deficiency.*

**Zinkpaste** *Riemser, Ger.*
Zinc oxide (p.1163·2).
*Skin disorders; skin ulcers; wounds.*

**Zink-Ratiopharm** *Ratiopharm, Ger.*
Zinc sulfate (p.1469·3).
*Zinc deficiency.*

**Zinksalbe** *CT, Ger.*
Zinc oxide (p.1163·2); cod-liver oil (p.1425·2); glycerol (p.1694·3).
*Wounds.*

**Zinksalbe Dialon** *Engelhard, Ger.*
Zinc oxide (p.1163·2).
*Skin disorders; wounds.*

**Zink-Sandoz** *Novartis Consumer, Ger.*
Zinc sulfate (p.1469·3).
*Zinc deficiency.*

**Zinkzalf** *Boots Healthcare, Neth.*
Zinc oxide (p.1163·2).
*Skin disorders.*

**Zinnat**
*GlaxoSmithKline, Austral.; GlaxoSmithKline, Austria; GlaxoSmithKline, Belg.; GlaxoSmithKline, Braz.; Etex, Chile; GlaxoSmithKline, Denm.; GlaxoSmithKline, Fin.; GlaxoSmithKline, Fr.; GlaxoSmithKline, Ger.; GlaxoSmithKline, Hong Kong; Glaxo Wellcome, Irl.; GlaxoSmithKline, Israel; GlaxoSmithKline, Ital.; GlaxoSmithKline, Malaysia; Glaxo Wellcome, Mex.; GlaxoSmithKline, Neth.; GlaxoSmithKline, NZ; GlaxoSmithKline, S.Afr.; GlaxoSmithKline, Singapore; GlaxoSmithKline, Spain; GlaxoSmithKline, Swed.; GlaxoSmithKline, Thai.; GlaxoSmithKline, UK.*
Cefuroxime axetil (p.184·1) or cefuroxime sodium (p.184·1).
Formerly known as Curoxime in *Fr.*
*Bacterial infections.*

**Zinnkraut-Tropfen** *Bio-Diat, Ger.*
Equisetum (p.1684·1).
*Urinary-tract disorders.*

**Zinocep** *Glaxo Allen, Ital.*
Cefuroxime sodium (p.184·1).
*Bacterial infections.*

**Zinopril** *Teuto, Braz.*
Lisinopril (p.946·3).
*Hypertension.*

**Zintona**
*Boehringer Ingelheim, Austria; Herbalist, Ger.; Chrisana, Switz.*
Ginger (p.1267·1).
*Digestive system disorders; gastric pain; motion sickness; vomiting.*

**Zinulin** *Sarabhai Piramal, India.*
Insulin zinc injection (porcine) (30% amorphous, 70% crystalline) (p.333·3).
*Diabetes mellitus.*

**Zinvit** *Vitaglow, Austral.†.*
Zinc sulfate (p.1469·3); magnesium sulfate (p.1228·2); vitamin B substances (p.1417·1).
*Herpes labialis; mouth ulcers; skin disorders; wounds; zinc deficiency.*

**Zinvit C** *Vitaglow, Austral.†.*
Zinc sulfate (p.1469·3); magnesium sulfate (p.1228·2); ascorbic acid (p.1460·2).
*Herpes labialis; mouth ulcers; skin disorders; wounds.*

**Zinvit G** *Vitaglow, Austral.†.*
Zinc sulfate (p.1469·3); magnesium sulfate (p.1228·2); vitamin B substances (p.1417·1).
*Skin disorders; zinc deficiency.*

**Zipos** *Alodial, Port.*
Cefuroxime axetil (p.184·1).
*Bacterial infections.*

**Zipra** *Columbia, Mex.*
Ciprofloxacin hydrochloride (p.188·2).
*Bacterial infections.*

**Ziprol** *Baldacci, Braz.*
Pantoprazole (p.1283·1).
*Peptic ulcer.*

**Zipzoc**
*Smith & Nephew, Denm.; Smith & Nephew, Fin.; Smith & Nephew, Irl.; Smith & Nephew Healthcare, UK.*
Zinc oxide (p.1163·2) impregnated stocking.
*Leg ulcers.*

**Zipzoc Salvstrumpa** *Smith & Nephew, Swed.*
Zinc oxide (p.1163·2).
Formerly known as Salvstrumpa.
*Skin ulcers; vascular disorders.*

**Ziradryl** *Parke, Davis, USA.*
Diphenhydramine hydrochloride (p.431·3); zinc oxide (p.1163·2); camphor (p.1665·3).
*Pruritus.*

**Ziremex** *Demo, Gr.*
Nimodipine (p.972·3).
*Neurological deficit following subarachnoid haemorrhage.*

**Zirkulin Beruhigungs-Tee** *Schulke & Mayr, Austria.*
Lupulus (p.1708·1).
*Restlessness; sleep disorders.*

**Zirpine** *Pinewood, Irl.*
Cetirizine hydrochloride (p.427·1).
*Allergic rhinitis; urticaria.*

**Zirtec** *UCB, Ital.*
Cetirizine hydrochloride (p.427·1).
*Conjunctivitis; rhinitis; urticaria.*

**Zirtek**
*UCB, Austria; UCB, Gr.; UCB, Irl.; UCB, UK.*
Cetirizine hydrochloride (p.427·1).
*Allergic conjunctivitis; allergic rhinitis; urticaria.*

**Zirvit** *Ativus, Braz.*
A range of vitamin and mineral preparations (p.1417·1).

**Zirvit Beta** *Ativus, Braz.*
Betacarotene (p.1422·3).
*Photosensitivity; vitamin A deficiency.*

**Zirvit E** *Ativus, Braz.*
Tocoferil acetate (p.1465·1).
*Vitamin E deficiency.*

**Zispin**
*Organon, Irl.; Organon, UK.*
Mirtazapine (p.307·3).
*Depression.*

**Zita** *Eastern Pharmaceuticals, UK.*
Cimetidine (p.1255·3).
*Gastrointestinal disorders associated with hyperacidity.*

**Zitazonium**
*Egis, Hong Kong; Egis, Malaysia; Egis, Thai.*
Tamoxifen citrate (p.584·1).
*Anovulatory infertility; breast cancer.*

**Zithromax**
*Pfizer, Austral.; Pfizer, Austria; Pfizer, Canad.; Pfizer, Chile; Pfizer, Fin.; Pfizer, Fr.; Mack, Illert., Ger.; Pfizer, Gr.; Pfizer, Hong Kong; Pfizer, Irl.; Pfizer, Israel; Pfizer, Malaysia; Pfizer, Neth.; Pfizer, NZ; Pfizer, Port.; Pfizer, S.Afr.; Pfizer, Singapore; Pfizer, Switz.; Pfizer, Thai.; Pfizer, UK; Pfizer, USA.*
Azithromycin (p.159·1).
*Bacterial infections.*

**Zitrix** *Metapharma, Ital.†.*
Propylene glycol cefatrizine (p.170·3).
*Bacterial infections.*

**Zitromax**
*Pfizer, Arg.; Pfizer, Belg.; Pfizer, Braz.; Pfizer, Denm.; Pfizer, Ital.; Pfizer, Spain.*
Azithromycin (p.159·1).
*Bacterial infections.*

**Zitroneo** *Neo Quimica, Braz.*
Azithromycin (p.159·1).
*Bacterial infections.*

**Zitumex** *Rafarm, Gr.*
Piroxicam (p.84·2).
*Dysmenorrhoea; gout; inflammation; musculoskeletal and joint disorders; pain.*

**Ziverone** *Rayere, Mex.*
Aciclovir (p.626·1).
*Herpesvirus infections.*

**Zix** *Lafi, Chile.*
Meloxicam (p.56·1).
*Inflammation; musculoskeletal and joint disorders; pain.*

**Ziz** *Chatfield Laboratories, UK.*
Promethazine hydrochloride (p.439·1).
*Insomnia.*

**Z-Kraft** *Hexal, Arg.*
Zinc sulfate (p.1469·3).
*Zinc deficiency.*

**Zleep** *Wockhardt, India.*
Zolpidem (p.729·2).
*Insomnia.*

**Z-Max** *Schering-Plough, Mex.*
Phentolamine mesilate (p.982·1).
*Erectile dysfunction.*

**ZN 220** *Covan, S.Afr.†.*
Zinc sulfate (p.1469·3).
*Wounds.*

**ZN Xampu** *Stiefel, Braz.*
Zinc (p.1469·2).
*Seborrhoea.*

**Zn-Fusin** *Pisa, Mex.*
Zinc sulfate (p.1469·3).

**ZNP**
*Stiefel, Arg.; Stiefel, Canad.; Stiefel, Chile; Stiefel, Fr.; Stiefel, Ital.; Stiefel, Mex.; Stiefel, USA.*
Pyrithione zinc (p.1156·2).
*Scalp disorders; seborrhoeic dermatitis.*

**Znupril** *Velka, Gr.*
Cetirizine hydrochloride (p.427·1).
*Allergic conjunctivitis; allergic rhinitis; pruritus.*

**Zobacide** *Garec, S.Afr.*
Metronidazole (p.607·2).
*Anaerobic bacterial infections; protozoal infections.*

**Zoben** *Raza, Malaysia; Pharmaniaga, Malaysia.*
Albendazole (p.101·2).
*Worm infections.*

**Zocor**
*Merck Sharp & Dohme, Arg.; Merck Sharp & Dohme, Austral.; Merck Sharp & Dohme, Belg.; Merck Sharp & Dohme, Braz.; Merck Frosst, Canad.; Merck Sharp & Dohme, Chile; Merck Sharp & Dohme, Denm.; Merck Sharp & Dohme, Fin.; Merck Sharp & Dohme-Chibret, Fr.; Dieckmann, Ger.; Vianex (Βιανεξ), Gr.; Merck Sharp & Dohme, Hong Kong; Merck Sharp & Dohme, Irl.; Neopharmed, Ital.; Merck Sharp & Dohme, Malaysia; Merck Sharp & Dohme, Mex.; Merck Sharp & Dohme, Neth.; Merck Sharp & Dohme, Norw.; Merck Sharp & Dohme, NZ†; Merck Sharp & Dohme, Port.; Merck Sharp & Dohme, S.Afr.; Merck Sharp & Dohme, Singapore; Merck Sharp & Dohme, Spain; Merck Sharp & Dohme, Switz.; Merck Sharp & Dohme, Thai.; Merck Sharp & Dohme, UK; Merck, USA.*
Simvastatin (p.997·1).
*Coronary atherosclerosis; hypercholesterolaemia; ischaemic heart disease.*

**Zocord**
*Merck Sharp & Dohme, Austria; Merck Sharp & Dohme, Swed.*
Simvastatin (p.997·1).
*Hypercholesterolaemia.*

**Zocord/ASA** *Merck Sharp & Dohme, Swed.*
Tablets, simvastatin (p.997·1); tablets, aspirin (p.15·1).
*Coronary atherosclerosis.*

**Zocovin** *TO-Chemicals, Thai.*
Aciclovir (p.626·1).
*Herpes simplex infections of the skin and mucous membranes.*

**Zodeac** *Econo Med, USA.*
Ferrous fumarate (p.1427·3); folic acid (p.1429·1); multivitamins and minerals (p.1417·1).
*Iron-deficiency anaemias.*

**Zodol** *Saval, Chile.*
Tramadol hydrochloride (p.94·3).
*Pain.*

**Zodorm** *Unipharm, Israel.*
Zolpidem (p.729·2).
*Insomnia.*

**Zodormdura** *Merck dura, Ger.*
Zolpidem tartrate (p.728·3).
*Sleep disorders.*

**Zodurat** *Pohl, Ger.*
Zopiclone (p.729·3).
*Sleep disorders.*

**Zofen** *Pharmaland, Thai.*
Pizotifen (p.470·3).
*Anorexia.*

**Zofenil**
*Menarini, Fr.*
Zofenopril calcium (p.1029·3).
*Hypertension.*

*Menarini, Irl.*
Zofenopril (p.1029·3).
*Hypertension; myocardial infarction.*

**Zoff**
*Note. This name is used for preparations of different composition.*
*Smith & Nephew, Austral.*
Dipropylene glycol methyl ether.
*Adhesive plaster remover.*

*Smith & Nephew Healthcare, UK.*
Trichloroethane (p.1477·3).
*Adhesive plaster removal.*

**Zoflut** *Cipla, India.*
Fluticasone propionate (p.1102·3).
*Inflammatory skin disorders.*

**Zoflux** *Libbs, Braz.*
Doxazosin mesilate (p.908·3).
*Benign prostatic hyperplasia; hypertension.*

**Zofora** *Pharmy, Fr.*
Piroxicam (p.84·2).
*Musculoskeletal, joint, and peri-articular disorders.*

**Zofran**
*GlaxoSmithKline, Arg.; GlaxoSmithKline, Austral.; GlaxoSmithKline, Austria; GlaxoSmithKline, Belg.; GlaxoSmithKline, Braz.; GlaxoSmithKline, Canad.; GlaxoSmithKline, Denm.; GlaxoSmithKline, Fin.; GlaxoSmithKline, Ger.; GlaxoSmithKline, Hong Kong; GlaxoSmithKline, Irl.; GlaxoSmithKline, Israel; GlaxoSmithKline, Ital.; GlaxoSmithKline, Malaysia; Glaxo Wellcome, Mex.; GlaxoSmithKline, Neth.; GlaxoSmithKline, Norw.; GlaxoSmithKline, NZ; Glaxo Wellcome, Port.; GlaxoSmithKline, S.Afr.; GlaxoSmithKline, Singapore; GlaxoSmithKline, Spain; GlaxoSmithKline, Swed.; GlaxoSmithKline, Switz.; GlaxoSmithKline, Thai.; GlaxoSmithKline, UK; Glaxo Wellcome, USA.*
Ondansetron (p.1281·1) or ondansetron hydrochloride (p.1281·1).
*Nausea and vomiting induced by cytotoxics and radiotherapy; postoperative nausea and vomiting.*

**Zofron** *Glaxo Wellcome, Gr.*
Ondansetron hydrochloride (p.1281·1).
*Chemotherapy or radiotherapy-induced nausea and vomiting.*

**Zoiral** *Aegis, Hong Kong.*
Clomipramine hydrochloride (p.289·3).
*Depression; obsessive-compulsive disorder; panic attacks; social phobias.*

**Zok-Zid**
*Pharmacia, Belg.; Pharmacia, Denm.*
Metoprolol succinate (p.957·1); hydrochlorothiazide (p.933·2).
*Hypertension.*

**Zolac**
*Xepa-Soul Pattinson, Hong Kong†; Xepa-Soul Pattinson, Malaysia.*
Bromocriptine mesilate (p.1200·3).
*Acromegaly; benign breast disorders; female infertility; galactorrhoea; hypogonadism; lactation inhibition; menstrual disorders; parkinsonism; prolactinomas.*

**Zoladex**
*AstraZeneca, Arg.; AstraZeneca, Austral.; AstraZeneca, Austria; AstraZeneca, Belg.; AstraZeneca, Braz.; AstraZeneca, Canad.; AstraZeneca, Chile; AstraZeneca, Denm.; AstraZeneca, Fin.; AstraZeneca, Fr.; AstraZeneca, Ger.; Astra-Zeneca, Gr.; AstraZeneca, Hong Kong; AstraZeneca, Irl.; Zeneca, Israel; AstraZeneca, Ital.; AstraZeneca, Malaysia; AstraZeneca, Mex.; AstraZeneca, Neth.; AstraZeneca, Norw.; AstraZeneca, NZ; AstraZeneca, Port.; Zeneca, S.Afr.; AstraZeneca, Singapore; AstraZeneca, Spain; AstraZeneca, Swed.; AstraZeneca, Switz.; AstraZeneca, Thai.; AstraZeneca, UK; Zeneca, USA.*
Goserelin acetate (p.1326·3).
*Breast cancer; endometriosis; female infertility; presurgical endometrial thinning; prostatic cancer; uterine fibroids.*

**Zolam** *Stadmed, India.*
Alprazolam (p.668·3).
*Anxiety; mixed anxiety depressive states.*

**Zolamid** *Faulding, Port.*
Midazolam hydrochloride (p.707·2).

**Zolamox** *Cazi, Braz.*
Acetazolamide (p.849·1).
*Glaucoma.*

**Zolanix** *Stiefel, Braz.*
Fluconazole (p.398·1).
*Fungal infections.*

**Zolapin** *BPL-Meizler, Braz.*
Clozapine (p.685·3).
*Psychoses.*

**Zolaten**
*Sigma, Austral.; Sigma, NZ.*
Aciclovir (p.626·1).
*Herpes labialis.*

**Zolben**
*Note. This name is used for preparations of different composition.*
*Sanofi Synthelabo, Braz.†.*
Albendazole (p.101·2).
*Worm infections.*

*Novartis, Chile; Sanopharm, Switz.*
Paracetamol (p.76·2).
*Fever; pain.*

**Zolben C** *Sanopharm, Switz.*
Paracetamol (p.76·2); ascorbic acid (p.1460·2).
*Fever; pain.*

**Zoldan-A** *Cryopharma, Mex.*
Danazol (p.1545·2).

**Zoldicam** *Rayere, Mex.*
Fluconazole (p.398·1).
*Fungal infections.*

**Zole** *Rexcel, India.*
Miconazole nitrate (p.405·3).
*Fungal and Gram-positive bacterial infections.*

**Zole-F** *Rexcel, India.*
Miconazole nitrate (p.405·3); fluocinolone acetonide (p.1101·2).
*Fungal and Gram-positive bacterial infections.*

**Zoleprim** *PP Lab, Thai.*
Co-trimoxazole (p.199·3).
*Bacterial infections.*

**Zoleptil** *Orion, UK.*
Zotepine (p.730·2).
*Schizophrenia.*

**Zoles** *Simoes, Braz.*
Mebendazole (p.108·2); tiabendazole (p.114·2).
*Worm infections.*

**Zolicef**
*Bristol-Myers Squibb, Austria; Apothecon, USA.*
Cefazolin sodium (p.170·3).
Lidocaine hydrochloride (p.1377·3) may be included in the intramuscular injection to alleviate the pain of injection.
*Bacterial infections.*

**Zolidan** *BPL-Meizler, Braz.*
Midazolam (p.707·1).
*Insomnia.*

**Zoliden** *Unipharma, Gr.*
Ranitidine hydrochloride (p.1285·2).
*Conditions where gastric acid reduction is beneficial; gastric hypersecretion including Zollinger-Ellison syndrome; peptic ulcer.*

**Zoliderm** *Raza, Malaysia; Pharmaniaga, Malaysia.*
Econazole nitrate (p.397·2).
*Fungal skin infections.*

**Zolidime** *Collins, Mex.*
Phenylbutazone (p.83·2); salicylamide (p.87·3); dexamethasone (p.1097·1); aluminium hydroxide (p.1249·2).
*Inflammation; musculoskeletal and joint disorders.*

**Zolidin** *Kener, Mex.†.*
Dipyrone (p.35·3).
*Fever; pain.*

**Zolief** *Genthon, Hong Kong.*
Zopiclone (p.729·3).
*Insomnia.*

**Zolim** *Schwarz, Ger.*
Mizolastine (p.437·3).
*Allergic conjunctivitis; allergic rhinitis; urticaria.*

**Zolin**
*Note. This name is used for preparations of different composition.*
*San Carlo, Ital.†.*
Cefazolin sodium (p.170·3).
Lidocaine hydrochloride (p.1377·3) is included in the intramuscular injection to alleviate the pain of injection.
*Bacterial infections.*
*Abigo, Swed.*
Oxymetazoline hydrochloride (p.1126·1).
*Rhinitis; sinusitis.*

**Zolina** *Llorens, Spain.*
Boric acid (p.1662·1); naphazoline hydrochloride (p.1124·3).
*Eye irritation.*

**Zoliparin** *Mann, Ger.*
Aciclovir (p.626·1).
*Herpes simplex eye infections.*

**Zolisint** *Benedetti, Ital.†.*
Cefazolin sodium (p.170·3).
Lidocaine hydrochloride (p.1377·3) is included in this preparation to alleviate the pain of injection.
*Bacterial infections.*

**Zolistam**
*Angelini, Ital.; Lepori, Port.*
Mizolastine (p.437·3).
*Allergic conjunctivitis; allergic rhinitis; urticaria.*

**Zolistan** *Novag, Spain.*
Mizolastine (p.437·3).
*Allergic rhinitis; urticaria.*

**Zolival**
*Reig Jofre, Spain†; Septa, Spain.*
Cefazolin sodium (p.170·3).
Formerly known as Cefabiot in *Spain*.
*Bacterial infections.*

**Zolken** *Kener, Mex.†.*
Itraconazole (p.401·3).
*Fungal infections.*

**Zolmic** *Delta, Braz.*
Fluconazole (p.398·1).
*Fungal infections.*

**Zolnod** *Rowex, Irl.*
Zolpidem tartrate (p.728·3).
*Insomnia.*

**Zoloft**
*Pfizer, Arg.; Roerig, Austral.; Pfizer, Braz.; Pfizer, Canad.; Pfizer, Denm.; Pfizer, Fin.; Pfizer, Fr.; Parke, Davis, Ger.; Pfizer, Ger.; Pfizer, Gr.; Pfizer, Hong Kong; Pfizer, Ital.; Pfizer, Malaysia; Pfizer, Neth.; Pfizer, Norw.; Pfizer, NZ; Pfizer, Port.; Pfizer, S.Afr.; Pfizer, Singapore; Pfizer, Swed.; Pfizer, Switz.; Pfizer, Thai.; Pfizer, USA.*
Sertraline hydrochloride (p.317·2).
*Depression; obsessive-compulsive disorder; panic disorder; post-traumatic stress disorder; premenstrual dysphoric disorder.*

**Zolpi-Lich** *Lichtenstein, Ger.*
Zolpidem tartrate (p.728·3).
*Sleep disorders.*

**Zolpinox** *Krewel, Ger.*
Zolpidem tartrate (p.728·3).
*Insomnia.*

**Zolpramex** *Sinteropico, Braz.†.*
Omeprazole (p.1278·2).
*Peptic ulcer.*

**Zolstatin** *Biochimico, Braz.; Aurantis, Braz.*
Fluconazole (p.398·1).
*Fungal infections.*

**Zoltec** *Pfizer, Braz.*
Fluconazole (p.398·1).
*Fungal infections.*

**Zoltenk** *Biotenk, Arg.*
Omeprazole (p.1278·2).
*Gastro-oesophageal reflux; peptic ulcer; Zollinger-Ellison syndrome.*

**Zolterol**
*CCM, Malaysia; CCM, Singapore.*
Diclofenac sodium (p.32·1).
*Musculoskeletal, joint, peri-articular, and soft-tissue disorders; pain.*

**Zoltren** *Teuto, Braz.*
Fluconazole (p.398·1).
*Fungal infections.*

**Zol-Triq** *Medley, Braz.†.*
Mebendazole (p.108·2).
*Worm infections.*

**Zoltum** *Aventis, Fr.*
Omeprazole (p.1278·2).
*Gastro-oesophageal reflux; peptic ulcer; Zollinger-Ellison syndrome.*

**Zolvera** *Rosemont, UK.*
Verapamil hydrochloride (p.1019·1).
*Angina pectoris; arrhythmias; hypertension.*

**Zomacton**
*Ferring, Austria; Ferring, Belg.; Ferring, Denm.; Ferring, Fin.; Ferring, Fr.; Ferring, Ger.; Chemipharma, Gr.; Ferring, Irl.; Ferring, Ital.; Ferring, Neth.; Ferring, Norw.; Ferring, Port.; Ferring, Spain; Ferring, Swed.; Ferring, UK.*
Somatropin (p.1327·2).
*Growth disorders in renal failure; growth hormone deficiency; Turner's syndrome.*

**Zomepral** *Laboratorios Chile, Chile.*
Omeprazole (p.1278·2).
*Gastro-oesophageal reflux; peptic ulcer; Zollinger-Ellison syndrome.*

**Zomera** *Novartis, Israel.*
Zoledronic acid (p.776·2).
*Hypercalcaemia of malignancy.*

**Zometa**
*Novartis, Arg.; Novartis, Austral.; Novartis, Braz.; Novartis, Canad.; Novartis, Chile; Novartis, Denm.; Novartis, Fin.; Novartis, Fr.; Novartis, Ger.; Novartis, Gr.; Novartis, Hong Kong; Novartis, Irl.; Novartis, Ital.; Novartis, Malaysia; Novartis, Norw.; Novartis, NZ; Novartis, Port.; Novartis, Singapore; Novartis, Spain; Novartis, Swed.; Novartis, Switz.; Novartis, Thai.; Novartis, UK; Novartis, USA.*
Zoledronic acid (p.776·2).
*Bone metastases; hypercalcaemia of malignancy; multiple myeloma.*

**Zometic** *Chemopharma, Chile.*
Zopiclone (p.729·3).
*Insomnia.*

**Zomig**
*AstraZeneca, Austral.; AstraZeneca, Austria; AstraZeneca, Belg.; AstraZeneca, Braz.; AstraZeneca, Canad.; AstraZeneca, Denm.; AstraZeneca, Fin.; AstraZeneca, Fr.; AstraZeneca, Hong Kong; AstraZeneca, Irl.; AstraZeneca, Israel; AstraZeneca, Ital.; Zeneca, Mex.; AstraZeneca, Neth.; AstraZeneca, Norw.; AstraZeneca, Port.; Zeneca, S.Afr.; AstraZeneca, Singapore; AstraZeneca, Spain; Astra, Swed.; AstraZeneca, Switz.; AstraZeneca, Thai.; AstraZeneca, UK; Zeneca, USA.*
Zolmitriptan (p.473·3).
*Migraine.*

**Zomigon**
*AstraZeneca, Arg.; Astra-Zeneca, Gr.*
Zolmitriptan (p.473·3).
*Migraine.*

**Zomigoro** *AstraZeneca, Fr.*
Zolmitriptan (p.473·3).
*Migraine.*

**Zomni** *Jean-Marie, Hong Kong.*
Zopiclone (p.729·3).
*Insomnia.*

**Zomorph** *Link, UK.*
Morphine sulfate (p.60·2).
*Pain.*

**Zon**
*Antula, Fin.; Antula, Swed.*
Ketoprofen (p.51·2).
*Musculoskeletal and joint disorders; sports injuries.*

**Zonal** *Galen, Mex.†.*
Fluconazole (p.398·1).
*Fungal infections.*

**Zonalon**
*Medicis, Canad.; Rafa, Israel; Medicis, USA.*
Doxepin hydrochloride (p.291·2).
*Pruritus.*

**Zonap** *Unichem, India.*
Zopiclone (p.729·3).
*Insomnia.*

**Zoncef** *AGIPS, Ital.*
Cefoperazone sodium (p.174·3).
Lidocaine hydrochloride (p.1377·3) is included in the intramuscular injection to alleviate the pain of injection.
*Gram-negative bacterial infections.*

**Zondar** *Niverpharm, Fr.*
Diacerein (p.30·1).
*Osteoarthritis.*

**Zone-A** *UAD, USA.*
Hydrocortisone acetate (p.1103·3); pramocaine (p.1382·2).

**Zonegran** *Elan, USA.*
Zonisamide (p.384·3).
*Epilepsy.*

**Zonite** *Menley & James, USA.*
Benzalkonium chloride (p.1168·3); edetic acid (p.1038·2); sodium acetate (p.1223·1); propylene glycol (p.1735·2); menthol (p.1711·3); thymol (p.1194·2).
*Vaginal disorders.*

**Zonivent** *Ashbourne, UK†.*
Beclometasone dipropionate (p.1091·1).
*Rhinitis.*

**Zoo Chews** *Hall, Canad.*
Multivitamin preparation (p.1417·1).

**Zoo Chews with Iron** *Hall, Canad.*
Multivitamin preparation with iron (p.1417·1).

**Zoodermina Cream** *Bajer, Arg.*
Vitamin A palmitate (p.1453·1) spermaceti; beeswax (p.1480·2).
*Emollient.*

**Zop** *Hexal, Ger.*
Zopiclone (p.729·3).
*Sleep disorders.*

**Zopam** *Pharmasant, Thai.*
Diazepam (p.690·1).
*Anxiety; insomnia; skeletal muscle spasm.*

**Zopax** *Cipla-Medpro, S.Afr.*
Alprazolam (p.668·3).
*Anxiety disorders; mixed anxiety depressive states; panic attacks.*

**Zophren** *GlaxoSmithKline, Fr.*
Ondansetron (p.1281·1) or ondansetron hydrochloride (p.1281·1).
*Nausea and vomiting.*

**Zopicalm** *Temmler, Ger.*
Zopiclone (p.729·3).
*Sleep disorders.*

**Zopicalma** *Ciclum, Spain.*
Zopiclone (p.729·3).
*Insomnia.*

**Zopiclodura** *Merck dura, Ger.*
Zopiclone (p.729·3).
*Sleep disorders.*

**Zopimed** *Parke-Med, S.Afr.*
Zopiclone (p.729·3).
*Insomnia.*

**Zopinox** *Orion, Fin.*
Zopiclone (p.729·3).
*Sleep disorders.*

**Zopi-Puren** *Alpharma-Isis, Ger.*
Zopiclone (p.729·3).
*Sleep disorders.*

**Zopitan** *Clonmel, Irl.*
Zopiclone (p.729·3).
*Insomnia.*

**Zopranol** *Guidotti, Ital.*
Zofenopril calcium (p.1029·3).
*Hypertension; myocardial infarction.*

**Zorac**
*Allergan, Austria; Allergan, Braz.; Bioglan, Fin.; Pierre Fabre, Fr.; Pierre Fabre Dermo Kosmetik, Ger.; Alvia (Αλβια), Gr.; Bioglan, Irl.; Pierre Fabre, Ital.; Pierre Fabre, Spain; Bioglan, Swed.; Pierre Fabre, Switz.; Allergan, UK.*
Tazarotene (p.1160·2).
*Psoriasis.*

**Zorail** *SAT, Spain.*
Enalapril maleate (p.909·2); nitrendipine (p.973·3).
*Hypertension.*

**Zorak** *Allergan, S.Afr.*
Tazarotene (p.1160·2).
*Psoriasis.*

**Zoral**
*DHA, Hong Kong; DHA, Malaysia; DHA, Singapore.*
Aciclovir (p.626·1).
*Herpesvirus infections.*

**Zoran** *Reddy, Singapore.*
Ranitidine hydrochloride (p.1285·2).
*Dyspepsia; gastro-oesophageal reflux; peptic ulcer; Zollinger-Ellison syndrome.*

**Zorax**
*Sunward, Malaysia; Sunward, Singapore.*
Aciclovir (p.626·1).
*Herpesvirus infections.*

**Zorbtive** *Serono, USA.*
Somatropin (p.1327·2).
*Short bowel syndrome.*

**Zorclone** *Ivax, Irl.*
Zopiclone (p.729·3).
*Insomnia.*

**Zordyl** *Julphar, UAE.*
Chlorhexidine (p.1173·2).
*Oral hygiene.*

**Zoref**
*Glaxo Allen, Ital.; Glaxo Wellcome, Port.*
Cefuroxime axetil (p.184·1).
*Bacterial infections.*

**Zorinax** *Xepa-Soul Pattinson, Singapore†.*
Ketoconazole (p.403·3).
*Dandruff; fungal infections; seborrhoeic dermatitis.*

**Zoroxin**
*Merck Sharp & Dohme, Austria; Merck Sharp & Dohme, Belg.; Merck Sharp & Dohme, Denm.*
Norfloxacin (p.238·3).
*Bacterial infections.*

**ZORprin** *Boots, USA.*
Aspirin (p.15·1).
*Fever; osteoarthritis; pain; rheumatoid arthritis.*

**Zoru** *E-Z-EM, Belg.*
Tartaric acid (p.1752·1); sodium bicarbonate (p.1223·2); dimethicone (p.1289·2).
*Gastrointestinal radiography.*

**Zost** *Allergan-Frumtost, Braz.†.*
Trifluridine (p.655·3).
*Herpes simplex eye infections.*

**Zostex** *Berlin-Chemie, Ger.*
Brivudine (p.629·2).
*Herpes zoster infections.*

**Zostrix**
*Link, Austral.; Medicis, Canad.; Rafa, Israel; AFT, NZ; Rodlen, USA.*
Capsaicin (p.24·2).
*Diabetic neuropathy; osteoarthritis; postherpetic neuralgia; rheumatoid arthritis.*

**Zostrum**
*Galderma, Ger.; Galderma, Irl.*
Idoxuridine (p.637·3) in dimethyl sulfoxide.
*Herpes simplex infections; herpes zoster.*

**Zosvir** *Elea, Arg.*
Famciclovir (p.633·2).
*Herpesvirus infections.*

**Zosyn**
*Wyeth Lederle, India; Lederle, USA.*
Piperacillin sodium (p.243·1); tazobactam sodium (p.264·3).
*Bacterial infections.*

**Zo-Tab** *Pacific, NZ†.*
Zopiclone (p.729·3).
*Insomnia.*

**Zotinar** *Cipan, Port.*
Desonide (p.1096·3).
*Skin disorders.*

**Zotinar-N** *Cipan, Port.*
Desonide (p.1096·3); neomycin sulfate (p.235·1).
*Infected skin disorders.*

**Zoto-HC** *Horizon, USA.*
Chloroxylenol (p.1177·2); pramocaine hydrochloride (p.1382·2); hydrocortisone (p.1103·3).
Formerly known as Xotic.
*Ear disorders.*

**Zoton**
*Wyeth, Austral.; Wyeth, Irl.; Neopharm, Israel; Wyeth Lederle, Ital.; Wyeth, NZ; Wyeth, UK.*
Lansoprazole (p.1269·3).
*Gastro-oesophageal reflux; peptic ulcer; Zollinger-Ellison syndrome.*

**Zotran** *Pharmacia, Chile.*
Alprazolam (p.668·3).
*Anxiety; panic attacks.*

**Zotrim** *Sigma, UK.*
Maté (p.1765·3); guarana (p.1765·3); damiana (p.1679·1).
*Slimming aid.*

**Zov800** *Wellcome, Port.*
Aciclovir (p.626·1).
*Herpesvirus infections.*

**Zovia** *Watson, USA.*
Ethinylestradiol (p.1553·2); etynodiol diacetate (p.1554·2).
28-Day packs also contain 7 inert tablets.
*Combined oral contraceptive.*

**Zoviplus** *Glaxo Wellcome, Denm.†.*
Aciclovir (p.626·1).
*Herpesvirus infections.*

**Zovir** *GlaxoSmithKline, Denm.*
Aciclovir (p.626·1).
*Herpesvirus infections.*

**Zovirax**
*GlaxoSmithKline, Arg.; GlaxoSmithKline, Austral.; GlaxoSmithKline, Austria; GlaxoSmithKline, Belg.; GlaxoSmithKline, Braz.; GlaxoSmithKline, Canad.; GlaxoSmithKline, Chile; GlaxoSmithKline, Fin.; GlaxoSmithKline, Fr.; Boehringer Ingelheim, Ger.; GlaxoSmithKline, Ger.; Glaxo Wellcome, Gr.; GlaxoSmithKline, Hong Kong; GlaxoSmithKline, India; Wellcome, Irl.; Warner-Lambert, Irl.; Wellcome, Israel; GlaxoSmithKline, Ital.; GlaxoSmithKline, Malaysia; Glaxo Wellcome, Mex.; GlaxoSmithKline, Neth.; GlaxoSmithKline, Norw.; GlaxoSmithKline, NZ; Wellcome, Port.; GlaxoSmithKline Consumer, Port.; GlaxoSmithKline, S.Afr.; GlaxoSmithKline, Singapore; GlaxoSmithKline, Spain; GlaxoSmithKline, Swed.; GlaxoSmithKline, Switz.; GlaxoSmithKline, Thai.; GlaxoSmithKline, UK; Biovail, USA; Glaxo Wellcome, USA.*
Aciclovir (p.626·1) or aciclovir sodium (p.626·1).
*Herpesvirus infections.*

**Zoxan** *Pfizer, Fr.*
Doxazosin mesilate (p.908·3).
*Benign prostatic hyperplasia.*

**Zoxil** *Xixia, S.Afr.*
Amoxicillin trihydrate (p.155·3).
*Bacterial infections.*

**Zoylex** *BPL-Meizler, Braz.*
Aciclovir (p.626·1).
*Herpesvirus infections.*

**ZP 11** *Revlon, Canad.*
Pyrithione zinc (p.1156·2).

**ZP Dermil** *Edol, Port.*
Pyrithione zinc (p.1156·2).
*Scalp disorders.*

**Z-Pak** *Pfizer, Canad.*
Azithromycin (p.159·1).
*Bacterial infections.*

**Z-Pam** *Ralab, S.Afr.†.*
Temazepam (p.723·2).
*Hypnotic.*

**Z-Plus** *Dormer, Canad.*
Pyrithione zinc (p.1156·2); menthol (p.1711·3).
*Seborrhoeic dermatitis.*

**ZSC** *Sigma, Austral.*
Zinc oxide (p.1163·2); starch (p.1449·1); chlorphenesin (p.396·1); talc (p.1159·1).
*Hyperhidrosis; nappy rash; skin irritation.*

**Zubes** *Ernest Jackson, UK.*
Menthol (p.1711·3); anise oil (p.1655·2).

**Zubes Blackcurrant** *Ernest Jackson, UK.*
Citric acid (p.1673·1); menthol (p.1711·3); anise oil (p.1655·2).

**Zubes Honey & Lemon** *Ernest Jackson, UK.*
Honey (p.1434·2); citric acid (p.1673·1); menthol (p.1711·3).

**Zuflax** *Richmond, Arg.*
Isoflurane (p.1301·1).
*General anaesthesia.*

**zuk Schmerzgel, zuk Schmerzsalbe** *Byk Gulden, Ger.; Roland, Ger.*
Glycol salicylate (p.44·3).

Formerly known as zuk rheuma.

*Musculoskeletal, joint, peri-articular, and soft-tissue disorders; neuralgia.*

**zuk thermo** Byk Gulden, Ger.; Roland, Ger.

Glycol salicylate (p.44·3); benzyl nicotinate (p.21·2).

*Musculoskeletal and joint disorders.*

**Zuledine** Demo, Gr.

Chlorpromazine hydrochloride (p.675·2).

*Agitation; psychoses.*

**Zuleptan** Bago, Chile.

Mirtazapine (p.307·3).

*Anxiety; depression; insomnia.*

**Zulex** Almirall, Spain.

Acamprosate calcium (p.668·1).

*Alcoholism.*

**Zumalgic** Sciencex, Fr.

Tramadol hydrochloride (p.94·3).

*Pain.*

**Zumba** Crefar, Port.

Yohimbine hydrochloride (p.1766·2).

*Erectile dysfunction.*

**Zumenon**
Solvay, Austral.; Solvay, Austria; Solvay, Belg.; Solvay, Fin.; Solvay, Neth.; Solvay, Port.; Solvay, Switz.; Solvay, UK.

Estradiol (p.1550·1).

*Menopausal disorders; osteoporosis.*

**Zumetil** 20th Century, Mex.†.

Methylthioninium chloride (p.1042·2).

**Zunden** Sankyo, Ital.†.

Piroxicam (p.84·2).

*Rheumatic disorders.*

**Zundic** Asofarma, Arg.

Amlodipine besilate (p.862·1).

*Angina pectoris; hypertension.*

**Zurcal**
Novartis, Arg.; Nycomed, Austria; Novartis, Braz.; Novartis, Chile; Novartis, Mex.; Novartis, Port.; Nycomed, Switz.

Pantoprazole sodium (p.1283·1).

*Gastritis; gastro-oesophageal reflux; peptic ulcer; Zollinger-Ellison syndrome.*

**Zurcale** Exel, Belg.

Pantoprazole sodium (p.1283·1).

*Gastro-oesophageal reflux; peptic ulcer.*

**Zurcazol** Nycomed, Gr.

Pantoprazole sodium (p.1283·1).

*Peptic ulcer; reflux oesophagitis.*

**Zurfix** Phoinix Pharm (Φοινιξ Φαρμ), Gr.

Ranitidine hydrochloride (p.1285·2).

*Conditions where gastric acid reduction is beneficial; gastric hypersecretion including Zollinger-Ellison syndrome; peptic ulcer.*

**Zurim** Atral-Vida, Port.

Allopurinol (p.412·2).

*Gout; hyperuricaemia.*

**Zurinel** Prater, Chile.

Atorvastatin (p.866·2).

**Zuvair** Reddy's, India.

Zafirlukast (p.807·1).

*Asthma.*

**Zwitsalax/N** Roche Nicholas, Neth.†.

Bisacodyl (p.1251·3).

*Constipation.*

**Zwitsanal** Roche, Neth.†.

Bismuth subnitrate (p.1252·2); zinc oxide (p.1163·2); lidocaine (p.1377·3).

*Haemorrhoids.*

**Zwitsavit-D** Roche Nicholas, Neth.†.

Calcium carbonate (p.1254·2); colecalciferol (p.1461·3).

*Calcium or vitamin D deficiency.*

**Z-Xtra** Magna, USA.

Mepyramine maleate (p.437·1); benzocaine (p.1370·3); zinc oxide (p.1163·2).

*Skin disorders.*

**Zyban**
GlaxoSmithKline, Austral.; GlaxoSmithKline, Austria; GlaxoSmithKline, Belg.; GlaxoSmithKline, Braz.; GlaxoSmithKline, Canad.; GlaxoSmithKline, Denm.; GlaxoSmithKline, Fr.; GlaxoSmithKline, Ger.; Glaxo Wellcome, Gr.; GlaxoSmithKline, Hong Kong; GlaxoSmithKline, India; GlaxoSmithKline, Irl.; GlaxoSmithKline, Israel; GlaxoSmithKline, Ital.; GlaxoSmithKline, Norw.; GlaxoSmithKline, NZ; Glaxo Wellcome, Port.; GlaxoSmithKline, Singapore; GlaxoSmithKline, Swed.; GlaxoSmithKline, Switz.; GlaxoSmithKline, UK; Glaxo Wellcome, USA.

Bupropion hydrochloride (p.287·2).

*Aid to smoking withdrawal.*

**Zycalcit** Cadila, India.

Calcitonin (salmon) (p.768·2).

*Hypercalcaemia of malignancy; metastatic bone pain; osteoporosis; Paget's disease of bone.*

**Zycel** Cadila, India.

Celecoxib (p.25·2).

*Osteoarthritis; rheumatoid arthritis.*

**Zyclir** Arrow, Austral.

Aciclovir (p.626·1).

*Herpesvirus infections; HIV infection.*

**Zyderm**
Collagen, Austral.; Collagen, Austria†; Collagen, Fr.†; Collagen, Ger.; McGhan, Ger.; McGhan, Hong Kong; TC Technocare, Israel†; Inamed, Singapore.

Collagen (bovine) (p.1674·3).

Lidocaine (p.1377·3) is included in this preparation to alleviate the pain of implantation.

*Skin contour defects.*

**Zydol**
Arrow, Austral.; Pharmacia, Irl.; Pharmacia, UK.

Tramadol hydrochloride (p.94·3).

*Pain.*

**Zydone** Endo, USA.

Hydrocodone tartrate (p.45·1); paracetamol (p.76·2).

*Pain.*

**Zydowin** Zydus, India.

Zidovudine (p.658·2).

*HIV infection.*

**Zyflo** Abbott, USA.

Zileuton (p.807·3).

*Asthma.*

**Zykinase** Cadila, India.

Streptokinase (p.1005·2).

*Thromboembolic disorders.*

**Zykolat-EDO** Mann, Ger.

Cyclopentolate hydrochloride (p.480·3).

*Production of mydriasis and cycloplegia.*

**Zylapour** Pharmanik (Φαρμανικ), Gr.

Allopurinol (p.412·2).

*Gout; hyperuricaemia associated with cancer chemotherapy; kidney stones.*

**Zylium** Farmasa, Braz.

Ranitidine hydrochloride (p.1285·2).

*Acid aspiration; gastro-oesophageal reflux; gastrointestinal haemorrhage; peptic ulcer; Zollinger-Ellison syndrome.*

**Zyllergy** Dexcel, Israel.

Cetirizine hydrochloride (p.427·1).

*Allergic rhinitis; urticaria.*

**Zylol** Teva, Israel.

Allopurinol (p.412·2).

*Gout; hyperuricaemia; uric acid nephropathy.*

**Zyloprim**
Sigma, Austral.; GlaxoSmithKline, Canad.; Glaxo Wellcome, Mex.; Glaxo Wellcome, NZ†; GlaxoSmithKline, S.Afr.; Faro, USA.

Allopurinol (p.412·2).

*Gout; hyperuricaemia; renal calculi.*

**Zyloric**
GlaxoSmithKline, Austria; GlaxoSmithKline, Belg.; GlaxoSmithKline, Braz.; GlaxoSmithKline, Chile; GlaxoSmithKline, Fin.; GlaxoSmithKline, Fr.; GlaxoSmithKline, Ger.; Glaxo Wellcome, Gr.; Sigma, Hong Kong; GlaxoSmithKline, India; Wellcome, Irl.; Wellcome, Israel; GlaxoSmithKline, Ital.; GlaxoSmithKline, Malaysia; GlaxoSmithKline, Neth.; GlaxoSmithKline, Norw.; Vitoria, Port.; GlaxoSmithKline, Singapore; Faes, Spain; GlaxoSmithKline, Swed.; GlaxoSmithKline, Switz.; GlaxoSmithKline, Thai.; GlaxoSmithKline, UK.

Allopurinol (p.412·2).

*Gout; hyperuricaemia; renal calculi.*

**Zymacap** Roberts, USA.

Multivitamin preparation (p.1417·1).

**Zyma-D2** Novartis Sante, Fr.

Ergocalciferol (p.1462·1).

*Vitamin D deficiency.*

**Zymaduo** Novartis Sante, Fr.

Sodium fluoride (p.1444·3); colecalciferol (p.1461·3).

*Dental caries prophylaxis; rickets.*

**Zymafluor**
Novartis Consumer, Austria; Novartis Sante, Fr.; Novartis Consumer, Ger.; Novartis, Israel; Novartis Consumer, Ital.; Novartis Consumer, Neth.; Novartis Consumer, Port.; Novartis Consumer, S.Afr.; Novartis Consumer, Spain; Novartis Consumer, Switz.; Novartis, Thai.

Sodium fluoride (p.1444·3).

*Dental caries prophylaxis.*

**Zymafluor D** Novartis Consumer, Ger.

Sodium fluoride (p.1444·3); colecalciferol (p.1461·3).

*Dental caries prophylaxis; rickets.*

**Zymamed** Novartis Consumer, Austria.

Diclofenac potassium (p.32·1).

*Fever; pain.*

**Zymar** Allergan, USA.

Gatifloxacin (p.216·2).

*Bacterial eye infections.*

**Zymase** Organon, USA†.

Pancrelipase (p.1725·3).

*Pancreatic enzyme deficiency.*

**Zymelin**
Nycomed, Denm.; Nycomed, Norw.

Xylometazoline hydrochloride (p.1132·2).

*Otitis; rhinitis; sinusitis.*

**Zymerol** Sons, Mex.†.

Cimetidine (p.1255·3).

**Zymine** Vindex, USA.

Triprolidine hydrochloride (p.442·3).

*Allergic conjunctivitis; allergic rhinitis; allergic skin disorders.*

**Zymizinc** Aguettant, Fr.

Zinc gluconate (p.1469·2).

*Zinc deficiency.*

**Zymoplex**
Note. This name is used for preparations of different composition.

Lophal, Fr.

Cellulase, amylase, and protease from *Aspergillus*; dimeticone (p.1289·2).

Formerly contained porcine pancreatic amylase, cellulase, amylase, and protease from *Aspergillus*, lipase from *Rhizopus*, and dimeticone.

*Dyspepsia.*

Genepharm, Gr.

Tamoxifen citrate (p.584·1).

*Breast cancer.*

Sanofi, Switz.

Pancreatic protease and amylase; enzymes of *Aspergillus oryzae*; amylase (p.1654·2); protease; cellulase (p.1669·1); lipase; dimethicone (p.1289·2).

*Dyspepsia; flatulence.*

**Zynace** Xepa-Soul Pattinson, Malaysia.

Enalapril maleate (p.909·2).

*Heart failure; hypertension.*

**Zynal** Korean Drug, Singapore.

Naproxen sodium (p.65·1).

*Gout; musculoskeletal, joint, and peri-articular disorders; pain.*

**Zynicor** Zydus, India.

Nicorandil (p.965·3).

*Angina pectoris.*

**Zynor** Ivax, Irl.

Cetirizine hydrochloride (p.427·1).

*Allergic rhinitis; pruritus; urticaria.*

**Zynox** Intramed, S.Afr.†.

Naloxone hydrochloride (p.1044·3).

*Opioid toxicity.*

**Zyntabac** GlaxoSmithKline, Spain.

Bupropion hydrochloride (p.287·2).

*Aid to smoking withdrawal.*

**Zyomet** Goldshield, UK.

Metronidazole (p.607·2).

*Rosacea.*

**Zyplast**
Luxurians, Arg.; Collagen, Austral.; Collagen, Austria†; Collagen, Fr.†; Collagen, Ger.; McGhan, Ger.; McGhan, Hong Kong; TC Technocare, Israel†; Inamed, Singapore.

Collagen (bovine) (p.1674·3).

Lidocaine (p.1377·3) is included in this preparation to alleviate the pain of injection.

*Skin contour defects.*

**Zyplo**
Pfizer, Braz.; Pfizer, Mex.

Levodropropizine (p.1119·3).

*Coughs.*

**Zyprexa**
Lilly, Arg.; Lilly, Austral.; Lilly, Austria; Lilly, Belg.; Lilly, Braz.; Lilly, Canad.; Lilly, Chile; Lilly, Denm.; Lilly, Fin.; Lilly, Fr.; Lilly, Ger.; Pharmaserve Lilly (Φαρμασερβ Λιλλυ), Gr.; Lilly, Hong Kong; Lilly, Irl.; Lilly, Israel; Lilly, Ital.; Lilly, Malaysia; Lilly, Mex.; Lilly, Neth.; Lilly, Norw.; Lilly, NZ; Lilly, Port.; Lilly, S.Afr.; Lilly, Singapore; Lilly, Spain; Lilly, Swed.; Lilly, Switz.; Lilly, Thai.; Lilly, UK; Lilly, USA.

Olanzapine (p.710·3).

*Psychoses.*

**Zyquin** Cadila, India.

Gatifloxacin (p.216·2).

*Bacterial infections.*

**Zyrantol** Leovan, Gr.

Ambroxol hydrochloride (p.1114·3).

*Respiratory disorders associated with viscous mucus.*

**Zyrazine** British Dispensary, Thai.

Cetirizine hydrochloride (p.427·1).

*Allergic conjunctivitis; allergic rhinitis; allergic skin disorders; insect bites.*

**Zyrcon** Condrugs, Thai.

Cetirizine hydrochloride (p.427·1).

*Allergic rhinitis; allergic skin disorders.*

**Zyrex** Masa, Thai.

Cetirizine hydrochloride (p.427·1).

*Allergic conjunctivitis; allergic rhinitis; allergic skin disorders.*

**Zyrlex** UCB, Swed.

Cetirizine hydrochloride (p.427·1).

*Allergic conjunctivitis; allergic rhinitis; pruritus; urticaria.*

**Zyrtec**
Rontag, Arg.; UCB, Austral.; UCB, Austria; UCB, Belg.; GlaxoSmithKline, Braz.; UCB, Canad.†; GlaxoSmithKline, Chile; UCB, Denm.; UCB, Fin.; UCB, Fr.; UCB, Ger.; UCB, Hong Kong; UCB, India; Dexcel, Israel†; UCB, Jpn; Sumitomo, Jpn; UCB, Malaysia; UCB, Mex.; UCB, Neth.; UCB, Norw.; Pharmabroker, NZ; UCB, Port.; UCB, S.Afr.; UCB, Singapore; UCB, Spain; UCB, Switz.; UCB, Thai.; Pfizer, USA.

Cetirizine hydrochloride (p.427·1).

*Allergic conjunctivitis; allergic rhinitis; allergic skin disorders; urticaria.*

**Zyrtec Decongestant** Pharmabroker, NZ.

Cetirizine hydrochloride (p.427·1); pseudoephedrine hydrochloride (p.1129·2).

*Allergic rhinitis; cold symptoms.*

**Zyrtec-D**
Rontag, Arg.; GlaxoSmithKline, Braz.; GlaxoSmithKline, Chile; UCB, Mex.; Pfizer, USA.

Cetirizine hydrochloride (p.427·1); pseudoephedrine hydrochloride (p.1129·2).

*Allergic rhinitis.*

**Zyrzine** Pharmasant, Thai.†.

Cetirizine hydrochloride (p.427·1).

*Allergic conjunctivitis; allergic skin disorders; rhinitis.*

**Zytaz** Cadila, India.

Ceftazidime (p.180·2).

*Bacterial infections.*

**Zytee** Raptakos, India.

Choline salicylate (p.26·2).

*Aphthous ulcers; denture irritation; teething pain.*

**Zytine** LSP, Thai.†.

Cetirizine hydrochloride (p.427·1).

*Allergic conjunctivitis; allergic skin disorders; rhinitis.*

**Zytofen** Progress, Thai.

Ketotifen fumarate (p.788·1).

*Asthma; hypersensitivity reactions.*

**Zytram**
Napp, NZ; Douglas, NZ; Zambon, Spain.

Tramadol hydrochloride (p.94·3).

*Pain.*

**Zytrim** Merckle, Ger.

Azathioprine (p.1349·1).

*Auto-immune disorders; organ transplant rejection.*

**Zyvox**
Pharmacia, Arg.; Pharmacia, Austral.; Pharmacia, Braz.; Pharmacia, Chile; Pharmacia, Hong Kong; Pharmacia, Irl.; Pharmacia, Israel; Pharmacia, NZ; Pharmacia, Singapore; Pharmacia, UK; Pharmacia Upjohn, USA.

Linezolid (p.226·3).

*Gram-positive bacterial infections.*

**Zyvoxam**
Pharmacia, Canad.; Pharmacia Upjohn, Mex.

Linezolid (p.226·3).

*Gram-positive bacterial infections.*

**Zyvoxid**
Pharmacia, Denm.; Pharmacia, Fin.; Pharmacia, Fr.; Pharmacia, Ital.; Pharmacia, Neth.; Pharmacia, Norw.; Pharmacia, Port.; Pharmacia, Spain; Pharmacia, Swed.; Pharmacia, Switz.

Linezolid (p.226·3).

*Gram-positive bacterial infections.*

# Directory of Manufacturers

The names and addresses of the manufacturers or distributors of the products and proprietary medicines mentioned in Martindale are listed below in alphabetical order of the abbreviated names used in Part 3.

**1A, Ger.** 1 A Pharma GmbH, Keltenring 1 + 3, 82041 Oberhaching, Germany.

**20th Century, Mex.** 20th Century, Mexico.

**2K, Denm.** 2K Pharma A/S, H P Christensens Vej 1, 3000 Helsingor, Denmark.

**3M, Arg.** 3M Argentina S.A.C.I.F.I.A., Los Arboles 842, 1686 Hurlingham, Buenos Aires, Argentina.

**3M, Austral.** 3M Pharmaceuticals P/L, P.O. Box 101, Pennant Hills, NSW 2120, Australia.

**3M, Belg.** 3M Pharma S.A., Hermeslaan 7, 1831 Diegem, Belgium.

**3M, Canad.** 3M Pharmaceuticals, P.O. Box 5757, London, Ontario, N6A 4T1, Canada.

**3M, Chile.** 3M Chile SA, Santa Isabel 1001, Santiago, Chile.

**3M, Denm.** 3M Pharma, Fabriksparken 15, 2600 Glostrup, Denmark.

**3M, Fin.** Soumen 3M Oy/3M Pharma, Lars Sonckin kaari 6, PL 90, 02601 Espoo, Finland.

**3M, Fr.** Laboratoires 3M Santé, Bd de l'Oise, 95029 Cergy-Pontoise cdx, France.

**3M, Ger.** 3M Medica, Hammfelddamm 11, 41460 Neuss, Germany.

**3M, Gr.** 3M SANTE, Greece.

**3M, Hong Kong.** 3M Hong Kong Ltd, 5/F Victoria Ctr, 15 Watson Rd, North Point, Hong Kong.

**3M, Irl.** See *United Drug, Irl.*

**3M, Israel.** 3M Israel Ltd, 91 Medinat Haehudim St, Herzliya 46120, Israel.

**3M, Ital.** 3M Italia S.p.A., Via S Bovio 3, Loc. S Felice, 20090 Segrate (MI), Italy.

**3M, Malaysia.** 3M Malaysia Sdn Bhd, Bangunan 3M, 6 Persiaran Tropicana, 47410 Petaling Jaya, Selangor, Malaysia.

**3M, Mex.** 3M Mexico S.A. de C.V., Av. Santa Fe No. 55, 01210 Mexico D.F., Mexico.

**3M, Neth.** 3M Pharma Nederland BV, Industrieweg 23, 2382 NW Zoeterwoude, Netherlands.

**3M, Norw.** 3M Pharma, Hvamv.6, Postboks 100, 2013 Skjetten, Norway.

**3M, NZ.** 3M Pharmaceuticals, C.P.O. Box 2201, Auckland, New Zealand.

**3M, Port.** See *Agostinho, Port.*

**3M, S.Afr.** 3M SA (Pty) Ltd, Buildings 12 and 13, The Woodlands Office Park, Woodlands Drive, Sandton 2128, South Africa.

**3M, Singapore.** 3M Singapore Pte Ltd, 9 Tagore Lane, S 7878822, Singapore.

**3M, Spain.** 3M España, Juan Ignacio Luca de Tena 19-25, 28027 Madrid, Spain.

**3M, Swed.** 3M Svenska AB, 191 89 Sollentuna, Sweden.

**3M, Switz.** 3M (Schweiz) AG, Eggstrasse 93, 8803 Rüschlikon, Switzerland.

**3M, Thai.** 3M Thailand Ltd, 12 Fl, Stern-Mit Tower, 159 Asoke Rd, Wattana, Bangkok 10110, Thailand.

**3M, UK.** 3M Health Care Ltd, Ashby Rd, Loughborough, Leicestershire, LE11 1EP, UK.

**3M, USA.** 3M Pharmaceuticals, 3M Center 275-2E-13, P.O. Box 33275, St Paul, MN 55133-3275, USA.

**3M Espe, Ger.** 3M ESPE AG, ESPE Platz, 82229 Seefeld, Germany.

**3-OL, Israel.** 3-OL, Israel.

**7 Oaks, USA.** 7 Oaks Pharmaceutical Corp., 161 Harry Stanley Drive, Easley, SC 29640, USA.

**A Natureza, Braz.** A Natureza Produtos Farmaceuticos Ltda, Av. P. Franca 84, Sao Paulo, SP, Brazil.

**Aaciphar, Belg.** Aaciphar S.A., Chaussee de la Hulpe 166, 1170 Brussels, Belgium.

**AAH, UK.** AAH Pharmaceuticals Ltd, Sapphire Court, Walsgrave Triangle Park, Coventry, Warwickshire, CV2 2TX, UK.

**aai, USA.** aaiPharma, 2320 Scientific Park Drive, Wilmington, NC 28405, USA.

**aar, Ger.** aar pharma GmbH & Co. KG, Alleestr. 11, 42853 Remscheid, Germany.

**AB, Ital.** AB Analitica S.r.l., Via Svizzeram16, 35127 Padua, Italy.

**Abana, USA.** See *Jones, USA.*

**Abatron, UK.** Abatron Ltd, Chapel St, Potton, Sandy, Bedfordshire, SG19 2PT, UK.

**Abbott, Arg.** Abbott Laboratories Argentina S.A., Sarmiento 1113, 1041 Buenos Aires, Argentina.

**Abbott, Austral.** Abbott Australasia P/L, P.O. Box 101, Cronulla, NSW 2230, Australia.

**Abbott, Austria.** Abbott GmbH, Perfektastrasse 86, A-1230 Vienna, Austria.

**Abbott, Belg.** Abbott S.A., Parc Scientific, Rue du Bosquet 2, 1348 Louvain-la-Neuve, Belgium.

**Abbott, Braz.** Abbott Laboratorios do Brasil Ltda, Caixa Postal No. 21111, 04601-970 Sao Paulo, SP, Brazil.

**Abbott, Canad.** Abbott Laboratories Ltd, P.O. Box 6150, Station A, Montreal, Quebec, H3C 3K6, Canada.

**Abbott, Chile.** Abbott Laboratories de Chile Ltda, El Salto 5380, Huechuraba, Santiago, Chile.

**Abbott, Denm.** Abbott Laboratories A/S, Smakkedalen 6, 2820 Gentofte, Denmark.

**Abbott, Fin.** Abbott Oy, Pihatörmä 1 A, 02240 Espoo, Finland.

**Abbott, Fr.** Abbott-France, 10 rue d'Arcueil, Silic 233, 94528 Rungis cdx, France.

**Abbott, Ger.** Abbott GmbH & Co. KG, Max-Planck-Ring 2, 65205 Wiesbaden, Germany.

**Abbott, Gr.** ABBOTT LABORATORIES (ΕΛΛΑΣ) ΑΒΕΕ, Λ. Βουλιαγμένης 512, 174 56 Αλιμος, Alimos, Greece.

**Abbott, Hong Kong.** Abbott Laboratories Ltd, 20/F AIA Tower, 183 Electric Rd, North Point, Hong Kong.

**Abbott, India.** Abbott Laboratories (India) Pvt Ltd, 17 R Kamani Marg, Mumbai 400 001, India.

**Abbott, Irl.** Abbott Laboratories, Ireland Ltd, 1 Broomhill Business Park, Tallaght, Dublin 24, Ireland.

**Abbott, Israel.** See *Promedico, Israel.*

**Abbott, Ital.** Abbott S.p.A., Via Pontina Km 52, 04010 Campoverde (Latina), Italy.

**Abbott, Malaysia.** Abbott Laboratories (M) Sdn Bdh, 22 Jln Pemaju U1/15, Seksyen U1, Hicom-Glenmarie Industrial Park, 40150 Shah Alam, Selangor, Malaysia.

**Abbott, Mex.** Abbott Laboratories de Mexico S.A. de C.V., Av. Coyoacan 1622, Col. del Valle, 03100 Mexico D.F., Mexico.

**Abbott, Neth.** Abbott BV, Postbus 727, 2132 WT Hoofddorp, Netherlands.

**Abbott, Norw.** Abbott Norge AS, Nesoyv.4, Postboks 123, 1361 Billingstad, Norway.

**Abbott, NZ.** Abbott Laboratories (NZ) Ltd, P.O. Box 35-128, Naenae, Lower Hutt, New Zealand.

**Abbott, Port.** Abbott Laboratórios, Lda, Rua Cidade de Cordova, 1, Alfragide, 2720 Amadora, Portugal.

**Abbott, S.Afr.** Abbott Laboratories South Africa (Pty) Ltd, P.O. Box 1616, Johannesburg 2000, South Africa.

**Abbott, Singapore.** Abbott Laboratories (S) Pte Ltd, 1 Maritime Square, 12-01 World Trade Centre, S 099253, Singapore.

**Abbott, Spain.** Abbott Laboratories, Josefa Valcarcel 48, 28027 Madrid, Spain.

**Abbott, Swed.** Abbott Scandinavia AB, Box 509, 169 29 Solna, Sweden.

**Abbott, Switz.** Abbott AG, Neuhofstrasse 23, Postfach, 6341 Baar, Switzerland.

**Abbott, Thai.** Abbott Laboratories Ltd, 2/4 Nai Lert Tower, 5th and 9th Floor, Wireless Rd, Lumpini, Pathumwan, Bangkok 10330, Thailand.

**Abbott, UK.** Abbott Laboratories Ltd, Abbott House, Norden Rd, Maidenhead, Berkshire, SL6 4XE, UK.

**Abbott, USA.** Abbott Laboratories, 100 Abbott Park Rd, Abbott Park, IL 60064-3500, USA.

**Abbott Nutrition, UK.** Abbott Nutrition, Division of Abbott Laboratories Ltd, Abbott House, Norden Rd, Maidenhead, Berkshire, SL6 4XE, UK.

**ABC, Ital.** ABC Farmaceutici, Istituto Biologico Chemioterapico S.p.A., Via Crescentino 25, 10154 Turin, Italy.

**ABC, Port.** See *Pierre Fabre, Port.*

**AB-Consult, Austria.** AB-Consult Handels-GmbH, Eichenstrasse 32, A-1120 Vienna, Austria.

**Abello, Ger.** Abello Deutschland Pharma GmbH, Postfach: 1320, 53310 Bornheim, Germany.

**Abello, Spain.** Abello, Josefa Valcarcel 38, 28027 Madrid, Spain.

**Abic, Hong Kong.** See *International Medical, Hong Kong.*

**Abic, Israel.** See *Teva, Israel.*

**Abic, Thai.** See *RX, Thai.*

**Abic-Teva, Thai.** See *RX, Thai.*

**Abigo, Denm.** Abigo A/S, Birkholmvej 28, Osted, 4000 Roskilde, Denmark.

**Abigo, Swed.** Abigo Medical AB, 436 32 Askim, Sweden.

**Abiogen, Ital.** Abiogen Pharma S.p.A., Via Meucci 36, 56014 Ospedaletto (PI), Italy.

**Able, USA.** Able Laboratories Inc., 6 Hollywood Court, South Plainfield, NJ 07080, USA.

**Abnoba, Ger.** Abnoba Heilmittel GmbH, Hohenzollernstr. 16, 75177 Pforzheim, Germany.

**ABZ, Ger.** AbZ-Pharma GmbH, Dr. Georg-Spohn-Str. 7, 89143 Blaubeuren, Germany.

**Ace, Neth.** Ace Pharmaceuticals, P.O. Box 1262, 3890 BB Zeewolde, Netherlands.

**Ache, Braz.** Ache Laboratorios Farmaceuticos S.A., Rodovia Presidente Dutra Km 222.2, 07034-904 Guarulhos, SP, Brazil.

**Acis, Ger.** acis Arzneimittelvertrieb GmbH, Bajuwarenring 14, 82041 Oberhaching, Germany.

**Aclimacao, Braz.** Aclimacao, Brazil.

**ACM, Fr.** Laboratoires ACM, 9 bis blvd Jean-Joures, 92100 Boulogne, France.

**Acme, USA.** Acme United Corp., 1931 Black Rock Turnpike, Fairfield, CT 06432, USA.

**ACO, Swed.** ACO AB, Box 501, Nasbypark, 183 25 Taby, Sweden.

**ACO Hud, Swed.** ACO Hud AB, Box 622, 194 26 Upplands Vasby, Sweden.

**Acorus, UK.** Acorus Therapeutics Ltd, High Crane Lodge, Hamsterley, County Durham, DL13 3QS, UK.

**ACP, Belg.** A.C.P. S.C, Rue Georges Moreau 174, 1070 Brussels, Belgium.

**ACRAF, Switz.** ACRAF AG, Case postale 1067, 1701 Fribourg-Moncor, Switzerland.

**Acro, Ital.** Acro S.r.l., Via Boccaccio 45, 20123 Milan, Italy.

**ACS, Austral.** ACS International PL, 20 Clarice Rd, Box Hill, South Victoria 3128, Australia.

**ACS Dobfar, Ital.** ACS Dobfar S.p.A., V.le Addetta 6/8/10, 20067 Tribiano, Italy.

**Actelion, Austral.** Actelion Pharmaceuticals Australia Pty Ltd, Level 2, Suite 48-50, 7 Narabang Way, Belrose, NSW 2085, Australia.

**Actelion, Irl.** See *Allphar, Irl.*

**Actelion, Switz.** Actelion Ltd, Gewerbestrasse 16, 4123 Allschwil, Switzerland.

**Actelion, UK.** Actelion Pharmaceuticals UK Ltd, 500 Chiswick High Rd, Chiswick, London, W4 5RG, UK.

**Actelion, USA.** See *Actelion, Switz.*

**Actipharm, Switz.** Actipharm SA, 42-4 rue Prevost-Martin, 1211 Geneva 9, Switzerland.

**Activa, Braz.** Activa, Rua Ministro Godoi 436, 05015-000 Sao Paulo, SP, Brazil.

**Acusan, Ger.** Acusan GmbH, Rheinstr. 219, 76532 Baden-Baden, Germany.

**Adam, Mon.** Laboratoires Adam, Les Flots Bleu, 16 rue du Gabian, BP 662, MC 98013, Monaco.

**Adams, Canad.** See *Pfizer Consumer, Canad.*

**Adams, Hong Kong.** See *LCH, Hong Kong.*

**Adams, Thai.** See *Pharmaland, Thai.*

**Adams, UK.** Adams Healthcare Ltd, Lotherton Way, Garforth, Leeds, South Yorkshire, LS25 2JY, UK.

**Adams, USA.** Adams Laboratories Inc., 14801 Sovereign Rd, Fort Worth, TX 76155-2645, USA.

**Adams Confectionery, UK.** Adams Confectionery, Division of Pfizer, Lambert Court, Chestnut Ave, Eastleigh, Hampshire, SO53 3ZQ, UK.

**Adcock Ingram, S.Afr.** Adcock Ingram Pharmaceuticals Ltd, Private Bag X69, Bryanston 2021, South Africa.

**Adcock Ingram, UK.** See *Lagap, UK.*

**Adcock Ingram Critical Care, S.Afr.** Adcock Ingram Critical Care, P.O. Box 6888, Johannesburg 2000, South Africa.

**Adcock Ingram Generics, S.Afr.** See *Adcock Ingram, S.Afr.*

**Adcock Ingram Self Medication, S.Afr.** See *Adcock Ingram, S.Afr.*

**Addenda, Ital.** Addenda, Italy.

**Addicare, Ger.** See *Hexal, Ger.*

**Adelco, Gr.** ADELCO ΧΡΩΜΑΤΟΥΡΓΙΑ ΑΘΗΝΩΝ Α.Ε., Πειραιώς 37, 183 46 Μοσχάτο, Moschato, Greece.

**Adesil, Arg.** Lab. Adesil S.A., Tabare 1033, 1437 Buenos Aires, Argentina.

**Adima, Switz.** Adima SA, Case postale 1065, 1701 Fribourg, Switzerland.

**Adipharm (Αδηφαρμ), Gr.** ΑΔΗΦΑΡΜ, Μάρνη 54, 104 37 Αθήνα, Athens, Greece.

**Adivar, Ital.** Angelini Distribuzioni Varie S.p.A., Viale Amelia 70, 00181 Rome, Italy.

**Adler, Austria.** Adler-Apotheke, Wahringer Strasse 149, A-1180 Vienna, Austria.

**Adler, Switz.** Adler Apotheke, Dr Urs Reinhard AG, Untertor 39, Postfach 1241, 8401 Winterthur, Switzerland.

**Adolphs, USA.** Adolphs, 75 Merritt Blvd, Trumbull, CT 06611, USA.

**ADP, Hong Kong.** See *Australian Medic-Care, Hong Kong.*

**Adrem, Canad.** Adrem Ltd, 2000 Ellesmere Rd, Unit 16, Scarborough, Ontario, M1H 2W4, Canada.

**Adria, USA.** See *Pharmacia, USA.*

**Adroka, Switz.** Adroka AG, Postfach, 4123 Allschwil, Switzerland.

**Advance, Hong Kong.** See *Loyal Advance, Hong Kong.*

**Advance, Singapore.** See *Wellchem, Singapore.*

**Advance, USA.** Advance, 2201-F 5th Avenue, Ronkonkoma, NY 11779, USA.

**Advance Diagnostic, Irl.** Advance Diagnostic Products Ltd, Church Rd, Greystones, Co. Wicklow, Ireland.

**Advanced, Singapore.** Advanced Medi Mart Pte Ltd, 53 Kim Keat Rd, 05-02C Mun Hean Building, S 328823, Singapore.

**Advanced Biotechnologies, Israel.** See *Rafa, Israel.*

**Advanced Care, USA.** Advanced Care Products, 199 Grandview Rd, Skillman, NJ 08558-9418, USA.

**Advanced Magnetics, Israel.** See *Dexxon, Israel.*

**Advanced Medical Optics, Austral.** See *Allergan, Austral.*

**Advanced Medical Optics, NZ.** Advanced Medical Optics, 401 Shortland St, Auckland, New Zealand.

**Advanced Medical Optics, UK.** See *Allergan, UK.*

**Advanced Nutritional Technology, USA.** Advanced Nutritional Technology Inc., 6988 Sierra Court, Dublin, CA 94568-2641, USA.

**Advanced Polymer, USA.** Advanced Polymer Systems, 123 Saginaw Drive, Redwood City, CA 94063, USA.

**Advanced Sterilization Products, USA.** Advanced Sterilization Products, a Johnson & Johnson Company, 33 Technology Drive, Irvine, CA 92618-9824, USA.

**Aegis, Hong Kong.** See *Universal, Hong Kong.*

**Aero, USA.** Aero Pharmaceuticals, 3620 Park Central Blvd, Pompano Beach, FL 33064, USA.

**Aeroceuticals, USA.** See *Graham-Field, USA.*

**Aerocid, Fr.** Laboratoires Aérocid, 248 bis, rue Gabriel-Peri, 94230 Cachan, France.

**Aesca, Austria.** Aesca GmbH, Badener Strasse 23, A-2514 Traiskirchen, Austria.

**Aesculapius, Ital.** Aesculapius Farmaceutici S.r.l., Via Cozzaglio 24, 25125 Brescia, Italy.

**AF, Mex.** A.F. Laboratorios, Aplicaciones Farmaceuticas S.A. de C.V., Heriberto Frias No. 1035, Col. del Valle, Delag. Benito Juarez, 03100 Mexico D.F., Mexico.

**AFI, Norw.** See *Nycomed, Norw.*

**AFOM, Ital.** AFOM Medical S.p.A., Via S Cristoforo 97, 20090 Trezzano S/Naviglio (MI), Italy.

**Afrox, S.Afr.** Afrox, Africa Oxygen Ltd, Gate C Sigma Rd, Industries West, Germiston, South Africa.

**AFT, NZ.** AFT Pharmaceuticals, P.O. Box 87-266, Meadowbank, Auckland, New Zealand.

**AGA, Denm.** See *AGA, Swed.*

**AGA, Swed.** AGA AB, 181 81 Lidingo, Sweden.

**Agamadon, Ger.** Agamadon Biol.-Pharm.-Praparate W. Hild Nachf., Postfach: 1565, 61215 Bad Nauheim, Germany.

**Age D'or, Singapore.** Age D'or Pte Ltd, 51 Ayer Rajah Crescent, 07-01/02, S 139948, Singapore.

**Agen, Austral.** Agen Biomedical Ltd, 11 Durbell St, Acacia Ridge, QLD 4110, Australia.

**Agepha, Austria.** Agepha GmbH, Gasselberg 53-54, A-8564 Gaisfeld, Austria.

**Agepharm, Fr.** Agepharm, Airspace, rue Gagarine, F33185 Le Haillan, France.

**AGEPS, Fr.** AGEPS, Agence Generale des Equipements et Produits de Sante, Etablissement Pharmaceutique des Hopitaux de Paris, 7 rue du Fer-a-Moulin, B.P. 09, 75221 Paris cdx 5, France.

**AGIPS, Ital.** AGIPS Farmaceutici S.r.l., Via Amendola 4, 16035 Rapallo (GE), Italy.

**Agis, Israel.** Agis Industries Ltd, 29 Lehi Street, Bnei Brak 51200, Israel.

**Agostinho, Port.** António Pacheco Agostinho, SA, Rua Rodrigues Sampaio 15, 1169-012 Lisbon, Portugal.

**Agouron, Canad.** Agouron Pharmaceuticals Canada Inc., 4 Robert Speck Parkway, Suite 240, Mississauga, Ontario, L4Z 1S1, Canada.

**Agouron, USA.** Agouron Pharmaceuticals Inc., 10350 North Torrey Pines Rd, La Jolla, CA 92037-1020, USA.

**Agpharm, Switz.** Agpharm AG, Postfach, 4123 Allschwil 1, Switzerland.

**Agropharm, UK.** Agropharm Ltd, Buckingham House, Church Rd, Penn, High Wycombe, Buckinghamshire, HP10 8LN, UK.

**Agua del Carmen, Spain.** Agua del Carmen, Avda Estanislao Figueras 4, 43003 Tarragona, Spain.

**Aguettant, Fr.** Laboratoires Aguettant, 1 rue Alexander-Fleming, 69007 Lyon, France.

**AHA, UK.** AHA Sales Services Ltd, 16a St Marys St, Wallingford, Oxfordshire, OX10 OEW, UK.

**Ahimsa, Arg.** Lab. Ahimsa S.A., Lima 369 Piso 6 Of. F, 1073 Buenos Aires, Argentina.

**AHP, Switz.** AHP (Schweiz) AG, Grafenauweg 10, 6301 Zug, Switzerland.

**Airflow, NZ.** Airflow Products, P.O. Box 1485, Wellington, New Zealand.

**Ajantha, Malaysia.** See *Ranbaxy, Malaysia.*

**AJC, Fr.** Laboratoires AJC, Usine de Fontaury, 16120 Chateauneuf, France.

**Ajinomoto, Thai.** See *Far East, Thai.*, and *Zuellig, Thai.*

**Akita, UK.** See *Manx, UK.*

**Akorn, Canad.** See *Dioptic, Canad.*

**Akorn, Israel.** See *Tradis-Gat, Israel.*

**Akorn, USA.** Akorn, Inc., 2500 Millbrook Drive, Buffalo Grove, IL 60089, USA.

**AkPharma, USA.** AkPharma Inc., P.O. Box 111, Pleasantville, NJ 08232, USA.

**Akripan, Austria.** Akripan GmbH, Johann-Wiesmayer-Gasse 17, A-2332 Hennersdorf, Austria.

**Akromed, S.Afr.** See *Wyeth, S.Afr.*

**Akzo, Braz.** Akzo Nobel Ltda, 10th Floor, Avenida Brigadeiro Faria Lima 1656, 01452-001 Sao Paulo, SP, Brazil.

**Alacan, Spain.** See *ASAC, Spain.*

**Albert-Roussel, Ger.** See *Aventis, Ger.*

**Alcala, Spain.** Alcala Farma, Ctra M-300 Km 29.920, Alcala de Henares, 28802 Madrid, Spain.

**Alchemy, S.Afr.** Alchemy Pharmaceuticals CC, 21 Dadoo Ave., Mackenzieville, Nigel 1490, South Africa.

**Alckamed, Ital.** Alckamed S.r.l., Via Benedetto Marcello 24, 20124 Milano, Italy.

**Alclin, S.Afr.** Alclin (Pty) Ltd, P.O. Box 1119, Harrismith 9880, South Africa.

**Alcon, Arg.** Alcon Laboratorios Argentina S.A., Estados Unidos 5335, 1667 Tortuguitas, Buenos Aires, Argentina.

**Alcon, Austral.** Alcon Laboratories (Australia) P/L, Private Bag 19, Frenchs Forest, NSW 1640, Australia.

**Alcon, Austria.** Alcon Ophthalmika GmbH, Mariahilferstrasse 121b, A-1060 Vienna, Austria.

**Alcon, Belg.** Alcon-Couvreur S.A., Rijksweg 14, 2870 Puurs, Belgium.

**Alcon, Braz.** Alcon Laboratorios do Brasil Ltda, Avenida Nossa Senhora da Assuncao 736, 05359-001 Sao Paulo, SP, Brazil.

**Alcon, Canad.** Alcon Canada Inc., 2665 Meadowpine Blvd, Mississauga, Ontario, L5N 6R8, Canada.

**Alcon, Chile.** Laboratorios Alcon Chile Ltda, Av. Los Leones 1459, Providencia, Santiago, Chile.

**Alcon, Denm.** Alcon Danmark ApS, Rodovre Parkvej 25, 2610 Rodovre, Denmark.

**Alcon, Fin.** Alcon Finland Oy, PL 13, 01641 Vantaa, Finland.

**Alcon, Fr.** Laboratoires Alcon, 4 rue Henri-Ste-Claire-Deville, 92563 Rueil-Malmaison, France.

**Alcon, Ger.** Alcon Pharma GmbH, Blankreutestr. 1, 79108 Freiburg, Germany.

**Alcon, Hong Kong.** Alcon Hong Kong Ltd, Suites 1201-2, 625 King's Rd, North Point, Hong Kong.

**Alcon, Irl.** See *Allphar, Irl.*

**Alcon, Israel.** See *Luxembourg, Israel.*

**Alcon, Ital.** Alcon Italia S.p.A., Viale Giulio Richard 1/B, 20143 Milan, Italy.

**Alcon, Jpn.** Alcon Japan Ltd, Koraku Kokusai Building, 1-5-3, Koraku, Bunkyo-Ku, Tokyo 112-0004, Japan.

**Alcon, Malaysia.** Alcon Laboratories (Malaysia) Sdn Bhd, 1001A & 1001D, 9th Floor, Block C Kompleks Kelana Centre Point, No 3 Jalan SS 7/19, Kelana Jaya, 47301 Petaling Jaya, Selangor, Malaysia.

**Alcon, Mex.** Alcon Laboratorios, S.A. de C.V., Jose Ma. Rico No. 418, Esq. Linares, Colonia Del Valle, 03100 Mexico D.F., Mexico.

**Alcon, Norw.** Alcon Norge AS, Eyvind Lychesv 10, Postboks 22, 1300 Sandvika, Norway.

**Alcon, NZ.** Alcon Laboratories Ltd, P.O. Box 14-562, Panmure, Auckland, New Zealand.

**Alcon, Port.** Alcon Portugal, Lda, Rua Castilho, 201-1, 1070-051 Lisbon, Portugal.

**Alcon, S.Afr.** Alcon Laboratories (South Africa) (Pty) Ltd, 261 Surrey Ave, Randburg, South Africa.

**Alcon, Singapore.** Alcon Pte Ltd, 159 Sin Ming Rd, 06-05 Amtech Building, S 575625, Singapore.

**Alcon, Swed.** Alcon Sverige AB, Box 12233, 102 26 Stockholm, Sweden.

**Alcon, Switz.** Alcon Pharmaceuticals Ltd, Bosch 69, Postfach 62, 6331 Hunenberg, Switzerland.

**Alcon, Thai.** Alcon Laboratories (Thailand) Ltd, 191 Silom Rd, 18 Fl, Silom Complex Building, Bangkok 10500, Thailand.

**Alcon, UK.** Alcon Laboratories (UK) Ltd, Pentagon Park, Boundry Way, Hemel Hempstead, Hertfordshire, HP2 7UD, UK.

**Alcon, USA.** Alcon Laboratories Inc., 6201 South Freeway, Fort Worth, TX 76134, USA.

**Alcon Cusi, Malaysia.** See *Alcon, Malaysia*, and *Summit, Malaysia.*

**Alcon Cusi, Spain.** Alcon Cusi, Camil Fabra 58, El Masnou, 08320 Barcelona, Spain.

**Alcon-Thilo, Ger.** See *Alcon, Ger.*

**Alcor, Spain.** Alcor, P Del Prado 14 1 C, 28014 Madrid, Spain.

**Aldo, Spain.** Aldo Union, Baronesa De Malda 73, Esplugas de Llobregat, 08950 Barcelona, Spain.

**Aldo-Union, Hong Kong.** See *Hong Kong Medical, Hong Kong.*

**Aldo-Union, Singapore.** See *Green Cross, Singapore.*

**Aldo-Union, Thai.** See *Greater Pharma, Thai.*

**Ale, Spain.** Ale Pedemonte, Pasaje Jaime Roig 26-8, 08028 Barcelona, Spain.

**Alembic, India.** Alembic Ltd, Alembic Rd, Vadodara 390 003, India.

**Alembic Products, UK.** Alembic Products Ltd, River Lane, Saltney, Chester, Cheshire, CH4 8RQ, UK.

**Aleph, Ital.** Aleph S.r.l., Via Liborio Coccetti 8, 06034 Foligno PG, Italy.

**Alergomed, Braz.** See *Daudt, Braz.*

**Alfa Biotech, Ital.** See *Wassermann, Ital.*

**Alfa Intes, Ital.** Industria Terapeutica Splendore - Oftalmoterapica ALFA, Via F.lli Bandiera 26, 80026 Casoria (NA), Italy.

**Alfa Wassermann, Thai.** See *Charoen, Thai.*

**Alfaco, Neth.** Alfaco, Baldschermweg 6B, 3821 AH Amersfoort, Netherlands.

**Algol, Fin.** Algol Oy, Lääkeosasto, Karapellontie 6, PL 13, 02611 Espoo, Finland.

**Alifarma, Ital.** Alifarma S.r.l., Via Piane 64, 47853 Coriano (RN), Italy.

**Aliud, Austria.** Aliud Pharma GmbH & Co. KG, Johann-Strauss-Gasse 7/5, A-1040 Vienna, Austria.

**Aliud, Ger.** Aliud Pharma GmbH & Co. KG, Gottlieb-Daimler-Str 19, 89150 Laichingen, Germany.

**ALK, Austria.** Alk-Abello Allergie-Service GmbH, Backermuhlweg 59, A-4030 Linz, Austria.

**ALK, Belg.** See *ALK, Neth.*

**ALK, Denm.** ALK-Abelló Danmark, Borups Alle 177, D4 (postboks 400), 2000 Frederiksberg, Denmark.

**ALK, Fin.** ALK-Abelló A/S, Liluodontie 17 B, 2. krs, 00980 Helsinki, Finland.

**ALK, Ital.** Alk-Abello S.p.A., Via Settembrini 60, 20020 Lainate (MI), Italy.

**ALK, Neth.** ALK-Abelló BV, Edisonbaan 26, 3430 BA Nieuwegein, Netherlands.

**ALK, Norw.** ALK Norge, Spireav. 6, Postboks 218 Okern, 0580 Oslo, Norway.

**ALK, Spain.** Alk Abello, Miguel Fleta 19, 28037 Madrid, Spain.

**ALK, Swed.** ALK Sverige AB, Smorhalevagen 3, 434 42 Kungsbacka, Sweden.

**ALK, UK.** ALK-Abelló (UK), 2 Tealgate, Hungerford, Berkshire, RG17 0YT, UK.

**ALK, USA.** ALK-Abelló Inc., 1700 Royston Lane, Round Rock, TX 78664, USA.

**Alk-Abello, NZ.** See *CSL, NZ.*

**Alkaloida, Thai.** See *Medline, Thai.*

**Alkapharm, Singapore.** See *Wellchem, Singapore.*

**Alkon (Αλκον), Gr.** ΑΛΚΟΝ ΑΕΒΕ, Κηφισίας 18, 151 25 Μαρούσι, Marousi, Greece.

**Alk-Scherax, Ger.** Alk-Scherax Arzneimittel GmbH, Sulldorfer Landstr. 128, 22589 Hamburg, Germany.

**Allen, Austria.** See *GlaxoSmithKline, Austria.*

**Allen, Gr.** ALLEN, Φιλλελήνων 34, 152 32 Χαλάνδρι, Chalandri, Greece.

**Allen, Mex.** Allen Laboratorios, S.A. de C.V., Av. Instituto Politecnico Nacional No. 4728, Col. Tlacamaca, Deleg. Gustavo A Madero, 07380 Mexico D.F, Mexico.

**Allen, Spain.** See *GlaxoSmithKline, Spain.*

**Allen & Hanburys, Austral.** See *GlaxoSmithKline, Austral.*

**Allen & Hanburys, Irl.** See *GlaxoSmithKline, Irl.*

**Allen & Hanburys, UK.** See *GlaxoSmithKline, UK.*

**Allens, UK.** Allens & Co. (Anglesey) Ltd, Freshwinds, Pentraeth, Isle of Anglesey, Gwynedd, LL75 8YF, UK.

**Allerbio, Fr.** Laboratoires Allerbio, 55270 Varennes-en-Argonne, France.

**Allerex, Canad.** Allerex Laboratory Ltd, P.O. Box 13307, Kanata, Ontario, K2K 1X5, Canada.

**Allergan, Arg.** Allergan-Loa S.A.I.C. y F., Rafaela 4831, 1407 Buenos Aires, Argentina.

**Allergan, Austral.** Allergan Australia P/L, 77 Ridge St, Gordon, NSW 2072, Australia.

**Allergan, Austria.** Pharm-Allergan GmbH, Wienerbergstrasse 11 Twin Tower, A-1100 Vienna, Austria.

**Allergan, Belg.** Allergan S.A., Meir 44 A, 2000 Antwerp, Belgium.

**Allergan, Braz.** See *Allergan-Frumtost, Braz.*

**Allergan, Canad.** Allergan Inc., 110 Cochrane Dr., Markham, Ontario, L3R 9S1, Canada.

**Allergan, Chile.** Laboratorios Alllergan Ltda, Vitacura 2736, Piso 15, Las Condes, Santiago, Chile.

**Allergan, Denm.** Allergan A/S, Produktionsvej 14, 2600 Glostrup, Denmark.

**Allergan, Fin.** Allergan Norden AB, Rajatorpantie 41 C, 01640 Vantaa, Finland.

**Allergan, Fr.** Allergan France, Font de l'Orme, av Dr Maurice-Donat, B.P. 442, 06254 Mougins, France.

**Allergan, Ger.** Pharm-Allergan GmbH, Pforzheimer Str.160, 76275 Ettlingen, Germany.

**Allergan, Gr.** Allergan, Greece.

**Allergan, Hong Kong.** Allergan Asia Ltd, Unit 3001 Metroplaza Tower 1, 223 Hing Fong Rd, Kwai Fong, N.T., Hong Kong.

**Allergan, India.** Allergan India Ltd, 9th Floor, North Block, Manipal Center, 47 Dickenson Road, Bangalore 560 042, India.

**Allergan, Irl.** Allergan Ltd, Pharmapark, California Heights, Dublin 20, Ireland.

**Allergan, Israel.** See *Tradis-Gat, Israel.*

**Allergan, Ital.** Allergan S.p.A., Via S Quasimodo 134/138, 00144 Rome EUR (Rome), Italy.

**Allergan, Jpn.** Allergan K.K., Toranomon 40 Mori Building, 13-1 Toranomon 5-Chome, Minato-ku, Tokyo 105-0001, Japan.

**Allergan, Malaysia.** See *Diethelm, Malaysia.*

**Allergan, Mex.** Allergan, S.A. de C.V., Mier y Perado No. 126, Col Del Valle, 03100 Mexico D.F., Mexico.

**Allergan, Norw.** See *Allergan, Swed.*

**Allergan, NZ.** Allergan Pharmaceuticals, P.O. Box 1873, Auckland 1, New Zealand.

**Allergan, Port.** Allergan S.A., Av. Do Forte 3 - Edif. Suecia IV, 1 Piso, 2795-504 Carnaxide, Portugal.

**Allergan, S.Afr.** Allergan Pharmaceuticals (Pty) Ltd, P.O. Box 3911, Halfway House 1685, South Africa.

**Allergan, Singapore.** See *JDH, Singapore.*

**Allergan, Spain.** Allergan, Avda Industria 24, Tres Cantos, 28760 Madrid, Spain.

**Allergan, Swed.** Allergan Norden AB, Business Campus, 194 81 Upplands Vasby, Sweden.

**Allergan, Switz.** Allergan AG, Feldmoosstrasse 6, 8853 Lachen, Switzerland.

**Allergan, Thai.** See *Maxim, Thai.*

**Allergan, UK.** Allergan Ltd, Crown Centre, Coronation Rd, Cressex Industrial Estate, High Wycombe, Buckinghamshire, HP12 3SH, UK.

**Allergan, USA.** Allergan Pharmaceuticals Inc., 2525 Dupont Dr., P.O. Box 19534, Irvine, CA 92623-9534, USA.

**Allergan Herbert, USA.** See *Allergan, USA.*

**Allergan-Frumtost, Braz.** Lab. Allergan Frumtost Ltda, Rua Dr. Cardoso de Melo 1855, 2 Andar, 04548-005 Sao Paulo, SP, Brazil.

**Allergomed, Switz.** Allergomed AG, Erlenstrasse 29, Postfach 117, 4106 Therwil, Switzerland.

**Allergopharma, Ger.** Allergopharma Joachim Ganzer KG, Hermann-Korner-Str. 52, 21465 Reinbek, Germany.

**Allergopharma, Switz.** See *Allergomed, Switz.*

**Allergy Therapeutics, Canad.** Allergy Therapeutics (Canada) Ltd, 1345 Fewster Drive, Mississauga, Ontario, L4W 2A5, Canada.

**Allergy Therapeutics, UK.** Allergy Therapeutics Ltd, Dominion Way, Worthing, West Sussex, BN14 8SA, UK.

**Allga, Austria.** Allga-Pharma Austria GmbH, Am Barentobel 215, A-6942 Krumbach, Austria.

**Alliance, Irl.** See *United Drug, Irl.*

**Alliance, S.Afr.** Alliance Pharmaceuticals Ltd, P.O. Box 261269, Excom 2023, South Africa.

**Alliance, UK.** Alliance Pharmaceuticals Ltd, Avonbridge House, Bath Rd, Chippenham, Wiltshire, SN15 2BB, UK.

**Alliance, USA.** Alliance Pharmaceuticals, 3040 Science Park Rd, San Diego, CA 92121, USA.

**Allmedica, Ger.** Allmedica Arzneimittel GmbH, Schillerstr. 4, 37269 Eschwege, Germany.

**Allmi-Care, UK.** Allmi-Care Ltd, U20 Lenton Business Centre, Lenton Boulevard, Nottingham, Nottinghamshire, NG7 2BY, UK.

**Allo Pro, Austria.** Allo Pro GmbH, Enzersdorfer Strasse 12A, A-2340 Modling, Austria.

**Allphar, Irl.** Allphar Services Ltd, Belgard Rd, Tallaght, Dublin 24, Ireland.

**Alltracel, Hong Kong.** See *Mekim, Hong Kong.*

**Alltracel, Irl.** Alltracel Pharma Ltd, Alltracel House, Church Place, Sallynoggin, Co. Dublin, Ireland.

**Almed, Switz.** Divapharma Chur AG, Abteilung Almed, Ankerstrasse 53, 8026 Zurich, Switzerland.

**Almi, Spain.** Almi, Alberto Alcocer 24, 28036 Madrid, Spain.

**Almirall, Belg.** Almirall Prodesfarma, Medialaan 32 B 4, 1800 Vilvoorde, Belgium.

**Almirall, Denm.** See *Lundbeck, Denm.*

**Almirall, Hong Kong.** See *Sincerity, Hong Kong.*

**Almirall, Neth.** Almirall, Netherlands.

**Almirall, Norw.** See *Lundbeck, Norw.*

**Almirall, Singapore.** See *Zyfas, Singapore.*

**Almirall, Spain.** Almirall Prodesfarma, Rda Gral Mitre 151, 08022 Barcelona, Spain.

**Alodial, Port.** Alodial Farmacêutica Lda, Sintra Business Park, Edificio 1 - Fraccao 1G, Abrunheira, 2710-089 Sintra, Portugal.

**Alonga, Spain.** See *Sanofi Synthelabo, Spain.*

**Alpes Chemie, Chile.** Alpes Chemie SA, Av. Pedro de Valdivia 1307, Providencia, Santiago, Chile.

**Alpha, Hong Kong.** See *Keller, Hong Kong.*

**Alpha, Israel.** See *Medogar, Israel.*

**Alpha, Mex.** Laboratorios Alpha S.A. de C.V., Heroes Ferrocarrileros No. 1325, Ferrocarril, 44440 Jalisco Guadalajara, Mexico.

**Alpha, NZ.** Alpha Pharmaceuticals Ltd, P.O. Box 705, Palmerston North, New Zealand.

**Alpha Therapeutic, Ger.** Alpha Therapeutic GmbH, Siemensstr. 18, Postfach: 1107, 63201 Langen, Germany.

**Alpha Therapeutic, Ital.** Alpha Therapeutic Italia SpA, Piazza Meda 3, Milan, Italy.

**Alpha Therapeutic, Malaysia.** Alpha Therapeutic (Malaysia) Sdn Bhd, 1202 Menara PJ, 18 Jln Persiaran Barat, 46050 Petaling Jaya, Selangor, Malaysia.

**Alpha Therapeutic, Singapore.** Alpha Therapeutic Asia Pte Ltd, 1 Maritime Square, 10-33A World Trade Centre, S 099253, Singapore.

**Alpha Therapeutic, Thai.** Alpha Therapeutic (Thailand) Ltd, 8 Fl, Liberty Square, 287 Silom Rd, Bangrak, Bangkok 10500, Thailand.

**Alpha Therapeutic, USA.** Alpha Therapeutic Corp., 2410 Lillyvale Ave, Los Angeles, CA 90032-3514, USA.

**Alphapharm, Austral.** Alphapharm P/L, P.O. Box 36, Camperdown, NSW 1450, Australia.

**Alphapharm, Hong Kong.** See *LCH, Hong Kong.*

**Alphapharm, Malaysia.** See *Summit, Malaysia*, and *Zuellig, Malaysia.*

**Alphapharm, Singapore.** See *Zuellig, Singapore.*

**Alpharma, Denm.** Alpharma ApS, Dalslandsgade 11 (postboks 1736), 2300 Copenhagen S, Denmark.

**Alpharma, Fin.** Alpharma Oy, Sinimäentie 10 B, 02630 Espoo, Finland.

**Alpharma, Fr.** Alpharma France, 40 rue Lecuyer, 93300 Aubervilliers, France.

**Alpharma, Hong Kong.** See *Primal, Hong Kong.*

**Alpharma, Malaysia.** See *Apex, Malaysia.*

**Alpharma, Mex.** Laboratorios Alpharma, S.A. de C.V., Boulevard Pipila No.1, Esq. Av. del Conscripto, Col. M.A. Camacho, Deleg. Miguel Hidalgo, 11610 Mexico D.F., Mexico.

**Alpharma, Norw.** Alpharma AS, Harbitzalleen 3, Postboks 158 Skoyen, 0212 Oslo, Norway.

**Alpharma, Port.** Alpharma ApS, Rua Virgilio Correira 11A, 1600-219 Lisbon, Portugal.

**Alpharma, Singapore.** See *Pharmed, Singapore*, and *Sime Darby, Singapore.*

**Alpharma, Swed.** Alpharma AB, 112 89 Stockholm, Sweden.

**Alpharma, Switz.** See *Dumex, Switz.*

**Alpharma, UK.** Alpharma Ltd, Whiddon Valley, Barnstaple, Devon, EX32 8NS, UK.

**Alpharma, USA.** Alpharma USPD Inc, 7205 Windsor Blvd, Baltimore, MD 21244, USA.

**Alpharma-Isis, Ger.** Alpharma-Isis Pharma GmbH & Co. KG, Elisabeth-Selbert-Str. 1, 40764 Langenfeld, Germany.

**Alphrema, Ital.** Alphrema S.r.l., Via Mascagni 2, 20020 Lainate (MI), Italy.

**Alpinamed, Switz.** Alpinamed AG, Pharmazeutische Produkte, 9306 Freidorf, Switzerland.

**Alpro, Spain.** See *Almirall, Spain.*

**Alps, S.Afr.** Alps, South Africa.

**Alra, USA.** Alra Laboratories Inc., 3850 Clearview Court, Gurnee, IL 60031, USA.

**Alsi, Canad.** Alsi Cie Ltee, 150 rue Seigneuriale, Beauport, Quebec, G1E 3B3, Canada.

**Alsitan, Ger.** Alsitan GmbH & Co. KG, Am Buhl 16-18, 86926 Greifenberg, Germany.

**Also, Ital.** Also S.p.A., Viale Monte Rosa 96, 20149 Milan, Italy.

**Altaire, USA.** Altaire Pharmaceuticals, Inc., 91 Colin Dr. 1, Holbrook, NY 11741, USA.

**Altana, Austral.** Altana Pharma Pty Ltd, Level 2, 71 Epping Rd, North Ryde, NSW 2113, Australia.

**Altana, Braz.** Altana Pharma Ltda, Rua do Estilo Barroco 721, Santo Amaro, 04709-011 Sao Paulo, SP, Brazil.

**Altana, Fr.** ALTANA Pharma S.A.S., 389 rue du Pressoir, 77350 le Mee-sur-Seine, France.

**Altana, Ger.** Altana Pharma Deutschland GmbH, Moltkestr. 4, 78467 Constance, Germany.

**Altana, Hong Kong.** Altana Pharma (HK), 608, 6/F, Devon House, Taikoo Place, Hong Kong.

**Altana, Malaysia.** Altana Pharma, 1 Jln SS 20/27, 47400 Petaling Jaya, Selangor, Malaysia.

**Altana, Mex.** Altana Pharma S.A. de C.V., Av Primero de Mayo No. 130, Col. San Andres Atoto, 53519 Naucalpan de Juarez., Mexico.

**Altana, Neth.** Altana, Netherlands.

**Altana, Spain.** Altana Pharma, Francisca Delgado 1, Parque Empresarial, Arryo de la Vega – Alcobendas, 28108 Madrid, Spain.

**Altana, Switz.** Altana Pharma Ltd, Bachstrasse 10, 8280 Kreuzlingen, Switzerland.

**Altana, UK.** Altana Pharma Ltd, Three Globeside Business Mark, Fieldhouse Lane, Marlow, Buckinghamshire, SL7 1HZ, UK.

**Altana, USA.** Altana Inc., 60 Baylis Rd, Melville, NY 11747, USA.

**Altana Consumer, Ger.** Altana Consumer Health GmbH, Bargkoppelweg 66, 22145 Hamburg, Germany.

**Alte Kreis, Austria.** Alte Kreis-Apotheke, Untere Hauptstrasse 1, A-7100 Neusiedl am See, Austria.

**Alter, Port.** Alter, SA, Estrada Marco do Grilo, Zemouto, 2830 Coina, Portugal.

**Alter, Spain.** Alter, Mateo Inurria 30, 28036 Madrid, Spain.

**Alterna, Ital.** Alterna Farmaceutici S.r.l., Via dei Pestagalli 7, 20138 Milan, Italy.

**Althin, Swed.** See *Baxter, Swed.*

**Altimed, Canad.** Altimed Pharma Inc., Division of Technilab Pharma Inc., 200 Natheson Bvld W, Suite 203, Mississauga, Ontario, L5R 3L7, Canada.

**Alva, USA.** Alva-Amco Pharmacal Inc., 7711 North Meremac Ave, Niles, IL 60714-3423, USA.

**Alvia (Αλβια), Gr.** ΑΛΒΙΑ ΑΕ, 18ο χλμ. Λ. Αθηνών-Μαραθώνος, 153 44 Παλλήνη, Pallini, Greece.

**Alza, Canad.** See *Janssen-Ortho, Canad.*

**Alza, Denm.** See *AstraZeneca, Denm.*

**Alza, Irl.** See *Cambridge, UK.*

**Alza, Singapore.** See *Faulding, Singapore.*

**Alza, USA.** Alza Corp., 1900 Charleston Ave, Mountain View, CA 94039, USA.

**AM, Arg.** Laboratorio A.M. Farma Activ, Italia 743, Santa Fe, Argentina.

**Amadeus, India.** Amadeus Biotech & Pharmaceuticals, Shreya House, 301/A Pereira Hill Rd, Andheri (E), Mumbai 400 099, India.

**AMBI, USA.** AMBI Pharmaceuticals Inc., 16206A Flight Path Drive, Brooksville, FL 34604-6875, USA.

**Ambix, USA.** Ambix Laboratories Inc., 210 Orchard St, Rutherford, NJ 07073, USA.

**Amcon, USA.** Amcon Laboratories, 40 North Rock Hill Rd, St Louis, MO 63119, USA.

**Amcron, Thai.** Amcron Enterprise Co. Ltd, 2711 Pattanakarn Rd, Suan Luang, Bangkok 10250, Thailand.

**Amdipharm, UK.** Amdipharm Plc, Regency House, Miles Gray Rd, Basildon, Essex, SS14 3AF, UK.

**Amenite, Arg.** Laboratorio Amenite, Caracas 4721, 1419 Buenos Aires, Argentina.

**American de Mexico, Mex.** Lab. American de Mexico S.A. de C.V., Av. Del Taller Retorno 7, Venustiano Carranza Jardmn Balbu, 15900 Mexico D.F., Mexico.

**American Health, Hong Kong.** See *Jebsen, Hong Kong.*

**American Lecithin, USA.** American Lecithin Co., 115 Hurley Rd, Unit 2B, Oxford, CT 06478, USA.

**American Medical, USA.** American Medical Industries, 28045 Ashley Circle 106, Libertyville, IL 60048, USA.

**American Pharmaceutical, USA.** American Pharmaceutical Partners Inc., 10866 Wiltshire Blvd, Suite 1270, Los Angeles, CA 90024, USA.

**American Red Cross, USA.** American Red Cross, 1616 Ft Myer Drive 17th Floor, Arlington, VA 22209-3100, USA.

**American Regent, USA.** American Regent, 1 Luitpold Drive, Shirley, NY 11967, USA.

**American Remedies, Malaysia.** See *Antah, Malaysia.*

**American Urologicals, USA.** American Urologicals Inc., 10031 Pines Blvd, Suite 216, Pembroke Pines, FL 33024, USA.

**Amersham, Austral.** Amersham Health Pty Ltd, Unit 4, 2 Eden Park Drive, North Ryde, NSW 2113, Australia.

**Amersham, Belg.** Amersham Health S.A., Koningin Astridlaan 49, 1780 Wemmel, Belgium.

**Amersham, Canad.** Amersham Health Canada Ltd, 1166 South Service Rd West, Oakville, Ontario, L6L 5T7, Canada.

**Amersham, Denm.** Amersham Health A/S, Slotsmarken 15, 2970 Horsholm, Denmark.

**Amersham, Fin.** Oy Amersham Health AB, Rajatorpantie 41 B, 01640 Vantaa, Finland.

**Amersham, Fr.** Amersham Health SA, 140 av Jean-Lolive, 93500 Pantin, France.

**Amersham, Ger.** See *Amersham Buchler, Ger.*

**Amersham, Ital.** See *Nycomed, Ital.*

**Amersham, Norw.** Amersham Health AS, Nycov. 2, Postboks 4220 Nydalen, 0401 Oslo, Norway.

**Amersham, NZ.** Amersham Health Ltd, Unit F, 156 Bush Rd, Albany, Auckland, New Zealand.

**Amersham, Spain.** Amersham Health, Ronda de Poniente, 12, Tres Cantos, 28760 Madrid, Spain.

**Amersham, Swed.** Amersham Health AB, Box 602, 16926 Solna, Sweden.

**Amersham, UK.** Amersham Health, The Grove Centre, White Lion Rd, Amersham, Buckinghamshire, HP7 9LL, UK.

**Amersham, USA.** Amersham Health Inc., 101 Carnegie Center, Princeton, NJ 08540-6231, USA.

**Amersham Buchler, Ger.** Amersham Buchler GmbH & Co. KG, Fraunhoferstr. 7, 85737 Ismaning b. Munich, Germany.

**Amerx, USA.** Amerx Health Care Corp., 1150 Cleveland St, Suite 410, Clearwater, FL 33755, USA.

**Ames, Irl.** See *Bayer Diagnostics, Irl.*

**Ames, Israel.** See *Bayer, Israel.*

**Amgen, Austral.** Amgen Australia P/L, P.O. Box 410, North Ryde, NSW 1670, Australia.

**Amgen, Austria.** Amgen GmbH, Prinz Eugen-Strasse 8-10, A-1040 Vienna, Austria.

**Amgen, Belg.** Amgen S.A., Ave Ariane 5, 1200 Brussels, Belgium.

**Amgen, Canad.** Amgen Canada Inc., 6755 Mississauga Rd, Suite 400, Mississauga, Ontario, L5N 7Y2, Canada.

**Amgen, Denm.** Amgen AB, Strandvejen 203, 2900 Hellerup, Denmark.

**Amgen, Fin.** Amgen AB, PL 75, 02201 Espoo, Finland.

**Amgen, Fr.** Amgen, 192 av Charles-de-Gaulle, 92200 Neuilly-sur-Seine, France.

**Amgen, Ger.** Amgen GmbH, Hanauer Str. 1, 80992 Munich, Germany.

**Amgen, Gr.** See *Genesis, Gr.*

**Amgen, Irl.** See *United Drug, Irl.*

**Amgen, Israel.** See *Megapharm, Israel.*

**Amgen, Ital.** Amgen Spa, Via E Tazzoli 6, 20154 Milan, Italy.

**Amgen, Neth.** Amgen Europe BV, Minervum 7061, 4817 ZG Breda, Netherlands.

**Amgen, Norw.** Amgen, Kronprinsensg 1, 0251 Oslo, Norway.

**Amgen, Port.** Amgen Biofarmaceutica, Lda, Tagus Park, Edificio Eastecnica, 2780-920 Porto Salvo, Portugal.

**Amgen, Spain.** Amgen, Muelle Barcelona S/N Ed, Sur 8 World Trade Centre, 08039 Barcelona, Spain.

**Amgen, Swed.** Amgen AB, Box 34107, 100 26 Stockholm, Sweden.

**Amgen, UK.** Amgen Ltd, 240 Cambridge Science Park, Milton Rd, Cambridge, Cambridgeshire, CB4 4WD, UK.

**Amgen, USA.** Amgen Inc., One Amgen Center Drive, Thousand Oaks, CA 91320-1799, USA.

**Amgros, Denm.** Amgros I/S, Dampfaergevej 22 (postboks 2593), 2100 Copenhagen O, Denmark.

**Amhof, Arg.** Lab. Amhof Maurino S.A., Nogoya 4811/15, 1407 Buenos Aires, Argentina.

**Amide, USA.** Amide Pharmaceuticals Inc., 101 East Main Street, Little Falls, NJ 07424, USA.

**Amido, Fr.** Laboratoires Amido, 37 av Gabriel-Peri, 92500 Rueil-Malmaison, France.

**Amino, Switz.** Amino AG, Althofstrasse 12, 5432 Neuenhof, Switzerland.

**Amirose, UK.** Amirose International, 249 Cranbrook Rd, Ilford, Essex, UK.

**Amnol, Ital.** Amnol Chimica Biologica S.r.l., C.so della Vittoria 12/b, 28100 Novara (NO), Italy.

**AMO, Austral.** Advanced Medical Optics, Level 1, 77 Ridge St, Gordon, NSW 2072, Australia.

**AMO, Singapore.** See *JDH, Singapore.*

**AMO, UK.** AMO (UK) Ltd, Jupiter House, Mercury Park, Wooburn Green, High Wycombe, Buckinghamshire, HP10 0HH, UK.

**Amphastar, USA.** Amphastar Pharmaceuticals Inc., 11570 6th St, Rancho Cucamonga, CA 91730, USA.

**Amrad, Austral.** See *Merck Sharp & Dohme, Austral.*

**Amrad, NZ.** See *CSL, NZ.*

**Amsa, Ital.** Amsa S.r.l., Passeggiata Ripetta 22, 00186 Rome, Italy.

**Amsco, USA.** See *Steris, USA.*

**Amternes, Denm.** Amternes Laegemiddelregistreringskontor I/S, Amstradsforeningen, Dampfaergevej 22 (postboks 2593), 2100 Copenhagen O, Denmark.

**Amuchina, Ital.** Amuchina S.p.A., Via Pontasso 13, 16015 Genoa (GE), Italy.

**Amway, Canad.** Amway Corp., 375 Exeter Rd, London, Ontario, N5Y 5V6, Canada.

**ANB, Malaysia.** See *Sime Darby, Malaysia.*

**ANB, Thai.** ANB Laboratories Co. Ltd, 39/1 Ram-Intra Rd, Kanayao, Bangkok 10230, Thailand.

**Anben, Fr.** Anben Pharma, 14 av P. Mendes-France, 67300 Schiltigheim, France.

**Anben, Israel.** See *Kivema, Israel.*

**Anben, Malaysia.** See *Antah, Malaysia.*

**Ancient, Austral.** Ancient Distributors, 2/16 Commercial Drive, Dandenong, VIC 3175, Australia.

**Andersen, Norw.** Jan F. Andersen A/S, Postboks 1132 Flattum, 3501 Honefoss, Norway.

**Andrae, Austria.** Andrae GmbH, Marinonigasse 2-6, A-1210 Vienna, Austria.

**Andre, India.** Andre Laboratories Pvt Ltd, 495/7 & 8 GIDC, Makarpura, Vadodara 390 101, India.

**Andreabal, Switz.** Andreabal AG, Rudolfstrasse 2, 4054 Basle, Switzerland.

**Andreu, Spain.** See *Roche, Spain.*

**Andromaco, Arg.** Laboratorios Andrómaco S.A.I.C.I., Ingeniero Huergo 1145, 1107 Buenos Aires, Argentina.

**Andromaco, Chile.** Laboratorios Andromaco SA, Av. Quilin 5273, Penalolen, Santiago, Chile.

**Andromaco, Mex.** Industria Farmaceutica Andromaco, S.A. de C.V., Andromaco No. 104, Col. Ampliacion Granada, Deleg. Miguel Hidalgo, 11520 Mexico D.F., Mexico.

**Andromaco, Port.** Laboratórios Andrómaco, Lda, Rua Alfredo da Silva 16, 2720-028 Amadora, Portugal.

**Andromaco, Spain.** See *Grunenthal, Spain.*

**Andrx, USA.** Andrx Pharmaceuticals Inc., 4001 SW 47th Ave, Fort Lauderdale, FL 33314, USA.

**Aneid, Port.** Aneid, Lda, Rua Jose Florindo, Quinta da Pedra, Bloco B, R/C A, 2750-401 Cascais, Portugal.

**Angelini, Hong Kong.** See *JDH, Hong Kong.*

**Angelini, Israel.** See *Rafa, Israel.*

**Angelini, Ital.** Aziende Chimiche Riunite Angelini Francesco S.p.A., Viale Amelia 70, 00181 Rome, Italy.

**Anglian, UK.** Anglian Pharma Plc, P.O. Box 161, Hitchin, Hertfordshire, SG4 7WE, UK.

**Anglo-French Drugs, India.** Anglo-French Drugs & Industries Ltd, 41, 3rd Cross, S.S.I. Area, V Block, Rajaji Nagar, Bangalore 560 010, India.

**Anglo-French Drugs, Thai.** Anglo-French Drugs.

**Anifer, Austria.** See *Hofmann, Austria.*

**Anika, Israel.** See *Rafa, Israel.*

**Anios, Fr.** Laboratoires Anios, Pave du Moulin, 59260 Lille-Hellemmes, France.

**Anmarate, S.Afr.** Anmarate (Pty) Ltd, P.O. Box 400, George 6530, South Africa.

**Anpharm (Ανφαρμ), Gr.** ΑΝΦΑΡΜ ΕΛΛΑΣ ΑΕ, Περικλεους 27, 152 32 Χαλάνδρι, Chalandri, Greece.

**Anpharm, UK.** See *Antigen, UK.*

**Ansell, Canad.** Ansell Canada Inc., 105 Lauder St, Cowansville, Quebec, J2K 2K8, Canada.

**Ansell, NZ.** Ansell International, P.O. Box 97-041, Auckland, New Zealand.

**Antah, Malaysia.** Antah Pharma Sdb Bhd, 3 Jln 19/1, 46300 Petaling Jaya, Selangor, Malaysia.

**Anthra, Israel.** See *Medison, Israel.*

**Antibioticos, Mex.** Antibioticos de Mexico S.A. de C.V., Las Flores No. 56,, Col. la Candelaria, Deleg. Coyoacan, 04380 Mexico D.F., Mexico.

**Antibioticos, Spain.** Antibioticos Farma, Ctra M-134 Km 1.5, Alcala de Henares, 28903 Madrid, Spain.

**Antigen, Hong Kong.** See *Universal, Hong Kong.*

**Antigen, Irl.** Antigen Pharmaceuticals Ltd, 54 Northumberland Rd, Dublin 4, Ireland.

**Antigen, Israel.** See *Trima, Israel.*

**Antigen, NZ.** See *Baxter, NZ.*

**Antigen, UK.** Antigen Pharmaceuticals Ltd, 82 Waterloo Rd, Southport, Merseyside, PR8 4QW, UK.

**Antipiol, Ital.** Laboratorio di Chimica Medica dell' Antipiol S.n.c., Via S. Benigno 26, 10154 Turin, Italy.

**Antistress, Switz.** Antistress AG, Gesellschaft fur Gesundheitsschutz, Fluhstrasse 30, 8640 Rapperswil, Switzerland.

**Antonetto, Ital.** Marco Antonetto S.p.A., Via Arsenale 29, 10121 Turin, Italy.

**Antonetto, Switz.** See *Corifel, Switz.*

**Antor, Gr.** ANTOR, Ομήρου 4, 151 26 Μαρουσι, Marousi, Greece.

**Antula, Fin.** See *Algol, Fin.*

**Antula, Swed.** Antula Healthcare AB, Odengatan 106, 113 22 Stockholm, Sweden.

**AOP Orphan, Austria.** AOP Orphan Pharmaceuticals AG, Graf Starhemberggasse 34/3, A-1040 Vienna, Austria.

**Apex, Malaysia.** Apex Pharmacy Sdn Bhd, 26-30 Jalan PJS 11/5, Bandar Sunway, 46150 Petaling Jaya, Selangor, Malaysia.

**Aplicare, USA.** Aplicare Inc., 50 E Industrial Rd, Branford, CT 06405, USA.

**Apodan, Denm.** Apodan A/S, Lergravsvej 63, 5, 2300 Copenhagen S, Denmark.

**Apogepha, Ger.** Apogepha Arzneimittel GmbH, Kyffhauserstr. 27, 01309 Dresden, Germany.

**Apolo, Arg.** Lab. Apolo S.A., Alem 2967, Santa Fe, Argentina.

**Apomedica, Austria.** Apomedica GmbH, Roseggerkai 3, A-8011 Graz, Austria.

**Apotex, Canad.** Apotex Inc., 4100 Weston Rd, Weston, Ontario, M9L 2Y6, Canada.

**Apotex, Denm.** See *Orphan, Denm.*

**Apotex, Gr.** See *Help, Gr.*

**Apotex, Hong Kong.** See *Hind Wing, Hong Kong.*

**Apotex, Malaysia.** See *Pharmaforte, Malaysia.*

**Apotex, NZ.** Apotex NZ Ltd, Private Bag 102-995, North Shore Mail Centre, Auckland, New Zealand.

**Apotex, S.Afr.** Apotex, South Africa.

**Apotex, Singapore.** See *Pharmaforte, Singapore.*

**Apotheca, Singapore.** Apotheca Marketing Pte Ltd, 63 Hillview Ave, 09-12 Lam Soon Industrial Building, S 669569, Singapore.

**Apothecary, USA.** Apothecary Products Inc., 11750 12th Ave S, Burnsville, MN 55337, USA.

**Apothecon, USA.** See *Bristol-Myers Squibb, USA.*

**Apothecus, Hong Kong.** See *Hind Wing, Hong Kong.*

**Apothecus, USA.** Apothecus Inc., 20 Audrey Ave, Oyster Bay, NY 11771, USA.

**Apotheke Erzengel Michael, Austria.** Apotheke zum Erzengel Michael, Sechshauser Strasse 9, A-1150 Vienna, Austria.

**Apotheke Gnadenmutter, Austria.** Apotheke zur Gnadenmutter, Hauptplatz 4, A-8630 Mariazell, Austria.

**Apotheke Heiligen Dreifaltigkeit, Austria.** Apotheke zur Heiligen Dreifaltigkeit, Kirchengasse 5, A-2460 Bruck a. d. Leitha, Austria.

**Apotheke Heiligen Josef, Austria.** Apotheke zum Heiligen Josef, Doblinger Hauptstrasse 64, A-1190 Vienna, Austria.

**Apotheke Heiligen Rupertus, Austria.** Apotheke zum Heiligen Rupertus, Maxglaner Hauptstrasse 13, A-5020 Salzburg, Austria.

**Apotheke Roten Krebs, Austria.** Apotheke zum Roten Krebs, Lichtensteg 4, A-1011 Vienna, Austria.

**Apotheke Tiroler Adler, Austria.** Apotheke zum Tiroler Adler, Museumstrasse 18, A-6020 Innsbruck, Austria.

**APP, Hong Kong.** See *LCH, Hong Kong.*

**Approved Prescription Services, UK.** Approved Prescription Services Ltd, Brampton Rd, Hampden Park, Eastbourne, East Sussex, BN22 9AG, UK.

**APS, Ger.** APS Pharma GmbH, Angelsrieder Feld 22, 82234 Wessling, Germany.

**APS, Port.** Farma-APS, Lda, Rua Jose Galhardo 3, 1750-131 Lisbon, Portugal.

**Apsen, Braz.** Apsen do Brasil Industria Quim. e Farm. Ltda, Rua La Paz 37/67, 04755-020 Sao Paolo, SP, Brazil.

**Aptus, NZ.** Aptus, P.O. Box 39-070, Wellington, New Zealand.

**Aqualab, Fr.** Laboratoires Aqualab, ZI Nord, B.P. 36, 470 av de Lossburg, 69480 Anse, France.

**Aquamaid, UK.** Aquamaid Co. Ltd, UK.

**Arab, Malaysia.** See *Antah, Malaysia.*

**Arcana, Austria.** Arcana Arzneimittel GmbH, Zimbagasse 5, A-1147 Vienna, Austria.

**Arcana, S.Afr.** Arcana (Pty) Ltd, P.O. Box 1998, Halfway House 1685, South Africa.

**Archifar, Thai.** See *TP, Thai.*

**Arco, USA.** Arco Pharmaceuticals Inc., 105 Orville Dr., Bohemia, NY 11716, USA.

**Arcola, USA.** Arcola Laboratories, P.O. Box 1200, Collegeville, PA 19426, USA.

**Arcolab, Switz.** Arcolab Ltd, 28 Chemin du Grand-Puits, 1217 Meyrin 2, Switzerland.

**Ardana, UK.** Ardana Bioscience Ltd, 58 Queen St, Edinburgh, EH2 3NS, UK.

**Arden, NZ.** Elizabeth Arden (NZ) Ltd, Private Bag 94104, Papatoetoe, South Auckland, New Zealand.

**Ardern, UK.** Ardern Healthcare Ltd, Pipers Brook Farm, Eastham, Tenbury Wells, Worcestershire, WR15 8NP, UK.

**Ardeypharm, Ger.** Ardeypharm GmbH, Loerfeldstr. 20, 58313 Herdecke, Germany.

**Ardix, Fr.** Ardix Médical, 27 rue du Pont, 92200 Neuilly-sur-Seine, France.

**Areu, Spain.** Areu, Ctra Madrid Valencia, Km 23.5, Arganda del Rey, 28500 Madrid, Spain.

**Argenfarma, Arg.** Lab. Argenfarma S.R.L., LLavallol 2649, 1417 Buenos Aires, Argentina.

**Argiletz, Fr.** Argiletz SA, 14 route d'Echampeu, 77440 Lizy-sur-Ourcq, France.

**ARI, Austral.** ARI, Division of ANSTO, Private Mail Bag 1, Menai, NSW 2234, Australia.

**Arion, Arg.** Lab. Arion S.R.L., Almafuerte 96, 2900 San Nicolas, Buenos Aires, Argentina.

**Aristegui, Spain.** See *Ifidesa Aristegui, Spain.*

**Aristo, India.** Aristo Pharmaceuticals Ltd, 23-A Shah Industrial Estate, Off Veea Desai Rd, Andheri (W), Mumbai 400 053, India.

**Ariston, Arg.** Quimica Ariston S.A.C.I.F., O'Connor 550/5, 1707 V. Sarmiento, Buenos Aires, Argentina.

**Ariston, Braz.** Ariston Industrias Quimicas e Farm. Ltda, Rua Adherbal Stresser 84, 05566-000 Sao Paulo, SP, Brazil.

**Arjo, Canad.** Arjo Canada Inc., 277 Cree Cres., Winnipeg, Manitoba, R3J 3X4, Canada.

**Arko, Ger.** Arko Pharma GmbH, Bajurwarenring 12, 82041 Oberhaching, Germany.

**Arkochim, Spain.** Arkochim España, Meneses 2, 28045 Madrid, Spain.

**Arkofarm, Ital.** Arkofarm S.r.l., Via Limone Piemonte 13/D, 18039 Ventimiglia (IM), Italy.

**Arkomedika, Fr.** See *Arkopharma, Fr.*

**Arkopharma, Belg.** Arkopharma, Edisonlaan 13, 1300 Wavre, Belgium.

**Arkopharma, Fr.** Laboratoires Arkopharma, B.P. 28, 06511 Carros cdx, France.

**Arkopharma, Israel.** See *Guri, Israel.*

**Arkopharma, Switz.** See *Naturpharma, Switz.*

**Arkopharma, UK.** Arkopharma UK Ltd, 6 Redlands Centre, Redlands, Coulsden, Surrey, CR5 2HT, UK.

**Arla, Fin.** Oy Arla Foods AB, PL 91, 00401 Helsinki, Finland.

**Arlex, Mex.** Arlex de México, S.A.deC.V., Puerto Acapulco No.35, Col. Piloto, Deleg. Alvaro Obregon, 01290 Mexico D.F., Mexico.

**Armour, Israel.** See *Aventis, Israel.*

**Armour, USA.** See *Aventis Behring, USA.*

**Armstrong, Arg.** Lab. Armstrong S.A.C.I.F., Joaquin V. Gonzalez 653, 1407 Buenos Aires, Argentina.

**Armstrong, Mex.** Armstrong Laboratorios de Mexico S.A. de C.V., Perifirico Sur No. 6677-1er Piso, Col. Ejidos de Tepepan, Deleg. Coyoacan, 16018 Mexico D.F., Mexico.

**Arnaldi-Uscio, Ital.** Colonia della Salute Carlo Arnaldi S.p.A., Via Carlo Arnaldi 6, 16030 Uscio (GE), Italy.

**Arrow, Austral.** Arrow Pharmaceuticals Ltd, P.O. Box 397, Surry Hills, NSW 2010, Australia.

**Ars Vitae, Switz.** Ars Vitae AG, Weingartenstrasse 9, 8803 Ruschilkon, Switzerland.

**Artegodan, Ger.** Artegodan GmbH, Wendlandstr. 1, 29439 Luchow, Germany.

**Artesan, Ger.** Artesan Pharma GmbH & Co. KG, Wendlandstr. 1, 29439 Luchow, Germany.

**Artesan, Switz.** See *Lubapharm Arlesheim, Switz.*

**Arteva, Ger.** Arteva Pharma GmbH, Leutstetenerstr. 10, 82131 Gauting, Germany.

**Artex, NZ.** Artex Ltd, P.O. Box 249, Waipukurau, New Zealand.

**Arthropharm, Austral.** Arthropharm P/L, 111 Bronte Rd, Bondi Junction, NSW 2022, Australia.

**Artsana, Ital.** Artsana S.p.A., Via Saldarini Catelli 1, 22070 Grandate (CO), Italy.

**Artu, Neth.** Artu Biologicals Europe BV, Vijzelweg 11, 8243 PM Lelystad, Netherlands.

**Arun, UK.** Arun Pharmaceuticals Ltd, Delta House, Southwood Cresent, Southwood, Farnborough, Hampshire, GU14 0NL, UK.

**A.S., UK.** A.S. Pharma Ltd, P.O. Box 181, Polegate, East Sussex, BN26 6WD, UK.

**ASAC, Spain.** A.S.A.C. Pharma, Sagitario 14, 03006 Alicante, Spain.

**Asahi, Jpn.** Asahi Chemical Industry Co. Ltd, 9-1 Kanda Mitoshirocho, Chiyoda-ku, Tokyo 101-8481, Japan.

**Ascent, USA.** Ascent Pediatrics Inc., 187 Ballardvale St, Suite B125, Wilmington, MA 01887, USA.

**Asche, Ger.** See *Asche Chiesi, Ger.*

**Asche Chiesi, Ger.** Asche Chiesi GmbH, Fischers Allee 49-59, 22763 Hamburg, Germany.

**Ascher, USA.** B.F. Ascher & Co., 15501 W 109th St, Lenexa, KS 66219, USA.

**Asconex, Ger.** Asconex Arzneimittelvertriebs GmbH, Kapellenstr. 18, 65606 Villmar, Germany.

**Ascot, Austral.** Ascot Pharmaceuticals, P.O. Box 79, Croydon, NSW 2132, Australia.

**Asens, Spain.** Asens, Alava 61, 08005 Barcelona, Spain.

**Asepta, Mon.** Laboratoires Asepta, 17 bd Prince-Hereditaire-Albert, MC 98000, Monaco.

**Ashbourne, UK.** Ashbourne Pharmaceuticals Ltd, Victors Barns, Hill Farm, Brixworth, Northamptonshire, NN6 9DQ, UK.

**Ashbury, Canad.** Ashbury Biologicals Inc., 349 Wildcat Rd, Toronto, Ontario, M3J 2S3, Canada.

**ASI, Israel.** ASI Pharma Ltd, 50 Bazel St, Herzliya Pituach, Israel.

**Asia Pharma, Malaysia.** Asia Pharma (M) Sdn Bhd, 31-1 Lorong Tiara 1A, Bandar Baru Klang, 41150 Klang, Selangor, Malaysia.

**Asian Pharm, Thai.** Asian Pharmaceutical Ltd Part, 9/4 Soi Wathanawong, Rajprarob Rd, Rajthavee, Bangkok 10400, Thailand.

**Asian TJD, Thai.** Asian TJD Enterprise Ltd, 90 Soi Ladprao 91 (Kesorn), Ledprao Rd, Wangthonglang Dist, Bangkok 10310, Thailand.

**Askit, UK.** Askit Laboratories Ltd, 47 Deerdykes View, Westfield, Cumbernauld, Glasgow, G68 9HN, UK.

**Asmopul, Arg.** Lab. Asmopul S.A., Independencia 4030, 1226 Buenos Aires, Argentina.

**Asofarma, Arg.** Lab. Asofarma S.A., Av. Cabildo 159, 1426 Buenos Aires, Argentina.

**Asofarma, Mex.** Asofarma de Mexico S.A. de C.V., Calz. Mexico-Xochimilco No. 43, Col. San Lorenzo Huipulco, Deleg. Tlalpan, 14370 Mexico D.F., Mexico.

**Aspen, Arg.** Lab. Aspen S.A., Remedios 3439/43, 1407 Buenos Aires, Argentina.

**Aspen, Austral.** Aspen Pharmacare Australia P/L, Suite 3, 36-46 Chandos St, St Leonards, NSW 2065, Australia.

**Aspen, Hong Kong.** See *Primal, Hong Kong.*

**Aspen, S.Afr.** Aspen Pharmacare (Pty) Ltd, P. O. Box 1587, Gallo Manor 2052, South Africa.

**Aspen Consumer, S.Afr.** See *Aspen, S.Afr.*

**Aspid, Mex.** Aspid, S.A. de C.V., Belgica No. 518, Col. Portales, 03300 Mexico D.F., Mexico.

**Assistance, Arg.** Assistance S.R.L., Av. Cordoba 950 Piso 13 A, 1954 Buenos Aires, Argentina.

**Associated Dental, UK.** Associated Dental Products Ltd, Purton, Swindon, Wiltshire, SN5 9HT, UK.

**Associated Hospital Supply, UK.** Associated Hospital Supply, Sherwood Rd, Aston Fields, Bromsgrove, Worcestershire, B60 3DR, UK.

**Associated Medical, Hong Kong.** Associated Medical Supplies Co. Ltd, Rm 1201, Fo Tan Industrial Ctr, 26 Au Pui Wan St, Fo Tan, N.T., Hong Kong.

**Asta, Gr.** See *Baxter, Gr.*

**Asta Medica, Austral.** Asta Medica Australasia P/L, P.O. Box 1305, Parramatta, NSW 2124, Australia.

**Asta Medica, Austria.** See *Viatris, Austria.*

**Asta Medica, Belg.** See *Viatris, Belg.*

**Asta Medica, Braz.** Asta Medica Ltda, Rua Santo Antonio 184 20° andar, 01314-900 Sao Paulo, SP, Brazil.

**Asta Medica, Canad.** Asta Medica Ltd, 25 Sheppard Ave W, Suite 1205, Toronto, Ontario, M2N 6S6, Canada.

**Asta Medica, Fin.** See *Viatria, Swed.*

**Asta Medica, Fr.** See *Viatris, Fr.*

**Asta Medica, Ger.** See *Baxter Oncology, Ger.*, and *Viatris, Ger.*

**Asta Medica, Hong Kong.** See *Unico, Hong Kong.*

**Asta Medica, Irl.** See *Viatris, UK.*

**Asta Medica, Israel.** See *Megapharm, Israel.*

**Asta Medica, Ital.** See *Viatris, Ital.*

**Asta Medica, Malaysia.** See *JDH, Malaysia*, and *Zuellig, Malaysia.*

**Asta Medica, Neth.** See *Viatris, Neth.*

**Asta Medica, Norw.** See *Viatria, Swed.*

**Asta Medica, NZ.** See *NZ Medical & Scientific, NZ.*

**Asta Medica, Port.** See *Viatris, Port.*

**Asta Medica, Singapore.** See *JDH, Singapore.*

**Asta Medica, Spain.** See *Viatris, Spain.*

**Asta Medica, Swed.** See *Viatria, Swed.*

**Asta Medica, Switz.** See *Viatris, Switz.*

**Asta Medica, Thai.** See *Zuellig, Thai.*

**Asta Medica, UK.** See *Viatris, UK.*

**Asta Medica, USA.** See *Muro, USA.*

**Asta Oncologia, Braz.** See *Asta Medica, Braz.*

**Aster, Braz.** Aster Produtos Medicos Ltda, Av. Independencia 2.541, 18001-970 Sorocaba, SP, Brazil.

**Astra, Austral.** See *AstraZeneca, Austral.*

**Astra, Austria.** See *AstraZeneca, Austria.*

**Astra, Belg.** See *AstraZeneca, Belg.*

**Astra, Canad.** See *AstraZeneca, Canad.*

**Astra, Denm.** See *AstraZeneca, Denm.*

**Astra, Ger.** See *AstraZeneca, Ger.*

**Astra, Gr.** ASTRA HELLAS AE, Θεοτοκοπούλου 4 & Αστροναυτών, 151 25 ,Μαρούσι, Marousi, Greece.

**Astra, Hong Kong.** See *AstraZeneca, Hong Kong.*

**Astra, Irl.** See *AstraZeneca, Irl.*

**Astra, Israel.** See *Teva, Israel.*

**Astra, Ital.** See *AstraZeneca, Ital.*

**Astra, Jpn.** See *AstraZeneca, Jpn.*

**Astra, Mex.** See *AstraZeneca, Mex.*

**Astra, Norw.** See *AstraZeneca, Norw.*

**Astra, Port.** See *AstraZeneca, Port.*

**Astra, S.Afr.** See *AstraZeneca, S.Afr.*

**Astra, Spain.** See *AstraZeneca, Spain.*

**Astra, Swed.** See *AstraZeneca, Swed.*

**Astra, Switz.** See *AstraZeneca, Switz.*

**Astra, USA.** See *AstraZeneca, USA.*

**Astra Tech, Denm.** Astra Tech A/S, Husby Alle 19, 2630 Taastrup, Denmark.

**Astra Tech, Fin.** Astra Tech Oy, Piispansilta 11, 02230 Espoo, Finland.

**Astra Tech, Norw.** Astra Tech AS, Luhrtoppen 2, Postboks 160, 1471 Lorenskog, Norway.

**Astra Tech, Swed.** Astra Tech AB, Box 14, 431 21 Molndal, Sweden.

**Astrapin, Ger.** See *Hameln, Ger.*

**AstraZeneca, Arg.** AstraZeneca Argentina S.A., Argerich 536, 1706 Haedo, Buenos Aires, Argentina.

**AstraZeneca, Austral.** Astrazeneca P/L, P.O. Box 131, North Ryde, NSW 1670, Australia.

**AstraZeneca, Austria.** AstraZeneca Österreich GmbH, Schwarzenbergplatz 7, A-1037 Vienna, Austria.

**AstraZeneca, Belg.** AstraZeneca Pharmaceuticals S.A., Rue Egide Van Ophem 110, 1180 Brussels, Belgium.

**AstraZeneca, Braz.** AstraZeneca do Brasil Ltda, Rod Raposo Tavares km 26.9, 06714-025 Cotia, SP, Brazil.

**AstraZeneca, Canad.** AstraZeneca Canada Inc., 1004 Middlegate Rd, Mississauga, Ontario, L4Y 1M4, Canada.

**AstraZeneca, Chile.** AstraZeneca de Chile Ltda, Francisco de Paula Taforo 1081, Nunoa, Santiago, Chile.

**AstraZeneca, Denm.** AstraZeneca A/S, Roskildevej 22, 2620 Albertslund, Denmark.

**AstraZeneca, Fin.** AstraZeneca Oy, Eteläinen Salmitie, PL 6, 02431 Masala, Finland.

**AstraZeneca, Fr.** AstraZeneca, 1 place Renault, 92844 Rueil-Malmaison cdx, France.

**AstraZeneca, Ger.** AstraZeneca GmbH, 22876 Wedel, Germany.

**Astra-Zeneca, Gr.** ASTRA-ZENECA, 21ο χλμ. Λ. Μαραθώνος, 190 09 Πικέρμι, Pikermi, Greece.

**AstraZeneca, Hong Kong.** AstraZeneca Hong Kong Ltd, 2301 Cosco Tower, Grand Millenium Plaza, 183 Queen's Rd Central, Hong Kong.

**AstraZeneca, India.** AstraZeneca Pharma India Ltd, P.O. Box 5039, Crescent Rd, Bangalore 560 001, India.

**AstraZeneca, Irl.** AstraZeneca, College Park House, 20 Nassau St, Dublin 2, Ireland.

**AstraZeneca, Israel.** See *Teva, Israel.*

**AstraZeneca, Ital.** AstraZeneca, Via F. Storxa - Palazzo Volta, 20080 Basiglio (MI), Italy.

**AstraZeneca, Jpn.** AstraZeneca K.K., 1-1-88 Oyodonaka, Kita-ku, Osaka 531-0076, Japan.

**AstraZeneca, Malaysia.** AstraZeneca Malaysia, P.O. Box 11221, 50740 Kuala Lumpur, Malaysia.

**AstraZeneca, Mex.** AstraZeneca S.A. de C.V., Super Avenida Lomas Verdes No. 67, 53120 Naucalpan de Juarez, Mexico.

**AstraZeneca, Neth.** AstraZeneca Pharmaceutica BV, Postbus 599, 2700 AN Zoetermeer, Netherlands.

**AstraZeneca, Norw.** AstraZeneca AS, Hoffsv 70 B, Postboks 200 Vinderen, 0319 Oslo, Norway.

**AstraZeneca, NZ.** AstraZeneca Ltd, P.O. Box 1301, Auckland, New Zealand.

**AstraZeneca, Port.** AstraZeneca - Produtos Farmaceuticos, Lda, Rua Humberto Madeira 7, Valejas, 2745 Barcarena, Portugal.

**AstraZeneca, S.Afr.** AstraZeneca Pharmaceuticals, Private Bag X30, Sunninghill 2157, South Africa.

**AstraZeneca, Singapore.** AstraZeneca Singapore Pte Ltd, 6 Temasek Boulevard, 06-01 Suntec Tower Four, S 038986, Singapore.

**AstraZeneca, Spain.** AstraZeneca Farmaceutica Spain, Parque Norte Ed Roble, C/Serrano Galvache 56, 28033 Madrid, Spain.

**AstraZeneca, Swed.** AstraZeneca Sverige AB, 151 85 Sodertalje, Sweden.

**AstraZeneca, Switz.** AstraZeneca AG, Grafenau 10, 6301 Zug, Switzerland.

**AstraZeneca, Thai.** AstraZeneca (Thailand) Ltd, 20 Fl, Phairojkijja Building, 400 Bangna-Trad Km 4, Bangkok 10260, Thailand.

**AstraZeneca, UK.** AstraZeneca UK Ltd, Horizon Place, 600 Capability Green, Luton, Bedfordshire, LU1 3LU, UK.

**AstraZeneca, USA.** AstraZeneca Pharmaceuticals LP, 1800 Concord Pike, P.O. Box 15437, Wilmington, DE 19850-5437, USA.

**Atache, Spain.** Atache, C/Sagitario 14, 03006 Alicante, Spain.

**Athena Neurosciences, USA.** See *Elan, USA.*

**Athenstaedt, Ger.** Athenstaedt Nachf. GmbH & Co. KG, Bocklinstr. 1, 80638 Munchen, Germany.

**Athenstaedt, Switz.** See *Drossapharm, Switz.*

**Athenstaedt & Redeker, Hong Kong.** See *Mekim, Hong Kong.*

**Athlon, USA.** Athlon Pharmaceuticals Inc., P.O. Box 3181, Ridgeland, MS 39158, USA.

**Athlone, Irl.** Athlone Laboratories, Ballymurray, Roscommon, Ireland.

**Atid, Ger.** See *Dexcel, Ger.*

**Ativus, Braz.** Ativus Farmaceutica Ltda, Rua Batista Parente 36, 03022-080 Sao Paulo, SP, Brazil.

**Atlantic, Hong Kong.** Atlantic Laboratories Ltd, Block A, 18/F, Wing Wah Industrial Bldg, 677 King's Rd, North Point, Hong Kong.

**Atlantic, Malaysia.** Atlantic Laboratories (M) Sdn Bhd, 14 & 16 Jln Angklung 33/20, Shah Alam Technology Park, Seksyen 33, 40400 Shah Alam, Selangor, Malaysia.

**Atlantic, Singapore.** Atlantic Pharmaceutical (S) Pte Ltd, 152 Paya Lebar Rd, 04-03 Citipoint Industrial Complex, S 409020, Singapore.

**Atlantic, Thai.** Atlantic Pharmaceutical Co. Ltd, 2038 Sukhumvit Rd, Bangkok 10250, Thailand.

**Atlantis, Mex.** Atlantis, S.A. de C.V., Tiburcio Montiel No. 16, San Miguel Chapultepec, 11850 Mexico D.F., Mexico.

**Atlas, Canad.** Laboratoire Atlas, 5750 Metropolitan E, Suite 200, St-Leonard, Quebec, H1S 1A7, Canada.

**Atley, USA.** Atley Pharmaceuticals Inc., 10511 Old Ridge Rd, Ashland, VA 23005, USA.

**Atral, Port.** Laboratóorios Atral, SA, Vala do Carregado, 2600-726 Castanheira do Ribatejo, Portugal.

**Atral-Vida, Port.** See *Atral, Port.*

**Atrix, UK.** Atrix Laboratories Ltd, St James House, Moon St, Bristol, BS2 8QY, UK.

**Atrix, USA.** Atrix Laboratories Inc., USA.

**Atzinger, Ger.** Dr. Atzinger Pharmazeutische Fabrik, Dr. Atzinger Str. 5, 94036 Passau, Germany.

**Auad, Braz.** Auad Quimica Ltda, Rodovia BR 153 Km 7.5, Trevo Sul, 74853-040 Goiania, GO, Brazil.

**Auden McKenzie, UK.** Auden McKenzie (Pharma Div.) Ltd, 30 Stadium Business Centre, North End Rd, Wembley, Middlesex, HA9 0AT, UK.

**Augot, Fr.** Laboratoires Augot, 26 rue de Beauregard, 03400 Yzeure, France.

**Aulo Gelio, Arg.** Aulo Gelio Argentina S.R.L., A. R. Bufano 1265, 1416 Buenos Aires, Argentina.

**Aura, USA.** Aura, USA.

**Aurantis, Braz.** See *Biochimico, Braz.*

**Aurora, Austral.** Aurora, Australia.

**Australasian Medical, Austral.** Austalasian Medical and Scientific Ltd, Unit 16, Artarmon Central, 54 Dickson Ave, Artarmon, NSW 2064, Australia.

**Australian Bodycare, UK.** Australian Bodycare Ltd, Danegate, Eridge Green, Tunbridge Wells, Kent, TN3 9JA, UK.

**Australian Medic-Care, Hong Kong.** Australian Medic-Care Co. Ltd, Room 3509, Metroplaza Tower 2, 223 Hing Fong Rd, Kwai Fong, Kwai Chung, Hong Kong.

**Austrodent, Austria.** Austrodent Handels-GmbH, Brandhofgasse 22, A-8010 Graz, Austria.

**Austroflex, Austria.** Austroflex Pharma, Schikanedergasse 12/8-10, A-1040 Vienna, Austria.

**Austroplant, Austria.** Austroplant-Arzneimittel GmbH, Richard-Strauss-Strasse 13, A-1232 Vienna, Austria.

**Auxilium, USA.** Auxilium Pharmaceuticals Inc., 160 W Germantown Pike, Suite D5, Norristown, PA 19401, USA.

**Avant Garde, Canad.** Avant-Garde Cosmetics Ltd, 3503 Griffith, St-Laurent, Quebec, H4T 1W5, Canada.

**Avantgarde, Ital.** Avantgarde S.p.A., Gruppo Sigma Tau, Via Treviso 4, 00040 Pomezia (Rome), Italy.

**Avene, Fr.** Avène, Laboratoires Dermatologiques, 45 place Abel-Gance, 92100 Boulogne, France.

**Aventis, Arg.** Aventis Pharma S.A., Av. Int. Tomkinso 2054, 1642 San Isidro, Buenos Aires, Argentina.

**Aventis, Austral.** Aventis Pharma P/L, Locked Bag 2067, Lane Cove, NSW 2066, Australia.

**Aventis, Austria.** Aventis Pharma GmbH, Altmannsdorfer Strasse 104, A-1121 Vienna, Austria.

**Aventis, Belg.** Aventis Pharma S.A., Bvld de la Plaine 9, 1050 Brussels, Belgium.

**Aventis, Braz.** Aventis Pharma Ltda, Avenida Marginal do Rio Pinheiros 5200, 04693-000 Sao Paulo, SP, Brazil.

**Aventis, Canad.** Aventis Pharma Inc., 2150 St-Elzear Blvd W, Laval, Quebec, H7L 4A8, Canada.

**Aventis, Chile.** Laboratorio Aventis Pharma SA, Hernando de Aguirre 268, Providencia, Santiago, Chile.

**Aventis, Denm.** Aventis Pharma A/S, Slotsmarken 13, 2970 Horsholm, Denmark.

**Aventis, Fin.** Aventis Pharma Oy, PL 96, Maistraatinportti 4 A, 00241 Helsinki, Finland.

**Aventis, Fr.** Laboratoires Aventis, 46 quai de la Rapee, Paris cdx 12, France.

**Aventis, Ger.** Aventis Pharma Deutschland GmbH, Konigsteiner Str. 10, 65812 Bad Soden am Ts, Germany.

**Aventis, Gr.** AVENTIS, Αυτοκρ. Νικολάου 2, 176 71 Αθήνα, Athens, Greece.

**Aventis, Hong Kong.** Aventis Pharma Ltd, 24/F DCH Commercial Ctr, 25 Westlands Rd, Quarry Bay, Hong Kong.

**Aventis, India.** Aventis Pharma Ltd, 54-A Sir Mathurdas Vasanji Rd, Andheri (E), Mumbai 400 093, India.

**Aventis, Irl.** Aventis Pharma (Ireland) Ltd, Lake Drive, 3400 City West, Naas Rd, Dublin 24, Ireland.

**Aventis, Israel.** Aventis Pharma, P.O. Box 8090, Netanya, Israel.

**Aventis, Ital.** Aventis S.p.A., Via G. Rossini 1/A, 20020 Lainate (MI), Italy.

**Aventis, Jpn.** Aventis Pharma Ltd, 2-17-51 Akasaka, Minato-ku, Tokyo 107-8465, Japan.

**Aventis, Malaysia.** Aventis Farma SA (Malaysia) Sdn Bhd, 74 Jln Universiti, 46200 Petaling Jaya, Selangor, Malaysia.

**Aventis, Mex.** Aventis Pharma S.A. de C.V., Av. Universidad No. 1738, Col. Coyoacan, 04000 Mexico D.F., Mexico.

**Aventis, Neth.** Aventis Pharma, Bijenvlucht 30, 3871 JJ Hoevelaken, Netherlands.

**Aventis, Norw.** Aventis Pharma AS, Vollsv. 2B, Postboks 393, 1326 Lysaker, Norway.

**Aventis, NZ.** Aventis Pharma Ltd, P.O. Box 34-010, Birkenhead, Auckland, New Zealand.

**Aventis, Port.** Aventis Pharma, Lda, Estrada Nacional 249, Km 15, 2725-397 Mem Martins, Portugal.

**Aventis, S.Afr.** Aventis Pharma (Pty) Ltd, Private Bag X207, Midrand 1683, South Africa.

**Aventis, Singapore.** Aventis Pharma Pte Ltd, 300 Beach Rd, 11-02/04 The Concourse, S 199555, Singapore.

**Aventis, Spain.** Aventis Pharma, Martinez Villergas 52, 28027 Madrid, Spain.

**Aventis, Swed.** Aventis Pharma AB, Box 47604, 117 94 Stockholm, Sweden.

**Aventis, Switz.** Aventis Pharma AG, Herostrasse 7, Postfach, 8048 Zurich, Switzerland.

**Aventis, Thai.** Aventis Pharma Ltd, 20 Fl, Lake Rajada Building, 193 Ratchadaphisek Rd, Klong Toey, Prakanong, Bangkok 10110, Thailand.

**Aventis, UK.** Aventis Pharma Ltd, Aventis House, 50 Kings Hill Ave, Kings Hill, West Malling, Kent, ME19 4AH, UK.

**Aventis, USA.** Aventis Pharmaceuticals, 300 Somerset Corporate Bvld, Bridgewater, NJ 08807-2854, USA.

**Aventis Behring, Austria.** See *Aventis, Austria.*

**Aventis Behring, Braz.** See *Aventis, Braz.*

**Aventis Behring, Denm.** See *Aventis Behring, Swed.*

**Aventis Behring, Fin.** See *Aventis Behring, Swed.*

**Aventis Behring, Fr.** Aventis Behring SA, 46 quai de la Rapee, 75012 Paris, France.

**Aventis Behring, Ger.** Aventis Behring GmbH, Postfach: 1230, 35002 Marburg (Lahn), Germany.

**Aventis Behring, Hong Kong.** See *Primal, Hong Kong.*

**Aventis Behring, Irl.** See *Aventis Behring, UK.*

**Aventis Behring, Israel.** See *Mediline, Israel.*

**Aventis Behring, Ital.** Aventis Behring S.p.A., P.le S Turr 5, 20149 Milan, Italy.

**Aventis Behring, Mex.** Aventis Behring S.A. de C.V., Calz. de Tlalpan No. 4255, Bosques de Tetlameya, 04730 Mexico D.F., Mexico.

**Aventis Behring, Neth.** See *Aventis Behring, Ger.*

**Aventis Behring, Norw.** See *Aventis, Norw.*, and *Aventis Behring, Swed.*

**Aventis Behring, Spain.** Aventis Behring, Via Augusta 252-260, 08017 Barcelona, Spain.

**Aventis Behring, Swed.** Aventis Behring AB, Berga Backe 2, 182 17 Danderyd, Sweden.

**Aventis Behring, Switz.** Aventis Behring AG, Herostrasse 7, 8048 Zurich, Switzerland.
**Aventis Behring, UK.** Aventis Behring Ltd, Aventis House, Market Place, Haywards Heath, West Sussex, RH16 1DB, UK.
**Aventis Behring, USA.** Aventis Behring, 1020 First Ave, King of Prussia, PA 19406, USA.
**Aventis Pasteur, Arg.** See *Aventis, Arg.*
**Aventis Pasteur, Austral.** Aventis Pasteur P/L, P.O. Box 7025, Baulkham Hills Business Centre, NSW 2153, Australia.
**Aventis Pasteur, Austria.** Aventis Pasteur GmBH, Richard-Strauss-Strasse 33, A-1230 Vienna, Austria.
**Aventis Pasteur, Belg.** Aventis Pasteur MSD S.A., Ave Jules Bordet 13, 1140 Brussels, Belgium.
**Aventis Pasteur, Braz.** Aventis Pasteur Soros e Vacinas S.A., Rua do Rocio 351 10° andar, 04552-905 Sao Paulo, SP, Brazil.
**Aventis Pasteur, Canad.** Aventis Pasteur, Connaught Campus, 1755 Steeles Ave. W, Toronto, Ontario, M2R 3T4, Canada.
**Aventis Pasteur, Chile.** See *Aventis, Chile.*
**Aventis Pasteur, Denm.** Aventis Pasteur MSD A/S, Toldbodgade 57, 1253 Copenhagen K, Denmark.
**Aventis Pasteur, Fin.** See *Aventis Pasteur, Denm.*
**Aventis Pasteur, Fr.** Aventis Pasteur Mérieux MSD, Halle Borie, 8 rue Jonas-Salk, 69367 Lyon cdx 07, France.
**Aventis Pasteur, Ger.** Aventis Pasteur MSD GmbH, Paul-Ehrlich-Str. 1, 69181 Leimen, Germany.
**Aventis Pasteur, Hong Kong.** See *Aventis, Hong Kong.*
**Aventis Pasteur, Irl.** See *Allphar, Irl.*
**Aventis Pasteur, Ital.** Aventis Pasteur MSD S.p.A., Via degli Aldobranddeschi 15, 00163 Rome, Italy.
**Aventis Pasteur, Malaysia.** See *Aventis, Malaysia.*
**Aventis Pasteur, Neth.** Aventis Pasteur MSD, Bovenkerkerweg 6-8, 1185 XE Amstelveen, Netherlands.
**Aventis Pasteur, Norw.** See *Aventis Pasteur, Denm.*
**Aventis Pasteur, Port.** See *UCB, Port.*
**Aventis Pasteur, Singapore.** See *Aventis, Singapore.*
**Aventis Pasteur, Spain.** Aventis Pasteur MSD, Edificio Cuzco IV, P de la Castellana 141, 28046 Madrid, Spain.
**Aventis Pasteur, Swed.** Aventis Pasteur MSD, Vretenvagen 10, 171 54 Solna, Sweden.
**Aventis Pasteur, Thai.** Aventis Pasteur (Thailand) Ltd, 4 Fl, VTT I Building, 3195/9 Rama IV Rd, Klong Toey, Bangkok 10110, Thailand.
**Aventis Pasteur, UK.** Aventis Pasteur MSD, Mallards Reach, Bridge Ave, Maidenhead, Berkshire, SL6 1QP, UK.
**Aventis Pasteur, USA.** Aventis Pasteur Inc, Discovery Drive, Swiftwater, PA 18370-0187, USA.
**Avon, Canad.** Avon Canada Inc., 5500 Trans Canada Hwy, Pointe-Claire, Quebec, H9R 1B6, Canada.
**AWD, Ger.** AWD.pharma GmbH & Co. KG, Leipziger Str. 7-13, 01097 Dresden, Germany.
**Axcan, Canad.** Axcan Pharma Inc., 597 Laurier Blvd, Mont St-Hilaire, Quebec, J3H 6C4, Canada.
**Axcan, Fr.** Axcan Pharma SA, Route de Bu, B.P. 41, 78550 Houdan, France.
**Axcan, Hong Kong.** See *C & L, Hong Kong.*
**Axcan, Israel.** See *Megapharm, Israel.*
**Axcan, USA.** Axcan Scandipharm, 22 Inverness Center Pkwy, Suite 310, Birmingham, AL 35242, USA.
**Ayerst, Israel.** See *Dexxon, Israel*, and *Neopharm, Israel.*
**Ayerst, USA.** See *Whitehall-Robins, USA*, and *Wyeth-Ayerst, USA.*
**Ayrton, UK.** Ayrton Saunders Ltd, Reeds Lane, Moreton, Wirral, CH46 1QW, UK.
**AyurCore, Singapore.** See *MD, Singapore.*
**Aza, Austral.** See *Lilly, Austral.*
**Azevedos, Port.** Laboratórios Azevedos, SA, Estrada Nacional 117-2, 2724-503 Amadora, Portugal.
**Azupharma, Ger.** Azupharma GmbH & Co., Dieselstr. 5, 70839 Gerlingen, Germany.
**Azupharma, Hong Kong.** See *Jebsen, Hong Kong.*
**BA Farma, Port.** Laboratorio B.A. Farma, Lda, R. Professor Sousa da Camara 207/211, 1070-803 Lisbon, Portugal.
**Bach, UK.** Bach Flower Remedies Ltd, Broadheath House, 83 Parkside, London, UK.
**Bacon, Arg.** Lab. Bacon, Uruguay 136, 1603 Villa Martelli, Buenos Aires, Argentina.
**Bad Heilbrunner, Ger.** Bad Heilbrunner Reform-Diat-Arznei GmbH & Co., Am Krebsenbach 5-7, 83670 Bad Heilbrunn, Germany.
**Baer, Ger.** Chemisch-pharmazeutische Fabrik Dr Baer KG GmbH & Co., Ehrwalder Str. 21, 81377 Munich, Germany.
**Bago, Arg.** Laboratorios Bagó S.A., Bernardo de Irigoyen 248, 1072 Buenos Aires, Argentina.
**Bago, Chile.** Laboratorios Bago SA, Av. Vicuna Mackenna 1835, Santiago, Chile.
**Baif, Ital.** Baif International Products, New York S.n.c., Via XX Setembre 20/68, 16121 Genoa, Italy.
**Bailleul, Fr.** Laboratoires Bailleul, 8 rue Laugier, 75017 Paris, France.
**Bailly, Fr.** Laboratoires Bailly SPEAB, 60 rue Peirre-Charron, 75008 Paris, France.
**Bajamar, USA.** Bajamar Chemical Co. Inc., 9609 Dielman Rock Island, St Louis, MO 63132, USA.
**Bajer, Arg.** Laboritorios Felipe Bajer S.A.I.C., Alfredo R. Bufano 1265, 1416 Buenos Aires, Argentina.
**Baker Cummins, Canad.** See *Alza, Canad.*
**Baker Cummins, USA.** See *Baker Norton, USA.*
**Baker Norton, Hong Kong.** See *Ivax, Hong Kong.*
**Baker Norton, Irl.** See *Ivax, Irl.*
**Baker Norton, USA.** Baker Norton Pharmaceuticals, 4400 Biscayne Blvd, Miami, FL 33137, USA.
**Baldacci, Braz.** Laboratorios Baldacci S.A., Rua Pedro de Toledo 520, 04039-001 Sao Paulo, SP, Brazil.
**Baldacci, Ital.** Laboratori Baldacci S.p.A., Via S. Michele degli Scalzi 73, 56100 Pisa, Italy.
**Baldacci, Port.** Farmoquimica Baldacci, SA, Rua Duarte Galvao 44, 1549-005 Lisbon, Portugal.
**Baldassari, Braz.** Baldassari, Brazil.
**Baliarda, Arg.** Lab. Baliarda S.A., Alberti 1283, 1247 Buenos Aires, Argentina.
**Ballay, USA.** Ballay Pharmaceuticals Inc., 200 Stillwater, P.O. Box 1356, Wimberley, TX 78676, USA.
**Balmar, NZ.** Balmar, New Zealand.
**Balneopharm, Ger.** See *Hanosan, Ger.*
**Bama, Spain.** Bama Geve, Avda Diagonal 456, 08006 Barcelona, Spain.
**Bamford, NZ.** W.M. Bamford & Co. Ltd, Private Bag 31-346, Lower Hutt, Wellington, New Zealand.
**Banana Boat, Canad.** The Banana Boat Company, 6363 Northam Drive, Mississauga, Ontario, L4V 1N5, Canada.
**Bang & Tegner, Denm.** Bang & Tegner, Vesterbrogade 149, 1620 Copenhagen V, Denmark.
**Bangkok Drug, Thai.** Bangkok Drug Co. Ltd, 874 Soi, 23 Rama 6 Rd, Rajthevee, Bangkok 10400, Thailand.
**Bangkok Lab & Cosmetic, Thai.** See *Bangkok Drug, Thai.*
**Banner, Hong Kong.** See *Well Favoured, Hong Kong.*
**Bano, Austria.** Mag. J. Bano chem. pharmazeutische Präparate, A-6580 St Anton/Arlberg 485, Austria.
**Banyu, Hong Kong.** See *Hing Ah, Hong Kong.*
**Banyu, Jpn.** Banyu Pharmaceutical Co. Ltd, 2-2-3 Nihonbashi Honcho, Chuo-ku, Tokyo 103-8416, Japan.
**Banyu, Thai.** See *Asian TJD, Thai.*
**Barcino, Spain.** Barcino, Tuset 1, 08006 Barcelona, Spain.
**Bard, Hong Kong.** See *US Summit, Hong Kong.*
**Bard, UK.** Bard Ltd, Forest House, Brighton Rd, Crawley, West Sussex, RH11 9BP, UK.
**Barnes Hind, Arg.** See *Maurino, Arg.*
**Barnes Hind, NZ.** See *Allergan, NZ.*
**Barr, USA.** Barr Laboratories Inc., 2 Quaker Rd, Pomona, NY 01970, USA.
**Barre-National, USA.** See *Alpharma, USA.*
**Barrenne, Braz.** Barrenne Industria Farmaceutica Ltda, Rua Antunes Maciel 68/86, Sao Cristovao, 20940-010 Rio de Janeiro, RJ, Brazil.
**Barry, Ital.** Barry Italia S.r.l., Via Sardegna 40, 20090 Fizzonasco Pieve Emanuele (MI), Italy.
**Bartor Pharmacal, USA.** Bartor Pharmacal Co., 70 High St, Rye, NY 10580, USA.
**BASF, Ger.** BASF Generics GmbH, Carl-Zeiss-Ring 3, 85737 Ismaning, Germany.
**Basi, Port.** See *Esteves Alves, Port.*
**Basics, Ger.** Basics GmbH, Hemmelrather Weg 201, 51377 Leverkusen, Germany.
**Basotherm, Ger.** See *Galderma, Ger.*
**Bastian, Ger.** Bastian-Werk GmbH, August-Exter-Str. 4, 81245 Munich, Germany.
**Bausch & Lomb, Arg.** Lab. Bausch & Lomb Argentina S.R.L., Av. Montevideo 160, 1019 Buenos Aires, Argentina.
**Bausch & Lomb, Austral.** Bausch & Lomb (Australia) P/L, Level 4, 113 Wicks Rd, North Ryde, NSW 2113, Australia.
**Bausch & Lomb, Belg.** Bausch & Lomb, Regent Building, 2600 Antwerp, Belgium.
**Bausch & Lomb, Braz.** Bausch & Lomb (BL) Industria Otica Ltda, Av. das Americas 500, Bl.14, Lj.106, Barra da Tijuca, 22640-100 Rio de Janeiro, RJ, Brazil.
**Bausch & Lomb, Canad.** Bausch & Lomb Canada Inc., 3762 Fourteenth Ave, 2nd Floor, Markham, Ontario, L3R 0G7, Canada.
**Bausch & Lomb, Fr.** See *Chauvin, Fr.*
**Bausch & Lomb, NZ.** Bausch & Lomb, New Zealand.
**Bausch & Lomb, S.Afr.** Bausch & Lomb (SA) (Pty) Ltd, P.O. Box 5435, Rivonia 2128, South Africa.
**Bausch & Lomb, Switz.** Bausch & Lomb Swiss AG, Sumpfstrasse 3, 6312 Steinhausen, Switzerland.
**Bausch & Lomb, Thai.** See *Zuellig, Thai.*
**Bausch & Lomb, UK.** Bausch & Lomb UK Ltd, 106-114 London Rd, Kingston-upon-Thames, Surrey, KT2 6TN, UK.
**Bausch & Lomb, USA.** Bausch & Lomb Pharmaceuticals, 8500 Hidden River Parkway, Tampa, FL 33637, USA.
**Bauxili, Spain.** Bauxili, Nueva 52, Igualada, 08700 Barcelona, Spain.
**Baxtar, Jpn.** Baxtar Ltd, 4 Banchi, 6 Bancho, Chiyoda-ku, Tokyo 102-8468, Japan.
**Baxter, Arg.** See *Baxter Immuno, Arg.*
**Baxter, Austral.** Baxter Healthcare P/L, P.O. Box 88, Toongabbie, NSW 2146, Australia.
**Baxter, Austria.** Baxter AG, Industriestrasse 67, A-1221 Vienna, Austria.
**Baxter, Belg.** Baxter S.A., Bvld de la Plaine 5, 1050 Brussels, Belgium.
**Baxter, Braz.** Baxter Hospitalar Ltda, Rua Eng. Francisco Pitta Brito 779, 04753-080 Sao Paulo Santo Amaro, SP, Brazil.
**Baxter, Canad.** Baxter Corporation, 4 Robert Speck Pkwy, Suite 700, Mississauga, Ontario, L4Z 3YA, Canada.
**Baxter, Chile.** Laboratorio Baxter/Asta Medica, General Salvo 68, Providencia, Santiago, Chile.
**Baxter, Denm.** Baxter A/S, Gydevang 43, 3450 Allerod, Denmark.
**Baxter, Fin.** Baxter Oy, Pakkalankuja 6, PL 46, 01511 Vantaa, Finland.
**Baxter, Fr.** Baxter SA, 6 av Louis-Pasteur, B.P. 56, 78311 Maurepas cdx, France.
**Baxter, Ger.** Baxter Deutschland GmbH, Edisonstr. 3-4, 85716 Unterschleissheim, Germany.
**Baxter, Gr.** BAXTER, Εθν. Μακαρίου 34, 163 41 Ηλιούπολη, Ilioupoli, Greece.
**Baxter, Hong Kong.** Baxter Healthcare Ltd, Rm 2006, MassMutual Tower, 38 Gloucester Rd, Wanchai, Hong Kong.
**Baxter, Irl.** Baxter Healthcare Ltd, 7 Deansgrange Industrial Estate, Blackrock, Dublin, Ireland.
**Baxter, Israel.** See *Teva, Israel.*
**Baxter, Ital.** Baxter S.p.A., Viale Tiziano 25, 00196 Rome, Italy.
**Baxter, Malaysia.** See *United Italian, Malaysia.*
**Baxter, Mex.** Baxter, S.A de C.V., Oklahoma No. 14-3er.piso, Col. Napoles, Deleg. Benito Juarez, 03810 Mexico D.F., Mexico.
**Baxter, Neth.** Baxter, Netherlands.
**Baxter, NZ.** Baxter Healthcare Ltd, P.O. Box 14-062, Panmure, Auckland, New Zealand.
**Baxter, Port.** Baxter, Lda, Urbanizacao Industrial Cabra Figa, Estrada Nacional 249/4, Lote 3, Cabra Figa, 2735 Rio de Mouro, Portugal.
**Baxter, Singapore.** See *United Italian, Singapore.*
**Baxter, Spain.** Baxter, C/ Dels Gremis 7, Polig. Inds. Vara de Cuart, 46014 Valencia, Spain.
**Baxter, Swed.** Baxter Medical AB, Box 63, 164 94 Kista, Sweden.
**Baxter, Switz.** Baxter AG, Mullerenstrasse 3, 8604 Volketswil., Switzerland.
**Baxter, Thai.** Baxter Healthcare (Thailand) Co. Ltd, 10 Fl, Grand Amarin Tower, 1550 New Petchburi Rd, Makasan, Rajthevi, Bangkok 10310.
**Baxter, UK.** Baxter Healthcare Ltd, Caxton Way, Thetford, Norfolk, IP24 3SE, UK.
**Baxter, USA.** Baxter Healthcare, One Baxter Parkway, Deerfield, IL 60015, USA.
**Baxter Anaesthesia, UK.** Baxter Anaesthesia, Unit 31, Wellington Business Park, Dukes Ride, Crowthorne, Berkshire, RG45 6LS, UK.
**Baxter BioScience, Ger.** Baxter Deutschland GmBH BioScience, Im Breitspiel 13, 69126 Heidelberg, Germany.
**Baxter BioScience, UK.** Baxter BioScience, Wallingford Rd, Compton, Newbury, Berkshire, RG20 7QW, UK.
**Baxter Healthcare, Switz.** See *Opopharma, Switz.*
**Baxter Immuno, Arg.** Baxter Immuno S.A., Entre Rios 1632, 1636 Olivos, Buenos Aires, Argentina.
**Baxter Oncology, Fr.** See *Baxter, Fr.*
**Baxter Oncology, Ger.** Baxter Oncology GmbH, Daimlerstr. 40, 60314 Frankfurt am Main, Germany.
**Baxter Oncology, Malaysia.** See *Zuellig, Malaysia.*
**Baxter Oncology, Singapore.** See *Zuellig, Singapore.*
**Baxter Oncology, UK.** Baxter Oncology, Wallingford Rd, Newbury, Berkshire, RG20 7QW, UK.
**Baxter-Hyland, Hong Kong.** See *Baxter, Hong Kong.*
**Baxter-Hyland, USA.** Baxter Hyland Immuno, 1627 Lake Cook Rd, Deerfield, IL 60015, USA.
**Bayer, Arg.** Bayer Argentina S.A., Ricardo Gutierrez 3652, 1605 Munro, Buenos Aires, Argentina.
**Bayer, Austral.** Bayer Australia Ltd (Pharmaceutical Business Group), P.O. Box 903, Pymble, NSW 2073, Australia.
**Bayer, Austria.** Bayer Austria GmbH, Am Heumarkt 10, Postfach 10, 1037 Vienna, Austria.
**Bayer, Belg.** Bayer S.A., Ave Louise 143, 1050 Brussels, Belgium.
**Bayer, Braz.** Bayer S.A., Caixa Postal 22523, 04798-970 Sao Paulo, SP, Brazil.
**Bayer, Canad.** Bayer Inc., 77 Belfield Rd, Toronto, Ontario, M9W 1G6, Canada.
**Bayer, Chile.** Bayer SA, Carlos Fernandez 260, San Joaquin, Santiago, Chile.
**Bayer, Denm.** Bayer Danmark A/S, Norgaardsvej 32, 2800 Lyngby, Denmark.
**Bayer, Fin.** Bayer Oy, Suomalaistentie 7, PL 13, 02270 Espoo, Finland.
**Bayer, Fr.** Bayer Pharma, 49-51 quai De Dion Bouton, 92815 Puteaux Cedex, France.
**Bayer, Ger.** Bayer Vital GmbH & Co. KG, 51368 Leverkusen, Germany.
**Bayer, Gr.** BAYER ΕΛΛΑΣ ΑΕΒΕ, Ακακιών 54α, Πολύδροσο, 151 25 Μαρούσι, Marousi, Greece.
**Bayer, Hong Kong.** Bayer China Co Ltd, 18/F Caroline Ctr, 28 Yun Ping Rd, Causeway Bay, Hong Kong.
**Bayer, India.** Bayer Pharmaceuticals Pvt Ltd, 1st Floor, Bayer Corporate Office, Kolshet Rd, Thane 400 607, India.
**Bayer, Irl.** Bayer Ltd, Chapel Lane, Swords, Dublin, Ireland.
**Bayer, Israel.** See *Agis, Israel.*
**Bayer, Ital.** Bayer S.p.A., Viale Certosa 126-130, 20156 Milan, Italy.
**Bayer, Jpn.** Bayer Yakuhin Ltd, 3-5-36 Miyahara, Yodogawa-ku, Osaka 532-8577, Japan.
**Bayer, Malaysia.** Bayer Malaysia, Wisma Zuellig Pharma, Lot 9, Jln. Bersatu 13/4, 46200 Petaling Jaya, Selangor, Malaysia.
**Bayer, Mex.** Bayer de Mexico S.A. de C.V., Division Farmaceutica, Blvd.M. de Cervantes Saavedra 259, 11520 Mexico D.F., Mexico.
**Bayer, Neth.** Bayer BV, Energieweg 1, 3641 RT Mijdrecht, Netherlands.
**Bayer, Norw.** Bayer AS, Brennav 18, Skyttafeltet, Nittedal, Postboks 114, 1483 Skytta, Norway.
**Bayer, NZ.** Bayer New Zealand Ltd, C.P.O. Box 2825, Auckland, New Zealand.
**Bayer, Port.** Bayer Portugal, SA, Apartado 666, 2795 Carnaxide, Portugal.
**Bayer, S.Afr.** Bayer (Pty) Ltd, P.O. Box 198, Isando 1600, South Africa.
**Bayer, Singapore.** Bayer (South East Asia) Pte Ltd, Pharmaceutical Division, 9 Benol Sector, S 629844, Singapore.
**Bayer, Spain.** Bayer, Calabria 268, 08029 Barcelona, Spain.
**Bayer, Swed.** Bayer AB, Box 5237, 402 24 Goteborg, Sweden.
**Bayer, Switz.** Bayer (Schweiz) AG, Pharma, Postfach, Grubenstrasse 6, 8045 Zurich, Switzerland.
**Bayer, Thai.** Bayer Thai Co. Ltd, 130/1 North Sathorn Rd, Silom, Bangrak, Bangkok 10500, Thailand.
**Bayer, UK.** Bayer plc, Pharmaceutical Division, Bayer House, Strawberry Hill, Newbury, Berkshire, RG13 1JA, UK.
**Bayer, USA.** Bayer Corp., 400 Morgan Lane, West Haven, CT 06516, USA.
**Bayer Biological, Hong Kong.** See *LCH, Hong Kong.*
**Bayer Consumer, Austral.** See *Bayer, Austral.*
**Bayer Consumer, Canad.** See *Bayer, Canad.*
**Bayer Consumer, Malaysia.** See *Bayer, Malaysia.*
**Bayer Consumer, Mex.** See *Bayer, Mex.*
**Bayer Consumer, Singapore.** See *Diethelm, Singapore.*
**Bayer Consumer, UK.** See *Bayer, UK.*
**Bayer Consumer, USA.** Bayer Consumer Care Division, 36 Columbia Rd, P.O. Box 1910, Morristown, NJ 07962-1910, USA.
**Bayer Diagnostici, Ital.** Bayer S.p.A., Divisione Diagnostici, Via Grosio 10, 20151 Milan, Italy.
**Bayer Diagnostics, Fr.** Bayer Diagnostics, Tour Horizon, 52 quai De Dion Bouton, 92807 Puteaux cdx, France.
**Bayer Diagnostics, Irl.** See *Cahill May Roberts, Irl.*
**Bayer Diagnostics, Irl.** Bayer Diagnostics, Chapel Lane, Swords, Co. Dublin, Ireland.
**Bayer Diagnostics, Mex.** Bayer de Mexico S.A. de C.V., Division Diagnosticos, Av. Col. del Valle No. 615, 1er piso, Col del Valle, 03100 Mexico D.F., Mexico.
**Bayer Diagnostics, UK.** See *Bayer, UK.*
**Baypharm, Austral.** See *Bayer, Austral.*
**BBC, Braz.** Brazilian Business Consultants, Avenida Brigadeiro Luis Antonio 1499, 01317-001 Sao Paulo, SP, Brazil.
**BC Lutz, Switz.** BCLutz Company Ltd, Pharmaceutical Products Switzerland, Dachslerenstrasse 11, P.O. Box, 8702 Zollikon, Switzerland.
**BCL, Switz.** See *BC Lutz, Switz.*
**BCM, UK.** BCM Ltd, Dio First 114, Nottingham, Nottinghamshire, NG90 2PR, UK.
**BCS, Fr.** See *CSP, Fr.*
**BDF, Mex.** See *Beiersdorf, Mex.*
**BDH, India.** BDH Industries Ltd, Nair Baug, Akurli Rd, Kandivli (E), Mumbai 400 101, India.
**BDI, USA.** BDI Pharmaceuticals, Inc., 9700 N Michigan Rd, Carmel, IN 46220, USA.
**Beach, USA.** Beach Pharmaceuticals, Division of Beach Products Inc., 5220 South Manhattan Ave, Tampa, FL 33611, USA.
**Beacon, UK.** Beacon Pharmaceuticals Ltd, 85 High St, Tunbridge Wells, Kent, TN1 1YG, UK.
**Beacons, Singapore.** Beacons Chemicals Pte Ltd, 21 Chin Bee Ave, S 619942, Singapore.

**Beaubour Nutrition, Fr.** Beaubour Nutrition, ZI La Canterie, B.P. 38, 37800 Sainte-Maure-de-Touraine, France.

**Beaufour, Fr.** Beaufour Ipsen Pharma, 24 rue Erlanger, 75781 Paris cdx 16, France.

**Beaufour, Switz.** See *Uhlmann-Eyraud, Switz.*

**Beaufour-Ipsen, Hong Kong.** See *JDH, Hong Kong.*

**Beaufour-Ipsen, Malaysia.** See *Antah, Malaysia.*

**Beaufour-Ipsen, Singapore.** See *Sime Darby, Singapore.*

**Beaufour-Ipsen, Switz.** See *Uhlmann-Eyraud, Switz.*

**Beaufour-Ipsen, Thai.** See *Pacific, Thai.*

**Beckerath, Ger.** M. v. Beckerath GmbH Pharmavertrieb, Leyentalstr. 78, 47799 Krefeld, Germany.

**Beckman, USA.** Beckman Coulter Inc, 1050 Page Mill Rd, Palo Alto, CA 94303, USA.

**Becton Dickinson, USA.** Becton Dickinson & Co., 1 Becton Drive, Franklin Lakes, NJ 07417, USA.

**Bedford, USA.** Bedford Laboratories, a Division of Ben Venue Laboratories Inc., 300 Northfield Rd, Bedford, OH 44146, USA.

**Beecham, Belg.** See *GlaxoSmithKline, Belg.*

**Beecham, Port.** See *GlaxoSmithKline, Port.*

**Beecham, Spain.** See *GlaxoSmithKline, Spain.*

**Beethoven, Ger.** Beethoven-Pharma Dr Wiemann GmbH, Steinthalstr. 1, 90455 Nurnberg, Germany.

**Befelka, Ger.** Befelka-Arzneimittel, Parkstr. 6 B, 49080 Osnabruck, Germany.

**Behring, Israel.** See *Mediline, Israel.*

**Behring, Neth.** See *Aventis, Neth.*

**Behringwerke, Israel.** See *Chemipharm, Israel.*

**Beiersdorf, Arg.** Beiersdorf S.A., Triunvirato 2902, 1427 Buenos Aires, Argentina.

**Beiersdorf, Austral.** Beiersdorf Australia Ltd, P.O. Box 139, North Ryde, NSW 2113, Australia.

**Beiersdorf, Austria.** Beiersdorf GmbH, Laxenburger Strasse 151, A-1101 Vienna, Austria.

**Beiersdorf, Canad.** See *Smith & Nephew, Canad.*

**Beiersdorf, Chile.** Beiersdorf SA, Lo Espejo 501, Maipu, Santiago, Chile.

**Beiersdorf, Ger.** Beiersdorf AG, Unnastr. 48, 20245 Hamburg, Germany.

**Beiersdorf, Irl.** Beiersdorf Ireland Ltd, First Floor, Block 8, St John's Court, Santry, Dublin 9, Ireland.

**Beiersdorf, Ital.** Beiersdorf S.p.A., Via Eraclito 30, 20128 Milan, Italy.

**Beiersdorf, Mex.** Beiersdorf Mexico S.A. de C.V., Poniente 116 No. 509, Col. Industrial Vallejo, 02300 Mexico D.F., Mexico.

**Beiersdorf, Port.** Beiersdorf Portuguesa, Lda, Rua Soeiro Pereira Gomes 59, 2746-952 Queluz, Portugal.

**Beiersdorf, Spain.** Beiersdorf, Ctra Mataro-Granollers Km 5.4, Argentona, 08310 Barcelona, Spain.

**Beiersdorf, Switz.** Beiersdorf AG, Aliothstrasse 40, 4142 Munchenstein, Switzerland.

**Beiersdorf, Thai.** Beirersdorf (Thailand) Co. Ltd, 12 Fl, Sathorn Thani Building 1, 90/30-33 North Sathorn Rd, Silom, Bangrak, Bangkok 10500, Thailand.

**Beiersdorf, UK.** Beiersdorf UK Ltd, Yeomans Drive, Blakelands, Milton Keynes, Buckinghamshire, MK14 5LS, UK.

**Beiersdorf, USA.** Beiersdorf Inc., Wilton Corporate Center, 187 Danbury Road, Wilton, CT 06897, USA.

**Beige, S.Afr.** See *Brunel, S.Afr.*

**Beldenta, Switz.** Beldenta-Anstalt, Birkenweg 6, FL-9490 Vaduz, Switzerland.

**Belfar, Braz.** Belfar Industria Farmaceutica, Rua Alair Marques Rodrigues 516, Santa Amelia, 031560-220 Belo Horizonte, MG, Brazil.

**Bell, India.** Bell Pharma, 75/C Government Industrial Estate, Kandivli (W), Mumbai 400 067, India.

**Bell, UK.** Bell, Sons & Co. (Druggists), P.O. Box 62, Tanhouse Lane, Widnes, Cheshire, WA8 0SA, UK.

**Bellon, Fr.** See *Aventis, Fr.*

**Belmac, Spain.** Belmac, C/Teide No 4, Planta Baja, Parque Empresarial La Marina, San Sebastian de los Reyes, 28700 Madrid, Spain.

**Belolab, Fr.** Belolab, 12 rue Tronchet, 75008 Paris, France.

**Bencard, Belg.** See *GlaxoSmithKline, Belg.*

**Bencard, Ger.** Bencard Allergie GmbH, Messerschmittstr 4, 80992 Munich, Germany.

**Bender, Austria.** Bender, Vienna, Austria.

**Bene, Ger.** bene-Arzneimittel GmbH, Herterichstr. 1, 81479 Munich, Germany.

**Bene-Chemie, Hong Kong.** See *Universal, Hong Kong.*

**Benedetti, Ital.** Benedetti S.p.A., Vicolo de' Bacchettoni 3, 51100 Pistoia (PT), Italy.

**Bengue, Irl.** See *Roche, Irl.*

**Benitol, Arg.** Laboratorios Benitol S.A.C.I., Felipe Vallese 3340/44, 1407 Buenos Aires, Argentina.

**Bennett, UK.** Bennett Natural Products, Wheelton, Chorley, Lancashire, PR6 8EP, UK.

**Berenguer Infale, Spain.** See *Almirall, Spain.*

**Bergamo, Braz.** Lab. Quim. Bergamo Ltda, Rua Rafael de Marco 43, 06765-000 Taboao da Serra, SP, Brazil.

**Bergamon, Ital.** Bergamon S.r.l., Via Farini 5, 00185 Rome, Italy.

**Bergen Brunswig, USA.** Bergen Brunswig, USA.

**Berk, Irl.** See *Blackhall, Irl.*

**Berk, UK.** See *Approved Prescription Services, UK.*

**Berlex, Canad.** Berlex Canada Inc., 2260, 32nd Ave, Lachine, Quebec, H8T 3H4, Canada.

**Berlex, NZ.** See *Schering, NZ.*

**Berlex, USA.** Berlex Laboratories Inc., 300 Fairfield Rd, Wayne, NJ 07470, USA.

**Berli, Thai.** Berli Jucker Public Co. Ltd, 99 Soi Rubia, Sukhumvit 42 Rd, Bangkok 10110, Thailand.

**Berlimed, Braz.** See *Schering, Braz.*

**Berlin Pharm, Singapore.** See *Polymedic, Singapore.*

**Berlin Pharm, Thai.** Berlin Pharmaceutical Industry Co. Ltd, 359 New Rd, Bangkok 10100, Thailand.

**Berlin-Chemie, Ger.** Berlin-Chemie AG, Glienicker Weg 125, 12489 Berlin, Germany.

**Berlipharm, Fr.** See *Schering, Fr.*

**Berman, Mex.** Berman Laboratorios S.A. de C.V., Laboratoristas No. 46, Col. Iztapalapa Sifon, 09400 Mexico D.F., Mexico.

**Berna, Belg.** Berna Products Belgium, Blvd du Souverain 207, bte. 3, 1160 Brussels, Belgium.

**Berna, Canad.** See *Berna, USA.*

**Berna, Denm.** See *Cortec, Denm.*

**Berna, Fin.** See *Cortec, Swed.*

**Berna, Hong Kong.** See *Keller, Hong Kong.*

**Berna, Ital.** Istituto Sieroterapico Berna S.r.l., Via Bellinzona 39, 22100 Como, Italy.

**Berna, Malaysia.** See *Diethelm, Malaysia.*

**Berna, Norw.** See *Cortec, Swed.*

**Berna, NZ.** See *Pharmabroker, NZ.*

**Berna, Port.** See *Vieira, Port.*

**Berna, Singapore.** See *Diethelm, Singapore.*

**Berna, Spain.** Berna, P Castellana 163, 28046 Madrid, Spain.

**Berna, Switz.** Berna Biotech Ltd, Rehhagstrasse 79, 3018 Berne, Switzerland.

**Berna, Thai.** See *Diethelm, Thai.*

**Berna, USA.** Berna Products Corp., 4216 Ponce de Leon Blvd, Coral Gables, FL 33146, USA.

**Berner, Fin.** Berner Oy, Lääkeryhmä, PL 15, 00131 Helsinki, Finland.

**Bernhauer, Austria.** Mr W Bernhauer OHG, Stadtplatz 7, A-4400 Steyr, Austria.

**Bersan, Ital.** Bersan Cosmetica Ipoallergenica S.r.l., Via delle Pervinche 10, 00171 Rome, Italy.

**Berta, Ital.** Berta S.r.l., Via Andrea Doria 7, 20124 Milan, Italy.

**Bertek, USA.** Bertek Pharmaceuticals Inc, P.O. Box 2006, Sugarland, TX 77478, USA.

**Bescansa, Spain.** Bescansa, Pl. Inds. Tambre-via Pasteur 8, Santiago de Compostela, 15890 La Coruna, Spain.

**Besins, Belg.** Besins International Belgique, Rue Grand-Bigard 128, 1620 Drogenbos, Belgium.

**Besins, Fr.** Laboratoires Besins International, 13 rue Perier, 92120 Montrouge, France.

**Besins, Ger.** See *Kade, Ger.*

**Besins, Hong Kong.** See *Bi Asian Pacific, Hong Kong,* and *JDH, Hong Kong.*

**Besins, Israel.** See *CTS, Israel.*

**Besins International, Israel.** See *CTS, Israel.*

**Besins-Iscovesco, Fr.** See *Besins, Fr.*

**Besins-Iscovesco, Israel.** See *CTS, Israel.*

**Besins-Iscovesco, Malaysia.** See *Wellchem, Malaysia.*

**Besins-Iscovesco, Singapore.** See *Pharmed, Singapore.*

**Best, Mex.** Laboratorios Best S.A. de C.V., Municipio Libre No. 199, Col. Benito Juarez Portales, 03300 Mexico D.F., Mexico.

**Beta, Arg.** Laboratorios Beta S.A., Av. San Juan 2266, 1232 Buenos Aires, Argentina.

**Beta, Canad.** Beta Brands, 100 Cumberland Ave, Hamilton, Ontario, L8M 1Z1, Canada.

**Beta, Ital.** Laboratorio Biologico Chemioterapico Beta S.r.l., Via IV Novembre 171/3, 25080 Prevalle, Italy.

**Beta, Spain.** See *AstraZeneca, Spain.*

**Beta, USA.** Beta Dermaceuticals, P.O. Box 691106, San Antonio, TX 78269-1106, USA.

**Beta Healthcare, UK.** Beta Healthcare, Standard House, Prospect Place, Lenton, Nottingham, Nottinghamshire, NG7 1RX, UK.

**Be-Tabs, S.Afr.** Be-Tabs Pharmaceuticals (Pty) Ltd, P.O. Box 43486, Industria 2042, South Africa.

**Betamadrileno, Spain.** Betamadrileño, Area Empresarial Andalucia, Sector 4 Parcela 28, Getafe, 28906 madrid, Spain.

**Betapharm, Ger.** Betapharm Arzneimittel GmbH, Kobelweg 95, 86156 Augsburg, Germany.

**Beutlich, USA.** Beutlich Pharmaceuticals, 1541 Shields Drive, Waukegan, IL 60085-8304, USA.

**Beximco, Singapore.** See *Advanced, Singapore.*

**BGA, Fr.** BGA Pharma, France.

**BHR, UK.** BHR Pharmaceuticals Ltd, 41 Centenary Business Centre, Hammond Close, Attleborough Fields, Nuneaton, Warkwickshire, CV11 6RY, UK.

**Bi Asian Pacific, Hong Kong.** Bi Asian Pacific Ltd, Flat B, 22/F, Tak Lee Commercial Building, 113-117 Wan Chai Rd, Wanchai, Hong Kong.

**Biagini, Ital.** See *Kedrion, Ital.*

**Bial, Port.** Laboratorios Bial (Portela & Co., SA), Av da Siderurgia Nacional, Apartado 19, 4745-457 Sao Mamede do Coronado, Portugal.

**Bial, Spain.** Bial-Industrial Farmaceutica, Alameda de Urquijo 27, Bilbao, 48008 Vizcaya, Spain.

**Bialfar, Port.** See *Bial, Port.*

**Bichsel, Switz.** Laboratorium Dr G Bichsel AG, Bahnhofstrasse 5a, 3800 Interlaken, Switzerland.

**Bieffe, Ital.** Bieffe Medital S.p.A., Via Nuova Provinciale, 23034 Grosotto (SO), Italy.

**Bieffe, Spain.** Bieffe Medital, C/Solsones 2 BJ Local 7, Parque "Mas Blau", El Trat Del LLobregat, 22666 Barcelona, Spain.

**Bieffe, Switz.** Bieffe Medital SpA, Via S Balestra 27, 6900 Lugano, Switzerland.

**Bier, Ital.** Bier Farmaceutici S.n.c. di Pepe G. E. Frattolino Rosa, Via Cupa Capodichino 19, 80144 Naples, Italy.

**Bifarma, Ital.** Bifarma Fitoterapici di Bignardi Sergio, Via Pallia 5, 20139 Milan, Italy.

**Bilgast, Ger.** Bilgast Arzneimittel Vertriebs GmbH, Unter den Rusten 36, 67578 Gimbsheim, Germany.

**Billiet, Arg.** Lab. Billiet & Cma. S.R.L., Soler 3564, 1425 Buenos Aires, Argentina.

**Bilosa, Austria.** Bilosa GmbH & Co. KG, Burgerstrasse 15, A-6020 Innsbruck, Austria.

**Binesa, Spain.** See *Pfizer, Spain.*

**Bio Merieux, UK.** Bio Merieux UK, Grafton Way, Basingstoke, Hampshire, RG22 6HY, UK.

**Bio Products, Malaysia.** See *Germax, Malaysia.*

**Bio Sidus, Thai.** See *Berli, Thai.*

**Bio Terapico Ralay, Spain.** Bio Terapico Ralay, Spain.

**Bio2, Fr.** Laboratoires Bio2, 99 bvd des Belges, 69006 Lyon, France.

**Biobasal, Switz.** Biobasal AG, Eulerstrasse 55, 4003 Basle, Switzerland.

**Biobras, Braz.** See *Novo Nordisk, Braz.*

**Bioceuticals, UK.** Bioceuticals Ltd, 26 Zennor Rd, London, SW12 0PS, UK.

**Biochem, India.** Biochem Pharmaceutical Industries, Aidun Building, John Crasto Lane, Mumbai 400 002, India.

**Biochem, Ital.** Biochem Immunosystems Italia S.p.A., Via Magnanelli 2, 40033 Casalecchio di Reno (BO), Italy.

**Biochemie, Austral.** Biochemie Australia P/L, Level 2, 11-17 Khartoum Rd, North Ryde, NSW 2113, Australia.

**Biochemie, Austria.** Biochemie GmbH, Brunner Strasse 59, A-1235 Vienna, Austria.

**Biochemie, Denm.** See *Orphan, Denm.*

**Biochemie, Fin.** See *Novartis, Fin.*

**Biochemie, Hong Kong.** See *Unipharm, Hong Kong.*

**Biochemie, Israel.** See *Pharmateam, Israel.*

**Biochemie, Malaysia.** Biochemie Marketing Office, LiFung Centre, Lot 6, Persiaran Perusahan, Seksyen 23, Kawasan Perusahaan Shah Alam, 40300 Shah Alam, Selangor, Malaysia.

**Biochemie, Norw.** See *Novartis, Norw.,* and *Swedish Orphan, Norw.*

**Biochemie, NZ.** See *CSL, NZ.*

**Biochemie, Singapore.** See *FP, Singapore.*

**Biochemie, Thai.** See *Novartis, Thai.*

**Biochimici, Ital.** Biochimici PSN S.p.A., Via Viadagola 30, 40050 Quarto Inferiore (BO), Italy.

**Biochimico, Braz.** Instituto Biochimico Ltda, Rod. Presidente Dutra km 310, 27580-000 Rio de Janeiro, RJ, Brazil.

**Bioclon, Mex.** Instituto Bioclon S.A. de C.V., Calz. de Tlalpan 4687, Coyoacan Toriello Guerra, 14050 Mexico D.F., Mexico.

**Bioclones, S.Afr.** Bioclones (Pty) Ltd, P.O. Box 784351, Sandton 2146, South Africa.

**Biocodex, Denm.** See *Biolac, Swed.*

**Biocodex, Fin.** See *Algol, Fin.*

**Biocodex, Fr.** Laboratoires Biocodex, 19 rue Barbès, 92126 Montrouge cdx, France.

**Biocodex, Hong Kong.** See *Primal, Hong Kong.*

**Biocom, Fr.** Laboratoires Biocom, 44 bd Saint-Jacques, 75014 Paris, France.

**Bioconcepts, Austral.** BioConcepts Pty Ltd, P.O. Box 1492, Eagle Farm, BC Qld 4009, Australia.

**Bioconcepts, UK.** Bioconcepts Ltd, P.O. Box 15, Havant, Hampshire, PO9 1RQ, UK.

**Biocontrol, Arg.** Biocontrol S.A., Fraga 1504, 1427 Buenos Aires, Argentina.

**Biocontrolfarm, Ital.** Biocontrolfarm s.n.c., Via dell'Epomeo 72, 80126 Naples, Italy.

**Biocrom, Arg.** Lab. Biocrom Esp. Med. S.A., Luis Viale 965, 1416 Buenos Aires, Argentina.

**Biocumed, Arg.** Lab. Biocumed S.A., Av. J. B. Justo 2781, 1414 Buenos Aires, Argentina.

**Biocur, Ger.** Biocur Arzneimittel GmbH, Otto-von-Guericke-Allee 1, 39179 Barleben, Germany.

**Biocure, Ital.** Biocure S.r.l., Via Friuli 88, 20135 Milan, Italy.

**Bioderma, Fr.** Bioderma, 75 cours Albert-Thomas, 69447 Lyon cdx 03, France.

**Bioderma, Ital.** See *SSL, Ital.*

**Biodiagnostics, Austral.** See *National Diagnostic, Austral.*

**Bio-Diat, Ger.** Bio-Diät-Berlin, Selerweg 43-45, 12169 Berlin, Germany.

**Biodim, Fr.** Biodim, 17 rue de l'Ancienne Mairie, 92100 Boulogne-Billiancourt, France.

**Biodiphar, Belg.** Biodiphar S.A., Rue des Trois Arbres 16 A, 1180 Brussels, Belgium.

**Biodue, Ital.** Biodue S.r.l., Via Benvenuto Cellini 67/69, 50020 Loc. Sambuca Val di Pesa (FI), Italy.

**Bioes, Fr.** Laboratoires Bioes, 38 bd Henri-Sellier, 92156 Suresnes cdx, France.

**Bioethical, Ital.** Bioethical S.r.l., Via Mariano Marchicelli 26, 00060 Formello (Rome), Italy.

**Bio-Familia, Switz.** bio-familia AG, Hochwertige Nahrungsmittel, 6072 Sachseln, Switzerland.

**Biofilm, USA.** Biofilm Inc., 3121 Scott St 1707 Vista, CA 92083-8323, USA.

**Bioflora, Austria.** Bioflora GmbH, Teichweg 2, A-5400 Hallein, Austria.

**Bioforce, Ger.** Bioforce GmbH, Bruhlstr. 15, 78465 Constance, Germany.

**Bioforce, Switz.** Bioforce AG, Postfach 76, 9325 Roggwil/TG, Switzerland.

**Bioforce, UK.** Bioforce UK Ltd, 2 Brewster Place, Irvine, Ayrshire, KA11 5DD, UK.

**Biofutura, Ital.** See *Sigma-Tau, Ital.*

**Biogal, Israel.** See *Teva, Israel.*

**Biogalenica, Spain.** Biogalenica, Ramon Trias Fargas 7-11 Ed, Marina Village, 08005 Barcelona, Spain.

**Biogalenique, Fr.** Laboratoires Biogalénique, 11 quai de la Rapee, 75601 Paris cdx 12, France.

**Biogam, Arg.** Biogam Argentina S.A., Av. Jujuy 1152, 1229 Buenos Aires, Argentina.

**Biogam, Switz.** See *Kart, Switz.,* and *Serolab, Switz.*

**Bio-Garten, Austria.** Bio-Garten GmbH, Triesterstrasse 14/1, A-2351 Wiener Neudorf, Austria.

**Biogen, Austral.** Biogen P/L, Suite 2601, Level 26, Miller St, North Sydney, NSW 2060, Australia.

**Biogen, Austria.** See *Biogen, Fr.*

**Biogen, Belg.** Biogen Belgium S.A., Rue des Colonies 11, 1000 Brussels, Belgium.

**Biogen, Canad.** Biogen Canada Inc., 3 Robert Speck Pkwy, Suite 300, Mississauga, Ontario, L4Z 2GS, Canada.

**Biogen, Denm.** Biogen Denmark A/S, Lyngbyvej 28, 2100 Copenhagen O, Denmark.

**Biogen, Fin.** Biogen Finland Oy, Äyritie 12, 01510 Vantaa, Finland.

**Biogen, Fr.** Biogen France SA, Le Capitole, 55 av. des Champs-Pierreux, 92012 Nanterre cdx, France.

**Biogen, Ger.** Biogen GmbH, Carl-Zeiss-Ring 6, 85737 Ismaning, Germany.

**Biogen, Gr.** Biogen, Greece.

**Biogen, Irl.** See *Biogen, UK.*

**Biogen, Israel.** See *Medison, Israel.*

**Biogen, Neth.** Biogen BV, Robijnlaan 8, 2132 WX Hoofddorp, Netherlands.

**Biogen, Norw.** Biogen Norway AS, Karenslyst alle 8b, 0278 Oslo, Norway.

**Biogen, NZ.** See *CSL, NZ.*

**Biogen, Swed.** Biogen Sweden AB, Kanaladgen 1 A, plan 2, 194 61 Upplands Vdsby, Sweden.

**Biogen, UK.** Biogen Ltd, 5d Roxborough Way, Foundation Park, Maidenhead, Berkshire, SL6 3UD, UK.

**Biogen, USA.** Biogen, 14 Cambridge Center, Cambridge, MA 02142, USA.

**Biogena, Ital.** Valetudo S.r.l., Divisione Biogena, Via Ghiaie 6, 24030 Presezzo (BG), Italy.

**Biogenetech, Thai.** Biogenetech Co. Ltd, Biopex Building, 749/12, Soi Watchannal, Off Soi Pradoo Sathupradit Rd, Bangphongphang, Yannawa, Bangkok 10120, Thailand.

**BioGenex, USA.** BioGenex Laboratories, 4600 Norris Canyon Rd, San Ramon, CA 94583, USA.

**Bioglan, Austral.** Bioglan Ltd, 8/10 Yalgar Rd, Yalgar Business Park, Kirrawee, NSW 2322, Australia.

**Bioglan, Denm.** See *Bioglan, Swed.*

**Bioglan, Fin.** See *Bioglan, Swed.*

**Bioglan, Ger.** Bioglan Pharma GmbH, Robert-Bosch-Str. 6, 35398 Giessen, Germany.

**Bioglan, Hong Kong.** See *Keller, Hong Kong.*

**Bioglan, Irl.** See *Bioglan, UK.*

**Bioglan, Israel.** See *Gamida-Medequip, Israel.*

**Bioglan, Malaysia.** See *United Italian, Malaysia.*

**Bioglan, Norw.** See *Bioglan, Swed.*

**Bioglan, Singapore.** See *Biomed, Singapore,* and *Pharmed, Singapore.*

**Bioglan, Swed.** Bioglan AB, Box 50310, 202 13 Malmo, Sweden.

**Bioglan, Thai.** See *Hua, Thai.*

**Bioglan, UK.** Bioglan Laboratories Ltd, 5 Hunting Gate, Hitchin, Hertfordshire, SG4 0TJ, UK.

**Bioglan, USA.** Bioglan Pharmaceuticals Co., 7 Great Valley Parkway, Suite 301, Malvern, PA 19355, USA.

**Biogyne, Fr.** Biogyne, Laboratoires groupe Poli, 183 rue de Courcelles, 75017 Paris, France.

**Bio-Health, UK.** Bio-Health Ltd, Culpeper Close, Medway City Estate, Rochester, Kent, ME2 4HU, UK.

**Biohorm, Spain.** See *Uriach, Spain.*

**Biohorma, Ital.** Biohorma Italia S.r.l., Via del Mare 32 N/1, 00040 Pomezia (RM), Italy.

**Bioiberica, Spain.** Bioiberica, Ctra N-II Km 680.6, Palafolls, 08389 Barcelona, Spain.

**Bioimmun, Ger.** BioImmunPharma GmbH, Im Dammwald 27, 61381 Friedrichsdorf, Germany.

**Bioindustria, Ital.** See *Pfizer, Ital.*

**Biokanol, Ger.** Biokanol Pharma GmbH, Kehler Str. 7, 76437 Rastatt, Germany.

**Biokosma, Braz.** Biokosma Ltda, Avenida Senador Cesar Lacerda, Vergueiro 1011, 13600-970 Araras, SP, Brazil.

**Biol, Arg.** Inst. Biolsgico Arg. S.A.I.C., J. E. Uriburu 153, 1027 Buenos Aires, Argentina.

**Biolab, Hong Kong.** See *Great Eastern, Hong Kong*, and *Mekim, Hong Kong.*

**Biolab, Malaysia.** See *Medispec, Malaysia.*

**Biolab, NZ.** Biolab Scientific, P.O. Box 102-922, North Shore Mail Centre, Auckland, New Zealand.

**Biolab, Singapore.** See *Indrugco, Singapore.*

**Biolab, Thai.** See *Biopharm, Thai.*

**Biolab Sanus, Braz.** Biolab Sanus Farmaceutica, Av. dos Bandeirantes 5386, Planalto Paulista, 04071-900 Sao Paulo, SP, Brazil.

**Biolac, Swed.** Biolac AB, Box 22057, 250 22 Helsingborg, Sweden.

**Biolatina, Chile.** Biolatina Chile SA, San Sebastian 2807, Las Condes, Santiago, Chile.

**Biolitec, UK.** Biolitec Pharma Ltd, Research Avenue South, Herriot Watt Research Park, Edinburgh, EH14 4AP, UK.

**Biologia, Braz.** Laboratorio Brasileiro de Biologia Ltda, Rua Allan Kardec 66, Engenho Novo, 20710-230 Rio de Janeiro, RJ, Brazil.

**Biological E, India.** Biological E. Ltd, 18/1&3, Azamabad, Hyderabad 500 020, India.

**Biologici Italia, Ital.** Biologici Italia Laboratories S.r.l., Via Cavour 41/3, 20026 Novate Milanese (MI), Italy.

**Biologiques de l'Ile-de-France, Fr.** See *Medix, Fr.*

**Biomatrix, Hong Kong.** See *Genzyme, Hong Kong.*

**Biomatrix, Israel.** See *Agis, Israel.*

**Biomatrix, Swed.** See *Genzyme, Denm.*

**Biomatrix, Switz.** Biomatrix (Schweiz) GmbH, Bahnhofstrasse 21, Postfach, 6301 Zug, Switzerland.

**Biomatrix, UK.** See *Genzyme, UK.*

**Biomed, Austral.** Biomed Australia Pty Ltd., Unit 3, 9 Packard Ave, Castle Hill, NSW 2154, Australia.

**Biomed, NZ.** Biomed Ltd, P.O. Box 44069, Pt Chevalier, Auckland, New Zealand.

**Biomed, Singapore.** Biomed Pte Ltd, 32 Kallang Pudding Rd, 07-06 Elite Industrial Building 1, S 349313, Singapore.

**Biomed, Spain.** Biomed, Aragon 178, Entreplanta, Palma de Mallorca, 07008 Mallorca, Spain.

**Biomed, Switz.** Biomed AG, Uberlandstrasse 199, Postfach, 8600 Dubendorf 1, Switzerland.

**Biomedica, Austral.** See *Keller, Austral.*

**Biomedica, Ger.** Biomedica Pharma-Produkte GmbH, Birkenweg 16, 63871 Heinrichsthal, Germany.

**Biomedica, Hong Kong.** See *Trendful, Hong Kong.*

**Biomedica, Ital.** Biomedica Foscama Industria Chimico Farmaceutica S.p.A., Via Morolense 87, 03013 Ferentino (FR), Italy.

**Biomedica, Thai.** See *Osotspa, Thai.*

**Biomedica-Chemica, Gr.** BIOMEDICA-CHEMICA AE, Γ. Λύρα 25, 145 64 Κ. Κηφισιά, K. Kiphisia, Greece.

**Bio-Medical, UK.** Bio-Medical Services Ltd, River View Rd, Beverley, North Humberside, HU17 0LD, UK.

**Biomedis, Hong Kong.** See *Unam, Hong Kong.*

**Biomedis, Malaysia.** See *Unam, Malaysia.*

**Biomedis, Singapore.** See *Far East, Singapore.*

**Biomedis, Thai.** See *Olic, Thai.*

**Biomerica, USA.** Biomerica Inc., 1533 Monrovia Ave, Newport Beach, CA 92663, USA.

**Bio-Merieux, Hong Kong.** See *Primal, Hong Kong.*

**Bio-Merieux, Spain.** bioMérieux España S.A., Manuel Tovar 36, 28034 Madrid, Spain.

**Biomet, Austral.** Biomet Australia Pty Ltd, 4/6-8 Byfield St, North Ryde, NSW 2113, Australia.

**Biomet, UK.** Biomet UK Ltd, Waterton Industrial Estate, Bridgend, South Wales, CF31 3XA, UK.

**Biomet Merck, Denm.** Biomet Merck ApS, Hattingvej 7, 8700 Horsens, Denmark.

**Biomet Merck, Ger.** Biomet Merck Deutschland GmbH, Gustav-Krone-Str. 2, 14167 Berlin, Germany.

**Biomet Merck, Norw.** Biomet Merck Norge AS, Sorkedalsv. 257, 0754 Oslo, Norway.

**Biomet Merck, UK.** See *Biomet, UK.*

**Biomo, Ger.** Biomo Pharma GmbH, Lendersbergstrasse 86, 53721 Siegburg, Germany.

**Bional, Ger.** Bional Pharma Deutschland GmbH & Co. KG, Heidsieker Heide 144, 33739 Bielefeld, Germany.

**Bionatec, Fr.** Laboratoires Bionatec, Parc de Sophia Antipolis, 774 route des Trois Moulins, 06600 Antibes, France.

**Bionax, Hong Kong.** Bionax Hong Kong Ltd, 2/F, Hong Kong Spinners Bldg, 800 Cheung Sha Wan Rd, Kowloon, Hong Kong.

**Bionax, Malaysia.** See *Diethelm, Malaysia*, and *JDH, Malaysia.*

**Bionax, Singapore.** Bionax Singapore Pte Ltd, 99 Bukit Timah Rd, Alfa Centre 03-06, S 229835, Singapore.

**Bionax, Thai.** Bionax (Thailand) Ltd, 10 Fl, Unit A, Lake Rajada Office Complex, 193/35 New Rachadapisek Rd, Kwaeng Klongtoey, Khet Klongtoey, Bangkok 10110, Thailand.

**Bioniche, Canad.** Bioniche Pharma, 151 Dundas St, Suite 507, London, Ontario, N6A 5R7, Canada.

**Bionorica, Ger.** Bionorica Arzneimittel GmbH, Kerschensteinerstr. 11-15, 92318 Neumarkt/Opf, Germany.

**Bionorica, Hong Kong.** See *Jacobson, Hong Kong.*

**Bionorica, Singapore.** See *MBD, Singapore.*

**Bionorica, Thai.** See *Zuellig, Thai.*

**Bio-Oil Research, Irl.** See *Allphar, Irl.*

**Bio-Oil Research, UK.** Bio-Oil Research Ltd, The Hawthorns, 64 Welsh Row, Nantwich, Cheshire, CW5 5EU, UK.

**Biopat, Spain.** See *Merck Sharp & Dohme, Spain.*

**Biopha, Fr.** Laboratoires Dermopharmaceutiques Biopha, 15 rue Ampere, 91748 Massy cdx, France.

**Biopharm, Hong Kong.** See *Great Eastern, Hong Kong*, and *Mekim, Hong Kong.*

**Biopharm, Thai.** Biopharm Chemicals Co. Ltd, 7 Fl, Bio House, 55 Sukhumvit 39, Bangkok 10110, Thailand.

**Biopharm, USA.** Bio-Pharm Inc, 10 H Runway Rd, Levittown, PA 19057, USA.

**Biopharma, Fr.** Biopharma, 29 rue du Pont, 92200 Neuilly-sur-Seine, France.

**Biopharma, Ital.** Biopharma S.r.l., Via delle Gerbere 20/22/30/32, 00040 Santa Palomba (RM), Italy.

**Bio-Pharmaceuticals, Malaysia.** Bio-Pharmaceuticals Sdn Bhd, C-5-8, Block C, Centre Point Business Park, 5 Jln 26/53, Seksyen 26, 400000 Shah Alam, Selangor, Malaysia.

**Biophausia, Denm.** See *Biophausia, Swed.*

**Biophausia, Ger.** See *Biophausia, Swed.*

**Biophausia, Norw.** See *Biophausia, Swed.*

**Biophausia, Swed.** BioPhausia AB, AR 4, 741 74 Uppsala, Sweden.

**Biophytarom, Fr.** Laboratoires Biophytarom, Cap 18, 43 rue de l'Evangile, 75886 Paris cdx 18, France.

**Bioprogress, Ital.** Bioprogress S.p.A., Via Aurelia 58, 00165 Rome, Italy.

**Bioprojet, Fr.** Bioprojet Pharma, 9 rue Rameau, 75002 Paris, France.

**Biopura, Port.** Biopura, Lda, Urbanizcao Industrial Ourreca, Rua Por do Sol 4, 2735 Cacem, Portugal.

**Bioquest, Ger.** BioQuest GmbH, Holtystr. 19, 30171 Hannover, Germany.

**Bioquimico, Arg.** Lab. Bioqummico Argentino S.R.L., Irala 1575, 1164 Buenos Aires, Argentina.

**Bioquimico, Mex.** Laboratorios Bioquimico Mexicano, S.A. de C.V, Lieja 8-8o. Piso, Col. Juarez, Deleg. Cuauhtemoc, 06600 Mexico D.F., Mexico.

**Bioren, Switz.** Bioren SA, 4 rue des iles, 2108 Couvet, Switzerland.

**Biores, Ital.** Biores Italia S.r.l., Via Vittorio Grassi 13, 00155 Rome, Italy.

**Bioresearch, Mex.** Bioresearch de Mexico S.A. de C.V., Calle San Luis Tlatilco No. 5, Fracc. Ind. San Luis Tlatilco, 53370 Naucalpan de Juarez, Mexico.

**Bioresearch, Spain.** Bioresearch, Avda de Burgos 91, Edif. 4, 28050 Madrid, Spain.

**Biorex, UK.** Biorex Laboratories Ltd, 2 Crossfield Chambers, Gladbeck Way, Enfield, Middlesex, EN2 7HT, UK.

**Biorga, Fr.** Laboratoires Biorga, 98 av de la Republique, 92400 Courbevoie, France.

**Biorga, Hong Kong.** See *CNW, Hong Kong.*

**Bios, Belg.** Bios-Coutelier S.A., Route de Lennik 437, 1070 Brussels, Belgium.

**Biosan, Ital.** Biosan S.r.l., Via Pisacane 26, 20016 Pero (MI), Italy.

**Biosano, Chile.** Laboratorios Biosano SA, Aeropuerto 9941, Cerrillos, Santiago, Chile.

**Bio-Sante, Canad.** Les Laboratoires Bio-Sante, 3564 Griffith St, St-Laurent, Quebec, H4C 1A7, Canada.

**Biosarto, Spain.** Biosarto, FOC 68-82, 08030 Barcelona, Spain.

**Biosaude, Port.** Biosaúe, Lda, Av. Duque d'Avila 193 - 8, 1050-082 Lisbon, Portugal.

**Bioscience, Thai.** Bioscience Co. Ltd, 4/15 Moo 5 Rama II Rd, Samae-Dam, Bangkhuntien, Bangkok 10150, Thailand.

**Bioser (Βιοσερ), Gr.** ΒΙΟΣΕΡ ΑΕ, Κανάρη 5, 141 22 Ν. Ηράκλειο, N. Irakleio, Greece.

**Biosintetica, Braz.** Laboratorios Biosintetica Ltda, Av das Nacoes Unidas 22.428, Jd. Jurubatuab, 04795-916 Sao Paulo, SP, Brazil.

**Biospray, Gr.** BIOSPRAY, Βικτ Ουγκώ 45, 104 37 Αθήνα, Athens, Greece.

**Biostam (Βιοσταμ), Gr.** ΒΙΟΣΤΑΜ Κ.ΜΠΟΥΓΙΑ & ΣΙΑ ΟΕ, Παπαδιαμαντοπούλου 66, 157 71 Ζωγραφου, Zographou, Greece.

**Biosyn, Ger.** biosyn Arzneimittel GmbH, Schorndorfer Str. 32, 70734 Fellbach, Germany.

**Biosyn, Switz.** See *Medinova, Switz.*

**Biotech, Austral.** See *Milton, Austral.*

**Biotech, S.Afr.** Biotech Laboratories (Pty) Ltd, P.O. Box 7115, Johannesburg 2000, South Africa.

**Bio-Tech, USA.** Bio-Tech Pharmacal, P.O. Box 1992, Fayetteville, AR 72702, USA.

**Biotechnology, Israel.** Biotechnology General Israel Ltd, Kiryat Weisman, Rehovot, Israel.

**Biotek, NZ.** Biotek, P.O. Box 14-323, Panmure, New Zealand.

**Biotekfarma, Ital.** Biotekfarma bkf S.r.l., Italy.

**Biotel, USA.** Biotel Corporation, 366 Madison Ave 1506, New York, NY 10017, USA.

**Biotenk, Arg.** Laboratorio Farmaceutico Biotenk S.A., Zuvirma 5747, 1439 Buenos Aires, Argentina.

**Biotest, Austria.** Biotest Pharmazeutika GmbH, Einsiedlergasse 58, Postfach 8, A-1053 Vienna, Austria.

**Biotest, Fin.** See *Leo, Fin.*

**Biotest, Ger.** Biotest Pharma GmbH, Landsteinerstr. 3-5, 63303 Dreieich, Germany.

**Biotest, Hong Kong.** See *Chong Lap, Hong Kong.*

**Biotest, Israel.** See *Margalit, Israel.*

**Biotest, Ital.** Biotest Italia S.r.l., Via L. da Vinci 43, 20090 Trezzano sul Naviglio (MI), Italy.

**Biotest, Malaysia.** See *Lazuli, Malaysia.*

**Biotest, Port.** See *Boehringer Ingelheim, Port.*

**Biotest, Singapore.** See *Summit, Singapore.*

**Biotest, Switz.** Biotest (Schweiz) AG, Schutzenstrasse 17, 5102 Rupperswil, Switzerland.

**Biotest, Thai.** See *Charoen, Thai.*

**Bio-Therabel, Belg.** See *Therabel, Belg.*

**Biotherapie, Fr.** See *Expanscience, Fr.*

**Biotherm, Canad.** Biotherm Canada, 2115 Crescent St, Montreal, Quebec, H3G 2C1, Canada.

**Biotrading, Ital.** Biotrading di Maurizio Mannone, Via Francesco Struppa 4, 91025 Marsala (TP), Italy.

**Bio-Transfusion, Fr.** Bio-Transfusion, France.

**Biotrends, Gr.** BIOTRENDS, Βορ Ηπείρου 65, 146 71 Ν. Ερυθραία, N. Erithraia, Greece.

**Biovac, S.Afr.** Biovac SA CC, P.O. Box 14374, Wadeville 1422, South Africa.

**Biovail, Canad.** Biovail Pharmaceuticals, 2480 Dunwin Drive, Mississauga, Ontario, L5L 1J9, Canada.

**Biovail, Denm.** See *Gea, Denm.*

**Biovail, USA.** Biovail Pharmaceuticals Inc., 170 Southport Drive, Morrisville, NC 27560, USA.

**Biovital, Austral.** Biovital P/L, 24/10 Yalgar Road, Kirrawee, NSW 2232, Australia.

**Biovitrum, Denm.** Biovitrum AB, Overgaden neden Vandet 7, 1414 Copenhagen K, Denmark.

**Biovitrum, Norw.** See *Biovitrum, Swed.*

**Biovitrum, Swed.** Biovitrum AB, Plasma Products, 112 76 Stockholm, Sweden.

**Bipharma, Neth.** Bipharma BV, Flevolaan 50, 1382 JZ Weesp, Netherlands.

**Birchwood, USA.** Birchwood Laboratories Inc., 7900 Fuller Rd, Eden Prairie, MN 53344, USA.

**Bird, USA.** Bird Products Corp., 1100 Bird Center Drive, Palm Springs, CA 92262, USA.

**Biscova, Ger.** Biscova-Arzneimittel, Fuhrenkamp 7, 29559 Wrestedt/Stederdorf, Germany.

**Bitelab, Fin.** Bitelab Oy, Paloheinäntie 62 b A, 00670 Helsinki, Finland.

**Bittermedizin, Ger.** Bittermedizin Arzneimittel Vertriebs-GmbH, Taku-Fort-Str. 20, 81827 Munich, Germany.

**Bittner, Austria.** Richard Bittner GmbH, A-9344 Weitensfeld 183, Austria.

**BL, Braz.** See *Bausch & Lomb, Braz.*

**Blackhall, Irl.** Blackhall Pharmaceutical Distributors Ltd, Saucertown, Swords, Dublin, Ireland.

**Blackmores, Austral.** Blackmores Ltd, P.O. Box 258, Balgowlah, NSW 2093, Australia.

**Blackmores, Thai.** Blackmores Ltd, 20B Mahanakorn Gypsum Building, 539/2 Sriayuddhaya Rd, Ratchathewi, Bangkok 10400, Thailand.

**Blackmores, UK.** Blackmores UK, 37 Rotasckild Rd, Chiswick, London, W4 5HT, UK.

**Blackwell, UK.** Blackwell Supplies Ltd, Medcare House, Centurion Close, Gillingham Business Park, Gillingham, Kent, ME8 0SB, UK.

**Blaine, USA.** Blaine Pharmaceuticals Co. Inc., 1515 Production Drive, Burlington, KY 41005, USA.

**Blair, USA.** See *Purdue Frederick, USA.*

**Blairex, USA.** Blairex Labs Inc., 3240 Indianapolis Rd, P.O. Box 2127, Columbus, IN 47202-2127, USA.

**Blake, UK.** Thomas Blake & Co., The Byre House, Fearby, Nr Masham, North Yorkshire, HG4 4NF, UK.

**Blansett, USA.** Blansett Pharmacal Co., Inc., P.O. Box 638, North Little Rock, AR 72115, USA.

**Blausiegel, Braz.** Blausiegel Industria e Comercio Ltda, Rodovia Raposo Tavares km 30.5 no.2833, 06705-030 Cotia Barro Branco, SP, Brazil.

**Bledina, Fr.** Bledina SA, B.P. 432, 69654 Villefranche-sur-Saone cdx, France.

**BLH, Thai.** BLH Trading Co. Ltd, 7/1 Wireless Rd, Bangkok 10330, Thailand.

**Blis, NZ.** Blis Technologies, P.O. Box 1229, Level 4, 31 Waring Taylor St, Wellington, New Zealand.

**Blistex, Canad.** Blistex Ltd, Canada.

**Blistex, Hong Kong.** See *Mekim, Hong Kong.*

**Blistex, Israel.** See *Mediline, Israel.*

**Blistex, USA.** Blistex Inc., 1800 Swift Drive, Oak Brook, IL 60523, USA.

**Block, Austria.** See *GlaxoSmithKline, Austria.*

**Block, Canad.** See *GlaxoSmithKline Consumer, Canad.*

**Block, Ger.** See *GlaxoSmithKline Consumer, Ger.*

**Block, USA.** See *GlaxoSmithKline Consumer, USA.*

**Blooms, Austral.** Blooms, Australia.

**BML, Austral.** BML Pharmaceuticals P/L, P.O. Box 31, Arncliffe, NSW 2205, Australia.

**BOC, UK.** BOC Gases, Priestly Rd, Worsley, Manchester, M28 2UT, UK.

**Boca, USA.** Boca Pharmacal Inc., 6601 Lyons Rd, Coconut Creek, FL 33073, USA.

**Bock, Ger.** Bock-Pharma GmbH, Odenwaldstr. 2, 64646 Heppenheim, Germany.

**Bode, Austria.** See *Bode, Ger.*

**Bode, Ger.** Bode Chemie Hamburg, Melanchthonstr. 27, 22525 Hamburg, Germany.

**Bodene, S.Afr.** See *Fresenius Kabi, S.Afr.*

**Body Research, Thai.** Body Research Co. Ltd, 72/2 Taksin Rd, Bukkalo Thonburi, Bangkok 10600, Thailand.

**Body Spring, Ital.** Body Spring S.r.l., Circ.ne Bran 40, 37013 Caprino V.se (VR), Italy.

**Boehringer de Angeli, Braz.** See *Boehringer Ingelheim, Braz.*

**Boehringer Ingelheim, Arg.** Boehringer Ingelheim S.A., Av. del Libertador 7208, 1429 Buenos Aires, Argentina.

**Boehringer Ingelheim, Austral.** Boehringer Ingelheim P/L, P.O. Box 1969, Macquarie Centre, North Ryde, NSW 2113, Australia.

**Boehringer Ingelheim, Austria.** Boehringer Ingelheim Austria GmbH, Dr Boehringer-Gasse 5-11, A-1121 Vienna, Austria.

**Boehringer Ingelheim, Belg.** Boehringer Ingelheim S.A., Vesalius Science Park, Ave Ariane 16, 1200 Brussels, Belgium.

**Boehringer Ingelheim, Braz.** Boehringer Ingelheim Do Brasil Quim. e Farm. Ltda, Av. Maria Coelho Aguiar 215, Bl. F. 3° andar, 05804-970 Sao Paulo, SP, Brazil.

**Boehringer Ingelheim, Canad.** Boehringer Ingelheim (Canada) Ltd, 5180 South Service Rd, Burlington, Ontario, L7L 5H4, Canada.

**Boehringer Ingelheim, Chile.** Boehringer Ingelheim, Carlos Fernandez 260, San Joaquin, Santiago, Chile.

**Boehringer Ingelheim, Denm.** Boehringer Ingelheim Danmark A/S, Strodamvej 52, 2100 Copenhagen O, Denmark.

**Boehringer Ingelheim, Fin.** Boehringer Ingelheim Finland Ky, Harmaaparrankuja 1, PL 57, 02101 Espoo, Finland.

**Boehringer Ingelheim, Fr.** Boehringer Ingelheim France, 37-9 rue Boissiere, 75116 Paris, France.

**Boehringer Ingelheim, Ger.** Boehringer Ingelheim Pharma GmbH & Co. KG, Binger Str. 173, 55216 Ingelheim, Germany.

**Boehringer Ingelheim, Gr.** BOEHRINGER ING AE, Ελληνικού 2, 167 77 Ελληνικό, Elliniko, Greece.

**Boehringer Ingelheim, Hong Kong.** Boehringer Ingelheim (Hong Kong) Ltd, Suite 1504-7, Great Eagle Ctr, 23 Harbour Rd, Wanchai, Hong Kong.

**Boehringer Ingelheim, Irl.** Boehringer Ingelheim Ltd, Corrig Court, Corrig Road, Sandyford Industrial Estate, Dublin 18, Ireland.

**Boehringer Ingelheim, Israel.** See *Teva, Israel.*

**Boehringer Ingelheim, Ital.** Boehringer Ingelheim Italia S.p.A., Via Lorenzini 8, 20139 Milan, Italy.

**Boehringer Ingelheim, Jpn.** Nippon Boehringer Ingelheim Co. Ltd, 3-10-1 Yato, Kawanishi-shi, Hyogo 666-0193, Japan.

**Boehringer Ingelheim, Malaysia.** Boehringer Ingelheim, Division Diethelm Malaysia Sdn Bhd, P.O. Box 3031, 47620 Subang Jaya, Selangor, Malaysia.

**Boehringer Ingelheim, Mex.** Boehringer Ingelheim Promeco, S.A. de C.V., Calle del Maiz No. 49, Col. Xaltocan, Deleg. Xochimilco, 16090 Mexico D.F., Mexico.

**Boehringer Ingelheim, Neth.** Boehringer Ingelheim BV, Berenkoog 28, 1822 BJ Alkmaar, Netherlands.

**Boehringer Ingelheim, Norw.** Boehringer Ingelheim Norway KS, Drengsrudbekken 25, Postboks 405, 1371 Asker, Norway.

**Boehringer Ingelheim, NZ.** Boehringer Ingelheim (NZ) Ltd, P.O. Box 76-216, Manukau City, Auckland, New Zealand.

**Boehringer Ingelheim, Port.** Boehringer Ingelheim, Lda, Av. Antonio Augusto de Aguiar 104, 1063-019 Lisbon, Portugal.

**Boehringer Ingelheim, S.Afr.** Boehringer Ingelheim (Pty) Ltd, Private Bag X3032, Randburg 2125, South Africa.

**Boehringer Ingelheim, Singapore.** See *Diethelm, Singapore.*

**Boehringer Ingelheim, Spain.** Boehringer Ingelheim, Prat d ela Riba S/N, Sector Turo de Can Matas, Sant Cugat del Valles, 08190 Barcelona, Spain.

**Boehringer Ingelheim, Swed.** Boehringer Ingelheim AB, Box 47608, 117 94 Stockholm, Sweden.

**Boehringer Ingelheim, Switz.** Boehringer Ingelheim (Schweiz) GmbH, Dufourstrasse 54, 4002 Basle, Switzerland.

**Boehringer Ingelheim, Thai.** Boehringer Ingelheim (Thai) Ltd, 12 Fl, Charn Issara Tower II, 2922/207-208 New Petchburi Rd, Bangkapi, Huay Kwang, Bangkok 10310, Thailand.

**Boehringer Ingelheim, UK.** Boehringer Ingelheim Ltd, Ellesfield Ave, Bracknell, Berkshire, RG12 4YS, UK.

**Boehringer Ingelheim, USA.** Boehringer Ingelheim Pharmaceuticals Inc., 900 Ridgebury Rd, P.O. Box 368, Ridgefield, CT 06877-0368, USA.

**Boehringer Ingelheim Consumer, Canad.** Boehringer Ingelhein (Canada) Ltd, Consumer Healthcare Division, 1781 W 75th Ave, Vancouver, British Columbia, V6P 6P2, Canada.

**Boehringer Ingelheim Promeco, Mex.** See *Boehringer Ingelheim, Mex.*

**Boehringer Ingelheim Self Medication, UK.** See *Boehringer Ingelheim, UK.*

**Boehringer Mannheim, Belg.** Boehringer Mannheim Belgium S.A., Avenue des Croix de Guerre 90, 1120 Brussels, Belgium.

**Boehringer Mannheim, Canad.** See *Roche, Canad.*

**Boehringer Mannheim, Fr.** See *Roche Diagnostics, Fr.*

**Boehringer Mannheim, Ger.** See *Roche, Ger.*

**Boehringer Mannheim, Irl.** See *Roche Diagnostics, UK.*

**Boehringer Mannheim, Israel.** See *Teva, Israel.*

**Boehringer Mannheim, Ital.** See *Roche, Ital.*

**Boehringer Mannheim, Neth.** See *Roche, Neth.*

**Boehringer Mannheim, Norw.** See *Roche, Norw.*

**Boehringer Mannheim, Port.** See *Roche, Port.*

**Boehringer Mannheim, S.Afr.** See *Roche, S.Afr.*

**Boehringer Mannheim, Spain.** See *Roche, Spain.*

**Boehringer Mannheim, Swed.** See *Roche, Swed.*

**Boehringer Mannheim, Switz.** See *Roche, Switz.*

**Boehringer Mannheim, USA.** See *Roche, USA.*

**Boehringer Mannheim Diagnostics, Irl.** See *Roche Diagnostics, UK.*

**Boehringer Mannheim Diagnostics, USA.** See *Roche, USA.*

**Boehringer Mannheim Roche, Spain.** See *Roche, Spain.*

**Boffi, Ital.** Eredi di Antonio Boffi S.n.c., Via Lorenzo Magalotti 6, 00197 Rome, Italy.

**Bohm, Spain.** Bohm, Molina Seca 23 Plg. Cobo Calleja, Fuenlabrada, 28947 Madrid, Spain.

**BOI, Spain.** Biologicos Organicos Industriales, Polig Ind Sur, Papiol, 08754 Barcelona, Spain.

**Boileau & Boyd, Irl.** Boileau & Boyd Ltd, Parkmore Estate, Walkinstown, Dublin 12, Ireland.

**Boiron, Canad.** Boiron Canada, 816 Guimond St, Longueil, Quebec, J4G 1T5, Canada.

**Boiron, Fr.** Boiron, 20 rue de la Liberation, 69110 Sainte-Foy-les-Lyon, France.

**Boiron, Port.** See *Prisfar, Port.*

**Boiron, Switz.** See *Serolab, Switz.*

**Bolder, Ger.** Bolder Arzneimittel GmbH & Co. KG, Koblenzer Str. 65, 50968 Cologne, Germany.

**Bonafarma, Port.** Bonafarma, SA, Apartado 197, Edificio JABA, Abrunheira, 2710-901 Sintra, Portugal.

**Bonapace, Thai.** Bonapace, Thailand.

**Boncour, Fr.** Laboratoires Boncour, 46 av. de Lattre-de-Tassigny, 94410 Saint-Maurice, France.

**Bone Care, USA.** Bone Care International, Bone Care Center, 1600 Aspen Commons, Middleton, WI 53562, USA.

**Boniscontro & Gazzone, Ital.** Laboratorio Prodotti Farmaceutici Boniscontro & Gazzone S.r.l., Via Tiburtina 1004, 00156 Rome, Italy.

**Bonne Bell, Canad.** Bonne Bell of Canada, 6711 Mississauga Rd, Ste 602, Mississauga, Ontario, L5N 2W3, Canada.

**Bonomelli, Ital.** Bonomelli S.r.l., Divisione Farmacia, Via Montecuccoli 1, 23843 Dolzago (LC), Italy.

**Boots, Austral.** See *Boots Healthcare, Austral.*

**Boots, Denm.** See *AstraZeneca, Denm.*

**Boots, Fin.** See *Alpharma, Fin.*

**Boots, Fr.** See *Knoll, Fr.*

**Boots, Ger.** See *Kanoldt, Ger.*

**Boots, Hong Kong.** See *Keller, Hong Kong.*

**Boots, Israel.** See *Teva, Israel.*

**Boots, Singapore.** The Boots Company (Far East) Pte Ltd, 180-B Bencoolen St, 09-03 The Bencoolen, S 189648, Singapore.

**Boots, Spain.** See *Boots Healthcare, Spain.*

**Boots, Switz.** See *Doetsch, Grether, Switz.*

**Boots, Thai.** See *Olic, Thai.*

**Boots, UK.** Boots the Chemists, Thane Rd, D90 East FO8, Nottingham, NG90 1BS, UK.

**Boots, USA.** See *Abbott, USA.*

**Boots Healthcare, Austral.** Boots Healthcare Australia P/L, Locked Bag 2067, North Ryde, NSW 2113, Australia.

**Boots Healthcare, Austria.** See *Boots Healthcare, Ger.*

**Boots Healthcare, Belg.** Boots Healthcare S.A., Koningin Astridlaan 164, 1780 Wemmel, Belgium.

**Boots Healthcare, Fr.** Laboratoires Boots Healthcare, 35 rue Baudin, 92300 Lavallois-Perret, France.

**Boots Healthcare, Ger.** Boots Healthcare Deutschland GmbH, Scholtzstr. 3, 21465 Reinbek, Germany.

**Boots Healthcare, Irl.** Boots Healthcare Ltd, Parkview House, Beech Hill Office Campus, Clonskeagh, Dublin 4, Ireland.

**Boots Healthcare, Ital.** Boots Healthcare S.p.A., Via Tarantelli 13/15, 22076 Mozzate (CO), Italy.

**Boots Healthcare, Malaysia.** Boots Trading (Malaysia) Sdn Bhd, Level 4, Wisma Samudra, 1 Jln Kontraktor U1/14, Hicom-Glenmarie Industrial Park, 40150 Shah Alam, Selangor, Malaysia.

**Boots Healthcare, Neth.** Boots Healthcare BV, Gooimeer 6-26, 1411 DD Naarden, Netherlands.

**Boots Healthcare, NZ.** Boots Healthcare New Zealand Ltd, P.O. Box 27-341, Wellington 1, New Zealand.

**Boots Healthcare, Port.** Boots Healthcare Portugal, Lda, Av. Duque d'Avila, 185, 1050 Lisbon, Portugal.

**Boots Healthcare, S.Afr.** Boots Healthcare (SA) (Pty) Ltd, P.O. Box 30178, Jet Park 1469, South Africa.

**Boots Healthcare, Spain.** Boots Healthcare, Doctor Zamenhof 36 Dup 2, 28027 Madrid, Spain.

**Boots Healthcare, Switz.** Boots Healthcare (Switzerland) AG, Hermal, Untermuli 11, 6300 Zug, Switzerland.

**Boots Piramal, India.** See *Nicholas Piramal, India.*

**Boots-Flint, USA.** See *Abbott, USA.*

**Borer, Thai.** Borer Chemie.

**Borg, UK.** Borg Medicare Ltd, P.O. Box 99, Hitchin, Hertfordshire, SG5 2GF, UK.

**Bottger, Ger.** Böttger GmbH, Paulsborner Str. 2, 10709 Berlin, Germany.

**Bouchara, Fr.** See *Bouchara-Recordati, Fr.*

**Bouchara, Port.** See *Neo-Farmaceutica, Port.*

**Bouchara, Singapore.** See *Pharmacon, Singapore.*

**Bouchara, Switz.** See *Actipharm, Switz.*, and *Interdelta, Switz.*

**Bouchara-Recordati, Fr.** Laboratoires Bouchara-Recordati, 68 rue Marjolin, 92302 Levallois-Perret, France.

**Bouchara-Recordati, Hong Kong.** See *Rich Plan, Hong Kong.*

**Boucher & Muir, Austral.** Boucher & Muir P/L, P.O. Box 333, North Sydney, NSW 2059, Australia.

**Bouhon, Ger.** Apotheker Walter Bouhon GmbH & Co. KG, Fuldaer Str. 10, 90427 Nurnberg, Germany.

**Bournonville, Belg.** Bournonville Pharma S.A., Ave De Messidor 330, 1180 Brussels, Belgium.

**Bournonville, Neth.** Bournonville Pharma BV, Nassaulaan 13, 2514 JS Den Haag, Netherlands.

**Bouty, Ital.** S.P.A. Italiana Laboratori Bouty, V.le Casiraghi 471, 20099 Sesto S Giovanni (MI), Italy.

**Bouzen, Arg.** Bouzen S.A.C.,I.F.A.F., Calle 36 No. 165/67, 1900 La Plata, Buenos Aires, Argentina.

**Bowman, USA.** Bowman Pharmaceuticals Inc., 119 Schroyer Ave SW, Canton, OH 44702, USA.

**Boyle, USA.** Boyle & Co. Pharmaceuticals, 1613 Chelsea Rd, San Marino, CA 91108, USA.

**BPL, Hong Kong.** See *JDH, Hong Kong.*

**BPL, India.** BPL Pharmaceuticals Pvt Ltd, 380/82 Sankersett Rd, Sankersett Smriti, Chira Bazar, Mumbai 400 002, India.

**BPL, Israel.** See *Kamada, Israel.*

**BPL, Singapore.** See *JDH, Singapore.*

**BPL, Thai.** See *Berli, Thai.*

**BPL, UK.** Bio Products Laboratory, Dagger Lane, Elstree, Hertfordshire, WD6 3BX, UK.

**BPL-Meizler, Braz.** See *Meizler, Braz.*

**BPR, Ital.** BPR International S.r.l., Via Valera 7, 20024 Garbagnate Milanese (MI), Italy.

**BPRL, Singapore.** See *Zyfas, Singapore.*

**BR Pharmaceuticals, UK.** BR Pharmaceuticals Ltd, 51a Broom Mill Estate, Coal Hill Lane, Farsley, Leeds, West Yorkshire, LS28 5NA, UK.

**Bracco, Canad.** Bracco Diagnostics Inc, Suite 103, Unit 11, 2600 Skymark Avenue, Mississauga, Ontario, L4W 5B2, Canada.

**Bracco, Denm.** See *Astra Tech, Denm.*

**Bracco, Israel.** See *Dexxon, Israel.*

**Bracco, Ital.** Bracco S.p.A., Via E. Folli 50, 20134 Milan, Italy.

**Bracco, Norw.** See *Astra Tech, Norw.*

**Bracco, Port.** See *Dario Correia, Port.*

**Bracco, Switz.** See *Sintetica, Switz.*, and *Uhlmann-Eyraud, Switz.*

**Bracco, UK.** Bracco UK Ltd, Bracco House, Mercury Park, Wycombe Lane, Wooburn Green, High Wycombe, Buckinghamshire, HP10 0HH, UK.

**Bracco, USA.** Bracco Diagnostics, 107 College Road East, Princeton, NJ 08540, USA.

**Bracey, UK.** Bracey's Pharmaceuticals, 209 Menlove Ave, Liverpool, Merseyside, L18 3EF, UK.

**Bradley, Canad.** Bradley Pharmaceuticals Inc., 1031 Meyerside Drive, Unit 12, Mississauga, Ontario, L5T 2H5, Canada.

**Bradley, Singapore.** See *MD, Singapore*, and *PMR, Singapore.*

**Bradley, USA.** See *Doak, USA.*

**Bradleys, NZ.** Bradleys Pharmaceuticals, 69 The Esplanade, Whangaparaoa, Hibiscus Coast, North Auckland, New Zealand.

**Brady, Austria.** Brady C. KG, Horlgasse 5, A-1092 Vienna, Austria.

**Bragg, UK.** J.L. Bragg (Ipswich) Ltd, 34 Boss Hall Rd, Ipswich, Suffolk, IP1 5BN, UK.

**Brahms, Ger.** BRAHMS Arzneimittel GmbH, Kreuzberger Ring 13, 65205 Wiesbaden, Germany.

**Braintree, Canad.** See *Source, Canad.*

**Braintree, USA.** Braintree Laboratories Inc., P.O. Box 850929, Braintree, MA 02185-0929, USA.

**Brandt, Switz.** See *Uhlmann-Eyraud, Switz.*

**Brasifa, Braz.** Sociedade Farmaceutica Brasifa Ltda, Rua Souto Carvalho 45, 23520-210 Rio de Janeiro, RJ, Brazil.

**Braskap, Braz.** Braskap Industria e Comercio S.A., Av. Conde Zepellin 3356, Eden, 18103-008 Sorocaba, SP, Brazil.

**Brasmedica, Braz.** Brasmedica S.A. Industrias Farmaceuticas, Avenida Miguel Stefano 2278, 04301-002 Sao Paulo, SP, Brazil.

**Brasterapica, Braz.** Brasterapica Industria Farmaceutica Ltda, Rua Bela Cintra 299 cj.71/72, 01415-000 Sao Paulo, SP, Brazil.

**Brauer, Austral.** Brauer Natural Medicine P/L, P.O. Box 234, Tanunda, SA 5352, Australia.

**Braun, Arg.** B. Braun Medical S.A., J. E. Uriburu 663 Pso. 7, 1027 Buenos Aires, Argentina.

**Braun, Austral.** B Braun Australia P/L, Norwest Business Park, 17 Lexington Drive, Bella Vista, NSW 2153, Australia.

**Braun, Austria.** Braun Austria GmbH, In den Langackern 5, A-2344 Maria Enzersdorf, Austria.

**Braun, Belg.** B. Braun Medical S.A., Woluwelaan 140 B, 1831 Diegem, Belgium.

**Braun, Braz.** Laboratorio B. Braun S.A., Avenida Dr Eugenio Borges 1092, Arsenal, 24751-000 Sao Goncalo, RJ, Brazil.

**Braun, Chile.** B Braun Medical SA, Calle Nueva 5319, Conchalf, Santiago, Chile.

**Braun, Denm.** B Braun Medical A/S, Halmtorvet 29, 1700 Copenhagen V, Denmark.

**Braun, Fin.** B. Braun Medical Oy, Niittyrinne 7, 02270 Espoo, Finland.

**Braun, Fr.** B Braun Medical SA, 204 av du Maljuin, B.P. 331, 92107 Boulogne cdx, France.

**Braun, Ger.** B. Braun Melsungen AG, Carl-Braun-Str. 1, 34212 Melsungen, Germany.

**Braun, Hong Kong.** B Braun Medical (HK) Ltd, 13-14/F Henan Bldg, 90 Jaffe Rd, Wanchai, Hong Kong.

**Braun, Irl.** B. Braun Medical Ltd, 3 Naas Rd Industrial Park, Dublin 12, Ireland.

**Braun, Israel.** Braun, Israel.

**Braun, Ital.** B. Braun Milano S.p.A., Via V. da Seregno 14, 20161 Milan, Italy.

**Braun, Norw.** B. Braun Medical A/S, Kjernasv 13 B, 3142 Vestskogen, Norway.

**Braun, Port.** B. Braun Medical, Lda, Estrada Consiglieri Pedroso 80, Queluz Park, Queluz de Baixo, 2745-533 Barcarena, Portugal.

**Braun, S.Afr.** B Braun (Pty) Ltd, P.O. Box 1787, Randburg 2125, South Africa.

**Braun, Singapore.** B Braun Singapore Pte Ltd, 460 Alexandra Rd, 34-03 PSA Building, S 119963, Singapore.

**Braun, Spain.** Braun Medical, Ctra Tarrasa 121, Rubi, 08191 Barcelona, Spain.

**Braun, Swed.** B. Braun Medical AB, Box 221, 167 22 Bromma, Sweden.

**Braun, Switz.** B. Braun Medical AG, Hospital Care, Postfach, 6020 Emmenbrucke, Switzerland.

**Braun, Thai.** B Braun (Thailand) Ltd, 12 Fl, Q-House Ploenchit Building, 598 Ploenchit Rd, Lumpini Pathumwan, Bangkok 10330, Thailand.

**Braun, UK.** B. Braun Medical Ltd, Thorncliffe Park Industrial Estate, Chapeltown, Sheffield, South Yorkshire, S35 2PW, UK.

**Braun, USA.** B. Braun Medical, 824 Twelfth Ave, Bethlehem, PA 18018, USA.

**Braun McGaw, Hong Kong.** See *LCH, Hong Kong.*

**Braun Melsungen, Ital.** See *Braun, Ital.*

**Braun Omnimed, S.Afr.** Braun Omnimed (Pty) Ltd, P.O. Box 2316, Randburg 2125, South Africa.

**Braun Surgical, Switz.** B. Braun Surgical AG, Postfach 427, 8212 Neuhausen, Switzerland.

**Bravir, Braz.** Bravir Industrial Ltda, Rua Simao Anotnio 1075, Cincao, 32371-610 Contagem, MG, Brazil.

**Bray, UK.** Bray Health & Leisure (Solport Ltd), 1 Regal Way, Faringdon, Oxfordshire, SN7 7BX, UK.

**Breathe Eazy, Austral.** Breathe Eazy Chest Rubs, 7 Melia Close, Medowie, NSW 2318, Australia.

**Breckenridge, USA.** Breckenridge Pharmaceutical Inc, 1141 South Rogers Circle, Suite 3, Boca Raton, FL 33487, USA.

**Bregenzer, Austria.** Herbert Bregenzer, Am Damm 20, A-6820 Frastanz, Austria.

**Brench, Ger.** Brench Pharma AG, Siegesstr. 26, 80802 Munich, Germany.

**Brenner-Efeka, Ger.** See *Wyeth, Ger.*

**Brenntag, Denm.** Brenntag Disinfection, Gl Strandv. 16, 2990 Niva, Denmark.

**Brenntag, Norw.** See *Brenntag, Denm.*

**Breves, Braz.** Bio Breves Industria Farmaceutica Ltda, Rua Barao de Petropolis 109, Rio Comprido, 20251-061 Rio de Janeiro, RJ, Brazil.

**Bride, Fr.** Laboratoires Bride, 263 c av de Laon, 51100 Reims, France.

**Bridoux, Fr.** Laboratoires Bridoux, 6 rue Salengro, 62160 Bully-les-Mines, France.

**Bright Future, Hong Kong.** Bright Future Pharmaceutical Laboratories Ltd, BF Pharmaceutical Ctr, 8 Wang Fu St, Yuen Long Industrial Estate, Yuen Long, N.T., Hong Kong.

**Brimms, Israel.** See *Trima, Israel.*

**Brioschi, Canad.** Brioschi Inc., 465 Fenmar Drive, Weston, Ontario, M9L 2R6, Canada.

**Bripharm, Irl.** See *United Drug, Irl.*

**Brissenco, S.Afr.** Brissenco, South Africa.

**Bristol, Canad.** See *Bristol-Myers Squibb, Canad.*

**Bristol, Jpn.** Bristol Pharmaceuticals K.K., 6-5-1 Nishi-Shinjuku, Shinjuku-ku, Tokyo 163-1328, Japan.

**Bristol-Myers, Austral.** See *Bristol-Myers Squibb, Austral.*

**Bristol-Myers, Spain.** Bristol Myers, Campus Empresarial Jose Ma Churruca, Almansa 101, 28040 Madrid, Spain.

**Bristol-Myers Products, USA.** See *Bristol-Myers Squibb, USA.*

**Bristol-Myers Squibb, Arg.** Bristol-Myers Squibb Argentina S.A., Monroe 801, 1428 Buenos Aires, Argentina.

**Bristol-Myers Squibb, Austral.** Bristol-Myers Squibb, Division of Bristol-Myers Australia P/L, P.O. Box 39, Noble Park, VIC 3174, Australia.

**Bristol-Myers Squibb, Austria.** Bristol-Myers Squibb GmbH, Columbusgasse 4, A-1100 Vienna, Austria.

**Bristol-Myers Squibb, Belg.** Bristol-Myers Squibb Belgium S.A., Waterloo Office Park, Building 1, Dreve Richelle 161 boite 23/24, 1410 Waterloo, Belgium.

**Bristol-Myers Squibb, Braz.** Bristol-Myers Squibb Brasil S.A., Rua Carlos Gomes 924, 04743-903 Sao Paulo, SP, Brazil.

**Bristol-Myers Squibb, Canad.** Bristol-Myers Squibb Canada Inc., 2365 Cote-de-Liesse Rd, Montreal, Quebec, H4N 2M7, Canada.

**Bristol-Myers Squibb, Chile.** Bristol-Myers Squibb, Av. Pte. Balmaceda 2174, Santiago, Chile.

**Bristol-Myers Squibb, Denm.** Bristol-Myers Squibb, Jaegersborgvej 64-66, 2800 Lyngby, Denmark.

**Bristol-Myers Squibb, Fin.** Oy Bristol-Myers Squibb (Finland) AB, Metsänneidonkuja 8, 02130 Espoo, Finland.

**Bristol-Myers Squibb, Fr.** Bristol-Myers Squibb, 3 rue Joseph-Monier, 92506 Rueill-Malmaison cdx, France.

**Bristol-Myers Squibb, Ger.** Bristol-Myers Squibb GmbH, Sapporobogen 6-8, 80809 Munich, Germany.

**Bristol-Myers Squibb, Gr.** BRISTOL-MYERS SQUIBB AEBE, Τατοΐου 102, 146 71 N. Ερυθραια, N. Erithraia, Greece.

**Bristol-Myers Squibb, Hong Kong.** Bristol-Myers Squibb (Hong Kong) Ltd, Unit 3001-2, 30/F, New York Life Tower, Windsor House, 311 Gloucester Rd, Causeway Bay, Hong Kong.

**Bristol-Myers Squibb, Irl.** Bristol-Myers Squibb Pharmaceuticals, Watery Lane, Swords, Co. Dublin, Ireland.

**Bristol-Myers Squibb, Israel.** Bristol-Myers Squibb Ltd, P.O. Box 3311, Petach Tikva, Israel.

**Bristol-Myers Squibb, Ital.** Bristol-Myers Squibb S.p.A., Via Virgilio Maroso 50, 00142 Rome, Italy.

**Bristol-Myers Squibb, Jpn.** See *Bristol, Jpn.*

**Bristol-Myers Squibb, Malaysia.** Bristol-Myers Squibb (Malaysia) Sdn Bhd, 16th Floor, Menara Lien Hoe, 8 Persiaran Tropicana, 47410 Petaling Jaya, Selangor, Malaysia.

**Bristol-Myers Squibb, Mex.** Bristol-Myers Squibb de Mexico S. de R.L. de C.V., Av. Revolucion No. 1267, Col. Tlacopac, Deleg. A. Obregon, 01040 Mexico D.F., Mexico.

**Bristol-Myers Squibb, Neth.** Bristol-Myers Squibb, Vijzelmolenlaan 9, 3447 GX Woerden, Netherlands.

**Bristol-Myers Squibb, Norw.** Bristol-Myers Squibb Norway Ltd, Sandviksv. 26, Postboks 464, 1322 Hovik, Norway.

**Bristol-Myers Squibb, NZ.** Bristol-Myers Squibb, P.O. Box 62663, Central Park, Aukland, New Zealand.

**Bristol-Myers Squibb, Port.** Bristol-Myers Squibb Farmacêutica Portuguesa, Lda, Edificio Fernao de Magalhaes, Quinta da Fonte, 2780-730 Paco De Arcos, Portugal.

**Bristol-Myers Squibb, S.Afr.** Bristol-Myers Squibb (Pty) Ltd, P.O. Box 1408, Bedfordview, 2008 Johannesburg, South Africa.

**Bristol-Myers Squibb, Singapore.** Bristol-Myers Squibb (S) Pte Ltd, 66-68 East Coast Rd, 04-00, S 428778, Singapore.

**Bristol-Myers Squibb, Spain.** See *Bristol-Myers, Spain.*

**Bristol-Myers Squibb, Swed.** Bristol-Myers Squibb AB, Box 15200, 167 15 Bromma, Sweden.

**Bristol-Myers Squibb, Switz.** Bristol-Myers Squibb AG, Neuhofstrasse 6, 6340 Baar, Switzerland.

**Bristol-Myers Squibb, Thai.** Bristol-Myers Squibb (Thailand) Ltd, Bristol-Myers Squibb Building, 10/10-11 Srinakarin Rd, Bangplee, Samutprakarn 10540, Thailand.

**Bristol-Myers Squibb, UK.** Bristol-Myers Squibb Pharmaceuticals Ltd, Bristol-Myers Squibb House, 141-149 Staines Road, Hounslow, Middlesex, TW3 3JA, UK.

**Bristol-Myers Squibb, USA.** Bristol-Myers Squibb, P.O. Box 4500, Princeton, NJ 08543-4500, USA.

**Bristol-Myers Squibb Oncology, USA.** See *Bristol-Myers Squibb, USA.*

**Britannia Health, UK.** Britannia Health Products Ltd, Forum House, 41-75 Brighton Rd, Redhill, Surrey, RH1 6YS, UK.

**Britannia Pharmaceuticals, Irl.** See *Clonmel, Irl.*

**Britannia Pharmaceuticals, UK.** Britannia Pharmaceuticals Ltd, 41-51 Brighton Rd, Redhill, Surrey, RH1 6YS, UK.

**BritHealth, UK.** BritHealth Limited, Weltech Centre, Ridgeway, Welwyn Garden City, Hertfordshire, AL7 2AA, UK.

**Britisfarma, Spain.** See *GlaxoSmithKline, Spain.*

**British Cod Liver Oils, Hong Kong.** See *Keller, Hong Kong.*

**British Dispensary, Thai.** British Dispensary, 31 Fl, Vongvanij Building, 100/103-108 Rama 9 Rd, Bangkok 10320, Thailand.

**British Pharmaceuticals, Austral.** See *Organon, Austral.*

**Britpharm, UK.** Britpharm Laboratories Ltd, Kramer Mews, London, SW5 9JL, UK.

**Broad, UK.** Broad Laboratories plc, UK.

**Brobel, Arg.** Lab. Brobel S.R.L., Cnel. Mendez 440, 1875 Wilde, Buenos Aires, Argentina.

**Brodie & Stone, UK.** Brodie & Stone Plc, 51 Calthorpe St, London, WC1X 0HH, UK.

**Bronchosirum, Canad.** Bronchosirum Inc. 15 JF Kennedy, Bur 10, St-Jerome, QC, J7Y 4B4, Canada.

**Bros, Gr.** BROS ΕΠΕ, Αυγής & Γαλήνης 15, 145 64 Νέα Κηφισσιά, Nea Kiphissia, Greece.

**Brothier, Fr.** Laboratoires Brothier, 41 rue de Neuilly, 92000 Nanterre, France.

**Brothier, Switz.** See *Uhlmann-Eyraud, Switz.*

**Brown & Burk, India.** Brown & Burk Pharmaceuticals Ltd, 303, A Wing, Queen's Corner Apartments, Bangalore 560 001, India.

**Brum, Spain.** Brum, Quevedo 4, Oviedo, 33012 Asturias, Spain.

**Brunel, S.Afr.** Brunel Laboratories (Pty) Ltd, P.O. Box 23103, Innesdale 0031, South Africa.

**Bruni, Ital.** Bruni Dr. Domenico (Farmacia), Via Anfossi 9, 20135 Milan, Italy.

**Bruno, Ital.** Bruno Farmaceutici S.p.A., Via Salvatore Quasimodo 136, 00144 Rome, Italy.

**Bruschettini, Hong Kong.** See *Jebsen, Hong Kong.*

**Bruschettini, Ital.** Bruschettini S.r.l., Via Isonzo 6, 16147 Genoa, Italy.

**Bruschettini, Switz.** See *Galenica, Switz.*

**Bryan, USA.** Bryan Corp., 4 Plympton St., Woburn, MA 01801, USA.

**BSM, Austria.** BSM Diagnostica GesmbH, Alser Strasse 25, A-1080 Vienna, Austria.

**BSN, Austral.** BSN Medical, 211 Wellington Rd, Clayton, Vic 3168, Australia.

**BSSAA, UK.** British Snoring & Sleep Apnoea Association Ltd, 2nd Floor Suite, 52 Albert Rd North, Reigate, Surrey, RH2 9EL, UK.

**BTG, USA.** BTG Pharmaceuticals, 70 Wood Ave South, Iselin, NJ 08830, USA.

**Bucaneve, Ital.** Bucaneve Medicinali S.r.l., Via Sercognani 15, 20156 Milan, Italy.

**Bucca, Spain.** Bucca, Juan Alvarez Mendizabal 43, 28008 Madrid, Spain.

**Buckley, Canad.** W.K. Buckley Ltd, 5230 Orbitor Drive, Mississauga, Ontario, L4W 5G7, Canada.

**Bull, Singapore.** See *Faulding, Singapore.*

**Bullivants, Austral.** Bullivants, Campus Pharmacy, The University of Queensland, Union Building, St. Lucia, QLD 4067, Australia.

**Bunker, Braz.** Bunker Industria Farmaceutica Ltda, Rua Anibal dos Anjos Carvalho 212, Cidade Dutra, 04810-050 Sao Paulo, SP, Brazil.

**Bushnell, India.** Walter Bushnell Ltd, Pragati Bhavan, 2nd Floor, Jai Singh Rd, New Delhi 110 001, India.

**Bustillos, Mex.** Laboratorios Bustillos, S.A. de C.V., Manuel Dublan No. 40, Col. Tacubaya, Deleg. Miguel Hidalgo, 11870 Mexico D.F., Mexico.

**Busto, Spain.** Busto, Paseo Del Deleite S/N, Aranjuez, Madrid, Spain.

**Butantan, Braz.** Instituto Butantan, Av. Vital Brazil 1500, 05503-900 Sao Paulo, SP, Brazil.

**Byk, Arg.** Byk Argentina S.A., Tronador 4890, 1430 Buenos Aires, Argentina.

**Byk, Austria.** Byk Österreich Pharma GmbH, Ketzergasse 200, A-1235 Vienna, Austria.

**Byk, Belg.** Byk Belga S.A., Rue Anatole France 115-121, 1030 Brussels, Belgium.

**Byk, Braz.** See *Altana, Braz.*

**Byk, Canad.** Byk Canada Inc., 1275 North Service Rd W, 7th Floor, Oakville, Ontario, L6M 3G4, Canada.

**Byk, Fr.** See *Altana, Fr.*

**Byk, Neth.** Byk Nederland BV, Weerenweg 29, 1161 AG Zwanenburg, Netherlands.

**Byk, Port.** Byk Portugal, Lda, Quinta da Fonte, Edificio Gil Eanes, Porto Salvo, 2780-730 Paco D'Arcos, Portugal.

**Byk, Switz.** See *Altana, Switz.*

**Byk Elmu, Spain.** See *Altana, Spain.*

**Byk Gulden, Denm.** See *Nycomed, Denm.*

**Byk Gulden, Ger.** See *Altana, Ger.*

**Byk Gulden, Hong Kong.** See *Altana, Hong Kong.*

**Byk Gulden, Ital.** Byk Gulden Italia S.p.A., Via Giotto 1, 20032 Cormano (MI), Italy.

**Byk Gulden, Mex.** See *Altana, Mex.*

**Byk Gulden, Norw.** See *Pharmacia, Norw.*

**Byk Gulden, Singapore.** See *Pacific Biosciences, Singapore.*

**Byk Gulden, Thai.** See *Zuellig, Thai.*

**Byk Leo, Spain.** Byk Leo Lab. Farm., Ctra N-III, Km 23, Arganda del Rey, 28500 Madrid, Spain.

**Byk Madaus, S.Afr.** Byk Madaus (Pty) Ltd, P.O. Box 3435, Halfway House 1685, South Africa.

**Byk Tosse, Ger.** See *Altana, Ger.*

**Bykomed, Port.** See *Byk, Port.*

**C & L, Hong Kong.** C & L Pharmaceutical Ltd, Unit A-C, 19/F Flourish Food Manufactory Ctr, 18 Tai Lee St, Yuen Long, N.T., Hong Kong.

**C & M, USA.** C & M Pharmacal Inc., 1721 Maplelane Ave, Hazel Park, MI 48030-1215, USA.

**C & RF, Ital.** C&RF S.r.l., Via Trinacria 34, 95030 Tremestieri Etneo (CT), Italy.

**Cabassi, Ital.** Cabassi & Giuriarti S.p.A., Via Uruguay 20/22, Z.I. Padua, 35127 Padua, Italy.

**Caber, Ital.** Farmaceutici Caber S.p.A., Via Cavour 11, 44022 Comacchio (FE), Italy.

**Cabon, Ital.** Cabon S.p.A., Via M. Gioia 168, 20125 Milan, Italy.

**Cabuchi, Arg.** Lab. Cabuchi S.A., Tucuman esq. San Juan, 5220 Jesus Marma, Cordoba, Argentina.

**CaDiGroup, Ital.** Ca.Di.Group S.r.l., Via Arturo Viligiardi 89, 00125 Rome, Italy.

**Cadila, India.** See *Zydus, India.*

**Cadila, Thai.** See *Pharmaland, Thai.*

**Cadila Pharma, India.** Cadila Pharmaceuticals Ltd, Cadila Corporate Campus, Sarkhej-Dholka Rd, Bhat, Ahmedabad 382 210, India.

**Cady, Ital.** Cady Paris by Caselli Alda, Vicolo della Neve 7, 40123 Bologna, Italy.

**Caesaro, Austria.** Caesaro Med GmbH, Raidenstrasse 46, A-4060 Leonding, Austria.

**Cahill May Roberts, Irl.** Cahill May Roberts Ltd, Chapelizod, Dublin 20, Ireland.

**Caldeira & Marques, Port.** Caldeira & Marques, Lda, Rua 25 de Abril, Lote 32-B, Brandoa, 2700-851 Amadora, Portugal.

**Caldeira & Metelo, Port.** Caldeira & Metelo, Lda, Rua 25 de Abril, Lote 26, loja, Brandoa, 2700-851 Amadora, Portugal.

**Calea, Austria.** Calea Austria Healthcare GmbH, Estermannstrasse 17, A-4020 Linz, Austria.

**Calgon Vestal, USA.** See *Steris, USA.*

**California Department of Health, USA.** California Department of Health, USA.

**Callegari, Ital.** Callegari S.p.A., Via Adamello 2/A, 43100 Parma, Italy.

**Calmante Vitaminado, Spain.** Calmante Vitaminado, Glorieta Perez Gimenez 1, Pol Ind de Chinales, 14080 Cordoba, Spain.

**Calmic, Irl.** See *GlaxoSmithKline, Irl.*

**Calmic, USA.** See *Wellcome, USA.*

**Cal-White, USA.** Cal-White Mineral Co., P.O. Box 7890, Klamath Falls, OR 97602, USA.

**Cambridge, Fr.** Cambridge Line, B.P. 18, 251 rue de la Gare, 44370 Varades, France.

**Cambridge, UK.** Cambridge Laboratories, Deltic House, Kingfisher Way, Silverlink Business Park, Wallsend, Tyne & Wear, NE28 9NX, UK.

**Cambridge Healthcare, UK.** Cambridge Healthcare Supplies Ltd, Unit 14D, Wendover Rd, Rackheath Industrial Estate, Rackheath, Norwich, NR13 6LH, UK.

**Camps, Spain.** Camps, Planeta 39, 08012 Barcelona, Spain.

**Cana, Gr.** CANA AE, Λ. Ηρακλείου 446, 141 22 N. Ηράκλειο, N Irakleio, Greece.

**Can-Am Care, USA.** Can Am Care Corp., Cimetra Industrial Park, P.O. Box 98, Chazy, NY 12921, USA.

**Canderm, Canad.** Canderm Pharma, 5353 Thimens Blvd, Saint-Laurent, Quebec, H4R 2H4, Canada.

**Candioli, Ital.** Istituto Candioli Profilattico & Farmaceutico S.p.A., Via Manzoni 2, 10092 Beinasco (TO), Italy.

**Cangene, Canad.** Cangene Corporation, 104 Chancellor Matheson Rd, Winnipeg, Manitoba, R3T 5Y3, Canada.

**Cangene, Israel.** See *Luxembourg, Israel.*

**Canonne, Braz.** Laboratorio Canonne Ltda, Avenida Canal do Anil 1263, 22765-430 Rio de Janeiro, RJ, Brazil.

**Cantabria, Spain.** Cantabria, Ctra de Cazona Adarzo S/N, Santander, 39011 Cantabria, Spain.

**Cantassium Co., UK.** The Cantassium Company, UK.

**Capellon, USA.** Capellon Pharmaceuticals Inc., 7462 Dogwood Drive, Fort Worth, TX 76118, USA.

**Capilares, Spain.** Productos Capilares, Lopez Bravo 78, Plg. Ind. Villalonquejar, 09080 Burgos, Spain.

**Capo Sole, Ital.** Capo Sole S.r.l., Via Edison 60, 20019 Settimo Milanese (MI), Italy.

**Caprice Greystoke, USA.** Caprice Greystoke, 1259 Activity Drive, Vista, CA 92083, USA.

**Caps, S.Afr.** Caps Pharmaceuticals (SA) (Pty) Ltd, P.O. Box 2801, Johannesburg 2000, South Africa.

**Caraco, USA.** Caraco Pharmaceutical Labs, 1150 Elijah McCoy Drive, Detroit, MI 48202, USA.

**Cardel, Fr.** See *Pharmacia, Fr.*

**Cardinal Health, USA.** Cardinal Health Inc., 7000 Cardinal Place, Dublin, OH 43017, USA.

**Cardinaux, Canad.** Cardinaux Enrg, 5420 Pasquier, Laval, QC, H7K 3K3, Canada.

**Care, USA.** Care Technologies Inc., P.O. Box 82, 10 Corbin Drive, Darien, CT 06820, USA.

**Careiatrics, Arg.** Careiatrics S.A., Dorrego 331, 1414 Buenos Aires, Argentina.

**Carinopharm, Ger.** Carinopharm GmbH, Rochusstr. 175-177, 53123 Bonn, Germany.

**Carlo Erba OTC, Ital.** See *Pharmacia, Ital.*

**Carlson, USA.** J.R. Carlson Laboratories Inc., 15 College Drive, Arlington Heights, IL 60004-1985, USA.

**Carmaran, Canad.** Carmaran, 1467 Cunard, Chomedey-Laval, QC, H7S 2H8, Canada.

**Carme, USA.** Carme Inc., 84 Galli, Novato, CA 94949, USA.

**Carnation, USA.** Carnation, 800 North Brand Blvd, Glendale, CA 91203, USA.

**Carnivora, Ger.** Carnivora-Forschungs-GmbH, Lobensteiner Str. 3, 96365 Nordhalben, Germany.

**Carnot, Mex.** Carnot Laboratorios, Productos Cientificos, S.A. de C.V., Nicolas San Juan No.1046, Col del Valle, Deleg. Benito Juarez, 03100 Mexico D.F., Mexico.

**Carnrick, USA.** See *Elan, USA.*

**Carolina, USA.** Carolina Medical Products Co., P.O. Box 147, Farmville, NC 27828, USA.

**Carrare, Fr.** Laboratoires Carrare, 1 rue Frederic-Bastiat, 75008 Paris, France.

**Carrington, USA.** Carrington Labs, 2001 Walnut Hill Lane, Irving, TX 75038, USA.

**Carter, NZ.** See *Wilson, NZ.*

**Carter Horner, Canad.** Carter Horner Inc., 6600 Kitimat Rd, Mississauga, Ontario, L5N 1L9, Canada.

**Carter Horner, Hong Kong.** See *US Summit, Hong Kong.*

**Carter Horner, Thai.** See *US Summit, Thai.*

**Carter-Wallace, Austral.** Carter Wallace (Australia) P/L, P.O. Box 216, Brookvale, NSW 2100, Australia.

**Carter-Wallace, Mex.** Carter Wallace, S.A. de C.V., Calz. de las Armas No. 110, Fracc. Industrial las Armas, 54080 Tlalnepantia, Mexico.

**Carter-Wallace, Switz.** See *Doetsch, Grether, Switz.*

**Carter-Wallace, UK.** Carter-Wallace Ltd, Wear Bay Rd, Folkestone, Kent, CT19 6PG, UK.

**Carter-Wallace, USA.** Carter Wallace, Half Acre Rd, P.O. Box 1001, Cranbury, NJ 08512-0181, USA.

**Cartilade, Arg.** Cartilade Arg. Farmacia Maure S.R.L., Av. Cabildo 499, 1426 Buenos Aires, Argentina.

**Casasco, Arg.** Lab. Casasco S.A.I.C., Carabobo 22, 1406 Buenos Aires, Argentina.

**Cascan, Ger.** Cascan GmbH & Co. KG, Industriestr. 32-36, 23843 Bad Oldesloe, Germany.

**Casen Fisons, Spain.** See *Casen Fleet, Spain.*

**Casen Fleet, Spain.** Casen Fleet, Autovia de Logrono Km 13.3, Utebo, 50180 Zaragoza, Spain.

**Casmar, Mex.** Corporacion Casmar S.A. de C.V., Zacatecas No. 208, Entrada por Yucatan No 66, Col. Roma, 06700 Mexico D.F., Mexico.

**Cassara, Arg.** Lab. Pablo Cassara S.R.L., Carhue 1096, 1408 Buenos Aires, Argentina.

**Cassella-med, Ger.** Cassella-med GmbH & Co. KG, Gereonsmuhlengasse 1, 50670 Cologne, Germany.

**Cassella-med, Switz.** Cassella-med AG, Steinentorstrasse 19, 4051 Basle, Switzerland.

**Cassenne, Fr.** See *Aventis, Fr.*

**Castlemead, UK.** Castlemead Healthcare Ltd, 2nd Floor, The Maltings, Bridge St, Hitchin, Hertfordshire, SG5 2DE, UK.

**Catalysis, Arg.** Catalysis Argentina S.A., Av. Raul S. Ortiz 1277, 1414 Buenos Aires, Argentina.

**Catarinense, Braz.** Laboratorio Catarinense S.A., Rua Doutor Joao Colin 1053, 89204-001 Joinville, SC, Brazil.

**Cavalheiro, Port.** See *Confar, Port.*

**Cazi, Braz.** Cazi Quimica Farmaceutica Industria e Comercio Ltda, Rua Antonio Lopes 17, 06600-000 Jandira, SP, Brazil.

**CCD, Fr.** Laboratoires CCD, 60 rue Pierre-Charron, 75008 Paris, France.

**CCM, Hong Kong.** See *Zuellig, Hong Kong.*

**CCM, Malaysia.** See *Upha, Malaysia.*

**CCM, Singapore.** See *FP, Singapore.*

**CCPC, Hong Kong.** See *Kai Yuen, Hong Kong.*

**CCS, Swed.** CCS Clean Chemical Sweden AB, Tunavagen 277 B, 781 73 Borlange, Sweden.

**Ceccarelli, Ital.** Ceccarelli Farmaceutici S.r.l., Via G. Caponsacchi 31, 50126 Florence, Italy.

**Cedar Health, UK.** Cedar Health Ltd, Pepper Rd, Bramhall Moor Lane, Hazel Grove, Stockport, Cheshire, SK7 5BW, UK.

**Cederroth, Spain.** Cederroth, Leon 26, Pol. Ind. Cobo Calleja, Fuenlabrada, 28947 Madrid, Spain.

**Cefak, Ger.** Cefak KG, Ostbahnhofstr. 15, 87437 Kempten, Germany.

**Celafar, Ital.** CE.LA.FAR S.r.l., Italy.

**Celgene, USA.** Celgene Corp., 7 Powder Horn Drive, Warren, NJ 07059, USA.

**Celia, Fr.** Celia Clinical Nutrition, Le Haute Montigne, 35370 Torce, France.

**Celina, Arg.** Lab. Celina, Charrua 3124, 1437 Buenos Aires, Argentina.

**Cell Pharm, Ger.** cell pharm Gesellschaft für pharmazeutische und diagnostische Präparate mbH, Feodor-Lynen-Str. 23, 30625 Hannover, Germany.

**Cell Therapeutics, UK.** Cell Therapeutics (UK) Ltd, 100 Pall Mall, London, SW1Y 5HP, UK.

**Cell Therapeutics, USA.** Cell Therapeutics, 501 Elliott Ave West, Suite 400, Seattle, WA 98119, USA.

**Cellegy, Austral.** Cellegy Australia P/L, Level 5, P.O. Box 474, Edgecliffe, NSW 2027, Australia.

**Celltech, Belg.** Celltech Pharma S.A., Rue des Colonies 11, 1000 Brussels, Belgium.

**Celltech, Fr.** Laboratoires Celltech Pharma, 6 pl Boulnois, 75017 Paris, France.

**Celltech, Ger.** Celltech Pharma GmbH & Co. KG, Bamlerstra. 1 B, 45141 Essen, Germany.

**Celltech, Hong Kong.** See *International Medical, Hong Kong.*

**Celltech, Irl.** Medeva Pharma Ltd, 25 Sandyford Office Park, Dublin 18, Ireland.

**Celltech, Singapore.** See *Ziwell, Singapore.*

**Celltech, Spain.** Celltech Pharma, Montalban 5, 2 Izda, 28014 Madrid, Spain.

**Celltech, UK.** Celltech Pharmaceuticals, 208 Bath Rd, Slough, Berks, SL1 3WE, UK.

**Celltech, USA.** Celltech Pharmaceuticals Co., 755 Jefferson Rd, Rochester, NY 14623, USA.

**Cenci, USA.** HR Cenci Labs Inc., P.O. Box 12524, Fresno, CA 93778-2524, USA.

**CeNeS, UK.** CeNeS Ltd, Compass House, Vision Park, Chivers Way, Histon, Cambridgeshire, CB4 9ZR, UK.

**Ceninter, Spain.** Ceninter, Roma 19, 28028 Madrid, Spain.

**Cenovis, Austral.** See *Mayne, Austral.*

**Centaur, India.** Centaur Laboratories Pvt Ltd, 279 New Ashirwad No. 5, Ram Mandir Rd, Goregaon West, Mumbai 400 104, India.

**Centeon, Austria.** See *Centeon, Ger.*

**Centeon, Denm.** See *Aventis Behring, Swed.*

**Centeon, Fin.** See *Aventis Behring, Swed.*

**Centeon, Ger.** See *Aventis Behring, Ger.*

**Centeon, Irl.** See *Aventis Behring, UK.*

**Centeon, Israel.** See *Mediline, Israel.*

**Centeon, Ital.** See *Aventis Behring, Ital.*

**Centeon, Mex.** See *Aventis Behring, Mex.*

**Centeon, Spain.** See *Aventis Behring, Spain.*

**Centeon, UK.** See *Aventis Behring, UK.*

**Centeon, USA.** See *Aventis Behring, USA.*

**Center, Israel.** See *Trupharm, Israel.*

**Center, USA.** Center Pharmaceuticals, 3620 Park Central Blvd North, Pompano Beach, FL 33064, USA.

**Centocor, Austria.** See *Centocor, Neth.*

**Centocor, Denm.** See *Lilly, Denm.*, and *Schering-Plough, Denm.*

**Centocor, Gr.** Centocor, Greece.

**Centocor, Israel.** See *Lilly, Israel.*

**Centocor, Neth.** Centocor Europe BV, Einsteinweg 101, 2333 CB Leiden, Netherlands.

**Centocor, Norw.** See *Lilly, Norw.*

**Centocor, USA.** Centocor, Inc., 200 Great Valley Pkwy, Malvern, PA 19355, USA.

**Centra, Ital.** Centra Medicamenta OTC S.r.l., Via N. Buonarroti 23, 20093 Cologno Monzese (MI), Italy.

**Centrafarm, Neth.** Centrafarm Services BV, Nieuwe Donk 9, 4879 AC Etten-Leur, Netherlands.

**Central, Irl.** Central Laboratories Ltd, 31 Ravensrock Rd, Sandyford Industrial Estate, Foxrock, Dublin 18, Ireland.

**Central, Thai.** Central Poly Trading Co. Ltd, 100/261 Moo 3, Saima Muang, Nonthaburi 11000, Thailand.

**Centrapharm, Belg.** Centrapharm S.A., Chaussee de Gand 615, 1080 Brussels, Belgium.

**Centrapharm, Fr.** Laboratoires Centrapharm, 35 rue de la Chapelle, 63450 Saint-Amant-Tallende, France.

**Centrapharm, Neth.** Centrapharm, Netherlands.

**Centrapharm, UK.** Centrapharm Ltd, Dale House, Suckley Road, Knightwick, Worcestershire, WR6 5QE.

**Centrum, Spain.** See *ASAC, Spain.*

**Century, USA.** Century Pharmaceuticals Inc., 10377 Hague Rd, Indianapolis, IN 46256-3399, USA.

**Ceom, Ital.** Ce.o.m. S.r.l., Via L/mare Colombo 323, 84124 Salerno, Italy.

**CEPA, Spain.** CEPA Schwartz Pharma, Po. de la Castellana 141-15, Edif. Cuzco IV, 28046 Madrid, Spain.

**Cephalon, Fr.** See *Lafon, Fr.*

**Cephalon, Ger.** Cephalon GmbH, Fraunhoferstr. 22, 82152 Martinsried, Germany.

**Cephalon, Irl.** See *Cephalon, UK.*

**Cephalon, UK.** Cephalon UK Ltd, 11-13 Frederick Sanger Rd, Surrey Research Park, Guildford, Surrey, GU2 5YD, UK.

**Cephalon, USA.** Cephalon Inc., 145 Brandywine Pkwy, West Chester, PA 19380, USA.

**Cernelle, Switz.** Cernelle SA, Natural Products, Chemin des tilleuls, 2108 Couvet, Switzerland.

**Cesam, Port.** Cesam, Lda, Rua de Ceuta 4, Piso, 2795-056 Linda-a-Velha, Portugal.

**Cesra, Ger.** Cesra Arzneimittelfabrik GmbH & Co. KG, Braunmattstr. 20, 76532 Baden-Baden, Germany.

**Cetem, Fr.** Laboratoires Cetem, 18 rue E. & H.-Rousselle, 75013 Paris, France.

**Cetus, Arg.** Lab. Cetus S.R.L., Querandmes 4275, 1183 Buenos Aires, Argentina.

**Cetylite, USA.** Cetylite Industries Inc., P.O. Box 90006, Pennsauken, NJ 08110-0700, USA.

**Ceuta, UK.** Ceuta Healthcare Ltd, Hill House, 41 Richmond Hill, Bournemouth, Dorset, BH2 6HS, UK.

**Ceutical, Hong Kong.** Ceutical Trading Co., Rm 24, 12/F, Goldfield Industrial Ctr, 1 Sui Wo Rd, Fo Tan, Shatin, N.T., Hong Kong.

**Cevallos, Arg.** Lab. Cevallos Salud S.R.L., Zapiola 2836/40, 1428 Buenos Aires, Argentina.

**CFL, India.** CFL Pharmaceuticals Ltd, 501/502 Sigma, Hiranandani Gardens, Powai, Mumbai 400 076, India.

**CGM, Ital.** CGM Farmaceutici Srl, Via E Gianturco 21, 80055 Portici, Italy.

**Chaix et du Marais, Fr.** Ste des Laboratoires Chaix et du Marais, 7 rue Labie, 75017 Paris, France.

**Charoen, Thai.** S Charoen Bhaesaj Trading Co. Ltd, 713-715-717 Mahachai Rd, Bangkok 10200, Thailand.

**Charoen Bhaesaj, Malaysia.** See *Propharm, Malaysia.*

**Charoen Bhaesaj, Thai.** Charoen Bhaesaj Lab Ltd, 209/56 Sol Chokchai 1, Phetkasem Rd, Bangkok 10160, Thailand.

**Charton, Canad.** See *Technilab, Canad.*

**Charwell, Israel.** See *Manon, Israel.*

**Charwell, Singapore.** See *JDH, Singapore.*

**Charwell Pharmaceuticals, UK.** Charwell Pharmaceuticals Ltd, Charwell House, Wilsom Rd, Alton, Hampshire, GU34 2TJ, UK.

**Chatelut, Fr.** Laboratoires Chatelut, 36170 St-Benoit-du-Sault, France.

**Chatfield Laboratories, UK.** Chatfield Laboratories, Kramer Mews, London, SW5 9JL, UK.

**Chattem, Canad.** Chattem (Canada) Inc., 2220 Argentia Rd, Mississauga, Ontario, L5N 2K7, Canada.

**Chattem, Singapore.** See *Green Cross, Singapore.*

**Chattem, USA.** Chattem Consumer Products, 1715 West 38th St, Chattanooga, TN 37409, USA.

**Chauvin, Fr.** Laboratoires Chauvin Bausch & Lomb, 416 rue Samuel-Morse, B.P. 1174, 34009 Montpellier cdx 1, France.

**Chauvin, Hong Kong.** See *Rich Plan, Hong Kong.*

**Chauvin, Irl.** See *Cahill May Roberts, Irl.*

**Chauvin, Israel.** See *Rekah, Israel.*

**Chauvin, Port.** Laboratorio Chauvin, Lda, Av. do Forte No.3, Edificio Suecia IV, Piso 0, 2795-504 Carnaxide, Portugal.

**Chauvin, Singapore.** See *Age D'or, Singapore.*

**Chauvin, Thai.** See *Neopharm, Thai.*

**Chauvin, UK.** Chauvin Pharmaceuticals Ltd, 106 London Rd, Kingston-Upon-Thames, Surrey, KT2 6TN, UK.

**Chauvin ankerpharm, Ger.** Chauvin ankerpharm GmbH, Francois-Mitterrand-Allee 1, 07407 Rudolstadt, Germany.

**Chauvin Novopharma, Switz.** See *Bausch & Lomb, Switz.*

**Chefaro, Belg.** Chefaro S.A., Venecoweg 26, 9810 Nazareth, Belgium.

**Chefaro, Fin.** See *Tamro, Fin.*

**Chefaro, Ger.** Deutsche Chefaro Pharma GmbH, Wirrigen 25, 45731 Waltrop, Germany.

**Chefaro, Israel.** See *Neopharm, Israel.*

**Chefaro, Neth.** Chefaro Nederland BV, Keileweg 8, 3029 BS Rotterdam, Netherlands.

**Chefaro, Spain.** Chefaro Española, Ed Roma Ronda de Dalt, Ctra Hospitalet 147, Cornella de Llobregat, 08940 Barcelona, Spain.

**Chefaro, UK.** Chefaro Proprietaries Ltd, 1 Tower Close, St Peters Industrial Park, Huntingdon, Cambridgeshire, PE18 7DR, UK.

**Chefaro Ardeval, Fr.** Laboratoires Chefaro-Ardeval, 2-4 rue de Chaintron, 92542 Montrouge cdx, France.

**Cheil, Singapore.** See *Zyfas, Singapore.*

**Chelsea, USA.** See *Watson, USA.*

**Chemedica, Fr.** Chemedica, B.P. 51, 74500 St-Gingolph, France.

**Chemedica, Ger.** TRB Chemedica AG Pharmavertrieb, Richard-Reitzner-Allee 1, 85540 Haar/Munich, Germany.

**Chemedica, Hong Kong.** TRB Chemedica Hong Kong Ltd, Rm 2104, 21/F CC Wu Building, 302-8 Hennessy Rd, Wanchai, Hong Kong.

**Chemedica, Malaysia.** See *Somedico, Malaysia.*

**Chemedica, Switz.** TRB Chemedica SA, Chemin St Marc 3, Case Postale 240, 1896 Vouvry, Switzerland.

**Chemedica, UK.** Chemedica, UK.

**Chemidex, UK.** Chemidex Pharma Ltd, Chemidex House, Egham Business Village, Crabtree Rd, Egham, Surrey, TW20 8RB, UK.

**Chemineau, Fr.** Laboratoires Chemineau, 93 rte de Monnaie, 37210 Vouvray, France.

**Cheminova, Spain.** Cheminova, Emilio Munoz 15, Madrid, Spain.

**Chemipal, Israel.** Chemipal, P.O. Box 8111, Netanya 42293, Israel.

**Chemipharm, Israel.** Chemipharm Ltd, Brodetzky 43, Tel Aviv, Israel.

**Chemipharma, Gr.** CHEMIPHARMA, Αγ. Κωνσταντίνου 40, 141 22 Ν. Ηράκλειο, N. Irakleio, Greece.

**Chemists Own, Austral.** See *Hunter, Austral.*

**Chemomedica, Austria.** Chemomedica Medizintechnik und Arzneimittel GmbH, Wipplingerstrasse 19, A-1013 Vienna, Austria.

**Chemopharma, Chile.** See *Sanitas, Chile.*

**Chemo-Pharma, India.** Chemo-Pharma Labs Ltd, Empire House, 214 D. N. Road, Fort, Mumbai 400 001, India.

**Chemosan, Austria.** See *Liebermann, Ger.*

**Chephasaar, Ger.** Chephasaar, Chem.-pharm. Fabrik GmbH, Muhlstr. 50, 66386 St Ingbert, Germany.

**Cheplapharm, Ger.** Cheplapharm Arzneimittel GmbH, Basler Str. 115, 79115 Freiburg i. Br., Germany.

**Chesebrough-Pond's, USA.** See *Unilever, USA.*

**Cheshire, UK.** Cheshire Cosmetics Ltd, Cromet House, 1 Gunco Lane, Macclesfield, Cheshire, SK11 7JX, UK.

**Chester, Canad.** See *Technilab, Canad.*

**Chew, Thai.** Chew Brothers & Co. Ltd Part, 1561/3 Petchburi Rd, New Extension, Makason, Bangkok 10310, Thailand.

**Chi Sheng, Thai.** See *Charoen, Thai.*

**Chibret, Denm.** See *Merck Sharp & Dohme, Denm.*

**Chibret, Ger.** See *Merck Sharp & Dohme, Ger.*

**Chibret, Port.** See *Merck Sharp & Dohme, Port.*

**Chibret, Spain.** See *Merck Sharp & Dohme, Spain.*

**Chiesi, Fr.** Chiesi SA, Imm. le Doublon, bat B, 11 av. Dubonnet, 92400 Courbevoie, France.

**Chiesi, Gr.** CHIESI HELLAS, Λ. Πεντέλης 1, 152 35 Βριλήσσια, Vrilissia, Greece.

**Chiesi, Hong Kong.** See *William, Hong Kong.*

**Chiesi, Ital.** Chiesi Farmaceutici S.p.A., Via Palermo 26/A, 43100 Parma, Italy.

**Chiesi, Malaysia.** See *Germax, Malaysia.*

**Chiesi, Singapore.** See *JDH, Singapore.*

**Chiesi, Spain.** Chiesi España, Berlin 38-48, 7 planta, 08029 Barcelona, Spain.

**Chiesi, Switz.** Chiesi SA, Via Franscini 17, 6900 Lugano, Switzerland.

**Chiesi, Thai.** See *Pacific, Thai.*

**Chilton, USA.** Chilton Labs Inc., 23 Fairfield Place, W Caldwell, NJ 07006, USA.

**Chimicor, Fr.** See *Chimicor, Ital.*

**Chimicor, Ital.** Chimicor S.r.l., Via Veneto 54, 36061 Bassano del Grappa (VI), Italy.

**Chinoin, Hung.** Chinoin Pharmaceutical and Chemical Works Ltd, P.O. Box 110, 1325 Budapest, Hungary.

**Chinoin, Mex.** Chinoin, Productos Farmaceuticos, S.A. de C.V., Lago Tanganica No. 18, Col. Granada, Deleg. Miguel Hidalgo, 11520 Mexico D.F., Mexico.

**Chinosolfabrik, Ger.** Chinosolfabrik (Zweigniederlassung der Riedel-de Haen AG), Wunstorfer Str. 40, 30926 Seelze, Germany.

**Chinta, Thai.** See *Square, Thai.*

**Chiron, Belg.** See *Chiron, Neth.*

**Chiron, Canad.** Chiron Canada Ltd, 3300 Cote-Vertu Bvld, Suite 403, St. Laurent, Quebec, H4R 2B7, Canada.

**Chiron, Denm.** See *Amgros, Denm.*

**Chiron, Fr.** Chiron France, 10 rue Chevreul, 92150 Suresnes, France.

**Chiron, Ger.** Chiron GmbH, Linprunstr. 16, 89335 Munich, Germany.

**Chiron, Hong Kong.** See *Hong Wo, Hong Kong.*

**Chiron, Irl.** See *Allphar, Irl.*, and *Cahill May Roberts, Irl.*

**Chiron, Israel.** See *Concept, Israel.*

**Chiron, Ital.** Chiron Italia S.r.l., Via Cimarosa 4, 20144 Milan, Italy.

**Chiron, Neth.** Chiron BV, Paasheuvelweg 30, 1105 BJ Amsterdam Zuidoost, Netherlands.

**Chiron, NZ.** See *Baxter, NZ.*

**Chiron, Singapore.** See *Pacific Biosciences, Singapore*, and *Sime Darby, Singapore.*

**Chiron, Spain.** Chiron Iberia, Edificio Dublin, Parque Emp. San Fernando, San Fernando de Henares, 28831 Madrid, Spain.

**Chiron, Thai.** See *Biogenetech, Thai.*

**Chiron, UK.** Chiron Corporation Ltd, Symphony House, 7 Cowley Business Park, High St, Cowley, Middlesex, UB8 2AD, UK.

**Chiron, USA.** Chiron Therapeutics, 4560 Horton St, Emeryville, CA 94608-2916, USA.

**Chiron Behring, Fin.** See *Chiron Behring, Ger.*

**Chiron Behring, Ger.** Chiron Behring GmbH & Co, Emil-von-Behring-Str. 76, 35041 Marburg, Germany.

**Chiron Behring, Malaysia.** See *Chiron Behring, Ger.*

**Chiron Behring, Norw.** See *Chiron Behring, Ger.*

**Chiron Vaccines, Ital.** Chiron Vaccines, Divisione Chiron S.p.A., Via Fiorentina 1, 53100 Siena, Italy.

**Chiron Vaccines, UK.** Chiron Vaccines Evans, Gaskill Rd, Speke, Liverpool, Merseyside, L24 9GR, UK.

**Chlorella, UK.** Chlorella Products Ltd, UK.

**Choay, Israel.** See *Promedico, Israel.*

**Choay, Port.** See *Sanofi Synthelabo, Port.*

**Chobet, Arg.** Soubeiran Chobet S.R.L., Ibera 5055, 1431 Buenos Aires, Argentina.

**Chong Kun Dang, Ital.** Chong Kun Dang Italia S.p.A., Fraz. Domodossolina, 28651 Borgo S Giovanni (LO), Italy.

**Chong Kun Dang, Singapore.** See *Zyfas, Singapore.*

**Chong Kun Dang, Thai.** See *Charoen, Thai.*

**Chong Lap, Hong Kong.** Chong Lap (HK) Co. Ltd, Rm 1215, Lippo Sun Plaza, 28 Canton Rd, Tsim Sha Tsui, Kowloon, Hong Kong.

**Choongwae, Hong Kong.** See *Vantone, Hong Kong.*

**Choongwae, Singapore.** See *Kyowa, Singapore.*

**Chowgule, India.** Chowgule & Co. (Hind) Ltd, Malhotra House, Opposite GPO, Walchand Hirachand Marg, Mumbai 400 001, India.

**CHR, Ger.** C.H.R. Heim Arzneimittel GmbH, Elisabethenstr. 34, 64283 Darmstadt, Germany.

**Chrisana, Switz.** Chrisana GmbH, Ruggenstrasse 17, 8903 Birmensdorf, Switzerland.

**Chrispa (Χρισπα), Gr.** ΧΡΙΣΠΑ ΑΛΦΑ ΑΕ, Μενάνδρου 58, 104 32 Αθήνα, Athens, Greece.

**Christiaens, Belg.** Christiaens Pharma S.A., Chaussee de Gand 615, 1080 Brussels, Belgium.

**Christiaens, Neth.** Christiaens BV, Nikkelstraat 5, 4823 AE Breda, Netherlands.

**Chugai, Denm.** See *Aventis, Denm.*

**Chugai, Ger.** Chugai Pharma Marketing Ltd, Lyoner Str. 15, 60528 Frankfurt/Main, Germany.

**Chugai, Hong Kong.** See *Tai Tong, Hong Kong.*

**Chugai, Jpn.** Chugai Pharmaceutical Co. Ltd, 2-1-9 Kyobashi, Chuo-ku, Tokyo 104-8301, Japan.

**Chugai, Norw.** See *Aventis, Norw.*

**Chugai, Thai.** See *Siam Pharm, Thai.*

**Chugai, UK.** Chugai Pharma UK, Mulliner House, Flanders Rd, Turnham Green, London, W4 1NN, UK.

**Ci & Di, Ital.** Ci & Di S.r.l., Via Cechov 48, 20151 Milan, Italy.

**Ciba, Canad.** See *Novartis, Canad.*

**Ciba, Ger.** See *Novartis, Ger.*

**Ciba, Gr.** See *Novartis, Gr.*

**Ciba, Ital.** See *Novartis, Ital.*

**Ciba, Switz.** See *Novartis, Switz.*, and *Novartis Consumer, Switz.*

**Ciba, USA.** See *Novartis, USA.*

**Ciba Consumer, USA.** See *Novartis, USA.*

**Ciba Vision, Austral.** Ciba Vision Australia P/L, Private Bag 100, Baulkham Hills Business Centre, Baulkham Hills, NSW 2153, Australia.

**Ciba Vision, Austria.** See *Novartis, Austria.*

**Ciba Vision, Braz.** See *Novartis, Braz.*

**Ciba Vision, Canad.** See *Novartis Ophthalmics, Canad.*

**Ciba Vision, Denm.** See *Novartis, Denm.*

**Ciba Vision, Fr.** See *Novartis, Fr.*

**Ciba Vision, Ger.** See *Novartis, Ger.*

**Ciba Vision, Hong Kong.** See *Novartis, Hong Kong.*

**Ciba Vision, Irl.** See *United Drug, Irl.*

**Ciba Vision, Israel.** See *Promedico, Israel.*

**Ciba Vision, Ital.** Ciba Vision S.r.l., gruppo Novartis, Via Enrico Mattei 17, 30020 Marcon (VE), Italy.

**Ciba Vision, Neth.** Ciba Vision, A Novartis Company, Postbus 3126, 4800 DC Breda, Netherlands.

**Ciba Vision, NZ.** See *Novartis, NZ.*

**Ciba Vision, Port.** See *Novartis, Port.*

**Ciba Vision, Singapore.** See *Novartis, Singapore.*

**Ciba Vision, Spain.** Ciba Vision, Marina 206, 08013 Barcelona, Spain.

**Ciba Vision, Swed.** See *Novartis, Swed.*

**Ciba Vision, Switz.** See *Novartis Ophthalmics, Switz.*

**Ciba Vision, Thai.** See *Zuellig, Thai.*

**Ciba Vision, USA.** Ciba Vision, a Novartis Company, 11460 Johns Creek Parkway, Duluth, GA 30097-1556, USA.

**Ciba-Geigy, Austria.** See *Novartis, Austria.*

**Ciba-Geigy, Belg.** See *Novartis, Belg.*

**Ciba-Geigy, Jpn.** Nihon Ciba-Geigy, 10-66 Bikocho, Takarazuka-shi, Japan.

**Ciba-Geigy, USA.** See *Novartis, USA.*

**Cibran, Braz.** Companhia Brasileira de Antibioticos Cibran, Rua da Quitanda 3, 4 andar, 20011-030 Rio de Janeiro, RJ, Brazil.

**CIC, Spain.** See *Schering, Spain.*

**Ciclum, Spain.** Ciclum Farma, Doctor Zamenhof 36, 28027 Madrid, Spain.

**Cielle, Ital.** Farma Cielle S.r.l., Via Michele Amari 15, 90139 Palermo, Italy.

**CIF, Braz.** Companhia Industrial Farmaceutica, Rua Figueira de Melo 301, 20941-001 Rio de Janeiro, RJ, Brazil.

**Cifarma, Braz.** Cifarma Cientmfica Farmaceutica Ltda, Av. das Industrias 3651, 33040-130 Belo Horizonte, MG, Brazil.

**Cilag, Hong Kong.** See *Janssen, Hong Kong*, and *Keller, Hong Kong.*

**Cilag, Mex.** Cilag de Mexico S.A. de C.V., Miguel Angel de Quevedo No. 247, Col. Romero de Terreros, Deleg. Coyoacan, 04310 Mexico D.F., Mexico.

**Cilag, UK.** See *Janssen-Cilag, UK.*

**Cimed, Braz.** Cimed Indzstria de Medicamentos Ltda, Rua Engenheiro Prudente 119, 01550-000 Sao Paulo Vila Monumento, SP, Brazil.

**Cimex, Hong Kong.** See *LCH, Hong Kong.*

**Cimex, Israel.** See *Taro, Israel.*

**Cimex, Singapore.** See *Pharma 2000, Singapore.*

**Cimex, Switz.** Cimex AG Pharmazeutika, Birsweg 2, 4253 Liesberg, Switzerland.

**Cinetic, Arg.** Cinetic Laboratories Argentina S.A., Av. Triunvirato 2734/6, 1427 Buenos Aires, Argentina.

**Cinfa, Spain.** Cinfa, Olaz-Chipi 10, Poligono Areta, Huarte-Pamplona, 31620 Navarra, Spain.

**Cipan, Port.** Cipan, SA, Vala do Carregado, Apartado 60, 2600-726 Castanheira do Ribatejo, Portugal.

**Cipla, Austral.** Cipla GenPharm Australia Pty Ltd, Kaybank Plaza, 33 Scarborough St, Southport, Qld 4215, Australia.

**Cipla, India.** Cipla Ltd, Mumbai Central, Mumbai 400 008, India.

**Cipla, Israel.** See *Margalit, Israel.*

**Cipla, Thai.** See *Zuellig, Thai.*

**Cipla-Medpro, S.Afr.** Cipla-Medpro (Pty) Ltd, Rosen Heights, Rosen Park, Bellville 7530, South Africa.

**Circle, USA.** Circle Pharmaceuticals Inc., 6788 Hawthorn Park Drive, Indianapolis, IN 46220, USA.

**CIS, Fr.** CIS bio International, B.P. 32, 91192 Gif-sur-Yvette cdx, France.

**CIS, Spain.** CIS España, Prim 5, 28004 Madrid, Spain.

**Clarben, Spain.** Clarben, Vallermoso 28, 28015 Madrid, Spain.

**Clariana, Spain.** Clariana Pico, Ctra Carlet Valencia Km 0.5, Carlet, 46240 Valencia, Spain.

**Clarins, Canad.** Clarins, 4757 Poirier Blvd, St-Laurent, Quebec, H4R 2A4, Canada.

**Clarmed, Ital.** Clarmed S.r.l., Via G Stephenson 94, 20157 Milan (MI), Italy.

**Clay Park, Hong Kong.** See *Hind Wing, Hong Kong.*

**Clement, Fr.** See *Clement-Thekan, Fr.*

**Clement Thionville, Fr.** Laboratoires Clément-Thionville, 6 rue Joffre, B.P. 60028, 57101 Thionville cdx, France.

**Clement-Thekan, Fr.** Laboratoires Clément-Thékan, 2-4 rue Chaintron, B.P. 850, 92542 Montrouge cdx, France.

**Climax, Braz.** Laboratorio Climax S.A., Rua Joaquim Tavora 822, 04015-011 Sao Paulo, SP, Brazil.

**Clinced, Austria.** Clinced Handelsgesellschaft mbH, Sandweg 8, A-8071 Gossendorf, Austria.

**CliniMed, UK.** CliniMed Ltd, Cavell House, Knaves Beech Way, Loudwater, High Wycombe, Buckinghamshire, HP10 9QY, UK.

**Clinique, Canad.** Clinique Laboratories, 121 Bloor St E, Toronto, Ontario, M4W 3M5, Canada.

**Clintec, Austria.** See *Baxter, Fr.*

**Clintec, Canad.** See *Baxter, Canad.*

**Clintec, Denm.** See *Baxter, Denm.*

**Clintec, Fr.** See *Nestle, Fr.*

**Clintec, Gr.** See *Baxter, Gr.*

**Clintec, Irl.** See *Baxter, Irl.*

**Clintec, Israel.** See *Teva, Israel.*

**Clintec, Ital.** See *Baxter, Ital.*

**Clintec, Thai.** See *Osotspa, Thai.*

**Clintec, USA.** See *Baxter, USA.*

**Clintex, Port.** Clintex, Lda, Rua Joao de Deus no 19, Venda Nova, 2700-487 Amadora, Portugal.

**Clissmann, Irl.** HE Clissmann, 44 Dartmouth Square, Dublin 6, Ireland.

**Clonmel, Irl.** Clonmel Healthcare Ltd, Waterford Rd, Clonmel, Co. Tipperary, Ireland.

**Clonmel, UK.** See *Clonmel, Irl.*

**CMS, Switz.** CMS Control & Monitoring Systems GmbH, Huslerstrasse 30, 5453 Remetschwill, Switzerland.

**CMS-Dental, Denm.** CMS-Dental ApS, Wildersgade 55, 1408 Copenhagen K, Denmark.

**CNW, Hong Kong.** CNW (Hong Kong) Ltd, Rm 606, 6/F, Fo Tan Industrial Ctr, 26-28 Au Pui Wan St, Fo Tan, Shatin, N.T., Hong Kong.

**COB, Belg.** COB & Cie S.A., Ave Albert Giraud 115, 1030 Brussels, Belgium.

**Cochon, Fr.** See *Tradiphar, Fr.*

**Codal Synto, Hong Kong.** See *CNW, Hong Kong, Hong Tai Hong, Hong Kong,* and *Star, Hong Kong.*

**Codal Synto, Malaysia.** See *Propharm, Malaysia.*

**Codal Synto, Thai.** See *Star, Thai.*

**Codali, Belg.** Codali S.A., Ave Henri Dunant 31, 1140 Brussels, Belgium.

**Codifra, Fr.** Laboratoires Codifra, 18 av. Dutarte, 78150 de Chesney, France.

**Codilab, Port.** Codilab, Indústria e Comércio de Produtos Farmacêuticos SA, Av. Marechal Gomes da Costa 19, 1800-255 Lisbon, Portugal.

**Colgate, Arg.** See *Colgate-Palmolive, Arg.*

**Colgate Oral, USA.** Colgate Oral Pharmaceuticals, 1 Colgate Way, Canton, MA 02021, USA.

**Colgate Oral Care, Austral.** Colgate Oral Care, P.O. Box 3964, Sydney, NSW 2001, Australia.

**Colgate-Hoyt, USA.** See *Colgate-Palmolive, USA.*

**Colgate-Palmolive, Arg.** Colgate-Palmolive Argentina S.A., Av. Antartida Argentina 2269, 1836 Llavallol, Buenos Aires, Argentina.

**Colgate-Palmolive, Austral.** See *Colgate Oral Care, Austral.*

**Colgate-Palmolive, Canad.** Colgate Palmolive Canada, 99 Vanderhoof Ave, Toronto, Ontario, M4G 2H6, Canada.

**Colgate-Palmolive, Denm.** Colgate Palmolive A/S, Postbox 93, 2600 Glostrup, Denmark.

**Colgate-Palmolive, Fr.** Colgate-Palmolive, 55 bd de la Mission-Marchand, 92401 Courbevoie cdx, France.

**Colgate-Palmolive, Ger.** Colgate-Palmolive GmbH, Liebigstr 2-20, 22113 Hamburg, Germany.

**Colgate-Palmolive, Ital.** Colgate Palmolive Italia S.r.l., Divisione Oral Pharmaceuticals, Via Giorgione 59/63, 00147 Rome, Italy.

**Colgate-Palmolive, Norw.** See *Colgate-Palmolive, Denm.*

**Colgate-Palmolive, Swed.** See *Colgate-Palmolive, Denm.*

**Colgate-Palmolive, Switz.** Colgate-Palmolive AG, Zurcherstrasse 68, 8800 Remetschwil, Switzerland.

**Colgate-Palmolive, UK.** Colgate-Palmolive Ltd, Guilford Business Park, Middleton Rd, Guildford, Surrey, GU2 5LZ, UK.

**Colgate-Palmolive, USA.** Colgate-Palmolive Co., 300 Park Ave, New York, NY 10022, USA.

**Coli, Ital.** Farmaceutici Coli S.r.l., Via Campobello 15, 00040 Pomezia (Rome), Italy.

**Coll, Spain.** Coll Farma, Napoles 166, 08013 Barcelona, Spain.

**Collado, Spain.** Collado, Spain.

**Collagen, Austral.** Collagen Biomedical P/L, Unit 1, Chullora Central, Chullora, NSW 2190, Australia.

**Collagen, Austria.** Collagen Vertrieb Biomed. Produkte GmbH, Esslinger Hauptstrasse 81-7, A-1228 Vienna, Austria.

**Collagen, Fr.** Collagen France, 113 rue Victor Hugo, 92300 Levallois Perret, France.

**Collagen, Ger.** Collagen Aesthetics, Hansaallee 201, 40549 Dusseldorf, Germany.

**Collagen, Ital.** Collagen Research Center S.r.l., Via Innocenzo XI 41, 00165 Rome, Italy.

**CollaGenex, UK.** CollaGenex International Ltd, The Old Stable Block, 7 Buttermarket, Thame, Oxfordshire, OX9 3EW, UK.

**CollaGenex, USA.** CollaGenex Pharmaceuticals Inc., 41 University Drive, Suite 200, Newtown, PA 18940, USA.

**Collins, Mex.** Productos Farmaceuticos Collins S.A. de C.V., Cipres No. 1677, Col. del Fresno, 44900 Guadalajara, Jal., Mexico.

**Collins Elixir, UK.** Collins Elixir Co., P.O. Box 33, Kingsbridge, Devon, TQ7 1YQ, UK.

**Coloplast, Arg.** Coloplast de Argentina S.A., Av. Alicia Moreau de Justo 1780, 1043 Buenos Aires, Argentina.

**Coloplast, Fr.** Laboratoires Coloplast, 58 rue Roger-Salengro, Peripole 126, 94126 Fontenay-sous-Bois cdx, France.

**Coloplast, Switz.** Coloplast AG, Eurobusiness Center, Euro 1, Blegistrasse 1, 6343 Rotkreuz, Switzerland.

**Coloplast, UK.** Coloplast Ltd, Peterborough Business Park, Peterborough, Cambridgeshire, PE2 0FX, UK.

**Coloplast, USA.** Coloplast Corp., 1955 West Oak Circle, Marietta, Georgia, GA 30062-2249, USA.

**Columbia, Fr.** See *Columbia, UK.*

**Columbia, Mex.** Laboratorios Columbia, S.A. de C.V., Calz. del Hueso No. 160, Col. Ejido de Santa Ursula Coapa, Deleg. Coyoacan, 04850 Mexico D.F., Mexico.

**Columbia, S.Afr.** Columbia Pharmaceuticals (Pty) Ltd, Middel Rd, Bardene Extension 32, Boksburg 1459, South Africa.

**Columbia, UK.** Columbia Laboratories Ltd, P.O. Box 24, Rye, East Sussex, TN31 7BF, UK.

**Columbia, USA.** Columbia Laboratories Inc., 2875 NE 191st St, 100 N Village Ave, Rockville Center, NY 11570, USA.

**Combe, Arg.** Lab. Combe, Zarraga 3922, 1427 Buenos Aires, Argentina.

**Combe, Canad.** See *Pinnacle, Canad.*

**Combe, Ger.** Combe Pharma Ltd, Rheinstr. 219, 76532 Baden-Baden, Germany.

**Combe, Israel.** See *Mediline, Israel.*

**Combe, Ital.** Combe Italia S.r.l., Via G C Procaccini 41, 20154 Milan, Italy.

**Combe, Spain.** Combe Europa, Orense 58, 28020 Madrid, Spain.

**Combe, UK.** Combe International Ltd, 4th Floor, AMP House, Dingwell Rd, Croydon, Surrey, CR9 2AU, UK.

**Combe, USA.** Combe Inc., 1101 Westchester Ave, White Plains, NY 10604, USA.

**Combustin, Ger.** Combustin Pharm. Präparate GmbH, Offinger Str. 7, 88525 Hailtingen/Bussen, Germany.

**Commerce, USA.** See *Del, USA.*

**Commonwealth Serum, Hong Kong.** See *LCH, Hong Kong.*

**Community Pharmacy, Thai.** Community Pharmacy Public Co. Ltd, 96/17 Moo 13, Khubon Rd, Kannayao, Bangkok 10230, Thailand.

**Compu, S.Afr.** CompuPharm (Pty) Ltd, P.O. Box 30599, Sunnyside 0132, South Africa.

**Concept, India.** Concept Pharmaceuticals Ltd, 167 C.S.T. Rd, Santacruz (E), Mumbai 400 098, India.

**Concept, Israel.** Concept for Pharmacy Ltd, P.O. Box 2105, Kfar Sava, Israel.

**Concord, UK.** Concord Pharmaceuticals Ltd, Melville House, High St, Dunmow, Essex, CM6 1AF, UK.

**Condrugs, Thai.** Condrugs International Co. Ltd, 51/507-508 Drive-in Square, Soi 1, Ladprao Rd, Klongjan, Bangkapi, Bangkok 10240, Thailand.

**Confar, Port.** Confar, Lda, Praca Natalia Correia 15, Damaia, 2720-414 Amadora, Portugal.

**Connaught, Canad.** See *Aventis Pasteur, Canad.*

**Connaught, Israel.** See *Dover, Israel.*

**Connaught, Norw.** See *Aventis Pasteur, Denm.*

**Connaught, NZ.** See *CSL, NZ.*

**Connell, Hong Kong.** Connell Bros Co. (HK) Ltd, Rm 601, 6/F Stanhope House, 738 King's Rd, North Point, Hong Kong.

**Connetics, USA.** Connetics, 3290 West Bayshore Rd, Palo Alto, CA 94303, USA.

**Consol, Ital.** Consol S.r.l., V.le E Ortolani, Z.I. Dragona, 00125 Acilia (RM), Italy.

**Consolidated Chemicals, Irl.** See *Whelehan, Irl.*

**Continental, Spain.** Continental Farmaceutica, Spain.

**Continental, USA.** Continental Consumer Products, 770 Forest, Suite B, Birmingham, MI 48009, USA.

**Continental Pharma, Belg.** Continental Pharma Inc., Ave de Tervuren 270-272 bte 24, 1150 Brussels, Belgium.

**Continental Pharma, Switz.** See *Vifor, Switz.*

**Continental Pharma, Thai.** See *Union Medical, Thai.*

**Continentales, Mex.** Farmacos Continentales S.A. de C.V., Mexico.

**Continental-Pharm, Thai.** Continental-Pharm Co Ltd, 85/5 Soi Prachoomporn, Chaengwattana Rd, Laksi, Bangkok, Thailand.

**Convatec, Austral.** Convatec Australia, Division of Bristol-Myers Squibb, P.O. Box 240, Noble Park, VIC 3174, Australia.

**Convatec, Canad.** Convatec Canada, Division of Bristol-Myers Squibb Inc., 555 Dr Frederick Philips St, Suite 110, St-Laurent, Quebec, H4M 2X4, Canada.

**Convatec, Fr.** See *Bristol-Myers Squibb, Fr.*

**Convatec, Irl.** See *Bristol-Myers Squibb, Irl.*

**Convatec, Israel.** See *Philtel, Israel.*

**Convatec, Ital.** See *Bristol-Myers Squibb, Ital.*

**Convatec, Port.** See *Bristol-Myers Squibb, Port.*

**Convatec, Switz.** See *Bristol-Myers Squibb, Switz.*

**Convatec, UK.** Harrington House, Milton Rd, Ickenham, Uxbridge, Middlesex, UB10 1DE, UK.

**Cook-Waite, USA.** See *Kodak, USA.*

**Coop. Farm., Ital.** Cooperativa Farmaceutica Soc. Coo. a.r.l. (CoFa Farmaceutici), Via Passione 8, 20122 Milan, Italy.

**Cooper, Fr.** Coopération Pharmaceutique Francaise, 77020 Melun cdx, France.

**Cooper (Κοπερ), Gr.** ΚΟΠΕΡ ΑΕ, Αριστοβούλου 64, 118 53 Πετραλώνα, Petralona, Greece.

**Cooperation Pharmaceutique, Fr.** See *Cooper, Fr.*

**Coopervision, Canad.** Coopervision Inc., 100 McPherson St, Markham, Ontario, L3R 3V6, Canada.

**Copernico, Ital.** Copernico Farmaceutici S.r.l., Viale Etiopia 8, 00199 Rome, Italy.

**Cophar, Switz.** Cophar SA, Route de Moncor 10, 1752 Villars-sur-Glane, Switzerland.

**Co-Pharma, UK.** Co-Pharma Ltd, Talbot House, Church Street, Rickmansworth, Hertfordshire, WD3 1DE, UK.

**Copley, USA.** Copley Pharmaceutical Inc., 25 John Road, Canton, MA 02021, USA.

**Cor Therapeutics, USA.** Cor Therapeutics Inc., 256 East Grand Ave., South San Francisco, CA 94080, USA.

**Coradol, Ger.** Coradol-Pharma GmbH, Ludwig-Erhard-Str. 10, 50129 Bergheim, Germany.

**Coraltis, Israel.** Coraltis Ltd, P.O. Box 168, Rosh Haayin 48091, Israel.

**corax, Ger.** corax pharma GmbH, Lendersbergstr. 86, 53721 Siegburg, Germany.

**Corbridge, Austral.** Corbridge Group, 3 Tait St, Smithfield, NSW 2164, Australia.

**Cord, Hong Kong.** See *Pan-Well, Hong Kong.*

**Cordoba, Arg.** Lab. Córdoba S.A., Rmo Negro 655, 6270 Huinca Renanco, Cordoba, Argentina.

**Corifel, Switz.** Corifel SA, Via Clemente Maraini 9, 6907 Lugano 7, Switzerland.

**Corixa, USA.** Corixa Corp., 1124 Columbia St, Suite 200, Seattle, WA 98104-2040, USA.

**Cork, Singapore.** Cork International Pte Ltd, 20 Toh Guan Rd, 08-02 Accord Distri Centre, S 608839, Singapore.

**Cortec, Denm.** Cortec Medical A/S, St Kongensgade 69, 1264 Copenhagen K, Denmark.

**Cortec, Swed.** Cortec Medical AB, Torggatan 4, 211 40 Malmo, Sweden.

**Cortecs, Irl.** See *Provalis, UK.*

**Cortecs, UK.** See *Provalis, UK.*

**Cortex, Ital.** Cortex Italia S.r.l., Via Vigoni 3, 20122 Milan, Italy.

**Cortunon, Canad.** Cortunon Inc., Canada.

**Corvi, Ital.** Camillo Corvi S.p.A., Via R Lepetit 8, 20020 Lainate (MI), Italy.

**Coryne de Bruynes, Mon.** Laboratoires Coryne de Bruynes, 1 rue du Gabian, Immeuble Le Thales, MC 98000, Monaco.

**Corypharma, Ital.** Corypharma S.r.l., Via Bellagamba s.n., 60035 Jesi (AN), Italy.

**Cos Farma, Ital.** Cos-Farma S.r.l., Via di Portonaccio 23/B, 00159 Rome, Italy.

**Cosan, Switz.** Cosan GmbH, Erlenwiesenstrasse 2, 8604 Volketswil ZH, Switzerland.

**Cosmair, Canad.** Cosmair Canada Inc., 4895 Hickmore, St-Laurent, Quebec, H4T 1K5, Canada.

**Cosmepharm, Gr.** Cosmepharm, Greece.

**Cosmetique Active, Switz.** Cosmétique Active (Suisse) SA, Industriestrasse 9, 5432 Neuenhof., Switzerland.

**Cosmochema, Ger.** Cosmochema Dr H.-H. Reckeweg GmbH, Dr Reckeweg-Str. 2-4, 76532 Baden-Baden, Germany.

**Cosmofarma, Port.** Cosmofarma, Lda (Laboratorios Cosmos), Rua do Arco Carvalhao 14, 1070 Lisbon, Portugal.

**Cosmopharm, Gr.** COSMOPHARM ΕΠΕ, Δρυός 1-3, 157 71 Ζωγράφου, Zographou, Greece.

**Costec, Arg.** Costec S.R.L. Esp. Dermatocosméticas, Av. Corrientes 1296 Piso 7 Dto.76, 1043 Buenos Aires, Argentina.

**Cotek, Singapore.** See *Zuellig, Singapore.*

**Coup, Gr.** COUP OE, Αγ. Βαρβάρας 53, 172 35, Δάφνη, Daphni, Greece.

**Couzian, Fr.** Laboratoires Gabriel Couzian, 1018 av. Tassigny, 71000 Macon, France.

**Covan, S.Afr.** See *Adcock Ingram, S.Afr.*

**Coventry, UK.** Coventry Chemicals Ltd, Woodhams Rd, Siskin Drive, Coventry, CV3 4FX, UK.

**Cow & Gate, Irl.** See *Nutricia, Irl.*

**Cow & Gate, Israel.** See *Guri, Israel.*

**Cow & Gate, UK.** See *Nutricia Clinical, UK.*

**Cox, Hong Kong.** See *Unipharm, Hong Kong.*

**Cox, Irl.** See *Alpharma, UK.*

**Cox, Singapore.** See *Pharmed, Singapore,* and *Sime Darby, Singapore.*

**Cox, UK.** See *Alpharma, UK.*

**CP, Israel.** See *Propharm, Israel.*

**CP Pharma, Switz.** CP Pharma (Schweiz) AG, Emil Frey-Strasse 85, Postfach 922, 4142 Munchenstein 1, Switzerland.

**CP Pharmaceuticals, Hong Kong.** See *Vantone, Hong Kong.*

**CP Pharmaceuticals, Irl.** See *CP Pharmaceuticals, UK.*

**CP Pharmaceuticals, UK.** CP Pharmaceuticals Ltd, Ash Rd North, Wrexham Industrial Estate, Wrexham, Clwyd, LL13 9UF, UK.

**CPC, Hong Kong.** See *Sheraton, Hong Kong.*

**CPF, Ger.** C.P.F, Chemisch-pharmazeutische Fabrik GmbH, Heinrich-Bocking-Str. 6-8, 66121 Saarbrucken, Germany.

**CPH, Port.** Companhia Portuguesa Higiene, SA, Rua do Entreposto Industrial No 3-2, Alfragide, 2720-442 Amadora, Portugal.

**Craveri, Arg.** Craveri S.A.I.C., Arengreen 830, 1405 Buenos Aires, Argentina.

**Crawford, UK.** Crawford Pharmaceuticals, Furtho House, 20 Towcester Rd, Old Stratford, Milton Keynes, Buckinghamshire, MK19 6AQ, UK.

**Crealko, Arg.** Crealko S.A., Paraguay 610 Piso 19, 1428 Buenos Aires, Argentina.

**Creative Brands, Austral.** Creative Brands P/L, P.O. Box 1435, Clayton South, VIC 3169, Australia.

**Crefar, Port.** Crefar, Lda, Rua da Madalena 171, 1100-032 Lisbon, Portugal.

**Creme d'Orient, Fr.** Laboratoires Crème d'Orient, 81 rue de l'Amiral-Roussin, 75015 Paris, France.

**Cress, Canad.** Cress Laboratories, P.O. Box 222, Kitchener, ON, N2G 3X9, Canada.

**Crinex, Fr.** Laboratoires Crinex, B.P. 337, 92541 Montrouge cdx, France.

**Crinos, Hong Kong.** See *Fandasy, Hong Kong.*

**Crinos, Ital.** Crinos Industria Farmacobiologica S.p.A., Piazza XX Settembre 2, 22079 Villaguardia (CO), Italy.

**Cris Flower, Ital.** Cris Flower International S.n.c., Via Livorno 61, 00162 Rome, Italy.

**Cristalia, Braz.** Cristalia Produtos Quimicos Farmaceuticos Ltda, Av. Nossa Senhora da Assuncao 574, Butanta, 05359-001 Sao Paulo, SP, Brazil.

**Crocus, Gr.** CROCUS, Αριστοτέλους 79-91, 104 34 Αθήνα, Athens, Greece.

**Croma, Austria.** Croma-Pharma GmbH, Industriezeile 6, A-2100 Leobendorf, Austria.

**Crombie, NZ.** Crombie and Price, P.O. Box 121, Oamaru, New Zealand.

**Crookes Healthcare, UK.** Crookes Healthcare Ltd, P.O. Box 57, Central Park, Lenton lane, Nottingham, Nottinghamshire, NG2 2LJ, UK.

**Crosara, Ital.** Laboratorio Farmaco Biologico Crosara S.p.A., Via Campobello 15, 00040 Pomezia (Rome), Italy.

**Cross, Swed.** Cross Pharma AB, Box 906, 170 09 Solna, Sweden.

**Crosslands, India.** See *Ranbaxy, India.*

**Crown, S.Afr.** Crown Laboratories Ltd, P.O. Box 100187, Moreleta Plaza 0167, South Africa.

**Cruciani, Ital.** Cruciani - Prodotti Crual, Via Edoardo Scarfoglio 5, 00159 Rome, Italy.

**Cruz, Spain.** Fernandez de la Cruz, Crta Sevilla Malaga Km 5.6, Alcala de Guadaira, 41500 Seville, Spain.

**Cryopharma, Mex.** Cryopharma, Pizzard y Salud, KM 22.5 Carretera Guadalajara Morelia, Jalisco Zuniga, 45640 Guadalajara, Jalisco, Mexico.

**CS, Fr.** Laboratoires CS Dermatologie, 35 rue d'Artois, 75008 Paris, France.

**CS, Port.** CS Portugal, Lda, Rua Joao de Deus 32, Venda Nova, 2700-488 Amadora, Portugal.

**CSC, Austria.** CSC Pharmaceuticals Handels-GmbH, Gewerbestrasse 18-20, A-2102 Bisamberg, Austria.

**CSL, Austral.** CSL Ltd, 45 Poplar Road, Parkville, VIC 3052, Australia.

**CSL, NZ.** CSL (NZ) Ltd, P.O. Box 62590, Central Park, Auckland 6, New Zealand.

**CSP, Fr.** See *ICN, Fr.*

**CT, Ger.** ct-Arzneimittel GmbH, Lengeder Str. 42A, 13407 Berlin, Germany.

**CT, Ital.** C.T., Laboratorio Farmaceutico S.r.l., Via D. Alighieri 69-71, 18038 Sanremo (IM), Italy.

**CTEX, USA.** See *Andrx, USA.*

**CTI, Israel.** See *CTS, Israel.*

**CTS, Israel.** C.T.S. Chemical Industries Ltd, 4 Haharosh St, Hod-Hasharon, Israel.

**Cubist, USA.** Cubist, USA.

**Cullen & Davison, Irl.** Cullen & Davison Ltd, Killenaule Rd, Fethard, Co Tipperary, Ireland.

**Cullen & Davison, UK.** See *Cullen & Davison, Irl.*

**Culver, Austral.** Alberto Culver (Aust) P/L, P.O. Box 253, Parramatta, NSW 2150, Australia.

**Cumberland, USA.** Cumberland Packing Corp., 35 Old Ridgefield Rd, P.O. Box 7688, Willton, CT 06897, USA.

**Cupal, UK.** See *SSL, UK.*

**Cuprocept, S.Afr.** Cuprocept SA, P.O. Box 400, New Germany 3620, South Africa.

**Curacel, Austral.** Curacel International P/L, Suite 14, 1645 Ipswich Rd, Rocklea, QLD 4106, Australia.

**Curaden, Ital.** Curaden Healthcare srl, Via Don Vercesi 18, 20152 Milan, Italy.

**Curamed, Austria.** See *Curamed, Ger.*

**Curamed, Ger.** CuraMED Pharma GmbH, Pforzheimer Str. 5, 76227 Karlsruhe, Germany.

**Curamed, Thai.** See *SPB, Thai.*

**Curasan, Austria.** See *Curasan, Ger.*

**Curasan, Ger.** curasan Pharma GmbH, Lindigstr. 4, 63801 Kleinostheim, Germany.

**Curatis, Ger.** Curatis Pharma GmbH, Karl-Wiechert-Allee 76, 30625 Hannover, Germany.

**Curex, Israel.** Curex, P.O. Box 8366, New Industry Area, Netanya, Israel.

**Cusi, Hong Kong.** See *Alcon, Hong Kong.*

**Cusi, Singapore.** See *Pharmaforte, Singapore.*

**Cusi, Spain.** See *Alcon Cusi, Spain.*

**Cussons, UK.** Cussons (UK) Ltd, Bird Hall Lane, Stockport, Cheshire, SK3 0N, UK.

**Cutter, Israel.** Cutter, Israel.

**Cutter, USA.** See *Bayer, USA.*

**Cuxson, Gerrard, Canad.** Cuxson Gerrard & Co. Ltd, 5775 Andover, Montreal, Quebec, H4T 1H6, Canada.

**Cuxson, Gerrard, UK.** Cuxson, Gerrard & Co. Ltd, 125 Broadwell Rd, Oldbury, Warley, West Midlands, B69 3BB, UK.

**Cyanamid, Ital.** See *Wyeth Lederle, Ital.*

**Cybermed, Austria.** CBM Cybermed AG & Co. KEG, Postfach 50, A-3402 Klosterneuburg, Austria.

**Cypress, USA.** Cypress Pharmaceutical, 135 Industrial Blvd, Madison, MS 39110, USA.

**Cypros, USA.** See *Questcor, USA.*

**CytoChemia, Ger.** CytoChemia AG, Im Burgerstock 7, 79241 Ihringen, Germany.

**Cytogen, Israel.** See *Megapharm, Israel.*

**Cytogen, USA.** Cytogen Corp., 600 College Rd East, Princeton, NJ 08540, USA.

**Cytosol, Israel.** See *Tzamal, Israel.*

**Cytosol, USA.** Cytosol Laboratories, 55 Messina Drive, Braintree, MA 02184, USA.

**DAB, Swed.** DAB Dental AB, Box 423, 194 04 Upplands Vasby, Sweden.

**Dabur, India.** Dabur Pharmaceuticals Ltd, Kaushambi, Ghaziabad 201 010, India.

**Dabur, Thai.** See *Bioscience, Thai.*

**Daewon, Hong Kong.** See *Health Care, Hong Kong.*

**Dagra, Port.** Dagra, Lda, Rua do Centro Cultural 13, 1700 Lisbon, Portugal.

**Daiichi, Hong Kong.** See *Hong Kong Medical, Hong Kong.*

**Daiichi, Jpn.** Daiichi Pharmaceutical Co. Ltd, 3-14-10 Nihonbashi, Chuo-ku, Tokyo 103-8234, Japan.

**Daiichi, Malaysia.** See *Kyowa, Malaysia.*

**Daiichi, Singapore.** See *Kyowa, Singapore.*

**Daiichi, Thai.** Daiichi Pharmaceutical (Thailand) Ltd, 10 Fl, Boonmitr Building, Silom Rd, Bangkok 10500, Thailand.

**Daiichi, USA.** Daiichi Pharmaceutical Corp., 11 Phillips Parkway, Montvale, NJ 07645, USA.

**Dainabot, Jpn.** Dainabot Co Ltd, Osaka Tokio Marine Building, 2-53, Shiromi 2-chome, Chuo-Ku, Osaka 540-0001, Japan.

**Dainippon, Jpn.** Dainippon Pharmaceutical Co. Ltd, 2-6-8 Dosho-machi, Chuo-ku, Osaka 541-8524, Japan.

**Daito, Jpn.** Daito Corp., 326 Yokamachi, Toyama-shi, Toyama 939-8221, Japan.

**Daker Farmasimes, Spain.** Daker Farmasimes, C/Trabajo S/N, Sant Just Desvern, 08960 Barcelona, Spain.

**Dakota, Braz.** Dakota Farmaceutica e Comercial Ltda, Rua Alexandre Gasparoni 68, Marechal Hermes, 21610-250 Rio de Janeiro, RJ, Brazil.

**Dales, Hong Kong.** See *Swiss Worldwide, Hong Kong.*

**Dallas, Arg.** Lab. Dallas S.A., Uriarte 2121/3, 1425 Buenos Aires, Argentina.

**Dallmann, Ger.** Dallmann & Co., Fabrik chem.-pharm. Präparate, Zehntenhofstr. 14-16, Postfach: 130307, 65091 Wiesbaden, Germany.

**Dal-Vita, Austral.** Dal-Vita Products Australia P/L, P.O. Box 477, Manly, NSW 1165, Australia.

**Damor, Ital.** Farmaceutici Damor S.p.A., Via E Scaglione 27, 80145 Naples, Italy.

**Danco, USA.** Danco Laboratories, P.O. Box 4816, New York, NY 10185, USA.

**Danes, Arg.** Lab. Danes Internacional, Division Grunenthal Argentina, Rivadavia 954 Piso 2, 1002 Buenos Aires, Argentina.

**Daniels, Canad.** David D Daniels Ltd, P.O. Box 9, 62 Boychuk Rd, Elliot Lake, Ontario, P5A 2S9, Canada.

**Daniels, Irl.** See *Boileau & Boyd, Irl.*

**Daniels, USA.** See *Jones, USA.*

**Danipharm, Denm.** Danipharm A/S, Englandsvej 350-356, 2770 Kastrup, Denmark.

**Danipharm, Hong Kong.** Danipharm Medic Team (Asia Pacific) Ltd, 206 Technology Plaza, 651 King's Rd, Quarry Bay, Hong Kong.

**Dankos, Singapore.** See *Zyfas, Singapore.*

**Dankos, Thai.** Dankos.

**Dannorth, Canad.** Dannorth Laboratories Inc., 225 Duncan Mill Rd, Suite 400, Toronto, Ontario, M3B 3K9, Canada.

**Dansk, Israel.** See *Promedico, Israel.*

**Dansk-Flama, Braz.** Dansk-Flama Instituto de Fisiologia Aplicada, Rua Barao de Petropolis 311, Rio Comprido, 20251-061 Rio de Janeiro, Brazil.

**Danval, Spain.** Danval, Avda de los Madronos 33, 28043 Madrid, Spain.

**Daquimed, Port.** Daquimed Lda, Rua Dr. Afonso Cordeiro 194 - 1, 4450-001 Matosinhos, Portugal.

**Dar Al Dawa, Hong Kong.** See *Primal, Hong Kong.*

**Darci, Belg.** Darci Pharma S.A., Route de Lennik 437, 1070 Brussels, Belgium.

**Darci, Fr.** See *UCB Healthcare, Fr.*

**Darier, Mex.** Laboratorios Dermatologicos Darier S.A. de C.V., Iglesia No. 2, Edif. E., Piso 13, Col. Tizapan de San Angel, 01090 Mexico D.F., Mexico.

**Dario Correia, Port.** Dario Correia, Lda, Rua Duque de Palmela 25, 1250 Lisbon, Portugal.

**Darrow, Braz.** Darrow Laboratorios S.A., Rua Marques de Olinda 69, 22251-040 Rio de Janeiro, RJ, Brazil.

**Dartmouth, USA.** Dartmouth Pharmaceuticals Inc., 38 Church Ave, Wareham, MA 02751, USA.

**Daudt, Braz.** Laboratorio Daudt Oliveira S.A., Rua Simoes da Mota 57, 21540-100 Rio de Janeiro, RJ, Brazil.

**Davi, Port.** Dávi Farmacêutica, Lda, Estrada da Barrosa, Elsopark, Arm. 8, Algueirao, 2725-193 Mem Martins, Portugal 1711 +351 21 9229720.

**David, India.** Albert David Ltd, 15 Chittaranjan Ave, Kolkata 700 072, India.

**Davigo, Belg.** Davigo s.a.r.l., Rue de l'Ourchet 17, 1367 Gerompont (Bomal), Belgium.

**Davis, Spain.** See *Pfizer, Spain.*

**Davis & Geck, UK.** See *Wyeth, UK.*

**Davur, Spain.** Davur S.L., Teide 4, Parque Empresarial la Marina, San Sebastian de los Reyes, 28700 Madrid, Spain.

**Day, Ital.** Day Farma S.a.s. di Franco Tovecci & C, Via Alessandro Manzoni 227, 80123 Naples, Italy.

**Dayton, USA.** Dayton Laboratories Inc., 7760 NW 56th St, Miami, FL 33166, USA.

**DB, Fr.** Laboratoires DB Pharma, 1 bis, rue du Cdt-Riviere, 94210 La Varenne-St-Hilaire, France.

**DB, Switz.** See *Uhlmann-Eyraud, Switz.*

**DBL, Austral.** See *Mayne, Austral.*

**DBL, NZ.** See *Baxter, NZ.*

**DBL, Thai.** See *Indochina Healthcare, Thai.*

**DC Labs, Canad.** DC Labs Ltd, 795 Pharmacy Ave, Toronto, Ontario, M1L 3K2, Canada.

**DCH, Hong Kong.** DCH Healthcare Products Ltd, 10th Floor, 20 Kai Cheung Rd, Kowloon Bay, Kowloon, Hong Kong.

**DDD, Hong Kong.** See *Trinity, Hong Kong.*

**DDD, Israel.** See *Chemipal, Israel.*

**DDD, Malaysia.** See *People's, Malaysia.*

**DDD, Singapore.** See *Indrugco, Singapore.*

**DDD, UK.** DDD Ltd, 94 Rickmansworth Rd, Watford, Hertfordshire, WD1 7JJ, UK.

**DDSA Pharmaceuticals, UK.** DDSA Pharmaceuticals Ltd, 310 Old Brompton Rd, London, SW5 9JQ, UK.

**De Angeli, Ital.** Istituto De Angeli Ph S.p.A., Via Lorenzini 8, 20139 Milan, Italy.

**De Mayo, Braz.** De Mayo Industrias Quimicas e Farmaceuticas Ltda, Rua Barao de Petropolis 109, 20251-016 Rio de Janeiro, RJ, Brazil.

**De Salute, Ital.** De Salute S.r.l., Via Cadore 7, 26015 Soresina (CR), Italy.

**De Witt, Austria.** See *De Witt, UK.*

**De Witt, Denm.** See *Ferring, Denm.*

**De Witt, Irl.** See *Mayrs, Irl.*

**De Witt, Norw.** See *Ferring, Norw.*

**De Witt, NZ.** See *Regional Health, NZ.*

**De Witt, UK.** E.C. De Witt & Co. Ltd, Tudor Rd, Manor Park, Runcorn, Cheshire, WA7 1SZ, UK.

**Debat, Denm.** See *Ipex, Swed.*

**Debat, Fr.** See *Fournier, Fr.*

**Debat, Hong Kong.** See *Wing Wai, Hong Kong.*

**Debat, Norw.** See *Ipex, Swed.*

**Debat, Thai.** See *Pacific, Thai.*

**Deca, Ital.** Laboratorio Chimico Deca S.r.l., Via Balzaretti 17, 20133 Milan, Italy.

**Declimed, Ger.** See *Desitin, Ger.*

**Decomed, Port.** Decomed Farmaceutica, Lda, Rua Sebastiao e Silva 56, 2745-838 Massama, Portugal.

**Defiante, Neth.** Defiante, Netherlands.

**Defuen, Arg.** Defuen S.A., Av. Dorrego 331, 1414 Buenos Aires, Argentina.

**Degab, Ger.** DeGAB GmbH & Co. KG, Regina-Protmann-Str. 16, 48159 Munster, Germany.

**Degorts, Mex.** Degort's Chemical S.A. de C.V., Alhambra No. 310, Col. Portales, 03300 Mexico D.F., Mexico.

**Degussa, UK.** Degussa Ltd, Winterton House, Winterton Way, Macclesfield, Cheshire, SK11 0LP, UK.

**Deklerht, USA.** Deklerht, USA.

**Del, Canad.** Del Pharmaceutics (Canada) Inc., 25 Morrow Rd, Barrie, Ontario, L4N 3V7, Canada.

**Del, Switz.** Del AG, Switzerland.

**Del, USA.** Del Pharmaceuticals Inc., 565 Broad Hallow Rd, Farmingdale, NY 11735, USA.

**Del Bel, Arg.** Lab. Del Bel S.R.L., Avellaneda 1523, 5000 Cordoba, Argentina.

**Del Saz & Filippini, Ital.** Farmaceutici Del Saz & Filippini S.r.l., Via Dei Pestagalli 7, 20138 Milan, Italy.

**Delagrange, Port.** See *Infar, Port.*

**Delalande, Port.** See *Confar, Port.*

**Delamac, Austral.** Delamac Pharmaceuticals P/L, P.O. Box 125, Spring Hill, Qld 4004, Australia.

**Delicias, Mex.** Delicias S.A. de C.V., Productos Alimenticios, Apartado Postal No. 376, Zona Industrial, 33000 Ciudad Delicias, Chih, Mexico.

**Delmont, USA.** Delmont Laboratories Inc., 715 Harvard Ave, Swarthmore, PA 19081, USA.

**Del-Ray, USA.** Del Ray Laboratories, 22 20th Ave NW, Birmingham, AL 35215, USA.

**Delta, Braz.** Instituto Terapeutico Delta Ltda, Rua Engenheiro Guilherme Cristiano Frendez 827, 03477-000 Sao Paulo, SP, Brazil.

**Delta, Fr.** Laboratoires Delta Pharm, B.P. 27, 22170 Chatelaudren, France.

**Delta, Ger.** See *DeltaSelect, Ger.*

**Delta, Irl.** Delta Laboratories Ltd, 26 Airfield Court, Dublin 4, Ireland.

**Delta, Port.** Laboratórios Delta, Lda, Rua Direita de Massama 148, 2745-751 Queluz, Portugal.

**Delta, Singapore.** See *Green Cross, Singapore.*

**Delta BKB, Ital.** Delta BKB S.r.l., V.le Emilio Po 224, 41100 Modena, Italy.

**delta pronatura, Ger.** delta pronatura Dr. Krauss & Dr. Beckmann GmbH & Co. KG, Kurt-Schumacher-Ring 15-17, 63329 Egelsbach, Germany.

**Delta West, Malaysia.** See *Pharmacia, Malaysia.*

**DeltaSelect, Ger.** DeltaSelect GmbH, Benzstr. 5, 72793 Pfullingen, Germany.

**Demo, Gr.** DEMO AEBE, 21ο χλμ. Εθνικής Οδού Αθηνών-Λαμίας 145 65 Κρυονέρι, Krioneri, Greece.

**Democal, Switz.** Democal AG, Postfach 1045, 1701 Fribourg-Moncor, Switzerland.

**Demopharm, Switz.** See *Democal, Switz.*

**Denamed, Norw.** Denamed AS, Stromsv. 48, 2010 Strommen, Norway.

**Dendron, UK.** See *DDD, UK.*

**Dendy, Austral.** Dendy Pharmaceuticals P/L, 44 Cromer St, East Brighton, VIC 3187, Australia.

**Denfleet, UK.** Denfleet International Ltd, 45 Essex St, London, WC2R 3JF, UK.

**Denk, Hong Kong.** See *Star, Hong Kong,* and *Universal, Hong Kong.*

**Denk, Singapore.** See *Luen Wah, Singapore.*

**Denolin, Belg.** Denolin S.A., Rue des Goujons 152, 1070 Brussels, Belgium.

**Dent, USA.** C.S. Dent & Co., 1820 Airport Exchange Bvld, Erlanger, KY 41018, USA.

**Dentaid, Chile.** Laboratorios Dentaid SA, Camino de la Colina 1432, Huechuraba, Santiago, Chile.

**Dentaid, Spain.** Dentaid, Parque Tecno del Valle, Ronda Can Fatjo 10, Cerdanyola, 08290 Barcelona, Spain.

**Dental Health Products, UK.** Dental Health Products Ltd, 60 Broughton Lane, Maidstone, Kent, ME15 9XS, UK.

**Dental Warehouse, S.Afr.** Dental Warehouse (Pty) Ltd, Private Bag X8, Wendywood 2144, South Africa.

**Dental-Kosmetik, Ger.** Dental-Kosmetik GmbH, Katharinestr. 4, 01099 Dresden, Germany.

**Dentinox, Ger.** Dentinox Gesellschaft für Pharmazeutische Präparate Lenk & Schuppan, Nunsdorfer Ring 19, 12277 Berlin, Germany.

**Dentinox, Switz.** See *Renapharm, Switz.*

**Dentox, UK.** Dentox Ltd, Hillmeadow, Lighthorne, Warwick, CV35 0AB, UK.

**Dentsply, Austral.** Dentsply (Australia) P/L, Private Bag 4, Abbotsford, VIC 3067, Australia.

**Dentsply, Braz.** Dentsply, Rua Alice Herve 86, Bingen, 25665-010 Petropolis, RJ, Brazil.

**Dentsply, Fin.** See *Tamro, Fin.*

**Dentsply, Fr.** Dentsply France, 17 rue Michael-Faraday, 78180 Montigny-le-Bretonneux, France.

**Dentsply, Ger.** Dentsply DeTrey GmbH, De-Trey-Strasse 1, 78467 Constance, Germany.

**Dentsply, Ital.** Dentsply Italia S.r.l., Via A Cavaglieri 26, 00173 Rome, Italy.

**Dentsply, UK.** Dentsply Ltd, Hamm Moor Lane, Addlestone, Weybridge, Surrey, KT15 2SE, UK.

**Denver, Arg.** Denver Farma S.A., Natalio Querido 2285, 1605 Munro, Buenos Aires, Argentina.

**Dep, Canad.** Dep Corporation, 966 Pantera Drive, Mississauga, Ontario, L4W 2S1, Canada.

**DEP, USA.** DEP Corp., 2101 East Via Arado, Rancho Dominguez, CA 90220, USA.

**Depofarma, Ital.** Depofarma S.r.l., Via Guindazzi 44/54, 80040 Pollena Trocchia (NA), Italy.

**Deproco, UK.** Deproco UK Ltd, Units R & S, Orchard Business Centre, St. Barnabas Close, Allington, Maidstone, Kent, ME16 0JZ, UK.

**DePuy, Ger.** DePuy Orthopädie GmbH, a Johnson & Johnson Company, Mellinweg 16, 66280 Sulzbach, Germany.

**DePuy, UK.** DePuy International Ltd, St Anthonys Rd, Leeds, West Yorkshire, LS11 8DT, UK.

**Derek, Singapore.** Derek Marketing Pte Ltd, Block 221 Henderson Rd, 05-12 Henderson Building, S 159557, Singapore.

**Dergam, Fr.** Laboratoires Dergam, 6 rue Saint-Nicolas, 75012 Paris, France.

**Derly, Spain.** Derly, Avenida de la Industria 30, Alcobendas, 28100 Madrid, Spain.

**Dermaclin, Mex.** Dermaclin S.A. de C.V., Rebsamen 747, Col. Narvarte, 03020 Mexico D.F., Mexico.

**Dermal, Israel.** See *Trupharm, Israel.*

**Dermal Laboratories, Irl.** See *Cahill May Roberts, Irl.*

**Dermal Laboratories, UK.** Dermal Laboratories Ltd, Tatmore Place, Gosmore, Hitchin, Hertfordshire, SG4 7QR, UK.

**Dermamend, UK.** Dermamend, UK.

**Dermapharm, Ger.** Dermapharm AG, Luise-Ullrich-Strasse 6, 82031 Grunwald, Germany.

**Dermapharm, Irl.** See *United Drug, Irl.*

**Dermapharm, UK.** See *Alliance, UK.*

**Dermatech, Austral.** Dermatech Laboratories, Unit 17, Prospect Highway, Seven Hills, NSW 2147, Australia.

**Dermatech, Singapore.** See *Sime Darby, Singapore.*

**Dermik, Canad.** Dermik Laboratories Canada Inc., 6205 Airport Rd, Building B, Suite 100, Mississauga, Ontario, L4V 1E1, Canada.

**Dermik, Hong Kong.** See *Health Care, Hong Kong.*

**Dermik, Israel.** See *Medibrands, Israel.*

**Dermik, Singapore.** See *JDH, Singapore.*

**Dermik, USA.** See *Aventis, USA.*

**DermoDuemila, Ital.** DermoDuemila Srl, P.le F.il Macedone 140, 00124 Casalpalocco (RM), Italy.

**Dermofarm, Spain.** Dermofarm, Can Sant Joan, Rubi, 08191 Barcelona, Spain.

**Dermofarma, Ital.** Dermofarma Italia S.r.l., Via Beata Francesca 10, 83100 Avellino, Italy.

**Dermol, USA.** Dermol Pharmaceuticals Inc., 3807 Roswell Rd, Marietta, GA 30062, USA.

**Dermopen, Braz.** Divisao Farmaceutica Dermopen Ltda, Rua Ida Romussi Gasparinetti 110, Parque Laguna, 06795-000 Taboao da Serra, SP, Brazil.

**Dermophil Indien, Fr.** Laboratoires du Dermophil Indien, B.P. 9, 61600 La Ferte-Mace, France.

**Dermophil Indien, Switz.** See *Uhlmann-Eyraud, Switz.*

**Dermoteca, Port.** Dermoteca, SA, Estrada Nacional 117, 2720 Alfragide, Portugal.

**Dermtek, Canad.** Dermtek Pharmaceuticals Ltd, 1600 Trans-Canada Highway, Suite 200, Dorval, Quebec, H9P 1H7, Canada.

**Desarrollo, Spain.** Desarrollo Farma y Cosmeticos, Pa de la Castellana 143, 28046 Madrid, Spain.

**Desatnik, S.Afr.** MI Desatnik, P.O. Box 39359, Booysens 2041, South Africa.

**Desbergers, Canad.** See *Technilab, Canad.*

**Desitin, Denm.** Desitin Pharma A/S, Nyhavn 43 B, 1051 Copenhagen K, Denmark.

**Desitin, Fin.** See *Tamro, Fin.*

**Desitin, Ger.** Desitin Arzneimittel GmbH, Weg beim Jager 214, 22335 Hamburg, Germany.

**Desitin, Hong Kong.** See *Jacobson, Hong Kong.*

**Desitin, Israel.** See *Megapharm, Israel.*

**Desitin, Malaysia.** See *Ranbaxy, Malaysia.*

**Desitin, Norw.** Desitin Pharma A/S, Niels Leuchsv. 99, 1359 Eiksmarka, Norway.

**Desitin, Singapore.** See *Zyfas, Singapore.*

**Desitin, Swed.** Desitin Pharma AB, Box 2064, 431 02 Molndal, Sweden.

**Desitin, Switz.** Desitin-Pharma GmbH, Oristalstrasse 87a, 4410 Liestal, Switzerland.

**Desma, Ger.** Desma GmbH, Rheinallee 122, 55120 Mainz, Germany.

**Desopharmex, Switz.** Desopharmex AG, Muttenzerstrasse 107, 4133 Pratteln 1, Switzerland.

**Dessau, Ger.** Pharma Dessau GmbH, Luxemburgstr. 8, 06846 Dessau, Germany.

**Deutsch Chinesische, Hong Kong.** Deutsch Chinesische Apotheke (Maple Inc.), 809, Wellborne Commercial Ctr, 8 Java Rd, North Point, Hong Kong.

**Deutsche, Chile.** See *Sanofi Synthelabo, Chile.*

**Deverge, Ital.** Devergè Medicina e Medicalizzazione S.r.l., C.so Casale 206, 10132 Turin, Italy.

**Devesa, Ger.** Devesa Dr Reingraber GmbH & Co. KG, Heinkelstr. 8a, 76461 Muggensturm, Germany.

**Devries, Israel.** Devries & Co. Ltd, 51 Ahad Ha'am St, Tel Aviv 65206, Israel.

**Dewitt, Malaysia.** See *JDH, Malaysia.*

**Dexa, Hong Kong.** See *Health Alliance, Hong Kong.*

**Dexa, Singapore.** See *Apotheca, Singapore.*

**Dexcel, Denm.** See *Vitaflo, Denm.*

**Dexcel, Ger.** Dexcel Pharma GmbH, Rontgenstr. 1, 63755 Alzenau, Germany.

**Dexcel, Israel.** See *Dexxon, Israel.*

**Dexcel, UK.** Dexcel Pharma Ltd, 1 Cottesbrooke Park, Heartlans Business Park, Daventry, Northamptonshire, NN11 5YI, UK.

**DexGen, USA.** DexGen Pharmaceuticals, P.O. Box 675, Manasquan, NJ 08736, USA.

**Dexo, Fr.** Laboratoires Dexo, 179 bureaux de la Colline, 92213 Saint-Cloud cdx, France.

**Dexo, Switz.** See *Actipharm, Switz.,* and *Uhlmann-Eyraud, Switz.*

**Dexo, Thai.** See *Pacific, Thai.*

**Dexter, Arg.** Dexter S.A.C.I. (Int'l), Humahuaca 4065, 1192 Buenos Aires, Argentina.

**Dexter, Spain.** Dexter Farmaceutica, Avda Virgen de Montserrat 215, 08026 Barcelona, Spain.

**Dexxon, Israel.** Dexxon, P.O. Box 50, Hadera 38100, Israel.

**Dey, USA.** Dey Laboratories, 2751 Napa Valley Corporate Drive, Napa, CA 94558, USA.

**Dey's, India.** Dey's Medical Stores (Manufacturing) Ltd, 62 Bondel Rd, Kolkata 700 087, India.

**DFL, Braz.** DFL Industria e ComErcio Ltda, Estrada do Guerengue 2059, Rio de Janeiro, RJ, Brazil.

**DHA, Hong Kong.** See *US Summit, Hong Kong.*

**DHA, Malaysia.** See *JDH, Malaysia.*

**DHA, Singapore.** Drug Houses of Australia (Asia) Pte Ltd, 2 Chia Ping Rd, 09-00 Haw Par Tiger Balm Building, S 619968, Singapore.

**DHN, Fr.** Laboratoires DHN, Nutrition Clinique, Le Haut-Montigne, 35370 Torce, France.

**DHU, Ger.** Deutsche Homöopathie-Union, Ottostr. 24, 76227 Karlsruhe, Germany.

**Diabact, Swed.** See *Orexo, Swed.*

**Diaco, Ital.** Laboratori Diaco Biomedicali S.p.A., Via Flavia 124, 34147 Trieste, Italy.

**Diadin, Ger.** Diadin-Gesellschaft Chemisches Laboratorium GmbH, Ludwig Merckle-Str. 3, 89143 Blaubeuren, Germany.

**Diafarm, Spain.** Diafarm, Avda Arraona 119-123, Barbera del Valles, 08210 Barcelona, Spain.

**Diamant, Fr.** See *Aventis, Fr.*

**Diamant, Port.** See *Aventis, Port.*

**Diamant, Singapore.** See *Zuellig, Singapore.*

**Diapit, Gr.** DIAPIT, Αγ. Κωνσταντίνου 6, 104 31 Αθήνα, Athens, Greece.
**Diatide, USA.** Diatide Inc., 9 Delta Dr., Londonderry, NH 03053, USA.
**Diba, Mex.** Laboratorios Diba, S.A., Escorza No. 728, 44190 Guadalajara, Jal, Mexico.
**Dibropharm, Ger.** Dibropharm GmbH Distribution & Co. KG, Kleine-Dollen-Str. 5, 76532 Baden-Baden, Germany.
**Dicamed, Swed.** Dicamed AB, Djupdalsvagen 24, 192 51 Sollentuna, Sweden.
**Dickinson, USA.** Dickinson Brands Inc., 31 East High St, East Hampton, CT 06424, USA.
**Dicofarm, Ital.** Dicofarm S.p.A., Via Vitorchiano 151, 00189 Rome, Italy.
**Dieckmann, Ger.** See *Merck Sharp & Dohme, Ger.*
**Diedenhofen, Ger.** Diedenhofen GmbH, Otto-von-Guericke-Str. 1, Postfach: 1252, 53730 St Augustin/Bonn, Germany.
**Diedenhofen, Thai.** See *Oui Heng, Thai.*
**Diele, Fr.** Diele Distripharma, 18 av Albert-Einstein, 93152 Le Blanc-Mesnil cdx, France.
**Diepal, Fr.** Diépal-NSA, B.P. 432, 69654 Villefranche-sur-Saone cdx, France.
**Diepha, Fr.** See *Diepharmex, Fr.*
**Diepharmex, Fr.** Laboratoires Diepharmex, 26 rue de l'Industrie, 92400 Corbevoie, France.
**Diet Erba, NZ.** See *NZ Distributors, NZ.*
**Dieterba, Ital.** Dieterba, Via Migliara 45, 04100 Latina, Italy.
**Dietetique et Sante, Fr.** See *Novartis Nutrition, Fr.*
**Diethelm, Malaysia.** Diethelm Malaysia Sdn Bhd, 74 Jln Universiti, 46200 Petaling Jaya, Selangor, Malaysia.
**Diethelm, Singapore.** Diethelm Singapore Pte Ltd, 34 Boon Leat Terrace, S 119866, Singapore.
**Diethelm, Thai.** Diethelm & Co. Ltd, Pharmaceutical Division, 280 New Rd, Bangkok 10100, Thailand.
**Difa, Ital.** Difa-Cooper S.p.A., Via Milano 160, 21042 Caronno Pertusella (VA), Italy.
**Diffucap, Braz.** Diffucap-Chemobras Quim Farm Ltda, Rua Goias 1232, 21380-010 Rio de Janeiro, RJ, Brazil.
**Diftersa, Spain.** Diftersa, Spain.
**Dimethaid, UK.** Dimethaid UK Ltd, Spectrum House, 20-26 Cursitor St, London, EC4A 1HY, UK.
**Dinafarma, Braz.** Laboratorio Dinafarma Ltda, Avenida Major Alvim 155, 12940-000 Atibaia, SP, Brazil.
**Diomed, UK.** Diomed Developments Ltd, UK.
**Dioptic, Canad.** Dioptic Laboratories, Division of Akorn Pharmaceuticals Canada Ltd, 1405 Denison St, Markham, Ontario, L3R 5V2, Canada.
**Discotrade, Israel.** See *Dexxon, Israel.*
**Discovery, UK.** Discovery Pharmaceuticals, The Old Vicarage, Market Place, Castle Donnington, Derbyshire, DE74 2JB, UK.
**Dispensapharm, Canad.** See *Pharmacia, Canad.*
**Disperga, Austria.** Dr C Szalagyl Disperga GmbH, Josefstadter Strasse 43, A-1080 Vienna, Austria.
**Dispolab, Chile.** Dispolab Farmaceutica SA, Santa Victoria 213, Providencia, Santiago, Chile.
**Disprofarma, Arg.** Disprofarma S.A., Virrey Cevallos 1643, 1135 Buenos Aires, Argentina.
**Disprovent, Arg.** Disprovent S.A., Cervantes 2950, 1417 Buenos Aires, Argentina.
**Dissolvurol, Mon.** Laboratoires Dissolvurol, Le Concorde, 11 rue du Gabian, MC 98000, Monaco.
**Dista, Austral.** See *Lilly, Austral.*
**Dista, Irl.** See *Lilly, Irl.*
**Dista, NZ.** See *Lilly, NZ.*
**Dista, Spain.** See *Lilly, Spain.*
**Dista, Switz.** See *Lilly, Switz.*
**Dista, UK.** See *Lilly, UK.*
**Dista, USA.** See *Lilly, USA.*
**Distri B3, Fr.** Laboratoires Distri B3, rue Max Planck, Technopole de Chateau-Gombert, 13013 Marseille, France.
**Distriborg, Fr.** Distriborg, 217 chem. du Grand-Revoyet, 69561 St-Genis-Laval, France.
**Distrifarma, Port.** Distrifarma, SA, Condominio Industrial Queluz Park, Estrada Consiglieri Pedroso 80 Lote 3, Queluz de Baixo, 2745-553 Barcarena, Portugal.
**Distriphar, UK.** See *Aventis, UK.*
**Distriquimica, Spain.** Distriquimica, Avd Mare de Due de Montserrat 221, 00081 Barcelona, Spain.
**Divapharma, Ger.** Divapharma-Knufinke Arzneimittel-werk GmbH, 12274 Berlin, Germany.
**Diviser Aquilea, Spain.** Diviser Aquilea, Pont Reixat 5, Saint Just Desvern, 08960 Barcelona, Spain.
**Dixon-Shane, USA.** Dixon-Shane Inc., 256 Geiger Rd, Philadelphia, PA 19115, USA.
**DJ, USA.** DJ Pharma Inc, 12730 High Bluff Bvld, Suite 160, San Diego, CA 92130, USA.
**DM, Braz.** DM Industria Farmaceutica Ltda, Av. Piracema 155, 06460-030 Barueri, SP, Brazil.
**DMG, Ger.** DMG Chemisch-Pharmazeutische Fabrik GmbH, Postfach: 530104, 22531 Hamburg, Germany.
**DMG, Ital.** DMG Italia S.r.l., Via Campello sul Clitunno 34, 00181 Rome, Italy.
**DNR, Arg.** Laboratorio DNR Farma SRL, Hipolito Vieytes 147, Villa Martelli, Buenos Aires, Argentina.
**Doak, Hong Kong.** See *International Medical, Hong Kong.*
**Doak, USA.** Doak Dermatologics, 383 Route 46 West, Fairfield, NJ 07004-2402, USA.
**DOC, Ital.** DOC Generici S.r.l., Via Manuzio 7, 20124 Milan, Italy.
**Doc Pharma, Belg.** Doc Pharma, Belgium.
**Docmed, S.Afr.** Docmed, South Africa.
**Docpharm, Ger.** Docpharm Arzneimittelvertrieb GmbH & Co. KGaA, Reetzstr. 83, 76327 Pfinztal, Germany.
**Docta, Spain.** Docta, Gran Via de les Corts, Catalanes 774, 08013 Barcelona, Spain.
**Doctum, Gr.** DOCTUM, 1ο χλμ. Λ. Παιανίας, 190 02 Παιανία, Paiania, Greece.
**Doerenkamp, Ger.** Doerenkamp GmbH, Gereonsmuhlengasse 3, 50670 Cologne, Germany.
**Doetsch, Grether, Switz.** Doetsch Grether AG, 4002 Basle, Switzerland.
**Dolisos, Belg.** Dolisos S.A., Rue Carli 5, 1140 Brussels, Belgium.
**Dolisos, Canad.** Dolisos, 1400 Hocquart St, St-Bruno, Quebec, J3V 6E1, Canada.
**Dolisos, Fr.** Laboratoires Dolisos, 45 place Abel Gance, 92100 Boulogne, France.
**Dolisos, Ital.** Laboratoires Dolisos Italia S.r.l., Via Pontina Vecchia km 34,200, 00040 Ardea (Rome), Italy.
**Dolorgiet, Denm.** See *Nordisk Ibu-Pharma, Denm.*
**Dolorgiet, Ger.** Dolorgiet GmbH & Co. KG, Otto-von-Guericke-Str. 1, 53754 St. Augustin/Bonn, Germany.
**Dolorgiet, Switz.** See *Mundipharma, Switz.*
**Dom, Spain.** Dom, Gallo 30, Esplugas de Llobregat, 08950 Barcelona, Spain.
**Dome, Switz.** See *Medinova, Switz.*
**Dome-Hollister-Stier, Fr.** Dome-Hollister-Stier, 6 rue Alexis-de-Tocqueville, 92180 Antony cdx, France.
**Dominguez, Arg.** Lab. Dominguez S.A., Av. La Plata 2552, 1437 Buenos Aires, Argentina.
**Dominion, Canad.** See *Pharmascience, Canad.*
**Dominion, India.** Dominion Chemical Industries Ltd, Hosur Rd, Bommanahalli, Bangalore 560 068, India.
**Dominion, Irl.** See *Dominion, UK.*
**Dominion, UK.** See *Pliva, UK.*
**Dompe, Ital.** Dompè Farmaceutici S.p.A., Via San Martino 12-12/A, 20122 Milan, Italy.
**Dompe Biogen, Switz.** Dompé-Biogen AG, Bahnhofstrasse 12, 6300 Zug, Switzerland.
**Dompe Biotec, Ital.** Dompè Biotec S.p.A., Via Santa Lucia 4, 20122 Milan, Italy.
**Doms, Switz.** See *Actipharm, Switz.*
**Doms-Adrian, Fr.** See *Bouchara-Recordati, Fr.*
**Doms-Adrian, Hong Kong.** See *Rich Plan, Hong Kong.*
**Don, Israel.** See *Manon, Israel.*
**Donell DerMedex, USA.** Donell DerMedex, 342 Madison Ave, Suite 1422, New York, NY 10173, USA.
**Dong, Singapore.** See *Pharmaforte, Singapore.*
**Dong Kook, Singapore.** See *Polymedic, Singapore,* and *Ziwell, Singapore.*
**Dong Kook, Thai.** See *Charoen, Thai.*
**Donini, Ital.** Donini S.r.l., Via Ecce Homo 18, 37054 Nogara (VR), Italy.
**Donmed, S.Afr.** Donmed Pharmaceuticals, P.O. Box 75907, Gardenview 2047, South Africa.
**DORC, Neth.** Dutch Ophthalmic Research Center International, Scheijdelveweg 2, 3214 VN Zuidland, Netherlands.
**Dormer, Canad.** Dormer Laboratories Inc., 91 Kelfield St, Unit 5, Rexdale, Ontario, M9W 5A3, Canada.
**Dorom, Ital.** Dorom S.r.l., Via Volturno 48, 20089 Quinto de Stampi Rozzano (MI), Italy.
**Dorwest, UK.** Dorwest Herbs Ltd, Shipton Gorge, Bridport, Dorset, DT6 4LP, UK.
**Dosa, Arg.** Lab. Dosa S.A., Girardot 1369, 1427 Buenos Aires, Argentina.
**Doskar, Austria.** Doskar Mag. Martin Pharm. Produkte, Schottenring 14, A-1010 Vienna, Austria.
**Douglas, Austral.** Douglas Pharmaceuticals Australia Ltd, P.O. Box 7004, Baulkham Hills Business Centre, Baulkham Hills, NSW 2153, Australia.
**Douglas, Hong Kong.** See *Hind Wing, Hong Kong.*
**Douglas, Israel.** See *Taro, Israel.*
**Douglas, Malaysia.** See *Schmidt, Malaysia.*
**Douglas, NZ.** Douglas Pharmaceuticals Ltd, P.O. Box 45-027, Aukland 8, New Zealand.
**Douglas, Singapore.** See *Grafton, Singapore.*
**Douglas, Thai.** See *JDH Borneo, Thai.*
**Dovalle, Braz.** Farmoterapica Dovalle Industria Quimica Farmaceutica Ltda, Rodovia SC 438 Km 3, 88708-080 Tubarao, SC, Brazil.
**Dover, Israel.** Dover Medical & Scientific Equipment Ltd, 11 Hamaalot St, Herzliya 46583, Israel.
**Dow, USA.** See *Bertek, USA.*
**Dow Corning, UK.** Dow Corning Ltd, Kings Court, 185 Kings Rd, Reading, Berkshire, RG1 4EX, UK.
**DP-Medica, Switz.** DP-Medica SA, Pharmazeutische Produkte, Case postale 238, Fribourg, Switzerland.
**Dr Janssen, Ger.** Dr. Werner Janssen Nachf. Chem.-pharm. Produkte GmbH, Grenzstr. 2, 53340 Meckenheim, Germany.
**Dr P, Ger.** Dr. P. Medizinische Dienste by Dr. Panzer GmbH, Gronauer Weg 45, 12207 Berlin, Germany.
**Draco, Swed.** See *AstraZeneca, Swed.*
**Drag, Chile.** Drag Pharma Invetec SA, Las Dalias 3193, Macul, Santiago, Chile.
**Dragenopharm, Israel.** See *Taro, Israel.*
**Drawer, Arg.** Lab. Drawer S.A., Dorrego 127, 1878 Quilmes, Buenos Aires, Argentina.
**Draxis, Canad.** Draxis Health Inc., 6870 Goreway Dr, Mississauga, Ontario, L4V 1P1, Canada.
**Dreiman, Spain.** See *Alcala, Spain.*
**Dreluso, Ger.** Dreluso Pharmazeutika, Dr Elten & Sohn GmbH, Marktplatz 5, 31840 Hessisch Oldendorf, Germany.
**Dresden, Ger.** Arzneimittelwerk Dresden GmbH, Meissner Str. 35, 01445 Radebeul, Germany.
**Dreveny, Austria.** Dr. Dreveny, Mag. pharm. & Co. OHG, Herrandgasse 7, A-8010 Graz, Austria.
**Drogasil, Braz.** Drogasil S.A., Avenida Corifeu de Azevedo Marques 3097, 05339-900 Sao Paulo, SP, Brazil.
**Drogenhansa, Austria.** Drogenhansa Bioreform GmbH, Haidestrasse 4, A-1110 Vienna, Austria.
**Droreth, Israel.** Matzkel I Droreth Ltd, 17 Lilienblum St, Tel Aviv 65132, Israel.
**Drossapharm, Israel.** See *Gilco, Israel.*
**Drossapharm, Switz.** Drossapharm SA, Drosselstrasse 47, 4059 Basle, Switzerland.
**Drug Research, Ital.** D.R. Drug Research S.r.l., Via F Turati 3, 22036 Erba (CO), Italy.
**Drug Research, Singapore.** See *Zyfas, Singapore.*
**Drug Trading, Canad.** Drug Trading Co. Ltd, 795 Pharmacy Ave, Scarborough, Ontario, M1L 3K2, Canada.
**Drugtech, Chile.** Laboratorio Drugtech, Av. Pedro de Valdivia 428, Providencia, Santiago, Chile.
**Du Pont, Belg.** Du Pont Pharma S.A., Centre Mercure, Rue de la Fusee 100, 1130 Brussels, Belgium.
**Du Pont, Canad.** See *Bristol-Myers Squibb, Canad.*
**Du Pont, Fr.** See *Bristol-Myers Squibb, Fr.*
**Du Pont, Ger.** Du Pont Pharma GmbH, Du Pont-Str. 1, 61352 Bad Homburg v.d.H., Germany.
**Du Pont, Hong Kong.** See *DCH, Hong Kong,* and *Keller, Hong Kong.*
**Du Pont, Irl.** See *United Drug, Irl.*
**Du Pont, Israel.** See *Teva, Israel.*
**Du Pont, Norw.** See *Meda, Norw.*
**Du Pont, Singapore.** See *Boots, Singapore.*
**Du Pont, Switz.** See *Opopharma, Switz.*
**Du Pont, USA.** DuPont Pharmaceuticals Co., Chestnut Run Plaza, Hickory Run, Wilmington, DE 19880-0723, USA.
**Duchesnay, Canad.** Duchesnay Inc., 2925 Industrial Blvd, Laval, Quebec, H7L 3W9, Canada.
**Ducray, Fr.** See *Pierre Fabre, Fr.*
**Ducto, Braz.** Lab. Ducto Ind. Farm. Ltda, Rua VPR 3 Quadra 2-A, Modulos 20/21 DAIA, 75133-600 Anapolis, GO, Brazil.
**Dumex, Ger.** See *Alpharma-Isis, Ger.*
**Dumex, Irl.** See *Alpharma, UK.*
**Dumex, Malaysia.** Dumex (Malaysia) Sdn Bhd, 1 Jln 205, 46050 Petaling Jaya, Selangor, Malaysia.
**Dumex, Norw.** See *Alpharma, Norw.*
**Dumex, NZ.** See *CSL, NZ.*
**Dumex, Port.** See *Alpharma, Port.*
**Dumex, Singapore.** Dumex, Representative Office, 9 Third Lok Yang Rd, S 628004, Singapore.
**Dumex, Switz.** See *Dumex-Alpharma, Switz.*
**Dumex, UK.** See *Alpharma, UK.*
**Dumex-Alpharma, Denm.** See *Alpharma, Denm.*
**Dumex-Alpharma, Fin.** See *Alpharma, Fin.*
**Dumex-Alpharma, Hong Kong.** See *Primal, Hong Kong.*
**Dumex-Alpharma, Singapore.** See *Sime Darby, Singapore.*
**Dumex-Alpharma, Swed.** See *Alpharma, Swed.*
**Dumex-Alpharma, Switz.** See *Medinova, Switz.*
**Dumex-Alpharma, Thai.** See *Stada, Thai.*
**Dumont, Arg.** Quim. Dumont Freres S.R.L., Saladillo 2452/68, 1440 Buenos Aires, Argentina.
**Duncan, Arg.** Laboratorios Duncan S.A., Av. San Martmn 6340/42, 1419 Buenos Aires, Argentina.
**Duncan, Spain.** See *GlaxoSmithKline, Spain.*
**Duncan, Flockhart, Irl.** See *GlaxoSmithKline, Irl.*
**Dunhall, USA.** Dunhall Pharmaceuticals Inc., Highway 59N, P.O. Box 100, Gravette, AR 72736, USA.
**Duomed, Switz.** Duomed AG, 9533 Kirchberg, Switzerland.
**Duopharm, Ger.** Duopharm GmbH, Grassingerstr. 9, 83043 Bad Aibling, Germany.
**Duopharma, Hong Kong.** See *Weston, Hong Kong.*
**Duphar, NZ.** See *Russells, NZ.*
**Duphar, Spain.** See *Solvay, Spain.*
**Duphar-Interfran, Thai.** See *Union Medical, Thai.*
**Dupomar, Arg.** Dupomar S.A.C.I.F., Av. Juan B. Justo 4840, 1416 Buenos Aires, Argentina.
**Dura, USA.** See *Elan, USA.*
**Durachemie, Ger.** See *Merck dura, Ger.*
**Duramed, USA.** Duramed Pharmaceuticals, 5040 Duramed Dr, Cincinnati, OH 45213, USA.
**Durascan, Denm.** DuraScan Medical Products AS, Svendborgvej 243, 5260 Odense S, Denmark.
**Durban, Spain.** Durban, Santos Zarate 20, 04004 Almeria, Spain.
**Durbin, UK.** Durbin Plc, 180 Northolt Rd, South Harrow, Middlesex, HA2 0LT, UK.
**Durex, Canad.** Durex Canada, Division of London International Group Ltd, 100 Courtland Ave, Concord, Ontario, L4K 3T6, Canada.
**Durex, USA.** Durex Consumer Products, 3585 Engineering Drive, Suite 200, Norcross, GA 30092, USA.
**DUSA, USA.** DUSA Pharmaceuticals Inc., 25 Upton, Wilmington, MA 01887, USA.
**Dutch Lady, Malaysia.** Dutch Lady Milk Industries Bhd, 13 Jln Semangat, 46200 Petaling Jaya, Selangor, Malaysia.
**Dutec, Austral.** Dutec Diagnostics P/L, P.O. Box 79, Croydon, NSW 2132, Australia.
**Dyckerhoff, Ger.** Dyckerhoff Pharma GmbH & Co., Robert-Perthel-Str. 49, 50739 Cologne, Germany.
**Dynacren, Ital.** Dynacren Laboratorio Farmaceutico del Dott. A. Francioni e di M. Gerosa S.r.l., Via P Nenni 12, Loc Malpensa, 28053 Castelletto Ticino (NO), Italy.
**Dynamed, S.Afr.** Dynamed, South Africa.
**Dynamit, Austria.** Dynamit Nobel Wien GmbH, A-8813 St Lamprecht, Austria.
**Dzwon, India.** Dzwon Remedies, 75/C Government Industrial Estate, Kandivli West, Mumbai 400 067, India.
**E. Merck, Denm.** See *Kemifarma, Denm.*
**E. Merck, Irl.** See *Merck, Irl.*
**E. Merck, UK.** See *Merck, UK.*
**E Pharma, Fr.** Laboratoires E Pharma, ZI Le Malcourlet, 03800 Gannat, France.
**Eagle, Austral.** Eagle Pharmaceuticals P/L, P.O. Box 927, Castle Hill, NSW 1765, Australia.
**East India Pharma, India.** East India Pharmaceutical Works Ltd, 6 Little Russel St, Kolkata 700 071, India.
**Eastern Pharmaceuticals, Irl.** See *Intra Pharma, Irl.*
**Eastern Pharmaceuticals, UK.** Eastern Pharmaceuticals Ltd, Coomb House, St. Johns Rd, Isleworth, Middlesex, TW7 6NA, UK.
**e+b, Austria.** See *e+b, Ger.*
**e+b, Ger.** e+b GmbH & Co. Pharma KG, Emil-Kemmer-Str. 33, 96103 Hallstadt, Germany.
**Eberth, Ger.** Dr. Friedrich Eberth Arzneimittel, Hohenburger Str. 39, 92289 Ursensollen, Germany.
**Eberth, Switz.** See *Uhlmann-Eyraud, Switz.*
**Ebewe, Austria.** Ebewe Pharma GmbH Nfg KG, Mondseestrasse 11, A-4866 Unterach am Attersee, Austria.
**Ebewe, Hong Kong.** See *Health Care, Hong Kong.*
**Ebewe, Thai.** See *Schumit, Thai.*
**Ebi, Switz.** Ebi-Pharm AG, Lindachstrasse 8c, 3038 Kirchlindach, Switzerland.
**Ebos, NZ.** Ebos Group Ltd, P.O. Box 302-161, North Harbour Postal Centre, Auckland, New Zealand.
**Echo, Ital.** Echo S.r.l., Via della Mattonaia 15, 50121 Florence, Italy.
**EciFarma, Chile.** EciFarma SA, Carmen Covarrubias 271, Nunoa, Santiago, Chile.
**Eco, S.Afr.** Eco Pharmaceuticals (Pty) Ltd, South Africa.
**Ecobi, Ital.** Farmaceutici Ecobi s.a.s., Via E. Bazzano 26, 16019 Ronco Scrivia (GE), Italy.
**Ecobrands, UK.** Ecobrands Ltd, 3 Adam & Eve Mews, London, W8 6UG, UK.
**Ecofarm, Ital.** Ecofarm Group Srl, Via F Vezzani 99/r, 16159 Genoa Rivarolo, Italy.
**Ecolab, Ger.** Ecolab Deutschland GmbH, Reisholzer Werftstr. 38-42, 40589 Dusseldorf, Germany.
**Econo Med, USA.** Econo Med Pharmaceuticals Inc., 4305 Sartin Rd, Burlington, NC 27217-7522, USA.
**Econolab, USA.** Econolab, P.O. Box 85543, Westland, MI 48185-0543, USA.
**Ecosol, Norw.** See *Andersen, Norw.*
**Ecosol, Switz.** Ecosol AG, Hohlstrasse 192, 8004 Zurich, Switzerland.
**ECR, Switz.** E.C. Robins Switzerland GmbH, Hinterbergstrasse 22, 6330 Cham, Switzerland.
**ECR, USA.** ECR Pharmaceuticals, P.O. Box 71600, Richmond, VA 23255, USA.
**Ecupharma, Ital.** Ecupharma S.r.l., Via Mazzini 20, 20123 Milan, Italy.
**Eczane, Arg.** Lab. Eczane Pharma S.A., Laprida 43, 1870 Avellaneda, Buenos Aires, Argentina.
**Eden, S.Afr.** See *Boots Healthcare, S.Afr.*
**Ederka, Mex.** Farmaceuticos Ederka S.A. de C.V., Calle 3 Num. 1, Fracc. Ind. Benito Juarez, 76130 Queretaro Qro, Mexico.

**Edigen, Spain.** Edigen, Ctra M-300 Km 29.92, Alcala de Henares, 28802 Madrid, Spain.
**Edmond Pharma, Ital.** Edmond Pharma S.r.l., Via dei Giovi 131, 20037 Paderno Dugnano (MI), Italy.
**Edochim, Ital.** Edochim S.r.l., Via Crescentino 31/A, 10154 Turin, Italy.
**Edol, Port.** Edol, SA, Av 25 de Abril 6-6A, Linda-a-Velha, 2795 Linda-a-Velha, Portugal.
**Edwards, Spain.** See *Baxter, Spain.*
**Edwards, USA.** Edwards Pharmaceuticals Inc., 111 Mulberry St, Ripley, MS 38663, USA.
**Efamol, Austral.** Efamol Ltd, P.O. Box 6745, Baulkham Hills BC, NSW 2153, Australia.
**Efamol, Canad.** Efamol Research Inc., Annapolis Valley Industrial Park, 15 Chipman Drive, P.O. Box 818, Kentville, Nova Scotia, B4N 4H8, Canada.
**Efamol, NZ.** See *Nutricia, NZ.*
**Efamol, UK.** Efamol Ltd, a Division of Nutricia, White Horse Business Park, Trowbridge, Wiltshire, BA14 0XQ, UK.
**Efarmes, Spain.** Efarmes, Sardenya 350, 08025 Barcelona, Spain.
**EF-EM-ES, Austria.** EF-EM-ES - Dr Smetana & Co., Scheidlstrasse 28, A-1180 Vienna, Austria.
**Effcon, USA.** Effcon Laboratories Inc., 1800 Sandy Plains Parkway, Marietta, GA 30066-7499, USA.
**Effik, Fr.** Laboratoires Effik, Burospace, 91571 Bievres cdx, France.
**Effik, Ital.** Effik Italia S.p.A., Via A Lincoln 7/a, 20092 Cinisello Balsamo (MI), Italy.
**Effik, Spain.** Effik, Antonio de Cabezon 27 5, Planta Ed Alfa Laval, 28034 Madrid, Spain.
**EG, Fr.** EG Labo (Laboratoire EuroGenerics), 12 rue Danjou, 92517 Boulogne-Billancourt cdx, France.
**EG, Ital.** EG S.p.A., Via Domenico Scarlatti 31, 20124 Milan, Italy.
**Egis, Hong Kong.** See *Mekim, Hong Kong.*
**EGIS, Hung.** EGIS Pharmaceuticals, Hungaria krt 179-187, 1146 Budapest, Hungary.
**Egis, Malaysia.** See *Pahang, Malaysia.*
**Egis, Singapore.** See *Sime Darby, Singapore.*
**Egis, Thai.** See *Medline, Thai.*
**Egis, UK.** Egis Pharmaceuticals Uk Ltd, 127 Shirland Rd, London, W9 2EP, UK.
**Ego, Austral.** Ego Pharmaceuticals P/L, 21-31 Malcolm Rd, Braeside, VIC 3195, Australia.
**Ego, Hong Kong.** See *Lision Hong, Hong Kong.*
**Ego, Malaysia.** See *Somedico, Malaysia.*
**Ego, NZ.** See *Douglas, NZ.*
**Ego, Singapore.** See *Grafton, Singapore.*
**EGS, Ger.** EGS Pharma Vertrieb, Schulstr. 38, 09125 Chemnitz, Germany.
**Ehlinger, Mex.** Ehlinger, Mexico.
**Ehrenhofer, Austria.** Dr. F. Ehrenhöfer GmbH, Triester Strasse 36, A-2620 Neunkirchen, Austria.
**Ehrmann, Austria.** Ehrmann Mag. pharm. Liselotte GmbH, Obertrumer Landstr. 7, A-5201 Seekirchen, Austria.
**Eifelfango, Ger.** Eifelfango GmbH & Co. KG, Ringener Str. 45, 53474 Bad Neuenahr-Ahrweiler, Germany.
**Eifelfango, Switz.** See *Agpharm, Switz.*
**Eight, Spain.** Eight Farmaceutica, Camino de Las Lenguas S/N, 28021 Madrid, Spain.
**Eiken, Jpn.** Eiken Chemical Co. Ltd, 5-26-20 Oji, Kita-ku, Tokyo 114-0002, Japan.
**Eisai, Fr.** Laboratoires Eisai, tour Manhattan, La Defense 2, 5-6 place de l'Iris, 92095 Paris-La-Defense, France.
**Eisai, Ger.** Eisai GmbH, Lyoner Str. 14, 60528 Frankfurt, Germany.
**Eisai, Hong Kong.** Eisai (Hong Kong) Co. Ltd, Rm 2008, Fortress Tower, 250 King's Rd, North Point, Hong Kong.
**Eisai, Jpn.** Eisai Co. Ltd, 4-6-10 Koishikawa, Bunkyo-ku, Tokyo 112-8088, Japan.
**Eisai, Malaysia.** Eisai (M) Sdn Bhd, 74 Jln Universiti, 46200 Petaling Jaya, Selangor, Malaysia.
**Eisai, Singapore.** Eisai Asia Regional Services Pte Ltd, 152 Beach Road, 11-04 Gateway East, S 189721, Singapore.
**Eisai, Thai.** Eisai (Thailand) Marketing Co. Ltd, 6 Fl, Diethelm Tower A, 93/1 Wireless Rd, Bangkok 10330, Thailand.
**Eisai, UK.** Eisai Ltd, 3 Shortlands, Hammersmith, London, W6 8EE, UK.
**Eisai, USA.** Eisai Inc., 500 Frank W Burr Blvd, Teaneck, NJ 07666, USA.
**El Monje, Arg.** Lab. El Monje Negro, Av. Maipu 1680 20 "A", 1672 San Martin Villa Lynch, Buenos Aires, Argentina.
**Eladon, UK.** Eladon Ltd, 63 High St, Bangor, Gwynedd, LL57 1NT, UK.
**Elaiapharm, Switz.** See *Interdelta, Switz.*
**Elan, Canad.** See *Draxis, Canad.*
**Elan, Denm.** See *Ipsen, Denm.*, and *Wyeth Lederle, Denm.*
**Elan, Fr.** Elan Pharma, 2 esplanade Grand-Siecle, CP 916, 78009 Versailles cdx, France.
**Elan, Ger.** Elan Pharma GmbH, Rosenkavalierplatz 8, 81925 Munich, Germany.
**Elan, Irl.** Elan Pharma (Ireland) Ltd, Unit E, Glencormack Business Park, Kilmacanogue, Co. Wicklow, Ireland.
**Elan, Ital.** See *Segix, Ital.*
**Elan, Spain.** Elan Pharma, Avda Alcalde Barnils 70, Edif Onada, Sant Cugat Del Valles, 08190 Barcelona, Spain.
**Elan, UK.** Elan Pharma Ltd, Abel Smith House, Gunnels Wood Rd, Stevenage, Hertfordshire, SG1 2FG, UK.
**Elan, USA.** Elan Phamaceuticals, 7475 Lusk Blvd, San Diego, CA 92121, USA.
**Elanco, Spain.** See *Lilly, Spain.*
**Elbea, Ital.** Elbea Pharma S.r.l., Via Q Sella 4, 20121 Milan, Italy.
**Elder, UK.** Don Elder Products Ltd, Unit 15, Chiltonian Industrial Estate, 203 Manor Lane, London, SE12 0TX, UK.
**Elea, Arg.** Laboratorio Elea S.A.C.I.F.yA., Sanabria 2353 Piso 1, 1417 Buenos Aires, Argentina.
**Electramed, Irl.** Electramed Ltd, U2 Kinsealy Business Park, Kinsealy, Co. Dublin, Ireland.
**Elerte, Fr.** Laboratoires des Réalisations Thérapeutiques Elerté, 181-3 rue Andre-Karman, B.P. 101, 93303 Aubervilliers cdx, France.
**Elfar, Spain.** Elfar Drag, Guzman el Bueno, 133 Edif, Britannia, 28003 Madrid, Spain.
**Elhoim, Arg.** Elhoim S.R.L., Independencia 2809 Piso 6 Dto. A, 1225 Buenos Aires, Argentina.
**Elisium, Arg.** Elisium S.A., Bacacay 1739, 1406 Buenos Aires, Argentina.
**Elkins-Sinn, USA.** See *Wyeth-Ayerst, USA.*
**Elofar, Braz.** Laboratorio Farmaceutico Elofar Ltda, Rua Tereza Cristina 67, 88075-970 Florianopolis, SC, Brazil.
**Elpen (Ελπεν), Gr.** ΕΛΠΕΝ ΑΕ, 21ο χλμ. Λ. Μαραθώνος, 190 09 Πικέρμι, Pikermi, Greece.
**Elpen, Singapore.** See *Green Cross, Singapore.*
**Elvetium, Arg.** Elvetium S.A., Catulo Castillo 2437, 1261 Buenos Aires, Argentina.
**Embil, Singapore.** See *Pharmaforte, Singapore.*
**Emerging Pharma, Malaysia.** Emerging Pharma Sdn Bhd, Phileo Damansara II, Lot 3A03, Block B, No 15, Jln 16/11, Off Jln Damansara, 46350 Petaling Jaya, Selangor, Malaysia.
**Emerging Pharma, Singapore.** See *Sime Darby, Singapore.*
**Emilio, Spain.** Emilio Romero, Spain.
**Emonta, Austria.** Emonta Pharma GmbH, Weidelstrasse 21, A-1100 Vienna, Austria.
**EMS, Braz.** EMS Natures Plus Farmaceutica Ltda, Rodovia SP 101, Km 08, 13186-481 Hortolandia, SP, Brazil.
**Enapharm, Swed.** Enapharm AB, Box 30, 745 21 Enkoping, Sweden.
**Endo, Canad.** See *Bristol-Myers Squibb, Canad.*
**Endo, USA.** Endo Pharmaceuticals Inc., 223 Wilmington West Chester Pike, Chadds Ford, PA 19317, USA.
**Engelhard, Ger.** Engelhard Arzneimittel GmbH & Co. KG, Herzbergstr. 3, 61138 Niederdorfelden, Germany.
**Engelhard, Hong Kong.** See *Unico, Hong Kong.*
**Engelhard, Malaysia.** See *Sime Darby, Malaysia.*
**Engelhard, Singapore.** See *Sime Darby, Singapore.*
**Engelhard, Switz.** See *Pharmakos, Switz.*
**Engelshof, Austria.** Engelshof-Apotheke, Leystrasse 19-21, A-1200 Vienna, Austria.
**English Grains, UK.** English Grains Ltd, Swains Park Industrial Estate, Park Rd, Overseal, Burton-on-Trent, Staffordshire, UK.
**Enila, Braz.** Laboratorio Enila S.A., Rua Viuva Claudio 355, 20970-030 Rio de Janeiro, RJ, Brazil.
**Ensinger, Ger.** Ensinger Mineral-Heilquellen GmbH, Horrheimer Strasse 28-36, 71665 Vaihingen-Ensingen, Germany.
**Enteris, Fr.** Laboratoires Enteris, 22 rue Vaugelas, 75015 Paris, France.
**Enviroderm, USA.** EnviroDerm Pharmaceuticals Inc., P.O. Box 32370, Louisville, KY 40232-2370, USA.
**Enzifarma, Port.** Enzifarma, Lda, Taguspark, Parque de Ciencia e Tecnologia, Nucleo Central 184, 2780 Oeiras, Portugal.
**Enzimas, Arg.** Enzimas S.A., San Rafael 1950, 6700 Lujan, Buenos Aires, Argentina.
**Enzon, USA.** Enzon, Inc., 40 Kingsbridge Rd, Piscataway, NJ 08854, USA.
**Enzpharma, NZ.** Enzpharma Ltd, P.O. Box 8167, Symond St, Auckland, New Zealand.
**Enzypharm, Austria.** Enzypharm GmbH, Piaristengasse 29, A-1080 Vienna, Austria.
**Enzypharm, Neth.** Enzypharm BV, Industrieweg 17, 3762 EG Soest, Netherlands.
**Eon, USA.** Eon Labs Manufacturing Inc., 227-15 North Conduit Ave, Laurelton, NY 11413, USA.
**Epicaris, Arg.** Lab. Epicaris S.A., Av. Piedrabuena 4190, 1439 Buenos Aires, Argentina.
**Epiderm, UK.** Epiderm Ltd, Copthorne House, Mill Lane, Burgh on Bain, Market Rasen, LN8 6JZ, UK.
**Epifarma, Ital.** Epifarma s.a.s., Via San Rocco 6, 85033 Episcopia (PZ), Italy.
**Epsilon, Spain.** See *AstraZeneca, Spain.*
**Equilibre Attitude, Fr.** Laboratoires Equilibre Attitude, B.P. 289, 06227 Vallauris cdx, France.
**Equity, S.Afr.** Equity Pharmaceuticals (Pty) Ltd, 1 Petunia St, Bryanston 1600, South Africa.
**ERA, Denm.** ERA Medical ApS, Storeholm 25, 2670 Greve, Denmark.
**Ercopharm, Denm.** Ercopharm A/S, Boegeskovvej 9, 3490 Kvistgaard, Denmark.
**Ercopharm, Switz.** See *Orion, Switz.*
**Ercopharm, Thai.** See *Pacific, Thai.*
**Erfa, Belg.** Erfa S.A., Rue des Cultivateurs 25, 1040 Brussels, Belgium.
**Erfa, Canad.** Erfa Canada Inc., 4545 Sherbrooke St W, Westmont, Quebec, H3Z 1E8, Canada.
**Erfar, Gr.** ERFAR, Μικάς Ασίας 2, 153 44 Παλλήνη, Pallini, Greece.
**Ergha, Irl.** See *Helsinn Birex, Irl.*
**Erjean, Fr.** Laboratoires Erjean, 9 rue de Sebastopol, B.P. 867, 31015 Toulouse cdx 6, France.
**Ern, Spain.** Laboratorios Ern S.A., C/ Pedro IV 499, 08020 Barcelona, Spain.
**Ernest Jackson, UK.** Ernest Jackson & Co. Ltd, 29 High St, Crediton, Devon, EX17 3AP, UK.
**Erol, Swed.** Erol AB, Box 95, 274 22 Skurup, Sweden.
**Erredici, Ital.** Erredici, Italy.
**Errekappa, Ital.** Errekappa Euroterapici S.p.A., Via C. Menotti 1/A, 20129 Milan, Italy.
**Escaned, Spain.** Escaned, Tomas Breton 46, 28045 Madrid, Spain.
**Esfar, Port.** Laboratórios Esfar, SA, Rua da Escola de Medicina Veterinaria 15-17, 1049-029 Lisbon, Portugal.
**Eshcol, Singapore.** See *Summit, Singapore.*
**ESI, USA.** ESI Lederle Inc., PO Box 41502, Philadelphia, PA 19101, USA.
**Esme, Arg.** Lab. Esme S.A.C.I., Uriarte 1686, 1414 Buenos Aires, Argentina.
**Esoform, Ital.** Esoform S.p.A., Viale del Lavoro 10, 45100 Rovigo, Italy.
**ESP, USA.** ESP Pharma Inc., 2035 Lincoln Highway, Suite 2150, Edison, NJ 08817, USA.
**Esparma, Ger.** esparma GmbH, Lange Gohren 3, 39171 Osterweddingen, Germany.
**Espe, Austria.** Espe HandelsGmbH, Marokkanergasse 9/8, A-1030 Vienna, Austria.
**Espe, Ger.** See *3M Espe, Ger.*
**Espe, Ital.** Espe Italia S.r.l., Via C Cantu 29, 20092 Cinisello Balsamo (MI), Italy.
**Espe, Switz.** Espe AG, Baumackerstrasse 46, Postfach 8360, 8050 Zurich, Switzerland.
**Esplanade, Austria.** Esplanade-Apotheke, Esplanade 18, A-4820 Bad Ischl, Austria.
**Esplanade, Fr.** Pharmaceutique de l'Esplanade, 34 route d'Ecully, B.P. 94, 69573 Dardilly cdx, France.
**Essential, NZ.** Simply Essential 2000 Ltd, 2 kamura St., Karitane, Otago, New Zealand.
**Esseti, Ital.** Esseti Farmaceutici S.p.A., Via Cavalli di Bronzo 41, 80046 S. Giorgio a Cremano (NA), Italy.
**Essex, Arg.** Lab. Essex S.A., Av. San Martin 1750, Florida, Buenos Aires, Argentina.
**Essex, Austral.** See *Schering-Plough, Austral.*
**Essex, Chile.** See *Schering-Plough, Chile.*
**Essex, Ger.** Essex Pharma GmbH, Thomas-Dehler-Str. 27, 81737 Munich, Germany.
**Essex, Ital.** Essex Italia S.p.A., Palazzo Borromini, 20090 Segrate (MI), Italy.
**Essex, Spain.** Farmaceutica Essex, Ctra Burgos Km 36, San Augustin De Guadalix, 28750 Madrid, Spain.
**Essex, Switz.** Essex Chemie AG, Postfach 2769, 6002 Lucerne, Switzerland.
**Essilor, Austria.** Essilor Austria GmbH, IZ NO Sud - Strasse 7/58c, A-2355 Wr. Neudorf, Austria.
**Estedi, Spain.** Estedi, Montseny 41, 08012 Barcelona, Spain.
**Estee Lauder, Canad.** Estee Lauder Cosmetics Ltd, 161 Commander Blvd, Agincourt, Ontario, M1S 3K9, Canada.
**Esteve, Port.** Esteve Farma Lda, Av do Forte 3, Edificio Suecia II, Piso 4 Ala A, 2795-504 Carnaxide, Portugal.
**Esteve, Spain.** Esteve, Avda Virgen Montserrat 221, 08041 Barcelona, Spain.
**Esteves Alves, Port.** José Esteves Alves, Lda, R. do Padrao 98, Apartado 464, 3002-906 Coimbra Codex, Portugal.
**Etajesa, Fr.** Etajesa, 14 av. Edouard-Vaillant, 93698 Pantin cdx, France.
**Etapharm, Austria.** Etapharm GmbH, Vormosergasse 3, 1190 Vienna, Austria.
**Etex, Chile.** Etex Farmaceutica Ltda, Av. Andres Bello 2687, Las Condes, Santiago, Chile.
**Ethex, Hong Kong.** See *Pan-Well, Hong Kong.*
**Ethex, USA.** Ethex Corp., 10888 Metro Court, St Louis, MO 63043-2413, USA.
**Ethical, Singapore.** See *Kyowa, Singapore.*
**Ethical Research, Irl.** See *Ethical Research, UK.*
**Ethical Research, UK.** Ethical Research Marketing, 3A Landgate, Rye, East Sussex, TN31 7LH, UK.
**Ethicals, Denm.** See *Kemifarma, Denm.*
**Ethicare, Austral.** Ethicare Pharmaceuticals P/L, P.O. Box 316, Applecross, WA 6953, Australia.
**Ethicon, Fr.** Ethicon SAS, 1 rue Camille-Desmoulins, TSA 81002, 92787 Issy-les-Mouline-aux cdx 9, France.
**Ethicon, Ger.** Ethicon GmbH & Co. KG, a Johnson & Johnson Company, Robert-Koch-Str. 1, 22851 Norderstedt, Germany.
**Ethicon, Ital.** Ethicon S.p.A., Via del Mare 56, 00040 Pratica di Mare Pomezia (Rome), Italy.
**Ethicon, UK.** Ethicon Ltd, P.O. Box 408, Bankhead Ave, Edinburgh, EH11 4HE, UK.
**Ethicus, Arg.** Lab. Ethicus, Argerich 687, 5501 Godoy Cruz, Mendoza, Argentina.
**Ethitek, USA.** Ethitek Pharmaceuticals Co., 7701 North Austin, Skokie, IL 60077, USA.
**Ethnor, India.** Ethnor Ltd, 30 Forjett St, Mumbai 400 036, India.
**Ethypharm, Austria.** See *Ethypharm, Fr.*
**Ethypharm, Denm.** See *Durascan, Denm.*
**Ethypharm, Fr.** Laboratoires Ethypharm SA, 194 bureaux de la Colline, 92213 St-Cloud, France.
**Ethypharm, Hong Kong.** See *Primal, Hong Kong.*
**Etris, Fr.** Etris, 14 rue de la Comète, 75007 Paris, France.
**Eu Rho, Ger.** Eu Rho Arznei GmbH, Kamen Karree 32-34, 59174 Kamen, Germany.
**Eucerin, Fr.** Laboratoires Dermatologiques Eucerin, 111 av. Victor-Hugo, 75116 Paris, France.
**Euderma, Ital.** Euderma S.p.A., Via Rigadara 27-29, 47852 Cerasolo di Coriano (FO), Italy.
**Euform, Fr.** Euform, 77 rue Marcel-Dassault, 92100 Boulogne, France.
**Eugal, Ital.** Laboratorio Chimico Farmaceutico Eugal S.r.l., Via Fabbriche 18, 15069 Serravalle Scrivia (AL), Italy.
**Eulactol, Austral.** Eulactol, Suite 3, 10 James St, Waterloo, NSW 2017, Australia.
**Eulactol, S.Afr.** Eulactol (Pty) Ltd, P.O. Box 3265, Randburg 2125, South Africa.
**Eumedica, Switz.** Eumedica Pharmaceuticals (Schweiz) AG, Peter Merian-Strasse 54, 4002 Basle, Switzerland.
**Euphar, Ital.** Euphar Group S.r.l., Via Gandine 4/6, 29100 Piacenza, Italy.
**Eurim, Ger.** Eurim-Pharm GmbH, Am Gänselehen 4-6, 83451 Piding, Germany.
**Euro Bio, Fr.** Euro. Bio. Serv., 1 mail des Catalpas, 78180 Montigny-le-Bretonneux, France.
**Eurocept, Neth.** Eurocept, Netherlands.
**Euroderm, Arg.** Euroderm laboratorios S.R.L., Emilio Mitre 1790/94, 1424 Buenos Aires, Argentina.
**Euroderm, Ital.** Euroderm S.r.l., V.le Italia 147, 19126 La Spezia, Italy.
**Euroderm-RDC, Ital.** Euroderm-RDC S.p.A., Via Enrico Fermi 50, 20019 Settimo Milanese (MI), Italy.
**Eurodrug, Hong Kong.** See *JDH, Hong Kong.*
**Eurodrug, Malaysia.** See *Apex, Malaysia.*
**Eurodrug, Singapore.** See *JDH, Singapore.*
**Eurodrug, Thai.** Eurodrug, 8B Fl, Ocean Tower 1, 170 New Ratchapisek Rd, Sukumvit 16 Klongtoey, Bangkok 10110, Thailand.
**Euroexim, Spain.** Euroexim, C/Emilio Munoz 15, 28037 Madrid, Spain.
**Eurofarma, Braz.** Eurofarma Laboratorios Ltda, Rua Barao do Triunfo 1440, 04602-005 Sao Paulo, SP, Brazil.
**Eurofarmaco, Ital.** Eurofarmaco S.r.l., Via Aurelia 58, 00166 Rome, Italy.
**Euro-Labor, Port.** See *Grunenthal, Port.*
**Euromed, Ital.** Euromed S.r.l., Via Napoli 101, Pianura, 80126 Naples, Italy.
**Euromedex, Fr.** Laboratoires Euromedex, 24 rue des Tuileries, B.P. 74684, Souffelweyersheim, 67458 Mundolschein cdx, France.
**Euromex, Mex.** Laboratorios Euromex S.A. de C.V., Unicornio No. 142, Col. Prado Churubusco, 04230 Mexico D.F., Mexico.
**Europharm, Austria.** Europharm, Jochen-Rindt-Strasse 23, A-1230 Vienna, Austria.
**Europharm, Hong Kong.** Europharm Laboratories Co. Ltd, 12-14 Dai Wang St, Tai Po Industrial Estate, Tai Po, N.T., Hong Kong.
**Euro-Pharma, Ital.** Euro-Pharma S.r.l., Via Filadelfia 126, 10137 Turin, Italy.
**Europharma, Spain.** See *Boehringer Ingelheim, Spain.*
**Europhta, Mon.** Laboratoires Europhta, Le Concorde, 11 rue du Gabian, MC 98000, Monaco.
**Eurospital, Ital.** Eurospital S.p.A., Via Flavia 122, 34147 Trieste, Italy.
**Eurosup, Ital.** Eurosup, Via Novara 4, 27030 Castello d'Agogna, Italy.
**Eurovita, Malaysia.** See *JDH, Malaysia.*
**Eurovita, Thai.** See *Diethelm, Thai.*
**Eutherapie, Belg.** Eutherapie Benelux S.A., Blvd International 57, 1070 Brussels, Belgium.
**Eutherapie, Fr.** Euthérapie, 27 rue du Pont, 92200 Neuilly-sur-Seine cdx, France.
**Evans, Fin.** See *Oriola, Fin.*
**Evans, Fr.** See *Celltech, Fr.*
**Evans, Irl.** See *Chiron Vaccines, UK.*
**Evans, Neth.** See *GlaxoSmithKline, Neth.*
**Evans, Norw.** See *Mericon, Norw.*
**Evans, Spain.** See *Celltech, Spain.*
**Evans Medical, Irl.** See *GlaxoSmithKline, Irl.*
**Evans Medical, Israel.** See *Mediline, Israel.*
**Everest, Canad.** Everest Pharmaceuticals Ltd, Canada.
**Everett, USA.** Everett Laboratories Inc., 29 Spring St, West Orange, NJ 07052, USA.
**Evers, Ger.** Pharmazeutische Fabrik Evers & Co. GmbH, Siemensstr. 4, 25421 Pinneberg, Germany.
**Evers, Hong Kong.** See *Pinneberg, Hong Kong.*
**Evers, Thai.** See *Sriprasit, Thai.*

**Eversil, Braz.** Eversil Produtos Farmaceuticos Industria e Comercio Ltda, Rua Agostinho Teixeira de Lima 344, 04826-230 Sao Paulo, SP, Brazil.

**Evisco, Ger.** Evisco-Pharma, Klosterplatz 6, 87509 Immenstadt, Germany.

**Excelentia, Arg.** Laboratorios Excelentia S.A., Santo Domingo 4088, 1437 Buenos Aires, Argentina.

**Exel, Belg.** Exel Pharma S.A., Chaussee de Gand 615, 1080 Brussels, Belgium.

**Exelgyn, Denm.** See *Exelgyn, Swed.*

**Exelgyn, Fin.** See *Exelgyn, Swed.*

**Exelgyn, Fr.** Exelgyn, 6 rue Christophe-Colomb, 75008 Paris, France.

**Exelgyn, Israel.** See *Lapidot, Israel.*

**Exelgyn, Norw.** See *Exelgyn, Swed.*

**Exelgyn, Spain.** See *Exelgyn, Fr.*

**Exelgyn, Swed.** Exelgyn, Box 1343, 181 25 Lidingo, Sweden.

**Exelgyn, UK.** Exelgyn Laboratories, P.O. Box 4511, Henley-on-Thames, Oxfordshire, RG9 5ZQ, UK.

**Exflora, Fr.** Laboratoires Exflora, 26 rue du Mont-Roti, 78550 Houdan, France.

**Exflora, Switz.** See *Uhlmann-Eyraud, Switz.*

**Expanpharm, Fr.** Laboratoires Expanpharm International, 60 rue Fessart, 92100 Boulogne, France.

**Expanpharm, Switz.** See *Uhlmann-Eyraud, Switz.*

**Expanscience, Fr.** Laboratoires Expanscience, 10 av. de l'Arche, 92400 Courbevoie, France.

**Expharma, Ital.** ExPharma S.r.l., Riviera Francia 3/A, 35127 Padua, Italy.

**Express Care, NZ.** Express Care Direct, New Zealand.

**Exterius, Ger.** Exterius Health Care GmbH, Robert-Koch-Str. 2, 51674 Wiehl, Germany.

**Extractum, Hung.** Extractum Pharma Rt, Foti St 56, 1047 Budapest, Hungary.

**Exxe, Ital.** Exxe Srl, Via Breda 120, 20126 Milan, Italy.

**E-Z-EM, Belg.** E-Z-EM Belgium S.A., Kiezelstraat 144, 3500 Hasselt, Belgium.

**E-Z-EM, Canad.** E-Z-EM Canada Inc., 11 065 L-H Lafontaine, Anjou, Quebec, H1J 2Z4, Canada.

**E-Z-EM, Israel.** See *Promedico, Israel.*

**E-Z-EM, Port.** See *Martins & Fernandes, Port.*

**E-Z-EM, UK.** E-Z-EM Ltd, 1230 High Rd, London, N20 0LH, UK.

**F5 Profas, Spain.** F5 Profas, Ed Indubuilding Goico, Via Los Poblados 17, 28033 Madrid, Spain.

**Fabop, Arg.** Lab. Fabop S.R.L., Av. Pueyrredsn 964, 2434 Arroyito, Cordoba, Argentina.

**Fabra, Arg.** Lab. Fabra S.R.L., Carlos Villate 5271, 1636 Olivos, Buenos Aires, Argentina.

**Fabrigen, Canad.** Fabrigen Inc., P.O. Box 507, Pierrefonds, Quebec, H9H 4M6, Canada.

**Face, Ital.** Face Laboratori Farmaceutici SpA, Via Albisola 49, 16163 Genova-Bolzaneto, Italy.

**Fada, Arg.** Fada Pharma S.A., Tabare 1641/9, 1437 Buenos Aires, Argentina.

**Fadim, Ital.** Fadim S.r.l., Via Milano 17, 20090 Cesano Boscone (MI), Italy.

**Faes, Spain.** Faes, Maximo Aguirre 14, Lejona, 48940 Vizcaya, Spain.

**Falk, Ger.** Dr. Falk Pharma GmbH, Leinenweberstr. 5, 79108 Freiburg, Germany.

**Falk, Hong Kong.** See *Jacobson, Hong Kong.*

**Falk, Malaysia.** See *JDH, Malaysia.*

**Falk, Neth.** See *Tramedico, Neth.*

**Falk, Norw.** See *Meda, Norw.*

**Falk, Port.** Dr. Falk Pharma Portugal Lda, Av. Jose Gomes Ferreira 11, Edificio Atlas II - 3 Piso, Sala 33, Miraflores, 1495-139 Alges, Portugal.

**Falk, Singapore.** See *JDH, Singapore.*

**Falk, Thai.** See *Zuellig, Thai.*

**Falqui, Ital.** Falqui Prodotti Farmaceutici S.p.A., Via Sabotino 19/2, 20135 Milan, Italy.

**FAMA, Ital.** F.A.M.A. Istituto Chimico Biologico S.r.l., Via A. Sauli 21, 20127 Milan, Italy.

**Family Planning Sales, UK.** Family Planning Sales Ltd, 28 Kelburne Rd, Cowley, Oxford, OX4 3SZ, UK.

**Fandasy, Hong Kong.** Fandasy Co. Ltd, Unit A, 18/F Federal Ctr, 77 Sheung On St, Chaiwan, Hong Kong.

**Fapromed, Arg.** Fapromed S.A., Gral. M.A. Rodrmguez 2830, 1416 Buenos Aires, Argentina.

**Far East, Singapore.** Far East Drug Co (Pte) Ltd, 1 Sophia Rd, 08-01 Peace Centre, S 228149, Singapore.

**Far East, Thai.** Far East Pharmaceutical Ltd Part, 92/1-2 Lanluang Rd, Bangkok 10100, Thailand.

**Faran, Gr.** ΦΑΡΑΝ ΑΒΕΕ, Αχαΐας & Τροιζηνίας, 145 64 Ν. Κηφισιά, N. Kiphisia, Greece.

**Farbo, Ital.** Farbo s.n.c. del dott. Donato Mele & C., Via Stelvio 12/18, 20021 Ospiate di Bollate (MI), Italy.

**Farco, Denm.** See *Tjellesen, Denm.*

**Farco, Ger.** Farco-Pharma GmbH Pharmazeutische Präparate, Mathias-Bruggen-Str. 82, 50829 Cologne, Germany.

**Farco, Hong Kong.** See *Sincerity, Hong Kong.*

**Farco, Irl.** See *Boileau & Boyd, Irl.*

**Farco, Israel.** See *CTS, Israel.*

**Farcoral, Mex.** Profesional Medica Farcoral S.A. de C.V., Circuito Norte No. 28, Unidad Guadalupe, 72560 Puebla, Pue., Mexico.

**Fardi, Spain.** Fardi, Grassot 16, 08025 Barcelona, Spain.

**Farex, Canad.** Laboratoire Farex Enrg, 5750 Metropolitan E Blvd, Bur 200, St-Leonard, Quebec, H1S 1A7, Canada.

**Fargim, Ital.** Far.g.im S.r.l., Via Cervignano 29, 95129 Catania, Italy.

**Fargin, Port.** See *Tecnifar, Port.*

**Faria, Braz.** Laboratorio Farmaceutico Faria Ltda, Rua Coronel Delfino Nonato de Faria 151, Sta Tereza, 36020-170 Juiz de Fora, MG, Brazil.

**Fariberica, Port.** Faribérica, SA, Estrada da Luz 90 - 9 D/E, 1600-160 Lisbon, Portugal.

**Farma Energy, Ital.** Farma Energy, Via Polia 36/38, 00178 Rome, Italy.

**Farma Lepori, Spain.** Farma Lepori, Osi 7-9, 08034 Barcelona, Spain.

**Farmabion, Spain.** See *Alter, Spain.*

**Farmabraz, Braz.** Farmabraz Beta Atalaia Farmaceutica Ltda, Rua Com. Joao C. de Almeida 36, 20770-100 Rio de Janeiro, RJ, Brazil.

**Farmacelsia, Spain.** Farmacelsia, A Ramallosa S/N, Santiago de Compostela, 15883 Coruna, Spain.

**Farmachimici, Ital.** Farmachimici S.r.l., Via Mercanti 36, 84121 Salerno, Italy.

**Farmaco, Mex.** Laboratorio de Productos Farmaceuticos y Biologicos Farmaco S.A., Jaime Nuno No. 112, Col. Guadalupe Inn, 01020 Mexico D.F., Mexico.

**Farmacologico Milanese, Ital.** Laboratorio Farmacologico Milanese S.r.l., Via Monterosso 273, 21042 Caronno Pertusella (VA), Italy.

**Farmacusi, Spain.** Farmacusi, Marina 16-18, Torre Mapfre 8 Planta, 08005 Barcelona, Spain.

**Farmades, Ital.** Farmades S.p.A., Via di Tor Cervara 282, 00155 Rome, Italy.

**Farmagan, Ital.** Farmagan S.A., Via Fosso del Canneto 34, 47891 Galazzano (Rep. San Marino), Italy.

**Farmaka, Ital.** Farmaka S.r.l., Via Vetreria 1, 22070 Grandate (CO), Italy.

**Farmalab, Braz.** Farmalab Industrias Quimicas e Farmaceuticas Ltda, Av. Brig. Faria Lima 1811, 12° andar, 01476-900 Sao Paulo, SP, Brazil.

**Farmalider, Spain.** Farmalider, C/ Aragoneses 9, Alcobendas, 28100 Madrid, Spain.

**Farmalight, Port.** Farmalight, Lda, Rua Padre Americo 18, Escritorio 1, 1600-548 Lisbon, Portugal.

**Farmaline, Thai.** Farmaline Co. Ltd, 48 Soi Urupong 1, Rama 6 Rd, Rajthevee, Bangkok 10400, Thailand.

**Farmanova, Ital.** Farmanova AFM S.r.l., Via Flaminia 287 Sc. A. int.10, 00196 Rome, Italy.

**Farmapros, Spain.** Farmapros, Aribau 180, 08036 Barcelona, Spain.

**Farmarekord, Ital.** Farmarekord S.r.l., Italy.

**Farmarin, Braz.** Farmarin Industria e Comercio Ltda, Brazil.

**Farmasa, Braz.** Laboratorio Americano de Farmacoterapia S/A, Rua Nova York 245, 04560-908 Sao Paulo, SP, Brazil.

**Farmasa, Mex.** Laboratorios Farmasa, S.A. de C.V., Bufalo No. 27, Col. del Valle, 03100 Mexico D.F., Mexico.

**Farmasan, Ger.** Farmasan Arzneimittel GmbH & Co., Pforzheimer Str. 5, 76227 Karlsruhe, Germany.

**Farmasan, Thai.** See *JDH Borneo, Thai.*

**Farmasierra, Spain.** Farmasierra, Ctra de Irun Km 26.2, San Sebastian de Los Reyes, 28100 Madrid, Spain.

**Farmasur, Spain.** Farmasur, Pol Store C/H 28-A, 41008 Seville, Spain.

**Farmatrading, Port.** Farmatrading, Lda, Travessa de Santa Catarina no 18, 1200-403 Lisbon, Portugal.

**Farmatre, Ital.** Farma 3 S.r.l., Via Solferino 42, 20036 Meda (MI), Italy.

**Farmavy, Braz.** Farmavy Industria Farmaceutica Ltda, Rua Vinte e Quatro de Maio 224/232, 20950-090 Rio de Janeiro, RJ, Brazil.

**Farmec, Ital.** Farmec S.n.c., Via W Flemming 7, 37026 Pescantina (VR), Italy.

**Farmed, Ital.** Farmed di Locatelli Ileano & C. S.a.s., Via C Colombo 82, 20036 Meda (MI), Italy.

**Farmedica, Braz.** Farmedica Industria Farmaceutica Ltda, Avenida Automovel Clube 1140, 25565-000 Joao de Meriti, RJ, Brazil.

**Farmetrusca, Ital.** Farmetrusca s.a.s. di C. Pini e C., Via G. di Vittorio, 50029 Tavarnuzze (FI), Italy.

**Farmigea, Ital.** Farmigea S.p.A., Via G.B. Oliva n. 8, 56121 Ospedaletto-Pisa, Italy.

**Farmila, Ital.** Farmila Farmaceutici Milano S.p.A., Via E. Fermi 50, 20019 Settimo Milanese (MI), Italy.

**Farminova, Port.** See *Pfizer, Port.*

**Farminvest, Ital.** Farminvest S.p.A., Strada Vicinale dei Moretti, 10090 Ivrea (TO), Italy.

**Farmion, Braz.** Farmion Laboratorio Brasileiro de Farmacologia Ltda, Avenida Celso dos Santos 579, 04658-240 Sao Paulo, SP, Brazil.

**Farmitalia Carlo Erba, UK.** See *Pharmacia, UK.*

**Farmoquimica, Braz.** Farmoquimica S.A., Av. Luis Carlos Prestes 410, 22775-030 Rio de Janeiro, RJ, Brazil.

**Farmorcore, Port.** Laboratórios Farmorcore, SA, Quinta da Francelha de Cima, 2685 Prior-Velho, Portugal.

**Farmoterapia, Arg.** Farmoterapia Internacional S.R.L., Alvear 231 Piso 1 of.1, 1640 Martinez, Buenos Aires, Argentina.

**Faro, USA.** Faro Pharmaceuticals Inc., 10607 Haddington 150, Houston, TX 77043, USA.

**Faromed, Austria.** Faromed GmbH, Johann Straussgasse 7/5, A-1040 Vienna, Austria.

**Fascino, Thai.** Fascino Pharmacy Groups, 99 Moo 2 Tumbon Bangtoey, Aumpeur Sampharn, Nakornphathom 73210, Thailand.

**Fate, UK.** Fate Special Foods, Unit E2, Brook Street Business Centre, Brook Street, Tipton, West Midlands, DY4 9DD, UK.

**Fater, Ital.** Fater S.p.A., Via Italica 101, 65127 Pescara, Italy.

**Fatol, Austria.** See *Fatol, Ger.*

**Fatol, Ger.** Fatol Arzneimittel GmbH, Robert-Koch-Str., 66578 Schiffweiler, Germany.

**Fatol, Hong Kong.** See *Mekim, Hong Kong.*

**Faulding, Austral.** See *Mayne, Austral.*

**Faulding, Denm.** See *Baxter, Denm.*

**Faulding, Hong Kong.** See *Mayne, Hong Kong.*

**Faulding, Israel.** See *Tzamal, Israel.*

**Faulding, Malaysia.** Faulding Pharmaceuticals (M) Sdn Bdh, Suite 201, 1st Floor, Wisma Glomac 3, Kompleks Kelana Centre Point, Jln SS 7/19, 47301 Petaling Jaya, Selangor, Malaysia.

**Faulding, NZ.** Faulding Pharmaceuticals (NZ) Ltd, P.O. Box 33-1668, Takapuna, Auckland, New Zealand.

**Faulding, Port.** Faulding Famacêutica, Lda, Rua Amilia Rodrigues, lote 4, 2750-228 Cascais, Portugal.

**Faulding, Singapore.** Faulding Pharmaceuticals, 70 Bendemeer Rd, 04-02 Hiap Huat House, S 339940, Singapore.

**Faulding, Thai.** See *Indochina Healthcare, Thai.*

**Faulding, USA.** Faulding USA, 650 From Rd, Mack-Cali Centre II, 5th Floor South, Paramus, NJ 07652, USA.

**Faulding Consumer, Austral.** See *Mayne, Austral.*

**Fawns & McAllan, Austral.** See *Sigma, Austral.*

**Fawns & McAllan, Hong Kong.** See *LCH, Hong Kong.*

**FD, Ital.** FD Farmaceutici S.r.l., Via Castello 15, 29019 San Giorgio Piacentino (PC), Italy.

**FDC, India.** FDC Ltd, 142-48 S.V. Rd, Jogeshwari (West), Mumbai 400 102, India.

**Febena, Ger.** Febena GmbH, Oskar-Jager-Str. 115, 50825 Cologne, Germany.

**Fecofar, Arg.** Fed. Arg. de Coop. Farm., Av. Pte. Peron 2742, 1754 San Justo, Buenos Aires, Argentina.

**Federfarma, Ital.** FederFARMA.CO SpA, Via Mecenate 90, 20138 Milan, Italy.

**Feldhoff, Ger.** W. Feldhoff & Comp. Arzneimittel GmbH, Hans-C.-Virz-Str. 2, 99867 Gotha, Germany.

**Felgentrager, Ger.** Dr. Felgenträger & Co. Öko-chem. und Pharma GmbH, Zerbster Str. 7a, 06862 Rodleben, Germany.

**Felo, Denm.** Felo ApS, Fensmarkvej 118, 4700 Naestved, Denmark.

**Felton, Austral.** Felton, Grimwade & Bickford P/L, P.O. Box 74, Oakleigh South, VIC 3167, Australia.

**Femagen, Austria.** Femagen Arzneimittel GmbH, Guntherstrasse 11, 1150 Vienna, Austria.

**Fenton, UK.** Fenton Pharmaceuticals Ltd, 4J Portman Mansions, Chiltern St, London, W1M 1LF, UK.

**Ferlito, Ital.** Ferlito Farmaceutici, Divisione Palmares S.p.A., Via E Ramarini 31-33, 00016 Monterotondo Scalo (RM), Italy.

**Ferlux, Fr.** Ferlux SA, 24 av. d'Aubiere, B.P. 151, 63804 Cournon d'Auvergne cdx, France.

**Fermentaciones y Sintesis, Spain.** Fermentaciones y Sintesis, Castellon 23, 28001 Madrid, Spain.

**Fermenti, Ital.** Istituto Italiano Fermenti S.p.A., Via B Quaranta 42, 20139 Milan, Italy.

**Ferndale, UK.** Ferndale Pharmaceuticals Ltd, Unit 605, Thorp Arch Estate, Wetherby, West Yorkshire, LS23 7BJ, UK.

**Ferndale, USA.** Ferndale Laboratories Inc., 780 West Eight Mile Rd, Ferndale, MI 48220, USA.

**Ferraton, Denm.** Ferraton Farmaceutisk Fabrik A/S, Kirkevejen 20, Teestrup, 4690 Haslev, Denmark.

**Ferraz, Lynce, Port.** Ferraz, Lynce, SA, Rua Consiglieri Pedroso 123, Queluz de Baixo, 2745-557 Barcarena, Portugal.

**Ferrer, Malaysia.** See *Wellmex, Malaysia.*

**Ferrer, Singapore.** See *Pharmacon, Singapore.*

**Ferrer, Spain.** Ferrer Farma, Gran Via Carlos III 94, 08028 Barcelona, Spain.

**Ferrier, Fr.** See *Arkopharma, Fr.*

**Ferring, Arg.** Ferring S.A., Venezuela 174, 1095 Buenos Aires, Argentina.

**Ferring, Austral.** Ferring Pharmaceuticals P/L, Suite 2B, Level 2, 802 Pacific Highway, Gordon, NSW 2072, Australia.

**Ferring, Austria.** Ferring Arzneimittel GmbH, Wienerbergstrasse 11, A-1100 Vienna, Austria.

**Ferring, Belg.** Ferring S.A., Hopmarkt 9 bus 3, 9300 Aalst, Belgium.

**Ferring, Braz.** Laboratorios Ferring Ltd, PCA Sao Marcos 624 1-andar, Vila Ida, 05455-050 Sao Paulo SP, Brazil.

**Ferring, Canad.** Ferring Inc., 200 Yorkland Blvd, Suite 800, Toronto, Ontario, M2J 5C1, Canada.

**Ferring, Chile.** See *Recalcine, Chile.*

**Ferring, Denm.** Ferring Laegemidler A/S, Kay Fiskers Plads 11, 2300 Copenhagen S, Denmark.

**Ferring, Fin.** Ferringlääkkeet Oy, Tähdenlennonkuja 1, PL 23, 02241 Espoo, Finland.

**Ferring, Fr.** Laboratoires Ferring SAS, 7 rue Jean-Baptiste-Clement, 94250 Gentilly, France.

**Ferring, Ger.** Ferring Arzneimittel GmbH, Wittland 11, 24109 Kiel, Germany.

**Ferring, Hong Kong.** Ferring Pharmaceuticals Ltd, Unit A, 9/F Garment Ctr, 576-586 Castle Peak Rd, Kowloon, Hong Kong.

**Ferring, India.** Ferring Pharmaceuticals Pvt Ltd, 403/404 Sigma, 4th Floor, Technology St, Central Ave, Hiranandani Gardens, Powai, Mumbai 400 076, India.

**Ferring, Irl.** See *United Drug, Irl.*

**Ferring, Israel.** See *Lapidot, Israel.*

**Ferring, Ital.** Ferring S.r.l., Via Senigallia 18/2, 20161 Milan, Italy.

**Ferring, Malaysia.** See *United Italian, Malaysia.*

**Ferring, Neth.** Ferring BV, Postbus 184, 2130 AD Hoofddorp, Netherlands.

**Ferring, Norw.** Ferring Legemidler AS, Postboks 4445 Torshov, 0403 Oslo, Norway.

**Ferring, NZ.** See *Pharmaco, NZ.*

**Ferring, Port.** Ferring Portuguesa, Lda, Rua Professor Henrique de Barros, Edificio Sagres, 8 - Sala A, 2685-338 Prior Velho, Portugal.

**Ferring, S.Afr.** Ferring (Pty) Ltd, P.O. Box 14358, Clubview 0014, South Africa.

**Ferring, Singapore.** See *United Italian, Singapore.*

**Ferring, Spain.** Ferring, Saturno 1, Edificio Saturno, Pozuelo de Alarcon, 28224 Madrid, Spain.

**Ferring, Swed.** Ferring AB, Box 30063, 200 61 Limhamn, Sweden.

**Ferring, Switz.** Ferring SA, Industriestrasse 50a, 8304 Wallisellen, Switzerland.

**Ferring, Thai.** See *Pacific, Thai.*

**Ferring, UK.** Ferring Pharmaceuticals UK, The Courtyard, Waterside Drive, Langley, Berkshire, SL3 6EZ, UK.

**Ferring, USA.** Ferring Pharmaceuticals Inc., 120 White Plains Rd, Suite 400, Tarrytown, NY 10591, USA.

**Ferro, Arg.** Lab. Ferro, Av. Mate de Luna 4333, 4000 S.M. de Tucuman, Tucuman, Argentina.

**Ferrosan, Denm.** Ferrosan A/S, Sydmarken 1-5, 2860 Sborg, Denmark.

**Ferrosan, Fin.** Oy Ferrosan AB, Kutojantie 11, 02630 Espoo, Finland.

**Ferrosan, Swed.** Ferrosan AB, Kungsgatan 23, 561 31 Huskvarna, Sweden.

**Fertin, Denm.** See *Meda, Denm.*

**Fertin, Norw.** See *Meda, Norw.*

**FertiPro, Irl.** See *Electramed, Irl.*

**Fher, Ital.** Fher, Divisione della Boehringer Ingelheim, Casella Postale, 50100 Florence, Italy.

**Fher, Spain.** See *Boehringer Ingelheim, Spain.*

**Fibertone, USA.** Fibertone Co., 14851 N Scottsdale Rd, Scottsdale, AZ 85254, USA.

**Fides, Ger.** See *FidesLine, Ger.*

**Fides, Spain.** See *Rottapharm, Spain.*

**Fides Ecopharma, Spain.** See *Rottapharm, Spain.*

**FidesLine, Ger.** FidesLine Biologische Heilmittel Heel GmbH, Dr.-Reckeweg-Str. 2-4, 76532 Baden-Baden, Germany.

**Fidex, Arg.** Prod. Farm. Fidex S.A., Gral. Savio Ruta 88 Km 9.5, 7601 Batan Mar del Plata, Buenos Aires, Argentina.

**Fidia, Hong Kong.** See *Hong Kong Medical, Hong Kong*, and *Chemedica, Hong Kong.*

**Fidia, Ital.** Fidia Farmaceutici S.p.A., Via Ponte della Fabbrica 3/A, 35031 Abano Terme (Padua), Italy.

**Fidia, Malaysia.** See *Somedico, Malaysia.*

**Fidia, Thai.** Fidia c/o Trans Bassan (Thailand) Ltd, 14 Fl, Q House Building, 66 Sukhumvit 21, Klongtoey, Bangkok 10110, Thailand.

**Fielding, USA.** Fielding Pharmaceutical Co., 2384 Centerline Ind. Dr., St Louis, MO 63146, USA.

**Filaxis, Arg.** Laboratorios Filaxis S.A., Panama 2121, 1640 Martinez, Buenos Aires, Argentina.

**Filorga, Fr.** Laboratoires Filorga, 18 rue de Miromesnil, 75008 Paris, France.

**Fimo, Ital.** F.I.M.O. S.r.l. Fabbrica Italiana Materiale Odontotecnico e Odontoiatrico, Via Edolo 40, 20125 Milan, Italy.

**Finadiet, Arg.** Finadiet S.A.C.I.F.I. Esp. Med., Hipolito Yrigoyen 3771, 1208 Buenos Aires, Argentina.

**Finderm, Ital.** Finderm Farmaceutici S.r.l. di Scaccia Fabbio e C., V.le Alcide De Gasperi 165, 95100 Catania, Italy.

**Fink, Ger.** See *GlaxoSmithKline Consumer, Ger.*

**Finmedical, Ital.** Finmedical S.r.l., Vicolo De Bacchettoni 1a, 51100 Pistoia, Italy.

**Finn Vita, Chile.** Laboratorio Finn Vita SA, Los Conquistadores 2178, Providencia, Santiago, Chile.

**Fiori, Ital.** Dr F & C Fiori S.n.c., Corso San Maurizio 35, 10124 Turin, Italy.
**FIRMA, Ital.** FIRMA-Fabbr. Ital. Ritrov. Medic. Aff. S.p.A., Via di Scandicci 37, 50143 Florence, Italy.
**First Horizon, USA.** First Horizon Pharmaceutical Corp., 6195 Shiloh Rd, Alpharetta, GA 30005, USA.
**Fischer, Israel.** Fischer Pharmaceuticals Ltd, P.O. Box 39071, Tel Aviv 61390, Israel.
**Fischer, USA.** Fischer Pharmaceuticals Inc., 7040 W Palmetto Park Rd 4, Suite 606, Boca Raton, FL 33433-3407, USA.
**Fisiopharma, Ital.** Fisiopharma S.r.l., Via Carnevali 116, 20158 Milan, Italy.
**Fiske, USA.** Fiske Industries, 527 Route 303, Orangeburg, NY 10962, USA.
**Fisons, Braz.** See *Aventis, Braz.*
**Fisons, Denm.** See *Aventis, Denm.*
**Fisons, Hong Kong.** See *Primal, Hong Kong.*
**Fisons, Irl.** See *Aventis, Irl.*
**Fisons, Israel.** See *Aventis, Israel.*
**Fisons, Singapore.** See *Aventis, Singapore.*
**Fisons, UK.** See *Aventis, UK.*
**Fisons, USA.** See *Celltech, USA.*
**Fitobucaneve, Ital.** Fitobucaneve S.r.l., Via Galvani 25/27, 20018 Sedriano (MI), Italy.
**Fitodorfarma, Ital.** Laboratorio Chimico Fitodorfarma S.a.s., Via Genova 28, 21052 Busto Arsizio (VA), Italy.
**Fitolife, Ital.** Laboratorio Fitolife S.r.l., Via Domiziana km 55, 80072 Arco Felice (NA), Italy.
**FL, Israel.** See *Neopharm, Israel.*
**Flanders, USA.** Flanders Inc., P.O. Box 39143, Northbridge Station, Charleston, SC 29407-9143, USA.
**FLAWA, Switz.** FLAWA Schweizer Verbandstoff- und Wattefabriken AG, Badstrasse 43, 9230 Flawil, Switzerland.
**Fleet, Austral.** C.B. Fleet Co. (Australia) P/L, P.O. Box 716, Braeside, VIC 3195, Australia.
**Fleet, Malaysia.** See *United Italian, Malaysia.*
**Fleet, NZ.** See *Baxter, NZ.*
**Fleet, Singapore.** See *JDH, Singapore.*
**Fleet, USA.** C.B. Fleet Co. Inc., 4615 Murray Pl., Lynchburg, VA 24506-1349, USA.
**Fleet-Dewitt, Hong Kong.** See *JDH, Hong Kong.*
**Fleming, USA.** Fleming & Co., 1733 Gilsinn Lane, Fenton, MO 63026-2918, USA.
**Flex-Power, USA.** Flex-Power, USA.
**Flopen, Braz.** Flopen, Brazil.
**Flora, Canad.** Flora Mfg & Dist. Ltd, 7400 Fraser Park Drive, Burnaby, BC, V5J 5B9, Canada.
**Florabio, Ger.** Florabio GmbH, Muhlstr. 5-7, 71106 Magstadt, Germany.
**Florafaun, Austral.** Florafaun P/L, P.O. Box 612, Balcatta, WA 6914, Australia.
**Flordis, Austral.** Flordis Pty Ltd, Level 2, 3 Carlingford Rd, Epping, NSW 2121, Australia.
**Florida, Arg.** Drogueria Florida S.R.L., Franklin D. Roosevelt 3430/2, 1430 Buenos Aires, Argentina.
**Floris, Israel.** Floris, Misgav 20179, Israel.
**Florizel, UK.** Florizel Ltd, P.O. Box 138, Stevenage, Hertfordshire, SG2 8YN, UK.
**Fluoritab, USA.** Fluoritab Corp., 8151 Brentwood Lane, Temperance, MI 48182-0507, USA.
**Flynn, Irl.** Flynn Pharma Ltd, Alton House, 4 Herbert St, Dublin 2, Ireland.
**Flynn, UK.** Flynn Pharma Ltd, 2nd Floor, The Maltings, Bridge St, Hitchin, Hertfordshire, SG5 2DE, UK.
**Fonten, Ital.** Fonten Farmaceutici S.r.l., Via dei Castelli Romani 22, 00040 Pomezia (RM), Italy.
**Fontovit, Braz.** Fontovit Laboratorios S.A., Rua Antonio das Chagas 862, 04714-001 Sao Paulo, Brazil.
**Food Supplement, UK.** Food Supplement Co. Ltd, Europa Park, Stoneclough Rd, Radcliffe, Manchester, M26 1GG, UK.
**Ford Medical, UK.** Ford Medical Associates Ltd, 2 Bridport Way, Braintree, Essex, CN7 9FJ, UK.
**Forder, Arg.** Forder Lab. Esp. Dermatologicas, Rivadavia 5747 Piso 5 Dto.A, 1406 Cdad., Buenos Aires, Argentina.
**Forest, Irl.** See *Forest Laboratories, UK.*
**Forest, Israel.** See *Pharmateam, Israel.*
**Forest Laboratories, UK.** Forest Laboratories Europe, Bourne Rd, Bexley, Kent, DA5 1NX, UK.
**Forest Laboratories, USA.** Forest Laboratories Inc., 909 Third Ave, New York, NY 10022, USA.
**Forest Pharmaceuticals, USA.** See *Forest Laboratories, USA.*
**Forley, UK.** Forley Ltd, 54 Hillbury Ave, Harrow, Middlesex, HA3 8EW, UK.
**Formenti, Ital.** Farmaceutici Formenti S.p.A., Via Correggio 43, 20149 Milan, Italy.
**Formula, NZ.** Formula Products, P.O. Box 36-443, Northcote, Auckland, New Zealand.
**Formulex, Israel.** See *Genmedix, Israel.*
**Fornet, Fr.** Laboratoires Fornet, 7/13 bd Paul-Emile-Victor, 92200 Neuilly-sur-Seine, France.
**Forster, Ger.** Dr Förster GmbH, Odenwaldstr. 15, 63263 Neu-Isenburg, Germany.
**Fortbenton, Arg.** Lab. Fortbenton Co. S.A., Escalada 133, 1407 Buenos Aires, Argentina.
**Forte, USA.** Forte Pharma, Laurelton, NY 11413, USA.
**Fortune, Hong Kong.** Fortune Pharmacal Co. Ltd, 14A/F Zung Fu Industrial Bldg, 1067 King's Rd, Hong Kong.
**Fouchard, Chile.** Laboratorio Fouchard SA, Monsenor Felix Cabrera 42, Of. 1, Providencia, Santiago, Chile.
**Fougera, USA.** E. Fougera Co., 60 Baylis Rd, Melville, NY 11747, USA.
**Fournier, Austria.** See *Fournier, Ger.*
**Fournier, Belg.** Fournier Pharma S.A., Rue des Trois Arbres 16b, 1180 Brussels, Belgium.
**Fournier, Canad.** Fournier Pharma Inc., 1010 Sherbrooke St W, 19th Floor, Montreal, Quebec, H3A 2R7, Canada.
**Fournier, Fr.** Laboratoires Fournier SA, 153 rue de Buzenval, 92380 Garches, France.
**Fournier, Ger.** Fournier Pharma GmbH, Justus-von-Liebig Str. 16, 66280 Sulzbach, Germany.
**Fournier, Gr.** FOURNIER (Γερολυματος), Γραντικού 7, 151 25 Μαρούσι, Marousi, Greece.
**Fournier, Hong Kong.** See *Wing Wai, Hong Kong,* and *Zuellig, Hong Kong.*
**Fournier, Irl.** Fournier Laboratories Ireland Ltd, Anngrove, Carrigtwohill, Co. Cork, Ireland.
**Fournier, Ital.** Fournier Farma S.p.A., Palazzo Caravaggio, Via Cassanese 224, 20090 Segrate (MI), Italy.
**Fournier, Malaysia.** See *Antah, Malaysia.*
**Fournier, Port.** Fournier Farmacêutica Portugal, Lda, Av Eng. Duarte Pacheco, Amoreiras, Torre 2 - 14B, 1070-103 Lisbon, Portugal.
**Fournier, Singapore.** See *Sime Darby, Singapore.*
**Fournier, Spain.** See *Fournier SA, Spain.*
**Fournier, Switz.** See *Searle, Switz.*
**Fournier, Thai.** See *Pacific, Thai.*
**Fournier, UK.** Fournier Pharmaceuticals Ltd, 19-20 Progress Business Centre, Whittle Parkway, Slough, Berkshire, SL1 6DQ, UK.
**Fournier SA, Spain.** Fournier SA, Ce Euronova 3, Rda Poniente 16, Tres Cantos, 28760 Madrid, Spain.
**Fox, UK.** C. H. Fox Ltd, 22 Tavistock St, London, WC2E 7PY, UK.
**FP, Singapore.** F.P. Marketing (S'Pore) Pte Ltd, 5 Pereira Rd, 04-03 Asiawide Industrial Building, S 368025, Singapore.
**Francia, Ital.** Francia Farmaceutici Industria Farmaco Biologica S.r.l., Via dei Pestagalli 7, 20138 Milan, Italy.
**Franco, Port.** See *Gestafarma, Port.*
**Franco-Indian, India.** Franco-Indian Pharmaceuticals Ltd, 20 Dr E Moses Rd, Mumbai 400 011, India.
**Franconpharm, Ger.** franconpharm Arzneimittel GmbH, Alexandrinenstr. 1, 96450 Coburg, Germany.
**Frandiet, Fr.** Frandiet SA, ZA des Savines, 101 rue Marc-Seguin, B.P. 315, 07503 Guilherand-Granges cdx, France.
**Frankin, Hong Kong.** Frankin Pharmaceutical Lab., 1/F, Block 1, Camelpaint Bldg, 60-62 Hoi Yuen Rd, Kwun Tong, Kowloon, Hong Kong.
**Frasca, Arg.** Frasca S.R.L., B. Blanca 1660, 1407 Buenos Aires, Argentina.
**Freda, Port.** Freda, SA, Quinta da Francelha de Cima, 2685 Prior Velho, Portugal.
**Freeda, USA.** Freeda Vitamins Inc., 36 E 41st St, New York, NY 10017-6203, USA.
**Frega, Canad.** See *Pharmalab, Canad.*
**Frere, Belg.** See *Arkopharma, Belg.*
**Fresenius, Belg.** See *Fresenius Kabi, Belg.*
**Fresenius, Braz.** See *Fresenius Kabi, Braz.*
**Fresenius, Fr.** See *Fresenius Kabi, Fr.*
**Fresenius, Ger.** See *Fresenius Kabi, Ger.*
**Fresenius, Hong Kong.** See *Fresenius Kabi, Hong Kong.*
**Fresenius, Israel.** See *Genmedix, Israel,* and *Promedico, Israel.*
**Fresenius, Switz.** See *Fresenius Kabi, Switz.*
**Fresenius, Thai.** See *Fresenius Kabi, Thai.*
**Fresenius Hemocare, Singapore.** See *Diethelm, Singapore.*
**Fresenius Kabi, Austria.** Fresenius Kabi Austria GmbH, Hafnerstrasse 36, A-8055 Graz, Austria.
**Fresenius Kabi, Belg.** Fresenius Kabi S.A., Molenberglei 7, 2627 Wilrijk, Belgium.
**Fresenius Kabi, Braz.** Fresenius Kabi Brazil Ltda, Rua Francisco Pereira Coutinho 347, 13088-100 Campinas, SP, Brazil.
**Fresenius Kabi, Denm.** Fresenius Kabi, Bredgade 71, 1260 Copenhagen K, Denmark.
**Fresenius Kabi, Fin.** Fresenius Kabi AB, Rajatorpantie 41 C, 01640 Vantaa, Finland.
**Fresenius Kabi, Fr.** Fresenius Kabi France, 5 place du Marivel, 92316 Sevres cdx, France.
**Fresenius Kabi, Ger.** Fresenius Kabi Deutschland GmbH, Else-Kroner-Str. 1, 61352 Bad Homburg v. d. H., Germany.
**Fresenius Kabi, Gr.** FRESENIUS-KABI, Μεσογείων 354, 153 41 Αγ. Παρασκευη, Ag. Paraskevi, Greece.
**Fresenius Kabi, Hong Kong.** Fresenius Kabi Hong Kong Ltd, Rm 5101-23, 51/F Sun Hung Kai Ctr, 30 Harbour Rd, Wanchai, Hong Kong.
**Fresenius Kabi, Irl.** Fresenius Kabi, Main St, Rush, Co. Dublin, Ireland.
**Fresenius Kabi, Ital.** Fresenius Kabi Italia S.p.A., Via Camagre 41, 37063 Isola della Scala (VR), Italy.
**Fresenius Kabi, Malaysia.** See *Antah, Malaysia.*
**Fresenius Kabi, Mex.** Laboratorios Frenesius Kabi Mexico S.A. de C.V., Av. Heroes Ferrocarrileros 1325, Sector Reforma, 44440 Guadalajara, Jalisco, Mexico.
**Fresenius Kabi, Neth.** Fresenius Kabi, Netherlands.
**Fresenius Kabi, Norw.** Fresenius Kabi Norge AS, Markedsavd., Gjerdrumsv. 12, 0486 Oslo, Norway.
**Fresenius Kabi, NZ.** See *Baxter, NZ.*
**Fresenius Kabi, Port.** Fresenius Kabi Pharma Portugal, Lda, Avenida do Forte 3, Edificio Suecia III, 2795-504 Carnaxide, Portugal.
**Fresenius Kabi, S.Afr.** Fresenius Kabi, P.O. Box 4156, Halfway House, South Africa.
**Fresenius Kabi, Singapore.** See *Diethelm, Singapore.*
**Fresenius Kabi, Spain.** Fresenius Kabi España, Marina 16-18, Pl 17, Torre Mapfre-Villa Olimpica, 08005 Barcelona, Spain.
**Fresenius Kabi, Swed.** Fresenius Kabi, 751 74 Uppsala, Sweden.
**Fresenius Kabi, Switz.** Fresenius Kabi (Schweiz) AG, Spichermatt 30, 6371 Stans, Switzerland.
**Fresenius Kabi, Thai.** Fresenius Kabi Thailand Ltd, The Millennia Building, 2403-4, 24th Floor, 62 Lungsuan Road, Lumpini, Patumwan, Bangkok 10330, Thailand.
**Fresenius Kabi, UK.** Fresenius Kabi Ltd, Building A, Hampton Court, Tudor Rd, Manor Park, Runcorn, Cheshire, WA7 1UF, UK.
**Fresenius Medical, Austral.** Fresenius Medical Care Australia P/L, 305 Woodpark Rd, Smithfield, NSW 2164, Australia.
**Fresenius Medical, Austria.** See *Fresenius Kabi, Ger.*
**Fresenius Medical, Denm.** Fresenius Medical Care Danmark A/S, Herstedvang 14, 2620 Albertslund, Denmark.
**Fresenius Medical, Fin.** Fresenius Medical Care Soumi Oy, Vattuniemenranta 2, 00210 Helsinki, Finland.
**Fresenius Medical, Ger.** See *Fresenius Kabi, Ger.*
**Fresenius Medical, Port.** Fresenius Medical Care, Lda, Rua da Boaviagem 35, Lugar de Crestins, Moreira, 4470 MAIA, Portugal.
**Fresenius Medical, Spain.** Fresenius Medical Care, Ctra Vallderiolf Km 0.4, La Roca Del Valles, 08430 Barcelona, Spain.
**Fresenius Medical, Switz.** See *Fresenius Kabi, Switz.*
**Fresenius-Klinik, Ger.** See *Fresenius Kabi, Ger.*
**Fresenius-Praxis, Ger.** See *Fresenius Kabi, Ger.*
**Fresh Ones, Arg.** Distribuidora Fresh ones S.A., Las Heras 4857, 1603 Villa Martelli, Buenos Aires, Argentina.
**Friesland, Hong Kong.** See *Keller, Hong Kong.*
**Friesland, Malaysia.** See *Dutch Lady, Malaysia.*
**Friesland, Singapore.** See *Diethelm, Singapore.*
**Frosst, Austral.** See *Merck Sharp & Dohme, Austral.*
**Frosst, Canad.** See *Merck Frosst, Canad.*
**Frosst, Port.** See *Merck Sharp & Dohme, Port.*
**Frosst, Spain.** See *Merck Sharp & Dohme, Spain.*
**Fruit of the Earth, Canad.** Fruit of the Earth, 110 Iron St, Etobicoke, Ontario, M9W 5L9, Canada.
**Fuca, Fr.** Laboratoires Fuca, 1 bis, rue de Plaisance, 94732 Nogent-sur-Marne cdx, France.
**Fucus, Arg.** Laboratorio Farmaciutico Argentino S.A., Santiago del Estero 3117, 1640 Martinez, Buenos Aires, Argentina.
**Fuji, Jpn.** Fuji Chemical Industry Co Ltd, 55 Yokohoonji, Kamiichi-machi, Toyama-Pref. 930-0397, Japan.
**Fuji, Swed.** Fuji Film Sverige AB, Box 23086, 104 35 Stockholm, Sweden.
**Fujirebio, Jpn.** Fujirebio Inc., FR Bldg, 62-5 Nihonbashi-Hamacho 2-chome, Chuo-ku, Tokyo 103-0007, Japan.
**Fujisawa, Austria.** Fujisawa GmbH, Linzerstrasse 221/E0.2, A-1140 Vienna, Austria.
**Fujisawa, Belg.** Fujisawa Belgian Branch, Sint-Maartenstraat 12A, 3000 Leuven, Belgium.
**Fujisawa, Canad.** Fujisawa Canada Inc., 625 Cochrane Drive, Suite 800, Markham, Ontario, L3R 9R9, Canada.
**Fujisawa, Denm.** Fujisawa Scandinavia AB, Carlsbergvej 24, 3400 Hillerod, Denmark.
**Fujisawa, Fin.** Fujisawa, Laivalahdenkaari 34, 00810 Helsinki, Finland.
**Fujisawa, Fr.** Fujisawa, 13 rue Gabriel, 78170 La Celle-Saint-Cloud, France.
**Fujisawa, Ger.** Fujisawa Deutschland GmbH, Berg-am-Laim-Str. 129, 81673 Munich, Germany.
**Fujisawa, Hong Kong.** Fujisawa Hong Kong Ltd, Unit 1015, Tower 1, Grand Century Place, 193 Prince Edward Rd West, Mongkok, Kowloon, Hong Kong.
**Fujisawa, Irl.** Fujisawa Pharma, 25 The Courtyard, Kilcarberry Business Park, Clondalkin, Dublin 22, Ireland.
**Fujisawa, Israel.** See *Teva, Israel.*
**Fujisawa, Ital.** Fujisawa r.l., C.so di Porta Romana 68, 20122 Milan, Italy.
**Fujisawa, Jpn.** Fujisawa Pharmaceutical Co. Ltd, 4-7 Doshomachi 3-chome, Chuo-ku, Osaka 541-8514, Japan.
**Fujisawa, Norw.** See *Fujisawa, Swed.*
**Fujisawa, Port.** Fujisawa SA, Av. Duque de Avila 185 -7, 1050-082 Lisbon, Portugal.
**Fujisawa, Spain.** Fujisawa SA, Avenida Bruselas 20, Edificio Gorbea IV, 28108 Alcobendas (Madrid), Spain.
**Fujisawa, Swed.** Fujisawa Scandinavia AB, Haraldsgatan 5, 413 14 Gothenburg, Sweden.
**Fujisawa, Thai.** See *Berli, Thai.*
**Fujisawa, UK.** Fujisawa Ltd, Fujisawa House, 62 London Rd, Staines, Middlesex, TW18 4HN, UK.
**Fujisawa, USA.** Fujisawa Healthcare Inc., 3 Parkway North Center, Deerfield, IL 60015-2548, USA.
**Fulford, India.** Fulford (India) Ltd, Eureka Towers, Mindspace, Link Rd, Malad (West), Mumbai 400 064, India.
**Fulton, Ital.** Fulton Medicinali S.p.A., Via Marconi 28/9, 20020 Arese, Italy.
**Fumedica, Ger.** Fumedica GmbH, Industriestr. 40, 44628 Herne, Germany.
**Fumouze, Fr.** Laboratoires Fumouze, Le Malesherbes, 110-114 rue Victor-Hugo, 92303 Levallois-Perret cdx, France.
**Fumouze, Israel.** See *Naveh, Israel.*
**Fund a Paiva, Braz.** Fund a Paiva, Brazil.
**Fund Trip, Hong Kong.** Fund Trip Pharmaceutical Ltd, B1220 Focal Industrial Ctr, 21 Man Lok St, Hunghom, Kowloon, Hong Kong.
**Funk, Spain.** See *Almirall, Spain.*
**Furp, Braz.** Furp, Rua Endres 1800, 07043-902 Guarulhos, SP, Brazil.
**Fuso, Hong Kong.** See *Hing Ah, Hong Kong,* and *Primal, Hong Kong.*
**Fuso, Jpn.** Fuso Pharmaceutical Industries Ltd, 2-3-11 Morinomiya, Joto-ku, Osaka 536-8523, Japan.
**Fustery, Mex.** See *Ivax, Mex.*
**G & W, USA.** G & W Laboratories Inc., 111 Coolidge St, South Plainfield, NJ 07080, USA.
**G Gam, Fr.** Laboratoires G Gam, Europarc, 33 rue Auguste-Perret, 94042 Cretell cdx, France.
**GABA, Belg.** GABA BV, Grote Steenweg 224 B2, 2600 Berchem, Belgium.
**GABA, Fr.** Laboratoires GABA, 86 rue du Dome, 92514 Boulogne cdx, France.
**GABA, Ger.** GABA GmbH, Berner Weg 7, 79539 Lorrach, Germany.
**GABA, Neth.** GABA BV, Bolderweg 1, 1332 AX Almere, Netherlands.
**GABA, Switz.** GABA AG, Pharmazeutische und kosmetische Praparate, Grabetsmattweg, 4106 Therwil, Switzerland.
**Gador, Arg.** Gador S.A., Darwin 429, 1414 Buenos Aires, Argentina.
**Galactina, Switz.** Galactina AG, Birkenweg 1-8, 3123 Belp, Switzerland.
**Galactopharm, Ger.** Galactopharm Hans Sanders, Sudstr. 10, 49751 Sogel, Germany.
**Galagen, USA.** GalaGen Inc., P.O. Box 64313, St Paul, MN 55164-0314, USA.
**Galderma, Arg.** Galderma Argentina S.A., San Lorenzo 3887, 1636 Olivos, Buenos Aires, Argentina.
**Galderma, Austral.** Galderma Australia P/L, P.O. Box 502, Frenchs Forest, NSW 2086, Australia.
**Galderma, Belg.** Galderma Belgilux S.A., Fountain Business Centre Bornem, Gebouw 5, bus 205, Van Kerckhovenstraat 110, 2880 Bornem, Belgium.
**Galderma, Braz.** Galderma Brasil Ltda, Av. Nacoes Unidas, 18001, 6th Floor, Vila Almeida, 04795-100 Sao Paulo, SP, Brazil.
**Galderma, Canad.** Galderma Canada Inc., 7300 Warden Ave, Suite 210, Markham, Ontario, L3R 9Z6, Canada.
**Galderma, Chile.** Galderma Chile Laboratorios Ltda, Europa 2066, Providencia, Santiago, Chile.
**Galderma, Denm.** Galderma Svenska, c/o Regus House, Lars Bjornsstraede 3, 1454 Copenhagen K, Denmark.
**Galderma, Fin.** Galderma, Aleksanterinkatu 17, 00100 Helsinki, Finland.
**Galderma, Fr.** Laboratoires Galderma, Tour Europlaza, La Defense 4, 20 av. Andre-Prothin, 92927 La Defense cdx, France.
**Galderma, Ger.** Galderma Laboratorium GmbH, Munzinger Str. 5, 79111 Freiburg i. Br., Germany.
**Galderma, Hong Kong.** Galderma Hong Kong Ltd, Unit 1303, 13/F CRE Building, 303 Hennessy Rd, Wanchai, Hong Kong.
**Galderma, India.** Galderma (India) Pvt Ltd, 23 Steelmade Industrial Estate, 2nd Floor, Marol Village, Andheri (E), Mumbai 400 059, India.
**Galderma, Irl.** See *Intra Pharma, Irl.*
**Galderma, Israel.** See *Luxembourg, Israel.*
**Galderma, Ital.** Galderma Italia S.p.A., C. Dir. Coleoni Pal. Sirio 3, 20041 Agrate Brianza (MI), Italy.
**Galderma, Malaysia.** See *Summit, Malaysia.*
**Galderma, Mex.** Galderma Mexico S.A. de C.V., Jose Maria Ibarraran No. 20, Col. San Jose Insurgentes, Delegacion Benito Juarez, 03900 Mexico D.F., Mexico.
**Galderma, Neth.** Galderma S.A., Avelingen-West 5, 4202 MS Gorinchem, Netherlands.

**Galderma, Norw.** See *Galderma, Swed.*

**Galderma, NZ.** See *Pacific, NZ.*

**Galderma, Port.** Laboratorios Galderma, SA, Av Duque d'Avila 185, 1050-082 Lisbon, Portugal.

**Galderma, S.Afr.** Galderma Laboratories SA (Pty) Ltd, P.O. Box 71150, Bryanston 2021, South Africa.

**Galderma, Singapore.** See *Summit, Singapore.*

**Galderma, Spain.** Galderma, C/ Agustin de Foxa 29 - 6 pl, 28036 Madrid, Spain.

**Galderma, Swed.** Galderma Nordic AB, Box 15028, 167 15 Bromma, Sweden.

**Galderma, Switz.** Galderma SA, World Trade Center, Ave de Gratta-Paille 1, Casa Postale 453, 1000 Lausanne 30 Grey, Switzerland.

**Galderma, Thai.** See *US Summit, Thai.*

**Galderma, UK.** Galderma (UK) Ltd, Galderma House, Church Lane, Kings Langley, Hertfordshire, WD4 8JP, UK.

**Galderma, USA.** Galderma Laboratories Inc., 14501 North Freeway, Fort Worth, TX 76177, USA.

**Galen, Ger.** Galenpharma, GmbH, Wittland 13, 24109 Kiel, Germany.

**Galen, Irl.** See *Allphar, Irl.*

**Galen, Mex.** See *Probiomed, Mex.*

**Galen, UK.** Galen Ltd, Seagoe Industrial Estate, Craigavon, Northern Ireland, BT63 5UA, UK.

**Galen, USA.** Galen, USA.

**Galena, Thai.** See *SPB, Thai.*

**Galenica, Gr.** GALENICA A.E., Αχιλλέως 2, 104 37 Αθήνα, Athens, Greece.

**Galenica, Switz.** Galenica Vertretungen AG, Untermattweg 8, 3001 Berne, Switzerland.

**Galenika, Ger.** See *Hetterich, Ger.*

**Galenogal, Braz.** See *Hertz, Braz.*

**Galephar, Fr.** Laboratoires Galephar, ZI de Krafft, bat B, 67150 Erstein, France.

**Galephar, Switz.** Galéphar SA, rue de la Servette 20, 1201 Geneva, Switzerland.

**Galien, Arg.** Lab. Galien S.A., Roque Perez 2543, 1430 Buenos Aires, Argentina.

**Gallia, Braz.** Gallia Farmaceutica Ltda, Av. Montese 840, 31560-150 Belo Horizonte, MG, Brazil.

**Gallia, Fr.** Laboratoires Gallia, B.P. 432, 69654 Villefranche-sur-Saone cdx, France.

**Galpharm, UK.** GalPharm International Ltd, Hugh House, Galpharm Way, Upper Cliffe Rd, Dodworth Business Park, Dodworth, Barnsley, South Yorkshire, S75 3SP, UK.

**Galpharma, Israel.** See *Luxembourg, Israel.*

**Gambar, Ital.** Laboratori Gambar S.r.l., Via Bolognola 45, 00138 Rome, Italy.

**Gambro, Denm.** Gambro A/S, Jydekrogen 8, 2625 Vallensbaek, Denmark.

**Gambro, Fin.** Oy Gambro AB, Sahaajankatu 24, PL 30, 00811 Helsinki, Finland.

**Gambro, Israel.** See *Teva, Israel.*

**Gambro, Spain.** Gambro, Avda de la Industria 16, Coslada, 28820 Madrid, Spain.

**Gambro, Swed.** Gambro, Box 10101, 220 10 Lund, Sweden.

**Gambro, USA.** Gambro Inc., 80810 W Collins Ave, Lakewood, CO 80215, USA.

**Gamida-Medequip, Israel.** Gamida-Medequip Ltd, 54 Harei Yehuda St, Savyon 56530, Israel.

**Ganassini, Ital.** Istituto Ganassini S.p.A. di Ricerche Biochimiche, Via Gaggia 16, 20139 Milan, Italy.

**Gandhour, Fr.** Laboratoires Gandhour, 1 bis, rue de Plaisance, 94732 Nogent-sur-Marne cdx, France.

**Gap, Gr.** GAP A.E., Αγησιλάου 46, 173 41 Αγ. Δημήτριος, Ag. Dimitrios, Greece.

**GAR, Singapore.** See *Innomed, Singapore.*

**Garant, Ital.** Laboratorio Chimico Garant S.r.l., Via Melchiorre Gioia 47, 20124 Milan, Italy.

**Garden House, Arg.** Lab. Garden House S.A., Estomba 1058/60, 1427 Buenos Aires, Argentina.

**Garec, S.Afr.** Garec Pharmaceuticals, P.O. Box 1123, Halfway House 1685, South Africa.

**Garnier, UK.** Laboratoires Garnier, Golden Ltd, P.O. Box 5, Pontyclun, Glamorgan, CF7 8XW, UK.

**Gaschler, Ger.** Pharma-Laboratorium S.M. Gaschler GmbH, Oeschlanderweg 17a, 88131 Lindau, Germany.

**Gastroenterologicos, Mex.** Gastroenterologicos S.A. de C.V., Viena 56, Del Carmen Coyoacan, Deleg. Coyoacan, 04100 Mexico D.F., Mexico.

**Gastropharm, Ger.** Gastropharm GmbH Arzneimittel, Geiststr. 1, 37073 Gottingen, Germany.

**Gate, USA.** Gate Pharmaceuticals, 1090 Horsham Rd, North Wales, PA 19454.

**Gautier, Arg.** Lab. Gautier S.A. Argentina, Terrada 1270, 1416 Buenos Aires, Argentina.

**Gazzoni, Ital.** Gazzoni S.r.l., Via Ilio Barontini 16/20, 40138 Bologna, Italy.

**GD, Ital.** GD Tecnologie Interdisciplinari Farmaceutiche S.r.l., Via Augusto Gaudenzi 29, 00163 Rome, Italy.

**Gea, Denm.** A/S GEA, Holger Danskes Vej 89, 2000 Frederiksberg, Denmark.

**Gea, Fin.** Oy Gea AB, Rajatorpantie 41, 01640 Vantaa, Finland.

**Gea, Norw.** GEA Farmaceutisk Fabrik AS, Stortorvet 10, 0155 Oslo, Norway.

**Gea, Swed.** GEA Farmaceutisk Fabrik AB, Berga Alle 1 E, 254 52 Helsingborg, Sweden.

**Gea, Switz.** See *Ecosol, Switz.*

**Gebauer, Canad.** See *Gebauer, USA.*

**Gebauer, Hong Kong.** See *Vantone, Hong Kong.*

**Gebauer, USA.** Gebauer Co., 9410 St Catherine Ave, Cleveland, OH 44104, USA.

**Gebro, Austria.** Gebro Pharma GmbH, A-6391 Fieberbrunn, Austria.

**Gebro, Spain.** Gebro Pharma, C/ Monestir 23, 08034 Barcelona, Spain.

**Gebro, Switz.** Gebro Pharma SA, Oristalstrasse 87a, 4410 Liestal, Switzerland.

**Gedeon Richter, Hong Kong.** See *Mekim, Hong Kong.*

**Gedeon Richter, Israel.** See *Trima, Israel.*

**Gedeon Richter, Malaysia.** See *Pahang, Malaysia.*

**Gedeon Richter, Singapore.** See *Sime Darby, Singapore.*

**Gedeon Richter, Thai.** See *Medline, Thai.*

**Gedis, Ital.** Gedis S.r.l., Via Vezzolano 15, 10153 Turin, Italy.

**Geigy, Ger.** See *Novartis, Ger.*

**Geigy, Switz.** See *Novartis, Switz.*, and *Novartis Consumer, Switz.*

**Geigy, USA.** See *Novartis, USA.*

**Geistlich, Irl.** Geistlich Pharma, 36 Lower Stephen Street, Dublin 2, Ireland.

**Geistlich, Singapore.** See *Diethelm, Singapore.*

**Geistlich, Switz.** Geistlich-Pharma AG, 6110 Wolhusen, Switzerland.

**Geistlich, UK.** Geistlich Pharma, Newton Bank, Long Lane, Chester, Cheshire, CH2 3PF, UK.

**Gelos, Spain.** Gelos, Joan XXIII 10, Esplugues de Llobregat, 08950 Barcelona, Spain.

**Gemardi, Thai.** See *Diethelm, Thai.*

**Gemballa, Braz.** Laboratorio Gemballa Ltda, Avenida Sete de Setembro 50, 89160-000 Rio do Sul, SC, Brazil.

**Gemelli, Denm.** Gemelli A/S, Nybrovej 110, 2800 Lyngby, Denmark.

**Gemepe, Arg.** Lab. GeMePe S.A., Jovellanos 886, 1267 Buenos Aires, Argentina.

**Geminis, Arg.** Géminis S.A., Flora 582, 1706 Haedo, Buenos Aires, Argentina.

**Geminis, Spain.** Geminis, Gran Via de las Corts, Catalanes 764, 08013 Barcelona, Spain.

**GenDerm, Canad.** See *Medicis, Canad.*

**GenDerm, USA.** See *Medicis, USA.*

**Genentech, USA.** Genentech Inc., 1 DNA Way, South San Francisco, CA 94080-4990, USA.

**Genepharm, Gr.** GENEPHARM A.E., 18ο χλμ. Λ. Μαραθώνος 153 51 Παλλήνη, Pallini, Greece.

**Genera, Switz.** Genera Pharma AG, Hilariweg 9, Postfach, 4501 Solothurn, Switzerland.

**General Dietary, UK.** General Dietary Ltd, P.O. Box 38, Kingston-upon-Thames, Surrey, KT2 7YP, UK.

**General Drugs, Thai.** General Drugs House Co. Ltd, 2-4 Soi Lard Prao 82, Bangkok 10310, Thailand.

**General Nutrition, Canad.** See *General Nutrition, USA.*

**General Nutrition, USA.** General Nutrition Inc., 300 6th Ave, Pittsburgh, PA 15222, USA.

**General Topics, Ital.** General Topics S.r.l., Localita Santigaro 32, 25010 S. Felice D/B (BS), Italy.

**Generfarma, Spain.** Generfarma, Los Centelles 7, 46006 Valencia, Spain.

**Genericon, Austria.** Genericon Pharma GmbH, Schlossplatz 1, A-8502 Lannach, Austria.

**Generics, Denm.** See *NM, Denm.*

**Generics, Israel.** See *Genmedix, Israel.*

**Generics, UK.** Generics (UK) Ltd, Albany Gate, Drakes Lane, Potters Bar, Hertfordshire, EN6 1AG, UK.

**Genesis, Gr.** GENESIS PHARMA AE, Φιλελλήνων 24, 152 32 Χαλάνδρι, Chalandri, Greece.

**Genesoft, USA.** Genesoft, USA.

**Genetics, Gr.** Genetics, Greece.

**Genetics Institute, Austria.** See *Baxter Bioscience, Ger.*

**Genetics Institute, Denm.** See *Baxter, Denm.*, *Pharmacia, Denm.*, and *Wyeth Lederle, Denm.*

**Genetics Institute, Switz.** See *AHP, Switz.*

**Genetics Institute, USA.** Genetics Institute, 35 Cambridge Park Drive, Cambridge, MA 02140, USA.

**Geneva, USA.** Geneva Pharmaceuticals, 506 Carnegie Center, Suite 400, Princeton, NJ 08540-6243, USA.

**Genevrier, Fr.** Laboratoires Génévrier, B.P. 47, 06901 Sophia Antipolis cdx, France.

**Genevrier, Singapore.** See *PMR, Singapore.*

**Geni, Spain.** Geni, Santa Susana 5, 28033 Madrid, Spain.

**Genmedix, Israel.** Genmedix Ltd, P.O. Box 8500, New Industrial Zone, Netanya, Israel.

**Geno, India.** Geno Pharmaceuticals Ltd, Pharmaceutical Complex, Karaswada, Mapusa, Goa 403 507, India.

**Genom, Braz.** Genom Farmaceutica Ltda, Av. Ceci 820, 06460-120 Barueri, SP, Brazil.

**Genop, S.Afr.** Genop Healthcare (Pty) Ltd, P.O. Box 3911, Halfway House 1685, South Africa.

**Genopharm, Fr.** Laboratoires Genopharm, Parc de l'Esplanade, 10 rue Enrico-Fermi, Saint-Thibault-des-Vignes, 77462 Lagny-sur-Marne cdx, France.

**Genove, Spain.** Genove, Feixa Llarga 105, L'hospitalet de Llobregat, 08902 Barcelona, Spain.

**Genpharm, Austral.** GenPharm Australia, 182 Alison Rd, Carrara, QLD 4211, Australia.

**Genpharm, Canad.** Genpharm Inc., 37 Advance Rd, Etobicoke, Ontario, M8Z 2S6, Canada.

**Genpharm, Israel.** See *Genmedix, Israel.*

**Genpharm, S.Afr.** Genpharm Pharmaceuticals CC, P.O. Box 607, Rivonia 2128, South Africa.

**Genpharm, USA.** Genpharm, USA.

**Genser, Arg.** Alimentos Genser S.A., Cucha Cucha 2542/48, 1416 Buenos Aires, Argentina.

**Gensia, Swed.** See *Gensia, UK.*

**Gensia, UK.** Gensia Automedics Ltd, Unit 31, Wellington Business Park, Dukes Ride, Crowthorne, Berkshire, RG45 6LS, UK.

**Gensia, USA.** See *Sicor, USA.*

**Genta, USA.** Genta Inc., Berkeley Heights, NJ 07922, USA.

**Genthon, Hong Kong.** See *International Medical, Hong Kong.*

**Gentili, Ital.** Istituto Gentili S.p.A., Via Mazzini 112, 56125 Pisa, Italy.

**Genus, UK.** Genus Pharmaceuticals, Benham Valence, Newbury, Berkshire, RG20 8LU, UK.

**Genzyme, Austral.** Genzyme Australasia P/L, P.O. Box 6207, Baulkham Hills Business Centre, Baulkham Hills, NSW 2153, Australia.

**Genzyme, Austria.** See *Genzyme, Neth.*

**Genzyme, Braz.** Genzyme do Brasil Ltda, Av Rio Branco 12, 11 Andar, 20090-000-Rio De Janeiro, RJ, Brazil.

**Genzyme, Canad.** Genzyme Canada Inc., 800-2700 Matheson Bvld E, East Tower, Mississauga, Ontario, L4W 4V9, Canada.

**Genzyme, Denm.** Genzyme A/S, Islands Brygge 57 st tv, 2300 Copenhagen S, Denmark.

**Genzyme, Fr.** Genzyme SAS, ZI des Beaux Soleils 9, Chaussee Jules Cesar, Bat 2, BP 225 Osny, 95523 Cergy-Pontoise Cedex, France.

**Genzyme, Ger.** Genzyme GmbH, Siemensstr. 5 b, 63263 Neu-Isenberg, Germany.

**Genzyme, Gr.** Genzyme, Greece.

**Genzyme, Hong Kong.** See *DCH, Hong Kong, Naturest, Hong Kong, Vantone, Hong Kong*, and *Zuellig, Hong Kong.*

**Genzyme, Irl.** See *Genzyme, UK.*

**Genzyme, Israel.** Genzyme Israel Ltd, P.O. Box 1188, Kfar Saba, Israel.

**Genzyme, Ital.** Genzyme Therapeutics S.r.l., Via Scaglia Est 144, 41100 Modena, Italy.

**Genzyme, Jpn.** Genzyme Japan, Izumiyamabuki-Cho Bldg, 333 Yamabuki-Cho, Shinjuku-Ku, Tokyo 162-0801, Japan.

**Genzyme, Neth.** Genzyme BV, Gooimeer 10, 1411 DD Naarden, Netherlands.

**Genzyme, Norw.** See *Nycomed, Norw.*

**Genzyme, Spain.** Genzyme, Damian Sanchez Lopez 3, San Sebastian de los Reyes, 28700 Madrid, Spain.

**Genzyme, Swed.** See *Genzyme, Denm.*

**Genzyme, Switz.** Genzyme Pharmaceuticals, Sygena Facility, Eichenweg 1, Postfach, 4410 Liestal, Switzerland.

**Genzyme, UK.** Genzyme Therapeutics Ltd, 4620 Kingsgate, Cascade Way, Oxford Business Park South, Oxford, Oxfordshire, OX4 2SU, UK.

**Genzyme, USA.** Genzyme Corp., One Kendall Square, Building 1400, Cambridge, MA 02139, USA.

**Gepepharm, Ger.** gepepharm GmbH, Lendersbergstr. 86, 53721 Siegburg, Germany.

**Gerard, Denm.** See *NM, Denm.*

**Gerard, Irl.** Gerard Laboratories, 2004A Orchard Ave, City West Business Campus, Naas Rd, Dublin 24, Ireland.

**Gerard, Israel.** See *Genmedix, Israel.*

**Gerard, Norw.** See *Norgesfarma, Norw.*

**Gerard House, UK.** Gerard House Ltd, UK.

**Gerber, Mex.** Productos Gerber S.A. de C.V., Epigmenio Gonzalez No. 59, Col. Industrial, 76150 Queretaro, Qro, Mexico.

**Gerbex, Canad.** Gerbex Inc. Produits, 331 Principale St, St-Thomas d'Aquin, Quebec, J0H 2A0, Canada.

**Gerda, Fr.** Laboratoires Gerda, 6 rue Childebert, 69002 Lyon, France.

**Geriatric Pharm. Corp., USA.** See *Roberts, USA.*

**Geritrex, USA.** Geritrex Corp., 144 Kingsbridge Rd East, Mt Vernon, NY 10550, USA.

**Gerlach, Ger.** Eduard Gerlach GmbH, Backerstr. 4-8, 32312 Lubbecke, Germany.

**German Remedies, India.** German Remedies Ltd, Shivsagar Estate 'A', Dr Annie Besant Rd, Worli, Mumbai 400 018, India.

**Germania, Austria.** Germania Pharmazeutika GmbH, Schuselkagasse 8, A-1150 Vienna, Austria.

**Germax, Malaysia.** Germax Sdn Bhd, P.O. Box 6514, Kampung Tunku, 47307 Petaling Jaya, Selangor, Malaysia.

**Germiphene, Canad.** Germiphene Corporation, 1379 Colborne St E, P.O. Box 1748, Brantford, Ontario, N3T 5V7, Canada.

**Germiphene, Israel.** Germiphene, Israel.

**Gerolimatos (Γερολυματος), Gr.** ΓΕΡΟΛΥΜΑΤΟΣ ΠΙΝ ΑΕΒΕ, Ασκληπιού 13, 145 68 Κρυονέρι Αττικής, Krioneri Attikis, Greece.

**Gerolymatos, Hong Kong.** See *Primal, Hong Kong.*

**Gerolymatos, Thai.** See *US Summit, Thai.*

**Gerot, Austria.** Gerot-Pharmazeutika GmbH, Arnethgasse 3, A-1160 Vienna, Austria.

**Gerot, Malaysia.** See *Germax, Malaysia.*

**Gerot, Singapore.** See *Green Cross, Singapore.*

**Gerot, Switz.** See *Orion, Switz.*

**Gestafarma, Port.** Sociedade Farmacêutica Gestafarma, Lda, Rua Dr. Alvaro de Castro 63-7, 1600-058 Lisbon, Portugal.

**Geva, Mex.** Laboratorios Geva S.A. de C.V., 9 Norte No. 401-103, Col. Centro, 72000 Puebla Pue, Mexico.

**Gewo, Ger.** Gewo Chemie GmbH, Schneidweg 5, 76534 Baden-Baden, Germany.

**Geyer, Braz.** Geyer Medicamentos SA, Rua Pelotas 280, 90220-110 Porto Alegre, RS, Brazil.

**Geymonat, Ital.** Geymonat S.p.A., Via S. Anna 2, 03012 Anagni (FR), Italy.

**Geymonat, Switz.** See *Lucchini, Switz.*

**Gezzi, Arg.** See *Hiperfarm, Arg.*

**Ghimas, Ital.** Ghimas S.p.A., Via R. Fucini 2, 40033 Casalecchio di Reno (BO), Italy.

**GHP, Thai.** General Hospital Products Public Co. Ltd, 75/1 Rama VI Rd, Bangkok 10400, Thailand.

**GiEnne, Ital.** GiEnne Pharma S.p.A., Groupe Therabel, Via Lorenteggio 270/A, 20152 Milan, Italy.

**Gifrer Barbezat, Fr.** Laboratoires Gifrer Barbezat, 4-10 rue Paul Bert, BP 165, 69153 Decines cdx, France.

**Gilbert, Fr.** Laboratoires Gilbert, av. du General-de-Gaulle, B.P.115, 14204 Herouville-Saint-Clair cdx, France.

**Gilco, Israel.** Gilco Pharm Ltd, P.O. Box 21665, Tel Aviv, Israel.

**Gilead, Austral.** Gilead Sciences Pty Ltd, Unit 2, 41 Stamford Rd, Oakleigh, VIC 3166, Australia.

**Gilead, Canad.** Gilead Sciences Canada Inc., Vancouver, Canada.

**Gilead, Denm.** See *Orphan, Denm.*

**Gilead, Fr.** Gilead Sciences, 100 Avenue de Suffren, 75015 Paris, France.

**Gilead, Ger.** Gilead Sciences GmbH, Fraunhoferstr. 22, 82152 Martinsried/Planegg, Germany.

**Gilead, Gr.** Gilead Sciences, Inc., 2 Rizountas and Thrakis Str., Helliniko, 167 77 Αθήνα, Athens, Greece.

**Gilead, Hong Kong.** See *JDH, Hong Kong.*

**Gilead, Irl.** Gilead Sciences Ltd, Stillorgan Industrial Park, Blackrock, Co. Dublin, Ireland.

**Gilead, Ital.** Gilead Sciences S.r.l., Via G Frua 16, 20146 Milan, Italy.

**Gilead, Neth.** Gilead Sciences BV, Postbus 1054, 1300 BB Almere, Netherlands.

**Gilead, Norw.** See *Swedish Orphan, Norw.*

**Gilead, NZ.** See *Baxter, NZ.*

**Gilead, Spain.** Gilead Sciences S.L., Agustin de Foxa 27, Planta 11, 28036 Madrid, Spain.

**Gilead, Thai.** See *Siam Pharm, Thai.*

**Gilead, UK.** Gilead Sciences Ltd, The Flowers Building, Granta Park, Abington, Cambridge, Cambridgeshire, CB1 6GT, UK.

**Gilead, USA.** Gilead Sciences Inc., 333 Lakeside Drive, Foster City, CA 94404, USA.

**Gillette, Arg.** Gillette Argentina, Gdor. Ugarte 3561, 1605 Munro, Buenos Aires, Argentina.

**Gilton, Braz.** Gilton do Brasil Industria Quimica e Farmaceutica Ltda, Rua Claudio Furquim 21/25, Tatuape, 03072-010 Sao Paulo, SP, Brazil.

**Gingi-Pak, Switz.** See *Beldenta, Switz.*

**Giovanardi, Ital.** Giovanardi Farmaceutici S.n.c. del Dr Benito Giovanardi e Figli, Via Sapeto 28, 16131 Genoa, Italy.

**Girard, Switz.** See *Uhlmann-Eyraud, Switz.*

**Gisand, Switz.** Gisand AG, Schlaflistrasse 14, 3013 Berne, Switzerland.

**Giscard, Arg.** Lab. Gastón Giscard S.R.L., Rivadavia 4178 Piso 1 Dto.A, 1205 Buenos Aires, Argentina.

**Giuliani, Ital.** Giuliani S.p.A., Via Palagi 2, 20129 Milan, Italy.

**Giuliani, Switz.** Giuliani SA, via Riviera 21, 6976 Castagnola-Lugano, Switzerland.

**Giulini, Israel.** See *Gramse, Israel.*

**Glades, USA.** Glades Pharmaceuticals, 500 Satellite Bvld, Suwanee, GA 30024, USA.

**Glaxo, Austria.** See *GlaxoSmithKline, Austria.*

**Glaxo, Jpn.** See *GlaxoSmithKline, Jpn.*

**Glaxo, USA.** See *GlaxoSmithKline, USA.*

**Glaxo Allen, Ital.** See *GlaxoSmithKline, Ital.*

**Glaxo Wellcome, Austral.** See *GlaxoSmithKline, Austral.*

**Glaxo Wellcome, Austria.** See *GlaxoSmithKline, Austria.*

**Glaxo Wellcome, Belg.** See *GlaxoSmithKline, Belg.*

**Glaxo Wellcome, Braz.** See *GlaxoSmithKline, Braz.*

**Glaxo Wellcome, Canad.** See *GlaxoSmithKline, Canad.*

**Glaxo Wellcome, Denm.** See *GlaxoSmithKline, Denm.*

**Glaxo Wellcome, Fin.** See *GlaxoSmithKline, Fin.*

**Glaxo Wellcome, Ger.** See *GlaxoSmithKline, Ger.*

**Glaxo Wellcome, Gr.** GLAXO-WELLCOME AEBE, Κηφισίας 266, 152 32 Χαλάνδρι, Chalandri, Greece.

**Glaxo Wellcome, Hong Kong.** See *GlaxoSmithKline, Hong Kong.*

**Glaxo Wellcome, Irl.** See *GlaxoSmithKline, Irl.*

**Glaxo Wellcome, Israel.** See *GlaxoSmithKline, Israel.*

**Glaxo Wellcome, Ital.** See *GlaxoSmithKline, Ital.*

**Glaxo Wellcome, Mex.** See *GlaxoSmithKline, Mex.*

**Glaxo Wellcome, Neth.** See *GlaxoSmithKline, Neth.*

**Glaxo Wellcome, Norw.** See *GlaxoSmithKline, Norw.*

**Glaxo Wellcome, NZ.** See *GlaxoSmithKline, NZ.*

**Glaxo Wellcome, Port.** See *GlaxoSmithKline, Port.*

**Glaxo Wellcome, S.Afr.** See *GlaxoSmithKline, S.Afr.*

**Glaxo Wellcome, Singapore.** See *GlaxoSmithKline, Singapore.*

**Glaxo Wellcome, Spain.** See *GlaxoSmithKline, Spain.*

**Glaxo Wellcome, Swed.** See *GlaxoSmithKline, Swed.*

**Glaxo Wellcome, Switz.** See *GlaxoSmithKline, Switz.*

**Glaxo Wellcome, Thai.** See *GlaxoSmithKline, Thai.*

**Glaxo Wellcome, UK.** See *GlaxoSmithKline, UK.*

**Glaxo Wellcome, USA.** See *GlaxoSmithKline, USA.*

**GlaxoSmithKline, Arg.** GlaxoSmithKline S.A., Carlos Casares 3690, 1644 Victoria, Buenos Aires, Argentina.

**GlaxoSmithKline, Austral.** GlaxoSmithKline, Pharmaceticals Division, P.O. Box 168, Boronia, VIC 3155, Australia.

**GlaxoSmithKline, Austria.** GlaxoSmithKline Pharma, Albert-Schweitzer-Gasse 6, A-1140 Vienna, Austria.

**GlaxoSmithKline, Belg.** GlaxoSmithKline, Rue du Tilleul 13, 1332 Genval, Belgium.

**GlaxoSmithKline, Braz.** GlaxoSmithKline S.A., Estrada dos Bandeirantes 8464, 22783-110 Rio de Janeiro, RJ, Brazil.

**GlaxoSmithKline, Canad.** GlaxoSmithKline, 7333 Mississauga Rd North, Mississauga, Ontario, L5N 6L4, Canada.

**GlaxoSmithKline, Chile.** GlaxoSmithKline, Av. Andres Bello 2687, Las Condes, Santiago, Chile.

**GlaxoSmithKline, Denm.** GlaxoSmithKline, Nykaer 68, 2605 Brondby, Denmark.

**GlaxoSmithKline, Fin.** GlaxoSmithKline Oy, Kurjenkellontie 5, PL 5, 02270, 02271 Espoo, Finland.

**GlaxoSmithKline, Fr.** Laboratoires GlaxoSmithKline, 100 rte de Versailles, 78163 Marly-le-Roi cdx, France.

**GlaxoSmithKline, Ger.** GlaxoSmithKline GmbH & Co, Theresienhohe 11, 80339 Munich, Germany.

**GlaxoSmithKline, Hong Kong.** GlaxoSmithKline, 23/F, Tower 6, The Gateway, 9 Canton Rd, Tsimshatsui, Hong Kong.

**GlaxoSmithKline, India.** GlaxoSmithKline Pharmaceuticals (India) Ltd, Dr Annie Besant Rd, Mumbai 400 025, India.

**GlaxoSmithKline, Irl.** GlaxoSmithKline, Grange Rd, Rathfarnham, Dublin 16, Ireland.

**GlaxoSmithKline, Israel.** GlaxoSmithKline, 1 Bazel St, Petach Tikva 49510, Israel.

**GlaxoSmithKline, Ital.** GlaxoSmithKline S.p.A., Via A. Fleming 2, 37135 Verona, Italy.

**GlaxoSmithKline, Jpn.** GlaxoSmithKline, 6-15 Sendagaya 4-Chome, Shibuya-ku, Tokyo 151-8566, Japan.

**GlaxoSmithKline, Malaysia.** GlaxoSmithKline Pharmaceutical Sdn Bhd, 7th and 8th floor, Lien Hoe Building, 8 Persiaran Tropicana, 47410 Petaling Jaya, Selangor, Malaysia.

**GlaxoSmithKline, Mex.** GlaxoSmithKline Mexico S.A. de C.V., Calz. Mexico-Xochimilco No. 4900, Deleg. Tlalpan, 14370 Mexico D.F., Mexico.

**GlaxoSmithKline, Neth.** GlaxoSmithKline BV, Huiz-Ter-Heide-Weg 62, 3705 LZ Zeist, Netherlands.

**GlaxoSmithKline, Norw.** GlaxoSmithKline A/S, Forskningsv. 2, Postboks 180 Vindern, 0319 Oslo, Norway.

**GlaxoSmithKline, NZ.** GlaxoSmithKline, Private Bag 10-6600, Downtown, Aukland, New Zealand.

**GlaxoSmithKline, Port.** GlaxoSmithKline, Rua Dr. Antonio Borges 3, Arquiparque, Miraflores, 1495-131 Alges, Portugal.

**GlaxoSmithKline, S.Afr.** GlaxoSmithKline SA (Pty) Ltd, P.O. Box 3388, Halfway House 1685, South Africa.

**GlaxoSmithKline, Singapore.** GlaxoSmithKline Pte Ltd, 150 Beach Road, 22-00 Gateway West, S 189720, Singapore.

**GlaxoSmithKline, Spain.** GlaxoSmithKline, Severo Ochoa 2, Tres Cantos, 28760 Madrid, Spain.

**GlaxoSmithKline, Swed.** GlaxoSmithKline AB, Box 263, 431 23 Molndal, Sweden.

**GlaxoSmithKline, Switz.** GlaxoSmithKline, Bahnhofstrasse 5, 3322 Schonbuhl, Switzerland.

**GlaxoSmithKline, Thai.** GlaxoSmithKline Thailand Ltd, 12 Fl, Wave Place, 55 Wireless Rd, Lumpini Patumwam, Bangkok 10330, Thailand.

**GlaxoSmithKline, UK.** GlaxoSmithKline, Stockley Park West, Uxbridge, Middlesex, UB11 1BT, UK.

**GlaxoSmithKline, USA.** GlaxoSmithKline, 5 Moore Drive, P.O. Box 13398, Research Triangle Park, NC 27709, USA.

**GlaxoSmithKline Consumer, Austral.** GlaxoSmithKline, Consumer Healthcare Division, 82 Hughes Ave, Ermington, NSW 2115, Australia.

**GlaxoSmithKline Consumer, Belg.** See *GlaxoSmithKline, Belg.*

**GlaxoSmithKline Consumer, Canad.** GlaxoSmithKline Consumer Healthcare, 2030 Bristol Circle, Oakville, Ontario, L6H 5V2, Canada.

**GlaxoSmithKline Consumer, Ger.** GlaxoSmithKline Consumer Healthcare GmbH & Co. KG, Bussmatten 1, 77815 Buhl, Germany.

**GlaxoSmithKline Consumer, Irl.** See *GlaxoSmithKline, Irl.*

**GlaxoSmithKline Consumer, Ital.** GlaxoSmithKline Consumer Healthcare S.p.A., Via Zambeletti, 20021 Branzate di Bollate (MI), Italy.

**GlaxoSmithKline Consumer, Malaysia.** GlaxoSmithKline Consumer Healthcare, Lot 89, Jalan Enggang, Ampang/Ulu Kelang Industrial Estate, 54200 Selangor, Selangor, Malaysia.

**GlaxoSmithKline Consumer, Mex.** GlaxoSmithKline Mexico, S.A. de C.V. (Div. Consumo), Av. Insurgentes Sur 1605, Deleg. Benito Juarez, 01020 Mexico D.F., Mexico.

**GlaxoSmithKline Consumer, NZ.** GlaxoSmithKline Consumer Healthcare Ltd, P.O. Box 62-043, Sylvia Park, 6A Pacific Rise, Mt Wellington, Auckland, New Zealand.

**GlaxoSmithKline Consumer, Port.** See *GlaxoSmithKline, Port.*

**GlaxoSmithKline Consumer, Swed.** See *GlaxoSmithKline, Swed.*

**GlaxoSmithKline Consumer, UK.** GlaxoSmithKline Consumer Healthcare, 980 Great West Rd, Brentford, Middlesex, TW8 9BD, UK.

**GlaxoSmithKline Consumer, USA.** GlaxoSmithKline Consumer Healthcare, 257 Cornelison Avenue, Jersey City, NJ 07302, USA.

**GlaxoSmithKline Sante, Fr.** See *GlaxoSmithKline, Fr.*

**Glenbrook, USA.** Glenbrook Laboratories, Division of Sterling Drug Inc., 90 Park Ave, New York, NY 10016, USA.

**Glenmark, India.** Glenmark Pharmaceuticals Ltd, 801-813, 8th Floor, Mahalaxmi Chambers, 22 Bhulabhai Desai Rd, Mumbai 400 026, India.

**Glenmark, Singapore.** See *Uni, Singapore.*

**Glenmark, Thai.** See *Union Medical, Thai.*

**Glenwood, Canad.** Glenwood Laboratories Canada Ltd, 2406 Speers Rd, Oakville, Ontario, L6L 5M2, Canada.

**Glenwood, Ger.** Glenwood GmbH, Riedener Weg 23, 82319 Starnberg, Germany.

**Glenwood, Hong Kong.** See *Mita, Hong Kong.*

**Glenwood, Switz.** See *Galenica, Switz.*

**Glenwood, UK.** Glenwood Laboratories Ltd, Jenkins Dale, Chatham, Kent, ME4 5RD, UK.

**Glenwood, USA.** Glenwood Inc., P.O. Box 5419, Englewood, NJ 07631, USA.

**Glicolabor, Braz.** Glicolabor Industria Farmaceutica Ltda, Avenida Presidente Castelo Branco 999, Lagoinha, 14095-000 Ribierao Preto, SP, Brazil.

**Global, USA.** Global Pharmaceuticals Inc., Castor & Kenesington Aves, Philadelphia, PA 19124, USA.

**Globopharm, Switz.** Globopharm AG, Seestrasse 200, 8700 Kusnacht, Switzerland.

**GN, Ger.** See *Biosyn, Ger.*

**GNLD, Austral.** GNLD International P/L, P.O. Box 419, Beenleigh, Qld 4207, Australia.

**GNR, Fr.** Laboratoires GNR-pharma, 49 av Georges-Pompidou, 92593 Levallois-Perret cdx, France.

**GNR, Ital.** GNR S.p.A., Strada Statale 233 km 20.5, 21040 Origgio (Va), Italy.

**GNR, Port.** See *Agostinho, Port.*

**Go Travel, UK.** Go Travel Products, UK.

**Gobbi, Arg.** Lab. Gobbi Novag S.A., F. Onsari 498, 1875 Wilde, Buenos Aires, Argentina.

**Godecke, Ger.** See *Pfizer, Ger.*

**Golaz, Switz.** Laboratoire Golaz SA, Case postale 1067, 1701 Fribourg-Moncor, Switzerland.

**Golden Pride, Canad.** Golden Pride, 60 Colonnade Rd, Nepean, Ontario, K2E 7J6, Canada.

**Goldham, Ger.** See *Sanochemia, Ger.*

**Goldline, USA.** See *Ivax, USA.*

**Goldplus, Singapore.** Goldplus Universal Pte Ltd, 8 Kaki Bukit Rd 2, 02-19/20 Ruby Warehouse Complex, S 417841, Singapore.

**Goldschmidt, Switz.** See *Desopharmex, Switz.*

**Goldshield, Denm.** See *Goldshield, UK.*

**Goldshield, Fin.** See *Goldshield, UK.*

**Goldshield, Ger.** See *Nordend, Ger.*

**Goldshield, Hong Kong.** See *DCH, Hong Kong,* and *Treasure Mountain, Hong Kong.*

**Goldshield, Irl.** See *Alphar, Irl.*

**Goldshield, Israel.** See *Pharmateam, Israel.*

**Goldshield, Neth.** See *Goldshield, UK.*

**Goldshield, Norw.** See *Goldshield, UK.*

**Goldshield, Singapore.** See *Orient, Singapore.*

**Goldshield, Swed.** See *Goldshield, UK.*

**Goldshield, UK.** Goldshield Pharmaceuticals Ltd, NLA Tower, 12-16 Addiscombe Rd, Croydon, Surrey, CR0 0XT, UK.

**Gomenol, Fr.** Laboratoires du Gomenol, 48 rue des Petites-Écuries, 75010 Paris, France.

**Goodys, USA.** See *GlaxoSmithKline Consumer, USA.*

**Gordon, Arg.** Lab. Gordon S.A.C.I.F.I.A., Malvinas Argentinas 3311, 1644 Victoria, Buenos Aires, Argentina.

**Gordon, USA.** Gordon Laboratories, 6801 Ludlow St, Upper Darby, PA 19082-1694, USA.

**Gothaplast, Ger.** Gothaplast Verbandpflasterfabrik GmbH, Postfach: 100131, 99851 Gotha/Thuringen, Germany.

**Gothia, Norw.** Gothia Medical AS, Ostre Aker v 205, Postboks 109 Kalbakken, 0902 Oslo, Norway.

**Gothia, Swed.** Gothia Läkemedel AB, Bolshedens Industrivag 20, 427 50 Billdal, Sweden.

**Goulart, Braz.** Laboratorios Goulart S.A., Rua Aguape 56, Parada de Lucas, 21010-080 Rio de Janeiro, Brazil.

**GP, UK.** GP Pharma Ltd, ARC Progress, Beckerings Park, Lidlington, Bedfordshire, MK43 0RD, UK.

**G.P. Laboratories, Austral.** See *Pfizer, Austral.*

**GPL, Switz.** GPL Ginsana Products Lugano SA, Tochterunternehmen der Pharmaton SA, Postfach, 6903 Lugano, Switzerland.

**Graf Fruttasan, Switz.** Graf Fruttasan AG, Untere Etzmatten 16, 4467 Rothenfluh/BL, Switzerland.

**Grafton, Singapore.** Grafton Pharmasia Pte Ltd, 66 Tannery Lane, 01-05A Sindo Building, S 347805, Singapore.

**Grafton, UK.** Grafton International, Birchbrook Park, Shenstone, Staffordshire, WS14 0DJ, UK.

**Graham-Field, USA.** Graham Field Health Products Inc., 2935 NE Parkway, Atlanta, GA 30360, USA.

**Gramon, Arg.** Laboratorios Gramón, Intendente Amaro Avalos 4208, 1605 Buenos Aires, Argentina.

**Gramse, Israel.** Gramse Pharmaceuticals Ltd, 56 Bialik St, Ramat Gan, Israel.

**Granado, Braz.** Casa Granado Lab. Farmacias e Drogarias S.A., Travessa do Comercio 17, 20010-080 Rio de Janeiro, RJ, Brazil.

**Grandel, Ger.** Dr Grandel GmbH, Pfladergasse 7-13, 86150 Augsburg, Germany.

**Grandel-Synpharma, Ger.** See *Grandel, Ger.*

**Grands Espaces, Fr.** Les Grands Espaces Therapeutiques, B.P. 6054, 34030 Montpellier cdx 01, France.

**Granions, Mon.** Laboratoires des Granions, 7 rue de l'Industrie, MC 98000, Monaco.

**Grans Remedy, NZ.** See *Essential, NZ.*

**Grasler, Ger.** gräsler pharma GmbH, Brunnleitenstr. 3, 82284 Grafrath, Germany.

**Gray, Arg.** Prod. Farmaciuticos Dr. Gray S.A.C.I., Thames 372 Piso 1, 1414 Buenos Aires, Argentina.

**Gray, USA.** See *Purdue Frederick, USA.*

**Great Eastern, Hong Kong.** Great Eastern Healthcare Ltd, 9/F, Blk A Kerry BCI Godown, 3 Kin Chuen St, Kwai Chung, N.T., Hong Kong.

**Great Eastern, Thai.** Great Eastern Drug Co. Ltd, 18 Fl, Thai Wah Tower, 21/52-54 South Sathorn Rd, Sathorn, Bangkok 10120, Thailand.

**Great Liaison, Hong Kong.** Great Liaison Ltd, Unit 608, Fibres & Fabrics Industrial Ctr, 7 Shing Yip St, Kwun Tong, Kowloon, Hong Kong.

**Great Southern, USA.** Great Southern Laboratories, 10863 Rockley Rd, Houston, TX 77099, USA.

**Great Year, Hong Kong.** Great Year Trading Co. Ltd, 18/F, 80 Gloucester Rd, Wanchai, Hong Kong.

**Greater Pharma, Thai.** Greater Pharma Ltd Part, 46, 46/1-2 Soi Charansanitwongs 40, Bangyikhan, Bangkok 10700, Thailand.

**Green Cross, Hong Kong.** See *Great Year, Hong Kong.*

**Green Cross, Malaysia.** See *Propharm, Malaysia.*

**Green Cross, Singapore.** Green Cross Pte Ltd, 63 Hillview Ave, 07-06 Lam Soon Industrial Building, S 669569, Singapore.

**Green Cross, Thai.** See *Charoen, Thai.*

**Green Cross Guangzhou, Singapore.** See *Alpha Therapeutic, Singapore.*

**Green Turtle Bay Vitamin Co., USA.** The Green Turtle Bay Vitamin Co., P.O. Box 642, Summit, NJ 07901, USA.

**Greenridge, Austral.** Greenridge Botanicals, 17 Freighter Ave, Queensland, Australia.

**Grelan, Jpn.** Grelan Pharmaceutical Co. Ltd, 6-6 Kofunacho, Nihonbashi, Chuo-ku, Tokyo 103-0024, Japan.

**Gricar, Ital.** Industria Chimico Farmaceutica Gricar Chemical S.r.l., Via S Giuseppe 18/20, 20047 Brugherio (MI), Italy.

**Grifols, Arg.** Grifols Argentina S.A., Ruta 202, No. 3462, 1611 Don Torcuato, Buenos Aires, Argentina.

**Grifols, Chile.** Grupo Grifols de Chile SA, Av. Americo Vespucio 2242, Conchali, Santiago, Chile.

**Grifols, Ger.** Grifols Deutschland GmbH, Siemensstr. 18, 63225 Langen, Germany.

**Grifols, Ital.** Grifols Italia S.p.A., Loc. La Fontina, Via Carducci 62d, 56010 Ghezzano (Pi), Italy.

**Grifols, Port.** Grifols Portugal, Lda, Rua de Sao Sebastiao, 2, Zona Ind. Cabra Figa, 2635-448 Rio de Mouro, Portugal.

**Grifols, Singapore.** See *Diethelm, Singapore.*

**Grifols, Spain.** Grifols, C/Can Guasch 2 Pol. Levante, Parets del Valles, 08150 Barcelona, Spain.

**Grifols, UK.** Grifols UK Ltd, 72 St Andrews Rd, Cambridge, CB4 1GS, UK.

**Grifols, USA.** Grifols America Inc., 8870-8880 NW 18th Terrace, Miami, FL 33172, USA.

**Grimberg, Arg.** Grimberg Dentales, Lerma 426, 1414 Buenos Aires, Argentina.

**Grimberg, Fr.** Laboratoires Grimberg, 19 rue Poliveau, 75005 Paris, France.

**Grin, Mex.** Laboratorios Grin S.A. de C.V., Rodriguez Saro 630, Col. Del Valle, 03100 Mexico D.F., Mexico.

**Grisi, Mex.** Laboratorios Grisi Hermanos, S.A., Division Farmaceutica, Calle Amores No. 1746, Col. del Valle, Deleg. Benito Juarez, 03100 Mexico D.F., Mexico.

**Grogg, Switz.** Grogg Pharma AG, Christoffelgasse 3, 3001 Berne, Switzerland.

**Gross, Braz.** Laboratorio Gross S.A., Rua Padre Ildefonso Penalba 389, 20775-020 Rio de Janeiro, RJ, Brazil.

**Grossman, Mex.** See *ICN, Mex.*

**Grossmann, Hong Kong.** See *Kai Cheong, Hong Kong.*

**Grossmann, Switz.** Dr Grossmann AG, Pharmaca, Hardstrasse 25, Postfach 914, 4127 Birsfelden/Basle, Switzerland.

**Grunenthal, Arg.** Grunenthal Argentina S.A., Rivadavia 954, 2do. Piso, 1002 Buenos Aires, Argentina.

**Grunenthal, Austria.** Grünenthal GmbH, Liebermannstrasse A01/501, A-2345 Brunn am Gebirge, Austria.

**Grunenthal, Belg.** Grünenthal, Lenneke Marelaan 8, 1932 Sint-Stevens-Woluwe, Belgium.

**Grunenthal, Chile.** Grunenthal Chilena Ltda, Av. Providencia 727, Providencia, Santiago, Chile.

**Grunenthal, Denm.** See *Pharmacia, Denm.*

**Grunenthal, Fr.** Grunenthal, 43 rue de Villiers, 92523 Neuilly-sur-Seine, France.

**Grunenthal, Ger.** Grünenthal GmbH Aachen, Zieglerstr. 6, 52078 Aachen, Germany.

**Grunenthal, Hong Kong.** Grunenthal (Hong Kong) Ltd, Rm 1503, 15/F Wing On Ctr, 111 Connaught Rd Central, Hong Kong.

**Grunenthal, Mex.** Grünenthal de Mexico S.A. de C.V., Periferico Sur No. 6677, Col. Ejidos de Tepepan, Deleg. Xochimilco, 16018 Mexico D.F., Mexico.

**Grunenthal, Norw.** See *Pharmacia, Norw.*

**Grunenthal, Port.** Grunenthal SA, Rua Alfredo da Silva no 16, 2720-028 Amadora, Portugal.

**Grunenthal, Spain.** Grunenthal, Doctor Zamenhof 36, 28027 Madrid, Spain.

**Grunenthal, Switz.** Grünenthal Pharma AG, 8756 Mitlodi/GL., Switzerland.

**Gry, Ger.** Gry-Pharma GmbH, Kandelstr. 10, 79199 Kirchzarten, Germany.

**Guardian, Canad.** See *Pharmascience, Canad.*

**Guardian, USA.** Guardian Laboratories, A division of United-Guardian Inc., 230 Marcus Blvd, Hauppauge, NY 11788, USA.

**Gubler, Switz.** Dr AW Gubler, Petersgraben 5, 4051 Basle, Switzerland.

**Guerbert, Spain.** Guerbert, Avda de Menendez Pelayo 61 1o D, 28009 Madrid, Spain.

**Guerbet, Austria.** See *Guerbet, Fr.*

**Guerbet, Braz.** Guerbet Produtos Radiologicos Ltda, Rua Andre Rocha 3000, 22710-561 Rio de Janeiro, RJ, Brazil.

**Guerbet, Denm.** Guerbet, Parallelvej 10, 2800 Lyngby, Denmark.

**Guerbet, Fin.** See *Alpharma, Fin.*

**Guerbet, Fr.** Laboratoires Guerbet, B.P. 50400, 95943 Roissy-Charles-de-Gaulle cdx, France.

**Guerbet, Ger.** Guerbet GmbH, Otto-Volger Str. 11, 65843 Sulzbach/Ts, Germany.

**Guerbet, Israel.** See *Promedico, Israel.*

**Guerbet, Ital.** Guerbet S.p.A., V.le Brigata Bisagno 2/18, 16129 Genoa, Italy.

**Guerbet, Neth.** Guerbet Nederland BV, Avelingen West 28c, 4202 MS Gorinchem, Netherlands.

**Guerbet, Norw.** See *Gothia, Norw.*

**Guerbet, Port.** See *Martins & Fernandes, Port.*

**Guerbet, Switz.** Guerbet AG, Winterthurerstrasse 92, 8006 Zurich, Switzerland.

**Gufic, India.** Gufic Ltd, Subhas Road-A, Vile Parle (E), Mumbai 400 057, India.

**Guidotti, Gr.** GUIDOTTI HELLAS, Δαμβέργη 7, 104 45 Αθήνα, Athens, Greece.

**Guidotti, Ital.** Laboratori Guidotti S.p.A., Via Livornese 897, 56010 Pisa La Vettola (PI), Italy.

**Guidotti, Spain.** See *Menarini, Spain.*

**Guieu, Fr.** Laboratoires Guieu France, France.

**Guieu, Ital.** Laboratori Guieu S.p.A., V.le Filippetti 37, 20122 Milan, Italy.

**Guigoz, Fr.** Guigoz, B.P. 900, 77446 Marne-la-Vallee cdx 2, France.

**Guigoz, Ital.** Guigoz, Divisione Dietici, Viale Richard 5, 20143 Milan, Italy.

**Guildford, USA.** Guildford Pharmaceuticals Inc., 6611 Tributary St, Baltimore, MD 21224, USA.
**Guilford, Israel.** See *Medison, Israel.*
**Gunnar Kjems, Denm.** Gunnar Kjems ApS, Peder Huitfeldts Straede 12, 1173 Copenhagen K, Denmark.
**Gunther, Braz.** Produtos Farmaceuticos Gunther do Brasil Ltda, Rua Joao Moura 1151, 05412-002 Sao Paulo, SP, Brazil.
**Guri, Israel.** Pharma Guri, P.O. Box 11, Rishon Lezion, Israel.
**Gynetics, Singapore.** See *Sime Darby, Singapore.*
**Gynetics, USA.** Gynetics Inc., P.O. Box 8509, Somerville, NJ 08876, USA.
**Gynopharm, Chile.** See *Recalcine, Chile.*
**Hackmey, Israel.** Hackmey Ltd, 31 Yavne St, Tel Aviv, Israel.
**Haemacure, Canad.** Haemacure Corp., 16771 ch. Ste-Marie, Kirkland, Quebec, H9H 5H3, Canada.
**Haffkine, India.** Haffkine Bio-Pharmaceutical Corp. Ltd, Acharya Donde Marg, Parel, Mumbai 400 012, India.
**Hal, Ger.** Hal Allergie GmbH, Kolner Landstr. 34 a, 40591 Dusseldorf, Germany.
**Hal, Neth.** Haarlems Allergenen Laboratorium BV, Parklaan 125, 2011 KT Haarlem, Netherlands.
**Halal, UK.** Halal Pharmaceuticals Ltd, 7 Oxford St, Manchester, M1 4WX, UK.
**Halewood, Thai.** See *Sriprasit, Thai.*
**Hall, Canad.** Hall Laboratories Ltd, 13060-89th Ave, Suite 207, Surrey, British Columbia, V3W 3B2, Canada.
**Haller, Braz.** Quimica Haller Ltda, Avenida Alem Paraiba 104, 21061-090 Rio de Janeiro, RJ, Brazil.
**Halsey, USA.** Halsey Drug Co, 695 N Perryville Rd, Rockford, IL 61107, USA.
**Hameln, Ger.** Hameln Pharmaceuticals GmbH, Langes Feld 13, 31789 Hameln, Germany.
**Hameln, Thai.** See *JDH Borneo, Thai.*
**Hamilton, Austral.** Hamilton Pharmaceuticals P/L, P.O. Box 7, Adelaide, SA 5001, Australia.
**Hamilton, Hong Kong.** See *Australian Medic-Care, Hong Kong.*
**Hamilton, Israel.** See *Trima, Israel.*
**Hamilton, NZ.** See *Medic, NZ.*
**Hanosan, Ger.** Hanosan GmbH, Hanosanstr. 1, 30826 Garbsen, Germany.
**Hansam, Irl.** See *United Drug, Irl.*
**Hansam, UK.** Hansam Healthcare Ltd, 60 Ondine Rd, London, SE15 4EB, UK.
**Hanseler, Ger.** Hänseler GmbH, Gottlieb-Daimler-Str. 1, 78467 Constance a. B., Germany.
**Hanseler, Switz.** Hänseler AG, Industriestrasse 35, 9100 Herisau, Switzerland.
**Hargell, Canad.** Hargell Ltd, 5050 Dufferin St, Suite 108, North York, Ontario, M3H 5T5, Canada.
**Harley Street Supplies, UK.** Harley Street Supplies, 55 Paddington St, London, W1M 3RQ, UK.
**Harn, Thai.** Harn Thai Pharma Ltd, 2121 New Petchburi Rd, Bangkok 10320, Thailand.
**Harras-Curarina, Ger.** Harras Pharma Curarina Arzneimittel GmbH, Am Harras 15, 81373 Munich, Germany.
**Hartmann, Fr.** Laboratoires Paul Hartmann, 18 rue des Goumiers, 67730 Chatenois, France.
**Hartmann, Ger.** Paul Hartmann AG Verbandstoff-Fabriken, Paul-Hartmann-Str. 12, 89522 Heidenheim (Brenz), Germany.
**Harvey Scruton, Israel.** See *Meditrend, Israel.*
**Harvey-Scruton, UK.** Harvey-Scruton Ltd, 4 Barker Lane, York, North Yorkshire, YO1 6JR, UK.
**Hassle, Swed.** Hässle Läkemedel AB, 431 83 Molndal, Sweden.
**Hauck, USA.** See *Roberts, USA.*
**Haupt, Switz.** Medidenta AG, Schachenstrasse 2, 9016 St Gallen, Switzerland.
**Hausmann, Irl.** See *Clonmel, Irl.*
**Hautel, Arg.** Hautel S.A., Warnes 829 Dto. A, 1414 Buenos Aires, Argentina.
**Haw Par, Canad.** Haw Par Brothers International Ltd, P.O. Box 4129, Vancouver, British Columbia, V6B 3Z6, Canada.
**Hawgreen, UK.** Hawgreen Ltd, P.O. Box 157, Hatfield, AL10 8ZP, UK.
**Hawthorn, USA.** See *Cypress, USA.*
**Hayes, Israel.** Hayes, Israel.
**Health & Diet Food Co., UK.** Health & Diet Food Co. Ltd, Europa Trading Estate, Stoneclough Road, Radcliffe, Manchester, M26 9HE, UK.
**Health & Medical, USA.** See *Graham-Field, USA.*
**Health Alliance, Hong Kong.** Health Alliance International Co. Ltd, Unit 1302-03, SUP Tower, 75 King's Rd, North Point, Hong Kong.
**Health Care, Hong Kong.** Health Care Products Ltd, 8/F Eastwood Ctr, 5A Kung Ngam Village Rd, Shaukeiwan, Hong Kong.
**Health Care Products, USA.** Health Care Products, 369 Bayview Ave, Amityville, NY 11701, USA.
**Health Chemical, Hong Kong.** See *Sun Hing, Hong Kong.*
**Health Imports, UK.** Health Imports Ltd, York House, York Street, Bradford, West Yorkshire, BD8 0HR, UK.
**Health Perception, UK.** Health Perception Ltd, Lakeside Business Park, Swan Lane, Sandhurst, Berkshire, GU47 7DN, UK.
**Health Tech, Hong Kong.** Health Tech Ltd, 5/F A-2 Loyong Court Commercial Bldg, 212-220 Lockhart Rd, Wanchai, Hong Kong.
**Health Vision, Hong Kong.** Health Vision Enterprise Ltd, Rm 2504, K Wah Ctr, 191 Java Rd, North Point, Hong Kong.
**Health World, Austral.** Health World Ltd, 8/663 Kingsford Smith Drive, Eagle Farm, QLD 4009, Australia.
**Health-Care, Gr.** Health Care, Greece.
**Healthcare Innovations, UK.** Healthcare Innovations, 930 High Rd, London, N12 9RT, UK.
**Healthcrafts, UK.** Healthcrafts Ltd, UK.
**Healtheries, NZ.** Healtheries of New Zealand Ltd, 505 Mount Wellington Highway, Mount Wellington, Auckland, New Zealand.
**Healthfirst, USA.** Healthfirst Corp., 22316 70th Ave W, Mountlake Terrace, WA 98043, USA.
**Healthline, USA.** Healthline Laboratories Inc., 2805 Danbar Dr., Green Bay, WI 54313, USA.
**Healthpoint, USA.** Healthpoint Medical, 2600 Airport Fwy, Fort Worth, TX 76111, USA.
**Hearst, Braz.** Hearst Laboratorios do Brasil Ltda, Avenida Actura 100, Vila Actura, 25225-210 Duque de Caxias, RJ, Brazil.
**Heber, Thai.** See *Pharmadica, Thai.*
**Hebert, Canad.** Distribution L Hebert, 15260 Notre-Dame St E, Montreal, Quebec, H1A 1W6, Canada.
**Hebron, Braz.** Hebron S.A. Industria Quimica e Farmaceutica, Rua Ribeiro de Brito 573, 6 andar, 51021-310 Recife, PE, Brazil.
**Heca, Neth.** Heca BV, Industrieweg 24, Postbus 39, 7957 SG De Wijk, Netherlands.
**Heck, Switz.** Heck Pharma SA, Studenmatt 9, 1791 Courtaman, Switzerland.
**Heel, Ger.** Biologische Heilmittel Heel GmbH, Dr.-Reckeweg-Str. 2-4, 76532 Baden-Baden, Germany.
**Heel, S.Afr.** Heel South Africe (Pty) Ltd, P.O. Box 890558, Lyndhurst 2106, South Africa.
**Heel, USA.** Heel Inc., 11600 Cochiti SE, Albuerquerque, NM 87123, USA.
**Hefa, Ger.** See *Sanavita, Ger.*
**Heilit, Ger.** Heilit Arzneimittel GmbH, Danziger Str. 5, 21465 Reinbek, Germany.
**Heinz, UK.** H.J. Heinz Co. Ltd, 6 Roundwood Ave, Stockley Park, Uxbridge, Middlesex, UB11 1HZ, UK.
**Heinz-Wattie, NZ.** Heinz-Wattie's Australasia Ltd, Private Bag 99-920, Newmarket, Auckland, New Zealand.
**Helago, Ger.** Helago-Pharma GmbH, Rheinallee 11, 53173 Bonn, Germany.
**Helapet, UK.** Helapet, UK.
**Helber, Mex.** Helber de Mexico S.A. de C.V., San Esteban 88, Santo Tomas Azcaptzalco, 02020 Mexico D.F., Mexico.
**Helena, USA.** Helena Laboratories, 1530 Lindbergh Dr, P.O. Box 752, Beaumont, TX 77707, USA.
**Helfarma, Port.** Helfarma, Lda, Rua Joao Chagas 53, 1495-072 Alges, Portugal.
**Helios, UK.** Helios Healthcare Ltd, P.O. Box 36, Old Warden, Biggleswade, SG18 9UP, UK.
**Helixor, Ger.** Helixor Heilmittel GmbH & Co., Fischermuhle 1, 72348 Rosenfeld, Germany.
**Help, Gr.** HELP ABEE, Βαλαωρίτου 4, 144 52 Μεταμόρφωση, Metamorphosi, Greece.
**Helsinn, Hong Kong.** See *Zuellig, Hong Kong.*
**Helsinn, Port.** Helsinn, Lda, Estrada Nacional 249/4 (Km 1.6), Abrunheira, Apartado 155, 2710-901 Sintra, Portugal.
**Helsinn Birex, Hong Kong.** See *Treasure Mountain, Hong Kong.*
**Helsinn Birex, Irl.** Helsinn Birex Pharmaceuticals Ltd, Damastown, Mulhuddart, Dublin 15, Ireland.
**Helvepharm, Switz.** Helvepharm AG, Walzmuhlestrasse 60, 8500 Frauenfeld, Switzerland.
**Hemasure, Denm.** HemaSure AS, Sauntesvej 13, 2820 Gentofte, Denmark.
**Hemasure, Swed.** See *Hemasure, Denm.*
**HemispheRx, USA.** HemispheRx, 1 Penn Center, 1617 John F Kennedy Blvd, Philadelphia, PA 19103, USA.
**Hemoderivados, Arg.** U.N.C. Hemoderivados, Agencia postal 4, 5000 Cordoba, Argentina.
**Hemopharm, Ger.** Hemopharm GmbH, Konigsteiner Str. 2, 61350 Bad Homburg v. d. H., Germany.
**Henk, Ger.** See *Dolorgiet, Ger.*
**Henkel, Austria.** Henkel Austria GmbH, Erdbergstrasse 29, A-1030 Vienna, Austria.
**Henkel, Ger.** See *Ecolab, Ger.*
**Henkel, Ital.** Henkel Ecolab S.p.A., Via Morozzo Della Rocca 6, 20123 Milan, Italy.
**Hennig, Ger.** Hennig Arzneimittel GmbH & Co. KG, Liebigstr. 1-2, 65439 Florsheim am Main, Germany.
**Henning, Ger.** Henning Berlin GmbH & Co. OHG, Potsdamer Str. 8, 10785 Berlin, Germany.
**Henning Walldorf, Ger.** Dr. Georg Friedrich Henning, Chemische Fabrik Walldorf GmbH, Robert-Bosch-Str. 62, 69190 Walldorf, Germany.
**Hepacholan, Braz.** Laboratorio Hepacholan S.A., Av. Manoel Monteiro de Araujo 1051, Vila Jaguara, 05113-020 Sao Paulo, SP, Brazil.
**Hepatoum, Fr.** Laboratoires Hepatoum, B.P. 5, 03270 Saint-Yorre, France.
**Heralds, Braz.** Herald's do Brasil Ltda, Av. Eugenio Borges 1060, 24751-000 Sao Goncalo, RJ, Brazil.
**Herbal, Israel.** See *Concept, Israel.*
**Herbal Concepts, UK.** Herbal Concepts Ltd, Liscombe Park, Soulbury, Buckinghamshire, LU7 0JL, UK.
**Herbal Laboratories, UK.** Herbal Laboratories Ltd, Pierpoint House, 1 Beach Rd, St Annes-on-Sea, Lancashire, FY8 2NR, UK.
**Herbaline, Ital.** Herbaline S.n.c. di Ugo Venara & C, Via dell'Artigianato 13, 13040 Rovasenda (VC), Italy.
**Herbalist, Ger.** Herbalist & Doc Gesundheitsgesellschaft mbH, Waldseeweg 6, 13467 Berlin, Germany.
**Herbamed, Switz.** Herbamed AG, Untere Au, 9055 Buhler, Switzerland.
**Herbapharm, Ger.** See *CytoChemia, Ger.*
**Herbarium, Braz.** Herbarium Laboratorio Botanico Ltda, Rua Maua 838, 80030-200 Curitiba, PR, Brazil.
**Herbaxt, Fr.** Laboratoires Herbaxt, Z.I. Nord, bat 5, 77200 Torcy, France.
**Herbert, Ger.** Herbert Arzneimittel GmbH, Kreuzberger Ring 13, 65205 Wiesbaden, Germany.
**Herbes Universelles, Canad.** Herbes Universelles, 7, 70e Ave O, Blainville, Quebec, J7C 1R7, Canada.
**Herbrand, Ger.** Dr Herbrand KG, Brambachstr. 31, 77723 Gengenbach, Germany.
**Herchemie, Austria.** Herchemie, Hasnerstrasse 7, A-9020 Klagenfurt, Austria.
**Heritage Consumer, Canad.** Heritage Consumer Products, 120 Harry Walker Parkway N, Newmarket, Ontario, L3Y 7B2, Canada.
**Heritage Consumer, USA.** Heritage Consumer Products, 141 South Ave, Suite 2, Fanwood, NJ 07023, USA.
**Hermal, Austria.** See *Hermal, Ger.*
**Hermal, Denm.** See *Merck, Denm.*
**Hermal, Ger.** Hermal Kurt Herrmann GmbH & Co., Scholtzstr. 3, 21465 Reinbek, Germany.
**Hermal, Hong Kong.** See *Keller, Hong Kong.*
**Hermal, Israel.** See *Neopharm, Israel.*
**Hermal, Malaysia.** See *Boots Healthcare, Malaysia.*
**Hermal, Norw.** See *Meda, Norw.*
**Hermal, Port.** See *Boots Healthcare, Port.*
**Hermal, Singapore.** See *Boots, Singapore.*
**Hermal, Thai.** See *Olic, Thai.*
**Hermes, Austria.** See *Hermes, Ger.*
**Hermes, Ger.** Hermes Arzneimittel GmbH, Georg-Kalb-Str. 5-8, 82049 Grosshesselohe/Munich, Germany.
**Herron, Austral.** Herron Pharmaceuticals P/L, P.O. Box 95, Brisbane Market, QLD 4106, Australia.
**Hertz, Braz.** Kley Hertz SA, Rua Comendador Azevedo 133, 90220-150 Porto Alegre, Rio Grande do Sul, Brazil.
**Herus, Braz.** Herus Industria Farmaceutica Ltda, Rua Sanches de Aguiar 200, V. Paulina, 03192-140 Sao Paulo, SP, Brazil.
**Herzpunkt, Ger.** See *Sebamed, Ger.*
**Hestag, Austria.** Hestag GmbH, Kreitnergasse 1-3, A-1171 Vienna, Austria.
**Hetterich, Ger.** Chemische Fabrik Dr. Hetterich GmbH & Co. KG, Gebhardtstr. 5, 90762 Furth/Bayern, Germany.
**Heumann, Ger.** Heumann Pharma GmbH, Sudwestpark 50, 90449 Nurnberg, Germany.
**Heumann, Hong Kong.** See *Fund Trip, Hong Kong.*
**Heumann, Switz.** See *Pharmacia, Switz.*
**Heumann, Thai.** See *Sang Udom, Thai.*
**Hevert, Ger.** Hevert-Arzneimittel GmbH & Co. KG, In der Weiherwiese 1, 55569 Nussbaum, Germany.
**Hexa, Arg.** Lab. Hexa S.A., Helguera 254/58, 1406 Buenos Aires, Argentina.
**Hexal, Arg.** Hexal Argentina S.A., Paseo Colon 221 Piso 7, 1063 Buenos Aires, Argentina.
**Hexal, Austral.** Hexal Australia P/L, Level 4, Suite 1-6, 100 Harris St, Pyrmont, NSW 2009, Australia.
**Hexal, Austria.** Hexal Pharma GmbH, Wilhelminenstrasse 91/II F, A-1160 Vienna, Austria.
**Hexal, Braz.** Hexal do Brasil, Av. Itaborai 1425, 04135-001 Sao Paulo, SP, Brazil.
**Hexal, Ger.** Hexal AG, Industriestr. 25, 83607 Holzkirchen, Germany.
**Hexal, Israel.** See *Trima, Israel.*
**Hexal, NZ.** Hexal New Zealand Pty Ltd, P.O. Box 100044, North Shore Mail Centre, Glenfield, Auckland, New Zealand.
**Hexal, S.Afr.** Hexal Pharma South Africa, 10 Fangio Rd, Mahogony Ridge, Westmean, Pinetown 3608, South Africa.
**Hexa-Medinova, Arg.** See *Hexa, Arg.*
**Heyl, Ger.** Heyl Chemisch-pharmazeutische Fabrik GmbH & Co. KG, Goerzallee 253, 14167 Berlin, Germany.
**Heyl, USA.** Heyl, USA.
**Higate, Arg.** Productos Higaté S.A., Jose Marma Bosch 5434, 1650 Villa Libertad, Buenos Aires, Argentina.
**High Chemical, USA.** High Chemical Co., 3901-A Nebraska St, Levittown, PA 19056, USA.
**Hikma, Port.** Hikma Farmacêutica (Portugal), Lda, Estrada do Rio da Mo 8, 8A e 8B Fervenca, 2705-906 Terrugem SNT, Portugal.
**Hilarys, Canad.** Hilary's Distribution Ltd, 330 Esna Park Drive, Unit 38, Markham, Ontario, L3R 1H3, Canada.
**Hill, USA.** Hill Dermaceuticals Inc., 2650 S. Mellonville Ave, Sanford, FL 32773, USA.
**Hillcross, UK.** See *AAH, UK.*
**Himmel, USA.** Himmel Pharmaceuticals Inc., P.O. Box 5479, Lake Worth, FL 33466, USA.
**Hind Wing, Hong Kong.** Hind Wing Co. Ltd, Unit No 1103B, 11/F, Block B, Seaview Estate, 2-8 Watson Rd, North Point, Hong Kong.
**Hing Ah, Hong Kong.** Hing Ah Pharma Co. Ltd, Unit No. 3,5,6, 12/F Prosperity Ctr, 25 Chong Yip St, Kwun Tong, Kowloon, Hong Kong.
**Hing Yip, Hong Kong.** Hing Yip Medicine Co., 2/F, Lo Ko House, 133 Gloucester Rd, Hong Kong.
**Hiperfarm, Arg.** Hiperfarm S.A., Guevara 1347, 1427 Buenos Aires, Argentina.
**Hipolabor, Braz.** Hipolabor Farmaceutica Ltda, Rodovia BR-262 4600, 31950-640 Sabara, MG, Brazil.
**Hisamitsu, Braz.** Hisamitsu Farmaceutica do Brasil Ltda, Avenida Fagundes Filho 191, 04304-010 Sao Judas, Brazil.
**Hisamitsu, Jpn.** Hisamitsu Seiyaku, 408 Daikanmachi, Tashiro, Tosu, Saga 841-8686, Japan.
**Hisamitsu, Malaysia.** See *Sime Darby, Malaysia.*
**Hisamitsu, NZ.** See *Pharmaco, NZ.*
**Hishiyama, Thai.** See *Union Medical, Thai.*
**HK Pharma, UK.** HK Pharma Ltd, P.O. Box 105, Hitchin, Hertfordshire, SG5 2GG, UK.
**Hobein, Ger.** Dr. Hobein & Co. Nachf. GmbH Arzneimittel, Grenzstr. 2, 53340 Meckenheim, Germany.
**Hobein, Hong Kong.** See *Universal, Hong Kong.*
**Hobein, Malaysia.** Hobein, Malaysia.
**Hochstetter, Chile.** Laboratorios Hochstetter SA, Dardignac 6, Santiago, Chile.
**Hoe, Malaysia.** Hoe Pharmaceuticals Sdn Bhd, Lot 10, Jalan Sultan Mohamed 6, Bandar Sultan Suleiman, 42000 Pelabuhan Klang, Selangor, Malaysia.
**Hoe, Singapore.** See *Summit, Singapore.*
**Hoechst, Fr.** See *Aventis, Fr.*
**Hoechst, Ger.** See *Aventis, Ger.*
**Hoechst, Ital.** See *Aventis, Ital.*
**Hoechst Marion Roussel, Austria.** See *Aventis, Austria.*
**Hoechst Marion Roussel, Belg.** See *Aventis, Belg.*
**Hoechst Marion Roussel, Braz.** See *Aventis, Braz.*
**Hoechst Marion Roussel, Canad.** See *Aventis, Canad.*
**Hoechst Marion Roussel, Denm.** See *Aventis, Denm.*
**Hoechst Marion Roussel, Fin.** See *Aventis, Fin.*
**Hoechst Marion Roussel, Ger.** See *Aventis, Ger.*
**Hoechst Marion Roussel, Gr.** HOECHST-MARION ROUSSEL ABEE, Λ. Κηφισσίας 32, Μέγαρο Ατρινα, 151 10 Μαρούσι, Marousi, Greece.
**Hoechst Marion Roussel, Hong Kong.** See *Aventis, Hong Kong.*
**Hoechst Marion Roussel, Irl.** See *Aventis, Irl.*
**Hoechst Marion Roussel, Israel.** See *Aventis, Israel.*
**Hoechst Marion Roussel, Ital.** See *Aventis, Ital.*
**Hoechst Marion Roussel, Jpn.** See *Aventis, Jpn.*
**Hoechst Marion Roussel, Mex.** See *Aventis, Mex.*
**Hoechst Marion Roussel, Neth.** See *Aventis, Neth.*
**Hoechst Marion Roussel, Norw.** See *Aventis, Norw.*
**Hoechst Marion Roussel, S.Afr.** See *Aventis, S.Afr.*
**Hoechst Marion Roussel, Singapore.** See *Aventis, Singapore.*
**Hoechst Marion Roussel, Spain.** See *Aventis, Spain.*
**Hoechst Marion Roussel, Swed.** See *Aventis, Swed.*
**Hoechst Marion Roussel, Switz.** See *Aventis, Switz.*
**Hoechst Marion Roussel, Thai.** See *Aventis, Thai.*
**Hoechst Marion Roussel, USA.** See *Aventis, USA.*
**Hoeport, Port.** See *Aventis, Port.*
**Hoernecke, Ger.** Carl Hoernecke GmbH, Halberstadter Chaussee 22, 39116 Magdeburg, Germany.
**Hoeveler, Austria.** Hoeveler Mag. & Co. GmbH, Mosham 40, A-4943 Geinberg, Austria.
**Hofmann, Austria.** Hofmann Pharma GmbH & Co. KG, St Oswaldweg 20, A-5081 Anif, Austria.

**Hofmann & Sommer, Ger.** Hofmann & Sommer GmbH & Co. KG, Lindenstr. 11, 07426 Konigsee, Germany.

**Hogapharm, Switz.** Hogapharm AG, Unterdorf 8, 6403 Kussnacht am Rigi, Switzerland.

**Hogil, USA.** Hogil Pharmaceutical Corporation, 2 Manhattanville Rd, Purchase, NY 10577, USA.

**Hokuriku, Jpn.** Hokuriku Seiyaku Co. Ltd, 37-1-1 Inokuchi, Katsuyama, Fukui 911-8555, Japan.

**Holista, Canad.** Holista Health Corp, 70 Glacier St, Coquitlam, British Columbia, V3K 5Y9, Canada.

**Holistica, Fr.** Laboratoires Holistica International, 465 chemin des Jalassieres, 13510 Eguilles, France.

**Hollborn, Ger.** Dr K Hollborn & Sohne GmbH & Co. KG, Brahestr. 13, 04347 Leipzig, Germany.

**Hollister-Stier, USA.** See *Bayer, USA.*

**Holloway, USA.** Holloway Pharmaceuticals Inc., USA.

**Holsten, Ger.** Holsten Pharma GmbH, Im Burgerstock 7, 79241 Ihringen, Germany.

**Homberger, Switz.** Laboratoire du Dr E Homberger SA, 10 place du Bourg-de-Four, 1204 Geneva, Switzerland.

**Home, Ital.** Home Products Italiana S.p.A., Via Puccini 3, 20121 Milan, Italy.

**Home Diagnostics, USA.** Home Diagnostics Inc., 2300 NW 55th Court, Fort Lauderdale, FL 33309, USA.

**Homeocan, Canad.** Homeocan, 3025, boul. de l'Assomption, Montreal, Quebec, H1N 2H2, Canada.

**Homme de Fer, Fr.** Laboratoires de l'Homme de Fer, 2 pl. de l'Homme de Fer, 67000 Strasbourg, France.

**Hommel, Ger.** Hommel Pharma GmbH & Co. KG, Rohrkamp 26, 59348 Luedinghausen, Germany.

**Hong Kong Medical, Hong Kong.** Hong Kong Medical Supplies Ltd, 7/F China Aerospace Centre, 143 Hoi Bun Rd, Kwun Tong, Hong Kong.

**Hong Tai Hong, Hong Kong.** Hong Tai Hong, Rua de Almirante, Costa Cabral No 68, 1/F, Flat B, Edificio Sun Flat, Macau.

**Hong Wo, Hong Kong.** Hong Wo Trading Co., Unit 1, 9/F, Wayson Commercial Building, 28 Connaught Rd West, Hong Kong.

**Hope, USA.** Hope Pharmaceuticals, 8260 E Gelding Drive, Suite 104, Scottsdale, AZ 85260, USA.

**Hor-Fer-Vit, Ger.** HorFerVit Pharma GmbH, H.-Brockmann Str. 81, 26131 Oldenburg, Germany.

**Horizon, UK.** Horizon Lifecare Ltd, Millbank House, 171-185 Ewell Rd, Surbiton, Surrey, KT6 6AX, UK.

**Horizon, USA.** See *First Horizon, USA.*

**Hormel, Hong Kong.** See *JDH, Hong Kong.*

**Hormel, Singapore.** See *JDH, Singapore.*

**Hormona, Mex.** Laboratorios Hormona S.A. de C.V., Blvd. M. Avila Camacho No.470, Col. San Andres Atoto, 53500 Naucalpan de Juarez, Mexico.

**Hormonas, Mex.** See *Hormona, Mex.*

**Hormosan, Ger.** Hormosan-Kwizda GmbH, Wilhelmshoher Str. 106, 60389 Frankfurt/Main, Germany.

**Horner, Canad.** See *Carter Horner, Canad.*

**Hosbon, Spain.** Hosbon, Ronda General Mitre 72-74, 08017 Barcelona, Spain.

**Hospal, Denm.** See *Gambro, Denm.*

**Hotz, Ger.** See *Riemser, Ger.*

**Houghs Healthcare, UK.** Houghs Healthcare Ltd, UK.

**Hovid, Hong Kong.** See *Wellgo, Hong Kong.*

**Hovid, Malaysia.** Hovid Sdn Bhd, 121 Jalan Kuala Kangsar, 30010 Ipoh, Perak, Malaysia.

**Hovid, Singapore.** See *Goldplus, Singapore.*

**Howmedica, Spain.** Howmedica Iberica, Manuel Tovar 35, 28034 Madrid, Spain.

**Howmedica, Switz.** Howmedica Jaquet Orthopedie SA, Case postale 725, 1212 Grand-Lancy 1/GE, Switzerland.

**Hoyer, Ger.** Hoyer-Madaus GmbH & Co. KG, Alfred-Nobel-Str. 10, 40789 Monheim, Germany.

**HPC, Switz.** HPC Harras Pharma Curarina, Worbstrasse 221, 3073 Gumligen, Switzerland.

**HRA, Denm.** See *Nycomed, Denm.*

**HRA, Fr.** Laboratoires HRA Pharma, 19 rue Frederick-Lemaitre, 75020 Paris, France.

**HRA, Norw.** See *Nycomed, Norw.*

**HSL, NZ.** Health Support Ltd, P.O. Box 44 027, Point Chevalier, Auckland, New Zealand.

**Hua, Thai.** B L Hua & Co. Ltd, 2 Somdej Chaopraya Rd, Klongsan, Bangkok 10600, Thailand.

**Hubert, UK.** Hubert A.C. Thomas & Co., Copperworks Rd, New Dock, Llanelli, Dyfed, SA15 2EN, UK.

**Huckaby, USA.** Huckaby Pharmacal Inc., 11802 Brinley Ave, Suite 201, Louisville, KY 40243, USA.

**Hudson, USA.** Hudson Corp., 90 Orville Drive, Bohemia, NY 11716, USA.

**Hughes & Hughes, UK.** Hughes & Hughes Ltd, Unit 1F, Lowmoor Industrial Estate, Tonedale, Wellington, Somerset, TA21 0AZ, UK.

**Humana, Braz.** Humana, Brazil.

**Humana, Ital.** Humana Italia S.p.A., Via Boscovich 55, 20124 Milan, Italy.

**Hunter, Austral.** Stephen Hunter P/L, 18 Lancaster St, Ingleburn, NSW 2265, Australia.

**Husler, Switz.** Franz Hüsler AG, Pharmazeutische Praparate, Chriesbaumstrasse 2, 8604 Volketswil, Switzerland.

**HWS OTC, Austria.** HWS-OTC-Service GmbH, Steindorf 65, A-5570 Mauterndorf, Austria.

**Hyde, Canad.** Hyde Pharmaceuticals, 20 Lewis St, Fort Eire, Ontario, L2A 5M6, Canada.

**Hyland, Hong Kong.** See *Baxter, Hong Kong.*

**Hyland, USA.** See *Baxter-Hyland, USA.*

**Hylands, Canad.** Hylands, 381-A, route 139, Sutton, Quebec, J0E 2K0, Canada.

**Hypofarma, Braz.** Hypofarma - Inst. Hypodermia e Farmacia SA, Rua Doutor Irineu Marcellini 303, 33805-330 Ribeirao das Neves, MG, Brazil.

**Hypoguard, Irl.** See *Hypoguard, UK.*

**Hypoguard, UK.** Hypoguard (UK) Ltd, Dock Lane, Melton, Woodbridge, Suffolk, IP12 1PE, UK.

**Hyrex, USA.** Hyrex Pharmaceuticals, 3494 Democrat Rd, P.O. Box 18385, Memphis, TN 38118-0385, USA.

**I Farmacologia, Spain.** Instituto Farmacologia Española, Aragoneses 2, Alcobendas, 28108 Madrid, Spain.

**Iasis, Gr.** IASIS CHEMIPHARMA, Αγ. Κωνσταντίνου 40, 151 24 Μαρουσι, Marousi, Greece.

**Iatric, USA.** Iatric Corp, 2330 S Industrial Park Drive, Tempe, AZ 85282-1893, USA.

**Ibefar, Braz.** Ibefar Inst. Brasileiro de Esp. Ftcas. Ltda, Rua Franca Pinto 1357, 04016-035 Sao Paulo, Brazil.

**Ibfarma, Braz.** Ibfarma Industria de Biotecnologio Farm. Ltda, Via Aratu QD 10, Lote 01-CIA, 43700-000 Simoes Filho, BA, Brazil.

**Ibi, Ital.** Istituto Biochimico Italiano Giovanni Lorenzini S.p.A., Via Tucidide 56, Torre 6, 20134 Milan, Italy.

**IBI, Thai.** See *Siam Pharm, Thai.*

**Ibirn, Ital.** Istituto Bioterapico Nazionale S.r.l., Via V. Grassi 9/11/13/15, 00155 Rome, Italy.

**IBIS, UK.** IBIS Products, Stevenage, Hertfordshire, SG1 4QG, UK.

**IBN, Ital.** IBN Instituto Biologico Nazionale S.r.l., Via Cavour 11, 44022 Comacchio (FE), Italy.

**IBP, Ital.** Istituto Biochimico Pavese Pharma S.p.A., Viale Certosa 10, 27100 Pavia, Italy.

**IBSA, Hong Kong.** See *Mekim, Hong Kong,* and *Sincerity, Hong Kong.*

**IBSA, Ital.** Ibsa Farmaceutici Italia S.r.l., Viale Bianca Maria 33, 20122 Milan, Italy.

**IBSA, Switz.** Institut Biochimique SA, Via al Ponte 13, 6903 Lugano, Switzerland.

**Icaro, Spain.** See *AstraZeneca, Spain.*

**ICC, Israel.** See *Rekah, Israel.*

**Ichthyol, Austria.** See *Ichthyol, Ger.*

**Ichthyol, Ger.** Ichthyol-Gesellschaft Cordes, Hermanni & Co. (GmbH & Co.) KG, Sportallee 85, 22335 Hamburg, Germany.

**Ichthyol, Switz.** See *Medinova, Switz.*

**ICI, India.** ICI India Ltd, Ennore Express Highway, Ennore, Chennai 600 057, India.

**ICIM, Ital.** ICIM International S.r.l., Via Peloritana 28, 20024 Garbagnate Milanese (MI), Italy.

**ICN, Arg.** ICN ARG S.A.I.C. y F., Teodoro Vilardebo 2855/65, 1417 Buenos Aires, Argentina.

**ICN, Austral.** ICN Pharmaceuticals Australasia Pty Ltd, 85 Saint Hilliers Rd, Auburn, NSW 2144, Australia.

**ICN, Austria.** ICN Pharmaceuticals Austria GmbH, Michael-Pracher-Strasse 25A/7, A-5020 Salzburg, Austria.

**ICN, Braz.** ICN Farmaceutica Ltda, Rua F. Geraldo Gomez 61, andar 10, CEP 04575-060, SP, Brazil.

**ICN, Canad.** ICN Canada Ltd, 1956 Bourdon St, Montreal, Quebec, H4M 1V1, Canada.

**ICN, Denm.** See *Medilink, Denm.*

**ICN, Fin.** See *ICN, Neth.*

**ICN, Fr.** ICN Pharmaceuticals France SA, 4 rue Jean-Rostand, Parc Club, 91893 Orsay cdx, France.

**ICN, Ger.** ICN Pharmaceuticals Germany GmbH, Bolongarostr. 82-84, 65929 Frankfurt/Main, Germany.

**ICN, Hong Kong.** See *JDH, Hong Kong.*

**ICN, Irl.** See *Allphar, Irl.*

**ICN, Israel.** ICN, Israel.

**ICN, Ital.** ICN Pharmaceuticals Italy S.r.l., C. Dir. Milano 2, Pal. Canova, 20090 Segrate (MI), Italy.

**ICN, Malaysia.** See *JDH, Malaysia.*

**ICN, Mex.** ICN Farmaceutica S.A de C.V, Calzada Tlalpan 2021, 04040 Mexico D.F, Mexico.

**ICN, Neth.** ICN Pharmaceuticals Holland BV, Stephensonstraat 45, 2723 RM Zoetermeer, Netherlands.

**ICN, Norw.** See *Medilink, Denm.*

**ICN, NZ.** See *Pacific, NZ.*

**ICN, Port.** ICN Portugal Lda, Avenida Marechal Gomes da Costa 19, 1804-806 Lisbon, Portugal.

**ICN, Singapore.** See *JDH, Singapore.*

**ICN, Spain.** ICN Iberica, Casanova 27-31, Corbera de Llobregat, 08757 Barcelona, Spain.

**ICN, Switz.** ICN Pharmaceuticals Switzerland AG, Ruhrbergstrasse 21, 4127 Birsfelden, Switzerland.

**ICN, Thai.** See *Diethelm, Thai.*

**ICN, UK.** ICN Pharmaceuticals Ltd, Cedarwood, Chineham Business Park, Crockford Lane, Basingstoke, Hampshire, RG24 8WG, UK.

**ICN, USA.** ICN Pharmaceuticals Inc., ICN Plaza, 3300 Hyland Ave, Costa Mesa, CA 92626, USA.

**Ico, Ital.** Ico Spa, Via Ferrarese 156/8, 40128 Bologna, Italy.

**ICT, Ital.** Istituto Chemioterapico S.p.A., Strada Bobbiese 108, 29100 Piacenza, Italy.

**Ideal, Fr.** Ideal, 65 rue Alexandre-Dumas, B.P. 53, 69513 Vaulx-en-Velin cdx, France.

**Ideal Health, UK.** Ideal Health Group Ltd, The Common, Potten End, Berkhamstead, Hertfordshire, HP4 2QF, UK.

**IDEC, USA.** IDEC Pharmaceuticals Corp., 11011 Torreyana Rd, San Diego, CA 92121, USA.

**Ideco, Ital.** Ideco Srl, Via L Braille 18, 39100 Bolzano, Italy.

**Iderne, Fr.** Laboratoires Michel Iderne, Parc d'activites Rosenmeer, 67560 Rosheim, France.

**IDI, Ital.** IDI Farmaceutici S.p.A., Via dei Castelli Romani 83/85, 00040 Pomezia (Rome), Italy.

**IDIS, UK.** IDIS World Medicines, 171-185 Ewell Rd, Surbiton, Surrey, KT6 6AX, UK.

**Ido, Fr.** Laboratoires Ido, 13 rue Commines, 75003 Paris, France.

**Iema, Ital.** Iema S.r.l., Via Adelasio 33, 24020 Ranica (BG), Italy.

**IFET (ΙΦΕΤ), Gr.** Ι.Φ.Ε.Τ., 18ο χλμ. Λ. Μαραθώνος, 153 44 Παλλήνη, Pallini, Greece.

**IFI, Ital.** Istituto Farmacoterapico Italiano S.p.A., Via Paolo Frisi 23, 00197 Rome, Italy.

**Ifidesa Aristegui, Spain.** Ifidesa Aristegui, Alameda de Urquijo 27 1, Bilbao, 48008 Vizcaya, Spain.

**Ifusa, Mex.** Laboratorios Ifusa S.A., Francisco Lorenzana Num. 20, Col. San Rafael, Deleg. Cuauhtemoc, 06470 Mexico D.F., Mexico.

**IG, Malaysia.** See *Medidata, Malaysia,* and *Pharmaniaga, Malaysia.*

**Igefarma, Braz.** See *Theraskin, Braz.*

**Iketon, Ital.** Iketon Farmaceutici S.r.l., Via Cassanese 224, 20090 Segrate (MI), Italy.

**Illa, Ger.** ILLA Healthcare GmbH, Burgermeister-Seidl-Str. 8, 82515 Wolfratshausen, Germany.

**IMA, Braz.** Instituto de Medicamentos e Alergia IMA Ltda, Rua Araujo Leitao 193, 20715-310 Rio de Janeiro, RJ, Brazil.

**I-Med, Canad.** I-Med Pharma Inc., 3869 Sources Blvd, Suite 200, Dollard des Ormeaux, Quebec, H9B 2A2, Canada.

**Imeks, Malaysia.** Imeks Pharma Sdn Bhd, 2 Jln 6/33B, MWE Commercial Park Kepong, 52000 Kuala Lumpur, Wilaya Persekutuan, Malaysia.

**Immodal, Austria.** Immodal Pharmaka GmbH, Bundesstrasse 44, A-6111 Volders, Austria.

**Immunex, USA.** Immunex Corp., 51 University St, Seattle, WA 98101, USA.

**Immuno, Austria.** See *Baxter, Austria.*

**Immuno, Belg.** See *Baxter, Belg.*

**Immuno, Braz.** Immuno Prod. Biologicos e Quimicos Ltda, Rua Adolfo Lutz 82, 22451-120 Rio de Janeiro, RJ, Brazil.

**Immuno, Canad.** See *Baxter, Canad.*

**Immuno, Fr.** See *Baxter, Fr.*

**Immuno, Ger.** See *Baxter BioScience, Ger.*

**Immuno, Hong Kong.** See *Mekim, Hong Kong.*

**Immuno, Irl.** See *Allphar, Irl.*

**Immuno, Israel.** See *Teva, Israel.*

**Immuno, Ital.** See *Baxter, Ital.*

**Immuno, Spain.** See *Baxter, Spain.*

**Immuno, Switz.** See *Baxter, Switz.*

**Immuno, UK.** See *Baxter, UK.*

**Immuno, USA.** See *Baxter-Hyland, USA.*

**Immunomedics, UK.** Immunomedics, UK.

**Immunomedics, USA.** Immunomedics, 300 American Rd, Morris Plains, NJ 07950, USA.

**Immunotec, Canad.** Immunotec Research, 292 Adrien-Patenaude, Vaudreuil-Dorion, Quebec, J7V 5V5, Canada.

**Immunotec, USA.** See *Immunotec, Canad.*

**IMO, Ital.** Istituto di Medicina Omeopatica S.p.A., Via Vincenzo Monti 6, 20123 Milan, Italy.

**Imperial, Malaysia.** See *Unam, Malaysia.*

**Imperial, Singapore.** See *Far East, Singapore.*

**Impharm, UK.** Impharm Nationwide Ltd, Valley House, Britannia Business Park, Union Rd, Bolton, Lancashire, BL2 2HP, UK.

**Implementos Plasticos, Mex.** Implementos Plasticos S.A., Mar de Kara Num. 14, Col. Popotla, Deleg. Miguel Hidalgo, 11400 Mexico DF, Mexico.

**IMS, Ital.** International Medical Service S.r.l., Via Lauretina 169, 00040 Pomezia (RM), Italy.

**IMS, USA.** See *Celltech, USA.*

**Imtix, Belg.** See *Imtix, Fr.*

**Imtix, Denm.** See *Sangstat, Neth.*

**Imtix, Fr.** Imtix-SangStat, 58 av Debourg, B.P. 7055, 69348 Lyon cdx 07, France.

**Imtix, Ger.** Imtix SangStat GmbH, Hockenheimer Str. 6, 69775 Ketsch, Germany.

**Imtix, Ital.** IMTIX-Sangstat S.r.l., Via Winckelmann 2, 20146 Milan, Italy.

**Imtix, Neth.** See *Sangstat, Neth.*

**Imtix, Spain.** Imtix Sangstat, Conte de Urgell 143, 08036 Barcelona, Spain.

**Imtix, Switz.** See *Pro Vaccine, Switz.*

**Imtix Sangstat, Israel.** See *Medison, Israel.*

**Imvi, Arg.** Lab. Imvi S.A. (Div. Humana), Olazabal 1665/71, 1428 Buenos Aires, Argentina.

**Inaf, Braz.** See *Eurofarma, Braz.*

**InAgra, USA.** InAgra, USA.

**Inamed, Singapore.** See *Pharmacon, Singapore.*

**Inava, Fr.** See *Pierre Fabre, Fr.*

**Incaico, Arg.** Lab. Incaico, Montiel 156, 1408 Buenos Aires, Argentina.

**Incomex, Mon.** Incomex, 9 av. Saint-Michel, MC 98000, Monaco.

**Indeco, Arg.** Laboratorio Indeco S.A., Jose Marmol 1924, 1602 Florida, Buenos Aires, Argentina.

**Indevus, USA.** Indevus Pharmaceuticals Inc., 99 Hayden Ave, Suite 200, Lexington, MA 02421, USA.

**Indian Drugs, India.** Indian Drugs & Pharmaceuticals Ltd, IDPL Complex, Dundahera, Delhi-Gurgaon Rd, Gurgaon 122 001, India.

**Indochina Healthcare, Thai.** Indochina Healthcare Ltd, 23 Fl Olympia Thai Tower, 444 Ratchadapisek Rd, Samsennok Huay Kwang, Bangkok 10320, Thailand.

**Indoco, India.** Indoco Remedies Ltd, Indoco House, 166 CST Rd, Santacruz (East), Mumbai 400 098, India.

**Indoco, Thai.** See *Union Medical, Thai.*

**Indrugco, Singapore.** Indrugco Pte Ltd, 221 Henderson Rd, 07-20 Henderson Building, S 159557, Singapore.

**Inexfa, Spain.** Inexfa, Ctra Nacional 340, Km 28, Orihuela, 03300 Alicante, Spain.

**Infabra, Braz.** Infabra Industria Farmaceutica Brasileira Ltda, Rua Conselheiro Mayrink 365, Jacare, 20960-140 Rio de Janeiro, RJ, Brazil.

**Infan, Mex.** Laboratorios Infan, S.A. de C.V., Calz de Tlalpan No. 4515, Col Toriello Guerra, 14050 Mexico D.F., Mexico.

**Infar, India.** Infar (India) Ltd, 38 J L Nehru Rd, Kolkata 700 071, India.

**Infar, Port.** Infar, Lda, Estrada de circunvalacao, Rameiras, Alges, 1495 Lisbon, Portugal.

**Infectopharm, Ger.** Infectopharm Arzneimittel und Consilium GmbH, Von-Humboldt-Str. 1, 64646 Heppenheim, Germany.

**Infirmarius-Rovit, Ger.** Pharmazeutische Fabrik Infirmarius-Rovit GmbH, Eislinger Str. 66, 73084 Salach, Germany.

**Infosint, Ital.** Infosint S.p.A., C. Dir. Colleoni, Pal. Pegaso 2, 20041 Agrate Brianza (MI), Italy.

**Infosint, Switz.** Infosint SA, 7744 Campocologno, Switzerland.

**Inga, India.** Inga Laboratories Pvt Ltd, Mahakali Rd, Andheri East, Mumbai 400 093, India.

**Inga, Malaysia.** See *Pahang, Malaysia.*

**Ingens, Arg.** Laboratorios Ingens S.A., Arcos 2646, 1428 Buenos Aires, Argentina.

**Ingram & Bell, Canad.** Ingram & Bell Inc., 20 Bond Ave, Don Mills, Ontario, M3B 1L9, Canada.

**Inibsa, Port.** Laboratórios Inibsa, SA, Sintra Business Park, Zona Industrial da Abrunheira, Edificio 1 - 2, 2710-089 Sintra, Portugal.

**Inibsa, Spain.** Inibsa, Ctra Sabadell Granollers Km 14.5, Llissa de Vall, 08185 Barcelona, Spain.

**Inkeysa, Spain.** Inkeysa, Juan XXIII 15, Esplugas de Llobregat, 08950 Barcelona, Spain.

**Inkine, USA.** InKine Pharmaceutical Company Inc., 1787 Sentry Pkwy, West Bldg 18, Suite 440, Blue Bell, PA 19422, USA.

**Inmunolab, Arg.** Inmunolab S.A., Avalos 782, 1427 Buenos Aires, Argentina.

**Innoledge, Hong Kong.** Innoledge International Ltd, 31 Mau Po Village, Clear Water Bay, Hong Kong.

**Innomed, Singapore.** Innomed, Singapore.

**Innotech, Fr.** Laboratoires Innotech International, Sté du groupe Innothéra, 7-9 av Francois-Vincent-Raspail, B.P. 32, 94111 Arcueil cdx, France.

**Innotech, Hong Kong.** See *Wing Wai, Hong Kong.*

**Innotech, Port.** See *Confar, Port.*

**Innotech, Singapore.** See *Indrugco, Singapore.*

**Innothera, Denm.** See *Meda, Denm.*

**Innothera, Fr.** Sté du groupe Innothéra Industries, 7-9 av Francois-Vincent-Raspail, B.P. 35, 94111 Arcueil cdx, France.

**Innothera, Norw.** See *Meda, Norw.*

**Innova, Ital.** See *Recordati, Ital.*

**Innovatec, Singapore.** See *MBD, Singapore.*

**InnoVisions, USA.** Innovisions Inc., USA.

**INO Therapeutics, Spain.** INO Therapeutics, Genova 17, 02800 Madrid, Spain.

**INO Therapeutics, USA.** INO Therapeutics Inc., 6th State Route 173, Clinton, NJ 08809, USA.

**Inova, Ger.** Inova-Global GbR H & S Klein, Kaiserstr. 127, 51145 Cologne, Germany.

**Inpa, Gr.** INPA AE, Πλ. Συντριβανίου 4, 546 21 Θεσσαλονίκη, Thessaloniki, Greece.

**Inpharma, Fin.** See *Oriola, Fin.*

**Inpharzam, Hong Kong.** See *Universal, Hong Kong.*

**Inpharzam, Switz.** Inpharzam AG, PO Box 200, 6814 Cadempino, Switzerland.

**INQ, Braz.** Instituto Nacional de Quimioterapia Ltda, Rua Antonio Foster 85, 04760-040 Sao Paulo, SP, Brazil.

**Instituto Farmacologico, Spain.** Instituto Farmacologico Español, Ramallosa-Teo, Santiago de Compostela, 15883 A Coruna, Spain.

**Intas, India.** Intas Pharmaceuticals Ltd, Chinubhai Center, Off Nehru Bridge, Ashram Rd, Ahmedabad -80 009, India.

**Intas, Thai.** See *Union Medical, Thai.*

**Integrity, USA.** Integrity Pharmaceutical Corp., 9084 Technology Drive, Fishers, IN 46038, USA.

**Interbelle, Arg.** Interbelle Cosmetic S.A., Sanabria 2353 Piso 1, 1417 Buenos Aires, Argentina.

**Intercare, Irl.** See *Mayrs, Irl.*

**Intercare, NZ.** InterCare Corp. Ltd, P.O. Box 18446, Glen Innes, Auckland, New Zealand.

**Intercare, UK.** Intercare Products Ltd, UK.

**Interdelta, Switz.** Interdelta SA, Case postale 460, 1701 Fribourg, Switzerland.

**Interfarma, Ital.** Interfarma Farmaceutici S.r.l., Via Vivaldi 16, 35030 Selvazzano Dentro (PD), Italy.

**Interferon Sciences, USA.** Interferon Sciences Inc., 783 Jersey Ave., New Brunswick, NJ 08901-3660, USA.

**Interlab, Braz.** Interlab, Brazil.

**Interlogim, Neth.** Interlogim Pharma Service BV, Beeldschermweg 6B, 3821 AH Amersfoort, Netherlands.

**Intermedica, Switz.** Intermedica SA, Pharmazeutische Produkte, Boulevard de Perolles 17, Case postale 238, 1701 Fribourg, Switzerland.

**Intermuti, Ger.** intermuti pharma GmbH, Alfred-Nobel-Str. 10, 40789 Monheim, Germany.

**International Dermatologicals, Canad.** International Dermatologicals Inc., 1940 Lonsdale Ave, Suite 217A, Vancouver, British Columbia, V7M 2K2, Canada.

**International Ethical, USA.** International Ethical Labs, Reparto Metropolitano, Rio Piedras, PR 00921, USA.

**International Lab Tech, USA.** International Laboratory Technology Corp, 3389 Sheridan St, Suite 149, Hollywood, FL 33021, USA.

**International Medical, Hong Kong.** International Medical Co. Ltd, Unit 715, 7/F, Block B, Seaview Estate, 2-8 Watson Rd, North Point, Hong Kong.

**International Pharmaceuticals, Thai.** International Pharmaceuticals Ltd, 38/2 Sukhumvit 63 (Soi Ekamal), Kwaeng Prakanong Nua, Khet Wattana, Bangkok 10110, Thailand.

**Interpharm, Austria.** Interpharm GmbH, Effingergasse 21, A-1160 Vienna, Austria.

**Interpharma, Spain.** Interpharma, Santa Rosa 6, Santa Coloma de Gramanet, 08921 Barcelona, Spain.

**Intersan, Ger.** Intersan GmbH, Einsteinstr. 30, 76275 Ettlingen, Germany.

**Intersan, Switz.** See *Uhlmann-Eyraud, Switz.*

**Intersero, Ger.** Intersero GmbH, Am Klingenweg 13, 65396 Walluf, Germany.

**INTES, Ital.** See *Alfa Intes, Ital.*

**Intra Pharma, Irl.** Intra Pharma Ltd, IntraVeno House, 86 Broomhill Road, Tallaght, Dublin 24, Ireland.

**Intramed, S.Afr.** Intramed, South Africa.

**Intrapharm, Irl.** See *United Drug, Irl.*

**Intrapharm, UK.** Intrapharm Laboratories Ltd, 60 Boughton Lane, Maidstone, Kent, ME15 9QS, UK.

**Intsel, Fr.** Laboratoires Intsel Chimos, Technopolis, 145 rue J.-J. Rousseau, 92138 Issy-les-Moulineaux cdx, France.

**Invamed, USA.** See *Geneva, USA.*

**Inverdia, Swed.** Inverdia AB, Vretenvagen 8, 171 54 Solna, Sweden.

**Inverness Medical, Austral.** Inverness Medical Asia Pacific Pty Ltd., 14 Orange Grove Mall, Windsor St, Richmond, NSW 2753, Australia.

**Inverni della Beffa, Ital.** See *Sanofi Synthelabo, Ital.*

**Invest Impex, Israel.** Invest Impex Ltd, 24 Hametzuda St, Azur 58001, Israel.

**Investi, Arg.** Lab. Investi Farma S.A., Lisandro de la Torre 2160, 1440 Buenos Aires, Argentina.

**Investigacion, Mex.** Investigacion Farmaceutica (IFA) S.A. de C.V, Calle 13-E No. 5 CIVAC, 62500 Jiutepec Mor., Mexico.

**Investigaciones Filosoficas y Cientificas, Mex.** Investigaciones Filosoficas y Cientificas S.A. de C.V., Tlacote No. 128, 76230 Juriquilla, Qro, Mexico.

**Invicta, Irl.** See *Pfizer, Irl.*

**Inwood, USA.** Inwood Laboratories, 321 Prospect St, Inwood, NY 11096, USA.

**Iocom, UK.** Iocom (UK) Ltd, Hope Mill, Skipton Rd, Barnoldswick, Lancashire, BB18 6EN, UK.

**Iodo Suma, Braz.** Laboratorio Iodo Suma Ltda, Rua Maximiliano Fraga 35, 36880-000 Muriae, MG, Brazil.

**Iodosan, Ital.** See *GlaxoSmithKline Consumer, Ital.*

**Iolab, Israel.** See *Concept, Israel.*

**Iolab, USA.** See *Bausch & Lomb, USA,* and *Ciba Vision, USA.*

**Ioltech, Fr.** Laboratoires Ioltech, av. Paul-Langevin, B.P. 5, 17053 La Rochelle cdx 9, France.

**Iomed, Hong Kong.** See *Pan-Well, Hong Kong.*

**Iomed, USA.** Iomed Laboratories, Inc., 2441 S 3850 W, Suite A, Salt lake City, UT 84120, USA.

**Ion, USA.** Ion Laboratories Inc., 7431 Pebble Drive, Fort Worth, TX 76118, USA.

**Ionios (Ιονιος), Gr.** ΙΟΝΙΟΣ ΦΑΡΜΑΚΕΥΤΙΚΗ ΕΠΕ, Σαραντaπήχου 15-17, 114 71 Αθήνα, Athens, Greece.

**Iopharm, USA.** Iopharm, 7549 Pebble Dr, Ft Worth, TX 76118, USA.

**Ioquin, Austral.** See *Alcon, Austral.*

**IPA, Ital.** International Pharmaceuticals Associated S.r.l., Via del Casale Cavallari 53, 00156 Rome, Italy.

**Ipca, India.** Ipca Laboratories Ltd, 63-E Kandivli Industrial Estate, Kandivli (W), Mumbai 400 067, India.

**IPCA, Singapore.** See *Zyfas, Singapore.*

**Ipex, Austria.** See *Ipex, Swed.*

**Ipex, Fin.** See *Tamro, Fin.*

**Ipex, Ger.** See *Ipex, Swed.*

**Ipex, Norw.** See *Ipex, Swed.*

**Ipex, Swed.** Ipex Medical AB, Box 120, 182 12 Danderyd, Sweden.

**IPFI, Ital.** IPFI Industria Farmaceutica S.r.l., Via Egadi 7, 20144 Milan, Italy.

**IPG, Ger.** IPG Pharm GmbH, Schenkendorfstr. 17, 22085 Hamburg, Germany.

**Iphym, Fr.** Laboratoires Iphym, chemin de la Sereine, 01700 Beynost, France.

**IPI, Port.** I.P.I. Portugal Lda, Av. de Berne No 30-4 B, 1050-042 Lisbon, Portugal.

**IPRAD, Fr.** Laboratoires IPRAD, 42-52 rue de l'Aqueduc, 75010 Paris, France.

**IPRAD-Sante, Fr.** IPRAD-Santé, 221 rue Lafayette, 75010 Paris, France.

**IPS, Neth.** IPS, Beeldschermweg 6b, 3821 AH Amersfoort, Netherlands.

**IPS, Spain.** IPS Farma, Sagasta 21, 28004 Madrid, Spain.

**Ipsen, Austral.** Ipsen Pty Ltd, Suite 42, Waverley Business Centre, 21 Aristoc Rd, Glen Waverley, VIC 3150, Australia.

**Ipsen, Austria.** See *Ipsen, Ger.*

**Ipsen, Belg.** Ipsen S.A., Maaltecenter Blok A, Derbystraat 201, 9051 Sint-Denijs-Westrem, Belgium.

**Ipsen, Denm.** Ipsen Scandinavia A/S, Park Alle 292, 2605 Brondby, Denmark.

**Ipsen, Fin.** See *Ipsen, Denm.*

**Ipsen, Ger.** Ipsen Pharma GmbH, Einsteinstr. 30, 76275 Ettlingen, Germany.

**Ipsen, Gr.** IPSEN ΕΠΕ, Π. Μαρινοπούλου 7, 174 56 Άλιμος, Alimos, Greece.

**Ipsen, Hong Kong.** See *JDH, Hong Kong.*

**Ipsen, Irl.** Ipsen Pharmaceuticals Ltd, 7 Upper Leeson St, Dublin 4, Ireland.

**Ipsen, Israel.** See *Medison, Israel.*

**Ipsen, Ital.** Ipsen S.p.A., Via A Figino 16, 20156 Milan, Italy.

**Ipsen, Norw.** See *Ipsen, Denm.*

**Ipsen, NZ.** See *NZ Medical & Scientific, NZ.*

**Ipsen, Port.** Ipsen Portugal, SA, Rua General Ferreira Martins, Edificio Eca de Queiroz 8-9B, Miraflores, 1495-137 Alges, Portugal.

**Ipsen, Spain.** Ipsen Pharma, Ctra Laurea Miro 395, Sant Feliu de Llobregat, 08980 Barcelona, Spain.

**Ipsen, Swed.** See *Ipsen, Denm.*

**Ipsen, Switz.** See *Salmon, Switz.,* and *Uhlmann-Eyraud, Switz.*

**Ipsen, UK.** Ipsen Ltd, 190 Bath Road, Slough, Berkshire, SL1 3XE, UK.

**Ipsen Biotech, Fr.** See *Beaufour, Fr.*

**Ipso, Ital.** Ipso-Pharma S.r.l., Via San Rocco 6, 85033 Episcopia (PZ), Italy.

**IQB, Braz.** Instituto de Quimica e Biologia S.A., Rua A 20, 24140-210 Niteroi, RJ, Brazil.

**IQFA, Mex.** Industrias Quimico Farmaceuticas Americanas S.A. de C.V., Lago Peypus No. 215, Col. Anahuac, Deleg. Miguel Hidalgo, 11320 Mexico D.F., Mexico.

**Iqfasa, Mex.** See *IQFA, Mex.*

**Iquinosa, Spain.** Iquinosa, Alpedrete 24, 28045 Madrid, Spain.

**IRBI, Ital.** See *Wyeth Lederle, Ital.*

**Irex, Fr.** Laboratoires Irex, Groupe Sanofi-Synthelabo, 11 rue Salomon-de-Rothschild, 92150 Suresnes, France.

**Irex, Port.** Irex Lda, Edificio Fernao de Magalhaes (Q 43), Quinta da Fonte, Lote 7-C, r/c Esq., Porto Salvo, 2780-730 Paco de Arcos, Portugal.

**Irisfarma, Spain.** See *Lilly, Spain.*

**Irmed, Ital.** Istituto Ricerche Mediche S.r.l., Via della Consortia 17, 37127 Verona-Avesa, Italy.

**Iromedica, Switz.** Iromedica AG, Haggenstrasse 45, 9014 St Gallen, Switzerland.

**ISA, Arg.** Instituto Seroterapico Argentino S.A.I.C., Larrazabal 1848, 1440 Buenos Aires, Argentina.

**Isdin, Port.** Isdin Lda, Rua da Ilha dos Amores, Lote 4.08.01,X, Parque das Nacoes - Zona Norte, Santa Maria dos Olivais, 1990-118 Lisbon, Portugal.

**Isdin, Spain.** Isdin, Av. Diagonal 520, 08006 Barcelona, Spain.

**ISF, Ital.** ISF S.p.A., Via Tiburtina 1040, 00156 Rome, Italy.

**ISI, Ital.** See *Kedrion, Ital.*

**Isis, Fr.** Laboratoires Isis, 13 rue de Montholon, 01005 Bourg-en-Bresse, France.

**Isis, UK.** Isis Products Ltd, Gough Lane, Bamber Bridge, Preston, Lancashire, PR5 6AQ, UK.

**Isis Puren, Ger.** See *Alpharma-Isis, Ger.*

**Islacan, Spain.** Islacan, Ctra General San Lorenzo 119, Las Palmas de Gran Canaria, 35018 Gran Canaria, Spain.

**ISM, Ital.** Ist. Sieroterapico Milanese S. Belfanti, Via Darwin 22, 20143 Milan, Italy.

**Iso, Ger.** Iso-Arzneimittel GmbH & Co. KG, Bunsenstr. 6-10, 76275 Ettlingen, Germany.

**Isomed, Spain.** Isomed, Alberto Alcocer 46 Bajo B, 28016 Madrid, Spain.

**Isopharm, Hong Kong.** See *CNW, Hong Kong.*

**Isramedcom, Israel.** Isramedcom Ltd, 1 Ha'omanut St, Poleg Industrial Park, Netanya 42504, Israel.

**Ist. Chim. Inter., Ital.** Istituto Chimico Internazionale Dr. Giuseppe Rende S.r.l., Via Salaria 1240, 00138 Rome, Italy.

**Istoria, Ital.** Istoria Farmaceutici S.p.A., Riviera Francia 3/A, 35127 Padua, Italy.

**Itaca, Braz.** Itaca Laboratorios Ltda, Rua das Oficinas 182, Engenho de Dentro, 20770-010 Rio de Janeiro, RJ, Brazil.

**Italchimici, Ital.** Italchimici S.p.A., Via Pontina Km 29000, No 5, 00040 Pomezia (RM), Italy.

**Italfar, Ital.** Italfar S.r.l., Via Matteotti 16, 00040 Pomezia (RM), Italy.

**Italfarmacia, Ital.** Italfarmacia S.r.l., P.zza Cesare De Cupis 15, 00155 Rome, Italy.

**Italfarmaco, Ital.** Italfarmaco S.p.A., Viale Fulvio Testi 330, 20126 Milan, Italy.

**Italfarmaco, Spain.** Italfarmaco, San Rafael 3, Alcobendas, 28100 Madrid, Spain.

**Italmex, Mex.** Italmex S.A., Calz. de Tlalpan Num. 3218, Col. Ejido Santa Ursula Coapa, Deleg. Coyoacan, 04910 Mexico D.F., Mexico.

**Italzama, Ital.** Italzama, Via Leonardo da Vinci 75, 00016 Monterotondo Scalo (RM), Italy.

**ITF, Chile.** Lab. ITF Farma Chile SA, Encomenderos 161, Of. 3 B, Las Condes, Santiago, Chile.

**ITF, Gr.** I.T.F. HELLAS AE, Αγαμέμνονος 13, 155 61 Χολαργός, Cholargos, Greece.

**ITF, Port.** ITF, Lda, Rua Consiglieri Pedroso no 123, Queluz de Baixo, 2745-557 Barcarena, Portugal.

**Ivamed, Ger.** IVAmed Arzneimittel GmbH, Brauereistr., 68723 Plankstadt, Germany.

**Ivax, Hong Kong.** Ivax Asia Ltd, Unit 3301, Hopewell Ctr, Wanchai, Hong Kong.

**Ivax, Irl.** IVAX Ireland, Unit 301, Waterford Industrial Estate, Waterford, Ireland.

**Ivax, Mex.** Ivax Pharmaceuticals Mexico S.A. de C.V., Calz de Tlalpan No. 3007, Col. Sta. Ursula Coapa (Pueblo), Deleg. Coyoacan, 04650 Mexico D.F., Mexico.

**Ivax, Singapore.** See *FP, Singapore,* and *Green Cross, Singapore.*

**Ivax, Swed.** IVAX Scandinavia AB, Box 386, 111 73 Stockholm, Sweden.

**Ivax, UK.** IVAX Pharmaceuticals UK Ltd, IVAX Quays, Albert Basin, Royal Docks, London, E16 2QJ, UK.

**Ivax, USA.** Ivax Corp., 4400 Biscayne Bvld, Miami, FL 33137, USA.

**Ivex, UK.** Ivex Pharmaceuticals, Division of the Galen Group, Old Belfast Rd, Millbrook, Larne, Co. Antrim, BT40 2SH, UK.

**IVF, Switz.** IVF Hartmann AG, 8212 Neuhausen am Rheinfall, Switzerland.

**IVP, Ital.** Istituto Vaccinogeno Pozzi S.p.A., Via Petriccio 27, 53100 Siena, Italy.

**Ivy Corp, USA.** Ivy Corporation, 23 Fairfield Pl., W. Caldwell, NJ 07006, USA.

**IXL, UK.** IXL Pharma Ltd, Manor House, Victors Barns, Brixworth, Northamptonshire, NN6 9DQ, UK.

**Jaapharm, Canad.** Jaapharm, 200 Trowers Rd, Unit 1, Woodbridge, Ontario, L4L 5Z7, Canada.

**Jaba, Port.** Jaba Farmacêutica, SA, Rua da Tapada Grande No. 2, Abrunheira, 2710-089 Sintra, Portugal.

**Jacobs, UK.** Jacobs Bakery Ltd, Long Lane, Aintree, Liverpool, Merseyside, L9 7BQ, UK.

**Jacobson, Hong Kong.** Jacobson Medical (Hong Kong) Ltd, 15/F China Trade Ctr, 122-124 Wai Yip St, Kwun Tong, Kowloon, Hong Kong.

**Jacobus, USA.** Jacobus Pharmaceutical Co. Inc., 37 Cleveland Lane, P.O. Box 5290, Princeton, NJ 08540, USA.

**Jacoby, Austria.** Jacoby Pharmazeutika AG, Teichweg 2, A-5400 Hallein-Kaltenhausen, Austria.

**Jagson, India.** Jagson Pal Pharmaceuticals Ltd, P.O. Box 4545, New Delhi 110 049, India.

**Jaldes, Fr.** Laboratoires Jaldes, 10 ac de Poussan, B.P. 30, 34770 Gigean cdx, France.

**Jamieson, Canad.** Jamieson Laboratories, 4025 Rhodes Drive, Windsor, Ontario, N8W 5B5, Canada.

**Jamieson, Hong Kong.** See *Universal, Hong Kong.*

**Janpharm, S.Afr.** Janpharm (Pty) Ltd, 15th Rd, Halfway House 1685, S. Africa.

**Janssen, Braz.** See *Janssen-Cilag, Braz.*

**Janssen, Hong Kong.** Janssen Pharmaceutica, Unit 1302-1307, Tower 1, Grand Century Place, 193 Prince Edward Rd West, Mongkok, Kowloon, Hong Kong.

**Janssen, Jpn.** Janssen-Kyowa Co. Ltd., Takanawadai Daiichi-Seimei Bldg. 1-5, Higashi-Gotanda 3-chome, Shinagawa-ku, Tokyo 141-8633, Japan.

**Janssen, Mex.** See *Janssen-Cilag, Mex.*

**Janssen, Thai.** See *Janssen-Cilag, Thai.*

**Janssen, USA.** Janssen Pharmaceutical Inc., 1125 Trenton-Harbourton Road, P.O. Box 200, Titusville, NJ 08560-0200, USA.

**Janssen-Cilag, Arg.** Janssen-Cilag Farmaceutica S.A., Mendoza 1259, 1428 Buenos Aires, Argentina.

**Janssen-Cilag, Austral.** Janssen-Cilag P/L, Locked Bag 2070, North Ryde, NSW 1670, Australia.

**Janssen-Cilag, Austria.** Janssen-Cilag Pharma Vertrieb GmbH, Pfarrgasse 75, A-1232 Vienna, Austria.

**Janssen-Cilag, Belg.** Janssen-Cilag S.A., Roderveldlaan 1, 2600 Berchem, Belgium.

**Janssen-Cilag, Braz.** Janssen-Cilag Farmaceutica Ltda, Av.das Nacoes Unidas 12992, 29 andar, 04578-000 Sao Paulo, SP, Brazil.

**Janssen-Cilag, Chile.** See *Grunenthal, Chile.*

**Janssen-Cilag, Denm.** Janssen-Cilag A/S, Hammerbakken 19, 3460 Birkerod, Denmark.

**Janssen-Cilag, Fin.** Janssen-Cilag Oy, Metsänneidonkuja 8, 02130 Espoo, Finland.

**Janssen-Cilag, Fr.** Janssen-Cilag SA, 1 rue Camille-Desmoulins, 92787 Issy-les-Moulineaux cdx 9, France.

**Janssen-Cilag, Ger.** Janssen-Cilag GmbH, Raiffeisenstr. 8, 41470 Neuss, Germany.

**Janssen-Cilag, Gr.** JANSSEN-CILAG AEBE, Λ. Ειρήνης 56, 151 21 Πεύκη, Pevki, Greece.

**Janssen-Cilag, India.** Janssen-Cilag, India.

**Janssen-Cilag, Irl.** Janssen-Cilag Ltd, Little Island, County Cork, Ireland.

**Janssen-Cilag, Israel.** Janssen Cilag, Division of J-C Health Care Ltd, Kibbutz Shefayim 60990, Israel.

**Janssen-Cilag, Ital.** Janssen-Cilag S.p.A., Via Michelangelo Buonarroti 23, 20093 Cologno Monzese (MI), Italy.

**Janssen-Cilag, Malaysia.** See *Zuellig, Malaysia.*

**Janssen-Cilag, Mex.** Janssen Cilag S.A. de C.V., Canoa No. 79, Col. Tizapan, San Angel, 01090 Mexico D.F., Mexico.

**Janssen-Cilag, Neth.** Janssen-Cilag BV, Dr. Paul Janssenweg 150, 5026 RH Tilburg, Netherlands.

**Janssen-Cilag, Norw.** Janssen-Cilag AS, Hoffsveien 1 D, 0275 Oslo, Norway.

**Janssen-Cilag, NZ.** Janssen-Cilag Pty Ltd, P.O. Box 9222, Newmarket, Auckland, New Zealand.

**Janssen-Cilag, Port.** Janssen Cilag Farmacêutica, Lda, Rue Consiglieri Pedroso 69 A/B, Queluz de Baixo, 2745 Bacarena, Portugal.

**Janssen-Cilag, S.Afr.** Janssen-Cilag (Pty) Ltd, P.O. Box 785939, Sandton 2146, South Africa.

**Janssen-Cilag, Singapore.** Janssen-Cilag, A Division of Johnson & Johnson Pte Ltd, 3 International Rd, Jurong, S 619619, Singapore.

**Janssen-Cilag, Spain.** Janssen-Cilag, Paseo de las Doce Estrellas 5-7, Campo de Naciones, 28042 Madrid, Spain.

**Janssen-Cilag, Swed.** Janssen-Cilag AB, Box 7073, 192 07 Sollentuna, Sweden.

**Janssen-Cilag, Switz.** Janssen-Cilag AG, Sihlbruggstrasse 111, 6341 Baar, Switzerland.

**Janssen-Cilag, Thai.** Janssen-Cilag Ltd, 1550 Grand Amarin Tower, 11th Floor, New Petchburi Road, Makasan, Rachtevee, Bangkok 10310, Thailand.

**Janssen-Cilag, UK.** Janssen-Cilag Ltd, P.O. Box 79, Saunderton, High Wycombe, Buckinghamshire, HP14 4HJ, UK.

**Janssen-Kyowa, Jpn.** See *Janssen, Jpn.*

**Janssen-Ortho, Canad.** Janssen-Ortho Inc., 19 Green Belt Drive, Toronto, Ontario, M3C 1L9, Canada.

**Japan Tobacco, Jpn.** Japan Tobacco Inc., 2-2-1 Toranomon, Minato-ku, Tokyo 105-8422, Japan.

**Jauntal, Austria.** Jauntal-Apotheke, Bleiburger Strasse 16, A-9141 Eberndorf, Austria.

**JAV, Thai.** J.A.V. Pharmar Co. Ltd, 1848 soi Jaransabitwong, 65 Jaransanitwong Rd, Bangbamru, Bangplad, Bangkok 10700, Thailand.

**JB Williams, USA.** J. B. Williams Co. Inc., 65 Harriston Road, Glen Rock, NJ 07452-3317, USA.

**JC Healthcare, Ital.** See *Janssen-Cilag, Ital.*

**JCP, Canad.** JCP Laboratories Inc., P.O. Box 403, St-Martin Branch, Laval, QC, H7S 2A4, Canada.

**JDH, Hong Kong.** JDH (Hong Kong) Ltd, 14/F, LiFung Ctr, 2 On Ping St, Siu Lek Yuen, Shatin, N.T., Hong Kong.

**JDH, Malaysia.** JDH Pharmaceutical Sdn Bhd, LiFung Centre, Lot 6, Persiaran Perusahaan Seksyen 23, Kawasan Perusahaan Shah Alam, 40300 Shah Alam, Selangor, Malaysia.

**JDH, Singapore.** JDH Pharmaceutical Division, 279 Jalan Ahmad Ibrahim, 03-01, S 639938, Singapore.

**JDH Borneo, Thai.** JDH Borneo (Thailand) Ltd, 2160/1 Ramkhamhaeng Rd, Hua Mark, Bangkapi, Bangkok 10240, Thailand.

**JE IL, Singapore.** See *Pharmaforte, Singapore.*

**Jean-Marie, Hong Kong.** Jean-Marie Pharmacal Co. Ltd, 1/F, 12 Dai Fu St, Tai Po Industrial Estate, Tai Po, N.T., Hong Kong.

**Jean-Marie, Singapore.** See *Grafton, Singapore.*

**Jebsen, Hong Kong.** Jebsen & Co. Ltd, 12/F, Scomber Bldg, 1 Yip Fat St, Wong Chuk Hang, Hong Kong.

**Jenapharm, Ger.** Jenapharm GmbH & Co. KG, Otto-Schott-Str. 15, 07745 Jena, Germany.

**Jenapharm, Hong Kong.** See *Jacobson, Hong Kong.*

**Jenapharm, Malaysia.** See *Imeks, Malaysia.*

**Jenapharm, Thai.** See *Berli, Thai.*

**Jergens, Canad.** Jergens Canada Ltd, 5805 Whittle Rd, Unit 6, Mississauga, Ontario, L4Z 2J1, Canada.

**Jergens, USA.** Andrew Jergens Co., 2535 Spring Grove Ave, Cincinnati, OH 45214, USA.

**Jessel, Fr.** Laboratoires Jessel-Végébom SA, 59 av. d'Iena, 75116 Paris, France.

**Jessup, UK.** Jessup Marketing, 27 Old Gloucester St, London, WC1N 3XX, UK.

**JHC Healthcare, UK.** JHC Healthcare Ltd, The Maltings, Bridge St, Hitchin, Hertfordshire, SG5 2DE, UK.

**Jin Yang, Hong Kong.** See *Health Care, Hong Kong.*

**J&J-Merck, USA.** J&J Merck Consumer Pharmaceuticals, Camp Hill Rd, Ft Washington, PA 19034, USA.

**JMI, USA.** See *Jones, USA.*

**Jodquellen, Ger.** Jodquellen AG, Ludwigstr. 14, 83646 Bad Tolz, Germany.

**Jofadel, Braz.** Jofadel Ind. Farmaceutica S.A., Av. Jose da Frota Vasconcelos 100, 37062-500 Varginha, MG, Brazil.

**Jofrain, Mex.** Establecimientos Jofrain S.A. de C.V., Calzada de Tlalpan 2621, 04610 Mexico D.F., Mexico.

**Johanser, Ger.** St. Johanser Naturmittelvertrieb GmbH, Starnberger Str. 15, 82131 Gauting, Germany.

**John Wyeth, India.** See *Wyeth Lederle, India.*

**Johnson, Canad.** S.C. Johnson and Son Ltd, 1 Webster St, P.O. Box 250, Brantford, Ontario, N3T 5R1, Canada.

**Johnson & Johnson, Arg.** Johnson & Johnson de Argentina S.A.C. e I., Avda. Madero 900 Piso 3, 1106 Buenos Aires, Argentina.

**Johnson & Johnson, Austral.** Johnson & Johnson Medical P/L, P.O. Box 134, North Ryde, NSW 2113, Australia.

**Johnson & Johnson, Austria.** Johnson & Johnson GmbH, Weisslhofweg 9, A-5400 Hallein, Austria.

**Johnson & Johnson, Braz.** Johnson e Johnson Industria e Comercio Ltda, Rua Gerivativa 207, 05501-900 Sao Paulo, SP, Brazil.

**Johnson & Johnson, Canad.** Johnson & Johnson/Merck Consumer Pharmaceuticals of Canada, 890 Woodlawn Rd W, Guelph, Ontario, N1K 1A5, Canada.

**Johnson & Johnson, Fr.** See *Ethicon, Fr.*

**Johnson & Johnson, Ger.** See *Ethicon, Ger.*

**Johnson & Johnson, Hong Kong.** See *Jacobson, Hong Kong.*

**Johnson & Johnson, Irl.** Johnson & Johnson (Ireland) Ltd, Belgard Rd, Tallaght, Dublin 24, Ireland.

**Johnson & Johnson, Israel.** Johnson & Johnson, Kibbutz Shefayim, Israel.

**Johnson & Johnson, Ital.** Johnson & Johnson Divisione Farmacia S.p.A., 00040 S. Palomba, Pomezia (Rome), Italy.

**Johnson & Johnson, NZ.** Johnson & Johnson (NZ) Ltd, P.O. Box 97-027, Wiri, South Auckland, New Zealand.

**Johnson & Johnson, Port.** Johnson & Johnson, Lda, Estrada Consiglieri Pedroso 69 A, Queluz de Baixo, 2745-555 Barcarena, Portugal.

**Johnson & Johnson, Singapore.** See *Diethelm, Singapore.*

**Johnson & Johnson, Spain.** Johnson Johnson, Ctra Madrid-Valencia Km 24.7, Arganda del Rey, 28500 Madrid, Spain.

**Johnson & Johnson, Swed.** Johnson & Johnson AB, Staffansvag 2, 191 84 Sollentuna, Sweden.

**Johnson & Johnson, Switz.** See *Uhlmann-Eyraud, Switz.*

**Johnson & Johnson, Thai.** Johnson & Johnson (Thailand) Co. Ltd, 106 Moo 4 Lat Krabang, Industrial Estate, Chalongkrung Rd, Lumplatew, Lat Krabang, Bangkok 10520, Thailand.

**Johnson & Johnson, UK.** Johnson & Johnson Ltd, Foundation Park, Rocksborough Way, Maidenhead, Berkshire, SL6 3UG, UK.

**Johnson & Johnson, USA.** Johnson & Johnson Consumer Products Co., 199 Grandview Rd, Skillman, NJ 08558-9418, USA.

**Johnson & Johnson Consumer, Belg.** Johnson & Johnson Consumer S.A., Rue de la Grenouillette 2 E, 1130 Brussels, Belgium.

**Johnson & Johnson Medical, Arg.** Johnson & Johnson Medical S.A., Monsenor Magliano 3061, 1642 San Isidro, Buenos Aires, Argentina.

**Johnson & Johnson Medical, Fr.** See *Ethicon, Fr.*

**Johnson & Johnson Medical, UK.** Johnson & Johnson Medical, Coronation Rd, Ascot, Berkshire, SL5 9EY, UK.

**Johnson & Johnson Medical, USA.** Johnson & Johnson Medical Inc., P.O. Box 90130, Arlington, TX 76004-0130, USA.

**Johnson & Johnson MSD Consumer, UK.** Johnson & Johnson MSD Consumer Pharmaceuticals, Enterprise House, Station Rd, Loudwater, High Wycombe, Buckinghamshire, HP10 9UF, UK.

**Johnson Wax, USA.** S.C. Johnson Wax, 1525 Howe St, Racine, WI 53403-5011, USA.

**Jolly-Jatel, Fr.** Laboratoires Jolly-Jatel, 28 av. Carnot, 78100 Saint-Germain-en-Laye, France.

**Jones, USA.** Jones Pharma Inc., 501 5th St, Bristol, TN 37620, USA.

**Jorba, Spain.** Jorba, Josefa Valcarcel 30, 28027 Madrid, Spain.

**Jouveinal, Canad.** Jouveinal Inc., 3339 Griffith St, St Laurent, Quebec, H4T 1W5, Canada.

**Jouveinal, Fr.** Laboratoires Jouveinal, 1 rue des Moissons, B.P. 100, 94265 Fresnes cdx, France.

**Jukunda, Ger.** Jukunda Naturarzneimittel Dr Ludwig Schmitt GmbH & Co. KG, Hofmarkstr. 35, 82152 Planegg, Germany.

**Julphar, UAE.** Gulf Pharmaceutical Industries, Julphar, P.O. Box 997, Ras Al Khaimah, United Arab Emirates.

**Juste, Spain.** Juste, Julio Camba 7, 28028 Madrid, Spain.

**Justesa Imagem, Braz.** Justesa Imagem, Brazil.

**Justesa Imagen, Arg.** Justesa Imagen Argentina S.A., Viamonte 1328 Piso 9, 1053 Buenos Aires, Argentina.

**Juventus, Spain.** Juventus, Julian Camarillo 37, 2873 Madrid, Spain.

**Juvex, Fr.** Laboratoires Juvex, B.P. 11, 36110 Levroux, France.

**Kabi, Swed.** See *Pharmacia, Swed.*

**Kabi Pharmacia, Israel.** See *Promedico, Israel.*

**Kabi Pharmacia, NZ.** See *Pharmacia, NZ.*

**Kabi Pharmacia, USA.** See *Pharmacia, USA.*

**KabiVitrum, UK.** See *Pharmacia, UK.*

**Kabivitrum, USA.** See *Pharmacia, USA.*

**Kade, Ger.** Dr Kade Pharmazeutische Fabrik GmbH, Rigistr. 2, 12277 Berlin, Germany.

**Kade, Hong Kong.** Kade, Hong Kong.

**Kai Cheong, Hong Kong.** Kai Cheong Medical Co Ltd, Unit 1001, Tower 1, Harbour Ctr, 1 Hok Cheung St, Hunghom, Kowloon, Hong Kong.

**Kai Yuen, Hong Kong.** Kai Yuen Pharmaceuticals Co., 8/F Ngai Wong Commercial Bldg, 11-13 Mongkok Rd, Kowloon, Hong Kong.

**Kaken, Hong Kong.** See *Hing Ah, Hong Kong.*

**Kaken, Jpn.** Kaken Pharmaceutical Co. Ltd, 2-28-8 Honkomagome, Bunkyo-ku, Tokyo 113-8650, Japan.

**Kaketsuken, Thai.** See *Berli, Thai.*

**Kalbe, Singapore.** See *Apotheca, Singapore,* and *Sime Darby, Singapore.*

**Kamada, Israel.** Kamada Ltd, Kiryat Weizmann, Rehovot, Israel.

**Kamp, Arg.** Distribuidor Kamp S.R.L., Diagonal Norte 825 Piso 4 of.45, 1035 Buenos Aires, Argentina.

**Kampel Martian, Arg.** Lab. Kampel Martian S.A., Av. del Libertador 6550, 5 piso, 1428 Buenos Aires, Argentina.

**Kanda, Braz.** Kanda Industria Farmaceutica Ltda, Rodovia BR 262 Km 12.3 A, 33010-970 Santa Luzia, MG, Brazil.

**Kanebo, Jpn.** Kanebo Ltd, 3-20-20 Kaigan, Minato-ku, Tokyo 108-8080, Japan.

**Kanion, Israel.** See *Chemipal, Israel.*

**Kanoldt, Ger.** Kanoldt Arzneimittel GmbH, Karl-Zeiss-Ring 3, 85737 Ismaning, Germany.

**Kappa, Fr.** Laboratoires Kappa Biotech, ZI Albasud, 82000 Montauban, France.

**Karicare, NZ.** See *Nutricia, NZ.*

**Karrer, Ger.** Hans Karrer GmbH, Messerschmittring 54, 86343 Konigsbrunn, Germany.

**Kart, Switz.** Laboratoires Kart SA, En Budron A 16, 1052 Le Mont-sur-Lausanne, Switzerland.

**Katadyn, Switz.** Katadyn Produkte AG, Wasseraufbereitung, Birkenweg 4, 8304 Wallisellen, Switzerland.

**Kato, Singapore.** See *JDH, Singapore.*

**Katsoupas, Gr.** Ch. Katsoupas (Ant. Kouskos O.E.), 48 Socratous Str., 104 31 Αθήνα, Athens, Greece.

**Kattwiga, Ger.** Pharm. Fabrik Kattwiga GmbH, Zur Grenze 30, 48529 Nordhorn, Germany.

**Kay, Canad.** Mary Kay Cosmetics Ltd, 2020 Meadowvale Blvd, Mississauga, Ontario, L5N 6Y2, Canada.

**Kayaku, Jpn.** Nippon Kayaku Co. Ltd, 1-11-2 Fujimi, Chiyoda-ku, Tokyo 102-8172, Japan.

**Kayaku, Malaysia.** See *JDH, Malaysia.*

**Kayaku, Singapore.** See *JDH, Singapore.*

**KBR, Ital.** K.B.R. S.r.l. Kroton Biologic Researches, Corso Vittorio Emanuele 73, 88074 Crotone (KR), Italy.

**Kedrion, Ital.** Kedrion S.p.A., 55020 Castelvecchio Pascoli (LU), Italy.

**Kee, India.** Kee Pharma Ltd, A-1 Community Centre, Naraina Industrial Area, Phase II, New Delhi 110028, India.

**Keene, USA.** Keene Pharmaceuticals Inc., P.O. Box 7, Keene, TX 76059-0007, USA.

**Kelemata, Ital.** Kelemata S.p.A., Via S Quintino 28, 10121 Turin, Italy.

**Keller, Austral.** Edward Keller Australia Pty Ltd, P.O. Box 888, Hallam, VIC 3803, Australia.

**Keller, Hong Kong.** Edward Keller Ltd, 21/F Southmark, 11 Yip Hing St, Wong Chuk Hang, Hong Kong.

**Kemifarma, Denm.** Kemifarma Holdings ApS, Jaegersborg Alle 51, 2920 Charlottenlund, Denmark.

**Kemiflor, Swed.** Kemiflor AB, Box 7245, 103 89 Stockholm, Sweden.

**Kemiprogress, Ital.** Kemiprogress S.r.l., Via Aurelia 58, 00165 Rome, Italy.

**Kemopharm, Thai.** Kemopharm Thailand Co. Ltd, 138 Soi Indamara 18, Vibhavadi Rangsit Rd, Bangkok 10400, Thailand.

**Kemyos, Ital.** Kemyos Biomedical Research S.r.l., Via Tre Cannelle 12, 00040 Pomezia (RM), Italy.

**Kendall, USA.** Kendall Health Care Products, 15 Hampshire St, Mansfield, MA 02048, USA.

**Kendall McGaw, USA.** See *Braun, USA.*

**Kendon, UK.** Kendon International Ltd, 8-14 Orsman Rd, London, N1 5QJ, UK.

**Kendrick, Mex.** Laboratorios Kendrick, S.A., Paseo de los Laureles No. 458-205, Col. Bosques de las Lomas, Deleg. Cuajimalpa, 05120 Mexico D.F., Mexico.

**Kener, Mex.** Laboratorios Kener S.A. de C.V., Calderon de la Barca No. 27, Col. Polanc, Deleg. Miduel Hidalgo, 11560 Mexico D.F, Mexico.

**Kenfarma, Spain.** Kenfarma, Ctra de Rubi 90-100, Sant Cugat del Valles, 28002 Barcelona, Spain.

**Kenral, Austral.** See *Pharmacia, Austral.*

**Kenral, Canad.** See *Altimed, Canad.*

**Kent, UK.** Kent Pharmaceuticals Ltd, Wotton Rd, Ashford, Kent, TN23 6LL, UK.

**Kenwood, Hong Kong.** See *International Medical, Hong Kong.*

**Kenwood, USA.** See *Doak, USA.*

**Kenyaku, Thai.** See *Asian TJD, Thai.,* and *Schumit, Thai.*

**Kerapharm, Fr.** Kerapharm, 123 bureaux dela Colline, 92213 St-Cloud cdx, France.

**Kerifarm, Spain.** Kerifarm, Spain.

**Kern, Spain.** Kern Pharma, Venus 72, Pol Ind Colon II, Terrassa, 08228 Barcelona, Spain.

**Kern, Switz.** E Kern AG, Pharmazeutische Krauterspezialitaten, Hauptstrasse 23, 8867 Niederurnen, Switzerland.

**Keryos, Ital.** Keryos SpA, P.zza della Repubblica 28, 20124 Milan, Italy.

**Kestrel, UK.** Kestrel Healthcare Ltd, Network House, Basing View, Basingstoke, Hampshire, RG21 4HG, UK.

**Keton, Mex.** Laboratorios Keton de Mexico S.A. de C.V., Lago Xochimilco No. 65, Col. Anahuac, Deleg. Miguel Hidalgo, 11320 Mexico D.F., Mexico.

**Key, Arg.** Key Pharma S.A., Av. San Martmn 1750, 1602 Florida, Buenos Aires, Argentina.

**Key, Austral.** Key Pharmaceuticals P/L, P.O. Box 121, Concord West, NSW 2138, Australia.

**Key, Canad.** See *Schering, Canad.*

**Key, Chile.** Key Company SA, Panamericana Norte 5369, Santiago, Chile.

**Key, Israel.** See *Luxembourg, Israel.*

**Key, Spain.** Key Pharma, P Castellana 143, 28046 Madrid, Spain.

**Key, USA.** See *Schering-Plough, USA.*

**Keyerson, Mex.** Casa Keyerson S.A. de C.V., Calzada del hueso 160, Ej. Sta.Ursula Coapa, 04850 Mexico D.F., Mexico.

**KG, Ital.** KG Italia S.r.l., Via Volturno 10/12, 50019 Sesto Fiorentino (FI), Italy.

**Khandelwal, India.** Khandelwal Laboratories Ltd, 79/87 D. Lad Path, Mumbai 400 033, India.

**Khol, Braz.** Khol, Brazil.

**Kin, Spain.** Kin, Granada 123, 08018 Barcelona, Spain.

**Kinder, Braz.** Laboratorio Kinder S.A., Rua VPR 1 Quadra 2-A, Modulo 5 DAIA, 75133-600 Anapolis, GO, Brazil.

**King, Irl.** King Pharmaceuticals Ltd, Donegal St, Ballybofey, County Donegal, Ireland.

**King, UK.** See *King, Irl.*

**King, USA.** King Pharmaceuticals Inc., 501 Fifth St, Bristol, TN 37620, USA.

**Kingswood, USA.** Kingswood Laboratories Inc., 10375 Hague Rd, Indianapolis, IN 46256, USA.

**Kinsmor, Canad.** Kinsmor Pharmaceuticals Canada Inc., 210 Binnington Court, Kingston, Ontario, K7M 8R6, Canada.

**Kirby, Arg.** See *Schering-Plough, Arg.*

**Kirin, Jpn.** Kirin Brewery Co. Ltd, Pharmaceutical Division, 6-26-1 Jingu-mae, Shibuya-ku, Tokyo 150-8011, Japan.

**Kirkman, USA.** Kirkman Labs Inc., 6400 SW Rosewood, Lake Oswego, OR 97035, USA.

**Kissei, Jpn.** Kissei Pharmaceutical Co. Ltd, 19-48 Yoshino, Matsumoto, Nagano 399-8710, Japan.

**Kite (Κιτε), Gr.** ΚΙΤΕ ΕΛΛΑΣ ΕΠΕ, Λ. Ιωανίας 166, 111 44 Κ. Πατησια, K. Patisia, Greece.

**Kivema, Israel.** Kivema Ltd, 33 Hachoresh St, Kfar Shmaryahu 46910, Israel.

**Kiwi, USA.** Kiwi Brands, Inc., 447 Old Swede Rd, Douglassville, PA 19518-1239, USA.

**KK, UK.** KK Toiletries Ltd, 2 Westgate, Skelmersdale, Lancashire, WN8 8AZ, UK.

**Klein, Ger.** Dr Gustav Klein, Steinenfeld 3, 77736 Zell am Harmersbach, Germany.

**Klemenz, Ger.** Klemenz GmbH, Hermann-Burkhardt-Str. 3, 72793 Pfullingen, Germany.

**Kleva, Gr.** KLEVA ΕΠΕ, Πάρνηθος 189, 136 71 Αχαρνές, Acharnes, Greece.

**Klever, Ger.** F. W. Klever GmbH, Hauptstr. 20, 84168 Aham/Ndb., Germany.

**KLI, USA.** KLI Corp., 1119 Third Ave SW, Carmel, IN 46032, USA.

**Klinge, Austria.** Klinge Pharma GmbH, Hietzinger Hauptstrasse 64, A-1132 Vienna, Austria.

**Klinge, Ger.** See *Fujisawa, Ger.*

**Klinge, Irl.** Klinge Pharmaceuticals & Co., The Mews, James Place, Dublin 2, Ireland.

**Klinge, Switz.** Klinge Pharma AG, Bachstrasse 10, 8280 Kreuzlingen, Switzerland.

**Klinger, Braz.** Laboratorios Klinger, Rua Assahy 45, Rudge Ramos, 09633-010 Sao Bernardo do Campo, SP, Brazil.

**Klonal, Arg.** Lab. Klonal, Lamadrid esq. T. de Alvear, 1878 Quilmes, Buenos Aires, Argentina.

**Kloster, S.Afr.** Kloster Pharmaceuticals (Pty) Ltd, P.O. Box 2734, Paarl 7620, South Africa.

**Klosterfrau, Austria.** Maria Clementine Martin Klosterfrau GmbH, Doerenkampgasse 11, A-1105 Vienna, Austria.

**Klosterfrau, Ger.** Maria Clementine Martin Klosterfrau Vertriebsgesellschaft mbH, 50606 Cologne, Germany.

**Klus, Switz.** Klus-Apotheke, F & Dr J Fröhlich-Decurtins, Hegibachstrasse 102, 8032 Zurich, Switzerland.

**Kneipp, Austria.** See *Kneipp, Ger.*

**Kneipp, Ger.** Kneipp-Werke, 97064 Wurzburg, Germany.

**Kneipp, Switz.** Kneipp (Schweiz) GmbH, Schwarzackerstrasse 2, 8304 Wallisellen, Switzerland.

**Knoll, Austral.** See *Abbott, Austral.*

**Knoll, Belg.** See *Abbott, Belg.*

**Knoll, Braz.** Knoll Produtos Quimicos e Farmaceuticos Ltda, Estrada dos Bandeirantes 2400, 27710-104 Rio de Janeiro, RJ, Brazil.

**Knoll, Canad.** See *Abbott, Canad.*

**Knoll, Fin.** See *Abbott, Fin.*

**Knoll, Fr.** See *Abbott, Fr.*

**Knoll, Ger.** See *Abbott, Ger.*

**Knoll, Hong Kong.** Knoll China, Division of BASF China Ltd, Tower 1, 9/F South Seas Ctr, 75 Mody Rd, Tsimshatsui East, Kowloon, Hong Kong.

**Knoll, India.** See *Abbott, India.*

**Knoll, Irl.** See *Knoll, UK.*

**Knoll, Ital.** See *Abbott, Ital.*

**Knoll, Mex.** Quimica Knoll de Mexico S.A. de C.V., La Candelaria No.186, Col. Atlantida, Deleg. Coyoacan, 04370 Mexico D.F., Mexico.

**Knoll, Neth.** Knoll BV, Hettenheuvelweg 41-43, 1101 BM Amsterdam, Netherlands.

**Knoll, Norw.** See *Knoll, Swed.*

**Knoll, Port.** Knoll Lusitana, Lda, Rua Alfredo da Silva 3 C/D, 1300-040 Lisbon, Portugal.

**Knoll, S.Afr.** Knoll Pharmaceuticals (SA) (Pty) Ltd, P.O. Box 3030, Halfway House 1685, South Africa.

**Knoll, Singapore.** See *Boots, Singapore,* and *Diethelm, Singapore.*

**Knoll, Spain.** See *Abbott, Spain.*

**Knoll, Swed.** See *Abbott, Swed.*

**Knoll, Switz.** See *Abbott, Switz.*

**Knoll, Thai.** See *Pacific, Thai.*

**Knoll, UK.** Knoll Ltd, 9 Castle Quay, Castle Boulevard, Nottingham, Nottinghamshire, NG7 1FW, UK.

**Knoll, USA.** See *Abbott, USA.*

**Knop, Chile.** Laboratorio Esp. Med. Knop Ltda, Av. Lib. Bdo. O'higgins 1671, Santiago, Chile.

**Kobayashi, Thai.** See *Charoen, Thai.*

**Koch, Austria.** Edmund Koch, Biol. Heilmittel, Herrenstrasse 2, A-4010 Linz, Austria.

**Kodak, USA.** Kodak Dental, 343 State St, Rochester, NY 14650, USA.

**Kohler, Austria.** Dr Köhler Pharma GmbH, Steckhovengasse 17, A-1130 Vienna, Austria.

**Kohler, Ger.** Dr Franz Köhler Chemie GmbH, Neue Bergstr. 3-7, 64665 Alsbach-Hahnlein, Germany.

**Kohler-Pharma, Ger.** Köhler Pharma GmbH, Neue Bergstr. 3-7, 64665 Alsbach, Germany.

**Kolassa, Austria.** Dr. Kolassa & Merz GmbH, Gastgebgasse 5-13, A-1230 Vienna, Austria.

**Kollerics, Austria.** Kollerics Helmut, Hauptstrasse 25, A-8061 St Radegund, Austria.

**Kolynos, Braz.** Kolynos do Brasil Ltda, Rua Rio Grande 752, 04018-002 Sao Paulo, Brazil.

**Komedic, Malaysia.** Komedic Sdn Bhd, 4 Jln PJS 11/14, Bandar Sunway, 46150 Petaling Jaya, Selangor, Malaysia.

**Kondon, USA.** Kondon Manufacturing, Croswell, MI 48422, USA.

**Koni-Cofarm, Chile.** Laboratorio Koni-Cofarm SA, Crescente Errazuriz 2077, Nunoa, Santiago, Chile.

**Konsyl, Israel.** See *Pharmateam, Israel.*

**Konsyl, USA.** Konsyl Pharmaceuticals, 4200 South Hulen, Suite 513, Fort Worth, TX 76109, USA.

**Kopkins, Braz.** Kopkins do Brasil Industria Ltda, Rua Borja Reis 279, 20745-100 Rio de Janeiro, RJ, Brazil.

**Kora, Irl.** KoRa Healthcare, Frans Maas House, Swords Business Park, Swords, Co. Dublin, Ireland.

**Korangi, Port.** Korangi S.A., Parque Empresarial Primovel Edificio A1, r/c Albarraque, 2635-595 Rio de Mouro, Portugal.

**Korea Pharma, Singapore.** See *Pharma 2000, Singapore,* and *Pharmaforte, Singapore.*

**Korea United, Singapore.** See *Kyowa, Singapore,* and *Ziwell, Singapore.*

**Korean Drug, Singapore.** See *Ziwell, Singapore.*

**Korean United, Malaysia.** See *Kyowa, Malaysia.*

**Korhispana, Spain.** Korhispana, PSJ Can Politic 17 3, Hospitalet de Llobregat, 08907 Barcelona, Spain.

**KOS, USA.** Kos Pharmaceutics Inc., 2 Oakwood Blvd, Suite 140, Hollywood, FL 33020, USA.

**Kotra, Malaysia.** Kotra Pharma (M) Sdn Bhd, No. 1 Jln TTC 12, Cheng Industrial Estate, 75250 Melaka, Melaka, Malaysia.

**Kotsopoulos (Κωτσοπουλος), Gr.** ΚΩΤΣΟΠΟΥΛΟΣ, Αριστοτέλους 11-15, 104 32 Αθήνα, Athens, Greece.

**Kottas-Heldenberg, Austria.** Kottas-Heldenberg Mag. R.u. Sohn, Bauernmarkt 24, A-1014 Vienna, Austria.

**Kowa, Jpn.** Kowa Co. Ltd, 3-4-14 Nihonbashi-Honcho, Chuo-ku, Tokyo 103-8433, Japan.

**Kramer, Switz.** Kramer Pharma AG, 46 ave des Boveresses, 1000 Lausanne 21, Switzerland.

**Kramer, USA.** Kramer Laboratories Inc., 8778 SW 8th St, Miami, FL 33174-9990, USA.

**Kreussler, Denm.** See *Felo, Denm.*

**Kreussler, Fin.** See *Tamro, Fin.*

**Kreussler, Fr.** Laboratoire Kreussler Pharma, 2 rue de la Haye, Le Dome, B.P. 10901, 95731 Roissy-Charles-de-Gaulle cdx, France.

**Kreussler, Ger.** Chemische Fabrik Kreussler & Co. GmbH, Rheingaustr. 87-93, 65203 Wiesbaden, Germany.

**Kreussler, Switz.** See *Globopharm, Switz.*

**Kreussler, Thai.** See *Berlin Pharm, Thai.*

**Krewel, Ger.** Krewel Meuselbach GmbH, Krewelstr. 2, 53783 Eitorf, Germany.

**Krewel, Switz.** See *Lubapharm, Switz.*

**KRKA, Singapore.** See *Uni, Singapore.*

**Kropf, Switz.** Dr A & M Kropf-Schenk, Apotheke & Laboratorium,, Promenade, 3780 Gstaad, Switzerland.

**Krugher, Ital.** See *KG, Ital.*

**Krugmann, Ger.** See *Mundipharma, Ger.*

**KSL, Canad.** KSL Laboratories, 117-260 West Esplanade, North Vancouver, British Columbia, V7M 3G7, Canada.

**Kuhnil, Singapore.** See *Pharmaforte, Singapore.*

**Kunzle, Switz.** Krauterpfarrer Kunzle AG, 6648 Minusio, Switzerland.

**Kur und Stadtapotheke, Austria.** Kur- und Stadtapotheke, Oberer Stadtplatz 5, A-6060 Hall in Tirol, Austria.

**Kuraray, Jpn.** Kuraray Co. Ltd, Shin-Hankyu Bldg, 1-12-39 Umeda, Kita-ku, Osaka 530-8611, Japan.

**KV, Hong Kong.** See *Hind Wing, Hong Kong.*

**Kwizda, Austria.** F. Joh. Kwizda, Effingergasse 21, A-1160 Vienna, Austria.

**Kyorin, Jpn.** Kyorin Pharmaceutical Co. Ltd, 2-5 Kanda-Surugadai, Chiyoda-ku, Tokyo 101-8311, Japan.

**Kyorin, Thai.** Kyorin.

**Kyowa, Hong Kong.** See *Tai Tong, Hong Kong.*

**Kyowa, Jpn.** Kyowa Hakko Kogyo Co. Ltd, 1-6-1 Ohtemachi, Chiyoda-ku, Tokyo 100-8185, Japan.

**Kyowa, Malaysia.** Kyowa Hakko (Malaysia) Sdn Bhd, 20 Jln SS 19/5, 47500 Subang Jaya, Selangor, Malaysia.

**Kyowa, Singapore.** Kyowa Hakko Industry (S) Pte Ltd, 300 Orchard Rd, The Heeren 12-04, S 238855, Singapore.

**Kyowa, Thai.** Kyowa Hakko (Thailand) Ltd, 101/11 Srinakarin Rd, Suanluang, Bangkok 10250, Thailand.

**Kyowa, UK.** Kyowa Hakko (UK) Ltd, 258 Bath Rd, Slough, Berkshire, SL1 4DX, UK.

**Kytta, Ger.** See *Wyeth, Ger.*

**LA, Arg.** Lab. Austral S.A., Av. Olascoaga 951, 8300 Neuquen, Argentina.

**Lab, Port.** Laboratórios Lab, Lda, Rua Escola de Medicina Veterinaria 15-17, 1049-029 Lisbon, Portugal.

**Lab Francais du Fractionnement, Fr.** Lab Francais du Fractionnement et des Biotechnologies, 3 av des Tropiques, B.P. 305, Les Ulis, 91958 Courtaboeuf cdx, France.

**Labatec, Switz.** Labatec-Pharma SA, Case postale 62, 31 rue du Cardinal-Journet, 1217 Meyrin 2, Switzerland.

**Labcatal, Canad.** Labcatal Inc., 3750 East Cremazie Blvd, Suite 408, Montreal, Quebec, H2A 1B6, Canada.

**Labcatal, Fr.** Laboratoires Labcatal, 7 rue Roger-Salengro, B.P. 305, 92541 Montrouge cdx, France.

**Labcatal, Switz.** See *Oligosol, Switz.*

**Labesfal, Port.** Labesfal, SA, Campo de Besteiros, 3465-051 Campo de Besteiros, Portugal.

**Labima, Belg.** Labima S.A., Ave Van Volxem 328, 1190 Brussels, Belgium.

**Labinca, Arg.** Labinca S.A., Cramer 4130, 1429 Buenos Aires, Argentina.

**Labitec, Spain.** Labitec, Lope de Rueda 46, 28009 Madrid, Spain.

**Labocean, Fr.** Laboratoires Labocean, ZI de Kerjean, 56500 Locmine, France.

**Labocor, Port.** Labocor, Lda, Largo Cidade de Vittoria 7, 2750 Cascais, Portugal.

**Labomed, Chile.** Instituto Farmaceutico Labomed SA, Lira 278, Santiago, Chile.

**Laboratories for Applied Biology, Hong Kong.** See *Swiss Worldwide, Hong Kong.*

**Laboratories for Applied Biology, Irl.** See *Boileau & Boyd, Irl.*

**Laboratories for Applied Biology, Malaysia.** See *Sime Darby, Malaysia.*

**Laboratories for Applied Biology, Singapore.** See *Sime Darby, Singapore.*

**Laboratories for Applied Biology, UK.** Laboratories for Applied Biology Ltd, 91 Amhurst Park, London, N16 5DR, UK.

**Laboratorio Farm., Israel.** See *Premopharm, Israel.*

**Laboratorios Chile, Chile.** Laboratorios Chile SA, Av. Marathon 1315, Nunoa, Santiago, Chile.

**Laborest, Ital.** See *Pharma-Natura, Ital.*

**Labormedica, Braz.** Labormedica Industrial Ltda, Rua Jose Guide 500, Distrito Industrial, 15035-500 Sao Jose do Rio Preto, SP, Brazil.

**Laborsil, Braz.** Laborsil Industria Farmaceutica Ltda, Rodovia 160 RN Km 22, 59290-000 Sao Goncalo do Amarante, RN, Brazil.

**Labortecne, Braz.** Labortecne Ltda, Av. Agamenon Magalhaes 180, Vila Popular, 53203-010 Olinda, PE, Brazil.

**Lacefa, Arg.** Lab. Lacefa S.A.I.C.A., Ladines 2263/7, 1419 Buenos Aires, Argentina.

**Lacer, Hong Kong.** See *CNW, Hong Kong.*

**Lacer, Spain.** Lacer, Sardenya 350, 08025 Barcelona, Spain.

**Lachartre, Fr.** See *Procter & Gamble, Fr.*

**Lachifarma, Ital.** Lachifarma S.r.l., Laboratorio Chimico Farmaceutico Salentino, S.S. 16, Zona Industriale, 73010 Zollino (LE), Italy.

**Laclede, Singapore.** See *MBD, Singapore.*

**Lacoer, Ger.** See *Laves, Ger.*

**Lactel, Fr.** Sté Lactel, ZI Les Touches, 53093 Laval cdx 9, France.

**Lacteol, Fr.** See *Axcan, Fr.*

**Lacteol, Hong Kong.** See *Silroc, Hong Kong.*

**Lacteol, Singapore.** See *Age D'or, Singapore.*

**Lacteol, Switz.** See *Uhlmann-Eyraud, Switz.*

**Lacteol, Thai.** See *Diethelm, Thai.*

**Laetitia, Ger.** Laetitia Naturprodukte Vertriebs GmbH, Elsasser Str. 4-6, 81667 Munich, Germany.

**Laevosan, Austria.** Laevosan-Pharma Gessellschaftmbh, Estermannstrasse 17, A-4020 Linz, Austria.

**Lafage, Arg.** Lab. Lafage S.R.L., J. E. Uriburu 61, 1027 Buenos Aires, Argentina.

**Lafare, Ital.** Laboratorio Farmaceutico Reggiano S.r.l., Via S.B. Cozzolino 77, 80056 Ercolano Resina (NA), Italy.

**Lafarmen, Arg.** Lafarmen S.A., Rioja 2163/69, 5500 Mendoza, Argentina.

**Lafayette, USA.** Lafayette Pharmaceuticals Inc., 526 North Earl Ave, Lafayette, IN 47904-2819, USA.

**Lafedar, Arg.** Lafedar, Lab. Federales Argentinos S.A., Valentmn Torra 4880, 3100 Entre Rios, Argentina.

**Lafepe, Braz.** Lafepe, Largo Dois Irmaos 1117, 52071-010 Recife, PE, Brazil.

**Lafi, Chile.** See *Recalcine, Chile.*

**Lafon, Denm.** See *Organon, Denm.*

**Lafon, Fr.** Laboratoires Lafon, 19 av. du Professeur Cadiot, B.P. 22, 94701 Maisons-Alfort cdx, France.

**Lafon, Hong Kong.** See *Worldwide, Hong Kong.*

**Lafon, Israel.** See *Medison, Israel.*

**Lafran, Fr.** Laboratoires Lafran, 1 rte des Stains, 94387 Bonneuil-sur-Marne cdx, France.

**Lagamed, S.Afr.** Lagamed (Pty) Ltd, South Africa.

**Lagap, Hong Kong.** See *Hind Wing, Hong Kong.*

**Lagap, Switz.** Lagap SA, Via San Gottardo 9, 6943 Vezia, Switzerland.

**Lagap, UK.** Lagap Pharmaceuticals Ltd, 37 Woolmer Way, Bordon, Hampshire, GU35 9QE, UK.

**Lagos, Arg.** Lagos Laboratorios Argentina S.R.L., Jorge Newbery 1829, 1426 Buenos Aires, Argentina.

**Lailan, Spain.** See *AstraZeneca, Spain.*

**Lainco, Spain.** Lainco, Avda Bizet 8-12, Rubi, 08191 Barcelona, Spain.

**Lake, USA.** Lake Consumer Products Inc., 7300 Corporate Woods Pkwy, Vernon Hills, IL 60061, USA.

**Lakeside, Mex.** Lakeside de Mexico S.A. de C.V., Cerrada de Bezares No. 9, Lomas de Bezares, 11000 Mexico D.F., Mexico.

**Lalco, Canad.** See *Nobel, Canad.*

**Lam Thong, Thai.** Lam Thong.

**Lamberts Healthcare, UK.** Lamberts Healthcare Ltd, 1 Lamberts Rd, Tunbridge Wells, Kent, TN2 3EQ, UK.

**Lampugnani, Ital.** Lampugnani Farmaceutici S.p.A., Via Gramsci 4, 20014 Nerviano (Milan), Italy.

**Lancome, Canad.** See *Cosmair, Canad.*

**Lander, Canad.** Lander Co. Canada Ltd, 275 Finchdene Square, Scarborough, Ontario, M1X 1C7, Canada.

**Landmark, Canad.** Landmark Medical Systems Inc, P. O. Box 64575, Unionville, Ontario, L3R 0M9, Canada.

**Lane, UK.** G.R. Lane Health Products Ltd, Sisson Rd, Gloucester, GL1 3QB, UK.

**Lannacher, Austria.** Lannacher Heilmittel GmbH, Schlossplatz 1, A-8502 Lannach, Austria.

**Lannacher, Denm.** See *Nordic Drugs, Denm.*

**Lannacher, Israel.** See *Taro, Israel.*

**Lannacher, Norw.** See *Nordic, Swed.*

**Lannett, USA.** Lannett Inc., 9000 State Rd, Philadelphia, PA 19136, USA.

**Laphal, Fr.** Laphal Industrie, Avenue de Provence, 13190 Allauch cdx, France.

**Laphal, Hong Kong.** See *C & L, Hong Kong,* and *Wing Wai, Hong Kong.*

**Lapidot, Israel.** A. Lapidot Pharmaceuticals Ltd, 8 Ha'shita St, Industry Park, Caesaria 38900, Israel.

**Laproquifar, Spain.** Laproquifar, Las Carolinas 13, 08012 Barcelona, Spain.

**L'Arguenon, Fr.** See *SERB, Fr.*

**Larkhall Laboratories, UK.** Larkhall Laboratories, White Horse Business Park, Trowbridge, Wiltshire, BA14 0XQ, UK.

**Lasa, Spain.** See *Ipsen, Spain.*

**La-Sante, Braz.** La-Sante Laboratorios Ltda, Rua Senador Nabuco 49, 24030-160 Rio de Janeiro, RJ, Brazil.

**Laser, USA.** Laser Inc., 2200 W 97th Place, P.O. Box 905, Crown Point, IN 46307, USA.

**Lauria, Arg.** Lauria, Merlino & Cía. S.C., Av. La Plata 340/44, 1235 Buenos Aires, Argentina.

**Laus, Spain.** Laus Farma, Gran via Cortes Catalanes 764, 08013 Barcelona, Spain.

**Laves, Ger.** Laves-Arzneimittel GmbH, Barbarastr. 14, 30952 Ronnenberg, Germany.

**Lavipharm, Gr.** See *Synthelabo Lavipharm, Gr.*

**Lavipharm, Israel.** See *Megapharm, Israel.*

**LAW, Ger.** See *Riemser, Ger.*

**Layton, USA.** Layton Bioscience Inc., 709 E Evelyn Ave, Sunnyvale, CA 94086, USA.

**Lazar, Arg.** Laboratorio Dr. Lazar & Cia. S.A., Av. Velez Sarsfield 5855, 1605 Carapachay, Buenos Aires, Argentina.

**Lazuli, Malaysia.** Lazuli Sdn Bhd, 18 Jln SS 5 A/9, 47301 Petaling Jaya, Selangor, Malaysia.

**LBS, Thai.** LBS Laboratory Ltd Part, 602 Soi Phanichanant, Sukhumvit 71 Rd, Bangkok 10110, Thailand.

**LCA, Fr.** Laboratoire LCA, 9 allee Promethee, 28000 Chartres, France.

**LCH, Hong Kong.** Luen Cheong Hong Ltd, 25/F, 200 Gloucester Rd, Wanchai, Hong Kong.

**LDA, Arg.** Lab. LDA, Alcaraz 5294, 1407 Buenos Aires, Argentina.

**LDM, Fr.** LDM Santé, 2 pl Edmond-Puyo, B.P. 129, 29600 Morlaix, France.

**Le Marchand, Fr.** Laboratoires Le Marchand, 2 bis rue Moussard, 28600 Luisant, France.

**Leader, Hong Kong.** Leader Pharmaceutical & Cosmetic Co. Ltd, 2/F, 42 Hankow Rd, Kowloon, Hong Kong.

**Lebeh, USA.** Lebeh, USA.

**Lectec, USA.** LecTec Corp., 10701 Red Circle Dr., Minnetonka, MN 55343, USA.

**LED, Fr.** Laboratoires d'Evolution Dermatologique, 7 rue d'Aguesseau, 75008 Paris, France.

**Lederle, Austral.** See *Wyeth, Austral.*

**Lederle, Fr.** See *Wyeth Lederle, Fr.*

**Lederle, Ger.** See *Wyeth, Ger.*

**Lederle, Hong Kong.** See *Wyeth, Hong Kong.*

**Lederle, Irl.** See *Wyeth, Irl.*

**Lederle, Israel.** See *Neopharm, Israel.*

**Lederle, Neth.** See *Wyeth, Neth.*

**Lederle, NZ.** See *Wyeth, NZ.*

**Lederle, S.Afr.** See *Wyeth, S.Afr.*

**Lederle, Switz.** See *AHP, Switz.*

**Lederle, UK.** See *Wyeth, UK.*

**Lederle, USA.** Lederle Professional Medical Services, N Middletown Rd, Pearl River, NY 10965-1299, USA.

**Lederle-Praxis, USA.** Lederle-Praxis Biologicals, 7326 E Evans Rd, Scottsdale, AZ 85260, USA.

**Ledi, Ital.** Laboratori Eudermici Italiani S.r.l., Via Augusto Gaudenzi 29, 00163 Rome, Italy.

**Lee, USA.** Lee Pharmaceuticals, 1434 Santa Anita Blvd, South Elmonte, CA 91733, USA.

**Lee-Adams, Canad.** Lee-Adams Laboratories, 8400 Darnley Rd, Montreal, Quebec, H4T 1M4, Canada.

**Leeming, USA.** See *Pfizer, USA.*

**Lefevre, Fr.** Laboratoires du Dr J. Lefèvre-Albrenor S.A., 82 rue National, 57350 Stiring-Wendel, France.

**Legere, USA.** Legere Pharmaceuticals, 7326 E. Evans Rd, Scottsdale, AZ 85260, USA.

**Legon, Ital.** Legon Farmaceutici S.r.l., Via Tronto 14, 00198 Rome, Italy.

**Legrand, Braz.** See *EMS, Braz.*

**Legras, Fr.** Laboratoires Legras, 114 Bis, rue Michel-Ange, 75016 Paris, France.

**Lehning, Fr.** Laboratoires Lehning, 1-3 rue du Petit-Marais, 57640 Sainte-Barbe, France.

**Leiras, Denm.** See *Ferring, Denm.,* and *Schering, Denm.*

**Leiras, Fin.** Oy Leiras Finland AB, PL 1406, 00101 Helsinki, Finland.

**Leiras, Israel.** See *Agis, Israel.*

**Leiras, Norw.** See *Schering, Norw.*

**Leiras, Singapore.** See *MBD, Singapore.*

**Leiras, Swed.** See *Schering, Swed.*

**Leiras, Thai.** See *Berli, Thai.*

**Lek, Hong Kong.** See *Hind Wing, Hong Kong.*

**Lek, Singapore.** See *FP, Singapore.*

**Lek, Thai.** See *RX, Thai.*

**Leman, Fr.** See *Proteika, Fr.*

**Lemery, Mex.** Lemery S.A. de C.V., Calle 1 No. 5-A Interior 101, Mabuel Avila Camacho, 11610 Mexico D.F., Mexico.

**Lemery, Thai.** See *Pharmaland, Thai.*

**Lemmon, USA.** See *Teva, USA.*

**Lemoine, Fr.** Laboratoires Lemoine, Imm le Doublon, bat B, 11 av. Dubonnet, 92400 Courbevoie, France.

**Lennod, USA.** Lennod, USA.

**Lennon, S.Afr.** See *SA Druggists, S.Afr.*

**Lensa, Spain.** Lensa, Potosi 2-4, 08030 Barcelona, Spain.

**Lentheric, UK.** Lentheric Ltd, Amertrans Park, Bushey Mill Lane, Watford, Hertfordshire, WD2 4JG, UK.

**Leo, Austria.** Leo Pharma GesellschafftmbH, Mariahilfer Strasse 123/4.OG, A-1060 Vienna, Austria.

**Leo, Belg.** Leo Pharma S.A., Excelsiorlaan 40-42, 1930 Zaventem, Belgium.

**Leo, Canad.** Leo Pharma Inc., 123 Commerce Valley Dr. E, Suite 400, Thornhill, Ontario, L3T 7W8, Canada.

**Leo, Denm.** Leo Pharma A/S, Industriparken 55, 2750 Ballerup, Denmark.

**Leo, Fin.** Leo Pharma Oy, Äyritie 12 B, 01510 Vantaa, Finland.

**Leo, Fr.** Laboratoires Leo, B.P. 311, 78054 St-Quentin-Yvelines cdx, France.

**Leo, Ger.** Leo Pharma GmbH, Frankfurter Str. 233, A3, 63263 Neu-Isenburg, Germany.

**Leo, Hong Kong.** See *Keller, Hong Kong.*

**Leo, Irl.** Leo Laboratories Ltd, 285 Cashel Rd, Dublin 12, Ireland.

**Leo, Israel.** See *Dexxon, Israel.*

**Leo, Malaysia.** See *Diethelm, Malaysia,* and *Summit, Malaysia.*

**Leo, Neth.** Leo Pharma BV, Hoge Mossen 16-20, 4822 NH Breda, Netherlands.

**Leo, Norw.** Leo Pharma AS, Postboks 193 Lilleaker, 0216 Oslo, Norway.

**Leo, NZ.** See *CSL, NZ.*

**Leo, Port.** Leo-Farmaceuticos, Lda, Av das Nacoes Unidas 27, 1600-531 Lisbon, Portugal.

**Leo, Singapore.** Leo Pharma Singapore, 19 Loyang Way, 06-29 Changi International Logistic Centre, S 508724, Singapore.

**Leo, Swed.** Leo Pharma AB, Box 404, 201 24 Malmo, Sweden.

**Leo, Switz.** Leo Pharmaceutical Products Sarath Ltd, Eggbuhlstrasse 28, 8052 Zurich, Switzerland.

**Leo, Thai.** See *Olic, Thai.*

**Leo, UK.** Leo Pharma, Longwick Rd, Princes Risborough, Buckinghamshire, HP27 9RR, UK.

**Leo (Λεο), Gr.** ΛΕΟ ΕΛΛΑΣ ΕΠΕ, Μ. Ασίας 1, Χαλάνδρι, Chalandri, Greece.

**Leofarma, Braz.** Leofarma Comercio e Industria Ltda, Avenida Getulio Vargas 645, 36700-000 Leopoldina, MG, Brazil.

**Leovan, Gr.** LEOVAN, Χρ. Τραπεζούντος 10, 167 77 Ελληνικό, Elliniko, Greece.

**Lepetit, Ital.** See *Aventis, Ital.*

**Lepori, Port.** L. Lepori, Lda, Rua Joao Chagas No. 53, 3 Piso, 1495-072 Alges, Portugal.

**Lerads, Fr.** Lerads, 11 rue Rontgen, 29000 Quimper, France.

**Lersan, Arg.** See *Pharmos, Arg.*

**Lesourd, Fr.** Laboratoires Gabriel Lesourd, 6 rue Ste-Isaure, 75018 Paris, France.

**Lessel, Braz.** See *Mepha, Braz.*

**Lesvi, Spain.** Lesvi, Polig Ind Can Pelegri, Argent 1, Castellbisbal, 08755 Barcelona, Spain.

**Leti, Spain.** Leti, Gran Via de las Corts, Catalanes 184, 08038 Barcelona, Spain.

**Leurquin, Fr.** Laboratoires Leurquin Mediolanum, 68/88 rue Ampere, 93330 Neuilly-sur-Marne, France.

**Leurquin, Hong Kong.** See *Innoledge, Hong Kong,* and *Silroc, Hong Kong.*

**Leurquin, Switz.** See *Uhlmann-Eyraud, Switz.*

**Lever, UK.** Lever Faberge, 3 St James Rd, Kingston-upon-Thames, Surrey, KT1 2BA, UK.

**Levofarma, Ital.** See *Uno, Ital.*

**Lexis, USA.** Lexis Laboratories, P.O. Box 202887, Austin, TX 78720, USA.

**Lexon, UK.** Lexon (UK) Ltd, 18 Oxleasow Rd, East Moons Moat, Redditch, Worcestershire, B98 0RE, UK.

**Leyh, Ger.** Leyh Pharma GmbH, Gewerbegebeit Baierstal, 98596 Trusetal, Germany.

**LG Chem, Thai.** See *Aventis Pasteur, Thai.*

**LG Pharm, Hong Kong.** See *Hind Wing, Hong Kong.*

**Liade, Spain.** Liade, Avda de Burgos 91, 28050 Madrid, Spain.

**Libbs, Braz.** Libbs Farmaceutica Ltda, Rua Josef Kryss 250, 01140-050 Sao Paulo, SP, Brazil.

**Libra, Braz.** Libra, Brazil.

**Libra, S.Afr.** Libra, South Africa.

**Lichtenheldt, Ger.** Lichtenheldt GmbH, Pharmazeutische Fabrik, Justus-Liebig-Weg 1, 23812 Wahlstedt, Germany.

**Lichtenstein, Ger.** Lichtenstein Pharmazeutica GmbH & Co., Industriestrasse 26, 56218 Mulheim-Karlich, Germany.

**Lichtwer, Austria.** See *Lichtwer, Ger.*

**Lichtwer, Canad.** Lichtwer Pharma, 145 Idema Road, Markham, Ontario, L3R 1A9, Canada.

**Lichtwer, Ger.** Lichtwer Pharma AG, Wallenroder Str. 8-10, 13435 Berlin, Germany.
**Lichtwer, Switz.** See *Adroka, Switz.*
**Lichtwer, UK.** Lichtwer Pharma UK, Regency House, Mere Park, Dedmere Rd, Marlow, Buckinghamshire, SL7 1FJ, UK.
**Liebermann, Austria.** See *Liebermann, Ger.*
**Liebermann, Ger.** Pharma Liebermann GmbH, Hauptstr. 27, 89423 Gundelfingen/Do., Germany.
**Lierac, Fr.** Laboratoires Liérac, 35 av Franklin-Roosevelt, 75008 Paris, France.
**Life, Ger.** Life Pharma GmbH, Frigenstr. 5, 67065 Ludwigshafen, Germany.
**Life, Israel.** See *Rekah, Israel.*
**Life Essence, UK.** See *Elder, UK.*
**Life Plus, UK.** Life Plus Europe Ltd, Martin House, Howard Rd, Eaton Socon, Cambridgeshire, PE19 3ET, UK.
**Lifebiotech, Switz.** LifeBiotech AG, Gattikerstrasse 5, Postfach, 8029 Zurich, Switzerland.
**Lifepharma, Ital.** Lifepharma S.p.A., Via dei Lavoratori 54, 20092 Cinisello Balsamo (MI), Italy.
**Lifeplan, UK.** Lifeplan Products, Elizabethan Way, Lutterworth, Leicestershire, LE17 4ND, UK.
**Liferpal, Mex.** Liferpal MD, S.A. de C.V., Refineria No. 1266, Col. Alamo Industrial, 44490 Guadalajara, Jal., Mexico.
**Lifescan, Fr.** Laboratoires Lifescan, Division d'Ortho-Clinical Diagnostics, 1 rue Camille-Desmoulins, TSA 40007, 92787 Issy-les-Moulineaux cdx 9, France.
**Lifescan, Irl.** See *Cahill May Roberts, Irl.*
**Lifescan, Port.** See *Johnson & Johnson, Port.*
**Lifescan, USA.** Lifescan, 1000 Gibraltar, Milpitas, CA 95035-6312, USA.
**Lifesign, USA.** LifeSign LLC, 71 Veronica Way, P.O. Box 218, Somerset, NJ 08875-0218, USA.
**Lifetech, Hong Kong.** Lifetech Enterprises Inc., 22/F, New World Tower II, 18 Queen's Rd Central, Hong Kong.
**Ligand, Canad.** See *Ligand, USA.*
**Ligand, USA.** Ligand Pharmaceuticals Inc., 10275 Science Center Dr, San Diego, CA 92121, USA.
**Lignaform, Mon.** Lignaform, 57 bd d'Italie, MC 98000, Monaco.
**Li-il, Ger.** Li-iL GmbH Arzneimittel, Leipziger Str. 300, 01139 Dresden, Germany.
**Lilly, Arg.** Eli Lilly Interamerica, Scalabrini Ortiz 3333 5 Piso, 1425 Buenos Aires, Argentina.
**Lilly, Austral.** Eli Lilly Australia P/L, 112 Wharf Rd, West Ryde, NSW 2114, Australia.
**Lilly, Austria.** Eli Lilly GmbH (Austria), Barichgasse 40-2, A-1030 Vienna, Austria.
**Lilly, Belg.** Eli Lilly Benelux S.A., Rue de l'Etuve 52 boite 1, 1000 Brussels, Belgium.
**Lilly, Braz.** Eli Lilly do Brasil Ltda, Avenida Morumbi 8264, 04703-002 Sao Paulo, SP, Brazil.
**Lilly, Canad.** Eli Lilly Canada Inc., 3650 Danforth Ave, Scarborough, Ontario, M1N 2E8, Canada.
**Lilly, Chile.** Eli Lilly de Chile Ltda, Carmencita 25, Of. 91, Las Condes, Santiago, Chile.
**Lilly, Denm.** Eli Lilly Denmark A/S, Nybrovej 110, 2800 Lyngby, Denmark.
**Lilly, Fin.** Oy Eli Lilly Finland AB, Rajatorpantie 41 C 3. krs, PL 16, 01641 Vantaa, Finland.
**Lilly, Fr.** Lilly France, 13 rue Pages, 92158 Suresnes Cdx, France.
**Lilly, Ger.** Lilly Deutschland GmbH, Saalburgstr. 153, 61350 Bad Homburg, Germany.
**Lilly, Hong Kong.** Eli Lilly Asia Inc., Suites 1706-11, 17th Floor, CITIC Tower, 1 Tim Mei Ave Central, Hong Kong.
**Lilly, (India).** E. Lilly (India) Ltd, Plot No. 92, Sector 32, Gurgaon 122 001, India.
**Lilly, Irl.** Eli Lilly & Co. (Ireland) Ltd, Hyde House, 65 Adelaide Rd, Dublin 2, Ireland.
**Lilly, Israel.** Eli Lilly Israel Ltd, P.O. Box 2160, Herzliya Pituah, Israel.
**Lilly, Ital.** Eli Lilly Italia S.p.A., Via Gramsci 731/733, 50019 Sesto Fiorentino (FI), Italy.
**Lilly, Jpn.** Eli Lilly Japan K.K., 7-1-5 Isogami-dori, Chuo-ku Kobe, Hyago 651-0086, Japan.
**Lilly, Malaysia.** Eli Lilly (M) Sdn Bhd, 18.1, 18th Floor, CP Tower, No. 11, Section 16/11, Pusat Dagang Seksyen 16, 46350 Petaling Jaya, Selangor, Malaysia.
**Lilly, Mex.** Eli Lilly y Compania de Mexico S.A. de C.V., Calz de Tlalpan No. 2024, Col Campestre Churubusco, Deleg. Coyoacan, 04200 Mexico D.F., Mexico.
**Lilly, Neth.** Eli Lilly Nederland, Grootschlag 1-5, 3991 RA Houten, Netherlands.
**Lilly, Norw.** Eli Lilly Norge A.S, Grensev. 99, Postboks 6090 Etterstad, 0601 Oslo, Norway.
**Lilly, NZ.** Eli Lilly & Co. (NZ) Ltd, P.O. Box 97-046, South Auckland Mail Centre, Wiri, Auckland, New Zealand.
**Lilly, Port.** Lilly Farma, Lda, Rua Dr Antonio Loureiro Borges 4, Piso 3, Arquiparque, Miraflores, 1495-131 Alges, Portugal.
**Lilly, S.Afr.** Eli Lilly (SA) (Pty) Ltd, Private Bag X119, Brynston 2021, South Africa.
**Lilly, Singapore.** Eli Lilly (S) Pte Ltd, 7 Temasek Boulevard, 15-01 Suntec City Tower 1, S 038987, Singapore.
**Lilly, Spain.** Lilly, Avda de la Industria 30, Alcobendas, 28108 Madrid, Spain.
**Lilly, Swed.** Eli Lilly Sweden AB, Box 30037, 104 25 Stockholm, Sweden.
**Lilly, Switz.** Eli Lilly (Suisse) SA, 16 Ch. des Coquelicots, Case postale 580, 1214 Vernier/GE, Switzerland.
**Lilly, Thai.** See *Diethelm, Thai.*
**Lilly, UK.** Eli Lilly & Co. Ltd, Lilly House, Priestley Rd, Basingstoke, Hampshire, RG24 9NL, UK.
**Lilly, USA.** Eli Lilly & Co., Lilly Corporate Center, Indianapolis, IN 46285, USA.
**Lina, UK.** Lina Trading Ltd, P.O. Box 2341, London, W1A 2NZ, UK.
**Linde, UK.** Linde, UK.
**Linderma, UK.** Linderma Ltd, Canon Bridge House, Canon Bridge, Madley, Herefordshire, HR2 9JF, UK.
**Lindopharm, Ger.** Lindopharm GmbH, Neustr. 82, 40721 Hilden, Germany.
**Lineafarm, Spain.** Lineafarm, Spain.
**Linfar, Arg.** Laboritories Linfar S.R.L., Emilio Casas Ocampo 2838, 5009 Altos de San Martin, Cordoba, Argentina.
**Link, Austral.** Link Medical Products P/L, P.O. Box 135, Avalon Beach, NSW 2107, Australia.
**Link, Irl.** See *Intra Pharma, Irl.*
**Link, NZ.** Link Pharmaceuticals, Level 20, ASB Bank Centre, 135 Albert St, Auckland, New Zealand.
**Link, UK.** Link Pharmaceuticals Ltd, Bishops Weald House, Albion Way, Horsham, West Sussex, RH12 1AH, UK.
**Linobion, Austria.** Linobion Chem.-pharm. Laboratorium, Kardinal-Nagl-Platz 1, A-1030 Vienna, Austria.
**Linson, Canad.** Linson Pharma Inc., 2365 Cote de Liesse, St-Laurent, Quebec, H4N 2M7, Canada.
**Linton, S.Afr.** M Linton, South Africa.
**Lioh, Canad.** LIOH. Inc., 5950 Cote de Liesse, Mont-Royal, Ontario, H4T 1E2, Canada.
**Liomont, Mex.** Laboratorios Liomont S.A. de C.V., Adolfo Lopez Mateos No.68, Deleg. Cuajimalpa, 05000 Mexico D.F., Mexico.
**Lipha, Denm.** See *Nycomed, Denm.*
**Lipha, Irl.** See *Merck, Irl.*
**Lipha, Ital.** See *Merck, Ital.*
**Lipha, Norw.** See *Biomet Merck, Norw.*
**Lipha, Switz.** See *Merck, Switz.*
**Lipha Sante, Fr.** See *Merck-Lipha, Fr.*
**Liphaderm, Fr.** See *Merck-Lipha, Fr.*
**Lipomed, Israel.** See *Margalit, Israel.*
**Lipomed, Switz.** Lipomed AG, Fabrikmattenweg 4, 4144 Arlesheim, Switzerland.
**Liposome, Gr.** LIPOSOME, Greece.
**Liposome Company, Austria.** See *Wyeth Lederle, Austria.*
**Liposome Company, Canad.** See *Liposome Company, USA.*
**Liposome Company, Hong Kong.** See *Zuellig, Hong Kong.*
**Liposome Company, Irl.** See *Central, Irl.*
**Liposome Company, Norw.** See *Wyeth Lederle, Norw.*
**Liposome Company, Singapore.** See *Summit, Singapore.*
**Liposome Company, Switz.** Liposome S.á.r.l., En Budron D5, 1052 Le Mont-sur-Lausanne, Switzerland.
**Liposome Company, USA.** See *Elan, USA.*
**Liptis, USA.** Liptis Pharmaceuticals Inc., New York, USA.
**Liquipharm, USA.** Liquipharm, 10716 McCune Avenue, Los Angeles, CA 90034, USA.
**Lisapharm, Fr.** Laboratoires Lisapharm, 9 Bis, bd Jean-Juares, 92100 Boulogne, France.
**Lisapharm, Israel.** See *Premopharm, Israel.*
**Lisapharma, Hong Kong.** See *Mekim, Hong Kong.*
**Lisapharma, Israel.** See *Premopharm, Israel.*
**Lisapharma, Ital.** Lisapharma S.p.A., Via Licinio 11, 22036 Erba (Como), Italy.
**Lisapharma, Singapore.** See *Zyfas, Singapore.*
**Lisapharma, Thai.** See *Charoen, Thai., SPB, Thai.,* and *Sriprasit, Thai.*
**Lisfarma, Braz.** See *Genzyme, Braz.*
**Lision Hong, Hong Kong.** Lision Hong, Flat G, 7/F, Valiant Industrial Ctr, 2-12 Au Pui Wan St, Fo Tan, N.T., Hong Kong.
**Lizofarm, Ital.** Lizofarm S.r.l., Via S. Gottardo 37, 20052 Monza (MI), Italy.
**Llano, Spain.** Llano, Spain.
**Llorens, Spain.** Llorens, Ciudad de Balaguer 7-11, 08022 Barcelona, Spain.
**Llorente, Spain.** Llorente, Ctra el Pardo Km 1, 28035 Madrid, Spain.
**Lloyd, Aimee, UK.** Lloyd, Aimee & Co. Ltd, Kingsend House, 44 Kingsend, Ruislip, Middlesex, HA4 7DA, UK.
**Locatelli, Ital.** Farmaceutici Locatelli S.r.l., Via Campobello 15, 00040 Pomezia (Rome), Italy.
**Lofarma, Ital.** Lofarma S.p.A., Viale Cassala 40, 20143 Milan, Italy.
**Lofthouse of Fleetwood, Canad.** Lofthouse of Fleetwood, 600 Alden Rd, Suite 102, Markham, Ontario, L3R 0E7, Canada.
**Logeais, Fr.** See *Chiesi, Fr.*
**Logeais, Hong Kong.** See *CNW, Hong Kong.*
**Loges, Ger.** Dr. Loges & Co. GmbH Arzneimittel, Schutzenstr. 5, 21423 Winsen, Germany.
**Loges, Hong Kong.** See *Lision Hong, Hong Kong.*
**Logistics, Belg.** Pharma Logistics, Demeurslaan 71, 1654 Huizingen, Belgium.
**Logogen, Spain.** Logogen, San Rafael 3, Alcobendas, 28108 Madrid, Spain.
**Lohmann, Ger.** Lohmann & Rauscher International GmbH & Co. KG, Westerwaldstr. 4, 56579 Rengsdorf, Germany.
**Lohmann, Ital.** Lohmann & Rauscher S.r.l., Via E. Fermi 4, 35030 Sarmeola di Rubano (PD), Italy.
**Lomapharm, Ger.** Lomapharm, Rudolf Lohmann GmbH KG, Langes Feld 5, 31860 Emmerthal, Germany.
**Lomapharm, Singapore.** See *Polymedic, Singapore.*
**London Drugs, Canad.** London Drugs Ltd, 12831 Horseshoe Place, Richmond, British Columbia, V7A 4X5, Canada.
**Lopes, Braz.** Lopes Produtos Farmaceuticos S.A., Rodovia BR 491, Km 5, Caixa Postal:62, 37002-970 Varginha, Brazil.
**Loprofar, Braz.** See *Lopes, Braz.*
**L'Oreal, Canad.** See *Cosmair, Canad.*
**Loren, Mex.** Laboratorios Farmaceuticos Loren S.A. de C.V., Km. 91 Carr. Federal Mexico-Puebla, Corredor Industrial Quetzalcoatl, 74160 Huejotzingo, Pue, Mexico.
**Lorex, Denm.** See *Pharmacia, Denm.*
**Lorex Synthelabo, Neth.** See *Sanofi Synthelabo, Neth.*
**Lorvic, Canad.** See *Prof. Pharm. Corp., Canad.*
**Lorvic, USA.** See *Young, USA.*
**Lotus, USA.** Lotus Biochemical Corp., P.O. Box 485, Bristol, TN 37620, USA.
**Loveridge, UK.** J.M. Loveridge PLC, Southbrook Rd, Southampton, Hampshire, SO15 1BH, UK.
**Loyal Advance, Hong Kong.** Loyal Advance Ltd, 8/F, B2-B4 Tsing Yi Industrial Ctr, Phase 1, Tsing Yi Island, N.T., Hong Kong.
**LPB, Ital.** LPB Istituto Farmaceutico S.p.A., S.S. Varesina km 20.5, 21040 Origgio (VA), Italy.
**LPC, UK.** LPC Medical (UK) Ltd, 2 Covent Garden Close, Luton, Bedfordshire, LU4 8QB, UK.
**LPN, Fr.** Laboratoire Pharmaceutique Noroit, 7 rue Jean-Baptiste Clement, 94250 Gentilly, France.
**LRC, Israel.** See *Promedico, Israel.*
**LRC Products, UK.** LRC Products Ltd, London International House, Turnford Place, Broxbourne, Hertfordshire, EN10 6LN, UK.
**LSI, USA.** LSI America Corp., 4732 Twin Valley Drive, Austin, TX 78731-3586, USA.
**LSP, Thai.** Lerd Singh Pharmaceutical Fact Ltd Part, 922 Sukhumvit 50, Prakanong, Klongtoey, Bangkok 10250, Thailand.
**LTM, Neth.** See *Vemedia, Neth.*
**LTS, Israel.** See *Teva, Israel.*
**Luar, Arg.** Qummica Luar S.R.L., Angel Carranza 1946, 1414 Buenos Aires, Argentina.
**Lubapharm, Switz.** Lubapharm SA, Ringstrasse 29, Postfach 434, 4106 Therwil, Switzerland.
**Lubapharm Arlesheim, Switz.** Lubapharm AG, Postfach 348, 4144 Arlesheim, Switzerland.
**Lubapharm Phlebologie, Switz.** See *Lubapharm, Switz.*
**Lucchini, Ital.** Lucchini Italiana S.r.l., Via S. Anna 2, 03012 Anagni (FR), Italy.
**Lucchini, Switz.** Laboratoire Lucchini SA, Case postale 1214, 1211 Geneva 26, Switzerland.
**Luchon, Fr.** Laboratoires de Luchon, 22 bd Dardenne, 31110 Luchon, France.
**Ludwig, Singapore.** See *Apotheca, Singapore.*
**Luen Wah, Malaysia.** Luen Wah Medical Co, No. 37G, 37-1F & 39-1F The Highway Centre, Jln 51/205, 46050 Petaling Jaya, Selangor, Malaysia.
**Luen Wah, Singapore.** Luen Wah Medical Co (S) Pte Ltd, 40 North Canal Rd, S 059296, Singapore.
**Luhr-Lehrs, Ger.** A Lühr-Lehrs Arzneimittel & Praventivprodukte, Hohler Weg 12, 53902 Bad Munstereifel-Berresheim, Germany.
**Luitpold, Belg.** See *Sankyo, Belg.*
**Luitpold, Braz.** See *Sankyo, Braz.*
**Luitpold, Ger.** See *Sankyo, Ger.*
**Luitpold, Ital.** See *Sankyo, Ital.*
**Luitpold, Neth.** See *Will-Pharma, Neth.*
**Lundbeck, Austral.** Lundbeck Australia P/L, Unit 1/10 Inglewood Place, Norwest Business Park, NSW 2153, Australia.
**Lundbeck, Austria.** Lundbeck-Arzneimittel GmbH, Brigittagasse 22-6, Postfach 201, A-1201 Vienna, Austria.
**Lundbeck, Belg.** Lundbeck S.A., Ave Moliere 225, 1050 Brussels, Belgium.
**Lundbeck, Canad.** Lundbeck Canada Inc., 413 St-Jacques St W, Suite FB-230, Montreal, Quebec, H2Y 1N9, Canada.
**Lundbeck, Denm.** Lundbeck Pharma A/S, Dalbergstroget 5, 2630 Taastrup, Denmark.
**Lundbeck, Fin.** Oy H. Lundbeck AB, Lemminkäisenkatu 14-18 B, 20520 Turku, Finland.
**Lundbeck, Fr.** Laboratoires Lundbeck, 37 av Pierre-1er-de-Serbie, 75008 Paris, France.
**Lundbeck, Ger.** Lundbeck GmbH & Co., Karnapp 25, 21079 Hamburg, Germany.
**Lundbeck, Gr.** LUNDBECK HELLAS AE, Λ. Κηφισίας 64, 151 25 Μαρούσι, Marousi, Greece.
**Lundbeck, Hong Kong.** Lundbeck Hong Kong, 35/F Central Plaza, 18 Harbour rd, Wanchai, Hong Kong.
**Lundbeck, India.** Lundbeck India Pvt Ltd, 6/A Richmond Rd, Bangalore 560 027, India.
**Lundbeck, Irl.** Lundbeck (Ireland) Ltd, 14 Deansgrange Industrial Estate, Blackrock, Dublin 11, Ireland.
**Lundbeck, Israel.** See *Lapidot, Israel.*
**Lundbeck, Ital.** Lundbeck Italia S.p.A., Via G Fara 35, 20124 Milan, Italy.
**Lundbeck, Malaysia.** See *JDH, Malaysia.*
**Lundbeck, Neth.** Lundbeck BV, Hettenheuvelweg 37, 1101 BM Amsterdam Z.O., Netherlands.
**Lundbeck, Norw.** H. Lundbeck A/S, Lysaker torg nr. 10, Postboks 361, 1326 Lysaker, Norway.
**Lundbeck, NZ.** See *Zuellig, NZ.*
**Lundbeck, Port.** Lundbeck Portugal Lda, Quinta da Fonte, Edificio Q54, Dom Jose, Piso 1, 2780-730 Paco de Arcos, Portugal.
**Lundbeck, S.Afr.** Lundbeck South Africa, P.O. Box 2357, Randburg 2125, South Africa.
**Lundbeck, Singapore.** Lundbeck Export A/S, Representative Office, 101 Thomson Road, No. 13-05 United Square, S 307591, Singapore.
**Lundbeck, Spain.** Lundbeck España, Avda Diagonal 605, 9-1a, 08028 Barcelona, Spain.
**Lundbeck, Swed.** H. Lundbeck AB, Box 23, 250 53 Helsingborg, Sweden.
**Lundbeck, Switz.** Lundbeck (Schweiz) AG, Cherstrasse 4, Postfach, 8152 Opfikon-Glattbrugg, Switzerland.
**Lundbeck, Thai.** See *Hua, Thai.*
**Lundbeck, UK.** Lundbeck Ltd, Sunningdale House, Caldecotte Lake Business Park, Caldecotte, Milton Keynes, MK7 8LF, UK.
**Lunsco, USA.** Lunsco Inc., 4657 Wurno Rd, Pulaski, VA 24301, USA.
**Luond, Switz.** Pharma Lüönd, Bahnhofstrasse 17-19, 8280 Kreuzlingen, Switzerland.
**Luper, Braz.** Luper Industria Farmaceutica Ltda, Rua Doutor Clementino 608, 03059-030 Sao Paulo, SP, Brazil.
**Lupin, India.** Lupin Ltd, 159 CST Rd, Kalina, Santacruz (E), Mumbai 400 098, India.
**Lupin, USA.** Lupin, USA.
**Lusofarmaco, Ital.** Istituto Luso Farmaco d'Italia S.p.A., Via Carnia 26, 20132 Milan, Italy.
**Lusofarmaco, Port.** See *GlaxoSmithKline, Port.*
**Lutsia, Fr.** See *Boots Healthcare, Fr.*
**Luvos, Ger.** Heilerde-Gesellschaft Luvos Just GmbH & Co., Postfach: 47, 61381 Friedrichsdorf, Germany.
**Luxembourg, Israel.** Luxembourg Pharmaceuticals Ltd, P.O. Box 1174, Lod, Israel.
**Luxurians, Arg.** Lab. Luxurians S.A., Joaquin V. Gonzalez 2569, 1417 Buenos Aires, Argentina.
**Lyka, India.** Lyka Hetero Healthcare Ltd, 408, 4th Floor, Sharda Chambers, 15 New Marine Lines, Mumbai 400 020, India.
**Lyocentre, Fr.** Laboratoires Lyocentre, 24 av Georges Pompidou, B.P. 429, 15004 Aurillac cdx, France.
**Lyron, Switz.** Lyron AG, Postfach 3538, 4002 Basle, Switzerland.
**Lysoform, Ger.** Lysoform Dr. Hans Rosemann GmbH, Kaiser-Wilhelm-Str. 133, 12247 Berlin, Germany.
**M & H, Malaysia.** See *Germax, Malaysia.*
**M & H, Thai.** M & H Manufacturing Co. Ltd, 27/2-3 Wireless Rd, Bangkok 10330, Thailand.
**Maabarot, Israel.** See *Trima, Israel.*
**Mabo, Spain.** Mabo Farma, Ctra M-300 Km, 30.5, Alcala de Henares, 28820 Madrid, Spain.
**Mac, India.** Mac Laboratories Pvt Ltd, Kirol, Vidyavihar, Mumbai 400 086, India.
**Mac, Ital.** Mac Pharma S.a.s., Via Onaro 22, 33037 Rio S Martino di Scorze (VE), Italy.
**Mack, Belg.** See *Vitalpharma, Belg.*
**Mack, Denm.** See *Kemifarma, Denm.*
**Mack, Hong Kong.** See *Keller, Hong Kong.*
**Mack, Israel.** See *Pfizer, Israel.*
**Mack, Malaysia.** See *Summit, Malaysia.*
**Mack, Singapore.** See *Summit, Singapore.*
**Mack, Switz.** See *Pfizer, Switz.*
**Mack, Thai.** See *Zuellig, Thai.*
**Mack, Illert., Ger.** See *Pfizer, Ger.*
**Macrophar, Thai.** Macrophar Co Ltd, 89 Soi Patanakarn 20, Yaek 4, Patanakarn Rd, Bangkok 10250, Thailand.
**Macsil, USA.** Macsil Inc., P.O. Box 29276, Philadelphia, PA 19125-0976, USA.
**Madariaga, Spain.** Madariaga, Electronica, 7, Poligono Urtinsa II, Alcorcon, 28923 Madrid, Spain.
**Madaus, Arg.** Lab. Dr. Madaus & Co., Av. Luis Marma Campos 585, 1426 Buenos Aires, Argentina.
**Madaus, Austria.** Madaus GmbH, Lienfeldergasse 91-93, A-1171 Vienna, Austria.
**Madaus, Belg.** Madaus Pharma S.A., Rue des Trois Arbres 16, 1180 Brussels, Belgium.
**Madaus, Denm.** See *2K, Denm.*
**Madaus, Fin.** See *Schering-Plough, Fin.*
**Madaus, Fr.** Laboratoires Madaus, 55 bis, quai de Grenelle, Immeuble Mercure III, 75015 Paris, France.
**Madaus, Ger.** Madaus AG, Ostmerheimer Str. 198, 51109 Cologne, Germany.
**Madaus, Hong Kong.** See *Trinity, Hong Kong.*

**Madaus, Israel.** Madaus, S.L.E., P.O. Box 8077, Netanya, Israel.

**Madaus, Ital.** Madaus S.r.l., Via Galvani 33, 39100 Bolzano, Italy.

**Madaus, Spain.** Madaus, FOC 68-82, 08038 Barcelona, Spain.

**Madaus, Thai.** See *Oui Heng, Thai.*

**Maeil, Hong Kong.** Maeil HK, 17A China Trade Ctr, 122-124 Wai Yip St, Kwun Tong, Kowloon, Hong Kong.

**Maersk, Austral.** Maersk Medical, NSW, Australia.

**Maersk, UK.** Maersk Medical Ltd, 27 Thornhill Rd, North Moons Moat, Redditch, Worcestershire, B98 9NL, UK.

**Maffioli, Ital.** Prodotti Dott. Maffioli S.a.s. di A. Labruzzo & C., Via Firenze 40, 20060 Trezzano Rosa (MI), Italy.

**Maggioni, Ital.** See *GlaxoSmithKline Consumer, Ital.*

**Magis, Ital.** Magis Farmaceutici S.p.A., Via Cacciamali 34-36-38, Zona Ind. (Loc. Noce), 25125 Brescia, Italy.

**Magistra, Switz.** Laboratoires Magistra SA, 28 Chemin du Grand-Puits, Case postale 122, 1217 Meyrin 2/Geneva, Switzerland.

**Magna, USA.** MAGNA Pharmaceuticals Inc., 11802 Brinley Ave, Suite 201, Louisville, KY 40243, USA.

**Mahakam Beta, Malaysia.** See *Somedico, Malaysia.*

**Mahdeen, Canad.** Mahdeen Mediceuticals, Division of Canmax Laboratories, 6600 Kennedy Rd, 4, Mississauga, Ontario, L5T 2M9, Canada.

**Maigal, Arg.** Lab. Maigal Corp., 12 de Octubre 1725, 1416 Buenos Aires, Argentina.

**Main Life, Hong Kong.** Main Life Corp. Ltd, 9/F, Winning Ctr, 46-48 Wyndham St Central, Hong Kong.

**Major, USA.** Major Pharmaceuticals, 31778 Enterprise Dr, Livonia, MI 48150, USA.

**Makara, Austria.** Makara Pharm GmbH, A-6234 Brandenberg 19C, Austria.

**Makros, Braz.** Makros Industria Farmaceutica Ltda, Rua Riachuelo 410, 20230-013 Rio de Janeiro, RJ.

**Malam, UK.** Malam Laboratories Ltd, 37 Oakwood Rise, Heaton, Bolton, BL1 5EE, UK.

**Malayan, Hong Kong.** See *Hind Wing, Hong Kong.*

**Malayan, Singapore.** See *Luen Wah, Singapore.*

**Malaysia Chemist, Singapore.** Malaysia Chemist Pte Ltd, 104 Boon Keng Rd, 04-01, S 339775, Singapore.

**Malesci, Ital.** Malesci Istituto Farmacobiologico S.p.A., Via Lungo l'Ema 7, 50015 Bagno a Ripoli (FI), Italy.

**Mallard, USA.** Mallard Medical Products, 81 Corbett Way, Eatontown, NJ 07724-2264, USA.

**Mallinckrodt, Arg.** Mallinckrodt Medical Argentina Ltda, Esmeralda 1072, 1007 Buenos Aires, Argentina.

**Mallinckrodt, Austral.** Mallinckrodt Australia P/L, P.O. Box 2442, Rowville, VIC 3178, Australia.

**Mallinckrodt, Austria.** Mallinckrodt Medical GmbH, Im Campus 21, Europaring F09402, A-2345 Brunn am Gebirge, Austria.

**Mallinckrodt, Braz.** Mallinckrodt Medical do Brasil Ltda, Avda Nacoes Unidas 13.797, Bloco III 20th Floor, Morumbi, 04794-000 Sao Paulo SP, Brazil.

**Mallinckrodt, Canad.** Mallinckrodt Canada Inc., 7500 Trans-Canada Highway, Pointe-Claire, Quebec, H9R 5H8, Canada.

**Mallinckrodt, Denm.** See *Tyco, Denm.*

**Mallinckrodt, Ger.** See *Tyco, Ger.*

**Mallinckrodt, Port.** See *Tyco, Port.*

**Mallinckrodt, Switz.** Mallinckrodt Schweiz AG, Obere Zäune, CH-8001 Zürich, Switzerland.

**Mallinckrodt, UK.** Mallinckrodt Medical UK Ltd, 10 Talisman Business Centre, London Rd, Bicester, Oxfordshire, OX6 0JX, UK.

**Mallinckrodt, USA.** Mallinckrodt Medical Inc., 3600 N. Second St, P.O. Box 5839, St Louis, MO 63134, USA.

**Malpharm, Hong Kong.** See *International Medical, Hong Kong.*

**Mandri, Spain.** Mandri, Pau Claris 182, 08037 Barcelona, Spain.

**Manetti Roberts, Ital.** L. Manetti H. Roberts & C. per Azioni, Via Baldanzese 177, 50041 Calenzano (FI), Italy.

**Mann, Ger.** Dr Gerhard Mann, Chem.-pharm. Fabrik GmbH, Brunsbutteler Damm 165-73, 13581 Berlin, Germany.

**Mann, Irl.** See *Pharma-Global, Irl.*

**Mann, Malaysia.** See *People's, Malaysia.*

**Mann, Neth.** See *Tramedico, Neth.*

**Mann, Singapore.** See *Indrugco, Singapore.*

**Mann, Thai.** See *Zuellig, Thai.*

**Manne, USA.** Manne, P.O. Box 825, Johns Island, SC 29457, USA.

**Manon, Israel.** Manon Ltd, P.O. Box 3905, Tel Aviv, Israel.

**Manor, UK.** Manor Drug Co. (Nottingham) Ltd., Manor House, Merlin Way, Quarry Hill Rd, Ilkeston, Derbyshire, DE7 4RA, UK.

**Manuell, Mex.** Laboratorios Manuell, S.A., Av. del Trabajo No. 237, Col Morelos, Deleg. Venustiano Carranza, 15270 Mexico D.F., Mexico.

**Manx, UK.** Manx Pharma Ltd, Manx House, Spectrum Business Estate, Bircholt Rd, Maidstone, Kent, ME15 9YP, UK.

**MAP, Fin.** MAP Medical Technologies Oy, Elmenttitie 27, 41160 Tikkakoski, Finland.

**Mar, Arg.** Laboratorios Mar S.A., Av. Gaona 3875, 1407 Buenos Aires, Argentina.

**Marano, Ital.** Marano Benito, Via E Vittorini, Villa Scalea, 90147 Palermo, Italy.

**Marbot, Switz.** Dr C Marbot AG, Amselweg 3, 3422 Kirchberg, Switzerland.

**Marcel, Canad.** Les Cosmetiques Marcel de Sevres, 1777 Lavoisier, Ste-Julie, Quebec, J3E 1Y6, Canada.

**Marcel, Mex.** Laboratorios Marcel S.A. de C.V., Calzada Gonzalez Gallo 1707, Jalisco, 44870 Guadalajara, Mexico.

**March, Thai.** March Pharmaceuticals Co. Ltd, 655 Praditmanutham Rd, Wangthonglang, Bangkok 10310, Thailand.

**Marco, Austral.** Marco D'Polo Importing & Merchandising, 12 Lancaster St, Ingleburn, NSW 2565, Australia.

**Marc-O, Canad.** Marc-O Inc. Produits, 3175 Girard St, Trois-Rivieres, Quebec, G8Z 2M5, Canada.

**Marco Viti, Ital.** Marco Viti Farmaceutici S.p.A., Via Galvani 10, 36066 Sandrigo (VI), Italy.

**Marcofina, Hong Kong.** See *C & L, Hong Kong.*

**Marcos Pedrilson, Braz.** Marcos Pedrilson Produtos Hospitalares Ltda, Rua Marechal Niemeyer 22, Botafogo, 22251-060 Rio de Janeiro, RJ, Brazil.

**Margalit, Israel.** Margalit, P.O. Box 16666, Tel Aviv, Israel.

**Marien, Austria.** See *Marien, Ger.*

**Marien, Ger.** Marien-Apotheke Prien am Chiemsee, Marktplatz 10, 83209 Prien, Germany.

**Marin, USA.** AG Marin Pharmaceuticals, 1730 N W 79th Avenue, Miami, FL 33126, USA.

**MarinEx, Hong Kong.** See *Mekim, Hong Kong.*

**Marion Merrell, Fr.** See *Aventis, Fr.*

**Marion Merrell, Spain.** See *Aventis, Spain.*

**Marion Merrell Dow, Port.** See *Aventis, Port.*

**Marion Merrell Dow, Singapore.** See *Aventis, Singapore.*

**Marion Merrell Dow, USA.** See *Aventis, USA.*

**Marjan, Braz.** Marjan Industria e Comercio Ltda, Rua Gibraltar 165, 04755-070 Sao Paulo, SP, Brazil.

**Markos-Mefar, Ital.** Markos-Mefar SpA, Via dei Prati 62, 25073 Bovezzo (BS), Italy.

**Marlin, USA.** Marlin Industries, P.O. Box 560, Grover Beach, CA 93483-0560, USA.

**Marlop, USA.** Marlop Pharmaceuticals Inc., 5704 Mosholu Ave, Bronx, NY 10471, USA.

**Marlyn, USA.** Marlyn Nutraceuticals Inc., 4404 E Ellwood, Phoenix, AZ 85040, USA.

**Marnel, USA.** Marnel Pharmaceuticals Inc., 206 Luke Drive, Lafayette, LA 70506, USA.

**Marrero, Spain.** Marrero Perez, General Bravo 39, Pol. Industrial, Telde, 35200 Las Palmas, Spain.

**Mars, UK.** Mars Ltd, Dundee Rd, Slough, Berkshire, SL1 4JX, UK.

**Marsam, USA.** Marsam Pharmaceuticals Inc., 311 Bonnie Circle, Corona, CA 92882, USA.

**Martin, Arg.** Drogueria Martin S.A., Roque Perez 2543, 1430 Buenos Aires, Argentina.

**Martin, Fr.** See *Martin-Johnson & Johnson, Fr.*

**Martin, Spain.** B Martin Pharma, Centro Empresarial el Planto, Ochandiano 6, 28023 Madrid, Spain.

**Martin, Switz.** See *Uhlmann-Eyraud, Switz.*

**Martin & Harris, India.** Martin & Harris, India.

**Martindale, Hong Kong.** See *LCH, Hong Kong.*

**Martindale Pharmaceuticals, UK.** Martindale Pharmaceuticals Ltd, Bampton Rd, Harold Hill, Romford, Essex, RM3 8UG, UK.

NOTE. There is no connection between Martindale, The Complete Drug Reference and Martindale Pharmaceuticals.

**Martinez Llenas, Spain.** Martinez Llenas, Afueras del Barrio de Santa Ines S/N, La Roca del Valles, 08430 Barcelona, Spain.

**Martin-Johnson & Johnson, Fr.** Laboratoires Martin-Johnson & Johnson-MSD, 1 rue Camille-Desmoulins, TSA 20005, 92797 Issy-les-Moulineaux cdx 9, France.

**Martins & Fernandes, Port.** A. Martins & Fernandes, SA, Rua Raul Mesnier du Ponsard 4-B, 1700 Lisbon, Portugal.

**Maruishi, Jpn.** Maruishi Pharmaceutical Co. Ltd, 2-4-2 Imazunaka, Tsurumi-ku, Osaka 538-0042, Japan.

**Maruko, Jpn.** Maruko Pharmaceutical Co. Ltd, 5-17 Kodama 1-Chome, Nishi-ku, Nagoya 451-0066, Japan.

**Marvecs, Ital.** Marvecs, Italy.

**Masa, Thai.** Masa Lab Co. Ltd, 50/25 Soi Thongpan 2, Takham Rd, Bangkunthien, Bangkok 10150, Thailand.

**Mascia Brunelli, Ital.** Mascia Brunelli S.p.A., Viale Monza 272, 20128 Milan, Italy.

**Mason, USA.** Mason Pharmaceuticals Inc., 6578 Willowbrae Way, Sacramento, CA 95831, USA.

**Masta, UK.** Masta Ltd, Moorfield Rd, Yeadon, Leeds, West Yorkshire, LS19 7BN, UK.

**Mastelli, Ital.** Mastelli S.r.l., Via Bussana Vecchia 32, 18032 Sanremo (IM), Italy.

**Master, Chile.** Laboratorio Farmaceutico Master SA, Av. Irarrazaval 2821, Torre A, Of. 1001, Santiago, Chile.

**Master Pharma, Ital.** Master Pharma S.r.l., Via Firenze 1, 43100 Parma, Italy.

**Masters, UK.** Masters International Ltd, Masters House, 5 Sandridge Close, Harrow, Middlesex, HA1 1XD, UK.

**Matara, Fr.** Laboratoires Matara, 162 rue d'Aguesseau, 92100 Boulogne, France.

**Mathieu, Canad.** JL Mathieu Cie Ltee, 1225 Volta St, Suite 100, Boucherville, Quebec, J4B 7M7, Canada.

**Matley, UK.** Matley Ltd, 34 Sloane Ave, London, SW3 3AX, UK.

**Matrix, USA.** See *Chiron, USA.*

**Mauermann, Ger.** Mauermann-Arzneimittel, Franz Mauermann oHG, Heinrich-Knote-Str. 2, 82343 Pocking, Germany.

**Maurer, Ger.** See *Sebamed, Ger.*

**Maurino, Arg.** Laboratorio Maurino Hnos., 9 de Julio 245, 1708 Moron, Buenos Aires, Argentina.

**Mavena, Ger.** Mavena GmbH, Haubachstrasse 33, 10585 Berlin, Germany.

**Mavena, Switz.** Mavena AG, Birkenweg 1-8, 3123 Belp, Switzerland.

**Maver, Chile.** Laboratorios Maver SA, Emilio Vaisse 574, Providencia, Santiago, Chile.

**Maver, Mex.** Productos Maver S.A. de C.V., Av. Oleoducto No. 2804, Fracc. Industrial El Alamo, 44490 Tlaquepaque, Jal., Mexico.

**Mavi, Ital.** Mavi Sud S.r.l., V.le dell'Industria 1, 04011 Aprilia (LT), Italy.

**Mavi, Mex.** Productos Mavi S.A. de C.V., Osa Menor 197, Col. Prado Churubusco, Deleg. Coyoacan, 04230 Mexico D.F., Mexico.

**Max Farma, Ital.** Max Farma, Via Pisacane 7, 20016 Pero (MI), Italy.

**Max Ritter, Switz.** Max Ritter Pharma SA, Switzerland.

**Maxfarma, Spain.** Maxfarma, Salamanca 13, 28020 Madrid, Spain.

**Maxi, Thai.** Maxi Medical Drug (Mahavej), 27 Paholyothin 41, Bangkok 10900, Thailand.

**Maxim, Thai.** Maxim Intercontinental Ltd Part, 640/56-57 Petchburi 22 Rd, Rajthevi, Bangkok 10400, Thailand.

**May & Baker, Canad.** See *Aventis, Canad.*

**May & Baker, UK.** May & Baker Pharmaceuticals, Rhone Poulenc Ltd, Rainham Rd South, Dagenham, Essex, RM10 7XS, UK.

**Maybelline, Canad.** Maybelline Canada Inc., 6727 Airport Rd, Suite 205, Mississauga, Ontario, L4V 1V2, Canada.

**Mayne, Austral.** Mayne Pharma P/L, Level 7, 369 Royal Parade, Parkville, VIC 3052, Australia.

**Mayne, Hong Kong.** Mayne Pharma (HK) Ltd, Unit 3A, 16/F Eastwood Ctr, 5A Kung Ngam Village Rd, Shaukeiwan, Hong Kong.

**Mayne, UK.** Mayne Pharma Plc, Queensway, Royal Leamington Spa, Warwickshire, CV31 3RW, UK.

**Mayne, USA.** See *Mayne, Austral.*

**Mayo, Mex.** Mayo, Mexico.

**Mayoly-Spindler, Fr.** Laboratoires Mayoly-Spindler, 6 av de l'Europe, 78400 Chatou, France.

**Mayoly-Spindler, Hong Kong.** See *Wing Wai, Hong Kong.*

**Mayoly-Spindler, Malaysia.** See *Antah, Malaysia.*

**Mayoly-Spindler, Singapore.** See *Polymedic, Singapore.*

**Mayoly-Spindler, Switz.** See *Uhlmann-Eyraud, Switz.*

**Mayoly-Spindler, Thai.** See *Charoen, Thai.*

**Mayrand, USA.** See *Merz, USA.*

**Mayrhofer, Austria.** Mayrhofer Pharmazeutika, Melissenweg 15, A-4021 Linz, Austria.

**Mayrs, Irl.** David Mayrs Ltd, Broombridge Industrial Estate, Dublin 11, Ireland.

**Mazal, Fr.** Laboratoires Mazal Pharmaceutique, 11 rue Rontgen, B.P. 1309, 29000 Quimper cdx, France.

**MBD, Singapore.** MBD Marketing (S) Pte Ltd, 371 Beach Rd, 03-30 KeyPoint, S 199597, Singapore.

**MBP, Ger.** Medical Biomaterial Products GmbH, Lederstr. 7, 19306 Neustadt-Glewe, Germany.

**MC, Ital.** MC S.r.l. Off. Prod. Presidi Medico Chirurgici, S.S. 106, 89040 Portigliola (RC), Italy.

**McGaw, NZ.** See *Biomed, NZ.*

**McGaw, USA.** See *Braun, USA.*

**McGaw Biomed, NZ.** See *Biomed, NZ.*

**McGhan, Ger.** McGhan Medical GmbH, Hansaallee 201, 40549 Dusseldorf, Germany.

**McGhan, Hong Kong.** See *Onstrong, Hong Kong.*

**McGloin, Austral.** J. McGloin P/L, P.O. Box 294, Kings Grove, NSW 2208, Australia.

**McGregor, USA.** McGregor Pharmaceuticals Inc., 8420 Ulmenton Rd, Suite 305, Largo, FL 34641, USA.

**McGuff, USA.** McGuff Co., 3524 W Lake Center Drive, Santa Ana, CA 92704, USA.

**McHenry, USA.** McHenry Labs Inc., 118 N Wells, Lee Building, Edna, TX 77957, USA.

**MCM, S.Afr.** MCM Health Care (Pty) Ltd, P.O. Box 501, Halfway House 1685, South Africa.

**McNeil, Hong Kong.** See *Jacobson, Hong Kong,* and *Janssen, Hong Kong.*

**McNeil, Israel.** See *Invest Impex, Israel.*

**McNeil, USA.** RA McNeil Co, 1210 E Dallas Rd, Chattanooga, TN 37405, USA.

**McNeil Consumer, Canad.** McNeil Consumer Healthcare, 890 Woodlawn Rd W., Guelph, Ontario, N1K 1A5, Canada.

**McNeil Consumer, USA.** McNeil Consumer & Specialty Pharmaceuticals, Camp Hill Rd, Fort Washington, PA 19034, USA.

**McNeil Pharmaceutical, USA.** McNeil Pharmaceutical, 1000 US Highway Route 202, P.O. Box 300, Raritan, NJ 08869-0602, USA.

**MCR, USA.** MCR American Pharmaceuticals, 16206 Flight Path Drive, Brooksville, FL 34604, USA.

**MD, Singapore.** MD Pharmaceuticals Pte Ltd, 896 Dunearn Rd, 04-03 Sime Darby Centre, S 589472, Singapore.

**MDA, Austral.** MDA Pharma, 28 Park St, Mona Vale, NSW 2103, Australia.

**MDI, S.Afr.** MDI, South Africa.

**MDM, Fr.** MDM, 9 rue Brezin, 75014 Paris, France.

**MDM, Ital.** MDM S.p.A., Via Volturno 29/B, 20052 Monza (MI), Italy.

**MDR, USA.** MDR Fitness Corp., 14101 NW 4th St, Sunrise, FL 33325, USA.

**MDS Diagnostics, NZ.** MDS Diagnostics, P.O. Box 24-162, Royal Oak, Auckland, New Zealand.

**ME Pharmaceuticals, USA.** ME Pharmaceuticals Inc., 2800 Southeast Parkway, Richmond, IN 47374, USA.

**Mead Johnson, Austral.** See *Bristol-Myers Squibb, Austral.*

**Mead Johnson, Braz.** See *Bristol-Myers Squibb, Braz.*

**Mead Johnson, Chile.** See *Bristol-Myers Squibb, Chile.*

**Mead Johnson, Fr.** See *Bristol-Myers Squibb, Fr.*

**Mead Johnson, Gr.** MEAD JOHNSON, Τατοϊου 102, 146 71 Ν. Ερυθραια, N. Erithraia, Greece.

**Mead Johnson, Hong Kong.** See *Bristol-Myers Squibb, Hong Kong.*

**Mead Johnson, Irl.** See *Bristol-Myers Squibb, Irl.*

**Mead Johnson, Israel.** Mead-Johnson, P.O. Box 8609, New Industrial Zone, Netanya, Israel.

**Mead Johnson, Ital.** See *Bristol-Myers Squibb, Ital.*

**Mead Johnson, Malaysia.** See *Bristol-Myers Squibb, Malaysia.*

**Mead Johnson, Mex.** See *Bristol-Myers Squibb, Mex.*

**Mead Johnson, NZ.** See *Bristol-Myers Squibb, NZ.*

**Mead Johnson, Port.** See *Bristol-Myers Squibb, Port.*

**Mead Johnson, Singapore.** See *Diethelm, Singapore.*

**Mead Johnson Laboratories, USA.** See *Bristol-Myers Squibb, USA.*

**Mead Johnson Nutritionals, Canad.** Mead Johnson Nutritionals, Division of Bristol-Myers Squibb Canada Inc., 333 Preston Ave, Suite 700, Ottawa, Ontario, K1S 5N4, Canada.

**Mead Johnson Nutritionals, Fin.** Mead Johnson Nutritionals, Metsänneidonkuja 8, 02130 Espoo, Finland.

**Mead Johnson Nutritionals, Thai.** Mead Johnson Nutritional Division, Bristol-Myers Squibb Building, 10/10-11 Srinakarin Rd, Bangkaew, Bangplee, Samutprakarn 10540, Thailand.

**Mead Johnson Nutritionals, UK.** See *Bristol-Myers Squibb, UK.*

**Mead Johnson Nutritionals, USA.** Mead Johnson Nutritionals, 2400 W Lloyd Expressway, Evansville, IN 47721-0001, USA.

**Meadow, UK.** Meadow Laboratories, 18 Avenue Rd, Chadwell Heath, Romford, Essex, RM6 4JF, UK.

**Mebo, Thai.** Mebo Co. Ltd, 341 Sukhumvit 101/1 Rd, Bangjak Prakanong, Bangkok 10260, Thailand.

**Meckel, Ger.** Meckel-Spenglersan GmbH, Steinfeldweg 13, 77815 Buhl, Germany.

**Med Immune, Hong Kong.** See *Abbott, Hong Kong.*

**Med. Prod. Panam., USA.** Medical Products Panamericana Inc., 647 W Flagler St, Miami, FL 33130, USA.

**Meda, Denm.** Meda AS, Marielundvej 46A, 2730 Herlev, Denmark.

**Meda, Fin.** Meda Oy, Liesikuja 7, 01600 Vantaa, Finland.

**Meda, Irl.** See *Meda, UK.*

**Meda, Norw.** Meda A/S, Bjerkas Industriomrade, 3470 Slemmestad, Norway.

**Meda, Swed.** Meda AB, Box 906, 170 09 Solna, Sweden.

**Meda, UK.** Meda Pharmaceuticals, Regus House, Herald Way, Pegasus Business Park, Castle Donington, Derbyshire, DE74 2TZ, UK.

**Medac, Ger.** medac Gesellschaft fur klinische Spezialpraparate mbH, Theaterstr. 6, 22880 Wedel, Germany.

**Medac, Gr.** Medac, Greece.

**Medac, UK.** Medac UK, 13 Lynedoch Crescent, Glasgow, G36 6EQ, UK.

**Medchem, S.Afr.** Medchem Pharmaceuticals (Pty) Ltd, P.O. Box 36014, Menlo Park 0102, South Africa.

**Medco, USA.** Medco Laboratories Inc., P.O. Box 864, Sioux City, IA 51102-0864, USA.
**Med-Derm, USA.** Med-Derm Pharmaceuticals, 524 Suncrest Dr., Gray, TN 37615, USA.
**Medea, Spain.** See *Reig Jofre, Spain.*
**Medecine Vegetale, Fr.** Laboratoires Médecine Végétale, 89 rue Salvador-Allende, 95870 Bezons, France.
**Medefield, Austral.** Medefield P/L, 6 Gundah Rd, Mt Kuring-Gai, NSW 2080, Australia.
**Medentech, Irl.** Medentech Ltd, Whitemill Industrial Estate, Whitemill Rd, Wexford, Ireland.
**Medentech, Israel.** See *Concept, Israel.*
**Medestea, Ital.** Medestea Internazionale S.r.l., Via Magenta 43, 10128 Turin, Italy.
**Medeva, Fr.** See *Celltech, Fr.*
**Medeva, Irl.** See *Celltech, Irl.*
**Medeva, Israel.** See *Margalit, Israel.*
**Medeva, Spain.** See *Celltech, Spain.*
**Medeva, Switz.** See *Lifebiotech, Switz.*
**Medeva, UK.** See *Celltech, UK.*
**Medeva, USA.** See *Celltech, USA.*
**Medgenix, Belg.** Medgenix Benelux S.A., Vliegveld 21, 8560 Wevelgem, Belgium.
**Medhel, Gr.** Medhel, Greece.
**Medi Challenge, S.Afr.** Medi Challenge (Pty) Ltd, 1st Floor, Barvic House North, 4 Burke St., Kensington B, Randburg 2125, South Africa.
**Medibase, Ital.** Medibase S.r.l., Via della Selva 4, 59021 Vaiano (PO), Italy.
**Medibel, Switz.** Laboratoire Medibel SA, Case postale 2631, 1211 Geneva 2 Cornavin, Switzerland.
**Medibial, Port.** See *Bial, Port.*
**Medibios, India.** Medibios Labs. Pvt Ltd, 107 Mangalam, Kulupwadi, Mumbai 400 066, India.
**Medibrands, Israel.** Medibrands, P.O. Box 531, Yokneam 20692, Israel.
**Medic, Braz.** Medic Industrial Farmaceutica Ltda, Rua Conselheiro Mayrink 362, 20960-140 Rio de Janeiro, RJ, Brazil.
**Medic, Denm.** Medic Team a/s, Blokken 31 (postboks 193), 3460 Birkerod, Denmark.
**Medic, NZ.** Medic Corp. Ltd, Private Bag, Lower Hutt, Wellington, New Zealand.
**Medica, Arg.** Cosmética Médica, Carabobo 13, 1406 Buenos Aires, Argentina.
**Medica, NZ.** Medica Pacifica Ltd, P.O.Box 24-421, Royal Oak, Auckland, New Zealand.
**Medica Korea, Hong Kong.** See *Health Care, Hong Kong.*
**Medica Korea, Singapore.** See *Zyfas, Singapore.*
**Medicafarm, Ital.** Medicafarm srl, Via Dronero 2, 10144 Turin, Italy.
**Medical, Arg.** Qummica Medical Arg. S.A.C.I., Int. Amaro Avalos 4208, 1605 Munro, Buenos Aires, Argentina.
**Medical, Port.** See *Gestafarma, Port.*
**Medical, Spain.** Medical, Manuel Concha Ruiz 1, 14012 Cordoba, Spain.
**Medical Developments, Austral.** Medical Developments Australia P/L, 7/56 Smith Rd, Springvale, VIC 3171, Australia.
**Medical Diagnostics, UK.** Medical Diagnostics Europe Ltd, The Surrey Technology Centre, Surrey, GU2 7YG, UK.
**Medical Industries, Austral.** Medical Industries Australia P/L, 148-52 Regent St, Redfern, NSW 2016, Australia.
**Medical Instruments, Switz.** Medical Instruments Corp., P.O. Box 706, 4502 Solothurn, Switzerland.
**Medical Ophthalmics, USA.** Medical Ophthalmics Inc., 40146 U.S. Hwy 19 N, Tarpon Springs, FL 34689, USA.
**Medical Research, Austral.** Medical Research P/L, P.O. Box 6025, Parramatta BC, NSW 2150, Australia.
**Medical Research, Hong Kong.** See *Jebsen, Hong Kong.*
**Medical Specialties, Austral.** Medical Specialties Australia P/L, 2 McCabe Place, Willoughby, NSW 2068, Australia.
**Medical Supply, Thai.** Medical Supply Co. Ltd, 101 Sribumpen Rd, Yannawa, Bangkok 10120, Thailand.
**Medicamed, Port.** Medicamed, SA, Edificio Olympus, Av D Afonso Henriques 1462, 4450 Matosinhos, Portugal.
**Medican, Canad.** Medican Pharma Inc., 1120 Victoria St N, Suite 203, Kitchener, Ontario, N2B 3T2, Canada.
**Medicap, Thai.** See *Neopharm, Thai.*
**Medice, Ger.** Medice, Chem.-pharm. Fabrik Pütter GmbH & Co. KG, Kuhloweg 37-9, 58638 Iserlohn, Germany.
**Medice, Switz.** See *Ridupharm, Switz.*
**Medichem, Hong Kong.** See *Unam, Hong Kong.*
**Medichem, Malaysia.** See *Unam, Malaysia.*
**Medichem, Singapore.** See *Far East, Singapore.*
**Medichemie, Switz.** Medichemie AG, Bruhlstrasse 50, 4107 Ettingen, Switzerland.
**Medichemie Bioline, Switz.** See *Medichemie, Switz.*
**Medichrom, Gr.** MEDICHROM ABEE, 26ο χλμ. Λ. Μαρκοπούλου, 190 03 Μαρκόπουλο, Markopoulo, Greece.
**Medici, Ital.** Lab. Farm. Dr Medici S.r.l., Localita Tor Maggiore-Santa Palomba, 00040 Pomezia (Rome), Italy.
**Medicine Supply, Thai.** Medicine Supply Co. Ltd, 767/4 Phaholyothin Rd, Samsennai, Phyathai, Bangkok 10400, Thailand.
**Medicines Company, USA.** The Medicines Company, 5 Sylvan Way, Suite 200, Parsippany, NJ 07054, USA.
**Medicis, Canad.** Medicis Canada Ltd, 355 McCaffrey St, St-Laurent, Quebec, H4T 1Z7, Canada.
**Medicis, USA.** Medicis Pharmaceutical Corp., 8125 N Hayden Dr., Scottsdale, AZ 85258, USA.
**Medico-Biological Laboratories, UK.** Medico-Biological Laboratories Ltd, Kingsend House, 44 Kingsend, Ruislip, Middlesex, HA4 7DA, UK.
**Medicone, USA.** Medicone Co., USA.
**Medicopharm, Austria.** Medicopharm Dr H Sorgo GmbH, Thimiggasse 25, A-1180 Vienna, Austria.
**Medicus, Gr.** MEDICUS AE, Βαλαωρίτου 4, 144 52 Μεταμόρφωση, Metamorphosi, Greece.
**Medidata, Malaysia.** Medidata Sdn Bhd, 36 Jln PJS 8/6, Sunway Mentari, 46150 Petaling Jaya, Selangor, Malaysia.
**Mediderm, Chile.** See *Recalcine, Chile.*
**Medidom, Switz.** Laboratoire Medidom SA, Ave de Champel 24, Case postale 13, 1211 Geneva 12, Switzerland.
**Medifa, Fr.** Medifa, 96-100 avenue de chateaudun, BP 3302, 41033 Blois cedex, France.
**Medifarma, Mex.** Grupo Medifarma S.A. de C.V., Cuancontle No. 7, Col. San Gregorio, Atlapulco Xochimilico, 16600 Mexico D.F., Mexico.
**Medifive, Thai.** Medifive Pharma Co. Ltd, 51/465-466 Drive-in Square, Soi 3 Ladprao Rd, Klongjan, Bangkok 10240, Thailand.
**Medifood, Ital.** Medifood Italia S.r.l., Via Balbi 31/1, 16126 Genoa, Italy.
**Medika, Ger.** Medika Lizenz Pharmaz. Praparate, Am Alten Weg 20, 82041 Oberhaching, Germany.
**Medika, Switz.** Medika AG, Industriestrasse 121, 4147 Aesch, Switzerland.
**Medikem, Fr.** Laboratoires Medikem, Le Cyrano, Rue Rагueneau, B.P. 517, 24100 Bergerac, France.
**Mediline, Israel.** Mediline Ltd, 1 Sha'ar Ha'ir, 22c Ben Gurion St, Herzliya, Israel.
**Medilink, Denm.** Medilink A/S, Somandshvile Park 1 A, 2960 Rungsted Kyst, Denmark.
**Medilink, Norw.** See *Medilink, Denm.*
**Medilink, Swed.** See *Medilink, Denm.*
**MediMar, UK.** MediMar Laboratories, Division of Digen Ltd, 65 High St, Wheatley, Oxford, Oxfordshire, OX33 1XT, UK.
**Medimex, Ger.** Medimex GmbH & Co. KG, Konigsreihe 22, 22041 Hamburg, Germany.
**Medimmune, Denm.** See *Schering-Plough, Denm.*
**Medimmune, Gr.** Medimmune, Greece.
**Medimmune, Israel.** See *Teva, Israel.*
**Medimmune, Norw.** See *Swedish Orphan, Norw.*
**Medimmune, USA.** Medimmune Inc., 35 West Watkins Mill Rd, Gaithersburg, MD 20878, USA.
**Medimpex, UK.** Medimpex UK Ltd, 127 Shirland Rd, London, W9 2EP, UK.
**Medimport, Mex.** Laboratorios Medimport S.A. de C.V., Via Lactea No. 29, Coyoacan Prado Churubusco, 04230 Mexico D.F., Mexico.
**Medinaturals, UK.** Medinaturals, 37 Limpsfield Rd, Sanderstead, Surrey, CR2 9LA, UK.
**Medinex, Canad.** Medinex Ltd, 2 boul. Crepeau, Saint-Laurent, Quebec, H4N 1M7, Canada.
**Medinfar, Port.** Laboratório Medinfar, SA, Rua Manuel Ribeiro da Pavia 1 - 1, Venda Nova, 2700 Amadora, Portugal.
**Medinova (Μεντινοβα), Gr.** MENTINOBA AE, Μενάνδρου 58, 104 32 Αθήνα, Athens, Greece.
**Medinova, Hong Kong.** See *Great Liaison, Hong Kong.*
**Medinova, Port.** See *Confar, Port.*
**Medinova, Singapore.** See *Diethelm, Singapore.*
**Medinova, Switz.** Medinova AG, Eggbuhlstrasse 14, 8052 Zurich, Switzerland.
**Medinovum, Fin.** See *Ratiopharm, Fin.*
**Mediolanum, Ital.** Mediolanum Farmaceutici S.p.A., Via S.G. Cottolengo 15, 20143 Milan, Italy.
**Medipha, Fr.** Medipha Sante SAS, 19 av. de Norvege, Les Fjords, Immeuble le Nobel, 91953 Courtaboeuf cdx, France.
**Medipharm, Chile.** Medipharm SA, Carrion 1398, Independencia, Santiago, Chile.
**Medipharm, Switz.** Medipharm SA, Emil Frey-Strasse 99, 4142 Munchenstein, Switzerland.
**Medipharma, Arg.** Laboratorios Medipharma S.A., Calle 143 1435 e/61 y 62, 1900 La Plata, Buenos Aires, Argentina.
**Medipharma, Ger.** Medipharma Homburg GmbH, Michelinstr. 10, 66424 Homburg, Germany.
**Medipharma, Hong Kong.** Medipharma Ltd, Hong Kong, Unit 2409, Tsuen Wan Industrial Ctr, 220-248 Texaco Rd, Tsuen Wan, N.T., Hong Kong.
**Medi-Physics, USA.** Medi-Physics Inc., Amersham Healthcare, 2636 S Clearbrook Drive, Arlington Heights, Il 60005, USA.
**Mediplant, Belg.** Mediplant, Belgium.
**Mediplants, Gr.** MEDIPLANTS, 2ο χλμ. Σερρών-Θεσσαλονίκης 621 00 Σέρρες, Serres, Greece.
**Mediplus, UK.** Mediplus Ltd, 37-39 Baker St, High Wycombe, Buckinghamshire, HP11 2RX, UK.
**Medirel, Switz.** Medirel SA, Redondello, 6982 Agno, Switzerland.
**Medis, Denm.** Medis-Danmark A/S, Havelse Molle 14, 3600 Frederikssund, Denmark.
**Medis, Israel.** Pharma Medis Co. Ltd, P.O. Box 2820, Holon, Israel.
**Medisa, Switz.** Medisa AG, Postfach 440, 6343 Rotkreuz, Switzerland.
**Medisan, Canad.** See *Pharmacia, Canad.*
**Medisculab, Ger.** See *Biosyn, Ger.*
**Medisense, Austral.** MediSense Products, Abbott Diagnostics Division, 666 Doncaster Rd, Doncaster, VIC 3108, Australia.
**Medisense, Canad.** See *Abbott, Canad.*
**Medisense, UK.** MediSense, Division of Abbott Laboratories, Mallory House, Vanwell Business Park, Maidenhead, Berkshire, SL6 4UD, UK.
**Medisint, Ital.** Medisint S.r.l., Via Settala 10, 20124 Milan, Italy.
**Medison, Israel.** Medison Pharma Ltd, P.O. Box 7090, Petach Tikva, Israel.
**Medispec, Malaysia.** Medispec (M) Sdn Bhd, No 55 & 57 Lorong Sempadan 2, Off Boundary Rd, 11400 Ayer Itam, Penang, Malaysia.
**Medisport, UK.** Medisport International Lts, 1 The Briars, Waterberry Drive, Waterlooville, Hampshire, PO7 7YH, UK.
**Medi-Test, Fr.** Medi-Test, Imm Azur, 4 rue Rene-Razel, 91400 Saclay, France.
**Meditrend, Israel.** Meditrend, 13 Kehilat Saloniki, Tel Aviv, Israel.
**Medivis, Ital.** Medivis S.r.l., Corso Italia 171, 95127 Catania, Italy.
**Mediwhite, Ital.** Mediwhite Srl, Via del Forte Bravetta 98, 00164 Rome, Italy.
**Medix, Fr.** Laboratoires Médix, 18 rue Saint-Mathieu, 78550 Houdan, France.
**Medix, Israel.** See *Genmedix, Israel.*
**Medix, Mex.** Productos Medix S.A. de C.V., Calz. del Hueso No. 39, Col. Ejido Santa Ursula Coapa, Deleg. Coyoacan, 04910 Mexico D.F., Mexico.
**Medix, Spain.** Medix, Alcala 431, 28027 Madrid, Spain.
**Medley, Braz.** Medley S.A. Industria Farmaceutica, Rua Macedo Costa 55, Jardim Santa Genebra, 13080-010 Campinas, SP, Brazil.
**Medline, Thai.** Medline Co. Ltd, 736-742 Pracha-U-Thit Rd, Huay Kwang, Bangkok 10320, Thailand.
**Medlogic, UK.** MedLogic Global Ltd, Western Wood Way, Langage Science Park, Plympton, Plymouth, Devon, PL7 5BG, UK.
**Mednostica, S.Afr.** Mednostica (Pty) Ltd, P.O. Box 36482, Menlo Park 0102, South Africa.
**Medochemie, Hong Kong.** See *Star, Hong Kong.*
**Medochemie, Malaysia.** See *Komedic, Malaysia.*
**Medochemie, Singapore.** See *Derek, Singapore.*
**Medochemie, Thai.** See *Medline, Thai.*
**Medogar, Israel.** Medogar, 16 Halapid St, Petach Tikva 49258, Israel.
**Medopharm, Ger.** Medopharm Arzneimittel GmbH & Co. KG, Grunwalderstr. 22, 79098 Freiburg, Germany.
**Medosan, Ital.** Medosan S.r.l., Industrie Biochimiche Riunite, Via di Cancelliera 12, 00040 Cecchina (RM), Italy.
**Medphano, Ger.** medphano Arzneimittel GmbH, Maienbergstr. 10, 15562 Rudersdorf, Germany.
**Medpointe, USA.** MedPointe Healthcare Inc., 265 Davdison Ave, Suite 300, Somerset, NJ 08873-4120, USA.
**Medpro, S.Afr.** See *Cipla-Medpro, S.Afr.*
**Medquimica, Braz.** Medquimica Industria Farmaceutica Ltda, Rua Otacilio Esteves da Silva 40, Granja Betania, 36045-000 Juiz de Fora, MG, Brazil.
**Medra, Austria.** Medra Handels-GmbH, Gastgebgasse 5-13, A-1230 Vienna, Austria.
**Medra, NZ.** Medra Services, P.O. Box 115, Feilding, New Zealand.
**Medtech, Canad.** Medtech Lab, 330 Esna Park Drive, Markham, Ontario, L3R 1H3, Canada.
**Medtech, USA.** Medtech Laboratories Inc., 3510 N Lake Creek, P.O. Box 1108, Jackson, WY 83011-1108, USA.
**Meduna, Ger.** Meduna Arzneimittel GmbH, Ernst-Grote-Str. 23, 30916 Isernhagen, Germany.
**Mega Vitamin, Austral.** Mega Vitamin Laboratories P/L, 5 Tahlee St, Burwood, NSW 2134, Australia.
**Megapha, Singapore.** Megapha Pte Ltd, 12 Arumugam Rd, 04-08A Cheng Chwee Huat Industrial Building, S 409958, Singapore.
**Megapharm, Israel.** Megapharm Ltd., 8 Hapnina (Nice Building), Kfar Saba, Israel.
**Meiji, Jpn.** Meiji Seika Kaisha Ltd, 2-4-16 Kyobashi, Chuo-ku, Tokyo 104-8002, Japan.
**Meiji, Malaysia.** See *Somedico, Malaysia.*
**Meiji, Singapore.** See *Pharma 2000, Singapore.*
**Meiji, Thai.** Thai Meiji Pharmaceutical Co. Ltd, 8 Fl, Regent House, 183 Rajdamri Rd, Bangkok 10330, Thailand.
**Mein, Spain.** See *Fresenius Kabi, Spain.*
**Meizler, Braz.** Meizler SA, Alameda Jura 149, Alphaville, 06455-010 Barueri, SP, Brazil.
**Mekim, Hong Kong.** Mekim Ltd, Room 905, Harbour Centre Tower 2, 8 Hok Cheung St, Hunghom, Kowloon, Hong Kong.
**Melisana, Belg.** Melisana S.A., Ave du Four a Briques 1, 1140 Brussels, Belgium.
**Melisana, Switz.** Melisana AG, Ankerstrasse 53, Postfach, 8026 Zurich, Switzerland.
**Mellin, Ital.** Mellin, Div. Dietetica Star, Via Matteotti 142, 20041 Agrate Brianza (MI), Italy.
**Melpoejo, Braz.** Laboratorio Melpoejo Ltda, Rua Inacio Gama 723, Bairro de Lourdes, 36070-420 Juiz de Fora, MG, Brazil.
**Menadier, Ger.** Menadier Heilmittel GmbH, Fischers Allee 49-59, 22763 Hamburg, Germany.
**Menarini, Arg.** Laboratorios Menarini Argentina S.A., Girardot 1689, 1427 Buenos Aires, Argentina.
**Menarini, Belg.** Menarini Benelux S.A., Belgicastraat 4, 1930 Zaventem, Belgium.
**Menarini, Fr.** Menarini France, 1 rue du Jura, Silic 528, 94633 Rungis cdx, France.
**Menarini, Gr.** MENARINI HELLAS A.E., Αν. Δαμβέργη 7, 104 45 Αθήνα, Athens, Greece.
**Menarini, Hong Kong.** See *Mekim, Hong Kong.*
**Menarini, Irl.** A. Menarini Pharmaceuticals Ireland Ltd, 72 York Rd, Dun Laoghaire, Dublin, Ireland.
**Menarini, Ital.** A. Menarini Industrie Farmaceutiche Riunite S.r.l., Via Sette Santi 3, 50131 Florence, Italy.
**Menarini, Malaysia.** See *Pharmaforte, Malaysia.*
**Menarini, Neth.** Menarini Farma Nederland, De Bleek 17, 3447 GV Woerden, Netherlands.
**Menarini, Port.** A. Menarini Portugal, Farmaceutica SA, Rua General Ferreira Martins 8 - 6 e 7, 1495-137 Alges, Portugal.
**Menarini, Singapore.** See *Pharmaforte, Singapore.*
**Menarini, Spain.** Menarini, Alfonso XII 587, Badalona, 08918 Barcelona, Spain.
**Menarini, Swed.** Menarini, Sweden.
**Menarini, Switz.** A Menarini AG, Eggbuhlstrasse 14, 8026 Zurich, Switzerland.
**Menarini, Thai.** See *Biopharm, Thai.*
**Menarini, UK.** A Menarini Pharmaceuticals UK Ltd, Menarini House, Mercury Park, Wycombe Lane, Woburn Green, Buckinghamshire, HP10 0HH, UK.
**Menarini Diagnostics, Port.** A. Menarini Diagnósticos Lda, Estrada Nacional 249, Lote 4 - 1, Aboboda, 2785-000 S. Domingos De Rana, Portugal.
**Mendelejeff, Ital.** Stabilimento Chimico Farmaceutico Mendelejeff S.r.l., Via Aurelia 58, 00165 Rome, Italy.
**Menley & James, USA.** Menley & James Laboratories Inc., 100 Tournament Drive, Horsham, PA 19044, USA.
**Mennen, USA.** See *Colgate-Palmolive, USA.*
**Mentholatum, Austral.** Mentholatum Australasia P/L, P.O. Box 398, Mulgrave North, VIC 3170, Australia.
**Mentholatum, Canad.** Mentholatum Co. of Canada Ltd, 20 Lewis St, Fort Erie, Ontario, L2A 5M6, Canada.
**Mentholatum, Israel.** See *Mediline, Israel.*
**Mentholatum, Singapore.** See *Diethelm, Singapore.*
**Mentholatum, UK.** The Mentholatum Co. Ltd, 1 Redwood Ave, Peel Park Campus, East Kilbride, Glasgow, G74 5PF, UK.
**Mentholatum, USA.** Mentholatum Inc., 707 Sterling Dr., Orchard Park, NY 14127, USA.
**Mepha, Braz.** Mepha Inv. Des. e Fab. Farm. Ltda, Est. dos Bandeirantes 4015, 22775-112 Rio de Janeiro, RJ, Brazil.
**Mepha, Hong Kong.** See *Ceutical, Hong Kong.*
**Mepha, Israel.** See *Gilco, Israel.*
**Mepha, Malaysia.** See *JDH, Malaysia,* and *Mepharm, Malaysia.*
**Mepha, Port.** Mepha, Lda, R. Elias Garcia 28 C, Venda Nova, Apartado 6617, 2701-355 Amadora, Portugal.
**Mepha, Singapore.** See *Megapha, Singapore.*
**Mepha, Switz.** Mepha Pharma AG, Postfach 445, 4147 Aesch/BL, Switzerland.
**Mepha, Thai.** See *Amcron, Thai.*
**Mepharm, Malaysia.** Mepharm (Malaysia) Sdn Bhd, 15 Jln Permal 2/1, Taman Subang Permal, 47500 Petaling Jaya, Selangor, Malaysia.
**Merck, Arg.** Merck Qummica Argentina S.A.I.C., Artilleros 2436, 1428 Buenos Aires, Argentina.
**Merck, Austria.** Merck GmbH, Zimbagasse 5, A-1147 Vienna, Austria.
**Merck, Belg.** Merck S.A., Brusselsesteenweg 288, 3090 Overijse, Belgium.
**Merck, Braz.** Merck S.A. Industrias Quimicas, Estrada dos Bandeirantes 1099, 22710-571 Rio de Janeiro, RJ, Brazil.
**Merck, Chile.** Merck Quimica Chilena Ltda, Francisco de Paula Taforo 1981, Nunoa, Santiago, Chile.
**Merck, Denm.** See *Biomet Merck, Denm.,* and *Nordic Drugs, Denm.*
**Merck, Fin.** Merck Oy, Niittyrinne 7, 02270 Espoo, Finland.
**Merck, Ger.** Merck KGaA, Frankfurter Str. 250, 64271 Darmstadt, Germany.

**Merck, Gr.** See *Galenica, Gr.*

**Merck, Hong Kong.** Merck Apotec Ltd, Unit 10-12, 22/F, Paul Y. Ctr, 51 Hung To Rd, Kwan Tung, Hong Kong.

**Merck, India.** Merck (India) Ltd, Shiv Sagar Estate 'A', Dr Annie Besant Rd, Worli, Mumbai 400 018, India.

**Merck, Irl.** Merck Pharmaceuticals Ltd, 2004A Orchard Ave, City West Business Campus, Naas Rd, Dublin 24, Ireland.

**Merck, Israel.** See *Neopharm, Israel.*

**Merck, Ital.** Merck S.p.A., Via G. Stephenson 94, 20157 Milan, Italy.

**Merck, Malaysia.** Merck (Malaysia) Sdn Bhd, 4 Jln U1/26, Section U1, Hicom Glenmarie Industrial Park, 40150 Shah Alam, Selangor, Malaysia.

**Merck, Mex.** Merck-Mexico S.A., Calle 5 Num 7, 53370 Naucalpan de Juarez, Mexico.

**Merck, Neth.** Merck Nederland BV, Basisweg 34, 1043 AP Amsterdam, Netherlands.

**Merck, Norw.** See *Biomet Merck, Norw.*

**Merck, Port.** Merck Farma e Quimica, SA, Rua Alfredo da Silva 3-C, Apartado 3185, 1304 Lisbon, Portugal.

**Merck, S.Afr.** See *Xixia, S.Afr.*

**Merck, Singapore.** Merck Pte Ltd, Pharmaceutical Division, 3 International Business Park, 02-01 Nordic European Centre, S 609927, Singapore.

**Merck, Spain.** Merck Farma Quimica, Poligono Merck, Mollet del Valles, 08100 Barcelona, Spain.

**Merck, Swed.** Merck AB, Pharma Division, Box 23033, 10435 Stockholm, Sweden.

**Merck, Switz.** Merck (Schweiz) AG, Ruchligstrasse 20, 8953 Dietikon, Switzerland.

**Merck, Thai.** Merck Ltd, 19 Fl, Emporium Tower, 622 Sukhumvit Rd, Klongton Klongtoey, Bangkok 10110, Thailand.

**Merck, UK.** E. Merck Pharmaceuticals Ltd, Harrier House, High St, West Drayton, Middlesex, UB7 7QG, UK.

**Merck, USA.** Merck & Co., 1 Merck Dr, White House Station, NJ 08889, USA.

**Merck Bago, Braz.** See *Merck, Braz.*

**Merck Consumer, Singapore.** See *Zuellig, Singapore.*

**Merck Consumer, UK.** See *Seven Seas, UK.*

**Merck dura, Ger.** Merck dura GmbH, Postfach: 100635, 64206 Darmstadt, Germany.

**Merck Frosst, Canad.** Merck Frosst Canada Inc., P.O. Box 1005, Pointe-Claire, Dorval, Quebec, H9R 4P8, Canada.

**Merck Medication Familiale, Fr.** See *Merck-Lipha, Fr.*

**Merck Sante, Malaysia.** See *Merck, Malaysia.*

**Merck Sharp & Dohme, Arg.** Merck Sharp & Dohme (Arg.) Inc., Av. del Libertador 1410, 1638 Vicente Lopez, Buenos Aires, Argentina.

**Merck Sharp & Dohme, Austral.** Merck Sharp & Dohme (Australia) P/L, P.O. Box 79, Granville, NSW 2142, Australia.

**Merck Sharp & Dohme, Austria.** Merck Sharp & Dohme GmbH, Donau-City Strasse 6, A-1220 Vienna, Austria.

**Merck Sharp & Dohme, Belg.** Merck Sharp & Dohme B.V., Chaussee de Waterloo 1135, 1180 Brussels, Belgium.

**Merck Sharp & Dohme, Braz.** Merck Sharp & Dohme Farma Ltda, Rua Alexandre Dumas 2510, 04717-004 Sao Paulo, SP, Brazil.

**Merck Sharp & Dohme, Canad.** See *Merck Frosst, Canad.*

**Merck Sharp & Dohme, Chile.** Merck Sharp & Dohme, Av. Americo Vespucio Sur 100, Of. 401, Las Condes, Santiago, Chile.

**Merck Sharp & Dohme, Denm.** Merck Sharp & Dohme, Smedeland 8, 2600 Glostrup, Denmark.

**Merck Sharp & Dohme, Fin.** Soumen MSD Oy, PL 46, 02151 Espoo, Finland.

**Merck Sharp & Dohme, Ger.** MSD Sharp & Dohme GmbH, Lindenplatz 1, 85540 Haar, Germany.

**Merck Sharp & Dohme, Hong Kong.** Merck Sharp & Dohme (Asia) Ltd, 26/F Caroline Ctr, 28 Yun Ping Rd, Causeway Bay, Hong Kong.

**Merck Sharp & Dohme, Irl.** See *Cahill May Roberts, Irl.*

**Merck Sharp & Dohme, Israel.** MSD Israel, P.O. Box 7121, Petach Tikva, Israel.

**Merck Sharp & Dohme, Ital.** Merck Sharp & Dohme (Italia) S.p.A., Via G. Fabbroni 6, 00191 Rome, Italy.

**Merck Sharp & Dohme, Malaysia.** Merck Sharp & Dohme Malaysia, 15th Floor Menara Merias, 1 Jln 19/3, 46300 Petaling Jaya, Selangor, Malaysia.

**Merck Sharp & Dohme, Mex.** Merck Sharp & Dohme de Mexico S.A. de C.V., Av. Division del Norte No. 3377, Col. Xotepingo, Deleg. Coyoacan, 04610 Mexico D.F., Mexico.

**Merck Sharp & Dohme, Neth.** Merck Sharp & Dohme BV, Postbus 581, 2003 PC Haarlem, Netherlands.

**Merck Sharp & Dohme, Norw.** MSD (Norge) A/S, Solbakken 1, Postboks 458 Brakeroya, 3002 Drammen, Norway.

**Merck Sharp & Dohme, NZ.** Merck Sharp & Dohme (NZ) Ltd, 109 Carlton Gore Road, Newmarket, Auckland, New Zealand.

**Merck Sharp & Dohme, Port.** Merck Sharp & Dohme, Lda, Edificio Vasco da Gama, Quinta da Fonte, Porto Slavo, 2780-730 Paco de Arcos, Portugal.

**Merck Sharp & Dohme, S.Afr.** Merck Sharp & Dohme (Pty) Ltd, Private Bag 3, Halfway House 1685, South Africa.

**Merck Sharp & Dohme, Singapore.** Merck Sharp & Dohme (IA) Corp, Singapore Branch, 300 Beach Road, 13-02 The Concourse, S 199555, Singapore.

**Merck Sharp & Dohme, Spain.** Merck Sharp & Dohme, Josefa Valcarcel 38, 28027 Madrid, Spain.

**Merck Sharp & Dohme, Swed.** Merck Sharp & Dohme (Sweden) AB, Box 7125, 191 07 Sollentuna, Sweden.

**Merck Sharp & Dohme, Switz.** Merck Sharp & Dohme-Chibret SA, Niederlassung von Merck & Co., Inc., USA, Schaffhauserstrasse 136, Postfach, 8152 Glattbrugg, Switzerland.

**Merck Sharp & Dohme, Thai.** See *BLH, Thai.*

**Merck Sharp & Dohme, UK.** Merck Sharp & Dohme Ltd, Hertford Rd, Hoddesdon, Hertfordshire, EN11 9BU, UK.

**Merck Sharp & Dohme, USA.** See *Merck, USA.*

**Merck Sharp & Dohme-Chibret, Fr.** Laboratoires Merck Sharp & Dohme-Chibret, 3 ave Hoche, 75114 Paris cdx 08, France.

**Merck-Belgolabo, Belg.** See *Merck, Belg.*

**Merck-Clevenot, Fr.** Laboratoires Merck-Clévenot, 5-9 rue Anquetil, 94736 Nogent-sur-Marne cdx, France.

**Merckle, Ger.** Merckle GmbH, Graf-Arco-Str. 3, 89079 Ulm, Germany.

**Merck-Lipha, Fr.** Merck Lipha Sante, 37 rue St-Romain, 69008 Lyon, France.

**Merck-Lipha, Hong Kong.** See *Merck, Hong Kong.*

**Merck-Lipha, Singapore.** See *Zuellig, Singapore.*

**Merck-Lipha, Switz.** See *Actipharm, Switz.*

**Merck-Theramex, Hong Kong.** See *Hind Wing, Hong Kong.*

**Meretek, USA.** Meretek Diagnostics Inc., 618 Grassmere Park Drive, Suite 20, Nashville, TN 37211, USA.

**Merial, Denm.** Merial Norden A/S, Gladsaxevej 378, 2860 Soborg, Denmark.

**Mericon, Norw.** Mericon AS, Postboks 1865 Gulset, 3705 Skien, Norway.

**Mericon, USA.** Mericon Industries Inc., 8819 N Pioneer Rd, Peoria, IL 61615, USA.

**Meridian, Israel.** See *Teva, Israel.*

**Merieux, Fr.** See *Aventis Pasteur, Fr.*

**Merind, India.** See *Wockhardt, India.*

**Merisant, Arg.** Merisant Argentina S.R.L., Dardo Rocha 2754 Piso 2 of.2, 1640 Martinez, Buenos Aires, Argentina.

**Merisant, Thai.** See *Diethelm, Thai.*

**Merlin, UK.** Merlin Pharmaceuticals Ltd, 11 Picardy Street, Belvedere, Kent, DA17 5QQ, UK.

**Mer-National, S.Afr.** See *Adcock Ingram, S.Afr.*

**Mertens, Arg.** Mertens S.A. Esp. Medicinales, Av. Montes de Oca 1731, 1271 Buenos Aires, Argentina.

**Merz, Denm.** See *Meda, Denm.*

**Merz, Fin.** See *Tamro, Fin.*

**Merz, Ger.** Merz Pharmaceuticals GmbH, Eckenheimer Landstr. 100-104, 60318 Frankfurt (Main), Germany.

**Merz, Hong Kong.** See *Weston, Hong Kong.*

**Merz, Israel.** See *Megapharm, Israel.*

**Merz, Malaysia.** See *Germax, Malaysia,* and *Summit, Malaysia.*

**Merz, Neth.** See *Aventis, Neth.*

**Merz, Singapore.** See *Green Cross, Singapore.*

**Merz, Switz.** See *Adroka, Switz.*

**Merz, USA.** Merz Pharmaceuticals, 4215 Tudor Lane (27410), P.O. Box 18806, Greensboro, NC 27419, USA.

**Meta, Canad.** Meta Pharmaceuticals, 155 Orenda Rd, Brantford, Ontario, L6W 1W3, Canada.

**Meta Fackler, Ger.** meta Biologische Heilmittel Fackler KG, Philipp-Reis-Str. 3, 31832 Springe, Germany.

**Metabolic Solutions, USA.** Metabolic Solutions Inc., 460 Amherst St, Nashua, NH 03063, USA.

**Metapharma, Canad.** See *Meta, Canad.*

**Metapharma, Ital.** Metapharma S.p.A., Viale delle Dalie 26, 00042 Anzio (RM), Italy.

**Methapharm, Canad.** Methapharm Inc., 131 Clarence St, Brantford, Ontario, N3T 2V6, Canada.

**Methapharm, USA.** Methapharm Inc., 2825 University Dr., Suite 240, Coral Springs, FL 33065, USA.

**Metochem, Austria.** Metochem-Pharma GmbH, Jochen-Rindt-Strasse 23, A-1230 Vienna, Austria.

**Metrika, USA.** Metrika Inc., 510 Oakmead Parkway, Sunnyvale, CA 94085-4022, USA.

**Met-Rx, USA.** Met-Rx Substrate Technology, 2112 Business Center Drive, Irvine, CA 92612-1001, USA.

**Meuse, Belg.** See *Therabel, Belg.*

**Mexin, India.** Mexin Medicaments Pvt Ltd, 142-AB Government Industrial Estate, Kandivli (W), Mumbai 400 067, India.

**Meyer Zall, S.Afr.** Meyer Zall Laboratories (Pty) Ltd, P.O. Box 218, Fontainbleau 2023, South Africa.

**Meyer-Haake, Ger.** Meyer-Haake Medizin- und Dentalhandels GmbH, Adrenaueralle 21, 61440 Oberursel, Germany.

**MGI, Israel.** See *Megapharm, Israel.*

**MGI, USA.** MGI Pharma Inc., 9900 Bren Rd East, Suite 300E, Opus Center, Minnentonka, MN 55343-9667, USA.

**Miba, Ital.** Miba Prodotti Chimici e Farmaceutici S.p.A., Via Falzarego 8, 20021 Ospiate di Bollate (MI), Italy.

**Michallik, Ger.** Fritz Osk. Michallik GmbH & Co., Kisslingweg 60, 75417 Muhlacker, Germany.

**Michaux, Belg.** Labo Michaux, Rue Ed. Schmidt 19, 6280 Gerpinnes, Belgium.

**Mickan, Ger.** Mickan Arzneimittel GmbH, Industriestr. 5, 76189 Karlsruhe, Germany.

**Micro, India.** Micro Labs Ltd, 3 Queens Rd, Bangalore 560 001, India.

**Microsules, Arg.** Microsules Argentina de S.C.I.I.A., Hipolito Yrigoyen 3773, 1208 Buenos Aires, Argentina.

**Microsules Bernabo, Arg.** Microsules y Bernabo S.A., Terrada 2346, 1416 Buenos Aires, Argentina.

**Midax, Ital.** Midax Italia S.r.l., Via Piave 5, 35010 San Pietro in Gu (PD), Italy.

**Midro, Ger.** Midro Lörrach GmbH, Barenfelser Str. 7, 79539 Lorrach, Germany.

**Midro, Israel.** See *Promedico, Israel.*

**Midro, Switz.** Midro Vertrieb AG, Palmenstrasse 1, 4055 Basle, Switzerland.

**Midy, Spain.** See *Sanofi Synthelabo, Spain.*

**Milana, Ital.** Milana S.r.l., Via Liborio Giuffre 50, 90127 Palermo, Italy.

**Milance, USA.** Milance, USA.

**Milano, Thai.** Milano Lab Ltd Part, 62 Soi Latphrao 94, Bangkok 10310, Thailand.

**Miles, Canad.** See *Bayer, Canad.*

**Miles, Ital.** See *Bayer Diagnostici, Ital.*

**Miles, USA.** See *Bayer, USA.*

**Miles Consumer Healthcare, USA.** See *Bayer, USA.*

**Miles Laboratories, USA.** See *Bayer, USA.*

**Milex, Canad.** See *Milex, USA.*

**Milex, USA.** Milex Products Inc., 4311 N Normandy, Chicago, IL 60634-1403, USA.

**Milk Industries, Israel.** See *Hackmey, Israel.*

**Millenium, USA.** Millenium Pharmaceuticals Inc., 75 Sidney St, Cambridge, MA 02139, USA.

**Miller, Braz.** Miller Industrial Farmaceutica Ltda, Rua Magalhaes de Castro 180, 20961-020 Rio de Janeiro, RJ, Brazil.

**Miller, USA.** Miller Pharmacal Group Inc., 350 Randy Rd, Unit 2, Carol Stream, IL 60188, USA.

**Millet Roux, Braz.** Produtos Farmaceuticos Millet Roux Ltda, Praia de Botafogo 440, 25 andar, 22250-040 Rio de Janeiro, RJ, Brazil.

**Milmet, India.** See *Sun, India.*

**Milo, Spain.** Milo, Av. Constitucion 18 E, Cuarte de Huerva, 50410 Zaragoza, Spain.

**Milte, Ital.** Milte Italia S.p.A., Via Tadino 29/A, 20124 Milan, Italy.

**Milte, Port.** Milte Portugal, SA, Av Marechal Gomes da Costa 19, 1800-255 Lisbon, Portugal.

**Milton, Austral.** Milton Pharmaceuticals P/L, 100 Antimony St, Carole Park, QLD 4300, Australia.

**Milupa, Austria.** Milupa GmbH, Postfach 2, A-5412 Puch, Austria.

**Milupa, Fr.** Milupa, 4 rue Joseph-Monier, 92859 Rueil-Malmaison cdx, France.

**Milupa, Hong Kong.** See *Connell, Hong Kong.*

**Milupa, Irl.** Milupa Ltd, Block 1, Deansgrange Business Park, Co. Dublin, Ireland.

**Milupa, Ital.** Milupa S.p.A., Via Lepetit 8, 20020 Lainate (MI), Italy.

**Milupa, Port.** Milupa Portuguesa, Lda, Zona Industrial, 2795 Carnaxide, Portugal.

**Milupa, Singapore.** Milupa, Singapore.

**Milupa, Switz.** Milupa SA, 1564 Domdidier, Switzerland.

**Milupa, UK.** Milupa Ltd, Division of Nutricia, Newmarket Ave, White Horse Business Park, Trowbridge, Wiltshire, BA14 0XQ, UK.

**Minancora, Braz.** Minancora & Cia Ltda, Rua do Principe 461, 89201-001 Joinville, SC, Brazil.

**Minerva (Μινερβα), Gr.** ΜΙΝΕΡΒΑ ΦΑΡΜΑΚΕΥΤΙΚΗ ΑΕ, Λ. Κηφισού 132, 121 31 Περιστέρι, Peristeri, Greece.

**Mini, Switz.** Bernardo Mini & Co, Loretostrasse 5, 6300 Zug, Switzerland.

**Mintlab, Chile.** Mintlab Co SA, Nueva Andres Bello 1940, Independencia, Santiago, Chile.

**MIP, Ger.** MIP Pharma GmbH, Kirkeler Str. 41, 66440 Blieskastel, Germany.

**Mipharm, Ital.** Mipharm S.p.A., Via B Quaranta 12, 20141 Milan, Italy.

**Miquel Garriga, Spain.** Miquel Garriga, Joaquin Costa 18, Montgat, 08390 Barcelona, Spain.

**Miquel Otsuka, Spain.** See *Otsuka, Spain.*

**Mirren, S.Afr.** Mirren (Pty) Ltd, P.O. Box 87607, Houghton 2041, South Africa.

**Misemer, USA.** See *Edwards, USA.*

**Mission, Austral.** Mission Pharmacal Australia Pty Ltd., Level 2, 294 New South Head Road, Double Bay, NSW 2028, Australia.

**Mission Pharmacal, Hong Kong.** See *International Medical, Hong Kong.*

**Mission Pharmacal, Malaysia.** See *Somedico, Malaysia.*

**Mission Pharmacal, Singapore.** See *Pharma 2000, Singapore.*

**Mission Pharmacal, USA.** Mission Pharmacal Co., 10999 IH 10 West, Suite 1000, San Antonio, TX 78230-1355, USA.

**MIT, Ger.** MIT Gesundheit GmbH, Flutstr. 74, 47533 Kleeve, Germany.

**Mita, Hong Kong.** Mita Pharmaceutical Co. Ltd, Rm 1208, 12/F, Phase 1, Metro Ctr, 32 Lam Hing St, Kowloon Bay, Kowloon, Hong Kong.

**Mitchell, UK.** Mitchell International Pharmaceuticals Ltd, Unit 7, Kingston House Estate, Portsmouth Road, Thames Ditton, Surrey, KT6 5QG, UK.

**Mitim, Ital.** Mitim S.r.l., Via Rodi 27, 25126 Brescia, Italy.

**Mitsubishi, Jpn.** See *Mitsubishi-Tokyo, Jpn.*

**Mitsubishi, Thai.** See *Diethelm, Thai.*

**Mitsubishi-Tokyo, Hong Kong.** See *Hing Ah, Hong Kong.*

**Mitsubishi-Tokyo, Jpn.** Mitsubishi-Tokyo Pharmaceuticals Inc., 2-6 Nihonbashi-Honcho 2-chome, Chuo-ku, Tokyo 103-8405, Japan.

**Mitsui, Jpn.** Mitsui Seiyaku, Asahi Building, 3-12-2 Nihonbashi, Chuo-ku, Tokyo, Japan.

**Miyarisan, Jpn.** Miyarisan Pharmaceutical Co., Ltd, 1-10-3 Kaminakazato, Kita-ku, Tokyo 114-0016, Japan.

**Mizar, Spain.** Mizar Farmaceutica, Gran Via Corts Catalanes 764, 08013 Barcelona, Spain.

**ML Laboratories, UK.** ML Laboratories Plc, Blaby Hall, Church St, Blaby, Leicestershire, LE8 4FA, UK.

**MM, India.** M.M. Labs., Mahalaxmi Chambers, 22 Bhulabhai Desai Rd, Mumbai 400 026, India.

**Mochida, Jpn.** Mochida Pharmaceutical Co. Ltd, 1-7 Yotsuya, Shinjuku-ku, Tokyo 160-8515, Japan.

**Modern Health Products, UK.** Modern Health Products Ltd, Sisson Rd, Gloucester, GL1 3QB, UK.

**Modi-Mundipharma, India.** Modi-Mundipharma Ltd, 1400 Modi Tower, 98 Nehru Place, New Delhi 110 019, India.

**Molar, UK.** Molar Ltd, The Close, West End, Wedmore, Somerset, MS28 4BN, UK.

**Molimin, Ger.** Molimin Arzneimittel GmbH, Emil-Kemmer-Str. 33, 96103 Hallstadt, Germany.

**Molnlycke, Fr.** Laboratoires Mölnlycke Health Care, ZAC du Moulin, av Clement-Ader, B.P. 42, 59118 Wambrechies cdx, France.

**Molnlycke, Ital.** Molnlycke Health Care srl, Via Marsala 40/c, 21013 Gallarate (VA), Italy.

**Molteni, Ital.** L. Molteni & C. dei F.lli Alitti S.p.A., S.S. 67, Fraz. Granatieri, 50018 Scandicci (FI), Italy.

**Mona Lisa, Israel.** See *Hackmey, Israel.*

**Monal, Fr.** See *Novartis, Fr.*

**Monarch, USA.** Monarch Pharmaceuticals, 355 Beecham St, Bristol, TN 37620, USA.

**Monchpharma, Ger.** Mönchpharma Arzneimittel GmbH, Genhulsen 35, 41179 Munchengladbach, Germany.

**Monico, Ital.** Monico S.p.A., Via Ponte di Pietra 7, 30173 Venezia-Mestre (VE), Italy.

**Monik, Spain.** Monik, Avda de la Playa 1, Conil de la Frontera, 11140 Cadiz, Spain.

**Monin, Fr.** Laboratoires Monin-Chanteaud, Parc Euromedecine II, rue de la Valsiere, 34099 Montpellier cdx 5, France.

**Monmouth, Irl.** See *Allphar, Irl.*

**Monmouth, UK.** See *Shire, UK.*

**Monoclonal Antibodies, USA.** See *Quidel, USA.*

**Monot, Fr.** See *Merck-Lipha, Fr.*

**Monsanto, Fr.** See *Pharmacia, Fr.*

**Monsanto, Ital.** Monsanto Italiana S.p.A., Via Walter Tobagi 8, 20089 Peschiera Borromeo (MI), Italy.

**Monsanto, Port.** See *Pharmacia, Port.*

**Monsanto, Spain.** See *Pharmacia, Spain.*

**Monserrat, Arg.** Monserrat y Eclair S.A., Virrey Cevallos 1625/7, 1135 Buenos Aires, Argentina.

**Montavit, Austria.** Montavit GmbH, Salzbergstrasse 96, A-6060 Absam, Austria.

**Montavit, Israel.** See *Lapidot, Israel.*

**Montavit, Neth.** See *Roussel, Neth.*

**Montavit, Thai.** Montavit.

**Montebello, Fr.** Montebello France SA, av.des Noelles, B.P. 216, 44505 La Baule cdx, France.

**Montefarmaco, Ital.** Montefarmaco S.p.A., Via G. Galilei 7, 20016 Pero (MI), Italy.

**Montpellier, Arg.** See *Disprofarma, Arg.*

**Moore, USA.** Moore Medical Corp., 389 John Downey Dr., P.O. Box 2740, New Britain, CT 06050, USA.

**Morado, Ital.** Morado S.p.A., Via Cacciamali 36, 25125 Brescia, Italy.

**Moraz, UK.** See *Impharm, UK.*

**Morrith, Spain.** Morrith, Valle de la Fuenfria 3, 28034 Madrid, Spain.

**Morson, Irl.** See *Cahill May Roberts, Irl.*

**Morton Grove, USA.** Morton Grove Pharmaceuticals Inc., 6451 West Main St, Morton Grove, IL 60053, USA.

**Morton Salt, USA.** Morton Salt, 123 N Wacker Dr., Chicago, IL 60606-1597, USA.

**Moskizol, Fr.** Laboratoires Moskizol, Allee de la Gare, 95570 Bouffemont, France.
**Motima, Fr.** Laboratoires Motima, 19 rue de Passy, 75016 Paris, France.
**MPF, Singapore.** See *Luen Wah, Singapore.*
**MPS, Austral.** MPS Laboratories (Australia) P/L, 8 Kinane Street, Brighton, VIC 3186, Australia.
**MSD Chibropharm, Ger.** See *Merck Sharp & Dohme, Ger.*
**MSO, Ger.** MedacSchering Onkologie GmbH (MSO), Nordliche Auffahrtsallee 44, 80638 Munich, Germany.
**Mt. Vernon, USA.** Mt. Vernon Foods Inc., 13246 Wooster Rd, Mt. Vernon, OH 43050-9726, USA.
**Much, Ger.** Much Pharma GmbH, Memeier Str. 30, 42781 Haan, Germany.
**Mucos, Austria.** Mucos Emulsions-GmbH, Leberstrasse 96, A-1110 Vienna, Austria.
**Mucos, Ger.** Mucos Pharma GmbH & Co., Malvenweg 2, 82538 Geretsried, Germany.
**Muller Goppingen, Ger.** Chemisch-Pharmazeutische Fabrik Göppingen Carl Müller, Apotheker, GmbH & Co. KG, Bahnhofstr. 33-35 & 40, 73033 Goppingen, Germany.
**Multichem, NZ.** Multichem, Private Bag 93527, Takapuna, Auckland, New Zealand.
**Multilan, Israel.** See *Neopharm, Israel.*
**Multi-Pro, Canad.** Distributions Multi-Pro Inc., 8480 Champ d'eau, St-Leonard, Quebec, H1P 1Y3, Canada.
**Mundipharma, Austral.** Mundipharma, P.O. Box 5214, Sydney, NSW 1044, Australia.
**Mundipharma, Austria.** Mundipharma GmbH, Apollogasse 16-18, A-1072 Vienna, Austria.
**Mundipharma, Fin.** Mundipharma Oy, Rajatorpantie 41 B, 01640 Vantaa, Finland.
**Mundipharma, Fr.** Mundipharma, 42 rue d'Aguesseau, 92100 Boulogne-Billancourt, France.
**Mundipharma, Ger.** Mundipharma GmbH, Mundipharma Str. 2, 65549 Limburg (Lahn), Germany.
**Mundipharma, Hong Kong.** See *Jacobson, Hong Kong.*
**Mundipharma, Irl.** Mundipharma Pharmaceutical Co., 54 Fitzwilliam Square, Dublin 2, Ireland.
**Mundipharma, Norw.** mundipharma AS, Postboks 218, 1326 Lysaker, Norway.
**Mundipharma, Singapore.** See *Cork, Singapore.*
**Mundipharma, Swed.** Mundipharma AB, Mölndalsvagen 26, 412 63 Goteborg, Sweden.
**Mundipharma, Switz.** Mundipharma Medical Co, St Alban-Rheinweg 74, 4006 Basle, Switzerland.
**Mundipharma, Thai.** See *JDH Borneo, Thai.*
**Mundogen, Spain.** Mundogen Farma, Maria Tubau 5, Edif Auge VI, 28050 Madrid, Spain.
**Munro, UK.** Munro Wholesale Medical Supplies Ltd, 10 Stroud Rd, Kelvin Industrial Estate, East Kilbride, G75 0YA, UK.
**Murat, Fr.** Laboratoires Murat, 160 rue de Paris, 92771 Boulogne-Billancourt, France.
**Murdock, USA.** Murdock, Madaus, Schwabe, P.O. Box 4000, Springville, UT 84663, USA.
**Muro, Israel.** See *Megapharm, Israel.*
**Muro, USA.** Muro Pharmaceutical Inc., 890 East St, Tewksbury, MA 01876-1496, USA.
**Musa, Braz.** Laboratorio Musa Rodolpho Jordano Ltda, Rua Pedra Dourada 110, Zona Industrial de Jacarepagua, 22780-082 Rio de Janeiro, Brazil.
**MVM, Fr.** Laboratoires MVM, 33 rue Vivienne, 75002 Paris, France.
**Mykal, UK.** Mykal Industries Ltd, Farnsworth House, Morris Close, Park Farm Industrial Estate, Wellingborough, Northamptonshire, NN8 6XF, UK.
**Myplan, UK.** Myplan Ltd, Old Colwall, Malvern, Worcestershire, WR13 6HF, UK.
**Myra, Singapore.** See *Far East, Singapore.*
**Myra, Thai.** See *Olic, Thai.*
**MZ, S.Afr.** MZ, South Africa.
**Nabi, USA.** Nabi Biopharmaceuticals, 5800 Park of Commerce Blvd NW, Boca Raton, FL 33487, USA.
**Nadeau, Canad.** See *Technilab, Canad.*
**Nadinola, Canad.** See *Hargell, Canad.*
**Naf, Arg.** Lab. Naf S.A., Lamadrid 1263/75, 1653 Villa Ballester, Buenos Aires, Argentina.
**Nagor, UK.** Nagor Ltd, P.O. Box 21, Douglas, Isle of Man, IM99 1AX, UK.
**Naina, Singapore.** Naina Mohamed & Sons Pte Ltd, 1 Ubi Crescent, 05-04 Number One Building, S 408563, Singapore.
**Nakorn, Thai.** See *TNP, Thai.*, and *V & V, Thai.*
**Nakornpatana, Thai.** Nakornpatana Pharm Co. Ltd, 495, 601/5-8 Soi Suthiporn, Prachasongkroh Rd, Dindaeng, Bangkok 10400, Thailand.
**NAM, Ger.** NAM Neukönigsförder Arzneimittel GmbH, Moorbeker Strasse 35, 26197 Grossenkneten, Germany.
**Napp, Irl.** See *Mundipharma, Irl.*
**Napp, NZ.** See *Douglas, NZ.*
**Napp, UK.** Napp Pharmaceuticals Ltd, Cambridge Science Park, Milton Rd, Cambridge, Cambridgeshire, CB4 0GW, UK.
**Narco-Med, Switz.** Narco-Med AG, Romanshornerstrasse 115, 8280 Kreuzlingen, Switzerland.
**Narval, Spain.** Narval Pharma, Av.America 37, 28002 Madrid, Spain.
**Nasmark, Canad.** Nasmark Inc., 5650 Tomken Rd, Unit 12, Mississauga, Ontario, L4W 4P1, Canada.
**Nastech, Israel.** See *Tzamal, Israel.*
**Nat Druggists, S.Afr.** National Druggists (Pty) Ltd, P.O. Box 3253, Durban 4000, South Africa.
**Nathura, Ital.** Nathura Srl, Via Meucci 14, 42027 Montecchio Emilia (RE), Italy.
**National Blood Centre, Thai.** National Blood Centre, Thai Red Cross Society, Thailand.
**National Care, Canad.** National Care Products, 251 Saulteaux Crescent, Winnipeg, Manitoba, R3J 3C7, Canada.
**National Diagnostic, Austral.** National Diagnostic Products (Australia) P/L, 7-9 Merriwa St, Gordon, NSW 2072, Australia.
**Nativelle, Switz.** See *Interdelta, Switz.*
**Natrahealth, UK.** Natrahealth, UK.
**Natren, USA.** Natren Inc., 3105 Willow Lane, Westlake Village, CA 91361, USA.
**Nattermann, Ger.** Nattermann, Division der Aventis Pharma Deutschland GmbH, Nattermannallee 1, 50829 Cologne, Germany.
**Nattermann, Spain.** Nattermann, Avda de Leganes 62, Alcorcon, 28925 Madrid, Spain.
**Natufarma, Arg.** Lab. Natufarma, Av. Cordoba 1745, 3080 Esperanza, Santa Fe, Argentina.
**Natural Health, Arg.** Natural Health S.A. grup. K. Parker, Sarachaga 4457, 1407 Buenos Aires, Argentina.
**Natural Life, Arg.** Natural Life S.A., Tucuman 3516, 1189 Buenos Aires, Argentina.
**Natural Touch, UK.** Natural Touch Ltd, 7 Dragoon House, Hussar Court, Brambles Farm, Waterlooville, Hampshire, PO7 7SE, UK.
**Naturarzneimittel, Ger.** Naturarzneimittel Regneri GmbH & Co. KG, Carl-Zeiss-Str. 4, 76275 Ettlingen, Germany.
**Nature's Bounty, USA.** Nature's Bounty Inc., 90 Orville Drive, Bohemia, NY 11716, USA.
**Natures Kiss, Austral.** Nature's Kiss Australia P/L, Level 4, 171 Clarence St, Sydney, NSW 2000, Australia.
**Naturest, Hong Kong.** Naturest Co. Ltd, Suite 2508, Bank of America Tower, 12 Harcourt Rd Central, Hong Kong.
**Naturland, Austria.** Naturland GmbH, St Veit-Gasse 56, A-1130 Vienna, Austria.
**Naturmed, Ital.** Naturmed 2000 S.r.l., Via Prov.le 33 (Resid. Oasi), 19030 Castelnuovo Magra (SP), Italy.
**Naturopathica, Austral.** Naturopathica, P.O. Box 7096, Sydney, NSW 2001, Australia.
**Naturopathica, UK.** Naturopathica, UK.
**Naturpharma, Switz.** Naturpharma SA, 5d route des Jeunes, Case postale 8, 1211 Geneva 26, Switzerland.
**Natus, Braz.** Laboratorios Farmaceuticos Natus Ltda, Rua Maxwell 116, Vila Isabel, 20541-100 Rio de Janeiro, RJ, Brazil.
**Natysal, Spain.** Naytsal, C/ Molino 2, Meco, 28880 Madrid, Spain.
**Naveh, Israel.** Naveh Pharmacy, 170 Arlozoroff St, Tel Aviv, Israel.
**NBF-Lanes, Ital.** N.B.F. Lanes S.r.l., Corso di Porta Vittoria 14, 20122 Milan, Italy.
**NBI, S.Afr.** NBI, South Africa.
**NBZ, India.** NBZ-Pharma Ltd, R-905 MIDC, Rabale, Navi Mumbai 400 701, India.
**NCSN, Ital.** NCSN Farmaceutici S.r.l., Via Svetonio 15, 00136 Rome, Italy.
**Neat Feat, NZ.** Neat Feat Products Ltd, P.O. Box 65256, Auckland, New Zealand.
**Nebo, Hong Kong.** See *Zuellig, Hong Kong.*
**Neckerman, Braz.** Neckerman Industria Farmaceutica Ltda, Rua das Peroberias 157, 05879-470 Sao Paulo, SP, Brazil.
**Nefox, Spain.** See *Pfizer, Spain.*
**Nefro, Austria.** Nefro Pharma Grosshandelsgmbh, An der Landesbahn 2-4, A-2100 Korneuburg, Austria.
**Negma, Belg.** See *Vitalpharma, Belg.*
**Negma, Fr.** Laboratoires Negma-Lerads, Imm Strasbourg, av de l'Europe, Toussus-le-Noble, 78771 Magny-les-Hameaux cdx, France.
**Negma, Israel.** See *Pharmateam, Israel.*
**Neiadas (Νειαδας), Gr.** ΝΕΙΑΔΑΣ & ΥΙΟΙ Α.Ε., Αγ. Μαρίνης 190 02 Παιανια, Paiania, Greece.
**Nella, UK.** Nella Pharmaceutical Products Ltd, Rockfield House, Darwen Rd, Bromley Cross, Bolton, Lancashire, BL7 9DX, UK.
**Nelson, UK.** A Nelson & Co. Ltd, Broadheath House, 83 Parkside, London, SW19 5LP, UK.
**Neo Dermos, Arg.** Neo Dermos S.R.L., Francisco Bilbao 1927, 1406 Buenos Aires, Argentina.
**Neo Laboratories, UK.** Neo Laboratories Ltd, UK.
**Neo Quimica, Braz.** Laboratorio Neo Quimica Comercio e Industria Ltda, Rua VPR 1 Quadra 2-A, Modulo 4 DAIA, 75133-600 Anapolis, GO, Brazil.
**Neocorp, Ger.** Neocorp AG, Am Weidenbach 6, 82362 Weilheim, Germany.
**Neo-Farmaceutica, Port.** Neo-Farmacêutica, Lda, Avenida da Republica 45, 1050-187 Portugal, Portugal.
**Neolab, Canad.** Neolab, 5476 Upper Lachine Rd, Montreal, Quebec, H4A 2A4, Canada.
**Neo-Life, Austral.** See *GNLD, Austral.*
**Neom, Fr.** Laboratoires Neom, 5 ave., 17 rue, B.P. 556, 06516 Carros cdx, France.
**Neopharm, Israel.** Neopharm Ltd, P.O. Box 3506, Petach Tikva, Israel.
**Neopharm, Thai.** Neopharm Co. Ltd, 5/26-27 Soi Udomsap, Baromrachonnanee Rd, Arunamarin, Bangkoknoi, Bangkok 10700, Thailand.
**Neopharma, Ger.** Neopharma GmbH & Co. KG, Kirchstr. 10, 83229 Aschau i. Chiemgau, Germany.
**Neo-Pharma, India.** Neo-Pharma Pvt Ltd, Kasturi Building, 5th Floor, J. Tata Rd, Mumbai 400 020, India.
**Neopharmed, Ital.** Neopharmed S.p.A., Via Vitorchiano 151, 00189 Rome, Italy.
**Neovita, Braz.** Instituto Farmoterapico Neovita Ltda, Rua Dr. Rodrigues Santana 80, 20910-240 Rio de Janeiro, RJ, Brazil.
**Nepalm, Fr.** Laboratoires Nepalm Sarl, 136 bis, av des Freres-Luminiere, 69008 Lyon, France.
**Nephron, USA.** Nephron Pharmaceuticals Corp., 4121 SW 34th St, Orlando, FL 32811, USA.
**Nephro-Tech, USA.** Nephro-Tech, Inc., P.O. Box 16106, Shawnee, KS 66203, USA.
**Nestle, Arg.** Nestlé Argentina S.A., Carlos Pellegrini 887, 1009 Buenos Aires, Argentina.
**Nestle, Austral.** Nestle Australia Ltd, 60 Bathurst St, Sydney, NSW 2000, Australia.
**Nestle, Braz.** Nestle Indl. e. Coml. Ltda, Av. das Nacoes Unidas 12495, 04578-902 Sao Paulo, SP, Brazil.
**Nestle, Canad.** Nestle Canada Inc., 25 Sheppard Ave W, North York, Ontario, M2N 6S8, Canada.
**Nestle, Fr.** Nestlé, 7 bd Pierre-Carle, B.P. 900, Noisiel, 77446 Marne-la-Vallee cdx 2, France.
**Nestle, Hong Kong.** Nestle Hong Kong Ltd, 28/F, PCCW Tower, Taikoo Place, 979 King's Rd, Quarry Bay, Hong Kong.
**Nestle, Israel.** See *Megapharm, Israel.*
**Nestle, Ital.** Nestlè Italiana S.p.A., Viale G. Richard 5, 20143 Milan, Italy.
**Nestle, Malaysia.** Nestle (Malaysia) Bhd, Nestle House, 4, Lorong Pesiaran, 46918 Petaling Jaya, Selangor, Malaysia.
**Nestle, Mex.** Nestle Mexico S.A. de C.V., Av Ejercito Nacional No. 453, Col. Granada, Deleg. Miguel Hidalgo, 11520 Mexico D.F., Mexico.
**Nestle, Norw.** A/S Nestlé Norge, Barnematavd., Postboks 595, 1301 Sandvika, Norway.
**Nestle, Port.** Nestlé Portugal, SA, Rua Alexandre Herculano 8-8A, 2795-010 Linda-a-Velha (Carnaxide-Oeiras), Portugal.
**Nestle, Singapore.** Nestle, Singapore.
**Nestle, Switz.** Nestlé Suisse AG, Case postale 352, 1800 Vevey, Switzerland.
**Nestle, Thai.** Nestle Products (Thailand) Inc, 18-21 Fl, Amarin Tower, 500 Ploenchit Rd, Pathumwan, Bangkok 10330, Thailand.
**Nestle, UK.** Nestlé UK Ltd, St George's House, Park Lane, Croydon, Surrey, CR9 1NR, UK.
**Nestle, USA.** Nestle Clinical Nutrition, 3 Parkway N, Suite 500, Deerfield, IL 60015, USA.
**Nestle Clinical, Irl.** See *Baxter, Irl.*
**Netpharma, Swed.** See *Ivax, Swed.*
**Nettopharma, Denm.** See *Nycomed, Denm.*
**Network Health & Beauty, UK.** Network Health & Beauty, Network House, 41 Invincible Rd, Farnborough, Hampshire, GU14 7QU, UK.
**Neuners, Austria.** Neuner's Kräuterprodukte GmbH, Oberndorf 60, A-6322 Kirchbichl, Austria.
**Neuraxpharm, Ger.** neuraxpharm Arzneimittel GmbH & Co. KG, Elisabeth-Selbert-Str. 23, 40764 Langenfeld, Germany.
**Neurex, USA.** See *Elan, USA.*
**Neurogard, Spain.** See *Merck Sharp & Dohme, Spain.*
**NeuroGenesis, USA.** NeuroGenesis/Matrix Tech. Inc., 120 Park Ave, League City, TX 77573, USA.
**Neuropharma, Arg.** Neuropharma, Pringles 10 Piso 3, 1183 Buenos Aires, Argentina.
**Neusc, Spain.** Neusc, Apartado de Correos 11, Vic, 08500 Barcelona, Spain.
**Neutrogena, Fr.** See *Ethicon, Fr.*
**Neutrogena, Israel.** See *Randi, Israel.*
**Neutrogena, UK.** See *Johnson & Johnson, UK.*
**Neutrogena, USA.** Neutrogena Corp., 5760 W 96th St, Los Angeles, CA 90045-5595, USA.
**Neutrogena Dermatologicals, USA.** See *Neutrogena, USA.*
**Neutron Technology, USA.** Neutron Technology Corp, 800 S Federal Way, Boise, ID 83707, USA.
**Neves, Port.** Laboratório J. Neves, Lda, Parque Industrial do Seixal, 2840 Paio Pires, Portugal.
**New England Nuclear, Austria.** New England Nuclear, Vienna, Austria.
**New Farma, Ital.** New Farma Soc. Coop. a.r.l., Via Guglielmino 62/D, 95030 Tremestieri (CT), Italy.
**New Research, Ital.** New Research S.r.l., P.za Don Luigi Sturzo 34, 04011 Aprilia (LT), Italy.
**New Ulros, Ital.** New Ulros S.r.l., Via delle Industrie 40, 35020 Albignasego (PD), Italy.
**New Vision, Canad.** New Vision Nutritionals Co., 3140 14th Ave NE, Suite 1, Calgary, Alberta, T2A 6J4, Canada.
**NewFaDem, Ital.** New.Fa.Dem. Srl Farmaceutici e Chimici, Via Ferrovie dello Stato 1, 80014 Giugliano (NA), Italy.
**Newlab, Braz.** Newlab Industria Farmaceutica Ltda, Av. Sebastiao Eugenio de Camrgo 59, 05360-010 Sao Paulo, SP, Brazil.
**Newport, Irl.** Newport Pharmaceuticals Ltd, Frank Maas House, Swords Business Park, Swords, Co. Dublin, Ireland.
**Newport Synthesis, Irl.** Newport Synthesis Ltd, Baldoyle Industrial Estate, Dublin 13, Ireland.
**Nexis, Spain.** Nexis Farmaceutica, Principe de Vergara 112, 28001 Madrid, Spain.
**Nexstar, Belg.** Nexstar Pharmaceuticals Inc., Laarstraat 16, 2610 Wilrijk, Belgium.
**Nexstar, Israel.** See *Neopharm, Israel.*
**Nexstar, USA.** NeXstar Pharmaceuticals Inc., 2860 Wilderness Place, Boulder, CO 80301, USA.
**Nezel, Spain.** See *Solvay, Spain.*
**NHS, Fr.** NHS, 1-7 rue du Jura, Silic 528, 94633 Rungis cdx, France.
**Niche, Denm.** Niche Pharma, Tvedangen 225, 2730 Herlev, Denmark.
**Niche, Irl.** Niche Generics Ltd, Unit 5, Baldoyle Industrial Estate, Dublin 13, Ireland.
**Niche, Singapore.** See *JDH, Singapore.*
**Niche, USA.** Niche Pharmaceuticals Inc, 200 N Oak St, P.O. Box 449, Roanoake, TX 76262.
**Nicholas, Fr.** See *Roche Nicholas, Fr.*
**Nicholas Piramal, India.** Nicholas Piramal India Ltd, 100 Centre Point, Dr. Ambedkar Rd, Parel, Mumbai 400 012, India.
**Nida, Singapore.** See *Advanced, Singapore.*
**Niddapharm, Ger.** NIDDApharm GmbH, Konrad-Adenauer-Allee 8-10, 61118 Bad Vilbel, Germany.
**Niedermaier, Ger.** Dr Niedermaier GmbH, Taufkirchner Str. 59, 85662 Hohenbrunn bei Munich, Germany.
**Nigy, Fr.** Laboratoires Nigy, 6 av de l'Europe, B.P. 51, 78401 Chatou cdx, France.
**Nigy, Singapore.** See *Polymedic, Singapore.*
**Nihon, Jpn.** Nihon Pharmaceutical Co. Ltd, 9-8 Higashikanda 1-chome, Chiyoda-ku, Tokyo 101-0031, Japan.
**Nikken, Jpn.** Nikken Chemicals Co., Ltd, 5-4-14 Tsukiji, Chuo-ku, Tokyo 104-8448, Japan.
**Nikkho, Braz.** Quimica E Farmaceutica Nikkho do Brasil Ltda, Rua Jaime Perdigao 431-435, 21920-240 Ilha do Governador, RJ, Brazil.
**Nion, USA.** Nion Corp., 15501 First St, Irwindale, CA 91706, USA.
**Ni-The, Gr.** NI-THE ΕΠΕ, Αγ. Αθανασίου 51, 190 02 Παιανία, Paiania, Greece.
**Niverpharm, Fr.** Laboratoires Niverpharm, ZI des Taupieres, rue Francis-Garnier, 58000 Nevers, France.
**NM, Denm.** NM Pharma A/S, Overgaden neden Vandet 7, 1414 Copenhagen K, Denmark.
**NM, Swed.** See *Pfizer, Swed.*
**NMC, USA.** NMC Labs, 70-36 83rd St, Glendale, NY 11385, USA.
**Nnodum, USA.** Nnodum Corp., 886 Clinton Springs Ave, Cincinnati, OH 45229, USA.
**Nobel, Canad.** Nobel Pharm Enrg, 2615 pl. Chasse, Montreal, Quebec, H1Y 2C3, Canada.
**Nobel, Ital.** Nobel Farmaceutici S.r.l., Via Tirbutina 1004, 00156 Rome, Italy.
**Noel, India.** Noel, India.
**Nogues, Fr.** Laboratoires Noguès, 43 rue de Neuilly, 92000 Nanterre, France.
**Nogues, Switz.** See *Uhlmann-Eyraud, Switz.*
**Noir, India.** Noir Pharmaceuticals Pvt Ltd, 380/82 J. Sankersett Rd, Sankersett Smriti, Chira Bazar, Mumbai 00 020, India.
**Nomad, UK.** Nomad Medical Ltd, 3-4 Wellington Terrace, Turnpike Lane, Hornsey, London, N8 0PX, UK.
**Nomax, USA.** Nomax Inc., 40 North Rock Hill Rd, St Louis, MO 63119, USA.
**Noos, Ital.** Noos S.r.l., Via Campello S/Clitunno 34/1, 00181 Rome, Italy.
**Nordend, Ger.** Nordend-Apotheke Dr. Wolfgang Hotz, Friedrich-Ebert-Platz 17, 64289 Darmstadt, Germany.
**Nordiatech, Denm.** NorDiaTech A/S, Baldersbuen 29 F, 2640 Hedehusene, Denmark.
**Nordic, Fr.** Nordic Pharma, France.
**Nordic, Swed.** Nordic Drugs AB, Box 300 35, 200 61 Limhamn, Sweden.
**Nordic, UK.** Nordic Pharma UK Ltd, Abbey House, Arlington Business Park, Theale, Reading, Berkshire, RG7 4SA, UK.
**Nordic Drugs, Denm.** Nordic Drugs, Niels Juels Gade 5, 1059 Copenhagen K, Denmark.
**Nordic Drugs, Fin.** Nordic Drugs AB, PL 16, 02241 Espoo, Finland.
**Nordic Healthcare, Denm.** Nordic Health-Care Products ApS, Niels Andersens Vej 66, 2900 Hellerup, Denmark.
**Nordisk Ibu-Pharma, Denm.** Nordisk Ibu-Pharma ApS, Rytterskolevej 7, 3230 Graested, Denmark.
**Nordmark, Thai.** See *Pacific, Thai.*
**Norgesfarma, Norw.** Norgesfarma AS, Skarersletta 45, Postboks 198, 1471 Lorenskog, Norway.
**Norgine, Austral.** Norgine P/L, 6/33 Ryde Rd, Pymble, NSW 2073, Australia.

**Norgine, Austria.** Norgine Pharma GmbH, Haidestrasse 4, A-1110 Vienna, Austria.

**Norgine, Belg.** Norgine S.A., Haasrode Research Park, Romeinsestraat 10, 3001 Heverlee, Belgium.

**Norgine, Denm.** See *Biolac, Swed.*

**Norgine, Fr.** Laboratoires Norgine Pharma, 23 av. de Neuilly, 75116 Paris, France.

**Norgine, Ger.** Norgine GmbH, Im Schwarzenborn 4, 35041 Marburg, Germany.

**Norgine, Hong Kong.** See *Treasure Mountain, Hong Kong.*

**Norgine, Irl.** See *United Drug, Irl.*

**Norgine, Ital.** Norgine Italia S.r.l., Via Panzini 13, 20145 Milan (MI), Italy.

**Norgine, Malaysia.** See *Apex, Malaysia.*

**Norgine, Neth.** Norgine BV, Hogehilweg 7, 1101 CA Amsterdam Zuid-Oost, Netherlands.

**Norgine, Norw.** See *Andersen, Norw.*

**Norgine, NZ.** See *CSL, NZ.*

**Norgine, S.Afr.** Norgine (Pty) Ltd, P.O. Box 781247, Sandton 2146, South Africa.

**Norgine, Singapore.** See *Grafton, Singapore.*

**Norgine, Spain.** Norgine de España, Alberto Bosch 9, 28014 Madrid, Spain.

**Norgine, Switz.** Norgine AG, Industriestrasse 11/13, 6243 Rotkreuz, Switzerland.

**Norgine, Thai.** See *Zuellig, Thai.*

**Norgine, UK.** Norgine Ltd, Chaplin House, Moorhall Rd, Harefield, Uxbridge, Middlesex, UB9 6NS, UK.

**Noriega, Spain.** Noriega, Spain.

**Norit, Austria.** See *Vemedia, Neth.*

**Norit, Gr.** Norit, Greece.

**Norit, Israel.** See *Droreth, Israel.*

**Norma (Νορμα), Gr.** ΝΟΡΜΑ ΕΛΛΑΣ ΑΕ, Μενάνδρου 54, 103 31 Αθήνα, Athens, Greece.

**Norma, UK.** Norma Chemicals Ltd, New Abbey Court, 51-53 Stert St, Abingdon, Oxfordshire, OX14 3HB, UK.

**Normal, Port.** Laboratório Normal, Lda, Rua do Centro Empresarial, Edificio 8, Quinta da Beloura, 2710-444 Sintra, Portugal.

**Norman, Canad.** See *Norman, USA.*

**Norman, USA.** Merle Norman Cosmetics, 9130 Bellanca Ave, Los Angeles, CA 90045, USA.

**Normon, Spain.** Normon, Nierenberg 10, 28002 Madrid, Spain.

**Norpharma, Denm.** Norpharma A/S, Slotsmarken 15, 2970 Horsholm, Denmark.

**Norstar, USA.** Norstar Consumer Products, 5517 Ninety-fifth Ave, Kenosha, WI 53144, USA.

**North American Vaccine, USA.** North American Vaccine Inc., 10150 Old Columbia Rd, Columbia, MD 21046, USA.

**Northern Research, USA.** Northern Research Laboratories Inc., 4225 White Bear Pkwy, Suite 600, St Paul, MN 55110, USA.

**Northia, Arg.** Esp. Medicinales Northia S.A.C.I.F.I.A., Madero 135, 1408 Buenos Aires, Argentina.

**Norton, Denm.** See *Pharmacodane, Denm.*

**Norton, Israel.** See *Promedico, Israel.*

**Norton, S.Afr.** Norton, South Africa.

**Norton, UK.** H.N. Norton & Co. Ltd, Gemini House, Flex Meadow, Harlow, Essex, CM19 5TJ, UK.

**Norton Healthcare, Denm.** See *United Nordic, Denm.*

**Norton Healthcare, Singapore.** See *FP, Singapore*, and *Green Cross, Singapore.*

**Norton Healthcare, UK.** See *Ivax, UK.*

**Norton Waterford, Irl.** See *Ivax, Irl.*

**Norwood, Canad.** Norwood Packaging Ltd, 8519-132nd St, R.R. 4, Surrey, British Columbia, V3W 4N8, Canada.

**Nostrum, Port.** Sociedade Nostrum, Lda, Rua da Escola de Medicina Veterinaria, 15/17, 1049-029 Lisbon, Portugal.

**Nostrum, Spain.** See *Pfizer, Spain.*

**Nourypharma, Ger.** Nourypharma GmbH, Mittenheimer Strasse 62, 85764 Oberschleissheim, Germany.

**Nourypharma, Neth.** Nourypharma Nederland BV, Wethouder van Eschstraat 1, 5342 AV Oss, Netherlands.

**Nourypharma, Switz.** See *Orion, Switz.*

**Nova Argentia, Ital.** Nova Argentia Industria Farmaceutica S.r.l., Via G. Pascoli 1, 20064 Gorgonzola (MI), Italy.

**Novag, Mex.** Novag Infancia S.A. de C.V., Claz. de Tlalpan No. 3417, Col. Sta. Ursula Coapa-Coyoacan, 04650 Mexico D.F., Mexico.

**Novag, Spain.** See *Ferrer, Spain.*

**Novalac, Fr.** Novalac, 209 rue de l'Universite, 75007 Paris, France.

**Novalis, Fr.** See *Wyeth Lederle, Fr.*

**Novamed, Braz.** See *EMS, Braz.*

**Novaquimica, Braz.** Novaquimica Sigma Pharma-Nature's Plus Ltda, Rodovia SP101 (Campinas a Monte Mor) Km 08, 13186-481 Hortolandia, SP, Brazil.

**Novartis, Arg.** Novartis Argentina S.A., Ramallo 1851, 1429 Buenos Aires, Argentina.

**Novartis, Austral.** Novartis Pharmaceuticals P/L, P.O. Box 101, North Ryde, NSW 1670, Australia.

**Novartis, Austria.** Novartis Pharma GmbH, Brunner Strasse 59, A-1235 Vienna, Austria.

**Novartis, Belg.** Novartis Pharma S.A., Telecom Gardens, Medialaan 40 bus 1, 1800 Vilvoorde, Belgium.

**Novartis, Braz.** Novartis Biociencias S.A., Avenida Professor Vicente Rao 90/120, Predio 156 3° ander, 04706-900 Sao Paulo, SP, Brazil.

**Novartis, Canad.** Novartis Pharmaceuticals Canada Inc., 385 Bouchard Blvd, Dorval, Quebec, H9S 1A9, Canada.

**Novartis, Chile.** Laboratorio Novartis Chile SA, Francisco meneses 1980, Nunoa, Santiago, Chile.

**Novartis, Denm.** Novartis Healthcare AS, Lyngbyvej 172, 2100 Copenhagen O, Denmark.

**Novartis, Fin.** Novartis Finland Oy, Metsänneidonkuja 10, 02130 Espoo, Finland.

**Novartis, Fr.** Novartis Pharma SAS, 2-4 rue Lionel-Terray, 92500 Rueil-Malmaison, France.

**Novartis, Ger.** Novartis Pharma GmbH, Roonstr. 25, 90429 Nurnberg, Germany.

**Novartis, Gr.** NOVARTIS A.E., 12o χλμ. Εθνικής, Οδού Αθηνών-Λαμίας 144 51 Μεταμόρφωση, Metamorphosi, Greece.

**Novartis, Hong Kong.** Novartis Pharmaceuticals (HK) Ltd, 37/F Windsor House, 311 Gloucester Rd, Causeway Bay, Hong Kong.

**Novartis, India.** Novartis India Ltd, Pharmaceutical Division, 6th Floor, Royal Insurance Building, 14 J. Tata Road, Mumbai 400 020, India.

**Novartis, Irl.** Novartis Ireland Ltd, Beech House, Beech Hill Office Campus, Clonskeagh, Dublin 4, Ireland.

**Novartis, Israel.** Novartis Ltd, Hasivim 23, Petach Tikva, Israel.

**Novartis, Ital.** Novartis Farma S.p.A., SS 233 (Varesina) km 20.5, 21040 Origgio (VA), Italy.

**Novartis, Jpn.** Novartis Pharma K.K., 4-17-30 Nishi-Azabu, Minato-ku, Tokyo 106-8618, Japan.

**Novartis, Malaysia.** Novartis Corporation (Malaysia) Sdn Bhd, Lot 9, Jln 26/1, Seksyen 26, Kawansan Perindustrian Hicom, 40400 Shah Alam, Selangor, Malaysia.

**Novartis, Mex.** Novartis Farmaceutica S.A. de C.V., Calz. de Tlalpan No. 1779, Col. San Diego Churubusco, Deleg. Coyoacan, 04120 Mexico D.F., Mexico.

**Novartis, Neth.** Novartis Pharma BV, Postbus 241, 6800 LZ Arnhem, Netherlands.

**Novartis, Norw.** Novartis Norge AS, Brynsalleen 4, Postboks 237 Okern, 0510 Oslo, Norway.

**Novartis, NZ.** Novartis New Zealand Ltd, Private Bag 19-999, Avondale, Auckland, New Zealand.

**Novartis, Port.** Novartis Farma, SA, Rua do Centro Empresarial, Edificio 8, Quinta da Beloura, 2710-444 Sintra, Portugal.

**Novartis, S.Afr.** Novartis South Africa (Pty) Ltd, P.O. Box 92, Isando 1600, South Africa.

**Novartis, Singapore.** Novartis (Singapore) Pte Ltd, Pharmaceutical Sector, 10 Hoe Chiang Road, 09-05/06 Keppel Towers, S 089315, Singapore.

**Novartis, Spain.** Novartis Farmaceutica, Gran Via Corts Catalanes 764, 08013 Barcelona, Spain.

**Novartis, Swed.** Novartis Sverige AB, Box 1150, 183 11 Taby, Sweden.

**Novartis, Switz.** Novartis Pharma Schweiz AG, Sudbahnhofstrasse 14 D, Postfach, 3001 Berne, Switzerland.

**Novartis, Thai.** Novartis (Thailand) Ltd, 159/30 Vibhavadi Rangsit Rd, Laksi, Bangkok 10210, Thailand.

**Novartis, UK.** Novartis Pharmaceuticals UK Ltd, Frimley Business Park, Frimley, Camberley, Surrey, GU16 5SG, UK.

**Novartis, USA.** Novartis Pharmaceuticals Corp., One Health Plaza, East Hanover, NJ 07936-1080, USA.

**Novartis Consumer, Austral.** Novartis Consumer Health Australasia P/L, P.O. Box 4499, Mulgrave, VIC 3170, Australia.

**Novartis Consumer, Austria.** See *Gebro, Austria.*

**Novartis Consumer, Belg.** Novartis Consumer Health S.A., Rue de Wand 209-213, 1020 Brussels, Belgium.

**Novartis Consumer, Canad.** Novartis Consumer Health Canada Inc., 2233 Argentia Rd, Suite 205, Mississauga, Ontario, L5N 2X7, Canada.

**Novartis Consumer, Ger.** Novartis Consumer Health GmbH, Zielstattstr. 40, 81379 Munich, Germany.

**Novartis Consumer, Irl.** Novartis Consumer Health, M & P House, Hammond Lane, Dublin 7, Ireland.

**Novartis Consumer, Israel.** See *Novartis, Israel.*

**Novartis Consumer, Ital.** Novartis Consumer Health S.p.A., Casella Postale 34, 21047 Saronno, Italy.

**Novartis Consumer, Neth.** Novartis Consumer Health Benelux, Postbus 2014, 4800 CA Breda, Netherlands.

**Novartis Consumer, Port.** Novartis Consumer Health, Lda, Av Poeta Mistral 2-2, 1069-172 Lisbon, Portugal.

**Novartis Consumer, S.Afr.** Novartis Consumer Health, Private Bag X10, Rivonia 2128, South Africa.

**Novartis Consumer, Spain.** See *Novartis, Spain.*

**Novartis Consumer, Switz.** Novartis Consumer Health Schweiz AG, Monbijoustrasse 118, 3001 Berne, Switzerland.

**Novartis Consumer, UK.** Novartis Consumer Health, Wimblehurst Rd, Horsham, West Sussex, RH12 4AB, UK.

**Novartis Consumer, USA.** Novartis Consumer Health Inc., 560 Morris Ave, Summit, NJ 07901-1312, USA.

**Novartis Nutrition, Canad.** Novartis Nutrition Corporation, 2233 Argentia Road, Suite 205, West Tower, Mississauga, Ontario, L5N 2X7, Canada.

**Novartis Nutrition, Fr.** Laboratoires Novartis Nutrition, B.P. 29, 31250 Revel, France.

**Novartis Nutrition, Hong Kong.** See *Novartis, Hong Kong.*

**Novartis Nutrition, Port.** See *Novartis Consumer, Port.*

**Novartis Nutrition, Singapore.** See *Zuellig, Singapore.*

**Novartis Nutrition, USA.** Novartis Nutrition Corp., 445 State St, Fremont, MN 49412, USA.

**Novartis Ophthalmics, Arg.** See *Novartis, Arg.*

**Novartis Ophthalmics, Austral.** See *Novartis, Austral.*

**Novartis Ophthalmics, Braz.** See *Novartis, Braz.*

**Novartis Ophthalmics, Canad.** See *Novartis, Canad.*

**Novartis Ophthalmics, Fr.** See *Novartis, Fr.*

**Novartis Ophthalmics, Ger.** See *Novartis, Ger.*

**Novartis Ophthalmics, Hong Kong.** See *Novartis, Hong Kong.*

**Novartis Ophthalmics, Irl.** See *Novartis, UK.*

**Novartis Ophthalmics, Malaysia.** See *Novartis, Malaysia.*

**Novartis Ophthalmics, Port.** See *Novartis, Port.*

**Novartis Ophthalmics, Singapore.** See *Novartis, Singapore.*

**Novartis Ophthalmics, Swed.** See *Novartis, Swed.*

**Novartis Ophthalmics, Switz.** Novartis Ophthalmics AG, Grenzstrasse 10, 8180 Bulach, Switzerland.

**Novartis Ophthalmics, UK.** See *Novartis, UK.*

**Novartis Ophthalmics, USA.** Novartis Ophthalmics Inc., 11695 Johns Creek Parkway, Duluth, GA 30097, USA.

**Novartis Sante, Fr.** Novartis Santé Familiale SA, 14 bd Richelieu, B.P. 440, 92845 Rueil-Malmaison cdx, France.

**Novavax, USA.** Novavax Inc., 8320 Guildford Rd, Suite C, Columbia, MD 21046, USA.

**Novaxa, Ital.** Novaxa S.p.A., Via Aquileja 49, 20092 Cinisello Balsamo (MI), Italy.

**Novaxo, Fr.** Laboratoires Novaxo, 100 rte de Versailles, 78163 Marly-le-Roi cdx, France.

**Noveal, Switz.** See *Uhlmann-Eyraud, Switz.*

**Novel, Ital.** Novel OTC S.r.l., Via M. Bandello 4/2, 20123 Milan, Italy.

**Noven, USA.** Noven Pharmaceuticals, 11960 SW 144th St, Miami, FL 33186, USA.

**Novipharm, Austria.** Novipharm GmbH, Klagenfurter Strasse 164, A-9210 Portschach, Austria.

**Novipharm, Ger.** Novipharm GmbH, Haidachstr. 29, 75181 Pforzheim, Germany.

**Novo Nordisk, Arg.** Novo Nordisk Pharma Argentina S.A., Av. Del Libertador 2740, 1636 Olivos, Buenos Aires, Argentina.

**Novo Nordisk, Austral.** Novo Nordisk Pharmaceuticals P/L, P.O. Box 6086, Parramatta Business Centre, NSW 2150, Australia.

**Novo Nordisk, Austria.** Novo-Nordisk Pharma GmbH, Erdbrgstrasse 52-60/3/16, A-1030 Vienna, Austria.

**Novo Nordisk, Belg.** Novo Nordisk Pharma S.A., Blvd International 55, 1070 Brussels, Belgium.

**Novo Nordisk, Braz.** Novo Nordisk Farmaceutica do Brasil Ltda, Av. Francisco Matarazzo 1.500, 12/14 andar, 05001-400 Sao Paulo, SP, Brazil.

**Novo Nordisk, Canad.** Novo Nordisk Canada Inc., 2700 Matheson Blvd E, 3rd Floor, West Tower, Mississauga, Ontario, L4W 4V9, Canada.

**Novo Nordisk, Denm.** See *Novo Nordisk, Swed.*

**Novo Nordisk, Fin.** Novo Nordisk Farma Oy, Itäuulentie 1, 02100 Espoo, Finland.

**Novo Nordisk, Fr.** Novo Nordisk Pharmaceutique SA, 32 rue de Bellevue, 92773 Boulogne-Billancourt cdx, France.

**Novo Nordisk, Ger.** Novo Nordisk Pharma GmbH, Brucknerstr. 1, 55127 Mainz, Germany.

**Novo Nordisk, Gr.** NOVO-NORDISK ΕΠΕ, Μεσογείων 518, 153 42 Αγία Παρασκευή, Agia-Paraskevi, Greece.

**Novo Nordisk, Hong Kong.** Novo Nordisk Hong Kong Ltd, Unit 507, 5/F, Trade Square, 681 Cheung Sha Wan Rd, Kowloon, Hong Kong.

**Novo Nordisk, Irl.** Novo-Nordisk Pharmaceuticals Ltd, 3/4 Upper Pembroke St, Dublin 2, Ireland.

**Novo Nordisk, Israel.** Novo Nordisk Ltd, 20 Hataas St, Kfar Saba 44425, Israel.

**Novo Nordisk, Ital.** Novo Nordisk Farmaceutici S.p.A., Via Elio Vitorini 129, 00144 Rome (RM), Italy.

**Novo Nordisk, Jpn.** Novo Nordisk Pharma Ltd, 5-7 Nihonbashi Ohdenma-cho, Chuo-ku, Tokyo 103-8575, Japan.

**Novo Nordisk, Malaysia.** Novo Nordisk Pharma Malaysia Sdn Bhd, Suite 5.08, Level 5, Wisma KT, 14 Jln 19/1, 46300 Petaling Jaya, Selangor, Malaysia.

**Novo Nordisk, Neth.** Novo Nordisk Farma, Postbus 443, 2400 AK Alphen aan den Rijn, Netherlands.

**Novo Nordisk, Norw.** Novo Nordisk Scandinavia AS, Hauger skolev. 16, Postboks 24, 1351 Rud, Norway.

**Novo Nordisk, NZ.** Novo Nordisk Pharmaceuticals Ltd, P.O. Box 51268, Pakuranga, Auckland, New Zealand.

**Novo Nordisk, Port.** Novo-Nordisk, Lda, Quinta da Fonte, Edifico D Jose Q54, Piso 1, 2780-730 Paco de Arcos, Portugal.

**Novo Nordisk, S.Afr.** Novo-Nordisk (Pty) Ltd, P.O. Box 783155, Sandton 2146, South Africa.

**Novo Nordisk, Singapore.** See *JDH, Singapore.*

**Novo Nordisk, Spain.** Novo Nordisk Pharma, Calereuga 102, 28033 Madrid, Spain.

**Novo Nordisk, Swed.** Novo Nordisk Scandinavia AB, Box 50587, 202 15 Malmo, Sweden.

**Novo Nordisk, Switz.** Novo Nordisk Pharma AG, Untere Heslibachstrasse 46, Postfach, 8700 Kusnacht/ZH, Switzerland.

**Novo Nordisk, Thai.** Novo Nordisk Pharma (Thailand) Ltd, 4 Fl, Sethiwan Tower, 139 Pan Rd, Silom, Bangkok 10500, Thailand.

**Novo Nordisk, UK.** Novo Nordisk Pharmaceuticals Ltd, Novo Nordisk House, Broadfield Park, Brighton Rd, Pease Pottage, Crawley, West Sussex, RH11 9RT, UK.

**Novo Nordisk, USA.** Novo Nordisk Pharmaceuticals Inc., 100 College Rd West, Suite 200, Princeton, NJ 08540-7810, USA.

**Novocol, USA.** See *Septodont, USA.*

**Novofarma, Arg.** Novofarma S.R.L., Juana Garcia 5008, 1407 Floresta, Buenos Aires, Argentina.

**Novogaleno, Ital.** Novogaleno S.r.l., Largo Sermoneta 24, 80123 Naples, Italy.

**Novogen, Austral.** Novogen Laboratories P/L, 140 Wicks Rd, North Ryde, NSW 2113, Australia.

**Novopharm, Canad.** Novopharm Ltd, 30 Novopharm Court, Toronto, Ontario, M1B 2K9, Canada.

**Novopharm, Hong Kong.** See *Primal, Hong Kong*, and *Unipharm, Hong Kong.*

**Novopharm, Singapore.** See *Green Cross, Singapore.*

**Novum, Belg.** Novum Pharma s.p.r.l., Xavier de Cocklaan 66 bus 3, 9830 Sint-Martins-Latem, Belgium.

**NPC, Fr.** Laboratoires NPC, 01290 Saint-Andre-d'Huiriat, France.

**Nucare, UK.** Nucare Plc, Raebarn House, 86 Northolt Rd, Harrow, Middlesex, HA2 0EL, UK.

**Nuclear, Spain.** See *Nucliber, Spain.*

**Nucliber, Spain.** Nucliber S.A., Hierro 9, 28045 Madrid, Spain.

**Numark, Canad.** See *Numark, USA.*

**Numark, UK.** Numark Management Ltd, 5/6 Fairway Court, Amber Close, Tamworth Business Park, Tamworth, Staffordshire, B77 4RP, UK.

**Numark, USA.** Numark Laboratories Inc., 164 North Field Ave, Edison, NJ 08818, USA.

**Nuova ICT, Ital.** Nuova ICT S.r.l., Via M Borsa 11, 26845 Codogno (LO), Italy.

**Nuovo ISM, Ital.** Nuovo Istituto Sieroterapico Milanese S.r.l., Barga, Castelvecchio Pascoli (LU), Italy.

**Nu-Pharm, Canad.** Nu-Pharm Inc., 50 Mural St, Units 1 & 2, Richmond Hill, Ontario, L4B 1E4, Canada.

**Nutergia, Fr.** Laboratoires Nutergia, B.P. 52, 12700 Capdenac, France.

**Nutraceuticals, UK.** Nutraceuticals Ltd, Wurtley House, 16 Eastbourne Rd, Hornsea, East Yorkshire, HU18 1QS, UK.

**Nutralife, UK.** Nutralife UK Ltd, Omicron House, Fircroft Way, Edenbridge, Kent, TN8 6EL, UK.

**Nutraloric, USA.** Nutraloric, 350 N Lantana, Unit G1, Camarillo, CA 93010, USA.

**Nutramax, USA.** NutraMax Laboratories Inc., 208 Lakeside Bvld, Edgewood, MD 21040, USA.

**Nutrasweet, NZ.** Nutrasweet Consumer Products, P.O. Box 3872, Auckland, New Zealand.

**Nutravite, Canad.** Nutravite, 1470 Leathead Rd, Unit 2, Kelowna, British Columbia, V1X 7J6, Canada.

**Nutricia, Austral.** Nutricia Australia P/L, P.O. Box 6745, Baulkham Hills Business Centre, NSW 2153, Australia.

**Nutricia, Canad.** Nutricia Canada Inc., 35 Webster St, Suite 103, Kentville, Nova Scotia, B4N 1N4, Canada.

**Nutricia, Fin.** Nutricia Oy, Linnankatu 26 A, 20100 Turku, Finland.

**Nutricia, Fr.** Nutricia, 4 rue Joseph-Monier, 92859 Rueil-Malmaison cdx, France.

**Nutricia, Hong Kong.** Nutricia (Asia-Pacific) Ltd, Suite 1505, 15/F Harcourt House, 39 Gloucester Rd, Wanchai, Hong Kong.

**Nutricia, Irl.** Nutricia Ireland Ltd, 18 Sandyford Business Centre, Burton Hall Rd, Dublin 18, Ireland.

**Nutricia, Ital.** Nutricia S.p.A., Via Lepetit 8, 20020 Lainate (MI), Italy.

**Nutricia, Malaysia.** See *Zuellig, Malaysia.*

**Nutricia, NZ.** Nutricia New Zealand, P.O. Box 62523, Central Park, Auckland 6, New Zealand.
**Nutricia, Port.** Nutricia Portugal, Lda, Zona Industrial de Carnaxide, 2795-491 Carnaxide, Portugal.
**Nutricia, Singapore.** See *Sime Darby, Singapore.*
**Nutricia, Thai.** See *Berli, Thai.*
**Nutricia Clinical, UK.** Nutricia Clinical Care, Nutricia Ltd, Newmarket Ave, White Horse Business Park, Trowbridge, Wiltshire, BA14 0XQ, UK.
**Nutricia Dietary, UK.** See *Nutricia Clinical, UK.*
**Nutricia-Bago, Arg.** Nutricia-Bagó S.A., Av. Panamericana y Gral. Savio, Parque Industrial OKS, 1619 Garin, Buenos Aires, Argentina.
**Nutricia-Luma Lindar, USA.** See *Mt. Vernon, USA.*
**Nutrifar, Ital.** Nutrifar S.r.l., Via Cadore 7, 26015 Soresina (CR), Italy.
**Nutrifarma, Mex.** Nutrifarma, Mexico.
**Nutrilab, Braz.** See *Farmoquimica, Braz.*
**Nutrimed, Fr.** Nutrimed Medic System, 6/10 rue Mirabeau, 75016 Paris, France.
**Nutri-Metics, Canad.** Nutri-Metics International (Can) Ltd, 3915-16 Ave SE, Calgary, Alberta, T2C 1V5, Canada.
**Nutri-Pharm, Austral.** Nutri-Pharm, P.O. Box 7313, Karingal Centre, VIC 3199, Australia.
**Nutripharm, USA.** Nutripharm Laboratories Inc., Salem Industrial Park, Building 5, Lebanon, NJ 08833, USA.
**Nutrisoy, USA.** NutriSoy International Inc., 424 S Kentucky Ave, Evansville, IN 47714, USA.
**Nutrition Care, Austral.** Nutrition Care, 25-7 Keysborough Ave, Keysborough, VIC 3173, Australia.
**Nutrition Medical, Israel.** See *Megapharm, Israel.*
**Nutri-Well, Hong Kong.** See *Winsor, Hong Kong.*
**Nutrovit, Braz.** Nutrovit, Brazil.
**Nycomed, Arg.** Nycomed Argentina, Adolfo Alsina 2954, 1205 Buenos Aires, Argentina.
**Nycomed, Austral.** See *Amersham, Austral.*
**Nycomed, Austria.** Nycomed Austria GmbH, St Peter-Strasse 25, A-4020 Linz, Austria.
**Nycomed, Belg.** See *Amersham, Belg.*
**Nycomed, Denm.** Nycomed Danmark A/S, Langebjerg 1, 4000 Roskilde, Denmark.
**Nycomed, Fin.** Oy Nycomed AB, Pasilanraitio 9, 4 krs, 00240 Helsinki, Finland.
**Nycomed, Fr.** Nycomed France SAS, 140 av. Jean Lolive, 93695 Pantin cdx, France.
**Nycomed, Ger.** See *Amersham Buchler, Ger.*
**Nycomed, Gr.** NYCOMED (FARMAZAC) A.E., Κηφισίας 196, 152 31 Χαλάνδρι, Chalandri, Greece.
**Nycomed, Hong Kong.** See *JDH, Hong Kong.*
**Nycomed, Irl.** See *Newport Synthesis, Irl.*
**Nycomed, Israel.** See *Medison, Israel.*
**Nycomed, Ital.** Nycomed Amersham Sorin S.r.l., Via Crescentino, 13040 Saluggia (VC), Italy.
**Nycomed, Neth.** Nycomed BV, Nikkelstraat 5, 4823 AE Breda, Netherlands.
**Nycomed, Norw.** Nycomed Pharma AS, Hagalokkv. 13, Postboks 205, 1372 Asker, Norway.
**Nycomed, Singapore.** See *FP, Singapore.*
**Nycomed, Swed.** Nycomed AB, Box 1215, 181 24 Lidingo, Sweden.
**Nycomed, Switz.** Nycomed AG, Moosacherstrasse 14, Au, 8820 Wadenswil, Switzerland.
**Nycomed, Thai.** See *Shiwa, Thai.*
**Nycomed, USA.** See *Amersham, USA.*
**Nycomed Amersham, Swed.** See *Amersham, Swed.*
**Nycomed Amersham, Switz.** See *Nycomed, Switz.*
**Nycomed Amersham, UK.** See *Amersham, UK.*
**Nycomed Imaging, Canad.** See *Amersham, Canad.*
**Nycomed Imaging, Denm.** See *Amersham, Denm.*
**Nycomed Imaging, Norw.** See *Amersham, Norw.*
**NZ Distributors, NZ.** New Zealand Distributors Ltd, P.O. BOX 41014, St Lukes, Auckland, New Zealand.
**NZ Medical & Scientific, NZ.** New Zealand Medical & Scientific Ltd, P.O. Box 24-138, Royal Oak, Auckland, New Zealand.
**Oakhurst, USA.** Oakhurst Co., 3000 Hempstead Turnpike, Levittown, NY 11756, USA.
**OBA, Denm.** OBA Pharma ApS, Kronprinsessegade 26 A (postboks 117), 1004 Copenhagen K, Denmark.
**Oberlin, Fr.** See *UPSA Conseil, Fr.*
**Ocean Health, Singapore.** Ocean Health (S) Pte Ltd, 42 Mactaggart Rd, 05-02, S 368086, Singapore.
**Oclassen, USA.** Oclassen Pharmaceuticals Inc., 100 Pelican Way, San Rafael, CA 94901, USA.
**Octapharma, Austria.** Octapharma Pharmazeutika, Oberlaaer Strasse 235, A-1100 Vienna, Austria.
**Octapharma, Fr.** Laboratoires Octapharma SA, 70-72 rue du Marechal-Foch, B.P. 33, 67381 Lingolsheim, France.
**Octapharma, Ger.** Octapharma Vertrieb von Plasmaderivaten GmbH, Bahnhofstr. 43, 40764 Langenfeld, Germany.
**Octapharma, Hong Kong.** See *Weston, Hong Kong.*
**Octapharma, Norw.** Octapharma AS, Furubakken, 2090 Hurdal, Norway.
**Octapharma, Swed.** Octapharma AB, Nordenflychtsadgen 55, 112 75 Stockholm, Sweden.
**Octapharma, Switz.** Octapharma AG, Seidenstrasse 2, Postfach 416, 8853 Lachen, Switzerland.
**Octapharma, UK.** Octapharma Ltd, 6 Elm Court, Copse Drive, Coventry, CV5 9RG, UK.
**Ocumed, USA.** Ocumed Inc., 119 Harrison Ave, Roseland, NJ 07068, USA.
**Ocusoft, USA.** Cynacon/OCuSOFT, 5311 Ave N, P.O. Box 429, Richmond, TX 77406-0429, USA.
**Odan, Canad.** Odan Laboratories Ltd, 255 Hymus Bvld, Pointe-Claire, Quebec, H9R 1G6, Canada.
**Odin, Spain.** See *AstraZeneca, Spain.*
**Odontofarma, Braz.** Laboratorio Odontofarma Ltda, Rua Claudio Furquim 21/25 1° And., Tatuape, 03072-010 Sao Paulo, SP, Brazil.
**Odontomed, Braz.** Laboratorio Odontomed Industria e Comercio Ltda, Avenida Bosque da Saude 1088, 04142-081 Sao Paulo, SP, Brazil.
**Odontopharm, Switz.** Odontopharm AG, Engestrasse 23, 3000 Bern 26, Switzerland.
**Odyssey, USA.** Odyssey Pharmaceuticals Inc, 72 DeForest Ave, East Hanover, NJ 07936, USA.
**Oenobiol, Fr.** Laboratoires Oenobiol, 59 bd Exelmans, 75781 Paris cdx 16, France.
**Ofar, Arg.** Dist. Ofar S.A., Salom 651, 1277 Buenos Aires, Argentina.
**OFF, Ital.** Officina Farmaceutica Fiorentina S.r.l. Istituto Biochimico, Quart. Varignano 12-14, 55049 Viareggio (Lucca), Italy.
**Offenbach, Mex.** Offenbach Mexicana S.A. de C.V., Acueducto No. 15, Col. Reforma Social, 11650 Mexico D.F., Mexico.
**Ofimex, Mex.** See *Aventis, Mex.*
**Oftalder, Port.** See *Edol, Port.*
**Oftalmiso, Spain.** Oftalmiso, Spain.
**Ogera, Switz.** Ogera AG, Lerzenstrasse 18, 8953 Dietikon, Switzerland.
**Ogna, Ital.** Giovanni Ogna & Figli S.p.A., Via Figini 41, 20053 Muggio (MI), Italy.
**Ohara, Jpn.** Ohara Chemical Industries Ltd, 43-1 Oharaichiba, Koka-cho, Koka-gun, Shiga 520-3433, Japan.
**Ohm, USA.** OHM Laboratories Inc., P.O. Box 7397, North Brunswick, NJ 08902, USA.
**Ohmeda, USA.** See *Baxter, USA.*
**Ohropax, Switz.** See *Uhlmann-Eyraud, Switz.*
**Ohta, Hong Kong.** See *Primal, Hong Kong.*
**Olan-Kemed, Thai.** Olan-Kemed Co. Ltd, 176 Ladprao Rd, Bangkok 10900, Thailand.
**Olbas, Ger.** See *Schoenenberger, Ger.*
**Olic, Thai.** Olic (Thailand) Ltd, 7 Fl, 2535 Sukhumvit Rd, Bangchak, Phrakanong, Bangkok 10250, Thailand.
**Oligosol, Switz.** Oligosol AG, Untermattweg 8, 3001 Berne, Switzerland.
**Olvos, Gr.** OLVOS SCIENCE A.E., Αχιλλέως 2, 104 37 Αθήνα, Athens, Greece.
**OM, Ger.** Deutsche OM Arzneimittel GmbH, Am Houiller Platz 17, 61381 Friedrichsdorf/Ts, Germany.
**OM, Hong Kong.** See *Primal, Hong Kong.*
**OM, Malaysia.** See *Pharmaforte, Malaysia.*
**OM, Port.** OM Portuguesa, SA, Rua da Industria no 2, Quinta Grande, 2720 Alfragide, Portugal.
**OM, Switz.** OM Pharma, 22 rue du Bois-du-Lan, 1217 Meyrin 2/Geneva, Switzerland.
**Omedir, Arg.** Laboratorios Omedir S.A., Corvalan 1983/85, 1440 Buenos Aires, Argentina.
**Omega, Arg.** Esp. Medicinales Omega, Serrano 985, 1414 Buenos Aires, Argentina.
**Omega, Canad.** Omega Laboratories Ltd, 11177 Hamon St, Montreal, Quebec, H3M 3E4, Canada.
**Omega, Irl.** Omega Diagnostics Ireland Ltd, Unit A6, Southern Cross Business Park, Boghall Rd, Bray, Co. Wicklow, Ireland.
**Omega, Spain.** See *Almirall, Spain.*
**Omegin, Ger.** Omegin Dr Schmidgall GmbH & Co. KG, Industriepark 210, 78244 Gottmadingen, Germany.
**Omida, Switz.** Omida AG, Homoopathische Heilmittel, Erlistrasse 2, 6403 Kussnacht a.R., Switzerland.
**Omisan, Ital.** Omisan Farmaceutici di Antonio Vona & C S.a.s, Via Tossicia 15, 00131 Rome, Italy.
**OMJ, Hong Kong.** See *Keller, Hong Kong.*
**Omni, UK.** Omni Nutraceuticals, UK.
**Omnii, USA.** Omnii Oral Pharmaceuticals, 1500 N Florida Mango Rd, Suite 1, West Palm Beach, FL 33409, USA.
**Omnimed, S.Afr.** See *Braun Omnimed, S.Afr.*
**Omni-Protech, India.** Omni-Protech Drugs Pvt Ltd, C-4, 13 Functional Elec. Est., Bhosari, Pune 411 026, India.
**Omrix, Israel.** Omrix Biopharmaceuticals Ltd, P.O. Box 619, Rehovot 76106, Israel.
**Omrix, Israel.** Omrix Biopharmaceuticals Ltd, P.O. Box 619, Rehovot, Israel.
**One Drop Only, Ger.** One Drop Only Chem.-pharm.-Vertriebs-GmbH, Stieffring 14, 13627 Berlin, Germany.
**Onkoworks, Ger.** Onkoworks Gesellschaft zur Herstellung und Vertrieb onkologischer Spezialpräparate mbH, Schallbruch 5, 42781 Haan/Rhld., Germany.
**Ono, Hong Kong.** See *Hing Yip, Hong Kong.*
**Ono, Jpn.** Ono Pharmaceutical Co. Ltd, 2-1-5 Doshomachi, Chuo-ku, Osaka 541-8526, Japan.
**Onstrong, Hong Kong.** Onstrong Ltd, Rm B, 11/F, Bright Growth Medical Ctr, 335 Nathan Rd, Kowloon, Hong Kong.
**Ony, Israel.** See *Rafa, Israel.*
**OP, Ital.** OP Pharma Srl, Via Torino 51, 20123 Milan, Italy.
**Opco, Denm.** Opco Pharma A/S, Messingvej 54, 8900 Randers, Denmark.
**Opfermann, Ger.** Opfermann Arzneimittel GmbH, Robert-Koch-Str. 2, 51674 Wiehl, Germany.
**Ophtapharma, Canad.** Ophtapharma Canada Inc., 1100 Cremazie E, Suite 708, Montreal, Quebec, H2P 2X2, Canada.
**Ophtha, Denm.** Ophtha A/S, Halmtorvet 29, 1700 Copenhagen V, Denmark.
**Ophtha, Norw.** See *Ophtha, Denm.*
**Opocalcium, Fr.** Laboratoires de l'Opocalcium, 20 rue Louis-Charles-Vernin, 77190 Dammarie-les-Lys, France.
**Opofarm, Braz.** See *ICN, Braz.*
**Opopharma, Switz.** Opopharma SA, Kirchgasse 42, 8001 Zurich, Switzerland.
**Optident, UK.** Optident Dental Products, International Development Centre, Valley Drive, Ilkley, West Yorkshire, LS29 8PB, UK.
**Optikem, USA.** Optikem International Inc., 2172 S Jason St, Denver, CO 80223, USA.
**Optima, UK.** Optima Health Ltd, 47/48 St Mary St, Cardiff, South Glamorgan, CF10 1AD, UK.
**Optimal, Hong Kong.** See *Health Tech, Hong Kong.*
**Optimapharma, Canad.** See *Taro, Canad.*
**Optimed, Ger.** Optimed Pharma GmbH, Alfred-Nobel-Str. 5, 50226 Frechen, Germany.
**Optimox, USA.** Optimox Corp., 2720 Monterey St, Suite 406, Torrance, CA 90503, USA.
**Opto-Pharm, Singapore.** Opto-Pharm, Singapore.
**Optopics, USA.** See *Nutramax, USA.*
**Optrex, India.** Optrex, India.
**Optrex, Malaysia.** See *Boots Healthcare, Malaysia.*
**Optrex, Singapore.** See *Boots, Singapore.*
**Opus, S.Afr.** Opus Pharmaceuticals (Pty) Ltd, P.O.Box 78618, Sandton 2146, South Africa.
**Opus, UK.** See *Trinity, UK.*
**OPW, Ger.** See *Altana, Ger.*
**Oral-B, Arg.** See *Gillette, Arg.*
**Oral-B, Austral.** Oral-B Laboratories P/L, 5 Caribbean Drive, Scoresby, VIC 3179, Australia.
**Oral-B, Canad.** Oral-B Laboratories Inc., Division of Gillette Canada, 4 Robert Speck Parkway, Suite 1000, Mississauga, Ontario, L4Z 4C5, Canada.
**Oral-B, Irl.** Oral-B Laboratories Ireland, Green Rd, Newbridge, Country Kildare, Ireland.
**Oral-B, Ital.** Oral-B Laboratories, Gillette Group Italy S.p.A., Business Unit Braun-Oral Care, Via Pirelli 18, 20124 Milan, Italy.
**Oral-B, Mex.** Oral-B, Gillette Oral Care, Inc., Electron 22, Parke Industrial Naucalpan, Naucalpan, 533370 Mexico D.F., Mexico.
**Oral-B, UK.** Oral-B Laboratories Ltd, c/o Gillette U.K. Ltd, Gillette Corner, Great West Rd, Isleworth, Middlesex, TW7 5NP, UK.
**Oral-B, USA.** Oral-B Laboratories Inc., Prudential Tower Building, Boston, MA 02199-8004, USA.
**Oraldent, UK.** Oraldent Ltd, Unit 11, Harvard Industrial Estate, Kimbolton, Cambridgeshire, PE28 0NJ, UK.
**Oramon, Ger.** Oramon Arzneimittel GmbH, Mittelstr. 18, 88471 Laupheim, Germany.
**OraPharma, USA.** OraPharma Inc., 732 Louis Dr., Warminster, PA 18974, USA.
**Orbis Consumer, UK.** Orbis Consumer Products Ltd, Unit 31, Northfields Industrial Estate, Beresford Ave, Wembley, Middlesex, HA0 1NW, UK.
**Orchid, Hong Kong.** See *Mekim, Hong Kong.*
**Ordesa, Spain.** Ordesa, Ctra del Prat 9-11, Sant Boi de Llobregat, 08830 Barcelona, Spain.
**Or-Dov, Austral.** Or-Dov Pharmaceuticals P/L, P.O. Box 172, Doncaster, VIC 3108, Australia.
**Orexo, Swed.** Orexo AB, Box 303, 751 05 Upsala, Sweden.
**Orfi, Spain.** See *Wyeth, Spain.*
**Organon, Arg.** Organon Argentina, Sucre 865, 1428 Buenos Aires, Argentina.
**Organon, Austral.** Organon (Australia) P/L, Private Bag 25, Lane Cove, NSW 2066, Australia.
**Organon, Austria.** Organon GmbH, Siebenbrunnengasse 21/D/IV, A-1050 Vienna, Austria.
**Organon, Belg.** Organon S.A., Crown Building, Chaussee de la Hulpe 166, 1170 Brussels, Belgium.
**Organon, Braz.** See *Akzo, Braz.*
**Organon, Canad.** Organon Canada Ltd, 200 Consillium Place, Suite 700, Scarborough, Ontario, M1H 3E4, Canada.
**Organon, Chile.** Organon Chile Ltda, Loreley 1582, La Reina, Santiago, Chile.
**Organon, Denm.** Organon AS, Literbuen 9, 2740 Skovlunde, Denmark.
**Organon, Fin.** Oy Organon AB, Maistraatinportti 2, PL 101, 00241 Helsinki, Finland.
**Organon, Fr.** Organon, 10 rue Godefroy, 92821 Puteaux cdx, France.
**Organon, Ger.** Organon GmbH, Mittenheimer Strasse 62, 85764 Oberschleissheim, Germany.
**Organon (Οργανον), Gr.** ΟΡΓΑΝΟΝ ΕΛΛΑΣ ΑΕΕ, Λ. Βουλιαγμένης 122, 167 77 Ελληνικό, Elliniko, Greece.
**Organon, Hong Kong.** Organon (HK) Ltd, 27/F, 88 Hing Fat St, Causeway Bay, Hong Kong.
**Organon, Irl.** See *United Drug, Irl.*
**Organon, Israel.** See *Neopharm, Israel.*
**Organon, Ital.** Organon Italia S.p.A., Via Ostilia 15, 00184 Rome, Italy.
**Organon, Jpn.** Nippon Organon K.K., 5-90 Tomobuchi-cho 1-chome, Miyakojima-ku, Osaka City 534-0016, Japan.
**Organon, Malaysia.** Organon (Malaysia) Sdn Bhd, No 29-1/3 Jln USJ9/5Q, Subang Business Centre, 47620 UEP Subang Jaya, Selangor, Malaysia.
**Organon, Mex.** Organon Mexicana S.A. de C.V., Calz. de Camarones No.134, Col. San Salvador Xochimanca, Deleg. Azcapotzalco, 02870 Mexico D.F., Mexico.
**Organon, Neth.** Organon Nederland BV, Griekenweg 25, 5342 PX Oss, Netherlands.
**Organon, Norw.** Organon AS, Johan Drengsrudsv. 52, Postboks 324, 1372 Asker, Norway.
**Organon, NZ.** See *Pharmaco, NZ.*
**Organon, Port.** Organon Portuguesa, Lda, Av. Conde Valbom 30, 1069-037 Lisbon, Portugal.
**Organon, Singapore.** See *Zuellig, Singapore.*
**Organon, Spain.** Organon Española, Ctra de Hospitalet 147-149, Ed Amsterdam, Citypark, R Del Dalt, Cornella de Llobregat, 08940 Barcelona, Spain.
**Organon, Swed.** Organon AB, Fiskhamnsgatan 6A, 414 58 Goteborg, Sweden.
**Organon, Switz.** Organon SA, Churerstrasse 160b, 8808 Pfaffikon/SZ, Switzerland.
**Organon, Thai.** Organon (Thailand) Ltd, 14 Fl, Ploenchit Center Building, 2 Sukhumvit Rd, Klongtoey, Bangkok 10110, Thailand.
**Organon, UK.** Organon Laboratories Ltd, Cambridge Science Park, Milton Rd, Cambridge, CB4 0FL, UK.
**Organon, USA.** Organon Inc., 375 Mount Pleasant Ave, West Orange, NJ 07052, USA.
**Organon Teknika, Austria.** See *Organon Teknika, Ger.*
**Organon Teknika, Canad.** Organon Teknika Inc., 5-75 Shields Court, Markham, Ontario, L3R 9T4, Canada.
**Organon Teknika, Denm.** See *Organon, Denm.*
**Organon Teknika, Ger.** See *Organon, Ger.*
**Organon Teknika, Hong Kong.** Organon Teknika China Ltd, Unit 2704, Vicwood Plaza, 199 Des Voeux Rd Central, Hong Kong.
**Organon Teknika, Irl.** See *United Drug, Irl.*
**Organon Teknika, Israel.** See *Tec-O-Pharm, Israel.*
**Organon Teknika, Ital.** See *Organon, Ital.*
**Organon Teknika, Mex.** See *Organon, Mex.*
**Organon Teknika, Neth.** Organon Teknika Nederland BV, Postbus 23, 5280 AA Boxtel, Netherlands.
**Organon Teknika, Norw.** See *Organon, Norw.*
**Organon Teknika, Spain.** See *Bio-Merieux, Spain.*
**Organon Teknika, USA.** Organon Teknika Corporation, 100 Rodophe St, Durham, NC 27712, USA.
**Orient, Hong Kong.** Orient Europharma, Rm 1711, 17/F Olympia Plaza, 225 King's Rd, North Point, Hong Kong.
**Orient, Malaysia.** Orient Europharma (M) Sdn Bhd, 33 Jln U1/30, Section U1, 40150 Shah Alam, Selangor, Malaysia.
**Orient, Singapore.** Orient Europharm Pte Ltd, 1 Sophia Rd, 06-13 Peace Centre, S 228149, Singapore.
**Oriental, Arg.** Oriental Farmaceutica I.C.I.F.A., G. Cossio 6160, 1408 Buenos Aires, Argentina.
**Oriola, Fin.** Oriola Oy, PL 8, 02101 Espoo, Finland.
**Orion, Austral.** Orion Laboratories P/L, 85 Briggs St, Welshpool, WA 6106, Australia.
**Orion, Austria.** See *Orion, Fin.*
**Orion, Denm.** Orion Pharma A/S, Bogeskovvej 9, 3490 Kvistgard, Denmark.
**Orion, Fin.** Orion-yhtymä Oyj, Orionintie 1, 02200 Espoo, Finland.
**Orion, Fr.** Orion Pharma, 85 rue Edouard-Vaillant, 92300 Levallois-Perret, France.
**Orion, Ger.** Orion Pharma GmbH, Notkestr. 9, 22607 Hamburg, Germany.
**Orion, Gr.** See *Organon (Οργανον), Gr.*
**Orion, Irl.** See *Allphar, Irl.*
**Orion, Israel.** See *Genmedix, Israel,* and *Rafa, Israel.*
**Orion, Malaysia.** See *Apex, Malaysia.*
**Orion, Norw.** Orion Pharma AS, Ulvenv 84, Postboks 52 Okern, 0508 Oslo, Norway.
**Orion, NZ.** See *Zuellig, NZ,* and *St Ives, NZ.*
**Orion, Singapore.** See *Pharmacon, Singapore.*

**Orion, Swed.** Orion Pharma AB, Box 334, 192 30 Sollentuna, Sweden.

**Orion, Switz.** Orion Pharma AG, Untermuli 11, 6300 Zug, Switzerland.

**Orion, Thai.** See *Harn, Thai.*

**Orion, UK.** Orion Pharma UK Ltd, 1st Floor Leat House, Overbridge Square, Hambridge Lane, Newbury, Berkshire, RG14 5UX, UK.

**Orion, USA.** See *Lifesign, USA.*

**OroClean, Switz.** OroClean-Chemie AG, Buelstrasse 17, 8330 Pfaffikon/ZH, Switzerland.

**Orphan, Austral.** Orphan Australia P/L, 48 Kangan Drive, Berwick, VIC 3806, Australia.

**Orphan, Austria.** See *Orphan, Fr.*

**Orphan, Denm.** Swedish Orphan AS, Wilders Plads, Bygning V, 1403 Copenhagen K, Denmark.

**Orphan, Fin.** Oy Swedish Orphan AB, Rajatorpantie 41C, 01640 Vantaa, Finland.

**Orphan, Fr.** Orphan Europe SARL, Imm Le Guillaumet, 92046 Paris-La Defense, France.

**Orphan, Ger.** Orphan Europe (Germany) GmbH, Max-Planck-Str. 6, 63128 Dietzenbach, Germany.

**Orphan, Ital.** Orphan Europe Italy S.r.l., Via Cellini 11, 20090 Segrate (MI), Italy.

**Orphan, Spain.** Orphan Europe, Calle Santa Eulelia, 236-242, L'Hospitalet de Llobregat, 08902 Barcelona, Spain.

**Orphan, UK.** Orphan Europe (UK) Ltd, 32 Bell St, Henley-on-Thames, Oxfordshire, RG9 2BH, UK.

**Orphan Medical, Canad.** See *Orphan Medical, USA.*

**Orphan Medical, Israel.** See *Tzamal, Israel.*

**Orphan Medical, USA.** Orphan Medical Inc., 13911 Ridgedale Drive, Suite 250, Minnetonka, MN 55305, USA.

**Orravan, Spain.** See *Reig Jofre, Spain.*

**Orsade, Spain.** Orsade, Avda Virgen de Montserrat 221, 08026 Barcelona, Spain.

**Ortec, USA.** Ortec International Inc., 3960 Broadway, New York, NY 10032, USA.

**Ortega, USA.** Ortega, USA.

**Ortho, Hong Kong.** See *Keller, Hong Kong, Janssen, Hong Kong,* and *Jacobson, Hong Kong.*

**Ortho, Israel.** See *CTS, Israel.*

**Ortho, Ital.** Ortho Clinical Diagnostics S.p.A., Div. LifeScan Italia, Via Chiese 74, 20126 Milan, Italy.

**Ortho, UK.** See *Cilag, UK.*

**Ortho Biotech, UK.** See *Janssen-Cilag, UK.*

**Ortho Biotech, USA.** Ortho Biotech Inc., 700 US Hwy 202, P.O. Box 670, Raritan, NJ 08869-0670, USA.

**Ortho Dermatological, Canad.** Ortho Dermatological, Division of Johnson & Johnson Inc., 7101 Notre-Dame E, Montreal, Quebec, H1N 2G4, Canada.

**Ortho Dermatological, USA.** Ortho Pharmaceutical Corp. Dermatological, 199 Grandview Rd, Skillman, NJ 08558, USA.

**Ortho Diagnostic, USA.** Ortho-Clinical Diagnostic Inc., 100 Indigo Creek Dr., Rochester, NJ 14626, USA.

**Ortho McNeil, USA.** See *Ortho Pharmaceutical, USA.*

**Ortho Pharmaceutical, USA.** Ortho Pharmaceutical Corp., 1000 Route 202, P.O. Box 300, Raritan, NJ 08869-0602, USA.

**Orthos, Mex.** Laboratorios Orthos S.A. de C.V., Iturbide 326, Puebla Patrimonio, 72450 Puebla, Mexico.

**Ortomed, Neth.** Ortomed BV, Postbus 1081, 3330 CB Zwijndrecht, Netherlands.

**Ortoquimica, Braz.** Ortoquimica Ind. Quimico Farmaceutica Ltda, Av. Magalhaes de Castro 800, 05502-001 Sao Paulo, SP, Brazil.

**Oshima, Arg.** Oshima S.R.L., Av. Maipu 3105, 1636 Olivos, Buenos Aires, Argentina.

**Osler, Fr.** Laboratoires Osler, 42 rue Monge, 75005 Paris, France.

**Osorio de Moraes, Braz.** Laboratorios Osorio de Moraes Ltda, Avenida Cardeal Eugenio Pacelli 2281, 32210-001 Contagem, MG, Brazil.

**Osoth, Thai.** Osoth Inter Laboratories, 757/10 Soi Pradoo 1, Sathupradit 8 Rd, Bangpongpang, Yannawa, Bangkok 10120, Thailand.

**Osotspa, Thai.** Osotspa Co. Ltd, 2100 Ram Khamhaeng Rd, Hua Mark, Bangkapi, Bangkok 10240, Thailand.

**Osteolab, Chile.** See *Recalcine, Chile.*

**OTC, Spain.** OTC Iberica, C/Monturiol, 2, Poligono Ind. Sur, 08026 Barcelona, Spain.

**OTC Consult, Denm.** OTC Consult ApS, H A Clausensvej 24, 2820 Gentofte, Denmark.

**OTL, Fr.** OTL Pharma SA, 15 rue de Turbigo, 75002 Paris, France.

**OTL, Spain.** See *OTL, Fr.*

**Otosan, Ital.** Otosan, Via degli Scavi 32, 47100 Forli, Italy.

**Otsuka, Hong Kong.** Otsuka Pharmaceutical (HK) Ltd, Rm 1404, Phase 1, Ming An Plaza, 8 Sunning Rd, Causeway Bay, Hong Kong.

**Otsuka, Jpn.** Otsuka Pharmaceutical Co. Ltd, 2-9 Kanda-Tsukasa-cho, Chiyoda-ku, Tokyo 101-8535, Japan.

**Otsuka, Malaysia.** See *Luen Wah, Malaysia.*

**Otsuka, Singapore.** See *Luen Wah, Singapore.*

**Otsuka, Spain.** Otsuka Pharmaceutical, Provenza 388, 08025 Barcelona, Spain.

**Otsuka, Thai.** See *Zuellig, Thai.*

**Otsuka, UK.** Otsuka Pharmaceutical Europe Ltd, 9th Floor, Commonwealth House, 2 Chalkhill Rd, Hammersmith, London, W6 8DW, UK.

**Otsuka, USA.** Otsuka America Pharmaceutical Inc, 2440 Research Blvd, Rockville, MD 20850, USA.

**Ottolenghi, Ital.** Dr. Ottolenghi & C. S.r.l., Via Cuneo 5, 10028 Trofarello (TO), Italy.

**OTW, Ger.** Organotherapeutische Werke GmbH (OTW), Carl-Zeiss-Str. 4, 76275 Ettlingen, Germany.

**Oui Heng, Thai.** Oui Heng Import Co. Ltd, 46, 46/2 Soi Charansanitwongs 40, Charansanwitwongs Rd, Bangkok 10700, Thailand.

**Outdoor Recreations, USA.** Outdoor Recreations, USA.

**Ovation, USA.** Ovation Pharm, One Overlook Pt, Suite 110, Lincolnshire, IL 60069, USA.

**Ovelle, Irl.** Ovelle Ltd, Industrial Estate, Coe's Rd, Dundalk, Co. Louth, Ireland.

**Oxford Pharmaceuticals, UK.** See *Masters, UK.*

**Oxo, Switz.** See *Doetsch, Grether, Switz.*

**Oxo, Thai.** Oxo Chemie (Thailand) Co. Ltd, 6 Fl, Asoke Towers Com Building, 213/14-15 Sukhumvit 21 Rd, Klongtoey Nua, Watana, Bangkok 10110, Thailand.

**Pabisch, Austria.** Pabisch GmbH, Baldassgasse 5, A-1217 Vienna, Austria.

**Pacific, Hong Kong.** See *LCH, Hong Kong.*

**Pacific, Israel.** See *Genmedix, Israel.*

**Pacific, NZ.** Pacific Pharmaceuticals Co. Ltd, P.O. Box 11-183, Ellerslie, Auckland, New Zealand.

**Pacific, Singapore.** See *Ziwell, Singapore,* and *Zuellig, Singapore.*

**Pacific, Thai.** Pacific Healthcare (Thailand) Co. Ltd, 229/1 South Sathorn Rd, Bangkok 10120, Thailand.

**Pacific Biosciences, Singapore.** Pacific Biosciences Pte Ltd, 3 Kaki Bukit Crescent, 05-03, S 416237, Singapore.

**Paddock, USA.** Paddock Laboratories Inc., 3940 Quebec Ave North, Minneapolis, MN 55427, USA.

**Padia, Ger.** Pädia Arzneimittel GmbH, Gruhlstr. 3, 50374 Erftstadt, Germany.

**Padma, Switz.** Padma AG, Wiesenstrasse 5, 8603 Schwerzenbach, Switzerland.

**Padro, Spain.** Padro, Gran Via Corts, Catalanes 764, 08013 Barcelona, Spain.

**Paedpharm, Austral.** Paedpharm P/L, P.O. Box 6533, East Perth, WA 6892, Australia.

**Paesel, Ger.** Paesel & Lorei GmbH & Co. Hauptniederlassung, Freihafen 8, 47138 Duisburg, Germany.

**Pahang, Malaysia.** Pahang Pharmacy Sdn Bhd, Lot 5979, Jln Teratai, Off Jln Meru, 41050 Klang, Selangor, Malaysia.

**Paines & Byrne, Irl.** See *Paines & Byrne, UK.*

**Paines & Byrne, NZ.** See *NZ Medical & Scientific, NZ.*

**Paines & Byrne, Thai.** See *Union Medical, Thai.*

**Paines & Byrne, UK.** Paines & Byrne Ltd, Yamanouchi House, Pyrford Rd, West Byfleet, Surrey, KT14 6RA, UK.

**Paladin, Canad.** Paladin Laboratories Inc., 6111 Royalmount Ave, Suite 102, Montreal, Quebec, H4T 2T4, Canada.

**Palex, Spain.** Grupo Palex, Juan Sebastian Bach, 12, 08021 Barcelona, Spain.

**Palisades, USA.** See *Glenwood, USA.*

**Palmares, Ital.** See *Ferlito, Ital.*

**Palmicol, Ger.** See *Riemser, Ger.*

**Palmolive Skincare, Austral.** See *Colgate Oral Care, Austral.*

**Pal-Pak, USA.** Pal-Pak Inc., 1201 Llberty St, P.O. Box 299, Allentown, PA 18105, USA.

**Pamex, Irl.** Pamex Ltd, 4 Richard St., Castlebar, Co. Mayo, Ireland.

**Pan American, USA.** Pan American Laboratories, P.O. Box 8950, Mandeville, LA 70470-8950, USA.

**Pan Quimica, Spain.** Pan Quimica Farmaceutica, Rufino Gonzalez 50, 28037 Madrid, Spain.

**Panacea, India.** Panacea Biotec Ltd, B-1 Extn. A-27,, Mohan Co-op. Industrial Estate, Mathura Rd, New Delhi 110 044, India.

**Panalab, Arg.** Lab. Panalab S.A. Argentina, Av. Del Libertador 6250 Piso 2, 1428 Buenos Aires, Argentina.

**Panax, Switz.** Panax Import, F Ruckstuhl & Co., Bergtalweg 2a, 9500 Wil, Switzerland.

**Panderma, Austria.** Panderma Arzneimittel GmbH, Braunlichgasse 40-42, A-2700 Wiener Neustadt, Austria.

**Pangeo, Israel.** See *Mediline, Israel.*

**Pannoc, Belg.** Pannoc Chemie S.A., Lammerdries 21, 2250 Olen, Belgium.

**Panpharma, Fr.** Laboratoires Panpharma, ZI du Clairay-Luitre, 35133 Fougeres, France.

**Panpharma, Hong Kong.** See *Universal, Hong Kong.*

**Pantafarm, Ital.** Pantafarm S.r.l., Via Pomintella 12, Parco Verde, 80049 Somma Vesuviana (NA), Italy.

**Pantheon, UK.** Pantheon Healthcare Ltd, Unit 7, 26 Chestnut Grove, Penge, London, SE20 8PS, UK.

**Pantofarma, Spain.** See *Almirall, Spain.*

**Pan-Well, Hong Kong.** Pan-Well Trading Co., 4/F, Flat D, Goldfield Bldg, 42-44 Connaught Rd West, Hong Kong.

**Panzera, Ital.** Farmaceutici G.B. Panzera S.r.l., Via De Sanctis 71, 20141 Milan, Italy.

**Papaellinas (Παπαελληνας), Gr.** ΠΑΠΑΕΛΛΗ-ΝΑΣ Κ. ΑΕΒΕ, 26ο χλμ. Λ. Μαρκοπουλου, 194 00 Μαρκοπουλο, Markopoulo, Greece.

**Par, USA.** Par Pharmaceutical Inc., One Ram Ridge Rd, Spring Valley, NY 10977, USA.

**Paradise, Canad.** Paradise Promotions, P. O. Box 3876, Garibaldi Highlands, British Columbia, V0N 1T0, Canada.

**Paragerm, Fr.** Laboratoires Paragerm, ZI 3$^{e}$ rue, B.P. 68, 06511 Carros cdx, France.

**Paraphar, Fr.** Laboratoires Paraphar, 10 rue Varet, 75015 Paris, France.

**Paraphar, Singapore.** See *Polymedic, Singapore.*

**Parapharm, Austria.** Parapharm Sanfte Medizin Arzneimittel-VertriebsgesmbH, Siriusstrasse 13, A-9020 Klagenfurt, Austria.

**Parggon, Mex.** Laboratorios Parggon S.A. de C.V., Manuel Cambre No. 2093, Chapultepec Country, 44610 Guadalajara, Jal., Mexico.

**Parisis, Spain.** Parisis, Juan de Juanes 8, 28007 Madrid, Spain.

**Parke, Davis, Arg.** See *Pfizer, Arg.*

**Parke, Davis, Austral.** See *Pfizer, Austral.*

**Parke, Davis, Austria.** Parke-Davis GmbH, Brunner Strasse 81, A-1230 Vienna, Austria.

**Parke, Davis, Belg.** See *Pfizer, Belg.*

**Parke, Davis, Braz.** See *Pfizer, Braz.*

**Parke, Davis, Canad.** See *Pfizer, Canad.*

**Parke, Davis, Chile.** Parke Davis, Av. Las Americas 173, Cerrillos, Santiago, Chile.

**Parke, Davis, Denm.** See *Pfizer, Denm.*

**Parke, Davis, Fin.** See *Pfizer, Fin.*

**Parke, Davis, Fr.** See *Pfizer, Fr.*

**Parke, Davis, Ger.** See *Pfizer, Ger.*

**Parke, Davis, Hong Kong.** See *Warner-Lambert, Hong Kong,* and *Zuellig, Hong Kong.*

**Parke, Davis, India.** See *Pfizer, India.*

**Parke, Davis, Irl.** See *Pfizer, Irl.*

**Parke, Davis, Israel.** See *Neopharm, Israel.*

**Parke, Davis, Ital.** Parke Davis S.p.A., Via C. Colombo 1, 20020 Lainate (Milan), Italy.

**Parke, Davis, Malaysia.** See *Pfizer, Malaysia.*

**Parke, Davis, Mex.** See *Warner-Lambert, Mex.*

**Parke, Davis, Neth.** See *Pfizer, Neth.*

**Parke, Davis, NZ.** See *Pfizer, NZ.*

**Parke, Davis, Port.** See *Pfizer, Port.*

**Parke, Davis, S.Afr.** See *Pfizer, S.Afr.*

**Parke, Davis, Singapore.** See *Age D'or, Singapore.*

**Parke, Davis, Spain.** See *Pfizer, Spain.*

**Parke, Davis, Swed.** See *Pfizer, Swed.*

**Parke, Davis, Switz.** See *Pfizer, Switz.*

**Parke, Davis, UK.** Parke-Davis & Co Ltd, Lambert Court, Chestnut Ave, Eastleigh, Hampshire, SO53 3ZQ, UK.

**Parke, Davis, USA.** Parke-Davis, 6 Century Dr., 2nd Floor, Parsippany, NJ 07054, USA.

**Parkedale, Hong Kong.** See *Keller, Hong Kong.*

**Parkedale, USA.** Parkedale Pharmaceuticals, 501 5th St, Bristol, TN 37620, USA.

**Parke-Med, S.Afr.** See *Pfizer, S.Afr.*

**Parkfields, UK.** Parkfields Sterile Supply Unit, Pond Lane, Parkfields, Wolverhampton, West Midlands, WV2 1HL, UK.

**Parmed, USA.** Parmed Pharmaceuticals Inc., 4220 Hyde Park Blvd, Niagara Falls, NY 14305, USA.

**Parnell, Irl.** See *Blackhall, Irl.*

**Parnell, USA.** Parnell Pharmaceuticals, Inc., P.O. Box 5130, Larkspur, CA 94977, USA.

**Parsenn, Switz.** Parsenn-Produkte AG, Abt. Pharmazeutik, Klus, 7240 Kublis, Switzerland.

**Parthenon, USA.** Parthenon Inc., 3311 West 2400 South, Salt Lake City, UT 84119, USA.

**Pasadena, USA.** See *Taylor, USA.*

**Pascal, USA.** Pascal Co. Inc., P.O. Box 1478, Bellevue, WA 98009, USA.

**Pascoe, Ger.** Pascoe Pharmazeutische Präparate GmbH, Schiffenberger Weg 55, 35394 Giessen, Germany.

**Pascual, Hong Kong.** See *Yik Kwan, Hong Kong.*

**Pasquali, Ital.** Pasquali S.r.l., Via L. Longo 39/41, 50019 Sesto Fiorentino (FI), Italy.

**Passauer, Ger.** Herbert J Passauer GmbH & Co. KG, Ebersstrasse 56, 10827 Berlin, Germany.

**Passion for Life, Singapore.** See *PMR, Singapore.*

**Passion for Life, UK.** Passion for Life Products Ltd, 21 Heathmans Rd, London, SW6 4TJ, UK.

**Pasteur, Chile.** Laboratorios Pasteur Ltda, Ignacio Serrano 568, Concepcion, Santiago, Chile.

**Pasteur Merieux, Austria.** See *Aventis Pasteur, Austria.*

**Pasteur Merieux, Belg.** See *Aventis Pasteur, Belg.*

**Pasteur Merieux, Braz.** See *Aventis Pasteur, Braz.*

**Pasteur Merieux, Denm.** See *Aventis Pasteur, Denm.*

**Pasteur Merieux, Fr.** See *Aventis Pasteur, Fr.*

**Pasteur Merieux, Ger.** See *Aventis Pasteur, Ger.*

**Pasteur Merieux, Hong Kong.** See *Aventis, Hong Kong.*

**Pasteur Merieux, Irl.** See *Allphar, Irl.*

**Pasteur Merieux, Israel.** See *Promedico, Israel.*

**Pasteur Merieux, Ital.** See *Aventis Pasteur, Ital.*

**Pasteur Merieux, Neth.** See *Aventis Pasteur, Neth.*

**Pasteur Merieux, Singapore.** See *Aventis, Singapore.*

**Pasteur Merieux, Swed.** See *Aventis Pasteur, Denm.*

**Pasteur Merieux, UK.** See *Aventis Pasteur, UK.*

**Pasteur Merieux, USA.** See *Aventis Pasteur, USA.*

**Pasteur Vaccins, Fr.** See *Aventis Pasteur, Fr.*

**Pastor Farina, Ital.** Pastor Farina S.r.l., Via Garibaldi 69, 22100 Como, Italy.

**Patentex, Ger.** Patentex GmbH, Marschnerstr. 8-10, 60318 Frankfurt/Main, Germany.

**Patentex, Switz.** See *Adroka, Switz.*

**Pathogenesis, Denm.** See *Orphan, Denm.*

**Pathogenesis, Gr.** Pathogenesis, Greece.

**Pathogenesis, Irl.** See *Pathogenesis, UK.*

**Pathogenesis, Norw.** See *Swedish Orphan, Norw.*

**Pathogenesis, UK.** See *Chiron, UK.*

**Pathogenesis, USA.** PathoGenesis Corp., 201 Elliott Ave West, Seattle, WA 98119, USA.

**Pautrat, Fr.** See *PPDH, Fr.*

**PCR, Ger.** PCR Arzneimittel GmbH, Wielandstr. 7, 53173 Bonn, Germany.

**PD, Thai.** Thai PD Chemicals Ltd, 2 Soi Chokchairuammitr, Viphavadee Rungsit Rd, Bangkok 10310, Thailand.

**PD Pharm, S.Afr.** PD Pharmaceuticals, P.O. Box 47448, Greyville, Durban 4023, South Africa.

**Peach, UK.** Peach Pharmaceuticals, 16 Parkstone Rd, Poole, Dorset, BH15 2PG, UK.

**Pearson, Ital.** Guglielmo Pearson S.r.l., Via delle Fabbriche 40-40a R, 16158 Genova-Voltri (GE), Italy.

**Peckforton, Irl.** See *Allphar, Irl.*

**Peckforton, UK.** Peckforton Pharmaceuticals Ltd, Crewe Hall, Crewe, Cheshire, CW1 6UL, UK.

**Pediamed, USA.** PediaMed Pharmaceuticals, 782 Springdale Drive, Suite 120, Exton, PA 19341, USA.

**Pediatrica, Malaysia.** See *Unam, Malaysia.*

**Pediatrica, Singapore.** See *Far East, Singapore.*

**Pediatrica, Thai.** See *Olic, Thai.*

**Pedinol, USA.** Pedinol Pharmacal Inc., 30 Banfi Plaza North, Farmingdale, NY 11735, USA.

**Pedi-Pak, Canad.** Pedi-Pak Products Canada Inc., 700 Lawrence Ave W, Ste 125, Toronto, ON, M6A 3B4, Canada.

**Peithner, Austria.** Dr Peithner KG nunmehr GmbH & Co., Richard-Strauss-Strasse 13, A-1232 Vienna, Austria.

**Pekana, Ger.** Pekana Naturheilmittel GmbH, Raiffeisenstr. 15, 88353 Kisslegg/Allgau, Germany.

**Peking-Boell, Ger.** Peking Royal Jelly Deutschland BOELL HandelsKontor, Am Kirchberg 3, 86666 Burgheim, Germany.

**Pelayo, Spain.** Pelayo, Tallers 16, 08001 Barcelona, Spain.

**Penederm, Canad.** See *Pharmascience, Canad.*

**Penederm, USA.** See *Bertek, USA.*

**Penn, Irl.** See *Central, Irl.*

**Penn, UK.** Penn Pharmaceuticals Ltd, Tafarnaubach Industrial Estate, Tredegar, Gwent, NP2 3AA, UK.

**Pennex, Israel.** See *Gramse, Israel.*

**Pensa, Spain.** Pensa, Av. Virgen de Montserrat 215, 08026 Barcelona, Spain.

**Penta, Ger.** Penta Arzneimittel GmbH, Hohenburger Strasse 39, 92289 Ursensollen, Germany.

**Pentaderm, Ital.** Pentaderm Industria Chimica e Farmaceutica S.r.l., Via Nazionale Pentimele 157, 89121 Reggio Calabria, Italy.

**Pentafarm, Spain.** Pentafarm, Galileo 250, 08028 Barcelona, Spain.

**Pentafarma, Chile.** Pentafarma SA, Av. Pocuro 1915, Providencia, Santiago, Chile.

**Pentafarma, Port.** Pentafarma, SA, Rua Professor Henrique de Barros, Edificio Sagres 5 A, 2685-338 Prior Velho, Portugal.

**Pentamedical, Ital.** Pentamedical S.r.l., Via G. Mazzini 1, 20021 Bollate (MI), Italy.

**People's, Malaysia.** People's Pharmacy (M) Sdn Bhd, 59-61 Jln Bendahara, 75100 Malacca, Malaysia.

**Perez Gimenez, Spain.** See *Calmante Vitaminado, Spain.*

**Pergam, Ital.** Pergam S.r.l., Via Gradisca 8, 20151 Milan, Italy.

**Periproducts, UK.** Periproducts Ltd, P.O. Box 176, Audit House, 260 Field End Rd, Ruislip, Middlesex, HA4 9YR, UK.

**Permamed, Switz.** Permamed AG, Ringstrasse 29, Postfach 360, 4106 Therwil, Switzerland.

**Permark, S.Afr.** See *Boots Healthcare, S.Afr.*

**Person & Covey, Canad.** Person & Covey Inc., 1031 Meyerside Drive, Unit 12, Mississauga, Ontario, L5T 2H5, Canada.

**Person & Covey, USA.** Person & Covey Inc., 616 Allen Ave, P.O. Box 25018, Glendale, CA 91221-5018, USA.

**Personal Care, USA.** Personal Care Group Inc., 1 Paragon Drive, Montvale, NJ 07645, USA.

**Perstorp, Austria.** See *Pharmacia, Austria.*

**Pertussin, USA.** Pertussin Laboratories, USA.

**Peter, Ital.** Peter Italia sas, Via Tommaso Silvestri 22, 00135 Rome, Italy.

**Peter Black, UK.** Peter Black Healthcare Ltd, William Nadin Way, Swadlincote, Derbyshire, DE11 0BB, UK.

**Peters, Fr.** Laboratoires Peters, ZI Les Vignes, 42 rue Benoit-Frachon, 93000 Bobigny cdx, France.

**Petrasch, Austria.** Petrasch-Pharma GmbH, Schlachthausstrasse 3, A-6850 Dornbirn, Austria.

**Petrus, Austral.** Petrus Pharmaceuticals, P.O. Box 41, Midland, Perth, WA 6936, Australia.

**Petsiavas (Πετσιαβας), Gr.** ΠΕΤΣΙΑΒΑΣ Ν. ΑΕ, Αγ. Αναργύρων 21, 145 64 Κ. Κηφισια, K. Kiphisia, Greece.

**PFC, Switz.** PFC Pharma Focus Consultants AG, Chriesbaumstrasse 2, 8604 Volketswil, Switzerland.

**Pfeiffer, USA.** Pfeiffer Company, 71 University Ave, P.O. Box 4447, Atlanta, GA 30302, USA.

**Pfizer, Arg.** Pfizer S.R.L., Virrey Loreto 2477, 1426 Buenos Aires, Argentina.

**Pfizer, Austral.** Pfizer P/L, P.O. Box 57, West Ryde, NSW 2114, Australia.

**Pfizer, Austria.** Pfizer Corporation Austria GmbH, Seidengasse 33-35, A-1070 Vienna, Austria.

**Pfizer, Belg.** Pfizer S.A., Rue Leon Theodor 102, 1090 Brussels, Belgium.

**Pfizer, Braz.** Laboratorios Pfizer Ltda, Rua Alexandre Dumas 1860, Chacara Santo Antonio, 04717-904 Sao Paulo, SP, Brazil.

**Pfizer, Canad.** Pfizer Canada Inc., P.O. Box 800, Pointe-Claire, Dorval, Quebec, H9R 4V2, Canada.

**Pfizer, Chile.** Laboratorio Pfizer de Chile SA, Av. Las Americas 173, Cerrillos, Santiago, Chile.

**Pfizer, Denm.** Pfizer ApS Danmark, Lautrupvang 8, 2750 Ballerup, Denmark.

**Pfizer, Fin.** Pfizer Oy, PL 45, 02601 Espoo, Finland.

**Pfizer, Fr.** Laboratoires Pfizer, 23-25 av. du Dr-Lannelongue, 75668 Paris cdx 14, France.

**Pfizer, Ger.** Pfizer GmbH, Pfizerstr. 1, 76139 Karlsruhe, Germany.

**Pfizer, Gr.** PFIZER HELLAS A.E, Αλκέτου 5, 116 33 Παγκρατι, Pankrati, Greece.

**Pfizer, Hong Kong.** Pfizer Corporation Hong Kong Ltd, 16/F Stanhope House, 738 King's Rd, North Point, Hong Kong.

**Pfizer, India.** Pfizer Ltd, 5 Patel Estate, S.V. Rd, Jogeshwari West, Mumbai 400 102, India.

**Pfizer, Irl.** Pfizer Pharmaceuticals, Parkway House, Ballymount Rd Lower, Dublin 12, Ireland.

**Pfizer, Israel.** Pfizer Pharmaceuticals Ltd, 9 Shenkar St, Herzliya Pituah, Israel.

**Pfizer, Ital.** Pfizer Italiana S.p.A., Via Valbondione 113, 00188 Rome, Italy.

**Pfizer, Jpn.** Pfizer Pharmaceutical Inc., 2-1-1 Nishi-shinjuku, Shinjuku-ku, Tokyo 163-0461, Japan.

**Pfizer, Malaysia.** Pfizer (Malaysia) Sdn Bhd, Lot 4, Jln 13/6, 46200 Petaling Jaya, Selangor, Malaysia.

**Pfizer, Mex.** Pfizer S.A. de C.V., Paseo de los Tamarindos No. 40, Bosque de las Lomas, 05120 Cuajimalpa, Mexico D.F., Mexico.

**Pfizer, Neth.** Pfizer BV, Roer 266, 2908 AA Capelle a/d Ijssel, Netherlands.

**Pfizer, Norw.** Pfizer AS, Strandv. 55, 1366 Lysaker, Norway.

**Pfizer, NZ.** Pfizer Laboratories Ltd, P.O. Box 3998, Auckland, New Zealand.

**Pfizer, Port.** Laboratórios Pfizer, Lda, Porto Zemouto, Coina, Apartado 30, 2830 Ciona, Portugal.

**Pfizer, S.Afr.** Pfizer Laboratories (Pty) Ltd, P.O. Box 783720, Sandton 2146, South Africa.

**Pfizer, Singapore.** Pfizer Pte Ltd, 200 Middle Rd, 06-00 Prime Centre, S 188980, Singapore.

**Pfizer, Spain.** Pfizer, Avda Europa 20B, Epmresarial La Moraleja, Alcobendas, 28108 Madrid, Spain.

**Pfizer, Swed.** Pfizer AB, Box 501, 183 25 Taby, Sweden.

**Pfizer, Switz.** Pfizer SA, Postfach, 8048 Zurich, Switzerland.

**Pfizer, Thai.** Pfizer International Corp, 19-20 Fl, Ploenchit Center Tower, 2 Sukhumvit Rd, Kwang Klongtoey, Khet Klongtoey, Bangkok 10110, Thailand.

**Pfizer, UK.** Pfizer Ltd, Walton Oaks, Dorking Rd, Tadworth, Surrey, KT20 7NS, UK.

**Pfizer, USA.** Pfizer Inc., 235 East 42nd St, New York, NY 10017-5755, USA.

**Pfizer Consumer, Austral.** See *Pfizer, Austral.*

**Pfizer Consumer, Belg.** See *Pfizer, Belg.*

**Pfizer Consumer, Canad.** Pfizer Consumer Healthcare, Division of Pfizer Canada Inc., 2200 Eglinton Ave E, Toronto, Ontario, M1L 2N3, Canada.

**Pfizer Consumer, Ger.** See *Pfizer, Ger.*

**Pfizer Consumer, Irl.** See *Pfizer, Irl.*

**Pfizer Consumer, Ital.** See *Pfizer, Ital.*

**Pfizer Consumer, Port.** See *Pfizer, Port.*

**Pfizer Consumer, S.Afr.** See *Pfizer, S.Afr.*

**Pfizer Consumer, Singapore.** See *Pfizer, Singapore.*

**Pfizer Consumer, Spain.** See *Pfizer, Spain.*

**Pfizer Consumer, UK.** Pfizer Consumer Healthcare, Dorking Rd, Walton Oaks, Walton-on-the-Hill, Surrey, KT20 7NS, UK.

**Pfizer Consumer, USA.** See *Pfizer, USA.*

**Pfizer Lambert, Spain.** See *Pfizer, Spain.*

**Pfizer Sante, Fr.** See *Pfizer, Fr.*

**Pfleger, Ger.** Dr R. Pfleger Chemische Fabrik GmbH, 96045 Bamberg, Germany.

**Pfleger, Israel.** See *Gramse, Israel.*

**Pfluger, Ger.** Homöopathisches Laboratorium A. Pflüger GmbH, Bielefelder Str. 17, 33378 Rheda-Wiedenbruck, Germany.

**Pfrimmer Nutricia, Switz.** See *Uhlmann-Eyraud, Switz.*

**PGM, Ger.** PGM Pharmazeutische Gesellschaft mbH & Co. Munchen, Furstenstr 6, 80333 Munich, Germany.

**Phamos, Ger.** Phamos Arzneimittel GmbH, Oberster Kamp 1c, 59069 Hamm/Westf., Germany.

**Pharbenia, Ital.** Pharbenia S.r.l., Societa del Gruppo Bayer, V'le Certosa 130, 20156 Milan, Italy.

**Pharbita, Israel.** See *Genmedix, Israel.*

**Pharbita, Singapore.** See *FP, Singapore.*

**Phardi, Switz.** Phardi AG, Bruhlstrasse 50, 4107 Ettingen, Switzerland.

**Pharma 2000, Fr.** Laboratoires Pharma 2000, Imm Strasbourg, av de l'Europe, Toussus-le-Noble, 78771 Magny-les-Hameaux cdx, France.

**Pharma 2000, Singapore.** Pharma 2000 Pte Ltd, 63 Hillview Ave, 03-07 Lam Soon Industrial Building, S 669569, Singapore.

**Pharma Biotech, Israel.** See *Medison, Israel.*

**Pharma Clal, Israel.** Pharma-Clal Ltd, P.O. Box 31, Bnei Brak, Israel.

**Pharma Dynamics, S.Afr.** Pharma Dynamics (Pty) Ltd, 1st Floor, Grapevine House, Steenberg Office Park, Silverwood Close, Cape Town 7945, South Africa.

**Pharma Force, Austria.** Pharma Force, Drogen-Pharmazeutica, S. Unterweger, Postfach 1, A-9131 Grafenstein, Austria.

**Pharma Investi, Chile.** Pharma Investi de Chile SA, Av. Andres Bello 1495, Providencia, Santiago, Chile.

**Pharma Italia, Ital.** Pharma Italia Laboratori Farmaceutici S.r.l., Via Vittor Pisani 93, 70033 Corato (BA), Italy.

**Pharma Line, Ital.** Pharma Line S.r.l., Via M Ricci 15, 60020 Palombina Nuova (AN), Italy.

**Pharma Nord, Fin.** Oy Pharma Nord AB, Rajatorpantie 41 C, 01640 Vantaa, Finland.

**Pharma Nord, Fr.** Pharma Nord/Pharma Trade Healthcare, Batiment D/6, 4 rue de la Grande-Ourse, B.P. 8383, 95805 Cergy-Pontoise cdx, France.

**Pharma Nord, Irl.** See *Electramed, Irl.*

**Pharma Nord, Malaysia.** See *Sun, Malaysia.*

**Pharma Nord, Norw.** Pharma Nord Norge AS, Syretsrnet 25, 3048 Drammen, Norway.

**Pharma Nord, Thai.** See *Biogenetech, Thai.*

**Pharma Nord, UK.** Pharma Nord UK Ltd, Telford Court, Morpeth, Northumberland, NE61 2DB, UK.

**Pharma Tek, USA.** Pharma-Tek Inc., P.O. Box 1148, Elmira, NY 14902, USA.

**Pharmabroker, NZ.** Pharmabroker Sales Ltd, P.O. Box 302 234, North Harbour Postal Centre, Auckland, New Zealand.

**Pharmacal, Fin.** Oy Pharmacal AB, Nilsiänkatu 8, 00510 Helsinki, Finland.

**Pharmacal, Switz.** See *Democal, Switz.*

**Pharmacaps, Mex.** Pharmacaps, Division de Gelcaps Exportadora de Mexico S.A. de C.V., Calle 7 No. 6, Fracc. Ind. Alce Blanco, 53370 Naucalpan de Juarez Edo. de Mexico, Mexico.

**Pharmacard, Switz.** Pharmacard Family Astral AG, 7 rue Pedro Maylan, 1211 Geneva 17, Switzerland.

**Pharmacare, Canad.** Pharmacare Ltd, 120 Harry Walker Parkway N, New Market, Ontario, L3Y 2B2, Canada.

**Pharmacare, Gr.** PHARMA-CARE AE, Α. Σπάτων 68, 153 44 Γέρακας, Gerakas, Greece.

**Pharmacare, Hong Kong.** Pharmacare, Hong Kong.

**Pharmacare, Malaysia.** See *Medidata, Malaysia,* and *Pharmaniaga, Malaysia.*

**Pharmaceutical Co, India.** The Pharmaceutical Co of India, Arun Chambers, J. Dadajee Rd, Tardeo, Mumbai 400 034, India.

**Pharmaceutical Enterprises, S.Afr.** Pharmaceutical Enterprises (Pty) Ltd, P.O. Box 201, Howard Place 7450, South Africa.

**Pharmaceutical Specialties, USA.** Pharmaceutical Specialties Inc., P.O. Box 6298, Rochester, MN 55903, USA.

**Pharmachem, UK.** M & A Pharmachem Ltd, Allenby Laboratories, Wigan Rd, Westhoughton, Bolton, BL6 2LA, UK.

**Pharmachemie, Belg.** Pharmachemie, Belgium.

**Pharmachemie, Denm.** See *Pharmachemie, Neth.*

**Pharmachemie, Israel.** See *Teva, Israel.*

**Pharmachemie, Malaysia.** See *United Italian, Malaysia.*

**Pharmachemie, Neth.** Pharmachemie BV, Swensweg 5, 2031 GA Haarlem, Netherlands.

**Pharmachemie, S.Afr.** Pharmachemie (Pty) Ltd, P.O. Box 7115, Johannesburg 2000, South Africa.

**Pharmachemie, Singapore.** See *FP, Singapore.*

**Pharmachemie, Thai.** See *Pacific, Thai.*

**Pharmachoice, S.Afr.** Pharmachoice (Pty) Ltd, P.O. Box 291, Fourways 2055, South Africa.

**Pharmacia, Arg.** Pharmacia Argentina S.A., Moreno 877 Piso 21, 1091 Buenos Aires, Argentina.

**Pharmacia, Austral.** Pharmacia Australia P/L, P.O. Box 46, Rydalmere, NSW 2116, Australia.

**Pharmacia, Austria.** Pharmacia Austria GmbH, Oberlaaer Strasse 251, A-1100 Vienna, Austria.

**Pharmacia, Belg.** Pharmacia S.A., Twin Squares, Culliganlaan 1C, 1831 Diegem, Belgium.

**Pharmacia, Braz.** Pharmacia Brasil Ltda, Avenida Chucri Zaidan 940, 7° andar, Condominio Market Place, Tower II, 04589-906 Sao Paulo, SP, Brazil.

**Pharmacia, Canad.** Pharmacia Canada Inc., 55 Standish Court, Suite 1200, Mississauga, Ontario, L5R 4E3, Canada.

**Pharmacia, Chile.** Pharmacia Corporation de Chile SA, Del Inca 4446, Pso 4, Las Condes, Santiago, Chile.

**Pharmacia, Denm.** Pharmacia AS, Overgaden neden Vandet 7, 1414 Copenhagen K, Denmark.

**Pharmacia, Fin.** Pharmacia Oy, Rajatorpantie 41, 01640 Vantaa, Finland.

**Pharmacia, Fr.** Pharmacia SAS, B.P. 210, 78051 St-Quentin-Yvelines cdx, France.

**Pharmacia, Ger.** Pharmacia GmbH, Am Wolfsmantel 46, 91058 Erlangen, Germany.

**Pharmacia, Hong Kong.** Pharmacia Asia Ltd, 18/F Allied Kajima Bldg, 138 Gloucester Rd, Wanchai, Hong Kong.

**Pharmacia, India.** Pharmacia India Pvt Ltd, S.C.O. 27, Sector 14, Gurgaon 122 001, India.

**Pharmacia, Irl.** Pharmacia Ltd, P.O. Box 1752, Airways Industrial Estate, Dublin 17, Ireland.

**Pharmacia, Israel.** See *Agis, Israel.*

**Pharmacia, Ital.** Pharmacia S.p.A., Via Robert Koch 1.2, 20152 Milan, Italy.

**Pharmacia, Malaysia.** Pharmacia Malaysia Sdn Bhd, Unit 7-1, Level 7, CP Tower, No. 11, Section 16/11, Jan Damansara, 46350 Petaling Jaya, Selangor, Malaysia.

**Pharmacia, Mex.** Pharmacia S.A. de C.V., Calz. de Tlalpan No. 2962, Col. Espartaco, 04870 Mexico D.F., Mexico.

**Pharmacia, Neth.** Pharmacia BV, Postbus 17, 34407 AA Woerden, Netherlands.

**Pharmacia, Norw.** Pharmacia Norge AS, Lilleakerv. 2 B, 0283 Oslo, Norway.

**Pharmacia, NZ.** Pharmacia, P.O. Box 11-282, Ellerslie, Auckland, New Zealand.

**Pharmacia, Port.** Pharmacia Lda, Av do Forte 3, Edificio Suecia II, 2795-505 Carnaxide, Portugal.

**Pharmacia, S.Afr.** Pharmacia South Africa, P.O. Box 41111, Craighall 2024, South Africa.

**Pharmacia, Singapore.** Pharmacia Singapore Pte Ltd, 101 Thomson Rd, 31-04/05 United Square, S 307591, Singapore.

**Pharmacia, Spain.** Pharmacia Spain, Ctra de Rub 90-100, Sant Cugat del Valles, 08190 Barcelona, Spain.

**Pharmacia, Swed.** Pharmacia Sverige AB, 112 87 Stockholm, Sweden.

**Pharmacia, Switz.** Pharmacia AG, Lagerstrasse 14, 8600 Dubendorf, Switzerland.

**Pharmacia, Thai.** Pharmacia (Thailand) Ltd, 6 Fl, White Group Building, 75 Soi Sangchan-Rubia, Sukhumvit 42, Sukhumvit Rd Prakanong, Klongtoey, Bangkok 10110, Thailand.

**Pharmacia, UK.** Pharmacia Ltd, Davy Ave, Knowlhill, Milton Keynes, Buckinghamshire, MK5 8PH, UK.

**Pharmacia, USA.** Pharmacia Corp., 100 Route 206 N, Peapack, NJ 07977, USA.

**Pharmacia Consumer, Canad.** Pharmacia Consumer Healthcare, 4737 Levy St, St-Laurent, Quebec, H4R 2P9, Canada.

**Pharmacia Upjohn, Austral.** See *Pharmacia, Austral.*

**Pharmacia Upjohn, Austria.** See *Pharmacia, Austria.*

**Pharmacia Upjohn, Belg.** See *Pharmacia, Belg.*

**Pharmacia Upjohn, Braz.** See *Pharmacia, Braz.*

**Pharmacia Upjohn, Canad.** See *Pharmacia, Canad.*

**Pharmacia Upjohn, Denm.** See *Pharmacia, Denm.*

**Pharmacia Upjohn, Fin.** See *Pharmacia, Fin.*

**Pharmacia Upjohn, Fr.** See *Pharmacia, Fr.*

**Pharmacia Upjohn, Ger.** See *Pharmacia, Ger.*

**Pharmacia-Upjohn, Gr.** PHARMACIA & UPJOHN A.E., Καλαβρύτων 2, 145 64, Ν. Κηφισσιά, N. Kiphissia, Greece.

**Pharmacia Upjohn, Hong Kong.** See *Pharmacia, Hong Kong.*

**Pharmacia Upjohn, India.** See *Pharmacia, India.*

**Pharmacia Upjohn, Irl.** See *Pharmacia, Irl.*

**Pharmacia Upjohn, Israel.** See *Agis, Israel.*

**Pharmacia Upjohn, Ital.** See *Pharmacia, Ital.*

**Pharmacia Upjohn, Mex.** See *Pharmacia, Mex.*

**Pharmacia Upjohn, Neth.** See *Pharmacia, Neth.*

**Pharmacia Upjohn, Norw.** See *Pharmacia, Norw.*

**Pharmacia Upjohn, NZ.** See *Pharmacia, NZ.*

**Pharmacia Upjohn, Port.** See *Pharmacia, Port.*

**Pharmacia Upjohn, S.Afr.** See *Pharmacia, S.Afr.*

**Pharmacia Upjohn, Singapore.** See *Pharmacia, Singapore.*

**Pharmacia Upjohn, Spain.** See *Pharmacia, Spain.*

**Pharmacia Upjohn, Swed.** See *Pharmacia, Swed.*

**Pharmacia Upjohn, Switz.** See *Pharmacia, Switz.*

**Pharmacia Upjohn, Thai.** See *Pharmacia, Thai.*

**Pharmacia Upjohn, UK.** See *Pharmacia, UK.*

**Pharmacia Upjohn, USA.** See *Pharmacia, USA.*

**Pharmacie Centrale des Hopitaux, Fr.** See *AGEPS, Fr.*

**Pharmacie Principale, Fr.** Pharmacie Principale Tours, 53 rue Nationale, 37011 Tours cdx, France.

**Pharmaco, NZ.** Pharmaco (NZ) Ltd, P.O. Box 4079, Auckland, New Zealand.

**Pharmaco, S.Afr.** Pharmaco Distribution (Pty) Ltd, P.O. Box 786522, Sandton 2146, South Africa.

**Pharmacobel, Belg.** Laboratoires Belges Pharmacobel S.A., Ave de Scheut 46-50, 1070 Brussels, Belgium.

**Pharmacodane, Denm.** PharmaCoDane ApS, Marielundvej 46A, 2730 Herlev, Denmark.

**Pharmacon, Braz.** See *Cristalia, Braz.*

**Pharmacon, Singapore.** Pharmacon (Pte) Ltd, 8 Kaki Bukit Rd, 04-27/28 Ruby Warehouse Complex, S 417841, Singapore.

**Pharmacos, Mex.** Pharmacos Exakta S.A. de C.V., Av. del Nino Obrero No. 651, Col. Chapalita Sur, 45040 Guadalajara, Jal., Mexico.

**Pharmacos Abug, Mex.** Pharmacos Abug S.A. de C.V., Lago Ginebra 359, Col. Cinco de Mayo, Deleg. Miguel Hidalgo, 11470 Mexico D.F., Mexico.

**Pharmacypria, Gr.** PHARMACYPRIA, Παστέρ 6, 115 21 Αθήνα, Athens, Greece.

**Pharmadass, UK.** Pharmadass Ltd, 16 Aintree Rd, Greenford, Middlesex, UB6 7LA, UK.

**Pharmadent, Fr.** Laboratoires Pharmadent, 45 rue Jean-Jaures, B.P. 143, 92304 Levallois-Perret cdx, France.

**PharmaDerm, USA.** PharmaDerm, 4126 Steve Reynolds Blvd, Norcross, GA 30093, USA.

**Pharmadeveloppement, Fr.** Pharma Développement, 40 rue des Bergers, 75015 Paris, France.

**Pharmadica, Thai.** Pharmadica Co. Ltd, 4 Fl, Pharmaland Building, 15/56 Moo 1 Soi Supapong, Srinakarin Rd, Nongborn Pravej, Bangkok 10260, Thailand.

**Pharmador, S.Afr.** See *Protea, S.Afr.*

**Pharmafar, Ital.** Pharmafar S.r.l., Corso V Emanuele II 82, 10121 Turin, Italy.

**Pharmafarm, Fr.** Laboratoires Pharmafarm, 13 av de la Porte d'Italie, 75648 Paris, France.

**Pharmafina, Chile.** See *Recalcine, Chile.*

**Pharmaforte, Malaysia.** Pharmaforte (M) Sdn Bhd, 2 Jln PJU 3/49, Sunway Damansara, 47810 Petaling Jaya, Selangor, Malaysia.

**Pharmaforte, Singapore.** Pharmaforte Singapore Pte Ltd, 6 Tagore Drive, 03-11 Tagore Industrial Building, S 787623, Singapore.

**Pharmafrica, S.Afr.** Pharmafrica (Pty) Ltd, P.O. Box 18397, Hillbrow 2038, South Africa.

**Pharmagalen, Ger.** See *Galen, Ger.*

**Pharmagenics, UK.** Pharmagenics Healthcare Ltd, 251 Walworth Rd, London, SE17 1RL, UK.

**Pharmagenix, UK.** Pharmagenix Ltd, Manx House, Spectrum Business Estate, Maidstone, Kent, ME15 9YP, UK.

**Pharmagenus, Spain.** See *Uriach, Spain.*

**Pharmagic, Ital.** PharmaGIC S.r.l., Via Gerano 5, 00156 Rome, Italy.

**Pharma-Global, Irl.** Pharma-Global Ltd, Hudson Rd, Sandycove, Co. Dublin, Ireland.

**Pharma-Global, UK.** Pharma-Global (UK) Ltd, SEQ Ltd, Nerin House, 26 Ridgeway St, Isle of Man, IM1 1EL, UK.

**Pharmakochimiki (Φαρμακοχημικη), Gr.** ΦΑΡΜΑΚΟΧΗΜΙΚΗ ΑΕ, Πηγάσου 18, 151 25 Μαρουσι, Marousi, Greece.

**Pharmakon, Ger.** Pharmakon Arzneimittel GmbH, Leininger Ring 65a, 67278 Bockenheim, Germany.

**Pharmakon, Switz.** Pharmakon SA, Burglistrasse 39, 8304 Wallisellen, Switzerland.

**Pharmakon, USA.** Pharmakon Laboratories Inc., 6050 Jet Port Industrial Blvd, Tampa, FL 33634, USA.

**Pharmakos, Switz.** Pharmakos AG, Lowenstrasse 59, 8001 Zurich, Switzerland.

**Pharmalab, Austral.** Pharmalab P/L, 332 Burns Bay Rd, Lane Cove, NSW 2066, Australia.

**Pharmalab, Canad.** Pharmalab (1982) Inc., 8750 boul. de-la-Rive-Sud, Levis, QC, G6V 6N6, Canada.

**Pharmaland, Thai.** Pharmaland (1982) Co. Ltd, Pharmaland Building, 15/56 Moo 1 Soi Supapong, Srinakarin Rd, Nongborn Pravej, Bangkok 10260, Thailand.

**Pharmalex (Φαρμαλεξ), Gr.** ΦΑΡΜΑΛΕΞ ΑΕΒΕ, Τσόχα 15-17, 115 10 Αθήνα, Athens, Greece.

**Pharmalink, Denm.** See *Pharmalink, Swed.*

**Pharmalink, Ger.** See *Pharmalink, Swed.*

**Pharmalink, Norw.** See *Pharmalink, Swed.*

**Pharmalink, Swed.** Pharmalink AB, Box 625, 194 26 Upplands Vasby, Sweden.

**Pharma-Natura, Ital.** Pharma Natura S.r.l., Via Vicinale di Parabiago, 20014 Nerviano (MI), Italy.

**Pharmanel, Gr.** PHARMANEL A.E., Λ. Μαραθώνος 106, 153 44 Γέρακας, Gerakas, Greece.

**Pharmanex, USA.** Pharmanex Inc., 74 W Center, Provo, UT 84601, USA.

**Pharmaniaga, Malaysia.** Pharmaniaga Bhd, P.O. Box 2030, Pusat Business Bukit Raja, 40800 Shah Alam, Selangor, Malaysia.

**Pharmanik (Φαρμανικ), Gr.** ΦΑΡΜΑΝΙΚ, Φυλής 137, 134 51 Καματερο, Kamatero, Greece.

**Pharmaplan, S.Afr.** Pharmaplan (Pty) Ltd, P.O. Box 7115, Johannesburg 2000, South Africa.

**Pharmapol, Ger.** Pharmapol Arzneimittelvertrieb-GmbH, Kaddenbusch 11, 25578 Dageling, Germany.

**Pharmarecord, Ital.** Pharmarecord S.r.l., Via Laurentina Km 24.730, 00040 Pomezia (Rome), Italy.

**Pharmasant, Thai.** See *Central, Thai.*

**Pharmascience, Canad.** Pharmascience Inc., 6111 Royalmount Ave, Suite 100, Montreal, Quebec, H4T 2T4, Canada.

**Pharmascience, Fr.** See *Expanscience, Fr.*

**Pharmascience, Hong Kong.** See *Hind Wing, Hong Kong,* and *Jacobson, Hong Kong.*

**Pharmascience, Malaysia.** See *Ranbaxy, Malaysia.*

**Pharmascience, Singapore.** See *JDH, Singapore.*

**Pharmascience, Spain.** Pharmascience, Pol Ind Los Olivos, C/Adaptacion 33, Getafe, 28906 Madrid, Spain.

**Pharmaselect, Austria.** Pharmaselect Handels GmbH, Hutteldorfer Strasse 63-65/8, A-1150 Vienna, Austria.

**Pharmaselect, Ger.** Pharmaselect GmbH, Am Sagewerk 13, 68526 Ladenburg, Germany.

**Pharmaserve, Singapore.** See *Polymedic, Singapore.*

**Pharmasette, Ital.** Pharmasette di Paolo Donati e C. S.a.s., Via Lusitania 15/A, 00183 Rome, Italy.

**Pharmashalom, Israel.** Pharmashalom Ltd, 21 Hamelaha St, Park Afek, Rosh Ha'ayin, Israel.

**Pharmastra, Fr.** Pharmastra, Usines Chimiques et Pharmaceutiques de Strasbourg, 40 rue du Canal, 67460 Souffelweyersheim, France.

**Pharmateam, Israel.** Pharmateam Marketing, P.O. Box 405, Jerusalem, Israel.

**Pharmateam, UK.** Pharmateam, UK.

**Pharmatel, Austral.** Pharmatel P/L, 3 Chilvers Rd, Thornleigh, NSW 2120, Australia.

**Pharmatel, Malaysia.** See *Imeks, Malaysia.*

**Pharmatel, NZ.** See *Bamford, NZ.*

**Pharmaten (Φαρματεν), Gr.** ΦΑΡΜΑΤΕΝ ΕΠΕ, Μενάνδρου 68, 104 37 Αθήνα, Athens, Greece.

**Pharmatex, Ital.** Pharmatex Italia S.r.l., Via Appiani 22, 20121 Milan, Italy.

**Pharmathen, Hong Kong.** See *Health Alliance, Hong Kong.*

**Pharmaton, Ger.** See *Boehringer Ingelheim, Ger.*

**Pharmaton, Israel.** See *Pharmashalom, Israel.*

**Pharmaton, Malaysia.** See *Boehringer Ingelheim, Malaysia.*

**Pharmaton, NZ.** Pharmaton, New Zealand.

**Pharmaton, S.Afr.** See *Swisspharm, S.Afr.*

**Pharmaton, Singapore.** See *Diethelm, Singapore.*

**Pharmaton, Switz.** Pharmaton SA, 6934 Bioggio, Switzerland.

**Pharmaton, Thai.** See *Boehringer Ingelheim, Thai.*

**Pharmatrix, Arg.** Pharmatrix, Div. de Therabel Pharma S.A., Arenales 259, 1704 Ramos Mejia, Buenos Aires, Argentina.

**Pharmavite, Canad.** Pharmavite Corp., 5230 Orbitor Drive, Mississauga, Ontario, L4W 5G7, Canada.

**Pharmax, Hong Kong.** See *Hind Wing, Hong Kong.*

**Pharmax, Irl.** See *Allphar, Irl.*

**Pharmax, Singapore.** See *Naina, Singapore.*

**Pharmax, UK.** See *Forest Laboratories, UK.*

**Pharmazam, Spain.** Pharmazam, Maresme 5, Pol. Ind. Urvasa, Sta Perpetua de Mogoda, 08130 Barcelona, Spain.

**Pharmco, S.Afr.** Pharmco Holdings Ltd., 16a Drake Ave, Eastleigh Ridge, Edenvale 1609, South Africa.

**Pharmed, Austria.** Pharmed, Sackstrasse 4, A-8011 Graz, Austria.

**Pharmed, India.** Pharmed Medicare, Pharmed Gardens, Whitefield Rd, Bangalore 560048, India.

**Pharmed, Singapore.** Pharmed Import & Export Pte Ltd, 149 Rochor Rd, BI-16/17/18 Fu Lu Shou Complex, S 188425, Singapore.

**Pharmedia (Φαρμεντια), Gr.** ΦΑΡΜΕΝΤΙΑ ΕΠΕ, Αιγαίου Πελάγους 2Β, 153 41 Αγ. Παρασκευή, Ag. Paraskevi, Greece.

**Pharmedica, S.Afr.** Pharmedica Laboratories (Pty) Ltd, P.O. Box 87, East London 5200, Cape Province, South Africa.

**Pharmel, Canad.** Pharmel Inc., 8699 8e Ave, Montreal, Quebec, H1Z 2X4, Canada.

**Pharmelle, USA.** Pharmelle LLC, 890 N Lafayette, Florissant, MO 63031, USA.

**Pharmeso, Switz.** Pharmeso AG, Hauptbahnhofstrasse 6, 4500 Solothurn, Switzerland.

**Pharmethic, Belg.** Pharmethic S.A., Rue de Vivier 89-93, 1050 Brussels, Belgium.

**Pharmex (Φαρμεξ), Gr.** ΦΑΡΜΕΞ ΑΕ, Αυλώνος 156, 104 43 Σεπολια, Sepolia, Greece.

**Pharmexco, UK.** Pharmexco Ltd, 5-6 Zennor Rd, London, SW12 0PS, UK.

**Pharmia, Fin.** Pharmia Oy, PL 387, 00101 Helsinki, Finland.

**Pharmics, USA.** Pharmics Inc., 2350 S Redwood Rd, Salt Lake City, UT 84119, USA.

**Pharminter, Fr.** Laboratoires Pharminter, 34 rue St-Romain, 69008 Lyon, France.

**Pharmion, Irl.** See *Allphar, Irl.*

**Pharmion, UK.** Pharmion Ltd, McClintock Building, Granta Park, Gt Abington, Cambridgeshire, CB1 6GX, UK.

**Pharmion, USA.** Pharmion Corp., 4865 Riverbend Rd, Boulder, CO 80301, USA.

**Pharmonta, Austria.** Pharmonta Mag. pharm. Dr Fischer, Montanastrasse 7, A-8112 Gratwein, Austria.

**Pharmos, Arg.** Pharmos S.A., Saladillo 2450, 1440 Buenos Aires, Argentina.

**Pharmus, Braz.** Pharmus Quimica e Farmaceutica SA, Lotes 1 a 5, Quadra L, Loteamento IV, Distrito Industrial, 55000-000 Caruaru, PE, Brazil.

**Pharmy, Fr.** Laboratoires Pharmy II, Strategy Center, 26 rue des Gaudines, 78100 Saint-Germain-en-Laye, France.

**Pharmygiene, Fr.** Laboratoires Pharmygiène-SCAT, 2-4 rue Chaintron, B.P. 850, 92542 Montrouge cdx, France.

**Pharno-Wedropharm, Ger.** Pharno-Wedropharm GmbH, Heinrichstrasse 3, 21244 Buchholz, Germany.

**Pharos, Singapore.** See *Polymedic, Singapore.*

**Phillips Yeast, UK.** Phillips Yeast Products Ltd, Park Royal Rd, London, NW10 7JX, UK.

**Philopharm, Ger.** Philopharm GmbH, Vor dem Groperntor 20, 06484 Quedlinburg, Germany.

**Philtel, Israel.** Philtel Pharmaceuticals Ltd, P.O. Box 8609, New Industrial Zone, Netanya, Israel.

**Phoenix, Arg.** Laboratorios Phoenix S.A.I.C.F., Humahuaca 4065, 1192 Buenos Aires, Argentina.

**Phoenix Health, UK.** Phoenix Health Ltd, UK.

**Phoenix-Elea, Arg.** See *Phoenix, Arg.*

**Phoinix Pharm (Φοινιξ Φαρμ), Gr.** ΦΟΙΝΙΞ ΦΑΡΜ ΕΠΕ, Αναβρυτής 5, 111 43 Αθήνα, Athens, Greece.

**Phonix, Ger.** Phönix Laboratorium GmbH, Benzstr. 10, 71149 Bondorf, Germany.

**Phos-Kola, Braz.** Laboratorio Phos-Kola Ltda, Rua das Laranjeiras 984, 49010-000 Aracaju, SE, Brazil.

**Photocure, Norw.** PhotoCure ASA, Hoffsvein, 0377 Oslo, Norway.

**Photocure, Swed.** See *Photocure, Norw.*

**PH&T, Ital.** PH&T S.p.A., Via L Ariosto 34, 20145 Milan, Italy.

**Phygiene, Fr.** Laboratoires Phygiène, 11-13 rue de la Loge, B.P. 100, 94265 Fresnes cdx, France.

**Phyteia, Switz.** Phyteia AG, Drosselstrasse 47, 4059 Basle, Switzerland.

**Phytocare, Austral.** Phytocare, Australia.

**Phytodiet, Fr.** Laboratoires Phytodiet, B.P. 68012, 57028 Metz cdx 01, France.

**Phytomed, Switz.** Phytomed AG, Tschamerie 25, 3415 Hasle/Burgdorf, Switzerland.

**Phytomedica, Fr.** Laboratoires Phytomedica, ZI Les Milles, B.P. 5000, Parc d'activites de Pichaury, 13791 Aix-en-Provence cdx 3, France.

**Phytopharma, Switz.** Phytopharma SA, Praz de Neirivue, 1666 Grandvillard, Switzerland.

**Phytoprevent, Fr.** Laboratoires Phytoprevent, 15 av. de Segur, 75007 Paris, France.

**Phytosolba, Fr.** Laboratoires Phytosolba, 89 rue Salvador-Allende, 95870 Bezons, France.

**Piam, Ital.** Vecchi & C. Piam di G. Assereto, E. Maragliano e C. S.a.p.a., Via Padre G. Semeria 5, 16131 Genoa, Italy.

**Piam, Singapore.** See *Zyfas, Singapore.*

**Picharn, Thai.** Picharn c/o The Picharn Co. Ltd, 53/43 Soi Amornphan 5, Viphavadi-Rangsit Rd, Jatujak, Bangkok 10900, Thailand.

**Pickles, UK.** J. Pickles & Sons, Beech House, 62 High St, Knaresborough, North Yorkshire, HG5 0EA, UK.

**Picot, Fr.** Laboratoires des Produits Picot, 189 quai Lucien-Lheureux, B.P. 83, 62102 Calais cdx, France.

**Picot, Switz.** See *Ridupharm, Switz.*

**Piemont, Ital.** Piemont-Farm Srl, Via Cirie 8, 10099 San Mauro, Italy.

**Pierre Fabre, Arg.** Pierre Fabre Argentina S.A., Marcelo T de Alvear 684, piso 7, 1058 Buenos Aires, Argentina.

**Pierre Fabre, Austral.** Pierre Fabre Medicament Australia Pty Ltd., Parkview Business Centre, 1 Maitland Place, Baulkham Hills, NSW 2153, Australia.

**Pierre Fabre, Austria.** See *Pierre Fabre, Fr.*

**Pierre Fabre, Belg.** Pierre Fabre Medicament Benelux, Paepsem Business Park, Ave Paepsem 8a, 1070 Brussels, Belgium.

**Pierre Fabre, Denm.** See *Pierre Fabre, Swed.*

**Pierre Fabre, Fin.** See *Algol, Fin.*

**Pierre Fabre, Fr.** Laboratoires Pierre Fabre, 45 place Abel-Gance, 92100 Boulogne, France.

**Pierre Fabre, Ger.** Pierre Fabre Pharma GmbH, Jechtinger Str. 13, 79111 Freiburg, Germany.

**Pierre Fabre, Gr.** PIERRE FABRE FARMAKA A.E., Πόντου 64, 115 27 Αθήνα, Athens, Greece.

**Pierre Fabre, Hong Kong.** See *Zuellig, Hong Kong.*

**Pierre Fabre, Israel.** See *Mediline, Israel.*

**Pierre Fabre, Ital.** Pierre Fabre Italia S.p.A., Via G.G. Winckelmann 1, 20146 Milan, Italy.

**Pierre Fabre, Malaysia.** See *Orient, Malaysia.*

**Pierre Fabre, Neth.** Pierre Fabre Benelux, Ijsselburcht 4, 6825 BP Arnhem, Netherlands.

**Pierre Fabre, Norw.** See *Pierre Fabre, Swed.*

**Pierre Fabre, Port.** Pierre Fabre Médicament Portugal, Lda, Rua Rodrigo da Fonseca 178 - 2 Esq, 1099-067 Lisbon, Portugal.

**Pierre Fabre, Singapore.** See *Orient, Singapore.*

**Pierre Fabre, Spain.** Pierre Fabre Iberica, Ramon Trias Fargas 7-11, Edifico Marina Village, 08005 Barcelona, Spain.

**Pierre Fabre, Swed.** Pierre Fabre Pharma Norden AB, Box 349, 192 30 Sollentuna, Sweden.

**Pierre Fabre, Switz.** Pierre Fabre (Suisse) SA, Route Sous-Riette 21, 1023 Crissier, Switzerland.

**Pierre Fabre, Thai.** See *Berli, Thai.*

**Pierre Fabre, UK.** Pierre Fabre Ltd, Hyde Abbey House, 23 Hyde St, Winchester, Hampshire, SO23 7DR, UK.

**Pierre Fabre, USA.** Pierre Fabre, USA.

**Pierre Fabre Dermo Kosmetik, Ger.** See *Pierre Fabre, Ger.*

**Pierre Fabre Dermo-Cosmetique, Arg.** See *Pierre Fabre, Arg.*

**Pierre Fabre Sante, Fr.** See *Pierre Fabre, Fr.*

**Pierrel, Ital.** Pierrel Farmaceutici S.p.A., Via Revere 16, 20123 Milan, Italy.

**Pietrasanta, Ital.** Pietrasanta Pharma S.r.l., Loc. S. Rocchino, 55054 Massarosa (LU), Italy.

**Piette, Belg.** Piette International S.A., Rue Grand-Bigard 128, 1620 Drogenbos, Belgium.

**Piette, Thai.** See *International Pharmaceuticals, Thai.*

**Pilkington Barnes-Hind, USA.** See *Wesley, USA.*

**Pilsensee, Ger.** Pilsensee-Apotheke GmbH, Gunteringer Strasse 2, 82229 Seefeld/Hechendorf, Germany.

**Pinewood, Irl.** Pinewood Laboratories Ltd, Unit 1, M50 Business Park, Ballymount, Dublin 24, Ireland.

**Pinewood, UK.** See *Pinewood, Irl.*

**Piniol, Switz.** Piniol AG, Erlistrasse 2, 6403 Kussnacht a.R., Switzerland.

**Pinnacle, Canad.** Pinnacle Pharmaceutics, 519 Dundas St E, Unit 8, Whitby, Ontario, L1N 2J5, Canada.

**Pinneberg, Hong Kong.** Pinneberg Ltd, 1404 Chiao Shang Bldg, 92-94 Queen's Rd Central, Hong Kong.

**Pint, Austria.** Pint Pharma GmbH, Heinr. v Buolgasse 18, A-1210 Vienna, Austria.

**Pint, Israel.** See *Gilco, Israel.*

**Pionneau, Fr.** Laboratoires Pionneau, 33870 Vayres, France.

**Piramal, India.** See *Nicholas Piramal, India.*

**Piraud, Switz.** Piraud AG, Switzerland.

**Pisa, Mex.** Laboratorios Pisa S.A. de C.V., Av. Espana No. 1840, 44190 Guadalajara, Jal., Mexico.

**Pizarro, Braz.** Pizarro Farmaceutica Ltda, Rua Lino Coutinho 1568, 04207-002 Sao Paulo Ipiranga, SP, Brazil.

**Pizzard, Mex.** See *Cryopharma, Mex.*

**Plan, Switz.** Laboratoires Plan SA, Chemin des Sellieres, 1219 Aire-Geneva, Switzerland.

**Planta, Canad.** Planta Dei Pharma, P.O. Box 415, Route 105, Nackawic, NB, E0H 1P0, Canada.

**Plantamed, Ger.** See *Bionorica, Ger.*

**Plantes et Medecines, Fr.** Laboratoires Plantes et Medecines, Le Payrat, 46000 Cahors, France.

**Plantes Tropicales, Fr.** Laboratoires de Plantes Tropicales, 24 rue Jouffroy d'Abbans, 75017 Paris, France.

**Plantina, Ger.** Plantina Biologische Arzneimittel AG, Konrad-Celtis-Str. 81, 81369 Munich, Germany.

**Plants, Ital.** Plants, Laboratorio della Dott.ssa Luisa Coletta, Viaria C, Zona Industriale, 98040 Giammoro (ME), Italy.

**Plasmon, Ital.** Plasmon Dietetici Alimentari S.p.A., Via Cascina Bel Casule 7, 20141 Milan, Italy.

**Plevifarma, Spain.** Plevifarma, Fernando Puig 58,60, 08023 Barcelona, Spain.

**Pliva, Irl.** See *United Drug, Irl.*

**Pliva, Ital.** Pliva, Italy.

**Pliva, Spain.** Pliva Pharma Iberia, Lopex de Hoyos 35, 28923 Madrid, Spain.

**Pliva, UK.** Pliva Pharma Ltd, Vision House, Bedford Rd, Petersfield, Hampshire, GU32 3QB, UK.

**Plough, Port.** See *Schering-Plough, Port.*

**Plumbland, Arg.** Plumbland Holdings Ltd, Callao 1355 Piso 4 A, 1023 Buenos Aires, Argentina.

**Plurisystem, Ital.** Plurisystem S.a.s. di Arippa Lionello & C., Via F Vezzani 99r, 16159 Genova-Rivarolo, Italy.

**PMC, Austral.** See *AstraZeneca, Austral.*

**PMR, Singapore.** PMR Associates, 791 North Bridge Rd, S 198759, Singapore.

**Poehlmann, Ger.** Dr Poehlmann & Co. GmbH, Postfach: 1365, 58303 Herdecke, Germany.

**Poehlmann, Switz.** See *Renapharm, Switz.*

**Poen, Arg.** Lab. Poen S.A.C.I.F.I., Bermudez 1004, 1407 Buenos Aires, Argentina.

**Pohl, Denm.** See *Meda, Denm.*

**Pohl, Ger.** G. Pohl-Boskamp GmbH & Co., Kieler Str. 11, 25551 Hohenlockstedt, Germany.

**Pohl, Hong Kong.** See *Health Vision, Hong Kong.*

**Pohl, Israel.** See *Megapharm, Israel.*

**Pohl, Neth.** See *Tramedico, Neth.*

**Pohl, Norw.** See *Meda, Norw.*

**Pohl, Switz.** See *Lubapharm, Switz.*

**Point of Care Diagnostics, NZ.** Point of Care Diagnostics, New Zealand.

**Poirier, Fr.** Laboratoires Pharm. Poirier, ZA La Haute-Limougere, B.P. 24, 37230 Fondettes, France.

**Polaris, Ital.** Polaris Biolab S.r.l., Via Wagner 8, 20145 Milan, Italy.

**Polcopharma, Austral.** Polcopharma, F. Polley & Co. Pty Ltd, P.O. Box 100, Epping, NSW 2121, Australia.

**Poli, Hong Kong.** See *International Medical, Hong Kong.*

**Poli, Ital.** Poli Industria Chimica S.p.A., Via Volturno 45-48, 20089 Quinto de Stampi-Rozzano (MI), Italy.

**Poli, Switz.** See *Adroka, Switz.*

**Polidis, Fr.** Ste Polidis, 7 rue Gallieni, 92500 Rueil-Malmaison, France.

**Polifarma, Ital.** Polifarma S.p.A., Via Tor Sapienza 138, 00155 Rome, Italy.

**Polipharm, Thai.** Polipharm Co. Ltd, 109 Mu 12 Bangna-Trat Rd, Bangpleeyai, Bangplee, Samutprakan 10540, Thailand.

**Polive, Fr.** Laboratoires Polivé SNC, 19-23 bd Georges-Clemenceau, 92400 Courbevoie, France.

**Poly, USA.** Poly Pharmaceuticals Inc., P.O. Box 93, Quitman, MS 39355, USA.

**Polychaco, Arg.** Polychaco S.A.I.C., Santiago del Estero 1162, 1075 Buenos Aires, Argentina.

**Polymedic, Singapore.** Polymedic Trading Enterprise Pte Ltd, 150 Kampong Ampat, 06-07 KA Centre, S 368324, Singapore.

**PolyMedica, USA.** PolyMedica Pharmaceuticals (USA) Inc., 11 State St, Woburn, MA 01801, USA.

**Polymer Technology, Canad.** Polymer Technology, 400 Matheson Blvd E, 28, Mississauga, Ontario, L4Z 1N8, Canada.

**Polymer Technology, USA.** Polymer Technology Corp., 1400 N Goodman, St Rochester, NY 14692, USA.

**Polypharm, Ger.** Polypharm GmbH, Bad Nauheimer Str. 4, 64289 Darmstadt, Germany.

**Pond's, Thai.** Pond's Chemical Thailand ROP, 79 MU 4 Ramindra Rd, Bangkhen, Bangkok 10220, Thailand.

**Pond's Chemical, Singapore.** See *Wellchem, Singapore.*

**Portex, UK.** Portex Ltd, Boundary Rd, Hythe, Kent, CT21 6JL, UK.

**Porton, Israel.** See *Medogar, Israel.*

**Pose, Thai.** Pose Health Care Ltd, 11 Fl, 3300/72 Elephant Building, Tower B, Phaholyothin Rd Ladyao, Chatuchak, Bangkok 10900, Thailand.

**Potter's, UK.** Potter's (Herbal Supplies) Ltd, Leyland Mill Lane, Wigan, Lancashire, WN1 2SB, UK.

**Pound International, UK.** Pound International Ltd, 109 Baker St, London, W1M 1FE, UK.

**Powderject, USA.** Powderject, USA.

**Poythress, USA.** See *ECR, USA.*

**PP Lab, Thai.** See *Picharn, Thai.*

**PPDH, Fr.** PPDH SA, 247 bis rue des Pyrenees, 75020 Paris, France.

**PQS, Spain.** PQS Farma, Ctra Madrid-Cadiz Km 554.4, Dos Hermanas, 41700 Seville, Spain.

**Praecis, USA.** Praecis Pharmaceuticals Inc., 830 Winter St, Waltham, MA 02451-1420, USA.

**Pras, Spain.** See *Prasfarma, Spain.*

**Prasco, USA.** Prasco Laboratories, 7155 E Kemper Rd, Cincinnati, OH 45249, USA.

**Prasfarma, Spain.** See *Almirall, Spain.*

**Prater, Chile.** Laboratorio Prater SA, Av. P Aguirre Cerda 5291, Cerrillos, Santiago, Chile.

**Prats, Spain.** Prats, Traversera del Dalt 44, 08024 Barcelona, Spain.

**PRC, Ital.** P.R.C. S.r.l., Via Conforti 42, 84083 Castel San Giorgio SA, Italy.

**Precifarma, Braz.** Precifarma Laboratorio Farmaceutico Ltda, Rua Correia de Lemos 153, 04041-001 Sao Paulo, SP, Brazil.

**Precimex, Mex.** Precimex S.A. de C.V., Calle 6 No. 2510, Zona Industrial, 44940 Guadalajara, Jal, Mexico.

**Pred, Fr.** Laboratoires Pred, Batiment 6, 79 av Aristide Briand, 94118 Arcueil cdx, France.

**Premier, S.Afr.** See *Rolab, S.Afr.*

**Premier, USA.** See *Advanced Polymer, USA.*

**Premopharm, Israel.** Premopharm (Israel) Ltd, P.O. Box 319, Ra'anana, Israel.

**Presselin, Ger.** Presselin-Arzneimittel GmbH & Co. KG, Heinkelstr. 8a, 76461 Muggensturm, Germany.

**Prestige, UK.** Prestige Brands (UK) Ltd, 3 Scotlands Drive, Farnham Common, Slough, Berkshire, SL2 3ES, UK.

**Preston, Arg.** Lab. Dr. Preston, Villarino 2318, 1276 Buenos Aires, Argentina.

**Prevention et Biologie, Fr.** Prévention et Biologie SA, 29-33 rue de Metz, 94170 Le Perreux, France.

**Prevision, Spain.** See *Bayer, Spain.*

**Prieto, Arg.** Laboratorio Prieto S.A., Maza 1869/73, 1240 Buenos Aires, Argentina.

**Prima, Braz.** Laboratorios Prima Ltda, Rua Juparana 62, 20510-040 Rio de Janeiro, RJ, Brazil.

**Prima, Thai.** Prima Pharm Co. Ltd, 1420/1 Srisuk Building, Paholythin 26 Ladyao, Chatuchak, Bangkok 10900, Thailand.

**Primal, Hong Kong.** Primal Chemical Co. Ltd, Flat A, 7/F, Hoi Bun Industrial Bldg, 6 Wing Yip St, Kwun Tong, Kowloon, Hong Kong.

**Primula, Arg.** Lab. Primula S.A., Andonaegui 1141, 1427 Buenos Aires, Argentina.

**Princeton, USA.** See *Bristol-Myers Squibb, USA.*

**Prisfar, Port.** Prisfar, SA, Rua Antero de Quentel 629, 4200 Porto, Portugal.

**Prism, UK.** Prism Healthcare, UK.

**Pro Doc, Canad.** Pro Doc Limitee, 2925 Industrial Blvd, Laval, Quebec, H7L 3W9, Canada.

**Pro Medica, Swed.** See *Schering-Plough, Swed.*

**Pro Vaccine, Switz.** Pro Vaccine AG, Grabenstrasse 42, 6301 Zug, Switzerland.

**Probifasa, Mex.** Probifasa S.A. de C.V., Calz. Mexico-Tacuba No. 1419, Col Argentina Pte., Deleg. Miguel Hidalgo, 11230 Mexico D.F., Mexico.

**Probiomed, Mex.** Probiomed, S.A. de C.V., Ejercito Nacional No. 499 4o. piso, Col. Granada, 11520 Mexico D.F., Mexico.

**Probios, Port.** Probios, Lda, Rua Joao Chagas 53-A, Escritorio 201, 1495-072 Alges, Portugal.

**Procare, Austral.** See *Biovital, Austral.*

**Proceane, Fr.** Laboratoires Proceane Ressources Marines, B.P. 88, 44503 La Baule cdx, France.

**Procter & Gamble, Arg.** Procter & Gamble Interamericanos Inc., Suipacha 664 Piso 2, 1008 Buenos Aires, Argentina.

**Procter & Gamble, Austral.** Procter & Gamble Australia P/L, Locked Bag 75, Parramatta, NSW 2124, Australia.

**Procter & Gamble, Austria.** Procter & Gamble Austria GmbH, Guglgasse 7-9, A-1030 Vienna, Austria.

**Procter & Gamble, Belg.** Procter & Gamble Pharmaceuticals S.A., Temselaan 100, 1853 Strombeek-Bever, Belgium.

**Procter & Gamble, Braz.** Procter & Gamble do Brasil S.A., Av. Maria Coelho Aguiar 251, Bloco E- Andares 4./5, Jd Sao Luiz, 05805-000 Paulo, SP, Brazil.

**Procter & Gamble, Canad.** Procter & Gamble Inc., P.O. Box 355, Station A, Toronto, Ontario, M5W 1C5, Canada.

**Procter & Gamble, Denm.** See *Roche, Denm.*

**Procter & Gamble, Fin.** See *Oriola, Fin.*

**Procter & Gamble, Fr.** Procter & Gamble Pharmaceuticals France, 96 av Charles-de-Gaulle, 92201 Neuilly-sur-Seine cdx, France.

**Procter & Gamble, Ger.** Procter & Gamble Pharmaceuticals Germany GmbH, Sulzbacher Str. 40, 65824 Schwalbach am Taunus, Germany.

**Procter & Gamble, Hong Kong.** See *Keller, Hong Kong.*

**Procter & Gamble, Irl.** See *Aventis, Irl.*, and *United Drug, Irl.*

**Procter & Gamble, Israel.** See *Neopharm, Israel.*

**Procter & Gamble, Ital.** Procter & Gamble Italia S.p.A., Viale C Pavese 385, 00144 Rome, Italy.

**Procter & Gamble, Mex.** Procter & Gamble de Mexico S.A. de C.V., Loma Florida 32, Lomas de Vistahermosa, Del. Cuajimalpa, 05100 Mexico D.F., Mexico.

**Procter & Gamble, Neth.** Procter & Gamble Pharmaceuticals, Watermanweg 100, 3067 GG Rotterdam, Netherlands.

**Procter & Gamble, Norw.** See *Roche, Norw.*

**Procter & Gamble, NZ.** Procter & Gamble NPD, Inc., 7th Floor, Acer Building, 10-12 Scotia Place, Auckland, New Zealand.

**Procter & Gamble, Spain.** Procter Gamble, Av. Del Partenon 16-18, Campo De Las Naciones, 28042 Madrid, Spain.

**Procter & Gamble, Swed.** Procter & Gamble Nordic Inc., filial Sverige, Box 273 03, 102 54 Stockholm, Sweden.

**Procter & Gamble, Switz.** Procter & Gamble AG, 47 rue de Saint-Georges, 1213 Petit-Lancy 1, Switzerland.

**Procter & Gamble, UK.** Procter & Gamble Pharmaceuticals UK Ltd, Lovett House, Lovett Rd, Staines, Middlesex, TW18 3AZ, UK.

**Procter & Gamble, USA.** Procter & Gamble, 1 or 2, Procter & Gamble Plaza, Cincinnati, OH 45201, USA.

**Procter & Gamble (H&B Care), UK.** Procter & Gamble (Health & Beauty Care) Ltd, The Heights, Brooklands, Weybridge, Surrey, KT13 0XP, UK.

**Procyte, USA.** ProCyte Corp., 8511 154th Ave NE, Bldg A, Redmond, WA 98052-3557, USA.

**Prodava, Arg.** Lab. Prodava S.A., Raulies 1970/8, 1427 Buenos Aires, Argentina.

**Prodemdis, Canad.** Prodemdis Enrg, 4355 Sir Wilfred Laurier Blvd, St-Hubert, Quebec, J3Y 3X3, Canada.

**Prodes, Spain.** See *Almirall, Spain.*

**Prodome, Braz.** Prodome Quimica e Farmaceutica Ltda, Rua 13 de Maio 1161, 13106-504 Campinas, SP, Brazil.

**Prodotti, Braz.** Prodotti Laboratorio Farmaceutico Ltda, Avenida Joao Dias 1084, Santo Amaro, 04724-001 Sao Paulo, SP, Brazil.

**Produfarma, Port.** Produfarma, Lda, Estrada de Benfica 403-B, 1500-077 Lisbon, Portugal.

**Produits Dentaires, Switz.** Produits Dentaires SA, 18 rue des Bosquets, 1800 Vevey, Switzerland.

**Proel, Gr.** PROEL, Δήλου 9, 121 34 Περιστέρι, Peristeri, Greece.

**Proethic, USA.** Proethic, USA.

**Prof. Pharm. Corp., Canad.** Professional Pharmaceutical Corporation, 9200 Cote-de-Liesse Blvd, Lachine, Quebec, H8T 1A1, Canada.

**Profarb, Braz.** Profarb Ltda, Rua Paschoal Bernardino 25, 36880-000 Muriae, MG, Brazil.

**Profarma, Thai.** See *International Pharmaceuticals, Thai.*

**Professional Health, Canad.** Professional Health Products, 4307-49 St, Innisfail, AB, T4G 1P3, Canada.

**Profile, UK.** Profile Therapeutics plc, Heath Place, Bognor Regis, West Sussex, PO22 9SL, UK.

**Proge, Ital.** Proge Farm S.r.l., Via Croce 4, 28065 Cerano (NO), Italy.

**Progest, Ital.** Progest Industria Chimica S.r.l., Salita Castel Giubileo 2, 00138 Rome, Italy.

**Progress, Thai.** See *Medicine Supply, Thai.*

**Pro-Health, NZ.** Pro-Health Products Ltd, P.O. Box 28-545, Remuera, Auckland, New Zealand.

**Prolabor, Braz.** Prolabor Saude Ocupacional Ltda, Rua Lavradio 511, 01154-020 Sao Paulo, SP, Brazil.

**Promeco, Mex.** See *Boehringer Ingelheim, Mex.*

**Promed, Ger.** See *AstraZeneca, Ger.*

**Promedica, Fr.** See *Chiesi, Fr.*

**Promedica, Ital.** See *Chiesi, Ital.*

**Promedica, Malaysia.** See *Antah, Malaysia.*

**Promedica, Thai.** See *Pacific, Thai.*

**Promedical, Ital.** Promedical S.r.l., Via G Greco 8, 90017 Santa Flavia (PA), Italy.

**Promedico, Israel.** ProMedico Ltd, 4 Baltimor St, Petach Tikva, Israel.

**Promedis, Belg.** Promedis, Belgium.

**Promefarm, Ital.** Promefarm S.r.l., Corso Indipendenza 6, 20129 Milan, Italy.

**Prometheus, USA.** Prometheus Laboratories Inc., 5739 Pacific Center Blvd, San Diego, CA 92121, USA.

**Prometic, Canad.** Prometic Pharma Inc., 1000 Raoul Charette, Joliette, Quebec, J6E 8S9, Canada.

**Prometic, USA.** See *Prometic, Canad.*

**Promonta, Ger.** See *Lundbeck, Ger.*

**Pro-Nat, Fr.** Pro-Nat SA, 28 rue Meslay, 75003 Paris, France.

**Pronova, USA.** Pronova, USA.

**Propan, S.Afr.** See *Adcock Ingram, S.Afr.*

**Propharm, Israel.** Propharm, P.O. Box 4066, Zichron Yaacov, Israel.

**Propharm, Malaysia.** Propharm (M) Sdn Bhd, 640-A, 4th Mile, Ipoh Rd, 51200 Kuala Lumpur, Wilayah Persekutuan, Malaysia.

**Propharma, Denm.** Propharma A/S, Industrivaenget 18, 4622 Havdrup, Denmark.

**Prospa, Ital.** Prospa Italia S.r.l., Via Modica 6, 20143 Milan (MI), Italy.

**Prospa, Port.** Prospa, SA, Rua do Proletariado 15C, 2795-648 Carnaxide, Portugal.

**Protea, S.Afr.** Protea Pharm (Pty) Ltd, P.O. Box 422, East London 5200, South Africa.

**Protec, UK.** Protec Health International Ltd, 5 Priory Court, Poulton, Cirencester, Gloucestershire, GL7 5JB, UK.

**Proteika, Fr.** Proteika SA, Lab de Dietetique Medicale, 2 av des Noelles, B.P. 216, 44505 La Baule cdx, France.

**Protein, Mex.** Protein S.A. de C.V., Anil No. 865, Col. Granjas Mexico, Deleg. Iztacalco, 08400 Mexico DF, Mexico.

**Protermex, Mex.** Protermex, Mexico.

**Protherics, USA.** Protherics, 1207 17th Ave S, Suite 103, Nashville, TN 37212, USA.

**Protidiet, Fr.** Protidiet, ZAE Migelane, B.P. 10, 33650 Saucats, France.

**Protiforme, Fr.** Protiforme, 49 av. de la Motte-Picquet, 75015 Paris, France.

**Protina, Ger.** Protina Pharmazeutische Gesellschaft mbH, Adalperostr. 90, 85737 Ismaning, Germany.

**Protina, Switz.** See *Doetsch, Grether, Switz.*

**Provalis, UK.** Provalis Healthcare, Newtech Square, Deeside Industrial Park, Deeside, Flintshire, CH5 2NT, UK.

**Proveedora Teknimex, Mex.** Proveedora Teknimex S.A. de C.V., Gerogia 15, Napoles, Deleg. Benito Juarez, 03810 Mexico D.F., Mexico.

**Provit, Mex.** Provit S.A. de C.V., Nino Artillero No. 500, C.U. Independencia, 50070 Toluca, Mexico.

**Provita, Austria.** Provita Pharma GmbH, Seidengasse 33-35, A-1070 Vienna, Austria.

**Provita, Ital.** Provita Industria Farmaceutica S.r.l., Via Dora 7, 00198 Rome, Italy.

**PS, Ital.** PS Pharma Srl, Via Tor Vergata 14, 00133 Rome, Italy.

**Psicofarma, Mex.** Laboratorio Psicofarma S.A. de C.V., Calz. de Tlalpan No. 4369, Col. Toriello Guerra, 14050 Mexico D.F., Mexico.

**PSM, NZ.** PSM Healthcare Ltd, P.O. Box 76-401, Manukau City, Auckland, New Zealand.

**Puebla, Arg.** Lab. Puebla S.R.L., Andres Lamas 2427, 5009 Barrio Escobar, Cordoba, Argentina.

**Puerto Galiano, Spain.** Puerto Galiano, Calle 'S', 4, Parque Europolis, Las Rozas, 28230 Madrid, Spain.

**Pulitzer, Ital.** Pulitzer Italiana S.r.l., Via Tiburtina 1004, 00156 Rome, Italy.

**Pulsion, Ger.** Pulsion Medical Systems GmbH, Stahlgruberring 28, 81829 Munich, Germany.

**Pulsion, Israel.** See *Concept, Israel.*

**Purdue, Canad.** Purdue Pharma, 575 Granite Court, Pickering, Ontario, L1W 3W8, Canada.

**Purdue, USA.** See *Purdue Frederick, USA.*

**Purdue Frederick, Canad.** See *Purdue, Canad.*

**Purdue Frederick, USA.** The Purdue Frederick Co., 100 Connecticut Ave, Norwalk, CT 06850-3590, USA.

**Purissimus, Arg.** Purissimus S.A., Juan F.Segum 4635, 1425 Buenos Aires, Argentina.

**Puritan Quartz, Thai.** Puritan Quartz.

**Qestmed, S.Afr.** Qestmed Ltd, Unit 2, Gazelle Place, Corporate Park, Old Pretoria Main Rd, Midrand 1685, South Africa.

**QHP, USA.** Quality Health Products Inc., P.O. Box 31, Yaphank, NY 11980, USA.

**QIF, Braz.** See *Hexal, Braz.*

**Q-Med, Ital.** Q-Med ICT Srl, Via Mario Borsa 11, 26845 Codogno (LO), Italy.

**Q-Med, Singapore.** Q-Med, Singapore.

**Qualicare, Switz.** Qualicare AG, Florenz-Strasse 7, 4142 Munchenstein, Switzerland.

**Qualiphar, Belg.** Qualiphar S.A., Rijksweg 9, 2880 Bornem, Belgium.

**Qualitest, USA.** Qualitest Products Inc., 1236 Jordan Rd, Huntsville, AL 35811, USA.

**Quality Formulations, USA.** Quality Formulations Inc., P.O. Box 827, Zachary, LA 70791-0827, USA.

**Quantum, USA.** Quantum Pharmics Ltd, USA.

**Quatromed, S.Afr.** Quatromed, South Africa.

**Queisser, Austria.** See *Queisser, Ger.*

**Queisser, Ger.** Queisser Pharma GmbH & Co., Schleswiger Str. 74, 24941 Flensburg, Germany.

**Quesada, Arg.** Lab. Bioqummica Aplicada Dr. Rafael Quesada S.R.L., Saavedra 363/77, 1704 Ramos Mejia, Buenos Aires, Argentina.

**Quest, Canad.** See *Boehringer Ingelheim, Canad.*

**Quest, Malaysia.** See *JDH, Malaysia.*

**Quest, UK.** Quest Vitamins Ltd, 8 Venture Way, Aston Science Park, Birmingham, B7 4AP, UK.

**Questcor, USA.** Questcor Pharmaceuticals Inc., 26118 Research Rd, Hayward, CA 94545, USA.

**Quidel, USA.** Quidel Corp., 10165 McKellar Court, La Jolla, CA 92037, USA.

**Quies, Fr.** Laboratoires Quies, 4 rue Ambroise-Croizat, 91120 Palaiseau, France.

**Quimedical, Port.** Quimedical Lda, Edificio Azevedos, Estrada Nacional 117, 2724-503 Amadora, Portugal.

**Quimica Medica, Spain.** La Quimica Medica, San Juan Bosco 55, 08017 Barcelona, Spain.

**Quimica y Farmacia, Mex.** Quimica y Farmacia, S.A. de C.V., Av. Pacifico No. 332, Col. Rosedal Coyoacan, 04330 Mexico D.F., Mexico.

**Quimifar, Spain.** Quimifar, Comadran 37, Pol Ind Can Salvatella, Barbera del Valles, 08210 Barcelona, Spain.

**Quimioterapica, Braz.** Quimioterapica Brasileira Ltda, Rua Sao Januario 712, Tubalina, 38400-410 Uberlandia, MG, Brazil.

**Quimpe, Spain.** Quimpe, Cruz 47-49, Alhaurin el Grande, 29120 Malaga, Spain.

**Quinoderm, Hong Kong.** See *Mekim, Hong Kong.*

**Quinoderm, Irl.** See *Boileau & Boyd, Irl.*

**Quinoderm, Switz.** See *Golaz, Switz.*

**Quinoderm, UK.** See *Adams, UK.*

**Quintessa, USA.** Quintessa Corp., P.O. Box 808, Lancaster, CA 93584, USA.

**Rabi & Solabo, Fr.** Laboratoires Rabi & Solabo, 67 rue Voltaire, 92150 Suresnes, France.

**Rachelle, USA.** Rachelle, USA.

**Radiol, Israel.** See *Devries, Israel.*

**Rafa, Israel.** Rafa Laboratories Ltd, P.O. Box 405, Jerusalem 91003, Israel.

**Rafarm, Gr.** RAFARM AE, Κορίνθου 12, 154 51 Ν. Ψυχικό, N. Psichiko, Greece.

**Raffo, Arg.** Lab. Raffo S.A., Av. Cabildo 159, 1426 Buenos Aires, Argentina.

**Raffo, Chile.** Laboratorios Raffo SA, Simon Bolivar2183, Nunoa, Santiago, Chile.

**Ram, USA.** Ram Laboratories, Division of Bradley Pharmaceuticals Inc., 3300 University Drive, Coral Springs, FL 33065, USA.

**Ramelco, Canad.** Ramelco Ltd, Subsidiary of Maltby Ltd, 306 Dawlish Ave, Toronto, Ontario, M4N 1J5, Canada.

**Ramini, Ital.** Ramini S.r.l., Via di Vallerano 96, 00128 Rome, Italy.

**Ramon Sala, Spain.** Ramon Sala, Paris 174, 08036 Barcelona, Spain.

**RAN, Ger.** R.A.N. Novesia AG Arzneimittel, Hurtgener Str. 6, 41464 Neuss/Rhein, Germany.

**Ranbaxy, Braz.** Ranbaxy S.P. Medicamentos Ltda, Avenida das Americas 1155, Sala 1201 a 1204, Barra da Tijuca, 22631-000 Rio de Janeiro, RJ, Brazil.

**Ranbaxy, India.** Ranbaxy Laboratories Ltd, 6 Devika Towers, Nehru Place, New Delhi 110 019, India.

**Ranbaxy, Malaysia.** Ranbaxy (Malayasia) Sdn Bhd, Peti 5, Wisma Selangon Dredging, 10th Floor, West Block, 142-C Jalan Ampang, 50450 Kuala Lumpur, Kuala Lumpur, Malaysia.

**Ranbaxy, S.Afr.** Ranbaxy (SA) (Pty) Ltd, P.O. Box 10458, Centurion 0046, South Africa.

**Ranbaxy, Singapore.** See *Zyfas, Singapore.*

**Ranbaxy, Thai.** Ranbaxy Unichem Co. Ltd, 3 Fl, Rm 314-8, Phayathai Building, 31 Phayathai Rd, Rajathevi, Bangkok 10400, Thailand.

**Ranbaxy, UK.** Ranbaxy (UK) Ltd, Consolidated Pneumatic House, 6th Floor, 97-107 Uxbridge Rd, Ealing, London, W5 5TL, UK.

**Ranbaxy, USA.** Ranbaxy Pharmaceuticals Inc., 600 College Rd E, Suite 2100, Princeton, NJ 08540, USA.

**Randall, Mex.** Randall Laboratories, S.A de C.V., Lago Rodolfo No. 58, 11520 Mexico D.F., Mexico.

**Randi, Israel.** Randi, P.O. Box 18148, Tel Aviv, Israel.

**Randob, USA.** Randob Laboratories Ltd, P.O. Box 440, Cornwall, NY 12518, USA.

**Ransom, UK.** William Ransom & Sons Plc, 104 Bancroft, Hitchin, Hertfordshire, SG5 1LY, UK.

**Rapide, Spain.** See *Baxter, Spain*, and *Bieffe, Spain.*

**Rappai, Switz.** Dr F. Rappai Pharmazeutika, Postfach, 8952 Schlieren-Zurich, Switzerland.

**Raptakos, India.** Raptakos Brett & Co. Ltd, 47 Dr Annie Besant Rd, Worli, Mumbai 400 025, India.

**Raptakos, Thai.** See *Union Medical, Thai.*

**Ratiopharm, Austria.** Ratiopharm Arzneimittel Vertriebs-GmbH, Albert-Schweitzer-Gasse 3, A-1140 Vienna, Austria.

**Ratiopharm, Fin.** ratiopharm Oy, PL 67, 02631 Espoo, Finland.

**Ratiopharm, Ger.** ratiopharm GmbH, Graf-Arco-Str. 3, 89079 Ulm/Donautal, Germany.

**Ratiopharm, Hong Kong.** See *CNW, Hong Kong*, and *Hong Tai Hong, Hong Kong.*

**Ratiopharm, Ital.** Ratiopharm Italia S.r.l., Via Accademia 26, 20131 Milan, Italy.

**Ratiopharm, Port.** Ratiopharm, Lda, Edificio Tejo, 6 piso, Rua Quinta do Pinheiro, 2790-143 Carnaxide, Portugal.

**Ratiopharm, Spain.** Ratiopharm, Rosario Pino 14-16, Ed Torre Rioja, 28020 Madrid, Spain.

**Ratiopharm, Swed.** Ratiopharm AB, Box 1265, 25221 Helsingborg, Sweden.

**Ratiopharm, UK.** Ratiopharm UK Ltd, 5 Jackson Close, Grove Rd, Cosham, Portsmouth, Hampshire, PO6 1UP, UK.

**Ravensberg, Ger.** Ravensberg GmbH, Schneckenburgstr. 46, 78467 Constance, Germany.

**Ravizza, Ital.** See *Abbott, Ital.*

**Rawleigh, Canad.** Rawleigh, 60 Colonnade Rd, Nepean, ON, K2E 7J6, Canada.

**Rayere, Mex.** Farmaceuticos Rayere S.A., Alambra 621, Benito Juarez Portales, 03300 Mexico D.F., Mexico.

**Raymos, Arg.** Lab. Raymos S.A.I.C., Vuelta de Obligado 2775, 1428 Buenos Aires, Argentina.

**Raza, Hong Kong.** See *Health Care, Hong Kong.*

**Raza, Malaysia.** Raza Manufacturing Bhd, 11A Jln P/1, Kawasan Perusahaan Bangi, 43650 Bandar Baru Bangi, Selangor, Malaysia.

**RCA, Ital.** Ricerca Cosmetica Avanzata S.r.l., Zona Industriale Loc. Penitro, 04023 Formia (LT), Italy.

**R&D, Canad.** See *R&D, USA.*

**R&D, USA.** R & D Laboratories Inc., 4640 Admiralty Way, Suite 710, Marina Del Rey, CA 90292-5608, USA.

**RDC, Ital.** See *Euroderm-RDC, Ital.*

**Realdyme, Fr.** Sté Réaldyme, 28700 Garancieres-en-Beauce, France.

**Reall, Switz.** Medical Concepts Reall-YS S.á.r.l, Ave Villardin 22, 1009 Pully, Switzerland.

**Realpharma, Ger.** realpharma Geschaftsbereich der Dolorgiet Arzneimittel, Otto-von-Guericke Str. 1, 53754 St Augustin, Germany.

**Recalcine, Chile.** Laboratorios Recalcine SA, San Eugenio 567, Santiago, Chile.

**Reccius, Chile.** Laboratrios Reccius Ltda, Pucara 5326, Nunoa, Santiago, Chile.

**Recherche Botanique, Fr.** Laboratoires de Recherche Botanique, 9 av. Guy-Petit, 64200 Biarritz, France.

**Recip, Denm.** See *Pharmacia, Denm.*

**Recip, Fin.** See *Algol, Fin.*

**Recip, Norw.** See *Weifa, Norw.*

**Recip, Swed.** Recip AB, Branningevagen 12, 120 54 Arsta, Sweden.

**Reckeweg, Ger.** Pharmazeutische Fabrik Dr. Reckeweg & Co. GmbH, Berliner Ring 32, 64625 Bensheim, Germany.

**Reckitt & Colman, Arg.** Reckitt & Colman Arg. S.A., Avda. Pueyrredon 2446 Pso. 2, 1118 Buenos Aires, Argentina.

**Reckitt & Colman, Austral.** See *Reckitt Benckiser, Austral.*

**Reckitt & Colman, Belg.** See *Reckitt Benckiser, Belg.*

**Reckitt & Colman, Hong Kong.** See *Reckitt Benckiser, Hong Kong.*

**Reckitt & Colman, Israel.** See *Meditrend, Israel.*

**Reckitt & Colman, S.Afr.** See *Reckitt Benckiser, S.Afr.*

**Reckitt & Colman, Singapore.** See *Reckitt Benckiser, Singapore.*

**Reckitt & Colman, UK.** See *Reckitt Benckiser, UK.*

**Reckitt & Colman, USA.** See *Reckitt Benckiser, USA.*

**Reckitt Benckiser, Austral.** Reckitt Benckiser Pharmaceuticals, P.O. Box 138, West Ryde, NSW 2114, Australia.

**Reckitt Benckiser, Belg.** Reckitt Benckiser, Allee de la Recherche 20, 1070 Brussels, Belgium.

**Reckitt Benckiser, Hong Kong.** Reckitt Benckiser Hong Kong Ltd, 1203-5 Allied Kajima Bldg, 138 Gloucester Rd, Hong Kong.

**Reckitt Benckiser, India.** Reckitt Benckiser (India) Ltd, Enkay Centre 2nd Floor, Vanijya Nikunj, Udyog Vihar Phase V, Gurgaon 1122 016, India.

**Reckitt Benckiser, Irl.** Reckitt Benckiser, Pharmapark, Chapelizod, Dublin 20, Ireland.

**Reckitt Benckiser, Malaysia.** Reckitt Benckiser (Overseas) Ltd, Unit No 1101, Level 11, Uptown 2, 2 Jln SS 21-37, Damansara Uptown, 47400 Petaling Jaya, Selangor, Malaysia.

**Reckitt Benckiser, Norw.** See *Nycomed, Norw.*

**Reckitt Benckiser, NZ.** Reckitt Benckiser Pharmaceuticals, Private Bag 93121, Henderson, Auckland, New Zealand.

**Reckitt Benckiser, S.Afr.** Reckitt Benckiser Pharmaceuticals (Pty) Ltd, P.O. Box 164, Isando 1600, South Africa.

**Reckitt Benckiser, Singapore.** Reckitt Benckiser (Singapore) Pte Ltd, 1 Fifth Ave, 04-06 Guthrie House, S 268802, Singapore.

**Reckitt Benckiser, Spain.** Reckitt Benckiser Espana, Paseo de Gracia 9, 08007 Barcelona, Spain.

**Reckitt Benckiser, Thai.** Reckitt Benckiser (Thailand) Ltd, 9 Fl, Vanissa Building, 29 Soi Chidlom, Ploenchit Rd, Patumwan, Bangkok 10330, Thailand.

**Reckitt Benckiser, UK.** Reckitt Benckiser plc, Dansom House, Hull, Humberside, HU8 7DS, UK.

**Reckitt Benckiser, USA.** Reckitt Benckiser, 1655 Valley Rd, P.O. Box 943, Wayne, NJ 07470-0943, USA.

**Reckitt Piramal, India.** See *Nicholas Piramal, India.*

**Reckitts, Irl.** Reckitt's (Ireland) Ltd, P.O. Box 730, Cloverhill Industrial Estate, Clondalkin, Dublin 22, Ireland.

**Recofarma, Ital.** See *Recordati, Ital.*

**Recon, Singapore.** See *Zyfas, Singapore.*

**Recordati, Hong Kong.** See *Unico, Hong Kong.*

**Recordati, Ital.** Recordati Industria Chimica e Farmaceutica S.p.a., Via Civitali 1, 20148 Milan, Italy.

**Recordati, Singapore.** See *MD, Singapore,* and *Orient, Singapore.*

**Recordati, Spain.** Recordati España SL, Isla de la Palma 37, San Sebastian de los Reyes, 30588 Madrid, Spain.

**Recsei, USA.** Recsei Laboratories, 330 S Kellogg, Building M, Goleta, CA 93117-3875, USA.

**Reddy, Singapore.** See *Zyfas, Singapore.*

**Reddy, Thai.** See *Neopharm, Thai.*

**Reddy's, India.** Dr. Reddy's Laboratories Ltd, 7-1-27 Ameerpet, Hyderabad 500 016, India.

**Redel, Ger.** See *Cesra, Ger.*

**Redino, Ger.** RedinoMedica GmbH, Pinganserstr. 40, 81369 Munich, Germany.

**Redi-Products, USA.** See *Aplicare, USA.*

**Redken, Canad.** Redken Laboratories Canada Ltd, 5160 Yonge St, North York, Ontario, M2N 6L9, Canada.

**Reed & Carnrick, Canad.** See *Block, Canad.*

**Reed & Carnrick, USA.** See *Schwarz, USA.*

**Reedco, USA.** Reedco, USA.

**Reese, USA.** Reese Pharmaceutical Co. Inc., 10617 Frank Ave, Cleveland, OH 44106, USA.

**Regal, Canad.** Regal Pharmaceuticals, Division of Bradcan Corp., 900 Harrington Court, Burlington, Ontario, L7N 3N4, Canada.

**Regenaplex, Ger.** Regenaplex Homöopathische Komplexmittel, Robert-Bosch-Str. 3, 78467 Constance, Germany.

**Regina, UK.** Regina Health Ltd, NLA Tower, 12-16 Addiscombe Rd, Croydon, Surrey, CR0 0XT, UK.

**Regional Health, Austral.** Regional Health Care Products Group, Medi-Consumables P/L, 3-11 Primrose Ave, Rosebery, NSW 2018, Australia.

**Regional Health, NZ.** Regional Health Ltd, P.O. Box 101-104, North Shore Mail Centre, Auckland, New Zealand.

**Regius, Braz.** Laboratorio Regius Ltda, Rua Doutor Ramiro D'Avila 57, 90620-050 Porto Alegre, RS, Brazil.

**Reig Jofre, Spain.** Reig Jofre, Gran Capitan 10, Sant Joan Despi, 08970 Barcelona, Spain.

**Reith & Petrasch, Ger.** Reith & Petrasch GmbH, Martstr. 1, 77834 Rheinmunster, Germany.

**Rekah, Israel.** Rekah Ltd, P.O. Bos 25, Azor, Israel.

**Rekawan, Ger.** See *Riemser, Ger.*

**Relax, Ital.** Relax Health Care S.r.l., Corso Sempione 36, 20154 Milan, Italy.

**Reliant, USA.** Reliant, USA.

**Relyo, Gr.** RELYO HELLAS ΕΠΕ, Φαβιέρου 48, 104 38 Αθήνα, Athens, Greece.

**REM, Braz.** REM, Brazil.

**Remedica, Hong Kong.** See *Health Care, Hong Kong,* and *Primal, Hong Kong.*

**Remedica, Malaysia.** See *JDH, Malaysia.*

**Remedica, Singapore.** See *JDH, Singapore.*

**Remedica, Thai.** See *Pharmadica, Thai.*

**Remedina, Gr.** REMEDINA, Γούναρη 23, 134 51 Καματερό, Kamatero, Greece.

**Remek, Gr.** REMEK A.E., Κωλέτη 3, 144 52 Μεταμόρφωση, Metamorphosi, Greece.

**Remexa, Mex.** Representaciones Mex-America S.A. de C.V.,, Diagonal 20 de Noviembre No. 264, Col. Obrera, Deleg. Cuauhtemoc, 06800 Mexico D.F., Mexico.

**Remidex, India.** Remidex Pharma Pvt Ltd, B-249/250 Industrial Estate, Peenya II Stage, Bangalore 560 058, India.

**Remir, Mex.** Industrial Farmaceutica Remir S.A., Xochicalco Norte No. 46-B, Col. Navarte, Deleg. Benito Juarez, 03020 Mexico D.F., Mexico.

**Renapharm, Switz.** Renapharm S.A., Rue du Château 3, 1636 Broc, Switzerland.

**Renapharma, Norw.** See *Renapharma, Swed.*

**Renapharma, Swed.** Renapharma AB, Box 938, 751 09 Uppsala, Sweden.

**Renaudin, Fr.** Laboratoires Renaudin, ZA Errobi, 64250 Itxassou, France.

**Rendell, NZ.** See *NZ Medical & Scientific, NZ.*

**Rendell, UK.** WJ Rendell Ltd, Ickleford Manor, Hitchin, Hertfordshire, SG5 3XE, UK.

**Rentschler, Austria.** See *Rentschler, Ger.*

**Rentschler, Ger.** Dr. Rentschler Arzneimittel GmbH & Co., Mittelstr. 18, 88471 Laupheim, Germany.

**Rentschler, Israel.** Rentschler, Israel.

**Rentschler, Singapore.** See *PMR, Singapore.*

**Repha, Ger.** Repha GmbH Biologische Arzneimittel, Alt-Godshorn 87, 30855 Langenhagen, Germany.

**RepliGen, USA.** RepliGen, USA.

**Reprefar, Port.** See *Pierre Fabre, Port.*

**Republic, USA.** Republic Drug Co., 175 Great Arrow, Suite 4, Buffalo, NY 14207, USA.

**Requa, USA.** Requa Inc., 1 Seneca Place, P.O. Box 4008, Greenwich, CT 06830, USA.

**Research Industries Corp., USA.** See *Research Medical, USA.*

**Research Labs, S.Afr.** Research Labs, South Africa.

**Research Medical, USA.** Research Medical Inc., 6864 South 300 West, Midvale, UT 84047, USA.

**Resinag, Israel.** See *Promedico, Israel.*

**Resinag, Switz.** Resinag AG, Oberer Steisteg 18, 6430 Schwyz, Switzerland.

**Respa, USA.** Respa Pharmaceuticals Inc., PO Box 88222, Carol Stream, IL 60188, USA.

**Restan, S.Afr.** Restan Laboratories (Pty) Ltd, Private Bag X69, Bryanston 2021, South Africa.

**Restiva, Ital.** See *Pfizer, Ital.*

**Retrain, Spain.** Retrain, Alfonso XII 587, Badalona, 08912 Barcelona, Spain.

**Retterspitz, Ger.** Retterspitz GmbH, Laufer Str. 17-19, 90571 Schwaig, Germany.

**Reuabuen, USA.** Reuabuen, USA.

**Reuffer, Mex.** Reuffer Laboratorios S.A. de C.V., Juan de Dios Arias 78, Cuauhtemoc Vista Alegre, 06860 Mexico D.F., Mexico.

**Reusch, Ger.** Pharma Reusch GmbH, Hallestr. 50, 53125 Bonn, Germany.

**Revlon, Canad.** Revlon Canada Inc., 2501 Stanfield Rd, Mississauga, Ontario, L4Y 1R9, Canada.

**Rex, NZ.** Rex Medical, P.O. Box 23-025, Papatoetoe, Auckland, New Zealand.

**Rexcel, India.** See *Ranbaxy, India.*

**Rhein, Mex.** Siegfried Rhein S.A. de C.V., Monte Elbruz No. 124 4o Piso, Col. Palmitas Polanco, 11560 Mexico D.F., Mexico.

**Rhenomed, Ger.** Rhenomed Arzneimittel GmbH, Luth.-Kirch.-Str. 69/71, Postfach: 130662, 47758 Krefeld, Germany.

**Rhodia, Braz.** Rhodia Farma Ltda, Avenida Nacoes Unidas 22 428, 04795-916 Sao Paulo, SP, Brazil.

**Rhodia, Israel.** Rhodia, Israel.

**Rhodiapharm, Canad.** See *Aventis, Canad.*

**Rhone-Poulenc Aventis, Ital.** See *Aventis, Ital.*

**Rhone-Poulenc Rorer, Austral.** See *Aventis, Austral.*

**Rhone-Poulenc Rorer, Austria.** See *Aventis, Austria.*

**Rhone-Poulenc Rorer, Belg.** See *Aventis, Belg.*

**Rhone-Poulenc Rorer, Canad.** See *Aventis, Canad.*

**Rhone-Poulenc Rorer, Denm.** See *Aventis, Denm.*

**Rhone-Poulenc Rorer, Fin.** See *Aventis, Fin.*

**Rhone-Poulenc Rorer, Fr.** See *Aventis, Fr.*

**Rhone-Poulenc Rorer, Ger.** See *Aventis, Ger.*

**Rhone-Poulenc Rorer, Gr.** RHONE-POULENC RORER AEBE, Μεσογείων 290, 155 62 Χολαργός, Cholargos, Greece.

**Rhone-Poulenc Rorer, Hong Kong.** See *Aventis, Hong Kong.*

**Rhone-Poulenc Rorer, Irl.** See *Aventis, Irl.*

**Rhone-Poulenc Rorer, Israel.** See *Aventis, Israel.*

**Rhone-Poulenc Rorer, Ital.** See *Aventis, Ital.*

**Rhone-Poulenc Rorer, Jpn.** See *Aventis, Jpn.*

**Rhone-Poulenc Rorer, Mex.** See *Aventis, Mex.*

**Rhone-Poulenc Rorer, Neth.** See *Aventis, Neth.*

**Rhone-Poulenc Rorer, Norw.** See *Aventis, Norw.*

**Rhone-Poulenc Rorer, Port.** See *Aventis, Port.*

**Rhone-Poulenc Rorer, S.Afr.** See *Aventis, S.Afr.*

**Rhone-Poulenc Rorer, Singapore.** See *Aventis, Singapore.*

**Rhone-Poulenc Rorer, Spain.** See *Aventis, Spain.*

**Rhone-Poulenc Rorer, Swed.** See *Aventis, Swed.*

**Rhone-Poulenc Rorer, Switz.** See *Aventis, Switz.*

**Rhone-Poulenc Rorer, Thai.** See *Aventis, Thai.*

**Rhone-Poulenc Rorer, UK.** See *Aventis, UK.*

**Rhone-Poulenc Rorer, USA.** See *Aventis, USA.*

**Rhone-Poulenc Sante, Thai.** See *Aventis, Thai.*

**Rhoxalpharma, Canad.** Rhoxalpharma Inc., 4600 Thimens Bvld, St-Laurent, Quebec, H4R 2B2, Canada.

**Ribex, Ital.** See *Pfizer, Ital.*

**Ribosepharm, Ger.** ribosepharm GmbH, Bergam-Laim-Str. 127, 81673 Munich, Germany.

**Rice Steele, Irl.** Rice Steele & Co. Ltd, Cookstown Industrial Estate, Tallaght, Dublin 24, Ireland.

**Rich Plan, Hong Kong.** Rich Plan International Ltd, Flat 9, 16/F, Block C, Wah Lok Industrial Ctr, 31-41 Shan Mei St, Fotan, Shatin, N.T., Hong Kong.

**Richard, Fr.** Laboratoires Richard, rue du Progres, ZI des Reys de Saulce, 26270 Saulce-sur-Rhone, France.

**Richards & Appleby, UK.** Richards & Appleby Ltd, Unit 3, Heads of the Valley Industrial Park, Rhymney, Gwent, NP2 5RL, UK.

**Richardson-Vicks, Israel.** Richardson-Vicks, Israel.

**Richardson-Vicks, USA.** See *Procter & Gamble, USA.*

**Richardson-Vicks Personal Care, USA.** See *Procter & Gamble, USA.*

**Richelet, Fr.** Laboratoires Richelet, 15 rue La Perouse, 75116 Paris, France.

**Richet, Arg.** Lab. Richet S.A., Terrero 1251/9, 1416 Buenos Aires, Argentina.

**Richlife, Hong Kong.** See *Jebsen, Hong Kong.*

**Richmond, Arg.** Lab. Richmond, Av. Elcano 4938, 1427 Buenos Aires, Argentina.

**Richmond, Canad.** See *Rivex, Canad.*

**Richmond Ophthalmics, Canad.** See *Rivex, Canad.*

**Richmond Pharmaceuticals, UK.** Richmond Pharmaceuticals Ltd, Coomb House, St Johns Rd, Isleworth, Middlesex, UK.

**Richter, Austria.** Richter Pharma, Feldgasse 19, A-4600 Wels, Austria.

**Richwood, USA.** See *Shire Richwood, USA.*

**Ricola, Canad.** Ricola, Canada.

**RID, USA.** R.I.D. Inc., 609 N Mednik Ave, Los Angeles, CA 90022-1320, USA.

**Rider, Chile.** Laboratorios Rider SA, Placer 1348, Santiago, Chile.

**Ridupharm, Switz.** Ridupharm, Emil Frey-Strasse 99, 4142 Munchenstein, Switzerland.

**Riedel-Zabinka, Braz.** Riedel Zabinka Produtos Quimicos e Farmaceuticos S.A., Avenida Bras de Pina 11/202, 21070-030 Rio de Janeiro, RJ, Brazil.

**Riel, Austria.** Riel GmbH & Co. KG, Gasselberg 53-54, A-8564 Krottendorf-Gaisfeld, Austria.

**Riemser, Ger.** Riemser Arzneimittel GmbH, An der Wiek 7, 17493 Greifswald/Insel Riems, Germany.

**Rigers, Mex.** Rigers, Mexico.

**Riker, Mex.** See *3M, Mex.*

**Rima, UK.** Rima Pharmaceuticals Ltd, 214-16 St James's Rd, Croydon, Surrey, CR0 2BW, UK.

**Rimsa, Mex.** Rimsa, Representaciones e Investigaciones Medicas S.A. de C.V., Av. Acoxpa No. 464, Prado Coapa, Deleg. Coyoacan, 14350 Mexico D.F., Mexico.

**Rio Preto, Braz.** Laboratorio Farmaceutico Rio Preto Ltda, Rua Professora Zulmira Salles 1318, 15030-150 Sao Jose do Rio Preto, SP, Brazil.

**Riom, Fr.** See *Organon, Fr.*

**Ripari-Gero, Ital.** Istituto Farmaco Biologico Ripari-Gero S.p.A., Via Montarioso 11, 53035 Monteriggioni (SI), Italy.

**Rising Pharmaceuticals, USA.** Rising Pharmaceuticals, 411 Sette Drive, Paramus, NJ 07652, USA.

**Ritsert, Ger.** Dr. E. Ritsert GmbH & Co. KG, Klausenweg 12, 69412 Eberbach, Germany.

**Ritter, Ger.** Walter Ritter GmbH & Co., Spaldingstr. 110 B, 20097 Hamburg, Germany.

**Ritter, Hong Kong.** See *JDH, Hong Kong, Mekim, Hong Kong,* and *Suburfarm, Hong Kong.*

**Ritter, Malaysia.** See *JDH, Malaysia.*

**Ritter, Singapore.** See *JDH, Singapore.*

**Ritter, Thai.** See *Osotspa, Thai.*

**Rius, Spain.** Rius Garriga, Pujadas 95, 08005 Barcelona, Spain.

**Riva, Canad.** Laboratoire Riva Inc., 660 Industrial Blvd, Blainville, Quebec, J7C 3V4, Canada.

**Rivadis, Fr.** Laboratoires Rivadis, B.P. 111, ZI de Louzy, 79103 Thouars cdx, France.

**River, Singapore.** See *MBD, Singapore.*

**River Foods, Austral.** River Foods, 1/3 Macquarie Drive, Thomastown, VIC 3074, Australia.

**Rivero, Arg.** Laboratorios Rivero, Avenida Boyaca 419, 1406 Buenos Aires, Argentina.

**Rivex, Canad.** Rivex Pharma Inc., 3-305 Industrial Parkway S, Aurora, Ontario, L4G 6X7, Canada.

**Rivex Ophthalmics, Canad.** See *Rivex, Canad.*

**Rivopharm, Switz.** Rivopharm SA, 6928 Manno, Switzerland.

**RMC, Canad.** RMC Group, 5080 Timberlea Blvd, Ste 42, Mississauga, Ontario, L4W 4M2, Canada.

**R+N, Gr.** R+N ΦΑΡΜΑΚΕΥΤΙΚΑ ΑΕΒΕ, Κατεχάκη 58, 115 25 Ν. Ψυχικό, N. Psichiko, Greece.

**Robapharm, Fr.** See *Pierre Fabre, Fr.*

**Robapharm, Spain.** Robapharm España, Ramon Trias Fargas 7-11, Edificio Marina Village, 08005 Barcelona, Spain.

**Robapharm, Switz.** Robapharm SA, Gewerbestrasse 18, 4123 Allschwil, Switzerland.

**Robert, Spain.** Robert, Gran via de Carlos III 98, 08028 Barcelona, Spain.

**Roberts, Canad.** See *Shire Biochem, Canad.*

**Roberts, Israel.** See *Medison, Israel,* and *Pharmateam, Israel.*

**Roberts, USA.** Roberts Pharmaceutical Corp., 4 Industrial Way West, Eatontown, NJ 07724, USA.

**Roberts & Sheppey, UK.** Roberts & Sheppey (Melrose) Ltd, Manor Farm House, Ickford, Aylesbury, Buckinghamshire, HP18 9JB, UK.

**Robins, Hong Kong.** See *US Summit, Hong Kong.*

**Robins, Israel.** See *Neopharm, Israel.*

**Robins, USA.** See *Whitehall-Robins, USA.*

**Robinson, UK.** Robinson Healthcare, Waterside, Walton, Chesterfield, Derbyshire, S40 1YF, UK.

**Robugen, Ger.** Robugen GmbH Pharmazeutische Fabrik, Alleenstr. 22-6, 73730 Esslingen, Germany.

**Robugen, Hong Kong.** See *Mekim, Hong Kong.*

**RoC, Belg.** See *Johnson & Johnson Consumer, Belg.*

**RoC, Fr.** See *Johnson & Johnson Medical, Fr.*

**RoC, UK.** See *Johnson & Johnson, UK.*

**Roche, Arg.** Productos Roche S.A.Q. e I., Rawson 3150, 1610 Ricardo Rojas Tigre, Buenos Aires, Argentina.

**Roche, Austral.** Roche Products P/L, P.O. Box 255, Dee Why, NSW 2099, Australia.

**Roche, Austria.** Roche Austria GmbH, Engelhorngasse 3, A-1211 Vienna, Austria.

**Roche, Belg.** Roche S.A., Rue Dante 75, 1070 Brussels, Belgium.

**Roche, Braz.** Produtos Roche Quimicos e Farmaceuticos S.A., Avenida Engenheiro Billings 1729, 05321-900 Sao Paulo, SP, Brazil.

**Roche, Canad.** Hoffmann-La Roche Ltd, 2455 Meadowpine Blvd, Mississauga, Ontario, L5N 6L7, Canada.

**Roche, Chile.** Productos Roche Ltda, Av. Quilin 3750, Macul, Santiago, Chile.

**Roche, Denm.** Roche A/S, Industriholmen 59, 2650 Hvidovre, Denmark.

**Roche, Ecud.** Roche Ecuador S.A., Casilla 171 106 185, Quito, Ecuador.

**Roche, Fin.** Roche Oy, Sinimäentie 10 A, PL 12, 02631 Espoo, Finland.

**Roche, Fr.** Produits Roche, 52 bd du Parc, 92521 Neuilly-sur-Seine cdx, France.

**Roche, Ger.** Hoffmann-La Roche AG, Emil-Barell-Str. 1, 79639 Grenzach-Wyhlen, Germany.

**Roche, Gr.** ROCHE HELLAS AE, Αλαμάνας 4 & Δελφών, 151 25 Μαρούσι, Marousi, Greece.

**Roche, Hong Kong.** Roche Hong Kong Ltd, 802 The Lee Gardens, 33 Hysan Ave, Causeway Bay, Hong Kong.

**Roche, Irl.** Roche Pharmaceuticals (Ireland) Ltd, 3004 Lake Drive, City West, Naas Rd, Dublin 24, Ireland.

**Roche, Israel.** Roche Pharmaceuticals (Israel) Ltd, P.O. Box 7543, Petach Tikva, Israel.

**Roche, Ital.** Roche S.p.A., Viale G.B. Stucchi 10, 20052 Monza (MI), Italy.

**Roche, Jpn.** Nippon Roche K.K., Nippon Roche Building, 6-1 Shiba 2-chome, Minato-ku, Tokyo 105-8532, Japan.

**Roche, Mex.** Grupo Roche Syntex de Mixico, S.A. de C.V., Cerrada de Bezares No. 9, Col. Lomas de Bezares, 11910 Mexico D.F., Mexico.

**Roche, Neth.** Roche Nederland BV, P.O. Box 42, 3640 AA Mijdrecht, Netherlands.

**Roche, Norw.** Roche Norge AS, Kristoffer Robinsv. 13, Postboks 41 Haugenstua, 0915 Oslo, Norway.

**Roche, NZ.** Roche Products (New Zealand) Ltd, P.O. Box 12-492, Penrose, Auckland, New Zealand.

**Roche, Port.** Roche Farmacêutica Química, Lda, Estrada Nacional 249, 2720-413 Amadora, Portugal.

**Roche, S.Afr.** Roche Products (Pty) Ltd, P.O. Box 129, Isando 1600, South Africa.

**Roche, Singapore.** Roche Singapore Pte Ltd, 1 Kim Seng Promenade, 15-07/12 Great World City, S 237994, Singapore.

**Roche, Spain.** Roche Farma, Josefa Valcarcel 42, 28027 Madrid, Spain.

**Roche, Swed.** Roche AB, Box 47327, 100 74 Stockholm, Sweden.

**Roche, Switz.** Roche Pharma (Schweiz) AG, Schonmattstrasse 2, 4153 Reinach, Switzerland.

**Roche, Thai.** Roche Thailand Ltd, 19 Fl, Rasa Tower, 555 Phaholyothin Rd, Chatuchak, Bangkok 10900, Thailand.

**Roche, UK.** Roche Products Ltd, 40 Broadwater Rd, Welwyn Garden City, Hertfordshire, AL7 3AY, UK.

**Roche, USA.** Roche Pharmaceuticals, 340 Kingsland St, Nutley, NJ 07110-1199, USA.

**Roche Consumer, Austral.** See *Roche, Austral.*

**Roche Consumer, Ger.** Roche Consumer Health Deutschland GmbH, Valterweg 24-5, 65817 Eppstein-Bremthal, Germany.

**Roche Consumer, Irl.** See *Roche, Irl.*

**Roche Consumer, Neth.** Roche Consumer Health, Meerenakkerplein 5-6, 5652 BJ Eindhoven, Netherlands.

**Roche Consumer, S.Afr.** See *Roche, S.Afr.*

**Roche Consumer, Singapore.** See *Roche, Singapore.*

**Roche Consumer, UK.** See *Roche, UK.*

**Roche Diagnostics, Austral.** Roche Diagnostics, P.O. Box 955, Castle Hill, NSW 1765, Australia.

**Roche Diagnostics, Canad.** Roche Diagnostics, Division of Hoffman-La Roche Ltd, 201 Armand-Frappier Bvld, Laval, Quebec, H7V 4A2, Canada.

**Roche Diagnostics, Fr.** Roche Diagnostics, 2 av. du Vercors, B.P. 59, 38242 Meylan cdx, France.

**Roche Diagnostics, Irl.** See *Roche Diagnostics, UK.*

**Roche Diagnostics, Israel.** See *Teva, Israel.*

**Roche Diagnostics, Ital.** See *Roche, Ital.*

**Roche Diagnostics, NZ.** Roche Diagnostics NZ Ltd, P.O. Box 62-089, Auckland, New Zealand.

**Roche Diagnostics, UK.** Roche Diagnostics Ltd, Bell Lane, Lewes, East Sussex, BN7 1LG, UK.

**Roche Nicholas, Fr.** Laboratoires Roche Nicholas, 33 Rue de l'Industrie, 74240 Gaillard, France.

**Roche Nicholas, Ger.** See *Roche Consumer, Ger.*

**Roche Nicholas, Hong Kong.** See *CNW, Hong Kong.*

**Roche Nicholas, Israel.** See *Devries, Israel.*

**Roche Nicholas, Neth.** See *Roche Consumer, Neth.*

**Roche Nicholas, Spain.** See *Roche, Spain.*

**Roche Products, USA.** Roche Products Inc., HC 01 Box 16626, Humaco, PR 00791-9711, Puerto Rico.

**Roche-Posay, Arg.** Lab. Pharmaceutique La Roche-Posay, Avenida Roque Saenz Pena 1155, 7 Piso, 1041 Buenos Aires, Argentina.

**Roche-Posay, Braz.** La Roche Posay, L'Oreal-Belocap. Divisao Cosmetica Ativa, Rua Sao Bento 8, 14 andar, 20090-010 Rio de Janeiro, RJ, Brazil.

**Roche-Posay, Fr.** Laboratoires Pharmaceutiques La Roche-Posay, B.P. 23, 86270 La Roche-Posay, France.

**Roche-Posay, Irl.** La Roche-Posay Cosmetique Active, Merchant's Hall, 25/26 Merchant's Quay, Dublin 8, Ireland.

**Roche-Posay, Switz.** See *Cosmetique Active, Switz.*

**Rodisma, Ger.** Rodisma-Med Pharma GmbH, Kolner Str. 48, 51149 Cologne, Germany.

**Rodleben, Ger.** Rodleben Pharma GmbH, Am Waldchen 19, 06862 Rosslau, Germany.

**Rodlen, USA.** Rodlen Laboratories, 100 Fairway Drive, Ste 134, Vernon Hills, IL 60061, USA.

**Roemmers, Arg.** Roemmers S.A.I.C.F., Fray Justo Sarmiento 2350, 1636 Olivos, Buenos Aires, Argentina.

**Roerig, Austral.** See *Pfizer, Austral.*

**Roerig, Chile.** See *Pfizer, Chile.*

**Roerig, USA.** See *Pfizer, USA.*

**Rogers, Canad.** Rogers Pharmaceuticals Ltd, 330 Marwood Drive, Oshawa, Ontario, L1H 8B4, Canada.

**Roha, Ger.** roha Arzneimittel GmbH, Rockwinkeler Heerstr. 100, 28355 Bremen, Germany.

**Roha, Hong Kong.** See *Hind Wing, Hong Kong.*

**Roha, Irl.** See *Pharma-Global, Irl.*

**Roha, Israel.** See *Dexxon, Israel.*

**Roha, Port.** See *Vivalife, Port.*

**Roha, Switz.** See *Adroka, Switz.*

**Rolab, S.Afr.** Rolab (Division of Novartis SA (Pty) Ltd), 72 Steel Rd, Spartan Kempton Park, South Africa.

**Roland, Ger.** See *Altana Consumer, Ger.*

**Rolfe, S.Afr.** See *Boots Healthcare, S.Afr.*

**Rolmex, Canad.** Rolmex International Inc., 8750 de-la-Rive-Sud Blvd, Levis, Quebec, G6V 6N6, Canada.

**Romark, USA.** Romark Laboratories, 6200 Courtney Campbell Causeway, Suite 880, Tampa, FL, USA.

**Romer, Mex.** Laboratorios Romer S.A. de C.V., Indiana No. 170, Col. Napoles, Deleg. Benito Juarez, 03810 Mexico D.F., Mexico.

**Romigal, Ger.** Romigal-Werk, Galileiplatz 2, 81679 Munich, Germany.

**Romilo, Canad.** See *St Laurent, Canad.*

**Romsa, Mex.** Romsa de Mexico S.A., Metalurgia No. 2820, P. Industrial el Alamo, 45560 Tlaquepaque, Jal., Mexico.

**Rontag, Arg.** Lab. Rontag S.A., Arcos 2626, 1428 Buenos Aires, Argentina.

**Rorer, UK.** See *Aventis, UK.*

**Rosa-Phytopharma, Fr.** Laboratoires Rosa-Phytopharma, 68 rue Jean-Jaques-Rousseau, 75001 Paris, France.

**Rosa-Phytopharma, Switz.** See *Golaz, Switz.*

**Rosch & Handel, Austria.** Rösch & Handel, Gudrunstrasse 150, A-1100 Vienna, Austria.

**Rosco, Denm.** A/S Rosco, Farmaceutisk Industri, Taastrupgaardsvej 30, 2630 Taastrup, Denmark.

**Rosco, Norw.** See *Andersen, Norw.*

**Rosemont, Thai.** See *Star, Thai.*

**Rosemont, UK.** Rosemont Pharmaceuticals Ltd, Rosemont House, Yorkdale Industrial Park, Braithwaite St, Leeds, West Yorkshire, LS11 9XE, UK.

**Rosen, Ger.** Rosen Pharma GmbH, Kirkeler Str. 41, 66440 Blieskastel, Germany.

**Rosken, Hong Kong.** See *Suburfarm, Hong Kong.*

**Rosken, Singapore.** See *JDH, Singapore.*

**Ross, Hong Kong.** See *Abbott, Hong Kong.*

**Ross, Israel.** See *Promedico, Israel.*

**Ross, USA.** Ross Products, Division of Abbott Laboratories Inc., 625 Cleveland Ave, Columbus, OH 43215-1724, USA.

**Roter, Thai.** Roter, Thailand.

**Roterpharma, Irl.** See *Allphar, Irl.*

**Rotexmedica, Ger.** Rotexmedica GmbH Arzneimittelwerk, Bunsenstr. 4, 22946 Trittau, Germany.

**Roth, Austria.** G Roth & Söhne Pharmazeutische Präparate GmbH, Wagnerstrasse 29, A-2371 Hinterbruhl, Austria.

**Rothpharma, Austria.** See *Roth, Austria.*

**Rotta, Hong Kong.** See *JDH, Hong Kong.*

**Rotta, Israel.** See *Teva, Israel.*

**Rotta, Ital.** See *Rottapharm, Ital.*

**Rotta, Malaysia.** See *Antah, Malaysia.*

**Rotta, Singapore.** See *Sime Darby, Singapore.*

**Rotta, Thai.** See *Diethelm, Thai.*

**Rottapharm, Chile.** See *Silesia, Chile.*

**Rottapharm, Fin.** See *Algol, Fin.*

**Rottapharm, Fr.** Laboratoires Rottapharm, 83-85 bd Vincent-Auriol, 75013 Paris, France.

**Rottapharm, Ger.** See *Opfermann, Ger.*

**Rottapharm, Irl.** Rottapharm Ireland, Damastown Industrial Park, Mulhuddart, Dublin 15, Ireland.

**Rottapharm, Ital.** Rottapharm S.r.l., Via Valosa di Sopra 9, 20052 Monza (MI), Italy.

**Rottapharm, Spain.** Rottapharm, Ctra Barcelona 2, Almacera, 46132 Valencia, Spain.

**Rottapharm, Switz.** Rottapharm BV, Swiss Branch, Via Cantonale 19, 6900 Lugano, Switzerland.

**Rougier, Canad.** See *Technilab, Canad.*

**Rougier, Hong Kong.** See *Pan-Well, Hong Kong.*

**Roussel, Fr.** See *Aventis, Fr.*

**Roussel, Neth.** See *Aventis, Neth.*

**Roussel, Port.** See *Aventis, Port.*

**Roussel, S.Afr.** See *Hoechst Marion Roussel, S.Afr.*

**Roussel, Spain.** See *Aventis, Spain.*

**Roussel Diamant, Fr.** See *Aventis, Fr.*

**Roux-Ocefa, Arg.** Lab. Roux-Ocefa S.A., Montevideo 79/81, 1019 Buenos Aires, Argentina.

**Rovi, Spain.** Rovi, Julian Camarillo 35, 28037 Madrid, Spain.

**Rowa, Ger.** Rowa Wagner GmbH & Co. KG Arzneimittelfabrik, Frankenforster Str. 77, 51427 Bergisch Gladbach, Germany.

**Rowa, Hong Kong.** See *Jacobson, Hong Kong.*

**Rowa, Irl.** Rowa Pharmaceuticals Ltd, Bantry, Co. Cork, Ireland.

**Rowa, Israel.** See *Megapharm, Israel.*

**Rowa, Malaysia.** See *JDH, Malaysia.*

**Rowa, Singapore.** See *JDH, Singapore.*

**Rowa, Thai.** See *JDH Borneo, Thai.*

**Rowa Wagner, Hong Kong.** See *Deutsch Chinesische, Hong Kong.*

**Rowex, Irl.** See *Rowa, Irl.*

**Roxane, USA.** Roxane Laboratories Inc., P.O. Box 16532, Columbus, OH 43228-6532, USA.

**Royal, Chile.** See *Alpes Chemie, Chile.*

**Royal Childrens Hospital, Austral.** Royal Children's Hospital, Melbourne Pharmacy Dept, Flemington Rd, Parkville, VIC 3052, Australia.

**Royton, Braz.** Royton Quimica Farmaceutica Ltda, Avenida Doutor Cardoso de Melo 1318, 04548-004 Sao Paulo, SP, Brazil.

**RPG, India.** RPG Life Sciences Ltd, Ceat Mahal 463, Dr A.B. Rd, Mumbai 400 025, India.

**RTA, Switz.** Laboratoire RTA SA, chemin du Signal 18, 1071 Chexbres, Switzerland.

**Rubiepharm, Ger.** RubiePharm Vertriebs GmbH, Bruder-Grimm-Str. 121, 36396 Steinau an der Strasse, Germany.

**Rubio, Singapore.** See *Zyfas, Singapore.*

**Rubio, Spain.** Rubio, Industria 29, Pol Ind Comte de Sert, Castellbisal, 08755 Barcelona, Spain.

**Rubio, Thai.** See *JDH Borneo, Thai.*

**Rudefsa, Mex.** See *Sanofi Synthelabo, Mex.*

**Rueckert, Thai.** See *Sriprasit, Thai.*

**Rugby, USA.** See *Watson, USA.*

**Rupertus, Austria.** St Rupertus-Apotheke, Markt 107, A-5090 Lofer, Austria.

**Rusch, Ital.** Rusch S.r.l., Via Torina 5, 20039 Varedo (MI), Italy.

**Rusch, UK.** Rüsch UK Ltd, PO Box 138, Cressex Industrial Estate, High Wycombe, Buckinghamshire, HP12 3NB, UK.

**Russ, USA.** See *UCB, USA.*

**Russells, NZ.** Russells Pharmaceuticals Ltd, P.O. Box 9591, Newmarket, Auckland, New Zealand.

**RX, Thai.** RX Company Ltd, 93/90 Soi Prachanukul 2, Ratchadapisek Rd, Bangsue, Bangkok 10800, Thailand.

**Rybar, Irl.** See *Cahill May Roberts, Irl.*

**Rydelle, Fr.** See *Fornet, Fr.*

**Rydelle, Ital.** Rydelle Laboratories Business, Johnson Wax S.p.A., P.le M. Burke 3, 20020 Arese (MI), Italy.

**Rydelle, USA.** See *Johnson Wax, USA.*

**Rye, Austral.** Rye Pharmaceuticals, Unit 1, Block F, 25-7 Paul St North, North Ryde, NSW 2113, Australia.

**Rye, Singapore.** See *PMR, Singapore.*

**Rystan, USA.** Rystan Co. Inc., c/o Integra LifeSciences Corp., 105 Morgan Lane, Plainsboro, NJ 08536, USA.

**S & K, Ger.** S & K Pharma, Schumann & Kohl GmbH, Bahnhofstr. 4-6, 66706 Perl, Germany.

**S Med, Austria.** S Med Handels GmbH, Braunerstrasse 3/17, A-1010 Vienna, Austria.

**SA Druggists, S.Afr.** South African Druggists Pharma, South Africa.

**Saba, Ital.** Saba, Via Salbertrand 21, 10146 Turin, Italy.

**Sabater, Spain.** See *Generfarma, Spain.*

**Sabex, Canad.** Sabex Inc., 145 Jules-Leger St, Boucherville, Quebec, J4B 7K8, Canada.

**Sabiluc, Fr.** Laboratoires Sabiluc, 61 rue Lavoisier, 14200 Herouville-Saint-Clair, France.

**Sabona, Ger.** Sabona GmbH, Gutenbergstr. 1, 83052 Bruckmuhl, Germany.

**Sabora, Fin.** Sabora Pharma Oy, Hiisimetsänkatu 40, 03600 Karkkila, Finland.

**SAD, Denm.** See *Amternes, Denm.*

**Safeline, S.Afr.** Safeline Pharmaceuticals (Pty) Ltd, 72 Steel Road, Spartan, Kempton Park 1619, South Africa.

**Safire, Hong Kong.** See *Hong Kong Medical, Hong Kong.*

**Sairaalapalvelu, Fin.** Soumen Sairaalapalvelu Oy, Vattuniemenranta 2, 00210 Helsinki, Finland.

**Salf, Ital.** Salf Laboratorio Farmacologico S.p.A., Via G. d'Alzano 12, 24122 Bergamo, Italy.

**Salitine, Ger.** Salitine Pharma Vertriebs GmbH, Heidelberger Str. 57a, 68519 Viernheim, Germany.

**Salix, USA.** Salix Pharmaceuticals Inc., 3600 W Bayshore Rd, Palo Alto, CA 94303-4237, USA.

**Salmon, Switz.** Salmon Pharma, St Jakobs-Strasse 110, Postfach, 4002 Basle, Switzerland.

**Salonpas, UK.** Salonpas (UK) Ltd, Unit B, 32a Eveline Rd, Mitchum, Surrey, CR4 3LE, UK.

**Salters, S.Afr.** See *Adcock Ingram, S.Afr.*

**Salts Healthcare, UK.** Salts Healthcare, Lord St, Birmingham, B7 4DS, UK.

**Salud, Spain.** Salud, Spain.

**Salus, Fr.** Salus France, B.P. 104 Principal, 83403 Hyeres cdx, France.

**Salus, Ital.** Salus Researches S.p.A., Via Aurelia 58, 00165 Rome, Italy.

**Salus, Mex.** Laboratorios Salus S.A. de C.V., KM 22.5 Carretera Guadalajara Morelia, Jalisco Zuniga, 45640 Guadalajara, Jalisco, Mexico.

**Salushaus, Ger.** Salus-Haus Dr. med. Otto Greither Nachf. GmbH & Co KG, Bahnhofstr. 24, 83052 Bruckmuhl/Mangfall (Obb.), Germany.

**Salusif, Port.** Salusif, Lda, Rua do Centro Cultural 10 r/c, 1700 Lisbon, Portugal.

**Salvat, Spain.** Salvat, Gall 30-36, Esplugas de Llobregat, 08950 Barcelona, Spain.

**Salzmann, Switz.** Salzmann Medico, Unterstrasse 52, 9001 St Gallen, Switzerland.

**Sam Chun Dang, Singapore.** See *Zyfas, Singapore.*

**Samakeephaesaj, Thai.** Samakeephaesaj (Union Drug Laboratories Co. Ltd), 2601 Sukhumvit Rd, Bangkok 10250, Thailand.

**Samarth, India.** Samarth Pharma Pvt Ltd, Ram Mandir Rd, Goregaon (W), Mumbai 400 104, India.

**Samchully, Singapore.** See *Zyfas, Singapore.*

**Samil, Ital.** Samil S.p.A., Via Piemonte 32, 00187 Rome, Italy.

**Samjin, Singapore.** See *Zyfas, Singapore.*

**Samnam, Singapore.** See *Pharmaforte, Singapore.*

**Sam-On, Israel.** Meditec/Sam-On Ltd, P.O. Box 1224, Bat-Yam 59602, Israel.

**SAN, Ital.** S.A.N. s.a.s., Viale Corsica 92, 50127 Florence, Italy.

**San Carlo, Ital.** S. Carlo Farmaceutici S.p.A., Via Procoio 28, 00065 Fiano Romano (RM), Italy.

**Sanabo, Austria.** Sanabo Wien GmbH, Brunner Strasse 59, A-1235 Vienna, Austria.

**Sanamed, Austria.** Sanamed GmbH, Rudolf Waisenhorngasse 32, A-1230 Vienna, Austria.

**Sanapharm, Ger.** SanaPharm Arzneimittel GmbH, Alexandrinenstr. 1, 96450 Coburg, Germany.

**Sanavita, Ger.** Sanavita Pharma Vertriebs GmbH & Co. KG, Am Bahnhof 1-3, 59368 Werne, Germany.

**Sancor, Arg.** Sancor, Tacuari 202 Piso 11, 1071 Buenos Aires, Argentina.

**Sanderson, Chile.** Laboratorio Sanderson SA, Carlos Fernandez 244, Santiago, Chile.

**Sandersons, UK.** Sandersons (Chemists) Ltd, 37 Oakwood Rise, Heaton, Bolton, BL1 5EE, UK.

**Sandipro, Belg.** Sandipro S.A., Chaussee de Gand 615, 1080 Brussels, Belgium.

**Sandoz, Canad.** Sandoz Canada Inc., Pharmaceutical Division, 385 boul. Bouchard, Dorval, Quebec, H9R 4P5, Canada.

**Sandoz, Fr.** See *Novartis, Fr.*

**Sandoz, Ger.** See *Novartis, Ger.*

**Sandoz, Ital.** See *Novartis, Ital.*

**Sandoz, UK.** See *Novartis, UK.*

**Sandoz Consumer, USA.** See *Novartis Consumer, USA.*

**Sandoz Nutrition, Canad.** Sandoz Nutrition Corporation, 1621 McEwen Dr., Unit 50, Whitby, Ontario, L1N 9A5, Canada.

**Sandoz Nutrition, USA.** See *Novartis Nutrition, USA.*

**Sandoz OTC, Switz.** See *Novartis Consumer, Switz.*

**Sanfer, Mex.** Laboratorios Sanfer S.A. de C.V., Calz. de Tlalpan No. 550, Col. Moderna, Deleg. Benito Juarez, 03510 Mexico D.F., Mexico.

**Sang, Thai.** Sang Thai, 148/19-21 Nanglinjee Rd, Tungmahamek, Bangkok 10120, Thailand.

**Sang Udom, Thai.** Sang Udom Pharmacy Lp, 24-26 Songsawad Rd, Samyek, Sampantawong, Bangkok 10100, Thailand.

**Sang-A, Malaysia.** See *Sun, Malaysia.*

**Sang-A Pharm, Singapore.** See *Sime Darby, Singapore.*

**Sangstat, Neth.** SANGSTAT BV, Bovenkerkerweg 6-8, 1185 XE Amstelveen, Netherlands.

**Sangstat, Singapore.** See *Summit, Singapore.*

**Sangstat, UK.** Imitix Sangstat (UK) Ltd, 42 Thames St, Windsor, Berkshire, SL4 1PR, UK.

**Sanico, Belg.** Sanico S.A., Industriezone 4, Veedijk 59, 2300 Turnhout, Belgium.

**Sanico, Switz.** See *Uhlmann-Eyraud, Switz.*

**Sanidom, Austria.** Sanidom Handels-GmbH, Sundlweg 2, A-8045 Graz, Austria.

**Saninter, Port.** Saninter, SA, Av Durque d'Avila no 193, 1050-082 Lisbon, Portugal.

**Sanitalia, Ital.** Sanitalia S.n.c. di Battaglia & C., Strada dei Tadini 5, 10131 Turin, Italy.

**Sanitas, Arg.** Instituto Sanitas Arg. SACIPQ y M., Saladillo 2452, 1440 Buenos Aires, Argentina.

**Sanitas, Chile.** Instituto Sanitas SA, Avda Americo Vespucio 1260, Quilicura, Santiago, Chile.

**Sanitas, Ital.** Sanitas Lab. Chimico Farmaceutico S.r.l., Via Guala 4, 15057 Tortona (AL), Italy.

**Sanitas, Port.** See *Menarini, Port.*

**Sankyo, Austria.** Sankyo Pharmazeutika Austria GmbH, Effingergasse 21, A-1160 Vienna, Austria.

**Sankyo, Belg.** Sankyo Pharma Belgium S.A., Parc Scientifique Fleming LLN, Rue Fond Jean Paques 5, 1348 Louvain-la-Neuve, Belgium.

**Sankyo, Braz.** Sankyo Pharma Brasil Ltda, Alameda Xingu 706, 06455-960 Alphaville-Barueri, SP, Brazil.

**Sankyo, Denm.** See *Gea, Denm.*

**Sankyo, Fin.** Oy Sankyo Pharma Finland AB, PL 1310, Salomonkatu 17 A 5. krs, 00101 Helsinki, Finland.

**Sankyo, Ger.** Sankyo Pharma GmbH, Zielstattstr. 9, 81379 Munich, Germany.

**Sankyo, Hong Kong.** See *Hing Ah, Hong Kong,* and *Keller, Hong Kong.*

**Sankyo, Ital.** Sankyo Pharma Italia S.p.A., Via Reno 5, 00198 Rome, Italy.

**Sankyo, Jpn.** Sankyo Co. Ltd, 3-5-1 Nihonbashi-Honcho 3-chome, Chuo-ku, Tokyo 103-8426, Japan.

**Sankyo, Neth.** See *Will-Pharma, Neth.*

**Sankyo, Norw.** See *Weifa, Norw.*

**Sankyo, NZ.** See *Wilson, NZ.*

**Sankyo, Port.** Sankyo Pharma Portugal, Lda, Av Infante D Henrique 328 E, 1800-223 Lisbon, Portugal.

**Sankyo, Singapore.** See *Diethelm, Singapore.*

**Sankyo, Spain.** Sankyo Pharma España, Acanto 22, 28045 Madrid, Spain.

**Sankyo, Switz.** Sankyo Pharma (Schweiz) AG, Industriestrasse 7, 8117 Fallanden, Switzerland.

**Sankyo, Thai.** Thai Sankyo Co. Ltd, 18 Fl, Tipco Tower, 118/1 Rama 6 Rd, Phayathai, Bangkok 10400, Thailand.

**Sankyo, UK.** Sankyo Pharma UK Ltd, Sankyo House, Repton Place, White Lion Rd, Amersham, Buckinghamshire, HP7 9LP, UK.

**Sankyo, USA.** Sankyo Pharma, Two Hilton Court, Parsippany, NJ 07054, USA.

**Sankyo Luitpold, Braz.** See *Sankyo, Braz.*

**Sanobia, Port.** Sanóbia, Lda, Rua Joaquim Paco d'Darcos 111, 1500-365 Lisbon, Portugal.

**Sanochemia, Austria.** Sanochemia Pharmazeutika AG, Boltzmanngasse 9a-11, A-1091 Vienna, Austria.

**Sanochemia, Ger.** Sanochemia Diagnostics Deutschland GmbH, Stresemannallee 4c, 41460 Neuss, Germany.

**Sanochemia, UK.** Sanochemia UK Ltd, Argentum, 510 Bristol Business Park, Coldharbour Lane, Bristol, Avon, BS16 1EJ, UK.

**Sanofi, Switz.** See *Sanofi Synthelabo, Switz.*

**Sanofi, USA.** See *Sanofi Synthelabo, USA.*

**Sanofi Omnimed, S.Afr.** See *Omnimed, S.Afr.*

**Sanofi Synthelabo, Arg.** Sanofi-Synthelabo de Argentina S.A., Coronel Amaro Avalos 4208, 1605 Munro, Buenos Aires, Argentina.

**Sanofi Synthelabo, Austral.** Sanofi-Synthelabo Australia P/L, Riverview Park, 16 Byfield St, North Ryde, NSW 2113, Australia.

**Sanofi Synthelabo, Austria.** Sanofi-Synthelabo GmbH, Koppstrasse 116, A-1160 Vienna, Austria.

**Sanofi Synthelabo, Belg.** Sanofi-Synthelabo S.A., Ave de la Metrologie 5, 1130 Brussels, Belgium.

**Sanofi Synthelabo, Braz.** Sanofi Synthelabo Farmaceutica Ltda, Av. Brasil 22.155, 21670-000 Rio de Janeiro, RJ, Brazil.

**Sanofi Synthelabo, Canad.** Sanofi-Synthelabo Inc., 90 Allstate Parkway, Markham, Ontario, L3R 6H3, Canada.

**Sanofi Synthelabo, Chile.** Sanofi Synthelabo de Chile, Coyancura 2283, Piso 13, Providencia, Santiago, Chile.

**Sanofi Synthelabo, Denm.** Sanofi-Synthelabo, Ringager 4 A, 2605 Brondby, Denmark.

**Sanofi Synthelabo, Fin.** Sanofi-Synthelabo Oy, Vattuniemenranta 2, 00210 Helsinki, Finland.

**Sanofi Synthelabo, Fr.** Sanofi Synthelabo France, 174 av. de France, 75013 Paris, France.

**Sanofi Synthelabo, Ger.** Sanofi-Synthelabo GmbH, Potsdamer Str. 8, 10785 Berlin, Germany.

**Sanofi Synthelabo, Gr.** SANOFI-SYNTHELABO, Λ. Παιανίας Μαρκοπούλου, 190 02 Παιανία, Paiania, Greece.

**Sanofi Synthelabo, Hong Kong.** Sanofi-Synthelabo HK Ltd, Rm 2507-2511, Windsor House, 311 Gloucester Rd, Causeway Bay, Hong Kong.

**Sanofi Synthelabo, Irl.** Sanofi Synthelabo Ireland Ltd, United Drug House, Belgard Rd, Tallaght, Dublin 24, Ireland.

**Sanofi Synthelabo, Israel.** See *CTS, Israel.*

**Sanofi Synthelabo, Ital.** Sanofi-Synthelabo S.p.A., Via GB Piranesi 38, 20137 Milan, Italy.

**Sanofi Synthelabo, Malaysia.** Sanofi-Synthelabo (Malaysia) Sdn Bhd, 3.02 Level 3 Wisma Academy, Lot 4A Jln 19/1, 46300 Petaling Jaya, Selangor, Malaysia.

**Sanofi Synthelabo, Mex.** Sanofi-Synthelabo de Mexico S.A. de C.V., Km 37.5 Autopista Mexico-Qro, 54730 Cuautitlan Izcalli, Mexico.

**Sanofi Synthelabo, Neth.** Sanofi Synthelabo, Govert Van Wijnkade 48, 3144 EG Maassluis, Netherlands.

**Sanofi Synthelabo, Norw.** Sanofi-Synthelabo AS, Leif Tronstads plass 4, Postboks 413, 1302 Sandvika, Norway.

**Sanofi Synthelabo, NZ.** Sanofi Synthelabo Australia Pty Ltd, Lincoln Manor Office Park, 291 Lincoln Rd, Henderson, Waitkere City, Auckland 8, New Zealand.

**Sanofi Synthelabo, Port.** Sanofi-Synthelabo, SA, Praca Duque de Saldanha no 1-4, 1050-094 Lisbon, Portugal.

**Sanofi Synthelabo, S.Afr.** Sanofi-Synthelabo (Pty) Ltd, Postnet Suite 24, Private Bag X23, Gallo Manor 2052, South Africa.

**Sanofi Synthelabo, Singapore.** Sanofi-Synthelabo Singapore Pte Ltd, 61 Stamford RD, 02-01 Stamford Court, S 178892, Singapore.

**Sanofi Synthelabo, Spain.** Sanofi Synthelabo, Avda Litoral Mar 12-14, 08005 Barcelona, Spain.

**Sanofi Synthelabo, Swed.** Sanofi-Synthelabo AB, Box 14142, 167 14 Bromma, Sweden.

**Sanofi Synthelabo, Switz.** Sanofi-Synthélabo (Suisse) AG, 11 Rue de Voyrot, 1217 Meyrin 1, Switzerland.

**Sanofi Synthelabo, Thai.** Sanofi-Synthelabo (Thailand) Ltd, 9-11 Fl, Gypsum Metropolitan Tower, 539/2 Sri-Ayudhya Rd, Phyathai, Rajthevee, Bangkok 10400, Thailand.

**Sanofi Synthelabo, UK.** Sanofi Synthelabo Ltd, 1 Onslow St, Guildford, Surrey, GU1 4YS, UK.

**Sanofi Synthelabo, USA.** Sanofi-Synthelabo Inc., 90 Park Ave, New York, NY 10016, USA.

**Sanofi Synthelabo OTC, Fr.** Sanofi Synthelabo OTC, 9 rue du President-Allende, 94258 Gentilly cdx, France.

**Sanofi Synthelabo OTC, Ital.** Sanofi-Synthelabo OTC S.p.A., Via Messina 38, 20154 Milan, Italy.

**Sanofi Torrent, India.** See *Torrent, India.*

**Sanofi Winthrop, Austria.** See *Sanofi Synthelabo, Austria.*

**Sanofi Winthrop, Belg.** See *Sanofi Synthelabo, Belg.*

**Sanofi Winthrop, Braz.** See *Sanofi Synthelabo, Braz.*

**Sanofi Winthrop, Canad.** See *Sanofi Synthelabo, Canad.*

**Sanofi Winthrop, Denm.** See *Sanofi Synthelabo, Denm.*

**Sanofi Winthrop, Fin.** See *Sanofi Synthelabo, Fin.*

**Sanofi Winthrop, Fr.** See *Sanofi Synthelabo, Fr.*

**Sanofi Winthrop, Ger.** See *Sanofi Synthelabo, Ger.*

**Sanofi Winthrop, Irl.** See *Sanofi Synthelabo, Irl.*

**Sanofi Winthrop, Israel.** See *CTS, Israel.*

**Sanofi Winthrop, Ital.** See *Sanofi Synthelabo, Ital.*

**Sanofi Winthrop, Mex.** See *Sanofi Synthelabo, Mex.*

**Sanofi Winthrop, Neth.** See *Sanofi Synthelabo, Neth.*

**Sanofi Winthrop, Norw.** See *Sanofi Synthelabo, Norw.*

**Sanofi Winthrop, NZ.** See *Sanofi Synthelabo, NZ.*

**Sanofi Winthrop, Port.** See *Sanofi Synthelabo, Port.*

**Sanofi Winthrop, Swed.** See *Sanofi Synthelabo, Swed.*

**Sanofi Winthrop, Switz.** See *Sanofi Synthelabo, Switz.*

**Sanofi Winthrop, USA.** See *Sanofi Synthelabo, USA.*

**Sanol, Ger.** Sanol GmbH, Alfred-Nobel-Str. 10, 40789 Monheim, Germany.

**Sanopharm, Switz.** Sanopharm AG, vicolo dei Ciossi 8, 6648 Minusio, Switzerland.

**Sanorania, Ger.** See *Lichtenstein, Ger.*

**Sanorania, Switz.** See *Medipharm, Switz.*

**Sanoreform, Ger.** Sanoreform GmbH, Loerfeldstrasse 20, 58313 Herdecke, Germany.

**Sanorell, Ger.** Sanorell Pharma GmbH & Co., Rechtmurgstr. 27, 72270 Baiersbronn, Germany.

**Sanova, Austria.** Sanova Pharma GmbH, Postfach 3, A-1110 Vienna, Austria.

**Sanova, Denm.** See *Tjellesen, Denm.*

**Sant Gall, Arg.** Sant Gall Friburg Q.C.I., Brasil 3131/3, 1260 Buenos Aires, Argentina.

**Santa, Gr.** SANTA N. ΜΠΑΛΑΝΟΣ ΑΒΕΕ, Λεωφ. Δημοκρατίας 145, 136 71 Αχαρνές, Acharnes, Greece.

**Sante Naturelle, Canad.** Sante Naturelle (AG) Ltee, 369 Charles Peguy, La Prairie, Quebec, J5R 3E8, Canada.

**Santen, Denm.** Santen, Roskildevej 48 A, 3400 Hillerod, Denmark.

**Santen, Fin.** Santen Oy, Niittyhaankatu 20, PL 33, 33721 Tampere, Finland.

**Santen, Hong Kong.** See *Hong Kong Medical, Hong Kong,* and *Leader, Hong Kong.*

**Santen, Israel.** Santen, Israel.

**Santen, Jpn.** Santen Pharmaceutical Co Ltd, 3-9-19 Shimoshinjo, Higashi-Yodogawa-ku, Osaka 533-8651, Japan.

**Santen, Norw.** Santen Norge, Sjosenteret Vallo, 3150 Tolvsrod, Norway.

**Santen, Singapore.** See *JDH, Singapore,* and *Luen Wah, Singapore.*

**Santen, Swed.** Santen Pharma AB, 171 45 Solna, Sweden.

**Santen, Thai.** See *Greater Pharma, Thai.*

**Santen, USA.** Santen Inc., 555 Gateway Drive, Napa, CA 94558, USA.

**Santiveri, Spain.** Santiveri, Encuny 8, 08038 Barcelona, Spain.

**Sanum-Kehlbeck, Ger.** Sanum-Kehlbeck GmbH & Co. KG, Hasseler Steinweg 9-12, 27318 Hoya, Germany.

**Sanus, Braz.** See *Biolab Sanus, Braz.*

**Sanval, Braz.** Sanval Comercio e Industria Ltda, Rua Lagrange 401, 04761-050 Sao Paulo, SP, Brazil.

**Sanwa, Jpn.** Sanwa Kagaku Kenkyusho Co Ltd, 35 Higashi-Sotobori-cho, Higashi-ku, Nagoya 461-8631, Japan.

**Saprochi, Israel.** See *Meditrend, Israel.*

**Saprochi, Switz.** Saprochi SA, Chemin de la Cretaux, Case postale 327, 1196 Gland/VD, Switzerland.

**Sarabhai Piramal, India.** Sarabhai Piramal Pharma Ltd, Dr Vikram Sarabhai Marg, Wadi Wadi, Vadodara 390 007, India.

**Sarget, Fr.** See *Viatris, Fr.*

**Saros, Spain.** Saros Laboratorios, FOC 68, 08038 Barcelona, Spain.

**SAT, Spain.** SAT (Servicio Aplicacion Terapeuticas), Avda Barcelona 69, Sant Joan Despi, 08970 Barcelona, Spain.

**Satori, Fr.** Laboratoires Satori International, Parc d'activite de Limonest, 540 allee des Hetres, 69760 Limonest, France.

**Saunier-Daguin, Fr.** Laboratoires Saunier-Daguin, 2 rue Marechal-Foch, 45370 Clery-St-Andre, France.

**Sauter, Austral.** See *Roche, Austral.*

**Savage, USA.** Savage Laboratories, Division of Atlanta Inc., 60 Baylis Road, Melville, NY 11747-2006, USA.

**Saval, Chile.** Laboratorio Saval SA, Oanamericana Norte 4600, Santiago, Chile.

**Savio, Ital.** Istituto Biochimico Nazionale Savio S.r.l., Via E. Bazzano 14, 16019 Ronco Scrivia (GE), Italy.

**Savoma, Ital.** Savoma Medicinali S.p.A., Via Baganza 2/A, 43100 Parma, Italy.

**Savoy, Singapore.** See *Polymedic, Singapore.*

**SBL, Denm.** See *Pasteur Merieux, Denm.*

**SBL, Norw.** SBL Vaccin Norge, C. J. Hansensv. 3 A, 2007 Kjeller, Norway.

**SBL, Swed.** SBL Vaccin AB, 105 21 Stockholm, Sweden.

**SBPA, Austral.** SBPA, Australia.

**Scan Lab, Thai.** See *Harn, Thai.*

**Scand Pharm, Swed.** Scandinavian Pharmaceuticals-Generics AB, Box 23033, 104 35 Stockholm, Sweden.

**Scandimed, Swed.** ScandiMed, Forskaregatan 1, 275 37 Sjobo, Sweden.

**Scandinavian Health Care, Norw.** Scandinavian Health Care AB, Grini Naeringspark 1, 1361 Osteras, Norway.

**Scandinavian Natural Health & Beauty, USA.** Scandinavian Natural Health & Beauty Products Inc., 13 North Seventh St, Perkasie, PA 18944, USA.

**Scandipharm, Israel.** See *Megapharm, Israel.*

**Scandipharm, USA.** Scandipharm Inc., 22 Inverness Center Pkwy, Suite 310, Birmingham, AL 35242, USA.

**Scanpharm, Hong Kong.** See *Winsor, Hong Kong.*

**SCAT, Denm.** See *Norpharma, Denm.*

**SCAT, Switz.** See *Doetsch, Grether, Switz.*

**Schaffer, USA.** Schaffer Laboratories, 1058 North Allen Ave, Pasadena, CA 91104, USA.

**Schaper & Brummer, Ger.** Schaper & Brümmer GmbH & Co. KG, Bahnhofstr. 35, 38259 Salzgitter (Ringelheim), Germany.

**Schaper & Brummer, Malaysia.** See *JDH, Malaysia.*

**Schaper & Brummer, Singapore.** See *Bionax, Singapore.*

**Schaper & Brummer, Thai.** See *Diethelm, Thai.*

**Scharper, Ital.** Scharper S.r.l., Via Milanese 20, 20099 Sesto San Giovanni (MI), Italy.

**Scheffler, Ger.** Dr Scheffler Nachf. GmbH & Co. KG, Senefelderstr. 44, 51469 Bergisch Gladbach, Germany.

**Scheffler, Ital.** Dott. Scheffler Italia Srl, Via Sicilia 5, 20098 San Giuliano Milanese (MI), Italy.

**Schein, Canad.** Schein Pharmaceutical Canada Inc., 77 Belfield Rd, Toronto, Ontario, M9W 1G6, Canada.

**Schein, UK.** Schein Rexodent, 25-7 Merrick Rd, Southall, Middlesex, UB2 4AU, UK.

**Schein, USA.** See *Watson, USA.*

**Scherax, Ger.** See *Alk-Scherax, Ger.*

**Scherer, Braz.** RP Scherer do Brasil Encapsulacoes Ltda, Av. Gerente Case 1277, 18087-370 Sorocaba, SP, Brazil.

**Scherer, Hong Kong.** See *Atlantic, Hong Kong, Star, Hong Kong, Unam, Hong Kong,* and *Winsor, Hong Kong.*

**Scherer, Ital.** R.P. Scherer S.p.A., Via Nettunese Km. 20,100, 04011 Aprilia (LT), Italy.

**Scherer, Malaysia.** See *Abbott, Malaysia.*

**Scherer, Singapore.** See *Luen Wah, Singapore.*

**Scherer, Thai.** See *Kemopharm, Thai., Osotspa, Thai., Sriprasit, Thai.,* and *Star, Thai.*

**Scherer, USA.** Scherer Laboratories Inc., 2301 Ohio Dr., Suite 234, Plano, TX 75093, USA.

**Schering, Arg.** Schering Argentina S.A.I.C., Monroe 1378, 1428 Buenos Aires, Argentina.

**Schering, Austral.** Schering P/L, 27-31 Doody Street, Alexandria, NSW 2015, Australia.

**Schering, Austria.** Schering Wien GmbH, Scheringgasse 2, A-1147 Vienna, Austria.

**Schering, Belg.** Schering S.A., J.E. Mommaertslaan 14, 1831 Diegem, Belgium.

**Schering, Braz.** Schering do Brasil Quim Farm Ltda, Rua Cancioneiro de Evora 383, 04708-010 Sao Paulo, SP, Brazil.

**Schering, Canad.** Schering Canada Inc., 3535 Trans-Canada Hwy, Pointe-Claire, Quebec, H9R 1B4, Canada.

**Schering, Chile.** Schering de Chile SA, General del Canto 421, CC 3926, Providencia, Santiago, Chile.

**Schering, Denm.** Schering AS, Herstedostervej 27-29, 2620 Albertslund, Denmark.

**Schering, Fin.** Schering Oy, Eerikinkatu 24, PL 179, 00101 Helsinki, Finland.

**Schering, Fr.** Schering, rue de Toufflers, B.P. 69, 59452 Lys-lez-Lannoy cdx, France.

**Schering, Ger.** Schering Deutschland GmbH, Max-Dohrn-Str. 10, 10589 Berlin, Germany.

**Schering, Hong Kong.** Schering (Hong Kong) Ltd, 15/Fl Henan Building, 90-92 Jaffe Rd, Wanchai, Hong Kong.

**Schering, Irl.** See *Clissmann, Irl.*

**Schering, Israel.** See *Agis, Israel.*

**Schering, Ital.** Schering S.p.A., Via E. Schering 21 (z. Marconi), 20090 Segrate (MI), Italy.

**Schering, Jpn.** Nihon Schering K.K., 6-64 Nishimiyahara 2-chome, Yodogawa-ku, Osaka 532-0004, Japan.

**Schering, Malaysia.** See *Zuellig, Malaysia.*

**Schering, Mex.** Schering Mexicana S.A. de C.V., Calz. Mexico Xochimilco No. 5019, Apartado Postal No. 22-111, 14370 Mexico D.F., Mexico.

**Schering, Neth.** Schering Nederland BV, Postbus 116, 1380 AC Weesp, Netherlands.

**Schering, Norw.** Schering Norge A/S, Ringv 3, Postboks 183, 1321 Stabekk, Norway.

**Schering, NZ.** Schering (NZ) Ltd, P.O. Box 101-691, North Shore Mail Centre, Auckland 10, New Zealand.

**Schering, Port.** Schering Lusitana, Lda, Estrada Nacional No 249, km 15, 2726-919 Mem Martins, Portugal.

**Schering, S.Afr.** Schering AG Germany, P.O. Box 5278, Halfway House 1685, South Africa.

**Schering, Singapore.** See *Zuellig, Singapore.*

**Schering, Spain.** Schering, Mendez Alvaro 55, 28045 Madrid, Spain.

**Schering, Swed.** Schering Nordiska AB, Box 912, 175 29 Jarfalla, Sweden.

**Schering, Switz.** Schering (Schweiz) AG, Blegistrasse 5, Postfach, 6341 Baar, Switzerland.

**Schering, Thai.** Schering (Bangkok) Ltd, P.O. Box 106, Laksi Post Office, Bangkok 10210, Thailand.

**Schering, UK.** Schering Health Care Ltd, The Brow, Burgess Hill, West Sussex, RH15 9NE, UK.

**Schering, USA.** See *Schering-Plough, USA.*

**Schering, USA.** See *Schering-Plough, USA.*

**Schering-Plough, Arg.** Schering-Plough S.A., Avenida San Martmn 1750, 1602 Florida, Buenos Aires, Argentina.

**Schering-Plough, Austral.** Schering-Plough P/L, Locked Bag 5011, Baulkham Hills Business Centre, NSW 2153, Australia.

**Schering-Plough, Austria.** See *Aesca, Austria.*

**Schering-Plough, Belg.** Schering-Plough S.A., Rue de Stalle 67, 1180 Brussels, Belgium.

**Schering-Plough, Braz.** Schering Plough, Rua Antonio das Chagas 1623 2° ander, 04714-0024 Sao Paulo, SP, Brazil.

**Schering-Plough, Canad.** Schering-Plough Healthcare Products Canada Inc., 6400 Northam Drive, Mississauga, Ontario, L4V 1J1, Canada.

**Schering-Plough, Chile.** Laboratorio Schering-Plough, Burgos 80, Las Condes, Santiago, Chile.

**Schering-Plough, Denm.** Schering-Plough A/S, Hvedemarken 12, 3520 Farum, Denmark.

**Schering-Plough, Fin.** Schering-Plough Oy, Riihitontuntie 14 A, PL 3, 02201 Espoo, Finland.

**Schering-Plough, Fr.** Schering-Plough, 92 rue Baudin, 92307 Levallois-Perret cdx, France.

**Schering-Plough, Gr.** SCHERING-PLOUGH ABEE, Αγ. Δημητρίου 63, 174 56 Άλιμος, Alimos, Greece.

**Schering-Plough, Hong Kong.** Schering-Plough, Division of SOL Ltd, 17/F Chinachem Exchange Square, 1 Hoi Wan St, Quarry Bay, Hong Kong.

**Schering-Plough, Irl.** See *Pharmacia, Irl.*

**Schering-Plough, Israel.** See *Trading, Israel.*

**Schering-Plough, Ital.** Schering Plough S.p.A., Palazzo Borromini, 20090 Segrate (MI), Italy.

**Schering-Plough, Malaysia.** Schering-Plough Sdn Bhd, Level 3-1, CP Tower, 11 Jln 16/11, Pusat Dagang Seksyen 16, 46350 Petaling Jaya, Selangor, Malaysia.

**Schering-Plough, Mex.** Schering-Plough S.A. de C.V., Av. 16 de Septiembre No. 301, Col. Xaltocan, Deleg. Xochimilco, 16090 Mexico D.F., Mexico.

**Schering-Plough, Neth.** Schering Plough BV, Maarssenbroeksedijk 4, 3542 DN Utrecht, Netherlands.

**Schering-Plough, Norw.** Schering-Plough A/S, Ankerv. 209, 1359 Eiksmarka, Norway.

**Schering-Plough, NZ.** Schering-Plough Pty Ltd, Private Bag 908, Upper Hutt, Wellington, New Zealand.

**Schering-Plough, Port.** Schering-Plough Farma, Lda, Casal Colaride, Agualva, Cacem. Apartado 28, 2736 Cacem Codex, Portugal.

**Schering-Plough, S.Afr.** Schering-Plough (Pty) Ltd, P.O. Box 46, Isando 1600, South Africa.

**Schering-Plough, Singapore.** See *Zuellig, Singapore.*

**Schering-Plough, Spain.** Schering Plough, Po de la Castellana 143, 28046 Madrid, Spain.

**Schering-Plough, Swed.** Schering-Plough AB, Box 27190, 102 52 Stockholm, Sweden.

**Schering-Plough, Thai.** Schering-Plough Ltd, 10 Fl, Maneeya Center Building, 518/5 Ploenchit Rd, Lumpini, Patumwan, Bangkok 10330, Thailand.

**Schering-Plough, UK.** Schering-Plough Ltd, Schering-Plough House, Shire Park, Welwyn Garden City, Herts, AL7 1TW, UK.

**Schering-Plough, USA.** Schering-Plough Corp., Galloping Hill Rd, Kenilworth, NJ 07033-0530, USA.

**Scheurich, Ger.** E. Scheurich Pharma GmbH, Strassburger Str. 77, Postfach: 1361, 77763 Appenweier, Germany.

**Schiapparelli, Ital.** Schiapparelli Farma S.r.l., Via Ragazzi del 99n.5, 40133 Bologna, Italy.

**Schiapparelli Searle, USA.** See *SCS, USA.*

**Schieffer, Ger.** See *Roche Consumer, Ger.*

Schieffer, Switz. Switzerland.

**Schlatter, Switz.** J.P. Schlatter SA, Boulevard de Perolles 17, Case postale 238, 1701 Fribourg, Switzerland.

**Schmid, Canad.** Julius Schmid Canada Ltd, 100 Courtland Ave, Concord, Ontario, L4K 3T6, Canada.

**Schmid, Israel.** Schmid, Israel.

**Schmid, USA.** See *Durex, USA.*

**Schmidgall, Austria.** Dr A & L Schmidgall, Wolfganggasse 45-7, A-1121 Vienna, Austria.

**Schmidt, Malaysia.** Schmidt Scientific Sdn Bhd, 5/F Wisma Domain, No 18A, Lot 318, Jln 51A/223, 46100 Petaling Jaya, Selangor, Malaysia.

**Schoenenberger, Ger.** Walther Schoenenberger GmbH & Co. KG, Muhlstr. 5-7, 71106 Magstadt, Germany.

**Scholl, Israel.** See *Dexxon, Israel.*

**Scholl, UK.** See *SSL, UK.*

**Schonenberger, Switz.** Schönenberger Pharma AG, Schachenstrasse 24, 5012 Schonenwerd, Switzerland.

**Schoning-Berlin, Ger.** Schöning Pharmazeutische Präparate GmbH & Co. KG, Porschestr. 22-24, 12107 Berlin, Germany.

**Schuck, Ger.** Schuck GmbH, Industriestr. 11, 90571 Schwaig b. Nurnberg, Germany.

**Schulke & Mayr, Austria.** Schülke & Mayr GmbH, Zieglergasse 8/3, A-1070 Vienna, Austria.

**Schulke & Mayr, Ger.** Schülke & Mayr GmbH, Robert-Koch-Str. 1, 22851 Norderstedt, Germany.

**Schulke & Mayr, Switz.** Schülke & Mayr AG, Obere Zaune 2, Postfach 865, 8025 Zurich, Switzerland.

**Schulke & Mayr, Thai.** See *Diethelm, Thai.*

**Schumit, Thai.** Schumit 1967 Co. Ltd, 13 Soi Latphrao 91, Latphrao Rd, Wangthonglaeng, Bangkok 10310, Thailand.

**Schupp, Ger.** Schupp GmbH & Co., Postfach: 840, 72238 Freudenstadt, Germany.

**Schur, Ger.** Schur Pharmazeutika GmbH & Co. KG, Schorlemerstr. 68, 40547 Dusseldorf, Germany.

**Schutz, Austria.** Maria Schutz Apotheke, Reinprechtsdorfer Strasse 2, A-1050 Vienna, Austria.

**Schwabe, Arg.** Schwabe S.A.C.I., Tte. Gral. Peron 1666, 1037 Buenos Aires, Argentina.

**Schwabe, Austria.** See *Austroplant, Austria.*

**Schwabe, Ger.** Dr Willmar Schwabe GmbH & Co., Willmar-Schwabe-Str. 4, 76227 Karlsruhe, Germany.

**Schwabe, Malaysia.** See *Antah, Malaysia.*

**Schwabe, Neth.** See *VSM, Neth.*

**Schwabe, Spain.** Dr W Schwabe, Pol Ind Francoli, Parcela 3, Nave 2, 43006 Tarragona, Spain.

**Schwabe, Switz.** Schwabe Pharma AG, Erlistrasse 2, Postfach, 6403 Kussnacht a.R., Switzerland.

**Schwabe Extracta, Ger.** See *Schwabe, Ger.*

**Schwartz, Fr.** Laboratoires Robert Schwartz, Parc d'Innovation, Illkirck, 67400 Strasbourg, France.

**Schwarz, Fr.** Laboratoires Schwarz Pharma, 235 av Le Jour-se-Leve, 92100 Boulogne-Billancourt, France.

**Schwarz, Ger.** Schwarz Pharma Deutschland GmbH, Alfred-Nobel-Str. 10, 40789 Monheim, Germany.

**Schwarz, Hong Kong.** Schwarz Pharma (HK) Ltd, Unit B, 24/F CMA Bldg, 64 Connaught Rd Central, Hong Kong.

**Schwarz, Irl.** See *Allphar, Irl.*

**Schwarz, Ital.** Schwarz Pharma S.p.A., Via Gadames 57, 20151 Milan, Italy.

**Schwarz, Malaysia.** See *Ranbaxy, Malaysia.*

**Schwarz, Norw.** See *Meda, Norw.*

**Schwarz, Singapore.** See *Zyfas, Singapore.*

**Schwarz, Switz.** See *Pharmacia, Switz.*

**Schwarz, Thai.** See *Berli, Thai.*

**Schwarz, UK.** Schwarz Pharma Ltd, Schwarz House, East St, Chesham, Buckinghamshire, HP5 1DG, UK.

**Schwarz, USA.** Schwarz Pharma Inc., P.O. Box 2038, Milwaukee, WI 53201, USA.

**Schwarzhaupt, Austria.** See *Schwarzhaupt, Ger.*

**Schwarzhaupt, Ger.** Kommanditgesellschaft Schwarzhaupt GmbH & Co., Sachsenring 37-47, 50677 Cologne, Germany.

**Schwarzhaupt, Hong Kong.** See *US Summit, Hong Kong.*

**Schwarzhaupt, Thai.** See *Pacific, Thai.*

**Schwarzkopf, Canad.** See *Dep, Canad.*

**Schwarzwalder, Ger.** Schwarzwälder Natur-Heilmittel, Marktplatz 4, 93183 Kallmunz, Germany.

**Schworer, Ger.** Pharma Schwörer GmbH, Goethestr. 29, 69257 Wiesenbach, Germany.

**Schwulst, S.Afr.** Geo Schwulst Laboratories (Pty) Ltd, P.O. Box 38481, Booysens 2016, South Africa.

**Sciclone, Ital.** Sciclone Pharmaceuticals Italy S.r.l., Via Lisbona n. 11, 00198 Rome, Italy.

**Sciclone, Malaysia.** See *Diethelm, Malaysia.*

**Sciclone, Singapore.** See *Zuellig, Singapore.*

**Sciclone, Thai.** See *Diethelm, Thai.*

**Scidia, Arg.** Scidia, Argentina.

**Sciencex, Fr.** Laboratoires Sciencex, 1 rue Edmond-Guillout, 75015 Paris, France.

**Scientific, S.Afr.** Scientific Pharmaceuticals (Pty) Ltd, P.O. Box 13119, Vorna Valley 1686, South Africa.

**Scientific Hospital Supplies, Austral.** Scientific Hospital Supplies, P.O. Box 6745, Baulkham Hills Business Centre, NSW 2153, Australia.

**Scientific Hospital Supplies, Irl.** Scientific Hospital Supplies (Ireland) Ltd, Block 1, Deansgrange Business Park, Co. Dublin, Ireland.

**Scientific Hospital Supplies, Israel.** See *Megapharm, Israel.*

**Scientific Hospital Supplies, NZ.** See *Nutricia, NZ.*

**Scientific Hospital Supplies, UK.** See *SHS, UK.*

**Scigen, Austral.** SciGen Ltd, Level 7, 2 Bligh St, Sydney, NSW 2000, Australia.

**Scigen, Hong Kong.** See *Zuellig, Hong Kong.*

**Scigen, Singapore.** SciGen Pte Ltd, 14 Science Park drive, 04-01A The Maxwell, S 118226, Singapore.

**Scios, USA.** Scios Inc., 820 W Maude Ave, Sunnyvale, CA 94086, USA.

**Scipharm, S.Afr.** Scipharm Ltd, P.O. Box 13119, Vorna Valley 1686, South Africa.

**Sclavo, Israel.** See *Promedico, Israel.*

**Sclavo, Ital.** Sclavo Diagnostics International S.p.A., Via Fiorentina 1, 53100 Siena, Italy.

**Scot, Israel.** See *Trupharm, Israel.*

**Scotia, Denm.** See *Norpharma, Denm.*

**Scotia, Hong Kong.** See *Health Care, Hong Kong.*

**Scotia, Irl.** See *Scotia, UK.*

**Scotia, NZ.** Scotia Pharmaceuticals (NZ) Ltd, P.O. Box 33-118, Takapuna, Auckland, New Zealand.

**Scotia, UK.** Scotia Pharmaceuticals Ltd, Scotia House, Castle Business Park, Stirling, Stirlingshire, FK9 4TZ, UK.

**Scott, Canad.** See *Lander, Canad.*

**Scott-Cassara, Arg.** Scott-Cassara, Galicia 3431/3, 1408 Buenos Aires, Argentina.

**Scot-Tussin, USA.** Scot-Tussin Pharmacal Co. Inc., 50 Clemence St, P.O. Box 8217, Cranston, RI 02920-0217, USA.

**SCS, USA.** SCS Pharmaceuticals, P.O. Box 5110, Chicago, IL 60680-5110, USA.

**SDA, USA.** SDA Laboratories, 280 Railroad Ave, Greenwich, CT 06830, USA.

**SDR, USA.** SDR Pharmaceuticals Inc., Andover, NJ 07821, USA.

**Sea-Band, UK.** Sea-Band Ltd, Lancaster Rd, Hinckley, Leicestershire, LE10 0AW, UK.

**Searle, Austral.** See *Pharmacia, Austral.*

**Searle, Belg.** See *Continental Pharma, Belg.*

**Searle, Braz.** See *Pharmacia, Braz.*

**Searle, Canad.** See *Pharmacia, Canad.*

**Searle, Denm.** See *Pfizer, Denm.*, and *Pharmacia, Denm.*

**Searle, Fin.** See *Pharmacia, Fin.*

**Searle, Hong Kong.** Monsanto Far East Ltd, Searle Division, 2/F, Cityplaza 3, 14 Taikoo Wan Rd, Hong Kong.

**Searle, Irl.** See *Pharmacia, Irl.*

**Searle, Israel.** See *Agis, Israel.*

**Searle, Ital.** See *Monsanto, Ital.*

**Searle, Mex.** See *Pharmacia, Mex.*

**Searle, Neth.** See *Pharmacia, Neth.*

**Searle, NZ.** See *Pharmacia, NZ.*

**Searle, Port.** See *Monsanto, Port.*

**Searle, S.Afr.** See *Pharmacia, S.Afr.*

**Searle, Singapore.** See *Pharmacia, Singapore.*

**Searle, Swed.** See *Pharmacia, Swed.*

**Searle, Switz.** See *Pharmacia, Switz.*

**Searle, Thai.** See *Zuellig, Thai.*

**Searle, UK.** See *Pharmacia, UK.*

**Searle, USA.** See *Pharmacia, USA.*

**Seatrace, USA.** Seatrace Pharmaceuticals, P.O. Box 363, Gadsden, AL 35902-0363, USA.

**Sebamed, Ger.** Sebamed GmbH & Co. KG, Binger Str. 80, 56154 Boppard/Bad Salzig, Germany.

**Sebapharma, Hong Kong.** See *Mekim, Hong Kong.*

**Sebapharma, Thai.** See *Oui Heng, Thai.*

**Seber, Port.** Seber Portuguesa Farmacêutica, SA, Rua Norberto de Oliveira 1-5, 2675-130 Povoa de St Adriao, Portugal.

**Sedabel, Braz.** Laboratorio Sedabel Ltda, Rodovia Washington Luiz 1308 Km 4.5, 25085-000 Duque de Caxias, RJ, Brazil.

**Sedar, Braz.** Sedar Industria Farmaceutica Ltda, Rodovia BR 101 Sul Km 18, Distr. Ind. dos Prazeres, 50950-000 Recife, PE, Brazil.

**Sedifa, Mon.** Laboratoires Sédifa, 4 av. Prince-Hereditaire-Albert, Fontvieille, MC 98000, Monaco.

**SEDR, Israel.** See *Rafa, Israel.*

**Sefarma, Ital.** Sefarma S.r.l., Via Robert Koch 1.2, 20152 Milan, Italy.

**Segix, Ital.** Segix Italia S.p.A., Via del Mare 36, 00040 Pomezia (RM), Italy.

**Seid, Spain.** Seid, Ctra Sabadell Granollers Km 15, Llissa de Vall, 08185 Barcelona, Spain.

**Selder, Mex.** Selder S.A. de C.V., Fernando Villalpando Num. 48, Col. Guadalupe Inn, Deleg. Alvaro Obregon, 01020 Mexico D.F., Mexico.

**Select, Ital.** Select Pharma S.p.A., Via Pontina 100, 04011 Aprilia (LT), Italy.

**Selena, Swed.** See *Selena Fournier, Swed.*

**Selena Fournier, Swed.** Selena Fournier AB, Box 1266, 172 25 Sundbyberg, Sweden.

**Self-Care Products, UK.** Self-Care Products Ltd, 30 Sycamore Rd, Amersham, Buckinghamshire, HP6 5DR, UK.

**Sella, Ital.** Sella A. Lab. Chim. Farm. S.r.l., Via Vicenza 2, 36015 Schio (Vicenza), Italy.

**Selmag, Switz.** Selmag-Weibel, Bergackerweg 4, 3054 Schupfen/BE, Switzerland.

**Selvi, Ital.** Selvi Laboratorio Bioterapico S.p.A., Via Procoio 28, 00065 Fiano Romano (RM), Italy.

**Selz, Ger.** Pharma Selz GmbH, Leininger Ring 65a, 67278 Bockenheim, Germany.

**Semar, Spain.** See *Sanofi Synthelabo, Spain.*

**Semper, Fin.** See *Arla, Fin.*

**Seneca, USA.** Seneca, USA.

**Senese, Ital.** Industria Farmaceutica Galenica Senese S.r.l., Via Cassia Nord 3, 53014 Monteroni d'Arbia (SI), Italy.

**Seng, Hong Kong.** See *Health Alliance, Hong Kong.*

**Seng, Thai.** See *Sang, Thai.*

**Senju, Jpn.** Senju Pharmaceutical Co. Ltd, 2-5-8 Hiranomachi, Chuo-ku, Osaka 541-0046, Japan.

**Senosiain, Mex.** Laboratorios Senosiain S.A. de C.V., Lago Silverio No. 177, Col. Anahuac, Miguel Hidalgo, 11320 Mexico D.F., Mexico.

**Seoul Pharma, Singapore.** See *Pharmaforte, Singapore.*

**Sepharma, Ital.** See *Sefarma, Ital.*

**Sephytal, Fr.** Sephytal SA, 6 av. Charles de Gaulle, 78150 Le Chesnay, France.

**Sepi, Ital.** Sepi Chimica Srl, Via V Grassi 9, 00155 Rome, Italy.

**Sepracor, USA.** Sepracor, 111 Locke Drive, Marlborough, MA 01752, USA.

**Septa, Spain.** Septa Chemifarma, Sierra Guadarrama 11, Pol. Ind. 2, San Fernando de Henares, 28850 Madrid, Spain.

**Septodont, Austral.** Specialites Septodont Pty Ltd., P.O. Box 288, Emu Plains, NSW 2750, Australia.

**Septodont, Denm.** See *CMS-Dental, Denm.*

**Septodont, Norw.** See *Denamed, Norw.*

**Septodont, Switz.** See *Odontopharm, Switz.*

**Septodont, USA.** Septodont Inc., P.O. Box 11926, Wilmington, DE 19850, USA.

**Sequus, Austria.** See *Sequus, UK.*

**Sequus, Israel.** See *Gamida-Medequip, Israel.*

**Sequus, UK.** Sequus Pharmaceuticals Inc., 10 Barley Mow Passage, London, W4 4PH, UK.

**Sequus, USA.** See *Alza, USA.*

**Serag-Wiessner, Ger.** Serag-Wiessner KG, Zum Kugelfang 8-12, 95119 Naila, Germany.

**SERB, Fr.** Laboratoires SERB, 53 rue Villiers de l'Isle Adam, 75020 Paris, France.

**Serch, Arg.** Lab. Serch S.R.L., Av. Arturo Illia 668, 1706 Haedo, Buenos Aires, Argentina.

**Serdex, Port.** See *Confar, Port.*

**Serdex, Thai.** See *Pacific, Thai.*

**Serdia, India.** Serdia Pharmaceuticals (India) Ltd, Serdia House, Off Dr S.S. Rao Rd, Parel, Mumbai 400 012, India.

**Sermmitr, Thai.** Sermmitr c/o The Sermmitr Co. Ltd, 82, 84 Arkarn 2, Ratchamnoen Ave, Bangkok 10200, Thailand.

**Serolab, Switz.** Serolab SA, En Marin, CP36, Ch. de la Vulliette 4, 1000 Lausanne 25, Switzerland.

**Serolam, Israel.** See *Trima, Israel.*

**Serono, Arg.** Serono Argentina S.A., Thames 158, 1642 San Isidro, Buenos Aires, Argentina.

**Serono, Austral.** Serono Australia P/L, Allambie Grove Business Park, 4/25 Frenchs Forest Rd (East), Frenchs Forest, NSW 2086, Australia.

**Serono, Austria.** Serono Austria GmbH, Widerhofergasse 3/24, A-1090 Vienna, Austria.

**Serono, Belg.** Serono Benelux S.A., Rue de l'Association 40-42, 1000 Brussels, Belgium.

**Serono, Braz.** Serono Produtos Farmaceuticos Ltda, Rua Dr Eduardo de Souza Aranha 387, 11° andar, 04543-121 Sao Paulo, SP, Brazil.

**Serono, Canad.** Serono Canada Inc., 1075 North Service Rd, Suite 100, Oakville, Ontario, L6M 2G2, Canada.

**Serono, Denm.** Serono Nordic, Aarhusgade 88, 7, 2100 Copenhagen O, Denmark.

**Serono, Fin.** Serono Nordic, Rajatorpantie 41 C, 01640 Vantaa, Finland.

**Serono, Fr.** Laboratoires Serono, L'Arche du Parc, 738 rue Yves-Kermen, 92658 Boulogne cdx, France.

**Serono, Ger.** Serono Pharma GmbH, Freisinger Str. 5, 85716 Unterschleissheim, Germany.

**Serono, Gr.** SERONO A.E., Κονίτσης 3-5, 151 25 Μαρούσι, Marousi, Greece.

**Serono, Hong Kong.** Serono Hong Kong Ltd, Rm 2004-6, 20/F, Alliance Building, 130-136 Connaught Rd Central, Hong Kong.

**Serono, Irl.** See *Allphar, Irl.*

**Serono, Israel.** See *ASI, Israel.*

**Serono, Ital.** Industria Farmaceutica Serono S.p.A., Via Casilina 125, 00176 Rome, Italy.

**Serono, Malaysia.** See *Antah, Malaysia.*

**Serono, Mex.** Serono de Mexico S.A. de C.V., Av. Insurgentes Sur No. 1898 Piso 16, Colonia Florida, 01030 Mexico D.F., Mexico.

**Serono, Neth.** Serono Benelux, Alexanderstraat 3-5, 2514 TJ The Hague, Netherlands.

**Serono, Norw.** Serono Nordic AB, Luhrtoppen 2, 1470 Lorenskog, Norway.

**Serono, NZ.** Serono, P.O. Box 45-027, Auckland, New Zealand.

**Serono, Port.** Serono, Lda, Rua Tierno Galvan 3, 16 piso-Esc.1, 1070-104 Lisbon, Portugal.

**Serono, S.Afr.** Serono South Africa (Pty) Ltd, P.O. Box 1877, Fourways 2055, South Africa.

**Serono, Singapore.** Serono Singapore Pte Ltd, 9 Temasek Boulevard, 24-01/03 Suntac City Tower 2, S 038989, Singapore.

**Serono, Spain.** Serono, Maria de Molina 40, 28006 Madrid, Spain.

**Serono, Swed.** Serono Nordic AB, Box 1803, 171 21 Solna, Sweden.

**Serono, Switz.** Serono Pharma Schweiz, Steinhauserstrasse 70, 6395 Zug, Switzerland.

**Serono, Thai.** Serono Thailand Co. Ltd, 4 Fl, S & B Tower, 68-68/6 Pan Rd, Silom, Bangrak, Bangkok 10500, Thailand.

**Serono, UK.** Serono UK Ltd, Bedfont Cross, Stanwell Rd, Feltham, Middlesex, TW14 8NX, UK.

**Serono, USA.** Serono Laboratories Inc., One Technology Place, Rockland, MA 02061, USA.

**Serotherapeutisches, Austria.** Serotherapeutisches Institut, Richard-Strauss-Strasse 33, A-1232 Vienna, Austria.

**Seroyal, Canad.** Seroyal International Inc., 44 E Beaver Creek Rd, Unit 17, Richmond Hill, Ontario, L4B 1G8, Canada.

**Serozym, Fr.** See *Grimberg, Fr.*

**SERP, Mon.** SERP, le Triton, 5 rue du Gabian, MC 98000, Monaco.

**Serpero, Ital.** Serpero Industria Galenica Milanese S.p.A., Via F. Serpero 2, 20060 Masate (MI), Italy.

**Serra Pamies, Spain.** Serra Pamies, Ctra de Castellvell 24, Reus, 43206 Tarragona, Spain.

**Serral, Mex.** Serral S.A. de C.V., Adolfo Prieto No. 1009, Col. del Valle, Deleg. Benito Juarez, 03100 Mexico D.F., Mexico.

**Serranita, Arg.** La Serranita, Lab. de Esp. Medic. y Cosmet., Calle 49 3752, 1653 Villa Ballester, Buenos Aires, Argentina.

**Sertex, Arg.** Laboratorio Sertex S.R.L., Brown 2862, 2000 Rosario, Buenos Aires, Argentina.

**Serturner, Ger.** Sertürner Arzneimittel GmbH, Wallenroder Str. 8-10, 13435 Berlin, Germany.

**Serum Institute, India.** Serum Institute of India Ltd, 501 Dalamal Tower, 211 Nariman Point, Mumbai 400 021, India.

**Serum-Werk Bernburg, Ger.** Serum-Werk Bernburg AG, Hallesche Landstr. 105 b, 06406 Bernburg, Germany.

**Servier, Arg.** Servier Argentina S.A., Av. Belgrano 1480, 1093 Buenos Aires, Argentina.

**Servier, Austral.** Servier Laboratories (Australia) P/L, P.O. Box 196, Hawthorn, VIC 3122, Australia.

**Servier, Austria.** Servier Pharma GmbH, Mariahilfe Strasse 20/5, A-1070 Vienna, Austria.

**Servier, Belg.** Servier Benelux S.A., Riverside Business Park, Blvd International 57, 1070 Brussels, Belgium.

**Servier, Braz.** Servier Do Brasil Ltda, Rua Mario Piragibe 23, Lins de Vasconcelos, 20720-320 Rio de Janeiro, RJ, Brazil.

**Servier, Canad.** Servier Canada Inc., 235 blvd Armand-Frappier, Laval, Quebec, H7V 4A7, Canada.

**Servier, Chile.** See *Grunenthal, Chile.*

**Servier, Denm.** Servier Danmark A/S, Roskildevej 39 A, 2000 Frederiksberg, Denmark.

**Servier, Fin.** Servier Finland Oy, Vanhankyläntie 44 C, PL 157, 04401 Järvenpää, Finland.

**Servier, Fr.** Laboratoires Servier, 22 rue Garnier, 92200 Neuilly-sur-Seine, France.

**Servier, Ger.** Servier Deutschland GmbH, Westendstr. 170, 80686 Munich, Germany.

**Servier, Gr.** SERVIER (ΣΕΡΒΙΕ) ΕΛΛΑΣ ΕΠΕ, Λ. Συγγρού 181, 171 21 Ν. Σμύρνη, N. Smirni, Greece.

**Servier, Hong Kong.** Servier Hong Kong Ltd, Rm 1901, 19/F The Lee Gardens, 33 Hysan Ave, Causeway Bay, Hong Kong.

**Servier, Irl.** Servier Laboratories (Ireland) Ltd, Nutley Buildings, Merrion Centre, Dublin 4, Ireland.

**Servier, Israel.** See *Teva, Israel.*

**Servier, Ital.** Servier Italia S.p.A., Via degli Aldobrandeschi 107, 00163 Rome, Italy.

**Servier, Malaysia.** See *Zuellig, Malaysia.*

**Servier, Neth.** Servier Nederland BV, Einsteinweg 82, 2333 CD Leiden, Netherlands.

**Servier, NZ.** Servier Laboratories (NZ) Ltd, P.O. Box 14673, Panmure, Auckland, New Zealand.

**Servier, Port.** Servier Portugal, Lda, Av Antonio Agusto de Aguiar 128, 1069-133 Lisbon, Portugal.

**Servier, S.Afr.** Servier Laboratories (SA) (Pty) Ltd, P.O. Box 930, Rivonia 2128, South Africa.

**Servier, Singapore.** Servier (S) Pte Ltd, 510 Thomson Rd, 09-02 SLF Complex, S 298135, Singapore.

**Servier, Spain.** Servier, Avda de Madronos 33, 28043 Madrid, Spain.

**Servier, Switz.** Servier (Suisse) SA, 21 rue de Veyrot, 1217 Meyrin 1, Switzerland.

**Servier, Thai.** Servier (Thailand) Ltd, 15 Fl, Ploenchit Center Building, 2 Sukhumvit Rd, Klongtoey, Bangkok 10110, Thailand.

**Servier, UK.** Servier Laboratories Ltd, Fulmer Hall, Windmill Rd, Fulmer, Slough, Buckinghamshire, SL3 6HH, UK.

**Servipharm, Hong Kong.** See *Unipharm, Hong Kong.*

**Servipharm, Israel.** Servipharm, Israel.

**Servipharm, Malaysia.** See *JDH, Malaysia.*

**Servipharm, Singapore.** See *FP, Singapore.*

**Servipharm, Switz.** Servipharm AG, Postfach, 4002 Basle, Switzerland.

**Servipharm, Thai.** See *Zuellig, Thai.*

**Sessa, Ital.** Sessa Carlo S.p.A., Viale Gramsci 212, 20099 Sesto S. Giovanni (MI), Italy.

**Seton, Irl.** See *SSL, Irl.*

**Seton, Israel.** See *Pharmateam, Israel.*
**Seton, NZ.** See *Pharmaco, NZ.*
**Seton, UK.** See *SSL, UK.*
**Seton Scholl, Austral.** See *SSL, Austral.*
**Seton Scholl, Fr.** See *SSL, Fr.*
**Seven Seas, Irl.** Seven Seas (Ireland) Ltd, 7 The Anchorage, Charlotte Quay, Dublin 4, Ireland.
**Seven Seas, Singapore.** See *Zuellig, Singapore.*
**Seven Seas, UK.** Seven Seas Ltd, Hedon Rd, Marfleet, Hull, HU9 5NJ, UK.
**Seven Stars, Thai.** See *Charoen, Thai.*
**Seyer, USA.** Seyer Pharmatec Inc., 413 St George Street, San Juan, PR 00936, USA.
**SFD, Port.** Sociedade Farmaceutica de Desenvolvimento, Lda, Rua Duque d'Avila no 193, 1050-082 Lisbon, Portugal.
**Shabba, Arg.** Lab. Shabba S.R.L., Dorrego 3246, 1650 San Martin, Buenos Aires, Argentina.
**Shaklee, Canad.** Shaklee Canada Inc., 952 Century Dr, Burlington, Ontario, L7L 5P2, Canada.
**Shalpharm, Israel.** See *Rekah, Israel.*
**Shanta, India.** Shanta Biotechnics Pvt Ltd, 3rd Floor, Serene Chambers, Road No.7, Banjara Hills, Hyderabad 500 021, India.
**Shantys, UK.** Shanty's Ltd, 3-4 Coppen Rd, Dagenham, Essex, RM8 1HU, UK.
**Sharpe, NZ.** See *Douglas, NZ.*
**Shepa, Gr.** SHEPA OE, Βερανζέρου 33, 104 32 Αθήνα, Athens, Greece.
**Shepherd, Canad.** Shepherd Pharmaceuticals Inc., 3332 Yonge St, P.O. Box 94018, Toronto, Ontario, M4N 3R1, Canada.
**Sheraton, Hong Kong.** Sheraton Worldwide Drugs Co. Ltd, 3/F Flat A & 6/F Flat B, Heep Cheung Commercial Bldg, 251 Temple St, Tsimshatsui, Kowloon, Hong Kong.
**Sherman, Israel.** Sherman, Israel.
**Sherman, USA.** Sherman Pharmaceuticals Inc., P.O. Box 1377, Mandeville, LA 70470-1377, USA.
**Sherwood, USA.** See *Kendall, USA.*
**Shield, Irl.** Shield Health Ltd, Unit 1, Thompson Business Park, Clane, Co. Kildare, Ireland.
**Shigaken, Singapore.** See *Luen Wah, Singapore.*
**Shin Poong, Singapore.** See *Zyfas, Singapore.*
**Shinfuso, Thai.** See *Asian TJD, Thai.*
**Shinnick, Austral.** Shinnick Pharmaceuticals, 6/6-18 Bridge Rd, Hornsby, NSW 2077, Australia.
**Shinyaku, Hong Kong.** See *Hing Ah, Hong Kong.*
**Shinyaku, Jpn.** Nippon Shinyaku Co. Ltd, 14 Nishinosho-Monguchi-cho, Kisshoin, Minami-ku, Kyoto 601-8550, Japan.
**Shinyaku, Malaysia.** See *Wellchem, Malaysia.*
**Shinyaku, Singapore.** See *Wellchem, Singapore.*
**Shinyaku, Thai.** See *Asian TJD, Thai.*
**Shionogi, Jpn.** Shionogi & Co. Ltd, 3-1-8 Doshomachi, Chuo-ku, Osaka 541-0045, Japan.
**Shionogi, USA.** Shionogi USA Inc., 3848 Carson St, Suite 206, Torrance, CA 90503, USA.
**Shire, Canad.** Shire Canada Inc., 400 Iroquois Shore Rd, Oakville, Ontario, L6H 1M5, Canada.
**Shire, Denm.** See *Meda, Denm.*
**Shire, Fr.** Shire France, 160 rue de Paris, 92771 Boulogne-Billancourt, France.
**Shire, Ger.** Shire Deutschland GmbH & Co. KG, Siegburger Str. 126, 50679 Cologne, Germany.
**Shire, Hong Kong.** See *JDH, Hong Kong.*
**Shire, Irl.** Shire Pharmaceuticals Ireland Ltd, Pharmapark, Chapelizod, Dublin 20, Ireland.
**Shire, Ital.** Shire Italia S.p.A., Via Provinciale Lucchese 70, 50019 Sesto Fiorentino (FI), Italy.
**Shire, Malaysia.** See *JDH, Malaysia.*
**Shire, Norw.** See *Meda, Norw.*
**Shire, Singapore.** See *JDH, Singapore.*
**Shire, Spain.** Shire Pharmaceuticals Iberica, Benito Gutierrez 26, 28008, Spain.
**Shire, UK.** Shire Pharmaceuticals Ltd, Hampshire International Business Park, Chineham, Basingstoke, Hampshire, RG24 8EP, UK.
**Shire Biochem, Canad.** Shire Biochem Inc., 275 Armand-Frappier Bvld, Laval, Quebec, H7V 4A7, Canada.
**Shire Biologics, Canad.** Shire Biologics, Division of Shire Biochem Inc., 2323 Parc Technologique Bvld, Sainte-Foy, Quebec, G1P 4R8, Canada.
**Shire Richwood, USA.** Shire Richwood Inc., 7900 Tanners Gate Dr., Suite 200, Florence, KY 41042, USA.
**Shiseido, Canad.** Shiseido Company Ltd, 486 Queen St E, Ste 212, Toronto, Ontario, M5A 1T7, Canada.
**Shiwa, Thai.** Shiwa Chemicals Co. Ltd, 34/1 Sukhumvit 39, (Soi Prompong), Bangkok 10110, Thailand.
**Shoppers Drug Mart, Canad.** Shoppers Drug Mart, 225 Yorkland Blvd, Willowdale, Ontario, M2J 4Y7, Canada.
**SHS, Fr.** SHS International Ltd, 4 passage St-Antoine, 92508 Rueil-Malmaison, France.
**SHS, Israel.** See *Megapharm, Israel.*
**SHS, Singapore.** See *Pharma 2000, Singapore.*
**SHS, UK.** SHS International Ltd, 100 Wavertree Boulevard, Liverpool, Merseyside, L7 9PT, UK.
**SHS, USA.** SHS N. America/Scientific Hospital Supplies, 9600 Medical Center Drive, Suite 102, Rockville, MD 20850, USA.
**Siam Bheasach, Thai.** See *Siam Pharm, Thai.*
**Siam Medicare, Thai.** Siam Medicare Co. Ltd, 77/37 Soi Senanikom 1, Phaholyothin Rd, Bangkok 10900, Thailand.
**Siam Pharm, Thai.** Siam Pharmaceutical Co. Ltd, 171/1 Soi Choke Chai Ruammitr, Vibhavadi-Rangsit Rd, Bangkok 10900, Thailand.
**Sibras, Braz.** Sibras Laboratorios Ltda, Avenida Pedro Adams Filho 2.340, 93320-000 Novo Hamburgo, RS, Brazil.
**Sicomed, Hong Kong.** See *Hong Kong Medical, Hong Kong.*
**Sicor, Ital.** Sicor S.p.A., Via Terrazzano 77, 20017 Rho (MI), Italy.
**Sicor, USA.** SICOR Inc., 19 Hughes, Irvine, CA 92718, USA.
**Sidefarma, Port.** Sidefarma, Lda, Rua da Guine, Prior Velho, 2685 Sacavem, Portugal.
**Sidepal, Braz.** Sidepal Industrial e Comercial Ltda, Av. Nova Cumbica 920/30, 7231000 Guarulhos, SP, Brazil.
**Sidmak, India.** Sidmak Laboratories (India) Ltd, National Highway No.8, Abrama, Valsad 396 001, India.
**Sidone, Braz.** Sidone Industria e Comercio Ltda., Rua Sao Francisco Xavier 930, 38412-080 Uberlandia, MG, Brazil.
**Sidroga, Switz.** Sidroga AG, Postfach, 4800 Zofingen, Switzerland.
**Sidus, Arg.** Laboratorios Sidus S.A., Av. del Libertador 742, 1638 Vicente Lopez, Buenos Aires, Argentina.
**Siegfried, Swed.** Siegfried, Nonnens vag 6, 451 50 Uddevalla, Sweden.
**Siegfried, Switz.** Siegfried CMS AG, 4800 Zofingen, Switzerland.
**Siegfried, Thai.** See *Diethelm, Thai.*
**Siemens, Ger.** Siemens & Co., Heilwasser und Quellenprodukte des Staatsbades Bad Ems GmbH & Co. KG, Arzbacher Str. 78, 56130 Bad Ems, Germany.
**Siemens, Switz.** See *Ecosol, Switz.*
**Sifarma, Ital.** Sifarma S.p.A., Via Brunelleschi 12, 20146 Milan, Italy.
**SIFI, Ital.** Società Industria Farmaceutica Italiana S.p.A., Via Ercole Patti 36, 95020 Lavinao-Aci S. Antonio (CY), Italy.
**SIFI, Singapore.** See *Green Cross, Singapore.*
**SIFRA, Ital.** See *Fresenius Kabi, Ital.*
**Sigma, Austral.** Sigma Pharmaceuticals P/L, 96 Merrindale Drive, Croydon, VIC 3136, Australia.
**Sigma, Braz.** See *Novaquimica, Braz.*
**Sigma, Hong Kong.** See *LCH, Hong Kong,* and *Treasure Mountain, Hong Kong.*
**Sigma, India.** Sigma Laboratories Ltd, 18 Subhash Rd, Vile Parle (E), Mumbai 400 057, India.
**Sigma, NZ.** See *Zuellig, NZ.*
**Sigma, UK.** Sigma Chemical Co. Ltd, P.O. Box 233, Watford, Hertfordshire, WD2 4EW, UK.
**Sigmapharm, Austria.** Sigmapharm Arzneimittel GmbH & Co KG, Leystrasse 129, A-1204 Vienna, Austria.
**Sigmapharm, Switz.** See *Ridupharm, Switz.*
**Sigma-Tau, Canad.** Sigma-Tau Pharmaceuticals Inc., 200 Ellesmere Rd, Unit 16, Scarborough, Ontario, M1H 2W4, Canada.
**Sigma-Tau, Fr.** Sigma-Tau France, 5 av. de Verdun, 94202 Ivry sur Seine, France.
**Sigma-Tau, Ger.** Sigma-Tau Arzneimittel GmbH, Am Wehrhahn 86, 40211 Dusseldorf, Germany.
**Sigma-Tau, Hong Kong.** See *Keller, Hong Kong,* and *Sino-Asia, Hong Kong.*
**Sigma-Tau, Ital.** Sigma Tau S.p.A., Via Pontina Km. 30,400, 00040 Pomezia (Rome), Italy.
**Sigma-Tau, Neth.** Sigma-Tau Ethifarma B.V., Postbus 10072, 9400 CB Assen, Netherlands.
**Sigma-Tau, Spain.** Sigma Tau, Pl. Ind. Azque C/Bolivia 15, Alcala de Henares, 28806 Madrid, Spain.
**Sigma-Tau, Switz.** Sigma-Tau Pharma AG, Luzernerstrasse 2, 4800 Zofingen, Switzerland.
**Sigma-Tau, USA.** Sigma-Tau Pharmaceuticals Inc., 800 S Frederick Ave, Suite 300, Gaithersburg, MD 20877, USA.
**Silanes, Mex.** Laboratorios Silanes S.A. de C.V., Amores No. 1304, Col. del Valle, Deleg. Benito Juarez, 03100 Mexico D.F., Mexico.
**Silarx, USA.** Silarx Pharmaceuticals Inc., 19 West St, Spring Valley, NY 10977, USA.
**Silesia, Chile.** Laboratorios Silesia SA, Av. Chile Espana 325, Santiago, Chile.
**Silhouette, Austria.** Silhouette International GmbH, Ellbognerstrasse 24, A-4020 Linz, Austria.
**Silom, Thai.** Silom Medical Co. Ltd, 35/3 Suparaj Soi 1, Phaholyothin Rd, Samsennai, Bangkok 10400, Thailand.
**Silroc, Hong Kong.** Silroc International (HK) Ltd, Unit C, 5/F, Skyline Tower, 18 Tong Mi Rd, Mongkok, Kowloon, Hong Kong.
**Silvestre, Braz.** Silvestre Labs. Quimica & Farmaceutica Ltda., Av. Vinte e Quatro S/N, 21941-590 Rio de Janeiro, RJ, Brazil.
**Simco, Switz.** See *Unipharma, Switz.*
**Sime Darby, Malaysia.** Sime Darby Marketing Sdn Bhd, F-F10, Mezzanine Fl, Lot PT 11101, Kompleks Sime Darby, Jln Kewajipan, 47600 Subang Jaya, Selangor, Malaysia.
**Sime Darby, Singapore.** Sime Darby Marketing, A Division of Sime Darby Singapore Ltd, 896 Dunearn Rd, 04-03 Sime Darby Centre, S 589472, Singapore.
**Simesa, Ital.** Simesa S.p.A., Via F. Sforza Palazzo Galileo, 20080 Basiglio (MI), Italy.
**Simoes, Braz.** Laboratorio Simoes Ltda, Rua Pereira de Almeida 102, 20260-100 Rio de Janeiro, RJ, Brazil.
**Simons, Ger.** Georg Simons GmbH, Bunsenstr. 5, 82152 Planegg/Martinsried, Germany.
**Sinbio, Fr.** See *Pierre Fabre, Fr.*
**Sincerity, Hong Kong.** Sincerity (Asia) Co. Ltd, 1/F, Blk E, Nam Pak Hong Bldg, 24 Bonham Strand W, Hong Kong.
**Sinclair, Irl.** See *Pinewood, Irl.*
**Sinclair, UK.** Sinclair Pharmaceuticals Ltd, Borough Rd, Godalming, Surrey, GU7 2AB, UK.
**Singer, Hong Kong.** See *Zuellig, Hong Kong.*
**Singer, Switz.** Pharma-Singer AG, Windeggstrasse 2, 8867 Niederurnen, Switzerland.
**Sino-Asia, Hong Kong.** Sino-Asia Pharmaceutical Supplies Ltd, 1 Fung Fai Terrace, Upper G/F, Village Rd, Happy Valley, Hong Kong.
**Sintactica, Ital.** Sintactica S.r.l., Strada Padana Superiore 1, 20060 Cassina de' Pecchi (MI), Italy.
**Sinterapico, Braz.** Laboratorio Sinterapico Industrial e Farmaceutico Ltda, Rua Olegario Cunha Lobo 25, 12940-000 Atibaia, SP, Brazil.
**Sintesa, Belg.** Sintesa S.A., Blvd de la Woluwe 34 Bte 11, 1200 Brussels, Belgium.
**Sintesina, Arg.** Sintesina S.A., Av. Pte. Arturo Illia 4194, 1613 Los Polvorines, Buenos Aires, Argentina.
**Sintetica, Switz.** Sintetica SA, Via Penate 5, casella postale 1764, 6850 Mendrisio, Switzerland.
**Sintofarm, Ital.** Sintofarm Farmaceutici S.p.A., Via Torri Bianche 1, 20059 Vimercate (MI), Italy.
**Sintofarma, Braz.** Laboratorios Sintofarma S.A., Rua Sergipe 120, 01243-000 Sao Paulo, SP, Brazil.
**Sipaco, Denm.** See *Niche, Denm.*
**Sipaco, Port.** Sipaco Internacional, Avda 5 de Outubro 267,6, 01600 Lisbon, Portugal.
**Sipaco, Spain.** See *Sipaco, Port.*
**Siphar, Switz.** Siphar SA, Casella postale 32, 6814 Cadempino, Switzerland.
**SIRC, Singapore.** See *Zyfas, Singapore.*
**Sirius, USA.** Sirius Laboratories Inc., 100 Fairway Drive, Suite 130, Vernon Hills, IL 60061, USA.
**Sirmeta, Austral.** Sirmeta, Australia.
**Sirval, Ital.** Società Italiana Ritrovati Val s.a.s., Via Maloia 8, 20158 Milan, Italy.
**Sisu, Canad.** Sisu Enterprises Ltd, 104A-3430 Brighton Ave, Burnaby, British Columbia, V5A 3H4, Canada.
**SIT, Ital.** Specialità Igienico Terapeutiche S.r.l., C.so Cavour 70, 27035 Mede (Pavia), Italy.
**Sivaderm, Arg.** Lab. Sivaderm S.A., Sarmiento 2171 Pso. 8 Dto.A, 1044 Buenos Aires, Argentina.
**SK, Singapore.** See *Wellchem, Singapore.*
**Skills, Ital.** Skills in Farmacia S.r.l., Piazza Buonarroti 32, 20145 Milan, Italy.
**Skinicles, Canad.** Skinicles Ltd, 150 Priscilla Ave, P.O. Box 1655, Toronto, Ontario, M6S 3W3, Canada.
**SkinMedica, USA.** SkinMedica Inc., 5909 Sea Lion Place, Ste H, Carlsbad, CA 92008, USA.
**SK-RIT, Belg.** See *SmithKline Beecham, Belg.*
**Skye, USA.** SkyePharma Inc., 10450 Science Center Drive, San Diego, CA 92121, USA.
**Slapak, Arg.** Lab. León Slapak Esp. Medicinales S.R.L., Alte. F.J. Segum 1167, 1416 Buenos Aires, Argentina.
**SLE, Israel.** See *Madaus, Israel.*
**Slimax, Austral.** Slimax, Australia.
**Slovakofarma, Singapore.** See *Sime Darby, Singapore.*
**Slovakofarma, Thai.** See *Medline, Thai.*
**SM, Thai.** SM Pharmaceutcal Co. Ltd, 82, 84 Arkarn 2, Ratchdamnoen Ave, Bangkok 10200, Thailand.
**SMA Nutrition, Irl.** See *Wyeth, UK.*
**Smaller, Spain.** See *ASAC, Spain.*
**SMB, Belg.** Laboratoires S.M.B. S.A., Rue de la Pastorale 26-28, 1080 Brussels, Belgium.
**SMB, Chile.** Laboratorios SMB Farma SA, Av. Bulnes 377, Dpto 305, Santiago, Chile.
**SMB, Thai.** See *Berlin Pharm, Thai.*
**Smetana, Austria.** See *EF-EM-ES, Austria.*
**Smith & Nephew, Austral.** Smith & Nephew P/L, P.O. Box 150, Clayton, VIC 3168, Australia.
**Smith & Nephew, Canad.** Smith & Nephew Inc., 4707 Levy St, St-Laurent, Quebec, H4R 2P9, Canada.
**Smith & Nephew, Denm.** Smith & Nephew A/S, Naerum Hovedgade 2, 2850 Naerum, Denmark.
**Smith & Nephew, Fin.** Smith & Nephew Oy, Rajatorpantie 41 C, 01640 Vantaa, Finland.
**Smith & Nephew, Fr.** Smith & Nephew SA, 25 bd Alexandre-Oyon, 72019 Le Mans cdx 2, France.
**Smith & Nephew, Ger.** Smith & Nephew GmbH, Max-Planck-Str. 103, 34253 Lohfelden, Germany.
**Smith & Nephew, Hong Kong.** Smith & Nephew Ltd, Unit 1318, 13/F Grandtech Ctr, 8 On Ping St, Siu Lek Yuen, Shatin, N.T., Hong Kong.
**Smith & Nephew, Irl.** Smith & Nephew Medical, Carraig Court, George's Ave, Blackrock, Co. Dublin, Ireland.
**Smith & Nephew, Ital.** Smith & Nephew S.r.l., Viale Colleoni 13, 20041 Agrate Brianza (MI), Italy.
**Smith & Nephew, Neth.** See *GlaxoSmithKline, Neth.*
**Smith & Nephew, Norw.** Smith & Nephew AS, Postboks 224, 1379 Nesbru, Norway.
**Smith & Nephew, NZ.** Smith & Nephew Ltd, P.O. Box 442, Auckland, New Zealand.
**Smith & Nephew, S.Afr.** Smith & Nephew Pharmaceuticals (Pty) Ltd, P.O. Box 92, Pinetown 3600, South Africa.
**Smith & Nephew, Singapore.** See *Zuellig, Singapore.*
**Smith & Nephew, Spain.** Smith Nephew, Fructous Gelabert 2-4, Sant Joan Despi, 08970 Barcelona, Spain.
**Smith & Nephew, Swed.** Smith & Nephew AB, Box 143, 431 22 Molndal, Sweden.
**Smith & Nephew, Switz.** Smith & Nephew AG, Glutz Blotzheim-Strasse 1, 4502 Solothurn, Switzerland.
**Smith & Nephew, Thai.** Smith & Nephew Ltd, 344/3 Soi Rongrien Yepun, Rama IX Rd, Bangapi, Huay Kwang, Bangkok 10320, Thailand.
**Smith & Nephew, UK.** See *Smith & Nephew Healthcare, UK.*
**Smith & Nephew, USA.** Smith & Nephew United, 11775 Starkey Rd, Largo, FL 33773-1970, USA.
**Smith & Nephew Healthcare, UK.** Smith & Nephew Healthcare Ltd, Healthcare House, Goulton St, Hull, HU3 4DJ, UK.
**Smith & Nephew SoloPak, USA.** See *SoloPak, USA.*
**Smith Kline & French, Port.** See *GlaxoSmithKline, Port.*
**SmithKline, Spain.** See *GlaxoSmithKline, Spain.*
**SmithKline Beecham, Austral.** See *GlaxoSmithKline, Austral.*
**SmithKline Beecham, Austria.** See *GlaxoSmithKline, Austria.*
**SmithKline Beecham, Belg.** See *GlaxoSmithKline, Belg.*
**SmithKline Beecham, Braz.** See *GlaxoSmithKline, Braz.*
**SmithKline Beecham, Canad.** See *GlaxoSmithKline, Canad.*
**SmithKline Beecham, Denm.** See *GlaxoSmithKline, Denm.*
**SmithKline Beecham, Fr.** See *GlaxoSmithKline, Fr.*
**SmithKline Beecham, Ger.** See *GlaxoSmithKline, Ger.*
**SmithKline Beecham, Gr.** SMITH KLINE-BEECHAM AEBE, Κόδρου 3, 155 32 Χαλάνδρι, Chalandri, Greece.
**SmithKline Beecham, Hong Kong.** See *GlaxoSmithKline, Hong Kong.*
**SmithKline Beecham, Irl.** See *GlaxoSmithKline, Irl.*
**SmithKline Beecham, Israel.** See *GlaxoSmithKline, Israel.*
**SmithKline Beecham, Ital.** See *GlaxoSmithKline, Ital.*
**SmithKline Beecham, Jpn.** See *GlaxoSmithKline, Jpn.*
**SmithKline Beecham, Mex.** See *GlaxoSmithKline Consumer, Mex.*
**SmithKline Beecham, Neth.** See *GlaxoSmithKline, Neth.*
**SmithKline Beecham, Norw.** See *GlaxoSmithKline, Norw.*
**SmithKline Beecham, NZ.** See *GlaxoSmithKline, NZ.*
**SmithKline Beecham, S.Afr.** See *GlaxoSmithKline, S.Afr.*
**SmithKline Beecham, Singapore.** See *GlaxoSmithKline, Singapore.*
**SmithKline Beecham, Spain.** See *GlaxoSmithKline, Spain.*
**SmithKline Beecham, Switz.** See *GlaxoSmithKline, Switz.*
**SmithKline Beecham, Thai.** See *GlaxoSmithKline, Thai.*
**SmithKline Beecham, UK.** See *GlaxoSmithKline, UK.*
**SmithKline Beecham, USA.** SmithKline Beecham Pharmaceuticals, 1 Franklin Plaza, P.O. Box 7929, Philadelphia, PA 19101, USA.
**SmithKline Beecham Consumer, Austral.** See *GlaxoSmithKline Consumer, Austral.*
**SmithKline Beecham Consumer, Belg.** See *GlaxoSmithKline, Belg.*
**SmithKline Beecham Consumer, Canad.** See *GlaxoSmithKline Consumer, Canad.*
**SmithKline Beecham Consumer, Irl.** See *GlaxoSmithKline, Irl.*
**SmithKline Beecham Consumer, Neth.** See *GlaxoSmithKline, Neth.*
**SmithKline Beecham Consumer, Switz.** SmithKline Beecham Consumer Healthcare AG, Brunnmattstrasse 5, Postfach, 3174 Thorishaus, Switzerland.
**SmithKline Beecham Consumer, UK.** See *GlaxoSmithKline, UK.*

**SmithKline Beecham Consumer, USA.** SmithKline Beecham Consumer Healthcare L.P., Unit of SmithKline Beecham Inc., P.O. Box 1467, Pittsburgh, PA 15230, USA.

**SmithKline Beecham OTC, Ger.** See *GlaxoSmithKline Consumer, Ger.*

**SmithKline Beecham Sante, Fr.** See *GlaxoSmithKline, Fr.*

**SmithKline Diagnostics, USA.** See *Beckman, USA.*

**SMTL, UK.** Surgical Materials Testing Laboratory, Princess of Wales Hospital, Coity Rd, Bridgend, Mid Glamorgan, CF31 1RQ, UK.

**SNBTS, UK.** Scottish National Blood Transfusion Service, Protein Fractionation Centre, Ellen's Glen Rd, Edinburgh, EH17 7QT, UK.

**Sobral, Braz.** Laboratorio Industrial Farmaceutico Sobral, Rua Bento Leao 25, Floriano Pl, Brazil.

**Socopharm, Fr.** Laboratoires Socopharm, Chemin de Marcy, 58800 Corbigny, France.

**Sodia, Fr.** Laboratoires Sodia, av. Robert Schuman, 51100 Reims, France.

**Sodilac, Fr.** See *Wyeth Lederle, Fr.*

**Sodip, Switz.** Sodip SA, 11 rue Alphonse-Large, 1217 Meyrin 1, Switzerland.

**Sofar, Ital.** Sofar Farmaceutici S.p.A., Via Firenze 40, 20060 Trezzano Rosa (MI), Italy.

**Sofex, Port.** Sofex Farmacêutica, Lda, Rua Sebastiao e Silva 25, Zona Industrial de Massama, 2745-838 Queluz, Portugal.

**SofLens, S.Afr.** See *Bausch & Lomb, S.Afr.*

**Sohan, Canad.** Sohan Chemicals Ltd, 70 Gibson Drive, Unit 14, Markham, ON, L3R 2Z3, Canada.

**Sojar, Arg.** Sojar S.A., Velez Sarsfield 870, 2013 Rosario, Santa Fe, Argentina.

**Solar, Canad.** Solar Cosmetics Labs Inc, 6845 Rexwood Rd, Unit 3-5, Mississauga, Ontario, L4V 1S5, Canada.

**Solco, Austria.** Solco Pharma Austria GmbH, Michael Pacher Strasse 25A/7, A-5020 Salzburg, Austria.

**Solco, Fin.** See *Oriola, Fin.*

**Solco, Ger.** See *ICN, Ger.*

**Solco, Hong Kong.** See *Kai Cheong, Hong Kong.*

**Solco, Ital.** Solco, Italy.

**Solco, Malaysia.** See *Pharmaforte, Malaysia.*

**Solco, Singapore.** See *Pharmaforte, Singapore.*

**Solco, Swed.** See *Solco, Ger.*

**Solco, Switz.** Solco Basel SA, Ruhrbergstrasse 21, 4127 Birsfelden, Switzerland.

**Solco, Thai.** See *Diethelm, Thai.*

**Soldan, Ger.** Dr. C. Soldan GmbH, Herderstr. 5-9, 90427 Nurnberg, Germany.

**Solea, Ital.** Solea S.a.s., Via Cassoli 22, 42100 Reggio Emilia, Italy.

**Solfran, Mex.** Laboratorios Solfran S.A., Altos Hornos No. 2721, Fracc. Ind. el Alamo, 44490 Tlaquepaque, Jal., Mexico.

**Solgar, UK.** See *Boots, UK.*

**Solgar, USA.** Solgar Vitamin Co. Inc., 500 Willow Tree Rd, Leonia, NJ 07605, USA.

**Solmer, Switz.** Solmer SA, Postfach 100, 6976 Castagnola-Suisse, Switzerland.

**SoloPak, USA.** SoloPak Pharmaceuticals Inc., 1845 Tonne Rd, Elk Grove Village, IL 60007-5125, USA.

**Solpro, Mex.** Solpro S.A. de C.V., Ciruelos No. 137, Local 26, Centro Comercial El Pinar, Jurica, 76100 Queretaro, Mexico.

**Soludia, Fr.** Laboratoires Soludia, Rte de Revel, 31450 Fourquevaux, France.

**Solus, India.** See *Ranbaxy, India.*

**Solvay, Austral.** Solvay Pharmaceuticals, Division of Solvay Biosciences P/L, Locked Bag 1070, Pymble, NSW 2073, Australia.

**Solvay, Austria.** Solvay Pharma GmbH, Donaustrasse 106, A-3400 Klosterneuburg, Austria.

**Solvay, Belg.** Solvay Pharma & Cie S.N.C., Blue Planet Building, Ave Bourgemestre E. Demunter 3, 1090 Brussels, Belgium.

**Solvay, Canad.** Solvay Pharma Inc., 50 Venture Drive, Scarborough, Ontario, M1B 3LG, Canada.

**Solvay, Denm.** Solvay Pharma ApS, Horkaer 32, 1, 2730 Herlev, Denmark.

**Solvay, Fin.** See *Algol, Fin.*

**Solvay, Fr.** Solvay Pharma, 42 rue Rouget-de-Lisle, B.P. 22, 92151 Suresnes cdx, France.

**Solvay, Ger.** Solvay Arzneimittel GmbH, Hans-Bockler-Allee 20, 30173 Hannover, Germany.

**Solvay, Gr.** SOLVAY PHARMA M.E.Π.E., Αγ. Δημητρίου 63, 174 56 Άλιμος, Alimos, Greece.

**Solvay, Hong Kong.** See *Keller, Hong Kong.*

**Solvay, India.** Solvay Pharma India Ltd, Suraj Prakash, 1st floor, 86 Shankar Ghanekar Marg, Prabhadevi, Mumbai 400 025, India.

**Solvay, Irl.** Solvay Healthcare Ltd, Belgard Rd, Tallaght, Dublin 24, Ireland.

**Solvay, Israel.** See *Agis, Israel.*

**Solvay, Ital.** Solvay Pharma S.p.A., Via della Liberta 30, 10095 Grugliasco (TO), Italy.

**Solvay, Malaysia.** See *Zuellig, Malaysia.*

**Solvay, Neth.** Solvay Pharma BV, C J Van Houtenlaan 36, 1381 CP Weesp, Netherlands.

**Solvay, Norw.** Solvay Pharma AS, Hamang Terrasse 55, Postboks 248, 1301 Sandvika, Norway.

**Solvay, NZ.** See *Russells, NZ.*

**Solvay, Port.** Solvayfarma, Lda, Av. Marechal Gomes da Costa 33, 1800-255 Lisbon, Portugal.

**Solvay, S.Afr.** Solvay Pharma (Pty) Ltd, P.O. Box 5278, halfway House 1685, South Africa.

**Solvay, Singapore.** See *Sime Darby, Singapore.*

**Solvay, Spain.** Solvay Pharma, Avda Diagonal 507-509, 08029 Barcelona, Spain.

**Solvay, Swed.** Solvay Pharma AB, Sisjo Kullegata 8, 421 32 Vastra Frolunda, Sweden.

**Solvay, Switz.** Solvay Pharma AG, Untermattweg 8, 3027 Bern, Switzerland.

**Solvay, Thai.** See *Berli, Thai.*

**Solvay, UK.** Solvay Healthcare, Mansbridge Rd, West End, Southampton, Hampshire, SO18 3JD, UK.

**Solvay, USA.** Solvay Pharmaceuticals Inc., 901 Sawyer Road, Marietta, GA 30062-2224, USA.

**Solvay Duphar, Swed.** See *Meda, Swed.*

**Solver, Ital.** Solver Pharma S.r.l., Via G. Revere 16, 20123 Milan, Italy.

**Soma, Switz.** Soma Pharma AG, Soma Medical, Ruessenstrasse 5A, 6340 Baar, Switzerland.

**Somedico, Malaysia.** Somedico Sdn Bhd, 68 Jln SS 21/39, Damansara Utama, 47400 Petaling Jaya, Selangor, Malaysia.

**Somerset, USA.** Somerset Pharmaceuticals Inc., 777 S Harbour Island Bvld, Suite 880, Tampa, FL 33602, USA.

**Sons, Mex.** Laboratorios Quimica Son's S.A. de C.V., Av. 23 Poniente No. 2302-A, 72410 Puebla, Pue., Mexico.

**Sooft, Ital.** Sooft Italia Srl, C.da Molino 17, 63025 Montegiorgio, Italy.

**Sophia, Mex.** Laboratorios Sophia S.A. de C.V., Hidalgo 737, 44290 Guadalajara, Mexico.

**Soria Natural, Spain.** Soria Natural, Pol Ind La Sacea 1, Garray, 42162 Soria, Spain.

**Sorin, Spain.** Sorin, Spain.

**Sorin-Maxim, Fr.** Laboratoires Sorin-Maxim, rue Claude-Bernard, 12700 Capdenac, France.

**SoSe, Ital.** So.Se. Pharm S.r.l., Via dei Castelli Romani 22, 00040 Pomezia (Rome), Italy.

**Source, Canad.** Source Medical Corp., 60 International Bvld, Toronto, Ontario, M9W 6J2, Canada.

**Sovedis, Fr.** Laboratoires Sovedis, 9 av. d'Arromanches, 94100 Saint-Maur des Fosses, France.

**Sovereign, UK.** Sovereign Medical, Sovereign House, Miles Gray Rd, Basildon, Essex, SS14 3FR, UK.

**SP, Denm.** See *Schering-Plough, Denm.*

**SP, Spain.** SP Biotech, Po Castellana 143, 28046 Madrid, Spain.

**SPA, Ital.** Società Prodotti Antibiotici S.p.A., Via Biella 8, 20143 Milan, Italy.

**Spagyros, Switz.** Spagyros AG, Tannackerstrasse 7, 3073 Gumlingen, Switzerland.

**Spaly, Spain.** Spaly Bioquimica, Avda de la Industria 30, Alcobendas, 28108 Madrid, Spain.

**Sparks, NZ.** David Sparks Ltd, P.O. Box 83-122, Edmonton, Auckland, New Zealand.

**SPB, Thai.** S.P.B. Pharma Co. Ltd, Apt 14B, Sathorn Park Place, 27/44 South Sathorn, Sathorn, Bangkok 10120, Thailand.

**Specia, Fr.** See *Aventis, Fr.*

**Spectropharm, Canad.** Spectropharm Dermatology, 6870 Goreway Drive, Mississauga, Ontario, L4V 1P1, Canada.

**Spedrog, Arg.** Spedrog Caillon S.A.I.y C., Alte. Fco. J. Segui 2106, 1416 Buenos Aires, Argentina.

**Speywood, Switz.** See *Opopharma, Switz.*

**Speywood, USA.** Speywood Pharmaceuticals Inc, 27 Maple St, Milford, MA 01757-3650, USA.

**Spineda, Arg.** Spineda, Pérez y Hnos., Zado 3735, 1431 Buenos Aires, Argentina.

**Spiphar, Belg.** Ets Spiphar S.P.R.L., Ave de la Couronne 114A, 1050 Brussels, Belgium.

**Spirig, Fr.** Laboratoires Spirig SA, 109 bd d'Haussonville, 54000 Nancy, France.

**Spirig, Singapore.** See *Summit, Singapore.*

**Spirig, Switz.** Spirig Pharma AG, Postfach 111, 4622 Egerkingen, Switzerland.

**Spitzner, Ger.** W. Spitzner, Arzneimittelfabrik GmbH, Bunsenstr. 6-10, 76275 Ettlingen, Germany.

**Sportbalm, Austral.** Sportbalm Australia P/L, 29 Woodland St, Strathmore, VIC 3041, Australia.

**Spreewald, Ger.** Spreewald Pharma GmbH, Obere Hardtstr. 18, 79114 Freiberg/Breisgau, Germany.

**Spyfarma, Spain.** Spyfarma, Ctra Sevilla Malaga Km 5.5 Km, Alcala de Guadaira, 41500 Seville, Spain.

**Square, Thai.** Pharma Square Co. Ltd, 5 Fortune Town, 4 Fl, Rm 22-26, Ratchadapisek Rd, Bangkok 103320, Thailand.

**Squibb, Canad.** See *Bristol-Myers Squibb, Canad.*

**Squibb, Spain.** Squibb, Josep Anselm Clave 95, Esplugues de Llobregat, 08950 Barcelona, Spain.

**Squibb, UK.** See *Bristol-Myers Squibb, UK.*

**Squibb, USA.** See *Bristol-Myers Squibb, USA.*

**Squibb Diagnostics, Canad.** See *Bristol-Myers Squibb, Canad.*

**Squibb Diagnostics, USA.** See *Bristol-Myers Squibb, USA.*

**Sriprasit, Thai.** Sriprasit Dispensary R O P, 617 Charoen Rath Rd, Klongsarn, Bangkok 10600, Thailand.

**SS, Jpn.** SS Pharmaceutical Co. Ltd, 2-12-4 Nihonbashi Hama-cho, Chuo-ku, Tokyo 103-0007, Japan.

**SSI, Swed.** SSI Sverige, Slagthuset, 211 20 Malmo, Sweden.

**SSL, Austral.** SSL International, 225 Beach Rd, Mordilloc, VIC 3195, Australia.

**SSL, Fr.** SSL Healthcare France SA, 49 av Georges-Pompidou, 92593 Levallois-Perret cdx, France.

**SSL, Hong Kong.** See *JDH, Hong Kong.*

**SSL, Irl.** SSL Healthcare Ireland Ltd, 86 Broomhill Rd, Tallaght, Dublin 24, Ireland.

**SSL, Ital.** SSL Healthcare Italia S.p.A., Via M. E. Lepido 178/5, 40132 Bologna, Italy.

**SSL, Malaysia.** Seton Scholl (Malaysia) Sdn Bhd, Level 5, Wisma Samudra, 1 Jln Kontraktor U1/14, Seksyen U1, Hicom Glenmarie Industrial Park, 40150 Shah Alam, Selangor, Malaysia.

**SSL, Norw.** See *SSL, Swed.*

**SSL, NZ.** SSL New Zealand Ltd, P.O. Box 100-091, North Shore Mail Centre, Auckland, New Zealand.

**SSL, Swed.** SSL Sverige AB, Box 1326, 171 26 Solna, Sweden.

**SSL, Switz.** SSL Healthcare Schweiz AG, Sternenhofstrasse 15A, Postfach 332, 4153 Reinach 1, Switzerland.

**SSL, Thai.** See *Diethelm, Thai.*, *JDH Borneo, Thai.*, and *Olic, Thai.*

**SSL, UK.** SSL International plc, Toft Hall, Knutsford, Chesire, WA16 9PD, UK.

**ST, Thai.** ST Pharma, 1937/16 Soi Ramkamhaeng 21, Banhkapi, Bangkok 10240, Thailand.

**St Ives, NZ.** St Ives Medical, P.O. Box 65-069, Auckland, New Zealand.

**St Laurent, Canad.** St Laurent Laboratoire, 1010 Berlier St, Laval, Quebec, H7L 3R9, Canada.

**St Valentinus Apotheke, Austria.** St Valentinus Apotheke, St Valentin, Austria.

**Stada, Austria.** Stada Arzneimittel GmbH, Heiligenstadter Strasse 52/2/8, A-1190 Vienna, Austria.

**Stada, Ger.** Stada Arzneimittel AG, Stadastr. 2-18, 61118 Bad Vilbel, Germany.

**Stada, Hong Kong.** Stada Pharmaceuticals (Asia) Ltd, 2208-2209 Paul Y Ctr, 51 Hung To Rd, Kwun Tong, Hong Kong.

**Stada, Malaysia.** See *Antah, Malaysia*, and *JDH, Malaysia.*

**Stada, Singapore.** See *JDH, Singapore.*

**Stada, Switz.** Stada Arzneimittel (Schweiz) AG, Route Andre-Piller 2, Case postale 76, 1762 Givisiez, Switzerland.

**Stada, Thai.** Stada Asiatic Co. Ltd, 41/18 Rama III Rd, Chongnonsee, Yannawa, Bangkok 10120, Thailand.

**Stada, USA.** STADA Pharmaceuticals Inc., 5 Cedar Brook Drive, Cranbury, NJ 08512, USA.

**Stadmed, India.** Stadmed Pvt Ltd, AA-21 Sector-I, Salt Lake City, Kolkata 700 064, India.

**Stafford, Mex.** See *GlaxoSmithKline Consumer, Mex.*

**Stafford-Miller, Austral.** Stafford Miller Ltd, P.O. Box 406, North Ryde, NSW 1670, Australia.

**Stafford-Miller, Braz.** See *GlaxoSmithKline, Braz.*

**Stafford-Miller, Fin.** See *Tamro, Fin.*

**Stafford-Miller, Fr.** See *GlaxoSmithKline, Fr.*

**Stafford-Miller, Hong Kong.** See *Trinity, Hong Kong.*

**Stafford-Miller, Irl.** See *Intra Pharma, Irl.*

**Stafford-Miller, Israel.** See *CTS, Israel.*

**Stafford-Miller, Ital.** See *GlaxoSmithKline Consumer, Ital.*

**Stafford-Miller, Mex.** See *GlaxoSmithKline Consumer, Mex.*

**Stafford-Miller, Norw.** See *Meda, Norw.*

**Stafford-Miller, NZ.** Stafford-Miller (NZ) Ltd, P.O. Box 100-490, Auckland, New Zealand.

**Stafford-Miller, Port.** See *GlaxoSmithKline, Port.*

**Stafford-Miller, Spain.** Stafford Miller, Pol. Ind. Malpica C/C 102-F, 50016 Zaragoza, Spain.

**Stafford-Miller, Switz.** See *Doetsch, Grether, Switz.*

**Stafford-Miller, UK.** See *GlaxoSmithKline, UK.*

**Stallergenes, Belg.** Stallergenes Belgium S.A., Chaussee de Louvain 277, 1410 Waterloo, Belgium.

**Stallergenes, Fr.** Stallergènes SA, 6 rue Alexis-de-Tocqueville, 92183 Antony cdx, France.

**Stallergenes, Ital.** Stallergenes Italia S.r.l., Via Portici 13, 21047 Saronno (VA), Italy.

**Stallergenes, Switz.** Stallergenes, 162 Rte de Boujean, 2500 Nienne 6, Switzerland.

**Stancare, India.** See *Ranbaxy, India.*

**Standard, Hong Kong.** See *Kai Yuen, Hong Kong.*

**Standard Drug, USA.** Standard Drug Company, 1279 N 7th St, Riverton, IL 62561, USA.

**Stanley, Canad.** Stanley Pharmaceuticals Ltd, Division of Vita Health Products Ltd, 117-260 West Esplanade, North Vancouver, British Columbia, V7M 3G7, Canada.

**Stanley, Israel.** See *Manon, Israel.*

**Star, Hong Kong.** Star Medical Supplies Ltd, Unit E, 1/F Hop Hing Industrial Bldg, 704 Castle Peak Rd, Lai Chi Kok, Kowloon, Hong Kong.

**Star, Thai.** Star Lab Co. Ltd, 542 Vipavadi Rangsit Rd, Din Dang, Bangkok 10400, Thailand.

**Star, USA.** Star Pharmaceuticals Inc., 1990 NW 44th St, Pompano Beach, FL 33064-8712, USA.

**Stark, Ger.** H. C. Stark GmbH Chemische Fabrik, Schneckenburgstr. 46, 78467 Constance, Germany.

**Statens Serum Institut, Denm.** Statens Serum Institut, Artillerivej 5, 2300 Copenhagen S, Denmark.

**Statens Serum Institut, Fin.** See *Statens Serum Institut, Denm.*

**Staufen, Ger.** Staufen-Pharma GmbH & Co., Bahnhofstr. 35, 73033 Goppingen, Germany.

**Stauffacher, Switz.** Stauffacher Apotheke, Dr Langer AG, Birmensdorferstrasse 1, 8004 Zurich, Switzerland.

**STD, Irl.** See *STD Pharmaceutical Products, UK.*

**STD Pharmaceutical Products, UK.** STD Pharmaceutical Products Ltd, Fields Yard, Plough Lane, Hereford, Herefordshire, HR4 0EL, UK.

**Stegropharm, Ger.** StegroPharm Arzneimittel GmbH, St.-Johann-Str. 8, 80999 Munich, Germany.

**Steierl, Ger.** Steierl Pharma GmbH, Muhlfelder Str. 48, 82211 Herrsching, Germany.

**Steigerwald, Ger.** Steigerwald Arzneimittelwerk GmbH, Havelstr. 5, 64295 Darmstadt, Germany.

**Steigerwald, Switz.** See *Hanseler, Switz.*

**Steiner, Ger.** Steiner & Co. Deutsche Arzneimittel Gesellschaft, Ostpreussendamm 72/74, 12207 Berlin, Germany.

**Stella, Belg.** Laboratoires Stella S.A., Rue des Pontons 25, 4032 Chenee, Belgium.

**Stella, Canad.** Stella Pharmaceutical Canada Inc., 407-220 Duncan Mill Rd, Don Mills, ON, M3B 3J5, Canada.

**Stellar, Canad.** Stellar International Inc., Stellar Healthcare, 235 Yorkland Bvld, Suite 300, Unit 16, North York, Ontario, M2J 4Y8, Canada.

**Stellar, USA.** Stellar Pharmacal Corp., 1990 NW 44th St, Pompano Beach, FL 33064-1278, USA.

**Step, Arg.** Step Argentina S.A., Saenz 314, 1832 Lomas de Zamora, Buenos Aires, Argentina.

**Sterfil, India.** Sterfil Laboratories, 101 Sterling Chambers, Mogra Village Lane, Andheri (E), Mumbai 400 069, India.

**Steris, USA.** Steris Laboratories Inc., 620 N 51st Ave, Phoenix, AZ 85043, USA.

**Sterling, India.** Sterling Lab., 57 Sipcot Industrial Complex, Hosur 635 126, India.

**Sterling, Port.** See *GlaxoSmithKline, Port.*

**Sterling, USA.** See *Sterling Health, USA.*

**Sterling Health, Austral.** See *GlaxoSmithKline, Austral.*

**Sterling Health, Spain.** See *GlaxoSmithKline, Spain.*

**Sterling Health, USA.** See *Bayer, USA.*

**Sterling Midy, Ital.** Sterling Midy S.p.A., Italy.

**Stern, Ger.** See *AstraZeneca, Ger.*

**Sterop, Belg.** Sterop, Avenue de Scheut 46-50, 1070 Brussels, Belgium.

**Sterwin, UK.** See *Sanofi Synthelabo, UK.*

**Stevia, Braz.** Inga Stevia Industrial Ltda, Rua Stevia 300, Pq. Ind. Bandeirantes, 87070-100 Maringa, PR, Brazil.

**Stewart Jackson, USA.** Stewart-Jackson Pharmacal, 4200 Lamar, Suite 103, Memphis, TN 38118, USA.

**Stiefel, Arg.** Stiefel Argentina S.A., Av. Federico Lacroze 3194, 1426 Buenos Aires, Argentina.

**Stiefel, Austral.** Stiefel Laboratories P/L, Unit 2, 10 Salisbury Road, Castle Hill, NSW 2154, Australia.

**Stiefel, Braz.** Laboratorios Stiefel Ltda, Rua Joao Cavalheiros Salem 1081/1301, 07243-580 Guarulhos, SP, Brazil.

**Stiefel, Canad.** Stiefel Canada Inc., 6635 Henri-Bourassa Blvd W, Montreal, Quebec, H4R 1E1, Canada.

**Stiefel, Chile.** Laboratorios Stiefel de Chile y Cia Ltda, Av. Americo Vespucio 1220, Penalolen, Santiago, Chile.

**Stiefel, Denm.** See *Ferring, Denm.*, and *OTC Consult, Denm.*

**Stiefel, Fin.** See *Bitelab, Fin.*

**Stiefel, Fr.** Laboratoires Stiefel (France), 6 Av. de L'Imperatrice Josephine, 92500 Reuil-Malmaison, France.

**Stiefel, Ger.** Stiefel Laboratorium GmbH, Muhlheimer Str. 231, 63075 Offenbach am Main, Germany.

**Stiefel, Gr.** See *Minerva (Μινερβα), Gr.*

**Stiefel, Hong Kong.** Stiefel Laboratories (Hong Kong) Ltd, 601B, 6F, Tower 2, Cheung Sha Wan Plaza, 833 Cheung Sha Wan Rd, Kowloon, Hong Kong.

**Stiefel, Irl.** See *Allphar, Irl.*

**Stiefel, Israel.** See *Agis, Israel.*

**Stiefel, Ital.** Stiefel Laboratories S.r.l., Via Calabria 15, 20090 Redecesio di Segrate (MI), Italy.

**Stiefel, Malaysia.** See *Diethelm, Malaysia.*

**Stiefel, Mex.** Stiefel Mexicana S.A. de C.V., Av. Uno No. 63, Col. San Pedro de los Pinos, Delegacion Benito Juarez, 03800 Mixico D.F., Mexico.

**Stiefel, Neth.** See *Bipharma, Neth.*

**Stiefel, Norw.** See *Scandinavian Health Care, Norw.*

**Stiefel, NZ.** See *Sparks, NZ.*

**Stiefel, Port.** Laboratórios Farmacêuticos Stiefel (Portugal), Lda, Av Maria Lamas, Lote 19, Bloco D, Piso 2, Serra das Minas, 2735 Rio de Mouro, Portugal.

**Stiefel, S.Afr.** Stiefel Laboratories SA (Pty) Ltd, P.O. Box 27114, Benrose 2011, South Africa.

**Stiefel, Singapore.** See *Diethelm, Singapore.*

**Stiefel, Spain.** Stiefel, Coto de Donana 11-13 Area, Andalucia Sector 1, Pinto, 28320 Madrid, Spain.
**Stiefel, Switz.** Stiefel Laboratorium AG, c/o Micucci Treuhand AG, Romertorstrasse 1, 8404 Winterthur, Switzerland.
**Stiefel, Thai.** Stiefel Laboratories (Thailand) Ltd, 33 Fl, Phaholyothin Place Building, 408/143 Phaholylothin Rd, Samsenni Phayathal, Bangkok 10400, Thailand.
**Stiefel, UK.** Stiefel Laboratories (UK) Ltd, Holtspur Lane, Wooburn Green, High Wycombe, Buckinghamshire, HP10 0AU, UK.
**Stiefel, USA.** Stiefel Laboratories Inc., 255 Alhambra Circle, Coral Gables, FL 33134, USA.
**Stomygen, Ital.** Gruppo Stomygen S.r.l., Via F. Jorini 69, 00149 Rome, Italy.
**Storz, Israel.** See *Isramedcom, Israel.*
**Storz, UK.** See *Wyeth, UK.*
**Stotzer, Switz.** Stotzer AG, Jura-Apotheke Bern, Breitenrainplatz 40, 3000 Bern 22, Switzerland.
**Strakan, UK.** Strakan Ltd, Buckholm Mill, Buckholm Mill Brae, Galashiels, Scotland, TD1 2HB, UK.
**Strallhofer, Austria.** Mag. Dr. Till Strallhofer, St-Veit-Gasse 56, A-1130 Vienna, Austria.
**Strand, Malaysia.** See *Pharmaniaga, Malaysia.*
**Strathmann, Ger.** Strathmann AG & Co., Sellhopsweg 1, 22459 Hamburg, Germany.
**Stratus, USA.** Stratus Pharmaceuticals Inc., 14377 SW 142nd St, P.O. Box 4632, Miami, FL 33186, USA.
**Streger, Mex.** Streger S.A., Km. 8 Antigua Carretera Xalapa-Coatepec, 91500 Consolapa-Coatepec, Ver., Mexico.
**Streuli, Switz.** G. Streuli & Co. AG, 8730 Uznach, Switzerland.
**Strickland, Canad.** See *Hargell, Canad.*
**Stroder, Ital.** Ist. Farmaco Biologico Stroder S.r.l., Via di Ripoli 207/V, 50126 Florence, Italy.
**Stroschein, Ger.** See *Strathmann, Ger.*
**Stuart, USA.** See *AstraZeneca, USA.*
**Stulln, Ger.** Pharma Stulln GmbH, Werksstr. 2, 92551 Stulln, Germany.
**Sturtevant, USA.** The F.C. Sturtevant Company, P.O. Box 607, Bronxville, NY 10708, USA.
**Substipharm, Fr.** Laboratoires Substipharm, 264 rue du Fbg-St-Honore, 75008 Paris, France.
**Suburfarm, Hong Kong.** Suburfarm Investment & Trading Co. Ltd, Medical Health Care Division, Unit 7A-B, 39/F Cable TV Tower, 9 Hoi Shing Rd, Tsuen Wan, N.T., Hong Kong.
**Sudmedica, Ger.** Südmedica GmbH, Ehrwalder Str. 21, 81377 Munich, Germany.
**Sudo, Singapore.** See *Pharma 2000, Singapore.*
**Sumitomo, Hong Kong.** See *Main Life, Hong Kong.*
**Sumitomo, Jpn.** Sumitomo Pharmaceuticals Co. Ltd, 2-2-8 Doshomachi, Chuo-ku, Osaka 541-8510, Japan.
**Summers, USA.** Summers Laboratories Inc., 103 G.P. Clement Dr., Collegeville, PA 19426, USA.
**Summit, Malaysia.** Summit Co (M) Sdn Bhd, Lot 6, Jln 19/1, 46300 Petaling Jaya, Selangor, Malaysia.
**Summit, Port.** See *Dario Correia, Port.*
**Summit, Singapore.** Summit Company (S) Ltd, 10 Pandan Crescent, 02-05 UE Tech Park, S 128466, Singapore.
**Summit, USA.** See *Novartis, USA.*
**Sun, Canad.** Sun Pharmaceutical Industries Inc., 1111 Flint Rd, Unit 23, Downsview, Ontario, M3J 3C7, Canada.
**Sun, India.** Sun Pharmaceutical Industries Ltd, Acme Plaza, Andheri Kurla Rd, Andheri (E), Mumbai 400 059, India.
**Sun, Malaysia.** Sun Pharmaceutical, 3A03, Block E, Phileo Damansara 1, Jln 16/11, 46350 Petaling Jaya, Selangor, Malaysia.
**Sun, Singapore.** See *Apotheca, Singapore.*
**Sun, Thai.** See *Pharmaland, Thai.*
**Sun Hing, Hong Kong.** Sun Hing Pharmaceutical Co. Ltd, Rm 1012, Blk 3, Nan Fung Ind City, 18 Tin Hau Rd, Tuen Mun, N.T., Hong Kong.
**Sunrise, Austral.** Sunrise Nutrition P/L, P.O. Box 355, Deepdene DC, VIC 3103, Australia.
**Sunspot, Austral.** Sunspot Products P/L, Level 3, Suite 303, 20 Bungan St, Mona Vale, NSW 2103, Australia.
**Sunstar, Jpn.** Sunstar Inc., 3-1 Asahi-machi, Takatsuki City, Osaka 569-1195, Japan.
**Suntory, Jpn.** Suntory Ltd, Dojimahama 2-1-40, Kita-ku, Osaka 530-8203, Japan.
**Sunward, Malaysia.** Sunward Pharmaceutical Sdn Bhd, 9 Jln Kempas 4, Taman Perinductrian, Tampoi Indah, 81200 Tampoi, Johor, Malaysia.
**Sunward, Singapore.** Sunward Pharmaceutical Pte Ltd, 11 Wan Lee Rd, Jurong, S 627943, Singapore.
**Super Mayoreo Naturista, Mex.** Super Mayoreo Naturista S.A. de C.V., Calle 3 No. 13 Local 4, Fracc. Industrial Alce Blanco, Naucalpan de Juarez, 53370 Mexico D.F., Mexico.
**SuperGen, Canad.** See *SuperGen, USA.*
**SuperGen, USA.** SuperGen Inc., 2 Annabel Lane, Suite 220, San Ramon, CA 94583, USA.
**Support, Braz.** Support Produtos Nutricionais Ltda, Vincente Pinzon 173, 2 andar, 04547-130 Sao Paulo, Brazil.
**Surf Ski International, UK.** Surf Ski International Ltd, UK.
**Surgicraft, UK.** Surgicraft Ltd, 16 The Oaks, Clews Road, Redditch, Worcestershire, B98 7ST, UK.
**Survival Technology, USA.** Survival Technology Inc., 2275 Research Blvd, Rockville, MD 20850, USA.
**Surya, Singapore.** See *Polymedic, Singapore.*
**Sussex, UK.** Sussex Pharmaceutical Ltd, Charlwoods Rd, East Grinstead, Sussex, RH19 2HL, UK.
**Sutton, Canad.** HJ Sutton Industries Ltd, 8701 Jane St, Unit C, Vaughan, Ontario, L4K 2M6, Canada.
**Suyog, India.** Suyog Pharmaceuticals Pvt Ltd, Plot No. T/46, MIDC, Tarapur, Boisar, Thane 401 506, India.
**SVR, Fr.** Laboratoires SVR Cosmétologie Médicale, ZAC de La Tremblaie, rue de la Mare-a-Blot, 91220 Le Plessis-Pate, France.
**SVR, Ital.** Laboritoires SVR-ZAC La Tremblaie, Via dei Cybo 5, 20127 Milan, Italy.
**Swedish Orphan, Irl.** See *Cahill May Roberts, Irl.*
**Swedish Orphan, Norw.** Swedish Orphan AS, Trollasv. 6, 1414 Trollasen, Norway.
**Swedish Orphan, Swed.** Swedish Orphan AB, Drottninggatan 98, 111 60 Stockholm, Sweden.
**Swiss Herbal, Canad.** Swiss Herbal Remedies Ltd, 35 Leek Cres, Richmond Hill, Ontario, L4B 4C2, Canada.
**Swiss Serum, Malaysia.** See *Diethelm, Malaysia.*
**Swiss Serum, Thai.** See *Diethelm, Thai.*
**Swiss Serum Institute, Israel.** See *Droreth, Israel.*
**Swiss Worldwide, Hong Kong.** Swiss Worldwide Ltd, 9C Ho King Bldg, 128 On Ling Rd, Yuen Long, Hong Kong.
**Swisshealth, UK.** SwissHealth, UK.
**Swisspharm, S.Afr.** Swisspharm (Pty) Ltd, South Africa.
**Sydenham, Mex.** Sydenham S.A. de C.V., Prolongacion Moctezuma 58, Romero de Terrenos, Coyoacan, 04310 Mexico D.F., Mexico.
**Sydney Ross, Braz.** See *GlaxoSmithKline, Braz.*
**Sylak, Swed.** Sylak AB, 436 32 Askim, Sweden.
**Symbiopharm, Ger.** SymbioPharm GmbH, Auf den Luppen, 35745 Herborn-Horbach, Germany.
**Synapse, Irl.** Synapse Medical, Unit 12, Keypoint Business Park, Rosemount Business Park Drive, Ballycoolin Rd, Dublin 11, Ireland.
**Synco, Hong Kong.** Synco (HK) Ltd, Blk D, 3/F, Sun View Industrial Bldg, 3 On Yip St, Chaiwan, Hong Kong.
**Syner-Med, UK.** Syner-Med (Pharmaceutical Products) Ltd, Beech House, 840 Brighton Rd, Purley, Surrey, CR8 2BH, UK.
**Synmedic, Switz.** Synmedic AG, Gernardstrasse 1, Postfach, 8036 Zurich, Switzerland.
**Synmosa, Singapore.** See *Zyfas, Singapore.*
**Synpharma, Austria.** Synpharma GmbH, Wiener Bundesstrasse 21 PF.4, A-5300 Hallwang bei Salzburg, Austria.
**Synpharma, Switz.** Synpharma AG, Postfach, 9240 Uzwil, Switzerland.
**Syntetic, Denm.** A/S Syntetic, Danisco Cultor, Edwin Rahrs Vej 38, 8220 Brabrand, Denmark.
**Syntex, Canad.** See *Roche, Canad.*
**Syntex, Ger.** See *Roche, Ger.*
**Syntex, Mex.** See *Roche, Mex.*
**Syntex, Spain.** Syntex Roche, C/Severo Ochoa 13, Leganes, 28914 Madrid, Spain.
**Syntex, Swed.** See *GlaxoSmithKline, Swed.*
**Syntex, Switz.** See *Uhlmann-Eyraud, Switz.*
**Syntex, UK.** See *Roche, UK.*
**Syntex, USA.** See *Roche, USA.*
**Synthelabo, Belg.** See *Sanofi Synthelabo, Belg.*
**Synthelabo, Fr.** See *Sanofi Synthelabo, Fr.*, and *Sanofi Synthelabo OTC, Fr.*
**Synthelabo, Ger.** See *Sanofi Synthelabo, Ger.*
**Synthelabo, Hong Kong.** See *Sanofi Synthelabo, Hong Kong.*
**Synthelabo, Israel.** See *Mediline, Israel.*
**Synthelabo, Ital.** See *Sanofi Synthelabo, Ital.*
**Synthelabo, Port.** See *Sanofi Synthelabo, Port.*
**Synthelabo, Spain.** See *Sanofi Synthelabo, Spain.*
**Synthelabo, Switz.** See *Sanofi Synthelabo, Switz.*
**Synthelabo Lavipharm, Gr.** SYNTHELABO-LAVIPHARM A.E., Αγ. Μαρίνας, 190 02 Παιανία, Paiania, Greece.
**Synthes, Austria.** Synthes GmbH, Karolingerstrasse 16, A-5035 Salzburg, Austria.
**Synthon, USA.** Synthon Pharmaceuticals Ltd, 6330 Quadrangle Drive, Suite 305, Chapel Hill, NC 27517, USA.
**Syosset, USA.** Syosset Laboratories Inc., 150 Eileen Way, Syosset, NY 11791, USA.
**Systopic, India.** Systopic Laboratories Ltd, 101 Pragati Chamber, Commercial Complex, Ranjit Nagar, New Dehli 110 008, India.
**Syxyl, Ger.** Syxyl GmbH & Co. KG, Gereonsmuhlengasse 5, 50670 Cologne, Germany.
**Szama, Arg.** Lab. Szama S.A., Lafuente 161, 1406 Buenos Aires, Argentina.
**T Man, Thai.** T Man Pharma Ltd, Part, 101/2 Soi Moungsakul, Bangkuntian, Bangkok 10150, Thailand.
**Tablets, India.** Tablets (India) Ltd, Jhaver Centre, IV Floor, 72 Marshalls Road, Chennai 600 008, India.
**Tack Fung, Hong Kong.** Tack Fung Medical Supplies Co., Rm 504, Tien Cheung Hong Bldg, 77-81 Jervois St Central, Hong Kong.
**Taco, Ger.** Taco-GmbH, Chem.-Pharm. Fabrik, Alte Heerstr. 76, 53757 St. Augustin, Germany.
**TAD, Ger.** TAD Pharma GmbH, Heinz-Lohmann-Str. 5, 27472 Cuxhaven, Germany.
**Taejoon, Singapore.** See *Pharmaforte, Singapore.*
**Tafir, Spain.** Tafir, Trifon Pedrero 4-6, 28019 Madrid, Spain.
**Tai Guk, Singapore.** See *Polymedic, Singapore.*
**Tai Tong, Hong Kong.** Tai Tong Co. Ltd, Rm 901-902, Alliance Bldg, 130-136 Connaught Rd Central, Hong Kong.
**Taiho, Jpn.** Taiho Pharmaceutical Co. Ltd, 1-27 Kanda-Nishiki-cho, Chiyoda-ku, Tokyo 101-8444, Japan.
**Taiho, Malaysia.** See *Luen Wah, Malaysia.*
**Taiho, Singapore.** See *Luen Wah, Singapore.*
**Takeda, Austria.** Takeda Pharma GmbH, Seidengasse 33-35/4, A-1070 Vienna, Austria.
**Takeda, Denm.** See *Lilly, Denm.*
**Takeda, Fr.** Laboratoires Takeda, 15 quai de Dion-Bouton, 92816 Puteaux cdx, France.
**Takeda, Ger.** Takeda Pharma GmbH, Viktoriaallee 3-5, 52066 Aachen, Germany.
**Takeda, Gr.** Takeda, Greece.
**Takeda, Hong Kong.** Takeda Chemical Industries Ltd, Unit 1801-2, 18/F Fook Lee Commercial Ctr, Town Place, 33 Lockhart Rd, Wanchai, Hong Kong.
**Takeda, Israel.** See *Promedico, Israel.*
**Takeda, Ital.** Takeda Italia Farmaceutici S.p.A., Via Elio Vittorini 129, 00144 Rome, Italy.
**Takeda, Jpn.** Takeda Chemical Industries Ltd, 4-1-1 Doshomachi, Chuo-ku, Osaka 540-8645, Japan.
**Takeda, Malaysia.** See *Luen Wah, Malaysia*, and *Zuellig, Malaysia.*
**Takeda, Norw.** See *Lilly, Norw.*
**Takeda, Singapore.** See *Luen Wah, Singapore.*
**Takeda, Switz.** Takeda Pharma AG, Alpenblickstrasse 26, 8853 Lachen, Switzerland.
**Takeda, Thai.** Takeda (Thailand) Ltd, 12A Fl, Si Ayutthaya Building, Si Ayutthaya Rd, 487/1 Ratchathewi, Bangkok 10400, Thailand.
**Takeda, UK.** Takeda UK Ltd, Takeda House, The Mercury Centre, Wycombe Lane, Wooburn Green, High Wycombe, Buckinghamshire, HP10 0HH, UK.
**Takeda, USA.** Takeda Pharmaceuticals America, 475 Half Day Rd, Suite 500, Lincolnshire, IL 60069, USA.
**Talcris, Arg.** Talcris S.A., Congreso 2160 PB. A, 1428 Buenos Aires, Argentina.
**Tamar, Israel.** Tamar, Israel.
**Tamilnadu Dadha, India.** See *Sun, India.*
**Tamro, Fin.** Tamro Distribution/Pharmakon, Rajatorpantie 41 B, PL 11, 01640 Vantaa, Finland.
**Tamustino, Braz.** See *Guerbet, Braz.*
**Tanabe, Hong Kong.** See *Primal, Hong Kong.*
**Tanabe, Jpn.** See *Mitsubishi-Tokyo, Jpn.*
**Tanabe, Malaysia.** See *Pharmaforte, Malaysia.*
**Tanabe, Singapore.** See *Pharmaforte, Singapore.*
**Tanabe, Thai.** See *Wellchem, Thai.*
**Tanki, Arg.** Tanki S.A., Erezcano 3161, 1437 Buenos Aires, Argentina.
**Tanning Research, Canad.** See *Tropic Suncare, Canad.*
**Tanning Research, USA.** Tanning Research Labs Inc., P.O. Box 265111, Daytone Beach, FL 32126-5111, USA.
**Tanta, Canad.** Tanta Pharmaceuticals Inc., 1009 Burns St East, Whitby, Ontario, L1N 6A6, Canada.
**TAP, USA.** TAP Pharmaceuticals Inc., 2355 Waukegan Rd, Deerfield, IL 60015, USA.
**Taphlan, Switz.** See *Serolab, Switz.*
**Taranis, Fr.** Taranis-dhn, Le Haut Montigne, 35370 Torce, France.
**Tarbis, Spain.** Tarbis Farma SL, Gran Via de Carlos III 94, 08028 Barcelona, Spain.
**Taro, Canad.** Taro Pharmaceuticals Inc., 130 East Drive, Bramalea, Ontario, L6T 1C3, Canada.
**Taro, Israel.** Taro Pharmaceutical International, Beit Italia, Euro Park, Yakum, Israel.
**Taro, Thai.** See *Union Medical, Thai.*
**Taro, UK.** Taro Pharmaceuticals (UK) Ltd, Riverside House, Station Rd, Bishops Stortford, Hertfordshire, CM23 3AJ, UK.
**Taro, USA.** Taro Pharmaceuticals USA Inc., 5 Skyline Drive, Hawthorne, NY 10532-9998, USA.
**Tau, Spain.** Tau, Mestre Joan Corrales 95-105, Esplugues Llobregat, 08950 Barcelona, Spain.
**Taurus, Ger.** Taurus Pharma GmbH, Berner Str. 40-42, 60437 Frankfurt, Germany.
**Taxandria, Neth.** Taxandria Pharmaceutica BV, Postbus 90241, 5000 LV Tilburg, Netherlands.
**Taylor, USA.** Taylor Pharmaceuticals, P.O. Box 5136, San Clemente, CA 92674-5136, USA.
**TC Technocare, Israel.** See *TP, Israel.*
**Teamm, USA.** Teamm Pharmaceuticals, 3000 Aerial Center Parkway, Suite 110, Morrisville, NC 27560, USA.
**Tecefarma, Spain.** Tecefarma, Guifre 724, Badalona, 08912 Barcelona, Spain.
**Technikon, S.Afr.** Technikon Laboratories, P.O. Box 150, Maraisburg 1700, South Africa.
**Technilab, Canad.** Technilab Pharma Inc., 17, 800 Lapointe St, Mirabel, Quebec, J7J 1P3, Canada.
**Technilab, Hong Kong.** See *Hind Wing, Hong Kong.*
**Techni-Pharma, Mon.** Techni-Pharma, 7 rue de l'Industrie, B.P. 717, MC 98014, Monaco.
**Technipro, Austral.** Technipro Marketing P/L, 13 Bourke St, North Parramatta, NSW 2150, Australia.
**Technostic, Austral.** Technostic Consulting Pty Ltd, 6735 Cutrock Rd, Lisarow, NSW 2250, Australia.
**Teclapharm, Ger.** Teclapharm GmbH, Heilgenthalar Str. 4, 21335 Luneburg, Germany.
**Tecnifar, Port.** Tecnifar, SA, Rua Tierno Galvan, Torre 3, 12 Piso, 1099-036 Lisbon, Portugal.
**Tecnimede, Port.** Tecnimede, SA, Rua Prof. Henrique de Barros, Edifmcio Sagres, 3 A, 2685-338 Prior Velho, Portugal.
**Tecnobio, Spain.** See *Almirall, Spain.*
**Tecnofarma, Chile.** Tecnofarma SA, Las Violetas 2169, Santiago, Chile.
**Tecnofarma, Mex.** Tecnofarma S.A. de C.V., Azafran No. 123, Col. Granjas Mexico, 08400 Mexico D.F., Mexico.
**Tecnonat, Arg.** Tecnonat S.A., 24 de Noviembre 368, 1170 Buenos Aires, Argentina.
**Tec-O-Pharm, Israel.** Tec-O-Pharm, P.O. Box 45054, Jerusalem 91450, Israel.
**Tedec Meiji, Israel.** See *Trima, Israel.*
**Tedec Meiji, Spain.** Tedec Meiji Farma, Ctra M-300, Km 30.5, Alcala De Henares, 28820 Madrid, Spain.
**Tedec-Meiji, Thai.** See *Meiji, Thai.*
**Teekanne, Austria.** Teekanne GmbH, Munchner Bundesstrasse 120, A-5021 Salzburg, Austria.
**Tegur, Mex.** Labs. Tegur de Mixico, S.A. de C.V., Calle Avena 513 /101, Iztacalco Granjas Mexico, 08400 Mexico D.F., Mexico.
**Teijin, Jpn.** Teijin Ltd, 2-1-1 Uchisaiwai-cho, Chiyoda-ku, Tokyo 100-8585, Japan.
**Teijin, Singapore.** See *Pharmacon, Singapore.*
**Teijin, Thai.** See *Berli, Thai.*
**Teikoku, Jpn.** Teikoku Hormone Mfg Co. Ltd, 2-5-1 Shibaura, Minato-ku, Tokyo 108-8532, Japan.
**Teikoku Seiyaku, Jpn.** Teikoku Seiyaku Co. Ltd, 567 Sanbonmatsu, Ochi-cho, Okawa-gun, Kagawa 769-2695, Japan.
**Tek, Thai.** See *Neopharm, Thai.*
**Teknofarma, Ital.** Teknofarma S.p.A., Strada Comunale da Bertolla alla Abbadia di Stura 14, 10156 Turin, Italy.
**Telluride, USA.** Telluride Pharm. Corp, 146 Flanders Drive, Hillsborough, NJ 08876-4656, USA.
**Tema, S.Afr.** Tema Medical (Pty) Ltd, P.O. Box 3467, Cramerview 2060, South Africa.
**Temis, Arg.** Lab. Temis Lostaló S.A., Zepita 3178, 1285 Buenos Aires, Argentina.
**Temmler, Denm.** See *Kemifarma, Denm.*
**Temmler, Ger.** Temmler Pharma GmbH & Co. KG, Temmlerstr. 2, 35039 Marburg/Lahn, Germany.
**Temmler, Israel.** See *Megapharm, Israel.*
**Temmler, Port.** See *Confar, Port.*
**Temmler, Thai.** See *JDH Borneo, Thai.*
**Tempo Scan Pacific, Malaysia.** See *Wellmex, Malaysia.*
**Tendem, Neth.** Tendem BV, Punterweg 30, 8042 PB Zwolle, Netherlands.
**Tender, Canad.** Tender Corp. Canada, 18 Alliance Blvd, Unit 10, Barrie, Ontario, L4M 5A5, Canada.
**Tender, Israel.** See *Meditrend, Israel.*
**Tentan, Switz.** Tentan AG, Brunnliweg 16, 4433 Ramlinsburg, Switzerland.
**Teofarma, Austria.** See *Teofarma, Ital.*
**Teofarma, Fr.** See *Teofarma, Ital.*
**Teofarma, Ger.** See *Teofarma, Ital.*
**Teofarma, Ital.** Teofarma, Via F.lli Cervi 5, 27100 Valle Salimbene (PV), Italy.
**Teofarma, Neth.** Teofarma, Netherlands.
**Teofarma, Port.** See *Teofarma, Ital.*
**Teofarma, Spain.** Teofarma Iberica, Alfonso XII 19, 08006 Barcelona, Spain.
**Teomed, Switz.** Teomed AG, Tumigerstrasse 71, Postfach 20, 8606 Greifensee, Switzerland.
**Terapeutico, Ital.** Laboratorio Terapeutico M.R. S.r.l., Via Domenico Veneziano 13, 50143 Florence, Italy.
**Terapia, Mex.** Terapia Infantil S.A. de C.V., Queretaro No. 131, Col. Roma, 06700 Mexico D.F., Mexico.
**Teravix, Port.** Teravix, Lda, Av Antonio Augusto de Aguiar 128, 1050 Lisbon, Portugal.
**Terme di Chianciano, Ital.** Terme di Chianciano S.p.A., Via delle Rose 12, 53042 Chianciano Terme (Siena), Italy.
**Terme di Montecatini, Ital.** Terme di Montecatini S.p.A., Viale Marconi 7, 51016 Montecatini Terme (PT), Italy.
**Terme di Salsomaggiore, Ital.** Terme di Salsomaggiore S.p.A., Via Roma 9, 43039 Salsomaggiore Terme (Parma), Italy.

**Terme di Tabiano, Ital.** Termi di Tabiano SpA, Viale Alle Terme 32, 43030 Tabiano (PR), Italy.

**Terme Sirmione, Ital.** Terme Sirmione S.p.A., Piazza Virgillio 1, 25010 Colombare di Sirmione (BS), Italy.

**Terra-Bio, Ger.** Terra-Bio-Chemie GmbH, Lindenbergstr. 5, 79199 Kirchzarten, Germany.

**Terrafor, Fr.** Laboratoires Terrafor, B.P. 62, 76302 Sotteville-les-Rouen cdx, France.

**Terralife, Austria.** Terralife Pharma GmbH, Moosham 29, A-5580 Unternberg, Austria.

**Terramin, Austria.** Terramin Pharma GmbH & Co. KEG, Maria Pfarr 135, A-5571, Austria.

**Terrapharm, Austria.** Terrapharm Pharm. Produktions- und Handels-GmbH, Braunlichgasse 40-42, A-2700 Wiener Neustadt, Austria.

**Terrier, Mex.** See *Columbia, Mex.*

**Tetido, Ital.** Te.Ti.Do di Brunelli Donata S.a.s., Via Bevanella 60, 48010 Savio (RA), Italy.

**Tetra, Israel.** Tetra Pharm, 10 Barshavski St, Rishon Lezion 75910, Israel.

**Teuto, Braz.** Laboratorio Teuto-Brasileiro Ltda, VP 7-D Modulo 11 Quadra 13, 75133-600 Anapolis, GO, Brazil.

**Teva, Canad.** Teva Neuroscience G.P.-S.E.N.C., 999 de Maisonneuve W, Suite 550, Montreal, Quebec, H3A 3L4, Canada.

**Teva, Denm.** See *Aventis, Denm.*

**Teva, Ger.** TEVA Generics GmbH, Kandelstrasse 10, 79199 Kirchzarten, Germany.

**Teva, Hong Kong.** See *International Medical, Hong Kong*, and *Primal, Hong Kong.*

**Teva, Israel.** Teva Pharmaceuticals Ind. Ltd, P.O. Box 8077, Kiryat Nordau, Netanya, Israel.

**Teva, Ital.** Teva Pharma Italia S.r.l., V.le G. Richard 7, 20143 Milan, Italy.

**Teva, Norw.** See *Aventis, Norw.*

**Teva, S.Afr.** Teva Pharmaceuticals (Pty) Ltd, P.O. Box 43419, Industria 2042, South Africa.

**Teva, Singapore.** See *Green Cross, Singapore.*

**Teva, Thai.** See *RX, Thai.*, and *Union Medical, Thai.*

**Teva, UK.** Teva Pharmaceuticals Ltd, Barclays House, 1 Gatehouse Way, Aylesbury, Buckinghamshire, HP19 8DB, UK.

**Teva, USA.** Teva Pharmaceuticals USA, 1090 Horsham Rd, North Wales, PA 19454-1090, USA.

**Teva Tuteur, Arg.** Teva Tuteur S.A., Av. Juan de Garay 848/50, 1153 Buenos Aires, Argentina.

**Textilease, USA.** Textilease Medique Products, 900 Lively Blvd, Wood Dale, IL 60191, USA.

**Thai Otsuka, Thai.** Thai Otsuka Pharmaceutical Co. Ltd, 11 Fl, Regent House Building, 183 Rajdamri Rd, Khwang Lumpini, Khet Pathumwan, Bangkok 10330, Thailand.

**Thaipharmed, Thai.** See *ST, Thai.*

**Thames, USA.** Thames Pharmacal Co. Inc., 2100 Fifth Ave, Ronkonkoma, NY 11779-6906, USA.

**The Forty-Two, Thai.** See *Siam Medicare, Thai.*

**Thea, Fr.** Laboratoires Théa, 12 rue Louis-Bleriot, 63016 Clermont-Ferrand cdx 2, France.

**Thea, Hong Kong.** See *Silroc, Hong Kong.*

**Thea, Ital.** Thea Farmaceutici S.r.l., Via Gioberti 1, 20123 Milan, Italy.

**Thea, Spain.** Thea, PG Sant Joan 91, 08007 Barcelona, Spain.

**Themis, India.** Themis Pharmaceuticals Ltd, 38 Suren Rd, Andheri (E), Mumbai 400 093, India.

**Themis Chemicals, India.** Themis Chemicals Ltd, 11/12 Udyognagar Industrial Estate, S.V. Rd, Goregaon (W), Mumbai 400 062, India.

**Thepenier, Switz.** See *Uhlmann-Eyraud, Switz.*

**Thera, Fr.** See *Alpharma, Fr.*

**Therabel, Belg.** Therabel Pharma S.A., Rue Egide Van Ophem 108, 1180 Brussels, Belgium.

**Therabel, Fr.** Laboratoires Thérabel Lucien Pharma, 123 rue Jules-Guesde, 92309 Levallois-Perret cdx, France.

**Therabel, Ital.** Therabel Pharma S.p.A., Via Lorenteggio 270/a, 20152 Milan, Italy.

**Therabel, Neth.** Therabel Pharma NV, Westblaak 89, 3012 KG Rotterdam, Netherlands.

**Therakos, USA.** Therakos Inc., 437 Creamery Way, Exton, PA 19341, USA.

**Theralab, Canad.** See *E-Z-EM, Canad.*

**Theramed, Canad.** Theramed Corp., 6891 Edwards Bvld, Mississauga, Ontario, L5T 2T9, Canada.

**Theramex, Ital.** Theramex S.p.A., Via Mancinelli 11, 20131 Milan, Italy.

**Theramex, Mon.** Laboratoires Théramex, 6 av. Prince-Hereditaire-Albert, B.P. 59, MC 98007, Monaco.

**Theranol-Deglaude, Fr.** See *DB, Fr.*

**Therapeutic-Ocean, Singapore.** See *Zuellig, Singapore.*

**Therapex, Canad.** See *E-Z-EM, Canad.*

**Therapharm, Austral.** See *AstraZeneca, Austral.*

**Therapharma, Thai.** See *Olic, Thai.*

**Theraplix, Fr.** See *Aventis, Fr.*

**Theraskin, Braz.** Theraskin, Marginal Direita da Anchieta Km 13.3, 09883-000 Sao Bernardo do Compo, SP, Brazil.

**Therasophia, Fr.** Therasophia, 630 route des Dolines, 06560 Valbonne, France.

**Theratech, Fr.** Laboratoires Theratech, 6 rue Dubais, 27000 Evreux, France.

**Theriaca, Ital.** Theriaca S.r.l., Palazzina C Int. 2, Via Pietroantonio Micheli 78, 00197 Rome, Italy.

**Therica, Fr.** See *Bailleul, Fr.*

**Thermalife, Austral.** Thermalife International Pharmaceuticals Ltd, Level 1, 284 Oxford St, Leederville, WA 6007, Australia.

**Ther-Rx, USA.** Ther-Rx Corp., 13622 Lakefront Dr., Earth City, MO 63045, USA.

**Therval, Fr.** Therval Medical, 29 rue du Pont, 92200 Neuilly-sur-Seine, France.

**Thiemann, Ger.** See *Celltech, Ger.*

**Thilo, Hong Kong.** See *Health Care, Hong Kong.*

**Thomae, Ger.** See *Boehringer Ingelheim, Ger.*

**Thompson, Austral.** See *Thompson, NZ.*

**Thompson, NZ.** Thompson Nutrition Ltd, 25 Constellation Drive, Mairangi Bay, Auckland, New Zealand.

**Thompson, UK.** Thompson Medical Co. Ltd, Riding Court, Riding Court Rd, Datchet, Slough, Berkshire, SL3 9JT, UK.

**Thompson, USA.** Thompson Medical Co. Inc., 777 S Flagler, West Palm Beach, FL 33401, USA.

**Thomson, Austral.** Richard Thomson P/L, Unit D1, 46-62 Maddox St, Alexandria, NSW 2065, Australia.

**Thornton & Ross, Irl.** See *Allphar, Irl.*

**Thornton & Ross, UK.** Thornton & Ross Ltd, Linthwaite Laboratories, Huddersfield, West Yorkshire, HD7 5QH, UK.

**Thuasne, Fr.** Thuasne SA, 118-120 rue Marius-Aufan, B.P. 243, 92300 Levallois-Perret, France.

**Thuna, Canad.** Thuna Herbal Remedies Ltd, 298 Danforth Ave, Toronto, Ontario, M4K 1N6, Canada.

**Tika, Norw.** See *AstraZeneca, Norw.*

**Tika, Swed.** See *AstraZeneca, Swed.*

**Tillomed, UK.** Tillomed Laboratories Ltd, 3 Howard Rd, Eaton Socon, St Neots, Cambridgeshire, PE19 3ET, UK.

**Tillotts, Hong Kong.** See *Associated Medical, Hong Kong.*

**Tillotts, Israel.** See *Tradis-Gat, Israel.*

**Tillotts, NZ.** See *Baxter, NZ.*

**Tillotts, Singapore.** See *Wellchem, Singapore.*

**Tillotts, Switz.** Tillotts Pharma AG, Hauptstrasse 27, 4417 Ziefen, Switzerland.

**Tillotts, Thai.** See *Union Medical, Thai.*

**Tilman, Belg.** Tilman, Zoning Industriel 15, 5377 Baillonville, Belgium.

**Time-Cap, Hong Kong.** See *Sheraton, Hong Kong.*

**Time-Cap, USA.** Time-Cap Labs Inc., 7 Michael Ave, Farmingdale, NY 11735, USA.

**Tipomark, Ital.** Tipomark S.r.l., Via Andrea Appiani 12, 20121 Milan, Italy.

**Tiroler, Austria.** Tiroler Steinölwerke OHG, A-6213 Pertisau am Achensee, Austria.

**Tisane Provencale, Switz.** See *Uhlmann-Eyraud, Switz.*

**Tishcon, Hong Kong.** See *International Medical, Hong Kong.*

**Tissot, Fr.** Laboratoires du Dr Tissot, 3 rue de Versailles, 78470 St-Remy-les-Chevreuse, France.

**Tjellesen, Denm.** E. Tjellesen A/S, Blokken 81, 3460 Birkerod, Denmark.

**TKT, Denm.** TKT Europe-5S, Overodvej 47 A, 1411 Copenhagen K, Denmark.

**TKT, Fr.** See *TKT, Swed.*

**TKT, Ger.** TKT 5 S Europe GmbH, Am Weissen Berg 21, 96193 Wachenroth, Germany.

**TKT, Israel.** See *Medison, Israel.*

**TKT, Spain.** TKT Europe 5S, Serrano 240, 5, 28016 Madrid, Spain.

**TKT, Swed.** TKT Europe-5S AB, Rinkebyvdgen 11 B, 182 36 Danderyd, Sweden.

**TNP, Thai.** TNP Health Care Co. Ltd, 94/7 Soi Yimprakrob, Ngamwongwan Rd, Nonthaburi 11000, Thailand.

**TO-Chemicals, Singapore.** See *Advanced, Singapore.*

**TO-Chemicals, Thai.** TO-Chemicals (1979) Ltd, 280 Soi Sabai Jai, Suthisarn Rd, Bangkok 10320, Thailand.

**Tocogino, Mex.** Laboratorios Tocogino S.A. de C.V., Chihuahua No. 185, Col. Roma, 06700 Mexico D.F., Mexico.

**Togal, Ger.** Togal-Werk AG, Ismaninger Str.105, 81675 Munich, Germany.

**Togal, Switz.** Togal-Werk SA, Via Val Gersa 4, 6900 Lugano-Massagno, Switzerland.

**Toho, Hong Kong.** See *Primal, Hong Kong.*

**Toho, Thai.** See *Diethelm, Thai.*

**Tokyo Tanabe, Hong Kong.** See *Hing Ah, Hong Kong.*

**Tonipharm, Fr.** Laboratoires Tonipharm, 3 rue des 4-Cheminees, 92514 Boulgne cdx, France.

**Topfer, Ger.** Töpfer GmbH, Heisingerstr. 6, 87463 Dietmannsried, Germany.

**Toray, Jpn.** Toray Industries Inc., 2-1 Nihonbashi-Muromachi 2-chome, Chuo-ku, Tokyo 103-8666, Japan.

**Torbet, Irl.** See *Allphar, Irl.*

**Torbet Laboratories, UK.** See *Typharm, UK.*

**Torfwerk Einfeld, Ger.** Torfwerk Einfeld Carl Hornung, Postfach: 2667, 24516 Neumunster, Germany.

**Torii, Hong Kong.** See *Hing Yip, Hong Kong.*

**Torlan, Spain.** LPD Torlan, Ctra Barcelona 135-B, Cerdenola del Valles, 08290 Barcelona, Spain.

**Torre, Ital.** Dr. A. Torre Farmaceutici S.r.l., Viale E. Forlanini 15, 20134 Milan, Italy.

**Torrens, Spain.** Torrens, Camino del Hospital S/N, Olesa de Bonevalls, 08739 Barcelona, Spain.

**Torrent, India.** Torrent Pharmaceuticals Ltd, Torrent House, Off Ashram Rd, Ahmedabad 380 009, India.

**Torrent, Thai.** See *Union Medical, Thai.*

**Torrex, Austria.** Torrex Pharma GmbH, Lange Gasse 76/12, A-1080 Vienna, Austria.

**Tosara, Irl.** See *Forest Laboratories, UK.*

**Tosara, UK.** See *Forest Laboratories, UK.*

**Tosi, Hong Kong.** See *Sincerity, Hong Kong.*

**Tosi, Ital.** Tosi Farmaceutici sas di Silvana Tosi & C, Via Mattei 24, 28100 Novara, Italy.

**Tosse, Ger.** E. Tosse & Co. mbH, Friedrich-Ebert-Damm 101, 22047 Hamburg, Germany.

**Toulade, Fr.** Laboratoires Toulade, av. du Docteur-Aubry, 76280 Criquetot-L'Esneval, France.

**Toyama, Jpn.** Toyama Chemical Co., Ltd, 3-2-5 Nishishinjuku, Shinjuku-ku, Tokyo 160-0023, Japan.

**Toyo, Hong Kong.** See *Hing Yip, Hong Kong.*

**TP, Israel.** TP Technology Pharmaceuticals Ltd, 24 Leichi St, Bnei Brak 51200, Israel.

**TP, Thai.** TP Drug Lab Co. Ltd, 67 Sukhumvit 62, Prakanong, Bangkok 10250, Thailand.

**Trading, Israel.** Trading Pharma A.G., 11 Haodem St, Petach Tikva, Israel.

**Tradiphar, Fr.** Laboratoires Tradiphar, 176 rue de l'Arbrisseau, 59000 Lille, France.

**Tradis-Gat, Israel.** Tradis-Gat, P.O. Box 7775, Petach Tikva, Israel.

**Trahan, Thai.** See *Diethelm, Thai.*

**Tramedico, Belg.** Tramedico S.A., Europark-Oost 34, PB 50, 9100 Sint-Niklaas, Belgium.

**Tramedico, Neth.** Tramedico BV, Postbus 192, 1380 AD Weesp, Netherlands.

**Trans Bussan, Switz.** trans bussan s.a., 12 Rue Michel-Servet, 1211 Geneva 12, Switzerland.

**Trans Canaderm, Canad.** See *Stiefel, Canad.*

**Trans Dermal, Austral.** Trans Dermal Pharmaceuticals Pty Ltd, Level 10, St Martins Tower, 31 Market St, Sydney, NSW 2000, Australia.

**Transcontinental, Braz.** Transcontinental, Brazil.

**Transdermal, UK.** Transdermal Ltd, Grimwade Ave, Croydon, Surrey, CR0 5DJ, UK.

**Transpen, UK.** Transpen, UK.

**Transphyto, Fr.** Laboratoires Transphyto, 12 rue Louis-Blériot, 63100 Clermont-Ferrand, France.

**Travel-Safe, UK.** Travel-Safe Products Ltd, Hippodrome House, Birchett Rd, Aldershot, Hampshire, GU11 1LZ, UK.

**Travenol, UK.** Travenol Laboratories Ltd, Caxton Way, Thetford, Norfolk, IP24 3SE, UK.

**TRB, Arg.** TRB Pharma S.A., Plaza 939, 1427 Buenos Aires, Argentina.

**TRB, Braz.** TRB Pharma Industria Quimica e Farmaceutica Ltda, Av. Giuseppina V. Di Napoli 1100, 13086-550 Campinas, SP, Brazil.

**TRB, Singapore.** See *Pharma 2000, Singapore.*

**Treasure Mountain, Hong Kong.** Treasure Mountain Development Co. Ltd, 19/F Chit Lee Commercial Bldg, 30-36 Shaukeiwan Rd, Hong Kong.

**Treiner, USA.** Treiner Co, USA.

**Tremedic, Swed.** Tremedic AB, Faktorvagen 13, 434 37 Kungsbacka, Sweden.

**Trendful, Hong Kong.** Trendful Development Ltd, Room 1217 China Merchants Tower, Shun Tak Ctr, 168-200 Connaught Rd Central, Hong Kong.

**Trenier, USA.** Trenier, USA.

**Trenka, Austria.** F Trenka Chemisch-Pharmazeutische Fabrik GmbH, Goldeggassee 5, A-1040 Vienna, Austria.

**Trenka, Israel.** See *Tetra, Israel.*

**Trenka, Malaysia.** See *Antah, Malaysia.*

**Trenka, Switz.** See *Uhlmann-Eyraud, Switz.*

**Trenka Difer, Ital.** Trenka Difer International S.r.l., Via della Zonta 2, 34122 Trieste, Italy.

**Trenker, Belg.** Laboratoires Pharmaceutiques Trenker S.A., Ave Dolez 480-482, 1180 Brussels, Belgium.

**Trenker, Thai.** See *JAV, Thai.*

**Treupha, Switz.** Treupha SA, Zurcherstrasse 59, 5401 Baden, Switzerland.

**Tri Tec, USA.** Tri Tec Labs, 1000 Robins Rd, Lynchburg, VA 24504-3558, USA.

**Triangle, USA.** See *Tri Tec, USA.*

**Trianon, Canad.** Trianon Laboratories Inc., 660 Industriel Blvd, Blainville, Quebec, J7C 3V4, Canada.

**Trima, Israel.** Trima, Kibbutz Ma'abarot, Israel.

**Trima, Singapore.** See *Green Cross, Singapore.*

**Trima, Thai.** See *Union Medical, Thai.*

**Tri-Med, USA.** Tri-Med Specialties Inc., 16309 W 108th Circle, Lenexa, KS 66219-1372, USA.

**Trimedal, Switz.** Trimedal AG, Postfach, 8306 Bruttisellen, Switzerland.

**Trimen, USA.** Trimen Laboratories Inc., USA.

**Trinity, Hong Kong.** Trinity Trading Co. Ltd, Unit 7A-B, 39/F Cable TV Tower, 9 Hoi Shing Rd, Tsuen Wan, N.T., Hong Kong.

**Trinity, UK.** Trinity Pharmaceuticals Ltd, The Old Exchange, 12 Compton Rd, Wimbledon, London, SW19 7QD, UK.

**Triomed, S.Afr.** Triomed (Pty) Ltd, P.O. Box 36679, Chempet 7442, South Africa.

**Tripharma, Switz.** Tripharma AG, 8730 Uznach, Switzerland.

**Triton, USA.** Triton Consumer Products, Inc., 561 West Golf, Arlington Heights, IL 60005, USA.

**Trofomed, Ital.** Trofomed S.r.l., Via IV Novembre 7, 70020 Cassano delle Murge (BA), Italy.

**Troikaa, India.** Troikaa Pharmaceuticals Ltd, Om Towers, Satellite Rd, Ahmedabad 380 015, India.

**Trommsdorff, Ger.** Trommsdorff GmbH & Co. KG Arzneimittel, Trommsdorffstr. 2-6, 52477 Alsdorf, Germany.

**Tropic Suncare, Canad.** Tropic Suncare Canada Ltd, P. O. Box 6249, Station D, London, Ontario, N5W 5S1, Canada.

**Tropon, Ger.** Tropon GmbH, Neurather Ring 1, 51063 Cologne, Germany.

**Trupharm, Israel.** Trupharm, 1 Haomanut St, Netanya, Israel.

**Truw, Ger.** Truw Arzneimittel Vertriebs GmbH, Ziethenstr. 8, 33330 Gutersloh, Germany.

**Truxton, USA.** C.O. Truxton Inc., 136 Harding Ave, Bellmawr, NJ 08099, USA.

**TS, Ital.** Farmacetici T.S. S.r.l., Via M. G. dell'Unita 2, 00046 Grottaferrata (Rome), Italy.

**Tsumura, Jpn.** Tsumura & Co., 12-7 Nibancho, Chiyoda-ku, Tokyo 102-8422, Japan.

**TTK, India.** TTK Healthcare Ltd, 91 Santhome High Road, Chennai 600 028, India.

**TTN, Thai.** TTN Thitiratsanon Co. Ltd, 157/9 Prannok Rd, Siriraj Bangkoknoi, Bangkok 10700, Thailand.

**Tubilux, Ital.** Tubilux Pharma S.p.A., Via Costarica 20/22, 00040 Pomezia (RM), Italy.

**Turimed, Switz.** Turimed SA, Hertistrasse 8, 8304 Wallisellen, Switzerland.

**Tussin, Ger.** Tussin Pharma GmbH, Menchestr. 22 A, 35274 Kirchhain, Germany.

**Tutogen, Ger.** Tutogen Medical GmbH, Industriestr. 6, 91077 Neunkirchen a. Br., Germany.

**Twardy, Austria.** See *Twardy, Ger.*

**Twardy, Ger.** Astrid Twardy GmbH, Liebigstr. 18, 65439 Florsheim/Main, Germany.

**Tyco, Denm.** Tyco Healthcare Danmark, Langebrogade 6 E, 4, 1411 Copenhagen K, Denmark.

**Tyco, Ger.** Tyco Healthcare Deutschland GmbH, Gewerbepark 1, 93333 Neustadt/Donau, Germany.

**Tyco, Port.** Tyco Healthcare Portugal Lda, Estrada do Outeiro de Polima, Lote 10, 1 Piso, Abssboda, 2785-521 S. Domingos de Rana, Portugal.

**Tyco, Spain.** Tyco Healthcare Spain S.L., Fructuos Gelabert 6, 8a Planta, 08970 Barcelona, Spain.

**Tyco, Swed.** Tyco Healthcare Norden AB, Box 710, 169 27 Solna, Sweden.

**Tyco, UK.** Tyco Healthcare, 154 Fareham Rd, Gosport, Hampshire, PO13 0AS, UK.

**Typen, Arg.** Typen S.A.I.C.F., Colombres 257, 1177 Buenos Aires, Argentina.

**Typharm, Irl.** See *Boileau & Boyd, Irl.*

**Typharm, UK.** Typharm Ltd, 14D Wendover Rd, Rackheath Industrial Estate, Norwich, Norfolk, NR13 6LH, UK.

**Tyrol, Austria.** Tyrol Pharma GmbH, Biochemiestrasse 10, A-6250 Kundl, Austria.

**Tyson, USA.** Tyson & Associates Inc., 12832 S Chadron Ave, Hawthorne, CA 90250-5525, USA.

**Tzamal, Israel.** Tzamal Pharma Ltd, 20 Hamgshimim, Kiryat Matalon, Petach Tikva, Israel.

**UAD, USA.** See *Forest Laboratories, USA.*

**UB Interpharm, Switz.** UB Interpharm SA, 36 av Cardinal-Mermillod, 1227 Carouge/GE, Switzerland.

**UCB, Austral.** UCB Pharma, A Division of UCB Australia P/L, 19 Potter St, Carigieburn, VIC 3064, Australia.

**UCB, Austria.** UCB Pharma GmbH, Brunnerstrasse 73/5, A-1210 Vienna, Austria.

**UCB, Belg.** UCB Pharma S.A., Route de Lennik 437, 1070 Brussels, Belgium.

**UCB, Canad.** See *UCB, USA.*

**UCB, Denm.** UCB Pharma, Postboks 2312, 1026 Copenhagen K, Denmark.

**UCB, Fin.** UCB Pharma Oy Finland, Ratavallintie 2, 00720 Helsinki, Finland.

**UCB, Fr.** UCB Pharma S.A., 21 rue de Neuilly, 92003 Nanterre, France.

**UCB, Ger.** UCB GmbH, Huttenstr. 205, 50170 Kerpen, Germany.

**UCB, Gr.** UCB PHARMA AE, Βουλιαγμένης 580, 164 52 Αργυρούπολη, Argiroupoli, Greece.

**UCB, Hong Kong.** UCB Pharma Ltd, Unit 1002-03, 10/F Guangdong Finance Building, 88 Connaught Rd West, Hong Kong.

**UCB, India.** UCB India Pvt Ltd, VIP House, 1st Floor, 88C Old Prabhadevi Rd, Mumbai 400 025, India.

**UCB, Irl.** See *United Drug, Irl.*

**UCB, Ital.** UCB Pharma S.p.A., Via Praglia 15, 10044 Pianezza (TO), Italy.

**UCB, Jpn.** UCB Japan Co. Ltd, 2-2 Kanda-Surugadai, Chiyoda-ku, Tokyo 101-0062, Japan.

**UCB, Malaysia.** UCB Asia Pacific Sdn Bhd, Suite 3.08, 3rd floor, Wisma Academy, 4A, Jln 19/1, 46300 Petaling jaya, Selangor, Malaysia.

**UCB, Mex.** UCB de Mexico S.A. de C.V., Homero No. 440, Piso 7, Col. Chapultepec Morales, 11570 Mexico D.F., Mexico.

**UCB, Neth.** UCB Pharma BV, Druivenstraat 5, 4816 KB Breda, Netherlands.

**UCB, Norw.** UCB Pharma AS, Brynsv. 96, 1352 Kolsas, Norway.

**UCB, Port.** UCB, Lda, Rua Gregorio Lopes, Lote 1597, 1400-195 Lisbon, Portugal.

**UCB, S.Afr.** UCB SA (Pty) Ltd, P.O. Box 31036, Braamfontein 2017, South Africa.

**UCB, Singapore.** UCB Singapore Pte Ltd, Singapore.

**UCB, Spain.** UCB Pharma, Ramon y Cajal 6, Molins de Rei, 08750 Barcelona, Spain.

**UCB, Swed.** UCB Pharma AB (Sweden), 212 25 Malmo, Sweden.

**UCB, Switz.** UCB-Pharma AG, Kreuzstrasse 60, 8008 Zurich, Switzerland.

**UCB, Thai.** UCB Pharma (Thailand) Ltd, 27 Fl, Panjathani Tower, 127/32 Nonsee Rd, Yannawa, Bangkok 10120, Thailand.

**UCB, UK.** UCB Pharma Ltd, 3 George St, Watford, Hertforshire, WD1 8UH, UK.

**UCB, USA.** UCB Pharma Inc., 1950 Lake Park Drive, Atlanta, GA 30080, USA.

**UCB Healthcare, Fr.** Laboratoire UCB Healthcare, 3-5 rue Diderot, 92003 Nanterre, France.

**UCI, Braz.** UCI-Farma Industria Farmaceutica Ltda, Rua Cruzeiro 374, 09725-310 Sao Bernardo do Campo, SP, Brazil.

**Ucyclyd, USA.** Ucyclyd Pharma Inc., 500 McCormic Dr., Suite J, Glen Burnie, MD 21061, USA.

**Ueno, Jpn.** Ueno Fine Chemicals Industry Ltd, 4-8 Koraibashi 2-chome, Chuo-ku, Osaka 541-8543, Japan.

**Uhlmann-Eyraud, Switz.** F. Uhlmann-Eyraud SA, 28 chemin du Grand-Puits, 1217 Meyrin 2/Geneva, Switzerland.

**Ulmer, USA.** Ulmer Pharmacal Co., 2440 Fernbrook Lane, Plymouth, MN 55447-9987, USA.

**Ultrapharm, UK.** Ultrapharm Ltd, 1,2,3 Centenary Business Park, Henley-on-Thames, Oxfordshire, RG9 1DS, UK.

**Unam, Hong Kong.** Unam Corp Ltd, 7/F Chiu Lung Bldg, 25 Chiu Lung St Central, Hong Kong.

**Unam, Malaysia.** Unam Corporation (M) Sdn Bhd, 11th Floor, Menara ING, 84 Jln Raja Chulan, 50200 Kuala Lumpur, Kuala Lumpur, Malaysia.

**Undra, Mex.** Undra, Mexico.

**Ungar, Austria.** Ungar-Apotheke zur Göttlichen Vorsehung, Ungargasse 14, A-1030 Vienna, Austria.

**Uni, Singapore.** Uni Drug House Pte Ltd, 61 Kaki Bukit Ave 1, 05-31 Shunli Industrial Park, S 417943, Singapore.

**Uniao Quimica, Braz.** Uniao Quimica Farmaceutica Nacional S.A., Avenida dos Bandeirantes 5386, 04071-900 Sao Paulo, SP, Brazil.

**Unibios, Spain.** Unibios, Spain.

**Unichem, India.** Unichem Laboratories Ltd, Prabhat Estate, S.V. Rd, Jogeshwari (W), Mumbai 400 102, India.

**Unichem, UK.** Unichem Ltd, Unichem House, Cox Lane, Chessington, Surrey, KT9 1SN, UK.

**Unico, Hong Kong.** Unico Health Care Products Ltd, Rm 1007, Tower B Seaview Estate, 2-8 Watson Rd, North Point, Hong Kong.

**Unico, USA.** Unico Inc., 1830 2nd Ave N, Lake Worth, FL 33461, USA.

**Unicure, India.** Unicure Remedies Pvt Ltd, F/25 Industrial Estate, Gorwa, Vadodara 390 016, India.

**Uniderm, Israel.** See *Promedico, Israel.*

**Uniderm, Ital.** Uniderm Farmaceutici S.r.l., P.le F. il Macedone 140, 001246 Casalpalocco (RM), Italy.

**Unifa, Port.** See *CPH, Port.*

**Unifarm, Ital.** Unifarm S.p.A., Via Provina 3, 38040 Ravina (TN), Italy.

**Unifarma, Spain.** See *Unipharma, Spain.*

**Unigreg, Irl.** See *Unigreg, UK.*

**Unigreg, UK.** Unigreg Ltd, Enterprise House, 181-9 Garth Rd, Morden, Surrey, SM4 4LL, UK.

**Unilever, Canad.** Unilever, 160 Bloor St. E, Suite 300, Toronto, Ontario, M4W 3W3, Canada.

**Unilever, USA.** Unilever HPC, 33 Benedict Place, Greenwich, CT 06830, USA.

**Unimed, India.** Unimed Technologies Pvt Ltd, Synergy House, Subhanpura, Gorwa Rd, Vadodara 390 016, India.

**Unimed, Israel.** See *Megapharm, Israel.*

**Unimed, USA.** Unimed Pharmaceuticals Inc., 2150 E. Lake Cook Road, Buffalo Grove, IL 60089-1862, USA.

**Unimedic, Swed.** Unimedic AB, Box 91, 864 21 Matfors, Sweden.

**Union, Singapore.** Union Chem & Pharm, Singapore.

**Union Medical, Thai.** Union Medical (Thailand) Co. Ltd, 513/199-200 Jaransanitwong Rd, Soi 37 Bangkoknoi, Bangkok 10700, Thailand.

**Unipack, Austria.** Unipack GmbH, Braunlichgasse 40-42, A-2700 Wiener Neustadt, Austria.

**Unipath, Israel.** See *Agis, Israel.*

**Unipath, UK.** Unipath Ltd, Priory Business Park, Bedford, Bedfordshire, MK44 6UP, UK.

**Unipharm, Hong Kong.** Unipharm Trading Co., Rm 634-635, Nan Fung Ctr, 264-298 Castle Peak Rd, Tsuen Wan, N.T., Hong Kong.

**Unipharm, Israel.** Unipharm Ltd, P.O. Box 21429, Tel Aviv, Israel.

**Unipharm, Singapore.** See *Green Cross, Singapore.*

**Unipharma, Gr.** UNI-PHARMA AE, 14ο χλμ. Εθνικής Οδού Αθηνών-Λαμίας Greece.

**Unipharma, Spain.** Unipharma, Mino 8, 08022 Barcelona, Spain.

**Unipharma, Switz.** Unipharma SA, Via Pian Scairolo 6, 6917 Barbengo, Switzerland.

**Unique, India.** Unique Pharmaceutical Laboratories, Neelam Centre, B Wing, 4th floor, Hind Cycle Rd, Worli, Mumbai 400 025, India.

**Unique, Thai.** See *Union Medical, Thai.*

**Uni-Sankyo, India.** Uni-Sankyo Ltd, 392 Sagar Society, Plot 84, Road No. 2, Banjara Hills, Hyderabad 500 034, India.

**Unison, Hong Kong.** See *Health Alliance, Hong Kong.*

**Unison, Malaysia.** See *Pahang, Malaysia.*

**Unison, Singapore.** See *Age D'or, Singapore.*

**Unison, Thai.** Unison Laboratories Co. Ltd, 160 Soi Onnuch, Sukhumvit Rd, Ladkrabang, Bangkok 10520, Thailand.

**Unitech, Irl.** Unitech Ltd, United Drug House, Belgard Rd, Tallaght, Dublin 24, Ireland.

**United American, Hong Kong.** See *Unam, Hong Kong.*

**United American, Malaysia.** See *Unam, Malaysia.*

**United American, Singapore.** See *Far East, Singapore.*

**United American, Thai.** See *Olic, Thai.*

**United Drug, Irl.** United Drug, United Drug House, Belgard Rd, Tallaght, Dublin 24, Ireland.

**United Drug, UK.** United Drug Distribution Group (UDG) Ltd, Amber Park, Berristow Lane, South Normanton, Derbyshire, DE55 2FH, UK.

**United Italian, Malaysia.** United Italian Trading (M) Sdn Bhd, P.O. Box 746, Jln Sultan, 46780 Petaling Jaya, Selangor, Malaysia.

**United Italian, Singapore.** United Italian Trading Corp Pte Ltd, 65 Upper Paya Lebar Rd, 06-03 Guang Ming Industrial Building, S 534817, Singapore.

**United Medical, Braz.** United Medical Ltda, Rua Jesuino Arruda 769, 9 andar, 04532-082 Sao Paulo, SP, Brazil.

**United Nordic, Denm.** United Nordic Pharma A/S, Hammervej 7, 2970 Horsholm, Denmark.

**United Therapeutics, Israel.** See *Rafa, Israel.*

**United Therapeutics, USA.** United Therapeutics Corp., Research Triangle Park, NC 27709, USA.

**Universal, Hong Kong.** Universal Pharmaceutical Lab Ltd, Eastern Ctr, G/F & 1/F, Unit 1-5, 1065 King's Rd, Quarry Bay, Hong Kong.

**Universal, S.Afr.** Universal Pharmaceuticals (Pty) Ltd, P.O. Box 33068, Jeppestown 2043, South Africa.

**Universales, Mex.** Productos Quimicos Universales S.A. de C.V., Alicante No. 127, Col. Alamos, 03400 Mexico D.F., Mexico.

**Uno, Ital.** Farma Uno S.r.l., Via Conforti 42, 84083 Castel San Giorgio (SA), Italy.

**Upha, Malaysia.** Upha Corporation (M) Sdn Bhd, Lot 2 & 4, Jln P/7, Section 13, Bangi Industrial Estate, 43650 Bandar Baru Bangi, Selangor, Malaysia.

**Upha, Singapore.** See *FP, Singapore*, and *Zuellig, Singapore.*

**Upjohn, UK.** See *Pharmacia, UK.*

**Upjohn, USA.** See *Pharmacia, USA.*

**UPSA, Fr.** Laboratoires UPSA, La Grande Arche Nord, 92044 Paris-La Defense cdx, France.

**UPSA, Hong Kong.** See *Wing Wai, Hong Kong.*

**Upsa, Ital.** Upsa S.p.A., Via Virgillio Maroso 50, 00142 Rome, Italy.

**UPSA Conseil, Fr.** See *Bristol-Myers Squibb, Fr.*

**Upsamedica, Belg.** See *Bristol-Myers Squibb, Belg.*

**Upsamedica, Ital.** See *Upsa, Ital.*

**Upsamedica, Spain.** Upsa Medica, C/Almansa, 101, 28040 Madrid, Spain.

**Upsamedica, Switz.** Upsamedica SA, Neuhofstrasse 6, 6341 Baar, Switzerland.

**Upsher Smith, Israel.** See *Meditrend, Israel.*

**Upsher-Smith, USA.** Upsher-Smith Laboratories Inc., 14905 23rd Ave North, Minneapolis, MN 55447-4709, USA.

**Upsifarma, Port.** Upsifarma, Lda, S. Domingos a Lapa 8, Letra H, 1200-835 Lisbon, Portugal.

**Uragme, Ital.** Uragme, Via A. Vivaldi 9, 00199 Rome, Italy.

**Urbion, Spain.** Urbion Farma, Avda Portugal, Parcela 85 Pol Allendeduero, Aranada de Duero, 09400 Burgos, Spain.

**Urgo, Belg.** See *Fournier, Belg.*

**Urgo, Fr.** Laboratoires Urgo, B.P. 157, 42 rue de Longvic, 21300 Chenove, France.

**Urgo, Ger.** See *Fournier, Ger.*

**Urgo, Israel.** See *Agis, Israel.*

**Uriach, Spain.** Uriach, Dega Bahi 59, 08026 Barcelona, Spain.

**Uriage, Fr.** Laboratoires Dermatologiques Uriage, 98 av de la Republique, 92400 Courbevoie, France.

**URL, USA.** United Research Laboratories, 1100 Orthodox St, Philadelphia, PA 19124, USA.

**Urocor, USA.** Urocor, USA.

**URPAC, Fr.** See *Beaufour, Fr.*

**Ursapharm, Ger.** Ursapharm Arzneimittel GmbH & Co. KG, Industriestr., 66129 Saarbrucken, Germany.

**Ursapharm, Israel.** Ursapharm, Israel.

**Ursapharm, Malaysia.** See *Pharmaforte, Malaysia.*

**Ursapharm, Neth.** Ursapharm Benelux BV, Postbus 376, 3770 AJ Barneveld, Netherlands.

**US Bio, Israel.** US Bio, Israel.

**US Bioscience, Denm.** See *Orphan, Denm.*, and *Schering-Plough, Denm.*

**US Bioscience, USA.** US Bioscience Inc., One Tower Bridge, 100 Front St, West Conshohocken, PA 19428, USA.

**US Pharmaceutical, USA.** US Pharmaceutical Corp., 2401-C Mellon Court, Decatur, GA 30035, USA.

**US Summit, Hong Kong.** U.S. Summit Co. Ltd, Unit A, 32/F, Manulife Tower, 169 Electric Rd, North Point, Hong Kong.

**US Summit, Thai.** US Summit Corp (Overseas), 52/184 Sukhapibai 3 Rd, Huamark, Bangkapi, Bangkok 10240, Thailand.

**US Surgical, USA.** Unites States Surgical Corp., 150 Glover Ave, Norwalk, CT, USA.

**Usana, Canad.** See *USANA, USA.*

**Usana, Hong Kong.** Usana Hong Kong Ltd, Unit 2504-06, 25/F, World Trade Centre, 280 Gloucester Rd, Causeway Bay, Hong Kong.

**USANA, USA.** USANA, Inc., 3838 West Parkway Blvd, Salt Lake City, UT 84120-6336, USA.

**Usmed, Braz.** Laboratorio Usmed Ltda, Rua Ana Ribeiro 164, Bairro Gloria, 32310-510 Contagem, MG, Brazil.

**USV, India.** USV Ltd, B.S. Devshi Marg, Govandi, Mumbai 400 088, India.

**USV, Israel.** USV, Israel.

**Utopian, Thai.** Utopian Co. Ltd, 602 Moo 3, Teparak Rd, Muang, Samuthprakarn 10270, Thailand.

**V & V, Thai.** V & V Bangkok, 94/7 Soi Yimprakrob, Ngamwongwan, Nonthaburi, Thailand.

**VAAS, Ital.** VAAS S.r.l., Via Siena 268, 47032 Capocolle di Bertinoro (FO), Italy.

**Vaccina, S.Afr.** Vaccina CC, P.O. Box 75804, Gardenview 2047, South Africa.

**Vachon, Canad.** Les Laboratoires Vachon Inc., 8700 de-la-Rive-Sud Blvd, Levis, Quebec, G6V 6N6, Canada.

**Vaillant, Ital.** Laboratori Italiani Vaillant S.r.l., Via Cavalieri V. Veneto 241, 21040 Cislago (VA), Italy.

**Valda, Canad.** See *Bayer, Canad.*

**Valda, Ital.** See *GlaxoSmithKline Consumer, Ital.*

**Valdecasas, Mex.** Laboratorios Valdecasas S.A., Av. Insurgentes Sur No. 4058, Deleg. Tlalpan, 14430 Mexico D.F., Mexico.

**Valeas, Ital.** Valeas S.p.A., Via Vallisneri 10, 20133 Milan, Italy.

**Valens, Ital.** Farma Valens S.r.l., Via Passopomo 5, 95101 Snata Venerina (CT), Italy.

**Valio, Fin.** Valio Oy, Meijeritie 6, PL 10, 00039 Valio, Finland.

**Valma, Chile.** Laboratorio Valma Ltda, Miguel de Atero 2883, Santiago, Chile.

**ValMed, USA.** ValMed Inc., 100 Otis St, Suite 4A, Northboro, MA 01532, USA.

**Valmo, Canad.** Lab. Valmo Enrg, 1000 Industriel Blvd, Chambly, Quebec, J3L 3H9, Canada.

**Valomed, Spain.** Valomed, San Rafael 3, Alcobendas, 28108 Madrid, Spain.

**Vana, Thai.** Vana Corp Ltd, 2038 Sukhumvit Rd, Bangkok 10250, Thailand.

**Vangard, USA.** Vangard Labs Inc., P.O. Box 1268, Glasgow, KY 42142-1268, USA.

**Vannier, Arg.** Lab. Vannier S.A., B. Quinquela Martin 2228, 1296 Buenos Aires, Argentina.

**Vantone, Hong Kong.** Vantone Medical Supplies Co. Ltd, Flat J, 10/F International Industrial Ctr, 2-8 Kwei Tei St, Fotan, N.T., Hong Kong.

**Varifarma, Arg.** Lab. Varifarma S.A., Ernesto de las Carreras 2469, 1643 Beccar, Buenos Aires, Argentina.

**Varos, Braz.** Varos Industria e Comercio de Produtos Farmaceuticos Ltda, Rua Viuva Lacerda 203, Botafogo, 22261-050 Rio de Janeiro, RJ, Brazil.

**Veafarm, Braz.** Laboratorio Veafarm Ltda, Rua Doutor Pena Forte Mendes 255, 01308-010 Sao Paulo, SP, Brazil.

**Vebas, Ital.** Vebas S.r.l., Via Benaco 1/3, 20098 San Giuliano Milanese (MI), Italy.

**Vectem, Spain.** Vectem, Wagner 22, Pol Ind Can Jardi, Rubi, 08191 Barcelona, Spain.

**Veda, Fr.** See *Zambon, Fr.*

**Vedim, Fr.** Laboratoires Vedim Pharma, 7 rue Diderot, 92003 Nanterre, France.

**Vedim, Ger.** See *UCB, Ger.*

**Vedim, Port.** Vedim Pharma, Lda, Rua Carlos Calisto 4-B, 1400-043 Lisbon, Portugal.

**Vedim, Spain.** Vedim Pharma, Avda de Barcelona 239, Molins de Rei, 08750 Barcelona, Spain.

**Vegetal, Ital.** Vegetal Progress S.r.l., Localita Novaro 8, 10070 Devesi di Cirie (TO), Italy.

**Veinfar, Arg.** Veinfar, Esp. Medicinales Larjan, Piedrabuena 4190, 1439 Buenos Aires, Argentina.

**Velka, Gr.** VELKA HELLAS A.E., Κορίνθου 12, 154 51 Ν. Ψυχικό, N. Psichiko, Greece.

**Vemedia, Neth.** See *Solvay, Neth.*

**Vent-3, Arg.** Lab. Vent-3, Ruta 9 4765, 5020 Ferreira, Cordoba, Argentina.

**Veripalvelu, Fin.** Soumen Punainen Risti Veripalvelu, Kivihaantie 7, 00310 Helsinki, Finland.

**Veritas, Braz.** Laboratorio Hanemaniano Veritas Ltda, Rua Barbosa 48, 21350-020 Rio de Janeiro, RJ, Brazil.

**Verla, Ger.** Verla-Pharm, Arzneimittelfabrik, Apotheker H.J.v. Ehrlich GmbH & Co. KG, Hauptstr. 98, 82327 Tutzing, Germany.

**Verman, Fin.** Oy Verman AB, Vanhankyläntie 44 B, PL 152, 04401 Järvenpää, Finland.

**Veron, Ger.** Veron Pharma Vertriebs-GmbH, Neuweg 30, 67697 Otterberg, Germany.

**Verum, USA.** Verum Pharmaceuticals, 1000 Park Forty Plaza, Suite 300, Research Triangle Park, NC 27713, USA.

**Vesta, S.Afr.** Vesta Medicines (Pty) Ltd, South Africa.

**Veyron-Froment, Fr.** Laboratoires Veyron et Froment, 30 rue Benedit, 13248 Marseille cdx 04, France.

**Vezedes, Fr.** Vézédès Sarl, 9 quai de Rotterdam, 68110 Illzach, France.

**VHB, India.** VHB Pharmaceuticals Pvt Ltd, 40-B/1 Shankar Smruti, Sir Bhalchandra Rd, Dadar (E), Mumbai 400 014, India.

**Via, Switz.** Via Marketing & Promotion SA, Via Ponte Tresa 7-7A, 6924 Sorengo, Switzerland.

**Viamedica, Spain.** Viamedica, Spain.

**Vianex (Βιανεξ), Gr.** ΒΙΑΝΕΞ ΑΕ, Λ. Τατοΐου, 146 10 Ν. Ερυθραια, N. Erithraia, Greece.

**Viatria, Swed.** Viatria AB, Kemistvagen 17, 183 79 Taby, Sweden.

**Viatris, Austria.** Viatris Pharma GmbH, Liesinger Flur-Gasse 2C, A-1230 Vienna, Austria.

**Viatris, Belg.** VIATRIS S.A., Rue de l'Etuve 77-81, 1000 Brussels, Belgium.

**Viatris, Fr.** Viatris, Av J.F. Kennedy, 33701 Merignac cdx, France.

**Viatris, Ger.** VIATRIS GmbH & Co. KG, Weismullerstr. 45, 60314 Frankfurt a.M., Germany.

**Viatris, Ital.** VIATRIS S.p.A., Via Zanella 3/5, 20133 Milan, Italy.

**Viatris, Neth.** Viatris BV, Verrijn Stuartweg 60, 1112 AX Diemen, Netherlands.

**Viatris, Port.** VIATRIS Farmaceutica SA, Rua do Centro Cultural 13, 1749-066 Lisbon, Portugal.

**Viatris, Spain.** Viatris Pharmaceuticals S.A.U., Avenida Fuentemar 27, Poligono Industrial de Coslada, 28820 Madrid, Spain.

**Viatris, Switz.** VIATRIS GmbH, Hegnaustrasse 60, 8602 Wangen, Switzerland.

**Viatris, UK.** VIATRIS Pharmaceuticals Ltd, Building 2000, Cambridge Research Park, Waterbeach, Cambridge, Cambridgeshire, CB5 9PD, UK.

**Vicente, Spain.** Vicente, Spain.

**Vichy, Canad.** See *Cosmair, Canad.*

**Vickmans, Hong Kong.** Vickmans Laboratories Ltd, 1/F Kai Yip Factory Building, 15 Sam Chuk St, San Po Kong, Kowloon, Hong Kong.

**Vida, Hong Kong.** Vida Laboratories Ltd, Unit 919 Vanta Industrial Ctr, 21 Tai Lin Pai Rd, Kwai Chung, N.T., Hong Kong.

**Vida, Port.** See *Atral, Port.*

**Vieira, Port.** Raul Vieira, Lda, Rua dos Correeiros 41, 1100 Lisbon, Portugal.

**Vifor, Denm.** See *Nordiatech, Denm.*

**Vifor, Gr.** See *Genesis, Gr.*, and *Nycomed, Gr.*

**Vifor, Hong Kong.** See *Hong Kong Medical, Hong Kong*, and *Keller, Hong Kong.*

**Vifor, Israel.** See *CTS, Israel.*

**Vifor, Malaysia.** See *Diethelm, Malaysia.*

**Vifor, Port.** See *Ferraz, Lynce, Port.*, and *Confar, Port.*

**Vifor, Singapore.** See *Diethelm, Singapore.*

**Vifor, Switz.** Vifor SA, Case Postale 1067, 1701 Fribourg-Moncor, Switzerland.

**Vifor, Thai.** See *Diethelm, Thai.*

**Vifor International, Switz.** Vifor (International) AG, Pharmazeutische Spezialitäten, Rechenstrasse 37, Postfach, 9001 St Gallen, Switzerland.

**Vifor Medical, Switz.** Vifor Medical SA, 9 route de Sorge, Case postale 161, 1023 Crissier, Switzerland.

**Vilardell, Spain.** Vilardell, Constitucion 66-8, Les Grases, San Feliu de Llobregat, 08980 Barcelona, Spain.

**Vilco, Gr.** VILCO, Πεύκων 121, 141 22 Ν. Ηράκλειο, N. Irakleio, Greece.

**Vinas, Spain.** Viñas, Provenza 386, 08025 Barcelona, Spain.

**Vinas, Switz.** See *Golaz, Switz.*

**Vindex, USA.** Vindex Pharmaceuticals, USA.

**Vingmed, Norw.** Vingmed AS, Fjordv. 1, Postboks 374, 1363 Hovik, Norway.

**Viofar, Gr.** VIOFAR ΕΠΕ, Ε. Αντιστάσεως & Τριφυλλίας, 136 71, Αχαρναι, Acharnai, Greece.

**Vir, Spain.** Vir, Laguna 42-4, Pol In Urtinsa II, Alcorcon, 28923 Madrid, Spain.

**Viranative, Swed.** ViraNative AB, Box 7979, 907 19 Umea, Sweden.

**Virco, Canad.** Virco Pharmaceuticals (Canada) Inc., 30 St Clair Ave W, Suite 400, Toronto, Ontario, M4V 3A1, Canada.

**Virgo Healthcare, Austral.** Virgo Healthcare, Unit 2, 85-7 Moore St, Leichhardt, NSW 2040, Australia.

**Virtus, Braz.** Virtu's Industria e Comercio Ltda, Avenida Sargento Geraldo Santana 660, 04674-000 Sao Paulo, SP, Brazil.

**Vision, USA.** Vision Pharmaceuticals Inc., P.O. Box 400, Mitchell, SD 57301-0400, USA.

**Vistapharm, USA.** VistaPharm, 4647 T Hwy 280 E, Suite 145, Birmingham, AL 35242, USA.

**Visufarma, Ital.** Visufarma S.r.l., Via Canino 21, 00191 Rome, Italy.

**Vita, Ital.** Laboratori Farmaceutici Vita S.r.l., Via Messina 38, 20154 Milan, Italy.

**Vita, Spain.** Grupo Vita, Avda de Barcelona 69, Sant Juan Despi, 08970 Barcelona, Spain.

**Vita Elan, Spain.** See *Elan, Spain.*

**Vita Health, Canad.** Vita Health Co. (1985) Ltd, 150 Beghin Ave, Winnipeg, Manitoba, R2J 3W2, Canada.

**Vita Health, Singapore.** Vita Health Laboratories Pte Ltd, Blk 1 Alexandra Distripark, 10-32/33/34 Pasir Panjang Rd, S 118478, Singapore.

**Vita Healthcare, UK.** Vita Healthcare Ltd, Palladium House, 1-4 Argyll St, London, W1V 2LD, UK.

**Vita Pharm, Canad.** Vita Pharm Canada Ltd, 2835 Kew Dr., Windsor, Ontario, N8T 3B7, Canada.

**Vitabalans, Fin.** Vitabalans Oy, Varastokatu 8, 13500 Hämeenlinna, Finland.

**Vitabiotics, Hong Kong.** See *Mekim, Hong Kong.*

**Vitabiotics, Irl.** See *Allphar, Irl.*

**Vitabiotics, UK.** Vitabiotics Ltd, 1 Beresford Ave, Wembley, Middlesex, HA0 1NU, UK.

**Vitae, Mex.** Vitae Laboratorios S.A. de C.V., Euclides No. 3214, Fracc. Vallarta San Jorge, 44690 Guadalajara, Jal., Mexico.

**Vitafarma, Spain.** Vitafarma, Florida 29, Hernani, 20120 Guipuzcoa, Spain.

**Vitaflo, Denm.** Vitaflo Scandinavia AB, Boks 144, 3400 Hillerod, Denmark.

**Vitaflo, Fin.** See *Tamro, Fin.*

**Vitaflo, Irl.** See *Allphar, Irl.*

**Vitaflo, Norw.** Vitaflo Norge, Carl Kjelsensv. 38, 0874 Oslo, Norway.

**Vitaflo, Swed.** Vitaflo Scandinavia AB, Box 53063, 400 14 Goteborg, Sweden.

**Vitaflo, UK.** Vitaflo Ltd, 11 Century Building, Brunswick Business Park, Liverpool, Merseyside, L3 4BL, UK.

**Vitaglow, Austral.** See *Blackmores, Austral.*

**Vita-Health, Hong Kong.** See *Great Liaison, Hong Kong,* and *Hind Wing, Hong Kong.*

**Vitalia, UK.** Vitalia Ltd, UK.

**Vitaline, Fin.** See *Sairaalapalvelu, Fin.*

**Vitaline, Norw.** See *Vingmed, Norw.*

**Vitaline, Swed.** Vitaline Scandinavia AB, Box 938, 751 03 Uppsala, Sweden.

**Vitaline, UK.** Vitaline Pharmaceuticals UK Ltd, 8 Ridge Way, Drakes Drive, Crendon Business Park, Long Crendon, Buckinghamshire, HP18 9BF, UK.

**Vitaline, USA.** Vitaline Corp., 385 Williamson Way, Ashland, OR 97520, USA.

**Vitality, USA.** Vitality Inc., 63 South Royal, Suite 801, Mobile, AL 36602, USA.

**Vitalpharma, Belg.** Vitalpharma S.A., Rue Egide Van Ophem 110, 1180 Brussels, Belgium.

**Vitamed, Braz.** Laboratorio Farmaceutico Vitamed Ltda, Rue Flavio Francisco Bellini 459, 95098-170 Caxias do Sul, RS, Brazil.

**Vitamed, Israel.** Vitamed Ltd, P.O. Box 114, Binyamina 30550, Israel.

**Vitaplex, Austral.** Vitaplex Products, P.O. Box 270, Gymea, NSW 2227, Australia.

**Vitasan, Austria.** Vitasan GmbH, Teichweg 2, A-5400 Hallein, Austria.

**Vitelle, Austral.** See *Mayne, Austral.*

**Viternat, Braz.** Viternat Laboratorios Ltda, Av Dr Luis Arrobas Martins 759, 04781-001 Sao Paulo, SP, Brazil.

**Vitex, Braz.** Vitex, Brazil.

**Vitorgan, Ger.** vitOrgan Arzneimittel GmbH, Brunnweisenstr. 21, 73760 Ostfildern, Germany.

**Vitoria, Port.** Laboratórios Vitória, SA, Rua Elias Garcia 28, Venda Nova, 2700-327 Amadora, Portugal.

**Vitrolife, Swed.** Vitrolife AB, Molndalsvagen 30, 412 63 Goteborg, Sweden.

**Vivalife, Port.** Vivalife Laboratorios Lda, Rotunda Nuno R. Santos, 2685 Portela de Sacavim, Portugal.

**Vivance, Fr.** Vivance SA, La Maison blanche, 71570 Romaneche-Thorins, France.

**Vivant, Mex.** Vivant, Mexico.

**Viviar, Spain.** Viviar, Pol Ind Pista de Ademuz, Autov Valencia-Liria Km 9.4, Paterna, 46980 Valencia, Spain.

**Vivus, Austria.** See *Vivus, USA.*

**Vivus, Norw.** See *Abbott, Norw.*

**Vivus, USA.** Vivus Inc, 605 East Fairchild Dr., Mountain View, CA 94043, USA.

**Vocate, Gr.** VOCATE, Γούναρη 150, 166 74 Γλυφάδα, Glyfada, Greece.

**Voco, Denm.** See *Voco, Ger.*

**Voco, Ger.** Voco GmbH, Postfach: 767, 27457 Cuxhaven, Germany.

**Volchem, Ital.** Volchem, Via E Dandolo 14, 35010 Grossa di Gazzo (PD), Italy.

**Volta, Chile.** Laboratorio Volta Ltda, Jose Miguel Carrera 14-A Complejo Ind., Los Libertadores Colina, Santiago, Chile.

**Vortech, USA.** Vortech Pharmaceuticals, 6851 Chase Rd, Dearborn, MI 48126, USA.

**Voyage, Fr.** Laboratoires Pharma Voyage, 29 av. de la Gare, 78310 Ciognieres, France.

**VSM, Neth.** VSM Geneesmiddelen BV, Postbus 9321, 1800 GH Alkmaar, Netherlands.

**Wabosan, Austria.** Wabosan Arzneimittelvertriebs GmbH, Anton Anderer Platz 6, A-1210 Vienna, Austria.

**Wakamoto, Hong Kong.** See *Tai Tong, Hong Kong.*

**Wakefield, USA.** Wakefield Pharmaceuticals, Inc., 310 Maxwell Rd, Suite 100, Alpharetta, GA 30004, USA.

**Wala, Ger.** Wala Heilmittel GmbH, Bosslerweg 2, 73087 Bad Boll/Eckwalden, Germany.

**Waldheim, Austria.** See *Sanochemia, Austria.*

**Walker, Arg.** Laboratorio Walker S.R.L., E. Zeballos 249, 2000 Rosario, Santa Fe, Argentina.

**Walker Laboratories, USA.** Walker Laboratories, 4200 Laclede Ave, St Louis, MO 63108, USA.

**Walker Pharmacal, USA.** See *Walker Laboratories, USA.*

**Wallace, India.** Wallace Pharmaceuticals Ltd, 101/2 Floral Deck Plaza, Off Central MIDC Rd, Andheri (East), Mumbai 400 093, India.

**Wallace, USA.** Wallace Laboratories, Division of Carter-Wallace Inc., P.O. Box 1001, Cranbury, NJ 08512, USA.

**Wallace Mfg Chem., UK.** Wallace Manufacturing Chemists Ltd, Wallace House, New Abbey Court, 51-53 Stert St, Abingdon, Oxfordshire, OX14 3HB, UK.

**Wallis, UK.** Wallis Laboratory, Laporte Way, Luton, Bedfordshire, LU4 8WL, UK.

**Wampole, Canad.** Wampole Canada Inc., 465 Milner Ave, Unit 1, Scarborough, Ontario, M1B 2K4, Canada.

**Wampole, USA.** Wampole Laboratories, Half Acre Rd, P.O. Box 1001, Cranbury, NJ 08512-0181, USA.

**Wander, Belg.** See *Novartis, Belg.*

**Wander, India.** Wander Ltd, Plot No. 21, Sector-19, Kopri Rd, Vashi, Navi Mumbai 400 703, India.

**Wander, Ital.** Wander S.p.A., Via Meucci 39, 20128 Milan, Italy.

**Wander Health Care, Switz.** Wander AG, Postfach, 3001 Bern, Switzerland.

**Wander OTC, Switz.** See *Novartis Consumer, Switz.*

**Wanskerne, UK.** Wanskerne Ltd, 31 High Cross Street, St Austell, Cornwall, PL25 4AN, UK.

**Warner Chilcott, USA.** Warner Chilcott Laboratories, Rockaway 80 Corporate Center, 100 Enterprise Drive, Suite 280, Rockaway, NJ 07866, USA.

**Warner-Lambert, Austral.** See *Pfizer, Austral.*

**Warner-Lambert, Braz.** See *Pfizer, Braz.*

**Warner-Lambert, Canad.** See *Pfizer Consumer, Canad.*

**Warner-Lambert, Denm.** See *Pfizer, Denm.*

**Warner-Lambert, Fr.** See *Pfizer, Fr.*

**Warner-Lambert, Ger.** See *Pfizer, Ger.*

**Warner-Lambert, Gr.** WARNER-LAMBERT AE, Δελφών & Αλαμάνας 1, 151 25 Μαρούσι, Marousi, Greece.

**Warner-Lambert, Hong Kong.** See *Pfizer, Hong Kong.*

**Warner-Lambert, Irl.** See *Pfizer, Irl.*

**Warner-Lambert, Israel.** See *Pfizer, Israel.*

**Warner-Lambert, Ital.** See *Pfizer, Ital.*

**Warner-Lambert, Mex.** See *Pfizer, Mex.*

**Warner-Lambert, Neth.** See *Pfizer, Neth.*

**Warner-Lambert, Norw.** See *Pfizer, Norw.*

**Warner-Lambert, NZ.** See *Pfizer, NZ.*

**Warner-Lambert, Port.** See *Pfizer, Port.*

**Warner-Lambert, Spain.** See *Pfizer, Spain.*

**Warner-Lambert, Swed.** See *Pfizer, Swed.*

**Warner-Lambert, Switz.** See *Pfizer, Switz.*

**Warner-Lambert, UK.** See *Parke, Davis, UK.*

**Warner-Lambert, USA.** See *Pfizer, USA.*

**Warner-Lambert Consumer, Belg.** See *Pfizer, Belg.*

**Warner-Lambert Consumer, Port.** See *Pfizer, Port.*

**Warner-Lambert Consumer, Switz.** See *Pfizer, Switz.*

**Warner-Wellcome, USA.** See *Warner-Lambert, USA.*

**Wassen, Ital.** Wassen Italia S.r.l., Via Canova 25, 20145 Milan, Italy.

**Wassen, UK.** Wassen International Ltd, 14 The Mole Business Park, Leatherhead, Surrey, KT22 7BA, UK.

**Wasserman, Spain.** See *Chiesi, Spain.*

**Wassermann, Ital.** Alfa Wassermann S.p.A., Contrada Sant'Emidio, 65020 Alanno (PE), Italy.

**Wassermann, Malaysia.** See *Antah, Malaysia, Emerging Pharma, Malaysia,* and *Zyfas, Malaysia.*

**Watson, USA.** Watson Laboratories Inc., 311 Bonnie Circle, Corona, CA 91720, USA.

**Watsons, Canad.** Watsons Pharmaceuticals, 3 Ontario St, Port Hope, Ontario, L1A 3T5, Canada.

**Waymar, Canad.** Waymar Pharmaceuticals Inc., 330 Marwood Drive, Unit 4, Oshawa, Ontario, L1H 8B4, Canada.

**Wayne, Mex.** Wayne S.A. de C.V., Lago Nargis 47, Col. Granada, Deleg. Miduel Hidalgo, 11520 Mexico D.F., Mexico.

**WE, USA.** WE Pharmaceuticals Inc, P.O. Box 1142, Ramona, CA 92065, USA.

**Weber & Weber, Ger.** Weber & Weber GmbH & Co. KG, Herrschinger Str. 33, 82266 Inning/Ammersee, Germany.

**Weider, UK.** Weider Nutrition Ltd, Forum House, Redhill, Surrey, RH1 6YS, UK.

**Weifa, Norw.** Weifa AS, Hausmannsg. 6, Postboks 9113 Gronland, 0133 Oslo, Norway.

**Weifa, Thai.** See *Harn, Thai.*

**Weimer, Ger.** See *Biokanol, Ger.*

**Weimer, Hong Kong.** See *Hong Kong Medical, Hong Kong.*

**Weimer, Switz.** Weimer Pharma AG, Diepold-Schillingstrasse 14a, 6004 Luzern, Switzerland.

**Weimer, Thai.** See *Schumit, Thai.*

**Weinco, Spain.** Weinco, Spain.

**Welcker-Lyster, Canad.** See *Technilab, Canad.*

**Weleda, Austria.** Weleda GmbH & Co. KG, Hosenedelgasse 27, A-1220 Vienna, Austria.

**Weleda, Fr.** Laboratoires Weleda, 9 rue Eugene-Jung, 68330 Huningue, France.

**Weleda, Ger.** Weleda AG-Heilmittelbetriebe, Mohlerstr. 3-5, 73525 Schwabisch Gmund, Germany.

**Weleda, Switz.** Weleda AG, Stollenrain 11, 4144 Arlesheim, Switzerland.

**Weleda, UK.** Weleda (UK) Ltd, Heanor Rd, Ilkeston, Derbyshire, DE7 8DR, UK.

**Welfer, Mex.** Welfer, Carr. Saltillo-Monterrey Km 13, 25900 R. Arizpe Coahuila, Mexico.

**Welfide, Malaysia.** See *Antah, Malaysia.*

**Welfide, Singapore.** See *Alpha Therapeutic, Singapore.*

**Well Favoured, Hong Kong.** Well Favoured Ltd, 9/F Henley Centre, 9-15 Bute St, Mongkok, Kowloon, Hong Kong.

**Wellchem, Malaysia.** Syarikat Wellchem Sdn Bdh, 928-929 Jln 17/38, 46400 Petaling Jaya, Selangor, Malaysia.

**Wellchem, Singapore.** Wellchem Pharmaceuticals Pte Ltd, 221 Henderson Rd, 04-15 Henderson Building, S 159557, Singapore.

**Wellchem, Thai.** Wellchem Pharmaceutical Co. Ltd, 99/287-288 Nonsee Rd, Yannawa, Bangkok 10120, Thailand.

**Wellcome, Canad.** See *GlaxoSmithKline, Canad.*

**Wellcome, Irl.** See *GlaxoSmithKline, Irl.*

**Wellcome, Israel.** See *GlaxoSmithKline, Israel.*

**Wellcome, Port.** See *GlaxoSmithKline, Port.*

**Wellcome, Spain.** See *GlaxoSmithKline, Spain.*

**Wellcome, Switz.** See *GlaxoSmithKline, Switz.*

**Wellcome, UK.** See *GlaxoSmithKline, UK.*

**Wellcome, USA.** See *GlaxoSmithKline, USA.*

**Wellcome Diagnostics, UK.** Wellcome Diagnostics, A Division of The Wellcome Foundation Ltd, Temple Hill, Dartford, DA1 5AH, UK.

**Wellgo, Hong Kong.** Wellgo Pharmaceutical Co. Ltd, Unit 03-08, 22/F Millenium City, 378 Kwun Tong Rd, Kwun Tong, Kowloon, Hong Kong.

**Wellmex, Malaysia.** Wellmex Sdn Bhd, 23-26 Jln Bidara 1, Taman Bidara, 68100 Batu Caves, Selangor, Malaysia.

**Wellspring, Canad.** Wellspring Pharmaceuticals Canada Corp., 400 Iroquois Shore Rd, Oakville, Ontario, L6H 1M5, Canada.

**Wellspring, USA.** Wellspring Pharmaceutical, 1430 Route 40, Colts Neck, NJ 07722, USA.

**Welt, Arg.** Lab. Welt S.A.I.C., Tronador 3030/2, 1430 Buenos Aires, Argentina.

**Welti, Switz.** Dr Heinz Welti AG, Althofstrasse 12, 5432 Neuenhof, Switzerland.

**Weltrap, Arg.** Lab. Weltrap S.A., Balcarce 1072, 2000 Rosario, Santa Fe, Argentina.

**Wenig, Austria.** Mr J W Wenig GmbH, Van der Nullgasse 22, A-1100 Vienna, Austria.

**Wernigerode, Austria.** See *Wernigerode, Ger.*

**Wernigerode, Ger.** Pharma Wernigerode GmbH, Dornbergsweg 35, 38855 Wernigerode/Harz, Germany.

**Wesley, USA.** Wesley Pharmacal Inc., 114 Railroad Drive, Ivyland, PA 18974, USA.

**Westbrook, UK.** Westbrook Lanolin Co., Argonaut Works, Laisterdyke, Bradford, BD4 8AU, UK.

**WestCan, Canad.** See *Vita Health, Canad.*

**West-Coast, Thai.** See *Union Medical, Thai.*

**Western Medical, USA.** Western Medical, USA.

**Western Research, USA.** Western Research Laboratories, 21602 North 21st Ave, Phoenix, AZ 85027, USA.

**Westlake, USA.** Westlake Laboratories Inc., 24700 Center Ridge Rd, Cleveland, OH 44145, USA.

**Westmont, Hong Kong.** See *Unam, Hong Kong.*

**Westmont, Malaysia.** See *Unam, Malaysia.*

**Westmont, Singapore.** See *Far East, Singapore.*

**Westmont, Thai.** See *Olic, Thai.*

**Weston, Hong Kong.** Weston Pharmaceutical Ltd, Unit 26, 8/F Tower A, Southmark, 11 Yip Hing St, Wong Chuk Hang, Hong Kong.

**Westward, Canad.** Westward Dist., Canada.

**Westwood, Singapore.** See *Diethelm, Singapore.*

**Westwood, USA.** See *Bristol-Myers Squibb, USA.*

**Westwood-Squibb, Canad.** See *Bristol-Myers Squibb, Canad.*

**Westwood-Squibb, USA.** See *Bristol-Myers Squibb, USA.*

**Whan In, Singapore.** See *MD, Singapore.*

**Whelehan, Irl.** Whelehan T.P. Son & Co. Ltd, North Rd, Finglas, Dublin 11, Ireland.

**White, Arg.** White Pharma S.A., Av. San Martmn 1750, 1602, Florida, Buenos Aires, Argentina.

**Whitehall, Austral.** Whitehall Laboratories Australia P/L, Private Mailbag 1, Punchbowl, NSW 2196, Australia.

**Whitehall, Belg.** Whitehall Benelux s.a., Rue du Bosquet 15, 1348 Louvain-la-Neuve, Belgium.

**Whitehall, Braz.** See *Wyeth, Braz.*

**Whitehall, Denm.** See *Whitehall, UK.*

**Whitehall, Fin.** See *Tamro, Fin.*

**Whitehall, Fr.** Whitehall, 80 av du General-de-Gaulle, 92031 Paris-La Defense cdx, France.

**Whitehall, Hong Kong.** Whitehall Hong Kong, Division of Wyeth (HK) Ltd, Rm 1401-1403, C C Wu Bldg, 302-308 Hennessy Rd, Wanchai, Hong Kong.

**Whitehall, Irl.** See *Wyeth, Irl.*

**Whitehall, Israel.** See *Neopharm, Israel.*

**Whitehall, Ital.** Whitehall Italia S.p.A., Via Puccini 3, 20121 Milan, Italy.

**Whitehall, Norw.** See *Wyeth Lederle, Norw.*

**Whitehall, NZ.** Whitehall, P.O. Box 12736, Penrose, Auckland, New Zealand.

**Whitehall, Port.** See *Wyeth Consumer, Port.*

**Whitehall, S.Afr.** See *Wyeth, S.Afr.*

**Whitehall, Singapore.** Whitehall, 22 Martin Rd, 02-01 King Sun Building, S 239058, Singapore.

**Whitehall, Swed.** See *Wyeth Lederle, Swed.*

**Whitehall, Thai.** Whitehall Thailand, 23 Fl, Silom Complex Building, 191 Silom Rd, Bangkok 10500, Thailand.

**Whitehall, UK.** See *Wyeth, UK.*

**Whitehall, USA.** See *Whitehall-Robins, USA.*

**Whitehall Consumer, Austral.** Whitehall Consumer Healthcare Pty Ltd, 17-19 Solent Circuit, Norwest Business Park, Baulkham Hills, NSW 2153, Australia.

**Whitehall-Much, Ger.** Whitehall-Much GmbH, Regina-Protmann-Str. 16, 48159 Munster, Germany.

**Whitehall-Robins, Canad.** Whitehall-Robins Inc., 5975 Whittle Rd, Mississauga, Ontario, L4Z 3M6, Canada.

**Whitehall-Robins, Mex.** See *Wyeth, Mex.*

**Whitehall-Robins, Switz.** Whitehall-Robins AG, Grafenauweg 10, 6301 Zug 7, Switzerland.

**Whitehall-Robins, USA.** Whitehall Robins Healthcare, Five Giralda Farms, Madison, NJ 07940-0871, USA.

**Wick, Ger.** Wick Pharma Zweigniederlassung der Procter & Gamble GmbH, Sulzbacher Str. 40, 65824 Schwalbach, Germany.

**Wider, Ger.** Dr. Wider GmbH & Co., Brennerstr. 48, Postfach: 1862, 71208 Leonberg, Germany.

**Widmer, Austria.** Louis Widmer GmbH, Itzlinger Hauptstrasse 34, A-5020 Salzburg, Austria.

**Widmer, Fin.** Louis Widmer Oy, Sömäisten rantatie 29, 00580 Helsinki, Finland.

**Widmer, Ger.** Louis Widmer GmbH, Grossmattstr. 11, 79618 Rheinfelden, Germany.

**Widmer, Switz.** Dermatologica Widmer, Laboratoires Louis Widmer AG, 8048 Zurich, Switzerland.

**Wiedemann, Ger.** Wiedemann Pharma GmbH, Pilotyweg 14, 82541 Munsing, Germany.

**Wieger, Fr.** Laboratoires Wieger, 209 rte de Schirmeck, 67200 Strasbourg, France.

**Wiener, Mex.** Wiener Codex S.A. de C.V., Av. Ninos Heroes de Chapultepec 125, Benito Juarez, 03440 Mexico D.F., Mexico.

**Wierhom, Arg.** Wierhom Pharma S.A., Sinclair 3139 Pso. 1 A, 1425 Buenos Aires, Argentina.

**Wigglesworth, UK.** Wigglesworth (1982) Ltd, Cunard Rd, North Acton, London, NW10 6PN, UK.

**Wild, Switz.** Dr Wild & Co. AG, Lange Gasse 4, 4002 Basle, Switzerland.

**William, Hong Kong.** William Pharm, 801-D Causeway Bay, Commercial Building, 1-5 Sugar St, Causeway Bay, Hong Kong.

**Williams, USA.** Williams T.E. Pharm. Inc., P.O. Box 340, Guthrie, OK 73044, USA.

**Willmar, Mex.** Laboratorios Willmar S.A. de C.V., Los Placeres 1030, Chapalita, 44510 Guadalajara, Jal., Mexico.

**Willmar, Thai.** See *JDH Borneo, Thai.*

**Will-Pharma, Austria.** See *Will-Pharma, Belg.*

**Will-Pharma, Belg.** Will-Pharma S.A., Rue du Manil 80, 1301 Wavre, Belgium.

**Will-Pharma, Neth.** Will-Pharma BV, Wilgenlaan 5, 1161 JK Zwanenburg, Netherlands.

**Willpharma, Thai.** See *Berli, Thai.*

**Willvonseder, Austria.** Willvonseder & Marchesani, Heinrich-v-Buol-Gasse 45, A-1211 Vienna, Austria.

**Wilson, NZ.** Wilson Consumer Products Ltd, P.O. Box 105125, Auckland, New Zealand.

**Windson, Braz.** Windson Produtos Quimicos e Farmaceuticos Ltda, Rua Doutor Nicolau de Souza Queiroz 136, 04105-000 Sao Paulo, SP, Brazil.

**Windsor, Irl.** See *Allphar, Irl.*

**Windsor, UK.** Windsor Healthcare Ltd, Ellesfield Ave, Bracknell, Berkshire, RG12 4YS, UK.

**Wing Wai, Hong Kong.** Wing Wai Trading Co., Unit E, 2/F Freder Ctr, 3 Mok Cheong St, Kowloon, Hong Kong.

**Win-Medicare, India.** See *Modi-Mundipharma, India.*

**Win-Medicare, Thai.** See *Union Medical, Thai.*

**Winsor, Hong Kong.** Winsor & Co., Rm 1707-1707A, Wu Sang House, 655 Nathan Rd, Kowloon, Hong Kong.

**Winthrop Consumer, USA.** See *Bayer Consumer, USA.*

**Winzer, Ger.** Dr Winzer Pharma GmbH, Brunsbutteler Damm 165-173, 13581 Berlin, Germany.

**Wisconsin Pharmacal, USA.** Wisconsin Pharmacal Co., 1 Repel Rd, Jackson, WI 53037, USA.

**Wise, UK.** Wise Pharmaceuticals Ltd, Unit 7, Hani Wells Business Park, Hardicker St, Manchester, M19 2RB, UK.

**Wockhardt, India.** Wockhardt Ltd, Wockhardt Towers, Bandra Kurla Complex, Bandra (East), Mumbai 400 051, India.

**Woelm, Ger.** Woelm Pharma GmbH & Co., Rhondorfer Str. 80, 53604 Bad Honnef, Germany.

**Woelm, Israel.** See *CTS, Israel.*

**Wolff, Ger.** Dr. August Wolff Arzneimittel GmbH & Co., Sudbrackstr. 56, 33611 Bielefeld, Germany.

**Wolfs, Belg.** Wolfs S.A., Industriepark West 68, 9100 Sint-Niklaas, Belgium.

**Women First, USA.** Women First Healthcare Inc., 12220 El Camino Real, Suite 400, San Diego, CA 92130, USA.

**Womens Capital, USA.** Women's Capital Corp., P.O. Box 5026, Bellevue, WA 98009, USA.

**Woods, Austral.** H.W. Woods P/L, P.O. Box 1005, Huntingdale, VIC 3166, Australia.

**Woodward, USA.** Woodward Laboratories, Inc., 11132 Winners Circle 100, Los Alamitos, CA 90720, USA.

**Worldwide, Hong Kong.** Worldwide Resources Pharmaceutical Ltd, Unit 14, 19/F Concordia Plaza, No 1 Science Museum Rd, TST East, Kowloon, Hong Kong.

**Worndli, Switz.** Labor Worndli, Postfach 53, 5300 Turgi, Switzerland.

**Worwag, Ger.** Wörwag Pharma GmbH & Co. KG, Calwer Str. 7, 71034 Boblingen, Germany.

**Wrigley, USA.** Wrigley, USA.

**Wunderpharm, Arg.** Laboratorio Wunderpharm S.R.L., Remedios 5322, 1440 Buenos Aires, Argentina.

**Wybert, Ger.** See *GABA, Ger.*

**Wyeth, Arg.** See *Wyeth-Whitehall, Arg.*

**Wyeth, Austral.** Wyeth Pharmaceuticals, Division of Wyeth Australia P/L, Locked Bag 5002, Baulkham Hills BC, NSW 2153, Australia.

**Wyeth, Belg.** Wyeth, Division of AHP Pharma, Parc Scientifique Einstein, Rue du Bosquet 15, 1348 Louvain-la-Neuve, Belgium.

**Wyeth, Braz.** Laboratorios Wyeth-Whitehall Ltda, Rua Alexandre Dumas 2200, 5th Floor, 04717-004 Sao Paulo, SP, Brazil.

**Wyeth, Chile.** Laboratorios Wyeth Inc., Los Tres Antonios 2526, Santiago, Chile.

**Wyeth, Denm.** See *Wyeth Lederle, Denm.*

**Wyeth, Ger.** Wyeth Pharma GmbH, Wienburgstr. 207, 48159 Munster, Germany.

**Wyeth, Gr.** WYETH HELLAS, Κύπρου 126 και 25ης Μαρτίου, 164 52 Αργυρούπολη, Argiroupoli, Greece.

**Wyeth, Hong Kong.** Wyeth (Hong Kong) Ltd, 22/F Oxford House, 979 King's Rd, Taikoo Place, Island East, Hong Kong.

**Wyeth, India.** See *Wyeth Lederle, India.*

**Wyeth, Irl.** Wyeth Laboratories Ltd, 765 South Circular Road, Dublin 8, Ireland.

**Wyeth, Israel.** See *Dexxon, Israel,* and *Neopharm, Israel.*

**Wyeth, Malaysia.** Wyeth (Malaysia) Sdn Bhd, 701 & 801 Block C (Menara Glomac), Kelana Business Centre, 97 Jln SS 7/2, Kelana Jaya, 47301 Petaling Jaya, Selangor, Malaysia.

**Wyeth, Mex.** Wyeth S.A. de C.V., Avenida 1 de mayo No. 127, Col. San Andres Atoto, 53500 Naucalpan, Mexico.

**Wyeth, Neth.** Wyeth Pharmaceuticals BV, Planetenweg 99, 2132 HL Hoofddorp, Netherlands.

**Wyeth, NZ.** Wyeth (NZ) Ltd, P.O. Box 12736, Penrose, Auckland, New Zealand.

**Wyeth, S.Afr.** Wyeth South Africa (Pty) Ltd, Private Bag X211, Midrand 1685, South Africa.

**Wyeth, Singapore.** Wyeth (S) Pte Ltd, 111 Somerset Rd, 11-01 Singapore Power Building, S 238164, Singapore.

**Wyeth, Spain.** Wyeth Orfi, Ctra Burgos, Km-23, Desvio Algete Km, 1, San Sebastian de Los Reyes, 28070 Madrid, Spain.

**Wyeth, Switz.** See *AHP, Switz.*

**Wyeth, UK.** Wyeth Laboratories, Huntercombe Lane South, Taplow, Maidenhead, Berkshire, SL6 0PH, UK.

**Wyeth Consumer, Chile.** Wyeth Consumer Healthcare, Del Inca 4446, Of. 201, Las Condes, Santiago, Chile.

**Wyeth Consumer, Irl.** See *Wyeth, Irl.*

**Wyeth Consumer, Malaysia.** See *Wyeth, Malaysia.*

**Wyeth Consumer, Neth.** See *Wyeth, Neth.*

**Wyeth Consumer, Port.** Wyeth Consumer, Home Products de Portugal Lda, Avenida do Forte No 3, Edifcio Suecia III, Piso 0 - Ala Direita, 2795-504 Carnaxide, Portugal.

**Wyeth Consumer, Singapore.** See *Wyeth, Singapore.*

**Wyeth Consumer, UK.** See *Wyeth, UK.*

**Wyeth Consumer, USA.** See *Wyeth-Ayerst, USA.*

**Wyeth Health, Austral.** See *Wyeth, Austral.*

**Wyeth Lederle, Austria.** Wyeth-Lederle Pharma GmbH, Storchengasse 1, A-1150 Vienna, Austria.

**Wyeth Lederle, Belg.** See *Wyeth, Belg.*

**Wyeth Lederle, Denm.** Wyeth Lederle, Produktionsvej 24, 2600 Glostrup, Denmark.

**Wyeth Lederle, Fin.** Wyeth Lederle Nordiska AB, Filial I Finland, Rajatorpantie 41 C, 01640 Vantaa, Finland.

**Wyeth Lederle, Fr.** Wyeth-Lederle, Le Wilson 2, 80 av du General-de-Gaulle, Puteaux, 92031 Paris-La Defense cdx, France.

**Wyeth Lederle, India.** Wyeth Lederle Ltd, RBC, Mahindra Towers, 4th Floor, Dr GM Bhosale Rd, Worli, Mumbai 400 018, India.

**Wyeth Lederle, Ital.** Wyeth Lederle S.p.A., Via Nettunense 90, 04011 Aprilia (LT), Italy.

**Wyeth Lederle, Jpn.** Wyeth Lederle Japan Ltd, Hattori Bldg, 5th Floor, 1-10-3 Kyobashi, Chuo-ku, Tokyo 104-0031, Japan.

**Wyeth Lederle, Norw.** Wyeth Lederle Norge, P.O. Box 313, Skoyen, 0213 Oslo, Norway.

**Wyeth Lederle, Port.** Wyeth Lederle Portugal (Farma), Lda, Rua Dr Antonio Loureiro Borges 2, Arquiparque-Miraflores, 1495-131 Alges, Portugal.

**Wyeth Lederle, Swed.** Wyeth Lederle Nordiska AB, Box 1822, 171 24 Solna, Sweden.

**Wyeth-Ayerst, Austral.** See *Wyeth, Austral.*

**Wyeth-Ayerst, Canad.** Wyeth-Ayerst Canada Inc., 1025 Marcel Laurin Blvd, St-Laurent, Quebec, H4R 1J6, Canada.

**Wyeth-Ayerst, Hong Kong.** See *Wyeth, Hong Kong.*

**Wyeth-Ayerst, Israel.** See *Dexxon, Israel,* and *Neopharm, Israel.*

**Wyeth-Ayerst, Thai.** Wyeth-Ayerst (Thailand) Ltd, 23 Fl, Silom Complex Building, 191 Silom Rd, Bangkok 10500, Thailand.

**Wyeth-Ayerst, USA.** Wyeth-Ayerst Laboratories, P.O. Box 8299, Philadelphia, PA 19101, USA.

**Wyeth-Whitehall, Arg.** Wyeth-Whitehall S.A., Ing. Enrique Butty 275, 1001 Buenos Aires, Argentina.

**Wyss, Switz.** Wyss Pharma AG, Riedstrasse 1, 6330 Cham, Switzerland.

**Wyvern, UK.** Wyvern Medical Ltd, P.O. Box 17, Ledbury, Herefordshire, HR8 2ES, UK.

**Xanodyne, USA.** Xanodyne Pharmacal Inc., 7310 Turfway Rd, Suite 490, Florence, KY 41042, USA.

**Xcel, USA.** Xcel Pharmaceuticals, 6363 Greenwich Drive, Suite 100, San Diego, CA 92122, USA.

**Xepa-Soul Pattinson, Hong Kong.** See *Tack Fung, Hong Kong.*

**Xepa-Soul Pattinson, Malaysia.** Xepa-Soul Pattinson (Malaysia) Sdn Bhd, 1-5 Cheng Industrial Estate, 75250 Melaka, Malaysia.

**Xepa-Soul Pattinson, Singapore.** See *Grafton, Singapore.*

**Xeragen, S.Afr.** Xeragen Laboratories (Pty) Ltd, P.O. Box 22316, Glenashley, South Africa.

**Xixia, S.Afr.** Xixia Pharmaceuticals (Pty) Ltd, P.O. Box 1998, Halfway House 1685, South Africa.

**Yabrofarma, Port.** See *Yamanouchi, Port.*

**Yamanouchi, Austria.** See *Yamanouchi, Ger.,* and *Yamanouchi, Neth.*

**Yamanouchi, Belg.** Yamanouchi Pharma B.V., Riverside Business Park, Blvd International 55 Boite 7, 1070 Brussels, Belgium.

**Yamanouchi, Denm.** Yamanouchi Pharma A/S, Naverland 4, 2600 Glostrup, Denmark.

**Yamanouchi, Fin.** See *Algol, Fin.*

**Yamanouchi, Fr.** Yamanouchi Pharma SA, 10 Place de La Coupole, P.O. Box 105, 94223 Charenton-Le-Pont Cedex, France.

**Yamanouchi, Ger.** Yamanouchi Pharma GmbH, Im Breitspiel 19, 69126 Heidelberg, Germany.

**Yamanouchi, Gr.** Yamanouchi, Greece.

**Yamanouchi, Irl.** See *United Drug, Irl.*

**Yamanouchi, Israel.** See *CTS, Israel.*

**Yamanouchi, Ital.** Yamanouchi Pharma S.p.A., Via delle Industrie 2, 20061 Carugate (MI), Italy.

**Yamanouchi, Jpn.** Yamanouchi Pharmaceutical Co. Ltd, 3-11 Nihonbashi-Honcho 2-chome, Chuo-ku, Tokyo 103-8411, Japan.

**Yamanouchi, Neth.** Yamanouchi Europe BV, Elisabethhof 19, 2353 EW Leiderdorp, Netherlands.

**Yamanouchi, Norw.** Yamanouchi Pharma AS, Solbraveien 47, 1383 Asker, Norway.

**Yamanouchi, NZ.** See *CSL, NZ.*

**Yamanouchi, Port.** Yamanouchi Farma, Lda, Edificio Cinema, Rua Jose Fontana, no 1, 2780-805 Paco de Arcos, Portugal.

**Yamanouchi, Spain.** Yamanouchi Pharma, Centro Empresarial EL Plantio, Calle Ochandiano 10, 28023 Madrid, Spain.

**Yamanouchi, Swed.** Yamanouchi Pharma AB, Ridspogatan 10, 213 77 Malmo, Sweden.

**Yamanouchi, Switz.** See *Doetsch, Grether, Switz.*

**Yamanouchi, Thai.** Yamanouchi (Thailand) Co. Ltd, 10 Fl, Wave Place, 55 Wireless Rd, Lumpini, Patumwan, Bangkok 10330, Thailand.

**Yamanouchi, UK.** Yamanouchi Pharma Ltd, Yamanouchi House, Pyrford Rd, West Byfleet, Weybridge, Surrey, KT14 6RA, UK.

**Yauquimia, Mex.** Yauquimia de Mexico S.A. de C.V., Purmsima 12 BIS, Yautepec Rancho Nuevo, 62731 Morelos, Mexico.

**Yauyip, Austral.** Yauyip P/L, Suite 503 Cliveden, 4 Bridge Street, NSW 2000, Australia.

**YF Chem, Thai.** See *Sriprasit, Thai.*

**Yik Kwan, Hong Kong.** Yik Kwan Pharmaceuticals Co. Ltd, Flat A10, 6/F Merit Industrial Ctr, 94 To Kwa Wan Rd, Kowloon, Hong Kong.

**Yorkshire Pharmaceuticals, UK.** Yorkshire Pharmaceuticals Ltd, KAM House, 87 Horton Grange Rd, Bradford, West Yorkshire, BD7 3AH, UK.

**Yoshitomi, Jpn.** Yoshitomi Pharmaceutical Industries Ltd, 6-9 Hiranomachi 2-chome, Chuo-ku, Osaka 541-0046, Japan.

**Yoshitomi, Malaysia.** See *Antah, Malaysia.*

**Young, Canad.** WF Young Inc., 1225 rue Volta, Boucherville, Quebec, J4B 7M7, Canada.

**Young, USA.** Young Dental Mfg, 13705 Shoreline Ct E, Earth City, MO 63045, USA.

**Young Again Nutrients, USA.** Young Again Nutrients, Magnolia, Texas, USA.

**Young Again Products, USA.** Young Again Products Inc., 3608-B Oleander Drive 310, Wilmington, NC 28403, USA.

**Youngflex, Canad.** Youngflex Manufacturing Inc., 60 Granton Drive, Unit 6, Richmond Hill, Ontario, L4B 1H7, Canada.

**Ysatfabrik, Ger.** Johannes Bürger Ysatfabrik GmbH, Herzog-Julius-Str. 81/83, 38667 Bad Harzburg, Germany.

**YSP, Malaysia.** Y.S.P. Industries (M) Sdn Bhd, 18 Jln Wan Kadir, Taman Dr Ismail, 60000 Kuala Lumpur, Wilayah Perskutuan, Malaysia.

**Yu Sheng, Singapore.** See *Polymedic, Singapore.*

**Yung Shin, Singapore.** Yung Shin Pharmaceutical (S) Pte Ltd, 8 Kaki Bukit Rd 2, 02-26 Ruby Warehouse Complex, S 417841, Singapore.

**Yung Shin, Thai.** See *Far East, Thai.*

**Yungjin, Singapore.** See *Zyfas, Singapore.*

**Yves Ponroy, Fr.** Laboratoires Yves Ponroy, 85612 Montaigu cdx, France.

**Yves Ponroy, Singapore.** See *Age D'or, Singapore.*

**Zafiro, Mex.** Laboratorios Zafiro S.A. de C.V., Circunvalacion Norte No. 56, Fracc. Las Fuentes, 45070 Zapopan, Jal., Mexico.

**Zambon, Austria.** See *Zambon, Ital.*

**Zambon, Belg.** Zambon S.A., Ave Bourgemestre E. Demunter 1 boite 9, 1090 Brussels, Belgium.

**Zambon, Braz.** Zambon Laboratorios Farmaceuticos Ltda, Rua Descampado 63, 04296-090 Sao Paulo, SP, Brazil.

**Zambon, Fr.** Laboratoires Zambon France, 13 rue Rene-Jaques, 92138 Issy-les-Moulineaux, France.

**Zambon, Ger.** Zambon GmbH, Heinrich-Hertz-Str. 13, 50170 Kerpen, Germany.

**Zambon, Hong Kong.** Zambon (HK) Ltd, Rm 4109-4110, 41/F China Resources Bldg, 26 Harbour Rd, Wanchai, Hong Kong.

**Zambon, Ital.** Zambon Italia S.r.l., Via Lillo del Duca 10, 20091 Bresso (MI), Italy.

**Zambon, Neth.** Zambon Nederland BV, Algolweg 9 A, 3821 BG Amersfoort, Netherlands.

**Zambon, Port.** Zambon, Lda, Rua Jorge Barradas 24 B, 1500-370 Lisbon, Portugal.

**Zambon, Singapore.** See *United Italian, Singapore.*

**Zambon, Spain.** Zambon, Maresme 5, Pol. Ind. Urvasa, Santa Perpetua de Mogoda, 08130 Barcelona, Spain.

**Zambon, Thai.** See *SM, Thai.*

**Zanfel, USA.** Zanfel Laboratories Inc., P.O. Box 349, Moreton, IL 61550, USA.

**Zarbi (Ζαρμπη), Gr.** ΖΑΡΜΠΗ Ε.Ι. & ΣΙΑ Ο.Ε., Κομνηνών 22, 114 72 Αθήνα, Athens, Greece.

**Zee, Canad.** Zee Medical Canada, 5919 3rd St SE, Calgary, Alberta, T2H 1K3, Canada.

**Zee, USA.** Zee Medical Inc., 22 Corporate Park, Irvine, CA 92606, USA.

**Zekides, Gr.** ΖΗΚΙΔΗΣ Ν., Greece.

**Zellaforte, Switz.** Zellaforte Vertriebsanstalt, Austrasse 52, FL-9490 Vaduz, Switzerland.

**Zeller, Israel.** See *Promedico, Israel.*

**Zeller, Port.** Zeller Farmacêutica, Lda, Rua Sebastiao da Silva 25, Zona Industrial de Massama, 2745 Queluz, Portugal.

**Zeller, Singapore.** See *Green Cross, Singapore.*

**Zeller, Switz.** Max Zeller Söhne AG, Pflanzliche Heilmittel, Seeblickstrasse 4, Postfach 29, 8590 Romanshorn, Switzerland.

**Zeneca, Austral.** See *AstraZeneca, Austral.*

**Zeneca, Austria.** See *AstraZeneca, Austria.*

**Zeneca, Belg.** See *AstraZeneca, Belg.*

**Zeneca, Denm.** See *AstraZeneca, Denm.*

**Zeneca, Ger.** See *AstraZeneca, Ger.*

**Zeneca, Hong Kong.** See *AstraZeneca, Hong Kong.*

**Zeneca, Irl.** See *Astra, Irl.*

**Zeneca, Israel.** See *Teva, Israel.*

**Zeneca, Ital.** See *AstraZeneca, Ital.*

**Zeneca, Mex.** See *AstraZeneca, Mex.*

**Zeneca, Neth.** See *AstraZeneca, Neth.*

**Zeneca, Norw.** See *AstraZeneca, Norw.*

**Zeneca, Port.** See *AstraZeneca, Port.*

**Zeneca, S.Afr.** See *AstraZeneca, S.Afr.*

**Zeneca, Spain.** See *AstraZeneca, Spain.*

**Zeneca, Swed.** See *AstraZeneca, Swed.*

**Zeneca, Switz.** See *AstraZeneca, Switz.*

**Zeneca, USA.** See *AstraZeneca, USA.*

**Zenith, UK.** Zenith Pharmaceuticals Ltd, P.O. Box 85, Abingdon, Oxfordshire, OX14 3UA, UK.

**Zenith Goldline, USA.** See *Ivax, USA.*

**Zeppenfeldt, Ger.** Zeppenfeldt Pharma GmbH, Weiler Str. 19-21, 79540 Lorrach, Germany.

**Zerboni, Mex.** Laboratorios Zerboni S.A. de C.V., Anahuac 147, Col. El Mirador, Ex-Hacienda de Coapa, 04950 Mexico D.F., Mexico.

**Zeroderma, UK.** Zeroderma Ltd, The Manor House, Victor Barns, Northampton Rd, Brixworth, Northamptonshire, NN6 9DQ, UK.

**Zest, Braz.** Zest Farmaceutica Ltda, Viuva Claudio 300, 20970-030 Rio de Janeiro, RJ, Brazil.

**Zeta, Ital.** Zeta Farmaceutici S.p.A., Via Galvani 10, 36066 Sandrigo (VI), Italy.

**Zeus, Braz.** Zeus Lifesciences Ltda, Rua Estados Unidos 242, 01427-000 Sao Paulo, SP, Brazil.

**Zeus, Ital.** Zeus Srl, Via dei Castelli Romani 22, 00040 Pomezia (Rome), Italy.

**Zicor, Fr.** Zicor, France.

**Ziethen, Ger.** Ziethen, Tengstr. 26, 80798 Munich, Germany.

**Zila, Canad.** Zila Pharmaceuticals Inc., 111 Flint Rd, Downsview, Ontario, M3J 3C7, Canada.

**Zila, USA.** Zila Pharmaceuticals Inc., 5227 N. 7th Street, Phoenix, AZ 85014-2817, USA.

**Zilliken, Ital.** Italy.

**Zilly, Ger.** Fritz Zilly GmbH, Eckbergstr. 18, 76534 Baden-Baden, Germany.

**Zimaia, Port.** Laboratório Zimaia, SA, Rua de Andaluz 38, 1050-006 Lisbon, Portugal.

**Zimmer, Ger.** Zimmer Chirurgie GmbH, Maria-Merian-Str. 7, 24145 Kiel, Germany.

**Ziwell, Singapore.** Ziwell Medical (S) Pte Ltd, 1 Ubi Crescent, 05-03 Number One Building, S 408563, Singapore.

**ZLB, Switz.** ZLB Bioplasma AG, Wankdorfstrasse 10, 3000 Berne 22, Switzerland.

**ZLB, UK.** ZLB Bioplasma UK Ltd, Breckland House, St Nicholas St, Thetford, Norfolk, IP24 1BT, UK.

**Zodiac, Braz.** Zodiac Prods. Farms. S.A., Rua Venancio Aires 417, 05024-030 Sao Paulo, SP, Brazil.

**Zoja, Hong Kong.** See *Deutsch Chinesische, Hong Kong.*

**Zoki, Thai.** See *Asian TJD, Thai.*

**Zollweiden, Switz.** Zollweiden Apotheke, Baselstrasse 71, 4142 Munchenstein, Switzerland.

**Zuellig, Hong Kong.** Zuellig Pharma Ltd, Suite 608, 6/F, Devon House, Taikoo Place, Quarry Bay, Hong Kong.

**Zuellig, Malaysia.** Zuellig Pharma Sdn Bhd, Level 2, Wisma Zuellig, 9 Jln Bersatu Jaya, 46200 Petaling Jaya, Selangor, Malaysia.

**Zuellig, NZ.** Zuellig Pharma, 316-318 Richmond Road, Grey Lynn, Auckland, New Zealand.

**Zuellig, Singapore.** Zuellig Pharma Pte Ltd, 19 Loyang Way, 08-20, S 508724, Singapore.

**Zuellig, Thai.** Zuellig Pharma Ltd, 8-9 Ploenchit Center, 2 Sukhumvit Rd, Kwang Klongtoey, Khet Klongtoey, Bangkok 10110, Thailand.

**Zurich, S.Afr.** Zurich, South Africa.

**Zurita, Braz.** Zurita Laboratorio Farmaceutico Ltda, Rua Domingos Graziano 104, 13600-000 Araras, SP, Brazil.

**Zyber, USA.** Zyber Pharmaceuticals, P.O. Box 40, Gonzales, LA 70707, USA.

**Zydus, India.** Zydus Cadila Group, Zydus Tower, Satellite Cross Roads, Ahmedabad 380 015, India.

**Zyfas, Malaysia.** The Zyfas Medical Co., 7 Jln Molek 3/10, Taman Molek, 81100 Johor Molek, Johor, Malaysia.

**Zyfas, Singapore.** Zyfas Medical Co, 102E Pasir Panjang Rd, 02-10/11 Citilink Warehouse Complex, S 118529, Singapore.

**Zyma, Belg.** See *Novartis Consumer, Belg.*

**Zyma, Fr.** See *Novartis Sante, Fr.*

**Zyma, Ger.** See *Novartis Consumer, Ger.*

**Zyma, Spain.** See *Novartis, Spain.*

**Zyma, Switz.** See *Novartis, Switz.,* and *Novartis Consumer, Switz.*

# General Index

Entries cover drugs (by monograph title, other approved names, synonyms, and chemical names), diseases (by disease treatment review title and associated terms), and proprietary preparations (by proprietary or brand name). They are arranged alphabetically in word-by-word order. Page references give both the page and column number as in 476·1, where 476 represents the page number and the figure 1 indicates that the entry will be found in column 1 of that page. There is no column number when the entry is in a table.


2-4-2, 1767·1
3-01003, 927·3
10-80-07, 407·2
27-400, 1351·2
42-548, 1589·1
43-715, 86·1
44, 1767·1
50:50, 1767·1
89-12, 1637·3
107, 1058·3
217, 1767·1
222, 1767·1
282, 1767·1
292, 1767·1
375, 1441·1
381, 1427·2
510, 1115·2
518, 1228·2
542, 1699·3
545, 1654·1
572, 1574·2
640/359, 184·1
642, 1767·1
666, 1506·3
692, 1767·1
905, 1479·1, 1479·3
924, 1734·1
925, 1175·3
926, 1176·2
1592, 625·2
2936, 990·3
5052, 1112·3
5058, 486·3
5190, 1115·1
27165, 1510·2
29866, 1124·1
33379, 1100·3
34977, 166·1
38253, 168·3
38489, 310·2
40045, 1370·3
40602, 168·3
41071, 168·2
46083, 170·3
46236, 905·3
47657, 158·2
47663, 271·2
52230, 408·1
64716, 188·1
66873, 168·1
83405, 169·3
106223, 169·3
177501, 770·2

**A**

A, 1289·2, 1421·1
2-5410-3A, 1063·3
3-A, 1767·1
4A65, 606·1
A-16, 1653·1
33A74, 1399·1
A-41-304, 1096·3
A-101, 710·3
A-200, 1767·1
A 313, 1767·1
A-2371, 580·2
A-4166, 343·3
A-4828, 590·2
A-5610, 425·2
A-8103, 580·1
A-8327, 264·3
A-16686, 249·1
A-19120, 978·3
A-27053, 880·2
A-29622, 634·2
A-32686, 990·3
A-35957, 1541·3
A-40664, 719·2
A-41300, 1541·3
A-46745, 1556·2
A-56268, 192·2
A-56619, 205·3
A-56620, 254·3
A-57135, 254·3
A-62254, 266·1
A-64077, 807·3
A-65006, 1269·3
A-71100, 348·3
A-73001, 795·3
A-84538, 653·2
A-157378.0, 649·3
A-195773, 185·1
A771726, 53·3
A Acido, 1767·1
17-1A Antibody, 550·2
A + B Balsam N, 1767·2
A Curitybina, 1767·2
A & D, 1767·2
A + D + E-Vicotrat, 1767·2
A and D Medicated, 1767·2
A & D Ointment, 1767·2
A + $D_3$-Vicotrat, 1767·2
A + E Thilo, 1767·2
A Grin, 1767·2
3A Ofteno, 1767·2
A Saude da Mulher, 1767·2
A Vogel Capsules a l'ail, 1767·2
A Vogel Capsules Polyvitaminees, 1767·2
A to Z, 1767·3
AA-149, 1757·2
AA-673, 781·1
AA-2414, 795·3
AA Cold, 1767·3
AAA, 1767·3
Aacidexam, 1767·3
Aacifemine, 1767·3
AA-HC Otic, 1767·3
Aar Brain N, 1767·3
Aar Gamma N, 1767·3
Aar Os, 1767·3
Aar Vir, 1767·3
Aarane, 1767·3
Aarane N, 1767·3
Aaron's Rod, 1764·1
AAS, 1767·4
AB, 1767·4
AB-08, 206·2
AB Antitusivo, 1767·4
AB FE, 1767·4
Abacateirol, 1767·4
Abacavir, 625·2
Abacavir Succinate, 625·2
Abacavir, Succinato de, 625·2
Abacavir Sulfate, 625·2
Abacavir, Sulfato de, 625·2
Abacavir Sulphate, 625·2
Abacin, 1767·4
Abacten, 1767·4
Abactrim, 1767·4
Abacus, 1767·4
Abaktal, 1767·4
Abalgin, 1767·4
Abamectin, 101·2
Abamectina, 101·2
Abaprim, 1768·1
Abarelix, 1319·1
Abba, 1768·1
Abbiofort, 1768·1
Abbocalcijex, 1768·1
Abbocillin-V, 1768·1
Abbocillin-VK, 1768·1
Abboderm, 1768·1
Abbodop, 1768·1
Abbokinase, 1768·1
Abbolipid, 1768·1
Abboplegisol, 1768·1
Abbosynagis, 1768·1
Abboticin, 1768·1
Abboticine, 1768·1
Abbott-34842, 1373·1
Abbott-35616, 685·1
Abbott-36581, 1116·2
Abbott-38579, 1337·3
Abbott-39083, 685·1
Abbott-41070, 1325·2
Abbott-43326, 880·3
Abbott-43818, 1331·1
Abbott-44089, 380·1
Abbott-44090, 380·1
Abbott-44747, 158·3
Abbott-45975, 1010·3
Abbott-46811, 180·2
Abbott-47631, 697·3
Abbott-48999, 177·2
Abbott-50192, 173·2
Abbott-50711, 380·1
Abbott-56268, 192·2
Abbott-56619, 205·3
Abbott-56620, 254·3
Abbott-61827, 272·2
Abbott-62254, 266·1
Abbott-64077, 807·3
Abbott-70569.1, 378·1
Abbott-73001, 795·3
Abbott-74187, 964·2
Abbott-84538, 653·2
Abbott-195773, 185·1
Abbottracurium, 1768·1
Abbottselsun, 1768·1
ABC, 1768·1
ABC 12/3, 785·1
ABC Warme-Pflaster, 1768·1
ABC Warme-Pflaster Sensitive, 1768·1
ABC Warme-Salbe, 1768·1
ABC to Z, 1768·1
ABCDin, 1768·1
Abciximab, 841·3
Abdijsiroop (Akker-Siroop), 1768·1
Abdine Cold Relief, 1768·1
Abdomilon N, 1768·1
Abdominol, 1768·1
Abdoscan, 1768·1
Abduce, 1768·2
Abecarnil, 668·1
Abecarnilo, 668·1
Abecidin A C D, 1768·2
Abedul, Hojas de, 1660·3
Abelcet, 1768·2
Abenol, 1768·2
Abentel, 1768·2
Aberel, 1768·2
Aberela, 1768·2
Aberten, 1768·2
Abesira, 1768·2
Abetimus Sodium, 1348·2
Abetol, 1768·2
Abflex, 1768·2
Abfuhr Herbagran, Kneipp— *see* Kneipp Abfuhr Herbagran, 2081·1
Abfuhr Tee N, Kneipp— *see* Kneipp Abfuhr Tee N, 2081·1
Abfuhrdragees, 1768·2
Abfuhrdragees Mild, 1768·2
Abfuhrtee, 1768·2
Abfuhrtee EF-EM-ES, 1768·2
Abfuhrtee N, 1768·2
Abfuhrtropfen, 1768·2
Abidec, 1768·2
Abietinarum, Pix, 1159·3
Abilify, 1768·2
Abine, 1768·2
Abinol, 1768·2
Abiocef, 1768·2
Abiolex, 1768·2
Abiostil, 1768·2
Abiotyl, 1768·2
Abiplatin, 1768·3
Abiposid, 1768·3
Abitilguanide Hydrochloride, 649·3
Abitren, 1768·3
Abitrexate, 1768·3
ABJ-538, 653·2
ABK, 158·3
Ablock, 1768·3
Ablock Plus, 1768·3
Abnobaviscum, 1768·3
ABOB, 649·3
Abóbora, 1677·3
Abolibe, 1768·3
Abopur, 1768·3
Abortion, Induced— *see* Termination of Pregnancy, 1512·2
ABPP, 532·2
Abrasive Agents, 1140·1
Abrasivos, 1140·1
Abrasone, 1768·3
Abrasone Rectal, 1768·3
Abreva, 1768·3
Abrilar, 1768·3
Abrin, 1645·1
Abrol, 1768·3
Abrolen, 1768·3
Abrolet, 1768·3
Abrus, 1645·1
*Abrus precatorius*, 1645·1
Abrus Seed, 1645·1
Abscess, Brain, 120·3
Abscess, Dental— *see* Mouth Infections, 136·1
Abscess, Liver, 120·3
Abscess, Lung— *see* Pneumonia, 141·3
Absence Seizures— *see* Epilepsy, 349·1
Absence Status Epilepticus— *see* Status Epilepticus, 352·1
Absenor, 1768·3
Absimed, 1768·3
Absint, 1768·3
Absinthii Herba, 1645·1
Absinthium, 1645·1
Absorbase, 1768·3
Absorber HFV, 1768·3
Absorbine Analgesic, 1768·3
Absorbine Antifungal, 1768·3
Absorbine Antifungal Foot Powder, 1768·3
Absorbine Arthritis, 1768·3
Absorbine Athletes Foot Care, 1768·3
Absorbine Jr, 1768·3
Absorbine Jr Antifungal, 1768·3
Absorbine Power Gel, 1768·3
Absorlent, 1768·3
Absorlent Plus, 1768·4
Abstem, 1768·4

Absten S, 1768·4
Abstensyl, 1768·4
ABT-001, 795·3
ABT-187, 964·2
ABT-358, 1462·1
ABT-378, 649·3
ABT-569, 378·1
ABT-773, 185·1
Abtrim, 1768·4
Abufene, 1768·4
Abuglib, 1768·4
Abutiroi, 1768·4
Abutol, 1768·4
AC-0137, 344·3
AC-137, 344·3
AC-1802, 864·2
AC-3810, 781·3
AC-4464, 1015·3
AC & C, 1768·4
AC Vascular, 1768·4
Aca, 1768·4
Acabel, 1768·4
Acac., 1576·2
Acacia, 1576·2
*Acacia senegal*, 1576·2
*Acacia seyal*, 1576·2
Acacia, Spray-dried, 1576·2
Acaciae Gummi, 1576·2
Acaciae Gummi Dispersione Desiccatum, 1576·2
Acacin, 1768·4
Acadesina, 842·2
Acadesine, 842·2
Acadione, 1768·4
Açafrão , 1058·2
Acalix, 1768·4
Acalka, 1768·4
Acamed, 1768·4
Acamol, 1768·4
Acamol Compuesto, 1768·4
Acamol Tsinun Day, 1768·4
Acamol Tsinun Night, 1768·4
Acamoli, 1768·4
Acamoli Cold, 1768·4
Acamprosate Calcium, 668·1
Acamprosato de Calcio, 668·1
Acamprosatum Calcicum, 668·1
Acamylophenine Hydrochloride, 1666·1
Acanol, 1768·4
Acantex, 1768·4
Acanthamoeba Infections— *see* Acanthamoeba Keratitis, 595·1
Acanthamoeba Keratitis, 595·1
*Acanthopanax senticosus*, 1744·1
Acarbosa, 328·3
Acarbose, 328·3
Acarcid, 1768·4
Acarcid Perles, 1768·4
Acardi, 1768·4
Acardust, 1769·1
Acarex, 1769·1
Acaricides, 1499·1
Acaril, 1769·1
Acarilbial, 1769·1
Acarosan, 1769·1
Acarsan, 1769·1
Acasmul, 1769·1
Acatar, 1769·1
ACB, 1769·1
ACC, 1769·1
ACC-9653, 361·3
ACC-9653-010, 361·3
Accolate, 1769·1
Accoleit, 1769·1
Accomin, 1769·1
Accomin Centrum, 1769·1
Accomin Vitamin, 1769·1
Accu-Check Advantage, 1769·1
Accu-Check III/Chemstrip BG, 1769·1
Accu-Chek, 1769·1
Accuhist, 1769·1
Accuhist DM Pediatric, 1769·1
Accuhist LA, 1769·1
Accuhist PDX, 1769·1
Accumulator Acid, 1750·3
Accuneb, 1769·1
Accupaque, 1769·1
AccuPeel, 1769·1
Accupep, 1769·2
Accupril, 1769·2
Accuprin, 1769·2
Accupro, 1769·2
Accupro Comp, 1769·2
Accupron, 1769·2
Accurbron, 1769·2
Accure, 1769·2
Accuretic, 1769·2
Accutane, 1769·2
Accutest Fecal, 1769·2
Accutest Multi-Drug, 1769·2
Accutin, 1769·2
Accutrend Cholesterol, 1769·2
Accutrend Colesterol, 1769·2
Accutrend GC, 1769·2
Accutrend Glucosa, 1769·2
Accutrend Glucose, 1769·2
Accutrend Trigliceridos, 1769·2
Accuvit, 1769·2
Accuzide, 1769·2
Accuzyme, 1769·2
ACD, 1769·2
ACD Whole Blood, 744·1
Ac-De, 1769·2
ACE Inhibitors, 809·1, 842·3
Acea, 1769·2
Acebrofylline, 1114·3
Acebutolol, 848·1
Acebutolol, Hidrocloruro de, 848·1
Acebutolol Hydrochloride, 848·1
Acebutololi Hydrochloridum, 848·1
Acecainida, Hidrocloruro de, 848·3
Acecainide Hydrochloride, 848·3
Acecamycin, 231·3
Acecarbromal, 668·2
Aceclidina, Hidrocloruro de, 1487·1
Aceclidine Hydrochloride, 1487·1
Aceclofar, 1769·2
Aceclofenac, 11·2
Aceclofenaco, 11·2
Aceclofenacum, 11·2
Acecol, 1769·2
Acecomb, 1769·2
Acecor, 1769·2
Acecromol, 1769·3
Acedera Común, 1749·1
Acediasulfona Sódica, 153·3
Acediasulfone Sodium, 153·3
Acedicone, 1769·3
Acediur, 1769·3
Acedoben, 640·2, 1645·2
Acedoben Potassium, 1645·2
Acedoben Sodium, 1645·2
Acef, 1769·3
Aceflan, 1769·3
Acéfyllinate d'Heptaminol, 786·3
Acefyllinate, Heptaminol, 786·3
Acefylline Piperazine, 780·1
Acefyllinum Heptaminolum, 786·3
Aceglutamida, 1645·2
Aceglutamida de Aluminio, 1248·1
Aceglutamide, 1645·2
Aceglutamide Aluminium, 1248·1
ACE-Hemmer, 1769·3
ACE-Hemmer Comp, 1769·3
Aceite Acalorico, 1769·3
Aceite de Ajonjoli, 1743·3
Aceite de Algodon, 1676·1
Aceite de Almendra, 1651·1
Aceite de Brea de Abedul, 1159·2
Aceite de Cártamo, 1443·3
Aceite de Coco, 1481·1
Aceite de Crotón, 28·2
Aceite de Girasol, 1451·1
Aceite de Hígado de Bacalao, 1425·2
Aceite de Hígado de Fletán, 1434·1
Aceite de Higado de Hipogloso, 1434·1
Aceite de Linaza, 1707·2
Aceite de Maíz, 1439·2
Aceite de Oliva, 1723·2
Aceite de Palma Refinado, 1481·3
Aceite de Quenopodio, 103·3
Aceite de Ricino, 1668·2
Aceite de Ricino Hidrogenado Polioxil 40, 1414·3
Aceite de Ricino Polioxil 35, 1414·3
Aceite de Ricino Sulfatado, 1575·3
Aceite de Soja, 1447·2
Aceite Esmeralda Moone, 1769·3
Aceite Geve Concentrado, 1769·3
Aceite Vegetal Hidrogenado, 1763·3
Aceite Yodado, 1063·2
Aceites de Ricino Hidrogenados y Polioxietilenados, 1414·3
Aceites de Ricino Polioxietilenados, 1414·3
Acekapton, 1769·3
Acel-Imune, 1769·3
Acelluvax, 1769·3
Acelluvax DTP, 1769·3
Acel-P, 1769·3
Acemanán, 1645·2
Acemannan, 1645·2
Acemedrox, 1769·3
Acemetacin, 11·3
Acemetacina, 11·3
Acemetadoc, 1769·3
Acemin, 1769·3
Acemix, 1769·3
Acemuc, 1769·3
Acemucol, 1769·3
Acemuk, 1769·3
Acemycin, 1769·3
Acenocoumarol, 848·3
Acenocumarin, 848·3
Acenocumarol, 848·3
Acenorm, 1769·3
Acenorm HCT, 1769·3
Acenox, 1769·3
Acenterine, 1769·3
Aceomel, 1769·4
Aceon, 1769·4
Aceoto, 1769·4
Aceoto Plus, 1769·4
Acephen, 1769·4
Acephlogont, 1769·4
Acephyllinate, Heptaminol, 786·3
Acepifylline, 780·1
Aceplus, 1769·4
Acepran, 1769·4
Acepress, 1769·4
Acepril, 1769·4
Aceprilex, 1769·4
Acepromazina, 668·3
Acepromazina, Maleato de, 668·3
Acepromazine, 668·3
Acepromazine Maleate, 668·3
Aceprometazina, 668·3
Aceprometazine, 668·3
Aceprometazine Maleate, 668·3
Acequide, 1769·4
Acequin, 1769·4
Aceratun, 1769·4
Acerbine, 1769·4
Acerbiol, 1769·4
Acerbon, 1769·4
Acercomp, 1769·4
Acerdil, 1769·4
Acerdil-D, 1769·4
Aceren, 1769·4
Aceril, 1769·4
Acerpes, 1770·1
Acertil, 1770·1
Acertol, 1770·1
Aces, 1770·1
Acesal, 1770·1
Acesal Calcium, 1770·1
Acesistem, 1770·1
Acestrol, 1770·1
Acesulfame K, 1420·3
Acesulfame Potassium, 1420·3
Acesulfamo Potásico, 1420·3
Acesulfamum Kalicum, 1420·3
Acet, 1770·1
Acet-2, 1770·1
Acet-3— *see* Acet-2, Acet-3, 1770·1
Acet Codeine, 1770·1
Aceta, 1770·1
Aceta with Codeine, 1770·1
Acetab, 1770·1
Acetabs, 1770·1
Acetacol, 1770·1
Acetadiazol, 1770·1
Acetadote, 1770·1
Acetafen, 1770·1
Aceta-Gesic, 1770·1
Acetaldehyde, 713·2
Acetalgine, 1770·1
Acetamide, 609·2
3-Acetamido-5-acetamidomethyl-2,4,6-triiodobenzoic Acid, 1063·2
5-Acetamido-2,6-anhydro-3,4,5-trideoxy-4-guanidino-D-*glycero*-D-*galacto*-non-2-enonic Acid, 658·1
4-Acetamidobenzaldehyde Thiosemicarbazone, 269·3
*p*-Acetamidobenzoic Acid, 1645·2
Acetamidocaproic Acid, Epsilon, 1646·2
(1→3)-*O*-(2-Acetamido-2-deoxy-β-D-glucopyranosyl)-(1→4)-*O*-β-D-glucopyranosiduronan, 1697·3
(−)-(*S*)-2-Acetamido-*N*-(3,4-dihydroxyphenethyl)-4-(methylthio)butyramide Bis(ethyl Carbonate) Ester, 906·3
6-Acetamidohexanoic Acid, 1646·2
5-Acetamido-*N*-(2-hydroxyethyl)-2,4,6-triiodoisophthalamic Acid, 1066·3
3-Acetamido-4-hydroxyphenylarsonic Acid, 600·2
4-Acetamidophenyl *O*-Acetylsalicylate, 20·3
4-Acetamidophenyl Diethylaminoacetate Hydrochloride, 85·3
4-Acetamidophenyl 2,2,2-Trichloroethyl Carbonate, 1756·2
(*p*-Acetamidophenyl)acetic Acid, 12·1
5-Acetamido-1,3,4-thiadiazole-2-sulphonamide, 849·1
2-[3-Acetamido-2,4,6-tri-iodo-5-(*N*-methylacetamido)benzamido]-2-deoxy-D-glucose, 1067·1
3-Acetamido-2,4,6-tri-iodo-5-(*N*-methylacetamido)benzoic Acid, 1067·1
5-Acetamido-2,4,6-tri-iodo-*N*-(methylcarbamoylmethyl)isophthalamic Acid, 1064·1
5-Acetamido-2,4,6-tri-iodo-*N*-methylisophthalamic Acid, 1065·3
Acetaminohydroxyphenylarsonsäure, 600·2
Acetaminophen, 76·2
Acetaminophen with Codeine, 1770·1
Acetamol, 1770·1
Acetan, 1770·1
Acetanilida, 11·3
Acetanilide, 11·3
Aceta-P, 1770·1
Acetapyrin-C, 1770·1
Acetar, 1770·1
Acetard, 1770·2
Acetarsol, 600·2
Acetarsol Lithium, 600·2
Acetarsol Sodium, 600·2
Acetarsone, 600·2
Acetasil, 1770·2
Acetasol, 1770·2
Acetasol HC, 1770·2
Acetat-Haemodialyse, 1770·2
Acetato de Alfadolona, 1296·3
Acetato de Amilo, 1471·2
Acetato de Betametasona, 1093·1
Acetato de Bisoxatina, 1253·2
Acetato de Buserelina, 1319·2
Acetato de Butilo, 1472·1
Acetato de Caspofungina, 395·3
Acetato de Ciproterona, 1544·1
Acetato de Clorhexidina, 1173·2
Acetato de Clormadinona, 1542·1
Acetato de Clostebol, 1543·2
Acetato de Cortisona, 1096·1
Acetato de Delmadinona, 1547·2
Acetato de Desmopresina, 1322·3
Acetato de Desoxicortona, 1097·1
Acetato de Dexametasona, 1097·1
Acetato de Diclorisona, 1099·3
Acetato de Etilo, 1474·3
Acetato de Flecainida, 916·2
Acetato de Fludrocortisona, 1100·1

Acetato de Flugestona, 1555·2
Acetato de Fluorometolona, 1102·2
Acetato de Fluprednideno, 1102·2
Acetato de Ganirelix, 1325·1
Acetato de Gonadorelina, 1325·2
Acetato de Goserelina, 1326·3
Acetato de Guanabenzo, 926·2
Acetato de Hidrocortisona, 1103·3
Acetato de Histrelina, 1329·3
Acetato de Isoflupredona, 1105·3
Acetato de Lanreotida, 1330·3
Acetato de Leuprorelina, 1331·1
Acetato de Lisina, 1439·2
Acetato de Mafenida, 228·2
Acetato de Medroxiprogesterona, 1557·2
Acetato de Megestrol, 1558·2
Acetato de Metenolona, 1559·2
Acetato de Metilprednisolona, 1106·1
Acetato de Nafarelina, 1332·3
Acetato de Nomegestrol, 1562·1
Acetato de Noretisterona, 1562·2
Acetato de Octreotida, 1333·1
Acetato de Orbofibrán, 977·2
Acetato de Oxifenisatina, 1282·3
Acetato de Parametasona, 1107·3
Acetato de Pirbuterol, 790·3
Acetato de Prednisolona, 1108·1
Acetato de Prednisona, 1109·3
Acetato de Prezatida Cúprica, 1156·1
Acetato de Sarasalina, 996·3
Acetato de Sermorelina, 1339·2
Acetato de Sodio, 1223·1
Acetato de Teriparatida, 775·2
Acetato de Trenbolona, 1573·2
Acetato de Zuclopentixol, 730·3
Acetato Ftalato de Polivinilo, 1581·1
Acetatocobalamin, 1458·2
(Acetato)phenylmercury, 1189·2
Acetazolam, 849·1
Acetazolamida, 849·1
Acetazolamida Sódica, 849·1
Acetazolamide, 849·1
Acetazolamide Sodium, 849·1
Acetazolamidum, 849·1
Acetazone Forte, 1770·2
Acetazone Forte C8, 1770·2
Acetcarbromal, 668·2
Acetec, 1770·2
Aceten, 1770·2
Acetensil, 1770·2
Acetensil Plus, 1770·2
Acetest, 1770·2
Acethiamine Hydrochloride, 1454·3
Acethydrocodone Hydrochloride, 1131·2
Acetiamina, Hidrocloruro de, 1454·3
Acetiamine Hydrochloride, 1454·3
Acetic Acid, 1645·2
Acetic Acid ($^{11}$C), 1523·1
Acetic Acid, Dilute, 1645·2
Acetic Acid, Glacial, 1645·2
Acetic Acid (6 Per Cent), 1645·2
Acetic Acid (33 Per Cent), 1645·2
Acetic Ether, 1474·3
Aceticil, 1770·2
Acetif, 1770·2
Acetilcarnitina, Hidrocloruro de, 1646·1
Acetilcisteína, 1112·3
Acetilcolina, Cloruro de, 1487·1
Acetildigoxina, 851·1
Acetildihidrocodeína, Hidrocloruro de, 1114·2
Acetileucina, 1646·1
Acetilsalicilato de Aluminio, 14·1
Acetilsalicilato de Lisina, 54·3
Acetilsalicílico, Ácido, 15·1
Acetilsulfafurazol, 260·1
(+)-(5*R*,6*S*)-3{[(*S*)-1-Acetimidoyl-3-pyrrolidinyl]thio}-6-[(*R*)-1-hydroxyethyl]-7-oxo-1-azabicyclo[3.2.0]hept-2-ene-2-carboxylic Acid, 241·3
Acetin, 1770·2
Acetocaustin, 1770·2
Acetocaustine, 1770·2
Acetofen, 1770·2
Acetofenido de Algestona, 1541·3
Acetoflux, 1770·2
Acetohexamida, 329·2
Acetohexamide, 329·2
Acetohidroxámico, Ácido, 1645·3
Acetohydroxamic Acid, 1645·3
Acetolit, 1770·2
Acetolyt, 1770·2
Acetomenadione, 1466·3
Acetomenaftona, 1466·3
Acetomenaph., 1466·3
Acetomenaphthone, 1466·3
Acetona, 1471·1
Acetonal, 1770·2
Acetone, 1471·1
Acetone-Chloroforme, 1176·3
Acetónido de Fluclorolona, 1100·1
Acetónido de Fluocinolona, 1101·2
Acetónido de Triamcinolona, 1110·2
Acetonitrile, 1471·1
Acetonitrilo, 1471·1
Acetonum, 1471·1
(±)-Acetonyl Methyl 1,4-Dihydro-2,6-dimethyl-4-(*o*-nitrophenyl)-3,5-pyridinedicarboxylate, 864·2
Aceto-*p*-phenetidide, 82·2
*p*-Acetophenetidide, 82·2
Acetophenetidin, 82·2
Acetopt, 1770·2
Acetorphan, 1285·2
Acetosal, 1770·2
Acetosulfaminum, 257·3
*N*-(5-Acetoxy-3-acetylthiopent-2-en-2-yl)-*N*-(4-amino-2-methylpyrimidin-5-ylmethyl)formamide Hydrochloride Monohydrate, 1454·3
2-Acetoxybenzoic Acid, 15·1
10-Acetoxy-9,10-dihydro-8,8-dimethyl-2-oxo-2*H*,8*H*-pyrano[2,3-*f*]chromen-9-yl 2-Methylbutyrate, 1653·3
*ent*-16α-Acetoxy-3β-dihydroxy-4β,8β,14α-trimethyl-18-nor-5β,10α-cholesta-(17*Z*)-17(20),24-dien-21-oic Acid Hemihydrate, 215·2
(+)-*cis*-3-Acetoxy-5-(2-dimethylaminoethyl)-2,3-dihydro-2-(4-methoxyphenyl)-1,5-benzothiazepin-4(5*H*)-one Hydrochloride, 900·1
(2-Acetoxyethyl)trimethylammonium Chloride, 1487·1
6-Acetoxy-1,4a,5,6,7,7a-hexahydro-1-isovaleryloxy-4-isovaleryloxymethylcyclopenta[*c*]pyran-7-spiro-2′-oxiran, 1762·2
1-(17β-Acetoxy-3α-hydroxy-2β-morpholino-5α-androstan-16β-yl)-1-allylpyrrolidinium Bromide, 1405·2
Acetoxyl, 1770·2
4-Acetoxymethyl-(1 or 6)-3-(acetoxy-3-methylbutyryloxy)-1,6,7,7a-tetrahydro-(6 or 1)-isovaleryloxycyclopenta[*c*]pyran-7-spiro-2′-oxiran, 1762·2
4-Acetoxymethyl-1,6-di-isovaleryloxy-1,6,7,7a-tetrahydrocyclopenta[*c*]pyran-7-spiro-2′-oxiran, 1762·2
3-Acetoxyphenol, 1156·3
1-(3α-Acetoxy-2β-piperidino-17β-propionyloxy-5α-androstan-16β-yl)-1-allylpiperidinium Bromide, 1405·2
(2-Acetoxypropyl)trimethylammonium Chloride, 1492·1
3-Acetoxyquinuclidine Hydrochloride, 1487·1
2-Acetoxy-4-trifluoromethylbenzoic Acid, 1017·3
8-Acetoxy-3,11,18-trihydroxy-16-ethyl-1,6,19-trimethoxy-4-methoxymethylaconitan-10-yl Benzoate, 1646·3
1-(4-Acetoxy-2,3,5-trimethylphenoxy)-3-isopropylaminopropan-2-ol, 955·3
Acetphenarsinum, 600·2
Acetphenolisatin, 1282·3
Acetuber, 1770·2
Aceturato de Diminazeno, 604·2
Acetyl Hydroperoxide, 1187·3
*N*-Acetyl Hydroxyacetamide, 1645·3
Acetyl Mandelic Acid, 228·3
Acetyl Sulfafurazole, 260·1
Acetyl Sulfamethoxypyridazine, 263·1
Acetyl Sulphafurazole, 260·1
$N^1$-Acetyl Sulphafurazole, 260·1
*N*-Acetyl Trovafloxacin, 274·3
Acetyl-alpha-methylfentanyl, 40·3
(+)-(7*S*,9*S*)-9-Acetyl-9-amino-7-[(2-deoxy-β-D-*erythro*-pentopyranosyl)oxy]-7,8,9,10-tetrahydro-6,11-dihydroxy-5,12-naphthacenedione, 527·3
5-Acetylamino-6-formylamino-3-methyluracil, 783·1
2-Acetylamino-L-glutaramic Acid, 1645·2
*N*-Acetylaminoglutethimide, 527·1
*N*-Acetyl-*p*-aminophenol, 76·2
Acetyl-5-aminosalicylic Acid, 1274·2
(8*S*-*cis*)-8-Acetyl-10-[(3-amino-2,3,6-trideoxy-α-L-*lyxo*-hexopyranosyl)]oxy-7,8,9,10-tetrahydro-6,8,11-trihydroxy-1-methoxy-5,12-naphthacenedione Hydrochloride, 545·3
(7*S*,9*S*)-9-Acetyl-7-(3-amino-2,3,6-trideoxy-α-L-*lyxo*-hexopyranosyloxy)-7,8,9,10-tetrahydro-6,9,11-trihydroxynaphthacene-5,12-dione Hydrochloride, 560·2
*N*-Acetyl-*N*-(3-amino-2,4,6-tri-iodophenyl)-2-methyl-β-alanine, 1063·2
*N*-(*N*-Acetyl-L-α-aspartyl)-L-glutamic Acid, 1702·2
Acetylated Wool Alcohols, 1483·1
1-(4-Acetylbenzenesulphonyl)-3-cyclohexylurea, 329·2
*N*-Acetyl-*p*-benzoquinoneimine, 76·3
Acetylbenzoylaconine, 1646·3
*N*-Acetyl-*N*′-(2-bromo-2-ethylbutyryl)urea, 668·2
3-{3-Acetyl-4-[3-(*tert*-butylamino)-2-hydroxypropoxy]phenyl}-1,1-diethylurea Hydrochloride, 881·3
Acetylcarbromal, 668·2
Acetyl-L-carnitine Chloride, 1646·1
Acetylcarnitine Hydrochloride, 1646·1
Acetylcholine Chloride, 1487·1
Acetylcholini Chloridum, 1487·1
Acetylcodone, 1770·3
Acetylcysteine, 1112·3
*N*-Acetyl-L-cysteine, 1112·3
Acetylcysteine, 1112·3
*N*-Acetyl-L-cysteine Salicylate, 1157·2
Acetylcysteine Sodium, 1113·1
Acetylcysteinum, 1112·3
*N*-Acetylcystine, 1113·2
(±)-*cis*-1-Acetyl-4-{4-[2-(2,4-dichlorophenyl)-2-imidazol-1-ylmethyl-1,3-dioxolan-4-ylmethoxy]phenyl}piperazine, 403·3
3β-[(*O*-3-*O*-Acetyl-2,6-dideoxy-β-D-*ribo*-hexopyranosyl-(1→4)-*O*-2,6-dideoxy-β-D-*ribo*-hexopyranosyl-(1→4)-2,6-dideoxy-β-D-*ribo*-hexopyranosyl)oxy]-12β,14-dihydroxy-5β,14β-card-20(22)-enolide, 851·1
3β-[(*O*-4-*O*-Acetyl-2,6-dideoxy-β-D-*ribo*-hexopyranosyl-(1→4)-*O*-2,6-dideoxy-β-D-*ribo*-hexopyranosyl-(1→4)-2,6-dideoxy-β-D-*ribo*-hexopyranosyl)oxy]-12β,14-dihydroxy-5β,14β-card-20(22)-enolide, 851·1
Acetyldigoxin, 851·1
α-Acetyldigoxin, 851·1
β-Acetyldigoxin, 851·1
Acetyldihydrocodeine Hydrochloride, 1114·2
Acetyldihydrocodeinone Hydrochloride, 1131·2
6-*O*-Acetyl-7,8-dihydro-3-*O*-methyl-6,7-didehydromorphine Hydrochloride, 1131·2
Acetyldimethylamine, 1474·1
Acetylene Tetrachloride, 1477·1
Acetylerythromycin Stearate, 208·1
$N^2$-Acetyl-L-glutamine, 1645·2
(1*S*,3*S*)-3-Acetyl-1,2,3,4,6,11-hexahydro-3,5,12-trihydroxy-10-methoxy-6,11-dioxonaphthacen-1-yl 3-Amino-2,3,6-trideoxy-α-L-*lyxo*-pyranoside Hydrochloride, 545·3
*N*′-{5-[(4-{[5-(Acetylhydroxyamino)pentyl]amino}-1,4-dioxobutyl)hydroxyamino]pentyl}-*N*-(5-aminopentyl)-*N*-hydroxy-butanediamide Monomethanesulphonate, 1033·1
(±)-3′-Acetyl-4′-(2-hydroxy-3-isopropylaminopropoxy)butyranilide, 848·1
3-Acetyl-4-hydroxy-6-methyl-2*H*-pyran-2-one, 1178·1
Acetylhydroxyproline, 1725·1
(−)-1-Acetyl-4-hydroxy-L-proline, 1725·1
Acetylin, 1770·3
Acetylisoniazid, 224·1
Acetylkitasamycin, 225·3
*N*-Acetyl-DL-leucine, 1646·1
Acetylleucine, 1646·1
*l*-α-Acetylmethadol, 54·1
*N*-Acetyl-5-methoxytryptamine, 1710·2
Acetyl-β-methylcholine Chloride, 1492·1
3-Acetyl-6-methyl-2*H*-pyran-2,4(3*H*)-dione, 1178·1
6-Acetylmorphine, 31·1
*N*-Acetylmuramide Glycanohydrolase Hydrochloride, 1717·2
4-(Acetyloxy)-*N*-[2,4-dibromo-6-[(cyclohexylmethylamino)methyl]phenyl]-3-methoxybenzamide Monohydrochloride, 1116·1
Acetylpenicillamine, 1049·1
Acetylphenetidin, 82·2
*N*-Acetylprocainamide Hydrochloride, 848·3
Acetylpromazine Maleate, 668·3
Acetylsal. Acid, 15·1
*O*-Acetylsalicylic Acid, 15·1
Acetylsalicylic Acid, 15·1
Acetylsalicylic Acid Guaiacol Ester, 1121·3
Acetylsalicylicum, Acidum, 15·1
Acetylspiramycin, 255·3
*N*-Acetylsuperoxide Dismutase, 92·3
*N*-[(*R*,*S*)-3-Acetylthio-2-benzylpropanoyl]glycine Benzyl Ester, 1285·2
(7α,17α)-7-(Acetylthio)-17-hydroxy-3-oxopregn-4-ene-21-carboxylic Acid γ-Lactone, 1003·1
*N*-[2-(3-Acetylthio-7-methoxycarbonylheptyldithio)-4-hydroxy-1-methylbut-1-enyl]-*N*-(4-amino-2-methylpyrimidin-5-ylmethyl)formamide, 1455·1
(±)-*N*-{2-[(Acetylthio)methyl]-1-oxo-3-phenylpropyl}glycine Phenylmethyl Ester, 1285·2
7α-Acetylthio-3-oxo-17α-pregn-4-ene-21,17β-carbolactone, 1003·1
Acetyltributyl Citrate, 1757·3
*O*-Acetyl-4-(trifluoromethyl)salicylic Acid, 1017·3
*N*-Acetylzonisamide, 385·2
Acetyst, 1770·3
Acevaltrate, 1762·2
Acevit, 1770·3
Acevor, 1770·3
Acexamic Acid, 1646·2
Acexámico, Ácido, 1646·2
Acezide, 1770·3
AC-FA, 1770·3
Acfol, 1770·3
Ac-globulin, 735·3
Achalasia— *see* Oesophageal Motility Disorders, 1246·3
Aches/Pains, 1770·3
Achillea, 1646·2
*Achillea millefolium*, 1646·2
Achillée Millefeuille, 1646·2
Achisane Troubles du Sommeil— *see* Actisane Troubles du Sommeil, 1774·1
Achlorhydria, 1699·2
Achondroplasia— *see* Growth Retardation, 1314·2
Achromide, 1770·3
Achromycin, 1770·3
Achromycin V, 1770·3
Achromycine, 1770·3
Aci Tip, 1770·3
Acibar, 1248·2
Aciben, 1770·3
Acic, 1770·3
Aciclin, 1770·3
Aciclo, 1770·3
Aciclobene, 1770·3
Aciclobeta, 1770·3
Aciclodan, 1770·3
Aciclomed, 1770·3
Aciclor, 1770·3
Aciclosina, 1770·3
Aciclostad, 1770·3
Aciclotyrol, 1770·3
Aciclovir, 626·1
Aciclovir Sódico, 626·1

Aciclovir Sodium, 626·1
Aciclovirum, 626·1
Acic-Ophtal, 1770·3
Acicvir, 1770·3
Acid A Vit, 1770·3
Acid Alpha Glucosidase, 1646·2
Acid Blue 1, 1750·3
Acid Blue 3, 1729·1
Acid Brilliant Green BS, 1057·3
Acid Calcium Phosphate, 1664·2
Acid Control, 1770·3
Acid Fuchsine, 1646·3
Acid α-Glucosidase, 1646·2
Acid β-Glucosidase, 1649·2
Acid Green S, 1057·3
Acid Halt, 1770·4
Acid Light Yellow 2G, 1058·3
Acid Magenta, 1646·3
Acid Maltase, 1646·2
Acid Mantle, 1770·4
Acid Modafinil, 1591·1
Acid Red 1, 1058·1
Acid Reducer, 1770·4
Acid Roseine, 1646·3
Acid Rubine, 1646·3
Acid. Sulph., 1750·3
Acid. Sulph. Dil., 1750·3
Acid Yellow 17, 1058·3
Acide Acetylsalicylique Comp. "Radix", 1770·4
Acide Clodronique, 770·2
Acide Neridronique, 773·2
Acide Zymonucléique, 1722·2
Aciderm, 1770·4
Acidern, 1770·4
Acidex, 1770·4
Acid-Eze, 1770·4
Acidin, 1770·4
Acidine, 1770·4
Acidion, 1770·4
Acidix, 1770·4
Acid-Lac, 1770·4
Ácido Acético, 1645·2
Ácido Acetohidroxámico, 1645·3
Ácido Acexámico, 1646·2
Ácido Alendrónico, 765·3
Ácido Algínico, 1576·3
Ácido Aminocaproico, 741·3
Ácido Arsanílico, 158·3
Ácido Ascórbico, 1460·2
Ácido Aspártico, 1422·3
Ácido Azelaico, 1142·3
Ácido Bórico, 1662·1
Ácido Cicloxílico, 1671·2
Ácido Cinamético, 1671·3
Ácido Clavulánico, 193·3
Ácido Clodrónico, 770·2
Ácido Dehidrocólico, 1679·2
Ácido del Limón, 1673·1
Ácido Edético, 1038·2
Ácido Esteárico, 1749·2
Ácido Etacrínico, 913·2
Ácido Etidrónico, 771·2
Ácido Flufenámico, 43·2
Ácido Fólico, 1429·1
Ácido Fosfórico, 1731·2
Ácido Fusídico, 215·2
Ácido Gadobénico, 1062·1
Ácido Gadopentético, 1062·2
Ácido Gadotérico, 1062·3
Ácido Gamolénico, 1690·2
Ácido Glutámico, 1433·2
Ácido Ibandrónico, 772·3
Ácido Incadrónico, 773·1
Ácido Iocetámico, 1063·2
Ácido Iodoxámico, 1064·1
Ácido Ioglícico, 1064·1
Ácido Iopanoico, 1065·1
Ácido Iotalámico, 1065·3
Ácido Iotróxico, 1066·1
Ácido Ioxáglico, 1066·2
Ácido Ioxitalámico, 1066·3
Ácido Isospaglúmico, 1702·2
Ácido Meclofenámico, 55·1
Ácido Medrónico, 773·2
Ácido Mefenámico, 55·2
Ácido Nalidíxico, 234·1
Ácido Neridrónico, 773·2
Ácido Nicotínico, 1441·1
Ácido Niflúmico, 67·1
Ácido Octanoico, 1723·1
Ácido Orótico, 1724·3
Ácido Ortóxibenzoico, 1157·1
Ácido Oxidrónico, 773·3
Ácido Oxolínico, 240·3
Ácido Pamidrónico, 773·3
Ácido Pipemídico, 243·1
Ácido Piromídico, 244·1
Ácido Quenodeoxicólico, 1670·1
Ácido Risedrónico, 774·3
Ácido Tiaprofénico, 93·3
Ácido Tienílico, 1012·2
Ácido Tiludrónico, 776·1
Ácido Timico, 1194·2
Ácido Tolfenámico, 94·2
Ácido Tranexámico, 760·3
Ácido Ursodeoxicólico, 1760·3
Ácido Valproico, 380·1
Ácido Zoledrónico, 776·2
Acidodermil, 1770·4
Acidofilofago, 1770·4
Acidophilus, 1770·4
Acidophilus Bifidus, 1770·4
Acidophilus Complex, 1770·4
Acidophilus Plus, 1770·4
Acidophilus Plus, Natures Own— *see* Natures Own Acidophilus Plus, 2153·2
Acidophilus Plus, Natures Way— *see* Natures Way Acidophilus Plus, 2153·3
Acidophilus Tablets, 1770·4
Ácidos de Alquitrán, 1193·3
Ácidos Grasos Omega 3, 976·1
Acidosis, 1770·4
Acidosis— *see* Metabolic Acidosis, 1217·2
Acidovert, 1771·1
Acidown, 1771·1
Acidrina, 1771·1
Acidrine, 1771·1
Acidum Aceticum Glaciale, 1645·2
Acidum Acetylsalicylicum, 15·1
Acidum Adipicum, 1648·1
Acidum Alginicum, 1576·3
Acidum Amidotrizoicum, 1060·1
Acidum 4-Aminobenzoicum, 1142·2
Acidum Aminocaproicum, 741·3
Acidum Arsenicosum Anhydricum, 1657·1
Acidum Ascorbicum, 1460·2
Acidum Asparticum, 1422·3
Acidum Benzoicum, 1169·3
Acidum Boricum, 1662·1
Acidum Caprylicum, 1723·1
Acidum Chenodeoxycholicum, 1670·1
Acidum Cinameticum, 1671·3
Acidum Citricum Anhydricum, 1673·1
Acidum Citricum Monohydricum, 1673·1
Acidum Clodronicum, 770·2
Acidum Edeticum, 1038·2
Acidum Etacrynicum, 913·2
Acidum Folicum, 1429·1
Acidum Fusidicum, 215·2
Acidum Glutamicum, 1433·2
Acidum Hydrochloridum, 1699·1
Acidum Hydrochloridum Concentratum, 1699·1
Acidum Hydrochloridum Dilutum, 1699·1
Acidum Hypophosphorosum, 1700·2
Acidum Iopanoicum, 1065·1
Acidum Ioxaglicum, 1066·2
Acidum Lacticum, 1704·1
Acidum Maleicum, 1709·2
Acidum Mefenamicum, 55·2
Acidum Mersalylicum, 952·2
Acidum Nalidixicum, 234·1
Acidum Neridronicum, 773·2
Acidum Nicotinicum, 1441·1
Acidum Nitricum, 1722·1
Acidum Nucleicum, 1722·2
Acidum Oleicum, 1481·3
Acidum Oxolinicum, 240·3
Acidum Phosphoricum Med Complex, 1771·1
Acidum Picrinicum Med Complex, 1771·1
Acidum Pipemidicum Trihydricum, 243·1
Acidum Salicylicum, 1157·1
Acidum Silicicum Colloidale, 1581·3
Acidum Sorbicum, 1192·3
Acidum Stearicum, 1749·2
Acidum Tannicum, 1751·2
Acidum Tartaricum, 1752·1
Acidum Tolfenamicum, 94·2
Acidum Tranexamicum, 760·3
Acidum Trichloraceticum, 1162·1
Acidum Undecylenicum, 410·3
Acidum Ursodeoxycholicum, 1760·3
Acidum Valproicum, 380·1
Acidumphos-Gastreu, 1771·1
Acid-X, 1771·1
Acidylina, 1771·1
Aciflux, 1771·1
Acifol, 1771·1
Acifolico, 1771·1
Aciforin, 1771·1
Acifugan, 1771·1
Acifur, 1771·1
Aciglumin, 1433·2
Acigon, 1771·1
Acihexal, 1771·1
Aci-Jel, 1771·1
Acilac, 1771·1
Acilax, 1771·1
Acilen, 1771·1
Acilin, 1771·1
Aciloc, 1771·1
Acimax, 1771·2
Acimed, 1771·2
Aci-Med, 1771·2
Acimethin, 1771·2
Acimol, 1771·2
Acimox, 1771·2
Acimox-Ex, 1771·2
Acimpil, 1771·2
Acinal, 1771·2
Acinil, 1771·2
Acintor, 1771·2
Acipem, 1771·2
Acipen, 1771·2
Acipen-V, 1771·2
Aciphex, 1771·2
Acipimox, 851·1
Aciril, 1771·2
Acirufan, 1771·2
Aci-Sanorania, 1771·2
Acistin, 1771·2
Acistrato de Eritromicina, 208·1
Acitab, 1771·2
Acitak, 1771·2
Aci-Tip, 1771·2
Acitop, 1771·2
Acitra, 1771·2
Acitretin, 1140·2
Acitretina, 1140·2
Acitretinum, 1140·2
Acitrom, 1771·2
Acival, 1771·2
Aciveral, 1771·2
Acivir, 1771·2
Ackee, 1700·2
Acks, 1771·3
Aclacin, 1771·3
Aclacinomycin A, 525·2
Aclaplastin, 1771·3
Aclarubicin, 525·2
Aclarubicin Hydrochloride, 525·2
Aclarubicina, Hidrocloruro de, 525·2
Aclav, 1771·3
Aclimafel, 1771·3
Aclin, 1771·3
Aclinda, 1771·3
Aclon Lievit, 1771·3
Aclonium, 1771·3
Aclophen, 1771·3
Acloral, 1771·3
Aclorisan, 1771·3
Aclosan, 1771·3
Aclosone, 1771·3
Aclotan, 1771·3
Aclotine, 1771·3
Aclovate, 1771·3
Aclovir, 1771·3
ACM 20, 1771·3
Acnacyl, 1771·3
Acnaid, 1771·3
Acnase, 1771·3
Acnaveen, 1771·3
Acne, 1133·3, 1771·3
Acne Blemish Cream, 1771·3
Acne Creme, 1771·3
Acne Creme Plus, 1771·4
Acne Derm, 1771·4
Acne Gel, 1771·4
Acne Hermal, 1771·4
Acne Lotion, 1771·4
Acne Lotion 10, 1771·4
Acne Mask, 1771·4
Acne Mask, Neutrogena— *see* Neutrogena Acne Mask, 2165·1
Acne Oral Spray, 1771·4
Acne & Pimple Gel, 1771·4
Acne Plus, 1771·4
Acne-Aid, 1771·4
Acnecide, 1771·4
Acneclear, 1771·4
Acneclin, 1771·4
Acnecolor, 1771·4
Acnecure, 1771·4
Acnederm, 1771·4
Acnederm Foaming Wash, 1771·4
Acnederm Wash, 1771·4
Acnefuge, 1771·4
Acne-Med Wolff Simplex, 1772·1
Acneryne, 1772·1
Acnesan, 1772·1
Acnesoap, 1772·1
Acnesol, 1772·1
Acnestop, 1772·1
Acnetrim, 1772·1
Acnetrol, 1772·1
Acnex, 1772·1
Acnexyl, 1772·1
Acnezaic, 1772·1
Acnidazil, 1772·1
Acnisal, 1772·1
Acnisdin, 1772·1
Acnisdin Retinoico, 1772·1
Acno, 1772·1
Acno Cleanser, 1772·1
Acnoil Free, 1772·1
Acnomel, 1772·1
Acnomel Acne Mask, 1772·1
Acnosan, 1772·1
Acnosil, 1772·1
Acnotex, 1772·2
AlcNOW, 1772·2
Acnoxin, 1772·2
Acnoxyl Abrasivo, 1772·2
Acnoxyl Gel Cuidado Intensivo, 1772·2
Acnoxyl Gel De Limpieza, 1772·2
Acnoxyl Gel Humectante, 1772·2
Acnoxyl Jabon, 1772·2
Acnoxyl Jabon Liquido, 1772·2
Acnoxyl Locion Tonica, 1772·2
Acnoxyl Shampoo Cabello Graso, 1772·2
Acnoxyl Stick Corrector, 1772·2
ACNU, 576·3, 1772·2
Acobiotic, 1772·2
Acocantherin, 977·3
Acocontin, 1772·2
Acodon, 1772·2
Acoflam, 1772·2
Acoin, 1772·2
*Acokanthera ouabaio*, 977·3
*Acokanthera schimperi*, 977·3
Acolitium, 1772·2
Acolyt, 1772·2
Acon, 1772·2
Acondicionador Labial, 1772·2
Aconeurin, 1772·2
Aconex, 1772·2
Aconit., 1646·3
Aconit Napel, 1646·3
Aconit Schmerzol, 1772·2
Aconite, 1646·3
Aconite Root, 1646·3
Aconiti Tuber, 1646·3

Acónito, 1646·3
Aconitum, 1772·2
Aconitum Med Complex, 1772·2
*Aconitum napellus*, 1646·3
Aconitum-Homaccord, 1772·2
Acordin, 1772·2
Acore Vrai, 1664·1
Acorus, 1772·2
*Acorus calamus*, 1664·1
Acotoss, 1772·2
Acovil, 1772·3
Acpan, 1772·3
Acqta, 1772·3
Acqua di Sirmione, 1772·3
Acqua Virginiana, 1772·3
Acquired Immunodeficiency Syndrome— *see* HIV Infection and AIDS, 621·3
Acraldehyde, 1647·1
Acrichinum, 606·3
Acridin, 1772·3
Acridina, Derivados, 1165·3
Acridine Derivatives, 1165·3
Acridine Orange, 1647·1
Acridinyl Anisidide, 527·3
4′-(Acridin-9-ylamino)methanesulphon-*m*-anisidide, 527·3
Acriflavine, 1165·3
Acriflavine Hydrochloride, 1165·3
Acriflavine, Neutral, 1165·3
Acriflavinii Dichloridum, 1165·3
Acriflavinii Monochloridum, 1165·3
Acriflavinio, Cloruro de, 1165·3
Acriflavinium Chloride, 1165·3
Acriflavinium Monochloride, 1165·3
Acriflex, 1772·3
Acrilamida, 1647·1
Acrinamine, 606·3
Acrinol, 1165·3
Acrisuxin, 1772·3
Acrivastina, 423·3
Acrivastine, 423·3
Acrocyanosis— *see* Raynaud's Syndrome, 833·3
Acrodermatitis Chronica Atrophicans— *see* Lyme Disease, 134·1
Acrolein, 1647·1
Acroleína, 1647·1
Acromax, 1772·3
Acromegaly— *see* Acromegaly and Gigantism, 1312·1
Acromicina, 1772·3
Acrosin, 1772·3
Acrosoxacin, 254·1
Acroxil, 1772·3
Acrylaldehyde, 1647·1
Acrylamide, 1647·1
Acrylarm, 1772·3
Acrylic Acid Polymers, 1577·2
Acrylic Aldehyde, 1647·1
Acrylonitrile-starch Copolymer, 1145·1
Acsacea, 1772·3
Ac-Sal, 1772·3
Acset, 1772·3
ACT, 1772·3
ACT-3, 1772·3
Acta, 1772·3
Actacel, 1772·3
Actacode, 1772·3
Actaea Rac, 1671·3
*Actaea racemosa*, 1671·3
Actagen, 1772·3
Actagen-C Cough, 1772·3
Actal, 1772·3
Actal Plus, 1772·4
Actan, 1772·4
Actapront, 1772·4
Actapulgite, 1772·4
Actarit, 12·1
Actebral, 1772·4
Acteoside, 1738·2
ACTH, 1322·1
ACTH Secretion, Excess— *see* Cushing's Syndrome, 1313·1
Acthar, 1772·4
Acthelea, 1772·4
Act-HIB, 1772·4
Act-HIB— *see* Pentacel, 2211·1
Act-HIB— *see* Pentacoq, 2211·1
Act-HIB DTP, 1772·4
Act-HIB Plus DPT, 1772·4
Act-HIB Polio, 1772·4
Acthrel, 1772·4
Acti 5, 1772·4
Acti Valda Diet, 1772·4
Acti-$B_{12}$, 1772·4
ActiBath, 1772·4
Actibil, 1772·4
Actibrush, 1772·4
ActiCal Plus, 1772·4
Acticalcin, 1773·1
Acticarbine, 1773·1
Actichlor, 1773·1
Acticillin, 1773·1
Acticin, 1773·1
Acticinco, 1773·1
Acticolin, 1773·1
Acticort, 1773·1
Acticrom, 1773·1
Actidil, 1773·1
Actidine, 1773·1
Actidose with Sorbitol, 1773·1
Actidose-Aqua, 1773·1
Actidox, 1773·1
Actidue, 1773·1
Actifed Preparations, 1773·1
Actifed Chesty Coughs, Multi-Action— *see* Multi-Action Actifed Chesty Coughs Expectorant, 2144·3
Actifed Compound— *see* Multi-Action Actifed Dry Coughs, 2144·3
Actifed Dry Coughs, Multi-Action— *see* Multi-Action Actifed Dry Coughs, 2144·3
Actifed Expectorant— *see* Multi-Action Actifed Chesty Coughs Expectorant, 2144·3
Actifed, Multi-Action— *see* Multi-Action Actifed, 2144·3
Actifedrin, 1773·3
Actifedrin Antitusivo, 1773·3
Actifen, 1773·3
Actiferrine, 1773·3
Actiferrine-F Nouvelle Formule, 1773·3
Actiferro, 1773·3
Actifluor, 1773·3
Actigall, 1773·3
Actigeron, 1773·3
Actigesic— *see* Actifed Cold & Fever, 1773·2
Actigrip, 1773·3
Actihaemyl, 1773·3
Actihist, 1773·3
Actihist Expectorant, 1773·3
Actihist-Co, 1773·3
Actil, 1773·3
Actilam, 1773·3
Actilax, 1773·3
Actilevol Orex, 1773·3
Actilife, 1773·3
Actilis, 1773·3
Actilyse, 1773·3
Actimag, 1773·4
Actiment, 1773·4
Actimidol, 1773·4
Actimmune, 1773·4
Actimol, 1773·4
Actimoxi, 1773·4
Actin, 1773·4
Actinac, 1773·4
Actinerval, 1773·4
Actinic Dermatitis, Chronic— *see* Light-induced Skin Reactions, 1136·3
Actinic Keratosis— *see* Basal Cell and Squamous Cell Carcinoma, 522·3
Actino-Hermal, 1773·4
*Actinomyces bovis*, 1703·3
Actinomycetales, 116·1
Actinomycetoma— *see* Mycetoma, 136·2
Actinomycin C, 545·1
Actinomycin $C_1$, 545·1
Actinomycin $C_2$, 545·1
Actinomycin $C_3$, 545·1
Actinomycin D, 545·1
Actinomycosis, 120·3
*Actinoplanes teichomyceticus*, 264·3
Actinoquinol Sodium, 1647·2
Actinospectacin, 255·2
Action, 1773·4
Action Chewable, 1773·4
Action Cold & Flu, 1773·4
Actiphos, 1773·4
Actiplas, 1773·4
Actipram, 1773·4
Actiprofen, 1773·4
Actiq, 1773·4
Actiquim, 1773·4
Actira, 1773·4
Actireuma, 1773·4
Actisac, 1773·4
Actisane Constipation Occasionnelle, 1773·4
Actisane Digestion, 1773·4
Actisane Douleurs Articulaires, 1773·4
Actisane Fatigue Passagere, 1773·4
Actisane Hemorroides, Jambes Lourdes, 1774·1
Actisane Minceur, 1774·1
Actisane Nervosite, 1774·1
Actisane Troubles Du Sommeil, 1774·1
Actisens, 1774·1
Actisite, 1774·1
Actiskenan, 1774·1
Actisorb, 1774·1
Actisorb Plus, 1774·1
Actisorb Silver, 1774·1
Actisoufre, 1774·1
Actisson, 1774·1
Actithiol, 1774·1
Actithiol Antihist, 1774·1
Actitonic, 1774·1
Activadone, 1774·1
Activarol, 1774·1
Activase, 1774·1
Activated Attapulgite, 1251·1
Activated Attapulgite, Colloidal, 1251·1
Activated Charcoal, 1030·2
Activated Dimethicone, 1289·2
Activated Dimethylpolysiloxane, 1289·2
Activated Factor VII, 750·3
Activated Glutaral, 1181·1
Activated Partial Thromboplastin Time, 735·3
Activated Protein C, 759·2
Activated Protein C Resistance— *see* Thromboembolic Disorders, 837·3
Activated Prothrombin Complex Concentrate, 752·2
Activator, 1774·1
Active C, 1774·1
Active Dry Lotion, 1774·1
Active Immunisation, 1605·1
Active Multi, 1774·1
Activella, 1774·1
Activelle, 1774·1
Activex 40 Plus, 1774·2
Activir, 1774·2
Activital, 1774·2
Activon, 1774·2
Activox, 1774·2
Actizyme, 1774·2
Actocortina, 1774·2
Actol, 1774·2
Actomin, 1774·2
Actomite, 1774·2
Actonel, 1774·2
Actonorm, 1774·2
Actophlem, 1774·2
Actopril, 1774·2
Actos, 1774·2
Actosolv, 1774·2
Actospect, 1774·2
Actovegin, 1774·2
Actraphane HM Preparations, 1774·2
Actrapid, 1774·3
Actrapid HM, 1774·3
Actrapid, Human— *see* Human Actrapid, 2049·2
Actrapid MC, 1774·3
Actron, 1774·3
Actron Compuesto, 1774·3
Actroneffix, 1774·3
Actualene, 1774·3
Actuss, 1774·3
Actymine, 1774·3
Actypral, 1774·3
Acuaderm, 1774·3
Acuafil, 1774·3
Acuafil Ofteno, 1774·3
Acuatim, 1774·3
Acubiron, 1774·3
Acucil, 1774·3
Acuco, 1774·3
Acudor, 1774·3
ACU-dyne, 1774·3
Acu-Erylate S, 1774·3
Acuflex, 1774·3
Acuflu-P, 1774·3
Acugesic, 1774·3
Acugesil, 1774·4
Acugest, 1774·4
Acugest Co, 1774·4
Acugest Expect, 1774·4
Acuilix, 1774·4
Acuitel, 1774·4
Acular, 1774·4
Aculare, 1774·4
Acularen, 1774·4
Aculfin, 1774·4
Aculoid, 1774·4
Acumet, 1774·4
Acumod, 1774·4
Acunaso, 1774·4
Acuode, 1774·4
Acuolens, 1774·4
Acu-Oxytet, 1774·4
Acupan, 1774·4
Acuphlem, 1774·4
Acupillin, 1774·4
Acuprel, 1774·4
Acupril, 1774·4
Acurate, 1774·4
Acuretic, 1774·4
Acusprain, 1774·4
Acustat, 1774·4
Acustop, 1774·4
Acustop Cataplasma, 1775·1
Acute Chest Syndrome— *see* Sickle-cell Disease, 734·3
Acute Respiratory Distress Syndrome, 1075·2
AcuTect, 1775·1
Acutil Fosforo, 1775·1
Acutrim, 1775·1
Acutussive, 1775·1
Acuzide, 1775·1
Acuzole, 1775·1
ACV, 1775·1
ACWY Vax, 1775·1
Acxen, 1775·1
ACY, 1775·1
Acycloguanosine, 626·1
Acyclostad, 1775·1
Acyclo-V, 1775·1
Acyclovir, 626·1
Acyclovir Sodium, 626·1
Acydona, 1775·1
Acyflox, 1775·1
Acylene, 1775·1
Acyprin, 1775·1
Acypront, 1775·1
Acyrax, 1775·1
Acyvir, 1775·1
AD-32, 590·3
AD-810, 384·3
AD-03055, 361·1
AD-4833, 344·1
AD Pabyrn, 1775·1
AD Shock, 1775·1
ADA, 1775·1
Adacel, 1775·1
Adaferin, 1775·1
Adagen, 1775·1
ADAH, 530·2
Adalat, 1775·1
Adalate, 1775·1

Adalgen, 1775·2
Adalgur, 1775·2
Adalgur N, 1775·2
Adalimumab, 12·1
Adalken, 1775·2
Adam, 1589·3
1-Adamantanamine Hydrochloride, 1197·2
Adamantanamines, 1196·1
(*RS*)-1-(Adamantan-1-yl)ethylamine Hydrochloride, 653·1
*N*-1-Adamantyl-2-(2-dimethylaminoethoxy)acetamide Hydrochloride, 656·1
6-[3-(1-Adamantyl)-4-methoxyphenyl]-2-naphthoic Acid, 1141·1
Adamon, 1775·2
Adancor, 1775·2
Adant, 1775·2
Adapalene, 1141·1
Adapaleno, 1141·1
Adapettes, 1775·2
Adapine, 1775·2
Adaptic, 1775·2
Adasept, 1775·2
Adaspor, 1775·2
Adato-Cel, 1775·2
Adato-Deca, 1775·2
Adato-Octa, 1775·2
Adato-Sil Ol, 1775·2
Adavite, 1775·2
Adax, 1775·2
Adaxil, 1775·2
A-D-C, 1775·2
ADC Fluor, 1775·2
ADCA, 530·2
Adcal, 1775·2
Adcal-$D_3$, 1775·2
Adco-Amoclav, 1775·2
Adco-Ciprin, 1775·2
Adco-Dermed, 1775·2
Adco-Dol, 1775·2
Adco-Flupain, 1775·3
Adco-Indogel, 1775·3
Adco-Kiddipayne, 1775·3
Adco-Linctopent, 1775·3
Adco-Liquilax, 1775·3
Adco-Loten, 1775·3
Adco-Muco Expect, 1775·3
Adco-Payne, 1775·3
Adco-Phenobarbitone Vitalet, 1775·3
Adcor, 1775·3
Adco-Retic, 1775·3
Adcortyl, 1775·3
Adcortyl with Graneodin, 1775·3
Adcortyl in Orabase, 1775·3
Adco-Sinal Co, 1775·3
Adco-Sodasol, 1775·3
Adco-Sufedrin, 1775·3
Adco-Tussend, 1775·3
Addamel, 1775·3
Addamel N, 1775·3
Addamel Novum, 1775·3
'Add-back' Therapy, 1325·3
Addel N, 1775·3
Addera, 1775·3
Adderall, 1775·3
Addex, 1775·3
Addex-THAM, 1775·3
Addigrip, 1775·4
Addi-K, 1775·4
Addiphos, 1775·4
Addison's Disease— *see* Adrenocortical Insufficiency, 1075·3
Additene, 1775·4
Additrace, 1775·4
Addivita, 1775·4
ADE 2 (Adedois), 1775·4
Adecaps, 1775·4
Adecur, 1775·4
Adecut, 1775·4
Adedois— *see* ADE 2 (Adedois), 1775·4
Adeflor M, 1775·4
Adeforte, 1775·4
Adefovir, 628·1
Adefovir Dipivoxil, 628·1
Adefovir, Dipivoxilo de, 628·1
Adeglos, 1775·4
Adegrip, 1775·4
Adegripan, 1775·4
Adehl, 1775·4
Adek, 1775·4
Adekin, 1775·4
Adekon, 1775·4
Adekon C, 1775·4
Adeks, 1775·4
Adel, 1775·4
Adelcort, 1775·4
Ad-Element, 1775·4
Adelfa, 1723·1
Adelfan-Esidrex, 1775·4
Adelheid-Jodquelle, Tolzer, 1775·4
Adelone, 1775·4
Adeloren, 1775·4
Adelphane, 1776·1
Adelphane-Esidrex, 1776·1
Adelphan-Esidrex, 1776·1
Adelphan-Esidrix, 1776·1
Ademethionine, 1647·2
Ademetionina, 1647·2
Ademetionine, 1647·2
Ademetionine Butanedisulfonate, 1647·2
Ademetionine Sulfate Tosilate, 1647·2
Adena C, 1776·1
Adenas, 1776·1
Adenil, 1776·1
Adenina, 1647·3
Adenine, 1647·3
Adenine Arabinoside, 657·1
Adenine Hydrochloride, 1647·3
Adeninum, 1647·3
Adenobeta, 1776·1
Adenocard, 1776·1
Adenocor, 1776·1
Adenoidal Hypertrophy, 1092·2
Adenoject, 1776·1
Adenoplex Forte, 1776·1
Adenoprostal, 1776·1
Adenosan, 1776·1
Adenoscan, 1776·1
Adenosina, 851·2
Adenosina, Fosfato de, 1647·3
Adenosina, Trifosfato de, 1648·1
Adenosine, 851·2
Adenosine Deaminase, 1729·2
Adenosine Deaminase Deficiency, 1729·2
Adenosine 5′-Monophosphate, 1647·3
Adenosine Phosphate, 1647·3
Adenosine 5′-(Tetrahydrogen Triphosphate), 1648·1
Adenosine Triphosphate, 1648·1
Adenosine 5′-Triphosphate, 1648·1
Adenosine Triphosphate, Disodium Salt, 1648·1
Adenosine Triphosphate Sodium, 1648·1
Adenosine-5′-(dihydrogen Phosphate), 1647·3
Adenosine-5′-phosphoric Acid, 1647·3
Adenosinum, 851·2
Adenosylcobalamin, 1459·1
*S*-Adenosyl-L-methionine, 1647·2
Adenovit, 1776·1
Adenyl, 1776·1
5′-Adenyldiphosphoric Acid, 1648·1
5′-Adenylic Acid, 1647·3
Adenylic Acid, Muscle, 1647·3
Adenylocrat, 1776·1
Adenylpyrophosphoric Acid, 1648·1
Adepal, 1776·1
Adepril, 1776·1
Adeps Lanae, 1483·1
Adeps Lanae cum Aqua, 1483·2
Adeps Lanae Hydrogenatus, 1483·2
Adeps Neutralis, 1481·1
Adeps Solidus, 1481·1
Adepsique, 1776·1
Adept, 1776·1
Adeptolon, 1776·1
Aderan, 1776·2
Aderm, 1776·2
Aderma Dermalibour, 1776·2
Aderma Epitheliale, 1776·2
Aderma Exomega, 1776·2
A-Derma Lait Ecran, 1776·2
A-Derma Pain Salicylique, 1776·2
Aderma Ultra High Protection, 1776·2
Adermicina, 1776·2
Adermicina A, 1776·2
Adermina, 1776·2
Adermine Hydrochloride, 1456·3
Adermykon, 1776·2
Adermykon-C, 1776·2
Aderofix D3, 1776·2
Aderogil D3, 1776·2
Aderogyl, 1776·2
Aderplus Spezial Dr Hagedorn, 1776·2
Adesinon-P, 1776·2
Adesipress-TTS, 1776·2
Adesitrin, 1776·2
Adex, 1776·2
Adexolin, 1776·2
Adexone, 1776·2
Adezan, 1776·2
Adezio, 1776·2
Adfen, 1776·2
AD-Furp, 1776·2
Adgyn Combi, 1776·2
Adgyn Estro, 1776·3
Adgyn Medro, 1776·3
ADH, 1342·2
ADH Deficiency— *see* Diabetes Insipidus, 1314·1
ADH, Inappropriate Secretion of— *see* Syndrome of Inappropriate ADH Secretion, 1318·3
ADH Resistance— *see* Diabetes Insipidus, 1314·1
Adhaegon, 1776·3
Adiantine, 1776·3
Adiaril, 1776·3
Adiazine, 1776·3
Adibal, 1776·3
Adiboran AD, 1776·3
Adicanil, 1776·3
Adiclair, 1776·3
Adiecal, 1776·3
Adiefim Calcium, 1776·3
Adifax, 1588·3
Adifen, 1776·3
Adifteper, 1776·3
Adilox, 1776·3
Adimod, 1776·3
Adinol, 1776·3
Adiod, 1776·3
Adios, 1776·3
Adipato de Dioctilo, 1504·2
Adipex, 1776·3
Adipex-P, 1776·3
Adiphenine, 1648·1
Adiphenine Hydrochloride, 1648·1
Adiphenini Hydrochloridum, 1648·1
Adipic Acid, 1648·1
Adípico, Ácido, 1648·1
Adipicum, Acidum, 1648·1
Adipine, 1776·3
Adipinsäure, 1648·1
Adipiodona, 1060·1
Adipiodona de Meglumina, 1060·1
Adipiodone, 1060·1
Adipiodone Meglumine, 1060·1
Adipodiet, 1776·3
Adiporell, 1776·3
Adiporetic, 1776·3
Adipost, 1776·3
3,3′-Adipoyldiaminobis(2,4,6-tri-iodobenzoic Acid), 1060·1
Adiro, 1776·3
Adisar, 1776·3
Adisterolo, 1776·3
Adistop, 1776·4
Adistop Lax, 1776·4
Adital, 1776·4
Adiugrip, 1776·4
Adiuvant, 1776·4
Adivon, 1776·4
Adizem, 1776·4
ADL, 1776·4
ADL-8-2698, 1250·2
*Adleria gallae-tinctoriae*, 1690·2
Admag, 1776·4
Admag-M, 1776·4
Admiral, 1776·4
Admon, 1776·4
Ad-Muc, 1776·4
ADN, 852·2, 1679·2, 1776·4
Adnax, 1776·4
Adnemic, 1776·4
Adnemic F, 1776·4
Ado C, 1776·4
Adocante Docura, 1776·4
Adocomp, 1776·4
Adocor, 1776·4
Adocyl C, 1776·4
Adofen, 1776·4
Adol, 1776·4
Adol Allergy Sinus, 1776·4
Adol Cold, 1776·4
Adol Compound, 1776·4
Adol Extra, 1776·4
Adol PM, 1776·4
Adol Sinus, 1776·4
Adolan, 1777·1
Adolcas, 1777·1
Adolkin, 1777·1
Adolonta, 1777·1
Adolorin, 1777·1
Adolorin ASS/Vit C, 1777·1
Adolphs Salt Substitute, 1777·1
Adolquir, 1777·1
Adoluron CC, 1777·1
Adona, 1777·1
Adonide, 1648·1
Adonidis, Herba, 1648·1
Adonis, 1648·1
Adonis Vernal, 1648·1
Adonis Vernalis, 1648·1
*Adonis vernalis*, 1648·1
Adoniskraut, 1648·1
Adop-Tar, 1777·1
Adoquick Vit C, 1777·1
Adormidera, Aceite de Semilla de, 1733·3
Adormidera, Fruto de, 1129·1
Adormix, 1777·1
Adovit C, 1777·1
Adoxa, 1777·1
Adprex, 1777·1
Adprin-B, 1777·1
ADR-033, 1018·1
ADR-529, 1036·1
Adrafinil, 1584·2
Adrafinilo, 1584·2
Adragante, Gomme, 1582·2
Adrebloc, 1777·1
Adrecort, 1777·1
Adrectal, 1777·1
Adreject, 1777·1
Adrekar, 1777·1
Adrenal Hyperplasia, Congenital— *see* Congenital Adrenal Hyperplasia, 1078·3
Adrenaline, 852·2
Adrenaline Acid Tartrate, 852·2
Adrenaline Bitartrate, 852·2
Adrenaline Borate, 854·3
Adrenaline Hydrochloride, 852·3
Adrenaline, Racemic, 854·2
Adrenaline Tartrate, 852·2
Adrenalini Bitartras, 852·2
Adrenalini Tartras, 852·2
Adrenalinii Tartras, 852·2
Adrenalinium Hydrogentartaricum, 852·2
Adrenalona, Hidrocloruro de, 1648·2
Adrenalone, 1648·1
Adrenalone Hydrochloride, 1648·2
Adrenam, 1777·1
Adrenergic Neurone Blockers, 809·1
Adrenochrome Monosemicarbazone, 745·1
Adrenocortical Insufficiency, 1075·3
Adrenocorticotrophic Hormone, 1322·1
Adrenocorticotrophin, 1322·1
Adrenol, 1777·1
Adrenoleucodystrophy, 1707·3
Adrenomyeloneuropathy— *see* Adrenoleucodystrophy, 1707·3
Adrenoplasma, 1777·1
Adrenor, 1777·1

Adrenoxil, 1777·1
Adrenoxyl, 1777·2
Adreson, 1777·2
Adrevil, 1777·2
Adrexan, 1777·2
Adrezon, 1777·2
Adriamycin, 547·3
Adriamycinol, 549·2
Adriblastin, 1777·2
Adriblastina, 1777·2
Adriblastine, 1777·2
Adrigyl, 1777·2
Adrim, 1777·2
Adrimedac, 1777·2
Adrinex, 1777·2
Adrocil, 1777·2
Adro-derm, 1777·2
Adronat, 1777·2
Adroxef, 1777·2
Adroyd, 1777·2
Adrucil, 1777·2
Adrusen, 1777·2
Ad-Sorb, 1777·2
Adsorbed Diphtheria Prophylactic, 1612·3
Adsorbed Diphtheria-Tetanus Prophylactic, 1613·1
Adsorbed Diphtheria–Tetanus–Whooping-cough Prophylactic, 1613·3
Adsorbed DT Coq, 1777·2
Adsorbed DT Vax, 1777·2
Adsorbocarpine, 1777·2
Adsorbonac, 1777·2
ADT, 1777·2
AD-Til, 1777·2
Aduar, 1777·2
Aducin, 1777·3
Adulax, 1777·3
Adult Chesty Cough, 1777·3
Adult Chesty Cough Non Drowsy, 1777·3
Adult Citrex, 1777·3
Adult Citrex Cal-Mag-D3, 1777·3
Adult Citrex Multivitamin + Ginseng + Omega 3, 1777·3
Adult Dry Cough, 1777·3
Adult Ideal Quota, 1777·3
Adult Meltus for Chesty Coughs & Catarrh, 1777·3
Adult Respiratory Distress Syndrome— *see* Acute Respiratory Distress Syndrome, 1075·2
AdultPatch, Trans-Ver-Sal— *see* Trans-Ver-Sal AdultPatch, 2341·2
Adumbran, 1777·3
Adurix, 1777·3
Adursal, 1777·3
Advair, 1777·3
Advance, 1777·3
Advanced Antioxidants Formula, 1777·3
Advanced Cardiac Life Support, 812·2
Advanced Formula Di-Gel, 1777·3
Advanced Formula Dristan— *see* Dristan Cold, 1955·1
Advanced Formula Multibionta, 1777·3
Advanced Formula Plax, 1777·3
Advanced Formula Tegrin, 1777·3
Advanced Formula Zenate, 1777·3
Advanced Relief Visine, 1777·3
Advanced-RF Natal Care, 1777·3
Advantage, 1777·3
Advantage 24, 1777·3
Advantan, 1777·3
Advate, 1777·4
Adventan, 1777·4
Advera, 1777·4
Adversuten, 1777·4
Advicor, 1777·4
Advil, 1777·4
Advil Allergy Sinus, 1777·4
Advil Cold, 1777·4
Advil Cold & Flu, 1777·4
Advil Cold & Sinus, 1777·4
Advil CS, 1777·4
Advil Mono, 1777·4
Advisor, 1777·4
AD-vitamin, 1777·4
AD-Vitan, 1777·4
Adynamic Ileus— *see* Decreased Gastrointestinal Motility, 1241·1
Adyston, 1777·4
AE-941, 525·3
Aedolac, 1777·4
Aegrosan, 1777·4
A-E-Mulsin, 1777·4
Aequalyre, 1777·4
Aequamen, 1777·4
Aequifusine, 1777·4
Aequiseral, 1777·4
Aequiton-P, 1777·4
A-E-R, 1777·4
Aer Medicinalis, 1236·3
Aer Medicinalis Artificiosus, 1236·3
Aerflu, 1777·4
Aerius, 1777·4
Aero Helpp Forte, 1778·1
Aero Itan, 1778·1
Aero Plus, 1778·1
Aero Red, 1778·1
Aero Red Antiacido, 1778·1
Aero Red Complex, 1778·1
Aero Red Eupeptico— *see* Aero Red Complex, 1778·1
Aeroaid, 1778·1
AeroBec, 1778·1
AeroBid, 1778·1
Aerobin, 1778·1
Aero-Bud, 1778·1
Aerocaine, 1778·1
Aerocef, 1778·1
Aerocid, 1778·1
Aero-Clenil, 1778·1
Aerocort, 1778·1
Aerocrom, 1778·1
Aeroderm, 1778·1
Aerodesin, 1778·1
Aerodigestive Tract Cancer— *see* Malignant Neoplasms of the Head and Neck, 517·3
Aerodine, 1778·1
Aerodiol, 1778·1
Aerodur, 1778·1
Aerodyne, 1778·1
Aerofagil, 1778·1
Aerofane, Natusor— *see* Natusor Aerofane, 2153·4
Aeroflat, 1778·2
Aeroflux, 1778·2
Aeroflux Edulito, 1778·2
Aerofreeze, 1778·2
Aerogal, 1778·2
Aerogastrol, 1778·2
Aerogel, 1778·2
AeroHist Plus, 1778·2
Aero-Jet, 1778·2
AeroKid, 1778·2
Aerolate, 1778·2
Aerolid, 1778·2
Aerolin, 1778·2
Aerolind, 1778·2
Aeromax, 1778·2
Aeromicrosona C, 1778·2
Aeromuc, 1778·2
Aeronix, 1778·2
Aero-Om, 1778·2
Aeropax, 1778·2
Aeropaxyn, 1778·2
Aero-Ped, 1778·2
Aerophobia— *see* Rabies, 1636·2
Aero-Plus, 1778·2
Aero-Sal, 1778·2
Aeroseb, 1778·2
Aeroseb-Dex, 1778·2
Aerosil, 1778·2
Aerosol Propellants, 1235·1
Aerosol Spitzner N, 1778·3
Aerosolv, 1778·3
Aerosoma, 1778·3
Aerosporin, 1778·3
Aerotamol, 1778·3
Aerotec, 1778·3
Aerotherm, 1778·3
Aerotide, 1778·3
Aerotina, 1778·3
Aerotrat, 1778·3
Aerovac, 1778·3
Aerovac G, 1778·3
Aerovacuna, 1778·3
Aerovent, 1778·3
Aerovial, 1778·3
Aeroxina, 1778·3
Aerozoin, 1778·3
AErrane, 1778·3
*Aeschrion excelsa*, 1737·2
Aescin, 1648·2
Aescorin Forte, 1778·3
Aescorin N, 1778·3
Aescosulf N, 1778·3
Aesculaforce, 1778·3
Aesculaforce N, 1778·3
AesculaMed, 1778·3
Aesculin, 1648·2
Aesculo Gel L, 1778·3
Aesculus, 1648·2
Aesculus Hippocastanum, 1648·2
*Aesculus hippocastanum*, 1648·2
Aesculus Med Complex, 1778·3
Aescusan, 1778·3
Aescuven, 1778·3
Aesim, 1778·3
Aesol, 1778·4
Aesrutal S, 1778·4
Aesrutan, 1778·4
Aet, 1778·4
Aetaphen. Tartrat., 977·3
Aethacridinium Lacticum, 1165·3
Aethaminalum, 713·2
Aethaminalum-Natrium, 713·3
Aethanolum, 1166·1
Aethaphenum Tartaricum, 977·3
Aether, 1474·2
Aether ad Narcosin, 1298·3
Aether Aethylicus, 1474·2
Aether Anaestheticus, 1298·3
Aether pro Narcosi, 1298·3
Aether Purissimus, 1298·3
Aether Solvens, 1474·2
Aetheroleum Chenopodii, 103·3
Aetheroleum Cinnamomi Zeylanici, 1672·2
Aetheroleum Citri, 1706·2
Aetheroleum Foeniculi, 1687·3
Aetheroleum Pelargonii, 1692·2
Aetheroleum Terebinthinae, 1760·1
Aethinyloestradiolum, 1553·2
Aethophyllinum, 785·1
Aethoxazorutin, 1688·2
Aethoxazorutoside, 1688·2
Aethoxybenzamidum, 37·2
Aethoxysclerol, 1778·4
Aethoxysklerol, 1778·4
Aethroma, 1778·4
Aethyldimethylmethanolum, 1471·2
Aethylis Acetas, 1474·3
Aethylis Biscoumacetas, 914·1
Aethylis Oleas, 1685·2
Aethylium Aceticum, 1474·3
Aethylium Chloratum, 1376·2
Aethylmorphinae Hydrochloridum, 37·3
Aethylmorphini Hydrochloridum, 37·3
Aethylum Hydroxybenzoicum, 1183·2
Aethynodiolum Diaceticum, 1554·2
Aetoxisclerol, 1778·4
Aetoxy Sklerol, 1778·4
Aezodent, 1778·4
AF, 1778·4
AF-102, 1488·3
222 AF, 1778·4
AF-438, 1126·1
AF-634, 1735·3
AF-864, 21·1
AF-983, 20·3
AF-1161, 319·1
AF-1890, 565·3
AF-1934, 20·3
AF-2071, 1092·3
AF-2139, 1679·1
AF Anacin, 1778·4
Afalpi Tiptipot, 1778·4
Afazol, 1778·4
Afazol Z, 1778·4
AF-102B, 1488·3
Afebrin, 1778·4
Afebryl, 1778·4
Afecton, 1778·4
Afeditab, 1778·4
Afeksin, 1778·4
Afelimomab, 1648·3
Afeme, 1778·4
Afenil, 1778·4
Afenoxin, 1779·1
Aferadol, 1779·1
Affectine, 1779·1
Affective Disorders, 278·1
Affex, 1779·1
AFI-$B_6$, 1779·1
AFI-B-Total, 1779·1
AFI-C, 1779·1
AFI-$D_2$, 1779·1
Afid Plus, 1779·1
AFI-E, 1779·1
A-Fil, 1779·1
Afilan, 1779·1
Afilite, 1779·1
Afipran, 1779·1
Aflamid, 1779·1
Aflamin, 1779·1
Aflamina, 1779·1
Aflarex, 1779·1
Aflat, 1779·1
Aflatoxinas, 1648·3
Aflatoxins, 1648·3
Aflen, 1779·1
Afloben, 1779·1
Aflocualona, 1386·3
Aflodac, 1779·1
Aflogen, 1779·1
Aflogine, 1779·1
Aflogol, 1779·1
Aflogos, 1779·1
Afloqualone, 1386·3
Afloxan, 1779·1
Afloyan, 1779·1
Aflubin, 1779·1
Aflukin C, 1779·1
Aflumycin, 1779·1
Afluon, 1779·1
Afluta, 1779·1
Afluvit, 1779·2
AFMU, 783·1
Afongan, 1779·2
Afonilum, 1779·2
Afonilum Novo, 1779·2
Afonina, 1779·2
Afonisan, 1779·2
Afopic, 1779·2
Aforinol, 1779·2
Afos, 1779·2
Afpred-1— *see* afpred-DEXA, 1779·2
Afpred-2— *see* afpred-THEO, 1779·2
Afpred-DEXA, 1779·2
Afpred-THEO, 1779·2
Afrazine, 1779·2
African Chillies, 1667·1
African Gold, 1779·2
African Prune, 1568·2
Afrin, 1779·2
Afrin Moisturizing Saline Mist, 1779·2
Afrin Natural, 1779·2
Afrin Saline Mist— *see* Afrin Moisturizing Saline Mist, 1779·2
Afrinex, 1779·2
Afrinex Infantil, 1779·2
Afrodor, 1779·2
Afrolate, 1779·2
Afron, 1779·2
Aftab, 1779·2
Aftach, 1779·2
Af-Taf, 1779·2
Aftagel, 1779·2
Aftajuventus, 1779·2
Aftasone, 1779·3
Aftasone B C, 1779·3
Aftate, 1779·3
After Bite, 1779·3
After Burn, 1779·3
After Sun, 1779·3

Afterburn, 1779·3
Afterburner, 1593·3
After-Work, 1779·3
Aftir Gel, 1779·3
Aftir Shampoo, 1779·3
Aftosium, 1779·3
Aftsinun, 1779·3
Aftsinun Veshiul, 1779·3
Afungil, 1779·3
AG-3, 880·2
AG-337, 576·3
AG-1343, 650·1
AG-1749, 1269·3
AG-58107, 1066·3
Agaffin, 1779·3
Agallas de Roble, 1690·2
Agalsidasa β, 1651·1
Agalsidase Alfa, 1651·1
Agalsidase Beta, 1651·1
Agamadon, 1779·3
Agamadon N, 1779·3
Agammaglobulinaemia— *see* Primary Antibody Deficiency, 1629·2
Agapurin, 1779·3
Agar, 1576·3
Agar-agar, 1576·3
Agaric, Deadly, 1717·3
Agaric, Fly, 1717·3
Agaricus Muscarius, 1717·3
Agarol, 1779·3
Agarol CM, 1779·3
Agarol Extra, 1779·3
Agarol Fibras Naturales, 1779·3
Agarol N, 1779·3
Agarol Plain, 1779·4
Agarol with Sennosides, 1779·4
Agarol Soft, 1779·4
Agaroletten, 1779·4
Agasten, 1779·4
Agastrin, 1779·4
Agathol, 1779·4
*Agathosma betulina*, 1663·1
*Agathosma crenulata*, 1663·1
AGB, 1779·4
Age Block, 1779·4
Agedin Plus, 1779·4
AG-EE-6232W, 344·3
AG-EE-623-ZW, 344·3
A-Gel, 1779·4
Agelan, 1779·4
Agelmin, 1779·4
A-gen 53, 1779·4
Agenerase, 1779·4
Agent Orange, 1510·3, 1681·1
Agermin, 1779·4
Ageroplas, 1779·4
Agerpen, 1779·4
Agerpen Mucolitico, 1779·4
Ageusia— *see* Taste Disorders, 682·2
Agevit, 1779·4
Agglad Ofteno, 1779·4
Aggrastat, 1779·4
Aggrastet, 1780·1
Aggrenox, 1780·1
Aggressive Behaviour— *see* Disturbed Behaviour, 665·1
Aggripal S1, 1780·1
Agilan, 1780·1
Agilex, 1780·1
Agilisin, 1780·1
Agilo, 1780·1
Agilona, 1780·1
Aginax, 1780·1
Agiobulk, 1780·1
Agiocur, 1780·1
Agiofibe, 1780·1
Agiofibra, 1780·1
Agiolax, 1780·1
Agiolax— *see* Manevac, 2113·4
Agiolax Ballast, 1780·1
Agiolax Mite, 1780·1
Agiolax Pico, 1780·1
Agiolind, 1780·1
Agiopic, 1780·1
AgioPico Plus, 1780·1
Agioten, 1780·1
Agipiu, 1780·1
Agiserc, 1780·1
Agisolvan, 1780·1
Agispor, 1780·1
Agispor Onychoset, 1780·1
Agisten, 1780·1
Agisten, Baby— *see* Baby Agisten, 1824·2
Agit, 1780·1
Agit Plus, 1780·2
Agitation— *see* Disturbed Behaviour, 665·1
*Agkistrodon rhodostoma*, 863·2
Aglio, 1691·1, 1780·2
Aglucide, 1780·2
Aglucil, 1780·2
Aglutella, 1780·2
AGN-190168, 1160·2
AGN-192013, 526·2
AGN-192024, 1514·1
Agnesin, 1780·2
AGN-190342-LF, 876·3
Agnocasto, 1649·1
Agnofem, 1780·2
Agnolyt, 1780·2
Agno-Sabona, 1780·2
Agnucaston, 1780·2
Agnuchol, 1780·2
Agnufemil, 1780·2
Agnukliman, 1780·2
Agnumens, 1780·2
Agnurell, 1780·2
Agnus Castus, 1649·1, 1780·2
Agnuside, 1649·1
Agofell, 1780·2
Agofenac, 1780·2
Agon, 1780·2
Agoprim, 1780·2
Agopton, 1780·2
Agoral, 1780·2
Agoraphobia— *see* Phobic Disorders, 663·3
Agorex, 1780·2
Agorhino, 1780·2
Agpisen, 1780·2
A/G-Pro, 1780·2
Agradil, 1780·2
A-Gram, 1780·2
Agranulocytosis, 740·2
Agrastat, 1780·2
Agreal, 1780·3
Agre-Gola, 1780·3
Agremol, 1780·3
Agrenox, 1780·3
Agrimel, 1780·3
Agrimonas N, 1780·3
Agrimonia, 1649·1
*Agrimonia eupatoria*, 1649·1
*Agrimonia odorata*, 1649·1
*Agrimonia procera*, 1649·1
Agrimoniae Herba, 1649·1
Agrimony, 1649·1
Agripalma, 1717·1
Agrippal, 1780·3
Agropyron, 1676·2
*Agropyron repens*, 1676·2
Agrumina, 1780·3
Agruvit, 1780·3
Agrylin, 1780·3
Agua, 1764·3
Agua del Carmen, 1780·3
Agua Inglesa, 1780·3
Agua Melisa Carminativa, 1780·3
Agua para Inyecciones, 1765·1
Agua Purificada, 1764·3
Agua Sulfatada Picrica, 1780·3
Aguala, 1780·3
Agudil, 1780·3
Agufam, 1780·3
Agurin, 1780·3
Agyr, 1780·3
Agyrax, 1780·3
AH-2250, 1371·1
AH-3232, 685·1
AH-3365, 791·3
AH-19065, 1285·2
AH 3 N, 1780·3
AHA, 1645·3
AH-5158A, 943·3
AHA Skin Lightening Gel, 1780·3
AHB-DBK, 158·3
AHButBP, 765·3
AH-chew, 1780·4
AH-chew D, 1780·4
AHD 2000, 1780·4
AHDP, 773·2
Ahecan, 1780·4
AHF, 735·3, 751·1, 1780·4
AHHexBP, 773·2
Ahiston, 1780·4
Ahiston Compound, 1780·4
AHP 200, 1780·4
AHP,BP, 774·2
17-AHPC, 1556·3
AHR-233, 1395·1
AHR-438, 1395·1
AHR-504, 482·3
AHR-619, 1587·2
AHR-3002, 1588·2
AHR-3018, 20·1
AHR-3053, 1116·2
AHR-3070-C, 1274·3
AHR-3096, 615·2
AHR-3219, 698·1
AHR-3260B, 1284·2
AHR-4698, 942·1
AHR-10282, 21·3
AHR-10282B, 21·3
A-Hydrocort, 1780·4
AIC, 544·3
AICA Orotate, 1724·2
AICA Riboside, 842·2
Aicamin, 1780·4
Aid III MSUD, 1780·4
Aida, 1780·4
Aidar, 1780·4
Aid-Lax, 1780·4
Aidol, 1780·4
AIDS— *see* HIV Infection and AIDS, 621·3
AIDS Dementia Complex— *see* HIV-associated Neurological Complications, 623·2
AIDS Immunoglobulins, 1607·3
AIDS Vaccines, 1607·3
AIDS-associated Diarrhoea— *see* HIV-associated Wasting and Diarrhoea, 623·2
AIDS-associated Malignancies— *see* HIV-associated Malignancies, 623·1
AIDS-associated Wasting— *see* HIV-associated Wasting and Diarrhoea, 623·2
AIDS-related Complex— *see* HIV Infection and AIDS, 621·3
AIDS-related Infections— *see* HIV-associated Infections, 623·1
AIDS-related Lymphomas, 510·3
Aigin, 1780·4
Aiglonyl, 1780·4
Aigremoine, 1649·1
Ail, 1691·1
Ailax, 1780·4
Aima-Calcin, 1780·4
Aimafix, 1780·4
Ainedif, 1780·4
Ainex, 1780·4
Ainscrid, 1780·4
Air Citronella, 1780·4
Air, Medical, 1236·3
Air, Medicinal, 1236·3
Air Salonpas, 1780·4
Air Sickness— *see* Nausea and Vomiting, 1245·2
Air, Synthetic, 1236·3
Air, Synthetic Medicinal, 1236·3
Airbeclosona, 1780·4
Airbronal, 1780·4
Aircort, 1780·4
Airest, 1780·4
Airol, 1781·1
Airomet, 1781·1
Airomir, 1781·1
Airsalbu, 1781·1
Air-Tal, 1781·1
Airtal, 1781·1
Airtal Difucrem, 1781·1
Airum, 1781·1
Airvitess, 1781·1
Air-X, 1781·1
Ait Makhlif, 1666·1
Ajaka, 1781·1
Ajan, 1781·1
Ajenjo, 1645·1
(17*R*,21*R*)-Ajmalan-17,21-diol, 856·1
Ajmalicine, 994·3
Ajmalina, 856·1
Ajmaline, 856·1, 994·3
Ajmaline Hydrochloride, 856·2
Ajmaline Phenobarbital, 856·2
Ajmalinine, 994·3
Ajmalinum, 856·1
Ajo, 1691·1
Ajoene, 1691·2
Ajolip, 1781·1
Ajomast, 1781·1
Ajomast Circulatorio, 1781·1
Ajuta, 1781·1
Akabar, 1781·1
Akacin, 1781·1
Akaderm N, 1781·1
Akamin, 1781·1
Akamon, 1781·1
Akarin, 1781·1
Akarpine, 1781·1
Akathisia— *see* Extrapyramidal Disorders, 677·1
Akatinol, 1781·1
Akatinol— *see* Axura, 1822·4
Ak-Beta, 1781·1
Ak-Chlor, 1781·1
Ak-Cide, 1781·1
Ak-Con, 1781·2
Ak-Dex, 1781·2
Ak-Dilate, 1781·2
AKE, 1781·2
Akee, 1700·2
Akeral, 1781·2
Akerat, 1781·2
Aker-tuba, 1510·1
Akevir, 1781·2
Akezol, 1781·2
Akfen, 1781·2
Ak-Fluor, 1781·2
Akhauma, 1781·2
Akicin, 1781·2
Akila Mains Et Peau, 1781·2
Akila Spray, 1781·2
Akildia, 1781·2
Akileine, 1781·2
Akilen, 1781·2
Akindex, 1781·2
Akindol, 1781·2
Akineton, 1781·2
Akinspray, 1781·2
Akipic, 1781·2
Akirol, 1781·2
Akistin, 1781·2
Akker-Siroop— *see* Abdijsiroop (Akker-Siroop), 1768·1
Aklonin, 1781·2
Ak-NaCl, 1781·2
Akne, 1781·3
Akne Cordes, 1781·3
Aknecin, 1781·3
Aknederm Ery, 1781·3
Aknederm N, 1781·3
Aknederm Neu, 1781·3
Aknederm Oxid, 1781·3
Ak-Nefrin, 1781·3
Aknefug Simplex, 1781·3
Aknefug-EL, 1781·3
Aknefug-Emulsion, 1781·3
Aknefug-liquid, 1781·3
Aknefug-oxid, 1781·3
Aknemago, 1781·3
Aknemin, 1781·3
Akne-Mycin, 1781·3
Aknemycin, 1781·3
Aknemycin Compositum, 1781·3
Aknemycin Plus, 1781·3
Ak-Neo-Dex, 1781·3
Akne-Puren, 1781·3

Aknereduct, 1781·3
Akneroxid, 1781·3
Aknex, 1781·3
Aknicare, 1781·3
Aknichthol, 1781·3
Aknichthol Creme, 1781·3
Aknichthol N, 1781·3
Aknilox, 1781·4
Aknin, 1781·4
Aknin-Mino, 1781·4
Aknin-N, 1781·4
Aknoral, 1781·4
Aknosan, 1781·4
Akorazol, 1781·4
Ak-Pentolate, 1781·4
Ak-Poly-Bac, 1781·4
Ak-Pred, 1781·4
AkPro, 1781·4
Akratol, 1781·4
Akrinor, 1781·4
Ak-Rinse, 1781·4
Ak-Rose, 1781·4
Akrotherm, 1781·4
Ak-Spore, 1781·4
Ak-Spore HC, 1781·4
Ak-Sulf, 1781·4
Akt-3, 1781·4
Akt-4, 1781·4
Ak-Taine, 1781·4
Aktiferrin, 1781·4
Aktiferrin Compositum, 1781·4
Aktiferrin N, 1781·4
Aktiferrin-F, 1781·4
Aktiosan, 1781·4
Aktipar, 1782·1
Aktiv Blasen- und Nierentee, 1782·1
Aktiv Husten- und Bronchialtee, 1782·1
Aktiv Leber- und Gallentee, 1782·1
Aktiv Milder Magen- und Darmtee, 1782·1
Aktiv Nerven- und Schlaftee, 1782·1
Aktivakid, 1782·1
Aktivanad, 1782·1
Aktivanad-N, 1782·1
Aktivin, 1782·1
Aktiv-Puder, 1782·1
AkTob, 1782·1
Akton, 1782·1
Ak-Tracin, 1782·1
Aktren, 1782·1
Ak-Trol, 1782·1
Akudol, 1782·1
Ak-Vernacon, 1782·1
Akwa Tears, 1782·1
AKZ, 1782·1
AL-20, 429·2
Al 110, 1782·1
AL-281, 1384·2
AL-02145, 864·1
AL-4862, 877·1
AL-6221, 1521·1
Ala, 1421·1
ALA, 527·2
5-ALA, 527·2
AL-1577A, 946·1
AL-3432A, 433·2
Alacepril, 856·2
Alacetan, 1782·2
Alacol DM, 1782·2
Alacor, 1782·2
Ala-Cort, 1782·2
Alacramyn, 1782·2
Alacta-NF, 1782·2
Ala-Gln, 1433·2
Alaidol, 1782·2
Alamag, 1782·2
Alamag Plus, 1782·2
Alamast, 1782·2
Alamil, 1782·2
Alamin, 1782·2
Álamo, Brotes de, 1733·3
Alanase, 1782·2
Alandiem, 1782·2
Alanina, 1421·1
Alanine, 1421·1
L-Alanine, 1421·1
Alaninum, 1421·1
Alant, 1119·3
Alant Camphor, 1119·3
Alant Starch, 1702·1
Alantoína, 1141·3
Alantolactone, 1119·3
Alantomicina Complex, 1782·2
*N*(2)-L-Alanyl-L-glutamine, 1421·1, 1433·2
D-Ala-peptide-T-amide, 651·3
Alapren, 1782·2
Alapril, 1782·2
Alapryl, 1782·2
Alasenn, 1782·2
Alastik, 1782·2
Alasulf, 1782·2
Alatrofloxacin Mesilate, 154·1
Alatrofloxacin Mesylate, 154·1
Alatrofloxacino, Mesilato de, 154·1
Alaun, 1652·1
Alavac-S, 1782·2
Alavert, 1782·2
Alavert Allergy & Sinus D, 1782·2
Alaxa, 1782·2
Alaxan, 1782·2
Alaxan PI, 1782·2
Alba, 1782·2
Alba-3, 1782·3
Albalon, 1782·3
Albalon Relief, 1782·3
Albalon-A, 1782·3
Albamycin, 1782·3
Albasol, 1782·3
Albasol A, 1782·3
Albassol, 1782·3
Albatel, 1782·3
Albay, 1782·3
Albay— *see* Albey, 1782·3
Albego, 1782·3
Alben, 1782·3
Albenda, 1782·3
Albendazol, 101·2
Albendazole, 101·2
Albendazole Sulfoxide, 101·3
Albendazolum, 101·2
Albendrox, 1782·3
Albendy, 1782·3
Albensil, 1782·3
Albentel, 1782·3
Albenza, 1782·3
Albenzonil, 1782·3
Albeoler, 1782·3
Alber T, 1782·3
Albert Tiafen, 1782·3
Albesine Biotic, 1782·3
Albetol, 1782·3
Albey, 1782·3
Albezole, 1782·3
Albicansan, 1782·3
Albicar, 1782·4
Albicon, 1782·4
Albicort, 1782·4
Albicort Compositum, 1782·4
Albicort Oticum, 1782·4
Albinism— *see* Pigmentation Disorders, 1137·2
Albintil, 1782·4
Albios, 1782·4
Albiotic, 1782·4
Albistat, 1782·4
Albistin, 1782·4
Albital, 1782·4
Albocresil, 1782·4
Alboral, 1782·4
Albothyl, 1782·4
Alboz, 1782·4
Albraton, 1782·4
Albucid, 1782·4
Albulin, 1782·4
Albumaid Preparations, 1782·4
Albuman, 1782·4
Albumar, 1782·4
Albumarc, 1782·4
Albumax, 1782·4
Albumex, 1782·4
Albumin, 740·3
Albumin Human, 740·3
Albumin, Human, 740·3
Albumin, Iodinated ($^{125}$I) Human, 1524·2
Albumin, Iodinated ($^{131}$I) Human, 1524·3
Albumin Solution, Human, 740·3
Albumin Tannate, 1248·1
Albumin, Technetium ($^{99m}$Tc), 1525·3
Albúmina, 740·3
Albúmina, Tanato de, 1248·1
Albuminar, 1782·4
Albumini Humani Solutio, 740·3
Albumosesilber, 1746·2
Albumyn, 1782·4
Albunex, 1782·4
Alburone, 1783·1
Albusol, 1783·1
Albustix, 1783·1
Albutamol, 1783·1
Albutannin, 1248·1
Albutein, 1783·1
Albuterol, 791·3
Albuterol Sulfate, 791·3
Albyl, 1783·1
Albyl Minor, 1783·1
Albyl-E, 1783·1
Albym-Test, 1783·1
ALCA, 1141·2
Alca-C, 1783·1
Alcacat, 1783·1
Alcachofa, 1678·3
Alcachôfra, 1678·3
Alcaçuz, 1270·2
Alcacyl, 1783·1
Alcacyl Instant, 1783·1
Alcafelol, 1783·1
Alcaine, 1783·1
Alcalinos Gelos, 1783·1
Alcalinos Vita, 1783·1
Alcalone Plus, 1783·1
Alcalosio, 1783·1
Alca-Luftal, 1783·1
Alcamag, 1783·1
Alcamex, 1783·1
Alcan, 1783·1
Alcanfor, 1665·3
Alcaphor, 1783·1
Alcaravea, 1667·2
Alcaravea, Aceite Esencial de, 1667·3
Alcaravia, 1667·2
Alcare, 1783·1
Alcasedine, 1783·1
Alcasol, 1783·2
Alcaten, 1783·2
Alcatex, 1783·2
Alcatira, Goma, 1582·2
Alcatrão Mineral, 1159·2
Alcelam, 1783·2
*Alchemilla arvensis*, 1729·1
Alchera, 1783·2
Alcinal, 1783·2
Alcinal New, 1783·2
Alcinal Plus, 1783·2
Alcinonide, 1103·2
Alcis, 1783·2
Alciton, 1783·2
Alclometasona, Dipropionato de, 1090·3
Alclometasone Dipropionate, 1090·3
Alcloxa, 1141·2
Alcobon, 1783·2
Alcobon— *see* Ancotil, 1799·3
Alcoderm, 1783·2
Alcodin, 1783·2
Alcohcan, 1783·2
Alcohocel, 1783·2
Alcohol, 1166·1
Alcohol, Absolute, 1166·1
Alcohol Bencílico, 1170·2
Alcohol Benzalconio, 1783·2
Alcohol, Benzyl, 1170·2
Alcohol Benzylicus, 1170·2
Alcohol Butílico, 1472·1
Alcohol Cetil, 1783·2
Alcohol Cetílico, 1480·3
Alcohol Cetilpi Cuve, 1783·2
Alcohol Cetoestearílico, 1480·2
Alcohol Cetylicus, 1480·3
Alcohol Cetylicus et Stearylicus, 1480·2
Alcohol Cetylicus et Stearylicus Emulsificans A, 1480·2
Alcohol Cetylicus et Stearylicus Emulsificans B, 1480·3
Alcohol CL Benz, 1783·2
Alcohol, Dehydrated, 1166·1
Alcohol, Denatured, 1185·3
Alcohol Diclorobencílico, 1178·3
Alcohol Estearílico, 1482·3
Alcohol, Ethyl, 1166·1
Alcohol Feniletílico, 1188·1
Alcohol Isobutílico, 1475·1
Alcohol Isopropílico, 1184·3
Alcohol, Isopropyl, 1184·3
Alcohol Isopropylicus, 1184·3
Alcohol, Methyl, 1475·2
Alcohol Miristilo, 1718·3
Alcohol Nicotinílico, Tartrato de, 966·2
Alcohol Oleico, 1481·3
Alcohol Oleicus, 1481·3
Alcohol (96 Per Cent), 1166·1
Alcohol Polivinílico, 1581·1
Alcohol Poten, 1783·2
Alcohol Potenciado, 1783·2
Alcohol Propílico, 1191·2
Alcohol Reforzado, 1783·2
Alcohol Sanit Cuve, 1783·2
Alcohol, Secondary Propyl, 1184·3
Alcohol Stearylicus, 1482·3
Alcohol Trichlorisobutylicus, 1176·3
Alcohol Withdrawal Syndrome— *see* Alcohol Withdrawal and Abstinence, 1166·2
Alcoholes Adipis Lanae, 1482·3
Alcoholes de Lana, 1482·3
Alcoholes Desnaturalizados, 1185·3
Alcoholia Lanae, 1482·3
Alcoholism— *see* Alcohol Withdrawal and Abstinence, 1166·2
Alcohols, Lanolin, 1482·3
Alcohols, Sulfated Fatty, 1574·1
Alcohols, Wool, 1482·3
Alcohols, Wool Wax, 1482·3
Alcohten, 1783·2
Alcojel, 1783·2
Alcolanum, 1482·3
Alcolex, 1783·2
Alcomicin, 1783·2
Alcon Adequad, 1783·2
Alcon AE, 1783·3
Alcon Eye Gel, 1783·3
Alcon Lagrimas, 1783·3
Alcontar, 1783·3
Alcool, 1166·1
Alcool Benzylique, 1170·2
Álcool Cetílico, 1480·3
Alcool Cetostearilico, 1480·2
Alcool Stéarylique, 1482·3
Alcopac Reforzado, 1783·3
Alcophyllex, 1783·3
Alcophyllin, 1783·3
Alcos-Anal, 1783·3
Alco-Screen, 1783·3
Alcover, 1783·3
Alcowipe, 1783·3
Alcoxidine, 1783·3
Alcur, 1783·3
Alcuronii Chloridum, 1398·3
Alcuronio, Cloruro de, 1398·3
Alcuronium Chloride, 1398·3
Alcusal, 1783·3
ALDA, 1141·2
Alda, 1783·3
Aldactacine, 1783·3
Aldactazide, 1783·3
Aldactazine, 1783·3
Aldactide, 1783·3
Aldactone, 1783·3
Aldactone Saltucin, 1783·3
Aldadiene Potassium, 984·2
Aldalix, 1783·3
Aldar, 1783·3
Aldara, 1783·3
Aldarone, 1783·4
Aldazida, 1783·4
Aldazide, 1783·4

Aldazine, 1783·4
Aldecin, 1783·4
Aldecina, 1783·4
Alder Buckthorn Bark, 1266·3
Aldesleukin, 562·3
Aldesleukina, 562·3
Aldic, 1783·4
Al-Dim, 1783·4
Aldioxa, 1141·2
Aldipin, 1783·4
Aldira, 1783·4
Aldo Asma, 1783·4
Aldo Otico, 1783·4
Aldoacne, 1783·4
Aldobronquial, 1783·4
Aldoclor, 1783·4
Aldocumar, 1783·4
Aldoderma, 1783·4
Aldoleo, 1783·4
Aldolor, 1783·4
Aldomet, 1783·4
Aldometil, 1783·4
Aldomin, 1783·4
Aldonar, 1783·4
Aldophosphamide, 541·3
Aldopren, 1783·4
Aldopur, 1784·1
Aldoretic, 1784·1
Aldoril, 1784·1
Aldoron, 1784·1
Aldo-Silverderma, 1784·1
Aldosomnil, 1784·1
Aldospirone, 1784·1
Aldospray Analgesico, 1784·1
Aldosterona, 1091·1
Aldosterone, 1091·1
Aldosterone Sodium Succinate, 1091·1
Aldotensin, 1784·1
Aldozone, 1784·1
Aldrox, 1784·1
Aldurazyme, 1784·1
Alec, 1784·1
Alecrim, Essência de, 1740·2
Aledin, 1784·1
Aledron, 1784·1
Aleevex, 1784·1
Alefacept, 1141·2
Alefexole Hydrochloride, 1215·3
Alegysal, 1784·1
Alembicol D, 1784·1
Alemelano, 1784·1
Alemtuzumab, 526·1
Al-En, 1784·1
Alenato, 1784·1
Alenbit, 1784·1
Alencast, 1784·1
Alendil, 1784·1
Alendronate Sodium, 765·3
Alendronato Sódico, 765·3
Alendronic Acid, 765·3
Alendrónico, Ácido, 765·3
Alendros, 1784·1
Alenic Alka, 1784·1
Alenic Alka, Extra Strength— *see* Extra Strength Alenic Alka, 1986·2
Alenstran, 1784·1
Alental, 1784·1
Alenzantyl, 1784·2
Aleot, 1784·2
Alepa, 1784·2
Alepam, 1784·2
Aleppo Galls, 1690·2
Aleprozil, 1784·2
Alepsal, 1784·2
Alepsal Compuesto, 1784·2
Alercortil, 1784·2
Alercrom, 1784·2
Alerdil, 1784·2
Aler-Dryl, 1784·2
Alerfedine, 1784·2
Alerfedine D, 1784·2
Alerfrin, 1784·2
Alerfur, 1784·2
Alerg, 1784·2
Alergaliv, 1784·2
Alergan, 1784·2
Alergenos, 1650·1
Alergi, 1784·2
Alergibon, 1784·2
Alergical, 1784·2
Alergical Expect, 1784·2
Alergiderm, 1784·2
Alergidryl, 1784·2
Alergiftalmina, 1784·2
Alergin, 1784·2
Alergist, 1784·2
Alergitanil, 1784·3
Alergitrat, 1784·3
Alergo Filinal, 1784·3
Alergo Glucalbet, 1784·3
Alergocrom, 1784·3
Alergoftal, 1784·3
Alergogel, 1784·3
Alergoliber, 1784·3
Alergolon, 1784·3
Alergomed, 1784·3
Alergoral, 1784·3
Alergosan, 1784·3
Alergotox, 1784·3
Alergotox Efedrina, 1784·3
Alergotox Expectorante, 1784·3
Alergotox Nasal, 1784·3
Alergotox Pastilhas, 1784·3
Alergovalle, 1784·3
Alergyo, 1784·3
Alerid, 1784·3
Alerjon, 1784·3
Alerken, 1784·3
Alerlisin, 1784·3
Alermine, 1784·3
Alermizol, 1784·3
Alernex, 1784·3
Alerpriv, 1784·3
Alerpriv D, 1784·3
Aler-Releaf, 1784·4
Alersan, 1784·4
Alertal, 1784·4
Alertec, 1784·4
Alertonic, 1784·4
Alertop, 1784·4
Alertrin, 1784·4
Alerzona, 1784·4
Alesion, 1784·4
Alesse, 1784·4
Aletir, 1784·4
Aletris Oligoplex, 1784·4
Aleucin, 1784·4
Aleudrina, 1784·4
Aleve, 1784·4
Alex, 1784·4
Alex Cough, 1784·4
Alex Paediatric, 1784·4
Alexan, 1784·4
Alexandria Senna, 1288·2
Alexandrian Senna, 1288·2
Alexandrian Senna Fruit, 1288·2
Alexia, 1784·4
Alexia D, 1784·4
Alexin, 1784·4
Alexitol Sódico, 1248·1
Alexitol Sodium, 1248·1
Alex-P, 1785·1
Aleztem, 1785·1
Alfa, 1785·1
Alfa Acid, 1785·1
Alfa C, 1785·1
Alfa Calcimax, 1785·1
Alfa D, 1785·1
Alfa Kappa, 1785·1
Alfabase, 1785·1
Alfabase 8, 1785·1
Alfabetal, 1785·1
Alfabios, 1785·1
Alfacaina, 1785·1
Alfacalcidol, 1461·2
Alfacalcidolum, 1461·2
Alfacid, 1785·1
Alfacort, 1785·1
Alfacortone, 1785·1
AlfaD, 1785·1
Alfad, 1785·1
Alfadelta, 1785·1
Alfadex, 1678·2
Alfadexum, 1678·2
Alfadil, 1785·1
Alfadolona, Acetato de, 1296·3
Alfadolone Acetate, 1296·3
Alfadoxin, 1785·1
Alfaferone, 1785·1
Alfaflor, 1785·1
Alfa-Fluorone, 1785·1
Alfagamma, 1785·1
Alfagen, 1785·1
Alfaken, 1785·1
Alfakinasi, 1785·2
Alfalfa, 1649·1
Alfalfa Sativa Compuesta, 1785·2
Alfalfa Tonic, 1785·2
Alfamox, 1785·2
Alfan, 1785·2
Alfanative, Interferon— *see* Multiferon, 2144·3
Alfaprostol, 1512·3
Alfapsin, 1785·2
Alfare, 1785·2
Alfarol, 1785·2
Alfasidasa β, 1651·1
Alfasin, 1785·2
Alfason, 1785·2
Alfast, 1785·2
Alfater, 1785·2
Alfatil, 1785·2
Alfavit, 1785·2
Alfavitil, 1785·2
Alfaxalona, 1296·3
Alfaxalone, 1296·3
Alfazema, Essência de, 1705·2
Alfazina, 1785·2
Alfazol, 1785·2
Alfener, 1785·2
Alfenta, 1785·2
Alfentanil Hydrochloride, 12·2
Alfentanili Hydrochloridum, 12·2
Alfentanilo, Hidrocloruro de, 12·2
Alferm, 1785·2
Alferon, 1785·2
Alferon N, 1785·2
Alferos, 1785·2
Alfetim, 1785·2
Alficetin, 1785·2
Alfin, 1785·2
Alfitar, 1785·2
Al-Flor, 1785·2
Alfoscerato de Colina, 1488·3
Alfospas, 1785·2
Alfuca, 1785·2
Alfuzosin Hydrochloride, 856·2
Alfuzosina, Hidrocloruro de, 856·2
Alfuzosini Hydrochloridum, 856·2
ALG, 1348·3
Algafan, 1785·3
Alganex, 1785·3
Algedol, 1785·3
Algedrox, 1785·3
Algefit, 1785·3
Algeldrate, 1249·2
Algenac, 1785·3
Algesal, 1785·3
Algesal Forte, 1785·3
Algesal Suractive, 1785·3
Algesalona, 1785·3
Algesalona E, 1785·3
Algestona, Acetofenido de, 1541·3
Algestone Acetophenide, 1541·3
Algexin, 1785·3
Algho, 1785·3
Algi, 1785·3
Algiasdin, 1785·3
Algi-Butazolon, 1785·3
Algice, 1785·3
Algicon, 1785·3
Algicote, 1785·4
Algi-Danilon, 1785·4
Algidente, 1785·4
Algiderm, 1785·4
Algiderma, 1785·4
Algidol, 1785·4
Algidrin, 1785·4
Algifemin, 1785·4
Algifen, 1785·4
Algifene, 1785·4
Algiflamanil, 1785·4
Algiflex, 1785·4
Algifor, 1785·4
Algi-Itamanil, 1785·4
Algik, 1785·4
Algikey, 1785·4
Algimate, 1785·4
Algimesil, 1785·4
Algin, 1577·1
Alginates, 1577·1
Alginato Cálcico, 745·1
Alginato de Propilenglicol, 1576·3
Alginato Sódico, 1577·1
Alginex, 1785·4
Alginflan, 1785·4
Alginic Acid, 1576·3
Alginor, 1785·4
Algin-Vek, 1786·1
Algio Nervomax, 1786·1
Algio Nervomax Fuerte, 1786·1
Algio-Bladuril, 1786·1
Algion, 1786·1
Algiopiret, 1786·1
Algioprofen, 1786·1
Algioprux, 1786·1
Algiospray, 1786·1
Algio-Truxa, 1786·1
Algioxib, 1786·1
Algipan, 1786·1
Algi-Ped, 1786·1
Algi-Peralgin, 1786·1
Algiprofen, 1786·1
Algi-Reumac, 1786·1
Algi-Reumatril, 1786·1
Algirona, 1786·1
Algisan, 1786·1
Algiseda, 1786·1
Algisedal, 1786·1
Algiseptico, 1786·1
Algispray, 1786·1
Algist, 1786·1
Algi-Tanderil, 1786·2
Algitec, 1786·2
Algitrin, 1786·2
Algizolin, 1786·2
Alglucerasa, 1649·1
Alglucerase, 1649·1
Algobene, 1786·2
Algoceanic, 1786·2
Algoced, 1786·2
Algocetil, 1786·2
Algocor, 1786·2
Algodão-Polvora , 1156·2
Algodoeiro, Oléo de, 1676·1
Algodon, Aceite de, 1676·1
Algodystrophy— *see* Complex Regional Pain Syndrome, 5·3
Algofen, 1786·2
Algofina, 1786·2
Algoflex Same, 1786·2
Algofren, 1786·2
Algogen, 1786·2
Algolider, 1786·2
Algolisina, 1786·2
Algolysin, 1786·2
Algonapril, 1786·2
Algo-Nevriton, 1786·2
Algophene, 1786·2
Algopirina, 1786·2
Algoplaque, 1786·2
Algopriv, 1786·2
Algo-Prolixan, 1786·2
Algosenac, 1786·2
Algosfar, 1786·2
Algostase, 1786·2
Algosteril, 1786·2
Algotropyl, 1786·3
Algoxam, 1786·3
Alho Rogoff, 1786·3
Alho-Arthrosan N, 1786·3
Alho-Sedosan, 1786·3
Alhucema, Aceite Esencial de, 1749·2
Alhucema, Esencia de, 1705·2

Alhydrate, 1786·3
Alhydrox, 1786·3
Ali Veg, 1786·3
Aliageusia— *see* Taste Disorders, 682·2
Aliamba, 1666·1
Alib, 1786·3
Alibendol, 1649·3
A-Lices, 1786·3
Alicura, 1786·3
Alidase, 1786·3
Alidol, 1786·3
Alidor, 1786·3
Aliflus, 1786·3
Aligest, 1786·3
Aligest Plus, 1786·3
Alikal, 1786·3
Alilestrenol, 1541·3
Alimemazina, Tartrato de, 423·3
Alimemazine Tartrate, 423·3
Alimentum, 1786·3
Alimix, 1786·3
Alimta, 1786·3
Alin, 1786·3
Alin Nasal, 1786·3
Alin Oftalmico, 1786·3
Alinamin B12, 1786·3
Alinamin-F, 1786·4
Alindapril Hydrochloride, 892·2
Alindrin, 1786·4
Alinia, 1786·4
Alinol, 1786·4
Alinor, 1786·4
Alinvit, 1786·4
Alipase, 1786·4
Alipride, 1786·4
Aliseum, 1786·4
Alisobumalum, 673·3
Alitest, 1786·4
Alitraq, 1786·4
Alitretinoin, 526·2
Alitretinoína, 526·2
Aliucillin, 1786·4
Aliudox, 1786·4
Aliviador, 1786·4
Alivian, 1786·4
Alivioderm, 1786·4
Aliviomas, 1786·4
Aliviosin, 1786·4
Alizaprida, Hidrocloruro de, 1248·1
Alizapride Hydrochloride, 1248·1
ALK, 1786·4
Alka, 1786·4
Alka XS Go, 1786·4
Alkafizz, 1786·4
Alkagin, 1786·4
Alkala N, 1787·1
Alkala T, 1787·1
Alkali-metal Soaps, 1574·1
Alkaline Glutaral, 1181·1
Alkalinising Agents, 1223·1
Alkalite D, 1787·1
Alkaloid F, 994·3
Alkaloidosum Opii Hydrochloridum, 74·3
Alkalosis, Metabolic— *see* Metabolic Alkalosis, 1217·3
Alkamine, 1787·1
Alka-Mints, 1787·1
Alkanil, 1787·1
Alka-Seltzer Preparations, 1787·1
Alka-Seltzer Effervescent Tablets, Extra Strength— *see* Extra Strength Alka-Seltzer Effervescent Tablets, 1986·2
Alka-Seltzer Effervescent Tablets, Original— *see* Original Alka-Seltzer Effervescent Tablets, 2192·3
Alka-Seltzer, Gold— *see* Gold Alka-Seltzer, 2029·3
Alkasid, 1787·2
Alkasol, 1787·2
Alkasol-P, 1787·2
Alkasolve, 1787·2
Alkavite, 1787·2
Alkekengi, 1731·3
Alkenide, 1787·2
Alkeran, 1787·2
Alkerana, 1787·2
Alket, 1787·2
Alkets, 1787·2
Alko Isol, 1787·2
Alkocean, 1787·2
Alkyl Aryl Sulfonates, 1574·1
Alkyl Benzoate, 1480·1
Alkyl (C12-15) Benzoate, 1480·1
Alkyl Carboxylates, 1574·1
Alkyl Ether Sulfates, 1574·1
Alkyl Gallates, 1168·1
Alkyl Sulfates, 1574·1
Alkyl Sulfates, Ethoxylated, 1574·1
Alkyl Sulfonates, 492·1, 1574·1
Alkylating Agents, 492·1
Alkylbenzyldimethylammonium Chlorides, 1168·3
Alkyloxan, 1787·2
All Clear, 1787·2
All In One Plus Grapefruit, 1787·2
All Pecium, 1787·2
Allamin, 1787·2
Allantoin, 1141·3
Allapinin, 945·1
Allbee, 1787·2
Allbee with C, 1787·2
Allbee C-550, 1787·2
Allbee C-800, 1787·2
Allbee C-800 Plus Iron, 1787·2
Allcock's Porous Capsicum Plaster, 1787·2
Alleal, 1787·2
Alledryl, 1787·2
Allegra, 1787·2
Allegra-D, 1787·3
Allegro, 1787·3
Allegron, 1787·3
Allens Chesty Cough, 1787·3
Allens Dry Tickly Cough, 1787·3
Allens Junior Cough, 1787·3
Allens Pine & Honey, 1787·3
Allent, 1787·3
Aller-Aide, 1787·3
Allerbiocid S, 1787·3
Allercalm, 1787·3
Aller-Chlor, 1787·3
Allercon, 1787·3
Allercreme, 1787·3
Allercrom, 1787·3
Allerdine, 1787·3
Allerdryl, 1787·3
Allerest, 1787·3
Allerest Allergy & Sinus Relief, 1787·3
Allerest, Children's— *see* Children's Allerest, 1882·4
Allerest Headache Strength, 1787·3
Allerest 12 Hour, 1787·3
Allerest 12 Hour Nasal, 1787·3
Allerest Maximum Strength, 1787·3
Allerest, No-Drowsiness— *see* No-Drowsiness Allerest, 2171·3
Allerest Sinus Pain Formula, 1787·3
Aller-Eze, 1787·3
Aller-Eze Plus, 1787·3
Allerfen, 1787·3
Allerfre, 1787·3
Allerfrim, 1787·4
Allerfrim with Codeine, 1787·4
Allergan, 1787·4
Allergan 211, 637·3
Allergan Enzymatic, 1787·4
Allergefon, 1787·4
Allergen, 1787·4
Allergen Immunotherapy, 1650·2
Allergen Products, 1650·1
Allergenid, 1787·4
Allergex, 1787·4
Allergie-Injektopas, 1787·4
Allergies, 1787·4
Allergika, 1787·4
Allergin, 1787·4
Allergipuran N, 1787·4
Allergocomod, 1787·4
Allergo-COMOD, 1787·4
Allergocrom, 1787·4
Allergodil, 1787·4
Allergodose— *see* Cromedil, 1912·2
Allergofact, 1787·4
Allergoid-HAL, 1787·4
Allergojovis, 1787·4
Allergokatt, 1787·4
Allergo-Loges, 1787·4
Allergopos N, 1787·4
Allergospasmin, 1787·4
Allergospasmine, 1787·4
Allergosyx, 1787·4
Allergotin, 1787·4
Allergoval, 1787·4
Allergovit, 1788·1
Allergy, 1788·1
Allergy— *see* Hypersensitivity, 419·2
Allergy Drops, 1788·1
Allergy Drops, Maximum Strength— *see* Maximum Strength Allergy Drops, 2116·3
Allergy Elixir, 1788·1
Allergy Eyes, 1788·1
Allergy, Food— *see* Food Allergy, 422·1
Allergy Formula, 1788·1
Allergy Formula, Children's— *see* Children's Allergy Formula, 1882·4
Allergy Hayfever Sinus Relief, Chemists Own— *see* Chemists Own Hayfever Sinus Relief, 1882·1
Allergy Relief, 1788·1
Allergy Relief, Nyal Plus+ — *see* Nyal Plus+ Allergy Relief, 2182·1
Allergy Sinus, 1788·1
Allergy Symptoms Relief— *see* Allergy Relief, 1788·1
Allergy Tablets, 1788·1
Allerief, 1788·1
Allerin, 1788·1
AllerMax, 1788·1
Allermed, 1788·1
Allernix, 1788·1
Allerphed, 1788·1
Allerphen, 1788·1
Allersan, 1788·1
Allerset, 1788·1
Allersil, 1788·1
Allersol, 1788·1
Aller-Tab, 1788·1
Allertac, 1788·1
AllerTek, 1788·2
AlleRx, 1788·2
Allerzil, 1788·2
Allethrin I, 1500·3
Allevyn, 1788·2
Allfen, 1788·2
Allfen-DM, 1788·2
Allgauer, 1788·2
Allicin, 1691·2
Alliin, 1691·2
All-in-One, Natures Way— *see* Natures Way All-in-One, 2153·3
Allio Vital, 1788·2
Alliocaps Oligoplex, 1788·2
Alliosan, 1788·2
Allium, 1691·1
*Allium cepa*, 1723·2
Allium Cepa Compose, 1788·2
Allium Plus, 1788·2
*Allium sativum*, 1691·2
All-Nite Cold Formula, 1788·2
Allnol, 1788·2
Allnortoxiferin Chloride, 1398·3
Allo, 1788·2
Allobarbital, 668·3
Allobarbitone, 668·3
Allo-basan, 1788·2
Allobenz, 1788·2
Allobeta, 1788·2
Alloboxal, 1788·2
Allocaine, 1383·2
Allochrysine, 1788·2
Alloclamide Hydrochloride, 1114·2
Allo.comp., 1788·2
Allodynia, 2·1
Allo-Efeka, 1788·2
Alloferin, 1788·2
Alloferine, 1788·2
Allohexal, 1788·2
Alloin, 1248·3
Allomalenic Acid, 1147·3
Allomaron, 1788·2
Allonol, 1788·2
Allopin, 1788·2
Allopur, 1788·2
Allo-Puren, 1788·3
Allopurinol, 412·2
Allopurinol Riboside, 414·2
Allopurinol Sodium, 413·3
Allopurinolum, 412·2
Alloril, 1788·3
Allorin, 1788·3
Allostad, 1788·3
Allo-300-Tablinen, 1788·3
Allotyrol, 1788·3
Alloxanthine, 413·2
Allpargin, 1788·3
All-Pro, 1788·3
Allpyral, 1788·3
Allpyral Pure Mite, 1788·3
Allpyral Special Grass, 1788·3
Allsan, 1788·3
Allstam, 1788·3
All-*rac*-α-Tocopherol, 1464·3
All-*rac*-α-Tocopheryl Acetate, 1465·1
Alltotal, 1788·3
Alltracel P, 1788·3
Alltracel S, 1788·3
Allume, 1652·1
Allura Red AC, 1056·1
Allural, 1788·3
Allurit, 1788·3
Allvoran, 1788·3
Allya, 1788·3
Allyl Isothiocyanate, 1718·2
Allylamine Antifungals, 386·1
6-Allyl-2-amino-5,6,7,8-tetrahydro-4*H*-thiazolo[4,5-*d*]azepine Dihydrochloride, 1215·3
Allylbarbital, 673·3
Allylbarbituric Acid, 673·3
5-Allyl-5-(2-bromoallyl)barbituric Acid, 671·3
17-Allyl-6-deoxy-7,8-dihydro-14-hydroxy-6-oxo-17-normorphine Hydrochloride Dihydrate, 1044·3
6-Allyl-6,7-dihydro-5*H*-dibenz[*c,e*]azepine Dihydrogen Phosphate, 866·2
1-Allyl-1-(3α,17β-dihydroxy-2β-morpholino-5α-androstan-16β-yl)pyrrolidinium Bromide 17-Acetate, 1405·2
1-Allyl-1-(3α,17β-dihydroxy-2β-piperidino-5α-androstan-16β-yl)piperidinium Bromide, 3-Acetate 17-Propionate, 1405·2
(8*R*)-6-Allyl-*N*-[3-(dimethylamino)propyl]-*N*-(ethylcarbamoyl)ergoline-8-carboxamide, 1203·3
(−)-(5*R*,14*S*)-9a-Allyl-4,5-epoxy-3,14-dihydroxymorphinan-6-one Hydrochloride Dihydrate, 1044·3
(−)-(5*R*,6*S*)-9a-Allyl-4,5-epoxymorphin-7-en-3,6-diol, 1044·2
1-[(6-Allylergolin-8β-yl)carbonyl]-1-[3-(dimethylamino)propyl]-3-ethylurea, 1203·3
Allylestrenol, 1541·3
17α-Allylestr-4-en-17β-ol, 1541·3
4-Allylguaiacol, 1686·2
(−)-(3*S*,4*R*,5*S*,8*R*,9*E*,12*S*,14*S*,15*R*,16*S*,-18*R*,19*R*,26a*S*)-8-Allyl-5,6,8,11,12,-13,14,15,16,17,18,19,24,25,26,26a-hexadecahydro-5,19-dihydroxy-3-{(*E*)-2-[(1*R*,3*R*,4*R*)-4-hydroxy-3-methoxycyclohexyl]-1-methylvinyl}-14,16,-dimethoxy-4,10,12,18-tetramethyl-15,19-epoxy-3*H*-pyrido[2,1-*c*][1,4]oxaazacyclotricosine-1,7,20,21(4*H*,23*H*)-tetrone Monohydrate, 1363·3
5-Allyl-*N*-(2-hydroxyethyl)-3-methoxysalicylamide, 1649·3
17α-Allyl-17β-hydroxy-19-norandrosta-4,9,11-trien-3-one, 1541·3
5-Allyl-5-(2-hydroxypropyl)barbituric Acid, 718·1
5-Allyl-5-isobutylbarbituric Acid, 673·3
5-Allyl-5-isopropylbarbituric Acid, 670·3
Allylisopropylmalonylurea, 670·3
4-Allyl-2-methoxyphenol, 1686·2
5-Allyl-5-(1-methylbutyl)barbituric Acid, 721·2

(±)-5-Allyl-1-methyl-5-(1-methylpent-2-ynyl)barbituric Acid, 1303·2
(*RS*)-3-Allyl-2-methyl-4-oxocyclopent-2-enyl (1*R*,3*R*)-2,2-Dimethyl-3-(2-methylprop-1-enyl)cyclopropanecarboxylate, 1500·3
(*S*)-3-Allyl-2-methyl-4-oxocyclopent-2-enyl (1*R*,3*R*)-2,2-Dimethyl-3-(2-methylprop-1-enyl)-cyclopropanecarboxylate, 1505·1
17-Allyl-17-normorphine, 1044·2
*N*-Allylnoroxymorphone Hydrochloride, 1044·3
Allyloestrenol, 1541·3
2-Allyloxy-4-chloro-*N*-(2-diethylaminoethyl)benzamide Hydrochloride, 1114·2
(±)-1-(β-Allyloxy-2,4-dichlorophenethyl)imidazole, 397·3
1-(*o*-Allyloxyphenoxy)-3-isopropylaminopropan-2-ol Hydrochloride, 978·1
1-(2-Allylphenoxy)-3-isopropylaminopropan-2-ol, 856·3
(±)-*N*-[(1-Allyl-2-pyrrolidinyl)methyl]-4-amino-5-(methylsulfamoyl)-*o*-anisamide, 465·3
*N*-(1-Allyl-2-pyrrolidinylmethyl)-6-methoxy-1*H*-benzotriazole-5-carboxamide Hydrochloride, 1248·1
*N*-[(1-Allyl-2-pyrrolidinyl)methyl]-5-sulphamoyl-2-veratramide, 727·2
Allylsenföl, 1718·2
3-Allylthiomethyl-6-chloro-3,4-dihydro-2*H*-1,2,4-benzothiadiazine-7-sulphonamide 1,1-Dioxide, 858·1
Allypropymal, 670·3
Alma, 1788·3
Almac, 1788·3
Almáciga, 1710·1
Almacone, 1788·3
Almag, 1788·3
Almagate, 1248·2
Almagato, 1248·2
Almagatum, 1248·2
Almagel, 1788·3
Almagel Plus, 1788·3
Almarion, 1788·3
Almarl, 1788·3
Almarytm, 1788·4
Almasal, 1788·4
Almasilate, 1248·2
Almasilato, 1248·2
Almax, 1788·4
Almaxane, 1788·4
Almebex Plus $B_{12}$, 1788·4
Almendra, Aceite de, 1651·1
Almendras Dulces, Aceite de, 1651·1
Almevax, 1788·4
Almide, 1788·4
Almidón, 1449·1
Almidón, Éteres de, 750·1
Almigastrico, 1788·4
Almigripe, 1788·4
Alminoprofen, 14·1
Alminoprofeno, 14·1
Alminox, 1788·4
Almiral, 1788·4
Almirid, 1788·4
Almiron, 1788·4
Almiron Pepti, 1788·4
Almíscar, 1718·2
Almitil, 1788·4
Almitrina, Dimesilato de, 1584·2
Almitrine Bismesylate, 1584·2
Almitrine Dimesilate, 1584·2
Almitrine Dimesylate, 1584·2
Almitrine Mesylate, 1584·2
Almizcle, 1718·2
Almodan, 1788·4
Almogran, 1788·4
Almond Oil, 1651·1
Almond Oil, Refined, 1651·1
Almond Oil, Virgin, 1651·1
Almond Oil, Volatile Bitter, 1659·3
Almora, 1788·4
Almorsan, 1788·4
Almotrex, 1788·4
Almotriptan Malate, 465·2
Almotriptán, Malato de, 465·2
Almyrol, 1788·4
Alna, 1788·4
Alnase, 1788·4
Alnax, 1788·4
Alnex, 1788·4
Alnok, 1788·4
ALO-1401-02, 873·1
ALO-4943A, 438·1
Alobarbital, 668·3
Aloclair, 1788·4
Aloclamida, Hidrocloruro de, 1114·2
Alocril, 1789·1
Alodan, 1789·1
Alodont, 1789·1
Alodorm, 1789·1
Aloe, 1248·2
Áloe, 1141·3, 1248·2
Aloe Barbadensis, 1248·2
*Aloe barbadensis*, 1141·3, 1248·2, 1645·2
Aloe Capensis, 1248·2
Aloe Complex, 1789·1
*Aloe ferox*, 1248·2
Aloe Grande, 1789·1
Aloe Gum, 1248·2
Aloe Vera, 1141·3
*Aloe vera*, 1645·2
Aloe Vera Plus, 1789·1
Aloe Vesta, 1789·1
Aloebel, 1789·1
Aloelax, 1789·1
Aloes, 1248·2
Aloes, Barbados, 1248·2
Aloes, Cape, 1248·2
Aloes, Curaçao, 1248·2
Alofedina, 1789·1
Alofresh, 1789·1
Alogesia, 1789·1
Aloglutamol, 1248·3
Aloid, 1789·1
Aloin, 1248·3
Aloína, 1248·3
Aloinophen, 1789·1
Alomen, 1789·1
Alomide, 1789·1
Alonet, 1789·1
Alongamicina Balsa, 1789·1
Alopam, 1789·1
Alopate, 1789·1
Alopecia, 1134·1
Aloperidin, 1789·1
Aloperidolo, 701·2
Alopexy, 1789·1
Alophen, 1789·1
Aloplastine, 1789·1
Alopon, 1789·2
Alopresin, 1789·2
Alopresin Diu, 1789·2
Aloprim, 1789·2
Alopurinol, 412·2
Alor, 1789·2
Alora, 1789·2
Aloral, 1789·2
Alorin, 1789·2
Aloset, 1789·2
Alosetron Hydrochloride, 1248·3
Alosfar, 1789·2
Alosol, 1789·2
Alostil, 1789·2
Alotano, 1299·3
Alovir, 1789·2
Alox, 1789·2
Aloxan Derma, 1789·2
Aloxi, 1789·2
Aloxidil, 1789·2
Al-Oxin, 1789·2
Aloxiprin, 14·1
Aloxiprina, 14·1
*Aloysia triphylla*, 1706·3
ALP-201, 213·1
Alpagelle, 1789·2
Alpare, 1789·2
Alpaz, 1789·2
1-Alpha, 1789·2
$Alpha_1$ Antitrypsin, 1651·2
$Alpha_1$ Antitrypsin Deficiency, 1651·3
Alpha Blockers, 809·2
Alpha Cade, 1789·2
Alpha D3, 1789·2
Alpha 5 DS, 1789·2
Alpha Fraction, 1789·2
Alpha Galactosidase A, 1651·1
Alpha Keri, 1789·2
Alpha Keri Silky Smooth, 1789·2
Alpha Keri Tar, 1789·3
Alpha Lipoic Acid, 1754·3
Alpha Septol, 1789·3
*d*-Alpha Tocoferil Acetate, 1465·1
*dl*-Alpha Tocoferil Acetate, 1465·1
*d*-Alpha Tocoferil Acid Succinate, 1465·1
*dl*-Alpha Tocoferil Acid Succinate, 1465·1
*dl*-Alpha Tocoferil Palmitate, 1465·3
Alpha Tocopherol, 1464·3
*d*-Alpha Tocopherol, 1464·3
*dl*-Alpha Tocopherol, 1464·3
Alpha Tocopherol, Natural, 1464·3
Alpha Tocopherol, Synthetic, 1464·3
Alpha Tocopherols, 1464·3
Alpha Tocopheryl Acetate, 1465·1
*d*-Alpha Tocopheryl Acetate, 1465·1
*dl*-Alpha Tocopheryl Acetate, 1465·1
Alpha Tocopheryl Acetate Concentrate (Powder Form), 1465·1
*d*-Alpha Tocopheryl Acid Succinate, 1465·1
*dl*-Alpha Tocopheryl Acid Succinate, 1465·1
Alpha Tocopheryl Hydrogen Succinate, 1465·1
*RRR*-Alpha Tocopheryl Hydrogen Succinate, 1465·1
Alpha UV, 1789·3
Alpha-adrenergic Antagonists, 809·2
Alpha-Amoxyclav, 1789·3
Alpha-amylases, 1654·2
Alphacade, Item— *see* Item Alphacade, 2069·3
Alphacaine, 1789·3
Alphacarotene, 1423·1
Alphacedre, 1789·3
Alpha-cellulose, 1578·3
Alphachloralose, 1501·2
Alpha-Chymocutan, 1789·3
Alpha-Chymotrase, 1789·3
Alphacin, 1789·3
Alphacortison, 1789·3
Alphacutanee, 1789·3
Alphacyclodextrin, 1678·2
Alpha-cypermethrin, 1502·3
Alpha-Depressan, 1789·3
Alphaderm, 1789·3
Alphadinal, 1789·3
Alphadine, 1789·3
Alphadolone Acetate, 1296·3
Alphadopa, 1789·3
Alphadrate, 1789·3
Alphaflam, 1789·3
Alphagan, 1789·3
Alphaglobin, 1789·3
Alpha-hydroxymidazolam, 708·1
Alpha-hypophamine, 1336·1
Alpha-L-iduronidase, 1705·1
Alphakeptol, 1789·3
Alphakeptol, Item— *see* Item Alphakeptol, 2069·3
Alphakinase, 1789·3
Alpha-linolenic Acid, 976·2
Alpha-Lipogamma, 1789·3
Alpha-Lipon, 1789·3
Alpha-lobeline Hydrochloride, 1589·1
Alphalox-D, 1789·4
Alpha-methyldopa, 953·2
Alpha-methylfentanyl, 40·3
Alpha-methylnoradrenaline, 955·1
Alpha-methylthiofentanyl, 40·3
Alphamox, 1789·4
Alphamox— *see* Pylorid-KA, 2247·2
Alphanate, 1789·4
Alphane, 1789·4
Alphanine, 1789·4
Alphaparin, 1789·4
Alphapress, 1789·4
Alphapril, 1789·4
$Alpha_1$-proteinase Inhibitor, 1651·2
Alphasone Acetophenide, 1541·3
Alphastria, 1789·4
*RRR*-Alpha-Tocopherol, 1464·3
*RRR*-Alpha-Tocopheryl Acetate, 1465·1
Alphatrex, 1789·4
Alphavase, 1789·4
Alpha-Vibolex, 1789·4
Alphaxalone, 1296·3
Alpha-Zedex, 1789·4
Alphazole, 1789·4
Alphazole, Item— *see* Item Alphazole, 2069·3
Alphazurine 2G, 1750·3
Alphexine, 1789·4
Alphintern, 1789·4
Alphosyl, 1789·4
Alphosyl 2 in 1, 1789·4
Alphosyl HC, 1789·4
Alphosyle, 1789·4
Alpicort, 1789·4
Alpicort F, 1789·4
Alpin, 1789·4
Alpina Gel a la Consoude, 1790·1
Alpina Gel a l'Arnica avec Spilanthes, 1790·1
Alpina Pommade au Souci, 1790·1
Alpirex, 1790·1
Alpiroprida, 465·3
Alpiropride, 465·3
Alplax, 1790·1
Alplax Digest, 1790·1
Alplax Net, 1790·1
Alpovex, 1790·1
Alpoxen, 1790·1
Alpralid, 1790·1
Alpratyrol, 1790·1
Alprax, 1790·1
Alpraz, 1790·1
Alprazig, 1790·1
Alprazolam, 668·3
Alprazolamum, 668·3
Alprenolol, 856·3
Alprenolol Benzoate, 856·3
Alprenolol, Benzoato de, 856·3
Alprenolol, Hidrocloruro de, 856·3
Alprenolol Hydrochloride, 856·3
Alprenololi Benzoas, 856·3
Alprenololi Hydrochloridum, 856·3
Alpress, 1790·1
Alprim, 1790·1
Alprocontin, 1790·1
Alpronax, 1790·1
Alprostadil, 1512·3
Alprostadil Alfadex, 1512·3
Alprostadilum, 1512·3
Alprostapint, 1790·1
Alprostar, 1790·1
Alprox, 1790·1
Alquen, 1790·1
Alquequenje, 1731·3
Alquimila Arvense, 1729·1
Alquitrán de Enebro, 1159·2
Alquitrán de Hulla, 1159·2
Alquitrán Vegetal, 1159·3
Alra, 1790·1
Alrac, 1790·1
Alramucil, 1790·1
Alramucil Instant Mix, 1790·1
Alrex, 1790·1
Alrheumun, 1790·1
Alrin, 1790·1
Alrof, 1790·2
ALRT-1057, 526·2
Alserine, 1790·2
Alsicur, 1790·2
Alsidexten, 1790·2
Alsidrine, 1790·2
Alsilax, 1790·2
Alsiline, 1790·2
Alsimine with Vitamins A & D, 1790·2
Alsiphene, 1790·2
Alsiroyal, 1790·2
Alsirub, 1790·2
Alsogil, 1790·2
Alsol, 1790·2
Alsol N, 1790·2

Alsoy, 1790·2
Alstat, 1790·2
Alsucral, 1790·2
Alsylax, 1790·2
Altace, 1790·2
Altacite, 1790·2
Altacite Plus, 1790·2
Altan, 1790·2
Altat, 1790·2
Altea, 1651·3
Altea (Specie Composta), 1790·2
Alteia, 1651·3
Altemol, 1790·2
Alten, 1790·2
Alteplasa, 857·1
Alteplase, 857·1
Alteplase for Injection, 857·1
Alteplasum ad Iniectabile, 857·1
Alteporina, 1790·2
Altergen, 1790·3
Alter-$H_2$, 1790·3
Altermon, 1790·3
Alterna, 1790·3
ALternaGEL, 1790·3
Alternus, 1790·3
Altersol, 1790·3
Altesona, 1790·3
Alth., 1651·3
Althaea, 1651·3
Althaea Complex, 1790·3
Althaea Folium, 1651·3
*Althaea officinalis*, 1651·3
Althaeae Radix, 1651·3
Althiazide, 858·1
Althrocin, 1790·3
Altiazem, 1790·3
Alticort, 1790·3
Alti-CPA, 1790·3
Altim, 1790·3
Alti-MPA, 1790·3
Altinac, 1790·3
Altior, 1790·3
Altizida, 858·1
Altizide, 858·1
Altocel, 1790·3
Altocor, 1790·3
Altodor, 1790·3
Altone, 1790·3
Altosone, 1790·3
Altracart II, 1790·3
Altramet, 1790·3
Altrenogest, 1541·3
Altretamina, 526·2
Altretamine, 526·2
Altruline, 1790·3
Altumomab Pentetate, Indium ($^{111}$In), 1524·1
Alu-3, 1790·3
Alubifar, 1790·3
Alubron-Saar, 1790·3
Alu-Cap, 1790·3
Alucid, 1790·4
Alucinol, 1790·4
Alucol, 1790·4
Alucol Silicona, 1790·4
Aluctyl, 1790·4
Aludal, 1790·4
Aludrox, 1790·4
Aludrox II, 1790·4
Aludrox AC, 1790·4
Aludrox Forte, 1790·4
Aludrox MH, 1790·4
Aludroxil, 1790·4
Alufibrate, 884·3
Alugel, 1790·4
Alugel Magnesiado, 1790·4
Alugelibys— *see* Alugel, 1790·4
Alugelibys Magnesiado— *see* Alugel Magnesiado, 1790·4
Aluin, 1652·1
Alukon, 1790·4
Alum, 1652·1
Alum, Ammonia, 1652·1
Alum, Ammonium, 1652·1
Alum, Chrome, 1670·2
Alum, Dried, 1652·1
Alum Milk, 1790·4
Alum, Potash, 1652·1
Alum, Potassium, 1652·1
Alumadrine, 1790·4
Alu-Mag, 1790·4
Alumag, 1791·1
Alumagall, 1791·1
Alumbre, 1652·1
Alumen, 1652·1
Aluminato de Bismuto, 1252·1
Aluminii Chloridum Hexahydricum, 1142·1
Aluminii Hydroxidum Hydricum ad Adsorptionem, 1249·2
Aluminii Magnesii Silicas, 1577·1
Aluminii Monostearas, 1574·1
Aluminii Oxidum, 1140·1
Aluminii Phosphas, 1250·1
Aluminii Phosphas Hydricus, 1250·1
Aluminii Sulfas, 1653·1
Aluminio, 1652·2
Aluminio, Acetato de, 1652·3
Aluminio, Cloreto de, 1142·1
Aluminio, Clorohidróxido de, 1142·1
Aluminio, Cloruro de, 1142·1
Aluminio, Glicinato de, 1249·1
Aluminio, Lactato de, 1653·1
Aluminio, Sulfato de, 1653·1
Aluminium, 1652·2
Aluminium Acetate, 1652·3
Aluminium Acetate, Basic, 1653·1
Aluminium Acetotartrate, 1652·3
Aluminium Aminoacetate, Basic, 1249·1
Aluminium Aspirin, 14·1
Aluminium Carbonate, Basic, 1249·1
Aluminium Chloratum, 1142·1
Aluminium Chlorhydrate, 1142·1
Aluminium Chlorhydroxyallantoinate, 1141·2
Aluminium Chloride, 1142·1
Aluminium Chloride, Basic, 1142·1
Aluminium Chloride Hexahydrate, 1142·1
Aluminium Chloride Hydroxide Hydrate, 1142·1
Aluminium Chlorohydrate, 1142·1
Aluminium Chlorohydrex Polyethylene Glycol, 1142·1
Aluminium Chlorohydrex Propylene Glycol, 1142·1
Aluminium Clofibrate, 884·3
Aluminium Dichlorohydrex Polyethylene Glycol, 1142·1
Aluminium Dichlorohydrex Propylene Glycol, 1142·1
Aluminium Dihydroxyallantoinate, 1141·2
Aluminium Fluoride, 1446·1
Aluminium Free Indigestion, 1791·1
Aluminium Glycinate, 1249·1
Aluminium Glycyrrhetate, 1264·3
Aluminium Glycyrrhetinate, 1264·3
Aluminium Hydroxide, 1249·2
Aluminium Hydroxide, Dried, 1249·2
Aluminium Hydroxide, Hydrated, for Adsorption, 1249·2
Aluminium Hydroxide-Magnesium Carbonate Co-dried Gel, 1250·1
Aluminium Hydroxycarbonate, 1249·1
Aluminium Kalium Sulfuricum, 1652·1
Aluminium Lactate, 1653·1
Aluminium Magnesium Carbonate Hydroxide Hydrate, 1267·3
Aluminium Magnesium Hydroxide, 1271·3
Aluminium Magnesium Silicate, 1251·1, 1577·1
Aluminium Magnesium Silicate Hydrate, 1248·2
Aluminium Metallicum, 1652·3
Aluminium Monopalmitate, 1574·1
Aluminium Monostearate, 1574·1
Aluminium Overload, 1035·1
Aluminium Oxide, 1140·1
Aluminium Oxide, Hydrated, 1140·1, 1249·2
Aluminium Oxidum Hydricum, 1249·2
Aluminium Phosphate, 1250·1
Aluminium Phosphate, Dried, 1250·1
Aluminium Phosphate, Hydrated, 1250·1
Aluminium Phosphide, 1500·1
Aluminium Polystyrene Sulfonate, 1053·3
Aluminium Potassium Sulphate, 1652·1
Aluminium Powder, 1652·2
Aluminium Sesquichlorohydrex Polyethylene Glycol, 1142·1
Aluminium Sesquichlorohydrex Propylene Glycol, 1142·1
Aluminium Silicate, 1250·2, 1268·3
Aluminium/Silicate, Hydrated, 1039·3
Aluminium Sodium Carbonate Hydroxide, 1261·2
Aluminium Sodium Silicate, 1250·2
Aluminium Subacetate, 1653·1
Aluminium Sulfate, 1653·1
Aluminium Sulfuricum, 1653·1
Aluminium Sulphate, 1653·1
Aluminium Trimagnesium Carbonate Heptahydroxide Dihydrate, 1248·2
Aluminium Trisulphate, 1653·1
Aluminium Zirconium Octachlorohydrate, 1142·1
Aluminium Zirconium Octachlorohydrex Gly, 1142·1
Aluminium Zirconium Pentachlorohydrate, 1142·1
Aluminium Zirconium Pentachlorohydrex Gly, 1142·1
Aluminium Zirconium Tetrachlorohydrate, 1142·1
Aluminium Zirconium Tetrachlorohydrex Gly, 1142·1
Aluminium Zirconium Trichlorohydrate, 1142·1
Aluminium Zirconium Trichlorohydrex Gly, 1142·1
Aluminiumoxid, Wasserhaltiges, 1249·2
Aluminon, 1757·3
Aluminosilicato Magnésico, 1577·1
Aluminum, 1652·2
Aluminum Acetate, 1652·3
Aluminum Acetylsalicylate, 14·1
Aluminum Aspirin, 14·1
Aluminum Bismuth Oxide, 1252·1
Aluminum Chlorhydroxide, 1142·1
Aluminum Chloride, 1142·1
Aluminum Chloride Hydroxide Hydrate, 1142·1
Aluminum Chlorohydrate, 1142·1
Aluminum Clofibrate, 884·3
Aluminum Hydroxide, 1249·2
Aluminum Hydroxide Gel, 1249·2
Aluminum Hydroxide Gel, Dried, 1249·2
Aluminum Hydroxychloride, 1142·1
Aluminum Magnesium Hydroxide Sulfate, 1271·3
Aluminum Monostearate, 1574·1
Aluminum Phosphate, 1250·1
Aluminum Phosphate Gel, 1250·2
Aluminum Phosphide, 1500·1
Aluminum Sulfate, 1653·1
Alumite, 1791·1
Alumpak, 1791·1
Alun, 1652·1
Alupent, 1791·1
Alupent Expectorant, 1791·1
Alupep, 1791·1
Alupir, 1791·1
Aluprim, 1791·1
Alurate, 1791·1
Alusil, 1791·1
Alusorb, 1791·1
Alu-Tab, 1791·1
Alutard, 1791·1
Alutard SQ, 1791·1
Alutop, 1791·1
Aluzime, 1791·1
Alvadermo Fuerte, 1791·1
Alvear, 1791·1
Alvear Complex, 1791·1
Alvear con Ginseng, 1791·1
Alvear Sport, 1791·1
Alvedon, 1791·1
Alvedrin, 1791·2
Alven, 1791·2
Alvent, 1791·2
Alveofact, 1791·2
Alveofen, 1791·2
Alveolex, 1791·2
Alveolitis, Cryptogenic Fibrosing— *see* Diffuse Parenchymal Lung Disease, 1079·3
Alveolitis, Extrinsic Allergic— *see* Diffuse Parenchymal Lung Disease, 1079·3
Alveoten, 1791·2
Alvercol, 1791·2
Alverina, Citrato de, 1250·2
Alverine Citrate, 1250·2
Alvesco, 1791·2
Alvesin, 1791·2
Alvidina, 1791·2
Alvimopan, 1250·2
Alvis, 1791·2
Alvityl, 1791·2
Alvium, 1791·2
Alvo Nasal, 1791·2
Alvofact, 1791·2
Alvogil, 1791·2
Alvogyl, 1791·2
ALX1-11, 774·3
Alxen, 1791·2
Alymphon, 1791·2
Alyostal, 1791·2
Alyrane, 1791·2
Alzaimax, 1791·2
Alzam, 1791·2
Alzaten, 1791·2
Alzen, 1791·2
Alzental, 1791·2
Alzheimer's Disease— *see* Dementia, 1484·1
Alzol, 1791·2
Alzolam, 1791·2
Alzomed-F, 1791·2
AM, 1791·3
AM-715, 238·3
AM-833, 213·2
AM-1155, 216·2
AM Treatment, 1791·3
Ama, 1791·3
AMA-1, 1622·3
AMA-1080, 166·3
Amabagyl, 1791·3
Amace-BP, 1791·3
Amacetam Sulphate, 1734·3
Amacin, 1791·3
Amacone, 1791·3
Amadol, 1791·3
Amagesan, 1791·3
Amalium, 1791·3
Amamelide, 1696·3
Aman, 1791·3
Am-An, 1791·3
Amande, Huile d', 1651·1
*Amanita*, 1663·2
*Amanita bisporigera*, 1717·3
*Amanita muscaria*, 1717·3
*Amanita pantherina*, 1717·3
*Amanita phalloides*, 1717·3
*Amanita verna*, 1717·3
*Amanita virosa*, 1717·3
α-Amanitin, 1717·3
β-Amanitin, 1717·3
γ-Amanitin, 1717·3
Amanta, 1791·3
Amantadina, Hidrocloruro de, 1197·2
Amantadina, Sulfato de, 1197·2
Amantadine Hydrochloride, 1197·2
Amantadine Sulfate, 1197·2
Amantadine Sulphate, 1197·2
Amantadini Hydrochloridum, 1197·2
Amantagamma, 1791·3
Amantan, 1791·3
Amantrel, 1791·3
Amaphen, 1791·3
Amaphen with Codeine, 1791·3
Amapola, Pétalos de, 1058·1
Amara, 1791·3
Amaranth, 1056·1
Amaranto, 1056·1
Amara-Tropfen, 1791·3
Amara-Tropfen-Pascoe, 1791·3
Amarel, 1791·3
Amarillo de Quinoleína, 1057·3
Amarillo 2G, 1058·3

Amarillo Ocaso FCF, 1058·2
Amaro Medicinale, 1791·3
Amaro Padil, 1791·3
Amarum, Sal, 1228·2
Amaryl, 1791·3
Amarylle, 1791·3
Amasulin, 1791·4
Amatine, 1791·4
Amatoxins, 1717·3
Amaurosis Fugax— *see* Stroke, 836·1
Amazyl, 1791·4
Ambacamp, 1791·4
Ambamida, 1791·4
Ambatrol, 1791·4
Ambaxino, 1791·4
Ambe 12, 1791·4
Amben, 1142·2, 1791·4
Ambenat, 1791·4
Ambene, 1791·4
Ambene Comp, 1791·4
Ambene N, 1791·4
Ambenonio, Cloruro de, 1487·3
Ambenonium Chloride, 1487·3
Ambenyl, 1791·4
Ambenyl Cough Syrup, 1791·4
Ambenyl-D, 1791·4
Amber Gold, 1791·4
Ambestigmini Chloridum, 1487·3
Ambezetal, 1791·4
Ambi 10, 1791·4
AMBI 60/580, 1791·4
AMBI 60/580/30, 1791·4
AMBI 1000/55, 1792·1
Ambi Skin Tone, 1792·1
Ambidrin, 1792·1
Ambien, 1792·1
Ambilan, 1792·1
Ambilan Bid, 1792·1
Ambiosol, 1792·1
Ambirix, 1792·1
AmBisome, 1792·1
Ambistryn-S, 1792·1
Ambi-Wolff, 1792·1
Ambiz, 1792·1
Amblyopia, Tobacco, 1459·1
Ambodil, 1792·1
Amboneural, 1792·1
Amboral, 1792·1
Ambotetra, 1792·1
Ambotonin, 1792·1
Ambra Med Complex, 1792·1
Ambra Oligoplex, 1792·1
Ambral, 1792·1
Ambramicina, 1792·1
Ambra-Sinto T, 1792·1
Ambre Solaire, 1792·1
Ambredin, 1792·1
Ambrexin, 1792·1
Ambril, 1792·1
Ambritan, 1792·1
Ambro, 1792·1
Ambrobene, 1792·1
Ambrobeta, 1792·2
Ambrobion, 1792·2
Ambrodoc, 1792·2
Ambrodoxy, 1792·2
Ambrofur, 1792·2
Ambrohexal, 1792·2
Ambroinfant, 1792·2
Ambrol, 1792·2
Ambrolan, 1792·2
Ambrolitic, 1792·2
Ambrolos, 1792·2
Ambrolytic, 1792·2
Ambromucil, 1792·2
Ambromyc, 1792·2
Ambropp, 1792·2
Ambro-Puren, 1792·2
Ambroten, 1792·2
Ambrotos, 1792·2
Ambrowel, 1792·2
Ambrox, 1792·2
Ambroxan, 1792·2
Ambroxol Acefyllinate, 1114·3
Ambroxol AL Comp, 1792·2
Ambroxol Comp, 1792·2
Ambroxol, Hidrocloruro de, 1114·3
Ambroxol Hydrochloride, 1114·3
Ambroxoli Hydrochloridum, 1114·3
Ambroxolvan, 1792·2
Ambucetamida, 1653·1
Ambucetamide, 1653·1
Ambucetamide Hydrochloride, 1653·2
Ambufen, 1792·2
Ambuphylline, 781·3
Ambutonium Bromide, 1653·2
AMCA, 760·3
*trans*-AMCHA, 760·3
Amchafibrin, 1792·2
Amciderm, 1792·2
Amcidil, 1792·2
Amcillin, 1792·2
Amcinafal, 1792·2
Amcinil, 1792·3
Amcinónida, 1091·1
Amcinonide, 1091·1
Amcinopol, 1091·1
Amclo, 1792·3
Amco, 1792·3
Amcopan, 1792·3
Amcopan Plus, 1792·3
Amcort, 1792·3
Amc-Puren, 1792·3
AMD, 1792·3
Amdinocillin, 228·3
Amdinocillin Pivoxil, 244·2
Amdipin, 1792·3
Amdox-Puren, 1792·3
Amebamagma, 1792·3
Ameblin, 1792·3
Amebyl, 1792·3
Amebysol, 1792·3
Amechol Chloride, 1492·1
Ameclina, 1792·3
Amedran, 1792·3
Amefin, 1792·3
Amefur, 1792·3
Ameisensäure, 1689·3
Ameixa, 1285·1
Ameixa Composto, Xarope Peitoral de— *see* Xarope Peitoral de Ameixa Composto, 2387·4
Amekrin, 1792·3
Amen, 1792·3
Amender, 1792·3
Amêndoas, Oleo de, 1651·1
Amendoim, Óleo de, 1656·1
Amenicil, 1792·3
Amenite A, 1792·3
Amenite Cap, 1792·3
Amenite E, 1792·3
Amenorrhoea, 1313·1
Amenox, 1792·3
Amerge, 1792·3
Americaine, 1792·3
Americaine Anesthetic, 1792·3
Americaine First Aid, 1792·3
Americaine Otic, 1792·4
American Dwarf Palm, 1569·1
American Ginseng, 1693·2
American Hellebore, 1764·1
American Mandrake, 1155·2
American Storax, 1749·3
American Veratrum, 1764·1
American Wormseed, Oil of, 103·3
Americet, 1792·4
Ameride, 1792·4
Amerifed, 1792·4
Amerigel, 1792·4
Amerituss AD, 1792·4
Amermycin, 1792·4
Amersan, 1792·4
Amerscan DMSA, 1792·4
Amerscan Hepatate, 1792·4
Amerscan Medronate, 1792·4
Amerscan Pentetate, 1792·4
Amerscan Pulmonate, 1792·4
Amerscan Stannous, 1792·4
Amertec, 1792·4
A-Methapred, 1792·4
Amethocaine, 1385·1
Amethocaine Hydrochloride, 1385·1
Amethopterin, 568·2
Ametic, 1792·4
Ametionin, 1792·4
Ametop, 1792·4
Ametricid, 1792·4
Ametriodinic Acid, 1063·2
Ametycine, 1792·4
Ameu, 1792·4
Amevive, 1792·4
Amezinio, Metilsulfato de, 858·2
Amezinium Methylsulphate, 858·2
Amezinium Metilsulfate, 858·2
Amfamox, 1792·4
Amfebutamone Hydrochloride, 287·2
Amfepramone Hydrochloride, 1587·1
Amfetamine, 1584·3
Amfetamine Aspartate, 1584·3
Amfetamine Phosphate, 1584·3
Amfetamine Sulfate, 1584·3
Amfetamine Sulphate, 1584·3
Amfetamini Sulfas, 1584·3
Amfetaminil, 1584·3
Amfetyline Hydrochloride, 1588·2
Amfipen, 1792·4
Amfostat, 1792·4
Amfotericina B, 391·2
AMG-073, 770·2
Amgenal Cough, 1793·1
Amgrip, 1793·1
AMI-25, 1061·3
AMI-121, 1061·3
Amias, 1793·1
Amicacil, 1793·1
Amicacina, 154·1
Amicalin, 1793·1
Amicaliq, 1793·1
Amicar, 1793·1
Amicasil, 1793·1
Amicel, 1793·1
Amicic, 1793·1
Amicilon, 1793·1
Amicin, 1793·1
Amicla, 1793·1
Amiclair, 1793·1
Amiclav, 1793·1
Amico, 1793·1
Amico-L, 1793·1
Amicose, 1793·1
Amicrobin, 1793·1
Amidal, 1793·1
Amidalin, 1793·1
Amidate, 1793·1
Amidazofen, 14·2
Amide Sulfonates, 1574·1
Amide Type Local Anaesthetics, 1367·1
Amidefrina, Mesilato de, 1115·1
Amidefrine Mesilate, 1115·1
Amidephrine Mesylate, 1115·1
Amidiaz, 1793·1
Amidine Hydrochloride, 57·2
({1-[*N*-(*p*-Amidinobenzoyl)-L-tyrosyl]-4-piperidyl}oxy)acetic Acid, 944·3
*N*-[(*R*)-({(2*S*)-2-[(*p*-Amidinobenzyl)carbamoyl]-1-azetidinyl}carbonyl)cyclohexylmethyl]glycine, 952·1
*N*-Amidino-3,5-diamino-6-chloropyrazine-2-carboxamide Hydrochloride Dihydrate, 858·2
*N*-Amidino-2-(2,6-dichlorophenyl)acetamide Hydrochloride, 927·2
$N^6$-Amidino-$N^2$-(3-mercaptopropionyl)-L-lysylglycyl-L-α-aspartyl-L-tryptophyl-L-prolyl-L-cysteinamide, Cyclic (1→6)-Disulfide, 912·2
6-Amidino-2-naphthyl *p*-Guanidinobenzoate Dimethanesulfonate, 1719·1
*N*-{[(3*S*)-1-(*p*-Amidinophenyl)-2-oxo-3-pyrrolidinyl]carbamoyl}-β-alanine Ethyl Ester Monoacetate Quadrantihydrate, 977·2
8-[3-(*m*-Amidinophenyl)-2-triazeno]3-amino-5-ethyl-6-phenylphenanthridinium Chloride, 606·1
*N'*-Amidinosulphanilamide, 260·3
Amido, 1449·1
Amidon, 1449·1
Amidona, 1793·1
Amidonal, 1793·1
Amidone Hydrochloride, 57·2
Amidopyrine, 14·2
Amidopyrine-Pyramidon, 14·2
Amidotrizoato de Meglumina, 1060·2
Amidotrizoato de Sodio, 1060·2
Amidotrizoic Acid, 1060·1
Amidotrizoic Acid Dihydrate, 1060·1
Amidotrizoico, Ácido, 1060·1
Amidox, 1793·1
Amidrin, 1793·1
Amieiro Negro, 1266·3
Amifenazol, Hidrocloruro de, 1584·3
Amifostina, 1031·3
Amifostine, 1031·3
Amigdagen, 1793·1
Amigdalol, 1793·1
Amigdamicin, 1793·2
Amigdobis, 1793·2
Amigesic, 1793·2
Ami-Hydrotride, 1793·2
Amikacin, 154·1
Amikacin Sulfate, 154·1
Amikacin Sulphate, 154·1
Amikacina, 154·1
Amikacina, Sulfato de, 154·1
Amikacini Sulfas, 154·1
Amikacinum, 154·1
Amikafur, 1793·2
Amikal, 1793·2
Amikalem, 1793·2
Amikan, 1793·2
Amikasol, 1793·2
Amikasons, 1793·2
Amikavi, 1793·2
Amikayect, 1793·2
Amikelina, Hidrocloruro de, 1653·2
Amikhelline Hydrochloride, 1653·2
Amikin, 1793·2
Amikine, 1793·2
Amiklin, 1793·2
Amilamont, 1793·2
Amilande, 1793·2
Amilasa, 1654·2
Amilco, 1793·2
Amil-Co, 1793·2
Amilene, 1793·2
Amilhydrozide, 1793·2
Amilide, 1793·2
Amilin, 1793·2
Amilit-IFI, 1793·2
Amilmaxco, 1793·2
Amilmetacresol, 1168·2
Amilo, 1449·1
Amilo, Azotito de, 1032·1
Amilo, Nitrito de, 1032·1
Amilo-basan, 1793·2
Amilocaína, Hidrocloruro de, 1370·2
Amilocomp Beta, 1793·2
Amiloferm, 1793·3
Amilohyd, 1793·3
Amilomer, 1653·2
Amiloral/HCT, 1793·3
Amiloretic, 1793·3
Amiloretik, 1793·3
Amilorid Comp, 1793·3
Amilorida, Hidrocloruro de, 858·2
Amiloride Composto, 1793·3
Amiloride Hydrochloride, 858·2
Amilorid/HCT, 1793·3
Amiloridi Hydrochloridum, 858·2
Amilostad HCT, 1793·3
Amiloxate, 1142·2
Amiloxato, 1142·2
Amilozid, 1793·3
Amimox, 1793·3
Amin 21 K, 1793·3
Aminacrine Hydrochloride, 1165·3
Aminaftona, 741·3
Aminaftone, 741·3
Amin-Aid, 1793·3
Aminaphthone, 741·3
Aminaphtone, 741·3
Aminarsonic Acid, 158·3
Aminazine, 675·2
Amindan, 1793·3
Amine Fluoride 297, 1442·3

Amine Soaps, 1574·1
Amineptina, Hidrocloruro de, 280·3
Amineptine Hydrochloride, 280·3
Aminess, 1793·3
Aminess-N, 1793·3
Amineurin, 1793·3
Aminic Acid, 1689·3
Amino, 1793·3
Amino 3, 1793·3
Amino Acid Metabolic Disorders, 1417·2
Amino Acids, 1417·1
Amino MS, 1793·3
Amino PG, 1793·3
Aminoacetic Acid, 1433·3
Aminoacridina, Hidrocloruro de, 1165·3
9-Aminoacridine Antimalarials, 444·1
Aminoacridine Hydrochloride, 1165·3
9-Aminoacridine Hydrochloride Monohydrate, 1165·3
4-*O*-[(2*R*,3*R*,4a*S*,6*R*,7*S*,8*R*,8a*R*)-3-Amino-6-(4-amino-4-deoxy-α-D-glucopyranosyloxy)-8-hydroxy-7-methylaminoperhydropyrano[3,2-*b*]pyran-2-yl]-2-deoxystreptamine, 158·2
4-Amino-1-(2-amino-*N*-methylacetamido)-1,4-dideoxy-3-*O*-(2,6-diamino-2,3,4,6,7-pentadeoxy-β-L-*lyxo*-heptopyranosyl)-6-*O*-methyl-L-*chiro*-inositol Sulphate, 158·3
4-*O*-[(2*R*,3*R*)-*cis*-3-Amino-6-aminomethyl-3,4-dihydro-2*H*-pyran-2-yl]-2-deoxy-6-*O*-(3-deoxy-4-*C*-methyl-3-methylamino-β-L-arabinopyranosyl)-1-*N*-ethylstreptamine Sulphate, 236·3
4-*O*-[(2*R*,3*R*)-*cis*-3-Amino-6-aminomethyl-3,4-dihydro-2*H*-pyran-2-yl]-2-deoxy-6-*O*-(3-deoxy-4-*C*-methyl-3-methylamino-β-L-arabinopyranosyl)streptamine Sulphate, 254·3
(−)-5-Amino-2-({(6*R*,7*R*)-7-[2-(2-amino-4-thiazolyl)glyoxylamido]-2-carboxy-8-oxo-5-thia-1-azabicyclo[4.2.0]oct-2-en-3-yl}methyl)-1-(2-hydroxyethyl)pyrazolium Hydroxide, Inner Salt, $7^2$-(*Z*)-(*O*-Methyloxime) Sulfate, 175·2
4-Amino-1-β-D-arabinofuranosylpyrimidin-2(1*H*)-one, 543·1
7-[(1*R*,5*S*,6*S*)-6-Amino-3-azabicyclo[3.1.0]hex-3-yl]-1-(2,4-difluorophenyl)-6-fluoro-1,4-dihydro-4-oxo-1,8-naphthyridine-3-carboxylic Acid Monomethanesulphonate, 274·3
(±)-*endo*-4-Amino-*N*-(1-azabicyclo[3.3.1]non-4-yl)-5-chloro-*o*-anisamide, 1287·3
(±)-α-Aminobenzeneacetic Acid 3-Methylbutyl Ester Hydrochloride, 487·3
*p*-Aminobenzenearsonic Acid, 158·3
4-Aminobenzenesulphonamide, 263·2
Aminobenzoate Potassium, 1733·3
Aminobenzoate Sodium, 1747·1
Aminobenzoato Potásico, 1733·3
Aminobenzoic Acid, 1142·2
4-Aminobenzoic Acid, 1142·2
Aminobenzoico, Ácido, 1142·2
3-Amino-1,2,4-benzotriazine 1,4-Dioxide, 588·3
*N*-4-Aminobenzoylaminoacetic Acid, 1653·2
*p*-Aminobenzoylglycine, 1653·2
2-(4-Aminobenzoyloxy)ethyldiethylammonium (6*R*)-6-(2-Phenylacetamido)penicillanate Monohydrate, 246·1
Aminobenzylpenicillin, 157·1
Aminobenzylpenicillin Sodium, 157·1
4-Amino-*N*-(1-benzyl-4-piperidyl)-5-chloro-*o*-anisamide, 1260·3
5-Amino-3,4′-bipyridyl-6(1*H*)-one, 862·3
5-Amino-1,3-bis(2-ethylhexyl)hexahydro-5-methylpyrimidine, 1182·1
Aminobisphosphonates, 766·3
4-Amino-5-bromo-*N*-(2-diethylaminoethyl)-*o*-anisamide, 1254·1
2-Amino-5-bromo-6-phenyl-4(3*H*)-pyrimidinone, 532·2
γ-Aminobutírico, Ácido, 1690·2
Aminobutyric Acid, 1690·2
4-Aminobutyric Acid, 1690·2
Aminocaproic Acid, 741·3
Aminocaproico, Ácido, 741·3
$N^5$-(Aminocarbonyl)-L-ornithine, 1425·2
1-({[4-(Aminocarbonyl)pyridinio]methoxy}methyl)-2-[(hydroxyimino)methyl]pyridinium Dichloride, 1032·2
Aminocarboxylic Acids, 1574·1
(3-Amino-3-carboxypropyl)dimethylsulphonium Chloride, 1714·1
(*S*)-5′-[(3-Amino-3-carboxypropyl)methylsulphonio]-5′-deoxyadenosine Hydroxide, Inner Salt, 1647·2
Aminocephalosporanic Acid, 117·2
Amino-Cerv, 1793·3
4-Amino-5-chloro-*N*-(2-diethylaminoethyl)-2-methoxybenzamide, 1274·3
(±)-4-Amino-5-chloro-2-ethoxy-*N*-{[4-(*p*-fluorobenzyl)-2-morpholinyl]methyl}benzamide Citrate Dihydrate, 1276·3
*cis*-4-Amino-5-chloro-*N*-{1-[3-(4-fluorophenoxy)propyl]-3-methoxy-4-piperidyl}-2-methoxybenzamide Monohydrate, 1259·2
(*RS*)-Amino-3-(4-chlorophenyl)butyric Acid, 1386·3
2-Amino-3-(4-chlorophenyl)propionic Acid, 1687·2
Aminocid, 1793·3
Aminocina, 1793·3
7-Aminoclonazepam, 359·2
*p*-Aminoclonidine Hydrochloride, 864·1
Aminocont, 1793·3
Aminocyclitols, 120·1
Aminocyclitols, Aminoglycosidic, 116·2
(6*R*)-6-(1-Aminocyclohexanecarboxamido)penicillanic Acid, 188·1
4-Amino-*N*-[1-(3-cyclohexen-1-ylmethyl)-4-piperidyl]-2-ethoxy-5-nitrobenzamide, 1259·2
{(1*S*,4*R*)-4-[2-Amino-6-(cyclopropylamino)-9*H*-purin-9-yl]cyclopent-2-enyl}methanol, 625·2
5-Amino-1-cyclopropyl-7-(*cis*-3,5-dimethylpiperazin-1-yl)-6,8-difluoro-1,4-dihydro-4-oxoquinoline-3-carboxylic Acid, 255·1
(−)-(3*S*)-10-(1-Aminocyclopropyl)-9-fluoro-2,3-dihydro-3-methyl-7-oxo-7*H*-pyrido[1,2,3-*de*]-1,4-benzoxazine-6-carboxylic Acid Methanesulfonate, 241·3
4-Amino-1-(2-deoxy-2,2-difluoro-β-D-ribofuranosyl)pyrimidin-2(1*H*)-one Hydrochloride, 558·1
2-Amino-2-deoxy-β-D-glucopyranose, 1694·1
6-*O*-(3-Amino-3-deoxy-α-D-glucopyranosyl)-4-*O*-(6-amino-6-deoxy-α-D-glucopyranosyl)-$N^1$-[(2*S*)-4-amino-2-hydroxybutyryl]-2-deoxystreptamine, 154·1
6-*O*-(3-Amino-3-deoxy-α-D-glucopyranosyl)-4-*O*-(6-amino-6-deoxy-α-D-glucopyranosyl)-2-deoxystreptamine Sulphate Monohydrate, 225·1
4-*O*-(6-Amino-6-deoxy-α-D-glucopyranosyl)-1-*N*-(3-amino-L-lactoyl)-2-deoxy-6-*O*-(3-deoxy-4-*C*-methyl-3-methylamino-β-L-arabinopyranosyl)streptamine, 222·2
6-*O*-(3-Amino-3-deoxy-α-D-glucopyranosyl)-2-deoxy-4-*O*-(2,6-diamino-2,6-dideoxy-α-D-glucopyranosyl)-D-streptamine Sulphate, 162·2
6-*O*-(3-Amino-3-deoxy-α-D-glucopyranosyl)-2-deoxy-4-*O*-(2,6-diamino-2,3,4,6-tetradeoxy-α-D-*erythro*-hexopyranosyl)-streptamine Sulphate, 205·2
6-*O*-(3-Amino-3-deoxy-α-D-glucopyranosyl)-2-deoxy-4-*O*-(2,6-diamino-2,3,6-trideoxy-α-D-*ribo*-hexopyranosyl)streptamine, 271·2
*O*-3-Amino-3-deoxy-α-D-glucopyranosyl-(1→4)-*O*-[2,6-diamino-2,3,4,6-tetradeoxy-α-D-*erythro*-hexopyranosyl-(1→6)]-*N*′-[(2*S*)-4-amino-2-hydroxybutyryl]-2-deoxy-L-streptamine Sulphate, 158·3
*O*-6-Amino-6-deoxy-L-glycero-D-galactoheptopyranosylidene-(1→2-3)-*O*-β-D-talopyranosyl-(1→5)-2-deoxy-$N^3$-methyl-D-streptamine, 105·3
Aminodeoxykanamycin Sulphate, 162·2
4-Amino-4-deoxy-10-methylpteroyl-L-glutamic Acid, 568·2
4-Amino-1-(2-deoxy-β-D-*erythro*-pentofuranosyl)-1,3,5-triazin-2(1*H*)-one, 546·2
*trans*-4-(2-Amino-3,5-dibromobenzylamino)cyclohexanol Hydrochloride, 1114·3
2-Amino-3,5-dibromobenzyl(cyclohexyl)methylamine, 1115·3
1-(4-Amino-3,5-dichlorophenyl)-2-*tert*-butylaminoethanol Hydrochloride, 784·2
2-[(4-Amino-2,6-dichlorophenyl)imino]imidazolidine Hydrochloride, 864·1
(*RS*)-5-Amino-1-(2,6-dichloro-4-trifluoromethylphenyl)-4-(trifluoromethylsulfinyl)pyrazole-3-carbonitrile, 1505·3
*O*-{4-Amino-4,6-dideoxy-*N*-[(1*S*,4*R*,5*S*,6*S*)-4,5,6-trihydroxy-3-hydroxymethylcyclohex-2-enyl]-α-D-glucopyranosyl}-(1→4)-*O*-α-D-glucopyranosyl-(1→4)-D-glucopyranose, 328·3
4-Amino-*N*-(2-diethylaminoethyl)benzamide Hydrochloride, 987·1
3-Amino-9,13b-dihydro-1*H*-dibenz[*c*,*f*]imidazo[1,5-*a*]azepine Hydrochloride, 433·3
2-Amino-1,9-dihydro-9-(2-hydroxyethoxymethyl)-6*H*-purin-6-one, 626·1
2-Amino-3,5-dihydro-7-(3-pyridylmethyl)-4*H*-pyrrolo[3,2-*d*]pyrimidin-4-one, 579·1
(−)-2-Amino-2-(3,4-dihydroxybenzyl)propionic Acid Sesquihydrate, 953·2
(*R*)-2-Amino-1-(3,4-dihydroxyphenyl)ethanol, 974·3
(−)-2-Amino-1-(3,4-dihydroxyphenyl)propan-1-ol, 1675·3
(−)-(6*R*)-2-Amino-6-[(1*R*,2*S*)-1,2-dihydroxypropyl]- 5,6,7,8-Tetrahydro-4(3*H*)-pteridinone Dihydrochloride, 1742·1
2-Amino-1-(2,5-dimethoxyphenyl)propan-1-ol Hydrochloride, 953·1
1-(4-Amino-6,7-dimethoxyquinazolin-2-yl)-4-(1,4-benzodioxan-2-ylcarbonyl)piperazine Methanesulphonate, 908·3
1-(4-Amino-6,7-dimethoxy-2-quinazolinyl)-4-butyrylhexahydro-1*H*-1,4-diazepine Monohydrochloride, 878·1
*N*-{3-[4-Amino-6,7-dimethoxyquinazolin-2-yl(methyl)amino]propyl}tetrahydro-2-furamide Hydrochloride, 856·2
1-(4-Amino-6,7-dimethoxyquinazolin-2-yl)-4-(tetrahydro-2-furoyl)piperazine Hydrochloride Dihydrate, 1010·3
1-Amino-3,5-dimethyladamantane Hydrochloride, 1711·2
3-Amino-7-dimethylamino-2-methylphenazathionium Chloride, 1757·1
3-Amino-7-dimethylamino-2-methylphenazine Hydrochloride, 1719·3
$N^{2.1}$,$N^{2'.1'}$-(2-Amino-4,6-dimethyl-3-oxo-3*H*-phenoxazine-1,9-diyldicarbonyl)bis[threonyl-D-valylprolyl(*N*-methylglycyl)(*N*-methylvaline) 1.5–3.1-Lactone], 545·1
Aminodrip, 1793·3
Aminoefedrison NF, 1793·4
2-Aminoethanesulphonic Acid, 1752·1
2-Aminoethanethiol, 1712·1
2-Aminoethanol, 1716·1
2-Aminoethanol Compound with Oleic Acid, 1716·1
4-Amino-2-(ethoxymethyl)-α,α-dimethyl-1*H*-imidazo[4,5-*c*]quinoline-1-ethanol, 652·1
(4*R*,5*S*)-5-[(2-Aminoethyl)amino]-$N^2$-(10,12-dimethyltetradecanoyl)-4-hydroxy-L-ornithyl-L-threonyl-*trans*-4-hydroxy-L-prolyl-(*S*)-4-hydroxy-4-(*p*-hydroxyphenyl)-L-threonyl-*threo*-3-hydroxy-L-ornithyl-*trans*-3-hydroxy-L-proline Cyclic (6→1)-Peptide Diacetate, 395·3
*N*-(2-Aminoethyl)-5-chloropicolinamide, 1205·2
3-(2-Aminoethyl)-1*H*-indol-5-ol, 1743·2
4-(2-Aminoethyl)phenol Hydrochloride, 1760·1
4-(2-Aminoethyl)pyrocatechol Hydrochloride, 907·1
(*RS*)-4-Amino-*N*-[(1-ethylpyrrolidin-2-yl)methyl]-5-(ethylsulfonyl)-*o*-anisamide, 669·3
4-Amino-*N*-[(1-ethyl-2-pyrrolidinyl)methyl]-5-(ethylsulphonyl)-2-methoxybenzamide, 669·3
Aminofenazona, 14·2
Aminofilin, 1793·4
Aminofilina, 780·2
Aminofilina Hidratada, 780·2
Aminoflex, 1793·4
Aminofluid, 1793·4
7-Aminoflunitrazepam, 698·3
6-Amino-2-fluoromethyl-3-*o*-tolylquinazolin-4(3*H*)-one, 1386·3
4-Amino-5-fluoropyrimidin-2(1*H*)-one, 399·3
Aminoform, 230·1
*N*-[4-(2-Amino-5-formyl-5,6,7,8-tetrahydro-4-hydroxypteridin-6-ylmethylamino)benzoyl]-L(+)-glutamic Acid, 1431·1
Aminofusin Hepar, 1793·4
Aminofusin L Kohlenhydratfrei, 1793·4
Aminofusin N, 1793·4
Aminofusin 10% Plus, 1793·4
L-(+)-2-Aminoglutaramic Acid, 1433·2
L-(+)-2-Aminoglutaric Acid, 1433·2
L-(+)-2-Aminoglutaric Acid Hydrochloride, 1433·2
Aminoglutethimide, 526·3
Aminoglutetimida, 526·3
Aminoglycosides, 116·1
Aminoglycosidic Aminocyclitols, 116·2
Aminogran, 1793·4
Aminogran Mineral Mixture, 1793·4
Aminoguanidine, 344·1
2-Amino-4-(guanidinooxy)butyric Acid, 1649·1
(2*S*)-2-Amino-5-guanidinopentanoic Acid (2*S*)-2-Aminobutanedioate, 1421·1
L-2-Amino-5-guanidinovaleric Acid, 1421·1
6-Amino-1,1a,2,8,8a,8b-hexahydro-8-(hydroxymethyl)-8a-methoxy-1,5-dimethylazirino[2′,3′:3,4]pyrrolo[1,2-*a*]-indole-4,7-dione Carbamate Ester, 581·1
6-Amino-1,1a,2,8,8a,8b-hexahydro-8-hydroxymethyl-8a-methoxy-5-methylazirino[2′,3′:3,4]pyrrolo[1,2-*a*]indole-4,7-dione Carbamate, 573·3
(1*S*,2*S*,9*S*,9a*R*)-7-Amino-2,3,5,8,9,9a-hexahydro-9a-methoxy-6-methyl-5,8-dioxo-1,2-epimino-1-*H*-pyrrolo[1,2-*a*]indol-9-ylmethyl Carbamate, 573·3
Aminohexane Diphosphonate, 773·2
6-Aminohexanoic Acid, 741·3
4-Amino-5-hexenoic Acid, 383·2
4-Aminohex-5-enoic Acid, 383·2
Aminohippurate Sodium, 1653·2
Aminohippuric Acid, 1653·2
*p*-Aminohippuric Acid, 1653·2
Aminohipúrico, Ácido, 1653·2
α-Aminohydrocinnamic Acid, 1443·1
4-Amino-2-hydroxybenzoic Acid, 154·3
4-Amino-1-hydroxybutane-1,1-diylbis(phosphonic Acid), 765·3
Aminohydroxybutylidene Diphosphonic Acid, 765·3
L-2-Amino-3-hydroxybutyric Acid, 1451·1
3-Amino-4-hydroxybutyric Acid, 353·3
4-Amino-3-hydroxybutyric Acid, 353·2
2-Amino-*N*-(β-hydroxy-2,5-dimethoxyphenethyl)acetamide Hydrochloride, 959·2
(6-Amino-1-hydroxyhexylidene)diphosphonic Acid, 773·2
L-2-Amino-3-(5-hydroxy-1*H*-indol-3-yl)propionic Acid, 311·1
2-Amino-2-(hydroxymethyl)propane-1,3-diol, 1758·2
2-Amino-2-hydroxymethylpropane-1,3-diol Gluconate Dihydroxyaluminate, 1248·3
5-((1*S*,2*S*)-2-{(2*R*,6*S*,9*S*,11*R*,12*R*,14a*S*,-15*S*,16*S*,20*S*,23*S*,25a*S*)-20-[(1*R*)-3-Amino-1-hydroxy-3-oxopropyl]-2,11,12,15-tetrahydroxy-6-[(1*R*)-1-hydroxyethyl]-16-methyl-5,8,14,19,22,25-hexaoxo-9-[(4-{5-[4-(pentyloxy)phenyl]isoxazol-3-yl}benzoyl)amino]tetracosahydro-1*H*-dipyrrolo[2,1-*c*:2′,1′-*l*][1,4,7,10,13,16]hexaazacyclohenicosin-23-yl}-1,2-dihydroxyethyl)-2-hydroxyphenyl Sodium Sulfate, 405·2
(6*R*,7*R*)-7-[(*R*)-2-Amino-2-(*p*-hydroxyphenyl)acetamido]-8-oxo-3-(1-propenyl)-5-thia-1-azabicyclo[4.2.0]oct-2-ene-2-carboxylic Acid Monohydrate, 179·2
(−)-*N*-[(2*S*,3*R*)-3-Amino-2-hydroxy-4-phenylbutyryl]-L-leucine, 590·3
2-Amino-1-(3-hydroxyphenyl)ethanol Hydrochloride, 975·3
(−)-2-Amino-1-(3-hydroxyphenyl)propan-1-ol Hydrogen Tartrate, 952·2

L-2-Amino-3-(4-hydroxyphenyl)propionic Acid, 1451·1
L-2-Amino-3-hydroxypropionic Acid, 1444·3
1*N*-(*S*-3-Amino-2-hydroxypropionyl)-gentamicin B, 222·2
Aminohydroxypropylidenebisphosphonate, 773·3
Aminohydroxypropylidenebisphosphonate Disodium, 773·3
3-Amino-1-hydroxypropylidenebis(phosphonic Acid), 773·3
*N*-[4-(2-Amino-4-hydroxypteridin-6-ylmethylamino)benzoyl]-L(+)-glutamic Acid, 1429·1
2-Amino-3-hydroxy-2′-(2,3,4-trihydroxybenzyl)propionohydrazide, 1200·2
Aminoima, 1793·4
5-Aminoimidazole-4-carboxamide, 544·3
5-Aminoimidazole-4-carboxamide Orotate Dihydrate, 1724·2
5-Aminoimidazole-4-carboxamide Ureidosuccinate, 1760·3
L-2-Amino-3-(1*H*-imidazol-4-yl)propionic Acid, 1434·2
*N*-(Aminoiminomethyl)-*N*-methylglycine, 1677·2
L-2-Amino-3-(indol-3-yl)propionic Acid, 320·3
4-Amino-1-isobutyl-1*H*-imidazo[4,5-*c*]quinoline, 638·1
α-Aminoisocaproic Acid, 1439·1
2-Amino-7-isopropyl-5-oxo-5*H*-[1]benzopyrano[2,3-*b*]pyridine-3-carboxylic Acid, 781·1
α-Aminoisovaleric Acid, 1451·2
(+)-(*R*)-4-Aminoisoxazolidin-3-one, 202·1
δ-Aminolaevulinic Acid, 527·2
5-Aminolaevulinic Acid, 527·2
Aminolaevulinic Acid Hydrochloride, 527·2
Aminoleban, 1793·4
Aminoleban EN, 1793·4
5-Aminolevulinic Acid, 527·2
Aminolevulinic Acid Hydrochloride, 527·2
5-Aminolevulinic Acid Hydrochloride, 527·2
5-Aminolevulínico, Ácido, 527·2
Aminoliv, 1793·4
Aminomal, 1793·4
Aminomega, 1793·4
Aminomel Preparations, 1793·4
Amino-Mel Preparations, 1793·4
L-2-Amino-3-mercaptopropionic Acid, 1426·3
L-2-Amino-3-mercaptopropionic Acid Hydrochloride Monohydrate, 1426·3
2-Amino-6-mercaptopurine, 588·2
Aminomercuric Chloride, 1152·1
3-Amino-*N*-(α-methoxycarbonylphenethyl)succinamic Acid, 1422·1
4-Amino-6-methoxy-1-phenylpyridazinium Methylsulphate, 858·2
Aminomethyl Chlorohydrocinnamic Acid, 1386·3
Aminomethylbenzoic Acid, 742·1
4-Aminomethylbenzoic Acid, 742·1
(±)-4-(Aminomethyl)-1-benzyl-2-pyrrolidinone, 1719·2
(*S*)-2-Amino-3-methylbutanoic Acid, 1451·2
(±)-8-[(4-Amino-1-methylbutyl)amino]-2,6-dimethoxy-4-methyl-5-[(α,α,α-trifluoro-*m*-tolyl)oxy]quinoline, 463·3
(*RS*)-8-(4-Amino-1-methylbutylamino)-6-methoxyquinoline Diphosphate, 456·2
({2-[(*R*)-2-Amino-3-methylbutyramido]-1,1-dimethylethyl}thio)acetic Acid 8-Ester with (3a*S*,4*R*,5*S*,6*S*,8*R*,9*R*,9a*R*,10*R*)-Octahydro-5,8-dihydroxy-4,6,9,10-tetramethyl-6-vinyl-3a,9-propano-3a*H*-cyclopentacycloocten-1(4*H*)-one, 275·1
(2*S*,5*R*,6*R*)-6-{(2*R*)-2-[(2*R*)-2-Amino-3-(methylcarbamoyl)propionamido]-2-(*p*-hydroxyphenyl)acetamido}-3,3-dimethyl-7-oxo-4-thia-1-azabicyclo[3.2.0]-heptane-2-carboxylic Acid, 158·3
β-Aminomethyl-*p*-chlorohydrocinnamic Acid, 1386·3
1-(Aminomethyl)cyclohexaneacetic Acid, 362·2
*trans*-4-(Aminomethyl)cyclohexanecarboxylic Acid, 760·3
(±)-*cis*-2-(Aminomethyl)-*N*,*N*-diethyl-1-phenylcyclopropanecarboxamide Hydrochloride, 307·3
(±)-2-Amino-*N*-(1-methyl-1,2-diphenylethyl)acetamide, 377·2
L-2-Amino-3-(2-methylenecyclopropyl)propionic Acid, 1700·2
4-Amino-10-methylfolic Acid, 568·2
6-Amino-2-methylheptan-2-ol Hydrochloride, 1697·1
4-Aminomethyl-5-hydroxy-6-methyl-3-pyridinemethanol Hydrochloride, 1456·3
2-Amino-1-methyl-4-imidazolidinone, 1677·2
(*S*)-3-(Aminomethyl)-5-methylhexanoic Acid, 376·2
(±)-7-[3-(Aminomethyl)-4-oxo-1-pyrrolidinyl]-1-cyclopropyl-6-fluoro-1,4-dihydro-4-oxo-1,8-naphthyridine-3-carboxylic Acid $7^4$-(*Z*)-(*O*-Methyloxime) Methanesulfonate, 216·3
2-Amino-2-methylpropan-1-ol 8-Bromotheophyllinate, 978·2
2-Amino-2-methylpropan-1-ol Theophyllinate, 781·3
2-Amino-6-methyl-5-(4-pyridylthio)-4(3*H*)-quinazolinone, 576·3
*N*-(4-Amino-2-methylpyrimidin-5-ylmethyl)-*N*-(2-benzoylthio-4-dihydroxyphosphinyloxy-1-methylbut-1-enyl)formamide, 1454·3
3-[(4-Amino-2-methylpyrimidin-5-yl)methyl]-1-(2-chloroethyl)-1-nitrosourea Hydrochloride, 576·3
3-(4-Amino-2-methylpyrimidin-5-ylmethyl)-5-(2-hydroxyethyl)-4-methylthiazolium Chloride Hydrochloride, 1455·1
3-(4-Amino-2-methylpyrimidin-5-ylmethyl)-5-(2-hydroxyethyl)-4-methylthiazolium Nitrate, 1455·1
*N*-(4-Amino-2-methylpyrimidin-5-ylmethyl)-*N*-(4-hydroxy-1-methyl-2-propyldithiobut-1-enyl)formamide, 1455·1
*N*-(4-Amino-2-methylpyrimidin-5-ylmethyl)-*N*-[4-hydroxy-1-methyl-2-(tetrahydrofurfuryldithio)but-1-enyl]formamide, 1454·3
*N*-(4-Amino-2-methylpyrimidin-5-ylmethyl)-*N*-[1-(2-oxo-1,3-oxathian-4-ylidene)ethyl]formamide, 1454·3
4-Amino-*N*-(4-methyl-2-thiazolyl)benzenesulfonamide, 263·1
L-2-Amino-4-(methylthio)butyric Acid, 1042·1
DL-2-Amino-4-(methylthio)butyric Acid, 1042·1
Aminomethylthiopurine, 588·3
L-2-Amino-3-methylvaleric Acid, 1438·2
L-2-Amino-4-methylvaleric Acid, 1439·1
Aminometilbenzoico, Ácido, 742·1
Amino-Min-D, 1793·4
Aminomix, 1793·4
Aminomux, 1794·1
Aminonaphthone, 741·3
(−)-13β-Amino-5,6,7,8,9,10,11α,12-octahydro-5α-methyl-5,11-methanobenzocyclodecen-3-ol, 30·1
Amino-Opti-C, 1794·1
Amino-Opti-E, 1794·1
5-Amino-4-oxopentanoic Acid, 527·2
{[(*S*)-2-(4-Amino-2-oxo-1(2*H*)-pyrimidinyl)-1-(hydroxymethyl)ethoxy]methyl}phosphonic Acid, 629·2
Aminopad, 1794·1
Aminopan, 1794·1
Aminoped, 1794·1
Aminopenicillanic Acid, 118·3
Aminopentamide, 481·3
Aminopentamide Sulfate, 481·3
Aminophenazone, 14·2
Aminophenazone Salicylate, 14·2
Aminophenazone-sulfonate Calcium, 36·1
Aminophenazone-sulfonate Magnesium, 36·1
*m*-Aminophenol, 155·1
4-Aminophenylarsonic Acid, 158·3
2-(4-Aminophenyl)-2-ethylglutarimide, 526·3
3-(4-Aminophenyl)-3-ethylpiperidine-2,6-dione, 526·3
4-[(4-Aminophenyl)(4-iminocyclohexa-2,5-dien-1-ylidene)-methyl]aniline, 1185·1
4-[(4-Aminophenyl)(4-iminocyclohexa-2,5-dien-1-ylidene)methyl]-2-methylaniline, 1185·1
(1*RS*,2*SR*)-2-Amino-1-phenylpropan-1-ol, 1127·3
*threo*-2-Amino-1-phenylpropan-1-ol, 1585·2
L-2-Amino-3-phenylpropionic Acid, 1443·1
Aminophylline, 780·2
Aminophylline Hydrate, 780·2
Aminophylline Hydrochloride, 781·1
Aminophyllinum, 780·2
Aminoplasmal, 1794·1
Aminoplasmal E Kohlenhydratfrei, 1794·1
Aminoplasmal Elektrolyt- und Kohlenhydratfrei, 1794·1
Aminoplasmal Hepa, 1794·1
Aminoplasmal PO, 1794·1
Aminoplex, 1794·1
Aminoplex 12, 1794·1
Aminoplex 24, 1794·1
Aminopropilona, 14·2
7-{(1*R*,5*S*,6*s*)-6-[(*S*)-2-((*S*)-2-Aminopropionamido)propionamido]-3-azabicyclo[3.1.0]hex-3-yl}-1-(2,4-difluorophenyl)-6-fluoro-1,4-dihydro-4-oxo-1,8-naphthyridine-3-carboxylic Acid Monomethanesulphonate, 154·1
Aminopropionic Acid, 1574·1
L-2-Aminopropionic Acid, 1421·1
Aminopropionitrile, 21·2
β-Aminopropionitrile, 21·2
3-Aminopropionitrile, 21·2
β-Aminopropionitrilo, 21·2
2-Aminopropiono-2′,6′-xylidide, 1014·1
(*S*)-2-Aminopropiophenone, 1585·2
(±)-*N*-[({4-[(3-Aminopropyl)amino]butyl}carbamoyl)hydroxymethyl]-7-guanidinoheptanamide Trihydrochloride, 1360·2
*S*-[2-(3-Aminopropylamino)ethyl] Dihydrogen Phosphorothioate, 1031·3
Aminopropylon, 14·2
Aminopropylone, 14·2
Aminopropylone Hydrochloride, 14·2
(±)-4-(2-Aminopropyl)phenol Hydrobromide, 1699·3
(+)-(*S*)-*m*-(2-Aminopropyl)phenol Tartrate, 923·2
1-(4-Amino-2-propylpyrimidin-5-ylmethyl)-2-methylpyridinium Chloride Hydrochloride, 600·3
Aminopt, 1794·1
Aminopterin, 497·3
6-Aminopurine, 1647·3
2-Aminopurine-6-thiol, 588·2
2-Aminopurine-6(1*H*)-thione, 588·2
2-[(6-Amino-1*H*-purin-8-yl)amino]ethanol, 1685·2
{[2-(6-Amino-9*H*-purin-9-yl)ethoxy]methyl}phosphonic Acid, 628·1
2[2-(2-Amino-9*H*-purin-9-yl)ethyl]trimethylene Diacetate, 633·2
{[(*R*)-2-(6-Amino-9*H*-purin-9-yl)-1-methylethoxy]methyl}phosphonic Acid Monohydrate, 655·1
4-Aminopyridine, 1491·2
Aminopyrine, 14·2
Aminopyrine-sulphonate Sodium, 35·3
(±)-7-(3-Amino-1-pyrrolidinyl)-8-chloro-1-cyclopropyl-6-fluoro-1,4-dihydro-4-oxo-3-quinolinecarboxylic Acid Hydrochloride, 194·2
(±)-7-(3-Amino-1-pyrrolidinyl)-1-(2,4-difluorophenyl)-6-fluoro-1,4-dihydro-4-oxo-1,8-naphthyridine-3-carboxylic Acid, 272·2
4-Aminoquinoline Antimalarials, 444·1
8-Aminoquinoline Antimalarials, 444·1
Aminoquinurida, Hidrocloruro de, 1168·2
Aminoquinuride Hydrochloride, 1168·2
Aminoram, 1794·1
Aminorell, 1794·1
5-Amino-1-(β-D-ribofuranosyl)imidazole-4-carboxamide, 842·2
6-Amino-9-β-D-ribofuranosyl-9*H*-purine, 851·2
6-Amino-9-β-D-ribofuranosylpurine 5′-(Dihydrogen Phosphate), 1647·3
4-Amino-1-β-D-ribofuranosyl-1,3,5-triazin-2(1*H*)-one, 529·2
Aminosalicilato Cálcico, 155·1
Aminosalicilato Sódico, 155·1
Aminosalicílico, Ácido, 154·3
Aminosalicylate Calcium, 155·1
Aminosalicylate Sodium, 155·1
Aminosalicylic Acid, 154·3
4-Aminosalicylic Acid, 154·3
5-Aminosalicylic Acid, 1273·2, 1292·2
5-Amino-2-salicylic Acid, 1273·2
Aminosalylnatrium, 155·1
Aminosalylum, 154·3
Aminosidin Sulphate, 612·3
Aminosidine Sulphate, 612·3
Aminosol, 1794·1
Aminosolut, 1794·1
Aminostab, 1794·1
Aminosteril, 1794·1
Aminosteril 15%, 1794·1
Aminosteril KE Elektrolyt- u. Kohlenhydratfrei M, 1794·1
Aminosteril KE Kohlenhydratfrei, 1794·1
Aminosteril N-Hepa, 1794·1
Aminosteril Plus, 1794·2
Aminostress, 1794·2
[Aminosuberic Acid 1,7]-Eel Calcitonin, 768·3
L-Aminosuccinic Acid, 1422·3
5-(Aminosulphonyl)-4-chloro-*N*-(2,6-dimethylphenyl)-2-hydroxy-benzamide, 1029·2
*cis*-3-(Aminosulphonyl)-4-chloro-*N*-(2,6-dimethyl-1-piperidinyl)benzamide, 888·2
Aminosyn, 1794·2
Aminoterapia, 1794·2
Aminoterapia M, 1794·2
*O*-2-Amino-2,3,4,6-tetradeoxy-6-(methylamino)-*a*-D-*erythro*-hexopyranosyl-(1→4)-*O*-[3-deoxy-4-*C*-methyl-3-(methylamino)-β-L-arabinopyranosyl-(1→6)]-2-deoxy-D-streptamine Hemipentasulphate, 231·3
(*S*)-2-Amino-4,5,6,7-tetrahydro-6-(propylamino)benzothiazole Dihydrochloride Monohydrate, 1212·2
(−)-{(*E*)-3-[(6*R*,7*R*)-7-[2-(5-Amino-1,2,4-thiadiazol-3-yl)glyoxylamido]-2-carboxy-8-oxo-5-thia-1-azabicyclo[4.2.0]oct-2-en-3-yl]allyl}(carbamoylmethyl)ethylmethylammonium Hydroxide, Inner Salt, $7^2$-(*Z*)-[*O*-(Fluoromethyl)oxime], 173·2
(−)-1-{[(6*R*,7*R*)-7-[2-(5-Amino-1,2,4-thiadiazol-3-yl)glyoxylamido]-2-carboxy-8-oxo-5-thia-1-azabicyclo[4.2.0]oct-2-en-3-yl]methyl}-1*H*-imidazo[1,2-*b*]pyridazin-4-ium Hydroxide Inner Salt, $7^2$-(*Z*)-(*O*-Methyloxime), Hydrochloride, 178·2
7-[2-(2-Amino-1,3-thiazol-4-yl)acetamido]-3-[1-(2-dimethylaminoethyl)-1*H*-tetrazol-5-ylthiomethyl]-3-cephem-4-carboxylic Acid Dihydrochloride, 177·2
(*Z*)-(2-Aminothiazol-4-yl){[(2*S*,3*S*)-2-carbamoyloxymethyl-4-oxo-1-sulphoazetidin-3-yl]carbamoyl}methyleneamino-oxyacetic Acid, Disodium Salt, 166·3
7-[2-(2-Amino-1,3-thiazol-4-yl)-4-carboxyisocrotonamide]-3-cephem-4-carboxylic Acid, 182·1
(*Z*)-7-[2-(2-Aminothiazol-4-yl)-2-(carboxymethoxyimino)acetamido]-3-vinyl-3-cephem-4-carboxylic Acid Trihydrate, 172·3
(*Z*)-(7*R*)-7-[2-(2-Aminothiazol-4-yl)-2-(1-carboxy-1-methylethoxyimino)acetamido]-3-(1-pyridiniomethyl)-3-cephem-4-carboxylate Pentahydrate, 180·2
(6*R*,7*R*)-7-[2-(2-Amino-4-thiazolyl)-glyoxylamido]-3-mercaptomethyl-8-oxo-5-thia-1-azabicyclo[4.2.0]oct-2-ene-2-carboxylate, $7^2$-(*Z*)-(*O*-Methyloxime), 2-Furoate (Ester), Monohydrochloride, 182·2
(−)-(6*R*,7*R*)-7-[2-(2-Amino-4-thiazolyl)glyoxylamido]-8-oxo-3-vinyl-5-thia-1-azabicyclo[4.2.0]oct-2-ene-2-carboxylic Acid, $7^2$-(*Z*)-Oxime, 171·3

7-{(2-Amino-1,3-thiazol-4-yl)-2-[(*Z*)-hydroxyimino]acetamido}-3-vinylcephem-4-carboxylic Acid, 171·3
(*Z*)-7-[2-(2-Aminothiazol-4-yl)-2-methoxyiminoacetamido]-3-(5-carboxymethyl-4-methylthiazol-2-ylthiomethyl)-3-cephem-4-carboxylic Acid, Disodium Salt, 174·1
(*Z*)-7-[2-(2-Aminothiazol-4-yl)-2-methoxyiminoacetamido]-3-[(2,5-dihydro-6-hydroxy-2-methyl-5-oxo-1,2,4-triazin-3-yl)thiomethyl]-3-cephem-4-carboxylic Acid, Disodium Salt, Sesquaterhydrate, 182·3
(*Z*)-7-[2-(2-Amino-1,3-thiazol-4-yl)-2-methoxyiminoacetamido]-3-methoxymethyl-3-cephem-4-carboxylic Acid, 178·3
(*Z*)-7-[2-(2-Aminothiazol-4-yl)-2-methoxyiminoacetamido]-3-methyl-3-cephem-4-carboxylic Acid, 172·3
7-{(2-Amino-1,3-thiazol-4-yl)-2-[(*Z*)-methoxyimino]acetamido}-3-(1-methylpyrrolidiniomethyl)-3-cephem-4-carboxylate Hydrochloride, 172·1
(*Z*)-(7*R*)-7-[2-(2-Aminothiazol-4-yl)-2-methoxyiminoacetamido]-3-[(1-methyl-1*H*-tetrazol-5-yl)thiomethyl]-3-cephem-4-carboxylic Acid Hydrochloride, 173·2
(*Z*)-7-[2-(2-Aminothiazol-4-yl)-2-methoxyiminoacetamido]-3-(1-pyrindiniomethyl)-3-cephem-4-carboxylate Sulphate, 178·2
{6*R*-[6α,7β(*Z*)]}-1-[(7-{[(2-Amino-4-thiazolyl)-(methoxyimino)acetyl]amino}-2-carboxy-8-oxo-5-thia-1-azabicyclo[4.2.0]oct-2-en-3-yl)methyl]-1-methylpyrrolidinium Chloride Monohydrochloride Monohydrate, 172·1
{6*R*-[6α,7β(*Z*)]}-1-[(7-{[(2-Amino-4-thiazolyl)-(methoxyimino)acetyl]amino}-2-carboxy-8-oxo-5-thia-1-azabicyclo[4.2.0]oct-2-en-3-yl)methyl]-5,6,7,8,-tetrahydroquinolinium Sulfate (1:1), 179·3
(*Z*)-2-{2-Aminothiazol-4-yl-[(2*S*,3*S*)-2-methyl-4-oxo-1-sulphoazetidin-3-ylcarbamoyl]methyleneamino-oxy}-2-methylpropionic Acid, 160·3
α-Aminotoluene-*p*-sulphonamide, 228·2
7-[2-(α-Amino-*o*-tolyl)acetamido]-3-(1-carboxymethyl-1*H*-tetrazol-5-ylthiomethyl)-3-cephem-4-carboxylic Acid, 175·2
Aminotool, 1794·2
Aminotox, 1794·2
Aminotrans, 1794·2
4-Amino-6-(trichlorovinyl)benzene-1,3-disulphonamide, 103·3
(2*R*,3*S*,4*S*,5*R*,6*R*,8*R*,10*R*,11*R*,12*S*,13*R*)-5-(3-Amino-3,4,6-trideoxy-*N*,*N*-dimethyl-β-D-*xylo*-hexopyranosyloxy)-3-(2,6-dideoxy-3-*C*,3-*O*-dimethyl-α-L-*ribo*-hexopyranosyloxy)-13-ethyl-6,11,12-trihydroxy-2,4,6,8,10,12-hexamethyl-9-oxotridecan-13-olide, 208·1
(8*S*,10*S*)-10-(3-Amino-2,3,6-trideoxy-α-L-*arabino*-hexopyranosyloxy)-8-glycolloyl-7,8,9,10-tetrahydro-6,8,11-trihydroxy-1-methoxynaphthacene-5,12-dione Hydrochloride, 550·2
(4″*R*)-22-*O*-(3-Amino-2,3,6-trideoxy-3-*C*-methyl-α-L-*arabino*-hexopyranosyl)-$N^{3''}$-[*p*-(*p*-chlorophenyl)benzyl]vancomycin, 240·2
(8*S*,10*S*)-10-{[3-Amino-2,3,6-trideoxy-4-*O*-(2*R*-tetrahydro-2*H*-pyran-2-yl)-α-L-*lyxo*-hexopyranosyl]oxy}-8-glycoloyl-7,8,9,10-tetrahydro-6,8,11-trihydroxy-1-methoxy-5,12-naphthacenedione, 580·1
7-Amino-4,5,6-triethoxy-3-(5,6,7,8-tetrahydro-4-methoxy-6-methyl-1,3-dioxolo[4,5-*g*]isoquinolin-5-yl)phthalide, 443·3
2-Amino-6-(trifluoromethoxy) Benzothiazole, 1738·3
30-Amino-3,14,25-trihydroxy-3,9,14,20,25-penta-azatriacontane-2,10,13,21,24-pentaone Methanesulphonate, 1033·1
2-(3-Amino-2,4,6-tri-iodobenzyl)butyric Acid, 1065·1
2-[*N*-(3-Amino-2,4,6-tri-iodophenyl)acetamidomethyl]-propionic Acid, 1063·2
Aminotril, 1794·2
Aminotripa, 1794·2
α-Amino-δ-ureidovaleric Acid, 1425·2
Aminovac, 1794·2
Aminoveinte, 1794·2
Aminoven, 1794·2
Aminoven Infant, 1794·2
Aminovenoes N-Paed, 1794·2
Aminovenos Infant— *see* Aminoven Infant, 1794·2
Aminovenos N-Pad— *see* Aminovenoes N-Paed, 1794·2
Aminovenos Pad, 1794·2
Aminovenos Pad— *see* Aminoven Infant, 1794·2
Aminovit con Carnosina, 1794·2
Aminoxidin, 1794·2
Aminoxidin Sulbactam, 1794·2
Aminozim, 1794·2
Aminozyme, 1794·2
Aminsane, 1794·2
Amiobal, 1794·2
Amiobeta, 1794·2
Amiocar, 1794·2
Amiod, 1794·2
Amiodacore, 1794·2
Amiodar, 1794·3
Amiodarex, 1794·3
Amiodarona, Hidrocloruro de, 859·2
Amiodarone, 859·2
Amiodarone Hydrochloride, 859·2
Amiodaroni Hydrochloridum, 859·2
Amiodura, 1794·3
Amiogamma, 1794·3
Amiohexal, 1794·3
Amiopia, 1794·3
Amiorel, 1794·3
Amiorel Compuesto DM, 1794·3
Amioxid, 1794·3
Amiparen, 1794·3
Amiphenazole Chloride, 1584·3
Amiphenazole Hydrochloride, 1584·3
Amiphos, 1794·3
Amipramizide, 858·2
Amipress, 1794·3
Amiretic, 1794·3
Amirone, 1794·3
Amisol, 1794·3
Amisulprida, 669·3
Amisulpride, 669·3
Amisulpridum, 669·3
Amitacon, 1794·3
Ami-Tex LA, 1794·3
Amithiazide, 1794·3
Amithiozone, 269·3
Amitone, 1794·3
Amitraz, 1500·2
Amitrex, 1794·3
Amitrid, 1794·3
Amitrip, 1794·3
Amitriptilina, 280·3
Amitriptilina, Embonato de, 280·3
Amitriptilina, Hidrocloruro de, 280·3
Amitriptyline, 280·3
Amitriptyline Embonate, 280·3
Amitriptyline Hydrochloride, 280·3
Amitriptyline Oxide, 285·3
Amitriptylini Hydrochloridum, 280·3
Amitriptylinoxide, 285·3
Amitrol, 1794·3
Amitron, 1794·3
Amivia, 1794·3
Amix, 1794·3
Amixen, 1794·3
Amixen Plus, 1794·4
Amixx, 1794·4
Amiyec, 1794·4
Amiyodazol, 1794·4
Amiyu, 1794·4
Amizal, 1794·4
Amizet 10, 1794·4
Amizet 10X, 1794·4
Amizide, 1794·4
AMK, 1794·4
Amlactin, 1794·4
AmLactin AP, 1794·4
Amlexanox, 781·1
Amloc, 1794·4
Amlodac, 1794·4
Amlodin, 1794·4
Amlodine, 1794·4
Amlodipine Besilate, 862·1
(*S*)-Amlodipine Besilate, 862·2
Amlodipine Besylate, 862·1
Amlodipine Maleate, 862·1
Amlodipini Besilas, 862·1
Amlodipino, Besilato de, 862·1
Amlopine, 1794·4
Amloprax, 1794·4
Amlopres, 1794·4
Amlor, 1794·4
Amlotens, 1794·4
Amlovasc, 1794·4
Ammeltz, 1794·4
*Ammi majus*, 1153·1
Ammi Visnaga Fruit, 1653·3
Ammidene, 1794·4
Ammiformin, 1794·4
Ammi-Indocin, 1794·4
Ammilazo, 1795·1
Amminac, 1795·1
Ammirox, 1795·1
Ammitram, 1795·1
Ammi-Votara, 1795·1
Ammoidin, 1152·1
Ammon. Cit., 1654·1
Ammonaps, 1795·1
Ammonia, 1653·3, 1654·1
0.880 Ammonia, 1654·1
Ammonia $(^{13}N)$, 1525·1
Ammonia Alum, 1652·1
Ammonia Caramel, 1057·1
Ammonia, Muriate of, 1115·2
Ammonia Solution, Concentrated, 1653·3
Ammonia Solution, Dilute, 1653·3
Ammonia Solution, Strong, 1653·3
Ammonia Water, 1653·3
Ammoniaca, 1653·3
Ammoniacum, 1653·3
Ammoniae Dilutus, Liquor, 1653·3
Ammoniae Fortis, Liquor, 1653·3
Ammoniae, Liquor, 1653·3
Ammoniae Solutio Concentrata, 1653·3
Ammoniaque Officinale, 1653·3
Ammoniated Mercury, 1152·1
Ammonii Chloridum, 1115·2
Ammonii Hydrogenocarbonas, 1115·1
Ammonii Sulfogyrodalas, 1148·2
Ammonio Methacrylate Copolymer, 1714·3
Ammonio Methacrylate Copolymer Dispersion, 1714·3
Ammonio Methacrylate Copolymer (Type A), 1714·3
Ammonio Methacrylate Copolymer (Type B), 1714·3
Ammonio Sulfoittiolato, 1148·2
Ammonium Acetate, 1115·1
Ammonium Alginate, 1577·1
Ammonium Alum, 1652·1
Ammonium Bicarbonate, 1115·1
Ammonium Biphosphate, 1654·2
Ammonium Bithiolicum, 1148·2
Ammonium Bitumenosulfonicum, 1148·2
Ammonium Bituminosulphonate, 1148·2
Ammonium Bromide, 1662·3
Ammonium Camphocarbonate, 1585·1
Ammonium Camphorate, 1115·2
Ammonium Carbamate, 1115·1
Ammonium Carbonate, 1115·1
Ammonium Chloratum, 1115·2
Ammonium Chloride, 1115·2
Ammonium Citrate, 1654·1
Ammonium Citrate, Iron and, 1427·2
Ammonium Dichromate, 1670·3
Ammonium Ferric Citrate, 1427·2
Ammonium Fluoride, 1446·1
Ammonium Glycyrrhizate, 1270·3
Ammonium Glycyrrhizinate, 1115·2
Ammonium Hydricum Solutum, 1653·3
Ammonium Hydrogen Carbonate, 1115·1
Ammonium Hydroxide, 1653·3
Ammonium Ichthosulphonate, 1148·2
Ammonium Lactate, 1142·3
Ammonium Laurilsulfate, 1574·3
Ammonium Mandelate, 228·3
Ammonium Molybdate, 1440·3
Ammonium Monofluorophosphate, 1446·3
Ammonium Phosphate, 1654·1
Ammonium Polystyrene Sulfonate, 1053·3
Ammonium Salicylate, 14·2
Ammonium Silicofluoride, 1446·3
Ammonium Soaps, 1574·1
Ammonium Sulfobituminosum, 1148·2
Ammonium Sulpho-Ichthyolate, 1148·2
Ammonium (2*R*,3*S*,4*S*,5*R*,6*S*)-Tetrahydro-2-hydroxy-6-{(*R*)-1-[(2*S*,5*R*,7*S*,8*R*,9*S*)-9-hydroxy-2,8-dimethyl-2-{(2*S*,2′*R*,3′*S*,5*R*,5′*R*)-octahydro-2-methyl-3′-[(2*R*,4*S*,5*S*,6*S*)-tetrahydro-4,5-dimethoxy-6-methyl-2*H*-pyran-2-yl]oxy}-5′-[(2*S*,3*S*,5*R*,6*S*)-tetrahydro-6-hydroxy-3,5,6-trimethyl-2*H*-pyran-2-yl](2,2′-bifuran-5-yl)-1,6-dioxaspiro[4.5]dec-7-yl]ethyl}-4,5-dimethoxy-3-methyl-2*H*-pyran-2-acetate, 606·1
Ammonium Tetrathiomolybdate, 1032·1
Ammoniumbituminosulfonat Hell, 1148·2
Ammoniumsulfobitol, 1148·2
Amnesteem, 1795·1
Amniex, 1795·1
Amniolina, 1795·1
Amnion, 1654·2
Amnios, 1654·2
Amnivent, 1795·1
AMO Endosol, 1795·1
Amo Resan, 1795·1
AMO Vitrax, 1795·1
Amobarbital, 670·1
Amobarbital Sódico, 670·1
Amobarbital Sodium, 670·1
Amobarbitalum, 670·1
Amobarbitalum Natricum, 670·1
Amobay, 1795·1
Amobiotic, 1795·1
Amobronc, 1795·1
Amocarzina, 102·3
Amocarzine, 102·3
Amocasin, 1795·1
Amocetin, 1795·1
Amocid, 1795·1
Amocillin, 1795·1
Amocla, 1795·1
Amoclan, 1795·1
Amoclav, 1795·1
Amoclav, Adco- — *see* Adco-Amoclav, 1775·2
Amoclavam, 1795·1
Amoclave, 1795·1
Amoclax, 1795·1
Amocol, 1795·1
Amodex, 1795·1
Amodiaquina, 446·3
Amodiaquina, Hidrocloruro de, 446·3
Amodiaquine, 446·3
Amodiaquine Hydrochloride, 446·3
Amodiaquine Quinone Imine, 447·1
Amodiaquini Hydrochloridum, 446·3
Amodivyr, 1795·2
Amoebiasis, 595·2
Amoebic Encephalitis, Granulomatous— *see* Disseminated Acanthamoeba Infection, 595·2
Amoebic Infections, 595·1
Amoebic Meningoencephalitis, Primary— *see* Primary Amoebic Meningoencephalitis, 595·3
Amofat, 1795·2
Amofil, 1795·2
Amoflamisan, 1795·2
Amoflux, 1795·2
Amohexal, 1795·2
Amoksiklav, 1795·2
Amol Heilkrautergeist N, 1795·2
Amolex, 1795·2
Amolgen, 1795·2
Amolin, 1795·2
Am-O-Lin, 1795·2
Amoníaco, Solución Diluida de, 1653·3
Amonio, Acetato de, 1115·1
Amonio, Bicarbonato de, 1115·1
Amonio, Carbonato de, 1115·1
Amonio, Cloruro de, 1115·2
Amopen, 1795·2
Amophar, 1795·2
Amor de Hortelano, 1673·2

Amoram, 1795·2
Amorion, 1795·2
Amorion— *see* Helipak A, 2038·2
Amorion— *see* Helipak K, 2038·2
Amorolfina, Hidrocloruro de, 391·1
Amorolfine, 391·1
Amorolfine Hydrochloride, 391·1
*Amorphophallus konjac*, 1693·3
Amosan, 1795·2
Amosite, 1658·1
Amosol, 1795·2
Amosulalol, Hidrocloruro de, 862·3
Amosulalol Hydrochloride, 862·3
Amosyt, 1795·2
Amotein, 1795·2
Amoval, 1795·2
Amoval Duo, 1795·2
Amox, 1795·2
Amoxa, 1795·2
Amoxal, 1795·2
Amoxanox, 781·1
Amoxapen, 1795·2
Amoxapina, 286·3
Amoxapine, 286·3
Amoxaren, 1795·2
Amoxcillin, 1795·3
Amox-G, 1795·3
Amox-G Bronquial, 1795·3
Amoxi, 1795·3
Amoxi Gobens, 1795·3
Amoxi Gobens Mucol, 1795·3
Amoxi Respiratorio, 1795·3
Amoxibacter, 1795·3
Amoxi-basan, 1795·3
Amoxibeta, 1795·3
Amoxibiocin, 1795·3
Amoxibiot, 1795·3
Amoxibron, 1795·3
Amoxicap, 1795·3
Amoxicilina, 155·3
Amoxicilina Sódica, 155·3
Amoxicilina Trihidrato, 155·3
Amoxicillin, 155·3
Amoxicillin Sodium, 155·3
Amoxicillin Trihydrate, 155·3
Amoxicillinum Natricum, 155·3
Amoxicillinum Trihydricum, 155·3
Amoxicina, 1795·3
Amoxiclav, 1795·3
Amoxi-Clavulan, 1795·3
Amoxicler, 1795·3
Amoxi-Cophar, 1795·3
Amoxid, 1795·3
Amoxidal, 1795·3
Amoxidal Duo, 1795·3
Amoxidal Respiratorio, 1795·3
Amoxidal Respiratorio Duo, 1795·3
Amoxidel, 1795·3
Amoxidel Bronquial, 1795·3
Amoxident, 1795·3
Amoxidil, 1795·3
Amoxi-Diolan, 1795·3
Amoxidoc, 1795·3
Amoxidura Plus, 1795·4
Amoxifar, 1795·4
Amoxifar Balsamico, 1795·4
Amoxifur, 1795·4
Amoxigran, 1795·4
Amoxigrand, 1795·4
Amoxigrand Bronquial, 1795·4
Amoxigrand Compuesto, 1795·4
Amoxi-Hefa, 1795·4
Amoxihexal, 1795·4
Amoxil, 1795·4
Amoxil— *see* Klacid HP 7, 2080·1
Amoxil— *see* Losec Helicopak, 2105·4
Amoxil— *see* Losec Hp 7, 2105·4
Amoxilan, 1795·4
Amoxillat, 1795·4
Amoxillat-Clav, 1795·4
Amoxillin, 1795·4
Amoximedical, 1795·4
Amoxi-Mepha, 1795·4
Amoximerck, 1795·4
Amoximex, 1795·4
Amoxin, 1795·4
Amoxin Comp, 1795·4
Amoxina, 1795·4
Amoxinovag, 1795·4
Amoxi-Ped, 1795·4
Amoxipen, 1795·4
Amoxipenil, 1795·4
Amoxipenil Bronquial, 1795·4
Amoxiplus, 1795·4
Amoxipoten, 1796·1
Amoxi-Puren, 1796·1
Amoxisol, 1796·1
Amoxistad, 1796·1
Amoxitab, 1796·1
Amoxi-Tablinen, 1796·1
Amoxitan, 1796·1
Amoxitenk, 1796·1
Amoxitenk Plus, 1796·1
Amoxitenk Respiratorio, 1796·1
Amoxivan, 1796·1
Amoxivet, 1796·1
Amoxi-Wolff, 1796·1
Amoxtiol, 1796·1
Amoxy, 1796·1
Amoxycillin, 155·3
Amoxycillin Sodium, 155·3
Amoxycillin Trihydrate, 155·3
Amoxyfizz, 1796·1
Amoxylin, 1796·1
Amoxypen, 1796·1
Amoxyplus, 1796·1
Amoxyvinco Mucolitico— *see* Halitol Mucolitico, 2035·2
AMP, 1647·3
A-5MP, 1647·3
Ampamet, 1796·1
Amparax, 1796·1
Ampat, 1796·1
Ampavit, 1796·1
Ampecyclal, 1796·1
Amperozida, 670·3
Amperozide, 670·3
Ampex, 1796·1
Ampexin, 1796·1
Amphetamine, 1584·3
Amphetamine Sulfate, 1584·3
Amphetamine Sulphate, 1584·3
Amphetaminil, 1584·3
Amphiboles, 1658·1
Amphisept, 1796·1
Amphisept E, 1796·1
Amphocil, 1796·1
Amphocycline, 1796·1
Amphodyn, 1796·2
Amphojel, 1796·2
Amphojel 500, 1796·2
Amphojel Plus, 1796·2
Ampholysine Plus, 1796·2
Ampholytic Surfactants, 1574·1
Ampho-Moronal, 1796·2
Ampho-Moronal V, 1796·2
Ampho-Moronal V L, 1796·2
Amphosca a l'Orchitine, 1796·2
Amphosca a l'Ovarine, 1796·2
Amphosca Orchitine, 1796·2
Amphosca Ovarine, 1796·2
Amphosept BV, 1796·2
Amphotec, 1796·2
Amphoteric Surfactants, 1574·1
Amphotericin, 391·2
Amphotericin A, 391·2
Amphotericin B, 391·2
Ampho-Vaccin Intestinal, 1796·2
Ampi, 1796·2
Ampibac, 1796·2
Ampibal, 1796·2
Ampi-Bis, 1796·2
Ampi-Bis Plus, 1796·2
Ampicap, 1796·2
Ampicidar, 1796·2
Ampiciflan, 1796·2
Ampicil, 1796·2
Ampicilase, 1796·2
Ampicilib, 1796·2
Ampicilina, 157·1
Ampicilina Sódica, 157·1
Ampicilina Trihidrato, 157·2
Ampicillin, 157·1, 157·2
Ampicillin, Anhydrous, 157·1
Ampicillin Benzathine, 158·1
Ampicillin Ethoxycarbonyloxyethyl Hydrochloride, 161·2
Ampicillin, Pivaloyloxymethyl Ester, 244·2
Ampicillin Sodium, 157·1
Ampicillin Trihydrate, 157·2
Ampicillinnatrium, 157·1
Ampicillinum, 157·1
Ampicillinum Anhydricum, 157·1
Ampicillinum Natricum, 157·1
Ampicillinum Trihydricum, 157·2
Ampicilon, 1796·2
Ampicimax, 1796·3
Ampicin, 1796·3
Ampicler, 1796·3
Ampicler com Probenecide, 1796·3
Ampiclox, 1796·3
Ampiclox-D, 1796·3
Ampicrom, 1796·3
Ampicyn, 1796·3
Ampidrat, 1796·3
Ampifar, 1796·3
Ampifar Balsamico, 1796·3
Ampifen, 1796·3
Ampigen, 1796·3
Ampigen SB, 1796·3
Ampigran, 1796·3
Ampigrand, 1796·3
Ampigrin, 1796·3
Ampilevel, 1796·3
Ampilin, 1796·3
Ampilisa, 1796·3
Ampillin, 1796·3
Ampilon, 1796·3
Ampilong, 1796·3
Ampilox, 1796·3
Ampilux, 1796·3
Ampimax, 1796·3
Ampimex, 1796·4
Ampina, 1796·4
Ampipen, 1796·4
Ampiplus, 1796·4
Ampiplus Simplex, 1796·4
Ampi-Quim, 1796·4
Ampiretard, 1796·4
Ampiroxicam, 14·2
Ampiset, 1796·4
Ampispectrin, 1796·4
Ampisuspen, 1796·4
Ampitab, 1796·4
Ampi-Tecno, 1796·4
Ampitenk, 1796·4
Ampitotal, 1796·4
Ampival, 1796·4
Ampixen, 1796·4
Ampizan, 1796·4
Amplacilina, 1796·4
Amplal, 1796·4
Amplamox, 1796·4
Amplavit, 1796·4
Amplexol, 1796·4
Ampliactil, 1796·4
Ampliar, 1796·4
Amplibenzatin Bronquial, 1796·4
Amplictil, 1796·4
Amplidermis, 1796·4
Amplifar, 1796·4
Ampligen, 1797·1
Amplimed, 1797·1
Ampliron, 1797·1
Amplital, 1797·1
Amplitor, 1797·1
Amplium, 1797·1
Amplium-G, 1797·1
Amplizer, 1797·1
Amplofen, 1797·1
Amplomicina, 1797·1
Amplospec, 1797·1
Amplotal, 1797·1
Amplozol, 1797·1
Amplus, 1797·1
Ampoxin, 1797·1
Ampoxin-LB, 1797·1
Ampra, 1797·1
Amprace, 1797·1
Amprenavir, 628·2
Amprexyl, 1797·1
Ampro, 1797·1
Amprolio, Hidrocloruro de, 600·3
Amprolium, 600·3
Amprolium Hydrochloride, 600·3
AMR-69, 1732·3
Amrinona, 862·3
Amrinona, Lactato de, 862·3
Amrinone, 862·3
Amrinone Lactate, 862·3
Amrubicin, 527·3
AMS, 1797·1
*m*-AMSA, 527·3
Amsa P-D, 1797·1
Amsacrina, 527·3
Amsacrine, 527·3
Amsapen, 1797·1
Amsidine, 1797·1
Amsidyl, 1797·2
Amsulosin Hydrochloride, 1009·2
Amsupros, 1797·2
AMT, 1797·2
Amtolmetin Guacil, 14·3
Amtolmetina Guacilo, 14·3
Amuchina, 1797·2
Amuchina Med, 1797·2
Amuclan, 1797·2
Amuclean, 1797·2
Amuctol, 1797·2
Amukin, 1797·2
Amukine, 1797·2
Amukine Med, 1797·2
A-Mulsin, 1797·2
A-Mulsion, 1797·2
Amuno, 1797·2
Amunovax, 1797·2
Amvey, 1797·2
Amvisc, 1797·2
AMX, 1797·2
Amxol, 1797·2
Amyben, 1797·2
Amycil, 1797·2
*Amycolatopsis coloradensis*, 159·1
*Amycolatopsis mediterranei*, 253·2
*Amycolatopsis orientalis*, 275·2
Amycor, 1797·2
Amycor Onychoset, 1797·2
Amydramine, 1797·2
Amydramine II, 1797·2
Amydramine Paediatric, 1797·2
Amygdalae Oleum Raffinatum, 1651·1
Amygdalae Oleum Virginale, 1651·1
Amygdalic Acid, 228·3
Amygdalin, 1704·3
Amygdol, 1797·2
Amygdorectol, 1797·2
Amygdospray, 1797·2
Amykon, 1797·3
Amyl Acetate, 1471·2
*iso*-Amyl Acetate, 1471·2
*n*-Amyl Acetate, 1471·2
*sec*-Amyl Acetate, 1471·2
Amyl Alcohol, Tertiary, 1471·2
Amyl Dimethylaminobenzoate, 1155·1
Amyl Nitrite, 1032·1
Amyl Salicylate, 14·3
Amylase, 1654·2
Amylatin, 1797·3
Amyleinii Chloridum, 1370·2
Amylene Hydrate, 1471·2
Amylin, 344·3
Amylis Nitris, 1032·1
Amylium Nitrosum, 1032·1
Amylmetacresol, 1168·2
Amylobarbitone, 670·1
Amylobarbitone Sodium, 670·1
Amylobarbitone, Soluble, 670·1
Amylocain. Hydrochlor., 1370·2
Amylocaine Hydrochloride, 1370·2
Amylodiastase, 1797·3
Amyloglucosidases, 1654·2
Amyloidosis, 567·1
Amylopectin, 1449·1
Amylose, 1449·1

Amylum, 1449·1
Amylum Marantae, 1422·1
Amylum Pregelificatum, 1449·1
Amyotrophic Lateral Sclerosis— *see* Motor Neurone Disease, 1739·1
Amytal, 1797·3
Amytril, 1797·3
Amze, 1797·3
Amzepril, 1797·3
AN 1, 1797·3
AN-021, 1395·3
AN-448, 1589·1
AN-1324, 333·1
ANA-756, 1009·3
Anabact, 1797·3
Anabar, 1797·3
Anabet, 1797·3
Anabol, 1797·3
Anabol-Hevert, 1797·3
Anabolic Steroids, 1527·2
Anaboline Depot, 1797·3
Anabol-loges, 1797·3
Anabron, 1797·3
Anacal, 1797·3
Anacalcit, 1797·3
Anacaps, 1797·3
Anacervix, 1797·3
Anacidol, 1797·3
Anacidron, 1797·3
Anacidron-H, 1797·3
Anacin, 1797·3
Anacin-3— *see* Aspirin Free Anacin, 1816·3
Anacin with Codeine, 1797·3
Anaclosil, 1797·4
Anacrodyne, 1797·4
Anacyclin, 1797·4
Anadekin, 1797·4
Anadent, 1797·4
Anadermin, 1797·4
Anadin, 1797·4
Anadin Cold Control, 1797·4
Anadin Cold Control Flu Strength, 1797·4
Anadin Extra, 1797·4
Anadin Ibuprofen, 1797·4
Anadin Paracetamol, 1797·4
Anadin Ultra, 1797·4
Anadol, 1797·4
Anador, 1797·4
Anadrol, 1797·4
Anadvil, 1797·4
Anadvil Rhume, 1797·4
Anaebell, 1797·4
Anaemia, Aplastic— *see* Aplastic Anaemia, 732·1
Anaemia, Fanconi's— *see* Aplastic Anaemia, 732·1
Anaemia, Folate-deficiency— *see* Megaloblastic Anaemia, 734·1
Anaemia, Haemolytic— *see* Haemolytic Anaemia, 733·1
Anaemia, Hypochromic, 732·1
Anaemia, Iron-deficiency— *see* Iron-deficiency Anaemia, 733·2
Anaemia, Megaloblastic— *see* Megaloblastic Anaemia, 734·1
Anaemia, Normochromic, 732·1
Anaemia, Normocytic-normochromic— *see* Normocytic-normochromic Anaemia, 734·2
Anaemia, Pernicious— *see* Megaloblastic Anaemia, 734·1
Anaemia of Prematurity— *see* Normocytic-normochromic Anaemia, 734·2
Anaemia of Renal Failure— *see* Normocytic-normochromic Anaemia, 734·2
Anaemia, Sideroblastic— *see* Sideroblastic Anaemia, 734·2
Anaemia, Vitamin $B_{12}$-deficiency— *see* Megaloblastic Anaemia, 734·1
Anaemias, 732·1
Anaemodoron, 1797·4
Anaerobex, 1797·4
Anaerobic Bacterial Infections, 121·1
Anaerobic Vaginosis— *see* Bacterial Vaginosis, 121·2
Anaeromet, 1797·4
Anaestalgin, 1797·4
Anaesthecomp N, 1797·4
Anaestherit, 1797·4
Anaesthesia, Balanced— *see* Anaesthetic Techniques, 1296·2
Anaesthesia, Dissociative— *see* Anaesthetic Techniques, 1296·2
Anaesthesia, General— *see* Anaesthesia, 1296·1
Anaesthesia, Induction of— *see* Anaesthesia, 1296·1
Anaesthesia, Infiltration— *see* Infiltration Anaesthesia, 1370·1
Anaesthesia, Intravenous Regional— *see* Intravenous Regional Anaesthesia, 1370·1
Anaesthesia, Local, 1369·1
Anaesthesia, Maintenance of— *see* Anaesthesia, 1296·1
Anaesthesia, Neuromuscular Blockade in— *see* Anaesthesia, 1397·1
Anaesthesia, Surface— *see* Surface Anaesthesia, 1370·2
Anaesthesia, Topical— *see* Surface Anaesthesia, 1370·2
Anaesthesia, Total Intravenous— *see* Anaesthetic Techniques, 1296·2
Anaesthesin, 1797·4
Anaesthesin N, 1797·4
Anaesthesin-Rivanol, 1797·4
Anaesthesinum, 1370·3
Anaesthesulf, 1798·1
Anaesthetic Compound No. 347, 1298·1
Anaesthetic Ear Drops, 1798·1
Anaesthetic Ether, 1298·3
Anaesthetics, General, 1295·1
Anaesthetics, Local, 1367·1
Anaesthol, 1798·1
Anafen, 1798·1
Anafertin, 1798·1
Anaflam, 1798·1
Anaflex, 1798·1
Ana-Flex, 1798·1
Anaflin, 1798·1
Anafortan, 1798·1
Anafranil, 1798·1
Anagastra, 1798·1
Anagen, 1798·1
Anagregal, 1798·1
Anagrelida, Hidrocloruro de, 1654·3
Anagrelide Hydrochloride, 1654·3
Ana-Guard, 1798·1
Anahelp, 1798·1
Anakinra, 14·3
Anakit, 1798·1
Ana-Kit, 1798·1
Anal Fissure, 1390·1
Analab, 1798·1
Analept, 1798·1
Analeric, 1798·1
Analfin, 1798·1
Analgen, 1798·1
Anal-Gen, 1798·2
Analgen-SA, 1798·2
Analgesia Creme, 1798·2
Analgesia in Intensive Care— *see* Intensive Care, 666·3
Analgesia, Patient-augmented— *see* Patient-controlled Analgesia, 3·3
Analgesia, Patient-controlled— *see* Patient-controlled Analgesia, 3·3
Analgesia, Pre-emptive— *see* Postoperative Analgesia, 4·1
Analgesic Adjuvants, 3·1
Analgesic Balm, 1798·2
Analgesic Ladder— *see* Cancer Pain, 5·1
Analgesic/Calmative, 1798·2
Analgesico Ut Asens Fn, 1798·2
Analgésicos Opiáceos, 71·2
Analgesics, 1·1
Analgesics Anti-inflammatory Drugs and Antipyretics, 1·1
Analgesics, Inhalational, 3·1
Analgesics, Opioids, 71·2
Analgesics, Topical, 4·3
Analgesil, 1798·2
Analgesin, 1798·2
Analgésine, 82·3
Analgex, 1798·2
Analgex C, 1798·2
Analgil, 1798·2
Analgilasa, 1798·2
Analgin, 1798·2
Analgin C-R, 1798·2
Analgina, 1798·2
Analgine, 1798·2
Analginum, 35·3
Analgiol, 1798·2
Analgiplus, 1798·2
Analgit, 1798·2
Analgosedan, 1798·2
Analip, 1798·3
Analka, 1798·3
Analmex, 1798·3
Analmorph, 1798·3
Analog LCP, 1798·3
Analog MSUD, 1798·3
Analog, MSUD— *see* MSUD Analog, 2142·2
Analog RVHB, 1798·3
Analog XLEU, 1798·3
Analog XLYS, 1798·3
Analog XLYS Low Try, 1798·3
Analog XMET, 1798·3
Analog, XMET— *see* XMET Analog, 2388·3
Analog XMET, Cys, 1798·3
Analog Xmet, Thre, Val, Isoleu— *see* Analog XMTVI, 1798·3
Analog XMTVI, 1798·3
Analog, XMTVI— *see* XMTVI Analog, 2388·3
Analog XP, 1798·3
Analog, XP— *see* XP Analog, 2388·4
Analog XP— *see* XP Analog LCP, 2388·4
Analog Xphen, Tyr, 1798·3
Analog XPTM, 1798·3
Analpan, 1798·3
Analpram-HC, 1798·3
Analsona, Neo— *see* Neo Analsona, 2156·1
Analter, 1798·3
Analtrix, 1798·3
Analux, 1798·3
Analverin, 1798·3
Analverin Composto, 1798·3
Analverin Plus, 1798·3
Anamai, 1798·3
AnaMantle HC, 1798·3
Anamine, 1798·3
Anamorph, 1798·3
*Ananas comosus*, 1662·3
*Ananas sativus*, 1662·3
Ananase, 1798·3
Ananase Forte, 1798·4
Anandron, 1798·4
Anapen, 1798·4
Anapenil, 1798·4
Anaphase, 1798·4
Anaphyl, 1798·4
Anaphylactic Shock, 855·2
Anaphylaxie-Besteck, 1798·4
Anaphylaxis— *see* Anaphylactic Shock, 855·2
Anaphylaxis, Idiopathic— *see* Urticaria and Angioedema, 1138·3
Anapirol, 1798·4
Anaplex, 1798·4
Anaplex DM, 1798·4
Anaplex HD, 1798·4
Anapolon, 1798·4
Anapres, 1798·4
Anapril, 1798·4
Anaprol, 1798·4
Anaprolina, 1798·4
Anaprox, 1798·4
Anapsique, 1798·4
Anapsyl, 1798·4
Anaptivan, 1798·4
Anapyon, 1798·4
Anara, 1798·4
Anarex, 1798·4
Anargil, 1798·4
Anaribes, 1799·1
Anaritide, 964·2
Anartril, 1799·1
Anartrit, 1799·1
Anasclerol, 1799·1
Anased, 1799·1
Anaseptil, 1799·1
Anasilpiel, 1799·1
Anasma, 1799·1
Anaspaz, 1799·1
Anassa, 1666·1
Anastase, 1799·1
Anasten, 1799·1
Anastil, 1799·1
Anastil N, 1799·1
Anastim con RTH, 1799·1
Anastrozol, 528·1
Anastrozole, 528·1
Anatac, 1799·1
Anatensol, 1799·1
Anatetall, 1799·1
Anatine, 1799·1
Anatopic, 1799·1
Anatoxal Di, 1799·1
Anatoxal Di Te, 1799·1
Anatoxal Di Te Berna, 1799·1
Anatoxal Di Te Per, 1799·1
Anatoxal Te, 1799·2
Anatoxal Te Di, 1799·2
Anatoxal-TE-Berna, 1799·2
Anatoxina Estafilococica, 1799·2
Anatrast, 1799·2
Anatuss, 1799·2
Anatuss DM, 1799·2
Anatuss LA, 1799·2
Anatyl, 1799·2
Anauran, 1799·2
Anaus, 1799·2
Anausin, 1799·2
Anavix, 1799·2
Anax, 1799·2
Anaxeryl, 1799·2
Anazo, 1799·2
Anbesol, 1799·2
Anbesol Baby, 1799·2
Anbesol, Baby— *see* Baby Anbesol, 1824·2
Anbesol, Maximum Strength— *see* Maximum Strength Anbesol, 2116·3
Anbifen, 1799·2
Anbikan, 1799·2
Anbikin, 1799·2
Anbin, 1799·2
Anbycin, 1799·2
Ancamin, 1799·3
Ancef, 1799·3
Anceron, 1799·3
Ancestim, 742·2
Ancet, 1799·3
Anchocalm, 1799·3
Anchoic Acid, 1142·3
Ancid, 1799·3
Ancivin, 1799·3
Anclomax, 1799·3
Anco, 1799·3
Ancobon, 1799·3
Ancoloxin, 421·1
Anconevron, 1799·3
Ancopir, 1799·3
Ancoren, 1799·3
Ancoron, 1799·3
Ancotil, 1799·3
Ancrod, 863·2
Ancylostomiasis— *see* Hookworm Infections, 99·2
Andante, 1799·3
Andantol, 1799·3
Andapsin, 1799·3
Andehist, 1799·3
Andehist DM, 1799·3
Andergin, 1799·3
Anderson-Fabry Disease, 1651·2
Andil, 1799·3
Andilex, 1799·3
Andion, 1799·3
Andociclina Balsamica, 1799·3
Andolba, 1799·4
Andolex, 1799·4
Andolex-C, 1799·4

Andolor, 1799·4
Andopan, 1799·4
Andoprim, 1799·4
Andornkraut, 1124·1
Andox, 1799·4
Andractim, 1799·4
Andre, 1799·4
Andreafol, 1799·4
Andregen, 1799·4
Andre-I-Kul, 1799·4
Andrews, 1799·4
Andrews Answer, 1799·4
Andrews Antacid, 1799·4
Andrews, Sais— *see* Sais Andrews, 2273·4
Andrews, Sal de— *see* Sal de Andrews, 2273·4
Andrews Tums Antacid, 1799·4
Andrioderma, 1799·4
Andriodermol, 1799·4
Andriol, 1799·4
Androbloc, 1799·4
Androcur, 1799·4
Androderm, 1799·4
Andro-Diane, 1800·1
Androdor, 1800·1
Androfemon, 1800·1
AndroGel, 1800·1
Androgenetic Alopecia— *see* Alopecia, 1134·1
Androgens, 1527·1
Android, 1800·1
Androlic, 1800·1
Androlip, 1800·1
Androlistica, 1800·1
Androlone-D, 1800·1
Andropatch, 1800·1
Andropel, 1800·1
Andropository, 1800·1
Androskat, 1800·1
Androstanazole, 1569·2
Androstanolo, 1541·3
Androstanolona, 1541·3
Androstanolone, 1541·3
Androstat, 1800·1
Androstenedione, 1542·1
Androst-4-ene-3,17-dione, 1542·1
Androstenodiona, 1542·1
Androsteron, 1800·1
Androsterone, 1571·2
Androtardyl, 1800·1
Androvite, 1800·1
Androxicam, 1800·1
Androxinon, 1800·1
Androxon, 1800·1
Androxyl, 1800·1
Andrumin, 1800·1
Andursil, 1800·1
Andursil N, 1800·1
Anebron, 1800·1
Anectine, 1800·1
Anekron, 1800·1
Anemagen, 1800·1
Anemagen OB, 1800·1
*Anemarrhena asphodeloides*, 1750·2
Anemet, 1800·2
Anemidox, 1800·2
Anemidox-Ferrum, 1800·2
Anemital, 1800·2
Anemix, 1800·2
Anemofer, 1800·2
Anemokol, 1800·2
*Anemone pulsatilla*, 1737·1
Anemul Mono, 1800·2
Anencephaly— *see* Neural Tube Defects, 1430·1
Anerex, 1800·2
Anergan, 1800·2
Anervan, 1800·2
Anesdente Do Bebe, 1800·2
Anespas, 1800·2
Anest Compuesto, 1800·2
Anestacon, 1800·2
Anestalcon, 1800·2
Anestesi Doble, 1800·2
Anestesia Loc Braun C/A, 1800·2
Anestesia Loc Braun S/A, 1800·2
Anestesia Topi Braun C/A, 1800·2
Anestesia Topi Braun S/A, 1800·2
Anestesico, 1800·2
Anestesiol, 1800·3
Anesthal, 1800·3
Anesthamine, 1370·3
Anesthesique Double, 1800·3
Anestina Braun, 1800·3
Anestocil, 1800·3
Aneth, 1680·2
Anethaine, 1800·3
Anethi, Oleum, 1680·2
Anethol, 1654·3
Anethole, 1654·3
*cis*-Anethole, 1655·2
*trans*-Anethole, 1655·2
Anethole Dithiolthione, 1655·1
Anethole Trithione, 1655·1
Anethum, 1680·2
*Anethum graveolens*, 1680·2
*Anethum sowa*, 1680·2
Anetin, 1800·3
Anetol, 1654·3
Anetol Tritiona, 1655·1
Aneural, 1800·3
Aneurin, 1800·3
Aneurine Hydrochloride, 1455·1
Aneurine Mononitrate, 1455·1
Aneurol, 1800·3
Anevrase, 1800·3
Anevrasi, 1800·3
Anew, 1800·3
Anew Day Force, 1800·3
Anew Luminosity, 1800·3
Anew Positivity, 1800·3
Anexa, 1800·3
Anexate, 1800·3
Anexsia, 1800·3
ANF, 964·2
Anfagladin, 1800·3
Anfenax, 1800·3
Anfepramona, Hidrocloruro de, 1587·1
Anfertil, 1800·3
Anfetamina, 1584·3
Anfetamina, Sulfato de, 1584·3
Anfetaminilo, 1584·3
Anflat, 1800·4
Anflene, 1800·4
Anfocort, 1800·4
Anfokali, 1800·4
Anfomicin, 1800·4
Anforicin B, 1800·4
Anfotericina B, 391·2
Anfoterin, 1800·4
Anfozan, 1800·4
Angass, 1800·4
Angass S, 1800·4
Ange, 1800·4
Angel, Destroying, 1717·3
Angel Dust, 784·2, 1730·3
Angel Hair, 1730·3
Angel Mist, 1730·3
Angelica, 1655·1
*Angelica acutiloba*, 1655·1
*Angelica archangelica*, 1655·1
*Angelica dahurica*, 1655·1
*Angelica polymorpha*, 1655·1
*Angelica pubescens*, 1655·1
Angelica Root, 1655·1
*Angelica sinensis*, 1655·1
Angelicae Radix, 1655·1
Angenol, 1800·4
Angettes, 1800·4
Angeze, 1800·4
Anghostan-100, 1800·4
Angiact, 1800·4
Angi-a-Mid, 1800·4
Angicon, 1800·4
Angicontin, 1800·4
Angicor, 1800·4
Angidil, 1800·4
Angidine, 1800·4
Angifebrine, 1800·4
Angifonil, 1800·4
Angil, 1800·4
Angileptol, 1800·4
Angilol, 1800·4
Angimon, 1800·4
Angina— *see* Angina Pectoris, 813·1
Angina MCC, 1800·4
Angina Pectoris, 813·1
Angina, Prinzmetal's— *see* Angina Pectoris, 813·1
Angina-Gastreu S R1, 1800·4
Anginamide, 1800·4
Anginasin N, 1801·1
Anginazol, 1801·1
Anginesin, 1801·1
Anginin, 1801·1
Anginine, 1801·1
Angino Tricin, 1801·1
Anginol, 1801·1
Anginol-Lidocaine, 1801·1
Anginomycin, 1801·1
Anginor, 1801·1
Angino-Rub, 1801·1
Anginotrat, 1801·1
Anginova, 1801·1
Anginovag, 1801·1
Anginovin H, 1801·1
Anginozetes, 1801·1
Angiocardyl N, 1801·1
Angiocine, 1801·1
Angiocis, 1801·1
Angio-Conray, 1801·1
Angiodarona, 1801·1
Angiodrox, 1801·1
Angioedema, Hereditary— *see* Hereditary Angioedema, 761·3
Angioedema— *see* Urticaria and Angioedema, 1138·3
Angiofilina, 1801·1
Angiofluor, 1801·1
Angioflux, 1801·1
Angioftal, 1801·2
Angiografin, 1801·2
Angiografin, Uro— *see* Uro Angiografin, 2361·4
Angiografina, 1801·2
Angiolingual, 1801·2
Angiolit, 1801·2
Angiolong, 1801·2
Angiomax, 1801·2
Angioneurina, 1801·2
Angioneurotic Oedema, Hereditary— *see* Hereditary Angioedema, 761·3
Angionorm, 1801·2
Angiopas, 1801·2
Angiophtal, 1801·2
Angiopine, 1801·2
Angioplasty— *see* Reperfusion and Revascularisation Procedures, 834·1
Angiopril, 1801·2
Angiorex, 1801·2
Angiosedante, 1801·2
Angiostrongyliasis, 97·3
Angiotensin II, 863·3
Angiotensin Amide, 863·3
Angiotensin II Receptor Antagonists, 809·2
Angiotensinamida, 863·3
Angiotensinamide, 863·3
Angiotensin-converting Enzyme Inhibitors, 809·1, 842·3
Angioton, 1801·2
Angioton S, 1801·2
Angiotrofin, 1801·2
Angiovist, 1801·2
Angiozem, 1801·2
Angipress, 1801·2
Angipress CD, 1801·2
Angised, 1801·2
Angispray, 1801·2
Angi-Spray, 1801·2
Angitak, 1801·2
Angitil, 1801·3
Angitrate, 1801·3
Angitrit, 1801·3
Angizem, 1801·3
Anglais, Sel, 1228·2
Anglix, 1801·3
Anglopen, 1801·3
Anglucid, 1801·3
Angocin Anti-Infekt N, 1801·3
Angocin Bronchialtropfen, 1801·3
Angocin Percutan, 1801·3
Angoron, 1801·3
Angostura, 1678·1
Angostura Bark, 1678·1
Angostura Bitters, 1678·1
Angoten, 1801·3
Angstrom Corpo, 1801·3
Angstrom Viso, 1801·3
Anguilce, 1801·3
Angular, 1801·3
Angurate Magentee, 1801·3
Angyton, 1801·3
*Anhalonium lewinii*, 1713·3
*Anhalonium williamsii*, 1713·3
Anhascha, 1666·1
Anhedonia, 278·1
Anhídrido Crómico, 1670·3
Anhidrot, 1801·3
Anhisnon, 1801·3
Anhista, 1801·3
Anhydroepitetracycline, 267·1
Anhydrol Forte, 1801·3
Anhydrotetracycline, 266·3
Anhydrous Citric Acid, 1673·1
Anhydrous Disodium Hydrogen Phosphate, 1231·1
Anhydrous Glucose, 1432·2
Anhydrous Lactose, 1438·3
Anhydrous Sodium Dihydrogen Phosphate, 1230·3
Anhydrous Sodium Sulfate, 1290·1
Anhydrous Sodium Sulphate, 1290·1
Anhypen, 1801·3
Anice, 1655·2
Anice (Specie Composta), 1801·3
Anidrosan, 1801·3
Anidulafungin, 395·1
Aniduv, 1801·3
Anifed, 1801·3
Anifer Fenchelhonig, 1801·3
Anifer Hustenbalsam, 1801·3
Anifer Hustentee, 1801·4
Anifer Hustentropfen, 1801·4
Anifer Krauterol, 1801·4
Aniflazime, 1801·4
Aniflazym, 1801·4
Anikef, 1801·4
Anilar, 1801·4
Anileridina, 15·1
Anileridina, Fosfato de, 15·1
Anileridina, Hidrocloruro de, 15·1
Anileridine, 15·1
Anileridine Hydrochloride, 15·1
Anileridine Phosphate, 15·1
Anilid, 1801·4
Anilina, 1471·2
Aniline, 1471·2
Aniline Green, 1185·2
Aniline Red, 1185·1
Anilusin, 1801·4
Animal Bites, Infections in— *see* Bites and Stings, 121·3
Animal Shapes, 1801·4
Animal Shapes + Iron, 1801·4
Animativ, 1801·4
Animex-On, 1801·4
Animic, 1801·4
Animine, 1801·4
Anionen-Spurenelement, 1801·4
Anionic Emulsifying Wax, 1481·1
Anionic Surfactants, 1574·1
Aniospray, 1801·4
Aniracetam, 1655·1
Anís, Aceite Esencial de, 1655·2
Anís, Esencia de, 1655·2
Anis, Essence d', 1655·2
Anís Estrellado, 1655·2
Anis Étoilé, 1655·2
Anís, Semilla de, 1655·2
Anis Verde, 1655·2
Anis Vert, 1655·2
Anisaldehyde, 1655·2
Anisan, 1801·4

Anise, 1655·2
Anise Fruit, 1655·2
Anise Fruit, Star, 1655·2
Anise Oil, 1655·2
Anise Oil, Star, 1655·2
Anise, Star, 1655·2
Aniseed, 1655·2
Aniseed Oil, 1655·2
Anisi Aetheroleum, 1655·2
Anisi Fructus, 1655·2
Anisi, Oleum, 1655·2
Anisi Stellati Aetheroleum, 1655·2
Anisi Stellati Fructus, 1655·2
Anisi Vulgaris, Fructus, 1655·2
Anisimol, 1801·4
Anisindiona, 863·3
Anisindione, 863·3
Anismus, 1390·1
Anisotropine Methobromide, 486·1
Anisotropine Methylbromide, 486·1
*p*-Anisoylated (Human) Lys-plasminogen Streptokinase Activator Complex (1:1), 863·3
Anisoylated Plasminogen Streptokinase Activator Complex, 863·3
Anistal, 1801·4
Anistreplasa, 863·3
Anistreplase, 863·3
Anisum Badium, 1655·2
Anisum Stellatum, 1655·2
*N*-*p*-Anisyl-*N'N'*-dimethyl-*N*-(2-pyridyl)ethylenediamine Hydrochloride, 437·1
*N*-*p*-Anisyl-*N'N'*-dimethyl-*N*-(pyrimidin-2-yl)ethylenediamine Hydrochloride, 442·2
Anitos, 1801·4
Anitrim, 1801·4
Anivy, 1801·4
Ankylosing Spondylitis— *see* Spondyloarthropathies, 11·1
Anlodibal, 1801·4
Anna, 1801·4
Annadine, 1801·4
Annatto, 1056·1
Anningzochin, 1801·4
Annoxen, 1801·4
Anodan-HC, 1801·4
Anodesyn, 1802·1
Anogenital Warts— *see* Warts, 1139·2
Anolor, 1802·1
Anoquan, 1802·1
Anoran, 1802·1
Anore Dolor, 1802·1
Anore Rheumatic N, 1802·1
Anore X N, 1802·1
Anorectics, 1583·1
Anoreine, 1802·1
Anoreine mit Lidocain, 1802·1
Anorexia, Cancer-related— *see* Cachexia, 1558·3
Anorfin, 1802·1
Anorsia, 1802·1
102 Anos, 1802·1
Anosedil, 1802·1
Anovate, 1802·1
Anovulatorio Micro-Dosis, 1802·1
Anovulatorios, 1802·1
Anoxant, 1802·1
Anoxic Seizures, 478·2
Anoxid, 1802·1
ANP, 964·2
ANP-246, 26·3
ANP-3260, 26·3
Anpec, 1802·1
Anplag, 1802·1
Anposel, 1802·1
Anpress, 1802·1
Anquil, 1802·1
Ansaid, 1802·1
Ansamicin, 249·1
Ansamycin, 249·1
Ansamycins, 117·1
Ansar, 1802·1
Ansatipin, 1802·1
Ansatipine, 1802·1
Anselol, 1802·1
Ansentron, 1802·2
Anseren, 1802·2
Ansial, 1802·2
Ansiderm, 1802·2
Ansienon, 1802·2
Ansieten, 1802·2
Ansietil, 1802·2
Ansilan, 1802·2
Ansilive, 1802·2
Ansilor, 1802·2
Ansimar, 1802·2
Ansiokey, 1802·2
Ansiolin, 1802·2
Ansiopax, 1802·2
Ansiotex, 1802·2
Ansitec, 1802·2
Ansiten, 1802·2
Ansium, 1802·2
Ansiven, 1802·2
Anso, 1802·2
Ansudor, 1802·2
Answer, 1802·2
Answer Now, 1802·2
Anta, 1802·2
Antabus, 1802·2
Antabuse, 1802·2
Antacal, 1802·2
Antacia, 1802·3
Antacid, 1802·3
Antacid Chewable Tablets, 1802·3
Antacid Liquid, 1802·3
Antacid, Liquid— *see* Liquid Antacid, 2099·4
Antacid Plus Antiflatulant, 1802·3
Antacid Plus Simethicon, Liquid— *see* Liquid Antacid Plus Simethicon, 2099·4
Antacid Suspension, 1802·3
Antacid Tablet, 1802·3
Antacide Suspension, 1802·3
Antacide Suspension avec Antiflatulent, 1802·3
Antacids, 1239·1
Antacidum, 1802·3
Antacidum OPT, 1802·3
Antacidum Rennie, 1802·3
Antacil, 1802·3
Antacsal, 1802·3
Antaderm, 1802·3
Antadine, 1802·3
Antadys, 1802·3
Antafit, 1802·3
Antagon, 1802·3
Antagon 1, 1802·3
Antagonil, 1802·3
Antagonista del Receptor de la Interleucina 1, 1701·3
Antagosan, 1802·3
Antak, 1802·4
Antalgic, 1802·4
Antalgil, 1802·4
Antalgin, 1802·4
Antalgo, 1802·4
Antalin, 1802·4
Antalisin, 1802·4
Antalon, 1802·4
Antalvic, 1802·4
Antalyre, 1802·4
Antanazol, 1802·4
Antanidina, 1802·4
Antarene, 1802·4
Antares, 1802·4
Antarol, 1802·4
Antassa, 1802·4
Antasten, 1802·4
Antasten-Privin, 1802·4
Antaxone, 1802·4
Antazallerge, 1802·4
Antazolina, Fosfato de, 424·2
Antazolina, Hidrocloruro de, 424·2
Antazolina, Mesilato de, 424·2
Antazolina, Sulfato de, 424·2
Antazoline Hydrochloride, 424·2
Antazoline Mesilate, 424·2
Antazoline Mesylate, 424·2
Antazoline Methanesulphonate, 424·2
Antazoline Phosphate, 424·2
Antazoline Sulfate, 424·2
Antazoline Sulphate, 424·2
Antazoline-V, 1802·4
Antazolini Hydrochloridum, 424·2
Antazolinium Chloride, 424·2
Antebor, 1802·4
Antebor $B_6$, 1802·4
Antebor N, 1802·4
Antecollis— *see* Spasmodic Torticollis, 1391·1
Antelepsin, 1802·4
Antelmina, 1802·4
Antemesyl, 1802·4
Antemin, 1802·4
Antemin Compositum, 1803·1
Anten, 1803·1
Antenex, 1803·1
Antepan, 1803·1
Antepar, 1803·1
Antepsin, 1803·1
Antergan, 1803·1
Anterior Pituitary Hormones, 1312·1
Anthel, 1803·1
Anthelios, 1803·1
Anthelios Stick, 1803·1
Anthelios T, 1803·1
Anthelmintics, 97·1
Anthelone, 1294·2
*Anthemis nobilis*, 1669·3
Antherpos, 1803·1
Anthex, 1803·1
Anthisan, 1803·1
Anthisan Plus, 1803·1
Anthocyanins, 1056·1
Anthophyllite, 1658·1
Anthozym, 1803·2
Anthozym N, 1803·2
9,10-Anthracenedicarboxaldehyde Bis(2-imidazolin-2-ylhydrazone) Dihydrochloride, 530·2
Anthraderm, 1803·2
Anthra-Derm, 1803·2
Anthraforte, 1803·2
Anthralin, 1146·1
Anthranol, 1803·2
Anthrascalp, 1803·2
Anthrax, 121·2
Anthrax Vaccines, 1608·1
Anthraxiton, 1803·2
Anthraxivore, 1803·2
*Anthriscus sylvestris*, 1765·1
Anti Anorex Triple, 1803·2
Anti B, 1803·2
Anti CD3, 1803·2
Anti Itch, 1803·2
Anti-Ac, 1803·2
Antiacid, 1803·2
Antiacide, 1803·2
Anti-Acido, 1803·2
Antiacido Eno, 1803·2
Antiacido Salud, 1803·2
Antiacil, 1803·2
Antiacne, 1803·2
Anti-Acne, 1803·2
Anti-Acne Control Formula, 1803·2
Anti-Acne Formula for Men, 1803·2
Anti-Acne Spot Treatment, 1803·2
Antiacneicos Ac-Sal, 1803·3
Antiacneicos Niacex, 1803·3
Antiadipositum X-112, 1803·3
Antiadipositum X-112 N, 1803·3
Antiadipositum X-112 S, 1803·3
Antiadiposo, 1803·3
Anti-Ageing Kalmia, 1803·3
Anti-Algos, 1803·3
Antiarrhythmics, 809·2
Anti-Asmatico, 1803·3
Anti-asthma Drugs, 777·1
Antiax, 1803·3
Antibacin, 1803·3
Antibacter, 1803·3
Antibacterials, 116·1
Antibex, 1803·3
Antibio-Aberel, 1803·3
Antibiocilina, 1803·3
Antibiocin, 1803·3
Antibiocort, 1803·3
Antibiofilus, 1803·3
Antibiopen, 1803·3
Antibiophilus, 1803·3
Antibiophilus— *see* Bacilor, 1825·1
Antibioptal, 1803·3
Antibio-Synalar, 1803·3
AntibiOtic, 1803·3
Antibi-Otic, 1803·3
Antibiotic 899, 277·3
Antibiotic 6640, 254·3
Antibiotic A-5283, 406·2
Antibiotic Cold Sore Ointment, 1803·3
Antibiotic Cream, 1803·3
Antibiotic Ointment, 1803·4
Antibiotic Simplex, 1803·4
Antibiotic-associated Colitis, 128·1
Antibiotics, 116·1
Antibiotics, Antineoplastic, 492·1
Antibiotique Onguent, 1803·4
Antibiotrex, 1803·4
Antibiotulle Lumiere, 1803·4
Antiblef Eczem, 1803·4
Antiblefarica, 1803·4
Antiblut, 1803·4
Antibody Deficiency, Primary— *see* Primary Antibody Deficiency, 1629·2
Antibody Fragments, Digoxin-specific, 1036·3
Antibron, 1803·4
Anticatarral, 1803·4
Anti-CD4 Monoclonal Antibodies, 1668·3
Anti-CD11a, 1146·3
Anticerumen, 1803·4
Antichloric, 1803·4
Anticholinergic Bronchodilators, 777·1
Anticholinergics, 475·1
Anticholinesterases, 1484·1
Anticholium, 1803·4
Anticoagulants, 810·1
Anticoagulants, Coumarin, 810·1
Anticoagulants, Direct, 810·1
Anticoagulants, Indanedione, 810·1
Anticoagulants, Indirect, 810·1
Anticold, 1803·4
Anticon, 1803·4
Anticonceptivos Hormonales, 1527·3
Anticongestiva, 1803·4
Anticorizza, 1803·4
Anticude, 1803·4
Anticuerpos Antiendotoxinas, 1615·2
Anticuerpos CD4, 1668·3
Anti-D, 1803·4
Anti-D Immunoglobulin for Intravenous Use, 1608·1
Anti-D Immunoglobulins, 1608·1
Anti-D ($Rh_0$) Immunoglobulin, 1608·1
Anti-Dandruff Shampoo, 1803·4
Antidep, 1803·4
Antidepressants, 278·1
Antidepressants, Tricyclic, 278·2, 285·2
Anti-Dessechement, 1803·4
Antidia, 1803·4
Antidiabéticos Biguanídicos, 329·2
Antidiabéticos Sulfonilureas, 346·1
Antidiabetics, 324·1
Antidiar, 1803·4
Anti-Diarrheal, 1803·4
Antidiarrhoeals, 1239·2
Antidifar, 1803·4
Antidin, 1803·4
Antidiuretic Hormone, 1342·2
Antidol, 1804·1
Antidoloroso Rudol, 1804·1
Antidote Anti-Digitale BM, 1804·1
Antidotes, 1030·1
Antidoto Arvin, 1804·1
Antidotum Thallii-Heyl, 1804·1
Antidrasi, 1804·1
Antidry, 1804·1
Antiedema, 1804·1
Antiemetics, 1239·2
Antiemorroidali, 1804·1
Antiepileptics, 349·1
Antiespasmodico, 1804·1
Antiestrias, 1804·1
Antietanol, 1804·1

Antifebrin, 11·3, 1804·1
Antifect, 1804·1
Antiflam, 1804·1
Anti-Flamme, 1804·1
Antiflog, 1804·1
Antiflogil, 1804·1
Antiflogol, 1804·1
Antifloxil, 1804·1
Antiflu, 1804·1
Antiflu Forte, 1804·1
Antiflu-Des, 1804·2
Antiflu-N-Forte, 1804·2
Antifoam A, 1289·2
Antifoam AF, 1289·2
Antifoam M— *see* Minifom, 2134·2
AntiFocal, 1804·2
AntiFocal N, 1804·2
Antifohnon-N, 1804·2
Antifungal, 1804·2
Antifungal Foot Deodorant, 1804·2
Antifungals, 386·1
Antifungol, 1804·2
Anti-GBM Nephritis— *see* Glomerular Kidney Disease, 1080·2
1-92 Antigen LFA-3 (Human) Fusion Protein with Human Immunoglobulin G1 (Hinge-$C_H$2-$C_H$3 γ1-Chain), 1141·2
Antígeno de Kveim, 1703·3
Antigeron, 1804·2
Anti-Geruchs, 1804·2
Antiglan, 1804·2
Antigout Drugs, 412·1
Antigoutteux Rezall, 1804·2
Antigreg, 1804·2
Antigrietun, 1804·2
Antigripal Compuesto, 1804·2
Anti-Gripe, 1804·2
Antigriphine, 1804·2
Antigripine, 1804·2
Antigrippine, 1804·2
Antigrippine a l'Aspirine, 1804·2
Antigrippine Midy, 1804·2
Anti-H, 1804·3
Antihaemophilic Factor, 735·3, 751·1
Antihemophilic Factor, 751·2
Antihemophilic Factor, Cryoprecipitated, 751·2
Anti-Hemorroidaires, 1804·3
Antihemorroidal, 1804·3
Anti-Hist, 1804·3
Antihist-1, 1804·3
Antihistamine Forte, 1804·3
Antihistamines, 419·1
Antihistaminico, 1804·3
Antihist-D, 1804·3
Anti-Homocysteine Factor, 1804·3
Antihydral, 1804·3
Antihydral M, 1804·3
Antihypertonicum Forte, 1804·3
Antihypertonicum S, 1804·3
Antihypertonicum-Weliplex, 1804·3
Antihypertonikum-Tropfen N, 1804·3
Anti-inflammatory Drugs, 1·1
Anti-inflammatory Drugs, Nonsteroidal, 67·3
Anti-inflammatory Hormone, 1103·3
Anti-inhibitor Coagulant Complex, 752·2, 1804·3
Anti-Inhibitor Coagulant Complex (Autoplex T), 1804·3
Anti-Kalium, 1804·3
Antikataraktikum N, 1804·3
Antikataraktikum N Oral, 1804·3
Antikatarata, 1804·3
Antikeloides Creme, 1804·3
Antil, 1804·3
Antilerg, 1804·4
Antilergal, 1804·4
Anti-leukotrienes, 777·1
Antilipid, 1804·4
Antilirium, 1804·4
Antilymphocyte Immunoglobulins, 1348·3
Antilymphocyte Serum, 1348·3
Antim. Pot. Tart., 103·1
Antim. Sod. Tart., 103·1
Antimalarials, 444·1
Antimalarinae Chlorhydras, 606·3
Antimast N, 1804·4
Antimast T, 1804·4
Antimet, 1804·4
Antimetabolites, 492·1
Antimic, 1804·4
Anti-Micot, 1804·4
Antimicotica Solforata, 1804·4
Antimicotico, 1804·4
Antimicrobial Preservatives, 1164·1
Antimigraine Drugs, 464·1
Antimigrin, 1804·4
Antiminth, 1804·4
Antimoniato de Meglumina, 600·3
Antimónico Potásico, Tartrato, 103·1
Antimónico Sódico, Tartrato, 103·1
Antimony Compounds, Pentavalent, 600·3
Antimony Compounds, Trivalent, 103·1
Antimony Meglumine, 600·3
Antimony Potassium Tartrate, 103·1
Antimony Sodium Dimercaptosuccinate, 103·1
Antimony Sodium *meso*-2,3-Dimercaptosuccinate, 103·1
Antimony Sodium Tartrate, 103·1
Antimuscarinic Bronchodilators, 777·1
Antimuscarinics, 475·1
Antimycobacterials, 117·1
Antimyk, 1804·4
Antimyopikum, 1804·4
Antinaus, 1804·4
Anti-Nauseant, 1804·4
Antineoplastics, 492·1
Antineoplaston A10, 528·2
Antineoplaston AS2.1, 528·2
Antineoplaston AS2.5, 528·2
Antinephrin M, 1804·4
Antinerveux Lesourd, 1804·4
Antineuralgica, 1804·4
Antineuralgicum (Rowo-633), 1804·4
Antineurina, 1804·4
Antinevralgico Dr Knapp, 1804·4
Antinevralgico Penegal, 1804·4
Antinicoticum Sine (Rowo-100), 1804·4
Antio, 1804·4
Antiobes, 1804·4
Antiobiocilina, 1804·4
Antiopiaz, 1804·4
Antiotic, 1805·1
Antiox, 1805·1
Antioxidans E, 1805·1
Antioxidant Forte Tablets, 1805·1
Antioxidant Nutrients, 1805·1
Antioxidant Tablets, 1805·1
Antioxidante Vital, 1805·1
Antioxirell, 1805·1
Anti-oxygens, 1164·2
Antipanin N, 1805·1
Antipanin P, 1805·1
Antiparkin, 1805·1
Antipasmol, 1805·1
Antipeol, 1805·1
Antiphlogistine, 1805·1
Antiphlogistine Rub A-535, 1805·1
Antiphlogistine Rub A-535 Capsaicin, 1805·1
Antiphlogistine Rub A-535 Ice, 1805·1
Antiphlogistine Rub A-535 No Odour, 1805·1
Anti-Phosphat, 1805·1
Anti-Phosphate, 1805·1
Antiphospholipid Antibody Syndrome— *see* Systemic Lupus Erythematosus, 1088·3
Anti-Plaque Chewing Gum, 1805·1
$\alpha_2$-Antiplasmin, 735·3
Antiplatelet Drugs, 810·2
Antipressan, 1805·1
Antiprex, 1805·1
Antiprotin, 1805·2
Antiprotozoals, 595·1
Antiprurit, 1805·2
Antipsichos, 1805·2
Antipsychotics, 663·1
Antipulmina, 1805·2
Antipyn, 1805·2
Antipyn Forte, 1805·2
Antipyretics, 1·1
Antipyrin, 82·3
Antipyrin Salicylate, 82·3
Antipyrine, 82·3
Antipyrino-Coffeinum Citricum, 82·3
Antireumina, 1805·2
Antirrinum, 1805·2
Anti-rugas C, 1805·2
Antis, 1805·2
Antiscabbia Candioli Al DDT Terapeutico, 1805·2
Antiscabiosum, 1805·2
Antisecretory Drugs, 1239·2
Antisense Agents, 498·2
Antisept, 1805·2
Antisepthic Hexil, 1805·2
Antiseptic Foot Balm, 1805·2
Antiseptic Lozenges, 1805·2
Antiseptic Mouthwash, 1805·2
Antiseptic Ointment, 1805·2
Antiseptic Skin Cream, 1805·2
Antiseptic Sore Throat Lozenges— *see* Antiseptic Throat Lozenges, 1805·2
Antiseptic Throat Lozenges, 1805·2
Antiseptico Hertz, 1805·2
Antiseptics, 1164·1
Antiseptin, 1805·2
Antiseptique Pastilles, 1805·2
Antiseptique-Calmante, 1805·3
Antisera, 1605·1
Antisettico Astringente Sedativo, 1805·3
Antisklerosin S, 1805·3
Anti-Smoking Tablets, 1805·3
Antisol, 1805·3
Antispa, 1805·3
Antispas, 1805·3
Antispasmin, 1805·3
Antispasmina, 1805·3
Antispasmina Colica, 1805·3
Antispasmodic Elixir, 1805·3
Antisseptico, 1805·3
Antistax, 1805·3
Antistina, 424·2
Antistina-Privin, 1805·3
Antistine-Privine, 1805·3
Antistin-Privin, 1805·3
Antistin-Privina, 1805·3
Antisuero contra el Veneno de Arañas, 1640·1
Antisuero contra el Veneno de Escorpión, 1638·3
Antisuero contra el Veneno de Garrapata, 1641·3
Antisuero contra el Veneno de la Medusa, 1621·3
Antisuero contra el Veneno de Serpiente, 1639·1
Antisuero contra el Veneno del Pez Piedra Estuarino, 1640·2
Antisuero de la Rabia, 1635·3
Antisueros, 1605·1
Anti-T Lymphocyte Immunoglobulin for Human Use, Animal, 1348·3
Antitensin, 1805·3
Antithrombin III, 735·3, 742·2
Antithrombin III Concentrate, Human, 742·2
Antithrombin III Deficiency— *see* Thromboembolic Disorders, 837·3
Antithrombin III Human, 742·2
Antithrombin, Major, 735·3, 742·2
Antithrombinum III Humanum Densatum, 742·2
Antithymocyte Gammaglobulin, 1348·3
Antithymocyte Globulin, 1348·3
Antithymocyte Immunoglobulin, 1348·3
Antithymocyte Serum, 1348·3
Antithyroid Drugs, 1594·3
Antitis, 1805·3
Antitoxikon, 1805·3
Antitoxinas Botulínicas, 1610·3
Antitoxinas de la Gangrena Gaseosa, 1615·3
Antitoxinas Diftéricas, 1612·2
Antitoxinas Tetánicas, 1640·2
Antitoxins, 1605·1
Antitrombina III, 742·2
Antitrypsin, Alpha$_1$, 1651·2
Antituss, 1805·3
Anti-Tuss, 1805·3
Antitussive Decongestant Antihistamine Syrup, 1805·3
Antitussivum Burger, 1805·4
Antitussivum Burger N, 1805·4
Antivenin, 1805·4
Antivenin (Crotalidae) Polyvalent, 1639·1
Antivenin (Latrodectus Mactans), 1640·1, 1805·4
Antivenin (Micrurus Fulvius), 1639·1
Antivenins, 1605·1
Antivenoms, 1605·1
Antiverrugas, 1805·4
Antivert, 1805·4
Anti-Ves, 1805·4
Antivipmyn, 1805·4
Antivirals, 618·1
Antivirax, 1805·4
Antivom, 1805·4
Antixerophthalmic Vitamin, 1451·2
Antizid, 1805·4
Antizine, 1805·4
Antizol, 1805·4
Antizona, 1805·4
Antocin, 1805·4
Antomiopic, 1805·4
Antopal, 1805·4
Antopar, 1805·4
Antoral, 1805·4
Antoril, 1805·4
Antoxidant Synergists, 1164·2
Antoxidants, 1164·1
Antoxymega, 1805·4
Antra, 1805·4
Antral, 1805·4
Antramups, 1805·4
Antran, 1805·4
Antranol, 1805·4
Antrapurol, 1261·1
Antrenyl, 1805·4
Antrex, 1805·4
Antrima— *see* Trimadiaz Antrima, 2346·3
Antrizine, 1805·4
Antrocol, 1805·4
Antroquoril, 1805·4
Antrypol, 615·3
Antu, 1500·2
Antup R, 1806·1
Anturan, 1806·1
Anturane, 1806·1
Antussan, 1806·1
Antussia, 1806·1
Antust, 1806·1
Antux, 1806·1
Anu-Aide, 1806·1
Anuar, 1806·1
Anucet, 1806·1
Anucort-HC, 1806·1
Anugesic, 1806·1
Anugesic-HC, 1806·1
Anulbet, 1806·2
Anulette, 1806·2
Anumed, 1806·2
Anumed HC, 1806·2
Anumedin, 1806·2
Anurin, 1806·2
Anusept, 1806·2
Anusol, 1806·2
Anusol Duo, 1806·3
Anusol Duo S, 1806·3
Anusol Plus, 1806·3
Anusol Plus HC— *see* Anusol-HC, Plus HC, 1806·3
Anusol-A, 1806·3
Anusol-HC, 1806·3
Anuzinc, 1806·3
Anuzinc HC, 1806·3
Anuzinc HC Plus, 1806·3
Anvitoff, 1806·3
Anvitol, 1806·3
Anxer, 1806·4
Anxicalm, 1806·4
Anxielax, 1806·4
Anxietum, 1806·4

Anxiety and Depressive Disorder, Mixed, 278·1
Anxiety Disorders, 663·1
Anxiety/Stress L72, 1806·4
Anxiolan, 1806·4
Anxiolit, 1806·4
Anxiolit Plus, 1806·4
Anxiolytic Sedatives Hypnotics and Antipsychotics, 663·1
Anxipress-D, 1806·4
Anxira, 1806·4
Anxirid, 1806·4
Anxium, 1806·4
Anxoral, 1806·4
Anxut, 1806·4
Anxyrex, 1806·4
Any, 1806·4
Anzac, 1806·4
Anzatax, 1806·4
Anzemet, 1806·4
Anzion, 1806·4
Anzopac, 1806·4
AO-33, 366·2
AO-128, 348·3
Aodrops, 1806·4
Aofen, 1806·4
Aoflow, 1806·4
A-O-Q10 MaxiPower Formula, 1806·4
Aorinyl, 1806·4
Aorten, 1806·4
Aosept, 1806·4
Aotal, 1806·4
Aova, 1807·1
AP, 1807·1
AP-12009, 528·2
AP Inyec Cloruro Potasic, 1807·1
APA, 1807·1
Apacef, 1807·1
Apacet, 1807·1
Apafant, 781·1
Apaflurane, 1236·2
Apagen, 1807·1
Apain, 1807·1
Apaisac, 1807·1
Apaisance, 1807·1
Apaisyl, 1807·1
Apalin, 1807·1
Apamid, 1807·1
Apamox, 1807·1
Apap, 1807·1
A-Par, 1807·1
A-Parkin, 1807·1
Aparoxal, 1807·1
Aparsonin N, 1807·1
Apasmil, 1807·1
Apasmo, 1807·1
Apasmo Compuesto, 1807·1
Apatate, 1807·1
Apatate with Fluoride, 1807·1
Apatef, 1807·1
Apatite, 1807·1
Apazone, 20·1
Apcitide, Technetium ($^{99m}$Tc), 1525·3
APD, 773·3
Apecitab, 1807·1
Apefer, 1807·1
Apegmone, 1807·2
Apekumarol, 1807·2
Apen, 1807·2
A-Pen, 1807·2
Apeplus, 1807·2
Aperamid, 1807·2
Aperdan, 1807·2
Apergan, 1807·2
Aperisan, 1807·2
Aperop, 1807·2
Apertia, 1807·2
Apetibe, 1807·2
Apetil, 1807·2
Apetin, 1807·2
Apetinil-Depo, 1807·2
Apetitol Forte, 1807·2
Apetrol, 1807·2
Apevitin BC, 1807·2
ApexiCon, 1807·2
APF, 1807·2
Aphanes, 1729·1
*Aphanes arvensis*, 1729·1
Aphenylbarbit, 1807·2
Aphilan, 1807·2
Aphloine P, 1807·2
Aphrodine Hydrochloride, 1766·2
Aphrodyne, 1807·2
Aphthasol, 1807·2
Aphthous Stomatitis— *see* Mouth Ulceration, 1245·1
Aphthous Ulcer— *see* Mouth Ulceration, 1245·1
Aphtiria, 1807·2
Aphtoral, 1807·2
Api Baby, 1807·3
Apifortyl, 1807·3
Apigenin-7-glucoside, 1669·3
Apihepar, 1807·3
Apilaxe, 1807·3
Apilcav, 1807·3
Apimid, 1807·3
Apio, 1669·1
Apiocolina, 1807·3
Apir Bicarbonato Sod, 1807·3
Apir Clorurado, 1807·3
Apir Cloruro Amonico, 1807·3
Apir Glucoibys, 1807·3
Apir Glucopotasico, 1807·3
Apir Glucosado, 1807·3
Apir Glucosalino, 1807·3
Apir Ringer, 1807·3
Apir Ringer Lactato, 1807·3
Apiretal, 1807·3
Apiretal Codeina, 1807·3
Apiroflex Clorurado, 1807·3
Apiroflex Glucosada, 1807·3
Apiroflex Glucosalina, 1807·3
Apirol, 1807·3
Apiron, 1807·3
Apis, 1807·3
Apis Mel, 1655·3
Apis Mellifera, 1655·3
*Apis mellifera*, 1434·2, 1480·2, 1655·3, 1740·3
Apis Mellifera ad Praeparationes Homoeopathicas, 1655·3
Apis Mellifica, 1655·3
Apis Salbe— *see* Arnica comp/Apis Salbe, 1812·2
Apiserum, 1807·3
Apiserum con Telergon 1, 1807·3
Apisgel, 1807·3
Apis-Homaccord, 1807·3
Apistress, 1807·3
Apium, 1669·1
Apixol, 1807·3
APL, 1807·3
Aplacasse, 1807·3
Aplace, 1807·3
Aplacid, 1807·4
Aplactin, 1807·4
Aplaket, 1807·4
Aplastic Anaemia, 732·1
A-Plex, 1807·4
Aplexil, 1807·4
Aplical, 1807·4
Aplical-D, 1807·4
Apligraf, 1807·4
Aplisol, 1807·4
Aplitest, 1807·4
Aplodan, 1807·4
Aplona, 1807·4
Aplonidine Hydrochloride, 864·1
Aplosyn-Otic, 1807·4
APM, 1422·1
Apnoea, Neonatal— *see* Neonatal Apnoea, 806·1
Apnoea of Prematurity— *see* Neonatal Apnoea, 806·1
Apnol, 1807·4
Apoacor, 1807·4
Apo-Alpraz, 1807·4
Apo-Amilzide, 1807·4
Apo-Amoxi, 1807·4
Apo-Ampi, 1807·4
Apo-Atenol, 1807·4
Apobase, 1807·4
Apo-C, 1807·4
Apo-Cal, 1807·4
Apocanda, 1807·4
Apocapen, 1807·4
Apo-Capto, 1807·4
Apocard, 1807·4
15-Apo-β-caroten-15-oic Acid, 1161·1
(13*Z*)-15-Apo-β-caroten-15-oic Acid, 1148·3
15-Apo-β-caroten-15-ol, 1451·2
Apo-Cepalex, 1807·4
Apo-Cephalex, 1807·4
Apo-Chlorax, 1808·1
Apociclina, 1808·1
Apocillin, 1808·1
Apo-Cloxi, 1808·1
Apocort, 1808·1
Apocortal, 1808·1
Apo-Cromolyn, 1808·1
Apocyclin, 1808·1
Apoderm, 1808·1
Apo-Diclo, 1808·1
Apo-Diltiaz, 1808·1
Apodorm, 1808·1
Apodoxin, 1808·1
Apodoxy, 1808·1
Apo-Doxy, 1808·1
Apo-Erythro, 1808·1
Apo-Feno, 1808·1
Apo-Feno-Micro, 1808·1
Apoferritin, 1427·2
Apofin, 1808·1
Apo-Gain, 1808·1
Apogastine, 1808·1
APO-go, 1808·1
APO-go Pen, 1808·1
Apohair, 1808·1
Apo-Hepat, 1808·1
Apo-Hexa, 1808·1
Apo-Hydro, 1808·1
Apo-Infekt, 1808·1
Apo-Ipravent, 1808·1
Apo-ISDN, 1808·1
Apo-K, 1808·2
Apo-Keto, 1808·2
Apokinon, 1808·2
Apokyn, 1808·2
Apolar, 1808·2
Apolar med Dekvalon, 1808·2
Apolato de Sodio, 1000·2
Apo-Levocarb, 1808·2
Apolide, 1808·2
Apollonset, 1808·2
Apo-Methazide, 1808·2
Apo-Methoprazine, 1808·2
Apo-Metoclop, 1808·2
Apomex, 1808·2
Apomin, 1808·2
Apomine, 1808·2
Apominolin, 1808·2
Apomorfina, Hidrocloruro de, 1199·1
Apomorphine Hydrochloride, 1199·1
Apomorphini Hydrochloridum, 1199·1
Apomoxyn, 1808·2
Aponacin, 1808·2
Apo-Nadol, 1808·2
Aponal, 1808·2
Apo-Napro-Na, 1808·2
Aponatura Preparations 1808·2
Apo-Nifed, 1808·3
Aponil, 1808·3
Apo-Norflox, 1808·3
Aponorm, 1808·3
Apo-Oflox, 1808·3
Apo-Paradex, 1808·3
Apo-Pen-VK, 1808·3
Apophage, 1808·3
Apo-Pindol, 1808·3
Apopiran, 1808·3
Apoplectal, 1808·3
Apoplectal N, 1808·3
Apo-Prazo, 1808·3
Apoprin, 1808·3
Apo-Pulm, 1808·3
A-Por, 1808·3
Aporex, 1808·3
Aporil, 1808·3
6aβ-Aporphine-10,11-diol Hydrochloride Hemihydrate, 1199·1
Apo-Salvent, 1808·3
Apo-Sulfatrim, 1808·4
Apo-Sulin, 1808·4
Apo-Tamox, 1808·4
Apotel, 1808·4
Apoterfin, 1808·4
Apo-Tetra, 1808·4
Apotheker Bauer's Preparations, 1808·4
Apotheker Ehrmanns Grippekapseln, 1808·4
Apotheker Hoyers Brennesseltonikum, 1808·4
Apo-Theo, 1808·4
Apotil, 1808·4
Apo-Timol, 1808·4
Apo-Timop, 1808·4
Apo-Triazide, 1808·4
Apo-Triazo, 1809·1
Apo-Trihex, 1809·1
Apo-Trimip, 1809·1
Apotrin, 1809·1
Apo-Tuss, 1809·1
Apoven, 1809·1
Apovent, 1809·1
Apo-Verap, 1809·1
Apox, 1809·1
Apozan, 1809·1
Apozepam, 1809·1
Appearex, 1809·1
Appedrine, 1809·1
Appelin-B12, 1809·1
Appetiser Mixture, 1809·1
Appeton, 1809·1
Appeton Weight Gain, 1809·1
Appetrol, 1809·1
Apple Acid, 1709·2
Apple, Bitter, 1260·3
Applicaine, 1809·1
APR, 864·1
APR Cream, 1809·1
Apra, 1809·1
Apraclonidina, Hidrocloruro de, 864·1
Apraclonidine Hydrochloride, 864·1
Apracur, 1809·1
Apracur Antifebril, 1809·1
Apracur Biotic, 1809·2
Apracur Bucofaringeo, 1809·2
Apracur Expectorante, 1809·2
Apracur Nasal, 1809·2
Apra-Gel, 1809·2
Apramicina, Sulfato de, 158·2
Apramycin, 158·2
Apramycin Sulfate, 158·2
Apramycin Sulphate, 158·2
Apranax, 1809·2
Apraz, 1809·2
Aprednislon, 1809·2
Aprepitant, 1250·3
Apresazide, 1809·2
Apresolin, 1809·2
Apresolina, 1809·2
Apresoline, 1809·2
Apressinum, 931·2
Apri, 1809·2
Aprical, 1809·2
Apricot Kernels, 1704·3
April, 1809·2
Aprindina, Hidrocloruro de, 864·2
Aprindine Hydrochloride, 864·2
Aprinol, 1809·2
Aprinox, 1809·2
Aprix-DN, 1809·2
Aprobarbital, 670·3
Aprobarbital Sodium, 671·1
Aprobarbitone, 670·3
Aprodine, 1809·2
Aprodine with Codeine, 1809·2
Aprofen, 1809·2
Aproten, 1809·2
Aprotinin, 742·3
Aprotinin Concentrated Solution, 742·3
Aprotinina, 742·3
Aprotininum, 742·3

Aprovel, 1809·2
Aprovel HCT, 1809·2
Aproxal, 1809·2
Aprozide, 1809·3
APS Balneum, 1809·3
APSAC, 863·3
Apsomol, 1809·3
Apsor, 1809·3
APT-070, 1675·2
Aptamil AR, 1809·3
Aptamil HA, 1809·3
Aptamil HA 2, 1809·3
Aptamil HA con LCP Milupan, 1809·3
APT-Ampicloxa, 1809·3
Aptiganel, 1655·3
Aptiganel Hydrochloride, 1655·3
Aptin, 1809·3
Aptin N, 1809·3
Aptine, 1809·3
Aptodin Plus, 1809·3
Apton, 1809·3
Aptus Amphetamine, 1809·3
Aptus Benzodiazepine, 1809·3
Aptus Cannabis, 1809·3
Aptus Cocaine, 1809·3
Aptus Methadone, 1809·3
Aptus Methamphetamine, 1809·3
Aptus Opiate, 1809·3
Apurin, 1809·3
Apurol, 1809·3
Apurone, 1809·3
Apuzin, 1809·3
Apydan, 1809·3
Apyrol, 1809·3
AQ-110, 806·3
Aq. pro Inj., 1765·1
Aqium Active Defence, 1809·3
Aqsia, 1809·3
Aqua, 1764·3
Aqua ad Iniectabilia, 1765·1
Aqua ad Injectionem, 1765·1
Aqua Ban, 1809·4
Aqua Ban Plus, 1809·4
Aqua Communis, 1764·3
Aqua Dermis, 1809·4
Aqua Ear, 1809·4
Aqua Emoform, 1809·4
Aqua Fontana, 1764·3
Aqua Fortis, 1722·1
Aqua Injectabilis, 1765·1
Aqua Lub, 1809·4
Aqua Potabilis, 1764·3
Aqua pro Injectione, 1765·1
Aqua pro Injectionibus, 1765·1
Aqua Purificata, 1764·3
Aqua Soap, 1809·4
Aqua Valde Purificata, 1764·3
AquaBalm, 1809·4
Aqua-Ban, Maximum Strength— *see* Maximum Strength Aqua-Ban, 2116·3
Aquabase, 1809·4
Aquacaps, 1809·4
Aquacare, 1809·4
Aquacel, 1809·4
Aquachloral, 1809·4
Aquacort, 1809·4
Aquaderm, 1809·4
Aquadon, 1809·4
Aquadrate, 1809·4
Aquae, 1809·4
Aquaear, 1809·4
Aquafilme, 1809·4
Aquafor, 1809·4
Aquaform, 1809·4
Aquagel, 1809·4
Aquagen SQ, 1809·4
Aqualan, 1809·4
Aqualane, 1809·4
Aqualarm, 1809·4
Aqualcium, 1810·1
Aqualette, 1810·1
Aqualibra, 1810·1
Aquamag, 1810·1
Aquamephyton, 1810·1
Aquamycetin-N, 1810·1
Aquanil, 1810·1
Aquanil HC, 1810·1
Aquaphilic, 1810·1
Aquaphor, 1810·1
Aquaphor Healing Ointment, 1810·1
Aquaphoril, 1810·1
Aquaphyllin, 1810·1
Aquapred, 1810·1
Aquareduct, 1810·1
Aquaretic, 1810·1
Aquarhine, 1810·1
Aquarid, 1810·1
Aquarius, 1810·1
Aquasalina, 1810·1
Aquasept, 1810·1
Aquasite, 1810·1
Aquasol, 1810·1
Aquasol A, 1810·1
Aquasol A+D, 1810·2
Aquasol E, 1810·2
Aquasport, 1810·2
Aquasteril, 1810·2
Aquasun, 1810·2
Aquasun Sports, 1810·2
Aquasun Stick, 1810·2
Aquatab C, 1810·2
Aquatab D, 1810·2
Aquatab DM, 1810·2
Aquatabs, 1810·2
Aquatain, 1810·2
AquaTar, 1810·2
AquaTears, 1810·2
Aquatensen, 1810·2
Aquaviron, 1810·2
Aquavit-E, 1810·2
Aqua-Vite Super Kelp, 1810·2
Aqucilina, 1810·2
Aqucilina D A, 1810·2
Aquedux, 1810·2
Aquella, 1810·2
Aqueous Charcodote, 1810·2
Aquilea, 1646·2
Aquim, 1810·2
Aquitol, 1810·2
Aquocobalamin, 1458·2
Aquo-Cytobion, 1810·2
Aquomin, 1810·3
Aquo-Trinitrosan, 1810·3
Aqupla, 1810·3
AR-12008, 1016·2
Ara-A, 657·1
Ara-AMP, 657·1
Arabine, 1810·3
9-β-D-Arabinofuranosyladenine 5′-(Dihydrogen Phosphate), 657·1
9-β-D-Arabinofuranosyladenine 5′-(Dihydrogen Phosphate) Disodium, 657·1
9-β-D-Arabinofuranosyladenine Monohydrate, 657·1
(*E*)-1-β-D-Arabinofuranosyl-5-(2-bromovinyl)uracil, 654·2
1-β-D-Arabinofuranosylcytosine, 543·1
*N*-(1-β-D-Arabinofuranosyl-1,2-dihydro-2-oxo-4-pyrimidinyl)docosanamide, 550·2
9-β-D-Arabinofuranosyl-2-fluoroadenine 5′-Dihydrogenphosphate, 553·2
1-β-D-Arabinofuranosyluracil, 543·3
Arabinosyl Hypoxanthine, 657·1
Arabinosyladenine Monophosphate, 657·1
Arabinosylcytosine, 543·1
Ara-C, 543·1
Aracaf, 1810·3
ARA-cell, 1810·3
Arachide, Huile d', 1656·1
Arachidis Oleum Hydrogenatum, 1656·1
Arachidis Oleum Raffinatum, 1656·1
Arachidonic Acid, 1511·1
Arachis Oil, 1656·1
Arachis Oil, Hydrogenated, 1656·1
Arachis Oil, Refined, 1656·1
Arachis, Oleum, 1656·1
Arachitol, 1810·3
Aracmyn Plus, 1810·3
Aracytin, 1810·3
Aracytine, 1810·3
Aradix, 1810·3
Aradois, 1810·3
Aradois H, 1810·3
Aragest, 1810·3
Aralast, 1810·3
Aralen, 1810·3
Aralia Med Complex, 1810·3
Aramexe, 1810·3
Aramin, 1810·3
Aramine, 1810·3
Arancia Dolce Essenza, 1724·1
Arándano, 1676·3
Arándano Rojo, 1676·3
Araneism— *see* Spider Bites, 1640·1
Aranesp, 1810·3
Aranidipine, 864·2
Aranidipino, 864·2
Aranidorm-S, 1810·3
Araniforce-forte, 1810·3
Aranisan-N, 1810·3
Araruta, 1422·1
Aratac, 1810·3
Aratan, 1810·3
Aratan D, 1810·3
Ara-U, 543·3
Arava, 1810·3
Arbekacin Sulfate, 158·3
Arbekacin Sulphate, 158·3
Arbekacina, Sulfato de, 158·3
Arbe-Plus, 1810·4
Arbid, 1810·4
Arbid N, 1810·4
Arbid-top, 1810·4
Arbil, 1810·4
Árbol de la Cera, 1659·2
Arbralene, 1810·4
Arbum, 1810·4
Arbutamina, Hidrocloruro de, 864·2
Arbutamine Hydrochloride, 864·2
Arbuz, 1810·4
ARC— *see* HIV Infection and AIDS, 621·3
Arca-Be, 1810·4
Arcablock, 1810·4
Arcablock Comp, 1810·4
Arca-Enzym, 1810·4
Arcafen, 1810·4
Arcalion, 1810·4
Arcana Expectorant, 1810·4
Arcanacycline, 1810·4
Arcanacysteine, 1810·4
Arcanafed, 1810·4
Arcanafenac, 1810·4
Arcanaflex, 1810·4
Arcanaflu, 1810·4
Arcanagesic, 1810·4
Arcanamycin, 1810·4
Arcanaprim, 1810·4
Arcasin, 1811·1
Arcavit A, 1811·1
Arcavit A/E, 1811·1
Arceligasol, 1811·1
Arcental, 1811·1
Archangelica, 1655·1
*Archangelica officinalis*, 1655·1
Archidex, 1811·1
Archifen, 1811·1
Architex, 1811·1
Arcid, 1811·1
Arcitumomab, Technetium ($^{99m}$Tc), 1526·1
Arclonac, 1811·1
Arco Pain, 1811·1
Arcobee with C, 1811·1
Arcoiran, 1811·1
Arcolan, 1811·1
Arcolane, 1811·1
Arco-Lase, 1811·1
Arco-Lase Plus, 1811·1
Arcosal, 1811·1
Arcostrong, 1811·1
Arcoxia, 1811·1
*Arctium lappa*, 1704·3
*Arctium majus*, 1704·3
*Arctostaphylos uva-ursi*, 1659·2
Arctuvan, 1811·1
Ardeparin Sodium, 864·3
Ardeparina Sódica, 864·3
Ardey-aktiv, 1811·1
Ardeyceryl P, 1811·1
Ardeycholan N, 1811·1
Ardeycordal N, 1811·1
Ardeydorm, 1811·1
Ardeydystin, 1811·1
Ardeyhepan N, 1811·2
Ardeysedon N, 1811·2
Ardeytropin, 1811·2
ARDF-26, 332·3
Ardin, 1811·2
Ardine, 1811·2
Ardine Bronquial, 1811·2
Ardineclav, 1811·2
Ardinex, 1811·2
Ardoral, 1811·2
ARDS— *see* Acute Respiratory Distress Syndrome, 1075·2
Arduan, 1811·2
Arec, Noix d', 1656·2
Areca, 1656·2
*Areca catechu*, 1656·2
Areca Nuts, 1656·2
Arecae Semen, 1656·2
Arecaidine, 1656·2
Arecamin, 1811·2
Arecoline, 1656·2
Aredia, 1811·2
Aredronet, 1811·2
Arekasame, 1656·2
Arelcant, 1811·2
Arelix, 1811·2
Arelix ACE, 1811·2
Arem, 1811·2
Aremin, 1811·2
Aremis, 1811·2
Arendal, 1811·2
Arestal, 1811·2
Arestin, 1811·2
Aretensin, 1811·2
Areuma, 1811·2
Areuzolin, 1811·2
Arfarel, 1811·2
Arfen, 1811·3
Arfen Plus, 1811·3
Arfloxina, 1811·3
Arflur, 1811·3
Arg, 1421·1
Argatroban, 864·3, 1811·3
Argeal, 1811·3
Argeflox, 1811·3
Argenpal, 1811·3
Argent, 1811·3
Argent. Nit., 1746·2
Argental, 1811·3
Argent-Eze, 1811·3
Argenti Acetas, 1746·1
Argenti Nitras, 1746·1
Argentine Haemorrhagic Fever Vaccines, 1609·2
Argentinian Haemorrhagic Fever— *see* Haemorrhagic Fevers, 618·2
Argentocromo, 1811·3
Argentofenol, 1811·3
Argentoproteinum, 1746·2
Argentoproteinum Mite, 1746·2
Argentum Med Complex, 1811·3
Argentum Metallicum, 1746·1
Argentum Nitricum, 1746·2
Argentum Proteinicum, 1746·2
Argentum Vitellinicum, 1746·2
Argesic, 1811·3
Argesic-SA, 1811·3
Argicilline, 1811·3
Argidam, 1811·3
Argiletz, 1811·3
Argin, 1811·3
Arginaid Extra, 1811·3
Arginina, 1421·1
Arginina, Glutamato de, 1421·1
Arginina, Hidrocloruro de, 1421·1
Arginina, Piroglutamato de, 1732·3
Arginine, 1421·1
L-Arginine, 1421·1
Arginine Acetylasparaginate, 1421·2
Arginine Aspartate, 1421·1
Arginine Butyrate, 735·1, 735·3

Arginine Citrate, 1421·2
Arginine Glutamate, 1421·1
L-Arginine L-Glutamate, 1421·1
Arginine Hydrochloride, 1421·1
L-Arginine Monohydrochloride, 1421·1
Arginine Oxoglurate, 1421·2
Arginine Pidolate, 1732·3
Arginine Pyroglutamate, 1732·3
L-Arginine DL-Pyroglutamate, 1732·3
Arginine Tidiacicate, 1421·2
Arginine Timonacicate, 1421·2
[8-Arginine]vasopressin, 1342·3
Arginini Aspartas, 1421·1
Arginini Hydrochloridum, 1421·1
Argininum, 1421·1
Arginotri-B, 1811·3
Argipidine, 864·3
Argipresina, 1342·3
Argipressin, 1342·3
Argipressin Tannate, 1342·3
Argirofedrina, 1811·3
Argirol, 1811·3
Argisone, 1811·3
Argital, 1811·3
Argivit, 1811·3
Argocian, 1811·3
Argotone, 1811·4
Argousier, 1742·2
Argun, 1811·4
Argyrol, Colirio de— *see* Colirio de Argyrol, 1899·4
Argyrophedrine, 1811·4
Arhemapectine Antihemorragique, 1811·4
Aria, 1811·4
Arial, 1811·4
Arianna, 1811·4
Ariboflavinosis, 1456·2
Aricept, 1811·4
Aricodiltosse, 1811·4
Aridil, 1811·4
Arifenicol, 1811·4
Arilin, 1811·4
Ariline, 1811·4
Arilvax, 1811·4
Arima, 1811·4
Arimidex, 1811·4
Aripax, 1811·4
Aripiprazole, 671·1
Aristaloe, 1811·4
Aristamed, 1811·4
Aristin-C, 1811·4
Aristo, 1811·4
Aristo L, 1811·4
Aristochol, 1811·4
Aristochol CC, 1812·1
Aristochol N, 1812·1
Aristocor, 1812·1
Aristocort, 1812·1
Aristoforat, 1812·1
Aristogyl, 1812·1
Aristolochate Sodium, 1656·3
Aristolochia, 1656·3
*Aristolochia*, 1656·3
*Aristolochia brasiliensis*, 1656·3
*Aristolochia clematitis*, 1656·3
*Aristolochia contorta*, 1656·3
*Aristolochia debilis*, 1656·3
*Aristolochia fangchi*, 1656·3
*Aristolochia manshuriensis*, 1656·3
*Aristolochia reticulata*, 1656·3
*Aristolochia ringens*, 1656·3
*Aristolochia serpentaria*, 1656·3
Aristolochic Acid, 1656·3
Aristomycin, 1812·1
Aristopramida, 1812·1
Aristospan, 1812·1
Aritmina, 1812·1
Arixtra, 1812·1
Arkamin, 1812·1
Arkamin-H, 1812·1
Arkocaps, 1812·1
Arkocapsulas Carbon Veg, 1812·1
Arkocapsulas Hiperico, 1812·1
Arkogelules, 1812·1
Arkonsol, 1812·1
Arkonutril MM, 1812·1
Arkophytum, 1812·1
Arkotonic, 1812·1
Arkovital, 1812·1
Arkovital C, 1812·1
Arlette 28, 1812·1
Arlevert, 1812·1
Arlexicam, 1812·1
Arlidin, 1812·1
Arlitene, 1812·1
ARM, 1812·1
Armaya, 1812·1
Armeniacae Semen, 1730·2
Armil, 1812·2
Arminol, 1812·2
Armocur, 1812·2
Armoglobulina, 1812·2
Armonil, 1812·2
Armonyl, 1812·2
Armoracia, 1697·3
*Armoracia rusticana*, 1697·3
ARN, 1738·2
Arnecrem, 1812·2
Arnela, 1812·2
Arnica, 1656·3
*Arnica chamissonis*, 1656·3
Arnica Comp, 1812·2
Arnica Flos, 1656·3
Arnica Flower, 1656·3
Arnica Hamamelis Compuesta, 1812·2
Arnica Kneipp Salbe, 1812·2
Arnica Komplex, 1812·2
Arnica Massage Balm, 1812·2
Arnica Med Complex, 1812·2
*Arnica montana*, 1657·1
Arnica Oligoplex, 1812·2
Arnica Plus, 1812·2
Arnicadol, 1812·2
Arnicaid, 1812·2
Arnicalm, 1812·2
Arnica-loges, 1812·2
Arnican, 1812·2
Arnicet, 1812·2
Arnicon, 1812·2
Arniflor, 1812·2
Arniflor-N, 1812·2
Arnigel, 1812·2
Arnika Plus, 1812·2
Arnikaderm, 1812·2
Arnikamill, 1812·2
Arnikatinktur, 1812·3
Arnileve, 1812·3
Arnilose, 1812·3
Arobon, 1812·3
Arocin, 1812·3
Arofexx, 1812·3
Arola Rosebalm, 1812·3
Arolac, 1812·3
Aroltex, 1812·3
Aromabyl, 1812·3
Aromacin, 1812·3
Aromadendrene, 1710·2
Aromasil, 1812·3
Aromasin, 1812·3
Aromasine, 1812·3
Aromasol, 1812·3
Aromatase Inhibitors, 492·1
Aronal Forte, 1812·3
Aropax, 1812·3
Aroselin, 1812·3
Arotinolol, Hidrocloruro de, 865·1
Arotinolol Hydrochloride, 865·1
Arovit, 1812·3
Aroxat, 1812·3
Aroxin, 1812·3
Arpamyl LP, 1812·3
Arpha, 1812·3
Arpha Hustensirup, 1812·3
Arphos, 1812·3
Arpicolin, 1812·4
Arpilon, 1812·4
Arpimycin, 1812·4
Arrest, Cardiac— *see* Advanced Cardiac Life Support, 812·2
Arrestin, 1812·4
Arret, 1812·4
Arrête-Boeuf, 1723·3
Arretin, 1812·4
Arrhythmias, Atrial— *see* Cardiac Arrhythmias, 816·1
Arrhythmias, Atrioventricular Junctional— *see* Cardiac Arrhythmias, 816·1
Arrhythmias, Cardiac— *see* Cardiac Arrhythmias, 816·1
Arrhythmias, Supraventricular— *see* Cardiac Arrhythmias, 816·1
Arrhythmias, Ventricular— *see* Cardiac Arrhythmias, 816·1
Arritlan, 1812·4
Arrowroot, 1422·1
Arrumalon, 1812·4
Arsacol, 1812·4
Arsanilato Sódico, 158·3
Arsanilic Acid, 158·3
Arsanílico, Ácido, 158·3
Arscolloid, 1812·4
Arseni Trioxydum, 1657·1
Arseniato de Sodio, 1747·1
Arsenic, 1657·1
Arsenic Anhydride, 1657·3
Arsenic Oxide, 1657·1
Arsenic Trihydride, 1658·1
Arsenic Trioxide, 1657·1
Arsenic, White, 1657·1
Arsénico, Trióxido de, 1657·1
Arsenicosum Anhydricum, Acidum, 1657·1
Arsenicum Album, 1657·1
Arsenii Trioxidum ad Praeparationes Homoeopathicae, 1657·1
Arsenious Acid, 1657·1
Arsenious Trioxide for Homoeopathic Preparations, 1657·1
Arsenous Oxide, 1657·1
Arsina, 1658·1
Arsine, 1658·1
Arsiquinoforme, 1812·4
Art, 1812·4
Artagen, 1812·4
Artal, 1812·4
Artamin, 1812·4
Artandyl, 1812·4
Artane, 1812·4
Artaxan, 1812·4
Arte Rautin Forte S, 1812·4
Arteannuin, 447·2
Artecom, 456·1
Artedin, 1812·4
Arteether, 447·2
Arteflene, 448·1
Artekin, 456·1
Artelac, 1812·4
Artelinic Acid, 448·1
Artemeter, 447·2
Artemether, 447·2
Artemetherum, 447·2
*Artemisia absinthium*, 1645·1
*Artemisia annua*, 447·3
*Artemisia cina*, 114·1
Artemisinin, 447·2
Artemisinin Derivatives, 447·2
Artemisinina, 447·2
Artemisinina, Derivados, 447·2
Artemisinine, 447·2
Artemisininum, 447·2
Artemotil, 447·2
Artemotilo, 447·2
Artemotilum, 447·2
Arteolol, 1812·4
Arteopilo, 1812·4
Arteoptic, 1812·4
Arterase, 1813·1
Arterenol, 1813·1
Arterenol Acid Tartrate, 974·3
*l*-Arterenol Bitartrate, 974·3
Artergin, 1813·1
Arteria-cyl Ho-Len-Complex, 1813·1
Arterial Disease, Occlusive— *see* Peripheral Vascular Disease, 831·2
Arterial Disease, Peripheral— *see* Peripheral Vascular Disease, 831·2
Arterial Disease, Vasospastic— *see* Raynaud's Syndrome, 833·3
Arterial Embolism, Peripheral— *see* Peripheral Arterial Thromboembolism, 830·3
Arterial Occlusion, Acute— *see* Peripheral Arterial Thromboembolism, 830·3
Arterial Thromboembolism— *see* Thromboembolic Disorders, 837·3
Arterial Thromboembolism, Peripheral— *see* Peripheral Arterial Thromboembolism, 830·3
Arterial Thrombosis— *see* Thromboembolic Disorders, 837·3
Arterial Thrombosis, Peripheral— *see* Peripheral Arterial Thromboembolism, 830·3
Arteriobrate, 1813·1
Arterioflexin, 1813·1
Arteriol, 1813·1
Arteriovinca, 1813·1
Arteritis, Cranial— *see* Giant Cell Arteritis, 1080·1
Arteritis, Giant Cell— *see* Giant Cell Arteritis, 1080·1
Arteritis, Takayasu's— *see* Takayasu's Arteritis, 1089·3
Arteritis, Temporal— *see* Giant Cell Arteritis, 1080·1
Arterium, 1813·1
Arterodiet, 1813·1
Arterosan, 1813·1
Arterosan Plus, 1813·1
Arte-Rutin C, 1813·1
Artesol, 1813·1
Artesunate, 447·2
Artesunate Sodium, 447·2
Artesunato Sódico, 447·2
Artesunatum, 447·2
Arteven, 1813·1
Artevil, 1813·1
Artex, 1813·1
Artexal, 1813·1
Artflex, 1813·1
Arth-A Oligocan, 1813·1
Artha-G, 1813·1
Arthaxan, 1813·1
Arth-B Oligocan, 1813·1
Arthotec, 1813·1
Arthrabas, 1813·1
Arthrease, 1813·1
Arthrex, 1813·1
Arthrex Duo, 1813·1
Arthrexin, 1813·1
Arthribosan B 31, 1813·1
Arthricare Double Ice, 1813·2
Arthri-Care, Extralife— *see* Extralife Arthri-Care, 1986·3
Arthricare Hand & Body, 1813·2
Arthricare Odor Free, 1813·2
Arthricare Triple Medicated, 1813·2
Arthricare Ultra, 1813·2
Arthrifid S, 1813·2
Arthriforte, 1813·2
Arthrirub, 1813·2
Arthrisan, 1813·2
Arthriselect, 1813·2
Arthriten, Maximum Strength— *see* Maximum Strength Arthriten, 2116·3
Arthritic Pain, 1813·2
Arthritic Pain Herbal Formula 1, 1813·2
Arthritic Pain L10, 1813·2
Arthritic Pain Relief, 1813·2
Arthritis, Aseptic— *see* Spondyloarthropathies, 11·1
Arthritis, Bacterial— *see* Bone and Joint Infections, 122·1
Arthritis, Enteropathic— *see* Spondyloarthropathies, 11·1
Arthritis Foundation Pain Reliever, 1813·2
Arthritis, Gouty— *see* Gout and Hyperuricaemia, 412·1
Arthritis Hot Creme, 1813·2
Arthritis, Infective— *see* Bone and Joint Infections, 122·1
Arthritis, Juvenile Chronic— *see* Juvenile Idiopathic Arthritis, 9·1
Arthritis, Juvenile Idiopathic— *see* Juvenile Idiopathic Arthritis, 9·1
Arthritis Pain Formula, 1813·2

Arthritis Pain Formula Aspirin Free, 1813·2
Arthritis, Psoriatic— see Spondyloarthropathies, 11·1
Arthritis, Reactive— see Bone and Joint Infections, 122·1
Arthritis, Reactive— see Spondyloarthropathies, 11·1
Arthritis Relief, 1813·2
Arthritis, Rheumatoid— see Rheumatoid Arthritis, 9·3
Arthritis, Septic— see Bone and Joint Infections, 122·1
Arthritis, Seronegative— see Spondyloarthropathies, 11·1
Arthrixyl N, 1813·2
Arthro Akut, 1813·2
Arthrocine, 1813·2
Arthrodeformat P, 1813·2
Arthrodestal N, 1813·2
Arthrodont, 1813·2
Arthrodynat N, 1813·2
Arthrodynat P, 1813·2
Arthrofen, 1813·2
Arthrokehlan A, 1813·3
Arthrokehlan U, 1813·3
Arthropan, 1813·3
Arthropas K, 1813·3
Arthrorell, 1813·3
Arthrose-Echtroplex, 1813·3
Arthrose-Gastreu R73, 1813·3
Arthrosenex AR, 1813·3
Arthrosetten H, 1813·3
Arthrosin, 1813·3
Arthrotabs, 1813·3
Arthrotec, 1813·3
Arthrotone, 1813·3
Arthroxen, 1813·3
Arthrum H, 1813·3
Arthryl, 1813·3
Articaina C/E, 1813·3
Articaína, Hidrocloruro de, 1370·3
Articaine Hydrochloride, 1370·3
Articaini Hydrochloridum, 1370·3
Artichaut, 1678·3
Artichoke, Globe, 1678·3
Artichoke Leaf, 1678·3
Articlox, 1813·3
Articolase, 1813·3
Articolase (W/glucosamine), 1813·3
Articulan, 1813·3
Articurell, 1813·3
Artifene, 1813·3
Artificial Lung Expanding Compound, 1736·2
Artificial Saliva, 1576·1
Artificial Tears, 1576·1, 1813·3
Artificial Tears Extra, PMS— see PMS-Artificial Tears Extra, 2224·3
Artificial Tears, PMS— see PMS-Artificial Tears, 2224·3
Artiflam, 1813·3
Artilane, Natusor— see Natusor Artilane, 2153·4
Artilog, 1813·3
Artin, 1813·3
Artinizona, 1813·3
Artinor, 1813·3
Artischocke Plus Legastol, 1813·4
Artisial, 1813·4
Artistry, 1813·4
Artocoron, 1813·4
Artofen, 1813·4
Artoid, 1813·4
Artok, 1813·4
Artonil, 1813·4
Artosin, 1813·4
Artotec, 1813·4
Artoxan, 1813·4
Artragel, 1813·4
Artragil, 1813·4
Artrait, 1813·4
Artren, 1813·4
Artrenac, 1813·4
Artrenac Pro, 1813·4
Artrex, 1813·4
Artri, 1813·4
Artribid, 1813·4
Artricam, 1813·4
Artriden, 1813·4
Artridol, 1813·4
Artril, 1814·1
Artrilan, 1814·1
Artrilase, 1814·1
Artrinid, 1814·1
Artrinovo, 1814·1
Artritol, 1814·1
Artriunic, 1814·1
Artrizona, 1814·1
Artrocaptin, 1814·1
Artrocur, 1814·1
Artrodar, 1814·1
Artrodesmol Extra, 1814·1
Artrodol, 1814·1
Artrodue, 1814·1
Artrofenac, 1814·1
Artrofene, 1814·1
Artroglobina, 1814·1
Artrogota, 1814·1
Artrol, Neo— see Neo Artrol, 2156·1
Artrolyt, 1814·1
Artromed, 1814·1
Artron, 1814·1
Artroplex, 1814·1
Artroreuma, 1814·1
Artrosal, 1814·1
Artrosan, 1814·1
Artrosil, 1814·2
Artrosilene, 1814·2
Artrotec, 1814·2
Artroxen, 1814·2
Artroxicam, 1814·2
Artruic, 1814·2
Arturic, 1814·2
Artyflam, 1814·2
Artz, 1814·2
Artzal, 1814·2
Aru C, 1814·2
Arubendol, 1814·2
Aruclonin, 1814·2
Arudel, 1814·2
Arufil, 1814·2
Arutimol, 1814·2
Arutrin, 1814·2
Arvekap, 1814·2
Arvenum, 1814·2
Arvin, 1814·2
Arwin, 1814·2
Arythmol, 1814·2
Arzepam, 1814·2
Arzide, 1814·2
Arzimol, 1814·3
Arzomicin, 1814·3
Arzomicina, 1814·3
AS/85, 1814·3
AS-101, 158·3
AS 101 VA N, 1814·3
AS-4370, 1276·3
AS-18908, 263·1
AS Cor, 1814·3
ASA, 1814·3
5-ASA, 1273·2
ASA-158/5, 1115·2
Asa Right Powder, 1814·3
Asa Tones, 1814·3
Asacol, 1814·3
Asacolitin, 1814·3
Asacolon, 1814·3
ASAD, 1814·3
Asadon, XMTVI— see XMTVI Asadon, 2388·3
Asafen, 1814·3
Asafen Nueva Formula, 1814·3
Asafetida, 1658·1
Asaflow, 1814·3
Asafoetida, 1658·1
Asalazin, 1814·3
Asalen, 1814·3
Asalex, 1814·3
Asalit, 1814·3
Asamax, 1814·3
Asant, 1658·1
Asaphen, 1814·3
Asarabacca, 1658·1
ASA-ratio, 1814·3
Asari, Rhizoma, 1658·1
Asarid, 1814·3
Ásaro Europeo, 1658·1
*Asarum europaeum*, 1658·1
Asarum Med Complex, 1814·3
Asasantin, 1814·3
Asasantine, 1814·4
ASAtard, 1814·4
Asaurex, 1814·4
Asawin, 1814·4
Asax, 1814·4
Asazine, 1814·4
Asba, 1814·4
Asbesto, 1658·1
Asbestos, 1658·1
Asbestosis— see Diffuse Parenchymal Lung Disease, 1079·3
Ascabiol, 1814·4
Ascal, 1814·4
Ascariasis, 97·3
Ascarical, 1814·4
Ascaridil, 1814·4
Ascaridol, 103·2
Ascaridole, 103·2
Ascarin, 1814·4
Ascarinase, 1814·4
Ascariobel, 1814·4
Ascaritor, 1814·4
Ascarobex, 1814·4
Ascarotrat, 1814·4
Ascaverm, 1814·4
Ascencyl, 1814·4
Ascensia, 1814·4
Ascensia Glucodisc, 1814·4
Ascites, 815·1
Asclepia Tuberosa, 1733·1
*Asclepias tuberosa*, 1733·1
Ascocid, 1814·4
Ascodyne, 1814·4
Ascofer, 1814·4
Ascomed, 1814·4
Ascomp with Codeine, 1814·4
*Ascophyllum nodosum*, 1742·3
Ascor, 1814·4
Ascorbate-2-sulfate, 1460·3
Ascorbato Cálcico, 1460·2
Ascorbato de Quinina, 1737·2
Ascorbato de Sodio, 1460·2
Ascorbato Sódico, 1460·2
Ascorbex, 1814·4
Ascorbic Acid, 1460·2
L-Ascorbic Acid, 1460·2
L-Ascorbic Acid 6-Hexadecanoate, 1168·2
L-Ascorbic Acid 6-Palmitate, 1168·2
Ascórbico, Ácido, 1460·2
Ascorbicum, Acidum, 1460·2
Ascorbilo, Palmitato de, 1168·2
Ascorbin, 1814·4
Ascorbisal, 1814·4
Ascorbyl Palmitate, 1168·2
Ascorbylis Palmitas, 1168·2
Ascorell, 1815·1
Ascortil, 1815·1
Ascortonyl, 1815·1
Ascorvit, 1815·1
Ascosal, 1815·1
Ascot, 1815·1
Ascotodin, 1815·1
AscoTop, 1815·1
Ascoxal, 1815·1
Ascredar, 1815·1
Ascriptin, 1815·1
Asdron, 1815·1
ASE-136BS, 206·1
Aselli, 1815·1
Asendin, 1815·1
Asendis, 1815·1
Asenlix, 1815·1
Asenta, 1815·1
ASEP, 1815·1
Asepsal, 1815·1
Aseptalum, 1815·1
Aseptic Surgical Wax, 1480·2
Aseptiderm, 1815·1
Aseptil, 1815·1
Aseptisol, 1815·1
Asepto 7— see Septisept, 2285·3
Aseptobron Preparations, 1815·2
Asepto-Glutaral, 1815·2
Aseptoman, 1815·2
Aseptone 1, 1815·2
Aseptone 2, 1815·2
Aseptone 5, 1815·2
Aseptone Quat, 1815·2
Aseptosyl, 1815·2
Aserbine, 1815·2
Asercit, 1815·2
Aseroprim, 1815·2
Asestor, 1815·2
Asfeina, 1815·2
Asgoviscum N, 1815·2
Ash, 1273·1
Ash, Soda, 1747·1
Ashbourne Emollient Medicinal Bath Oil, 1815·2
Ashton & Parsons Infants Powders, 1815·2
Asialax, 1815·2
Asialum, 1815·3
Asiamox, 1815·3
Asian Ginseng, 1693·2
Asianbron, 1815·3
Asiatapp, 1815·3
Asiatic Acid, 1144·3
Asiaticoside, 1144·3
Asiazole, 1815·3
Asiazole-TN, 1815·3
Asic, 1815·3
Asig, 1815·3
Asilone, 1815·3
Asilone Heartburn, 1815·3
Asilone Windcheaters, 1815·3
Asimil B12, 1815·3
Asinis, 1815·3
Asiolex, 1815·3
Asipral, 1815·3
Asisdun, 1815·3
Askina, 1815·3
Askina Biofilm, 1815·3
Askina Sorb, 1815·3
Askit, 1815·3
ASL, 1815·3
ASL-279, 907·1
ASL-601, 848·3
ASL-603, 876·2
ASL-8052, 913·1
Aslanvital, 1815·3
Aslavital, 1815·4
Asmabec, 1815·4
Asmabiol, 1815·4
Asmacortone, 1815·4
Asmafen, 1815·4
Asmafin, 1815·4
Asmaflu, 1815·4
Asmafort, 1815·4
Asmalene, 1815·4
Asmalergin, 1815·4
Asmaline, 1815·4
Asmaliv, 1815·4
Asmalix, 1815·4
Asmanex, 1815·4
Asmanoc, 1815·4
Asmanon, 1815·4
Asmapax, 1815·4
Asmapen, 1815·4
Asmaral-K, 1815·4
Asmasal, 1815·4
Asmasal Expectorant, 1815·4
Asmasolon, 1815·4
Asmatec, 1815·4
Asmaten, 1815·4
Asmaten, Natusor— see Natusor Asmaten, 2153·4
Asmatil, 1815·4
Asmatiron, 1815·4
Asmatol, 1815·4
Asmaven, 1815·4
Asmavent, 1815·4
Asmavent-B, 1816·1
Asmax, 1816·1
Asmen, 1816·1

Asmeren, 1816·1
Asmeton, 1816·1
Asmifen, 1816·1
Asmodrin, 1816·1
Asmofen, 1816·1
Asmol, 1816·1
Asmo-Lavi, 1816·1
Asmopul, 1816·1
Asmoquinol, 1816·1
Asmosterona, 1816·1
Asmotone Plus, 1816·1
Asmovent, 1816·1
Asmovent Expectorant, 1816·1
Aso DDI, 1816·1
Asodal, 1816·1
Asodocel, 1816·1
Asoflut, 1816·1
Asofurtal, 1816·1
Asoifos, 1816·1
Asolmicina, 1816·1
A-Solmicina-C, 1816·1
Asomutan, 1816·1
Asonacor, 1816·1
Asotax, 1816·1
Asotecan, 1816·1
Asoteron, 1816·1
Asotrex, 1816·2
Asovon, 1816·2
Asovorin, 1816·2
Asoxima, Cloruro de, 1032·2
Asoxime Chloride, 1032·2
Asp, 1422·3
ASP, 1816·2
Aspac, 1816·2
Aspagin, 1816·2
Aspalgin, 1816·2
Asparaginasa, 528·3
Asparaginase, 528·3
L-Asparaginase, 528·3
L-Asparagine Amidohydrolase, 528·3
Asparagine Monohydrate, 1422·1
L-Asparagine Monohydrate, 1422·1
[1-Asparagine,5-valine]angiotensin II, 863·3
Asparaginum Monohydricum, 1422·1
Asparagus-P, 1816·2
Aspargininum, 1421·1
Aspart, Insulin, 334·3, 340·3
Aspartame, 1422·1
Aspartame Acesulfame, 1422·2
Aspartamins, 1816·2
Aspartamo, 1422·1
Aspartamum, 1422·1
Aspartatol, 1816·2
Asparten, 1816·2
Aspartic Acid, 1422·3
L-Aspartic Acid, 1422·3
Aspártico, Ácido, 1422·3
Aspartina, 1816·2
Aspartono, 1816·2
*N*-L-α-Aspartyl-L-phenylalanine, 1-Methyl Ester, 1422·1
A-Spas, 1816·2
Aspaserine B6 Tranq, 1816·2
Aspasmine, 1816·2
Aspasmon N, 1816·2
Aspav, 1816·2
Aspec, 1816·2
Aspecton, 1816·2
Aspecton Eukaps, 1816·2
Aspecton N, 1816·2
Aspecton-Balsam, 1816·2
Aspectonetten N, 1816·2
Aspegic, 1816·2
Aspellin, 1816·2
Aspent, 1816·2
Aspercreme, 1816·2
Aspergilloma— *see* Aspergillosis, 386·1
Aspergillosis, 386·1
*Aspergillus flavus*, 1648·3
*Aspergillus fumigatus*, 605·2
*Aspergillus melleus*, 1735·2
*Aspergillus niger*, 1669·1
*Aspergillus oryzae*, 1654·2
*Aspergillus parasiticus*, 1648·3
Aspergum, 1816·3
Aspergun, 1816·3
Asperivo, 1816·3
Aspex, 1816·3
Asphaline, 1816·3
Aspi-C, 1816·3
Aspic, Huile Essentielle d', 1749·2
Aspicot, 1816·3
Aspidium, 108·2
Aspidium Oleoresin, 108·2
Aspidol, 1816·3
Aspiglicina, 1816·3
Aspilets, 1816·3
Aspinfantil, 1816·3
Aspiration, Acid— *see* Aspiration Syndromes, 1240·1
Aspiration Pneumonia— *see* Pneumonia, 141·3
Aspiration Syndromes, 1240·1
Aspiricor, 1816·3
Aspirin, 15·1
Aspirin Aluminium, 14·1
Aspirin Backache, 1816·3
Aspirin C, 1816·3
Aspirin + C, 1816·3
Aspirin Cardio, 1816·3
Aspirin Forte, 1816·3
Aspirin Free Anacin, 1816·3
Aspirin Free Anacin PM, 1816·3
Aspirin Free Excedrin, 1816·3
Aspirin Free Excedrin Dual, 1816·3
Aspirin Free Pain Relief, 1816·3
Aspirin DL-Lysine, 54·3
Aspirin Plus C, 1816·3
Aspirin with Stomach Guard, 1816·3
Aspirina, 1816·3
Aspirina 03, 1816·3
Aspirina 05, 1816·4
Aspirina 05— *see* Aspirina 03 and 05, 1816·3
Aspirina C, 1816·4
Aspirina Complex, 1816·4
Aspirina Forte, 1816·4
Aspirina Plus, 1816·4
Aspirine, 1816·4
Aspirine C, 1816·4
Aspirine Duo, 1816·4
Aspirine pH8, 1816·4
Aspirine Protect, 1816·4
Aspirine Vitamine C, 1816·4
Aspirinetas, 1816·4
Aspirinetta, 1816·4
Aspirinetta C, 1816·4
Aspirin-Free Bayer Select Allergy Sinus, 1816·4
Aspirin-Free Bayer Select Head & Chest Cold, 1816·4
Aspirin-paracetamol Ester, 20·3
Aspirisan, 1816·4
Aspirisucre, 1816·4
Aspi-Rub, 1816·4
Aspisin, 1816·4
Aspisol, 1816·4
Aspitopic, 1816·4
Asplenism, Infection Prophylaxis— *see* Spleen Disorders, 146·3
Asplin, 1816·4
Asporin 0.5, 1816·4
Asporin 2, 1816·4
Aspoxicilina, 158·3
Aspoxicillin, 158·3
Asprimox, 1816·4
Aspro, 1816·4
Aspro C, 1817·1
Aspro + C, 1817·1
Aspro mit Vitamin C, 1817·1
Aspro Vitamine C, 1817·1
Asproaccel, 1817·1
Aspylin, 1817·1
ASS, 1817·1
ASS + C, 1817·1
ASS OPT, 1817·1
ASS, Togal— *see* Togal ASS, 2336·1
Assal, 1817·1
Assalix, 1817·1
Assan, 1817·1
Assan-Thermo, 1817·1
ASSbene, 1817·1
Assenzio, 1645·1
Assenzio (Specie Composta), 1817·1
Assepium, 1817·1
Assepium Balsamico, 1817·1
Asseptobron, 1817·1
Assieme, 1817·1
Assist, 1817·1
Assist Energetico, 1817·1
Assist Reintegratore, 1817·1
Assival, 1817·1
ASS-Kombi, 1817·1
Assocort, 1817·1
Assogen, 1817·1
Assoral, 1817·1
Assplant, 1817·1
Assume Maleate— *see* Avandia, 1821·2
Assy Espuma, 1817·2
Assyuni, 1666·1
Asta-3746, 480·2
Asta C-4898, 900·1
Astahis, 1817·2
Astaplatin, 1817·2
Astat, 1817·2
Astelin, 1817·2
Astem, 1817·2
Astemina, 1817·2
Astemizol, 424·2
Astemizole, 424·2
Astemizolum, 424·2
Astenol, 1817·2
Astenolit, 1817·2
Astergyl, 1817·2
Asteriodine, 1817·2
Astesen, 1817·2
Astezol, 1817·2
Asthalin, 1817·2
Asthalin Expectorant, 1817·2
Asthamsian, 1817·2
Asthavent, 1817·2
Asthenal, 1817·2
Asthenopin, 1817·2
Asthma, 777·2, 1817·2
Asthma & Catarrh Relief, 1817·2
Asthma 23 D, 1817·2
Asthma Efeum, 1817·2
Asthma H, 1817·2
Asthma 6-N, 1817·2
Asthma T, 1817·2
Asthma-Bomin H, 1817·2
AsthmaHaler Mist, 1817·2
Asthma-Hilfe, 1817·2
Asthmakhell N, 1817·3
Asthmalgine, 1817·3
Asthmalitan, 1817·3
Asthmalyticum-Ampullen N (Rowo-210), 1817·3
AsthmaNefrin, 1817·3
Asthma-Spray, 1817·3
Asthmatee EF-EM-ES, 1817·3
Asthmavowen-N, 1817·3
Asthmaxine, 1817·3
Asthmino, 1817·3
Asthmo-Kranit Mono, 1817·3
Asthmolin, 1817·3
Asthmolysin, 1817·3
Asthmoprotect, 1817·3
Asthmotrat, 1817·3
Astho-Med, 1817·3
Asticol, 1817·3
Astidin, 1817·3
Astifat, 1817·3
Astin, 1817·3
Astmazol, 1817·3
Astomera, 1817·3
Astone, 1817·3
Astonin, 1817·3
Astonin H, 1817·3
Astra-1512, 1382·3
Astra-1572, 1438·1
Astracaine, 1817·3
*Astragalus*, 1582·2
*Astragalus gummifer*, 1582·2
Astramorph, 1817·3
Astramorph PF, 1817·3
Astratonil, 1817·3
Astreptine, 1817·3
Astressane, 1817·4
Astrexine, 1817·4
Astriderm, 1817·4
Astrin, 1817·4
Astringel, Natusor— *see* Natusor Astringel, 2153·4
Astrix, 1817·4
Astrocast, 1817·4
Astrocytoma— *see* Malignant Neoplasms of the Brain, 513·2
Astroglide, 1817·4
Astromicin Sulfate, 158·3
Astromicin Sulphate, 158·3
Astromicina, Sulfato de, 158·3
Astronautal, 1817·4
Astudal, 1817·4
Astyl, 1817·4
Astymin-3, 1817·4
Astymin Forte, 1817·4
Asucrose, 1817·4
[Asu$^{1,7}$]-E-CT, 768·3
Asulblan, 1817·4
Asumalife, 1817·4
Asverin, 1817·4
Asystole— *see* Advanced Cardiac Life Support, 812·2
AT III, 1817·4
AT-III, 742·2,
AT 10, 1817·4
AT-17, 1118·3
AT-101, 941·1
AT-327, 1131·3
AT-877, 914·3
AT-2101, 1698·1
AT-2266, 207·2
AT-4140, 255·1
Atacand, 1817·4
Atacand HCT, 1817·4
Atacand Plus, 1817·4
Atacand-D, 1817·4
AtacandZid, 1817·4
Ataclor, 1817·4
Atacoly, 1817·4
Atagripe, 1817·4
Atalin, 1818·1
Ataline, 1818·1
Atamet, 1818·1
Atamir, 1818·1
Atano, 1818·1
Atapec, 1818·1
Atapryl, 1818·1
Atapulgita, 1251·1
Atarax, 1818·1
Ataraxone, 1818·1
Atarin, 1818·1
Atarone, 1818·1
Atarviton, 1818·1
Atasol Preparations, 1818·1
Atassol, 1818·1
Atatosse Balsamico, 1818·1
Atazanavir Sulfate, 629·1
Atazanavir Sulphate, 629·1
Atazid, 1818·1
ATC, 1756·2
Atd, 1818·1
Ate, 1818·1
Ate Lich, 1818·1
Ate Lich Comp, 1818·1
Atebemyxine, 1818·1
Ateben, 1818·1
Atebeta, 1818·1
Atecard, 1818·1
Atecard-D, 1818·1
Atecor, 1818·1
Atedurex, 1818·1
Atege, 1818·2
Atehexal, 1818·2
Atehexal Comp, 1818·2
Atel, 1818·2
Atel C, 1818·2
Atel N, 1818·2
Atelec, 1818·2
Atem, 1818·2
Atemaron N R30, 1818·2
Atemperator, 1818·2

Atemur, 1818·2
Atenase, 1818·2
Atenativ, 1818·2
Atenblock, 1818·2
Atendol, 1818·2
Ateneo, 1818·2
Atenet, 1818·2
Atenetic, 1818·2
Atenfar, 1818·2
Ateni, 1818·2
AteNif Beta, 1818·2
Ate-Nife, 1818·2
Atenigron, 1818·2
Atenil, 1818·2
Atenix, 1818·2
AtenixCo, 1818·3
Ateno, 1818·3
Ateno Comp, 1818·3
Ateno-basan, 1818·3
Ateno-basan Comp., 1818·3
Atenobene, 1818·3
Atenobene Comp, 1818·3
Atenoblock, 1818·3
Atenoblok, 1818·3
Atenoblok Co, 1818·3
Atenodan, 1818·3
Atenogamma, 1818·3
Atenogamma Comp, 1818·3
Atenogen, 1818·3
Atenol, 1818·3
Atenolan, 1818·3
Atenolan Comp, 1818·3
Atenolol, 865·2
Atenolol AL Comp, 1818·3
Atenolol Comp, 1818·3
Atenololum, 865·2
Atenomel, 1818·3
Atenomerck, 1818·3
Atenomerck Comp, 1818·3
Atenopress, 1818·3
Atenor, 1818·3
Atenoric, 1818·3
Atenos, 1818·3
Atenotyrol, 1818·3
Atenotyrol Comp, 1818·3
Atens, 1818·4
Atens H, 1818·4
Atenses, 1818·4
Atensin, 1818·4
Atensina, 1818·4
Atenual, 1818·4
Atepadene, 1818·4
Atepodin, 1818·4
Ateran, 1818·4
Aterax, 1818·4
Atereal, 1818·4
Aterina, 1818·4
Ateriosan, 1818·4
Aterkey, 1818·4
Atermin, 1818·4
Ateroclar, 1818·4
Ateroid, 1818·4
Ateroide, 1818·4
Ateroxide, 1818·4
Atesifar, 1818·4
Atevirdine Mesilate, 629·1
Atevirdine Mesylate, 629·1
At-Eze, 1818·4
ATG, 1348·3, 1818·4
Atgam, 1818·4
ATG-S, 1818·4
Athelmin, 1818·4
Athenol, 1819·1
Athera, 1819·1
Ätherisches Muskatöl, 1722·3
Athero, 1819·1
Atherogenesis— *see* Atherosclerosis, 815·2
Atherosclerosis, 815·2
Athimbin P, 1819·1
Athimil, 1819·1
Athletes Foot, 1819·1
Athlete's Foot— *see* Skin Infections, 390·1
Athletes Foot Antifungal, 1819·1
Athletes Foot Cream, 1819·1
Athlete's Foot Preparations, Scholl— *see* Scholl Athlete's Foot Preparations, 2279·2
Athlete's Foot, Scholl— *see* Scholl Athlete's Foot, 2279·2
Athos, 1819·1
Athrofen, 1819·1
Athru-Derm, 1819·1
Athymil, 1819·1
ATI-01, 1736·2
ATI-02, 1736·2
Atiflan, 1819·1
Atilan, 1819·1
Atinac, 1819·1
A-Tinic, 1819·1
Atinorm, 1819·1
Atipamezol, Hidrocloruro de, 1032·3
Atipamezole, 1032·3
Atipamezole Hydrochloride, 1032·3
Atiramin, 1819·1
Atirosin, 1819·1
Atisuril, 1819·1
Atiten, 1819·1
Ativan, 1819·1
Ativit, 1819·1
Atizor, 1819·1
Atkinson & Barker's Gripe Mixture, 1819·1
ATL-1251, 1287·3
Atlansil, 1819·1
Atlizumab, 1757·1
Atma, 1819·1
Atmadisc, 1819·1
Atmocol, 1819·2
Atmos, 1819·2
Atoactive, 1819·2
Atock, 1819·2
Atodel, 1819·2
Atoderm, 1819·2
Atolant, 1819·2
Atolone, 1819·2
Atomase, 1819·2
Atomic Enema, 1819·2
Atomide, 1819·2
Atomo Desinflamante C, 1819·2
Atomo Desinflamante Depor, 1819·2
Atomo Desinflamante Familiar, 1819·2
Atomo Desinflamante G, 1819·2
Atomo Desinflamante Geldic, 1819·2
Atomoderma A, 1819·2
Atomoderma A-D, 1819·2
Atomoderma A-E, 1819·2
Atomoderma Plus, 1819·2
Atomoxetine Hydrochloride, 1585·1
Atonic Seizures— *see* Epilepsy, 349·1
Atopic, 1819·2
Atopic Eczema— *see* Eczema, 1135·1
Atopil, 1819·2
Atorva, 1819·2
Atorvastan, 1819·2
Atorvastatin Calcium, 866·1
Atorvastatina Cálcica, 866·1
Atosiban, 1319·1
Atosiban Acetate, 1319·1
Atosil, 1819·2
Atossion, 1819·2
Atossisclerol Kreussler, 1819·2
Atovacuona, 601·3
Atovaquone, 601·3
Atoxecar, 1819·3
ATP, 1648·1, 1819·3
ATR, 477·1
Atractil, 1819·3
Atracur, 1819·3
Atracurio, Besilato de, 1399·1
Atracurium Besilate, 1399·1
Atracurium Besylate, 1399·1
Atralcilina, 1819·3
Atralidon, 1819·3
Atralmicina, 1819·3
Atrasentan, 522·1
*Atrax robustus* Antiserum, 1640·1
*Atrax robustus* Antivenin, 1640·1
*Atrax robustus* Antivenom, 1640·1
Atretol, 1819·3
Atrial Arrhythmias— *see* Cardiac Arrhythmias, 816·1
Atrial Fibrillation— *see* Cardiac Arrhythmias, 816·1
Atrial Flutter— *see* Cardiac Arrhythmias, 816·1
Atrial Natriuretic Factor, 964·2
Atrial Natriuretic Peptide, 964·2
Atrial Premature Beats— *see* Cardiac Arrhythmias, 816·1
Atrial Tachycardia— *see* Cardiac Arrhythmias, 816·1
Atrican, 1819·3
Atridox, 1819·3
Atrilon, 1819·3
Atrimon, 1819·3
Atriopeptidase Inhibitors, 964·2
Atriopeptin, 964·2
Atrioventricular Block— *see* Cardiac Arrhythmias, 816·1
Atrioventricular Dissociation— *see* Cardiac Arrhythmias, 816·1
Atrioventricular Junctional Arrhythmias— *see* Cardiac Arrhythmias, 816·1
Atriscal, 1819·3
Atrisol, 1819·3
Atrisolon, 1819·3
Atrium, 1819·3
Atrival, 1819·3
Atro Grin, 1819·3
Atrobel, 1819·3
Atrodual, 1819·3
Atrohist Pediatric, 1819·3
Atrohist Plus, 1819·3
Atrombin, 1819·3
Atromicin, 1819·3
Atromid, Neo— *see* Neo Atromid, 2156·1
Atromidin, 1819·3
Atromid-S, 1819·3
Atronase, 1819·4
Atrop, 1819·4
Atrop. Methonit., 477·1
Atrop. Sulph., 477·1
*Atropa belladonna*, 479·1
AtroPen, 1819·4
Atrophic Thyroiditis— *see* Hypothyroidism, 1595·3
Atrophic Vaginitis— *see* Menopausal Disorders, 1540·2
Atropina, 476·3
Atropina, Metilbromuro de, 476·3
Atropina, Metilnitrato de, 477·1
Atropina, Sulfato de, 477·1
Atropine, 476·3
Atropine Borate, 478·3
Atropine, Chibro- — *see* Chibro-Atropine, 1882·3
Atropine and Demerol, 1819·4
Atropine Methobromide, 476·3
Atropine Methonitrate, 477·1
Atropine Methylbromide, 476·3
Atropine Oxide Hydrochloride, 478·3
Atropine Sulfate, 477·1
Atropine Sulphate, 477·1
Atropini Methonitras, 477·1
Atropini Sulfas, 477·1
Atropinol, 1819·4
Atropinum, 476·3
Atropion, 1819·4
Atropisol, 1819·4
Atropocil, 1819·4
Atropt, 1819·4
Atrosept, 1819·4
Atrospan, 1819·4
Atrotil, 1819·4
Atrovent, 1819·4
Atrovent Beta, 1819·4
Atrovent Comp, 1819·4
Atroveran, 1819·4
Atrovex, 1819·4
ATS, 1819·4
Atse, 1819·4
Atta, 1819·4
Attafur, 1819·4
Attain, 1819·4
Attapulgite, 1251·1
Attapulgite, Activated, 1251·1
Attapulgite, Colloidal Activated, 1251·1
Attar of Rose, 1740·2
Attenta, 1819·4
Attention Deficit Hyperactivity Disorder— *see* Hyperactivity, 1583·1
Attenuvax, 1820·1
Aturgyl, 1820·1
Atus, 1820·1
Atusil, 1820·1
Atuss DM, 1820·1
Atuss-12 DM, 1820·1
Atuss-12 DX, 1820·1
Atuss EX, 1820·1
Atuss G, 1820·1
Atuss HD, 1820·1
Atuxane, 1820·1
AT-V, 1820·1
Atypical Antipsychotics, 663·1
Atypical Mycobacterial Infections— *see* Opportunistic Mycobacterial Infections, 137·2
Ätzkali, 1734·2
Ätznatron, 1747·3
15AU81, 1521·2
AU 4 Regeneresen, 1820·1
Aubeline, 1820·1
Aubépine, 1677·1
Aubril, 1820·1
Aucusik, 1820·1
Audax, 1820·1
Audazol, 1820·1
Audicort, 1820·1
Audifluor, 1820·1
Audione, 1820·1
Audispray, 1820·1
Auditol, 1820·1
Augelit, 1820·1
Augenkraft, 1820·1
Augentonicum, 1820·1
Augentonikum N, 1820·1
Augentropfen Mucokehl D5, 1820·2
Augentropfen Stulln, 1820·2
Augentropfen Stulln Mono, 1820·2
Augmaxil, 1820·2
Augmentan, 1820·2
Augmentation of Labour— *see* Labour Induction and Augmentation, 1511·1
Augmentin, 1820·2
Augmentin Bid, 1820·2
Augmentin-Duo, 1820·2
Augmentine, 1820·2
Aulcer, 1820·2
Aulin, 1820·2
Aulo Gelio Pie, 1820·2
Aulo Gelio Repelente, 1820·2
Aunativ, 1820·2
Aunativ S.D., 1820·2
Aunée, 1119·3
Auralgan, 1820·2
Auralgicin, 1820·2
Auralyt, 1820·2
Auram, 1820·2
Auramin, 1820·2
Auranofin, 19·1
Auranofina, 19·1
Aurantii Amari Epicarpium et Mesocarpium, 1723·3
Aurantii Amari Floris Aetheroleum, 1719·2
Aurantii Amari Flos, 1723·3
Aurantii Deterpenatum, Oleum, 1724·2
Aurantii Dulcis Aetheroleum, 1724·1
Aurantin, 1820·2
Auraphene-B, 1820·2
Aurasept, 1820·2
Auratek HCG, 1820·2
Aureciclina, 1820·2
Aurecil, 1820·2
Aurene, 1820·3
Aureocort, 1820·3
Aureocrem, 1820·3
Aureodelf, 1820·3
Aureodermil, 1820·3
Aureolic Acid, 580·2
Aureomicina, 1820·3
Aureomix, 1820·3

Aureomycin, 1820·3
Aureomycin N, 1820·3
Aureomycine, 1820·3
Aureotan, 1820·3
Auricid, 1820·3
Auricularum, 1820·3
Auriculin, 964·2
Auricum, 1820·3
Auriderm Corps, 1820·3
Auridonal, 1820·3
Aurigen, 1820·3
Aurigoutte, 1820·3
Aurisan, 1820·3
Auristan, 1820·3
Aurita-Bronchialtee, 1820·3
Aurita-Erkaltungstee, 1820·3
Aurita-Leber-Galletee, 1820·3
Aurita-Nerventee, 1820·3
Aurita-Nieren-Blasentee, 1820·3
Aurita-Verdauungstee, 1820·3
Auritricin, 1820·3
Auro, 1820·4
Auroanalin N, 1820·4
Aurochobet, 1820·4
Auroclim, 1820·4
Auro-Dri, 1820·4
Auroguard Otic, 1820·4
Auroken, 1820·4
Aurolate, 1820·4
Auromyose, 1820·4
Aurone, 1820·4
Aurone Forte, 1820·4
Auroplatin, 1820·4
Auroplatin— *see* Cimicifuga comp, 1887·1
Aurorex, 1820·4
Aurorix, 1820·4
Aurosulfo, 1820·4
Aurosyx N, 1820·4
1-Aurothio-D-glucopyranose, 19·3
Aurothioglucose, 19·3
Aurothiopolypeptide, 45·1
(Aurothio)succinic Acid, 88·2
Aurotioglucosa, 19·3
Aurotiomalato de Sodio, 88·2
Aurotioprol, 20·1
Aurotiosulfato de Sodio, 90·1
Auroto, 1820·4
Aurum, 1695·3
Aurum Met., 1695·3
Aurum-Gastreu S R2, 1820·4
Aurumheel, 1820·4
Auscap, 1820·4
Auscard, 1820·4
Ausclav, 1820·4
Ausentron, 1820·4
Ausgem, 1820·4
Ausobronc, 1820·4
Ausomina, 1820·4
Auspril, 1820·4
Ausran, 1820·4
Aussie Tan, 1820·4
Aussie Tan Pre-Tan, 1820·4
Aussie Tan Skin Moisturiser, 1821·1
Aussie Tan Sunstick, 1821·1
Austral-Balm, 1821·1
Australian Tea Tree Oil, 1710·2
Austrapen, 1821·1
Austrialens, 1821·1
Austrian Digitalis, 894·2
Austrian Foxglove, 894·2
Austroflex, 1821·1
Austrophyllin, 1821·1
Austrorinse, 1821·1
Austrosept, 1821·1
Austyn, 1821·1
Aut, 1821·1
Autan, 1821·1
Autdol, 1821·1
Aution Sticks 10EA, 1821·1
Autohaler, 1821·1
Autohelios, 1821·1
Auto-immune Hepatitis— *see* Chronic Active Hepatitis, 1078·1
Autoimmune Thrombocytopenic Purpura— *see* Idiopathic Thrombocytopenic Purpura, 1082·1
Autonic, 1821·1
Autoplasme Vaillant, 1821·1
Autoplex, 1821·1
Autoplex T, 1821·1
Autoplex T— *see* Anti-Inhibitor Coagulant Complex (Autoplex T), 1804·3
Autoprothrombin, 735·3
Autosterile, 1821·1
Autrin, 1821·1
Autrinic Compuesto, 1821·1
Autritis, 1821·1
Auxergyl $D_3$, 1821·1
Auxergyl D3, 1821·1
Auxiloson, 1821·1
Auxina A + E, 1821·1
Auxina A Masiva, 1821·2
Auxina Complejo B, 1821·2
Auxina E, 1821·2
Auxitrans, 1821·2
Auxofer, 1821·2
Auxxil, 1821·2
AV-42810, 633·2
Avadene, 1821·2
Avafontan, 1821·2
Avafortan, 1821·2
Avage, 1821·2
Avail, 1821·2
Avala, 1821·2
Avaldrian, 1821·2
Avalide, 1821·2
Avalin, 1821·2
Avallone, 1821·2
Avalon, 1821·2
Avalox, 1821·2
Avamigran, 1821·2
Avamigran N, 1821·2
Avance, 1821·2
Avancel, 1821·2
Avancort, 1821·2
Avandamet, 1821·2
Avandia, 1821·2
Avant, 1821·3
Avant Garde Shampoo, 1821·3
Avantrin, 1821·3
Avanza, 1821·3
Avapena, 1821·3
Avapro, 1821·3
Avapro HCT, 1821·3
Avar, 1821·3
Avastin, 1821·3
Avaxim, 1821·3
Avazinc, 1821·3
AVC, 1821·3
Avecyde, 1821·3
Avedorm, 1821·3
Avedorm Duo, 1821·3
Avedorm N, 1821·3
Aveendix, 1821·3
Aveeno Preparations, 1821·3
Aveenocream, 1821·4
Aveenoderm, 1821·4
Avelon, 1821·4
Avelox, 1821·4
Aven, 1658·2
Avena, 1658·2
Avena Complex, 1821·4
Avena Med Complex, 1821·4
Avena Rihom Komplex, 1821·4
*Avena sativa*, 1658·2
Avena Sativa Comp, 1821·4
Avenaforce, 1821·4
Avene Antirougeurs, 1821·4
Avene Creme Protectrice, 1821·4
Avene Ecran, 1821·4
Avene Ecran Extreme, 1821·4
Avene Ecran Jour, 1821·4
Avene Ecran Tres Haute Protection, 1821·4
Avene Lait Protecteur— *see* Avene Creme Protectrice and Lait Protecteur, 1821·4
Avene 50 Proteccion Extrema, 1821·4
Avene 20 Proteccion Total, 1821·4
Avenin, 1658·2
Aveno, 1821·4
Avenoc, 1821·4
Aventyl, 1821·4
Avermectins, 106·2
Averpan, 1821·4
Avertex, 1822·1
Averuk Bruciaporri, 1822·1
Avesoap, 1822·1
Aviane, 1822·1
Avibon, 1822·1
A-Vicon, 1822·1
A-Vicotrat, 1822·1
Avidin, 1423·2
Avigilen, 1822·1
Avil, 1822·1
Avil Decongestant, 1822·1
Avil Expectorant, 1822·1
Avilac, 1822·1
Avilamicina, 159·1
Avilamycin, 159·1
Avinal-Ex, 1822·1
Avintac, 1822·1
Avinza, 1822·1
Aviptadil, 1763·2
Avipur, 1822·1
Aviral, 1822·1
Avirase, 1822·1
Avirax, 1822·1
Avirex-T, 1822·1
Avirin, 1822·1
Avirostat, 1822·1
Avirox, 1822·1
Avishot, 1822·1
Avita, 1822·1
A-Vita, 1822·1
A-Vitamiini, 1822·1
A-vitamin, 1822·2
Avitcid, 1822·2
A-Vite, 1822·2
A-Vitel, 1822·2
A-Vitel E, 1822·2
Avitene, 1822·2
A-Vitex, 1822·2
Avitol, 1822·2
Avitracid, 1822·2
Avix, 1822·2
Avixis, 1822·2
Avlocardyl, 1822·2
Avloclor, 1822·2
Avlosulfon, 1822·2
Avobenzona, 1142·3
Avobenzone, 1142·3
Avoca, 1822·2
Avoca Menthol Cone, 1822·2
Avocin, 1822·2
Avodart, 1822·2
Avomine, 1822·2
Avon Footworks, 1822·2
Avon Techniques Anti-Dandruff, 1822·2
Avonex, 1822·2
Avopàrcin, 159·1
Avoparcina, 159·1
Avorax, 1822·2
AVP, 1342·3
Avril, 1822·2
Avural, 1822·2
Avyclor, 1822·2
Avyplus, 1822·2
Avysal, 1822·3
AW-105-843, 406·2
Awesome Animals, 1822·3
A-60386X, 1736·2
Axacef, 1822·3
Axagon, 1822·3
Axal, 1822·3
Axasol, 1822·3
Axcil, 1822·3
Axel, Locion— *see* Locion Axel, 2102·2
Axelorax, 1822·3
Axelvin, 1822·3
Axepim, 1822·3
Axer, 1822·3
Axerophtholum, 1451·2
Axert, 1822·3
Axetine, 1822·3
Axiago, 1822·3
Axid, 1822·3
Axilin, 1822·3
Aximad, 1822·3
Axion, 1822·3
Axis, 1822·3
Axistal, 1822·3
Axocet, 1822·3
Axocillin, 1822·3
Axofor, 1822·3
Axol, 1822·3
Axonyl, 1822·3
Axoren, 1822·3
Axotide, 1822·3
Axsain, 1822·3
Axtin, 1822·4
Axura, 1822·4
Axyol, 1822·4
AY-4166, 343·3
AY-5312, 1173·3
AY-5710, 1271·3
AY-6108, 157·1
AY-6608, 1729·3
AY-20385, 607·2
AY-22989, 1363·1
AY-022989, 1363·1
AY-24031, 1325·2
AY-24236, 37·3
AY-24269, 990·3
AY-25650, 1341·2
AY-27255, 1764·2
AY-61123, 884·3
AY-62014, 289·1
AY-62021, 730·3
AY-62022, 1557·1
AY-64043, 989·3
Ayahuasca, 1696·3
Aydolid, 1822·4
Aydolid Codeina, 1822·4
Ayercillin, 1822·4
Aygestin, 1822·4
Ayoral, 1822·4
Ayoral Simple, 1822·4
Ayr-5, 1822·4
Ayr Saline, 1822·4
Ayrementol, 1822·4
Ayrton's Antiseptic, 1822·4
Ayrton's Chilblain, 1822·4
Ayton, 1822·4
Aywet, 1822·4
Az, 1822·4
AZ 15, 1822·4
AZ Junior, 1822·4
Az Ofteno, 1822·4
AZ Protezione Completa, 1822·4
AZ Protezione Gengive, 1822·4
AZ Tartar Control, 1822·4
AZ Verde, 1822·4
(3*R*)-1-Azabicyclo[2.2.2]oct-3-yl (1*S*)-1-Phenyl-3,4-dihydroisoquinoline-2(1*H*)-carboxylate, 489·2
1-(3-Azabicyclo[3.3.0]oct-3-yl)-3-*p*-tolylsulphonylurea, 332·1
1-(3-Azabicyclo[3.3.0]oct-3-yl)-3-tosylurea, 332·1
Azacitidina, 529·2
Azacitidine, 529·2
Azacort, 1096·2
Azacortid, 1822·4
Azactam, 1822·4
5-Azacytidine, 529·2
5-Aza-2′-deoxycytidine, 546·2
Azadirachta, 1658·2
*Azadirachta indica*, 1658·2
Azadose, 1822·4
Azafalk, 1823·1
Azafrán, 1058·2
Azafrán, Estigmas de, 1058·2
Azahar, Aceite Esencial de, 1719·2
Azahar, Esencia de, 1719·2
Azahexal, 1823·1
Azamedac, 1823·1
Azameno, 1823·1
Azamethiphos, 1500·2
Azamethonium Bromide, 866·2
Azametifós, 1500·2
Azamun, 1823·1
Azanidazol, 602·3
Azanidazole, 602·3
Azanplus, 1823·1

Azantac, 1823·1
Azaperona, 671·2
Azaperone, 671·2
Azaperone for Veterinary Use, 671·2
Azaperonum, 671·2
Azapetine Phosphate, 866·2
Azapress, 1823·1
Azapropazona, 20·1
Azapropazone, 20·1
Azapropazone Dihydrate, 20·1
Azaron, 1823·1
Azasan, 1823·1
Azasetrón, Hidrocloruro de, 1251·1
Azasetron Hydrochloride, 1251·1
Azatadina, Maleato de, 425·1
Azatadine Maleate, 425·1
Azathiodura, 1823·1
Azathioprine, 1349·1
Azathioprine Sodium, 1350·1
Azathioprinum, 1349·1
Azatioprina, 1349·1
Azatrilem, 1823·1
Azatyl, 1823·1
Azectol, 1823·1
Azeda-Brava, 1749·1
Azedavit, 1823·1
Azeite, 1723·2
Azelaic Acid, 1142·3
Azelaico, Ácido, 1142·3
Azelan, 1823·1
Azelast, 1823·1
Azelastina, Hidrocloruro de, 425·2
Azelastine Hydrochloride, 425·2
Azelastini Hydrochloridum, 425·2
Azelcream, 1823·1
Azelderm, 1823·1
Azelex, 1823·1
Azelnidipine, 866·2
Azenil, 1823·1
Azep, 1823·1
Azepam, 1823·1
Azepine Phosphate, 866·2
Azerodol, 1823·1
Azerty, 1823·1
Azetavir, 1823·1
Azi, 1823·1
Aziac, 1823·1
Aziclav, 1823·1
Azida Sódica, 1191·3
Azidamfenicol, 159·1
Azidamphenicol, 159·1
Azidanfenicol, 159·1
Azidoamphenicol, 159·1
Azidobenzylpenicillin Sodium, 159·1
Azidocillin Potassium, 159·1
Azidocillin Sodium, 159·1
Azidodeoxythymidine, 658·2
3′-Azido-3′-deoxythymidine, 658·2
2-Azido-*N*-[(α*R*,β*R*)-β-hydroxy-α-hydroxymethyl-4-nitrophenethyl]acetamide, 159·1
Azidothymidine, 658·2
Aziliv, 1823·1
Azilline, 1823·2
Azimax, 1823·2
Azime, 1823·2
Azimilida, Hidrocloruro de, 866·3
Azimilide Dihydrochloride, 866·3
Azimilide Hydrochloride, 866·3
Azimix, 1823·2
Azinc, 1823·2
Azintamida, 1658·3
Azintamide, 1658·3
Azinthiamide, 1658·3
Aziram, 1823·2
Aziridinylbenzoquinone, 546·3
Azithral, 1823·2
Azithromycin, 159·1
Azithromycinum, 159·1
Azitrax, 1823·2
Azitrix, 1823·2
Azitrocin, 1823·2
Azitrom, 1823·2
Azitromax, 1823·2
Azitromicina, 159·1
Azitromin, 1823·2
Azitron, 1823·2
Azitronal, 1823·2
Azitroxil, 1823·2
Aziwok, 1823·2
Azlocilina Sódica, 160·2
Azlocillin, 160·2
Azlocillin Sodium, 160·2
Azmacort, 1823·2
Azmasol, 1823·2
Azoazol, 1823·2
Azobenzene-2,4-diamine Hydrochloride Citrate, 1670·3
Azodisal Sodium, 1278·1
Azoflune, 1823·2
Azo-Gen, 1823·2
Azol, 1823·2
Azole Antifungals, 386·1
Azolin, 1823·2
Azoline, 1823·2
Azolinic Acid, 188·1
Azolmen, 1823·2
Azomid, 1823·2
Azomycin, 1823·2
Azomyr, 1823·3
Azona, 1823·3
Azone, 1481·2
Azonutril, 1823·3
Azophenum, 82·3
Azopi, 1823·3
Azopine, 1823·3
Azopt, 1823·3
Azor, 1823·3
Azoran, 1823·3
Azorubine, 1057·1
Azorubrum, 1056·2
Azosemida, 866·3
Azosemide, 866·3
Azo-Standard, 1823·3
Azostix, 1823·3
Azotato de Estricnina, 1750·1
Azote, 1236·3
Azote, Protoxyde d', 1304·3
Azotic Acid, 1722·1
Azotine, 1823·3
Azotito de Amilo, 1032·1
Azoto Protossido, 1304·3
Azovan Blue, 1658·3
Azovanum Caeruleum, 1658·3
Azo-Wintomylon, 1823·3
AZQ, 546·3
AZT, 658·2, 1349·1
Aztemin, 1823·3
Azthreonam, 160·3
Aztil, 1823·3
Aztreonam, 160·3
Azuben, 1823·3
Azubronchin, 1823·3
Azucalcit, 1823·3
Azucaps, 1823·3
Azúcar, 1450·1
Azúcar Invertido, 1434·3
Azucimet, 1823·3
Azuder, 1823·3
Azudoxat, 1823·3
Azudoxat Comp, 1823·3
Azufibrat, 1823·3
Azufracid, 1823·3
Azufre, 1158·2
Azuglucon, 1823·3
Azul Brillante FCF, 1056·2
Azul de Evans, 1658·3
Azul de Metileno, 1042·2
Azul de Prusia, 1051·2
Azul Metile, 1823·3
Azul Patente V, 1729·1
Azul Sulfán, 1750·3
Azulen, 1823·4
Azulenal, 1823·4
Azulene, 1658·3, 1823·4
Azulene Sodium Sulfonate, 1658·3
Azuleno, 1658·3
Azulfidine, 1823·4
Azulfin, 1823·4
Azulina, 1823·4
Azulipont, 1823·4
Azulon, 1823·4
Azumetop, 1823·4
Azumetop HCT, 1823·4
Azunaftil, 1823·4
Azunol, 1823·4
Azupamil, 1823·4
Azupanthenol, 1823·4
Azupentat, 1823·4
Azuperamid, 1823·4
Azuprostat, 1823·4
Azuprostat Sabal, 1823·4
Azuprostat Urtica, 1823·4
Azur, 1823·4
Azur Compositum, 1823·4
Azur Compositum SC, 1823·4
Azuranit, 1823·4
Azuril, 1823·4
Azutranquil, 1823·4
Azutrimazol, 1823·4
Azym, 1823·4

## B

B-1, 589·3
B1-12-15, 1823·4
3B, 1824·1
5B706, 632·2
B-6, 1824·1
B15, 1824·1
B-436, 1735·1
B-518, 540·2
B-577, 38·1
B-663, 197·1
B-1312, 878·1
B-2360, 266·2
B-4130, 1063·2
B-9302-107, 791·3
B-10610, 1064·1
B-15000, 1064·3
B-19036, 1062·1
B-19036/7, 1062·1
$B_{12}$ Ankermann, 1824·1
3B Beer Belly Buster, Bioglan— *see* Bioglan 3B Beer Belly Buster, 1843·4
B Chabre, 1824·1
B Complex, 1824·1
B-100 Complex, 1824·1
B Complex 500, 1824·1
B Complex with C, 1824·1
B Complex C 550, 1824·1
B Complex Fosforilado, 1824·1
B Complex, Multi— *see* Multi B Complex, 2144·2
B Complex Plus C, 1824·1
$B_{12}$ Compositum, 1824·1
B Compound, 1824·1
$B_{12}$ Depot-Hevert, 1824·1
B12 Depot-Rotexmedica, 1824·1
$B_{12}$ Depot-Vicotrat, 1824·1
$B_{1/6}$ Effekton, 1824·1
B12 Ehrl, 1824·1
$B_{12}$ Fol-Vicotrat, 1824·1
B Forte, 1824·1
B Hormone, 1332·2
B 12-L 90, 1824·1
B & O Supprettes No. 15A, 1824·1
B & O Supprettes No. 16A, 1824·1
B Plus C, 1824·1
B12 Rotexmedica, 1824·1
B Six, 1824·1
B12 Steigerwald, 1824·1
B Stress C Plus Iron & Vitamins, 1824·1
B Stress Select, 1824·1
B Totum, 1824·1
$B_1$ Vicotrat, 1824·1
$B_6$ Vicotrat, 1824·1
$B_{12}$ Vicotrat, 1824·1
B Virol, 1824·1
Ba-168, 1041·2
Ba-253, 790·3
Ba-598BR, 482·3
BA-679, 806·2
Ba-679BR, 806·2
Ba-16038, 526·3
21401-Ba, 1757·3
Ba-21401, 1757·3
Ba-29837, 1033·1
Ba-33112, 1033·1
Ba-34276, 306·1
Ba-34647, 1386·3
Ba-39089, 978·1
Ba-41166/E, 250·2
Babcon, 1824·2
Babee, 1824·2
Babefen Sus, 1824·2
Babesiosis, 595·3
Babic, 1824·2
Babiforton, 1824·2
Babigoz Crema Protettiva, 1824·2
Babix, 1824·2
Babix-Inhalat N, 1824·2
Babix-Wundsalbe N, 1824·2
Baby AF, 1824·2
Baby Agisten, 1824·2
Baby Anbesol, 1824·2
Baby Block, 1824·2
Baby Cough, 1824·2
Baby Cough with Antihistamine, 1824·2
Baby Cough Syrup, 1824·2
Baby Fact B, 1824·2
Baby Gel, 1824·2
Baby Gripe, 1824·2
Baby Liberol, 1824·2
Baby Luuf, 1824·2
Baby Orajel, 1824·2
Baby Orajel Tooth and Gum Cleanser, 1824·2
Baby Paste, 1824·2
Baby Paste + Chamomile, 1824·2
Baby Sebamed, 1824·2
Baby Shield, 1824·3
BabyBIG, 1824·3
Babycare, 1824·3
Babycheck-Plus, 1824·3
Baby-Drax, 1824·3
Babyfort, 1824·3
Babygella, 1824·3
Babygencal, 1824·3
Babyglos, 1824·3
Babylax, 1824·3
Baby-Line, 1824·3
Babypasmil, 1824·3
Babypiril, 1824·3
Baby-Rinolo, 1824·3
Babys Own Gripe Water, 1824·3
Babys Own Infant Drops, 1824·3
Babys Own Ointment, 1824·3
Babys Own Teething Gel, 1824·3
Babysan, 1824·3
Babysiton, 1824·3
Babysteril, 1824·3
Baby-Transpulmin, 1824·3
Babyzim, 1824·3
B-A-C, 1824·3
Bac Resistente, 1824·3
Bac Septin, 1824·3
Bac Septin Balsamico, 1824·3
Bacacil, 1824·3
Bacagen, 1824·3
Bacalao, Aceite de Hígado de, 1425·2
Bacalhau, Óleo de, 1425·2
Bacampicilina, Hidrocloruro de, 161·2
Bacampicillin Hydrochloride, 161·2
Bacampicillini Hydrochloridum, 161·2
Bacampicin, 1824·4
Bacampicine, 1824·4
Bacard, 1824·4
Bacard Antiseptic, 1824·4
Bacasint, 1824·4
Bacattiv, 1824·4
Bacca Spinae Cervinae, 1254·1
Baccae Juniperi, 1703·1
Baccae Myrtilli, 1718·3
Baccalin, 1824·4
Baccidal, 1824·4
Bacfar, 1824·4
Bacfar Balsamico, 1824·4
Bacferol, 1824·4
Bacgen, 1824·4
Bacgen Balsamico, 1824·4
Bach Rescue Remedy, 1824·4
Bacibact, 1824·4
Bacicoline, 1824·4
Bacicoline-B, 1824·4
Bacid, 1824·4

Baciderma, 1824·4
Bacifim, 1824·4
Bacifurane, 1824·4
Bacigen, 1824·4
Baciguent, 1824·4
Baciguent Plus Pain Reliever, 1824·4
Baci-IM, 1824·4
Bacillary Angiomatosis— *see* Cat Scratch Disease, 123·1
Bacillary Dysentery— *see* Shigellosis, 130·1
Bacillary Lepromin, 1707·1
Bacillin, 1824·4
Bacillocid Rasant, 1824·4
Bacillocid Spezial, 1824·4
Bacillol, 1825·1
Bacillol AF, 1825·1
Bacillol Plus, 1825·1
Bacillotox, 1825·1
*Bacillus anthracis*, 1608·1
*Bacillus brevis*, 220·2, 275·1
Bacillus Calmette-Guérin Vaccine, 1609·2
Bacillus Calmette-Guérin Vaccine, Percutaneous, 1609·2
Bacillus Calmette-Guérin Vaccines, 1609·2
*Bacillus licheniformis*, 161·3
*Bacillus polymyxa*, 120·2, 198·3, 245·1
*Bacillus subtilis*, 161·3, 1654·2, 1751·1
Bacilor, 1825·1
Bacimex, 1825·1
Bacimycin, 1825·1
Bacimyxin, 1825·1
Bacin, 1825·1
Bacineo, 1825·1
Bacisporin, 1825·1
Bacitin, 1825·1
Bacitopic, 1825·1
Bacitopic Compuesto, 1825·1
Bacitracin, 161·3
Bacitracin Zinc, 161·3
Bacitracina, 161·3
Bacitracina Zinc, 161·3
Bacitracina-Neo, 1825·1
Bacitracins Zinc Complex, 161·3
Bacitracinum, 161·3
Bacitracinum Zincum, 161·3
Bacitrin Hidrocortis, Neo— *see* Neo Bacitrin Hidrocortis, 2156·1
Bacitrin, Neo— *see* Neo Bacitrin, 2156·1
Back Pain, Low— *see* Low Back Pain, 7·1
Backache, 1825·1
Backache with Arnica, 1825·1
Backache Ledum, 1825·1
Backache Maximum Strength Relief, 1825·1
Backache Relief, 1825·1
Back-Aid, 1825·1
Back-Ese M, 1825·1
BackOsamine, 1825·1
Baclo, 1825·1
Baclofen, 1386·3
Baclofeno, 1386·3
Baclofenum, 1386·3
Baclohexal, 1825·1
Baclon, 1825·2
Baclopar, 1825·2
Baclosal, 1825·2
Baclospas, 1825·2
Bacmin, 1825·2
Bacnutri, 1825·2
Bacocil, 1825·2
Bacotan, 1825·2
Bacpiryl, 1825·2
Bacprotin, 1825·2
Bacris, 1825·2
Bacrocin, 1825·2
Bac-Sulfitrin, 1825·2
Bacta, 1825·2
Bactacin, 1825·2
Bactedene, 1825·2
Bactelan, 1825·2
Bacteomycine, 1825·2
Bacteracin, 1825·2
Bacteracin Balsamico, 1825·2
Bacteraemia— *see* Septicaemia, 144·3
Bacterial, 1825·2
Bacterial Arthritis— *see* Bone and Joint Infections, 122·1
Bacterial Conjunctivitis— *see* Eye Infections, 127·2
Bacterial Endocarditis— *see* Endocarditis, 125·2
Bacterial Endophthalmitis— *see* Eye Infections, 127·2
Bacterial Eye Infections— *see* Eye Infections, 127·2
Bacterial Infections, Anaerobic— *see* Anaerobic Bacterial Infections, 121·1
Bacterial Infections in Immunocompromised Patients— *see* Infections in Immunocompromised Patients, 131·2
Bacterial Keratitis— *see* Eye Infections, 127·2
Bacterial Meningitis— *see* Meningitis, 134·3
Bacterial Prostatitis— *see* Urinary-tract Infections, 153·1
Bacterial Vaginosis, 121·2
Bacterian, 1825·2
Bacterianos D, 1825·2
Bactericidal Permeability Increasing Protein, 1658·3
Bacterinil, 1825·2
Bacterion, 1825·2
Bacteriuria— *see* Urinary-tract Infections, 153·1
Bacterix, 1825·2
Bacternil, 1825·2
Bacterol, 1825·2
Bacteroskin, 1825·2
Bacticef, 1825·2
Bacticel, 1825·2
Bacticil, 1825·3
Bacti-Cleanse, 1825·3
Bacticlor, 1825·3
Bacticort, 1825·3
Bacticort Complex, 1825·3
Bactidan, 1825·3
Bactide, 1825·3
Bactident, 1825·3
Bactidol, 1825·3
Bactidox, 1825·3
Bactidron, 1825·3
Bactifor, 1825·3
Bactigras, 1825·3
Bactil, 1825·3
Bactilen, 1825·3
Bactilina, 1825·3
Bactine, 1825·3
Bactine Antiseptic, 1825·3
Bactine First Aid Antibiotic Plus Anesthetic, 1825·3
Bactine Pain Relieving Cleansing, 1825·3
Bactio Rhin, 1825·3
Bactio Rhin Prednisolona, 1825·3
Bactisubtil, 1825·3
Bacti-Uril, 1825·3
Bactiver, 1825·3
Bactocef, 1825·3
Bactocill, 1825·3
Bactocin, 1825·4
Bactoderm, 1825·4
Bactofen, 1825·4
Bactoflox, 1825·4
Bactomicin, 1825·4
Bactopumon, 1825·4
Bactoreduct, 1825·4
Bactoscrub, 1825·4
Bactosept, 1825·4
BactoShield, 1825·4
Bactosone Retard, 1825·4
Bactox, 1825·4
Bactox Balsamico, 1825·4
Bactracid, 1825·4
Bactrazine, 1825·4
Bactren, 1825·4
Bactrex, 1825·4
Bactrian, 1825·4
Bactricin, 1825·4
Bactricin Balsamico, 1825·4
Bactrim, 1825·4
Bactrim Balsamico, 1825·4
Bactrim Compositum, 1825·4
Bactrimel, 1826·1
Bactrisan, 1826·1
Bactrisan Balsamico, 1826·1
Bactrizol, 1826·1
Bactroban, 1826·1
Bactroneo, 1826·1
Bactropin, 1826·1
Bactropin Balsamico, 1826·1
Bactyl, 1826·1
Bactylisine, 1826·1
Bac-Xolid, 1826·1
Bac-Zidim, 1826·1
Baczole, 1826·1
Badeol, 1826·1
Badiana, 1655·2
Badiane de Chine, 1655·2
Badoh, 1723·2
Badoh Negro, 1723·2
Badyket, 1826·1
Bafucin, 1826·1
Bagnisan Med Heilbad, 1826·1
Bagno Oculare, 1826·1
Bagobutam, 1826·1
Bagociletas con Anestesia, 1826·1
Bagociletas sin Anestesia, 1826·1
Bagoderm, 1826·1
Bagohepat, 1826·1
Bagomicina, 1826·1
Bagovit A, 1826·1
Bagovit A Plus, 1826·1
Bagovit Avant Piel, 1826·2
Bagovit-A, 1826·2
Bagren, 1826·2
Baical Skullcap Root, 1746·3
Baicurina, 1826·2
Bain Antirhumatismal, 1826·2
Bain contre les Refroidissements, 1826·2
Bain de Bouche Lipha, 1826·2
Bain de Soleil Preparations, 1826·2
Bain Extra-doux Dermatologique, 1826·2
Bain Extra-doux Dermatologique Nouvelle Formule, 1826·2
Bains Romains, 1826·3
Bainto, 1826·3
Bajaten, 1826·3
Bajaten D, 1826·3
Bajiaolian, 1155·3
Bajumol, 1826·3
Bakam, 1826·3
Bakanasan Einschlaf, 1826·3
Bakanasan Entwasserungs, 1826·3
Bakanasan Leber-Galle, 1826·3
Baking Soda, 1223·2
Baklinger, 1826·3
Baknyl, 1826·3
Bakteriostat "Herbrand", 1826·3
Baktobod, 1826·3
Baktobod N, 1826·3
Baktonium, 1826·3
Bakumondo-to, Tsumura— *see* Tsumura Bakumondo-to, 2351·1
BAL, 1037·1, 1826·3
Bal Tar, 1826·3
Balad, 1826·3
Balance ACE, 1826·3
Balance Elastin E, 1826·3
Balanced Anaesthesia— *see* Anaesthetic Techniques, 1296·2
Balanced B, 1826·3
Balanced B Complex Plus Vitamins C & E, 1826·3
Balanced C Complex, 1826·3
Balanced E, 1826·3
Balanced Irrigating Salt Solution, 1826·3
Balanced Ratio Cal-Mag, 1826·3
Balanced Salt Solution, 1826·3
Balancid, 1826·3
Balancid Novum, 1826·3
Balans, 1826·4
Balantidiasis, 596·1
Balbek, 1826·4
B-Alcerin, 1826·4
Balcor, 1826·4
Balcoran, 1826·4
Baldin-CE, 1826·4
Baldmin, 1826·4
Baldness— *see* Alopecia, 1134·1
Baldracin, 1826·4
Baldrian, 1826·4
Baldrian AMA, 1826·4
Baldrian Dispert Compositum, 1826·4
Baldrian + Hopfen, Kneipp— *see* Kneipp Baldrian + Hopfen, 2081·1
Baldrian Pflanzensaft Nerventrost, Kneipp— *see* Kneipp Baldrian Pflanzensaft Nerventrost, 2081·2
Baldrian-Dispert, 1826·4
Baldrian-Dispert Nacht, 1826·4
Baldrian-Elixier, 1826·4
Baldrian-Krautertonikum, 1826·4
Baldrianox S, 1826·4
Baldrianwurzel, 1762·2
Baldrinetten, 1826·4
Baldriparan, 1826·4
Baldriparan Beruhigungs, 1826·4
Baldriparan N, 1826·4
Baldriparan N Stark, 1826·4
Baldriparan pour la Nuit, 1826·4
Baldriparan Stark, 1826·4
Baldrisedon, 1826·4
Baldrisedon Mono, 1826·4
Baldurat, 1826·4
Balepton, 1826·4
Balgifen, 1826·4
Baliartrin, 1826·4
Balidon, 1826·4
Balin, 1827·1
Balisa, 1827·1
Balisa VAS, 1827·1
Balkis, 1827·1
Balkis Spezial, 1827·1
Ballism, 664·1
Balm, 1711·1
Balm of Gilead, 1827·1
Balm of Gilead Buds, 1733·3
Balm Oil, 1711·2
Balmandol, 1827·1
Balmex, 1827·1
Balmex Baby, 1827·1
Balmex Emollient, 1827·1
Balminil Preparations, 1827·1
Balmosa, 1827·2
Balmox, 1827·2
Balneoconzen N, 1827·2
Balneogel, 1827·2
Balneol, 1827·2
Balneovit, 1827·2
Balnetar, 1827·2
Balneum, 1827·2
Balneum F, 1827·2
Balneum Hermal, 1827·2
Balneum Hermal F, 1827·2
Balneum Hermal Forte, 1827·2
Balneum Hermal Plus, 1827·2
Balneum Intensiv, 1827·2
Balneum Intensiv Plus, 1827·2
Balneum mit Teer, 1827·2
Balneum Plus, 1827·2
Balneum Surgras, 1827·3
Balneum with Tar, 1827·3
Balnostim Bad N, 1827·3
Balodin, 1827·3
Balofloxacin, 162·2
Balofloxacino, 162·2
Balpril, 1827·3
Bals. Peruv., 1730·2
Balsabit, 1827·3
Balsalazida Sódica, 1251·2
Balsalazide Disodium, 1251·2
Balsalazide Sodium, 1251·2
Balsalazine Disodium, 1251·2
Balsam, Peru, 1730·2
Balsam, Peruvian, 1730·2
Balsam, Tolu, 1131·3
Balsamico (Unguento), 1827·3
Balsamicum, 1827·3
Balsamin, 1827·3
Balsamina Kroner, 1827·3
Balsamo Analgesic Karmel, 1827·3
Balsamo Analgesico, 1827·3
Balsamo Analgesico con Fenilbutazona, 1827·3

Balsamo Analgesico Labesfal, 1827·3
Balsamo Analgesico Sanitas, 1827·3
Balsamo Bengue, 1827·3
Balsamo Branco, 1827·3
Bálsamo de Tolú, 1131·3
Bálsamo del Perú, 1730·2
Balsamo Ifusa, 1827·3
Balsamo Italstadium, 1827·3
Balsamo Kneipp, 1827·3
Balsamo Leon, 1827·3
Balsamo Midalgan, 1827·3
Balsamo Nostrum, 1827·3
Balsamo Primi Denti, 1827·3
Balsamo Sifcamina, 1827·3
Balsamorhinol, 1827·3
Balsamum Peruvianum, 1730·2
Balsamum Styrax Liquidus, 1749·3
Balsamum Tolutanum, 1131·3
Balsan, 1827·3
Balsandin, 1827·4
Balsasulf, 1827·4
Balsatux, 1827·4
Balsedrina, 1827·4
Balseptol, 1827·4
Balsibron, 1827·4
Balsibron-C, 1827·4
Balsiprin, 1827·4
Balsoclase, 1827·4
Balsoclase Antitussivum, 1827·4
Balsoclase Compositum, 1827·4
Balsoclase Expectorans, 1827·4
Balsoclase-E, 1827·4
Balsofumine, 1827·4
Balsofumine Mentholee, 1827·4
Balsolene, 1827·4
Balsoprim, 1827·4
Balta Intimo, 1827·4
Balta-Crin Tar, 1827·4
Baltar, 1827·4
Balto Foot Balm, 1827·4
Balurol, 1827·4
Balzide, 1827·4
Bamalite, 1827·4
Bambalacha, 1666·1
Bambec, 1827·4
Bambermicina, 162·2
Bambermycin, 162·2
Bambermycins, 162·2
Bambia, 1666·1
Bambudil, 1828·1
Bambuterol, Hidrocloruro de, 781·2
Bambuterol Hydrochloride, 781·2
Bambuteroli Hydrochloridum, 781·2
Bametán, Sulfato de, 866·3
Bamethan Nicotinate, 866·3
Bamethan Succinate, 866·3
Bamethan Sulfate, 866·3
Bamethan Sulphate, 866·3
Bamifilina, Hidrocloruro de, 781·3
Bamifix, 1828·1
Bamifylline Hydrochloride, 781·3
Bamipina, 425·3
Bamipine, 425·3
Bamipine Hydrochloride, 425·3
Bamipine Lactate, 425·3
Bamipine Salicylate, 425·3
Bamixol, 1828·1
Bamycor, 1828·1
Bamyl, 1828·1
Bamyl Koffein, 1828·1
Bamyl S, 1828·1
Bamyl S Koffein, 1828·1
Bamyxin, 1828·1
Ban Pain, 1828·1
Banadroxin, 1828·1
Banadyne-3, 1828·1
Banalg, 1828·1
Banan, 1828·1
Banana Boat Preparations, 1828·1
Banatin, 1828·2
Bancap HC, 1828·2
Bancroftian Filariasis— *see* Lymphatic Filariasis, 100·1
Band Aid Spruhpflaster, 1828·2
Band-Aid Antibiotic, 1828·2
Band-Aid Corn Remover, 1828·2
Bandol, 1828·2
Bandotan, 1828·2
Bandrobon, 1828·2
Banedif, 1828·2
Banedif Oftalmico, 1828·3
Banedif Oftalmico con Prednisolona, 1828·3
Baneocin, 1828·3
Baneopol, 1828·3
Banflex, 1828·3
Bangi-Aku, 1666·1
Bango, 1666·1
Bangue, 1666·1
Banholeum, 1828·3
Banholeum Composto, 1828·3
Banholeum Gel, 1828·3
Banidor, 1828·3
Banimax, 1828·3
Banish II, 1828·3
Banishing Cream, 1828·3
*Banisteria caapi*, 1696·3
Banisterine, 1696·3
Banlice, 1828·3
Banner Protein, 1828·3
Bano Liquido con Eucalipto, 1828·3
Bano Ocular, 1828·3
Banocide, 1828·3
Banocin, 1828·3
Banoclus, 1828·3
Banoftal, 1828·3
Banophen Allergy, 1828·3
Banophen Decongestant, 1828·3
Banotu, 485·2
Ban-Sol, 1828·3
Bansor, 1828·3
Bantel, 1828·3
Bantenol, 1828·3
Banthine, 1828·3
BAPN, 21·2
BAQD-10, 1178·1
Baquiloprim, 162·2
Baquiloprima, 162·2
Baralgin, 1828·3
Baralgin M, 1828·3
Baralgina M, 1828·3
Baran-mild N, 1828·3
Baratol, 1828·4
Barazan, 1828·4
Barba de Capuchino, 1762·1
Barbados Aloes, 1248·2
Barbaloin, 1248·2, 1248·3
Barbamin, 1828·4
Barbamylum, 670·1
Barbated Skullcap Herb, 1746·3
Barbexaclona, 353·3
Barbexaclone, 353·3
Barbidonna, 1828·4
Barbital, 671·2
Barbital Sódico, 671·2
Barbital Sodium, 671·2
Barbitalum, 671·2
Barbitalum Natricum, 671·2
Barbitone, 671·2
Barbitone Sodium, 671·2
Barbitone, Soluble, 671·2
Barbitron, 1828·4
Barbiturate Withdrawal Syndrome, 670·2
Barbiturates, 663·1
Barbloc, 1828·4
Barbusco, 1510·1
Barc, 1828·4
Barcan, 1828·4
Bardana, 1704·3
Bardanae Radix, 1704·3
Bardane (Grande), 1704·3
Bärentraubenblätter, 1659·2
Barex, 1828·4
Barexal, 1828·4
Baricon, 1828·4
Baridium, 1828·4
Barigraf, 1828·4
Barigraf Tac, 1828·4
Barii Sulfas, 1061·1
Barii Sulphas, 1061·1
Barilux, 1828·4
Barilux Brausetabletten, 1828·4
Bario, 1659·1
Bario, Cal con Hidróxido de, 1659·1
Bario Dif, 1828·4
Bario Llorente, 1828·4
Bariofarma, 1828·4
Bariogel, 1828·4
Bariopacin, 1828·4
Bariotest, 1828·4
Baripril, 1828·4
Baripril Diu, 1828·4
Baritop, 1828·4
Barium, 1659·1
Barium Carbonate, 1659·1
Barium Hydroxide Lime, 1659·1
Barium Hydroxide Octahydrate, 1659·1
Barium Med Complex, 1828·4
Barium Sulfate, 1061·1
Barium Sulfide, 1659·1
Barium Sulfuricum, 1061·1
Barium Sulphate, 1061·1
Barley, Malted Grain of, 1439·2
Barmicil, 1828·4
Barnetil, 1828·4
Barnidipine Hydrochloride, 866·3
Barnidipino, Hidrocloruro de, 866·3
Barnotil, 1828·4
Baro-cat, 1829·1
Barokaton, 1829·1
Baropac, 1829·1
Baros, 1829·1
*Barosma betulina*, 1663·1
*Barosma crenulata*, 1663·1
Barosmin, 1688·2
Barosperse, 1829·1
Barotonal, 1829·1
Baroxal, 1829·1
Barpil, 1829·1
Barrett's Oesophagus— *see* Gastro-oesophageal Reflux Disease, 1242·3
Barrier Cream, 1829·1
Barriere, 1829·1
Barriere-HC, 1829·1
Barrycidal, 1829·1
Bartelin N, 1829·1
Bartelin Nico, 1829·1
Bartter's Syndrome, 1220·1
Barytgen, 1829·1
Baryum (Sulfate de), 1061·1
Basab, 1829·1
Basal Cell Carcinoma— *see* Basal Cell and Squamous Cell Carcinoma, 522·3
Basal-H-Insulin, 1829·1
Basaljel, 1829·1
Basan, 1829·1
Bascardial, 1829·1
Basdene, 1829·1
Bas-Dextrano, 1829·1
Basedow's Disease— *see* Hyperthyroidism, 1594·3
Baseler Haussalbe, 1829·1
Basen, 1829·1
Baserin, 1829·1
Bases, 1479·1
Basic Aluminium Acetate, 1653·1
Basic Aluminium Aminoacetate, 1249·1
Basic Aluminium Carbonate, 1249·1
Basic Aluminium Chloride, 1142·1
Basic Bismuth Carbonate, 1252·1
Basic Bismuth Gallate, 1252·2
Basic Bismuth Nitrate, 1252·2
Basic Bismuth Salicylate, 1252·1
Basic Butylated Methacrylate Copolymer, 1714·3
Basic Fuchsin, 1185·1
Basic Magenta, 1185·1
Basic Phenylmercury Nitrate, 1189·2
Basic Quinine Hydrobromide, 460·2
Basic Quinine Hydrochloride, 460·2
Basic Quinine Sulphate, 460·2
Basic Zinc Carbonate, 1144·1, 1163·2
Basicaina, 1829·1
Basilan, 1829·1
Basilicao, 1829·2
Basiliximab, 1351·1
Basinal, 1829·2
Basireuma, 1829·2
Basiron, 1829·2
Basisches Wismutgallat, 1252·2
Basisches Wismutkarbonat, 1252·1
Basisches Wismutnitrat, 1252·2
Basiter, 1829·2
Basiton, 1829·2
B1-ASmedic, 1829·2
B2-ASmedic, 1829·2
B6-ASmedic, 1829·2
$B_{12}$-ASmedic, 1829·2
Basocef, 1829·2
Basocin, 1829·2
Basodexan, 1829·2
Basofortina, 1829·2
Basoplex, 1829·2
Basoquin, 1829·2
Basotar, 1829·2
Bassado, 1829·2
Bastard Saffron, 1444·1
Basti-Cal, 1829·2
Basticrat, 1829·2
Bastilong, 1829·2
Basti-Mag, 1829·2
Bastiverit, 1829·2
Bastoncino, 1829·2
Basuco, 1373·3
Bat, 1829·2
Bateral, 1829·2
Bath E45, 1829·2
Batimastat, 529·2
Batinel, 1829·2
Batistol, 1829·2
Batixim, 1829·2
Batmen, 1829·2
Batrafen, 1829·2
Batramycin, 1829·3
Batramycine, 1829·3
Batrax, 1829·3
Batrevac, 1829·3
Batrizol, 1829·3
Batroxobin, 743·3
Batroxobina, 743·3
Battery Acid, 1750·3
Baudry, 1829·3
Baume, 1829·3
Baume Analgesique, 1829·3
Baume Analgesique Medicamente, 1829·3
Baume Aroma, 1829·3
Baume Bengue, 1829·3
Baume Dalet, 1829·3
Baume de Chine Temple of Heaven Blanc, 1829·3
Baume de Tolu, 1131·3
Baume du Chalet, 1829·3
Baume du Pérou, 1730·2
Baume du San Salvador, 1730·2
Baume Esco, 1829·3
Baume Esco Forte, 1829·3
Baume Saint-Bernard, 1829·3
Baunilha, 1762·3
Bausch & Lomb Preparations, 1829·3
Bauxol, 1829·4
BAX-1515, 1751·1
BAX-1526, 1671·1
BAX-2739Z, 781·3
BAX-3084, 1307·3
Baxan, 1829·4
Baxapril, 1829·4
Baxedin, 1829·4
Baxidin, 1829·4
Baxi-K, 1829·4
Baxil, 1829·4
Baxo, 1829·4
Bay-10-3356, 1743·2
Bay-12-8039, 233·1
Bay-38-9456, 1763·1
Bay-56-6854, 213·1
Bay-1500, 951·3
Bay-2353, 110·1
Bay-5097, 396·2
Bay-9002, 110·1
Bay-a-1040, 966·2
Bay-b-4231, 333·1
Bay-d-1107, 38·1
Bay-e-5009, 973·3
Bay-e-6905, 160·2

Bay-e-6975, 396·2
Bay-e-9736, 972·3
Bay-f-1353, 231·1
Bay-f-4975, 11·3
Bay-g-5421, 328·3
Bay-h-4502, 395·1
Bay-h-5757, 105·2
Bay-i-3930, 1438·3
Bay-k-5552, 973·2
Bay-m-1099, 343·2
Bay-NTN-33893, 1506·2
Bay-o-9867, 188·2
Bay-q-3939, 188·2
Bay-q-7821, 703·1
Bay-Va-1470, 1766·1
Bay-Va-9391, 1723·1
Bay-Vh-5757, 105·2
Bay-Vi-9142, 617·3
Bay-Vl-1704, 1502·3
Bay-Vp-2674, 207·3
Bay-w-3356, 1743·2
Bay-W-6228, 881·3
Bay-w-6240, 751·2
Bay Leaf Oil, 1659·1
Bay Oil, 1659·1
Bay Rum, 1659·2
Bayaspirina, 1829·4
Bayaspirina C, 1829·4
Bayberry, 1659·2
Bayberry Bark, 1659·2
Baycaron, 1829·4
Baycidal, 1829·4
Baycillin, 1829·4
Baycip, 1829·4
Baycol, 1829·4
Baycuten, 1829·4
Baycuten N, 1829·4
Bayer-205, 615·3
Bayer-1420, 1305·3
Bayer-2502, 611·2
Bayer-5360, 607·2
Bayer-9053, 1509·1
Bayer-21199, 1502·2
Bayer-29493, 1505·2
Bayer 52910, 159·1
Bayer A-128, 742·3
Bayer Extra Strength Back & Body Pain, 1829·4
Bayer Low Adult Strength, 1829·4
Bayer Plus, Extra Strength— *see* Extra Strength Bayer Plus, 1986·2
Bayer Select Preparations, 1829·4
Bayer Select Allergy Sinus, Aspirin-Free— *see* Aspirin-Free Bayer Select Allergy Sinus, 1816·4
Bayer-L-1359, 109·2
Bayers Tonic, 1830·1
Baygam, 1830·1
Baygon, 1830·1
BayHep, 1830·1
BayHep B, 1830·1
Baylotensin, 1830·1
Baymycard, 1830·1
Bayolin, 1830·1
Bayotensin, 1830·1
Baypen, 1830·1
Baypresol, 1830·1
Baypress, 1830·1
BayRab, 1830·1
BayRho-D, 1830·1
Bayro, 1830·1
Bayro Termo, 1830·1
Bayrogel, 1830·1
Bayro-Therm, 1830·1
BayTet, 1830·1
Baythion EC, 1830·2
Bazalin, 1830·2
Bazooka, 1373·3
Bazoton, 1830·2
Bazuctril, 1830·2
Bazuka, 1830·2
BB-94, 529·2
BB-882, 1707·2
BB-2516, 565·3
BB Fleet, 1830·2
BB Test, 1830·2
BBdent Gel Topico, 1830·2
BB-K8, 154·1, 1830·2
BC, 1830·2
BC-48, 1488·3
BC-51, 1489·2
BC-105, 470·3
*levo*-BC-2627, 23·3
BC 500, 1830·2
BC Cold-Sinus, 1830·2
BC 500 with Iron, 1830·2
BC Multi Symptom Cold Powder, 1830·2
BCAD 2, 1830·2
B-Caroteno, 1830·2
B-C-Bid, 1830·2
BCG ad Immunocurationem, 1609·2
BCG for Immunotherapy, 1609·2
BCG Vaccine, 1609·2
BCG Vaccine, Freeze-dried, 1609·2
BCG Vaccine, Percut., 1609·2
BCG Vaccines, 1609·2
BCM, 1830·2
BCNU, 535·1
B-Combin, 1830·2
B-Complex, 1830·2
B-Complex Threshold, 1830·2
B-Cool, 1830·2
B-Cool, New— *see* New B-Cool, 2165·4
BCX-34, 579·1
BCX-2600, 377·3
BD-40A, 786·1
BDF-5895, 962·3
BDF-5896, 962·3
BDH-1298, 1558·2
B-Dol, 1830·2
Be-1293, 1029·2
BE-5895, 962·3
Beacolux, 1830·2
Beacolytic, 1830·2
Beacon K, 1830·2
Beacons, 1830·2
Beactafed, 1830·2
Beafemic, 1830·2
Beaflu-Plus, 1830·2
Beagenco, 1830·3
Beagenta, 1830·3
Beaglobe, 1830·3
Beagocrine, 1830·3
Beagyne, 1830·3
Beahexol, 1830·3
Beakopectin, 1830·3
Beamat, 1830·3
Beamodium, 1830·3
Beamoken A, 1830·3
Beamotil, 1830·3
Beamoxy, 1830·3
Be-Ampicil, 1830·3
Beano, 1830·3
Beapen, 1830·3
Beaphenicol, 1830·3
Beapizide, 1830·3
Bear Essentials, 1830·3
Bear Grass, 1766·2
Bearax, 1830·3
Bearberry, 1659·2
Bearberry Leaf, 1659·2
Bearberry Leaves, 1659·2
Beatacycline, 1830·3
Beatafed, 1830·3
Beatafed Compound, 1830·3
Beathricin, 1830·3
Beatifen, 1830·3
Beatizem, 1830·3
Beatoconazole, 1830·3
Beatolin, 1830·3
Beatolin Expectorant, 1830·3
Beatrolol, 1830·3
*Beauveria nivea*, 1351·2
Beavate, 1830·3
Beavate N, 1830·4
Beazyme, 1830·4
Bebedermis, 1830·4
Bebegel, 1830·4
Bebelac EC, 1830·4
Bebelac FL, 1830·4
Beben, 1830·4
Beben Clorossina, 1830·4
Bebesales, 1830·4
Bebia, 1830·4
Bebidol, 1830·4
Bebimix, 1830·4
Bebulin, 1830·4
Bebulin TIM 3, 1830·4
Bebulin TIM 4, 1830·4
Bebulin VH, 1830·4
Bebyderm, 1830·4
Bec, 1830·4
Becacort, 1830·4
Becadexamin, 1830·4
Becalm, Heath & Heather— *see* Heath & Heather Becalm, 2037·3
Becaltrin, 1830·4
Became, 1830·4
Becantex, 1830·4
Becantosse, 1830·4
Becaplermin, 1143·1, 1679·1
Becaplermina, 1143·1
Becaps, 1830·4
Becardin, 1830·4
Becarin, 1830·4
Because, 1830·4
Bece, 1831·1
Becede, 1831·1
Becenun, 1831·1
Becetamol, 1831·1
Beceze, 1831·1
Bechilar, 1831·1
Bechlomin, 1831·1
Becilan, 1831·1
Beclamida, 353·3
Beclamide, 353·3
Beclase, 1831·1
Beclasma, 1831·1
Beclate, 1831·1
Beclate-C, 1831·1
Beclate-N, 1831·1
Beclazone, 1831·1
Beclo Aqua, 1831·1
Beclo Asma, 1831·1
Beclo Rino, 1831·1
Beclo Siozwo, 1831·1
Beclodisk, 1831·1
Becloforte, 1831·1
Beclogen, 1831·1
Beclohale, 1831·1
Beclojet, 1831·1
Beclomet, 1831·1
Beclometasona, Dipropionato de, 1091·1
Beclometasone Dipropionate, 1091·1
Beclometasone Dipropionate Monohydrate, 1091·1
Beclometasone Salicylate, 1092·2
Beclometasoni Dipropionas, 1091·1
Beclomethasone Dipropionate, 1091·1, 1091·2
Beclomin, 1831·1
Beclonarin, 1831·1
Beclonasal, 1831·2
Beclonato, 1831·2
Beclone, 1831·2
Beclophar, 1831·2
Beclo-Rhino, 1831·2
Beclorhinol, 1831·2
Beclosema, 1831·2
Beclosol, 1831·2
Beclosona, 1831·2
Beclotaide, 1831·2
Beclotamol, 1831·2
Becloturmant, 1831·2
Beclovent, 1831·2
Beco, 1831·2
Becocent, 1831·2
Becodisk, 1831·2
Becodisks, 1831·2
Becof, 1831·2
Becolim, 1831·2
Becoloxin, 1831·2
Becombion, 1831·2
Becomplex, 1831·2
Becomplina Fuerte, 1831·2
Beconase, 1831·2
Beconase Allergy, 1831·2
Beconase Aquosum, 1831·2
Beconase Hayfever, 1831·3
Beconasol, 1831·3
Becoplex Ido, 1831·3
Becortin, 1831·3
Becosol, 1831·3
Becosules, 1831·3
Becosym, 1831·3
Becotal, 1831·3
Becotide, 1831·3
Becotide A, 1831·3
Becovit, 1831·3
Becovitan, 1831·3
Becozym, 1831·3
Becozym NF, 1831·3
Becozym-C, 1831·3
Becozyme, 1831·3
Becozyme C, 1831·3
Becozyme C Forte, 1831·3
Becozyme-S, 1831·3
Bectam, 1831·3
Bed Wetting, 1831·3
Bed Wetting— *see* Nocturnal Enuresis, 475·3
Bed Wetting Relief, 1831·3
Bedelix, 1831·3
Bediatil, 1831·3
Bedin, 1831·3
Bedix, 1831·3
Bedix-D, 1831·3
Bedocil, 1831·3
Bedodeka, 1831·4
Bedodeka Antineuralgica, 1831·4
Bedorma, 1831·4
Bedovit Pharmaton, 1831·4
Bedoxine, 1831·4
Bedoyecta, 1831·4
Bedoyecta Tri, 1831·4
Bedoz, 1831·4
Bedoze, 1831·4
Bedozil, 1831·4
Bedranol, 1831·4
Bee Glue, 1735·2
Bee, Honey, 1655·3
Bee Venom, 1655·3
Beech Nut Cough Drops, 1831·4
Beecham Preparations, 1831·4
Beef Tapeworm Infections— *see* Taeniasis, 101·1
Beefolic, 1832·1
Beehive Balsam, 1832·1
Beeline, 1832·1
Beelith, 1832·1
Beepen-VK, 1832·1
Beer Belly Buster, Bioglan 3B— *see* Bioglan 3B Beer Belly Buster, 1843·4
Beer Caramel, 1057·1
Beespan, 1832·1
Beeswax, White, 1480·1
Beeswax, Yellow, 1480·2
Beet Red, 1056·2
Beetle, Blistering, 1666·3
Beetrion, 1832·1
Beetroot Red, 1056·2
Bee-Zee, 1832·1
Befact, 1832·1
Befelka-Oel, 1832·1
Befelka-Tinktur, 1832·1
Befenio, Hidroxinaftoato de, 103·2
Beferon, 1832·1
Befibrat, 1832·1
Befimat, 1832·1
Befizal, 1832·1
Beflavine, 1832·1
Befloxatona, 287·1
Befloxatone, 287·1
Befol, 1832·1
Beforplex, 1832·1
Befort, 1832·1
Befunolol, Hidrocloruro de, 867·1
Befunolol Hydrochloride, 867·1
Begadon, 1832·1
Begalin, 1832·1
Begalin-P, 1832·1
Begesic, 1832·1
Beglan, 1832·2
Beglunina, 1832·2

Begrivac, 1832·2
Begrocit, 1832·2
Behaviour, Disturbed— *see* Disturbed Behaviour, 665·1
Behçet's Disease— *see* Behçet's Syndrome, 1076·2
Behçet's Syndrome, 1076·2
Behenato de Glicerilo, 1411·3
Behenoyl Cytarabine, 550·2
Behenoylcytosine Arabinoside, 550·2
Behenyl Alcohol, 632·1
Behepan, 1832·2
Behexine, 1832·2
Beiklin, 1832·2
Bejel— *see* Syphilis, 148·2
Bekanamicina, Sulfato de, 162·2
Bekanamycin Sulfate, 162·2
Bekanamycin Sulphate, 162·2
Bekanamycini Sulfas, 162·2
Bekfan, 1832·2
Bekidiba, 1832·2
Bekidiba Dex, 1832·2
Beknol, 1832·2
Beko, 1832·2
Bekunis Preparations, 1832·2
Belacid, 1832·2
Belacodid, 1832·2
Belagin, 1832·3
Belara, 1832·3
Be-Lax, 1832·3
Belbar, 1832·3
Belcetin, 1832·3
Belcid, 1832·3
Belcomycine, 1832·3
Beleño, 485·2
Belep, 1832·3
Belestar, 1832·3
Belexa, 1832·3
Belfactrin, 1832·3
Bel-Gel, 1832·3
Belglos, 1832·3
Beliam, 1832·3
Belidral, 1832·3
Belifax, 1832·3
Belisina, 1832·3
Belisir, 1832·3
Belivon, 1832·3
Bell Diono Resolvent, 1832·3
Bell Pentolate, 1832·3
Bell Pino-Atrin, 1832·3
Bell Resolvent, 1832·3
Bellacane, 1832·3
BellaCarotin Mono, 1832·3
Belladol, 1832·3
Belladona, 479·1
Belladone, 479·1
Belladonna, 479·1
Belladonna Herb, 479·1
Belladonna Herb, Powdered, 479·1
Belladonna Herb, Prepared, 479·1
Belladonna Leaf, 479·1
Belladonna Med Complex, 1832·3
Belladonna, Prepared, 479·1
Belladonnae Folium, 479·1
Belladonnae Pulvis Normatus, 479·1
Belladonna-Homaccord, 1832·3
Belladonnysat Burger, 1832·3
Bellafit N, 1832·3
Bellafoline— *see* Bellergal-S, 1832·4
Bellagotin, 1832·4
Bellahist-D, 1832·4
Bellamine, 1832·4
Bellanorm, 1832·4
Bellanox, 1832·4
Bellatal, 1832·4
Bellatard, 1832·4
Bellatotal, 1832·4
Belle Cream, 1832·4
Bellergal, 1832·4
Bellergal Retardado, 1832·4
Bellergal-S, 1832·4
Bellergil, 1832·4
Belloform Nouvelle Formule, 1832·4
Belloid, 1832·4
Bells Muscle Rub, 1832·4
Bell's Palsy, 1076·3
Belmacina, 1832·4
Belmalax, 1832·4
Belmalen, 1832·4
Belmalen Plus, 1832·4
Belmalip, 1832·4
Belmazol, 1832·4
Belmirax, 1832·4
Belnif, 1832·4
Beloc, 1832·4
Beloc Comp, 1833·1
Beloc COR, 1833·1
Beloc-Zok, 1833·1
Beloc-Zok Comp, 1833·1
Beloken, 1833·1
Belomet, 1833·1
Belpen, 1833·1
Bel-Phen-Ergot S, 1833·1
Beltrax Uno, 1833·1
Belupan, 1833·1
Belustine, 1833·1
Belzer Solution, 414·2, 851·3
Bemaz, 1833·1
Bemedrex, 1833·1
Bemegrida, 1585·2
Bemegride, 1585·2
Bemegridum, 1585·2
Bemetizida, 867·1
Bemetizide, 867·1
Bemetrazole, 1833·1
Bemetson, 1833·1
Bemicin, 1833·1
Beminal, 1833·1
Beminal C Fortis, 1833·1
Beminal Fortis, 1833·1
Beminal with Iron and Liver, 1833·1
Beminal Plus, 1833·1
Beminal Z, 1833·1
Bemiparin Sodium, 867·1
Bemofil, 1833·1
Bemolan, 1833·1
Bemon, 1833·1
Bemonalcool, 1833·1
Bemplas, 1833·1
Bena, 1833·1
Benace, 1833·1
Benacilina, 1833·1
Benacne, 1833·2
Benacticina, Hidrocloruro de, 287·1
Benactiv, 1833·2
Benactyzine Hydrochloride, 287·1
Benactyzine Methobromide, 485·3
Benaday, 1833·2
Benaderma, 1833·2
Benaderma com Calamina, 1833·2
Benadon, 1833·2
Benadryl Preparations, 1833·2
Benadryl— *see* Emergent-Ez, 1967·2
Benagol, 1833·4
Benagol Collutorio, 1833·4
Benagol Mentolo-Eucaliptolo, 1833·4
Benagol Vitamina C, 1833·4
Benal, 1833·4
Benalapril, 1833·4
Benalcon, 1833·4
Benalet, 1833·4
Benalgis, 1833·4
Benalix, 1833·4
Benapen, 1833·4
Benaprost, 1833·4
Be-Natal— *see* Prenatal, 2232·4
Benatoss, 1833·4
Benaxima, 1833·4
Benaxona, 1833·4
Benazepril, Hidrocloruro de, 867·2
Benazepril Hydrochloride, 867·2
Benazeprilat, 867·2
Bencard Skin Testing Solutions, 1833·4
Bencelin, 1833·4
Bencelin Combinado, 1833·4
Benceno, 1471·3
Bencenosulfonato de Mesoridazina, 706·3
Bencetonio, Cloruro de, 1169·2
Benciclano, Fumarato de, 867·3
Bencid, 1833·4
Bencidamina, Hidrocloruro de, 21·1
Bencilo, Benzoato de, 1500·2
Bencilo, Isotiocinato de, 1659·3
Bencilpenicilina, 163·2
Bencilpenicilina Potásica, 163·2
Bencilpenicilina Sódica, 163·2
Benciltiouracilo, 1596·1
Benciodarona, 415·1
Benclamin, 1833·4
Bencole, 1833·4
Bencyclane Acefyllinate, 867·3
Bencyclane Fumarate, 867·3
Bencyclane Hydrogen Fumarate, 867·3
Benda, 1833·4
Bendacort, 1092·3
Bendalina, 1833·4
Bendamustine Hydrochloride, 529·3
Bendapar, 1833·4
Bendazac, 20·3
Bendazac Lysine, 20·3
Bendazaco, 20·3
Bendazaco de Lisina, 20·3
Bendazol Hydrochloride, 1659·2
Bendectin, 420·3
Bendex, 1833·4
Bendigon N, 1833·4
Bendiocarb, 1500·2
Bendracol, 1834·1
Bendrax, 1834·1
Bendrofluaz., 867·3
Bendrofluazide, 867·3
Bendroflumethiazide, 867·3
Bendroflumethiazidum, 867·3
Bendroflumetiazida, 867·3
Bendzon, 1834·1
Benecid, 1834·1
Benectrin, 1834·1
Benectrin Balsamico, 1834·1
Benecut, 1834·1
Benedaxol, 1834·1
Benedorm, 1834·1
Benefiber, 1834·1
Benefix, 1834·1
Beneflora, 1834·1
Beneflur, 1834·1
Benegel, 1834·1
Benegrip, 1834·1
Benemid, 1834·1
Benemide, 1834·1
Benera, 1834·1
Beneroc, 1834·1
Benerva, 1834·1
Benestan, 1834·1
Benethamine Penicillin, 162·3
Benetoss, 1834·1
Benetussin, 1834·1
Beneuran, 1834·2
Beneuran Compositum, 1834·2
Beneuran Vit B-Komplex, 1834·2
Beneurol, 1834·2
Beneuron Forte, 1834·2
Benevat, 1834·2
Benevolus, 1834·2
Benevran, 1834·2
Benexate Hydrochloride, 1251·2
Benexate Hydrochloride Betadex, 1251·2
Benexato, Hidrocloruro de, 1251·2
Benexol, 1834·2
Benexol B1 B6 B12, 1834·2
Benexol B12, 1834·2
Benfast, 1834·2
Benflogin, 1834·2
Benflorene, 1834·2
Benflumelol, 453·3
Benflumetol, 453·3
Benfluorex, Hidrocloruro de, 868·1
Benfluorex Hydrochloride, 868·1
Benfluorexi Hydrochloridum, 868·1
Benflux, 1834·2
Benfofen, 1834·2
Benfogamma— *see* Imilgamma, 2057·4
Benfotiamina, 1454·3
Benfotiamine, 1454·3
Ben-Gay Preparations, 1834·2
Benglau, 1834·3
Bengue's Balsam, 1834·3
Benhex, 1834·3
Benhexachlor, 1506·3
Benical, 1834·3
Benicar, 1834·3
Benicar HCT, 1834·3
Beni-cur, 1834·3
Benidipine Hydrochloride, 868·1
Benidipino, Hidrocloruro de, 868·1
Benign Intracranial Hypertension— *see* Raised Intracranial Pressure, 833·1
Benign Prostatic Hyperplasia, 1555·1
Benisan, 1834·3
Benistina, 1834·3
Benium, 1834·3
Benjamin, Gum, 1751·1
Benjoim, 1751·1
Benjoin du Laos, 1744·1
Benjuí, Bálsamo de, 1751·1
Benjuí de Siam, 1744·1
Benn, 1834·3
Bennasone, 1834·3
Bennatuss, 1834·3
Benne Oil, 1743·3
Benocten, 1834·3
Benodent, 1834·3
Benodent CLX, 1834·3
Benodent Gel Gengivale, 1834·3
Benomilo, 1500·2
Benomyl, 1500·2
Benoquin, 1834·3
Benoral, 1834·3
Benorilate, 20·3
Benorilato, 20·3
Benormal, 1834·3
Benorylate, 20·3
Benosid, 1834·3
Benotrin, 1834·3
Benovate, 1834·3
Benoxaprofen, 21·1
Benoxaprofeno, 21·1
Benoxid, 1834·3
Benoxinat SE, 1834·3
Benoxinate, 1834·3
Benoxinate Hydrochloride, 1382·1
Benoxinato, 1834·3
Benoxygel, 1834·3
Benoxyl, 1834·4
Benpen, 1834·4
Benperidol, 671·2
Benperidolum, 671·2
Benpine, 1834·4
Benproperina, 1115·2
Benproperine, 1115·2
Benproperine Embonate, 1115·2
Benproperine Phosphate, 1115·2
Benquil, 1834·4
Bens, 1834·4
Bensal HP, 1834·4
Benserazida, Hidrocloruro de, 1200·2
Benserazide, 1200·2
Benserazide Hydrochloride, 1200·2
Benserazidi Hydrochloridum, 1200·2
Bensolmin, 1834·4
Bensulf, 1834·4
Bensulfoid, 1834·4
Bentasil, 1834·4
Bentasil Black Currant, 1834·4
Bentasil Eucalyptus, 1834·4
Bentasil Licorice with Echinacea, 1834·4
Bentasil Menthol, 1834·4
Bentazepam, 671·3
Bentelan, 1834·4
Bentiamin, 1834·4
Bentiromida, 1659·2
Bentiromide, 1659·2
Bentonine, 1834·4
Bentonita, 1577·2
Bentonite, 1577·2
Bentonite, Purified, 1577·2
Bentonitum, 1577·2
Bentophyto, 1834·4
Bentoquatam, 1143·1
Bentos, 1834·4
Bentyl, 1834·4
Bentylol, 1834·4
Benur, 1834·4
Ben-u-ron, 1834·4
Benursil, 1834·4

Benuryl, 1834·4
Benutrex 1000, 1834·4
Benylan, 1834·4
Benylin Preparations, 1835·1
Benza, 1835·3
Benzac, 1835·3
Benzac Eritromicina, 1835·3
Benzac-AC, 1835·3
Benzacine, 1585·3
BenzaClin, 1835·3
Benzac-W, 1835·3
Benzaderm, 1835·3
Benzagel, 1835·3
Benzaknen, 1835·3
Benzalc, 1835·3
Benzalconio, Cloreto de, 1168·3
Benzalconio Cloruro, 1168·3
Benzalconio, Cloruro de, 1168·3
Benzalcream, 1835·3
Benzaldehído, 1659·3
Benzaldehyde, 1659·3
Benzalkonii Chloridum, 1168·3
Benzalkonium Bromide, 1168·3
Benzalkonium Chloratum, 1168·3
Benzalkonium Chloride, 1168·3
Benzalkonium Saccharinate, 1169·1
DL-α-Benzamido-*p*-[2-(diethylamino)ethoxy]-*N,N*-dipropylhydrocinnamamide Hydrochloride, 1757·1
(±)-4-Benzamido-*N,N*-dipropylglutaramic Acid, 1284·3
3-Benzamidopropionic Acid, 165·3
Benzamycin, 1835·3
Benzamycine, 1835·3
Benzanil Compuesto, 1835·3
Benzanil Simple, 1835·3
Benzantine H, 1835·3
Benzapen G, 1835·3
Benzasal, 21·1
Benzashave, 1835·3
Benzatec, 1835·3
Benzathine Benzylpenicillin, 162·3
Benzathine, Cloxacillin, 198·2
Benzathine Penicillin, 162·3
Benzathine Phenoxymethylpenicillin, 163·2
Benzathini Benzylpenicillinum, 162·3
Benzatina Bencilpenicilina, 162·3
Benzatina Fenoximetilpenicilina, 163·2
Benzatron, 1835·3
Benzatropina, Mesilato de, 479·2
Benzatropine Hydrochloride, 479·3
Benzatropine Mesilate, 479·2
Benzatropine Methanesulfonate, 479·2
Benzazoline Hydrochloride, 1015·1
Benzbromarona, 414·3
Benzbromarone, 414·3
Benzbromaronum, 414·3
Benzchlorpropamide, 353·3
Benzcurine Iodide, 1403·2
Benzecilin, 1835·4
Benzedrex, 1835·4
Benzemul, 1835·4
Benzene, 1471·3
1,2-Benzenedicarboxaldehyde, 1189·3
Benzene-1,2-dicarboxylic Acid Diethyl Ester, 1473·2
Benzene-1,3-diol, 1156·3
1,4-Benzenediol, 1148·1
Benzenemethanol, 1170·2
Benzene-1,2,3-triol, 1156·2
Benzene-1,3,5-triol, 1731·1
2,2′,2″-(Benzene-1,2,3-triyltrioxy)tris(tetraethylammonium) Tri-iodide, 1403·2
Benzet, 1835·4
Benzetacil, 1835·4
Benzetacil Combinado, 1835·4
Benzetacil Compuesta, 1835·4
Benzethacil, 162·3
Benzethonii Chloridum, 1169·2
Benzethonium Chloride, 1169·2
Benzevit, 1835·4
Benzfetamina, Hidrocloruro de, 1585·2
Benzfetamine Hydrochloride, 1585·2
Benzhexol Hydrochloride, 490·2
Benzhydramine, 431·3
Benzhydramine Citrate, 431·3
Benzhydramine Di(acefyllinate), 431·3
Benzhydramine Hydrochloride, 431·3
1-Benzhydryl-4-cinnamylpiperazine, 428·3
*N*-(2-Benzhydrylethyl)-α-methylbenzylamine Hydrochloride, 915·1
2-Benzhydrylethyl(α-methylphenethyl)amine, 1735·1
4-Benzhydrylidene-1,1-dimethylpiperidinium Methylsulphate, 481·3
1-Benzhydryl-4-methylpiperazine, 429·3
2-Benzhydryloxy-*NN*-dimethylethylamine, 431·3
4-Benzhydryloxy-1-methylpiperidine Hydrochloride, 432·3
(1*R*,3*r*,5*S*)-3-Benzhydryloxytropane Methanesulphonate, 479·2
1-[3-(4-Benzhydrylpiperazin-1-yl)propyl]benzimidazolin-2-one, 438·1
Benzibel, 1835·4
Benziflex, 1835·4
Benzihex, 1835·4
Benzilol, 1835·4
3-Benziloyloxy-1,1-dimethylpiperidinium Bromide, 485·3
4-Benziloyloxy-1,1-dimethylpiperidinium Bromide, 487·2
1-(2-Benziloyloxyethyl)-1-ethylpiperidinium Bromide, 487·3
3-Benziloyloxy-1-ethyl-1-methylpiperidinium Bromide, 487·3
(*RS*)-2-Benziloyloxymethyl-1,1-dimethylpyrrolidinium Methylsulphate, 488·2
3-Benziloyloxy-1-methylquinuclidinium Bromide, 480·2
3α-Benziloyloxynortropane-8-spiro-1′-pyrrolidinium Chloride, 491·2
Benzilpenicillina Benzatinica, 162·3
3-(Benzimidazol-2-yl)propionic Acid, 1735·2
(1*S*,2*S*)-(2-{[3-(2-Benzimidazolyl)propyl]methylamino}ethyl)-6-fluoro-1,2,3,4-tetrahydro-1-isopropyl-2-naphthyl Methoxyacetate Dihydrochloride, 959·1
Benzin, 1471·3
Benzina, 1471·3
Benzindamine Hydrochloride, 21·1
Benzine, 1471·3
Benzinum Medicinale, 1476·3
Benziodarone, 415·1
Benzirin, 1835·4
1,2-Benzisothiazolin-3-one 1,1-Dioxide, 1443·2
*cis*-*N*-{4-[4-(1,2-Benzisothiazol-3-yl)-1-piperazinyl]butyl}-1,2-cyclohexanedicarboximide Hydrochloride, 714·1
5-{2-[4-(1,2-Benzisothiazol-3-yl)-1-piperazinyl]ethyl}-6-chloro-2-indolinone, 728·1
Benzitrat, 1835·4
Benznidazol, 602·3
Benznidazole, 602·3
Benznidazolum, 602·3
Benzoates, 1169·3
Benzoato de Alprenolol, 856·3
Benzoato de Alquilo, 1480·1
Benzoato de Bencilo, 1500·2
Benzoato de Benzilo, 1500·2
Benzoato de Betametasona, 1093·1
Benzoato de Denatonio, 1679·2
Benzoato de Estradiol, 1550·1
Benzoato de Metronidazol, 607·2
Benzoato de Rizatriptán, 471·1
Benzoato Sódico, 1169·3
Benzoatos, 1169·3
Benzoax, 1835·4
Benzobarbital, 353·3
Benzobarbitone, 353·3
Benzoben, 1835·4
Benzocaína, 1370·3
Benzocaine, 1370·3
Benzocaine Hydrochloride, 1371·1
Benzocaine PD, 1835·4
Benzocainum, 1370·3
Benzocan, 1835·4
Benzodent, 1835·4
Benzoderm Myco, 1835·4
Benzodiazepine Withdrawal Syndrome, 690·2
Benzodiazepines, 663·1
Benzodiazepines, Intermediate-acting, 695·2
Benzodiazepines, Long-acting, 695·2
Benzodiazepines, Short-acting, 695·3
(1,4-Benzodioxan-6-ylmethyl)guanidine, 926·2
1-(1,4-Benzodioxan-2-ylmethyl)guanidine Sulphate, 927·3
1,3-Benzodioxole-5-carboxaldehyde, 1509·1
Benzododecinio, Bromuro de, 1170·2
Benzododecinium Bromide, 1170·2
Benzododecinium Chloride, 1170·2
Benzoë, 1751·1
Benzoe Tonkinensis, 1744·1
Benzoesäure, 1169·3
Benzoesäurebenzylester, 1500·2
6-Benzofenona, 1143·1
α-(Benzofuran-2-yl)-α-(4-chlorophenyl)methanol, 889·1
Benzogen Ferri, 1835·4
Benzo-Ginestryl, 1835·4
Benzo-Ginoestril, 1835·4
Benzo-Gynoestryl, 1835·4
Benzoic Acid, 1169·3
Benzoic Acid (2*S*-*cis*)-{1-[4-(3-Amino-2,3,6-trideoxy-α-L-*lyxo*-hexopyranosyloxy)-1,2,3,4,6,11-hexahydro-2,5,12-trihydroxy-7-methoxy-6,11-dioxonaphthacen-2-yl]ethylidene}hydrazide Hydrochloride, 594·3
Benzoic Acid Compound Ointment— *see* Whitfields (Benzoic Acid Compound) Ointment, 2385·4
Benzoic Acid Sulphimide, 1443·2
Benzoic Sulfimide, 1443·2
Benzoico, Ácido, 1169·3
Benzoicum, Acidum, 1169·3
Benzoin, 1744·1, 1751·1
Benzoin, Gum, 1751·1
Benzoin, Siam, 1744·1
Benzoin, Sumatra, 1751·1
Benzol, 1471·3, 1835·4
Benzole, 1471·3
Benzolum, 1471·3
Benzomel, 1835·4
Benzomix, 1835·4
Benzonal, 353·3, 1835·4
Benzonalum, 353·3
Benzonatate, 1115·3
Benzonatato, 1115·3
Benzononatine, 1115·3
Benzophenone-3, 1154·3
Benzophenone-4, 1158·3
Benzophenone-6, 1143·1
Benzophenone-8, 1145·3
Benzophenone-10, 1154·2
Benzopin, 1835·4
Benzoporphyrin Derivative, 591·1
2*H*-1-Benzopyran-2-one, 1676·2
1,2-Benzopyrone, 1676·2
5,6-Benzo-α-pyrone, 1676·2
Benzoral, 1835·4
Benzosulphimide, 1443·2
Benzotal, 1835·4
Benzotal Balsamico, 1836·1
(±)-4-(2-Benzothiazolylmethylamino)-α-[(4-fluorophenoxy)methyl]-1-piperidineethanol, 1741·2
(*S*)-1-{4-[1,3-Benzothiazol-2-yl(methyl)amino]piperidino}-3-(3,4-difluorophenoxy)propan-2-ol, 950·2
(±)-1-(1-Benzo[*b*]thien-2-ylethyl)-*N*-hydroxyurea, 807·3
Benzotizan, 1836·1
Benzotran, 1836·1
4,4′-(3*H*-2,1-Benzoxathiol-3-ylidene)diphenol *S,S*-Dioxide, 1730·3
Benzoxazocine, 66·2
1-(1,2-Benzoxazol-3-yl)methanesulphonamide, 384·3
Benzoxiquine, 1170·2
Benzoxiquine Salicylate, 1170·2
Benzoxonio, Cloruro de, 1170·2
Benzoxonium Chloride, 1170·2
Benzoyl Metronidazole, 607·2
Benzoyl Peroxide, 1143·2
Benzoyl Peroxide, Hydrous, 1143·2
*N*-Benzoyl-β-alanine, 165·3
(±)-5-Benzoyl-2,3-dihydro-1*H*-pyrrolizine-1-carboxylic Acid, 52·1
Benzoylecgonine, 1375·3
*N*-(1-Benzoylethyl)-*NN*-diethylammonium Chloride, 1587·1
1-Benzoyl-5-ethyl-5-phenylbarbituric Acid, 353·3
5-Benzoyl-4-hydroxy-2-methoxybenzenesulphonic Acid, 1158·3
Benzoylis Peroxidum, 1143·2
*m*-Benzoyl-*N*-(4-methyl-2-pyridyl)hydratropamide, 84·1
(*RS*)-2-(3-Benzoylphenyl)propionic Acid, 51·2
6-Benzoyl-5,6,7,8-tetrahydropyrido[4,3-*c*]pyridazin-3-ylhydrazone Monomethanesulfonate, 910·3
*O*-Benzoylthiamine Disulphide, 1454·3
*S*-Benzoylthiamine *O*-Monophosphate, 1454·3
2-(5-Benzoyl-2-thienyl)propionic Acid, 93·3
4-(*N*-Benzoyl-L-tyrosylamino)benzoic Acid, 1659·2
Benzoyt, 1836·1
Benzperidol, 671·2
Benzperox, 1836·1
Benzphetamine Hydrochloride, 1585·2
Benzquercin, 1688·2
Benzquercina, 1688·2
Benzthiazide, 868·1
Benztiazida, 868·1
Benztrop, 1836·1
Benztropine Mesylate, 479·2
Benzum, 1836·1
Benzydamine Hydrochloride, 21·1
Benzydamine Salicylate, 21·1
Benzydroflumethiazide, 867·3
Benzyl Alcohol, 1170·2, 1170·3
Benzyl Benz., 1500·2
Benzyl Benzoate, 1500·2
Benzyl Carbinol, 1188·1
Benzyl (8*S*,10*S*)-(1,6-Dimethylergolin-8-ylmethyl)carbamate, 1211·2
Benzyl Hydroxybenzoate, 1183·2
Benzyl 4-Hydroxybenzoate, 1183·2
Benzyl Isothiocyanate, 1659·3
Benzyl Mustard Oil, 1659·3
Benzyl Nicotinate, 21·2
Benzyl Parahydroxybenzoate, 1183·2
Benzyl Pyridine-3-carboxylate, 21·2
Benzyl Salicylate *trans*-4-(Guanidinomethyl)cyclohexanecarboxylate Hydrochloride, 1251·2
2-(*N*-Benzylanilino)ethyl (±)-1,4-Dihydro-2,6-dimethyl-4-(*m*-nitrophenyl)-5-phosphononicontinate Hydrochloride, Cyclic 2,2-Dimethyltrimethylene Ester, 909·2
2-Benzylbenzimidazole Hydrochloride, 1659·2
(α*R*,γ*S*,2*S*)-α-Benzyl-2-(*tert*-butylcarbamoyl)-γ-hydroxy-*N*-[(1*S*,2*R*)-2-hydroxy-1-indanyl]-4-(3-pyridylmethyl)-1-piperazinevaleramide Sulfate (1:1), 638·2
$N^1$-{(1*S*,2*R*)-1-Benzyl-3-[(3*S*,4a*S*,8a*S*)-3-(*tert*-butylcarbamoyl)perhydroisoquinolin-2-yl]-2-hydroxypropyl}-$N^2$-(2-quinolylcarbonyl)-L-aspartamide, 653·3
*N*′-(2-Benzylcarbamoylethyl)isonicotinohydrazide, 310·2
Benzyl(2-chloroethyl)(1-methyl-2-phenoxyethyl)amine Hydrochloride, 981·2
2-Benzyl-4-chlorophenol, 1177·3
*N*-Benzyl-3-chloropropionamide, 353·3
3-(1-Benzylcycloheptyloxy)-*NN*-dimethylpropylamine Hydrogen Fumarate, 867·3
Benzyldiethyl-2-[4-(1,1,3,3-tetramethylbutyl)phenoxy]ethylammonium Chloride Monohydrate, 1187·1
Benzyldiethyl(2,6-xylylcarbamoylmethyl)ammonium Benzoate Monohydrate, 1679·2
(5′*S*,8*R*)-5′-Benzyl-9,10-dihydro-12′-hydroxy-2′-methyl-3′,6′,18-trioxoergotaman, 465·3
(5′*S*,8*R*)-5′-Benzyl-9,10-dihydro-12′-hydroxy-2′-methyl-3′,6′,18-trioxoergotaman Methanesulphonate, 465·3

6-Benzyl-2,3-dihydro-2-thioxopyrimidin-4(1*H*)-one, 1596·1
3-Benzyl-3,4-dihydro-6-trifluoromethyl-2*H*-1,2,4-benzothiadiazine-7-sulphonamide 1,1-Dioxide, 867·3
*N*-((1*S*)-1-Benzyl-2-{[(1*R*)-1-(dihydroxyboranyl)-3-methylbutyl]amino}-2-oxoethyl)pyrazinecarboxamide, 532·1
(+)-(1*S*,2*R*)-1-Benzyl-3-dimethylamino-2-methyl-1-phenylpropyl Propionate, 28·3
(1*R*,2*S*)-1-Benzyl-3-dimethylamino-2-methyl-1-phenylpropyl Propionate Naphthalene-2-sulphonate Monohydrate, 1124·1
2-Benzyl-1,3-dimethylguanidine Sulphate, 872·3
(+)-*N*-Benzyl-*N*,α-dimethylphenethylamine Hydrochloride, 1585·2
Benzyldimethyl(2-phenoxyethyl)ammonium 3-Hydroxy-2-naphthoate, 103·2
*N*-Benzyl-*N′N′*-dimethyl-*N*-(2-pyridyl)ethylenediamine Dihydrogen Citrate, 442·3
Benzyldimethyltetradecylammonium Chloride, 1186·3
Benzyldimethyl(2-{2-[4-(1,1,3,3-tetramethylbutyl)phenoxy]ethoxy}ethyl)ammonium Chloride, 1169·2
Benzyldimethyl-2-{2-[4-(1,1,3,3-tetramethylbutyl)-*o*-tolyloxy]ethoxy}ethylammonium Chloride Monohydrate, 1186·1
Benzyldodecylbis(2-hydroxyethyl)ammonium Chloride, 1170·2
Benzyl(dodecylcarbamoylmethyl)dimethylammonium Chloride, 1185·3
Benzyldodecyldimethylammonium Bromide, 1170·2
Benzyldodecyldimethylammonium Chloride, 1170·2
1-Benzyl-3-ethyl-6,7-dimethoxyisoquinoline Hydrochloride, 1717·2
8-Benzyl-7-[2-(*N*-ethyl-*N*-2-hydroxyethylamino)ethyl]theophylline Hydrochloride, 781·3
5-Benzyl-3-furylmethyl (1*RS*,3*RS*)-(1*RS*,3*SR*)-2,2-Dimethyl-3-(2-methylprop-1-enyl)cyclopropanecarboxylate, 1509·3
Benzylhexadecyldimethylammonium Chloride, 1172·1
(6a*R*,9*R*,10a*R*)-*N*-[(2*R*,5*S*,10a*S*,10b*S*)-5-Benzyl-10b-hydroxy-2-isopropyl-3,6-dioxooctahydro-8*H*-[1,3]oxazolo[3,2-*a*]pyrrolo[2,1-*c*]pyrazin-2-yl]-7-methyl-4,6,6a,7,8,9,10,10a-octahydroindolo[4,3-*fg*]quinoline-9-carboxamide Methanesulphonate, 1680·1
$N^1$-[(1*S*,3*S*,4*S*)-1-Benzyl-3-hydroxy-5-phenyl-4-(1,3-thiazol-5-ylmethoxycarbonylamino)pentyl]-$N^2$-{[(2-isopropyl-1,3-thiazol-4-yl)methyl](methyl)carbamoyl}-L-valinamide, 653·2
2-Benzyl-2-imidazoline Hydrochloride, 1015·1
*N*-Benzyl-*N*-(2-imidazolin-2-ylmethyl)aniline Hydrochloride, 424·2
(1-Benzyl-1*H*-indazol-3-yloxy)acetic Acid, 20·3
3-(1-Benzyl-1*H*-indazol-3-yloxy)-*NN*-dimethylpropylamine Hydrochloride, 21·1
Benzylis Benzoas, 1500·2
*N*-Benzyl-*N*-(3-isobutoxy-2-pyrrolidin-1-ylpropyl)aniline Hydrochloride Monohydrate, 868·1
6-Benzyl-2-mercaptopyrimidin-4-ol, 1596·1
2-[Benzyl(methyl)amino]ethyl Methyl 1,4-Dihydro-2,6-dimethyl-4-(3-nitrophenyl)pyridine-3,5-dicarboxylate Hydrochloride, 965·1
2′-Benzyl-5-methylisoxazole-3-carbohydrazide, 300·3
*N*-Benzyl-*N*-(1-methyl-4-piperidyl)aniline, 425·3
Benzylmethylprop-2-ynylamine Hydrochloride, 978·3
(±)-*cis*-*N*-(1-Benzyl-2-methyl-3-pyrrolidinyl)-5-chloro-4-(methylamino)-*o*-anisamide, 710·1
*N*-Benzyl-2-(2-nitroimidazol-1-yl)acetamide, 602·3
[2-(Benzyloxymethyl)-6-(carboxylatomethyl-κ*O*)-3,9-bis(carboxymethyl-κ*O*)-3,6,9-triazaundecanedioato-$\kappa^3N^{3,6,9}\kappa^2$-$O^{1,11}$] Gadolinium (III), 1062·1
4-Benzyloxyphenol, 1154·2
Benzylparaben, 1183·2
Benzylpenicillin, 163·2
Benzylpenicillin, Benzathine, 162·3
Benzylpenicillin Novocaine, 246·1
Benzylpenicillin Potassium, 163·2
Benzylpenicillin, Procaine, 246·1
Benzylpenicillin Sodium, 163·2
Benzylpenicillinum Benzathinum, 162·3
Benzylpenicillinum Kalicum, 163·2
Benzylpenicillinum Natricum, 163·2
Benzylpenicillinum Procainum, 246·1
Benzylpenicilloyl Polylysine Concentrate, 1729·2
Benzylpenicilloyl-polylysine, 1729·2
Benzyl(phenethyl)ammonium (6*R*)-6-(2-Phenylacetamido)penicillanate, 162·3
2-(2-Benzylphenoxy)-*NN*-dimethylethylamine Dihydrogen Citrate, 439·1
1-[2-(2-Benzylphenoxy)-1-methylethyl]piperidine, 1115·2
(±)-2-(4-Benzylpiperidino)-1-(4-hydroxyphenyl)propan-1-ol Tartrate, 938·1
(±)-($R^*$)-3-[($R^*$)-1-Benzyl-3-piperidyl]methyl 1,4-Dihydro-2,6-dimethyl-4-(*m*-nitrophenyl)-3,5-pyridinedicarboxylate Hydrochloride, 868·1
(±)-2-[(1-Benzyl-4-piperidyl)methyl]-5,6-dimethoxy-1-indanone Hydrochloride, 1489·2
(*S*)-2-(1-Benzyl-4-piperidyl)-2-phenylglutarimide, 481·1
(+)-(3′*S*,4*S*)-1-Benzyl-3-pyrrolidinyl Methyl 1,4-Dihydro-2,6-dimethyl-4-(*m*-nitrophenyl)-3,5-pyridinedicarboxylate Hydrochloride, 866·3
Benzylsenföl, 1659·3
5-Benzyl-1,2,3,4-tetrahydro-2-methyl-γ-carboline, 436·3
3-Benzylthiomethyl-6-chloro-2*H*-1,2,4-benzothiadiazine-7-sulphonamide 1,1-Dioxide, 868·1
(4*S*)-1-[(2*S*)-3-(Benzylthio)-2-methylpropionyl]-4-(phenylthio)-L-proline, 1029·3
Benzylthiouracil, 1596·1
6-Benzyl-2-thiouracil, 1596·1
Benzyme, 1836·1
Beocid Puroptal, 1836·1
Beof, 1836·1
Beofenac, 1836·1
Beofta, 1836·1
Be-Oxytet, 1836·1
Bepanten, 1836·1
Bepanthen, 1836·1
Bepanthen Plus, 1836·1
Bepanthene, 1836·1
Bepanthene Plus, 1836·1
Bepantol, 1836·1
Beparine, 1836·1
Bepeben, 1836·1
Bepeno, 1836·2
Bepeno-G, 1836·2
Bepep, 1836·2
Bephen, 1836·2
Bephenium Hydroxynaphthoate, 103·2
Beplex, 1836·2
Beplexaron, 1836·2
Beplex-Zee, 1836·2
Beplus, 1836·2
Bepotastina, 425·3
Bepotastine, 425·3
Bepridil, Hidrocloruro de, 868·1
Bepridil Hydrochloride, 868·1
Beprogel, 1836·2
Beprogent, 1836·2
Beprogenta, 1836·2
Beprosalic, 1836·2
Beprosone, 1836·2
Beptazine, 1836·2
Beptazine-H, 1836·2
Bequidril, 1836·2
Bequipecto, 1836·2
Bequium, 1836·2
Beractant, 1736·2
Beramicina, 1836·2
Beramikin, 1836·2
Beramin, 1836·2
Beraprost Sódico, 1514·1
Beraprost Sodium, 1514·1
Berazole, 1836·2
Berberell, 1836·2
Berberil Dry Eye, 1836·2
Berberil N, 1836·2
Berberina, 1659·3
Berberine, 1659·3
Berberine Chloride, 1659·3
Berberine Sulfate, 1659·3
Berberine Tannate, 1659·3
*Berberis*, 1659·3
Berberis Complex, 1836·2
Berberis Cosmoplex, 1836·2
Berberis Med Complex, 1836·2
Berberis Oligoplex, 1836·2
Bercetina, 1836·2
Berciclina, 1836·3
Berciclina Enzimatica, 1836·3
Berclomine, 1836·3
Berenil, 604·2
Berex, 1836·3
Bergagyn, 1836·3
Bergamol, 1836·3
Bergamon Sapone, 1836·3
Bergamot Essence, 1659·3
Bergamot Oil, 1659·3
Bergamota, Aceite Esencial de, 1659·3
Bergamottae, Oleum, 1659·3
Bergapten, 1154·1
Berger's Disease— *see* Glomerular Kidney Disease, 1080·2
Berggeist, 1836·3
Bergon, 1836·3
Beriate, 1836·3
Beriate P, 1836·3
Beri-beri, 1455·2
Beribumin, 1836·3
Bericard, 1836·3
Beriglobin, 1836·3
Beriglobin P, 1836·3
Beriglobina, 1836·3
Beriglobina Anti D-P, 1836·3
Beriglobina P, 1836·3
Berigripina, 1836·3
Berinert, 1836·3
Berinert HS, 1836·3
Berinert P, 1836·3
Berinin, 1836·3
Berinin HS, 1836·3
Berinin P, 1836·3
Beriplast, 1836·3
Beriplast P, 1836·3
Beriplex, 1836·4
Beriplex PN, 1836·4
Berirab, 1836·4
Berirab-P, 1836·4
Berivine, 1836·4
Berkamil, 1836·4
Berkolol, 1836·4
Berlactone, 1836·4
Berlex, 1836·4
Berlicetin, 1836·4
Berlicort, 1836·4
Berlin Blue, 1051·2
Berlinsulin H 20/80, 1836·4
Berlinsulin H 30/70— *see* Berlinsulin H 20/80, 30/70, 1836·4
Berlinsulin H Basal, 1836·4
Berlinsulin H Normal, 1836·4
Berlison, 1836·4
Berlithion, 1836·4
Berlocid, 1836·4
Berlocombin, 1836·4
Berlofen, 1836·4
Berloque Dermatitis, 1154·1
Berlosin, 1836·4
Berlthyrox, 1836·4
Bermacia, 1836·4
Bernadine, 1836·4
Bernice, 1373·3
Berniter, 1836·4
Berocca Preparations, 1836·4
Beroccal, 1837·1
Berodual, 1837·1
Berodualin, 1837·1
Berofin, 1837·1
Berofor, 1837·1
Beromin, 1837·1
Beromun, 1837·1
Berotec, 1837·1
Berotec Solvens, 1837·1
Berovent, 1837·1
Berplex, 1837·1
Bersen, 1837·1
Bertocil, 1837·1
Berubi, 1837·1
Beruhigungs-Bad Spezial, Kneipp— *see* Kneipp Beruhigungs-Bad spezial, 2081·2
Besaprin, 1837·2
Besedan, 1837·2
Besemax, 1837·2
Besenol, 1837·2
Beserol, 1837·2
Beserol-S, 1837·2
Besidin, 1837·2
Bésilate de Cisatracurium, 1399·1
Besilato de Amlodipino, 862·1
Besilato de Atracurio, 1399·1
Besilato de Cisatracurio, 1399·1
Besitran, 1837·2
Besix, 1837·2
Besone, 1837·2
Besone-N, 1837·2
Besopartin, 1837·2
Bespar, 1837·2
Bessasone, 1837·2
Best EPA, 1837·2
Bestafen, 1837·2
Bestatin, 590·3, 1837·2
Bestcall, 1837·2
Bestelar, 1837·2
Bester Complex, 1837·2
Bestocin, 1837·2
Bestozyme, 1837·2
Bestrol, 1837·2
Bestron, 1837·2
Be-Supra, 1837·2
BET, 1093·1
Beta, 1837·3
Beta 21, 1837·3
Beta A-C, 1837·3
Beta Adenil, 1837·3
$Beta_2$ Agonists, 777·1
Beta Alcanforado, 1837·3
Beta Blockers, 810·3, 868·1
Beta C E with Selenium, 1837·3
Beta Carotene, 1422·3
Beta Long, 1837·3
Beta Micoter, 1837·3
Beta Nicardia, 1837·3
Beta Ophtiole, 1837·3
Beta Plus Vitamins C, E & Selenium, 1837·3
Beta Prostate, 1837·3
Beta Romero, 1837·3
$Beta_2$ Stimulants, 777·1
Beta Tocopherols, 1464·3
*Beta vulgaris*, 1450·1
Beta-Ace Tablets, 1837·3
Beta-Adalat, 1837·3
Beta-Adalate, 1837·3
Beta-adrenoceptor Blocking Drugs, 868·1
Beta-aminopropionitrile, 21·2
Beta-aminopropionitrile Fumarate, 21·2
Beta-amylases, 1654·2
Beta-apo-8′-carotenal, 1056·1
Beta-apo-8′-carotenoic Acid, Ethyl Ester, 1056·1
Betabactyl, 1837·3
Betabion, 1837·3
Betabioptal, 1837·3
Betabiotic, 1837·3
Betabloc, 1837·3
Be-Tabs Antacid, 1837·3
Beta-C, 1837·3
Betacap, 1837·4
Betacar, 1837·4
Beta-Cardone, 1837·4
Betacarotene, 1422·3
Betacaroteno, 1422·3
Betacarotenum, 1422·3
Betacarpin, 1837·4
Betacef, 1837·4

Betacept, 1837·4
Betachek, 1837·4
Betacin, 1837·4
Betaclar, 1837·4
Betaclomin, 1837·4
Betaclopramide, 1837·4
Betacod— *see* Painamol Plus, 2200·4
Betacomplesso, 1837·4
Betacort, 1837·4
Betacorten, 1837·4
Betacorten-G, 1837·4
Betacortone, 1837·4
Betacortone S, 1837·4
BetaCreme, 1837·4
Betacyanins, 1056·2
Betaderm, 1837·4
Betaderma, 1837·4
Betadermic, 1837·4
Betades, 1837·4
Betadex, 1678·2
Betadexamethasone, 1093·1
Betadexum, 1678·2
Betadine, 1837·4
Betadine First Aid Antibiotics + Moisturizer, 1838·1
Betadine, Garze Disinfettanti Alla Pomata— *see* Garze Disinfettanti alla Pomata Betadine, 2016·1
Betadine Plus First Aid Antibiotics & Pain Reliever, 1838·1
Betadine-AD, 1838·1
Beta-Dipo, 1838·1
Betadipresan, 1838·1
Betadipresan Diu, 1838·1
Betadiur, 1838·1
Betadona, 1838·1
Betadorm-A, 1838·1
Betadrenol, 1838·1
Betadur CR, 1838·1
Betadur CR, Half— *see* Half Betadur CR, 2035·2
Betaeffe Complex, 1838·1
Betaeffe Plus, 1838·1
Beta-endorphin, 73·3
Betafact, 1838·1
Betafed, 1838·1
Betaferon, 1838·1
Betaflex, 1838·1
Betafloroto, 1838·1
Betaform Habitat, 1838·1
Betagalen, 1838·1
Betagan, 1838·1
Betagard, 1838·1
Betagen, 1838·1
Betagentam, 1838·2
Betagesic, 1838·2
Betagon, 1838·2
Betahistina, Hidrocloruro de, 1660·1
Betahistina, Mesilato de, 1660·1
Betahistine, 1660·1
Betahistine Dihydrochloride, 1660·1
Betahistine Hydrochloride, 1660·1
Betahistine Mesilate, 1660·1
Betahistine Mesylate, 1660·1
Betahistini Mesilas, 1660·1
Beta-hydroxyfentanyl, 40·3
Beta-hydroxy-3-methylfentanyl, 40·3
Beta-Hypophamine, 1342·2
Betaimune, 1838·2
Betaína, 1660·1
Betaína, Hidrocloruro de, 1660·2
Betaine, 1660·1
Betaine Digestive Aid, 1838·2
Betaine Glucuronate, 1660·2
Betaine Hydrochloride, 1660·2
Betaines, Long-chain, 1574·1
Betaisodona, 1838·2
Betaisodona, SP— *see* SP Betaisodona, 2301·2
Beta-Isoket, 1838·2
Betaject, 1838·2
Beta-lactamase Inhibitors, 119·1
Betalevedim, 1838·2
Betalgil, 1838·2
Betalin, 1838·2
Beta-lipotrophin, 73·3
Betaliver, 1838·2
Betalix, 1838·2
Betaloc, 1838·2
Betaloc Comp, 1838·2
Betalol, 1838·2
Betama-EN, 1838·2
Betamann, 1838·2
Betamatil, 1838·2
Betamatil con Neomicina, 1838·2
Betamaze, 1838·2
Betamed, 1838·2
Betamesol, 1838·2
Betametagen, 1838·2
Betametasona, 1093·1
Betametasona, Acetato de, 1093·1
Betametasona, Benzoato de, 1093·1
Betametasona, Dipropionato de, 1093·1
Betametasona, Fosfato Sódico de, 1093·1
Betametasona, Valerato de, 1093·2
Betameth, 1838·2
Betamethason Plus, 1838·3
Betamethasone, 1093·1
Betamethasone Acetate, 1093·1
Betamethasone 21-Acetate, 1093·1
Betamethasone Adamantoate, 1093·3
Betamethasone Benzoate, 1093·1
Betamethasone 17α-Benzoate, 1093·1
Betamethasone Butyrate Propionate, 1093·3
Betamethasone Dipropionate, 1093·1
Betamethasone 17α,21-Dipropionate, 1093·1
Betamethasone Disodium Phosphate, 1093·1
Betamethasone 21-(Disodium Phosphate), 1093·1
Betamethasone Phosphate, 1093·3
Betamethasone Salicylate, 1093·3
Betamethasone Sodium Phosphate, 1093·1, 1093·2
Betamethasone Valerate, 1093·2
Betamethasone 17α-Valerate, 1093·2
Betamethasone Valero-acetate, 1093·3
Betamethasoni Acetas, 1093·1
Betamethasoni Dipropionas, 1093·1
Betamethasoni Natrii Phosphas, 1093·1
Betamethasoni Valeras, 1093·2
Betamethasonum, 1093·1
Betameth-N, 1838·3
Beta-(2-methoxyphenoxy)-lactic Acid, 1122·1
Betamican, 1838·3
Betamida, 1838·3
Betamil-M, 1838·3
Betamin, 1838·3
Betamine, 1838·3
Betamipron, 165·3
Betam-Ophtal, 1838·3
Betamox, 1838·3
Betamycin, 1838·3
Beta-N, 1838·3
Betanaftol, 103·2
Betanaphthol, 103·2
Betanaphthyl Benzoate, 103·2
Betanecol, Cloruro de, 1487·3
Betanidina, Sulfato de, 872·3
Betanidine Sulfate, 872·3
Betanidine Sulphate, 872·3
Betanidini Sulfas, 872·3
Betanine, 1056·2
Betanoid, 1838·3
Betanoid N, 1838·3
Betanol, 1838·3
Beta-oestradiol, 1550·1
Beta-oestradiol Benzoate, 1550·1
Beta-Ophtiole, 1838·3
Betapace, 1838·3
Betapam, 1838·3
Betapect, 1838·3
Betapen, 1838·3
Betaperamide, 1838·3
Betaphlem, 1838·3
Betapindol, 1838·3
Betaplex, 1838·3
Betapred, 1838·3
Betapresin, 1838·3
Betapress, 1838·3
Betapressin, 1838·3
Betapressine, 1838·3
Betaprofen, 1838·4
Beta-Prograne, 1838·4
Beta-Prograne, Half— *see* Half Beta-Prograne, 2035·2
Betaprol, 1838·4
Betaprospan, 1838·4
Betapyn, 1838·4
Betapyr, 1838·4
Betarelix, 1838·4
Betaren, 1838·4
Betaretic, 1838·4
Betartrinovo, 1838·4
Beta-S, 1838·4
BetaSalbe, 1838·4
Betasan, 1838·4
Betascor B12, 1838·4
Betasedar, 1838·4
Betasel, 1838·4
Betaselen, 1838·4
Betasemid, 1838·4
Betasept, 1838·4
Betaseptic, 1838·4
Betaserc, 1838·4
Betaseron, 1838·4
Betasit Plus, 1838·4
Betasleep, 1838·4
Betasoda, 1838·4
Betasol, 1838·4
Beta-Sol, 1838·4
Betasone, 1839·1
Betasone-G, 1839·1
Betasone-G 12 Horas, 1839·1
Betaspan, 1839·1
Beta-Stulln, 1839·1
Betasyn, 1839·1
Betatab, 1839·1
Beta-Tablinen, 1839·1
Betatene, 1839·1
Betathiazid, 1839·1
Betathiazid A, 1839·1
Beta-Tim, 1839·1
Betaton, 1839·1
Betaton with Ginseng, 1839·1
Betatop, 1839·1
Betatrex, 1839·1
Betatul, 1839·1
Beta-Turfa, 1839·1
Beta-Val, 1839·1
Betavert, 1839·1
Betavite, 1839·1
Betavix, 1839·1
Beta-Wolff, 1839·1
Betaxin, 1839·1
Betaxina, 1839·1
Betaxolol, Hidrocloruro de, 873·1
Betaxolol Hydrochloride, 873·1
Betaxololi Hydrochloridum, 873·1
Betaxon, 1839·1
Betazim, 1839·1
Betazok, 1839·2
Betazol Cort, 1839·2
Betazon, 1839·2
Betazone, 1839·2
BETE, 1839·2
Betel, 1656·2
Betel Nuts, 1656·2
Betel Pepper, 1656·2
Betel Quid, 1656·2
Betelvine, 1656·2
Bethacil, 1839·2
Bethanechol Chloride, 1487·3
Bethanidine Sulfate, 872·3
Bethanidine Sulphate, 872·3
Bethasone, 1839·2
Bethasone-N, 1839·2
Betiatide, Technetium ($^{99m}$Tc), 1526·1
Betim, 1839·2
Betimol, 1839·2
Betinex, 1839·2
Betinjectol, 1839·2
Betiral, 1839·2
Betistine, 1839·2
Betitotal, 1839·2
Betlife, 1839·2
Betnasol, 1839·2
Betnelan, 1839·2
Betnelan-V, 1839·2
Betnelan-VC, 1839·2
Betnelan-VN, 1839·2
Betnesalic, 1839·2
Betnesol Preparations, 1839·2
Betneval, 1839·3
Betneval-Neomycine, 1839·3
Betnor, 1839·3
Betnovat Preparations, 1839·3
Betnovate Preparations, 1839·3
Betoid, 1839·4
Betolvex, 1839·4
Betolvidon, 1839·4
Betonin, 1839·4
Betonvit, 1839·4
Betoptic, 1839·4
Betoptic S, 1839·4
Betoptima, 1839·4
Betoquin, 1839·4
Betosalic, 1839·4
Betosone, 1839·4
Betosone-CE, 1839·4
Be-Total, 1839·4
Betozone, 1839·4
Betrat B, 1839·4
Betres AP, 1839·4
Betriphos-C, 1839·4
Betrivit, 1839·4
Betron R, 1839·4
Betsol Z, 1839·4
Betsona, 1839·4
Betsuril, 1839·4
Bettamousse, 1839·4
Better Cholesterol, 1839·4
Better Prostate, 1839·4
*Betula alba*, 1159·2
*Betula pendula*, 1159·2, 1660·3
*Betula pubescens*, 1159·2, 1660·3
*Betula verrucosa*, 1159·2
Betulac, 1839·4
Betulae Albae, Oleum, 1159·2
Betulae Empyreumaticum, Oleum, 1159·2
Betulae Folium, 1660·3
Betulae, Pix, 1159·2
Betulae, Pyroleum, 1159·2
Betulae Pyroligneum, Oleum, 1159·2
Betuline, 1840·1
Betulla (Specie Composta), 1840·1
Be-Uric, 1840·1
Beurises, 1840·1
Beurre de Cacao, 1482·3
Bevacizumab, 529·3
Bevantolol, Hidrocloruro de, 873·2
Bevantolol Hydrochloride, 873·2
Beverages, Xanthine-containing, 1765·2
Bevicomplex, 1840·1
Beviplex, 1840·1
Beviplex Forte, 1840·1
Bevispas, 1840·1
Bevit Forte, 1840·1
Be-Vital— *see* Viteral, 2382·2
Bevitamel, 1840·1
Bevitin, 1840·1
Bevitine, 1840·1
Bevitol, 1840·1
Bevitotal Comp, 1840·1
Bevoren, 1840·1
Bewon, 1840·1
Bex, 1840·1
Bexarotene, 529·3
Bexaroteno, 529·3
Bex-Hepar, 1840·1
Bexicortil, 1840·1
Bexid, 1840·1
Bexident, 1840·1
Bexidermil, 1840·1
Bexine, 1840·1
Bexinor, 1840·1
Bexon, 1840·1
Bextra, 1840·1
Bexxar, 1840·1
Beza, 1840·2
Bezabeta, 1840·2

Bezacur, 1840·2
Bezadoc, 1840·2
Bezafibrate, 873·2
Bezafibrato, 873·2
Bezafibratum, 873·2
Bezafisal, 1840·2
Bezagamma, 1840·2
Bezagen, 1840·2
Beza-Lande, 1840·2
Bezalex, 1840·2
Bezalip, 1840·2
Bezalip Mono, 1840·2
Bezamerck, 1840·2
Bezamil, 1840·2
Bezapham, 1840·2
Beza-Puren, 1840·2
Bezastad, 1840·2
Bezitramida, 21·2
Bezitramide, 21·2
BFE-60, 867·1
B-Feron, 1840·2
BFI, 1840·2
BG-8301, 562·2
BG-8967, 875·2
BG-9273, 1141·2
BG-9712, 1141·2
B-G Prot, 1840·2
BGB Norflox, 1840·2
Bgramin, 1840·2
$BH_4$, 1742·1
BHA, 1171·2
BH-AC, 550·2
Bhang, 1666·1
Bhangaku, 1666·1
Bheng, 1666·1
B-Hex, 1840·2
B12-Horfervit, 1840·2
BHT, 1171·3
B-HT-920, 1215·3
BI-61.012, 760·1
BI-71.052, 747·2
Biactol Antibacterial Facewash, 1840·2
Biactol Liquid, 1840·2
Biaferone, 1840·2
Biafine, 1840·2
Biaflu, 1840·2
Biaflu-Zonale SU, 1840·3
Bi-Aglut, 1840·3
Bialcol, 1840·3
Bialerge, 1840·3
Bialminal, 1840·3
Bialzepam, 1840·3
Biamotil, 1840·3
Biamotil-D, 1840·3
Bianco Val, 1840·3
Biancospino, 1677·1
Biapenem, 165·3
Biartac, 1840·3
Biatos, 1840·3
Biavax II, 1840·3
Biaven, 1840·3
Biaxin, 1840·3
Biaxin— *see* Hp-Pac, 2048·4
Biaxin— *see* Prevpac, 2234·3
Biaxsig, 1840·3
Biazolina, 1840·3
Bibenzonio, Bromuro de, 1115·3
Bibenzonium Bromide, 1115·3
Bibivit Light, 1840·3
Bibol Leloup, 1840·3
BIBR-277, 1010·1
BIBR-277-SE, 1010·1
Bibrocathin, 1660·2
Bibrocathol, 1660·2
Bibrocatol, 1660·2
Bibrokatol, 1660·2
Bica, 1840·3
Bicaflac, 1840·3
Bicain, 1840·3
Bicalutamida, 530·1
Bicalutamide, 530·1
Bicam, 1840·3
Bicaprost, 1840·3
Bicarbonate, 1223·1
Bicarbonato, 1223·1
Bicarbonato de Potasio, 1223·1
Bicarbonato de Sodio, 1223·2
Bicarnat, 1840·3
Bicarnitine Chloride, 1424·1
BiCart, 1840·3
Bicavine, 1840·3
Bicbag, 1840·3
Bicetil, 1840·3
Bicholate, 1840·4
Bicidal Plus, 1840·4
Bicide, 1840·4
Bicillin, 1840·4
Bicillin A-P, 1840·4
Bicillin C-R, 1840·4
Bicillin L-A, 1840·4
Biciron, 1840·4
Bicisate, Technetium ($^{99m}$Tc), 1526·1
Bicitra, 1840·4
Bi-Citrol, 1840·4
Biclar, 1840·4
Biclin, 1840·4
Biclinocilline, 1840·4
Biclopan, 1840·4
Bicloruro de Mercurio, 1712·3
Biclotimol, 1171·1
Biclotymol, 1171·1
BiCNU, 535·1, 1840·4
Bicobon, 1840·4
Bicofen, 1840·4
Bicold, 1840·4
Bicomplex, 1840·4
Biconcor, 1840·4
Bicor, 1840·4
Bicozene, 1840·4
Bicromil, 1840·4
1-(Bicyclo[2.2.1]hept-5-en-2-yl)-1-phenyl-3-piperidinopropan-1-ol, 479·3
Bicyclohexylammonium Fumagillin, 605·2
Bidanzen, 1840·4
Bidiabe, 1840·4
Bidien, 1841·1
Bidor, 1841·1
Bidrolar, 1841·1
Bidrostat, 1841·1
Biduret, 1841·1
Biebrich Scarlet R Medicinal, 1191·3
Bienfait Total, 1841·1
Bienterico, 1841·1
Bier's Block— *see* Intravenous Regional Anaesthesia, 1370·1
Bietanautine, 431·3
Bi-Euglucon, 1841·1
Bi-Euglucon M, 1841·1
Bifardol S, 1841·1
Bifazol, 1841·1
Bifebral, 1841·1
Bifemelane, 1660·2
Bifemelano, 1660·2
Bifen, 1841·1
Bifena, 1841·1
Bifenac, 1841·1
*Bifidobacterium bifidum*, 1704·2
Bifidosa, 1841·1
Bifilact, 1841·1
Bifinorma, 1841·1
Bifiteral, 1841·1
Bifix, 1841·1
Bifized, 1841·1
Bifluorid, 1841·1
Bifokey, 1841·1
Bifomyk, 1841·1
Bifon, 1841·1
Bifonal, 1841·1
Bifonazol, 395·1
Bifonazole, 395·1
Bifonazolum, 395·1
Bifort, 1841·1
Bifosa, 1841·2
Bifosfonatos, 766·3
Bifril, 1841·2
Big V, 1841·2
Big V Baby, 1841·2
Big V Cough Lozenge, 1841·2
Big V Kids, 1841·2
Bigaradier, 1723·3
Bigasan, 1841·2
Bigenol, 1841·2
Bigetric, 1841·2
Bigonist, 1841·2
Bigpen, 1841·2
Biguanide Antidiabetics, 329·2
Biguanide Antimalarials, 444·1
Bigumalum, 457·1
Bikalm, 1841·2
Biklin, 1841·2
Bil 13, 1841·2
Bil 13 Enzimatico, 1841·2
Bilagit Mono, 1841·2
Bilagol, 1841·2
Bilamide, 1841·2
Bilan, 1841·2
Bilaten, 1841·2
Bilatin, 1841·2
Bilatin Fischol, 1841·2
Bilaxil, 1841·2
Bilberry, 1718·3
Bilberry Formula, 1841·2
Bilberry Fruit, Dried, 1718·3
Bilberry Fruit, Fresh, 1718·3
Bilberry Plus, 1841·2
Bilberry Plus Eye Health, 1841·3
Bilduretic, 1841·3
Bile Acids and Salts, 1660·3
Bile-acid Binding Resins, 811·3
Bile-acid Sequestrants, 811·3
Bileco, 1841·3
Bilem, 1841·3
Bilenor, 1841·3
Bilenzima, 1841·3
Biletan, 1841·3
Biletan Enzimatico, 1841·3
Bilgast Echinac, 1841·3
Bilharzia Vaccines, 1638·2
Bilharziasis— *see* Schistosomiasis, 100·3
Biliares, Ácidos Y Sales, 1660·3
Biliary Calculi— *see* Gallstones, 1761·3
Biliary Cirrhosis, Primary— *see* Primary Biliary Cirrhosis, 1761·2
Biliary Colic— *see* Biliary and Renal Colic, 4·3
Biliary-tract Infections, 121·3
Bilicanta, 1841·3
Bilicante, 1841·3
Bilicura Forte, 1841·3
Bilidren, 1841·3
Biliepar, 1841·3
Bilifel, 1841·3
Bilifluine, 1841·3
Biliflux, 1841·3
Bilifuge, 1841·3
Biligrama, 1841·3
Bili-Labstix, 1841·3
Bilina, 1841·3
Biliosan Compuesto, 1841·3
Bilipax, 1841·3
Bilipeptal Mono, 1841·3
Biliranin, 1841·3
Bilisan C3, 1841·3
Bilisan Duo, 1841·3
Biliscopin, 1841·3
Bilisegrol, 1841·3
Bilkaby, 1841·4
Billerol, 1841·4
Biloban, 1841·4
Bilobene, 1841·4
Biloina, 1841·4
Bilol, 1841·4
Bilopaque, 1841·4
Biloptin, 1841·4
Bilron, 1841·4
Bilsan, 1841·4
Bilsenkraut, 485·2
Biltricide, 1841·4
Biluen Enzimatico, 1841·4
Bilugen, 1841·4
Bim, 1841·4
BIM-21003, 1341·2
BIM-23014C, 1330·3
Bimatoprost, 1514·1
Bimicot, 1841·4
Bi-Miotic, 1841·4
Bimixin, 1841·4
Bimolin, 1841·4
Binaldan, 1841·4
μ-(2,2′-Binaphthalene-3-sulphonyloxy)bis(phenylmercury), 1182·2
Bindazac, 20·3, 1841·4
Bi-Nerisona, 1841·4
Binifibrate, 875·1
Binifibrato, 875·1
Biniwas, 1841·4
Binoctrin, 1841·4
Binodian, 1841·4
Binopen, 1841·4
Binordiol, 1841·4
Binospan Composto, 1841·4
Binotal, 1841·4
Binotine, 1841·4
Binotine Balsamico, 1842·1
Binovum, 1842·1
B-Insulin, 1842·1
Binvex, 1842·1
Bio², 1842·1
Bio-200, 1842·1
Bio Ace, 1842·1
Bio Ace Excell, 1842·1
Bio Acidophilus, 1842·1
Bio C, 1842·1
Bio Cabal, 1842·1
Bio E, 1842·1
Bio Enhaced Natural E, 1842·1
Bio Equisan, 1842·1
Bio Espectrum, 1842·1
Bio Eutrical, 1842·1
Bio Flora, 1842·1
Bio Gelin, 1842·1
Bio Grip C, 1842·1
Bio Grip Plus, 1842·1
Bio Magnesium, 1842·1
Bio Slim Silueta, 1842·1
Bio Star, 1842·1
Bio Tarbun, 1842·1
Bio Tears, 1842·1
Bio Zinc, 1842·1
Bio-Acerola C Complex, 1842·1
Bioact-D, 1842·1
Bioactiv Preparations, 1842·1
Bioage Peripheral, Bioglan— *see* Bioglan Bioage Peripheral, 1843·4
Bioagil, 1842·2
Bioaler, 1842·2
Bioaletrina, 1500·3
Bioallethrin, 1500·3
Bio-Amoksiclav, 1842·2
Bio-Antioxydant, 1842·2
Bioarginina, 1842·2
Bio-Arscolloid, 1842·2
Bio-Ascorbate, 1842·2
Biobalm, 1842·2
Bioband, 1842·2
Biobase, 1842·2
Biobase-G, 1842·2
Biobees, 1842·2
Bio-Biol, 1842·2
Bio-C, 1842·2
Bio-C A Vogel, 1842·2
Bio-C Complex, 1842·2
Biocadmio, 1842·2
Biocalcin, 1842·2
Biocalcio, 1842·2
Biocalcium, 1842·2
Bio-Calcium + $D_3$, 1842·2
Bio-Calcium + $D_3$ + K, 1842·2
Biocalm, 1842·2
Biocalron, 1842·2
Biocalyptol, 1842·2
Bio-Caps, 1842·2
Biocarbo, 1842·2
Biocarbon, 1842·3
Biocarde, 1842·3
Biocarn, 1842·3
Biocarnil, 1842·3
Biocarotine, 1842·3
Biocatalase, 1842·3
Bioceanat, 1842·3
Biocebe, 1842·3
Biocef, 1842·3
Bio-Cest, 1842·3
Biochanin A, 1737·3

Biochetasi, 1842·3
Biochin, 1842·3
Bio-Chrome, 1842·3
Bio-Chromium, 1842·3
Bio-Ci, 1842·3
Biociclin, 1842·3
Biocid, 1842·3
Biocidan, 1842·3
Biocil, 1842·3
Biocilin, 1842·3
Biocin, 1842·3
Biocine Test, 1842·4
Biocine Test PPD, 1842·4
Biocitronil, 1842·4
Bioclaril, 1842·4
Bioclate, 1842·4
Bioclavid, 1842·4
Bioclin Kera, 1842·4
Bioclin Sebo Care, 1842·4
Bioclox, 1842·4
Biocobal, 1842·4
Biocodone, 1842·4
Biocol, 1842·4
Bioconseils, 1842·4
Biocord, 1842·4
Biocort, 1842·4
Biocortin, 1842·4
Biocoryl, 1842·4
Biocos, 1842·4
BioCox, 1842·4
Biocream, 1842·4
Biocrinal, 1842·4
Biocrist, 1842·4
Bio-Cuivre, 1842·4
Bio-C-Vitamin, 1842·4
Biocyclin, 1842·4
BioCyst, 1842·4
Bio-Dac, 1842·4
Biodalgic, 1843·1
Biodan, 1843·1
Bioday, 1843·1
Bio-Delta Cortilen, 1843·1
Bioderm, 1843·1
Biodermatin, 1843·1
Biodexan, 1843·1
Biodexin, 1843·1
Biodezil, 1843·1
Biodif, 1843·1
Biodinam, 1843·1
Biodine, 1843·1
Bio-Disc, 1843·1
Biodone, 1843·1
Biodone Forte, 1843·1
Biodophilus, 1843·1
Biodoxi, 1843·1
Biodramina, 1843·1
Biodramina Cafeina, 1843·1
Biodrop, 1843·1
Biodroxil, 1843·1
Bio-Dyne— *see* Preparation H, 2233·1
Bio-E, 1843·1
Bio-E-Vitamin, 1843·1
Bio-Energol Plus, 1843·1
Bioenterine, 1843·1
Bioequiseto, 1843·1
Bioesse Plus, 1843·1
Biofanal, 1843·1
Biofax, 1843·1
Biofaxil, 1843·1
Biofem, 1843·2
Biofenac, 1843·2
Bio-Fer, 1843·2
Bioferal, 1843·2
Bioferina, 1843·2
Bioferon, 1843·2
Bioferon Hepakit, 1843·2
Bioferro, 1843·2
Biofiber, 1843·2
Biofibra, 1843·2
Biofigado, 1843·2
Biofilm, 1843·2
Biofim, 1843·2
Bioflac, 1843·2
Bioflam, 1843·2
Bioflavonoids, 1688·2
Bioflex, 1843·2
Bioflogil, 1843·2
Bioflor, 1843·2
Bio-Flora, 1843·2
Bioflorin, 1843·2
Bioflox, 1843·2
Biofloxin, 1843·2
Biofluor, 1843·2
Biofluor Sensitive, 1843·2
Bioflusin, 1843·3
Bioflutin-N, 1843·3
Biofolic, 1843·3
Bioform, 1843·3
Biofreeze, 1843·3
Biofructose, 1843·3
Biofurex, 1843·3
Biofurin, 1843·3
Biofuroso, 1843·3
Biogam, 1843·3
Biogaracin, 1843·3
Biogardol, 1843·3
Bio-Garten Entschlackungstee, 1843·3
Bio-Garten Tee Preparations, 1843·3
Bio-Garten Tropfen Preparations, 1843·3
Biogaze, 1843·4
Biogel, 1843·4
Biogelat Erkaltungs & Grippe, 1843·4
Biogelat Herzstarkungs, 1843·4
Biogelat Leberschutz, 1843·4
Biogelat Schlaf, 1843·4
Biogena Dermo, 1843·4
Biogenis, 1843·4
Biogenis One-a-Day, 1843·4
Biogenol, 1843·4
Biogesic, 1843·4
Bioget, 1843·4
BioGinkgo, 1843·4
Bioglan Preparations, 1843·4
Bioglufer, 1844·2
Bioglusil, 1844·2
Biogreen, 1844·2
Biogrip Forte, 1844·2
Biogyl, 1844·2
Biohepax, 1844·2
Bio-Hep-B, 1844·2
Biohisdex DM, 1844·2
Biohisdine DM, 1844·2
Biohist, 1844·2
Biohist-LA, 1844·2
Bio-H-Tin, 1844·2
Biohulin Preparations, 1844·2
Bio-Insulin Preparations, 1844·3
Bioiodine, 1844·3
Biojad, 1844·3
Biokacin, 1844·3
Biokids, 1844·3
Bioklysm, 1844·3
Biokosma Embrocation, 1844·3
Biokosma Medizinalbad, 1844·3
Biokosma Red Point-Massagecreme, 1844·3
Biokur, 1844·3
Biol Preo, 1844·3
Biolac, 1844·3
Biolactine, 1844·3
Biolactona, 1844·3
Biolactus, 1844·3
Biolactyl, 1844·3
Biolan Tar, 1844·3
Biolane, 1844·3
Biolau, 1844·4
Biolavan, 1844·4
Biolax, 1844·4
Biolecit H3, 1844·4
Biolectra Calcium, 1844·4
Biolectra Magnesium, 1844·4
Biolectra Zink, 1844·4
Bioleine, 1844·4
BIOLF-62, 635·3
Biolid, 1844·4
Biolina, 1844·4
Biolix, 1844·4
Biological Response Modifiers, 492·1
Bio-Logos, 1844·4
Biolon, 1844·4
Biolone, 1844·4
Biolucchini, 1844·4
Biomag, 1844·4
Biomag Vital, 1844·4
Biomagnesin, 1844·4
Bio-Magnesium, 1844·4
Bio-Marine Plus, 1844·4
Biomega-3, 1844·4
Biometalle II-Heyl, 1844·4
Biometalle III-Heyl, 1844·4
Biometrox, 1844·4
Biomida, 1844·4
Biomina, 1844·4
Biomineral, 1844·4
Biomineral 5-Alfa, 1845·1
Bio-Mineral Formula, 1845·1
Biomineral One, 1845·1
Biomineral Plus, 1845·1
Biomineral Unghie, 1845·1
Biominol A, 1845·1
Biominol A D, 1845·1
Biomisen, 1845·1
Biomitin, 1845·1
Biomo-lipon, 1845·1
Biomona, 1845·1
Biomont, 1845·1
Biomox, 1845·1
Biomoxil, 1845·1
Biomunil, 1845·1
Bion Tears, 1845·1
Bionafil, 1845·1
Bionagre Plus E, 1845·1
Bionagrol, 1845·1
Bionagrol Plus, 1845·1
Bionaril, 1845·1
Bionet, 1845·1
Bioneural B12, 1845·1
Bioneuryl, 1845·1
Bionicard, 1845·1
Bionif, 1845·1
Bionobal, 1845·1
Bionocalcin, 1845·1
Bionolip, 1845·1
Bionorm, 1845·1
Bionoxol, 1845·1
Bionutrin, 1845·2
Biopasal Fibra, 1845·2
Biopause, 1845·2
Biopaxel, 1845·2
Biopental, 1845·2
Bioperazone, 1845·2
Bioperidolo, 1845·2
Biophil, 1845·2
Biophylin, 1845·2
Biopim, 1845·2
Biopiper, 1845·2
Bioplak, 1845·2
Bioplant-Kamillenfluid, 1845·2
Bioplasma FDP, 1845·2
Bioplatino, 1845·2
Bioplex, 1845·2
Bioplus, 1845·2
Biopram, 1845·2
Bioprim, 1845·2
Bioprofol, 1845·2
Bioprol, 1845·2
Bioprotus, 1845·2
Bioptic, 1845·2
Bioptic DX, 1845·2
Bioptimum, 1845·2
Biopto-E, 1845·2
Biopulmin, 1845·2
Biopyr, 1845·2
Bioquidan, 1845·2
Bioquil, 1845·3
Bioquin, 1845·3
Bio-Quinon Q10 Super, 1845·3
Bio-Quinone, 1845·3
Bioral, 1845·3
Bioralin, 1845·3
Bioran, 1845·3
Biordin, 1845·3
Bio-Real, 1845·3
Bio-Real Complex, 1845·3
Bio-Real Plus, 1845·3
Bioreform Preparations, 1845·3
Bio-Regenerat S 3, 1845·3
Bioregime, 1845·3
Bioregime Fort, 1845·3
Bioregime SlimKit, 1845·3
Biorenal, 1845·3
Biorenyn, 1845·3
Bioreucam, 1845·3
Bioreunil, 1845·3
Biorevit Solar 15, 1845·4
Biorganic Geri, 1845·4
Biorgasept, 1845·4
Biorinil, 1845·4
Bio-Ritmo, 1845·4
Biormon, 1845·4
Biorphen, 1845·4
Biorrub, 1845·4
Biortho, 1845·4
Biosal, 1845·4
Biosan E, 1845·4
Biosan Zink, 1845·4
Bioscalin, 1845·4
Bioscefal, 1845·4
Bioscina, 1845·4
Bioscina Composta, 1845·4
Biosedon S, 1845·4
Bio-Sel, 1845·4
Bioselenium, 1845·4
Bio-Selenium, 1845·4
Biosern, 1845·4
Biosil, 1845·4
Biosint, 1845·4
Biosol A, 1845·4
Biosol B, 1845·4
Biosonide, 1845·4
Biosorb, 1845·4
Biosorbin MCT, 1845·4
Biosor-C, 1845·4
Biosoviran, 1846·1
Bio-Sport, 1846·1
Biostan, 1846·1
Biostatine, 1846·1
Biostim, 1846·1
Biostin, 1846·1
Biostop, 1846·1
Bio-Strath Preparations, 1846·1
Biosun, 1846·1
Biosurgery, 1151·3
Bio-Tab, 1846·1
Biotaer, 1846·1
Biotaer Gamma, 1846·1
Biotaer Nasal, 1846·1
Biotaer Nebulizable, 1846·1
Biotaer Ultrason Nebulizable, 1846·1
Biotamoxal, 1846·1
Biotanica Feminine, 1846·2
Biotanica Ginsemag, 1846·2
Biotanica Nocturn, 1846·2
Biotanica Pro Energy, 1846·2
Biotanica Regenerance, 1846·2
Biotanica Uricalm, 1846·2
Biotarson N, 1846·2
Biotarson O, 1846·2
Biotase, 1846·2
Biotassina, 1846·2
Biotax, 1846·2
Biotaxime, 1846·2
Biotazol, 1846·2
Biotecan, 1846·2
Biotel Kidney, 1846·2
Biotene, 1846·2
Biotene Dry Mouth, 1846·2
Biotene Oralbalance, 1846·2
Biotens, 1846·2
Biotenzol, 1846·2
Bioteral, 1846·2
Bioterona, 1846·2
Biotherm Preparations, 1846·2
Biothymus, 1846·3
Biothymus DS, 1846·3
Biothymus F Urto, 1846·3
Biothymus M Urto, 1846·3
Biotic, 1846·3
Bioticaps, 1846·3
Bioticic, 1846·3
Biotin, 1423·2
Biotina, 1423·2
Biotin-Asmedic, 1846·3
Biotinum, 1423·2

Bioton, 1846·3
Biotone, 1846·3
Biotonico Fontoura, 1846·3
Biotonus, 1846·3
Biototal, 1846·3
Biotrefon L, 1846·3
Biotrefon Plus, 1846·3
Biotrexate, 1846·3
Biotricina, 1846·3
Biotril, 1846·3
Biotrivin, 1846·3
Biotrixina, 1846·3
Biotron, 1846·4
Biotropic, 1846·4
Bio-Tropin, 1846·4
Biotropin, 1846·4
Biotuss, 1846·4
Biotyage, 1846·4
Biovac HB, 1846·4
Bio-Vagin, 1846·4
Biovancomin, 1846·4
Biovelbin, 1846·4
Biovent, 1846·4
Biovicerin, 1846·4
Biovigor, 1846·4
Biovir, 1846·4
Biovit, 1846·4
Biovit-A, 1846·4
Biovital, 1846·4
Biovital Aktiv, 1846·4
Biovital Classic, 1846·4
Biovital Forte N— *see* Biovital Aktiv, 1846·4
Biovital Ginseng, 1846·4
Biovital N, 1846·4
Biovital N— *see* Biovital Classic, 1846·4
Biovital Weissdorn, 1846·4
Biovital Weissdorn Tonikum, 1846·4
Bio-Vitas, 1846·4
Bioxan, 1846·4
Bioxel, 1846·4
Bioxifeno, 1847·1
Bioxilina, 1847·1
Bioxilina Plus, 1847·1
Bioxima, 1847·1
Bioximicina, 1847·1
Bioximil, 1847·1
BioXtra, 1847·1
BioXtra Programme, 1847·1
Bioxyol, 1847·1
Bioyetin, 1847·1
Biozac, 1847·1
Bio-Zinc, 1847·1
Biozole, 1847·1
Biozolene, 1847·1
Biozolin, 1847·1
Biozoral, 1847·1
Bipasmin, 1847·1
Bipasmin Composto, 1847·1
Bipasmin Compuesto, 1847·1
Bipasmin Compuesto NF, 1847·1
Bipectinol, 1847·1
Bipencil, 1847·1
Bipensaar, 1847·1
Biperiden, 479·3
Biperiden Hydrochloride, 479·3
Biperiden Lactate, 479·3
Biperideni Hydrochloridum, 479·3
Biperideno, 479·3
Biperideno, Hidrocloruro de, 479·3
Biperideno, Lactato de, 479·3
Biphasic Insulins, 334·2
Biphasil, 1847·1
Biphaston, 1847·1
Biphenamine Hydrochloride, 1163·1
Biphenyl, 1681·2
Biphenylacetic Acid, 39·2
2-Biphenylol, 1187·2
Biphenyl-4-ylacetic Acid, 39·1
1-(α-Biphenyl-4-ylbenzyl)imidazole, 395·1
4-(Biphenyl-4-yl)-4-oxobutyric Acid, 39·1
3-(3-Biphenyl-4-yl-1,2,3,4-tetrahydro-1-naphthyl)-4-hydroxycoumarin, 1504·1
Biphosphonates, 766·3
Biplatrix, 1847·1
Bipodial, 1847·1
Bipolar Disorder, 278·2
BIPP, 1184·2
Bipranix, 1847·1
Bipreterax, 1847·1
Bipro, 1847·1
Bi-Profenid, 1847·2
Bipronyl, 1847·2
Biquin, 1847·2
Biquinate, 1847·2
Bi-Qui-Nol, 1847·2
Birac, 1847·2
Biral, 1847·2
Birch Leaf, 1660·3
Birch Tar Oil, 1159·2
Bird Fanciers' Lung— *see* Diffuse Parenchymal Lung Disease, 1079·3
BI-RG-587, 650·2
BIRG-0587, 650·2
Birkenblätter, 1660·3
Birkenblatter Pflanzensaft, Kneipp— *see* Kneipp Birkenblatter Pflanzensaft, 2081·2
Birkenteer, 1159·2
Birley's, 1847·2
Birobin, 1847·2
Birodogyl, 1847·2
Birofenid, 1847·2
Biron, 1847·2
Biroxol, 1847·2
BIRR-004, 655·3
Birvac, 1847·2
(−)-α-Bisabolol, 1707·1
(*OC*-6-43)-Bis(acetato)amminedichloro(cyclohexylamine)platinum, 583·2
Bis(2-acetoxybenzoato-*O'*)hydroxyaluminium, 14·1
(2*S*,5*R*,7*S*,10*R*,13*S*)-10,20-Bis(acetoxy)-2-benzoyloxy-1,7-dihydroxy-9-oxo-5,20-epoxytax-11-en-13-yl (3*S*)-3-Benzoylamino-3-phenyl-D-lactate, 577·3
Bisacodilo, 1251·3
Bisacodyl, 1251·3
Bisacodyl Tannex, 1251·3
Bisacodylum, 1251·3
Bisacolax, 1847·2
Bisalax, 1847·2
Bisa-Lax, 1847·2
1,3-Bis(4-amidinophenyl)triazene Bis(*N*-acetylglycinate), 604·2
Bis(2-aminoethyl) *p*-[(4,6-Diamino-*s*-triazin-2-yl)amino]dithiobenzenearsonite, 109·2
*N*,*N'*-Bis(2-Aminoethyl)-1,2-ethanediamine Dihydrochloride, 1055·2
1,3-Bis(4-amino-2-methyl-6-quinolyl)urea Dihydrochloride, 1168·2
Bis(4-aminophenyl) Sulphone, 202·2
Bisantrene Hydrochloride, 530·2
Bisantreno, Hidrocloruro de, 530·2
Bisatin, 1282·3
2,5-Bis(aziridin-1-yl)-3-(2-hydroxy-1-methoxyethyl)-6-methyl-*p*-benzoquinone Carbamate, 535·1
Bisbentiamina, 1454·3
Bisbentiamine, 1454·3
1,4-Bis(3-bromopropionyl)piperazine, 580·1
1,3-Bis(3-butoxy-2-hydroxypropyl)-5-ethyl-5-phenylbarbituric Acid Dicarbamate Ester, 697·2
{*N'*,*N''*-Bis(carboxymethyl)-*N'*,*N''*-[(aceto)iminodiethylene]diglycinato-*O*,*O'*,*O''*,*N*,*N'*,*N''*}gadolinium(3+), 1062·2
*p*-[Bis(carboxymethylmercapto)arsino]benzamide, 114·1
{*N*,*N*-Bis[2-({(carboxymethyl)[(2-methoxyethyl)carbamoyl]methyl}amino)-ethyl]glycinato(3-)}gadolinium, 1063·1
[*N*,*N*-Bis(2-{(carboxymethyl)[(methylcarbamoyl)methyl]amino}ethyl)glycinato(3-)]gadolinium, 1062·1
Biscasil, 1847·2
1,3-Bis(4-chlorobenzylideneamino)guanidine Hydrochloride, 615·2
Bis(2-chloroethyl) 3-Chloro-4-methylcoumarin-7-yl Phosphate, 105·2
5-[Bis(2-chloroethyl)amino]-1-methyl-2-benzimidazolebutyric Acid Hydrochloride, 529·3
2-[Bis(2-chloroethyl)amino]perhydro-1,3,2-oxazaphosphorinan 2-Oxide Monohydrate, 540·2
4-Bis(2-chloroethyl)amino-L-phenylalanine, 566·1
4-[4-Bis(2-chloroethyl)aminophenyl]butyric Acid, 536·1
(±)-2-({2-[Bis(2-chloroethyl)amino]tetrahydro-2*H*-1,3,2-oxazaphosphorin-4-yl}thio)ethanesulphonic Acid *P-cis* Oxide, 565·3
Bis(2-chloroethyl)methylamine Hydrochloride, 537·1
1,3-Bis(2-chloroethyl)-1-nitrosourea, 535·1
Bis(2-chloroethyl)sulphide, 1679·3
Bis[2-(4-chlorophenoxy)-2-methylpropionato]hydroxyaluminium, 884·3
1,3-Bis[1-(7-chloro-4-quinolyl)-4'-piperazinyl]propane, 456·1
Biscotto Plasmon, 1847·2
Bisco-Zitron, 1847·2
Biscumacetato de Etilo, 914·1
Bisdesethylchloroquine, 450·2
Bis(diethylthiocarbamoyl) Disulfide, 1681·3
Bis[4,5-dihydroxybenzene-1,3-disulphonato(4−)-$O^4$,$O^5$]antimonate(5−) Pentasodium Heptahydrate, 103·1
*N*,*N'*-Bis(2,3-dihydroxypropyl)-5-[*N*-(2,3-dihydroxypropyl)acetamido]-2,4,6-tri-iodoisophthalamide, 1064·2
*N*,*N'*-Bis(2,3-dihydroxypropyl)-5-[*N*-(2-hydroxyethyl)glycolamido]-2,4,6-tri-iodoisophthalamide, 1066·2
*N*,*N'*-Bis(2,3-dihydroxypropyl)-5-(3-hydroxy-2-hydroxymethylpropionamido)-2,4,6-tri-iodo-*N*,*N'*-dimethylisophthalamide, 1063·1
*N*,*N'*-Bis(2,3-dihydroxypropyl)-5-[*N*-(2-hydroxy-3-methoxypropyl)acetamido]-2,4,6-tri-iodoisophthalamide, 1065·1
*N*,*N'*-Bis(2,3-dihydroxypropyl)-5-[2-(hydroxymethyl)hydracrylamido]-2,4,6-triiodo-*N*,*N'*-dimethylisophthalamide, 1063·1
*N*,*N'*-Bis(2,3-dihydroxypropyl)-2,4,6-triiodo-5-(2-methoxyacetamido)-*N*-methylisophthalamide, 1065·2
*N*,*N'*-Bis(2,3-dihydroxypropyl)-2,4,6-triiodo-5-(*N*-methylglycolamido)-isophthalamide, 1064·3
3,6-Bis(dimethylamino)acridine, 1647·1
4-[4,4'Bis(dimethylamino)benzhydrylidene]cyclohexa-2,5-dien-1-ylidenedimethylammonium Chloride, 1186·1
Bis{6-dimethylamino-2-[2-(2,5-dimethyl-1-phenylpyrrol-3-yl)vinyl]-1-methylquinolinium} 4,4'-Methylenebis(3-hydroxy-2-naphthoate), 113·3
(4*S*,4a*S*,5a*R*,12a*S*)4,7-Bis(dimethylamino)-1,4,4a,5,5a,6,11,12a-octahydro-3,10,12,12a-tetrahydroxy-1,11-dioxonaphthacene-2-carboxamide, 231·3
3,7-Bis(dimethylamino)phenazathionium Chloride Trihydrate, 1042·2
Biseko, 1847·2
Biselic, 1847·2
Biseptine, 1847·2
Biserirte Magnesia, 1847·2
Biserol-Potassium, 1847·2
(1*RS*,1'*RS*)-1,1'-[(2*RS*,2'*SR*)-Bis(6-fluorochroman-2-yl)]-2,2'-iminodiethanol, 964·3
4-[4,4-Bis(4-fluorophenyl)butyl]-*N*-ethylpiperazine-1-carboxamide, 670·3
8-[4,4-Bis(4-fluorophenyl)butyl]-1-phenyl-1,3,8-triazaspiro[4.5]decan-4-one, 701·1
1-{1-[4,4-Bis(4-fluorophenyl)butyl]-4-piperidyl}benzimidazolin-2-one, 715·1
Bis(D-gluconato-$O^1$,$O^2$) Copper, 1425·3
Bis(D-gluconato-$O^1$,$O^2$) Manganese, 1440·1
Bishydroxycoumarin, 894·2
Bis(2-hydroxyethyl)amine, 1681·1
(*S*)-*N*,*N'*-Bis[2-hydroxy-1-(hydroxymethyl)ethyl]-2,4,6-tri-iodo-5-lactamidoisophthalamide, 1064·3
1,7-Bis(4-hydroxy-3-methoxyphenyl)hepta-1,6-diene-3,5-dione, 1057·2
9-[(1*R*,2*R*,3*S*)-2,3-Bis(hydroxymethyl)cyclobutyl]guanine, 649·3
2,2-Bis(hydroxymethyl)propane-1,3-diol, 1283·2
2,2-Bis(hydroxymethyl)propane-1,3-diol Tetranicotinate, 965·3
2,2-Bis(hydroxymethyl)propane-1,3-diol Tetranitrate, 979·1
*N*,*N'*-Bis(hydroxymethyl)urea, 1187·2
2,2-Bis(4-hydroxyphenyl)-1,4-benzoxazin-3(2*H*,4*H*)-one Diacetate, 1253·2
3,3-Bis(4-hydroxyphenyl)indolin-2-one, 1282·3
3,3-Bis(4-hydroxyphenyl)phthalide, 1284·1
Bis(*p*-hydroxyphenyl)pyridyl-2-methane, 1251·3, 1289·3
Bis[1-hydroxypyridine-2(1*H*)-thionato]zinc, 1156·2
Bisibutiamine, 1455·1
Bisil, 1847·2
1,3-Bis[3-(2-imidazolin-2-yl)phenyl]urea Dipropionate, 606·1
9-{(*R*)-2-[(Bis{[(isopropoxycarbonyl)oxy]methoxy}phosphinyl)methoxy]propyl}adenine Fumarate (1:1), 655·1
Biskapect, 1847·3
Bislan, 1847·3
Bism. Carb., 1252·1
Bism. Subgall., 1252·2
Bism. Subnit., 1252·2
Bisma Rex, 1847·3
Bismag, 1847·3
Bisma-Rex, 1847·3
Bismatrol, 1847·3
Bismed, 1847·3
2'-[2,3-Bis(methoxycarbonyl)guanidino]-5'-phenylthio-2-methoxyacetanilide, 105·2
3,4-Bis(*p*-methoxyphenyl)-5-isoxazoleacetic Acid, 60·1
2,6-Bis(1-methylethyl)phenol, 1305·3
(−)-(*R*)-1-[4,4-Bis(3-methyl-2-thienyl)-3-butenyl]nipecotic Acid Hydrochloride, 378·1
Bismofalk, 1847·3
Bismofarma, 1847·3
Bismolan, 1847·3
Bismolan H Corti, 1847·3
Bismolan N, 1847·3
Bismopepsin, 1847·3
Bismorectal, 1847·3
Bismubell, 1847·3
Bismu-Jet, 1847·3
Bismultin, 1847·3
Bismurectol, 1847·3
Bismutal, 1847·3
Bismuth Aluminate, 1252·1
Bismuth Carbonate, 1252·1
Bismuth Carbonate, Basic, 1252·1
Bismuth Citrate, 1252·1
Bismuth Citrate, Ranitidine, 1287·2
Bismuth Compounds, 1252·1
Bismuth Hydroxide Nitrate Oxide, 1252·2
Bismuth and Iodoform Paste— *see* OxBipp, 2198·2
Bismuth, Magistery of, 1252·2
Bismuth Nitrate, Basic, 1252·2
Bismuth Nitrate, Heavy, 1252·2
Bismuth Oxide, 1252·1
Bismuth Oxycarbonate, 1252·1
Bismuth Oxygallate, 1252·2
Bismuth Oxynitrate, 1252·2
Bismuth Oxysalicylate, 1252·1
Bismuth Resorcinol Compounds, 1253·2
Bismuth Salicylate, 1252·1
Bismuth Salicylate, Basic, 1252·1
Bismuth (Sous-Nitrate de) Léger, 1252·2
Bismuth (Sous-Nitrate de) Lourd, 1252·2
Bismuth Subcarbonate, 1252·1, 1252·2
Bismuth Subcitrate, Colloidal, 1252·2
Bismuth Subgallate, 1252·2
Bismuth Subnitrate, 1252·2
Bismuth Subnitrate, Heavy, 1252·2
Bismuth Subnitrate and Iodoform Paste, 1184·2
Bismuth Subsalicylate, 1252·1
Bismuth Tetrabrompyrocatechinate, 1660·2
Bismuth Trioxide, 1252·1
Bismuth Tulasne, 1847·3
Bismuth, White, 1252·2
Bismuthi Subcarbonas, 1252·1
Bismuthi Subgallas, 1252·2

Bismuthi Subnitras, 1252·2
Bismuthi Subnitras Levis, 1252·2
Bismuthi Subsalicylas, 1252·1
Bismuthum, 1253·2
Bismuthyl Nitrate, 1252·2
Bismutila, Carbonato de, 1252·1
Bismutilo, Nitrato de, 1252·2
Bismuto, Compuestos de, 1252·1
Bismuto, Subazotato de, 1252·2
Bismutrex, Ranitidine, 1287·2
Bismutylum Carbonicum, 1252·1
Bismylate, 1847·3
Bisnortilidate, 94·1
Bisnortilidine, 94·1
Biso, 1847·3
Biso Lich, 1847·3
Bisobeta, 1847·3
Bisobloc, 1847·3
Bisocor, 1847·3
Bisodol, 1847·4
Bisodol Extra— *see* Bisodol Wind Relief, 1847·4
Bisodol Extra Strong Mint Tablets, 1847·4
Bisodol Heartburn Relief, 1847·4
Bisodol Wind Relief, 1847·4
Bisogamma, 1847·4
Bisohexal, 1847·4
Bisolapid, 1847·4
Bisolax, 1847·4
Bisolbruis, 1847·4
Bisolgrip, 1847·4
Bisolgrip T, 1847·4
Bisolnasal, 1847·4
Bisolol, 1847·4
Bisolrapid, 1847·4
Bisolspray, 1847·4
Bisoltab, 1847·4
Bisoltus, 1847·4
Bisolvex, 1847·4
Bisolvomycin, 1847·4
Bisolvon Preparations, 1847·4
Bisolvonat, 1848·1
Bisolvonat Mono, 1848·1
Bisomerck, 1848·1
Bisomerck Plus, 1848·1
Bisopine, 1848·1
Bisopral, 1848·1
Bisoprolol Fumarate, 875·1
Bisoprolol, Fumarato de, 875·1
Bisoprolol Hemifumarate, 875·1
Bisoprolol-HCT, 1848·1
Biso-Puren, 1848·1
Bisotyrol, 1848·1
Bisoxatin Acetate, 1253·2
Bisoxatin Diacetate, 1253·2
Bisoxatina, Acetato de, 1253·2
Bispan, 1848·1
Bis-Pectin, 1848·1
Bisphonal, 1848·1
Bisphosphonates, 766·3
9-[2-({Bis[(pivaloyloxy)methoxy]phosphinyl}methoxy)ethyl]adenine, 628·1
Bispyridostigmine Bromide, 1489·2
Bistatin V, 1848·1
Bisteron, 1848·1
Bistrepen, 1848·1
2,8-Bis(trifluoromethyl)-4-quinoline Carboxylic Acid, 455·2
(*RS*)-[2,8-Bis(trifluoromethyl)-4-quinolyl]-(*SR*)-(2-piperidyl)methanol Hydrochloride, 453·3
2,2′-Bis(1,6,7-trihydroxy-3-methyl-5-isopropylnaphthalene-8-carboxaldehyde), 1695·3
Bistropamide, 491·1
Bistryl, 1848·1
Bisuisan, 1848·1
Bisulfato de Clopidogrel, 888·3
Bisulfito Potásico, 1193·1
Bisulfito Sódico, 1193·1
Bisulfito Sódico de Menadiona, 1466·3
Bisval, 1848·2
Bitartarato de Colina, 1424·3
Bitartrate de Dextromoramide, 28·2
Bitartrato de Epinefrina, 852·2
Bitartrato de Mercaptamina, 1712·1
Bitartrato de Norepinefrina, 974·3
Bitartrato de Prajmalio, 984·3
Bite & Itch Lotion, 1848·2
Bite Rx, 1848·2
Bitecain AA, 1848·2
Bitensil, 1848·2
Bitensil Diu, 1848·2
Bites, Infections in— *see* Bites and Stings, 121·3
Bites, Snake— *see* Snake Bites, 1639·2
Bites, Spider— *see* Spider Bites, 1640·1
Bithiolate Ammonique, 1148·2
Bithionol, 103·3
Bithionol Oxide, 103·3
Bithyol, 1148·2
Bi-Tildiem, 1848·2
Bitionol, 103·3
Bitolterol Mesilate, 781·3
Bitolterol, Mesilato de, 781·3
Bitolterol Mesylate, 781·3
Bitrex, 1186·1, 1679·2
Bitter Almond Oil, 1651·1
Bitter Almond Oil, Volatile, 1659·3
Bitter Apple, 1260·3
Bitter Cucumber, 1260·3
Bitter Fennel, 1687·2
Bitter-Fennel Fruit Oil, 1687·3
Bitter Orange, 1723·3
Bitter-orange Epicarp and Mesocarp, 1723·3
Bitter-orange Flower, 1723·3
Bitter-orange Flower Oil, 1719·2
Bitter Orange Oil, 1723·3
Bitter-orange Peel, Dried, 1723·3
Bitter Root, 1692·2
Bitter Wood, 1737·2
Bitteridina, 1848·2
Bitterklee, 1712·1
Bittersüss, 1683·1
Bittersweet, 1683·1
Bituelve, 1848·2
Bituminol, 1148·2
Bivacyn, 1848·2
Bivalem, 1848·2
Bivalirudin, 875·2
Bivalirudina, 875·2
Bi-Vaspit, 1848·2
Bivate, 1848·2
Biviol, 1848·2
Biviraten, 1848·2
Bivitasi, 1848·2
Bivitox, 1848·2
Bivorilan, 1848·2
Bixin, 1056·1
Biznaga, Fruto de la, 1653·3
B-Ject, 1848·2
BK, 1848·2
BK HC, 1848·2
B-kombin, 1848·2
BL22, 508·2
BL-191, 979·3
BL-700B, 1653·2
BL-5617, 790·3
BL-4162a, 1654·3
BL-4162A, 1654·3
B-Laboterol, 1848·2
Black BN, Brilliant, 1056·2
Black Catechu, 1661·1
Black Cherry Bark, 1765·2
Black Cherry Bark, Wild, 1765·2
Black Cohosh, 1671·3
Black Currant, 1661·1
Black Currant Leaf, 1661·1
Black Currant Seed Oil, 1661·1
Black Fluids, 1193·3
Black Forest Herbal Tea, 1848·2
Black Henna, 1696·3
Black Mint, 1283·2
Black Mustard, 1718·2
Black Nightshade, 1661·2
Black PN, 1056·2
Black PN, Brilliant, 1056·2
Black Sampson, 1683·2
Black Seed, 1848·2
Black Snakeroot, 1671·3
Black Widow Spider Antiserum, 1640·1
Black Widow Spider Antivenin, 1640·1
Black Widow Spider Antivenom, 1640·1
Black-Draught, 1848·2
Blackheads— *see* Acne, 1133·3
Blackmores B Plus C, 1848·2
Blackmores Bio, 1848·2
Blackmores Exec B's, 1848·2
Blackmores Naturetime, 1848·2
Blackmores Pregnancy & Breastfeeding Formula, 1848·3
Blackmores for Women Bio Iron, 1848·3
Blackmores for Women PMT, 1848·3
Blackmores for Women Total Calcium, 1848·3
Blackoids du Docteur Meur, 1848·3
Blacor, 1848·3
Bladder Cancer— *see* Malignant Neoplasms of the Bladder, 512·3
Bladder Cherry, 1731·3
Bladder Disorders— *see* Micturition Disorders, 475·3
Bladder Infections— *see* Urinary-tract Infections, 153·1
Bladder Irritation, 1848·3
Bladder, Unstable— *see* Urinary Incontinence and Retention, 476·1
Bladder Wrack, 1742·3
Bladderon, 1848·3
Bladderwrack, 1742·3
Blader, 1848·3
Bladex, 1848·3
Bladuril, 1848·3
Blaeberry, 1718·3
Blairex Lens Lubricant, 1848·3
Blanc de Zinc, 1163·2
Blancaler, 1848·3
Blandonal, 1848·3
Blanel, 1848·3
Blanoxan, 1848·3
Blasen- und Nierentee, 1848·3
Blasen- und Nieren-Tee, Kneipp— *see* Kneipp Blasen- und Nieren-Tee, 2081·2
Blasen-Nieren-Tee Stada, 1848·3
Blasen-Tee, 1848·3
Blasentee EF-EM-ES, 1848·3
Blastocarb, 1848·3
Blastocystis Hominis Infection, 596·1
Blastoestimulina, 1848·3
Blastolem, 1848·3
Blastomycosis, 386·3
Blastomycosis, South American— *see* Paracoccidioidomycosis, 389·1
Blaston, 1848·3
Blastop, 1848·3
Blastovin, 1848·4
Blaubimax, 1848·4
Blaubumin, 1848·4
Blauferon, 1848·4
Blauinfuion, 1848·4
Blavin, 1848·4
Blazing Star, 1696·3
Bleaches, 1192·2
Bleaching Powder, 1175·3
Bledilait, 1848·4
Bleduran, 1848·4
Blef-10, 1848·4
Blefamide, 1848·4
Blefamide SF, 1848·4
Blefamide SOP, 1848·4
Blefarida, 1848·4
Blefarolin, 1848·4
Blefarosan, 1848·4
Blefcon, 1848·4
Blemaren N, 1848·4
Blemerase, 1848·4
Bleminol, 1848·4
Blemish Control, 1848·4
Blemix, 1848·4
Blenamax, 1848·4
Blend-a-Med Periochip, 1848·4
Blendera, 1848·4
Blendox, 1848·4
Blenox, 1848·4
Blenoxane, 1849·1
Bleo, 1849·1
Bleo-cell, 1849·1
Bleocin, 1849·1
Bleocris, 1849·1
Bleolem, 1849·1
Bleomicina, Sulfato de, 530·2
Bleomycin $A_2$, 530·2
Bleomycin A5 Hydrochloride, 530·2
Bleomycin $B_2$, 530·2
Bleomycin $B_4$, 530·2
Bleomycin Hydrochloride, 530·2
Bleomycin, Indium ($^{111}$In), 1524·1
Bleomycin Sulfate, 530·2
Bleomycin Sulphate, 530·2
Bleomycini Sulfas, 530·2
Bleo-S, 1849·1
Bleph-10, 1849·1
Blephagel, 1849·1
Blephamide, 1849·1
Blepharitis— *see* Eye Disorders, 1224·2
Blepharitis— *see* Eye Infections, 127·2
Blepharospasm, 1390·1
Blephasol, 1849·1
Blessed Thistle, 1673·3
Blexit, 1849·1
Blezamont, 1849·1
Blifamol, 1849·1
*Blighia sapida*, 1700·2
Blink, 1849·1
Blinkene, 1849·1
Blinx, 1849·1
Blio, 1849·1
Blis K12 Throat Guard, 1849·1
Blisprotex, 1849·1
BlisterGard, 1849·1
Blistering Beetle, 1666·3
Blistex Preparations, 1849·1
Blisteze— *see* Blistex Relief Cream, 1849·2
Blistik, 1849·2
Blis-To-Sol, 1849·2
Bliz, 1849·2
Blizer, 1849·2
Blocacid, 1849·3
Blocadren, 1849·3
Blocamicina, 1849·3
Blocan, 1849·3
Blocanol, 1849·3
Blocar, 1849·3
Blocatril, 1849·3
Blocotenol, 1849·3
Blocotenol Comp, 1849·3
Blodex, 1849·3
Bloken, 1849·3
Blokium, 1849·3
Blokium B12, 1849·3
Blokium Cox, 1849·3
Blokium Diu, 1849·3
Blokium Flex, 1849·3
Blokium Gesic, 1849·3
Bloktus, 1849·3
Blonax, 1849·3
Blond Psyllium, 1268·1
Blood, 743·3
Blood Cells, Red, 759·3
Blood Clotting Factors, 735·3
Blood Coagulation Factors, 735·3
Blood Fluke Infections, 97·1
Blood Products Plasma Expanders and Haemostatics, 732·1
Blood Substitutes, Perfluorocarbon, 1730·1
Blood, Whole, 743·3
Bloodroot, 1741·3
Blootec, 1849·3
Blopresid, 1849·3
Blopress, 1849·3
Blopress D, 1849·3
Blopress 16 Mg + 12,5 Mg, 1849·4
Blopress Plus, 1849·4
β-Bloqueantes, 868·1
Blosyn, 1849·4
Blotex, 1849·4
Blow, 1373·3
Blox, 1849·4
Bloxang, 1849·4
Blox-D, 1849·4
BL-P-1322, 170·2
BL-S578, 167·2
BL-S640, 170·3
BL-S786, 175·2

Blu di Metilene, 1042·2
Bluboro, 1849·4
Bluco, 1849·4
Bluderm, 1849·4
Blue, 1849·4
Blue AC, Patent, 1056·2
Blue 1, Acid, 1750·3
Blue 3, Acid, 1729·1
Blue Asbestos, 1658·1
Blue, Azovan, 1658·3
Blue, Berlin, 1051·2
Blue Cohosh, 1661·2
Blue Collyrium, 1849·4
Blue Copperas, 1426·1
Blue Drops, Vicks— *see* Vicks Blue Drops, 2375·2
Blue EGS, 1056·2
Blue, Evans, 1658·3
Blue FCF, Brilliant, 1056·2
Blue Flag, 1702·1
Blue Flag Root Compound, 1849·4
Blue Galls, 1690·2
Blue O, Toluidine, 1757·1
Blue, Prussian, 1051·2
Blue Stone, 1426·1
Blue, Sulfan, 1750·3
Blue, Sulphan, 1750·3
Blue V, Patent, 1729·1, 1750·3
Blue Vitriol, 1426·1
Blue VRS, 1750·3
Blue X, 1700·3
Huesteril, 1849·4
Bluetest, 1849·4
Blum, 1849·4
Blumel, 1849·4
Blumen, 1849·4
Blumen, Colirio— *see* Colirio Blumen, 1899·4
Blumol, 1849·4
Blunorm, 1849·4
Blustark, 1849·4
Blutegel, 945·1
Blutquick Forte, 1849·4
Blutquick Forte S, 1849·4
BM-06.011, 770·2
BM-06.019, 747·2
BM-06.022, 995·2
BM-21.0955, 772·3
BM-02001, 866·3
BM-02015, 1015·3
BM-14190, 881·1
BM-15075, 873·2
BM-15275, 964·1
BM-22145, 942·1
BM-51052, 880·2
B-66256M, 1018·1
BM-Accutest, 1849·4
BM-Hopitest, 1849·4
BMOI-004, 955·3
BMP, 768·1
BMP-3, 768·2
BMP-7, 768·2
BMS-180194, 649·3
BMS-181158, 1151·3
BMS-181173, 1360·2
BMS-181339-01, 577·3
BMS-182751, 583·2
BMS-186091, 1142·3
BMS-186295, 940·1
BMS-186716, 976·1
BMS-186716-01, 976·1
BMS-200980, 945·1
BMS-206584-01, 216·2
BMS-217380-01, 587·3
BMS-232632, 629·1
BMS-232632-05, 629·1
BM-Tests, 1849·4
BMY-13754, 309·2
BMY-13805-1, 701·1
BMY-25182, 171·2
BMY-26517, 790·3
BMY-26538-01, 1654·3
BMY-27857, 654·2
BMY-28100, 179·2
BMY-28100-03-800, 179·2
BMY-28142, 172·1
BMY-28167, 179·2
BMY-30056, 1111·3
BMY-33419, 587·3
BMY-40481, 551·3
BMY-40900, 630·3
BMY-41606, 1342·2
BMY-42215-1, 1360·2
BMY-45594, 583·2
BN, 1850·1
BN 53, 1850·1
(±)-BN-1270, 883·2
BN-52014, 1341·2
BN-52020, 1693·1
BN-52021, 1693·1
BN-52022, 1693·1
BN-52023, 1693·1
BN-52024, 1693·1
BN-52030, 1330·3
BN-52063, 1693·1
BNAG, 1489·2
BN-B759V, 635·3
BNIL, 1850·1
BNP, 964·2
BNX, 1382·1
BO-714, 1672·3
Bo-Cal, 1850·1
Bocasan, 1850·1
Bocatriol, 1850·1
Bockshornsame, 1688·1
Bocytin, 1850·1
Bodaril, 1850·1
Bodigarde, 1850·1
Bodisan, 1850·1
Bodivitin, 1850·1
Body, 1850·1
Body Lice— *see* Pediculosis, 1499·1
Body Rox, 1850·1
Body Smarts, 1850·1
Body Wash, 1850·1
Bodyguard, 1850·1
*Boerhaavia diffusa*, 1737·1
*Boerhaavia repens*, 1737·1
Boestrol, 1850·1
Boflavin, 1850·1
Boforsin, 1674·3
Bog Myrtle, 1661·2
Bogbean, 1712·1
Bogbean Leaf, 1712·1
Bogil, 1850·1
Bo-Gum, 1850·1
Bogumil-tassenfertiger Milder Abfurtee, 1850·1
Boi K, 1850·1
Boi K Aspartico, 1850·1
Boil Ease, 1850·2
Boiled Oil, 1707·2
Bokey EMC, 1850·2
Bolchipen, 1850·2
Bolcitol, 1850·2
Boldex, 1850·2
Boldi Folium, 1661·2
Boldigan, 1850·2
Boldina He, 1850·2
Boldine, 1661·2
Boldine Dimethyl Ether, 1121·3
Boldo, 1661·2, 1850·2
Boldo Jurubeba, 1850·2
Boldo Leaf, 1661·2
Boldo Leaves, 1661·2
Boldo N "Hanosan", 1850·2
Boldobeba, 1850·2
Boldocynara, 1850·2
Boldoflorine, 1850·2
Boldolaxin, 1850·2
Boldopeptan, 1850·2
Boldosal, 1850·2
Boletic Acid, 1147·3
Bolinan, 1850·2
Bolisegna, 1850·2
Bolivian Haemorrhagic Fever— *see* Haemorrhagic Fevers, 618·2
Bolivian Leaf, 1373·3
Boljuprima, 1850·2
Bollinol, 1850·2
Bolo, 1850·2
Bolsa de Pastor, 1744·1
Boltin, 1850·2
Bolus Alba, 1268·3
Bolus Eucalypti Comp, 1850·2
Bolutol, 1850·3
Bolvidon, 1850·3
B-OM, 1850·3
B-OM Forte, 1850·3
Boma, 1850·3
Bomacorin, 1850·3
Bomagall Forte S, 1850·3
Bomagall Mono, 1850·3
Bomaklim, 1850·3
Bomapect, 1850·3
Bomex, 1850·3
Bomexin, 1850·3
Bomix, 1850·3
Bonactin, 1850·3
Bonadoxina, 1850·3
Bonalen, 1850·3
Bonalfa, 1850·3
Bonamina, 1850·3
Bonamine, 1850·3
Bonapetit, 1850·3
Bonar, 1850·3
Bonasanit, 1850·3
Bonased-L, 1850·3
Bonatol-R, 1850·3
Bonavit, 1850·3
Bonazin, 1850·3
Boncordin, 1850·3
Bondil, 1850·3
Bondiol, 1850·3
Bondormin, 1850·3
Bondronat, 1850·3
Bone Cancer— *see* Malignant Neoplasms of the Bone, 513·1
Bone Cements, 1714·3
Bone Cysts, 1077·1
Bone Disease, Hyperparathyroid— *see* Renal Osteodystrophy, 764·3
Bone Disease, Metastatic— *see* Malignant Neoplasms of the Bone, 513·1
Bone and Joint Infections, 122·1
Bone Marrow Transplantation— *see* Haematopoietic Stem Cell Transplantation, 1344·3
Bone Mineralisation, Impaired— *see* Osteomalacia, 762·3
Bone Modulating Drugs, 762·1
Bone Morphogenetic Proteins, 762·2, 768·1
Bone Pain— *see* Cancer Pain, 5·1
Bone Plus, 1850·4
Bone Sarcoma, 524·3
Bo-Ne-Ca, 1850·4
Bonefos, 1850·4
Bonemass, 1850·4
Boneset, 1661·3, 1675·2
Bongreen, 1850·4
Boniderma, 1850·4
Bonidon, 1850·4
Bonifen, 1850·4
Bonine, 1850·4
Boniva, 1850·4
Bonjela, 1850·4
Bonjela Teething Gel, 1850·4
Bon-Ker, 1850·4
Bonlax, 1850·4
Bonmax, 1850·4
Bonney's Blue, 1171·1, 1186·2
Bonningtons Irish Moss, 1850·4
Bonocef, 1850·4
Bonomint, 1850·4
Bon-One, 1850·4
Bonserin, 1850·4
Bontoss, 1850·4
Bontril, 1850·4
Bonyl, 1850·4
Boost, 1851·1
Boostrix, 1851·1
Boots Preparations, 1851·1
B.O.P., 1851·1
Bopindolol Hydrogen Malonate, 875·3
Bopindolol Malonate, 875·3
Bopindolol, Malonato de, 875·3
Boplatex, 1851·1
Boracap, 1851·2
Boracelle, 1851·2
Boracic Acid, 1662·1
Boracough, 1851·2
Boradren, 1851·2
Boradrine, 1851·2
Borafen, 1851·2
Borage, 1661·3
Borage Oil, 1661·3
*Borago officinalis*, 1661·3
Borakid, 1851·2
Boralina, 1851·2
Boraline, 1851·2
Boramycin, 1851·2
Borato de Fenilmercurio, 1189·2
Borato de Sodio, 1851·2
Borax, 1661·3
Borax Glycerin, 1662·1
Borax, Honey of, 1662·1
Borax, Purified, 1661·3
Borbalan, 1851·2
Bordeaux B, 1056·2
Bordeaux S, 1056·1
*Bordetella pertussis*, 1613·3, 1631·2
Borea, 1851·2
Boric Acid, 1662·1
Boric Acid Solution, Chlorinated Lime and, 1175·3
Boripharm Granules— *see* Granules Boripharm, 2031·1
Born, 1851·2
Bornan-2-one, 1665·3
Bornaprina, Hidrocloruro de, 480·1
Bornaprine Hydrochloride, 480·1
Borneol, 1740·2
Borneol Acetate, 1662·2
Borneol Salicylate, 21·2
Bornilene, 1851·2
Bornilo, Acetato de, 1662·2
Bornosan-Entwasserungsdragees, 1851·2
Bornosan-Leberschutz, 1851·2
Bornyl Acetate, 1662·2, 1740·2
Bornyl Salicylate, 21·2
6-[(1*R*,2*S*,4*S*)-Born-2-yl]-3,4-xylenol, 277·3
Borocaina, 1851·2
Borocaina Gola, 1851·2
Borocarpin-S, 1851·2
Borocell, 1851·2
Boroclarine, 1851·2
Borofair Otic, 1851·2
Borofax, 1851·2
Boronex, 1851·2
Boropak, 1851·2
Boro-Scopol, 1851·2
Borossigeno Plus Stomatologico, 1851·2
Borostyrol, 1851·3
Borostyrol N, 1851·3
Borotartrato Potásico, 1734·1
Borraginol-N, 1851·3
Borraja, 1661·3
Borraja, Aceite de, 1661·3
Borreliosis, Lyme— *see* Lyme Disease, 134·1
Borsäure, 1662·1
Bortezomib, 532·1
Borymycin, 1851·3
Bosconar, 1851·3
Bosentan, 875·3
Bosentano, 875·3
Bosisto's Eucalyptus Inhalant, 1851·3
Bosisto's Eucalyptus Rub, 1851·3
Bosisto's Eucalyptus Spray, 1851·3
Bosporon, 1851·3
Boston, 1851·3
Boston Advance, 1851·3
*Boswellia carteri*, 1690·1
*Boswellia glabra*, 1690·1
*Boswellia sacra*, 1690·1
*Boswellia serrata*, 1690·1
Botaderm, 1851·3
Botamycin-N, 1851·3
Botanica Hayfever, 1851·3
Botastin, 1851·3
*Bothrops atrox*, 743·3
*Bothrops jararaca*, 743·3, 1010·3
*Bothrops moojeni*, 743·3
Botox, 1851·3

Botropase, 1851·3
Bot/Ser, 1610·3
Bottom Better, 1851·3
Botulinum A Toxin, 1388·3
Botulinum A Toxin–Haemagglutinin Complex, 1389·3
Botulinum Antitoxin, 1610·3
Botulinum Antitoxin, Mixed, 1610·3
Botulinum B Toxin, 1388·3
Botulinum F Toxin, 1389·3
Botulinum Toxin Type A for Injection, 1388·3
Botulinum Toxins, 1388·3
Botulism, 1611·1
Botulism Antitoxin, 1610·3
Botulism Antitoxins, 1610·3
Boucren, 1851·3
Bouillet, 1851·3
Bouillon Blanc, 1764·1
Bouleau, 1660·3
Bounty Bears, 1851·3
Bourbon Vanilla, 1762·3
Bourdaine, 1266·3
Bourget, 1851·3
Bourrache, 1661·3
Boutonneuse— *see* Spotted Fevers, 147·1
BOV, 1750·3
Bovactant, 1736·2
Bovine Colostrum, 1611·1
Bovine Fibrinolysin, 916·2
Bovine Growth Hormone, Methionyl, 1327·2
Bovine Growth Hormone, Synthetic, 1327·2
Bovine Insulin, 333·3, 334·1
Bovine Skin, 1158·1
Bovine Somatotrophin, 1329·3
Bovine Somatotropin, 1329·3
Bovine Superoxide Dismutase, 92·2
Bovisan, 1851·3
Bowa, 1851·3
Bowen's Disease— *see* Basal Cell and Squamous Cell Carcinoma, 522·3
Box Jellyfish Antiserum, 1621·3
Box Jellyfish Antivenin, 1621·3
Box Jellyfish Sting, 1621·3
Boxazin Plus C, 1851·4
Boxocalm, 1851·4
Boxol, 1851·4
Boxolip, 1851·4
Boyol Salve, 1851·4
BOZ Ointment, Gold Cross— *see* Gold Cross BOZ Ointment, 2029·3
Bozaktral, 1851·4
BP-400, 439·1
BPD, 591·1
B2036-PEG, 1337·2
$BPF_{9a}$, 1010·3
BPL, 1191·2
B-Platin, 1851·4
B-Plex, 1851·4
B-Plex C, 1851·4
B-Plus, 1851·4
BQ-22-708, 910·3
BQL, 1851·4
BR-700, 43·1
Braccopiral, 1851·4
Brachiapas S, 1851·4
Brachont, 1851·4
Bradelmin, 1851·4
Bradimox, 1851·4
Bradoral, 1851·4
Bradosol, 1851·4
Bradosol Plus, 1851·4
Bradyarrhythmias— *see* Cardiac Arrhythmias, 816·1
Bradyl, 1851·4
Brady's-Magentropfen, 1851·4
Bragg's Medicinal Charcoal, 1851·4
*Brahea serrulata*, 1569·1
Brain Abscess— *see* Abscess, Brain, 120·3
Brain Injury— *see* Spinal Cord Injury, 1088·2
Brain N, Aar— *see* Aar Brain N, 1767·3
Brain Natriuretic Peptide, 964·2
Brain Tumours— *see* Malignant Neoplasms of the Brain, 513·2
Brain Tumours, Metastatic— *see* Malignant Neoplasms of the Brain, 513·2
Brainal, 1851·4
Brain-derived Neurotrophic Factor, 1739·1
Brainox, 1851·4
Braintop, 1851·4
Bralix, 1851·4
Brallobarbital, 671·3
Brallobarbital Calcium, 671·3
Bralobarbital, 671·3
Bramedil, 1851·4
Bramedil Compuesto, 1851·4
Bramin-hepa, 1852·1
Bran, 1253·2
Bran, Wheat, 1253·2
BranchAmin, 1852·1
Brand- u. Wundgel-Medice N, 1852·1
Brand- und Wund-Gel Eu Rho, 1852·1
Brandiazin, 1852·1
Branigen, 1852·1
Branitil, 1852·1
Branolind N, 1852·1
Brasivil, 1852·1
Brasivol, 1852·1
Brassel, 1852·1
*Brassica alba*, 1718·2
*Brassica campestris*, 1737·3
*Brassica juncea*, 1718·2
*Brassica napus*, 1737·3
*Brassica nigra*, 1718·2
*Brassica sinapioides*, 1718·2
Bratenol, 1852·1
Braudeide, 1852·1
Brauneria, 1683·2
Braunoderm, 1852·1
Braunol, 1852·1
Braunosan, 1852·1
Braunosan H Plus, 1852·1
Braunovidon, 1852·1
Bravavir, 654·2
Bravelle, 1852·1
Braxan, 1852·1
Brazepam, 1852·1
Brazil Wax, 1668·1
Brazilian Ginseng, 1693·1
Brea de Enebro, 1159·2
Brea de Hulla, 1159·2
Brea de Pino, 1159·3
Brea Vegetal, 1159·3
Breacol, 1852·1
Breacol Decongestant & Cough Suppressant, 1852·1
Breas y Aceites de Brea, 1159·2
Breast Cancer— *see* Malignant Neoplasms of the Breast, 514·1
Breast Cancer, Male— *see* Malignant Neoplasms of the Male Breast, 515·2
Breast Cancer, Prophylaxis— *see* Prophylaxis of Breast Cancer, 515·1
Breast Pain— *see* Mastalgia, 1546·3
Breath Holding Attacks— *see* Anoxic Seizures, 478·2
Breathe Eazy Chest Rub, 1852·1
Breathe Free, 1852·1
Breathe More, 1852·1
Breatheze, 1852·2
Breathquality-UBT, 1852·2
Brechnuss, 1722·3
Brechweinstein, 103·1
Bredon, 1852·2
Breezee Mist Antifungal, 1852·2
Brefar, 1852·2
Brefus, 1852·2
Brek, 1852·2
Brelomax, 1852·2
Bremagan Flu, 1852·2
Bremax, 1852·2
Bremicina, 1852·2
Bremide, 1852·2
Breminal, 1852·2
Bremon, 1852·2
Brenazol, 1852·2
Brenda-35 ED, 1852·2
Brennessel, Kneipp Pflanzen- Dragees— *see* Kneipp Pflanzen-Dragees Brennessel, 2081·3
Brennesselkraut Pflanzensaft Kneippianum, Kneipp— *see* Kneipp Brennesselkraut Pflanzensaft Kneippianum, 2081·2
Brennesseltonikum, 1852·2
Brenoxil, 1852·2
Brentacort, 1852·2
Brentan, 1852·2
Breonesin, 1852·2
Brequinar Sódico, 1351·2
Brequinar Sodium, 1351·2
Bres, 1852·2
Bresal, 1852·2
Bresben, 1852·2
Bresec, 1852·2
Breston, 1852·2
Brethaire, 1852·2
Brethine, 1852·3
Bretilio, Tosilato de, 876·2
Bretylate, 1852·3
Bretylium Tosilate, 876·2
Bretylium Tosylate, 876·2
Bretylol, 1852·3
Breva, 1852·3
Brevafen, 1852·3
Brevex, 1852·3
Brevibloc, 1852·3
Brevicon, 1852·3
Brevilon, 1852·3
Brevimytal, 1852·3
Brevinaze, 1852·3
Brevinor, 1852·3
Brevital, 1852·3
Brevoxyl, 1852·3
Brewers Yeast, 1852·3
Brewers' Yeast, 1469·1
Brewers Yeast with Garlic, 1852·3
Brexecam, 1852·3
Brexicam, 1852·3
Brexic-DT, 1852·3
Brexidol, 1852·3
Brexin, 1852·3
Brexin LA, 1852·3
Brexine, 1852·4
Brexinil, 1852·4
Brexivel, 1852·4
Brexodin, 1852·4
Brexon, 1852·4
Brexonase, 1852·4
Brexotide, 1852·4
Brexovent, 1852·4
Brezal, 1852·4
BRI, 1067·3
Briazide, 1852·4
Bricalin, 1852·4
Bricanyl, 1852·4
Bricanyl Comp, 1852·4
Bricanyl Composto, 1852·4
Bricanyl EX, 1852·4
Bricanyl Expectorant, 1852·4
Bricarex, 1852·4
Bridotrim, 1852·4
Briem, 1852·4
Brier Fruit, 1740·1
Brietal, 1852·4
Briklin, 1852·4
Brilliant Black BN, 1056·2
Brilliant Black PN, 1056·2
Brilliant Blue FCF, 1056·2
Brilliant Green, 1171·1
Brilliant Ponceau 4RC, 1057·3
Brilliant Scarlet, 1057·3
Brimonidina, Tartrato de, 876·3
Brimonidine Tartrate, 876·3
Brimopress, 1852·4
Brinaldix, 1852·4
Brinerdin, 1852·4
Brinerdina, 1852·4
Brinerdine, 1852·4
Brintenal, 1853·1
Brintoverilte, 1853·1
Brinzolamida, 877·1
Brinzolamide, 877·1
Briocor, 1853·1
Briofil, 1853·1
Briogen, 1853·1
Brionil, 1853·1
Brionot, 1853·1
Brioschi, 1853·1
Briovitan, 1853·1
Briovitase, 1853·1
Briscocough, 1853·1
Briscopyn, 1853·1
Briserin N, 1853·1
Brisfirina, 1853·1
Brisfirina Balsamica, 1853·1
Brismucol, 1853·1
Brisomax, 1853·1
Brisoral, 1853·1
Brisovent, 1853·1
Brispen, 1853·1
Bristaciclina, 1853·1
Bristaciclina Dental, 1853·1
Bristacol, 1853·1
Bristaflam, 1853·1
Bristamox, 1853·1
BrisTaxol, 1853·1
Bristopen, 1853·1
Britacil, 1853·1
Britaject, 1853·2
Britamox, 1853·2
Britane, 1853·2
Britapen, 1853·2
Britaxol, 1853·2
British Anti-Lewisite, 1037·1
British Army Foot Powder, 1853·2
British Gum, 1427·1
Britlofex, 1853·2
Brittle Bone Syndrome— *see* Osteogenesis Imperfecta, 762·3
Brivudina, 629·2
Brivudine, 629·2
Brixia, 1853·2
Brixoral, 1853·2
Brizolina, 1853·2
BRL-1241, 230·3
BRL-1341, 157·1
BRL-1621, 198·2
BRL-1702, 205·2
BRL-2039, 213·3
BRL-2064, 166·2
BRL-2288, 270·2
BRL-2333, 155·3
BRL-2333AB-B, 155·3
BRL-3475, 166·3
BRL-4910A, 233·1
BRL-4910F, 233·2
BRL-14151, 193·3
BRL-14151K, 193·3
BRL-14777, 63·3
BRL-17421, 266·1
BRL-24924A, 1287·3
BRL-26921, 863·3
BRL-29060, 311·2
BRL-29060A, 311·2
BRL-34915, 890·3
BRL-38705, 105·2
BRL-39123, 651·2
BRL-39123-D, 651·2
BRL-42810, 633·2
BRL-43694A, 1267·1
BRL-49653-C, 345·2
BRN-5030440, 1731·1
Broad Spectrum Sunblock, 1853·2
Brocide, 1505·1
Brocil, 1853·2
Brocolan, 1853·2
Brodifac, 1853·2
Brodifacoum, 1500·3
Brodifacum, 1500·3
Brodil, 1853·2
Brodimoprim, 165·3
Brodimoprima, 165·3
Brofaromina, 287·2
Brofaromine, 287·2
Brofed, 1853·2
Broflex, 1853·2
Brogal, 1853·2
Brogal Compositum, 1853·2
Brogal-T, 1853·2

Brolamfetamine, 1593·3
Brolamina, 1853·2
Brolene, 1853·2
Brolene Cool Eyes, 1853·2
Brol-eze, 1853·2
Brolin, 1853·2
Broluidan, 1853·2
Bromadine-DM, 1853·2
Bromadiolona, 1501·1
Bromadiolone, 1501·1
Bromalex, 1853·2
Bromalgina, 1853·3
Bromaline, 1853·3
Bromaline Plus, 1853·3
Bromam, 1853·3
Broman, 1853·3
Bromanate, 1853·3
Bromarest DX, 1853·3
Bromatane DX, 1853·3
Bromatanil, 1853·3
Bromatapp, 1853·3
Bromato Potásico, 1734·1
Bromavon, 1853·3
Bromax, 1853·3
Bromaz, 1853·3
Bromazanil, 1853·3
Bromaze, 1853·3
Bromazep, 1853·3
Bromazepam, 671·3
Bromazepamum, 671·3
Bromazepan, 1853·3
Bromazina, Hidrocloruro de, 425·3
Bromazine Hydrochloride, 425·3
Bromazolo, 1853·3
Bromchlophos, 1507·3
Bromchlorophen, 1171·1
Bromchlorophene, 1171·1
Bromed, 1853·3
Bromelaína, 1662·2
Bromelains, 1662·2
Bromelin, 1853·3
Bromelins, 1662·2
Bromergon, 1853·3
Bromesep Elixir, 1853·3
Bromesep Expectorant, 1853·3
Bromex, 1853·3
Bromexidryl, 1853·3
Bromexina, 1115·3
Bromfed, 1853·3
Bromfed-DM, 1853·4
Bromfed-PD, 1853·4
Bromfenac Sodium, 21·3
Bromfenaco Sódico, 21·3
Bromfenex, 1853·4
Bromfeniramina, Maleato de, 426·1
Bromfenofos, 103·3
Bromhexina, 1115·3
Bromhexina, Hidrocloruro de, 1115·3
Bromhexine, 1115·3
Bromhexine Compound, 1853·4
Bromhexine Hydrochloride, 1115·3
Bromhexini Hydrochloridum, 1115·3
Bromhidrato de Escopolamina, 483·3
Bromhidrato de Hidroxianfetamina, 1699·3
Bromhist, 1853·4
Bromhist-DM, 1853·4
Bromhistop, 1853·4
Bromidem, 1853·4
Bromides, 1662·3
Bromidol, 1853·4
Bromidrastina, 1853·4
Bromidrato de Hiosciamina, 485·1
Bromifen, 1853·4
Bromil, 1853·4
Bromi-Lotion, 1853·4
Brominated Salicylanilides, 1171·2
Bromindione, 416·3
Bromine, 1663·1
Bromiramin, 1853·4
Bromism, 1662·3
Bromisoval, 672·1
Bromisovalerylurea, 672·1
Bromisovalum, 672·1
Bromixen, 1853·4
Bromo, 1663·1
Bromo Madelon, 1853·4
Bromo Seltzer, 1853·4
Bromo Seltzer Effervescent Granules, 1853·4
2-(4-Bromobenzhydryloxy)-*NN*-dimethylethylamine Hydrochloride, 425·3
(2-Bromobenzyl)ethyldimethylammonium Toluene-4-sulphonate, 876·2
3-[3-(4′-Bromobiphenyl-4-yl)-3-hydroxy-1-phenylpropyl]-4-hydroxycoumarin, 1501·1
3-[3-(4′-Bromobiphenyl-4-yl)-1,2,3,4-tetrahydro-1-naphthyl]-4-hydroxycoumarin, 1500·3
5-Bromo-*N*-(4-bromophenyl)-2-hydroxybenzamide, 1171·2
Bromocal, 1853·4
Bromocalcio, 1853·4
Bromochlorodifluoromethane, 1235·1
Bromochlorodimethylhydantoin, 1178·2
(±)-*trans*-7-Bromo-6-chloro-3-[3-(3-hydroxy-2-piperidyl)acetonyl]quinazolin-4(3*H*)-one Hydrobromide, 605·3
Bromochlorophane, 1171·1
7-Bromo-5-(2-chlorophenyl)-1,3-dihydro-2*H*-1,4-benzodiazepin-2-one, 715·1
5-Bromo-*N*-(4-chlorophenyl)-2-hydroxybenzamide, 395·2
2-Bromo-4-(2-chlorophenyl)-9-methyl-6*H*-thieno[3,2-*f*][1,2,4]triazolo[4,3-*a*][1,4]diazepine, 672·1
Bromochlorosalicylanilide, 395·2
5-Bromo-4′-chlorosalicylanilide, 395·2
(*RS*)-2-Bromo-2-chloro-1,1,1-trifluoroethane, 1299·3
Bromoclorodifluorometano, 1235·1
Bromoclorofeno, 1171·1
Bromoclorosalicilanilida, 395·2
Bromocod N, 1853·4
Bromocrel, 1853·4
Bromocriptina, Mesilato de, 1200·3
Bromocriptine Mesilate, 1200·3
Bromocriptine Mesylate, 1200·3
Bromocriptine Methanesulphonate, 1200·3
Bromocriptini Mesilas, 1200·3
Bromocryptine Mesylate, 1200·3
5-Bromo-1-(2-deoxy-β-D-ribofuranosyl)pyrimidine-2,4(1*H*,3*H*)-dione, 532·2
Bromodeoxyuridine, 532·2
5-Bromo-2′-deoxyuridine, 532·2
*p*-Bromo-*N*-[(*E*)-({2-[({2-[(diaminomethylene)amino]-4-thiazolyl}methyl)thio]ethyl}amino)methylene]benzenesulfonamide, 1264·3
*O*-4-Bromo-2,5-dichlorophenyl *O*,*O*-Dimethyl Phosphorothioate, 1501·1
Bromodiethylacetylurea, 674·1
7-Bromo-1,3-dihydro-5-(2-pyridyl)-1,4-benzodiazepin-2-one, 671·3
4-Bromo-2,5-dimethoxyamfetamine, 1593·3
Bromodiphenhydramine Hydrochloride, 425·3
Bromo-DMA, 1593·3
Bromodol, 1853·4
Bromo-DOM, 1593·3
2-Bromo-α-ergocryptine Mesylate, 1200·3
2-Bromoergocryptine Monomethanesulfonate, 1200·3
*N*-(2-Bromo-2-ethylbutyryl)urea, 674·1
α-Bromo-β-(4-ethylphenyl)stilbene, 1542·1
Bromofenofos, 103·3
2-Bromo-6-fluoro-*N*-(1-imidazolin-2-yl)aniline, 721·2
10-Bromo-11b-(2-fluorophenyl)-2,3,7,11b-tetrahydrooxazolo[3,2-*d*][1,4]benzodiazepin-6(5*H*)-one, 702·3
Bromofós, 1501·1
1-Bromoheptadecafluorooctane, 1730·1
Bromohexal, 1853·4
(5′*S*)-2-Bromo-12′-hydroxy-2′-(1-methylethyl)-5′-(2-methylpropyl)-ergotaman-3′,6′,18-trione Methanesulphonate, 1200·3
5-Bromo-6-(2-imidazolin-2-ylamino)quinoxaline D-Tartrate, 876·3
Bromo-Kin, 1854·1
Bromolactin, 1854·1
Bromolactobionato de Calcio, 674·1
Bromomethane, 1507·2
4-(7-Bromo-5-methoxy-2-benzofuranyl)piperidine, 287·2
4-Bromo-2,5-methoxyphenylethylamine, 1593·3
2-(4-Bromo-α-methylbenzhydryloxy)-*NN*-dimethylethylamine Hydrochloride, 433·2
*N*-(2-Bromo-3-methylbutyryl)urea, 672·1
7-Bromo-5-methylquinolin-8-ol, 617·1
2-Bromo-2-nitropropane-1,3-diol, 1171·2
Bromopar, 1854·1
Bromophar, 1854·1
Bromophen TD, 1854·1
Bromophenophos, 103·3
(±)-3-(4-Bromophenyl)-*NN*-dimethyl-3-(2-pyridyl)propylamine Hydrogen Maleate, 426·1
4-[4-(*p*-Bromophenyl)-4-hydroxypiperidino]-4′-fluorobutyrophenone, 672·1
5-Bromo-2-phenyl-indan-1,3-dione, 416·3
Bromophos, 1501·1
Bromopirin, 1854·1
Bromoprid, 1854·1
Bromoprida, 1254·1
Bromopride, 1254·1
Bromopride Hydrochloride, 1254·1
Bromosalicilanilidas, 1171·2
Bromosalicylic Acid, 1157·2
Bromosedan, 1854·1
Bromoson, 1854·1
Bromotec, 1854·1
Bromotiren, 1854·1
Bromotuss with Codeine, 1854·1
4-(6-Bromoveratryl)-4-{2-[2-(6,6-dimethyl-2-norpinyl)ethoxy]ethyl}morpholinium Bromide, 1732·1
Bromovinylarauracil, 654·2
(*E*)-5-(2-Bromovinyl)-2′-deoxyuridine, 629·2
Bromoxon, 1854·1
Bromped, 1854·1
Bromperidol, 672·1
Bromperidol Decanoate, 672·1
Bromperidol, Decanoato de, 672·1
Bromperidol Lactate, 672·1
Bromperidoli Decanoas, 672·1
Bromperidolum, 672·1
Bromphen DX Cough, 1854·1
Bromphenex, 1854·1
Brompheniramine Cough, 1854·1
Brompheniramine DC Cough, 1854·1
Brompheniramine Maleate, 426·1
Brompheniramini Maleas, 426·1
Bromphenphos, 103·3
Brom-PP, 1854·1
Brompton Cocktail, 5·2
Brom-Ramine Compound, 1854·1
Bromsalans, 1171·2
Bromselon, 1854·1
Bromso, 1854·1
Bromso-Ex, 1854·1
Bromsulfophthalein Sodium, 1750·3
Bromsulphthalein Sodium, 1750·3
Bromtine, 1854·1
Bromtussia, 1854·1
Bromtussia DC, 1854·2
Bromtussin, 1854·2
Bromuc, 1854·2
Bromum, 1663·1
Bromurex, 1854·2
Bromuro de Bibenzonio, 1115·3
Bromuro de Butropio, 480·1
Bromuro de Cetrimonio, 1173·1
Bromuro de Ciclonio, 480·2
Bromuro de Cimetropio, 480·2
Bromuro de Clidinio, 480·2
Bromuro de Demecario, 1488·3
Bromuro de Distigmina, 1489·2
Bromuro de Domifeno, 1179·1
Bromuro de Emepronio, 482·1
Bromuro de Fenpiverinio, 1688·1
Bromuro de Fentonio, 482·2
Bromuro de Flutropio, 482·3
Bromuro de Glicopirronio, 482·3
Bromuro de Ipratropio, 787·1
Bromuro de Mepenzolato, 485·3
Bromuro de Metantelinio, 485·3
Bromuro de Metilbenacticio, 485·3
Bromuro de Metilo, 1507·2
Bromuro de Neostigmina, 1492·2
Bromuro de Otilonio, 1725·1
Bromuro de Oxifenonio, 487·2
Bromuro de Oxitropio, 790·3
Bromuro de Pancuronio, 1404·3
Bromuro de Pinaverio, 1732·1
Bromuro de Pipecuronio, 1405·2
Bromuro de Pipenzolato, 487·3
Bromuro de Piridostigmina, 1496·1
Bromuro de Prifinio, 488·2
Bromuro de Propantelina, 489·1
Bromuro de Rapacuronio, 1405·2
Bromuro de Rocuronio, 1405·2
Bromuro de Timepidio, 489·3
Bromuro de Tiotropio, 806·2
Bromuro de Tiquizio, 1757·1
Bromuro de Tonzonio, 1757·2
Bromuro de Vecuronio, 1409·3
Bromuro de Xenitropio, 491·3
Bromuros, 1662·3
Bromvalerylurea, 672·1
Bromvaletone, 672·1
Bromxin, 1854·2
Bromxine, 1854·2
Bromylum, 672·1
Bron 6, 1854·2
Bronalide, 1854·2
Bronalin Decongestant, 1854·2
Bronalin Dry Cough, 1854·2
Bronalin Expectorant, 1854·2
Bronalin Junior, 1854·2
Broncal, 1854·2
Broncalene, 1854·2
Broncalene Nourisson, 1854·2
Broncard, 1854·2
Broncasma, 1854·2
Broncasmin Composto, 1854·2
Broncatar, 1854·2
Broncelix, 1854·2
Bronch Eze, 1854·2
Bronchalene, 1854·3
Bronchalin, 1854·3
Bronchalis-Heel, 1854·3
Bronchathiol, 1854·3
Bronchenolo, 1854·3
Bronchenolo Antiflu, 1854·3
Bronchette, 1854·3
Bronchex, 1854·3
Bronchial, 1854·3
Bronchial Balsam, Jacksons— *see* Jackson's Bronchial Balsam, 2070·2
Bronchial Cough, 1854·3
Bronchial Mixture, 1854·3
Bronchialbalsam, 1854·3
Bronchialtee N, 1854·3
Bronchiase, 1854·3
Bronchicough, 1854·3
Bronchicum Preparations, 1854·3
Bronchi-Do, 1854·4
Bronchiflu, 1854·4
Bronchil, 1854·4
Bronchilet, 1854·4
Bronchilin, 1854·4
Bronchilon, 1854·4
Bronchiolitis Obliterans Organising Pneumonia— *see* Diffuse Parenchymal Lung Disease, 1079·3
Bronchi-Pertu, 1854·4
Bronchiplant, 1854·4
Bronchiplant Light, 1854·4
Bronchipret, 1854·4
Bronchisaft, 1854·4
Bronchisan, 1854·4
Bronchiselect, 1854·4
Bronchithym, 1854·4
Bronchitis, 122·2
Bronchitis— *see* Chronic Obstructive Pulmonary Disease, 779·2
Bronchitten, 1854·4
Bronchitten Forte K, 1854·4
Broncho D, 1854·4
Broncho Fertiginhalat, 1854·4
Broncho Inhalat, 1854·4
Broncho Munal, 1854·4
Broncho Rub, 1855·1

Broncho Saline, 1855·1
Bronchobactan, 1855·1
Bronchobel, 1855·1
Bronchobest, 1855·1
Bronchocal, 1855·1
Bronchocedin N, 1855·1
Bronchocort, 1855·1
Bronchocux, 1855·1
Bronchocyst, 1855·1
Bronchodermine, 1855·1
Bronchodex D, 1855·1
Bronchodex DM, 1855·1
Bronchodex Pastilles, 1855·1
Bronchodex Pastilles Antiseptiques, 1855·1
Bronchodex Pediatrique, 1855·1
Bronchodex Vapo, 1855·1
Bronchodil, 1855·1
Bronchodilators and Anti-asthma Drugs, 777·1
Bronchodine, 1855·1
Bronchodual, 1855·1
Bronchodurat Eucalyptusol, 1855·1
Bronchodurat N, 1855·1
Broncho-Euphyllin, 1855·1
Broncho-Fips, 1855·1
Bronchofluid, 1855·1
Bronchofluid N, 1855·1
Bronchoforton, 1855·2
Bronchoforton Kinderbalsam, 1855·2
Bronchoforton-Solinat, 1855·2
Broncho-Grippol-DM, 1855·2
Bronchohexal, 1855·2
Broncho-Kid, 1855·2
Bronchokod, 1855·2
Bronchol, 1855·2
Bronchol N, 1855·2
Broncholate, 1855·2
Broncholate Forte, 1855·2
Broncholate Plus, 1855·2
Broncholine, 1855·2
Bronchomed, 1855·2
Bronchopan DM, 1855·2
Bronchoparat, 1855·2
Broncho-pectoralis, 1855·2
Bronchoped, 1855·2
Bronchophylline, 1855·2
Bronchoplus, 1855·2
Bronchoprex, 1855·2
Bronchoprex Expectorant, 1855·3
Bronchopront, 1855·3
Bronchopulmonary Dysplasia, 1077·2
Bronchorectine au Citral, 1855·3
Bronchoretard, 1855·3
Broncho-Rivo, 1855·3
Bronchosan, 1855·3
Bronchosan Nouvelle Formule, 1855·3
Bronchosedal, 1855·3
Broncho-Sern, 1855·3
Bronchosirum, 1855·3
Bronchosolvin, 1855·3
Bronchospasmin, 1855·3
Bronchospasmine, 1855·3
Bronchospect, 1855·3
Bronchospray, 1855·3
Bronchostad Hustenloser, 1855·3
Bronchostop, 1855·3
Bronchostop Sine, 1855·3
Bronchosyl, 1855·3
Bronchosyx N, 1855·3
Broncho-Tulisan Eucalyptol, 1855·4
Bronchotussine, 1855·4
Broncho-Tyrosolvetten, 1855·4
Broncho-Vaxom, 1855·4
Bronchowern, 1855·4
Bronchozone, 1855·4
Bronchyteine, 1855·4
Bronchytuc, 1855·4
Broncimucil, 1855·4
Broncivent, 1855·4
Bronclear, 1855·4
Broncleer, 1855·4
Broncleer with Codeine, 1855·4
Broncmel, 1855·4
Bronco Aseptilex, 1855·4
Bronco Aseptilex Fuerte, 1855·4
Bronco Asmo, 1855·4
Bronco Asmol, 1855·4
Bronco Bactifor, 1855·4
Bronco Biotaer, 1855·4
Bronco Cilimox, 1855·4
Bronco Etersan, 1855·4
Bronco Lizom, 1855·4
Bronco Medical, 1855·4
Bronco Pensusan, 1855·4
Bronco Sergo, 1856·1
Bronco Tonic, 1856·1
Bronco-Amoxil, 1856·1
Broncocalmine, 1856·1
Broncoclar, 1856·1
Broncodeina, 1856·1
Bronco-Dex, 1856·1
Broncodiazina, 1856·1
Broncodil, 1856·1
Broncodual, 1856·1
Broncodual Compuesto, 1856·1
Broncofenil, 1856·1
Broncofisin, 1856·1
Broncofluid, 1856·1
Broncoflux, 1856·1
Broncoformo Muco Dexa, 1856·1
Broncokin, 1856·1
Broncol, 1856·1
Broncolex, 1856·1
Broncoliber, 1856·1
Broncolin, 1856·1
Broncomed, 1856·1
Broncomega, 1856·2
Broncomicin Bals, 1856·2
Broncomnes, 1856·2
Broncomucil, 1856·2
Bronconait, 1856·2
Bronconovag, 1856·2
Bronco-Ped, 1856·2
Broncopinol, 1856·2
Broncoplus, 1856·2
Bronco-Polimoxil, 1856·2
Broncopul, Natusor— *see* Natusor Broncopul, 2153·4
Broncopulmin, 1856·2
Broncopulmo, 1856·2
Broncoral, 1856·2
Broncorema, 1856·2
Broncorinol Etats Grippaux, 1856·2
Broncorinol Expectorant, 1856·2
Broncorinol Maux de Gorge, 1856·2
Broncorinol Rhinites, 1856·2
Broncorinol Rhume, 1856·2
Bug Proof, 1858·4
Bugazon, 1858·4
Bugbane, 1671·3
Bugesic, 1858·4
Bugrane, Racine de, 1723·3
Bugs Bunny, 1858·4
Bulbo de Escila, 1130·3
Bulboid, 1858·4
Bulboshap, 1858·4
Bulgarolax, 1858·4
Bulk, 1858·4
Bulk Laxatives, 1239·3
Bulk-forming Laxatives, 1239·3
Bulking Agents, 1239·3
Bullfrog, 1858·4
Bullfrog for Kids, 1858·4
Bullfrog Sport, 1858·4
Bullous Pemphigoid— *see* Pemphigus and Pemphigoid, 1137·1
Bullrich Salz, 1858·4
Bumadizona Cálcica, 21·3
Bumadizone Calcium, 21·3
Bumaflex N, 1858·4
Bumed, 1858·4
Bumedyl, 1858·4
Bumetanida, 877·2
Bumetanide, 877·2
Bumetanidum, 877·2
Bumex, 1858·4
Buminate, 1858·4
Bumps and Bruises, 1859·1
Bumps 'N Falls, 1859·1
Bunafon, 1859·1
Bunazosin Hydrochloride, 878·1
Bunazosina, Hidrocloruro de, 878·1
Bunil, 1859·1
Bunion Salve, 1859·1
Bunitrolol, Hidrocloruro de, 878·1
Bunitrolol Hydrochloride, 878·1
*l*-Bunolol Hydrochloride, 946·2
(−)-Bunolol Hydrochloride, 946·2
BUP-4, 489·1
Bupafen, 1859·1
Bupap, 1859·1
Buparvacuona, 603·1
Buparvaquone, 603·1
Buphenine Hydrochloride, 1663·2
Buphenyl, 1859·1
Bupiabbott, 1859·1
Bupiabbott Plus, 1859·1
Bupibil, 1859·1
Bupicain, 1859·1
Bupicaina, 1859·1
Bupiforan, 1859·1
Bupinex, 1859·1
Bupinostrum Adrenalina, 1859·1
Bupisen, 1859·1
Bupisolver, 1859·1
Bupivacaína, Hidrocloruro de, 1371·1
*S*(−)-Bupivacaine, 1377·1
Bupivacaine, Carbonated, 1369·2, 1372·1
Bupivacaine Hydrochloride, 1371·1
Bupivacaini Hydrochloridum, 1371·1
Bupixamol, 1859·1
Bupogesic, 1859·1
Bupranolol, Hidrocloruro de, 878·1
Bupranolol Hydrochloride, 878·1
Buprenex, 1859·1
Buprenorfina, 21·3
Buprenorfina, Hidrocloruro de, 21·3
Buprenorphine, 21·3
Buprenorphine Hydrochloride, 21·3
Buprenorphini Hydrochloridum, 21·3
Buprenorphinum, 21·3
Buprex, 1859·1
Buprine, 1859·1
Bupropión, Hidrocloruro de, 287·2
Bupropion Hydrochloride, 287·2
Bupyl, 1859·1
Buram, 1859·1
Burana, 1859·2
Burana-C, 1859·2
Buraton 10 F, 1859·2
Burdeos B, 1056·2
Burdock, 1704·3
Burdock Root, 1704·3
Burgerstein Geriatrikum, 1859·2
Burgerstein S, 1859·2
Burgerstein TopVital, 1859·2
Burgodin, 1859·2
Burinax, 1859·2
Burinex, 1859·2
Burinex A, 1859·2
Burinex K, 1859·2
Burinex med Kaliumklorid, 1859·2
Burkitt Cell Leukaemia— *see* Acute Lymphoblastic Leukaemia, 506·1
Burkitt's Lymphoma, 511·1
Burmicin, 1859·2
Burn Cream, 1859·2
Burn Healing Cream, 1859·2
Burnaid, 1859·2
Burnaid First Aid Burn Gel, 1859·2
Burn-A-Sept, 1859·2
Burnet, 1663·2
Burneze, 1859·2
Burnocaine, 1859·2
Burnol Plus, 1859·2
Burns, 1134·2
Burns Cream, 1859·2
Burns, Eye, 1461·1
Burns, Eye— *see* Eye Disorders, 1224·2
Burns, Infections in— *see* Skin Infections, 146·2
Burnshield Gel, 1859·2
Burnt Sugar, 1056·3
Buro Derm, 1859·2
Buronil, 1859·2
Buro-Sol, 1859·2
Burow's, 1859·2
Burow's Preparations, 1653·1
Burro Di Cacao, 1482·3
Bursitis— *see* Soft-tissue Rheumatism, 11·1
Burten, 1859·2
Buruli Ulcer— *see* Opportunistic Mycobacterial Infections, 137·2
Busala, 1859·3
Busansil, 1859·3
Buscalm, 1859·3
Buscalma, 1859·3
Buscapina, 1859·3
Buscapina Compositum, 1859·3
Buscapina Compositum N, 1859·3
Buscofen, 1859·3
Buscolysin, 1859·3
Busconet, 1859·3
Buscono, 1859·3
Buscopamol, 1859·3
Buscopan, 1859·3
Buscopan Compositum, 1859·3
Buscopan Compositum N, 1859·3
Buscopan Composto, 1859·3
Buscopan Plus, 1859·3
Buscoveran Composto, 1859·3
Busepan, 1859·3
Buserelin, 1319·2
Buserelin Acetate, 1319·2
Buserelina, Acetato de, 1319·2
Buserelinum, 1319·2
Bush Formula, 1859·3
Bushi, 1859·3
Busidril, 1859·3
Busilvex, 1859·3
Busina, 1859·3
Businessman's Trip, 1680·3
Busonid, 1859·3
Busopin, 1859·4
Busp, 1859·4
Buspanil, 1859·4
Buspar, 1859·4
Buspimen, 1859·4
Buspirex, 1859·4
Buspirol, 1859·4
Buspirona, Hidrocloruro de, 672·2
Buspirone Hydrochloride, 672·2
Buspisal, 1859·4
Buspril, 1859·4
Busprina, 1859·4
Busprina-S, 1859·4
Busserole, 1659·2
Bussulfam, 532·2
Bustab, 1859·4
Bustrix, 1859·4
Busulfan, 532·2
Busulfano, 532·2
Busulfanum, 532·2
Busulfex, 1859·4
Busulphan, 532·2
Buta, 1859·4
Buta Pee Dee, 1859·4
Buta Rut B12, 1859·4
Butabarbital, 721·2
Butabarbital Sodium, 721·2
Butabarbitone, 721·2
Butacain. Sulph., 1372·3
Butacaína, Sulfato de, 1372·3
Butacaine Sulfate, 1372·3
Butacaine Sulphate, 1372·3
Butacort, 1859·4
Butacortelone, 1859·4
Butacote, 1859·4
Butadion, 1859·4
Butadione, 83·2
Butafen, 1859·4
Butafosfan, 1231·3
Butahale, 1859·4
Butalamina, Hidrocloruro de, 878·2
Butalamine Hydrochloride, 878·2
Butalbital, 673·3
Butalen, 1859·4
Butalin, 1859·4
Butaline, 1859·4
Butaliret, 1859·4
Butalitab, 1859·4
Butamben, 1373·1
Butamben Picrate, 1373·1

Butamidum, 348·1
Butamine, 1860·1
Butamir, 1860·1
Butamirate Citrate, 1116·2
Butamirato, Citrato de, 1116·2
Butamol, 1860·1
Butamyrate Citrate, 1116·2
Butane, 1235·1
*n*-Butane, 1235·1
1,4-Butanediol, 1308·3
Butane-1,4-diol Di(methanesulphonate), 532·2
Butane-1,2,3,4-tetrol Tetranitrate, 913·1
Butanil, 1860·1
Butanimide, 1750·2
Butano, 1235·1
*n*-Butanol, 1472·1
Butan-1-ol, 1472·1
Butan-2-one, 1476·2
Butaparin, 1860·1
Butapirin, 1860·1
Buta-Proxyvon, 1860·1
Butarion, 1860·1
Butartrol, 1860·1
Butasona, 1860·1
Butasona RL, 1860·1
Butavate, 1860·1
Butayonacol, 1860·1
Butazil, 1860·1
Butazolidin, 1860·1
Butazolidina, 1860·1
Butazolidine, 1860·1
Butazolon, 1860·1
Butazona, 1860·1
Butazone, 1860·1
Butazonil, 1860·1
Butcher's Broom, 1741·1
Butenafina, Hidrocloruro de, 395·2
Butenafine Hydrochloride, 395·2
*cis*-Butenedioic Acid, 1709·2
*trans*-Butenedioic Acid, 1147·3
Buteridol, 1860·1
Butesin Picrate, 1860·1
Butetamate Citrate, 1116·2
Butetamato, Citrato de, 1116·2
Butethal, 673·3
Butethamate Citrate, 1116·2
Butethamate Dihydrogen Citrate, 1116·2
Butetisalicilato de Metilo, 59·2
Butex, 1860·2
Buthiazide, 878·2
Butibel, 1860·2
Butibufén Sódico, 23·3
Butibufen Sodium, 23·3
Buticina, 1860·2
Buticrem, 1860·2
Butidiona, 1860·2
Butil Éster de la Fluocortina, 1102·1
Butilamin, 1860·2
Butilamina, 1472·1
Butilaminobenzoato, 1373·1
Butilaminobenzoato, Picrato de, 1373·1
Butilhidroquinona Terciaria, 1193·3
Butilhidroxianisol, 1171·2
Butilhidroxitolueno, 1171·3
Butilidrossianisolo, 1171·2
Butilparabeno, 1183·2
Butilparabeno Sódico, 1183·3
Butimerin, 1860·2
Butin, 1860·2
Butinat, 1860·2
Butinolina, Fosfato de, 1663·3
Butinoline Phosphate, 1663·3
Butiral, 1860·2
Butiran, 1860·2
Butirato de Clobetasona, 1095·3
Butirato de Hidrocortisona, 1104·1
Butisol, 1860·2
Buti-Spirobene, 1860·2
Butix, 1860·2
Butizida, 878·2
Butizide, 878·2
Buto Asma, 1860·2
Butobarbital, 673·3
Butobarbitalum, 673·3
Butobarbitone, 673·3
Butoconazol, Nitrato de, 395·2
Butoconazole Nitrate, 395·2
Butoforme, 1373·1
Butohaler, 1860·2
Buton, 1860·2
Butopiroxinilo, 1501·1
Butopyronoxyl, 1501·1
Butorfanol, Tartrato de, 23·3
Butorphanol Tartrate, 23·3
Butosali, 1860·2
Butosol, 1860·2
Butotal, 1860·2
Butotal B, 1860·2
Butovent, 1860·2
Butoxicaína, Hidrocloruro de, 1373·1
Butóxido de Piperonilo, 1509·2
(−)-(1*R*,3*r*,5*S*)-8-(4-Butoxybenzyl)-3-[(*S*)-tropoyloxy]tropanium Bromide, 480·1
Butoxycaine Hydrochloride, 1373·1
Butoxycaini Hydrochloridum, 1373·1
1-(3-Butoxy-2-carbamoyloxypropyl)-5-ethyl-5-phenylbarbituric Acid, 698·2
2-Butoxy-*N*-(2-diethylaminoethyl)cinchoninamide, 1373·2
2-Butoxy-*N*-(2-diethylaminoethyl)quinoline-4-carboxamide, 1373·2
5-[2-(2-Butoxyethoxy)ethoxymethyl]-6-propyl-1,3-benzodioxole, 1509·2
Butoxyethyl Nicotinate, 66·3
2-Butoxyethyl Nicotinate, 66·3
1-Butoxy-3-phenoxy-2-propanol, 1687·1
4-[3-(4-Butoxyphenoxy)propyl]morpholine Hydrochloride, 1382·2
2-(4-Butoxyphenyl)acetohydroxamic Acid, 21·3
4′-Butoxy-3-piperidinopropiophenone Hydrochloride, 1376·2
Butriptilina, Hidrocloruro de, 289·1
Butriptyline Hydrochloride, 289·1
Butropio, Bromuro de, 480·1
Butropium Bromide, 480·1
Butterbur, 1663·3
Buttercup Infant Cough Syrup, 1860·2
Buttercup Lozenges, 1860·2
Buttercup Pol'N'Count, 1860·2
Buttercup Syrup, 1860·2
Buttercup Syrup (Blackcurrant Flavour), 1860·2
Buttercup Syrup (Honey and Lemon Flavour), 1860·3
Butterfly Weed, 1733·1
Butt-Out, 1860·3
Butyl, 1860·3
Butyl Acetate, 1472·1
*n*-Butyl Acetate, 1472·1
*tert*-Butyl {(1*S*,2*S*)-2-[(2*S*,5*R*,7*S*,10*R*,13*S*)-4-Acetoxy-2-benzoyloxy-1,7,10-trihydroxy-9-oxo-5,20-epoxytax-11-en-13-yloxycarbonyl]-2-hydroxy-1-phenylethyl}carbamate, 547·1
Butyl Alcohol, 1472·1
*n*-Butyl Alcohol, 1472·1
Butyl Aminobenzoate, 1373·1
Butyl 4-Aminobenzoate, 1373·1
Butyl Aminobenzoate Picrate, 1373·1
Butyl 2-Cyanoacrylate, 1678·1
Butyl 3,4-Dihydro-2,2-dimethyl-4-oxo-2*H*-pyran-6-carboxylate, 1501·1
Butyl 6α-Fluoro-11β-hydroxy-16α-methyl-3,20-dioxopregna-1,4-dien-21-oate, 1102·1
Butyl Hydroxybenzoate, 1183·2
Butyl 4-Hydroxybenzoate, 1183·2
Butyl Hydroxybenzoate, Sodium, 1183·3
Butyl Nitrite, 1663·3
Butyl Parahydroxybenzoate, 1183·2
Butyl Parahydroxybenzoate, Sodium, 1183·3
Butyl Phthalate, 1503·1
Butylamine, 1472·1
*n*-Butylamine, 1472·1
2-*tert*-Butylamino-1-*o*-chlorophenylethanol Hydrochloride, 806·3
(±)-2-(*tert*-Butylamino)-3′-chloropropiophenone Hydrochloride, 287·2
1-*tert*-Butylamino-3-(6-chloro-*m*-tolyloxy)propan-2-ol Hydrochloride, 878·1
(*S*)-1-*tert*-Butylamino-3-(2-cyclopentylphenoxy)propan-2-ol Hemisulfate, 979·1
2-*tert*-Butylamino-1-(3,5-dihydroxyphenyl)ethanol Sulphate, 797·2
(*RS*)-5-(2-*tert*-Butylamino-1-hydroxyethyl)-*m*-phenylene Bis(dimethylcarbamate) Hydrochloride, 781·2
4-[2-(*tert*-Butylamino)-1-hydroxyethyl]-*o*-phenylene Di-*p*-toluate Methanesulphonate, 781·3
2-*tert*-Butylamino-1-(4-hydroxy-3-hydroxymethylphenyl)ethanol, 791·3
2-*tert*-Butylamino-1-(5-hydroxy-6-hydroxymethyl-2-pyridyl)ethanol Acetate, 790·3
2-*tert*-Butylamino-1-(5-hydroxy-6-hydroxymethyl-2-pyridyl)ethanol Dihydrochloride, 790·3
2-Butylamino-1-(4-hydroxyphenyl)ethanol Sulfate, 866·3
2-(3-*tert*-Butylamino-2-hydroxypropoxy)benzonitrile Hydrochloride, 878·1
5-(3-*tert*-Butylamino-2-hydroxypropoxy)-3,4-dihydroquinolin-2(1*H*)-one Hydrochloride, 880·3
(±)-1-{*p*-[3-(*tert*-Butylamino)-2-hydroxypropoxy]phenyl}-3-cyclohexylurea, 1009·2
(2*R*,3*S*)-5-(3-*tert*-Butylamino-2-hydroxypropoxy)-1,2,3,4-tetrahydronaphthalene-2,3-diol, 963·1
(−)-5-(3-*tert*-Butylamino-2-hydroxypropoxy)-1,2,3,4-tetrahydronaphthalen-1-one Hydrochloride, 946·2
(±)-5-[2-{[3-(*tert*-Butylamino)-2-hydroxypropyl]thio}-4-thiazolyl]-2-thiophenecarboxamide Hydrochloride, 865·1
1-Butylamino-1-methylethylphosphinic Acid, 1231·3
(*R*)-$\alpha^1$-[(*tert*-Butylamino)methyl]-4-hydroxy-*m*-xylene-α,α′-diol Hydrochloride, 788·2
(±)-1-(*tert*-Butylamino)-3-[(2-methylindol-4-yl)oxy]propan-2-ol Benzoate Malonate, 875·3
(*S*)-1-*tert*-Butylamino-3-(4-morpholino-1,2,5-thiadiazol-3-yloxy)propan-2-ol Maleate, 1012·2
3-Butylamino-4-phenoxy-5-sulphamoylbenzoic Acid, 877·2
(±)-1-(*tert*-Butylamino)-3-(thiochroman-8-yloxy)propan-2-ol Hydrochloride, 1011·1
Butylated Hydroxyanisole, 1171·2
Butylated Hydroxytoluene, 1171·3
2-Butylbenzofuran-3-yl 4-(2-Diethylaminoethoxy)-3,5-di-iodophenyl Ketone, 859·2
α-Butylbenzyl Alcohol, 1687·2
(*RS*)1-(4-*tert*-Butylbenzyl)-4-(4-chlorobenzhydryl)piperazine Dihydrochloride, 426·3
*N*-(*p*-*tert*-Butylbenzyl)-*N*-methyl-1-naphthalenemethylamine Hydrochloride, 395·2
4-*tert*-Butylbenzyl(methyl)(1-naphthalenemethyl)amine Hydrochloride, 395·2
1-Butylbiguanide, 330·3
(*S*)-*N*-[(α*S*)-α-{(1*R*)-2-[(3*S*,4a*S*,8a*S*)-3-(*tert*-Butylcarbamoyl)octahydro-2(1*H*)-isoquinolyl]-1-hydroxyethyl}phenethyl]-2-quinaldamidosuccinamide, 653·3
(*E*)-2-Butyl-1-(*p*-carboxybenzyl)-α-2-thenylimidazole-5-acrylic Acid Methanesulfonate, 912·1
*N*-Butyl-4-chloro-2-hydroxybenzamide, 395·2
4-*tert*-Butyl-2-chloro-mercuriphenol, 1185·3
*N*-Butyl-4-chlorosalicylamide, 395·2
2-Butyl-4-chloro-1-[*p*-(*o*-1*H*-tetrazol-5-ylphenyl)benzyl]imidazole-5-methanol Potassium, 947·2
*trans*-2-(4-*tert*-Butylcyclohexylmethyl)-3-hydroxy-1,4-naphthoquinone, 603·1
(3*S*,4a*S*,8a*S*)-*N*-*tert*-Butyldecahydro-2-[(2*R*,3*R*)-3-(3-hydroxy-*o*-toluamido)-2-hydroxy-4-(phenylthio)butyl]isoquinoline-3-carboxamide Monomethanesulphonate, 650·1
Butyldeoxynojirimycin, 1715·2
*n*-Butyl-deoxynojirimycin, 1715·2
(±)-2-*sec*-Butyl-4-[4-(4-{4-[(2$R^*$,4$S^*$)-2-(2,4-dichlorophenyl)-2-(1*H*-1,2,4-triazol-1-ylmethyl)-1,3-dioxolan-4-ylmethoxy]phenyl}-piperazin-1-yl)phenyl]-2,4-dihydro-1,2,4-triazol-3-one, 401·3
2-*sec*-Butyl-4-[4-(4-{4-[(2*RS*,4*SR*)-2-(2,4-difluorophenyl)-2-(1*H*-1,2,4-triazol-1-ylmethyl)-1,3-dioxolan-4-ylmethoxy]phenyl}piperazin-1-yl)phenyl]-2,4-dihydro-1,2,4-triazol-3-one, 408·1
2-(4-*tert*-Butyl-2,6-dimethylbenzyl)-2-imidazoline Hydrochloride, 1132·2
4′-*tert*-Butyl-4-[4-(diphenylmethoxy)piperidino]butyrophenone, 433·1
1-*tert*-Butyl-4,4-diphenylpiperidine, 1203·3
4-Butyl-1,2-diphenylpyrazolidine-3,5-dione, 83·2
5-Butyl-5-ethylbarbituric Acid, 673·3
5-*sec*-Butyl-5-ethylbarbituric Acid, 721·2
2-*tert*-Butylhydroquinone, 1193·3
Butylhydroquinone, Tertiary, 1193·3
Butylhydroxitoluenum, 1171·3
Butylhydroxyanisole, 1171·2
Butylhydroxyanisolum, 1171·2
*p*-*tert*-Butyl-*N*-[6-(2-hydroxyethoxy)-5-(*o*-methoxyphenoxy)-2-(2-pyrimidinyl)-4-pyrimidinyl]benzenesulfonamide, 875·3
4-Butyl-4-hydroxymethyl-1,2-diphenylpyrazolidine-3,5-dione Hydrogen Succinate (Ester), 93·1
(2*R*,3*R*,4*R*,5*S*)-1-Butyl-2-(hydroxymethyl)piperidine-3,4,5-triol, 1715·2
4-Butyl-1-(4-hydroxyphenyl)-2-phenylpyrazolidine-3,5-dione Monohydrate, 76·1
Butylhydroxytoluene, 1171·3
16α,17α-Butylidenedioxy-11β,21-dihydroxypregna-1,4-diene-3,20-dione, 1094·2
1,5-(Butylimino)-1,5-dideoxy-D-glucitol, 1715·2
Butylin, 1860·3
Butylis Parahydroxybenzoas, 1183·2
Butylis Paraoxybenzoas, 1183·2
2-(3-Butyl-1-isoquinolyloxy)-*NN*-dimethylethylamine Hydrochloride, 1384·2
Butylmethoxydibenzoylmethane, 1142·3
4-*tert*-Butyl-4′-methoxydibenzoylmethane, 1142·3
2-*tert*-Butyl-4-methoxyphenol, 1171·2
2-*sec*-Butyl-2-methyltrimethylene Dicarbamate, 951·2
*N*-*tert*-Butyl-3-oxo-4-aza-5α-androst-1-ene-17β-carboxamide, 1554·2
*tert*-Butyloxycarbonyl-[β-Ala$^{13}$]gastrin-(13-17)-pentapeptide Amide, 1729·3
Butylparaben, 1183·2
Butylparaben Sodium, 1183·3
1-(4-*tert*-Butylphenyl)-4-[4-(α-hydroxybenzhydryl)piperidino]butan-1-ol, 441·1
(±)-*p*-[4-(*p*-*tert*-Butylphenyl)-2-hydroxybutoxy]benzoic Acid, 946·3
1-(*p*-*tert*-Butylphenyl)-3-(*p*-methoxyphenyl)-1,3-propanedione, 1142·3
4-Butyl-1-phenylpyrazolidine-3,5-dione, 60·1
(*S*)-1-Butyl-2-piperidylformo-2′,6′-xylidide, 1377·1
(±)-(1-Butyl-2-piperidyl)formo-2′,6′-xylidide Hydrochloride Monohydrate, 1371·1
Butylscopolamine Bromide, 483·3
*N*-Butylscopolammonium Bromide, 483·3
Butylscopolamonii Bromidum, 483·3
(6-*O*-*tert*-Butyl-D-serine)-des-10-glycinamidegonadorelin Ethylamide, 1319·2
(α*S*)-α-[(α*S*)-α-[(*tert*-Butylsulfonyl)methyl]hydrocinnamamido]-*N*-[(1*S*,2*R*,3*S*)-1-(cyclohexylmethyl)-3-cyclopropyl-2,3-dihydroxypropyl]imidazole-4-propionamide, 994·3
*N*-(Butylsulfonyl)-4-[4-(4-piperidyl)butoxy]-L-phenylalanine Hydrochloride Monohydrate, 1013·3
1-Butyl-3-sulphanilylurea, 330·3
2-Butyl-3-[*p*-(*o*-1*H*-tetrazol-5-ylphenyl)benzyl]-1,3-diazaspiro[4.4]non-1-en-4-one, 940·1
*N*-(5-*tert*-Butyl-1,3,4-thiadiazol-2-yl)benzenesulphonamide, 333·1
2-(4-Butylthiobenzhydrylthio)ethyldimethylamine Hydrochloride, 674·1
1-Butyl-3-*p*-tolylsulphonylurea, 348·1
1-Butyl-3-tosylurea, 348·1

(2*R*,4a*R*,5a*R*,6*S*,7*S*,8*R*,9*S*,9a*R*,10a*S*)-2-Butyl-4a,7,9-trihydroxy-6,8-bis(methylamino)perhydropyrano[2,3-*b*][1,4]benzodioxin-4-one Sulphate Pentahydrate, 274·2
1-Butyric Acid-7-(L-2-aminobutyric Acid)-26-L-aspartic Acid-27-L-valine-29-L-alaninecalcitonin (Salmon), 768·3
1-Butyric Acid-2-[3-(*p*-methoxyphenyl)-L-alanine]oxytocin, 1320·2
γ-Butyrobetaine, 1424·1
*Butyrospermum parkii*, 1482·1
Butyrum Cacao, 1482·3
Butyvinal, 727·2
Buvacaina, 1860·3
Buventol, 1860·3
Buxamin, 353·2
Buxon, 1860·3
Buzepida, Metioduro de, 480·2
Buzepide Metiodide, 480·2
Buzpel, 1860·3
BV-araU, 654·2
B-Vasc, 1860·3
BVAU, 654·2
BVDU, 629·2
B-Vesil, 1860·3
BVK Roche Plus C, 1860·3
BW-49-210, 603·2
BW-50-63, 458·1
BW-56-72, 272·2
BW-56-158, 412·2
BW-323, 287·2
BW-759, 635·3
BW-57322, 1349·1
BW-33A, 1399·1
BW-A566C, 601·3
BW-A509U, 658·2
BW-A770U, 540·2
BW-A938U, 1403·1
BWB-759U, 635·3
BW-B1090U, 1403·3
BW-430C, 363·3
BW-467-C-60, 872·3
BW-546C88, 1752·1
BW-566C, 601·3
BW-566C80, 601·3
BW-589C, 1759·3
BW-720C, 603·1
BW-825C, 423·3
BW-72U, 272·2
BW-248U, 626·1
BW-301U, 580·1
BW-509U, 658·2
BW-759U, 635·3
BW-51W, 1399·1
BW-51W89, 1399·1
BW-524W91, 632·3
1BX, 277·3
BX-661A, 1251·2
BY-217, 791·3
BY-1023, 1283·1
Byclomine, 1860·3
Bye Bye Bite, 1860·3
Bye Bye Burn, 1860·3
BYK-20869, 791·3
Bykomycin, 1860·3
Byl, 1860·3
By-Madol, 1860·3
Bymeniere, 1860·3
By-Mycin, 1860·3
Byodin, 1860·3
Byodinoral, 1860·3
By-Vertin, 1860·3
BZ-55, 330·3

## C

C, 1373·3, 1426·3
C1, 550·2
4-C-32, 1011·2
C-20, 1860·3
53-32C, 1011·2
C061, 1725·1
C68-22, 912·2
C-78, 806·3
C-84-04, 1755·1
C-86, 1860·3
183C91, 473·3
C-225, 536·1
C-238, 1395·2
311C90, 473·3
C500, 1860·3
546C88, 1752·1
566C, 601·3
566C80, 601·3
589C, 1759·3
589C80, 1759·3
776C85, 550·2
C-1000, 1860·3
C-1000-C, 1873·3
C-3000, 1860·3
C-5581H, 439·1
C-5720, 25·1
C Calcio, 1860·3
C2 with Codeine, 1860·3
$C_1$ Esterase Inhibitor, 1675·2
C1 Esterase Inhibitor, Complement, 1675·2
C Factors "1000" Plus, 1860·4
C Forte, 1860·4
C1 Inattivatore Umano, 1860·4
C Mon, 1860·4
C Monovit, 1860·4
C Pal, 1860·4
C Plus E Natural, 1860·4
C Rose Hips, 1860·4
C Supa + Bioflavonoids, 1860·4
CA2, 50·1
Ca-1022, 330·3
Ca Lac, 1860·4
Caa-40, 1702·2
Caapi, 1696·3
Caas, 1860·4
CAB-2001, 1160·3
C-50005/A-Ba, 986·3
Cabal, 1860·4
Cabaser, 1860·4
Cabaseril, 1860·4
Cabastine, 435·2
Cabdrivers Expectorant, Original— *see* Original Cabdrivers Expectorant, 2192·3
Cabdrivers Sugar-Free Linctus, 1860·4
Cabergolina, 1203·3
Cabergoline, 1203·3
Ca-C, 1860·4
Ca-C— *see* Sandoz Calcium + Vitamine C, 2277·1
Cacahuete, Aceite de, 1656·1
Cacao, Beurre de, 1482·3
Cacao, Burro di, 1482·3
Cacao Butter, 1482·3
Cacao, Butyrum, 1482·3
Cacao, Manteca de, 1482·3
Cacao, Oleum, 1482·3
Cacao Powder, 1754·3
Cacau, Licor de— *see* Licor de Cacau, 2095·3
Cacau, Manteiga de, 1482·3
Caceff, 1860·4
Cachectin, 590·2
Cachexia, 1558·3
Cachexia, AIDS-associated— *see* HIV-associated Wasting and Diarrhoea, 623·2
Cachexia, Cancer-related— *see* Cachexia, 1558·3
Cachexon, 1860·4
Cacit, 1860·4
Cacit— *see* Didrokit, 1937·3
Cacit— *see* Didronel PMO, 1937·3
Cacit D3, 1860·4
Cacit mit Vitamin $D_3$, 1860·4
Cacit Vitamina D3, 1860·4
Cacit Vitamine $D_3$, 1860·4
Cacital, 1860·4
Cactinomycin, 545·1
Cactus, 1669·2, 1713·3
Cactus Compositum, 1860·4
*Cactus grandiflorus*, 1669·2
CaD, 1860·4
Ca-D, Sandoz— *see* Sandoz Ca-D, 2276·4
Cade Oil, 1159·2
Cadencial Plus, 1861·1
Cadens, 1861·1
Cadevit, 1861·1
Cadex, 1861·1
Cadexcin-N, 1861·1
Cadexomer Iodine, 1172·1
Cadexomer-Iodine, 1172·1
Cadexómero Yodado, 1172·1
Cadi, Pix, 1159·2
Cadicon, 1861·1
Cadifen, 1861·1
Cadimasol, 1861·1
Cadimint, 1861·1
Cadinene, 1159·2
Cadinol, 1861·1
Cadinum, Oleum, 1159·2
Cadinyl, 1861·1
Cadiphylate, 1861·1
Cadisper C, 1861·1
Caditar, 1861·1
Cadmio, 1663·3
Cadmium, 1663·3
Cadmium Sulfate, 1663·3
Cadmium Sulfide, 1663·3
Cadolac, 1861·1
Cadralazina, 878·2
Cadralazine, 878·2
Cadramine, 1861·1
Cadramine-V, 1861·1
Cadraten, 1861·1
Cadrilan, 1861·1
Cadron, Chibro- — *see* Chibro-Cadron, 1882·3
Cadrox, 1861·1
Caduet, 1861·1
Cadvion, 1861·1
Cadyoil, 1861·1
C-A-E, 1861·1
Caedax, 1861·1
Caelyx, 1861·1
Caerulein, 1669·2
Caeruleum, Azovanum, 1658·3
Caeruleum, Sulphanum, 1750·3
*Caesalpinia spinosa*, 1751·2
Caext, 1861·2
Cafadol, 1861·2
Cafalena, 1861·2
Cafatine, 1861·2
Cafatine-PB, 1861·2
Cafcit, 1861·2
Cafedrina, Hidrocloruro de, 878·2
Cafedrine Hydrochloride, 878·2
Cafeína, 782·1
Cafeína, Citrato de, 782·1
Cafeína Hidrato, 782·1
Caféine, 782·1
Cafergot, 1861·2
Cafergot N, 1861·2
Cafergot-PB, 1861·2
Cafestol, 1765·2
Cafetrate, 1861·2
Caffalgina, 1861·2
Caffedrine, 1861·2
Caffeine, 782·1
Caffeine, Anhydrous, 782·1
Caffeine Citrate, 782·1
Caffeine Citrate, Phenazone and, 82·3
Caffeine, Citrated, 782·1
Caffeine Hydrate, 782·1
Caffeine Monohydrate, 782·1
Caffeine and Sodium Benzoate, 783·2
Caffeine and Sodium Iodide, 783·2
Caffeine and Sodium Salicylate, 783·2
Caffeine Withdrawal Support, 1861·2
Cafiaspirina, 1861·2
Cafinitrina, 1861·2
Caginal, 1861·2
Caina G, 1861·2
Cajeput Oil, 1664·1
Cajuput Essence, 1664·1
Cajuput Oil, 1664·1, 1672·1
Cajuputi, Oleum, 1664·1
Cajuputol, 1672·1
Cal-500, 1861·2
Cal Alkyline, 1861·2
Cal C, Bioglan— *see* Bioglan Cal C, 1843·4
Cal Clorada, 1175·3
Cal, Cloruro de, 1175·3
Cal D, 1861·2
Cal Gel, 1861·2
Cal Mag Plus Vitamin D, 1861·2
Cal Mo Dol, 1861·2
CAL Ocean, 1861·2
Cal Sodada, 1747·1
Cal Sulfurada, 1158·2
Calaband, 1861·2
Calabar Bean, 1494·1
Calabaza, Semillas de, 1677·3
Calabren, 1861·3
Caladaryl Panal, 1861·3
Caladerm, 1861·3
Caladryl, 1861·3
Caladryl Clear, 1861·3
Caladryl Incoloro, 1861·3
Cala-gen, 1861·3
Cal-Aid, 1861·3
Calais, 1861·3
Calamatum, 1861·3
Calamina, 1144·1, 1861·3
Calamina Composta, 1861·3
Calamine, 1144·1
Calamine Antihistamine, 1861·3
Calamine Lotion, 1861·3
Calamine-D, 1861·4
Cálamo Aromático, 1664·1
Calamox, 1861·4
Calamus, 1664·1
Calamus Oil, 1664·1
Calamus Rhizome, 1664·1
Calamycin, 1861·4
Calamyn— *see* Calamina Composta, 1861·3
Calan, 1861·4
Calanda, 1861·4
Calanif, 1861·4
Calanol, 1861·4
Cal-Antagon, 1861·4
Calapro, 1861·4
Calaptin, 1861·4
Calasthetic, 1861·4
Calatrim, 1861·4
Calatrim Cum Sulphur, 1861·4
Calax, 1861·4
Calbion, 1861·4
Calbisan, 1861·4
Calburst, 1861·4
Calc. Carb., 1254·3
Calc. Cyclam., 1426·2
Calc. Fluor., 1423·3
Calc. Phos., 1227·1
Calcanate, 1861·4
Cal-Car, 1861·4
Calcarb with Vitamin D, 1861·4
Calcarea Carbonica, 1254·3
Calcarea Fluorica, 1423·3
Calcarea Phosphorica, 1227·1
Calcaria Absorbens, 1747·1
Calcaria Chlorata, 1175·3
Calcaria Compositio, 1747·1
Calcascorbin, 1861·4
Calcedon, 1861·4
Calcefor, 1861·4
Calcefor Cap, 1861·4
Calcefor D, 1861·4
Calceos, 1861·4
Calcet, 1861·4
Calcet Plus, 1861·4
Calcetat, 1862·1
Calcette, 1862·1
Calcevita, 1862·1
Calchan, 1862·1
Calchek, 1862·1
Calchew, 1862·1
Calci, 1862·1
Calcia, 1862·1
Calciben, 1862·1
Calcibind, 1862·1
Calcibon, 1862·1
Calcibronat, 1862·1
CalciCaps, 1862·1
CalciCaps with Iron, 1862·1
CalciCaps M-Z, 1862·1
Calcicard, 1862·1
Calcichell, 1862·1

Calcichew, 1862·1
Calci-Chew, 1862·1
Calcichew $D_3$, 1862·1
Cálcico, Fluoruro, 1423·3
Calciday, 1862·1
Calcidia, 1862·1
Calcidiol, 1461·2
Calcidon, 1862·1
Calcidose, 1862·1
Calcidose Vitamine D, 1862·1
Calcidrine, 1862·1
Calcidrink, 1862·1
Calcifar, 1862·2
Calcifediol, 1461·2
Calcifediolum, 1461·2
Calciferol, 1462·1, 1862·2
Calciferol B12, 1862·2
Calciferol Composto, 1862·2
Calcifluol, 1862·2
Calcifluor, 1862·2
Calcifolin, 1862·2
Calcifort, 1862·2
Calciforte, 1862·2
Calcigamma, 1862·2
Calcigard, 1862·2
Calcigen D, 1862·2
Calcigenol, 1862·2
Calcigenol B12, 1862·2
Calcigenol Irradiado, 1862·2
Calcigran, 1862·2
Calci-Gry, 1862·2
Calcihep, 1862·2
Calcihexal, 1862·2
Calcii Ascorbas, 1460·2
Calcii Carbonas, 1254·2
Calcii Chloridum, 1225·1
Calcii Chloridum Dihydricum, 1225·1
Calcii Chloridum Hexahydricum, 1225·1
Calcii Dobesilas, 1664·2
Calcii et Hydrogenii Phosphas, 1225·2
Calcii Folinas, 1431·1
Calcii Glucoheptonas, 1225·2
Calcii Gluconas, 1225·2
Calcii Glycerophosphas, 1225·2
Calcii Hydrogenophosphas, 1225·2
Calcii Hydrogenophosphas Anhydricus, 1225·2
Calcii Hydrogenophosphas Dihydricus, 1225·2
Calcii Hydroxidum, 1664·3
Calcii Hypochloris, 1175·3
Calcii Lactas, 1225·3
Calcii Lactas Pentahydricus, 1225·3
Calcii Lactas Trihydricus, 1225·3
Calcii Levofolinas Pentahydricus, 1431·1
Calcii Levulinas Dihydricum, 1225·3
Calcii Pantothenas, 1442·3
Calcii Para-aminosalicylas, 155·1
Calcii Saccharas, 1665·1
Calcii Stearas, 1574·1
Calcii Sulfas, 1665·1
Calcii Sulfas Hemihydricus, 1665·1
Calciject, 1862·3
Calcijex, 1862·3
Calcilac KT, 1862·3
Calcilat, 1862·3
Calcilean, 1862·3
Calciless, 1862·3
Calcilin, 1862·3
Calcilin Compositum, 1862·3
Calcilo XD, 1862·3
Calcilos, 1862·3
Calcimagon, 1862·3
Calcimagon-D3, 1862·3
Calcimar, 1862·3
Calcimax, 1862·3
Calcimax D3, 1862·3
Calcimed, 1862·3
Calcimed $D_3$, 1862·3
Calcimega, 1862·3
Calcimex, 1862·3
Calcimimetics, 765·2
Calci-Mix, 1862·3
Calcimon, 1862·3
Calcimonta, 1862·3
Calcimore, 1862·3
Calcinatal, 1862·3
Calcined Gypsum, 1665·1
Calcinil, 1862·3
Calcinol, 1862·3
Calcinosis Cutis— *see* Polymyositis and Dermatomyositis, 1086·2
Calcio, 1225·1
Calcio 20, 1862·4
Calcio 520, 1862·4
Calcio, Acetato de, 1225·1
Calcio Cit, 1862·4
Calcio Cit Simple, 1862·4
Calcio, Citrato de, 1225·1
Cálcio, Cloreto de, 1225·1
Calcio, Cloruro de, 1225·1
Calcio Cm, 1862·4
Calcio 20 Complex, 1862·4
Calcio Day D, 1862·4
Calcio Dobetin, 1862·4
Calcio 20 Emulsion, 1862·4
Calcio, Fosfato de, 1225·3
Calcio 20 Fuerte, 1862·4
Calcio Geve D Y C, 1862·4
Calcio, Glicerofosfato de, 1225·2
Calcio, Glubionato de, 1225·1
Calcio, Glucoheptonato de, 1225·2
Calcio, Gluconato de, 1225·2
Calcio, Gluconato Lactato de, 1225·3
Calcio, Hidrogenofosfato de, 1225·2
Calcio, Lactato de, 1225·3
Calcio, Lactato Sódico de, 1226·1
Calcio, Lactobionato de, 1225·3
Calcio, Levulinato de, 1225·3
Calcio Masticable, 1862·4
Calcio Nil, 1862·4
Calcio Nil Forte, 1862·4
Calcio, Pidolato de, 1226·1
Calcio, Silicato de, 1226·1
Calcio Vitam D3, 1862·4
Calcio Vitaminado, 1862·4
Calcio Vitaminado B12, 1862·4
Calciobion, 1862·4
Calcioday-D, 1862·4
Calciodie, 1862·4
Calcioedetato de Sodio, 1051·3
Calciofix, 1862·4
Calciokatabios, 1862·4
Calciomed— *see* Lubical, 2107·1
Calcional, 1862·4
Calciopen, 1863·1
Calciopiu, 1863·1
Calcior, 1863·1
Calcioral, 1863·1
Calcioral D3, 1863·1
Calcioretard, 1863·1
Calciosan, 1863·1
Calciosint, 1863·1
Calcioton, 1863·1
Calciovit Puro, 1863·1
Calciovit Urto, 1863·1
Calciovital Irradiado, 1863·1
Calciozim, 1863·1
Calciparin, 1863·1
Calciparina, 1863·1
Calciparine, 1863·1
Calci-Ped, 1863·1
Calcipen, 1863·1
Calciplex, 1863·1
Calciplus, 1863·1
Calcipor, 1863·1
Calcipot, 1863·1
Calcipot C, 1863·1
Calcipot $D_3$, 1863·1
Calcipotriene, 1144·1
Calcipotriol, 1144·1
Calciprat, 1863·1
Calciprat $D_3$, 1863·1
Calcipulpe, 1863·1
Calci-Rav, 1863·2
Calciretard, 1863·2
Calcirol, 1863·2
Calcisan, 1863·2
Calcisan B + C, 1863·2
Calcisan C, 1863·2
Calcisan D, 1863·2
Calcisorb, 1863·2
Calcitab, 1863·2
Calcitab D, 1863·2
Calcitar, 1863·2
Calcitare, 1863·2
Calcite, 1863·2
Calcite D, 1863·2
Calcitol, 1863·2
Calcitonin, 1863·2
Calcitonin, [Aminosuberic Acid 1,7]-Eel, 768·3
Calcitonin Gene-related Peptide, 878·3
Calcitonin (Human), 768·2
Calcitonin (Pork), 768·2
Calcitonin (Salmon), 768·2
Calcitonina, 1863·2
Calcitonina (Cerdo), 768·2
Calcitonina (Humana), 768·2
Calcitonina (Salmón), 768·2
Calcitoninas, 768·2
Calcitonin-human, 768·2
Calcitonins, 768·2
Calcitonin-salmon, 768·2
Calcitoninum Salmonis, 768·2
Calcitoran, 1863·2
Calcitran B12, 1863·2
Calcitrans, 1863·2
Calcitrat, 1863·2
Cal-Citrate, 1863·2
Calcitridin, 1863·2
Calcitriol, 1461·2
Calcitriolum, 1461·2
Calcitugg, 1863·2
Calcium, 1225·1
Calcium 600, 1863·2
Calcium 3-Acetamido-1-propanesulphate, 668·1
Calcium Acetate, 1225·1
Calcium Acetylsalicylate, 25·1
Calcium Acetylsalicylate Carbamide, 25·1
Calcium Acexamate, 1646·2
Calcium AL, 1863·2
Calcium Alginate, 745·1, 1577·1
Calcium Amidotrizoate, 1061·1
Calcium 4-Amino-2-hydroxybenzoate Trihydrate, 155·1
Calcium Aminosalicylate, 155·1
Calcium Antagonists, 810·3
Calcium Ascorbate, 1460·2
Calcium Benzosulphimide, 1443·3
Calcium Beta, 1863·3
Calcium Bis[2-(acetoxy)benzoate]—urea, 25·1
Calcium 1,4-Bis(2-ethylhexyl) Sulphosuccinate, 1262·1
Calcium Borogluconate, 1225·2
Calcium Braun, 1863·3
Calcium Bromide Lactobionate Hexahydrate, 674·1
Calcium Bromolactobionate, 674·1
Calcium C, 1863·3
Calcium Carbaspirin, 25·1
Calcium Carbimide, 1664·2
Calcium Carbimide, Citrated, 1664·2
Calcium Carbonate, 1254·2, 1255·3
Calcium Carbonate, Precipitated, 1254·2
Calcium Carboxymethylcellulose, 1577·3
Calcium Chewable, 1863·3
Calcium Chloratum, 1225·1
Calcium Chloride, 1225·1
Calcium Chloride Dihydrate, 1225·1
Calcium Chloride Hexahydrate, 1225·1
Calcium 3-(4-Chlorophenyl)-1-phenylpyrazol-4-ylacetate, 54·2
Calcium Citrate, 1225·1
Calcium Clear, 1863·3
Calcium Clofibrate, 885·1
Calcium compositum N, Kneipp— *see* Kneipp Calcium compositum N, 2081·2
Calcium Copperedetate, 1425·3
Calcium Corbiere, 1863·3
Calcium Corbiere Vitamine CDPP, 1863·3
Calcium Cyanamide, 1664·2
Calcium Cyanide, 1506·2
Calcium Cyclamate, 1426·2
Calcium Cyclohexanesulfamate, 1426·2
Calcium 5-(Cyclohex-1-enyl)-5-ethylbarbiturate, 689·2
Calcium *N*-Cyclohexylsulphamate Dihydrate, 1426·2
Calcium D, 1863·3
Calcium $D_3$, 1863·3
Calcium D Sauter, 1863·3
Calcium Dago, 1863·3
Calcium Di[2-(acetyloxy)benzoate], 25·1
Calcium α-(4-Diethylaminophenyl)-α-(4-diethyliminiocyclohexa-2,5-dienylidene)-5-hydroxytoluene-2,4-disulphonate, 1729·1
Calcium Dihydrogen Phosphate, 1664·2
Calcium Dihydrogenphosphoricum, 1664·2
Calcium 2,5-Dihydroxybenzenesulphonate, 1664·2
Calcium D-(+)-4-(2,4-Dihydroxy-3,3-dimethylbutyramido)butyrate Hemihydrate, 1664·3
Calcium (*RS*)-2,3-Dihydroxypropyl Phosphate, 1225·2
Calcium 3-(3-Dimethylaminomethyleneamino-2,4,6-tri-iodophenyl)propionate, 1065·2
Calcium Diorthosilicate, 1226·1
Calcium 2-(1,2-Diphenylhydrazinocarbonyl)hexanoate Hemihydrate, 21·3
Calcium Disodium Edathamil, 1051·3
Calcium Disodium Edetate, 1051·3
Calcium Disodium Ethylenediaminetetraacetate, 1051·3
Calcium Disodium Versenate, 1051·3
Calcium Di(undec-10-enoate), 410·3
Calcium Dobesilate, 1664·2
Calcium Dobesilate Monohydrate, 1664·2
Calcium Docuphen, 1863·3
Calcium Doxybenzylate, 1664·2
Calcium EDTA, 1051·3
Calcium Eifelfango, 1863·3
Calcium (1*R*,2*S*)-1,2-Epoxypropylphosphonate Monohydrate, 214·2
Calcium and Ergocalciferol Tablets, 1863·3
Calcium [Ethylenediaminetetra-acetato-{4—}-*N*,*N'*,*O*,*O'*]copper (II) Dihydrate, 1425·3
Calcium 5-Ethyl-5-(1-methylbutyl)barbiturate, 713·3
Calcium Factor, 1863·3
Calcium Fluoride, 1423·3
Calcium (β*R*,δ*R*)-2-(*p*-Fluorophenyl)-β,δ-dihydroxy-5-isopropyl-3-phenyl-4-(phenylcarbamoyl)pyrrole-1-heptanoic Acid (1:2) Trihydrate, 866·1
Calcium Folinate, 1431·1
Calcium Folinate-SF, 1431·1
Calcium Formate, 1689·3
Calcium Forte D, 1863·3
Calcium Fosforylcholine, 1690·1
Calcium Fresenius, 1863·3
Calcium Galactogluconate Bromide, 674·1
Calcium 4-*O*-β-D-Galactopyranosyl-D-gluconate Dihydrate, 1225·3
Calcium Glubionate, 1225·1
Calcium D-Glucarate Tetrahydrate, 1665·1
Calcium Gluceptate, 1225·2
Calcium Glucoheptonate, 1225·2
Calcium Gluconate, 1225·2
Calcium D-Gluconate Lactobionate Monohydrate, 1225·1
Calcium Gluconate Lactobionate Monohydrate, 1225·1
Calcium D-Gluconate Monohydrate, 1225·2
Calcium Gluconicum— *see* Calcium Eifelfango, 1863·3
Calcium Gluconogalactogluconate Monohydrate, 1225·1
Calcium Glycerinophosphate, 1225·2
Calcium Glycerophosphate, 1225·2
Calcium Glycerylphosphate, 1225·2
Calcium Glycinate, Theophylline, 805·2
Calcium Glyconate, 1225·2
Calcium Gold Keratinate, 45·1
Calcium Guaiacolglycolate, 1122·1
Calcium Guaiacolsulfonate, 1131·1
Calcium Guaifenesin, 1122·2
Calcium Heparin, 927·3
Calcium Heumann, 1863·3
Calcium Hexal, 1863·3
Calcium Homopantothenate, 1664·3
Calcium Hopantenate, 1664·3

Calcium Hydrate, 1664·3
Calcium Hydrogen Orthophosphate, 1225·2
Calcium Hydrogen Phosphate, 1225·2
Calcium Hydrogen Phosphate, Anhydrous, 1225·2
Calcium Hydrogen Phosphate Dihydrate, 1225·2
Calcium Hydrophosphoricum, 1225·2
Calcium Hydroxide, 1664·3
Calcium Hydroxide Phosphate, 1226·1
Calcium 2-Hydroxy-1-(hydroxymethyl)ethyl Phosphate, 1225·2
Calcium 2-Hydroxypropionate, 1225·3
Calcium Hypochlorite, 1175·3
Calcium Hypochlorosum, 1175·3
Calcium Iodide, 1116·2
Calcium Iopodate, 1065·2
Calcium Ipodate, 1065·2
Calcium Lactate, 1225·3
Calcium Lactate Gluconate, 1225·3
Calcium Lactate Pentahydrate, 1225·3
Calcium Lactate Trihydrate, 1225·3
Calcium Lactobionate, 1225·3
Calcium Lactobionate Dihydrate, 1225·3
Calcium Laevulate, 1225·3
Calcium Laevulinate, 1225·3
Calcium Leucovorin, 1431·1
Calcium Levofolinate, 1431·1
Calcium Levofolinate Pentahydrate, 1431·1
Calcium Levulinate, 1225·3
Calcium Levulinate Dihydrate, 1225·3
Calcium Magnesium Plus, 1863·3
Calcium Mandelate, 228·3
Calcium Mefolinate, 1431·3
Calcium Mercaptoacetate, 1160·3
Calcium Mercaptoacetate Trihydrate, 1160·3
Calcium Metasilicate, 1226·1
Calcium Metrizoate, 1067·2
Calcium 600Mg, 1863·3
Calcium Monofluorophosphate, 1446·3
Calcium Monohydrogen Phosphate, 1225·2
Calcium Novartis, 1863·3
Calcium Novobiocin, 239·2
Calcium Octadecanoate, 1574·1
Calcium Oleate, 1574·3
Calcium Orotate, 1724·3
Calcium Orthophosphate, 1225·3
Calcium Oxide, 1664·3
Calcium 5-Oxopyrrolidine-2-carboxylate, 1226·1
Calcium 4-Oxovalerate Dihydrate, 1225·3
Calcium Oxydatum, 1664·3
Calcium Oyster Shell, 1863·3
Calcium Palmitate, 1574·2
Calcium Pangamate, 1727·2
Calcium Pantothenate, 1442·3
Calcium Pantothenate, Racemic, 1443·1
Calcium PAS, 155·1
Calcium Pentetate, 1050·1
Calcium (±)-2-(3-Phenoxyphenyl)propionate Dihydrate, 39·2
Calcium Phosphate, 1225·3
Calcium Phosphate, Acid, 1664·2
Calcium Phosphate, Dibasic, 1225·2
Calcium Phosphate, Monobasic, 1664·2
Calcium Phosphate, Precipitated, 1225·3
Calcium, Phosphate Tertiaire de, 1225·3
Calcium Phosphate, Tribasic, 1226·1
Calcium Pidolate, 1226·1
Calcium Plus, 1863·3
Calcium Polycarbophil, 1284·2
Calcium Polystyrene Sulfonate, 1032·3
Calcium Polystyrene Sulphonate, 1032·3
Calcium Polysulfides, 1158·2
Calcium Propionate, 408·1
Calcium Pyroglutamate, 1226·1
Calcium Receptor Agonists, 765·2
Calcium Resonium, 1863·3
Calcium Rich Rolaids, 1863·4
Calcium Saccharate, 1665·1
Calcium D-Saccharate, 1665·1
Calcium Saccharin, 1443·3
Calcium Salicylate, Theobromine and, 798·2
Calcium Salicylate, Theophylline, 805·2
Calcium Sennoside A, 1289·1
Calcium Sennoside B, 1289·1
Calcium Silicate, 1226·1
Calcium Sodium Lactate, 1226·1
Calcium Stada, 1863·4
Calcium Stanley, 1863·4
Calcium Stearate, 1574·1
Calcium Sulfate, 1158·2, 1665·1
Calcium Sulfate Dihydrate, 1665·1
Calcium Sulfuricum ad Usum Chirurgicum, 1665·1
Calcium Sulphate, 1665·1
Calcium Sulphate, Dried, 1665·1
Calcium Sulphide, 1158·2
Calcium Sulphuricum Ustum, 1665·1
Calcium Tetrahydrogen Diorthophosphate Monohydrate, 1664·2
Calcium Thioglycollate, 1160·3
Calcium Thiosulfate, 1158·2
Calcium Trisilicate, 1226·1
Calcium Trisodium DTPA, 1050·1
Calcium Trisodium Nitrilodiethylenedinitrilopenta-acetate, 1050·1
Calcium Trisodium Pentetate, 1050·1
Calcium Truw, 1863·4
Calcium Undecenoate, 410·3
Calcium Undecylenate, 410·3
Calcium Unison, 1863·4
Calcium Valproate, 382·2
Calcium Verla, 1863·4
Calcium Verla D, 1863·4
Calcium and Vitamin D Tablets— *see* Calcium and Ergocalciferol Tablets, 1863·3
Calcium Vitis, 1863·4
Calcium Von CT, 1863·4
Calcium-C, Sandoz— *see* Sandoz Calcium-C, 2277·1
Calcium-channel Blockers, 810·3
Calcium-D-Redoxon, 1863·4
Calcium-D-Sandoz, 1863·4
Calcium-D3-Sandoz, 1863·4
Calcium-dura, 1863·4
Calcium-dura Vit $D_3$, 1863·4
Calcium-EAP, 1863·4
Calciumedetate, Sodium, 1051·3
Calcium-entry Blockers, 810·3
Calcium-Rougier, 1863·4
Calcium-Rutinion, 1863·4
Calcium-Sandoz, 1863·4
Calcium-Sandoz C, 1864·1
Calcium-Sandoz F, 1864·1
Calcium-Sandoz Forte, 1864·1
Calcium-Sandoz Forte D, 1864·1
Calcium-Sandoz— *see* Sandoz Calcium, 2276·4
Calcium-Sandoz + Vit C, 1864·1
Calcium-Sandoz + Vitamin C, 1864·1
Calcium-Sandoz + Vitamina C, 1864·1
Calcium-Sorbisterit, 1864·1
Calciumvit, 1864·1
Calciumvit Infantil, 1864·1
Calcival, 1864·1
Calcivit, 1864·1
Calcivit D, 1864·2
Calcivit F, 1864·2
Calcivitase, 1864·2
Calcivorin, 1864·2
Calcivorin D, 1864·2
Calco, 1864·2
Calcort, 1864·2
Calcos Vitamine $D_3$, 1864·2
Cal-C-Tose, 1864·2
Calcufel Aqua, 1864·2
Calculi, Biliary— *see* Gallstones, 1761·3
Calculi H, 1864·2
Calculi, Renal— *see* Renal Calculi, 936·2
Calculina, 1864·2
Calcusan, 1864·2
Cal-C-Vita, 1864·2
Cal-C-Vita Fluor, 1864·2
Cal-D3, 1864·2
Caldar-D, 1864·2
Cal-De, 1864·2
Caldease, 1864·2
CaldeCort, 1864·2
Calderol, 1864·2
Caldesene, 1864·2
Caldeval, 1864·2
Caldine, 1864·2
Caldomine-DH, 1864·2
Cal-D-or, 1864·3
Caldramine, 1864·3
Cal-D-Vita, 1864·3
Calel-D, 1864·3
Calendaderm, 1864·3
Calendolon, 1864·3
Calendula, 1665·2
Calendula +, 1864·3
Calendula Concreta, 1864·3
Calendula Echinacea Comp, 1864·3
Calendula Flower, 1665·2
Calendula Nappy Change Cream, 1864·3
*Calendula officinalis*, 1665·2
Calendula Oil, 1665·2
Calendulae Flos, 1665·2
Calendulene, 1864·3
Calendumed, 1864·3
Calfactant, 1736·2
Calfate, 1864·3
Calferon— *see* Calciferol Composto, 1862·2
Calfolex, 1864·3
Calfolin, 1864·3
Calfosina, 1864·3
Calfovit D3, 1864·3
Calgayan, 1864·3
Calgel, 1864·3
Calibral, 1864·3
Calicheamicin, 558·3
Calicida Indiano, 1864·3
Caliderm, 1864·3
Califig, 1864·3
Calimal, 1864·3
Calinat, 1864·3
Calinofen, 1864·3
Calista, 1864·3
Calisvit, 1864·4
Cal-Lac, 1864·4
Callicida, 1864·4
Callicida 2, 1864·4
Callicida Brujo, 1864·4
Callicida Brum, 1864·4
Callicida Cor Pik, 1864·4
Callicida Durcall, 1864·4
Callicida Globodermis, 1864·4
Callicida Gras, 1864·4
Callicida Rojo, 1864·4
Callicida Salve, 1864·4
Callicida Unguento Morri— *see* Unguento Morry, 2358·1
Callicrein, 1703·2
Callimon, 1864·4
Callivoro Marthand, 1864·4
Callix, 1864·4
Callofin, 1864·4
*Calloselasma rhodostoma*, 863·2
Callus Removal, Scholl— *see* Scholl Callus Removal, 2279·3
Callus Salve, 1864·4
Calm Life, HRI— *see* HRI Calm Life, 2048·4
Calma, 1864·4
Calmaben, 1864·4
Calmaderm, 1864·4
Calmador, 1864·4
Cal-Mag, 1864·4
Cal-Mag Citrate with Vitamin D & Zinc, 1865·1
Calmag D, 1865·1
CalMag Plus, 1865·1
Cal-Mag Plus Vitamin D, 1865·1
Cal-Mag Vitamin C & Zinc, 1865·1
Cal-Mag with Vitamin D & Zinc, 1865·1
Cal-Mag & Vitamins C & D, 1865·1
Calmag Zn, 1865·1
Calman, 1865·1
Calmanervin, 1865·1
Calmant Martou, 1865·1
Calmante Creosotado, 1865·1
Calmante de Aftas, 1865·1
Calmante de Denticion, 1865·1
Calmante Vitaminado P G, 1865·1
Calmante Vitaminado PG Efervescente, 1865·1
Calmante Vitaminado Rinver, 1865·1
Calmanticold, 1865·1
Calmanticold Vit C, 1865·1
Calmantina, 1865·1
Calmapax, 1865·1
Calmapele, 1865·1
Calmapica, 1865·1
Calmapir, 1865·1
Calmapir-P, 1865·1
Calmaril, 1865·1
Calmarum, 1865·1
Calmatel, 1865·1
Calmatoss, 1865·2
Calmaven, 1865·2
Calmaverine, 1865·2
Calmax, 1865·2
Calmaxid, 1865·2
Calmazin, 1865·2
Calmday, 1865·2
Calmerphan, 1865·2
Calmerphan-L, 1865·2
Calmese, 1865·2
Calmesine, 1865·2
Calmettes, 1865·2
Calmex, 1865·2
Calmine, 1865·2
Calminex Atleta, 1865·2
Calminex H, 1865·2
Calmiphase, 1865·2
Calmiplan, 1865·2
Calmiton, 1865·2
Calmixene, 1865·2
Calmo, 1865·2
Calmobrul, 1865·2
Calmociteno, 1865·2
Calmoflorine, 1865·2
Calmogel, 1865·2
Calmogenol, 1865·3
Calmol, 1865·3
Calmomusc, 1865·3
Calmonex, 1865·3
Calmophytum, 1865·3
Calmopirin, 1865·3
Calmoplex, 1865·3
Calmoroide, 1865·3
Calmose, 1865·3
Calmosedan, 1865·3
Calmosine, 1865·3
Calmovarin, 1865·3
Calmpose, 1865·3
Calms, 1865·3
Calms Forte, 1865·3
Calmtabs, 1865·3
Calm-U, 1865·3
Calmurid, 1865·3
Calmurid Comp, 1865·3
Calmurid HC, 1865·3
Calmuril, 1865·3
Calmuril-Hydrokortison, 1865·3
Calm-X, 1865·3
Calmydone, 1865·3
Calmylin Preparations, 1865·3
Cal-Nate, 1865·4
Calner, 1865·4
Calnisan, 1865·4
Calnit, 1865·4
Calociclina, 1865·4
Calogen, 1865·4
Calomel, 1712·3
Calomelanos, 1712·3
Calonat, 1865·4
Calope, 1865·4
Caloreen, 1865·4
Calostro Bovino, 1611·1
Calotrat, 1865·4
Calox, 1865·4
Calpan, 1865·4
Calparine, 1865·4
Calperos, 1865·4
Calperos $D_3$, 1866·1
Calphosan, 1866·1
Calphron, 1866·1
Calpix, 1866·1
Cal-Plus, 1866·1

CalplusD3, 1866·1
Calpol, 1866·1
Calpol Extra, 1866·1
Calporo, 1866·1
Calpred, 1866·1
Calpres, 1866·1
Calprimum, 1866·1
Calprofen, 1866·1
Calron, 1866·1
Calrub, 1866·1
Cal-Rutina, 1866·1
Calsalettes, 1866·1
Calsan, 1866·1
Calsein, 1866·1
Calshake, 1866·1
Calsip, 1866·1
Calslot, 1866·1
Calsorp, 1866·1
Calsum Forte, 1866·1
Cal-Sup, 1866·1
Calsyn, 1866·1
Calsynar, 1866·1
Calsynar Lyo, 1866·2
Caltab, 1866·2
Caltabs, 1866·2
Caltheon, 1866·2
Caltine, 1866·2
Caltoson Balsamico, 1866·2
Caltrate Preparations, 1866·2
Caltrec, 1866·2
Caltren, 1866·2
Caltro, 1866·2
Caltusine, 1866·2
Calumba, 1665·2
Calumba Root, 1665·2
Calvakehl, 1866·2
Calvepen, 1866·2
Calvidin, 1866·3
Calvita, 1866·3
Calvita B12, 1866·3
Calx, 1664·3
Calx Chlorata, 1175·3
Calx Chlorinata, 1175·3
Calx Sodica, 1747·1
Calx Sulphurata, 1158·2
Calx Usta, 1664·3
Calypsol, 1866·3
Calyptol, 1866·3
Calyptol Inhalante, 1866·3
Cam, 1866·3
CAM, 1866·3
Cama Arthritis Pain Reliever, 1866·3
Camalox, 1866·3
Camalox— *see* Maaloxan Ca, 2109·4
Camazepam, 674·1
Camazol, 1866·3
Cambem, 1866·3
Cambendazole, 103·3
Camboacy, 1866·3
Camcolit, 1866·3
Camegel, 1866·3
*Camellia sinensis*, 1765·3
*Camellia thea*, 1765·3
Cameo, 1866·3
Camil, 1866·3
Camilia, 1866·3
Camiline, 1866·3
Camilofina, Hidrocloruro de, 1666·1
Caminol, 1866·3
Camoderm, 1866·3
Camomila, 1866·3
Camomile Allemande, 1669·3
Camomilina C, 1866·4
Camomilla, 1669·3
Camomilla (Specie Composta), 1866·4
Camomille (Grande), 469·1
Camoquin, 1866·4
Camostat Mesilate, 1665·2
Camostat, Mesilato de, 1665·2
Camostat Mesylate, 1665·2
Camoxin, 1866·4
Campanyl, 1866·4
Campathyl, 1866·4
Campath-1, 526·1
Campath-1G, 526·1
Campath-1H, 526·1
Campden Tablets, 1193·3
Campel, 1866·4
2-Camphanone, 1665·3
Camphene, 1740·2, 1760·1
Camphoderm N, 1866·4
Camphodionyl, 1866·4
Campho-Phenique, 1866·4
Campho-Phenique Antibiotic Plus Pain Reliever Ointment, 1866·4
Camphopin, 1866·4
Campho-Pneumine, 1866·4
Camphor, 1665·3, 1740·2
D-Camphor, 1665·3
Camphor Linctus Compound, 1866·4
Camphor, Natural, 1665·3
D-Camphor (Natural), 1665·3
Camphor, Racemic, 1665·3
Camphor, Synthetic, 1665·3
Camphora, 1665·3
Camphorated Parachlorophenol, 1187·3
Camphoscapine, 1125·3
Camphre Compose, 1866·4
Camphre Droit (Natural), 1665·3
Camphre du Japon (Natural), 1665·3
Camphrice du Canada, 1866·4
Campicilin, 1866·4
Campral, 1866·4
Campto, 1866·4
Camptosar, 1866·4
*Camptotheca acuminata*, 564·3
Camptothecin, 564·3
Campylobacter Enteritis, 128·3
Campylobacter Jejuni Vaccines, 1611·1
Camsilato de Etamifilina, 785·1
Camylofin Dihydrochloride, 1666·1
Camylofin Hydrochloride, 1666·1
Camylofin Noramidopyrine Mesilate, 1666·1
Camylofin Sodium, 1666·1
Canadine, 1866·4
Canadiol, 1866·4
Canalba, 1866·4
Cáñamo Indiano, 1666·1
Canapa, 1666·1
Canary Yellow, 1057·3
Canasa, 1866·4
Canasone, 1867·1
Canavanine, 1649·1
Canazol, 1867·1
Canazol-BE, 1867·1
Cancer, 499·1
Cancer Pain, 5·1
Cancer Vaccines, 1611·2
Cancidas, 1867·1
Candacide, 1867·1
Candacort, 1867·1
Candalba, 1867·1
Candaspor, 1867·1
Candazol, 1867·1
Candazole, 1867·1
Candelilla Wax, 1480·2
Canderel, 1867·1
Canderme, 1867·1
Candermil, 1867·1
Candermyl, 1867·1
Candesar, 1867·1
Candesartan Cilexetil, 878·3
Candesartán Cilexetilo, 878·3
Candibene, 1867·1
Candicidin, 395·3
Candicidina, 395·3
Candicort, 1867·1
Candid, 1867·1
Candida Yeast, 1867·1
Candiden, 1867·1
Candiderm, 1867·1
Candidiasis, 386·3
Candidine, 1867·1
Candidosis— *see* Candidiasis, 386·3
Candimon, 1867·1
Candimyc, 1867·1
Candinox, 1867·1
Candio, 1867·1
Candio E comp N— *see* Candio-Hermal Plus, 1867·1
Candio-Hermal Plus, 1867·1
Candiplas, 1867·1
Candipres, 1867·1
Candistat, 1867·1
Candistatin, 1867·2
Canditral, 1867·2
Candizol, 1867·2
Candizole, 1867·2
Candizole-T, 1867·2
Candle Berry Bark, 1659·2
Candoral, 1867·2
Candoxatrilat, 879·1
Candoxatril, 879·1
Candoxatrilo, 879·1
Candyl, 1867·2
Candyl-D, 1867·2
Cane Sugar, 1450·1
Canef, 1867·2
Canela, 1672·2
Canela, Aceite Esencial de, 1672·2
Canela de la China, Aceite de, 1668·2
Canela do Ceilão , 1672·2
Canela, Esencia de, 1672·2
Canephron, 1867·2
Canephron N, 1867·2
Canephron Novo, 1867·2
Canephron S, 1867·2
Canescine, 892·3
Canesten Preparations, 1867·2
Canesten, Gine— *see* Gine Canesten, 2024·2
Canestene, 1867·2
Canex, 1867·2
Canfocarbonato de Amonio, 1585·1
Canfomenol, 1867·2
Cânfora, 1665·3
Canfosalicilica, 1867·2
Cangonha, 1666·1
Canhama, 1666·1
Canifug, 1867·2
Canker Sores— *see* Mouth Ulceration, 1245·1
Cankerol, 1867·2
Cannab., 1666·1
Cannabidiol, 1666·1
Cannabinol, 1666·1
Cannabis, 1666·1
Cannabis Indica, 1666·1
*Cannabis sativa*, 1666·1
Cannacoro, 1666·1
Cannelle de Ceylan, Essence de, 1672·2
Cannelle Dite de Ceylan, 1672·2
Canoderm, 1867·2
Canol, 1867·3
Cánola, Aceite de, 1666·3
Canola Oil, 1666·3
Canovex, 1867·3
Canrenoate Potassium, 984·2
Canrenoato de Potasio, 984·2
Canrenol, 1867·3
Canrenona, 879·1
Canrenone, 879·1, 1004·1
Canscreen, 1867·3
Cansilato de Trimetafán, 1017·3
Canstat, 1867·3
Cantabilin, 1867·3
Cantabiline, 1867·3
Cantadrill, 1867·3
Cantalene, 1867·3
Cantamac, 1867·3
Cantamega, 1867·3
Cantapollen, 1867·3
Cantáridas, 1666·3
Cantaridina, 1667·1
Cantassium Discs, 1867·3
Cantavite with FF, 1867·3
Cantaxantina, 1056·3
Canthacur, 1867·3
Canthacur-PS, 1867·3
Cantharides, 1666·3
Cantharidin, 1667·1
Cantharis, 1666·3
Cantharis Med Complex, 1867·3
*Cantharis vesicatoria*, 1667·1
Cantharone, 1867·3
Cantharone Plus, 1867·3
Canthaxanthin, 1056·3
Cantil, 1867·3
Cantipal, 1867·3
Cantopal, 1867·3
Cantril, 1867·3
Canusal, 1867·3
Can-Yac, 1666·1
Caolax, 1867·3
Caolín, 1268·3
Caomet, 1867·3
Caopecfar, 1867·3
Caosina, 1867·3
Caosina D, 1867·3
Caoutchouc, 1741·1
CAP, 1578·2
Capace, 1867·3
Capadex, 1867·3
Caparin, 1867·4
Capasal, 1867·4
Capastat, 1867·4
CAPD, 1867·4
CAPD/DPCA, 1867·4
Cape Aloes, 1248·2
Cape Gooseberry, 1731·3
Capecitabina, 533·2
Capecitabine, 533·2
Capel, 1867·4
Capent, 1867·4
Caper Spurge, 1686·3
Caperase, 1668·3
Capergyl, 1867·4
Capex, 1867·4
Capginvit, 1867·4
Capibaryne, 1867·4
Capilarema, 1867·4
Capill, 1867·4
Capillarema, 1867·4
Capillariasis, 98·1
Capillaron, 1867·4
Capillary Leak Syndrome, Systemic— *see* Systemic Capillary Leak Syndrome, 798·2
Capillon, 1867·4
Capiloton, 1867·4
Capim-Limão, Essência de, 1706·3
Capistan, 1867·4
Capital with Codeine, 1867·4
Capitis, 1867·4
Capitrol, 1867·4
Capiven, 1867·4
Caplenal, 1867·4
Capocard, 1867·4
Caposan, 1867·4
Caposten, 1867·4
Capoten, 1867·4
Capotena, 1868·1
Capotril, 1868·1
Capozid, 1868·1
Capozide, 1868·1
Capramin, 1868·1
Capreomicina, Sulfato de, 166·1
Capreomycin I, 166·1
Capreomycin IA, 166·1
Capreomycin IB, 166·1
Capreomycin II, 166·1
Capreomycin IIA, 166·1
Capreomycin IIB, 166·1
Capreomycin Disulfate, 166·1
Capreomycin Sulfate, 166·1
Capreomycin Sulphate, 166·1
Capricin, 1868·1
Capril, 1868·1
Caprilate, 1868·1
Caprilon, 1868·1
Caprimida, 1868·1
Caprimida D, 1868·1
Caprin, 1868·1
Caprisana, 1868·1
Caprisset, 1868·1
Caproamin, 1868·1
Caproato de Fluocortolona, 1102·1
Caproato de Gestonorona, 1556·2
Caproato de Hidroxiprogesterona, 1556·3
Caproato de Prednisolona, 1108·1
Caprofides Hemostatico, 1868·1
Caprolisin, 1868·1

Capromab Pendetide, Indium ($^{111}$In), 1524·1
Capromycin Sulphate, 166·1
Capros, 1868·1
Caprylic Acid, 1723·1
Caprysin, 1868·1
Capsaicin, 24·2
Capsaicin, Synthetic, 67·2
Capsaicina, 24·2
Capsamol, 1868·1
Capsanthin, 1056·1
Capsella, 1744·1
*Capsella bursa-pastoris*, 1744·1
Capsic, 1868·1
Capsic., 1667·1
Capsici Fructus, 1667·1
Capsicin, 1667·1, 1868·1
Capsicof, 1868·1
Capsicum, 1667·1
*Capsicum*, 24·2
*Capsicum annuum*, 1667·1
Capsicum + Arthri-Cream, 1868·2
Capsicum Farmaya, 1868·2
*Capsicum fruiscons*, 1667·1
Capsicum Frutescens, 1667·1
*Capsicum frutescens*, 1667·1
Capsicum, Japanese, 1667·1
Capsicum, Japanese, Honka Variety, 1667·1
Capsicum, Old Louisiana Sport, 1667·1
Capsicum Oleoresin, 1667·1
Capsidol, 1868·2
Capsin, 1868·2
Capsina, 1868·2
Capsiplast, 1868·2
Capso, 1868·2
Capsoid, 1868·2
Capsolin, 1868·2
Capson, 1868·2
Capsulas Handel, 1868·2
Capsules Laxatives Nattermann Nr. 13, 1868·2
Capsules-vital, 1868·2
Capsuvac, 1868·2
Capsyl, 1868·2
Captagon, 1868·2
Captaton, 1868·2
Captea, 1868·2
Capti, 1868·2
Captil, 1868·2
Captimer, 1868·2
Captin, 1868·2
Captirex, 1868·2
Capto, 1868·2
Capto Comp, 1868·2
Capto Plus, 1868·2
Capto-basan, 1868·2
Captobeta, 1868·2
Captobeta Comp, 1868·3
Capto-Co, 1868·3
Captocomp, 1868·3
Captodan, 1868·3
Captodiame Hydrochloride, 674·1
Captodiamine Hydrochloride, 674·1
Captodiamo, Hidrocloruro de, 674·1
Captodoc, 1868·3
Captodoc Comp, 1868·3
Capto-dura Cor, 1868·3
Capto-dura M, 1868·3
Captoflux, 1868·3
Captogamma, 1868·3
Captogamma HCT, 1868·3
Captohexal, 1868·3
Captohexal Comp, 1868·3
Captol, 1868·3
Captolane, 1868·3
Captomax, 1868·3
Captomed, 1868·3
Captomerck, 1868·3
Captomin, 1868·3
Capton, 1868·3
Capton Diet, 1868·3
Captopiril, 1868·3
Captoplus, 1868·3
Captopril, 879·2
Captopril Comp, 1868·3
Captopril Compositum, 1868·3
Captopril HCT, 1868·3
Captopril Plus, 1868·3
Captoprilum, 879·2
Captor, 1868·3
Captoreal, 1868·3
Captoretic, 1868·4
Captor-HCT, 1868·4
Captoser, 1868·4
Captosina, 1868·4
Captosol, 1868·4
Captosol Comp, 1868·4
Captostad, 1868·4
Captotec, 1868·4
Captotec + HCT, 1868·4
Captotyrol, 1868·4
Captral, 1868·4
Captril, 1868·4
Captrizin, 1868·4
Captus, 1868·4
Capuchin Cress, 1659·3
Capucine, 1659·3
Capurate, 1868·4
Capval, 1868·4
Capxidin, 1868·4
Capzasin-P, 1868·4
CAR, 1488·1
Car Sickness— *see* Nausea and Vomiting, 1245·2
Car Ti Buron, 1868·4
Carac, 1868·4
Carace, 1868·4
Carace Plus, 1868·4
Caradrin, 1868·4
Carafate, 1868·4
Caraguata, Xarope de— *see* Xarope de Caraguata, 2387·3
Caramel, 1056·3
Caramel, Ammonia, 1057·1
Caramel, Beer, 1057·1
Caramel, Caustic, 1057·1
Caramel, Caustic Sulfite, 1057·1
Caramel, Plain, 1057·1
Caramel, Soft-drink, 1057·1
Caramel, Spirit, 1057·1
Caramel, Sulfite Ammonia, 1057·1
Caramelle alle Erbe Digestive, 1868·4
Caramelo, 1056·3
Caramelos Agua del Carmen, 1868·4
Caramelos Antibioticos, 1868·4
Caramelos Antibioticos Bucoangin, 1868·4
Caramelos Balsam, 1869·1
Caramelos Oriental, 1869·1
Caramelos Vit C, 1869·1
Caramels, 1057·1
Caramifeno, Edisilato de, 1116·2
Caramiphen Edisilate, 1116·2
Caramiphen Edisylate, 1116·2
Caramiphen Hydrochloride, 1116·2
Carampicillin, 161·2
Caranda Wax, 1668·1
Carasel, 1869·1
Caraway, 1667·2
Caraway Fruit, 1667·2
Caraway Oil, 1667·3
Caraway, Powdered, 1667·2
Caraway Seed, 1667·2
Carazolol, 880·2
Carba, 1869·1
Carbabeta, 1869·1
Carbac, 1869·1
Carbacephems, 117·3
Carbach., 1488·1
Carbachol, 1488·1
Carbacholine, 1488·1
Carbacholum, 1488·1
Carbacholum Chloratum, 1488·1
Carbacide, 1869·1
Carbacol, 1488·1
Carbactive, 1869·1
Carbactol Retard, 1869·1
Carbaderme, 1869·1
Carbadox, 166·1
Carbadura, 1869·1
Carbaflux, 1869·1
Carbagamma, 1869·1
Carbagen, 1869·1
Carbager-Plus, 1869·1
Carbaglu, 1869·1
Carbagramon, 1869·1
Carbaica, 1869·1
Carbalan, 1869·1
Carbalax, 1869·1
Carbaldrate, 1261·2
Carbamaldehyde, 1474·3
Carbamann, 1869·1
Carbamat, 1869·1
Carbamate Insecticides, 1501·1
Carbamato de Clorfenesina, 1392·2
Carbamazepina, 353·3
Carbamazepine, 353·3
Carbamazepine-10,11-epoxide, 357·1
Carbamazepinum, 353·3
Carbamid + VAS, 1869·1
Carbamidated Quinine Dihydrochloride, 1737·2
Carbamide, 1162·2
Carbamide Creme, 1869·1
Carbamide Peroxide, 1195·3
Carbamide + VAS, 1869·1
Carbamidine Hydrochloride, 1492·1
Carbamidum Phenylaceticum, 367·3
Carbamol, 1187·2
Carbamox, 1869·1
(7*S*)-7-[(4-Carbamoylcarboxymethylene-1,3-dithietan-2-yl)carboxamido]-7-methoxy-3-[(1-methyl-1*H*-tetrazol-5-yl)thiomethyl]-3-cephem-4-carboxylic Acid, 177·1
(7*S*)-7-[(4-Carbamoylcarboxymethylene-1,3-dithietan-2-yl)carboxamido]-7-methoxy-3-[(1-methyl-1*H*-tetrazol-5-yl)thiomethyl]-3-cephem-4-carboxylic Acid, Disodium Salt, 177·1
Carbamoylcefaloridine, 168·2
*O*-Carbamoylcholine Chloride, 1488·1
3-Carbamoyl-4-*O*-deacetyl-3-de(methoxycarbonyl)vincaleukoblastine Sulfate, 593·3
(3-Carbamoyl-3,3-diphenylpropyl)di-isopropylmethylammonium Iodide, 485·2
(3-Carbamoyl-3,3-diphenylpropyl)ethyldimethylammonium Bromide, 1653·2
1-(3-Carbamoyl-3,3-diphenylpropyl)-1-methylperhydroazepinium Iodide, 480·2
1-(3-Carbamoyl-3,3-diphenylpropyl)-1-methylpiperidinium Bromide, 1688·1
*N*-Carbamoyl-L-glutamic Acid, 1668·1
(2-Carbamoyloxyethyl)trimethylammonium Chloride, 1488·1
(*Z*)-3-Carbamoyloxymethyl-7-[2-(2-furyl)-2-methoxyiminoacetamido]-3-cephem-4-carboxylic Acid, 184·1
(2-Carbamoyloxypropyl)trimethylammonium Chloride, 1487·3
Carbamoylphenoxyacetic Acid, 87·3
(2-Carbamoylphenoxy)acetic Acid, 87·3
(7*R*)-3-(4-Carbamoyl-1-pyridiniomethyl)-7-[2-(2-thienyl)acetamido]-3-cephem-4-carboxylate, 168·2
1-(3-Carbamoylpyridinio)-β-D-ribofuranoside 5-(Adenosine-5′-pyrophosphate), 1719·1
(2*S*)-*N*[(1*S*)-1-[[(2*S*)-2-Carbamoyl-1-pyrrolidinyl]carbonyl]-3-methylbutyl]-6-oxopipecolamide, 1337·2
Carbamylmethylcholine Chloride, 1487·3
$N^{\delta}$-Carbamylornithine, 1425·2
4-Carbamylphenyl Bis[carboxymethylthio]arsenite, 114·1
Carbapenems, 117·3
Carbaril, 1501·2
Carbarilo, 1501·2
Carbaryl, 1501·2
Carbasalate Calcium, 25·1
Carbasalato Cálcico, 25·1
Carbasalatum Calcicum, 25·1
Carbasalatum Calcium, 25·1
Carbaspirin Calcium, 25·1
Carbastat, 1869·1
Carbatil, 1869·1
Carbatrol, 1869·2
Carbaval, 1869·2
Carbazene, 1869·2
Carbazep, 1869·2
Carbazilquinone, 535·1
Carbazina, 1869·2
Carbazochrome, 745·1
Carbazochrome Dihydrate, 745·1
Carbazochrome Salicylate, 745·1
Carbazochrome Sodium Sulfonate, 745·1
Carbazocromo, 745·1
1-(Carbazol-4-yloxy)-3-isopropylaminopropan-2-ol, 880·2
1-Carbazol-4-yloxy-3-[2-(2-methoxyphenoxy)ethylamino]propan-2-ol, 881·1
Carbazotic Acid, 1758·1
Carbecin, 1869·2
Carbellon, 1869·2
Carbem, 1869·2
*Carbenia benedicta*, 1673·3
Carbenicilina Sódica, 166·2
Carbenicillin Disodium, 166·2
Carbenicillin Indanyl Sodium, 166·3
Carbenicillin Phenyl Sodium, 166·3
Carbenicillin Sodium, 166·2
Carbenicillinum Natricum, 166·2
Carbenin, 1869·2
Carbenoxolona Sódica, 1254·3
Carbenoxolone Sodium, 1254·3
Carbetapentane, 1126·2
Carbetapentane Citrate, 1126·2
Carbetocin, 1320·2
Carbetocina, 1320·2
Carbex, 1869·2
Carbi, 1869·2
Carbicalcin, 1869·2
Carbidol, 1869·2
Carbidopa, 1204·3
Carbidopum, 1204·3
Carbilev, 1869·2
Carbimazol, 1596·2
Carbimazole, 1596·2
Carbimazolum, 1596·2
Carbimida Cálcica, 1664·2
Carbimide, 1664·2
Carbinib, 1869·2
Carbinoxamina, Maleato de, 426·3
Carbinoxamine Compound, 1869·2
Carbinoxamine Maleate, 426·3
Carbinoxamine Polistirex, 426·3
Carbiset, 1869·2
Carbistad, 1869·2
Carbium, 1869·2
Carbloc, 1869·2
Carbo, 1869·2
Carbo Activatus, 1030·2
Carbo Konigsfeld, 1869·2
Carbo Ligni, 1031·1
Carbo Veg, 1869·2
Carbobel, 1869·2
Carbocain, 1869·2
Carbocaina, 1869·2
Carbocaine, 1869·3
Carbocaine with Neo-Cobefrin, 1869·3
Carbocal, 1869·3
Carbocal D, 1869·3
Carbocalcitonin, 768·3
Carbocin, 1869·3
Carbocisteína, 1116·2
Carbocisteína Sódica, 1116·3
Carbocisteine, 1116·2
Carbocisteine Lysine, 1116·3
Carbocisteine Sodium, 1116·3
Carbocisteinum, 1116·2
Carbocit, 1869·3
Carbocromen Hydrochloride, 880·2
Carbocromeno, Hidrocloruro de, 880·2
Carbocuona, 535·1
Carbocysteine, 1116·2
Carbocysteine Sodium, 1116·3
Carbodec, 1869·3
Carbodec DM, 1869·3
Carbodex DM, 1869·3
Carbo-Dome, 1869·3
Carbofan, 1869·3
Carboflex, 1869·3
Carbofos, 1507·1
Carbogasol, 1869·3
Carbogasol Antiacido, 1869·3
Carbogasol Digestivo, 1869·3

Carbogasol Forte, 1869·3
Carbohydrate-Free Mixture, 1869·3
Carbohydrates, 1417·1
Carbo-Levedo, 1869·3
Carbolevure, 1869·3
Carbolic Acid, 1188·1
Carbolidine Hydrochloride, 1756·3
Carbolim, 1869·3
Carbolit, 1869·3
Carbolith, 1869·3
Carbolithium, 1869·4
Carbolitium, 1869·4
Carbomer 934, 1577·3
Carbomer 934P, 1577·3
Carbomer 940, 1577·3
Carbomer 941, 1577·3
Carbomer 1342, 1577·3
Carbomer Copolymer, 1577·3
Carbomer Interpolymer, 1577·3
Carbomera, 1577·2
Carbómeros, 1577·2
Carbomers, 1577·2
Carbomix, 1869·4
Carbomox, 1869·4
Ca-R-Bon, 1869·4
Carbon-11, 1523·1
Carbon-13, 1667·3
Carbon-14, 1523·1
Carbón Adsorbente, 1030·2
Carbon Bisulphide, 1472·1
Carbon Black, 1058·3
Carbon Dioxide, 1235·2
Carbon Dioxide, Solid, 1235·2
Carbon Disulfide, 1472·1
Carbon Disulphide, 1472·1
Carbon Monoxide, 1235·2
Carbon Monoxide $(^{11}C)$, 1523·1
Carbon., Pix, 1159·2
Carbon Tabs, 1869·4
Carbon Tetrachloride, 1472·2
Carbón Vegetal, 1058·3
Carbonated Bupivacaine, 1369·2, 1372·1
Carbonated Lidocaine, 1369·2, 1379·2
Carbonated Lignocaine— *see* Xylocaine, 2389·2
Carbonated Prilocaine, 1369·2
Carbonato Básico de Aluminio, 1249·1
Carbonato de Bismutila, 1252·1
Carbonato de Calcio, 1254·2
Carbonato de Propileno, 1476·3
Carbonato de Sodio Anhidro, 1747·1
Carbonato de Sodio Decahidratado, 1747·2
Carbonato de Sodio Monohidratado, 1747·2
Carbonato Sódico de Dihidroxialuminio, 1261·2
Carbondifer, 1869·4
Carbone Composto, 1869·4
Carbonei Dioxidum, 1235·2
Carbonei Dioxydum, 1235·2
Carbonei Sulfidum, 1472·1
Carbonesia, 1869·4
Carbonet, 1869·4
Carboneum Bisulfuratum, 1472·1
Carboneum Sulfuratum, 1472·1
Carbonex, 1869·4
Carbonic Acid Diamide, 1162·2
Carbonic Acid Gas, 1235·2
Carbonic Anhydrase Inhibiting Diuretics, 811·2
Carbonic Anhydride, 1235·2
Carbonic Dichloride, 1731·1
Carbonis Detergens, Liquor, 1159·2
Carbonis, Pix, 1159·2
Carbono 11, 1523·1
Carbono 13, 1667·3
Carbono 14, 1523·1
Carbonpectate, 1869·4
Carbonyl Chloride, 1731·1
Carbophagix, 1869·4
Carbophos, 1869·4
Carboplat, 1869·4
Carboplatin, 533·3
Carboplatino, 533·3
Carboplatinum, 533·3
Carbopols, 1577·2
Carboprost, 1514·2
Carboprost Methyl, 1514·2
Carboprost Trometamol, 1514·2
Carboprost Tromethamine, 1514·2
Carboquone, 535·1
Carboron, 1869·4
Carbosan, 1869·4
Carbosen, 1869·4
Carboseptol, 1869·4
Carbosin, 1869·4
Carbosint, 1869·4
Carbosol, 1869·4
Carbosorb, 1869·4
Carbosorb S, 1869·4
Carbospare, 1869·4
Carbospect, 1869·4
Carbostesin, 1870·1
Carbosulfan, 1501·2
Carbosylane, 1870·1
Carbosymag, 1870·1
Carbotec, 1870·1
Carboticon, 1870·1
Carbotiol, 1870·1
Carbotop, 1870·1
Carbovir, 660·2
Carbovir Triphosphate, 625·3
Carboxine, 1870·1
Carboxine-PSE, 1870·1
Carboxtie, 1870·1
*p*-Carboxybenzenesulfonamide, 228·2
α-Carboxybenzylpenicillin Sodium, 166·2
2-(2-Carboxy-4-cyano-5-[*N*,*N*-di(carboxymethyl)amino]thiophen-3-yl) Acetic Acid Distrontium Salt, 775·2
1-Carboxy-4,5-dihydroxy-1,3-cyclohexylene Bis(3,4-dihydroxycinnamate), 1678·3
(*Z*)-(*S*)-6-Carboxy-6-[(*S*)-2,2-dimethylcyclopropanecarboxamido]hex-5-enyl-L-cysteine, Monosodium Salt, 188·1
5-[4-(2-Carboxyethylcarbamoyl)phenylazo]salicylic Acid, Disodium Salt, Dihydrate, 1251·2
4-(2-Carboxyethyl)phenyl *trans*-4-Aminomethylcyclohexanecarboxylate Hydrochloride, 1255·2
4-(2-Carboxyethyl)phenyl Tranexamate Hydrochloride, 1255·2
6-{[(4*R*,5*S*,6*S*)-2-Carboxy-6-[(1*R*)-1-hydroxyethyl]-4-methyl-7-oxo-1-azabicyclo[3.2.0]hept-2-en-3-yl]thio}-6,7-dihydro-5*H*-pyrazolo[1,2-*a*]-*s*-triazol-4-ium Hydroxide, Inner Salt, 165·3
(7*R*)-7-[2-Carboxy-2-(4-hydroxyphenyl)acetamido]-7-methoxy-3-(1-methyl-1*H*-tetrazol-5-ylthiomethyl)-1-oxa-3-cephem-4-carboxylic Acid, Disodium Salt, 225·3
(3-Carboxy-2-hydroxypropyl)trimethylammonium Acetate (Ester) Chloride, 1646·1
(3-Carboxy-2-hydroxypropyl)trimethylammonium Hydroxide, Inner Salt, 1423·3
(*R*)-(3-Carboxy-2-hydroxypropyl)trimethylammonium Hydroxide, Inner Salt, 1423·3
4-Carboxyl-4-(*N*-phenylpropionamido)-1-piperidine Propionic Acid Dimethyl Ester Monohydrate, 86·1
3-Carboxymefenamic Acid, 55·3
{3-[2-(Carboxymethoxy)benzamido]-2-methoxypropyl}hydroxymercury, 952·2
9-Carboxymethoxymethylguanine, 627·1
Carboxymethylamylum Natricum, 1582·1
Carboxymethylamylum Natricum A, 1582·1
Carboxymethylamylum Natricum B, 1582·1
Carboxymethylamylum Natricum C, 1582·2
Carboxymethylcellulose, 1577·3
Carboxymethylcellulose Calcium, 1577·3
Carboxymethylcellulose Sodium, 1577·3, 1578·1
Carboxymethylcellulose Sodium 12, 1578·1
Carboxymethylcellulose Sodium, Crosslinked, 1578·1
Carboxymethylcellulose Sodium, Low-Substituted, 1578·1
Carboxymethylcellulose Sodium, Microcrystalline Cellulose and, 1578·3
Carboxymethylcellulosum Natricum, 1577·3
*S*-Carboxymethyl-L-cysteine, 1116·2
1-Carboxymethyl-3-[1-ethoxycarbonyl-3-phenyl-(1*S*)-propylamino]-2,3,4,5-tetrahydro-1*H*-1(3*S*)-benzazepin-2-one Hydrochloride, 867·2
(Carboxymethyl)trimethylammonium Hydroxide Inner Salt, 1660·1
(Carboxymethyl)trimethylammonium Hydroxide Inner Salt Hydrochloride, 1660·2
Carboxynalidixic Acid, 234·3
(6*R*)-6-(2-Carboxy-2-phenylacetamido)penicillanic Acid, 166·2
Carboxyphenylacetamidopenicillanic Acid, Disodium Salt, 166·2
(2*R*,3*S*)-*N*-Carboxy-3-phenylisoserine, *N*-*tert*-Butyl Ester, 13-Ester with 5β-20-Epoxy-1,2α,4,7β,10β,13α-hexahydroxytax-11-en-9-one 4-Acetate 2-Benzoate, 547·1
*N*-{*N*-[(*S*)-1-Carboxy-3-phenylpropyl]-L-alanyl}-L-proline Dihydrate, 909·3
*N*-{*N*-[(*S*)-1-Carboxy-3-phenylpropyl]-L-lysyl}-L-proline Dihydrate, 946·3
Carboxypolymethylene, 1577·2
Carboxyprimaquine, 456·3
3β-(3-Carboxypropionyloxy)-11-oxo-olean-12-en-30-oic Acid, Disodium Salt, 1254·3
Carboxyquinolones, 119·1
Carboxysulfamidochrysoidine, 258·1
Carboxythienylacetamidomethoxypenicillanic Acid, 266·1
(6*S*)-6-[2-Carboxy-2-(3-thienyl)acetamido]-6-methoxypenicillanic Acid, 266·1
Carboxythienylacetamidomethoxypenicillanic Acid, Disodium Salt, 266·1
Carboxyvinyl Polymers, 1577·2
Carboyoghurt, 1870·1
Carbromal, 674·1
Carbutamida, 330·3
Carbutamide, 330·3
Carcinil, 1870·1
Carcinoid Syndrome— *see* Carcinoid Tumours and Other Secretory Neoplasms, 504·1
Cardace, 1870·1
Cardace Comp, 1870·1
Cardactona, 1870·1
Cardalept, 1870·1
Cardalin, 1870·1
Cardamom, 1667·3
Cardamom Fruit, 1667·3
Cardamom Oil, 1668·1
Cardamom Seed, 1667·3
Cardamomi, 1667·3
Cardamomo, Aceite Esencial de, 1668·1
Cardamomo, Fruto del, 1667·3
Cardanat, 1870·1
Cardaxen, 1870·1
Cardaxen Plus, 1870·1
Cardcal, 1870·1
Cardcor, 1870·1
Cardec, 1870·1
Cardec DM, 1870·1
Cardec-S, 1870·1
Cardegic, 1870·1
Cardeloc, 1870·2
Cardem, 1870·2
Cardenalin, 1870·2
Cardene, 1870·2
Cardenol, 1870·2
Cardensiel, 1870·2
Cardepine, 1870·2
Cardeymin, 1870·2
Card-Floe II, 1870·2
Cardiac Arrest— *see* Advanced Cardiac Life Support, 812·2
Cardiac Arrhythmias, 816·1
Cardiac Depressants, 809·2
Cardiac Glycosides, 811·1
Cardiac Inotropes, 811·1
Cardiac Life Support, Advanced— *see* Advanced Cardiac Life Support, 812·2
Cardiace, 1870·2
Cardiacton, 1870·2
Cardiacum PMD, 1870·2
Cardiaforce, 1870·2
Cardiagen, 1870·2
Cardiagen— *see* Kreislauftropen, 2083·4
Cardiagen HCT, 1870·2
Cardialgine, 1870·2
Cardiavis N, 1870·2
Cardiax, 1870·2
Cardiazem, 1870·2
Cardiazidine, 1870·2
Cardiazol-Dicodid, 1870·2
Cardiazol-Paracodina, 1870·2
Cardibisana, 1870·2
Cardibloc, 1870·2
Cardiblok, 1870·2
Cardicon, 1870·2
Cardicor, 1870·2
Cardif Beta, 1870·2
Cardifen, 1870·2
Cardiject, 1870·2
Cardil, 1870·3
Cardilat, 1870·3
Cardilate, 1870·3
Cardilate MR, 1870·3
Cardiloc, 1870·3
Cardilol, 1870·3
Cardimet, 1870·3
Cardin, 1870·3
Cardinit, 1870·3
Cardinol, 1870·3
Cardinorm, 1870·3
Cardinorma, 1870·3
Cardioace, 1870·3
Cardioaspirin, 1870·3
Cardioaspirina, 1870·3
Cardioaspirine, 1870·3
Cardiobil, 1870·3
Cardiobron, 1870·3
Cardiocalm, 1870·3
Cardiocap, 1870·3
Cardiocor, 1870·3
Cardiodisco, 1870·3
Cardiodopa, 1870·3
Cardiodoron, 1870·3
Cardiofort, 1870·3
Cardiofrik, 1870·4
Cardiogen, 1870·4
Cardiogenic Shock— *see* Shock, 835·1
Cardiogoxin, 1870·4
Cardio-Green, 1870·4
Cardioguard, 1870·4
Cardiol, 1870·4
Cardiolan, 1870·4
Cardiolen, 1870·4
Cardiolite, 1870·4
Cardio-Longoral, 1870·4
Cardi-Omega 3, 1870·4
Cardiomin, 1870·4
Cardiomyopathies, 818·2
Cardionatrin, 964·2
Cardionil, 1870·4
Cardionorm, 1870·4
Cardionox, 1870·4
Cardiopina, 1870·4
Cardiopine, 1870·4
Cardio-Plantina, 1870·4
Cardioplegia, 1870·4
Cardioplegia A, 1870·4
Cardioplegia Concentrate, 1870·4
Cardioplegin N, 1870·4
Cardiopril, 1870·4
Cardioprotect, 1870·4
Cardiopulmonary Resuscitation— *see* Advanced Cardiac Life Support, 812·2
Cardioquin, 1870·4
Cardioquine, 1870·4
Cardioreg, 1870·4
Cardioregis, 1870·4
Cardiorex, 1871·1
Cardiorona, 1871·1
Cardiosedantol, 1871·1
Cardioselect N, 1871·1
Cardiosolupsan, 1871·1
Cardiostenol, 1871·1
Cardioten, 1871·1
Cardioton, 1871·1

Cardiotone, 1871·1
Cardiotonicum (Rowo-15), 1871·1
Cardiovas, 1871·1
Cardiovasc, 1871·1
Cardiovascular Drugs, 809·1
Cardiovascular Risk Reduction, 819·1
Cardioxane, 1871·1
Cardioxin, 1871·1
Cardip, 1871·1
Cardiphyt, 1871·1
Cardipin, 1871·1
Cardiplant, 1871·1
Cardipril, 1871·1
Cardiprin, 1871·1
Cardirenal, 1871·1
Cardirene, 1871·1
Cardiser, 1871·1
Cardispan, 1871·1
Cardium, 1871·1
Cardizem, 1871·1
Cardo Santo, 1673·3
Cardol, 1871·1
Cardopar, 1871·1
Cardopax, 1871·2
Cardoral, 1871·2
Cardoxan, 1871·2
Cardoxin, 1871·2
Cardoxone, 1871·2
Cards HCG-Urine, 1871·2
Carduben, 1871·2
Cardular, 1871·2
Cardules, 1871·2
Cardules Plus, 1871·2
Carduokatt N, 1871·2
Cardura, 1871·2
Carduran, 1871·2
*Carduus benedictus*, 1673·3
*Carduus marianus*, 1043·3
Carduus-monoplant, 1871·2
Cardyl, 1871·2
Care 55+ Multi, 1871·2
Careflu, 1871·2
Carencil, 1871·2
Carencyl, 1871·2
Car-3-ene, 1760·1
Carentil, 1871·2
Caresel, 1871·2
Caress, 1871·2
Carexan, 1871·2
Careza, 1871·2
Carfecilina Sódica, 166·3
Carfecillin Sodium, 166·3
Carfentanil Citrate, 25·1
Carfentanilo, Citrato de, 25·1
Carfosid, 1871·2
Carginine, 1871·2
Carglumic Acid, 1668·1
Carglutamic Acid, 1668·1
Cargosil, 1871·2
Cari, Oleum, 1667·3
Cariamyl, 1871·2
Cariban, 1871·2
Carica, 1266·3
*Carica papaya*, 1671·1, 1727·3
Caricef, 1871·2
Caril, 1871·3
Carilax, 1871·3
Carin, 1871·3
Carindacilina Sódica, 166·3
Carindacillin Sodium, 166·3
Carinose, 1871·3
Cariomix, 1871·3
Carisano, 1871·3
Cariso-Co, 1871·3
Carisoma, 1871·3
Carisoma Compound, 1871·3
Carisoprodol, 1392·1
Carisoprodolum, 1392·1
Caristop, 1871·3
Caritasone, 1871·3
Caritec, 1871·3
Carito Mono, 1871·3
Carl Baders Divinal, 1871·3
Carli, 1871·3
Carloc, 1871·3
Carloxan, 1871·3
Carlytene, 1871·3
Carmapine, 1871·3
Carmatis, 1871·3
Carmazin, 1871·3
Carmellose, 1577·3
Carmellose Calcium, 1577·3
Carmellose Sodium, 1577·3
Carmellose Sodium, Low-substituted, 1578·1
Carmellosum Calcicum, 1577·3
Carmellosum Natricum, 1577·3
Carmellosum Natricum Conexum, 1578·1
Carmellosum Natricum, Substitutum Humile, 1578·1
Carmelosa, 1577·3
Carmelosa Cálcica, 1577·3
Carmelosa Sódica, 1577·3
Carmen, 1871·3
Carmian, 1871·3
Carmicide, 1871·3
Carmicina, 1871·3
Carmín, 1057·1
Carminagal N, 1871·3
Carminative, 1871·3
Carminative Tea, 1871·4
Carminativo Ibys, 1871·4
Carminativo Juventus, 1871·4
Carminativum Babynos, 1871·4
Carminativum-Hetterich N, 1871·4
Carminativum-Pascoe, 1871·4
Carmine, 1057·1
Carmine, Indigo, 1700·3
Carminetum, 1871·4
Carminex, 1871·4
Carminic Acid, 1057·1
Carmint, 1871·4
Carmitol, 1871·4
Carmofur, 535·1
Carmoisina, 1057·1
Carmoisine, 1057·1
Carmol, 1871·4
Carmol HC, 1871·4
Carmol Magen-Galle-Darm, 1871·4
Carmubris, 1871·4
Carmustina, 535·1
Carmustine, 535·1
Carmustinum, 535·1
Carnabol, 1871·4
Carnation, 1871·4
Carnauba Wax, 1668·1
Carneferrol, 1871·4
Carnicor, 1871·4
Carnidazol, 603·1
Carnidazole, 603·1
Carnigen, 1871·4
Carnitene, 1871·4
Carnitina, 1423·3
Carnitine, 1423·3
D-Carnitine, 1424·2
DL-Carnitine, 1424·1
L-Carnitine, 1423·3
Carnitine Hydrochloride, 1424·1
Carnitine Orotate, 1424·1, 1724·3
Carnitolo, 1871·4
Carnitop, 1871·4
Carnitor, 1871·4
Carnivora VF, 1871·4
Carnizin, 1872·1
Carnot Colutorio, 1872·1
Carnot Topico, 1872·1
Carnotprim, 1872·1
Carnovis, 1872·1
Carnum, 1872·1
Carob Bean Gum, 1579·1
Carob Gum, 1579·1
Carobel, 1872·1
Caroçuda, 1666·1
Carofril, 1872·1
Carogil, 1872·1
Caroid, 1872·1
Carominthe, 1872·1
Carony Bark, 1678·1
Carotaben, 1872·1
β,β-Carotene, 1422·3
β-Carotene, All-*trans*, 1422·3
β,β-Carotene-4,4′-dione, 1056·3
β,ε-Carotene-3,3′-diyl Dipalmitate, 1765·3
Carotenes, 1056·1
Carotenoids, 1056·1
Carotenoplos, 1872·1
Carotenos, 1872·1
Carotin, 1872·1
Caroube, Gomme de, 1579·1
Caroverina, 1668·1
Caroverine, 1668·1
Caroverine Hydrochloride, 1668·1
Carovit, 1872·1
Carovit Forte, 1872·1
Carovit Melanin, 1872·1
Carovit Repair, 1872·1
Carpal Tunnel Syndrome— *see* Soft-tissue Rheumatism, 11·1
Carpantin, 1872·1
Carperitida, 880·2
Carperitide, 880·2
Carphedon, 1731·1
Carpilo, 1872·1
Carpin, 1872·1
Carpina, Isopto— *see* Isopto Carpina, 2068·3
Carpine, 1872·1
Carpipramina, Hidrocloruro de, 674·2
Carpipramine Hydrochloride, 674·2
Carpo-Miotic, 1872·1
Carprofen, 25·1
Carprofeno, 25·1
Carrageenan, 1578·2
ι-Carrageenan, 1578·2
κ-Carrageenan, 1578·2
λ-Carrageenan, 1578·2
Carrageenin, 1578·2
Carragenina, 1578·2
Carraghénates, 1578·2
Carrasyn, 1872·1
Carreldon, 1872·1
Carrier, 1872·1
Carrot, Wild, 1765·1
Carsuquin, 1872·1
Cartan, 1872·2
Carteabak, 1872·2
Carteol, 1872·2
Carteolol, Hidrocloruro de, 880·3
Carteolol Hydrochloride, 880·3
Carteololi Hydrochloridum, 880·3
Carteopil, 1872·2
Carter Petites Pilules, 1872·2
Carters, 1872·2
Carters Little Pills, 1872·2
Carthamex, 1872·2
Carthami Oleum Raffinatum, 1443·3
*Carthamus tinctorius*, 1443·3
Cartia, 1872·2
Carticaine Hydrochloride, 1370·3
Cartidont, 1872·2
Cartilade, 1872·2
Cartilag, 1872·2
Cartilago Compuesto, 1872·2
Cartisorb, 1872·2
Cartivix, 1872·2
Cartrax, 1872·2
Cartrol, 1872·2
Carudol, 1872·2
Carui, Oleum, 1667·3
Carum, 1667·2
*Carum carvi*, 1667·2
Carumonam Sódico, 166·3
Carumonam Sodium, 166·3
Carvasin, 1872·2
Carvedilol, 881·1
Carvedilolum, 881·1
Carvi, Fructus, 1667·2
Carvi, Oleum, 1667·3
Carvicum, 1872·2
Carvil, 1872·2
Carvipress, 1872·2
Carvis, 1872·2
Carvit, 1872·2
Carvomin, 1872·2
Carvomin Magentropfen mit Pomeranze, 1872·2
Carvone, 1283·2, 1667·3, 1680·2, 1749·1
Carvone, Hydrated, 1130·2
Carylderm, 1872·3
Caryolysine, 1872·3
Caryoph., 1673·2
β-Caryophyllene, 1706·2, 1760·1
Caryophyllene Oxide, 1760·1
Caryophylli Floris Aetheroleum, 1673·3
Caryophylli Flos, 1673·2
Caryophylli, Oleum, 1673·3
Caryophyllum, 1673·2
Carzem, 1872·3
Carzenida, 1668·2
Carzenide, 1668·2
Carzepine, 1872·3
Carzilasa, 1872·3
Carzodelan, 1872·3
CAS-276, 961·3
Casacol, 1872·3
Casalm, 1872·3
Casanthranol, 1255·1
Casantranol, 1255·1
Casbol, 1872·3
Cascade, 1872·3
Cascalax, 1872·3
Cascapride, 1872·3
Cascara, 1255·1
Cascara Sagrada, 1255·1
Cascara Sagrada Puler, 1872·3
Cascara Sagrada Sanaplex, 1872·3
Cascararinde, 1255·1
Cascara-Salax, 1872·3
Cascaroside A, 1255·1
Cascor, 1872·3
Casec, 1872·3
Caseical, 1872·3
Caseincal, 1872·3
Casenfilus, 1872·3
Casfen, 1872·3
Casilan, 1872·3
Casodex, 1872·3
CASOIL, 1668·2
Caspacil, 1872·3
Caspiselenio, 1872·3
Caspofungin Acetate, 395·3
Caspofungina, Acetato de, 395·3
Casprin, 1872·4
Cassadan, 1872·4
Cassava Starch, 1449·2
Cassella-4489, 880·2
*Cassia acutifolia*, 1288·2
*Cassia angustifolia*, 1288·2
Cassia Bark, 1668·2
*Cassia fistula*, 1255·2
Cassia Oil, 1668·2
Cassia Pulp, 1255·2
*Cassia senna*, 1288·2
Cassiae, Oleum, 1668·2
Cassis, 1661·1
Cast— *see* Strabismus, 1487·1
Castaderm, 1872·4
Castanha de India Composta, 1872·4
Castaño de Indias, 1648·2
Castanospermine, 660·2
Castel, 1872·4
Castellani mit Miconazol, 1872·4
Castellani's Paint, 1185·2
Casticin, 1649·1
Castile Soap, 1575·2
Castilium, 1872·4
Castindia, 1872·4
Castor Oil, 1668·2
Castor Oil, Hydrogenated, 1668·2
Castor Oil, Sulfated, 1575·3
Castor Oil, Sulfonated, 1575·3
Castor Oil, Sulphated, 1575·3
Castor Oil, Virgin, 1668·2
Castor Oils, Polyethoxylated, 1414·3
Castor Oils, Polyoxyethylene, 1414·3
Castor Oils, Polyoxyl, 1414·3
Castor Oils, Polyoxyl Hydrogenated, 1414·3
Castoria, 1872·4
Castufemin, 1872·4
Cat Scratch Disease, 123·1
Catabex, 1872·4
Catabex Expectorans, 1872·4
Catabina, 1872·4

Catabina Expectorante, 1872·4
Catabolin, 1701·3
Cataclot, 1872·4
Catacol, 1872·4
Cataflam, 1872·4
Catalasa, 1668·3
Catalase, 1668·3
Catalgem, 1872·4
Catalgine, 1872·4
Catalgix, 1872·4
Catalgix C, 1872·4
Catalin, 1872·4
Catalin Sodium, 1732·2
Catalip, 1872·4
Catamenial Epilepsy— *see* Epilepsy, 349·1
Catamin, 1872·4
Catanac, 1872·4
Cataplexy— *see* Narcoleptic Syndrome, 1583·2
Catapres, 1872·4
Catapres Diu, 1872·4
Catapresan, 1873·1
Catapressan, 1873·1
Cataren, 1873·1
Cataridol, 1873·1
Catarrh, 1873·1
Catarrh Cream, 1873·1
Catarrh Mixture, 1873·1
Catarrh Pastilles, 1873·1
Catarrh Tablets, 1873·1
Catarrh-eeze, 1873·1
Catarrh-Ex, 1873·1
Catarrosan, 1873·1
Catarrosine, 1873·1
Catarstat, 1873·1
Catazyme-P, 1873·1
CAT-Barium (E-Z-CAT), 1873·1
Catechol-*O*-methyltransferase Inhibitors, 1196·1
Catechu, 1668·3
Catechu, Black, 1661·1
Catechu, Pale, 1668·3
Catenulin Sulphate, 612·3
Caterol, 1873·1
Catex, 1873·1
Catha, 1585·2
*Catha edulis*, 1585·2
*Catharanthus roseus*, 591·2, 592·2
Cathartics, 1239·3
Cathejell, 1873·1
Cathejell with Lidocaine, 1873·1
Cathejell mit Lidocain, 1873·1
Cathejell N, 1873·1
Cathejell S, 1873·1
Catheter Care— *see* Injection Site and Catheter Care, 1165·2
Catheter Preparation, 1873·1
Catheter-associated Bladder Infections— *see* Urinary-tract Infections, 153·1
Catheter-associated Infections— *see* Intensive Care, 132·2
Cathine, 1585·2
Cathine Hydrochloride, 1585·2
Cathinone, 1585·2
Catina, 1585·2
Catinona, 1585·2
Cationic Surfactants, 1172·3
Catiz Plus, 1873·2
Catlep, 1873·2
Cato-Bell, 1873·2
Catona, 1873·2
Catonet, 1873·2
Catonin, 1873·2
Catoplin, 1873·2
Catoprol, 1873·2
Catorid, 1873·2
Catovit, 1873·2
Catovit N, 1873·2
Catrix, 1873·2
Catrix Correction, 1873·2
Catrix Lip, 1873·2
Catuaba, 1873·2
Catuama, 1873·2
Caucasian Snowdrop, 1491·2
Caucho, 1741·1
Caudal Block— *see* Central Nerve Block, 1370·1
Caulófilo, 1661·2
Caulophyllum, 1661·2
Caulophyllum Complex, 1873·2
*Caulophyllum thalictroides*, 1661·2
Causalgia— *see* Complex Regional Pain Syndrome, 5·3
Causalon, 1873·2
Causalon Bronquial, 1873·2
Causalon Gesic, 1873·2
Causalon Grip, 1873·2
Causalon Pro, 1873·2
Causat, 1873·2
Causat B12 N, 1873·2
Causat N, 1873·2
Caustic Caramel, 1057·1
Caustic Potash, 1734·2
Caustic Soda, 1747·3
Caustic Sulfite Caramel, 1057·1
Caustinerf Forte, 1873·2
Cauterex, 1873·2
Cauteridol, 1873·2
Caved-S, 1873·3
Caveril, 1873·3
Caverject, 1873·3
Caverta, 1873·3
Caviamina, 1873·3
CaviD, 1873·3
Cavilon, 1873·3
Cavinton, 1873·3
Cavirox, 1873·3
Cavirox Junior, 1873·3
Cavit-D3, 1873·3
Cavodan, 1873·3
Cavodine, 1873·3
Cavumox, 1873·3
Caye Balsam, 1873·3
Cayenne Pepper, 1667·1
Cayenne Plus, 1873·3
Cayeput, Aceite Esencial de, 1664·1
Caziderm, 1873·3
Cazigeran, 1873·3
Cazmar, 1873·3
Cazole, 1873·3
2-CB, 1593·3
16-64 CB, 668·3
CB-154, 1200·3
CB-311, 1327·2
CB-313, 575·1
CB-337, 952·1
CB-1314, 1714·3
CB-1348, 536·1
CB-1678, 440·3
CB-2041, 532·2
CB-3007, 566·1
CB-3025, 566·1
CB-3026, 566·1
CB-4261, 724·1
4306-CB, 685·1
4311-CB, 685·1
CB-8053, 269·2
CB-8089, 671·2
8102-CB, 781·3
CB-8102, 781·3
CB-8129, 418·3
C-48401-Ba, 1103·3
CBA-93626, 26·3
CBDCA, 533·3
C-C2470, 397·2
CCA, 1707·2
C-Calcium, 1873·3
CCI-4725, 1095·2
CCI-5537, 1095·3
CCI-15641, 184·1
CCI-18781, 1102·3
CCK, 1727·2, 1873·3
CCK Flunarizina, 1873·4
CCK-OP, 1746·2
CCK-PZ, 1727·2
CCN, 1373·3
CC-Nefro, 1873·4
CCNU, 565·2, 1873·4
CCRG-81045, 587·1
CCT, 1454·3
CD59, 1675·2
CD-271, 1141·1
CD4 Antibodies, 1668·3
CDCA, 1670·1
CDC/NIIMALVAC-1, 1622·3
CDDD-5604, 1105·3
CDDP, 538·1
C-Destrosio, 1873·4
CDHP, 586·3
CD4mAb, 1668·3
C-Dose, 1873·4
CDP-571, 1743·2
CDP-771, 558·3
CDP-Choline, 1672·3
CDT, 1873·4
CE-264, 1114·2
CE-746, 1121·1
C7E3, 841·3
C7E3 Fab, 841·3
Ceanel, 1873·4
CEA-Scan, 1873·4
Cebedex, 1873·4
Cebedexacol, 1873·4
Cebemyxine, 1873·4
Cebenicol, 1873·4
Cebera, 1873·4
Cebesine, 1873·4
Cebexin, 1873·4
Cebid, 1873·4
Cebiolon, 1873·4
Cebion Preparations, 1873·4
Cebiopirina, 1874·1
Cebolla, 1723·2
Cebolla Albarrana, 1130·3
Cebralat, 1874·1
Cebran, 1874·1
Cebrilin, 1874·1
Cebrocal, 1874·1
Cebrofort, 1874·1
Cebrotex, 1874·1
Cebroton, 1874·1
Cebrotonin, 1874·1
Cebutid, 1874·1
Cec, 1874·1
Cecap, 1874·1
Cecenu, 1874·1
Ceclor, 1874·1
Ceclorbeta, 1874·1
Cecon, 1874·1
Cecrisina, 1874·1
Ced Compl, 1874·1
Cedax, 1874·1
Cedelate, 1874·1
Cedilanid, 1874·1
Cedilanide, 1874·1
Cedine, 1874·1
Cedium, 1874·1
Cedixen, 1874·1
Cedocard, 1874·1
Cedol, 1874·2
Cedozelin, 1874·2
Cedril, 1874·2
Cedril Strumenti, 1874·2
Cedrin, 1874·2
Cedrol, 1874·2
Cedrox, 1874·2
Cedur, 1874·2
Ceelin, 1874·2
CeeNU, 1874·2
Ceerexin, 1874·2
Ceezinc, 1874·2
Cef...— *see also under* Ceph...
CEF-3, 1874·2
CEF-4, 1874·2
Cefa Resan, 1874·2
Cefaben, 1874·2
Cefabene, 1874·2
Cefabiot, 1874·2
Cefabiot— *see* Zolival, 2395·1
Cefabiozim, 1874·2
Cefabol, 1874·2
Cefabrina, 1874·2
Cefabronchin, 1874·2
Cefacar, 1874·2
Cefacar Mucolitico, 1874·2
Cefacene, 1874·2
Cefacet, 1874·2
Cefachol, 1874·3
Cefacidal, 1874·3
Cefacile, 1874·3
Cefacilina, 1874·3
Cefacilina Bronquial, 1874·3
Cefacin-M, 1874·3
Cefaclor, 167·1
Cefaclorum, 167·1
Cefacolin, 1874·3
Cefacor, 1874·3
Cefacure, 1874·3
Cefacynar, 1874·3
Cefade, 1874·3
Cefadel, 1874·3
Cefadian, 1874·3
Cefadin, 1874·3
Cefadol, 1874·3
Cefadolor, 1874·3
Cefadolor H, 1874·3
Cefadrex, 1874·3
Cefadril, 1874·3
Cefadrin, 1874·3
Cefadrox, 1874·3
Cefadroxil, 167·2
Cefadroxil Monohydrate, 167·2
Cefadroxilo, 167·2
Cefadroxilum Monohydricum, 167·2
Cefadroxon, 1874·3
Cefadyn, 1874·3
Cefadysbasin, 1874·3
Cefafloria, 1874·3
Cefagastrin, 1874·3
Cefager, 1874·3
Cefagil, 1874·3
Cefagon, 1874·3
Cefagran, 1874·4
Cefakava, 1874·4
Cefakes, 1874·4
Cefakliman, 1874·4
Cefakliman Mono, 1874·4
Cefakliman N, 1874·4
Cefaktivon, 1874·4
Cefalan, 1874·4
Cefaldina, 1874·4
Cefalektin, 1874·4
Cefalen, 1874·4
Cefalex, 1874·4
Cefalexan, 1874·4
Cefalexgobens, 1874·4
Cefalexi, 1874·4
Cefalexin, 168·1
Cefalexin Hydrochloride, 168·1
Cefalexin Lysine, 168·2
Cefalexin Monohydrate, 168·1
Cefalexin Sodium, 168·2
Cefalexina, 168·1
Cefalexina, Hidrocloruro de, 168·1
Cefalexinum Monohydricum, 168·1
Cefalin, 1874·4
Cefaline Hauth, 1874·4
Cefaline-Pyrazole, 1874·4
Cefalium, 1874·4
Cefaliv, 1874·4
Cefallone, 1874·4
Cefalmin, 1874·4
Cefaloject, 1874·4
Cefalom, 1874·4
Cefalomicina, 1874·4
Cefalonio, 168·2
Cefalonium, 168·2
Cefalor, 1874·4
Cefaloridina, 168·3
Cefaloridine, 168·3
Cefaloridinum, 168·3
Cefalot, 1874·4
Cefalotin Sodium, 168·3
Cefalotina Sódica, 168·3
Cefalotinum Natricum, 168·3
Cefaluffa, 1874·4
Cefalver, 1874·4
Cefalymphat, 1874·4
Cefam, 1875·1
Cefamadar, 1875·1
Cefamandol, 169·3
Cefamandol, Nafato de, 169·3
Cefamandol Sódico, 169·3

Cefamandole, 169·3
Cefamandole Formate Sodium, 169·3
Cefamandole Nafate, 169·3
Cefamandole Sodium, 169·3
Cefamar, 1875·1
Cefamezin, 1875·1
Cefamig, 1875·1
Cefamiso, 1875·1
Cefamox, 1875·1
Cefamusel, 1875·1
Cefanal, 1875·1
Cefanalgin, 1875·1
Cefanephrin, 1875·1
Cefanex, 1875·1
Cefangipect, 1875·1
Cefanorm, 1875·1
Cefaperos, 1875·1
Cefapirin Sodium, 170·2
Cefapirina Sódica, 170·2
Cefapirinum Natricum, 170·2
Cefaporex, 1875·1
Cefapoten, 1875·1
Cefapulmon Mono, 1875·1
Cefarheumin N, 1875·1
Cefarheumin S, 1875·1
Cefariston, 1875·1
Cefasabal, 1875·1
Cefascillan, 1875·1
Cefasedativ, 1875·1
Cefasel, 1875·1
Cefasept, 1875·1
Cefasept Mono, 1875·1
Cefasin, 1875·2
Cefasliymarin, 1875·2
Cefaspasmon N, 1875·2
Cefasporina, 1875·2
Cefassin, 1875·2
Cefastad, 1875·2
Cefasulfon N, 1875·2
Cefatec, 1875·2
Cefatenk, 1875·2
Cefatox, 1875·2
Cefatrex, 1875·2
Cefatrix, 1875·2
Cefatrizina, 170·3
Cefatrizine, 170·3
Cefatrizine Propylene Glycol, 170·3
Cefavale, 1875·2
Cefavora, 1875·2
Cefawell, 1875·2
Cefa-Wolff, 1875·2
Cefax, 1875·2
Cefaxicina, 1875·2
Cefaxim, 1875·2
Cefaxon, 1875·2
Cefaxona, 1875·2
Cefaxone, 1875·2
Cefazil, 1875·2
Cefazillin, 1875·2
Cefazima, 1875·2
Cefazink, 1875·2
Cefazol, 1875·2
Cefazolin, 170·3
Cefazolin Dibenzylamine, 171·2
Cefazolin Sodium, 170·3
Cefazolina, 170·3
Cefazolina Sódica, 170·3
Cefazolinum Natricum, 170·3
Cefazone, 1875·2
Cefbuperazone, 171·2
Cefbuperazone Sodium, 171·2
Cefcapene Pivoxil Hydrochloride, 171·3
Cefdinir, 171·3
Cef-Diolan, 1875·2
Cefditoren Pivoxil, 172·1
Cefec, 1875·2
Cefedrin N— *see* Cefadrin, 1874·3
Cefen, 1875·3
Cefepima, Hidrocloruro de, 172·1
Cefepime Hydrochloride, 172·1
Ceferro, 1875·3
Cefetamet, 172·3
Cefetamet Pivaloyloxymethyl Hydrochloride, 172·3
Cefetamet Pivoxil Hydrochloride, 172·3
Cefexin, 1875·3
Cefimix, 1875·3
Cefin, 1875·3
Cefine, 1875·3
Cefiran, 1875·3
Cefirex, 1875·3
Cefiton, 1875·3
Cefixima, 172·3
Cefixime, 172·3
Cefiximum, 172·3
Cefixoral, 1875·3
Cefizox, 1875·3
Cefkor, 1875·3
Ceflacid, 1875·3
Ceflax, 1875·3
Ceflexin, 1875·3
Ceflin, 1875·3
Ceflour, 1875·3
Cefluprenam, 173·2
Ceflux, 1875·3
Cefmandol, 1875·3
Cefmandoli Nafas, 169·3
Cefmenoxima, Hidrocloruro de, 173·2
Cefmenoxime Hemihydrochloride, 173·2
Cefmenoxime Hydrochloride, 173·2
Cefmetazol, 173·3
Cefmetazol Sódico, 173·3
Cefmetazole, 173·3
Cefmetazole Sodium, 173·3
Cefmetazon, 1875·3
Cefminox Sódico, 174·1
Cefminox Sodium, 174·1
Cefnax, 1875·3
Cefobacter, 1875·3
Cefobid, 1875·3
Cefobis, 1875·3
Cefociclin, 1875·3
Cefoclin, 1875·3
Cefodie, 1875·3
Cefodime, 1875·3
Cefodizima Sódica, 174·1
Cefodizime Sodium, 174·1
Cefodox, 1875·4
Cefofix, 1875·4
Cefogen, 1875·4
Cefoger, 1875·4
Cefogram, 1875·4
Cefok, 1875·4
Cefol, 1875·4
Cefomic, 1875·4
Cefomycin, 1875·4
Cefoneg, 1875·4
Cefonicid Sódico, 174·2
Cefonicid Sodium, 174·2
Cefoper, 1875·4
Cefoperazona Sódica, 174·3
Cefoperazone A, 175·1
Cefoperazone Sodium, 174·3
Cefoperazonum Natricum, 174·3
Cefoplus, 1875·4
Cefoprim, 1875·4
Ceforal, 1875·4
Ceforan, 1875·4
Ceforanida, 175·2
Ceforanide, 175·2
Ceforanide Lysinate, 175·2
Ceforanide Lysine, 175·2
Cefortam, 1875·4
Cefoselis Sulfate, 175·2
Cefoselis Sulphate, 175·2
Cefosint, 1875·4
Cefosporen, 1875·4
Cefosporin, 1875·4
Cefossin, 1875·4
Cefossin H— *see* Cefassin, 1875·2
Cefotan, 1875·4
Cefotax, 1875·4
Cefotaxima Sódica, 175·3
Cefotaxime Sodium, 175·3
Cefotaximum Natricum, 175·3
Cefotetan, 177·1
Cefotetán Disódico, 177·1
Cefotetan Disodium, 177·1
Cefotex, 1875·4
Cefotiam Hexetil Hydrochloride, 177·2
Cefotiam, Hidrocloruro de, 177·2
Cefotiam Hydrochloride, 177·2
Cefotrizin, 1875·4
Cefovis, 1876·1
Cefovit, 1876·1
Cefoxan, 1876·1
Cefoxin, 1876·1
Cefoxitin Sodium, 177·2
Cefoxitina Sódica, 177·2
Cefoxitinum Natricum, 177·2
Cefozone, 1876·1
Cefozopran Hydrochloride, 178·2
Cefpiramida, 178·2
Cefpiramida Sódica, 178·2
Cefpiramide, 178·2
Cefpiramide Sodium, 178·2
Cefpiroma, Sulfato de, 178·2
Cefpirome Sulfate, 178·2
Cefpirome Sulphate, 178·2
Cefpodoxima Proxetilo, 178·3
Cefpodoxime Proxetil, 178·3
Cefprenam, 173·2
Cefprozil, 179·2
Cefprozilo, 179·2
Cefquinome Sulfate, 179·3
Cefquinome Sulphate, 179·3
Cefra, 1876·1
Cefrabiotic, 1876·1
Cefraden, 1876·1
Cefradil, 1876·1
Cefradina, 179·3
Cefradine, 179·3
Cefradinum, 179·3
Cefradur, 1876·1
Cefral, 1876·1
Cefril, 1876·1
Cefrin, 1876·1
Cefrom, 1876·1
Cefron, 1876·1
Cefspan, 1876·1
Cefsulodin Sodium, 180·2
Cefsulodina Sódica, 180·2
Ceft, 1876·1
Ceftaran, 1876·1
Ceftazidima, 180·2
Ceftazidime, 180·2
Ceftazidime Arginine, 180·3
Ceftazidime Sodium, 180·3
Ceftazidimum, 180·2
Ceftazidon, 1876·1
Ceftazin, 1876·1
Ceften, 1876·1
Cefteram Pivoxil, 181·3
Ceftezol Sódico, 182·1
Ceftezole Sodium, 182·1
Ceftibuten, 182·1
Ceftibuteno, 182·1
Ceftidin, 1876·1
Ceftim, 1876·1
Ceftin, 1876·1
Ceftina, 1876·1
Ceftiofur Hydrochloride, 182·2
Ceftiofur Sódico, 182·2
Ceftiofur Sodium, 182·2
Ceftix, 1876·1
Ceftizon, 1876·1
Ceftizoxima Sódica, 182·2
Ceftizoxime Sodium, 182·2
Cefton, 1876·1
Ceftoral, 1876·2
Ceftrat, 1876·2
Ceftrex, 1876·2
Ceftriax, 1876·2
Ceftriaxona Sódica, 182·3
Ceftriaxone Sodium, 182·3
Ceftriaxonum Natricum, 182·3
Ceftriaz, 1876·2
Ceftrilem, 1876·2
Ceftrinal, 1876·2
Ceftriphin, 1876·2
Cefudura, 1876·2
Cefuhexal, 1876·2
Cefulton, 1876·2
Cefumax, 1876·2
Cefunk, 1876·2
Cefur, 1876·2
Cefuracet, 1876·2
Cefurax, 1876·2
Cefurex, 1876·2
Cefurim, 1876·2
Cefurin, 1876·2
Cefuro-Puren, 1876·2
Cefurox, 1876·2
Cefuroxima, 184·1
Cefuroxima Axetilo, 184·1
Cefuroxima Sódica, 184·1
Cefuroxime, 184·1
Cefuroxime Axetil, 184·1
Cefuroxime Sodium, 184·1
Cefuroximum Axetili, 184·1
Cefuroximum Natricum, 184·1
Cefurox-Reu, 1876·2
Cefurox-Wolff, 1876·2
Cefuzime, 1876·2
Cefxin, 1876·2
Cefxitin, 1876·2
Cefzil, 1876·2
Cefzon, 1876·2
Ceglution, 1876·2
Cegripe, 1876·3
Cegrovit, 1876·3
Cehafolin, 1876·3
Cehapark, 1876·3
Cehasol, 1876·3
Ceklin, 1876·3
Celacefato, 1578·2
Celamine, 1876·3
Celance, 1876·3
Celandine, Greater, 1695·3
Celanide, 945·1
Celanidum, 945·1
Celapram, 1876·3
Celco, 1876·3
Celcox, 1876·3
Celebra, 1876·3
Celebrex, 1876·3
Celecoxib, 25·2
Celectol, 1876·3
Celemax, 1876·3
Celemin, 1876·3
Celen, 1876·3
Celenid, 1876·3
Celery, 1669·1
Celesdepot, 1876·3
Celesemine, 1876·3
Celestamil, 1876·3
Celestamin, 1876·3
Celestamine, 1876·3
Celestamine N, 1876·3
Celestamine NS, 1876·4
Celestamine-F, 1876·4
Celestamine-L, 1876·4
Celestan, 1876·4
Celestan Depot, 1876·4
Celestan, Solu— *see* Solu-Celestan, 2298·1
Celestan Solubile, 1876·4
Celestan-V, 1876·4
Celestan-V, Sulmycin mit— *see* Sulmycin mit Celestan-V, 2312·1
Celestene, 1876·4
Celestene Chronodose, 1876·4
Celestial Seasonings, 1876·4
Celestoderm, 1876·4
Celestoderm cum Chinoform, 1876·4
Celestoderm cum Garamycin, 1876·4
Celestoderm Gentamicina, 1876·4
Celestoderm met Neomycine, 1876·4
Celestoderm-V, 1876·4
Celestoderm-V with Garamycin, 1876·4
Celestoderm-V with Neomycin, 1876·4
Celestoform, 1876·4
Celeston, 1876·4
Celeston Bifas, 1876·4
Celeston Chronodose, 1877·1
Celeston Med Chinoform, 1877·1
Celeston Valerat, 1877·1
Celeston Valerat Comp, 1877·1
Celeston Valerat Med Chinoform, 1877·1
Celeston Valerat Med Gentamicin, 1877·1
Celestone, 1877·1
Celestone Chronodose, 1877·1
Celestone Cronodose, 1877·1
Celestone M, 1877·1

Celestone S, 1877·1
Celestone Soluspan, 1877·1
Celestone V, 1877·1
Celestone VG, 1877·1
Celevac, 1877·1
Celex, 1877·1
Celexa, 1877·1
Celexin, 1877·1
Celfax, 1877·1
Celib, 1877·1
Celidonia, 1695·3
Celidonia Menor, 1732·1
Ce-Limo, 1877·1
Ce-Limo Plus 10 Vitamine, 1877·1
Ce-Limo-Calcium, 1877·1
Celin, 1877·1
Celipro, 1877·1
Celiprolol, Hidrocloruro de, 881·3
Celiprolol Hydrochloride, 881·3
Celiprololi Hydrochloridum, 881·3
Celit, 1877·2
Celkalm, 1877·2
Cellacefate, 1578·2
Cellacephate, 1578·2
Cellasene, 1877·2
Cellavie, 1877·2
Cellblastin, 1877·2
CellCept, 1877·2
Cellcristin, 1877·2
Cellferon, 1877·2
Cellidrin, 1877·2
Cellidrine, 1877·2
Cellmustin, 1877·2
Cellobexon, 1877·2
Cellobiose, 1669·1
Celloid Compounds Magcal Plus, 1877·2
Celloid Compounds Sodical Plus, 1877·2
Celloids Preparations, 1877·2
Celltop, 1877·2
Cellufresh, 1877·2
Cellugel, 1877·2
Cellular Formula, 1877·2
Cellulase, 1669·1
Cellulin Retinale, 1877·2
Cellulitis— *see* Skin Infections, 146·2
Cellulolytic Enzymes, 1669·1
Cellulone, 1877·2
Cellulosa Microgranulare, 1578·3
Cellulose, 1578·3
Cellulose Acetate Phthalate, 1578·2
Cellulose, Dispersible, 1578·3
Cellulose Ethyl Ether, 1579·1
Cellulose Gel, 1578·3
Cellulose Gum, 1577·3
Cellulose Gum, Modified, 1578·1
Cellulose, Microcrystalline, 1578·3
Cellulose, Microcrystalline, and Carboxymethylcellulose Sodium, 1578·3
Cellulose Nitrate, 1156·2
Cellulose, Oxidised, 757·1
Cellulose, Oxidized, 757·1
Cellulose, Oxidized Regenerated, 757·2
Cellulose Powder, 1578·3
Cellulose, Powdered, 1578·3
Cellulose Sodium Phosphate, 1052·1
Cellulose Tetranitrate, 1156·3
Cellulosi Acetas Phthalas, 1578·2
Cellulosi Pulvis, 1578·3
Cellulosic Acid, 757·1
Cellulosum Acetylphthalicum, 1578·2
Cellulosum Microcrystallinum, 1578·3
Celluson, 1877·2
Celluspan, 1877·3
Celluvisc, 1877·3
Cellvital, 1877·3
Celmoleukin, 562·3
Celnium, 1877·3
Celobar, 1877·3
Celocurin, 1877·3
Celocurine, 1877·3
Celoftal, 1877·3
Celol, 1877·3
Celontin, 1877·3
Celophthalum, 1578·2
Celucrem, 1877·3
Cel-U-Jec, 1877·3
Celulasa, 1669·1
Celulase, 1877·3
Celulase con Neomicina, 1877·3
Celulase Plus, 1877·3
Celulosa, 1578·3
Celulosa Dispersable, 1578·3
Celulosa en Polvo, 1578·3
Celulosa, Fosfato Sódico de, 1052·1
Celulosa Microcristalina, 1578·3
Celulosa Oxidada, 757·1
Celulose, 1877·3
Celumax, 1877·3
Celupan, 1877·3
Celuvital, 1877·3
Celvista, 1877·3
Cemac B12, 1877·3
Cemado, 1877·3
Cemaflavone, 1877·3
Cemalyt, 1877·3
Cemaquin, 1877·3
Cementin, 1877·3
Cemetol, 1877·3
Cemidin, 1877·4
Cemidon, 1877·4
Cemidon B6, 1877·4
Cemina, 1877·4
Cemirit, 1877·4
Cemol, 1877·4
Cenacert, 1877·4
Cenafed, 1877·4
Cenafed Plus, 1877·4
Cenai, 1877·4
Cena-K, 1877·4
Cenalfan, 1877·4
Cenalfan Plus, 1877·4
Cenat, 1877·4
Cencamet, 1877·4
Cencopan, 1877·4
Cendalon, 1877·4
Ceneo, 1877·4
Cenestin, 1877·4
Cenevit, 1877·4
Cenilene, 1877·4
Cenizas de Soda, 1747·1
Cenlidac, 1877·4
Cennlacs, 1877·4
Cenogen Ultra, 1877·4
Cenogen-OB, 1877·4
Cenol, 1877·4
Cenolate, 1877·4
Cenpine, 1877·4
Centa Vite, 1877·4
Centabel, 1877·4
Centagin, 1877·4
Centany, 1877·4
Centapp, 1877·4
Centáurea Menor, 1669·2
Centaurea (Specie Composta), 1878·1
Centaurii Minoris Herba, 1669·2
*Centaurium erythraea*, 1669·2
*Centaurium minus*, 1669·2
*Centaurium umbellatum*, 1669·2
Centaury, 1669·2
Centchroman, 1564·3
Centella, 1144·3
*Centella asiatica*, 1144·3
Centella Complex, 1878·1
Centella Queen Complex, 1878·1
Centella Queen Reductora, 1878·1
Centellae Asiaticae Herba, 1144·3
Centellase, 1878·1
Centella-Vit, 1878·1
Center-Al, 1878·1
Centerfen, 1878·1
Centeril H, 1878·1
Centica, 1878·1
Centilux, 1878·1
CenTNF, 50·1
Centra Acid, 1878·1
Centra Acid Plus, 1878·1
Centrac, 1878·1
Centracetam, 1878·1
Centracol, 1878·1
Centracol DM, 1878·1
Centracol Pediatrique, 1878·1
Central Nerve Block, 1370·1
Central Pain— *see* Central Post-stroke Pain, 5·3
Centralgine, 1878·1
Centralgol, 1878·1
Centrally Acting Antihypertensives, 811·2
Centramin, 1878·1
Centramina, 1878·1
Centratuss DM, 1878·1
Centratuss DM Expectorant, 1878·1
Centratuss DM-D, 1878·1
Centrax, 1878·1
Centromicina, 1878·1
Centron, 1878·2
Centrophene, 1878·2
Centrophenoxine Hydrochloride, 1710·1
Centrovite, 1878·2
Centrum, 1878·2
Centural Gold, 1878·2
Centurion A–Z, 1878·2
Centyl, 1878·2
Centyl K, 1878·2
Centyl K, Low— *see* Low Centyl K, 2106·3
Centyl Med Kaliumklorid, 1878·2
Ceolat, 1878·2
Ceolat Compositum, 1878·2
Ceo-Two, 1878·2
Ceoxil, 1878·2
Ceoxx, 1878·2
CEP-151, 1338·3
CEP-1538, 1591·1
Cepa Med Complex, 1878·2
Cepacaina, 1878·2
Cepacaine, 1878·2
Cepacilina, 1878·2
Cepacilina 633, 1878·2
Cepacol Preparations, 1878·2
Cepacol, Childrens— *see* Childrens Cepacol, 1882·4
Cepadont, 1878·3
Cepadyne, 1878·3
Cepal, 1878·3
Cepasium, 1878·3
Cepastat, 1878·3
Cepastat Cherry, 1878·4
Cepazine, 1878·4
Cepevit, 1878·4
Cepexin, 1878·4
Ceph...— *see also under* Cef...
CEPH, 1015·1
Cephadol, 1878·4
Cephadroxil, 167·2
Cephaëline, 605·1
Cephaeline, 1122·3
*Cephaelis acuminata*, 1122·3
*Cephaelis ipecacuanha*, 1122·3
Cephalalgia, Histaminic— *see* Cluster Headache, 464·1
Cephalen, 1878·4
Cephalex, 1878·4
Cephalexin, 168·1
Cephalexin Hydrochloride, 168·1
Cephalexyl, 1878·4
Cephalgan, 1878·4
Cephalobene, 1878·4
Cephalodoc, 1878·4
Cephalonium, 168·2
Cephaloplant, 1878·4
Cephaloridine, 168·3
Cephalosporin C, 117·2
Cephalosporins, 117·2
*Cephalosporium acremonium*, 117·2
Cephalotaxine 2-(Methoxycarbonylmethyl)-2,6-dihydroxy-5-methylheptanoate, 558·3
*Cephalotaxus harringtonia*, 558·3
Cephalothin Sodium, 168·3
Cephamandole, 169·3
Cephamandole Nafate, 169·3
Cephamandole Sodium, 169·3
Cephamycin C, 117·3
Cephamycins, 117·3
Cephanmycin, 1878·4
Cephanol, 1878·4
Cephapirin Benzathine, 170·2
Cephapirin Sodium, 170·2
Cephaxin, 1878·4
Cephazolin, 170·3
Cephazolin Sodium, 170·3
Ceph-Biocin, 1878·4
Cephem Antibacterials, 117·2
Cephin, 1878·4
Cephoral, 1878·4
Cephos, 1878·4
Cephradine, 179·3
Cephulac, 1878·4
Cephyl, 1878·4
Cepifran, 1878·4
Cepim, 1878·4
Cepimex, 1878·4
Ceplac, 1878·4
Cepodem, 1878·4
Ceporacin, 1878·4
Ceporan, 1878·4
Ceporex, 1878·4
Ceporexin, 1879·1
Ceporexine, 1879·1
Ceposil, 1879·1
Cepral, 1879·1
Ceprandal, 1879·1
Ceprater, 1879·1
Ceprazol, 1879·1
Ceprimax, 1879·1
Ceprin, 1879·1
Ceprofen, 1879·1
Ceprotin, 1879·1
Ceprovit, 1879·1
Ceptaz, 1879·1
Cepton, 1879·1
Cequinyl, 1879·1
Cera Alba, 1480·1
Cêra Amarela, 1480·2
Cera Amarilla, 1480·2
Cera Blanca, 1480·1
Cêra Branca, 1480·1
Cera Carnauba, 1668·1
Cera Coperniciae, 1668·1
Cera de Abejas, 1480·1
Cera de Abejas Amarilla, 1480·2
Cera de Carnauba, 1668·1
Cera de Ésteres Cetílicos, 1480·3
Cera Emulsificans, 1481·1
Cera Emulsionante, 1481·1
Cera Flava, 1480·2
Cera Lanae, 1483·1
Cera Microcristalina, 1481·3
Ceractiv, 1879·1
Ceradolan, 1879·1
Ceralan, 1879·1
Ceralip, 1879·1
Ceramide Glucosidase, 1649·1
Cerasorb, 1879·1
Cerasus, 1058·1
Cerat., 1579·1
Cerat Inalterable, 1879·1
Ceratonia, 1579·1
Ceratonia Gum, 1579·1
*Ceratonia siliqua*, 1579·1
Cerax, 1879·1
Cerazet, 1879·1
Cerazette, 1879·1
Cerbon, 1879·1
Cercon, 1879·1
Cere, 1879·1
Cerebokan, 1879·2
Cerebral Infarction— *see* Stroke, 836·1
Cerebral Oedema, High-altitude— *see* High-altitude Disorders, 822·2
Cerebral-Do, 1879·2
Cerebramed, 1879·2
Cerebrex, 1879·2
Cerebrino, 1879·2
Cerebroad, 1879·2
Cerebroforte, 1879·2
Cerebrol, 1879·2
Cerebrol Sans Codeine, 1879·2
Cerebrolysin, 1879·2
Cerebrolysin— *see* Ambotonin, 1792·1
Cerebropan, 1879·2
Cerebrotonin, 1879·2
Cerebrovascular Accident— *see* Stroke, 836·1
Cerebrovascular Disease, 820·2

Cerebrovascular Insufficiency— *see* Cerebrovascular Disease, 820·2
Cerebroxine, 1879·2
Cerebryl, 1879·2
Cerebyx, 1879·2
Ceredase, 1879·2
Cereginkgo, 1879·2
Ceregumil, 1879·2
Cerekinon, 1879·2
Cerelac, 1879·2
Cerella, 1879·2
Cereloid, 1879·2
Cereluc, 1879·2
Ceremin, 1879·2
Cereneu, 1879·2
Cereon, 1879·2
Cerepar, 1879·3
Cerepar N, 1879·3
Cereron, 1879·3
Cerestabon, 1879·3
Cerestar, 1879·3
Ceretec, 1879·3
Cereus, 1669·2
Cerevisiae Fermentum Siccatum, 1469·1
Cerevon, 1879·3
Cerexin, 1879·3
Cerezyme, 1879·3
Cergem, 1879·3
Cergodun, 1879·3
Ceridal, 1879·3
Cerina, 1879·3
Ceri-Nutrina, 1879·3
Ceris, 1879·3
Cerise Rouge, 1058·1
Cerium Nitrate, 1144·3
Cerium Oxalate, 1255·2
Cerivastatin Sodium, 881·3
Cerivastatina Sódica, 881·3
Cerivikehl, 1879·3
1709-CERM, 438·1
CERM-1978, 868·1
CERM-3024, 1132·3
CERM-10202, 96·3
Cermox, 1879·3
Cernevit, 1879·3
Cernilton, 1879·3
Cernitin GBX— *see* Prostaflor, 2241·4
Cernitin T— *see* Prostaflor, 2241·4
Cernitin T-60— *see* Cernilton, 1879·3
Cerofene, 1879·3
Cerose DM, 1879·3
Cerotto Bertelli Arnikos, 1879·3
Cerous Nitrate, 1144·3
Cerous Oxalate, 1255·2
Cerovite, 1879·3
Cerox, 1879·3
Ceroxmed Steril, 1879·3
Cerson, 1879·3
Certagen, 1879·3
Certagen Senior, 1879·3
Certalac, 1879·3
Certa-Vite, 1879·4
Certified Decongestant, 1879·4
Certified Ice, 1879·4
Certified Nasal, 1879·4
Certiva, 1879·4
Certobil, 1879·4
Certomycin, 1879·4
Certonal, 1879·4
Certoparin, 882·1
Certoparin Sodium, 882·1
Certoparina Sódica, 882·1
Certovermil, 1879·4
Certuss, 1879·4
Ceru Spray, 1879·4
Cerubidin, 1879·4
Cerubidine, 1879·4
Cerucal, 1879·4
Cerulein, 1669·2
Ceruleinum, 1700·3
Ceruletida, 1669·2
Ceruletide, 1669·2
Ceruletide Diethylamine, 1669·2
Cerulisina, 1879·4
Cerulyse, 1879·4
Cerumenex, 1879·4
Cerumenex N, 1879·4
Cerumenol, 1879·4
Cerumenol— *see* Cerumol, 1879·4
Cerumex, 1879·4
Cerumin, 1879·4
Cerumol, 1879·4
Cerutil, 1880·1
Ceruxim, 1880·1
Cervagem, 1880·1
Cervageme, 1880·1
Cervasta, 1880·1
Cerveja, Fermento de, 1469·1
Cervekanin, 1880·1
Cervep, 1880·1
Cervical Cancer— *see* Malignant Neoplasms of the Cervix, 515·3
Cervical Dystonia— *see* Spasmodic Torticollis, 1391·1
Cervical Ripening— *see* Labour Induction and Augmentation, 1511·1
Cervicitis, 123·2
Cervidil, 1880·1
Cervilan, 1880·1
Cervilane, 1880·1
Cervinca, 1880·1
Cerviprime, 1880·1
Cerviprost, 1880·1
Cervitec, 1880·1
Cervonic Acid, 976·2
Cervoxan, 1880·1
Cervusen, 1880·1
CES, 1880·1
Cesamet, 1880·1
Cesbron, 1880·1
Cesol, 1880·1
Cesoline, 1880·1
Cesplon, 1880·1
Cesplon Plus, 1880·1
Cesradyston, 1880·1
Cesran, 1880·1
Cesrasanol, 1880·1
Cessagripe, 1880·1
Cessatosse, 1880·2
Cessaverm, 1880·2
Cestode Infections, 97·1
Cestop, 1880·2
Cestop B, 1880·2
Cestox, 1880·2
Ceta, 1880·2
Ceta Plus, 1880·2
Ceta Sulfa, 1880·2
Cetabon, 1880·2
Cetacaine, 1880·2
Cetacort, 1880·2
Cetafeine, 1880·2
Cetafrin, 1880·2
Cetal, 1880·2
Cetalconio, Cloruro de, 1172·1
Cetalkonium Bromide, 1172·1
Cetalkonium Chloride, 1172·1
Cetam, 1880·2
Cetamide, 1880·2
Cetamine, 1880·2
Cetampril, 1880·2
Cetan, 1880·2
Cetanol, 1480·3
Cetanorm, 1880·2
Cetaphil, 1880·2
Cetaphil Daily Facial, 1880·2
Cetapred, 1880·2
Cetapril, 1880·2
Cetasil, 1880·2
Cetavlex, 1880·2
Cetavlon, 1880·3
Cetaxim, 1880·3
Cetaz, 1880·3
Cetazin, 1880·3
Cetearyl Alcohol, 1480·2
Cetebe, 1880·3
Cetexonio, Bromuro de, 1172·1
Cethexonium Bromide, 1172·1
Cethromycin, 185·1
Ceti, 1880·3
Cetidura, 1880·3
Cetiedil Citrate, 882·1
Cetiedil, Citrato de, 882·1
Cetihis, 1880·3
Cetildrops, 1880·3
Cetilpiridinio, Cloruro de, 1173·1
Cetilsan, 1880·3
Cetimil, 1880·3
Cetina, 1880·3
Cetiprin, 1880·3
Cetiprin Novum, 1880·3
Cetiram, 1880·3
Cetirizina, Hidrocloruro de, 427·1
Cetirizine Dihydrochloride, 427·1
Cetirizine Hydrochloride, 427·1
Cetirizini Dihydrochloridum, 427·1
Cetirlan, 1880·3
Cetirocol, 1880·3
Cetiva AE, 1880·3
Cetobemidone Hydrochloride, 51·1
Cetobemidoni Hydrochloridum, 51·1
Cetobeta, 1880·3
Cetocort, 1880·3
Cetoestearilsulfato de Sodio, 1574·2
Cetoglutaran, 1880·3
Cetohexal, 1880·3
Cetomacrogol 1000, 1412·2
Cetomed, 1880·3
Cetona Plus, 1880·3
Cetonax, 1880·3
Cetoneo, 1880·3
Cetonil, 1880·3
Cetoquina Y, 1880·3
Cetornan, 1880·4
Cetostearyl Alc., 1480·2
Cetostearyl Alcohol, 1480·2, 1480·3
Cetostearyl Alcohol (Type A), Emulsifying, 1480·2
Cetostearyl Alcohol (Type B), Emulsifying, 1480·3
Cetoteron, 1880·4
Cetovinca, 1880·4
Cetoxil, 1880·4
Cetoxol, 1880·4
Cetozan, 1880·4
Cetozol, 1880·4
Cetozone, 1880·4
Cetraben, 1880·4
Cetraben Bath Oil, 1880·4
Cetralon, 1880·4
Cetraria Salbe, 1880·4
Cetraxal, 1880·4
Cetraxal Plus, 1880·4
Cetraxate Hydrochloride, 1255·2
Cetraxato, Hidrocloruro de, 1255·2
Cetrazil, 1880·4
Cetrexidin, 1880·4
Cetriderm con Triclosan, 1880·4
Cetrilan, 1880·4
Cetriler, 1880·4
Cetriler D, 1880·4
Cetrimed, 1880·4
Cetrimida, 1172·1
Cetrimide, 1172·1
Cetrimide Solution, Strong, 1172·2
Cetrimidum, 1172·1
Cetrimonio, Bromuro de, 1173·1
Cetrimonium Bromide, 1172·1, 1173·1
Cetrimonium Chloride, 1173·1
Cetrimonium Tosilate, 1173·1
Cetrin, 1880·4
Cetrine, 1880·4
Cetrinets, 1880·4
Cetrinox, 1880·4
Cetrisan, 1880·4
Cetriwal, 1880·4
Cetrizet, 1880·4
Cetrizin, 1880·4
Cetrolac, 1881·1
Cetron, 1881·1
Cetrorelix Acetate, 1320·2
Cetrorelix Embonate, 1320·3
Cetrotide, 1881·1
Cetuximab, 536·1
Cetyl Alcohol, 1480·3
Cetyl Esters Wax, 1480·3
Cetylamine Hydrofluoride, 1434·2
Cetylanum, 1481·1
Cetylcide II, 1881·1
Cetylcide-G, 1881·1
Cetylpyridinii Chloridum, 1173·1
Cetylpyridinium Chloride, 1173·1
Cetylstearylalkohol, 1480·2
Cetylstearylschwefelsaures Natrium, 1574·2
Cetyltrimethylammonium Bromide, 1173·1
Cetylyre, 1881·1
Cetynol, 1881·1
Cevaderm, 1881·1
Cevalin, 1881·1
Cevanil, 1881·1
Cevi-Bid, 1881·1
Cevicort, 1881·1
Cevi-drops, 1881·1
Cevi-Fer, 1881·1
Cevigen, 1881·1
Cevimelina, Hidrocloruro de, 1488·3
Cevimeline Hydrochloride, 1488·3
Cevinolon, 1881·1
Cevirin, 1881·1
Ceviron, 1881·1
Cevita, 1881·1
Cevi-Tabs, 1881·1
Cevitamic Acid, 1460·2
Cevitol, 1881·1
Ceviton, 1881·1
Cewin, 1881·1
Cexidal Otico, 1881·1
Ceylon Cinnamon, 1672·2
Ceylon Cinnamon Bark Oil, 1672·2
Ceylonzimt, 1672·2
Cezane, 1881·1
Cezin, 1881·1
Cezolin, 1881·1
Cezox, 1881·2
CF Vite, 1881·2
CFC-11, 1236·1
CFC-12, 1236·1
CFC-114, 1235·3
CFCs, 1235·3
C-Film, 1881·2
C-Flox, 1881·2
C-Floxacin, 1881·2
CG, 1320·3
C-G, 1881·2
CG-315, 94·3
CG-5501, 216·2
CGA-18809, 1500·2
CGA-23654, 110·2
CGA-50439, 1502·3
CGA-72662, 1503·1
CGA-157419, 1505·3
CGA-179246, 110·1
CGA-184699, 1507·1
CGA-192357, 1502·3
CG-315E, 94·3
CGP-6140, 102·3
CGP-14458, 1111·3
CGP-30694, 550·1
CGP-32349, 557·1
CGP-33101, 377·3
CGP-39393, 892·3
CGP-42446, 776·2
CGP-48933, 1018·3
CGP-11305A, 287·2
CGP-23339A, 773·3
CGP-25827A, 786·1
CGP-42446A, 776·2
CGP-23339AE, 773·3
CGP-57-148B, 562·1
CGP-7760B, 986·3
CGP-42446B, 776·2
CGP-45840B, 32·1
CGP-2175C, 956·3
CGP-2175E, 957·1
CGP-7174E, 180·2
CGP-14221E, 177·2
CGP-18684/E, 878·2
CGP-21690E, 1725·2
CGRP, 878·3
CGS-16949, 553·1
CGS-19755, 1743·1
CGS-20267, 565·1
CGS-14824A, 867·2
CGS-16949A, 553·1

CGS-9343B, 1294·3
CGT, 1881·2
CH-846, 1764·2
CH-3565, 1195·2
Chá, 1765·3
Chagas' Disease— *see* American Trypanosomiasis, 600·1
Chalena, 1881·2
Chalk, 1255·3
Chalk, Precipitated, 1254·2
Chalk, Prepared, 1255·3
Chamaelirium, 1696·3
*Chamaelirium luteum*, 1696·3
*Chamaemelum nobile*, 1669·3
*Chamaesyce hirta*, 1686·3
Chamazulene, 1646·2, 1658·3, 1669·3
Chamillamont, 1881·2
Chamo S, 1881·2
Chamoca M, 1881·2
Chamomile, 1669·3
Chamomile Blend, 1881·2
Chamomile Flower, Roman, 1669·3
Chamomile Flowers, 1669·3
Chamomile, German, 1669·3
Chamomile, Hungarian, 1669·3
Chamomilla, 1669·3
Chamomilla Comp, 1881·2
*Chamomilla recutita*, 1669·3
Chamomillae Anthodium, 1669·3
Chamomillae, Flos, 1669·3
Chamomillae Romanae Flos, 1669·3
Chamomillae Vulgaris, Flos, 1669·3
Championyl, 1881·2
Champuacid, 1881·2
Chancroid, 123·2
Channel Black, 1058·3
Chanoclavine, 1723·2
Chantaline, 1881·2
Chanvre, 1666·1
Chap Stick, 1881·2
Chaparral, 1670·1
Chapstick Preparations, 1881·2
Charabs, 1881·3
Charac, 1881·3
Charac Tol, 1881·3
Charas, 1666·1
Charbon de Belloc, 1881·3
Charcoaid, 1881·3
Charcoal, Activated, 1030·2
Charcoal, Decolorising, 1030·2
Charcoal Plus, 1881·3
Charcoal, Vegetable, 1031·1
Charcoal, Wood, 1031·1
Charcocaps, 1881·3
Charcodote, 1881·3
Charcodote Aqueous, 1881·3
Charcodote, Aqueous— *see* Aqueous Charcodote, 1810·2
Charcotabs, 1881·3
Chardon Bénit, 1673·3
Charlie, 1373·3
Charlieu Anti-Poux, 1881·3
Charlieu Topic, 1881·3
Charlieu Topicrem, 1881·3
Charris, 1666·1
Chase Coldsorex, 1881·3
Chase Kolik Gripe Water, 1881·3
Chase Kolik Gripe Water Alcohol-Free, 1881·3
Chaste Tree, 1649·1
Chaste Tree Fruit, 1649·1
Chaux, Chlorure de, 1175·3
Chaux Sodée, 1747·1
Chaux Vive, 1664·3
Chebil, 1881·3
Check-Mate, 1881·3
Chefarine 4, 1881·3
Chefir, 1881·3
Cheiranthol, 1881·3
Chek-Stix, 1881·3
Chelated Bone Meal, 1881·3
Chelated Cal-Mag, 1881·4
Chelated Cal-Mag Plus Vitamin, 1881·4
Chelated Dol Mite, 1881·4
Chelated Dolomite, 1881·4
Chelated Solamins, 1881·4
Chelated Zinc, 1881·4
Chelators, 1030·1
Chelators Antidotes and Antagonists, 1030·1
Chelatran, 1881·4
Chelidonii Herba, 1695·3
Chelidonium, 1695·3
Chelidonium Compose, 1881·4
*Chelidonium majus*, 1695·3
Chelidophyt, 1881·4
Chelintox, 1881·4
Chemacin, 1881·4
Chemcard, 1881·4
Chemet, 1881·4
Chemical Burns, Eye, 1461·1
Chemical Burns, Eye— *see* Eye Disorders, 1224·2
Chemically Defined Elemental Diet, 1417·3
Chemicetina, 1881·4
Chemiofurin, 1881·4
Chemionazolo, 1881·4
Chemisolv, 1881·4
Chemists Own Chesty Cough, 1881·4
Chemists Own Chesty Mucus Cough, 1881·4
Chemists Own Clozole, 1881·4
Chemists Own Cold & Allergy, 1881·4
Chemists Own Cold & Flu Day/Night, 1881·4
Chemists Own Cold & Flu Relief, 1881·4
Chemists Own Cold Sore, 1881·4
Chemists Own Coldeze, 1881·4
Chemists Own Cough Suppressant, 1881·4
Chemists Own De Worm, 1881·4
Chemists Own Decongestant Nasal Spray, 1882·1
Chemists Own Diarrhoea Mixture, 1882·1
Chemists Own Diarrhoea Relief, 1882·1
Chemists Own Difenacol, 1882·1
Chemists Own Dolased— *see* Dolased Day/Night Pain Relief, 1948·1
Chemists Own Dry Cough, 1882·1
Chemists Own Dry Raspy Cough, 1882·1
Chemists Own Expectalix, 1882·1
Chemists Own Hayfever Sinus Relief, 1882·1
Chemists Own Junior Cough & Cold, 1882·1
Chemists Own Kiddicol, 1882·1
Chemists Own Natural Laxative with Softener, 1882·1
Chemists Own Pain, 1882·1
Chemists Own Pain & Fever, 1882·1
Chemists Own Peetalix, 1882·1
Chemists Own Period Pain Tablets, 1882·1
Chemists Own Phescode, 1882·1
Chemists Own Sinus Relief, 1882·1
Chemists Own Sinus-Pain Relief, 1882·1
Chemists Own Ultra Sun, 1882·1
Chemists Own Zapazole, 1882·1
Chemisulide, 1882·1
Chemitrim, 1882·1
Chemix, 1882·1
Chemopent, 1882·1
Chemoprim, 1882·1
Chemotherapy-induced Nausea and Vomiting— *see* Nausea and Vomiting, 1245·2
Chemotrim, 1882·2
Chemstrip Tests, 1882·2
Chemydur, 1882·2
Chemyparin, 1882·2
Chendol, 1882·2
Chêne, Écorce de, 1722·3
Chenic Acid, 1670·1
Chenodeoxycholic Acid, 1660·3, 1670·1
Chenodiol, 1670·1
Chenofalk, 1882·2
Chenofalk, Ursofalk + — *see* Ursofalk + Chenofalk, 2363·2
*Chenopodium ambrosioides*, 103·3
Chenopodium Oil, 103·3
Chephapyrin N, 1882·2
Cheracap, 1882·2
Cheracap S, 1882·2
Cheracol Preparations, 1882·2
Cheripex, 1882·3
Cherry Bark, Wild, 1765·2
Cherry Bark, Wild Black, 1765·2
Cherry, Bladder, 1731·3
Cherry Chest Rub— *see* Chest Rub, 1882·3
Cherry, Ground, 1731·3
Cherry Juice, 1058·1
Cherry, Red, 1058·1
Cherry, Sour, 1058·1
Cherry Stalks, 1058·1
Cherry, Sweet, 1058·1
Cherry, Winter, 1731·3
Chest Cold Complex— *see* Chest Cold Relief, 1882·3
Chest Cold Relief, 1882·3
Chest Mixture, 1882·3
Chest Rub, 1882·3
Chest Rub, Sigma Relief— *see* Sigma Relief Chest Rub, 2289·3
Chest Syndrome, Acute— *see* Sickle-cell Disease, 734·3
Chesty Cough, Chemists Own— *see* Chemists Own Chesty Cough, 1881·4
Chesty Cough, Nyal Plus+ — *see* Nyal Plus+ Chesty Cough, 2182·1
Chesty Cough Relief, 1882·3
Chesty Mucus Cough, Chemists Own— *see* Chemists Own Chesty Mucus Cough, 1881·4
Chetocaina Cloridrata, 1377·1
Chetofen, 1882·3
Chetotest, 1882·3
Chew-E, 1882·3
Chewette C, 1882·3
Chewies, 1882·3
Chewy C, 1882·3
CHF-1194, 84·2
Chiana, 1882·3
Chibretico, 1882·3
Chibro Uvelina, 1882·3
Chibro-Amuno 3, 1882·3
Chibro-Atropine, 1882·3
Chibro-Boraline, 1882·3
Chibro-Cadron, 1882·3
Chibro-Kerakain, 1882·3
Chibro-Pilocarpine, 1882·3
Chibro-Proscar, 1882·3
Chibro-Timoptol, 1882·3
Chibroxin, 1882·3
Chibroxine, 1882·3
Chibroxol, 1882·3
Chickenpox— *see* Varicella-zoster Infections, 621·1
Chiclida, 1882·3
Chicovit Pharmaton, 1882·3
Chiendent, 1676·2
Chiggerex, 1882·3
Chigger-Tox, 1882·4
Chikungunya— *see* Haemorrhagic Fevers, 618·2
Chilblain Formula, 1882·4
Chilblains Cream, 1882·4
Chilblains— *see* Raynaud's Syndrome, 833·3
Child Chesty Cough, 1882·4
Child Chew C, 1882·4
Child Formula, 1882·4
Childrens Advil Cold, 1882·4
Children's Allerest, 1882·4
Children's Allergy Formula, 1882·4
Childrens Appetite Tonic, 1882·4
Children's Calcium With Minerals, 1882·4
Childrens Cepacol, 1882·4
Childrens Cherry Sucrets, 1882·4
Childrens Chewable, 1882·4
Childrens Chewable Vita-Mins, 1882·4
Childrens Chewables, 1882·4
Children's Choice, 1882·4
Childrens Coltalin with Vit $B_1$, 1882·4
Childrens Diarrhoea Mixture, 1882·4
Childrens Dynafed Jr, 1882·4
Childrens Feverhalt, 1882·4
Children's Formula Cough, 1882·4
Children's Kaopectate, 1882·4
Childrens Mapap, 1882·4
Childrens Motion Sickness Liquid, 1882·4
Childrens Motrin Cold, 1882·4
Childrens Multi, 1882·4
Children's Multivitamins, 1882·4
Children's Nostril, 1882·4
Childrens Nyquil, 1882·4
Childrens Panadol, 1883·1
Childrens Panadol Cold & Flu, 1883·1
Childrens Panadol Cold Relief Elixir, 1883·1
Childrens Panadol Drops for Infants, 1883·1
Childrens Sudafed Cold & Cough, 1883·1
Childrens Sudafed Nasal Decongestant, 1883·1
Children's SunKist Multivitamins Complete, 1883·1
Children's SunKist Multivitamins + Extra C, 1883·1
Children's SunKist Multivitamins + Iron, 1883·1
Children's Tylenol, 1883·1
Children's Tylenol Cold Multi-Symptom, 1883·1
Children's Tylenol Cold Multi-Symptom Plus Cough, 1883·1
Children's Tylenol Cold Plus Cough, 1883·1
Childrevit, 1883·1
Chile Saltpetre, 1192·2
Chillies, 1667·1
Chillies, African, 1667·1
Chilvax, 1883·1
Chimar, 1883·1
Chimax, 1883·1
Chimodil, 1883·1
Chimono, 1883·1
China Diarrhea L107, 1883·1
China Eisenwein, 1883·1
China Green, 1185·2
China Med Complex, 1883·1
China White, 40·3
China-Balsam, 1883·1
Chinacin-T, 1883·1
Chinacrina, 606·3
Chinae Cortex, 1671·3
China-Eisenwein, 1883·1
China-Homaccord, 1883·2
China-Oel, 1883·2
China-Ol, 1883·2
Chinarinde, 1671·3
Chinclonac, 1883·2
Chinese Angelica, 1655·1
Chinese Blistering Beetle, 1667·1
Chinese Cantharides, 1667·1
Chinese Cinnamon Oil, 1668·2
Chinese Cucumber, 655·3
Chinese Lantern, 1731·3
Chinese Rhapontica, 1287·3
Chinese Rhubarb, 1287·3
Chinese Seasoning, 1441·1
Chinethazonum, 991·2
Chingaminum, 448·2
Chingazol, 1883·2
Chinidini Sulfas, 991·3
Chinidinsulfate, 991·3
Chinidinum, 991·3
Chinidinum Sulfuricum, 991·3
Chinina, 460·1
Chinini Bromidum, 460·2
Chinini Dihydrochloridum, 460·1
Chinini Hydrochloridum, 460·2
Chinini Sulfas, 460·2
Chininii Chloridum, 460·2
Chininium Chloratum, 460·2
Chininum, 460·1
Chininum Bisulfuricum, 460·1
Chininum Dihydrochloricum Carbamidatum, 1737·2
Chininum Hydrochloricum, 460·2
Chininum Sulfuricum, 460·2
Chinisocainum Hydrochloride, 1384·2
Chinoform, 196·3
Chinoidina, 1883·2
Chinosol, 1883·2
Chinosol S Vaseline, 1883·2
Chinosolum, 1700·1
Chinta, 1883·2
Chintaral, 1883·2

Chinteina, 1883·2
Chira, 1666·1
Chirocaine, 1883·2
Chiroflu, 1883·2
Chirofossat N, 1883·2
Chiromas, 1883·2
Chiron Barrier Cream, 1883·2
Chironair Odour Control Liquid, 1883·2
*Chironex fleckeri* Antiserum, 1621·3
*Chironex fleckeri* Antivenin, 1621·3
*Chironex fleckeri* Sting— *see* Box Jellyfish Sting, 1621·3
Chiroplexan H, 1883·2
Chitin, 1694·1
Chitodine, 1883·2
Chito-Lafarmen, 1883·2
Chiton, 1883·2
Chitosamine, 1694·1
Chitosan C, 1883·2
Chitosano, 1883·2
Chittem Bark, 1255·1
Chlamydial Infections, 123·3
Chlamydial Lymphogranuloma— *see* Lymphogranuloma Venereum, 134·2
Chlamydial Neonatal Conjunctivitis— *see* Neonatal Conjunctivitis, 136·3
Chlo-Amine, 1883·2
Chloasma— *see* Pigmentation Disorders, 1137·2
Chlobax, 1883·2
Chloment, 1883·2
Chlomide, 1883·2
Chlomy-P, 1883·2
Chlophedianol Hydrochloride, 1117·1
Chlor-3, 1883·2
Chloracetamide, 1176·3
Chloracil, 1883·3
Chloractil, 1883·3
Chloraethyl "Dr Henning", 1883·3
Chlorafed, 1883·3
Chloral Betaine, 684·1
Chloral Hydrate, 684·1
Chloraldurat, 1883·3
Chlorali Hydras, 684·1
Chloralosane, 1501·2
Chloralose, 1501·2
α-Chloralose, 1501·2
Chlorambucil, 536·1
Chlorambucilum, 536·1
Chloram-D, 1883·3
Chloramex, 1883·3
Chloramidum, 1194·3
Chloramine, 1194·3, 1883·3
Chloramine T, 1194·3
Chloraminophene, 536·1, 1883·3
Chloraminum, 1194·3
Chloramiphene Citrate, 1542·2
Chlorammonic, 1883·3
Chloramno, 1883·3
Chloramon, 1883·3
Chloramphenicol, 185·1
Chloramphenicol Arginine Succinate, 187·1
Chloramphenicol Cinnamate, 187·1
Chloramphenicol Glycinate, 187·1
Chloramphenicol Glycinate Sulfate, 187·1
Chloramphenicol Hydrogen Succinate, 187·1
Chloramphenicol Palmitate, 185·1
Chloramphenicol α-Palmitate, 185·1
Chloramphenicol Palmitoylglycolate, 187·1
Chloramphenicol Pantothenate, 187·1
Chloramphenicol Sodium Succinate, 185·1
Chloramphenicol α-Sodium Succinate, 185·1
Chloramphenicol Steaglate, 187·1
Chloramphenicol Stearate, 187·1
Chloramphenicoli Natrii Succinas, 185·1
Chloramphenicoli Palmitas, 185·1
Chloramphenicols, 117·3
Chloramphenicolum, 185·1
Chloramsaar N, 1883·3
Chloranautine, 431·1
Chloranfenicol, 185·1
Chloranic, 1883·3
Chlorasept, 1883·3
Chloraseptic Lozenges, 1883·3
Chloraseptic Sore Throat Spray, 1883·3
Chloraseptic Sore Throat, Vicks— *see* Vicks Chloraseptic Sore Throat, 2375·2
Chloraseptic, Vicks Children's— *see* Vicks Children's Chloraseptic, 2375·2
Chloraseptic, Vicks— *see* Vicks Chloraseptic, 2375·2
Chloraseptine, 1883·3
Chlorasol, 1883·3
Chlorazin, 1883·3
Chlorazol, 1883·3
Chlorbutanol, 1176·3
Chlorbutanolum, 1176·3
Chlorbutinum, 536·1
Chlorbutol, 1176·3
Chlorcarpipramine Hydrochloride, 683·1
Chlorcinnazine Dihydrochloride, 429·2
Chlorcol, 1883·3
Chlorcyclizine Dibunate, 427·3, 1130·3
Chlorcyclizine Hydrochloride, 427·2
Chlorcyclizini Hydrochloridum, 427·2
Chlorcyclizinium Chloride, 427·2
Chlordane, 1501·3
Chlordantoin, 396·2
Chlordesmethyldiazepam, 689·3
Chlordex GP, 1883·3
Chlordiazepoxide, 674·2
Chlordiazepoxide Hydrochloride, 674·2
Chlordiazepoxidi Hydrochloridum, 674·2
Chlordiazepoxidum, 674·2
Chlordrine, 1883·3
Chloresium, 1883·3
Chlorestrol, 1883·3
Chlorethazine Hydrochloride, 537·1
Chlorethyl, 1376·2, 1883·3
Chlorethylphenamide, 353·3
Chloretone, 1176·3
Chlorex-A, 1883·3
Chlorfenvinphos, 1502·2
Chlorformin, 1883·3
Chlorgest, 1883·4
Chlorhex, 1883·4
Chlorhexamed, 1883·4
Chlorhex-C, 1883·4
Chlorhexidine, 1173·2
Chlorhexidine Acetate, 1173·2
Chlorhexidine Diacetate, 1173·2
Chlorhexidine Digluconate, 1173·2
Chlorhexidine Digluconate Solution, 1173·2
Chlorhexidine Dihydrochloride, 1173·3
Chlorhexidine Gluconate, 1173·2
Chlorhexidine Gluconate Solution, 1173·2
Chlorhexidine Hydrochloride, 1173·3
Chlorhexidini Diacetas, 1173·2
Chlorhexidini Digluconatis Solutio, 1173·2
Chlorhexidini Dihydrochloridum, 1173·3
Chlorhexseptic, 1883·4
Chlorhist, 1883·4
Chlorhist Baby Cough, 1883·4
Chlorhist Cough, 1883·4
Chlorhistan, 1883·4
Chlorhydrate d'Amyléine, 1370·2
Chlorhydrate de Codéthyline, 37·3
Chlorhydrate de Québrachine, 1766·2
Chlorhydroxyquinoline, 220·3
Chloride of Lime, 1175·3
Chloridrato de Cocaína, 1373·3
Chloridrato de Fenazopiridina, 83·1
Chloriguane Hydrochloride, 457·1
Chlorimipramine Hydrochloride, 289·3
Chlorinated Insecticides, 1501·3
Chlorinated Lime, 1175·3
Chlorinated Lime and Boric Acid Solution, 1175·3
Chlorinated Soda Solution, Surgical, 1175·3
Chlorine, 1175·3
Chlorine Dioxide, 1176·2
Chlorispray, 1883·4
Chlorkalk, 1175·3
Chlorkresolum, 1177·1
Chlorleate, 1883·4
Chlorleate Expectorant, 1883·4
Chlormadinone Acetate, 1542·1
Chlormeprazine, 716·2
Chlormeprazine Edisylate, 716·2
Chlormeprazine Maleate, 716·3
Chlormeprazine Mesylate, 716·3
Chlormerodrin, 952·2
Chlor-Mes D, 1883·4
Chlormethazanone, 675·1
Chlormethiazole, 683·1
Chlormethiazole Edisylate, 683·1
Chlormethiazole Ethanedisulphonate, 683·1
Chlormethine Hydrochloride, 537·1
Chlormezanone, 675·1
Chlormezanonum, 675·1
Chlormidazole Hydrochloride, 396·1
Chlormixin, 1883·4
Chlornamol, 1883·4
Chlornicol, 1883·4
Chloroacetaldehyde, 561·2
Chloroacetamide, 1176·3
2-Chloroacetamide, 1176·3
Chloroacetic Acid, 1154·2
Chloroacetophenone, 1670·1
2-Chloroacetophenone, 1670·1
*N*-(3-Chloroallyl)hexaminium Chloride, 1176·3
1-(3-Chloroallyl)-3,5,7-triaza-1-azoniaadamantane Chloride, 1176·3
4-Chloroaniline, 457·2, 1173·3
3-(4-Chloroanilino)-10-(4-chlorophenyl)-2,10-dihydro-2-phenazin-2-ylideneisopropylamine, 197·1
(±)-α-(*p*-Chlorobenzamido)-1,2-dihydro-2-oxo-4-quinolinepropionic Acid, 1287·3
2-[4-(2-*p*-Chlorobenzamidoethyl)phenoxy]-2-methylpropionic Acid, 873·2
1-(4-Chlorobenzenesulphonyl)-3-propylurea, 330·3
1-(4-Chlorobenzenesulphonyl)-3-(pyrrolidin-1-yl)urea, 333·1
1-(4-Chlorobenzhydryl)-4-cinnamylpiperazine Dihydrochloride, 429·2
1-(4-Chlorobenzhydryl)-4-(3-methylbenzyl)piperazine Dihydrochloride, 436·3
1-(4-Chlorobenzhydryl)-4-methylpiperazine Hydrochloride, 427·2
1-(4-Chlorobenzhydryl)perhydro-4-methyl-1,4-diazepine Dihydrochloride, 434·3
2-[4-(4-Chlorobenzhydryl)piperazin-1-yl]ethoxyacetic Acid, 427·1
2-{2-[4-(4-Chlorobenzhydryl)piperazin-1-yl]ethoxy}ethanol 4,4′-Methylenebis(3-hydroxy-2-naphthoate), 434·3
6-Chloro-2*H*-1,2,4-benzothiadiazine-7-sulphonamide 1,1-Dioxide, 882·1
Chlorobenzoxazolinone, 1392·3
5-Chlorobenzoxazol-2(3*H*)-one, 1392·3
2-{2-[1-(4-Chlorobenzoyl)-5-methoxy-2-methylindol-3-yl]acetamido}-2-deoxy-D-glucose, 44·3
[1-(4-Chlorobenzoyl)-5-methoxy-2-methylindol-3-yl]acetic Acid, 47·3
3-{4-[2-(1-*p*-Chlorobenzoyl-5-methoxy-2-methylindol-3-ylacetoxy)ethyl]piperazin-1-yl}propyl 4-Benzamido-*N*,*N*-dipropylglutaramate Dimaleate, 85·2
*O*-[(1-*p*-Chlorobenzoyl-5-methoxy-2-methylindol-3-yl)acetyl]glycolic Acid, 11·3
1-[1-(4-Chlorobenzyl)benzimidazol-2-ylmethyl]pyrrolidinium (6*R*)-6-(2-Phenylacetamido)penicillanate, 194·1
2-(4-Chlorobenzyl)-3-(dimethylaminomethyl)butan-2-ol Hydrochloride, 1117·1
*N*-(4-Chlorobenzyl)-*N′N′*-dimethyl-*N*-(2-pyridyl)ethylenediamine Hydrochloride, 427·3
4-(*p*-Chlorobenzyl)-2-(hexahydro-1-methyl-1*H*-azepin-4-yl)-1(2*H*)-phthalazinone Monohydrochloride, 425·2
α-(*o*-Chlorobenzylidene) Malonitrile, 1677·3
1-(4-Chlorobenzyl)-2-methylbenzimidazole Hydrochloride, 396·1
(+)-*N*-(2-Chlorobenzyl)-α-methylphenethylamine Hydrochloride, 1585·3
1-(1-{*o*-[(*m*-Chlorobenzyl)oxy]phenyl}vinyl)imidazole Hydrochloride, 397·1
1-(4-Chlorobenzyl)-2-(pyrrolidin-1-ylmethyl)benzimidazole Hydrochloride, 429·2
1-[1-(2-Chlorobenzyl)pyrrol-2-yl]-2-(di-*sec*-butyl)aminoethanol 4-Hydroxybenzoate, 96·3
5-(2-Chlorobenzyl)-4,5,6,7-tetrahydrothieno[3,2-*c*]pyridine Hydrochloride, 1011·2
7-Chlorobicyclo[3.2.0]hepta-2,6-dien-6-yl Dimethyl Phosphate, 1506·1
Chlorobutanol, 1176·3
Chlorobutanol, Anhydrous, 1176·3
Chlorobutanol Hemihydrate, 1176·3
Chlorobutanolum, 1176·3
(±)-2-(6-Chlorocarbazol-2-yl)propionic Acid, 25·1
Chlorochin, 1883·4
Chlorochinium Phosphoricum, 448·2
Chlorochinum Diphosphoricum, 448·2
5′-Chloro-4′-(4-chloro-α-cyanobenzyl)-3,5-di-iodosalicyl-*o*-toluidide, 104·1
3-[5-Chloro-α-(4-chloro-β-hydroxyphenethyl)-2-thenyl]-4-hydroxycoumarin, 1013·2
6-Chloro-3-chloromethyl-3,4-dihydro-2-methyl-2*H*-1,2,4-benzothiadiazine-7-sulphonamide 1,1-Dioxide, 953·2
5-Chloro-*N*-(2-chloro-4-nitrophenyl)-2-hydroxybenzamide, 110·1
3-Chloro-4-(3-chloro-2-nitrophenyl)pyrrole, 408·1
3′-Chloro-4′-(4-chlorophenoxy)-3,5-di-iodosalicylanilide, 114·1
7-Chloro-5-(2-chlorophenyl)-1,3-dihydro-2*H*-1,4-benzodiazepin-2-one, 689·3
7-Chloro-5-(2-chlorophenyl)-1,3-dihydro-3-hydroxy-1,4-benzodiazepin-2-one, 704·1
(*RS*)-7-Chloro-5-(2-chlorophenyl)-1,3-dihydro-3-hydroxy-1-methyl-1,4-benzodiazepin-2-one, 705·2
8-Chloro-6-(2-chlorophenyl)-1-methyl-4*H*-[1,2,4]triazolo[4,3-*a*][1,4]benzodiazepine, 725·3
10-Chloro-11b-(2-chlorophenyl)-2,3,7,11b-tetrahydro-3-methyloxazolo[3,2-*d*][1,4]benzodiazepin-6(5*H*)-one, 707·1
10-Chloro-11b-(2-chlorophenyl)-2,3,7,11b-tetrahydro-oxazolo[3,2-*d*][1,4]benzodiazepin-6(5*H*)-one, 685·3
1-(4-Chloro-3-{[3-chloro-5-(trifluoromethyl)-2-pyridyl]oxy}phenyl)-3-(2,6-difluorobenzoyl)urea, 1505·3
Chlorocort, 1883·4
Chlorocresol, 1177·1
*p*-Chloro-*m*-cresol, 1177·1
Chlorocresolum, 1177·1
*N*,*N′*-(2-Chloro-5-cyano-*m*-phenylene)dioxamic Acid, 1707·3
7-Chloro-5-(cyclohex-1-enyl)-1,3-dihydro-1-methyl-2*H*-1,4-benzodiazepin-2-one, 724·1
6-Chloro-3-cyclopentylmethyl-3,4-dihydro-2*H*-1,2,4-benzothiadiazine-7-sulphonamide 1,1-Dioxide, 890·3
(*S*)-6-Chloro-4-(cyclopropylethynyl)-1,4-dihydro-4-(trifluoromethyl)-2*H*-3,1-benzoxazin-2-one, 632·2
7-Chloro-1-(cyclopropylmethyl)-1,3-dihydro-5-phenyl-2*H*-1,4-benzodiazepin-2-one, 716·2
7-Chloro-6-demethyl-6-deoxy-5β-hydroxy-6-methylenetetracycline, 229·1
7-Chloro-6-demethyltetracycline, 204·3
2-Chlorodeoxyadenosine, 539·3
2-Chloro-2′-deoxyadenosine, 539·3
2-Chloro-9-(2-deoxy-2-fluoro-β-D-arabinofuranosyl)-9*H*-purin-6-amine, 540·2
Chlorodeoxylincomycin Hydrochloride, 194·2
(7*S*)-Chloro-7-deoxylincomycin Hydrochloride, 194·2
2-[(8-Chlorodibenzo[*b*,*f*]-thiepin-10-yl)oxy]-*N*,*N*-dimethylethylamine, 730·2
(*Z*)-2-{4-[3-(2-Chloro-10*H*-dibenzo[*b*,*e*]thiin-10-ylidene)propyl]piperazin-1-yl}ethanol, 730·3
6-Chloro-3-dichloromethyl-3,4-dihydro-2*H*-1,2,4-benzothiadiazine-7-sulphonamide 1,1-Dioxide, 1017·2
5-Chloro-6-(2,3-dichlorophenoxy)-2-(methylthio)benzimidazole, 115·2
5-Chloro-2-(2,4-dichlorophenoxy)phenol, 1195·2
2-Chloro-1-(2,4-dichlorophenyl)vinyl Diethyl Phosphate, 1502·2

7-Chloro-1-(2-diethylaminoethyl)-5-(2-fluorophenyl)-1,3-dihydro-1,4-benzodiazepin-2-one, 700·3
6-Chloro-9-(4-diethylamino-1-methylbutylamino)-2-methoxyacridine Dihydrochloride Dihydrate, 606·3
7-Chloro-4-(4-diethylamino-1-methylbutylamino)quinoline, 448·2
2′-Chloro-2-[2-[(diethylamino)methyl]imidazol-1-yl]-5-nitrobenzophenone, 1722·2
21-Chloro-6α,9-difluoro-11β,17-dihydroxy-16β-methylpregna-1,4-diene-3,20-dione 17-Propionate, 1111·3
Chlorodifluoroethane, 1236·1
1-Chloro-1,1-difluoroethane, 1236·1
Chlorodifluoromethane, 1236·1
2-Chloro-1-(difluoromethoxy)-1,1,2-trifluoroethane, 1298·1
2-Chloro-2-(difluoromethoxy)-1,1,1-trifluoroethane, 1301·1
2-Chloro-6α,9-difluoro-11β,17,21-trihydroxy-16α-methylpregna-1,4-diene-3,20-dione, 1103·3
6-Chloro-3,4-dihydro-2*H*-1,2,4-benzothiadiazine-7-sulphonamide 1,1-Dioxide, 933·2
1′-[3-(3-Chloro-10,11-dihydro-5*H*-dibenz[*b,f*]azepin-5-yl)propyl][1,4′-bipiperidine]-4′-carboxamide Dihydrochloride Monohydrate, 683·1
3-(3-Chloro-10,11-dihydro-5*H*-dibenz[*b,f*]azepin-5-yl)propyldimethylamine Hydrochloride, 289·3
(±)-1′-[3-(3-Chloro-10,11-dihydro-5*H*-dibenz[*b,f*]azepin-5-yl)propyl]hexahydrospiro[imidazo[1,2-*a*]pyridine-3(2*H*),4′-piperidin]-2-one, 710·1
7-Chloro-2,3-dihydro-2,2-dihydroxy-5-phenyl-1*H*-1,4-benzodiazepine-3-carboxylic Acid, 685·1
11-Chloro-8,12b-dihydro-2,8-dimethyl-12b-phenyl-4*H*-[1,3]oxazino[3,2-*d*][1,4]benzodiazepine-4,7(6*H*)-dione, 703·1
(±)-[2-Chloro-4-(4,5-dihydro-3,5-dioxo-*as*-triazin-2(3*H*)-yl)phenyl]-(*p*-chlorophenyl)acetonitrile, 603·1
6-Chloro-1β,2β-dihydro-17α-hydroxy-3′*H*-cyclopropa[1,2]pregna-1,4,6-triene-3,20-dione Acetate, 1544·1
7-Chloro-1,3-dihydro-3-hydroxy-1-methyl-5-phenyl-1,4-benzodiazepin-2-one, 723·2
7-Chloro-1,3-dihydro-3-hydroxy-5-phenyl-1,4-benzodiazepin-2-one, 712·2
6-Chloro-3,4-dihydro-3-isobutyl-2*H*-1,2,4-benzothiadiazine-7-sulphonamide 1,1-Dioxide, 878·2
6-Chloro-3,4-dihydro-3-(α-methylbenzyl)-2*H*-1,2,4-benzothiadiazine-7-sulphonamide 1,1-Dioxide, 867·1
7-[(3-Chloro-6,11-dihydro-6-methyldibenzo[*c,f*][1,2]thiazepin-11-yl)amino]heptanoic Acid *S,S*-Dioxide, 318·2
7-Chloro-2,3-dihydro-1-methyl-2-oxo-5-phenyl-1*H*-1,4-benzodiazepin-3-yl Dimethylcarbamate, 674·1
(±)-6-Chloro-3,4-dihydro-4-methyl-3-oxo-*N*-3-quinuclidinyl-2*H*-1,4-benzoxazine-8-carboxamide Hydrochloride, 1251·1
7-Chloro-2,3-dihydro-1-methyl-5-phenyl-1*H*-1,4-benzodiazepine, 706·1
7-Chloro-1,5-dihydro-1-methyl-5-phenyl-1,5-benzodiazepine-2,4(3*H*)-dione, 358·2
7-Chloro-1,3-dihydro-1-methyl-5-phenyl-2*H*-1,4-benzodiazepin-2-one, 690·1
8-Chloro-6,11-dihydro-11-{1-[(5-methyl-3-pyridyl)methyl]-4-piperidylidene}-5*H*-benzo[5,6]cyclohepta[1,2-*b*]pyridine, 440·3
6-Chloro-3,4-dihydro-2-methyl-3-(2,2,2-trifluoroethylthiomethyl)-2*H*-1,2,4-benzothiadiazine-7-sulphonamide 1,1-Dioxide, 984·2
6-Chloro-3,4-dihydro-3-(norborn-5-en-2-yl)-2*H*-1,2,4-benzothiadiazine-7-sulphonamide 1,1-Dioxide, 891·1
*S*-[(6-Chloro-2,3-dihydro-2-oxo-1,3-oxazolo[4,5-*b*]pyridin-3-yl)methyl] *O,O*-Dimethyl Phosphorothioate, 1500·2
7-Chloro-1,3-dihydro-5-phenyl-2*H*-1,4-benzodiazepin-2-one, 710·3
7-Chloro-1,3-dihydro-5-phenyl-1-(prop-2-ynyl)-2*H*-1,4-benzodiazepin-2-one, 715·3
7-Chloro-1,3-dihydro-5-phenyl-1-(2,2,2-trifluoroethyl)-1,4-benzodiazepin-2-one, 701·2
8-Chloro-6,11-dihydro-11-(4-piperidylidene)-5*H*-benzo[5,6]cyclohepta[1,2-*b*]pyridine, 431·1
5-Chlorodihydropyrimidine, 586·3
6-Chloro-3,4-dihydro-3-trichloromethyl-2*H*-1,2,4-benzothiadiazine-7-sulphonamide 1,1-Dioxide Potassium, 1010·1
6-Chloro-3,4-dihydro-3-(2,2,2-trifluoroethylthiomethyl)-2*H*-1,2,4-benzothiadiazine-7-sulphonamide 1,1-Dioxide, 911·3
4′-Chloro-3,5-dimethoxy-4-(2-morpholinoethoxy)benzophenone, 1124·3
2-Chloro-α-(2-dimethylaminoethyl)benzyl Alcohol Hydrochloride, 1117·1
(4*S*,4a*S*,5a*S*,6*S*,12a*S*)-7-Chloro-4-dimethylamino-1,4,4a,5,5a,6,11,12a-octahydro-3,6,10,12,12a-pentahydroxy-1,11-dioxonaphthacene-2-carboxamide, 204·3
(4*S*,4a*S*,5a*S*,6*S*,12a*S*)-7-Chloro-4-dimethylamino-1,4,4a,5,5a,6,11,12a-octahydro-3,6,10,12,12a-pentahydroxy-6-methyl-1,11-dioxonaphthacene-2-carboxamide, 187·3
(4*S*,4a*R*,5*S*,5a*R*,6*S*,12a*S*)-7-Chloro-4-dimethylamino-1,4,4a,5,5a,6,11,12a-octahydro-3,5,10,12,12a-pentahydroxy-6-methylene-1,11-dioxonaphthacene-2-carboxamide, 229·1
6-Chloro-3-(1,2-dimethylbutyl)-3,4-dihydro-2*H*-1,2,4-benzothiadiazine-7-sulphonamide 1,1-Dioxide, 951·2
4-Chloro-3,5-dimethylphenol, 1177·2
4-Chloro-*N*-(2,6-dimethylpiperidino)-3-sulphamoylbenzamide, 888·2
1-Chloro-2,4-dinitrobenzene, 1680·3
2-{*p*-[(*Z*)-4-Chloro-1,2-diphenyl-1-butenyl]phenoxy}-*N,N*-dimethylethylamine Citrate, 589·2
2-[4-(2-Chloro-1,2-diphenylvinyl)phenoxy]triethylamine Dihydrogen Citrate, 1542·2
1-Chloro-2,3-epoxypropane, 1474·2
Chloroethane, 1376·2
3-(2-Chloroethoxy)-9α-fluoro-11β,21-dihydroxy-16α,17α-isopropylidenedioxy-20-oxopregna-3,5-diene-6-carbaldehyde 21-Acetate, 1103·2
3-(2-Chloroethyl)-2-[bis(2-chloroethyl)amino]tetrahydro-2*H*-1,3,2-oxazaphosphorine-2-oxide, 590·2
3-(2-Chloroethyl)-2-(2-chloroethylamino)perhydro-1,3,2-oxazaphosphorinane 2-Oxide, 561·1
1-(2-Chloroethyl)-3-cyclohexyl-1-nitrosourea, 565·2
Chloroethylene, 1764·3
1-(2-Chloroethyl)-3-(4-methylcyclohexyl)-1-nitrosourea, 583·2
5-(2-Chloroethyl)-4-methyl-1,3-thiazole, 683·1
5-(2-Chloroethyl)-4-methylthiazole Ethane-1,2-disulphonate, 683·1
2-[3-(2-Chloroethyl)-3-nitrosoureido]-2-deoxy-D-glucopyranose, 538·1
1-Chloro-3-ethylpent-1-en-4-yn-3-ol, 697·3
7-Chloro-2-ethyl-1,2,3,4-tetrahydro-4-oxoquinazoline-6-sulphonamide, 991·2
Chlorofenotano, 1502·1
Chlorofluorocarbons, 1235·3
9α-Chloro-6α-fluoro-11β,21-dihydroxy-16α-methylpregna-1,4-diene-3,20-dione 21-Pivalate, 1096·1
21-Chloro-9α-fluoro-11β,17α-dihydroxy-16β-methylpregna-1,4-diene-3,20-dione 17-Propionate, 1095·2
4-(4′-Chloro-5-fluoro-2-hydroxybenzhydrylideneamino)butyramide, 377·2
21-Chloro-9α-fluoro-11β-hydroxy-16α,17α-isopropylidenedioxypregn-4-ene-3,20-dione, 1103·2
21-Chloro-9α-fluoro-17α-hydroxy-16β-methylpregna-1,4-diene-3,11,20-trione 17-Butyrate, 1095·3
2-{[(2-Chloro-6-fluorophenyl)amino]-5-methylphenyl}acetic Acid, 54·3
7-Chloro-5-(2-fluorophenyl)-2,3-dihydro-3-hydroxy-2-oxo-1*H*-1,4-benzodiazepine-1-propionitrile, 683·1
7-Chloro-5-(2-fluorophenyl)-1,3-dihydro-1-methyl-2*H*-1,4-benzodiazepin-2-one, 698·2
7-Chloro-5-(2-fluorophenyl)-1,3-dihydro-1-(2,2,2-trifluoroethyl)-1,4-benzodiazepine-2-thione, 718·2
1-(2-{4-[5-Chloro-1-(*p*-fluorophenyl)indol-3-yl]piperidino}ethyl)-2-imidazolidinone, 721·3
*N*-(3-Chloro-4-fluorophenyl)-7-methoxy-6-[3-(morpholin-4-yl)propoxy]quinazolin-4-amine, 557·3
8-Chloro-6-(2-fluorophenyl)-1-methyl-4*H*-imidazo[1,5-*a*][1,4]benzodiazepine, 707·1
(6*R*)-6-[3-(2-Chloro-6-fluorophenyl)-5-methylisoxazole-4-carboxamido]penicillanic Acid, 213·3
Chloroform, 1296·3
Chloroformium Anesthesicum, 1296·3
Chloroformum, 1296·3
Chloroformum Pro Narcosi, 1296·3
Chloroformyl Chloride, 1731·1
4-Chloro-*N*-furfuryl-5-sulphamoylanthranilic Acid, 919·3
Chlorogenium, 1195·1
Chloroguanide Hydrochloride, 457·1
Chlorohex, 1883·4
4-Chloro-*N*-(*endo*-hexahydro-4,7-methanoisoindolin-2-yl)-3-sulphamoylbenzamide, 1018·1
Chlorohistol, 1883·4
4-Chloro-17β-hydroxyandrost-4-en-3-one Acetate, 1543·2
(5*R**)-5-[(α*S**)-*o*-Chloro-α-hydroxybenzyl]-4-methoxy-2(5*H*)-furanone, 366·2
5-Chloro-3-{2-[4-(2-hydroxyethyl)piperazin-1-yl]-2-oxoethyl}benzothiazolin-2-one Hydrochloride, 94·1
(*Z*)-7-[(1*R*,2*R*,3*R*,5*R*)-5-Chloro-3-hydroxy-2-[(*E*)-(3*R*)-3-hydroxy-4,4-dimethyl-1-octenyl]cyclopentyl]-5-heptenoic Acid, 1520·3
6-Chloro-4-hydroxy-2-methyl-*N*-2-pyridyl-2*H*-thieno[2,3-*e*][1,2]-thiazine-3-carboxamide 1,1-Dioxide, 54·2
2-Chloro-5-(1-hydroxy-3-oxoisoindolin-1-yl)benzenesulphonamide, 882·3
6-Chloro-17-hydroxypregna-4,6-diene-3,20-dione Acetate, 1542·1
6-Chloro-17α-hydroxypregna-1,4,6-triene-3,20-dione Acetate, 1547·2
4-Chloro-5-(2-imidazolin-2-ylamino)-6-methoxy-2-methylpyrimidine, 962·3
5-Chloro-*N*-(2-imidazolin-2-yl)-2,1,3-benzothiadiazol-4-ylamine Hydrochloride, 1395·3
4-Chloro-2,2′-iminodibenzoate Disodium, 1707·2
Chloroiodoquine, 196·3
5-Chloro-7-iodoquinolin-8-ol, 196·3
4-Chloro-2-isopropyl-5-methylphenol, 1177·2
4′-Chloro-*N*-(1-isopropyl-4-piperidyl)-2-phenylacetanilide Hydrochloride, 947·2
Chloro-Magnesion, 1883·4
Chloromethane, 1476·2
1-{4-[2-(5-Chloro-2-methoxybenzamido)ethyl]benzenesulphonyl}-3-cyclohexylurea, 331·2
7-Chloro-2-methoxy-10-[3,5-bis(pyrrolidinomethyl)-4-hydroxyanilino]benzo-[*b*]-1,5-naphthyridine Phosphate, 460·1
(3*S*,4*R*,5*S*,8*R*,9*E*,12*S*,14*S*,15*R*,16*S*,18*R*,19*R*,26a*S*)-3-{(*E*)-2-[(1*R*,3*R*,4*S*)-4-Chloro-3-methoxycyclohexyl]-1-methylvinyl}-8-ethyl-5,6,8,11,12,13,14,15,16,17,18,19,-24,25,26,26a-hexadecahydro-5,19-dihydroxy-14,16-dimethoxy-4,10,12,18-tetramethyl-15,19-epoxy-3*H*-pyrido[2,1-*c*][1,4]oxaazacyclotricosine-1,7,20,-21(4*H*,23*H*)-tetrone, 1155·1
7-Chloro-2-methylamino-5-phenyl-3*H*-1,4-benzodiazepine 4-Oxide, 674·2
2-(4-Chloro-α-methylbenzhydryloxy)-*NN*-dimethylethylamine Hydrochloride, 428·3
(+)-(2*R*)-2-{2-[(*R*)-4-Chloro-α-methylbenzhydryloxy]ethyl}-1-methylpyrrolidine Hydrogen Fumarate, 429·1
7-Chloro-3-methyl-2*H*-1,2,4-benzothiadiazine 1,1-Dioxide, 893·2
*O*-3-Chloro-4-methyl-7-coumarinyl *O,O*-Diethyl Phosphorothioate, 1502·2
4-Chloro-*N*-(2-methylindolin-1-yl)-3-sulphamoylbenzamide, 938·2
5-Chloro-2-methyl-4-isothiazolin-3-one, 1185·1
5-Chloro-2-methyl-3(2*H*)-isothiazolone, 1185·1
5-Chloro-6′-methyl-3-[*p*-(methylsulfonyl)phenyl]-2,3′-bipyridine, 38·2
3′-Chloro-2′-[*N*-methyl-*N*-(morpholinocarbonylmethyl)aminomethyl]benzanilide Hydrochloride, 1121·3
1-Chloro-3-(2-methyl-5-nitroimidazol-1-yl)propan-2-ol, 612·2
4-Chloro-3-methylphenol, 1177·1
6-Chloro-4-methyl-4-phenyl-3,1-benzoxazin-2-yl(ethyl)amine Hydrochloride, 698·1
1-{2-[(*p*-Chloro-α-methyl-α-phenylbenzyl)oxy]ethyl}hexahydro-1*H*-azepine Hydrochloride, 441·1
8-Chloro-1-methyl-6-phenyl-4*H*-1,2,4-triazolo[4,3-*a*][1,4]benzodiazepine, 668·3
8-Chloro-11-(4-methylpiperazin-1-yl)-5*H*-dibenzo[*b,e*][1,4]diazepine, 685·3
2-Chloro-11-(4-methylpiperazin-1-yl)dibenzo[*b,f*][1,4]thiazepine, 685·2
2-Chloro-11-(4-methylpiperazin-1-yl)dibenz[*b,f*][1,4]oxazepine, 705·2
2-Chloro-10-[3-(4-methylpiperazin-1-yl)propyl]phenothiazine, 716·2
9α-Chloro-16β-methylprednisolone Dipropionate, 1091·1
4-Chloro-$N^1$-methyl-$N^1$-(tetrahydro-2-methylfurfuryl)benzene-1,3-disulphonamide, 951·3
4-Chloro-*N*-(2-morpholinoethyl)benzamide, 308·2
Chloromycetin, 1883·4
Chloromycetin Ear Drops, 1883·4
2-[(4-Chloro-1-naphthyl)methyl]-2-imidazoline Hydrochloride, 1117·1
Chloronguent, 1883·4
4-Chloro-3-oxoandrost-4-en-17β-yl Acetate, 1543·2
5-Chloro-1-{1-[3-(2-oxobenzimidazolin-1-yl)propyl]-4-piperidyl}benzimidazolin-2-one, 1263·2
(6*R*,7*S*)-3-Chloro-8-oxo-7-D-phenylglycylamino-1-azabicyclo[4.2.0]oct-2-ene-2-carboxylic Acid Monohydrate, 228·1
Chloropect, 1884·1
Chloroph, 1884·1
Chlorophacinone, 1501·3
5-{3-[*N*-(Chlorophenacyl)-*N*-methylamino]propyl}-10,11-5*H*-dihydrodibenz[*b,f*]azepine Hydrochloride, 305·3
4-Chlorophenol, 1187·3
Chlorophenothane, 1502·1
3-(2-Chlorophenothiazin-10-yl)-*NN*-diethylpropylamine Hydrochloride, 675·1
3-(2-Chlorophenothiazin-10-yl)propyldimethylamine, 675·1
2-{4-[3-(2-Chlorophenothiazin-10-yl)propyl]piperazin-1-yl}ethanol, 714·2
2-{4-[3-(2-Chlorophenothiazin-10-yl)propyl]piperazin-1-yl}ethyl Decanoate, 714·2
2-{4-[3-(2-Chlorophenothiazin-10-yl)propyl]piperazin-1-yl}ethyl Heptanoate, 714·2
2-(4-Chlorophenoxy)-*N*-(2-diethylaminoethyl)acetamide, 26·3
Chlorophenoxyethanol, 1189·1
[2-(*p*-Chlorophenoxy)ethyl]dodecyldimethylammonium Bromide, 1178·3
(±)-(*Z*)-7-{(1*S*,2*R*,3*R*,5*S*)-2-[(2*S*)-3-(3-Chlorophenoxy)-2-hydroxypropylthio]-3,5-dihydroxycyclopentyl}hept-5-enoic Acid, 1519·2
1-(*p*-Chlorophenoxy)-1-imidazol-1-yl-3,3-dimethyl-2-butanone, 396·2
Chlorophenoxyisobutyric Acid, 885·1
2-(4-Chlorophenoxy)-2-methylpropionic Acid Ester with 1,3-Dinicotinoyloxypropan-2-ol, 875·1
3-(4-Chlorophenoxy)propane-1,2-diol, 396·1
3-(4-Chlorophenoxy)propane-1,2-diol 1-Carbamate, 1392·2
DL-3-(*p*-Chlorophenyl)alanine, 1687·2
2-[2-(4-Chlorophenyl)benzoxazol-5-yl]propionic Acid, 21·1
1-{2-[(*p*-Chloro-α-phenylbenzyl)oxy]ethyl}piperidine Fendizoate, 1117·2

(2-{4-[(R)-p-Chloro-α-phenylbenzyl]-1-piperazinyl}ethoxy)acetic Acid, 435·3
p-Chlorophenylbiguanide, 457·2
2-[trans-4-(4-Chlorophenyl)cyclohexyl]-3-hydroxy-1,4-naphthoquinone, 601·3
1-[4-(4-Chlorophenyl)-2-(2,6-dichlorophenylthio)butyl]imidazole Mononitrate, 395·2
1-(4-Chlorophenyl)-3-(3,4-dichlorophenyl)urea, 1195·1
(±)-4-Chlorophenyl[2,6-dichloro-4-(2,3,4,5-tetrahydro-3,5-dioxo-1,2,4-triazin-2-yl)phenyl]acetonitrile, 603·2
1-(4-Chlorophenyl)-3-(2,6-difluorobenzoyl)urea, 1504·1
5-(4-Chlorophenyl)-2,5-dihydro-3H-imidazo[2,1-a]isoindol-5-ol, 1589·1
(±)-3-(p-Chlorophenyl)-1,3-dihydro-6-methylfuro[3,4-c]pyridin-7-ol, 883·2
6-(2-Chlorophenyl)-2,4-dihydro-2-(4-methylpiperazin-1-ylmethylene)-8-nitroimidazo[1,2-a][1,4]benzodiazepin-1-one Methanesulphonate Monohydrate, 704·1
5-(2-Chlorophenyl)-1,3-dihydro-7-nitro-1,4-benzodiazepin-2-one, 359·1
(±)-3-(4-Chlorophenyl)-NN-dimethyl-3-(2-pyridyl)propylamine Hydrogen Maleate, 427·3
(±)-α-[(E)-4-(o-Chlorophenyl)-1,3-dithiolan-2-ylidene]imidazole-1-acetonitrile, 405·2
5-(2-Chlorophenyl)-7-ethyl-1,3-dihydro-1-methyl-2H-thieno[2,3-e]-1,4-diazepin-2-one, 685·2
4-(2-Chlorophenyl)-2-ethyl-9-methyl-6H-thieno[3,2-f]-s-triazolo[4,3-a][1,4]diazepine, 698·1
5-(4-Chlorophenyl)-6-ethylpyrimidine-2,4-diyldiamine, 458·1
1-{[5-(p-Chlorophenyl)furfurylidene]amino}-3-[4-(4-methyl-1-piperazinyl)-butyl]hydantoin Dihydrochloride, 866·3
(7R)-3-Chloro-7-(α-D-phenylglycylamino)-3-cephem-4-carboxylic Acid Monohydrate, 167·1
4-(4-p-Chlorophenyl-4-hydroxypiperidino)-NN-dimethyl-2,2-diphenylbutyramide Hydrochloride, 1271·1
4-[4-(4-Chlorophenyl)-4-hydroxypiperidino]-4′-fluorobutyrophenone, 701·2
(±)-1-(p-Chlorophenyl)-α-isobutyl-N,N-dimethylcyclobutanemethylamine Hydrochloride Monohydrate, 1593·1
1-(4-Chlorophenyl)-5-isopropylbiguanide Hydrochloride, 457·1
(±)-2-(2-Chlorophenyl)-2-methylaminocyclohexanone Hydrochloride, 1302·1
(6R)-6-[3-(2-Chlorophenyl)-5-methylisoxazole-4-carboxamido]penicillanic Acid, 198·2
2-(4-Chlorophenyl)-3-methylperhydro-1,3-thiazin-4-one 1,1-Dioxide, 675·1
4-{3-[4-(o-Chlorophenyl)-9-methyl-6H-thieno[3,2-f]-s-triazolo[4,3-a][1,4]diazepin-2-yl]propionyl}morpholine, 781·1
2-[2-(4-Chlorophenyl)-2-phenylacetyl]indane-1,3-dione, 1501·3
2-[1-(4-Chlorophenyl)-1-phenylethoxy]-N,N-dimethyl-1-propanamine Citrate, 485·3
[4-(4-Chlorophenyl)-2-phenylthiazol-5-yl]acetic Acid, 43·1
m-Chlorophenylpiperazine, 310·1, 320·1
2-{3-[4-(3-Chlorophenyl)piperazin-1-yl]propyl}-4,5-diethyl-2,4-dihydro-3H-1,2,4-triazol-3-one Hydrochloride, 292·1
2-{3-[4-(3-Chlorophenyl)piperazin-1-yl]propyl}-5-ethyl-2,4-dihydro-4-(2-phenoxyethyl)-1,2,4-triazol-3-one Monohydrochloride, 309·2
2-[3-(4-m-Chlorophenylpiperazin-1-yl)propyl]-1,2,4-triazolo[4,3-a]pyridin-3(2H)-one Hydrochloride, 319·1
(RS)-[O-1-(4-Chlorophenyl)pyrazol-4-yl O-Ethyl S-Propyl Phosphorothioate], 1509·2
{[(p-Chlorophenyl)thio]methylene}diphosphonic Acid, 776·1
8-Chloro-6-phenyl-4H-1,2,4-triazolo[4,3-a]-1,4-benzodiazepine, 697·3
Chlorophyl Liquid "Schuh", 1884·1
Chlorophyll, 1057·1, 1884·1
Chlorophyll A, 1057·1
Chlorophyll B, 1057·1
Chlorophyllin Copper Complex Sodium, 1057·1
Chlorophyllin Salbe "Schuh", 1884·1
Chlorophyllins, 1057·1
Chloropicrin, 1502·1, 1507·3
2-Chloro-11-(piperazin-1-yl)dibenz-[b,f][1,4]oxazepine, 286·3
Chloroplatinic Acid, 1670·2
Chloropotassuril, 1884·1
Chloroprocaine Hydrochloride, 1373·1
N-(3-Chloropropyl)-α-methylphenethylamine Hydrochloride, 1589·2
Chloroptic, 1884·1
Chloropyramine Hydrochloride, 427·3
N[1]-(6-Chloropyrazinyl)sulfanilamide, 258·1
N[1]-(6-Chloropyridazin-3-yl)sulphanilamide, 258·1
2-[(6-Chloro-3-pyridazinyl)thio]-N,N-diethylacetamide, 1658·3
1-[(6-Chloro-3-pyridinyl)methyl]-4,5-dihydro-N-nitro-1H-imidazol-2-amine, 1506·2
2-[4-Chloro-α-(2-pyridyl)benzyloxy]-NN-dimethylethylamine Hydrogen Maleate, 426·3
(+)-4-{[(S)-p-Chloro-α-2-pyridylbenzyl]oxy}-1-piperidinebutyric Acid, 425·3
6-(5-Chloro-2-pyridyl)-6,7-dihydro-7-oxo-5H-pyrrolo[3,4-b]pyrazin-5-yl 4-Methylpiperazine-1-carboxylate, 729·3
Chloroquine, 448·2
Chloroquine Hydrochloride, 448·2
Chloroquine Phosphate, 448·2
Chloroquine Sulfate, 448·2
Chloroquine Sulphate, 448·2
Chloroquini Diphosphas, 448·2
Chloroquini Phosphas, 448·2
Chloroquini Sulfas, 448·2
5-Chloroquinolin-8-ol, 397·1
4-(7-Chloro-4-quinolylamino)-2-(diethylaminomethyl)phenol, 446·3
4-(7-Chloro-4-quinolylamino)-2-(diethylaminomethyl)phenol Dihydrochloride Dihydrate, 446·3
4-(7-Chloro-4-quinolylamino)pentyldiethylamine, 448·2
2-{N-[4-(7-Chloro-4-quinolylamino)pentyl]-N-ethylamino}ethanol Sulphate, 452·3
Chlorosin, 1884·1
4-Chloro-5-sulfamoyl Anthranilic Acid, 921·1
4-Chloro-5-sulphamoylsalicylo-2′,6′-xylidide, 1029·2
Chlorotenoxicam, 54·2
4-Chlorotestosterone Acetate, 1543·2
7-Chlorotetracycline, 187·3
6-Chloro-2,3,4,5-tetrahydro-1-(p-hydroxyphenyl)-1H-3-benzazepine-7,8-diol Methanesulfonate, 915·3
7-Chloro-1,2,3,4-tetrahydro-2-methyl-4-oxo-3-o-tolylquinazoline-6-sulphonamide, 956·2
10-Chloro-2,3,7,11b-tetrahydro-2-methyl-11b-phenyloxazolo[3,2-d][1,4]benzodiazepin-6(5H)-one, 712·3
7-Chloro-1,2,3,4-tetrahydro-4-oxo-2-phenylquinazoline-6-sulphonamide, 916·2
Chlorotetrahydroxy[(2-hydroxy-5-oxo-2-imidazolin-4-yl)ureato]dialuminium, 1141·2
2-Chloro-5-(1H-tetrazol-5-yl)-4-(2-thenylamino)benzenesulphonamide, 866·3
Chlorotheophylline, Benzhydryloxymethylpiperidine Salt, 439·1
Chlorotheophylline, Diphenhydramine Salt, 431·1
Chlorotheophylline, Diphenylpyraline Salt, 439·1
Chlorotheophylline, Promethazine Salt, 439·2
Chlorothiazide, 882·1
Chlorothiazide Sodium, 882·2
Chlorothiazidum, 882·1
(Z)-3-(2-Chlorothioxanthen-9-ylidene)-NN-dimethylpropylamine, 682·3
Chlorothymol, 1177·2
6-Chlorothymol, 1177·2
2-(3-Chloro-o-toluidino)nicotinic Acid, 26·3
N-(3-Chloro-o-tolyl)anthranilic Acid, 94·2
Chlorotracin, 1884·1
Chlorotrianisene, 1542·1
(+)-6-[4-Chloro-α-(1,2,4-triazol-1-yl)benzyl]-1-methyl-1H-benzotriazole, 594·3
2-Chloro-1-(2,4,5-trichlorophenyl)vinyl Dimethyl Phosphate, 1510·2
1-Chloro-2,2,2-trifluoroethyl Difluoromethyl Ether, 1301·1
2-Chloro-1,1,2-trifluoroethyl Difluoromethyl Ether, 1298·1
2-Chloro-N-([{4-(trifluoromethoxy)phenyl}amino]carbonyl)benzamide, 1510·3
4-(4-Chloro-3-trifluoromethylphenyl)-1-[3-(p,p′-difluorobenzhydryl)propyl]piperidin-4-ol, 713·2
N-[2-Chloro-4-(trifluoromethyl)phenyl]DL-valine, Cyano(3-phenoxyphenyl)methyl Ester, 1505·3
7α-Chloro-11β,17α,21-trihydroxy-16α-methylpregna-1,4-diene-3,20-dione 17,21-Dipropionate, 1090·3
9α-Chloro-11β,17α,21-trihydroxy-16β-methylpregna-1,4-diene-3,20-dione 17,21-Dipropionate, 1091·1
6-Chloro-11β,17α,21-trihydroxypregna-1,4,6-triene-3,20-dione, 1096·1
(2S,4′R)-7-Chloro-2′,4,6-trimethoxy-4′-methylspiro[benzofuran-2(3H),3′-cyclohexene]-3,6′-dione, 400·3
Chlorotris(4-methoxyphenyl)ethylene, 1542·1
1-(α-2-Chlorotrityl)imidazole, 396·2
β-Chlorovinyl Ethyl Ethynyl Carbinol, 697·3
Chloroxylenol, 1177·2
4-Chloro-3,5-xylenol, 1177·2
Chlorozotocin, 538·1
Chlorphed-LA, 1884·1
Chlorphedrine SR, 1884·1
Chlorphen, 1884·1
Chlorphenamine Maleate, 427·3
Chlorphenamine Polistirex, 428·2
Chlorphenamine Tannate, 428·2
Chlorphenamini Maleas, 427·3
Chlorphenesin, 396·1
Chlorphenesin Carbamate, 1392·2
Chlorpheniramine Maleate, 427·3
Chlorpheno, 1884·1
Chlorphenothanum, 1502·1
Chlorphenoxamide, 603·1
Chlorphenoxamine Hydrochloride, 428·3
Chlor-Pro, 1884·1
Chlorproethazine Hydrochloride, 675·1
Chlorproguanil Hydrochloride, 452·1
Chlorpromanyl, 1884·1
Chlorpromasit, 1884·1
Chlorpromazine, 675·1
Chlorpromazine Embonate, 675·1
Chlorpromazine Hydrochloride, 675·2
Chlorpromazine 4,4′-Methylenebis(3-hydroxy-2-naphthoate), 675·1
Chlorpromazine Pamoate, 675·1
Chlorpromazini Hydrochloridum, 675·2
Chlorpromed, 1884·1
Chlorpropamide, 330·3
Chlorpropamidum, 330·3
Chlorprophenpyridamine Maleate, 427·3
Chlorprothixene, 682·3
Chlorprothixene Acetate, 682·3
Chlorprothixene Citrate, 682·3
Chlorprothixene Hydrochloride, 682·3
Chlorprothixene Lactate, 682·3
Chlorprothixene Mesilate, 682·3
Chlorprothixene Mesylate, 682·3
Chlorprothixene-sulfoxide, 682·3
Chlorprothixene-sulfoxide-N-oxide, 682·3
Chlorprothixeni Hydrochloridum, 682·3
Chlorprothixenium Mesylicum, 682·3
Chlorpyramine, 1884·1
Chlorpyrifos, 1502·1
Chlorpyrimine, 1884·1
Chlorquin, 1884·1
Chlorquinaldol, 187·3
Chlorquinol, 220·3
Chlor-Rest, 1884·1
Chlorsig, 1884·1
Chlortalidone, 882·3
Chlortalidonum, 882·3
Chlortenoxicam, 54·2
Chlortestosterone Acetate, 1543·2
Chlortetracycline, 187·3
Chlortetracycline Bisulfate, 187·3
Chlortetracycline Bisulphate, 187·3
Chlortetracycline Hydrochloride, 187·3
Chlortetracyclini Hydrochloridum, 187·3
Chlorthalidone, 882·3
Chlortralim, 1884·1
Chlor-Trimeton, 1884·1
Chlor-Trimeton Allergy Sinus, 1884·1
Chlor-Trimeton 4 Hour Relief, 1884·1
Chlor-Trimeton 12 Hour Relief, 1884·1
Chlor-Tripolon, 1884·1
Chlor-Tripolon Decongestant, 1884·2
Chlor-Tripolon ND, 1884·2
Chlorumagene, 1884·2
Chlorure de Chaux, 1175·3
Chlorure de Magnésium Cristallisé, 1228·1
Chlorure de Sodium, 1233·3
Chlorvescent, 1884·2
Chlorzide, 1884·2
Chlorzox, 1884·2
Chlorzoxazone, 1392·3
Chlotride, 1884·2
Choanol N, 1884·2
Chocaton, 1884·2
Chocolate, 1482·3, 1754·3
Chocolate Brown FK, 1056·2
Chocolate Brown HT, 1056·3
Chocovite, 1884·2
Chofabol, 1884·2
Chofitol, 1884·2
Chofranina, 1884·2
Choice DM, 1884·2
Chol 4000, 1884·2
Cholac, 1884·2
Cholacid, 1884·2
Cholagogum F, 1884·2
Cholagogum N, 1884·2
Cholagutt, 1884·2
Cholagutt-N, 1884·2
Cholaktol, 1884·2
Cholal Modificado, 1884·2
Cholangitis— see Biliary-tract Infections, 121·3
Cholangitis— see Gallstones, 1761·3
Cholan-HMB, 1884·2
Cholapret, 1884·2
Chol-Arbuz N, 1884·2
Cholarist, 1884·3
Cholasitrol, 1884·3
Cholasyn, 1884·3
Cholasyn II, 1884·3
Cholax, 1884·3
Choldestal, 1884·3
Chol-Do, 1884·3
Cholebine, 1884·3
Cholebrin, 1884·3
Cholebrine, 1884·3
Cholecalciferol, 1461·3
Cholecalciferol Concentrate (Oily Form), 1461·3
Cholecalciferol Concentrate (Powder Form), 1461·3
Cholecalciferol Concentrate (Water-dispersible Form), 1461·3
Cholecalciferol Solution, 1461·3
Cholecalciferoli Pulvis, 1461·3
Cholecalciferolum, 1461·3
Cholecalciferolum in Aqua Dispergibile, 1461·3
Cholecalciferolum Densatum Oleosum, 1461·3
Cholecis, 1884·3
Chole-cyl Ho-Len-Complex, 1884·3
Cholecysmon, 1884·3
Cholecystitis— see Biliary-tract Infections, 121·3
Cholecystitis— see Gallstones, 1761·3
Cholecystokinin, 1727·2
Choledocholithiasis— see Gallstones, 1761·3
Choledyl, 1884·3
Choledyl Expectorant, 1884·3
Cholegerol, 1884·3

Cholelithiasis— *see* Gallstones, 1761·3
Choleodoron, 1884·3
Cholera— *see* Cholera and other Vibrio Infections, 128·3
Cholera Vaccine, 1611·2
Cholera Vaccine, Freeze-dried, 1611·2
Cholera Vaccines, 1611·2
Cholesolvin, 1884·3
Cholestabyl, 1884·3
Cholest-5-en-3β-ol, 1480·3
Cholesterin, 1480·3
Cholesterol, 1480·3
Cholesterol Reducing Plan, 1884·3
Cholesterol Support, 1884·3
Cholesterolum, 1480·3
Cholesteryl Benzoate, 1481·1
Cholestin, 1884·3
Cholest-X L112, 1884·3
Cholestyramine, 889·3
Cholestyramine Resin, 889·3
Choletec, 1884·3
Cholex, 1884·3
Chol-Grandelat, 1884·3
Cholhepan, 1884·3
Cholhepan N, 1884·3
Choliatron, 1884·3
Cholic Acid, 1660·3
Cholidase, 1884·3
Choline Acid Tartrate, 1424·3
Choline Alfoscerate, 1488·3
Choline Bitartrate, 1424·3
Choline Chloride, 1424·3
Choline Chloride Carbamate, 1488·1
Choline Chloride Succinate, 1406·2
Choline Cytidine-5′-pyrophosphate, 1672·3
Choline Dihydrogen Citrate, 1424·3
Choline Esters, 1484·1
Choline Glycerophosphate, 1488·3
Choline Magnesium Trisalicylate, 26·2
Choline Orotate, 1424·3, 1724·3
Choline Salicylate, 26·2
Choline Salicylate Solution, 26·2
Choline Theophyllinate, 784·2
Cholinergic Agonists, 1484·1
Cholinesterase Inhibitors, 1484·1
Cholinii Chloridum, 1424·3
Cholinii Tartras, 1424·3
Cholinogo, 1884·3
Cholinoid, 1884·4
Cholinomimetics, 1484·1
Cholipin, 1884·4
Cholit-Ursan, 1884·4
Chol-Kugeletten Neu, 1884·4
Chol-Less, 1884·4
Cholofalk, 1884·4
Chologon, 1679·2
Cholografin, 1884·4
Cholonerton, 1884·4
Cholosan, 1884·4
Cholosom Phyto N, 1884·4
Cholosom SL, 1884·4
Cholosom-Tee, 1884·4
Choloxin, 1884·4
Cholspasmin, 1884·4
Cholspasmin Phyto, 1884·4
Cholspasminase N, 1884·4
Chol-Spasmoletten, 1884·4
Cholstat, 1884·4
Chol-Truw S, 1884·4
Chomelanum, 1884·4
*Chondodendron tomentosum*, 1409·2
Chondroitin 4-Sulfate, 1670·2
Chondroitin Sulfate B, 892·2
Chondroitin Sulfate B Sodium, 892·2
Chondroitin Sulfate–Iron Complex, 1425·1
Chondroitin Sulfate Sodium, 1670·2
Chondroitin Sulphate–Iron Complex, 1425·1
Chondroitin Sulphate Sodium, 1670·2
Chondroitinsulphatase, 1755·1
Chondrosarcoma— *see* Bone Sarcoma, 524·3
Chondrosteo, 1884·4
Chondrosulf, 1884·4
*Chondrus crispus*, 1578·2
Chondrus Extract, 1578·2
Chooz, 1884·4
Chophytol, 1884·4
Chopnut, 1494·1
Choragon, 1884·4
Chorea, 664·2
Chorex, 1884·4
Chorigon, 1885·1
Choriocarcinoma— *see* Gestational Trophoblastic Tumours, 505·1
Choriogonadotrophin, 1320·3
Choriogonadotropin Alfa, 1320·3
Choriomon, 1885·1
Chorion, 1654·2
Chorionic Gonadotrophin, 1320·3
Chorionic Gonadotropin, 1320·3
Chorioretinitis— *see* Uveitis, 1090·1
Choroiditis— *see* Uveitis, 1090·1
Choron, 1885·1
Chotachand, 994·3
Cho/Vac, 1611·2
Cho/Vac, Dried, 1611·2
Chributan, 1885·1
Christmas Disease— *see* Haemorrhagic Disorders, 737·3
Christmas Factor, 735·3, 752·2
Chromagen, 1885·1
Chromagen FA, 1885·1
Chromagen Forte, 1885·1
Chromagen OB, 1885·1
Chroma-Pak, 1885·1
Chromargon, 1885·1
Chromatophore Hormone, 1332·2
Chrome, 1885·1
Chrome Alum, 1670·2
Chromelin Complexion Blender, 1885·1
ChromeMate— *see* Cromotex, 1912·3
Chromic Acid, 1670·3
Chromic Anhydride, 1670·3
Chromic Chloride, 1425·1
Chromic Chloride ($^{51}$Cr), 1523·2
Chromic Phosphate ($^{32}$P), 1525·1
Chromium, 1425·1
Chromium-51, 1523·2
Chromium Edetate ($^{51}$Cr), 1523·2
Chromium Orotate, 1724·3
Chromium Picolinate, 1425·1
Chromium Potassium Sulfate, 1670·2
Chromium Potassium Sulphate, 1670·2
Chromium Trichloride, 1425·1
Chromium Trioxide, 1670·3
Chromium Tripicolinate, 1425·1, 1670·3
Chromoblastomycosis, 387·2
Chromocarb Diethylamine, 1670·3
Chromomycosis— *see* Chromoblastomycosis, 387·2
Chromonar Hydrochloride, 880·2
Chronadalate, 1885·1
Chronexan, 1885·1
Chronic Actinic Dermatitis— *see* Light-induced Skin Reactions, 1136·3
Chronic Fatigue Syndrome— *see* Depression, 279·1
Chronic Obstructive Pulmonary Disease, 779·2
Chronocard N, 1885·1
Chronocorte, 1885·1
Chrono-Indocid, 1885·1
Chronophyllin, 1885·1
Chronovera, 1885·1
Chronulac, 1885·1
Chrysanthème Insecticide, 1509·3
Chrysanthemic Acid, 1509·3
Chrysanthemin, 1718·3
*Chrysanthemum cinerariaefolium*, 1509·3
*Chrysanthemum vulgare*, 1751·3
Chrysazin, 1261·1
Chrysocor, 1885·1
Chrysoidine Hydrochloride Citrate, 1670·3
Chrysoidine Y, 1670·3
Chrysotile, 1658·1
Chuanxiong, 1750·2
Chuker, 1885·1
Chuna, 1664·3
Chur Ganja, 1666·1
Churg-Strauss Syndrome, 1078·3
Churrus, 1666·1
Chus, 1666·1
Chutras, 1666·1
Chutsao, 1666·1
CHX-10, 566·1
CHX-100, 566·1
CHX-3673, 781·1
CHX Dental Gel, 1885·1
Chylomicronaemia— *see* Hyperlipidaemias, 823·1
Chymex, 1885·1
Chymodiactin, 1885·1
Chymodiactine, 1885·1
Chymol, 1885·1
Chymopapain, 1671·1
Chymotrypsin, 1671·2
α-Chymotrypsin, 1671·2
Chymotrypsinum, 1671·2
CI-107, 1342·3
CI-366, 360·1
CI-395, 1730·3
CI-406, 1565·2
CI-440, 43·2
CI-473, 55·2
CI-581, 1302·1
CI-583, 55·1
CI-634, 1310·2
CI-673, 657·1
CI-705, 707·1
CI-716, 728·3
CI-718, 671·3
CI-719, 923·1
CI-775, 873·2
CI-808, 657·1
CI-808 Sodium, 657·1
CI-825, 579·2
CI-845, 984·1
CI-871, 1732·1
CI-874, 1700·3
CI-879, 1734·3
CI-880, 527·3
CI-888, 791·1
CI-898, 410·2
CI-904, 546·3
CI-906, 991·1
CI-912, 384·3
CI-919, 207·2
CI-925, 961·2
CI-945, 362·2
CI-960, 194·2
CI-970, 1497·2
CI-978, 255·1
CI-981, 866·1
CI-982, 361·3
CI-983, 171·3
CI-991, 348·2
CI-1003, 615·3
CI-1008, 376·2
CI-1009, 96·3
CI-9148, 1712·2
CI-75610, 1692·1
CI Acid Blue 9, 1056·2
CI Acid Red 17, 1056·2
CI Acid Red 27, 1056·1
CI Acid Red 87, 1057·2
CI Acid Red 93, 1740·1
CI Acid Red 94, 1740·1
CI Acid Violet 19, 1646·3
CI Acid Yellow 3, 1057·3
CI Acid Yellow 73, 1689·1
CI Basic Blue 9, 1042·2
CI Basic Blue 17, 1757·1
CI Basic Green 1, 1171·1
CI Basic Green 4, 1185·2
CI Basic Orange 2, 1670·3
CI Basic Red 5, 1719·3
CI Basic Violet 1, 1186·2
CI Basic Violet 3, 1186·1
CI Basic Violet 14, 1185·1
CI Direct Blue 14, 1758·3
CI Direct Blue 53, 1658·3
CI Direct Red 28, 1675·3
CI Food Black 1, 1056·2
CI Food Blue 1, 1700·3
CI Food Blue 2, 1056·2
CI Food Blue 5, 1729·1
CI Food Brown 1, 1056·2
CI Food Brown 3, 1056·3
CI Food Green 4, 1057·3
CI Food Orange 8, 1056·3
CI Food Red 3, 1057·1
CI Food Red 7, 1057·3
CI Food Red 9, 1056·1
CI Food Red 10, 1058·1
CI Food Red 14, 1057·2
CI Food Red 17, 1056·1
CI Food Yellow 3, 1058·2
CI Food Yellow 4, 1058·2
CI Food Yellow 5, 1058·3
CI Food Yellow 13, 1057·3
CI Mordant Yellow 5, 1278·1
CI Natural Green 3, 1057·1
CI Natural Red 4, 1057·1, 1057·2
CI Natural Yellow 3, 1058·3
CI Natural Yellow 6, 1058·2
CI No.— *see under* Colour Index No.
CI Pigment Blue 27, 1051·2
CI Pigment White 6, 1160·3
CI Solvent Red 24, 1191·3
Ciagen, 1885·2
Cialis, 1885·2
Ciamemazina, 689·2
Cianhídrico, Ácido, 1506·1
Cianoacrilato, Adhesivos de, 1678·1
Cianocobalamina, 1458·2
Cianomin, 1885·2
Cianon B12, 1885·2
Cianotrat, 1885·2
Cianotrat-Dexa, 1885·2
Ciapar, 1885·2
Ciarbiot, 1885·2
Ciatyl-Z, 1885·2
Ciba Vision Cleaner For Sensitive Eyes, 1885·2
Cibacalcin, 1885·2
Cibacalcina, 1885·2
Cibacalcine, 1885·2
Cibace, 1885·2
Cibacen, 1885·2
Cibacene, 1885·2
Cibadrex, 1885·2
Cibaflam, 1885·2
Cibalena A, 1885·2
Cibalgin Compositum N, 1885·2
Cibalgina Due Fast, 1885·2
Cibenol, 1885·2
Cibenzolina, 883·1
Cibenzoline, 883·1
Cibis, 1885·2
Ciblex, 1885·2
Ciblor, 1885·2
Cibral, 1885·2
Cibramicina, 1885·3
Cibronal, 1885·3
Cica-Care, 1885·3
Cicaderma, 1885·3
Cicafissan, 1885·3
Cicalfate, 1885·3
Cicamosa, 1885·3
Cicapost, 1885·3
Cicatral, 1885·3
Cicatrene, 1885·3
Cicatrex, 1885·3
Cicatricial Pemphigoid— *see* Pemphigus and Pemphigoid, 1137·1
Cicatrin, 1885·3
Cicatrina, 1885·3
Cicatrizan, 1885·3
Cicatrol, 1885·3
Cicatryl, 1885·3
Cicatul, 1885·3
Ciclacilina, 188·1
Ciclacillin, 188·1
Cicladol, 1885·3
Ciclafast, 1885·3
Ciclamato de Calcio, 1426·2
Ciclamato de Sodio, 1426·2
Ciclámico, Ácido, 1426·2
Ciclamil, 1885·3
Ciclandelato, 890·3
Ciclavix, 1885·4
Ciclesonide, 1095·2
Cicletanina, Hidrocloruro de, 883·2

Cicletanine, 883·2
Cicletanine Hydrochloride, 883·2
Ciclidon, 1885·4
Ciclidrol, 1130·2
Ciclinalgin, 1885·4
Cicliomenol, 1177·3
Ciclisan, 1885·4
Ciclizina, 429·3
Ciclizina, Hidrocloruro de, 429·3
Ciclizina, Lactato de, 429·3
Ciclizina, Tartrato de, 429·3
Ciclo, 1885·4
Ciclobarbital, 689·2
Ciclobarbital Cálcico, 689·2
Ciclobarbital Calcium, 689·2
Ciclobenzaprina, Hidrocloruro de, 1393·1
Ciclobiotico, 1885·4
Ciclobutirol Sódico, 1678·2
Ciclochem, 1885·4
Ciclocris, 1885·4
Ciclocur, 1885·4
Cicloderm, 1885·4
Cicloderm-C, 1885·4
Ciclodextrinas, 1678·2
Ciclodrina, Hidrocloruro de, 480·3
Ciclofalina, 1885·4
Ciclofenilo, 1544·1
Cicloferon, 1885·4
Ciclofosfamida, 540·2
Ciclohexal, 1885·4
Ciclohexano, 1472·3
Ciclohexilpropionato de Nandrolona, 1561·2
Cicloheximida, 1502·1
Cicloheximide, 1502·1
Ciclolux, 1885·4
Ciclomestril, 1885·4
Ciclomex, 1885·4
Ciclon, 1885·4
Ciclonio, Bromuro de, 480·2
Ciclonium Bromide, 480·2
Ciclopenal, 1885·4
Ciclopentiazida, 890·3
Ciclopentolato, Cloridrato de, 480·3
Ciclopentolato, Hidrocloruro de, 480·3
Ciclopirox, 396·1
Ciclopirox, Aminoethanol Salt, 396·1
Ciclopirox Olamina, 396·1
Ciclopirox Olamine, 396·1
Ciclopiroxolamine, 396·1
Ciclopiroxum, 396·1
Cicloplant, 1885·4
Ciclople, 1885·4
Cicloplegicedol, 1885·4
Cicloplegico, 1885·4
Cicloplejic, 1885·4
Cicloplejico, 1885·4
Cicloplejico, Colircusi— *see* Colircusi Cicloplejico, 1899·4
Cicloprimogyna, 1885·4
Ciclopropano, 1297·1
Ciclor, 1885·4
Cicloral, 1885·4
Cicloserina, 202·1
Ciclosmida, 1885·4
Ciclospasmol, 1885·4
Ciclosporin, 1351·2
Ciclosporina, 1351·2
Ciclosporinum, 1351·2
Ciclotal, 1885·4
Ciclotetryl, 1886·1
Ciclotiazida, 891·1
Ciclotos, 1886·1
Ciclotran, 1886·1
Ciclovalona, 1678·2
Cicloven, 1886·1
Cicloviral, 1886·1
Ciclovular, 1886·1
Ciclovulon, 1886·1
Cicloxal, 1886·1
Cicloxilic Acid, 1671·2
Cicloxílico, Ácido, 1671·2
Cicnor, 1886·1
Ciconazol, 1886·1
Cicotiamina, 1454·3
Cidalin, 1886·1
Cidegol C, 1886·1
Cideox, 1886·1
Cidermex, 1886·1
Cidetox, 1886·1
Cidex, 1886·1
Cidex OPA, 1886·1
Cidezyme, 1886·1
Cidilin, 1886·1
Cidine, 1886·1
Cidofovir, 629·2
Cidofovir Diphosphate, 629·3
Cidomel, 1886·1
Cidomycin, 1886·1
Cidoten, 1886·1
Cidoten V, 1886·1
Cidoten Rapilento, 1886·1
Cidra, Esencia de, 1706·2
Cidrin, 1886·1
Ciella, 1886·1
Cif Candioli, 1886·2
Cifenline, 883·1
Cifespasmo, 1886·2
Cifespasmo Compuesto, 1886·2
Ciflan, 1886·2
Cifloc, 1886·2
Ciflogex, 1886·2
Ciflolan, 1886·2
Ciflox, 1886·2
Cifloxin, 1886·2
Cifloxtron, 1886·2
Ciflutrina, 1502·3
Cifran, 1886·2
Cifrantil, 1886·2
Cigamet, 1886·2
Ciganclor, 1886·2
Cig-Ridettes, 1886·2
Ciguatera Poisoning, 951·1
Cihalotrina, 1502·3
Cikavit, 1886·2
CIL, 1886·2
Cila, 1130·3
Cilab, 1886·2
Cilamin, 1886·2
Cilamox, 1886·2
Cilansetron, 1255·3
Cilantro, Aceite Esencial de, 1676·1
Cilantro, Fruto del, 1676·1
Cilastatin Sodium, 188·1
Cilastatina Sódica, 188·1
Cilastatinum Natricum, 188·1
Cilatron, 1886·2
Cilaxoral, 1886·2
Cilazapril, 883·3
Cilazaprilat, 883·3
Cilazaprilum, 883·3
Cilclar, 1886·2
Cildox, 1886·2
Cilergil, 1886·2
Cilest, 1886·2
Cileste, 1886·2
Cilestoderme, 1886·2
Cilex, 1886·3
Cilfer-12-F, 1886·3
Cilferon-A, 1886·3
Ciliar, 1886·3
Ciliary Neurotrophic Factor, 1671·3
Cilicaine, 1886·3
Cilicaine Syringe, 1886·3
Cilicaine V, 1886·3
Cilicaine VK, 1886·3
Cilinafosal, 1886·3
Cilinafosal DHD Estrep, 1886·3
Cilinafosal Hidrocort, 1886·3
Cilinafosal Neomicina, 1886·3
Cilinase, 1886·3
Cilinavagin Neomicina, 1886·3
Cilinon, 1886·3
Cilipen, 1886·3
Cillimicina, 1886·3
Cilnidipine, 884·1
Cilnidipino, 884·1
Cilodex, 1886·3
Cilopen VK, 1886·3
Ciloprin, 1886·3
Ciloprin cum Anaesthetico, 1886·3
Ciloprine Ca, 1886·3
Ciloprost, 1518·2
Ciloprost Tromethamine, 1518·2
Ciloquin, 1886·3
Cilostazol, 884·1
Cilox, 1886·3
Ciloxacin, 1886·3
Ciloxan, 1886·3
Cilpen, 1886·3
Cilpier, 1886·3
Cilroton, 1886·4
Cim, 1886·4
Cimaas, 1886·4
Cimadronic Acid, 773·1
Cimag, 1886·4
Cimagen, 1886·4
Cimal, 1886·4
Cimascal, 1886·4
Cimascal D, 1886·4
Cime, 1886·4
Cimebec, 1886·4
Cimebeta, 1886·4
Cimecard, 1886·4
Cimecodan, 1886·4
Cimedine, 1886·4
Cimedul, 1886·4
Cimefer, 1886·4
Cimegripe, 1886·4
Cimehexal, 1886·4
Cimeldine, 1886·4
Cimelide, 1886·4
Cimelin, 1886·4
Cimemerck, 1886·4
Cimeno, 28·2
Cimephil, 1886·4
Cimet, 1886·4
Cimeta, 1886·4
Cimetag, 1887·1
Cimetase, 1887·1
Cimetid, 1887·1
Cimetidan, 1887·1
Cimetidina, 1255·3
Cimetidine, 1255·3
Cimetidine Hydrochloride, 1255·3
Cimetidini Hydrochloridum, 1255·3
Cimetidinum, 1255·3
Cimetil, 1887·1
Cimetimax, 1887·1
Cimetin, 1887·1
Cimetina, 1887·1
Cimetinax, 1887·1
Cimetine, 1887·1
Cimetival, 1887·1
Cimet-P, 1887·1
Cimetrin, 1887·1
Cimetropio, Bromuro de, 480·2
Cimetropium Bromide, 480·2
Cimex, 1887·1
Cimex Sirop contre la Toux, 1887·1
Cimexyl, 1887·1
Cimi, 1887·1
Cimiazol, 1502·3
Cimicifuga, 1671·3
Cimicifuga Comp, 1887·1
Cimicifuga Med Complex, 1887·1
Cimicifuga Oligoplex, 1887·1
*Cimicifuga racemosa*, 1671·3
*Cimicifuga* spp., 1671·3
Cimidine, 1887·1
Cimifemine, 1887·1
Cimipax, 1887·1
Cimisan, 1887·1
CimLich, 1887·1
Cimlok, 1887·1
Cimogal, 1887·1
Cimulcer, 1887·1
Cinabel, 1887·2
Cinacalcet Hydrochloride, 770·2
Cinacris, 1887·2
Cinactiv, 1887·2
Cinadine, 1887·2
Cinaflan, 1887·2
Cinageron, 1887·2
Cinalong, 1887·2
Cinamato de Etilo, 1685·2
Cinametic Acid, 1671·3
Cinamético, Ácido, 1671·3
Cinámico, Ácido, 1177·3
Cinaran, 1887·2
Cinarina, 1678·3
Cinarix, 1887·2
Cinarizina, 428·3
Cinarizina-Cinarin, 1887·2
Cinaro Bilina, 1887·2
Cinaryl, 1887·2
Cinaziere, 1887·2
Cinazon, 1887·2
Cinazyn, 1887·2
Cincain, 1887·2
Cincaini Chloridum, 1373·2
Cincainum, 1373·2
Cinchocaine, 1373·2
Cinchocaine Benzoate, 1373·3
Cinchocaine Hydrochloride, 1373·2
Cinchocaini Hydrochloridum, 1373·2
Cinchona, 1671·3
*Cinchona*, 460·1
Cinchona Bark, 1671·3
Cinchona Bark, Red, 1671·3
*Cinchona calisaya*, 1671·3
*Cinchona ledgeriana*, 1671·3
*Cinchona pubescens*, 1671·3
*Cinchona succirubra*, 1671·3
Cinchonae Cortex, 1671·3
Cinchonae Succirubrae Cortex, 1671·3
Cinchonidine, 1672·1
Cinchonine, 1672·1
Cinchophen, 1024·1
Cinclamina, 1887·2
Cincocaína, 1373·2
Cincocaína, Hidrocloruro de, 1373·2
Cincofarm, 1887·2
Cinco-Fu, 1887·2
Cincopal, 1887·2
Cincordil, 1887·2
Cincuental, 1887·2
Cineol, 1672·1
Cineole, 1283·2, 1672·1, 1710·2, 1740·2
Cineolum, 1672·1
Cinepazet Maleate, 884·2
Cinepazet, Maleato de, 884·2
Cinepazic Acid Ethyl Ester Maleate, 884·2
Cinepazida, Maleato de, 884·2
Cinepazide Maleate, 884·2
Cinergil, 1887·2
Cinerin I, 1509·3
Cinerin II, 1509·3
Cinerine, 1887·2
Cinet, 1887·2
Cinetic, 1887·2
Cinetol, 1887·2
Cinfacromin, 1887·2
Cinfamar, 1887·2
Cinfamar Cafeina, 1887·3
Cinfatos, 1887·3
Cinfatos Complex, 1887·3
Cinfatos Expectorante, 1887·3
Cinfloxine, 1887·3
Cinifa, 1887·3
Cinitaprida, 1259·2
Cinitapride, 1259·2
Cinitapride Acid Tartrate, 1259·2
Cinkef-U, 1887·3
Cinna, 1887·3
Cinnabene, 1887·3
Cinnacet, 1887·3
Cinnageron, 1887·3
Cinnam., 1672·2
Cinnam. Oil, 1672·2
Cinnamaldehyde, 1668·2, 1672·2
Cinnamed, 1887·3
Cinnamedrine, 1672·2
Cinnamedrine Hydrochloride, 1672·2
Cinnamic Acid, 1177·3
Cinnamomi Cassiae Aetheroleum, 1668·2
Cinnamomi Cassiae, Oleum, 1668·2
Cinnamomi Cortex, 1672·2
Cinnamomi, Oleum, 1668·2, 1672·2
Cinnamomi Zeylanici, Aetheroleum, 1672·2
*Cinnamomum aromaticum*, 1668·2
*Cinnamomum camphora*, 1665·3
*Cinnamomum cassia*, 1668·2

*Cinnamomum verum*, 1672·2
*Cinnamomum zeylanicum*, 1672·2
Cinnamon, 1672·2
Cinnamon Bark, 1668·2, 1672·2
Cinnamon Bark Oil, Ceylon, 1672·2
Cinnamon, Ceylon, 1672·2
Cinnamon Leaf Oil, Ceylon, 1672·2
Cinnamon Oil, 1672·2
Cinnamon Oil, Chinese, 1668·2
Cinnamoni Zeylanicii Corticus Aetheroleum, 1672·2
(±)-(*E*)-Cinnamyl 2-Methoxyethyl 1,4-Dihydro-2,6-dimethyl-4-(*m*-nitrophenyl)-3,5-pyridinedicarboxylate, 884·1
Cinnamyl-cocaine, 1373·3
*trans*-1-Cinnamyl-4-(4,4′-difluorobenzhydryl)piperazine Dihydrochloride, 434·1
*N*-Cinnamylephedrine, 1672·2
*N*-Cinnamylephedrine Hydrochloride, 1672·2
Cinnamylic Acid, 1177·3
(*E*)-*N*-Cinnamyl-*N*-methyl(1-naphthylmethyl)amine Hydrochloride, 406·2
Cinnar, 1887·3
Cinnarizine, 428·3
Cinnarizinum, 428·3
Cinnaron, 1887·3
Cinnarplus, 1887·3
Cinnaza, 1887·3
Cinnipirine, 1887·3
Cinnoxicam, 85·1
Cinobac, 1887·3
Cinobactin, 1887·3
Cinocil, 1887·3
Cinoflax, 1887·3
Cinolazepam, 683·1
Cinon, 1887·3
Cinopal, 1887·3
Cinotec, 1887·3
Cinoxacin, 188·1
Cinoxacino, 188·1
Cinoxate, 1145·1
Cinoxato, 1145·1
Cinoxen, 1887·3
Cinquefoil, Erect, 1757·2
Cinquerix, 1887·3
Cinrizine, 1887·3
Cintigo, 1887·3
Cintilan, 1887·4
Cinton, 1887·4
Ciocar, 1887·4
Cional, 1887·4
Cional S— *see* Dynexan Zahnfleischtropfen, 1960·2
Cipadur, 1887·4
Cipalat, 1887·4
Cipamox, 1887·4
Cipanfeno, 1887·4
Cipasid, 1887·4
Cipermetrina, 1502·3
Cipex, 1887·4
Cipflocin, 1887·4
Cipide, 1887·4
Cipionato de Estradiol, 1550·1
Cipionato de Hidrocortisona, 1104·1
Cipionato de Oxabolona, 1565·1
Cipionato de Testosterona, 1569·3
Ciplactin, 1887·4
Ciplar, 1887·4
Ciplar-H, 1887·4
Ciplatec, 1887·4
Ciplazin, 1887·4
Ciplin, 1887·4
Ciplox, 1887·4
Cipobacter, 1887·4
Cipofix, 1887·4
Ciprain, 1887·4
Cipralan, 1887·4
Cipralex, 1887·4
Cipram, 1887·4
Cipramil, 1887·4
Ciprenit Otico, 1887·4
Ciprex, 1888·1
Cipridanol, 1888·1
Cipride, 1888·1
Cipril, 1888·1
Cipril-H, 1888·1
Ciprin, 1888·1
Ciprin, Adco- — *see* Adco-Ciprin, 1775·2
Cipro, 1888·1
Cipro HC, 1888·1
Ciprobac, 1888·1
Ciprobay, 1888·1
Ciprobay HC, 1888·1
Ciprobeta, 1888·1
Ciprobid, 1888·1
Ciprobiot, 1888·1
Ciprobiotic, 1888·1
Cipro-Cent, 1888·1
Ciprocep, 1888·1
Ciprocin, 1888·1
Ciprocina, 1888·1
Ciprocinonida, 1095·2
Ciprocinonide, 1095·2
Ciprocort, 1888·1
Ciprocort D, 1888·1
Ciprocort L, 1888·1
Ciprodex, 1888·1
Ciprodexol, 1888·2
Ciprodine, 1888·2
Ciprodura, 1888·2
Ciprofar, 1888·2
Ciprofarma, 1888·2
Ciprofibrate, 884·2, 884·3
Ciprofibrato, 884·2
Ciprofibratum, 884·2
Ciprofin, 1888·2
Ciproflox, 1888·2
Ciprofloxacin, 188·2
Ciprofloxacin Hydrochloride, 188·2
Ciprofloxacin Hydrochloride Monohydrate, 188·2
Ciprofloxacin Lactate, 188·3
Ciprofloxacini Hydrochloridum, 188·2
Ciprofloxacino, 188·2
Ciprofloxacino, Hidrocloruro de, 188·2
Ciprofloxacino, Lactato de, 188·3
Ciprofloxacinum, 188·2
Ciprofur, 1888·2
Ciprogamma, 1888·2
Ciprogen, 1888·2
Ciprogis, 1888·2
Ciproglen, 1888·2
Ciproheptadina, Hidrocloruro de, 430·1
Ciprohexal, 1888·2
Ciprok, 1888·2
Ciprol, 1888·2
Ciprolet, 1888·2
Cipro-Lich, 1888·2
Ciprolisina, 1888·2
Ciprom-H, 1888·2
Cipromycin, 1888·2
Cipronal, 1888·2
Cipro-Otico, 1888·2
Ciproplex, 1888·2
Ciproquinol, 1888·2
Ciproser, 1888·2
Ciprospes, 1888·2
Ciprosun, 1888·2
Ciprotenk, 1888·2
Ciproterona, Acetato de, 1544·1
Ciproval, 1888·2
Ciproviron, 1888·2
Ciprovit Calcio, 1888·3
Ciprovit Energizante, 1888·3
Ciprovit Magnesico, 1888·3
Ciprowin, 1888·3
Cipro-Wolff, 1888·3
Ciproxan, 1888·3
Ciproxil, 1888·3
Ciproxin, 1888·3
Ciproxin HC, 1888·3
Ciproxina, 1888·3
Ciproxine, 1888·3
Ciproxin-Hydrocortison, 1888·3
Ciproxino, 1888·3
Ciproxyl, 1888·3
Ciqfadin, 1888·3
Circanetten, 1888·3
Circanol, 1888·3
Circavite-T, 1888·3
Circles, 698·3
Circo-Maren, 1888·3
Circonyl, 1888·3
Circonyl N, 1888·3
Circovenil, 1888·3
Circovenil Fuerte, 1888·3
Circularine, 1888·3
Circulation, 1888·3
Circulatonic, 1888·3
Circumax, 1888·4
Circupon, 1888·4
Circupon RR, 1888·4
Circusil, Natusor— *see* Natusor Circusil, 2153·4
Circuvit, 1888·4
Circuvit E, 1888·4
Cire Blanche, 1480·1
Cire Jaune, 1480·2
Cirflo, Bioglan— *see* Bioglan Cirflo, 1843·4
Cirflox-G, 1888·4
Ciriax, 1888·4
Ciriax Otic, 1888·4
Cirkan, 1888·4
Cirkan a la Prednacinolone, 1888·4
Cirku Sed, 1888·4
Cirkufemal, 1888·4
Cirkulin Baldrian, 1888·4
Cirkuprostan, 1888·4
Cirkused, 1888·4
Ciromazina, 1503·1
Cirrhosis, Primary Biliary— *see* Primary Biliary Cirrhosis, 1761·2
Cirrhotic Ascites— *see* Ascites, 815·1
Cirrus, 1888·4
Ciruela, 1285·1
Cirulan, 1888·4
Cirulaxia, 1888·4
Cisaken, 1888·4
Cisalone, 1888·4
Cisap, 1888·4
Cisapan, 1888·4
Cisapin, 1888·4
Cisaprida, 1259·2
Cisapride, 1259·2
Cisapride Monohydrate, 1259·2
Cisapride Tartrate, 1259·2
Cisapridi Tartras, 1259·2
Cisapridum, 1259·2
Cisatec, 1888·4
Cisatracurio, Besilato de, 1399·1
Cisatracurium Besilate, 1399·1
Cisatracurium Besylate, 1399·1
Cisday, 1888·4
Cis-Gry, 1888·4
Cishexal, 1888·4
Cisordinol, 1888·4
Cisplatex, 1889·1
Cisplatin, 538·1
Cisplatina, 538·1
Cisplatino, 538·1
Cis-platinum, 538·1
Cisplatinum, 538·1
Cisplatyl, 1889·1
Cispride, 1889·1
Cistalgan, 1889·1
Cistalgina, 1889·1
Cistamine, 1889·1
Cisteína, 1426·3
Cisteína, Hidrocloruro de, 1426·3
Cisticid, 1889·1
Cistidil, 1889·1
Cistimax, 1889·1
Cistina, 1426·3
Cistobil, 1889·1
Cistofuran, 1889·1
Cistomid, 1889·1
Cistopax, 1889·1
Cistoquine Plus, 1889·1
Cistosan, 1889·1
Cistus Canadensis Oligoplex, 1889·1
Citab, 1889·1
Citadura, 1889·1
Citagenin, 1889·1
Cital, 1889·1
Citalgan, 1889·1
Citalopram, 289·1
Citalopram, Hidrobromuro de, 289·1
Citalopram, Hidrocloruro de, 289·1
Citalopram Hydrobromide, 289·1
Citalopram Hydrochloride, 289·1
*S*-Citalopram Oxalate, 292·1
Citalor, 1889·1
Citaloxan, 1889·1
Citanest Preparations, 1889·1
Citarabina, 543·1
Citavi, 1889·2
Citavir, 1889·2
Citax F, 1889·2
Citemul S, 1889·2
Citicef, 1889·2
Citicil, 1889·2
Citiclor, 1889·2
Citicolina, 1672·3
Citicoline, 1672·3
Citicoline Sodium, 1672·3
Citidel, 1889·2
Citidine, 1889·2
Citidoline, 1672·3
Citifar, 1889·2
Citiflux, 1889·2
Citilat, 1889·2
Citimid, 1889·2
Citinoides, 1889·2
Citioato, 1503·1
Citiolase, 1889·2
Citiolona, 1672·3
Citiolone, 1672·3
Cition, 1889·2
Citireuma, 1889·2
Citivir, 1889·2
Citizem, 1889·2
Citoburol, 1889·2
Citocaina, 1889·2
Citocartin, 1889·2
Citochol, 1889·3
Citocinas, 1678·3
Citocromo C, 1678·3
Citodon, 1889·3
Citodox, 1889·3
Citofolin, 1889·3
Citofur, 1889·3
Citogel, 1889·3
Cito-Guakalin, 1889·3
Citoken T, 1889·3
Citomid, 1889·3
Citoneurin, 1889·3
Citoneuron, 1889·3
Citonina, 1889·3
Citopam, 1889·3
Citoplatino, 1889·3
Citorsal, 1889·3
Citosin, 1889·3
Citostal, 1889·3
Citovirax, 1889·3
Citra pH, 1889·3
Citracal, 1889·3
Citracal + D, 1889·3
Citracal Plus with Magnesium, 1889·3
Citral, 1711·1
Citralax— *see* X-Prep Bowel Evacuant Kit-2, 2388·4
Citralite, 1889·3
Citralka, 1889·3
Citramag, 1889·3
Citramar, 1889·4
Citramar D, 1889·4
Citranacea, 1889·4
Citrarginine, 1889·4
Citrated Caffeine, 782·1
Citrated Calcium Carbimide, 1664·2
Citrato Ácido de Sodio, 1223·2
Citrato Amónico Férrico, 1427·2
Citrato de Alverina, 1250·2
Citrato de Bismuto, 1252·1
Citrato de Bismuto y Ranitidina, 1287·2
Citrato de Butamirato, 1116·2
Citrato de Butetamato, 1116·2
Citrato de Carfentanilo, 25·1
Citrato de Cetiedil, 882·1
Citrato de Clomifeno, 1542·2
Citrato de Deptropina, 430·3
Citrato de Dietilcarbamazina, 104·1
Citrato de Difenhidramina, 431·3

Citrato de Etoheptacina, 37·2
Citrato de Feniltoloxamina, 439·1
Citrato de Fentanilo, 40·1
Citrato de Isoaminilo, 1123·3
Citrato de Mecloxamina, 485·3
Citrato de Morantel, 110·1
Citrato de Mosaprida, 1276·3
Citrato de Orfenadrina, 486·1
Citrato de Oxolamina, 1126·1
Citrato de Pentoxiverina, 1126·2
Citrato de Potasio, 1223·1
Citrato de Proxazol, 1735·3
Citrato de Sildenafilo, 1744·2
Citrato de Sodio, 1223·2
Citrato de Sufentanilo, 90·2
Citrato de Tamoxifeno, 584·1
Citrato de Tandospirona, 723·2
Citrato de Tripelenamina, 442·3
Citrato Espresso Gabbiani, 1889·4
Citrato Espresso S. Pellegrino, 1889·4
Citravescent, 1889·4
Citravite, 1889·4
Citrec, 1889·4
Citredici UBT Kit, 1889·4
Citrex, 1889·4
Citrex Vitamin E, 1889·4
Citri, Aetheroleum, 1706·2
Citri, Oleum, 1706·2
Citri Slim+Trim, 1889·4
Citric Acid, 1673·1
Citric Acid, Anhydrous, 1673·1
Citric Acid, Hydrous, 1673·1
Citric Acid Monohydrate, 1673·1
Cítrico Anhidro, Ácido, 1673·1
Cítrico Monohidrato, Ácido, 1673·1
Citricum Anhydricum, Acidum, 1673·1
Citricum Monohydricum, Acidum, 1673·1
Citrihexal, 1889·4
Citrimax, 1889·4
Citrisource, 1889·4
Citrizan, 1889·4
Citrizan Antibiotico, 1889·4
Citro Jod, 1889·4
Citrocarbonate, 1889·4
Citrocholine, 1889·4
Citrocil, 1889·4
Citrocit, 1889·4
Citroepatina, 1889·4
Citro-Flav, 1889·4
Citroflavona, 1890·1
Citroflavona Mag, 1890·1
Citroftalmina, 1890·1
Citroftalmina VC, 1890·1
Citrokehl, 1890·1
Citrolider, 1890·1
Citrolith, 1890·1
Citro-Mag, 1890·1
Citromed, 1890·1
Citromed 80, 1890·1
Citromed 85— *see* Citromed 80 and 85, 1890·1
Citromed Chirurgico, 1890·1
Citromed Chlor, 1890·1
Citromed Soap, 1890·1
Citromedics Disinfettante, 1890·1
Citromedics Pronto, 1890·1
Citromel, 1890·1
Citron, 1890·1
Citron Chaud, 1890·1
Citron Chaud DM, 1890·1
Citron, Essence de, 1706·2
Citronela, Aceite Esencial de, 1673·2
Citronella Oil, 1673·2
Citronellae Aetheroleum, 1673·2
Citronellae, Oleum, 1673·2
Citronellal, 1673·2
Citronellol, 1673·2, 1740·2
Citronellyl Acetate, 1673·2
Citronenöl, 1706·2
Citronensäure, 1673·1
Citropepsin, 1890·1
Citropiperazina, 1890·1
Citroplex, 1890·1
Citroplus, 1890·1
Citrosan, 1890·1
Citrosil, 1890·1
Citrosil Alcolico Azzuro, 1890·1
Citrosil Alcolico Bruno, 1890·1
Citrosil Alcolico Incolore, 1890·1
Citrosil Nubesan, 1890·2
Citrosil Sapone, 1890·2
Citro-Soda, 1890·2
Citrosodina, 1890·2
Citrosodine, 1890·2
Citrosteril Preparations, 1890·2
Citrosystem, 1890·2
Citrotein, 1890·2
Citrovenot, 1890·2
Citrovit, 1890·2
Citrovorum Factor, 1431·1
Citrucel, 1890·2
Citrulina, 1425·2
Citrulline, 1425·2
Citrulline Malate, 1425·2
*Citrullus colocynthis*, 1260·3
*Citrus aurantium*, 1719·2, 1723·3, 1724·1
*Citrus bergamia*, 1660·1
Citrus C with Acerola, 1890·2
*Citrus limon*, 1706·2
*Citrus × limon*, 1706·2
*Citrus limonum*, 1706·2
*Citrus sinensis*, 1724·1
Citrus-flav C, 1890·2
Citsav, 1890·2
Cituridina, 1890·2
Ciuk, 1890·2
Civeran, 1890·2
Civicor, 1890·2
Civigel, 1890·2
Ciwujia, 1744·1
Cizoren, 1890·2
CJ-91B, 1278·1
CL-68, 1096·1
C-L90, 1890·2
CL-369, 1302·1
CL-399, 1310·2
CL-1388R, 926·3
CL-10304, 741·3
CL-12625, 406·2
CL-14377, 568·2
CL-34433, 1110·2
CL-34699, 1091·1
CL-36467, 703·2
CL-39743, 703·2
CL-40881, 211·3
CL-61965, 1110·2
CL-62362, 705·2
CL-65336, 760·3
CL-67772, 286·3
CL-71563, 705·2
CL-78116, 615·2
CL-82204, 39·1
CL-83544, 39·1
CL-106359, 1110·2
CL-112302, 21·3
CL-118532, 1341·2
CL-184116, 580·3
CL-186815, 165·3
CL-216942, 530·2
CL-227193, 243·1
CL-232315, 575·2
CL-273703, 606·1
CL-284635, 172·3
CL-284846, 727·3
CL-287389, 972·2
CL-297939, 875·1
CL-298741, 264·3
CL-301423, 110·1
CL-307579, 264·3
CL-318952, 591·1
CL Tre, 1890·2
Claben, 1890·2
Clabin, 1890·3
Clacef, 1890·3
Cladribina, 539·3
Cladribine, 539·3
Claforan, 1890·3
Clafordil, 1890·3
Claim, 1890·3
Clairo Tea, 1890·3
Clairodermyl, 1890·3
Clamarvit, 1890·3
Clamentin, 1890·3
Clamiben, 1890·3
Clamicin, 1890·3
Clamide, 1890·3
Clamist, 1890·3
Clamonex, 1890·3
Clamox, 1890·3
Clamoxin, 1890·3
Clamoxyl, 1890·3
Clamoxyl Mucolitico, 1890·3
Clamycin, 1890·3
Clanzoflat, 1890·3
Clanzol, 1890·3
Claradol, 1890·3
Claradol Cafeine, 1890·3
Claradol Codeine, 1890·4
Claragine, 1890·4
Claral, 1890·4
Claral Plus, 1890·4
Claramax, 1890·4
Claramid, 1890·4
Claratyne, 1890·4
Claratyne Decongestant, 1890·4
Claravis, 1890·4
Claraxim, 1890·4
Clarema, 1890·4
Clarens, 1890·4
Claribid, 1890·4
Claricort, 1890·4
Clariderm, 1890·4
Claridon, 1890·4
Clariflu, 1890·4
Clarifriol, 1890·4
Claril, 1890·4
Clarilerg, 1890·4
Clarimac, 1890·4
Clarimax, 1890·4
Clarimid, 1890·4
Clarimir, 1890·4
Clarimir F, 1890·4
Clarinase, 1890·4
Clarineo, 1890·4
Clarinex, 1890·4
Claripel, 1891·1
Claripex AL, 1891·1
Clarisco, 1891·1
Claritab, 1891·1
Clariteyes, 1891·1
Clarithromycin, 192·2
Clarithromycinum, 192·2
Claritin, 1891·1
Claritin Allergic Congestion Relief, 1891·1
Claritin Extra, 1891·1
Claritin Eye Allergy Relief, 1891·1
Claritin Skin Itch Relief, 1891·1
Claritin-D, 1891·1
Claritine, 1891·1
Claritone, 1891·1
Claritromicina, 192·2
Clarityn, 1891·1
Clarityne, 1891·1
Clarityne Cort, 1891·1
Clarityne D, 1891·1
Clarix, 1891·1
Claroft, 1891·1
Claroftal, 1891·1
Clarograf, 1891·1
Clarover, 1891·1
Clarvisan, 1891·1
Clarvisol, 1891·1
Clarvisor, 1891·2
Clarvix, 1891·2
Clasifel, 1891·2
Classic Swiss One, 1891·2
Clasteon, 1891·2
Clastidin, 1891·2
Clastoban, 1891·2
Clatromicin, 1891·2
Claudemor, 1891·2
Claudicat, 1891·2
Clauparest, 1891·2
Clavamel, 1891·2
Clavamox, 1891·2
Claventin, 1891·2
Clavepen, 1891·2
Claversal, 1891·2
*Claviceps purpurea*, 1685·1
Clavigrenin, 1891·2
Clavinex, 1891·2
Clavinex Duo, 1891·2
Clavo, 1673·2
Clavo, Aceite Esencial de, 1673·3
Clavo, Esencia de, 1673·3
Clavoxil, 1891·2
Clavoxilina Bid, 1891·2
Clavucar, 1891·2
Clavucid, 1891·2
Clavulanate Potassium, 193·3
Clavulanato Potásico, 193·3
Clavulanic Acid, 193·3
Clavulánico, Ácido, 193·3
Clavulin, 1891·2
Clavulox, 1891·3
Clavulox Duo, 1891·3
Clavumox, 1891·3
Clavurion, 1891·3
Clazuril, 603·1
Clazuril for Veterinary Use, 603·1
Clazurilo, 603·1
Clazurilum, 603·1
Cleactor, 1891·3
Clean & Clear Preparations, 1891·3
Clean Hair, 1891·3
Clean Skin Anti Acne, 1891·3
Clean Skin Face Wash, 1891·3
Clean-AC, 1891·3
Clean-AF, 1891·3
Cleanal, 1891·3
Cleanance, 1891·3
Cleancef, 1891·3
Cleaner No 4, 1891·3
Clean-N-Soak, 1891·3
Cleanomed, 1891·4
Cleansing Herbs, 1891·4
Cleanxate, 1891·4
Clear Away, 1891·4
Clear By Design, 1891·4
Clear Complexion, HRI— *see* HRI Clear Complexion, 2048·4
Clear Cough, 1891·4
Clear Ear, 1891·4
Clear Eyes, 1891·4
Clear Eyes ACR, 1891·4
Clear Eyes CLR, 1891·4
Clear Pore, 1891·4
Clear Skin, NeoCeuticals— *see* NeoCeuticals Clear Skin, 2157·3
Clear Total Lice Elimination System, 1891·4
Clear Tussin 30, 1891·4
ClearAc, 1891·4
ClearAc Cleanser, 1891·4
Clearamed, 1891·4
Clearasil Preparations, 1891·4
Clearblue, 1892·1
Clearblue Easy, 1892·1
Clearblue One Step, 1892·1
Clearex, 1892·1
Clearex Cover Up, 1892·1
Clear-Flex Formula, 1892·1
Clearine, 1892·1
Clearon, 1892·1
Clearplan, 1892·1
Clearplan Easy, 1892·1
Clearplan One Step, 1892·1
Clearsing, 1892·2
Clearskin Preparations, 1892·2
Clearsol, 1892·2
Clearsore, 1892·2
Clear-View, 1892·2
Clearview HCG, 1892·2
Cleavers, 1673·2
Clebofex, 1892·2
Clebopride, Malato de, 1260·3
Clebopride, 1260·3
Clebopride Malate, 1260·3
Clebopridi Malas, 1260·3
Cleboril, 1892·2
Clebudan, 1892·2
Clebutec, 1892·2
Cledist, 1892·2
Cleensheen, 1892·2

Clefamide, 603·1
Clemastina, Fumarato de, 429·1
Clemastine Fumarate, 429·1
Clemastini Fumaras, 429·1
Clematis III Oligoplex, 1892·2
Clembroxol, 1892·2
Clembumar, 1892·2
Clemental, 1892·2
Clements Iron, 1892·2
Clements Tonic, 1892·2
Clemenzil ST, 1892·2
Clemizol, Hidrocloruro de, 429·2
Clemizol Penicilina, 194·1
Clemizole Benzylpenicillin, 194·1
Clemizole Hexachlorophene, 429·2
Clemizole Hydrochloride, 429·2
Clemizole Penicillin, 194·1
Clemizole Sodium Sulfate, 429·2
Clemizole Undecylate, 429·2
Clenasma, 1892·2
Clenbuterol, Hidrocloruro de, 784·2
Clenbuterol Hydrochloride, 784·2
Clenia, 1892·3
Cleniderm, 1892·3
Clenil, 1892·3
Clenil Compositum, 1892·3
Clenil "Forte Jet", 1892·3
Clenilexx, 1892·3
Clenoliximab, 1668·3
Clen-Zym, 1892·3
Cleocin, 1892·3
Cleocin T, 1892·3
Cleregil, 1892·3
Cleridium, 1892·3
Clerz, 1892·3
Clerz Moisturising Drops, 1892·3
Clesidren, 1892·3
Cletonol, 1892·3
Clever, 1892·3
Cleveral, 1892·3
Cleveron, 1892·3
Clevian, 1892·3
Clevosan, 1892·3
Clexane, 1892·3
Cliacil, 1892·3
Cliane, 1892·3
Clibium, 1892·3
Clidets, 1892·4
Clidinio, Bromuro de, 480·2
Clidinium Bromide, 480·2
Clifemin, 1892·4
Clifordin, 1892·4
Climabelle, 1892·4
Climacilin, 1892·4
Climacteron, 1892·4
Climadan, 1892·4
Climaderm, 1892·4
Climadil, 1892·4
Climagest, 1892·4
Climara, 1892·4
Climara Duo, 1892·4
ClimaraPro, 1892·4
Climarest, 1892·4
Climaston, 1892·4
Climatidine, 1892·4
Climatrol E, 1892·4
Climatrol Ht, 1892·4
Climatrol Ht Continuo, 1892·4
Climaval, 1892·4
Climaxol, 1892·4
Climbazole, 396·2
Climbazole, Hegor— *see* Hegor Climbazole, 2037·4
Climen, 1892·4
Climene, 1893·1
Climesse, 1893·1
Climil-80, 1893·1
Climil Complex, 1893·1
Climil Gel, 1893·1
Climodien, 1893·1
Climopax, 1893·1
Climopax Cyclo, 1893·1
Clinac, 1893·1
Clinac BPO, 1893·1
Clinadil, 1893·1
Clinadil Compositum, 1893·1
Clinadol, 1893·1
Clinadryl, 1893·1
Clinafloxacin Hydrochloride, 194·2
Clinafloxacino, Hidrocloruro de, 194·2
Clinagel, 1893·1
Clinal, 1893·1
Clinasol, 1893·1
Clinda, 1893·1
Clindabeta, 1893·1
Clindac, 1893·1
Clindacin, 1893·1
Clindacne, 1893·1
Clinda-Derm, 1893·2
Clindagel, 1893·2
Clindahexal, 1893·2
Clindal, 1893·2
ClindaMax, 1893·2
Clindamicina, Fosfato de, 194·2
Clindamicina, Hidrocloruro de, 194·2
Clindamicina, Hidrocloruro del Palmitato de, 194·2
Clindamin C, 1893·2
Clindamycin, 194·2
Clindamycin 2-(Dihydrogen Phosphate), 194·2
Clindamycin Hydrochloride, 194·2
Clindamycin Palmitate Hydrochloride, 194·2
Clindamycin 2-Palmitate Hydrochloride, 194·2
Clindamycin Phosphate, 194·2
Clindamycini Hydrochloridum, 194·2
Clindamycini Phosphas, 194·2
Clindarix, 1893·2
Clinda-saar, 1893·2
Clindastad, 1893·2
Clindatech, 1893·2
Clindaz, 1893·2
Clindazyn, 1893·2
Clindets, 1893·2
Clindex, 1893·2
Clindopax, 1893·2
Clinensol, 1893·2
Clinesfar, 1893·2
Clinfar, 1893·2
Clinic A Retinol Vital Day, 1893·2
Clinical Program Thickened Juice, 1893·2
Cliniderm, 1893·2
Clinifeed, 1893·2
Clinigel, 1893·2
Clinikold, 1893·2
Clinimet, 1893·2
Clinimix, 1893·2
Clinimycin, 194·2, 1893·2
Clinique Acne Spot Treatment, 1893·2
Clinisorb, 1893·3
Clinistix, 1893·3
Clinit N, 1893·3
Clinitar, 1893·3
Clinitek HCG, 1893·3
Clinitek Microalbumin, 1893·3
Clinitest, 1893·3
Clinium, 1893·3
Clinoderm, 1893·3
Clinofar, 1893·3
Clinofem, 1893·3
Clinofibrate, 884·3
Clinofibrato, 884·3
Clinofug D, 1893·3
Clinofug Gel, 1893·3
Clinogel, 1893·3
Clinoleic, 1893·3
Clinomel, 1893·3
Clinopront, 1893·3
Clinoril, 1893·3
Clinovir, 1893·3
Clin-Sanorania, 1893·3
Clintopic, 1893·3
Clinutren, 1893·4
Clinvit, 1893·4
Clinwas, 1893·4
Clio-Betnovate, 1893·4
Cliochinolum, 196·3
Cliogan, 1893·4
Clioquinol, 196·3
Clioquinolum, 196·3
Cliovyl, 1893·4
Clipper, 1893·4
Clipto, 1893·4
Cliptol, 1893·4
Cliptol Sport, 1893·4
C-Lisa, 1893·4
Clisemina, 1893·4
Clisflex, 1893·4
Clisin, 1893·4
Clisma Bieffe Medital, 1893·4
Clisma Fleet, 1893·4
Clisma-Lax, 1893·4
Clistin, 1893·4
Clitaxel, 1893·4
*Clitocybe*, 1717·3
Clivarin, 1893·4
Clivarina, 1893·4
Clivarine, 1893·4
Clivasol, 1893·4
Clivers, 1673·2
Clivoten, 1893·4
$Cl_2MBP$, 770·2
$Cl_2MDP$, 770·2
Clo-5, 1893·4
Clo Zinc, 1893·4
Clobasol, 1893·4
Clobasone, 1893·4
Clobatos, 1894·1
Clobazam, 358·2
Clobazamum, 358·2
Clobegalen, 1894·1
Clobemix, 1894·1
Clobendian, 1894·1
Clobenfurol, 889·1
Cloben-G, 1894·1
Clobenzorex, Hidrocloruro de, 1585·3
Clobenzorex Hydrochloride, 1585·3
Clobeplus, 1894·1
Clobesol, 1894·1
Clobesol LA, 1894·1
Clobeson, 1894·1
Clobet, 1894·1
Clobetasol Propionate, 1095·2
Clobetasol, Propionato de, 1095·2
Clobetasona, Butirato de, 1095·3
Clobetasone Butyrate, 1095·3
Clobetasoni Butyras, 1095·3
Clobetate, 1894·1
Clobex, 1894·1
Cloburate, 1894·1
Clobutinol, Hidrocloruro de, 1117·1
Clobutinol Hydrochloride, 1117·1
Clob-X, 1894·1
Clocapramina, Hidrocloruro de, 683·1
Clocapramine Hydrochloride, 683·1
Clocim, 1894·1
Clocinizina, Hidrocloruro de, 429·2
Clocinizine Hydrochloride, 429·2
Cloconazole Hydrochloride, 397·1
Clocortolona, Pivalato de, 1096·1
Clocortolone Caproate, 1096·1
Clocortolone Pivalate, 1096·1
Clocream, 1894·1
Clocreme, 1894·1
Clodantoin, 396·2
Clodantoína, 396·2
Clodavan, 1894·1
Cloderm, 1894·1
Clodron, 1894·1
Clodronate Disodium, 770·2
Clodronate Sodium, 770·2
Clodronato Disódico, 770·2
Clodronic Acid, 770·2
Clodrónico, Ácido, 770·2
Clody, 1894·1
Cloel, 1894·1
Clo-Far, 1894·1
Clofarabine, 540·2
Clofaren, 1894·1
Clofazimina, 197·1
Clofazimine, 197·1
Clofaziminum, 197·1
Clofec, 1894·1
Clofedanol, Hidrocloruro de, 1117·1
Clofedanol Hydrochloride, 1117·1
Clofeme, 1894·1
Clofen, 1894·1
Clofenac, 1894·2
Clofenak, 1894·2
Clofend, 1894·2
Clofenotane, 1502·1
Clofenotano, 1502·1
Clofenoxine Hydrochloride, 1710·1
Clofenpyride Hydrochloride, 965·3
Clofenvinfos, 1502·2
Clofert, 1894·2
Clofexamida, 26·3
Clofexamide, 26·3
Clofexamide Hydrochloride, 26·3
Clofexamidephenylbutazone, 26·3
Clofexan, 1894·2
Clofezona, 26·3
Clofezone, 26·3
Clofibrate, 884·3
Clofibrate, Aluminium, 884·3
Clofibrate, Calcium, 885·1
Clofibrate, Etofylline, 914·2
Clofibrate, Magnesium, 885·1
Clofibrato, 884·3
Clofibrato de Aluminio, 884·3
Clofibrato de Calcio, 885·1
Clofibrato de Etofilina, 914·2
Clofibrato de Magnesio, 885·1
Clofibratum, 884·3
Clofibric Acid, 885·1
Clofoctol, 198·1
Clofon, 1894·2
Clofozine, 1894·2
Clofranil, 1894·2
Clogar, 1894·2
Clogen, 1894·2
Cloisone, 1894·2
Clo-Kit, 1894·2
Clomaderm, 1894·2
Clomag, 885·1
Clomazen, 1894·2
Clomethiazole, 683·1
Clomethiazole Edisilate, 683·1
Clomethiazole Edisylate, 683·1
Clometiazol, 683·1
Clometiazol, Edisilato de, 683·1
Clometocilina Potásica, 198·1
Clometocillin Potassium, 198·1
Clomhexal, 1894·2
Clomicin, 1894·2
Clomid, 1894·2
Clomidazole Hydrochloride, 396·1
Clomifen, 1894·2
Clomifene Citrate, 1542·2
Clomifeni Citras, 1542·2
Clomifeno, 1894·2
Clomifeno, Citrato de, 1542·2
Clomihexal, 1894·2
Clomin, 1894·2
Clomiphene Citrate, 1542·2
Clomipramina, Hidrocloruro de, 289·3
Clomipramine Hydrochloride, 289·3
Clomipramini Hydrochloridum, 289·3
Clomivid, 1894·2
Clomycin, 1894·2
Clonagin, 1894·2
Clonalgin, 1894·2
Clonalgin Compuesto, 1894·2
Clonalin, 1894·2
Clonamox, 1894·3
Clonamp, 1894·3
Clonapam, 1894·3
Clonasten, 1894·3
Clonax, 1894·3
Clonazepam, 359·1
Clonazepamum, 359·1
Clonazine, 1894·3
Clonazolina, Hidrocloruro de, 1117·1
Clonazoline Hydrochloride, 1117·1
Clondepryl, 1894·3
Clonea, 1894·3
Clonesina, 1894·3
Clonex, 1894·3
Clonfolic, 1894·3
Clonic Seizures— *see* Epilepsy, 349·1
Clonidina, Hidrocloruro de, 885·2
Clonidine, 885·2

Clonidine Hydrochloride, 885·2
Clonidini Hydrochloridum, 885·2
Clonidinum, 885·2
Clonid-Ophtal, 1894·3
Clonidural, 1894·3
Clonilix, 1894·3
Clonistada, 1894·3
Clonix, 1894·3
Clonixil, 1894·3
Clonixin, 26·3
Clonixin Lysine, 26·3
Clonixino, 26·3
Clonnirit, 1894·3
Clonodifen, 1894·3
Clonofilin, 1894·3
Clonorax, 1894·3
Clonorchiasis— *see* Liver Fluke Infections, 99·3
Clonovate, 1894·3
Clonoxifen, 1894·3
Clont, 1894·3
Clonteric, 1894·3
Clonuretic, 1894·3
Clopamida, 888·2
Clopamide, 888·2
Clopamon, 1894·3
Clopan, 1894·3
α-Clopenthixol, 730·3
*cis*-Clopenthixol, 730·3
Z-Clopenthixol, 730·3
Cloperastina, Fendizoato de, 1117·2
Cloperastina, Hidrocloruro de, 1117·2
Cloperastine Fendizoate, 1117·2
Cloperastine Hydrochloride, 1117·2
Cloperastine Hydroxyphenylbenzoyl Benzoic Acid, 1117·2
Cloperastine Phendizoate, 1117·2
Clophenoxate Hydrochloride, 1710·1
Clopidogrel Bisulfate, 888·3
Clopidogrel, Bisulfato de, 888·3
Clopidogrel Bisulphate, 888·3
Clopidogrel Hydrogen Sulphate, 888·3
Clopidol, 603·1
Clopindol, 603·1
Clopine, 1894·3
Clopirim, 1894·3
Clopixol, 1894·3
Cloponone, 1177·3
Clopra, 1894·4
Clopradone Hydrochloride, 292·1
Clopram, 1894·4
Cloprane, 1894·4
Cloprednol, 1096·1
Clopress, 1894·4
Cloprostenol Sódico, 1514·3
Cloprostenol Sodium, 1514·3
Clopsine, 1894·4
Cloptison, 1894·4
Cloptison-N, 1894·4
CloraCEF, 1894·4
Clorad, 1894·4
Cloradex, 1894·4
Cloradryn, 1894·4
Clorafen, 1894·4
Clorafenil, 1894·4
Cloral Betaína, 684·1
Cloral Betaine, 684·1
Cloral, Hidrato de, 684·1
Cloral Hydrate, 684·1
Cloralosa, 1501·2
Cloram Hemidexa, 1894·4
Cloram Zinc, 1894·4
Clorambucilo, 536·1
Cloramed, 1894·4
Cloramfen, 1894·4
Cloramfeni, 1894·4
Cloramfenil, 1894·4
Cloramina, 1194·3
Clorampast, 1894·4
Cloran, 1894·4
Cloran Otico, 1894·4
Clorana, 1894·4
Cloranfe, 1894·4
Cloranfe Hemidex— *see* Cloram Hemidexa, 1894·4
Cloranfenic, 1894·4
Cloranfenic Zinc— *see* Cloram Zinc, 1894·4
Cloranfenicol, 185·1
Cloranfenicol, Palmitato de, 185·1
Cloranfenicol, Succinato Sódico de, 185·1
Cloranfenil, 1895·1
Cloranpectina, 1895·1
Cloraseptic, 1895·1
Clorato de Potasio, 1747·2
Clorato Potásico, 1734·2
Cloraxene, 1895·1
Clorazepate Dipotassium, 685·1
Clorazepate Monopotassium, 685·1
Clorazepato de Dipotasio, 685·1
Clorazepato Monopotásico, 685·1
Clorazepic Acid, 685·1
Clorazépico, Ácido, 685·1
Clorazin, 1895·1
Clorazolam, 725·3
Clorciclizina, Hidrocloruro de, 427·2
Clorcin-Ped, 1895·1
Clorcorticil, 1895·1
Clordano, 1501·3
Clordesmethyldiazepam, 689·3
Clordiazepóxido, 674·2
Clordiazepóxido, Hidrocloruro de, 674·2
Clordil, 1895·1
Clordispenser, 1895·1
Clordox, 1895·1
Cloretilo Chemirosa, 1895·1
Cloreto de Aluminio, 1142·1
Cloreto de Benzalconio, 1168·3
Cloreto de Cálcio, 1225·1
Cloreto de Magnésio, 1228·1
Cloreto de Potássio, 1232·2
Cloreto de Sódio, 1233·3
Cloreto Mercúrico, 1712·3
Cloreto Mercuroso, 1712·3
Clorevan, 1895·1
Clorexan, 1895·1
Clorexan Ferri, 1895·1
Clorexident, 1895·1
Clorexident Ortodontico, 1895·1
Clorfenamina, Maleato de, 427·3
Clorfene, 1177·3
Clorfenesina, 396·1
Clorfenesina, Carbamato de, 1392·2
Clorfenil, 1895·1
Clorfenoxamina, Hidrocloruro de, 428·3
Clorfibrase, 1895·1
Clorfriol, 1895·1
Clorgiline, 316·1
Clorhexidina, 1173·2
Clorhexidina, Acetato de, 1173·2
Clorhexidina, Gluconato de, 1173·2
Clorhexidina, Hidrocloruro de, 1173·3
Clorhexitulle, 1895·1
Clorhidrato de Euftalmina, 482·1
Clorhídrico, Ácido, 1699·1
Cloricromen, 889·1
Cloricromeno, 889·1
Cloridarol, 889·1
Cloridrato de Adifenina, 1648·1
Cloridrato de Amilorida, 858·2
Cloridrato de Bromexina, 1115·3
Cloridrato de Ciclopentolato, 480·3
Cloridrato de Daunorrubicina, 545·3
Cloridrato de Dicicloverina, 481·2
Cloridrato de Doxorrubicina, 547·3
Cloridrato de Emetina, 604·3
Cloridrato de Levamizol, 107·2
Cloridrato de Metildopato, 953·2
Cloridrato de Naloxona, 1044·3
Cloridrato de Profenamina, 488·3
Cloridrato de Protamina, 1050·3
Cloridrato de Triexilfenidila, 490·2
Clorimet-Z, 1895·1
Clorina, 1895·1
Cloritines, 1895·1
Clor-K-Zaf, 1895·1
Clormadinona, Acetato de, 1542·1
Clormetina, Hidrocloruro de, 537·1
Clormezanona, 675·1
Clormidazol, Hidrocloruro de, 396·1
Cloro, 1175·3
Cloroacetamida, 1176·3
Cloroacetofenona, 1670·1
*N*-(3-Cloroalil)hexaminio, Cloruro de, 1176·3
Cloroboral, 1895·1
Clorobutanol, 1176·3
Clorocil, 1895·1
Clorocresol, 1177·1
Clorodifluoroetano, 1236·1
Clorodifluorometano, 1236·1
Clorofacinona, 1501·3
Clorofene, 1177·3
Clorofeno, 1177·3
Clorofila, 1057·1
Clorofluorocarbonos, 1235·3
Cloroformo, 1296·3
Cloromi-T, 1895·1
Clorophene, 1177·3
Clorophene Sodium, 1177·3
Cloropicrina, 1502·1
Cloropiramina, Hidrocloruro de, 427·3
Cloroplatínico, Ácido, 1670·2
Cloroprocaína, Hidrocloruro de, 1373·1
Cloroquina, 448·2
Cloroquina, Fosfato de, 448·2
Cloroquina, Hidrocloruro de, 448·2
Cloroquina, Sulfato de, 448·2
Clorosan, 1895·2
Clorotalidona, 882·3
Clorotiazida, 882·1
Clorotiazida Sódica, 882·2
Clorotimol, 1177·2
Clorotir, 1895·2
Clorotrianiseno, 1542·1
Cloro-Trimeton, 1895·2
Cloroxilenol, 1177·2
Clorozotocina, 538·1
Clorpactin, 1895·2
Clorpactin WCS-90, 1895·2
Clorpamina, 1895·2
Clorpirifós, 1502·1
Clorpres, 1895·2
Clorprimeton, 1895·2
Clorproetazina, Hidrocloruro de, 675·1
Clorproguanil, Hidrocloruro de, 452·1
Clorpromaz, 1895·2
Clorpromazina, 675·1
Clorpromazina, Embonato de, 675·1
Clorpromazina, Hidrocloruro de, 675·2
Clorpropamida, 330·3
Clorprotixeno, 682·3
Clorprotixeno, Hidrocloruro de, 682·3
Clorprotixeno, Mesilato de, 682·3
Clorquinaldol, 187·3
Clorsulon, 103·3
Clortalidona, 882·3
Clortalil, 1895·2
Clortanol, 1895·2
Clortetraciclina, 187·3
Clortetraciclina, Hidrocloruro de, 187·3
Clortil, 1895·2
Cloruro de Acetilcolina, 1487·1
Cloruro de Acriflavinio, 1165·3
Cloruro de Alcuronio, 1398·3
Cloruro de Aluminio, 1142·1
Cloruro de Ambenonio, 1487·3
Cloruro de Amonio, 1115·2
Cloruro de Bencetonio, 1169·2
Cloruro de Benzalconio, 1168·3
Cloruro de Benzoxonio, 1170·2
Cloruro de Cal, 1175·3
Cloruro de Calcio, 1225·1
Cloruro de Cetalconio, 1172·1
Cloruro de Cetilpiridinio, 1173·1
Cloruro de Colina, 1424·3
Cloruro de Decualinio, 1178·1
Cloruro de Doxacurio, 1403·1
Cloruro de Edrofonio, 1490·3
Cloruro de Etilo, 1376·2
Cloruro de Isometamidio, 606·1
Cloruro de Metacolina, 1492·1
Cloruro de Metilbencetonio, 1186·1
Cloruro de Metilo, 1476·2
Cloruro de Metilrosanilina, 1186·1
Cloruro de Metiltioninio, 1042·2
Cloruro de Miripirio, 1186·3
Cloruro de Miristalconio, 1186·3
Cloruro de Mivacurio, 1403·3
Cloruro de Obidoxima, 1046·3
Cloruro de Octafonio, 1187·1
Cloruro de Suxametonio, 1406·2
Cloruro de Tolonio, 1757·1
Cloruro de Trospio, 491·2
Cloruro de Tubocurarina, 1409·2
Clorxil, 1895·2
Clorzoxazona, 1392·3
Closantel, 104·1
Closantel Sodium, 104·1
Closantel Sodium Dihydrate for Veterinary Use, 104·1
Closcript, 1895·2
Closecs, 1895·2
Closin, 1895·2
Closina, 1895·2
Clospipramine, 710·1
Clostebol Acetate, 1543·2
Clostebol, Acetato de, 1543·2
Clostedal, 1895·2
Clostet, 1895·2
Clostilbegyt, 1895·2
Clostridiopeptidase A, 1675·1
*Clostridium botulinum*, 1610·3
Clostridium Difficile Colitis— *see* Antibiotic-associated Colitis, 128·1
*Clostridium histolyticum*, 1675·1
*Clostridium novyi*, 1615·3
*Clostridium perfringens*, 1615·3, 1632·3
*Clostridium septicum*, 1615·3
*Clostridium tetani*, 1640·2, 1640·3, 1641·1
CloSYS II— *see* Retardent, 2260·2
CloSYS II— *see* Retardex, 2260·2
Clotam, 1895·2
Clotan, 1895·2
Clotassio, 1895·2
Clotest, 1895·2
Clothiapine, 685·2
Clotiapina, 685·2
Clotiapine, 685·2
Clotiazepam, 685·2
Cloton, 1895·2
Clotramid, 1895·2
Clotrason, 1895·2
Clotrasone, 1895·2
Clotreme, 1895·2
Clotren, 1895·2
Clotri, 1895·3
Clotri OPT, 1895·3
Clotricin, 1895·3
Clotri-Denk, 1895·3
Clotrifug, 1895·3
Clotrigalen, 1895·3
Clotrihexal, 1895·3
Clotrimaderm, 1895·3
Clotrimazol, 396·2
Clotrimazole, 396·2
Clotrimazolum, 396·2
Clotrimin, 1895·3
Clotrimin-B, 1895·3
Clotrimix, 1895·3
Clotrinolon, 1895·3
Clotrizan, 1895·3
Clotting Factors, Blood, 735·3
Clou de Girofle, 1673·2
Cloudy Ammonia, 1654·1
Cloval, 1895·3
Cloval Compuesto, 1895·3
Clovate, 1895·3
Clove, 1673·2
Clove Oil, 1673·3
Cloves, 1673·2
Clovin, 1895·3
Clovir, 1895·3
Clovira, 1895·3
Clovirax, 1895·3
Clox, 1895·3
Cloxa, 1895·3
Cloxacap, 1895·3
Cloxacilina, 198·2
Cloxacilina Benzatina, 198·2
Cloxacilina Sódica, 198·2
Cloxacillin, 198·2
Cloxacillin Benzathine, 198·2

Cloxacillin, Dibenzylethylenediamine Salt, 198·2
Cloxacillin Sodium, 198·2
Cloxacillinum Natricum, 198·2
Cloxalin, 1895·3
Cloxam, 1895·3
Cloxan, 1895·3
Cloxanbin, 1895·3
Cloxapan, 1895·3
Cloxapen, 1895·3
Cloxasian, 1895·4
Cloxazolam, 685·3
Cloxgen, 1895·4
Cloxifenol, 1195·2
Cloxil, 1895·4
Cloxillin, 1895·4
Cloximar Duo, 1895·4
Cloxin, 1895·4
Cloxipen, 1895·4
Cloxiquine, 397·1
Cloxydin, 1895·4
Cloxyquin, 397·1
Clozal, 1895·4
Clozan, 1895·4
Clozanil, 1895·4
Clozapina, 685·3
Clozapine, 685·3
Clozapinum, 685·3
Clozaril, 1895·4
Clozole, 1895·4
Clozole, Chemists Own— *see* Chemists Own Clozole, 1881·4
CLS-2210, 1664·2
Clupanodonic Acid, 976·2
Clusivol, 1895·4
Clusivol Composto, 1895·4
Cluster Headache, 464·1
Cluyer, 1895·4
CLY-503, 997·1
Clysmol, 1895·4
Clyss-Go, 1895·4
CM-31-916, 182·2
CM-6912, 698·1
CM-8252, 1254·1
CM-9155, 1100·1
CMA-676, 558·3
CMC, 1577·3
CMD, 1895·4
C-Mox, 1895·4
CMP, 1895·4
CMV Immunoglobulin, 1895·4
CMV Iveegam, 1895·4
CMW, 1895·4
CMW mit Gentamicin, 1895·4
C-Mycin, 1895·4
CN, 1670·1
CN-25, 1896·1
CN-100, 96·3
CN-3123, 199·3
CN-10395, 360·1
CN-25253-2, 1730·3
CN-27554, 43·2
CN-35355, 55·2
CN-38703, 707·1
CN-52372-2, 1302·1
CN-54521-2, 1310·2
C-Naryl, 1896·1
C'Nergil, 1896·1
Cnicus Benedictus, 1673·3
*Cnicus benedictus*, 1673·3
CNP, 964·2
CNS-1102, 1655·3
CNTF, 1671·3
Co Amoxin, 1896·1
Co Bucal, 1896·1
Co Fluocin Fuerte, 1896·1
$CO_2$ Granulat, 1896·1
Co Hepa B12, 1896·1
CoA, 1674·3
Co-Acetan, 1896·1
CoActifed, 1896·1
Coadvil— *see* Advil Cold & Sinus, 1777·4
Coagulation, 735·3
Coagulation Cascade, 735·3
Coagulation Factor VIII, Human, 751·1
Coagulation Factor VIII (rDNA), Human, 751·2
Coagulation Factor IX, Human, 752·2
Coagulation Factors, Blood, 735·3
Coagulation Pathways, 735·3
Coagulopathies, Complex Acquired— *see* Haemorrhagic Disorders, 737·3
Coal Tar, 1159·2
Coal Tar, Crude, 1159·2
Coal Tar, Prepared, 1159·2
Coalgan, 1896·1
Coalip, 1896·1
Coaltar Saponine le Beuf, 1896·1
Co-amilofruse, 858·2, 919·3
Co-Amilorid, 1896·1
Co-amilozide, 858·2, 933·2
Coamox, 1896·1
Co-Amoxi, 1896·1
Co-amoxiclav, 155·3, 193·3
Co-Apap, 1896·1
CoAprovel, 1896·1
Coarol, 1896·1
Coartem, 1896·1
CoASH, 1674·3
Co-Atenolol, 1896·1
Cobactin, 1896·1
Cobadex Forte, 1896·1
Cobaforte, 1896·1
Cobaglobal, 1896·1
Cobalamins, 1458·2
Cobalatec, 1896·1
Cobaldoze, 1896·2
Cobalin-H, 1896·2
Cobalplex, 1896·2
Cobalt-57, 1523·2
Cobalt-58, 1523·2
Cobalt Chloride, 1674·1
Cobalt Edetate, 1036·2
Cobalt EDTA, 1036·2
Cobalt [Ethylenediaminetetra-acetato(4–)-*N,N′,O,O′*]cobalt(II), 1036·2
Cobalt Oxide, 1674·1
Cobalt Sulfate, 1674·1
Cobalt Tetracemate, 1036·2
Cobalti, 1896·2
Cobalto 57, 1523·2
Cobalto 58, 1523·2
Cobalto, Cloruro de, 1674·1
Cobalto, Óxido de, 1674·1
Cobaltous Chloride, 1674·1
Cobamamide, 1459·1
Cobamet, 1896·2
Cobamin, 1458·2, 1896·2
Cobamol, 1896·2
Cobantril, 1896·2
Cobanzyme, 1896·2
Cobavital, 1896·2
Cobaxid, 1896·2
Cobederm-H, 1896·2
Cobefen, 1896·2
Co-beneldopa, 1200·2, 1205·2
Cobenexol Forte, 1896·2
Cobenexol Fuerte, 1896·2
Cobenzil Compuesto, 1896·2
Co-Betaloc, 1896·2
Cobidec N, 1896·2
Cobiona, 1896·2
Cobirolyte, 1896·2
Cobotiaxina, 1896·2
Cobre, 1425·3
Cobre, Cloruro de, 1425·3
Cobre, Gluconato de, 1425·3
Cobre, Oleato de, 1502·2
Cobre, Sulfato de, 1426·1
Co-bucafAPAP, 76·2, 673·3, 782·1
Coca, 1373·3
Coca, Hoja de, 1373·3
Coca Leaves, 1373·3
Cocaethylene, 1375·3
Cocaína, 1373·3
Cocaína, Chloridrato de, 1373·3
Cocaína, Hidrocloruro de, 1373·3
Cocaine, 1373·3
Cocaine Hydrochlor., 1373·3
Cocaine Hydrochloride, 1373·3
Cocaine Sulfate, 1374·1
Cocaine Withdrawal Syndrome— *see* Withdrawal, 1375·2
Cocaini Hydrochloridum, 1373·3
Cocainium Chloratum, 1373·3
Co-Captopril, 1896·2
Co-Captral, 1896·2
Cocarboxylase, 1455·2
Co-careldopa, 1204·3, 1205·2
Co-Carnetina B12, 1896·2
*Coccidioides immitis*, 1674·1
Coccidioidin, 1674·1
Coccidioidina, 1674·1
Coccidioidomycosis, 387·3
Coccidiosis, 596·2
Coccila, 1896·2
Coccine Nouvelle, 1057·3
Coccionella, 1057·2
Cocculine, 1896·2
Cocculus Oligoplex, 1896·2
Cocculus-Homaccord, 1896·2
Coccus, 1057·2
Coccus Cacti, 1057·2
Cochineal, 1057·2
Cochineal Red A, 1057·3
Cochinilla, 1057·2
*Cochlearia armoracia*, 1697·3
Cocillana, 1117·2, 1896·2
Cocillana Co, 1896·3
Cocillana Compound, 1896·3
Cocillana-Etyfin, 1896·3
Co-Cillin, 1896·3
Cocktail Reale, 1896·3
Co-climasone, 396·2, 1093·1
Coco, Aceite de, 1481·1
Cocoa Butter, 1482·3
Cocoa Powder, 1754·3
Co-codamol, 27.1, 76·2
Co-Codamol, 1896·3
Co-codAPAP, 27·1, 76·2
Co-codaprin, 15·1, 27·1
Cocois, 1896·3
Cocois, Oleum, 1481·1
Coconut Butter, 1481·1
Coconut Oil, 1481·1
Coconut Oil, Refined, 1481·1
*Cocos nucifera*, 1440·3, 1481·1
Cocos Raffinatum, Oleum, 1481·1
Cocosis, Oleum, 1481·1
Cocydal, 1896·3
Cocyntal, 1896·3
Co-cyprindiol, 1544·1, 1553·2
Cod Efferalgan, 1896·3
Cod Liver Oil, 1425·2
COD N 70, 1896·3
Codabrol, 1896·3
Cod-Acamol Forte, 1896·3
Codaewon, 1896·3
Co-Dafalgan, 1896·3
Codafen Continus, 1896·3
Codalax, 1896·3
Codal-DH, 1896·3
Codal-DM, 1896·3
Codalgin, 1896·3
Codalgin Plus, 1896·3
Coda-Med, 1896·3
Codamine, 1896·3
Codant, 1896·3
Co-danthramer, 1261·1, 1414·2
Co-danthrusate, 1261·1, 1262·2
Codapane, 1896·4
Codaphed, 1896·4
Codaphed Plus, 1896·4
Codecarboxylase, 1456·3
Codedrill, 1896·4
Codef, 1896·4
Codegest Expectorant, 1896·4
Codehist DH, 1896·4
Codehydrogenase I, 1719·1
Codeína, 27·1
Codeína, Fosfato de, 27·1
Codeína, Hidrocloruro de, 27·1
Codeína, Sulfato de, 27·1
Codeine, 27·1
Codeine Acefyllinate, 28·1
Codeine Camsilate, 28·1
Codeine Contin, 1896·4
Codeine Hydrobromide, 28·1
Codeine Hydrochloride, 27·1
Codeine Hydrochloride Dihydrate, 27·1
Codeine Phosphate, 27·1
Codeine Phosphate Hemihydrate, 27·1
Codeine Phosphate Sesquihydrate, 27·1
Codeine Polistirex, 28·1
Codeine Sulfate, 27·1
Codeine Sulphate, 27·1
Codeini Hydrochloridum Dihydricum, 27·1
Codeini Phosphas, 27·1
Codeini Phosphas Hemihydricus, 27·1
Codeini Phosphas Sesquihydricus, 27·1
Codeinii Phosphas, 27·1
Codeinol, 1896·4
Codeinum, 27·1
Codeipar, 1896·4
Codeisan, 1896·4
Codelasa, 1896·4
Codella, 1896·4
Codelum, 1896·4
Codenfan, 1896·4
Codepect, 1896·4
Codergine, 1896·4
Codergocrina, Mesilato de, 1674·1
Co-dergocrine Esilate, 1674·2
Codergocrine Mesilate, 1674·1
Co-dergocrine Mesilate, 1674·1
Co-dergocrine Mesylate, 1674·1
Co-dergocrine Methanesulphonate, 1674·1
Codergocrini Mesilas, 1674·1
Coderit, 1896·4
Codesan Comp, 1896·4
Codesan N, 1896·4
Codesia, 1896·4
Codesic, 1896·4
Codethyline, 1896·4
Codéthyline, Chlorhydrate de, 37·3
Codetilina-Eucaliptolo He, 1897·1
Codetol, 1897·1
Codetol PM, 1897·1
Codetricine, 1897·1
Codetricine Vitamine C, 1897·1
Codeverin, 1897·1
Codex, 1897·1
Codexine-R, 1897·1
Cod-Guaiacol, 1897·1
Codi OPT, 1897·1
Codical, 1897·1
Codicaps, 1897·1
Codicaps Mono, 1897·1
Codicaps N, 1897·1
Codicet, 1897·1
Codiclear DH, 1897·1
Codicompren, 1897·1
Codicontin, 1897·1
Codidol, 1897·1
Codiforton, 1897·1
Codigesic, 1897·1
Co-Dilatrend, 1897·1
Codilergi, 1897·1
Codimal DH, 1897·1
Codimal DM, 1897·1
Codimal PH, 1897·1
Codimin, 1897·1
Codimol, 1897·1
Co-Diovan, 1897·1
Co-Diovane, 1897·1
Codipar, 1897·2
Codipertussin, 1897·2
Codiphen, 1897·2
Codipront, 1897·2
Codipront cum Expectorans, 1897·2
Codipront Mono, 1897·2
Codipront N, 1897·2
Codis, 1897·2
Codisal Forte, 1897·2
Coditard, 1897·2
Codivis, 1897·2
Codivite, 1897·2
Cod-liver Oil, 1425·2
Cod-liver Oil (Type A), 1425·2
Cod-liver Oil (Type B), 1425·2
Codocalyptol, 1897·2
Codoforme, 1897·2
Codol, 1897·2

Codoliprane, 1897·2
Codomex Orange, 1897·2
Codomex Purple, 1897·2
Codomill, 1897·2
Codoplex, 1897·2
Codotusil, 1897·3
Codotussyl Expectorant, 1897·3
Codotussyl Maux de Gorge, 1897·3
Codotussyl Toux Seche, 1897·3
Codox, 1897·3
Codral Preparations, 1897·3
Codrinan, 1897·3
Coduretas Gragenil, 1897·3
Co-dydramol, 35·1, 76·2
Codyl, 1897·3
Coease, 1897·3
Coedieci, 1897·3
Co-Efferalagan, 1897·3
Coeliac Disease, 1417·3
Coeliac Sprue— see Coeliac Disease, 1417·3
Co-Enaran, 1897·3
Coenrelax, 1897·3
Coentro, 1676·1
Coenzima A, 1674·3
Coenzyme A, 1674·3
Coenzyme I, 1719·1
Coenzyme Q10, 1760·2
Coenzyme R, 1423·2
Coergot, 1897·4
Co-erynsulfisox, 208·1, 260·1
Coex, 1897·4
Cofasol, 1897·4
Cofbron, 1897·4
Cofed, 1897·4
Cofena, 1897·4
Cofendyl, 1897·4
Coffalon N, 1897·4
*Coffea arabica*, 1765·3
*Coffea canephora*, 1765·3
*Coffea liberica*, 1765·3
Coffee, 1765·3
Coffee, Instant, 1765·3
Coffeemed N, 1897·4
Coffeinum, 782·1
Coffeinum Citricum, 782·1
Coffeinum Monohydricum, 782·1
Coffekapton, 1897·4
Coffetylin, 1897·4
Coffo Selt, 1897·4
Coff-Rest, 1897·4
Coff-Up, 1897·4
Coficold-Ped, 1897·4
Cofi-Tabs, 1897·4
Co-Flem, 1897·4
Co-fluampicil, 157·1, 213·3
Co-flumactone, 937·2, 1003·1
Cofrel, 1897·4
Cofron, 1897·4
Cofsed, 1897·4
Cogalactoisomerasa Sódica, 1674·3
Cogalactoisomerase Sodium, 1674·3
Cogan's Syndrome, 1078·3
Co-Gel, 1897·4
Cogenate, 1897·4
Cogentin, 1897·4
Cogentinol, 1897·4
Co-Gesic, 1897·4
Cogetine, 1897·4
Cogitum, 1898·1
Cognex, 1898·1
Cognitiv, 1898·1
Cognito, 1898·1
Cohemin, 1898·1
Co-Hist, 1898·1
Cohistan, 1898·1
Cohistan Expectorant, 1898·1
Cohoba, 1663·2, 1680·3
Cohortan, 1898·1
Cohortan Antibiotico, 1898·1
Cohosh, Black, 1671·3
Cohosh, Blue, 1661·2
Co-hycodAPAP, 45·1, 76·2
Co-Hypert, 1898·1
Co-I, 1719·1
Co-Inhibace, 1898·1
Coke, 1373·3
Cokenzen, 1898·1
Col Apestosa, 1746·3
Cola, 1765·3
*Cola acuminata*, 1765·3
Cola de Caballo, 1684·1
Cola, Gotu, 1144·3
*Cola nitida*, 1765·3
Cola Seeds, 1765·3
Cola Tonic, 1898·1
Colace, 1898·1
Colace Infant/Child, 1898·1
Colachofra, 1898·1
Coladren, 1898·1
Colagain, 1898·1
Colagenan, 1898·1
Colagenasa, 1675·1
Colágeno, 1674·3
Colagolen, 1898·1
Colagotil, 1898·1
Colambil, 1898·1
Colamin, 1898·1
Colaspase, 528·3
Colatan, 1898·1
Colatus, 1898·2
Co-Lav, 1898·2
Colax, 1898·2
Colax-C, 1898·2
Colax-S, 1898·2
Colazal, 1898·2
Colazid, 1898·2
Colazide, 1898·2
ColBenemid, 1898·2
Colbiocin, 1898·2
Colbuzer, 1898·2
Colcaps, 1898·2
Colchicina, 415·1
Colchicine, 415·1
Colchicine Amide, 415·1
Colchicinum, 415·1
Colchico, 416·3
*Colchicum*, 415·1
Colchicum, 416·3
*Colchicum autumnale*, 416·3
Colchicum Med Complex, 1898·2
Colchily, 1898·2
Colchimax, 1898·2
Colchique, 416·3
Colchiquim, 1898·2
Colchis, 1898·2
Colchysat, 1898·2
Colcine, 1898·2
Colcleer, 1898·2
Cold & Allergy, 1898·2
Cold & Allergy, Chemists Own— see Chemists Own Cold & Allergy, 1881·4
Cold & Allergy Relief, 1898·2
Cold & Catarrh, Modern Herbals— see Modern Herbals Cold & Catarrh, 2138·2
Cold, Common— see Common Cold, 618·1
Cold & Congestion, Modern Herbals— see Modern Herbals Cold & Congestion, 2138·2
Cold Control, 1898·2
Cold Cream Avene, 1898·2
Cold Cream Naturel, 1898·3
Cold Cream Salicyle, 1898·3
Cold Decongestant, 1898·3
Cold & Flu Day/Night, Chemists Own— see Chemists Own Cold & Flu Day/Night, 1881·4
Cold & Flu (Non-Drowsy) Tablets, 1898·3
Cold & Flu, Nyal Plus+ Day & Night— see Nyal Plus+ Day & Night Cold & Flu, 2182·1
Cold & Flu, Nyal Plus+ — see Nyal Plus+ Cold & Flu, 2182·1
Cold and Flu Relief, 1898·3
Cold & Flu Relief, Chemists Own— see Chemists Own Cold & Flu Relief, 1881·4
Cold & Flu Tablets, 1898·3
Cold & Flu Tablets Non Drowsy, 1898·3
Cold Max, 1898·3
Cold Medication D, 1898·3
Cold Medication Daytime Relief, 1898·3
Cold Medication N, 1898·3
Cold Medication Nighttime Relief, 1898·3
Cold Powders, Real Lemon— see Real Lemon Cold Powders, 2252·4
Cold Relief, 1898·3
Cold Relief Daytime, 1898·3
Cold Relief Night-Time, 1898·3
Cold Sore, 1898·3
Cold Sore Balm, 1898·3
Cold Sore, Chemists Own— see Chemists Own Cold Sore, 1881·4
Cold Sore Lotion, 1898·3
Cold Sore Relief, 1898·4
Cold Sore Tablets, 1898·4
Cold Sores— see Herpes Simplex Infections, 620·2
Cold Sores, Fever Blisters, 1898·4
Cold Tablets with Zinc, 1898·4
Colda, 1898·4
Coldacrom, 1898·4
Coldadolin, 1898·4
Coldagrippin, 1898·4
Coldan, 1898·4
Coldangin, 1898·4
Coldargan, 1898·4
Coldastop, 1898·4
Coldate, 1898·4
Coldec D, 1898·4
Coldec DM, 1898·4
Cold-eeze, 1898·4
Coldenza, 1898·4
Colderina, 1898·4
Coldetab, 1898·4
Coldex, 1898·4
Coldeze, Chemists Own— see Chemists Own Coldeze, 1881·4
Cold-Gard, 1898·4
Coldil, 1898·4
Coldin, 1898·4
Cold-insoluble Globulin, 1688·1
Coldistan, 1898·4
Coldistop, 1899·1
Coldloc, 1899·1
Coldloc-LA, 1899·1
Coldoff, 1899·1
Coldophthal, 1899·1
Coldosian, 1899·1
Coldrex, 1899·1
Coldrex C, 1899·1
Coldrex Day/Night, 1899·1
Coldrex Flu, 1899·1
Coldrex Head & Chest Cold, 1899·1
Coldrex Head Cold, 1899·1
Coldrex, Hot— see Hot Coldrex, 2048·3
Coldrex Night Relief, 1899·1
Coldrin, 1899·1
Coldrine, 1899·1
Colds & Flu, Natures Own— see Natures Own Colds & Flu, 2153·2
Coldstat, 1899·1
Coldvac, 1899·1
Coldy, 1899·1
Coleb, 1899·1
Colebrina, 1899·1
Colecalciferol, 1461·3
Colecalciferol Concentrate (Oily Form), 1461·3
Colecalciferol Concentrate (Powder Form), 1461·3
Colecalciferol Concentrate (Water-dispersible Form), 1461·3
Coledis, 1899·2
Coledos, 1899·2
Colegraf, 1899·2
Colemin, 1899·2
Colenon, 1899·2
Coléoptères Hétéromères, Insects, 1666·3
Colepren, 1899·2
Colerin, 1899·2
Colerin-F, 1899·2
Colese, 1899·2
Colesevelam, Hidrocloruro de, 889·2
Colesevelam Hydrochloride, 889·2
Colesom, 1899·2
Colestase, 1899·2
Colesterinex, 1899·2
Colesterol, 1480·3
Colesthexal, 1899·2
Colestid, 1899·2
Colestilan, 889·2
Colestimide, 889·2
Colestipol, Hidrocloruro de, 889·2
Colestipol Hydrochloride, 889·2
Colestiramina, 889·3
Colesto Cero, 1899·2
Colestyr, 1899·2
Colestyramine, 889·3
Colestyraminum, 889·3
Colesvir, 1899·2
*Coleus forskohlii*, 1674·3
Colevix, 1899·2
Colex, 1899·2
Colextrán, Hidrocloruro de, 890·3
Colextran Hydrochloride, 890·3
Colfed-A, 1899·2
Colforsin, 1674·3
Colforsin Daropate Hydrochloride, 1674·3
Colforsina, 1674·3
Colfosceril Palmitate, 1736·2
Colfoscerilo, Palmitato de, 1736·2
Colfur, 1899·2
Colgen, 1899·2
Colgout, 1899·2
Colhidrol, 1899·2
Coliacron, 1899·2
Colibiogen, 1899·2
Colic, 1899·2
Colic, Infant— see Gastrointestinal Spasm, 1242·2
Colic, Intestinal— see Gastrointestinal Spasm, 1242·2
Colic Pain— see Biliary and Renal Colic, 4·3
Colic Relief, 1899·2
Colicon, 1899·2
Colicort, 1899·3
Colief, 1899·3
Colifagina S, 1899·3
Coli-Fagina S, 1899·3
Colifilm, 1899·3
Colifoam, 1899·3
Colifossim, 1899·3
Colimax, 1899·3
Colimet, 1899·3
Colimex, 1899·3
Colimicina, 1899·3
Colimil, 1899·3
Colimix, 1899·3
Colimune, 1899·3
Colimycin, 1899·3
Colimycine, 1899·3
Colin, 1899·3
Colina, 1899·3
Colina, Alfoscerato de, 1488·3
Colina, Cloruro de, 1424·3
Colina Spezial, 1899·3
Colinex, 1899·3
Colinsan, 1899·3
Colinvintol, 1899·4
Coli-Om, 1899·4
Coliopan, 1899·4
Coliper, 1899·4
Coliquifilm, 1899·4
Coliracin, 1899·4
Colircusi Anestesi Doble— see Anestesi Doble, 1800·2
Colircusi Anestesico, 1899·4
Colircusi Cicloplejico, 1899·4
Colircusi Gentadexa, 1899·4
Colircusi Iodine-Thio-Calcic, 1899·4
Coliri Llorens Clor Hem— see Cloram Hemidexa, 1894·4
Colirid, 1899·4
Colirio Blumen, 1899·4
Colirio de Argyrol, 1899·4
Colirio Helios, 1899·4
Colirio Legrand, 1899·4
Colirio Llorens Sulfacet— see Sulfacet, 2311·2
Colirio Llorens Vasodexa— see Vasodexa, 2368·3
Colirio Moura Brasil, 1899·4
Colirio Sulvi, 1899·4
Colirio Teuto, 1899·4

Colirio Vima, 1899·4
Coliriocilina, 1899·4
Coliriocilina Adren Astr, 1899·4
Coliriocilina Espectro, 1899·4
Coliriocilina Gentam, 1899·4
Coliriocilina Homatrop, 1899·4
Coliriocilina Prednisona, 1899·4
Colistimetato de Sodio, 199·1
Colistimethate Sodium, 199·1
Colistimethatum Natrium, 199·1
Colistin Sulfate, 198·3
Colistin Sulphate, 198·3
Colistin Sulphomethate Sodium, 199·1
Colistina, Sulfato de, 198·3
Colistineméthanesulfonate Sodique, 199·1
Colistini Sulfas, 198·3
Colistop, 1899·4
Colistoral, 1899·4
Colitis, Amoebic— *see* Amoebiasis, 595·2
Colitis, Antibiotic-associated— *see* Antibiotic-associated Colitis, 128·1
Colitis, Clostridium Difficile— *see* Antibiotic-associated Colitis, 128·1
Colitis, Collagenous— *see* Collagenous Colitis, 1240·2
Colitis, Haemorrhagic— *see* Escherichia Coli Enteritis, 129·1
Colitis, Pseudomembranous— *see* Antibiotic-associated Colitis, 128·1
Colitis, Ulcerative— *see* Inflammatory Bowel Disease, 1243·3
Colitofalk, 1899·4
Colitromin, 1899·4
Colix, 1900·1
Colizin, 1900·1
Colizole, 1900·1
Collafilm, 1900·1
Collagen, 1674·3
Collagenase, 1675·1
Collagenous Colitis, 1240·2
Collatamp G, 1900·1
Collaven, 1900·1
Collazin, 1900·1
Colle du Japon, 1576·3
Colleofer, 1900·1
Colli, 1900·1
Collins Elixir, 1900·1
Collins Elixir Decongesant Pasilles, 1900·1
Collins Elixir Pastilles, 1900·1
Collinsonia, 1749·3
*Collinsonia canadensis*, 1749·3
Collinsonia del Canadá, 1749·3
Collirio Alfa, 1900·1
Collirio Alfa Antistaminico, 1900·1
Collirium Geymonat, 1900·1
Collis Browne's, 1900·1
Collodyne, 1900·1
Colloid Plasma Expanders, 835·2
Colloidal 75, 1900·1
Colloidal Activated Attapulgite, 1251·1
Colloidal Anhydrous Silica, 1581·3
Colloidal Bismuth Subcitrate, 1252·2
Colloidal Gold ($^{198}$Au), 1523·3
Colloidal Hydrated Silica, 1581·3
Colloidal Oatmeal, 1658·2
Colloidal Silica, 1581·3
Colloidal Silicon Dioxide, 1581·3
Colloidal Silver Iodide, 1746·1
Colloidal Sulfur, 1158·2
Colloidine, 1900·1
Collomack, 1900·1
Collosol, 1900·1
Colloxylinum, 1156·2
Collubiazol, 1900·1
Collu-Blache, 1900·1
Collubleu, 1900·1
Colludol, 1900·1
Collu-Hextril, 1900·1
Collunosol-N, 1900·2
Collunovar, 1900·2
Collupressine, 1900·2
Collustan, 1900·2
Collylarm, 1900·2
Collypan, 1900·2
Collyre Alpha, 1900·2
Collyre Bleu, 1900·2
Collyre Bleu Laiter, 1900·2
Collyrex, 1900·2
Collyria, 1900·2
Collyrium, 1900·2
Collyrium Fresh, 1900·2
Collyrium for Fresh Eyes, 1900·2
Colmax, 1900·2
Colme, 1900·2
Colobolina, 1900·2
Colobolina D, 1900·2
Colocarb, 1900·2
ColoCare, 1900·2
Colocinto, 1260·3
Colocynth, 1260·3
Colocynth Pulp, 1260·3
Colocynthis, 1260·3
Colodium, 1900·2
Colofac, 1900·2
Colofiber, 1900·2
Colofoam, 1900·2
Colofonia, 1675·1
Cololyt, 1900·2
Colomba Spezial, 1900·2
Colombo, 1665·2
Colominte, 1900·3
Colominthe, 1900·3
Colomycin, 1900·3
Colonic Cancer— *see* Malignant Neoplasms of the Gastrointestinal Tract, 516·2
Colonic Lavage Powder, 1900·3
Colonic Pseudo-obstruction— *see* Decreased Gastrointestinal Motility, 1241·1
Colonlytely, 1900·3
Colonlytely— *see* Colonprep, 1900·3
Colonorm, 1900·3
Colonorm N, 1900·3
Colonprep, 1900·3
Colonsteril, 1900·3
Colony-stimulating Factors, 754·2
Colopeg, 1900·3
Coloph., 1675·1
Colophane, 1675·1
Colophonium, 1675·1
Colophony, 1675·1
Colophos, 1900·3
Coloplast OAD (Sween), 1900·3
Colo-Pleon, 1900·3
Colo-Prep, 1900·3
Colopriv, 1900·3
Colopten, 1900·3
Coloquinte, 1260·3
Coloquintidas, 1260·3
Colorectal Cancer— *see* Malignant Neoplasms of the Gastrointestinal Tract, 516·2
Colo-Rectal Test, 1900·3
Colosan Mite, 1900·3
Colosan Plus, 1900·3
Coloscreen, 1900·3
Colosina, 1900·3
Colosoft, 1900·3
Colo-Sol, 1900·3
Colospa, 1900·3
Colospan, 1900·3
Colostrum, 1900·3
Colostrum, Bovine, 1611·1
Colotal, 1900·3
Colour Index No. 11270, 1670·3
Colour Index No. 14130, 1278·1
Colour Index No. 14720, 1057·1
Colour Index No. 15985, 1058·2
Colour Index No. 16035, 1056·1
Colour Index No. 16180, 1056·2
Colour Index No. 16185, 1056·1
Colour Index No. 16255, 1057·3
Colour Index No. 18050, 1058·1
Colour Index No. 18965, 1058·3
Colour Index No. 19140, 1058·2
Colour Index No. 20285, 1056·3
Colour Index No. 22120, 1675·3
Colour Index No. 23850, 1758·3
Colour Index No. 23860, 1658·3
Colour Index No. 26105, 1191·3
Colour Index No. 28440, 1056·2
Colour Index No. 40850, 1056·3
Colour Index No. 42000, 1185·2
Colour Index No. 42040, 1171·1
Colour Index No. 42045, 1750·3
Colour Index No. 42051, 1729·1
Colour Index No. 42090, 1056·2
Colour Index No. 42510, 1185·1
Colour Index No. 42535, 1186·2
Colour Index No. 42555, 1186·1
Colour Index No. 42685, 1646·3
Colour Index No. 44090, 1057·3
Colour Index No. 45350, 1689·1
Colour Index No. 45380, 1057·2
Colour Index No. 45430, 1057·2
Colour Index No. 45435, 1740·1
Colour Index No. 45440, 1740·1
Colour Index No. 47005, 1057·3
Colour Index No. 50040, 1719·3
Colour Index No. 52015, 1042·2
Colour Index No. 52040, 1757·1
Colour Index No. 73015, 1700·3
Colour Index No. 75100, 1058·2
Colour Index No. 75300, 1057·2
Colour Index No. 75470, 1057·1, 1057·2
Colour Index No. 75810, 1057·1
Colour Index No. 77510, 1051·2
Colour Index No. 77520, 1051·2
Colour Index No. 77891, 1160·3
Colouring Agents, 1056·1
Coloxyl, 1900·3
Coloxyl with Senna, 1900·4
Colpacid, 1900·4
Colpagex N, 1900·4
Colpanist, 1900·4
Colpatrin, 1900·4
Colpermin, 1900·4
Colphen, 1900·4
Colpist, 1900·4
Colpistar, 1900·4
Colpistatin, 1900·4
Colpocin-T, 1900·4
Colpogyn, 1900·4
Colpolase, 1900·4
Colposeptine, 1900·4
Colpotrofin, 1900·4
Colpotrofine, 1900·4
Colpotrophine, 1900·4
Colpovis, 1900·4
Colpro, 1900·4
Colpron, 1900·4
Colprone, 1900·4
Colpuril, 1900·4
Colsanac, 1901·1
Colser, 1901·1
Colsor, 1901·1
Colsprin, 1901·1
Colstat, 1901·1
Coltalin with Vit $B_1$, 1901·1
Coltalin with Vit $B_1$, Childrens— *see* Childrens Coltalin with Vit $B_1$, 1882·4
Coltapaste, 1901·1
Colterol, 781·3
Colther, 1901·1
Coltix, 1901·1
Coltramyl, 1901·1
Coltrax, 1901·1
Coltsfoot, 1117·2
Colubiazol, 1901·1
Colufase, 1901·1
Columbia Antiseptic Powder, 1901·1
Columina, 1901·1
Colutoide, 1901·1
Coly-Mycin M, 1901·1
Coly-Mycin S Otic, 1901·1
Colyrazul, 1901·1
CoLyte, 1901·1
Colza, Aceite de, 1737·3
Colza Oil, 1737·3
Comafusin Hepar, 1901·1
Co-magaldrox, 1249·2, 1272·2
Comagis, 1901·1
Comalose-R, 1901·1
Comat, 1901·1
Combacid, 1901·2
Combactam, 1901·2
Combact-HIB, 1901·2
Combantrin, 1901·2
Combantrin-1, 1901·2
Combantrin-1 with Mebendazole, 1901·2
Combaren, 1901·2
Combetasi, 1901·2
Combeylax— *see* Hydrafuca, 2050·4
Combi-Cal, 1901·2
Combid, 1901·2
Combiderm, 1901·2
Combiflam, 1901·2
Combifusin, 1901·2
Combilosung, 1901·2
Combina, 1901·2
Combina 2, 1901·2
Combina 3, 1901·2
Combina Glucose, 1901·2
Combinacion PI, 1901·2
Combinacion Rubin-Calcagno, 1901·2
Combined Oral Contraceptives, 1527·3
Combinovita, 1901·2
Combinplex, 1901·2
Combion-B, 1901·2
CombiPatch, 1901·2
Combiplasmal, 1901·2
Combipres, 1901·2
Combipresan, 1901·2
Combiron, 1901·2
Combisartan, 1901·3
Combiseven, 1901·3
Combistix, 1901·3
Combithyrex, 1901·3
Combitora, 1901·3
Combitorax, 1901·3
Combitrex, 1901·3
Combivax, 1901·3
Combivent, 1901·3
Combivir, 1901·3
Combivitol, 1901·3
Combizym, 1901·3
Combizym Compositum, 1901·3
Combizym Composto, 1901·3
Combreti Folium, 1703·3
Combretum, 1703·3
*Combretum altum*, 1703·3
*Combretum micranthum*, 1703·3
*Combretum raimbaultii*, 1703·3
Combudoron, 1901·3
Combunex, 1901·3
Combur Tests, 1901·3
Comburic, 1901·4
Combustin Heilsalbe, 1901·4
Combutol, 1901·4
Comenter, 1901·4
Co-Mepril, 1901·4
Co-methiamol, 76·2, 1042·1
Cometon, 1901·4
Comfarol Plus, Hexal— *see* Hexal Comfarol Plus, 2043·3
Comfeel, 1901·4
Comfeel Plus, 1901·4
Comfeel Purilon, 1901·4
Comfeel Seasorb, 1901·4
Comfort, 1901·4
Comfort Eye Drops, 1901·4
Comfort Tears, 1901·4
Comfortcare Dual Action, 1901·4
Comfortcare GP, 1901·4
Comfortcare Wetting & Soaking, 1901·4
Comfortine, 1901·4
Comfrey, 1675·2
Comfrey Plus, 1901·4
Comfrey Root, 1675·2
Comfy, 1901·4
Comhist LA, 1902·1
Co-Micardis, 1902·1
Comilorid, 1902·1
Comital L, 1902·1
Comizial, 1902·1
*Commiphora molmol*, 1718·3
Commit, 1902·1
Common Cold, 618·1
Common Nasturtium, 1659·3
Common Oak, 1722·3
Common Oleander, 1723·1
Common Stinging Nettle for Homoeopathic Preparations, 1762·1
Comoprin, 1902·1

Compact, 1902·1
Compact Sorb, 1902·1
Compactin, 958·1
Compagel, 1902·1
Compagen, 1902·1
Companion 2, 1902·1
Compaz, 1902·1
Compazine, 1902·1
Compendium, 1902·1
Compensal, 1902·1
Compensan, 1902·1
Compete, 1902·1
Competitive Muscle Relaxants, 1397·1
Competitive Neuromuscular Blockers, 1397·1
Complamin, 1902·1
Complamin Spezial, 1902·1
Complamina, 1902·1
Complan, 1902·1
Compleat, 1902·1
Compleat Modified, 1902·1
Complegel Novo, 1902·1
Complegil, 1902·1
Complejo B, 1902·1
Complejo Coagulante Antiinhibidor Del Factor VIII, 752·2
Complejo de Hierro Succinil-proteína, 1438·1
Complejo Polisacárido Hierro, 1443·2
Complement Blockers, 1675·2
Complement C1 Esterase Inhibitor, 1675·2
Complement C1 Esterase Inhibitor Deficiency— *see* Hereditary Angioedema, 761·3
Complementa, 1902·1
Complenatal FF, 1902·1
Complesso B, 1902·1
Completax Plus, 1902·2
Complete, 1902·2
Complete All-In-One, 1902·2
Complete Comfort Plus, 1902·2
Complete Multi Pre- and Post-Natal, 1902·2
Complete Multi-Adult, 1902·2
Complete Protein Remover, 1902·2
Complete Solution, 1902·2
Compleven, 1902·2
Complevit, 1902·2
Complevit Pediatrico, 1902·2
Complevitan, 1902·2
Complex 15, 1902·2
Complex 75, 1902·2
Complex B, 1902·2
Complexan B, 1902·2
Complexe B Compose, 1902·2
Complexe Preparations, 1902·2
Complexo B, 1902·2
Complidermol, 1902·2
Comploment Continus, 1902·2
Complutine, 1902·2
Comply, 1902·2
Compocillin, 1902·2
Composto Anticelulitico, 1902·2
Composto Emagrecedor, 1902·2
Compound 22-708, 910·3
Compound 254, 159·1
Compound 347, 1298·1
Compound 469, 1301·1
Compound 1080, 1510·1
Compound 1081, 1505·3
Compound 4047, 1507·1
Compound 5071, 1558·2
Compound 5107, 684·1
Compound 5411, 1065·1
Compound 25398, 1303·2
Compound 33006, 329·2
Compound 33355, 1559·2
Compound 35483, 891·1
Compound 37231, 592·2
Compound 49510, 1462·1
Compound 64716, 188·1
Compound 79891, 611·1
Compound 81929, 905·3
Compound 83405, 169·3
Compound 83846, 864·2
Compound 90459, 21·1
Compound 99170, 864·2
Compound 99638, 167·1
Compound 109514, 1277·1
Compound 112531, 593·3
Compound A, 1308·1
Compound B, 1308·1
Compound E Acetate, 1096·1
Compound F, 1103·3
Compound Inhalation of Menthol, 1902·3
Compound Mastic Paint, 1710·1
Compound Q, 655·3
Compound Thymol Glycerin, 1194·3
Compound V, 1902·3
Compound W, 1902·3
Compound W Plus, 1902·3
Compound-S, 658·2
Compoz Night-time Sleep Aid, 1902·3
Compralgyl, 1902·3
Compralsol, 1902·3
Comprecin, 1902·3
Comprimes Analgesiques No 534, 1902·3
Comprimes Analgesiques "S", 1902·3
Comprimes contre la Toux, 1902·3
Comprimes Gynecologiques Pharmatex, 1902·3
Comprimes pour l'Estomac, 1902·3
Comprimes Somniferes Formule 533, 1902·3
Comprimes Somniferes "S", 1902·3
Compro, 1902·3
Compuestos de Antimonio Pentavalente, 600·3
Compuestos de Antimonio Trivalente, 103·1
Compufen, Hexal— *see* Hexal Compufen, 2043·3
Compu-Gel, 1902·3
Computed Tomography, 1059·1
Computer Eye Drops, 1902·3
Computer Eye Drops, Bausch & Lomb— *see* Bausch & Lomb Computer Eye Drops, 1829·3
Comstrong, 1902·3
Comtan, 1902·3
Comtaplex, 1902·3
Comtess, 1902·3
COMT-inhibitors, 1196·1
Comtrex, 1902·3
Comtrex Allergy-Sinus, 1902·3
Comtrex Day & Night Maximum Strength, 1902·3
Comtrex Day & Night Multi-Symptom, 1902·3
Comtrex Hot Flu Relief, 1902·4
Comtrex Liqui-Gels, 1902·4
Comvax, 1902·4
Conacid, 1902·4
Conadyl, 1902·4
Conamic, 1902·4
Conan, 1902·4
Conazine, 1902·4
Conazol, 1902·4
Conazole, 1902·4
Conbutol, 1902·4
Concatag, 1902·4
Concavit, 1902·4
Conceive, 1902·4
Conceive Ovulation Predictor, 1902·4
Conceive Pregnancy, 1902·4
Concentrado Acido, 1902·4
Concentrado Basico, 1902·4
Concentrated Cleaner, 1902·4
Concentrated Milk of Magnesia-Cascara, 1902·4
Concentrin, 1902·4
Conceplan M, 1902·4
Concept, 1902·4
Concerta, 1902·4
Conchae Comp., 1902·4
Conchivit, 1902·4
Concor, 1902·4
Concor Plus, 1902·4
Concordin, 1903·1
Condelone, 1903·1
Condil, 1903·1
Condiment, Non-brewed, 1645·3
Conditioning Solution, 1903·1
Condiuren, 1903·1
Condral, 1903·1
Condress, 1903·1
Condro Sorb, 1903·1
Condrofer, 1903·1
Condroitina, 1903·1
Condrosamina, 1903·1
Condrosulf, 1903·1
Condrotec, 1903·1
Conducat, 1903·1
Conductasa, 1903·1
Conducton, 1903·1
Condurango, 1675·3
Condurango Bark, 1675·3
Condyline, 1903·1
Condylomata Acuminata— *see* Warts, 1139·2
Condylox, 1903·1
Conectol, 1903·1
Conef, 1903·1
Coneflower, 1683·2
Conevit, 1903·1
Conex, 1903·1
Conex with Codeine, 1903·1
Conexine, 1903·1
Confer, 1903·1
Conferma 3 Plus, 1903·1
Confetti Lassativi CM, 1903·1
Confetto CM, 1903·1
Confiance, 1903·2
Confiance Donna, 1903·2
Confidelle, 1903·2
Confidelle Progress, 1903·2
Confidol, 1903·2
Confirm, 1903·2
Confit, 1903·2
Confludin N, 1903·2
Confobos, 1903·2
Conformal, 1903·2
Conformil, 1903·2
Confor-Tar, 1903·2
Confortel, 1903·2
Confortid, 1903·2
Congest, 1903·2
Congest Aid, 1903·2
Congestac, 1903·2
Congestaid, 1903·2
Congestant, 1903·2
Congestant D, 1903·2
Congestex, 1903·2
Congest-Eze, 1903·2
Congestion Relief, 1903·2
Congex, 1903·2
Congo Red, 1675·3
Conidrin, 1903·2
Coniel, 1903·2
Coniuncti Estrogeni, 1543·2
Conjonctyl, 1903·2
Conjugated Estrogens, 1543·2
Conjugated Estrogens, A, Synthetic, 1543·3
Conjugated Estrogens, B, Synthetic, 1543·3
Conjugated Oestrogens, 1543·2
Conjugated Oestrogens, A, Synthetic, 1543·3
Conjugated Oestrogens, B, Synthetic, 1543·3
Conjugen, 1903·2
Conjuncain-EDO, 1903·2
Conjunctilone, 1903·2
Conjunctilone-S, 1903·2
Conjunctisan-A, 1903·3
Conjunctisan-B, 1903·3
Conjunctivitis, Allergic— *see* Conjunctivitis, 421·3
Conjunctivitis, Bacterial— *see* Eye Infections, 127·2
Conjunctivitis, Neonatal— *see* Neonatal Conjunctivitis, 136·3
Conjuntin, 1903·3
Conjunto Soramin Hipercalorico, 1903·3
Conjuvac, 1903·3
Conkers, 1648·2
Conludag, 1903·3
Conmel, 1903·3
Connettivina, 1903·3
Connettivina Plus, 1903·3
*Conocybe*, 1717·3, 1736·1
Conotrane, 1903·3
Conova, 1903·3
Conpin, 1903·3
Conpremin, 1903·3
Conpremin Pak, 1903·3
Conpremin Pak Plus, 1903·3
Conprim, 1903·3
Conrax, 1903·3
Conray Preparations, 1903·3
Consec, 1903·3
Consept Step 1, 1903·3
Consept Step 2, 1903·3
Consil, 1903·3
Consil Clean, 1903·4
Consinut, 1903·4
Consolda Vermelha, 1757·2
Consolidae Radix, 1675·2
Consolin, 1903·4
Constilac, 1903·4
Constilax, 1903·4
Constipal, 1903·4
Constipation, 1240·2, 1903·4
Constipation L106, 1903·4
Constrilia, 1903·4
Constulose, 1903·4
Consudine, 1903·4
Consuelda, 1675·2
Consupren, 1903·4
Contac Preparations, 1903·4
Contaclair, 1904·1
Contact, 1904·1
Contact Eyes, 1904·1
Contact Laxatives, 1239·3
Contact Lens Care, 1164·2
Contactol, 1904·1
Contafilm, 1904·1
Contalax, 1904·1
Conta-Lens Wetting, 1904·1
Contalgin, 1904·1
Contaren, 1904·1
Contefur, 1904·1
Contem, 1904·1
ConTE-PAK, 1904·2
Conthram, 1904·2
Contiabe, 1904·2
Contigen, 1904·2
Contilen, 1904·2
Contimit, 1904·2
Continucor, 1904·2
Contiphyllin, 1904·2
Contopharma, 1904·2
Contra Combustiones, 1904·2
Contracep, 1904·2
Contraception, 1535·3
Contraception, Emergency— *see* Emergency Contraception, 1536·1
Contraception, Postcoital— *see* Emergency Contraception, 1536·1
Contraceptive Vaccines, 1611·3
Contraceptives, Hormonal, 1527·3
Contraceptives, Implantable, 1527·3
Contraceptives, Injectable, 1527·3
Contraceptives, Intra-uterine, Progestogen-releasing, 1527·3
Contraceptives, Oral, 1527·3
Contraceptives, Postcoital, 1527·3
Contraceptives, Transdermal, 1527·3
Contraceptives, Vaginal, 1527·3
Contracid, 1904·2
Contracide, 1904·2
Contra-Coff, 1904·2
Contractubex, 1904·2
Contradol, 1904·2
Contraforte, 1904·2
Contralgen, 1904·2
Contralmor, 1904·2
Contralorin, 1904·2
Contralum Ultra, 1904·2
Contramal, 1904·2
Contramareo, 1904·2
Contramutan, 1904·2
Contraneural, 1904·2
Contraneural Forte— *see* Contraneural Paracetamol/Codeine, 1904·2

Contraneural Paracetamol/Codeine, 1904·2
Contrasmina, 1904·3
Contraspasmin, 1904·3
Contrast Media, 1059·1
Contrasthenyl, 1904·3
Contrathion, 1904·3
Contravert $B_6$, 1904·3
Contre-Coups de l'Abbe Perdrigeon, 1904·3
Contre-Douleurs, 1904·3
Contre-Douleurs C, 1904·3
Contre-Douleurs P, 1904·3
Contre-Douleurs Plus, 1904·3
Contreet, 1904·3
Contrelmin, 1904·3
Contrheuma, 1904·3
Contrheuma Bad L, 1904·3
Contrheuma V + T Bad N, 1904·3
Contrheuma-Gel Forte N, 1904·3
Contrin, 1904·3
Control, 1904·3
Control K, 1904·3
Controlip, 1904·3
Controloc, 1904·3
Controloc— *see* Klacid HP 7, 2080·1
ControlRx, 1904·3
Controlvas, 1904·4
Contromet, 1904·4
Contugesic, 1904·4
Contumax, 1904·4
Contusil, 1904·4
Contusin, 1904·4
Contuss, 1904·4
Contuxin, 1904·4
Convacard, 1904·4
Conva-cyl Ho-Len-Complex, 1904·4
Convalaria, 1675·3
Convallaria, 1675·3
*Convallaria majalis*, 1675·3
Convallarin, 1675·3
Convallatoxin, 1675·3
Convallatoxoloside, 1675·3
Convallocor, 1904·4
Convallocor-SL, 1904·4
Convalloside, 1675·3
Convastabil, 1904·4
Convectal, 1904·4
Conventional Insulins, 334·2
Conversion Disorders— *see* Conversion and Dissociative Disorders, 696·2
Convertal, 1904·4
Converten, 1904·4
Convertin, 1904·4
Convifer C/Hierro, 1904·4
Conviron-TR, 1904·4
Convulex, 1904·4
Convulsan, 1904·4
Convulsions— *see* Epilepsy, 349·1
Convulsions, Febrile— *see* Febrile Convulsions, 353·1
Convulsofin, 1904·4
Cool Eyes, Brolene— *see* Brolene Cool Eyes, 1853·2
Coolips, 1904·4
Cool-Mint Listerine, 1904·4
Cooper AR, 1904·4
Cooper Tears, 1904·4
Co-oxycodAPAP, 75·2, 76·2
COP-1, 1693·3
Copal, 1904·4
Copalchi, 1669·2, 1676·3
Copaltra, 1669·2, 1905·1
Copamide, 1905·1
Copan, 1905·1
Copastin, 1905·1
Copaxone, 1905·1
Cope, 1905·1
Copegus, 1905·1
Copena, 1905·1
Copercilex, 1905·1
*Copernicia cerifera*, 1668·1
Coperniciae, Cera, 1668·1
Cophene No. 2, 1905·1
Cophene XP, 1905·1
Cophene-X, 1905·1
Co-phenotrope, 477·1, 1261·3
Cophenylcaine, 1905·1
Cophylac, 1905·1
6 Copin, 1905·1
Copinal, 1905·1
Copiron, 1905·1
Coplexina, 1905·1
Copolymer 1, 1693·3
Copolyvidone, 1581·2
Copolyvidonum, 1581·2
Copovan, 1905·1
Copovidona, 1581·2
Copovidone, 1581·2
Copovidonum, 1581·2
Copper, 1425·3
Copper Chloride, 1425·3
Copper Chlorophyll Complex, 1057·1
Copper Chlorophyllin Complex, 1057·1
Copper Gluconate, 1425·3
Copper D-Gluconate (1:2), 1425·3
Copper for Homoeopathic Preparations, 1425·3
Copper Methionate, 1426·1
Copper Naphthenate, 397·1
Copper Oleate, 1502·2
Copper Oxide, 1426·1
Copper Phaeophytins, 1057·1
Copper Solution Reagent Tablets— *see* Clinitest, 1893·3
Copper Sulfate, 1426·1
Copper Sulph., 1426·1
Copper Sulphate, 1426·1
Copper Sulphate, Anhydrous, 1426·1
Copper Sulphate Pentahydrate, 1426·1
Copper (II) Sulphate Pentahydrate, 1426·1
Copper Usnate, 1762·1
Copperas, Blue, 1426·1
Copperas, Green, 1428·2
Copperas, White, 1469·3
Coppertone Preparations, 1905·1
Coppertone Waterbabies— *see* Water Babies, 2385·2
Co-prenozide, 890·3, 978·1
Co-Pressotec, 1905·3
Coprine, 1717·3
*Coprinus atramentarius*, 1717·3
Co-proxamol, 28·3, 76·2
Co-proxAPAP, 28·3, 76·2
Coptin, 1905·3
Copyrkal N, 1905·3
Co-Pyronil, 1905·3
Co-Q-10, 1905·3
Coquelicot, 1058·1
Coquelusedal, 1905·3
Coquelusedal Paracetamol, 1905·3
Coquevit, 1905·3
CoQuinone, 1905·3
Cor Mio, 1905·3
Cor Pulmonale— *see* Chronic Obstructive Pulmonary Disease, 779·2
Cor Tensobon, 1905·3
Coraben, 1905·3
Coracten, 1905·3
Coradol, 1905·3
Coradur, 1905·4
Coral, 1905·4
Coralen, 1905·4
Coralgesic, 1905·4
Coralmyn, 1905·4
Coralzul, 1905·4
Coramedan, 1905·4
Coramil, 1905·4
Coramine Glucose, 1905·4
Corangin, 1905·4
Corangin Nitrokapseln, 1905·4
Corangin Nitrospray— *see* Corangin Nitrokapseln and Nitrospray, 1905·4
Corangine, 1905·4
Coras, 1905·4
Corase, 1905·4
Coraspir, 1905·4
Corathiem, 1905·4
Coratol, 1905·4
Corazem, 1905·4
Corazet, 1905·4
Corazol, 1592·1
Corbadrina, 1675·3
Corbadrine, 1675·3
Corbar, 1905·4
Corbar M, 1905·4
Corbar S, 1905·4
Corbeta, 1905·4
Corbetazine, 1905·4
Corbeton, 1905·4
Corbin, 1905·4
Corbionax, 1905·4
Corbis, 1905·4
Corcanfol, 1905·4
Corciclen, 1905·4
Cordalin, 1906·1
Cordanum, 1906·1
Cordapur Novo, 1906·1
Cordarex, 1906·1
Cordarone, 1906·1
Cordarone X, 1906·1
Cordes Beta, 1906·1
Cordes BPO, 1906·1
Cordes Estriol, 1906·1
Cordes Nystatin Soft, 1906·1
Cordes VAS, 1906·1
Cordesin, 1906·1
Cordiaminum, 1591·2
Cordiax, 1906·1
Cordicant, 1906·1
Cordichin, 1906·1
Cordil, 1906·1
Cordilan, 1906·1
Cordilat, 1906·1
Cordilox, 1906·1
Cordinal, 1906·1
Cordiodoron, 1906·1
Cordipatch, 1906·1
Cordipin, 1906·1
Cordipina, 1906·1
Cordiplast, 1906·1
Cordisol, 1906·2
Corditrine, 1906·2
Cordium, 1906·2
Cordodopa, 1906·2
Cordran, 1906·2
Cordycepic Acid, 950·2
*Cordyline*, 1710·2
Cordymax, 1906·2
Coreg, 1906·2
Corega, 1906·2
Coreine, 1906·2
Co-Renitec, 1906·2
Co-Reniten, 1906·2
Corenza C, 1906·2
Coreptil, 1906·2
Coretec, 1906·2
Corethium, 1906·2
Corex, 1906·2
Corex Dx, 1906·2
Corfen-DM, 1906·2
Corflo, 1906·2
Corgard, 1906·2
Corgaretic, 1906·2
Corguttin N Plus, 1906·2
Coriand., 1676·1
Coriander, 1676·1
Coriander Fruit, 1676·1
Coriander Oil, 1676·1
Coriander Seed, 1676·1
Coriandri Aetheroleum, 1676·1
Coriandri Fructus, 1676·1
Coriandri, Oleum, 1676·1
*Coriandrum sativum*, 1676·1
Coric, 1906·2
Coric Plus, 1906·2
Coricide Le Diable, 1906·2
Coricidil-D, 1906·3
Coricidin, 1906·3
Coricidin D, 1906·3
Coricidin Expec, 1906·3
Coricidin F, 1906·3
Coricidin Fuerte, 1906·3
Coricidin HBP Chest Congestion & Cough, 1906·3
Coricidin Maximum Strength Sinus Headache, 1906·3
Coricidin Non-Drowsy, 1906·3
Coricidin Pediatrico NF, 1906·3
Coricidin Sinus Headache, 1906·3
Coridil, 1906·3
Corifeo, 1906·3
Corifin, 1906·3
Corifina, 1906·3
Corilax, 1906·3
Corilin F, 1906·3
Corilisina, 1906·3
Corindocomb, 1906·3
Corindolan, 1906·4
Corinfar, 1906·4
Coriodal, 1906·4
Coriogonadotropina Alfa, 1320·3
Corion, 1906·4
Coriosta Vitaltonikum N, 1906·4
Coriovaccine, 1906·4
Corisol, 1906·4
Coristex-DH, 1906·4
Coristina D, 1906·4
Coristina R, 1906·4
Coristina Reforcada, 1906·4
Coristine-DH, 1906·4
Coritab, 1906·4
Coritensil, 1906·4
Coritex, 1906·4
Coritussal, 1906·4
Corium, 1906·4
Coriver, 1906·4
Corizina, 1906·4
Corizzina, 1906·4
Cor-L 90 N, 1906·4
Corlan, 1906·4
Cor-loges, 1906·4
Corlopam, 1906·4
Cormagnesin, 1907·1
Cormax, 1907·1
Cormelian, 1907·1
Corn, Callus Plaster Preparation, Scholl— *see* Scholl Corn, Callus Plaster Preparation, 2279·3
Corn & Callus Removal Liquid, Scholl— *see* Scholl Corn & Callus Removal Liquid, 2279·3
Corn Huskers, 1907·1
Corn Oil, 1439·2
Corn Removal, Scholl— *see* Scholl Corn Removal, 2279·3
Corn Removing Liquid, 1907·1
Corn Salve, 1907·1
Corn Salve, Scholl— *see* Scholl Corn Salve, 2279·3
Corn Silk, 1676·1
Corn Starch, 1449·1
Corn Sugar Gum, 1582·3
Cornaron, 1907·1
Corneal Inflammation— *see* Dry Eye, 1576·1
Corneal Ulceration— *see* Dry Eye, 1576·1
Cornel, 1907·1
Corneregel, 1907·1
Cornezuelo del Centeno, 1685·1
Corni Limp, 1907·1
Cornina, 1907·1
Cornina Hornhaut, 1907·1
Cornina Huhneraugen, 1907·1
Cornkil, 1907·1
Corocrat, 1907·1
Coroday, 1907·1
Corodil, 1907·1
Corodil Comp, 1907·1
Corodin, 1907·1
Corodin D, 1907·1
Corodoc S, 1907·1
Corodyn, 1907·1
Corogal, 1907·1
Corolater, 1907·1
Corolin, 1907·1
Coromert, 1907·1
Coronar, 1907·1
Coronarine, 1907·1
Coronary Angioplasty, Percutaneous Transluminal— *see* Reperfusion and Revascularisation Procedures, 834·1
Coronary Artery Bypass Surgery— *see* Reperfusion and Revascularisation Procedures, 834·1

Coronary Artery Disease— *see* Atherosclerosis, 815·2
Coronary Heart Disease— *see* Atherosclerosis, 815·2
Coronary Syndromes, Acute— *see* Angina Pectoris, 813·1
Coronator, 1907·1
Coronex, 1907·1
Coro-Nitro, 1907·1
Coronorm, 1907·2
Coronovo, 1907·2
Coronur, 1907·2
Coropres, 1907·2
Cororell, 1907·2
Corosan, 1907·2
Corotal, 1907·2
Corotenol, 1907·2
Corotrend, 1907·2
Corotrop, 1907·2
Corotrope, 1907·2
Coroval, 1907·2
Coroval B, 1907·2
Coroverlan, 1907·2
Corovliss, 1907·2
Corozell, 1907·2
Corpamil, 1907·2
Corpea, 1907·2
Corpendol, 1907·2
Corplus, 1907·2
Corpotasin CL, 1907·2
Corpril, 1907·2
Corprilor, 1907·2
Corpus Luteum Hormone, 1566·2
Corque, 1907·2
Correctol, 1907·2
Correctol Stool Softener, 1907·3
Corrigast, 1907·3
Corrosive Sublimate, 1712·3
Corsalbene, 1907·3
Cor-Select, 1907·3
Corsifar, 1907·3
Corsodyl, 1907·3
CorSotalol, 1907·3
Corsym, 1907·3
Cortacet, 1907·3
Cortafrin, 1907·3
Cortafriol C, 1907·3
Cortafriol Complex, 1907·3
Cor-Tagrip, 1907·3
Cortagrip, 1907·3
Cortagrip D, 1907·3
Cortaid, 1907·3
Cortaid with Aloe, 1907·3
Cortal, 1907·3
Cortal for Adults, 1907·3
Cortal for Children, 1907·3
Cortalen C, 1907·3
Cortaler Novo, 1907·4
Cortamed, 1907·4
Cortamide, 1907·4
Cortancyl, 1907·4
Cortane-B, 1907·4
Cortanest, 1907·4
Cortanest Plus, 1907·4
Cortapaisyl, 1907·4
Cortasm, 1907·4
Cortate, 1907·4
Cortatrigen, 1907·4
Cortax, 1907·4
Cortazac, 1092·3
Cort-Dome, 1907·4
Cortef, 1907·4
Cortef Feminine Itch, 1907·4
Cortegripan, 1907·4
Cortenem, 1907·4
Cortenema, 1907·4
Corteroid, 1907·4
Corteroid Gesic, 1907·4
Corteroid Retard, 1907·4
Corteza de Cerezo Silvestre, 1765·2
Corteza de Frángula, 1266·3
Corteza de Roble, 1722·3
Corteza de Sauce, 87·3
Corteza Suprarrenal, 1110·1
Corti Biciron N, 1907·4
Corti Jaikal, 1907·4
Corti-Arscolloid, 1908·1
Cortibiotique, 1908·1
Cortic, 1908·1
Corticaine, 1908·1
Cortical, 1908·1
Corticel, 1908·1
Corticetine, 1908·1
Corticil T, 1908·1
Corticin, 1908·1
Corti-Clyss, 1908·1
Corticoderm, 1908·1
Corticoliberin, 1321·3
Corticorelin, 1321·3
Corticorelin Trifluoroacetate, 1321·3
Corticorelin Triflutate, 1321·3
Corticorelina, 1321·3
Corticorten, 1908·1
Corticosteroids, 1068·1
Corticosterone, 1110·1
Corticosterone— *see* Sinsurrene, 2292·3
Corticotrophin, 1322·1
$\alpha^{1-24}$-Corticotrophin, 1340·2
$\beta^{1-24}$-Corticotrophin, 1340·2
Corticotrophin-releasing Hormone, 1321·3
Corticotrophin-(1–24)-tetracosapeptide, 1340·2
Corticotropin, 1322·1
Corticotropina, 1322·1
Corticotropin-releasing Factor, 1321·3
Corticotropinum, 1322·1
Corticotulle Lumiere, 1908·1
Corticreme, 1908·1
Cortidax, 1908·1
Cortidene, 1908·1
Cortiderma, 1908·1
Cortidex, 1908·1
Cortidexason, 1908·1
Cortidexason Comp, 1908·1
Cortidro, 1908·1
Corti-Dynexan, 1908·1
Cortiespec, 1908·1
Cortifenol H, 1908·1
Corti-Flexiole, 1908·1
Cortifluid N, 1908·1
Corti-Fluoral, 1908·2
Cortifoam, 1908·2
Cortiglanden, 1908·2
Cortigrin, 1908·2
Cortigrip, 1908·2
Cortigrip Dia/Noche, 1908·2
Cortigripe, 1908·2
Cortilate, 1908·2
Cortilona, 1908·2
Cortilona Compuesta, 1908·2
Cortiment, 1908·2
Cortimycin, 1908·2
Cortimycine, 1908·2
Cortimyk, 1908·2
Cortimyxin, 1908·2
Cortin, 1097·1
Cort-Inal, 1908·2
*Cortinarius*, 1717·3
Cortine Naturelle, 1908·2
Cortinorex, 1908·2
Cortiphenol H, 1908·2
Cortiprex, 1908·2
Cortipyren B, 1908·2
Cortirel, 1908·2
Cortirell, 1908·2
Cortiron, 1908·2
Cortisal, 1908·3
Cortisdin Urea, 1908·3
Cortisol, 1103·3
Cortisol Acetate, 1103·3
Cortisol Butyrate, 1104·1
Cortisol Cypionate, 1104·1
Cortisol Hemisuccinate, 1104·1
Cortisol Sodium Phosphate, 1104·1
Cortisol Sodium Succinate, 1104·1
Cortisol Valerate, 1104·2
Cortisolona, 1908·3
Cortison Chemicet Topica, 1908·3
Cortison Chemicetina, 1908·3
Cortison Kemicetin, 1908·3
Cortison Kemicetine, 1908·3
Cortisona, Acetato de, 1096·1
Cortisonal, 1908·3
$\Delta^1$-Cortisone, 1109·3
Cortisone Acetate, 1096·1
Cortisoni Acetas, 1096·1
Cortispec, 1908·3
Cortisporin, 1908·3
Cortisporin-TC, 1908·3
Cortistamin L, 1908·3
Cortistamin NF, 1908·3
Cortisteron, 1908·3
Cortiston, 1908·3
Cortisumman, 1908·3
Cortisyl, 1908·3
Cortival, 1908·3
Cortivazol, 1096·2
Cortivent, 1908·3
Cortizone, 1908·3
Cortizul, 1908·3
Cortobenzolone, 1093·3
Cortobion, 1908·4
Cortoderm, 1908·4
Cortoftal, 1908·4
Cortogen, 1908·4
Cortola-m, 1908·4
Cortone, 1908·4
Cortop, 1908·4
Cortopic, 1908·4
Cortopin, 1908·4
Cortoquinol, 1908·4
Cortos, 1908·4
Corto-Tavegil, 1908·4
Cortril, 1908·4
Cortropin, 1908·4
Cortrosina, 1908·4
Cortrosyn, 1908·4
Cortuss, 1908·4
Coruno, 1908·4
Corus, 1908·4
Corus H, 1908·4
Coruzol, 1908·4
Corvasal, 1908·4
Corvatard, 1908·4
Corvaton, 1908·4
Cor-Vel, 1909·1
Cor-Vel N, 1909·1
Corvert, 1909·1
Corvipas, 1909·1
Corvo, 1909·1
Corwin, 1909·1
Coryaid, 1909·1
Coryfin C, 1909·1
Corylophyline, 1694·2
Corymunun, 1909·1
*Corynanthe yohimbi*, 1766·2
*Corynebacterium diphtheriae*, 1612·2, 1612·3, 1742·2
Corynebacterium Parvum, 540·2
*Corynebacterium parvum*, 540·2
Corynine Hydrochloride, 1766·2
Coryphen, 1909·1
Coryx, 1909·1
Coryzalia, 1909·1
Corzide, 1909·1
Cosaar, 1909·1
Cosaar Plus, 1909·1
Cosaldon, 1909·1
Cosaldon A, 1909·1
Cosalgesic, 1909·1
Co-Salt, 1909·1
Cosamin, 1909·1
Cosavil, 1909·1
Cosbiol, 1482·2
Coscopin, 1909·1
Coscopin BR, 1909·1
Coscopin Plus, 1909·1
Cose-Anal, 1909·2
Cosig, 1909·2
Co-simalcite, 1267·3, 1289·2
Coslan, 1909·2
Coslyte, 1909·2
Cosmaxil, 1909·2
Cosmegen, 1909·2
Cosmegen, Lyovac— *see* Lyovac Cosmegen, 2109·1
Cosmetar-S, 1909·2
Cosmiciclina, 1909·2
Cosmofer, 1909·2
Cosmopril, 1909·2
Coso, 1909·2
Cosome, 1909·2
Cosopt, 1909·2
Cospanon, 1909·2
Co-spironozide, 933·2, 1003·1
Cost, 1909·2
Costi, 1909·2
Costop, 1909·2
Cosudex, 1909·2
Cosuric, 1909·2
Cosylan, 1909·2
Cosyntropin, 1340·2
Cosyr, 1909·2
Cosyr (Reformulated), 1909·2
Cotamox, 1909·3
Cotareg, 1909·3
Co-Tareg, 1909·3
Cotaryl, 1909·3
Co-Tasian, 1909·3
Cotazym, 1909·3
Cotazym S Forte, 1909·3
Co-tenidone, 865·2, 882·3
Cotenol, 1909·3
Cotenolol, 1909·3
Cotenomel, 1909·3
Cotesifar, 1909·3
Cotet, 1909·3
Co-tetroxazine, 199·3
Cothilyne, 1909·3
Cotibin Compuesto, 1909·3
Cotibin Dia y Noche, 1909·3
Cotibin Flu, 1909·3
Cotina, 1909·3
Cotinazin, 1909·3
Cotinine, 1721·1
Co-Tioctan, 1909·3
Cotofin, 1909·3
Cotone Emostatico, 1909·3
Cotrane, 1909·3
Cotrazol, 1909·3
Cotren, 1909·3
Co-triamterzide, 933·2, 1016·2
Cotribene, 1909·3
Cotridin, 1909·3
Cotridin Expectorant, 1909·4
Cotrifamol, 199·3
Co-trifamole, 199·3
Cotrim, 1909·4
Co-trimazine, 199·3
Cotrimazol, 1909·4
Cotrim-Diolan, 1909·4
Co-Trimed, 1909·4
Cotrimel, 1909·4
Cotrimhexal, 1909·4
Cotrimoxazol, 199·3
Co-trimoxazole, 199·3
Cotrimox-Wolff, 1909·4
Cotrimstada, 1909·4
Co-trim-Tablinen, 1909·4
Cotrisan, 1909·4
Cotristad, 1909·4
Cotrizol-G, 1909·4
Cotron, 1909·4
Cotton Oil, 1676·1
Cottonseed Oil, 1676·1, 1695·3
Cottonseed Oil, Hydrogenated, 1676·1
Co-Tuss V, 1909·4
Cotussin, 1909·4
Co-Tylenol, 1909·4
Couch Grass Rhizome, 1676·2
Couch-grass, 1676·2
Cough, 1112·1
Cough & Cold, 1909·4
Cough, Cold & Allergy Relief, 1909·4
Cough & Cold L52, 1909·4
Cough Control Sucrets, 1909·4
Cough Drops, 1909·4
Cough Drops, Vicks— *see* Vicks Cough Drops, 2375·2
Cough Elixir, 1909·4
Cough & Flu Syrup, 1909·4
Cough Formula Comtrex, 1909·4
Cough, Hylands— *see* Hylands Cough, 2052·3

Cough L64, 1909·4
Cough Lozenges, 1909·4
Cough Medicine, Gold Cross— *see* Gold Cross Cough Medicine, 2029·3
Cough Mixture, Modern Herbals— *see* Modern Herbals Cough Mixture, 2138·2
Cough N Cold Syrup, 1909·4
Cough Relief, 1910·1
Cough Silencers, Vicks— *see* Vicks Cough Silencers, 2375·2
Cough Suppressant, Chemists Own— *see* Chemists Own Cough Suppressant, 1881·4
Cough Suppressant Syrup DM, 1910·1
Cough Suppressants, 1112·1
Cough Suppressants Expectorants Mucolytics and Nasal Decongestants, 1112·1
Cough Syrup, 1910·1
Cough Syrup with Codeine, 1910·1
Cough Syrup DM, 1910·1
Cough Syrup DM Decongestant, 1910·1
Cough Syrup DM Decongestant for Children, 1910·1
Cough Syrup DM Decongestant Expectorant, 1910·1
Cough Syrup DM Expectorant, 1910·1
Cough Syrup DM-D-E, 1910·1
Cough Syrup DM-E, 1910·1
Cough Syrup Expectorant, 1910·1
Cough Syrup with Guaifenesin & Dextromethorphan, 1910·1
Cough Syrup with Honey, 1910·1
Coughcod, 1910·1
Cough-eeze, 1910·1
Cough-EN, 1910·1
Coughlax, 1910·1
Coughmin, 1910·1
Coughnadryl, 1910·1
Coughwort, 1117·2
Cough-X, 1910·1
Couldina, 1910·1
Couldina C, 1910·1
Couldina Instant, 1910·2
Coumadin, 1910·2
Coumadine, 1910·2
Coumafos, 1502·2
Coumaphos, 1502·2
Coumarin, 1676·2
Coumarin Anticoagulants, 810·1
Coumatetralyl, 1502·3
Counterpain, 1910·2
Counterpain Cool, 1910·2
Courge, Semence de, 1677·3
Coutarea Latiflora, 1676·3
*Coutarea latiflora*, 1669·2
COV, 1750·3
Co-Vals, 1910·2
Covamet, 1910·2
Covan, 1910·2
Covancaine, 1910·2
Covance, 1910·2
Covangesic, 1910·2
Covarex, 1910·2
Covastin, 1910·2
Covatine, 1910·2
Covaxis, 1910·2
Covera, 1910·2
Coverene, 1910·2
Covermark, 1910·2
Coversum, 1910·2
Coversum Combi, 1910·2
Coversyl, 1910·2
Coversyl Plus, 1910·2
Co-Vibedoze, 1910·2
Co-vidarabine, 579·2
Covidarabine, 579·2
Covitasa B12, 1910·2
Covite, 1910·2
Covochol, 1910·2
Covocort, 1910·3
Covomycin, 1910·3
Covomycin-D, 1910·3
Covonia Bronchial Balsam, 1910·3
Covonia for Children, 1910·3
Covonia Mentholated, 1910·3
Covonia Night-Time, 1910·3
Covonia Throat Spray, 1910·3
Covorit, 1910·3
Covosan, 1910·3
Covospor, 1910·3
Covostet, 1910·3
Covosulf, 1910·3
Covotop, 1910·3
Cow Clover, 1737·3
Cow & Gate Formula-S, 1910·3
Cow & Gate Pepti-Junior, 1910·3
Cow Parsley, 1765·1
Cowberry, 1676·3
Cows' Milk, Intolerance to— *see* Food Intolerance, 1448·2
Cowslip, 1735·1
Cox-189, 54·3
Coxa-cyl Ho-Len-Complex, 1910·3
Coxanturenasi, 1910·3
Coxel, 1910·3
Coxflam, 1910·3
*Coxiella burnetii*, 1635·3
Coxiro, 1910·3
Coxtenk, 1910·3
Coxxil, 1910·3
Cozaar, 1910·3
Cozaar Comp, 1910·3
Cozaar Plus, 1910·4
Cozaarex, 1910·4
Cozaarex D, 1910·4
Co-zidocapt, 879·2, 933·2
Cozole, 1910·4
CP-15-639-2, 166·2
CP-20, 1033·1
CP-10188, 1687·2
CP-10423-16, 113·2
CP-12009-18, 110·1
CP-12252-1, 725·2
CP-12299-1, 985·1
CP-12574, 617·1
CP-14445-16, 111·1
CP-15464-2, 166·3
CP-15467-61, 301·1
CP-16171, 84·2
CP-16533-1, 1019·1
CP-24314-1, 790·3
CP-24314-14, 790·3
CP-28720, 332·2
CP-34089, 1520·3
CP-45634, 345·3
CP-45899, 257·2
CP-45899-2, 257·2
CP-49952, 264·2
CP-51974-1, 317·2
CP-51974-01, 317·2
CP-52640, 174·3
CP-52640-2, 174·3
CP-52640-3, 174·3
CP-62993, 159·1
CP-65703, 14·2
CP-76136, 202·2
CP-76136-27, 202·2
CP-88059, 728·1
CP-88059-1, 728·1
CP-88059/27, 728·1
CP-99219, 274·3
CP-99219-27, 274·3
CP-116517-27, 154·1
CP-526555-18, 1763·2
CP Tannic, 1910·4
CPC-211, 1747·2
CPD, 1910·4
CPD Whole Blood, 744·1
CPDA-1 Whole Blood, 744·1
C-Pela, 1910·4
CP3H, 277·3
CPHPC, 567·1
CPL, 185·1
C-Platin, 1910·4
C-Plus, 1910·4
CPM PSE MSC, 1910·4
CPM/PE/MSC, 1910·4
C-Poretta, 1910·4
CPS, 62·2
CPS Pulver, 1910·4
CPT, 1910·4
CPT-11, 564·1
CR-242, 1284·3
CR-604, 85·2
CR-662, 1131·3
CR-1505, 1271·3
CR Gas, 1676·3
Crab Lice— *see* Pediculosis, 1499·1
Crack, 1373·3
Cracoa B, 1910·4
Cradocap, 1910·4
Craegium, 1910·4
Crafilm, 1910·4
Cralonin, 1910·4
Cralsanic, 1910·4
Cramigen, 1910·4
Cramp— *see* Muscle Spasm, 1386·1
Cramp, Haemodialysis-induced— *see* Haemodialysis-induced Cramp, 1221·2
Cramp, Haemodialysis-induced— *see* Muscle Spasm, 1386·1
Cramp, Writer's— *see* Dystonias, 1209·3
Crampex, 1910·4
Crampiton, 1910·4
Cranberry, 1676·3
Cranberry, American, 1677·1
Cranberry Complex, 1910·4
Cranberry, European, 1677·1
Cranberry Liquid Preparation, 1676·3
Cranbiotic Super, Bioglan— *see* Bioglan Cranbiotic Super, 1843·4
Cranio-cyl Ho-Len-Complex, 1910·4
Crank, 1589·2
Cranoc, 1910·4
Crasnitin, 1910·4
Crataegan, 1910·4
Crataegi Folium Cum Flore, 1677·1
Crataegi Fructus, 1677·1
Crataegisan, 1910·4
Crataegitan, 1911·1
Crataegol, 1911·1
Crataegus, 1677·1
Crataegus Complex, 1911·1
*Crataegus laevigata*, 1677·1
Crataegus Med Complex, 1911·1
*Crataegus monogyna*, 1677·1
*Crataegus oxyacantha*, 1677·1
Crataegutt, 1911·1
Crataegysat F, 1911·1
Crataelanat, 1911·1
Cratae-Loges, 1911·1
Crataepas, 1911·1
Crataezyma, 1911·1
Cratecor, 1911·1
Cratenox, 1911·1
Cratimon, 1911·1
Craun, 1911·1
Cravinho, 1673·2
Craviscum Mono, 1911·1
Cravit, 1911·1
Cravo-da-Índia, 1673·2
Cravo-Espin, 1911·1
CRD-401, 900·1
Creacal, 1911·1
Creagin, 1911·1
Cream E45, 1911·1
Cream E45— *see* E45, 1960·4
Cream of Tartar, Purified, 1284·3
Cream of Tartar, Soluble, 1734·1
Creamy Tar, 1911·1
Creanolona, 1911·1
Creasote, 1117·2
Creatile, 1911·1
Creatina, Fosfato de, 1677·2
Creatine, 1677·2
Creatine Monohydrate, 1677·2
Creatine Phosphate, 1677·2
Creatine Phosphoric Acid, 1677·2
Creatinina, 1677·2
Creatinine, 1677·2
Creatinolfosfate Sodium, 1677·3
Creatinolfosfato Sódico, 1677·3
Creatyl, 1911·1
Creavit, 1911·1
Crebiocén, 1703·3
Crecil, 1911·1
Credaxol, 1911·1
Creeping Eruption— *see* Cutaneous Larva Migrans, 98·1
Crelo Blanco, 1911·1
Crema Axel, 1911·1
Crema Blanca, 1911·1
Crema Coloreada de Proteccion Total, 1911·2
Crema Compensadora Avene, 1911·2
Crema Contracepti Lanzas, 1911·2
Crema de Magnesia, 1911·2
Crema de Ordene, 1911·2
Crema de Proteccion Extrema 50B, 1911·2
Crema Facial De Dia AHA Formula 405, 1911·2
Crema Facial De Noche AHA Formula 405, 1911·2
Crema Invisible de Proteccion Total, 1911·2
Crema Para Pieles Intolerantes Avene, 1911·2
Cremaffin, 1911·2
Cremalax, 1911·2
Cremalgin, 1911·2
Crema-U, 1911·2
Creme Anti-Rides Auto-Bronzante, 1911·2
Creme au Melilot Composee, 1911·2
Creme Auto-Bronzant, 1911·2
Creme Autobronzante Visage, 1911·2
Creme de Base, 1911·2
Creme des 3 Fleurs D'Orient, 1911·2
Creme Ecran Total, 1911·2
Creme Gordo Barral, 1911·2
Creme Haute Protection, 1911·2
Creme Laser Hidrante, 1911·2
Creme Protectrice, 1911·2
Creme Rap, 1911·3
Creme Solaire Anti-Rides, 1911·3
Creme Solaire Bronzage, 1911·3
Creme Solaire Bronzage Rapide, 1911·3
Creme Solaire Bronzage Securite, 1911·3
Creme Solaire Bronzage Securite Special, 1911·3
Creme Solaire Ecran Special Visage, 1911·3
Creme Solaire Haute Protection, 1911·3
Creme Universal, 1911·3
Cremederme, 1911·3
Cremicort-H, 1911·3
Creminem, 1911·3
Creminem-B, 1911·3
Cremirit, 1911·3
Cremisona, 1911·3
Cremol-P, 1911·3
Cremol-Ritter, 1911·3
Cremophor EL, 1414·3
Cremosan, 1911·3
Cremsol, 1911·3
Cremsor N, 1911·3
Crenodyn, 1911·3
Creo Grippe, 1911·3
Creodermol, 1911·3
Creolina, 1911·3
Creon, 1911·3
Creo-Rectal, 1911·4
Creosedin, 1911·4
Creosol, 1159·2
Creosota, 1117·2
Creosotal, 1117·2
Creosote, 1117·2
Creosote Bush, 1670·1
Creosote Carbonate, 1117·2
Creosote, Wood, 1117·2
Creosoto Composto, 1911·4
Creo-Terpin, 1911·4
Crescicalcio, 1911·4
Crescom, 1911·4
Cresol, 1177·3
Cresol, Crude, 1178·1
Cresol and Soap Solution, 1178·1
Cresolox, 1911·4
Cresols, 1193·3
*m*-Cresolsulphonic Acid-formaldehyde, 756·1
Cresolum Crudum, 1178·1
Cresophene, 1911·4
Cresoxydiol, 1394·3
Crest, Sensitivity Protection— *see* Sensitivity Protection Crest, 2285·1
Crestanon, 1911·4

Crestomycin Sulphate, 612·3
Crestor, 1911·4
Cresylate, 1911·4
Cresylic Acid, 1177·3
Cresylic Acids, 1193·3
Creta, 1255·3
Creta Preparada, 1254·2
Cretinism, Endemic— *see* Iodine Deficiency Disorders, 1599·1
Cretinism— *see* Hypothyroidism, 1595·3
Creutzfeldt-Jakob Disease, Disinfection Procedures— *see* Disinfection in Creutzfeldt-Jakob Disease, 1164·3
Crevet, 1911·4
CRF, 1321·3
CRH, 1321·3, 1911·4
Criam, 1911·4
Crilanomer, 1145·1
Crilanómero, 1145·1
Crilem, 1911·4
Crima, 1911·4
Crimanex, 1911·4
Crimean Congo Haemorrhagic Fever— *see* Haemorrhagic Fevers, 618·2
Crimean-Congo Haemorrhagic Fever Immunoglobulins, 1612·1
Crinalsofex, 1911·4
Criniton, 1911·4
Crino Cordes, 1911·4
Crino Cordes N, 1911·4
Crinohermal Fem, 1911·4
Crino-Kaban N, 1911·4
Crinone, 1911·4
Crinopex, 1911·4
Crinoren, 1911·4
Crinoretic, 1911·4
Crinotar, 1911·4
Criofluorano, 1235·3
Criostat SD 2, 1912·1
Criotonal, 1912·1
Cripar, 1912·1
Criptamine, 1912·1
Criptón 81M, 1525·1
CRI-regen, 1912·1
Crisabon, 1912·1
Crisacide, 1912·1
Crisafeno, 1912·1
Crisantaspase, 528·3
Crisapla, 1912·1
Crisasma, 1912·1
Crisazet, 1912·1
Crisdazol, 1912·1
Crislaxo, 1912·1
Crismol, 1912·1
Crisnatol Mesilate, 540·2
Crisnatol, Mesilato de, 540·2
Crisnatol Mesylate, 540·2
Crisofimina, 1912·1
Crisoidina, Hidrocloruro Del Citrato de, 1670·3
Crisomet, 1912·1
Cristaclar, 1912·1
Cristal, 1912·1
Cristalcrom, 1912·1
Cristales de Sosa, 1747·2
Cristalmina, 1912·1
Cristalomicina, 1912·1
Cristalpen, 1912·1
Cristan, 1912·1
Cristerona, 1912·1
Cristopal, 1912·1
Criten, 1912·1
Criticare HN, 1912·1
Critichol, 1912·2
Crivion, 1912·2
Crixivan, 1912·2
CRL-40048, 1584·2
CRL-40476, 1591·1
Cro 50, 1912·2
Croben, 1912·2
Crocetins, 1058·2
Croci Stigma, 1058·2
Crocidolite, 1658·1
Crocin, 1912·2
Crocines, 1058·2
Croconazol, Hidrocloruro de, 397·1
Croconazole Hydrochloride, 397·1
Crocus, 1058·2
*Crocus sativus*, 1058·2
CroFab, 1912·2
Croferron, 1912·2
Croglina, 1912·2
Crohn's Disease— *see* Inflammatory Bowel Disease, 1243·3
Croix Blanche, 1912·2
Crolidin, 1912·2
Crolix, 1912·2
Crolom, 1912·2
Crom 80, 1912·2
Cromabak, 1912·2
Cromadoses, 1912·2
Cromakalim, 890·3
Cromal, 1912·2
Cromantal, 1912·2
Cro-Man-Zin, 1912·2
Cromatonbic B12, 1912·2
Cromatonbic Ferro, 1912·2
Cromatonbic Folinico, 1912·2
Cromatonferro, 1912·2
Cromedil, 1912·2
Cromer Orto, 1912·2
Cromese, 1912·2
Cromex, 1912·2
Cromezin, 1912·3
Cromifusin, 1912·3
Cromo, 1425·1, 1912·3
Cromo 51, 1523·2
Cromo, Alumbre de, 1670·2
Cromo Asma, 1912·3
Cromo, Picolinato de, 1425·1
Cromo, Tricloruro de, 1425·1
Cromo, Trióxido de, 1670·3
Cromocarbo, Dietilamina de, 1670·3
Cromocato, 1912·3
Cromocur, 1912·3
Cromodyn, 1912·3
Cromoftol, 1912·3
Cromogen, 1912·3
Cromogen, Steri-Neb— *see* Steri-Neb Cromogen, 2306·4
Cromoglicate, Sodium, 795·3
Cromoglicato de Sodio, 795·3
Cromoglicin, 1912·3
Cromoglin, 1912·3
Cromoglycate, Sodium, 795·3
Cromohexal, 1912·3
Cromol, 1912·3
Cromolerg, 1912·3
Cromolergin UD, 1912·3
Cromolind, 1912·3
Cromolyn, 1912·3
Cromolyn Sodium, 795·3
Cromophtal, 1912·3
Crom-Ophtal, 1912·3
Cromopp, 1912·3
Cromoptic, 1912·3
Cromosan, 1912·3
Cromoseptil Plus, 1912·3
Cromosoft, 1912·3
Cromosol Ophta, 1912·3
Cromosol UD, 1912·3
Cromotex, 1912·3
Cromovisus, 1912·3
Cromoxin K, 1912·3
Cromozil, 1912·4
Cromunal, 1912·4
Cromycin, 1912·4
Cronacol, 1912·4
Cronal, 1912·4
Cronase, 1912·4
Cronasma, 1912·4
Cronassial, 1912·4
Cronavit, 1912·4
Croneparina, 1912·4
Cronizat, 1912·4
Cronobe, 1912·4
Cronocaps, 1912·4
Cronocef, 1912·4
Cronocol, 1912·4
Cronocorteroid, 1912·4
Cronodine, 1912·4
Cronoferril, 1912·4
Cronogeron, 1912·4
Cronol, 1912·4
Cronolax, 1912·4
Cronolevel, 1912·4
Cronomet, 1912·4
Cronopen, 1912·4
Cronopen Balsamico, 1912·4
Cronoplex, 1912·4
Cronovera, 1912·4
Croscarmellose Sodium, 1578·1
Croscarmelosa Sódica, 1578·1
Crospovidona, 1581·2
Crospovidone, 1581·2
Crospovidonum, 1581·2
Crosslinked Carboxymethylcellulose Sodium, 1578·1
Crosslinked Haemoglobin, 755·3
Crotalaria, 1677·3
Crotam, 1145·1
Crotamitex, 1912·4
Crotamiton, 1145·1
Crotamitonum, 1145·1
Croton Oil, 28·2
*Croton sublyratus*, 1284·2
*Croton tiglium*, 28·2
Crotonis, Oleum, 28·2
Crotorax, 1912·4
Crotorax-HC, 1912·4
Croup, 1079·1
Crowne, 1913·1
Crucial, 1913·1
Cruex, 1913·1
Crusca, 1253·2
Cruscasohn, 1913·1
Crushed Linseed, 1707·2
Crusken, 1913·1
Cruzzy, 1913·1
Cruzzy Antiparassitario, 1913·1
Cruzzy Shampoo Potenziato Alla Sumitrina, 1913·1
Cryobutol, 1913·1
Cryocriptina, 1913·1
Cryofluorane, 1235·3
Cryogenine Plus, 1913·1
Cryogesic, 1913·1
Cryometasona, 1913·1
Cryoperacid, 1913·1
Cryopina, 1913·1
Cryoprecipitate, 752·1
Cryoprecipitated Antihemophilic Factor, 751·2
Cryopril, 1913·1
Cryosolona, 1913·1
Cryotol, 1913·1
Cryo-Tropin, 1913·1
Cryoval, 1913·1
Cryovin, 1913·1
Cryoxifeno, 1913·1
Cryozol, 1913·1
Cryptococcal Meningitis— *see* Cryptococcosis, 387·3
Cryptococcosis, 387·3
Cryptocur, 1913·1
Cryptogenic Fibrosing Alveolitis— *see* Diffuse Parenchymal Lung Disease, 1079·3
Cryptorchidism, 1313·1
Cryptosporidiosis, 596·2
Crysanal, 1913·1
Cryselle, 1913·1
Cryst. I.Z.S, 334·2
Crystacide, 1913·1
Crystacit, 1913·1
Crystal, 1589·2, 1730·3
Crystal Clear, 1913·1
Crystal Meth, 1589·2
Crystal Violet, 1186·1
Crystalline Cellulose, 1578·3
Crystalline Penicillin G, 163·2
Crystallinic Acid, 239·2
Crystallized Trypsin, 1758·3
Crystalloid Plasma Expanders, 835·2
Crystamine, 1913·1
Crystapen, 1913·2
Crysti 1000, 1913·2
Crysticillin, 1913·2
Crystodigin, 1913·2
Crytion, 1913·2
Crytioro, 1913·2
CS-045, 348·2
CS-370, 685·3
CS-386, 707·1
CS-443, 165·3
CS-500, 958·1
CS-511, 977·2
CS-514, 984·3
CS-600, 54·3
CS-622, 1010·2
CS-684, 1284·1
CS-807, 178·3
CS-866, 975·3
CS-905, 866·2
CS-1170, 173·3
CS Gas, 1677·3
CS Spray, 1677·3
CSA, 1670·2
CSAG-144, 1273·1
C-Sik, 1913·2
C-Soft, 1913·2
C-Solve, 1913·2
CST, 1913·2
CT-848, 1725·2
CT-1101, 1698·1
CT Ointment, 1913·2
CT Pommade, 1913·2
CT Shampoo, 1913·2
CTAB, 1173·1
C-Tabs, 1913·2
C-Tanna 12D, 1913·2
C-Tard, 1913·2
C-Tron Calcium, 1913·2
C/T/S, 1913·2
CTX, 54·2, 175·3
C-type Natriuretic Peptide, 964·2
Cuadel, 1913·2
Cuait D, 1913·2
Cuait N, 1913·2
Cuantil, 1913·2
Cuasia, 1737·2
Cuasia, Leño de, 1737·2
Cuatroderm, 1913·2
Cuatroepi, 1913·2
Cuatromin, 1913·2
Cube Root, 1510·1
Cubicin, 1913·2
Cubison, 1913·2
Cubitan, 1913·2
Cucumber, Bitter, 1260·3
Cucumber, Chinese, 655·3
Cucurbita, 1677·3
Cucurbita Compuesta, 1913·2
*Cucurbita pepo*, 1677·3
Cuerpo Amarillo Fuerte, 1913·2
Cuidaderma, 1913·2
Cuivre (Sulfate de), 1426·1
Culat, 1913·3
Cullens Headache Powders, 1913·3
Cultivo BCG, 1913·3
Culture Care, 1913·3
Culturelle LCG, 1913·3
Cumafós, 1502·2
Cumarin, 1676·2
Cumarina, 1676·2
Cumatetralilo, 1502·3
Cumatil L, 1913·3
Cumin des Prés, 1667·2
Cunesin, 1913·3
Cunil, 1913·3
CuNova T, 1913·3
Cunticina, 1913·3
Cupanol, 1913·3
Cupanol— *see* Medinol, 2119·2
Cuplaton, 1913·3
Cuplex, 1913·3
Cupressin, 1913·3
Cupri Sulfas, 1426·1
Cupri Sulphas, 1426·1
Cupric Chloride, 1425·3
Cupric Sulfate, 1426·1
Cuprid— *see* Syprine, 2317·2
Cupridium, 1913·3
Cuprifusin, 1913·3

Cuprimine, 1913·3
Cupripen, 1913·3
Cuprocept CCL, 1913·3
Cuproedetato Cálcico, 1425·3
Cuprofen, 1913·3
Cuprofen Plus, 1913·3
Cuprosodio, 1913·3
Cuprosodio Plus, 1913·3
Cuproxoline, 1426·1
Cuprum ad Praeparationes Homoeopathicae, 1425·3
Cuprum Met., 1426·1
Cuprum Metallicum, 1426·1
Cura, 1913·3
Curaçao Aloes, 1248·2
Curacid, 1913·3
Curacit, 1913·3
Curacleanse, 1913·3
Curacne, 1913·4
Curadent, 1913·4
Curaderm, 1913·4
Curadon, 1913·4
Curadona, 1913·4
Curafil, 1913·4
Curakalos, 1913·4
Curam, 1913·4
Curandron, 1913·4
Curantyl N, 1913·4
Curapic, 1913·4
Curare, 1409·2
Curarina Miro, 1913·4
Curarine, 1913·4
Curash Anti-Rash, 1913·4
Curash Baby Wipes, 1913·4
Curash Babycare, 1913·4
Curash Medicated, 1913·4
Curastatin, 1913·4
Curasten, 1913·4
Curatane, 1913·4
Curatin, 1913·4
Curativ, 1913·4
Curatoderm, 1913·4
Curaven, 1913·4
Curazink, 1913·4
Curban, 1913·4
Cúrcuma, 1058·3
*Curcuma longa*, 1058·3
*Curcuma xanthorrhiza*, 1759·3
Curcuma Zanthorrhiza, 1759·3
Curcumae Javanicae, 1759·3
Curcumae Xanthorrhizae Rhizoma, 1759·3
Curcumen, 1913·4
Curcumin, 1057·2
Curcumina, 1057·2
Curcu-Truw, 1913·4
Curd Soap, 1575·2
Curel, 1914·1
Curethyl, 1914·1
Curine, 1914·1
Curinflam, 1914·1
Curisept, 1914·1
Curlem, 1914·1
Curling Factor, 400·3
Curly Dock, 1766·1
Curocef, 1914·1
Curol, 1914·1
Curon-B, 1914·1
Curosurf, 1914·1
Curoveinyl, 1914·1
Curoxim, 1914·1
Curoxima, 1914·1
Curoxime, 1914·1
Curoxime— *see* Zinnat, 2394·1
Curpol, 1914·1
Curyken, 1914·1
Curzon, Gerard House— *see* Gerard House Curzon, 2022·1
Cusate, 1914·1
Cuscutine, 1914·1
Cushing's Disease— *see* Cushing's Syndrome, 1313·1
Cushing's Syndrome, 1313·1
Cusicrom, 1914·1
Cusigel, 1914·1
Cusimolol, 1914·1
Cusiter, 1914·1
Cusiviral, 1914·1
Cusparia, 1678·1
Cusparia Bark, 1678·1
Custey, 1914·1
Custodial, 1914·1
Custodiol, 1914·1
Customed, 1914·1
Custoplex, 1914·1
Cutacelan, 1914·1
Cutaclin, 1914·2
Cutacnyl, 1914·2
Cutaderm, 1914·2
Cutaneous Larva Migrans, 98·1
Cutaneous T-cell Lymphomas, 511·2
Cutanil, 1914·2
Cutaninfant, 1914·2
Cutanit, 1914·2
Cutanplast, 1914·2
Cutanum, 1914·2
Cutar, 1914·2
Cutasept, 1914·2
Cutch, 1661·1
Cutemol, 1914·2
Cutemul, 1914·2
Cuteral, 1914·2
Cuterpes, 1914·2
Cuticura, 1914·2
Cutiderm, 1914·2
Cutidermin, 1914·2
Cuti-Do, 1914·2
Cutifitol, 1914·2
Cutimian, 1914·2
Cutimix, 1914·2
Cutinova, 1914·2
Cutinova Alginate, 1914·2
Cutiphile, 1914·2
Cutisan, 1914·2
Cutisanol, 1914·2
Cutistad, 1914·2
Cutivat, 1914·2
Cutivate, 1914·2
Cuttle Fish, 1743·2
Cuvalit, 1914·3
Cuvefilm, 1914·3
Cuxabrain, 1914·3
Cuxafenon, 1914·3
Cuxanorm, 1914·3
CV-205-502, 1213·1
CV-2619, 1700·3
CV-3317, 892·2
CV-4093, 950·2
CV-11974, 878·3
C-vimin, 1914·3
C-Vit, 1914·3
CVP, 1914·3
CVP B1 B6 B12, 1914·3
CVP Duo, 1914·3
CVP Flebo, 1914·3
CVP Forte, 1914·3
C-Will, 1914·3
Cx-3, 1914·3
Cx-4, 1914·3
Cx-5, 1914·3
CX Powder, 1914·3
CY-39, 1736·1
CY-116, 741·3
CY-153, 1646·2
CY-216, 963·3
Cyamemazine, 689·2
Cyamemazine Tartrate, 689·2
Cyamepromazine, 689·2
*Cyamopsis tetragonolobus*, 333·2
Cyanamide, 1664·2
Cyanide, 1506·1
Cyanide Antidote Package, 1914·3
Cyanides, 1506·2
Cyanidin Chloride, 1677·1
Cyanidin-3-glucoside Chloride, 1718·3
Cyaninoside, 1703·2
Cyanoacrylate Adhesives, 1678·1
*R*-α-Cyanobenzyl-6-*O*-β-D-glucopyranosiduronic Acid, 1704·3
*R*-α-Cyanobenzyl-6-*O*-β-D-glucopyranosyl-β-D-glucopyranoside, 1704·3
Cyanocobalamin, 1458·2
Cyanocobalamin ($^{57}$Co), 1523·2
Cyanocobalamin ($^{58}$Co), 1523·2
Cyanocobalaminum, 1458·2
(*E*)-α-Cyano-*N*,*N*-diethyl-3,4-dihydroxy-5-nitrocinnamamide, 1205·1
(*E*)-2-Cyano-3-(3,4-dihydroxy-5-nitrophenyl)-*N*,*N*-diethylacrylamide, 1205·1
1-(3-Cyano-3,3-diphenylpropyl)-4-phenylpiperidine-4-carboxylic Acid, 1261·2
1-(3-Cyano-3,3-diphenylpropyl)-4-piperidinopiperidine-4-carboxamide, 84·1
*N*-2-Cyanoethylamphetamine Hydrochloride, 1588·3
α-Cyano-4-fluoro-3-phenoxybenzyl 3-(β,4-Dichlorostyryl)-2,2-dimethylcyclopropanecarboxylate, 1505·3
(*RS*)-α-Cyano-4-fluoro-3-phenoxybenzyl (1*RS*,3*RS*;1*RS*,3*SR*)-3-(2,2-Dichlorovinyl)-2,2-dimethylcyclopropanecarboxylate, 1502·3
(−)-*trans*-1-[*cis*-4-Cyano-4-(*p*-fluorophenyl)cyclohexyl]-3-methyl-4-phenylisonipecotic Acid Hydrochloride, 435·2
Cyanoject, 1914·3
Cyanokit, 1914·3
2-Cyano-1-methyl-3-[2-(5-methylimidazol-4-ylmethylthio)ethyl]guanidine, 1255·3
(6*R*,7*S*)-7-{2-[(Cyanomethyl)thio]acetamido}-7-methoxy-3-{[(1-methyl-1*H*-tetrazol-5-yl)thio]methyl}-8-oxo-5-thia-1-azabicyclo-[4.2.0]oct-2-ene-2-carboxylic Acid, 173·3
1-[3-(2-Cyanophenothiazin-10-yl)propyl]piperidin-4-ol, 714·1
(*RS*)-α-Cyano-3-phenoxybenzyl (*RS*)-2-(4-Chlorophenyl)-3-methylbutyrate, 1505·2
(*RS*)-α-Cyano-3-phenoxybenzyl (*Z*)-(1*RS*,3*RS*)-3-(2-Chloro-3,3,3-trifluoropropenyl)-2,2-dimethylcyclopropanecarboxylate, 1502·3
(*S*)-α-Cyano-3-phenoxybenzyl (1*R*,3*R*)-3-(2,2-Dibromovinyl)-2,2-dimethylcyclopropanecarboxylate, 1503·1
(*RS*)-α-Cyano-3-phenoxybenzyl (1*RS*,3*RS*)-(1*RS*,3*RS*)-3-(2,2-Dichlorovinyl)-2,2-dimethylcyclopropanecarboxylate, 1502·3
(*SR*)-α-Cyano-3-phenoxybenzyl (1*RS*,3*RS*)-3-(2,2-Dichlorovinyl)-2,2-dimethylcyclopropanecarboxylate, 1502·3
3′-(3-Cyanopyrazolo[1,5-*a*]pyrimidin-7-yl)-*N*-ethylacetanilide, 727·3
(±)-2-Cyano-1-(4-pyridyl)-3-(1,2,2-trimethylpropyl)guanidine, 983·1
(*RS*)-4′-Cyano-α′,α′,α′-trifluoro-3-(4-fluorophenylsulphonyl)-2-hydroxy-2-methylpropiono-*m*-toluidide, 530·1
Cyater, 1914·3
Cybutol, 1914·3
CYC, 480·3
Cycin, 1914·3
Cyclabil, 1914·3
Cyclacillin, 188·1
Cyclacur, 1914·3
Cycladol, 1914·3
Cyclafem, 1914·4
Cyclam. Acid, 1426·2
Cyclamate Calcium, 1426·2
Cyclamate Sodium, 1426·2
Cyclamic Acid, 1426·2
Cyclan, 1914·4
Cyclandelate, 890·3
Cycleane, 1914·4
Cyclen, 1914·4
Cyclergine, 1914·4
Cyclessa, 1914·4
(±)-Cycletanide, 883·2
Cyclic-HPMPC, 630·1
Cyclidox, 1914·4
Cyclidrol, 1130·2
Cyclimorph, 1914·4
Cyclimycin, 1914·4
Cyclinex, 1914·4
Cyclitis— *see* Uveitis, 1090·1
Cyclivex, 1914·4
Cyclizine, 429·3
Cyclizine Hydrochloride, 429·3
Cyclizine Lactate, 429·3
Cyclizine Tartrate, 429·3
Cyclizini Hydrochloridum, 429·3
Cyclo 3, 1914·4
Cyclo 3 Fort, 1914·4
Cyclobarbital, 689·2
Cyclobarbital Calcium, 689·2
Cyclobarbitalum, 689·2
Cyclobarbitalum Calcicum, 689·2
Cyclobarbitone, 689·2
Cyclobarbitone Calcium, 689·2
Cyclobenzaprine Hydrochloride, 1393·1
Cyclobiol, 1914·4
Cycloblastin, 1914·4
Cycloblastine, 1914·4
*cis*-[*trans*-1,2-Cyclobutanebis(methylamine)][(*S*)-lactato-*O*$^1$,*O*$^1$]platinum, 565·1
Cyclo{-[4-(*E*)-but-2-enyl-*N*,4-dimethyl-L-threonyl]-L-homoalanyl-(*N*-methylglycyl)-(*N*-methyl-L-leucyl)-L-valyl-(*N*-methyl-L-leucyl)-L-alanyl-D-alanyl-(*N*-methyl-L-leucyl)-(*N*-methyl-L-leucyl)-(*N*-methyl-L-valyl)-}, 1351·2
17-Cyclobutylmethyl-7,8-dihydro-14-hydroxy-17-normorphine Hydrochloride, 64·2
(−)-(5*R*,6*S*,14*S*)-9a-Cyclobutylmethyl-4,5-epoxymorphinan-3,6,14-triol Hydrochloride, 64·2
(−)-17-(Cyclobutylmethyl)morphinan-3,14-diol Hydrogen Tartrate, 23·3
Cyclobutyrol Betaine, 1678·2
Cyclobutyrol Calcium, 1678·2
Cyclobutyrol Nicotinamide, 1678·2
Cyclobutyrol Sodium, 1678·2
$S^1$,$S^6$-Cyclo[$N^6$-carbamimidoyl-$N^2$-(3-sulfanylpropanoyl)-L-lysylglycyl-L-α-aspartyl-L-tryptophyl-L-prolyl-L-cysteinamide], 912·2
Cyclocarbothiamine, 1454·3
Cyclo-cell, 1914·4
Cyclocort, 1914·4
Cyclocur, 1914·4
Cycloderm, 1914·4
α-Cyclodextrin, 1678·2
β-Cyclodextrin, 1678·2
α-Cyclodextrin Alprostadil, 1512·3
Cyclodextrins, 1678·2
Cyclodolum, 490·2
Cyclodox, 1914·4
Cyclodrine Hydrochloride, 480·3
Cyclofem, 1558·1, 1914·4
Cyclofemina, 1914·4
Cyclofenil, 1544·1
Cyclogest, 1914·4
Cycloguanil, 457·2
Cycloguanil Embonate, 457·3
Cyclogyl, 1914·4
Cyclo-α-(1→4)-D-heptaglucopyranoside, 1678·2
[(Cycloheptylamino)methylene]diphosphonic Acid, 773·1
(7*R*)-7-(α-D-Cyclohexa-1,4-dienylglycylamino)-3-methyl-3-cephem-4-carboxylic Acid, 179·3
Cyclohexane, 1472·3
[(1*R*,2*R*)-1,2-Cyclohexanediamine-*N*,*N*′][oxalato(2-)-*O*,*O*′]platinum, 577·1
1-(Cyclohexanespiro-2′-[1′,3′]dioxolan-4′-ylmethyl)guanidine Sulphate, 926·3
Cyclohex-1-ene-1,2-dicarboximidomethyl (1*RS*,3*RS*)-(1*RS*,3*SR*)-2,2-Dimethyl-3-(2-methylprop-1-enyl)cyclopropanecarboxylate, 1510·2
5-(Cyclohex-1-enyl)-1,5-dimethylbarbituric Acid, 703·1
5-(Cyclohex-1-enyl)-5-ethylbarbituric Acid, 689·2
Cycloheximide, 1502·1
Cyclohexylamine, 1426·3
2-Cyclohexylcarbonyl-1,2,3,6,7,11b-hexahydropyrazino[2,1-*a*]isoquinolin-4-one, 112·2
2-Cyclohexylcarbonyl-1,2,3,4,6,7,8,12b-octahydropyrazino[2,1-*a*][2]benzazepin-4-one, 105·2
(2a*E*,4*E*,5′*S*,6*S*,6′*S*,7*S*,8*E*,11*R*,13*R*,15*S*,17a*R*,20a*R*,20b*S*)-6′-Cyclohexyl-7-[(2,6-dideoxy-3-*O*-methyl-α-L-*arabino*-hexopyranosyl)oxy]-3′,4′,5′,6,6′,7,10,11,14,15,20a,-20b-dodecahydro-20b-hydroxy-5′,6,8,19-tetramethylspiro(11,15-methano-2*H*,13*H*,17*H*-furo[4,3,2-*p*,*q*][2,6]benzodioxacyclooctadecin-13,2′-[2*H*]pyran)-17,20(17a*H*)-dione 20-Oxime, 114·1

1-Cyclohexyl-3-{4-[2-(3,4-dihydro-7-methoxy-4,4-dimethyl-1,3-dioxo-2(1*H*)-isoquinolyl)ethyl]benzenesulphonyl}urea, 332·3
6-Cyclohexyl-1-hydroxy-4-methyl-2-pyridone, 396·1
6-Cyclohexyl-1-hydroxy-4-methyl-2-pyridone, 2-Aminoethanol Salt, 396·1
(3-Cyclohexyl-3-hydroxy-3-phenylpropyl)triethylammonium Chloride, 490·2
2,2′-[Cyclohexylidenebis(4-phenyleneoxy)]bis[2-methylbutyric Acid], 884·3
4,4′-(Cyclohexylidenemethylene)bis(phenyl Acetate), 1544·1
2-Cyclohexyl-4-iodo-3,5-xylenol, 1177·3
2-(α-Cyclohexylmandeloyloxy)ethyldiethylmethylammonium Bromide, 487·2
2-Cyclohexyl-1-methylethyl-(methyl)amine, 1592·3
1-Cyclohexyl-3-{*p*-[2-(5-methylisoxazole-3-carboxamido)ethyl]benzenesulphonyl}urea, 333·1
(±)-4-Cyclohexyl-α-methyl-1-naphthaleneacetic Acid, 96·3
(4*S*)-4-Cyclohexyl-1-{[(*RS*)-2-methyl-1-(propionyloxy)propoxy](4-phenylbutyl)phosphinylacetyl}-L-proline Sodium, 919·1
1-Cyclohexyl-3-{4-[2-(5-methylpyrazine-2-carboxamido)ethyl]benzenesulphonyl}urea, 332·2
1-Cyclohexyl-1-phenyl-3-piperidinopropan-1-ol Hydrochloride, 490·2
1-Cyclohexyl-1-phenyl-3-(pyrrolidin-1-yl)propan-1-ol Hydrochloride, 488·2
*N*-Cyclohexylsulphamic Acid, 1426·2
6-[4-(1-Cyclohexyl-1*H*-tetrazol-5-yl)butoxy]-3,4-dihydrocarbostyril, 884·1
1-Cyclohexyl-3-*p*-tolylsulphonylurea, 333·1
1-Cyclohexyl-3-tosylurea, 333·1
Cyclomaltohexaose, 1678·2
Cyclomandol, 1914·4
Cyclomed, 1915·1
Cyclo-Meff, 1915·1
Cyclomen, 1915·1
Cyclo-Menorette, 1915·1
Cyclomethicone, 1482·1
Cyclo{[(2*S*,4*R*,6*E*)-4-methyl-2-(methylamino)-3-oxo-6-octenoyl]-L-valyl-*N*-methylglycyl-*N*-methyl-L-leucyl-L-valyl-*N*-methyl-L-leucyl-L-alanyl-D-alanyl-*N*-methyl-L-leucyl-*N*-methyl-L-leucyl-*N*-methyl-L-valyl}, 591·1
Cyclominol, 1915·1
Cyclomydril, 1915·1
Cyclonamine, 749·3
Cyclone, 1730·3
CycloOstrogynal, 1915·1
Cyclopam, 1915·1
Cyclopentacycloheptene, 1658·3
Cyclopentanone 2α,3α-Epithio-5α-androstan-17β-yl Methyl Acetal, 1559·1
Cyclopenthiaz., 890·3
Cyclopenthiazide, 890·3
Cyclopentol, 1915·1
Cyclopentolate Hydrochloride, 480·3
Cyclopentolati Hydrochloridum, 480·3
Cyclopentyl 3-{2-Methoxy-4-[(*o*-tolylsulfonyl)carbamoyl]benzyl}-1-methylindole-5-carbamate, 807·1
1-Cyclopentyl-3-[*p*-(2-*o*-anisamidoethyl)benzenesulphonyl]urea, 333·1
16α,17α-Cyclopentylidenedioxy-9α-fluoro-11β,21-dihydroxypregna-1,4-diene-3,20-dione 21-Acetate, 1091·1
3-(α-Cyclopentylmandeloyloxy)-1,1-dimethylpyrrolidinium Bromide, 482·3
17β-(3-Cyclopentyl-1-oxopropoxy)androst-4-en-3-one, 1569·3
3-Cyclopentyloxyestra-1,3,5(10)-triene-16α,17β-diol, 1568·2
3-Cyclopentyloxy-19-nor-17α-pregna-1,3,5(10)-trien-20-yn-17β-ol, 1568·2
3-[*N*-(4-Cyclopentyl-1-piperazinyl)formimidoyl]rifamycin, 253·3
Cyclophosphamide, 540·2
Cyclophosphamidum, 540·2
Cyclophosphanum, 540·2
Cycloplegia— *see* Mydriasis and Cycloplegia, 476·2
CycloPolar, 1915·1
Cyclo-Premarin-MPA, 1915·1
Cyclo-Premella, 1915·1
Cyclo-Premella ST, 1915·1
Cyclo-Progynon, 1915·1
Cyclo-Progynova, 1915·1
Cyclo-Progynova 1 Mg, 1915·1
Cyclo-Progynova 2 Mg, 1915·1
Cyclopropane, 1297·1
(6α,11β,16α)-21-[(Cyclopropylcarbonyl)oxy]-6,9-difluoro-11-hydroxy-16,17-[(1-methylethylidene)-bis(oxy)]-pregna-1,4-diene-3,20-dione, 1095·2
11-Cyclopropyl-5,11-dihydro-4-methyl-6*H*-dipyrido[3,2-*b*:2′,3′-*e*]-[1,4]diazepin-6-one, 650·2
1-Cyclopropyl-7-(*cis*-3,5-dimethyl-1-piperazinyl)-5,6,8-trifluoro-1,4-dihydro-4-oxo-3-quinolinecarboxylic Acid, 240·2
1-Cyclopropyl-7-(4-ethylpiperazin-1-yl)-6-fluoro-1,4-dihydro-4-oxoquinoline-3-carboxylic Acid, 207·3
(±)-1-Cyclopropyl-6-fluoro-1,4-dihydro-8-methoxy-7-[3-(methylamino)piperidino]-4-oxo-3-quinolinecarboxylic Acid, 162·2
(±)-1-Cyclopropyl-6-fluoro-1,4-dihydro-8-methoxy-7-(3-methyl-1-piperazinyl)-4-oxo-3-quinolinecarboxylic Acid Sesquihydrate, 216·2
1-Cyclopropyl-6-fluoro-1,4-dihydro-8-methoxy-7-[(4a*S*,7a*S*)-octahydro-6*H*-pyrrolo[3,4-*b*]pyridin-6-yl]-4-oxo-3-quinolinecarboxylic Acid Hydrochloride, 233·1
1-Cyclopropyl-6-fluoro-1,4-dihydro-7-[(1*S*,4*S*)-5-methyl-2,5-diazabicyclo[2.2.1]hept-2-yl]-4-oxo-3-quinolinecarboxylic Acid Monomethanesulphonate, 202·2
(±)-1-Cyclopropyl-6-fluoro-1,4-dihydro-5-methyl-7-(3-methyl-1-piperazinyl)-4-oxo-3-quinolinecarboxylic Acid Monohydrochloride, 220·3
1-Cyclopropyl-6-fluoro-1,4-dihydro-4-oxo-7-piperazin-1-ylquinoline-3-carboxylic Acid, 188·2
(3*R*,5*S*,6*E*)-7-[2-Cyclopropyl-4-(*p*-fluorophenyl)-3-quinolyl]-3,5-dihydroxy-6-heptenoic Acid, 984·1
3-(Cyclopropylmethoxy)-*N*-(3,5-dichloro-4-pyridyl)-4-(difluoromethoxy)benzamide, 791·3
(−)-(*S*)-1-{*p*-[2-(Cyclopropylmethoxy)ethyl]phenoxy}-3-isopropylaminopropan-2-ol Hydrochloride, 946·1
1-{4-[2-(Cyclopropylmethoxy)ethyl]phenoxy}-3-isopropylaminopropan-2-ol Hydrochloride, 873·1
(6*R*,7*R*,14*S*)-17-Cyclopropylmethyl-7,8-dihydro-7-(1-hydroxy-1-methylethyl)-6-*O*-methyl-6,14-ethano-17-normorphine Hydrochloride, 1037·3
(6*R*,7*R*,14*S*)-17-Cyclopropylmethyl-7,8-dihydro-7-[(1*S*)-1-hydroxy-1,2,2-trimethylpropyl]-6-*O*-methyl-6,14-ethano-17-normorphine, 21·3
(5*R*)-9a-Cyclopropylmethyl-3,14-dihydroxy-4,5-epoxymorphinan-6-one, 1046·1
17-(Cyclopropylmethyl)-4,5α-epoxy-3,14-dihydroxymorphinan-6-one, 1046·1
(2*S*)-2-[(−)-(5*R*,6*R*,7*R*,14*S*)-9a-Cyclopropylmethyl-4,5-epoxy-3-hydroxy-6-methoxy-6,14-ethanomorphinan-7-yl]-3,3-dimethylbutan-2-ol, 21·3
2-[(−)-(5*R*,6*R*,7*R*,14*S*)-9a-Cyclopropylmethyl-4,5-epoxy-3-hydroxy-6-methoxy-6,14-ethanomorphinan-7-yl]propan-2-ol Hydrochloride, 1037·3
8-(Cyclopropylmethyl)-6β,7β-epoxy-3α-hydroxy-1α*H*,5α*H*-tropanium Bromide, (−)-(*S*)-Tropate, 480·2
(5*R*)-9a-Cyclopropylmethyl-4,5-epoxy-6-methylenemorphinan-3,14-diol, 1044·1
17-(Cyclopropylmethyl)-4,5α-epoxy-6-methylenemorphinan-3,14-diol, 1044·1
(5*Z*,7*E*,22*E*,24*S*)-24-Cyclopropyl-9,10-secochola-5,7,10(19),22-tetraene-1α,3β,24-triol, 1144·1
*N*-Cyclopropyl-1,3,5-triazine-2,4,6-triamine, 1503·1
Cyclorax, 1915·1
Cyclorel, 1915·1
Cyclorine, 1915·1
Cyclosa, 1915·1
D-Cycloserin, 202·1
Cycloserine, 202·1, 1915·1
L-Cycloserine, 202·2
Cycloserinum, 202·1
Cycloson, 1915·1
Cyclospasmol, 1915·1
Cyclosporiasis, 596·3
Cyclosporin, 1351·2
Cyclosporin A, 1351·2
Cyclosporine, 1351·2
Cyclostin, 1915·1
Cycloteriam, 1915·2
Cyclothiazide, 891·1
Cyclothymia, 278·1
Cyclovalone, 1678·2
Cyclovax, 1915·2
Cycloven Forte N, 1915·2
Cyclovir, 1915·2
Cycloviran, 1915·2
Cycloxan, 1915·2
Cycobemin, 1458·2
Cycofed, 1915·2
Cycotiamine, 1454·3
Cycrin, 1915·2
Cydec, 1915·2
Cydec DM, 1915·2
Cydoxmine-B, 1915·2
Cyflox, 1915·2
Cyfluthin, 1502·3
Cyfluthrin, 1502·3
Cy-Gesic, 1915·2
Cyhalothrin, 1502·3
Cyhalothrin, Lambda, 1502·3
Cyheptine, 1915·2
Cyklo-F, 1915·2
Cyklokapron, 1915·2
Cykrina, 1915·2
Cylert, 1915·2
Cylex, 1915·2
Cyllind, 1915·2
Cylocide, 1915·2
Cyltabs, 1915·2
Cymalon, 1915·2
*Cymbopogon citratus*, 1706·3
*Cymbopogon flexuosus*, 1706·3
Cymene, 28·2
*p*-Cymene, 28·2, 1710·2, 1740·2
Cymerin, 1915·2
Cymerion, 1915·2
Cymevan, 1915·2
Cymeven, 1915·3
Cymevene, 1915·3
Cymex, 1915·3
Cymiazole, 1502·3
Cymine, 1915·3
*p*-Cymol, 28·2
Cyna Bilisan, 1915·3
Cynacur, 1915·3
Cynafol, 1915·3
Cynara, 1678·3
*Cynara scolymus*, 1678·3
Cynarex, 1915·3
Cynarin, 1678·3
Cynarine, 1678·3
Cynarix, 1915·3
Cynarix Comp, 1915·3
Cynarix N, 1915·3
Cynaro Bilina, 1915·3
Cynarobil, 1915·3
Cynarol, 1915·3
Cynaron, 1915·3
Cynarzym N, 1915·3
Cynatrop, 1915·3
Cyndal, 1915·3
Cyndal HD, 1915·3
Cyne, 1915·3
*Cynips gallae-tinctoriae*, 1690·2
Cynomel, 1915·3
Cynomycin, 1915·3
Cynoplus, 1915·3
Cynosbati Fructus, 1740·1
Cynosbati Pseudofructus, 1740·1
Cynovit, 1915·3
Cynt, 1915·3
Cyntex, 1915·3
Cyomin, 1915·3
Cyotic, 1915·4
Cypermethrin, 1502·3
Cypermethrin, Alpha, 1502·3
Cypermethrin, Zeta, 1502·3
Cypex, 1915·4
Cyprid, 1915·4
Cyprodemanol, 1585·3
Cyprodenate, 1585·3
Cyprogin, 1915·4
Cyproheptadine Acefyllinate, 430·3
Cyproheptadine Acetylaspartate, 430·3
Cyproheptadine Aspartate, 430·3
Cyproheptadine Cyclamate, 430·3
Cyproheptadine Hydrochloride, 430·1, 430·2
Cyproheptadine Orotate, 430·3, 1724·3
Cyproheptadine, Pyridoxal Phosphate Salt, 430·3
Cyproheptadine 7-Theophyllineacetate, 430·3
Cyproheptadini Hydrochloridum, 430·1
Cypron, 1915·4
Cyprone, 1915·4
Cyprono, 1915·4
Cyprosian, 1915·4
Cyprostat, 1915·4
Cyprostol, 1915·4
Cyproterone Acetate, 1544·1
Cyproteroni Acetas, 1544·1
Cyral, 1915·4
Cyress, 1915·4
Cyriamine, 1915·4
Cyromazine, 1503·1
Cyrpon, 1915·4
Cys, 1426·3
Cys Hydrochloride, 1426·3
Cysporin, 1915·4
Cystadan, 1915·4
Cystadane, 1915·4
Cystagon, 1915·4
Cysteamine, 1712·1
Cysteamine Bitartrate, 1712·1
Cysteamine Hydrochloride, 1712·2
Cysteine, 1113·2, 1426·3
L-Cysteine, 1426·3
Cysteine Hydrochloride, 1426·3
Cysteine Hydrochloride Monohydrate, 1426·3
L-Cysteine Hydrochloride Monohydrate, 1426·3
Cysteini Hydrochloridum Monohydricum, 1426·3
Cystel Antipelliculaire, 1915·4
Cystel Shampooing Antiseborrheique, 1915·4
Cystemme, 1915·4
Cystex, 1915·4
Cystibosin B 48, 1915·4
Cystic Fibrosis, 123·3
Cysticercosis, 98·1
Cystichol, 1915·4
Cysticide, 1915·4
Cystine, 1426·3
L-Cystine, 1426·3
Cystine $B_6$, 1915·4
Cystinex, 1916·1
Cystinol, 1916·1
Cystinol Akut, 1916·1
Cystinol Long, 1916·1
Cystinosis, 1712·2
Cystinum, 1426·3
Cystinuria, 1049·2
Cystiselect N, 1916·1
Cystistat, 1916·1
Cystit, 1916·1
Cystitis, Bacterial— *see* Urinary-tract Infections, 153·1
Cystitis, Haemorrhagic— *see* Haemorrhagic Cystitis, 1180·2
Cystitis, Haemorrhagic, Prophylaxis, 1041·3
Cystitis, Interstitial— *see* Interstitial Cystitis, 1473·3
Cystitis Juniperus, 1916·1
Cystitis Relief, 1916·1
Cystium Solidago, 1916·1
Cystium-wern, 1916·1
Cysti-Z, 1916·1
Cysto Fink, 1916·1

Cysto Fink Mono, 1916·1
Cystocalm, 1916·1
Cysto-Caps Chassot, 1916·1
Cysto-Conray, 1916·1
Cysto-cyl Ho-Len-Complex, 1916·1
Cystofem, 1916·1
Cysto-Gastreu S R18, 1916·1
Cystografin, 1916·1
Cystoid Macular Oedema— *see* Postoperative Inflammatory Ocular Disorders, 70·3
Cystoleve, 1916·1
Cysto-Myacyne N, 1916·1
Cystonorm, 1916·1
Cystopurin, 1916·1
Cysto-Saar, 1916·1
Cystosol, 1916·1
Cystospaz, 1916·1
Cystospaz-M, 1916·1
Cysto-Urgenin, 1916·1
Cystrin, 1916·2
Cysts, Bone— *see* Bone Cysts, 1077·1
Cytacon, 1916·2
Cytadren, 1916·2
Cytagon, 1916·2
Cytamen, 1916·2
Cytarabine, 543·1
Cytarabine Hydrochloride, 543·1
Cytarabine Ocfosfate, 544·1
Cytarabinum, 543·1
Cytarbel, 1916·2
Cytarine, 1916·2
Cyteal, 1916·2
Cytelium, 1916·2
Cythioate, 1503·1
Cytidine Diphosphate Choline, 1672·3
Cytidine Diphosphocholine, 1672·3
Cytidine 5′-{Sodium *P′*-[2-(Trimethylammonio)-ethyl] Hydrogen Diphosphate}, Inner Salt, 1672·3
Cytine, 1916·2
Cytisine, 1704·1
*Cytisus laburnum*, 1704·1
*Cytisus scoparius*, 1742·2
Cyto-Bifidus, 1916·2
Cytobion, 1916·2
Cytoblastin, 1916·2
Cytochrome C, 1678·3
Cytochrome C Solution, 1678·3
Cytocristin, 1916·2
CytoGam, 1916·2
Cytoglobin, 1916·2
Cytokines, 1678·3
Cytolog, 1916·2
Cytomegalovirus Immunoglobulins, 1612·1
Cytomegalovirus Infections, 619·2
Cytomegalovirus Vaccines, 1612·1
Cytomel, 1916·2
Cytophosphan, 1916·2
Cytoprotective Drugs, 1240·1
Cytosar, 1916·2
Cytosar-U, 1916·2
Cytosine Arabinoside, 543·1
Cytotec, 1916·2
Cytotect, 1916·3
Cytotoxic Drugs, 492·1
Cytotoxic Urotoxicity, 1041·3
Cytovene, 1916·3
Cytovis— *see* Alexan, 1784·4
Cytoxan, 1916·3
Cytozyme, 760·2
Cytra-2, 1916·3
Cytra-3, 1916·3
Cytra-K, 1916·3
Cytra-LC, 1916·3
Cytur Test, 1916·3
Cytuss HC, 1916·3
Cyzine, 1916·3


## D


D, 1422·3
2,4-D, 1503·2
D 4, 1916·3
D-25, 397·3
D-41, 656·1
D-138, 1563·2
D-145, 1711·2
D-204, 1916·3
D-206, 718·1
D-248, 1916·3
D-254, 1129·1
D-300, 1916·3
D-326, 1916·3
D-365, 1019·1
467$D_3$, 1383·3
D-563, 978·2
D-600, 922·3
722-D, 984·1
D-775, 703·1
D-1694, 582·1
D-1959, 791·2
D-2083, 1096·3
D-7093, 1041·2
D-9998, 43·3
D-18506, 573·2
D-19466, 565·1
D-20761, 1320·2
D & C Red No. 22, 1057·2
D & C Yellow No. 8, 1689·1
D & C Yellow No. 10, 1057·3
D Dimethicone, 1289·2
D Epifrin, 1916·3
D Sucril, 1916·3
$D_3$ Vicotrat, 1916·3
DA II, 1916·3
DA-398, 36·3
DA-688, 1267·1
DA-1773, 1289·3
DA-2370, 43·1
DA-3177, 480·2
DA Chewable, 1916·3
$DAB_{486}$ Interleukin-2, 1701·3
Daben, 1916·3
Dabenzol, 1916·3
Dabetil, 1916·3
Dabex, 1916·3
Dabex G, 1916·3
$DAB_{389}$IL2, 546·3
Da-boa, 1666·1
Dabonal, 1916·3
Dabonal Plus, 1916·3
Dabroson, 1916·3
DAC, 546·2
Dacam, 1916·4
Dacam RL, 1916·4
Dacarb, 1916·4
Dacarbaziba, 1916·4
Dacarbazina, 544·2
Dacarbazine, 544·2
Dacarbazinum, 544·2
Dacatic, 1916·4
Dacef, 1916·4
Dacha, 1666·1
Dacin-F, 1916·4
Dacisteína de Metilo, 1124·2
Dacisteine, 1124·2
Daclin, 1916·4
Dacliximab, 1359·3
Daclizumab, 1359·3
Dacmozen, 1916·4
Dacoren, 1916·4
Dacortin, 1916·4
Dacortin H, 1916·4
Dacovo, 1916·4
Dacplat, 1916·4
Dacrin, 1916·4
Dacrine, 1916·4
Dacrio Gel, 1916·4
Dacriogel, 1916·4
Dacriose, 1916·4
Dacriosol, 1916·4
Dacrodil, 1916·4
Dacrolux, 1916·4
Dacryne, 1916·4
Dacryoboraline, 1916·4
Dacryolarmes, 1916·4
Dacryoseptil— *see* Dacryne, 1916·4
Dacryoserum, 1916·4
Dacten, 1916·4
Dactil OB, 1917·1
Dactinomicina, 545·1
Dactinomycin, 545·1
*Dactylopius coccus*, 1057·2
Dacudoses, 1917·1
DADPS, 202·2
Daewo, 1917·1
Dafalgan, 1917·1
Dafalgan Codeine, 1917·1
Daflon, 1917·1
Daflon 500, 1917·1
Dafloxen, 1917·1
Dafloxen F, 1917·1
Dafne, 1917·1
Dafnegil, 1917·1
Dafnegil Neo, 1917·1
Dafnegin, 1917·1
Daforin, 1917·1
Daga, 1917·1
Dagan, 1917·1
Dagenan, 1917·1
Dagga, 1666·1
Dago, Calcium— *see* Calcium Dago, 1863·3
Dagol, 1917·1
Dagotil, 1917·1
Dagra Fluor, 1917·1
Dagracycline, 1917·1
Dagragel, 1917·1
Dagramycine, 1917·1
Dagravit, 1917·1
Dagravit A, 1917·1
Dagravit A Forte, 1917·2
Dagravit A-E, 1917·2
Dagravit A-E Forte, 1917·2
Dagravit B-Complex, 1917·2
Dagravit B-Complex Forte, 1917·2
Dagravit Totaal 8, 1917·2
Dagravit Total, 1917·2
Dagravit Total 8, 1917·2
Dagrilan, 1917·2
Dagynil, 1917·2
*Dahlia variabilis*, 1702·1
Dahllite, 1700·1
Dai Natha, 1917·2
Daidzein, 1448·2, 1737·3
Daiet B, 1917·2
Daigaku, New— *see* New Daigaku, 2165·4
Dai-kenchu-to, Tsumura— *see* Tsumura Dai-kenchu-to, 2351·1
Dailat, 1917·2
Daily, 1917·2
Daily Balance, 1917·2
Daily Benefits, 1917·2
Daily Care— *see* Desitin Creamy, 1930·2
Daily Conditioning, 1917·2
Daily Fatigue Relief, 1917·2
Daily Gold Pack, 1917·2
Daily Menopause Relief, 1917·2
Daily Multi, 1917·2
Daily Overwork & Mental Fatigue Relief, 1917·2
Daily Plus, Bioglan— *see* Bioglan Daily Plus, 1843·4
Daily Plus Max, Bioglan— *see* Bioglan Daily Plus Max, 1844·1
Daily Protection Moisturizer, 1917·2
Daily Tension & Strain Relief, 1917·2
Daily-Vite, 1917·2
Daimeton, 1917·2
Dairy Ease, 1917·2
Dairyaid, 1917·2
Daiv, 1917·2
Daivobet, 1917·2
Daivonex, 1917·2
Dakar, 1917·3
Dakin, 1917·3
Dakincooper, 1917·3
Dakin's Solution, 1175·3
Daktacort, 1917·3
Daktacort HC, 1917·3
Daktagold, 1917·3
Daktar, 1917·3
Daktarin, 1917·3
Daktarin Gold, 1917·3
Daktazol, 1917·3
Daktodor, 1917·3
Daktozin, 1917·3
Dal, 1917·3
Dalacin Preparations, 1917·3
Dalacin-C, 1917·3
Dalacine, 1917·4
Dalacine T, 1917·4
Dalagis T, 1917·4
Dalalgan Codeina, 1917·4
Dalalone, 1917·4
Dalam, 1917·4
Dalamon, 1917·4
Dalamon Inyectable, 1917·4
Dalanated Insulin, 334·2
Dalcap, 1917·4
Dalcept, 1917·4
Dalcipran, 1917·4
Dal-E, 1917·4
Dalet Med Balsam, 1917·4
Dalfaz, 1917·4
Dalfopristin, 248·1
Dalfopristin Mesilate, 248·1
Dalfopristin Mesylate, 248·1
Dalfopristina, Mesilato de, 248·1
Dalgan, 1917·4
Dalgen, 1917·4
Dalgex, 1917·4
Dalidome, 1917·4
Dalinar, 1917·4
Dalisol, 1917·4
Dalivit, 1917·4
Dallamizol-D, 1917·4
Dallapasmo, 1917·4
Dallergy, 1918·1
Dallergy-D, 1918·1
Dallergy-JR, 1918·1
Dalmacol, 1918·1
Dalmadorm, 1918·1
Dalmane, 1918·1
Dalmasin, 1918·1
Dalmatian Insect Flowers, 1509·3
Dalminette, 1918·1
Dalparan, 1918·1
Dalsin, 1918·1
Dalsy, 1918·1
Dalteparin Sodium, 891·1
Dalteparina Sódica, 891·1
Dalteparinum Natricum, 891·1
Daltroid, 1918·1
Dalun, 1918·1
Dalys, 1918·1
Dalzolston, 1918·1
Dam, 1918·1
Dama-Lax, 1918·1
Damason-P, 1918·1
Damax, 1918·1
Damiana, 1679·1
Damiana and Kola Tablets, 1918·1
Damiana and Saw Palmetto Elixir— *see* Elixir Damiana and Saw Palmetto, 1965·4
Damiana-Sarsaparilla Formula, 1918·1
Damiclin, 1918·1
Damide, 1918·1
Daminate, 1918·1
Daminozida, 1503·1
Daminozide, 1503·1
Damira, 1918·1
Damixa, 1918·1
Damosal, 1918·2
Damoxicil, 1918·2
Damoxicil Mucolitico, 1918·2
Damoxy, 1918·2
Dampo, 1918·2
Dampo bij Droge Hoest, 1918·2
Dampo Mucopect, 1918·2
Dampo Solvopect, 1918·2
DAN-216, 669·3
Danalem, 1918·2
Danantizol, 1918·2
Danaparoid Sodium, 891·2
Danaparoide Sódico, 891·2
Danatrol, 1918·2
Danazant, 1918·2
Danazol, 1545·2
Dancimin-C, 1918·2
Dancor, 1918·2
Dandelion Root, 1751·3
Dandrazol, 1918·2
Dandrid, 1918·2

Dandruff Control Pert 2 in 1, 1918·2
Dandruff— *see* Seborrhoeic Dermatitis, 1138·3
Dandruff Shampoo Plus Conditioner, 1918·2
Dandruff Treatment Shampoo, 1918·2
Daneral, 1918·2
Danferane, 1918·2
Dan-Gard, 1918·2
Danilax, 1918·2
Danilon, 1918·2
Danitin, 1918·2
Danka, 1918·2
Danlax, 1918·2
Danlox, 1918·3
Danocrine, 1918·3
Danofloxacin Mesilate, 202·2
Danofloxacin Mesylate, 202·2
Danofloxacino, Mesilato de, 202·2
Danogar, 1918·3
Danogen, 1918·3
Danokrin, 1918·3
Danol, 1918·3
Danovag, 1918·3
Danovir, 1918·3
Danruf, 1918·3
Danssan, 1918·3
Dantalin, 1918·3
Dantamacrin, 1918·3
Dan-Tar Plus, 1918·3
Dantenk, 1918·3
Danthron, 1261·1
D-Antihist, 1918·3
Dantrium, 1918·3
Dantrolen, 1918·3
Dantrolene Sodium, 1393·3
Dantroleno Sódico, 1393·3
Dantron, 1261·1
Danubial, 1918·3
Dany, 1918·3
Danzen, 1918·3
Danzyme, 1918·3
Daohair-S, 1918·3
Daonil, 1918·3
Daonil, Hemi- — *see* Hemi-Daonil, 2039·1
Daonil, Semi- — *see* Semi-Daonil, 2284·2
Daono, 1918·3
Dapa, 1918·4
Dapacin Cold, 1918·4
Dapamax, 1918·4
Dapa-Tabs, 1918·4
Dapaz, 1918·4
Dapiprazol, Hidrocloruro de, 1679·1
Dapiprazole Hydrochloride, 1679·1
Dapotum, 1918·4
Dapropterin Hydrochloride, 1742·1
Daprox, 1918·4
Daps, 1918·4
Dapsoderm-X, 1918·4
Dapsona, 202·2
Dapsone, 202·2
Dapsonum, 202·2
Daptacel, 1918·4
Daptaral, 1918·4
Daptomicina, 204·2
Daptomycin, 204·2
Daptril, 1918·4
Darakte-Bang, 1666·1
Daralix, 1918·4
Daram, 1918·4
Daramal, 1918·4
Daramal-Paludrine, 1918·4
Daranide, 1918·4
Daraprim, 1918·4
Daraprin, 1918·4
Darax, 1918·4
Darbalan, 1918·4
Darbalan Plus, 1918·4
Darbepoetin Alfa, 745·2
Darbepoetina Alfa, 745·2
Darcipireno, 1918·4
Dardex, 1918·4
Dardum, 1918·4
Darebon, 1918·4
Daren, 1918·4
Dari, 1919·1
Daricon, 1919·1
Darier's Disease, 1134·3
Darifenacin, 481·1
Darifenacina, 481·1
Dariseb, 1919·1
Darkene, 1919·1
Darleton, 1919·1
Darlin, 1919·1
Darmen Salt, 1919·1
Darmol, 1919·1
Darmol Bisacodyl, 1919·1
Darmol Lactulose, 1919·1
Darmol Pico, 1919·1
Daro, 1919·1
Daro Hoofdpijnpoeders, 1919·1
Daro Thijm, 1919·1
Darob, 1919·1
Darocet, 1919·1
Darocillin, 1919·1
Darolan Hoestprikkeldempende, 1919·1
Darolan Slijmplossende, 1919·1
Daromide, 1919·1
Daronda, 1919·1
Darosed, 1919·1
Darrow-Liq, 1919·1
Darrowped, 1919·1
Dart, 1919·1
Dartrox, 1919·1
Daruma, 1919·1
Darvocet, 1919·2
Darvocet-N, 1919·2
Darvon, 1919·2
Darvon Compound, 1919·2
Darvon Simple, 1919·2
Darvon-N, 1919·2
Darvon-N Compuesto, 1919·2
Darzitil, 1919·2
Darzitil Plus, 1919·2
Darzitil SB, 1919·2
Dasc, 1919·2
Dasen, 1919·2
Daskil, 1919·2
Daskyl, 1919·2
Daslin, 1919·2
Dasmetrol, 1919·2
Dasolin, 1919·2
Dasten, 1919·2
Dastonil, 1919·2
Dastosin, 1919·2
Dastusin, 1919·2
Dasuglor, 1919·2
Datisan, 1919·2
Datolan, 1919·2
Datril, 1919·2
DaTSCAN, 1919·2
Datura, 489·2
Datura Herb, 489·2
Datura Leaf, 489·2
*Datura metel*, 489·2
*Datura meteloides*, 1723·2
*Datura stramonium*, 489·2
Dauci Herba, 1765·1
Daucus, 1765·1
*Daucus carota*, 1765·1
Daunoblastin, 1919·2
Daunoblastina, 1919·2
Daunocin, 1919·3
Daunomycin Hydrochloride, 545·3
Daunorubicin Citrate, 545·3
Daunorubicin Citrate Liposome, 545·3
Daunorubicin Hydrochloride, 545·3
Daunorubicina, Hidrocloruro de, 545·3
Daunorubicini Hydrochloridum, 545·3
Daunorubicinol, 546·1
DaunoXome, 1919·3
Daurocina, 1919·3
Dauxona, 1919·3
Davedax, 1919·3
D'Aveia, 1919·3
Daverium, 1919·3
Davicaina, 1919·3
David Morton's Quintessential, 1919·3
Davilla, 1919·3
Davilose, 1919·3
Davimicina, 1919·3
Davinefrina, 1919·3
Davistar, 1919·3
Davitamon AD, 1919·3
Davitamon AD Fluor, 1919·3
Davitamon E, 1919·3
Davitamon Fem, 1919·3
Davitamon Fluor, 1919·3
Davixolol, 1919·3
Daxon, 1919·3
Daxotel, 1919·3
Day Cold Comfort, 1919·3
Day & Night, 1919·3
Day & Night Cold & Flu, 1919·3
Day & Night Nurse, 1919·3
Day Nurse, 1919·4
Day Time Liquigels, 1919·4
Dayalets, 1919·4
Dayalets + Iron, 1919·4
Dayalets Plus Iron, 1919·4
Dayamin, 1919·4
Dayamineral, 1919·4
Daycef, 1919·4
Dayhist, 1919·4
Dayhist-1, 1919·4
Daypro, 1919·4
Dayquil, 1919·4
DayQuil Allergy Relief, Vicks— *see* Vicks DayQuil Allergy Relief, 2375·2
Dayquil Sinus and Pain Relief, 1919·4
DayQuil Sinus Pressure & Pain Relief, Vicks— *see* Vicks DayQuil Sinus Pressure & Pain Relief, 2375·2
DayQuil, Vicks— *see* Vicks DayQuil, 2375·2
Days, 1919·4
Daytime Cold & Flu, 1919·4
Dayto Himbin, 1919·4
Dayto Sulf, 1919·4
Dayvit, 1919·4
Daywear, 1919·4
Dazamide, 1919·4
Dazen, 1919·4
Dazid, 1919·4
Dazine, 1919·4
Dazocan, 1919·4
Dazol, 1919·4
Dazolin, 1919·4
DBcAMP, 1663·2
DBD, 573·3
DBI, 1920·1
DBI AP, 1920·1
DBM, 573·2
DBP, 1503·1
DBV, 330·3
DC Softgels, 1920·1
DC Vin, 1920·1
DCA, 1747·2
D-Calsor, 1920·1
DCCK, 1920·1
DCMX, 1178·3
DCNU, 538·1
D-Coate, 1920·1
D-Cure, 1920·1
DD-01, 490·1
DD-3480, 725·2
DDA, 1502·2
DDAVP, 1322·3, 1920·1
DDC, 657·1
DdC, 657·1
DdCyd, 657·1
DDD, 1920·1
*o,p'*DDD, 575·1
DDE, 1502·2
*o,p'*-DDE, 575·2
DDI, 630·3
DdI, 630·3
DdIno, 630·3
DDP, 538·1
*cis*-DDP, 538·1
DDS, 202·2
DDT, 1502·1
DDTC, 1038·2
DDVP, 1503·2
D2E7, 12·1
DE-019, 1663·2
De A A Zinc Grossesse, 1920·1
De Icin, 1920·1
De Icol, 1920·1
de STAT, 1920·1
De Witt's Preparations, 1920·1
De Witt's, Pilulas— *see* Pilulas De Witt's, 2220·1
De Worm, Chemists Own— *see* Chemists Own De Worm, 1881·4
Deacetyl-lanatoside C, 893·1
25-Deacetylrifabutin, 250·1
25-*O*-Deacetylrifampicin, 252·2
25-Deacetylrifapentine, 253·3
Deacetylvinorelbine, 594·2
Deacos, 1920·2
Deacura, 1920·2
17-Deacylnorgestimate, 1562·1
Deadly Agaric, 1717·3
Deadly Nightshade, 479·1
DEAE-dextran Hydrochloride, 890·3
Deafort, 1920·2
Deaftol Avec Lidocaine, 1920·2
Dealan, 1920·2
Dealgic, 1920·2
*N*-Dealkylbuprenorphine, 22·3
Dealyd, 1920·2
[1-Deamino,8-D-arginine]vasopressin, 1322·3
Deamino-oxytocin, 1322·3
Deanacaps, 1920·2
Deanol, 1585·3
Deanol Aceglumate, 1585·3
Deanol Acetamidobenzoate, 1585·3
Deanol Benzilate, 1585·3
Deanol Benzilate Hydrochloride, 1585·3
Deanol Bisorcate, 1585·3
Deanol 4-Chlorophenoxyacetate Hydrochloride, 1710·1
Deanol Cyclohexylpropionate, 1585·3
Deanol Diphenylglycolate, 1585·3
Deanol Hemisuccinate, 1585·3
Deanol Orotate, 1724·3
Deanol Pidolate, 1585·3
Deanol Tartrate, 1585·3
Deanxit, 1920·2
Death Cap, 1717·3
Deavynfar, 1920·2
Deb, 1920·2
Debacterol, 1920·2
Debax, 1920·2
Debefenium, 1920·2
Debei, 1920·2
Debeina, 1920·2
Debekacyl, 1920·2
Debela, 1920·2
Debelex, 1920·2
Debendox, 420·3
Debeone, 1920·2
Debequin, 1920·2
Debequin-C, 1920·2
Debisor, 1920·2
Deblaston, 1920·2
Debonal, 1920·2
Debridat, 1920·2
Debridat B, 1920·2
Debril, 1920·3
Debrisan, 1920·3
Debrisoquin Sulfate, 891·3
Debrisoquina, Sulfato de, 891·3
Debrisoquine Sulfate, 891·3
Debrisoquine Sulphate, 891·3
Debrisorb, 1920·3
Debrox, 1920·3
Debrum, 1920·3
Debrumyl, 1920·3
Debtan, 1920·3
Dec, 1920·3
DEC, 1920·3
Deca, 1920·3
Decabutin, Neo— *see* Neo Decabutin, 2156·2
Decacalcium Dihydroxide Hexakis(orthophosphate), 1699·3
Decacef, 1920·3
Decadran, 1920·3
Decadran Neomicina, 1920·3
Decadron Preparations, 1920·3

Decadronal, 1920·4
Deca-Durabol, 1920·4
Deca-Durabolin, 1920·4
Decafar, 1920·4
Decagen, 1920·4
Decahist-DM, 1920·4
(3*R*,5a*S*,6*R*,8a*S*,9*R*,10*S*,12*R*,12a*R*)-Decahydro-10-ethoxy-3,6,9-trimethyl-3,12-epoxy-12*H*-pyrano[4,3-*j*]-1,2-benzodioxepin, 447·2
(3*R*,5a*S*,6*R*,8a*S*,9*R*,10*S*,12*R*,12a*R*)-Decahydro-10-methoxy-3,6,9-trimethyl-3,12-epoxy-12*H*-pyrano[4,3-*j*]-1,2-benzodioxepin, 447·2
(3*S*,7*R*)-3,4,5,6,7,8,9,10,11,12-Decahydro-7,14,16-trihydroxy-3-methyl-1*H*-2-benzoxacyclotetradecin-1-one, 1573·3
(3*R*,5a*S*,6*R*,8a*S*,9*R*,10*S*,12*R*,12a*R*)-Decahydro-3,6,9-trimethyl-3,12-epoxy-12*H*-pyrano-[4,3-*j*]-1,2-benzodioxepin-10-ol Hydrogen Succinate, 447·2
(3*R*,5a*S*,6*R*,8a*S*,9*R*,10*S*,12*R*,12a*R*)-Decahydro-3,6,9-trimethyl-3,12-epoxy-12*H*-pyrano-[4,3-*j*]-1,2-benzodioxepin-10-ol Hydrogen Succinate Sodium, 447·2
Decaject, 1920·4
Decal, 1920·4
Decalcit, 1920·4
Decalinium Chloride, 1178·1
Decalogiflox, 1920·4
Decaltrex, 1920·4
Decamethrin, 1503·1
2-Deca(3-methylbut-2-enylene)-5,6-dimethoxy-3-methyl-*p*-benzoquinone, 1760·2
*N*,*N*-Decamethylenebis(4-amino-2-methylquinolinium Chloride), 1178·1
*N*,*N*′-Decamethylenebis(*N*,*N*,*N*-trimethyl-3-methylcarbamoyloxyanilinium) Dibromide, 1488·3
2,2′-(Decamethylenedithio)diethanol, 1011·2
Decaminum, 1178·1
Decan, 1920·4
Decanal, 1724·1, 1724·2
Decanedioic Acid, 1157·3
Decaneurabol, 1920·4
Decanoato de Bromperidol, 672·1
Decanoato de Flufenazina, 699·3
Decanoato de Flupentixol, 699·1
Decanoato de Haloperidol, 701·3
Decanoato de Nandrolona, 1561·2
Decanoato de Perfenazina, 714·2
Decanoato de Testosterona, 1570·1
Decanoato de Zuclopentixol, 730·3
Deca-Noralone, 1920·4
Decapeptyl, 1920·4
Decaprednil, 1921·1
Decaquinon, 1921·1
8-Decarboxamido-8-(3,3-diethylureido)-D-lysergamide Maleate, 1210·3
Decaris, 1921·1
Deca-Scab, 1921·1
Decasept N, 1921·1
Decasona, 1921·1
Decasone, 1921·1
Decaspiride, 786·1
Decaspray, 1921·1
Decatylen, 1921·1
Decatylene, 1921·1
Decatylene Neo, 1921·1
Decaugh, 1921·1
Decaven, 1921·1
Deca-Vi-Sol, 1921·1
Decavit, 1921·1
Decdan, 1921·1
Decdan-N, 1921·1
Decentan, 1921·1
De-Chlor Preparations, 1921·1
3-Dechloroethyl-ifosfamide, 561·2
Decho, 1921·2
Decholin, 1921·2
Decidex, 1921·2
Decidex Compuesto, 1921·2
Decidex Plus, 1921·2
Decilina, 1921·2
Decipar, 1921·2
Decitabina, 546·2
Decitabine, 546·2
Decitriol, 1921·2
Decliten, 1921·2
Decloban, 1921·2
Declomycin, 1921·2
Declovir, 1921·2
Decme, 1921·2
Decocort, 1921·2
Decoderm Preparations, 1921·2
Decofam Cough, 1921·2
Decofed, 1921·2
Decohistine DH, 1921·2
Decolgen, 1921·3
Decolorising Charcoal, 1030·2
Decomit, 1921·3
Decon, 1921·3
Deconamine, 1921·3
Deconamine CX, 1921·3
Deconex 50FF, 1921·3
Deconex 53IN, 1921·3
Decongest, 1921·3
Decongestabs, 1921·3
Decongestant, 1921·3
Decongestant Antihistamine, Nyal Plus+ — *see* Nyal Plus+ Decongestant Antihistamine, 2182·2
Decongestant Antihistaminic Syrup, 1921·3
Decongestant Expectorant, 1921·3
Decongestant Nasal Mist, 1921·3
Decongestant Nasal Spray, 1921·3
Decongestant Nasal Spray, Chemists Own— *see* Chemists Own Decongestant Nasal Spray, 1882·1
Decongestant Nose Drops, 1921·3
Decongestant, Nyal Plus+ — *see* Nyal Plus+ Decongestant, 2182·2
Decongestant SR, 1921·3
Decongestant Tablets, 1921·3
Decongex Plus, 1921·3
Decongex Plus Expectorante, 1921·3
Deconhist LA, 1921·3
Decono, 1921·4
Deconomed, 1921·4
Deconsal II, 1921·4
Deconsal Pediatric, 1921·4
Deconsal Sprinkle, 1921·4
Decontractyl, 1921·4
Decontractyl New, 1921·4
Decontril, 1921·4
Decoquinate, 603·2
Decoquinato, 603·2
Decorenone, 1921·4
Decorex, 1921·4
Decorpa, 1921·4
Decortilen, 1921·4
Decortin, 1921·4
Decortin H, 1921·4
Decortone Acetate, 1097·1
Decos, 1921·4
Decosil, 1921·4
Decostriol, 1921·4
Decozol, 1921·4
Decrelip, 1921·4
Decresco, 1921·4
Decrin, 1921·4
Dectaflur, 1427·1
Dectancyl, 1921·4
Decualinio, Cloruro de, 1178·1
Decubal, 1921·4
Decurin, 1921·4
*N*-Decyl-*N*,*N*-demethyl-1-decanaminium Chloride, 1178·3
Decylenes, 1921·4
Dedaleira, Folha de, 894·2
$4^{A}$-*O*-De(2,6-dideoxy-3-*C*-methyl-α-L-*ribo*-hexopyranosyl)-20-deoxo-20-(*cis*-3,5-dimethyl-piperidino)tylosin, 271·2
Dedile, 1921·4
Dediol, 1921·4
Dedolor, 1921·4
Dedostryl, 1922·1
Dedralen, 1922·1
Dedrei, 1922·1
Dedrogyl, 1922·1
Deep Preparations, 1922·1
Deep Freeze, 1922·1
Deep Freeze Cold Gel, 1922·1
Deep Heat Preparations, 1922·1
Deep Heating Preparations, 1922·1
Deep Relief, 1922·1
Deep-Down Rub, 1922·1
Deep-vein Thrombosis— *see* Venous Thromboembolism, 839·1
Deer Musk, 1718·2
DEET, 1503·3
Deetipat, 1922·1
Defalan Insulin, 334·2
Defanac, 1922·1
Defanyl, 1922·1
Defarol, 1922·1
Defatig, 1922·1
Defaxina, 1922·1
DeFed, 1922·1
Defencid, 1922·1
Defen-LA, 1922·1
Deferiprona, 1033·1
Deferiprone, 1033·1
Deferoxamina, Mesilato de, 1033·1
Deferoxamine Mesilate, 1033·1
Deferoxamine Mesylate, 1033·1
Deferoxamini Mesilas, 1033·1
Defibrase, 1922·1
Defibrotida, 892·1
Defibrotide, 892·1
Deficical B12, 1922·1
Defiltran, 1922·1
Definity, 1922·2
Defirin, 1922·2
Defix, 1922·2
Deflam, 1922·2
Deflamat, 1922·2
Deflamm, 1922·2
Deflamol, 1922·2
Deflamon, 1922·2
Deflamox, 1922·2
Deflan, 1922·2
Deflanil, 1922·2
Deflaren, 1922·2
Deflazacort, 1096·2
Deflogen, 1922·2
Deflogix, 1922·2
Deflox, 1922·2
Defluin, 1922·2
Defluin Plus, 1922·2
Defluina, 1922·2
Defluina N, 1922·2
Defomil, 1922·2
Deftan, 1922·2
Defungo, 1922·2
Degabina, 1922·2
DeGalin, 1922·2
De-Gas, 1922·2
Degas, 1922·2
Degas Extra, 1922·3
Degas Infant Drops, 1922·3
Degenerative Joint Disease— *see* Osteoarthritis, 9·2
Degest, 1922·3
Degest 2, 1922·3
Deglycyrrhizinised Liquorice, 1270·3
Deglymidodrine, 959·2
Degona, 1922·3
Degoran, 1922·3
Degoran C, 1922·3
Degoran Cold & Flu, 1922·3
Degoran Cough, 1922·3
Degoran Plus, 1922·3
Degorflan, 1922·3
Degran, 1922·3
Degranol, 1922·3
DEHA, 1504·2
Dehidrobenzperidol, 1922·3
Dehidrocólico, Ácido, 1679·2
Dehistine, 1922·3
Dehydral, 1922·3
Dehydrated Alcohol, 1166·1
Dehydro Sanol Tri, 1922·3
Dehydro Tri Mite, 1922·3
Dehydroacetic Acid, 1178·1
Dehydroandrosterone, 1565·3
Dehydro-aripiprazole, 671·1
Dehydrobenzperidol, 1922·3
7-Dehydrocholesterol, 1461·3
Dehydrocholesterol, Activated, 1461·3
Dehydrocholic Acid, 1660·3, 1679·2
1,2-Dehydrocortisone, 1109·3
Dehydroemetine Hydrochloride, 603·2
2,3-Dehydroemetine Hydrochloride, 603·2
Dehydroepiandrosterone, 1565·3
Dehydroepiandrosterone Enanthate, 1565·3
Dehydroepiandrosterone Sulphate Sodium, 1566·1
1,2-Dehydrohydrocortisone, 1108·1
11-Dehydro-17-hydroxycorticosterone Acetate, 1096·1
Dehydroisoandrosterone, 1565·3
Dehydroprogesterone, 1549·2
6-Dehydro-*retro*-progesterone, 1549·2
6-Dehydro-9β,10α-progesterone, 1549·2
Dehydrosertindole, 722·1
Dehydrostilbestrol, 1547·3
1-Dehydrotestololactone, 587·3
Deiten, 1922·3
Dekamega, 1922·3
Dekamin, 1922·3
Dekar 2, 1922·3
Dekatin, 1922·3
Dekinet, 1922·4
Dekka, 1922·4
Dekristol, 1922·4
DEL-1267, 1274·3
Del Aqua, 1922·4
Delabarre, 1922·4
De-Lact, 1922·4
Delagil, 1922·4
Delak, 1922·4
Delaket, 1922·4
Delakete, 1922·4
Delakmin, 1922·4
Delalande Diarrhee— *see* Ercestop, 1974·2
Delapride, 1922·4
Delapril, Hidrocloruro de, 892·2
Delapril Hydrochloride, 892·2
Delatestryl, 1922·4
Delavirdina, Mesilato de, 630·2
Delavirdine Mesilate, 630·2
Delavirdine Mesylate, 630·2
Delbiase, 1922·4
Delbulasa, 1922·4
Delcoprep, 1922·4
Delecit, 1922·4
Delegol, 1922·4
Delepsine, 1922·4
Deleptin, 1922·4
Delestrogen, 1922·4
Deletus, 1922·4
Deletus A, 1922·4
Deletus D, 1922·4
Deletus P, 1922·4
Delfen, 1922·4
Delfos, 1922·4
Delgacin Fibras, 1923·1
Delgafen, 1923·1
Delgamer, 1923·1
Delical, 1923·1
Delicate Skin Pasta, 1923·1
Delidose, 1923·1
Delimmun, 1923·1
Delimon, 1923·1
Delin, 1923·1
Delinar, 1923·1
Delipoderm, 1923·1
Deliproct, 1923·1
Delirex, 1923·1
Delirium— *see* Disturbed Behaviour, 665·1
Delirium— *see* Psychoses, 665·1
Delirium Tremens— *see* Alcohol Withdrawal and Abstinence, 1166·2
Delitan, 1923·1
Delitex N, 1923·1
Delitroxin, 1923·1
Deliver, 1923·1
Delix, 1923·1
Delix Plus, 1923·1
Delixi, 1923·1
Delixir, 1923·1
Del-Lend, 1923·1
Dellova, 1923·1

Delmadinona, Acetato de, 1547·2
Delmadinone Acetate, 1547·2
Delmuno, 1923·1
Del-Mycin, 1923·1
Delonal, 1923·1
Delorazepam, 689·3
Delos, 1923·1
Delph Sun Lotion, 1923·1
Delphi, 1923·1
Delphicol, 1923·1
Delphicort, 1923·2
Delphimix, 1923·2
Delphinac, 1923·2
Delpral, 1923·2
Delrosa, 1923·2
Delsacid, 1923·2
Delsym, 1923·2
Delta 80, 1923·2
Delta Charcoal, 1923·2
Delta 80 Plus, 1923·2
Delta Tocopherols, 1464·3
Delta Tomanil B12, 1923·2
Deltacef, 1923·2
Deltacid, 1923·2
Deltacid Plus, 1923·2
Deltacina, 1923·2
Delta-Cortef, 1923·2
Deltacortene, 1923·2
Deltacortisone, 1109·3
Deltacortril, 1923·2
Delta-D, 1923·2
Deltadehydrocortisone, 1109·3
Delta-Diona, 1923·2
Deltaflan, 1923·2
Deltaflogin, 1923·2
Delta-Hadensa, 1923·2
Deltahydrocortisone, 1108·1
Deltalaf, 1923·2
Deltalipid, 1923·2
Deltamethrin, 1503·1
Deltametrina, 1503·1
Deltamid, 1923·2
Deltamidrina, 1923·3
Deltamitren, 1923·3
Deltanoids, 1463·3
Deltapio, 1923·3
Deltaran, 1923·3
Deltaren, 1923·3
Deltarhinol-Mono, 1923·3
Deltarinolo, 1923·3
Deltasone, 1923·3
Deltasoralen, 1923·3
Deltastab, 1923·3
Delta-Tritex, 1923·3
Deltavac, 1923·3
Deltavagin, 1923·3
Deltavit, 1923·3
Deltazen, 1923·3
Deltisan, 1923·3
Deltison, 1923·3
Deltisona B, 1923·3
Delto-cyl Ho-Len-Complex, 1923·3
Deltrox, 1923·3
Delufen, 1923·3
Delursan, 1923·3
Delvas, 1923·3
Del-Vi-A, 1923·3
Demac, 1923·3
Demadex, 1923·3
Démanol, 1585·3
Demazin Preparations, 1923·3
Dembrexina, 1117·3
Dembrexine, 1117·3
Dembrexine Hydrochloride, 1117·3
Dembroxol, 1117·3
Demdec, 1923·4
Demecario, Bromuro de, 1488·3
Demecarium Bromide, 1488·3
Demeclociclina, 204·3
Demeclociclina, Hidrocloruro de, 204·3
Demeclocycline, 204·3
Demeclocycline Calcium, 205·1
Demeclocycline Hydrochloride, 204·3
Demeclocycline Magnesium, 205·1
Demeclocyclini Hydrochloridum, 204·3
Demegestona, 1547·2
Demegestone, 1547·2
De-menthasin, 1923·4
Dementholised Mint Oil, 1715·2
Dementia, 1484·1
Dementia— *see* Psychoses, 665·1
Dementia, HIV-associated— *see* HIV-associated Neurological Complications, 623·2
Demergin, 1923·4
Demerol, 1923·4
4-Demethoxydaunorubicin Hydrochloride, 560·2
Demethylazelastine, 425·2
Demethylchlortetracycline, 204·3
Demethylcitalopram, 289·1
(4″-*R*)-5-*O*-Demethyl-25-de(1-methylpropyl)-4″-deoxy-4″-(methylamino)-25-(1-methylethyl)avermectin $A_{1a}$, 1504·3
5-*O*-Demethyl-25-de(1-methylpropyl)-25-(1-methylethyl)-22,23-dihydroavermectin $A_{1a}$, 105·3
6-Demethyl-6-deoxy-7-dimethylaminotetracycline, 231·3
(6*R*,15*S*)-5-*O*-Demethyl-28-deoxy-25-[(*E*)-1,3-dimethylbut-1-enyl]-6,28-epoxy-23-oxomilbemycin B (*E*)-23-*O*-Methyloxime, 110·1
6-Demethyl-6-deoxy-5β-hydroxy-6-methylenetetracycline, 230·1
(4″-*R*)-5-*O*-Demethyl-4″-deoxy-4″-(methylamino)avermectin $A_{1a}$, 1504·3
Demethyldiazepam, 710·3
5-*O*-Demethyl-22,23-dihydroavermectin $A_{1a}$, 105·3
4′-Demethylepipodophyllotoxin 9-[4,6-*O*-(*R*)-Ethylidene-β-D-glucopyranoside], 551·3
4′-Demethylepipodophyllotoxin 9-(4,6-*O*-Ethylidene-β-D-glucopyranoside) 4′-(Dihydrogen Phosphate), 551·3
6-Demethylgriseofulvin, 401·2
*N*-Demethyl-*N*-heptylphysostigmine, 1491·2
*N*-Demethylvancomycin, 239·2
56-Demethylvancomycin, 239·2
Demetil, 1923·4
Demetrin, 1923·4
Demex, 1923·4
Demiax, 1923·4
Demineralised Water, 1764·3
Demi-Regroton, 1923·4
Demix, 1923·4
Demo Preparations, 1923·4
Demo-Cineol, 1924·1
Democyl, 1924·1
Demodek, 1924·1
Demodenal, 1924·1
Demodenal Compositum, 1924·1
Demoderhin, 1924·1
Demodon Neo, 1924·1
Demogripal, 1924·1
Demogripal C, 1924·1
Demolaxin, 1924·1
Demolibral, 1924·1
Demolox, 1924·1
Demonatur Preparations, 1924·1
Demopart, 1924·1
DemoPectol, 1924·1
Demoplas, 1924·1
Demoprin Nouvelle Formule, 1924·2
Demostan, 1924·2
Demostan N, 1924·2
Demosvelte N, 1924·2
Demotest, 1924·2
Demotherm Pommade contre le Rhumatisme, 1924·2
Demotidini Hydrochloridum, 689·3
Demotussil, 1924·2
Demotussol, 1924·2
Demovarin, 1924·2
Demoven N, 1924·2
Demovit, 1924·2
Demovit C, 1924·2
Demoxepam, 674·3
Demoxitocina, 1322·3
Demoxytocin, 1322·3
Dempol, 1924·2
Demser, 1924·2
Demulcin, 1924·2
Demulen, 1924·2
Demusin, 1924·2
Demyelinating Neuropathy, Acute Idiopathic— *see* Guillain-Barré Syndrome, 1630·2
Demyelination, Osmotic— *see* Hyponatraemia, 1220·3
Denacen, 1924·2
Denaclof, 1924·2
Denan, 1924·2
Denapril, 1924·2
Denatonio, Benzoato de, 1679·2
Denatonium Benzoate, 1186·1, 1679·2
Denatured Alcohol, 1185·3
Denatured Ethanol, 1185·3
Denavir, 1924·2
Denaxpren, 1924·2
Denazox, 1924·2
Dencorub, 1924·2
Dencorub Anti-Inflammatory, 1924·2
Dencorub Arthritis, 1924·2
Dencorub Arthritis Ice, 1924·3
Dencorub Extra Strength, 1924·3
Dencorub Pain Relieving Cream, 1924·3
Denerel, 1924·3
Denex, 1924·3
Dengue Fever— *see* Haemorrhagic Fevers, 618·2
Dengue Fever Vaccines, 1612·2
Deniban, 1924·3
Denileucina Diftitox, 546·3
Denileukin Difitox, 546·3
Denileukin Diftitox, 546·3
Denim, 1924·3
Deniren, 1924·3
Denisoline, 1924·3
Denium, 1924·3
Denkacort, 1924·3
De-Nol, 1924·3
De-Noltab, 1924·3
Denopamina, 892·2
Denopamine, 892·2
Denoral, 1924·3
Denorex, 1924·3
Denorex Daily, 1924·3
Denorex Herbal, 1924·3
Denorex Plus, 1924·3
Denosol, 1924·3
Denpru, 1924·3
Denquel, 1924·3
Densical, 1924·3
Densical D, 1924·3
Densical Vitamine $D_3$, 1924·4
Denson, 1924·4
Densopax, 1924·4
Denta Plus, 1924·4
DentaGel, 1924·4
Dentagesic, 1924·4
Dental Abscess— *see* Mouth Infections, 136·1
Dental Caries— *see* Mouth Infections, 136·1
Dental Caries Prophylaxis, 1445·3
Dental Caries Vaccines, 1612·2
Dental Pain Relief, Boots— *see* Boots Dental Pain Relief, 1851·1
Dental Sedation, 666·2
Dentalgar, 1924·4
Dentaliv, 1924·4
Dentalivio, 1924·4
Dental-Phenjoca, 1924·4
Dental-Type Silica, 1581·3
Dentan, 1924·4
Dentapaine, 1924·4
Dentaton Antisettico, 1924·4
Dentecalcio, 1924·4
Dentex, 1924·4
Denticare, 1924·4
Dentigoa, 1924·4
Dentikrisos, 1924·4
Dentilin, Resina Carbolica— *see* Resina Carbolica Dentilin, 2259·1
Dentin, 1924·4
Dentinale, 1924·4
Dentinox, 1924·4
Dentinox Colic Drops, 1924·4
Dentinox Cradle Cap, 1924·4
Dentinox N, 1924·4
Dentinox Teething Gel, 1924·4
Dentipatch, 1925·1
Dentispray, 1925·1
Dentogen, 1925·1
Dentohexine, 1925·1
Dentol Topico, 1925·1
Dentolamina, 1925·1
Dentolina Plus, 1925·1
Dentomicin, 1925·1
Dentomycin, 1925·1
Dentophar, 1925·1
Dentosan Preparations, 1925·1
Dentosedina, 1925·1
Dentovax, 1925·1
Dentoxil, 1925·1
Dent's Extra Strength Toothache Gum, 1925·1
Dent's Maximum Strength Toothache Drops, 1925·1
Dentsiblen, 1925·1
Dentyl pH, 1925·2
Denubil, 1925·2
Denulcer, 1925·2
Denvar, 1925·2
Denvercrem, 1925·2
Denyl, 1925·2
Denzo, 1925·2
Deo, 1925·2
Deolin, 1925·2
Deopens, 1925·2
Deopid, 1925·2
Deotrin, 1925·2
9-Deoxo-9a-aza-9a-methyl-9a-homoerythromycin A Dihydrate, 159·1
(9*S*)-9-Deoxo-11-deoxy-9,11-{imino[(1*R*)-2-(2-methoxyethoxy)-ethylidene]oxy}erythromycin, 206·1
9-Deoxo-16,16-dimethyl-9-methylene-prostaglandin $E_2$, 1519·2
De-1-(5-oxo-L-proline)-de-2-L-glutamine-5-methionine-caerulein, 1746·2
Deoxycholic Acid, 1660·3
Deoxycoformycin, 579·2
2′-Deoxycoformycin, 579·2
11-Deoxycorticosterone Acetate, 1097·1
Deoxycorticosterone Pivalate, 1097·1
Deoxycorticosterone Trimethylacetate, 1097·1
Deoxycortone Acetate, 1097·1
Deoxycortone Pivalate, 1097·1
Deoxycortone Trimethylacetate, 1097·1
2-Deoxy-6-*O*-(3-deoxy-4-*C*-methyl-3-methylamino-β-L-arabinopyranosyl)-4-*O*-(2,6-diamino-2,3,4,6-tetradeoxy-D-*glycero*-hex-4-enopyranosyl)streptamine Sulphate, 254·3
2-Deoxy-4-*O*-(2,6-diamino-2,6-dideoxy-α-D-glucopyranosyl)-5-*O*-[3-*O*-(2,6-diamino-2,6-dideoxy-β-L-idopyranosyl)-β-D-ribofuranosyl]streptamine Sulphate, 215·1
2′-Deoxy-2′,2′-difluorocytidine Hydrochloride, 558·1
2′-Deoxy-2′,2′-difluorouridine, 558·2
6-Deoxy-7,8-dihydro-14-hydroxy-3-*O*-methyl-6-oxomorphine Hydrochloride, 75·2
6-Deoxy-7,8-dihydro-14-hydroxy-6-oxomorphine Hydrochloride, 76·1
6-Deoxy-7,8-dihydro-6-oxomorphine Hydrochloride, 45·2
*l*-Deoxyephedrine, 1124·1
*d*-Deoxyephedrine Hydrochloride, 1589·2
2′-Deoxy-5-ethyluridine, 632·1
2-Deoxy-2-fluoro-$^{18}$F-α-D-glucopyranose, 1523·3
2′-Deoxy-5-fluorouridine, 553·1
5′-Deoxy-5-fluorouridine, 547·3
Deoxyharringtonine, 558·3
6-Deoxy-5β-hydroxytetracycline Monohydrate, 206·2
2′-Deoxy-5-iodocytidine, 637·3
2′-Deoxy-5-iodouridine, 637·3
3-[6-*O*-(6-Deoxy-α-L-mannopyranosyl)-β-D-glucopyranosyloxy]-3′,4′,5,7-tetrahydroxyflavylium Chloride, 1703·2
6-Deoxy-L-mannose, 1738·1
1-Deoxy-1-methylamino-D-glucitol Antimonate, 600·3

*O*-2-Deoxy-2-methylamino-α-L-glucopyranosyl-(1→2)-*O*-5-deoxy-3-*C*-formyl-α-L-lyxofuranosyl-(1→4)-$N^3$,$N^3$-diamidino-D-streptamine, 256·1
*O*-2-Deoxy-2-methylamino-α-L-glucopyranosyl-(1→2)-*O*-5-deoxy-3-*C*-hydroxymethyl-α-L-lyxofuranosyl-(1→4)-$N^1$,$N^3$-diamidino-D-streptamine Sulphate, 205·3
2-Deoxy-2-(3-methyl-3-nitrosoureido)-D-glucopyranose, 584·1
6-Deoxy-3-*O*-methyl-6-oxomorphine Hydrogen Tartrate Hemipentahydrate, 45·1
(*R*)-3-(2-Deoxy-β-D-*erythro*-pentofuranosyl)-3,6,7,8-tetrahydroimidazo[4,5-*d*][1,3]diazepin-8-ol, 579·2
1-(2-Deoxy-β-D-ribofuranosyl)-5-fluoropyrimidine-2,4(1*H*,3*H*)-dione, 553·1
1-(2-Deoxy-β-D-ribofuranosyl)-5-methyluracil, 1755·3
1-(2-Deoxy-β-D-ribofuranosyl)-1,2,3,4-tetrahydro-5-methylpyrimidine-2,4-dione, 1755·3
Deoxyribonuclease, 1119·1
Deoxyribonuclease I, 1119·1
Deoxyribonuclease, Streptococcal, 1749·3
Deoxyribonucleic Acid, 1679·2
Deoxyspergualin Hydrochloride, 1360·2
15-Deoxyspergualin Hydrochloride, 1360·2
(−)-2′-Deoxy-3′-thiacytidine, 648·2
2′-Deoxy-5-trifluoromethyluridine, 655·3
Depacon, 1925·2
Depade, 1925·2
Depain Plus, 1925·2
Depakene, 1925·2
Depakin, 1925·2
Depakin Chrono, 1925·2
Depakine, 1925·2
Depakine Chrono, 1925·2
Depakine Crono, 1925·2
Depakote, 1925·2
Depalept, 1925·2
Depalept Chrono, 1925·2
Depallethrin, 1500·3
Depamag, 1925·2
Depamide, 1925·2
DepAndro, 1925·2
DepAndrogyn, 1925·2
Deparon, 1925·3
Depas, 1925·3
Depen, 1925·3
DepGynogen, 1925·3
Depicor, 1925·3
Depiderm, 1925·3
Depin, 1925·3
Depixol, 1925·3
Depizide, 1925·3
Deplecat, 1925·3
DepMedalone, 1925·3
Depnil, 1925·3
Depnon, 1925·3
Depo Moderin, 1925·3
Depo-Clinovir, 1925·3
Depocon, 1925·3
DepoCyt, 1925·3
DepoCyte, 1925·3
Depofin, 1925·3
Depogen, 1925·3
Depo-Gestin, 1925·3
Depoject, 1925·3
Depolan, 1925·3
Depolarising Muscle Relaxants, 1397·1
Depolarising Neuromuscular Blockers, 1397·1
Depolut, 1925·3
Depolymerised Heparins, 949·2
Depo-Medrate, 1925·3
Depo-Medrol Preparations, 1925·3
Depo-Medrone, 1925·4
Depo-Medrone with Lidocaine, 1925·4
Depon, 1925·4
Depon Maximum, 1925·4
Depo-Nisolone, 1925·4
Deponit, 1925·4
Depopred, 1925·4
Depo-Prodasone, 1925·4
Depo-Progesno, 1925·4
Depo-Progesta, 1925·4
Depo-Progevera, 1925·4
Depo-Provera, 1925·4
Depo-Ralovera, 1925·4
Depostat, 1925·4
Deposteron, 1925·4
Depotest, 1925·4
Depo-Testadiol, 1926·1
Depotestogen, 1926·1
Depot-Hal, 1926·1
Depot-H-Insulin, 1926·1
Depot-H15-Insulin, 1926·1
Depot-Insulin, 1926·1
Depot-Insulin S, 1926·1
Depotrone, 1926·1
Depot-Thrombophob-N, 1926·1
Deprakine, 1926·1
Deprakine Depot, 1926·1
Depramina, 1926·1
Deprancol, 1926·1
Depraser, 1926·1
Deprax, 1926·1
Deprece, 1926·1
Deprefax, 1926·1
Deprelio, 1926·1
Deprenyl, 1214·1
L-Deprenyl, 1214·1
Deprenyl, 1926·1
Depreotide, Technetium ($^{99m}$Tc), 1526·1
Depress, 1926·1
Depressan, 1926·1
Depression, 279·1
Depression, Manic— *see* Bipolar Disorder, 278·2
Deprexan, 1926·1
Deprexen, 1926·1
Deprexin, 1926·1
Deprilan, 1926·2
Deprilept, 1926·2
Deprimil, 1926·2
Deprocid, 1926·2
Deprodona, 1096·3
Deprodone, 1096·3
Deprodone Propionate, 1096·3
Deproic, 1926·2
Deproist Expectorant with Codeine, 1926·2
Depronal, 1926·2
*N*-Depropylpropafenone, 989·2
Deproxin, 1926·2
Deprozol, 1926·2
Depsonil, 1926·2
Depsonil-DZ, 1926·2
Depten, 1926·2
Deptran, 1926·2
Deptropina, Citrato de, 430·3
Deptropine Citrate, 430·3
Deptropini Citras, 430·3
Depuran, 1926·2
Depuratif Des Alpes, 1926·2
Depuratif Parnel, 1926·2
Depuratif Richelet, 1926·2
Depurativo, 1926·2
Depurativo Richelet, 1926·2
Depuratum, 1926·2
Depurfat, 1926·2
Depurol, 1926·2
Depygon, 1926·2
Depyrel, 1926·2
Deq, 1926·3
Dequacaine, 1926·3
Dequa-Coff, 1926·3
Dequa/Delin, 1926·3
Dequadin, 1926·3
Dequadin C, 1926·3
Dequadin Complex, 1926·3
Dequadin Mouth Paint, 1926·3
Dequa-Flu, 1926·3
Dequafungan, 1926·3
Dequalid, 1926·3
Dequalinetten, 1926·3
Dequalinii Chloridum, 1178·1
Dequalinium, 1926·3
Dequalinium Chloride, 1178·1
Dequalinium Salicylate, 1178·2
Dequalinium Undecenoate, 1178·2
Dequamed, 1926·3
Dequasept, 1926·3
Dequasine, 1926·3
Dequaspray, 1926·3
Dequavagyn, 1926·3
Dequin, 1926·3
Dequonal, 1926·3
Dequosangola, 1926·3
Deralbine, 1926·3
Deralin, 1926·3
Deralin, Slow— *see* Slow Deralin, 2295·1
Deratin, 1926·3
Derbac-C, 1926·3
Derbac-C— *see* Carylderm, 1872·3
Derbac-M, 1926·3
Dercolina, 1926·4
Dercome, 1926·4
Dercusan, 1926·4
Dercut, 1926·4
Dereme, 1926·4
Derifil, 1926·4
Deril, 1926·4
Derilate, 1926·4
Derinase Plus, 1926·4
Derinox, 1926·4
Deriphyllin, 1926·4
Deripil, 1926·4
Derivatio H, 1926·4
Derivoco, 1926·4
Derivon, 1926·4
Derm Hydralin, 1926·4
Derma Care, 1926·4
Derma Keri, 1926·4
Derma Viva, 1926·4
Dermabase, 1926·4
Dermabaz, 1926·4
Dermabel, 1926·4
Dermabiotico, 1926·4
Dermablend, 1926·4
Dermabond, 1926·4
Dermac, 1926·4
Dermac Crema, 1926·4
Dermac Jabon, 1927·1
Dermacalm-d, 1927·1
Dermacare, 1927·1
Derma-Care, 1927·1
Dermacerium, 1927·1
Dermacetin-Ped, 1927·1
Dermachrome, 1927·1
Dermacide, 1927·1
Dermacne, 1927·1
Dermacoat, 1927·1
Dermacol, 1927·1
Dermacolor, 1927·1
Dermacombin, 1927·1
Dermacort, 1927·1
Dermacreme, 1927·1
Dermacure, 1927·1
Dermacyd, 1927·1
Dermadex, 1927·1
Dermadex NN, 1927·1
Dermadine, 1927·1
Dermadrate, 1927·1
Dermaflex, 1927·1
Dermaflogil, 1927·2
Dermaflor, 1927·2
Dermaglos, 1927·2
Dermaglos Plus, 1927·2
Dermagor, 1927·2
Dermagor Ecran Solar, 1927·2
Dermagor-Antitranspirante, 1927·2
Dermagraft, 1927·2
Derm-Aid, 1927·2
Dermal C, 1927·2
Dermal Care, 1927·2
Dermal G, 1927·2
Dermal SA, 1927·2
Dermalar, 1927·2
Dermalibour, 1927·2
Dermalife, 1927·2
Dermalife Plus, 1927·2
Dermalisan, 1927·2
Dermallerg, 1927·2
Dermalo, 1927·2
Dermalog, 1927·2
Dermalog-C, 1927·2
Derma-loges N, 1927·3
Dermamina, 1927·3
Dermamist, 1927·3
Dermamycin, 1927·3
Derma-Mykotral, 1927·3
Dermana, 1927·3
Dermana Pasta, 1927·3
DermaNail, 1927·3
Dermanatur, 1927·3
Derman-Oil, 1927·3
Dermaor, 1927·3
Derma-Pax, 1927·3
Dermapro, 1927·3
Dermarell, 1927·3
Dermaren, 1927·3
Dermarest, 1927·3
Dermarest Dri-Cort, 1927·3
Dermarest Dricort Anti-Itch, 1927·3
Dermarest Plus, 1927·3
Dermase, 1927·3
Dermaseb, 1927·3
Dermasept Antifungal, 1927·3
Dermasil, 1927·3
Derma-Smoothe/FS, 1927·3
Dermasol, 1927·3
Dermasole, 1927·3
Dermasole DP, 1927·3
Dermasole N, 1927·3
Dermasone, 1927·4
Dermaspraid Antiseptique, 1927·4
Dermaspraid Demangeaison, 1927·4
Dermaspray, 1927·4
Dermaspray Demangeaison, 1927·4
Dermasten, 1927·4
Dermatan Sulfate, 892·2
Dermatan Sulfate Sodium, 892·2
Dermatán, Sulfato de, 892·2
Dermatan Sulphate, 892·2
Dermatan Sulphate Sodium, 892·2
Dermatar, 1927·4
Dermatech Liquid, 1927·4
Dermatech Wart Treatment, 1927·4
Dermatitis, Atopic— *see* Eczema, 1135·1
Dermatitis, Berloque, 1154·1
Dermatitis, Chronic Actinic— *see* Light-induced Skin Reactions, 1136·3
Dermatitis Herpetiformis, 1134·3
Dermatitis Relief, 1927·4
Dermatitis, Seborrhoeic— *see* Seborrhoeic Dermatitis, 1138·3
Dermatix, 1927·4
Dermatodoron, 1927·4
Dermatofides, 1927·4
Dermatol, 1927·4
Dermatological Drugs and Sunscreens, 1133·1
Dermatomyositis— *see* Polymyositis and Dermatomyositis, 1086·2
Dermatop, 1927·4
Dermatophytoses— *see* Skin Infections, 390·1
Dermatosis, Pigmented Purpuric— *see* Non-infective Skin Disorders, 401·2
Dermatovate, 1927·4
Dermatrans, 1927·4
Derm'attive, 1927·4
Derm'attive Solaire, 1927·4
Dermaval, 1927·4
Dermaveen, 1927·4
DermaVeen Preparations, 1927·4
DermaVite, 1928·1
Dermax, 1928·1
Dermazellon, 1928·1
Dermazin, 1928·1
Dermazinc, 1928·1
Dermazine, 1928·1
Dermazol, 1928·1
Dermazole, 1928·1
Dermazon, 1928·1
Dermdryl, 1928·1
Der-med, 1928·1
Dermed, Adco- — *see* Adco-Dermed, 1775·2
Dermedal, 1928·1
Dermenet, 1928·1
Dermeol, 1928·1
Dermestril, 1928·1
Dermex, 1928·1
Dermeze, 1928·1

Derm-Freeze, 1928·1
Dermic, 1928·1
Dermichthol, 1928·1
Dermicin, 1928·1
Dermicon, 1928·1
Dermi-cyl, 1928·1
Dermi-cyl Allerg, 1928·1
Dermi-cyl Ho-Lens-Complex, 1928·1
Dermi-cyl Schrunden, 1928·1
Dermidex, 1928·2
Dermifun, 1928·2
Dermil, 1928·2
Dermilan, 1928·2
Dermilia Flebozin, 1928·2
Dermilon, 1928·2
Dermimade Bacitracina, 1928·2
Dermimade Cloranfenicol, 1928·2
Dermimade Hidrocortisona, 1928·2
Derminiol, 1928·2
Derminovag, 1928·2
Dermirex, 1928·2
Dermirit, 1928·2
Dermisdin, 1928·2
Dermisone Beclo, 1928·2
Dermisone Epitelizante, 1928·2
Dermisone Tri Antibiotic, 1928·2
Dermitina, 1928·2
Dermizan, 1928·2
Dermizol, 1928·2
Dermizol G, 1928·2
Dermizol Trio, 1928·2
Dermo 6, 1928·2
Dermo Base Grassa, 1928·2
Dermo Base Magra, 1928·2
Dermo H Infantil— *see* Dermo Halibut Infantil, 1928·2
Dermo Halibut Infantil, 1928·2
Dermo Hubber, 1928·2
Dermo Lassar, 1928·2
Dermo Posterisan, 1928·2
Dermo Silanols, 1928·2
Dermo WAS, 1928·3
Dermoangiopan, 1928·3
Dermobacter, 1928·3
Dermobarrina, 1928·3
Dermobase, 1928·3
Dermobel, 1928·3
Dermo-Bell, 1928·3
Dermobene, 1928·3
Dermobet, 1928·3
Dermobeta, 1928·3
Dermobion, 1928·3
Dermobios, 1928·3
Dermobiotico, 1928·3
Dermobras, 1928·3
Dermocaine, 1928·3
Dermocal, 1928·3
Dermocalm, 1928·3
Dermocica, 1928·3
Dermocinetic, 1928·3
Dermocortal, 1928·3
Dermocrem, 1928·3
Dermocreme, 1928·3
Dermocridin, 1928·3
Dermocuivre, 1928·3
Dermodan, 1928·3
Dermodex, 1928·3
Dermodis, 1928·4
Dermodrin, 1928·4
Dermofenac, 1928·4
Dermofibrin C, 1928·4
Dermofilm, 1928·4
Dermofix, 1928·4
Dermofug, 1928·4
Dermofytol, 1928·4
Dermogaze, 1928·4
Dermogen, 1928·4
Dermoglos, 1928·4
Dermoil, 1928·4
Dermojela, 1928·4
Dermojuventus, 1928·4
Dermokin, 1928·4
Dermol, 1928·4
Dermol HC, 1928·4
Dermolate, 1928·4
Dermolin, 1928·4
Dermomycin, 1928·4
Dermomycose Liquido, 1928·4
Dermomycose Talco, 1928·4
Dermon, 1928·4
Dermopan, 1928·4
Dermoper, 1928·4
Dermoperative, 1928·4
Dermophil Indien, 1929·1
Dermophil Indien Nouvelle Formule, 1929·1
Dermoplast, 1929·1
Dermoplex Antifungal, 1929·1
Dermoplex Antiseptic, 1929·1
Dermoplex Calamine, 1929·1
Dermoprolyn, 1929·1
Dermoquinol, 1929·1
Dermorelle, 1929·1
Dermoretin, 1929·1
Dermosa Aureomicina, 1929·1
Dermosa Hidrocortisona, 1929·1
Dermosalic, 1929·1
Dermosed, 1929·1
Dermoseptic, 1929·1
Dermoskin, 1929·1
Dermoskin C, 1929·1
Dermosol, 1929·1
Dermosolon, 1929·1
Dermosona, 1929·1
Dermo-Steril, 1929·1
Dermo-Sulfuryl, 1929·1
Dermovagisil, 1929·1
Dermoval, 1929·1
Dermovan, 1929·2
Dermovat, 1929·2
Dermovate, 1929·2
Dermovate-NN, 1929·2
Dermovit, 1929·2
Dermovitamina, 1929·2
Dermowas, 1929·2
Dermowund, 1929·2
Dermox, 1929·2
Dermoxin, 1929·2
Dermoxinale, 1929·2
Dermoxyl, 1929·2
Derms, 1929·2
Dermtex HC with Aloe, 1929·2
Dermum, 1929·2
Dermuspray, 1929·2
Dermycose, 1929·2
Derobin Skin, 1929·2
Deroctyl, 1929·3
Derofen Miel, 1929·3
Deronga Heilpaste, 1929·3
Deroxat, 1929·3
Derozin, 1929·3
Derris, 1510·1
*Derris elliptica*, 1510·1
Derrumal, 1929·3
Derso TCC, 1929·3
Dertrase, 1929·3
Dertrin, 1929·3
Dervin, 1929·3
Derzid, 1929·3
Derzid-C, 1929·3
DES, 1548·1
Desacetyl Vinblastine Amide Sulfate, 593·3
Desacetylalacepril, 856·2
Desacetylcefalotin, 169·2
Desacetylcefotaxime, 176·1
Desacetyldiltiazem, 901·3
Desacetyl-lanatoside C, 893·1
17-Desacetylrocuronium, 1406·1
Desacetylvinblastine, 592·1
Desacil, 1929·3
Désaglybuzole, 333·1
Des-alanyl-1, Serine-125 Human Interleukin-2, 562·3
Desalark, 1929·3
Desalex, 1929·3
Desalfa, 1929·3
*N*-Desalkylflurazepam, 700·3, 718·2
*N*-Desalkyl-2-oxoquazepam, 718·2
Desamethasone, 1097·1
Desamin Same, 1929·3
2,1-Desamino-4,1-desthio-$O^{4,2}$-methyl[1-homocysteine]oxytocin, 1320·2
Desamino-oxytocin, 1322·3
Desamix Effe, 1929·3
Desamix-Neomicina, 1929·3
Desamon, 1929·3
Desanden, 1929·3
Desarell, 1929·3
Desarrol, 1929·3
Desatura, 1929·3
Desbenzoylindomethacin, 48·3
Desbly, 1929·3
Desbutylhalofantrine, 452·3
Descaling Agents, 1689·3
Descarbamylcefoxitin, 177·3
Descarboethoxyloratadine, 431·1
Desclidium, 1929·3
Descon, 1929·4
Descon AP, 1929·4
Descon Expectorante, 1929·4
Desconasal, 1929·4
Desconex, 1929·4
Descongestan, 1929·4
Descongestivo Cuve Nasal, 1929·4
Desconphar, 1929·4
Descutan, 1929·4
Desderman N, 1929·4
Desdol, 1929·4
Desec, 1929·4
Deselex, 1929·4
Desenex, 1929·4
Desenex Antifungal, Maximum Strength— *see* Maximum Strength Desenex Antifungal, 2116·3
DesenexMax, 1929·4
Desenfriol Preparations, 1929·4
Desenfriolito, 1929·4
Desenfriolito Con Paracetamol, 1930·1
Desenfriol-Ito Plus, 1930·1
Desenfriol-Ito TF, 1930·1
Desensib, 1930·1
Desensibilizante Chauvin, 1930·1
Desensitisation, 1650·2
Desentol, 1930·1
Deseril, 1930·1
Deserila, 1930·1
Desernil, 1930·1
Deserpidina, 892·3
Deserpidine, 892·3
Deserril, 1930·1
Desert Fever— *see* Coccidioidomycosis, 387·3
Desert Pure Calcium, 1930·1
Desert Rheumatism— *see* Coccidioidomycosis, 387·3
Desethylamiodarone, 861·2
Desethylamodiaquine, 447·1
*N*-Desethyloxybutynin, 487·1
Desethylzaleplon, 727·3
Desfatigan, 1930·1
Desfatin, 1930·1
Desferal, 1930·1
Desferin, 1930·1
Desferrioxamine Mesilate, 1033·1
Desferrioxamine Mesylate, 1033·1
Desferrioxamine Methanesulphonate, 1033·1
Desflam, 1930·1
Desfluorotriamcinolone Acetonide, 1096·3
Desflurane, 1297·2
Desflurano, 1297·2
Desfrin, 1930·1
Desglucolanatoside C, 851·1
Desglymidodrine, 959·2
Deshidroacetato Sódico, 1178·1
Deshidroacético, Ácido, 1178·1
Deshidroemetina, Hidrocloruro de, 603·2
Desicort, 1930·1
Desidoxepin, 1930·1
Desifluvoxamin, 1930·1
Desiken, 1930·1
Desinflam, 1930·1
Desinflam Biotic, 1930·1
Desinflex, 1930·1
Desintan P, 1930·1
Desintex, 1930·1
Desintex Infantile, 1930·1
Desintex-Choline, 1930·1
Desinvag, 1930·2
Desiperiden, 1930·2
Desipramina, Hidrocloruro de, 290·2
Desipramine, 300·1
Desipramine Hydrochloride, 290·2
Desipramini Hydrochloridum, 290·2
Desirel, 1930·2
Desirudin, 892·3
Desirudina, 892·3
Desisulpid, 1930·2
Desiticlopidin, 1930·2
Desitin, 1930·2
Desitin Creamy, 1930·2
Desitin Daily Care, 1930·2
Desitin Nappy Rash Ointment, 1930·2
Desitin with Zinc Oxide, 1930·2
Desitur, 1930·2
Desketo, 1930·2
Deslanoside, 893·1
Deslanosídeo, 893·1
Deslanósido, 893·1
Deslanosidum, 893·1
Deslor, 1930·2
Desloratadina, 431·1
Desloratadine, 431·1
Deslorelin, 1322·3
Deslorelina, 1322·3
Desmanol, 1930·2
Desmanol G, 1930·2
11-Desmethoxyreserpine, 892·3
Desmethylastemizole, 425·1
Desmethylchlordiazepoxide, 674·3
Desmethylchlorphenamine, 428·1
*N*-Desmethylchlorprothixene-sulfoxide, 682·3
*N*-Desmethylclobazam, 358·3
Desmethylclomipramine, 289·3
*N*-Desmethylclozapine, 688·2
Desmethyldiazepam, 674·3, 695·2, 710·3, 716·2
*N*-Desmethyldiazepam, 710·3
Desmethyldothiepin, 291·1
Desmethyldoxepin, 291·2
*N*-Desmethylflunitrazepam, 698·3
Desmethylimipramine Hydrochloride, 290·2
Desmethylindomethacin, 48·3
Desmethylmaprotiline, 306·2
*N*-Desmethylmesuximide, 366·2
Desmethylmethadone Hydrochloride, 1125·2
Desmethylmianserin, 307·2
6-*O*-Desmethylnaproxen, 65·3
Desmethylofloxacin, 239·3
Desmethylpantoprazole, 1283·1
*N*-Desmethylpheniramine, 438·3
*N*-Desmethylpromethazine, 439·3
*l*-(−)-Desmethylselegiline, 1214·3
*N*-Desmethylsertraline, 317·3
Desmethylsibutramine, 1593·2
*N*-Desmethylsildenafil, 1745·1
*N*-Desmethyltamoxifen, 585·3
*O*-Desmethyltramadol, 95·2
Desmethyltrimipramine, 320·3
*N*-Desmethylvenlafaxine, 322·3
*O*-Desmethylvenlafaxine, 322·3
*N*-Desmethylzolmitriptan, 473·3
*N*-Desmethylzopiclone, 730·1
Desmin, 1930·2
Desmogalen, 1930·2
Desmoline, 1930·2
Desmopresina, 1322·3
Desmopresina, Acetato de, 1322·3
Desmopressin, 1322·3
Desmopressin Acetate, 1322·3
Desmopressinum, 1322·3
Desmospray, 1930·2
Desmotabs, 1930·2
Desmycosin, 274·3
Desobesi-M, 1930·2
Desocol, 1930·2
Desocort, 1930·2
Desoform, 1930·3
Desogen, 1930·3

Desogestrel, 1547·2
Desol, 1930·3
Desolett, 1930·3
Desolone, 1096·3
Desomedine, 1930·3
Deson, 1930·3
Desonax, 1930·3
Desonida, 1096·3
Desonide, 1096·3
Desonide Pivalate, 1096·3
Desonide Sodium Phosphate, 1096·3
Desonol, 1930·3
Desoplus, 1930·3
Desorelle, 1930·3
Desoren, 1930·3
DesOwen, 1930·3
Desoxi, 1930·3
Desoxicortona, Acetato de, 1097·1
Desoxicortona, Pivalato de, 1097·1
Desoxil, 1930·3
Desoximetasona, 1096·3
Desoximetasone, 1096·3
Desoxirribonucleico, Ácido, 1679·2
Desoxycorticosterone Acetate, 1097·1
Desoxycorticosterone Pivalate, 1097·1
Desoxycorticosterone Trimethylacetate, 1097·1
Desoxycortone Acetate, 1097·1
Desoxycortone Enantate, 1097·1
Desoxycortone Phenylpropionate, 1097·1
Desoxycortone Pivalate, 1097·1
Desoxycortone Sodium Hemisuccinate, 1097·1
Desoxycortoni Acetas, 1097·1
L-Desoxyephedrine, 1124·1
*d*-Desoxyephedrine Hydrochloride, 1589·2
Desoxymethasone, 1096·3
6-Desoxy-6-methylene-naltrexone, 1044·1
6-Desoxy-6-methylene-naltrexone Hydrochloride, 1044·1
Desoxyn, 1930·3
Desoxynorephedrine, Racemic, 1584·3
Desoxypentose Nucleic Acid, 1679·2
Desoxyribonuclease, 1119·1
Desoxyribonucleic Acid, 1679·2
Desoxyribose Nucleic Acid, 1679·2
Despacilina, 1930·3
Despamen, 1930·3
Desparasil, 1930·3
Despex, 1930·3
Despigmentante, 1930·3
Desquam, 1930·3
Desquaman, 1930·3
De-squaman N, 1930·3
Desquamative Interstitial Pneumonia— *see* Diffuse Parenchymal Lung Disease, 1079·3
Desquam-X, 1930·3
Dessolets, 1930·3
Destamin, 1930·3
Destap, 1930·3
DeSTAT 3, 1930·4
Destilbenol, 1930·4
Destolit, 1930·4
Destoxican, 1930·4
Destrobac, 1930·4
Destroying Angel, 1717·3
Destroying Angel, White, 1717·3
63-Desulfohirudin, 892·3
Desulphatohirudin, 892·3
Desuric, 1930·4
Desyrel, 1930·4
DET, 1680·3
DET MS, 1930·4
DET MS Spezial, 1930·4
Detajmium Bitartrate, 893·1
Detamol, 1930·4
Detane, 1930·4
Detantol, 1930·4
Detaxtran Hydrochloride, 890·3
Detebencil, 1930·4
Deteclo, 1930·4
Detect Baby, 1930·4
Detemes, 1930·4
Detemir, Insulin, 334·3, 340·3
Detensiel, 1930·4
Detensor, 1930·4
Detergent, 1574·1
Detergil, 1930·4
DETF, 109·2
Dethamycin, 1930·4
Dethaphrine, 1930·4
Deticene, 1930·4
Detilem, 1930·4
Detimedac, 1930·4
Detoch, 1930·4
Detomidina, Hidrocloruro de, 689·3
Detomidine Hydrochloride, 689·3
Detomidine Hydrochloride for Veterinary Use, 689·3
Detox, 1931·1
Detox Thuja, 1931·1
Detoxalgine, 1931·1
Detoxergon, 1931·1
Detoxicon, 1931·1
Detraine, 1931·1
Detrixin, 1931·1
Detrol, 1931·1
Detrunorm, 1931·1
Detrusan, 1931·1
Detrusitol, 1931·1
Detrusor Hyperreflexia— *see* Urinary Incontinence and Retention, 476·1
Detrusor Instability— *see* Urinary Incontinence and Retention, 476·1
Detsel, 1931·1
Dettol Preparations, 1931·1
Dettolin, 1931·1
Dettonjab, 1931·2
Detulin, 1931·2
Deturgylone, 1931·2
Detuss, 1931·2
Deucoaler, 1931·2
Deucodol, 1931·2
Deucotos, 1931·2
Deucoval, 1931·2
Deursil, 1931·2
Devaron, 1931·2
Develanid, 1931·2
Develin, 1931·2
Deverol, 1931·2
Deverol mit Thiazid, 1931·2
Devil's Claw, 28·2
Devils Claw Plus, 1931·2
Devil's Claw Root, 28·2
Devil's Dung, 1658·1
Devincal, 1931·2
Devitol, 1931·2
Devitre, 1931·2
Devix, 1931·2
Devorfungi, 1931·2
Devrom, 1931·2
Dewax, 1931·2
Dex, 1931·2
Dex4 Glucose, 1931·2
Dexa, 1931·2
Dexa Aminofilin, 1931·2
Dexa ANB, 1931·2
Dexa Biciron, 1931·2
Dexa in der Ophtiole, 1931·2
Dexa Fenic, 1931·2
Dexa Loscon Mono, 1931·3
Dexa Polyspectran, 1931·3
Dexa Tavegil, 1931·3
Dexa Teosona, 1931·3
Dexa Vasoc, 1931·3
Dexa-Allvoran, 1931·3
Dexabene, 1931·3
Dexabion, 1931·3
Dexa-Brachialin N, 1931·3
Dexacap, 1931·3
Dexacidin, 1931·3
Dexacin, 1931·3
Dexacine, 1931·3
Dexa-Citoneurin, 1931·3
Dexa-clinit, 1931·3
Dexaclor, 1931·3
Dexacloran, 1931·3
Dexacobal, 1931·3
Dexacollyre, 1931·3
Dexacort, 1931·3
Dexacortal, 1931·3
Dexacortin, 1931·3
Dexacortin-K, 1931·3
Dexacortisone, 1931·3
Dexacrinin, 1931·4
Dexa-Cronobe, 1931·4
Dexadermil, 1931·4
Dexador, 1931·4
Dexadoze, 1931·4
DexaEDO, 1931·4
Dexa-Effekton, 1931·4
Dexafarm, 1931·4
Dexafed Cough, 1931·4
Dexafenicol, 1931·4
Dexaflam, 1931·4
Dexaflam N, 1931·4
Dexaflan, 1931·4
Dexafrin, 1931·4
Dexafurazon, 1931·4
Dexagalen, 1931·4
Dexagel, 1931·4
Dexagenta, 1931·4
Dexa-Gentamicin, 1931·4
Dexagenta-POS, 1931·4
Dexagil, 1931·4
Dexagrane, 1931·4
Dexagrin, 1931·4
Dexa-Helvacort, 1931·4
Dexahexal, 1931·4
Dexalergin, 1931·4
Dexalgen, 1932·1
Dexalin, 1932·1
Dexalocal, 1932·1
Dexalocal-F, 1932·1
Dexalone, 1932·1
DexAlone, 1932·1
Dexaltin, 1932·1
Dexam Constric, 1932·1
Dexambutol, 1932·1
Dexambutol-INH, 1932·1
Dexamed, 1932·1
Dexameral, 1932·1
Dexameson, 1932·1
Dexametasona, 1097·1
Dexametasona, Acetato de, 1097·1
Dexametasona, Fosfato de, 1097·2
Dexametasona, Fosfato Sódico de, 1097·2
Dexametasona, Isonicotinato de, 1097·2
Dexametasona, Metasulfobenzoato Sódico de, 1097·2
Dexametasone, 1097·1
Dexametax, 1932·1
Dexameth, 1932·1
Dexamethasone, 1097·1
Dexamethasone Acetate, 1097·1
Dexamethasone 21-Acetate, 1097·1
Dexamethasone Acetate Monohydrate, 1097·1
Dexamethasone 21-(Dihydrogen Phosphate), 1097·2
Dexamethasone 21-(Disodium Orthophosphate), 1097·2
Dexamethasone Hemisuccinate, 1098·2
Dexamethasone Isonicotinate, 1097·2
Dexamethasone 21-Isonicotinate, 1097·2
Dexamethasone Linoleate, 1098·2
Dexamethasone Palmitate, 1098·2
Dexamethasone Phenpropionate, 1098·2
Dexamethasone Phosphate, 1097·2
Dexamethasone Phosphate Sodium, 1097·2
Dexamethasone Pivalate, 1098·2
Dexamethasone Propionate, 1098·2
Dexamethasone Sodium Metasulfobenzoate, 1097·2
Dexamethasone Sodium Metasulphobenzoate, 1097·2
Dexamethasone Sodium Phosphate, 1097·2
Dexamethasone Sodium Succinate, 1098·2
Dexamethasone 21-(Sodium *m*-Sulphobenzoate), 1097·2
Dexamethasone Tebutate, 1098·2
Dexamethasone Troxundate, 1098·2
Dexamethasone Valerate, 1098·2
Dexamethasoni Acetas, 1097·1
Dexamethasoni Natrii Phosphas, 1097·2
Dexamethasonum, 1097·1
Dexametonal, 1932·1
Dexamfetamine Saccharate, 1586·3
Dexamfetamine Sulfate, 1585·3
Dexamfetamine Sulphate, 1585·3
Dexamicin, 1932·1
Dexamin, 1932·1
Dexaminoglutethimide, 527·1
Dexaminor, 1932·1
Dexamol Preparations, 1932·1
Dexamonozon, 1932·2
Dexamonozon N, 1932·2
Dexamphetamine Sulphate, 1585·3
Dexamphetamini Sulfas, 1585·3
Dexamycin, 1932·2
Dexamytrex, 1932·2
Dexamytrex Ophtiole, 1932·2
Dexa-Neuriberi, 1932·2
Dexaneurin, 1932·2
Dexanevral, 1932·2
Dexanfetamina, Sulfato de, 1585·3
Dexanil, 1932·2
Dexano, 1932·2
Dex-Antihist, 1932·2
Dexa-P, 1932·2
Dexaphen-SA, 1932·2
Dexa-Phlogont L, 1932·2
Dexapolyfra— *see* Framyxone, 2009·3
Dexa-Polyspectran, 1932·2
Dexapos, 1932·2
Dexa-POS, 1932·2
Dexaprof D, 1932·2
Dexa-ratiopharm, 1932·2
Dexa-Rhinaspray, 1932·2
Dexa-Rhinaspray Duo, 1932·2
Dexa-Rhinospray, 1932·3
Dexa-Rhinospray M, 1932·3
Dexa-Rhinospray N, 1932·3
Dexasalyl, 1932·3
Dexasil, 1932·3
Dexa-sine, 1932·3
Dexa-Siozwo, 1932·3
Dexason, 1932·3
Dexasone, 1932·3
Dexasporin, 1932·3
Dexatam, 1932·3
Dexatopic, 1932·3
Dexatrim, 1932·3
Dexatrim Plus Vitamin C, 1932·3
Dexatrim Plus Vitamins, 1932·3
Dexaval Preparations, 1932·3
Dexa-Vastrictol, 1932·3
Dexavison, 1932·3
Dexazen, 1932·4
Dexazona, 1932·4
Dexbenzetimide Hydrochloride, 481·1
Dexbromfeniramina, Maleato de, 426·1
Dexbrompheniramine Maleate, 426·1
Dexchloramine, 1932·4
Dexchlorphenamine Maleate, 427·3
Dexchlorpheniramine Maleate, 427·3
Dexchlorpheniramine Tannate, 428·2
Dexchlorpheniramini Maleas, 427·3
Dexclor, 1932·4
Dexclorfeniramina, Maleato de, 427·3
Dexcophan, 1932·4
Dexcophan Cough, 1932·4
Dexedrine, 1932·4
Dexef, 1932·4
Dexefrin, 1932·4
Dexelle, 1932·4
Dexemel, 1932·4
Dexeryl, 1932·4
Dexetimida, Hidrocloruro de, 481·1
Dexetimide, 481·1
Dexetimide Hydrochloride, 481·1
Dexfenfluramina, Hidrocloruro de, 1586·3
Dexfenfluramine Hydrochloride, 1586·3
DexFerrum, 1932·4
Dexibuprofen, 46·1
Dexicam, 1932·4
Dexicar, 1932·4
Dexide, 1932·4
Deximune, 1932·4
Dexipan, 1932·4
Dexir, 1932·4
Dexiron, 1932·4
Dexit, 1932·4
Dexi-Tuss, 1932·4

Dexium, 1932·4
Dexiven, 1932·4
Dexketoprofen Trometamol, 51·2
Dexketoprofeno Trometamol, 51·2
Dexlerg, 1932·4
Dexloxiglumide, 1271·3
Dexmedetomidina, Hidrocloruro de, 689·3
Dexmedetomidine Hydrochloride, 689·3
Dexmethsone, 1932·4
Dexmethylphenidate Hydrochloride, 1587·1
Dexmin, 1932·4
Dexne, 1933·1
Dexnon, 1933·1
Dexnorgestrel, 1563·2
Dexnorgestrel Acetime, 1563·2
Dexo, 1933·1
Dexodin, 1933·1
Dexodon, 1933·1
Dexofan, 1933·1
Dexofen, 1933·1
Dexol, 1933·1
Dexolan, 1933·1
Dexoline, 1933·1
Dexolix, Chemists Own— *see* Chemists Own Dry Raspy Cough, 1882·1
Dexomon, 1933·1
Dexon, 1933·1
Dexona, 1933·1
Dexona Eye/Ear, 1933·1
Dexoph, 1933·1
DexOptifen, 1933·1
Dexorange, 1933·1
Dexosyn-C, 1933·1
Dexosyn-N, 1933·1
Dex-Otic, 1933·1
DexPak, 1933·1
Dex-Panol, 1933·1
Dexpanol, 1933·1
Dexpantenol, 1727·2
Dexpanthenol, 1727·2
Dexpanthenolum, 1727·2
Dexpin, 1933·2
Dexrazoxane, 1036·1
Dexrazoxano, 1036·1
Dexsal, 1933·2
Dexsol, 1933·2
Dexsotalol, 1002·2
Dexsul, 1933·2
Dextasona, 1933·2
Dexthasol, 1933·2
Dextolyte-E, 1933·2
Dextoma, 1933·2
Dexton, 1933·2
Dextracin, 1933·2
Dextralpha, 1933·2
Dextran 1, 745·2
Dextran 1 for Injection, 745·2
Dextran 40, 745·3
Dextran 40 for Injection, 745·3
Dextran 60, 746·1
Dextran 60 for Injection, 746·1
Dextran 70, 746·2
Dextran 70 for Injection, 746·2
Dextran 75, 747·1
Dextran 110, 747·1
Dextran 2-(Diethylamino)ethyl Ether Hydrochloride, 890·3
Dextran 2,3-Dihydroxypropyl 2-Hydroxy-1,3-propanediyl Ether, 1145·2
Dextran Sulfate, 1679·2
Dextran Sulfate Potassium, 1679·2
Dextran Sulfate Sodium, 1679·2
Dextran Sulphate, 1679·2
Dextran Sulphate Sodium, 1679·2
Dextrano, Sulfato de, 1679·2
Dextranomer, 1145·2
Dextranómero, 1145·2
Dextranum 1, 745·2
Dextranum 40, 745·3
Dextranum 70, 746·2
Dextranum 75, 747·1
Dextranum 110, 747·1
Dextrarine Phenylbutazone, 1933·2
Dextrates, 1579·1
Dextratos, 1579·1
Dextrevit, 1933·2
Dextricea, 1933·2
Dextrin, 1427·1
Dextrina, 1427·1
Dextrinum, 1427·1
Dextrinum Album, 1427·1
Dextro, 1933·2
Dextro Amphetamine Sulphate, 1585·3
Dextro BS, 1933·2
Dextro Calcium Pantothenate, 1442·3
Dextro + Dipirona, 1933·2
Dextro GG, 1933·2
Dextro OG-T, 1933·2
Dextro Plus, 1933·2
Dextroamphetamine Sulfate, 1585·3, 1586·1
Dextrocalmine, 1933·2
Dextrodip, 1933·2
Dextrodiphenopyrine, 28·2
Dextrodyl, 1933·2
Dextrolyte, 1933·2
Dextrolyte-G, 1933·2
Dextrolyte-M, 1933·2
Dextrolyte-P, 1933·2
Dextromethorphan, 1117·3
Dextromethorphan Hydrobromide, 1117·3
Dextromethorphan Hydrobromide Monohydrate, 1117·3
Dextromethorphan Polistirex, 1118·2
Dextromethorphani Hydrobromidum, 1117·3
Dextrometorfano, 1117·3
Dextrometorfano, Hidrobromuro de, 1117·3
Dextromine, 1933·3
Dextromoramida, 28·2
Dextromoramida, Tartrato de, 28·2
Dextromoramide, 28·2
Dextromoramide Acid Tartrate, 28·2
Dextromoramide, Bitartrate de, 28·2
Dextromoramide Hydrogen Tartrate, 28·2
Dextromoramide Tartrate, 28·2
Dextromoramidi Tartras, 28·2
Dextro-Pantothenyl Alcohol, 1727·2
Dextropirac, 1933·3
Dextropropoxifeno, 28·3
Dextropropoxifeno, Hidrocloruro de, 28·3
Dextropropoxifeno, Napsilato de, 28·3
Dextropropoxyphene, 28·3
Dextropropoxyphene Hydrochloride, 28·3
Dextropropoxyphene Naphthalene-2-sulphonate Monohydrate, 28·3
Dextropropoxyphene Napsilate, 28·3
Dextropropoxyphene Napsylate, 28·3
Dextropropoxypheni Hydrochloridum, 28·3
Dextroral, 1933·3
Dextrorfano, 1679·3
Dextrorphan, 1118·1, 1679·3
Dextrorphan Hydrochloride, 1679·3
Dextrose, 1432·2
Dextrose, Anhydrous, 1432·2
Dextrostat, 1933·3
Dextrostix, 1933·3
Dextrosulphenidol, 269·2
Dextrosum Anhydricum, 1432·2
Dextrosum Monohydridicum, 1432·2
Dextrothyroxine Sodium, 893·2
Dextrotiroxina Sódica, 893·2
Dextrotos, 1933·3
Dextrovitase, 1933·3
Dexylin, 1933·3
Dezacor, 1933·3
Dezartal, 1933·3
Dezepan, 1933·3
Dezocina, 30·1
Dezocine, 30·1
Dezol, 1933·3
Dezor, 1933·3
Dezoral, 1933·3
DF-526, 1119·3
DF 118, 1933·3
DF Multi-Symptom, 1933·3
DFdU, 558·2
D-Feda II, 1933·3
D-Fluoretten, 1933·3
DFMO, 604·2
DFN, 1933·3
DFP, 1490·1
5-DFUR, 547·3
DG-6, 1933·3
DG-6 Iodopovidona, 1933·3
DG-5128, 343·2
D-Gam, 1933·3
D-Gluconic Acid, Iron (3+) Sodium Salt, 1444·3
DH-581, 986·3
DHA, 976·1, 1145·2
Dhabesol, 1933·3
Dhacillin, 1933·3
Dhacodine, 1933·3
Dhacold, 1933·3
Dhacopan, 1933·3
Dhacort, 1933·3
Dhactulose, 1933·4
DHAD, 575·2
Dhaflu, 1933·4
Dhalgesic, 1933·4
Dhalumag, 1933·4
Dhamol, 1933·4
Dhamotil, 1933·4
Dhaperazine, 1933·4
Dharmendra Antigen, 1707·1
DHA-S, 1566·1
Dhasedyl, 1933·4
Dhasedyl DM, 1933·4
Dhasolone, 1933·4
Dhatalin, 1933·4
Dhatifen, 1933·4
Dhatracin, 1933·4
Dhatrin, 1933·4
DHC, 1933·4
DHC Continus, 1933·4
DHC Plus, 1933·4
DHE, 603·2, 1933·4
DHEA, 1565·3
DHEAS, 1566·1
DHEP, 33·3
DHPG, 635·3
DHS Sal, 1933·4
DHS Tar, 1933·4
DHS Tar Gel, 1933·4
DHS Zinc, 1933·4
DHT, 1933·4
Di Anatoxal, 1933·4
Di Bella Regimen, 1335·1
Di Dolko, 1933·4
Di Retard, 1933·4
Di Te Anatoxal, 1933·4
Di Te, Anatoxal— *see* Anatoxal Di Te, 1799·1
Di Te Per Anatoxal, 1934·1
Di Te Per, Anatoxal— *see* Anatoxal Di Te Per, 1799·1
Dia-Aktivanad-N, 1934·1
DiaB Gel, 1934·1
Diabact UBT, 1934·1
Diabamyl, 1934·1
Dia-BASF, 1934·1
Diabecontrol, 1934·1
Diabeedol, 1934·1
Diabemet, 1934·1
Diabemide, 1934·1
Diabemin, 1934·1
Diaben, 1934·1
Diabene, 1934·1
Diabenol, 1934·1
Diabenor, 1934·1
Diabenyl T, 1934·1
Diabenyl-Rhinex, 1934·1
Diabeside, 1934·1
Diabesin, 1934·1
Diabesor, 1934·1
Diabestat, 1934·1
DiaBeta, 1934·1
Diabetamide, 1934·1
Diabetan S, 1934·1
Diabetase, 1934·1
Diabetes Insipidus, 1314·1
Diabetes Mellitus, 324·1
Diabetes-Gastreu S R40— *see* Acidum-phos-Gastreu, 1771·1
Diabetex, 1934·1
Diabetic Diarrhoea— *see* Diabetic Complications, 326·2
Diabetic Foot Disease— *see* Diabetic Complications, 326·2
Diabetic Gastroparesis— *see* Diabetic Complications, 326·2
Diabetic Ketoacidosis— *see* Diabetic Emergencies, 328·2
Diabetic Nephropathy— *see* Diabetic Complications, 326·2
Diabetic Neuropathy— *see* Diabetic Complications, 326·2
Diabetic Neuropathy, Pain of— *see* Diabetic Neuropathy, 6·1
Diabetic Patients, Hypertension in— *see* Hypertension, 825·1
Diabetic Retinopathy— *see* Diabetic Complications, 326·2
Diabetic Tussin, 1934·1
Diabetic Tussin DM, 1934·1
Diabetic Tussin EX, 1934·1
Diabetiks, 1934·1
Diabetisource Com Nutrishield, 1934·1
Diabetmin, 1934·1
Diabe-Tuss DM, 1934·2
Diabex, 1934·2
Diabexan, 1934·2
Diabexil, 1934·2
Diabiclor, 1934·2
Diabiformine, 1934·2
Diabines, 1934·2
Diabinese, 1934·2
Diabitex, 1934·2
Diaborale, 1934·2
Diabrezide, 1934·2
Diabur-5000, 1934·2
Diabur-Test 5000, 1934·2
Diacard, 1934·2
Diacare, 1934·2
Diaceplex, 1934·2
Diaceplex Simple, 1934·2
Diacerein, 30·1
Diacereína, 30·1
Diacerhein, 30·1
3,5-Diacetamido-2,4,6-tri-iodobenzoic Acid, 1060·1
α,5-Diacetamido-2,4,6-tri-iodo-*m*-toluic Acid, 1063·2
Diacetato de Diflorasona, 1099·3
Diacetato de Etinodiol, 1554·2
Diacetato de Propilenglicol, 1415·3
Diacetato de Sodio, 1191·3
Diacetato de Triamcinolona, 1110·2
Diacetazotol, 1178·2
Diacethiamine Hydrochloride, 1454·3
Diacetilmorfina, Hidrocloruro de, 30·2
Diacetolol, 848·2
1,1′-(3α,17β-Diacetoxy-5α-androstan-2β,16β-ylene)bis(1-methylpiperidinium) Dibromide, 1404·3
Diacetoxydiphenylisatin, 1282·3
1-(3α,17β-Diacetoxy-2β-piperidino-5α-androstan-16β-yl)-1-methylpiperidinium Bromide, 1409·3
Diacetyl Monoxime, 1050·3
Diacetylaminoazotoluene, 1178·2
4-Diacetylamino-2′,3-dimethylazobenzene, 1178·2
Diacetylated Monoglycerides, 1411·2
*N,N*-Diacetylcystine, 1113·2
Diacetyldiphenolisatin, 1282·3
Diacetylhydrazine, 224·1
9,3″-Diacetylmidecamycin, 231·3
Diacetylmorphine Hydrochloride, 30·2
Diacetylrhein, 30·1
Dia-Chek, 1934·2
Diaclaron, 1934·2
Diaclide, 1934·2
Diacol, 1934·2
Dia-Colon, 1934·2
Diacor, 1934·2
Diacron, 1934·2
Diactal, 1934·2
Di-Actane, 1934·2
Diacure, 1934·2
Diacure Plus, 1934·3
Diacylglycerols, 1412·1
Diadermina, 1934·3

Diadicon, 1934·3
Diadin M, 1934·3
Di-Adreson-F, 1934·3
Diadupsan, 1934·3
Dia-Eptal, 1934·3
Diaethanolamin, 1681·1
Diaethazinium Chloratum, 481·3
Diaformin, 1934·3
Diafuran, 1934·3
Diafusor, 1934·3
Diagesil, 1934·3
Diaglucide, 1934·3
Diaglyk, 1934·3
Diagnosis, 1934·3
Diagnostic Skin Testing Kit, 1934·3
Diagran, 1934·3
Diagran Minerale, 1934·3
Diagrin, 1934·3
Diahalt, 1934·3
Diah-Limit, 1934·3
Dialacid, 1934·3
Dialamine, 1934·3
Dialar, 1934·3
Dialens, 1934·3
Dialgin, 1934·3
Dialgine Forte, 1934·3
Dialgirex, 1934·3
Dialibra, 1934·3
Dialine, 1934·4
Dialisis Perit, 1934·4
Dialisol, 1934·4
Diallyl Disulfide, 1691·2
Diallylbarbitone, 668·3
Diallylbarbituric Acid, 668·3
5,5-Diallylbarbituric Acid, 668·3
*NN*′-Diallylbisnortoxiferinium Dichloride, 1398·3
*NN*′-Diallyl-6-[4-(4,4′-difluorobenzhydryl)piperazin-1-yl]-1,3,5-triazine-2,4-diyldiamine Bis(methanesulphonate), 1584·2
Diallylmalonylurea, 668·3
Diallylnortoxiferine Dichloride, 1398·3
Diallyltoxiferine Chloride, 1398·3
Diallymalum, 668·3
Dialoc, 1934·4
Dialon, 1934·4
Dialster, 1934·4
Dialudon, 1934·4
Dialume, 1934·4
Dialvit, 1934·4
Dialycare, 1934·4
Dialysis, Peritoneal, 1221·3
Dialysis Procedures, 1221·3
Dialysis Solutions, 1221·1
Dialysol Acide, 1934·4
Dialysol Bicarbonate, 1934·4
Dialytan H, 1934·4
Dialyte, 1934·4
Diamaze, 1934·4
Diamba, 1666·1
Diameb, 1934·4
Diamet, 1934·4
Diamexon, 1934·4
Diamfenetida, 104·1
Diamfenetide, 104·1
Diamfenetidum, 104·1
Diamicron, 1934·4
Diamin, 1934·4
3,6-Diaminoacridine Sulphate Dihydrate, 1165·3
2,4-Diamino-5-(4-bromo-3,5-dimethoxybenzyl)pyrimidine, 165·3
Diaminocillina, 1934·4
2,4-Diamino-6-(2,5-dichlorophenyl)-*S*-triazine Maleate, 1267·3
*O*-2,6-Diamino-2,6-dideoxy-β-L-idopyranosyl-(1→3)-*O*-β-D-ribofuranosyl-(1→5)-*O*-[2-amino-2-deoxy-α-D-glucopyranosyl-(1→4)]-2-deoxystreptamine Sulphate, 612·3
2,4-Diamino-6-(2,5-dimethoxybenzyl)-5-methylpyrido[2,3-*d*]pyrimidine Mono(2-hydroxyethanesulphonate), 580·1
Diaminodiphenylsulfone, 202·2
6,9-Diamino-2-ethoxyacridine Lactate, 1165·3
L-2,6-Diaminohexanoic Acid, 1439·1
L-2,6-Diaminohexanoic Acid Acetate, 1439·2
L-2,6-Diaminohexanoic Acid Hydrochloride, 1439·2
3,6-Diamino-10-methylacridinium Chloride 3,6-Diaminoacridine Monohydrochloride, 1165·3
3,6-Diamino-10-methylacridinium Chloride Hydrochloride 3,6-Diaminoacridine Dihydrochloride, 1165·3
3-[2-(Diaminomethyleneamino)thiazol-4-ylmethylthio]-*N*-sulphamoylpropionamidine, 1265·2
(2*S*)-2,4-Diamino-4-oxobutanoic Acid Monohydrate, 1422·1
2,6-Diamino-4-piperidinopyrimidine 1-Oxide, 960·1
3,4-Diaminopiridina, 1489·1
Di(α-aminopropionic)-β-disulphide, 1426·3
*N*-{4-[(2,4-Diamino-6-pteridinylmethyl)methylamino]benzoyl}-L-glutamic Acid, 568·2
*N*-(*p*-{1-[(2,4-Diamino-6-pteridinyl)methyl]propyl}benzoyl)-L-glutamic Acid, 550·1
3,4-Diaminopyridine, 1489·1
Diaminopyrimidine Antibacterials, 119·3
Diaminopyrimidine Antimalarials, 444·1
3,5-Diamino-2-(*p*-sulfamoylphenylazo) Benzoic Acid, 258·1
2-[4-(4,6-Diamino-1,3,5-triazin-2-ylamino)phenyl]-1,3,2-dithiarsolan-4-ylmethanol, 606·1
α,δ-Diaminovaleric Acid, 1442·3
L-2,5-Diaminovaleric Acid, 1442·3
Diamitex, 1934·4
*cis*-Diammine(cyclobutane-1,1-dicarboxylato)platinum, 533·3
*cis*-Diamminedichloroplatinum, 538·1
*cis*-Diammine(glycolato-$O^1$,$O^2$)platinum, 576·2
Diammonium Hydrogen Orthophosphate, 1654·1
Diammonium Hydrogen Phosphate, 1654·1
Diamond Green B, 1185·2
Diamond Green G, 1171·1
Diamorf, 1934·4
Diamoril, 1934·4
Diamorphine Hydrochloride, 30·2
Diamox, 1934·4
Diamphenethide, 104·1
Diamplicil, 1934·4
Dianben, 1934·4
Diane, 1934·4
Diane-35 ED, 1934·4
Dianeal, 1935·1
Dianette, 1935·1
Dianhydrogalactitol, 573·3
1,4:3,6-Dianhydro-D-glucitol, 941·1
1,4:3,6-Dianhydro-D-glucitol 2,5-Dinitrate, 941·1
1,4:3,6-Dianhydro-D-glucitol 5-Nitrate, 942·1
Dianicotyl, 1935·1
Dianid, 1935·1
Diano, 1935·1
Dianoct, 1935·1
Dianormax, 1935·1
Di-Antalvic, 1935·1
Dianthon, 1261·1
Diapam, 1935·1
Diapanil, 1935·1
Diaparene Corn Starch, 1935·1
Diaparene Diaper Rash, 1935·1
Diapatol, 1935·1
Diaper Guard, 1935·1
Diaper Rash, 1935·1
Diaphal, 1935·1
Diaphenylsulfone, 202·2
Diapid, 1935·1
Diapine, 1935·1
Diapo, 1935·1
Diapool, 1935·1
Diaquitte, 1935·2
Diarcalm, 1935·2
Diaren, 1935·2
Diarent, 1935·2
Diaretyl, 1935·2
Diarex, 1935·2
Diareze, 1935·2
Diarfin, 1935·2
Diargal, 1935·2
Diarigoz, 1935·2
Diaril, 1935·2
Diarim, 1935·2
Diarlac, 1935·2
Diarlop, 1935·2
Diarman, 1935·2
Diaro, 1935·2
Diarodil, 1935·2
Diarona, 1935·2
Diaront Mono, 1935·2
Diarresec, 1935·2
Diarrest, 1935·2
Diarrest RF, 1935·2
Diarret, 1935·2
Diarrex, 1935·2
Diarr-Eze, 1935·2
Diarrhea Relief, 1935·2
Diarrheel S, 1935·2
Diarrhoea, 1241·1
Diarrhoea, Antibiotic-associated— *see* Antibiotic-associated Colitis, 128·1
Diarrhoea Complex, 1935·2
Diarrhoea, Diabetic— *see* Diabetic Complications, 326·2
Diarrhoea, HIV-associated— *see* HIV-associated Wasting and Diarrhoea, 623·2
Diarrhoea, Infective— *see* Gastro-enteritis, 127·3
Diarrhoea Mixture, Chemists Own— *see* Chemists Own Diarrhoea Mixture, 1882·1
Diarrhoea Relief, Chemists Own— *see* Chemists Own Diarrhoea Relief, 1882·1
Diarrhoea Relief Tablets, 1935·2
Diarrhoea, Travellers'— *see* Gastro-enteritis, 127·3
Diarrhoea, Viral— *see* Gastro-enteritis, 618·2
Diarrhoesan, 1935·2
Diarrhoesan SC, 1935·3
Diarril, 1935·3
Diarrocalmol, 1935·3
Diarsed, 1935·3
Diarsenic Trioxide, 1657·1
Diarstop, 1935·3
Diarzero, 1935·3
Diasatin, 1282·3
Diascan, 1935·3
Diascreen Tests, 1935·3
Diasec, 1935·3
Diasectral, 1935·3
Diasef, 1935·3
Diaseptyl, 1935·3
Diasgest, 1935·3
Diasorb, 1935·3
Diastabol, 1935·3
Diastase, 1654·2
Diastat, 1935·3
Diastix, 1935·3
Diastone, 1935·4
Diastop, 1935·4
Diatabs, 1935·4
Diatec, 1935·4
Diatelan, 1935·4
Diatex, 1935·4
Diathynil, 1935·4
Diatil, 1935·4
Diatin, 1935·4
Diatol, 1935·4
Diatolil, 1935·4
Diatomaceous Earth, 1581·3
Diatomite, 1581·3
Diatracin, 1935·4
Diatrizoate Meglumine, 1060·2
Diatrizoate Sodium, 1060·2
Diatrizoic Acid, 1060·1
Diatrum, 1935·4
Diatussin, 1935·4
Diatx, 1935·4
Diatx Fe, 1935·4
Diaval, 1935·4
Diaveridina, 603·2
Diaveridine, 603·2
Dia-Vite, 1935·4
Diawern, 1935·4
Diaz, 1935·4
Diazelong, 1935·4
Diazemuls, 1935·4
Diazep, 1935·4
Diazepam, 690·1
Diazepamum, 690·1
Diazepan, 1935·4
Diazicuona, 546·3
Diazinon, 1504·2
Diaziquone, 546·3
Diazol, 1935·4
Diazolen, 1935·4
Diazolinum, 436·3
Diazon, 1935·4
Diazoxide, 893·2
Diazóxido, 893·2
Diazoxidum, 893·2
Diba, 1935·4
Dibacilina, 1935·4
Dibagesic, 1935·4
Diban, 1936·1
Dibapec Compuesto, 1936·1
Dibaprim, 1936·1
Dibasic Ammonium Phosphate, 1654·1
Dibasic Calcium Phosphate, 1225·2
Dibasic Magnesium Phosphate Trihydrate, 1228·1
Dibasic Potassium Phosphate, 1230·3
Dibasic Sodium Phosphate, 1231·1
Dibasona, 1936·1
Dibasul, 1936·1
Dibaterr, 1936·1
Dibazol, 1659·2
Dibecon, 1936·1
Dibekacin Sulfate, 205·2
Dibekacin Sulphate, 205·2
Dibekacina, Sulfato de, 205·2
Dibelet, 1936·1
Dibendril, 1936·1
Dibendyl, 1936·1
Dibendyl Forte CD, 1936·1
Dibent, 1936·1
Dibenyline, 1936·1
5*H*-Dibenz[*b,f*]azepine-5-carboxamide, 353·3
2-[4-(3-5*H*-Dibenz[*b,f*]azepin-5-ylpropyl)piperazin-1-yl]ethanol Dihydrochloride, 311·1
Dibenzepin Hydrochloride, 290·3
Dibenzepina, Hidrocloruro de, 290·3
Dibenzheptropine Citrate, 430·3
3-(5*H*-Dibenzo[*a,d*]cyclohepten-5-ylidene)-*NN*-dimethylpropylamine Hydrochloride, 1393·1
4-(5*H*-Dibenzo[*a,d*]cyclohepten-5-ylidene)-1-methylpiperidine Hydrochloride Sesquihydrate, 430·1
3-(5*H*-Dibenzo[*a,d*]cyclohept-5-enyl)propyl(methyl)amine Hydrochloride, 316·2
Dibenzoilmetano, 1145·2
2-[2-(4-Dibenzo[*b,f*][1,4]thiazepin-11-yl-1-piperazinyl)ethoxy]ethanol Fumarate (2:1) Salt, 718·2
3-(Dibenzo[*b,e*]thiepin-11-ylidene)propyldimethylamine Hydrochloride, 291·1
3-(Dibenzo[*b,e*]thiepin-11(6*H*)-ylidene)tropane Hydrochloride, 491·1
Dibenz[*b,f*][1,4]oxazepine, 1676·3
(*E*)-3-(Dibenz[*b,e*]oxepin-11-ylidene)propyldimethylamine Hydrochloride, 291·2
Dibenzoyl Peroxide, 1143·2
Dibenzoylmethane, 1145·2
4,6-Dibenzyl-4,6-diaza-1-thioniatricyclo[6.3.0.$0^{3,7}$]undecan-5-one 2-Oxobornane-10-sulphonate, 1017·3
*N,N*′-Dibenzylethylenediammonium Bis[(6*R*)-6-(2-phenoxyacetamido)penicillanate], 163·2
*NN*′-Dibenzylethylenediammonium Bis[(6*R*)-6-(2-phenylacetamido)penicillanate], 162·3
Dibenzyline, 1936·1
(+)-1,3-Dibenzylperhydro-2-oxothieno[1′,2′:1,2]thieno[3,4-*d*]-imidazol-5-ium 2-Oxobornane-10-sulphonate, 1017·3
Dibenzyran, 1936·1
Dibertil, 1936·1
Dibetasol, 1936·1

Dibetid, 1936·1
Dibetop, 1936·1
Dibetop Q, 1936·1
Dibilan F, 1936·1
Dibional, 1936·1
Dibistic, 1936·1
Diblocin, 1936·1
Dibondrin, 1936·1
Dibotermin Alfa, 768·1
Dibro-Be Mono, 1936·1
3,5-Dibromo-*N*-(4-bromophenyl)-2-hydroxybenzamide, 1171·2
Dibromochloropropane, 1503·1
1,2-Dibromo-3-chloropropane, 1503·1
Dibromocloropropano, 1503·1
1,6-Dibromo-1,6-dideoxy-D-galactitol, 573·3
1,6-Dibromo-1,6-dideoxy-D-mannitol, 573·2
Dibromodulcitol, 573·3
1,2-Dibromoethane, 1505·1
4′,6′-Dibromo-α-[(*trans*-4-hydroxycyclohexyl)amino]-2-thiophene-carboxy-*o*-toluidide, 1125·2
3,5-Dibromo-4-hydroxyphenyl 2-Ethylbenzofuran-3-yl Ketone, 414·3
3,5-Dibromo-2-hydroxy-*N*-phenylbenzamide, 1171·2
Dibromol, 1936·1
Dibromomannitol, 573·2
Dibromopropamidine Isethionate, 1178·2
5,7-Dibromoquinolin-8-ol, 165·3
*trans*-4-[(3,5-Dibromosalicyl)amino]cyclohexanol, 1117·3
3,5-Dibromosalicylanilide, 1171·2
4′,5-Dibromosalicylanilide, 1171·2
Dibromotirosina, 1597·3
3,3′-Dibromo-4,4′-trimethylenedioxydibenzamidine Bis(2-hydroxyethanesulphonate), 1178·2
Dibromotyrosine, 1597·3
3,5-Dibromo-L-tyrosine, 1597·3
Dibrompropamidina, Isetionato de, 1178·2
Dibrompropamidine Isetionate, 1178·2
Dibromsalan, 1171·2
Dibromuro de Diquat, 1504·3
Dibromuro de Etileno, 1505·1
Dibroxin, 1936·1
Dibtrigen, 1936·1
Dibucaine, 1373·2
Dibucaine Hydrochloride, 1373·2
Dibucaine Number— *see* Plasma Cholinesterase Deficiency, 1408·1
Dibucainium Chloride, 1373·2
Dibufen, 1936·2
Dibunafon, 1936·2
Dibunato de Sodio, 1130·2
Dibutamide, 1653·1
3,4-Dibutoxy-3-cyclobutene-1,2-dione, 1158·1
Dibutyl Benzene-1,2-dicarboxylate, 1503·1
Dibutyl Phthalate, 1503·1
Dibutyl Sebacate, 1679·3
(*RS*)-3-Dibutylamino-1-(1,3-dichloro-6-trifluoromethyl-9-phenanthryl)propan-1-ol Hydrochloride, 452·2
2-Dibutylamino-2-(4-methoxyphenyl)acetamide, 1653·1
3-Dibutylaminopropyl 4-Aminobenzoate Sulphate, 1372·3
2,6-Di-*tert*-butyl-*p*-cresol, 1171·3
Dibutylis Phthalas, 1503·1
*NN*-Dibutyl-*N*′-(3-phenyl-1,2,4-oxadiazol-5-yl)ethylenediamine Hydrochloride, 878·2
Dibutyryl Cyclic AMP Sodium, 1663·2
DIC, 544·2
1,5-Dicaffeoylquinic Acid, 1678·3
Dicainum, 1385·1
Dical, 1936·2
Di-Calcii-Plex, 1936·2
Dicalcium, 1936·2
Dicalcium Orthophosphate, 1225·2
Dicalcium Phosphate, 1225·2
Dical-D, 1936·2
Dicalm, 1936·2
Dicalmir, 1936·2
Dicalys 11, 1936·2
Dicalys 17, 1936·2
Dicap, 1936·2
3-(3,3′-Dicarboxy-4,4′-dihydroxybenzhydrylidene)-6-oxocyclohexa-1,4-diene-1-carboxylic Acid, Triammonium Salt, 1757·3
Dicavin, 1936·2
Dicentril, 1936·2
Dicepin B6, 1936·2
Dicetel, 1936·2
Dicfafena, 1936·2
Dichloralphenazone, 697·1
Dichlorbenzol, 1728·3
Dichlordimethylhydantoin, 1178·2
Dichlorisone Acetate, 1099·3
Dichloroacetic Acid, 1304·2, 1747·2
1-(Dichloroacetyl)-1,2,3,4-tetrahydroquinolin-6-ol 2-Furoic Acid Ester, 615·2
2-(2,6-Dichloroanalino)phenylacetoxyacetic Acid, 11·2
2-(2,6-Dichloroanilino)-2-imidazoline, 885·2
[*o*-(2,6-Dichloroanilino)phenyl]acetate Glycolic Acid Ester, 11·2
[2-(2,6-Dichloroanilino)phenyl]acetic Acid, 32·1
4-(2,6-Dichloroanilino)-3-thiopheneacetic Acid, 36·2
(±)-4-(3,4-Dichlorobenzamido)-*N*-(3-methoxypropyl)-*N*-pentylglutaramic Acid, 1271·3
1,2-Dichlorobenzene, 1724·3
1,4-Dichlorobenzene, 1728·3
4,5-Dichlorobenzene-1,3-disulphonamide, 894·1
Dichlorobenzyl Alcohol, 1178·3
2,4-Dichlorobenzyl Alcohol, 1178·3
(2,6-Dichlorobenzylideneamino)guanidine Acetate, 926·2
Dichlorobenzylidine Antimalarials, 444·1
1-(2,4-Dichlorobenzyl)indazole-3-carboxylic Acid, 565·3
2-(2,4-Dichlorobenzyl)-4-(1,1,3,3-tetramethylbutyl)phenol, 198·1
1,1-Dichloro-2,2-bis(*p*-chlorophenyl)ethylene, 1502·2
(±)-1-{2,4-Dichloro-β-[(7-chlorobenzo[*b*]thien-3-yl)methoxy]phenethyl}imidazole Nitrate, 408·1
1-[2,4-Dichloro-β-(4-chlorobenzyloxy)phenethyl]imidazole, 397·1
(±)-1-[2,4-Dichloro-β-(4-chlorobenzyloxy)phenethyl]imidazole Nitrate, 397·2
1-[2,4-Dichloro-β-(4-chlorobenzyl)thiophenethyl]imidazole Nitrate, 408·2
(*RS*)-2,2-Dichloro-*N*-[4-chloro-α-(chloromethyl)phenacyl]acetamide, 1177·3
(*Z*)-1-{2,4-Dichloro-β-[2-(*p*-chlorophenoxy)ethoxy]-α-methylstyryl}imidazole Nitrate, 407·2
1,1-Dichloro-2-(2-chlorophenyl)-2-(4-chlorophenyl)ethane, 575·1
2,7-Dichloro-9-[(4-chlorophenyl)methylene]-α-[(dibutylamino)methyl]-9*H*-fluorene-4-methanol, 453·3
1-[2,4-Dichloro-β-(2-chloro-3-thenyloxy)phenethyl]imidazole, 409·3
2-[4-(2,2-Dichlorocyclopropyl)phenoxy]-2-methylpropionic Acid, 884·2
1,3-Dichloro-α-[2-(dibutylamino)ethyl]-6-trifluoromethyl-9-phenanthrene-methanol Hydrochloride, 452·2
1-[2,4-Dichloro-β-(2,4-dichlorobenzyloxy)phenethyl]imidazole, 405·2
1-[2,4-Dichloro-β-(2,6-dichlorobenzyloxy)phenethyl]imidazole, 401·3
1,6-Dichloro-1,6-dideoxy-β-D-fructofuranosyl 4-Chloro-4-deoxy-α-D-galactopyranoside, 1450·1
Dichlorodiethylsulfide, 1679·3
Dichlorodiethylsulphide, 1679·3
2,2-Dichloro-1,1-difluoroethyl Methyl Ether, 1304·1
Dichlorodifluoromethane, 1236·1
2,2-Dichloro-1,1-difluoro-1-methoxyethane, 1304·1
(±)-1-(2,4-Dichloro-10,11-dihydro-5*H*-dibenzo[*a*,*d*]cyclohepten-5-yl)imidazole, 397·1
(±)-[2,6-Dichloro-4-(4,5-dihydro-3,5-dioxo-*as*-triazin-2(3*H*)-yl)phenyl](*p*-fluorophenyl)acetonitrile, 606·1
6,7-Dichloro-1,5-dihydroimidazo[2,1-*b*]quinazolin-2(3*H*)-one Hydrochloride, 1654·3
9α,21-Dichloro-11β,17-dihydroxy-16α-methylpregna-1,4-diene-3,20-dione 17-(2-Furoate), 1107·2
9α,11β-Dichloro-17α,21-dihydroxypregna-1,4-diene-3,20-dione 21-Acetate, 1099·3
1,3-Dichloro-5,5-dimethylhydantoin, 1178·2
1,3-Dichloro-5,5-dimethylimidazolidine-2,4-dione, 1178·2
2,4-Dichloro-3,5-dimethylphenol, 1178·3
3,5-Dichloro-2,6-dimethylpyridin-4-ol, 603·1
Dichlorodiphenyltrichloroethane, 1502·1
1,2-Dichloroethane, 1505·1
2,2-Dichloro-*N*-(2-ethoxyethyl)-*N*-[4-(4-nitrophenoxy)benzyl]acetamide, 605·2
[2,3-Dichloro-4-(2-ethylacryloyl)phenoxy]acetic Acid, 913·2
(*S*)-3,5-Dichloro-*N*-(1-ethylpyrrolidin-2-ylmethyl)-2-hydroxy-6-methoxybenzamide, 719·2
9α,11β-Dichloro-6α-fluoro-21-hydroxy-16α,17α-isopropylidenedioxypregna-1,4-diene-3,20-dione, 1100·1
2,2-Dichloro-*N*-[(α*S*,β*R*)-α-(fluoromethyl)-β-hydroxy-4-methanesulfonylphenethyl]acetamide, 213·3
(*RS*)-*N*-[2,5-Dichloro-4-(1,1,2,3,3,3-hexafluoropropoxy)phenylcarbamoyl]-2,6-difluorobenzamide, 1507·1
1-[2,5-Dichloro-4-(1,1,2,3,3,3-hexafluoropropoxy)phenyl]-3-(2,6-difluorobenzoyl)urea, 1507·1
2,2-Dichloro-*N*-(2-hydroxyethyl)-*N*-[4-(4-nitrophenoxy)benzyl]acetamide, 603·1
(α*R*,β*R*)-2,2-Dichloro-*N*-(β-hydroxy-α-hydroxymethyl-4-methylsulphonylphenethyl)acetamide, 269·2
2,2-Dichloro-*N*-[(α*R*,β*R*)-β-hydroxy-α-hydroxymethyl-4-nitrophenethyl]acetamide, 185·1
2,6-Dichloro-*N*-(imidazolidin-2-ylidene)aniline, 885·2
2,6-Dichloro-$N^1$-imidazolidin-2-ylidene-*p*-phenylenediamine Hydrochloride, 864·1
2′,4′-Dichloro-2-imidazol-1-ylacetophenone (*Z*)-*O*-(2,4-Dichlorobenzyl)oxime Mononitrate, 407·3
*O*-2,5-Dichloro-4-iodophenyl *O*,*O*-Dimethyl Phosphorothioate, 1506·3
Dichloroisocyanuric Acid, 1191·3
Dichlorometaxylenol, 1178·3
Dichloromethane, 1473·1
Dichloromethane Diphosphonate Disodium, 770·2
3,4-Dichloro-α-methoxybenzylpenicillin Potassium, 198·1
2,2′-Dichloro-*N*-methyldiethylamine Hydrochloride, 537·1
Dichloromethylene Diphosphonate Disodium, 770·2
(Dichloromethylene)diphosphonic Acid, 770·2
[2,3-Dichloro-4-(2-methylene-1-oxobutyl)phenoxy]acetic Acid, 913·2
5,7-Dichloro-2-methylquinolin-8-ol, 187·3
2′,5-Dichloro-4′-nitrosalicylanilide, 110·1
Dichlorophen, 104·1
Dichlorophenoxyacetic Acid, 1503·2
2,4-Dichlorophenoxyacetic Acid, 1503·2
2-[1-(2,6-Dichlorophenoxy)ethyl]-2-imidazoline Hydrochloride, 1041·2
4,6-Dichloro-3-[(*E*)-2-(phenylcarbamoyl)vinyl]indole-2-carboxylic Acid, 1691·3
Dichlorophenylcarbinol, 1178·3
1-(3,4-Dichlorophenyl)-5-isopropylbiguanide Hydrochloride, 452·1
(6*R*)-6-[3-(2,6-Dichlorophenyl)-5-methylisoxazole-4-carboxamido]penicillanic Acid, 205·2
7-{4-[4-(2,3-Dichlorophenyl)-piperazin-1-yl]butoxy}-3,4-dihydroquinolin-2(1*H*)-one, 671·1
*cis*-1-{[2-(2,4-Dichlorophenyl)-4-[(2-propynyloxy)methyl]-1,3-dioxolan-2-yl]methyl}-1*H*-imidazole Hydrochloride, 407·3
(1*S*,4*S*)-4-(3,4-Dichlorophenyl)-1,2,3,4-tetrahydro-1-naphthyl(methyl)amine Hydrochloride, 317·2
(±)-1-[2,4-Dichloro-β-{[*p*-(phenylthio)benzyl]oxy}phenethyl]imidazole Mononitrate, 397·3
6-(2,3-Dichlorophenyl)-1,2,4-triazine-3,5-diyldiamine, 363·3
1-{4-[[2-(2,4-Dichlorophenyl)-*r*-2-(1*H*-1,2,4-triazol-1-ylmethyl)-1,3-dioxolan-*c*-4-yl]methoxy]phenyl}-4-isopropylpiperazine, 409·3
Dichloropropane, 1473·1
1,2-Dichloropropane, 1473·1
5,7-Dichloroquinolin-8-olchloroxine5-chloroquinolin-8-olcloxyquin, 220·3
4-(Dichlorosulphamoyl)benzoic Acid, 1181·2
Dichlorotetrafluoroethane, 1235·3
1,2-Dichloro-1,1,2,2-tetrafluoroethane, 1235·3
Dichlorotetraiodofluorescein, 1740·1
Dichlorotetraiodofluorescein, Dipotassium Salt, 1740·1
Dichlorotetraiodofluorescein, Disodium Salt, 1740·1
[2,3-Dichloro-4-(2-thenoyl)phenoxy]acetic Acid, 1012·2
*N*-(2,6-Dichloro-*m*-tolyl)anthranilic Acid, 55·1
1,3-Dichloro-1,3,5-triazine-2,4,6(1*H*,-3*H*,5*H*)-trione Sodium, 1191·3
2,2-Dichlorovinyl Dimethyl Phosphate, 1503·2
Dichloroxylenol, 1178·3
2,4-Dichloro-3,5-xylenol, 1178·3
Dichlorphenamide, 894·1
Dichlor-Stapenor, 1936·2
Dichlorvos, 109·3, 1503·2
Dichlotride, 1936·2
Dichophanum, 1502·1
Dichysterol, 1461·3
Diciclovenina, Cloridrato de, 481·2
Diciclovenina, Hidrocloruro de, 481·2
Dicillin, 1936·2
Dicinone, 1936·2
Dicitrate, 1936·2
Dicitratobismutato Tripotásico, 1252·2
Dickflüssiges Paraffin, 1479·1
DICL, 32·1
Diclac, 1936·3
Dicladox, 1936·3
Diclamina, 1936·3
Diclanil, 1936·3
Diclax, 1936·3
Diclaxol, 1936·3
Diclazuril, 603·2
Diclazuril for Veterinary Use, 603·2
Diclazurilo, 603·2
Diclazurilum, 603·2
Diclectin, 1936·3
Diclen, 1936·3
Diclex, 1936·3
Diclo, 1936·3
Diclo P, 1936·3
Diclo-B, 1936·3
Diclo-basan, 1936·3
Diclobene, 1936·3
Diclocil, 1936·3
Diclocillin, 1936·3
Diclocular, 1936·3
Diclodan, 1936·3
Diclo-Denk, 1936·3
Dicloderm Forte, 1936·3
Diclo-Divido, 1936·3
Diclodoc, 1936·3
Diclodol, 1936·3
Diclofan, 1936·3
Diclofen, 1936·4
Diclofenac, 32·1
Diclofenac Diethylamine, 32·1
Diclofenac Diethylammonium, 32·1
Diclofenac Epolamine, 33·3
Diclofenac Hydroxyethylpyrrolidine, 33·3
Diclofenac Potassium, 32·1
Diclofenac Sodium, 32·1
Diclofenaco, 32·1
Diclofenaco Dietilamina, 32·1

Diclofenaco Potásico, 32·1
Diclofenaco Sódico, 32·1
Diclofenacum Kalicum, 32·1
Diclofenacum Natricum, 32·1
Diclofenamida, 894·1
Diclofenamide, 894·1
Diclofenamide Sodium, 894·1
Diclofenamidum, 894·1
Diclofenax, 1936·4
Diclofenbeta, 1936·4
Diclofetamol, 1936·4
Diclofibrate, 997·1
Dicloflam, 1936·4
Dicloflex, 1936·4
Dicloftal, 1936·4
Dicloftil, 1936·4
Diclogea, 1936·4
Diclogel, 1936·4
Diclogenom, 1936·4
Diclogenta, 1936·4
Diclogesic, 1936·4
Diclogesic Relax, 1936·4
Diclogrand, 1936·4
Diclogrun, 1936·4
Diclohexal, 1936·4
Diclokin, 1936·4
Diclolan, 1936·4
Diclomar, 1936·4
Diclomar Flex, 1936·4
Diclomax, 1936·4
Diclomel, 1936·4
Diclomelan, 1936·4
Diclomerck, 1936·4
Diclometin, 1936·4
Diclomex, 1936·4
Diclomin, 1936·4
Diclomol, 1937·1
Diclon, 1937·1
Diclonac, 1937·1
Diclondazolic Acid, 565·3
Diclonina, Hidrocloruro de, 1376·2
Diclophenac Sodium, 32·1
Diclophlogont, 1937·1
Dicloplast, 1937·1
Diclo-Puren, 1937·1
Dicloral, 1937·1
Dicloralfenazona, 697·1
Dicloran, 1937·1
Dicloran-A, 1937·1
Diclorektal, 1937·1
Diclorengel, 1937·1
Dicloreum, 1937·1
Diclorisona, Acetato de, 1099·3
Diclorisone Acetate, 1099·3
Dicloroacetato de Sodio, 1747·2
Diclorodifluorometano, 1236·1
Diclorodimetilhidantoína, 1178·2
Diclorofeno, 104·1
Diclorofenoxiacético, Ácido, 1503·2
Dicloroisocianurato Sódico, 1191·3
Diclorometano, 1473·1
Dicloropropano, 1473·1
Dicloruro de Etileno, 1505·1
Dicloruro de Paraquat, 1508·1
Diclorvós, 1503·2
Diclo-saar, 1937·1
Diclosian, 1937·1
Diclosifar, 1937·1
Dicloson, 1937·1
Diclo-Spondyril, 1937·1
Diclostad, 1937·1
Diclosyl, 1937·1
Diclo-Tablinen, 1937·1
Diclotard, 1937·1
Diclotec, 1937·1
Diclo-Tecno, 1937·1
Diclotride, 1937·2
Diclovit, 1937·2
Diclovol, 1937·2
Diclowal, 1937·2
Diclox, 1937·2
Dicloxacilina, 205·2
Dicloxacilina Sódica, 205·2
Dicloxacillin, 205·2
Dicloxacillin Sodium, 205·2
Dicloxacillinum Natricum, 205·2
Dicloxia, 1937·2
Dicloxin, 1937·2
Dicloxman, 1937·2
Dicloxno, 1937·2
Dicloxsig, 1937·2
Diclozip, 1937·2
Dicobalt Edetate, 1036·2
Dicobalt Trioxide, 1674·1
Dicobalto, Edetato de, 1036·2
Dicodid, 1937·2
Dicodid, Cardiazol- — *see* Cardiazol-Dicodid, 1870·2
Dicodin, 1937·2
Dicodral, 1937·2
Dicofan, 1937·2
Dicofarm, 1937·2
Dicoflor, 1937·2
Dicogel, 1937·2
Dicoman, 1937·2
Dicomin, 1937·2
Diconal, 1937·2
Diconpin, 1937·2
Dicopac, 1937·2
Dicophane, 1502·1
Dicoplus, 1937·2
Dicorantil, 1937·2
Dicortal, 1937·2
Dicorten, 1937·2
Dicorvin, 1937·2
Dicorynan, 1937·2
Dicoumarin, 894·2
Dicoumarol, 894·2
Dicresulene Polymer, 756·1
Dicton, 1937·2
Dicumarol, 894·2
2-(2,2-Dicyclohexylethyl)piperidine Hydrogen Maleate, 980·2
Dicyclomine Hydrochloride, 481·2
2-[(Dicyclopropylmethyl)amino]-2-oxazoline Phosphate, 996·1
Dicycloverine Hydrochloride, 481·2
Dicycloverini Hydrochloridum, 481·2
Dicynene, 1937·3
Dicynone, 1937·3
Didamega, 1937·3
Didanosina, 630·3
Didanosine, 630·3
Didecildimetilamonio, Cloruro de, 1178·3
Didecyldimethylammonium Chloride, 1178·3
3′,4′-Didehydro-4′-deoxy-8′-norvincaleukoblastine Ditartrate, 594·1
7,8-Didehydro-4,5-epoxy-3-ethoxy-17-methylmorphinan-6-ol Hydrochloride Dihydrate, 37·3
7,8-Didehydro-4,5-epoxy-3-methoxy-17-methylmorphinan-6-ol Monohydrate, 27·1
7,8-Didehydro-4,5-epoxy-17-methylmorphinan-3,6-diol, 60·1
2,3-Didehydro-L-*threo*-hexono-1,4-lactone, 1460·2
9,10-Didehydro-*N*-[(*S*)-2-hydroxy-1-methylethyl]-6-methylergoline-8β-carboxamide Hydrogen Maleate, 1684·1
9,10-Didehydro-*N*-[1-(hydroxymethyl)propyl]-1,6-dimethylergoline-8β-carboxamide, 469·3
9,10-Didehydro-*N*-[(*S*)-1-(hydroxymethyl)propyl]-6-methylergoline-8β-carboxamide Hydrogen Maleate, 1714·2
3-(9,10-Didehydro-6-methylergolin-8α-yl)-1,1-diethylurea Hydrogen Maleate, 1210·3
2,3-Didehydro-6′,7′,10,11-tetramethoxyemetan Dihydrochloride, 603·2
Di-Delamine, 1937·3
3,10-Di(demethoxy)-3-glucopyranosyloxy-10-methylthiocolchicine, 1395·2
Didemnin A, 546·3
Didemnin B, 546·3
Didemnin C, 546·3
Didemnina B, 546·3
Dideoxyadenosine Triphosphate, 631·3
Dideoxycytidine, 657·1
2′,3′-Dideoxycytidine, 657·1
(9*S*,13*S*,14*S*)-6,18-Dideoxy-7,8-dihydro-3-*O*-methylmorphine, 1117·3
(2*R*,3*S*,4*S*,5*R*,6*R*,8*R*,10*R*,11*R*,12*S*,13*R*)-3-(2,6-Dideoxy-3-*C*,3*O*-dimethyl-α-L-*ribo*-hexopyranosyloxy)-11,12-dihydroxy-6-methoxy-2,4,6,8,10,12-hexamethyl-9-oxo-5-(3,4,6-trideoxy-3-dimethylamino-β-D-*xylo*-hexopyranosyloxy)pentadecan-13-olide, 192·2
(1*R*,2*R*,3*R*,6*R*,7*S*,8*S*,9*R*,10*R*,12*R*,13*S*,15*R*,17*S*)-7-(2,6-Dideoxy-3-*C*,3-*O*-dimethyl-α-L-*ribo*-hexopyranosyloxy)-3-ethyl-2,10-dihydroxy-15-(2-methoxyethoxymethyl)-2,6,8,10,12,17-hexamethyl-9-(3,4,6-trideoxy-3-dimethylamino-β-L-*xylo*-hexopyranosyloxy)-4,16-dioxa-14-azabicyclo[11.3.1]heptadecan-5-one, 206·1
(2*R*,3*S*,4*R*,5*R*,8*R*,10*R*,11*R*,12*S*,13*S*,14*R*)-13-(2,6-Dideoxy-3-*C*-3-*O*-dimethyl-α-L-*ribo*-hexopyranosyloxy)-2-ethyl-3,4,10-trihydroxy-3,5,6,8,10,12,14-heptamethyl-11-(3,4,6-trideoxy-3-dimethylamino-β-D-*xylo*-hexopyranosyloxy)-1-oxa-6-azacyclopentadecan-15-one Dihydrate, 159·1
3β-[(*O*-2,6-Dideoxy-β-D-*ribo*-hexopyranosyl-(1→4)-*O*-2,6-dideoxy-β-D-*ribo*-hexopyranosyl-(1→4)-2,6-dideoxy-β-D-*ribo*-hexopyranosyl)oxy]-12β,14β-dihydroxy-5β-card-20(22)-enolide, 895·2
3β-[(*O*-2,6-Dideoxy-β-D-*ribo*-hexopyranosyl-(1→4)-*O*-2,6-dideoxy-β-D-*ribo*-hexopyranosyl-(1→4)-2,6-dideoxy-β-D-*ribo*-hexopyranosyl)oxy]-14β-hydroxy-5β-card-20(22)-enolide, 894·3
3,4-Dideoxy-4-{[2-hydroxy-1-(hydroxymethyl)ethyl]amino}-2-*C*-(hydroxymethyl)-*D*-epi-inositol, 348·3
Dideoxyinosine, 630·3
2′,3′-Dideoxyinosine, 630·3
3′,4′-Dideoxykanamycin B, 205·2
(4*R*,5*S*,6*S*,7*R*,9*R*,10*R*,16*R*)-(11*E*,13*E*)-6-[(*O*-2,6-Dideoxy-3-*C*-methyl-α-L-*ribo*-hexopyranosyl)-(1→4)-(3,6-dideoxy-3-dimethylamino-β-D-glucopyranosyl)oxy]-7-formylmethyl-4-hydroxy-5-methoxy-9,16-dimethyl-10-[(2,3,4,6-tetradeoxy-4-dimethylamino-D-*erythro*-hexopyranosyl)oxy]oxacyclohexadeca-11,13-dien-2-one, 255·3
3β-[(*O*-2,6-Dideoxy-4-*O*-methyl-D-*ribo*-hexopyranosyl-(1→4)-*O*-2,6-dideoxy-D-*ribo*-hexopyranosyl-(1→4)-2,6-dideoxy-D-*ribo*-hexopyranosyl)oxy]-12β,14-dihydroxy-5β,14β-card-20(22)-enolide, 955·2
(2*R*,3*S*,4*R*,5*S*,6*S*,8*R*,10*R*,11*S*,12*R*,13*R*)-3-(2,6-Dideoxy-3-*O*-methyl-α-L-*arabino*-hexopyranosyloxy)-8,9-epoxymethano-11-hydroxy-2,4,6,10,12,13-hexamethyl-9-oxo-5-(3,4,6-trideoxy-3-dimethylamino-β-D-*xylo*-hexopyranosyloxy)tridecan-13-olide Phosphate, 240·2
1-(2,3-Dideoxy-β-D-*glycero*-pent-2-enofuranosyl)thymine, 654·2
1,2-Dideoxy-1-[(*R*)-3,6,7,8-tetrahydro-8-hydroxyimidazo[4,5-*d*][1,3]diazepin-3-yl]-D-*erythro*-pentofuranose, 579·2
Didesethylchloroquinine, 450·2
Didesmethylchlorphenamine, 428·1
*N*-Didesmethylpheniramine, 438·3
*N*,*O*-Didesmethylvenlafaxine, 322·3
DIDMOAD Syndrome— *see* Diabetes Insipidus, 1314·1
Didor, 1937·3
Didralin, 1937·3
Didrex, 1937·3
Didrica, 1937·3
Didrocal, 1937·3
Didrogesteron, 1549·2
Didrogesterona, 1549·2
Didrogyl, 1937·3
Didrokit, 1937·3
Didro-Kit, 1937·3
Didronate, 1937·3
Didronate Calcium, 1937·3
Didronate + Calcium, 1937·3
Didronate + Calsium, 1937·3
Didronel, 1937·3
Didronel— *see* Didrokit, 1937·3
Didronel— *see* Didronel PMO, 1937·3
Didronel Kit, 1937·3
Didronel PMO, 1937·3
Didropyridinum, 718·1
Didrovaltrate, 1762·2
Dieldrin, 1503·3
Dieldrina, 1503·3
Diele, 1937·3
Diemalnatrium, 671·2
Diemalum, 671·2
Diemil, 1937·3
Diemon, 1937·3
Dienestrol, 1547·3
Dienestrol Diacetate, 1548·1
Dienestrolum, 1547·3
Dienoestrol, 1547·3
Dienoestrolum, 1547·3
Dienogest, 1548·1
Dienpax, 1937·3
Diente de León, 1751·3
Dientrin, 1937·3
Diergo, 1937·4
Diergospray, 1937·4
Diertina, 1937·4
Diertine, 1937·4
Di-Ertride, 1937·4
Diesan, 1937·4
Diesel, 1937·4
Diespor, 1937·4
Diestet, 1937·4
Diet Ayds, 1937·4
Diet Complet, 1937·4
Diet Sucaryl, 1937·4
Dietacil, 1937·4
Dietamina, 1937·4
Diétamiphylline Camphosulfonate, 785·1
Dietary Fibre, 1253·3
Dietasal, 1937·4
Dietazina, Hidrocloruro de, 481·3
Dietene, 1937·4
Diethamphenazole, 905·3
Diethanolamine, 1681·1
Diethazine Hydrochloride, 481·3
Diethion, 1505·1
Diethizine, 1937·4
1-(3,4-Diethoxybenzylidene)-6,7-diethoxy-1,2,3,4-tetrahydroisoquinoline, 1683·1
6,7-Diethoxy-1-(3,4-diethoxybenzyl)isoquinoline Hydrochloride, 1685·2
2-(Diethoxyphosphinothioyloxyimino)-2-phenylacetonitrile, 1509·1
(2-Diethoxyphosphinylthioethyl)trimethylammonium Iodide, 1490·2
Diethyl 2,5-Bis-(1-aziridinyl)-3,6-dioxo-1,4-cyclohexadiene-1,4-dicarbamate, 546·3
Diethyl 4-{2-[(*tert*-Butoxycarbonyl)vinyl]phenyl}-1,4-dihydro-2,6-dimethylpyridine-3,5-dicarboxylate, 944·2
(±)-Diethyl {1-[3-(2-Chloroethyl)-3-nitrosoureido]ethyl}phosphonate, 557·2
Diethyl 2-(Dimethoxyphosphinothioylthio)succinate, 1507·1
Diethyl Ether, 1298·3, 1474·2
*O*,*O*-Diethyl *O*-(2-Isopropyl-6-methylpyrimidin-4-yl) Phosphorothioate, 1504·2
Diethyl Naphthalimido-oxyphosphonate, 110·1
Diethyl *p*-Nitrophenyl Phosphate, 1494·1
*O*,*O*-Diethyl *O*-4-Nitrophenyl Phosphorothioate, 1508·2
Diethyl Phthalate, 1473·2
*O*,*O*-Diethyl *O*-3,5,6-Trichloro-2-pyridyl Phosphorothioate, 1502·1
Diethylamine, 1682·3
Diethylamine Salamidacetate, 87·3
Diethylamine Salicylate, 34·1
2-Diethylaminoaceto-2′,6′-xylidide, 1377·3
4-(4-Diethylaminobenzhydrylidene)cyclohexa-2,5-dien-1-ylidenediethylammonium Hydrogen Sulphate, 1171·1
4-(Diethylamino)but-2-ynyl (*RS*)-2-Cyclohexyl-2-hydroxy-2-phenylacetate Hydrochloride, 486·3
4-Diethylaminobut-2-ynyl α-Cyclohexylmandelate Hydrochloride, 486·3
3-Diethylaminobutyranilide Hydrochloride, 1382·1
Diethylaminoethanol, 1383·2, 1587·1
2-Diethylaminoethanol, 1587·1
Diethylaminoethanol Hydrochloride, 1587·1
Diethylaminoethanol Malate, 1587·1
2-[2-(Diethylamino)ethoxy]-benzanilide Hydrochloride, 1741·3

2-(2-Diethylaminoethoxy)ethyl 2-Ethyl-2-phenylbutyrate Dihydrogen Citrate, 1126·1
2-(2-Diethylaminoethoxy)ethyl 2-Phenylbutyrate Dihydrogen Citrate, 1116·2
2-[2-(Diethylamino)ethoxy]ethyl 1-Phenylcyclopentanecarboxylate, 1126·2
9-(2-Diethylaminoethoxy)-4-hydroxy-7-methyl-5*H*-furo[3,2-*g*][1]benzopyran-5-one Hydrochloride, 1653·2
2′-(2-Diethylaminoethoxy)-3-phenylpropiophenone Hydrochloride, 914·1
2-Diethylaminoethyl 4-Aminobenzoate Hydrochloride, 1383·2
2-Diethylaminoethyl 4-Amino-3-butoxybenzoate Hydrochloride, 1382·1
2-Diethylaminoethyl 4-Amino-2-chlorobenzoate Hydrochloride, 1373·1
2-Diethylaminoethyl 3-Amino-4-propoxybenzoate Hydrochloride, 1384·1
2-Diethylaminoethyl 4-Amino-2-propoxybenzoate Hydrochloride, 1384·1
2-Diethylaminoethyl Benzilate Hydrochloride, 287·1
2-Diethylaminoethyl Bicyclohexyl-1-carboxylate Hydrochloride, 481·2
2-Diethylaminoethyl Diphenylacetate, 1648·1
2-Diethylaminoethyl 2,2-Diphenylvalerate Hydrochloride, 1735·2
2-Diethylaminoethyl 4-Ethoxybenzoate Hydrochloride, 1382·2
2-Diethylaminoethyl 2-(1-Hydroxycyclopentyl)-2-phenylacetate Hydrochloride, 480·3
2-Diethylaminoethyl 2-Hydroxy-3-phenylbenzoate Hydrochloride, 1163·1
2-Diethylaminoethyl 3-(1-Naphthyl)-2-tetrahydrofurfurylpropionate Hydrogen Oxalate, 964·1
Diethylaminoethyl Penicillin G Hydroiodide, 242·1
2-Diethylaminoethyl (6*R*)-6-(2-Phenylacetamido)penicillanate Hydriodide, 242·1
2-Diethylaminoethyl 2-Phenylbutyrate Citrate, 1116·2
2-(Diethylamino)ethyl α-Phenylcyclohexaneacetate Hydrochloride, 482·1
2-Diethylaminoethyl 1-Phenylcyclopentane-1-carboxylate Ethane-1,2-disulphonate, 1116·2
2-Diethylaminoethyl 3-Phenylsalicylate Hydrochloride, 1163·1
1-(2-Diethylaminoethylamino)-4-hydroxymethylthioxanthen-9-one Methanesulphonate, 105·3
2-Diethylaminoethyl-(*p*-butoxybenzoate) Hydrochloride, 1373·1
4′-[(2-Diethylaminoethyl)carbamoyl]acetanilide Hydrochloride, 848·3
Diethylaminoethyl-dextran Hydrochloride, 890·3
7-(2-Diethylaminoethyl)-1,3-dimethylxanthine Camphor-10-sulphonate, 785·1
1-[2-(Diethylamino)ethyl]-3-(*p*-methoxybenzyl)-2(1*H*)-quinoxalinone, 1668·1
*N*-(2-Diethylaminoethyl)-2-methoxy-5-methylsulphonylbenzamide Hydrochloride, 725·1
10-(2-Diethylaminoethyl)phenothiazine Hydrochloride, 481·3
5-[2-(Diethylamino)ethyl]-3-phenyl-1,2,4-oxadiazole, 1126·1
(26*R*,27*S*)-26-{[2-(Diethylamino)-ethyl]sulfonyl}-26,27-dihydrovirginiamycin $M_1$ Methanesulphonate, 248·1
(3*R*,4*R*,5*E*,10*E*,12*E*,14*S*,26*R*,26a*S*)-26-{[2-(Diethylamino)ethyl]sulfonyl}-8,9,-14,15,24,25,26,26a-octahydro-14-hydroxy-3-isopropyl-4,12-dimethyl-3*H*-21,18-nitrilo-1*H*,22*H*-pyrrolo[2.1-*c*][1,8,4,19]dioxadiazacyclotetracosine-1,7,16,22(4*H*,17*H*)-tetrone Methanesulphonate, 248·1
7-(2-Diethylaminoethyl)theophylline Camphor-10-sulphonate, 785·1
4-[3-(Diethylamino)-2-hydroxypropyl]ajmalinium Hydrogen Tartrate Monohydrate, 893·1
2-Diethylamino-1-methylethyl *cis*-1-Hydroxy(bicyclohexyl)-2-carboxylate, 1740·1
*O*-2-Diethylamino-6-methylpyrimidin-4-yl *O,O*-Dimethyl Phosphorothioate, 1509·2
7-Diethylamino-5-methyl-1,2,4-triazolo[1,5-*a*]pyrimidine, 1016·2
3-Diethylamino-1-phenylpropyl Benzoate Hydrochloride, 1383·3
(*RS*)-α-Diethylaminopropiophenone Hydrochloride, 1587·1
2-Diethylaminopropiophenone Hydrochloride, 1587·1
3-Diethylaminopropyl 2-Phenylbicyclo[2.2.1]heptane-2-carboxylate Hydrochloride, 480·1
*N*-(3-Diethylaminopropyl)-*N*-indan-2-ylaniline Hydrochloride, 864·2
10-(2-Diethylaminopropyl)phenothiazine Hydrochloride, 488·3
2-Diethylamino-2′,4′,6′-trimethylacetanilide Hydrochloride, 1385·3
Diethylammonium 2,5-Dihydroxybenzenesulphonate, 749·3
5,5-Diethylbarbituric Acid, 671·2
Diethylcarbam. Cit., 104·1
Diethylcarbamazine Acid Citrate, 104·1
Diethylcarbamazine Citrate, 104·1
Diethylcarbamazine *N*-Oxide, 104·3
Diethylcarbamazini Citras, 104·1
Diethyldithiocarbamate, 1682·3
Diethylene Dioxide, 1474·2
Diethylene Ether, 1474·2
Diethylene Glycol, 1685·3
Diethylene Glycol Monolaurate, 1411·2
Diethylene Glycol Mono-oleate, 1411·2
Diethylene Glycol Monopalmitostearate, 1411·2
Diethylene Glycol Monostearate, 1411·2
Diéthylène Glycol (Stéarate de), 1411·2
Diethylene Glycol Stearates, 1411·2
Diethylenetriamine Penta-acetic Acid, 1062·2
Diethylenetriamine Penta-acetic Acid Bismethylamide, 1062·1
Diethylenetriamine Penta-acetic Acid Complex, Gadolinium and, 1062·2
Diethylenetriamine-*NNN*′*N*″*N*″-penta-acetic Acid, 1050·1
Diethylenglycoli Monopalmitostearas, 1411·2
Diethyleni Glycoli Stearas, 1411·2
4,4′-(1,2-Diethylethylene)diphenol, 1556·3
*N,N*-Diethylglycine Ester with Paracetamol, 85·3
(6a*R*,9*R*)-*NN*-Diethyl-4,6,6a,7,8,9-hexahydro-7-methylindolo[4,3-*fg*]quinoline-9-carboxamide, 1708·2
Di-(2-ethylhexyl)adipate, 1504·2
Diethyl(2-hydroxyethyl)methylammonium Bromide Benzilate, 485·3
4,4′-(1,2-Diethylidene-1,2-ethanediyl)bisphenol, 1547·3
(*E,E*)-4,4′-[Di(ethylidene)ethylene]diphenol, 1547·3
*NN*-Diethyl-*N*′-indan-2-yl-*N*′-phenyltrimethylenediamine Hydrochloride, 864·2
Diethylis Phthalas, 1473·2
(+)-*NN*-Diethyl-D-lysergamide, 1708·2
Diethylmalonylurea, 671·2
*N*-(β,β-Diethyl-*m*-methoxyphenethyl)-4-hydroxybutyramide, 36·2
*N,N*-Diethyl-3-methylbenzamide, 1503·3
1,1-Diethyl-3-(6-methylergolin-8α-yl) Urea, 1216·1
Diethylmethyl{2-[(α-methyl-α-5-norbornen-2-ylbenzyl)oxy]ethyl}ammonium Bromide, 480·2
Diethylmethyl[2-(3-methyl-2-phenylvaleryloxy)ethyl]ammonium Bromide, 491·3
Diethylmethyl{2-[4-(2-octyloxybenzamido)benzoyloxy]ethyl}ammonium Bromide, 1725·1
Diethylmethyl{2-[4-(4-phenylthiophenyl)-3*H*-1,5-benzodiazepin-2-ylthio]ethyl}ammonium Iodide, 1756·2
*NN*-Diethyl-4-methylpiperazine-1-carboxamide Dihydrogen Citrate, 104·1
Diethylmethyl[2-(xanthen-9-ylcarbonyloxy)ethyl]ammonium Bromide, 485·3
*N,N*-Diethylnicotinamide, 1591·2
(±)-*N,N*-Diethyl-N′-[(3*R**,4a*R**,10a*S**)-1,2,3,4,4a,5,10,10a-octahydro-6-hydroxy-1-propylbenzo[*g*]quinolin-3-yl]sulfamide Hydrochloride, 1213·1
*N,N*-Diethyl-2-[4-(phenylmethyl)phenoxy]-ethanamine Hydrochloride, 587·3
*NN*-Diethyl-3-(1-phenylpropyl)-1,2,4-oxadiazole-5-ethanamine Citrate, 1735·3
Diethylpropion Hydrochloride, 1587·1
*N,N*-Diethylpyridine-3-carboxamide, 1591·2
3,3-Diethylpyridine-2,4(1*H*,3*H*)-dione, 718·1
(*E*)-αβ-Diethylstilbene-4-4′-diol, 1548·1
(*E*)-αα′-Diethylstilbene-4,4′-diol Bis(dihydrogen Phosphate), 1555·3
(*E*)-αβ-Diethylstilbene-4,4′-diol Dipropionate, 1548·1
Diethylstilbestrol, 1548·1
Diethylstilbestrol Diphosphate, 1555·3
Diethylstilbestrol Dipropionate, 1548·1
Diethylstilbestrolum, 1548·1
Diethylstilboestrol, 1548·1
(*S*)-4,11-Diethyl-3,4,12,14-tetrahydro-4-hydroxy-3,14-dioxo-1*H*-pyrano[3′,4′:6′,7′]-indolizino[1,2-*b*]quinolin-9-yl [1,4′-Dipiperidine]-1′-carboxylate Hydrochloride Trihydrate, 564·1
1,8-Diethyl-1,3,4,9-tetrahydropyrano[3,4-*b*]indol-1-ylacetic Acid, 37·3
Diethyltoluamide, 1503·3
*NN*-Diethyl-*m*-toluamide, 1503·3
Diethyltoluamidum, 1503·3
Diethyltryptamine, 1680·3
*N,N*-Diethylvanillamide, 1588·1
(*E*)-4,4′-(1,2-Diethylvinylene)bis(phenyl Dihydrogen Orthophosphate), 1555·3
Dietil, 1937·4
Dietilaminoetanol, 1587·1
Dietilcarbamazina, Citrato de, 104·1
Dietilestilbestrol, 1548·1
Dietilestilbestrol, Dipropionato de, 1548·1
Dietiltoluamida, 1503·3
Dietmann, 1937·4
Dietoman, 1937·4
Dieutrim, 1937·4
Dievril, 1937·4
Diezime, 1937·4
Dif Vitamin A Masivo, 1937·4
Difarben, 1937·4
Difaterol, 1937·4
Difebarbamate, 697·2
Difebarbamato, 697·2
Difedram, 1937·4
Difelene, 1938·1
Difemanilo, Metilsulfato de, 481·3
Difemerina, Hidrocloruro de, 481·3
Difemerine Hydrochloride, 481·3
Difemic, 1938·1
Difen, 1938·1
Difena, 1938·1
Difenac, 1938·1
Difenacol, Chemists Own— *see* Chemists Own Difenacol, 1882·1
Difenacoum, 1504·1
Difenacum, 1504·1
Difenadiona, 1504·3
Difenan, 1938·1
Difenciprona, 1145·3
Difene, 1938·1
Difenet, 1938·1
Difenhidramina, 431·3
Difenhidramina, Citrato de, 431·3
Difenhidramina, Di(acefilinato) de, 431·3
Difenhidramina, Hidrocloruro de, 431·3
Difenhistat, 1938·1
Difenidol, Hidrocloruro de, 1261·1
Difenidol Hydrochloride, 1261·1
Difenidrin, 1938·1
Difenilo, 1681·2
Difenilpiralina, Hidrocloruro de, 432·3
Difeno, 1938·1
Difenol, 1938·1
Difenoxilato, Hidrocloruro de, 1261·3
Difenoxilic Acid, 1261·2
Difenoxin, 1261·2
Difenoxin Hydrochloride, 1261·2
Difenoxina, Hidrocloruro de, 1261·2
Difenoxylic Acid Hydrochloride, 1261·2
Diferbest, 1938·1
Diferin, 1938·1
Difexon, 1938·1
Differin, 1938·1
Differine, 1938·1
Difflam Preparations, 1938·1
Difflam-C, 1938·2
Diffu-K, 1938·2
Diffumal, 1938·2
Diffuse Parenchymal Lung Disease, 1079·3
Diffusyl, 1938·2
Difilina Asmorax, 1938·2
Difiram, 1938·2
Difix, 1938·2
Diflamil, 1938·2
Diflerix, 1938·2
Diflonid, 1938·2
Diflorasona, Diacetato de, 1099·3
Diflorasone Diacetate, 1099·3
Difloxacin Hydrochloride, 205·3
Difloxacino, Hidrocloruro de, 205·3
Diflubenzuron, 1504·1
Diflucan, 1938·2
Diflucortolona, Valerato de, 1099·3
Diflucortolone, 1099·3
Diflucortolone Pivalate, 1099·3
Diflucortolone 21-Pivalate, 1099·3
Diflucortolone Valerate, 1099·3
Diflucortolone 21-Valerate, 1099·3
Difludol, 1938·2
Difluid, 1938·2
Diflunisal, 34·1
Diflunisal Arginine, 34·3
Diflunisalum, 34·1
6-{2-[4-(4,4′-Difluorobenzhydrylidene)piperidino]ethyl}-7-methyl[1,3]thiazolo[3,2-*a*]pyrimidin-5-one, 721·1
4-[3-(4,4′-Difluorobenzhydryl)propyl]piperazin-1-ylaceto-2′,6′-xylidide, 946·3
1-{1-[3-(4,4′-Difluorobenzhydryl)propyl]-4-piperidyl}benzimidazolin-2-one, 715·1
1-(2,6-Difluorobenzyl)-1*H*-1,2,3-triazole-4-carboxamide, 377·3
Difluorodichloromethane, 1236·1
6α,9α-Difluoro-11β,21-dihydroxy-16α,17α-isopropylidenedioxypregna-1,4-diene-3,20-dione, 1101·2
6α,9α-Difluoro-11β,21-dihydroxy-16α,17α-isopropylidenedioxypregna-1,4-diene-3,20-dione 21-Acetate, 1101·3
6α,9α-Difluoro-11β,21-dihydroxy-16α-methylpregna-1,4-diene-3,20-dione, 1099·3
Difluoroetano, 1236·2
Difluoroethane, 1236·2
1,1-Difluoroethane, 1236·2
6,8-Difluoro-1-(2-fluoroethyl)-1,4-dihydro-7-(4-methyl-1-piperazinyl)-4-oxo-3-quinolinecarboxylic Acid, 213·2
(6α,11β,16α)-6,9-Difluoro-11-hydroxy-16,17-[(1-methylethylidene)bis(oxy)]-21-(1-oxopropoxy)-pregna-1,4-diene-3,20-dione, 1110·1
6α,9α-Difluoro-16α-hydroxyprednisolone Acetonide, 1101·2
Difluoromethoxyacetic Acid, 1304·2
5-Difluoromethoxybenzimidazol-2-yl 3,4-Dimethoxy-2-pyridylmethyl Sulphoxide, 1283·1
(±)-2-Difluoromethyl 1,2,2,2-Tetrafluoroethyl Ether, 1297·2
α-Difluoromethylornithine Hydrochloride, 604·2
2-(Difluoromethyl)-DL-ornithine Monohydrochloride Monohydrate, 604·2
7*R*-7-[2-(Difluoromethylthio)acetamido]-3-[1-(2-hydroxyethyl)-1*H*-tetrazol-5-ylthiomethyl]-7-methoxy-1-oxa-3-cephem-4-carboxylic Acid Sodium, 213·2
Difluorophate, 1490·1
2-(2,4-Difluorophenyl)-1,3-bis(1*H*-1,2,4-triazol-1-yl)propan-2-ol, 398·1
(*RS*)-1-(2,4-Difluorophenyl)-6-fluoro-1,4-dihydro-7-(3-methylpiperazin-1-yl)-4-oxoquinoline-3-carboxylic Acid, 266·1
(2*R*,3*S*)-2-(2,4-Difluorophenyl)-3-(5-fluoropyrimidin-4-yl)-1-(1,2,4-triazol-1-yl)butan-2-ol, 411·2

[R-(R*,R*)]-α-(2,4-Difluorophenyl)-α[1-(methylsulphonyl)ethyl]-1H-1,2,4-triazole-1-ethanol, 400·3
5-(2,4-Difluorophenyl)salicylic Acid, 34·1
4-{p-[4-(p-{[(3R,5R)-5-(2,4-Difluorophenyl)tetrahydro-5-(1H-1,2,4-triazol-1-ylmethyl)-3-furyl]methoxy}phenyl)-1-piperazinyl]phenyl}-1-[(1S,2S)-1-ethyl-2-hydroxypropyl]-Δ²-1,2,4-triazolin-5-one, 407·3
6α,9α-Difluoro-11β,17α,21-trihydroxy-16β-methylpregna-1,4-diene-3,20-dione 17,21-Diacetate, 1099·3
6α,9α-Difluoro-11β,17α,21-trihydroxypregna-1,4-diene-3,20-dione 21-Acetate 17-Butyrate, 1100·1
(RS)-1-(2,4′-Difluorotrityl)imidazole, 400·3
Difluprednate, 1100·1
Difluprednato, 1100·1
Diflusal, 1938·2
Diflux, 1938·2
Difmecor, 1938·2
Difmedol, 1938·2
Difmetre, 1938·2
Difmetus Compositum, 1938·2
Difnal, 1938·2
Difnan, 1938·2
Diformil, 1938·2
Diformiltricina, 1938·3
Diformin, 1938·3
Difosfato de Primaquina, 456·2
Difosfen, 1938·3
Difosfocin, 1938·3
Difosfonal, 1938·3
Difosquin, 1938·3
Difoxacil, 1938·3
Dif-Per-Tet-All, 1938·3
Difrarel, 1938·3
Difrarel E, 1938·3
Difrin, 1938·3
Diftavax, 1938·3
Dif-Tet-All, 1938·3
Difur, 1938·3
Difuran, 1938·3
Difusil, 1938·3
Digacin, 1938·3
Digallic Acid, 1751·2
Digaol, 1938·3
Digaril, 1938·3
Digassim, 1938·3
Digastril, 1938·3
Digecap, 1938·3
Digecap-Zimatico, 1938·3
Digedryl, 1938·3
Digeflash, 1938·3
Di-Gel, 1938·4
Di-Gel Forte, 1938·4
Digelax, 1938·4
Digene, 1938·4
Digenil, 1938·4
Digenor Plus, 1938·4
Digenorflat, 1938·4
Digenormotil, 1938·4
Digenormotil Plus, 1938·4
Digepepsin, 1938·4
Digeplex, 1938·4
Digeplex-T, 1938·4
Digeplus, 1938·4
Digerall, 1938·4
Digerent, 1938·4
Digerex, 1938·4
Digerfit, 1938·4
Digervin, 1938·4
Digesan, 1938·4
Di-Gesic, 1938·4
Digesnorma, 1938·4
Digespar, 1938·4
Digesplen, 1939·1
Digesprid, 1939·1
Digess, 1939·1
Digest, 1939·1
Digest Plus, 1939·1
Digestaid, 1939·1
Digestal, 1939·1
Digestar, 1939·1
Digestbem, 1939·1
Digestelact, 1939·1
Digestif Marga, 1939·1
Digestif Rennie, 1939·1
Digestif-Ara, 1939·1
Digestil, 1939·1
Digestin, 1939·1
Digestina, 1939·1
Digestinas Super, 1939·1
Digestion L114, 1939·1
Digestive, 1939·1
Digestive Aid, 1939·1
Digestive Enzymes, Natures Own— *see* Natures Own Digestive Enzymes, 2153·2
Digestive Rennie, 1939·1
Digestive Zyme, Bioglan— *see* Bioglan Digestive Zyme, 1844·1
Digestivo Antonetto, 1939·1
Digestivo Giuliani, 1939·1
Digestivo Rennie, 1939·1
Digestivum-Hetterich S, 1939·2
Digest-Merz, 1939·2
Digestodoron, 1939·2
Digestol, 1939·2
Digestol Sanatorium, 1939·2
Digestomen, 1939·2
Digestomen Complex, 1939·2
Digeston, 1939·2
Digestopan, 1939·2
Digestosan, 1939·2
Digestovital, 1939·2
Digestron, 1939·2
Digest-X Yucca L110, 1939·2
Digezanol, 1939·2
Digezin, 1939·2
Digezyme, 1939·2
Digherbal, 1939·2
Digi-Aldopur, 1939·2
Digibind, 1939·2
Digidot, 1939·2
DigiFab, 1939·2
Digifar, 1939·2
Digimed, 1939·2
Digimerck, 1939·2
Digit. Fol., 894·2
Digit. Leaf, 894·2
Digital, Hoja de, 894·2
Digitale, Feuille de, 894·2
Digitale Pourprée, 894·2
Digitalin, 1680·1
Digitalin, Amorphous, 1680·1
Digitalina, 1680·1
Digitaline, 1939·2
Digitaline Cristallisée, 894·3
Digitalinum Purum Germanicum, 1680·1
Digitalis, 894·2
Digitalis Antidot, 1939·3
Digitalis Antidote, 1939·3
Digitalis, Austrian, 894·2
Digitalis Folium, 894·2
*Digitalis lanata*, 894·2, 895·2
Digitalis Lanata, Hoja de, 894·2
Digitalis Lanata Leaf, 894·2
Digitalis Lanatae Folium, 894·2
Digitalis Leaf, 894·2
*Digitalis purpurea*, 894·2, 1680·1
Digitalis Purpureae Folium, 894·2
Digitalysat Scilla-Digitaloid, 1939·3
Digitoxin, 894·3
Digitoxina, 894·3
Digitoxinum, 894·3
Digitoxoside, 894·3
Digitrin, 1939·3
Diglexol, 1939·3
Diglycerides of Food Fatty Acids, Self-emulsifying, 1412·2
Di-glycerides, Mono- and, 1413·2
Diglycol Stearate, 1411·2
Dignobeta, 1939·3
Dignobroxol, 1939·3
Dignodolin, 1939·3
Dignofenac, 1939·3
Dignoflex, 1939·3
Dignokonstant, 1939·3
Dignometoprol, 1939·3
Dignonitrat, 1939·3
Dignoretik, 1939·3
Dignotrimazol, 1939·3
Dignover, 1939·3
Dignowell, 1939·3
Digocard-G, 1939·3
Digomal, 1939·3
Digophton, 1939·3
Digosin, 1939·3
Digostada, 1939·3
Digotab, 1939·3
Digox, 1939·3
Digoxigenin, 898·3
Digoxil, 1939·3
Digoxin, 895·2
Digoxin "Didier", 1939·3
Digoxin Immune Fab (Ovine), 1036·3
Digoxina, 895·2
Digoxin-specific Antibody Fragments, 1036·3
Digoxinum, 895·2
Digoxosidum, 895·2
Digton, 1939·3
Dihaematoporphyrin Ether, 580·3
Dihexazine, 430·3
Dihexiverina, Hidrocloruro de, 481·3
Dihexiverine Hydrochloride, 481·3
Dihexyverine Hydrochloride, 481·3
Dihidralazina, Sulfato de, 899·3
Dihidrocloruro de Flurazepam, 700·3
Dihidrocloruro de Mitoguazona, 573·3
Dihidrocloruro de Trientina, 1055·2
Dihidrocodeína, Fosfato de, 34·3
Dihidrocodeína, Tartrato de, 34·3
Dihidroergocriptina, Mesilato de, 1680·1
Dihidroergocristina, Mesilato de, 1680·1
Dihidroergotamina, 465·3
Dihidroergotamina, Mesilato de, 465·3
Dihidroergotamina, Tartrato de, 466·1
Dihidroestreptomicina, Sulfato de, 205·3
Dihidrotaquisterol, 1461·3
Dihidroxiacetona, 1145·2
Dihidroxidibutiléter, 1680·2
Dihomo-γ-linolenic Acid, 1511·1
Di-Hydan, 1939·3
Dihydergot, 1939·3
Dihydergot Plus, 1939·4
Dihydral, 1939·4
Dihydralazine Hydrochloride, 900·1
Dihydralazine Mesilate, 900·1
Dihydralazine Sulfate, 899·3
Dihydralazine Sulphate, 899·3
Dihydralazine Sulphate, Hydrated, 900·1
Dihydralazine Tartrate, 900·1
Dihydralazini Sulfas Hydricus, 899·3
Dihydralazinum Sulfuricum, 899·3
Dihydrallazine Sulphate, 899·3
Dihydroartemisinin, 447·3, 448·1
Dihydroartemisinin Ethyl Ether, 447·2
Dihydroartemisinin Hemisuccinate Sodium, 447·2
Dihydroartemisinin Methyl Ether, 447·2
2-(2,3-Dihydro-1,4-benzodioxin-2-yl)-2-imidazoline Hydrochloride, 1700·2
1-(2,3-Dihydro-1,4-benzodioxin-2-ylmethyl)guanidine Sulphate, 927·3
1-(2,3-Dihydro-1,4-benzodioxin-6-yl)-3-(3-phenyl-1-pyrrolidinyl)-1-propanone, 990·3
(S)-1-[2-(2,3-Dihydro-5-benzofuranyl)ethyl]-α,α-diphenyl-3-pyrrolidineacetamide, 481·1
3-(6,12-Dihydrobenzofuro[3,2-c][1]benzoxepin-6-ylidene)-NN-dimethylpropylamine Hydrogen Fumarate, 470·2
Dihydrochinidin Hydrochloride, 937·3
Dihydrochinin Hydrobromide, 1699·3
Dihydrocodeine Acid Tartrate, 34·3
Dihydrocodeine Bitartrate, 34·3
Dihydrocodeine Hydrochloride, 35·2
Dihydrocodeine Hydrogen Tartrate, 34·3
Dihydrocodeine Phosphate, 34·3
Dihydrocodeine Polistirex, 35·2
Dihydrocodeine Tartrate, 34·3
Dihydrocodeine Thiocyanate, 35·2
Dihydrocodeini Hydrogenotartras, 34·3
Dihydrocodeinone Acid Tartrate, 45·1
Dihydrocodeinone Enol Acetate Hydrochloride, 1131·2
DiHydro-CP, 1939·4
9,10-Dihydro-8a,10a-diazoniaphenanthrene Dibromide, 1504·3
3-(10,11-Dihydro-5H-dibenz[b,f]azepin-5-yl)propyldimethylamine, 300·1
3-(10,11-Dihydro-5H-dibenz[b,f]azepin-5-yl)propyl(methyl)amine Hydrochloride, 290·2
1-[3-(10,11-Dihydro-5H-dibenz[b,f]azepin-5-yl)propyl]-4-piperidinopiperidine-4-carboxamide Dihydrochloride Monohydrate, 674·2
7-[(10,11-Dihydro-5H-dibenzo[a,d]cyclohepten-5-yl)amino]heptanoic Acid Hydrochloride, 280·3
3-(10,11-Dihydro-5H-dibenzo[a,d]cyclohepten-5-ylidene)propyldimethylamine, 280·3
3-(10,11-Dihydro-5H-dibenzo[a,d]cyclohepten-5-ylidene)propyl(methyl)amine Hydrochloride, 310·2
(±)-3-(10,11-Dihydro-5H-dibenzo[a,d]cyclohepten-5-yl)-2-methylpropyldimethylamine Hydrochloride, 289·1
(1R,3r,5S)-3-(10,11-Dihydro-5H-dibenzo[a,d]cyclohepten-5-yloxy)tropane Dihydrogen Citrate, 430·3
Dihydrodiethylstilboestrol, 1556·3
Dihydrodigoxigenin, 898·3
Dihydrodigoxin, 898·3
9,10-Dihydro-4,5-dihydroxy-9,10-dioxo-2-anthroic Acid Diacetate, 30·1
5,6-Dihydro-9,10-dimethoxybenzo[g]-1,3-benzodioxolo[5,6-a]quinolizinium, 1659·3
3-(9,10-Dihydro-10,10-dimethyl-9-anthrylidene)propyldimethylamine Hydrochloride, 306·3
2,3-Dihydro-2,2-dimethylbenzofuran-7-yl (Dibutylaminothio)methylcarbamate, 1501·2
10,11-Dihydro-N,N-dimethyl-5H-dibenzo[a,d]cycloheptene-Δ$^{5,\gamma}$-propylamine, 280·3
N-(2,3-Dihydro-1,5-dimethyl-3-oxo-2-phenyl-1H-pyrazol-4-yl)-2-(dimethylamino)propanamide, 14·2
3,7-Dihydro-1,3-dimethylpurine-2,6(1H)-dione, 798·3
3,7-Dihydro-3,7-dimethylpurine-2,6(1H)-dione, 798·2
3,10-Dihydro-7,8-dimethyl-10-(D-*ribo*-2,3,4,5-tetrahydroxypentyl)benzopteridine-2,4-dione, 1456·1
5,8-Dihydro-2,4-dimethyl-8-[p-(o-1H-tetrazol-5-ylphenyl)benzyl]pyrido[2,3-d]pyrimidin-7(6H)-one, 1009·3
17α-Dihydroequilin Sulfate, Sodium, 1543·2
17β-Dihydroequilin Sulfate, Sodium, 1543·2
Dihydroergocornine Mesilate, 1674·1
Dihydroergocristine Mesilate, 1680·1
Dihydroergocristine Mesylate, 1680·1
Dihydroergocristine Methanesulphonate, 1680·1
Dihydroergocristini Mesilas, 1680·1
Dihydroergocryptine Mesilate, 1680·1
Dihydroergocryptine Mesylate, 1680·1
Dihydroergocryptine Methanesulphonate, 1680·1
Dihydroergokryptine Mesylate, 1680·1
Dihydroergotamine, 465·3
Dihydroergotamine Mesilate, 465·3
Dihydroergotamine Mesylate, 465·3
Dihydroergotamine Methanesulphonate, 465·3
Dihydroergotamine Tartrate, 466·1
Dihydroergotamini Mesilas, 465·3
Dihydroergotamini Tartras, 466·1
Dihydroergotoxine Mesylate, 1674·1
Dihydroergotoxine Methanesulphonate, 1674·1
3-(9,10-Dihydro-9,10-ethanoanthracen-9-yl)propyl(methyl)amine, 306·1
Dihydrofolliculin, 1550·1
Dihydrogen [N-{(2S)-2-[Bis(carboxymethyl)amino]-3-(p-ethoxyphenyl)propyl}-N-{2-[bis(carboxymethyl)amino]ethyl}glycinato(5-)]gadolinate(2-), 1063·1

Dihydrogen [(±)-4-Carboxy-5,8,11-tris(carboxymethyl)-1-phenyl-2-oxa-5,8,11-triaza-tridecan-13-oato(5-)]gadolinate(2-), 1062·1
Dihydrogenated Ergot Alkaloids, 1674·1
DiHydro-GP, 1939·4
3,4-Dihydroharmine, 1696·3
Dihydrohelenalin Tiglate, 1657·1
10,11-Dihydro-10-hydroxy-carbamazepine, 367·1
7,8-Dihydro-14-hydroxycodeinone Hydrochloride, 75·2
(±)-*trans*-3,4-Dihydro-3-hydroxy-2,2-dimethyl-4-(2-oxopyrrolidin-1-yl)-2*H*-chromene-6-carbonitrile, 890·3
1,2-Dihydro-4-hydroxy-*N*,1-dimethyl-2-oxo-3-quinolinecarboxanilide, 583·2
3,7-Dihydro-7-(2-hydroxyethyl)-1,3-dimethyl-1*H*-purine-2,6-dione, 785·1
2-[2,3-Dihydro-7-hydroxy-2-(4-hydroxy-3-methoxyphenyl)-3-(hydroxymethyl)-5-benzofuranyl]-3,5,7-trihydroxy-4-chromanone, 1043·3
(6*R*,7*R*,14*R*)-7,8-Dihydro-7-(1*R*-1-hydroxy-1-methylbutyl)-6-*O*-methyl-6,14α-ethenomorphine Hydrochloride, 38·3
7,8-Dihydro-14-hydroxymorphinone Hydrochloride, 76·1
3′-{(1*R*)-1-[(6*R*)-5,6-Dihydro-4-hydroxy-2-oxo-6-phenethyl-6-propyl-2*H*-pyran-3-yl]propyl}-5-(trifluoromethyl)-2-pyridinesulfonanilide, 655·3
1,2-Dihydro-12-hydroxysenecionan-11,16-dione Hydrogen Tartrate, 488·2
13-Dihydroidarubicin, 560·2
1,2-Dihydro-5-imidazo[1,2-*a*]pyridin-6-yl-6-methyl-2-oxonicotinonitrile Hydrochloride, 976·1
1,6-Dihydro-6-iminopurine, 1647·3
Dihydrolevobunolol, 946·2
8α,9*R*-10,11-Dihydro-6′-methoxycinchonan-9-ol Hydrobromide, 1699·3
(8*R*,9*S*)-10,11-Dihydro-6′-methoxycinchonan-9-ol Hydrochloride, 937·3
*trans*-1-{2-[4-(3,4-Dihydro-7-methoxy-2,2-dimethyl-3-phenyl-2*H*-1-benzopyran-4-yl)phenoxy]ethyl}pyrrolidine, 1564·3
(+)-10,11-Dihydro-5-methyl-5*H*-dibenzo[*a*,*d*]-cyclohepten-5,10-imine Maleate, 1683·1
1,3-Dihydro-1-methyl-7-nitro-5-phenyl-1,4-benzodiazepin-2-one, 710·1
1,6-Dihydro-2-methyl-6-oxo[3,4′-bipyridine]-5-carbonitrile, 959·2
(±)-10,11-Dihydro-α-methyl-10-oxodibenzo[*b*,*f*]thiepin-2-acetic Acid, 96·3
3,4-Dihydro-3-methyl-4-oxoimidazo[5,1-*d*][1,2,3,5]tetrazine-8-carboxamide, 587·1
1-{[3-(3,4-Dihydro-5-methyl-4-oxo-7-propylimidazo[5,1-*f*]-*as*-triazin-2-yl)-4-ethoxyphenyl]sulfonyl}-4-ethylpiperazine, 1763·1
1-{[3-(6,7-Dihydro-1-methyl-7-oxo-3-propyl-1*H*-pyrazolo[4,3-*d*]pyrimidin-5-yl)-4-ethoxyphenyl]sulfonyl}-4-methylpiperazine Citrate, 1744·2
*N*-{5-[3,4-Dihydro-2-methyl-4-oxoquinazolin-6-ylmethyl(methyl)amino]-2-thenoyl}-L-glutamic Acid, 582·1
5,11-Dihydro-11-(4-methylpiperazin-1-ylacetyl)pyrido[2,3-*b*][1,4]benzodiazepin-6-one Dihydrochloride Monohydrate, 488·1
(±)-3,4-Dihydro-1-methyl-1-(2-piperidinoethyl)-2(1*H*)-napthalenone, 1125·2
9,10-Dihydro-4-(1-methylpiperidin-4-ylidene)-4*H*-benzo[4,5]cyclohepta[1,2-*b*]thiophene, 470·3
6,11-Dihydro-11-(1-methyl-4-piperidylidene)-5*H*-benzo[5,6]cyclohepta[1,2-*b*]pyridine Dimaleate, 425·1
4,5-Dihydro-6-[2-(*p*-methyoxyphenyl)-5-benzimidazolyl]-5-methyl-3(2*H*)-pyridazinone, 983·1
Dihydromorphine, 35·2
Dihydromorphinone Hydrochloride, 45·2
Dihydrone Hydrochloride, 75·2
1,3-Dihydro-7-nitro-5-phenyl-2*H*-1,4-benzodiazepin-2-one, 710·1
10,11-Dihydro-10-oxo-5*H*-dibenz[*b*,*f*]azepine-5-carboxamide, 366·3
4-[4-(2,3-Dihydro-2-oxo-3-propionyl-1*H*-benzimidazol-1-yl)piperidino]-2,2-diphenylbutyronitrile, 21·2
(12*Z*,14*E*,24*E*)-(2*S*,16*S*,17*S*,18*R*,19*R*,20*R*,21*S*,22*R*,23*S*)-1,2-Dihydro-5,6,9,17,19-pentahydroxy-23-methoxy-2,4,12,16,18,20,22-heptamethyl-8-(4-methylpiperazin-1-yliminomethyl)-1,11-dioxo-2,7-(epoxypentadeca-[1,11,13]trienimino)naphtho[2,1-*b*]furan-21-yl Acetate, 250·2
3,3′,3″,3‴-(7,8-Dihydroporphyrin-5,10,15,20-tetrayl)tetraphenol, 586·3
2,3-Dihydro-6-propyl-2-thioxopyrimidin-4(1*H*)-one, 1603·1
1,7-Dihydro-6*H*-purine-6-thione Monohydrate, 567·2
1,5-Dihydro-4*H*-pyrazolo[3,4-*d*]pyrimidin-4-one, 412·2
Dihydroqinghaosu Ethyl Ether, 447·2
Dihydroqinghaosu Hemisuccinate Sodium, 447·2
Dihydroqinghaosu Methyl Ether, 447·2
Dihydroquinidine Hydrochloride, 937·3
Dihydroquinine Hydrobromide, 1699·3
10,11-Dihydro-5-(quinuclidin-3-yl)-5*H*-dibenz[*b*,*f*]azepine, 316·3
6,9-Dihydro-9-β-D-ribofuranosyl-1*H*-purin-6-one, 1701·2
Dihydrorofecoxib, 87·2
Dihydrospirenone, 1549·1
Dihydrostilboestrol, 1556·3
Dihydrostreptomycin Sulfate, 205·3
Dihydrostreptomycin Sulphate, 205·3
Dihydrostreptomycin Sulphate for Veterinary Use, 205·3
Dihydrostreptomycini Sulfas, 205·3
Dihydrotachysterol, 1461·3
Dihydrotestosterone, 1541·3, 1571·2
7,8-Dihydro-5,10,15,20-tetrakis(3-hydroxyphenyl)porphyrin, 586·3
Dihydrotheelin, 1550·1
*N*-(5,6-Dihydro-4*H*-1,3-thiazin-2-yl)-2,6-xylidine, 1765·3
2,3-Dihydro-2-thioxo-6-methylpyrimidin-4(1*H*)-one, 1602·3
3,4-Dihydro-6-trifluoromethyl-2*H*-1,2,4-benzothiadiazine-7-sulphonamide 1,1-Dioxide, 937·2
Dihydroxyacetone, 1145·2
Dihydroxyaluminium Sodium Carbonate, 1261·2
Dihydroxyaluminum Allantoinate, 1141·2
Dihydroxyaluminum Aminoacetate, 1249·1
Dihydroxyaluminum Sodium Carbonate, 1261·2
Dihydroxyanthracenedione Dihydrochloride, 575·2
1,8-Dihydroxy-9(10*H*)-anthracenone, 1146·1
1,8-Dihydroxyanthraquinone, 1261·1
1,8-Dihydroxyanthrone, 1146·1
(*R*)-10,11-Dihydroxy-6a-aporphine Hydrochloride Hemihydrate, 1199·1
*m*-Dihydroxybenzene, 1156·3
2,5-Dihydroxybenzoic Acid Ethanolamide, 1692·2
2,5-Dihydroxybenzoic Acid Methyl Ester, 59·2
(+)-2-(3,4-Dihydroxybenzyl)-2-hydrazinopropionic Acid Monohydrate, 1204·3
1,4-Dihydroxy-5,8-bis[2-(2-hydroxyethylamino)ethylamino]anthraquinone Dihydrochloride, 575·2
Dihydroxybusulphan, 590·2
(2*R*,3*R*)-2,3-Dihydroxybutane-1,4-dioic Acid, 1752·1
(±)-7-{4-[(*Z*)-2,3-Dihydroxy-2-butenyl]-1-piperazinyl}-6-fluoro-1-methyl-4-oxo-1*H*,4*H*-[1,3]thiazeto[3,2-*a*]quinoline-3-carboxylic Acid Cyclic Carbonate, 246·3
3α,7α-Dihydroxy-5β-cholan-24-oic Acid, 1670·1
3α,7β-Dihydroxy-5β-cholan-24-oic Acid, 1760·3
1α,24-Dihydroxycholecalciferol, 1158·3
1,25-Dihydroxycholecalciferol, 1461·2
1α,25-Dihydroxycholecalciferol, 1461·2
3,4-Dihydroxy-3-cyclobutene-1,2-dione, 1158·1
Dihydroxydibutylether, 1680·2
8′,10′-Dihydroxydihydroergotamine, 466·2
2,2′-Dihydroxy-4,4′-dimethoxybenzophenone, 1143·1
(+)-7′,12′-Dihydroxy-6,6′-dimethoxy-2,2′,2′-trimethyltubocuraranium Dichloride Pentahydrate, 1409·2
(+)-(*R*)-3-(2,4-Dihydroxy-3,3-dimethylbutyramido)propionic Acid, 1442·3
Dihydroxydimethyldiphenylmethanedisulphonic Acid Polymer, 756·1
5,5-Dihydroxy-6,6-dimethyl-3,3-dithiodimethylenebis(4-pyridylmethanol) Dihydochloride Monohydrate, 1737·2
(5*Z*,13*E*)-(8*R*,11*R*,12*R*,15*R*)-11,15-Dihydroxy-16,16-dimethyl-9-methyleneprosta-5,13-dienoic Acid, 1519·2
1,25-Dihydroxyergocalciferol, 1462·3
3,16α-Dihydroxyestra-1,3,5(10)-trien-17-one Diacetate, 1556·3
4,17β-Dihydroxyestr-4-en-3-one 17-(β-Cyclopentylpropionate), 1565·1
Dihydroxyethylrutoside, 1688·2
(*Z*)-7-{(1*R*,2*R*,3*R*,5*S*)-3,5-Dihydroxy-2-[(*E*)-(3*S*)-3-hydroxy-3-methyloct-1-enyl]cyclopentyl}hept-5-enoic Acid, 1514·2
{10-[(1*RS*,2*SR*)-2,3-Dihydroxy-1-(hydroxymethyl)propyl]-1,4,7,10-tetraazacyclododecane-1,4,7-triacetato(3-)}gadolinium, 1062·1
(*Z*)-7-{(1*R*,2*R*,3*R*,5*S*)-3,5-Dihydroxy-2-[(*E*)-(3*S*)-3-hydroxyoct-1-enyl]cyclopentyl}hept-5-enoic Acid, 1514·3
Dihydroxy[(2-hydroxy-5-oxo-2-imidazolin-4-yl)ureato]aluminium, 1141·2
5,7-Dihydroxy-3-(4-hydroxyphenyl)-4*H*-1-benzopyran-4-one, 1692·1
(*Z*)-7-{(1*R*,2*R*,3*R*,5*S*)-3,5-Dihydroxy-2-[(1*E*,3*S*)-3-hydroxy-5-phenyl-1-pentenyl]cyclopentyl}-*N*-ethyl-5-heptenamide, 1514·1
(*R*)-2,4-Dihydroxy-*N*-(3-hydroxypropyl)-3,3-dimethylbutyramide, 1727·2
(±)-(*Z*)-7-{(1*R*,2*R*,3*R*,5*S*)-3,5-Dihydroxy-2-[(*E*)-(3*RS*)-3-hydroxy-4-(3-thienyloxy)but-1-enyl]cyclopentyl}hept-5-enoic Acid, 1521·1
11β,21-Dihydroxy-16α,17α-isopropylidenedioxypregna-1,4-diene-3,20-dione, 1096·3
3,4-Dihydroxymandelic Acid, 854·1
11β,17α-Dihydroxy-21-mercaptopregn-4-ene-3,20-dione 21-Pivalate, 1110·1
2,2′-Dihydroxy-4-methoxybenzophenone, 1145·3
Dihydroxymethyl Carbamide, 1187·2
3′,4′-Dihydroxy-2-(methylamino)acetophenone, 1648·1
3,4-Dihydroxy-4′-methyl-5-nitrobenzophenone, 1216·1
11α,17β-Dihydroxy-17β-methyl-3-oxoandrosta-1,4-diene-2-carbaldehyde, 1555·3
11β,17-Dihydroxy-21-(4-methyl-1-piperazinyl)pregna-1,4-diene-3,20-dione, 1105·3
17α,21-Dihydroxy-16β-methylpregna-1,4-diene-3,11,20-trione, 1106·1
11β,21-Dihydroxy-2′-methyl-5′β*H*-pregna-1,4-dieno[17,16-*d*]oxazole-3,20-dione 21-Acetate, 1096·2
3,4-Dihydroxy-5-nitrophenyl(4-methylphenyl)methanone, 1216·1
*l*-3,4-Dihydroxynorephedrine, 1675·3
Dihydroxy(octadecanoato-*O*-)aluminium, 1574·1
Dihydroxyoestrin, 1550·1
Dihydroxyoestrin Dipropionate, 1550·1
Dihydroxyoestrin Monobenzoate, 1550·1
1α,25-Dihydroxy-22-oxavitamin $D_3$, 1462·1
(5*Z*,13*E*)-(8*R*,11*R*,12*R*,15*S*)-11,15-Dihydroxy-9-oxoprosta-5,13-dienoic Acid, 1515·1
(*E*)-(8*R*,11*R*,12*R*,15*S*)-11,15-Dihydroxy-9-oxoprost-13-enoic Acid, 1512·3
(4*R*,5*R*)-4,5-Dihydroxy-$N^2$-{[4″-(pentyloxy)-*p*-terphenyl-4- Yl]carbonyl}-L-ornithyl-L-threonyl-*trans*-4-hydroxy-L-prolyl-(*S*)-4-hydroxy-4-(*p*-hydroxyphenyl)-L-threonyl-L-threonyl-(3*S*,4*S*)-3-hydroxy-4-methyl-L-proline Cyclic (6→1)-Peptide, 395·1
1-((4*R*,5*R*)-4,5-Dihydroxy-$N^2$-{[4″-(pentyloxy)(1,1′:4′,1″-terphenyl)-4-yl]carbonyl}-L-ornithine)-echinocandin B, 395·1
(*Z*)-7-[(1*R*, 2*R*,3*R*,5*S*)-3,5-Dihydroxy-2-[(*E*)-2-[2-(phenoxymethyl)-1,3-dioxolan-2-yl]vinyl]cyclopentyl]-5-heptenoic Acid, 1518·1
*erythro*-(3,4-Dihydroxyphenyl) (2-Piperidyl)methanol Hydrobromide, 791·3
Dihydroxyphenylacetic Acid, 1208·3
Dihydroxyphenylalanine, 1205·2
(−)-3-(3,4-Dihydroxyphenyl)-L-alanine, 1205·2
*p*,γ-Dihydroxyphenylbutazone, 84·1
2-(3,4-Dihydroxyphenyl)chroman-3,4,5,7-tetrol, 1688·2
2-(3,4-Dihydroxyphenyl)-5,7-dihydroxy-4-oxo-4*H*-chromen-3-yl 6-*O*-(α-L-Rhamnosyl)-β-D-glucoside, 1688·2
1-(3,5-Dihydroxyphenyl)-2-(4-hydroxy-α-methylphenethylamino)ethanol, 785·2
1-(3,5-Dihydroxyphenyl)-2-(4-hydroxy-α-methylphenethylamino)ethanol Hydrobromide, 785·2
Dihydroxyphenylisatin, 1282·3
1-(3,4-Dihydroxyphenyl)-2-isopropylaminobutan-1-ol, 787·3
1-(3,4-Dihydroxyphenyl)-2-isopropylaminoethanol, 940·2
1-(3,5-Dihydroxyphenyl)-2-isopropylaminoethanol Sulphate, 790·2
1-(3,4-Dihydroxyphenyl)-2-[4-(2-methoxyphenyl)piperazin-1-yl]ethanol, 983·3
(−)-3-(3,4-Dihydroxyphenyl)-2-methyl-L-alanine Sesquihydrate, 953·2
(*R*)-1-(3,4-Dihydroxyphenyl)-2-methylaminoethanol, 852·2
(−)-*threo*-3-(3,4-Dihydroxyphenyl)-L-serine, 1204·3
DL-*threo*-3,4-Dihydroxyphenylserine, 1205·1
L-*threo*-3,4-Dihydroxyphenylserine, 1204·3
2-(3,4-Dihydroxyphenyl)-3,5,7-trihydroxy-4*H*-1-benzopyran-4-one, 1688·2
2-(3,4-Dihydroxyphenyl)-3,5,7-trihydroxy-4-oxo-4*H*-chromen-3-yl Rutinoside Trihydrate, 1688·2
Dihydroxyphthalophenone, 1284·1
*erythro*-3,4-Dihydroxy-α-(2-piperidyl)benzyl Alcohol Hydrobromide, 791·3
11β,17α-Dihydroxypregna-1,4-diene-3,20-dione, 1096·3
17α,21-Dihydroxypregna-1,4-diene-3,11,20-trione, 1109·3
3α,21-Dihydroxy-5α-pregnane-11,20-dione 21-Acetate, 1296·3
17α,21-Dihydroxypregn-4-ene-3,11,20-trione 21-Acetate, 1096·1
Dihydroxyprogesterone Acetophenide, 1541·3
1,3-Dihydroxypropan-2-one, 1145·2
Dihydroxypropoxymethylguanine, 635·3
9-(1,3-Dihydroxy-2-propoxymethyl)guanine, 635·3
2,3-Dihydroxypropyl *N*-(7-Chloro-4-quinolyl)anthranilate, 44·3
2,3-Dihydroxypropyl *N*-(8-Trifluoromethyl-4-quinolyl)anthranilate, 43·2
*N*-(2,3-Dihydroxypropyl)-5-[*N*-(2,3-dihydroxypropyl)acetamido]-*N*′-(2-hydroxyethyl)-2,4,6-triidoisophthalamide, 1066·3
1-(2,3-Dihydroxypropyl)-3,5-di-iodo-4-pyridone, 1065·3
7-(2,3-Dihydroxypropyl)-1,3-dimethylxanthine, 784·3
3-(2,3-Dihydroxypropyl)-2-methyl-4(3*H*)-quinazolinone, 35·3
7-(2,3-Dihydroxypropyl)theophylline, 784·3
Dihydroxypropyltheophyllinum, 784·3
3′,6′-Dihydroxyspiro[isobenzofuran-1(3*H*),9′(9*H*)xanthen]-3-one, 1689·1
Dihydroxy(stearato)aluminium, 1574·1
1α,24-Dihydroxyvitamin $D_3$, 1158·3
1α,25-Dihydroxyvitamin $D_3$, 1461·2
Dihytamin, 1939·4
Dihyzin, 1939·4
Diidergot, 1939·4
3,3′-Di-2-imidazolin-2-ylcarbanilide Dipropionate, 606·1
Diiodohidroxiquinoleína, 603·3
Diiodohydroxyquin, 603·3
Di-iodohydroxyquinoline, 603·3
Diiodohydroxyquinoline, 603·3

2,6-Diiodo-4-nitrophenol, 105·1
3,5-Di-iodo-4-pyridone, 1065·3
Di-iodopyridone Acetate, 1067·3
5,7-Di-iodoquinolin-8-ol, 603·3
Diiodotirosina, 1597·3
Diiodotyrosine, 1597·3
L-Di-iodotyrosine, 1594·1
3,5-Di-iodo-L-tyrosine Dihydrate, 1597·3
Di-iodoxychinolinum, 603·3
Diiodoxyquinoléine, 603·3
*p*-Diisobutilfenoxipolietoxietanol, 1411·2
Diisobutylphenoxyethoxyethyldimethylbenzylammonium Chloride, 1169·2
*p*-Di-isobutyl-phenoxypolyethoxyethanol, 1411·2
Diisopromina, Hidrocloruro de, 1261·2
Diisopromine Hydrochloride, 1261·2
Di-isopromine Hydrochloride, 1261·2
Diisopropanolamina, 1680·2
Diisopropanolamine, 1680·2
Diisopropanolamine Felbinac, 39·1
Diisopropilamina, Dicloroacetato de, 900·1
Di-isopropyl Adipate, 1481·2
Diisopropyl 1,3-Dithiole-$\Delta^{2,\alpha}$-malonate, 1709·3
Di-isopropyl Fluorophosphate, 1490·1
Di-isopropyl Phosphorofluoridate, 1490·1
Diisopropyl Sebacate, 1157·3
Di-isopropylamine Dichloroacetate, 900·1
Di-isopropylamine Dichloroethanoate, 900·1
2′-(2-Di-isopropylaminoethoxy)butyrophenone Hydrochloride, 1377·1
(+)-(*R*)-2-{α-[2-(Diisopropylamino)ethyl]benzyl}-*p*-cresol Tartrate, 489·3
*N*-[2-(Diisopropylamino)ethyl]-2-oxo-1-pyrrolidineacetamide Sulphate, 1734·3
4-Di-isopropylamino-2-phenyl-2-(2-pyridyl)butyramide, 903·3
Di-isopropylammonium Dichloroacetate, 900·1
*NN*-Di-isopropyl-3,3-diphenylpropylamine Hydrochloride, 1261·2
Di-isopropylfluorophosphonate, 1490·1
2,3:4,5-Di-*O*-isopropylidene-β-D-fructopyranose Sulphamate, 378·3
Di-isopropylmethyl[2-(xanthen-9-ylcarbonyloxy)ethyl]ammonium Bromide, 489·1
2,6-Di-isopropylphenol, 1305·3
Dijex, 1939·4
Dikacine, 1939·4
Dikalii Clorazepas, 685·1
Dikalii Phosphas, 1230·3
6,15-Diketo-13,14-dihydro-prostaglandin $F_{1\alpha}$, 1517·2
Dilabar, 1939·4
Dilabar Diu, 1939·4
Dilacard, 1939·4
Dilaclan, 1939·4
Dilacor, 1939·4
Dilacoran, 1939·4
Dilacoron, 1939·4
Diladel, 1939·4
Dilaescol, 1939·4
Dilaflux, 1939·4
Dilafurane, 1939·4
Dilamax, 1939·4
Dilamet, 1939·4
Dilamol, 1939·4
Dilanacin, 1939·4
Dilanorm, 1939·4
Dilantin, 1940·1
Dilantin with Phenobarbital, 1940·1
Dilaplus, 1940·1
Dilapres, 1940·1
Dilar, 1940·1
Dilarmine, 1940·1
Dilartan, 1940·1
Dilarterial, 1940·1
Dilatam, 1940·1
Dilatol, 1940·1
Dilatol-Chinin, 1940·1
Dilatrane, 1940·1
Dilatrat, 1940·1
Dilatrate, 1940·1
Dilatrend, 1940·1
Dilaudid, 1940·1
Dilaudid Cough, 1940·1
Dilaudid-Atropin, 1940·1
Dilazep, Hidrocloruro de, 900·1
Dilazep Hydrochloride, 900·1
Dilbloc, 1940·1
Dilcard, 1940·1
Dilcardia, 1940·1
Dilclor, 1940·1
Dilcontin, 1940·1
Dilcor, 1940·1
Dilcoran, 1940·2
Dilem, 1940·2
Dilena, 1940·2
Diletan, 1940·2
Dilevalol, 943·3
Dilfar, 1940·2
Diligan, 1940·2
Dilinct, 1940·2
Diliter, 1940·2
Dilithium Carbonate, 301·1
Dilizem, 1940·2
Dill, 1680·2
Dill Fruit, 1680·2
Dill Oil, 1680·2
Dill Seed Oil, European, 1680·2
Dilmin, 1940·2
Diloc, 1940·2
Dilocaine, 1940·2
Dilomil, 1940·2
Dilongo, 1940·2
Dilor, 1940·2
Dilor-G, 1940·2
Dilospir, 1940·2
Dilostop, 1940·2
Dilosyn, 1940·2
Dilosyn Expectorant, 1940·2
Dilotab, 1940·2
Dilox, 1940·2
Diloxanida, Furoato de, 604·1
Diloxanide Furoate, 604·1
Diloxin, 1940·3
Dilpral, 1940·3
Dilrene, 1940·3
Dilsal, 1940·3
Dilsana, 1940·3
Dil-Sanorania, 1940·3
Dilta, 1940·3
Diltabeta, 1940·3
Diltahexal, 1940·3
Diltam, 1940·3
Diltan, 1940·3
Diltapham, 1940·3
Diltaretard, 1940·3
Diltec, 1940·3
Diltelan, 1940·3
Diltenk, 1940·3
Dilti, 1940·3
Diltia, 1940·3
Diltiacor, 1940·3
Diltiagamma, 1940·3
Diltiamax, 1940·3
Diltiamerck, 1940·3
Diltiangina, 1940·3
Diltiastad, 1940·3
Diltiazem, Hidrocloruro de, 900·1
Diltiazem Hydrochloride, 900·1
Diltiazem Malate, 900·1
Diltiazemi Hydrochloridum, 900·1
Diltiem, 1940·3
Diltikard, 1940·3
Diltin, 1940·3
Diltipress, 1940·3
Diltiuc, 1940·3
Diltiwas, 1940·3
Diltix, 1940·3
Diltizem, 1940·3
Diltotal, 1940·4
Dilubrin, 1940·4
Dilucid, 1940·4
Dilucort, 1940·4
Dilum, 1940·4
Diluplex, 1940·4
Dilusol, 1940·4
Dilusol AHA, 1940·4
Dilute Acetic Acid, 1645·2
Dilute Ammonia Solution, 1653·3
Dilute Ethanols, 1166·1
Dilute Hydrogen Peroxide Solution, 1182·2
Dilute Sodium Hypochlorite Solution, 1192·1
Dilute Sulphuric Acid, 1750·3
Diluted Acetic Acid, 1645·3
Diluted Alcohol, 1166·1
Diluted Hydrochloric Acid, 1699·1
Diluted Isosorbide Dinitrate, 941·1
Diluted Nitroglycerin, 923·2
Diluted Phosphoric Acid, 1731·2
Dilutional Hyponatraemia— *see* Hyponatraemia, 1220·3
Dilutol, 1940·4
Dilydrin, 1940·4
Dilydrine Retard, 1940·4
Dilzanol, 1940·4
Dilzatyrol, 1940·4
Dilzem, 1940·4
Dilzene, 1940·4
Dilzen-G, 1940·4
Dilzereal, 1940·4
Dilzicardin, 1940·4
Dima, 1940·4
Dimac, 1940·4
Dimacol, 1940·4
Dimafit, 1940·4
Dimagrasi, 1940·4
Dimagrasicell, 1940·4
Dimagress, 1940·4
Dimagrir Triac, 1940·4
Dimaleato de Pirisudanol, 1732·3
Dimalosio, 1940·4
Dimanin R, 1940·4
Dim-Antos, 1940·4
Dimaphen, 1940·4
Dimate, 1941·1
Dimaval, 1941·1
Dimaxin, 1941·1
Dimayon, 1941·1
Dimecaina, 1941·1
Dimeclofenone, 1124·3
Dimecrotic Acid, 1680·3
Dimedrolum, 431·3
Dimeflina, Hidrocloruro de, 1587·2
Dimefline Hydrochloride, 1587·2
Dimefor, 1941·1
Dimegan, 1941·1
Dimeglumine Gadopentetate, 1062·2
Dimeglumine Iodipamide, 1060·1
Dimeglumine Iodoxamate, 1064·1
Dimeglumine Iotroxate, 1066·1
Dimelor, 1941·1
Dimemorfan Phosphate, 1118·3
Dimemorfano, Fosfato de, 1118·3
Dimen, 1941·1
Dimenate, 1941·1
Dimenformon, 1941·1
Dimenhidrinato, 431·1
Dimenhydrinate, 431·1
Dimenhydrinatum, 431·1
Dimeno, 1941·1
Dimepranol, 640·2
Dimepranol Acedoben, 640·2
Dimepropion Hydrochloride, 1714·1
Dimercaprol, 1037·1
Dimercaprolum, 1037·1
($R^*$,$S^*$)-2,3-Dimercapto-butanedioic Acid, 1054·2
2,3-Dimercaptopropanesulfonate, Sodium, 1055·3
2,3-Dimercaptopropan-1-ol, 1037·1
*meso*-2,3-Dimercaptosuccinic Acid, 1054·2
Dimertest, 1941·1
Dimesilato de Almitrina, 1584·2
Dimesna, 1041·3
Dimesul, 1941·1
Dimetabs, 1941·1
Dimetamfenol Hydrochloride, 1037·3
Dimetane Preparations, 1941·1
Dimetapp Preparations, 1941·2
Dimethicone, 1482·1
Dimethicone, Activated, 1289·2
Dimethicream, 1941·4
Dimethindene Maleate, 431·2
Dimethisoquin Hydrochloride, 1384·2
Dimethisoquinium Chloride, 1384·2
Dimethoate, 1504·1
Dimethothiazine Mesylate, 431·3
Dimethoxanate Hydrochloride, 1119·1
Dimethoxane, 1681·1
2,5-Dimethoxy-4-bromoamfetamine, 1593·3
*N*-(3,4-Dimethoxycinnamoyl)anthranilic Acid, 806·3
6,7-Dimethoxy-1-(3,4-dimethoxybenzyl)isoquinoline, 1728·1
6,7-Dimethoxy-1-(3,4-dimethoxybenzyl)isoquinoline Hydrochloride, 1728·1
2,5-Dimethoxy-4-metamfetamine, 1593·3
Dimethoxymethane, 1680·3
5-[3,5-Dimethoxy-4-(2-methoxyethoxy)-benzyl]pyrimidine-2,4-diyldiamine, 269·2
2,4-Dimethoxy-β-methylcinnamic Acid, 1680·3
4,9-Dimethoxy-7-methyl-5*H*-furo[3,2-*g*]chromen-5-one, 1653·3
5-(4,5-Dimethoxy-2-methylphenyl)methyl-2,4-pyrimidinediamine, 240·2
5,6-Dimethoxy-2-methyl-3-[2-(4-phenylpiperazin-1-yl)ethyl]indole, 713·1
(*RS*)-$N^4$-[2,6-Dimethoxy-4-methyl-5-(3-trifluoromethylphenoxy)quinolin-8-yl]pentane-1,4-diamine, 463·3
Dimethoxyphenecillin Sodium, 230·3
(−)-(*R*)-α-{[(3,4-Dimethoxyphenethyl)amino]methyl}-*p*-hydroxybenzyl Alcohol, 892·2
1-(3,4-Dimethoxyphenethylamino)-3-*m*-tolyloxypropan-2-ol Hydrochloride, 873·2
5-[*N*-(3,4-Dimethoxyphenethyl)-*N*-methylamino]-2-(3,4-dimethoxyphenyl)-2-isopropylvaleronitrile Hydrochloride, 1019·1
5-[*N*-(3,4-Dimethoxyphenethyl)-*N*-methylamino]-2-(3,4,5-trimethoxyphenyl)-2-isopropylvaleronitrile Hydrochloride, 922·3
Dimethoxyphenyl Penicillin Sodium, 230·3
1-(3,4-Dimethoxyphenyl)-5-ethyl-7,8-dimethoxy-4-methyl-5*H*-2,3-benzodiazepine, 725·3
{5*R*-[5α,5aβ,8aα,9β(*R*$^*$)]}-5-[3,5-Dimethoxy-4-(phosphonooxy)phenyl]-9-[(4,6-*O*-ethylidene-β-D-glucopyranosyl)oxy]-5,8,8a,9-tetrahydrofuro-[3′,4′:6,7]naphtho[2,3-*d*]-1,3-dioxol-6(5a*H*)-one, 551·3
$N^1$-(2,6-Dimethoxypyrimidin-4-yl)sulphanilamide, 259·2
$N^1$-(5,6-Dimethoxypyrimidin-4-yl)sulphanilamide, 259·3
6,7-Dimethoxy-2-[4-(tetrahydrofuran-2-carbonyl)piperazin-1-yl]quinazolin-4-ylamine Hydrochloride Dihydrate, 1010·3
(3*S*)-6,7-Dimethoxy-3-[(5*R*)-5,6,7,8-tetrahydro-4-methoxy-6-methyl-1,3-dioxolo[4,5-*g*]isoquinolin-5-yl]phthalide, 1125·3
6,7-Dimethoxy-3-(5,6,7,8-tetrahydro-6-methyl-1,3-dioxolo[4,5-*g*]isoquinolin-5-yl)isobenzofuran-1(3*H*)-one Hydrochloride, 1698·3
Dimethpyrindene Maleate, 431·2
Dimethyl Benzene-1,2-dicarboxylate, 1504·1
Dimethyl (3*S*,8*S*,9*S*,12*S*)-9-Benzyl-3,12-di-*tert*-butyl-8-hydroxy-4,11-dioxo-6-(*p*-2-pyridylbenzyl)-2,5,6,10,13-pentaazatetradecanedioate Sulfate (1:1), 629·1
Dimethyl Carbinol, 1184·3
Dimethyl 1,2-Dibromo-2,2-dichloroethyl Phosphate, 1507·3
Dimethyl 1,4-Dihydro-2,6-dimethyl-4-(2-nitrophenyl)pyridine-3,5-dicarboxylate, 966·2
Dimethyl Ether, 1236·1
Dimethyl Fumarate, 1147·3
Dimethyl Ketone, 1471·1
Dimethyl {2-[2-(2-Methoxyacetamido)-4-(phenylthio)phenyl]imidocarbonyl}dicarbamate, 105·2
*O,O*-Dimethyl *S*-Methylcarbamoylmethyl Phosphorodithioate, 1504·1
Dimethyl (1-Methyl-2-phenothiazin-10-ylethyl)amine, 439·1
*O,O*-Dimethyl *O*-4-Methylthio-*m*-tolyl Phosphorothioate, 1505·2

*O,O*-Dimethyl *O*-4-Nitro-*m*-tolyl Phosphorothioate, 1505·2
Dimethyl Oxide, 1236·1
Dimethyl Phthalate, 1504·1
*O,O*-Dimethyl Phthalimidomethyl Phosphorodithioate, 1509·1
Dimethyl Silicone Fluid, 1482·1
Dimethyl Sulfide, 1473·3
Dimethyl Sulfone, 1473·3
Dimethyl Sulfoxide, 1473·2
*O,O*-Dimethyl *O*-(4-Sulphamoylphenyl) Phosphorothioate, 1503·1
Dimethyl Sulphoxide, 1473·2
Dimethyl 2,2,2-Trichloro-1-hydroxyethylphosphonate, 109·2
Dimethyl Tubocurarine Iodide, 1403·3
Dimethylacetamide, 1474·1
*NN*-Dimethylacetamide, 1474·1
Dimethylacetamidum, 1474·1
*N'*-(3,3-Dimethylacroyl)sulphanilamide, 259·2
3,5-Dimethyl-1-adamantanamine Hydrochloride, 1711·2
Dimethylaminoantipyrine, 14·2
[4-(4-Dimethylaminobenzhydrylidene)cyclohexa-2,5-dienylidene]dimethylammonium Chloride, 1185·2
*N*-{(6*R*,9*S*,10*R*,13*S*,15a*S*,18*R*,22*S*,24a*S*)-22-[*p*-(Dimethylamino)benzyl]-6-ethyldocosahydro-10,23-dimethyl-5,8,12,15,17,21,24-heptaoxo-13-phenyl-18-{[(3*S*)-3-quinuclidinylthio]methyl}-12*H*-pyrido[2,1-*f*]pyrrolo[2,1-*l*][1,4,7,10,13,16]-oxapentaazacyclononadecin-9-yl}-3-hydroxy-picolinamide Methanesulphonate, 248·2
2-Dimethylamino-1,1-dimethylethyl Benzilate Hydrochloride, 481·3
4-Dimethylamino-1,5-dimethyl-2-phenyl-4-pyrazolin-3-one, 14·2
(−)-(3*S*,6*S*)-6-(Dimethylamino)-4,4-diphenyl-3-heptanol Acetate Hydrochloride, 54·1
(±)-6-Dimethylamino-4,4-diphenylheptan-3-one Hydrochloride, 57·2
(−)-6-Dimethylamino-4,4-diphenylheptan-3-one Hydrochloride, 54·1
6-Dimethylamino-4,4-diphenylhexan-3-one Hydrochloride, 1125·2
2-Dimethylaminoethanol, 1585·3
*N*-[4-(2-Dimethylaminoethoxy)benzyl]-3,4,5-trimethoxybenzamide Hydrochloride, 442·2
*N*-{*p*-[2-(Dimethylamino)ethoxy]benzyl}veratramide Hydrochloride, 1268·2
2-(2-Dimethylaminoethoxy)ethyl Phenothiazine-10-carboxylate Hydrochloride, 1119·1
4-(2-Dimethylaminoethoxy)-5-isopropyl-2-methylphenyl Acetate Hydrochloride, 962·2
(*E*)-α-{*p*-[2-(Dimethylamino)ethoxy]phenyl}-α′-ethyl-3-stilbenol, 550·1
2-(2-Dimethylaminoethoxy)-*N*-(tricyclo[3.3.1.1$^{3,7}$]dec-1-yl)acetamide Hydrochloride, 656·1
2-Dimethylaminoethyl 4-Butylaminobenzoate, 1385·1
2-Dimethylaminoethyl 4-Chlorophenoxyacetate Hydrochloride, 1710·1
2-Dimethylaminoethyl 2-(1-Hydroxycyclopentyl)-2-phenylacetate Hydrochloride, 480·3
2-Dimethylaminoethyl 5-Hydroxy-4-hydroxymethyl-6-methyl-3-pyridylmethyl Succinate Maleate, 1732·3
10-(2-Dimethylaminoethyl)-5,10-dihydro-5-methyl-dibenzo[*b,e*][1,4]diazepin-11-one Hydrochloride, 290·3
(−)-4-Dimethylamino-1-ethyl-2,2-diphenylpentyl Acetate, 54·1
2-(Dimethylamino)ethyldiphenyl(2-propynyloxy)acetate Hydrochloride, 487·3
3-(2-Dimethylaminoethyl)indole, 1680·3
3-(2-Dimethylaminoethyl)indol-4-ol, 1736·1
3-(2-Dimethylaminoethyl)indol-5-ol, 1663·2
3-(2-Dimethylaminoethyl)indol-4-yl Dihydrogen Phosphate, 1736·1
3-(2-Dimethylaminoethyl)indol-5-yl-*N*-methylmethanesulphonamide Succinate, 471·2
(*S*)-4-{3-[2-(Dimethylamino)ethyl]indol-5-ylmethyl}-1,3-oxazolidin-2-one, 473·3
1-[({3-[2-(Dimethylamino)ethyl]indol-5-yl}methyl)sulfonyl]pyrrolidine Malate (1:1), 465·2
(−)-*m*-[(*S*)-1-(Dimethylamino)ethyl]phenyl Ethylmethylcarbamate, 1497·1
(2*S*,3*S*)-5-(2-Dimethylaminoethyl)-2,3,4,5-tetrahydro-2-(4-methoxyphenyl)-4-oxo-1,5-benzothiazepin-3-yl Acetate Hydrochloride, 900·1
3-[2-(Dimethylamino)ethyl]-5-(1*H*-1,2,4-triazol-1-ylmethyl)indole Monobenzoate, 471·1
4-Dimethylamino-2-isopropyl-2-phenylpentanonitrile, 1123·3
4-Dimethylamino-2-isopropyl-2-phenylvaleronitrile Dihydrogen Citrate, 1123·3
(±)-2-(Dimethylamino)-1-{[*o*-(*m*-methoxyphenethyl)phenoxy]methyl}ethyl Hydrogen Succinate Hydrochloride, 996·3
(*RS*)-1-(2-Dimethylamino-1-*p*-methoxyphenylethyl)cyclohexanol Hydrochloride, 321·3
3-(3-Dimethylaminomethyleneamino-2,4,6-tri-iodophenyl)propionic Acid, 1065·2
(*S*)-10-Dimethylaminomethyl-4-ethyl-4,9-dihydroxy-1*H*-pyrano[3′,4′:6,7]indolizino[1,2*b*]quinoline-3,14(4*H*,12*H*)-dione Hydrochloride, 589·1
*N*-[2-({5-[(Dimethylamino)methyl]furfuryl}thio)-ethyl]-*N′*-methyl-2-nitro-1,1-ethenediamine, Compound with Bismuth(3+) Citrate (1:1), 1287·2
*N*-[2-({5-[(Dimethylamino)methyl]furfuryl}thio)ethyl]-2-nitro-*N′*-piperonyl-1,1-ethenediamine Hydrochloride, 1277·2
8-Dimethylaminomethyl-7-methoxy-3-methyl-2-phenylchromen-4-one Hydrochloride, 1587·2
(±)-*trans*-2-Dimethylaminomethyl-1-(3-methoxyphenyl)cyclohexanol Hydrochloride, 94·3
1-(Dimethylaminomethyl)-1-methylpropyl Benzoate Hydrochloride, 1370·2
4-[4-(Dimethylamino)-*N*-methyl-L-phenylalamine]-5-(*cis*-5-{[(*S*)-1-azabicyclo[2.2.2]oct-3-ylthio]methyl}-4-oxo-L-2-piperidinecarboxylic acid)-virginiamycin $S_1$ Methanesulphonate, 248·2
10-(3-Dimethylamino-2-methylpropyl)phenothiazine 5,5-Dioxide, 438·2
10-(3-Dimethylamino-2-methylpropyl)phenothiazine-2-carbonitrile, 689·2
5-Dimethylamino-9-methyl-2-propylpyrazolo[1,2-*a*][1,2,4]benzotriazine-1,3(2*H*)-dione, 20·1
5-(8-Dimethylamino-7-methyl-5-quinolylmethyl)pyrimidin-2,4-diyldiamine, 162·2
*N*-[2-(2-Dimethylaminomethylthiazol-4-ylmethylthio)ethyl]-*N′*-methyl-2-nitrovinylidenediamine, 1277·2
4*S*,4a*R*,5*S*,5a*R*,6*S*,12a*S*-4-Dimethylamino-1,4,4a,5,5a,6,11,12a-octahydro-3,5,6,10,12,12a-hexahydroxy-6-methylene-1,11-dioxonaphthacene-2-carboxamide, 241·1
(4*S*,4a*S*,5a*S*,6*S*,12a*S*)-4-Dimethylamino-1,4,4a,5,5a,6,11,12a-octahydro-3,6,10,12,12a-pentahydroxy-6-methyl-1,11-dioxonaphthacene-2-carboxamide, 266·2
(4*S*,4a*R*,5*S*,5a*R*,6*S*,12a*S*)-4-Dimethylamino-1,4,4a,5,5a,6,11,12a-octahydro-3,5,10,12,12a-pentahydroxy-6-methyl-1,11-dioxonaphthacene-2-carboxamide Monohydrate, 206·2
(4*S*,4a*R*,5*S*,5a*R*,6*R*,12a*S*)-4-Dimethylamino-1,4,4a,5,5a,6,11,12a-octahydro-3,5,10,12,12a-pentahydroxy-6-methylene-1,11-dioxonaphthacene-2-carboxamide, 230·1
Dimethylaminophenazone, 14·2
4-Dimethylaminophenol Hydrochloride, 1037·3
2-Dimethylamino-2-phenylbutyl 3,4,5-Trimethoxybenzoate Hydrogen Maleate, 1758·1
11β-(4-Dimethylaminophenyl)-17β-hydroxy-17α-prop-1-ynylestra-4,9-dien-3-one, 1560·2
2-Dimethylamino-1-phenylpropan-1-ol Hydrochloride, 1124·2
(±)-1-(Dimethylamino)-2-propanol, 640·2
2-Dimethylaminopropiophenone Hydrochloride, 1714·1
10-(2-Dimethylaminopropyl)-*NN*-dimethylphenothiazine-2-sulphonamide Methanesulphonate, 431·3
1-(3-Dimethylaminopropyl)-1-(4-fluorophenyl)-1,3-dihydroisobenzofuran-5-carbonitrile, 289·1
(+)-(*S*)-1-[3-(Dimethylamino)propyl]-1-(*p*-fluorophenyl)-5-phthalancarbonitrile Oxalate, 292·1
11-[(*Z*)-3-(Dimethylamino)propylidene]-6,11-dihydrodibenz[*b,e*]oxepin-2-acetic Acid Hydrochloride, 438·1
10-(2-Dimethylaminopropyl)phenothiazin-2-yl Methyl Ketone, 668·3
10-(3-Dimethylaminopropyl)phenothiazin-2-yl Methyl Ketone, 668·3
10-(3-Dimethylaminopropyl)phenothiazin-2-yl Methyl Ketone Hydrogen Maleate, 668·3
1-[10-(2-Dimethylaminopropyl)phenothiazin-2-yl]propan-1-one, 440·3
α-[2-(Dimethylamino)propyl]-α-phenylbenzeneacetamide, 481·3
*N*-Dimethylaminosuccinamic Acid, 1503·1
4-Dimethylamino-*O*-tolylphosphinic Acid, 1231·3
Dimethylarsinic Acid, 1657·3
Dimethylbenzene, 1478·2
(*R*)-*N*,α-Dimethylbenzeneethanamine, 1124·1
*Co*α-[α-(5,6-Dimethylbenzimidazolyl)]-*Co*β-cyanocobamide, 1458·2
*Co*α-[α-(5,6-Dimethylbenzimidazolyl)]-*Co*β-hydroxocobamide, 1458·2
*N*,α-Dimethyl-1,3-benzodioxole-5-ethanamine, 1589·3
*p*,α-Dimethylbenzyl Alcohol, 1680·3
*p*,α-Dimethylbenzyl Alcohol Nicotinate, 1680·3
4-(2,3-Dimethylbenzyl)imidazole Monohydrochloride, 689·3
1,1-Dimethylbiguanide Hydrochloride, 342·3
1,1′-Dimethyl-4,4′-bipyridyldiylium Ion, 1508·1
*N*-[*N*-(3,3-Dimethylbutyl)-L-α-aspartyl]-L-phenylalanine 1-Methyl Ester, 1441·1
*N,N*-Dimethylcarbamoylmethyl 4-(4-Guanidinobenzoyloxy)phenylacetate Methanesulphonate, 1665·2
3-Dimethylcarbamoyloxy-1-methylpyridinium Bromide, 1496·1
3-(Dimethylcarbamoyloxy)trimethylanilinium Ion, 1492·2
(4*R*,5*S*,6*S*)-3-[(3*S*,5*S*)-5-Dimethylcarbamoylpyrrolidin-3-ylthio]-6-[(*R*)-1-hydroxyethyl]-4-methyl-7-oxo-1-azabicyclo[3.2.0]hept-2-ene-2-carboxylic Acid Trihydrate, 229·1
(+)-*O,O′*-Dimethylchondrocurarine Di-iodide, 1403·3
(±)-*N*-α-Dimethylcyclo-hexaneethylamine, 1592·3
(−)-*N*,α-Dimethylcyclohexaneethylamine with 5-Ethyl-5-phenylbarbituric Acid, 353·3
D-3,3-Dimethylcysteine, 1046·3
Dimethyl{3-(10,11-dihydro-5*H*-dibenz[*b,f*]-azepin-5-yl-2-methyl)propyl}amine, 320·2
(−)-[(*S*)-2,2-Dimethyl-1,3-dioxolan-4-yl]methyl *p*-((*S*)-2-Hydroxy-3-{[2-(4-morpholinecarboxamido)ethyl]amino}propoxy)hydrocinnamate Hydrochloride, 945·1
Dimethyldiphenylene Disulphide, 1152·1
(−)-*N,N*-Dimethyl-1,2-diphenylethylamine Hydrochloride, 53·1
Dimethylethyl Carbinol, 1471·2
3*S*[2(2*S**,3*S**),3α,4aβ,8aβ]-*N*-(1,1-Dimethylethyl)decahydro-2-2-hydroxy-3-[(3-hydroxy-2-methylbenzoyl)amino]-4-(phenylthio)butyl-3-isoquinolinecarboxamide Monomethanesulphonate, 650·1
2-(1,1-Dimethylethyl)-4-methoxyphenol, 1171·2
1-[4-(1,1-Dimethylethyl)phenyl]-3-(4-methoxyphenyl)-1,3-propanedione, 1142·3
Dimethylformamide, 1474·1
*NN*-Dimethylformamide, 1474·1
*N*-3,5-Dimethyl-gludantan, 1711·2
(*E*)-6,6-Dimethylhept-2-en-4-ynl(methyl)-(1-naphthylmethyl)amine, 408·2
(±)-(6a*R*,10a*R*)-3-(1,1-Dimethylheptyl)-6a,7,8,9,10,10a-hexahydro-1-hydroxy-6,6-dimethyl-6*H*-benzo[*c*]chromen-9-one, 1277·1
1,5-Dimethylhex-4-enyl(methyl)amine Hydrochloride, 1702·1
1,5-Dimethylhexylamine, 975·3
(*RS*)-1,3-Dimethyl-7-(2-hydroxypropyl)purine-2,6(3*H*,1*H*)-dione, 791·2
Dimethylhydroxypyridone, 1033·1
1,2-Dimethyl-3-hydroxypyrid-4-one, 1033·1
Dimethylis Sulfoxidum, 1473·2
1,4-Dimethyl-7-isopropylazulene, 1696·2
*N*[1]-(3,4-Dimethylisoxazol-5-yl)sulphanilamide, 260·1
*N*-(3,4-Dimethylisoxazol-5-yl)-*N*-sulphanilylacetamide, 260·1
Dimethylmethane, 1238·2
(−)-*NN*-Dimethyl-3-(2-methoxyphenothiazin-10-yl)-2-methylpropylamine, 703·2
*NN*-Dimethyl-5-[2-(1-methylamino-2-nitrovinylamino)ethylthiomethyl]furfurylamine, 1285·2
(*RS*)-Dimethyl[2-(2-methylbenzhydryloxy)ethyl]amine Dihydrogen Citrate, 486·1
(*RS*)-Dimethyl[2-(2-methylbenzhydryloxy)ethyl]amine Hydrochloride, 486·1
(2*S*,3*R*)-3-{(*S*)-[2,2-Dimethyl-1-(methylcarbamoyl)propyl]carbamoyl}-2-hydroxy-5-methylhexanohydroxamic Acid, 565·3
4,4-Dimethyl-1-[(3,4-methylenedioxy)phenyl]-1-penten-3-ol, 377·3
(±)-*cis*-2,6-Dimethyl-4-[2-methyl-3-(*p*-*tert*-pentylphenyl)propyl]morpholine, 391·1
*NN*-Dimethyl-2-methyl-3-(phenothiazin-10-yl)propylamine Tartrate, 423·3
(*Z*)-*NN*-Dimethyl-9-[3-(4-methylpiperazin-1-yl)propylidene]thioxanthene-2-sulphonamide, 725·2
*NN*-Dimethyl-10-[3-(4-methylpiperazin-1-yl)propyl]phenothiazine-2-sulphonamide Dimethanesulphonate, 724·1
*NN*-Dimethyl-2-[α-methyl-α-(2-pyridyl)benzyloxy]ethylamine Hydrogen Succinate, 432·3
2,4-Dimethyl-*N*-(3-methyl-2(3*H*)-thiazolylidene)benzenamine, 1502·3
*N,N*-Dimethyl-2-(6-methyl-2-*p*-tolylimidazo[1,2-*a*]pyridin-3-yl)acetamide Hemitartrate, 728·3
(+)-3,9a-Dimethylmorphinan Phosphate, 1118·3
1,2-Dimethyl-5-nitroimidazole, 604·1
(2*Z*,6*E*)-2-[(3*E*)-4,8-Dimethyl-3,7-nonadienyl]-6-methyl-2,6-octadiene-1,8-diol, 1284·1
3,7-Dimethylocta-2,6-dienyl 5,9,13-Trimethyltetradeca-4,8,12-trienoate, 1267·1
*N*[1]-(4,5-Dimethyl-1,2-oxazol-3-yl)sulfanilamide, 264·1
*N*[1]-(4,5-Dimethyloxazol-2-yl)sulphanilamide, 263·2
3-{(2*R*)-2-[(1*S*,3*S*,5*S*)-3,5-Dimethyl-2-oxocyclohexyl]-2-hydroxyethyl}glutarimide, 1502·1
3,7-Dimethyl-1-(5-oxohexyl)xanthine, 979·3
(2*S*,5*R*,6*R*)-3,3-Dimethyl-7-oxo-6-(2-phenylacetamido)-4-thia-1-azabicyclo[3.2.0]heptane-2-carboxylic Acid, 163·2
*N*-(2,3-Dimethyl-5-oxo-1-phenyl-3-pyrazolin-4-yl)nicotinamide, 66·3
(2*S*,5*R*)-3,3-Dimethyl-7-oxo-4-thia-1-azabicyclo[3.2.0]heptane-2-carboxylic Acid 4,4-Dioxide, 257·2
3-Dimethyl-7-oxo-4-thia-1-azabicyclo[3.2.0]heptane-2-carboxylic Acid Monohydrate, 243·1
(−)-(*R*)-*N*,α-Dimethylphenethylamine, 1124·1
α,α-Dimethylphenethylamine, 1592·2
(+)-*N*,α-Dimethylphenethylamine Hydrochloride, 1589·2

*NN*-Dimethyl-3-phenothiazin-10-ylpropylammonium Chloride, 717·3
*N*-(2,6-Dimethylphenyl)-*N'*-[imino(methylamino)methyl]urea Hydrochloride, 1270·2
(+)-3,4-Dimethyl-2-phenylmorpholine Hydrogen Tartrate, 1592·1
*N,N*-Dimethyl-α-(3-phenylpropyl)veratrylamine Hydrochloride, 1764·2
1,5-Dimethyl-2-phenyl-4-pyrazolin-3-one, 82·3
(±)-*cis*-2,6-Dimethyl-α-phenyl-α-2-pyridyl-1-piperidinebutanol Hydrochloride, 984·1
*NN*-Dimethyl-3-phenyl-3-(2-pyridyl)propylamine, 438·3
*N*,2-Dimethyl-2-phenylsuccinimide, 366·2
*NN*-Dimethyl-3-phenyl-3-*p*-tolylpropylamine Hydrochloride, 442·2
2,4'-Dimethyl-3-piperidinopropiophenone Hydrochloride, 1396·3
Dimethylpolysiloxane, 1482·1
Dimethylpolysiloxane, Activated, 1289·2
6,17α-Dimethylpregna-4,6-diene-3,20-dione, 1557·1
*N,N*-Dimethyl-2-(*N*-propylcrotonamido)butyramide, 1592·3
(*S*)-2',6'-Dimethyl-1-propylpiperidine-2-carboxanilide Hydrochloride Monohydrate, 1384·2
(−)-(*R*)-*N*,α-Dimethyl-*N*-(prop-2-ynyl)phenethylamine Hydrochloride, 1214·1
16,16-Dimethyl-*trans*-$\Delta^2$-prostaglandin $E_1$ Methyl Ester, 1518·1
*NN*-Dimethyl-1-(pyrido[3,2-*b*][1,4]benzothiazin-10-ylmethyl)ethylamine Hydrochloride, 435·2
*NN*-Dimethyl-3-(pyrido[3,2-*b*][1,4]benzothiazin-10-yl)propylamine Hydrochloride Monohydrate, 718·1
*NN*-Dimethyl-2-{3-[1-(2-pyridyl)ethyl]-1*H*-inden-2-yl}ethylamine Hydrogen Maleate, 431·2
*NN*-Dimethyl-*N'*-(2-pyridyl)-*N'*-(3-thenyl)ethylenediamine Hydrochloride, 442·1
3,3-Dimethyl-*N*-{4-[4-(2-pyrimidinyl)-1-piperazinyl]butyl}glutarimide Hydrochloride, 701·1
$N^1$-(2,6-Dimethylpyrimidin-4-yl)sulphanilamide, 264·1
$N^1$-(4,6-Dimethylpyrimidin-2-yl)sulphanilamide, 259·2
Dimethylpyrindene Maleate, 431·2
7,8-Dimethyl-10-(1'-D-ribityl)isoalloxazine, 1456·1
*NN*-Dimethylserotonin, 1663·2
Dimethylsiloxane, 1482·1
2-{4-[3-(2-Dimethylsulphamoylphenothiazin-10-yl)propyl]piperazin-1-yl}ethanol, 716·1
$N^1$-[3-(Dimethylsulphonio)propyl]bleomycinamide, 530·2
4,4'-(2,3-Dimethyltetramethylene)bis(benzene-1,2-diol), 1187·1
*meso*-4,4'-(2,3-Dimethyltetramethylene)dipyrocatechol, 566·1
Dimethylthianthrene, 1152·1
2,7-Dimethylthianthrene, 1152·1
5-(3,3-Dimethyltriazeno)imidazole-4-carboxamide, 544·2
Dimethyl{2-[5-(1*H*-1,2,4-triazol-1-ylmethyl)indol-3-yl]ethyl}amine Monobenzoate, 471·1
2,2'-Dimethyl-2,2'-[5-(1*H*-1,2,4-triazol-1-ylmethyl)-1,3-phenylene]bis(propiononitrile), 528·1
3,5-Dimethyltricyclo[3.3.1.1.$^{3,7}$]decan-l-amine Hydrochloride, 1711·2
*NN*-Dimethyl-3-(2-trifluoromethylphenothiazin-10-yl)propylamine, 727·1
5,5-Dimethyl-3-(α,α,α-trifluoro-4-nitro-*m*-tolyl)-imidazolidine-2,4-dione, 576·2
(2*E*,4*E*,6*Z*,8*E*)-3,7-Dimethyl-9-(2,6,6-trimethyl-1-cyclohexen-1-yl)-2,4,6,8-nonatetraenoic Acid, 526·2
(2*Z*,4*E*,6*E*,8*E*)-3,7-Dimethyl-9-(2,6,6-trimethylcyclohex-1-enyl)nona-2,4,6,8-tetraenoic Acid, 1148·3
3,7-Dimethyl-9-(2,6,6-trimethylcyclohex-1-enyl)nona-2,4,6,8-*all-trans*-tetraenoic Acid, 1161·1
3,7-Dimethyl-9-(2,6,6-trimethylcyclohex-1-enyl)nona-2,4,6,8-tetraen-1-ol, 1451·2
Dimethyltryptamine, 1680·3
*N,N*-Dimethyltryptamine, 1680·3
Dimethyltubocurarine Iodide, 1403·3
1,3-Dimethyluric Acid, 804·1
Dimethylxanthine, 783·1
1,3-Dimethylxanthine, 798·3
3,7-Dimethylxanthine, 798·2
2,2-Dimethyl-5-(2,5-xylyloxy)valeric Acid, 923·1
Dimeticonas, 1482·1
Dimeticone, 1482·1
Dimeticonum, 1482·1
Dimetigal, 1941·4
Dimetil Sulfóxido, 1473·2
Dimetilacetamida, 1474·1
4-Dimetilaminofenol, Hidrocloruro de, 1037·3
Dimetilformamida, 1474·1
Dimetiltriptamina, 1680·3
Dimetiltubocurarinio, Ioduro de, 1403·3
Dime-Time, 1941·4
Dimetindene Maleate, 431·2
Dimetindeni Maleas, 431·2
Dimetindeno, Maleato de, 431·2
Dimetin-F, 1941·4
Dimetirol, 1941·4
Dimetoato, 1504·1
Dimetofrina, Hidrocloruro de, 902·3
Dimetofrine Hydrochloride, 902·3
Dimetophrine Hydrochloride, 902·3
Dimetotiazina, Mesilato de, 431·3
Dimetotiazine Mesilate, 431·3
Dimetoxanato, Hidrocloruro de, 1119·1
Dimetoximetano, 1680·3
Dimetridazol, 604·1
Dimetridazole, 604·1
Dimetriose, 1941·4
Dimetrose, 1941·4
Dimevamida, 481·3
Dimevamide, 481·3
Dimevamide Sulfate, 481·3
Dimex, 1941·4
Dimezin, 1941·4
Dimicaps, 1941·4
Dimicin, 1941·4
Dimicina, 1941·4
DiMill, 1941·4
Diminazene Aceturate, 604·2
Diminazeno, Aceturato de, 604·2
Diminex, 1941·4
Diminex Antitusigeno, 1941·4
Diminex Balsamico, 1941·4
Diminon, 1941·4
Diminual, 1941·4
Diminut, 1941·4
Dimirel, 1941·4
Dimiril, 1941·4
Dimitone, 1941·4
Dimodan, 1941·4
Dimol, 1941·4
Dimophebumine Hydrochloride, 1764·2
Dimophen, 1942·1
Dimophen DC, 1942·1
Dimor, 1942·1
Dimorf, 1942·1
Dimotane, 1942·1
Dimotane Co, 1942·1
Dimotane Expectorant, 1942·1
Dimotane Plus, 1942·1
Dimotapp, 1942·1
Dimotapp Expectorant, 1942·1
Dimpilato, 1504·2
Dimpylate, 1504·2
DIM-SA, 1054·2
Dina, 1942·1
Dinabac, 1942·1
Dinac, 1942·1
Dinacode, 1942·1
Dinacode Avec Codeine, 1942·1
Dinacode N, 1942·1
Dinaflex, 1942·1
Dinaflex Duo, 1942·1
Dinagen, 1942·1
Dinalexin, 1942·1
Dinamotonic, 1942·1
Dinapres, 1942·1
Dinasepte, 1942·1
Dinate, 1942·2
Dinaton, 1942·2
Dinatrii Edetas, 1037·3
Dinatrii Phosphas, 1231·1
Dinatrii Phosphas Anhydricus, 1231·1
Dinatrii Phosphas Dihydricus, 1231·1
Dinatrii Phosphas Dodecahydricus, 1231·1
Dinavir, 1942·2
Dinavital Ginseng, 1942·2
Dinavital Q10, 1942·2
Dinavital Vascular, 1942·2
Dinaxil, 1942·2
Dinaxil Capilar, 1942·2
Dinaxin, 1942·2
Dinazide, 1942·2
Dindevan, 1942·2
Dinefec, 1942·2
Di-Neumobron, 1942·2
Dineurin, 1942·2
3,6-Di-*O*-nicotinoylmorphine Hydrochloride, 66·3
1,3-Dinicotinoyloxypropan-2-ol, 2-(4-Chlorophenoxy)-2-methylpropionic Acid Ester with, 875·1
Diniket, 1942·2
Dinill, 1942·2
Dinintel, 1942·2
Dinisor, 1942·2
Dinistenile, 1942·2
Dinit, 1942·2
Dinitolmida, 604·2
Dinitolmide, 604·2
Dinitrato de Isosorbida, 941·1
2,4-Dinitrochlorobenzene, 1680·3
2,4-Dinitroclorobenceno, 1680·3
Dinitro-*o*-cresol, 1504·2
4,6-Dinitro-*o*-cresol, 1504·2
Dinitrofenol, 1504·2
Dinitrogen Oxide, 1304·3
Dinitrogenii Oxidum, 1304·3
3,5-Dinitro-2'-(5-nitrofurfurylidene)salicylohydrazide, 611·2
Dinitrophenol, 1504·2
2,4-Dinitrophenol, 1504·2
Dinitrotoluamide, 604·2
3,5-Dinitro-*o*-toluamide, 604·2
Dinnefords Teejel, 1942·2
Dinobroxol, 1942·2
Dinoprost, 1514·3
Dinoprost Trometamol, 1514·3
Dinoprost Tromethamine, 1514·3
Dinoprostona, 1515·1
Dinoprostone, 1515·1
Dinoprostonum, 1515·1
Dinoprostum Trometamoli, 1514·3
Dinostral, 1942·2
Dinoven, 1942·2
Dintoina, 1942·2
Dintoinale, 1942·2
Dinul, 1942·2
Dio, 1942·2
Dioalgo, 1942·3
Diocaine, 1942·3
Diocalm Dual Action, 1942·3
Diocalm Junior— *see* Diocalm Replenish, 1942·3
Diocalm Replenish, 1942·3
Diocalm Ultra, 1942·3
Diocam, 1942·3
Diocaps, 1942·3
Diocarpine, 1942·3
Diochloram, 1942·3
Diocimex, 1942·3
Diocla, 1942·3
Dioctosal, 1942·3
Dioctyl, 1942·3
Dioctyl Adipate, 1504·2
Dioctyl Calcium Sulfosuccinate, 1262·1
Dioctyl Calcium Sulphosuccinate, 1262·1
Dioctyl Potassium Sulfosuccinate, 1262·1
Dioctyl Potassium Sulphosuccinate, 1262·1
Dioctyl Sodium Sulfosuccinate, 1262·2
Dioctyl Sodium Sulphosuccinate, 1262·2
Diodarone, 1942·3
Dioderm, 1942·3
Diodex, 1942·3
Diodine, 1942·3
Diodolina, 1942·3
Diodoquin, 1942·3
Dioeze, 1942·3
Diofen, 1942·3
Diofluor, 1942·3
Diogent, 1942·3
Diolamina, 1681·1
Diolamine, 1681·1, 1758·2
Diolamine Fusidate, 216·2
Diolamine Laurilsulfate, 1574·3
Diolaxil, 1942·3
Diolin, 1942·3
Diomicete, 1942·3
Diomycin, 1942·3
Diondel, 1942·3
Dionephrine, 1942·4
Dionina, 1942·4
Dionina— *see* Mindol-Merck, 2134·1
Diono Resolvent, Bell— *see* Bell Diono Resolvent, 1832·3
Dionosil, 1942·4
Dioparine, 1942·4
Diopentolate, 1942·4
Diophenyl-T, 1942·4
Diopine, 1942·4
Diopred, 1942·4
Diopteаrs, 1942·4
Dioptec, 1942·4
Diopticon, 1942·4
Diopticon A, 1942·4
Dioptimyd, 1942·4
Dioptrol, 1942·4
Dioralyte, 1942·4
Dioralyte Effervescent, 1942·4
Dioralyte Relief, 1942·4
Dioralyte Rice, 1942·4
Dioran, 1942·4
Diosma, 1663·1
Diosmectal, 1942·4
Diosmetin 7-Rutinoside, 1688·2
Diosmil, 1942·4
Diosmin, 1688·2
{$\mu_7$-[(Diosmin Heptasulfato)(7-)]}tetracontahydroxytetradecaaluminium, 1264·1
Diosmina, 1688·2
Diosminil, 1942·4
Diosminum, 1688·2
Diospor HC, 1942·4
Diosporin, 1942·4
Diostate, 1942·4
Diosulf, 1942·4
Diosven, 1942·4
Diotrope, 1942·4
Diotroxin, 1942·4
Diotul, 1942·4
Diotyrosine, 1597·3
Diovan, 1943·1
Diovan Comp, 1943·1
Diovan D, 1943·1
Diovan HCT, 1943·1
Diovane, 1943·1
Diovenor, 1943·1
Diovol, 1943·1
Diovol EX, 1943·1
Diovol Forte, 1943·1
Diovol Forte DGL, 1943·1
Diovol Plus, 1943·1
Diovol Plus AF, 1943·1
Dioxadol, 1943·1
Dioxaflex, 1943·1
Dioxaflex B12, 1943·1
Dioxaflex Forte, 1943·1
Dioxaflex Gesic, 1943·2
Dioxaflex Plus, 1943·2
Dioxan, 1474·2
*S,S'*-1,4-Dioxan-2,3-diyl Bis(*O,O*-diethyl Phosphorodithioate), 1504·2
Dioxane, 1474·2
1,4-Dioxane, 1474·2
Dioxano, 1474·2
1-(1,4-Dioxaspiro[4.5]dec-2-ylmethyl)guanidine Sulphate, 926·3

Dioxathion, 1504·2
Dioxation, 1504·2
Dioxetedrina, Hidrocloruro de, 1119·1
Dioxethedrin Hydrochloride, 1119·1
Dioxethedrine Hydrochloride, 1119·1
Dioxibenzona, 1145·3
Dioxicolagol, 1943·2
Dióxido de Azufre, 1193·2
Dióxido de Carbono, 1235·2
Dióxido de Silicio, 1581·3
Dióxido de Silicio Coloidal, 1581·3
Dióxido de Titanio, 1160·3
Dioxinas, 1681·1
Dioxins, 1681·1
(1*R*,1′*R*,2*R*,2′*R*)-2,2′-(3,11-Dioxo-4,10-dioxatridecamethylene)bis(1,2,3,4-tetrahydro-6,7-dimethoxy-2-methyl-1-veratrylisoquinolinium) Dibenzenesulfonate, 1399·1
2,2′-(3,11-Dioxo-4,10-dioxatridecamethylene)bis(1,2,3,4-tetrahydro-6,7-dimethoxy-2-methyl-1-veratrylisoquinolinium) Di(benzenesulphonate), 1399·1
2,5-Dioxo-4,4-diphenylimidazolidin-1-ylmethyl Phosphate Disodium, 361·3
2,5-Dioxoimidazolidin-4-ylurea, 1141·3
7-(1,3-Dioxolan-2-ylmethyl)theophylline, 785·1
3,20-Dioxopregn-4-en-17α-yl Hexanoate, 1556·3
Dioxopromethazine Hydrochloride, 440·1
Dioxyanthrachinonum, 1261·1
Dioxyanthranol, 1146·1
Dioxybenzolum, 1156·3
Dioxybenzone, 1145·3
DIPA-DCA, 900·1
1,2-Dipalmitoyl-*sn*-glycero(3)phosphocholine, 1736·2
Dipalmitoylphosphatidylcholine, 1736·2
Dipasic, 1943·2
Dipatropin, 1943·2
Dipaverina, 1943·2
Dipazide, 1943·2
Dipedyne, 1943·2
Dipen, 1943·2
Dipentum, 1943·2
Dipep, 1943·2
Dipeptamin, 1943·2
Dipeptiven, 1943·2
Diperflox, 1943·2
Dipergon, 1943·2
Diperil, 1943·2
Diperocaine Hydrochloride, 1376·2
Diperodón, Hidrocloruro de, 1376·2
Diperodon Hydrochloride, 1376·2
Diperpen, 1943·2
Dipervina, 1943·2
Dipezona, 1943·2
Diphacinone, 1504·3
Diphamine, 1943·2
Diphantoine, 1943·2
Diphemanil Methylsulfate, 481·3
Diphemanil Methylsulphate, 481·3
Diphemanil Metilsulfate, 481·3
Diphemin, 1943·2
Diphen AF, 1943·2
Diphen Cough, 1943·2
Diphenadione, 1504·3
Diphenamill, 1943·2
Diphenazol, 1943·2
Diphencyprone, 1145·3
Diphenetholine Bromide, 1115·3
Diphenhist, 1943·2
Diphenhydramine, 431·3
Diphenhydramine Bis(theophyllin-7-ylacetate), 431·3
Diphenhydramine Citrate, 431·3
Diphenhydramine Compound Linctus, 1943·2
Diphenhydramine Constrictor, 1943·3
Diphenhydramine Di(acefyllinate), 431·3
Diphenhydramine Di(acephyllinate), 431·3
Diphenhydramine Hydrochloride, 431·3
Diphenhydramine Methylbromide, 432·2
Diphenhydramine Methylsulfomethylate, 432·2
Diphenhydramine Metilsulfate, 432·2
Diphenhydramine Monoacefyllinate, 431·3
Diphenhydramine Polistirex, 432·2
Diphenhydramine Salicylate, 432·2
Diphenhydramine Tannate, 431·3
Diphenhydramine Teoclate, 431·1
Diphenhydramine Theoclate, 431·1
Diphenhydramini Hydrochloridum, 431·3
Diphenhydraminium Chloride, 431·3
Diphenidol Hydrochloride, 1261·1
Diphenin, 370·2
Diphenmethanil Methylsulphate, 481·3
Diphenoxylate Hydrochloride, 1261·3
Diphenoxylati Hydrochloridum, 1261·3
Diphenoxylic Acid, 1261·2
Diphenoxylic Acid Hydrochloride, 1261·2
Di-phenthane-70, 104·1
Diphenyl, 1681·2
2-(Diphenylacetyl)indan-1,3-dione, 1504·3
(*Z*)-2-[4-(1,2-Diphenylbut-1-enyl)phenoxy]ethyldimethylamine Citrate, 584·1
2,3-Diphenylcyclopropenone-1, 1145·3
(±)-2-(2,2-Diphenylcyclopropyl)-2-imidazoline, 883·1
[2-(1,2-Diphenylethoxy)ethyl]trimethylammonium Bromide, 1115·3
3-(2,2-Diphenylethyl)-5-(2-piperidinoethyl)-1,2,4-oxadiazole Hydrochloride, 1129·1
Diphenylhydantoin, 370·2
5,5-Diphenylhydantoin, 370·2
5,5-Diphenylimidazolidine-2,4-dione, 370·2
(*R*)-3-(Diphenylmethoxy)-1-[3,4-(methylenedioxy)phenetyl]piperidene, 491·3
3-[1-(Diphenylmethyl)-3-azetidinyl] 5-Isopropyl (±)-2-Amino-1,4-dihydro-6-methyl-4-(*m*-nitrophenyl)-3,5-pyridinedicarboxylate, 866·2
3-Diphenylmethylene-1,1-diethyl-2-methylpyrrolidinium Bromide, 488·2
(*E*)-1-(Diphenylmethyl)-4-(3-phenylprop-2-enyl)piperazine, 428·3
2-[4-(Diphenylmethyl)-1-piperazinyl]ethyl Methyl (±)-1,4-Dihydro-2,6-dimethyl-4-(*m*-nitrophenyl)-3,5-pyridinedicarboxylate Dihydrochloride, 950·2
2-[(Diphenylmethyl)sulfinyl]acetamide, 1591·1
2-[(Diphenylmethyl)sulfinyl]acetohydroxamic Acid, 1584·2
2,2′-[(4,5-Diphenyloxazol-2-yl)imino]diethanol, 905·3
3-(4,5-Diphenyloxazol-2-yl)propionic Acid, 75·1
1,2-Diphenyl-4-(2-phenylsulphinylethyl)pyrazolidine-3,5-dione, 417·3
5,5-Diphenyl-3-[(phosphonooxy)methyl]-2,4-imidazolidinedione, Disodium Salt, 361·3
α,α-Diphenyl-2-piperidinemethanol Hydrochloride, 1592·3
1,1-Diphenyl-4-piperidinobutan-1-ol Hydrochloride, 1261·1
2,2-Diphenyl-4-piperidinobutyramide Hydrochloride, 1687·3
2,2-Diphenyl-4-piperidinobutyramide Methyl Bromide, 1688·1
5,5-Diphenyl-2-(2-piperidinoethyl)-1,3-dioxolan-4-one, 1732·1
(±)-4,4-Diphenyl-6-piperidinoheptan-3-one Hydrochloride Monohydrate, 35·3
1,1-Diphenyl-3-piperidinopropan-1-ol Methanesulphonate, 1395·2
1,3-Diphenyl-1,3-propanedione, 1145·2
1-(3,3-Diphenylpropyl)cyclohexamethyleneimine Hydrochloride, 1736·1
(±)-2-[(3,3-Diphenylpropyl)methylamino]-1,1-dimethylethyl Methyl 1,4-Dihydro-2,6-dimethyl-4-(*m*-nitrophenyl)-3,5-pyridinedicarboxylate Hydrochloride, 946·1
Diphenylpyraline, 432·3
Diphenylpyraline Hydrochloride, 432·3
Diphenylpyraline Teoclate, 439·1
Diphenylpyraline Theoclate, 439·1
1,1-Diphenyl-4-pyrrolidino-1′-yl But-2-yn-1-ol Phosphate, 1663·3
α,α-Diphenyl-3-quinuclidinemethanol Hydrochloride, 440·3
Diphereline, 1943·3
Diphesatin, 1282·3
Diphexamide Iodomethylate, 480·2
Diphlogen, 1943·3
Diphos, 1943·3
Diphosphonates, 766·3
Diphosphopyridine Nucleotide, 1719·1
Diphtheria, 125·1
Diphtheria Antitoxin, 1612·2
Diphtheria Antitoxins, 1612·2
Diphtheria Formol Toxoid, 1612·3
Diphtheria Prophylactic, Adsorbed, 1612·3
Diphtheria, Tetanus, and Haemophilus Influenzae Vaccines, 1613·3
Diphtheria, Tetanus, and Hepatitis B Vaccines, 1613·3
Diphtheria, Tetanus, and Hepatitis (rDNA) Vaccine (Adsorbed), 1613·3
Diphtheria, Tetanus, Pertussis (Acellular, Component) and Haemophilus Type B Conjugate Vaccine (Adsorbed), 1614·2
Diphtheria, Tetanus, Pertussis (Acellular, Component), Hepatitis B (rDNA), Poliomyelitis (Inactivated) and Haemophilus Type B Conjugate Vaccine (Adsorbed), 1614·3
Diphtheria, Tetanus, Pertussis (Acellular, Component) and Hepatitis B (rDNA) Vaccine (Adsorbed), 1614·3
Diphtheria, Tetanus, Pertussis (Acellular, Component), Poliomyelitis (Inactivated) and Haemophilus Type B Conjugate Vaccine (Adsorbed), 1615·1
Diphtheria, Tetanus, Pertussis (Acellular, Component) and Poliomyelitis (Inactivated) Vaccine (Adsorbed), 1615·1
Diphtheria, Tetanus and Pertussis (Acellular, Component) Vaccine (Adsorbed), 1613·3
Diphtheria, Tetanus, Pertussis, and Haemophilus Influenzae Vaccines, 1614·2
Diphtheria, Tetanus, Pertussis, Haemophilus Influenzae, and Hepatitis B Vaccines, 1614·3
Diphtheria, Tetanus, Pertussis, Hepatitis B, Poliomyelitis, and Haemophilus Influenzae Vaccines, 1614·3
Diphtheria, Tetanus, Pertussis, and Hepatitis B Vaccines, 1614·3
Diphtheria, Tetanus, Pertussis, Poliomyelitis, and Haemophilus Influenzae Vaccines, 1615·1
Diphtheria, Tetanus, Pertussis, Poliomyelitis, and Hepatitis B Vaccines, 1615·2
Diphtheria, Tetanus, Pertussis, Poliomyelitis (Inactivated) and Haemophilus Type B Conjugate Vaccine (Adsorbed), 1615·1
Diphtheria, Tetanus, Pertussis and Poliomyelitis (Inactivated) Vaccine (Adsorbed), 1615·1
Diphtheria, Tetanus, Pertussis, and Poliomyelitis Vaccines, 1615·1
Diphtheria, Tetanus and Pertussis Vaccine (Adsorbed), 1613·3
Diphtheria, Tetanus, and Pertussis Vaccines, 1613·3
Diphtheria, Tetanus, and Poliomyelitis Vaccines, 1615·2
Diphtheria, Tetanus, and Rubella Vaccines, 1615·2
Diphtheria and Tetanus Toxoids Adsorbed, 1613·1
Diphtheria and Tetanus Vaccine (Adsorbed), 1613·1
Diphtheria and Tetanus Vaccine (Adsorbed) for Adults and Adolescents, 1613·1
Diphtheria and Tetanus Vaccines, 1613·1
Diphtheria Toxin for Schick Test, 1742·2
Diphtheria Toxoids Adsorbed for Adult Use, Tetanus and, 1613·1
Diphtheria Vaccine (Adsorbed), 1612·3
Diphtheria Vaccine (Adsorbed) for Adults and Adolescents, 1612·3
Diphtheria Vaccines, 1612·3
Diphtheria-Tetanus Prophylactic, Adsorbed, 1613·1
Diphtheria–Tetanus–Whooping-cough Prophylactic, Adsorbed, 1613·3
Diphyllobothriasis, 98·1
Dipidolor, 1943·3
Dipigrand, 1943·3
Dipimax, 1943·3
Dipine, 1943·3
Dipipanona, Hidrocloruro de, 35·3
Dipipanone Hydrochloride, 35·3
2,2′,2″,2‴-[(4,8-Dipiperidinopyrimido[5,4-*d*]pyrimidine-2,6-diyl)dinitrilo]tetraethanol, 903·1
Dipiperon, 1943·3
Dipiperon R-3345, 1943·3
Dipiraxil, 1943·3
Dipirex, 1943·3
Dipiridamol, 903·1
Dipiritiona, 1146·1
Dipirol, 1943·3
Dipiron, 1943·3
Dipironax, 1943·3
Dipivalyl Adrenaline Hydrochloride, 1681·2
Dipivalyl Epinephrine, 1681·2
Dipivalyl Epinephrine Hydrochloride, 1681·2
Dipivefrin, 1681·2
Dipivefrin Hydrochloride, 1681·2
Dipivefrina, Hidrocloruro de, 1681·2
Dipivefrine, 1681·2
Dipivefrine Hydrochloride, 1681·2
Dipivefrini Hydrochloridum, 1681·2
Dipivoxilo de Adefovir, 628·1
Diplexil, 1943·3
Diplexil-R, 1943·3
Diplovax, 1943·3
Dipni, 1943·3
Dipofen, 1943·3
Dipoquin, 1943·3
Diposef, 1943·3
Dipot, 1943·3
Dipotassium Bis{μ-[2,3-dihydroxybutanedioato(4-)-$O^1,O^2:O^3,O^4$]}-diantimonate(2-) Trihydrate, 103·1
Dipotassium Bis[μ-tartrato(4-)]diantimonate(2-) Trihydrate, 103·1
Dipotassium Clorazepate, 685·1
Dipotassium Hydrogen Orthophosphate, 1230·3
Dipotassium Hydrogen Phosphate, 1230·3
Dipotassium Phosphate, 1230·3
Dipotassium Pyrosulphite, 1193·1
Diprazinum, 439·1
Diprenorfina, Hidrocloruro de, 1037·3
Diprenorphine Hydrochloride, 1037·3
Dipres, 1943·3
Diprifusor, 1307·1
Diprin, 1943·3
Diprivan, 1943·3
Dipro AS, 1943·4
Diprobase, 1943·4
Diprobath, 1943·4
Diprobet, 1943·4
Diprobeta, 1943·4
Diprocel, 1943·4
Diprocualona, 35·3
Diproderm, 1943·4
Diprodol, 1943·4
Diprofilina, 784·3
Diprofol, 1943·4
Diproform, 1943·4
Diproforte, 1943·4
Diprofos, 1943·4
Diprogen, 1943·4
Diprogenta, 1943·4
Diprolen, 1943·4
Diprolene, 1943·4
Diprolene Glycol, 1943·4
Di-Promal, 1943·4
Diprophos, 1943·4
Diprophylline, 784·3
Diprophyllinum, 784·3
Dipropimazine, 718·1
Dipropionato de Alclometasona, 1090·3
Dipropionato de Beclometasona, 1091·1
Dipropionato de Betametasona, 1093·1
Dipropionato de Dietilestilbestrol, 1548·1
Dipropionato de Estradiol, 1550·1
Dipropionato de Imidocarbo, 606·1
Dipropylacetamide, 380·1
4-[2-(Dipropylamino)ethyl]-2-indolinone Hydrochloride, 1213·3
Dipropylene Glycol Salicylate, 44·3
Dipropyline Citrate, 1250·2
4-(Dipropylsulphamoyl)benzoic Acid, 416·3

Dipropyltryptamine, 1680·3
Diproqualone, 35·3
Diproqualone Camsilate, 35·3
Diproquin, 1943·4
Diprosalic, 1943·4
Diprosept, 1944·1
Diprosis, 1944·1
Diprosone, 1944·1
Diprosone Depot, 1944·1
Diprosone G, 1944·1
Diprosone Neomycine, 1944·1
Diprosone Y, 1944·1
Diprospan, 1944·1
Diprospan G, 1944·1
Diprostene, 1944·1
Diprotop, 1944·1
Diprox, 1944·1
Dip/Ser, 1612·2
Dipsin, 1944·1
Dipulmin, 1944·1
Dip/Vac/Ads(Adults), 1612·3
Dip/Vac/Ads(Child), 1612·3
Dipxapen, 1944·1
Dipydol, 1944·1
Dipyridamole, 903·1
Dipyridamolum, 903·1
Dipyridan, 1944·1
Dipyrin, 1944·1
Dipyrithione, 1146·1
Dipyrone, 35·3, 36·1
21-[4-(2,6-Di-1-pyrrolidinyl-4-pyrimidinyl)-1-piperazinyl]-16α-methylpregna-1,4,9(11)-triene-3,20-dione Monomethanesulfonate Hydrate, 1013·2
Diquat Dibromide, 1504·3
Dirahist, 1944·1
Direct Anticoagulants, 810·1
Directim, 1944·1
Direktan, 1944·1
Dirfaben, 1944·1
Dirijo, 1666·1
Dirine, 1944·1
Dirinol, 1944·1
Dirithromycin, 206·1
Dirithromycinum, 206·1
Diritromicina, 206·1
Diroquine, 1944·1
Dirosea, 1944·1
Diroseal, 1944·2
Dirox, 1944·2
Dirret, 1944·2
Dirtop, 1944·2
Dirythmin, 1944·2
Dirytmin, 1944·2
Disaccharides, 1417·1
Disalcid, 1944·2
Disalgil, 1944·2
Disalgyl, 1944·2
Disalpin, 1944·2
Disalunil, 1944·2
Disanal, 1944·2
Disbuspan, 1944·2
Discase, 1944·2
Dis-Cinil Complex, 1944·2
Dis-Cinil Ilfi, 1944·2
Disclar, 1944·2
Disclo-Gel, 1944·2
Disclo-Plaque, 1944·2
Disclo-Tabs, 1944·2
Discmigon, 1944·2
Disco Biscuits, 1589·3
Disco-cyl Ho-Len-Complex, 1944·2
Discone, Bioglan— *see* Bioglan Discone, 1844·1
Discorid, 1944·2
Discotrine, 1944·2
Discover, 1944·2
Discover One Step, 1944·2
Discover Onestep, 1944·2
Discover Onestep Ovulation Prediction, 1944·2
Discretal, 1944·2
Discromil, 1944·2
Discus Compositum, 1944·2
Disdolen, 1944·3
Disdolen Codeina, 1944·3
Disebrin, 1944·3
Disel, 1944·3
Disel Hidrocortisona, 1944·3
Disento, 1944·3
Disento PF, 1944·3
Diseon, 1944·3
Diseptil, 1944·3
Diseptyl, 1944·3
Diserim, 1944·3
Diserinal, 1944·3
Disfil, 1944·3
Disflatyl, 1944·3
Disfruta, 1944·3
Disgren, 1944·3
Disifelit, 1944·3
Disinal, 1944·3
Disinclor, 1944·3
Disinfectants, 1164·1
Disinfectants and Preservatives, 1164·1
Disintyl, 1944·3
Disipal, 1944·3
Disipan, 1944·3
Diskin, 1944·3
Diskinebyl, 1944·3
Dislax, 1944·3
Dislembral, 1944·3
Dislep, 1944·4
Dislipina, 1944·4
Dislipor, 1944·4
Disman Sobres, 1944·4
Dismaren, 1944·4
Dismenol N, 1944·4
Dismenol Neu, 1944·4
Dismifen, 1944·4
Dismolan, 1944·4
Dismozon Pur, 1944·4
Disnal, 1944·4
Disne Asmol, 1944·4
Disneumon Pernasal, 1944·4
D-Iso, 1944·4
Disobrom, 1944·4
Disocor, 1944·4
Disoderme, 1944·4
Disodium 5-Acetamido-4-hydroxy-3-phenylazonaphthalene-2,7-disulphonate, 1058·1
Disodium *N*-{*p*-[2-(2-Amino-4,7-dihydro-4-oxo-1*H*-pyrrolo[2,3-*d*]pyrimidin-5-yl)ethyl]benzoyl}-L-glutamate, 579·1
Disodium 3-Amino-1-hydroxypropylidenebisphosphonate Pentahydrate, 773·3
Disodium Aminohydroxypropylidenediphosphonate, 773·3
Disodium 5,5′-Azodisalicylate, 1278·1
Disodium 3,3′-[Biphenyl-4,4′-diylbis(azo)]bis[4-aminonaphthalene-1-sulphonate], 1675·3
Disodium 3-[Bis(2-chloroethyl)-carbamoyloxy]estra-1,3,5(10)-trien-17β-yl Orthophosphate, 551·1
Disodium Bis{μ-[2,3-dihydroxybutanedioato(4-)-$O^1$,$O^2$:$O^3$,$O^4$]}diantimonate(2-), 103·1
Disodium 4′,4″-Bis(*N*-ethyl-3-sulphonatobenzylamino)triphenylmethylium-2-sulphonate, 1056·2
Disodium Bis{μ-[L-(+)-tartrato(4-)]}diantimonate(2-), 103·1
Disodium Calcium Tetracemate, 1051·3
Disodium (6*R*)-6-[2-Carboxy-2-(3-thienyl)acetamido]penicillanate, 270·2
Disodium Clodronate, 770·2
Disodium Cromoglycate, 795·3
Disodium [(Cycloheptylamino)methylene]diphosphonate, 773·1
Disodium 4,4′-(2,4-Diamino-5-methyl-1,3-phenylenebisazo) Dibenzenesulphonate, 1056·2
Disodium 4,4′-(2,4-Diamino-1,3-phenylenebisazo) Dibenzenesulphonate, 1056·2
Disodium 4,4′-(4,6-Diamino-1,3-phenylenebisazo) Dibenzenesulphonate, 1056·2
Disodium 2,7-Dibromo-4-hydroxymercurifluorescein, 1185·3
Disodium 2,5-Dichloro-4-[5-hydroxy-3-methyl-4-(4-sulphonatophenylazo)pyrazol-1-yl]benzenesulphonate, 1058·3
Disodium (Dichloromethylene)diphosphonate Tetrahydrate, 770·2
Disodium 7,12-Diethenyl-3,8,13,17-tetramethyl-21*H*,23*H*-porphine-2,18-dipropanoate, 1735·3
Disodium Dihydrogen {[(*p*-Chlorophenyl)thio]methylene}diphosphonate Hemihydrate, 776·1
Disodium Dihydrogen Ethylenediaminetetra-acetate Dihydrate, 1037·3
Disodium Dihydrogen (1-Hydroxyethylidene)diphosphonate, 771·2
Disodium Dihydrogen (1-Hydroxy-2-imidazol-1-ylethylidene)diphosphonate Tetrahydrate, 776·2
Disodium Dihydrogen Methylenediphosphonate, 773·2
Disodium 4,4′-(2,4-Dihydroxy-5-hydroxymethyl-1,3-phenylenebisazo)di(naphthalene-1-sulphonate), 1056·3
Disodium 3,3′-Dioxo-2,2′-bi-indolinylidene-5,5′-disulphonate, 1700·3
Disodium 4,4′-Dioxo-5,5′-(2-hydroxytrimethylenedioxy)di(4*H*-chromene-2-carboxylate), 795·3
Disodium Edathamil, 1037·3
Disodium Edetate, 1037·3
Disodium EDTA, 1037·3
Disodium Enoxolone Succinate, 1254·3
Disodium (1*R*,2*S*)-1,2-Epoxypropylphosphonate, 214·3
Disodium 9-Ethyl-6,9-dihydro-4,6-dioxo-10-propyl-4*H*-pyrano[3,2-*g*]quinoline-2,8-dicarboxylate, 789·3
Disodium Etidronate, 771·2
Disodium Fluorescein, 1689·1
Disodium Fumarate, 1147·3
Disodium Guanosine-5′-monophosphate, 1681·3
Disodium Guanylate, 1681·3
Disodium Hydrogen Citrate, 1223·2
Disodium Hydrogen Orthophosphate, 1231·1
Disodium Hydrogen Phosphate, 1231·1
Disodium Hydrogen Phosphate, Anhydrous, 1231·1
Disodium Hydrogen Phosphate Dihydrate, 1231·1
Disodium Hydrogen Phosphate Dodecahydrate, 1231·1
Disodium 3-Hydroxyestra-1,3,5(10)-triene-16α,17β-diyl Disuccinate, 1552·3
Disodium 6-Hydroxy-5-(6-methoxy-4-sulphonato-*m*-tolylazo)naphthalene-2-sulphonate, 1056·1
Disodium (Hydroxymethylene)diphosphonate, 773·3
Disodium 3-Hydroxy-4-(1-naphthylazo)naphthalene-2,7-disulphonate, 1056·2
Disodium 4-Hydroxy-3-(4-sulphonato-1-naphthylazo)naphthalene-1-sulphonate, 1057·1
Disodium 6-Hydroxy-5-(4-sulphonatophenylazo)naphthalene-2-sulphonate, 1058·2
Disodium Incadronate, 773·1
Disodium Indigotin-5,5′-disulphonate, 1700·3
Disodium Inosinate, 1681·3
Disodium Inosine-5′-monophosphate, 1681·3
Disodium Medronate, 773·2
Disodium Methylene Diphosphonate, 773·2
Disodium Monomethylarsonate Hexahydrate, 1748·1
Disodium Oxidronate, 773·3
Disodium (4-Oxo-2-phenyl-4*H*-chromene-5,7-diyldioxy)diacetate, 1688·2
Disodium Pamidronate, 773·3
Disodium (*OC*-6-22)-Pentakis(cyano-*C*)nitrosylferrate Dihydrate, 1000·2
Disodium Phosphate, 1231·1
Disodium Phosphate, Anhydrous, 1231·1
Disodium Phosphate Dihydrate, 1231·1
Disodium Phosphate Dodecahydrate, 1231·1
Disodium Phosphorofluoridate, 1446·2
Disodium 4,4′-(2-Pyridylmethylene)di(phenyl Sulphate), 1289·3
Disodium Pyrosulphite, 1193·1
Disodium Selenate, 1444·1
Disodium Silibinin Dihemisuccinate, 1043·3
Disodium Tetraborate, 1661·3
Disodium 4,5,6,7-Tetrabromophenolphthalein-3′,3″-disulphonate, 1750·3
Disodium 5,5′-(4,5,6,7-Tetrabromophthalidylidene)bis(2-hydroxybenzenesulphonate), 1750·3
Disodium Tetracemate, 1037·3
Disodium Thiosulfate Pentahydrate, 1053·3
Disodium Tiludronate, 776·1
Disodium[(ethylenedinitrilo)tetraacetato]calciate(2–) Hydrate, 1051·3
Diso-Duriles, 1944·4
Disofarin, 1944·4
Disofenin, Technetium $(^{99m}Tc)$, 1526·1
Disofenol, 105·1
Disofrin, 1944·4
Disofrol, 1944·4
Disogel, 1944·4
Disogram, 1944·4
Disol, 1944·4
Di-Solvente, 1944·4
Disomet, 1944·4
Disonorm, 1944·4
Disopam, 1944·4
Disophenol, 105·1
Disophrol, 1944·4
Disopiramida, 903·3
Disopiramida, Fosfato de, 903·3
Disopranil, 1945·1
Disoprivan, 1945·1
Disoprofol, 1305·3
Disopyramide, 903·3
Disopyramide Phosphate, 903·3
Disopyramidi Phosphas, 903·3
Disopyramidum, 903·3
Disotat, 1945·1
Disotate, 1945·1
Disothiazide, 1945·1
Disotron, 1945·1
Dispaclonidin, 1945·1
Dispacromil, 1945·1
Dispadex Comp, 1945·1
Dispagent, 1945·1
Dispasan, 1945·1
Dispasmol, 1945·1
Dispatenol, 1945·1
Dispatim, 1945·1
Dispello, 1945·1
Dispeptal, 1945·1
Dispeptrin, 1945·1
Disperbarium, 1945·1
Dispercarpine, 1945·1
Disperin, 1945·1
DisperMox, 1945·1
Dispersible Cellulose, 1578·3
Displata, 1945·1
Display, 1945·1
Dispneitrat, 1945·1
Dispon, 1945·1
Dispril, 1945·1
Disprin, 1945·1
Disprin CV, 1945·1
Disprin Direct, 1945·1
Disprin Extra, 1945·2
Disprin Forte, 1945·2
Disprin, Junior— *see* Junior Disprin, 2072·2
Disprina, 1945·2
Disprol, 1945·2
Dispromil, 1945·2
Disques Coricides, 1945·2
Disseminated Intravascular Coagulation, 737·1
Dissenten, 1945·2
Dissociative Disorders— *see* Conversion and Dissociative Disorders, 696·2
Dissolursil, 1945·2
Dissolvurol, 1945·2
Dissulfiramo, 1681·3
Distaclor, 1945·2
Distalene, 1945·2
Distalgesic, 1945·2
Distalgic, 1945·2
Distamine, 1945·2
Distaph, 1945·2

Distaquaine V-K, 1945·2
Distasil, 1945·2
Distaxid, 1945·2
Distenil, 1945·2
Distensan, 1945·2
Disteril, 1945·2
Distex, 1945·2
Distickstoffmonoxid, 1304·3
Distigmina, Bromuro de, 1489·2
Distigmine Bromide, 1489·2
Distilbene, 1945·2
Distilled Water, 1764·3
Distinon, 1945·2
Distobram, 1945·2
Distonal, 1945·2
Distovagal, 1945·2
Distraneurin, 1945·3
Distraneurine, 1945·3
Disturbed Behaviour, 665·1
Di-Su-Frone, 1945·3
Disulfiram, 1681·3
Disulfiramum, 1681·3
Disulfuro de Carbono, 1472·1
Disulone, 202·2, 1945·3
Disupril, 1945·3
Diswart, 1945·3
DIT, 1594·1
DIT1-2, 1945·3
Ditanrix, 1945·3
Ditaven, 1945·3
Ditaven Comp, 1945·3
Ditavene, 1945·3
Ditayod, 1945·3
Ditazol, 905·3
Ditazole, 905·3
DiTe Anatoxal, 1945·3
DiTe Booster, 1945·3
Ditec, 1945·3
Di-Te-Kik, 1945·3
Di-Te-Ki-Pol, 1945·3
Ditemer, 1945·3
Ditenate N, 1945·3
Ditenside, 1945·3
Ditensor, 1945·3
DiTePer Anatoxal, 1945·3
Di-Te-Per Anatoxal, 1945·3
DiTePerPol Vaccin, 1945·3
Di-Te-Pol, 1945·3
Diteutrin, 1945·4
Dithiazid, 1945·4
Dithiazide, 1945·4
3-[Di-(2-thienyl)methylene]-5-methoxy-1,1-dimethylpiperidinium Bromide Monohydrate, 489·3
3-[Di(2-thienyl)methylene]-1-methylpiperidine 2-(4-Hydroxybenzoyl)benzoate, 1131·3
*trans*-3-(Di-2-thienylmethylene)octahydro-5-methyl-2*H*-quinolizinium Bromide, 1757·1
L-3,3′-Dithiobis(2-aminopropionic Acid), 1426·3
*NN*′-{Dithiobis[2-(2-benzoyloxyethyl)-1-methylvinylene]}bis[*N*-(4-amino-2-methylpyrimidin-5-ylmethyl)formamide], 1454·3
(*R*)-*NN*′-[Dithiobis(ethyleneiminocarbonylethylene)]bis(2,4-dihydroxy-3,3-dimethylbutyramide), 978·3
*NN*′-{Dithiobis[2-(2-isobutyryloxyethyl)-1-methylvinylene]}bis[*N*-(4-amino-2-methylpyrimidin-5-ylmethyl)formamide], 1455·1
Dithiocarb Sodium, 1038·2
β,β′-Dithiodialanine, 1426·3
2,2′-Dithiodipyridine 1,1′-Dioxide, 1146·1
Dithiol, 1945·4
5-(1,2-Dithiolan-3-yl)valeric Acid, 1754·3
Dithiosalicylic Acid, 1146·1
Dithranol, 1146·1
Dithranol Triacetate, 1146·2
Dithranolum, 1146·1
Dithrasal, 1945·4
Dithrocream, 1945·4
Ditiocarb Sodium, 1038·2
Ditiocarbo Sódico, 1038·2
Ditionito de Sodio, 1747·3
Ditiosalicílico, Ácido, 1146·1
Ditizem, 1945·4
Ditoin, 1945·4
Ditolyl Disulfide, 1152·1
Ditomed, 1945·4
Ditonal, 1945·4
Ditonal N, 1945·4
Ditopax, 1945·4
Ditopax-F, 1945·4
Ditral, 1945·4
Ditran, 1945·4
Ditranol, 1146·1
Ditrazini Citras, 104·1
Ditrei, 1945·4
Ditrenil, 1945·4
Ditrim, 1945·4
Ditripentat-Heyl, 1945·4
Ditropan, 1945·4
Ditropan XL— *see* Lyrinel XL, 2109·2
Ditropine, 1945·4
Ditterolina, 1945·4
Ditum, 1945·4
Diu-60, 867·1
Diu Rauwiplus, 1946·1
Diu Venostasin, 1946·1
Diu-Atenolol, 1946·1
Diube, 1946·1
Diubeloc, 1946·1
Diucardin, 1946·1
Diucomb, 1946·1
Diucontin-K, 1946·1
Diulo, 1946·1
Diu-melusin, 1946·1
Diumide-K Continus, 1946·1
Diupres, 1946·1
Diupress, 1946·1
Diuprol, 1946·1
Diuprotect, 1946·1
Diurace, 1946·1
Diural, 1946·1
Diuramid, 1946·1
Diuramin, 1946·1
Diurana, 1946·1
Diurapid, 1946·1
Diurek, 1946·1
Diuremid, 1946·1
Diurene, 1946·1
Diurepina, 1946·1
Diuresal, 1946·1
Diurese, 1946·2
Diuresix, 1946·2
Diuret, 1946·2
Diuretabs, 1946·2
Diuretic, 1946·2
Diuretics, 811·2
Diuretics, Carbonic Anhydrase Inhibiting, 811·2
Diuretics, High-ceiling, 811·2
Diuretics, Loop, 811·2
Diuretics, Osmotic, 811·2
Diuretics, Potassium-sparing, 811·2
Diuretics, Thiazide, 811·2
Diuretikum Verla, 1946·2
Diuretil, 1946·2
Diuret-P, 1946·2
Diurevit Mono, 1946·2
Diurex, 1946·2
Diurexan, 1946·2
Diurezin, 1946·2
Diurid, 1946·2
Diurigen, 1946·2
Diuril, 1946·2
Diurin, 1946·2
Diurinat, 1946·2
Diurisa, 1946·2
Diurit, 1946·2
Diurix, 1946·2
Diurolan, 1946·2
Diursan, 1946·2
Diutec, 1946·2
Diutensat, 1946·2
Diutensat Comp, 1946·2
Diutensen-R, 1946·2
Diutropan, 1946·3
Diuzine, 1946·3
Divacuna DT, 1946·3
Divalol W, 1946·3
Divalproex Sodium, 380·1
2,6-Divanillylidenecyclohexanone, 1678·2
Divanon, 1946·3
Divaril, 1946·3
Divarius, 1946·3
Divascan, 1946·3
Divegal, 1946·3
Divelol, 1946·3
Divermil, 1946·3
Diverticular Disease, 1241·3
Diverticulitis— *see* Diverticular Disease, 1241·3
Diverticulosis— *see* Diverticular Disease, 1241·3
Divial, 1946·3
Divical, 1946·3
Divicil, 1946·3
Dividol, 1946·3
Divigel, 1946·3
Diviminol Hydroxybenzoate, 96·3
Divina, 1946·3
Divina Plus, 1946·3
Divinyl Glycol, 1284·2
Divinylbenzene, 1733·2
Divinylbenzene with Styrene Copolymer, Sulfonated, Sodium Salt, 1053·2
Diviplus, 1946·3
Diviseq, 1946·3
Divistiramina, 905·3
Divistyramine, 905·3
Divitren, 1946·3
Diviva, 1946·3
Dixamonum Bromidum, 485·3
Dixarit, 1946·3
Dixen, 1946·3
Dixeran, 1946·4
Dixi-35, 1946·4
Dixidrol, 1946·4
Dixiflen, 1946·4
Dixirazina, 697·2
Dixocillin, 1946·4
Dixonal, 1946·4
Dixyrazine, 697·2
Diyomex, 1946·4
Diyosul, 1946·4
Diyowil, 1946·4
Dizan, 1946·4
Dizem, 1946·4
Dizepam, 1946·4
Dizinil, 1946·4
Dizmiss, 1946·4
Dizocilpina, Maleato de, 1683·1
Dizocilpine Maleate, 1683·1
Dizolam, 1946·4
Dizolvin, 1946·4
Dizziness— *see* Vertigo, 423·2
DJ-1550, 263·2
Djamba, 1666·1
DJN-608, 343·3
Djoma, 1666·1
DK-7419, 864·3
DkhMDF, 770·2
DL-473, 253·3
DL-832, 1121·3
DL-8280, 239·3
D-Lisin, 1946·4
DL-458-IT, 1096·2
DL-473-IT, 253·3
DL-507-IT, 264·3
DLPA, 1946·4
DM-9384, 1719·2
DM Cough Syrup, 1946·4
DM Cough Syrup Decongestant, 1946·4
DM Cough Syrup Expectorant, 1946·4
DM Creme, 1946·4
DM E Suppressant Expectorant, 1946·4
DM Expectorant Cough, 1946·4
DM Gel, 1946·4
DM Plus, 1946·4
DM Plus Decongestant, 1946·4
DM Plus Decongestant Expectorant, 1946·4
DM Plus Expectorant, 1947·1
DM Sans Sucre, 1947·1
DM Syrup— *see* DM Plus, 1946·4
DM Termo, 1947·1
DMAA, 1711·2
DMAC, 1474·1
4-DMAP, 1037·3, 1947·1
DMax, 1947·1
DM-D Expectorant Cough & Cold, 1947·1
D-Methylphenidate Hydrochloride, 1587·1
DMF, 1474·1
DMG-B15, 1947·1
DMI, 290·2
DML, 1947·1
DML Facial, 1947·1
DML Forte Con Pantenol, 1947·1
DMP, 1504·1
DMP-115, 1067·2
DMP-266, 632·2
D-MPH, 1587·1
DMPS, 1055·3
DMSA, 1054·2
DMSC, 206·2
DMSO, 1473·2
DMT, 1680·3
D-Mulsin, 1947·1
D/N PR, 1947·1
DNA, 1679·2
Dnaren, 1947·1
DNase I, 1119·1
DNCB, 1680·3
DNCG, 1947·1
DNOC, 1504·2
DO-6, 1707·2
Doak-Oil, 1947·1
Doans, 1947·1
Doans Backache Pills, 1947·1
Doans PM, Extra Strength— *see* Extra Strength Doans PM, 1986·2
DOB, 1593·3
Dobacen, 1947·1
Dobendan, 1947·1
Dobesifar, 1947·1
Dobesilato de Calcio, 1664·2
Dobesin, 1947·1
Dobesix, 1947·1
Dobetin, 1947·1
Dobetin Con Vitamina B1, 1947·1
Dobetin Totale, 1947·1
Dobica, 1947·1
Dobil, 1947·2
Dobiron, 1947·2
Doblexan, 1947·2
Dobren, 1947·2
Dobriciclin, 1947·2
Dobtan, 1947·2
Dobucard, 1947·2
Dobucor, 1947·2
Dobuject, 1947·2
Dobupal, 1947·2
Dobutabbott, 1947·2
Dobutal, 1947·2
Dobutam, 1947·2
Dobutamina, Hidrocloruro de, 905·3
Dobutamine Hydrochloride, 905·3
Dobutamini Hydrochloridum, 905·3
Dobutil, 1947·2
Dobutina, 1947·2
Dobuton, 1947·2
Dobutrex, 1947·2
Doc, 1947·2
Docaine, 1947·2
Docard, 1947·2
Docarpamina, 906·3
Docarpamine, 906·3
Docatone, 1947·2
Docdol, 1947·2
Doce Vida, 1947·2
Docetaxel, 547·1
Docetril, 1947·2
Docgel, 1947·2
Docidrazin, 1947·2
Dociretic, 1947·2
Dociteren, 1947·2
Dociton, 1947·3
Dock, Curly, 1766·1
Dock, Sour, 1766·1
Docline, 1947·3
Doclis, 1947·3
Doconexent, 976·1

Doconexento, 976·1
Docosahexaenoic Acid, 976·1
Docosahexa-4,7,10,13,16,19-enoic Acid, 976·1
*n*-Docosanol, 632·1
Docosanol, 632·1
1-Docosanol, 632·1
Docostyl, 1947·3
Docosyl Alcohol, 632·1
Docrub, 1947·3
Docsed, 1947·3
Doctar, 1947·3
Docticam, 1947·3
Doctodermis, 1947·3
Doctofril Antiinflamat, 1947·3
Doctogaster, 1947·3
Doctomitil, 1947·3
Doctril, 1947·3
Doctrim, 1947·3
Docusate Calcium, 1262·1
Docusate Potassium, 1262·1
Docusate Sodium, 1262·2
Docusates, 1262·1
Docusato Cálcico, 1262·1
Docusato Potásico, 1262·1
Docusato Sódico, 1262·2
Docusatos, 1262·1
Docusatum Natricum, 1262·2
Docusoft, 1947·3
Docusoft Plus, 1947·3
Docusol, 1947·3
Dodds, 1947·3
Dodds Back Ease, 1947·3
Dodecafluoropentane, 1067·2
Dodecahydro-7,14-methano-2*H*,6*H*-dipyrido[1,2-*a*:1′,2′-*e*][1,5]diazocine Sulphate Pentahydrate, 1749·1
Dodecahydrosqualene, 1482·2
(3*R*,4a*R*,5*S*,6*S*,6a*S*,10*S*,10a*R*,10b*S*)-Dodecahydro-5,6,10,10b-tetrahydroxy-3,4a,7,7,10a-pentamethyl-3-vinyl-1*H*-naphtho[2,1-*b*]pyran-1-one, 5-Acetate, 1674·3
Dodecarbonium Chloride, 1185·3
Dodecatol N, 1947·3
Dodecavit, 1947·3
Dodeclonium Bromide, 1178·3
Dodecyl Gallate, 1168·1
Dodecyl 3,4,5-Trihydroxybenzoate, 1168·1
1-Dodecylazacycloheptan-2-one, 1481·2
Dodecyldimethyl-2-phenoxyethylammonium Bromide, 1179·1
1-Dodecylhexahydro-2*H*-azepin-2-one, 1481·2
α-Dodecyl-ω-hydroxypoly(oxyethylene), 1412·3
Dodecylis Gallas, 1168·1
Dodecyltrimethylammonium Bromide, 1172·2
Dodemox, 1947·3
Dodepar, 1947·3
Doderlein Med, 1947·3
Dodesept, 1947·3
Dodesept Gefarbt, 1947·3
Dodesept N, 1947·3
Dodicin, 1574·1
Do-Do ChestEze, 1947·3
Do-Do Expectorant Linctus, 1947·4
Doederlein, 1947·4
Dofedrin, 1947·4
Dofen, 1947·4
Doferol, 1947·4
Dofetilida, 906·3
Dofetilide, 906·3
Dofisan, 1947·4
Doflex, 1947·4
Dog Rose, 1740·1
Dog Rose Fruits, 1740·1
Dogistin, 1947·4
Dogmatil, 1947·4
Dogmatyl, 1947·4
Dogoxine, 1947·4
Dogs Grass, 1676·2
Dohyfral Vitamine AD3, 1947·4
DOK, 1947·4
Doketrol, 1947·4
Dokka, 1666·1
Doktacillin, 1947·4
Dolac, 1947·4
Dolacet, 1947·4
Dolak, 1947·4
Dolal, 1947·4
Dolalgial, 1947·4
Dolamin, 1947·4
Dolan, 1947·4
Dolanaest, 1947·4
Dolanet, 1947·4
Dolantin, 1947·4
Dolantina, 1947·4
Dolantine, 1947·4
Dolaren, 1948·1
Dolased Analgesic Calmative, 1948·1
Dolased Day/Night Pain Relief, 1948·1
Dolasetron Mesilate, 1262·3
Dolasetrón, Mesilato de, 1262·3
Dolasetron Mesylate, 1262·3
Dolaut, 1948·1
Dolcevita, 1948·1
Dolcidium, 1948·1
Dolcin, 1948·1
Dolcol, 1948·1
Dolcontin, 1948·1
Dolcopin, 1948·1
Dolcor, 1948·1
Dolcoxx, 1948·1
Dolean, 1948·1
Dolectran, 1948·1
Dolefin Paracetamol, 1948·1
Dolemicin, 1948·1
Dolenon, 1948·1
Dolenso, 1948·1
Doleron, 1948·1
Doleside, 1948·1
Dolestan, 1948·1
Dolestan Forte Comp, 1948·1
Dolestine, 1948·1
Dolex, 1948·1
Dolexaderm H, 1948·1
Dolexamed N, 1948·2
Dolflam, 1948·2
Dolflash, 1948·2
Dolgan, 1948·2
Dolgenal, 1948·2
Dolgesic, 1948·2
Dolgesic Codeina, 1948·2
Dolgic, 1948·2
Dolgic LQ, 1948·2
Dolgit, 1948·2
Dolgit-Diclo, 1948·2
Dolgosin, 1948·2
Doli Rhume, 1948·2
Dolib, 1948·2
Dolibu, 1948·2
Dolical, 1948·2
Dolicoccil, 1948·2
Dolidermil, 1948·2
Dolidon, 1948·2
Dolifebril, 1948·2
Dolilux, 1948·2
Dolinac, 1948·2
Doline, 1948·2
Dolipranе, 1948·2
Dolirelax, 1948·2
Dolisedal, 1948·2
Dolistamine, 1948·2
Dolitabs, 1948·2
Dolitravel, 1948·2
Dolium, 1948·2
Dolkin, 1948·3
Dolko, 1948·3
Dolmatil, 1948·3
Dolmed, 1948·3
Dolmen, 1948·3
Dolmex, 1948·3
Dolmigral, 1948·3
Dol-Mite, 1948·3
Dolmitin, 1948·3
Dolmix, 1948·3
Dolnaxen, 1948·3
Dolnefort, 1948·3
Dolnix, 1948·3
Dolnot, 1948·3
Dolo Demotherm, 1948·3
Dolo Mobilat, 1948·3
Dolo Neos, 1948·3
Dolo Nervobion, 1948·3
Dolo Nervobion 10000, 1948·3
Dolo Sanol, 1948·3
Dolo Target, 1948·3
Dolo Tomanil, 1948·3
Doloana, 1948·3
Dolo-Arthrodynat, 1948·3
Dolo-Arthrosenex, 1948·3
Dolo-Arthrosenex N, 1948·3
Dolo-Arthrosenex Sine Heparino, 1948·4
Dolo-Arthrosetten H, 1948·4
Doloatrixen, 1948·4
Dolobene, 1948·4
Dolobid, 1948·4
Dolobis, 1948·4
Doloc, 1948·4
Dolocalma, 1948·4
Dolocibal, 1948·4
Dolocid, 1948·4
DoloCitran C, 1948·4
Dolocod, 1948·4
Doloctaprin, 1948·4
Doloctaprin Plus, 1948·4
Dolo-cyl, 1948·4
Dolocyl, 1948·4
Dolodens, 1948·4
Dolodent, 1948·4
Doloderm, 1948·4
Dolo-Dismenol, 1948·4
Dolo-Dobendan, 1948·4
Dolodoc, 1948·4
Dolofar, 1948·4
Dolofarma, 1949·1
Dolofast, 1949·1
Dolofenac, 1949·1
Doloflex, 1949·1
Dolofort, 1949·1
Dolofrix, 1949·1
Dolofur, 1949·1
Dologel, 1949·1
Dologen, 1949·1
Dologesic, 1949·1
Dologex, 1949·1
Dologyne, 1949·1
Doloject, 1949·1
Dolokapton, 1949·1
Dolo-Ketazon, 1949·1
Dolokey, 1949·1
Dolol, 1949·1
Dolomedil, 1949·1
Dolo-Menthoneurin, 1949·1
Dolo-Menthoneurin CreSa, 1949·1
Dolomin, 1949·1
Dolomine, 1949·1
Dolomite, 1949·1
Dolomo, 1949·1
Dolomo TN, 1949·1
Dolonase, 1949·1
Dolonerv, 1949·1
Doloneuro, 1949·2
Dolo-Neurobion, 1949·2
Dolo-Neurobion Forte, 1949·2
Dolo-Neurobion N, 1949·2
Dolo-Neurobionta, 1949·2
Dolonex, 1949·2
Dolono, 1949·2
Dolonovag, 1949·2
Dolo-Octirona, 1949·2
Dolo-Pangavit, 1949·2
Dolopharm, 1949·2
Dolophine, 1949·2
DoloPosterine N, 1949·2
Doloproct, 1949·2
Doloproct Comp, 1949·2
Dolo-Prolixan, 1949·2
Dolo-Puren, 1949·2
Dolopyrine, 1949·2
Dolorac, 1949·2
Doloreduct, 1949·2
Dolorelax, 1949·2
Dolorex, 1949·3
Dolorex Neo, 1949·3
Dolorgiet, 1949·3
Dolor-loges, 1949·3
Dolormin, 1949·3
Dolorol, 1949·3
Dolorol Forte, 1949·3
Dolorsan-Balsam, 1949·3
Dolorsin, 1949·3
Dolorsyn, 1949·3
Dolorub, 1949·3
Dolo-Rubriment H, 1949·3
Dolosal, 1949·3
Dolosarto, 1949·3
Dolospam, 1949·3
Dolo-Spedifen, 1949·3
Dolostop, 1949·3
Dolosul, 1949·3
Dolotandax, 1949·3
Dolotard, 1949·3
Dolotec, 1949·3
Doloteffin, 1949·3
Dolotemp, 1949·3
Dolo-Tiaminal, 1949·3
Dolotol 12, 1949·3
Dolotor, 1949·4
Dolotren, 1949·4
Dolo-Veniten, 1949·4
Doloverina, 1949·4
Dolovin, 1949·4
DoloVisano M, 1949·4
DoloVisano Salbe, 1949·4
Dolo-Voltaren, 1949·4
Doloxene, 1949·4
Doloxene Co, 1949·4
Doloxene Compound, 1949·4
Doloxene-A, 1949·4
Doloxtren, 1949·4
Dolpasse, 1949·4
Dolpic Forte, 1949·4
Dolpocetmol, 1949·4
Dolprin, 1949·4
Dolprofen, 1949·4
Dolprone, 1949·4
Dolpyc, 1949·4
Dolquine, 1949·4
Dolsed, 1949·4
Dolsinal, 1949·4
Doltard, 1949·4
Dolten, 1949·4
Dol-u-ron, 1950·1
Doluvital, 1950·1
Dolval, 1950·1
Dolvan, 1950·1
Dolver, 1950·1
Dolviran, 1950·1
Dolviran N, 1950·1
Dolxen, 1950·1
Dolzam, 1950·1
Dolzycam, 1950·1
DOM, 1593·3
Doma Grip, 1950·1
Doma Grip NF, 1950·1
Domar, 1950·1
Domeboro, 1950·1
Domenal, 1950·1
Domenan, 1950·1
Domeni, 1950·1
Dome-Paste, 1950·1
Domer, 1950·1
Domerdon, 1950·1
Domes, 1950·1
Domex, 1950·1
Domical, 1950·1
Domicap, 1950·1
Domicetina, 1950·1
Domidone, 1950·2
Domifeno, Bromuro de, 1179·1
Domiken, 1950·2
Domilium, 1950·2
Domin, 1950·2
Dominal, 1950·2
Dominans, 1950·2
Dominium, 1950·2
Domiodol, 1119·1
Domiphen Bromide, 1179·1
Domnamid, 1950·2
Domol, 1950·2
Dompel, 1950·2
Dompenyl, 1950·2

Dompeon, 1950·2
Domper, 1950·2
Domperamol, 1950·2
Domperdone, 1950·2
Domperidona, 1263·2
Domperidona, Maleato de, 1263·2
Domperidone, 1263·2
Domperidone Maleate, 1263·2
Domperidoni Maleas, 1263·2
Domperidonum, 1263·2
Domper-M, 1950·2
Domperol, 1950·2
Dompil, 1950·2
Dom-Polienzim, 1950·2
Domstal, 1950·2
Domutussina, 1950·2
Domuvar, 1950·2
Dona, 1950·2
Dona 200-S, 1950·2
Donajuanita, 1666·1
Donalg, 1950·2
Donamet, 1950·2
Donaprox, 1950·2
Donaren, 1950·2
Donataxel, 1950·2
Donatiol, 1950·2
Donatussin, 1950·3
Donatussin DC, 1950·3
Doncef, 1950·3
Donegal, 1950·3
Doneka, 1950·3
Doneka Plus, 1950·3
Donepezil Hydrochloride, 1489·2
Donepezilo, Hidrocloruro de, 1489·2
Doneurin, 1950·3
Dong Quai, 1655·1
Dong Quai Complex, 1950·3
Donicer, 1950·3
Donix, 1950·3
Donna, 1950·3
Donnagel, 1950·3
Donnagel-PG, 1950·3
Donnalix, 1950·3
Donnamar, 1950·3
Donnatab, 1950·3
Donnatal, 1950·3
Donnazyme, 1950·3
Donobid, 1950·3
Donodol, 1950·3
Donodol Compuesto, 1950·3
Donomix, 1950·3
Donorest, 1950·3
Donormyl, 1950·4
Donovanosis— *see* Granuloma Inguinale, 131·1
Dontisolon D, 1950·4
Dontopivalone, 1950·4
Dontuxin, 1950·4
Donulide, 1950·4
Donum, 1950·4
L-Dopa, 1205·2
Dopabane, 1950·4
DOPAC, 1208·3
Dopacard, 1950·4
Dopacris, 1950·4
Dopa-decarboxylase Inhibitors, 1196·1
Dopadura C, 1950·4
Dopaflex, 1950·4
Dopagon, 1950·4
Dopagrand, 1950·4
Dopagyt, 1950·4
Dopamed, 1950·4
Dopamet, 1950·4
Dopametil, 1950·4
Dopamex, 1950·4
Dopamina, Hidrocloruro de, 907·1
Dopamine Agonists, 1196·1
Dopamine Hydrochloride, 907·1
Dopaminergics, 1196·1
Dopaminex, 1950·4
Dopamini Hydrochloridum, 907·1
Dopar, 1950·4
Doparid, 1950·4
Dopasian, 1950·4
Dopatral, 1950·4
Dopatropin, 1950·4
Dopegyt, 1950·4
Dopergin, 1950·4
Dopergine, 1950·4
Dopexamina, Hidrocloruro de, 908·2
Dopexamine Hydrochloride, 908·2
Dopicar, 1950·4
Dopin, 1951·1
Dopinga, 1951·1
Dopmin, 1951·1
Dopo Pik, 1951·1
Doppelherz Energie-Tonikum N, 1951·1
Doppelherz Ginseng Aktiv, 1951·1
Doppelherz Magenstarkung, 1951·1
Doppelherz Melissengeist, 1951·1
Doppelherz Tonikum, 1951·1
Doppel-Spalt Compact, 1951·1
Dopram, 1951·1
Dopress, 1951·1
Doprit, 1951·1
Doproct, 1951·1
Dops, 1951·1
Dopsan, 1951·1
Doqua, 1951·1
Doraine, 1951·1
Doral, 1951·1
Doralem, 1951·1
Doralese, 1951·1
Doralgina, 1951·1
Doralin, 1951·1
Doralon, 1951·1
Doramectin, 105·1
Doramectina, 105·1
Doran, 1951·2
Doraplax, 1951·2
Dorbantil, 1951·2
Dorbid, 1951·2
Dorcalor, 1951·2
Dorcol Children's Cold Formula, 1951·2
Dorcol Children's Cough Syrup, 1951·2
Dorcol Children's Decongestant, 1951·2
Dordendril, 1951·2
Dordente, 1951·2
Dore Immun, 1951·2
Doregrippin, 1951·2
Dorehydrin, 1951·2
Dorenasin, 1951·2
Dorend, 1951·2
Doreperol N, 1951·2
Doretrim, 1951·2
Dorex, 1951·2
Dorf, 1951·2
Dorfen, 1951·2
Dorflan, 1951·2
Dorflex, 1951·2
Dorgen, 1951·2
Dori, 1951·2
Dorib, 1951·2
Doribel, 1951·2
Dorical, 1951·2
Doricin, 1951·2
Dorico, 1951·2
Doricoflu, 1951·2
Doricum, 1951·3
Doridamina, 1951·3
Doridina, 1951·3
Doridone, 1951·3
Doriflan, 1951·3
Doril, 1951·3
Dorilan, 1951·3
Dorilax, 1951·3
Doriman, 1951·3
Dorithricin, 1951·3
Dorithricin Limone, 1951·3
Dorithricin Original, 1951·3
Dorival, 1951·3
Dorixina, 1951·3
Dorixina B1 B6 B12, 1951·3
Dorixina Relax, 1951·3
Dorken, 1951·3
Dorless, 1951·3
Dorm, 1951·3
Dormalon, 1951·3
Dormarist, 1951·3
Dorme, 1951·3
Dormeasan, 1951·3
Dormelox, 1951·3
Dormen, 1951·3
Dormer 211, 1951·3
Dormex, 1951·4
Dormicum, 1951·4
Dormid, 1951·4
Dormideiras, 1129·1
Dormidina, 1951·4
Dormi-Gastreu S R14, 1951·4
Dormigoa N, 1951·4
Dormilam, 1951·4
Dormilona, 1666·1
Dormin, 1951·4
Dorminoctil, 1951·4
Dormiphen, 1951·4
Dormiplant, 1951·4
Dormire, 1951·4
Dormium, 1951·4
Dormodor, 1951·4
Dormonid, 1951·4
Dormonoct, 1951·4
Dormo-Puren, 1951·4
Dormo-Sern, 1951·4
Dormosol, 1951·4
Dormosyx, 1951·4
Dormoverlan, 1951·4
Dormplus, 1951·4
Dormutil N, 1951·4
Dornal, 1951·4
Dornasa Alfa, 1119·1
Dornase Alfa, 1119·1
Dorner, 1951·4
Dorocoff-ASS Plus, 1951·4
Dorocoff-Paracetamol, 1951·4
Dorofen, 1951·4
Dorona, 1952·1
Dorox, 1952·1
Dorpane, 1952·1
Dorpiel, 1952·1
Dorpinol, 1952·1
Dorpiren, 1952·1
Dorscopena, 1952·1
Dorsedin, 1952·1
Dorserol, 1952·1
Dorsiflex, 1952·1
Dorsof T, 1952·1
Dorspan, 1952·1
Dorvan, 1952·1
Dorveran, 1952·1
Doryl, 1952·1
Doryx, 1952·1
Dorzoflax, 1952·1
Dorzolamida, Hidrocloruro de, 908·3
Dorzolamide Hydrochloride, 908·3
Dorzone, 1952·1
Dos Dias N, 1952·1
DOS Softgel, 1952·1
Dosaflex, 1952·1
Dosalax, 1952·1
Dosamont, 1952·1
Dosan, 1952·1
Dosanac, 1952·1
Dosate, 1952·1
Dosberotec, 1952·1
Doscafis, 1952·1
Doses-O-Son, 1952·2
Dosier, 1952·2
Dosil, 1952·2
Dosil Enzimatico, 1952·2
Dosin, 1952·2
Dosiseptine, 1952·2
Dosmalfate, 1264·1
Dosodos, 1952·2
Dosoxygenee, 1952·2
Dospan Pento, 1952·2
Dospir, 1952·2
Doss, 1952·2
Dossiciclina Iclato, 206·2
Dostein, 1952·2
Dostil, 1952·2
Dostinex, 1952·2
Dosulepin Hydrochloride, 291·1
Dosulepina, Hidrocloruro de, 291·1
Dosulepini Hydrochloridum, 291·1
Dosulfin Bronquial, 1952·2
Dosulfin Fuerte, 1952·2
Dosyklin, 1952·2
Dotalsec, 1952·2
Dotarem, 1952·2
Dotest, 1952·2
Dothapax, 1952·2
Dothep, 1952·2
Dothiepin Hydrochloride, 291·1
Dotur, 1952·2
Double Action Indigestion Mixture— *see* Indigestion Relief Liquid, 2059·4
Double Action Indigestion Tablets— *see* Indigestion Relief Tablets, 2059·4
Double Check, 1952·2
Double-Action Toothache Kit, 1952·2
Doublebase, 1952·3
Doublecap, 1952·3
Double-Tussin DM, 1952·3
Douce-Amère, 1683·1
Douglas Protein Plus, 1952·3
Doulax, 1952·3
Douleurs & Fievre, 1952·3
Douzabox, 1952·3
Doval, 1952·3
Dovate, 1952·3
Dovavixin, 1952·3
Doven, 1952·3
Doveri, 1952·3
Doves, 1589·3
Dovobet, 1952·3
Dovonex, 1952·3
Doxacard, 1952·3
Doxacor, 1952·3
Doxacurio, Cloruro de, 1403·1
Doxacurium Chloride, 1403·1
Doxacyne, 1952·3
Doxadura, 1952·3
Doxagamma, 1952·3
Doxakne, 1952·3
Doxal, 1952·3
Doxaloc, 1952·3
Doxam, 1952·3
Doxamil, 1952·3
Doxapram, Hidrocloruro de, 1587·2
Doxapram Hydrochloride, 1587·2
Doxaprami Hydrochloridum, 1587·2
Doxapril, 1952·3
Doxa-Puren, 1952·3
Doxasin, 1952·3
Doxasyn, 1952·3
Doxate-C, 1952·4
Doxatensa, 1952·4
Doxate-S, 1952·4
Doxazobene, 1952·4
Doxazomerck, 1952·4
Doxazosin Mesilate, 908·3
Doxazosin Mesylate, 908·3
Doxazosin Methanesulphonate, 908·3
Doxazosina, Mesilato de, 908·3
Doxederm, 1952·4
Doxemina, 1952·4
Doxepia, 1952·4
Doxepin Hydrochloride, 291·2
Doxepina, Hidrocloruro de, 291·2
Doxepini Hydrochloridum, 291·2
Doxercalciferol, 1462·1
Doxergan, 1952·4
Doxetal, 1952·4
Doxi Crisol, 1952·4
Doxi Sergo, 1952·4
Doxibiot, 1952·4
Doxibiotic, 1952·4
Doxican, 1952·4
Doxiciclina, 206·2
Doxiciclina Cálcica, 206·2
Doxiciclina Fosfatex, 206·2
Doxiciclina, Hiclato de, 206·2
Doxiclat, 1952·4
Doxidan, 1952·4
Doxifen, 1952·4
Doxifluridina, 547·3
Doxifluridine, 547·3
Doxil, 1952·4
Doxilamina, Succinato de, 432·3
Doxilin, 1952·4
Doximal, 1952·4
Doximed, 1952·4
Doximucol, 1952·4

Doximycin, 1952·4
Doxin, 1952·4
Doxina, 1952·4
Doxinate, 1952·4
Doxine, 1953·1
Doxi-Om, 1953·1
Doxiproct, 1953·1
Doxiproct Mit Dexamethason, 1953·1
Doxiproct Plus, 1953·1
Doxitab, 1953·1
Doxiten, 1953·1
Doxiten Bio, 1953·1
Doxiten Enzimatico, 1953·1
Doxithal, 1953·1
Doxitin, 1953·1
Doxium, 1953·1
Doxivenil, 1953·1
Doxmil, 1953·1
DOXO-cell, 1953·1
Doxocris, 1953·1
Doxofilina, 785·1
Doxofylline, 785·1
Doxolbran, 1953·1
Doxolem, 1953·1
Doxorbin, 1953·1
Doxorrubicina, Cloridrato de, 547·3
Doxorubicin, 547·3
Doxorubicin Citrate Complex, 547·3
Doxorubicin Hydrochloride, 547·3
Doxorubicina, Hidrocloruro de, 547·3
Doxorubicini Hydrochloridum, 547·3
Doxorubicinol, 549·2
Doxorubin, 1953·1
Doxotec, 1953·1
Doxsig, 1953·1
Doxtie, 1953·1
Doxtran, 1953·1
Doxy, 1953·1
Doxy-1, 1953·1
Doxy-100, 1953·2
Doxy Comp, 1953·2
Doxy Komb, 1953·2
Doxy Lindoxyl, 1953·2
Doxy M, 1953·2
Doxy Plus, 1953·2
Doxy-basan, 1953·2
Doxybene, 1953·2
Doxybiocin, 1953·2
Doxycap, 1953·2
Doxychel, 1953·2
Doxycillin, 1953·2
Doxycin, 1953·2
Doxycline, 1953·2
Doxycycline, 206·2
Doxycycline Calcium, 206·2
Doxycycline Fosfatex, 206·2
Doxycycline Hyclate, 206·2
Doxycycline Hydrochloride, 206·2
Doxycycline Hydrochloride Hemiethanolate Hemihydrate, 206·2
Doxycycline Monohydrate, 206·2
Doxycyclini Hyclas, 206·2
Doxycyclinum, 206·2
Doxycyl, 1953·2
Doxy-Dagra, 1953·2
Doxyderm, 1953·2
Doxyderma, 1953·2
Doxy-Diolan, 1953·2
Doxydoc, 1953·2
Doxy-duramucal, 1953·2
Doxydyn, 1953·2
Doxyfene, 1953·2
Doxyferm, 1953·2
Doxyfim, 1953·2
Doxygram, 1953·2
Doxyhexal, 1953·2
Doxy-HP, 1953·2
Doxylag, 1953·2
Doxylamine Hydrogen Succinate, 432·3
Doxylamine Succinate, 432·3
Doxylamini Hydrogenosuccinas, 432·3
Doxylaminium Succinate, 432·3
Doxylan, 1953·3
Doxylar, 1953·3
Doxylets, 1953·3
Doxylin, 1953·3
Doxyline, 1953·3
Doxymerck, 1953·3
Doxymono, 1953·3
Doxymycin, 1953·3
Doxy-N-Tablinen, 1953·3
Doxy-P, 1953·3
Doxypal-DR, 1953·3
Doxypalu, 1953·3
Doxypol, 1953·3
Doxy-Puren, 1953·3
Doxysol, 1953·3
Doxysolvat, 1953·3
Doxystad, 1953·3
Doxy-Tablinen, 1953·3
Doxytec, 1953·3
Doxytem, 1953·3
Doxytrex, 1953·3
Doxytrim, 1953·3
Doxy-Wolff, 1953·3
Doxy-Wolff Mucolyt, 1953·3
Doyle, 1953·3
Dozbe, 1953·3
Dozebion, 1953·3
Dozelin Junior, 1953·3
Dozelin Lisina, 1953·3
Dozeneurin, 1953·3
Dozic, 1953·4
Dozile, 1953·4
Dozol, 1953·4
D-P, 1953·4
DP, 1953·4
Dp, 1953·4
DP-178, 633·1
DP Barrier Cream, 1953·4
DP Hand Rub, 1953·4
DP Hydrocortisone, 1953·4
DP Lotion - HC, 1953·4
DP Lubricating Gel, 1953·4
DP Warm Up, 1953·4
D-Pam, 1953·4
DPCA, 1953·4
DPCA 2, 1953·4
DPE, 1681·2, 1953·4
D-Penamine, 1953·4
DPH, 1953·4
DPN, 1719·1, 1953·4
DPN, Reduced, 1719·1
DPPC, 1736·2
DPPE, 587·3
DPT, 1680·3
DPT Merieux, 1953·4
DPT-Impfstoff, 1953·4
DPT-Vaccinol, 1953·4
DQM, 1953·4
DR-3305, 1683·2
DR-3355, 225·3
Dr Calm, 1953·4
Dr Dermi-Heal, 1953·4
Dr Ernst Richter's Abfuhrtee, 1953·4
Dr. Ernst Richter's Abfuhrtee-Filterbeutel, 1954·1
Dr Ernst Richter's Abfuhrtee-tassenfertig, 1954·1
Dr Grandel Brennessel Vital Tonikum, 1954·1
Dr Grandel Granobil, 1954·1
Dr. Hotz Vollbad, 1954·1
Dr Janssens Teebohnen, 1954·1
Dr Schmidgall Halsweh, 1954·1
Dr Scholl's Athlete's Foot, 1954·1
Dr Scholl's Callus Removers, 1954·1
Dr Scholl's Clear Away, 1954·1
Dr Scholl's Corn Removers, 1954·1
Dr Scholl's Corn/Callus Remover, 1954·1
Dr Scholl's Cracked Heel Relief, 1954·1
Dr Scholl's Wart Remover, 1954·1
Dr Selby, 1954·1
Dr Smiths, 1954·1
Dr Wiemanns Rheumatonikum, 1954·1
Dracanyl, 1954·1
Dracodermalin, 1954·1
Dracontiasis— *see* Dracunculiasis, 98·1
*Dracontium foetidum*, 1746·3
Dracunculiasis, 98·1
Dracylic Acid, 1169·3
Drafilyn-Z, 1954·1
Draganon, 1954·1
Dragee Vauban, 1954·1
Dragees Antirhumatismales, 1954·1
Dragees aux Figues avec du Sene, 1954·1
Dragees contre la Toux No 536, 1954·1
Dragees contre les Maux de Tete, 1954·1
Dragees contre les Maux de Voyage No 537, 1954·1
Dragees Fuca, 1954·1
Dragees Laxatives No 510, 1954·1
Dragees Neunzehn, 1954·2
Dragees Neunzehn Senna, 1954·2
Dragees pour la Detente Nerveuse, 1954·2
Dragees pour le Coeur et les Nerfs, 1954·2
Dragees pour le Sommeil Nouvelle Formule, 1954·2
Dragees pour Reins et Vessie S, 1954·2
Dragees Vegetales Rex, 1954·2
Dragon Balm, 1954·2
Dragon, Gum, 1582·2
Dragosil, 1954·2
Drainactil, 1954·2
Draituss-Ped, 1954·2
Dralen, 1954·2
Dralinsa, 1954·2
Dramamine, 1954·2
Dramamine II, 1954·2
Dramamine-compositum, 1954·2
Dramanate, 1954·2
Dramavit, 1954·2
Dramavit B6, 1954·2
Dramigel, 1954·2
Dramin, 1954·2
Dramin B-6, 1954·2
Dramin B-6 DL, 1954·2
Dramine, 1954·2
Dramnate, 1954·2
Dranat, 1954·2
Drapix, 1954·2
Drapolene, 1954·3
Dravyr, 1954·3
Draxon, 1954·3
Drazine, 1954·3
DRC-1201, 1063·2
Dreemon, 1954·3
Dreierlei, 1954·3
Drei-Pflanzen-Dragees N, Kneipp— *see* Kneipp Drei-Pflanzen-Dragees N, 2081·2
Dreisacarb, 1954·3
Dreisafer, 1954·3
DreisaFol, 1954·3
Dreisavit, 1954·3
Dreisavit N, 1954·3
Drenalin, 1954·3
Drenian, 1954·3
Drenidra, 1954·3
Dreniformio, 1954·3
Drenison, 1954·3
Drenison N, 1954·3
Drenison Neomicina, 1954·3
Dren'it, 1954·3
Drenocol, 1954·3
Drenoflux, 1954·3
Drenol, 1954·3
Drenomade, 1954·3
Drenotosse, 1954·3
Drenovac, 1954·3
Drenoxol, 1954·3
Drenur, 1954·3
Drenural, 1954·3
Drepatil, 1954·4
Dresan, 1954·4
Dresan Biotic, 1954·4
Dresplan, 1954·4
Driclor, 1954·4
Dridase, 1954·4
Dridol, 1954·4
Dri/Ear, 1954·4
Dried Aluminium Hydroxide, 1249·2
Dried Aluminium Phosphate, 1250·1
Dried Aluminum Hydroxide Gel, 1249·2
Dried Bilberry, 1718·3
Dried Bitter-Orange Peel, 1723·3
Dried Calcium Sulfate, 1665·1
Dried Calcium Sulphate, 1665·1
Dried Epsom Salts, 1228·2
Dried Factor VII Fraction, 750·3
Dried Factor VIII Fraction, 751·1
Dried Factor IX Fraction, 752·2
Dried Ferrous Sulfate, 1428·3
Dried Ferrous Sulphate, 1428·3
Dried Lemon Peel, 1706·2
Dried Magnesium Sulphate, 1228·2
Dried Prothrombin Complex, 752·2
Dried Yeast, 1469·1
Dried/Cho/Vac, 1611·2
Dried/Tub/Vac/BCG, 1609·2
Dried/Typhoid/Vac, 1642·2
Drifen, 1954·4
DriHist, 1954·4
Driken, 1954·4
Drilix, 1954·4
Drill, 1954·4
Drill Expectorant, 1954·4
Drill Mucolitico, 1954·4
Drill Rhinites, 1954·4
Drill Tosse Seca, 1954·4
Drill Toux Seche, 1954·4
Drilyna, 1954·4
Drimen, 1954·4
*Drimia indica*, 1130·3
*Drimia maritima*, 991·1, 1130·3
Drimnorth, 1954·4
Drimpam, 1954·4
Drin, 1954·4
Drina, 1954·4
Drioquilen, 1954·4
Driptane, 1954·4
Drisdol, 1954·4
Drisi-Ven, 1954·4
Drisofal, 1955·1
Dristal Cold, 1955·1
Dristan Preparations, 1955·1
Dristan Cold, Maximum Strength— *see* Maximum Strength Dristan Cold, 2116·4
Dristancito, 1955·2
Drithocreme, 1955·2
Dritho-Scalp, 1955·2
Drivermide, 1955·2
Drix, 1955·2
Drix Abfuhr-Dragees, 1955·2
Drix Bisacodyl, 1955·2
Drixin, 1955·2
Drixine, 1955·2
Drixine Nasal, 1955·2
Drixomed, 1955·2
Drixora, 1955·2
Drixoral Preparations, 1955·2
Drixtab, 1955·3
Drize, 1955·3
Droal, 1955·3
Drocef, 1955·3
Droclina, 1955·3
Drocode Bitartrate, 34·3
Drocon-CS, 1955·3
Drofaron, 1955·3
Drofaxil, 1955·3
Drofenina, Hidrocloruro de, 482·1
Drofenine Hydrochloride, 482·1
Drogenil, 1955·3
Drogimed, 1955·3
Drolasona, 1955·3
Droleptan, 1955·3
Droloxifene, 550·1
Droloxifeno, 550·1
Dromadol, 1955·3
Dromos, 1955·3
Dronabinol, 1264·2
Dronal, 1955·3
Dronate-OS, 1955·3
2-Drop Corn Remedy, Scholl— *see* Scholl 2-Drop Corn Remedy, 2279·3
Dropcina, 1955·3
Droperdal, 1955·3
Droperidol, 697·2
Droperidolum, 697·2
Droperol, 1955·3
Dropgel, 1955·3
Dropicine, 1955·3
Dropid, 1955·3
Dropilton, 1955·3

Dropovit, 1955·4
Dropropizina, 1119·3
Dropropizine, 1119·3
Dropstar, 1955·4
Droptimol, 1955·4
Dropyal, 1955·4
Drosana Femicin— *see* Femicin, 1991·1
Drosana Hyperflorin, 1955·4
Drosana Resiston, 1955·4
Drosera, 1683·1
Drosera Komplex, 1955·4
*Drosera rotundifolia*, 1683·1
Droserae Herba, 1683·1
Droserapect, 1955·4
Drosera-Weliplex, 1955·4
Drosetux, 1955·4
Drosinula, 1955·4
Drosithym-N, 1955·4
Drospirenona, 1549·1
Drospirenone, 1549·1
Drossadin, 1955·4
Drossanose, 1955·4
Drossa-Nose, 1955·4
Drosten, 1955·4
Drosyn, 1955·4
Drotaverina, 1683·1
Drotaverine, 1683·1
Drotaverine Hydrochloride, 1683·1
Drotin, 1955·4
Drotrecogin Alfa (Activated), 759·2
Drovitol, 1955·4
Droxaine, 1955·4
Droxaryl, 1955·4
Droxel, 1955·4
Droxia, 1955·4
Droxicam, 36·2
Droxidopa, 1204·3
Droxil, 1955·4
Droximag, 1955·4
Droxitop, 1955·4
Droxiurea, 1955·4
Droxivit, 1955·4
Droxol, 1955·4
Droxyl, 1956·1
Drufusan N, 1956·1
Druisel, 1956·1
Dry Antiperspirant Foot Spray, Scholl— *see* Scholl Dry Antiperspirant Foot Spray, 2279·3
Dry Cough, Chemists Own— *see* Chemists Own Dry Cough, 1882·1
Dry Cough, Nyal Plus+ — *see* Nyal Plus+ Dry Cough, 2182·2
Dry Cough Syrup, 1956·1
Dry Eye, 1576·1
Dry Eyes, 1956·1
Dry Hacking Cough & Head Congestion, Vicks Pediatric Formula 44D— *see* Vicks Pediatric Formula 44D Dry Hacking Cough & Head Congestion, 2375·4
Dry Hacking Cough, Vicks— *see* Vicks Dry Hacking Cough, 2375·2
Dry Ice, 1235·2
Dry Mouth, 1576·2
Dry Raspy Cough, Chemists Own— *see* Chemists Own Dry Raspy Cough, 1882·1
Drylin, 1956·1
Drynalken, 1956·1
Drynalquin, 1956·1
Drynisan, 1956·1
*Dryopteris filix-mas*, 108·2
Dryptal, 1956·1
Drysol, 1956·1
Drytergent, 1956·1
Drytex, 1956·1
Dryvax, 1956·1
DS-36, 263·2
DS-103-282, 1395·3
DS Emulsion, 1956·1
DS-103-282-ch, 1395·3
D-Seb, 1956·1
DSP, 1097·2
D-S-S, 1956·1
DSS, 1262·2
D-Stop, 1956·1
D-Stress, 1956·1
D4T, 654·2
DT-327, 888·2
DT-5621, 1663·2
DT Bis, 1956·1
DT Coq, 1956·1
DT Coq, Adsorbed— *see* Adsorbed DT Coq, 1777·2
DT Polio, 1956·1
DT Vax, 1956·1
DT Vax, Adsorbed— *see* Adsorbed DT Vax, 1777·2
D-40TA, 697·3
D-Tabs, 1956·1
DTap-IPV, 1956·1
D-Tato, 1956·1
DTC, 1038·2
DTCoq/DTP, 1956·1
DTCP— *see* Pent-HIBest, 2211·3
DTI, 1956·1
DTIC, 544·2, 1956·1
DTIC-Dome, 1956·2
DT-Impfstoff, 1956·2
DTM, 1956·2
DTP, 1956·2
DTPA, 1050·1
DTPA, Calcium Trisodium, 1050·1
DTPer/Vac/Ads, 1613·3
DTP-Merieux, 1956·2
DTP-Rix, 1956·2
DTPT, 1455·1
D-Tracetten, 1956·2
DT-reduct, 1956·2
DT-Rix, 1956·2
D-Trp LHRH-PEA, 1322·3
D-Tussin, 1956·2
DT/Vac/Ads(Adult), 1613·1
DT/Vac/Ads(Child), 1613·1
DT-Vaccinol, 1956·2
D.T.Vax Adsorbe, 1956·2
DU-1219, 856·2
DU-1227, 856·2
DU-21220, 1739·2
DU-23000, 298·2
Duac, 1956·2
Duac Once Daily, 1956·2
Duact, 1956·2
Duadacin, 1956·2
Duadacin Extra Strength Cold & Flu, 1956·2
Duafen, 1956·2
Dual Action Cough Drops, Vicks Victors— *see* Vicks Victors Dual Action Cough Drops, 2376·1
Dual Antigen, 1956·2
Dualgan, 1956·2
Dualid, 1956·2
Dualid S, 1956·2
Dualizol, 1956·2
Dual-Lax Extra Strong, 1956·2
Dual-Lax Normal Strength, 1956·2
Dualten, 1956·2
Duan, 1956·2
Duaneo, 1956·2
Duaneo Mit Codein, 1956·3
Dubam, 1956·3
Dube, 1956·3
Dublon, 1956·3
Ducene, 1956·3
Duchenne Muscular Dystrophy— *see* Muscular Dystrophies, 1083·3
Duciclon, 1956·3
Ductal Carcinoma in Situ— *see* Malignant Neoplasms of the Breast, 514·1
Ductelmin, 1956·3
Ductogel, 1956·3
Ductomet, 1956·3
Ductopan, 1956·3
Ductopril, 1956·3
Ductoveran, 1956·3
Ductus Arteriosus, Patent— *see* Patent Ductus Arteriosus, 49·2
Duebien, 1956·3
Duet, 1956·3
Dueva, 1956·3
Dufaston, 1956·3
Dufine, 1956·3
Duflemina, 1956·3
Duinum, 1956·3
Dukoral, 1956·3
Dularell Classic, 1956·3
Dularell— *see* Dularell Classic, 1956·3
Dularell N, 1956·3
Dulax, 1956·3
Dulcamara, 1683·1
Dulcamarae Caulis, 1683·1
Dulcamara-Homaccord, 1956·3
Dulceril, 1956·3
Dulcilarmes, 1956·3
Dulciphak, 1956·3
Dulcivit, 1956·3
Dulco Laxo, 1956·3
Dulcodruppels, 1956·3
Dulcolan, 1956·3
Dulcolax, 1956·4
Dulcolax Liquid, 1956·4
Dulcolax NP, 1956·4
Dulcolax Picosulphate, 1956·4
Dulconatur, 1956·4
Dulcosol, 1956·4
Dulinas, 1956·4
Dull-C, 1956·4
Duloxetina, Hidrocloruro de, 291·3
Duloxetine Hydrochloride, 291·3
Dul-X, 1956·4
Dumesil, 1956·4
Dumex Lactose-Free, 1956·4
Dumex Plus, 1956·4
Dumicoat, 1956·4
Dumin, 1956·4
Dumirox, 1956·4
Dumocalcin, 1956·4
Dumocyclin, 1956·4
Dumolid, 1956·4
Dumovit C, 1956·4
Dumovital, 1956·4
Dumoxin, 1956·4
Dumozol, 1956·4
Dumping Syndrome, 1242·1
Dumyrox, 1956·4
Duna, 1956·4
Dunason, 1957·1
Duncan, 1957·1
Duncankil, 1957·1
Dung, Devil's, 1658·1
Dünnflüssiges Paraffin, 1479·1
Dunox, 1957·1
Duo Celloids Preparations, 1957·1
Duo Decadron, 1957·1
Duo Gobens, 1957·1
Duo Minoxi, 1957·1
Duo Vizerul, 1957·1
Duobact, 1957·1
Duobar, 1957·1
Duo-C, 1957·2
Duocal, 1957·2
Duocet, 1957·2
Duocort, 1957·2
Duoctrin, 1957·2
Duoctrin Balsamico, 1957·2
Duoctrin Enterico, 1957·2
Duo-CVP, 1957·2
Duo-Cyp, 1957·2
Duo-Decadron, 1957·2
Duodenal Ulcer— *see* Peptic Ulcer Disease, 1246·3
Duoderm, 1957·2
Duodexa N, 1957·2
Duodil, 1957·2
Duo-Extolen, 1957·2
Duofem, 1957·2
Duofer, 1957·2
Duofer Fol, 1957·2
Duofilm, 1957·2
Duoflam, 1957·2
Duoflam Gel, 1957·3
Duoflam Plus, 1957·3
Duoflex, 1957·3
Duoform Novo, 1957·3
Duoforte, 1957·3
Duogas, 1957·3
Duogastral, 1957·3
Duogink, 1957·3
Duokapton, 1957·3
Duolax, 1957·3
Duolaxan, 1957·3
Duolin, 1957·3
Duolip, 1957·3
Duolube, 1957·3
Duoluton, 1957·3
Duoluton-L, 1957·3
Duolys A, 1957·3
Duolys B, 1957·3
Duomet, 1957·3
Duonalc, 1957·3
Duonalc-E, 1957·3
Duonasa, 1957·3
Duonate, 1957·3
DuoNeb, 1957·3
Duo-Ormogyn, 1957·3
Duopack, 1957·3
Duoplant, 1957·4
Duoplant Gel, 1957·4
Duoran, 1957·4
Duorol, 1957·4
Duo-Scabil, 1957·4
Duotec, 1957·4
Duoton, 1957·4
Duo-Trach Kit, 1957·4
Duotric, 1957·4
Duova, 1957·4
Duoval, 1957·4
Duovax, 1957·4
Duovent, 1957·4
Duoventrin, 1957·4
Duoventrinetten N, 1957·4
Duovir, 1957·4
Duovisc, 1957·4
Duovitan, 1957·4
Duozol, 1957·4
DuP-753, 947·2
DuP-785, 1351·2
Duphalac, 1957·4
Duphaston, 1957·4
Duphaston— *see* Femapak, 1990·4
Duplamin, 1958·1
Duplex, 1958·1
Duplex T, 1958·1
Duplexcillina, 1958·1
Duplexil, 1958·1
Duplicalcio, 1958·1
Duplicalcio 150, 1958·1
Duplicalcio B12, 1958·1
Duplicalcio Hidraz, 1958·1
Duplide, 1958·1
Duplobar, 1958·1
Duplocitrin, 1958·1
Duplo-Penicillin, 1958·1
Duplotrast, 1958·1
Duplotrast Z, 1958·1
Duponil, 1958·1
Dura AL, 1958·1
Dura AX, 1958·1
Duraampicillin, 1958·1
Durabezur, 1958·1
Durabiotic, 1958·1
Durabolin, 1958·1
Durabronchal, 1958·1
Duracain, 1958·1
Duracaine, 1958·1
Duracare, 1958·1
Duracebrol, 1958·2
Duracef, 1958·2
Duracetamol, 1958·2
Duraclean, 1958·2
Duraclon, 1958·2
Duracoll, 1958·2
Duracoron, 1958·2
Duracreme, 1958·2
Duracroman, 1958·2
Duradermal, 1958·2
Duradiuret, 1958·2
Duradoce, 1958·2
Duradox, 1958·2
Duradoxal, 1958·2
Duradrin, 1958·2
Duraerythromycin, 1958·2
Durafenat, 1958·2
Duraflor, 1958·2
Duraflu, 1958·2

Durafungol, 1958·2
Durafurid, 1958·2
Duragel, 1958·2
Duragentamicin, 1958·2
Duragesic, 1958·2
Dura-Gest, 1958·2
Duraglucon N, 1958·2
DuraH2, 1958·3
Durahist, 1958·3
Dura-Ibu, 1958·3
DuraIbuprofen, 1958·3
Durakne, 1958·3
Duralex, 1958·3
Duralgin, 1958·3
Duralipon, 1958·3
Duralith, 1958·3
Duralmor, 1958·3
Duralone, 1958·3
Duralopid, 1958·3
Duralozam, 1958·3
DuraMCP, 1958·3
Duramipress, 1958·3
Duramist Plus, 1958·3
Duramonitat, 1958·3
Duramorph, 1958·3
Duramucal, 1958·3
Duran, 1958·3
Duranest, 1958·3
Duranifin, 1958·3
Duranifin Sali, 1958·3
Duranil, 1958·3
Duranitrat, 1958·3
Durapaediat, 1958·3
Durapatite, 1699·3
Durapen, 1958·3
Durapen Balsamico, 1958·3
Durapenicillin, 1958·3
Durapental, 1958·3
Duraphat, 1958·4
Duraphyllin, 1958·4
Durapindol, 1958·4
Durapirenz, 1958·4
Durapirox, 1958·4
Durapitrop, 1958·4
Duraprednisolon, 1958·4
Duraprox, 1958·4
Durarese, 1958·4
Durasal, 1958·4
Durascreen, 1958·4
Durasilymarin, 1958·4
Durasina, 1958·4
Durasolets, 1958·4
Durasoptin, 1958·4
Duraspiron, 1958·4
Duraspiron-comp, 1958·4
Duratamoxifen, 1958·4
Dura-Tap/PD, 1958·4
Duratears, 1958·4
Duratears Naturale, 1958·4
Duratenol, 1958·4
Duratenol Comp, 1959·1
Durater, 1959·1
Duratest, 1959·1
Durateston, 1959·1
Duratestrin, 1959·1
Durathate, 1959·1
Duratimol, 1959·1
Duration, 1959·1
Duratirs, 1959·1
Duratocin, 1959·1
Duratuss, 1959·1
Duratuss DM, 1959·1
Duratuss G, 1959·1
Duratuss GP, 1959·1
Duratuss HD, 1959·1
Duraultra, 1959·1
Dura-Vent, 1959·1
Dura-Vent/A, 1959·1
Dura-Vent/DA, 1959·1
Duravolten, 1959·1
Durazanil, 1959·1
Durazepam, 1959·1
Durazidum, 1959·1
Durazina, 1959·1
Dura-Zok, 1959·1
Durbis, 1959·1
Durekal, 1959·2
Dur-Elix, 1959·2
Dur-Elix— *see* Duro-Tuss Mucolytic, 1959·3
Dur-Elix Plus, 1959·2
Duremesan, 1959·2
Duremid, 1959·2
Durex Sensilube, 1959·2
Duricef, 1959·2
Duride, 1959·2
Durijo, 1666·1
Durin, 1959·2
Durmast Oak, 1722·3
Durobac, 1959·2
Duroferon, 1959·2
Duroferon Vitamin, 1959·2
Durogesic, 1959·2
Duro-K, 1959·2
Durolax, 1959·2
Durolax X-Pack, 1959·2
Durolax SP, 1959·2
Duromine, 1959·2
Duronitrin, 1959·2
Durotan, 1959·2
Duro-Tuss, 1959·2
Duro-Tuss Cold & Allergy, 1959·2
Duro-Tuss Cough Lozenges, 1959·2
Duro-Tuss Decongestant, 1959·2
Duro-Tuss Expectorant, 1959·3
Duro-Tuss Lozenges, 1959·3
Duro-Tuss Mucolytic, 1959·3
Duro-Tuss Mucolytic Cough Liquid, 1959·3
Duro-Tuss Sinus, 1959·3
Durvitan, 1959·3
Dusil, 1959·3
Dusodril, 1959·3
Duspatal, 1959·3
Duspatalin, 1959·3
Duspatin, 1959·3
Dust, 1730·3
Dutacor, 1959·3
Dutasterida, 1549·2
Dutasteride, 1549·2
Dutch Liquid, 1505·1
Duteplasa, 909·2
Duteplase, 909·2
Dutimelan, 1959·3
Dutonin, 1959·3
Dutross, 1959·3
Duvadilan, 1959·3
Duvaxan, 1959·3
Duvig, 1959·3
Duvium, 1959·3
Duvoid, 1959·3
Duxaril, 1959·3
Duxil, 1959·3
Duxima, 1959·3
Duxor, 1959·3
DV-1006, 1255·2
D-Vi-Sol, 1959·4
D-Vital, 1959·4
D-Void, 1959·4
DW-61, 482·2
DW-62, 1587·2
Dwarf Nettle, 1762·1
Dwarf Pine Needle Oil, 1737·1
Dwarf Tapeworm Infections— *see* Hymenolepiasis, 99·2
Dwarfism— *see* Growth Retardation, 1314·2
D-Worm, 1959·4
DX-88, 761·3
DXM, 1117·3
Dyazide, 1959·4
Dycholium, 1959·4
Dycill, 1959·4
Dyclocaine Hydrochloride, 1376·2
Dyclocaini Chloridum, 1376·2
Dyclone, 1959·4
Dyclonine Hydrochloride, 1376·2
Dydrogesterone, 1549·2
Dyflex-G, 1959·4
Dyflos, 1490·1
Dy-G, 1959·4
Dygratyl, 1959·4
Dyka-D, 1959·4
Dykatuss Co, 1959·4
Dyline GG, 1959·4
Dylix, 1959·4
Dymadon, 1959·4
Dymadon Co, 1959·4
Dymadon Forte, 1959·4
Dymelor, 1959·4
Dymenate, 1959·4
Dymion, 1959·4
Dymotil, 1959·4
Dyna Jets, 1959·4
Dyna-Ampcil, 1959·4
Dynabac, 1959·4
Dynabolon, 1959·4
Dynacide, 1959·4
Dynacil, 1959·4
Dynacil Comp, 1960·1
Dynacin, 1960·1
Dynacirc, 1960·1
Dynacold, 1960·1
Dynadol, 1960·1
Dynafed Asthma Relief, 1960·1
Dynafed EX, 1960·1
Dynafed, Maximum Strength— *see* Dynafed Plus, 1960·1
Dynafed Plus, 1960·1
Dynafed Pseudo, 1960·1
Dynafemme, 1960·1
Dynagastrin, 1960·1
Dyna-Hex, 1960·1
Dynalert, 1960·1
Dynametron, 1960·1
Dynamin, 1960·1
Dynamisan, 1960·1
Dynamo, 1960·1
Dynamogen, 1960·1
Dynamucil, 1960·1
Dynapayne, 1960·1
Dynapen, 1960·1
Dynaphos-C, 1960·1
Dynaspor, 1960·1
Dynasprin, 1960·1
Dynastat, 1960·2
Dynatra, 1960·2
Dynavital, 1960·2
Dynazole, 1960·2
Dynef, 1960·2
Dynergum, 1960·2
Dyneric, 1960·2
Dynese, 1960·2
Dynexan, 1960·2
Dynexan Herpescreme, 1960·2
Dynexan Mundgel, 1960·2
Dynexan Zahnfleischtropfen, 1960·2
Dynofen, 1960·2
Dynorm, 1960·2
Dynorm Plus, 1960·2
Dynorphins, 73·3
Dynos, 1960·2
Dynothel, 1960·2
Dynoxytet, 1960·2
Dyphylline, 784·3
Dyphylline-GG, 1960·2
Dyprotex, 1960·2
Dyrade-M, 1960·2
Dyrenium, 1960·2
Dyrenium Compositum, 1960·2
Dyrexan-OD, 1960·2
Dyrosol, 1960·2
Dysalfa, 1960·3
Dysbetalipoproteinaemia, Familial— *see* Hyperlipidaemias, 823·1
Dyscornut, 1960·3
Dysentery, Amoebic— *see* Amoebiasis, 595·2
Dysentery, Bacillary— *see* Shigellosis, 130·1
Dysentery Vaccines, 1638·3
Dysetrin, 1960·3
Dysfunctional Uterine Bleeding— *see* Menorrhagia, 1567·3
Dysfur-M, 1960·3
Dysgeusia— *see* Taste Disorders, 682·2
Dyskinebyl, 1960·3
Dyskinesia, Tardive— *see* Extrapyramidal Disorders, 677·1
Dyskinon, 1960·3
Dyslipidaemias— *see* Hyperlipidaemias, 823·1
Dysman, 1960·3
Dysmen, 1960·3
Dysmen-500, 1960·3
Dysmen Forte, 1960·3
Dysmenalgit, 1960·3
Dysmenorrhoea, 6·1
Dysmenorrhoe-Gastreu S R75, 1960·3
*Dysosma pleianthum*, 1155·3
Dyspagon, 1960·3
Dyspamet, 1960·3
Dyspen, 1960·3
Dyspepsia, 1242·1
Dysphagia, Dystonic— *see* Dystonias, 1209·3
Dysphonia— *see* Dystonias, 1209·3
Dysphoric Disorder, Premenstrual— *see* Premenstrual Syndrome, 1551·3
Dyspne-Inhal, 1960·3
Dyspnoea, 74·1
Dysport, 1960·3
Dysthymia, 278·1
Dysto-L 90 N, 1960·3
Dystolise, 1960·3
Dysto-loges, 1960·3
Dysto-lux, 1960·3
Dystonal, 1960·3
Dystonia, Cervical— *see* Spasmodic Torticollis, 1391·1
Dystonias, 1209·3
Dystonic Reactions, Drug-induced— *see* Extrapyramidal Disorders, 677·1
Dystophan, 1960·3
Dystrol, 1960·3
Dystrophies, Muscular— *see* Muscular Dystrophies, 1083·3
Dystrophy, Reflex Sympathetic— *see* Complex Regional Pain Syndrome, 5·3
Dysurgal, 1960·3
Dysurgal N, 1960·3
Dytac, 1960·3
Dytan, 1960·3
Dytan-D, 1960·4
Dyta-Urese, 1960·4
Dytenzide, 1960·4
Dyterene, 1960·4
Dytide, 1960·4
Dytide H, 1960·4
Dytuss, 1960·4
Dyzole, 1960·4
DZL-221, 1719·2
D-Zol, 1960·4

## E

E, 1433·2, 1589·3
E5, 1615·2
7E3, 841·3
E45, 1960·4
E100, 1057·2
E101, 1456·1
E102, 1058·2
E104, 1057·3
E110, 1058·2
E120, 1057·1, 1057·2
E122, 1057·1
E123, 1056·1
E124, 1057·3
E127, 1057·2
E128, 1058·1
E129, 1056·1
E131, 1729·1
E132, 1700·3
E133, 1056·2
E140, 1057·1
E-141, 749·3
E141, 1057·1
E142, 1057·3
E150a, 1057·1
E150d, 1057·1
E151, 1056·2
E153, 1058·3
E154, 1056·2
E155, 1056·3

E160a, 1056·1
E160(a), 1422·3
E160d, 1056·1
E161(g), 1056·3
E162, 1056·2
E163, 1056·1
E170, 1254·2
E171, 1160·3
E172, 1057·3
E173, 1652·2
E174, 1746·1
E175, 1695·3
E180, 1057·3
E200, 1192·3
E202, 1192·3
205E, 1664·2
E210, 1169·3
E211, 1169·3
E214, 1183·2
E215, 1183·3
E216, 1183·3
E217, 1183·3
E218, 1183·3
E219, 1183·3
E220, 1193·2
E221, 1193·1
E222, 1193·1
E223, 1193·1
E224, 1193·1
E228, 1193·1
E230, 1681·2
E231, 1187·2
E232, 1187·2
E233, 114·2
E234, 237·2
E235, 406·2
E236, 1689·3
E237, 1689·3
E238, 1689·3
E239, 230·1
E250, 1052·3
E251, 1192·2
E252, 1190·1
E260, 1645·2
E261, 1232·1
E262, 1191·3, 1223·1
E263, 1225·1
E270, 1704·1
E280, 407·3
E281, 408·1
E282, 407·3
E283, 407·3
E284, 1662·1
E285, 1661·3
E290, 1235·2
E296, 1709·2
E297, 1147·3
E300, 1460·2
E301, 1460·2
E302, 1460·2
E304, 1168·2
E306, 1464·3
E307, 1464·3
E310, 1168·1
E311, 1168·1
E312, 1168·1
E320, 1171·2
E321, 1171·3
E322, 1706·1
E325, 1223·2
E326, 1704·1
E327, 1225·3
E330, 1673·1
E331, 1223·2
E332, 1223·1
E334, 1752·1
E335, 1290·1
E336, 1232·2, 1284·3
E337, 1284·3
E338, 1731·2
E339, 1230·3, 1231·1
E340, 1230·3
E341, 1225·2, 1225·3, 1664·2
E353, 1752·1
E363, 1748·3
E380, 1654·1
E385, 1051·3
E400, 1576·3
E401, 1577·1
E404, 745·1
E405, 1576·3
E406, 1576·3
E407, 1578·2
E410, 1579·1
E412, 333·2
E413, 1582·2
E414, 1576·2
E415, 1582·3
E416, 1290·2
E420, 1446·3
E421, 950·2
E422, 1694·3
E425, 1693·3
E432, 1415·1
E433, 1415·2
E434, 1415·1
E435, 1415·1
E440, 1580·3
E442, 1706·1
E452, 1734·3, 1748·2
E459, 1678·2
E460, 1578·3
E461, 1580·2
E462, 1579·1
E463, 1579·2
E464, 1579·3
E466, 1577·3
E468, 1578·1
E471, 1413·2
E473, 1416·3
E477, 1415·3
E491, 1416·2
E492, 1416·3
E493, 1416·1
E494, 1416·1
E495, 1416·2
E500, 1223·2, 1747·1, 1747·2
E501, 1223·1
E503, 1115·1
E504, 1272·1
E507, 1699·1
E508, 1232·2
E509, 1225·1
E511, 1228·1
E513, 1750·3
E514, 1290·1
E515, 1232·2
E516, 1665·1
E520, 1653·1
E522, 1652·1
E524, 1747·3
E525, 1734·2
E526, 1664·3
E527, 1653·3
E528, 1272·2
E529, 1664·3
E530, 1272·3
E551, 1581·3
E552, 1226·1
E553(a), 1272·3, 1580·2
E554, 1250·2
E558, 1577·2
E559, 1268·3
E576, 1747·3
E577, 1232·2
E578, 1225·2
E579, 1428·1
E585, 1428·2
E-600, 1494·1
E-614, 1018·1
E620, 1433·2
E621, 1441·1
E627, 1681·3
E631, 1681·3
E640, 1433·3
E-643, 878·1
E650, 1469·2
E-0659, 425·2
E-671, 1293·3
E900, 1482·1
E901, 1480·1, 1480·2
E902, 1480·2
E903, 1668·1
E904, 1743·3
E905, 1481·3
E920, 1426·3
E939, 1236·1
E941, 1236·3
E942, 1304·3
E943a, 1235·1
E944, 1238·2
E948, 1236·3
E950, 1420·3
E951, 1422·1
E952, 1426·2
E953, 1438·3
E954, 1443·2, 1443·3
E957, 1451·1
E965, 1439·3
E966, 1269·1
E967, 1469·1
E999, 1416·1
E-1000, 1142·2
E-1077, 173·2
E1105, 1717·2
E1201, 1581·2
E1505, 1757·3
E1518, 410·2
E1520, 1735·2
E-2020, 1489·2
E-2663, 1659·2
E3100, 1467·1
E-3174, 948·1
E-3340, 947·2
E-3810, 1285·1
E-5166, 1156·1
E-6010, 961·3
E-9002, 110·1
E45, Bath— *see* Bath E45, 1829·2
E45, Cream— *see* Cream E45, 1911·1
E45 Itch Relief, 1960·4
E Mal, 1960·4
E Plus, 1960·4
E Radicaps, 1960·4
E45 Sun, 1960·4
E45 Sun Block, 1960·4
E45, Wash— *see* Wash E45, 2385·2
Ea-0167, 1467·1
EA-3547, 1676·3
EACA, 741·3
Eaca Balsamico, 1960·4
EAEC, 129·2
Eagle-vine Bark, 1675·3
Eanox, 1960·4
EAP-61, 1960·4
Ear Clear, 1960·4
Ear Clear for Swimmer's Ear, 1960·4
Ear Infections— *see* Otitis Externa, 138·1
Ear Infections— *see* Otitis Media, 138·1
Ear Wax Removal, 1262·3
Earache, 1960·4
Earache Pain, 1960·4
EarCalm, 1960·4
Earclear, 1960·4
Ear-Dry, 1960·4
Earex, 1961·1
Earex Plus, 1961·1
Ear-Eze, 1961·1
Early Bird, 1961·1
Early Golden-rod, 1748·3
EarSol, 1961·1
EarSol-HC, 1961·1
Earth, Diatomaceous, 1581·3
Earth, Purified Infusorial, 1581·3
Earth, Purified Siliceous, 1581·3
Earth-nut Oil, 1656·1
EAS, 1961·1
Ease Pain Away, 1961·1
Easiko, 1961·1
Easistix BG, 1961·1
Easistix UG, 1961·1
Easprin, 1961·1
Easy Bronz, Bioglan— *see* Bioglan Easy Bronz, 1844·1
Easy Gel, 1961·1
Easylax, 1961·1
Eatan N, 1961·1
Eaton-Lambert Myasthenic Syndrome, 1485·1
Eau de Javel, 1192·2
Eau Oxygénée, Soluté Officinal d', 1182·2
Eau Potable, 1764·3
Eau Pour Préparations Injectables, 1765·1
Eau Precieuse, 1961·1
Eau-de-vie de France avec Huile de Pin Nain du Tirol, 1961·1
Eavit, 1961·1
Eavit Plus, 1961·1
Eazamine Hydrochloride, 481·3
E150b, 1057·1
E160b, 1056·1
E161b, 1056·1
E553(b), 1159·1
EB-644, 1461·2
E927b, 1162·2
E943b, 1236·2
EB-1089, 583·3
Ebamin, 1961·1
E-Base, 1961·1
Ebastel, 1961·1
Ebastel D, 1961·1
Ebastina, 433·1
Ebastine, 433·1
Ebastinum, 433·1
Ebefen, 1961·1
Ebenol, 1961·1
Eberconazol, 397·1
Eberconazole, 397·1
Ebersept, 1961·1
Ebertuss, 1961·1
Ebexid, 1961·1
Ebixa, 1961·1
Ebrantil, 1961·2
Ebromin, 1961·2
Ebromin-P, 1961·2
Ebrotidina, 1264·3
Ebrotidine, 1264·3
Ebselen, 1683·2
Ebseleno, 1683·2
Ebufac, 1961·2
Eburdent, 1961·2
Eburdent F, 1961·2
Eburnal, 1961·2
(3α,16α)-Eburnamenin-14(15*H*)-one, 1764·2
(−)-Eburnamonine, 1764·2
3α,16α-Eburnamonine, 1764·2
Eburnate, 1961·2
Eburnoxin, 1961·2
Eburos, 1961·2
E150c, 1057·1
E160c, 1056·1
EC + Complex, 1961·2
Ecabet Sódico, 1264·3
Ecabet Sodium, 1264·3
Ecabil, 1961·2
Ecadiu, 1961·2
Ecadotril, 964·2, 1285·2
Ecafast, 1961·2
Ecamannan, 1961·2
Ecamsule, 1146·3
Ecanol, 1961·2
Ecapresan, 1961·2
Ecapril, 1961·2
Ecaprilat, 1961·2
Ecarazine Hydrochloride, 1015·1
Ecasil, 1961·2
Ecasolv, 1961·2
Ecaten, 1961·2
Ecax, 1961·2
Ecazide, 1961·2
Eccarvit Plus, 1961·2
Eccelium, 1961·2
Eccoxolac, 1961·2
Ecee2, 1961·2
Ecee Plus, 1961·2
Echan, 1961·2
Echifit, 1961·3
Echiherb, 1961·3
Echina Pro, 1961·3
Echinacea, 1683·2, 1961·3
Echinacea 4000, 1961·3
Echinacea ACE Plus Zinc, 1961·3

Echinacea ACE + Zinc, 1961·3
Echinacea Akut, 1961·3
*Echinacea angustifolia*, 1683·2
Echinacea Angustifolia, 1683·2
Echinacea & Antioxidants, 1961·3
Echinacea Comp, 1961·3
Echinacea Complex, 1961·3
Echinacea Herbal Plus Formula, 1961·3
Echinacea L40, 1961·3
Echinacea Lozenge, 1961·3
Echinacea Med Complex, 1961·3
Echinacea Oligoplex, 1961·3
*Echinacea pallida*, 1683·2
Echinacea Pallida, 1683·2
Echinacea Plus, 1961·3
*Echinacea purpurea*, 1683·2
Echinacea Purpurea Root, 1683·2
Echinacea Ro-Plex (Rowo-415), 1961·3
Echinacea Urtinktur, 1961·3
Echinacea-Complex, 1961·3
Echinacea-Cosmoplex, 1961·3
Echinacin, 1961·3
Echinaforce, 1961·3
EchinaMed, 1961·3
Echinapur, 1961·3
Echinarell, 1961·3
Echinart, 1961·3
Echinasyx, 1961·3
Echinatur, 1961·3
Echine, 1961·3
Echinococcosis, 98·1
Echnatol, 1961·3
Echnatol $B_6$, 1961·3
Echocontrast Agents, 1059·3
Echo-enhancers, 1059·3
Echothiophate Iodide, 1490·2
Echovist, 1961·4
Echte Sodener Mineral-Pastillen, 1961·4
Echtes Goldrutenkraut, 1748·3
Echtroferment-N, 1961·4
Echtronerval-N, 1961·4
Echtrosept-N, 1961·4
Echtrovit, 1961·4
Echtrovit-K, 1961·4
Eciclean, 1961·4
Eclampsia— *see* Eclampsia and Pre-eclampsia, 352·3
Eclamptic Seizure— *see* Eclampsia and Pre-eclampsia, 352·3
Eclaran, 1961·4
Eclipse Lip and Face, 1961·4
Eclipsol, 1961·4
Eclorion, 1961·4
ECMO, 1237·3
Ecnagel, 1961·4
Ecnagel E, 1961·4
Ecnagel PB, 1961·4
Eco Mi, 1961·4
Ecobec, 1961·4
Ecocain, 1961·4
Ecocillin, 1961·4
Ecocort, 1961·4
Ecodax, 1961·4
Ecodergin, 1961·4
Ecoderm, 1961·4
Ecodipine, 1961·4
Ecodolor, 1961·4
Ecodurex, 1962·1
Ecoendocilli Testimonia, 1962·1
Ecofenac, 1962·1
Ecofermenti, 1962·1
Ecofibra, 1962·1
Ecoflorina, 1962·1
Ecofol, 1962·1
Ecolicin, 1962·1
Ecomucyl, 1962·1
Econ, 1962·1
Econac, 1962·1
Econacort, 1962·1
Econazine, 1962·1
Econazol, Nitrato de, 397·2
Econazole, 397·1
Econazole Nitrate, 397·2
Econazole Sulfosalicylate, 397·2
Econazoli Nitras, 397·2
Econazolum, 397·1
Economycin, 1962·1
Econopred, 1962·1
Ecopace, 1962·1
Ecophane, 1962·1
Ecoprin, 1962·1
Ecoprofen, 1962·1
Écorce de Chêne, 1722·3
Ecorex, 1962·1
Ecos, 1962·1
Ecosette, 1962·1
Ecoshampoo, 1962·1
Ecosporina, 1962·1
Ecosprin, 1962·1
Ecostatin, 1962·1
Ecosteril, 1962·2
Ecostigmine Iodide, 1490·2
Ecotam, 1962·2
Ecothiopate Iodide, 1490·2
Ecotiopato, Ioduro de, 1490·2
Ecotrin, 1962·2
Ecoval, 1962·2
Ecoval con Neomicina, 1962·2
Ecovent, 1962·2
Ecovist, 1962·2
Eco-Vita-Min, 1962·2
Ecran Anti-Solaire, 1962·2
Ecran Extreme, 1962·2
Ecran Lutsia, 1962·2
Ecran Teinte, 1962·2
Ecran Total, 1962·2
Ecrans Anti-Solaires, 1962·2
Ecreme, 1962·2
Ecstasy, 1589·3
Ecstasy, Liquid, 1308·3
Ectaprim, 1962·2
*Ecteinascidia turbinata*, 589·3
Ecteinascidin-743, 589·3
Ectinex, 1962·2
Ectiva, 1962·2
Ectodyne, 1962·2
Ectofus, 1962·2
Ectopal, 1962·2
Ectoparasiticides, 1499·1
Ectopic Beats— *see* Cardiac Arrhythmias, 816·1
Ectopic Ossification, 762·2
Ectopic Pregnancy, 572·2
Ectosone, 1962·2
Ectren, 1962·2
Ectrin, 1962·2
Ectrin Balsamico, 1962·2
Ecuamon, 1962·2
Eculizumab, 1675·2
Ecur Test, 1962·2
Ecur Test and Leucocytes, 1962·2
Ecural, 1962·3
Eczema, 1135·1, 1962·3
Eczema Cream, 1962·3
Eczema L87, 1962·3
Eczema Ointment, 1962·3
Eczo-Wokadine, 1962·3
Ed A-Hist, 1962·3
ED Tuss HC, 1962·3
Edamina, 1686·1
Edamine, 1686·1
Edamox, 1962·3
Edaravone, 909·2
Edason, 1962·3
Edathamil, 1038·2
Edathamil, Calcium Disodium, 1051·3
Edathamil, Disodium, 1037·3
Edatrexate, 550·1
Edatrexato, 550·1
EDB, 1505·1
Eddia, 1962·3
Ede, 1962·3
Ede 6, 1962·3
Edecril, 1962·3
Edecrin, 1962·3
Edecrina, 1962·3
Edefen, 1962·3
Edemax, 1962·3
Edemox, 1962·3
Edenil, 1962·3
Edenol, 1962·3
Ederal, 1962·3
Ederphyt, 1962·3
Edetate Calcium Disodium, 1051·3
Edetate, Chromium ($^{51}$Cr), 1523·2
Edetate, Cobalt, 1036·2
Edetate, Dicobalt, 1036·2
Edetate Disodium, 1037·3
Edetate, Sodium Calcium, 1051·3
Edetate Trisodium, 1037·3
Edetato de Dicobalto, 1036·2
Edetato Disódico, 1037·3
Edetato Trisódico, 1037·3
Edetic Acid, 1038·2
Edético, Ácido, 1038·2
Edeticum, Acidum, 1038·2
Edeven, 1962·3
Edex, 1962·3
Edhanol, 1962·3
EDHEA, 1565·3
Edicin, 1962·4
Edifaringen, 1962·4
Edigastrol, 1962·4
Ediluna, 1962·4
Edinol, 1962·4
Ed-in-Sol, 1962·4
Edirel, 1962·4
Edisilato de Caramifeno, 1116·2
Edisilato de Clometiazol, 683·1
Edisilato de Proclorperazina, 716·2
Ediston, 1962·4
Edmilla, 1962·4
Edmonton Protocol, 1347·3
Ednyt, 1962·4
Edobacomab, 1615·2
Edodekin Alfa, 1701·3
Edolfene, 1962·4
Edolglau, 1962·4
Edoltar, 1962·4
Edolzine, 1962·4
Edoxil, 1962·4
Edoxil Mucolitico, 1962·4
Edoxudina, 632·1
Edoxudine, 632·1
EDP-Evans Dermal Powder, 1962·4
Edrecolomab, 550·2
EDRF, 974·1
Edrigyl, 1962·4
Edrofonio, Cloruro de, 1490·3
Edronax, 1962·4
Edrophonii Chloridum, 1490·3
Edrophonium Bromide, 1491·1
Edrophonium Chloride, 1490·3
E-Drops, 1962·4
ED-SPAZ, 1962·4
EDTA, 1038·2
EDTA, Calcium, 1051·3
EDTA, Cobalt, 1036·2
EDTA, Disodium, 1037·3
ED-TLC, 1962·4
EDTMP, Samarium ($^{153}$Sm), 1525·2
EDU, 632·1
Edual, 1962·4
Eductyl, 1962·4
Edul K-200, 1962·4
Eduprim, 1962·4
Eduprim Mucolitico, 1962·4
Edurid, 1962·4
Edusan Fte Rectal, 1962·4
Edym Sedante, 1963·1
E160e, 1056·1
Eel Calcitonin, 768·3
EE3ME, 1559·2
$EE_3ME$, 1559·2
EES, 1963·1
Eetless, 1963·1
EF-4, 1687·1
EF-9, 586·3
EF-12, 1687·1
EF-27, 1687·1
E160f, 1056·1
EFA Steri, 1963·1
Efabetic, 1963·1
Efacal, 1963·1
Efadermin, 1963·1
Efagel, 1963·1
Efalex, 1963·1
Efalex Focus, 1963·1
Efalith, 1963·1
Efalizumab, 1146·3
Efamarine, 1963·1
Efamast, 1963·1
Efamax, 1963·1
Efamol, 1963·1
Efamol Fortify, 1963·1
Efamol G, 1963·1
Efamol Plus Coenzyme Q10, 1963·1
Efamol PMP, 1963·1
Efamol Safflower & Linseed, 1963·1
Efanatal, 1963·1
Efaprost, 1963·1
Efargen, 1963·1
Efasit N, 1963·1
Efatime, 1963·2
Efavir, 1963·2
Efavirenz, 632·2
Efavite, 1963·2
Efcorlin, 1963·2
Efcortelan, 1963·2
Efcortesol, 1963·2
Efectin, 1963·2
Efederm, 1963·2
Efedra, 1119·3
Efedrina, 1120·1
Efedrina, Hidrocloruro de, 1120·1
Efedrina, Sulfato de, 1120·1
Efedronal, 1963·2
Efedrosan, 1963·2
Efektolol, 1963·2
Efemida, 1963·2
Efemolin, 1963·2
Efemolina, 1963·2
Efemoline, 1963·2
Efensol, 1963·2
E-Ferol, 1415·2
Eferox, 1963·2
Efetonina— *see* Sciroppo Merck all'Efetonina, 2279·4
Efexor, 1963·2
Effaclar, 1963·2
Effacne, 1963·2
Effagel, 1963·2
Effalpha, 1963·2
Effcal, 1963·2
Effective Strength Cough Formula, 1963·3
Effective Strength Cough Formula Liquid With Decongestant, 1963·3
Effectsal, 1963·3
Effederm, 1963·3
Effekton, 1963·3
Efferalgan, 1963·3
Efferalgan C, 1963·3
Efferalgan Codeine, 1963·3
Efferalgan Vit C, 1963·3
Efferalgan Vitamine C, 1963·3
Efferalganodis, 1963·3
Efferbalgine, 1963·3
Effercal, 1963·3
Effercal D3, 1963·3
Effercet, 1963·3
Effercitrate, 1963·3
Effer-K, 1963·3
Effersol, 1963·3
Effersyllium, 1963·3
Efferzyme, 1963·3
Effetre, 1963·3
Effexor, 1963·3
Efficlean, 1963·3
Effico, 1963·3
Efficort, 1963·3
Effidigest, 1963·3
Effidrate, 1963·4
Effiplen, 1963·4
Effiprev, 1963·4
Efflumidex, 1963·4
Efflumycin, 1963·4
Effort Angina— *see* Angina Pectoris, 813·1
Effortil, 1963·4
Effortil Comp, 1963·4
Effortil Plus, 1963·4
Effusions, Malignant— *see* Malignant Effusions, 512·2
Efherol, 1963·4

Efical, 1963·4
Efidac 24 Chlorpheniramine, 1963·4
Efidac 24 Pseudoepehdrine, 1963·4
Efiken, 1963·4
Efimag, 1963·4
Efisol S, 1963·4
Efixano, 1963·4
Eflevar, 1963·4
Eflone, 1963·4
Eflornithine Hydrochloride, 604·2
Eflornitina, Hidrocloruro de, 604·2
Efluvium Anti-caspa, 1963·4
Efluvium Anti-seborreico, 1963·4
Efodil, 1963·4
Efodine, 1963·4
Efonidipine Hydrochloride, 909·2
Eformoterol Fumarate, 786·1
Efortil, 1963·4
Efrane, 1963·4
Efridol, 1963·4
Efrin, 1963·4
Efrina, Poen— *see* Poen Efrina, 2225·1
Efriviral, 1963·4
Eftab, 1964·1
Eftapan, 1964·1
Eftapan Tetra, 1964·1
Eftazid, 1964·1
Eftiar Decalin, 1964·1
Eftiar Octane, 1964·1
Efudex, 1964·1
Efudix, 1964·1
Efurix, 1964·1
Efxine, 1964·1
Egacene, 1964·1
Egarone, 1964·1
Egarone Oximetazolina, 1964·1
Egazil, 1964·1
EGB-761, 1692·3
E-Gems, 1964·1
E-Gen-C, 1964·1
Egery, 1964·1
EGF-URO, 1294·2
Eggs, 723·2
Egibren, 1964·1
Egicalm, 1964·1
EGIS-2062, 441·1
Eglandin, 1964·1
Églantier, 1740·1
Eglidon, 1964·1
Eglonyl, 1964·1
Egmovit, 1964·1
Ego Skin Cream, 1964·1
Egocort, 1964·1
Egoderm, 1964·1
Egogyn, 1964·2
Egogyn 30, 1964·2
Egomycol, 1964·2
Egopsoryl TA, 1964·2
Egosona, 1964·2
Egotussano, 1964·2
Egozinc, 1964·2
Egozite Baby, 1964·2
Egozite Baby Cream, 1964·2
Egozite Cradle Cap, 1964·2
Egozite Protective Baby Lotion, 1964·2
EGYT-341, 725·3
EGYT-2062, 441·1
EH Retard, 1964·2
EHB-776, 634·2
EHDP, 771·2
EHEC, 129·2
Ehlifena, 1964·2
Ehlifung, 1964·2
Ehlindopa, 1964·2
Ehliten, 1964·2
Ehlixacin, 1964·2
Ehrenhofer-Salbe, 1964·2
Ehrlichiosis, 125·1
Ehrmann's Entschlackungstee, 1964·2
EI-546, 1746·3
Eibisch, 1651·3
Eichenrinde, 1722·3
Eicosan, 1964·3
Eicosanoids, 1511·1
Eicosapen, 1964·3
Eicosapentaenoic Acid, 976·2, 1511·1
Eicosapenta-5,8,11,14,17-enoic Acid, 976·2
Eicosatetraenoic Acid, 976·2, 1511·1
Eicosatrienoic Acid, 1511·1
Eicovis, 1964·3
EIEC, 129·2
Eifel, 1964·3
Eifelfango-Neuenahr, 1964·3
EinsAlpha, 1964·3
Einschlafkapseln, 1964·3
Einschlaf-Kapseln Biologisch, 1964·3
Eiquinon, 1964·3
Eisen-Diasporal, 1964·3
Eisendragees-ratiopharm, 1964·3
Eisen(II)-Gluconat, 1428·1
Eisen(II)-Sulfat, 1428·2
Eisenkapseln, 1964·3
Eisen-Sandoz, 1964·3
Eisenzucker, 1438·2
Eisessig, 1645·2
EK Burger, 1964·3
Ekanin, 1964·3
Ekilid, 1964·3
Eksalb, 1964·3
Eksalb Simplex, 1964·3
Ektebin, 1964·3
Ektogan, 1964·3
Ektoselene, 1964·3
Ektrofil, 1964·3
Ekuba, 1964·3
Ekvacillin, 1964·3
Ekxine, 1964·3
Ekzemase, 1964·3
Ekzemsalbe F, 1964·3
Ekzevowen, 1964·3
EL-466, 984·1
EL-857, 158·2
EL-857/820, 158·2
EL-870, 271·2
EL-970, 1491·2
EL-1035, 1124·2
EL Diet, 1964·3
Elacto, 1964·3
Elacur, 1964·4
Elacutan, 1964·4
*Elaeis guineensis*, 1440·3, 1481·3
Elafax, 1964·4
Elagen, 1964·4
Elageno OS, 1964·4
Elaidyl Alcohol, 1481·3
Elamax, 1964·4
ELA-Max— *see* L-M-X4, 2101·4
Elan, 1964·4
Elana, 1964·4
Elana Mono, 1964·4
Elandur, 1964·4
Elan-Forte, 1964·4
Elantan, 1964·4
Elanver, 1964·4
Elase, 1964·4
Elase-Chloromycetin, 1964·4
Elaspol, 1964·4
Elastab, 1964·4
Elastase Inhibitor, 1651·2
Elatrol, 1964·4
Elatrolet, 1964·4
Elavil, 1964·4
Elavil Plus, 1964·4
Elawox, 1964·4
Elazor, 1964·4
Elbat, 1964·4
Elbrol, 1964·4
Elcal, 1964·4
Elcal I, 1964·4
Elcal-D, 1964·4
Elcarn, 1965·1
Elcatonin, 768·3
Elcatonina, 768·3
Elcimen, 1965·1
Elcion, 1965·1
Elcoman, 1965·1
Elcometrine, 1549·3
Elcrit, 1965·1
ELD-950, 1683·3
Eldepryl, 1965·1
Elder Flower, 1741·3
Eldercaps, 1965·1
Elderin, 1965·1
Eldertonic, 1965·1
Eldicet, 1965·1
Eldisin, 1965·1
Eldisine, 1965·1
Eldopaque, 1965·1
Eldoquin, 1965·1
Eldox, 1965·1
Elebloc, 1965·1
Eléboro Blanco, 1764·1
Eléboro Verde, 1764·1
Elecampane, 1119·3
Elecampane Camphor, 1119·3
EleCare, 1965·1
Electopen, 1965·1
Electopen Balsam Retard, 1965·1
Electopen Retard, 1965·1
Electral, 1965·1
Electric Blue Headlice, 1965·1
Electrobion, 1965·1
Electrocortin, 1091·1
Electrolade, 1965·1
Electrolit, 1965·1
Electrolit Pediatrico, 1965·2
Electrolysed Acid Water, 1164·3
Electrolytes, 1217·1
Electromechanical Dissociation— *see* Advanced Cardiac Life Support, 812·2
Electrona, 1965·2
Electropak, 1965·2
Electrorice, 1965·2
Eledoisin, 1683·3
Eledoisin Trifluoroacetate, 1683·3
Eledoisina, 1683·3
Elegelin, 1965·2
Elem, 1965·2
Elemental 028, 1965·2
Elemental Diets, 1417·3, 1418·2
Elemental Zinc, 1965·2
Elenol, 1965·2
Elental, 1965·2
Elentol, 1965·2
Eleparon, 1965·2
Elephant Tranquilliser, 1730·3
Elephantiasis— *see* Lymphatic Filariasis, 100·1
Elepril, 1965·2
Elepsin, 1965·2
Elequine, 1965·2
Elestat, 1965·2
Eletriptan Hydrobromide, 467·1
*Elettaria cardamomum*, 1667·3
Eleu, 1965·2
Eleu-Kokk, 1965·2
Eleuphrat, 1965·2
Eleuthero, 1744·1
Eleutherococci Radix, 1744·1
Eleutherococcus, 1744·1
*Eleutherococcus senticosus*, 1744·1
Eleutheroforce, 1965·2
Eleutherokokk, 1965·2
Eleutherokokk-Aktiv-Kapseln SenticoMega, 1965·2
Eleutheroside B, 1744·1
Eleutheroside E, 1744·1
Eleu-Twardypharm, 1965·2
Eleval, 1965·2
Elevat, 1965·2
Elevit, 1965·2
Elevit Geriatrico, 1965·2
Elevit Pronatal, 1965·2
Elevit Vitamine $B_9$, 1965·2
Elex, 1965·2
Elex E, 1965·2
Elfanex, 1965·3
Elfer, 1965·3
Elferri, 1965·3
Elferri-Z, 1965·3
Elgadil, 1965·3
Elgam, 1965·3
Elgydium, 1965·3
Elgydium Bicarbonate, 1965·3
Elgyfluor, 1965·3
Elgyfluor Junior, 1965·3
Elian, 1965·3
Elibet, 1965·3
Elica, 1965·3
Elicodil, 1965·3
Elicor, 1965·3
Elidel, 1965·3
Elidiur, 1965·3
Eligard, 1965·3
Elimicin, 1722·3
Elimin, 1965·3
Elimite, 1965·3
Elimitona, 1965·3
Elina, 1965·3
Elinap, 1965·3
Elingrip, 1965·3
Elios, 1965·3
Elisir Depurativo Ambrosiano, 1965·3
Elisir Terpina, 1965·3
Elisor, 1965·3
Elissan, 1965·4
Elitan, 1965·4
Elitar, 1965·4
Elite, 1965·4
Elitek, 1965·4
Eliten, 1965·4
Elitiran, 1965·4
Elitos, 1965·4
Elitos Et, 1965·4
Elityran, 1965·4
Eliur, 1965·4
Elixifilin, 1965·4
Elixine, 1965·4
Elixir 914, 1965·4
Elixir Americano, 1965·4
Elixir Bonjean, 1965·4
Elixir Contre La Toux Weleda, 1965·4
Elixir Damiana and Saw Palmetto, 1965·4
Elixir de Inhame, 1965·4
Elixir de Maracuja Composto, 1965·4
Elixir de Marinheiro, 1965·4
Elixir de Passiflora, 1965·4
Elixir Fortifiant, 1965·4
Elixir Grez, 1965·4
Elixir Paregorico, 1965·4
Elixir Rebleuten, 1965·4
Elixir Spark, 1965·4
Elixofilina, 1965·4
Elixomin, 1965·4
Elixophyllin, 1965·4
Elixophyllin-GG, 1966·1
Elixophyllin-KI, 1966·1
Elizabeth Arden Suncare, 1966·1
Elkamol, 1966·1
Elkapin, 1966·1
Elkin, 1966·1
ELKO, 1966·1
Elkostop, 1966·1
Elkotheran, 1966·1
Ellanco, 1966·1
Ellatun, 1966·1
Ell-Cranell, 1966·1
Ell-Cranell Alpha, 1966·1
Ell-Cranell Dexa, 1966·1
Elle-care, 1966·1
Elleci, 1966·1
Ellence, 1966·1
Elleste Duet Conti, 1966·1
Elleste-Duet, 1966·1
Elleste-Solo, 1966·1
Elle-Test, 1966·1
Ellimans, 1966·1
Elliots B, 1966·1
Ellsurex, 1966·1
Elm, 1747·1
Elm Bark, 1747·1
Elm Bark, Slippery, 1747·1
Elm, Slippery, 1747·1
Elmego, 1966·1
Elmetacin, 1966·1
Elmetin, 1966·1
Elmetrin, 1966·1
Elmex, 1966·1
Elmex Sensitive, 1966·2
Elmiron, 1966·2
Elmogan, 1966·2
Elmuten, 1966·2
Elo-admix, 1966·2
Eloamin, 1966·2

Elobact, 1966·2
Elocin, 1966·2
Elocom, 1966·2
Elocon, 1966·2
Elocor, 1966·2
Elocort, 1966·2
Elofuran, 1966·2
Eloglucose, 1966·2
Elohaes, 1966·2
Elohast, 1966·2
Elohes, 1966·2
Eloisin, 1966·2
Elolipid, 1966·2
ELO-MEL, 1966·3
Elomet, 1966·3
Elongal, 1966·3
ELO-oral, 1966·3
Elopram, 1966·3
Elorgan, 1966·3
Elorheo, 1966·3
Elosalic, 1966·3
Elotin, 1966·3
Elotrace, 1966·3
Elotrans, 1966·3
Eloverlan, 1966·3
Elovol, 1966·3
Eloxatin, 1966·3
Eloxatine, 1966·3
Elozell, 1966·3
Elozell Spezial, 1966·3
Elozima, 1966·3
Elpi, 1966·3
Elpi Lip, 1966·3
Elroquil N, 1966·3
Elsilimomab, 1701·3
Elspar, 1966·3
Elstatin, 1966·3
Eltair, 1966·3
Elteans, 1966·3
Eltenac, 36·2
Eltenaco, 36·2
Elthyrone, 1966·4
Eltocin, 1966·4
Eltor, 1966·4
Eltroxin, 1966·4
Eltroxine, 1966·4
Elucent Skin Refining Day Cream, 1966·4
Eludril, 1966·4
Eludril— *see* Aphtoral, 1807·2
Elugan, 1966·4
Elugel, 1966·4
Elum, 1966·4
Elusanes, 1966·4
Elusanes Espino Albar, 1966·4
Elutit-Calcium, 1966·4
Elutit-Natrium, 1966·4
Elva, 1666·1
Elvecis, 1966·4
Elvefocal, 1966·4
Elvenavir, 1966·4
Elvesil, 1966·4
Elvorine, 1966·4
Elymoclavine, 1723·2
*Elymus repens*, 1676·2
E-Lyte, 1966·4
Elyzol, 1966·4
Elzogram, 1966·4
Elzym, 1966·4
EM Eukal, 1966·4
Emadine, 1966·4
Emaftol, 1967·1
Emagel, 1967·1
Emagrevit, 1967·1
Emagrex, 1967·1
Emamectin, 1504·3
Emamectina, 1504·3
Emanthal, 1967·1
Emantid, 1967·1
Emasex A, 1967·1
Emasex-N, 1967·1
Emazian B12, 1967·1
EMB, 1967·1
Embalming Fluid, 1730·3
EMBAY-8440, 112·2
Embelia, 105·1
*Embelia ribes*, 105·1
*Embelia robusta*, 105·1
*Embelia tsjeriamcottam*, 105·1
Embelic Acid, 105·1
Embelin, 105·1
Embeline, 1967·1
Embial, 1967·1
EMB-INH, 1967·1
Emblon, 1967·1
Embol, 1967·1
Embolex, 1967·1
Embolex NM, 1967·1
Embolism— *see* Thromboembolic Disorders, 837·3
Embolism, Peripheral Arterial— *see* Peripheral Arterial Thromboembolism, 830·3
Embolism, Pulmonary— *see* Venous Thromboembolism, 839·1
Embonato de Amitriptilina, 280·3
Embonato de Clorpromazina, 675·1
Embonato de Hidroxizina, 434·3
Embonato de Imipramina, 300·1
Embonato de Oxantel, 111·1
Embonato de Pirantel, 113·2
Embonato de Pirvinio, 113·3
Embonato de Promazina, 717·3
Embramina, Hidrocloruro de, 433·2
Embramine Hydrochloride, 433·2
Embramine Teoclate, 433·2
Embraminium Chloratum, 433·2
Embrex, 1967·1
Embrocacion Gras, 1967·1
Embropax, 1967·1
Embutramida, 36·2
Embutramide, 36·2
Emconcor, 1967·1
Emconcor Comp, 1967·1
Emcor, 1967·1
Emcoretic, 1967·1
Emcredil, 1967·2
Emcyt, 1967·2
EMD-9806, 1734·3
EMD-33512, 875·1
Emdalen, 1967·2
Emdar, 1967·2
Emecort, 1967·2
Emedal, 1967·2
Emedastina, Fumarato de, 433·2
Emedastine Difumarate, 433·2
Emedastine Fumarate, 433·2
Emediba, 1967·2
Emedrin N, 1967·2
Emedyl, 1967·2
Emelis, 1967·2
Emend, 1967·2
Eme-Ped, 1967·2
Emepronio, Bromuro de, 482·1
Emepronio, Carragenato de, 482·1
Emepronium Bromide, 482·1
Emepronium Carrageenate, 482·1
Emeproton, 1967·2
Emerald Green, 1171·1
Emercol, 1967·2
Emercreme No 4, 1967·2
Emereze Plus, 1967·2
Emergen, 1967·2
Emergency Contraception, 1536·1
Emergent-Ez, 1967·2
Emersal, 1967·2
Emesafene, 1967·2
Emesan, 1967·2
Emeset, 1967·2
Emeside, 1967·2
Emesis— *see* Nausea and Vomiting, 1245·2
Emet. Hydrochlor., 604·3
Emetal, 1967·2
Emetic, 1967·2
Emetina, Cloridrato de, 604·3
Emetina, Hidrocloruro de, 604·3
Emetine, 1122·3
Emetine Dihydrochloride, 604·3
Emetine Hydrochloride, 604·3
Emetine Hydrochloride Heptahydrate, 604·3
Emetine Hydrochloride Pentahydrate, 605·1
Emetini Chloridum, 604·3
Emetini Hydrochloridum Heptahydricum, 604·3
Emetostop, 1967·2
Emetrol, 1967·3
Em-eukal, 1967·3
Em-eukal Forte N, 1967·3
Em-eukal Husten- Und Brusttee, 1967·3
Em-eukal Mono, 1967·3
Emex, 1967·3
Emflam, 1967·3
Emflam Plus, 1967·3
Emflex, 1967·3
Emforal, 1967·3
Emgecard, 1967·3
Emgel, 1967·3
Emgesan, 1967·3
Emican, 1967·3
Emicilin, 1967·3
Emidoxin, 1967·3
Emidoxyn, 1967·3
Emidrat, 1967·3
Emifol, 1967·3
Emiken, 1967·3
E-Mil, 1967·3
Emilace, 1967·3
Eminase, 1967·3
Emistin, 1967·3
Emitex, 1967·4
Emivox, 1967·4
Emizol, 1967·4
Emko, 1967·4
Emla, 1967·4
Emlapatch, 1967·4
Emlyte, 1967·4
Emlyte-S, 1967·4
Emmenoiasi, 1967·4
Emmenovis, 1967·4
Emmetipi, 1967·4
Emmolate— *see* Dermalo, 1927·2
Emoantitossina, 1967·4
Emoclot, 1967·4
Emo-Cort, 1967·4
Emocrat Forte, 1967·4
Emodella, 1967·4
Emoderm, 1967·4
Emoferrina, 1967·4
Emoflux, 1967·4
Emoform, 1967·4
Emoform, Aqua— *see* Aqua Emoform, 1809·4
Emoform Gencives, 1967·4
Emoform Nouvelle Formule, 1967·4
Emoform, Pronto— *see* Pronto Emoform, 2240·2
Emoform Sensibles, 1967·4
Emoform-F Au Fluor, 1967·4
Emoform-Tat, 1968·1
Emoklar, 1968·1
Emol, 1968·1
Emolan, 1968·1
Emolan Bloqueador Solar, 1968·1
Emolan H, 1968·1
Emolan Protector Solar, 1968·1
Emollia, 1968·1
Emollient Medicinal Bath Oil, Ashbourne— *see* Ashbourne Emollient Medicinal Bath Oil, 1815·2
Emolytar, 1968·1
Emonapride, 710·1
Emonorm, 1968·1
Emopads, 1968·1
Emopon, 1968·1
Emopremarin, 1968·1
Emoren, 1968·1
Emorril, 1968·1
Emortrofine, 1968·1
Emorzim, 1968·1
Emosint, 1968·1
Emotion, 1968·1
Emotival, 1968·1
Emoton, 1968·1
Emotonico, 1968·1
Emotpin, 1968·1
Emovat, 1968·1
Emovate, 1968·1
Emovis, 1968·1
Emoxiron, 1968·2
Empacod, 1968·2
Empaped, 1968·2
Empapol, 1968·2
Empecid, 1968·2
Empecid Cort, 1968·2
Emperal, 1968·2
Emphysema— *see* Chronic Obstructive Pulmonary Disease, 779·2
Empirin, 1968·2
Empirin with Codeine, 1968·2
Emplasto Monopolis, 1968·2
Emplastro Salonpas, 1968·2
Emplatre Croix D, 1968·2
Emportal, 1968·2
Empracet, 1968·2
Emprazil-A, 1968·2
Empynase, 1968·2
Emquin, 1968·2
EMS Expectorante, 1968·2
Emscab, 1968·2
Emser Preparations, 1968·2
Emsilat, 1968·3
Emsogen, 1968·3
Emsyn, 1968·3
Emtec-30, 1968·3
Emthexat, 1968·3
Emthexate, 1968·3
Emtricitabina, 632·3
Emtricitabine, 632·3
Emtriva, 1968·3
Emuclens, 1968·3
Emucream, 1968·3
Emulave, 1968·3
Emulax, 1968·3
Emuliquen Laxante, 1968·3
Emuliquen Simple, 1968·3
Emulsan, 1968·3
Emulsao de Lipidos, 1968·3
Emulsao Scott, 1968·3
Emulsao Universal, 1968·3
Emulsiderm, 1968·3
Emulsif. Wax, 1481·1
Emulsifiers, 1411·1
Emulsifying Agents, 1576·1
Emulsifying Wax, 1481·1
Emulsifying Wax, Anionic, 1481·1
E-Mulsin, 1968·3
Emulsoil, 1968·3
Emu-V, 1968·3
E-Mycin, 1968·3
En, 1968·3
EN-141, 224·3
EN-313, 961·3
EN-15304, 1044·3
EN-1639A, 1046·1
EN-1733A, 709·3
EN-2234A, 64·2
Ena, 1968·3
ENA-713, 1497·1
Enabeta, 1968·4
Enac, 1968·4
Enacard, 1968·4
EnAce, 1968·4
EnAce-D, 1968·4
Enada, 1968·4
Enadil, 1968·4
Enadiol, 1968·4
Enadiol CC, 1968·4
Enadiol MP, 1968·4
Enadura, 1968·4
Enahexal, 1968·4
Enal, 1968·4
Enalabal, 1968·4
Enalabene, 1968·4
Enaladex, 1968·4
Enaladil, 1968·4
Enalafel, 1968·4
Enalagamma, 1968·4
Enalamed, 1968·4
Enalapril, 909·2
Enalapril Comp, 1968·4
Enalapril Maleate, 909·2
Enalapril, Maleato de, 909·2
Enalaprilat, 909·3

Enalaprilat Dihydrate, 909·3
Enalapril/HCT, 1968·4
Enalaprili Maleas, 909·2
Enalaprilic Acid, 909·3
Enaldun, 1968·4
Enalind, 1968·4
Enallynymalnatrium, 1303·2
Enaloc, 1968·4
Enaloc Comp, 1968·4
Enalprin, 1968·4
Enalten, 1968·4
Enalten D, 1968·4
Enalten DN, 1968·4
Enam, 1968·4
Enaminoleban, 1969·1
Enangel, 1969·1
Enantato de Estradiol, 1550·1
Enantato de Flufenazina, 699·3
Enantato de Metenolona, 1559·3
Enantato de Noretisterona, 1562·2
Enantato de Perfenazina, 714·2
Enantato de Prasterona, 1565·3
Enantato de Testosterona, 1570·1
Enanton, 1969·1
Enantone, 1969·1
Enantone-Gyn, 1969·1
Enantyum, 1969·1
Enap, 1969·1
Enap HL, 1969·1
Enap-Co, 1969·1
Enapren, 1969·1
Enapress, 1969·1
Enapril, 1969·1
Enaprotec, 1969·1
Ena-Puren, 1969·1
Enaran, 1969·1
Enaril, 1969·1
Enasifar, 1969·1
Enatec, 1969·1
Enatec F, 1969·1
Enatia, 1969·1
Enatral, 1969·1
Enatrial, 1969·1
Enatus, 1969·1
Enatyrol, 1969·1
Enbrel, 1969·1
Enbucrilate, 1678·1
Encainida, Hidrocloruro de, 910·3
Encainide Hydrochloride, 910·3
Encare, 1969·1
Encaskin Cream, 1969·1
Encaskin Creme, 1969·2
Encaskin Detergente, 1969·2
Encaskin Liquid Detergent, 1969·2
Encebrin, 1969·2
Encefabol, 1969·2
Encegam, 1969·2
Encelin, 1969·2
Encephabol, 1969·2
Encephalitis, Amoebic, Granulomatous— *see* Disseminated Acanthamoeba Infection, 595·2
Encephalitis Vaccine (Inactivated), Tick-borne, 1642·1
Encephalitis, Viral— *see* Encephalitis, 618·2
Encephalopathy, Glycine— *see* Nonketotic Hyperglycinaemia, 1750·2
Encephalopathy, Hepatic— *see* Hepatic Encephalopathy, 1243·2
Encephalopathy, Portal Systemic— *see* Hepatic Encephalopathy, 1243·2
Encephalopathy, Wernicke's— *see* Wernicke-Korsakoff Syndrome, 1455·3
Encepur, 1969·2
Encetrop, 1969·2
Encialina, 1969·2
Enclomifene, 1542·2
Encorate, 1969·2
Encypalmed, 1969·2
End Lice, 1969·2
Endace, 1969·2
Endacil, 1969·2
Endafed, 1969·2
Endagen-HD, 1969·2
Endak, 1969·2
Endal, 1969·2
Endal Expectorant, 1969·2
Endal HD, 1969·2
Endalbumin, 1969·2
Endal-HD, 1969·2
Endal-HD Plus, 1969·2
Endantadine, 1969·2
Endcol Preparations 1969·3
En-De-Kay, 1969·3
Endep, 1969·3
Endermyl, 1969·3
Endial, 1969·3
Endiaron, 1969·3
Endium, 1969·3
Endoamylases, 1654·2
Endobil, 1969·3
Endobon, 1969·3
Endobulin, 1969·3
Endobuline, 1969·3
Endocaina, 1969·3
Endocal, 1969·3
Endocarditis, Bacterial— *see* Endocarditis, 125·2
Endocarditis, Fungal— *see* Endocarditis, 388·1
Endocarditis, Q Fever— *see* Q Fever, 143·3
Endocet, 1969·3
Endocodone, 1969·3
Endocorion, 1969·3
Endocrine Tumours, Pancreatic— *see* Carcinoid Tumours and Other Secretory Neoplasms, 504·1
Endocris, 1969·3
Endod, 1504·3
Endodan, 1969·3
Endofalk, 1969·3
Endofolin, 1969·3
Endogel Esteril, 1969·3
Endogenous Pyrogen, 1701·3
Endogest, 1969·3
Endol, 1969·3
Endolac, 1969·4
Endolipid, 1969·4
Endolipide, 1969·4
Endolor, 1969·4
Endomethasone, 1969·4
Endomethazone, 1969·4
Endometrial Cancer— *see* Malignant Neoplasms of the Endometrium, 516·1
Endometrin, 1969·4
Endometriosis, 1546·2
Endometritis, 126·3
Endomicina, 1969·4
Endomina, 1969·4
Endomyometritis— *see* Endometritis, 126·3
Endone, 1969·4
Endoneutralio, 1969·4
Endopancrine 40, 1969·4
Endopancrine 100, 1969·4
Endopancrine Protamine, 1969·4
Endopancrine Zinc Protamine, 1969·4
Endo-Paractol, 1969·4
Endophleban, 1969·4
Endophthalmitis, Bacterial— *see* Eye Infections, 127·2
Endophthalmitis, Fungal— *see* Eye Infections, 388·1
Endoprost, 1969·4
Endorem, 1969·4
Endorphins, 73·3
Endosalil, 1969·4
Endoscopes, Disinfection of— *see* Disinfection of Endoscopes, 1164·3
Endoscopy, Premedication and Sedation in— *see* Endoscopy, 666·2
Endosgel, 1969·4
Endosporine, 1969·4
Endospray, 1969·4
Endosulfan, 1504·3
Endotelon, 1969·4
Endothelium-derived Relaxing Factor, 974·1
Endotoxin Antibodies, 1615·2
Endotoxin Antisera, 1615·2
Endotropina, 1969·4
Endotussin, 1969·4
Endoxan, 1969·4
Endoxana, 1970·1
Endralazina, Mesilato de, 910·3
Endralazine Mesilate, 910·3
Endralazine Mesylate, 910·3
Endrate, 1970·1
Endrin, 1504·3
Endrine, 1970·1
Endrine Doux, 1970·1
Endrine Mild, 1970·1
Endronax, 1970·1
End-stage Renal Disease— *see* Chronic Renal Failure, 1222·1
Enduron, 1970·1
Enduronil, 1970·1
Enduronyl, 1970·1
Enduxan, 1970·1
Eneas, 1970·1
Enebro, 1703·1
Enebro, Aceite Esencial de, 1703·1
Enecat, 1970·1
Enelbin-Paste N, 1970·1
Enelbin-Salbe N, 1970·1
Eneldo, 1680·2
Eneldo, Aceite Esencial de, 1680·2
Enelfa, 1970·1
Enema Casen, 1970·1
Enema Cooper, 1970·1
Enemac, 1970·1
Enemol, 1970·1
Ener-B, 1970·1
Enerbody, 1970·1
Enercal Plus, 1970·1
Enercomplex, 1970·1
Enerday, 1970·1
Ener-E, 1970·1
Ener-G, 1970·1
Energeia, 1970·2
Energen, 1970·2
Energex Fort, 1970·2
Energiclin, 1970·2
Energil C, 1970·2
Energisan, 1970·2
Energitum, 1970·2
Energivit, 1970·2
Energizante, 1970·2
Energona, 1970·2
Energoplex, 1970·2
Energy Alfa, 1970·2
Energy Plus, 1970·2
Energyn-T, 1970·2
Energysor, 1970·2
Enerjets, 1970·2
Ener-Mix, 1970·2
Enertonic, 1970·2
Enervit, 1970·2
Enervon-C, 1970·2
Enervon-C Plus, 1970·2
Enetege, 1970·2
Enfalac Preparations, 1970·2
Enfamil Preparations, 1970·3
Enflurane, 1298·1
Enflurano, 1298·1
Enfluthane, 1970·3
Enforan, 1970·3
Enfran, 1970·3
Enfuvirtida, 633·1
Enfuvirtide, 633·1
En-Ga-Lax, 1970·3
Engerix, 1970·3
Engerix-B, 1970·3
English Lavender, 1705·1
Engov, 1970·3
Engystol, 1970·3
Engystol N, 1970·3
Enhancin, 1970·3
Enhexymalnatrium, 703·1
Enhexymalum, 703·1
Eni, 1970·3
Enicul, 1970·3
Enidazol, 1970·3
Enidin, 1970·3
Eniflex, 1970·3
Enilconazol, 397·3
Enilconazole, 397·3
Enilconazole for Veterinary Use, 397·3
Enilconazolum, 397·3
Eniluracil, 550·2
Eniluracilo, 550·2
Enimal, 703·1
Enirant, 1970·3
Enison, 1970·4
Enit, 1970·4
Enjomin, 1970·4
Enjoy, 1970·4
Enkephalins, 73·3
Enlinea, 1970·4
Enlirane, 1970·4
Enlive, 1970·4
Enlon, 1970·4
Enlon-Plus, 1970·4
Eno, 1970·4
Eno, Sal de Fruta— *see* Sal de Fruta Eno, 2273·4
Enocitabina, 550·2
Enocitabine, 550·2
Enofosforina Vigor, 1970·4
Enomdan, 1970·4
Enomine, 1970·4
Enorden, 1970·4
Enoton, 1970·4
Enoval, 1970·4
Enoxacin, 207·2
Enoxacino, 207·2
Enoxaparin Sodium, 910·3
Enoxaparina Sódica, 910·3
Enoxaparinum Natricum, 910·3
Enoxen, 1970·4
Enoximona, 911·1
Enoximone, 911·1
Enoxin, 1970·4
Enoxolona, 36·2
Enoxolona de Aluminio, 1264·3
Enoxolone, 36·2
Enoxolone Aluminium, 1264·3
Enoxolone Aluminum, 1264·3
Enoxolonum, 36·2
Enoxor, 1970·4
Enper, 1970·4
Enphenemalum, 366·3
Enpott, 1970·4
Enpovax HDC, 1970·4
Enpresse, 1970·4
Enprin, 1970·4
Enrich, 1970·4
Enrofloxacin, 207·3
Enrofloxacino, 207·3
Enromic, 1971·1
Ensinger Schiller-Quelle Heilwasser, 1971·1
Ensini, 1971·1
Ensulizol, 1147·1
Ensulizole, 1147·1
Ensure, 1971·1
Ensure— *see* Ez-HBT, 1987·1
Ensure Plus, 1971·1
ENT, 1971·1
ENT-25567, 110·1
ENT-25841, 1510·2
Entacapona, 1205·1
Entacapone, 1205·1
Entacyl, 1971·1
Entalgic, 1971·1
Entamizole, 1971·1
Entecet, 1971·1
Entera, 1971·1
Enteral 400, 1971·1
Enteramine, 1743·2
Enterasin, 1971·1
Entercal, 1971·1
Enterex, 1971·1
Enteric Fever— *see* Typhoid and Paratyphoid Fever, 152·2
Enteritis, Campylobacter— *see* Campylobacter Enteritis, 128·3
Enteritis, Escherichia Coli— *see* Escherichia Coli Enteritis, 129·1
Enteritis, Necrotising— *see* Necrotising Enterocolitis, 129·2
Enteritis, Salmonella— *see* Salmonella Enteritis, 129·3
Enteritis, Shigella— *see* Shigellosis, 130·1

Enteritis, Yersinia— *see* Yersinia Enteritis, 130·2
Entermid, 1971·1
Entero Heractrin, 1971·1
Entero Micinovo, 1971·1
Entero VU, 1971·1
Enterobacilli, 1971·1
Enterobacticel, 1971·1
Enterobene, 1971·1
Enterobiasis, 99·1
Enterobion, 1971·1
Enterocare, 1971·1
Enterocid, 1971·1
Enterocir, 1971·1
Enterocler, 1971·2
Enterococcal Infections, 126·3
Enterocolitis, Necrotising— *see* Necrotising Enterocolitis, 129·2
Enterodina, 1971·2
Entero-Diyod, 1971·2
Enterodrip, 1971·2
Enterodyne, 1971·2
Enterofigon, 1971·2
Enteroftal, 1971·2
Enterogermina, 1971·2
Enterogil, 1971·2
Enterol, 1971·2
Enterol con Nifuroxacida, 1971·2
Enterolidon, 1971·2
Enterolyte, 1971·2
Enteromicina, 1971·2
Enteromix, 1971·2
Enteromucilage, 1971·2
Enterone, 1971·2
Enteronorm, 1971·2
Enteropathic Arthritis— *see* Spondyloarthropathies, 11·1
Enteropathy, Gluten-sensitive— *see* Coeliac Disease, 1417·3
Enteropathyl, 1971·2
Enteropen, 1971·2
Enteroplant, 1971·2
Enteropride, 1971·2
Entero-Quinol, 1971·2
Enterosan, 1971·2
Enteroseven, 1971·2
Enterosilicona, 1971·2
Enterostop, 1971·3
Entero-Teknosal, 1971·3
Enterotonus, 1971·3
Enterovaccino ISI (Antitifico), 1971·3
Enterovaccino Nuovo ISM, 1971·3
Enterovit, 1971·3
Enterozol, 1971·3
Entertainer's Secret, 1971·3
Enterum, 1971·3
Entex, 1971·3
Entex HC, 1971·3
Entex LA, 1971·3
Entex PSE, 1971·3
Entianthe, 1971·3
Entir, 1971·3
Entocir, 1971·3
Entocord, 1971·3
Entocort, 1971·3
Entodiba, 1971·3
Entom, 1971·3
Entom Nature, 1971·3
Entonox, 1971·3
Entoplus, 1971·3
Entosorbine-N, 1971·3
Entox-P, 1971·3
Entrarin, 1971·4
Entrition, 1971·4
Entrobar, 1971·4
Entrocalm, 1971·4
Entrocalm Replace, 1971·4
Entrodyn, 1971·4
Entrolate, 1971·4
Entrolax, 1971·4
Entrophen, 1971·4
Entrotabs, 1971·4
Entrozyme Plain, 1971·4
Entrydil, 1971·4
Entschlackender Abfuhrtee EF-EM-ES, 1971·4
Entschlackungs-Tee, Kneipp— *see* Kneipp Entschlackungs-Tee, 2081·2
ENTsol, 1971·4
Entsufón Sódico, 1683·3
Entsufon Sodium, 1683·3
Entumin, 1971·4
Entumin— *see* Etumin/Entumin, 1980·4
Entumine, 1971·4
Enturen, 1971·4
Entuss Expectorant, 1971·4
Entuss-D, 1971·4
Entuss-D Jr, 1971·4
Entwasserungs-Tabletten, 1971·4
Entzundungstropfen, 1971·4
Enuclen, 1971·4
Enuclene, 1971·4
Enulid, 1971·4
Enulose, 1971·4
EnurAid, 1971·4
Enuresis, Nocturnal— *see* Nocturnal Enuresis, 475·3
Enuretine, 1971·4
Enuroplant, 1971·4
Envas, 1972·1
Enveloppements ECR, 1972·1
Enviro-Stress, 1972·1
Enxak, 1972·1
Enxôfre, 1158·2
Enzacamene, 1147·1
Enzacameno, 1147·1
Enzace, 1972·1
Enzaprost, 1972·1
Enziagil Magenplus, 1972·1
Enzianwurzel, 1692·2
Enzicoba, 1972·1
Enzipan, 1972·1
Enziprid, 1972·1
Enzivital, 1972·1
Enzogenol, 1972·1
Enzone, 1972·1
Enzyflat, 1972·1
Enzym Novo, Hevert— *see* Hevert Enzym Novo, 2042·4
Enzymatic Cleaner, 1972·1
Enzyme, 1972·1
Enzyme Digest, 1972·1
Enzyme Plus, 1972·1
Enzymet, 1972·1
Enzym-Harongan, 1972·1
Enzym-Lefax, 1972·1
Enzym-Wied, 1972·1
Enzynorm, 1972·1
Enzynorm Forte, 1972·1
Enzyplex, 1972·1
Eogran, 1972·1
Eoline, 1972·1
Eolus, 1972·2
Eosin, 1057·2
Eosin Y, 1057·2
Eosina, 1057·2
Éosine Disodique, 1057·2
Eosinophilic Fasciitis, 1258·3
Eosinophilic Granuloma— *see* Histiocytic Syndromes, 505·2
E.P., 1972·2
EPA, 976·2
EPAB, 1376·3
Epabetina, 1972·2
Epa-Bon, 1972·2
Epacalcica, 1972·2
Epacaps, 1972·2
Epacrosil, 1972·2
Epadel, 1972·2
Epaderm, 1972·2
Epadoren, 1972·2
Epagest, 1972·2
Epagogo, 1972·2
Epailis, 1972·2
Epalat EPS, 1972·2
Epalfen, 1972·2
Epalrestat, 331·1
Epamin, 1972·2
Epanutin, 1972·2
Epaplex 40, 1972·2
Epaq, 1972·2
Eparema, 1972·2
Eparema-Levul, 1972·2
Eparex, 1972·2
Epargriseovit, 1972·2
Eparical, 1972·2
Eparinlider, 1972·2
Eparinovis, 1972·2
Eparmefolin, 1972·3
Eparsil, 1972·3
Eparven, 1972·3
Epasan 30% Omega 3, 1972·3
Epasol, 1972·3
Epativan B6, 1972·3
Epatovis, 1972·3
Epatoxil, 1972·3
Epa-Treis, 1972·3
Epaxal, 1972·3
EPC-272, 161·2
EP&C Essence, 1972·3
EPEC, 129·1
EPEG, 551·3
Epelin, 1972·3
Eperisona, Hidrocloruro de, 1394·3
Eperisone Hydrochloride, 1394·3
Ephed 20th, 1972·3
Ephedra, 1119·3
*Ephedra*, 1129·2
*Ephedra equisetina*, 1119·3
*Ephedra gerardiana*, 1119·3
*Ephedra intermedia*, 1119·3
*Ephedra nebrodensis*, 1119·3
*Ephedra sinica*, 1119·3
Ephedrina, 1120·1
Ephedrinae Hydrochloridum, 1120·1
Ephedrine, 1120·1
(−)-Ephedrine, 1120·1
*d*-Ψ-Ephedrine, 1129·2
Ephedrine, Anhydrous, 1120·1
Ephedrine Camsilate, 1120·3
Ephedrine Chloride, 1120·1
Ephedrine Hemihydrate, 1120·1
Ephedrine Hydrochloride, 1120·1
Ephedrine Hydrochloride, Racemic, 1120·1
Ephedrine Levulinate, 1120·3
Ephedrine Sulfate, 1120·1
Ephedrine Sulphate, 1120·1
Ephedrine Tannate, 1120·3
Ephedrini Hydrochloridum, 1120·1
Ephedrinium Chloratum, 1120·1
Ephedrinum, 1120·1
*l*-Ephedrinum Hydrochloricum, 1120·1
Ephedroides, 1972·3
Ephedronguent, 1972·3
Ephedyl, 1972·3
Ephelia, 1972·3
Ephepect, 1972·3
Ephepect-Blocker-Pastillen N, 1972·3
Ephepect-Pastillen N, 1972·3
Ephydion, 1972·3
Ephydrol, 1972·3
Ephynal, 1972·3
Epi EZ, 1972·3
Epi-Aberel, 1972·4
4′-Epiadriamycin Hydrochloride, 550·2
Epianal, 1972·4
Epi-C, 1972·4
Epicef, 1972·4
Epi-Cell, 1972·4
Epichlorohydrin, 1474·2
Epiclodina, 1972·4
Epiclorhidrina, 1474·2
Epicol, 1972·4
Epicol NF, 1972·4
Epicol Pediatrico, 1972·4
Epicondylitis, Humeral— *see* Soft-tissue Rheumatism, 11·1
Epicordin, 1972·4
Epicrin, 1972·4
Epicriptine Mesilate, 1674·1
Epident, 1972·4
Epidermal Growth Factor, 1294·2
Epidermal Growth Factor, Human, 1294·2
Epidermal Thymocyte Activating Factor, 562·2
Epidermil, 1972·4
Epidermolysis Bullosa, 1135·3
Epidex, 1972·4
Epididymitis, 127·1
Epidona, 1972·4
Epidosin, 1972·4
Epidoxo, 1972·4
4′-Epidoxorubicin Hydrochloride, 550·2
Epidropal, 1972·4
Epidural Block— *see* Central Nerve Block, 1370·1
Epiestrol, 1972·4
Epiferol, 1972·4
Epifil, 1972·4
Epifoam, 1972·4
Epifrin, 1972·4
Epigen, 1972·4
Epiglottitis, 127·1
Epiglu, 1972·4
Epiject, 1972·4
Epikebir, 1972·4
Epikur, 1972·4
Epilactose, 1269·1
Epilan, 1973·1
Epilan-D, 1973·1
Epilantin, 1973·1
Epilantine, 1973·1
Epilem, 1973·1
Epilenil, 1973·1
Epilepsy, 349·1
Epilepsy, Status Epilepticus— *see* Status Epilepticus, 352·1
Epilex, 1973·1
Epilim, 1973·1
Epilim Chrono, 1973·1
E-Pilo, 1973·1
Epi-Lyt, 1973·1
Epimaz, 1973·1
Epi-Monistat, 1973·1
Epinal, 1973·1
Epinastina, Hidrocloruro de, 433·3
Epinastine Hydrochloride, 433·3
Epinat, 1973·1
Epinefrina, 852·2
Epinefrina, Bitartrato de, 852·2
Epinefrina, Hidrocloruro de, 852·3
Epinephrine, 852·2
Epinephrine Acid Tartrate, 852·2
Epinephrine Bitartrate, 852·2
Epinephrine Hydrochloride, 852·3
Epinephrine Hydrogen Tartrate, 852·2
Epinephrinum, 852·2
Epinephryl Borate, 854·3
Epinine, 937·3
Epinitril, 1973·1
Epione, 1973·1
Epipak, 1973·1
Epipen, 1973·1
Epi-Pevaryl, 1973·1
Epi-Pevaryl Heilpaste, 1973·1
Epi-Pevaryl Pv, 1973·1
Epipevisone, 1973·1
Epiphane, 1973·1
Epiphane 7, 1973·1
Epiphysan, 1973·1
Epiplaie Epitege, 1973·2
Epipodophyllotoxin, 551·3
Epiprocto, 1973·2
Epipropane, 1973·2
EpiQuin, 1973·2
Epirenamine, 852·2
Epirenamine Bitartrate, 852·2
Epirizol, 36·3
Epirizole, 36·3
Epirubicin Hydrochloride, 550·2
Epirubicina, Hidrocloruro de, 550·2
Epirubicini Hydrochloridum, 550·2
Epirubicinol, 550·3
Episcleritis— *see* Scleritis, 1088·1
Episcorit, 1973·2
Episec, 1973·2
Episoft, 1973·2
Episol, 1973·2
Epistaxol, 1973·2
Epitaloe, 1973·2
Epitege, Epiplaie— *see* Epiplaie Epitege, 1973·2
Epiteliol-C, 1973·2
Epitelizante, 1973·2

4-Epitetracycline, 266·2
Epitetracycline Hydrochloride, 266·2
Epitezan, 1973·2
Epithea, 1973·2
Epithelial, 1973·2
Epitheliale, 1973·2
Epithiazide, 911·3
Epitizida, 911·3
Epitizide, 911·3
Epitol, 1973·2
Epitomax, 1973·2
Epitopic, 1973·2
Epitril, 1973·2
Epival, 1973·2
Epivir, 1973·2
Epixian, 1973·2
Epizon, 1973·2
Eplerenone, 911·3
Eplonat, 1973·2
EPN, 852·2
EPO, 747·2
E.P.O. & E, 1973·2
Epo + Maxepa + Vitamin E Herbal Plus Formula 8, 1973·3
Epocan, 1973·3
Epocelin, 1973·3
EPOCH, 747·2
Epocler, 1973·3
Epoetin Alfa, 747·2
Epoetin Beta, 747·2
Epoetin Delta, 747·2
Epoetin Gamma, 747·2
Epoetin Omega, 747·2
Epoetinas, 747·1
Epoetins, 747·1
Epogam, 1973·3
Epogen, 1973·3
Epogin, 1973·3
Epokelan, 1973·3
Epomax, 1973·3
Epomediol, 1683·3
Epopa, 1973·3
Epopen, 1973·3
Epoprostenol, 1516·3
Epoprostenol Sódico, 1516·3
Epoprostenol Sodium, 1516·3
Eposal, 1973·3
Eposerin, 1973·3
Eposid, 1973·3
Eposido, 1973·3
Eposin, 1973·3
Epostane, 1683·3
Epostano, 1683·3
Epotin, 1973·3
Epoxide, 1973·3
Epoxitin, 1973·3
(−)-(1*S*,3*s*,5*R*,6*R*,7*S*,8*r*)-6,7-Epoxy-8-butyl-3-[(*S*)-tropoyloxy]tropanium Bromide, 483·3
4α,5α-Epoxy-3,17β-dihydroxy-4β,17α-dimethyl-5α-androst-2-ene-2-carbonitrile, 1683·3
(−)-(5*R*,6*S*,14*S*)-4,5-Epoxy-3,14-dihydroxy-9a-methylmorphinan-6-one Hydrochloride, 76·1
11β,18-Epoxy-18,21-dihydroxypregn-4-ene-3,20-dione, 1091·1
(5*Z*,13*E*)-(8*R*,9*S*,11*R*,12*R*,15*S*)-6,9-Epoxy-11,15-dihydroxyprosta-5,13-dienoic Acid, 1516·3
4-(1,2-Epoxy-1,6-dimethylhex-4-enyl)-5-methoxy-1-oxaspiro[2.5]oct-6-yl Hydrogen Deca-2,4,6,8-tetraenedioate, 605·2
6,7-Epoxy-8-ethyl-3-[(*S*)-tropoyloxy]tropanium Bromide, 790·3
(2*R*)-2-[(−)-(5*R*,6*R*,7*R*,14*R*)-4,5-Epoxy-3-hydroxy-6-methoxy-9a-methyl-6,14-ethenomorphinan-7-yl]pentan-2-ol Hydrochloride, 38·3
4,5α-Epoxy-14-hydroxy-3-methoxy-17-methylmorphinan-6-one 1,4-Benzenedicarboxylate (2:1) Salt, 75·2
(−)-(5*R*,6*S*,14*S*)-4,5-Epoxy-14-hydroxy-3-methoxy-9a-methylmorphinan-6-one Hydrochloride, 75·2
9-[(2*E*)-4-[(2*S*,3*R*,4*R*,5*S*)-5-[(2*S*,3*S*,4*S*,5*S*)-2,3-Epoxy-5-hydroxy-4-methylhexyl]tetrahydro-3,4-dihydroxypyran-2-yl]-3-methylbut-2-enoyloxy]nonanoic Acid, 233·1
(−)-(5*R*)-4,5-Epoxy-3-hydroxy-9a-methylmorphinan-6-one Hydrochloride, 45·2
6β,7β-Epoxy-3β-hydroxy-8-methyl-1α*H*,5α*H*-tropanium Bromide Di-2-thienylglycolate, 806·2
4α,5α-Epoxy-17β-hydroxy-3-oxoandrostane-2α-carbonitrile, 1757·3
9,11α-Epoxy-17-hydroxy-3-oxo-17α-pregn-4-ene-7α,21-dicarboxylic Acid γ-Lactone Methyl Ester, 911·3
1,8-Epoxy-4-isopropyl-1-methylcylohexane-2,6-diol, 1683·3
1,8-Epoxy-*p*-menthane, 1672·1
Epoxymethamine Bromide, 483·3
4,5-Epoxy-3-methoxy-17-methylmorphinan-6-ol Hydrogen Tartrate, 34·3
(−)-(5*R*)-4,5-Epoxy-3-methoxy-9a-methylmorphinan-6-one Hydrogen Tartrate Hemipentahydrate, 45·1
4,5-Epoxy-3-methoxy-9a-methylmorphinan-6-yl Acetate Hydrochloride, 1114·2
(−)-(5*R*)-4,5-Epoxy-3-methoxy-9a-methylmorphin-6-en-6-yl Acetate Hydrochloride, 1131·2
4,5-Epoxy-17-methylmorphinan-3,6-diyl Diacetate Hydrochloride Monohydrate, 30·2
(−)-(5*R*,6*S*)-4,5-Epoxy-9a-methylmorphin-7-en-3,6-diyl Dinicotinate Hydrochloride, 66·3
(−)-(1*S*,3*s*,5*R*,6*R*,7*S*)-6,7-Epoxy-8-methyl-3-[(*S*)-tropoyloxy]tropanium Bromide, 483·3
(−)-(1*S*,3*s*,5*R*,6*R*,7*S*)-6,7-Epoxy-8-methyl-3-[(*S*)-tropoyloxy]tropanium Nitrate, 483·3
(1*R*,2*S*)-1,2-Epoxypropylphosphonic Acid, 214·2, 214·3
(−)-(1*S*,3*S*,5*R*,6*R*,7*S*)-6,7-Epoxytropan-3-yl (*S*)-Tropate Hydrobromide Trihydrate, 483·3
(−)-(1*S*,3*s*,5*R*,6*R*,7*S*,8*s*)-6,7-Epoxy-3[(*S*)-tropoyloxy] Tropane, 483·3
Eppy, 1973·3
EPR, 1973·3
Epratuzumab, 551·1
Eprazinona, Hidrocloruro de, 1121·1
Eprazinone Hydrochloride, 1121·1
Epresat, 1973·3
Eprex, 1973·3
Epril, 1973·4
E-Prime, 1973·4
Eprinomectin, 105·2
Eprinomectina, 105·2
Eprodine, 1973·4
Eprofil, 1973·4
Eprosartan Mesilate, 912·1
Eprosartán, Mesilato de, 912·1
Eprosartan Mesylate, 912·1
Eprozinol, Hidrocloruro de, 1121·1
Eprozinol Hydrochloride, 1121·1
Epsicaprom, 1973·4
Epsidox, 1973·4
Epsilat, 1973·4
Epsilon Acetamidocaproic Acid, 1646·2
Epsilon Aminocaproic Acid, 741·3
Epsin, 1973·4
Epsiprantel, 105·2
Epsitron, 1973·4
Epsoclar, 1973·4
Epsodil, 1973·4
Epsolin, 1973·4
Epsom Salts, 1228·2
Epsom Salts, Dried, 1228·2
Epstein-Barr Virus Infections, 620·1
Epstein-Barr Virus Vaccines, 1615·3
Ept Stick Test, 1973·4
Eptacog Alfa (Activated), 750·3
Eptadone, 1973·4
Eptastatin Sodium, 984·3
Eptastigmina, 1491·2
Eptastigmine, 1491·2
Eptico, 1973·4
Eptifibatida, 912·2
Eptifibatide, 912·2
Eptoin, 1973·4
Eptotermin Alfa, 768·2
Epulor, 1973·4
Epuram, 1973·4
Equagesic, 1973·4
Equal, 1973·4
Equalactin, 1973·4
Equanil, 1973·4
Equanox, 1973·4
Equasym, 1973·4
Equiday, 1973·4
Equiday E, 1973·4
Equiderm, 1973·4
Equidral, 1973·4
Equilase, 1668·3
Equilet, 1974·1
Equilibra, 1974·1
Equilibrane, 1974·1
Equilibrin, 1974·1
Equilibrium, 1974·1
Equilibrium Creme Anti-transpirante, 1974·1
Equilid, 1974·1
Equilin, 1549·3
Equilin Sulfate, Sodium, 1543·2, 1549·3
Equilina, 1549·3
Equilium, 1974·1
Equilon, 1974·1
Equilon Herbal, 1974·1
Equin, 1974·1
Equinacea, 1974·1
Equinácea, 1683·2
Equinorm, 1974·1
Equipax, 1974·1
Equipur, 1974·1
Equirex, 1974·1
Equisedin, 1974·1
Equiseti Herba, 1684·1
Equiseto, 1684·1
Equisetum, 1684·1
*Equisetum arvense*, 1684·1
*Equisetum hiemale*, 1684·1
Equisetum Stem, 1684·1
Equisil N, 1974·1
Equi-Sleep, 1974·1
Equitam, 1974·1
Equiton, 1974·1
Eqvalan— *see* Mectizan, 2118·1
ER-115, 723·2
ER-4111, 1489·2
ER Cream, 1974·1
Era, 1974·1
Eracillin, 1974·1
Eracine, 1974·1
Eradacil, 1974·2
Eradix, 1974·2
Eralga, 1974·2
Eramox, 1974·2
Eramycin, 1974·2
Erantin, 1974·2
Eranz, 1974·2
Erasis, 1974·2
Erasol, 1974·2
Erathrom, 1974·2
Eraverm, 1974·2
Eraxil, 1974·2
Erbazid, 1974·2
Erbazide, 1974·2
Erbesil, 1974·2
Erbitux, 1974·2
Erbium-169, 1523·2
Erbonda Noche, 1974·2
Erbrumina de Perindopril, 980·2
Ercaf, 1974·2
Ercal, 1974·2
Ercar, 1974·2
Ercefuryl, 1974·2
Erceryl, 1974·2
Ercestop, 1974·2
Ercestopyl, 1974·2
Ercevit, 1974·2
Erco-Fer, 1974·2
Erco-Fer Vitamin, 1974·2
Ercolax, 1974·2
Ercoquin, 1974·2
Ercorax Roll-on, 1974·2
Ercoril, 1974·3
Ercotina, 1974·3
Erdnussöl, 1656·1
Erdopect, 1974·3
Erdosteína, 1121·1
Erdosteine, 1121·1
Erdotin, 1974·3
Erdrauchkraut, 1690·1
Erect Cinquefoil, 1757·2
Erectile Dysfunction, 1745·2
Eremfat, 1974·3
Eres N, 1974·3
Erevan, 1974·3
Erfolgan, 1974·3
Erg XXI, 1974·3
Ergamisol, 1974·3
Ergenyl, 1974·3
Ergenyl Chrono, 1974·3
Ergine, 1723·2
Ergix, 1974·3
Ergo Sanol Spezial N, 1974·3
Ergobasine Maleate, 1684·1
Ergobel, 1974·3
Ergobelan, 1974·3
Ergocaf, 1974·3
Ergocalciferol, 1462·1
Ergocalciferol Tablets, Calcium and— *see* Calcium and Ergocalciferol Tablets, 1863·3
Ergocalciferolum, 1462·1
Ergocalm, 1974·3
Ergoclavin, 1974·3
Ergocornine, 1685·2
Ergocris, 1974·3
Ergocristine, 1685·2
Ergocryptine, 1685·2
Ergodavur, 1974·3
Ergodesit, 1974·3
Ergodilat, 1974·3
Ergodose, 1974·3
Ergodryl, 1974·3
Ergodryl Mono, 1974·3
Ergofar, 1974·4
Ergoffin, 1974·4
Ergofit, 1974·4
Ergo-Fort, 1974·4
Ergohepat B12, 1974·4
Ergohydrine, 1974·4
Ergokapton, 1974·4
Ergokoffin, 1974·4
Ergo-Kranit, 1974·4
Ergo-Kranit Mono, 1974·4
Ergolefrin, 1974·4
Ergolin, 1974·4
Ergoloid Mesylates, 1674·1
Ergo-Lonarid PD, 1974·4
Ergomar, 1974·4
Ergomed, 1974·4
Ergomemor, 1974·4
Ergometrina, Maleato de, 1684·1
Ergometrine, 1685·1
Ergometrine Maleate, 1684·1
Ergometrine Tartrate, 1684·3
Ergometrinhydrogenmaleat, 1684·1
Ergometrini Maleas, 1684·1
Ergomicon, 1974·4
Ergomimet, 1974·4
Ergomimet Plus, 1974·4
Ergonef, 1974·4
Ergonovina, Maleato de, 1684·1
Ergonovine Bimaleate, 1684·1
Ergonovine Maleate, 1684·1
Ergont, 1974·4
Ergoplus, 1974·4
Ergoram, 1974·4
Ergosanol a la Cafeine, 1974·4
Ergosanol Special, 1974·4
Ergosanol Special a la Cafeine, 1974·4
Ergosia, 1974·4
Ergosterol, Irradiated, 1462·1
Ergostetrine Maleate, 1684·1
Ergot, 1685·1
Ergot Alkaloids, Dihydrogenated, 1674·1
Ergot Alkaloids, Hydrogenated, 1674·1
Ergotab, 1974·4
Ergotam, 1975·1

Ergotamina, Tartrato de, 467·2
Ergotamine Tartrate, 467·2
Ergotamine Withdrawal Syndrome— *see* Dependence, 468·1
Ergotamini Tartras, 467·2
Ergotan, 1975·1
Ergotocine Maleate, 1684·1
Ergotonine, 1975·1
Ergotop, 1975·1
Ergotox, 1975·1
Ergotoxina, 1685·2
Ergotoxine, 1685·1, 1685·2
Ergotoxine Esilate, 1685·2
Ergotoxine Phosphate, 1685·2
Ergotrate, 1975·1
Ergotyl, 1975·1
Ergovasan, 1975·1
Ergovis, 1975·1
Ergoxina, 1975·1
Ergybiol, 1975·1
Ergymag, 1975·1
Ergyphilus, 1975·1
Eribec, 1975·1
Eriber, 1975·1
Eribiotic, 1975·1
Eribus, 1975·1
Ericin, 1975·1
Ericosol, 1975·1
Eridamin, 1975·1
Eridan, 1975·1
Eridosis, 1975·1
Eriflogin, 1975·1
Erifoscin, 1975·1
Erifostine, 1975·1
Eriglobin, 1975·1
Erigrand, 1975·1
Eriken, 1975·1
Eril, 1975·1
Erimicin, 1975·1
Erimicina, 1975·2
Erimit, 1975·2
Erimycin, 1975·2
Eriodictyon, 1121·2
*Eriodictyon californicum*, 1121·2
Erios, 1975·2
Erisol, 1975·2
Erisuspen, 1975·2
Eritina, 1975·2
Eritolat, 1975·2
Eritos, 1975·2
Eritrax, 1975·2
Eritrerba, 1975·2
Eritrex, 1975·2
Eritrex A, 1975·2
Eritril, 1975·2
Eritrin, 1975·2
Eritritilo, Tetranitrato de, 913·1
Eritrityl Tetranitrate, 913·1
Eritrobron, 1975·2
Eritrocin, 1975·2
Eritrocina, 1975·2
Eritrocist, 1975·2
Eritrocitos, 759·3
Eritroderm, 1975·2
Eritrofar, 1975·2
Eritrofarm, 1975·2
Eritrofarmin, 1975·2
Eritrogen, 1975·2
Eritrogobens, 1975·2
Eritrolat, 1975·2
Eritromax, 1975·2
Eritromed, 1975·2
Eritromicina, 208·1, 1975·2
Eritromicina, Acistrato de, 208·1
Eritromicina, Estearato de, 208·2
Eritromicina, Estolato de, 208·1
Eritromicina, Etilsuccinato de, 208·1
Eritromicina, Gluceptato de, 208·2
Eritromicina, Lactobionato de, 208·2
Eritromicina, Propionato de, 208·2
Eritropiu, 1975·2
Eritroquim, 1975·3
Eritrosima, 1975·3
Eritrosina, 1057·2
Eritrosol, 1975·3
Eritroveinte, 1975·3
Eritrovier, 1975·3
Eritrovit B12, 1975·3
Eritrowel, 1975·3
Erjean, 1975·3
Erkaltungsbad, 1975·3
Erkaltungs-Bad, Kneipp— *see* Kneipp Erkaltungs-Bad, 2081·2
Erkaltungsbad Spezial, Kneipp— *see* Kneipp Erkaltungsbad Spezial, 2081·2
Erkaltungsbalsam, 1975·3
Erkaltungsbalsam Forte Salbe, 1975·3
Erkaltungs-Balsam N, Kneipp— *see* Kneipp Erkaltungs-Balsam N, 2081·2
Erkaltungsbalsam-ratiopharm E Salbe, 1975·3
Erkaltungs-Saft Fur Die Nacht, Wick— *see* Wick Erkaltungs-Saft fur die Nacht, 2385·4
Erkaltungstee, 1975·3
Erkaltungs-Tee, Kneipp— *see* Kneipp Erkaltungs-Tee, 2081·2
Erladexone, 1975·3
Erlecit, 1975·3
Erliten, 1975·3
Erlivin, 1975·3
Erlmetin, 1975·3
Erloric, 1975·3
Erlotyl, 1975·3
Erlvirax, 1975·3
Ermofan, 1975·3
Ermsech, 1975·3
Ermycin, 1975·3
Ermysin, 1975·3
Ernex, 1975·4
Ernodasa, 1975·4
ERO, 1975·4
Ero Test, 1975·4
Erocap, 1975·4
Erogran, 1975·4
Erole Forte, 1975·4
Erole-C, 1975·4
Eromel, 1975·4
Eromel-S, 1975·4
Eromycin, 1975·4
Erosfil, 1975·4
Erotab, 1975·4
Eroxade, 1975·4
Erpalfa, 1975·4
Erpecalm, 1975·4
Erradic, 1975·4
Erreclor, 1975·4
Erremox, 1975·4
Errevit Combi, 1975·4
Errevit Forte Gamma, 1975·4
Errolon, 1975·4
Errolon A, 1975·4
Ertaczo, 1975·4
Ertapenem Sodium, 207·3
Erthiol, 1975·4
Erucic Acid, 1707·3, 1737·3
Erva do Norte, 1666·1
Erva Maligna, 1666·1
Ervemin, 1975·4
Ervevax, 1975·4
Ervin, 1975·4
Erwinase, 1976·1
*Erwinia carotovora*, 528·3
*Erwinia chrysanthemi*, 528·3
Erxetilan, 1976·1
Ery, 1976·1
Eryacne, 1976·1
Eryacnen, 1976·1
Eryaknen, 1976·1
Eryase, 1976·1
Erybesan, 1976·1
Erybeta, 1976·1
Erybid, 1976·1
Erybros, 1976·1
Eryc, 1976·1
Erycette, 1976·1
Erycin, 1976·1
Erycinum, 1976·1
Erycocci, 1976·1
Erycytol, 1976·1
Eryderm, 1976·1
Erydermec, 1976·1
Ery-Diolan, 1976·1
Eryfer, 1976·1
Eryfer Comp, 1976·1
Eryfluid, 1976·2
Erygel, 1976·2
Eryhexal, 1976·2
Erylar, 1976·2
Erylik, 1976·2
Erymax, 1976·2
Ery-Max, 1976·2
Erymin, 1976·2
Erymycin, 1976·2
Erynite, 979·1
Eryped, 1976·2
Ery-Ped, 1976·2
Eryplast, 1976·2
Erypo, 1976·2
Ery-Reu, 1976·2
Erysafe, 1976·2
Erysec, 1976·2
Ery-Set, 1976·2
Erysidoron, 1976·2
Erysil, 1976·2
Erysipelas— *see* Skin Infections, 146·2
Erysol, 1976·2
Erysolvan, 1976·2
Eryson, 1976·2
Erystad, 1976·2
Erystamine-K, 1976·2
Erystat, 1976·2
Erystrat, 1976·2
Ery-Tab, 1976·2
Erytab, 1976·2
Erytab-S, 1976·3
Eryteal, 1976·3
Erythema Migrans— *see* Lyme Disease, 134·1
Erythema Multiforme, 1135·3
Erythermalgia— *see* Raynaud's Syndrome, 833·3
Eryth-mycin, 1976·3
Erythra-Derm, 1976·3
*Erythraea centaurium*, 1669·2
Erythrina Mulungu, 1717·2
*Erythrina verna*, 1717·2
Erythritol Tetranitrate, 913·1
Erythrityl Tetranitrate, 913·1
Erythro, 1976·3
Erythrocin, 1976·3
Erythrocin Neo, 1976·3
Erythrocine, 1976·3
Erythrocytosis, 806·1
Erythroderm, 1976·3
Erythroforte, 1976·3
Erythrogel, 1976·3
Erythrogenat, 1976·3
Erythrogram, 1976·3
Erythro-Hefa, 1976·3
Erythrohydrobupropion, 288·2
Erythrol, 1976·3
Erythrol Nitrate, 913·1
Erythrol Tetranitrate, 913·1
Erythromelalgia— *see* Raynaud's Syndrome, 833·3
Erythromid, 1976·3
Erythromycin, 208·1
Erythromycin A, 208·1
Erythromycin 2′-Acetate Stearate, 208·1
Erythromycin Acistrate, 208·1
Erythromycin Estolate, 208·1
Erythromycin Ethyl Succinate, 208·1
Erythromycin Ethylsuccinate, 208·1
Erythromycin 2′-(Ethylsuccinate), 208·1
Erythromycin Gluceptate, 208·2
Erythromycin Gluceptate, Sterile, 208·2
Erythromycin Glucoheptonate, 208·2
Erythromycin Lactobionate, 208·2
Erythromycin Lactobionate, Sterile, 208·2
Erythromycin 9-{*O*-[(2-Methoxyethoxy)-methyl]oxime}, 254·2
Erythromycin Mono(4-*O*-β-D-galactopyranosyl-D-gluconate), 208·2
Erythromycin Octadecanoate, 208·2
Erythromycin Phosphate, 211·1
Erythromycin Propanoate, 208·2
Erythromycin Propionate, 208·2
Erythromycin 2′-Propionate, 208·2
Erythromycin 2′-Propionate Dodecyl Sulphate, 208·1
Erythromycin Propionate Lauryl Sulfate, 208·1
Erythromycin Propionate Lauryl Sulphate, 208·1
Erythromycin Salnacedin, 211·1
Erythromycin Stearate, 208·2
Erythromycin Thiocyanate, 211·1
Erythromycini Estolas, 208·1
Erythromycini Ethylsuccinas, 208·1
Erythromycini Lactobionas, 208·2
Erythromycini Stearas, 208·2
Erythromycinum, 208·1
Erythromycylamine, 206·1
Erythroped, 1976·3
Erythropoietin, 747·1
Erythropoietin Concentrated Solution, 747·1
Erythrosine, 1057·2
Erythrosine BS, 1057·2
Erythrosine Sodium, 1057·2
Erythro-Teva, 1976·3
*Erythroxylum*, 1373·3
*Erythroxylum coca*, 1373·3
*Erythroxylum truxillense*, 1373·3
Erytop, 1976·3
Erytran, 1976·3
Erytrociclin, 1976·3
Eryval, 1976·3
Eryzole, 1976·3
ES-132, 1115·3
ES Bronchial Mixture, 1976·3
Esacinone, 1976·3
Esafosfina, 1976·3
Esafosfina Glutammica, 1976·3
Esaglut, 1976·4
Esalfon, 1976·4
Esalfon-D, 1976·4
Esametilentetrammina, 230·1
Esametone, 1976·4
Esammina, 230·1
Esanic, 1976·4
Esapent, 1976·4
Esarondil, 1976·4
Esavir, 1976·4
Esbelcaps, 1976·4
Esbelt, 1976·4
Esbeltex, 1976·4
Esbeltrat, 1976·4
Esbericard, 1976·4
Esbericard Novo, 1976·4
Esbericum, 1976·4
Esberitop, 1976·4
Esberitox Mono, 1976·4
Esberitox N, 1976·4
Esberiven, 1976·4
Esberiven Fort, 1976·4
Escabin, 1976·4
Escabron, 1976·4
Escacin, 1976·4
Escalgin sans Codeine, 1976·4
Escalol 507— *see* Totalbloc Maximum Protection, 2339·1
Escancil, 1976·4
Escandine, 1976·4
Escapin-N, 1976·4
Escar T, 1977·1
Escar T-Neomicina, 1977·1
Escaramujo, 1740·1
Escarbicida, 1977·1
Escarine, 1977·1
Escarol, 1977·1
Escatitona, 1977·1
Escherichia Coli Enteritis, 129·1
*Escherichia coli* J5, 1615·2
Escherichia Coli Vaccines, 1615·3
Escila, 1130·3
Escila, Bulbo de, 1130·3
Escila India, 1130·3
Escin, 1648·2
Escina Forte, 1977·1
Escina Omega, 1977·1
Escinogel, 1977·1
Escitalopram Oxalate, 292·1
Esclama, 1977·1

Esclebin, 1977·1
Esclerobion, 1977·1
Esclerovitan, 1977·1
Esclerovitan A O, 1977·1
Esclerovitan Antioxidante, 1977·1
Esclerovitan E, 1977·1
Esclim, 1977·1
Esclima, 1977·1
Escodarone, 1977·1
Escogripp sans Codeine, 1977·1
Esconitro, 1977·1
Escophylline, 1977·1
Escopolamina, 483·3
Escopolamina, Bromhidrato de, 483·3
Escopolamina, Butilbromuro de, 483·3
Escopolamina, Hidrobromuro de, 483·3
Escopolamina, Metilbromuro de, 483·3
Escopolamina, Metilnitrato de, 483·3
Escoprim, 1977·1
Escor, 1977·1
Escoretic, 1977·1
Escotussin, 1977·1
Escozem, 1977·1
Escualano, 1482·2
Escudo, 1977·1
Esculeol P, 1977·1
Esculin, 1648·2
Esculoside, 1648·2
Escumycin, 1977·1
Escutelaria, 1746·3
Esdepaletrina, 1505·1
Esdepallethrine, 1505·1
ESE, 1977·1
Esedril, 1977·1
Eselan, 1977·1
Eselin, 1977·2
Esencia de Alhucema, 1705·2
Esencia de Anís, 1655·2
Esencia de Azahar, 1719·2
Esencia de Canela, 1672·2
Esencia de Cidra, 1706·2
Esencia de Clavo, 1673·3
Esencia de Espliego, 1705·2
Esencia de Eucalipto, 1686·2
Esencia de Hinojo, 1687·3
Esencia de Melisa, 1711·2
Esencia de Nuez Moscada, 1722·3
Esencia de Quenopodio Vermifuga, 103·3
Esencia de Romero, 1740·2
Esencia de Rosa, 1740·2
Esencia de Tomillo, 1755·3
Esencia de Trementina, 1760·1
Eseridina, Salicilato de, 1491·2
Eseridine Salicylate, 1491·2
Eserine, 1494·1
Eserine Aminoxide Salicylate, 1491·2
Eserine Oxide Salicylate, 1491·2
Eserine Salicylate, 1494·1
Eserine Sulphate, 1494·2
Eserini Salicylas, 1494·1
Eserini Sulfas, 1494·2
Eseroline, 1494·2
Esfenvalerate, 1505·2
Esforza, 1977·2
Esgic, 1977·2
Esgic-Plus, 1977·2
Esgipyrin, 1977·2
Esgipyrin DS, 1977·2
Esidrex, 1977·2
Esidrix, 1977·2
Esilgan, 1977·2
Esilresorcina, 1182·1
Esimil, 1977·2
Esiteren, 1977·2
Eskacef— *see* Julphacef, 2072·1
Eskaflam, 1977·2
Eskalith, 1977·2
Eskamel, 1977·2
Eskapar, 1977·2
Eskazine, 1977·2
Eskazole, 1977·2
Esketamine Hydrochloride, 1302·2
Esketamini Hydrochloridum, 1302·2
Eskim, 1977·2
Eskold, 1977·2
Eskold Expectorant, 1977·2
Eskornade, 1977·2
Esmacen, 1977·2
Esmalorid, 1977·2
Esme Topico, 1977·2
Esmedent Con Fluor, 1977·2
Esmeron, 1977·2
Esmolol, Hidrocloruro de, 913·1
Esmolol Hydrochloride, 913·1
Eso Preparations, 1977·3
Esoalcolico Incolore, 1977·3
Esocetic, 1977·3
Esodar, 1977·3
Esodrox, 1977·3
Esofenol 60, 1977·3
Esofenol Ferri, 1977·3
Esofex, 1977·3
Esoform Preparations, 1977·3
Eso-Jod, 1977·4
Esol, 1977·4
Esolut, 1977·4
E-Solve, 1977·4
Esomeprazol Magnésico, 1265·1
Esomeprazole Magnesium, 1265·1
Esomeprazole Sodium, 1265·1
Esonide, 1977·4
Esopral, 1977·4
Esorid, 1977·4
Esosan, 1977·4
Esosan Casa, 1977·4
Esosan Pronto, 1977·4
Esoterica Preparations, 1977·4
Esotran, 1977·4
Esotropia— *see* Strabismus, 1487·1
Esoxid, 1977·4
Espabion, 1977·4
Espa-butyl, 1977·4
Espacil, 1977·4
Espacil Compuesto, 1977·4
Espadol, 1977·4
Espa-dorm, 1977·4
Espa-formin, 1977·4
Espa-lepsin, 1977·4
Espa-lipon, 1977·4
Espa-moxin, 1977·4
Espar, 1977·4
Esparfloxacino, 255·1
Esparil, 1977·4
Esparon, 1978·1
Esparteína, Sulfato de, 1749·1
Espasal, 1978·1
Espasantral, 1978·1
Espasevit, 1978·1
Espasmacid, 1978·1
Espasmalgon, 1978·1
Espasmo Preparations, 1978·1
Espasmobel, 1978·1
Espasmocron, 1978·1
Espasmodid Composto, 1978·1
Espasmofin, 1978·1
Espasmolex, 1978·2
Espasmo-Ped, 1978·2
Espasmosan, 1978·2
Espasmosan Composto, 1978·2
Espasmotropin, 1978·2
Espa-Valept, 1978·2
Espaven, 1978·2
Espaven Alcalino, 1978·2
Espaven Enzimatico, 1978·2
Espaven MD, 1978·2
Espaven Pediatrico, 1978·2
Especies Calmantes, 1978·2
Espectinomicina, 255·2
Espectinomicina, Hidrocloruro de, 255·2
Espectocural, 1978·2
Espectral, 1978·2
Espectral Balsamico, 1978·2
Espectrin, 1978·2
Espectrosira, 1978·2
Espeden, 1978·2
Esperal, 1978·2
Espercil, 1978·2
Espermicida Preserv, 1978·2
Esperson, 1978·2
Esperson N, 1978·2
Espesil, 1978·2
Espidifen, 1978·2
Espin, 1978·2
Espino Cerval, 1254·1
Espiramicina, 255·3
Espiran, 1978·2
Espirapril, Hidrocloruro de, 1003·1
Espiride, 1978·2
Espirolona, 1978·3
Espironolactona, 1003·1
Espirulina, 1749·2
Espledol, 1978·3
Espliego, Esencia de, 1705·2
Espo, 1978·3
Espongostan, 1978·3
Espotabs, 1978·3
Esprenit, 1978·3
Esprit, 1978·3
Esprit Sensor, 1978·3
Espritin, 1978·3
Espumisan, 1978·3
Espundia— *see* Leishmaniasis, 597·2
Esquila, 1509·3
Esracain, 1978·3
Esradin, 1978·3
Esrar, 1666·1
Essamin, 1978·3
Essaven Preparations, 1978·3
Essavenon, 1978·3
Esseldon, 1978·3
Essen, 1978·3
Essen Enzimatico, 1978·3
Essence Algerienne, 1978·3
Essence d'Anis, 1655·2
Essence de Cannelle de Ceylan, 1672·2
Essence de Citron, 1706·2
Essence de Genièvre, 1703·1
Essence de Girofle, 1673·3
Essence de Menthe Poivrée, 1283·2
Essence de Muscade, 1722·3
Essence de Niaouli, 1719·3
Essence de Pin de Montagne, 1737·1
Essence de Romarin, 1740·2
Essence de Térébenthine, 1760·1
Essence d'Eucalyptus Rectifiée, 1686·2
Essence of Mustard, 1718·2
Essence of Orange, 1724·1
Essence of Portugal, 1724·1
Essência de Alecrim, 1740·2
Essência de Alfazema, 1705·2
Essência de Capim-Limão , 1706·3
Essência de Flor de Laranjeira, 1719·2
Essência de Funcho, 1687·3
Essência de Hortelã-Pimenta , 1283·2
Essência de Laranja, 1724·1
Essência de Limão , 1706·2
Essência de Moscada, 1722·3
Essência de Tomilho, 1755·3
Essential 50+, 1978·3
Essential Amino Acids, 1417·1
Essential B, 1978·3
Essential Balance, 1978·4
Essential Fatty Acids, 1417·1
Essential Oils, 1763·3
Essential ProPlus, 1978·4
Essential Thrombocythaemia— *see* Primary Thrombocythaemia, 509·1
Essentiale, 1978·4
Essentiale N, 1978·4
Essentiale-L, 1978·4
Essentielle Aminosauren, 1978·4
Essex, 1978·4
Essigsäure, 1645·2
Essigsaure Tonerde-Salbe, 1978·4
Essitol, 1978·4
Est...— *see also under* Oest...
EST, 1978·4
Establix, 1978·4
Estac, 1978·4
Estafan, 1978·4
Estafiloide, 1978·4
Estafiloquinasa, 1005·2
Estalis, 1978·4
Estalis Continuous, 1978·4
Estalis Sekvens, 1978·4
Estalis Sequens, 1978·4
Estalis Sequi, 1978·4
Estandron P, 1978·4
Estandron Prolongado, 1978·4
Estaño, 1756·3
Estanol, Ésteres de, 1448·3
Estanozolol, 1569·2
Estaprol, 1978·4
Estar, 1979·1
Estavudina, 654·2
Estazolam, 697·3
Esteaglato de Prednisolona, 1108·2
Estearato de Calcio, 1574·1
Estearato de Eritromicina, 208·2
Estearato de Magnesio, 1574·2
Estearato de Sodio, 1574·3
Estearato de Sorbitán, 1416·2
Estearato de Zinc, 1575·3
Esteárico, Ácido, 1749·2
Estearilfumarato de Sodio, 1575·1
Estecina, 1979·1
Esteclin, 1979·1
Esteclin Bac, 1979·1
Estelle, 1979·1
Esteprim, 1979·1
Estepronina, 1130·3
Ester Aces, 1979·1
Ester C EVC, 1979·1
Éster Dibutílico del Ácido Escuárico, 1158·1
Ester Type Local Anaesthetics, 1367·1
Esterasine, 1979·1
Esterbiol, 1979·1
Ester-C, 1979·1
Ester-C Plus, 1979·1
Ester-C Plus Multi-Mineral, 1979·1
Ésteres de Sacarosa, 1416·3
Ésteres del Macrogol, 1413·2
Ésteres del Sorbitán, 1416·1
Estericlean, 1979·1
Esterified Estrogens, 1549·3
Esterified Oestrogens, 1549·3
Esterofundina, 1979·1
Esterol, 1979·1
Esterol Plus, 1979·1
Esteromicin, 1979·1
Esteronide, 1979·1
Esteviósido, 1449·3
Estibocaptato de Sodio, 103·1
Estibofeno, 103·1
Estibogluconato de Sodio, 600·3
Estigmas de Azafrán, 1058·2
Estigyn, 1979·1
Estilomicin, 1979·1
Estilsona, 1979·1
Estima, 1979·1
Estimulocel, 1979·1
Estinyl, 1979·1
Estiripentol, 377·3
Estival, 1979·1
Estivan, 1979·1
Esto, 1979·2
Estolato de Eritromicina, 208·1
Estomafitino, 1979·2
Estomagel, 1979·2
Estomaplus, 1979·2
Estomazil, 1979·2
Estomepe, 1979·2
Estomil, 1979·2
Estomina, 1979·2
Estomycin, 1979·2
Estomycin Sulphate, 612·3
Estopause, 1979·2
Estopein, 1979·2
Estoraque, 1749·3
Estoraque Líquido, 1749·3
Estovyn-T, 1979·2
Estrabeta, 1979·2
Estrace, 1979·2
Estracomb, 1979·2
Estracomb TTS, 1979·2
Estracombi, 1979·2
Estracutan, 1979·2
Estracyt, 1979·2
Estradelle, 1979·2
Estraderm, 1979·2
Estraderm— *see* Estracomb, 1979·2
Estraderm— *see* Estracombi, 1979·2
Estraderm— *see* Estrapak, 1979·3

Estraderm TTS, 1979·3
Estraderm TTS— *see* Estracomb, 1979·2
Estraderm TTS— *see* Estracombi, 1979·2
Estradiol, 1550·1
Estradiol Benzoate, 1550·1
Estradiol, Benzoato de, 1550·1
Estradiol Cipionate, 1550·1
Estradiol, Cipionato de, 1550·1
Estradiol Cypionate, 1550·1
Estradiol Dipropionate, 1550·1
Estradiol, Dipropionato de, 1550·1
Estradiol Enantate, 1550·1
Estradiol, Enantato de, 1550·1
Estradiol Enanthate, 1550·1
Estradiol, Fenilpropionato de, 1550·2
Estradiol Hemihydrate, 1550·1
Estradiol, Hexahidrobenzoato de, 1550·1
Estradiol Hexahydrobenzoate, 1550·1
Estradiol Phenylpropionate, 1550·2
17α-Estradiol Sulfate, Sodium, 1543·2
Estradiol Undecylate, 1551·2
Estradiol Valerate, 1550·2
Estradiol, Valerato de, 1550·2
Estradioli Benzoas, 1550·1
Estradioli Valeras, 1550·2
Estradiolum, 1550·1
Estradot, 1979·3
Estradurin, 1979·3
Estradurine, 1979·3
Estrafemol, 1979·3
Estragest, 1979·3
Estragest— *see* Estracomb, 1979·2
Estragest— *see* Estracombi, 1979·2
Estragest TTS— *see* Estracomb, 1979·2
Estragest TTS— *see* Estracombi, 1979·2
Estragole, 1655·2
Estramon, 1979·3
Estramonio, 489·2
Estramustina, Fosfato Sódico de, 551·1
Estramustine Phosphate Sodium, 551·1
Estramustine Sodium Phosphate, 551·1
Estranova CC, 1979·3
Estranova E, 1979·3
Estranova 30 Simple, 1979·3
Estrapak, 1979·3
Estrapatch, 1979·3
Estrapronicate, 1552·3
Estrapronicato, 1552·3
Estrarona, 1979·3
Estrasorb, 1979·3
Estratab, 1979·3
Estratest, 1979·3
Estra-1,3,5(10)-triene-3,17β-diol, 1550·1
Estra-1,3,5(10)-triene-3,17β-diol 3-Benzoate, 1550·1
Estra-1,3,5(10)-triene-3,17β-diol 3-[Bis(2-chloroethyl)carbamate] 17-(Disodium Phosphate), 551·1
Estra-1,3,5(10)-triene-3,17β-diol 17-Cyclohexanecarboxylate, 1550·1
Estra-1,3,5(10)-triene-3,17β-diol 17-(3-Cyclopentylpropionate), 1550·1
Estra-1,3,5(10)-triene-3,17β-diol Dipropionate, 1550·1
Estra-1,3,5(10)-triene-3,17β-diol 17-Heptanoate, 1550·1
Estra-1,3,5(10)-triene-3,17β-diol 17-(3-Phenylpropionate), 1550·2
Estra-1,3,5(10)-triene-3,17β-diol 17-Valerate, 1550·2
Estra-1,3,5(10)-triene-3,16α,17β-triol, 1552·3
Estrefen, 1979·3
Estregur, 1979·3
Estrena, 1979·3
Estreptocarbocaftiazol, 1979·3
Estreptodornasa, 1749·3
Estreptoenterol, 1979·3
Estreptomicina, 256·1
Estreptomicina, Hidrocloruro de, 256·1
Estreptomicina, Sulfato de, 256·2
Estreptoquinasa, 1005·2
Estreptozocina, 584·1
Estreva, 1979·3
Estrex, 1979·3
Estriagel, 1979·4
Estricnina, 1750·1
Estricnina, Azotato de, 1750·1
Estricnina, Hidrocloruro de, 1750·1
Estricnina, Nitrato de, 1750·1
Estricnina, Sulfato de, 1750·1
Estrifam, 1979·4
Estring, 1979·4
Estriol, 1552·3
Estriol Sodium Succinate, 1552·3
Estriol Succinate, 1552·3
Estriol, Succinato de, 1552·3
Estriol, Succinato Sódico de, 1552·3
Estriolum, 1552·3
Estrocare, 1979·4
Estroclim, 1979·4
Estrodose, 1979·4
Estrofantina, 1009·1
Estrofem, 1979·4
Estrofem N, 1979·4
Estrogel, 1979·4
EstroGel, 1979·4
Estrogen Replacement Therapy, 1536·3
Estrogeni Coniuncti, 1543·2
Estrogenon, 1979·4
Estrógenos Conjugados, 1543·2
Estrógenos Esterificados, 1549·3
Estrogens, A, Synthetic Conjugated, 1543·3
Estrogens, B, Synthetic Conjugated, 1543·3
Estrogens, Conjugated, 1543·2
Estrogens, Esterified, 1549·3
Estro-Logic, 1979·4
Estromustine, 551·2
Estrona, 1553·1
Estronar, 1979·4
Estroncio 89, 1525·2
Estroncio, Cloruro de, 1749·3
Estrone, 1553·1
Estrone Sulfate, Sodium, 1543·2, 1549·3
Estronorm, 1979·4
Estro-Pause, 1979·4
Estropipate, 1553·1
Estropipato, 1553·1
Estroplus, 1979·4
Estroquin, 1979·4
Estrostep, 1979·4
Estrostep Fe, 1979·4
Estroxyn, 1979·4
Estulic, 1979·4
Esucos, 1979·4
Esvit C, 1979·4
Eszopiclone, 730·1
ET-394, 1171·2
ET-495, 1212·2
ET-743, 589·3
Eta Biocortilen, 1979·4
Eta Biocortilen VC, 1979·4
Eta Cortilen, 1979·4
Etabus, 1980·1
Etaconil, 1980·1
Etacridina, Lactato de, 1165·3
Etacril, 1980·1
Etacrinato Sódico, 913·3
Etacrínico, Ácido, 913·2
Etacrynate Sodium, 913·3
Etacrynic Acid, 913·2
Etacrynicum, Acidum, 913·2
Etacrynsäure, 913·2
Etaden, 1685·2
Etadiona, 360·1
ETAF, 562·2
Etafedrina, Hidrocloruro de, 1121·2
Etafedrine Hydrochloride, 1121·2
Etafenona, Hidrocloruro de, 914·1
Etafenone Hydrochloride, 914·1
Etalpha, 1980·1
Etambutol, Hidrocloruro de, 211·3
Etamifilina, Camsilato de, 785·1
Etamiphylline, 785·1
Etamiphylline Camsilate, 785·1
Etamiphylline Camsylate, 785·1
Etamiphylline Dehydrocholate, 785·1
Etamiphylline Hydrochloride, 785·1
Etamiphylline Methiodide, 785·1
Etamivan, 1588·1
Etamphyllin Camsylate, 785·1
Etamsilato, 749·3
Etamsylate, 749·3
Etamsylatum, 749·3
Etamucin, 1980·1
Etanautine, 431·3
Etanercept, 36·3
Etanicozid B6, 1980·1
Etanidazol, 551·2
Etanidazole, 551·2
Etanoico, 1645·2
Etanolamida del Ácido Gentísico, 1692·2
Etapiam, 1980·1
Etaretin, 1980·1
Etasisen, 1980·1
Etaverina, Hidrocloruro de, 1685·2
Etaverol, 1980·1
Etaxene, 1980·1
Etclorvinol, 697·3
ETDR, 1980·1
Etec, 1980·1
ETEC, 129·2
Etec 1000, 1980·1
Etenzamida, 37·2
Etenzamide, 37·2
Eter, 1474·2
Éter Anestésico, 1298·3
Éter Cetoestearílico de Polioxil 20, 1412·2
Éter de Petróleo, 1476·3
Éter Dimetílico, 1236·1
Éter Disolvente, 1474·2
Éter Metilterbutílico, 1475·3
Éter Oleílico de Polioxil 10, 1413·1
Éter Puríssimo, 1298·3
Eterciclina, 1980·1
Éteres Cetoestearílicos de Macrogol, 1412·2
Éteres Láuricos de Macrogol, 1412·3
Éteres Monometílicos de Macrogol, 1413·1
Éteres Oleílicos de Macrogol, 1413·1
Etermol, 1980·1
Etermol Antitusivo, 1980·1
Eternex, 1980·1
Etfariol, 1980·1
Ethacid, 1980·1
Ethacridine Lactate, 1165·3
Ethacridine Lactate Monohydrate, 1165·3
Ethacridini Lactas, 1165·3
Ethacrynate Sodium, 913·3
Ethacrynic Acid, 913·2
Ethaden, 1685·2
Ethadione, 360·1
Etham, 1980·1
Ethambutol Hydrochloride, 211·3
Ethambutoli Hydrochloridum, 211·3
Ethamicort, 1103·3
Ethaminal Sodium, 713·3
Ethamivan, 1588·1
Ethamolin, 1980·1
Ethamsylate, 749·3
Ethanedial, 1181·1
Ethane-1,2-diol, 1685·3
1,2-Ethanedione, 1181·1
Ethanenitrile, 1471·1
Ethanoic Acid, 1645·2
Ethanol, 1166·1
Ethanol (96 Per Cent), 1166·1
Ethanol, Anhydrous, 1166·1
Ethanol, Denatured, 1185·3
Ethanolamine, 1716·1
Ethanolamine Oleate, 1716·1
Ethanols, Dilute, 1166·1
Ethanolum, 1166·1
Ethanolum Anhydricum, 1166·1
Ethasyl, 1980·1
Ethatyl, 1980·1
Ethaverine Hydrochloride, 1685·2
Ethaverine Sulfamate, 1685·2
Ethbutol, 1980·1
Ethchlorvynol, 697·3
*E*-Ethchlorvynol, 697·3
EtheDent, 1980·1
*trans*-18-Ethenyl-4,4a-dihydro-3,4-bis(methoxycarbonyl)-4a,8,14,19-tetramethyl-23*H*,25*H*-benzo[*b*]porphine-9,13-dipropanoic Acid Monomethyl Ester, 591·1
1-Ethenylpyrrolidin-2-one, 1581·2
Ethenzamide, 37·2
Etheophyl, 1980·1
Ether, 1298·3, 1474·2
Ether, Anaesthetic, 1298·3
Ether Anesthesicus, 1298·3
Ether de Kay, 1121·2
Ether, Ethyl, 1474·2
Ether, Hydrochloric, 1376·2
Ether, Petroleum, 1476·3
Éther Rectifié, 1474·2
Ether, Solvent, 1474·2
Ethereal Oils, 1763·3
Etherified Starches, 750·1
Ethezyme, 1980·1
Ethibloc, 1980·2
Ethical Nutrients Preparations, 1980·2
Ethicholine, 1980·2
Ethicoline, 1980·2
Ethimil, 1980·2
Ethinyl Estradiol, 1553·2
Ethinylestradiol, 1553·2
Ethinylestradiolum, 1553·2
Ethinylestrenol, 1557·1
Ethinylnortestosterone, 1562·2
Ethinyloestradiol, 1553·2
17α-Ethinyloestradiol 3-Cyclopentyl Ether, 1568·2
Ethinyloestradiol-3-methyl Ether, 1559·2
Ethiodized Oil, 1063·2
Ethiodol, 1980·2
Ethiofos, 1031·3
Ethion, 1505·1
Ethionamide, 212·3
Ethionamide Hydrochloride, 213·1
Ethionamidum, 212·3
Ethipramine, 1980·2
Ethisterone, 1545·3
Ethmozine, 1980·2
Ethocaine Hydrochloride, 1383·2
Ethoform, 1370·3
Éthoforme, 1370·3
Ethoheptazine Citrate, 37·2
Ethohexadiol, 1505·1
Ethopabate, 605·1
Ethopropazine Hydrochloride, 488·3
Ethosuximide, 360·1
Ethotoin, 361·1
Ethoxazorutin, 1688·2
Ethoxazorutoside, 1688·2
4′-Ethoxyacetanilide, 82·2
Ethoxybenzamide, 37·2
2-Ethoxybenzamide, 37·2
(2*S*,3a*S*,7a*S*)-1-{*N*-[(*S*)-1-Ethoxycarbonylbutyl]-L-alanyl}perhydroindole-2-carboxylic Acid, 980·2
2-[2-(Ethoxycarbonylmethylthio)ethyl]thiazolidine-4-carboxylic Acid, 1123·3
*N*-Ethoxycarbonyl-3-morpholinosydnonimine, 961·3
4-[1-(Ethoxycarbonyloxy)ethoxy]-2-methyl-$N^2$-pyridyl-2*H*-1,2-benzothiazine-3-carboxamide 1,1-Dioxide, 14·2
1-(Ethoxycarbonyloxy)ethyl (6*R*)-6-(α-D-Phenylglycylamino)penicillanate Hydrochloride, 161·2
(11β,17α)-17-[(Ethoxycarbonyl)oxy]-11-hydroxy-3-oxoandrosta-1,4-diene-17-carboxylic Acid Chloromethyl Ester, 1105·3
(*S*)-7-{*N*-[(*S*)-1-Ethoxycarbonyl-3-phenylpropyl]-L-alanyl}-1,4-dithia-7-azaspiro[4.4]nonane-8-carboxylic Acid Hydrochloride, 1003·1
(*S*)-3-{*N*-[(*S*)-1-Ethoxycarbonyl-3-phenylpropyl]-L-alanyl}-1-methyl-2-oxoimidazoline-4-carboxylic Acid Hydrochloride, 938·2
(2*S*,3a*S*,6a*S*)-1-{*N*-[(*S*)-1-Ethoxycarbonyl-3-phenylpropyl]L-alanyl}perhydrocyclopenta[*b*]pyrrole-2-carboxylic Acid, 994·1
(2*S*,3a*R*,7a*S*)-1-{*N*-[(*S*)-1-Ethoxycarbonyl-3-phenylpropyl]-L-alanyl}perhydroindole-2-carboxylic Acid, 1016·1

N-{N-[(S)-1-Ethoxycarbonyl-3-phenylpropyl]-L-alanyl}-L-proline, 909·2
N-{N-[(S)-1-Ethoxycarbonyl-3-phenylpropyl]-L-alanyl}-L-proline Hydrogen Maleate, 909·2
(3S)-2-{N-[(S)-1-Ethoxycarbonyl-3-phenylpropyl]-L-alanyl}-1,2,3,4-tetrahydro-isoquinoline-3-carboxylic Acid Hydrochloride, 991·1
(1S,9S)-9-[(S)-1-Ethoxycarbonyl-3-phenylpropylamino]-10-oxoperhydropyridazino[1,2-a][1,2]diazepine-1-carboxylic Acid Monohydrate, 883·3
(3S-{2[$R^*$($R^*$)],3$R^*$})-2-(2-{[1-(Ethoxycarbonyl)-3-phenylpropyl]amino}-1-oxopropyl)-1,2,3,4-tetrahydro-6,7-dimethoxy-3-isoquinoline-carboxylic Acid Hydrochloride, 961·2
{(3S)-3-[(1S)-1-Ethoxycarbonyl-3-phenylpropylamino]-2,3,4,5-tetrahydro-2-oxo-1H-1-benzazepin-1-yl}acetic Acid Hydrochloride, 867·2
(+)-(2S,6R)-6-{[(1S)-1-Ethoxycarbonyl-3-phenylpropyl]amino}tetrahydro-5-oxo-2-(2-thienyl)-1,4-thiazepine-4(5H)-acetic Acid Hydrochloride, 1010·2
6-Ethoxy-1,2-dihydro-2,2,4-trimethylquinoline, 1179·1
α-[(p-Ethoxy-β,β-dimethylphenethyl)oxy]-m-phenoxytoluene, 1505·2
2-Ethoxyethyl p-Methoxycinnamate, 1145·1
1-(2-Ethoxyethyl)-2-(hexahydro-4-methyl-1H-1,4-diazepin-1-yl)benzimidazole Fumarate (1:2), 433·2
3-Ethoxy-4-hydroxybenzaldehyde, 1685·3
(3-{[4-(3-Ethoxy-2-hydroxypropoxy)phenyl]amino}-3-oxopropyl)dimethylsulphonium p-Toluenesulphonate, 797·2
(±)-(2-{[p-(3-Ethoxy-2-hydroxypropoxy)phenyl]carbamoyl}ethyl)dimethylsulphonium p-Toluenesulphonate, 797·2
(+)-2-Ethoxy-α-{[(S)-α-isobutyl-o-piperidinobenzyl]carbamoyl}-p-toluic Acid, 344·3
Ethoxylated Alkyl Sulfates, 1574·1
Ethoxylated Glycerol, Trihydroxystearate Ester of, 1414·3
Ethoxylated Glycerol, Triricinoleate Ester of, 1414·3
Ethoxylated Lanolin, 1483·3
Ethoxylated Wool Alcohols, 1483·1
5-[2-Ethoxy-5-(4-methylpiperazin-1-ylsulfonyl)phenyl]-1,6-dihydro-1-methyl-3-propylpyrazolo[4,3-d]pyrimidin-7-one Citrate, 1744·2
3-[4-(β-Ethoxyphenethyl)piperazin-1-yl]-2-methylpropiophenone Dihydrochloride, 1121·1
2-Ethoxyphenol, 1122·2
(±)-(2RS)-2-[(αRS)-α-(2-Ethoxyphenoxy)benzyl]morpholine Methanesulphonate, 316·3
(−)-(R)-5-(2-{[2-(o-Ethoxyphenoxy)-ethyl]amino}-propyl)-2-methoxybenzenesulfonamide Hydrochloride, 1009·2
2-(2-Ethoxyphenoxymethyl)morpholine Hydrochloride, 323·3
3-(2-Ethoxyphenoxy)propane-1,2-diol, 1122·1
N-(4-Ethoxyphenyl)acetamide, 82·2
Ethoxyphenyldiethylphenylbutylamine Hydrochloride, 1685·2
1-(4-Ethoxyphenyl)-N,N-diethyl-3-phenylbutylamine Hydrochloride, 1685·2
(S)-2-Ethoxy-4-{[1-(o-piperidinophenyl)-3-methylbutyl]carbamoylmethyl}benzoic Acid, 344·3
Ethoxyquin, 1179·1
Ethrane, 1980·2
Ethychlordiphene, 605·2
Ethyl (3R,4R,5S)-4-Acetamido-5-amino-3-(1-ethylpropoxy)-1-cyclohexene-1-carboxylate Phosphate (1:1), 651·1
Ethyl Acetate, 1474·3
Ethyl Alcohol, 1166·1
Ethyl (3S)-3-{3-[(p-Amidinophenyl)carbamoyl]propionamido}-4-pentynoate Monohydrochloride, 1029·2
Ethyl Aminobenzoate, 1370·3
Ethyl 4-Aminobenzoate, 1370·3
Ethyl 3-Aminobenzoate Methanesulphonate, 1385·3
Ethyl (−)-2-Amino-2-(3,4-dihydroxybenzyl)propionate Hydrochloride, 953·2
Ethyl 2-Amino-6-(4-fluorobenzylamino)-3-pyridylcarbamate Maleate, 43·3
Ethyl L-2-Amino-3-mercaptopropionate Hydrochloride, 1121·2
Ethyl 1-(4-Aminophenethyl)-4-phenylpiperidine-4-carboxylate, 15·1
Ethyl Apovincaminate, 1764·2
Ethyl Apovincaminoate, 1764·2
Ethyl Biscoumacetate, 914·1
Ethyl Bis(4-hydroxycoumarin-3-yl)acetate, 914·1
Ethyl (±)-4-[Bis(2-hydroxypropyl)amino]benzoate, 1157·1
Ethyl (S)-2-{[(S)-1-(Carboxymethyl-2-indanylcarbamoyl)ethyl]amino}-4-phenylbutyrate Hydrochloride, 892·2
Ethyl (2S,3aR,7aS)-1-{(S)-N-[(S)-1-Carboxy-3-phenylpropyl]alanyl}hexahydro-2-indolinecarboxylate, 1016·1
Ethyl Chloride, 1376·2
Ethyl ({8-Chloro-3-[2-(diethylamino)ethyl]-4-methyl-2-oxo-2H-1-benzopyran-7-yl}oxy)acetate, 889·1
Ethyl 4-(8-Chloro-5,6-dihydro-11H-benzo[5,6]cyclohepta[1,2-b]pyridin-11-ylidene)piperidine-1-carboxylate, 436·1
Ethyl 7-Chloro-5-(2-fluorophenyl)-2,3-dihydro-2-oxo-1H-1,4-benzodiazepine-3-carboxylate, 698·1
Ethyl p-Chlorophenoxyisobutyrate, 884·3
Ethyl 2-(4-Chlorophenoxy)-2-methylpropionate, 884·3
Ethyl Cinnamate, 1685·2
Ethyl Clofibrate, 884·3
Ethyl 1-(3-Cyano-3,3-diphenylpropyl)-4-phenylpiperidine-4-carboxylate Hydrochloride, 1261·3
Ethyl N-{(R)-Cyclohexyl[((2S)-2-{[4-(hydroxycarbamimidoyl)benzyl]carbamoyl}-1-azetidinyl)carbonyl]methyl}glycinate, 952·1
Ethyl Cysteine Hydrochloride, 1121·2
Ethyl 6-Decyloxy-7-ethoxy-4-hydroxyquinoline-3-carboxylate, 603·2
Ethyl Deoxyuridine, 632·1
Ethyl 3-(2-Diethylaminoethyl)-4-methylcoumarin-7-yloxyacetate Hydrochloride, 880·2
Ethyl Dihydroxypropyl PABA, 1157·1
(±)-Ethyl trans-2-Dimethylamino-1-phenylcyclohex-3-ene-1-carboxylate Hydrochloride Hemihydrate, 94·1
Ethyl N-Dimethylphosphoramidocyanidate, 1719·2
Ethyl 6-[(4,4-Dimethylthiochroman-6-yl)ethynyl]nicotinate, 1160·2
Ethyl (3α,16α)-Eburnamenine-14-carboxylate, 1764·2
Ethyl Ethanoate, 1474·3
Ethyl Ether, 1298·3, 1474·2
Ethyl 3-{6-[Ethyl(2-hydroxypropyl)amino]pyridazin-3-yl}carbazate, 878·2
Ethyl 8-Fluoro-5,6-dihydro-5-methyl-6-oxo-4H-imidazo[1,5-a][1,4]benzodiazepine-3-carboxylate, 1038·3
Ethyl Gallate, 1168·1
Ethyl Green, 1171·1
Ethyl 4-(6-Guanidinohexanoyloxy)benzoate Methanesulphonate, 1690·1
Ethyl Hydrogen Fumarate, 1147·3
(−)-3-Ethyl Hydrogen (R)-3,4-Thiazolidinedicarboxylate, 1131·1
Ethyl (Z)-[(1-{N-[(p-Hydroxyamidino)benzoyl]-L-alanyl}-4-piperidyl)oxy] Acetate, 996·3
Ethyl Hydroxybenzoate, 1183·2
Ethyl 2-Hydroxybenzoate, 37·3
Ethyl 4-Hydroxybenzoate, 1183·2
Ethyl 1-(3-Hydroxy-3-phenylpropyl)-4-phenylpiperidine-4-carboxylate Hydrochloride, 83·2
Ethyl 10-(4-Iodophenyl)undecanoate, 1064·1
Ethyl Iodophenylundecylate, 1064·1
Ethyl Lactate, 1147·1
Ethyl Loflazepate, 698·1
Ethyl 3-Methoxy-15-apo-ϕ-caroten-15-oate, 1147·1
Ethyl (all-trans)-9-(4-Methoxy-2,3,6-trimethylphenyl)-3,7-dimethylnona-2,4,6,8-tetra-enoate, 1147·1
3-Ethyl 5-Methyl 2-(2-Aminoethoxymethyl)-4-(2-chlorophenyl)-1,4-dihydro-6-methylpyridine-3,5-dicarboxylate Monobenzenesulphonate, 862·1
Ethyl Methyl 4-(2,3-Dichlorophenyl)-1,4-dihydro-2,6-dimethylpyridine-3,5-dicarboxylate, 914·3
Ethyl Methyl 1,4-Dihydro-2,6-dimethyl-4-(3-nitrophenyl)pyridine-3,5-dicarboxylate, 973·3
Ethyl Methyl Ketone, 1476·2
R-(+)-Ethyl 1-(α-Methylbenzyl)imidazole-5-carboxylate, 1299·1
Ethyl N-Methyl-N-[α-(2-methylimidazo[4,5-c]pyridin-1-yl)tosyl]-L-leucinate, 1707·2
Ethyl (3-Methyl-4-oxo-5-piperidinothiazolidin-2-ylidene)acetate, 914·2
Ethyl 1-Methyl-4-phenylperhydroazepine-4-carboxylate Dihydrogen Citrate, 37·2
Ethyl 1-Methyl-4-phenylpiperidine-4-carboxylate Hydrochloride, 80·2
Ethyl 3-Methyl-2-thioxo-4-imidazoline-1-carboxylate, 1596·2
Ethyl [10-(3-Morpholinopropionyl)phenothiazin-2-yl]carbamate, 961·3
Ethyl Nicotinate, 37·2
Ethyl Oleate, 1685·2
Ethyl Orthoformate, 1121·2
Ethyl Oxide, 1474·2
Ethyl Parahydroxybenzoate, 1183·2
Ethyl Phenyl Carbinol, 1731·1
Ethyl (E)-3-Phenylprop-2-enoate, 1685·2
Ethyl Phthalate, 1473·2
Ethyl 3-(Phthalazin-1-yl)carbazate Hydrochloride Monohydrate, 1015·1
Ethyl p-Piperidinoacetylaminobenzoate, 1376·3
Ethyl Propionate, 1761·3
Ethyl Salicylate, 37·3
Ethyl 3,5,6-Tri-O-benzyl-D-glucofuranoside, 1757·3
Ethyl 3,4,5-Trihydroxybenzoate, 1168·1
Ethyl 4-(3,4,5-Trimethoxycinnamoyl)piperazin-1-ylacetate Hydrogen Maleate, 884·2
Ethyl Vanillin, 1685·3
Ethyladrianol Hydrochloride, 914·1
(R)-4-(Ethylamino)-3,4-dihydro-2-(3-methoxypropyl)-2H-thieno[3,2-e]-1,2-thiazine-6-sulfonamide 1,1-Dioxide, 877·1
(4S,6S)-4-(Ethylamino)-5,6-dihydro-6-methyl-4H-thieno[2,3-b]thiopyran-2-sulphonamide 7,7-Dioxide Hydrochloride, 908·3
α-(1-Ethylaminoethyl)protocatechuyl Alcohol Hydrochloride, 1119·1
2-Ethylamino-1-(3-hydroxyphenyl)ethanol Hydrochloride, 914·1
1-[3-(Ethylamino)-2-pyridyl]-4-[(5-methoxyindol-2-yl)carbonyl]piperazine Monomethanesulfonate, 629·1
2-Ethylamino-2-(2-thienyl)cyclohexanone Hydrochloride, 1310·2
Ethylamphetamine Hydrochloride, 1588·1
Ethylbenzhydramine, 431·3
2-Ethylbenzofuran-3-yl 4-Hydroxy-3,5-diiodophenyl Ketone, 415·1
α-Ethylbenzyl Alcohol, 1731·1
Ethylcellulose, 1579·1
Ethylcellulosum, 1579·1
2-(N-Ethylcrotonamido)-N,N-dimethylbutyramide, 1592·3
N-Ethylcrotono-o-toluidide, 1145·1
Ethyldicoumarol, 914·1
(RS)-1-Ethyl-6,8-difluoro-1,4-dihydro-7-(3-methylpiperazin-1-yl)-4-oxoquinoline-3-carboxylic Acid Hydrochloride, 227·2
(3S,4R)-3-Ethyldihydro-4-[(1-methyl-1H-imidazol-5-yl)methyl]furan-2(3H)-one, 1494·3
1-Ethyl-1,4-dihydro-7-methyl-4-oxo-1,8-naphthyridine-3-carboxylic Acid, 234·1
1-Ethyl-1,4-dihydro-4-oxo-1,3-dioxolo[4,5-g]cinnoline-3-carboxylic Acid, 188·1
5-Ethyl-5,8-dihydro-8-oxo-1,3-dioxolo[4,5-g]quinoline-7-carboxylic Acid, 240·3
8-Ethyl-5,8-dihydro-5-oxo-2-(piperazin-1-yl)pyrido[2,3-d]pyrimidine-6-carboxylic Acid, 243·1
1-Ethyl-1,4-dihydro-4-oxo-7-(4-pyridyl)quinoline-3-carboxylic Acid, 254·1
8-Ethyl-5,8-dihydro-5-oxo-2-(pyrrolidin-1-yl)pyrido[2,3-d]pyrimidine-6-carboxylic Acid, 244·1
Ethyldimethyl(1-methyl-3,3-diphenylpropyl)ammonium Bromide, 482·1
3-Ethyl-5,5-dimethyl-2,4-oxazolidinedione, 360·1
(+)-(R)-α-Ethyl-N,N-dimethyl-α-{[(3,4,5-trimethoxybenzyl)oxy]methyl}benzylamine, 1266·3
(6R)-6-[R-2-(4-Ethyl-2,3-dioxopiperazine-1-carboxamido)-2-phenylacetamido]penicillanic Acid Monohydrate, 243·1
7-[(2R,3S)-2-(4-Ethyl-2,3-dioxopiperazin-1-ylcarboxamido)-3-hydroxybutyramido]-7-methoxy-3-(1-methyl-1H-tetrazol-5-ylthiomethyl)-3-cephem-4-carboxylic Acid., 171·2
N-Ethyl-3,3′-diphenyldipropylamine Citrate, 1250·2
2-Ethyl-3,3-diphenyl-5-methylpyrrolidine, 58·2
Éthyldithiourame, 1681·3
Ethylendiaminum, 1686·1
Ethylene Alcohol, 1685·3
Ethylene Chlorohydrin, 1179·1
Ethylene Dibromide, 1505·1
Ethylene Dichloride, 1505·1
Ethylene Fluoride, 1236·2
Ethylene Glycol, 1685·3
Ethylene Glycol Monolaurate, 1411·3
Ethylene Glycol Monomethyl Ether, 1475·2
Ethylene Glycol Mono-oleate, 1411·3
Ethylene Glycol Monopalmitostearate, 1411·3
Ethylene Glycol Monosalicylate, 44·3
Ethylene Glycol Monostearate, 1411·3
Ethylene Glycol Stearate, 1411·3
Éthylène Glycol (Stéarate d'), 1411·3
Ethylene Glycol Stearates, 1411·3
Ethylene Oxide, 1179·1
1,1′-Ethylene-2,2′-bipyridyldiylium Dibromide, 1504·3
(S,S)-N,N′-Ethylenebis(2-aminobutan-1-ol) Dihydrochloride, 211·3
4,4′-Ethylenebis[1-(hydroxymethyl)-2,6-piperazinedione] Bis(isobutyl Carbonate), 583·3
NN′-Ethylenebis(3-methylaminopropyl 3,4,5-Trimethoxybenzoate) Dihydrochloride, 931·2
Ethylenediamine, 1686·1
Ethylenediamine Hydrate, 1686·1
Ethylenediamine, Theophylline and, 780·2
Ethylenediamine Thioctate, 1754·3
Ethylenediaminetetra-acetate, Calcium Disodium, 1051·3
Ethylenediaminetetra-acetate, Disodium Dihydrogen, 1037·3
Ethylenediaminetetra-acetate, Trisodium Hydrogen, 1037·3
Ethylenediaminetetra-acetic Acid, 1038·2
2,2′-Ethylenedi-iminobis(ethylamine) Dihydrochloride, 1055·2
Ethyleneglycol Monophenylether, 1189·1
Ethyleneimine Compounds, 492·1
Ethylenglycoli Monopalmitostearas, 1411·3
Ethylenglycoli Monostearas, 1411·3
Ethyleni Glycoli Stearas, 1411·3
Ethylephedrine Hydrochloride, 1121·2
Ethylestrenol, 1554·1
17α-Ethylestr-4-en-17β-ol, 1554·1
6-[(3R,4S,5S,7R)-7-{(2S,3S,5S)-5-Ethyl-5-[(2R,5R,6S)-5-ethyltetrahydro-5-hydroxy-6-methyl-2H-pyran-2-yl]tetrahydro-3-methyl-2-furyl}4-hydroxy-3,5-dimethyl-6-oxononyl]-2-hydroxy-m-toluic Acid, 606·1
1-Ethyl-6-fluoro-1,4-dihydro-7-(4-methyl-1-piperazinyl)-4-oxo-3-quinolinecarboxylic Acid Methanesulphonate Dihydrate, 241·3
1-Ethyl-6-fluoro-1,4-dihydro-4-oxo-7-(1-piperazinyl)-1,8-naphthyridine-3-carboxylic Acid, 207·2

1-Ethyl-6-fluoro-1,4-dihydro-4-oxo-7-(piperazin-1-yl)quinoline-3-carboxylic Acid, 238·3
Ethylguaiacol, 1159·2
(±)-4′-[4-(Ethylheptylamino)-1-hydroxybutyl]methanesulfonanilide Fumarate (2:1), 938·1
Ethylhexabital, 689·2
Ethylhexadecyldimethylammonium Ethyl Sulphate, 1185·2
(2*S*,3*R*,11b*S*)-3-Ethyl-1,3,4,6,7,11b-hexahydro-9,10-dimethoxy-2-[(1*R*)-1,2,3,4-tetrahydro-6,7-dimethoxy-1-isoquinolylmethyl]-2*H*-benzo[*a*]quinolizine Dihydrochloride Heptahydrate, 604·3
(3a*S*,4*R*,7*R*,9*R*,10*R*,11*R*,13*R*,15*R*,15a*R*)-4-Ethyl-3a,7,9,11,13,15-hexamethyl-11-{[3-(quinolin-3-yl)prop-2-enyl]oxy}-10-{[3,4,6-trideoxy-3-(dimethylamino)-β-D-*xylo*-hexopyranosyl]oxy}octahydro-2*H*-oxacyclotetradecino[4,3-*d*]oxazole-2,6,8,14(1*H*,7*H*,9*H*)-tetrone, 185·1
Ethylhexanediol, 1505·1
2-Ethylhexane-1,3-diol, 1505·1
2-Ethylhexyl 2-Cyano-3,3-diphenylacrylate, 1154·3
2-Ethylhexyl α-Cyano-β-phenylcinnamate, 1154·3
2-Ethylhexyl 4-(Dimethylamino)benzoate, 1155·1
2-Ethylhexyl Salicylate, 1154·3
2-Ethylhexyl-*p*-methoxycinnamate, 1154·3
7-Ethyl-10-hydroxycamptothecin, 564·3
(+)-7-Ethyl-10-hydroxycamptothecine 10-[1,4′-Bipiperidine]-1′-carboxylate Hydrochloride Trihydrate, 564·1
13β-Ethyl-17β-hydroxy-18,19-dinor-17α-pregna-4,15-dien-20-yn-3-one, 1556·1
13β-Ethyl-17β-hydroxy-18,19-dinor-17α-pregna-4,9,11-trien-20-yn-3-one, 1556·2
(±)-13-Ethyl-17β-hydroxy-18,19-dinor-17α-pregn-4-en-20-yn-3-one, 1563·2
(−)-13β-Ethyl-17β-hydroxy-18,19-dinor-17α-pregn-4-en-20-yn-3-one, 1563·2
13-Ethyl-17-hydroxy-18,19-dinor-17α-pregn-4-en-20-yn-3-one Oxime, 1562·1
17α-Ethyl-17β-hydroxyestr-4-en-3-one, 1562·2
16β-Ethyl-17β-hydroxyestr-4-en-3-one, 1565·2
13β-Ethyl-3-hydroxyimino-18,19-dinor-17α-pregn-4-en-20-yn-17β-yl Acetate, 1563·2
13-Ethyl-17-hydroxy-11-methylene-18,19-dinor-17α-pregn-4-en-20-yn-3-one, 1554·1
2-Ethyl-2-hydroxymethylpropane-1,3-diol Trinitrate, 989·3
Ethyl(3-hydroxyphenyl)dimethylammonium Chloride, 1490·3
(2*RS*)-*N*-Ethyl-3-hydroxy-2-phenyl-*N*-(pyridin-4-ylmethyl)propanamide, 491·1
1,1′-Ethylidenebis(tryptophan), 321·1
(5*S*,5a*R*,8a*S*,9*R*)-9-(4,6-*O*-Ethylidene-β-D-glucopyranosyloxy)-5,8,8a,9-tetrahydro-5-(4-hydroxy-3,5-dimethoxyphenyl)-isobenzofuro[5,6-*f*][1,3]benzodioxol-6(5a*H*)-one, 551·3
2-Ethylidine-1,5-dimethyl-3,3-diphenylpyrrolidine, 58·2
4-(2-Ethyl-2-indanyl)imidazole, 1032·3
Ethylis Acetas, 1474·3
Ethylis Aminobenzoas, 1370·3
Ethylis Biscoumacetas, 914·1
Ethylis Chloridum, 1376·2
Ethylis Oleas, 1685·2
Ethylis Parahydroxybenzoas, 1183·2
Ethylis Paraoxybenzoas, 1183·2
5-Ethyl-5-isopentylbarbituric Acid, 670·1
Ethylmercury, 1713·2
4-[Ethyl(4-methoxy-α-methylphenethyl)amino]butyl Veratrate Hydrochloride, 1273·1
(*all-trans*)-*N*-Ethyl-9-(4-methoxy-2,3,6-trimethylphenyl)-3,7-dimethyl-2,4,6,8-nonatetraenamide, 1154·2
(−)-2-(Ethylmethylamino)-1-phenylpropan-1-ol Hydrochloride, 1121·2
5-Ethyl-5-(1-methylbutyl)barbituric Acid, 713·2
13β-Ethyl-11-methylene-18,19-dinor-17α-pregn-4-en-20-yn-17β-ol, 1547·2
3-Ethyl-3-methylglutarimide, 1585·2
1-({*p*-[2-(3-Ethyl-4-methyl-2-oxo-3-pyrroline-1-carboxamido)ethyl]phenyl}sulfonyl)-3-(*trans*-4-methylcyclohexyl)urea, 332·2
3-(3-Ethyl-1-methylperhydroazepin-3-yl)phenol Hydrochloride, 56·3
*N*-Ethyl-α-methylphenethylamine Hydrochloride, 1588·1
5-Ethyl-1-methyl-5-phenylbarbituric Acid, 366·3
*N*-Ethyl-*N*-(2-methylphenyl)-2-butenamide, 1145·1
5-Ethyl-3-methyl-5-phenylhydantoin, 366·2
4-Ethyl-4-methylpiperidine-2,6-dione, 1585·2
4′-Ethyl-2-methyl-3-piperidinopropiophenone Hydrochloride, 1394·3
2-Ethyl-2-methylsuccinimide, 360·1
4-{2-[2-Ethyl-3′-methyl-5′-(tetrahydro-6-hydroxy-6-hydroxymethyl-3,5-dimethylpyran-2-yl)perhydro-2,2′-bifuran-5-yl]-9-hydroxy-2,8-dimethyl-1,6-dioxaspiro[4.5]dec-7-yl}3-methoxy-2-methylpentanoic Acid, 611·1
*N*-Ethyl-α-methyl-3-trifluoromethylphenethylamine Hydrochloride, 1588·2
(*S*)-*N*-Ethyl-α-methyl-3-trifluoromethylphenethylamine Hydrochloride, 1586·3
2-Ethyl-3-methylvaleramide, 727·2
Ethylmorphine, 37·3
Ethylmorphine Camphorate, 37·3
Ethylmorphine Camsilate, 37·3
Ethylmorphine Hydrochloride, 37·3
3-*O*-Ethylmorphine Hydrochloride Dihydrate, 37·3
Ethylmorphini Hydrochloridum, 37·3
Ethylmorphinium Chloride, 37·3
1-Ethyl-4-(2-morpholinoethyl)-3,3-diphenyl-2-pyrrolidinone Hydrochloride Monohydrate, 1587·2
Ethylnorgestrienone, 1556·2
Ethylnorphenylephrine Hydrochloride, 914·1
(3a*S*,4*R*,7*R*,9*R*,10*R*,11*R*,13*R*,15*R*,15a*R*)-4-Ethyloctahydro-11-methoxy-3a,7,9,11,13,15-hexamethyl-1-{4-[4-(3-pyridyl)imidazol-1-yl]butyl}-10-{[3,4,6-trideoxy-3-(dimethylamino)-β-D-*xylo*-hexopyranosyl]oxy}-2*H*-oxacyclotetradecino[4,3-*d*][1,3]oxazole-2,6,8,14(1*H*,7*H*,9*H*)-tetrone, 265·2
Ethyloestrenol, 1554·1
*N*-{1-[2-(4-Ethyl-5-oxo-2-tetrazolin-1-yl)ethyl]-4-(methoxymethyl)-4-piperidyl}propionanilide Hydrochloride, 12·2
Ethylparaben, 1183·2
5-(1-Ethylpentyl)-3-(trichloromethylthio)hydantoin, 396·2
5-(1-Ethylpentyl)-3-(trichloromethylthio)imidazolidine-2,4-dione, 396·2
Ethylphenacemide, 367·3
5-Ethyl-5-phenylbarbituric Acid, 367·3
5-Ethyl-5-phenylbarbituric Acid with (−)-*N*,α-Dimethylcyclohexaneethylamine, 353·3
*N*-Ethyl-3-phenylbicyclo[2.2.1]hept-2-ylamine Hydrochloride, 1588·2
*N*-Ethyl-1-phenylcyclohexylamine, 1730·3
2-Ethyl-2-phenylglutarimide, 701·2
3-Ethyl-5-phenylhydantoin, 361·1
5-Ethyl-5-phenylhydantoin, 366·2
1-(*m*-Ethylphenyl)-1-methyl-3-(1-naphthyl)guanidine, 1655·3
5-Ethyl-5-phenylperhydropyrimidine-4,6-dione, 376·3
3-Ethyl-3-phenylpiperidine-2,6-dione, 701·2
1-Ethyl-3-piperidyl Diphenylacetate Hydrochloride, 487·3
Ethylpipethanate Bromide, 487·3
(±)-2-(*N*-Ethylpropylamino)-butyro-2′,6′-xylidide, 1376·3
2-Ethylpyridine-4-carbothioamide, 212·3
(±)-5-{*p*-[2-(5-Ethyl-2-pyridyl)ethoxy]benzyl}-2,4-thiazolidinedione Hydrochloride, 344·1
*N*-Ethyl-*N*-(4-pyridylmethyl)tropamide, 491·1
*N*-(1-Ethylpyrrolidin-2-ylmethyl)-5-ethylsulphonyl-2-methoxybenzamide Hydrochloride, 723·1
*N*-(1-Ethylpyrrolidin-2-ylmethyl)-2-methoxy-5-sulphamoylbenzamide, 722·2
Ethylsalicylamide, 37·2
$N^1$-Ethylsissomicin, 236·3
1-[2-(Ethylsulphonyl)ethyl]-2-methyl-5-nitroimidazole, 617·1
*N*-Ethyltenamfetamine, 1593·3
3-Ethyl-1,6,7,11b-tetrahydro-9,10-dimethoxy-2-(1,2,3,4-tetrahydro-6,7-dimethoxy-1-isoquinolylmethyl)-4*H*-benzo[*a*]quinolizine Dihydrochloride, 603·2
2-(6-{5-[2-(5-Ethyltetrahydro-5-hydroxy-6-methylpyran-2-yl)-15-hydroxy-2,10,12-trimethyl-1,6,8-trioxadispiro[4.1.5.3]pentadec-13-en-9-yl]-2-hydroxy-1,3-dimethyl-4-oxoheptyl}tetrahydro-3,5-dimethylpyran-2-yl)butyric Acid, 611·1
3-Ethyl-1,5,6,7-tetrahydro-2-methyl-5-(morpholinomethyl)indol-4-one Hydrochloride, 709·3
7-Ethyltheophylline Amphetamine Hydrochloride, 1588·2
2-Ethylthioisonicotinamide, 212·3
2-Ethylthio-10-[3-(4-methylpiperazin-1-yl)-propyl]phenothiazine, 442·1
*N*-Ethyl-*N*-*o*-tolylcrotonamide, 1145·1
(1α,14α,16β)-20-Ethyl-1,14,16-trimethoxyaconitane-4,8,9-triol 4-[2-(Acetylamino)benzoate] Hydrobromide, 945·1
(3*s*,6*R*,7*S*,8*r*)-8-Ethyl-3-[(*S*)-tropoyloxy]-6,7-epoxytropanium Bromide, 790·3
Ethynodiol Diacetate, 1554·2
17α-Ethynylestra-1,3,5(10)-triene-3,17β-diol, 1553·2
5-Ethynyluracil, 550·2
Ethyol, 1980·2
Etiaxil, 1980·2
Etibi, 1980·2
Etidocaína, Hidrocloruro de, 1376·3
Etidocaine, 1376·3
Etidocaine Hydrochloride, 1376·3
Etidrate, 1980·2
Etidron, 1980·2
Etidronate Disodium, 771·2
Etidronate, Rhenium ($^{186}$Re), 1525·1
Etidronato Disódico, 771·2
Etidronic Acid, 771·2
Etidrónico, Ácido, 771·2
Etifenin, Technetium ($^{99m}$Tc), 1526·1
Etifollin, 1980·3
Etifoxin Hydrochloride, 698·1
Etifoxina, Hidrocloruro de, 698·1
Etifoxine Hydrochloride, 698·1
Etil, 1980·3
Etil Adrianol, 1980·3
Etilamfetamine Hydrochloride, 1588·1
Etilcelulosa, 1579·1
Etilcisteína, Hidrocloruro de, 1121·2
Etildopanan, 1980·3
Etilefrina, Hidrocloruro de, 914·1
Etilefrine Hydrochloride, 914·1
Etilefrine Polistirex, 914·1
Etilefrini Hydrochloridum, 914·1
Etilenglicol, 1685·3
Etiles, 1980·3
Etilestrenol, 1554·1
Etilmorfina, Hidrocloruro de, 37·3
Etilo, Biscumacetato de, 914·1
Etilo, Cloruro de, 1376·2
Etilparabeno, 1183·2
Etilsulfato de Mecetronio, 1185·2
Etiltox, 1980·3
Etilvanilina, 1685·3
Etimonis, 1980·3
Etindrax, 1980·3
Etinilestradiol, 1553·2
Etinodiol, Diacetato de, 1554·2
Etiocholanolone, 1571·2
Etión, 1505·1
Etionamida, 212·3
Etionamide, 212·3
Etioven, 1980·3
Etiplus, 1980·3
Etiproston Trometamol, 1518·1
Etiproston Tromethamine, 1518·1
Eti-Puren, 1980·3
*S*-Etiracetam, 366·1
Etizem, 1980·3
Etizolam, 698·1
Etmoren, 1980·3
Etnoderm, 1980·3
ETO CS, 1980·3
Etobromuro de Pipetanato, 487·3
Etocin, 1980·3
Etocoderm, 1980·3
Etocovit, 1980·3
Etocris, 1980·3
Etodolac, 37·3
Etodolaco, 37·3
Etodolacum, 37·3
Etodolic Acid, 37·3
Etofamida, 605·2
Etofamide, 605·2
Etofen, 1980·3
Etofenamate, 38·1
Etofenamato, 38·1
Etofenamatum, 38·1
Etofenprox, 1505·2
Etofibrate, 914·2
Etofibrato, 914·2
Etofilina, 785·1
Etofilina, Clofibrato de, 914·2
Etofylline, 785·1
Etofylline Clofibrate, 914·2
Etofylline Nicotinate, 785·1
Etofyllinum, 785·1
Eto-Gry, 1980·3
Etoheptacina, Citrato de, 37·2
Etohexadiol, 1505·1
Etoina, 1980·3
Etomedac, 1980·3
Etomidate, 1299·1
Etomidato, 1299·1
Etomidatum, 1299·1
Etomine, 1980·3
E-Tonil, 1980·3
Etono, 1980·3
Etonogestrel, 1554·1
Etonox, 1980·3
Etopabato, 605·1
Etopan, 1980·3
Etoperidona, Hidrocloruro de, 292·1
Etoperidone Hydrochloride, 292·1
Etophylate, 1980·3
Etopofos, 1980·3
Etopophos, 1980·3
Etopos, 1980·4
Etoposide, 551·3
Etoposide Phosphate, 551·3
Etopósido, 551·3
Etoposidum, 551·3
Etopul, 1980·4
Etorfina, Hidrocloruro de, 38·3
Etoricoxib, 38·2
Etorphine Hydrochloride, 38·3
Etosid, 1980·4
Etosin, 1980·4
Etosuximida, 360·1
Etotoína, 361·1
Etoxazorutósido, 1688·2
Etoxifenildietilfenilbutilamina, Hidrocloruro de, 1685·2
Etoxiquina, 1179·1
Etoxisclerol, 1980·4
Etozolin, 914·2
Etozolina, 914·2
ETP, 587·2
Etrafon, 1980·4
Etramon, 1980·4
Etrane, 1980·4
Etrat, 1980·4
Etrat Sportgel, 1980·4
Etrat Sportsalbe MPS, 1980·4
Etretin, 1140·2
Etretinate, 1147·1
Etretinato, 1147·1
Etro, 1980·4
Etro Balsamico, 1980·4
E-Trocima-P, 1980·4
Etrogran, 1980·4
Etrolate, 1980·4
Etronil, 1980·4
Etrosteron, 1980·4
Etrotab, 1980·4

ETS-2%— *see* Erythra-Derm, 1976·3
ETTN, 989·3
Ettriol Trinitrate, 989·3
Etumina, 1980·4
Etumine, 1980·4
Etumin— *see* Etumin/Entumin, 1980·4
Etynodiol Diacetate, 1554·2
Etyofil, 1980·4
Etyprenaline Hydrochloride, 787·3
Etyzem, 1980·4
EU-1806, 964·1
EU-4200, 1212·2
EU-5306, 241·3
Eubetal, 1980·4
Eubetal Antibiotico, 1980·4
Eubetal Biotic, 1981·1
Eubine, 1981·1
Eubiol, 1981·1
Eubiolac, 1981·1
Euboral, 1981·1
Eubos, 1981·1
Eubucal, 1981·1
Eucabal, 1981·1
Eucabal-Balsam S, 1981·1
Eucafluid N, 1981·1
Eucalcic, 1981·1
Eucalin, 1981·1
Eucaliptan, 1981·1
Eucalipto, Aceite Esencial de, 1686·2
Eucalipto Composto, 1981·1
Eucalipto, Esencia de, 1686·2
Eucaliptol, 1672·1, 1981·1
Eucaliptol Composto, 1981·1
Eucalyptamint, 1981·1
Eucalypti Aetheroleum, 1686·2
Eucalypti Folium, 1686·1
Eucalypti, Oleum, 1686·2
Eucalyptine, 1981·1
Eucalyptine Le Brun, 1981·1
Eucalyptine Pholcodine Le Brun, 1981·2
Eucalyptol, 1672·1
Eucalyptospirine, 1981·2
Eucalyptospirine Lact, 1981·2
Eucalyptrol L, 1981·2
*Eucalyptus globulus*, 1686·1, 1686·2
Eucalyptine Pholcodine, 1981·2
Eucalyptus Leaf, 1686·1
Eucalyptus Oil, 1672·1, 1686·2
*Eucalyptus polybractea*, 1686·2
Eucalyptus Rectifiée, Essence d', 1686·2
*Eucalyptus smithii*, 1686·2
Eucalyptusblätter, 1686·1
Eucalytux, 1981·2
Eucament, 1981·2
Eucamenth, 1981·2
Eucanol, 1981·2
Eucar, 1981·2
Eucarbon, 1981·2
Eucarbon— *see* Carbondifer, 1869·4
Eucardic, 1981·2
Eucardina, 1981·2
Eucardion, 1981·2
Eucarnil, 1981·2
Eucatropina, Hidrocloruro de, 482·1
Eucatropine Hydrochloride, 482·1
Eucatropinium Chloride, 482·1
Eucerin Preparations, 1981·2
Eucerinum, 1981·3
Euceta, 1981·3
Euceta avec Camomille et Arnica, 1981·3
Euceta mit Kamille, 1981·4
Euceta Pic, 1981·4
Euchessina, 1981·4
Euchessina CM, 1981·4
Euci, 1981·4
Eucid, 1981·4
Eucil, 1981·4
Eucillin, 1981·4
Euciton, 1981·4
Euciton Complex, 1981·4
Euclorina, 1981·4
Eucol, 1981·4
Eucoprost, 1981·4
Eucor, 1981·4
Eucorten, 1981·4
Eucycline, 1981·4
Eudal-SR, 1981·4
Eudemine, 1981·4
Eudent con Glysan, 1981·4
Euderm, 1981·4
Eudermal Pasta, 1981·4
Eudermal Sapone allo Zolfo pH 5, 1981·4
Eudermico, 1981·4
Eudextran, 1981·4
Eudigestio, 1981·4
Eudigox, 1981·4
Eudipar, 1981·4
Eudolene, 1981·4
Eudon, 1982·1
Eudorlin, 1982·1
Eudorlin Extra, 1982·1
EUDR, 632·1
Eudur, 1982·1
Eudyna, 1982·1
Eufans, 1982·1
Eufenil, 1982·1
Eufermen, 1982·1
Eufibron, 1982·1
Eufidol, Magnesium- — *see* Magnesium-Eufidol, 2112·1
Eufilin, 1982·1
Eufilina, 1982·1
Eufimenth N Mild, 1982·1
Eufimenth-Balsam N, 1982·1
Euflat I, 1982·1
Euflat-E, 1982·1
Euflavina, 1165·3
Euflavine, 1165·3
Euflex, 1982·1
Euflux-N, 1982·1
Eufor, 1982·1
Euforbia, 1686·3
Eufrasia, 1686·3
Euftalmina, Clorhidrato de, 482·1
Eufusin, 1982·1
Eugalac, 1982·1
Eugalan Topfer Forte, 1982·1
Eugen., 1686·2
*Eugenia caryophyllus*, 1673·2
Eugenic Acid, 1686·2
Eugenol, 1673·3, 1686·2
Eugenol-Guaiacolo Composto, 1982·1
Eugenolum, 1686·2
Eugerial, 1982·1
Eugerminal, 1982·1
Eugiron, 1982·1
Euglamin, 1982·1
Euglim, 1982·1
Euglucan, 1982·1
Euglucon, 1982·2
Euglucon, Semi- — *see* Semi-Euglucon, 2284·2
Euglucon N, 1982·2
Euglucon N, Semi- — *see* Semi-Euglucon N, 2284·2
Euglusid, 1982·2
Eugrippine, 1982·2
Eugune, 1982·2
Eugusal, 1982·2
Eugynol, 1982·2
Eugynon, 1982·2
Eugynon 30, 1982·2
Eugynon 250, 1982·2
Euhypnos, 1982·2
Euipnos, 1982·2
Euka, 1982·2
Eukalisan Forte, 1982·2
Eukalisan N, 1982·2
Eukamillat, 1982·2
Eukavan, 1982·2
Euketos, 1982·2
Euky Bear Preparations, 1982·2
Eulactol, 1982·2
Eulactol Antifungal, 1982·2
Eulatin N, 1982·2
Eulatin NN, 1982·3
Eulexin, 1982·3
Eulexine, 1982·3
Eulip, 1982·3
Eulitop, 1982·3
Eulux, 1982·3
Eulyptan, 1982·3
Eu-Med, 1982·3
Eumetic, 1982·3
Eumetinex, 1982·3
Euminz, 1982·3
Eumol, 1982·3
Eumosone, 1982·3
Eumotol, 1982·3
Eumovate, 1982·3
Eumovate Eye Drops— *see* Cloburate, 1894·1
EuMunil, 1982·3
Eumycetoma— *see* Mycetoma, 388·3
Eunades, 1982·3
Eunasin, 1982·3
Eunerpan, 1982·3
Eunova, 1982·3
Euonymus, 1265·2
*Euonymus atropurpureus*, 1265·2
Eupantol, 1982·3
Eupatal, 1982·3
Eupatol, 1982·3
Eupatorin, 1449·3
*Eupatorium*, 1656·3
Eupatorium Oligoplex, 1982·3
Eupatorium Perfoliatum, 1661·3
*Eupatorium perfoliatum*, 1661·3
*Eupatorium purpureum*, 1695·3
Eupeclanic, 1982·3
Eupen, 1982·3
Eupen Bronquial, 1982·3
Eupept, 1982·4
Eupeptina, 1982·4
Euphidra G2 Radical, 1982·4
Euphon, 1982·4
Euphon N, 1982·4
Euphorbia, 1686·3
*Euphorbia antisyphilitica*, 1480·2
Euphorbia Complex, 1982·4
*Euphorbia hirta*, 1686·3
*Euphorbia humifusa*, 1686·3
*Euphorbia lathyrus*, 1686·3
*Euphorbia maculata*, 1686·3
*Euphorbia pekinensis*, 1686·3
*Euphorbia pilulifera*, 1686·3
Euphorbium Compositum, 1982·4
Euphorbium Compositum S, 1982·4
Euphorbium Compositum-Nasentropfen SN, 1982·4
Euphrasia, 1686·3
*Euphrasia officinalis*, 1686·3
*Euphrasia rostkoviana*, 1686·3
Euphyllin, 1982·4
Euphyllina, 1982·4
Euphylline, 1982·4
Euphyllinum, 780·2
Euphylong, 1982·4
Euphytose, 1982·4
Euplix, 1982·4
Eupneron, 1982·4
Eupnol, 1982·4
Eupragin, 1982·4
Eupres, 1982·4
Eupressin, 1982·4
Eupressin H, 1982·4
Eupressyl, 1982·4
Euproct, 1982·4
Euproctol, 1982·4
Euproctol N, 1983·1
Euprotin, 1983·1
Euquinina, 460·1
Euquinine, 460·1
Euradal, 1983·1
Euralben, 1983·1
Eurax, 1983·1
Eurax-Hydrocortisone, 1983·1
Euraxil, 1983·1
Euraxil Hidrocort, 1983·1
Eureceptor, 1983·1
Eurelix, 1983·1
Euretico, 1983·1
Eurex, 1983·1
Eurhyton, 1983·1
Eurifam, 1983·1
Euritmin, 1983·1
Euritsin, 1983·1
Eurixor, 1983·1
Eurobiol, 1983·1
Eurocal D3, 1983·1
Eurocefix, 1983·1
Eurocoal, 1983·1
Eurocolor, 1983·1
Eurocolor Post Solar, 1983·1
Eurocolor Sin Sol, 1983·1
Euroderm-A, 1983·1
Eurodin, 1983·1
Eurofer, 1983·1
Euroflash, 1983·1
Euroflu, 1983·1
Eurogel, 1983·2
Eurogesic Gel, 1983·2
Eurolase, 1983·2
Eurolat, 1983·2
Eurolol, 1983·2
Euromicina, 1983·2
Euromucil, 1983·2
Euronac, 1983·2
European Goldenrod, 1748·3
European Opium, 74·3
European Viper Venom Antiserum, 1639·1
Europiel, 1983·2
Europranolol, 1983·2
Europrazosin, 1983·2
Europrotec P, 1983·2
Europrotec Post Solar, 1983·2
Europrotec Ultra, 1983·2
Eurosan, 1983·2
Euroton, 1983·2
Eurotretin, 1983·2
Eurovan, 1983·2
Eurovir, 1983·2
Euroxi, 1983·2
Eurozyme, 1983·2
Eurythmic, 1983·2
Eusaprim, 1983·2
Eusedon Mono, 1983·2
Euserpina Cellulite, 1983·2
Euskin, 1983·2
Eusol, 1175·3
Eusovit, 1983·2
Euspirax, 1983·2
Eustidil, 1983·2
Eutalgic, 1983·2
Eutecaina, 1983·2
Euthyral, 1983·2
Euthyrox, 1983·3
Eutirox, 1983·3
Eutiz, 1983·3
Eutocol, 1983·3
Eutrodin, 1983·3
Eutrofic, 1983·3
Eutrofic Forte Gel Despigmentante, 1983·3
Eutroid, 1983·3
Eutroxsig, 1983·3
Eutys-Kili, 1983·3
Euvaderm, 1983·3
Euvaderm N, 1983·3
Euvalon, 1983·3
Euvanol, 1983·3
Euvax-B, 1983·3
Euvaxon, 1983·3
Euvegal Balance, 1983·3
Euvegal Entspannungs- und Einschlafdragees, 1983·3
Euvegal Entspannungs- und Einschlaftropfen, 1983·3
Euvegal Forte, 1983·3
Euvegal N, 1983·3
Euvifor, 1983·3
Euvitan, 1983·3
Euvitol, 1983·3
Euxat, 1983·3
Euzymina Lisina I, 1983·3
Euzymina Lisina II, 1983·4
Evacode, 1983·4
Evac-Q-Kwik, 1983·4
Evac-Q-Kwik Suppository, 1983·4
Evac-Q-Mag, 1983·4
Evac-Q-Tabs, 1983·4
Evacream, 1983·4
Evacrine, 1983·4
Evacuante, 1983·4
Evacuol, 1983·4

Evadene, 1983·4
Evadermin, 1983·4
Evadol, 1983·4
Evafer, 1983·4
Evafilm, 1983·4
Evagelin, 1983·4
Evagrip, 1983·4
Evalgan, 1983·4
Evalin, 1983·4
Evalon, 1983·4
Evalose, 1983·4
Evamilk, 1983·4
Evana, 1983·4
Evanor, 1983·4
Evanor-D, 1983·4
Evans Blue, 1658·3
Evapause, 1983·4
Evaphol, 1983·4
Evaplan, 1983·4
Evarose, 1983·4
Evasen Crema, 1984·1
Evasen Dischetti, 1984·1
Evasen Liquido, 1984·1
Evasidol, 1984·1
Evasprin, 1984·1
Evastel, 1984·1
Evatest, 1984·1
Evatest One Step, 1984·1
Evavit, 1984·1
Evazol, 1984·1
EVC, 1984·1
Eve, 1593·3, 1984·1
Evelea, 1984·1
Evening Gold, 1984·1
Evening Primrose, 1686·3
Evening Primrose Oil, 1686·3
Evercid, 1984·1
Ever-fit Cardio, 1984·1
Ever-Fit Plus, 1984·1
Evergin, 1984·1
Everolimus, 1360·1
Everon, 1984·1
Everone, 1984·1
Eversun, 1984·1
Evestrel, 1984·1
Eviantrina, 1984·1
Evicer, 1984·1
E-Vicotrat, 1984·1
E-Vicotrat + Magnesium, 1984·1
Evicyl, 1984·1
E-vidon, 1984·1
Eviepar, 1984·1
Eviletten N, 1984·1
Evilin, 1984·1
Evimal, 1984·2
E-vimin, 1984·2
Evina, 1984·2
Evinopon, 1984·2
Eviol, 1984·2
Eviol-A, 1984·2
Evion, 1984·2
Eviprostat, 1984·2
Eviprostat N, 1984·2
Eviprostat-S, 1984·2
Evisco Mistel Urtinktur, 1984·2
Evisco Misteltropfen N, 1984·2
Evista, 1984·2
Evit, 1984·2
Evitas, 1984·2
Evitex, 1984·2
Evitex A E Fuerte, 1984·2
Evitina, 1984·2
Evitocor, 1984·2
Evitocor Plus, 1984·2
Evitol, 1984·3
E-Vitum, 1984·3
Evo-Conti, 1984·3
Evolis, 1984·3
Evónimo, 1265·2
*Evonymus atropurpurea*, 1265·2
Evopad, 1984·3
Evoprim, 1984·3
Evoquin, 1984·3
Evorel, 1984·3
Evorel Conti, 1984·3
Evorel Micronor, 1984·3
Evorel Pak, 1984·3
Evorel Sequi, 1984·3
Evorelconti, 1984·3
Evo-Sequi, 1984·3
Evoxac, 1984·3
Evra, 1984·3
Evril, 1984·3
Ewadyl, 1984·3
Ewing's Sarcoma— *see* Bone Sarcoma, 524·3
EX-10-781, 1124·3
EX-4355, 290·2
Exabrol, 1984·3
Exacol, 1984·3
Exacor, 1984·3
Exact, 1984·3
ExacTech, 1984·3
Exacyl, 1984·3
Exafenil, 1984·3
Exafil, 1984·3
Ex'ail, 1984·3
Exalamin, 1984·3
Exaler, 1984·4
Exalgin, 1984·4
Exaliver, 1984·4
Exalver, 1984·4
Exametazime, Technetium ($^{99m}$Tc), 1526·1
Examicyn, 1984·4
Examida, 1984·4
Examolin, 1984·4
Exangina N, 1984·4
Exarex, 1984·4
Exastrin, 1984·4
Exasul, 1984·4
Exatech, 1984·4
Exaverm, 1984·4
Exavir, 1984·4
Exavit, 1984·4
Exazen, 1984·4
Exbenzol, 1984·4
Excedrin Preparations, 1984·4
Excedrin, Aspirin Free— *see* Aspirin Free Excedrin, 1816·3
Excegran, 1984·4
Excel ET, 1984·4
Excelcur MF1, 1984·4
Excelsior, 1984·4
Excillin, 1984·4
Excipial, 1984·4
Excipial U, 1984·4
Excivit, 1984·4
Excough, 1984·4
Exdol, 1985·1
Exe-Cort, 1985·1
Executive B, 1985·1
Executive Formula, Natures Way— *see* Natures Way Executive Formula, 2153·3
Exel, 1985·1
Exelderm, 1985·1
Exelmin, 1985·1
Exelon, 1985·1
Exemestane, 552·3
Exemestano, 552·3
Exempla, 1985·1
Exenatide, 325·1
Exendin-4, 325·1
Exertial, 1985·1
Exetin-A, 1985·1
Exeu, 1985·1
Exflam, 1985·1
Exflem, 1985·1
Exfoliac, 1985·1
Exfolium, 1985·1
Exgest LA, 1985·1
Exhirud, 1985·1
Ex-Histine, 1985·1
Exibral, 1985·1
Exidine, 1985·1
Exido, 1985·1
Exidol, 1985·1
Exil, 1985·1
Exipan, 1985·1
Exiplon, 1985·1
Exirel, 1985·1
Exisulind, 552·3
Exit, 1985·1
Exitop, 1985·2
Ex-Lax Preparations, 1985·2
Ex-Lax, Maximum Relief— *see* Maximum Relief Ex-Lax, 2116·3
Exlutena, 1985·2
Exluton, 1985·2
Exlutona, 1985·2
Exmykehl, 1985·2
Exna, 1985·2
Exneural, 1985·2
Exoamylases, 1654·2
Exocaine, 1985·2
Exocin, 1985·2
Exocine, 1985·2
Exodalina, 1985·2
Exoderil, 1985·2
Exofat, 1985·2
Exo'Fat, 1985·2
Exofur, 1985·2
*Exogonium purga*, 1268·3
Exolise, 1985·2
Exolit, 1985·2
Exolyt, 1985·2
Exomega, 1985·3
Exomega, Aderma— *see* Aderma Exomega, 1776·2
Exomuc, 1985·3
Exorex, 1985·3
Exormin, 1985·3
Exorvit, 1985·3
Exorvit VM, 1985·3
Exoseptoplix, 1985·3
Exostrept, 1985·3
Exosurf, 1985·3
Exova, 1985·3
Exovir, 1985·3
44 Exp, 1985·3
EXP-105-1, 1197·2
EXP-126, 653·1
EXP-999, 1276·3
EXP-3174, 948·1
Expafusin, 1985·3
Expahes, 1985·3
Expal, 1985·3
Expanden, 1985·3
Expandol— *see* Expandox, 1985·3
Expandox, 1985·3
Expanfen, 1985·3
Expec, 1985·3
Expectal N, 1985·3
Expectal-Balsam, 1985·3
Expectalin, 1985·3
Expectalin with Codeine, 1985·3
Expectalix, Chemists Own— *see* Chemists Own Expectalix, 1882·1
Expectal-Tropfen, 1985·3
Expectamin, 1985·3
Expectil, 1985·3
Expectobron, 1985·4
Expectocilin, 1985·4
Expectocilin Balsamico, 1985·4
Expectofar, 1985·4
Expectol, 1985·4
Expectolu, 1985·4
Expectomel, 1985·4
Expectoral, 1985·4
Expectoran Codein, 1985·4
Expectorant Cough Formula, 1985·4
Expectorant Cough Syrup, 1985·4
Expectorant and Decongestant Cough Syrup, 1985·4
Expectorant Syrup, 1985·4
Expectorants, 1112·1
Expectosan Hierbas y Miel, 1985·4
Expectotussin C, 1985·4
Expectovac, 1985·4
Expectuss, 1985·4
Expectussin, 1985·4
Expectysat N, 1985·4
Expeflen, 1985·4
Expelinct, 1985·4
Expergesic, 1985·4
Expicin, 1985·4
Expigen, 1985·4
Expiran, 1985·4
Expit, 1985·4
Exposis, 1986·1
Exprep, 1986·1
Expressed Mustard Oil, 1718·2
Expressed Oils, 1763·3
Expron, 1986·1
Expros, 1986·1
Expulin Preparations, 1986·1
Expuryl, 1986·1
Exputex, 1986·1
Exrheudon OPT, 1986·1
Exrhinin, 1986·1
Exsel, 1986·1
Exsiccated Ferrous Sulphate, 1428·3
Exsiccated Sodium Carbonate, 1747·1
Exsiccated Sodium Sulphate, 1290·1
Ext. D & C Red No. 5, 1740·1
Ext. D & C Red No. 6, 1740·1
Ext. D & C Red No. 11, 1058·1
Extencilline, 1986·1
Extendryl, 1986·1
Exteny, 1986·1
Exterol, 1986·1
Extin N, 1986·1
Extiser Q, 1986·1
Extosen, 1986·1
Extovyl, 1986·1
Extra Action Cough, 1986·1
Extra Once A Day, 1986·1
Extra Power Pain Reliever, 1986·1
Extra Strength Acetaminophen with Codeine, 1986·1
Extra Strength Alenic Alka, 1986·2
Extra Strength Alka-Seltzer Effervescent Tablets, 1986·2
Extra Strength Allergy Sinus, 1986·2
Extra Strength Analgesic, 1986·2
Extra Strength Bayer Plus, 1986·2
Extra Strength Cold Medication Daytime Relief, 1986·2
Extra Strength Cold Medication Nightime, 1986·2
Extra Strength Cold Medication Nighttime Relief, 1986·2
Extra Strength Cough Syrup Expectorant, 1986·2
Extra Strength Doans PM, 1986·2
Extra Strength Genaton, 1986·2
Extra Strength Maalox Antacid/Anti-Gas, 1986·2
Extra Strength Mintox Plus, 1986·2
Extra Strength Multi-Symptom PMS Relief, 1986·2
Extra Strength Pyrroxate, 1986·2
Extra Strength Sinus and Congestion Relief, 1986·2
Extra Strength Sinus Medication, 1986·2
Extra Strength Tylenol Headache Plus, 1986·2
Extra Strength Tylenol PM, 1986·2
Extra Strength Vicks Cough Drops, 1986·2
Extra Strong Formula 12, 1986·2
Extraboline, 1986·2
Extra-Brite, Extralife— *see* Extralife Extra-Brite, 1986·3
Extracorporeal Membrane Oxygenation, 1237·3
Extracorporeal Photochemotherapy, 1153·2
Extracorporeal PUVA, 1153·2
Extracort, 1986·2
Extracort Rhin Sine, 1986·2
Extracort Tinktur, 1986·2
Extracto de Malta, 1439·2
Extracto de Mejillón de Labios Verdes, 1696·1
Extractos de Ovario, 1565·1
Extractos Testiculares, 1569·3
Extractum Bynes, 1439·2
Extractum Concentratum Opii, 74·3
Extrafer, 1986·2
Extralife Preparations, 1986·3
Extranase, 1986·3
Extraneal, 1986·3
Extrapan, 1986·3
Extraplus, 1986·3
Extrapyramidal Disorders, 664·1
Extrapyramidal Disorders, Drug-induced— *see* Extrapyramidal Disorders, 677·1

Extrasystoles— *see* Cardiac Arrhythmias, 816·1
Extrato Hepatico Composto, 1986·3
Extrato Hepatico Vitaminado, 1986·3
Extravite, 1986·3
Extravits, 1986·3
Extur, 1986·3
Exuracid, 1986·3
Exviral, 1986·4
Exzem Oil, 1986·4
Eye Dew, 1986·4
Eye Drops, 1986·4
Eye Drops Extra, 1986·4
Eye Eze, 1986·4
Eye Formula Euphr, 1986·4
Eye Health Herbal Plus Formula 4, 1986·4
Eye Infections, Bacterial— *see* Eye Infections, 127·2
Eye Infections, Fungal— *see* Eye Infections, 388·1
Eye Mo, 1986·4
Eye Mo 36, 1986·4
Eye Mo Moist, 1986·4
Eye Scrub, 1986·4
Eye Vites, 1986·4
Eye Wash, 1986·4
Eyebrex, 1986·4
Eyebright, 1686·3
Eye-Care, Extralife— *see* Extralife Eye-Care, 1986·3
Eyecon, 1986·4
Eye-Crom— *see* Hay-Crom, 2037·1
Eyedex, 1986·4
Eye-Gene, 1986·4
Eye-Gene Soft, 1986·4
Eyelube, 1986·4
Eye-Lube-A, 1986·4
Eye-Sed, 1986·4
Eyesine, 1986·4
Eyestil, 1986·4
Eye-Stream, 1986·4
Eyetobrin, 1986·4
EyeVit, 1986·4
Eyevite, 1986·4
Eyewash, 1986·4
Eye-Zine, 1987·1
Eykosacol, 1987·1
EZ Detect, 1987·1
EZ HP, 1987·1
E-Z-Cat, 1987·1
E-Z-CAT— *see* CAT-Barium (E-Z-CAT), 1873·1
Ezede, 1987·1
Ezetimibe, 914·2
Ezetrol, 1987·1
E-Z-Gas II, 1987·1
Ez-HBT, 1987·1
E-Z-HD, 1987·1
E-Z-HD— *see* Microbar-HD (E-Z-HD), 2130·3
Ezipol, 1987·1
Ezon-T, 1987·1
Ezopen, 1987·1
Ezopta, 1987·1
Ezosina, 1987·1
E-Z-Paque, 1987·1

**F**

F, 1443·1
1 + 1-F, 1987·1
F-4, 602·3
F9, 1987·1
F080, 1987·1
F-368, 1393·3
F-440, 1393·3
F-2207, 307·3
F-3616, 1264·1
F-6066, 1544·1
F 99 Sulgan N, 1987·1
Fa-402, 482·2
FAB, 1987·1
F(ab), 1036·3
FAB Co, 1987·1
Fab (Ovine), Digoxin Immune, 1036·3
FAB Tri-Cal, 1987·1
Fabopxicam, 1987·1
Fabracin, 1987·1
Fabralgina, 1987·1
Fabramicina, 1987·1
Fabrapride, 1987·2
Fabrazol, 1987·2
Fabrazyme, 1987·2
Fabroven, 1987·2
Fabry Disease, 1651·2
Fabubac, 1987·2
Fabudol, 1987·2
Fabulaxol, 1987·2
Fabutin, 1987·2
Face Foundation, 1987·2
Face Zone, 1987·2
Facelit, 1987·2
Faces Only, 1987·2
Facetin-D, 1987·2
Facicam, 1987·2
Facilgest, 1987·2
Facilit, 1987·2
Facitor, 1987·2
Faclor, 1987·2
Facogen, 1987·2
Facort, 1987·2
Facovit, 1987·2
Fact Plus, 1987·2
Factane, 1987·2
Facteur Thymique Serique, 1756·1
Faction, 1987·2
Factioneye, 1987·2
Factive, 1987·2
Factodin, 1987·3
Factofer, 1987·3
Factofer B12, 1987·3
Factor I, 735·3, 753·2
Factor II, 735·3, 752·2
Factor IIa, 760·1
Factor III, 735·3, 760·2
Factor IV, 735·3
Factor V, 735·3
Factor VI, 735·3
Factor VII, 735·3, 750·3, 752·2
Factor VIIa, 750·3
Factor VII, Activated, 750·3
Factor VII Coagulationis Humanus, 750·3
Factor VII Fraction, Dried, 750·3
Factor VII, Human Coagulation, 750·3
Factor VIII, 735·3, 751·1
Factor VIII Coagulationis Humanus, 751·1
Factor VIII Coagulationis Humanus (AD-Nr), 751·2
Factor VIII Deficiency— *see* Haemorrhagic Disorders, 737·3
Factor VIII Fraction, Dried, 751·1
Factor VIII Inhibitor Bypassing Fraction, 752·2
Factor VIII (rDNA), 751·2
Factor VIII-related Antigen, 735·3
Factor IX, 735·3, 752·2
Factor IX Coagulationis Humanus, 752·2
Factor IX Complex, 752·3
Factor IX Deficiency— *see* Haemorrhagic Disorders, 737·3
Factor IX Fraction, Dried, 752·2
Factor X, 735·3, 752·2
Factor XI, 735·3
Factor XI Deficiency— *see* Haemorrhagic Disorders, 737·3
Factor XII, 735·3
Factor XIII, 735·3, 753·1
Factor AF2, 1987·3
Factor AG, 1987·3
Factor AG Antiacido, 1987·3
Factor AG Antiespasmodico, 1987·3
Factor Antigripal, 1987·3
Factor, Antihaemophilic, 735·3
Factor, Curling, 400·3
Factor de Necrosis Tumoral, 590·2
Factor Dermico, 1987·3
Factor, Melanocyte-stimulating-hormone-releasing, 1332·2
Factor Neurotrófico Ciliar, 1671·3
Factorine, 1987·3
Factors, Blood Clotting, 735·3
Factors, Blood Coagulation, 735·3
Factors, Hypothalamic, 1312·1
Factoss, 1987·3
Factrel, 1987·3
Factus, 1987·3
Fa-Cyl, 1987·3
Facyl M, 1987·3
FAD, 1456·2
FAD Ophthalmic Soln, 1987·3
Fadacaina, 1987·3
Fadaespasmol, 1987·3
Fadafilina, 1987·3
Fadaflumaz, 1987·3
Fadalefrina, 1987·3
Fadalivio, 1987·3
Fadametasona, 1987·3
Fadamine, 1987·3
Fadanasal, 1987·3
Fadastigmina, 1987·3
Fade Cream, 1987·3
Fadiamone, 1987·3
Fadig, 1987·3
Fadina, 1987·3
Fadine, 1987·3
Fadol, 1987·4
Fadrozol, Hidrocloruro de, 553·1
Fadrozole Hydrochloride, 553·1
Fadul, 1987·4
Faecal Impaction— *see* Constipation, 1240·2
Faecal Softeners, 1239·3
Faelac, 1987·4
Faenum-Graecum, 1688·1
Faex Siccata, 1469·1
Faexojodan, 1987·4
Fagastril, 1987·4
Fagatrim, 1987·4
Fagizol, 1987·4
Fagolipo, 1987·4
*Fagopyrum esculentum*, 1688·2
Fagorutin Buchweizen, 1987·4
Fagorutin Rosskastanien-Balsam N, 1987·4
Fagorutin Ruscus, 1987·4
Fagus, 1987·4
Fagusan, 1987·4
Faifloc, 1987·4
Fairgenol, 1987·4
Fairy ADE, 1987·4
Faktu, 1987·4
Faktu Akut, 1987·4
Falacid, 1987·4
Falcigo, 1987·4
Falcol, 1987·4
Falecalcitriol, 1462·1
Falexol, 1987·4
Falgos, 1987·4
Falibaryt— *see* Barilux, 1828·4
Falicard, 1987·4
Falimint, 1987·4
Falithrom, 1987·4
Falitonsin, 1987·4
Falkamin, 1987·4
Falmonox, 1988·1
Falot, 1988·1
Falquigut, 1988·1
Falquilax, 1988·1
False Blusher, 1717·3
False Hellebore, 1648·1
False Saffron, 1444·1
False Unicorn, 1696·3
Faltium, 1988·1
Falvin, 1988·1
Famciclovir, 633·2
Famcod, 1988·1
Famel Preparations, 1988·1
Famethacin— *see* Betacin, 1837·4
Famfur, 1505·2
Famidal, 1988·1
Famidal Ad, 1988·1
Familial Mediterranean Fever, 416·2
Family Medic First Aid Treatment, 1988·1
Family Medicated Sunburn Relief, 1988·1
Famine, 1988·1
Fam-Lax, 1988·1
Fam-Lax Senna, 1988·1
Famo, 1988·1
Famobeta, 1988·1
Famoc, 1988·1
Famocid, 1988·1
Famodil, 1988·1
Famodine, 1988·2
Famodine, Vida— *see* Vida Famodine, 2376·2
Famokey, 1988·2
Famolta, 1988·2
Famonerton, 1988·2
Famonox, 1988·2
Famophos, 1505·2
Famopril, 1988·2
Famopsin, 1988·2
Famoset, 1988·2
Famotab, 1988·2
Famotal, 1988·2
Famotec, 1988·2
Famotid, 1988·2
Famotidina, 1265·2
Famotidine, 1265·2
Famotidine *S*-Oxide, 1266·1
Famotidinum, 1265·2
Famotil, 1988·2
Famotin, 1988·2
Famowal, 1988·2
Famox, 1988·2
Famoxal, 1988·2
Famoxil, 1988·2
Famphur, 1505·2
Fampin, 1988·2
Fampridina, 1491·2
Fampridine, 1491·2
Famprofazona, 38·3
Famprofazone, 38·3
Famstim, 1988·2
Famtac, 1988·2
Famtuss, 1988·2
Famucaps, 1988·2
Famulan, 1988·2
Famulcer, 1988·2
Famvir, 1988·2
Fanaletas, 1988·3
Fanalgic, 1988·3
Fanalgin, 1988·3
Fanasil, 1988·3
Fanaxal, 1988·3
Fanciadazol, 1988·3
Fanclomax, 1988·3
Fanconi's Anaemia— *see* Aplastic Anaemia, 732·1
Fandall, 1988·3
Fangan, 1988·3
Fangji, 1656·3
Fangopress, 1988·3
Fango-Rubriment, 1988·3
Fangotherm, 1988·3
Fanhdi, 1988·3
Fanolyte, 1988·3
Fanosin, 1988·3
Fanox, 1988·3
Fansamac, 1988·3
Fansia, 1988·3
Fansidar, 1988·3
Fansidol, 1988·3
Fansimef, 1988·3
Fantomalt, 1988·3
Fantrodol, 1988·3
2-F-ara-AMP, 553·2
Faradil, 1988·3
Faradil Enzimatico, 1988·3
Faradil Novo, 1988·3
Farakil, 1988·3
Faraxen, 1988·3
Farbee with Vitamin C, 1988·4
Farbovil, 1988·4
Farcef, 1988·4
Farcolan, 1988·4
Farco-Oxicyanid-Tupfer, 1988·4
Farco-Tril, 1988·4
Farco-Uromycin, 1988·4
Farcyclin, 1988·4
Fardixon, 1988·4
Fardolpin, 1988·4
Farecef, 1988·4
Farecillin, 1988·4
Fareclox, 1988·4
Farelo, 1253·2
Faremicin, 1988·4

Faremid, 1988·4
Fareston, 1988·4
Faretrizin, 1988·4
Fárfara, 1117·2
Fargan, 1988·4
Farganesse, 1988·4
Fargestium, 1988·4
Farial, 1988·4
Farin Gola, 1988·4
Faringesic, 1988·4
Faringina, 1988·4
Faringotricina, 1988·4
Farinol, Natusor— *see* Natusor Farinol, 2153·4
Farizym, 1988·4
Farlac, 1988·4
Farlin, 1988·4
Farludiol, 1989·1
Farludiol Ciclo, 1989·1
Farlupost, 1989·1
Farlutal, 1989·1
Farlutal Estrogeno, 1989·1
Farlutale, 1989·1
Farlutes, 1989·1
Farmabroxol, 1989·1
Farmacetamol, 1989·1
Farmacola, 1989·1
Fármacos Antiinflamatorios No Esteroideos, 67·3
Farmacrom, 1989·1
Farmadiuril, 1989·1
Farmaflebon, 1989·1
Farmagola, 1989·1
Farmagripine, 1989·1
Farmalcohol, 1989·1
Farmalex, 1989·1
Farmaproina, 1989·1
Farmeban, 1989·1
Farmers' Lung— *see* Diffuse Parenchymal Lung Disease, 1079·3
Farmiblastina, 1989·1
Farmicam, 1989·1
Farmicetina, 1989·1
Farmidal S, 1989·1
Farmifeno, 1989·1
Farmigras, 1989·1
Farmin, 1989·1
Farmistin, 1989·1
Farmitrexat, 1989·1
Farmiz, 1989·2
Farmorrubicina, 1989·2
Farmorubicin, 1989·2
Farmorubicina, 1989·2
Farmorubicine, 1989·2
Farmospasmina, 1989·2
Farmotal, 1989·2
Farmotex, 1989·2
Farmoxil, 1989·2
Farm-X, 1989·2
Farm-X Duo, 1989·2
Farm-X Ginecologico, 1989·2
Farnerate, 1989·2
Farnezone, 1989·2
Farnitin, 1989·2
Farnitran, 1989·2
Farnwurzel, 108·2
Farocid, 1989·2
Farom, 1989·2
Faropenem Daloxate, 213·1
Faropenem Sódico, 213·1
Faropenem Sodium, 213·1
Faros, 1989·2
Farpectol, 1989·2
Farpik, 1989·2
Farpresse, 1989·2
Fartoxol, 1989·2
Fartricon, 1989·2
Fartussin, 1989·2
Farvicett, 1989·2
Farviran, 1989·2
Farxen, 1989·2
Fasarax, 1989·2
Fasax, 1989·2
Fasciitis— *see* Soft-tissue Rheumatism, 11·1
Fasciitis, Eosinophilic— *see* Eosinophilic Fasciitis, 1258·3
Fasciitis, Necrotising— *see* Necrotising Fasciitis, 136·2
Fascioliasis— *see* Liver Fluke Infections, 99·3
Fasciolopsiasis— *see* Intestinal Fluke Infections, 99·2
Fase, 1989·3
Faselut, 1989·3
Fasidine, 1989·3
Fasigin, 1989·3
Fasigin N, 1989·3
Fasigyn, 1989·3
Fasigyn Nistatina, 1989·3
Fasigyn VT, 1989·3
Fasigyne, 1989·3
Faslodex, 1989·3
Fasolan, 1989·3
Faspic, 1989·3
Fast Powder, 1989·3
Fast-Acting Mylanta, 1989·3
Fastenyl, 1989·3
Fastfen, 1989·3
Fastin, 1989·3
Fastium, 1989·3
Fastjekt, 1989·3
Fastum, 1989·3
Fasturtec, 1989·3
Fasudil, Hidrocloruro de, 914·3
Fasudil Hydrochloride, 914·3
Fasulide, 1989·3
Fasupond, 1989·3
Fat, Hard, 1481·1
Fat Ponceau R, 1191·3
Fate Low Protein, 1989·3
Fatec, 1989·3
Father John's Medicine Plus, 1989·4
Fatidin, 1989·4
Fatigan Bronquial, 1989·4
Fatigue, 1989·4
Fatigue L5, 1989·4
Fatol, 1989·4
Fatori 8Y, 1989·4
Fatoril, 1989·4
Fats, 1417·1
Fat-Solv, 1989·4
Fatty Acids, Essential, 1417·1
Fatty Alcohols, Sulfated, 1574·1
Fatty Oils, Vegetable, 1763·3
Faulbaumrinde, 1266·3
Faulcris, 1989·4
Faulcurium, 1989·4
Fauldetic, 1989·4
Fauldexato, 1989·4
Fauldoxo, 1989·4
Faulplatin, 1989·4
Faulviral, 1989·4
Faustan, 1989·4
Fave Di Fuca, 1989·4
Faverin, 1989·4
Favistan, 1989·4
Favorex, 1989·4
Favoxil, 1989·4
Favus— *see* Skin Infections, 390·1
FAW-76, 20·3
Fawodin, 1989·4
Faxet, 1989·4
Fazol, 1989·4
Fazol G, 1989·4
Fazolin, 1989·4
Fazoplex, 1989·4
FB-5097, 396·2
FBA-1420, 1305·3
FBA-1500, 951·3
FBB-4231, 333·1
FBC, 1989·4
FBC Plus, 1989·4
FBIC, 1989·4
5-FC, 399·3
FC-1157a, 589·2
FC-3001, 93·3
FCE-20124, 316·3
FCE-21336, 1203·3
FCE-24304, 552·3
FCF-89, 583·2
FD & C Blue No. 1, 1056·2
FD & C Blue No. 2, 1700·3
FD & C Red No. 2, 1056·1
FD & C Red No. 3, 1057·2
FD & C Red No. 40, 1056·1
FD & C Yellow No. 5, 1058·2
FD & C Yellow No. 6, 1058·2
18F-FDG, 1989·4
FDP, 1990·1
F-dUMP, 553·2
$Fe^{50}$, 1990·1
Fealin, 1990·1
Febantel, 105·2
Febarbamate, 698·2
Febarbamato, 698·2
Febichol, 1990·1
Febmil, 1990·1
Febracyl, 1990·1
Febralgin, 1990·1
Febran, 1990·1
Febranine, 1990·1
Febratic, 1990·1
Febrax, 1990·1
Febrectal, 1990·1
Febrectal Simple— *see* Febrectal, 1990·1
Febrectol, 1990·1
Febricol, 1990·1
Febrideine, Ordov— *see* Ordov Febrideine, 2192·1
Febridol, 1990·1
Febrigesic, Ordov— *see* Ordov Febrigesic, 2192·1
Febrigrip, 1990·1
Febrile Convulsions, 353·1
Febrile Seizures— *see* Febrile Convulsions, 353·1
Febrim, 1990·1
Febrimicina, 1990·1
Febrinal, 1990·1
Febro-cyl Ho-Len-Complex, 1990·1
Febronyl, 1990·1
Febs, 1990·1
Febupen, 1990·1
Febuprol, 1687·1
Febuproll, 1687·1
Fecinole, 1990·1
Fecol, 1990·1
Fecontin-F, 1990·2
Fecontin-Z, 1990·2
Fectri, 1990·2
Fectrim, 1990·2
Fedac, 1990·2
Fedac Compound, 1990·2
Fedip, 1990·2
Fedolen, 1990·2
Fedotozina, 1266·3
Fedotozine, 1266·3
Fedra, 1990·2
Fedrilate, 1121·2
Fedrilato, 1121·2
Fedrilatum, 1121·2
Feel Naturale, 1990·2
Feel Perfecte, 1990·2
Feen-A-Mint, 1990·2
Fefol, 1990·2
Fefol-Z, 1990·2
FegaCoren, 1990·2
FegaCoren N, 1990·2
Fegatex, 1990·2
Fegenor, 1990·2
Fegran, 1990·2
Feiba, 1990·2
Feiba S-TIM 4, 1990·2
Feiba TIM 4, 1990·2
Felaxen, 1990·2
Felbamate, 361·1
Felbamato, 361·1
Felbamyl, 1990·3
Felbatol, 1990·3
Felbinac, 39·1
Felbinac Diisopropanolamine, 39·1
Felbinaco, 39·1
Felcam, 1990·3
Felce Maschio, 108·2
Feldegel, 1990·3
Felden, 1990·3
Feldene, 1990·3
Feldexican, 1990·3
Feldox, 1990·3
Felexin, 1990·3
Felfar, 1990·3
Feliberal, 1990·3
Felicium, 1990·3
Felidon Neu, 1990·3
Felipresina, 1324·2
Felis, 1990·3
Felison, 1990·3
Felix, 1990·3
Felixene, 1990·3
Felixsan, 1990·3
Feller, 1990·3
Fellesan, 1990·3
Felnan, 1990·3
Felo, 1990·3
Felobits, 1990·3
Felocor, 1990·3
Feloday, 1990·3
Felodipine, 914·3
Felodipino, 914·3
Felodipinum, 914·3
Felodur, 1990·3
Felogard, 1990·3
Felo-Puren, 1990·3
Felotens, 1990·4
Felrox, 1990·4
Felsol, 1990·4
Felsol Neo, 1990·4
Felxicam, 1990·4
Felypressin, 1324·2
Fem-1, 1990·4
Fem 7, 1990·4
Fem 7 Combi, 1990·4
Fem 7 Sequi, 1990·4
Fem pH, 1990·4
Femalon, 1990·4
Femanest, 1990·4
Femanor, 1990·4
Femapak, 1990·4
Femapirin, 1990·4
Femaplus Spezial Dr Hagedorn, 1990·4
Femaprin, 1990·4
Femar, 1990·4
Femara, 1990·4
Femasekvens, 1990·4
Femaston, 1990·4
Fematab, 1990·4
Fematrix, 1990·4
Fematrix— *see* Femapak, 1990·4
Femavit, 1990·4
FemCal, 1990·4
Femcet, 1990·4
Fêmea, 1666·1
Femease, 1991·1
Femen, 1991·1
Femepen, 1991·1
Femerital, 1991·1
Femeron, 1991·1
Femex, 1991·1
Femexin, 1991·1
FemHRT, 1991·1
Femiane, 1991·1
Femibel, 1991·1
Femibion, 1991·1
Femicin, 1991·1
Femicur N, 1991·1
Femi-cyl Ho-Len-Complex, 1991·1
Femiderm, 1991·1
Femidol, 1991·1
Femigel, 1991·1
Femigoa, 1991·1
Femikliman Uno, 1991·1
Femilar, 1991·1
Femilla N, 1991·1
Femina, 1991·1
Feminalin, 1991·1
Feminax, 1991·1
Femin-Do, 1991·1
Feminease, 1991·1
Femineo, 1991·1
Feminesse, 1991·1
Feminex, 1991·1
Feminine Herbal Complex, 1991·1

Feminique, 1991·2
Feminique with Iron and Calcium, 1991·2
Feminoflex, 1991·2
Feminol, 1991·2
Feminon A, 1991·2
Feminon C, 1991·2
Feminon N, 1991·2
Feminosan, 1991·2
Feminova, 1991·2
Feminova Plus, 1991·2
Feminova-T, 1991·2
Feminvit, 1991·2
Femipak, 1991·2
Femiplexe, 1991·2
Femiplus, 1991·2
Femipres, 1991·2
Femipres Plus, 1991·2
Femiron, 1991·2
Femiron Multi-Vitamins and Iron, 1991·2
Femisan, 1991·2
Femisana, 1991·2
Femisana H, 1991·2
Femit, 1991·2
Femixol, 1991·2
Femizol-M, 1991·2
Femme, 1991·2
Fem-Mono, 1991·2
Femnet, 1991·2
Femodeen, 1991·2
Femoden, 1991·2
Femoden ED, 1991·2
Femodene, 1991·2
Femodene ED, 1991·3
Femodette, 1991·3
Femogex, 1991·3
Femoston, 1991·3
Femoston 1/5, 1991·3
Femoston Conti, 1991·3
Femoston Mono, 1991·3
Femovan, 1991·3
FemPatch, 1991·3
Femphascyl, 1991·3
Femphascyl Conti, 1991·3
Femplan-MA, 1991·3
Fempress, 1991·3
Fempress Plus, 1991·3
Femranette Mikro, 1991·3
Femring, 1991·3
Femsept, 1991·3
FemseptCombi, 1991·3
FemSeven, 1991·3
FemSeven Combi, 1991·3
FemSeven Conti, 1991·3
FemSeven Sequi, 1991·3
FemSieben, 1991·3
Femstal, 1991·3
Femstat, 1991·3
FemTab, 1991·3
FemTab Continuous, 1991·3
FemTab Sequi, 1991·3
Femtran, 1991·3
Femulen, 1991·4
Fen...— *see also under* Phen...
Fenac, 1991·4
Fenacemida, 367·3
Fenacetina, 82·2
Fenactol, 1991·4
Fenadine, Vida— *see* Vida Fenadine, 2376·2
Fenadium, 1991·4
Fenadol, 1991·4
Fenaflan, 1991·4
Fenagel, 1991·4
Fenalgin, 1991·4
Fenam, 1991·4
Fenamazida, Hidrocloruro de, 487·3
Fenamic, 1991·4
Fenamide, 1991·4
Fenamin, 1991·4
Fenamine, 1991·4
Fenamon, 1991·4
Fenantoin, 1991·4
Fenaplus, 1991·4
Fenaplus-MR, 1991·4
Fenaren, 1991·4
Fenarol-S, 1991·4
Fenasil, 1991·4
Fenason, 1991·4
Fenasprate, 20·3
Fenasten, 1991·4
Fenatrop, 1991·4
Fenatrop-A, 1991·4
Fenax, 1991·4
Fenazepam, 715·1
Fenazil, 1991·4
Fenazocina, Hidrobromuro de, 82·2
Fenazona, 82·3
Fenazona Salicilato, 82·3
Fenazona y Citrato de Cafeína, 82·3
Fenazopiridina, Cloridrato de, 83·1
Fenazopiridina, Hidrocloruro de, 83·1
Fenazoxine, 66·2
Fenbendazol, 105·2
Fenbendazole, 105·2
Fenbendazole for Veterinary Use, 105·2
Fenbid, 1991·4
Fenbufen, 39·1
Fenbufenum, 39·1
Fenburil, 1992·1
Fencamfamin Hydrochloride, 1588·2
Fencanfamina, Hidrocloruro de, 1588·2
Fenchel, 1687·2
Fenchelsaft N, 1992·1
Fencibutirol, 1687·1
Fenciclidina, Hidrocloruro de, 1730·3
Fenclonina, 1687·2
Fenclonine, 1687·2
Fendazol, 1992·1
Fender, 1992·1
Fendibina, 1992·1
Fendilina, Hidrocloruro de, 915·1
Fendiline Hydrochloride, 915·1
Fendimetrazina, Tartrato de, 1592·1
Fendin, 1992·1
Fendiprazol, 1992·1
Fendizoato de Cloperastina, 1117·2
Fendyl, 1992·1
Fenelzina, Sulfato de, 312·1
Fenemal, 1992·1
Fenergan, 1992·1
Fenergan Expectorante, 1992·1
Fenergan Topico, 1992·1
Fenesin, 1992·1
Fenesin DM, 1992·1
Fenethylline Hydrochloride, 1588·2
Feneticilina Potásica, 242·1
Fenetilina, Hidrocloruro de, 1588·2
Feneturida, 367·3
Fenetylline Hydrochloride, 1588·2
Fenfedrin, 1992·1
Fenfluramina, Hidrocloruro de, 1588·2
Fenfluramine Hydrochloride, 1588·2
Fenformina Cloridrato, 344·1
Fenformina, Hidrocloruro de, 344·1
Fengam, 1992·1
Feniben, 1992·1
Fenicarbazida, 83·2
Feniclor, 1992·1
Fenicol, 1992·1
Fenicol, Isopto— *see* Isopto Fenicol, 2068·3
Fenidantal, 1992·1
Fenidantoin S, 1992·1
Fenidex, 1992·1
Fenidina, 1992·1
Fenigramon, 1992·1
Feniken, 1992·1
Fenilacetato de Sodio, 1748·2
Fenilalanina, 1443·1
Fenilbutazona, 83·2
Fenilbutirato de Sodio, 1748·2
Fenilefrina, 1126·3
Fenilefrina, Bitartrato de, 1126·3
Fenilefrina, Hidrocloruro de, 1126·3
Fenil-Livre, 1992·1
Fenilmercurio, Acetato de, 1189·2
Fenilmercurio, Borato de, 1189·2
Fenilmercurio, Nitrato de, 1189·2
Fenilmercurio, Sales, 1189·2
Fenilpropanol, 1731·1
Fenilpropanolamina, 1127·3
Fenilpropanolamina, Hidrocloruro de, 1127·3
Fenilpropionato de Estradiol, 1550·2
Fenilpropionato de Nandrolona, 1561·3
Fenilpropionato de Testosterona, 1570·1
Feniltoloxamina, Citrato de, 439·1
Fenil-V, 1992·1
Fenindamina, Tartrato de, 438·2
Fenindiona, 981·1
Fenindione, 981·1
Fenint, 1992·1
Fenipencil, 1992·1
Fenipentol, 1687·2
Fenipentol Hemisuccinate, 1687·2
Fenipentol Sodium Hemisuccinate, 1687·2
Feniramina, 438·3
Feniramina, Aminosalicilato de, 438·3
Feniramina, Maleato de, 438·3
Fenisal, 1992·2
Fenisec, 1992·2
Fenisol, 1992·2
Fenistil, 1992·2
Fenital, 1992·2
Fenitenk, 1992·2
Fenitoína, 370·2
Fenitoína Sódica, 370·2
Feniton, 1992·2
Fenitron, 1992·2
Fenitrothion, 1505·2
Fenitrotión, 1505·2
Fenizolan, 1992·2
Fenizzard, 1992·2
Fenmetrazina, Hidrocloruro de, 1592·2
Fenn, 1992·2
Fennel, 1687·2
Fennel, Bitter, 1687·2
Fennel, Bitter, Fruit Oil, 1687·3
Fennel Fruit, 1687·2
Fennel Oil, 1687·3
Fennel Seed, 1687·2
Fennel, Sweet, 1687·2
Fennings Childrens Cooling Powders, 1992·2
Fennings Little Healers— *see* Jacksons Little Healers, 2070·2
Feno, 1992·2
Fenobarbital, 367·3
Fenobarbital Sódico, 367·3
Fenobeta, 1992·2
Fenobrate, 1992·2
Fenoclof, 1992·2
Fenocris, 1992·2
Fenocriz, 1992·2
Fenodid, 1992·2
Fenofibrate, 915·2
Fenofibrato, 915·2
Fenofibratum, 915·2
Fenofibric Acid, 915·2
Fenogal, 1992·2
Fenogar, 1992·2
Fenogel, 1992·2
Fenogreco, 1688·1
Fenoket, 1992·2
Fenokomp 39, 1992·2
Fenol, 1188·1
Fenoldopam Mesilate, 915·3
Fenoldopam, Mesilato de, 915·3
Fenoldopam Mesylate, 915·3
Fenolftaleína, 1284·1
Fenolftaleina Compuesta, 1992·2
Fenolip, 1992·2
Fenolsolfonftaleina, 1730·3
Fenolsulfonftaleína, 1730·3
Fenomel, 1992·3
Fenoperidina, Hidrocloruro de, 83·2
Fenopraine Hydrochloride, 988·3
Fenoprofen Calcium, 39·2
Fenoprofeno Cálcico, 39·2
Fenopron, 1992·3
Fenoptic, 1992·3
Fenorit, 1992·3
Fenospen, 1992·3
Fenostad, 1992·3
Fenoterol, 785·2
Fenoterol, Hidrobromuro de, 785·2
Fenoterol Hydrobromide, 785·2
Fenoteroli Hydrobromidum, 785·2
Fenotricin, 1992·3
Fenotrina, 1509·1
Fenouil, 1687·2
Fenouil Amer, 1687·2
Fenoverina, 1687·3
Fenoverine, 1687·3
Fenox, 1992·3
Fenoxazolina, Hidrocloruro de, 1121·3
Fenoxazoline Hydrochloride, 1121·3
Fenoxazoline, Prednisolone Compound with, 1129·1
Fenoxcillin, 1992·3
Fenoxene, 1992·3
Fenoxibenzamina, Hidrocloruro de, 981·2
Fenoxietanol, 1189·1
Fenoxiisopropanol, 1189·2
Fenoximetilpenicilina, 242·1
Fenoximetilpenicilina Cálcica, 242·1
Fenoximetilpenicilina Potásica, 242·1
Fenoximetilpenicilina Potássica, 242·1
Fenoximone, 911·1
Fenoxypen, 1992·3
Fenozan, 1992·3
Fenpaed, 1992·3
Fenpic, 1992·3
Fenpipramida, Hidrocloruro de, 1687·3
Fenpipramide Hydrochloride, 1687·3
Fenpipramide Methobromide, 1688·1
Fenpipramide Methylbromide, 1688·1
Fenpiverinio, Bromuro de, 1688·1
Fenpiverinium Bromide, 1688·1
Fenprobamato, 715·1
Fenprocomón, 981·3
Fenproporex, 1588·3
Fenproporex Diphenylacetate, 1589·1
Fenproporex, Hidrocloruro de, 1588·3
Fenproporex Hydrochloride, 1588·3
Fenproporex Resinate, 1589·1
Fenquizona Potásica, 916·2
Fenquizone, 916·2
Fenquizone Potassium, 916·2
Fenretinida, 553·1
Fenretinide, 553·1
Fensaide, 1992·3
Fensaide-P, 1992·3
Fensedyl, 1992·3
Fensel, 1992·3
Fenspin, 1992·3
Fenspir, 1992·3
Fenspirida, Hidrocloruro de, 786·1
Fenspiride Hydrochloride, 786·1
Fensum, 1992·3
Fensuximida, 370·1
Fentabbott, 1992·3
Fenta-Hameln, 1992·3
Fentalim, 1992·3
Fentanest, 1992·3
Fentanilo, 40·1
Fentanilo, Citrato de, 40·1
Fentanyl, 40·1
Fentanyl Citrate, 40·1
Fentanyli Citras, 40·1
Fentanylum, 40·1
Fentatienil, 1992·3
Fentax, 1992·3
Fentazin, 1992·3
Fentermina, 1592·2
Fentermina, Hidrocloruro de, 1592·2
Fenthion, 1505·2
Fentiazac, 43·1
Fentiazac Calcium, 43·1
Fentiazaco, 43·1
Fenticlor, 397·3
Fenticloro, 397·3
Fenticonazol, Nitrato de, 397·3
Fenticonazole Nitrate, 397·3
Fenticonazoli Nitras, 397·3
Fentiderm, 1992·3
Fentigyn, 1992·4
Fentión, 1505·2
Fentizol, 1992·4
Fentolamina, Mesilato de, 982·1
Fentonii Bromidum, 482·2
Fentonio, Bromuro de, 482·2
Fentonium Bromide, 482·2

Fentos, 1992·4
Fentrinol, 1992·4
Fentul, 1992·4
Fenugreek, 1688·1
Fenugrene, 1992·4
Fenulin, 1992·4
Fenuril, 1992·4
Fenuril-Hydrokortison, 1992·4
Fenvalerate, 1505·2
Fenvalerato, 1505·2
Fenwal ACD, 1992·4
Fenyramidol, 372·2, 1024·1
Feocyte, 1992·4
Feofol, 1992·4
FeoGen, 1992·4
Feosol, 1992·4
Feospan, 1992·4
Feostat, 1992·4
Fepalitan, 1992·4
Feparil, 1992·4
Fepradinol, 43·1
Fepradinol Hydrochloride, 43·1
Feprapax, 1992·4
Feprazona, 43·1
Feprazone, 43·1
Feprazone Piperazine, 43·2
Fepron, 1992·4
Fer Sucré, Oxyde de, 1438·2
Fer UCB, 1992·4
Feraken, 1992·4
Feratab, 1992·4
Fercayl, 1992·4
Fercovit, 1992·4
Ferdek, 1992·4
Ferdromaco, 1992·4
Feredetato Sódico, 1444·3
Ferfolic SV, 1993·1
Fer-gen-sol, 1993·1
Fergon, 1993·1
Feridex, 1993·1
Ferifer, 1993·1
Ferig, 1993·1
Ferin, 1993·1
Ferinsol, 1993·1
Fer-In-Sol, 1993·1
Fer-Iron, 1993·1
Ferlactis, 1993·1
Ferlasin, 1993·1
Ferlatum, 1993·1
Ferlea, 1993·1
Ferli-6, 1993·1
Ferlis B12, 1993·1
Ferlixir, 1993·1
Ferlixit, 1993·1
Ferlor AF, 1993·1
Fermalac, 1993·1
Fermalac Vaginal, 1993·1
Fermasian, 1993·1
Fermate, 1993·1
Fermathron, 1993·1
Fermavisc, 1993·1
Fermentmycin, 1993·1
Fermento de Cerveja, 1469·1
Fermento Duodenal, 1993·1
Fermentol, 1993·1
Fermenturto-Lio, 1993·2
Fermetone Composto, 1993·2
Fernadin, 1993·2
Fernore, 1993·2
Ferodan, 1993·2
Fero-Folic, 1993·2
Fero-folic-500, 1993·2
Feroglobin, 1993·2
Fero-Grad, 1993·2
Fero-Grad Vitamine C, 1993·2
Fero-Gradumet, 1993·2
Feromiel, 1993·2
Feron, 1993·2
Ferona, 1993·2
Ferosof, 1993·2
Ferotrinsic, 1993·2
Ferplex, 1993·2
Ferplus-B, 1993·2
Ferquifa $B_{12}$, 1993·2
Ferr. Perchlor., 1688·1
Ferradol, 1993·2
Ferralet Plus, 1993·2
Ferranem, 1993·2
Ferranim, 1993·2
Ferranin, 1993·3
Ferranin Complex, 1993·3
Ferranina, 1993·3
Ferranina Fol, 1993·3
Ferrascorbin, 1993·3
Ferrematos, 1993·3
Ferremon, 1993·3
Ferretab, 1993·3
Ferretab Comp, 1993·3
Ferretab Compuesto, 1993·3
Ferretts, 1993·3
Ferreux (Sulfate), 1428·2
Ferrex, 1993·3
Ferrex Forte, 1993·3
Ferrex Forte Plus, 1993·3
Ferrex PC, 1993·3
Ferrex Plus, 1993·3
Ferri Chloridum Hexahydricum, 1688·1
Ferric Ammonium Citrate, 1427·2
Ferric Chloride, 1688·1
Ferric Chloride ($^{59}$Fe), 1524·3
Ferric Chloride Hexahydrate, 1688·1
Ferric Citrate ($^{59}$Fe), 1524·3
Ferric Ferrocyanide, 1051·2
Ferric Hexacyanoferrate (II), 1051·2
Ferric Hydroxide and Isomaltose Complex, 1437·3
Ferric Hydroxide Sucrose, 1438·2
Ferric Oxide, 1057·3
Ferric Oxide, Saccharated, 1438·2
Ferric Pyrophosphate, 1427·2
Ferric Sodium Gluconate, 1444·3
Ferric Subsulfate Solution, 1428·3
Férrico, Cloruro, 1688·1
Férrico, Pirofosfato, 1427·2
Ferricum Citricum Ammoniatum, 1427·2
Ferricure, 1993·3
Ferri-Emina, 1993·3
Ferrifol, 1993·3
Ferrifol-3, 1993·3
Ferrifol B12, 1993·3
Ferrigot, 1993·3
Ferrimed, 1993·3
Ferrimed DS, 1993·3
Ferrin, 1993·3
Ferrioxamine, 1034·2
Ferripel-3, 1993·3
Ferriprox, 1993·3
Ferriseltz, 1993·4
Ferriseptil, 1993·4
Ferristene, 1061·3
Ferristeno, 1061·3
Ferrister, 1993·4
Ferritamin, 1993·4
Ferritin, 1427·2
Ferritin Complex, 1993·4
Ferritin Oti, 1993·4
Ferritina, 1427·2
Ferrlecit, 1993·4
Ferrlecit 2, 1993·4
Ferro, 1993·4
Ferro-12, 1993·4
Ferro 66, 1993·4
Ferro Complex, 1993·4
Ferro Drops L, 1993·4
Ferro F-500 Gradumet, 1993·4
Ferro Folic, 1993·4
Ferro Folico, 1993·4
Ferro Sanol, 1993·4
Ferro Sanol Comp, 1993·4
Ferro Sanol Duodenal, 1993·4
Ferro Sanol Gyn, 1993·4
Ferro Semar, 1993·4
Ferro Vitaminico, 1993·4
Ferro-Agepha, 1993·4
Ferroben, 1993·4
Ferro-Be-Sian, 1993·4
Ferrobet, 1994·1
Ferrocal, 1994·1
Ferrocap F, 1994·1
Ferro-C-Calcium, 1994·1
Ferrocebrina, 1994·1
Ferrocel, 1994·1
Ferrochelate, 1994·1
Ferrochelate-Z, 1994·1
Ferrocholinate, 1427·3
Ferrocitol, 1994·1
Ferrocolinato, 1427·3
Ferrocomplex, 1994·1
Ferrocur, 1994·1
Ferrocutid, 1994·1
Ferrocyte, 1994·1
Ferrodix, 1994·1
Ferro-Dok, 1994·1
Ferro-Folgamma, 1994·1
Ferrofolin, 1994·1
Ferrofolin Simplex, 1994·1
Ferro-Folsan, 1994·1
Ferro-Folsan— *see* Folsana, 2006·2
Ferrofran, 1994·1
Ferrogamma, 1994·1
Ferrogels Forte, 1994·1
Ferrograd, 1994·1
Ferrograd C, 1994·1
Ferrograd Fol, 1994·2
Ferrograd Folic, 1994·2
Ferrograd Folico, 1994·2
Ferro-Gradumet, 1994·2
Ferrogyn, 1994·2
Ferroin, 1994·2
FERROinfant N, 1994·2
FERROinfant Neu, 1994·2
Ferrokapsul, 1994·2
Ferrokatabios, 1994·2
Ferroklinge, 1994·2
Ferrol-Cal, 1994·2
Ferromalt, 1994·2
Ferromaltose, 1437·3
Ferromas, 1994·2
Ferromax, 1994·2
Ferrometion, 1994·2
Ferromex, 1994·2
Ferromia, 1994·2
Ferromina, 1994·2
Ferromyn, 1994·2
Ferromyn S, 1994·2
Ferronil, 1994·2
Ferroplex, 1994·2
Ferroplex-frangula, 1994·2
Ferropolichondrum, 1425·1
Ferropro, 1994·2
Ferroprotina, 1994·2
Ferro-Retard, 1994·2
Ferrosanol Duodenal, 1994·2
Ferrosi Fumaras, 1427·3
Ferrosi Gluconas, 1428·1
Ferrosi Sulfas Exsiccatus, 1428·3
Ferrosi Sulfas Heptahydricus, 1428·2
Ferrosi Tartras, 1429·1
Ferrosig, 1994·2
Ferroso, Ascorbato, 1427·3
Ferroso, Aspartato, 1427·3
Ferroso, Cloruro, 1427·3
Ferroso de Glicina, Sulfato, 1428·2
Ferroso Desecado, Sulfato, 1428·3
Ferroso, Fumarato, 1427·3
Ferroso, Gluceptato, 1428·1
Ferroso, Gluconato, 1428·1
Ferroso, Lactato, 1428·2
Ferroso, Oxalato, 1428·2
Ferroso, Succinato, 1428·2
Ferroso, Sulfato, 1428·2
Ferroso, Tartrato, 1429·1
Ferrosprint, 1994·3
Ferrostrane, 1994·3
Ferrotab, 1994·3
Ferrotabs, 1994·3
Ferrotemp, 1994·3
Ferro-Terapina, 1994·3
Ferrotonico, 1994·3
Ferrotonico B12, 1994·3
Ferrototal, 1994·3
Ferrotrat, 1994·3
Ferrotrat B12, 1994·3
Ferro-Tre, 1994·3
Ferrotron, 1994·3
Ferrous Aminoacetosulphate, 1428·2
Ferrous Ascorbate, 1427·3
Ferrous Aspartate, 1427·3
Ferrous Chloride, 1427·3
Ferrous Citrate ($^{59}$Fe), 1524·3
Ferrous Fumarate, 1427·3
Ferrous Gluceptate, 1428·1
Ferrous Glucoheptonate, 1428·1
Ferrous Gluconate, 1428·1
Ferrous Glycine Sulfate, 1428·2
Ferrous Glycine Sulphate, 1428·2
Ferrous Lactate, 1428·2
Ferrous Orotate, 1724·3
Ferrous Oxalate, 1428·2
Ferrous Succinate, 1428·2
Ferrous Sulfate, 1428·2
Ferrous Sulfate, Dried, 1428·3
Ferrous Sulfate Monohydrate, 1428·3
Ferrous Sulfate Tetrahydrate, 1428·3
Ferrous Sulphate, 1428·2
Ferrous Sulphate, Dried, 1428·3
Ferrous Sulphate, Exsiccated, 1428·3
Ferrous Sulphate Heptahydrate, 1428·2
Ferrous Tartrate, 1429·1
Ferroven, 1994·3
Ferrovin-Chinaeisenwein, 1994·3
Ferrovin-Eisenelixier, 1994·3
Ferrum, 1434·3, 1994·3
Ferrum Ad Praeparationes Homoeopathicae, 1434·3
Ferrum Fol, 1994·3
Ferrum Fol Hausmann, 1994·3
Ferrum H, 1994·3
Ferrum Hausmann, 1994·3
Ferrum Oxalicum Oxydulatum, 1428·2
Ferrum Oxydatum Saccharatum, 1438·2
Ferrum Phosphoricum Comp, 1994·3
Ferrum Polyisomaltose, 1437·3
Ferrum Sesquichloratum, 1688·1
Ferrum Sulfuricum Oxydulatum, 1428·2
Ferrum Verla, 1994·4
Ferrum-Quarz, 1994·4
Ferrumvit, 1994·4
Fersaday, 1994·4
Fersamal, 1994·4
Fertibion, 1994·4
Fertilan, 1994·4
Fertility Day, 1994·4
Fertility Score, 1994·4
Fertinex, 1994·4
Fertinic, 1994·4
Fertinorm, 1994·4
Fertodur, 1994·4
Fertomcidina-U, 1994·4
Fertomid, 1994·4
Ferucarbotran, 1061·3
*Ferula*, 1658·1
Ferumat, 1994·4
Ferumoxides, 1061·3
Ferumóxidos, 1061·3
Ferumoxsil, 1061·3
Ferval, 1994·4
Fervex, 1994·4
Fervex Rhume, 1994·4
Fervical, 1994·4
Fervit, 1994·4
Ferxal, 1994·4
Ferybar, 1994·4
Fesema, 1994·4
Fesovit, 1994·4
Fess, 1994·4
Festal N, 1995·1
Fe-Tinic, 1995·1
Fe-Tinic Forte, 1995·1
Feto Macho, 108·2
Feto-Longoral, 1995·1
Fetrin, 1995·1
Fetrival, 1995·1
Feudoftal, 1995·1
Feuille de Digitale, 894·2
Feuille de Saule, 1995·1
Feuilles de Sauge, 1741·2
Fevamol, 1995·1
Fevarin, 1995·1
Fever— *see* Fever and Hyperthermia, 8·2
Fever Blisters— *see* Herpes Simplex Infections, 620·2
Fever & Inflammation Relief, 1995·1

Fever, Post-immunisation— *see* Fever and Hyperthermia, 8·2
Feverall, 1995·1
Feverfen, 1995·1
Feverfew, 469·1
Feverhalt, Childrens— *see* Childrens Feverhalt, 1882·4
Feverwort, 1661·3
Fevital Simplex, 1995·1
Fexicam, 1995·1
Fexin, 1995·1
Fexiron, 1995·1
Fexofen, 1995·1
Fexofenadina, Hidrocloruro de, 433·3
Fexofenadine Hydrochloride, 433·3
Fezona, 1995·1
FF-106, 23·3
FG-5111, 706·1
FG-5606, 670·3
FG-7051, 311·2
FGF Tabs, 1995·1
FGN-1, 552·3
Fhbc, 1995·1
FI-106, 547·3
FI-5852, 1565·1
FI-6146, 480·2
FI-6337, 1211·2
FI-6339, 545·3
FI-6341, 1103·2
FI-6714, 1719·3
FI-6934, 1669·2
Fiacin, 1995·1
Fialetta Odontalgica Dr Knapp, 1995·1
Fiamelis, 1995·1
Fibalip, 1995·1
Fiberall, 1995·1
Fibercon, 1995·1
Fiberform, 1995·1
Fiberform Mix, 1995·1
Fibergy, 1995·1
Fiberlan, 1995·2
Fiber-Lax, 1995·2
FiberNorm, 1995·2
Fibersource, 1995·2
Fibion, 1995·2
Fiblaferon, 1995·2
Fibonel, 1995·2
Fiboran, 1995·2
Fibra Light, 1995·2
Fibra Line, 1995·2
Fibrabene, 1995·2
Fibracap, 1995·2
Fibracol, 1995·2
Fibraflex, 1995·2
Fibraguar, 1995·2
Fibral, 1995·2
Fibralime, 1995·2
Fibramucil, 1995·2
Fibrasan, 1995·2
Fibrase, 1995·2
Fibrase SA, 1995·2
Fibrasol, 1995·2
Fibrates, 811·3
Fibrax, 1995·2
Fibre, Dietary, 1253·3
Fibre Dophilus, 1995·2
Fibre Plus, 1995·2
Fibre, Water-insoluble, 1253·2
Fibre, Water-soluble, 1253·2
Fibreline, 1995·2
Fibrepur, 1995·2
Fibresource, 1995·3
Fibre-Vit, 1995·3
Fibrex Hot Drink, 1995·3
Fibrex Tabletten, 1995·3
Fibrexin, 1995·3
Fibrezym, 1995·3
Fibrillation, Atrial— *see* Cardiac Arrhythmias, 816·1
Fibrillation, Ventricular— *see* Advanced Cardiac Life Support, 812·2
Fibrillation, Ventricular— *see* Cardiac Arrhythmias, 816·1
Fibrimol, 1995·3
Fibrin, 753·1
Fibrin Foam, Human, 753·2
Fibrin Glue, 753·2, 1995·3
Fibrin Glue— *see* Tissucol, 2334·4
Fibrin Glue— *see* Tissucol Duo Quick, 2334·4
Fibrin Sealant Kit, 753·1
Fibrina, 753·1
Fibrinase, 916·2
Fibrini Glutinum, 753·1
Fibrinogen, 735·3, 753·2
Fibrinogen, Human, 753·2
Fibrinogen, Iodinated ($^{125}$I) Human, 1524·2
Fibrinógeno, 753·2
Fibrinogenum Humanum, 753·2
Fibrinol, 1995·3
Fibrinolisina (Humana), 916·2
Fibrinolysin, 916·2
Fibrinolysin, Bovine, 916·2
Fibrinolysin (Human), 916·2
Fibrinolysis, 735·3
Fibrinomer, 1995·3
Fibrin-stabilising Factor, 753·1
Fibrit, 1995·3
Fibroblast Growth Factor, 1679·1
Fibroblast Interferon, 645·3
Fibrocid, 1995·3
Fibrocide, 1995·3
Fibrocit, 1995·3
Fibrocol, 1995·3
Fibrocystic Breast Disease— *see* Mastalgia, 1546·3
Fibroderm, 1995·3
Fibrogammin, 1995·3
Fibrogammin P, 1995·3
Fibroids, 1326·1
Fibrol, 1995·3
Fibrolan, 1995·3
Fibrolax, 1995·3
Fibrolax Complex, 1995·3
Fibrolip, 1995·3
Fibromucil, 1995·3
Fibromyalgia— *see* Soft-tissue Rheumatism, 11·1
Fibronectin, 1688·1
Fibronectina, 1688·1
Fibronevrina, 1995·3
Fibroquel, 1995·3
Fibroral, 1995·3
Fibrorelax, 1995·3
Fibros, 1995·3
Fibrosarcoma— *see* Bone Sarcoma, 524·3
Fibrosine, 1995·3
Fibrosing Alveolitis, Cryptogenic— *see* Diffuse Parenchymal Lung Disease, 1079·3
Fibrosis, Pulmonary, Idiopathic— *see* Diffuse Parenchymal Lung Disease, 1079·3
Fibrositis— *see* Soft-tissue Rheumatism, 11·1
Fibrospes, 1995·4
Fibrovein, 1995·4
Fibro-Vein, 1995·4
Fibrovit, 1995·4
Fibroxyn, 1995·4
Fibsol, 1995·4
Fibyrax, 1995·4
Ficaire, 1732·1
Ficaria Ranunculoides, 1732·1
Ficaria Verna, 1732·1
Fichtennadel Franzbranntwein, Kneipp— *see* Kneipp Fichtennadel Franzbranntwein, 2081·2
Fichtensirup N, 1995·4
Ficortril, 1995·4
Ficus, 1266·3
*Ficus carica*, 1266·3
Fideine, 1995·4
Fidium, 1995·4
Fiebrolito, 1995·4
Fienamina, 1995·4
Fiery Jack, 1995·4
Fig, 1266·3
Figadobil, 1995·4
Figadosan, 1995·4
Figalol, 1995·4
Figatil, 1995·4
Figen, 1995·4
Figozant, 1995·4
FIII Hc, 1995·4
Fijacid, 1995·4
Fil Olor, 1995·4
Filair, 1995·4
Filarial Nematode Infections, 97·1
Filariasis, Lymphatic— *see* Lymphatic Filariasis, 100·1
Filartros, 1995·4
Filcrin, 1995·4
File, 1995·4
Fileen, 1996·1
Filena, 1996·1
Filesna, 1996·1
Filgen, 1996·1
Filginase, 1996·1
Filgrastim, 753·3
Filibon, 1996·1
Filicin, 108·2
Filicine, 1996·1
Filide, 1996·1
Filigel, 1996·1
Filinasma, 1996·1
*Filipendula ulmaria*, 1710·1
Filipendulae Ulmariae, 1710·1
Filivir, 1996·1
Filix Mas, 108·2
Filmagene, 1996·1
Filmcel, 1996·1
Filmexil, 1996·1
Filmogen Same, 1996·1
Filnarine, 1996·1
Filocot, 1996·1
Filoderma, 1996·1
Filoderma Plus, 1996·1
Filogargan, 1996·1
Filogaster, 1996·1
Filoklin, 1996·1
Filosfil, 1996·1
Filotempo, 1996·1
Filotricin A, 1996·1
Filter Oil Free, 1996·1
Filter OTC, 1996·1
Filtrax, 1996·2
Fimdor, 1996·2
Fin-A, 1996·2
Finaber, 1996·2
Finac, 1996·2
Finacea, 1996·2
Finacilen, 1996·2
Finagrip, 1996·2
Finalgon, 1996·2
Finalgon N Schmerzpflaster, 1996·2
Finalop, 1996·2
Finamicina, 1996·2
Finan, 1996·2
Finap, 1996·2
Finaplac, 1996·2
Finasept, 1996·2
Finasterida, 1554·2
Finasteride, 1554·2
Finasteridum, 1554·2
Finasterin, 1996·2
Finastid, 1996·2
Finastil, 1996·2
Finaten, 1996·2
Finater, 1996·2
Finatux, 1996·2
Fincar, 1996·2
Fincoid, 1996·2
Findaler, 1996·2
Findaler-D, 1996·2
Findeclin, 1996·2
Findedol, 1996·2
Findol, 1996·2
Findol N, 1996·2
Findor, 1996·2
Finedal, 1996·2
Finelium, 1996·3
Fineural N, 1996·3
Finevin, 1996·3
Finex, 1996·3
Finfo, 1996·3
Fingerhutblatt, 894·2
Fingers & Toes, Bioglan— *see* Bioglan Fingers & Toes, 1844·1
Fingras, 1996·3
Finidol, 1996·3
Finigas, 1996·3
Finil, 1996·3
Finimal, 1996·3
Finimal, Kinder— *see* Kinder Finimal, 2079·3
Fininha, 1666·1
Finipect, 1996·3
Finiweh, 1996·3
Finlepsin, 1996·3
Finn, 1996·3
Finn Cristal, 1996·3
Finnferon-Alpha, 1996·3
Finote, 1666·1
Finoxi, 1996·3
Finprob, 1996·3
Finprostat, 1996·3
Finrexin, 1996·3
Fintal, 1996·3
Fintaxim, 1996·3
Finuret, 1996·3
Fioricet, 1996·3
Fioricet with Codeine, 1996·3
Fiorinal, 1996·3
Fiorinal C, 1996·4
Fiorinal Codeina, 1996·4
Fiorinal with Codeine, 1996·4
Fioritina, 1996·4
Fiormil, 1996·4
Fiorpap, 1996·4
Fiortal, 1996·4
Fiortal with Codeine, 1996·4
Fiosen Plus, 1996·4
Fiosen-A, 1996·4
Fiotan, 1996·4
Fioton, 1996·4
FiProFLAX, 1996·4
Fipronil, 1505·3
Fipronilo, 1505·3
Firac, 1996·4
Firac Plus, 1996·4
Firin, 1996·4
Firmacef, 1996·4
Firmacort, 1996·4
Firmavit, 1996·4
Firmel, 1996·4
Firon, 1996·4
Fironetta, 1996·4
First Choice, 1996·4
First Response, 1996·4
Fisalamine, 1273·2
Fisamox, 1996·4
Fish Factor, 1996·4
Fish Odour Syndrome, 1417·3
Fish Oil, Rich in Omega-3-Acids, 976·2
Fish Poison Bark, 1702·3
Fish Tank Granuloma— *see* Opportunistic Mycobacterial Infections, 137·2
Fish Tapeworm Infections— *see* Diphyllobothriasis, 98·1
Fishaphos, 1996·4
Fisherman's Friend, 1996·4
Fisherman's Friend Original, 1996·4
Fisherman's Friend Zinc, 1996·4
Fisher's Phospherine, 1997·1
Fishogar, 1997·1
Fisifax, 1997·1
Fisifer Folico, 1997·1
Fisiobil, 1997·1
Fisiodar, 1997·1
Fisiofer, 1997·1
Fisiogastrol, 1997·1
Fisiolimp, 1997·1
Fisiologica, 1997·1
Fisiologico, 1997·1
Fisiologico Bieffe M, 1997·1
Fisiologico Braun, 1997·1
Fisiologico Farmacelsia, 1997·1
Fisiologico Isoton, 1997·1
Fisiologico Mein, 1997·1
Fisiologico Vitulia, 1997·1
Fisioren, 1997·1
Fisiotens, 1997·1
Fisohex, 1997·1
Fisopred, 1997·1

Fisostigmina, 1494·1
Fisostigmina, Salicilato de, 1494·1
Fisostigmina, Sulfato de, 1494·2
Fissan, 1997·1
Fissan-Silberpuder, 1997·1
Fissan-Zinkschuttelmixtur, 1997·1
Fit, Epileptic— *see* Epilepsy, 349·1
Fitacnol, 1997·1
Fitato Sódico, 1052·3
Fitaxal, 1997·1
Fito Stomygen, 1997·1
Fitocalmin, 1997·1
Fitocrem, 1997·1
Fitocreme, 1997·1
Fitoderme, 1997·1
Fitodorf Alghe Marine, 1997·2
Fitodorf Rabarbaro, 1997·2
Fitoestimulina, 1997·2
Fitogen, 1997·2
Fitokey Ginkgo, 1997·2
Fitokey Harpagophytum, 1997·2
Fitolaca, 1733·1
Fitolax, 1997·2
Fitolinea, 1997·2
Fitomenadiona, 1467·1
Fitonal, 1997·2
Fitosonno, 1997·2
Fitostimoline, 1997·2
Fitostress, 1997·2
Fitosvelt, 1997·2
Fitotos, 1997·2
Fittig, 1997·2
Fitton, 1997·2
Fittydent, 1997·2
Fitzecalm, 1997·2
Fitzgerald Factor, 735·3
Fivasa, 1997·2
Fivefluro, 1997·2
Fiverocil, 1997·2
Fivoflu, 1997·2
Fixateur Phospho-calcique, 1997·2
Fixca, 1997·2
Fixed Oils, 1763·3
Fixed-drug Eruptions— *see* Drug-induced Skin Reactions, 1134·3
Fixical, 1997·2
Fixical Vitamine $D_3$, 1997·2
Fixim, 1997·2
Fixime, 1997·2
Fixobel— *see* Calox, 1865·4
Fixoten, 1997·2
Fixx, 1997·2
Fizz, 1997·2
Fizziclean, 1997·3
FK-027, 172·3
FK-037, 175·2
FK-235, 972·2
FK-463, 405·2
FK-482, 171·3
FK-506, 1363·3
FK-749, 182·2
FKS-508, 1488·3
FL-113, 773·2
FL-1039, 244·2
FL-1060, 228·3
FLA-870, 719·2
Flacar, 1997·3
Fladex, 1997·3
Flag, Blue, 1702·1
Flag, Sweet, 1664·1
Flagass, 1997·3
Flagass Baby, 1997·3
Flagenase, 1997·3
Flagenase 400, 1997·3
Flagenol, 1997·3
Flagentyl, 1997·3
Flaginazol, 1997·3
Flagosil, 1997·3
Flagyl, 1997·3
Flagyl— *see* Losec Helicopak, 2105·4
Flagyl Comp, 1997·3
Flagyl Compak, 1997·3
Flagyl Nistatina, 1997·3
Flagyl-F, 1997·3
Flagystatin, 1997·3
Flagystatin V, 1997·3
Flake, 1373·3
Flamadene, 1997·3
Flamanan, 1997·3
Flamar, 1997·3
Flamarene, 1997·3
Flamaret, 1997·3
Flamar-MX, 1997·3
Flamatak, 1997·3
Flamatec, 1997·3
Flamatrol, 1997·4
Flamazine, 1997·4
Flamazine C, 1997·4
Flamecid, 1997·4
Flameril, 1997·4
Flamic, 1997·4
Flamicina, 1997·4
Flamide, 1997·4
Flamin, 1997·4
Flamin 400, 1997·4
Flaminase, 1997·4
Flamirex, 1997·4
Flammacerium, 1997·4
Flammazine, 1997·4
Flamon, 1997·4
Flamostat, 1997·4
Flamrase, 1997·4
Flanakin, 1997·4
Flanamox, 1997·4
Flanaren, 1997·4
Flanax, 1997·4
Flancox, 1997·4
Flanders Buttocks, 1997·4
Flanid, 1997·4
Flanil, 1997·4
Flanizol, 1997·4
Flankol, 1998·1
Flanoquin, 1998·1
Flantadin, 1998·1
Flanzen, 1998·1
Flapex, 1998·1
Flapex E, 1998·1
Flar, 1998·1
Flarex, 1998·1
Flaspas, 1998·1
Flatex, 1998·1
Flatol, 1998·1
Flatoril, 1998·1
Flatugel, Vida— *see* Vida Flatugel, 2376·2
Flatulence Gastulence, 1998·1
Flatulex, 1998·1
Flatuol, Kneipp— *see* Kneipp Flatuol, 2081·2
Flatworm Infections, 97·1
Flaval, 1998·1
Flavamed Halstabletten, 1998·1
Flavan, 1998·1
Flavangin, 1998·1
Flavaspidic Acid, 108·2
Flavedon, 1998·1
Flaveric, 1998·1
Flavettes, 1998·1
Flavettes Neuroforte, 1998·1
Flaviastase, 1998·1
Flavicina, 1998·1
Flavine Adenine Dinucleotide, 1456·2
Flavine Mononucleotide, 1456·2
Flavinol, 1998·1
Flavion, 1998·2
Flavis, 1998·2
Flavit, 1998·2
Flavit-AV, 1998·2
Flavix, 1998·2
Flavodate Disodium, 1688·2
Flavodate Sodium, 1688·2
Flavodato Sódico, 1688·2
Flavodrei, 1998·2
Flavogin, 1998·2
Flavon, 1998·2
Flavone 500, 1998·2
Flavonex, 1998·2
Flavonoid Complex, 1998·2
Flavonoid Compounds, 1688·2
Flavonoides, 1688·2
Flavons, 1998·2
Flavophospholipol, 162·2
Flavoquine, 1998·2
Flavorin, 1998·2
Flavorola C, 1998·2
Flavo-Spa, 1998·2
Flavostat, 1998·2
Flavoton, 1998·2
Flavovenyl, 1998·2
Flavoxate Hydrochloride, 482·2
Flavoxato, Hidrocloruro de, 482·2
Flavo-Zinc, 1998·2
Flaxedil, 1998·2
Flaxin, 1998·2
Flaxseed, 1707·2
Flaxseed Oil, 1707·2
Flea Seed, 1268·1
Flebeside, 1998·2
Flebil, 1998·2
Flebior, 1998·2
Flebitol, 1998·2
Flebo Stop, 1998·3
Flebobag Fisio, 1998·3
Flebobag Glucosa, 1998·3
Flebobag Glucosal, 1998·3
Flebobag Ring Lact, 1998·3
Flebocortid, 1998·3
Fleboderma, 1998·3
Flebogamma, 1998·3
Flebon, 1998·3
Flebopex, 1998·3
Fleboplast Fisio, 1998·3
Fleboplast Glucosa, 1998·3
Fleboplast Glucosal, 1998·3
Fleboplast Levulosa, 1998·3
Fleboplast Plurisal, 1998·3
Flebopom, 1998·3
Fleboside, 1998·3
Flebosmil, 1998·3
Flebostasin, 1998·3
Fleboton, 1998·3
Flebotrat, 1998·3
Flebotropin, 1998·3
Flebovis, 1998·3
Flebozin, 1998·3
Flebs, 1998·3
Flecaine, 1998·3
Flecainida, Acetato de, 916·2
Flecainide Acetate, 916·2, 916·3
Flecainidi Acetas, 916·2
Flecatab, 1998·3
Flecor-N, 1998·3
Flectadol, 1998·4
Flector, 1998·4
Fleet Preparations, 1998·4
Flemex, 1999·1
Flemex Jat, 1999·1
Flemex-AC, 1999·1
Flemeze, 1999·1
Flemgo, 1999·1
Flemina, 1999·1
Fleminosan, 1999·1
Flemizyme, 1999·1
Flemlite, 1999·1
Flemoxin, 1999·1
Flemoxine, 1999·1
Flemoxon, 1999·1
Flemun, 1999·1
Flenalgin, 1999·1
Flenid, 1999·1
Flenin, 1999·1
Flenverme, 1999·1
Flepin X-3, 1999·1
Flerox, 1999·1
Fleroxacin, 213·2
Fleroxacino, 213·2
Flerudin, 1999·1
Fletanol, 1999·1
Fletcher Factor, 735·3
Fletchers Arachis Oil Retention Enema, 1999·1
Fletchers Castoria, 1999·1
Fletchers Enemette, 1999·1
Fletchers Phosphate Enema, 1999·2
Fletchers Sore Mouth Medicine, 1999·2
Fleur de Rose, 1058·1
Fleurs de Sureau, 1741·3
Fleurs d'Orient, Creme des 3— *see* Creme des 3 Fleurs d'Orient, 1911·2
Flevic, 1999·2
Flexafen, 1999·2
Flexagen, 1999·2
Flexagil, 1999·2
Flexal Brennessel, 1999·2
Flexal Vitamin E, 1999·2
Flex-All, 1999·2
Flex-all 454, 1999·2
Flexall 454, Maximum Strength— *see* Maximum Strength Flexall 454, 2116·4
Flexamina, 1999·2
Flexaphen, 1999·2
Flexar, 1999·2
Flexase, 1999·2
Flex-Care, 1999·2
Flexdor, 1999·2
Flexelite, 1999·2
Flexen, 1999·2
Flexeril, 1999·2
Flexeze, 1999·2
Flexfree, 1999·2
Flexiban, 1999·2
Flexicamin, 1999·2
Flexicamin A, 1999·2
Flexicamin B12, 1999·3
Flexicamin Crema, 1999·3
Flexican, 1999·3
Flexidin, 1999·3
Flexidol, 1999·3
Flexidon, 1999·3
Flexidone, 1999·3
Flexifer, 1999·3
Flexi-loges, 1999·3
Flexin, 1999·3
Flexin Continus, 1999·3
Flexirox, 1999·3
Flexital, 1999·3
Flexitec, 1999·3
Flexium, 1999·3
Flexocutan N, 1999·3
Flexogyne, 1999·3
Flexoject, 1999·3
Flexon, 1999·3
Flexono, 1999·3
Flexotard, 1999·3
Flex-Power Performance Sports, 1999·3
Flextoss, 1999·3
Flextra, 1999·3
Flexurat, 1999·3
Flezol, 1999·4
Flicum, 1999·4
Flies, Russian, 1666·3
Flindix, 1999·4
Flint, 1999·4
Flintstones, 1999·4
Flipal, 1999·4
Flivas, 1999·4
Flixoderm, 1999·4
Flixonase, 1999·4
Flixotaide, 1999·4
Flixotide, 1999·4
Flixovate, 1999·4
FLN, 1689·1
FLO-1347, 725·1
Flobac, 1999·4
Flobacin, 1999·4
Flocalcitriol, 1462·1
Flocet, 1999·4
Flociprin, 1999·4
Flo-Coat, 1999·4
Flocofil, 1999·4
Flocoumafen, 1505·3
Flocoumafene, 1505·3
Floctafenic Acid, 43·2
Floctafenina, 43·2
Floctafenine, 43·2
Flocumafeno, 1505·3
Flocur, 1999·4
Flodeneu, 1999·4
Flodermol, 1999·4
Flodil, 1999·4
Flodol, 1999·4
Flogan, 1999·4
Flogecyl, 1999·4
Flogen, 2000·1
Flogencyl, 2000·1

Flogene, 2000·1
Flogesic, 2000·1
Flogiatrin, 2000·1
Flogiatrin B12, 2000·1
Flogiftalmina, 2000·1
Flogilid, 2000·1
Floginax, 2000·1
Flogin-Ped, 2000·1
Flogiren, 2000·1
Flogo Rosa, 2000·1
Flogobene, 2000·1
Flogocan, 2000·1
Flogocefal, 2000·1
Flogocid, 2000·1
Flogocid NN, 2000·1
Flogocort, 2000·1
Flogodisten, 2000·1
Flogofenac, 2000·1
Flogofin, 2000·1
Flogogin, 2000·1
Flogojet, 2000·1
Flogoken, 2000·1
Flogol-gel, 2000·1
Flogonac, 2000·2
Flogoprofen, 2000·2
Flogoral, 2000·2
Flogosan, 2000·2
Flogosine, 2000·2
Flogostop, 2000·2
Flogoter, 2000·2
Flogotisol, 2000·2
Flogovis, 2000·2
Flogovis IdroGel, 2000·2
Flogovital, 2000·2
Flogovital NF, 2000·2
Flogoxen, 2000·2
Flogozen, 2000·2
Flogozyme, 2000·2
Flohale, 2000·2
Flolan, 2000·2
Flolid, 2000·2
Flomax, 2000·2
Flomed, 2000·2
Flomox, 2000·2
Flomoxef Sodium, 213·2
Flonase, 2000·2
Flonital, 2000·2
Flonorm, 2000·2
Flopen, 2000·2
Flopropiona, 1689·1
Flopropione, 1689·1
Flor del Pelitre, 1509·3
Florabio Mann-Feigen-Sirup mit Senna, 2000·3
Florabio Naturreiner Heilpflanzensaft, 2000·3
Floradix, 2000·3
Floradix Krauterblut, 2000·3
Floradix Maskam, 2000·3
Floradix Multipretten N, 2000·3
Floralac, 2000·3
Floralax, 2000·3
Floralaxative, 2000·3
Floraquin, 2000·3
Florate, 2000·3
Floratil, 2000·3
Florax, 2000·3
Floraxina, 2000·3
Florbiox, 2000·3
Floregin, 2000·3
Floregin Composto, 2000·3
Florelax, 2000·3
Florelax Stomaco, 2000·3
Florerbe Lassativa, 2000·3
Flores de Zinc, 1163·2
Floresse, 2000·3
Florexal, 2000·3
Florfenicol, 213·3
Florgynal, 2000·3
Floriabene— *see* Cefafloria, 1874·3
Florical, 2000·3
Floridine, 2000·3
Floridral, 2000·3
Florigien, 2000·3
Florilax, 2000·4
Florinef, 2000·4
Florinefe, 2000·4
Florisan, 2000·4
Florisan N, 2000·4
Florisene, 2000·4
Florissamol, 2000·4
Florlax, 2000·4
Florocycline, 2000·4
Floroglucinol, 1731·1
Florone, 2000·4
Floropipamide, 716·1
Florvite, 2000·4
Flos Chamomillae, 1669·3
Flos Chamomillae Vulgaris, 1669·3
Flos Rosae, 1058·1
Flosa, 2000·4
Flosef, 2000·4
Flosequinan, 918·2
Flosine, 2000·4
Flossac, 2000·4
Flotac, 2000·4
Flotina, 2000·4
Flotiran, 2000·4
Flotrin, 2000·4
Flovent, 2000·4
Flow-Care, Extralife— *see* Extralife Flow-Care, 1986·3
Flowers of Sulfur, 1158·2
Flowmega, 2000·4
Flox, 2000·4
Floxacillin, 213·3
Floxacin, 2000·4
Floxacipron, 2000·4
Floxager, 2000·4
Floxakin, 2000·4
Floxal, 2001·1
Floxalin, 2001·1
Floxamicin, 2001·1
Floxan, 2001·1
Floxanor, 2001·1
Floxantina, 2001·1
Floxapen, 2001·1
Floxaquil, 2001·1
Floxatral, 2001·1
Floxatrat, 2001·1
Floxedol, 2001·1
Floxelena, 2001·1
Floxen, 2001·1
Floxenor, 2001·1
Flox-ex, 2001·1
Floxicam, 2001·1
Floxid, 2001·1
Floxil, 2001·1
Floxin, 2001·1
Floxinol, 2001·1
Floxinon, 2001·1
Floxlevo, 2001·1
Floxsig, 2001·1
Floxstat, 2001·1
Floxur, 2001·1
Floxuridina, 553·1
Floxuridine, 553·1
Floxuridine Monophosphate, 555·2
Floxyfral, 2001·1
Flu-21, 2001·2
Flu, Cold & Cough Medicine, 2001·2
Flu & Fever Relief, 2001·2
Flu, Hylands— *see* Hylands Flu, 2052·3
Flu Oph, 2001·2
Fluad, 2001·2
Fluagel, 2001·2
Flu-Amp, 2001·2
Fluanisona, 698·2
Fluanisone, 698·2
Fluanxol, 2001·2
Fluarix, 2001·2
Fluaton, 2001·2
Fluazuron, 1505·3
Flubason, 2001·2
Flubendazol, 105·2
Flubendazole, 105·2
Flubendazolum, 105·2
Flubenisolone, 1093·1
Flubenisolonum, 1093·1
Flubenol— *see* Fluvermal, 2004·4
Flubilar, 2001·2
Flubiotic NF, 2001·2
Flubuperone Hydrochloride, 706·1
Flucacid, 2001·2
Flucalin, 2001·2
Flucam, 2001·2
Flucanol, 2001·2
Flucazol, 2001·2
Flucef, 2001·2
Fluciderm, 2001·2
Fluciderm-N, 2001·2
Flucil, 2001·2
Flucillin, 2001·2
Flucin, 2001·3
Flucinal, 2001·3
Flucinar, 2001·3
Flucinom, 2001·3
Flucinome, 2001·3
Flucistein, 2001·3
Flucitosina, 399·3
Fluclomix, 2001·3
Fluclon, 2001·3
Fluclorolona, Acetónido de, 1100·1
Fluclorolone Acetonide, 1100·1
Flucloronide, 1100·1
Fluclox, 2001·3
Flucloxa, 2001·3
Flucloxacilina, 213·3
Flucloxacilina Magnésica, 213·3
Flucloxacilina Sódica, 213·3
Flucloxacillin, 213·3
Flucloxacillin Magnesium, 213·3
Flucloxacillin Sodium, 213·3
Flucloxacillinum Natricum, 213·3
Flucloxil, 2001·3
Flucloxin, 2001·3
Fluclox-Reu, 2001·3
Flucol, 2001·3
Flucoltrix, 2001·3
Flucon, 2001·3
Fluconal, 2001·3
Fluconax, 2001·3
Fluconazol, 398·1
Fluconazole, 398·1
Fluconeo, 2001·3
Flucort, 2001·3
Flu-Cortanest, 2001·3
Flucort-C, 2001·3
Flucort-H, 2001·3
Flucort-MZ, 2001·3
Flucort-N, 2001·3
Flucoxan, 2001·3
Flucozal, 2001·3
Flucozen, 2001·3
Flucozole, 2001·3
Flucreme NM, 2001·3
Fluctin, 2001·3
Fluctine, 2001·4
Flucur, 2001·4
Flucytosine, 399·3
Flucytosinum, 399·3
Fludac, 2001·4
Fludactil, 2001·4
Fludactil Co, 2001·4
Fludactil Expectorant, 2001·4
Fludan, 2001·4
Fludan Codeina, 2001·4
Fludapamide, 2001·4
Fludara, 2001·4
Fludarabina, Fosfato de, 553·2
Fludarabine Monophosphate, 553·2
Fludarabine Phosphate, 553·2
Fludarene, 2001·4
Fludecate, 2001·4
Fluden, 2001·4
Fludent, 2001·4
Fludeoxyglucose ($^{18}F$), 1523·3
Fludestrin, 2001·4
Fludeten, 2001·4
Fludex, 2001·4
Fludiazepam, 698·2
Fludilat, 2001·4
Fluditec, 2001·4
Fludizol, 2001·4
Fludocel, 2001·4
Fludren, 2001·4
Fludrocortisona, Acetato de, 1100·1
Fludrocortisone Acetate, 1100·1
Fludrocortisoni Acetas, 1100·1
Fludronef, 2001·4
Fludrop, 2002·1
Fludroxicortida, 1100·3
Fludroxycortide, 1100·3
Fluend, 2002·1
Fluental, 2002·1
Fluenzen, 2002·1
Flufenal, 2002·1
Flufenamic Acid, 43·2
Flufenámico, Ácido, 43·2
Flufenan, 2002·1
Flufenazina, 699·3
Flufenazina, Decanoato de, 699·3
Flufenazina, Enantato de, 699·3
Flufenazina, Hidrocloruro de, 699·3
Fluforte, 2002·1
Fluforte N, 2002·1
Flufran, 2002·1
Flugen, 2002·1
Flugeral, 2002·1
Flugestona, Acetato de, 1555·2
Flugestone Acetate, 1555·2
Flui-Amoxicillin, 2002·1
Fluibil, 2002·1
Fluibron, 2002·1
Fluibrox, 2002·1
Fluid Loss, 2002·1
Fluidabak, 2002·1
Fluidasa, 2002·1
Fluid-Care, Extralife— *see* Extralife Fluid-Care, 1986·3
Fluide Hydratant Matifiant, 2002·1
Fluide Hydratant Quotidien, 2002·1
Fluide Multi-Confort, 2002·1
Fluide Multi-Regenerant Lift Jour, 2002·1
Fluide Protecteur Jeunesse des Mains, 2002·1
Fluidema, 2002·1
Fluiden, 2002·1
Fluidin, 2002·2
Fluidin Adulto, 2002·2
Fluidin Antiasmatico, 2002·2
Fluidin Infantil, 2002·2
Fluidin Mucolitico NF, 2002·2
Fluidin Nocturno, 2002·2
Flui-DNCG, 2002·2
Fluidox, 2002·2
Fluidrenol, 2002·2
Fluifort, 2002·2
Fluilast, 2002·2
Fluimare, 2002·2
Fluimucil, 2002·2
Fluimucil Antibiotic, 2002·2
Fluimucil Antibiotico, 2002·2
Fluimucil Biotic, 2002·2
Fluimucil Solucao Nasal, 2002·2
Fluindiona, 918·2
Fluindione, 918·2
Fluinol, 2002·2
Fluir, 2002·2
Fluirespir, 2002·2
Fluisedal, 2002·3
Fluisedal sans Promethazine, 2002·3
Fluitoss, 2002·3
Fluiven, 2002·3
Fluixol, 2002·3
Fluizan, 2002·3
Flukazol, 2002·3
Fluke Infections, 97·1
Fluke Infections, Blood, 97·1
Fluke Infections, Intestinal— *see* Intestinal Fluke Infections, 99·2
Fluke Infections, Liver— *see* Liver Fluke Infections, 99·3
Fluke Infections, Lung— *see* Lung Fluke Infections, 99·3
Fluken, 2002·3
Flukenol, 2002·3
Flukit, 2002·3
Flukiver, 104·1
Flulem, 2002·3
Flulium, 2002·3
Flulone, 2002·3
Flumach, 2002·3
Flumadine, 2002·3

Flumage, 2002·3
Flumanovag, 2002·3
Flumarc, 2002·3
Flumarin, 2002·3
Flumark, 2002·3
Flumasalen, 2002·3
Flumates, 2002·3
Flumazen, 2002·3
Flumazenil, 1038·3
Flumazenil ($^{11}$C), 1523·1
Flumazenilum, 1038·3
Flumazepil, 1038·3
Flumed, 2002·3
Flumequina, 214·2
Flumequine, 214·2
Flumequinum, 214·2
Flumetasona, Pivalato de, 1101·1
Flumetasone Pivalate, 1101·1
Flumetasoni Pivalas, 1101·1
Flumethasone Pivalate, 1101·1
Flumethasone 21-Pivalate, 1101·1
Flumethasone Trimethylacetate, 1101·1
Flumetholon, 2002·3
Flumethrin, 1505·3
Flumetol, 2002·3
Flumetol Antibiotico, 2002·3
Flumetol NF, 2002·4
Flumetol Semplice, 2002·4
Flumetrina, 1505·3
Flumex, 2002·4
Flumex N, 2002·4
Flumid, 2002·4
Flumil, 2002·4
Flumil Antibiotico, 2002·4
Flumil Antidoto, 2002·4
Fluminex, 2002·4
FluMist, 2002·4
Flumoxal, 2002·4
Flumural, 2002·4
Flunagen, 2002·4
Flunal, 2002·4
Flunal-Neo, 2002·4
Flunarin, 2002·4
Flunarium, 2002·4
Flunarizina, Hidrocloruro de, 434·1
Flunarizine Dihydrochloride, 434·1
Flunarizine Hydrochloride, 434·1
Flunarizini Dihydrochloridum, 434·1
Flunase, 2002·4
Flunavert, 2002·4
Flunaza, 2002·4
Flunazine, 2002·4
Flunazol, 2002·4
Flunco, 2002·4
Fluneurin, 2002·4
Fluni, 2002·4
Flunibeta, 2002·4
Flunidor, 2002·4
Flunigar, 2002·4
Fluniget, 2002·4
Flunimerck, 2002·4
Fluninoc, 2003·1
Flunipam, 2003·1
Flunir, 2003·1
Flunisolida, 1101·1
Flunisolide, 1101·1
Flunisolide Hemihydrate, 1101·1
Flunitec, 2003·1
Flunitop, 2003·1
Flunitrazepam, 698·2
Flunitrazepamum, 698·2
Flunixin Meglumine, 43·3
Flunixino Meglumina, 43·3
Flunolone, 2003·1
Flunolone-V, 2003·1
Flunox, 2003·1
Flunoxaprofen, 43·3
Flunoxaprofeno, 43·3
Fluo Fenic, 2003·1
Fluo Grin, 2003·1
Fluo Vasoc, 2003·1
Fluocal com Pectina, 2003·1
Fluo-calc, 2003·1
Fluocalcic, 2003·1
Fluocaril Preparations, 2003·1
Fluocid Forte, 2003·1
Fluocim, 2003·1
Fluocinolide, 1101·3
Fluocinolona, Acetónido de, 1101·2
Fluocinolone Acetonide, 1101·2
Fluocinolone Acetonide 21-Acetate, 1101·3
Fluocinolone Acetonide Dihydrate, 1101·2
Fluocinoloni Acetonidum, 1101·2
Fluocinónida, 1101·3
Fluocinonide, 1101·3
Fluoclox, 2003·1
Fluocortan, 2003·1
Fluocortin Butyl, 1102·1
Fluocortina, Butil Éster de la, 1102·1
Fluocortolona, 1102·1
Fluocortolona, Caproato de, 1102·1
Fluocortolona, Pivalato de, 1102·1
Fluocortolone, 1102·1
Fluocortolone Caproate, 1102·1
Fluocortolone Hexanoate, 1102·1
Fluocortolone 21-Hexanoate, 1102·1
Fluocortolone Pivalate, 1102·1
Fluocortolone 21-Pivalate, 1102·1
Fluocortolone Trimethylacetate, 1102·1
Fluocortoloni Pivalas, 1102·1
Fluodel, 2003·1
Fluodent, 2003·1
Fluoderm, 2003·2
Fluodermo Fuerte, 2003·2
Fluodonil, 2003·2
Fluodont, 2003·2
Fluodontyl, 2003·2
Fluodrazin F, 2003·2
Fluo-Fenicol, 2003·2
Flu-Off, 2003·2
Fluoftal, 2003·2
Fluogel, 2003·2
Fluogen, 2003·2
Fluogum, 2003·2
Fluohexal, 2003·2
Fluohydric Acid, 1699·2
Fluomint, 2003·2
Fluomint— *see* Mint-Lysoform, 2135·1
Fluomit, 2003·2
Fluomix Same, 2003·2
Fluomycin N, 2003·2
Fluon, 2003·2
Fluonid, 2003·2
Fluonid-N, 2003·2
Fluopate, 2003·2
Fluopiram, 2003·2
Fluoplexe, 2003·2
Fluopromazine, 727·1
Fluopromazine Hydrochloride, 727·1
Fluor, 2003·2
Flúor 18, 1523·3
Fluor Microsol, 2003·2
Fluor Verde, 2003·2
Fluoracaine, 2003·2
Fluor-A-Day, 2003·2
Fluoralfa, 2003·2
Fluorandrenolone, 1100·3
Fluordent, 2003·3
Fluore Stain Strips, 2003·3
Fluorescein, 1689·1
Fluorescein Dilaurate, 1689·1
Fluorescein Natrium, 1689·1
Fluorescein Sodium, 1689·1
Fluorescein, Soluble, 1689·1
Fluoresceína, 1689·1
Fluoresceína, Dilaurato de, 1689·1
Fluoresceína Sódica, 1689·1
Fluoresceinum Natricum, 1689·1
Fluorescite, 2003·3
Fluorets, 2003·3
Fluorette, 2003·3
Fluoretten, 2003·3
Fluorex, 2003·3
Fluorex Plus, 2003·3
Fluorexidina, 2003·3
Fluorhídrico, Ácido, 1699·2
Fluorhinose, 2003·3
Fluoric Acid, 1699·2
Fluoricum Acidum, 1699·3
Fluoridation, 1445·3
Fluoride, Sodium, 1444·3
Fluoridrops, 2003·3
Fluorigard, 2003·3
Fluorigard Gel-Kam, 2003·3
Fluorigard Ortho, 2003·3
Fluoril, 2003·3
Fluorilette, 2003·3
Fluori-Methane, 2003·3
Fluor-In, 2003·3
Fluorinated Piperazinyl Quinolones, 119·2
Fluorindione, 918·2
Fluorine-18, 1523·3
Fluorinse, 2003·3
Fluor-I-Strip, 2003·3
Fluor-I-Strip AT, 2003·3
Fluoritab, 2003·3
Fluoritabs, 2003·3
Fluornatrium, 2003·3
Fluoroacetamida, 1505·3
Fluoroacetamide, 1505·3
Fluoroacetato Sódico, 1510·1
2-Fluoro-ara-AMP, 553·2
3-{2-[4-(6-Fluoro-1,2-benzisoxazol-3-yl)piperidino]ethyl}-6,7,8,9-tetrahydro-2-methylpyrido[1,2-*a*]pyrimidin-4-one, 719·2
3-{2-[4-(4-Fluorobenzoyl)piperidino]ethyl}quinazoline-2,4(1*H*,3*H*)-dione, 943·1
1-[3-(4-Fluorobenzoyl)propyl]-4-piperidinopiperidine-4-carboxamide, 716·1
1-{1-[3-(4-Fluorobenzoyl)propyl]-4-piperidyl}benzimidazolin-2-one, 671·2
1-{1-[3-(4-Fluorobenzoyl)propyl]-1,2,3,6-tetrahydro-4-pyridyl}-benzimidazolin-2-one, 697·2
2-{1-[1-(4-Fluorobenzyl)-1*H*-benzimidazol-2-yl]-4-piperidyl(methyl)amino}pyrimidin-4(1*H*)-one, 437·3
1-(4-Fluorobenzyl)-2-{[1-(4-methoxyphenethyl)-4-piperidyl]amino}benzimidazole, 424·2
Fluorobioptal, 2003·3
2-(2-Fluorobiphenyl-4-yl)propionic Acid, 43·3
Fluorocaine, 2003·3
Fluorocalciforte, 2003·3
Fluorocarbon 134A, 1236·2
Fluorocare, 2003·3
6-α-Fluoroclobetasol Propionate, 1111·3
5-Fluorocytosine, 399·3
Fluorodeoxyglucose ($^{18}$F), 1523·3
5-Fluoro-2′-deoxyuridine, 553·1
(±)-9-Fluoro-6,7-dihydro-8-(4-hydroxypiperidino)-5-methyl-1-oxo-1*H*,5*H*-benzo[*ij*]quinolizine-2-carboxylic Acid, 233·3
9-Fluoro-2,3-dihydro-3-methyl-10-(4-methyl-1-piperazinyl)-7-oxo-7*H*-pyrido[3,2,1-*ij*][4,1,2]benzoxadiazine-6-carboxylic Acid, 228·3
(−)-(*S*)-9-Fluoro-2,3-dihydro-3-methyl-10-(4-methyl-1-piperazinyl)-7-oxo-7*H*-pyrido[1,2,3-*de*]-1,4-benzoxazine-6-carboxylic Acid, 225·3
(±)-9-Fluoro-2,3-dihydro-3-methyl-10-(4-methyl-1-piperazinyl)-7-oxo-7*H*-pyrido[1,2,3-*de*]-1,4-benzoxazine-6-carboxylic Acid, 239·3
9-Fluoro-6,7-dihydro-5-methyl-1-oxo-1*H*,5*H*-pyrido[3,2,1-*ij*]quinoline-2-carboxylic Acid, 214·2
9-Fluoro-2,3-dihydro-10-[4-methylpiperazin-1-yl]-7-oxo-7*H*-pyrido[1,2,3-*de*]-1,4-benzothiazine-6-carboxylic Acid Hydrochloride, 254·3
6α-Fluoro-11β,21-dihydroxy-16α,17α-isopropylidenedioxypregna-1,4-diene-3,20-dione, 1101·1
9α-Fluoro-11β,21-dihydroxy-16α,17α-isopropylidenedioxypregna-1,4-diene-3,20-dione, 1110·2
9α-Fluoro-11β,21-dihydroxy-16α,17α-isopropylidenedioxypregna-1,4-diene-3,20-dione 21-(3,3-Dimethylbutyrate), 1110·2
6α-Fluoro-11β,21-dihydroxy-16α,17α-isopropylidenedioxypregn-4-ene-3,20-dione, 1100·3
9α-Fluoro-11β,17β-dihydroxy-17α-methylandrost-4-en-3-one, 1555·3
6α-Fluoro-11β,21-dihydroxy-16α-methylpregna-1,4-diene-3,20-dione, 1102·1
9α-Fluoro-11β,17α-dihydroxy-6α-methylpregna-1,4-diene-3,20-dione, 1102·2
9α-Fluoro-11β,21-dihydroxy-16α-methylpregna-1,4-diene-3,20-dione, 1096·3
9α-Fluoro-11β,17α-dihydroxypregn-4-ene-3,20-dione 17-Acetate, 1555·2
Fluorodopa ($^{18}$F), 1523·3
(8*S*)-8-Fluoroerythromycin Mono(ethyl Butanedioate) Ester, 214·2
(8*r*)-8-(2-Fluoroethyl)-3α-hydroxy-1α*H*,5α*H*-tropanium Bromide Benzilate, 482·3
6-Fluoro-1-(*p*-fluorophenyl)-1,4-dihydro-7-(4-methyl-1-piperazinyl)-4-oxo-3-quinolinecarboxylic Acid Hydrochloride, 205·3
1-[*o*-Fluoro-α-(*p*-fluorophenyl)-α-phenylbenzyl]imidazole, 400·3
Fluoroformylon, 1103·2
Fluorogel, 2003·4
5-Fluoro-*N*-hexyl-3,4-dihydro-2,4-dioxo-1-(2*H*)-pyrimidinecarboxamide, 535·1
9α-Fluorohydrocortisone 21-Acetate, 1100·1
6α-Fluoro-16α-hydroxyhydrocortisone 16,17-Acetonide, 1100·3
5-Fluoro-1-[(2*R*,5*S*)-2-(hydroxymethyl)-1,3-oxathiolan-5-yl]cytosine, 632·3
9α-Fluoro-16α-hydroxyprednisolone, 1110·2
4′-Fluoro-4-(4-hydroxy-4-*p*-tolylpiperidino)butyrophenone Hydrochloride, 710·1
4′-Fluoro-4-[4-hydroxy-4-(3-trifluoromethylphenyl)piperidino]butyrophenone, 727·1
Fluoromebendazole, 105·2
Fluorometholone, 1102·2
Fluorometholone Acetate, 1102·2
Fluorometholone 17-Acetate, 1102·2
4′-Fluoro-4-[4-(2-methoxyphenyl)piperazin-1-yl]butyrophenone, 698·2
*S*-Fluoromethyl 6α,9α-Difluoro-11β,17α-dihydroxy-16α-methyl-3-oxoandrosta-1,4-diene-17β-carbothioate 17-Propionate, 1102·3
Fluoromethyl 2,2,2-Trifluoro-1-(trifluoromethyl)ethyl Ether, 1307·3
6α-Fluoro-16α-methyl-1-dehydrocorticosterone, 1102·1
5-Fluoro-2-methyl-1-[(*Z*)-*p*-(methylsulfonyl)benzylidene]indene-3-acetic Acid, 552·3
(*Z*)-[5-Fluoro-2-methyl-1-(4-methylsulphinylbenzylidene)inden-3-yl]acetic Acid, 91·2
7-Fluoro-1-methyl-3-methylsulphinyl-4-quinolone, 918·2
4′-Fluoro-4-(4-methylpiperidino)butyrophenone Hydrochloride, 706·1
9α-Fluoro-16α-methylprednisolone, 1097·1
9α-Fluoro-16β-methylprednisolone, 1093·1
6α-Fluoro-16α-methylprednisolone 21-Acetate, 1107·3
Fluorometolona, 1102·2
Fluorometolona, Acetato de, 1102·2
*N*-{[(*S*)-3-(3-Fluoro-4-morpholinophenyl)-2-oxo-5-oxazolidinyl]methyl}acetamide, 226·3
Fluoro-Ophtal, 2003·4
Fluor-Op, 2003·4
5-(2-Fluorophenyl)-1,3-dihydro-1-methyl-7-nitro-1,4-benzodiazepin-2-one, 698·2
4-(*o*-Fluorophenyl)-6,8-dihydro-1,3,8-trimethylpirazole[3,4-*e*][1,4]diazepin-7(1*H*)-one Monohydrochloride, 728·3
(3*R*,4*S*)-1-(*p*-Fluorophenyl)-3-[(3*S*)-3-(*p*-fluorophenyl)-3-hydroxypropyl]-4-(*p*-hydroxyphenyl)-2-azetidinone, 914·2
2-(4-Fluorophenyl)indan-1,3-dione, 918·2
(*E*)-(3*R*,5*S*)-7-{4-(4-Fluorophenyl)-6-isopropyl-2-[methyl(methylsulfonyl)amino]pyrimidin-5-yl}-3,5-dihydroxyhept-6-enoic Acid Calcium (2:1), 996·2
(+)-2-(*p*-Fluorophenyl)-α-methyl-5-benzoxazoleacetic Acid, 43·3
3-[((2*R*,3*S*)-3-(*p*-Fluorophenyl)-2-{[(α*R*)-α-methyl-3,5-bis(trifluoromethyl)benzyl]oxy}morpholino)methyl]-$\Delta^2$-1,2,4-triazolin-5-one, 1250·3
*N*-[3-(4-*p*-Fluorophenylpiperazin-1-yl)-1-methylpropyl]nicotinamide, 438·1
(−)-*trans*-5-(4-*p*-Fluorophenyl-3-piperidylmethoxy)-1,3-benzodioxole, 311·2

Fluoroplat, 2003·4
Fluoroplex, 2003·4
Fluoropoen, 2003·4
Fluoropos, 2003·4
6α-Fluoroprednisolone, 1102·3
9α-Fluoroprednisolone Acetate, 1105·3
4′-Fluoro-4-[4-(2-pyridyl)piperazin-1-yl]butyrophenone, 671·2
5-Fluoropyrimidine-2,4(1*H*,3*H*)-dione, 554·2
Fluoroquinolones, 119·2
Fluororinil, 2003·4
Fluoros, 2003·4
Fluorosol, 2003·4
(*S*)-6-Fluorospiro(chroman-4,4′-imidazolidine)-2′,5′-dione, 345·3
Fluorosulfato, Metilo de, 1714·1
5-Fluoro-1-(tetrahydro-2-furyl)pyrimidine-2,4(1*H*,3*H*)-dione, 586·2
5-Fluoro-1-(tetrahydro-2-furyl)uracil, 586·2
9α-Fluoro-11β,16α,17α,21-tetrahydroxypregna-1,4-diene-3,20-dione, 1110·2
4′-Fluoro-4-[4-(2-thioxo-1-benzimidazolinyl)piperidino]butyrophenone, 725·2
Fluorotirosina, 1598·1
Fluorotrichloromethane, 1236·1
9α-Fluoro-11β,17α,21-trihydroxy-16-methylenepregna-1,4-diene-3,20-dione 21-Acetate, 1102·2
9α-Fluoro-11β,17α,21-trihydroxy-16α-methylpregna-1,4-diene-3,20-dione, 1097·1
9α-Fluoro-11β,17α,21-trihydroxy-16β-methylpregna-1,4-diene-3,20-dione, 1093·1
6α-Fluoro-11β,17α,21-trihydroxy-16α-methylpregna-1,4-diene-3,20-dione 21-Acetate, 1107·3
6α-Fluoro-11β,17α,21-trihydroxypregna-1,4-diene-3,20-dione, 1102·3
9α-Fluoro-11β,17α,21-trihydroxypregna-1,4-diene-3,20-dione 21-Acetate, 1105·3
9α-Fluoro-11β,17α,21-trihydroxypregn-4-ene-3,20-dione 21-Acetate, 1100·1
Fluorotyrosine, 1598·1
3-Fluorotyrosine, 1598·1
Fluorotyrosinum, 1598·1
Fluorouracil, 554·2
5-Fluorouracil, 554·2
5-Fluorouracil Deoxyriboside, 553·1
Fluorouracilo, 554·2
Fluorouracilum, 554·2
5-Fluorouridine Monophosphate, 555·2
Fluorox, 2003·4
Fluorthyrin, 2003·4
Fluortop, 2003·4
Fluortyrosine, 1598·1
Fluoruro Estañoso, 1448·3
Fluoruro Sódico, 1444·3
Fluorvas, 2003·4
Fluor-Vigantoletten, 2003·4
Fluorvitin, 2003·4
Fluoselgine, 2003·4
Fluosept, 2003·4
Fluosilicato Sódico, 1446·3
Fluostigmine, 1490·1
Fluotec, 2003·4
Fluotest, 2003·4
Fluothane, 2003·4
Fluotic, 2003·4
Fluotrat, 2003·4
Fluo-Vaso, 2003·4
Fluovitef, 2003·4
Fluox, 2003·4
Fluoxa, 2003·4
Fluoxac, 2003·4
Fluox-basan, 2003·4
Fluoxemerck, 2004·1
Fluoxeren, 2004·1
Fluoxetina, Hidrocloruro de, 292·1
Fluoxetine Hydrochloride, 292·1
Fluoxetini Hydrochloridum, 292·1
Fluoxgamma, 2004·1
Fluoxibene, 2004·1
Fluoxifar, 2004·1
Fluoximesterona, 1555·3
Fluoxin, 2004·1
Flu-Oxinate, 2004·1
Fluoxine, 2004·1
Fluoxiprednisolonum, 1110·2
Fluoxistad, 2004·1
Fluoxityrol, 2004·1
Fluox-Puren, 2004·1
Fluoxymesterone, 1555·3
Fluoxytil, 2004·1
Flupamesone, 1111·1
Flupar, 2004·1
Flupazine, 2004·1
Flupenthixol Decanoate, 699·1
*cis*-Flupenthixol Decanoate, 699·1
(*Z*)-Flupenthixol Decanoate, 699·1
Flupenthixol Dihydrochloride, 699·1
Flupenthixol Hydrochloride, 699·1
*cis*-Flupentixol, 699·2
*trans*-Flupentixol, 699·2
α-Flupentixol, 699·2
β-Flupentixol, 699·2
(*E*)-Flupentixol, 699·2
(*Z*)-Flupentixol, 699·2
Flupentixol Decanoate, 699·1
Flupentixol, Decanoato de, 699·1
Flupentixol Dihydrochloride, 699·1
Flupentixol, Hidrocloruro de, 699·1
Flupentixol Hydrochloride, 699·1
Flupentixoli Dihydrochloridum, 699·1
Fluphenazine, 699·3
Fluphenazine Decanoate, 699·3
Fluphenazine Enantate, 699·3
Fluphenazine Enanthate, 699·3
Fluphenazine Heptanoate, 699·3
Fluphenazine Hydrochloride, 699·3
Fluphenazine Sulfoxide, 700·1
Fluphenazini Decanoas, 699·3
Fluphenazini Enantas, 699·3
Fluphenazini Hydrochloridum, 699·3
Flupid, 2004·1
Flupidol, 2004·1
Flupirtina, Maleato de, 43·3
Flupirtine Gluconate, 43·3
Flupirtine Maleate, 43·3
Fluprednidene Acetate, 1102·2
Flupredenideno, Acetato de, 1102·2
Fluprednisolona, 1102·3
Fluprednisolone, 1102·3
Fluprednylidene 21-Acetate, 1102·2
Flupress, 2004·1
Fluprim Tosse, 2004·1
Fluprosin, 2004·1
Fluprost, 2004·1
Flura, 2004·1
Flurablastin, 2004·1
Fluracedyl, 2004·1
Fluracil, 2004·1
Flurandrenolide, 1100·3
Flurandrenolone, 1100·3
Flurate, 2004·1
Fluraz, 2004·1
Flurazepam, 700·3
Flurazepam, Dihidrocloruro de, 700·3
Flurazepam Dihydrochloride, 700·3
Flurazepam Hydrochloride, 700·3
Flurazepam, Monohidrocloruro de, 700·3
Flurazepam Monohydrochloride, 700·3
Flurazepami Monohydrochloridum, 700·3
Flurbid, 2004·1
Flurbiprofen, 43·3
Flurbiprofen Axetil, 44·2
Flurbiprofen Sodium, 44·1
Flurbiprofeno, 43·3
Flurbiprofeno Sódico, 44·1
Flurbiprofenum, 43·3
Flurekain, 2004·1
Fluress, 2004·2
Flurets, 2004·2
Fluricin, 2004·2
Flurinol, 2004·2
Flurithromycin Ethyl Succinate, 214·2
Flurizic, 2004·2
Fluroblastin, 2004·2
Fluroblastine, 2004·2
Fluro-Ethyl, 2004·2
Flurofen, 2004·2
Flurogestone Acetate, 1555·2
Flurolon, 2004·2
Flurop, 2004·2
Fluropropiofenone, 1689·1
Fluroptic, 2004·2
Flurosyn, 2004·2
Flurox, 2004·2
Flurozin, 2004·2
Flurpax, 2004·2
Flusac, 2004·2
Flusan, 2004·2
Fluscand, 2004·2
Flusemide, 2004·2
Fluseminal, 2004·2
Flusenil, 2004·2
Fluserin, 2004·2
Flushield, 2004·2
Flusin, 2004·2
Flusin C, 2004·2
Flusin DM, 2004·3
Flusin S, 2004·3
Flusol, 2004·3
Flusolgen, 2004·3
Flusolv, 2004·3
Flusona, 2004·3
Flusonal, 2004·3
Fluspi, 2004·3
Fluspiral, 2004·3
Fluspirilene, 701·1
Fluspirileno, 701·1
Fluspirilenum, 701·1
Flusporan, 2004·3
Fluss 40, 2004·3
Flussorex, 2004·3
Flu-Stat, 2004·3
Flusten, 2004·3
Fluta, 2004·3
Flutabene, 2004·3
Flutacan, 2004·3
Flutaide, 2004·3
Flutamex, 2004·3
Flutamida, 556·2
Flutamide, 556·2
Flutamidum, 556·2
Flutamin, 2004·3
Flutan, 2004·3
Flutandrona, 2004·3
Flutaplex, 2004·3
Flutastad, 2004·3
Flutax, 2004·3
Flutec, 2004·3
Flutenal, 2004·3
Flutenal Gentamicina, 2004·3
Flutenal Sali, 2004·3
Flutepan, 2004·4
Flutex, 2004·4
Flutex Cough Linctus, 2004·4
Flutex Decon-S, 2004·4
Flutiamik, 2004·4
Fluticasona, Propionato de, 1102·3
Fluticasone Propionate, 1102·3
Fluticasoni Propionas, 1102·3
Flutide, 2004·4
Flutin, 2004·4
Flutinase, 2004·4
Flutine, 2004·4
Flutivate, 2004·4
Flutol, 2004·4
Flutox, 2004·4
Flutrax, 2004·4
Flutraz, 2004·4
Flutrimazol, 400·3
Flutrimazole, 400·3
Flutrimazolum, 400·3
Flutropio, Bromuro de, 482·3
Flutropium Bromide, 482·3
Flutter, Atrial— *see* Cardiac Arrhythmias, 816·1
Flu/Vac, 1620·2
Flu/Vac/SA, 1620·2
Flu/Vac/Split, 1620·2
Fluvaleas, 2004·4
Fluvalinate, 1505·3
Fluvalinato, 1505·3
Fluvastatin Sodium, 918·2
Fluvastatina Sódica, 918·2
Fluvax, 2004·4
Fluvean, 2004·4
Fluvermal, 2004·4
Fluvert, 2004·4
Fluvet, 2004·4
Fluvic, 2004·4
Fluviral, 2004·4
Fluvirin, 2004·4
Fluvirine, 2005·1
Fluvium, 2005·1
Fluvohexal, 2005·1
Fluvosol, 2005·1
Fluvoxadura, 2005·1
Fluvoxamina, Maleato de, 298·2
Fluvoxamine Maleate, 298·2
Fluvoxin, 2005·1
Flux, 2005·1
Fluxacil, 2005·1
Fluxacina, 2005·1
Fluxadir, 2005·1
Fluxal, 2005·1
Fluxantin, 2005·1
Fluxapril, 2005·1
Fluxarten, 2005·1
Fluxedan, 2005·1
Fluxema, 2005·1
Fluxene, 2005·1
Fluxet, 2005·1
Fluxetil, 2005·1
Fluxetin, 2005·1
Fluxifarm, 2005·1
Fluxil, 2005·1
Fluximesterona, 1555·3
Fluxinam, 2005·1
Fluxine, 2005·1
Fluxocor, 2005·1
Fluxol, 2005·1
FluxoMed, 2005·1
Fluxoten, 2005·2
Fluxpiren, 2005·2
Fluxum, 2005·2
Fluxus, 2005·2
Fluzac, 2005·2
Fluzal, 2005·2
Fluzerit, 2005·2
Fluzine, 2005·2
Fluzix, 2005·2
Fluzol, 2005·2
Fluzone, 2005·2
Fluzor, 2005·2
Fly Agaric, 1717·3
Fly, Spanish, 1666·3
Flynoken A, 2005·2
FM7 E, 2005·2
F-MA 11, 1250·1
FML, 2005·2
FML Neo, 2005·2
FML Neo Liquifilm, 2005·2
FML-S, 2005·2
FMN, 1456·2
FMP, 2005·2
FMP-1, 1622·3
FNZ, 2005·2
Foamicon, 2005·2
Foban, 2005·2
Fobancort, 2005·2
Fobidon, 2005·2
Focal Glomerulosclerosis— *see* Glomerular Kidney Disease, 1080·2
Focal Seizures— *see* Epilepsy, 349·1
Focalin, 2005·2
Focam, 2005·2
Focus, 2005·3
Focus Care All-in-One, 2005·3
Focus Care One Step, 2005·3
Foeniculi, Aetheroleum, 1687·3
Foeniculi Amari Fructus, 1687·2
Foeniculi Amari Fructus Aetheroleum, 1687·3
Foeniculi Dulcis Fructus, 1687·2
Foeniculi, Oleum, 1687·3
Foeniculin, 1655·2
Foeniculum, 1687·2
*Foeniculum vulgare*, 1687·2, 1687·3
Foenugraeci, Semen, 1688·1
Fohn- und Wettertropfen N, 2005·3
Fohnetten N, 2005·3
Foie de Soufre, 1158·3

Foille, 2005·3
Foille Insetti, 2005·3
Foille Scottature, 2005·3
Foille Sole, 2005·3
Foipan, 2005·3
Fokalepsin, 2005·3
Fokeston, 2005·3
Fokkra, 1666·1
Fol Sang, 2005·3
Folacid, 2005·3
Folacin, 1429·1, 2005·3
Folacin 12, 2005·3
Folarell, 2005·3
Folaren, 2005·3
Fol-Asmedic, 2005·3
Folate-deficiency Anaemia— *see* Megaloblastic Anaemia, 734·1
Folatine, 2005·3
Folavit, 2005·3
Folaxin, 2005·3
Folcane, 2005·3
Folcodal, 2005·3
Folcodex, 2005·3
Folcodina, 1128·3
Folcofen, 2005·4
Folcress, 2005·4
Folcur, 2005·4
Foldan, 2005·4
Folderm, 2005·4
Folderm Pomada, 2005·4
Foldox, 2005·4
Foldoxx, 2005·4
Foledrina, Sulfato de, 982·3
Folepar B12, 2005·4
Folergot-DF, 2005·4
Folex, 2005·4
Folgamma, 2005·4
Folgamma Mono, 2005·4
Folgard, 2005·4
Folha de Dedaleira, 894·2
Foli Doce, 2005·4
Folia Bucco, 1663·1
Folia Trifoli Fibrini, 1712·1
Foliamin, 2005·4
Foliben, 2005·4
Folic Acid, 1429·1
Folic Acid Plus, 2005·4
Folic Plus, 2005·4
Folicalgyn, 2005·4
Folicare, 2005·4
FOLI-cell, 2005·4
Folicil, 2005·4
Fólico, Ácido, 1429·1
Folicombin, 2005·4
Folicorin, 2005·4
Folicron, 2005·4
Folicum, 2005·4
Folicum, Acidum, 1429·1
Folidan, 2005·4
Folidar, 2006·1
Folifer, 2006·1
Foliferron, 2006·1
Foligan, 2006·1
Foliglobin, 2006·1
Foliment, 2006·1
Folimet, 2006·1
Folin, 2006·1
Folina, 2006·1
Folinac, 2006·1
Folinato, 2006·1
Folinato Cálcico, 1431·1
Folinemic Ferro, 2006·1
Folinfabra, 2006·1
Folingrav, 2006·1
Folinic Acid, 1431·1
Folínico, Ácido, 1431·1
Folinoral, 2006·1
Folinovo, 2006·1
Folinsyre, 1429·1
Folinvit, 2006·1
Foliper, 2006·1
Foliplus, 2006·1
Foli-Rivo, 2006·1
Folisanin, 2006·1
Folitab, 2006·1
Folitabs, 2006·1
Folitropina, 1324·2
Folitropina Alfa, 1324·2
Folitropina Beta, 1324·2
Folium, 2006·1
Folivit, 2006·1
Folix, 2006·1
Folix-Mater, 2006·1
Folizol, 2006·2
Follegon, 2006·2
Follicle Stimulating Hormone-releasing Factor, 1325·1
Follicle-stimulating Hormone, 1324·2, 1330·1
Follicular Hormone, 1553·1
Follicular Hormone Hydrate, 1552·3
Follicular Lymphoma— *see* Non-Hodgkin's Lymphomas, 510·1
Folliculin, 1553·1
Folliculitis— *see* Skin Infections, 146·2
Folliculitis, Seborrhoeic— *see* Seborrhoeic Dermatitis, 1138·3
Follimin, 2006·2
Follimon, 2006·2
Follinett, 2006·2
Follistim, 2006·2
Follistrel, 2006·2
Follitrin, 2006·2
Follitropin Alfa, 1324·2
Follitropin Beta, 1324·2
Folmigor, 2006·2
Folsan, 2006·2
Folsana, 2006·2
Foltene, 2006·2
Foltene Research Anticaspa, 2006·2
Foltran, 2006·2
FOLTX, 2006·2
Folverlan, 2006·2
Folvite, 2006·2
Fomagrippin N, 2006·2
Fomene, 2006·2
Fomentil, 2006·2
Fomepizol, 1039·2
Fomepizole, 1039·2
Fominobén, Hidrocloruro de, 1121·3
Fominoben Hydrochloride, 1121·3
Fomivirsen Sodium, 634·1
Fomivirseno Sódico, 634·1
Fomocaine Hydrochloride, 1376·3
Fomos, 2006·2
Fon Wan Preparations, 2006·2
Fonazine Mesylate, 431·3
Foncitril, 2006·3
Fondaparin Sodium, 918·3
Fondaparinux Sódico, 918·3
Fondaparinux Sodium, 918·3
Fonderyl, 2006·3
Fondril, 2006·3
Fondril HCT, 2006·3
Fondur, 2006·3
Fonergin, 2006·3
Fonergine, 2006·3
Fonergoral, 2006·3
Fonexel, 2006·3
Fongamil, 2006·3
Fongarex, 2006·3
Fongeryl, 2006·3
Fongitar, 2006·3
Fonicef, 2006·3
Fonicid, 2006·3
Fonigen, 2006·3
Fonisal, 2006·3
Fonlipol, 2006·3
Fonofos, 2006·3
Fontego, 2006·3
Fontex, 2006·3
Fontol, 2006·3
Fontolax, 2006·3
Fonto-Vit B6, 2006·3
Fonto-Vit C, 2006·3
Fonto-Vit E, 2006·4
Fonx, 2006·4
Fonzac, 2006·4
Fonzylane, 2006·4
Food Allergy, 422·1
Food Hypersensitivity— *see* Food Allergy, 422·1
Food Intolerance, 1448·2
Food Poisoning— *see* Gastro-enteritis, 127·3
Fool's Mushroom, 1717·3
Foot Disease, Diabetic— *see* Diabetic Complications, 326·2
Foot Zeta, 2006·4
Footworks, 2006·4
For Gas, 2006·4
For Kids Only, 2006·4
For Liver, 2006·4
For Men, 2006·4
For Peripheral Circulation Herbal Plus Formula 5, 2006·4
For the Post-Menopausal Years, 2006·4
For Women Active Woman Formula, 2006·4
For Women Multi Plus EPO, 2006·4
Foracet, 2006·4
Foracort, 2006·4
Foradil, 2006·4
Foradile, 2006·4
Foral, 2006·4
Forane, 2006·4
Forane— *see* Isoflurane, 2068·1
Forapin, 2006·4
Forapin E, 2006·4
Foraseq, 2006·4
Forbrand, 2006·4
Forcaltonin, 2007·1
Forcan, 2007·1
Forcapil, 2007·1
Forcemil, 2007·1
Forceval, 2007·1
Forceval Protein, 2007·1
Forcicline, 2007·1
Forcil, 2007·1
Forcilen, 2007·1
Forclina, 2007·1
Forcremol, 2007·1
Ford Fibre, 2007·1
Ford Pills, 2007·1
Fordilen, 2007·1
Fordiuran, 2007·1
Fordrim, 2007·1
Fordtran, 2007·1
Forehead-C, 2007·1
Forene, 2007·1
Forenium, 2007·1
Foresight, 2007·1
Foresight Iron Formula, 2007·1
Forexin, 2007·1
Forgenac, 2007·1
Forget Me Drug, 698·3
Forget Me Pill, 698·3
Forgrip, 2007·1
Foric, 2007·1
Forilin, 2007·1
Forimycin, 2007·1
Foristal, 2007·1
Forken, 2007·1
Forknow, 2007·1
Forlax, 2007·2
Forli, 2007·2
Formadon, 2007·2
Formal, 1680·3
Formaldehído, Solución, 1179·3
Formaldehído Sulfoxilato Sódico, 1192·1
Formaldehyde, 230·2, 1179·3
Formaldehyde Dimethyl Acetal, 1680·3
Formaldehyde Solution, 1179·3
Formaldehyde Solution (35 Per Cent), 1179·3
Formaldehyde-sulphathiazole, 214·2
Formaldehydi Solutio, 1179·3
Formalin, 1179·3
Formalyde, 2007·2
Formamida, 1474·3
Formamide, 1474·3
Formance, 2007·2
Formasan, 2007·2
Format, 2007·2
Formebolona, 1555·3
Formebolone, 1555·3
Formedico, 2007·2
Formel 44 Plus Hustenloser, Wick— *see* Wick Formel 44 Plus Hustenloser, 2385·4
Formel 44 Plus Hustenstiller, Wick— *see* Wick Formel 44 Plus Hustenstiller, 2386·1
Formel 44, Wick— *see* Wick Formel 44, 2385·4
Formestane, 557·1
Formestano, 557·1
Formic Acid, 1180·2, 1689·3
Formicain, 2007·2
Fórmico, Ácido, 1689·3
Formidium, 2007·2
*N*-Formimidoyl Thienamycin, 221·1
Formin, 2007·2
Formine, 230·1
Formisoton, 2007·2
Formistin, 2007·2
Formitonicum, 2007·2
Formitrol, 2007·2
Formocarbine, 2007·2
Formocortal, 1103·2
Formo-Cresol Mitis, 2007·2
Formoftil, 2007·2
Formol, 1179·3
Formomicin, 2007·2
Formononetin, 1737·3
Formosulfathiazole, 214·2
Formosulfatiazol, 214·2
Formosulphathiazole, 214·2
Formoterol Fumarate, 786·1
Formoterol Fumarate Dihydrate, 786·1
Formoterol, Fumarato de, 786·1
Formoteroli Fumaras Dihydricus, 786·1
Formula 2, 2007·2
Formula II Especial, 2007·2
Formula IV, 2007·2
Formula 28, 2007·2
Formula 33 SE, 2007·3
Formula 44, 2007·2
Formula 44, Vicks— *see* Vicks Formula 44, 2375·3
Formula 44 Cough Control Discs, Vicks— *see* Vicks Formula 44 Cough Control Discs, 2375·3
Formula 44D, 2007·2
Formula 44D Dry Hacking Cough & Head Congestion, Vicks Pediatric— *see* Vicks Pediatric Formula 44D Dry Hacking Cough & Head Congestion, 2375·4
Formula 44E, 2007·2
Formula 44E, Vicks Pediatric— *see* Vicks Pediatric Formula 44E, 2375·4
Formula 44M, 2007·3
Formula 44M Multi-Symptom Cough & Cold, Vicks Pediatric— *see* Vicks Pediatric Formula 44M Multi-Symptom Cough & Cold, 2375·4
Formula 44M Pediatric, 2007·3
Formula 405, 2007·2
Formula 405, Le Pont Tratamiento Ungueal— *see* Le Pont Tratamiento Ungueal Formula 405, 2090·2
Formula A-C-E & Selenium, 2007·2
Formula B Plus, 2007·2
Formula CDC, 2007·2
Formula CI, 2007·2
Formula E, 2007·2
Formula EM, 2007·2
Formula Forte Senior, 2007·3
Formula Four, Bioglan— *see* Bioglan Formula Four, 1844·1
Formula Gly, 2007·3
Formula Gyn, 2007·3
Formula O, 2007·3
Formula OSG, 2007·3
Formula OSX, 2007·3
Formula S, 2007·3
Formula-S, 2007·3
Formula-S, Cow & Gate— *see* Cow & Gate Formula-S, 1910·3
Formula Stress, 2007·3
Formula VM, 2007·3
Formula VM-75, 2007·3
Formulaexpec, 2007·3
Formulat Biosoya, 2007·3
Formulat Pregel, 2007·3

Formulation R, 2007·3
Formulatus, 2007·3
Formule de L'Abbe Chaupitre Preparations, 2007·3
Formule de L'Abbe Chaupitre No 5— *see* Hivernum, 2047·3
Formule 115 DM, 2007·3
Formule No 203 Profil, 2007·3
Formule No 204 Profil, 2007·3
Formule W, 2007·3
Formulex, 2007·3
Formulix, 2007·3
Formuly-Piel, 2007·3
4-Formyl-amino-antipyrine, 36·1
Formyldienolone, 1555·3
α-(2-Formyl-3-hydroxyphenoxy)-*p*-toluic Acid, 1759·3
*N*-Formyl-L-leucine, Ester with (3*S*,4*S*)-3-Hexyl-4-[(2*S*)-2-hydroxytridecyl]-2-oxetanone, 1724·2
7-(Formylmethyl)-4,10-dihydroxy-5-methoxy-9,16-dimethyl-2-oxo-oxacyclohexadeca-11,13-dien-6-yl 3,6-Dideoxy-4-*O*-(2,6-dideoxy-3-*C*-methyl-α-L-*ribo*-hexopyranosyl)-3-(dimethylamino)-β-D-glucopyranoside 4′-Acetate 4″-Isovalerate, 224·3
7-(Formylmethyl)-4,10-dihydroxy-5-methoxy-9,16,-dimethyl-2-oxo-oxacyclohexadeca-11,13-dien-6-yl 3,6-Dideoxy-4-*O*-(2,6-dideoxy-3-*C*-methyl-α-L-*ribo*-hexopyranosyl)-3-(dimethylamino)-β-D-glucopyranoside 4′,4″-Dipropionate, 231·3
[(4*R*,5*S*,6*S*,7*R*,9*R*,10*R*,11*E*,13*E*,16*R*)-7-(Formylmethyl)-4,10-dihydroxy-5-methoxy-9,16-dimethyl-2-oxooxacyclohexadeca-11,13-dien-6-yl]-3,6-dideoxy-4-*O*-(2,6-dideoxy-3-*C*-methyl-α-L-*ribo*-hexopyranosyl)-3-(dimethylamino)-β-D-glucopyranoside 4″-Butyrate 3″-Propionate, 254·1
2-Formyl-1-methylpyridinium Chloride Oxime, 1050·1
*N*-Formylpenicillamine, 163·3
Formylrifampicin, 252·2
5-Formyltetrahydropteroylglutamic Acid, 1431·1
Formyxan, 2007·3
Forpyn, 2007·3
Forsalil, 2007·3
Forscolin, 1674·3
Forskolin, 1674·3
Forsteo, 2007·3
Forta, 2007·3
Forta B, 2007·3
Fortacet, 2007·4
Fortacil, 2007·4
Fortagesic, 2007·4
Fortakehl, 2007·4
Fortal, 2007·4
Fortal Vision, 2007·4
Fortalgesic, 2007·4
Fortalgex GH, 2007·4
Fortalidon P, 2007·4
Fortalis, 2007·4
Fortam, 2007·4
Fortamines 10, 2007·4
Fortamol, 2007·4
Fortaneurin, 2007·4
Fortapal, 2007·4
Fortasec, 2007·4
Fortathrin, 2007·4
Fortavil, 2007·4
Fortax, 2007·4
Fortaz, 2007·4
Fortcinolona, 2007·4
Fortecortin, 2007·4
Fortefog, 2007·4
Fortel, 2007·4
Fortemethrin— *see* Fortefog, 2007·4
Forten, 2007·4
Fortenac, 2007·4
Forteo, 2007·4
Fortepen, 2008·1
Forterra, 2008·1
Fortevital, 2008·1
Fortfen, 2008·1
Forthane, 2008·1
Fortical, 2008·1
Fortical— *see* Polycal, 2226·4
Forticine, 2008·1
Forticol, 2008·1
Forticreme, 2008·1
Forticrin, 2008·1
Fortidrink, 2008·1
Fortifer, 2008·1
Fortifresh, 2008·1
Fortijuice, 2008·1
Fortilut, 2008·1
Fortimel, 2008·1
Fortimicin, 2008·1
Fortimicin A Sulphate, 158·3
Fortini, 2008·1
Fortini Multi Fibre, 2008·1
Fortinol, 2008·1
Fortipine, 2008·1
Fortiplex, 2008·1
Fortipudding, 2008·1
Fortisip, 2008·1
Fortison— *see* Nutrison, 2181·3
Fortistress, 2008·1
Fortolin, 2008·1
Fortonal, 2008·1
Fortovase, 2008·1
Fortplex, 2008·2
Fortradol, 2008·2
Fortral, 2008·2
Fortralin, 2008·2
Fortrans, 2008·2
Fortravel, 2008·2
Fortum, 2008·2
Fortumset, 2008·2
Fortwin, 2008·2
Fortyplan, 2008·2
Fortzaar, 2008·2
Forverm, 2008·2
Forvital, 2008·2
Forzaar, 2008·2
Forzid, 2008·2
Fosalan, 2008·2
Fosamax, 2008·2
Fosamprenavir Calcium, 634·1
Foscald3, 2008·2
Foscan, 2008·2
Foscarnet Sódico, 634·2
Foscarnet Sodium, 634·2
Foscarnet Sodium Hexahydrate, 634·2
Foscarnetum Natricum Hexahydricum, 634·2
Foscavir, 2008·2
Foscovir, 2008·3
Fosfalugel, 2008·3
Fosfalumina, 2008·3
Fosfamid, 1504·1
Fosfarsile Forte, 2008·3
Fosfarsile Junior, 2008·3
Fosfaserin, 2008·3
Fosfaseron, 2008·3
Fosfatan, 2008·3
Fosfatidilcolina, 1731·1
Fosfatidilserina, 1731·2
Fosfato, 1230·3
Fosfato de Adenosina, 1647·3
Fosfato de Aluminio, 1250·1
Fosfato de Amonio, 1654·1
Fosfato de Anileridina, 15·1
Fosfato de Antazolina, 424·2
Fosfato de Butinolina, 1663·3
Fosfato de Clindamicina, 194·2
Fosfato de Cloroquina, 448·2
Fosfato de Dexametasona, 1097·2
Fosfato de Dihidrocodeína, 34·3
Fosfato de Dimemorfano, 1118·3
Fosfato de Disopiramida, 903·3
Fosfato de Fludarabina, 553·2
Fosfato de Iproniazida, 300·3
Fosfato de Oleandomicina, 240·2
Fosfato de Oseltamivir, 651·1
Fosfato de Oxolamina, 1126·1
Fosfato de Poliestradiol, 1565·3
Fosfato de Potasio, Dihidrógeno, 1230·3
Fosfato de Potasio, Hidrógeno, 1230·3
Fosfato de Primaquina, 456·2
Fosfato de Rilmenidina, 996·1
Fosfato de Sodio, 1231·1
Fosfato de Sodio, Dihidrógeno, 1230·3
Fosfato de Sodio, Hidrógeno, 1231·1
Fosfato de Vidarabina, 657·1
Fosfato Monocálcico, 1664·2
Fosfato Sódico de Betametasona, 1093·1
Fosfato Sódico de Dexametasona, 1097·2
Fosfato Sódico de Estramustina, 551·1
Fosfato Sódico de Hidrocortisona, 1104·1
Fosfato Sódico de Prednisolona, 1108·1
Fosfato Sódico de Riboflavina, 1456·1
Fosfato Tricalcico, 1225·3
Fosfenitoína Sódica, 361·3
Fosfestrol, 1555·3
Fosfestrol Disodium, 1556·1
Fosfestrol Sódico, 1555·3
Fosfestrol Sodium, 1555·3
Fosfitone, 2008·3
Fosfo Plus, 2008·3
Fosfo-Acutil, 2008·3
Fosfoadital, 2008·3
Fosfo-Astenil, 2008·3
Fosfocaps, 2008·3
Fosfocil, 2008·3
Fosfocin, 2008·3
Fosfocina, 2008·3
Fosfocine, 2008·3
Fosfocreatine, 1677·2
Fosfocreatinina, 1689·3
Fosfocreatinine, 1689·3
Fosfocreatinine Sodium, 1689·3
Fosfocrisolo, 2008·3
Fosfo-Dom, 2008·3
Fosfoevac, 2008·3
Fosfoglicopeptical, 1693·3
Fosfoglutina B6, 2008·3
Fosfoguaiacol, 2008·3
Fosfomicina, 214·2
Fosfomik, 2008·3
Fosfomycin, 214·2
Fosfomycin Calcium, 214·2
Fosfomycin Sodium, 214·3
Fosfomycin Trometamol, 214·3
Fosfomycin Tromethamine, 214·3
Fosfomycinum Calcicum, 214·2
Fosfomycinum Natricum, 214·3
Fosfomycinum Trometamol, 214·3
Fosfor, 2008·3
Fosforal, 2008·4
Fosfórico, Ácido, 1731·2
Fosforil Calcium, 2008·4
Fosforilasi, 2008·4
Fosforilcolina, 1690·1
Fosforina, 2008·4
Fósforo, 1731·2
Fósforo 32, 1525·1
Fosforylcholine, 1690·1
Fosfosal, 44·2
Fosfosoda, 2008·4
Fosfo-Soda Fleet, 2008·4
Fosfosol, 2008·4
Fosfosol Stress, 2008·4
Fosfostilben, 2008·4
Fosfotonico, 2008·4
Fosfoutipi Vitaminico, 2008·4
Fosfovita, 2008·4
Fosfree, 2008·4
Fosfuro de Aluminio, 1500·1
Fosgeno, 1731·1
Fosgluten Reforzado, 2008·4
Fosgluten Super Reforcado, 2008·4
Fosicomb, 2008·4
Fosicombi, 2008·4
Fosicomp, 2008·4
Foside, 2008·4
Fosinil, 2008·4
Fosinopril Sódico, 919·1
Fosinopril Sodium, 919·1
Fosinoprilat, 919·1
Fosinorm, 2008·4
Fosinorm Comp, 2008·4
Fosipres, 2008·4
Fositen, 2008·4
Fositens, 2008·4
Fositens Plus, 2008·4
Foslainco, 2008·4
Fosmet, 1509·1
Fosmicin, 2008·4
Fosmicin-S, 2009·1
Fospartan Ginseng, 2009·1
Fosphenytoin Sodium, 361·3
Fossil Tree, 1692·3
Fossyol, 2009·1
Fostex Preparations, 2009·1
Fostimon, 2009·1
Fostril, 2009·1
Fosval, 2009·1
Fosvital, 2009·1
Fotax, 2009·1
Fotemustina, 557·2
Fotemustine, 557·2
Fotexina, 2009·1
Fotil, 2009·1
Fotocollyre, 2009·1
Fotocrem 8, 2009·1
Fotocrem P, 2009·1
Fotocrem Ultra, 2009·1
Fotocrem-P, 2009·1
Fotofil, 2009·1
Fotoprotector Preparations, 2009·1
Fotoprotectores, 2009·2
Fotoral, 2009·2
Fotorretin, 2009·2
Fototar, 2009·2
Fotrec DHA, 2009·2
Fouadin, 103·1
Fougère Mâle, 108·2
Fourneau-309, 615·3
Fournox, 2009·2
Four-Ton, 2009·2
Fovas, 2009·2
Fovysat, 2009·2
Fowlers, 2009·2
Foxetin, 2009·2
Foxglove, Austrian, 894·2
Foxglove Leaf, 894·2
Foxglove Leaf, Woolly, 894·2
Foxil, 2009·2
Foxim, 1509·1
Foximin, 2009·2
Foxin, 2009·2
Foxinon, 2009·2
Foxolin, 2009·2
Foxtil, 2009·2
Foy, 2009·2
FOY-305, 1665·2
Foziretic, 2009·2
Fozitec, 2009·2
FP 20, 2009·2
FPL-670, 795·3
FPL-59002, 789·3
FPL-60278, 908·2
FPL-12924AA, 377·2
FPL-60278AR, 908·2
FPL-59002KC, 789·3
FPL-59002KP, 789·3
FR-13749, 182·2
FR-17027, 172·3
FR-900506, 1363·3
Fracción Proteica Del Plasma, 758·2
Fracidin, 2009·2
Fractal, 2009·2
Fractar— *see* Pentrax, 2211·4
Fractionated Palm Kernel Oil, 1481·3
Frademicina, 2009·3
Fradilen, 2009·3
Fradiomycin Sulfate, 235·1
Frador, 2009·3
Fragador, 2009·3
Fragmentos de Anticuerpos Específicos Antidigoxina, 1036·3
Fragmin, 2009·3
Fragmine, 2009·3
Fragonal, 2009·3
Fragrant Agrimony, 1649·1
Frakidex, 2009·3
Frakitacine, 2009·3
Framboise, 1057·3
Frambuesa, 1057·3
Frambuesa, Hoja de, 1737·3
Framecef, 2009·3
Framicetina, Sulfato de, 215·1
Framil, 2009·3
Framin, 2009·3

Framybiotal, 2009·3
Framycetin Sulfate, 215·1
Framycetin Sulphate, 215·1
Framycetini Sulfas, 215·1
Framyxone, 2009·3
*Francisella tularensis*, 1642·1
Francital, 2009·3
*Frangula alnus*, 1266·3
Frangula Bark, 1266·3
*Frangula purshiana*, 1255·1
Frangulae Cortex, 1266·3
Frangulina, 2009·3
Franidipine Hydrochloride, 950·2
Frankincense, 1690·1
Frankincense, Indian, 1690·1
Franol, 2009·3
Franol Expectorant, 2009·3
Franol Plus, 2009·3
Franolyn Expectorant, 2009·3
Franolyn Sedative, 2009·3
Franzbranns, 2009·4
Franzbranntwein, 2009·4
Franzbranntwein, Klosterfrau— *see* Klosterfrau Franzbranntwein, 2081·1
Franzbranntwein Latschenkiefer, Klosterfrau— *see* Klosterfrau Franzbranntwein Latschenkiefer, 2081·1
Franzbranntwein Mit Fichtennadelol, 2009·4
Fraurs, 2009·4
Fravitan, 2009·4
Fraxidol, 2009·4
Fraxiforte, 2009·4
*Fraxinus ornus*, 1273·1
Fraxiparin, 2009·4
Fraxiparina, 2009·4
Fraxiparine, 2009·4
Fraxodi, 2009·4
Frazim, 2009·4
Frazoline, 2009·4
FRC-8653, 884·1
FreAmine, 2009·4
FreAmine III, 2009·4
FreAmine 3% Electrolitos, 2009·4
FreAmine HBC, 2009·4
FreAmine Hepatico, 2009·4
Frebac, 2009·4
Frebini, 2009·4
Fre-bre, 2009·4
Frecuental, 2009·4
Fredcina, 2009·4
Fredol, 2009·4
Fredyr, 2009·4
Free & Clear, 2009·4
Freebase, 1373·3
Freecad, 2010·1
Freedavite, 2010·1
Freedox, 2010·1
Freeflex Cloruro Sodico, 2010·1
Freeflex Ringer Lactato, 2010·1
Freenal, 2010·1
Freesept, 2010·1
Freezone, 2010·1
Freimax, 2010·1
Freka-cid, 2010·1
Freka-Clyss, 2010·1
Frekaderm, 2010·1
Freka-Derm, 2010·1
Freka-Drainjet, 2010·1
Freka-Drainjet Purisole, 2010·1
Freka-Nol, 2010·1
Freka-Sept 80, 2010·1
Freka-Steril, 2010·1
FrekaVit, 2010·1
Fremet, 2010·1
Frenacol, 2010·1
Frenactil, 2010·1
Frenadol, 2010·1
Frenadol Complex, 2010·1
Frenadol PS, 2010·1
Frenal, 2010·2
Frenal Compositum, 2010·2
Frenal Rinologico, 2010·2
Frenaler, 2010·2
Frenaler-D, 2010·2
Frenaseltz, 2010·2
Frenasma, 2010·2
Frenatus, 2010·2
French Chalk, Purified, 1159·1
French Psyllium, 1268·1
Frendox, 2010·2
Frenopect, 2010·2
Frenotos, 2010·2
Frenotos Muc, 2010·2
Frenotosse, 2010·2
Frenotossil, 2010·2
Frenovex, 2010·2
Frenurin, 2010·2
Frerichs Maldifassi, 2010·2
Frescansol, 2010·2
Fresco, 2010·2
Fresenius OPD, 2010·2
Fresenizol, 2010·2
Fresh Bilberry, 1718·3
Fresh Tears, 2010·2
FreshBurst Listerine, 2010·2
Freshmel, 2010·2
Freshmel Tos, 2010·2
Fresium High Energy— *see* Entera, 1971·1
Fresofol, 2010·2
Fresubin, 2010·2
Freudal, 2010·2
FRG-8813, 1269·3
Frialgina, 2010·3
Friax, 2010·3
Friccex, 2010·3
Friction Rub, 2010·3
Fridalit, 2010·3
Frigol, 2010·3
Frigoplasma, 2010·3
Frilen, 2010·3
Friliver, 2010·3
Frinova, 2010·3
Friobax, 2010·3
Frionex, 2010·3
Frionex Plus, 2010·3
Friosmin N, 2010·3
Fripi, 2010·3
Friral, 2010·3
Frisin, 2010·3
Frisium, 2010·3
Frisogrow, 2010·3
Frisol, 2010·3
Frisolac, 2010·3
Frisolona, 2010·3
Frisomum, 2010·3
Frisosoy, 2010·3
Frisovom, 2010·3
Fristamin, 2010·3
Frivent, 2010·3
Frixio, 2010·3
Frixodon, 2010·3
Frixopel, 2010·4
Froben, 2010·4
Froidir, 2010·4
Fromentyl, 2010·4
Frone, 2010·4
Frontal, 2010·4
Froop, 2010·4
Froop Co, 2010·4
Fropenem Sodium, 213·1
Frosinor, 2010·4
Frost Cream, 2010·4
Frostsalbe, 2010·4
Frotin, 2010·4
Frova, 2010·4
Frovatriptan, 469·2
Frovatriptan Succinate, 469·2
Frovex, 2010·4
Froxal, 2010·4
Frozen Shoulder— *see* Soft-tissue Rheumatism, 11·1
Frubiase, 2010·4
Frubiase Calcium, 2010·4
Frubiase Calcium Forte 500, 2010·4
Frubiase Calcium T, 2010·4
Frubienzym, 2010·4
Frubilurgyl, 2010·4
Frubiose Calcium, 2010·4
Frubiose Vitamine D, 2010·4
Frubizin, 2010·4
Frubizin Forte, 2010·4
Frucalde, 2010·4
Fru-Co, 2010·4
Fructal, 2011·1
Fructan, 2011·1
Fructines, 2011·1
Fructofin, 2011·1
β-D-Fructofuranosyl-α-D-glucopyranoside, 1450·1
β-D-Fructofuranosyl-α-D-glucopyranoside Octakis (Hydrogen Sulphate) Aluminium Complex, 1290·2
Fructogenase, 2011·1
Fructopiran, 2011·1
D-(−)-Fructopyranose, 1431·3
Fructosa, 1431·3
Fructose, 1431·3
D-Fructose, 1431·3
Fructosil, 2011·1
Fructosum, 1431·3
Fructus Agni Casti, 1649·1
Fructus Anisi Vulgaris, 1655·2
Fructus Carvi, 1667·2
Fructus Rubi Idaei, 1057·3
Frudemisan, 2011·1
Frugelletten, 2011·1
Fruhjahrs-Elixier Ohne Alkohol, 2011·1
Fruit du Pavot, 1129·1
Fruit of the Earth Preparations, 2011·1
Fruit Sugar, 1431·3
Fruitatives, 2011·1
Fruity Chews, 2011·1
Frumax, 2011·2
Frumeron, 2011·2
Frumil, 2011·2
Frunalia, 2011·2
Frusamil, 2011·2
Frusehexal, 2011·2
Frusemek, 2011·2
Frusemide, 919·3
Frusene, 2011·2
Frusenex, 2011·2
Frusid, 2011·2
Frusol, 2011·2
Frut, 2011·2
Fruta Milagrosa, 1715·2
Frutalax, 2011·2
Frutarine, 2011·2
Frutasal Knop, 2011·2
Frutin, 2011·2
Fruto de Adormidera, 1129·1
Fruto de Hinojo, 1687·2
Fruto del Cilantro, 1676·1
Frutoplex, 2011·2
Frutovena, 2011·2
Frutovitam, 2011·2
Fruttasan, 2011·2
Fruttocal, 2011·2
Fruver, 2011·2
Fruxucre, 2011·2
FS— *see* Capex, 1867·4
FS-069, 1067·2
FSF, 735·3, 753·1
FSH, 1324·2
FSME-Bulin, 2011·2
FSME-Immun, 2011·2
$F_3T$, 655·3
FT-81, 867·3
FT-207, 586·2
F-Tab, 2011·2
Ftalato de Dibutilo, 1503·1
Ftalato de Dietilo, 1473·2
Ftalato de Dimetilo, 1504·1
Ftalato de Hipromelosa, 1579·3
Ftalilsulfatiazol, 242·3
Ftazidime, 2011·2
FTC, 632·3
FTC-(−), 632·3
(−)-FTC, 632·3
FTDA, 2011·2
$F_3TDR$, 655·3
Ftivazide, 215·2
Ftivazidum, 215·2
Ftorafur, 586·2
Ftoral, 2011·3
Ftoralon, 2011·3
Ftorocort, 2011·3
FTS, 1756·1
5-FU, 554·2
Fuca, 2011·3
Fuca N, 2011·3
Fucafibres, 2011·3
Fucerox, 2011·3
Fuchsin, Basic, 1185·2
Fuchsine, 1185·1
Fuchsine, Acid, 1646·3
Fucibet, 2011·3
Fucicort, 2011·3
Fucidin, 2011·3
Fucidin H, 2011·3
Fucidin Hydrocortisone, 2011·3
Fucidine, 2011·3
Fucidine H, 2011·3
Fucidine Plus, 2011·3
Fucidin-Hydrocortison, 2011·3
Fucithalmic, 2011·3
Fuclode, 2011·3
Fucon, 2011·3
Fucsina, 1185·1
Fucsina Ácida, 1646·3
Fucsina Fenica, 2011·3
Fucus, 1742·3, 2011·3
Fucus Composto, 2011·3
Fucus Compuesto, 2011·3
Fucus Especial, 2011·4
*Fucus serratus*, 1742·3
Fucus vel Ascophyllum, 1742·3
*Fucus vesiculosus*, 1742·3
Fucusor, 2011·4
Fudermex, 2011·4
Fudimun, 2011·4
Fudirine, 2011·4
Fudone, 2011·4
Fudosteine, 1121·3
FUDR, 547·3, 553·1, 2011·4
Fugacar, 2011·4
Fugaten, 2011·4
Fugentin, 2011·4
Fugerel, 2011·4
Fugisept, 2011·4
Fulcin, 2011·4
Fulcin S, 2011·4
Fulcine, 2011·4
Fulcro, 2011·4
Fulgium, 2011·4
Ful-Glo, 2011·4
Fulgram, 2011·4
Fulgram 400, 2011·4
Fuling, 1750·2
Full Marks, 2011·4
Full Service Sunblock, 2011·4
Fullcilina, 2011·4
Fullcilina Duo, 2011·4
Fullcilina Plus, 2011·4
Fuller's Earth, 1039·3
Full-Fort, 2011·4
Fullgrip T, 2011·4
Fullvita Multivitaminas E Minerais, 2011·4
Fulmicoton, 1156·2
Fulsed, 2011·4
Fulsivin, 2012·1
Fulvestrant, 557·3
Fulvicin, 2012·1
Fulvina, 2012·1
Fulvistatin P/G, 2012·1
Fulzoltec, 2012·1
Fumaderm, 2012·1
Fumafer, 2012·1
Fumagilina, 605·2
Fumagillin, 605·2
Fumarato de Benciclano, 867·3
Fumarato de Bisoprolol, 875·1
Fumarato de Clemastina, 429·1
Fumarato de Disoproxilo de Tenofovir, 655·1
Fumarato de Emedastina, 433·2
Fumarato de Formoterol, 786·1
Fumarato de Ibutilida, 938·1
Fumarato de Ketotifeno, 788·1
Fumarato de Oxetorona, 470·2
Fumarato de Quetiapina, 718·2
Fumarato de Tiamulina, 270·2

Fumarato de Xamoterol, 1029·1
Fumaria, 1690·1
*Fumaria officinalis*, 1690·1
Fumaric Acid, 1147·3
Fumárico, Ácido, 1147·3
Fumarol, 2012·1
Fumasil, 2012·1
Fumatinic, 2012·1
Fumavit, 2012·1
Fuming Sulfuric Acid, 1750·3
Fumitory, 1690·1
Fumo Brabo, 1666·1
Fumo de Caboclo, 1666·1
Funa, 2012·1
Funazole, 2012·1
Funcenal, 2012·1
Funchicorea, 2012·1
Funcho, 1687·2
Funcho, Essência de, 1687·3
Funcort, 2012·1
Functional Dyspepsia— *see* Dyspepsia, 1242·1
Fundamin, 2012·1
Fundamin-E, 2012·1
Fundan, 2012·1
Funduscein, 2012·1
Funga, 2012·1
Fungal Endocarditis— *see* Endocarditis, 388·1
Fungal Eye Infections— *see* Eye Infections, 388·1
Fungal Infections in Immunocompromised Patients— *see* Infections in Immunocompromised Patients, 388·2
Fungal Meningitis— *see* Meningitis, 388·3
Fungal Nail Infections— *see* Skin Infections, 390·1
Fungal Peritonitis— *see* Peritonitis, 389·1
Fungal Respiratory-tract Infections— *see* Respiratory-tract Infections, 390·1
Fungal Skin Infections— *see* Skin Infections, 390·1
Fungamizol, 2012·1
Funganiline, 2012·1
Fungarest, 2012·1
Fungata, 2012·1
Fungating Tumours— *see* Skin Infections, 146·2
Fungazol, 2012·1
Fungederm, 2012·1
Fungex, 2012·1
Fungi B, 2012·2
Fungibacid, 2012·2
Fungicida, 2012·2
Fungicide, 2012·2
Fungicides, 1499·1
Fungicidin, 406·3
Fungicil, 2012·2
Fungicon, 2012·2
Fungicrem, 2012·2
Fungiderm, 2012·2
Fungiderm Comp, 2012·2
Fungiderm-B, 2012·2
Fungiderm-K, 2012·2
Fungidermo, 2012·2
Fungidexan, 2012·2
Fungifax, 2012·2
Fungifos, 2012·2
Fungilin, 2012·2
Fungi-M, 2012·2
Fungimax, 2012·2
Fungimon, 2012·2
Fungi-Nail, 2012·2
Funginox, 2012·2
Fungiquim, 2012·2
Fungireduct, 2012·2
Fungirox, 2012·2
Fungisan, 2012·2
Fungisdin, 2012·3
Fungisil, 2012·3
Fungisil-T, 2012·3
Fungistat, 2012·3
Fungisten, 2012·3
Fungium, 2012·3
Fungizid, 2012·3
Fungizon, 2012·3
Fungizona, 2012·3
Fungizone, 2012·3
Fungo, 2012·3
Fungo Hubber, 2012·3
Fungocina, 2012·3
Fungocop, 2012·3
Fungocort, 2012·3
Fungodermol, 2012·3
Fungoid, 2012·3
Fungoid AF, 2012·3
Fungoid HC, 2012·3
Fungol, 2012·3
Fungopirox, 2012·3
Fungoral, 2012·3
Fungos, 2012·3
Fungotox, 2012·3
Fungowas, 2012·3
Funguard, 2012·3
Fungur M, 2012·3
Fungusol, 2012·4
Fungustatin, 2012·4
Fungusteril, 2012·4
Funida, 2012·4
Funnel-web Spider Antiserum, 1640·1
Funnel-web Spider Antivenin, 1640·1
Funnel-web Spider Antivenom, 1640·1
Funzal, 2012·4
Furabid, 2012·4
Furacilinum, 238·2
Furacin, 2012·4
Furacine, 2012·4
Furacin-S, 2012·4
Furacin-Sol, 2012·4
Furadantin, 2012·4
Furadantina, 2012·4
Furadantine, 2012·4
Furadantine MC, 2012·4
Furadoine, 2012·4
Furadoninum, 237·2
Furagrand, 2012·4
Fural, 2012·4
Furaltadona, Hidrocloruro de, 215·2
Furaltadone Hydrochloride, 215·2
Furamid, 2012·4
Furamide, 2012·4
Furanthril, 2012·4
Furantoina, 2012·4
Furanton, 2012·4
Furanvit, 2012·4
4-(2-Furanylcarbonyl)-α-methylbenzeneacetic Acid, 44·3
Furasept, 2012·4
Furasian, 2012·4
Furazanol— *see* Mycoapaisyl, 2146·4
Furazidin, 215·2
Furazidine, 215·2
Furazolidona, 605·2, 2012·4
Furazolidone, 605·2
Furazolin, 2012·4
Furazolon, 2012·4
Furazosin Hydrochloride, 985·1
Furcellaran, 1578·2
Furdiuren, 2013·1
Furedan, 2013·1
Furese, 2013·1
Furesin, 2013·1
Furesis, 2013·1
Furesis Comp, 2013·1
Furetic, 2013·1
Furex, 2013·1
(±)-2-(Furfurylsulfinyl)-*N*-[(*Z*)-4-{[4-(piperidinomethyl)-2-pyridyl]oxy}-2-butenyl]acetamide, 1269·3
Furide, 2013·1
Furil, 2013·1
Furine, 2013·1
Furion, 2013·1
Furital, 2013·1
Furix, 2013·1
Furmidal, 2013·1
Furmide, 2013·1
Furo, 2013·1
Furo-Aldopur, 2013·1
Furoato de Diloxanida, 604·1
Furoato de Mometasona, 1107·2
Furobactina, 2013·1
Furo-basan, 2013·1
Furo-BASF, 2013·1
Furobeta, 2013·1
Furocloran, 2013·1
Furocombin, 2013·1
Furodermal, 2013·1
Furodermil, 2013·1
Furodrix, 2013·1
Furogamma, 2013·1
Furohexal, 2013·1
Furoic, 2013·1
Furolacton, 2013·1
Furolin, 2013·2
Furomed, 2013·2
Furomil, 2013·2
Furomin, 2013·2
Furon, 2013·2
Furonet, 2013·2
Furonex, 2013·2
Furopectin, 2013·2
Furopenem, 213·1
Furo-Puren, 2013·2
Furorese, 2013·2
Furorese Comp, 2013·2
Furosal, 2013·2
Furosan, 2013·2
Furoscand, 2013·2
Furosem, 2013·2
Furosemid Comp, 2013·2
Furosemida, 919·3
Furosemida Composta, 2013·2
Furosemide, 919·3
Furosemidum, 919·3
Furosetron, 2013·2
Furosifar, 2013·2
Furosix, 2013·2
Furospir, 2013·2
Furo-Spirobene, 2013·2
Furostad, 2013·2
Furoter, 2013·2
Furotricina, 2013·2
Furotyrol, 2013·2
Furovite, 2013·2
Furoxim, 2013·2
Furoxime, 2013·2
Furoxona, 2013·2
Furoxone, 2013·2
2-[4-(2-Furoyl)piperazin-1-yl]-6,7-dimethoxyquinazolin-4-ylamine Hydrochloride, 985·1
Furozix, 2013·2
Furprofen, 44·3
Furprofeno, 44·3
Fursemida, 2013·2
Fursol, 2013·3
Fursultiamina, 1454·3
Fursultiamine, 1454·3
Furtenk, 2013·3
Furtulon, 2013·3
Furunculosis— *see* Skin Infections, 146·2
Furunkulosin, 2013·3
Fusafungina, 215·2
Fusafungine, 215·2
Fusain Noir Pourpré, 1265·2
Fusalar, 2013·3
Fusaloyos, 2013·3
Fusanidazol, 2013·3
*Fusarium lateritium*, 215·2
Fusepina, 2013·3
Fusid, 2013·3
Fusidane Antibacterials, 120·2
Fusidate Sodium, 215·2
Fusidato Sódico, 215·2
Fusidic Acid, 215·2
Fusídico, Ácido, 215·2
Fusidicum, Acidum, 215·2
*Fusidium coccineum*, 215·2
Fusimed, 2013·3
Fusimed B, 2013·3
Fusitop, 2013·3
Fusiwal, 2013·3
Fustaren, 2013·3
Fustermicina, 2013·3
Fustermid, 2013·3
Fustermizol, 2013·3
Fuston, 2013·3
FUT-175, 1719·1
Futasole, 2013·3
Futasone, 2013·3
Futraful, 2013·3
Futroken, 2013·3
Futura, 2013·3
Futuran, 2013·3
Future E, 2013·3
Fuviron, 2013·3
Fuxen, 2013·3
Fuxol, 2013·3
Fuzeon, 2013·3
Fuzoltec, 2013·3
Fuzotyl, 2013·4
FX Passage, 2013·4
Fybogel, 2013·4
Fybogel Mebeverine, 2013·4
Fybozest, 2013·4
Fymnal, 2013·4
Fynnon Salt, 2013·4
Fysiofer, 2013·4
Fysionorm, 2013·4
Fysioquens, 2013·4
Fytate, Sodium, 1052·3
Fytic Acid, 1052·3, 1701·2
Fytosid, 2013·4
FZ-588, 214·3


## G


G, 1433·3
G-1— *see* Tencet, 2323·4
G-4, 104·1
G-11, 1181·2
G-137, 982·3
G-204, 2013·4
G-248, 2013·4
G-3139, 577·1
G-5668, 1592·3
G-7333, 996·3
G-11021, 857·1
G-11035, 857·1
G-11044, 857·1
G-23350, 848·3
G-27202, 76·1
G-28315, 417·3
G-30320, 197·1
G-32883, 353·3
G-33040, 311·1
G-33182, 882·3
G-34586, 289·3
G-35020, 290·2
G-704650, 765·3
G Tril, 2013·4
GA, 1719·2
GA-242, 1434·2
GA-297, 1442·3
Gab, 2013·4
GABA, 1690·2
Gaba, 2013·4
Gabacet, 2013·4
Gaballon, 2013·4
Gabapentin, 362·2
Gabapentina, 362·2
Gabatril, 2013·4
Gabax, 2013·4
Gabbromicina, 2013·4
Gabbroral, 2013·4
Gabecon M, 2013·4
Gabexate Mesilate, 1690·1
Gabexate Mesylate, 1690·1
Gabexato, Mesilato de, 1690·1
Gabil, 2013·4
Gabimex, 2013·4
Gabimex Plus, 2013·4
Gabisedil, 2013·4
Gabitran, 2013·4
Gabitril, 2014·1
Gabob, 353·2
Gabomade, 2014·1
Gabormon, 2014·1
Gabrene, 2014·1
Gabrilen, 2014·1
Gabunat, 2014·1
Gacida, 2014·1
Gadobenate Dimeglumine, 1062·1
Gadobenato de Meglumina, 1062·1
Gadobenic Acid, 1062·1

Gadobénico, Ácido, 1062·1
Gadobutrol, 1062·1
Gadodiamida, 1062·1
Gadodiamide, 1062·1
Gadograf, 2014·1
Gadolinium and Diethylenetriamine Pentaacetic Acid Complex, 1062·2
Gadolinium-DTPA, 1062·2
Gadopentetate Dimeglumine, 1062·2
Gadopentetate Meglumine, 1062·2
Gadopentetato de Meglumina, 1062·2
Gadopentetic Acid, 1062·2
Gadopentético, Ácido, 1062·2
Gadopril, 2014·1
Gadoterate Meglumine, 1062·3
Gadoterato de Meglumina, 1062·3
Gadoteric Acid, 1062·3
Gadotérico, Ácido, 1062·3
Gadoteridol, 1062·3
Gadoversetamide, 1063·1
Gadovist, 2014·1
Gadoxetic Acid, 1063·1
Gadral, 2014·1
Gaduol, 2014·1
*Gadus morhua*, 1425·2
GA-EPO, 747·2
Gaiarsol, 2014·1
Galacordin, 2014·1
Galactin, 1337·3
Galactogil, 2014·1
Galactomin, 2014·1
D-Galactopyranose, 1063·1
4-*O*-β-D-Galactopyranosyl-D-fructose, 1269·1
4-*O*-(β-D-Galactopyranosyl)-D-glucitol, 1269·1
Galactorrhoea— *see* Hyperprolactinaemia, 1315·2
Galactosa, 1063·1
Galactose, 1063·1
D-Galactose, 1063·1
Galactose Factor, Animal, 1724·3
α-D-Galactosidase, 1651·1
β-Galactosidase, 1756·2
β-D-Galactosidase, 1756·2
α-Galactosidase A, 1651·1
α-D-Galactoside Galactohydrolase, 1651·1
β-D-Galactoside Galactohydrolase, 1756·2
β-Galactosido-sorbitol, 1269·1
Galactosum, 1063·1
Galake, 2014·1
Galama Entschlackungselixier, 2014·1
Galamila, 2014·1
Galamina, Trietioduro de, 1403·2
Galanol GLX, 2014·1
Galanol Gold, 2014·1
Galantamina, Hidrobromuro de, 1491·2
Galantamine Hydrobromide, 1491·2
Galantase, 2014·1
Galanthamine Hydrobromide, 1491·2
Galanthamini Hydrobromidum, 1491·2
*Galanthus woronowii*, 1491·2
Galaren, 2014·1
Galato de Dodecilo, 1168·1
Galato de Etilo, 1168·1
Galato de Octilo, 1168·1
Galato de Propilo, 1168·1
Galatos de Alquilo, 1168·1
Galcdexan, 2014·1
Galciclina, 2014·1
Galcodine, 2014·1
Galebiron, 2014·2
Galecin, 2014·2
Galedol, 2014·2
Galemin, 2014·2
Galenamet, 2014·2
Galenamox, 2014·2
Galenat Kamill N, 2014·2
Galenavowen, 2014·2
Galenpamil, 2014·2
Galenphol, 2014·2
Galentromicina, 2014·2
*Galerina autumnalis*, 1717·3
*Galerina marginata*, 1717·3
*Galerina venenata*, 1717·3
Galfer, 2014·2
Galfer FA, 2014·2
Galfloxin, 2014·2
Galidrin, 2014·2
Galii Aparinis Herba, 1673·2
Galinocort, 2014·2
Galio 67, 1523·3
Galio, Nitrato de, 772·2
*Galipea officinalis*, 1678·1
Galirene, 2014·2
Galium, 1673·2
Galium Complex, 2014·2
Galivert, 2014·2
Gall, 1690·2
Galla, 1690·2
Gallamine Triethiodide, 1403·2
Gallamini Triethiodidum, 1403·2
Gallamone Triethiodide, 1403·2
Galläpfel, 1690·2
Galle, Noix de, 1690·2
Galle- und Leber-Tee N, Kneipp— *see* Kneipp Galle- und Leber-Tee N, 2081·2
Galleb S, 2014·2
Galle-Donau, 2014·2
Gallemolan Forte, 2014·2
Gallemolan G, 2014·2
Gallen- und Lebertee EF-EM-ES, 2014·2
Gallenja, 2014·2
Gallenperlen, 2014·2
Gallesyn, 2014·2
Gallesyn Neu, 2014·2
Gallexier, 2014·3
Gallia HA, 2014·3
Gallia Lactofidus, 2014·3
Gallia Soja, 2014·3
Galliagene, 2014·3
Gallic Acid, 1168·1, 1696·3
Gallifugo, 2014·3
Gallith, 2014·3
Gallium-67, 1523·3
Gallium Citrate ($^{67}$Ga), 1523·3
Gallium Nitrate, 772·2
Gallo Merz, 2014·3
Gallo Merz N, 2014·3
Gallo Merz Spasmo, 2014·3
Gallobeta, 2014·3
Gallogen, 2014·3
Gallogran, 2014·3
Gallopamil Hydrochloride, 922·3
Gallopas, 2014·3
Galloselect, 2014·3
Galloselect M, 2014·3
Gallotannic Acid, 1690·2, 1751·2
Galloway's Cough Syrup, 2014·3
Galls, 1690·2
Galls, Aleppo, 1690·2
Galls, Blue, 1690·2
Gallstones, 1761·3
Gall-wasp, 1690·2
Galmarin, 2014·3
Galmax, 2014·3
Galopamilo, Hidrocloruro de, 922·3
Galopran, 2014·3
Galpamol, 2014·3
Galpharm Flu Relief, 2014·3
Galphol— *see* Galenphol, 2014·2
Galprofen, 2014·3
Galpseud, 2014·3
Galpseud— *see* Galsud, 2014·3
Galpseud Plus, 2014·3
Galsud, 2014·3
Galtamicina, 2014·4
Galusan, 2014·4
Galutec, 2014·4
Gama Venina, 2014·4
Gamactrin, 2014·4
Gamafine, 2014·4
Gamalat, 2014·4
Gamalate B6, 2014·4
Gamaline-V, 2014·4
Gamanil, 2014·4
Gamatol, 2014·4
Gamavate, 2014·4
Gamax, 2014·4
Gambex, 2014·4
Gambier, 1668·3
Gambir, 1668·3
Gambrolys, 2014·4
Gambrosol, 2014·4
Gamespir, 2014·4
Gamibetal, 2014·4
Gamibetal Complex, 2014·4
Gamibetal Compositum, 2014·4
Gamibetal Plus, 2014·4
Gamikal, 2014·4
Gamimune, 2014·4
Gamimune N, 2015·1
Gamma Anti D, 2015·1
Gamma Antihep B, 2015·1
Gamma Antitenos, 2015·1
Gamma Antitetanos, 2015·1
Gamma Benzene Hexachloride, 1506·3
Gamma EPA, 2015·1
Gamma Glob Antihepa B, 2015·1
Gamma Marine, 2015·1
Gamma N, Aar— *see* Aar Gamma N, 1767·3
Gamma Oil, 2015·1
Gamma Oil Marine, 2015·1
Gamma Oryzanol, 1725·1
Gamma Tocopherols, 1464·3
Gamma-aminobutyric Acid, 1690·2
Gamma-amylases, 1654·2
Gamma-BHC, 1506·3
Gammabulin, 2015·1
Gammabulin A, 2015·1
Gamma-butyrolactone, 1308·3
Gammacarotene, 1423·1
Gammacur, 2015·1
Gammaderm, 2015·1
Gammadin, 2015·1
Gammagard, 2015·1
Gammagard SD, 2015·1
Gammaglob, 2015·1
Gammaglob Anti D, 2015·1
Gammaglob Antihep B P BE, 2015·1
Gammaglob Antite, 2015·1
Gammaglobulin, 2015·1
Gammaglobulin, Antithymocyte, 1348·3
Gammaglobulin SPR, 2015·1
Gammaglobulina, 2015·1
Gamma-HCH, 1506·3
Gamma-hydroxybutyrate, 1308·3
Gamma-hydroxybutyrate, Sodium, 1308·3
Gammakine, 2015·1
Gammalon, 2015·1
Gamma-Men, 2015·1
Gammamida Complex, 2015·1
Gammanorm, 2015·2
Gammanova, 2015·2
Gamma-OH, 2015·2
GammaOil Premium, 2015·2
Gammaphos, 1031·3
Gammaplus, 2015·2
Gammar, 2015·2
Gammariza, 2015·2
Gammar-P, 2015·2
Gamma-Scab, 2015·2
Gammatet, 2015·2
Gamma-Tet P, 2015·2
Gammatetanos, 2015·2
Gamma-Venin, 2015·2
Gamma-Venin P, 2015·2
Gammavit, 2015·2
Gammonativ, 2015·2
Gamolenic Acid, 1690·2
Gamolénico, Ácido, 1690·2
Gamonil, 2015·2
Gamophen, 2015·2
Gamulin Rh, 2015·2
Gamunex, 2015·2
Ganaprofene, 2015·2
Ganaton, 2015·2
Ganavit, 2015·2
Ganazolo, 2015·2
Gancao, 1750·2
Ganciclovir, 635·3
Ganciclovir Sódico, 635·3
Ganciclovir Sodium, 635·3
Gancivir, 2015·2
Ganda, 2015·2
Gandhour, 2015·2
Gandia, 1666·1
Gandin, 2015·2
Ganga, 1666·1
Ganglion Blockers, 811·2
Gangliosides, 1691·1
Gangliósidos, 1691·1
Gangrene, Gas— *see* Gas Gangrene, 127·3
Ganidin NR, 2015·2
Ganirelix Acetate, 1325·1
Ganirelix, Acetato de, 1325·1
Ganite, 2015·3
Gani-Tuss NR, 2015·3
Gani-Tuss-DM NR, 2015·3
Ganja, 1666·1
Ganjila, 1666·1
Ganor, 2015·3
Gantanol, 2015·3
Gantil, 2015·3
Gantin, 2015·3
Gantrim, 2015·3
Gantrimex, 2015·3
Gantrisin, 2015·3
Ganvirax, 2015·3
Ganvirel, 2015·3
Ganvirel Duo, 2015·3
Gaopathyl, 2015·3
Gaoptol, 2015·3
Gaosedal Codeine, 2015·3
Gapeworm Infections— *see* Syngamosis, 101·1
Gaproxen, 2015·3
Garacin, 2015·3
Garacol, 2015·3
Garacoll, 2015·3
Garalen, 2015·3
Garalone, 2015·3
Garamicina, 2015·3
Garamicina-V, 2015·3
Garamycin, 2015·3
Garanil, 2015·3
Garaouich, 1666·1
Garapepsin, 2015·3
Garasone, 2015·3
Garatec, 2015·3
Garawiche, 1666·1
Garceptol, 2015·4
Garcinol Max, 2015·4
Garde Gomas, 2015·4
Garde Jarabe, 2015·4
Garden Burnet, 1663·2
Garden Rhubarb, 1288·1
Garden Sorrel, 1749·1
Garden Thyme, 1755·2
Gardenal, 2015·4
Gardenale, 2015·4
Gardoton, 2015·4
GA-301-Redskin 301, 2015·4
Garfield, 2015·4
Garg L, Pastillas Antisep— *see* Pastillas Antisep Garg L, 2207·3
Garg M, Pastillas Antisep— *see* Pastillas Antisep Garg M, 2207·3
Gargaletas, 2015·4
Gargaril, 2015·4
Gargarisma zum Gurgeln, 2015·4
Gargarol, 2015·4
Gargaron, 2015·4
Gargilon, 2015·4
Gargocetil, 2015·4
Gargol, 2015·4
Gargosedans, 2015·4
Gargotan, 2015·4
Gargotrat, 2015·4
Garia, 2015·4
Garlic, 1691·1, 1691·2
Garlic Allium Complex, 2015·4
Garlic for Homoeopathic Preparations, 1691·2
Garlic, Horseradish, A & C Capsules, 2015·4
Garlic and Horseradish + C Complex, 2015·4
Garlic Oil, 1691·2
Garlic Powder, 1691·1
Garlimega, 2015·4
Garlix, 2016·1
Garlodex, 2016·1

Garmastan, 2016·1
Garoarsch, 1666·1
Garoin, 2016·1
Garonsept, 2016·1
Gartech, 2016·1
Gartricin, 2016·1
Garydol, 2016·1
Garze Disinfettanti alla Pomata Betadine, 2016·1
Gas Ban, 2016·1
Gas Ban DS, 2016·1
Gas CR, 1676·3
Gas CS, 1677·3
Gas Gangrene, 127·3
Gas, Hylands— *see* Hylands Gas, 2052·3
Gas, Laughing, 1304·3
Gas Mostaza, 1679·3
Gas Relief, 2016·1
Gasam, 2016·1
Gasbrand-Antitoxin, 2016·1
Gascoal, 2016·1
Gascop, 2016·1
Gasec, 2016·1
Gaseofin, 2016·1
Gases, 1235·1
Gases, Liquefied, 1235·1
Gases Nerviosos, 1719·2
Gas-gangrene Antitoxin, Mixed, 1616·1
Gas-gangrene Antitoxin (Novyi), 1615·3
Gas-gangrene Antitoxin (Oedematiens), 1615·3
Gas-gangrene Antitoxin (Perfringens), 1615·3
Gas-gangrene Antitoxin (Septicum), 1615·3
Gas-gangrene Antitoxins, 1615·3
Gaslon N, 2016·1
Gasmilen, 2016·1
Gas-MM, 2016·1
Gasmol, 2016·1
Gasmotin, 2016·1
Gas-Nep, 2016·1
Gasoline, 1476·3
Gasorbol, 2016·1
Gasorbol Plus, 2016·2
Gaspiren, 2016·2
Gas/Ser, 1616·1
Gassi, 2016·2
Gastab, 2016·2
Gastec, 2016·2
Gasteel, 2016·2
Gaster, 2016·2
Gasterogen, 2016·2
Gastidin, 2016·2
Gastidine, 2016·2
Gastop, 2016·2
Gastopride, 2016·2
Gastracol, 2016·2
Gastral, 2016·2
Gastralgin, 2016·2
Gastralgine, 2016·2
Gastralon N, 2016·2
Gastralsan, 2016·2
Gastran, 2016·2
Gastranil, 2016·2
Gastrarctin N, 2016·2
Gastrat, 2016·2
Gastrax, 2016·3
Gastrec, 2016·3
Gastregan, 2016·3
Gastrex, 2016·3
Gastrial, 2016·3
Gastrib, 2016·3
Gastribien, 2016·3
Gastric Cancer— *see* Malignant Neoplasms of the Gastrointestinal Tract, 516·2
Gastric MALT Lymphoma, 511·1
Gastric Mucin, 1579·1
Gastric Ulcer— *see* Peptic Ulcer Disease, 1246·3
Gastric Varices— *see* Variceal Haemorrhage, 1716·1
Gastricalm, 2016·3
Gastricard, 2016·3
Gastricholan-L, 2016·3
Gastricin, 2016·3
Gastricumeel, 2016·3
Gastricur, 2016·3
Gastricure, 2016·3
Gastride, 2016·3
Gastridin, 2016·3
Gastridina, 2016·3
Gastridin-E, 2016·3
Gastrifam, 2016·3
Gastrifom, 2016·3
Gastril, 2016·3
Gastri-L 90 N, 2016·3
Gastrimagal, 2016·4
Gastrimet, 2016·4
Gastrimet Enzimatico, 2016·4
Gastrimut, 2016·4
Gastrimuto, 2016·4
Gastrin-Do, 2016·4
Gastrinol, 2016·4
Gastrinoma— *see* Carcinoid Tumours and Other Secretory Neoplasms, 504·1
Gastrion, 2016·4
Gastri-P, 2016·4
Gastripan, 2016·4
Gastriselect, 2016·4
Gastritol, 2016·4
Gastrium, 2016·4
Gastriveran, 2016·4
Gastri-Vyr, 2016·4
Gastro, 2016·4
Gastro Gobens, 2016·4
Gastro H2, 2016·4
Gastroalgine, 2016·4
Gastrobario, 2016·4
Gastrobene, 2016·4
Gastrobid Continus, 2017·1
Gastrobion, 2017·1
Gastrobitan, 2017·1
Gastrobon, 2017·1
Gastrobul, 2017·1
Gastrocaine, 2017·1
Gastrocalm, 2017·1
Gastrocaps A, 2017·1
Gastroccult, 2017·1
Gastrocol, 2017·1
Gastrocote, 2017·1
Gastrocrom, 2017·1
Gastrocure, 2017·1
Gastrocynesine, 2017·1
Gastrodenol, 2017·1
Gastrodin, 2017·1
Gastrodina, 2017·1
Gastrodine, 2017·1
Gastrodomina, 2017·1
Gastrodue, 2017·1
Gastrodyn, 2017·1
Gastrodyn Comp, 2017·1
Gastro-enteritis, Bacterial— *see* Gastro-enteritis, 127·3
Gastro-enteritis, Campylobacter— *see* Campylobacter Enteritis, 128·3
Gastro-enteritis, Escherichia Coli— *see* Escherichia Coli Enteritis, 129·1
Gastro-enteritis, Protozoal— *see* Gastro-enteritis, 596·3
Gastro-enteritis, Salmonella— *see* Salmonella Enteritis, 129·3
Gastro-enteritis, Shigella— *see* Shigellosis, 130·1
Gastro-enteritis, Viral— *see* Gastro-enteritis, 618·2
Gastro-enteritis, Yersinia— *see* Yersinia Enteritis, 130·2
Gastroenterol, 2017·1
Gastrofilm, 2017·1
Gastroflat, 2017·1
Gastrofloral, 2017·2
Gastroflux, 2017·2
Gastrofrenal, 2017·2
Gastrofusine, 2017·2
Gastrogard-R, 2017·2
Gastroge, 2017·2
Gastrogel, 2017·2
Gastrogenol, 2017·2
Gastroglutal, 2017·2
Gastrografin, 2017·2
Gastrografina, 2017·2
Gastrografine, 2017·2
Gastrointestinal Cancer— *see* Malignant Neoplasms of the Gastrointestinal Tract, 516·2
Gastrointestinal Disorder, Functional— *see* Irritable Bowel Syndrome, 1244·3
Gastrointestinal Drugs, 1239·1
Gastrointestinal Motility, Decreased— *see* Decreased Gastrointestinal Motility, 1241·1
Gastrointestinal Spasm, 1242·2
Gastrokin, 2017·2
Gastrol, 2017·2
Gastrol S, 2017·2
Gastrol TC, 2017·2
Gastrolav, 2017·2
Gastrolem, 2017·2
Gastrolen, 2017·2
Gastrolen, Natusor— *see* Natusor Gastrolen, 2154·1
Gastrolene, 2017·3
Gastrolets, 2017·3
Gastroliber, 2017·3
Gastroloc, 2017·3
Gastroluft, 2017·3
Gastrolux, 2017·3
Gastrolyte, 2017·3
Gastrolyte-R, 2017·3
Gastrom, 2017·3
Gastromag, 2017·3
Gastromax, 2017·3
Gastromet, 2017·3
Gastromiro, 2017·3
Gastromol, 2017·3
Gastron, 2017·3
Gastron Fuerte, 2017·3
Gastronerton, 2017·3
Gastronol, 2017·3
Gastronorm, 2017·3
Gastro-oesophageal Reflux Disease, 1242·3
Gastropaque, 2017·3
Gastroparesis, Diabetic— *see* Diabetic Complications, 326·2
Gastro-Pasc, 2017·3
Gastropax, 2017·3
Gastropeache Susp, 2017·4
Gastropect, 2017·4
Gastropen, 2017·4
Gastro-Pepsin, 2017·4
Gastropin, 2017·4
Gastropiren, 2017·4
Gastroplant, 2017·4
Gastroplex, 2017·4
Gastroplus, 2017·4
Gastroprotect, 2017·4
Gastropulgit, 2017·4
Gastropulgite, 2017·4
Gastrosan, 2017·4
Gastrosecur, 2017·4
Gastrosed, 2017·4
Gastrosedol, 2017·4
Gastrosedyl, 2017·4
Gastrosil, 2017·4
Gastrosine, 2017·4
Gastrostad, 2017·4
Gastrostop, 2017·4
Gastro-Stop, 2017·4
Gastrotem, 2017·4
Gastrotest, 2018·1
Gastro-Timelets, 2018·1
Gastrotranquil, 2018·1
Gastrovegetalin, 2018·1
Gastrovison, 2018·1
Gastrozac, 2018·1
Gastrozepin, 2018·1
Gastrozepina, 2018·1
Gastrozepine, 2018·1
Gastrozol, 2018·1
Gastrulcer, 2018·1
Gastyl, 2018·1
Gasulsol, 2018·1
Gasva, 2018·1
Gas-X, 2018·1
Gasyran, 2018·1
Gaszym, 2018·1
Gat Globulina Antitimocitaria, 2018·1
Gatiflo, 2018·1
Gatifloxacin, 216·2
Gatifloxacino, 216·2
Gatinar, 2018·1
Gattilier, Fruit de, 1649·1
Gatuña, 1723·3
Gaucher Disease, 1649·2
Gauja, 1666·1
Gaurit— *see* Indobene, 2060·1
Gavestinel, 1691·3
Gavicid, 2018·1
Gavilast, 2018·1
Gavilimomab, 1360·2
Gaviscon Preparations, 2018·1
Gaviscon, Infant— *see* Infant Gaviscon, 2061·1
Gaviz, 2018·3
Gayuba, 1659·2
Gaz Away, 2018·3
Gazyme, 2018·3
GB, 1719·2
GB Tablets, 2018·3
GBE-761, 1692·3
GBH, 1308·3
GBL, 1308·3
GBN, 2018·3
GD, 1719·2
$G_{D1a}$, 1691·1
$G_{D1b}$, 1691·1
Gd-BOPTA, 1062·1
GdDTPA-BMA, 1062·1
Gd-EOB-DTPA, 1063·1
G-Dil, 2018·3
GDP-Ex, 2018·3
GE, 2018·3
Geangin, 2018·3
Geasalol, 2018·3
Geavir, 2018·3
Gebleichtes Wachs, 1480·1
Gebrannter Gips, 1665·1
Gebrannter Kalk, 1664·3
Gebrozil, 2018·3
Gedol, 2018·3
Gedun, 2018·3
Gee-Gee, 2018·3
Geepenil, 2018·3
Gefarnate, 1267·1
Gefarnato, 1267·1
Geffer, 2018·3
Gefina, 2018·3
Gefitinib, 557·3
Gegorvit, 2018·3
Gegrip, 2018·3
Gehwol Fungizid, 2018·3
Gehwol Huhneraugen Pflaster, 2018·3
Gehwol Huhneraugen Tinktur, 2018·4
Gehwol Nagelpilz, 2018·4
Gehwol Schalpaste, 2018·4
Gel 4000, 2018·4
Gel a la Consoude, 2018·4
Gel a l'Acetotartrate d'Alumine Defresne, 2018·4
Gel Antiinflamatorio, 2018·4
Gel Carpina, 2018·4
Gel Creme Protector, 2018·4
Gel de Calamine, 2018·4
Gel Kam, 2018·4
Gel Rubefiant, 2018·4
Gel Solaire Bronzage, 2018·4
Gel Solaire Bronzage Securite, 2018·4
Gel Solaire Bronzage Securite Special Sport, 2018·4
Gelacet, 2018·4
Gelacet N, 2018·4
Gelacid, 2018·4
Gelafundin, 2018·4
Gelafundina, 2018·4
Gelafusal-N in Ringeracetat, 2018·4
Gelamel, 2018·4
Gelan Plus, 2018·4
Gelasim, 2018·4
Gelaspon, 2018·4
Gelastypt, 2018·4
Gelatin, 754·3
Gelatin, Hydrolysed, 755·2
Gelatin, Succinylated, 755·2
Gelatin, Type A, 754·3
Gelatin, Type B, 754·3

Gelatina, 754·3
Gélatine, Sucre de, 1433·3
Gelbes Quecksilberoxyd, 1712·3
Gelbes Wachs, 1480·2
Gelbiotic, 2018·4
Gelbiotic Plus, 2019·1
Gelcain, 2019·1
Gelcen, 2019·1
Gelclair, 2019·1
Gelcosal, 2019·1
Gelcotar, 2019·1
Geldene, 2019·1
Geldrox Plus, 2019·1
Gelee Solaire Haute Protection, 2019·1
Gelenkja, 2019·1
Gelerit, 2019·1
Gelestra, 2019·1
Gelfilm, 2019·1
Gelflex, 2019·1
Gelfoam, 2019·1
Gelhist, 2019·1
Gelicain, 2019·1
Gelictar, 2019·1
Gelictar Fort, 2019·1
Gelidina, 2019·1
*Gelidium cartilagineum*, 1576·3
Gelifundol, 2019·1
Gelimag, 2019·1
Geliofil, 2019·1
Geliperm, 2019·1
Gelisyn, 2019·1
Gel-Kam, 2019·1
Gel-Larmes, 2019·2
Gellodex, 2019·2
Gelmax, 2019·2
Gelmicin, 2019·2
Geloalumin, 2019·2
Geloboll, 2019·2
Gelobronchial, 2019·2
Gelocast, 2019·2
Gelocatil, 2019·2
Gelocatil Codeina, 2019·2
Geloderm, 2019·2
Gelodiet, 2019·2
Gelodrin, 2019·2
Gelodrox, 2019·2
Gelodual, 2019·2
Gelodurat, 2019·2
Gelofalk, 2019·2
Gelofeno, 2019·2
Geloflex, 2019·2
Gelofrix, 2019·2
Gelofusin, 2019·2
Gelofusine, 2019·2
Gelogastrine, 2019·2
Gelogel, 2019·2
Gelol, 2019·2
Gelolagar, 2019·2
Gelomyrtol, 2019·2
Gelonasal, 2019·2
Gelonevral, 2019·3
Gelonic, 2019·3
Gelonic Forte, 2019·3
Gelonida, 2019·3
Gelonida NA, 2019·3
Gelopectose, 2019·3
Geloplasma, 2019·3
Gelora, 2019·3
Geloril, 2019·3
Gelosa, 1576·3
Gélose, 1576·3
Gelostretch, 2019·3
Gelotricar, 2019·3
Gelotrisin, 2019·3
Gelovit, 2019·3
Gelovital, 2019·3
Gelox, 2019·3
Gelpan, 2019·3
Gelparine, 2019·3
Gel-Phan, 2019·3
Gelpirin, 2019·3
Gelpirin-CCF, 2019·3
Gelplex, 2019·3
Gelsemine, 1691·3
Gelsemium, 1691·3
Gelsemium Comp, 2019·3
Gelsemium Oligoplex, 2019·3
Gelsemium Root, 1691·3
*Gelsemium sempervirens*, 1691·3
Gelsica, 2019·3
Gelsolets, 2019·3
GelTears, 2019·3
Gel-Tin, 2019·3
Gelucystine, 2019·3
Gelufene, 2019·4
Gelum, 2019·4
Gelumag, 2019·4
Gelumaline, 2019·4
Gelumen, 2019·4
Gelumina, 2019·4
Geluprane, 2019·4
Gelusil Preparations, 2019·4
Gely, 2019·4
Gem, 2019·4
Gemalt, 2019·4
Gemcitabina, Hidrocloruro de, 558·1
Gemcitabine Hydrochloride, 558·1
Gemcite, 2019·4
Gemd, 2019·4
Gemeprost, 1518·1
Gemfi, 2020·1
Gemfibril, 2020·1
Gemfibromax, 2020·1
Gemfibrozil, 923·1
Gemfibrozilo, 923·1
Gemfolid, 2020·1
Gemhexal, 2020·1
Gemicina, 2020·1
Gemifloxacin Mesilate, 216·3
Gemifloxacin Mesylate, 216·3
Gemifloxacino, Mesilato de, 216·3
Gemini, 2020·1
Gemipasmol, 2020·1
Gemitin, 2020·1
Gemitin con Prednisolona, 2020·1
Gemizol, 2020·1
Gemlipid, 2020·1
Gemnpid, 2020·1
Gemtro, 2020·1
Gemtuzumab Ozogamicin, 558·3
Gemtuzumab Ozogamicina, 558·3
Gemtuzumab Zogamicin, 558·3
Gemvites, 2020·1
Gemzar, 2020·1
Gemzil, 2020·1
Gen H-B-Vax, 2020·1
Genac, 2020·1
Genacol, 2020·1
Genaconazol, 400·3
Genaconazole, 400·3
Genahist, 2020·1
Genalen, 2020·1
Genalfa, 2020·1
Genalgen, 2020·1
Genalin, 2020·1
Genamin, 2020·2
Genapap, 2020·2
Genaphed, 2020·2
Genaprost, 2020·2
Genasal, 2020·2
Genasoft Plus Softgels, 2020·2
Genaspor, 2020·2
Genaton, 2020·2
Genaton, Extra Strength— *see* Extra Strength Genaton, 1986·2
Genatrop, 2020·2
Genatropine, 2020·2
Genatuss, 2020·2
Genatuss DM, 2020·2
Genavit, 2020·2
Gen-Beclo, 2020·2
Gen-bee with C, 2020·2
Gencalc, 2020·2
Gencardia, 2020·2
Gencefal, 2020·2
Genciana, 1692·2
Genciana, Raiz de, 1692·2
Gencifrice Baume 1re Dents, 2020·2
Gencin, 2020·2
Gencolax, 2020·2
Gencold, 2020·2
Gen-Cromolyn, 2020·2
Gencydo, 2020·2
Gendazel, 2020·2
Gendecon, 2020·2
Gene Therapy, 1691·3
Genebs, 2020·2
Genecalcin, 2020·2
Genefadrone, 2020·3
Genemicin, 2020·3
Generaid, 2020·3
General Anaesthesia— *see* Anaesthesia, 1296·1
General Anaesthetics, 1295·1
Generalised Seizures— *see* Epilepsy, 349·1
Generators, 1522·2
Genercin, 2020·3
Generet, 2020·3
Energin, 2020·3
Generix-T, 2020·3
Generlog, 2020·3
Generman, 2020·3
Genes Vit, 2020·3
Genesa, 2020·3
Geneserine, 2020·3
Genesis, 2020·3
Genêt, 1742·2
Genêt À Balai, 1742·2
Genevis, 2020·3
Genevis D2, 2020·3
Genexal, 2020·3
Geneye Extra, 2020·3
Gen-Formula, 2020·3
Gengibre, 1267·1
Gengigel, 2020·3
Gengisyl, 2020·3
Gengivario, 2020·3
Gengivarium, 2020·3
Gen-Glybe, 2020·3
Gengraf, 2020·3
GenHevac B, 2020·3
Geniad, 2020·3
Geniceral, 2020·3
Genièvre, 1703·1
Genièvre, Essence de, 1703·1
Genimox, 2020·3
Genin, 2020·3
Geniol, 2020·3
Geniol AP, 2020·4
Geniol Flex, 2020·4
Geniol SC Sin Cafeina, 2020·4
Geniolito, 2020·4
Geniol-P, 2020·4
Genisol, 2020·4
Genista, Planta, 1742·2
Genistein, 1692·1
Genisteol, 1692·1
Genite, 2020·4
Genitoflox, 2020·4
Genitopen, 2020·4
Gen-K, 2020·4
Genkova, 2020·4
Gen-Lac, 2020·4
Genlac, 2020·4
Genlip, 2020·4
Gen-Medroxy, 2020·4
Genocin, 2020·4
Genocolan, 2020·4
Genogris, 2020·4
Genola, 2020·4
Genolaxante, 2020·4
Genoptic, 2020·4
Genora 0.5/35, 2020·4
Genora 1/50, 2020·4
Genora 1/35— *see* Genora 0.5/35 and 1/35, 2020·4
Genoral, 2020·4
Genoscopolamine, 2020·4
Genotonorm, 2020·4
Genotropin, 2020·4
Genovox, 2021·1
Genox, 2021·1
Genoxal, 2021·1
Genoxal Trofosfamida, 2021·1
Genoxen, 2021·1
Genozil, 2021·1
Genozym, 2021·1
Genpril, 2021·1
Genprin, 2021·1
Genprol, 2021·1
Genquin, 2021·1
Genrex, 2021·1
Genrex-B, 2021·1
Gensan, 2021·1
Genser Sweet, 2021·1
Gensil, 2021·1
Gensumycin, 2021·1
Genta, 2021·1
Genta Gobens, 2021·1
Gentabac, 2021·1
Gentabilles, 2021·1
Gentac, 2021·1
Gentacarnot, 2021·1
Gentacidin, 2021·1
Gentacin, 2021·1
Gentacoll, 2021·1
Gentacort, 2021·2
Gentadexa, 2021·2
Gentadexa, Colircusi— *see* Colircusi Gentadexa, 1899·4
Gentagran, 2021·2
Gentak, 2021·2
Gental, 2021·2
Gental-F, 2021·2
Gentalline, 2021·2
Gentalodina, 2021·2
Gentalyn, 2021·2
Gentalyn Beta, 2021·2
Gentamed, 2021·2
Gentamedical, 2021·2
Gentamen, 2021·2
Gentamicin C1, 217·1
Gentamicin C1a, 217·1
Gentamicin C2, 217·1
Gentamicin C2a, 217·1
Gentamicin C2b, 217·1
Gentamicin $C_{2B}$ Sulphate, 231·3
Gentamicin Sulfate, 217·1
Gentamicin Sulphate, 217·1
Gentamicina, Sulfato de, 217·1
Gentamicini Sulfas, 217·1
Gentamil, 2021·2
Gentamina, 2021·2
Gentamival, 2021·2
Gentamytrex, 2021·2
Gentanacin, 2021·2
Genta-Oph, 2021·2
Gentapat, 2021·2
Gentapharma, 2021·2
Gentaplex, 2021·2
Gentaplus, 2021·2
Gentarim, 2021·2
Gentaron, 2021·2
Gentasol, 2021·2
Gentasone, 2021·3
Gentasporin, 2021·3
Gentatenk, 2021·3
Gentatrim, 2021·3
Gentavasor, 2021·3
Gentavivant, 2021·3
Gentax, 2021·3
Gentaxil, 2021·3
Gentazaf Z, 2021·3
Genteal, 2021·3
Genteal Lubricant, 2021·3
Genteal Moisturising, 2021·3
Gentiabron, 2021·3
Gentialoquin, 2021·3
Gentian, 1692·2
Gentian, Japanese, 1692·2
Gentian Root, 1692·2
Gentian Violet, 1186·1
Gentiana, 1692·2
*Gentiana lutea*, 1692·2
*Gentiana scabra*, 1692·2
Gentianae Radix, 1692·2
Gentibioptal, 2021·3
Genticin, 2021·3
Genticina, 2021·3
Genticol, 2021·3
Genticyn, 2021·3
Genticyn B Eye/Ear, 2021·3
Genticyn Eye/Ear, 2021·3

Genticyn HC, 2021·3
Gentipress, 2021·3
Gentiran, 2021·3
Gentisato de Metilo, 59·2
Gentisato de Sodio, 90·1
Gentisato Sodico, 90·1
Gentisic Acid, 17·3
Gentisic Acid Ethanolamide, 1692·2
Gentisone HC, 2021·3
Gentisuric Acid, 17·3
Gentlax, 2021·3
Gentle C with Bioflavonoids, 2021·3
Gentlees, 2021·4
Gent-L-Tip, 2021·4
Gentocelina, 2021·4
Gentocil, 2021·4
Gentoler, 2021·4
Gentomil, 2021·4
Gent-Ophtal, 2021·4
Gentos, 2021·4
Gentralay, 2021·4
Gentran 40, 2021·4
Gentran 70, 2021·4
Gentrisone, 2021·4
Gentus, 2021·4
Gentussiin, 2021·4
Genu-cyl Ho-Len-Complex, 2021·4
Genuine Australian Eucalyptus Drops, 2021·4
Genurat, 2021·4
Genurin, 2021·4
Genurin-S, 2021·4
Genuxal, 2021·4
Gen-Xene, 2021·4
Genziana, 1692·2
Genziana (Specie Composta), 2021·4
Geo Vit H3, 2021·4
Geocillin, 2021·4
Geodon, 2021·4
Geo-magnit, 2021·4
Geomicina, 2021·4
Geomycine, 2021·4
Geopen, 2022·1
Geophagol, 2022·1
Georkacina, 2022·1
Gepan, 2022·1
Gepefrina, Tartrato de, 923·2
Gepefrine Tartrate, 923·2
Gepeprostin, 2022·1
Gepirona, Hidrocloruro de, 701·1
Gepirone Hydrochloride, 701·1
Gepromi, 2022·1
GER-11, 344·1
Geracin, 2022·1
Geralen, 2022·1
Geram, 2022·1
Geramet, 2022·1
Geramox, 2022·1
Geranial, 1673·2, 1706·2, 1724·1
Geranii, Oleum, 1692·2
Geranil, 2022·1
Geranine 2G, 1058·1
Geranio, Aceite Esencial de, 1692·2
Geraniol, 1673·2, 1692·2
Geranium Oil, 1692·2
Geranium Oil, Rose, 1692·2
Geranyl Acetate, 1673·2, 1706·2
Geranyl Farnesylacetate, 1267·1
Geranylgeranylacetone (5*E*, 9*E*,13*E* Isomer), 1293·3
Gerard 99, 2022·1
Gerard House Preparations, 2022·1
Geratam, 2022·2
Geratar, 2022·2
Geravim, 2022·2
Geravitine, 2022·2
Gerax, 2022·2
Gerbin, 2022·2
Gerbstoff, 1751·2
Gercid Forte, 2022·2
Geref, 2022·2
Gereinigter Honig, 1434·2
Gerelax, 2022·2
Geri, 2022·2
Geriac, 2022·2
Geriaforce, 2022·2
Gerial B12, 2022·2
Gerialong, 2022·2
Geriaplasma, 2022·2
Geriaton, 2022·2
Geriatric, 2022·2
Geriatric Pharmaton, 2022·2
Geriatrie-Mulsin, 2022·2
Geriavit, 2022·2
Geriavite, 2022·2
Gericaps, 2022·2
Gericarb, 2022·2
Gericellulase— *see* Gustase, 2033·2
Gericellulase— *see* Gustase Plus, 2033·2
Gericin, 2022·3
Gericomplex, 2022·3
Geriflox, 2022·3
Gerigoa, 2022·3
Geri-Kan H3, 2022·3
Gerilase— *see* Gustase, 2033·2
Gerilase— *see* Gustase Plus, 2033·2
Gerilide, 2022·3
Gerimal, 2022·3
Gerimax Preparations, 2022·3
Gerimed, 2022·3
Gerin, 2022·3
Gerinap, 2022·3
Geriot, 2022·3
Geripan, 2022·3
Geri-Plus, 2022·3
Geriprotase— *see* Gustase, 2033·2
Geriprotase— *see* Gustase Plus, 2033·2
Geriso, 2022·3
Geritol, 2022·3
Geritol Complete, 2022·3
Geritol Extend, 2022·3
Geriton, 2022·3
Geritonic, 2022·3
Gerivent, 2022·3
Gerivit, 2022·3
Gerivite, 2022·4
Gerivites, 2022·4
Gerivix, 2022·4
Germacid, 2022·4
Germacort, 2022·4
German Chamomile, 1669·3
Germanin, 2022·4
Germanio, 1692·2
Germanium, 1692·2
Germ-Cell Cancer, Ovarian— *see* Malignant Neoplasms of the Ovary, 520·2
Germ-cell Cancer, Testicular— *see* Malignant Neoplasms of the Testis, 523·1
Germentin, 2022·4
Germic, 2022·4
Germicidin, 2022·4
Germisdin Antiseptico, 2022·4
Germisdin Higiene Intima, 2022·4
Germolene, 2022·4
Germolene First Aid, 2022·4
Germoloids, 2022·4
Germoloids HC, 2022·4
Germose, 2022·4
Germosept, 2022·4
Germozero, 2022·4
Germozero Dermo, 2022·4
Germozero Hospital, 2022·4
Germozero Plus, 2022·4
Gernebcin, 2022·4
Gernel, 2022·4
Gero H3, 2022·4
Gero H3 Aslan, 2023·1
Geroaslan H3, 2023·1
Geroderm, 2023·1
Geroderm Zolfo, 2023·1
Gerodorm, 2023·1
Geroforte, 2023·1
Gerogelat, 2023·1
Gerolin, 2023·1
Gerontamin, 2023·1
Gerontex, 2023·1
Gerontin, 2023·1
Geroplus, 2023·1
Gerosenil, 2023·1
Geroten, 2023·1
Gerotrex H3, 2023·1
Gerovital, 2023·1
Gerovital H3, 2023·1
Geroxalen, 2023·1
Geroxicam, 2023·1
Gerozac, 2023·1
Gerskin, 2023·1
Gertac, 2023·1
Gertalgin, 2023·1
Gertemycin, 2023·1
Gertocalm, 2023·1
Gervaken, 2023·1
GES 45, 2023·1
Gesamtnahrlosung, 2023·1
Gesicain, 2023·2
Gesidine, 2023·2
Gesiprox, 2023·2
Geslutin, 2023·2
Gêsso, 1665·1
Gestadinona, 2023·2
Gestaferron, 2023·2
Gestafortin, 2023·2
Gestageno, 2023·2
Gestagens, 1527·2
Gestakadin, 2023·2
Gestamater, 2023·2
Gestamestrol N, 2023·2
Gestamine, 2023·2
Gestanon, 2023·2
GestaPolar, 2023·2
Gestapuran, 2023·2
Gestarelle, 2023·2
Gestatest, 2023·2
Gestational Diabetes— *see* Diabetes Mellitus, 324·1
Gestational Trophoblastic Tumours, 505·1
Gestavit, 2023·2
Gester, 2023·2
Gesterol, 2023·2
Gestid, 2023·2
Gestiferrol, 2023·2
Gestinol, 2023·2
Gestodene, 1556·1
Gestodeno, 1556·1
Gestone, 2023·2
Gestonorona, Caproato de, 1556·2
Gestonorone Caproate, 1556·2
Gestoral, 2023·2
Gestrelan, 2023·2
Gestrinona, 1556·2
Gestrinone, 1556·2
Gestronol Hexanoate, 1556·2
Getrocknete Schilddrüse, 1604·2
Gets-It, 2023·2
Getting Roached, 698·3
Getup, 2023·3
Gevatran, 2023·3
Gevilon, 2023·3
Gevirol, 2023·3
Gevrabon, 2023·3
Gevral Preparations, 2023·3
Gevramycin, 2023·3
Gevramycin Topica, 2023·3
Gewacalm, 2023·3
Gewacyclin, 2023·3
Gewadal, 2023·3
Gewaglucon, 2023·3
Gewamol, 2023·3
Gewapurol, 2023·3
Gewazem, 2023·3
Gewodin, 2023·3
Gewodine, 2023·3
Gewürznelke, 1673·2
Gewusst wie Darmtee, 2023·3
Gewusst wie Entschlackungstee, 2023·3
Gewusst wie Gruner Fastentee, 2023·3
Gewusst wie Husten-Bronchialtee, 2023·3
Gewusst wie Leber-Gallentee, 2023·3
Gewusst wie Magentee Mild, 2023·4
Gewusst wie Nerven-Schlaftee, 2023·4
Geyderm, 2023·4
Geyderm Sepsi, 2023·4
Geyfritz, 2023·4
Gezon, 2023·4
GF-196960, 1751·1
G-Farlutal, 2023·4
G-Fen, 2023·4
GF-I115, 637·3
GFN Phenylephrine, 2023·4
GFN PSE DM, 2023·4
GFN/DM, 2023·4
GFN/DM/PE, 2023·4
GFN/PSE, 2023·4
GG-167, 658·1
GG-745, 1549·2
GH, 1327·2
GHB, 1308·3
GHRF, 1339·2
GHRH, 1339·2, 2023·4
GH-RIF, 1339·3
GHRIH, 1339·3
GI, 2023·4
GI-87084B, 86·1
GI-198745, 1549·2
Giamebil, 2023·4
Gianda, 2023·4
Giant Cell Arteritis, 1080·1
Giarcid, 2023·4
Giardiasis, 596·3
Giardil, 2023·4
Giarlam, 2023·4
Gibicef, 2023·4
Gibifer, 2023·4
Gibiflu, 2023·4
Gibilon, 2023·4
Gibinap, 2023·4
Gibixen, 2024·1
Gichtex, 2024·1
Gichtex Plus, 2024·1
Giflorex, 2024·1
Gigantism— *see* Acromegaly and Gigantism, 1312·1
Gigasept, 2024·1
Gigasept AF, 2024·1
Gigasept FF, 2024·1
Gigasept Med, 2024·1
Gigatrom, 2024·1
Gilemal, 2024·1
Gilex, 2024·1
Gillazyme, 2024·1
Gillazyme Plus, 2024·1
Gilles de la Tourette's Syndrome— *see* Tics, 664·2
Gilt, 2024·1
Gilucor, 2024·1
Giludop, 2024·1
Gilurytmal, 2024·1
Gilurytmal, Neo- — *see* Neo-Gilurytmal, 2158·4
Gilustenon, 2024·1
Gimabrol, 2024·1
Gimalxina, 2024·1
Gimestat, 586·3
Gin Pain, 2024·1
Ginal Cent, 2024·1
Ginal Gel, 2024·1
Ginarsan, 2024·1
Ginatex, 2024·1
Ginatren, 2024·1
Ginbiloba, 2024·1
Gincaps, 2024·1
Gincare, 2024·1
Gincoben, 2024·1
Gincola, 2024·1
Gincolin, 2024·2
Ginconazol, 2024·2
Gincosan, 2024·2
Gine Canesten, 2024·2
Gine Heyden, 2024·2
Gine Zalain, 2024·2
Gineburno, 2024·2
Ginec, 2024·2
Ginecofuran, 2024·2
Ginecopast, 2024·2
Ginecoside, 2024·2
Ginecrin, 2024·2
Ginedak, 2024·2
Ginedazol Dual, 2024·2
Ginedermofix, 2024·2
Ginedisc, 2024·2
Ginedisc 50 Plus, 2024·2
Gineflor, 2024·2
Ginejuvent, 2024·2
Ginelea, 2024·2

Ginelea T, 2024·2
Ginemaxim, 2024·2
Ginenorm, 2024·2
Ginesal, 2024·2
Gineseptina, 2024·2
Ginesse, 2024·2
Ginestatin, 2024·2
Ginetris, 2024·2
Ginevit, 2024·2
Ginex, 2024·3
Ginexin-F, 2024·3
Gingelly Oil, 1743·3
Gingembre, 1267·1
Ginger, 1267·1
Ginger, Unbleached, 1267·1
Gingeron, 2024·3
Ginger-Vite Forte, Bioglan— *see* Bioglan Ginger-Vite Forte, 1844·1
Gingicain D, 2024·3
Gingilacer, 2024·3
Gingiloba, 2024·3
Gingilone, 2024·3
Gingi-Pak, 2024·3
Gingisan, 2024·3
Gingium, 2024·3
Gingivan, 2024·3
Gingivitis, Acute Necrotising Ulcerative— *see* Mouth Infections, 136·1
Gingivitis— *see* Mouth Infections, 136·1
Gingivitol N, 2024·3
Gingo A, 2024·3
Gingobeta, 2024·3
Gingohexal, 2024·3
Gingol, 2024·3
Gingopret, 2024·3
Gingosol, 2024·3
Gingo-Ther, 2024·3
Gingviton, 2024·3
Ginil, 2024·3
Ginkan, 2024·3
Ginkapran, 2024·3
Ginkgo, 1692·3
Ginkgo Biloba, 1692·3
*Ginkgo biloba*, 1693·1
Ginkgo Biloba Comp, 2024·4
Ginkgo Biloba Plus, 2024·4
Ginkgo Complex, 2024·4
Ginkgo Leaf, 1692·3
Ginkgo Plus, 2024·4
Ginkgo Plus Herbal Plus Formula 10, 2024·4
Ginkgo Plus Vivo-Livo, 2024·4
Ginkgobakehl, 2024·4
Ginkgoforce, 2024·4
Ginkgolide A, 1693·1
Ginkgolide B, 1693·1
Ginkgolide C, 1693·1
Ginkgolide J, 1693·1
Ginkgolide M, 1693·1
Ginkgolides, 1693·1
Ginkgólidos, 1693·1
Ginkgo-PS, 2024·4
Ginkgorell, 2024·4
Ginkoba, 2024·4
Ginkoba M/E, 2024·4
Ginkobil, 2024·4
Ginkocer, 2024·4
Ginkodilat, 2024·4
Ginkoftal, 2024·4
Ginkogink, 2024·4
Ginkoplus, 2024·4
Ginkopur, 2024·4
Ginkor, 2024·4
Ginkor Fort, 2024·4
Ginkoret, 2024·4
Ginkosen, 2024·4
Ginkovital, 2024·4
Gino Clotrimix, 2024·4
Gino Conazol, 2024·4
Gino Loprox, 2024·4
Gino Monipax, 2024·4
Gino Pletil, 2024·4
Gino Tralen, 2024·4
Gino-Canesten, 2025·1
Ginocap, 2025·1
Gino-Cauterex, 2025·1
Ginoday, 2025·1
Ginoden, 2025·1
Ginoderm, 2025·1
Gino-Fibrase, 2025·1
Ginoflorax, 2025·1
Ginolax, 2025·1
Gino-Lotremine, 2025·1
Ginomains, 2025·1
Ginometrim, 2025·1
Ginometrim Oral, 2025·1
Ginomineral, 2025·1
Ginomizol, 2025·1
Gino-Panflogin, 2025·1
Ginopil, 2025·1
Ginoplan, 2025·1
Ginorectol, 2025·1
Ginosutin, 2025·1
Ginosutin M, 2025·1
Ginotarin, 2025·1
Gino-Teracin, 2025·1
Gino-Travogen, 2025·1
Ginotrax, 2025·1
Gino-Trosyd, 2025·1
Ginovagin, 2025·1
Ginoven, 2025·1
Ginoxil, 2025·1
Ginoxil Ecoschiuma, 2025·1
Ginroy, 2025·1
Ginsactiv, 2025·1
Ginsana, 2025·1
Ginsana Ton, 2025·2
Ginsatonic, 2025·2
Ginsavit, 2025·2
Ginsenetten, Kneipp— *see* Kneipp Ginsenetten, 2081·2
Ginseng, 1693·1
Ginseng, American, 1693·2
Ginseng, Asian, 1693·2
Ginseng, Brazilian, 1693·1
Ginseng King, The— *see* The Ginseng King, 2328·2
Ginseng Med Complex, 2025·2
Ginseng Radix, 1693·1
Ginseng, Red, 1693·1
Ginseng, Russian, 1693·1, 1744·1
Ginseng, Siberian, 1693·1, 1744·1
Ginseng-Complex "Schuh", 2025·2
GinsengSure, 2025·2
Ginsenosides, 1693·1
Ginsex, 2025·2
Ginsroy, 2025·2
Ginsynergy, Bioglan— *see* Bioglan Ginsynergy, 1844·1
Gintonal, 2025·2
Ginurovac, 2025·2
Ginvapast, 2025·2
Ginzing, 2025·2
Ginzing E, 2025·2
Ginzing G, 2025·2
Gipzide, 2025·2
Girha "Schuh", 2025·2
Girheulit HM, 2025·2
Girl, 1373·3
Girofle, Essence de, 1673·3
Giroflier, 1673·2
Giroflox, 2025·2
Gi-Sen, 2025·2
Gitaloxin, 894·2
Gitoxin, 894·2
Gittalun, 2025·2
Gityl, 2025·2
Giusquiamo, 485·2
Givalex, 2025·2
Givitol, 2025·2
GI-198745X, 1549·2
GL-701, 1565·3
GL Enzyme, 1698·2
GLA, 1690·2
GLA-130, 2025·2
GLA-Plus Vitamin E, 2025·3
Glaan, 2025·2
Glacial Acetic Acid, 1645·2
Gladase, 2025·2
Gladem, 2025·2
Gladiaton, 2025·2
Gladius, 2025·2
Gladixol, 2025·3
Gladixol N, 2025·3
Gladlax, Gerard House— *see* Gerard House Gladlax, 2022·1
Glafemak, 2025·3
Glafenina, 44·3
Glafenine, 44·3
Glafenine Hydrochloride, 44·3
Glafornil, 2025·3
Glakay, 2025·3
Glamidolo, 2025·3
Glamin, 2025·3
Glandicin, 2025·3
Glandol, 2025·3
Glandosane, 2025·3
Glandulae-F-Gastreu R20, 2025·3
Glandulae-M-Gastreu R19, 2025·3
Glandular Fever— *see* Epstein-Barr Virus Infections, 620·1
Glaphenine, 44·3
Glargine, Insulin, 334·3, 340·3
Glass, Soluble, 1748·3
Glass, Water, 1748·3
Glatim, 2025·3
Glatiramer Acetate, 1693·3
Glatiramer, Acetato de, 1693·3
Glauber's Salt, 1290·1
Glaucadrine, 2025·3
Glaucina, 1121·3
Glaucine, 1121·3
*d*-Glaucine, 1121·3
*dl*-Glaucine, 1121·3
*d*-Glaucine Hydrobromide, 1121·3
*d*-Glaucine Hydrochloride, 1121·3
*dl*-Glaucine Phosphate, 1121·3
*Glaucium flavum*, 1121·3
Glaucocare, 2025·3
Glaucocarpine, 2025·3
Glaucocin, 2025·3
Glaucofrin, 2025·3
Glaucol, 2025·3
Glaucoma— *see* Glaucoma and Ocular Hypertension, 1485·1
Glaucon, 2025·3
Glauconex, 2025·3
Glauconide, 2025·3
Glauco-Oph, 2025·3
Glaucosan, 2025·3
Glaucostat, 2025·4
Glauco-Stulln, 2025·4
Glaucotat, 2025·4
Glaucotensil, 2025·4
Glaucotensil T, 2025·4
Glaucotensil TD, 2025·4
Glaucothil, 2025·4
GlaucTabs, 2025·4
Glaudrops, 2025·4
Glaufrin, 2025·4
Glauko Biciron, 2025·4
Glaumetax, 2025·4
Glaumid, 2025·4
Glaunorm, 2025·4
Glau-opt, 2025·4
Glaupax, 2025·4
Glausine, 2025·4
Glausolets, 2025·4
Glautarakt, 2025·4
Glauteolol, 2025·4
Glautimol, 2025·4
Glavamin, 2025·4
Glaveral, 2025·4
Glavit, 2025·4
Glaxal Base, 2025·4
Glazidim, 2025·4
*Glechoma hederacea*, 1696·2
Gleevec, 2026·1
Glefos, 2026·1
Gleitgelen, 2026·1
Gleitmittel, 2026·1
Glemaz, 2026·1
Glemicid, 2026·1
Glencamide, 2026·1
Glenol, 2026·1
Gleptoferron, 1432·1
Glevomicina, 2026·1
Gliadel, 2026·1
Gliadin, 1694·2
Glial-cell-derived Neurotrophic Factor, 1739·2
Glianimon, 2026·1
Gliatilin, 2026·1
Glib, 2026·1
Gli-basan, 2026·1
Glibediab, 2026·1
Glibemid, 2026·1
Gliben, 2026·1
Gliben F, 2026·1
Gliben-Azu, 2026·1
Glibenbeta, 2026·1
Glibenclamida, 331·2
Glibenclamide, 331·2
Glibenclamidum, 331·2
Glibenclamon, 2026·1
Glibendoc, 2026·1
Glibenese, 2026·1
Glibenhexal, 2026·1
Glibenil, 2026·1
Gliben-Puren N, 2026·1
Glibenval, 2026·1
Glibesifar, 2026·1
Glibesyn, 2026·2
Glibetic, 2026·2
Glibexil, 2026·2
Glibic, 2026·2
Glibomet, 2026·2
Gliboral, 2026·2
Glibornurida, 331·3
Glibornuride, 331·3
Glib-ratiopharm, 2026·2
Glibuzol, 333·1
Glicacil, 2026·2
Glicalox, 2026·2
Glicamin, 2026·2
Glicel, 2026·2
Glicemin, 2026·2
Glicermina, 2026·2
Glicerofosfórico, Ácido, 1695·2
Glicerol, 1694·3
Glicerol Iodado, 1122·3
Glicerol, Palmitoestearato de, 1695·2
Glicerolax, 2026·2
Glicerolo Microclismi, 2026·2
Glicerotens, 2026·2
Glicero-Valerovit, 2026·2
Gliciclamida, 333·1
Gliciclamide, 333·1
Glicima, 2026·2
Glicina, 1433·3
Glicinal, 2026·2
Gliclazida, 332·1
Gliclazide, 332·1
Gliclazidum, 332·1
Gliclopiramida, 333·1
Glico Test, 2026·2
Glico Urine B, 2026·2
Glicobase, 2026·2
Glicoben, 2026·2
Glicoderm, 2026·2
Glicodin, 2026·2
Glicofisiologica, 2026·2
Glico-Fita, 2026·2
Glicofosfopeptical, 1693·3
Glicofurol, 1474·3
Glicol Propilênico, 1735·2
Glicolato Sódico de Almidón, 1582·1
Glicólico, Ácido, 1147·3
Gliconorm, 2026·2
Glicopirronio, Bromuro de, 482·3
Glicorest, 2026·2
Glicorp, 2026·2
Glicosado, 2026·2
Glicoxem, 2026·3
Glicron, 2026·3
Glidanil, 2026·3
Glide, 2026·3
Glidiab, 2026·3
Glifage, 2026·3
Glifarcal, 2026·3
Gliformin, 2026·3
Glifortex, 2026·3
Glifosato, 1505·3
Glikeyer, 2026·3

Glimbal, 2026·3
Glimel, 2026·3
Glimepil, 2026·3
Glimepirida, 332·2
Glimepiride, 332·2
Glimesec, 2026·3
Glimial, 2026·3
Glimicron, 2026·3
Glimide, 2026·3
Glimidina Sódica, 333·2
Glimidstada, 2026·3
Glimiton, 2026·3
Glinate, 2026·3
Glineon, 2026·3
Glinor, 2026·3
Glinorboral, 2026·3
Glioblastoma Multiforme— *see* Malignant Neoplasms of the Brain, 513·2
Glioma— *see* Malignant Neoplasms of the Brain, 513·2
Glionil, 2026·3
Glios, 2026·3
Gliosartan, 2026·3
Glioten, 2026·3
Gliotenzide, 2026·3
Glioxal, 1181·1
Glipentide, 333·1
Glipep, 2026·3
Glipgen, 2026·3
Glipicontin, 2026·3
Glipid, 2026·4
Glipiscand, 2026·4
Glipizida, 332·2
Glipizide, 332·2
Glipizidum, 332·2
Gliplex, 2026·4
Glipressina, 2026·4
Gliptide, 2026·4
Gliquidona, 332·3
Gliquidone, 332·3
Glisentida, 333·1
Glisentide, 333·1
Glisolamida, 333·1
Glisolamide, 333·1
Glisoxepid, 333·1
Glisoxepida, 333·1
Glisoxepide, 333·1
Glisuret, 2026·4
Glitisol, 2026·4
Glitral, 2026·4
Glivec, 2026·4
Glix, 2026·4
Gliza, 2026·4
Glizide, 2026·4
Glizone, 2026·4
Gln, 1433·2
Globac-Z, 2026·4
Globenicol, 2026·4
Globentyl, 2026·4
Globocef, 2026·4
Globoid, 2026·4
Globovit, 2026·4
Globuce, 2026·4
Globuli Preparations, 2026·4
Globulin, Antithymocyte, 1348·3
Globulin $G_1$ Hydrochloride, 1717·2
Globulina Lloren Anti RH, 2026·4
Globuman, 2026·4
Globuman Hepatite A, 2026·4
Globuman Hepatitis A, 2027·1
Globuman iv CMV, 2027·1
Globuren, 2027·1
Gloceda, 2027·1
Glofil, 2027·1
Glogama Antihepatitis B, 2027·1
Glomerular Kidney Disease, 1080·2
Glomerulonephritis— *see* Glomerular Kidney Disease, 1080·2
Glomerulopathy— *see* Glomerular Kidney Disease, 1080·2
Glomerulosclerosis, Focal— *see* Glomerular Kidney Disease, 1080·2
Glomycin, 241·1
Glonoin, 923·2, 2027·1
Glonoinum, 2027·1
Glopir, 2027·1
Glorixone, 2027·1
Glossderm, 2027·1
Glossithiase, 2027·1
Glossware & Brush, 2027·1
Glossyfin, 2027·1
Glotil, 2027·1
Glotone, 2027·1
Glottyl, 2027·1
Glovan, 2027·1
GLP-1, 325·1
GLQ-223, 655·3
Glu, 1433·2
Glu Hydrochloride, 1433·2
Gluben, 2027·1
Glubionato de Calcio, 1225·1
Gluborid, 2027·1
GlucaGen, 2027·1
Glucagon, 1039·3
Glucagon, Human, 1039·3
Glucagon-like Peptide 1, 325·1
Glucagonoma— *see* Carcinoid Tumours and Other Secretory Neoplasms, 504·1
Glucagonum, 1039·3
Glucagonum Humanum, 1039·3
Glucal, 2027·1
Glucal B12, 2027·1
Glucalbott Rth, 2027·1
Glucalcium, 2027·1
Glucamet, 2027·2
Glucametacin, 44·3
Glucametacina, 44·3
Glucaminol, 2027·2
Glucanet, 2027·2
Glucantim, 2027·2
Glucantime, 2027·2
Gluceptate, Technetium ($^{99m}$Tc), 1526·1
Gluceptato de Eritromicina, 208·2
Gluceride, 2027·2
Glucerna, 2027·2
Glucidoral, 2027·2
Glucinan, 2027·2
D-Glucitol, 1446·3
Glucoamylases, 1654·2
Glucobay, 2027·2
Glucobene, 2027·2
Glucobiosa, 1669·1
Glucobon, 2027·2
Glucocalcium, 2027·2
Gluco-Calcium, 2027·2
Glucocard, 2027·2
β-Glucocerebrosidase, 1649·2
β-Glucocerebrosidase, Macrophage-targeted, 1649·1
Glucocerebrosidosis— *see* Gaucher Disease, 1649·2
Glucochaux, 2027·2
Glucochloral, 1501·2
Gluco-Cinta, 2027·2
Glucocorticoids, 1068·1
Glucocron, 2027·2
Glucodex, 2027·2
Glucodiab, 2027·2
Glucodin, 2027·2
Glucoferro, 2027·2
Glucoferro K, 2027·2
Glucofilm, 2027·2
Glucoflex-R, 2027·2
Glucoformin, 2027·2
Glucofrangulin A, 1266·3
Glucogenase, 1654·2
Glucoheptonato de Calcio, 1225·2
Glucohex, 2027·3
Glucohexal, 2027·3
Glucoles-500, 2027·3
Glucolin, 2027·3
Glucolip, 2027·3
Glucolon, 2027·3
Glucolyte, 2027·3
Glucoman, 2027·3
Glucomanano, 1693·3
Glucomannan, 1693·3
Glucomed, 2027·3
Glucomen, 2027·3
Glucomet, 2027·3
Glucometer, 2027·3
Glucometer Elite, 2027·3
Glucometer Esprit, 2027·3
Glucomide, 2027·3
Glucomin, 2027·3
Glucomol, 2027·3
Glucomore, 2027·3
Gluconate, Technetium ($^{99m}$Tc), 1526·1
Gluconato de Clorhexidina, 1173·2
Gluconato de Sodio, 1747·3
Gluconic Acid 6-[Bis(diisopropylamino)acetate], 1727·2
Gluconil, 2027·3
Gluconorm, 2027·3
Glucophage, 2027·3
Glucopirida, 2027·3
Glucoplasmal, 2027·3
Glucoplex, 2027·3
Glucoplurisalina, 2027·3
Glucopolielectrol, 2027·3
Glucopotasica, 2027·3
Glucopotasico, 2027·4
Glucoprotamine, 1180·3
Glucoproteína de Klebsiella Pneumoniae, 1703·3
D-(+)-Glucopyranose, 1432·2
β-D-Glucopyranose Aerodehydrogenase, 1694·2
D-(+)-Glucopyranose Monohydrate, 1432·2
3-[(*O*-β-D-Glucopyranosyl-(1→4)-*O*-3-acetyl-2,6-dideoxy-β-D-*ribo*-hexopyranosyl-(1→4)-*O*-2,6-dideoxy-β-D-*ribo*-hexopyranosyl-(1→4)-*O*-2,6-dideoxy-β-D-*ribo*-hexopyranosyl)oxy]-12,14-dihydroxy-3β,5β,12β-card-20(22)-enolide, 945·1
3-[(*O*-β-D-Glucopyranosyl-(1→4)-*O*-2,6-dideoxy-β-D-*ribo*-hexopyranosyl-(1→4)-*O*-2,6-dideoxy-β-D-*ribo*-hexopyranosyl-(1→4)-*O*-2,6-dideoxy-β-D-*ribo*-hexopyranosyl)oxy]-12,14-dihydroxy-3β,5β,12β-card-20(22)-enolide, 893·1
α-D-Glucopyranosyl-1,4-D-glucitol, 1439·3
4-*O*-α-D-Glucopyranosyl-β-D-glucopyranose, 1440·1
4-*O*-β-D-Glucopyranosyl-D-glucose, 1669·1
6-β-D-Glucopyranosyloxy-7-hydroxycoumarin, 1648·2
Glucor, 2027·4
Glucoremed, 2027·4
Gluco-Rite, 2027·4
Glucosa, 1432·2
Glucosa Anhidra, 1432·2
Glucosa Monohidrato, 1432·2
Glucosa Oxidasa, 1694·2
Glucosa, Pruebas de, 1694·2
Glucosada, 2027·4
Glucosado, 2027·4
Glucosado Vitulia, Suero— *see* Suero Glucosado Vitulia, 2310·3
Glucosalin, 2027·4
Glucosalina, 2027·4
Glucosalina Modific, 2027·4
Glucosaline, 2027·4
Glucosalino, 2027·4
Glucosalino Vitulia, Suero— *see* Suero Glucosalino Vitulia, 2310·4
Glucosamina, 1694·1
Glucosamine, 1694·1
Glucosamine Hydriodide, 1694·1
Glucosamine Hydrochloride, 1694·1
Glucosamine Sulfate, 1694·1
Glucosamine Sulfate Potassium Chloride, 1694·1
Glucosamine Sulfate Sodium Chloride, 1694·1
Glucosaminoglycans, Sulfated, 810·2
Glucosan, 2027·4
Glucose, 1432·2
D-Glucose, 1432·2
Glucose, Anhydrous, 1432·2
Glucose, Liquid, 1432·2
Glucose, Liquid, Spray-dried, 1432·2
Glucose Monohydrate, 1432·2
D-Glucose Monohydrate, 1432·2
Glucose Nutramigen— *see* Nutramigen, 2180·4
Glucose Oxidase, 1694·2
Glucose Syrup, Hydrogenated, 1439·3
Glucose Tests, 1694·2
GlucoSelene, 2027·4
Glucose-6-phosphate Dehydrogenase Deficiency— *see* Haemolytic Anaemia, 733·1
Glucoseral, 2027·4
α-Glucosidasa, 1646·2
Glucosidase, Acid Alpha, 1646·2
Glucosmon, 2027·4
Glucostad, 2027·4
Glucosteril, 2027·4
Glucostix, 2027·4
Glucostrip, 2027·4
Glucosulfa, 2027·4
Glucosum Anhydricum, 1432·2
Glucosum Monohydridicum, 1432·2
β-D-Glucosyl-*N*-acylsphingosine Glucohydrolase, 1649·1, 1649·2
Glucosylceramidase, 1649·1, 1649·2
(D-Glucosylthio)gold, 19·3
Gluco-Tablinen, 2027·4
Glucotard, 2027·4
Glucotem, 2027·4
Glucotide, 2027·4
Glucotouch, 2027·4
Glucotrend, 2027·4
Glucotrol, 2027·4
Glucovance, 2027·4
Glucoven, 2027·4
Glucoven Infant, 2027·4
Glucovenos Pad— *see* Glucoven infant, 2027·4
Glucovitan Ginseng, 2028·1
Glucozide, 2028·1
Glucuronato de Trimetrexato, 410·2
Glucurono-2-amino-2-deoxyglucoglucan Sulphate, 1009·2
Glue Ear— *see* Otitis Media, 138·1
Glufcaps, 2028·1
Glufer-C, 2028·1
Glufor, 2028·1
Gluformin, 2028·1
Glukacel, 2028·1
Gluketur, 2028·1
Gluketurtest, 2028·1
Gluko, 2028·1
Glukolyt, 2028·1
Glukoreduct, 2028·1
Glukos-El, 2028·1
Glukotest, 2028·1
Glukovital, 2028·1
Glukurtest, 2028·1
Glulisine, Insulin, 340·3
Glumal, 2028·1
Glumet, 2028·1
Glumida, 2028·1
Gluparin, 2028·1
Glu-Phos, 2028·1
Glupitel, 2028·1
Glupozide, 2028·1
Glurenor, 2028·1
Glurenorm, 2028·1
GLURP, 1622·3
Gluside, 1443·2
Glustress, 2028·1
Gluta Complex, 2028·1
Glutabeina A, 2028·1
Glutabeina E, 2028·1
Glutacerebro, 2028·1
Glutacid, 2028·1
Glutacyl Vitaminado, 2028·2
Glutaferro, 2028·2
Glutafin, 2028·2
Glutamag Vitamine, 2028·2
Glutamato de Arginina, 1421·1
Glutamato Magnésico, Hidrobromuro de, 1709·2
Glutamato Monosódico, 1441·1
Glutamed, 2028·2
Glutamic Acid, 1433·2
L-Glutamic Acid, 1433·2
Glutamic Acid, 1433·2
L-Glutamic Acid 5-Amide, 1433·2
Glutamic Acid Hydrochloride, 1433·2
Glutámico, Ácido, 1433·2
Glutámico, Hidrocloruro del Ácido, 1433·2
Glutamin, 2028·2
Glutamin Fosforo, 2028·2

Glutamine, 1433·2
L-Glutamine, 1433·2
Glutaminic Acid, 1433·2
*N*-(*N*-L-γ-Glutamyl-L-cysteinyl)glycine, 1040·3
Glutanil, 2028·2
Glutaral, 1180·3
Glutaral Concentrate, 1180·3
Glutaral Disinfectant Solution, 1180·3
Glutaraldehyde, 1180·3
Glutaraldehyde Solution, Strong, 1180·3
Glutarex, 2028·2
Glutargin, 2028·2
Glutaric Dialdehyde, 1180·3
Glutaricaciduria, 1043·1
Glutarin, 2028·2
Glutarol, 2028·2
Glutarsin E, 2028·2
Glutasan, 2028·2
Glutasedan, 2028·2
Glutasey, 2028·2
Glutasorb, 2028·2
Glutathione, 1040·3
Glutathione Sodium, 1040·3
Glutatión, 1040·3
Glutaven, 2028·2
Glutavigon, 2028·2
Glutelins, 1694·2
Gluten, 1694·2
Glutenin, 1694·2
Gluten-sensitive Enteropathy— *see* Coeliac Disease, 1417·3
Glutethimide, 701·2
Glutethimidum, 701·2
Glutetimida, 701·2
Glutetimide, 701·2
Gluthion, 2028·2
Gluti-Agil Mono, 2028·2
Glutilage, 2028·2
Glutisal, 2028·2
Glutofac, 2028·2
Glutose, 2028·2
Glutoxil, 2028·2
Glutril, 2028·2
Gluzo, 2028·2
Gluzolyte, 2028·2
Gly, 1433·3
Gly Derm Super Sunblock, 2028·3
Glyade, 2028·3
Glyate, 2028·3
Glybenclamide, 331·2
Glybenzcyclamide, 331·2
Glyburide, 331·2
Glybutamide, 330·3
Glybuzole, 333·1
Glycemin, 2028·3
Glycemirex, 2028·3
Glyceol, 2028·3
Glycérides Semi-synthétiques Solides, 1481·1
Glycerin, 1694·3
Glycerine, 1694·3
Glycerol, 1694·3
Glycerol Dibehenate, 1411·3
Glycerol Distearate, 1411·3
Glycerol Esters, 1411·1
Glycerol, Iodinated, 1122·3
Glycerol Monolinoleate, 1412·1
Glycerol Mono-oleates, 1412·1
Glycerol Monostearate 40-55, 1412·1
Glycérol (Monostéarate de), 1412·1
Glycerol Triacetate, 410·2
Glyceroli Dibehenas, 1411·3
Glyceroli Distearas, 1411·3
Glyceroli Monolinoleas, 1412·1
Glyceroli Monostearas, 1412·1
Glyceroli Trinitratis, 923·2
Glycerolum, 1694·3
Glycerolum Triacetas, 410·2
Glycerophosphoric Acid, 1695·2
Glycerosteril, 2028·3
Glycerotone, 2028·3
Glyceryl Aminobenzoate, 1151·2
Glyceryl 1-(4-Aminobenzoate), 1151·2
Glyceryl Behenate, 1411·3
Glyceryl Dinitrates, 924·3
Glyceryl Di-octanoate, 1715·3
Glyceryl Distearate, 1411·3
Glyceryl Guaiacolate, 1122·1
Glyceryl Mono-decanoate, 1715·3
Glyceryl Monolinoleate, 1412·1
Glyceryl Mononitrates, 924·3
Glyceryl Mono-octanoate, 1715·3
Glyceryl Monooleate, 1412·1
Glyceryl Mono-oleate, 1412·1
Glyceryl Monopalmitate, 1412·1
Glyceryl Monostearate, 1412·1
Glyceryl Monostearate, Self-emulsifying, 1412·2
Glyceryl PABA, 1151·2
Glyceryl Palmitostearate, 1695·2
Glyceryl Triacetate, 410·2
Glyceryl Trierucate, 1707·3
Glyceryl Trinitrate, 923·2
Glyceryl Trinitrate Solution, 923·2
Glyceryl Trioleate, 1707·3
Glycerylguayacolum, 1122·1
Glycerylguethol, 1122·1
Glycerylphosphoric Acid, 1695·2
L-α-Glycerylphosphorylcholine, 1488·3
Glyceryl-T, 2028·3
Glycifer, 2028·3
Glycilax, 2028·3
(Glycinato-*N,O*)dihydroxyaluminium Hydrate, 1249·1
Glycine, 1433·3
Glycine Betaine, 1660·1
Glycine Encephalopathy— *see* Nonketotic Hyperglycinaemia, 1750·2
*Glycine hispida*, 1447·2
Glycine Hydrochloride, 1434·1
*Glycine max*, 1447·2
*Glycine soja*, 1447·2
Glycinexylidide, 1379·1
Glycinum, 1433·3
Glyciphage, 2028·3
Glycirenan, 2028·3
Glyclazide, 332·1
Glyclopyramide, 333·1
Glycobal, 2028·3
Glycobiarsol, 1253·2
Glycochenodeoxycholic Acid, 1660·3
Glycocholic Acid, 1660·3
Glycocoll, 1433·3
Glycocoll Betaine, 1660·1
Glycocortison, 2028·3
Glycocortisone H, 2028·3
Glycodiazine, 333·2
Glycofed, 2028·3
Glycofurol, 1474·3
Glycofurol 75, 1474·3
Glycogen Storage Disease Type I, 1449·3
Glycogen Storage Disease Type II, 1646·2
Glycogen Storage Disease Type V, 1450·2
Glycogen Storage Diseases— *see* Glycogen Storage Disease Type I, 1449·3
Glycol, 1685·3
Glycol Esters, 1411·1
Glycol Salicylate, 44·3
Glycolande N, 2028·3
Glycolic Acid, 1147·3
(8*S*,10*S*)-8-Glycoloyl-7,8,9,10-tetrahydro-6,8,11-trihydroxy-1-methoxy-10-{[2,3,6-trideoxy-3-(2,2,2-trifluoroacetamido)-α-L-*lyxo*-hexopyranosyl]oxy}-5,12-naphthacenedione $8^2$-Valerate, 590·3
Glycomin, 2028·3
Glycon, 2028·3
Glyconon, 2028·3
Glycopeptides, 118·1
Glycophos, 2028·3
Glycoplex, 2028·3
Glycoprep, 2028·3
Glycoprep-C, 2028·3
Glycoprep-C— *see* Prep Kit-C, 2233·1
1–453-Glycoprotein ICAM-1 (Human Reduced), 655·3
Glycoprotein IIb/IIIa-receptor Antagonists, 810·3
Glycopyrrolate, 482·3
Glycopyrronium Bromide, 482·3
Gly-Coramin, 2028·3
Glycoran, 2028·4
Glycosaminoglycan Polysulfate Compounds, 810·2, 931·1
Glycosphingolipids, 1691·1
Glycostigmin, 2028·4
Glycosum, 1432·2
Glyco-Thymoline, 2028·4
Glycotuss, 2028·4
Glycotuss-dM, 2028·4
Glycovit, 2028·4
Glycron, 2028·4
Glycyclamide, 333·1
Glycyl-L-glutamine, 1433·2, 1433·3
*N*-[*N*-(*N*-Glycylglycyl)glycyl]lypressin, 1340·1
Glycylpressin, 2028·4
Glycyrrhetic Acid, 36·2
Glycyrrhetinic Acid, 36·2, 1270·3
Glycyrrhiza, 1270·2
Glycyrrhiza Complex, 2028·4
*Glycyrrhiza glabra*, 1270·2
*Glycyrrhiza uralensis*, 1270·3, 1750·2
Glycyrrhizinic Acid, 1270·3
Glyderm, 2028·4
Glydiazinamide, 332·2
Glyfucan, 2028·4
Glygen, 2028·4
Gly-Gln, 1433·2
Glyguetol, 1122·1
Glykola, 2028·4
Glykresin, 1394·3
Glymax, 2028·4
Glymese, 2028·4
Glymidine, 333·2
Glymidine Sodium, 333·2
Glynase, 2028·4
Glynase, Mini- — *see* Mini-Glynase, 2134·2
Glyoktyl, 2028·4
Glyoxal, 1181·1
Gly-Oxide, 2028·4
Glyoxyldiureide, 1141·3
Glyphenarsine, 617·3
Glyphosate, 1505·3
Glyphyllin, 2028·4
Glyphyllinum, 784·3
Glypressin, 2028·4
Glypressine, 2028·4
Glyprin, 2028·4
Glyquin, 2028·4
Glyquin-XM, 2029·1
Gly-Rectal, 2029·1
Glysan, 2029·1
Glysan, Eudent Con— *see* Eudent con Glysan, 1981·4
Glysennid, 2029·1
Glyset, 2029·1
Glyteol Balsamico, 2029·1
Glytop, 2029·1
Glytoss, 2029·1
Glytrin, 2029·1
Glytuss, 2029·1
Glyvenol, 2029·1
Glyzide, 2029·1
Glyzip, 2029·1
$G_{M1}$, 1691·1
GM-CSF, 756·2
GMS, 1412·1
G-Myticin, 2029·1
GN-1600, 864·3
Gnaoui, 1666·1
Gnathostomiasis, 99·1
GNC, 2029·1
GNC Herbal Laxative, 2029·1
GNO, 2029·1
GNO CP, 2029·1
Gnostocardin, 2029·1
Gnostol, 2029·1
Gnostoval, 2029·1
GnRH, 1325·1
GNT, 217·1
Go-560, 698·2
Gö-687, 914·2
Gö 1261-C, 94·1
Go Kit, 2029·1
Go Kit Plus, 2029·1
Goanna Preparations, 2029·1
Gobab, 353·3
Gobanal, 2029·2
Gobbicaina, 2029·2
Gobbidona, 2029·2
Gobbizolam, 2029·2
Gobemicina, 2029·2
Gobemicina Retard, 2029·2
Gobens Trim, 2029·2
Gobrosan, 2029·2
Gocce Antonetto, 2029·2
Gocce Lassative Aicardi, 2029·2
Goccemed, 2029·2
Gocox-3, 2029·2
Gocox Compound, 2029·2
Godabion B6, 2029·2
Godal, 2029·2
Godamed, 2029·2
Goddards Embrocation, 2029·2
GOE-3450, 362·2
Goeckerman Regimen, 1160·1
Go-Evac, 2029·2
Gofreely, 2029·2
Goitre, Diffuse Non-toxic— *see* Goitre and Thyroid Nodules, 1594·1
Goitre, Endemic— *see* Iodine Deficiency Disorders, 1599·1
Goitre and Thyroid Nodules, 1594·1
Goitre, Toxic Nodular— *see* Hyperthyroidism, 1594·3
Gola Action, 2029·2
Golac, 2029·2
Golacetin, 2029·2
Goladin, 2029·2
Golamed, 2029·2
Golamed Due, 2029·2
Golamed Oral, 2029·2
Golamixin, 2029·3
Golan, 2029·3
Golapiol, 2029·3
Golapiol C, 2029·3
Golasan, 2029·3
Golasept, 2029·3
Golaseptine, 2029·3
Golasol, 2029·3
Golatux, 2029·3
Golaval, 2029·3
Gold, 1695·3
Gold-50, 2029·3
Gold-198, 1523·3
Gold Alka-Seltzer, 2029·3
Gold ($^{198}$Au), Colloidal, 1523·3
Gold Cross Antihistamine Elixir, 2029·3
Gold Cross BOZ Ointment, 2029·3
Gold Cross Cough Medicine, 2029·3
Gold Cross Gluco-lyte, 2029·3
Gold Cross Skin Basics Zinc Cream, 2029·3
Gold Cross Vaporiser Fluid, 2029·3
Gold Dust, 1373·3
Gold Keratinate, 45·1
Gold Keratinate, Calcium, 45·1
Gold Sodium Thiomalate, 88·2
Gold Sodium Thiosulphate, 90·1
Gold Thioglucose, 19·3
Gold Thiomalic Acid, 88·2
Goldar, 2029·3
Gold-bloom, 1665·2
Goldcare, 2029·3
Golden Chain, 1703·3
Golden Eye Drops, 2029·3
Golden Eye Ointment, 2029·3
Golden Rain, 1703·3
Golden Rod, 1748·3
Golden Seal, 1698·3
Golden Seal Compound, Gerard House— *see* Gerard House Golden Seal Compound, 2022·1
Golden Seal Digestive, HRI— *see* HRI Golden Seal Digestive, 2048·4
Golden Senecio, 1743·1
Golden Star, 2029·3
Goldenrod, 1748·3
Goldenrod, European, 1748·3
Goldenseal, 1698·3
Goldenseal Rhizome, 1698·3
Goldgeist, 2029·3
Goldgesic, 2029·3

Gold-Komplex, 2029·3
Goldrutenkraut, 1748·3
Goldtropfen N, 2029·3
Goldtropfen S, 2029·3
Goldtropfen-Hetterich, 2029·3
Golfer's Elbow— *see* Soft-tissue Rheumatism, 11·1
GoLytely, 2029·3
Goma Alcatira, 1582·2
Goma Arábiga, 1576·2
Goma de Garrofín, 1579·1
Goma de Tragacanto, 1582·2
Goma de Xantana, 1582·3
Goma Esterculia, 1290·2
Goma Guar, 333·2
Goma Laca, 1743·3
Gomec, 2029·4
Gomenol, 1719·3, 2029·4
Gomenoleo, 2029·4
Gomenol-Syner-Penicilline, 2029·4
Gomiliximab, 507·3
Gomme Adragante, 1582·2
Gomme Arabique, 1576·2
Gomme de Caroube, 1579·1
Gomme de Sénégal, 1576·2
Gomme Laque, 1743·3
Gon, 2029·4
Gonablok, 2029·4
Gonacor, 2029·4
Gonadoliberin, 1325·1
Gonadorelin, 1325·1
Gonadorelin Acetate, 1325·2
Gonadorelin Hydrochloride, 1325·2
Gonadorelina, 1325·1
Gonadorelina, Acetato de, 1325·2
Gonadorelina, Hidrocloruro de, 1325·2
Gonadorelinum, 1325·1
Gonadotrafon LH— *see* Gonasi HP, 2029·4
Gonadotraphon LH, 2029·4
Gonadotrofina Coriónica, 1320·3
Gonadotrophin, Chorionic, 1320·3
Gonadotrophin-releasing Hormone, 1325·1
Gonadotrophins, 1312·1
Gonadotrophins, Menopausal, Human, 1330·1
Gonadotrophinum Chorionicum, 1320·3
Gonadotropin, Chorionic, 1320·3
Gonadotropina Menopáusica Humana, 1330·1
Gonadotropinum Chorionicum, 1320·3
Gonadotropyl C, 2029·4
Gonak, 2029·4
Gonakor, 2029·4
Gonal-F, 2029·4
Gonapeptyl, 2029·4
Gonaplex, 2029·4
Gonasi HP, 2029·4
Gonasone, 2029·4
Gonaxine, 2029·4
Gondonar, 2029·4
Gongo, 1666·1
Gonic, 2029·4
Gonif, 2029·4
Gonioscopic, 2029·4
Goniosoft, 2029·4
Goniosol, 2029·4
Gonne Balm, 2029·4
Gonocilin, 2029·4
Gonococcal Infections— *see* Gonorrhoea, 130·2
Gonococcal Neonatal Conjunctivitis— *see* Neonatal Conjunctivitis, 136·3
Gonococcal Vaccines, 1616·1
Gonoform, 2029·4
Gonol, 2029·4
*Gonolobus condurango*, 1675·3
Gonorcin, 2030·1
Gonorrels, 2030·1
Gonorrhoea, 130·2
Gonorrhoea Vaccines, 1616·1
Gonotrop F, 2030·1
Goodnight, 2030·1
Goodnight Formula, 2030·1
Goodnight StopSnore, 2030·1
Goodpasture's Syndrome— *see* Glomerular Kidney Disease, 1080·2
Goodypops, 2030·1
Goody's Headache Powders, 2030·1
Goon, 1730·3
Go-On, 2030·1
Gooseberry, Cape, 1731·3
Goosegrass, 1673·2
Go-Pain, 2030·1
Go-Pain P, 2030·1
Gopten, 2030·1
Gordobalm, 2030·1
Gordochom, 2030·1
Gordofilm, 2030·1
Gordogesic, 2030·1
Gorgonium, 2030·1
Gormel, 2030·1
Goserelin, 1326·3
Goserelin Acetate, 1326·3
Goserelina, Acetato de, 1326·3
Goserelinum, 1326·3
Gosha-jinki-gan, Tsumura— *see* Tsumura Gosha-jinki-gan, 2351·1
Gosipol, 1695·3
Gossypii Oleum Hydrogenatum, 1676·1
Gossypii Seminis, Oleum, 1676·1
Gossypium Collodium, 1156·2
*Gossypium hirsutum*, 1676·2
Gossypol, 1695·3
Gota Cebrina, 2030·1
Gota Kola, 1144·3
Gotabiotic, 2030·1
Gotabiotic D, 2030·1
Gotabiotic F, 2030·1
Gotadex, 2030·1
Gotalax, 2030·1
Gotalgic, 2030·1
Gotas Binelli, 2030·1
Gotas Digestivas, 2030·2
Gotas Hepaticas, 2030·2
Gotas Nican, 2030·2
Gotas Otologicas, 2030·2
Gotas Ototilan, 2030·2
Gotas Preciosas, 2030·2
Gotas Zimaia, 2030·2
Gotavit, 2030·2
Gothaplast Capsicum-Warmepflaster, 2030·2
Gothaplast Rheumamed AC, 2030·2
Gotil-AD, 2030·2
Gotinal, 2030·2
Gotir, 2030·2
Gotu Cola, 1144·3
Gotu Kola, 1144·3, 2030·2
Goudron de Bouleau, 1159·2
Goudron de Cade, 1159·2
Goudron de Houille, 1159·2
Goudron Végétal, 1159·3
Gout— *see* Gout and Hyperuricaemia, 412·1
Goutichine, 2030·2
Goutnil, 2030·2
Gouttes aux Essences, 2030·2
Gouttes contre la Toux "S", 2030·2
Gouttes contre le Rhume des Foins, 2030·2
Gouttes Dentaires, 2030·2
Gouttes Homeopathiques contre le Rhume des Foins, 2030·2
Gouttes Nasales, 2030·2
Gouttes Nasales N, 2030·2
Gouttes pour le Coeur et les Nerfs Concentrees, 2030·2
Gouttes pour Mal d'Orreilles, 2030·2
Gouty Arthritis— *see* Gout and Hyperuricaemia, 412·1
Goval, 2030·2
Goxil, 2030·3
Gozah, 1666·1
Gozid, 2030·3
GP, 2030·3
GP-1-110, 842·2
GP-1-110-0, 842·2
GP-2-121-3, 864·2
GP-121, 1730·3
GP-45840, 32·1
GP-47680, 366·3
G6PD Deficiency— *see* Haemolytic Anaemia, 733·1
G-Press, 2030·3
GR-2/234, 1296·3
GR-2/925, 1095·2
GR-2/1214, 1095·3
GR-2/1574, 1296·3
GR-412, 1178·3
GR-20263, 180·2
GR-33343G, 795·1
GR-38032, 1281·1
GR-38032F, 1281·1
GR-43175C, 471·2
GR-43175X, 471·2
GR-43659X, 944·2
GR-68755C, 1248·3
GR-85548A, 470·1
GR-85548X, 470·1
GR-92132X, 348·2
GR-106642X, 1236·2
GR-109714X, 648·2
GR-121167X, 658·1
GR-122311X, 1287·2
Gracial, 2030·3
*Gracilaria confervoides*, 1576·3
Gradient, 2030·3
Gradin del D Andreu, 2030·3
Grafco Batonnets de Bois, 2030·3
Grafin, 2030·3
Graft-versus-host Disease— *see* Haematopoietic Stem Cell Transplantation, 1344·3
Gragenil— *see* Coduretas Gragenil, 1897·3
Grahni Sherdool, 1666·1
Graine de Moutarde Noire, 1718·2
Grains de Vals, 2030·3
Grains de Vals Nouvelle Formule, 2030·3
Graisse de Suint Purifiée, 1483·1
Gral, 2030·3
Grama, 1676·2
Gramal, 2030·3
Gramalil, 2030·3
Gramaxin, 2030·3
Gramcal, 2030·3
Gramcilina, 2030·3
Gramibiotic, 2030·3
Gramicidin, 220·2, 220·3
Gramicidin A1, 220·2
Gramicidin A2, 220·2
Gramicidin B1, 220·2
Gramicidin C1, 220·2
Gramicidin C2, 220·2
Gramicidin D, 220·2
Gramicidin (Dubos), 220·2
Gramicidin S, 220·3
Gramicidina, 220·2
Gramicidinum, 220·2
Gramicortil, 2030·3
Gramidil, 2030·3
Gramigna (Specie Composta), 2030·3
Graminflor, 2030·3
Graminis Citrati, Oleum, 1706·3
Graminis Rhizoma, 1676·2
Gramipan, 2030·3
Gramixina, 2030·3
Grammicin, 2030·3
Grammixin, 2030·3
Gramoce A, 2030·4
Gramoneg, 2030·4
Gramostim, 2030·4
Grampenil, 2030·4
Grampenil Bronquial, 2030·4
Gramplus, 2030·4
Gram-Val, 2030·4
Gran, 2030·4
Granado, 112·1
Granamon, 2030·4
Granati Cortex, 112·1
Granatrinde, 112·1
Granatum, 112·1
Grand Mal— *see* Epilepsy, 349·1
Grandaxin, 2030·4
Graneodin, 2030·4
Graneodin Expectorante, 2030·4
Graneodin N, 2030·4
Graneodin-Tos, 2030·4
Grani di Vals, 2030·4
Granicip, 2030·4
Granions, 2030·4
Granisetrón, Hidrocloruro de, 1267·1
Granisetron Hydrochloride, 1267·1
Granitron, 2030·4
Granobil, 2030·4
Granocol, 2030·4
Granocyte, 2030·4
Granoleina, 2030·4
Granon, 2030·4
Granoton, 2030·4
Grans Remedy, 2031·1
Granu Fink Kurbiskern, 2031·1
Granu Fink Kurbiskern N, 2031·1
Granu Fink Prosta, 2031·1
Granudoxy, 2031·1
Granuflex, 2031·1
Granugel, 2031·1
Granugen, 2031·1
Granulating Agents, 1576·1
Granulax, 2031·1
Granulderm, 2031·1
Granulen, 2031·1
Granules Boripharm Preparations, 2031·1
Granulex, 2031·1
Granulocyte-macrophage Colony-stimulating Factor, 756·2
Granulocytic Leukaemia, Chronic— *see* Chronic Myeloid Leukaemia, 507·3
Granulokine, 2031·1
Granuloma, Eosinophilic— *see* Histiocytic Syndromes, 505·2
Granuloma Inguinale, 131·1
Granulomatosis, Wegener's— *see* Wegener's Granulomatosis, 1090·2
Granulomatous Vasculitis— *see* Vasculitic Syndromes, 1090·1
GranuMed, 2031·1
Gran-Verm, 2031·1
Granvit, 2031·1
Grape Bark, 1117·2
Grape Sugar, 1432·2
Gras, Embrocacion— *see* Embrocacion Gras, 1967·1
Grasa Sólida, 1481·1
Grasmin, 2031·1
Grassolind Neutral, 2031·1
Graten, 2031·1
Gratusminal, 2031·1
Gravel Root, 1695·3
Gravergol, 2031·1
Graves' Disease— *see* Hyperthyroidism, 1594·3
Graves' Ophthalmopathy— *see* Hyperthyroidism, 1594·3
Gravibinan, 2031·1
Gravibinon, 2031·2
Gravidex, 2031·2
Gravidinona, 2031·2
Gravi-Fol, 2031·2
Gravigard, 2031·2
Gravigen Plus, 2031·2
Gravindex, 2031·2
Gravistat, 2031·2
Gravitamon, 2031·2
Gravitest, 2031·2
Gravitest Crual, 2031·2
Gravol, 2031·2
Grayxona, 2031·2
GRD, 2031·2
Great Mullein, 1764·1
Greatbloc, 2031·2
Greater Burnet, 1663·2
Greater Celandine, 1695·3
Greater-Gloxa, 2031·2
Greatofen, 2031·2
Greefe, 1666·1
Greek Hay, 1688·1
Greek Sage, 1741·2
Green, Aniline, 1185·2
Green Antiseptic Mouthwash & Gargle, 2031·2
Green B, Diamond, 1185·2
Green B, Wool, 1057·3
Green, Brilliant, 1171·1
Green BS, Acid Brilliant, 1057·3
Green, China, 1185·2
Green Copperas, 1428·2

Green Diet, 2031·2
Green, Emerald, 1171·1
Green, Ethyl, 1171·1
Green G, Diamond, 1171·1
Green G, Malachite, 1171·1
Green Hellebore, 1764·1
Green Hellebore Rhizome, 1764·1
Green, Indocyanine, 1701·1
Green, Lissamine, 1057·3
Green, Malachite, 1185·2
Green S, 1057·3
Green S, Acid, 1057·3
Green Soap, 1575·2
Green, Solid, 1171·1
Green Veratrum, 1764·1
Green Vitriol, 1428·2
Green-A KGCC, 2031·2
Green-lipped Mussel, 1696·1
Greenosan, 2031·2
Grefen, 2031·2
Gregoderm, 2031·2
Gregovite C, Uniflu &— *see* Uniflu & Gregovite C, 2358·4
Gregovite C, Uniflu with— *see* Uniflu with Gregovite C, 2358·4
Greini, 2031·2
Grenadier, 112·1
Grenadille, 1729·1
Grenfung, 2031·2
Grenin, 2031·2
Grenis, 2031·2
Grenis-cipro, 2031·2
Grenovix, 2031·2
Greosin, 2031·2
Grepafloxacin Hydrochloride, 220·3
Grepafloxacino, Hidrocloruro de, 220·3
Gretivit, 2031·2
G-Revm, 2031·3
Grexin, 2031·3
GRF, 1339·2
GRF(1-29)$NH_2$, 1339·2
GRF(1-40), 1339·2
GRF(1-44), 1339·2
GRF-44, 1339·2
Gricin, 2031·3
Grietalgen, 2031·3
Grietalgen Hidrocort, 2031·3
Grifa, 1666·1
Grifed, 2031·3
Grifenol, 2031·3
Griffonia Simplicifolia, 1696·1
Grifoalpram, 2031·3
Grifobutol, 2031·3
Grifociprox, 2031·3
Grifoclobam, 2031·3
Grifocriptina, 2031·3
Grifodilzem, 2031·3
Grifoftal, 2031·3
Grifoftal-D, 2031·3
Grifogemzilo, 2031·3
Grifonimod, 2031·3
Grifonitren, 2031·3
Grifoparkin, 2031·3
Grifopril, 2031·3
Grifopril-D, 2031·3
Grifotaxima, 2031·3
Grifotenol, 2031·3
Grifotriaxona, 2031·3
Grifulin, 2031·3
Grifulvin, 2031·3
Grifulvin V, 2031·3
Grilinctus, 2031·3
Grilinctus-BM, 2031·4
Grindelia, 1696·1
*Grindelia camporum*, 1696·1
*Grindelia humilis*, 1696·1
*Grindelia robusta*, 1696·1
*Grindelia squarrosa*, 1696·1
Grindocin, 2031·4
Grinevel, 2031·4
Grinflux, 2031·4
Grinsil, 2031·4
Grinsil Clavulanico, 2031·4
Grinsil Duo, 2031·4
Grinsil Respiratorio, 2031·4
Griottier, 1058·1
Gripakin, 2031·4
Gripalgine, 2031·4
Gripanil, 2031·4
Gripanil C, 2031·4
Gripasan Compuesto, 2031·4
Gripasan Nueva Formula, 2031·4
Gripavac, 2031·4
Gripcaps C, 2031·4
Gripe Mixture, 2031·4
Gripe Water, 2031·4
Gripefago C, 2031·4
Gripefin, 2031·4
Gripen, 2031·4
Gripenil, 2031·4
Gripeonil, 2031·4
Gripetral, 2031·4
Gripexin Limonada Caliente, 2032·1
Gripexin Nueva Formula Compuesto, 2032·1
Gripexin Nueva Formula C/Pseudoefedrina, 2032·1
Gripidor, 2032·1
Gripin C, 2032·1
Gripion, 2032·1
Gripionex, 2032·1
Gripol C, 2032·1
Gripol C Capuride, 2032·1
Gripol Composto, 2032·1
Gripol Composto Xarope, 2032·1
Gripomatine, 2032·1
Griponal, 2032·1
Griponia, 2032·1
Gripotermon, 2032·1
Gripotul, Natusor— *see* Natusor Gripotul, 2154·1
Gripp Heel, 2032·1
Grippal, 2032·1
Grippalgine N, 2032·1
Grippalin, 2032·1
Grippalin & C, 2032·1
Grippefloran, 2032·1
Grippe-Gastreu S R6, 2032·1
Grippetee Dr Zeidler, 2032·1
Grippetee EF-EM-ES, 2032·1
Gripp-Heel, 2032·1
Grippin-Merz, 2032·2
Grippinon, 2032·2
Grippogran, 2032·2
Grippon, 2032·2
Grippostad C, 2032·2
Grippostad Gute Nacht-Saft, 2032·2
Grippostad Heissgetrank, 2032·2
Gripps, 2032·2
Gripsay, 2032·2
Griptol, 2032·2
Grisactin, 2032·2
Grise, 2032·2
Grisefuline, 2032·2
Griseo, 2032·2
Griseocrem, 2032·2
Griseoful, 2032·2
Griseofulvin, 400·3
Griseofulvina, 400·3
Griseofulvinum, 400·3
Griseomed, 2032·2
Griseoplus, 2032·2
Griseostatin, 2032·2
Grisetin, 2032·2
Grisetin con Carnitina, 2032·2
Grisflavin, 2032·2
Grisical, 2032·2
Grisol, 2032·2
Grisomicon, 2032·2
Grisovin, 2032·2
Grisovin FP, 2032·3
Grisovina FP, 2032·3
Gris-PEG, 2032·3
Grisuvin, 2032·3
Grivin, 2032·3
Grodurex, 2032·3
Grofenac, 2032·3
Gromazol, 2032·3
Groprim, 2032·3
Grosella Negra (Casis), 1661·1
Grotanat, 2032·3
Ground Cherry, 1731·3
Ground Ivy, 1696·1
Ground-nut Oil, 1656·1
Group B Streptococcal Infection, Perinatal— *see* Perinatal Streptococcal Infections, 139·3
Grovixim, 2032·3
Growgen-GM, 2032·3
Growject, 2032·3
Growth Factor, Epidermal, 1294·2
Growth Factor, Human Epidermal, 1294·2
Growth Hormone, 1327·2
Growth Hormone Deficiency— *see* Growth Retardation, 1314·2
Growth Hormone, Human, 1327·2
Growth Hormone, Methionyl Bovine, 1327·2
Growth Hormone, Methionyl Human, 1327·2
Growth Hormone, Methionyl Porcine, 1327·2
Growth Hormone Resistance— *see* Growth Retardation, 1314·2
Growth Hormone Secretion, Excessive— *see* Acromegaly and Gigantism, 1312·1
Growth Hormone, Synthetic Bovine, 1327·2
Growth Hormone-releasing Factor (Human), 1339·2
Growth Hormone-releasing Factor (Human)-(1-29)-peptide Amide, 1339·2
Growth Hormone-releasing Hormone, 1339·2
Growth-hormone-release-inhibiting Hormone, 1339·3
Growth-hormone-releasing Peptide-6, 1339·2
Growth Retardation, 1314·2
Gruben, 2032·3
Grumivit, 2032·3
Gruncef, 2032·3
Grune Salbe "Schmidt" N, 2032·3
Grunicina, 2032·3
Grunlicht Dreierlei Tropfen, 2032·3
Grunlicht Hingfong Essenz, 2032·3
Grunlicht Magenbalsam Tropfen, 2032·3
Gruntin Tropfen, 2032·3
GS-95, 442·1
GS-0393, 628·1
GS-504, 629·2
GS-0504, 629·2
GS-0840, 628·1
GS-930, 630·1
GS-1278, 655·1
GS-2876, 230·1
GS-2989, 229·1
GS-3065, 206·2
GS-3159, 166·2
GS-4104/002, 651·1
GS-4331/05, 655·1
GS-6244, 166·1
GSH, 1040·3
G-Strophanthin, 977·3
GT31-104HB, 889·2
GT-41, 532·2
GT-92, 480·3
GT-1012, 984·3
GT16-026A, 1051·2
G-Tase, 2032·3
$G_{TIb}$, 1691·1
G.Test, 2032·3
GTN, 923·2
Guabenxan, 926·2
Guabenxan Sulfate, 926·2
Guabza, 1666·1
Guacetisal, 1121·3
Guafen, 2032·3
Guaiac, 1696·2
Guaiacalcium Complex, 2032·3
Guaiacol, 1122·1, 1159·2
*p*-Guaiacol, 1151·3
Guaiacol Carbonate, 1122·1
Guaiacol Cinnamate, 1122·1
Guaiacol Ethylglycolate, 1122·1
Guaiacol Glycerol Ether, 1122·1
Guaiacol Phenylacetate, 1122·1
Guaiacol Phenylbutyrate, 1122·1
Guaiacum, 1696·2
*Guaiacum officinale*, 1696·2
Guaiacum Resin, 1696·2
*Guaiacum sanctum*, 1696·2
Guaiacum Wood, 1696·2
Guaiacyl Glyceryl Ether, 1122·1
Guaiaspir, 2032·3
Guaiazulene, 1658·3, 1696·2
Guaietolin, 1122·1
Guaifed, 2032·4
Guaifed-PD, 2032·4
Guaifenesin, 1122·1
Guaifenesin Calcium, 1122·2
Guaifenesin DAC, 2032·4
Guaifenesin DM, 2032·4
Guaifenesin PSE, 2032·4
Guaifenesina, 1122·1
Guaifenesinum, 1122·1
Guaifenex Preparations, 2032·4
Guaimax-D, 2032·4
Guaimesal, 1122·2
Guaipax, 2032·4
Guaiphenesin, 1122·1
Guaiphenesin Carbamate, 1395·1
Guaitab, 2032·4
Guaivent, 2032·4
Guai-Vent/PSE, 2032·4
Guajabronc, 2032·4
Guajacol, 1122·1
Guajacolum Glycerolatum, 1122·1
Guajakharz, 1696·2
Guanabenz Acetate, 926·2
Guanabenzo, Acetato de, 926·2
Guanadrel Sulfate, 926·3
Guanadrel, Sulfato de, 926·3
Guanadrel Sulphate, 926·3
Guanethidine Hemisulfate, 927·1
Guanethidine Monosulfate, 926·3
Guanethidine Monosulphate, 926·3
Guanethidini Monosulfas, 926·3
Guanetidina, Monosulfato de, 926·3
Guanfacina, Hidrocloruro de, 927·2
Guanfacine Hydrochloride, 927·2
Guanidina, Hidrocloruro de, 1492·1
Guanidine Hydrochloride, 1492·1
4-Guanidino-2,4-dideoxy-2,3-dehydro-*N*-acetylneuraminic Acid, 658·1
$N^1$-4-(Guanidobutyl)bleomycinamide, 530·2
Guanilato Disódico, 1681·3
Guanor, 2032·4
Guanosine 5′-(Disodium Phosphate), 1681·3
Guanoxan Sulfate, 927·3
Guanoxan Sulphate, 927·3
Guanoxano, Sulfato de, 927·3
Guanylate Cyclase Inhibitors, 145·2
Guapi Bark, 1117·2
Guar, 333·2
Guar Flour, 333·2
Guar Galactomannan, 333·2
Guar Gum, 333·2
Guar Verlan, 2032·4
Guarana, 1765·3, 2032·4
Guaranace, 2032·4
Guaranine, 782·1, 1765·3
Guarasex, 2032·4
Guaratuaba, 2032·4
Guarcol, 2032·4
Guarem, 2032·4
Guastil, 2032·4
Guaxan, 2033·1
Guayacol, 1122·1
Guayalin-Plus, 2033·1
Guayazuleno, 1696·2
Guayetolina, 1122·1
Guaza, 1666·1
Gubamine, 2033·1
Guemusin, 2033·1
Guep'Away, 2033·1
Guethol, 1122·2
Guethol Carbonate, 1122·2
Guethol Nicotinate, 1122·2
Guethural, 2033·1
Guetol, 1122·2
Gugecin, 2033·1
Gui, 1715·3
GuiaCough CF, 2033·1
GuiaCough PE, 2033·1

Guiatex, 2033·1
Guiatex LA, 2033·1
Guiatex PSE, 2033·1
Guiatuss, 2033·1
Guiatuss CF, 2033·1
Guiatuss PE, 2033·1
Guiatussin with Codeine Expectorant, 2033·1
Guiatussin DAC, 2033·1
Guiatussin with Dextromethorphan, 2033·1
Guigoz Hypoallergenique, 2033·1
Guigoz Soja, 2033·1
Guigoz Transit, 2033·1
Guillain-Barré Syndrome, 1630·2
Guimauve, 1651·3
Guinea-worm Infection— *see* Dracunculiasis, 98·1
Gulf War Syndrome— *see* Nerve Gas Poisoning, 1496·3
L-Guluronic Acid, 1576·3
Gum Acacia, 1576·2
Gum Arabic, 1576·2
Gum Asafetida, 1658·1
Gum Benjamin, 1751·1
Gum Benzoin, 1751·1
Gum, British, 1427·1
Gum, Carob, 1579·1
Gum, Carob Bean, 1579·1
Gum, Cellulose, 1577·3
Gum, Cellulose, Modified, 1578·1
Gum, Ceratonia, 1579·1
Gum, Corn Sugar, 1582·3
Gum Dragon, 1582·2
Gum, Guar, 333·2
Gum, Jaguar, 333·2
Gum, Karaya, 1290·2
Gum, Locust Bean, 1579·1
Gum Myrrh, 1718·3
Gum Opium, 74·2
Gum Plant, 1696·1
Gum, Starch, 1427·1
Gum, Sterculia, 1290·2
Gum Tragacanth, 1582·2
Gum, Xantham, 1582·3
Gum, Xanthan, 1582·3
Gumbaral, 2033·1
Gumbix, 2033·1
Gum-Ese, 2033·1
Gumilk, 2033·1
Gummi Africanum, 1576·2
Gummi Arabicum, 1576·2
Gummi Mimosae, 1576·2
Gummi Plasticum, 1696·2
Gumweed, 1696·1
Guncotton, Soluble, 1156·2
Gunevax, 2033·1
Gunjah, 1666·1
Gunza, 1666·1
Gupisone, 2033·1
Gurfi Fibras, 2033·1
Gurfix, 2033·2
Gurgellosung Chauvin, 2033·2
Gurgellosung-ratiopharm, 2033·2
Gurgol, 2033·2
Guronsan, 2033·2
Gusperimús, Hidrocloruro de, 1360·2
Gusperimus Hydrochloride, 1360·2
Gusperimus Trihydrochloride, 1360·2
Gustase, 2033·2
Gustase Plus, 2033·2
Gutalax, 2033·2
Gutapercha, 1696·2
Gutnacht, 2033·2
Gutron, 2033·2
Gutt. Perch., 1696·2
Gutta Percha, 1696·2
Guttacor, 2033·2
Guttacor-Balsam N, 2033·2
Guttae 20 Hustentropfen N, 2033·2
Guttalax, 2033·2
Guttanotte, 2033·2
Guttaplast, 2033·2
GV-150526X, 1691·3
G-well, 2033·2
GW-433908G, 634·1
GX, 2033·2
GX-1048, 944·2
GX E, 2033·2
Gyalme, 2033·2
Gydrelle, 2033·2
Gydrelle Phyto, 2033·2
*Gymnopilus*, 1717·3
Gynaecomastia, 1546·3
Gynae-CVP, 2033·2
Gynaemine, 2033·3
Gynalpha, 2033·3
Gynamon, 2033·3
Gynasan, 2033·3
Gynaseptol, 2033·3
Gynasol, 2033·3
Gynatren, 2033·3
Gynatrol, 2033·3
Gynax-N, 2033·3
Gynazole, 2033·3
Gynebo, 2033·3
Gynecon, 2033·3
Gynecort, 2033·3
Gynecure, 2033·3
Gynefix, 2033·3
Gynegella P, 2033·3
Gynelle 375, 2033·3
Gyne-Lotremin, 2033·3
Gyne-Lotrimin, 2033·3
Gyne-Moistrin, 2033·3
Gynera, 2033·3
Gynergen Comp, 2033·3
Gynergene, 2033·3
Gynergene Cafeine, 2033·3
Gynerium, 2033·3
Gynescal, 2033·3
Gynesten-B, 2033·3
Gynestin, 2033·3
Gynestrel, 2033·4
Gyne-Sulf, 2033·4
Gyne-T, 2033·4
Gynezol, 2033·4
Gyn-Hydralin, 2033·4
Gynintim Film, 2033·4
Gynipral, 2033·4
Gyno Icaden, 2033·4
Gyno Iruxol, 2033·4
Gyno Oceral, 2033·4
Gyno Zalain, 2033·4
Gynocanesten, 2033·4
Gyno-Canesten, 2033·4
Gyno-Canestene, 2033·4
Gynocastus, 2033·4
Gynoco, 2033·4
Gyno-Daktar, 2033·4
Gyno-Daktarin, 2033·4
Gynodal, 2033·4
Gynodian Depot, 2033·4
Gynodiol, 2033·4
Gynofen 35, 2033·4
Gynoflor, 2033·4
Gyno-Flor E, 2033·4
Gynofug, 2033·4
Gyno-Fungistat, 2033·4
Gyno-Fungix, 2033·4
Gynokadin, 2034·1
Gynol, 2034·1
Gynol II, 2034·1
Gyno-Liderman, 2034·1
Gynomax, 2034·1
Gyno-Mikozal, 2034·1
Gyno-Monistat, 2034·1
Gyno-Mycel, 2034·1
Gyno-Myfungar, 2034·1
Gynomyk, 2034·1
Gyno-Mykotral, 2034·1
Gyno-Neuralgin, 2034·1
Gyno-Pevaryl, 2034·1
Gynoplix, 2034·1
Gynoplix Theraplix, 2034·1
Gynoplus, 2034·1
Gynormal, 2034·1
Gynosoja, 2034·1
Gynospasmine, 2034·1
Gynospor, 2034·1
Gynostat, 2034·1
Gynosyl, 2034·1
Gyno-Tardyferon, 2034·1
Gyno-Terazol, 2034·1
Gyno-Travogen, 2034·1
Gyno-Trimaze, 2034·1
Gyno-Trosyd, 2034·1
Gynova, 2034·1
Gynovin, 2034·2
Gynovite Plus, 2034·2
GynPolar, 2034·2
Gypsum, 1665·1
Gypsum, Calcined, 1665·1
Gypsum Siccatum, 1665·1
Gyrablock, 2034·2
Gyracon, 2034·2
Gyrol, 2034·2
*Gyromitra*, 1717·3
Gyromitrins, 1717·3
Gyrosan, 2034·2
Gy-Sol, 2034·2

**H**

H, 1434·2
H1, 2034·2
H56/28, 856·3
H73-3293, 1420·3
H-80/62, 986·3
H-93/26, 957·1
H133/22, 986·3
H-154/82, 914·3
H-168/68, 1278·2
H199/18, 1265·1
H-212/91, 878·3
H-319/68, 952·1
H-376/95, 952·1
H-610, 1588·2
H-814, 1588·2
H-990, 1126·1
H-3452, 1544·1
H-3625, 1096·2
H-4723, 358·2
H-8351, 878·2
H-8352, 1754·3
$H_2$-antagonists, 1239·3
H 2 Blocker, 2034·2
H Tussan, 2034·2
4-HA, 1151·3
HA-1077, 914·3
HA-1A, 1615·2
Haarlem, Huile de— *see* Huile de Haarlem, 2049·1
HAART, 622·2
HABA-Dibekacin, 158·3
Habas de Soja, 1447·2
Habitrol, 2034·2
Habstal-Cor N, 2034·2
Habstal-Nerv N, 2034·2
Habstal-Pulm N, 2034·2
HAC, 2034·2
Hacdil-S, 2034·2
Hachemina Fuerte, 2034·2
Hachiche, 1666·1
Hachimi-jio-gan, Tsumura— *see* Tsumura Hachimi-jio-gan, 2351·1
Hacks, 2034·2
Hacks Blackcurrant, 2034·2
Hactos, 2034·2
Hadarax, 2034·2
Hadensa, 2034·2
Hadiel, 2034·2
H-Adiftal, 2034·2
H-Adiftetal, 2034·2
Hadlinol, 2034·2
Haelan, 2034·2
Haem Arginate, 1040·3
Haem Derivatives, 1040·3
Haem Up, 2034·3
Haemaccel, 2034·3
Haemanal, 2034·3
Haemangioma, 1081·2
Haemate, 2034·3
Haemate HS, 2034·3
Haemate P, 2034·3
Haematicum Glausch, 2034·3
Haematin, 1040·3
Haematopoietic Growth Factors, 754·2
Haematopoietin-1, 1701·3
Haematoporphyrin, 1696·2
Haemin, 1040·3
Haemin Arginate, 1040·3
Haem-iron, 1435·3
Haemiton, 2034·3
Haemiton Compositum, 2034·3
Haemo Duoform, 2034·3
Haemochromatosis— *see* Iron Overload, 1035·2
Haemochromatosis— *see* β-Thalassaemia, 735·2
Haemocoagulase, 743·3
Haemocompletttan, 2034·3
Haemocompletttan-P, 2034·3
Haemocortin, 2034·3
Haemoctin SDH, 2034·3
Haemoctin SDM, 2034·3
Haemodiafiltration, 1221·3
Haemodialysis, 1221·3
Haemodialysis-induced Cramp, 1221·2
Haemodialysis-induced Cramp— *see* Muscle Spasm, 1386·1
Haemodyn, 2034·3
Haemo-Exhirud, 2034·3
Haemo-Exhirud Bufexamac, 2034·3
Haemofiltration, 1221·3
Haemofusin, 2034·3
Haemoglobin, 755·2
Haemoglobin, Crosslinked, 755·3
Haemoglobin Glutamer, 755·2
Haemoglobin-based Oxygen Carrier-201, 755·2
Haemoglobinopathies, 734·3
Haemoglukotest 20-800, 2034·3
Haemo-Glukotest 20-800, 2034·3
Haemolan, 2034·3
Haemolytic Anaemia, 733·1
Haemolytic Disease of the Newborn, 1608·2
Haemolytic-uraemic Syndrome— *see* Thrombotic Microangiopathies, 758·1
Haemomac, 2034·4
Haemophilia A— *see* Haemorrhagic Disorders, 737·3
Haemophilia B— *see* Haemorrhagic Disorders, 737·3
Haemophilia, Classical— *see* Haemorrhagic Disorders, 737·3
Haemophilus Influenzae, Diphtheria, and Tetanus Vaccines, 1613·3
Haemophilus Influenzae, Diphtheria, Tetanus, and Pertussis Vaccines, 1614·2
Haemophilus Influenzae, Diphtheria, Tetanus, Pertussis, and Poliomyelitis Vaccines, 1615·1
Haemophilus Influenzae and Hepatitis B Vaccines, 1616·3
Haemophilus Influenzae Infections, 131·1
Haemophilus Influenzae Meningitis— *see* Meningitis, 134·3
Haemophilus Influenzae and Poliomyelitis Vaccines, 1616·3
Haemophilus Influenzae Vaccines, 1616·1
Haemophilus Type B Conjugate Vaccine, 1616·1
Haemophilus Type B Conjugate Vaccine (Adsorbed), Diphtheria, Tetanus, Pertussis (Acellular, Component) and, 1614·2
Haemophilus Type B Conjugate Vaccine (Adsorbed), Diphtheria, Tetanus, Pertussis (Acellular, Component), Hepatitis B (rDNA), Poliomyelitis (Inactivated) and, 1614·3
Haemophilus Type B Conjugate Vaccine (Adsorbed), Diphtheria, Tetanus, Pertussis (Acellular, Component), Poliomyelitis (Inactivated) and, 1615·1
Haemophilus Type B Conjugate Vaccine (Adsorbed), Diphtheria, Tetanus, Pertussis, Poliomyelitis (Inactivated) and, 1615·1
Haemopressin, 2034·4
Haemoproct, 2034·4
Haemoprotect, 2034·4
Haemo-Red Formula, 2034·4
Haemorrhage, Alveolar, Diffuse— *see* Respiratory Disorders, 1087·1
Haemorrhage, Intracerebral— *see* Stroke, 836·1
Haemorrhage, Neonatal Intraventricular— *see* Neonatal Intraventricular Haemorrhage, 740·1

Haemorrhage, Periventricular— *see* Neonatal Intraventricular Haemorrhage, 740·1
Haemorrhage, Postpartum— *see* Postpartum Haemorrhage, 1684·3
Haemorrhage, Subarachnoid— *see* Stroke, 836·1
Haemorrhage, Variceal— *see* Variceal Haemorrhage, 1716·1
Haemorrhagic Colitis— *see* Escherichia Coli Enteritis, 129·1
Haemorrhagic Cystitis, 1180·2
Haemorrhagic Cystitis, Prophylaxis, 1041·3
Haemorrhagic Disease of the Newborn— *see* Vitamin K Deficiency Bleeding, 1468·2
Haemorrhagic Disorders, 737·3
Haemorrhagic Fever with Renal Syndrome Vaccines, 1617·1
Haemorrhagic Fevers, Viral— *see* Haemorrhagic Fevers, 618·2
Haemorrhagic Stroke— *see* Stroke, 836·1
Haemorrhoid Cream, 2034·4
Haemorrhoids, 1243·1
Haemosiderin, 1436·1
Haemosiderosis— *see* Iron Overload, 1035·2
Haemosol, 2034·4
Haemosolvate, 2034·4
Haemosolvex, 2034·4
Haemostasis, 735·3
Haemostatics, 732·1
Haemovex 4, 2034·4
Haemovex 8, 2034·4
Haemovital, 2034·4
Haenal, 2034·4
HAES Esteril, 2034·4
HAES, Serag- — *see* Serag-HAES, 2286·1
HAES-Rheopond, 2034·4
HAES-steril, 2034·4
HAES-sterile, 2034·4
Hafif, 2034·4
Hageman Factor, 735·3
Hagevir, 2034·4
Haimabig, 2034·4
Haimacig, 2034·4
Haima-D, 2034·4
Haimaferone, 2034·4
Haimalbumin, 2034·4
Haima-Parot, 2034·4
Haimapertus, 2034·4
Haimarab, 2034·4
Haimaserum, 2034·4
Haima-Tetanus, 2034·4
Haimaven, 2034·4
Haimazig, 2035·1
Haiprex, 2035·1
4 Hair, 2035·1
Hair Booster, 2035·1
Hair Nutrition, 2035·1
Hair & Scalp, 2035·1
Hair and Skin Formula, 2035·1
Hairclin, 2035·1
Hairgaine, 2035·1
Hairgrow, 2035·1
Hairplus, 2035·1
Hairscience, 2035·1
Hairscience Antidandruff, 2035·1
Hairscience Conditioner, 2035·1
Hairscience Shampoo, 2035·1
HairVit, 2035·1
Hairy-cell Leukaemia, 508·2
Halamid, 2035·1
Halazepam, 701·2
Halazona, 1181·2
Halazone, 1181·2
Halbmond, 2035·1
Halcicomb, 2035·1
Halciderm, 2035·1
Halciderm Combi, 2035·1
Halcinónida, 1103·2
Halcinonide, 1103·2
Halcion, 2035·1
Haldid, 2035·1
Haldol, 2035·1
Halenol, 2035·1
Haley's M-O, 2035·2
Half Betadur CR, 2035·2
Half Beta-Prograne, 2035·2
Half Capozide, 2035·2
Half Inderal, 2035·2
Half Securon, 2035·2
Half Sinemet, 2035·2
Halfan, 2035·2
Halfprin, 2035·2
Haliborange, 2035·2
Haliborange Calcium Plus Vitamin D, 2035·2
Haliborange Halibonbons, 2035·2
Haliborange High Strength Vitamin C, 2035·2
Haliborange Multivitamins, 2035·2
Halibut, 2035·2
Halibut Hidrocortisona, 2035·2
Halibut Multivit, 2035·2
Halibut-liver Oil, 1434·1
Halicar, 2035·2
Halita, 2035·2
Halitol, 2035·2
Halitol— *see* Britamox, 1853·2
Halitol Mucolitico, 2035·2
Halitran, 2035·2
Halivite, 2035·2
Halloo-Wach N, 2035·2
Halls, 2035·2
Halls Mentholyptus, 2035·3
Halls Sugar Free Mentho-Lyptus, 2035·3
Halls Zinc Defense, 2035·3
Halls-Plus Maximum Strength, 2035·3
Halo, 2035·3
Haloanisone, 698·2
Halobetasol Propionate, 1111·3
Halodin, 2035·3
Halofantrina, Hidrocloruro de, 452·2
Halofantrine Hydrochloride, 452·2
Halofantrini Hydrochloridum, 452·2
Halofed, 2035·3
Halofuginona, Hidrobromuro de, 605·3
Halofuginone Hydrobromide, 605·3
Halog, 2035·3
Halog Neomycine, 2035·3
Halog Tri, 2035·3
Halogabide, 377·2
Halogedol, 2035·3
Halogenated Hydroxyquinolines, 120·2
Halomed, 2035·3
Halometasona, 1103·3
Halometasone, 1103·3
Halometasone Monohydrate, 1103·3
Halomethasone, 1103·3
Halomycetin, 2035·3
Halon 1211, 1235·1
Haloneural, 2035·3
Halonix, 2035·3
Halo-P, 2035·3
Haloper, 2035·3
Haloperidol, 701·2
Haloperidol Decanoate, 701·3
Haloperidol, Decanoato de, 701·3
Haloperidol Lactate, 702·1
Haloperidoli Decanoas, 701·3
Haloperidolum, 701·2
Haloperil, 2035·3
Halopidol, 2035·3
Halopol, 2035·3
Haloprogin, 401·2
Haloprogina, 401·2
Halopyramine Hydrochloride, 427·3
Haloral, 2035·3
Hal-oral, 2035·3
Halotano, 1299·3
Halotestin, 2035·3
Halotex, 2035·3
Halothane, 1299·3
Halothanum, 1299·3
Halotussin, 2035·3
Halotussin-DM, 2035·3
Haloxazolam, 702·3
Haloxon, 105·2
Halozen, 2035·3
Halquinol, 220·3
Halquinols, 220·3
Halset, 2035·3
Halset Plus Dexpanthenol, 2035·4
Haltran, 2035·4
Halycitrol, 2035·4
Hamadin, 2035·4
Hamamelidis, 1696·3
Hamamelis, 1696·3
Hamamelis Complex, 2035·4
Hamamelis Compose, 2035·4
Hamamelis Leaf, 1696·3
*Hamamelis virginiana*, 1696·3
Hamamelis-Homaccord, 2035·4
Hamamilla, 2035·4
Hamasana, 2035·4
Hamatopan, 2035·4
Hamatopan F, 2035·4
Hametum, 2035·4
Hametum-N, 2035·4
HAMFL, 2035·4
Hamilton Preparations, 2035·4
Hamitan, 2036·1
Hamoagil Plus, 2036·1
Hamo-Europuran N, 2036·1
Hamofiltrasol, 2036·1
Hamo-ratiopharm, 2036·1
Hamo-ratiopharm N, 2036·1
Hamorrhoidal-Zapfchen, 2036·1
Hamos N, 2036·1
Hamos-Tropfen-S, 2036·1
Hamovannad, 2036·1
Hamo-Vibolex, 2036·1
Hamoxillin, 2036·1
Hamp, 1666·1
Hand Cream with Sunscreen, 2036·1
Handexin, 2036·1
Hand-Schüller-Christian Disease— *see* Histiocytic Syndromes, 505·2
Hanfkraut, 1666·1
Hanotoxin N, 2036·1
Hanp, 2036·1
Hansamed Spray, 2036·2
Hansaplast Antimicotico, 2036·2
Hansaplast Descongestionante, 2036·2
Hansaplast Footcare, 2036·2
Hansaplast Herbal Heat Plaster, 2036·2
Hansaplast Hornhaut-Pflaster, 2036·2
Hansaplast Huhneraugen-Pflaster, 2036·2
Hansaplast Spruhpflaster, 2036·2
Hansen's Disease— *see* Leprosy, 133·1
Hansepran, 2036·2
Hantavirus Pulmonary Syndrome, 618·3
Hantina, 2036·2
Haouzi, 1666·1
HAPA-B, 222·2
Hapilux, 2036·2
Happinose, 2036·2
Hard Fat, 1481·1
Hard Paraffin, 1479·1
Hard Soap, 1575·2
Hardhack, 1749·3
Haricon, 2036·2
Haridol, 2036·2
Harmalina, 1696·3
Harmaline, 1696·3
Harmina, 1696·3
Harmine, 1696·3
Harmogen, 2036·2
Harmomed, 2036·2
Harmonet, 2036·2
Harmonette, 2036·2
Harmonise, 2036·2
Harmosin, 2036·2
Harnal, 2036·2
Harnsauretropfen F, 2036·2
Harnsauretropfen N, 2036·2
Harntee 400, 2036·2
Harntee 450, 2036·2
Harntee STADA, 2036·2
Harntee-Steiner, 2036·3
Harongan, 2036·3
Harpadol, 2036·3
Harpagin, 2036·3
Harpagocid, 2036·3
Harpagofito Orto, 2036·3
Harpagoforte Asmedic, 2036·3
HarpagoMega, 2036·3
Harpagophyti Radix, 28·2
Harpagophyton, 28·2
Harpagophytum, 28·2
Harpagophytum Complex, 2036·3
Harpagophytum Procumbens, 28·2
*Harpagophytum procumbens*, 28·2
*Harpagophytum zeyheri*, 28·2
Harpagoside, 28·2
Harpagosinol, Natusor— *see* Natusor Harpagosinol, 2154·1
Harringtonine, 558·3
Hart, 2036·3
Hartfett, 1481·1
Hartiosen, 2036·3
Hartmannsche, 2036·3
Hartparaffin, 1479·1
Hartshorn and Oil, 1654·1
Hartsorb, 2036·3
Harzer Hustenelixier, 2036·3
Harzer Hustenloser, 2036·3
Harzol, 2036·3
Hascisc, 1666·1
Hashimoto's Thyroiditis— *see* Hypothyroidism, 1595·3
Hashish, 1666·1
Hasis, 1666·1
Hasji's, 1666·1
Hasjisj, 1666·1
Hassapirin Puro, 2036·3
Haszysz, 1666·1
HA-Tabletten N, 2036·3
H-Atetal, 2036·3
Hauhechelwurzel, 1723·3
Hautfunktionstropfen S, 2036·3
Hautplus N Dr Hagedorn, 2036·3
Haut-Vital N, 2036·3
Havlane, 2036·3
Havpur, 2036·3
Havrix, 2036·3
Haw, 1677·1
Hawaiian Tropic Preparations, 2036·3
Hawkmide, 2037·1
Hawkperan, 2037·1
Hawthorn Berries, 1677·1
Hawthorn, English, 1677·1
Hawthorn Leaf and Flower, 1677·1
Hawthorn Leaf with Flower, 1677·1
Haxixe, 1666·1
Hay Fever, 2037·1
Hay Fever— *see* Rhinitis, 422·3
Hay Fever Relief, 2037·1
Hay Fever & Sinus Relief, 2037·1
Hayclear, 2037·1
Hay-Crom, 2037·1
Hayfebrol, 2037·1
Hayfever & Allergy Relief, 2037·1
Hayfever Eye Drops, 2037·1
Hayfever Relief, 2037·1
Hayfever & Sinus Relief, 2037·1
Hayfever Sinus Relief, Chemists Own— *see* Chemists Own Hayfever Sinus Relief, 1882·1
Hayleve, 2037·1
Haymine, 2037·1
Hazelwort, 1658·1
HB-419, 331·2
HB Vac, 2037·1
HBF-386, 545·1
H-BIG, 2037·1
HbOC, 1616·2
HBOC-201, 755·2
HBOC-301, 755·3
H-B-Vax, 2037·1
H-B-Vax II, 2037·1
H-B-Vax, Gen— *see* Gen H-B-Vax, 2020·1
HB-Vax-DNA, 2037·2
HBVaxPro, 2037·2
HBW-023, 945·2
H-C, 2037·2
Hc45, 2037·2
HC-803, 1268·2
HC-1528, 603·2
HC-20511, 788·1
HC Bidex, 2037·2
HC Derma-Pax, 2037·2

HCB, 1506·1
HCFCs, 1236·1
HCFU, 535·1
HCG, 1320·3
HCH, 1506·3
HCOR, 1103·3
HCT, 2037·2
HCT-Beta, 2037·2
HCT-ISIS, 2037·2
HD, 2037·2
HD 85, 2037·2
HD 200 Plus, 2037·2
HDCV, 2037·2
HDPC, 573·2
HE-69, 1360·3
4Head, 2037·2
Head Cold Relief, 2037·2
Head Lice— *see* Pediculosis, 1499·1
Head and Neck Cancer— *see* Malignant Neoplasms of the Head and Neck, 517·3
Head & Shoulders, 2037·2
Head & Shoulders Intensive Treatment, 2037·2
Headache, 6·2
Headache, Analgesic-induced— *see* Analgesic-induced Headache, 464·1
Headache, Chronic Daily— *see* Analgesic-induced Headache, 464·1
Headache, Cluster— *see* Cluster Headache, 464·1
Headache, Combination— *see* Tension-type Headache, 465·1
Headache Complex, 2037·2
Headache, Episodic Tension-type— *see* Tension-type Headache, 465·1
Headache, Hylands— *see* Hylands Headache, 2052·3
Headache & Migraine, 2037·2
Headache, Mixed— *see* Tension-type Headache, 465·1
Headache, Muscle-contraction— *see* Tension-type Headache, 465·1
Headache, Post-dural Puncture— *see* Post-dural Puncture Headache, 1368·1
Headache, Rebound— *see* Analgesic-induced Headache, 464·1
Headache Relief, 2037·2
Headache Tablets, 2037·2
Headache, Tension-type— *see* Tension-type Headache, 465·1
Headgen, 2037·2
Headmaster, 2037·2
Headrin Extra Strength, 2037·2
Heads Shampoo, 2037·2
Headway, 2037·2
Heaf Test, 1759·1
Heafusine, 2037·2
Heal Aid Plus, 2037·2
Heal-all, 1749·3
Healex, 2037·2
Healing Cream, 2037·2
Healon, 2037·2
Healon Yellow, 2037·3
Healonid, 2037·3
HealthAid AquaFall— *see* HealthAid Boldo-Plus, 2037·3
HealthAid Boldo-Plus, 2037·3
HealthAid FemmeVit PMS Formula, 2037·3
Healtheries Musseltone, 2037·3
Healtheries Musseltone & Glucosamine, 2037·3
Healthy Feet, 2037·3
Heart Attack— *see* Myocardial Infarction, 828·2
Heart Disease, Coronary— *see* Atherosclerosis, 815·2
Heart Disease, Ischaemic— *see* Atherosclerosis, 815·2
Heart Disease, Rheumatic— *see* Rheumatic Fever, 144·2
Heart Failure, 820·3
Heart Transplantation, 1345·2
Heart Valves, Prosthetic— *see* Valvular Heart Disease, 838·2
Heartburn & Indigestion Liquid, 2037·3
Heartburn Relief, 2037·3
Heat Cream, 2037·3
Heat Rub, 2037·3
Heat Stroke— *see* Fever and Hyperthermia, 8·2
Heath & Heather Becalm, 2037·3
Heath & Heather Inner Fresh Tablets, 2037·3
Heath & Heather Quiet Night, 2037·3
Heath & Heather Skin Tablets, 2037·3
Heath & Heather Water Relief Tablets, 2037·3
Heavy Bismuth Nitrate, 1252·2
Heavy Kaolin, 1268·3
Heavy Liquid Petrolatum, 1479·1
Heavy Metals, Poisoning, 1050·1
Hebagam IM, 2037·3
Heberbiovac HB, 2037·3
Hebermin, 2037·3
Hebert Caramelos, 2037·3
Hebrin, 2037·3
Hebsbulin-IH, 2037·3
Hebucol, 2037·3
HEC, 2037·3
HECL, 1233·3, 1579·2
Heclivir, 2037·4
Hecrosine B12, 2037·4
Hectonona, 2037·4
Hectorol, 2037·4
Hedazol, 2037·4
Hedelix, 2037·4
Hederix, 2037·4
Hedex, 2037·4
Hedex Extra, 2037·4
Hedex Ibuprofen, 2037·4
Hedonin, 2037·4
Heduline, 2037·4
Heelbalm, Vesagex— *see* Vesagex Heelbalm, 2373·4
Heemex, 2037·4
Heer-More, 2037·4
Heet, 2037·4
Hefaclor, 2037·4
Hefasolon, 2037·4
Hegon, 2037·4
Hegor, 2037·4
Hegor Antipoux, 2037·4
Hegor Climbazole, 2037·4
Hegrimarin, 2037·4
Heidelbeere, 1718·3
Heidi, 2037·4
Heilbuttleberöl, 1434·1
Heilerde, Luvos— *see* Luvos Heilerde, 2108·3
Heilit, 2037·4
Heilit Rheuma-Olbad, 2037·4
Heitrin, 2037·4
Hekabetol, 2037·4
Hekbilin Kapseln, 2037·4
Heksavit, 2038·1
Helago-Pflege-Oel, 2038·1
Helarium, 2038·1
Helastop, 2038·1
Helberina, 2038·1
Helcon, 2038·1
Helecho Macho, 108·2
Heleniene, 1765·3
Helenil, 2038·1
Helenin, 1119·3
Helenio, 1119·3
Helfergin, 2038·1
Helianthi Annui Oleum, 1451·1
Helianthi Annui Oleum Raffinatum, 1451·1
Helianthi, Oleum, 1451·1
*Helianthus annuus*, 1451·1
Helianthus Comp, 2038·1
*Helianthus tuberosus*, 1702·1
Helicidina, 1122·2
Helicidine, 1122·2
Heliclar, 2038·1
Heliclear, 2038·1
Helicobacter Pylori Infection— *see* Peptic Ulcer Disease, 1246·3
Helicobacter Pylori Vaccines, 1617·1
Helicocin, 2038·1
Helicodid, 2038·1
Helicokit, 2038·1
Helicopac, 2038·1
Helicosec, 2038·1
Helicosol— *see* Ez-HBT, 1987·1
Helicostad, 2038·1
Helidac, 2038·1
Helifenicol, 2038·1
Heli-Kit, 2038·1
Heliklar, 2038·1
HeliMet, 2038·1
Helimox, 2038·1
Helio, 1236·1
Helioban, 2038·1
Heliobloc, 2038·1
Heliobloc Fort, 2038·1
Helioblock, 2038·2
Heliofilm, 2038·2
Heliopar, 2038·2
Helios, Colirio— *see* Colirio Helios, 1899·4
Heliotropin, 1509·1
Heliox, 1236·1
Helipak A, 2038·2
Helipak K, 2038·2
Helipak T, 2038·2
Heliphenicol, 2038·2
Heliplant, 2038·2
Helipur, 2038·2
Helipur H Plus, 2038·2
Helipur H Plus N, 2038·2
Helirad, 2038·2
Helis, 2038·2
Helisal, 2038·2
Heli-Sal, 2038·2
Heliton, 2038·2
Helium, 1236·1
Helix I, 2038·2
Helixate, 2038·2
Helixinum, 1122·2
Helixor, 2038·2
Helixor A— *see* Helixor, 2038·2
Helixor M— *see* Helixor, 2038·2
Helixor P— *see* Helixor, 2038·2
Hellebore, American, 1764·1
Hellebore, European, 1764·1
Hellebore, False, 1648·1
Hellebore, Green, 1764·1
Hellebore Rhizome, Green, 1764·1
Hellebore Rhizome, White, 1764·1
Hellebore White, 1764·1
Helmazan, 2038·2
Helmex, 2038·3
Helmib, 2038·3
Helmiben, 2038·3
Helmicin, 2038·3
Helmidrax, 2038·3
Helmifar, 2038·3
Helmine, 2038·3
Helmintal, 2038·3
Helmintox, 2038·3
Helminzole, 2038·3
Helmi-Ped, 2038·3
Helmisons, 2038·3
Helmizil, 2038·3
Helmizol, 2038·3
Helo-acid, 2038·3
Helonias, 1696·3
Helonias Compound, Gerard House— *see* Gerard House Helonias Compound, 2022·1
*Helonias dioica*, 1696·3
Helopanflat, 2038·3
Helopanflat N, 2038·3
Helopanzym, 2038·3
Helopyrin, 2038·3
Heloua, 1666·1
Helpin, 2038·3
Helporigin, 2038·3
Helposol, 2038·3
Helpp, 2038·3
Helvamox, 2038·3
Helvecin, 2038·3
Helvedoclyn, 2038·3
Helvedstensstifter, 2038·3
Helvegeron, 2038·3
Helvemycin, 2038·3
Helveprim, 2038·3
Helver Sal, 2038·4
Helvevir, 2038·4
Hem Anth, 2038·4
Hem Fe, 2038·4
Hemabate, 2038·4
Hema-Chek, 2038·4
Hema-Combistix, 2038·4
Hemafer, 2038·4
Hemafer Fol, 2038·4
Hemagene Tailleur, 2038·4
Hemamina, 2038·4
Hemarate, 2038·4
Hemarexin, 2038·4
Hemaspan, 2038·4
Hemastix, 2038·4
Hematest, 2038·4
Hematiase B12, 2038·4
Hematin, 1040·3
Hematinic, 2038·4
Hematinic Plus, 2038·4
Hematiron, 2038·4
Hematon, 2038·4
Hematone, 2038·4
Hematoporfirina, 1696·2
Hematrine, 2038·4
Hemax, 2039·1
Hemax-Eritron, 2039·1
HEMC, 1579·2
Hemcort HC, 2039·1
Heme Arginate, 1040·3
Heme Derivatives, 1040·3
Hemedonine, 2039·1
Hemeran, 2039·1
Hemerven, 2039·1
HemeSelect, 2039·1
Hemestal, 2039·1
Hemetiken, 2039·1
Hemiballism— *see* Ballism, 664·1
Hemibe, 2039·1
Hemicellulase, 1669·1
Hemicraneal, 2039·1
Hemi-Daonil, 2039·1
Hemifacial Spasm, 1390·3
Hemigoxine Nativelle, 2039·1
Hemin, 1040·3
Hemineurin, 2039·1
Heminevrin, 2039·1
Hemiphos, 2039·1
Hemipralon, 2039·1
Hemisulfato de Proflavina, 1165·3
Hemo, 2039·1
Hemo 141, 2039·1
Hemo, Derivados Del Grupo, 1040·3
Hemo Derminiol, 2039·1
Hemoaenus, 2039·1
Hemoal, 2039·1
Hemobion, 2039·1
Hemocalcin, 2039·1
Hemocane, 2039·2
Hemoccult, 2039·2
Hemoce, 2039·2
Hemocheck, 2039·2
Hemocid, 2039·2
Hemoclar, 2039·2
Hemocoagulase, 743·3
Hemocol, 2039·2
Hemocromo, 2039·2
Hemocyte, 2039·2
Hemocyte Plus, 2039·2
Hemocyte-F, 2039·2
Hemocyte-V, 2039·2
Hemo-Cyto-Serum, 2039·2
Hemodex, 2039·2
Hemodotti, 2039·2
Hemodren Compuesto, 2039·2
Hemodren Simple, 2039·2
Hemofactor, Bioglan— *see* Bioglan Hemofactor, 1844·1
Hemofactor HT, 2039·2
Hemofer, 2039·2
Hemoferrol, 2039·2
Hemofibrine Spugna, 2039·2
Hemofil, 2039·2
Hemofil HT, 2039·2
Hemofil M, 2039·2
Hemofiltracion E2, 2039·3
Hemofiltracion E3— *see* Hemofiltracion E2 and E3, 2039·3

Hemofiltracion E4, 2039·3
Hemofiltracion E5— *see* Hemofiltracion E4 and E5, 2039·3
Hemofiltracion HF 01, 2039·3
Hemofiltracion HF 02, 2039·3
Hemofiltracion HF 11, 2039·3
Hemofiltracion HF 23— *see* Hemofiltracion HF 11 and HF 23, 2039·3
Hemofiltrasol, 2039·3
Hemofiltrationslosning 401, 2039·3
Hemofissural, 2039·3
Hemofluss, 2039·3
Hemogenin, 2039·3
Hemoglobin Glutamer, 755·2
Hemoglobin Glutamer-200 (Bovine), 755·3
Hemoglobin Glutamer-250 (Bovine), 755·2
Hemoglobina, 755·2
Hemohes, 2039·3
Hemo-Ice, 2039·3
Hemolax, 2039·3
Hemoleven, 2039·3
Hemoluol, 2039·3
Hemon, 2039·3
Hemonet, 2039·3
Hemo-Ped, 2039·3
Hemoplex, 2039·3
Hemoray, 2039·3
Hemorhin, 2039·3
Hemorid, 2039·3
Hemorid For Women, 2039·3
Hemorrane, 2039·4
Hemorrhoid Ointment, 2039·4
Hemorrhoids, Hylands— *see* Hylands Hemorrhoids, 2052·3
Hemorrogel, 2039·4
Hemorroidex, 2039·4
Hemorrol, 2039·4
Hemosan, 2039·4
Hemosedan, 2039·4
Hemoset A, 2039·4
Hemoset A Glucos, 2039·4
Hemosin-K, 2039·4
Hemosol B0, 2039·4
Hemosol Bicar, 2039·4
Hemo-Somaton, 2039·4
Hemo-Somaton with Vitamin C, 2039·4
Hemostatico Antisep Asen, 2039·4
Hemotene, 2039·4
Hemototal, 2039·4
Hemovas, 2039·4
Hemovasal, 2039·4
Hemovirtu's, 2039·4
Hemovirtu's Pomada, 2039·4
Hemovit, 2039·4
Hemp, Indian, 1666·1
Hem-Prep, 2039·4
Hemril, 2039·4
Hemril-HC, 2039·4
Hemsi, 2040·1
Hemsyl, 2040·1
Henbane, 485·2
10-Hendecenoic Acid, 410·3
Heneicosapentaenoic Acid, 976·2
Henetix, 2040·1
Henexal, 2040·1
Henna, 1696·3
Henna Leaf, 1696·3
Hen-Nab, 1666·1
Henoch-Schönlein Purpura— *see* Hypersensitivity Vasculitis, 1081·3
Henofin, 2040·1
HEOD, 1503·3
Hep A/Vac, 1617·1
Hep B/Vac, 1618·1
Hep Lok, 2040·1
Hepa, 2040·1
Hepa Factor, 2040·1
Hepabene, 2040·1
Hepabig, 2040·1
Hepabil, 2040·1
Hepabionta, 2040·1
Hepabuzone, 2040·1
Hepacal, 2040·1
Hepacalmina, 2040·1
Hepacap, 2040·1
Hepaccine-B, 2040·1
Hepachofril, 2040·1
Hepachofril Solution, 2040·1
Hepacholan, 2040·1
Hepacholine, 2040·1
Hepacitol, 2040·1
Hepacitron, 2040·1
Hepaclem, 2040·1
Hepacoban B12, 2040·1
Hepacomplet B12 Triple, 2040·1
Hepactiv, 2040·1
Hepacur, 2040·1
Hepadial, 2040·1
Hepadif, 2040·1
Hepadigenor, 2040·2
Hepadoddi, 2040·2
Hepaduran V, 2040·2
Hepa-Factor, 2040·2
Hepaflex, 2040·2
Hepafol-F, 2040·2
Hepagallin N, 2040·2
Hepa-Gastreu S R7, 2040·2
Hepa-Gel, 2040·2
HepaGel, 2040·2
Hepagrisevit Forte-N, 2040·2
Hepagrume, 2040·2
Hepal, 2040·2
Hepa-L 90 N, 2040·2
Hepalac, 2040·2
Hepalean, 2040·2
Hepalean-Lok, 2040·2
Hepalin, 2040·2
Hepalipon N, 2040·2
Hepa-Loges, 2040·2
Hepa-Merz, 2040·2
Hepa-Merz KT, 2040·2
Hepa-Merz Lact, 2040·2
Hepa-Merz Sil, 2040·2
Hepamig, 2040·2
Hepanephrol, 2040·2
Hepanisan, 2040·2
Hepanutrin, 2040·3
Hepaplus, 2040·3
Hepar 10%, 2040·3
Hepar HM, 2040·3
Hepar 202 N, 2040·3
Hepar Pasc Mono, 2040·3
Hepar SL, 2040·3
Hepar Sulfuris, 1158·3
Hepar Sulph., 1158·3
Hepar Sulphuris, 1158·3
Heparan Sulfate, 1009·1
Heparan Sulfate Sodium, 1009·1
Heparan Sulphate, 1009·1
Heparano N, 2040·3
Heparegen, 2040·3
Heparexine, 2040·3
Hepargitol, 2040·3
Hepar-Hevert, 2040·3
Heparin, 927·3
Heparin Calcium, 927·3
Heparin Cofactor, 742·2
Heparin Cofactor I, 742·2
Heparin Comp, 2040·3
Heparin Kombi-Gel, 2040·3
Heparin Plus, 2040·3
Heparin Sodium, 928·1
Heparin, Standard, 927·3
Heparin, Unfractionated, 927·3
Heparin Whole Blood, 744·1
Heparina, 927·3
Heparina Cálcica, 927·3
Heparina Massae Molecularis Minoris, 949·2
Heparina Sódica, 928·1
Heparinas de Bajo Peso Molecular, 949·2
Heparinoides, 931·1
Heparinoids, 810·2, 931·1
Heparinol, 2040·3
Heparins, Low-molecular Mass, 949·2
Heparinum, 927·3
Heparinum Calcicum, 927·3
Heparinum Natricum, 928·1
Heparitin Sulfate, 1009·1
Heparmin, 2040·3
Heparon, 2040·3
Heparos, 2040·3
Hepar-Pasc, 2040·3
Hepar-Pasc Duo, 2040·3
Hepar-Pasc N, 2040·3
Hepar-POS, 2040·3
Heparstad, 2040·3
Heparsyx N, 2040·3
Heparth, 2040·3
Hepa-S, 2040·3
Hepa-Salbe, 2040·3
Hepasedan, 2040·3
Hepasil Composto, 2040·3
Hepasol, 2040·3
Hepasules, 2040·4
Hepasulfol, 2040·4
Hepasulfol-AA, 2040·4
Hepatalgina, 2040·4
Hepatamine, 2040·4
Hepatect, 2040·4
Hepathromb, 2040·4
Hepathrombin, 2040·4
Hepathrombine, 2040·4
Hepatic Amoebiasis— *see* Amoebiasis, 595·2
Hepatic Cancer— *see* Malignant Neoplasms of the Liver, 518·3
Hepatic Encephalopathy, 1243·2
Hepatic-Aid, 2040·4
Hepatic-Aid II, 2040·4
Hepaticum Novo, 2040·4
Hepaticum-Lac-Medice, 2040·4
Hepaticum-Medice H, 2040·4
Hepatilon, 2040·4
Hepationina, 2040·4
Hepatitis, 618·3
Hepatitis A and B Vaccines, 1620·1
Hepatitis A Immunoglobulin, Human, 1617·1
Hepatitis A Immunoglobulins, 1617·1
Hepatitis A (Inactivated) and Hepatitis B (rDNA) Vaccine (Adsorbed), 1620·1
Hepatitis A and Typhoid Vaccines, 1620·1
Hepatitis A Vaccine, Inactivated, 1617·1
Hepatitis A Vaccine (Inactivated, Adsorbed), 1617·1
Hepatitis A Vaccine (Inactivated, Virosome), 1617·1
Hepatitis A Vaccines, 1617·1
Hepatitis, Auto-immune— *see* Chronic Active Hepatitis, 1078·1
Hepatitis B and Haemophilus Influenzae Vaccines, 1616·3
Hepatitis B Immune Globulin, 1617·3
Hepatitis B Immunoglobulin, Human, 1617·2
Hepatitis B Immunoglobulin for Intravenous Administration, Human, 1617·3
Hepatitis B Immunoglobulins, 1617·2
Hepatitis B (rDNA), Poliomyelitis (Inactivated) and Haemophilus Type B Conjugate Vaccine (Adsorbed), Diphtheria, Tetanus, Pertussis (Acellular, Component), 1614·3
Hepatitis B (rDNA) Vaccine (Adsorbed), Diphtheria, Tetanus, and, 1613·3
Hepatitis B (rDNA) Vaccine (Adsorbed), Diphtheria, Tetanus, Pertussis (Acellular, Component) and, 1614·3
Hepatitis B (rDNA) Vaccine (Adsorbed), Hepatitis A (Inactivated) and, 1620·1
Hepatitis B Vaccine (rDNA), 1618·1
Hepatitis B Vaccines, 1618·1
Hepatitis B Virus Vaccine Inactivated, 1618·1
Hepatitis, Chronic Active— *see* Chronic Active Hepatitis, 1078·1
Hepatitis Infection, Disinfection Procedures— *see* Disinfection in Hepatitis and HIV Infection, 1165·1
Hepatitis, Viral— *see* Hepatitis, 618·3
Hepativax, 2040·4
Hepato Diet, 2040·4
Hepato Fardi, 2040·4
Hepatobe, 2040·4
Hepatobyl, 2040·4
Hepatocatalase, 1668·3
Hepatocellular Carcinoma— *see* Malignant Neoplasms of the Liver, 518·3
Hepatocler, 2040·4
Hepatodirectol, 2040·4
Hepatodoron, 2040·4
Hepato-Drainol, 2040·4
Hepatofalk, 2041·1
Hepatofalk Neu, 2041·1
Hepatofalk Planta, 2041·1
Hepatofalk Planta N, 2041·1
Hepato-Flux, 2041·1
Hepatogenol, 2041·1
Hepatoglobine, 2041·1
Hepatolenticular Degeneration— *see* Wilson's Disease, 1049·3
Hepatophil, 2041·1
Hepatoregius, 2041·1
Hepatorell, 2041·1
Hepatorell H Leber-Spezifikum, 2041·1
Hepatos, 2041·1
Hepatos B12, 2041·1
Hepatotal Family, 2041·1
Hepatotris, 2041·1
Hepatoum, 2041·1
Hepatoxane, 2041·1
Hepatron C, 2041·1
Hepatyrix, 2041·2
Hepavax-Gene, 2041·2
Hepavesical, Natusor— *see* Natusor Hepavesical, 2154·1
Hepa-Vibolex, 2041·2
Hepavirmo, 2041·2
Hepavit, 2041·2
Hepavite, 2041·2
Hepavitose, 2041·2
Hepax, 2041·2
Hep-Flush, 2041·2
Hepflush, 2041·2
Hep-Forte, 2041·2
Hepirax, 2041·2
Heplant, 2041·2
Hep-Lock, 2041·2
Heplok, 2041·2
Hepofilina, 2041·2
Heprecomb, 2041·2
Hep-Rinse, 2041·2
Hepro, 2041·2
Hepsal, 2041·2
Hepsera, 2041·2
Heptachlor, 1506·1
1,4,5,6,7,8,8-Heptachloro-3a,4,7,7a-tetrahydro-4,7-methanoindene, 1506·1
Heptacloro, 1506·1
Heptadon, 2041·2
Heptafluoropropane, 1236·2
1,1,1,2,3,3,3-Heptafluoropropane, 1236·2
Heptalac, 2041·2
Heptaminol, 1697·1
Heptaminol, Acefilinato de, 786·3
Heptaminol Acefyllinate, 786·3
Heptaminol Acephyllinate, 786·3
Heptaminol Adenosine Phosphate, 1697·1
Heptaminol, Hidrocloruro de, 1697·1
Heptaminol Hydrochloride, 1697·1
Heptaminol Theophylline Ethanoate, 786·3
Heptaminol Theophylline-7-acetate, 786·3
Heptaminoli Hydrochloridum, 1697·1
Hept-A-Myl, 2041·2
Heptan, 2041·2
Heptane, 1476·3
Heptane-1,7-dicarboxylic Acid, 1142·3
Heptar, 2041·2
Heptenofós, 1506·1
Heptenophos, 1506·1
Heptovir, 2041·3
Heptylon, 2041·3
Hepuman, 2041·3
Hepuman B, 2041·3
Her, 1373·3
HER-2 Monoclonal Antibody, 589·3
Heracillin, 2041·3
Heracline, 2041·3
Heractrin, 2041·3
Heralvent, 2041·3
Herb and Honey Cough Elixir, 2041·3
Herba Adonidis, 1648·1
Herba Bursae Pastoris, 1744·1
Herba Centellae, 1144·3
Herba Columbariae, 1764·1
Herba Equiseti, 1684·1

Herba Fumariae, 1690·1
Herba Herniariae, 1697·1
Herba Lactucae Virosae, 1765·2
Herba Lippiae Citriodorae, 1706·3
Herba Marrubii, 1124·1
Herba Rorellae, 1683·1
Herba Rumicis Acetosae, 1749·1
Herba Scutellariae Barbatae, 1746·3
Herba Verbenae, 1764·1
Herba Verbenae Odoratae, 1706·3
Herba Virgaureae, 1748·3
Herbaccion Preparations, 2041·3
Herbadon, 2041·3
Herbagola, 2041·3
Herbagyn, 2041·3
Herbal, 2041·3
Herbal Anxiety Formula, 2041·3
Herbal Arthritis Formula, 2041·3
Herbal Booster, 2041·4
Herbal Capillary Care, 2041·4
Herbal Cleanse, 2041·4
Herbal Cold & Flu Relief, 2041·4
Herbal Cold Relief, 2041·4
Herbal Cough Expectorant, 2041·4
Herbal Digestive Formula, 2041·4
Herbal Diuretic Formula, 2041·4
Herbal Essence Anti-Dandruff, 2041·4
Herbal Expectorant, 2041·4
Herbal Eye Care Formula, 2041·4
Herbal Headache Relief, 2041·4
Herbal Indigestion Naturtabs, 2041·4
Herbal Laxative, 2041·4
Herbal Laxative, Jacksons— *see* Jacksons Herbal Laxative, 2070·2
Herbal Liver Formula, 2041·4
Herbal Nerve, 2041·4
Herbal Pain Relief, 2041·4
Herbal PMS Formula, 2041·4
Herbal Premens, 2041·4
Herbal Sleep Aid, 2041·4
Herbal Sleep Formula, 2041·4
Herbal Stress Relief, 2041·4
Herbal Support for Active Lifestyles, 2041·4
Herbal Support for Men Over 45, 2041·4
Herbal Support for Stressful Lifestyles, 2041·4
Herbal Support for Women Over 45, 2042·1
Herbal Throat, 2042·1
Herb-a-Lax, 2042·1
Herbalax, 2042·1
Herbalax Forte, 2042·1
Herbalene, Lustys— *see* Lustys Herbalene, 2108·2
HerbAllerg, 2042·1
Herbaneurin, 2042·1
Herbapharm Rical, 2042·1
Herbatar, 2042·1
Herbatar Plus, 2042·1
Herbatorment, 2042·1
Herbavit, 2042·1
Herbe, 2042·1
Herbelax, 2042·1
Herbelix, 2042·1
Herbesan, 2042·1
Herbesan Instantane, 2042·1
Herbesser, 2042·1
Herb-Fibe, 2042·1
Herbheal Ointment, 2042·1
Herbicides, 1499·1
Herbogesic, 2042·1
Herbolax, 2042·1
Herbopyrine, 2042·1
Herborex, 2042·1
Herbulax, 2042·1
Herceptin, 2042·1
Herden, 2042·2
Hereditary Angioedema, 761·3
Hereditary Angioneurotic Oedema— *see* Hereditary Angioedema, 761·3
Herisan, 2042·2
Herivyl, 2042·2
Herklin, 2042·2
Hermal, 2042·2
Hermalind, 2042·2
Hermes ASS, 2042·2
Hermes ASS Plus, 2042·2
Hermes Cevitt, 2042·2
Hermes Cevitt + Calcium, 2042·2
Hermes Drix Abfuhr-Tee, 2042·2
Hermin, 2042·2
Hermixsofex, 2042·2
Hermocil, 2042·2
Hermodotti, 2042·2
Hermolepsin, 2042·2
Herniaria, 1697·1
*Herniaria glabra*, 1697·1
*Herniaria hirsuta*, 1697·1
Herniariae, Herba, 1697·1
Herniary, 1697·1
Herniated Disc— *see* Low Back Pain, 7·1
Hernia-Tee, 2042·2
Hernidisc, 2042·2
Herniol, 2042·2
Heroid, 2042·2
Heroin Hydrochloride, 30·2
Heroin, Synthetic, 40·3
Herolan Aerosol, 2042·2
Herpecin-L, 2042·2
Herpenon, 2042·2
Herpes B Virus Infection— *see* Herpesvirus Simiae Infections, 621·1
Herpes Encephalitis— *see* Herpes Simplex Infections, 620·2
Herpes, Genital— *see* Herpes Simplex Infections, 620·2
Herpes Labialis— *see* Herpes Simplex Infections, 620·2
Herpes, Ocular— *see* Herpes Simplex Infections, 620·2
Herpes Simiae Infection— *see* Herpesvirus Simiae Infections, 621·1
Herpes Simplex Infections, 620·2
Herpes Simplex Vaccines, 1620·1
Herpes Soothing Cream, 2042·2
Herpes Zoster— *see* Varicella-zoster Infections, 621·1
Herpesan, 2042·2
Herpes-Gastreu R68, 2042·2
Herpes-Gel, 2042·2
Herpesil, 2042·2
Herpesine, 2042·2
Herpesnil, 2042·2
Herpesvirus Infections, 619·2
Herpesvirus Simiae Infections, 621·1
*Herpesvirus varicellae*, 1643·2
Herpetad, 2042·2
Herpetrol, 2042·2
Herpex, 2042·3
Herphonal, 2042·3
Herpid, 2042·3
Herpidu, 2042·3
Herpilem, 2042·3
Herplex, 2042·3
Herplex-D, 2042·3
Herpofug, 2042·3
Herpolips, 2042·3
Herpomed, 2042·3
Herposicc, 2042·3
Herpotern, 2042·3
Herpoviric, 2042·3
Herron Baby Teething Gel, 2042·3
Herten, 2042·3
Herviros, 2042·3
Herz ASS, 2042·3
Herz- und Kreislauf-Tee, Kneipp— *see* Kneipp Herz- und Kreislauf-Tee, 2081·2
Herz- und Kreislauftonikum Bioflora, 2042·3
HerzASS, 2042·3
Herzkur, 2042·3
Herz-Punkt Starkungstonikum mit Ginseng N, 2042·3
Herz-Punkt Vitaltonikum N, 2042·3
Herz-Starkung N, 2042·3
Herztropfen CM, 2042·3
Herz-Tropfen Eu Rho, 2042·3
Herztropfen Truw Gold, 2042·3
HES, 750·1
Hespan, 2042·3
Hespander, 2042·3
Hespercorbin, 2042·3
Hesperidin, 1688·2
Hesperidin Methyl Chalcone, 1688·2
Hesperidina, 1688·2
Hesteril, 2042·4
Hetaclox, 2042·4
Hetacloxacin, 2042·4
Hetaflur, 1434·2
Hetastarch, 750·1
Heteroid, 2042·4
Heterophyiasis— *see* Intestinal Fluke Infections, 99·2
Heterotopic Ossification— *see* Ectopic Ossification, 762·2
Hetrazan, 2042·4
Hetrogalen, 2042·4
Hettytropin, 2042·4
Heumann Abfurhtee Solubilax N, 2042·4
Heumann Beruhigungstee Tenerval N, 2042·4
Heumann Blasen- und Nierentee Solubitrat S, 2042·4
Heumann Bronchialtee Solubifix, 2042·4
Heumann Leber- und Gallentee Solu-Hepar S, 2042·4
Heumann Magentee Solu-Vetan, 2042·4
Heumann's Bronchialtee, 2042·4
Heupack Herbatherm N, Kneipp— *see* Kneipp Heupack Herbatherm N, 2081·2
Heuschnupfenmittel, 2042·4
Heuschnupfenmittel DHU, 2042·4
Heusin, 2042·4
Hevac B, 2042·4
*Hevea brasiliensis*, 1741·1
Hevert Enzym Novo, 2042·4
Hevert-Aktivon Mono, 2042·4
Hevert-Blasen-Nieren-Tee N, 2042·4
Hevert-Card Forte, 2042·4
Hevert-Carmin Symbio, 2042·4
Hevert-Dorm, 2042·4
Hevert-Entwasserungs-Tee, 2042·4
Hevert-Enzym Plus, 2042·4
Hevert-Erkaltungs-Tee, 2043·1
Hevert-Gall S, 2043·1
Hevert-Gicht-Rheuma-Tee Comp, 2043·1
Hevertigon, 2043·1
Hevert-Mag, 2043·1
Hevert-Magen-Galle-Leber-Tee, 2043·1
Hevert-Migrane, 2043·1
Hevert-Nerv Plus Eisen, 2043·1
Hevert-Nier II, 2043·1
Hevertnier Complex, 2043·1
Hevertnier Spasmo, 2043·1
Hevertogyn, 2043·1
Hevertolax Duo, 2043·1
Hevertolax Phyto, 2043·1
Hevertopect N, 2043·1
Hevertoplex 147— *see* Secale (Hevertoplex 147), 2281·1
Hevertotox, 2043·1
Hevertoval Mono, 2043·1
Hevertozym, 2043·1
Hevert-Vitan N, 2043·1
Hewallergia, 2043·1
Heweberberol-Tee, 2043·1
Hewechol Artischockendragees, 2043·1
Hewedolor Preparations, 2043·1
Hewedormir, 2043·1
Hewedormir Doxyl Intens, 2043·1
Hewedormir Forte— *see* Hewedormir doxyl intens, 2043·1
Heweformica, 2043·2
Heweginkgo, 2043·2
Hewekliman, 2043·2
Hewekzem Novo N, 2043·2
Hewelymphon N, 2043·2
Hewenephron Duo, 2043·2
Heweneural, 2043·2
Hewepsychon Duo, 2043·2
Hewepsychon Mono, 2043·2
Hewepsychon Uno, 2043·2
Hewerheum N, 2043·2
Hewesabal Comp, 2043·2
Hewesabal Mono, 2043·2
Heweselen, 2043·2
Hewethyreon, 2043·2
Hewetraumen, 2043·2
Heweurat, 2043·2
Heweven P 3, 2043·2
Heweven P 7, 2043·2
Heweven Phyto, 2043·2
Hewletts, 2043·2
Hexaammonium Molybdate Tetrahydrate, 1440·3
Hexa-Blok, 2043·2
Hexabotin, 2043·2
Hexabrix, 2043·2
Hexacetónido de Triamcinolona, 1110·2
Hexachlorobenzene, 1506·1
1α,2α,3β,4α,5α,6β-Hexachlorocyclohexane, 1506·3
(1*R*,4*S*,5*S*,8*R*)-1,2,3,4,10,10-Hexachloro-6,7-epoxy-1,4,4a,5,6,7,8,8a-octahydro-1,4:5,8-dimethanonaphthalene, 1503·3
Hexachloroethane, 1474·3
(1*R*,4*S*,4a*S*,5*S*,6*S*,7*R*,8*R*,8a*R*)-1,2,3,4,10,10-Hexachloro-1,4,4a,5,6,7,8,8a-octahydro-6,7-epoxy-1,4:5,8-dimethanonaphthalene, 1504·3
Hexachlorophane, 1181·2
Hexachlorophene, 1181·2
Hexachlorophene Sodium, 1181·3
Hexachloroplatinic Acid Hexahydrate, 1670·2
1,4,5,6,7,7-Hexachloro-8,9,10-trinorborn-5-en-2,3-ylenebismethylene Sulphite, 1504·3
Hexaclorobenceno, 1506·1
Hexacloroetano, 1474·3
Hexaclorofeno, 1181·2
Hexacortone, 2043·2
Hexacroman, 2043·2
Hexadecadrol, 1097·1
(3*S*,6*R*,7*E*,9*R*,10*R*,12*R*,14*S*,15*E*,17*E*,19*E*,21*S*,23*S*,26*R*,27*R*,34a*S*)-9,10,12,13,14,21,22,23,24,25,26,27,32,33,34,34a-Hexadecahydro-9,27-dihydroxy-3-{(1*R*)-2-[(1*S*,3*R*,4*R*)-4-(2-hydroxyethoxy)-3-methoxycyclohexyl]-1-methylethyl}-10,21-dimethoxy-6,8,12,14,20,26-hexamethyl-23,27-epoxy-3*H*-pyrido[2,1-*c*][1,4]oxa-azacyclohentriacontine-1,5,11,28,29(4*H*,6*H*,31*H*)-pentone, 1360·1
(3*S*,6*R*,7*E*,9*R*,10*R*,12*R*,14*S*,15*E*,17*E*,19*E*,21*S*,23*S*,26*R*,27*R*,34a*S*)-9,10,12,13,14,21,22,23,24,25,26,27,32,33,34,34a-Hexadecahydro-9,27-dihydroxy-3-{(1*R*)-2-[(1*S*,3*R*,4*R*)-4-hydroxy-3-methoxycyclohexyl]-1-methylethyl}-10,21-dimethoxy-6,8,12,14,20,26-hexamethyl-23,27-epoxy-3*H*-pyrido[2,1-*c*][1,4]oxaazacyclohentriacontine-1,5,11,28,29(4*H*,6*H*,31*H*)-pentone, 1363·1
(6*R*,7*R*,8*R*,9*S*,10*R*,13*S*,14*S*,15*S*,16*S*,17*S*)-1,3′,4′,6,6a,7,8,9,10,11,12,13,14,15,15a,16-Hexadecahydro-10,13-dimethylspiro-[17*H*-dicyclopropa[6,7:15,16]cyclopenta[*a*]phenanthrene-17,2′(5′*H*)-furan]-3,5′(2*H*)-dione, 1549·1
Hexadecanoic Acid 1-Methylether Ester, 1481·2
1-Hexadecanol, 1480·3
Hexadecyl Alcohol, 1480·3
Hexadecylamine Hydrofluoride, 1434·2
Hexadecyl(2-hydroxycyclohexyl)dimethylammonium Bromide, 1172·1
Hexadecyl[2-(*N*-*p*-methoxybenzyl-*N*-pyrimidin-2-ylamino)ethyl]dimethylammonium Bromide, 1757·2
Hexadecylphosphocholine, 573·2
1-Hexadecylpyridinium Chloride Monohydrate, 1173·1
Hexadecyltrimethylammonium Bromide, 1173·1
Hexadecyltrimethylammonium Chloride, 1173·1
Hexa-Defital, 2043·2
Hexa-Defital NF, 2043·2
(*E*,*E*)-Hexa-2,4-dienoic Acid, 1192·3
Hexadilat, 2043·2
Hexadiphane Hydrochloride, 1736·1
Hexadrol, 2043·2
Hexafen, 2043·2
Hexafene, 2043·3
Hexafluid, 2043·3
Hexafluorocalcitriol, 1462·1
1,1,1,3,3,3-Hexafluoro-2-(fluoromethoxy)-propane, 1307·3
Hexafluoroisopropanol, 1308·2

α,α,α,α′,α′,α′-Hexafluoro-3-oxo-4-aza-5α-androst-1-ene-17β-carboxy-2′,5′-xylidide, 1549·2
(+)-(5*Z*,7*E*)-26,26,26,27,27,27-Hexafluoro-9,10-secocholesta-5,7,10(19)-triene-1α,3β,25-triol, 1462·1
Hexagastron, 2043·3
Hexaglucon, 2043·3
Hexahidrobenzoato de Estradiol, 1550·1
Hexahydroadiphenine Hydrochloride, 482·1
Hexahydrobenzene, 1472·3
Hexahydrodesoxyephedrine, 1592·3
Hexahydro-3aα,7aα-dimethyl-4β,7β-epoxyisobenzofuran-1,3-dione, 1667·1
(2*R**,6*R**,11*R**)-1,2,3,4,5,6-Hexahydro-6,11-dimethyl-3-(3-methylbut-2-enyl)-2,6-methano-3-benzazocin-8-ol, 79·3
(3*R*,5*R*)-7-{(1*S*,2*S*,6*R*,8*S*,8a*R*)-1,2,6,7,8,8a-Hexahydro-2,6-dimethyl-8-[(*S*)-2-methylbutyryloxy]-1-naphthyl}-3-hydroxyheptan-5-olide, 949·1
1,2,3,4,5,6-Hexahydro-6,11-dimethyl-3-phenethyl-2,6-methano-3-benzazocin-8-ol Hydrobromide Hemihydrate, 82·2
(1*S*,3*R*,7*S*,8*S*,8a*R*)-1,2,3,7,8,8a-Hexahydro-3,7-dimethyl-8-{2-[(2*R*,4*R*)-tetrahydro-4-hydroxy-6-oxo-2*H*-pyran-2-yl]ethyl}-1-naphthyl 2,2-Dimethylbutyrate, 997·1
(*E*)-(3a*S*,4*R*,5*R*,6a*S*)-Hexahydro-5-hydroxy-4-[(*E*)-(3*S*,4*RS*)-3-hydroxy-4-methyl-1-octen-6-ynyl]-$\Delta^{2(1H),\delta}$-pentalenevaleric Acid, 1518·2
({(1*R*,2*R*,3a*S*,9a*S*)-2,3,3a,4,9,9a-Hexahydro-2-hydroxy-1-[(3*S*)-3-hydroxyoctyl]-1*H*-benz[*f*]inden-5-yl}oxy)acetic Acid, 1521·2
(5*R*,5a*R*,8a*R*,9*R*)-5,5a,6,8,8a,9-Hexahydro-9-hydroxy-5-(3,4,5-trimethoxyphenyl)furo[3′4′:6,7]naphtho[2,3-*d*]-1,3-dioxol-6-one, 1155·3
1,3,4,6,7,11b-Hexahydro-3-isobutyl-9,10-dimethoxybenzo-[*a*]quinolizin-2-one, 1752·2
(2*R*,6a*S*,12a*S*)-1,2,6,6a,12,12a-Hexahydro-2-isopropenyl-8,9-dimethoxychromeno[3,4-*b*]furo[2,3-*h*]chromen-6-one, 1510·1
Hexahydro-1-(5-isoquinolylsulfonyl)-1*H*-1,4-diazepine Hydrochloride, 914·3
(4a*S*,6*R*,8a*S*)-4a,5,9,10,11,12-Hexahydro-3-methoxy-11-methyl-6*H*-benzofuro[3a,3,2-*ef*][2]benzazepin-6-ol Hydrobromide, 1491·2
1,2,3,4,10,14b-Hexahydro-2-methyldibenzo[*c*,*f*]pyrazino[1,2-*a*]azepine Hydrochloride, 306·3
(−)-*N*-{[(*S*)-Hexahydro-1-methyl-2,6-dioxo-4-pyrimidinyl]carbonyl}-L-histidyl-L-prolinamide, 1340·1
(6*R*,12a*R*)-2,3,6,7,12,12a-Hexahydro-2-methyl-6-[3,4-(methylenedioxy)phenyl]pyrazino[1′,2′:1,6]pyrido[3,4-*b*]indole-1,4-dione, 1751·1
2,3,3a,4,5,6-Hexahydro-8-methyl-1*H*-pyrazino[3,2,1-*jk*]carbazole, 316·2
(*RS*)-1,2,3,4,10,14b-Hexahydro-2-methylpyrazino-[2,1-*a*]pyrido[2,3-*c*][2]benzazepine, 307·3
(1*S*,7*S*,8*S*,8a*R*)-1,2,3,7,8,8a-Hexahydro-7-methyl-8-{2-[(2*R*,4*R*)-tetrahydro-4-hydroxy-6-oxo-2*H*-pyran-2-yl]ethyl}-1-naphthyl (*S*)-2-Methylbutyrate, 958·1
*cis*-5-(Hexahydro-2-oxo-1*H*-thieno[3,4-*d*]imidazol-4-yl)valeric Acid, 1423·2
1,3,6,7,8,9-Hexahydro-5-phenyl-2*H*-[1]benzothieno[2,3-*e*]-1,4-diazepin-2-one, 671·3
(3a*S*)-2,3,3a,4,5,6-Hexahydro-2-[(3*S*)-3-quinuclidinyl]-1*H*-benz[*de*]isoquinolin-1-one Hydrochloride, 1282·3
Hexahydrothymol, 1711·3
2-{Hexahydro-4-[3-(2-trifluoromethylphenothiazin-10-yl)propyl]-1,4-diazepin-1-yl}ethanol Dihydrochloride, 703·1
(4a*S*,9a*S*)-2,3,4,4a,9,9a-Hexahydro-2,4a,9-trimethyl-1,2-oxazino[6,5-*b*]indol-6-yl-methylcarbamate Salicylate, 1491·2
(3a*S*,8a*R*)-1,2,3,3a,8,8a-Hexahydro-1,3a,8-trimethylpyrrolo[2,3-*b*]indol-5-yl Heptylcarbamate, 1491·2
(3a*S*,8a*R*)-1,2,3,3a,8,8a-Hexahydro-1,3a,8-trimethylpyrrolo[2,3-*b*]indol-5-yl Methylcarbamate, 1494·1
Hexakapron, 2043·3
Hexal Comfarol Plus, 2043·3
Hexal Compufen, 2043·3
Hexal Konazol Shampoo, 2043·3
Hexalacton, 2043·3
Hexalectol, 2043·3
Hexalen, 2043·3
Hexalense, 2043·3
Hexalid, 2043·3
Hexalyse, 2043·3
Hexamarium Bromide, 1489·2
Hexamet, 2043·3
Hexamethylenamine, 230·1
Hexamethylene, 1472·3
*N*,*N*′-Hexamethylenebis[2-amino-1-(3,4-dihydroxyphenyl)ethanol] Dihydrochloride, 786·3
*N*,*N*′-Hexamethylenebis[4-(2-amino-1-hydroxyethyl)pyrocatechol] Dihydrochloride, 786·3
1,1′-Hexamethylenebis[5-(4-chlorophenyl)biguanide] Diacetate, 1173·2
1,1′-Hexamethylenebis[5-(4-chlorophenyl)biguanide] Digluconate, 1173·2
1,1′-Hexamethylenebis[5-(4-chlorophenyl)biguanide] Dihydrochloride, 1173·3
(±)-α,α′-[Hexamethylenebis(iminomethylene)]-bis[3,4-dihydroxybenzyl Alcohol] Sulfate (1:1), 786·3
3,3′-[*N*,*N*′-Hexamethylenebis(methylcarbamoyloxy)]bis(1-methylpyridinium Bromide), 1489·2
4,4′-(Hexamethylenedioxy)dibenzamidine Bis(2-hydroxyethanesulphonate), 1181·3
Hexamethylenetetramine, 230·1
Hexamethylenetetramine Hippurate, 230·2
Hexamethylenetetramine Mandelate, 230·2
Hexamethylmelamine, 526·2
Hexamethylpararosaniline Chloride, 1186·1
2,6,10,15,19,23-Hexamethyltetracosane, 1482·2
$N^2$,$N^2$,$N^4$,$N^4$,$N^6$,$N^6$-Hexamethyl-1,3,5-triazine-2,4,6-triamine, 526·2
Hexamic Acid, 1426·2
Hexamidina, Isetionato de, 1181·3
Hexamidine Diisetionate, 1181·3
Hexamidine Isethionate, 1181·3
Hexamidine Isetionate, 1181·3
Hexamidini Diisetionas, 1181·3
Hexamidinum, 376·3
Hexamine, 230·1
Hexamine Amygdalate, 230·2
Hexamine Hippurate, 230·2
Hexamine Mandelate, 230·2
Hexamon, 2043·3
Hexamycin, 2043·3
Hexane, 1476·3
*n*-Hexane, 1475·1
Hexane, Solvent, 1476·3
Hexanedioic Acid, 1648·1
2,5-Hexanedione, 1475·1
Hexanicit, 2043·3
Hexanios G+R, 2043·3
Hexanitrat, 2043·3
Hexanium, 2043·3
*n*-Hexano, 1475·1
Hexanoestrol, 1556·3
2-Hexanone, 1476·1
Hexan-2-one, 1476·1
Hexanurat, 2043·3
Hexaphane, 2043·3
Hexaphenyl, 2043·3
Hexapindol, 2043·3
Hexapneumine, 2043·3
Hexapress, 2043·4
Hexaquart L, 2043·4
Hexaquart Plus, 2043·4
Hexaquart S, 2043·4
Hexaquine, 2043·4
Hexaretic, 2043·4
Hexarone, 2043·4
Hexaseptine, 2043·4
Hexasodium 8,8′-{Carbonylbis[imino-3,1-phenylenecarbonylimino(4-methyl-3,1-phenylene)carbonylimino]}bis(1,3,5-naphthalenetrisulfonate), 615·3
Hexasoptin, 2043·4
Hexaspray, 2043·4
Hexastarch, 750·2
Hexastat, 2043·4
Hexatin, 2043·4
Hexatrione, 2043·4
Hexavac, 2043·4
Hexavitamin, 2043·4
Hexavitamins, 2043·4
Hexazide, 2043·4
Hexemalcalcium, 689·2
Hexemalum, 689·2
Hexenalum, 703·1
Hexene, 2043·4
Hexestrol, 1556·3
Hexetidina, 1182·1
Hexetidine, 1182·1
Hexetidinum, 1182·1
Hexiben Plus, 2043·4
Hexicide, 1506·3
Hexide, 2043·4
Hexident, 2043·4
Hexidin, 2044·1
Hexifluor, 2044·1
Hexil, 2044·1
Hexilenglicol, 1697·1
Hexilium, 2044·1
Hexilresorcinol, 1182·1
Hexinawas, 2044·1
Hexit, 2044·1
Hexobarbital, 703·1
Hexobarbital Sódico, 703·1
Hexobarbital Sodium, 703·1
Hexobarbitalum, 703·1
Hexobarbitalum Natricum, 703·1
Hexobarbitone, 703·1
Hexobarbitone Sodium, 703·1
Hexobarbitone, Soluble, 703·1
Hexobendina, Hidrocloruro de, 931·2
Hexobendine Hydrochloride, 931·2
Hexobion, 2044·1
Hexoestrol, 1556·3
Hexogen, 2044·1
Hexo-Imotryl, 2044·1
Hexokain, 2044·1
Hexol, 2044·1
Hexoll, 2044·1
Hexolvon, 2044·1
Hexomedin, 2044·1
Hexomedin N, 2044·1
Hexomedine, 2044·1
Hexone, 1476·2
Hexopal, 2044·1
Hexoprenalina, Hidrocloruro de, 786·3
Hexoprenalina, Sulfato de, 786·3
Hexoprenaline Hydrochloride, 786·3
Hexoprenaline Sulfate, 786·3
Hexoprenaline Sulphate, 786·3
Hexoral, 2044·1
Hexoraletten N, 2044·1
Hextril, 2044·1
Hextriletten, 2044·1
Hexyl Nicotinate, 45·1
*n*-Hexyl Nicotinate, 45·1
4-Hexylbenzene-1,3-diol, 1182·1
1-Hexylcarbamoyl-5-fluorouracil, 535·1
1-Hexyl-3,7-dimethylxanthine, 979·2
Hexylene Glycol, 1697·1
(*S*)-1-[(2*S*,3*S*)-3-Hexyl-4-oxo-oxetan-2-yl-methyl]dodecyl *N*-Formyl-L-leucinate, 1724·2
3-[4-(Hexyloxy)-1,2,5-thiadiazol-3-yl]-1,2,5,6-tetrahydro-1-methylpyridine, 1498·3
Hexylresorc, 1182·1
Hexylresorcinol, 1182·1
Hexylresorcinolum, 1182·1
1-Hexyltheobromine, 979·2
HF, 2044·1
HF-1854, 685·3
HF-1927, 290·3
HF-2159, 685·2
HFA-227, 1236·2
HFA-134a, 1236·2
HFAs, 1236·2
HF-BIC35+HF-EL010, 2044·1
HF-BIC35+HF-EL210, 2044·1
HFC-227, 1236·2
HFC-134a, 1236·2
HFC-152a, 1236·2
HFCs, 1236·2
HFIP, 1308·2
HFRS Vaccine, 1617·1
81723-Hfu, 270·2
HFZ, 703·1
HGF, 1039·3
HGH, 1327·2
HGP-1, 1105·3
HH-184, 718·1
HH-197, 1116·2
HHT, 2044·2
HI-6, 1032·2
Hi B Plus C, Natures Way— *see* Natures Way Hi B Plus C, 2153·3
Hi Potency B Compound, 2044·2
Hi Potency Cal, 2044·2
Hi Potency KIB$_6$, 2044·2
Hi Potency Multi-Mineral, 2044·2
Hi Potency Stress B with C, 2044·2
Hialid, 2044·2
Hialuronato Sódico, 1697·3
Hialurónico, Ácido, 1697·3
Hialuronidasa, 1698·2
Hib Infections— *see* Haemophilus Influenzae Infections, 131·1
HIB Merieux, 2044·2
Hib Vaccines, 1616·1
HIB-DPT, 2044·2
HIB-DT, 2044·2
Hibenzato de Tipepidina, 1131·3
Hiberix, 2044·2
Hiberix— *see* Tritanrix HB/Hiberix, 2349·1
Hibernal, 2044·2
HIBest, 2044·2
HIBest— *see* Pent-HIBest, 2211·3
Hibicet, 2044·2
Hibicet Concentraat, 2044·2
Hibicet Hospital Concentrate, 2044·2
Hibicet Verdunning, 2044·2
Hibiclens, 2044·2
Hibicol, 2044·2
Hibicrick, 2044·2
Hibident, 2044·2
Hibidil, 2044·2
Hibiguard, 2044·2
Hibimax, 2044·2
Hibiscrub, 2044·2
Hibisol, 2044·3
Hibisprint, 2044·3
Hibistat, 2044·3
Hibital, 2044·3
Hibitane, 2044·3
Hibitane Menta, 2044·3
Hibitane Teinture, 2044·3
Hibizene, 2044·3
Hibon, 2044·3
Hiboquad, 2044·3
Hibor, 2044·3
HibTITER, 2044·3
Hib/Vac, 1616·1
HIB-Vaccinol, 2044·3
Hicantona, Mesilato de, 105·3
Hicarlex, 2044·3
Hiccup, 682·1
Hicee, 2044·3
Hicin, 2044·3
Hiclato de Doxiciclina, 206·2
Hicomp, 2044·3
Hiconcil, 2044·3
Hiconcil-NS, 2044·4
Hi-Cor, 2044·4
Hicoseen, 2044·4
Hicoton, 2044·4
Hidalone, 2044·4
Hidantal, 2044·4
Hidantil, 2044·4
Hidantina, 2044·4
Hidantina Composta, 2044·4
Hidantoina, 2044·4
Hiderm, 2044·4
Hidil, 2044·4
Hidine, 2044·4
Hidomin, 2044·4
Hidonac, 2044·4

Hidra, 2044·4
Hidra Plus, 2044·4
Hidrabene, 2044·4
Hidrafil, 2044·4
Hidrafix, 2044·4
Hidrafix 90, 2044·4
Hidral, 2044·4
Hidralazina, Hidrocloruro de, 931·2
Hidralma, 2044·4
Hidramox, 2044·4
Hidramox-M, 2044·4
Hidrangea, 1698·3
Hidra-Ped, 2044·4
Hidrapel, 2045·1
Hidraplus, 2045·1
Hidrasal, 2045·1
Hidrasec, 2045·1
Hidrasix, 2045·1
Hidraste, 1698·3
Hidrastina, Hidrocloruro de, 1698·3
Hidrastis, 1698·3
Hidratagel, 2045·1
Hidratant, 2045·1
Hidratante Enriquecida, 2045·1
Hidratante Ligera, 2045·1
Hidratante VG, 2045·1
Hidratante VV, 2045·1
Hidrato de Amileno, 1471·2
Hidratoderme, 2045·1
Hidratoil Free, 2045·1
Hidrazida, 2045·1
Hidrazina, Sulfato de, 1699·1
Hidrenox A, 2045·1
Hidrion, 2045·1
Hidrium, 2045·1
Hidroaltesona, 2045·1
Hidroazer, 2045·1
Hidrobromuro de Aspartato Magnésico, 706·1
Hidrobromuro de Citalopram, 289·1
Hidrobromuro de Dextrometorfano, 1117·3
Hidrobromuro de Fenazocina, 82·2
Hidrobromuro de Fenoterol, 785·2
Hidrobromuro de Galantamina, 1491·2
Hidrobromuro de Halofuginona, 605·3
Hidrobromuro de Hidroxianfetamina, 1699·3
Hidrobromuro de Nalorfina, 1044·2
Hidrobromuro de Rimiterol, 791·3
Hidroc Cloranf, 2045·1
Hidroc Neomic, 2045·1
Hidrocil, 2045·1
Hidrocilina, 2045·1
Hidrocin, 2045·1
Hidrocisdin, 2045·1
Hidroclorofluorocarbonos, 1236·1
Hidroclorotiazida, 933·2
Hidroclorozil, 2045·1
Hidrocloruro de Acebutolol, 848·1
Hidrocloruro de Acecainida, 848·3
Hidrocloruro de Aceclidina, 1487·1
Hidrocloruro de Acetato de Roxatidina, 1288·1
Hidrocloruro de Acetiamina, 1454·3
Hidrocloruro de Aclarubicina, 525·2
Hidrocloruro de Adrenalona, 1648·2
Hidrocloruro de Alfentanilo, 12·2
Hidrocloruro de Alfuzosina, 856·2
Hidrocloruro de Alizaprida, 1248·1
Hidrocloruro de Aloclamida, 1114·2
Hidrocloruro de Alprenolol, 856·3
Hidrocloruro de Amantadina, 1197·2
Hidrocloruro de Ambroxol, 1114·3
Hidrocloruro de Amifenazol, 1584·3
Hidrocloruro de Amikelina, 1653·2
Hidrocloruro de Amilorida, 858·2
Hidrocloruro de Amineptina, 280·3
Hidrocloruro de Aminoacridina, 1165·3
Hidrocloruro de Aminoquinurida, 1168·2
Hidrocloruro de Amiodarona, 859·2
Hidrocloruro de Amitriptilina, 280·3
Hidrocloruro de Amodiaquina, 446·3
Hidrocloruro de Amorolfina, 391·1
Hidrocloruro de Amosulalol, 862·3
Hidrocloruro de Amprolio, 600·3
Hidrocloruro de Anagrelida, 1654·3
Hidrocloruro de Anfepramona, 1587·1
Hidrocloruro de Anileridina, 15·1
Hidrocloruro de Antazolina, 424·2
Hidrocloruro de Apraclonidina, 864·1
Hidrocloruro de Aprindina, 864·2
Hidrocloruro de Arbutamina, 864·2
Hidrocloruro de Arginina, 1421·1
Hidrocloruro de Arotinolol, 865·1
Hidrocloruro de Articaína, 1370·3
Hidrocloruro de Atipamezol, 1032·3
Hidrocloruro de Azasetrón, 1251·1
Hidrocloruro de Azelastina, 425·2
Hidrocloruro de Azimilida, 866·3
Hidrocloruro de Bacampicilina, 161·2
Hidrocloruro de Bambuterol, 781·2
Hidrocloruro de Bamifilina, 781·3
Hidrocloruro de Barnidipino, 866·3
Hidrocloruro de Befunolol, 867·1
Hidrocloruro de Benacticina, 287·1
Hidrocloruro de Benazepril, 867·2
Hidrocloruro de Bencidamina, 21·1
Hidrocloruro de Benexato, 1251·2
Hidrocloruro de Benfluorex, 868·1
Hidrocloruro de Benidipino, 868·1
Hidrocloruro de Benserazida, 1200·2
Hidrocloruro de Benzfetamina, 1585·2
Hidrocloruro de Bepridil, 868·1
Hidrocloruro de Betahistina, 1660·1
Hidrocloruro de Betaxolol, 873·1
Hidrocloruro de Bevantolol, 873·2
Hidrocloruro de Biperideno, 479·3
Hidrocloruro de Bisantreno, 530·2
Hidrocloruro de Bornaprina, 480·1
Hidrocloruro de Bromazina, 425·3
Hidrocloruro de Bromhexina, 1115·3
Hidrocloruro de Brovanexina, 1116·1
Hidrocloruro de Bucindolol, 877·1
Hidrocloruro de Buclizina, 426·3
Hidrocloruro de Bufenina, 1663·2
Hidrocloruro de Buflomedil, 877·2
Hidrocloruro de Bunazosina, 878·1
Hidrocloruro de Bunitrolol, 878·1
Hidrocloruro de Bupivacaína, 1371·1
Hidrocloruro de Bupranolol, 878·1
Hidrocloruro de Buprenorfina, 21·3
Hidrocloruro de Bupropión, 287·2
Hidrocloruro de Buspirona, 672·2
Hidrocloruro de Butalamina, 878·2
Hidrocloruro de Butenafina, 395·2
Hidrocloruro de Butriptilina, 289·1
Hidrocloruro de Cafedrina, 878·2
Hidrocloruro de Camilofina, 1666·1
Hidrocloruro de Captodiamo, 674·1
Hidrocloruro de Carbocromeno, 880·2
Hidrocloruro de Carpipramina, 674·2
Hidrocloruro de Carteolol, 880·3
Hidrocloruro de Cefalexina, 168·1
Hidrocloruro de Cefepima, 172·1
Hidrocloruro de Cefmenoxima, 173·2
Hidrocloruro de Cefotiam, 177·2
Hidrocloruro de Celiprolol, 881·3
Hidrocloruro de Cetirizina, 427·1
Hidrocloruro de Cetraxato, 1255·2
Hidrocloruro de Cevimelina, 1488·3
Hidrocloruro de Cicletanina, 883·2
Hidrocloruro de Ciclizina, 429·3
Hidrocloruro de Ciclobenzaprina, 1393·1
Hidrocloruro de Ciclopentolato, 480·3
Hidrocloruro de Cincocaína, 1373·2
Hidrocloruro de Ciprofloxacino, 188·2
Hidrocloruro de Ciproheptadina, 430·1
Hidrocloruro de Cisteína, 1426·3
Hidrocloruro de Citalopram, 289·1
Hidrocloruro de Clemizol, 429·2
Hidrocloruro de Clenbuterol, 784·2
Hidrocloruro de Clinafloxacino, 194·2
Hidrocloruro de Clindamicina, 194·2
Hidrocloruro de Clobenzorex, 1585·3
Hidrocloruro de Clobutinol, 1117·1
Hidrocloruro de Clocapramina, 683·1
Hidrocloruro de Clofedanol, 1117·1
Hidrocloruro de Clomipramina, 289·3
Hidrocloruro de Clonazolina, 1117·1
Hidrocloruro de Clonidina, 885·2
Hidrocloruro de Clonizina, 429·2
Hidrocloruro de Cloperastina, 1117·2
Hidrocloruro de Clorciclizina, 427·2
Hidrocloruro de Clordiazepóxido, 674·2
Hidrocloruro de Clorfenoxamina, 428·3
Hidrocloruro de Clorhexidina, 1173·3
Hidrocloruro de Clormetina, 537·1
Hidrocloruro de Clormidazol, 396·1
Hidrocloruro de Cloropiramina, 427·3
Hidrocloruro de Cloroprocaína, 1373·1
Hidrocloruro de Cloroquina, 448·2
Hidrocloruro de Clorproetazina, 675·1
Hidrocloruro de Clorproguanil, 452·1
Hidrocloruro de Clorpromazina, 675·2
Hidrocloruro de Clorprotixeno, 682·3
Hidrocloruro de Clortetraciclina, 187·3
Hidrocloruro de Colesevelam, 889·2
Hidrocloruro de Colestipol, 889·2
Hidrocloruro de Colextrán, 890·3
Hidrocloruro de Croconazol, 397·1
Hidrocloruro de Dapiprazol, 1679·1
Hidrocloruro de Daunorubicina, 545·3
Hidrocloruro de Delapril, 892·2
Hidrocloruro de Demeclociclina, 204·3
Hidrocloruro de Deshidroemetina, 603·2
Hidrocloruro de Desipramina, 290·2
Hidrocloruro de Detomidina, 689·3
Hidrocloruro de Dexetimida, 481·1
Hidrocloruro de Dexfenfluramina, 1586·3
Hidrocloruro de Dexmedetomidina, 689·3
Hidrocloruro de Dextropropoxifeno, 28·3
Hidrocloruro de Dibenzepina, 290·3
Hidrocloruro de Dicicloverina, 481·2
Hidrocloruro de Diclonina, 1376·2
Hidrocloruro de Dietazina, 481·3
Hidrocloruro de Difemerina, 481·3
Hidrocloruro de Difenhidramina, 431·3
Hidrocloruro de Difenidol, 1261·1
Hidrocloruro de Difenilpiralina, 432·3
Hidrocloruro de Difenoxilato, 1261·3
Hidrocloruro de Difenoxina, 1261·2
Hidrocloruro de Difloxacino, 205·3
Hidrocloruro de Dihexiverina, 481·3
Hidrocloruro de Diisopromina, 1261·2
Hidrocloruro de Dilazep, 900·1
Hidrocloruro de Diltiazem, 900·1
Hidrocloruro de Dimeflina, 1587·2
Hidrocloruro de Dimetofrina, 902·3
Hidrocloruro de Dimetoxanato, 1119·1
Hidrocloruro de Dioxetedrina, 1119·1
Hidrocloruro de Diperodón, 1376·2
Hidrocloruro de Dipipanona, 35·3
Hidrocloruro de Dipivefrina, 1681·2
Hidrocloruro de Diprenorfina, 1037·3
Hidrocloruro de Dobutamina, 905·3
Hidrocloruro de Donepezilo, 1489·2
Hidrocloruro de Dopamina, 907·1
Hidrocloruro de Dopexamina, 908·2
Hidrocloruro de Dorzolamida, 908·3
Hidrocloruro de Dosulepina, 291·1
Hidrocloruro de Doxapram, 1587·2
Hidrocloruro de Doxepina, 291·2
Hidrocloruro de Doxorubicina, 547·3
Hidrocloruro de Drofenina, 482·1
Hidrocloruro de Duloxetina, 291·3
Hidrocloruro de Eflornitina, 604·2
Hidrocloruro de Embramina, 433·2
Hidrocloruro de Encainida, 910·3
Hidrocloruro de Eperisona, 1394·3
Hidrocloruro de Epinastina, 433·3
Hidrocloruro de Epinefrina, 852·3
Hidrocloruro de Epirubicina, 550·2
Hidrocloruro de Eprazinona, 1121·1
Hidrocloruro de Eprozinol, 1121·1
Hidrocloruro de Esmolol, 913·1
Hidrocloruro de Espectinomicina, 255·2
Hidrocloruro de Espirapril, 1003·1
Hidrocloruro de Estreptomicina, 256·1
Hidrocloruro de Etafedrina, 1121·2
Hidrocloruro de Etafenona, 914·1
Hidrocloruro de Etambutol, 211·3
Hidrocloruro de Etaverina, 1685·2
Hidrocloruro de Etidocaína, 1376·3
Hidrocloruro de Etifoxina, 698·1
Hidrocloruro de Etilefrina, 914·1
Hidrocloruro de Etoperidona, 292·1
Hidrocloruro de Etorfina, 38·3
Hidrocloruro de Eucatropina, 482·1
Hidrocloruro de Fadrozol, 553·1
Hidrocloruro de Fasudil, 914·3
Hidrocloruro de Fenazopiridina, 83·1
Hidrocloruro de Fencanfamina, 1588·2
Hidrocloruro de Fenciclidina, 1730·3
Hidrocloruro de Fendilina, 915·1
Hidrocloruro de Fenetilina, 1588·2
Hidrocloruro de Fenfluramina, 1588·2
Hidrocloruro de Fenformina, 344·1
Hidrocloruro de Fenilefrina, 1126·3
Hidrocloruro de Fenilpropanolamina, 1127·3
Hidrocloruro de Fenmetrazina, 1592·2
Hidrocloruro de Fenoperidina, 83·2
Hidrocloruro de Fenoxazolina, 1121·3
Hidrocloruro de Fenoxibenzamina, 981·2
Hidrocloruro de Fenpipramida, 1687·3
Hidrocloruro de Fenproporex, 1588·3
Hidrocloruro de Fenspirida, 786·1
Hidrocloruro de Fentermina, 1592·2
Hidrocloruro de Fexofenadina, 433·3
Hidrocloruro de Flavoxato, 482·2
Hidrocloruro de Flufenazina, 699·3
Hidrocloruro de Flunarizina, 434·1
Hidrocloruro de Fluoxetina, 292·1
Hidrocloruro de Flupentixol, 699·1
Hidrocloruro de Fominobén, 1121·3
Hidrocloruro de Furaltadona, 215·2
Hidrocloruro de Galopamilo, 922·3
Hidrocloruro de Gemcitabina, 558·1
Hidrocloruro de Gepirona, 701·1
Hidrocloruro de Gonadorelina, 1325·2
Hidrocloruro de Granisetrón, 1267·1
Hidrocloruro de Grepafloxacino, 220·3
Hidrocloruro de Guanfacina, 927·2
Hidrocloruro de Gusperimús, 1360·2
Hidrocloruro de Halofantrina, 452·2
Hidrocloruro de Heptaminol, 1697·1
Hidrocloruro de Hexobendina, 931·2
Hidrocloruro de Hexoprenalina, 786·3
Hidrocloruro de Hidralazina, 931·2
Hidrocloruro de Hidrocodona, 45·1
Hidrocloruro de Hidrocortamato, 1103·3
Hidrocloruro de Hidromorfona, 45·2
Hidrocloruro de Hidroxizina, 434·3
Hidrocloruro de Homoclorciclizina, 434·3
Hidrocloruro de Homofenazina, 703·1
Hidrocloruro de Ibopamina, 937·3
Hidrocloruro de Idarubicina, 560·2
Hidrocloruro de Idazoxano, 1700·2
Hidrocloruro de Imidapril, 938·2
Hidrocloruro de Imipramina, 300·1
Hidrocloruro de Indanazolina, 1122·3
Hidrocloruro de Indeloxazina, 1700·3
Hidrocloruro de Indenolol, 939·1
Hidrocloruro de Indoramina, 939·2
Hidrocloruro de Ipsapirona, 703·1
Hidrocloruro de Irinotecán, 564·1
Hidrocloruro de Isoetarina, 787·3
Hidrocloruro de Isometepteno, 1702·1
Hidrocloruro de Isoprenalina, 940·2
Hidrocloruro de Isotipendil, 435·2
Hidrocloruro de Isoxsuprina, 1702·2
Hidrocloruro de Itoprida, 1268·2
Hidrocloruro de Ketamina, 1302·1
Hidrocloruro de Ketocaína, 1377·1
Hidrocloruro de Labetalol, 943·3
Hidrocloruro de Lefetamina, 53·1
Hidrocloruro de Lercanidipino, 946·1
Hidrocloruro de Levamisol, 107·2
Hidrocloruro de Levobetaxolol, 946·1
Hidrocloruro de Levobunolol, 946·2
Hidrocloruro de Levobupivacaína, 1377·1
Hidrocloruro de Levocabastina, 435·2
Hidrocloruro de Levomepromazina, 703·2
Hidrocloruro de Levometadona, 54·1
Hidrocloruro de Levosalbutamol, 788·2
Hidrocloruro de Lidamidina, 1270·2
Hidrocloruro de Lidocaína, 1377·3
Hidrocloruro de Lincomicina, 226·2
Hidrocloruro de Linsidomina, 946·3
Hidrocloruro de Lisina, 1439·2
Hidrocloruro de Lobelina, 1589·1
Hidrocloruro de Lofepramina, 305·3
Hidrocloruro de Lofexidina, 1041·2
Hidrocloruro de Lomefloxacino, 227·2

Hidrocloruro de Loperamida, 1271·1
Hidrocloruro de Lorcainida, 947·2
Hidrocloruro de Loxapina, 705·2
Hidrocloruro de Manidipino, 950·2
Hidrocloruro de Maprotilina, 306·1
Hidrocloruro de Mebeverina, 1273·1
Hidrocloruro de Mecamilamina, 951·3
Hidrocloruro de Mecisteína, 1124·1
Hidrocloruro de Meclofenoxato, 1710·1
Hidrocloruro de Meclozina, 436·3
Hidrocloruro de Medetomidina, 706·1
Hidrocloruro de Mefenorex, 1589·2
Hidrocloruro de Mefloquina, 453·3
Hidrocloruro de Melitraceno, 306·3
Hidrocloruro de Melperona, 706·1
Hidrocloruro de Memantina, 1711·2
Hidrocloruro de Mepacrina, 606·3
Hidrocloruro de Mepiramina, 437·1
Hidrocloruro de Mepivacaína, 1381·2
Hidrocloruro de Meptazinol, 56·3
Hidrocloruro de Mercaptamina, 1712·2
Hidrocloruro de Metaciclina, 230·1
Hidrocloruro de Metadona, 57·2
Hidrocloruro de Metanfepramona, 1714·1
Hidrocloruro de Metanfetamina, 1589·2
Hidrocloruro de Metformina, 342·3
Hidrocloruro de Metildopato, 953·2
Hidrocloruro de Metilfenidato, 1590·2
Hidrocloruro de Metixeno, 485·3
Hidrocloruro de Metizolina, 1124·3
Hidrocloruro de Metoclopramida, 1274·3
Hidrocloruro de Metodilazina, 437·2
Hidrocloruro de Metoxamina, 953·1
Hidrocloruro de Metoxifenamina, 1124·2
Hidrocloruro de Mianserina, 306·3
Hidrocloruro de Mibefradil, 959·1
Hidrocloruro de Midazolam, 707·2
Hidrocloruro de Midodrina, 959·2
Hidrocloruro de Milnaciprán, 307·3
Hidrocloruro de Minociclina, 231·3
Hidrocloruro de Mitoxantrona, 575·2
Hidrocloruro de Moexipril, 961·2
Hidrocloruro de Molindona, 709·3
Hidrocloruro de Moperona, 710·1
Hidrocloruro de Moracizina, 962·1
Hidrocloruro de Moroxidina, 649·3
Hidrocloruro de Moxaverina, 1717·2
Hidrocloruro de Moxifloxacino, 233·1
Hidrocloruro de Moxisilita, 962·2
Hidrocloruro de Nadoxolol, 963·3
Hidrocloruro de Nafazolina, 1124·3
Hidrocloruro de Naftifina, 406·2
Hidrocloruro de Nalbufina, 64·2
Hidrocloruro de Nalmefeno, 1044·1
Hidrocloruro de Nalorfina, 1044·2
Hidrocloruro de Naloxona, 1044·3
Hidrocloruro de Naltrexona, 1046·1
Hidrocloruro de Naratriptán, 470·1
Hidrocloruro de Nebivolol, 964·3
Hidrocloruro de Nefazodona, 309·2
Hidrocloruro de Nefopam, 66·2
Hidrocloruro de Neticonazol, 406·3
Hidrocloruro de Nicardipino, 965·1
Hidrocloruro de Nicofibrato, 965·3
Hidrocloruro de Nicomorfina, 66·3
Hidrocloruro de Nifekalant, 972·2
Hidrocloruro de Nimustina, 576·3
Hidrocloruro de Niperotidina, 1277·2
Hidrocloruro de Norepinefrina, 975·1
Hidrocloruro de Norfenefrina, 975·3
Hidrocloruro de Normetadona, 1125·2
Hidrocloruro de Nortriptilina, 310·2
Hidrocloruro de Noscapina, 1125·3
Hidrocloruro de Octacaína, 1382·1
Hidrocloruro de Octenidina, 1187·2
Hidrocloruro de Olopatadina, 438·1
Hidrocloruro de Olprinona, 976·1
Hidrocloruro de Ondansetrón, 1281·1
Hidrocloruro de Opipramol, 311·1
Hidrocloruro de Orfenadrina, 486·1
Hidrocloruro de Oxeladina, 1126·1
Hidrocloruro de Oxibuprocaína, 1382·1
Hidrocloruro de Oxibutinina, 486·3
Hidrocloruro de Oxicodona, 75·2
Hidrocloruro de Oxifedrina, 978·2
Hidrocloruro de Oxifenciclimina, 487·2
Hidrocloruro de Oxilofrina, 977·3
Hidrocloruro de Oximetazolina, 1126·1
Hidrocloruro de Oximorfona, 76·1
Hidrocloruro de Oxitetraciclina, 241·1
Hidrocloruro de Oxomemazina, 438·2
Hidrocloruro de Oxprenolol, 978·1
Hidrocloruro de Parconazol, 407·3
Hidrocloruro de Paretoxicaína, 1382·2
Hidrocloruro de Pargilina, 978·3
Hidrocloruro de Paroxetina, 311·2
Hidrocloruro de Pentazocina, 79·3
Hidrocloruro de Petidina, 80·2
Hidrocloruro de Pilsicainida, 983·1
Hidrocloruro de Pioglitazona, 344·1
Hidrocloruro de Pipamperona, 716·1
Hidrocloruro de Pipazetato, 1129·1
Hidrocloruro de Piperidolato, 487·3
Hidrocloruro de Pipradrol, 1592·3
Hidrocloruro de Pirbuterol, 790·3
Hidrocloruro de Pirenzepina, 488·1
Hidrocloruro de Piridoxina, 1456·3
Hidrocloruro de Piritinol, 1737·2
Hidrocloruro de Pirlimicina, 244·1
Hidrocloruro de Pirmenol, 984·1
Hidrocloruro de Pitofenona, 1732·3
Hidrocloruro de Pivampicilina, 244·2
Hidrocloruro de Pivmecilinam, 244·2
Hidrocloruro de Pramipexol, 1212·2
Hidrocloruro de Pramiverina, 1734·3
Hidrocloruro de Pramocaína, 1382·2
Hidrocloruro de Prazosina, 985·1
Hidrocloruro de Prenalterol, 986·3
Hidrocloruro de Prenoxdiazina, 1129·1
Hidrocloruro de Prilocaína, 1382·3
Hidrocloruro de Proadifeno, 1735·2
Hidrocloruro de Procaína, 1383·2
Hidrocloruro de Procainimida, 987·1
Hidrocloruro de Procarbazina, 581·2
Hidrocloruro de Procaterol, 791·1
Hidrocloruro de Prociclidina, 488·2
Hidrocloruro de Profenamina, 488·3
Hidrocloruro de Proguanil, 457·1
Hidrocloruro de Prolintano, 1592·3
Hidrocloruro de Promazina, 717·3
Hidrocloruro de Prometazina, 439·1
Hidrocloruro de Propacetamol, 85·3
Hidrocloruro de Propafenona, 988·3
Hidrocloruro de Propanocaína, 1383·3
Hidrocloruro de Propilhexedrina, 1592·3
Hidrocloruro de Propiomazina, 440·3
Hidrocloruro de Propiverina, 489·1
Hidrocloruro de Propoxicaína, 1384·1
Hidrocloruro de Propranolol, 989·3
Hidrocloruro de Protipendilo, 718·1
Hidrocloruro de Protriptilina, 316·2
Hidrocloruro de Proximetacaína, 1384·1
Hidrocloruro de Prozapina, 1736·1
Hidrocloruro de Pseudoefedrina, 1129·2
Hidrocloruro de Quinagolida, 1213·1
Hidrocloruro de Quinapril, 991·1
Hidrocloruro de Quinisocaína, 1384·2
Hidrocloruro de Raloxifeno, 1568·3
Hidrocloruro de Ramosetrón, 1285·2
Hidrocloruro de Ranitidina, 1285·2
Hidrocloruro de Ranolazina, 994·2
Hidrocloruro de Remacemida, 377·2
Hidrocloruro de Remifentanilo, 86·1
Hidrocloruro de Reproterol, 791·2
Hidrocloruro de Rimantadina, 653·1
Hidrocloruro de Ritodrina, 1739·2
Hidrocloruro de Robenidina, 615·2
Hidrocloruro de Ropinirol, 1213·3
Hidrocloruro de Ropivacaína, 1384·2
Hidrocloruro de Salverina, 1741·3
Hidrocloruro de Sapropterina, 1742·1
Hidrocloruro de Sarafloxacino, 254·3
Hidrocloruro de Sarpogrelato, 996·3
Hidrocloruro de Selegilina, 1214·1
Hidrocloruro de Sertralina, 317·2
Hidrocloruro de Setastina, 441·1
Hidrocloruro de Sevelámero, 1051·2
Hidrocloruro de Sibutramina, 1593·1
Hidrocloruro de Sotalol, 1001·3
Hidrocloruro de Sultoprida, 723·1
Hidrocloruro de Tacrina, 1497·2
Hidrocloruro de Talipexol, 1215·3
Hidrocloruro de Tamsulosina, 1009·2
Hidrocloruro de Tebacón, 1131·2
Hidrocloruro de Temocapril, 1010·2
Hidrocloruro de Tenildiamina, 442·1
Hidrocloruro de Teodrenalina, 1754·3
Hidrocloruro de Terazosina, 1010·3
Hidrocloruro de Terbinafina, 408·2
Hidrocloruro de Tertatolol, 1011·1
Hidrocloruro de Tetracaína, 1385·1
Hidrocloruro de Tetraciclina, 266·2
Hidrocloruro de Tetramisol, 114·1
Hidrocloruro de Tetrizolina, 1131·2
Hidrocloruro de Tiagabina, 378·1
Hidrocloruro de Tiamina, 1455·1
Hidrocloruro de Tiaprida, 725·1
Hidrocloruro de Tiaramida, 94·1
Hidrocloruro de Ticlopidina, 1011·2
Hidrocloruro de Tiletamina, 1310·2
Hidrocloruro de Tilidina, 94·1
Hidrocloruro de Tioridazina, 724·2
Hidrocloruro de Tiotixeno, 725·2
Hidrocloruro de Tirofibán, 1013·3
Hidrocloruro de Tiropramida, 1757·1
Hidrocloruro de Tizanidina, 1395·3
Hidrocloruro de Tocainida, 1014·1
Hidrocloruro de Todralazina, 1015·1
Hidrocloruro de Tolazolina, 1015·1
Hidrocloruro de Tolicaína, 1385·3
Hidrocloruro de Tolperisona, 1396·3
Hidrocloruro de Tolpropamina, 442·2
Hidrocloruro de Tomoxetina, 1585·1
Hidrocloruro de Tonzilamina, 442·2
Hidrocloruro de Topotecán, 589·1
Hidrocloruro de Tramadol, 94·3
Hidrocloruro de Tramazolina, 1131·3
Hidrocloruro de Trazodona, 319·1
Hidrocloruro de Tretoquinol, 806·3
Hidrocloruro de Trifluoperazina, 726·3
Hidrocloruro de Trifluperidol, 727·1
Hidrocloruro de Triflupromazina, 727·1
Hidrocloruro de Trihexifenidilo, 490·2
Hidrocloruro de Trimecaína, 1385·3
Hidrocloruro de Trimetazidina, 1018·1
Hidrocloruro de Trimetobenzamida, 442·2
Hidrocloruro de Tripelenamina, 442·3
Hidrocloruro de Triprolidina, 442·3
Hidrocloruro de Tromantadina, 656·1
Hidrocloruro de Tropatepina, 491·1
Hidrocloruro de Tropisetrón, 1293·3
Hidrocloruro de Tulobuterol, 806·3
Hidrocloruro de Urapidil, 1018·1
Hidrocloruro de Valaciclovir, 656·1
Hidrocloruro de Valganciclovir, 656·3
Hidrocloruro de Vancomicina, 275·2
Hidrocloruro de Venlafaxina, 321·3
Hidrocloruro de Verapamilo, 1019·1
Hidrocloruro de Vetrabutina, 1764·2
Hidrocloruro de Viloxazina, 323·3
Hidrocloruro de Viquidil, 1764·3
Hidrocloruro de Xemilofibán, 1029·2
Hidrocloruro de Xenisalato, 1163·1
Hidrocloruro de Xilazina, 1766·1
Hidrocloruro de Xilometazolina, 1132·2
Hidrocloruro de Yohimbina, 1766·2
Hidrocloruro de Zipeprol, 1132·3
Hidrocloruro de Zolazepam, 728·3
Hidrocloruro de Zorubicina, 594·3
Hidrocloruro de Zuclopentixol, 730·3
Hidrocloruro del Ácido Glutámico, 1433·2
Hidrocloruro del Palmitato de Clindamicina, 194·2
Hidrocodona, Hidrocloruro de, 45·1
Hidrocodona, Tartrato de, 45·1
Hidrocol, 2045·1
Hidrocortamato, Hidrocloruro de, 1103·3
Hidrocorte, 2045·1
Hidrocortin, 2045·1
Hidrocortisona, 1103·3
Hidrocortisona, Acetato de, 1103·3
Hidrocortisona, Butirato de, 1104·1
Hidrocortisona, Cipionato de, 1104·1
Hidrocortisona, Fosfato Sódico de, 1104·1
Hidrocortisona, Hidrogenosuccinato de, 1104·1
Hidrocortisona, Succinato Sódico de, 1104·1
Hidrocortisona, Valerato de, 1104·2
Hidrofall, 2045·1
Hidrofenil, 2045·1
Hidroferol, 2045·1
Hidroflumetiazida, 937·2
Hidrofluorocarbonos, 1236·2
Hidrofugal, 2045·2
Hidrofugal Forte, 2045·2
Hidrogel, 2045·2
Hidrogeno, Solución de Bióxido de, 1182·2
Hidrogenosuccinato de Hidrocortisona, 1104·1
Hidrogenosuccinato de Metilprednisolona, 1106·1
Hidrogenosuccinato de Prednisolona, 1108·1
Hidrogenotartrato de Rivastigmina, 1497·1
Hidrolac, 2045·2
Hidro-Lact, 2045·2
Hidrolyte, 2045·2
Hidromagma, 2045·2
Hidromens, 2045·2
Hidromorfona, Hidrocloruro de, 45·2
Hidrona, 2045·2
Hidroneo, 2045·2
Hidronovag Complex, 2045·2
Hidroperioduro de Tetraglicina, 1194·1
Hidropid, 2045·2
Hidroplus, 2045·2
Hidroplus CL, 2045·2
Hidroplus Nieve, 2045·2
Hidropolicin, 2045·2
Hidropolivit, 2045·2
Hidropolivit Mineral, 2045·2
Hidropril, 2045·2
Hidroquilaude, 2045·2
Hidroquin, 2045·2
Hidroquinidina, Hidrocloruro de, 937·3
Hidroquinina, Hidrobromuro de, 1699·3
Hidroquinona, 1148·1
Hidroral, 2045·2
Hidroronol, 2045·2
Hidroronol T, 2045·2
Hidrosaluretil, 2045·2
Hidrosam T, 2045·2
Hidrosol, 2045·2
Hidrotalcita, 1267·3
Hidrotisona, 2045·2
Hidrowil, 2045·2
Hidroxianfetamina, Bromhidrato de, 1699·3
Hidroxianfetamina, Hidrobromuro de, 1699·3
Hidroxiapatito, 1699·3
Hidroxibenzoato de Viminol, 96·3
Hidroxicarbamida, 559·1
Hidroxicarbamida, Mesilato de, 562·1
Hidroxicloroquina, Sulfato de, 452·3
Hidroxicobalamina, 1458·2
Hidroxid, 2045·3
Hidróxido Cálcico, 1664·3
Hidróxido de Aluminio, 1249·2
Hidróxido de Aluminio y Carbonato de Magnesio Desecado, Gel de, 1250·1
Hidróxido de Sodio, 1747·3
Hidróxido Potásico, 1734·2
Hidroxiestrona, Diacetato de, 1556·3
Hidroxietilcelulosa, 1579·2
Hidroxietilmetilcelulosa, 1579·2
Hidroxil B12 B6 B1, 2045·3
Hidroximetilnicotinamida, 1700·1
Hidroxina, 2045·3
Hidroxinaftoato de Befenio, 103·2
Hidroxiprogesterona, Caproato de, 1556·3
Hidroxipropilcelulosa, 1579·2
Hidroxiquinolina, Sulfato de, 1700·1
Hidroxizina, Embonato de, 434·3
Hidroxizina, Hidrocloruro de, 434·3
Hidroxogel, 2045·3
Hidyn H, 2045·3
Hiedra Terrestre, 1696·1
Hierba Luisa, 1706·3
Hierba Mora, 1661·2
Hierba Santa, 1121·2
Hierco, 2045·3
Hierro, 1434·3

Hierro 59, 1524·3
Hierro Dextrano, 1436·1
Hierro Polimaltosa, 1437·3
Hierro Sacarosa, 1438·2
Hierro Sorbitol, 1438·1
Hierro y Sulfato de Condroitina, Complejo de, 1425·1
Hierroquick, 2045·3
Hifamonil, 2045·3
Hifamonil Crema, 2045·3
Higan, 2045·3
Higesan, 2045·3
High Molecular Weight Kininogen, 735·3
High Potency Cal-Mag Plus, 2045·3
High Potency Lightening Serum, 2045·3
High Potency N-Vites, 2045·3
High-altitude Disorders, 822·2
High-ceiling Diuretics, 811·2
Highly Purified Insulins, 334·2
Higienex, 2045·3
Higigripe, 2045·3
Higo, 1266·3
Higromicina B, 105·3
Higroton, 2045·3
Higroton Reserpina, 2045·3
Higrotona, 2045·3
Higrotona Reserpina, 2045·3
Higroton-Res, 2045·3
Hijuven, 2045·3
Hill's Balsam Chesty Cough, 2045·3
Hill's Balsam Chesty Cough for Children, 2045·3
Hill's Balsam Chesty Cough Pastilles, 2045·3
Hill's Balsam Dry Cough, 2045·3
Hill's Balsam Extra Strong, 2045·3
Hill's Balsam Nasal Congestion Pastilles, 2045·3
Himalayan Rhubarb, 1287·3
Hima-Pasta Nouvelle Formule, 2045·4
Himbeer, 1057·3
Himecromona, 1700·1
Himega, 2045·4
Himelan, 2045·4
Himus, 2045·4
Hincomox, 2045·4
Hingfong-Essenz Hofmanns, 2045·4
Hinojo, 1687·2
Hinojo, Aceite Esencial, 1687·3
Hinojo, Esencia de, 1687·3
Hinojo, Fruto de, 1687·2
Hinox, 2045·4
H-Insulin, 2045·4
Hiosciamina, 485·1
Hiosciamina, Bromidrato de, 485·1
Hiosciamina, Hidrobromuro de, 485·1
Hiosciamina, Sulfato de, 485·1
Hiosinotil, 2045·4
Hiosinotil Compuesto, 2045·4
Hiospan, 2045·4
Hiospan Composto, 2045·4
Hioxyl, 2045·4
Hipalen, 2045·4
Hipax, 2045·4
Hipecor, 2045·4
Hipeksal, 2045·4
Hipen, 2045·4
Hipenox, 2045·4
Hiper Diet, 2045·4
Hiperbiotico, 2045·4
Hiperbiotico Retard, 2045·4
Hipercol, 2045·4
Hiperdipina, 2045·4
Hiperex, 2045·4
Hiperflex, 2045·4
Hipericin, 2045·4
Hiperico, 2045·4
Hipérico, 299·1
Hiperikan, 2045·4
Hiperil, 2045·4
Hiperlex, 2045·4
Hiperlex Plus, 2045·4
Hiperogyn, 2046·1
Hipersac, 2046·1
Hipersex, 2046·1
Hiperson, 2046·1
Hiperson-D, 2046·1
Hipersteno, 2046·1
Hipertenol, 2046·1
Hipertex, 2046·1
Hipertil, 2046·1
Hipertin, 2046·1
Hiperton, 2046·1
Hipfix, 2046·1
Hipnodem, 2046·1
Hipnopento, 2046·1
Hipnosedon, 2046·1
Hipoartel, 2046·1
Hipoartel H, 2046·1
Hipoartel Plus, 2046·1
Hipocatril, 2046·1
Hipoclorito Sódico, 1192·1
Hipocol, 2046·1
Hipoderme, 2046·1
Hipodermon, 2046·1
Hipodex, 2046·1
Hipodor, 2046·1
Hipofagin S, 2046·1
Hipofisina, 2046·1
Hipófisis Pulverizada (Neurohipófisis), 1337·3
Hipofosforoso, Ácido, 1700·2
Hipoge, 2046·1
Hipoglicina A, 1700·2
Hipoglos, 2046·1
Hipoglos Cicatrizante, 2046·2
Hipoglos con Hidrocortisona, 2046·2
Hipoglos Oftalmico, 2046·2
Hipoglos Plus, 2046·2
Hipogloso, Aceite de Higado de, 1434·1
Hipoglucin, 2046·2
Hipokinon, 2046·2
Hipolixan, 2046·2
Hiposan, 2046·2
Hiposcler, 2046·2
Hiposterol, 2046·2
Hiposul, 2046·2
Hipoten, 2046·2
Hipotensil, 2046·2
Hipotermal, 2046·2
Hipotest, 2046·2
Hipotosse, 2046·2
Hipovastin, 2046·2
Hi-Po-Vites, 2046·2
Hippoglossi, Oleum, 1434·1
*Hippoglossus*, 1434·1
*Hippophae rhamnoides*, 1742·2
Hippophan, 2046·2
Hippramine, 2046·2
Hippuric Acid, 1170·1, 1477·2
Hipress, 2046·2
Hiprex, 2046·2
Hipromelosa, 1579·3
Hips, 1740·1
Hipten, 2046·2
Hipurato de Metenamina, 230·2
Hiremon, 2046·2
Hirsutism, 1545·1
Hirtonin, 2046·2
Hirucreme, 2046·2
Hirudex, 2046·2
Hirudin, 931·2
Hirudina, 931·2
Hirudine, 931·2
Hirudo, 945·1
*Hirudo medicinalis*, 945·1
*Hirudo nipponica*, 945·1
Hirudoid, 2046·2
Hirulog, 875·2
His, 1434·2
Hiscifed, 2046·3
Hiscolgen, 2046·3
Hisdane, 2046·3
Hisfedin, 2046·3
Hismacon, 2046·3
Hismadrin, 2046·3
Hismanal, 2046·3
Hismizol, 2046·3
Hisno, 2046·3
Hisnot, 2046·3
Hisocel, 2046·3
Hisof, 2046·3
Hisoplex com Glicose, 2046·3
Hispamicina Retard, 2046·3
Hisprin, 2046·3
Histabloc, 2046·3
Histac, 2046·3
Histaclar, 2046·3
Histacon, 2046·3
Histacyl Compositum, 2046·3
Histacylettes, 2046·3
Histadane, 2046·3
Histade, 2046·3
Histadestal, 2046·3
Histadex, 2046·3
Histadin, 2046·3
Histadoxylamine Succinate, 432·3
Histafed, 2046·4
Histafed Comp, 2046·4
Histafed Expectorant, 2046·4
Histafen, 2046·4
Histafilin, 2046·4
Histafren, 2046·4
Histagesic Modified, 2046·4
Histaglobin, 2046·4
Histaglobulin, 2046·4
Histajodol N, 2046·4
Histak, 2046·4
Histalen, 2046·4
Histaler, 2046·4
Histalerg, 2046·4
Histalerg Profen, 2046·4
Histalet, 2046·4
Histalet X, 2046·4
Histalet Forte, 2046·4
Histalgane, 2046·4
Histalgane Mite, 2046·4
Histalino, 2046·4
Histalix, 2046·4
Histalix-C, 2046·4
Histaloc, 2046·4
Histalon, 2046·4
Histalor, 2047·1
Histamed, 2047·1
Histamed Compound, 2047·1
Histamen, 2047·1
Histamin, 2047·1
Histamina, 1697·1
Histamina, Fosfato de, 1697·2
Histamina, Hidrocloruro de, 1697·1
Histamine, 1697·1
Histamine Acid Phosphate, 1697·2
Histamine Dihydrochloride, 1697·1
Histamine Diphosphate, 1697·2
Histamine $H_1$-receptor Antagonists, 419·1
Histamine $H_2$-receptor Antagonists, 1239·3
Histamine Hydrochloride, 1697·1
Histamine Phosphate, 1697·2
Histamini Dihydrochloridum, 1697·1
Histamini Phosphas, 1697·2
Histaminic Cephalalgia— *see* Cluster Headache, 464·1
Histamino Corteroid L, 2047·1
Histaminos, 2047·1
Histamix, 2047·1
Histan, 2047·1
Histantil, 2047·1
Histaoph, 2047·1
Histaplus, 2047·1
Histaser, 2047·1
Histatab Plus, 2047·1
Histatapp, 2047·1
Histaterfen, 2047·1
Histatex, 2047·1
Hista-Vadrin, 2047·1
Hista-Vent DA, 2047·1
Histaverin, 2047·1
Histax, 2047·1
Histaxin, 2047·1
Histazine, 2047·1
Histema, 2047·1
Histenol Cold, 2047·1
Histenol-Forte, 2047·1
Histergan, 2047·1
Histerone, 2047·1
Histex, 2047·1
Histex CT, 2047·2
Histex HC, 2047·2
Histex PD, 2047·2
Histex SR, 2047·2
Histiacil NF, 2047·2
Histica, 2047·2
Histidanol, 2047·2
Histidina, 1434·2
Histidine, 1434·2
L-Histidine, 1434·2
Histidine Hydrochloride, 1434·2
Histidine Hydrochloride Monohydrate, 1434·2
L-Histidine Hydrochloride Monohydrate, 1434·2
Histidine Monohydrochloride, 1434·2
8-L-Histidine-α-L-iduronidase, 1705·1
Histidini Hydrochloridum Monohydricum, 1434·2
Histidinium Chloride, 1434·2
Histidinum, 1434·2
Histilos, 2047·2
Histimet, 2047·2
Histin, 2047·2
Histine DM, 2047·2
Histiness, 2047·2
Histinex D, 2047·2
Histinex DM, 2047·2
Histinex HC, 2047·2
Histinex PV, 2047·2
Histiocytic Syndromes, 505·2
Histiocytoma— *see* Bone Sarcoma, 524·3
Histiocytosis X— *see* Histiocytic Syndromes, 505·2
Histiocytosis, Langerhans-cell— *see* Histiocytic Syndromes, 505·2
Histoacryl, 2047·2
Histodil, 2047·2
Histodor, 2047·2
Histodor Expectorant, 2047·2
Histodryl, 2047·2
Histo-Fluine P, 2047·2
Histofreezer, 2047·2
Histol, 2047·2
Histolyn-CYL, 2047·2
Histop, 2047·3
Histopen, 2047·3
Histophtal, 2047·3
*Histoplasma capsulatum*, 1697·2
Histoplasmin, 1697·2
Histoplasmina, 1697·2
Histoplasmosis, 388·1
Histor-D, 2047·3
Histor-D Timecelles, 2047·3
Histosal, 2047·3
Histrelin, 1329·3
Histrelin Acetate, 1329·3
Histrelina, Acetato de, 1329·3
Histussin D, 2047·3
Histussin HC, 2047·3
Hitocobamin, 2047·3
Hitrechol, 2047·3
HIV Immunoglobulins, 1607·3
HIV Infection and AIDS, 621·3
HIV Infection, Disinfection Procedures— *see* Disinfection in Hepatitis and HIV Infection, 1165·1
HIV Infection Prophylaxis, 623·3
HIV Vaccines, 1607·3
HIV-associated Diarrhoea— *see* HIV-associated Wasting and Diarrhoea, 623·2
HIV-associated Infections, 623·1
HIV-associated Malignancies, 623·1
HIV-associated Neurological Complications, 623·2
HIV-associated Wasting and Diarrhoea, 623·2
Hi-Vegi-Lip, 2047·3
Hivensteril, 2047·3
Hivernum, 2047·3
Hives, 2047·3
Hives— *see* Urticaria and Angioedema, 1138·3
Hivid, 2047·3
Hivirux, 2047·3
Hivirux Complex, 2047·3
Hivita, 2047·3
Hivita Childvita, 2047·3
Hivita Liquivita, 2047·3

Hivotex, 2047·3
Hixizine, 2047·3
Hizaar, 2047·3
Hizin, 2047·3
Hjertealbyl, 2047·3
Hjertemagnyl, 2047·3
HK-256, 1129·1
HL-362, 1674·3
HL-1050, 397·3
HMD, 1565·2
HMDP, 773·3
HMG, 1330·1, 2047·3
HMG Massone, 2047·3
HMG-CoA Reductase Inhibitors, 811·3
H-Mide, 2047·3
HMM, 526·2
HMR-3647, 265·2
HMR-4396, 747·2
HMS, 2047·4
HMWK, 735·3
HN2, 537·1
HN-078, 806·3
HN 25, 2047·4
HN RL, 2047·4
HOA, 609·2
Hobaticam, 2047·4
Hobatolex, 2047·4
Hobatstress, 2047·4
Hochdisperses Silicumdioxid, 1581·3
Hochu-ekki-to, Kanebo— *see* Kanebo Hochu-ekki-to, 2074·2
Hochu-ekki-to, Tsumura— *see* Tsumura Hochu-ekki-to, 2351·1
Hocimin, 2047·4
Hocura-Spondylose Novo, 2047·4
Hodernal, 2047·4
Hodgkin's Disease, 509·2
Hoe-18-680, 36·2
Hoe-39-893d, 979·1
Hoe-045, 1370·3
Hoe-062, 1288·1
Hoe-095K, 1420·3
Hoe-118, 983·3
Hoe-280, 239·3
Hoe-296, 396·1
Hoe-296b, 396·1
Hoe-304, 1096·3
Hoe-471, 1325·1
Hoe-490, 332·2
Hoe-498, 994·1
Hoe-760, 1288·1
Hoe-766, 1319·2
Hoe-777, 1107·3
Hoe-881V, 105·2
Hoe-893d, 979·1
HOE-901, 334·3
Hoe-02982, 1506·1
Hoe-36801, 698·1
Hoechst-10582, 1125·2
Hoechst-12512, 1735·1
Hoecutin Olbad, 2047·4
Hoecutin Olbad F, 2047·4
Hoemarin Derma, 2047·4
Hoemarin Rheuma, 2047·4
Hoepixin Bad N, 2047·4
Hoepixin N, 2047·4
Hoevenol, 2047·4
Hoevenol A, 2047·4
Hofcomant, 2047·4
Hofels White Willow and Burdock, 2047·4
Hoffmannstropfen, 2047·4
Hog, 1730·3
Hoggar N, 2047·4
Hoigné's Syndrome, 246·2
Hoja de Coca, 1373·3
Hoja de Digital, 894·2
Hoja de Menta, 1283·2
Hokunalin, 2047·4
Holadren, 2047·4
Hold DM, 2047·4
Holfungin, 2047·4
Holgyeme, 2047·4
Holofusine, 2047·4
Holomagnesio, 2047·4
Holomagnesio Antioxidante, 2048·1
Holomagnesio B6, 2048·1
Holomagnesio Ginseng, 2048·1
Holopon, 2048·1
Holoxan, 2048·1
Holoxan Uromitexan, 2048·1
Holoxane, 2048·1
Holsten Aktiv, 2048·1
Holunderblüten, 1741·3
Holy Thistle, 1673·3
HOM, 483·2
Homa, 2048·1
Homasedin, 2048·1
Homatr. Hydrobrom., 483·2
Homatrocil, 2048·1
Homatrop, 2048·1
Homatropil, 2048·1
Homatropina, 483·2
Homatropina, Hidrobromuro de, 483·2
Homatropina, Metilbromuro de, 483·2
Homatropine, 483·2
Homatropine Hydrobromide, 483·2
Homatropine Methobromide, 483·2
Homatropine Methylbromide, 483·2
Homatropini Hydrobromidum, 483·2
Homatropini Methylbromidum, 483·2
Homatropinium Bromide, 483·2
Homatropinum Bromatum, 483·2
Homberg, Sal Sedativa de, 1662·1
Homebake, 27·2
Homeoaftyl, 2048·1
Homeocoksinum, 2048·1
Homeodent, 2048·1
Homeodose Preparations, 2048·1
Homeofortil, 2048·1
Homeofortin III, 2048·1
Homeogene 9, 2048·1
Homeogene 46, 2048·1
Homeomunil, 2048·1
Homeoplasmina, 2048·1
Homeoplasmine, 2048·1
Homeoptic, 2048·1
Homeovox, 2048·1
Hominex, 2048·1
Homo, 2048·1
Homocalmefyba, 2048·1
Homochlorcyclizine Hydrochloride, 434·3
Homocisteon Compuesto, 2048·1
Homoclomin, 2048·2
Homoclorciclizina, Hidrocloruro de, 434·3
Homocystinuria— *see* Amino Acid Metabolic Disorders, 1417·2
Homoderma, 2048·2
Homofenazina, Hidrocloruro de, 703·1
Homofenazine Hydrochloride, 703·1
Homoharringtonina, 558·3
Homoharringtonine, 558·3
Homomenthyl Salicylate, 1148·1
D-Homo-17a-oxaandrosta-1,4-diene-3,17-dione, 587·3
Homopafen, 2048·2
Homopan, 2048·2
Homosalate, 1148·1
Homosalato, 1148·1
Homosismin, 2048·2
Homovanillic Acid, 1208·3
Honey Bee, 1655·3
Honey Bee for Homoeopathic Preparations, 1655·3
Honey of Borax, 1662·1
Honey, Clarified, 1434·2
Honey Lemon Cough Lozenges, 2048·2
Honey & Molasses, 2048·2
Honey, Purified, 1434·2
Honey, Strained, 1434·2
Honeycold, 2048·2
Honeyflu, 2048·2
Honeygola, 2048·2
Honeytuss, 2048·2
Hongosan, 2048·2
Hongoseril, 2048·2
Honguil, 2048·2
Honguil Plus, 2048·2
Honsa, 2048·2
Honvan, 2048·2
Honvol, 2048·2
Honzil, 2048·2
Hookworm Infections, 99·2
Hop Strobile, 1708·1
Hopacem, 2048·2
Hopantenato Cálcico, 1664·3
Hopfenzapfen, 1708·1
Hopram, 2048·2
Hopranolol, 2048·2
Hops, 1708·1
Hordenol, 2048·2
*Hordeum distichon*, 1439·2
*Hordeum vulgare*, 1439·2
Horehound and Aniseed Cough Mixture, 2048·2
Horestyl, 2048·2
Horex, 2048·2
Horf, 2048·2
Horizem, 2048·2
Hormo Hepatico, 2048·2
Hormocervix, 2048·3
Hormodausse, 2048·3
Hormodausse Plus Calcium and Vitamin D, 2048·3
Hormodiol, 2048·3
Hormodose, 2048·3
Hormoginase, 2048·3
Hormolax, 2048·3
Hormonal Contraceptives, 1527·3
Hormone Multicap, 2048·3
Hormone Replacement Therapy, 1536·2
Hormonin, 2048·3
Horon, 2048·3
Horse Chestnut, 1648·2
Horse Radish and Garlic Tablets, 2048·3
Horse Tranquilliser, 1730·3
Horse-chestnut, 1648·2
Horseradish, 1697·3
Horsetail, 1684·1
Horsley's Wax, 1480·2
Hortelã-Pimenta , 1283·2
Hortelã-Pimenta, Essência de, 1283·2
Horton's Syndrome— *see* Cluster Headache, 464·1
Horvilan N, 2048·3
Hosboral, 2048·3
Hosboral Bronquial, 2048·3
Hospidermin, 2048·3
Hospisept, 2048·3
Hostacyclin, 2048·3
Hostacycline, 2048·3
Hostan, 2048·3
Hosterona, 2048·3
Hostid, 2048·3
Hostop, 2048·3
Hot Coldrex, 2048·3
Hot Lemon, 2048·3
Hot Lemon Relief, 2048·3
Hot Thermo, 2048·3
Hotemin, 2048·3
Houblon, 1708·1
12 Hour Antihistamine Nasal Decongestant, 2048·4
12 Hour Cold, 2048·4
Household Ammonia, 1654·1
Housemaid's Knee— *see* Soft-tissue Rheumatism, 11·1
Hova, 2048·4
Hova Expectorant, 2048·4
Hovaletten N, 2048·4
Hovalin, 2048·4
Hovasin, 2048·4
Hovid Q10 Plus, 2048·4
Hovite, 2048·4
Hox Alpha, 2048·4
$H_2$Oxyl, 2048·4
1HP, 277·3
HP-209, 37·2
HPB, 2048·4
H-Peran, 2048·4
HpGRF-40, 1339·2
HPMC-Ophtal, 2048·4
HPMPC, 629·2
HPP, 412·2
Hp-Pac, 2048·4
4-HPR, 553·1
HPRM, 1579·3
HPTH 1-34, 775·2
HQ-495, 1386·3
HQMME, 1151·3
HR-158, 704·1
HR-221, 174·1
HR-355, 225·3
HR-376, 358·2
HR-756, 175·3
HR-810, 178·2
H-R Lubricating Jelly, 2048·4
HrBMP-2, 768·1
HrBMP-7, 768·2
HRF, 2048·4
HRI Calm Life, 2048·4
HRI Clear Complexion, 2048·4
HRI Golden Seal Digestive, 2048·4
HRI Night, 2048·4
HRI Water Balance, 2048·4
HRT, 1536·3
HR-111V, 179·3
HS-592, 429·1
H-Sal, 2048·4
HSP-2986, 1734·3
HSR-803, 1268·2
HSR-902, 1757·1
HSV Infections— *see* Herpes Simplex Infections, 620·2
5-HT, 1743·2
5-$HT_3$ Antagonists, 1239·2
5-$HT_3$-receptor Antagonists, 1239·2
HT903, 2048·4
H-Tab, 2048·4
HTF-919, 1293·2
5-HTP, 311·1
H-Tronin, 2048·4
H-Tuss-D, 2049·1
Hu1124, 1146·3
Huanghuahaosu, 447·2
Huanuco Leaf, 1373·3
Huapi Bark, 1117·2
Hubber, Neo— *see* Neo Hubber, 2156·3
Huberdilat, 2049·1
Huberdoxina, 2049·1
Hubergrip, 2049·1
Hubermizol, 2049·1
Huberplex, 2049·1
Huckleberry, 1718·3
Huflattich, 1117·2
Huile Analgesique Polar-Bar— *see* Huile Analgesique "Temple of Heaven" contre les Maux de Tete, 2049·1
Huile Analgesique "Temple of Heaven" contre les Maux de Tete, 2049·1
Huile d'Amande, 1651·1
Huile d'Arachide, 1656·1
Huile de Bain Therapeutique, 2049·1
Huile de Foie de Morue, 1425·2
Huile de Haarlem, 2049·1
Huile de Lin, 1707·2
Huile de Maïs, 1439·2
Huile de Millepertuis A. Vogel (Huile de St. Jean), 2049·1
Huile de Noyaux, 1651·1
Huile de Ricin, 1668·2
Huile de Silicone, 1482·1
Huile de St. Jean— *see* Huile de millepertuis A. Vogel (huile de St. Jean), 2049·1
Huile de Tournesol, 1451·1
Huile de Vaseline Épaisse, 1479·1
Huile de Vaseline Fluide, 1479·1
Huile d'Oeillette, 1733·3
Huile Essentielle d'Aspic, 1749·2
Huile Essentielle de Lavande, 1705·2
Huile Essentielle de Menthe Crépue, 1749·1
Huile Gomenolee, 2049·1
Huile Po-Ho A. Vogel, 2049·1
Huile Solaire Bronzage, 2049·1
Humacart 3/7, 2049·1
Humaject Preparations, 2049·1
Humal, 2049·1
Humalog, 2049·1
Humalog Mix, 2049·2
Humalog Mix 25, 2049·1
Humalog NPL, 2049·2
Human Actrapid, 2049·2
Human Actrapid— *see* Actrapid, 1774·3
Human Albumin, 740·3
Human Albumin, Iodinated ($^{125}$I), 1524·2

Human Albumin, Iodinated ($^{131}$I), 1524·3
Human Albumin Solution, 740·3
Human Anti-D Immunoglobulin, 1608·1
Human Anti-D Immunoglobulin for Intravenous Administration, 1608·1
Human Antithrombin III Concentrate, 742·2
Human Calcitonin, 768·2
Human Chorionic Gonadotrophin, 1320·3
Human Coagulation Factor VII, 750·3
Human Coagulation Factor VIII, 751·1
Human Coagulation Factor VIII (rDNA), 751·2
Human Coagulation Factor IX, 752·2
Human Epidermal Growth Factor, 1294·2
Human Fibrin Foam, 753·2
Human Fibrinogen, 753·2
Human Fibrinogen, Iodinated ($^{125}$I), 1524·2
Human Growth Hormone, 1327·2
Human Growth Hormone, Methionyl, 1327·2
Human Hepatitis A Immunoglobulin, 1617·1
Human Hepatitis B Immunoglobulin, 1617·2
Human Hepatitis B Immunoglobulin for Intravenous Administration, 1617·3
Human Immunodeficiency Virus Infection— *see* HIV Infection and AIDS, 621·3
Human Insulatard— *see* Insulatard, 2063·3
Human Insulin, 334·1
Human Insultard, 2049·2
Human Interstitial-cell-stimulating Hormone, 1332·1
Human Measles Immunoglobulin, 1623·1
Human Menopausal Gonadotrophins, 1330·1
Human Mixtard, 2049·2
Human Mixtard— *see* Mixtard 10, 20, 30, 40, and 50, 2137·2
Human Monotard, 2049·2
Human Monotard— *see* Monotard, 2140·2
Human Normal Immunoglobulin, 1627·2
Human Normal Immunoglobulin for Intravenous Administration, 1627·2
Human Papilloma Virus Vaccines, 1620·2
(1-34) Human Parathormone, 775·2
Human Parathormone (1-34), 775·2
(1-34) Human Parathyroid Hormone, 775·2
Human Parathyroid Hormone (1-34), 775·2
Human Plasma for Fractionation, 757·3
Human Plasma (Pooled and Treated for Virus Inactivation), 757·3
Human Prothrombin Complex, 752·2
Human PTH (1-34), 775·2
Human Rabies Immunoglobulin, 1635·3
Human Rubella Immunoglobulin, 1637·3
Human Skin Equivalent, Bioengineered, 1158·1
Human Tetanus Immunoglobulin, 1640·3
Human Ultratard— *see* Ultratard, 2357·2
Human Varicella Immunoglobulin, 1643·1
Human Varicella Immunoglobulin for Intravenous Administration, 1643·1
Human Velosulin— *see* Velosulin, 2370·2
Humana AR, 2049·2
Humana Disanal, 2049·2
Humana HA, 2049·2
Humana Sinelac, 2049·2
Humanalbin, 2049·2
Humanilusin, 2049·2
Humanised Anti-Tac Antibody, 1359·3
Humaplus Preparations, 2049·2
Humate-P, 2049·2
Humatin, 2049·2
Humatrope, 2049·2
Humatro-Pen, 2049·2
Humavent, 2049·2
Humectante, 2049·2
Humectante Bucal, 2049·2
Humectol, 2049·2
Humedia, 2049·2
Humegon, 2049·2
Humektan, 2049·2
Humeral Epicondylitis— *see* Soft-tissue Rheumatism, 11·1
Humex, 2049·3
Humex Expectorant, 2049·3
Humex Mal de Gorge sans Sucre, 2049·3
Humex Rhume, 2049·3
Humibid, 2049·3
Humibid DM, 2049·3
Huminsulin Preparations, 2049·3
Humira, 2049·3
HuMist Nasal Mist, 2049·3
Humoferon, 2049·3
Humopin N, 2049·3
Humorap, 2049·3
Humorsol, 2049·3
Humoryl, 2049·3
Humotet— *see* Tetabulin, 2327·1
Humoxal, 2049·4
Humulin Preparations, 2049·4, *see* also Humaject Preparations, 2049·1
Humulina Preparations, 2050·1
Humuline Preparations, 2050·1
Humulus, 1708·1
*Humulus lupulus*, 1708·1
Humutard, 2050·1
Humutard Ultra, 2050·1
Hungarian Chamomile, 1669·3
Huntington's Chorea— *see* Chorea, 664·2
Huntington's Disease— *see* Chorea, 664·2
Hurricaine, 2050·1
Hursini, 1666·1
Hurtleberry, 1718·3
Hustagil, 2050·1
Hustagil Erkaltungsbalsam, 2050·1
Hustagil Inhalationsol, 2050·2
Hustagil Thymian-Hustensaft, 2050·2
Hustagil Thymiantropfen, 2050·2
Hustazol, 2050·2
Hustazol-C, 2050·2
Husten ACC, 2050·2
Husten- und Bronchial-Tee, Kneipp— *see* Kneipp Husten- und Bronchial-Tee, 2081·2
Husten- und Fieber-Saft, 2050·2
Hustensaft Weleda, 2050·2
Hustensaft-Dr Schmidgall, 2050·2
Hustenstiller, 2050·2
Hustenstiller N, 2050·2
Hustentabs, 2050·2
Husties, 2050·2
Hustosol, 2050·2
Hutrope, 2050·2
HVA, 1208·3
HVM, 2050·2
HWA-285, 989·3
HWA-486, 53·2
Hyaff— *see* Hyalofill, 2050·2
Hyaff— *see* Hyalogran, 2050·2
Hya-ject, 2050·2
Hyalart, 2050·2
Hyalase, 2050·2
Hyalcrom, 2050·2
Hyal-Drop, 2050·2
Hyalein, 2050·2
Hyalgan, 2050·2
Hyalistil, 2050·2
Hyalofill, 2050·2
Hyalogran, 2050·2
Hyalosidase, 1698·2
Hyalozima, 2050·2
Hyal-System, 2050·2
Hyaludermin, 2050·3
Hyalugel, 2050·3
Hyaluronan, 1697·3
Hyaluronate Sodium, 1697·3
Hyaluronic Acid, 1697·3
Hyaluronidase, 1698·2
Hyaluronidasum, 1698·2
Hyanac, 2050·3
Hyanit N, 2050·3
Hya-Ophtal, 2050·3
Hyasol, 2050·3
Hyason, 2050·3
Hyate:C, 2050·3
Hy-Bio, 2050·3
Hybloc, 2050·3
Hybolin, 2050·3
Hybridil, 2050·3
Hybutyl, 2050·3
Hycal, 2050·3
Hycamtin, 2050·3
Hycanthone Mesilate, 105·3
Hycanthone Mesylate, 105·3
Hyceral, 2050·3
Hycibex, 2050·3
Hycocin, 2050·3
HycoClear Tuss, 2050·3
Hycodan, 2050·3
Hycomine, 2050·3
Hycomine Compound, 2050·3
Hycomycin, 2050·3
Hycor, 2050·3
Hycort, 2050·4
Hycortin, 2050·4
Hycotuss, 2050·4
Hydac, 2050·4
Hydal, 2050·4
Hydantin, 2050·4
Hydatid Disease— *see* Echinococcosis, 98·1
Hydeltrasol, 2050·4
Hyderax, 2050·4
Hydergin, 2050·4
Hydergina, 2050·4
Hydergine, 2050·4
Hyderm, 2050·4
Hydiphen, 2050·4
Hydoftal, 2050·4
Hydol, 2050·4
Hydopa, 2050·4
Hydra, 2050·4
Hydra Form Day, 2050·4
Hydra Perfecte, 2050·4
Hydrabak, 2050·4
Hydracillin, 2050·4
Hydracort, 2050·4
Hydracuivre, 2050·4
Hydraderm, 2050·4
Hydrafuca, 2050·4
Hydragel, 2051·1
Hydragenic, 2051·1
Hydralazine Hydrochloride, 931·2
Hydralazini Hydrochloridum, 931·2
Hydralift Day, 2051·1
Hydralin, 2051·1
Hydrallazine Hydrochloride, 931·2
Hydralyte, 2051·1
Hydramine Cream, 2051·1
Hydramine Expectorant, 2051·1
Hydramox, 2051·1
Hydran, 2051·1
Hydrangea, 1698·3
*Hydrangea arborescens*, 1698·3
Hydranorme, 2051·1
Hydrap-ES, 2051·1
Hydraphase XL, 2051·1
Hydraphen, 1182·2
Hydraplus, 2051·1
Hydrapres, 2051·1
Hydrares, 2051·1
Hydrarg., 1713·1
Hydrarg. Perchlor., 1712·3
Hydrarg. Subchlor., 1712·3
Hydrargaphen, 1182·2
Hydrargyri Aminochloridum, 1152·1
Hydrargyri Dichloridum, 1712·3
Hydrargyri Oxidum Flavum, 1712·3
Hydrargyri Oxydum Flavum, 1712·3
Hydrargyri Perchloridum, 1712·3
Hydrargyri Subchloridum, 1712·3
Hydrargyri Subchloridum Praecipitatum, 1712·3
Hydrargyrosi Chloridum, 1712·3
Hydrargyrum, 1713·1
Hydrargyrum Amidochloratum, 1152·1
Hydrargyrum Ammoniatum, 1152·1
Hydrargyrum Bichloratum, 1712·3
Hydrargyrum Chloratum (Mite), 1712·3
Hydrargyrum Depuratum, 1713·1
Hydrargyrum Phenyloboricum, 1189·2
Hydrargyrum Praecipitatum Album, 1152·1
Hydrasense, 2051·1
Hydrasor, 2051·1
Hydrasorb, 2051·1
Hydrast., 1698·3
Hydrastine Hydrochloride, 1698·3
Hydrastis, 1698·3
*Hydrastis canadensis*, 1698·3
Hydrastis Complex, 2051·1
Hydrastis Rhizoma, 1698·3
Hydrastis Salbe N, 2051·1
Hydrate, 2051·1
Hydrated Aluminium Oxide, 1249·2
Hydrated Silica, Colloidal, 1581·3
Hydrated Zinc Carbonate, 1163·2
Hydrating B5 Gel, 2051·1
Hydrax, 2051·1
Hydrazide, 2051·1
Hydra-zide, 2051·1
Hydrazine Hydrate, 1699·1
Hydrazine Sulfate, 1699·1
Hydrazine Sulphate, 1699·1
(−)-L-α-Hydrazino-3,4-dihydroxy-α-methylhydrocinnamic Acid Monohydrate, 1204·3
1-Hydrazinophthalazine Hydrochloride, 931·2
Hydrea, 2051·1
Hydrene, 2051·2
Hydrex, 2051·2
Hydrigoz, 2051·2
Hydrinate, 2051·2
Hydrine, 2051·2
Hydrisalic, 2051·2
Hydrisea, 2051·2
Hydrisinol, 2051·2
Hydro Cobex, 2051·2
Hydro Cordes, 2051·2
Hydro DP, 2051·2
Hydro PC, 2051·2
Hydro-Adreson, 2051·2
Hydroagisten, 2051·2
Hydrobromic Acid, 1663·1
Hydrocal, 2051·2
Hydrocare Preparations, 2051·2
Hydro-Cebral, 2051·2
Hydrocerin, 2051·2
Hydrocet, 2051·3
Hydrochinin Hydrobromide, 1699·3
Hydrochinonum, 1148·1
Hydrochloric Acid, 1699·1
Hydrochloric Acid, Concentrated, 1699·1
Hydrochloric Acid, Dilute, 1699·1
Hydrochloric Ether, 1376·2
Hydrochlorides of Mixed Opium Alkaloids, 74·3
Hydrochloridum Acidum, 1699·1
Hydrochlorofluorocarbons, 1236·1
Hydrochlorothiazide, 933·2
Hydrochlorothiazidum, 933·2
Hydrocil Instant, 2051·3
Hydroclean, 2051·3
Hydroclonazone, 2051·3
Hydrocobamine, 2051·3
Hydrocodeine Bitartrate, 34·3
Hydrocodeine Phosphate, 34·3
Hydrocodeinon, 2051·3
Hydrocodone, 27·3
Hydrocodone Acid Tartrate, 45·1
Hydrocodone Bitartrate, 45·1
Hydrocodone CP, 2051·3
Hydrocodone GF, 2051·3
Hydrocodone HD, 2051·3
Hydrocodone Hydrochloride, 45·1
Hydrocodone PA, 2051·3
Hydrocodone Polistirex, 45·1
Hydrocodone and Sulfonated Diethenylbenzene-ethenylbenzene Copolymer Complex, 45·1
Hydrocodone Tartrate, 45·1
Hydrocodoni Bitartras, 45·1
Hydrocoll, 2051·3
Hydrocomp, 2051·3
Hydroconchinine Hydrochloride, 937·3
Hydrocone Bitartrate, 45·1
Hydrocort, 2051·3
Hydrocort Mild, 2051·3
Hydrocortamate Hydrochloride, 1103·3
Hydrocortancyl, 2051·3
Hydrocortimycin, 2051·3

Hydrocortisone, 1103·3
$\Delta^1$-Hydrocortisone, 1108·1
Hydrocortisone Aceponate, 1105·1
Hydrocortisone Acetate, 1103·3, 1104·1
Hydrocortisone 21-Acetate, 1103·3
Hydrocortisone Bendazac, 1092·3
Hydrocortisone Buteprate, 1104·1
Hydrocortisone Butyrate, 1104·1
Hydrocortisone 17α-Butyrate, 1104·1
Hydrocortisone Butyrate Propionate, 1104·1
Hydrocortisone 17-Butyrate 21-Propionate, 1104·1
Hydrocortisone Cipionate, 1104·1
Hydrocortisone Comp, 2051·3
Hydrocortisone Cyclopentylpropionate, 1104·1
Hydrocortisone 21-(3-Cyclopentylpropionate), 1104·1
Hydrocortisone Cypionate, 1104·1
Hydrocortisone Diethylaminoacetate Hydrochloride, 1103·3
Hydrocortisone 21-(Disodium Orthophosphate), 1104·1
Hydrocortisone Glycyrrhetinate, 1105·1
Hydrocortisone Hemisuccinate, 1104·1
Hydrocortisone Hydrogen Succinate, 1104·1
Hydrocortisone 21-(Hydrogen Succinate), 1104·1
Hydrocortisone Probutate, 1104·1
Hydrocortisone Propionate, 1105·1
Hydrocortisone Sodium Phosphate, 1104·1
Hydrocortisone Sodium Succinate, 1104·1
Hydrocortisone 21-(Sodium Succinate), 1104·1
Hydrocortisone Succinate, 1104·1
Hydrocortisone Valerate, 1104·2
Hydrocortisone 17-Valerate, 1104·2
Hydrocortisoni Acetas, 1103·3
Hydrocortisoni Hydrogenosuccinas, 1104·1
Hydrocortisonum, 1103·3
Hydrocortistab, 2051·3
Hydrocortisyl, 2051·3
Hydrocortone, 2051·3
Hydrocotyle, 1144·3
*Hydrocotyle asiatica*, 1144·3
Hydrocream, 2051·3
Hydro-Crysti-12, 2051·3
Hydrocutan, 2051·3
Hydrocutan Mild, 2051·3
Hydrocyanic Acid, 1506·1
Hydroderm, 2051·3
Hydroderm HC, 2051·4
Hydrodermed, 2051·4
Hydrodexan, 2051·4
HydroDiuril, 2051·4
Hydrodolasetron, 1263·1
Hydroflumethiazide, 937·2
Hydroflumethiazidum, 937·2
Hydrofluoric Acid, 1699·2
Hydrofluoric Acid Antidote, 2051·4
Hydrofluorocarbons, 1236·2
Hydrofluroalkanes, 1236·2
Hydroflux, 2051·4
Hydroform, 2051·4
Hydro-Funga, 2051·4
Hydrog. Perox. Soln, 1182·2
Hydrogalen, 2051·4
Hydrogen-3, 1526·2
Hydrogen Arsenide, 1658·1
Hydrogen Breath Test, 1269·2
Hydrogen Cyanide, 1506·1
Hydrogen Dioxide Solution, 1182·2
Hydrogen Fluoride, 1490·1, 1699·2
Hydrogen [$N^2$-(*N*-Glycyl-L-histidyl)-L-lysinato][$N^2$-(*N*-glycyl-L-histidyl)-L-lysinato(2–)]cuprate(1–) Diacetate, 1156·1
Hydrogen Peroxide, 1182·2
Hydrogen Peroxide Concentrate, 1182·3
Hydrogen Peroxide Solution, 1182·2
Hydrogen Peroxide Solution, Dilute, 1182·2
Hydrogen Peroxide Solution (3 Per Cent), 1182·2
Hydrogen Peroxide Solution (6 Per Cent), 1182·2
Hydrogen Peroxide Solution (27 Per Cent), 1182·3
Hydrogen Peroxide Solution (30 Per Cent), 1182·3
Hydrogen Peroxide Solution, Strong, 1182·3
Hydrogen Peroxide Solution (10-Volume), 1182·2
Hydrogen Peroxide Solution (20-Volume), 1182·2
Hydrogen Peroxide Solution (100-Volume), 1182·3
Hydrogen Peroxide Topical Solution, 1182·2
Hydrogen Sulfide, 1236·2
Hydrogen Sulphide, 1236·2
Hydrogen [1,4,7,10-Tetraazacyclododecane-1,4,7,10-tetraaceto(4–)]gadolinate(1–), 1062·3
Hydrogen [1,4,7,10-Tetrakis(carboxylatomethyl)-1,4,7,10-tetra-azacyclododecane-$\kappa^4N$]gadolinate(1–), 1062·3
Hydrogenated Castor Oil, 1668·2
Hydrogenated Castor Oils, Polyoxyl, 1414·3
Hydrogenated Cottonseed Oil, 1676·1, 1676·2
Hydrogenated Ergot Alkaloids, 1674·1
Hydrogenated Glucose Syrup, 1439·3
Hydrogenated High Maltose-glucose Syrup, 1439·3
Hydrogenated Lanolin, 1483·2
Hydrogenated Maltose, 1439·3
Hydrogenated Oil, 1763·3
Hydrogenated Polyoxyl Castor Oil, 1414·3
Hydrogenated Soybean Oil, 1447·2
Hydrogenated Vegetable Oil, 1763·3
Hydrogenated Wool Fat, 1483·1
Hydrogenii Peroxidati, Solutio, 1182·3
Hydrogenii Peroxidi, Liquor, 1182·2
Hydrogenii Peroxidum, 1182·2, 1182·3
Hydrogesic, 2051·4
Hydro-GP, 2051·4
Hydroheal Algin, 2051·4
Hydroheal Colloid, 2051·4
Hydroheal Gel, 2051·4
α-Hydro-ω-hydroxypoly(oxyethylene)poly(oxypropylene)poly(oxyethylene) Block Copolymer, 1414·1
Hydrol, 2051·4
Hydrolac, 2051·4
Hydro-Less, 2051·4
Hydrolid, 2051·4
Hydro-long, 2051·4
Hydrolotion, 2051·4
Hydrolysed Gelatin, 755·2
Hydromedin, 2051·4
Hydromet, 2051·4
Hydromol, 2051·4
Hydromorph, 2051·4
Hydromorphone Hydrochloride, 45·2
Hydromorphoni Hydrochloridum, 45·2
Hydromox, 2052·1
Hydromycin, 2052·1
Hydron CP, 2052·1
Hydron EX, 2052·1
Hydron KGS, 2052·1
Hydron PSC, 2052·1
Hydronet, 2052·1
Hy-Drop, 2052·1
Hydropane, 2052·1
Hydropel, 2052·1
Hydroperite, 1195·3
Hydroperoxyeicosatetraenoic Acids, 1511·1
Hydrophed, 2052·1
Hydrophil, 2052·1
Hydrophilic, 2052·1
Hydrophobia— *see* Rabies, 1636·2
Hydroplus, 2052·1
Hydropres, 2052·1
Hydroquinidine Alginate, 937·3
Hydroquinidine Hydrochloride, 937·3
Hydroquinine Hydrobromide, 1699·3
Hydroquinone, 1148·1
Hydroquinone Monobenzyl Ether, 1154·2
Hydroquinone Monomethyl Ether, 1151·3
Hydro-rapid, 2052·1
Hydros G, 2052·1
HydroSaluric, 2052·1
Hydro-Serp, 2052·1
Hydroserpine, 2052·1
Hydrosil, 2052·1
HydroSkin, 2052·1
Hydrosol Polyvitamin BON, 2052·1
Hydrosol Polyvitamine, 2052·1
Hydrosol Polyvitamine BON, 2052·1
Hydrosone, 2052·1
Hydrotalcite, 1267·3
HydroTex, 2052·1
Hydrotricine, 2052·1
Hydrotrix, 2052·1
Hydro-Tussin DM, 2052·1
Hydro-Tussin HD, 2052·1
Hydrous Benzoyl Peroxide, 1143·2
Hydrous Citric Acid, 1673·1
Hydrous Lanolin, 1483·2
Hydrous Tripiperazine Dicitrate, 111·2
Hydrous Wool Fat, 1483·1
HydroVal, 2052·2
Hydro-Wolff, 2052·2
Hydroxin, 2052·2
Hydroxocobalamin, 1458·2
Hydroxocobalamin Acetate, 1458·2
Hydroxocobalamin Chloride, 1458·2
Hydroxocobalamin Sulfate, 1458·2
Hydroxocobalamin Sulphate, 1458·2
Hydroxocobalamini Acetas, 1458·2
Hydroxocobalamini Chloridum, 1458·2
Hydroxocobalamini Sulfas, 1458·2
Hydroxocobalaminum, 1458·2
*N*-Hydroxy MDA, 1593·3
4′-Hydroxyacetanilide, 76·2
Hydroxyacetic Acid, 1147·3
8-Hydroxyacetyl (8*S*,10*S*)-10-[(3-Amino-2,3,6-trideoxy-α-L-*lyxo*-hexopyranosyl)oxy]-6,8,11-trihydroxy-1-methoxy-7,8,9,10-tetrahydronaphthacene-5,12-dione, 547·3
3-Hydroxyacetyldaunorubicin, 547·3
Hydroxyaethyltheophyllinum, 785·1
β-Hydroxyalanine, 1444·3
α-Hydroxyalprazolam, 669·1
Hydroxyamfetamine Hydrobromide, 1699·3
1-Hydroxy-9-aminotetrahydroacridine, 1498·1
Hydroxyamoxapine, 705·3
7-Hydroxyamoxapine, 287·1
8-Hydroxyamoxapine, 287·1
Hydroxyamphetamine Hydrobromide, 1699·3
*N*-Hydroxyamylobarbital, 670·3
3′-Hydroxyamylobarbital, 670·3
17β-Hydroxy-5α-androstan-3-one, 1541·3
4-Hydroxyandrostenedione, 557·1
4-Hydroxyandrost-4-ene-3,17-dione, 557·1
3β-Hydroxyandrost-5-en-17-one, 1565·3
17β-Hydroxyandrost-4-en-3-one, 1569·3
17β-Hydroxyandrost-4-en-3-one Cyclopentanepropionate, 1569·3
17β-Hydroxyandrost-4-en-3-one Decanoate, 1570·1
3β-Hydroxyandrost-5-en-17-one Heptanoate, 1565·3
17β-Hydroxyandrost-4-en-3-one Heptanoate, 1570·1
3β-Hydroxyandrost-5-en-17-one Hydrogen Sulphate Sodium, 1566·1
17β-Hydroxyandrost-4-en-3-one 4-Methylpentanoate, 1570·1
17β-Hydroxyandrost-4-en-3-one 3-Phenylpropionate, 1570·1
17β-Hydroxyandrost-4-en-3-one Propionate, 1570·1
17β-Hydroxyandrost-4-en-3-one Undecanoate, 1570·1
*p*-Hydroxyanisole, 1151·3
Hydroxyanisole, Butylated, 1171·2
Hydroxyapatite, 762·1, 1699·3
4-Hydroxyatomoxetine, 1585·1
8-Hydroxyazapropazone, 20·2
2-Hydroxybenzamide, 87·3
Hydroxybenzene, 1188·1
2-Hydroxybenzenecarbodithioic Acid, 1146·1
*o*-(*p*-Hydroxybenzenesulfonamido)hippuric Acid Pivalate, 1746·3
Hydroxybenzoates, 1183·2
*p*-Hydroxybenzoic Acid, 1184·2
2-Hydroxybenzoic Acid, 1157·1
2-Hydroxybenzoic Acid 1,7,7-Trimethylbicyclo[2.2.1]hept-2-yl Ester, 21·2
4-Hydroxy-1,3-benzoxathiol-2-one, 1160·3
6-Hydroxy-1,3-benzoxathiol-2-one, 1160·3
*O*-(2-Hydroxybenzoyl)salicylic Acid, 88·1
2-Hydroxybiphenyl, 1187·2
4-Hydroxy-biphenylbutyric Acid, 39·2
3-Hydroxy-4,5-bis(hydroxymethyl)-2-methylpyridine 2-(Theophyllin-7-yl)ethyl Sulphate, 791·2
3-Hydroxy-4,5-bis(hydroxymethyl)-2-picoline Hydrochloride, 1456·3
1-[(2*S*,3*R*)-2-Hydroxyborn-3-yl]-3-*p*-tolylsulphonylurea, 331·3
1-[(2*S*,3*R*)-2-Hydroxyborn-3-yl]-3-tosylurea, 331·3
6-β-Hydroxybudesonide, 1094·2
Hydroxybupropion, 288·2
Hydroxybutanedioic Acid, 1709·2
Hydroxybutyloxide, 1680·2
Hydroxy-Cal, 2052·2
Hydroxycarbamide, 559·1
Hydroxycarbamidum, 559·1
8-Hydroxycarteolol, 880·3
Hydroxychloroquine Sulfate, 452·3
Hydroxychloroquine Sulphate, 452·3
6-Hydroxychlorzoxazone, 1393·1
1α-Hydroxycholecalciferol, 1461·2
25-Hydroxycholecalciferol, 1461·2
14-Hydroxyclarithromycin, 193·1
3β-Hydroxycompactin Sodium, 984·3
17-Hydroxycorticosterone, 1103·3
4-Hydroxycyclophosphamide, 541·3
15β-Hydroxycyproterone, 1544·3
14-Hydroxydaunomycin, 547·3
4-Hydroxydebrisoquine, 892·1
2-(10-Hydroxydecyl)-5,6-dimethoxy-3-methyl-*p*-benzoquinone, 1700·3
Hydroxydesmethylloxapine, 705·3
3-Hydroxydiazepam, 723·2
Hydroxydiclofenac, 33·1
8′-β-Hydroxydihydroergotamine, 466·2
25-Hydroxydihydrotachysterol, 1462·3
4-Hydroxy-3,5-dimethoxy-α-[(methylamino)methyl]benzyl Alcohol Hydrochloride, 902·3
(*RS*)-$N^1$-(β-Hydroxy-2,5-dimethoxyphenethyl)glycinamide Hydrochloride, 959·2
17β-Hydroxy-7α,17-dimethylestr-4-en-3-one, 1560·1
(±)-α-{[(2-Hydroxy-1,1-dimethylethyl)amino]methyl}benzyl Alcohol, 43·1
2-Hydroxy-*N*-(2,6-dimethylphenyl)nicotinamide, 51·1
11β-Hydroxy-16α,17α-dimethyl-17β-propionylandrosta-1,4-dien-3-one, 1110·1
3-Hydroxy-1,2-dimethyl-4-pyridone, 1033·1
4-Hydroxy-*NN*-dimethyltryptamine, 1736·1
5-Hydroxy-*NN*-dimethyltryptamine, 1663·2
Hydroxydiphenoxylic Acid, 1261·3
*o*-Hydroxydiphenyl, 1187·2
11-Hydroxydronabinol, 1264·2
5-Hydroxyemedastine, 433·2
6-Hydroxyemedastine, 433·2
*p*-Hydroxyephedrine Hydrochloride, 977·3
13-Hydroxyepirubicin, 550·3
1α-Hydroxyergocalciferol, 1462·1
25-Hydroxyergocalciferol, 1462·3
4-Hydroxyestazolam, 697·3
3-Hydroxyestra-1,3,5(10),7-tetraen-17-one, 1549·3
3-Hydroxyestra-1,3,5(10)-triene-16α,17β-diyl Di(hydrogen Succinate), 1552·3
3-Hydroxyestra-1,3,5(10)-trien-17-one, 1553·1
17β-Hydroxyestra-4,9,11-trien-3-one Acetate, 1573·2
17β-Hydroxyestr-4-en-3-one, 1561·2
17β-Hydroxyestr-4-en-3-one Cyclohexylpropionate, 1561·2
17β-Hydroxyestr-4-en-3-one Decanoate, 1561·2

17β-Hydroxyestr-4-en-3-one Dodecanoate, 1561·2
17β-Hydroxyestr-4-en-3-one 3-Phenylpropionate, 1561·3
17β-Hydroxyestr-4-en-3-one Sodium Sulphate, 1561·3
17β-Hydroxyestr-4-en-3-one Undecanoate, 1561·3
Hydroxyestrone Diacetate, 1556·3
Hydroxyethanoic Acid, 1147·3
β-Hydroxyethoxy-acetic Acid, 1474·2
2-(2-Hydroxyethoxy)ethyl *N*-(ααα-Trifluoro-*m*-tolyl)anthranilate, 38·1
4-(2-Hydroxyethoxy)-3-methoxycinnamic Acid, 1671·3
*N*-{6-(2-Hydroxyethoxy)-5-(*o*-methoxyphenoxy)-2-[2-(1*H*-tetrazol-5-yl)-4-pyridyl]-4-pyrimidinyl}-5-isopropyl-2-pyridinesulfonamide, 1011·1
9-[(2-Hydroxyethoxy)methyl]guanine, 626·1
9-[(2-Hydroxyethoxy)methyl]guanine Hydrochloride, L-Valine Ester, 656·1
Hydroxyethyl Cellulose, 1579·2
2-Hydroxyethyl Ether Starch, 750·1
(±)-1-Hydroxyethyl 2-Ethoxy-1-[*p*-(*o*-1*H*-tetrazol-5-ylphenyl)benzyl]-7-benzimidazolecarboxylate, 878·3
Hydroxyethyl Methylcellulose, 1579·2
Hydroxyethyl Salicylate, 44·3
2-Hydroxyethyl Salicylate, 44·3
Hydroxyethyl Starch, 750·1
2-Hydroxyethylamine, 1716·1
2-Hydroxyethylamine Compound with Oleic Acid, 1716·1
2-(2-Hydroxyethylcarbamoyl)-3-methylquinoxaline 1,4-Dioxide, 1723·1
Hydroxyethylcellulose, 1579·2
Hydroxyethylcellulosum, 1579·2
*N*-(2-Hydroxyethyl)cinnamamide, 1394·3
7-(2-Hydroxyethyl)-1,3-dimethylxanthine, 785·1
1-(2-Hydroxyethyl)-2-hydroxymethyl-5-nitroimidazole, 609·2
(2*R*,3*R*,4*R*,5*S*)-1-(2-Hydroxyethyl)-2-(hydroxymethyl)piperidine-3,4,5-triol, 343·2
1-Hydroxyethylidenedi(phosphonic Acid), 771·2
(*Z*)-(2*R*,5*R*)-3-(2-Hydroxyethylidene)-7-oxo-4-oxa-1-azabicyclo[3.2.0]heptane-2-carboxylic Acid, 193·3
2,2′-(2-Hydroxyethylimino)bis[*N*-(αα-dimethylphenethyl)-*N*-methylacetamide], 1382·1
(5*R*,6*S*)-6-[(*R*)-1-Hydroxyethyl]-3-(2-iminomethylaminoethylthio)-7-oxo-1-azabicyclo[3.2.0]hept-2-ene-2-carboxylic Acid Monohydrate, 221·1
Hydroxyethylis Salicylas, 44·3
Hydroxyethylmethylcellulose, 1579·2
Hydroxyethylmethylguanidine Phosphate, Sodium Salt, 1677·3
*N*-(2-Hydroxyethyl)-2-nitroimidazole-1-acetamide, 551·2
6-[(2-{(2-Hydroxyethyl)[3-(*p*-nitrophenyl)propyl]amino}ethyl)amino]-1,3-dimethyluracil Hydrochloride, 972·2
2,2′-(3-[*N*-(2-Hydroxyethyl)octadecylamino]propylimino)diethanol Dihydrofluoride, 1442·3
*N*-(2-Hydroxyethyl)oxamic Acid, 609·2
*N*-(2-Hydroxyethyl)palmitamide, 1725·3
10-{3-[4-(2-Hydroxyethyl)piperidino]propyl}-*NN*-dimethylphenothiazine-2-sulphonamide, 716·1
10-{3-[4-(2-Hydroxyethyl)piperidino]propyl}phenothiazin-2-yl Methyl Ketone, 716·1
7-(β-Hydroxyethyl)rutoside, 1688·2
Hydroxyethylrutosides, 1688·2
(2-Hydroxyethyl)tetradecylammonium Lactate, 1186·3
Hydroxyéthylthéophylline, 785·1
7-(2-Hydroxyethyl)theophylline, 785·1
*N*-(2-Hydroxyethyl)-2,4,6-tri-iodo-5-[2′,4′,6′-tri-iodo-3′-(*N*-methylacetamido)-5′-methylcarbamoylhippuramido]isophthalamic Acid, 1066·2
2-Hydroxyethyltrimethylammonium Chloride, 1424·3
(2-Hydroxyethyl)trimethylammonium Chloride Dihydrogen Phosphate, 1690·1
2-Hydroxyethyltrimethylammonium Hydrogen Tartrate, 1424·3
(2-Hydroxyethyl)trimethylammonium Iodide Benzilate, 486·1
(2-Hydroxyethyl)trimethylammonium Salicylate, 26·2
6β-Hydroxyflunisolide, 1101·1
7-Hydroxyfluphenazine, 700·1
2-Hydroxyflutamide, 556·3
(*Z*)-7-{(1*R*,2*R*,3*R*)-3-Hydroxy-2-[(*E*)-(3*R*)-3-hydroxy-4,4-dimethyloct-1-enyl]-5-methylenecyclopentyl}hept-5-enoic Acid, 1519·2
(±)-*p*-{1-Hydroxy-4-[4-(hydroxydiphenylmethyl)-piperidino]butyl}-α-methylhydratropic Acid Hydrochloride, 433·3
5-Hydroxy-7-(2-hydroxyethoxy)-2-[3,4-bis(2-hydroxyethoxy)phenyl]-4-oxo-4*H*-chromen-3-yl Rutinoside, 1688·3
7-{2-Hydroxy-3-[(2-hydroxyethyl)methylamino]propyl}theophylline Nicotinate, 1029·1
(±)-*erythro*-8-Hydroxy-5-(1-hydroxy-2-isopropylaminobutyl)quinolin-2(1*H*)-one Hydrochloride, 791·1
(±)-8-Hydroxy-5-[(1*R**,2*S**)-1-hydroxy-2-isopropylaminobutyl]-2-quinolone Hydrochloride, 791·1
(±)-2′-Hydroxy-5′-[(*RS*)-1-hydroxy-2-{[(*RS*)-*p*-methoxy-α-methylphenethyl]amino}ethyl]formanilide Fumarate, 786·1
5-Hydroxy-2-(3-hydroxy-4-methoxyphenyl)-4-oxo-4*H*-chromen-7-yl Rutinoside, 1688·2
4-Hydroxy-3-[4-hydroxy-3-(3-methylbut-2-enyl)benzamido]-8-methylcoumarin-7-yl 3-*O*-Carbamoyl-5,5-di-*C*-methyl-α-L-lyxofuranoside, 239·2
9-[4-Hydroxy-3-(hydroxymethyl)butyl]guanine, 651·2
17β-Hydroxy-2-hydroxymethylene-17α-methyl-5α-androstan-3-one, 1565·2
9-[2-Hydroxy-1-(hydroxymethyl)ethoxymethyl]guanine, 635·3
3-Hydroxy-5-hydroxymethyl-2-methylpyridine-4-carboxaldehyde 5′-Phosphate, 1456·3
(*E*)-7-{(1*R*,2*R*,3*R*)-3-Hydroxy-2-[(*E*)-(3*S*,5*S*)-3-hydroxy-5-methyl-1-nonenyl]-5-oxocyclopentyl}-2-heptenoic Acid, 1519·2
5-Hydroxy-2-hydroxymethyl-4-pyrone, 1151·2
7-{(1*R*,2*R*,3*R*)-3-Hydroxy-2-[(*E*)-(3*S*)-3-hydroxyoct-1-enyl]-5-oxocyclopentyl}heptanoic Acid, 1512·3
(*Z*)-7-{(1*R*,2*R*,3*R*)-3-Hydroxy-2-[(*E*)-(3*S*)-3-hydroxyoct-1-enyl]-5-oxocyclopentyl}hept-5-enoic Acid, 1515·1
(*Z*)-5-{(3a*R*,4*R*,5*R*,6a*S*)-5-Hydroxy-4-[(*E*)-(3*S*)-3-hydroxyoct-1-enyl]perhydrocyclopenta[*b*]furan-2-ylidene}valeric Acid, 1516·3
(*Z*)-7-{(1*R*,2*R*,3*R*)-3-Hydroxy-2-[(*E*)-(3*R*)-3-hydroxy-4-phenoxybut-1-enyl]-5-oxocyclopentyl}-*N*-(methylsulphonyl)hept-5-enamide, 1520·3
*N*-{2-[2-Hydroxy-3-(4-hydroxyphenoxy)propylamino]ethyl}morpholine-4-carboxamide Fumarate, 1029·1
6-Hydroxy-2-(*p*-hydroxyphenyl)benzo[*b*]thien-3-yl-*p*-(2-piperidinoethoxy)phenyl Ketone Hydrochloride, 1568·3
(*R*)-4-(1-Hydroxy-2-[4-(4-hydroxyphenyl)butylamino]ethyl)pyrocatechol Hydrochloride, 864·2
(1-Hydroxy-2-imidazol-1-ylethylidene)diphosphonic Acid, 776·2
2-Hydroxyiminomethyl-1-methylpyridinium, 1050·1
2-[2-Hydroxy-3-(2-indol-3-yl-1,1-dimethylethylamino)propoxy]benzonitrile Hydrochloride, 877·1
4-Hydroxy-3-iodo-5-nitrobenzonitrile, 110·3
[4-(4-Hydroxy-3-iodophenoxy)-3,5-di-iodophenyl]acetic Acid, 1604·3
(2*S*,3*R*)-*N*[1]-Hydroxy-3-isobutyl-*N*[4]-[(*S*)-α-(methylcarbamoyl)phenethyl]-2-(2-thienylthiomethyl)succinamide, 529·2
4′-(1-Hydroxy-2-isopropylaminoethyl)methanesulphonanilide Hydrochloride, 1001·3
7-[2-Hydroxy-3-(isopropylamino)propoxy]-2-benzofuranyl Methyl Ketone Hydrochloride, 867·1
8-[2-Hydroxy-3-(isopropylamino)propoxy]-3-chromanol 3-Nitrate, 973·2
2-{*p*-[2-Hydroxy-3-(isopropylamino)propoxy]phenyl}acetamide, 865·2
4-(2-Hydroxy-3-isopropylaminopropoxy)-2,3,6-trimethylphenyl Acetate, 955·3
3-Hydroxy-1-isopropyl-5,6-indolinedione 5-Semicarbazone, 469·2
Hydroxyitraconazole, 402·3
Hydroxylamine Dapsone, 204·1
*N*-Hydroxylaminoglutethimide, 527·1
Hydroxylapatite, 1699·3
3-Hydroxylevobupivacaine, 1377·1
5-Hydroxyl-lansoprazole, 1270·1
Hydroxyloxapine, 705·3
Hydroxyloxapine-*N*-oxide, 705·3
Hydroxylucanthone Methanesulphonate, 105·3
5′-*O*-{3-Hydroxy-3-[2-(2-mercaptoethylcarbamoyl)ethylcarbamoyl]-2,2-dimethylpropyl}adenosine-3′-dihydrogenphosphate-5′-trihydrogendiphosphate, 1674·3
7-Hydroxymethotrexate, 571·2
4-Hydroxy-3-methoxybenzaldehyde, 1763·1
2-Hydroxy-4-methoxybenzophenone, 1154·3
4-Hydroxy-3-methoxymandelic Acid, 854·1
2-Hydroxy-4-methoxy-4′-methylbenzophenone, 1154·2
(±)-5-(1-Hydroxy-2-{[2-(*o*-methoxyphenoxy)ethyl]amino}ethyl)-*o*-toluenesulphonamide Hydrochloride, 862·3
2-Hydroxy-3-(2-methoxyphenoxy)propyl Carbamate, 1395·1
(±)-4-[2-Hydroxy-3-(*o*-methoxyphenoxy)propyl]-1-piperazineaceto-2′,6′-xylidide Dihydrochloride, 994·2
*N*-[(4-Hydroxy-3-methoxyphenyl)methyl]nonanamide, 67·2
3-Hydroxymethyl Mefenamic Acid, 55·3
Hydroxymethyl 2-Propylvalerate Pivalate, 380·1
*erythro*-*p*-Hydroxy-α-[1-(methylamino)ethyl]benzyl Alcohol Hydrochloride, 977·3
3-(1-Hydroxy-2-methylaminoethyl)methanesulphonanilide Methanesulphonate, 1115·1
(*RS*)-4-[1-Hydroxy-2-(methylamino)ethyl]-*o*-phenylene Dipivalate Hydrochloride, 1681·2
17β-Hydroxy-17α-methylandrosta-1,4-dien-3-one, 1559·3
17β-Hydroxy-1α-methyl-5α-androstan-3-one, 1559·1
17β-Hydroxy-17α-methylandrost-4-en-3-one, 1559·3
17β-Hydroxy-1-methyl-5α-androst-1-en-3-one Acetate, 1559·2
17β-Hydroxy-1-methyl-5α-androst-1-en-3-one Heptanoate, 1559·3
(5′*S*)-12′-Hydroxy-2′-methyl-5′-benzylergotaman-3′,6′,18-trione Tartrate, 467·2
(+)-(5*Z*,7*E*,20*S*)-20-(3-Hydroxy-3-methylbutoxy)-9,10-secopregna-5,7,10(19)-triene-1α,3β-diol, 1462·1
Hydroxymethylcimetidine, 1257·3
7-Hydroxy-4-methylcoumarin, 1700·1
3-(Hydroxymethyl)-5,5-diphenylhydantoin, Disodium Phosphate (Ester), 361·3
(Hydroxymethylene)diphosphonic Acid, 773·3
17β-Hydroxy-11-methylene-18-homo-19-nor-17α-pregn-4-en-20-yn-3-one, 1554·1
2-Hydroxymethylethisterone, 1545·3
17-Hydroxymethylethisterone, 1545·3
*N*-[(*S*)-2-Hydroxy-1-methylethyl]-D-lysergamide Hydrogen Maleate, 1684·1
4-(1-Hydroxy-1-methylethyl)-2-propyl-1-{[2′-(1*H*-tetrazol-5-yl)[1,1′-biphenyl]-4-yl]methyl}-1*H*-imidazole-5-carboxylic Acid, 975·3
3-Hydroxy-3-methylglutaric Acid, 952·1
3-Hydroxy-1-methyl-5,6-indolinedione Semicarbazone, 745·1
4-Hydroxy-2-methyl-*N*-(5-methyl-2-thiazolyl)-2*H*-1,2-benzothiazine-3-carboxamide 1,1-Dioxide, 56·1
1-Hydroxymethyl-3-methyl-2-thiourea, 1187·1
2-Hydroxy-3-methylnaphtho-1,4-hydroquinone 2-(4-Aminobenzoate), 741·3
Hydroxymethylnicotinamide, 1700·1
*N*-Hydroxymethylnicotinamide, 1700·1
(7*R*)-7-[(*R*)-2-(4-Hydroxy-6-methylnicotinamido)-2-(4-hydroxyphenyl)acetamido]-3-(1-methyl-1*H*-tetrazol-5-ylthiomethyl)-3-cephem-4-carboxylic Acid, 178·2
Hydroxymethylnitrofurantoin, 237·2
3-Hydroxymethyl-1-(5-nitrofurfurylideneamino)hydantoin, 237·2
17-Hydroxy-6-methyl-19-norpregna-4,6-diene-3,20-dione Acetate, 1562·1
17β-Hydroxy-7α-methyl-19-nor-17α-pregn-5(10)-en-20-yn-3-one, 1572·3
17β-Hydroxy-17α-methyl-2-oxa-5α-androstan-3-one, 1565·1
(−)-1-[(2*R*,5*S*)-2-(Hydroxymethyl)-1,3-oxathiolan-5-yl]cytosine, 648·2
[(7-Hydroxy-4-methyl-2-oxo-2*H*-1-benzopyran-6-yl)oxy]acetate Sodium, 1714·1
[1-Hydroxy-3-(methylpentylamino)propylidene]diphosphonic Acid, 772·3
3-Hydroxymethylphenazone, 82·3
7-[2-(β-Hydroxy-α-methylphenethylamino)ethyl]theophylline Hydrochloride, 878·2
L-3-(β-Hydroxy-α-methylphenethylamino)-3′-methoxypropiophenone Hydrochloride, 978·2
4-Hydroxy-α-methylphenylalanine, 956·1
5-[1-Hydroxy-2-(1-methyl-3-phenylpropylamino)ethyl]salicylamide Hydrochloride, 943·3
17α-Hydroxy-6-methylpregna-4,6-diene-3,20-dione Acetate, 1558·2
11β-Hydroxy-6α-methylpregn-4-ene-3,20-dione, 1106·1
17α-Hydroxy-6α-methylpregn-4-ene-3,20-dione Acetate, 1557·2
11β-Hydroxy-6α-methylprogesterone, 1106·1
*N*-[(*S*)-1-(Hydroxymethyl)propyl]-D-lysergamide Hydrogen Maleate, 1714·2
*N*-[1-(Hydroxymethyl)propyl]-1-methyl-D-lysergamide, 469·3
3-Hydroxymethylpyridine, 966·1
*N*-Hydroxymethylpyridine-3-carboxamide, 1700·1
3-Hydroxy-*N*-methylpyridinium, 1496·2
4-Hydroxy-2-methyl-*N*-(2-pyridyl)-2*H*-1,2-benzothiazine-3-carboxamide 1,1-Dioxide, 84·2
6-Hydroxymethyl-2-pyridylmethyl 2-(4-Chlorophenoxy)-2-methylpropionate, 984·1
4-Hydroxy-2-methyl-*N*-(2-pyridyl)-2*H*-thieno[2,3-*e*][1,2]thiazine-3-carboxamide 1,1-Dioxide, 93·1
α-(4-Hydroxy-2-methyl-5-sulfobenzyl)-ω-(4-hydroxy-5-sulfo-*o*-tolyl)poly[(4-hydroxy-2-methyl-5-sulfo-*m*-phenylene)methylene], 1190·1
5-(Hydroxymethyl)-3-*m*-tolyl-2-oxazolidinone, 318·2
(5′*S*)-12′-Hydroxy-2′-methyl-3′,6′,18-trioxo-5-benzylergotaman (+)-Tartrate, 467·2
8-Hydroxymianserin, 307·2
1-Hydroxymidazolam, 708·1
9-Hydroxyminocycline, 232·3
Hydroxymycin Sulphate, 612·3
Hydroxynalidixic Acid, 234·3
2-Hydroxy-1,4-naphthoquinone, 1705·2
Hydroxynaphthoquinone Antimalarials, 444·1
3-Hydroxy-4-(1-naphthyloxy)butyramide Oxime Hydrochloride, 963·3
Hydroxynefazodone, 310·1
4-Hydroxy-3-nitrophenylarsonic Acid, 1740·3
(*RS*)-4-Hydroxy-3-[1-(4-nitrophenyl)-3-oxobutyl]coumarin, 848·3
Hydroxynorephedrine Bitartrate, 952·2

17β-Hydroxy-19-nor-17α-pregna-4,9,11-trien-20-yn-3-one, 1564·3
17α-Hydroxy-19-norpregn-4-ene-3,20-dione Hexanoate, 1556·2
17β-Hydroxy-19-nor-17α-pregn-4-en-3-one, 1562·2
17β-Hydroxy-19-nor-17α-pregn-4-en-20-yn-3-one, 1562·2
17β-Hydroxy-19-nor-17α-pregn-5(10)-en-20-yn-3-one, 1563·1
17β-Hydroxy-19-nor-17α-pregn-4-en-20-yn-3-one Acetate, 1562·2
17β-Hydroxy-19-nor-17α-pregn-4-en-20-yn-3-one Heptanoate, 1562·2
10-Hydroxynortriptyline, 310·3
16α-Hydroxyoestrone Diacetate, 1556·3
Hydroxy-omeprazole, 1280·1
17-Hydroxy-3-oxo-19-nor-17α-pregna-4,9-diene-21-nitrile, 1548·1
3β-Hydroxy-11-oxo-olean-12-en-30-oic Acid, 36·2
3β-Hydroxy-11-oxo-olean-12-en-30-oic Acid, Aluminium Salt, 1264·3
Hydroxyoxophenylbutylcoumarin, Sodium Salt, 1022·2
17-Hydroxy-3-oxo-17α-pregna-4,6-diene-21-carboxylic Acid γ-Lactone, 879·1
4-Hydroxy-2-oxo-1-pyrrolidineacetamide, 1725·2
6α-Hydroxypaclitaxel, 578·2
4-Hydroxyphenazone, 82·3
γ-Hydroxyphenbutazone, 84·1
4-Hydroxyphenethylamine Hydrochloride, 1760·1
*erythro*-2-(4-Hydroxyphenethylamino)-1-(4-hydroxyphenyl)propan-1-ol Hydrochloride, 1739·2
2-[6-(β-Hydroxyphenethyl)-1-methyl-2-piperidyl]acetophenone Hydrochloride, 1589·1
(*S*)-1-(4-Hydroxyphenoxy)-3-isopropylaminopropan-2-ol Hydrochloride, 986·3
*N*-(4-Hydroxyphenyl)acetamide, 76·2
2-Hydroxy-2-phenylacetic Acid, 228·3
{6*R*-[6α,7β(*R**)]}-7-[(Hydroxyphenylacetyl)amino]-3-{[(1-methyl-1*H*-tetrazol-5-yl)thio]methyl}-8-oxo-5-thia-1-azabicyclo[4.2.0]oct-2-ene-2-carboxylic Acid, 169·3
Hydroxyphenylbutazone, 76·1
(*RS*)-5-{1-Hydroxy-2-[6-(4-phenylbutoxy)hexylamino]ethyl}salicyl Alcohol 1-Hydroxy-2-naphthoate, 795·1
*cis*-2-Hydroxy-2-phenylcyclohexanecarboxylic Acid, 1671·2
2-(1-Hydroxy-4-phenylcyclohexyl)butyric Acid, 1687·1
[((2*S*)-2-{[(3*R*,4*R*)-4-(3-Hydroxyphenyl)-3,4-dimethylpiperidin-1-yl]methyl}-3-phenylpropanoyl)amino]acetic Acid, 1250·2
(7*R*)-7-(α-D-4-Hydroxyphenylglycylamino)-3-methyl-3-cephem-4-carboxylic Acid Monohydrate, 167·2
(6*R*)-6-[α-D-(4-Hydroxyphenyl)glycylamino]penicillanic Acid, 155·3
7-(D-4-Hydroxyphenylglycylamino)-3-[(*E*)prop-1-enyl]cephem-4-carboxylic Acid Monohydrate, 179·2
(7*R*)-7-(α-D-4-Hydroxyphenylglycylamino)-3-(1*H*-1,2,3-triazol-4-ylthiomethyl)-3-cephem-4-carboxylate Propylene Glycol, 170·3
(7*R*)-7-(α-D-4-Hydroxyphenylglycylamino)-3-(1*H*-1,2,3-triazol-4-ylthiomethyl)-3-cephem-4-carboxylic Acid, 170·3
(1*R*)-1-(3-Hydroxyphenyl)-2-methylaminoethanol, 1126·3
(*RS*)-1-(4-Hydroxyphenyl)-2-(methylamino)ethanol, 977·3
1-(4-Hydroxyphenyl)-2-(1-methyl-2-phenoxyethylamino)propan-1-ol Hydrochloride, 1702·2
1-(4-Hydroxyphenyl)-2-(1-methyl-3-phenylpropylamino)propan-1-ol Hydrochloride, 1663·2
1-(4-*m*-Hydroxyphenyl-1-methyl-4-piperidyl)propan-1-one Hydrochloride, 51·1
(±)-4-{2-[3-(4-Hydroxyphenyl)-1-methylpropylamino]ethyl}pyrocatechol Hydrochloride, 905·3
5-(4-Hydroxyphenyl)-5-phenylhydantoin, 375·1
4-Hydroxy-3-(1-phenylpropyl)coumarin, 981·3
4-Hydroxyphenylretinamide, 553·1
4-[3-Hydroxy-3-phenyl-3-(2-thienyl)propyl]-4-methylmorpholinium Iodide, 489·3
4-[3-Hydroxy-3-phenyl-3-(2-thienyl)propyl]-4-methyl-morpholinium Methylsulphate, 489·3
3-Hydroxyphenyltrimethylammonium, 1493·1
1-[(*S*)-3-Hydroxy-2-(phosphonomethoxy)propyl]-cytosine, 629·2
Hydroxypiperaquine, 444·1
10-[3-(4-Hydroxypiperidino)propyl]phenothiazine-2-carbonitrile, 714·1
5′-Hydroxypiroxicam, 85·1
16-α-Hydroxyprednisolone, 1094·2
16-Hydroxyprednisolone 16,17-Acetonide, 1096·3
3α-Hydroxy-5α-pregnane-11,20-dione, 1296·3
21-Hydroxypregn-4-ene-3,20-dione 21-Acetate, 1097·1
17α-Hydroxypregn-4-ene-3,20-dione Hexanoate, 1556·3
21-Hydroxypregn-4-ene-3,20-dione 21-Pivalate, 1097·1
Hydroxyprogesterone Acetate, 1557·1
Hydroxyprogesterone Caproate, 1556·3
Hydroxyprogesterone Enantate, 1557·1
Hydroxyprogesterone Hexanoate, 1556·3
5-Hydroxypropafenone, 989·2
2-Hydroxypropane-1,2,3-tricarboxylic Acid, 1673·1
2-Hydroxy-1,2,3-propanetricarboxylic Acid Triethyl Ester, 1757·3
2-Hydroxypropionic Acid, 1704·1
4-*N*-(*N*-Hydroxypropionylanilino) Piperidine, 41·1
17β-[(*S*)-2-Hydroxypropionyl]-17α-methylestra-4,9-dien-3-one, 1573·3
4-Hydroxypropranolol, 990·1
Hydroxypropyl Cellulose, 1579·2
Hydroxypropyl Cellulose, Low-substituted, 1579·3
Hydroxypropyl Methylcellulose, 1579·3
Hydroxypropyl Methylcellulose Phthalate, 1579·3
3-Hydroxypropyl Nicotinate 2-(4-Chlorophenoxy)-2-methylpropionate, 996·1
2′-(2-Hydroxy-3-propylaminopropoxy)-3-phenylpropiophenone Hydrochloride, 988·3
α-Hydroxypropylbenzene, 1731·1
Hydroxypropylbetadex, 1678·2
Hydroxypropylbetadexum, 1678·2
Hydroxypropylcellulose, 1579·2
Hydroxypropylcellulosum, 1579·2
2-Hydroxypropyl-β-cyclodextrin, 1678·2
7-(2-Hydroxypropyl)-1,3-dimethylxanthine, 791·2
Hydroxypropylmethylcellulose, 1579·3
(±)-[10-(2-Hydroxypropyl)-1,4,7,10-tetraazacyclododecane-1,4,7-triacetato(3−)]gadolinium, 1062·3
7-(2-Hydroxypropyl)theophylline, 791·2
(−)-3-[(3-Hydroxypropyl)thio]-L-alanine, 1121·3
5-Hydroxypyrazinoic Acid, 247·3
[1-Hydroxy-2-(3-pyridinyl)ethylidene]diphosphonic Acid, 774·3
5-[α-Hydroxy-α-(2-pyridyl)benzyl]-7-[α-(2-pyridyl)benzylidene]-8,9,10-trinorborn-5-ene-2,3-dicarboximide, 1507·3
4-Hydroxy-4′-(2-pyridylsulphamoyl)azobenzene-3-carboxylic Acid, 1291·1
Hydroxyquinoline Benzoate, 1700·1
Hydroxyquinoline Borate, 1700·1
Hydroxyquinoline Hydrofluoride, 1700·1
Hydroxyquinoline, Indium ($^{111}$In), 1523·3
Hydroxyquinoline Iodochloride, 1700·1
Hydroxyquinoline Salicylate, 1700·1
Hydroxyquinoline Silicofluoride, 1700·1
Hydroxyquinoline Sulfate, 1700·1
Hydroxyquinoline Sulphate, 1700·1
Hydroxyquinoline Sulphate, Potassium, 1734·2
Hydroxyquinolines, Halogenated, 120·2
Hydroxyquinone Methyl Ether, 1151·3
*all-trans*-4′-Hydroxyretinanilide, 553·1
14-Hydroxy-3β-(α-L-rhamnopyranosyloxy)-14β-bufa-4,20,22-trienolide, 990·3
5-Hydroxy-1-β-D-ribofuranosylimidazole-4-carboxamide, 1360·3
9-Hydroxyrisperidone, 720·1
4′-Hydroxysalicylanilide, 1725·1
Hydroxystearin Sulfate, 1575·3
Hydroxysuccinic Acid, 1709·2
3-Hydroxytamoxifen, 550·1
*N*-Hydroxytenamfetamine, 1593·3
Hydroxytetrabenazine, 1752·2
Hydroxytetracycline, 241·1
5β-Hydroxytetracycline, 241·1
4-Hydroxy-3-(1,2,3,4-tetrahydro-1-naphthyl)coumarin, 1502·3
4-Hydroxy-3-[1,2,3,4-tetrahydro-3-[4-(4-trifluoromethylbenzyloxy)phenyl]-1-naphthyl]coumarin, 1505·3
(±)-*all-rac*-5-{*p*-[(6-Hydroxy-2,5,7,8-tetramethyl-2-chromanyl)methoxy]benzyl}-2,4-thiazolidinedione, 348·2
11-Hydroxy-6,7,10,12-tetramethyl-1-oxo-10-vinylperhydro-3a,7-pentanoinden-8-yl (2-Diethylaminoethylthio)acetate Hydrogen Fumarate, 270·2
5-Hydroxythiabendazole, 114·3
Hydroxytoluene, Butylated, 1171·3
2-Hydroxy-*p*-toluenesulfonic Acid, Polymer with Formaldehyde, 1190·1
Hydroxytriamterene Sulfate, 1017·1
3-Hydroxy-4-trimethylammoniobutyrate, 1423·3
(*R*)-3-Hydroxy-4-trimethylammoniobutyrate, 1423·3
4-Hydroxy-α,α,4-trimethylcyclohexanemethanol Monohydrate, 1131·1
5,5′-[(2-Hydroxytrimethylene)bis(acetylimino)]bis[*N*,*N*′-bis(2,3-dihydroxypropyl)-2,4,6-triiodoisophthalamide], 1063·3
*NN*-(2-Hydroxytrimethylene)bis(trimethylammonium) Di-iodide, 1603·1
17β-Hydroxy-19,21,24-trinorchola-4,9,11,22-tetraen-3-one, 1541·3
5-Hydroxytryptamine, 1743·2
L-5-Hydroxytryptophan, 311·1
3-Hydroxytyramine Hydrochloride, 907·1
3-Hydroxy-L-tyrosine, 1205·2
Hydroxyurea, 559·1
1α-Hydroxyvitamin $D_2$, 1462·1
1α-Hydroxyvitamin $D_3$, 1461·2
25-Hydroxyvitamin $D_3$, 1461·2
Hydroxyzine Embonate, 434·3
Hydroxyzine Hydrochloride, 434·3
Hydroxyzine Pamoate, 434·3
Hydroxyzini Hydrochloridum, 434·3
Hydrozide, 2052·2
Hydrozide Plus, 2052·2
Hydrozole, 2052·2
Hyetellose, 1579·2
Hyfac, 2052·2
Hyfac AHA, 2052·2
Hyfac Plus, 2052·2
Hyflex, 2052·2
Hy-GAG, 2052·2
Hygeol, 2052·2
Hygienist, 2052·2
Hygienist Pavimenti E Piastrelle, 2052·2
Hygine In, 2052·2
Hygiodermil, 2052·2
Hygraphen, 1182·2
Hygromycin B, 105·3
Hygroton, 2052·2
Hygroton-Reserpina, 2052·2
Hygroton-Reserpine, 2052·2
Hy-KXP, 2052·2
*Hyla caerulea*, 1669·2
Hylaform, 2052·2
Hylak, 2052·2
Hylak Forte, 2052·2
Hylak Forte N, 2052·3
Hylak N, 2052·3
Hylak Plus, 2052·3
Hylakombun, 2052·3
Hylands Preparations, 2052·3
Hylans, 1697·3
Hylase, 2052·3
Hylashield, 2052·3
Hylo-COMOD, 2052·3
Hylo-Comod, 2052·3
Hylocomod, 2052·3
Hylorel, 2052·3
Hylutin, 2052·3
Hymecromone, 1700·1
Hymecromone Sodium, 1700·2
Hymecromonum, 1700·1
Hymed, 2052·3
Hymenolepiasis, 99·2
Hymetellose, 1579·2
Hyneurin, 2052·3
Hynidase, 2052·3
HYO, 483·3
Hyomide, 2052·3
Hyoscal, 2052·3
Hyoscine, 479·1, 483·3, 485·2, 489·2
Hyoscine Borate, 484·2
Hyoscine Butylbromide, 483·3
Hyoscine Hydrobromide, 483·3
Hyoscine Hydrochloride, 484·2
Hyoscine Methobromide, 483·3
Hyoscine Methonitrate, 483·3
Hyoscine Methylbromide, 483·3
Hyoscine Methylnitrate, 483·3
Hyoscine Oxide Hydrobromide, 484·2
Hyoscine-*N*-butyl Bromide, 483·3
Hyoscine-*N*-(cyclopropylmethyl) Bromide, 480·2
Hyoscini Butylbromidum, 483·3
Hyoscini Hydrobromidum, 483·3
Hyoscy., 485·2
Hyoscyami, 485·2
Hyoscyamine, 479·1, 485·1, 489·2
*l*-Hyoscyamine, 485·1
(−)-Hyoscyamine, 485·1
(±)-Hyoscyamine, 476·3
Hyoscyamine Bromhydrate, 485·1
Hyoscyamine Hydrobromide, 485·1
Hyoscyamine Sulfate, 485·1
Hyoscyamine Sulphate, 485·1
Hyoscyamini Sulfas, 485·1
Hyoscyaminum Sulfuricum, 485·1
Hyoscyamus, 485·2
Hyoscyamus Leaf, 485·2
*Hyoscyamus niger*, 485·2
Hyosmed, 2052·3
Hyosophen, 2052·3
Hyospan, 2052·3
Hyospasmol, 2052·3
Hyostan, 2052·3
Hyozin, 2052·3
Hypace, 2052·3
Hypadil, 2052·3
Hypam, 2052·3
Hypan, 2052·3
Hypanthium Rosae, 1740·1
Hypaque, 2052·3
Hypaque 60%, 2052·4
Hypaque 76%, 2052·4
Hypaque-76— *see* Hypaque-M, Hypaque-76, 2052·4
Hypaque-M, 2052·4
Hypen, 2052·4
Hyperab, 2052·4
Hyperactivity, 1583·1
Hyperalgesia, 2·1
Hyperamine, 2052·4
Hyperammonaemia, 1421·2
Hyperbaric Oxygen, 1237·2
Hypercal, 2052·4
Hypercalcaemia, 1218·1
Hypercalcaemia of Malignancy, 1218·1
Hypercalcaemia, Vitamin-D Mediated— *see* Vitamin D-mediated Hypercalcaemia, 1218·2
Hypercalcio, 2052·4
Hypercapnia— *see* Respiratory Failure, 1237·3
Hypercard, 2052·4
Hypercholesterolaemia— *see* Hyperlipidaemias, 823·1
Hypercidin, 2052·4
Hypercrit, 2052·4
Hyperdine, 2052·4
Hyperdix, 2052·4
Hyperemesis Gravidarum— *see* Nausea and Vomiting, 1245·2

Hypereosinophilic Syndrome, 552·2
Hyperesa, 2052·4
Hyperforat, 2052·4
Hyperforat-forte, 2052·4
Hyperforin, 299·2, 299·3
Hypergel, 2052·4
Hyperglycaemia— *see* Diabetes Mellitus, 324·1
Hyperglycaemic Nonketotic Coma, Hyperosmolar— *see* Diabetic Emergencies, 328·2
Hyperglycaemic State, Hyperosmolar— *see* Diabetic Emergencies, 328·2
Hyperglycinaemia, Nonketotic— *see* Nonketotic Hyperglycinaemia, 1750·2
HyperHAES, 2052·4
HyperHep, 2052·4
HyperHep— *see* BayHep B, 1830·1
Hyperhes, 2052·4
Hyperhidrosis, 1136·1
Hypericaps, 2052·4
Hypericettes, 2052·4
Hyperici Herba, 299·1
Hypericin, 299·1
Hyperico, 2052·4
Hypericum, 299·1
Hypericum for Homoeopathic Preparations, 299·1
Hypericum Oil, 299·3
*Hypericum perforatum*, 299·1
Hypericum Perforatum ad Praeparationes Homoeopathicas, 299·1
Hyperiforce, 2052·4
Hyperiforce Comp, 2052·4
Hyperiforte, 2052·4
Hyperilex, 2053·1
HyperiMed, 2053·1
Hyperimerck, 2053·1
Hyperimmune Bovine Colostrum, 1611·1
Hyperiplant, 2053·1
Hyperium, 2053·1
Hyperkalaemia, 1219·2
Hyperkalaemic Periodic Paralysis, 1219·3
Hyperkeratosis— *see* Keratinisation Disorders, 1136·2
Hyperkinesis— *see* Hyperactivity, 1583·1
Hyperkinetic Syndrome— *see* Hyperactivity, 1583·1
Hyperlipen, 2053·1
Hyperlipidaemias, 823·1
Hyperlipoproteinaemias— *see* Hyperlipidaemias, 823·1
Hyperlite, 2053·1
Hyperlyte, 2053·1
Hypermagnesaemia, 1218·3
Hypermol, 2053·1
Hypernatraemia, 1220·2
Hypernol, 2053·1
Hyperoside, 1660·3, 1665·2, 1677·1, 1717·1, 1748·3
Hyperosmolar Hyperglycaemic Nonketotic Coma— *see* Diabetic Emergencies, 328·2
Hyperosmolar Hyperglycaemic State— *see* Diabetic Emergencies, 328·2
Hyperosmotic Laxatives, 1239·3
Hyperoxaluria, Primary— *see* Primary Hyperoxaluria, 1457·3
Hyperparathyroid Bone Disease— *see* Renal Osteodystrophy, 764·3
Hyperparathyroidism, 765·1
Hyperpathia, 2·1
Hyperphen, 2053·1
Hyperphosphataemia, 1219·1
Hyperpigmentation— *see* Pigmentation Disorders, 1137·2
Hyperprolactinaemia, 1315·2
Hyperprotidine, 2053·1
Hyperpur, 2053·1
Hyperpyrexia— *see* Fever and Hyperthermia, 8·2
Hyperpyrexia, Malignant— *see* Malignant Hyperthermia, 1394·2
HyperRab— *see* BayRab, 1830·1
Hyperretic, 2053·1
Hypersensitivity, Food— *see* Food Allergy, 422·1
Hypersensitivity Reactions— *see* Hypersensitivity, 419·2
Hypersensitivity Syndrome— *see* Drug-induced Skin Reactions, 1134·3
Hypersensitivity Vasculitis, 1081·3
Hypersol, 2053·1
Hypersol B, 2053·1
Hyperstat, 2053·1
Hypertension, 825·1
Hypertension in Diabetic Patients— *see* Hypertension, 825·1
Hypertension, Intracranial— *see* Raised Intracranial Pressure, 833·1
Hypertension, Isolated Systolic— *see* Hypertension, 825·1
Hypertension, Ocular— *see* Glaucoma and Ocular Hypertension, 1485·1
Hypertension in Pregnancy— *see* Hypertension, 825·1
Hypertension, Pulmonary— *see* Pulmonary Hypertension, 832·1
Hypertension in Renal Disease— *see* Hypertension, 825·1
Hypertension, Renovascular— *see* Hypertension, 825·1
Hypertensive Crises— *see* Hypertension, 825·1
Hyper-Tet, 2053·1
Hyper-Tet— *see* BayTet, 1830·1
Hyperthermia— *see* Fever and Hyperthermia, 8·2
Hyperthermia, Malignant— *see* Malignant Hyperthermia, 1394·2
Hyperthyroidism, 1594·3
Hypertonalum, 2053·1
Hypertorr, 2053·1
Hypertriglyceridaemia— *see* Hyperlipidaemias, 823·1
Hyperuricaemia— *see* Gout and Hyperuricaemia, 412·1
Hyperval, 2053·1
Hypery, 2053·1
Hyphed, 2053·1
Hy-Phen, 2053·1
Hyphylline, 784·3
Hypnagogic Hallucinations— *see* Narcoleptic Syndrome, 1583·2
Hypnasmine, 2053·1
Hypnodorm, 2053·1
Hypnol, 2053·1
Hypnomidate, 2053·1
Hypnor, 2053·1
Hypnorex, 2053·2
Hypnotex, 2053·2
Hypnotics, 663·1
Hypnovel, 2053·2
Hypo Tears, 2053·2
Hypoca, 2053·2
Hypocaina, 2053·2
Hypocalcaemia, 1218·3
Hypochlorous Acid, 1164·3
Hypochondriasis, 664·3
Hypochromic Anaemia, 732·1
Hypochylin, 2053·2
Hypodermoclysis, 1698·2
Hypodyn, 2053·2
Hypogammaglobulinaemia— *see* Primary Antibody Deficiency, 1629·2
Hypogeusia— *see* Taste Disorders, 682·2
Hypoglycaemia, Insulin-induced, 335·3
Hypoglycin A, 1700·2
Hypogonadism, 1316·1
Hypoguard, 2053·2
Hypoguard Supreme Plus, 2053·2
Hypokalaemia, 1219·3
Hypokalaemic Nephropathy— *see* Hypokalaemia, 1219·3
Hypokalaemic Periodic Paralysis, 1220·1
Hypol, 2053·2
Hypolac, 2053·2
Hypolar Retard, 2053·2
Hypomagnesaemia, 1219·1
Hypomania, 278·1
Hypomed, 2053·2
Hypomide, 2053·2
Hyponatraemia, 1220·3
Hypoparathyroidism, 765·2
Hypopharyngeal Carcinoma— *see* Malignant Neoplasms of the Head and Neck, 517·3
Hypophosphataemia, 1219·2
Hypophosphataemic Rickets, X-linked— *see* Osteomalacia, 762·3
Hypophosphatasia— *see* Osteomalacia, 762·3
Hypophosphorosum, Acidum, 1700·2
Hypophosphorous Acid, 1700·2
Hypophysis Cerebri Pars Posterior, 1337·3
Hypophysis Sicca, 1337·3
Hypopigmentation— *see* Pigmentation Disorders, 1137·2
Hyposedon N, 2053·2
Hyposensitisation, 1650·2
Hyposplenism, Infection Prophylaxis— *see* Spleen Disorders, 146·3
Hypostamin, 2053·2
Hypostamine, 2053·2
Hypotears, 2053·2
Hypotears E, 2053·2
Hypotears PF, 2053·2
Hypotears Plus, 2053·2
Hypoten, 2053·3
Hypotens, 2053·3
Hypotension, 828·1
Hypotension, Neurally Mediated— *see* Hypotension, 828·1
Hypotension, Orthostatic— *see* Orthostatic Hypotension, 1100·2
Hypotension, Postural— *see* Orthostatic Hypotension, 1100·2
Hypotensor, 2053·3
Hypothalamic Factors, 1312·1
Hypothalamic and Pituitary Hormones, 1312·1
Hypothalamic Regulatory Hormones, 1312·1
Hypothyroid Coma— *see* Hypothyroidism, 1595·3
Hypothyroidism, 1595·3
Hypothyroidism, Congenital— *see* Hypothyroidism, 1595·3
Hypothyroidism, Neonatal— *see* Hypothyroidism, 1595·3
Hypothyroidism, Subclinical— *see* Hypothyroidism, 1595·3
Hy-Po-Tone, 2053·3
Hypotonie-Gastreu R44, 2053·3
Hypovase, 2053·3
Hypovolaemic Shock— *see* Shock, 835·1
Hypoxaemia— *see* Respiratory Failure, 1237·3
Hypoxanthine Arabinoside, 657·1
Hypoxanthine Riboside, 1701·2
Hypren, 2053·3
Hypren Plus, 2053·3
Hyprenan, 2053·3
HypRho-D, 2053·3
HypRho-D— *see* BayRho-D, 1830·1
Hyprolose, 1579·2
Hypromellose, 1579·3
Hypromellose Phthalate, 1579·3
Hypromellosi Phthalas, 1579·3
Hypromellosum, 1579·3
Hyprosia, 2053·3
Hyprosin, 2053·3
Hyprosol, 2053·3
Hypurin Preparations, 2053·3
Hyrexin, 2053·3
Hyrin, 2053·3
Hyruan, 2053·3
Hyrvalan, 2053·3
Hysan, 2053·3
Hyseke, 2053·3
Hyskon, 2053·3
Hysone, 2053·3
Hysopan, 2053·4
Hy-Spa, 2053·4
Hysteria— *see* Conversion and Dissociative Disorders, 696·2
Hysterical Paralysis— *see* Conversion and Dissociative Disorders, 696·2
Hysticlar, 2053·4
Hytacand, 2053·4
Hytakerol, 2053·4
Hyteneze, 2053·4
Hythalton, 2053·4
Hytic, 2053·4
Hytinic, 2053·4
Hytisone, 2053·4
Hytone, 2053·4
Hytos Plus, 2053·4
Hytrast, 2053·4
Hytrin, 2053·4
Hytrin BPH, 2053·4
Hytrine, 2053·4
Hytrinex, 2053·4
Hytuss, 2053·4
Hyzaar, 2053·4
Hyzan, 2053·4
Hyzum N, 2053·4

**I**

I, 1438·2
I-612, 996·1
I-653, 1297·2
Ial, 2053·4
Ialect, 2053·4
Ialugen, 2053·4
Ialugen Plus, 2053·4
Ialum, 2054·1
Ialurex, 2054·1
Ialuset, 2054·1
Iamara, 1722·3
Iamin, 2054·1
Iamin Hydrating Gel, 2054·1
Iba-Cide, 2054·1
Ibacitabina, 637·3
Ibacitabine, 637·3
Ibamoxil, 2054·1
Ibandronate Sodium, 772·3
Ibandronato Sódico, 772·3
Ibandronic Acid, 772·3
Ibandrónico, Ácido, 772·3
Ibaril, 2054·1
Ibaril Med Salicylsyra, 2054·1
Ibaril Med Salicylsyre, 2054·1
Ibarin, 2054·1
Ibdazol, 2054·1
Ibenon, 2054·1
Ibenzmethyzin Hydrochloride, 581·2
Ibercal, 2054·1
Iberet, 2054·1
Iberet-Folic, 2054·1
Iberin Folico, 2054·1
Iberogast, 2054·1
Iberol, 2054·1
Iberol Folico, 2054·1
Iberol Simple, 2054·2
Ibexone, 2054·2
Ibiamox, 2054·2
Ibidomide Hydrochloride, 943·3
Ibifen, 2054·2
Ibilex, 2054·2
Ibimicyn, 2054·2
Ibimycin, 2054·2
Ibis, 2054·2
Iboflam, 2054·2
Ibogaina, 1700·2
Ibogaine, 1700·2
Ibopain, 2054·2
Ibopamina, Hidrocloruro de, 937·3
Ibopamine, 937·3
Ibopamine Hydrochloride, 937·3
Ibotenic Acid, 1717·3
Ibritumomab Tiuxetan, 560·1
Ibritumomab Tiuxetan, Indium ($^{111}$In), 1524·1
Ibritumomab Tiuxetan, Yttrium ($^{90}$Y), 1526·3
Ibrofen, 2054·2
Ibrufhalal, 2054·2
IBS Relief, 2054·2
IB-Stat, 2054·2
Ibtrim, 2054·2
Ibu Preparations, 2054·2
Ibualgic, 2054·2
Ibu-Attritin, 2054·2
Ibubest, 2054·2
Ibubeta, 2054·2
Ibu-Buscapina, 2054·2
Ibucler, 2054·2
Ibudilast, 786·3
Ibudol, 2054·2
Ibudolofrix, 2054·2
Ibudolor, 2054·2

Ibudristan, 2054·2
Ibudros, 2054·3
Ibufabra, 2054·3
Ibufac, 2054·3
Ibufem, 2054·3
Ibufen, 2054·3
Ibufen-L, 2054·3
Ibufix, 2054·3
Ibuflam, 2054·3
Ibuflamar-P, 2054·3
Ibuflex, 2054·3
Ibufran, 2054·3
Ibufug, 2054·3
Ibugan, 2054·3
Ibugel, 2054·3
Ibugesic, 2054·3
Ibugesic Plus, 2054·3
Ibugesic-M, 2054·3
Ibuhexal, 2054·3
Ibu-Lady, 2054·3
Ibulan, 2054·3
Ibular, 2054·3
Ibuleve, 2054·3
Ibuloid, 2054·3
Ibumac, 2054·3
Ibumar, 2054·3
Ibumar Migra, 2054·3
Ibumax, 2054·3
Ibumed, 2054·3
Ibumerck, 2054·4
Ibumetin, 2054·4
Ibumousse, 2054·4
Ibunet, 2054·4
Ibu-Novalgina, 2054·4
Ibupax, 2054·4
Ibupen, 2054·4
Ibuphlogont, 2054·4
Ibupirac, 2054·4
Ibupirac Compuesto, 2054·4
Ibupirac Fem, 2054·4
Ibupirac Flex, 2054·4
Ibupirac Migra, 2054·4
Ibupiretas, 2054·4
Ibupril, 2054·4
Ibuprin, 2054·4
Ibuprof, 2054·4
Ibuprofan, 2054·4
Ibuprofen, 45·3, 46·1
*R*-(−)-Ibuprofen, 46·3
*S*-(+)-Ibuprofen, 46·1
Ibuprofen Aminoethanol, 47·1
Ibuprofen Guaiacol, 47·1
Ibuprofen Isobutanolammonium, 47·1
Ibuprofen Lysine, 47·1
Ibuprofen Meglumine, 47·1
Ibuprofen Pyridoxine, 47·1
Ibuprofen Sodium, 47·1
Ibuprofeno, 45·3
Ibuprofenum, 45·3
Ibuprohm, 2054·4
Ibupron, 2054·4
Ibuprox, 2054·4
Ibuproxam, 47·2
Ibu-Proxyvon, 2054·4
Ibu-ratiopharm, 2054·4
Iburem, 2054·4
Iburen, 2054·4
Ibureumin, 2054·4
Ibusal, 2054·4
Ibuscent, 2054·4
Ibusi, 2054·4
Ibusifar, 2054·4
Ibuslow, 2055·1
Ibu-Slow, 2055·1
Ibuspray, 2055·1
Ibustrin, 2055·1
Ibusumal, 2055·1
Ibu-Tab, 2055·1
Ibutab, 2055·1
Ibutad, 2055·1
Ibutenk, 2055·1
Ibu-Tetralgin, 2055·1
Ibutilida, Fumarato de, 938·1
Ibutilide Fumarate, 938·1
Ibutin, 2055·1
Ibutop, 2055·1
Ibutop Cuprofen, 2055·1
Ibutop Ralgex, 2055·1
Ibu-Vivimed, 2055·1
Ibux, 2055·1
Ibuxin, 2055·1
Ibuzidine, 2055·1
IC-351, 1751·1
IC Green, 2055·1
Icaden, 2055·1
Icaps, 2055·1
Icaps Plus, 2055·1
Icar, 2055·1
Icar Prenatal, 2055·1
Icar-C Plus, 2055·1
Icatibant, 761·3, 844·1
Icavex, 2055·1
Icaz, 2055·1
ICC-1132, 1622·3
Ice, 1589·2
Ice Cool Stress & Tension Relief, 2055·1
Ice, Dry, 1235·2
Ice Gel, 2055·2
Ice Gel Therapy, 2055·2
Ice Hockey Lung— *see* Respiratory Disorders, 1087·1
Ice Lipbalm, 2055·2
Icespray, 2055·2
Icetazol, 2055·2
Ic-Gel, 2055·2
ICG-Pulsion, 2055·2
Ichor— *see* Ixor, 2070·1
Ichthalgan, 2055·2
Ichthalgan Forte, 2055·2
Ichthammol, 1148·2
Ichthammolum, 1148·2
Ichtho-Bad, 2055·2
Ichtho-Bellol, 2055·2
Ichtho-Bellol Compositum S, 2055·2
Ichtho-Cadmin, 2055·2
Ichtho-Cortin, 2055·2
Ichthocortin, 2055·2
Ichthoderm, 2055·2
Ichth-Oestren, 2055·2
Ichtholan, 2055·2
Ichtholan Spezial, 2055·2
Ichtholan T, 2055·2
Ichthopaste, 2055·2
Ichthoseptal, 2055·2
Ichthosin, 2055·2
Ichthosulphol, 1148·2
Ichthraletten, 2055·2
Ichthyol, 1148·2, 2055·2
Ichthyolammonium, 1148·2
Ichthyol-Natrium Hell, 1148·3
*Ichthyomethia piscipula*, 1702·3
Ichthyosis, 1136·1
Ichtopur, 2055·2
Icht-Oral, 2055·2
Ichtyosoft, 2055·2
ICI-9073, 1190·1
ICI-28257, 884·3
ICI-32525, 263·2
ICI-35868, 1305·3
ICI-45520, 989·3
ICI-46474, 584·1
ICI-46683, 111·2
ICI-48213, 1544·1
ICI-50123, 1729·3
ICI-50627, 114·1
ICI-55052, 607·2
ICI-58834, 323·3
ICI-59118, 582·2
ICI-59623, 107·2
ICI-66082, 865·2
ICI-80996, 1514·3
ICI-118587, 1029·1
ICI-118630, 1326·3
ICI-156834, 177·1
ICI-176334, 530·1
ICI-182780, 557·3
ICI-194660, 229·1
ICI-204219, 807·1
ICI-204636, 718·2
ICI-213689, 229·2
ICI-D1033, 528·1
ICI-D1694, 582·1
ICN-1229, 652·1
Icodextrin, 1427·1
Icodextrina, 1427·1
Icodial, 2055·3
Icol, 2055·3
Icolamida, 2055·3
Icoplax, 2055·3
Icoran, 2055·3
Icosapent, 976·2
Icosapento, 976·2
ICRF-159, 582·2
ICRF-187, 1036·1
ICS-205-930, 1293·3
ICSH, 1332·1
Ictage 6, 2055·3
Ictan, 2055·3
Ictasol, 1148·3
Icthaband, 2055·3
Ictholin, 2055·3
Ictiol, 1148·2
Ictiomen, 2055·3
Ictom 3, 2055·3
Ictotest, 2055·3
Ictyane, 2055·3
Ictyoderm, 2055·3
Icy Hot, 2055·3
ID-540, 698·2
Id Sedin, 2055·3
Ida, 2055·3
Ida-D, 2055·3
Idalon, 2055·3
Idalprem, 2055·3
Idamycin, 2055·3
Idaptan, 2055·3
Idarac, 2055·3
Idaralem, 2055·3
Idarrux, 2055·3
Idarubicin Hydrochloride, 560·2
Idarubicina, Hidrocloruro de, 560·2
Idarubicinol, 560·2
Idasal Nebulizador, 2055·3
Idazole, 2055·4
Idazoxan Hydrochloride, 1700·2
Idazoxano, Hidrocloruro de, 1700·2
Idc, 2055·4
IDDM— *see* Diabetes Mellitus, 324·1
Ideal Quota, Adult— *see* Adult Ideal Quota, 1777·3
Idealid, 2055·4
Idebenona, 1700·3
Idebenone, 1700·3
IDEC-102, 582·3
IDEC-129, 560·1
IDEC-152, 507·3
IDEC-C2B8, 582·3
IDEC-CE9.1, 10·2
IDEC-Y2B8, 560·1
Idecortex, 2055·4
Ideogrip, 2055·4
Ideolaxyl, 2055·4
Ideolider, 2055·4
Ideos, 2055·4
Iderpes, 2055·4
Idesole, 2055·4
Idesole Plus, 2055·4
Idicin, 2055·4
Idina, 2055·4
Idiopathic Anaphylaxis— *see* Urticaria and Angioedema, 1138·3
Idiopathic Dilated Cardiomyopathy— *see* Cardiomyopathies, 818·2
Idiopathic Pulmonary Fibrosis— *see* Diffuse Parenchymal Lung Disease, 1079·3
Idiopathic Rapidly Progressive Glomerulonephritis— *see* Glomerular Kidney Disease, 1080·2
Idiopathic Thrombocytopenic Purpura, 1082·1
Idle, 2055·4
IDM Solution, 2055·4
I-Doc, 2055·4
Ido A 50, 2055·4
Ido-C, 2055·4
Ido-E, 2055·4
Idom, 2055·4
Idomed, 2055·4
Idon, 2055·4
Idopamil, 2055·4
Idotrim, 2055·4
Idotyl, 2055·4
Idovit, 2055·4
Idoxuridina, 637·3
Idoxuridine, 637·3
Idoxuridinum, 637·3
IDR, 2055·4
Idracemi, 2055·4
Idracemi Eparina, 2056·1
Idralazina, 931·2
Idraste, 1698·3
Idratante Samil, 2056·1
Idril N Sine, 2056·1
Idro P2, 2056·1
Idrocet, 2056·1
Idrocilamida, 1394·3
Idrocilamide, 1394·3
Idrocol, 2056·1
Idrogeno Soluzione, Perossido d', 1182·3
Idrolac, 2056·1
Idrolax, 2056·1
Idrolone, 2056·1
Idroneomicil, 2056·1
Idropan B, 2056·1
Idroplurivit, 2056·1
Idropulmina, 2056·1
Idroquark, 2056·1
Idroskin, 2056·1
Idroskin C, 2056·1
Idrossocobalamina, 1458·2
Idrostamin, 2056·1
Idrovel, 2056·1
Idrum, 2056·1
IDU, 637·3
Iducher, 2056·1
Iducol, 2056·1
Iducutit, 2056·1
Idulamine, 2056·1
Idulanex, 2056·1
Idulea, 2056·1
Idu-Phor— *see* Jodosan, 2071·2
5-IDUR, 637·3
Iduridin, 2056·1
α-L-Iduronidase, 1705·1
Idustatin, 2056·1
Iduviran, 2056·1
Iduvo, 2056·1
Iecatec, 2056·2
Iecoris Aselli Oleum, 1425·2
Ietepar, 2056·2
Ifa Dex, 2056·2
Ifa Diety, 2056·2
Ifa Norex, 2056·2
Ifa Reducing S, 2056·2
Ifabla, 2056·2
Ifacap, 2056·2
Ifacil, 2056·2
Ifacur, 2056·2
Ifadac, 2056·2
Ifadox, 2056·2
Ifamet, 2056·2
Ifamit, 2056·2
Ifarab, 2056·2
Ifavac, 2056·2
Ifavin, 2056·2
Ifavor, 2056·2
Ifaxol, 2056·2
Ifecin, 2056·2
Ifemed, 2056·2
Ifenec, 2056·2
Ifenprodil Tartrate, 938·1
Ifenprodil, Tartrato de, 938·1
Ifersol, 2056·2
Ifex, 2056·2
Ificipro, 2056·2
Ifipef, 2056·2
Ifiral, 2056·2
IFN-α, 640·3
IFN-β, 645·3
IFN-γ, 647·2
IFO-cell, 2056·2
Ifocid, 2056·2
Ifocris, 2056·2
Ifolem, 2056·2
Ifomida, 2056·2

Ifos, 2056·2
Ifosfamida, 561·1
Ifosfamide, 561·1
Ifosfamidum, 561·1
Ifosmixan, 2056·3
Ifoxan, 2056·3
Ifuchol, 2056·3
Ifumelus, 2056·3
Ifupasil, 2056·3
Ifupeptol Magnesiado, 2056·3
Ifutemp, 2056·3
IFX, 2056·3
Ig Gamma, 2056·3
Ig Tetano, 2056·3
Ig Vena N, 2056·3
IgA Nephropathy— *see* Glomerular Kidney Disease, 1080·2
Igamad, 2056·3
Igantet, 2056·3
Igantibe, 2056·3
Igantid, 2056·3
Igbo, 1666·1
IgeE, 2056·3
I-Gesic, 2056·3
IGF-I, 1338·3
IGF-II, 1339·1
IGFs, 1338·3
IgG, 2056·3
Igitur-antirheumatische, 2056·3
Igitur-Rheumafluid, 2056·3
I-Glo, 2056·3
Ignatia, 1722·3
Ignatia Amara, 1722·3
Ignatia-Homaccord, 2056·3
IgRho, 2056·3
Igril, 2056·3
Igroseles, 2056·3
Igroton, 2056·3
Igroton-Lopresor, 2056·3
Igroton-Reserpina, 2056·3
Iguassina, 2056·3
IHD, 2056·4
Iiyalgon, 2056·4
IK-2, 632·1
Ikaclomin, 2056·4
Ikacor, 2056·4
Ikaflux, 2056·4
Ikapress, 2056·4
Ikaran, 2056·4
Ikatin, 2056·4
Ikatral, 2056·4
Ikatral Periferico, 2056·4
Ikeriane, 2056·4
Ikestatina, 2056·4
Iketoncid, 2056·4
Ikobel, 2056·4
Ikolan, 2056·4
Ikoplex Preparations, 2056·4
Ikorel, 2056·4
Iktorivil, 2056·4
IL-1, 1701·3
IL-2, 562·2
IL-3, 755·3
IL-4, 1701·3
IL-4R, 778·3
IL-6, 1701·3
IL-6 Antibody, 1701·3
IL-12, 1701·3
IL-5902, 255·3
IL-6001, 320·2
IL-6302, 431·3
IL-17803A, 848·1
IL-19552, 716·1
IL-22811, 56·3
Ilagane, 2056·4
Ila-med M, 2056·4
Ildamen, 2056·4
Ilduc, 2056·4
Ile, 1438·2
Iletin Lente, 2056·4
Iletin NPH, 2056·4
Iletin II Pork Lente, 2056·4
Iletin II Pork NPH, 2056·4
Iletin II Pork Regular, 2056·4
Iletin Regular, 2056·4
Ileus— *see* Decreased Gastrointestinal Motility, 1241·1
*Ilex paraguensis*, 1765·3
Ilgem, 2056·4
Ilgen, 2056·4
IL-1i, 1701·3
Iliaclor, 2056·4
Iliadin, 2057·1
Iliocin, 2057·1
Ilio-Funkton, 2057·1
Ilja Rogoff, 2057·1
Ilja Rogoff Forte, 2057·1
*Illicium verum*, 1655·2
Illings Bozner Maycur-Tee, 2057·1
Ilman, 2057·1
Iloban, 2057·1
Ilocin, 2057·1
Ilocit, 2057·1
Ilodecakin, 1700·3
Ilodecakina, 1700·3
Ilomedin, 2057·1
Ilomedine, 2057·1
Ilon Abszess, 2057·1
Ilopan, 2057·1
Ilopan-Choline, 2057·1
Iloprost, 1518·2
Iloprost Trometamol, 1518·2
Iloprost Tromethamine, 1518·2
Ilosin, 2057·1
Ilosone, 2057·1
Iloticina, 2057·1
Iloticina, Neo— *see* Neo Iloticina, 2156·3
Ilotrex, 2057·1
Ilotycin, 2057·1
Ilotycin TS, 2057·1
Ilotycin-A, 2057·1
Ilozyme, 2057·1
IL-1ra, 1701·3
Ilsatec, 2057·1
I-Lube, 2057·1
Ilube, 2057·1
Iluminoderm, 2057·2
Iluminoderm Lips, 2057·2
Iluminoderm Plus, 2057·2
Ilvico, 2057·2
Ilvico Grippal, 2057·2
Ilvico Mit Vitamin C, 2057·2
Ilvico N, 2057·2
Ilvinax, 2057·2
Ilvispect, 2057·2
Ilvitus, 2057·2
I-L-X, 2057·2
I-L-X $B_{12}$, 2057·2
IM 75, 2057·2
Imacillin, 2057·2
Imacol, 2057·2
Imacort, 2057·2
Imadrax, 2057·2
Imagent, 2057·2
Imagent GI, 2057·2
Imagopaque, 2057·2
Imanance, 2057·2
Imanol, 2057·2
Imap, 2057·3
Imaplus, 2057·3
Imatinib Mesilate, 562·1
Imatinib Mesylate, 562·1
Imavermil, 2057·3
Imazin, 2057·3
Imazol, 2057·3
Imazol Comp, 2057·3
Imbak, 2057·3
Imbrilon, 2057·3
Imbun, 2057·3
Imciromab Pentetate, Indium ($^{111}$In), 1524·1
IMD, 2057·3
Imda, 2057·3
Imdex, 2057·3
Imdur, 2057·3
Imecol, 2057·3
Imecromone, 1700·1
Imedeen, 2057·3
Imediat N, 2057·3
Imegul, 2057·3
Imepas, 2057·3
Imeron, 2057·3
Imeson, 2057·3
Imet, 2057·3
IMET-3393, 529·3
Imex, 2057·3
Imexim, 2057·3
Imferon, 2057·3
Imflac, 2057·3
IMI-28, 550·2
IMI-30, 560·2
Imidacloprid, 1506·2
Imidamine Hydrochloride, 424·2
Imidamine Mesylate, 424·2
Imidamine Phosphate, 424·2
Imidamine Sulphate, 424·2
Imidapril, Hidrocloruro de, 938·2
Imidapril Hydrochloride, 938·2
Imidaprilat, 938·2
Imidazol, Cetoglutarato de, 773·1
Imidazole Antifungals, 386·1
Imidazole Carboxamide, 544·2
Imidazole Cetoglutarate, 773·1
Imidazole α-Ketoglutarate, 773·1
Imidazole Oxoglurate, 773·1
Imidazole 2-Oxoglutarate, 773·1
Imidazole Salicylate, 47·2
(±)-2-[α-(2-Imidazolin-2-ylmethyl)benzyl]pyridine, 343·2
3-[*N*-(2-Imidazolin-2-ylmethyl)-*p*-toluidino]phenol Methanesulphonate, 982·1
2-(Imidazol-4-yl)ethylamine, 1697·1
(*E*)-*p*-(Imidazol-1-ylmethyl)cinnamic Acid, 1725·2
Imidazyl, 2057·3
Imidazyl Antistaminico, 2057·3
Imidil, 2057·4
Imidin K, 2057·4
Imidin N, 2057·4
Imidocarb Dipropionate, 606·1
Imidocarb Hydrochloride, 606·1
Imidocarbo, Dipropionato de, 606·1
Imidurea, 1184·2
Imiglucerasa, 1649·2
Imiglucerase, 1649·2
Imigran, 2057·4
Imigrane, 2057·4
Imiject, 2057·4
Imilgamma, 2057·4
Imin, 2057·4
Iminase, 2057·4
2,2′-Iminobisethanol, 1681·1
1,1′-Iminobis(propan-2-ol), 1680·2
2-Imino-5-phenyl-4-oxazolidinone, 1591·2
*N*-[Imino(phosphonoamino)-methyl]-*N*-methylglycine, 1677·2
Iminourea Hydrochloride, 1492·1
Imipem, 2057·4
Imipemide, 221·1
Imipenem, 221·1
Imipenemum, 221·1
Imipra, 2057·4
Imipram. Hydrochlor., 300·1
Imipramina, 300·1
Imipramina, Embonato de, 300·1
Imipramina, Hidrocloruro de, 300·1
Imipramine, 300·1
Imipramine Embonate, 300·1
Imipramine Hydrochloride, 300·1
Imipramine Oxide Hydrochloride, 300·2
Imipramine Pamoate, 300·1
Imipramini Chloridum, 300·1
Imipramini Hydrochloridum, 300·1
Imipraminoxide Hydrochloride, 300·2
Imiquimod, 638·1
Imitrex, 2057·4
Imizine, 300·1
Imizol, 2057·4
Immediat, 2057·4
Immignost, 2057·4
Immobilon, 38·3
Immubron, 2057·4
ImmuCyst, 2057·4
Immucytal, 2057·4
Immudynal, 2057·4
Immugrip, 2057·4
Immukin, 2057·4
Immukine, 2057·4
Immulem, 2057·4
Immumil, 2058·1
Immunace, 2058·1
Immun-Aid, 2058·1
Immunate, 2058·1
Immune Formula, 2058·1
Immune Globulin, 1627·2
Immune Globulin, Hepatitis B, 1617·3
Immune Globulin, Pertussis, 1631·2
Immune Globulin, Rabies, 1635·3
Immune Globulin, $Rh_o$ (D), 1608·1
Immune Globulin, Tetanus, 1640·3
Immune Globulin, Vaccinia, 1643·1
Immune Globulin, Varicella-Zoster, 1643·2
Immune Interferon, 647·2
Immune RNA, 1738·2
Immune-complex Nephritis— *see* Glomerular Kidney Disease, 1080·2
Immunex CRP, 2058·1
Immunine, 2058·1
Immunisation, 1605·1
Immunja, 2058·1
Immunocal, 2058·1
Immunocompromised Patients, Bacterial Infections in— *see* Infections in Immunocompromised Patients, 131·2
Immunocompromised Patients, Fungal Infections in— *see* Infections in Immunocompromised Patients, 388·2
Immunocompromised Patients, Protozoal Infections in— *see* Infections in Immunocompromised Patients, 597·1
Immunocompromised Patients, Viral Infections in— *see* Infections in Immunocompromised Patients, 624·2
Immunodeficiency Disease, Severe Combined, 1729·2
Immunoendocig, 2058·1
Immunoendozig, 2058·1
Immunoglobulin A, 1628·3
Immunoglobulin, Antithymocyte, 1348·3
Immunoglobulin, Human Normal, 1627·2
Immunoglobulin, Human Normal, for Intravenous Administration, 1627·2
Immunoglobulin, Human Rubella, 1637·3
Immunoglobulin for Human Use, Animal, Anti-T Lymphocyte, 1348·3
Immunoglobulins, 1605·2
Immunoglobulins, AIDS, 1607·3
Immunoglobulins, Anti-D, 1608·1
Immunoglobulins, Antilymphocyte, 1348·3
Immunoglobulins, Crimean-Congo Haemorrhagic Fever, 1612·1
Immunoglobulins, Cytomegalovirus, 1612·1
Immunoglobulins, Hepatitis A, 1617·1
Immunoglobulins, Hepatitis B, 1617·2
Immunoglobulins, HIV, 1607·3
Immunoglobulins, Measles, 1623·1
Immunoglobulins, Mumps, 1626·3
Immunoglobulins, Normal, 1627·2
Immunoglobulins, Pertussis, 1631·2
Immunoglobulins, Pseudomonas, 1635·2
Immunoglobulins, Rabies, 1635·3
Immunoglobulins, Respiratory Syncytial Virus, 1637·2
Immunoglobulins, Rubella, 1637·3
Immunoglobulins, Tetanus, 1640·3
Immunoglobulins, Tick-borne Encephalitis, 1642·1
Immunoglobulins, Vaccinia, 1643·1
Immunoglobulins, Varicella-Zoster, 1643·1
Immunoglobulinum Anti-T Lymphocytorum ex Animale ad Usum Humanum, 1348·3
Immunoglobulinum Humanum Anti-D, 1608·1
Immunoglobulinum Humanum Anti-D ad Usum Intravenosum, 1608·1
Immunoglobulinum Humanum Hepatitidis A, 1617·1
Immunoglobulinum Humanum Hepatitidis B, 1617·2
Immunoglobulinum Humanum Hepatitidis B ad Usum Intravenosum, 1617·3
Immunoglobulinum Humanum Morbillicum, 1623·1

Immunoglobulinum Humanum Normale, 1627·2
Immunoglobulinum Humanum Normale ad Usum Intravenosum, 1627·2
Immunoglobulinum Humanum Rabicum, 1635·3
Immunoglobulinum Humanum Rubellae, 1637·3
Immunoglobulinum Humanum Tetanicum, 1640·3
Immunoglobulinum Humanum Varicellae, 1643·1
Immunoglobulinum Humanum Varicellae ad Usum Intravenosum, 1643·1
ImmunoHBs, 2058·1
Immunokine, 2058·1
Immunomega, 2058·1
Immunomorb, 2058·1
Immunoparot, 2058·1
Immunopertox, 2058·1
Immunopret, 2058·1
Immunoprin, 2058·1
Immunorho, 2058·1
Immunoros, 2058·1
Immunosera, 1605·1
Immunoserum Botulinicum, 1610·3
Immunoserum Contra Venena Viperarum Europaearum, 1639·1
Immunoserum Diphthericum, 1612·2
Immunoserum Gangraenicum (Clostridium Novyi), 1615·3
Immunoserum Gangraenicum (Clostridium Perfringens), 1615·3
Immunoserum Gangraenicum (Clostridium Septicum), 1615·3
Immunoserum Gangraenicum Mixtum, 1616·1
Immunoserum Tetanicum ad Usum Humanum, 1640·2
Immunosuppressants, 1344·1
Immunotetan, 2058·1
Immunotrofina, 2058·1
Immunovac, 2058·1
Immunovir, 2058·1
Immunozig, 2058·1
Immunozima, 2058·1
Immutone, 2058·1
Immuwash, 2058·1
Imocap, 2058·1
Imoclone, 2058·1
Imocur, 2058·1
Imodium, 2058·2
Imodium Advanced, 2058·2
Imodium med Simethicon, 2058·2
Imodium Plus, 2058·2
Imogam, 2058·2
Imogam Rabia, 2058·2
Imogam Rabies, 2058·2
Imogam Rage, 2058·2
Imogam Tetano, 2058·2
Imosec, 2058·2
Imossel, 2058·2
Imosselduo, 2058·2
Imotab, 2058·2
Imotoran, 2058·2
Imovane, 2058·2
Imovax Preparations, 2058·2
Imovax, Rabies- — *see also* Rabies-Imovax, 2249·4
Imovexil, 2058·3
Imox, 2058·3
Imox-Clo, 2058·3
Imozop, 2058·3
Impact, 2058·3
Impaction, Faecal— *see* Constipation, 1240·2
Impaction, Oesophageal— *see* Oesophageal Motility Disorders, 1246·3
Impalamycin, 2058·3
Impalud, 2058·3
Impedil, 2058·3
Impelium, 2058·3
Impetex, 2058·3
Impetigo— *see* Skin Infections, 146·2
Impidol, 2058·3
Implanon, 2058·3
Implementor, 2058·3
Impletol, 2058·3
Implicane, 2058·3
Impore, 2058·3
Importal, 2058·3
Imposergon, 2058·3
Imposit N, 2058·3
Impotence— *see* Erectile Dysfunction, 1745·2
Impregon, 2058·3
Impresso, 2058·4
Impril, 2058·4
Impromen, 2058·4
Improntal, 2058·4
Improved Analgesic, 2058·4
Improved Once A Day, 2058·4
Improved Versal, 2058·4
Improvil, 2058·4
Impugan, 2058·4
IMS, 1186·1
Imtrate, 2058·4
Imuderm, 2058·4
Imudon, 2058·4
Imufor, 2058·4
Imuger, 2058·4
Imugins, 2058·4
Imukin, 2058·4
Imunen, 2058·4
Imuneprim, 2058·4
Imuno Max-gel, 2058·4
Imunoferon, 2058·4
Imunonutril, 2058·4
Imunoparvum, 2058·4
Imunovir, 2058·4
Imunoxa, 2058·4
Imunoxa Complex, 2058·4
Imuprel, 2059·1
Imuprin, 2059·1
Imuran, 2059·1
Imurek, 2059·1
Imurel, 2059·1
Imusporin, 2059·1
Imuvac, 2059·1
Imuvit, 2059·1
In A Wink, 2059·1
In A Wink Allergy, 2059·1
In A Wink Moisturing, 2059·1
Inabrin, 2059·1
Inabutol Forte, 2059·1
Inac, 2059·1
Inacid, 2059·1
Inacol, 2059·1
Inactivated Hepatitis A Vaccine, 1617·1
Inactivated Poliomyelitis Vaccines, 1633·3
Inadine, 2059·1
Inadol, 2059·1
INAH, 222·2
Inalacor, 2059·1
Inalador Vick, 2059·1
Inaladuo, 2059·1
Inalar, 2059·1
Inalcort, 2059·1
Inalgon Neu, 2059·2
Inalintra, 2059·2
Inalobel, 2059·2
Inalone A— *see* Becotide A, 1831·3
Inalpin, 2059·2
Inamide, 2059·2
Inamrinone, 862·3
Inapas, 2059·2
Inapsin, 2059·2
Inapsine, 2059·2
Inarub, 2059·2
Inaspir, 2059·2
Inastmol, 2059·2
Inatrex Balsamico, 2059·2
Inazid, 2059·2
Incad, 2059·2
Incadronato Disódico, 773·1
Incadronic Acid, 773·1
Incadrónico, Ácido, 773·1
Inca's Gold, 2059·2
Incena, 2059·2
Incidal, 2059·2
Incidal-OD, 2059·2
Incidin, 2059·2
Incidin Extra, 2059·2
Incidin Extra N, 2059·2
Incidin M Spray Extra, 2059·2
Incidin Perfekt, 2059·2
Incidin Plus, 2059·2
Incidin Spezial, 2059·2
Incidine, 2059·2
Incidur, 2059·2
Incidur Spray, 2059·3
Incontinence, Urinary— *see* Urinary Incontinence and Retention, 476·1
Incontinol, 2059·3
Inconturina, 2059·3
Incoril, 2059·3
Incremin, 2059·3
Incremin con Hierro, 2059·3
Incremin Iron, 2059·3
Incremin with Iron, 2059·3
Incremin with Vitamin C, 2059·3
Incutin, 2059·3
Ind. Podoph., 1155·2
Indacar, 2059·3
Indaco, 2059·3
Indaflex, 2059·3
Indahexal, 2059·3
Indalapril Hydrochloride, 892·2
Indalgin, 2059·3
Indalix, 2059·3
Indalone, 1501·1
Indamol, 2059·3
Indanazolina, Hidrocloruro de, 1122·3
Indanazoline Hydrochloride, 1122·3
Indanedione Anticoagulants, 810·1
Indanorm, 2059·3
*cis*-4-{1-[(*S*)-2-(Indan-5-yloxycarbonyl)-3-(2-methoxyethoxy)propyl]cyclopentylcarbonylamino}cyclohexanecarboxylic Acid, 879·1
Indapamida, 938·2
Indapamide, 938·2
Indapamide Hemihydrate, 939·1
Indapamidum, 938·2
Indapress, 2059·3
Inda-Puren, 2059·3
Indarzona-N, 2059·3
Indeloxazina, Hidrocloruro de, 1700·3
Indeloxazine Hydrochloride, 1700·3
Indenolol, Hidrocloruro de, 939·1
Indenolol Hydrochloride, 939·1
Indenyloxyisopropylaminopropanol Hydrochloride, 939·1
(±)-2-[(Inden-7-yloxy)methyl]morpholine Hydrochloride, 1700·3
Inderal, 2059·3
Inderal Comp, 2059·4
Inderal, Half— *see* Half Inderal, 2035·2
Inderalici, 2059·4
Inderetic, 2059·4
Inderex, 2059·4
Inderide, 2059·4
Inderm, 2059·4
Indermil, 2059·4
Indian Blistering Beetle, 1667·1
Indian Brandee, 2059·4
Indian Dill, 1680·2
Indian Frankincense, 1690·1
Indian Hemp, 1666·1
Indian Liquorice, 1645·1
Indian Melissa Oil, 1706·3
Indian Olibanum, 1690·1
Indian Opium, 74·3
Indian Pennywort, 1144·3
Indian Plantago, 1268·1
Indian Podophyllum, 1155·2
Indian Podophyllum Rhizome, 1155·2
Indian Psyllium, 1268·1
Indian Rhubarb, 1287·3
Indian Saffron, 1058·3
Indian Squill, 1130·3
Indian Tobacco, 1589·1
Indian Tragacanth, 1290·2
Indian Verbena Oil, 1706·3
Indianische Frauenwurzel, 2059·4
Indiaral, 2059·4
India-Rubber, 1741·1
Indican, 2059·4
Indicarminum, 1700·3
Indicatest, 2059·4
Indigestion, 2059·4
Indigestion— *see* Dyspepsia, 1242·1
Indigestion Complex, 2059·4
Indigestion and Flatulence, 2059·4
Indigestion and Flatulence Tablets, 2059·4
Indigestion Mixture, 2059·4
Indigestion Relief, 2059·4
Indigestion Relief Liquid, 2059·4
Indigestion Relief Tablets, 2059·4
Indigestion Tablets, 2059·4
Indigo Carmine, 1700·3
Indigon, 2059·4
Indigotina, 1700·3
Indigotindisulfonate Sodium, 1700·3
Indigotine, 1700·3
Indilea, 2059·4
Indinavir Sulfate, 638·2
Indinavir, Sulfato de, 638·2
Indinavir Sulphate, 638·2
Indinax, 2059·4
Indio 111, 1523·3
Indio 113M, 1524·1
Indirect Anticoagulants, 810·1
Indische-hennepkruid, 1666·1
Indisk Hampa, 1666·1
Indispensable Amino Acids, 1417·1
Indium-111, 1523·3
Indium ($^{111}$In) Altumomab Pentetate, 1524·1
Indium ($^{111}$In) Bleomycin, 1524·1
Indium ($^{111}$In) Capromab Pendetide, 1524·1
Indium Chloride ($^{111}$In), 1524·1
Indium ($^{111}$In) Hydroxyquinoline, 1523·3
Indium ($^{111}$In) Ibritumomab Tiuxetan, 1524·1
Indium ($^{111}$In) Imciromab Pentetate, 1524·1
Indium ($^{111}$In) Pentetate, 1523·3
Indium ($^{111}$In) Pentetreotide, 1524·1
Indium ($^{111}$In) Satumomab Pendetide, 1524·1
Indium-113m, 1524·1
Indium ($^{113m}$In) Colloid, 1524·1
Indium ($^{113m}$In) Pentetate, 1524·1
Indivina, 2060·1
Indo, 2060·1
Indo Framan, 2060·1
Indo Top, 2060·1
Indoarginine, 49·1
Indobene, 2060·1
Indobiotic, 2060·1
Indobloc, 2060·1
Indo-bros, 2060·1
Indobufen, 939·1
Indobufen Sodium, 939·1
Indocaf, 2060·1
Indocalm, 2060·1
Indocap, 2060·1
Indocarsil, 2060·1
Indochron, 2060·1
Indocid, 2060·1
Indocid, Chrono- — *see* Chrono-Indocid, 1885·1
Indocid Colirio, 2060·1
Indocid PDA, 2060·1
Indocin, 2060·1
Indocolir, 2060·1
Indocollirio, 2060·1
Indocollyre, 2060·1
Indocontin, 2060·2
Indocyanine Green, 1701·1
Indofeno, 2060·2
Indoflam, 2060·2
Indoftol, 2060·2
Indogel, Adco- — *see* Adco-Indogel, 1775·3
Indogesic, 2060·2
Indohexal, 2060·2
Indolar SR, 2060·2
Indolgina, 2060·2
Indolin, 2060·2
*N*-[1-(2-Indol-3-ylethyl)-4-piperidyl]benzamide Hydrochloride, 939·2
1-(Indol-4-yloxy)-3-isopropylaminopropan-2-ol, 983·2
Indom, 2060·2

Indoman, 2060·2
Indomax, 2060·2
Indomed, 2060·2
Indomee, 2060·2
Indomelan, 2060·2
Indomen, 2060·2
Indo-Mepha, 2060·2
Indomet, 2060·2
Indometacin, 47·3
Indometacin Farnesil, 49·1
Indometacin Sodium, 47·3
Indometacina, 47·3
Indometacina Sódica, 47·3
Indometacinum, 47·3
Indometacinum-mp, 2060·2
Indomethacin, 47·3
Indomethacin Sodium, 47·3
Indomethacin Sodium Trihydrate, 47·3
Indometin, 2060·2
Indomet-ratiopharm, 2060·2
Indomet-ratiopharm M, 2060·2
Indomisal, 2060·2
Indomod, 2060·2
Indon, 2060·2
Indonet, 2060·3
Indonilo, 2060·3
Indono, 2060·3
Indo-paed, 2060·3
Indo-Phlogont, 2060·3
Indophtal, 2060·3
Indoptic, 2060·3
Indoptol, 2060·3
Indoramin Hydrochloride, 939·2
Indoramina, Hidrocloruro de, 939·2
Indorektal, 2060·3
Indosan, 2060·3
Indospray, 2060·3
Indostad, 2060·3
Indo-Tablinen, 2060·3
Indotard, 2060·3
Indotec, 2060·3
Indotex, 2060·3
Indotrin, 2060·3
Indovis, 2060·3
Indoxen, 2060·3
Induced Abortion— *see* Termination of Pregnancy, 1512·2
Inducmina, 2060·3
Inductal, 2060·3
Induction of Anaesthesia— *see* Anaesthesia, 1296·1
Induction of Labour— *see* Labour Induction and Augmentation, 1511·1
Inductol, 2060·3
InductOs, 2060·3
Induken, 2060·3
Indulfan, 2060·3
Indulfan Plus, 2060·3
Indurgan, 2060·3
Indusil, 2060·3
Indusil T, 2060·3
Industrial Methylated Spirit, 1186·1
Industrial Methylated Spirit (Ketone-free), 1186·1
Industrial Methylated Spirits, 1185·3
Ineltano, 2060·3
Inesfay, 2060·4
Inespecin, 2060·4
Inexbron, 2060·4
Inexbron Mucolitico, 2060·4
Inexfal, 2060·4
Inexium, 2060·4
INF, 2060·4
INF-1837, 43·2
INF-3355, 55·2
INF-4668, 55·1
Infacol, 2060·4
Infa-C-Vit, 2060·4
Infaderm, 2060·4
Infadrops, 2060·4
Infafren Simple, 2060·4
Infalgina, 2060·4
Infalivina, 2060·4
Infalyte, 2060·4
Infanolyte, 2060·4
Infanrix Preparations, 2060·4
Infanrix Polio— *see* Infanrixtetra, 2061·1
Infanrix Polio-Hib— *see also* Infanrix-quinta, 2061·1
Infanrixhexa, 2061·1
Infanrixquinta, 2061·1
Infanrixtetra, 2061·1
Infant Calm, 2061·1
Infant Colic— *see* Gastrointestinal Spasm, 1242·2
Infant Gaviscon, 2061·1
Infant, Gaviscon— *see* Gaviscon Infant, 2018·2
Infant Multiple Vitamin, 2061·1
Infant Tonic, 2061·1
Infantaire, 2061·1
Infantile Malignant Osteopetrosis— *see* Osteopetrosis, 1085·2
Infantile Spasms— *see* Epilepsy, 349·1
Infantol, 2061·1
Infantoss, 2061·1
Infants, Pain in— *see* Choice of Analgesics in Children, 3·2
Infant's Tylenol, 2061·1
Infants Tylenol Cold Decongestant & Fever Reducer, 2061·1
Infantussin N, 2061·1
Infapain, 2061·1
Infapain Forte, 2061·2
Infarction, Cerebral— *see* Stroke, 836·1
Infarction, Myocardial— *see* Myocardial Infarction, 828·2
Infasoy, 2061·2
Infasoy Progress, 2061·2
Infasurf, 2061·2
Infa-Tardyferon, 2061·2
Infatrini, 2061·2
Infazinc, 2061·2
Infecteracin, 2061·2
Infectious Mononucleosis— *see* Epstein-Barr Virus Infections, 620·1
Infectious Polyneuropathy, Acute— *see* Guillain-Barré Syndrome, 1630·2
InfectoBicillin, 2061·2
InfectoBicillin H, 2061·2
InfectoCef, 2061·2
InfectoCillin, 2061·2
Infectoclont, 2061·2
Infectocortikrupp, 2061·2
Infectodiarrstop GG, 2061·2
InfectoDyspept, 2061·2
Infectoflam, 2061·2
InfectoFlu, 2061·2
InfectoFos, 2061·2
Infectogripp— *see* InfectoFlu, 2061·2
InfectoKrupp, 2061·2
InfectoMox, 2061·2
InfectoMycin, 2061·2
InfectoPedicul, 2061·2
Infectoroxit, 2061·2
InfectoSoor, 2061·2
Infectoss, 2061·2
InfectoStaph, 2061·2
InfectoTop, 2061·2
InfectoTrimet, 2061·2
Infectracina, 2061·3
Infectrin, 2061·3
Infectrin Balsamico, 2061·3
INFeD, 2061·3
Infekt-Komplex Ho-Fu-Complex, 2061·3
Infenol, Natusor— *see* Natusor Infenol, 2154·1
Infepan, 2061·3
Inferax, 2061·3
Infergen, 2061·3
Inferil, 2061·3
Inferno, 489·2
Infertility, 1316·1
Infesol, 2061·3
Infex, 2061·3
Infibran, 2061·3
Infi-China, 2061·3
Infidyston, 2061·3
Infi-Echinacea, 2061·3
Infifer, 2061·3
Infihepan, 2061·3
Infiltran B12, 2061·3
Infiltration Anaesthesia, 1370·1
Infi-Lymphect, 2061·3
Infiossan, 2061·3
Infi-Symphytum, 2061·3
Infi-tract, 2061·3
Infla-Ban, 2061·3
Inflaced, 2061·3
Inflacor, 2061·3
Infladase, 2061·3
Infladerm, 2061·3
Infladoren, 2061·4
Inflalid, 2061·4
Inflam, 2061·4
Inflamac, 2061·4
Inflamase, 2061·4
Inflamase IdroGel, 2061·4
Inflamate, 2061·4
Inflamax, 2061·4
Inflamene, 2061·4
Inflammatory Bowel Disease, 1243·3
Inflammatory Polyneuropathy, Acute Idiopathic— *see* Guillain-Barré Syndrome, 1630·2
Inflammide, 2061·4
Inflanac, 2061·4
Inflanan, 2061·4
Inflanaze, 2061·4
Inflanefran, 2061·4
Inflanegent, 2061·4
Inflanox, 2061·4
Inflaren, 2061·4
Inflax, 2061·4
Inflazone, 2061·4
Inflexal, 2061·4
Inflexal S, 2061·4
Infliximab, 50·1
Infloran, 2061·4
Infloxa, 2061·4
Influ-A, 2061·4
Influaforce, 2061·4
Influamin, 2062·1
Influbene, 2062·1
Influbene C, 2062·1
Influbene N, 2062·1
Infludo, 2062·1
Influenza, 624·2
Influenza and Tetanus Vaccines, 1641·3
Influenza Vaccine (Split Virion, Inactivated), 1620·2
Influenza Vaccine (Surface Antigen, Inactivated), 1620·2
Influenza Vaccine (Surface Antigen, Inactivated, Virosome), 1620·2
Influenza Vaccine (Whole Virion, Inactivated), 1620·2
Influenza Vaccines, 1620·2
Influenza Virus Vaccine, 1620·3
Influenzine, 2062·1
Influex, 2062·1
Influk, 2062·1
Influpiol C, 2062·1
Influpozzi, 2062·1
Influrem, 2062·1
Influsplit, 2062·1
Influsplit SSW, 2062·1
Influtruw, 2062·1
Influtux, 2062·1
Influvac, 2062·1
Influvac S, 2062·1
Influvac Sub-Unit, 2062·1
Influvidon, 2062·1
Influvirus, 2062·1
Influvit, 2062·1
Influ-Zinc, 2062·1
Influ-Zinc Gola, 2062·1
Inf-Oph, 2062·1
Infosan, 2062·1
Infostat, 2062·1
Infraline, 2062·1
Inframin, 2062·1
Infrarub, 2062·1
Infree, 2062·2
Infrotto Ultra, 2062·2
Infufer, 2062·2
Infukoll, 2062·2
Infukoll HES, 2062·2
Infukoll M 40, 2062·2
Infumal, 2062·2
Infumix, 2062·2
Infumorph, 2062·2
Infusorial Earth, Purified, 1581·3
Infuvite, 2062·2
Ingafol, 2062·2
Ingagen-M, 2062·2
Ingastri, 2062·2
Ingelan, 2062·2
Ingram Regimen, 1160·1
Ingro, 2062·2
Ingrown Toe Nail Salve, 2062·2
Ingwer, 1267·1
INH, 222·2
Inhacort, 2062·2
Inhadrina, 2062·2
Inhalador, 2062·2
Inhalador Medex, 2062·2
Inhalante Yatropan, 2062·2
Inhalation Analgesics, 3·1
Inhalene, 2062·2
Inhaler, Vicks— *see* Vicks Inhaler, 2375·3
Inhalosam, 2062·2
Inhelthran, 2062·2
Inhepar, 2062·2
Inhibac, 2062·2
Inhibace, 2062·3
Inhibace Comp, 2062·3
Inhibace Plus, 2062·3
Inhibidor de la C1 Esterasa, 1675·2
Inhibidor de la $\alpha_1$- Proteinasa, 1651·2
Inhibidores de la ECA, 842·3
Inhibidores del Complemento, 1675·2
Inhibin, 1701·2, 2062·3
Inhibina, 1701·2
Inhibisam, 2062·3
Inhibitron, 2062·3
Inhibostamin, 2062·3
Inhiston, 2062·3
Inibace, 2062·3
Inibace Plus, 2062·3
Inib-Dor, 2062·3
Inibex S, 2062·3
Inibina, 2062·3
Inicox, 2062·3
Inimur, 2062·3
Inimur Myko, 2062·3
Inipomp, 2062·3
Iniprol, 2062·3
Inistolin Antitusivo Ped, 2062·3
Inistolin Expectoran Ped, 2062·3
Iniston, 2062·3
Iniston Antitusivo, 2062·3
Iniston Expectorante, 2062·3
Initard— *see* Mixtard, 2137·2
Initiss, 2062·3
Initiss Plus, 2062·3
Injectio Lymphatica N EKF, 2062·3
Injection Site Disinfection— *see* Injection Site and Catheter Care, 1165·2
Ink Cap, 1717·3
Inkamil, 2062·3
Inmunoartro, 2062·3
Inmunobalt, 2062·4
Inmunoferon, 2062·4
Inmunoglobulinas, 1605·2
Inmunoglobulinas Anti-D, 1608·1
Inmunoglobulinas Antilinfocitarias, 1348·3
Inmunoglobulinas contra el Citomegalovirus, 1612·1
Inmunoglobulinas contra el Sarampión, 1623·1
Inmunoglobulinas contra el SIDA, 1607·3
Inmunoglobulinas contra el Tétanos, 1640·3
Inmunoglobulinas contra el Virus de la Vacuna, 1643·1
Inmunoglobulinas contra el Virus de la Varicela Zóster, 1643·1
Inmunoglobulinas contra el Virus Sincitial Respiratorio, 1637·2
Inmunoglobulinas contra la Fiebre Hemorrágica de Congo-Crimea, 1612·1
Inmunoglobulinas contra la Hepatitis A, 1617·1
Inmunoglobulinas contra la Hepatitis B, 1617·2

Inmunoglobulinas contra la Parotiditis, 1626·3
Inmunoglobulinas contra la Rabia, 1635·3
Inmunoglobulinas contra la Rubéola, 1637·3
Inmunoglobulinas contra la Tos Ferina, 1631·2
Inmunoglobulinas contra Pseudomonas, 1635·2
Inmunoglobulinas de la Encefalitis Transmitida Por Garrapatas, 1642·1
Inmunoglobulinas Inespecíficas, 1627·2
Inmunogrip, 2062·4
Inmunol, 2062·4
Inmupen, 2062·4
Inmutag, 2062·4
Inner Fresh Tablets, Heath & Heather— *see* Heath & Heather Inner Fresh Tablets, 2037·3
Innersource, 2062·4
Inno Rheuma, 2062·4
Innobrand, 2062·4
InnoGel Plus, 2062·4
Innohep, 2062·4
InnoLet N, 2062·4
InnoLet R, 2062·4
InnoLet 30R, 2062·4
Innomel, 2062·4
InnoPran, 2062·4
Innova Cd, 2062·4
Innovace, 2062·4
Innovar, 2062·4
Innozide, 2062·4
Inobesin, 2062·4
Inocar, 2062·4
Inocar Plus, 2062·4
Inocor, 2062·4
*Inocybe*, 1717·3
Inofer, 2063·1
Inoflox, 2063·1
Inolaxine, 2063·1
Inolaxol, 2063·1
Inolimomab, 1360·3
Inolin, 2063·1
INOmax, 2063·1
Inongan, 2063·1
Inopamil, 2063·1
Inopin, 2063·1
Inosina, 1701·2
Inosinato Disódico, 1681·3
Inosine, 640·2, 1701·2
Inosine Dimepranol Acedoben Complex, 640·2
Inosine 5′-(Disodium Phosphate), 1681·3
Inosine 2-Hydroxypropyldimethylammonium 4-Acetamidobenzoate (1:3), 640·2
Inosine Pranobex, 640·2
Inosiplex, 640·2
Inosital, 2063·1
Inositol, 1701·2
*i*-Inositol, 1701·2
*meso*-Inositol, 1701·2
*myo*-Inositol, 1701·2
*myo*-Inositol Hexakis(dihydrogen) Phosphate, Nonasodium Salt, 1052·3
*meso*-Inositol Hexanicotinate, 939·3
*myo*-Inositol Hexanicotinate, 939·3
Inositol Niacinate, 939·3
Inositol Nicotinate, 939·3
Inotan, 2063·1
Inotop, 2063·1
Inotrex, 2063·1
Inotropes, Cardiac, 811·1
Inotropin, 2063·1
Inotropisa, 2063·1
Inotyol, 2063·1
Inova, 2063·1
Inoval, 2063·1
Inovan, 2063·1
Inovapar, 2063·1
Inovec, 2063·1
Inoven, 2063·1
Inpanol, 2063·1
Inpront, 2063·2
Ins-316, 1760·3
Insacial, 2063·2
Insadol, 2063·2
Insect Ecran, 2063·2
Insect Flowers, 1509·3
Insect Repellents, 1499·1
Insectes Coléoptères Hétéromères, 1666·3
Insecticidas Clorados, 1501·3
Insecticidas del Grupo de los Carbamatos, 1501·1
Insecticidas Organofosforados, 1507·3
Insecticides, 1499·1
Insecticides, Carbamate, 1501·1
Insecticides, Chlorinated, 1501·3
Insecticides, Organochlorine, 1501·3
Insecticides, Organophosphate, 1507·3
Insecticides, Organophosphorus, 1507·3
Insecticides, Pyrethroid, 1509·3
Insektenblüten, 1509·3
Insensye, 2063·2
Insertec, 2063·2
Inside, 2063·2
Insidon, 2063·2
Insig, 2063·2
Insogen, 2063·2
Insogen Plus, 2063·2
Insom, 2063·2
Insoma, 2063·2
Insomin, 2063·2
Insomnal, 2063·2
Insomn-Eze, 2063·2
Insomnia, 667·2, 2063·2
Insomnia, Hylands— *see* Hylands Insomnia, 2052·3
Insomnia Passiflora, 2063·2
Insomnium, 2063·2
Inspirol Halsschmerztabletten, 2063·2
Inspirol Heilpflanzenol, 2063·2
Inspirol Mundwasser Konzentrat, 2063·2
Inspirol P, 2063·2
Inspiryl, 2063·2
Inspra, 2063·2
Instacare, 2063·2
Instacyl, 2063·2
Insta-Glucose, 2063·2
Instana, 2063·2
Instant Rub, 2063·3
Instantine, 2063·3
Instaret, 2063·3
Instat, 2063·3
Instenon, 2063·3
Instillagel, 2063·3
Instrunet, 2063·3
Instru-Safe, 2063·3
Instruzyme, 2063·3
Insuflen, 2063·3
Insulatard, 2063·3
Insulatard HM, 2063·3
Insulatard Human, 2063·3
Insulatard MC, 2063·3
Insulatard NPH, 2063·3
Insulex, 2063·3
Insulin, 333·3, 334·1
Insulin 2, 2063·3
Insulin Aspart, 334·1, 334·3, 340·3
Insulin Basal, 2063·3
Insulin, Biphasic, 334·2
Insulin, Biphasic Isophane, 334·2
Insulin, Bovine, 333·3, 334·1
Insulin, Dalanated, 334·2
Insulin Defalan, 334·2
Insulin Detemir, 334·3, 340·3
Insulin Glargine, 334·3, 340·3
Insulin Glulisine, 340·3
Insulin Human, 334·1
Insulin, Human, 334·1
Insulin Infusat, 2063·3
Insulin, Isophane, 334·2
Insulin, Isophane Protamine, 334·2
Insulin Komb 25/75, 2063·3
Insulin Lente, 334·2
Insulin Lente MC, 2063·3
Insulin Lispro, 334·1, 334·3, 340·2
Insulin Lyhyt, 2063·3
Insulin, Neutral, 334·2
Insulin (NPH), Isophane, 334·2
Insulin Pitka, 2063·3
Insulin, Porcine, 333·3, 334·1
Insulin, Protamine Zinc, 334·2
Insulin Rapid, 2063·3
Insulin Reaction, 2063·3
Insulin, Regular, 334·2
Insulin S, 2063·3
Insulin Semilente, 334·2
Insulin SNC, 2063·3
Insulin, Soluble, 334·2
Insulin, Sulfated, 334·2
Insulin Ultralente, 334·2
Insulin, Unmodified, 334·2
Insulin Zinc Suspension, Extended, 334·2
Insulin Zinc Suspension, Prompt, 334·2
Insulin Zinc Suspensions, 334·2
Insulina, 333·3
Insulin-dependent Diabetes Mellitus— *see* Diabetes Mellitus, 324·1
Insuline Semi Tardum, 2063·4
Insuline Tardum MX, 2063·4
Insuline Ultra Tardum, 2063·4
Insulin-like Growth Factor Binding Protein-3, 1339·1
Insulin-like Growth Factor I (Human), 1338·3
Insulin-like Growth Factors, 1338·3
Insulinoma— *see* Carcinoid Tumours and Other Secretory Neoplasms, 504·1
Insulinotropin, 325·1
Insulins, Conventional, 334·2
Insulins, Highly Purified, 334·2
Insulins, Monocomponent, 334·2
Insulins, Purified, 334·2
Insulins, Single-peak, 334·2
Insulin-tolerance Test, 341·3
Insulinum, 333·3
Insulinum Aspartum, 334·1
Insulinum Lisprum, 334·1
Insultard, Human— *see* Human Insultard, 2049·2
Insuman Preparations, 2063·4
Insup, 2063·4
Insuvac, 2063·4
Insuven, 2063·4
Intacglobin, 2063·4
Intal, 2063·4
Intapan, 2063·4
Intard, 2063·4
Intaxel, 2063·4
Inteflora, 2063·4
Integral Lepromin, 1707·1
Integrelin, 912·2
Integrilin, 2064·1
Integrobe, 2064·1
Inteligen, 2064·1
Inteligen Ginseng, 2064·1
Intensain, 2064·1
Intensive Care, Infection Control in— *see* Intensive Care, 132·2
Intensive Care, Neuromuscular Blockade in— *see* Intensive Care, 1398·1
Intensive Care, Sedation and Analgesia in— *see* Intensive Care, 666·3
Inter IF, 2064·1
Interacton, 2064·1
Interbion, 2064·1
Interceed, 2064·1
Intercron, 2064·1
Intercyton, 2064·1
Interderm, 2064·1
Interferon-α, 640·3
Interferon-β, 645·3
Interferon-γ, 647·2
Interferon Alfa, 640·3
Interferon Alfa-2 Concentrated Solution, 640·3
Interferon Alfa-2a, 640·3
Interferon Alfa-2b, 640·3
Interferon Alfa-n1, 640·3
Interferon Alfa-n3, 640·3
Interferon Alfacon-1, 640·3
Interferon Alfanative— *see* Multiferon, 2144·3
Interferon Beta, 645·3
Interferon Beta-1a, 645·3
Interferon Beta-1b, 645·3
Interferon, Fibroblast, 645·3
Interferon Gamma, 647·2
Interferon Gamma-1b, 647·2
Interferon Gamma-1b Concentrated Solution, 647·2
Interferon Gamma-2a, 647·2
Interferon, Immune, 647·2
Interferon, Leucocyte, 640·3
Interferon, Lymphoblastoid, 640·3
Interferoni Alfa-2 Solutio Concentrata, 640·3
Interferoni Gamma-1b Solutio Concentrata, 647·2
Interleucina 1, 1701·3
Interleucina 2, 562·2
Interleucina 3, 755·3
Interleukin-1, 1701·3
Interleukin-1α, 1701·3
Interleukin-1β, 1701·3
Interleukin-1 Inhibitors, 1701·3
Interleukin-1 Receptor Antagonists, 1701·3
Interleukin-2, 562·2
Interleukin-2 Fusion Toxins, 1701·3
Interleukin-3, 755·3
Interleukin-4, 1701·3
Interleukin-4 Receptor, 778·3
Interleukin-6, 496·3, 1701·3
Interleukin-6 Antibodies, 1701·3
Interleukin-6 Receptor Monoclonal Antibody, 1757·1
Interleukin-10, 1700·3, 1701·3
Interleukin-11, 757·1, 1701·3
Interleukin-12, 1701·3
Interleukins, 1701·3
Intermax-Alpha, 2064·1
Intermedin, 1332·2
Intermedina, 1332·2
Intermedin-inhibiting Factor, 1332·3
Intermittent Claudication— *see* Peripheral Vascular Disease, 831·2
Intersept, 2064·1
Interstitial Cystitis, 1473·3
Interstitial Lung Disease— *see* Diffuse Parenchymal Lung Disease, 1079·3
Intestamin, 2064·1
Intestinal Amoebiasis— *see* Amoebiasis, 595·2
Intestinal Colic— *see* Gastrointestinal Spasm, 1242·2
Intestinal Fluke Infections, 99·2
Intestinal Nematode Infections, 97·1
Intestinal Pseudo-obstruction— *see* Decreased Gastrointestinal Motility, 1241·1
Intestinal Transplantation, 1346·1
Intestinol, 2064·1
Intesul, 2064·1
Intetrix, 2064·1
Intetrix P, 2064·1
Inthacine, 2064·1
Intianhamppu, 1666·1
Intim, 2064·1
Intimide, 2064·1
Intocel, 2064·1
Intra-abdominal Infections— *see* Peritonitis, 140·1
Intracef, 2064·1
Intracerebral Haemorrhage— *see* Stroke, 836·1
Intracranial Hypertension, Benign— *see* Raised Intracranial Pressure, 833·1
Intracranial Pressure, Raised— *see* Raised Intracranial Pressure, 833·1
Intradermi, 2064·1
Intradermi Fluid N, 2064·1
Intradermi N, 2064·2
Intradermo Cort Ant Fung, 2064·2
Intrafat, 2064·2
Intrafer, 2064·2
Intrafusin, 2064·2
Intrafusin E, 2064·2
Intragam, 2064·2
Intraglobin, 2064·2
Intraglobin F, 2064·2
Intrait de Marron d'Inde P, 2064·2
Intralgin, 2064·2
Intralgis, 2064·2
Intralipid, 2064·2
Intralipide, 2064·2
Intralipos, 2064·2
Intramin, 2064·2

Intramin G, 2064·2
Intrasil, 2064·2
Intrasite, 2064·2
Intrasol, 2064·2
Intrastigmina, 2064·3
Intra-uterine Devices, Progestogen-releasing, 1527·3
Intraval, 2064·3
Intraval Sodium, 2064·3
Intravenous Anaesthesia, Total— *see* Anaesthetic Techniques, 1296·2
Intravenous Regional Anaesthesia, 1370·1
Intraventricular Haemorrhage, Neonatal— *see* Neonatal Intraventricular Haemorrhage, 740·1
Intra-Vite B Group Plus Ascorbic Acid, 2064·3
Intrazig, 2064·3
Intrazolina, 2064·3
Intricon, 2064·3
Intrimun, 2064·3
Introcin, 2064·3
Introlan, 2064·3
Introlite, 2064·3
Intron A, 2064·3
Intron A— *see* Rebetron, 2252·4
Intron A Peg, 2064·3
Intron A/Rebetol, 2064·3
IntronA, 2064·3
Introna, 2064·3
Intropin, 2064·3
Intsangu, 1666·1
Int-*rac*-α-Tocopherolum, 1464·3
Int-*rac*-α-Tocopherylis Acetas, 1465·1
Intubation— *see* Anaesthesia, 1397·1
Inula, 1119·3
Inula Camphor, 1119·3
*Inula helenium*, 1119·3
Inulac, 2064·3
Inulin, 1702·1
Inulina, 1702·1
Inutest, 2064·3
Invanz, 2064·3
Invasive Mole— *see* Gestational Trophoblastic Tumours, 505·1
Inveoxel, 2064·3
Inversine, 2064·3
Invert Sugar, 1434·3
Invertos, 2064·3
Invex, 2064·3
Invigan, 2064·4
Invirase, 2064·4
Invoigin, 2064·4
Invoril, 2064·4
Invozide, 2064·4
Inxibir, 2064·4
Inyesprin, 2064·4
Inza, 2064·4
Inzelloval, 2064·4
Inzitan, 2064·4
Inzolen, 2064·4
Iobenguane ($^{123}$I), 1524·1
Iobenguane ($^{131}$I), 1524·3
Iobid DM, 2064·4
Iobitridol, 1063·1
Iocare, 2064·4
Iocare Balanced Salt Solution, 2064·4
Iocare BSS, 2064·4
Iocetamic Acid, 1063·2
Iocetámico, Ácido, 1063·2
Iocon, 2064·4
Iodal, 2064·4
Iodamida, 1063·2
Iodamida de Meglumina, 1063·2
Iodamida Sódica, 1063·2
Iodamide, 1063·2
Iodamide Meglumine, 1063·2
Iodamide Sodium, 1063·2
Iodarsolo B12, 2064·4
Iodato Potásico, 1598·1
Iodax, 2064·4
Iode, 1598·1, 2064·4
Iodepol, 2064·4
Iodermol, 2064·4
Iodesin, 2064·4
Iodetal, 2064·4
Iodeto de Potassio, 1598·1, 2065·1
Iodeto de Potassio Composto, 2065·1
Iodeto de Potassio Composto, Xarope de— *see* Xarope de Iodeto de Potassio Composto, 2387·3
Iodeto de Potassium Composto, 2065·1
Iodeto de Sódio, 1598·1
Iodeton, 2065·1
Iodetoss, 2065·1
Iodex, 2065·1
Iodex com Salicilato de Metila, 2065·1
Iodex with Methyl Salicylate, 2065·1
Iodiflor, 2065·1
Iodina, 2065·1
Iodinated ($^{125}$I) Fibrinogen, 1524·2
Iodinated Glycerol, 1122·3
Iodinated ($^{125}$I) Human Albumin, 1524·2
Iodinated ($^{131}$I) Human Albumin, 1524·3
Iodinated ($^{125}$I) Human Fibrinogen, 1524·2
Iodinated ($^{131}$I) Norcholesterol, 1524·3
Iodinated Povidone, 1190·3
Iodine, 1598·1
Iodine-123, 1524·1
Iodine-125, 1524·2
Iodine-131, 1524·2
Iodine Deficiency Disorders, 1599·1
Iodine-Thio-Calcic, Colircusi— *see* Colircusi Iodine-Thio-Calcic, 1899·4
Iodipamide, 1060·1
Iodipamide Meglumine, 1060·1
Iodised Oil, 1063·2
Iodisis, 2065·1
Iodixanol, 1063·3
Iodo, 1598·1
Iodo 123, 1524·1
Iodo 125, 1524·2
Iodo 131, 1524·2
Iodoasept, 2065·1
Iodobec, 2065·1
*m*-Iodobenzylguanidine ($^{123}$I), 1524·1
*m*-Iodobenzylguanidine ($^{131}$I), 1524·3
Iodocaffeine, 783·2
Iodocaine, 2065·1
Iodochlorhydroxyquin, 196·3
Iodochlorhydroxyquinoline, 196·3
Iodocid, 2065·1
4′-Iodo-4′-deoxydoxorubicin, 567·1
Iododesoxycytidine, 637·3
Iodofenfós, 1506·3
Iodofenphos, 1506·3
Iodoflex, 2065·1
Iodoform, 1184·2
Iodoform Paste, Bismuth and— *see* OxBipp, 2198·2
Iodoformo, 1184·2
Iodogorgoic Acid, 1597·3
Iodoheparinate Sodium, 1748·1
Iodoheparinato de Sodio, 1748·1
Iodomax, 2065·1
2-Iodomethyl-1,3-dioxolan-4-ylmethanol, 1119·1
Iodomethylnorcholestenol ($^{131}$I), 1524·3
6β-Iodomethyl-19-norcholest-5(10)-en-3β-ol ($^{131}$I), 1524·3
Iodopanoic Acid, 1065·1
Iodopen, 2065·1
Iodophendylate, 1064·1
Iodophil Viscous, 2065·1
Iodophores, 1191·1
Iodopropylidene Glycerol, 1122·3
3-Iodoprop-2-ynyl 2,4,5-Trichlorophenyl Ether, 401·2
Iodopulmin, 2065·1
Iodoquinol, 603·3
Iodosan Collutorio, 2065·1
Iodosorb, 2065·1
Iodosteril, 2065·1
Iodo-Suma, Xarope— *see* Xarope Iodo-Suma, 2387·4
Iodoten, 2065·1
Iodotiazol, 2065·2
Iodotope, 2065·2
Iodouracil, 637·3
Iodo-Vit, 2065·2
Iodoxamate Meglumine, 1064·1
Iodoxamato de Meglumina, 1064·1
Iodoxamic Acid, 1064·1
Iodoxámico, Ácido, 1064·1
Iodum, 1598·1
Ioduro Cálcico, 1116·2
Ioduro de Ecotiopato, 1490·2
Ioduro de Isopropamida, 485·2
Ioduro de Pralidoxima, 1050·1
Ioduro de Prolonio, 1603·1
Ioduro de Tibezonio, 1756·2
Ioduro de Tiemonio, 489·3
Ioduro Potásico, 1598·1
Ioduro Sódico, 1598·1
Iofed, 2065·2
Iofendilato, 1064·1
Iofendylate, 1064·1
Ioflupane ($^{123}$I), 1524·1
Iofoscal, 2065·2
Ioglicate Meglumine, 1064·1
Ioglicate Sodium, 1064·2
Ioglicato de Meglumina, 1064·1
Ioglicato Sódico, 1064·2
Ioglicic Acid, 1064·1
Ioglícico, Ácido, 1064·1
Iohexol, 1064·2
Iohexolum, 1064·2
Iohist D, 2065·2
Iohist DM, 2065·2
Ioimbina Composta, 2065·2
Ioiro, 2065·2
Iol, 2065·2
Iolin, 2065·2
Iolin NPH, 2065·2
Iolin Regular, 2065·2
Iomeprol, 1064·3
Iomeron, 2065·2
Ionamin, 2065·2
Ionamine, 2065·2
Ionarthrol, 2065·2
Ionax Astringent, 2065·2
Ionax Foam, 2065·2
Ionax P, 2065·2
Ionax Scrub, 2065·2
Ionax T, 2065·2
Ionet, 2065·2
Ionil, 2065·3
Ionil Champu, 2065·3
Ionil P, 2065·3
Ionil Plus, 2065·3
Ionil Rinse, 2065·3
Ionil-T, 2065·3
Ionil-T Plus, 2065·3
Ionimag, 2065·3
Ionitan, 2065·3
Ionosteril, 2065·3
Ion-Sol, 2065·3
Ionyl, 2065·3
Iopamidol, 1064·3
Iopamidolum, 1064·3
Iopamiro, 2065·3
Iopamiron, 2065·3
Iopanchol, 2065·3
Iopanoic Acid, 1065·1
Iopanoico, Ácido, 1065·1
Iopanoicum, Acidum, 1065·1
Iopentol, 1065·1
Iophen, 2065·3
Iophendylate, 1064·1
Iopidine, 2065·3
Iopidol, 1065·3
Iopidona, 1065·3
Iopimax, 2065·3
Iopodato Cálcico, 1065·2
Iopodato de Sodio, 1065·2
Iopodic Acid, 1065·2
Iopódico, Ácido, 1065·2
Iopromida, 1065·2
Iopromide, 1065·2
Iopydol, 1065·3
Iopydone, 1065·3
Ior T3, 2065·3
Iosal II, 2065·3
Iosalide, 2065·4
Iosciamina Solfato, 485·1
Ioscina Bromidrato, 483·3
Iosopan, 2065·4
Iosopan Plus, 2065·4
Iotalamato de Meglumina, 1065·3
Iotalamato de Sodio, 1065·3
Iotalamic Acid, 1065·3
Iotalámico, Ácido, 1065·3
Iotalamicum, Acidum, 1065·3
Iothalamate Meglumine, 1065·3
Iothalamate Sodium, 1065·3
Iothalamic Acid, 1065·3
Iotrol, 1066·1
Iotrolan, 1066·1
Iotrolum, 1066·1
Iotrovist, 2065·4
Iotroxate Meglumine, 1066·1
Iotroxato de Meglumina, 1066·1
Iotroxic Acid, 1066·1
Iotróxico, Ácido, 1066·1
Iotussin HC, 2065·4
Ioversol, 1066·2
Ioxaglate Meglumine, 1066·2
Ioxaglate Sodium, 1066·2
Ioxaglato de Meglumina, 1066·2
Ioxaglato Sódico, 1066·2
Ioxaglic Acid, 1066·2
Ioxáglico, Ácido, 1066·2
Ioxaglicum, Acidum, 1066·2
Ioxilan, 1066·3
Ioxitalamate Meglumine, 1066·3
Ioxitalamate Sodium, 1066·3
Ioxitalamato de Meglumina, 1066·3
Ioxitalamato Sódico, 1066·3
Ioxitalamic Acid, 1066·3
Ioxitalámico, Ácido, 1066·3
Ioxithalamic Acid, 1066·3
IP-302, 1672·3
IP-631, 491·2
Ipacef, 2065·4
Ipacid, 2065·4
Ipagastril, 2065·4
Ipalat, 2065·4
Ipamicina, 2065·4
Ipamix, 2065·4
Iparen, 2065·4
Ipatox, 2065·4
Ipatrizina, 2065·4
Ipaviran, 2065·4
Ipavit, 2065·4
Ipazone, 2065·4
Ipcacin Kid, 2065·4
Ipcamox, 2065·4
Ipcazide, 2065·4
IPD-1151T, 797·2
Ipeca, 1123·2, 2065·4
Ipecac, 1122·3
Ipecac, Powdered, 1123·1
Ipecacuana, 1122·3
Ipecacuanha, 1122·3
Ipecacuanha, Matto Grosso, 1122·3
Ipecacuanha, Prepared, 1122·3
Ipecacuanha Root, 1122·3
Ipecacuanhae Pulvis Normatus, 1122·3
Ipecacuanhae Radix, 1122·3
Ipecavom, 2065·4
Ipecine Hydrochloride, 604·3
Ipecol, 2065·4
Ipercortis, 2065·4
Iperisan, 2065·4
Iperiton, 2065·4
Iperix, 2065·4
Iperplasin, 2065·4
Iperten, 2066·1
Ipertrofan, 2066·1
Ipervital, 2066·1
Ipesandrine, 2066·1
Ipesil, 2066·1
Ipetitrin, 2066·1
Iphosphamide, 561·1
Ipnopen, 2066·1
Ipnovel, 2066·1
Ipoazotal, 2066·1
Ipoazotal Complex, 2066·1
Ipocalcin, 2066·1
Ipocol, 2066·1
Ipocromo, 2066·1
Ipodate Calcium, 1065·2
Ipodate Sodium, 1065·2
Ipodic Acid, 1065·2
Ipofisi Posteriore, 1337·3

Ipogen, 2066·1
Ipoglusan, 2066·1
Ipogras, 2066·1
Ipol, 2066·1
Ipolab, 2066·1
Ipolipid, 2066·1
Ipomex, 2066·1
Ipomoea, 1267·3
*Ipomoea orizabensis*, 1267·3
*Ipomoea purga*, 1268·3
*Ipomoea purpurea*, 1723·2
Ipomoea Resin, 1267·3
Ipomoea Root, 1267·3
*Ipomoea tricolor*, 1723·2
*Ipomoea violacea*, 1723·2
Iposeb, 2066·1
Ippi Verde, 2066·1
Ipra, 2066·1
Iprabon, 2066·1
Iprabron, 2066·1
Ipradol, 2066·1
Iprafen, 2066·1
Ipragocce, 2066·1
Ipral, 2066·2
Ipraneo, 2066·2
Ipratrin, 2066·2
Ipratropii Bromidum, 787·1
Ipratropio, Bromuro de, 787·1
Ipratropium Bromide, 787·1
Ipravent, 2066·2
Iprazochrome, 469·2
Ipren, 2066·2
Ipri V, 2066·2
Ipriflavona, 773·2
Ipriflavone, 773·2
Ipriosten, 2066·2
Iprivask, 2066·2
Iproben, 2066·2
Iprogel, 2066·2
Iproniazid Phosphate, 300·3
Iproniazida, Fosfato de, 300·3
Iprosten, 2066·2
Iproveratril Hydrochloride, 1019·1
Ipsapirona, Hidrocloruro de, 703·1
Ipsapirone Hydrochloride, 703·1
Ipsatol, 2066·2
Ipsatol Cough Formula Liquid for Children and Adults, 2066·2
Ipser Europe, 2066·2
Ipsilon, 2066·2
Ipson, 2066·2
Ipsovir, 2066·2
Ipstyl, 2066·2
IPV, 2066·2
IPV Merieux, 2066·2
IPV-Virelon, 2066·2
Ipvent, 2066·2
Iqfacilina, 2066·2
Iqfadina, 2066·2
Iqfamicina, 2066·2
Iqfasol, 2066·2
Irban, 2066·2
Irban Plus, 2066·2
Irbesartan, 940·1
Ircon, 2066·3
Ircon-FA, 2066·3
Iremofar, 2066·3
Irenat, 2066·3
Irenax, 2066·3
Irene, 2066·3
Irenor, 2066·3
Iressa, 2066·3
Irfen, 2066·3
Irgaman, 2066·3
Irgamid, 2066·3
Irgasan— *see* Solyptol, 2299·1
Irgasan DP-300— *see* Daewo, 1917·1
Irgasan DP 300— *see* Ippi Verde, 2066·1
Irgasan DP 300— *see* Irgaman, 2066·3
Irgasan DP 300— *see* Levaknel, 2094·1
Iricalcin, 2066·3
Iricil, 2066·3
Iricil Plus, 2066·3
Iridina Due, 2066·3
Iridina Light, 2066·3
Iridocyclitis— *see* Uveitis, 1090·1
Iridus, 2066·3
Iridux, 2066·3
Irigal, 2066·3
Irilens, 2066·3
Iriniozol, 2066·3
Irinogen, 2066·3
Irinotecán, Hidrocloruro de, 564·1
Irinotecan Hydrochloride, 564·1
Irinotel, 2066·3
Iris Med Complex, 2066·3
Iris Versicolor, 1702·1
*Iris versicolor*, 1702·1
Iris Virginica, 1702·1
Irish Moss, 1578·2
Irish Moss Extract, 1578·2
Iri-Sol, 2066·3
Iristamina, 2066·3
Iritis— *see* Uveitis, 1090·1
Irix, 2066·3
Irix Lagrimas, 2066·3
Irocombivit, 2066·3
Irocopar c C, 2066·3
Irocophan, 2066·4
Iromin, 2066·4
Iromin-Chinin-C, 2066·4
Iromin-G, 2066·4
Iron, 1434·3
Iron-59, 1524·3
Iron and Ammonium Citrate, 1427·2
Iron (II) Chloride Tetrahydrate, 1427·3
Iron Complex, 2066·4
Iron Compound, 2066·4
Iron Dextran, 1436·1
Iron Dextran Injection, 1436·1
Iron (II) Di(D-gluconate), 1428·1
Iron Gluconate, 1444·3
Iron for Homoeopathic Preparations, 1434·3
Iron (III) Hydroxide-sucrose Complex, 1438·2
Iron Lactate, 1428·2
Iron Overload, 1035·2
Iron Oxide, Saccharated, 1438·2
Iron Perchloride, 1688·1
Iron Plus, 2066·4
Iron Poisoning, 1035·3
Iron Polymaltose, 1437·3
Iron Proteinsuccinylate, 1438·1
Iron Protoxalate, 1428·2
Iron Pyrophosphate, 1427·2
Iron Saccharate, 1438·2
Iron Sesquichloride, 1688·1
Iron (III) Sodium Ethylenediaminetetra-acetate Monohydrate, 1444·3
Iron Sorbitex, 1438·1
Iron Sorbitex Injection, 1438·1
Iron Sorbitol, 1438·1
Iron Sorbitol Injection, 1438·1
Iron Succinyl-Protein Complex, 1438·1
Iron Sucrose, 1438·2
Iron Sucrose Injection, 1438·2
Iron Sulphate, 1428·2
Iron (II) Sulphate Heptahydrate, 1428·2
Iron Trichloride, 1688·1
Ironax, 2066·4
Iron-deficiency Anaemia, 733·2
Iron-Dextran Complex, 1436·1
Ironfer, 2066·4
Ironorm, 2066·4
Iron-Sorbitol-Citric Acid Complex, 1438·1
Irontona, 2066·4
Iroplex, 2066·4
Irospan, 2066·4
Irovel, 2066·4
Iroviton-Irocombivit, 2066·4
Iroviton-Irocovit-C, 2066·4
Irradial, 2066·4
Irriclens, 2066·4
Irrigacion CLNA, 2066·4
Irrigor, 2066·4
Irritable Bowel Syndrome, 1244·3
Irritos, 2066·4
Irritren, 2066·4
Irrodan, 2066·4
IRS 19, 2066·4
Irsogladina, Maleato de, 1267·3
Irsogladine Maleate, 1267·3
Irtan, 2067·1
Irtonin, 2067·1
Irudil, 2067·1
Iruxol, 2067·1
Iruxol Mono, 2067·1
Iruxol N, 2067·1
Iruxol Neo, 2067·1
Iruxolum Mono, 2067·1
IS-499, 488·2
IS 5 Mono, 2067·1
Isacilin, 2067·1
Isadol, 2067·1
Isairon, 2067·1
Isangina, 2067·1
Isangu, 1666·1
Isaphenin, 1282·3
Isavir, 2067·1
Isaxion, 2067·1
Iscador, 2067·1
Ischaemia, Myocardial— *see* Angina Pectoris, 813·1
Ischaemic Attack, Transient— *see* Stroke, 836·1
Ischaemic Heart Disease— *see* Atherosclerosis, 815·2
Ischaemic Stroke— *see* Stroke, 836·1
Ischelium, 2067·1
Ischelium Papaverina, 2067·1
Ischemol, 2067·1
Ischemol A, 2067·1
Isclofen, 2067·1
Iscover, 2067·1
Isdibudol, 2067·1
Isdin Extrem, 2067·1
Isdin Infantil, 2067·1
Isdinex, 2067·2
Isdinium, 2067·2
ISDN, 941·1
Isdol, 2067·2
I-Sense, 2067·2
Isepacin, 2067·2
Isepacine, 2067·2
Isepalline, 2067·2
Isepamicin, 222·2
Isepamicin Sulfate, 222·2
Isepamicin Sulphate, 222·2
Isepamicina, 222·2
Isepamicina, Sulfato de, 222·2
Isephca S, 2067·2
Iset, 2067·2
Isetionato de Dibrompropamidina, 1178·2
Isetionato de Hexamidina, 1181·3
Isetionato de Pentamidina, 613·2
Isetionato de Piritrexima, 580·1
Isetionato de Propamidina, 1191·2
ISF-2469, 878·2
ISF-2522, 1725·2
ISF 09338, 2067·2
Isib, 2067·2
Isi-Calcin, 2067·2
Isicom, 2067·2
Isiferone, 2067·2
Isiflu V, 2067·2
Isiflu Zonale, 2067·2
ISI-F/2/ST, 2067·2
Isigrip Zonale, 2067·2
Isilung, 2067·2
Isimet, 2067·2
Isimoxin, 2067·2
Isis-2922, 634·1
Isisfen, 2067·2
Isitab, 2067·2
Isiven, 2067·2
Iskaemyl, 2067·2
Iskedyl, 2067·2
Iskemil, 2067·2
Isketam, 2067·2
Iskevert, 2067·2
Iski, 2067·2
Islamint, 2067·3
Isla-Mint, 2067·2
Isla-Mint Herbal, 2067·3
Isla-Moos, 2067·3
Islet-cell Transplantation— *see* Pancreatic Transplantation, 1347·3
Islet-cell Tumours— *see* Carcinoid Tumours and Other Secretory Neoplasms, 504·1
Islopir, 2067·3
Islotin, 2067·3
Isly, 2067·3
Ismelin, 2067·3
Ismeline, 2067·3
Ismexin, 2067·3
Ismigen, 2067·3
Ismipur, 2067·3
IS-5-MN, 942·1
Ismo, 2067·3
Ismotic, 2067·3
Ismox, 2067·3
Iso, 2067·3
Iso Mack, 2067·3
Iso Triraupin, 2067·3
Isoacne, 2067·3
Isoajmaline, 994·3
Isoaminile, 1123·3
Isoaminile Citrate, 1123·3
Isoaminile Cyclamate, 1123·3
Isoaminilo, 1123·3
Isoaminilo, Citrato de, 1123·3
Isoamyl Dimethylaminobenzoate, 1155·1
Isoamyl *p*-Methoxycinnamate, 1142·2
Isoamyl Nitrite, 1032·1
Isoamyl Salicylate, 14·3
ISO-Augentropfen C, 2067·3
Iso-B, 2067·3
Isobac, 2067·3
Isobar, 2067·3
Iso-Betadine, 2067·3
Isobin, 2067·3
Isobinate, 2067·3
6-(Isoborn-2-yl)-3,4-xylenol, 277·3
Isobranch, 2067·3
Isobromindiona, 416·3
Isobromindione, 416·3
Isobutane, 1236·2
Isobutano, 1236·2
Isobutanol, 1475·1
Isobutil, 2067·3
Isobutyl Alcohol, 1475·1
Isobutyl 2-Cyanoacrylate, 1678·1
Isobutyl Methyl 1,4-Dihydro-2,6-dimethyl-4-(2-nitrophenyl)pyridine-3,5-dicarboxylate, 973·2
4-Isobutylhydratropohydroxamic Acid, 47·2
Isobutylhydrochlorothiazide, 878·2
2-(4-Isobutylphenyl)propionic Acid, 45·3
*O*-Isobutyrylthiamine Disulphide, 1455·1
Isocaine, 2067·3
Isocainide Hydrochloride, 947·2
Isocal, 2067·4
Isocaproato de Testosterona, 1570·1
Isocar, 2067·4
Isocaramidine Sulphate, 891·3
Isocarboxazid, 300·3
Isocarboxazida, 300·3
Isocard, 2067·4
Iso-Card, 2067·4
Isocardide, 2067·4
Isocef, 2067·4
IsoCell, 2067·4
Isocet, 2067·4
Isochinol, 2067·4
Isochron, 2067·4
Isocillin, 2067·4
Isoclar, 2067·4
Isoclor, 2067·4
Isoclor Expectorant, 2067·4
Isocolan, 2067·4
Isocom, 2067·4
Isoconazol, 401·3
Isoconazol, Nitrato de, 401·3
Isoconazole, 401·3
Isoconazole Nitrate, 401·3
Isoconazoli Nitras, 401·3
Isoconazolum, 401·3
Isocord, 2067·4
Isocort, 2067·4
Isoday, 2067·4
Isoderm, 2067·4

Isodex, 2067·4
Isodilan, 2067·4
Isodine, 2067·4
Isodinit, 2067·4
Isodiur, 2067·4
Isodol, 2067·4
Isodril, 2067·4
Isodrine Sulphate, 982·3
Isodrink, 2068·1
Isodur, 2068·1
*d*-Isoephedrine, 1129·2
Iso-Eremfat, 2068·1
Isoergine, 1723·2
Isoess, 2068·1
Isoetam, 2068·1
Isoetarina, Hidrocloruro de, 787·3
Isoetarina, Mesilato de, 788·1
Isoetarine, 787·3
Isoetarine Hydrochloride, 787·3
Isoetarine Mesilate, 788·1
Isoetharine, 787·3
Isoetharine Hydrochloride, 787·3
Isoetharine Mesylate, 788·1
Isoetharine Methanesulphonate, 788·1
Isoflupredona, Acetato de, 1105·3
Isoflupredone Acetate, 1105·3
Isoflurane, 1301·1, 2068·1
Isoflurano, 1301·1
Isofluranum, 1301·1
Isoflurofato, 1490·1
Isoflurophate, 1490·1
Isoforine, 2068·1
Isofort, 2068·1
Isofra, 2068·1
Isoftal, 2068·1
Isogaine, 2068·1
Isogel, 2068·1
Isogen, 2068·1
Isoginkgo, 2068·1
Isoglaucon, 2068·1
Isogrow, 2068·1
Isogutt, 2068·1
Isogutt Akut, 2068·1
Isogyn, 2068·1
Isoharringtonine, 558·3
Isohes, 2068·1
Isohexal, 2068·1
Isoket, 2068·1
Isokin, 2068·1
Isokin-300, 2068·1
Isokin-T Forte, 2068·1
Isolan, 2068·1
Isoleucina, 1438·2
Isoleucine, 1438·2
L-Isoleucine, 1438·2
Isoleucinum, 1438·2
Isolin, 2068·1
Isoliv, 2068·2
D-Isolysergic Acid Amide, 1723·2
Isolyt, 2068·2
Isolyte, 2068·2
Isomalt, 1438·3
Isomalta, 1438·3
Isomaltitol, 1438·3
Isomaltose and Ferric Hydroxide Complex, 1437·3
Isomaltum, 1438·3
Isomel, 2068·2
Isomenthone, 1283·2
Isomerine, 2068·2
Isomerine N, 2068·2
Isomet, 2068·2
Isometamidio, Cloruro de, 606·1
Isometamidium, 606·1
Isometamidium Chloride, 606·1
Isometepteno, Hidrocloruro de, 1702·1
Isometepteno, Mucato de, 1702·1
Isometheptene Galactarate, 1702·1
Isometheptene Hydrochloride, 1702·1
Isometheptene Mucate, 1702·1
Isomide, 2068·2
Isomil, 2068·2
Isomil DF, 2068·2
Isomil SF, 2068·2
Isomol, 2068·2
Isomon, 2068·2
Isomonat, 2068·2
Isomonit, 2068·2
Isomonoreal, 2068·2
Isomyrtine, 2068·2
Isonefrine, 2068·2
Isonex, 2068·2
Isoniac, 2068·2
Isoniazid, 222·2
Isoniazid Aminosalicylate, 224·2
Isoniazid Mesylate, 230·1
Isoniazid Methanesulfonate, 230·1
Isoniazid Sodium Glucuronate, 224·2
Isoniazida, 222·2
Isoniazidum, 222·2
Isonicotinato de Dexametasona, 1097·2
Isonicotinic Acid, 224·1
Isonicotinic Acid Hydrazide, 222·2
Isonicotinohydrazide, 222·2
2-Isonicotinoylhydrazinomethanesulphonic Acid, 230·1
Isonicotinuric Acid, 224·1
Isonicotinyl Glycine, 224·1
Isonicotinylhydrazide, 222·2
Isonicotinylhydrazine, 222·2
Isonitril, 2068·2
Isonixin, 51·1
Isonixino, 51·1
Isontyn, 2068·2
Isopamil, 2068·2
Isopap, 2068·2
Isopaque, 2068·2
Isopaque Cysto, 2068·2
Isopen, 2068·3
Isopentyl 2-(2-Diethylaminoethylamino)-2-phenylacetate Dihydrochloride, 1666·1
Isopentyl 5,6-Dihydro-7,8-dimethyl-4,5-dioxo-4*H*-pyrano[3,2-*c*]quinoline-2-carboxylate, 791·2
Isopentyl 4-Dimethylaminobenzoate, 1155·1
Isopentyl *p*-Methoxycinnamate, 1142·2
Isopentyl Nitrite, 1032·1
Isopentyl Salicylate, 14·3
Isophane Insulin, 334·2
Isophane Insulin, Biphasic, 334·2
Isophane Insulin (NPH), 334·2
Isophane Protamine Insulin, 334·2
Isophosphamide, 561·1
Isophyllen, 2068·3
Isoplasmal G, 2068·3
Isopregnenone, 1549·2
Isoprenalina, 940·2
Isoprenalina, Hidrocloruro de, 940·2
Isoprenalina, Sulfato de, 940·2
Isoprenaline, 940·2
Isoprenaline Hydrochloride, 940·2
Isoprenaline Sulfate, 940·2
Isoprenaline Sulphate, 940·2
Isoprenalini Hydrochloridum, 940·2
Isoprenalini Sulfas, 940·2
Isoprinosina, 2068·3
Isoprinosine, 640·2, 2068·3
Isoprochin P, 2068·3
Isoprodian, 2068·3
Isopront, 2068·3
Isopropamida, Ioduro de, 485·2
Isopropamide Bromide, 485·2
Isopropamide Iodide, 485·2
Isopropanol, 1184·3
Isopropildibenzoilmetano, 1148·3
1-[4-(2-Isopropoxyethoxymethyl)phenoxy]-3-isopropylaminopropan-2-ol Fumarate, 875·1
7-Isopropoxyisoflavone, 773·2
2-Isopropoxyphenyl Methylcarbamate, 1509·2
Isopropyl Alcohol, 1184·3
Isopropyl 6-(Benzyloxy)-4-(methoxymethyl)-9*H*-pyrido(3,4-*b*)indole-3-carboxylate, 668·1
Isopropyl 2-[4-(4-Chlorobenzoyl)phenoxy]-2-methylpropionate, 915·2
Isopropyl (*Z*)-7-{(1*R*,2*R*,3*R*,5*S*)-3,5-Dihydroxy-2-[(3*R*)-3-hydroxy-5-phenylpentyl]cyclopentyl}-5-heptenoate, 1519·1
Isopropyl (*Z*)-7-((1*R*,2*R*,3*R*,5*S*)-3,5-Dihydroxy-2-{(1*E*,3*R*)-3-hydroxy-4-[(α,α,α-trifluoro-*m*-tolyl)oxy]-1-butenyl}cyclopentyl)-5-heptenoate, 1521·1
Isopropyl (+)-(*Z*)-7-[(1*R*,2*R*,3*R*,5*S*)-3,5-Dihydroxy-2-(3-oxodecyl)cyclopentyl]-5-heptenoate, 1521·3
Isopropyl (*E*)-3-[(Ethylamino)(methoxy)phosphinothio-oxy]but-2-enoate, 1509·2
Isopropyl Hexadecanoate, 1481·2
Isopropyl Lanolate, 1483·3
Isopropyl Laurate, 1481·2
Isopropyl Linoleate, 1481·2
Isopropyl Lunoprostone, 1521·3
Isopropyl 2-Methoxyethyl 1,4-Dihydro-2,6-dimethyl-4-(3-nitrophenyl)pyridine-3,5-dicarboxylate, 972·3
Isopropyl 11-Methoxy-3,7,11-trimethyldodeca-2(*E*),4(*E*)-dienoate, 1507·2
Isopropyl Methyl 4-(2,1,3-Benzoxadiazol-4-yl)-1,4-dihydro-2,6-dimethylpyridine-3,5-dicarboxylate, 942·2
5-Isopropyl 3-Methyl 2-Cyano-1,4-dihydro-6-methyl-4-(*m*-nitrophenyl)-3,5-pyridinedicarboxylate, 972·2
Isopropyl Methylphosphonofluoridate, 1719·2
Isopropyl Myristate, 1481·2
Isopropyl Palmitate, 1481·2
Isopropyl Tetradecanoate, 1481·2
Isopropyl 2-(Thiazol-4-yl)-1*H*-benzimidazol-5-ylcarbamate, 103·3
Isopropyl Unoprostone, 1521·3
Isopropylacetone, 1476·2
4-Isopropylamino-2,3-dimethyl-1-phenyl-3-pyrazolin-5-one, 86·1
(±)-1-Isopropylamino-3-[4-(2-methoxyethyl)phenoxy]propan-2-ol, 956·3
1-Isopropylamino-3-(2-methylindol-4-yloxy)propan-2-ol Sulfate, 952·2
(±)-1-Isopropylamino-3-(1-naphthyloxy)propan-2-ol Hydrochloride, 989·3
Isopropylaminophenazone, 86·1
1-[3-(Isopropylamino)-2-pyridyl]-4-[(5-methanesulfonamidoindol-2-yl)carbonyl]piperazine Monomethanesulfonate, 630·2
Isopropylantipyrine, 85·3
Isopropylantipyrinum, 85·3
Isopropylarterenol, 940·2
Isopropylarterenol Hydrochloride, 940·2
Isopropylarterenol Sulphate, 940·2
(−)-*N*-[(*trans*-4-Isopropylcyclohexyl)carbonyl]-D-phenylalanine, 343·3
Isopropyldibenzoylmethane, 1148·3
4-Isopropyl-2,3-dimethyl-1-phenyl-3-pyrazolin-5-one, 85·3
*N*-Isopropyl-4,4-diphenylcyclohexylamine Hydrochloride, 1734·3
*N*-Isopropylethylnoradrenaline Hydrochloride, 787·3
*N*-Isopropylethylnoradrenaline Mesylate, 788·1
Isopropylicus, Alcohol, 1184·3
2,3-Isopropylidenedioxyphenyl Methylcarbamate, 1500·2
16α,17α-Isopropylidenedioxypregn-4-ene-3,20-dione, 1541·3
4,4′-(Isopropylidenedithio)bis(2,6-di-*tert*-butylphenol), 986·3
Isopropylis Myristas, 1481·2
Isopropylis Palmitas, 1481·2
2′-Isopropylisonicotinohydrazide Phosphate, 300·3
Isopropylmeprobamate, 1392·1
Isopropylmetacresol, 1194·2
4-Isopropyl-1-methylbenzene, 28·2
2-Isopropyl-5-methylcyclohexanol, 1711·3
1-Isopropyl-4-methyl-2,3-dioxabicyclo[2.2.2]oct-5-ene, 103·2
*N*-Isopropyl-α-(2-methylhydrazino)-*p*-toluamide Hydrochloride, 581·2
4-Isopropyl-2-methyl-3-[methyl(α-methylphenethyl)aminomethyl]-1-phenyl-3-pyrazolin-5-one, 38·3
2-Isopropyl-5-methylphenol, 1194·2
2-(2-Isopropyl-5-methylphenoxymethyl)-2-imidazoline Hydrochloride, 1132·1
1-Isopropyl-7-methyl-4-phenylquinazolin-2(1*H*)-one, 86·1
Isopropylnoradrenaline, 940·2
Isopropylnoradrenaline Hydrochloride, 940·2
Isopropylnoradrenaline Sulphate, 940·2
Isopropylphenazone, 85·3
2-(2-Isopropylphenoxymethyl)-2-imidazoline Hydrochloride, 1121·3
1-(2-Isopropylpyrazolo[1,5-*a*]pyridin-3-yl)-2-methyl-1-propanone, 786·3
13-Isopropyl-12-sulphopodocarpa-8,11,13-trien-15-oic Acid Pentahydrate, Sodium Salt, 1264·3
*N*-Isopropylterephthalamic Acid, 581·3
4-Isopropyltoluene, 28·2
1-Isopropyl-3-(4-*m*-toluidinopyridine-3-sulphonyl)urea, 1015·3
*N*-Isopropyl-*N*(β,3,5-trihydroxyphenethyl)ammonium Sulphate, 790·2
(1*R*,3*r*,5*S*,8*r*)-8-Isopropyl-3-[(±)-tropoyloxy]tropanium Bromide Monohydrate, 787·1
Isoproterenol, 940·2
Isoproterenol Hydrochloride, 940·2
Isoproterenol Sulfate, 940·2
Isoptin, 2068·3
Isoptin Plus, 2068·3
Isoptina, 2068·3
Isoptine, 2068·3
Isoptino, 2068·3
Isopto Preparations, 2068·3
Isoptomax, 2068·4
Isopuramin, 2068·4
Iso-Puren, 2068·4
Isopyrin, 86·1, 222·2
Isoradin, 2068·4
Isoram, 2068·4
Isorauwolfine, 994·3
Isorbid, 2068·4
Isordil, 2068·4
Isorel, 2068·4
Isorem, 2068·4
Isoren, 2068·4
Isorifam, 2068·4
Isoritmon, 2068·4
Isorythm, 2068·4
Isosal, 2068·4
Isoselect, 2068·4
Isosifar, 2068·4
Isosorbida, 941·1
Isosorbida, Dinitrato de, 941·1
Isosorbida, Mononitrato de, 942·1
Isosorbide, 941·1
Isosorbide Concentrate, 941·1
Isosorbide Dinitrate, 941·1
Isosorbide Dinitrate, Diluted, 941·1
Isosorbide Mononitrate, 942·1
Isosorbide Mononitrate, Diluted, 942·1
Isosorbide-5-mononitrate, 942·1
Isosorbidi Dinitras, 941·1
Isosorbidi Mononitras, 942·1
Isosource, 2068·4
Isosource (Nutrodrip), 2068·4
Isospaglumic Acid, 1702·2
Isospaglúmico, Ácido, 1702·2
Isosporiasis, 597·1
Isostad, 2068·4
Isostenase, 2069·1
Isosteril, 2069·1
Isosulfan Blue, 1750·3
Isotamine, 2069·1
Isotard, 2069·1
Isotard MC, 2069·1
Isotein HN, 2069·1
Isoten, 2069·1
Isotenk, 2069·1
Isotetracycline, 266·3
Isothane, 2069·1
Isothazine Hydrochloride, 488·3
Isothiazolinones, 1185·1
Isothiocyanato-l-propene, 1718·2
Isothipendyl Hydrochloride, 435·2
Isotiazolinonas, 1185·1
Isotipendil, Hidrocloruro de, 435·2
Isotol, 2069·1
Isotone Kochsalz, 2069·1
Isotonic, 2069·1
Isotrate, 2069·1
Isotretinoin, 1148·3

Isotretinoína, 1148·3
Isotretinoinum, 1148·3
Isotrex, 2069·1
Isotrex Eritromicina, 2069·1
Isotrex Gel, 2069·1
Isotrexin, 2069·1
Isotrexol, 2069·1
Isotrim, 2069·1
Iso-Triraupin, 2069·1
Isovaleric Acid, 1762·2
Isovir, 2069·1
Isovist, 2069·1
Isovorin, 2069·1
Isovue, 2069·1
Isox, 2069·2
Isoxan, 2069·2
Isoxazolyl Penicillins, 118·3
Isoxsuprina, Hidrocloruro de, 1702·2
Isoxsuprine Hydrochloride, 1702·2
Isoxsuprine Resinate, 1702·3
Isoxsuprini Hydrochloridum, 1702·2
I-Soyalac, 2069·2
Isozid, 2069·2
Isozid Comp N, 2069·2
Isozid-compositum— *see* Isozid comp N, 2069·2
Isozid-H, 2069·2
Ispagel, 2069·2
Ispaghula, 1268·1
Ispaghula Husk, 1268·1
Ispaghula Seed, 1268·1
Ispágula, 1268·1
Ispenoral, 2069·2
Isquebral, 2069·2
Isquelium, 2069·2
Isradipine, 942·2
Isradipino, 942·2
Isradipinum, 942·2
Issium, 2069·2
Istamex, 2069·2
Istamyl, 2069·2
Isteropac, 2069·2
Isteropac ER, 2069·2
Isticilline, 2069·2
Istin, 2069·2
Istivac, 2069·2
Istix, 2069·2
Istopar, 2069·2
Istopril, 2069·2
Istotosal, 2069·2
Isudrine, 2069·2
Isugran, 2069·2
Isuhuman Preparations, 2069·2
Isuprel, 2069·3
IT SD-T, 2069·3
Itagil, 2069·3
Itaiflex, 2069·3
Italdermol, 2069·3
Italmicin, 2069·3
Italnik, 2069·3
Italon, 2069·3
Italprid, 2069·3
Ital-Ultra, 2069·3
Italviron, 2069·3
Itan, 2069·3
Itapredin, 2069·3
Itavastatin, 984·1
Itax Antipoux, 2069·3
Itax Preventif, 2069·3
ITC, 2069·3
Itching— *see* Pruritus, 1137·3
Itch-X, 2069·3
ITE B12 Forte, 2069·3
Item Alphacade, 2069·3
Item Alphakeptol, 2069·3
Item Alphazole, 2069·3
Item Antipoux, 2069·4
Iteol-3, 2069·4
Iteor, 2069·4
Iterium, 2069·4
ITF-282, 1438·1
Itinerol $B_6$, 2069·4
Itobarbital, 673·3
Itodal, 2069·4
Itoprida, Hidrocloruro de, 1268·2
Itopride Hydrochloride, 1268·2
Itorex, 2069·4
Itoxaril, 2069·4
Itra, 2069·4
Itracon, 2069·4
Itraconazol, 401·3
Itraconazole, 401·3
Itraconazolum, 401·3
Itracotan, 2069·4
Itranax, 2069·4
Itraspor, 2069·4
Itravil, 2069·4
Itrazol, 2069·4
Itrin, 2069·4
Itrio 90, 1526·3
Itrop, 2069·4
5-IUDR, 637·3
Iuniperi Pseudo-fructus, 1703·1
Iuvacor, 2069·4
Ivacin, 2069·4
Ivadal, 2069·4
I-Valex, 2069·4
Ivaliten, 2069·4
Ivamix, 2069·4
Ivarest, 2069·4
Iveegam, 2069·4
Iveegam, CMV— *see* CMV Iveegam, 1895·4
Ivel, 2069·4
Ivel Schlaf, 2069·4
Ivelip, 2069·4
Ivemix, 2070·1
Ivepaque, 2070·1
Ivermectin, 105·3
Ivermectin Component $H_2B_{1a}$, 105·3
Ivermectin Component $H_2B_{1b}$, 105·3
Ivermectina, 105·3
Ivhebex, 2070·1
Ividol, 2070·1
Ivofol, 2070·1
Ivomec— *see* Mectizan, 2118·1
Ivoran Pilot, 2070·1
Ivracain, 2070·1
Ivy Block, 2070·1
Ivy Dry, 2070·1
Ivy Dry, Super— *see* Super Ivy Dry, 2313·3
Ivy-Chex, 2070·1
Ivy-Rid, 2070·1
Iwamet, 2070·1
Iwazin, 2070·1
Ixana, 2070·1
Ixel, 2070·1
Ixense, 2070·1
*Ixodes holocyclus* Antiserum, 1641·3
*Ixodes holocyclus* Antivenin, 1641·3
*Ixodes holocyclus* Antivenom, 1641·3
Ixor, 2070·1
Ιχωρ— *see* Ixor, 2070·1
Ixoten, 2070·1
Ixprim, 2070·1
Iyafin, 2070·1
Izac, 2070·1
Izacef, 2070·1
Izadima, 2070·1
Izatax, 2070·1
Izerin, 2070·1
Izilox, 2070·2
Izo, 2070·2
Izofran, 2070·2
I.Z.S, 334·2
I.Z.S., Amorph, 334·2
I.Z.S., Cryst., 334·2


## J


Jaa Pyral, 2070·2
Jaaps Health Salt, 2070·2
Jaba $B_{12}$, 2070·2
Jabastatina, 2070·2
Jabasulide, 2070·2
Jabobip, 2070·2
Jabon Antiseptico Asens, 2070·2
Jabón Blando, 1575·2
Jabonacid, 2070·2
Jabonoil, 2070·2
Jack and Jill Preparations, 2070·2
Jacksonian Epilepsy— *see* Epilepsy, 349·1
Jackson's Preparations, 2070·2
Jacksons Childrens Cough Pastilles— *see* Potters Children's Cough Pastilles, 2229·3
Jactuss, 2070·2
Jacutin, 2070·2
Jacutin N, 2070·2
Jadelle, 2070·2
Jadit, 2070·2
Jaguar Gum, 333·2
Jaikal, 2070·3
Jaikin N, 2070·3
Jakava, 2070·3
Jalap, 1268·3
Jalap Resin, 1268·3
Jalap Root, 1268·3
Jalap Root, Orizaba, 1267·3
Jalap Tuber, 1268·3
Jalap, Vera Cruz, 1268·3
Jalapa, 1268·3
Jalapa Comp, 2070·3
Jalapa Composta, 2070·3
Jalapenharz, 1268·3
Jalapenwurzel, 1268·3
Jalea Real, 1740·3
Jalovis, 2070·3
Jaluran, 2070·3
Jamaica Dogwood, 1702·3
Jamaica Quassia, 1737·2
Jamaican Sarsaparilla, 2070·3
Jamaican Vomiting Sickness, 1700·2
Jamestown Weed, 489·2
Jamylene, 2070·3
Janacin, 2070·3
Janjah, 1666·1
Jantoven, 2070·3
Japan Freeze-Dried Tuberculin, 2070·3
Japanese Angelica, 1655·1
Japanese Capsicum, 1667·1
Japanese Capsicum, Honka Variety, 1667·1
Japanese Encephalitis Vaccines, 1621·2
Japanese Gentian, 1692·2
Japanese Isinglass, 1576·3
Japanese Valerian, 1762·2
Japanol, 2070·3
Japomin, 2070·3
Jaquedryl, 2070·3
Jaquesan, Natusor— *see* Natusor Jaquesan, 2154·1
Jaquesor, 2070·3
Jarabe Bago, 2070·3
Jarabe Manceau, 2070·3
Jarabe Manzanas Siken, 2070·3
Jarabe Palto Compuesto con Miel, 2070·3
Jarisch-Herxheimer Reaction, 163·3
Jarisch-Herxheimer Reaction— *see* Relapsing Fever, 143·3
Jarsin, 2070·3
Jasicholin N, 2070·3
Jasimenth CN, 2070·3
Jasmine, 2070·3
Jasmine Root, Yellow, 1691·3
Jasmolin I, 1509·3
Jasmolin II, 1509·3
Jatamansin, 2070·3
*Jateorhiza columba*, 1665·2
*Jateorhiza palmata*, 1665·2
Jatiphaladya Churna, 1666·1
Jatroneural, 2070·3
Jatropur, 2070·3
Jatrosom N, 2070·3
Jatrox, 2070·3
Jaune de Quinoléine, 1057·3
Jaune Orangé S, 1058·2
Jaune Soleil, 1058·2
Jaune Tartrique, 1058·2
Java Tea, 1702·3
Javanese Turmeric, 1759·3
Javel, Eau de, 1192·2
JB-11, 410·2
JB-8181, 290·2
JD-96, 727·2
JD-177, 741·3
Jea, 1666·1
Jecobiase, 2070·4
Jecohepat, 2070·4
Jecopeptol, 2070·4
Jecoris Aselli, Oleum, 1425·2
Jecoris Hippoglossi, Oleum, 1434·1
Jectocos, 2070·4
Jectocos Plus, 2070·4
Jectofer, 2070·4
Jedipin, 2070·4
Jekovit, 2070·4
Jellin, 2070·4
Jellin Polyvalent, 2070·4
Jellin-Neomycin, 2070·4
Jelliproct, 2070·4
Jellisoft, 2070·4
Jellisoft-Neomycin, 2070·4
Jellyfish Antivenins, 1621·3
Jellyfish Sting, 1645·3
Jellyfish Sting— *see* Box Jellyfish Sting, 1621·3
Jellyfish Venom Antisera, 1621·3
Jelonet, 2070·4
Jemalt 13+13, 2070·4
Jemizym, 2070·4
Jenabroxol, 2070·4
Jenabroxol Comp, 2070·4
Jenacard, 2070·4
Jenacillin V, 2070·4
Jenacillin A, 2070·4
Jenacillin O, 2070·4
Jenacyclin, 2070·4
Jenacysteine, 2070·4
Jenafenac, 2070·4
Jenamazol, 2070·4
Jenametidin, 2071·1
Jenamoxazol, 2071·1
Jenampin, 2071·1
Jenapamil, 2071·1
Jenapirox, 2071·1
Jenaprofen, 2071·1
Jenapurinol, 2071·1
Jenaspiron, 2071·1
Jenasteron, 2071·1
Jenatacin, 2071·1
Jenatenol, 2071·1
Jenateren Comp, 2071·1
Jenest, 2071·1
Jengibre, 1267·1
Jenoquine, 2071·1
Jenoxifen, 2071·1
Jephagynon, 2071·1
Jephoxin, 2071·1
Jeprolol, 2071·1
Jequirity Bean, 1645·1
Jessamine, 1691·3
Jestryl, 2071·1
Jesuit's Bark, 1671·3
Jet, 1302·3
Jet Lag, 1710·3, 2071·1
Jet Lag— *see* Insomnia, 667·2
Jetepar, 2071·1
Jetomisol-P, 2071·1
Jets, 2071·1
JE-Vaccine, 2071·1
JE-Vax, 2071·1
Jevity, 2071·1
Jezil, 2071·1
JF-1, 1044·1
JHP Rodler, 2071·1
Jiffy Toothache Drops, 2071·1
Jimson Weed, 489·2
Jin Bu Huan, 1703·1
Jinda, 2071·1
Jinofloxacin, 233·3
Jintsam, 1693·1
JL-1078, 481·3
JM-8, 533·3
JM-83, 577·1
JM-216, 583·2
JO-1016, 1110·1
Jodetten, 2071·2
Jodfenphos, 1506·3
Jodgamma, 2071·2
Jodid, 2071·2
Jodieci, 2071·2
Jodix, 2071·2
Jodlauge, Tolzer, 2071·2
Jodminerase, 2071·2
Jodo Calcio Vitaminico, 2071·2

Jodobac, 2071·2
Jodocur, 2071·2
Jodoform, 2071·2
Jodogard, 2071·2
Jodonorm, 2071·2
Jodoplex, 2071·2
Jodosan, 2071·2
Jodthyrox, 2071·2
Jodum, 1598·1
Joe Pye Weed, 1695·3
Joggers, 2071·2
Johanicum, 2071·2
Johanniskraut, 299·1
John Plunketts Protective Day Cream, 2071·2
John Plunketts Super Wrinkle Cream, 2071·2
John Plunketts Vita-Pore, 2071·2
Johnson & Johnson Burn Cream, 2071·2
Johnson & Johnson First Aid Ointment, 2071·2
Johnson's Preparations, 2071·2
Joint, 2071·3
Joint Action, 2071·3
Joint Disease, Degenerative— *see* Osteoarthritis, 9·2
Joint Disorders, Musculoskeletal and— *see* Soft-tissue Rheumatism, 11·1
Joint Failure— *see* Osteoarthritis, 9·2
Joint Infections, Bone and— *see* Bone and Joint Infections, 122·1
Joint Mobility, Bioglan— *see* Bioglan Joint Mobility, 1844·1
Joint & Muscle Complex, 2071·3
Joint & Muscle Oral Spray, 2071·3
Joint & Muscle Relief Cream, 2071·3
Joint & Muscle Tablets— *see* Joint & Muscle Oral Spray and Tablets, 2071·3
Joint Support, 2071·3
Jointace, 2071·3
Joint-e-Licious, 2071·3
Jolivette, 2071·3
Jomax, 2071·3
Jomethid, 2071·4
Jonac, 2071·4
Jonctum, 2071·4
Jonil T, 2071·4
Jonosteril, 2071·4
Jopamiro, 2071·4
Jopinol, 2071·4
Jorkil, 2071·4
Josacine, 2071·4
Josalid, 2071·4
Josamicina, 224·3
Josamicina, Propionato de, 224·3
Josamina, 2071·4
Josamy, 2071·4
Josamycin, 224·3
Josamycin Propionate, 224·3
Josamycin 10-Propionate, 224·3
Josamycini Propionas, 224·3
Josamycinum, 224·3
Josaxin, 2071·4
Joshua Tree, 1766·2
Josir, 2071·4
Jossalind, 2071·4
Jour Apres Jour, 2071·4
Jouvence, 2071·4
Jouvence de l'Abbe Soury, 2071·4
Joy-Rides, 2071·4
Joysun, 2071·4
Joyzol, 2071·4
JP-428, 786·1
JP-992, 868·1
JP Tone, 2071·4
Jsoskleran, 2071·4
Jsostoma S, 2071·4
Juaflor, 2071·4
Juana, 1666·1
Juanola, Pastillas— *see* Pastillas Juanola, 2207·4
JuBronchan C, 2071·4
JuCholan S, 2071·4
JuCor, 2071·4
Jucurba, 2071·4
JuCystan S, 2071·4
JuDorm, 2071·4
JuGrippan, 2072·1
JuGrippan S, 2072·1
JuHepan, 2072·1
Jukunda Melissen-Krautergeist, 2072·1
Jukunda Rotol, 2072·1
Julab, 2072·1
JuLax, 2072·1
JuLax S, 2072·1
JuLax-M, 2072·1
Juliet, 2072·1
Julmentin, 2072·1
Julphacef, 2072·1
Julphamox, 2072·1
Julphapen, 2072·1
Jumble Beads, 1645·1
JuMenstran, 2072·1
Jumex, 2072·1
Jumexal, 2072·1
Jumexil, 2072·1
Junamac, 2072·1
Junel Fe, 2072·1
JuNeuron S, 2072·1
Jungborn, 2072·1
Jungle Formula Insect Repellent, 2072·1
Jungle Formula Insect Repellent Plus U.V. Sunscreens, 2072·1
Jungle Formula Sting Relief Cream, 2072·1
Junifen, 2072·1
Junik, 2072·1
Junin Haemorrhagic Fever Vaccines, 1609·2
Junior Citrex, 2072·1
Junior Citrex Cal-Mag-D3, 2072·1
Junior Cough & Cold, Chemists Own— *see* Chemists Own Junior Cough & Cold, 1882·1
Junior Disprin, 2072·2
Junior Ideal Quota, 2072·2
Junior Kao-C, 2072·2
Junior Strength Cold DM, 2072·2
Junior Strength Tylenol, 2072·2
Junior Time C, 2072·2
Juniormen, 2072·2
Juniorvit, 2072·2
Juniper, 1703·1
Juniper Berry, 1703·1
Juniper Berry Oil, 1703·1
Juniper Fruit, 1703·1
Juniper Oil, 1703·1
Juniper Tar, 1159·2
Juniper Tar Oil, 1159·2
Juniperi Aetheroleum, 1703·1
Juniperi, Baccae, 1703·1
Juniperi Empyreumaticum, Oleum, 1159·2
Juniperi Fructus, 1703·1
Juniperi Galbulus, 1703·1
Juniperi, Oleum, 1703·1
Juniperi, Pix, 1159·2
Juniperi, Pyroleum, 1159·2
*Juniperus communis*, 1703·1
*Juniperus oxycedrus*, 1159·2
Juniperus-Komplex-Injektopas, 2072·2
Junisana, 2072·2
Junivite, 2072·2
Juno Junipah, 2072·2
JuPhlebon S, 2072·2
Jurubileno, 2072·2
Jusline 70/30, 2072·2
Jusline N, 2072·2
Jusline R, 2072·2
Jusprin, 2072·2
Jusquiame, 485·2
Jusquiame Noire, 485·2
Just One Per Day, 2072·2
Justar, 2072·2
Justebarin, 2072·2
Justegas, 2072·2
Justelax, 2072·2
Justogen Mono, 2072·2
Justor, 2072·2
Justum, 2072·2
Jutussin N R8, 2072·2
Jutussin Neo, 2072·2
Juvela, 2072·2
Juvenile Chronic Arthritis— *see* Juvenile Idiopathic Arthritis, 9·1
Juvenile Idiopathic Arthritis, 9·1
Juvenile Myoclonic Epilepsy— *see* Epilepsy, 349·1
Juvenile Osteopetrosis— *see* Osteopetrosis, 1085·2
Juvenile-onset Huntington's Chorea— *see* Chorea, 664·2
Juvenit, 2072·3
Juvental, 2072·3
Juvepirine, 2072·3
Juvitan, 2072·3
JuViton, 2072·3
Juwoment Sport, 2072·3


## K


K, 1302·3, 1439·1
K1, 2072·3
K5 Hair Tincture, 2072·3
K + 8, 2072·3
K-10, 2072·3
K + 10, 2072·3
K12 Throat Guard, Blis— *see* Blis K12 Throat Guard, 1849·1
K-17, 1752·3
K-38, 333·1
K-50, 2072·3
K-85, 976·2
K-351, 973·2
K-364, 615·2
K-386, 333·1
K-430, 605·2
K 1000 T, 2072·3
K-3917, 723·2
K-3920, 939·1
K-4024, 332·2
K-9147, 410·1
K-9321, 851·1
K-11941, 1512·3
K-12148, 946·3
K-21060E, 550·1
K-748364A, 615·2
K + Care, 2072·3
K Thrombin, 2072·3
Kabala, 2072·3
Kaban, 2072·3
Kabanimat, 2072·3
Kabi-2165, 891·1
Kabi-2234, 489·3
Kabiglobulin, 2072·3
Kabikinase, 2072·3
KabiMix, 2072·3
KabiMix Basal, 2072·3
Kabiven, 2072·3
Kacerutin, 2072·4
KA-Cilone, 2072·4
Kacinth, 2072·4
Kadalex, 2072·4
KadeFungin, 2072·4
Kadeöl, 1159·2
Kadian, 2072·4
Kadiur, 2072·4
Kadol, 2072·4
Kadolax, 2072·4
Kaergona Hidrosoluble, 2072·4
Kafa, 2072·4
Kafedrin Hydrochloride, 878·2
Kahweol, 1765·2
Kainever, 2072·4
Kaion Retard, 2072·4
Kaizem, 2072·4
Kajel, 2072·4
Kajos, 2072·4
Kakaobutter, 1482·3
Kakkon-to, Tsumura— *see* Tsumura Kakkon-to, 2351·1
Kal Sept, 2072·4
Kala, 2072·4
Kala-azar— *see* Leishmaniasis, 597·2
Kalaf, 2072·4
Kalaz D3, 2072·4
Kalbeten, 2072·4
Kal-Cee, 2072·4
Kalci-300, 2072·4
Kalcidon, 2072·4
Kalcikidz, 2072·4
Kalcipos, 2072·4
Kalcipos-D, 2072·4
Kalcitena, 2072·4
Kaldil Diet, 2072·4
Kaldor, 2072·4
Kaleorid, 2073·1
Kaletra, 2073·1
Kalgaron, 2073·1
Kalgut, 2073·1
Kali Mag, 2073·1
Kalicet, 2073·1
Kalicitrine, 2073·1
Kalidinogenasa, 1703·2
Kaliglutol, 2073·1
Kalii Acetas, 1232·1
Kalii Chloridum, 1232·2
Kalii Citras, 1223·1
Kalii Clavulanas, 193·3
Kalii Clavulanas Dilutus, 193·3
Kalii Dihydrogenophosphas, 1230·3
Kalii Hydrogenocarbonas, 1223·1
Kalii Hydrogenotartras, 1284·3
Kalii Hydroxidum, 1734·2
Kalii Hydroxydum, 1734·2
Kalii Iodetum, 1598·1
Kalii Iodidum, 1598·1
Kalii Jodidum, 1598·1
Kalii Metabisulfis, 1193·1
Kalii Natrii Tartras, 1284·3
Kalii Nitras, 1190·1
Kalii Perchloras, 1602·3
Kalii Permanganas, 1190·2
Kalii Sorbas, 1192·3
Kalii Stibyli Tartras, 103·1
Kalii Sulfas, 1232·2
Kalii Sulfidum, 1158·3
Kalii Tartras, Stibii Et, 103·1
Kaliject, 2073·1
Kaliklora Jod Med, 2073·1
Kalimate, 2073·1
Kalinor, 2073·1
Kalinorm, 2073·1
Kalinor-retard P, 2073·1
Kaliolite, 2073·1
Kalioral, 2073·1
Kalisol, 2073·1
Kalisteril, 2073·1
Kali-Sterop, 2073·1
Kalitabs, 2073·1
Kalitrans, 2073·1
Kalitrans Retard, 2073·1
Kalium Preparations, 2073·1
Kalium Chloratum, 1232·2
Kalium Chloricum, 1734·2
Kalium Guajacolsulfonicum, 1131·1
Kalium Hydrotartaricum, 1284·3
Kalium Hydroxydatum, 1734·2
Kalium Hypermanganicum, 1190·2
Kalium Iodatum, 1598·1
Kalium Jodatum, 1598·1
Kalium Natrium Tartaricum, 1284·3
Kalium Nitricum, 1190·1
Kalium Permanganicum, 1190·2
Kalium Sulfuricum, 1232·2
Kalius, 2073·2
Kalk, Gebrannter, 1664·3
Kalkurenal Goldrute, 2073·2
Kalléone, 1703·2
Kallidinogenase, 1703·2
Kallikrein, 1703·2
Kallmann's Syndrome— *see* Hypogonadism, 1316·1
Kalloplast, 2073·2
Kalma, 2073·2
Kalmafta, 2073·2
Kalmalin, 2073·2
Kalm-B, 2073·2
Kalmiren, 2073·2
Kalmocaps, 2073·2
Kalms, 2073·2
Kalmus, 1664·1
Kaloplasmal, 2073·2
Kaloplasmal E, 2073·2
Kalopsis, 2073·2
Kalostop, 2073·2
Kalovowen, 2073·2

Kalpastic, 2073·2
Kalpress, 2073·2
Kalpress Plus, 2073·2
Kalsimin, 2073·2
Kalspare, 2073·2
Kalten, 2073·2
Kalter, 2073·2
Kaltiazem, 2073·2
Kaltin MF, 2073·2
Kaltocarb, 2073·3
Kaltostat, 2073·3
Kaltrim, 2073·3
Kaluril, 2073·3
Kalyamon B12, 2073·3
Kalymin, 2073·3
Kalzana, 2073·3
Kalzonorm, 2073·3
Kam Rho-D, 2073·3
Kamacaine, 2073·3
Kaman, 2073·3
Kamfeine, 2073·3
Kamfer, 1665·3
Kamidex, 2073·3
Kamil Blue, 2073·3
Kamillan Plus, 2073·3
Kamillan Supra, 2073·3
Kamillat, 2073·3
Kamille N, 2073·3
Kamillen, 2073·3
Kamillen-Bad, 2073·4
Kamillenbad Intradermi, 2073·4
Kamillen-Bad N Ritsert, 2073·4
Kamillen-Bad-Robugen, 2073·4
Kamillenblüten, 1669·3
Kamillencreme N, 2073·4
Kamillenextract, 2073·4
Kamillen-Heel, 2073·4
Kamillin, 2073·4
Kamillin Medipharm, 2073·4
Kamillobad, 2073·4
Kamilloderm, 2073·4
Kamillofluid, 2073·4
Kamillomed, 2073·4
Kamillosan Preparations, 2073·4
Kamiloderm, 2073·4
Kamilon, 2073·4
Kamilotract, 2073·4
Kamiltract Baby, 2073·4
Kamina, 2073·4
Kami-shoyo-san, Tsumura— *see* Tsumura Kami-shoyo-san, 2351·1
Kamistad, 2073·4
Kamistad N, 2074·1
Kamol, 2074·1
Kamonga, 1666·1
Kamoxin, 2074·1
KamRho-D, 2074·1
Kamu Jay, 2074·1
Kamu Jay Multi Complex, 2074·1
Kamycine, 2074·1
Kanab, 1666·1
Kanacil, 2074·1
Kanacitrin, 2074·1
Kanacolirio, 2074·1
Kanacyl, 2074·1
Kanadrex, 2074·1
Kanafosal, 2074·1
Kanafosal Predni, 2074·1
Kanakion, 2074·1
Kanamicina, Sulfato Ácido de, 224·3
Kanamicina, Sulfato de, 225·1
Kanamycin A Sulphate, 225·1
Kanamycin Acid Sulfate, 224·3
Kanamycin Acid Sulphate, 224·3
Kanamycin B Sulphate, 162·2
Kanamycin Bisulfate, 225·2
Kanamycin Monosulphate, 225·1
Kanamycin Sulfate, 225·1
Kanamycin Sulphate, 225·1
Kanamycin Tannate, 225·2
Kanamycini Monosulfas, 225·1
Kanamycini Sulfas Acidus, 224·3
Kanamytrex, 2074·1
Kanapat, 2074·1
Kanapomada, 2074·1
Kana-Stulln, 2074·1
Kanavit, 2074·1
Kanazima, 2074·1
Kanazone, 2074·1
Kanbine, 2074·1
Kancin, 2074·1
Kancin-Gap, 2074·1
Kancin-L, 2074·1
Kandicin, 2074·1
Kandistat, 2074·1
Kandril, 2074·2
Kanebo Hochu-ekki-to, 2074·2
Kanebo Ninjin-yoei-to, 2074·2
Kanebo Sairei-to, 2074·2
Kanebo Sho-saiko-to, 2074·2
Kanendos, 2074·2
Kanescin, 2074·2
Kaneuron, 2074·2
Kangen, 2074·2
Kanibel, 2074·2
Kanin, 2074·2
Kank-A, 2074·2
Kank-Eze, 2074·2
Kan-Mycin, 2074·2
Kanolone, 2074·2
Kan-Ophtal, 2074·2
Kanormal, 2074·2
Kanrenol, 2074·2
Kantrex, 2074·2
Kantrexil, 2074·2
Kao, 2074·2
Kaobrol, 2074·2
Kao-C, Junior— *see* Junior Kao-C, 2072·2
Kaochlor, 2074·2
Kaodene, 2074·2
Kaodene Non-Narcotic, 2074·2
Kaogel, 2074·2
Kaolin, 1268·3
Kaolin, Heavy, 1268·3
Kaolin, Light, 1268·3
Kaolin, Light (Natural), 1268·3
Kaologeais, 2074·3
Kaomagma, 2074·3
Kaomagma with Pectin, 2074·3
Kaomuth, 2074·3
Kaomycin, 2074·3
Kaon, 2074·3
Kaon-Cl, 2074·3
Kao-Paverin, 2074·3
Kaopectal, 2074·3
Kaopectal-N, 2074·3
Kaopectate, 2074·3
Kaopectate II, 2074·3
Kaopectate Advanced Formula, 2074·3
Kaopectate, Children's— *see* Children's Kaopectate, 1882·4
Kaopectate Maximum Strength, 2074·3
Kaopectin, 2074·3
Kaoprompt-H, 2074·3
Kao-Pront, 2074·3
Kao-Spen, 2074·3
Kaostase, 2074·3
Kaostase Suspension, 2074·3
Kaostatex, 2074·3
Kaosyl, 2074·3
Kaotalil, 2074·3
Kapabloc, 2074·3
Kapake, 2074·3
Kapanol, 2074·4
Kaparlon-S, 2074·4
Kapectin Forte, 2074·4
Kaplon, 2074·4
Kapodin, 2074·4
Kaposalt, 2074·4
Kaposi's Sarcoma, 524·3
Kaptin, 2074·4
Kaptin II, 2074·4
Kaput, 2074·4
Kara, 2074·4
Karacil, 2074·4
Karaya, 1290·2
Karaya Bismuth, 2074·4
Karaya Gum, 1290·2
Karayal, 2074·4
Karbac, 2074·4
Karbaderm, 2074·4
Karbasal, 2074·4
Karbasalin, 2074·4
Karbolytt, 2074·4
Karbons, 2074·4
Karbromal, 674·1
Kardegic, 2074·4
Karden, 2074·4
Kardiamed, 2074·4
Kardil, 2074·4
Kardion, 2074·4
Kardioplex, 2074·4
Kardobenediktenkraut, 1673·3
Kardopal, 2074·4
Karelyne, 2074·4
Karex, 2074·4
Karfedon, 1731·1
Kariax, 2074·4
Karicare Preparations, 2074·4
Karidina, 2075·1
Karidium, 2075·1
Karigel, 2075·1
Karigel-N, 2075·1
Karil, 2075·1
Karile, 2075·1
Karilexina, 2075·1
Karin, 2075·1
Karison, 2075·1
Kariva, 2075·1
Karlit, 2075·1
Karmel Balsamo— *see* Balsamo Analgesic Karmel, 1827·3
Karmel, Balsamo Analgesic— *see* Balsamo Analgesic Karmel, 1827·3
Karoyan S, 2075·1
Karpura Rasa, 1666·1
Karrer, 2075·1
Kartal, 2075·1
Karvea, 2075·1
Karvezide, 2075·2
Karvisin, 2075·2
Karvol, 2075·2
Karvol Plus, 2075·2
Kary Uni, 2075·2
Kas, 2075·2
Ka-Sabona, 2075·2
Kas-Bah, 2075·2
Kasele, 2075·2
Kaskadil, 2075·2
Kasmal, 2075·2
Kastipron, 2075·2
Kat, 1585·2
KAT-256, 1117·1
Kata, 2075·2
Katabios, 2075·2
Katadolon, 2075·2
Katagrip, 2075·2
Katalem, 2075·2
Katapekt, 2075·2
Katar, 2075·2
Katasma, 2075·2
Kataval, 2075·2
Katayama Fever— *see* Schistosomiasis, 100·3
Katemfe, 1451·1
Kath, 1585·2
Kathon CG, 1185·1
Katifen, 2075·2
Katin, 2075·2
Kation, 2075·3
Kationen, 2075·3
Katoderm, 2075·3
Katogel, 2075·3
Katomed, 2075·3
Katopril, 2075·3
Katosilver, 2075·3
Katovit, 2075·3
Katoxyn, 2075·3
Katrim, 2075·3
Katrim Balsamico, 2075·3
Katrum, 2075·3
Katsin, 2075·3
Kattwiderm, 2075·3
Kattwigast, 2075·3
Kattwigripp, 2075·3
Kattwilact, 2075·3
Kattwilon N, 2075·3
Katulcin-R, 2075·3
Katulcin-Rupha, 2075·3
Kava, 1703·2
Kavacur, 2075·3
Kavaform, 2075·3
Kavaform N, 2075·3
Kavain Harras N, 2075·3
Kavain Harras Plus, 2075·3
Kavakan, 2075·3
Kava-Kava, 1703·2
Kavalac, 2075·3
Kava-Phyton, 2075·3
Kavasedon, 2075·3
Kavasol, 2075·3
Kavatino, 2075·3
Kavavit, 2075·3
Kavepenin, 2075·4
Kaveri, 2075·4
Kavetten, 2075·4
Kavipen, 2075·4
Kavit, 2075·4
Kavitanum, 1466·3
Kavitol, 2075·4
Kavosan, 2075·4
Kavosporal Comp, 2075·4
Kavosporal Forte, 2075·4
Kawaform, 2075·4
Kawain, 1703·2
Kawasaki Disease, 1629·3
Kay Ciel, 2075·4
Kay-Cee-L, 2075·4
Kayexalate, 2075·4
Kayexalate Calcium, 2075·4
Kayexalate Sodium, 2075·4
Kaytwo, 2075·4
Kazak, 2075·4
Kazinal, 2075·4
KB-2413, 433·2
K-Biofen, 2075·4
K-C, 2075·4
KC-404, 786·3
KC-9147, 410·1
KC-9946, 1255·3
K-Cil, 2075·4
KCl-retard, 2075·4
K.C.M.C, 2075·4
Kdiron, 2075·4
KDM, 162·2
K-Dur, 2075·4
Keal, 2075·4
Kebir, 2075·4
Kebirtecan, 2075·4
Kebuzona, 51·1
Kebuzone, 51·1
Kebuzone Sodium, 51·1
Keciflox, 2075·4
Kedacillin, 2075·4
Kedacillina, 2075·4
Keduo, 2076·1
Keduril, 2076·1
Keefloxin, 2076·1
Keep Alert, 2076·1
Keep Clear Anti-Dandruff Shampoo, 2076·1
Keets, 1302·3
Kefaclor, 2076·1
Kefadim, 2076·1
Kefadol, 2076·1
Kefalex, 2076·1
Kefalexin, 2076·1
Kefalotin, 2076·1
Kefamin, 2076·1
Kefandol, 2076·1
Kefazim, 2076·1
Kefazin, 2076·1
Kefazol, 2076·1
Kefazon, 2076·1
Kefdole, 2076·1
Kefen, 2076·1
Kefentech, 2076·1
Kefexin, 2076·1
Keflaxina, 2076·1
Keflex, 2076·1
Keflin, 2076·1
Keflin Neutral, 2076·1
Keflor, 2076·1
Kefloridina, 2076·1

Kefloridina Mucolitico, 2076·2
Kefol, 2076·2
Kefolor, 2076·2
Keforal, 2076·2
Kefox, 2076·2
Kefoxin, 2076·2
Kefoxina, 2076·2
Kefspor, 2076·2
Keftab, 2076·2
Keftid, 2076·2
Keftriaxon, 2076·2
Kefurim, 2076·2
Kefurion, 2076·2
Kefurox, 2076·2
Kefzim, 2076·2
Kefzol, 2076·2
Keimax, 2076·2
Keimicina, 2076·2
Keishi-bukuryo-gan, Tsumura— *see* Tsumura Keishi-bukuryo-gan, 2351·1
Kela, 2076·2
Kelac, 2076·2
Kelaplus, 2076·2
Kelatin, 2076·2
Kelatine, 2076·2
Kelavitam, 2076·2
Kelbium, 2076·2
Kelefusin, 2076·2
Kelfer, 2076·2
Kelfiprim, 2076·2
Kelfizina, 2076·2
Kelfizine W, 2076·3
Keli-med, 2076·3
Kelina, 1653·3
Keliximab, 1668·3
Kelnac, 2076·3
Keloc, 2076·3
Kelo-Cote, 2076·3
Kelocyanor, 2076·3
Kelofibrase, 2076·3
Kelosal, 2076·3
Kelosoft, 2076·3
Kelp, 1742·3
Kelp Plus 3, 2076·3
Kelsef, 2076·3
Kelsopen, 2076·3
Keltican N, 2076·3
Kelual, 2076·3
Kelual Zinc, 2076·3
Keluamid, 1151·2
Keluamida, 1151·2
Kemadren, 2076·3
Kemadrin, 2076·3
Kemanat, 2076·3
Kemeol, 2076·3
Kemerhine, 2076·3
Kemerhinose, 2076·3
Kemicetin, 2076·3
Kemicetina, 2076·3
Kemicetine, 2076·3
Kemicetine Antiozena, 2076·3
Kemicetine Otological, 2076·3
Kemocarb, 2076·4
Kemodyn, 2076·4
Kemoplat, 2076·4
Kemphor, 2076·4
Kempi, 2076·4
Kemsol, 2076·4
Kemstro, 2076·4
Kemzid, 2076·4
Kenacomb, 2076·4
Kenacombin Novum, 2076·4
Kenacort Preparations, 2076·4
Kenacutan, 2076·4
Kenaderm, 2076·4
Kenadion, 2076·4
Kenaject, 2076·4
Kenalcol, 2076·4
Kenalin, 2077·1
Kenalog Preparations, 2077·1
Kenalone, 2077·1
Kenalyn, 2077·1
Kenapril, 2077·1
Kenaprol, 2077·1
Kenaprox, 2077·1
Kenazol, 2077·1
Kenazole, 2077·1
Kenciclen, 2077·1
Kendazol, 2077·1
Kendix, 2077·1
Kendural, 2077·1
Kendural C, 2077·1
Kendural-Fol-500, 2077·1
Kendural-Plus, 2077·1
Kenedril, 2077·1
Kenefen, 2077·1
Kenergon, 2077·1
Kenesil, 2077·2
Kenhancer, 2077·2
Keno, 2077·2
Kenoid, 2077·2
Kenoket, 2077·2
Kenolan, 2077·2
Kenona, 2077·2
Kenonel, 2077·2
Kenopril, 2077·2
Kenoral, 2077·2
Kensodic, 2077·2
Kenspa, 2077·2
Kenstatin, 2077·2
Kentacef, 2077·2
Kentadin, 2077·2
Kentamol, 2077·2
Kentosanil, 2077·2
Kentovase, 2077·2
Kenvestin, 2077·2
Kenwood Therapeutic Liquid, 2077·2
Kenya-Mox, 2077·2
Kenzen, 2077·2
Kenzoflex, 2077·2
Kenzolol, 2077·2
Kenzomyl, 2077·2
Keoxifene Hydrochloride, 1568·3
Kephalodoron, 2077·2
Kepinol, 2077·2
Keppra, 2077·2
Keppur, 2077·2
Kepra, 2077·2
Keprobiozol, 2077·3
Keprodol, 2077·3
Kepsidol, 2077·3
Keptan Compuesto, 2077·3
Keracianina, 1703·2
Keracnyl, 2077·3
Keracyanin, 1703·2
Kerafilm, 2077·3
Keraflex, 2077·3
Keral, 2077·3
Keralac Plus, 2077·3
Keralin, 2077·3
Keraliss 14, 2077·3
Keralyt, 2077·3
Keranon, 2077·3
Kerapil, 2077·3
Kerarer, 2077·3
Kerasal, 2077·3
Keratinase, 1703·3
Keratinisation Disorders, 1136·2
Keratinocyte Growth Factor, 1679·1
Keratisdin, 2077·3
Keratitis, Acanthamoeba— *see* Acanthamoeba Keratitis, 595·1
Keratitis, Bacterial— *see* Eye Infections, 127·2
Keratitis, Fungal— *see* Eye Infections, 388·1
Kerato Biciron, 2077·3
Keratoconjunctivitis Sicca— *see* Dry Eye, 1576·1
Keratocynesine, 2077·3
Keratolip, 2077·3
Keratosane, 2077·3
Keratoses— *see* Keratinisation Disorders, 1136·2
Keratosis, 2077·3
Keratosis, Actinic— *see* Basal Cell and Squamous Cell Carcinoma, 522·3
Keratosis Follicularis— *see* Darier's Disease, 1134·3
Keratosis Forte, 2077·3
Keratospor, 2077·3
Keratotal, 2077·3
Keratyl, 2077·3
Keri Preparations, 2077·3
Keri Silky Smooth, Alpha— *see* Alpha Keri Silky Smooth, 1789·2
Keri Soap, 2077·4
Kerion— *see* Skin Infections, 390·1
Kerlocal, 2077·4
Kerlofin, 2077·4
Kerlon, 2077·4
Kerlone, 2077·4
Kernit, 2077·4
Kernosan Elixir, 2077·4
Kernosan Heidelberger Poudre, 2077·4
Kernosan Huile de Massage, 2077·4
Keroderm, 2077·4
Kerodex, 2077·4
Keromask, 2077·4
Kerosene, 1475·1
Kerosine, 1475·1
Kerpet, 2077·4
*Kerria lacca*, 1743·3
Kertyol, 2077·4
Kertyol-S, 2077·4
Kesan, 2077·4
Keshan Disease, 1444·1
Kesint, 2077·4
Kess, 2077·4
Kess Complex, 2077·4
Kessar, 2077·4
Kest, 2077·4
Kestin, 2077·4
Kestine, 2077·4
Kestomatine, 2078·1
Kestomatine Baby, 2078·1
Kestomatine Bebe, 2078·1
Kestomicol, 2078·1
Kestrone, 2078·1
Keta, 2078·1
Keta-Hameln, 2078·1
Ketalar, 2078·1
Ketalgesic, 2078·1
Ketalgine, 2078·1
Ketalin, 2078·1
Ketamina, Hidrocloruro de, 1302·1
Ketamine Hydrochloride, 1302·1
*S*-Ketamine Hydrochloride, 1302·2
Ketamini Hydrochloridum, 1302·1
Ketanest, 2078·1
Ketanine, 2078·1
Ketanov, 2078·1
Ketanserin, 943·1
Ketanserin Tartrate, 943·1
Ketanserina, Tartrato de, 943·1
Ketanserinol, 943·1
Ketartrium, 2078·1
Ketas, 2078·1
Ketasma, 2078·1
Ketava, 2078·1
Ketazol, 2078·1
Ketazolam, 703·1
Ketazon, 2078·1
Ketazon Flex, 2078·1
Ketek, 2078·1
Keten, 2078·1
Ketensin, 2078·2
Ketesse, 2078·2
Ketidin, 2078·2
Ketifen, 2078·2
Ketil, 2078·2
Ketina, 2078·2
Ketlur, 2078·2
Ketmin, 2078·2
Keto, 2078·2
Ketoacidosis, Diabetic— *see* Diabetic Emergencies, 328·2
Ketobemidone Hydrochloride, 51·1
Ketocaína, Hidrocloruro de, 1377·1
Ketocaine Hydrochloride, 1377·1
Ketocev, 2078·2
Ketocid, 2078·2
Ketocine, 2078·2
Ketocon, 2078·2
Ketoconazol, 403·3
Ketoconazole, 403·3
Ketoconazolum, 403·3
Ketoderm, 2078·2
3-Keto-Desogestrel, 1554·1
Keto-Diabur Test, 2078·2
Keto-Diabur Test 5000, 2078·2
Ketodiaburtest 5000, 2078·2
Ketodiastix, 2078·2
Keto-Diastix, 2078·2
Ketodol, 2078·2
Ketodur, 2078·2
Ketof, 2078·2
Ketofar, 2078·2
Ketofen, 2078·2
Ketofene, 2078·2
Ketoflam, 2078·2
Ketoftil, 2078·3
Ketogan, 2078·3
Ketogan Novum, 2078·3
Ketogel, 2078·3
α-Ketoglutarate, 1433·3
Ketohair, 2078·3
Ketohexal, 2078·3
Ketohydroxyoestrin, 1553·1
Ketoisdin, 2078·3
Ketokid, 2078·3
Ketolan, 2078·3
Ketolar, 2078·3
Ketolist, 2078·3
Ketomed, 2078·3
Ketomex, 2078·3
Ketomicol, 2078·3
Ketomizol, 2078·3
Ketonal, 2078·3
Ketonan, 2078·3
Ketonazol, 2078·3
Ketonazole, 2078·3
Ketone, 2078·3
Ketonex, 2078·3
Ketonic, 2078·3
Ketonil, 2078·3
Ketop, 2078·3
Ketopharm, 2078·3
Ketophenylbutazone, 51·1
Ketoplus, 2078·3
Ketoprofen, 51·2
Ketoprofen Lysine, 52·1
Ketoprofen Sodium, 52·1
Ketoprofeno, 51·2
Ketoprofenum, 51·2
6-Keto-prostaglandin $F_{1\alpha}$, 1517·2
Ketoral, 2078·3
Ketorax, 2078·3
Ketorin, 2078·3
Ketorolac Trometamol, 52·1
Ketorolac Tromethamine, 52·1
Ketorolaco Trometamol, 52·1
Ketoscilium, 482·2
Ketoselect, 2078·3
Ketosil, 2078·3
Ketosolan, 2078·4
Ketoson, 2078·4
Ketosteril, 2078·4
Ketostix, 2078·4
Ketotab, 2078·4
Ketotard, 2078·4
Ketotifen Fumarate, 788·1
Ketotifen Hydrogen Fumarate, 788·1
Ketotifeni Hydrogenofumaras, 788·1
Ketotifeno, Fumarato de, 788·1
Ketotisin, 2078·4
Ketotop, 2078·4
Ketotriose, 1145·2
Ketovail, 2078·4
Ketovite, 2078·4
Ketozal, 2078·4
Ketozip, 2078·4
Ketozol, 2078·4
Ketozole, 2078·4
Ketrax, 2078·4
Ketrel, 2078·4
Ketrizin, 2078·4
Ketum, 2078·4
Ketur-Test, 2078·4
Keuschlamm, 1649·1
Keval, 2078·4
Kevatril, 2078·4
Kevis, 2078·4
Kevopril, 2078·4
Kew Tree, 1692·3

Kexelate, 2078·4
Kexidil, 2078·4
K-Exit, 2078·4
Keyerpril, 2078·4
Keylyte, 2078·4
Key-Plex, 2079·1
Key-Pred, 2079·1
Key-Pred-SP, 2079·1
Kezepin, 2079·1
Kezer, 2079·1
Kezon, 2079·1
Kezoral, 2079·1
K-Flebo, 2079·1
K-Fosfosteril, 2079·1
KG-2413, 433·2
K-G Elixir, 2079·1
KGS-PE, 2079·1
KH3, 2079·1
KH3 Powel, 2079·1
KH3-Vit, 2079·1
Khanh-Chha, 1666·1
Khanje, 1666·1
Khartoum Senna, 1288·2
Khat, 1585·2
Khella, 1653·3
Khellah, 1653·3
Khellangan N, 2079·1
Khellin, 1653·3
Khelline, 1653·3
Khellinum, 1653·3
Kiadon, 2079·1
Kiatrium, 2079·1
Kid Kare Childrens Cough/Cold, 2079·1
Kid Kare Pediatric Nasal Decongestant, 2079·1
Kidbar, 2079·1
Kiddi, 2079·1
Kiddi Choo, 2079·1
Kiddi Nouvelle Formule— *see* Kiddi, 2079·1
Kiddi Pharmaton, 2079·1
Kiddicol, Chemists Own— *see* Chemists Own Kiddicol, 1882·1
Kiddicrom, 2079·1
Kiddie Vite, 2079·1
Kiddiekof, 2079·2
Kiddipayne, Adco- — *see* Adco-Kiddipayne, 1775·3
Kiddyflu, 2079·2
Kid-Eeze, 2079·2
Kidmin, 2079·2
Kidney Cancer— *see* Malignant Neoplasms of the Kidney, 518·1
Kidney Disease, Glomerular— *see* Glomerular Kidney Disease, 1080·2
Kidney Failure— *see* Acute Renal Failure, 1221·3
Kidney Failure— *see* Chronic Renal Failure, 1222·1
Kidney Stones— *see* Renal Calculi, 936·2
Kidney Transplantation, 1346·2
Kidrolase, 2079·2
Kid's Bumps, 2079·2
Kid's Colic, 2079·2
Kids' Earache, 2079·2
Kids Sunblock, 2079·2
Kids' Teething, 2079·2
KIE, 2079·2
Kieselguhr, Purified, 1581·3
KI-Expectorante, 2079·2
Kif, 1666·1
Kif Ktami, 1666·1
Kikelaio EF 3, 2079·2
Kilios, 2079·2
Kilkof, 2079·2
Killer Weed, 1730·3
Killgrip, 2079·2
Killit, 2079·2
Killpan, 2079·2
Kilmicen, 2079·2
Kilnits, 2079·2
Kilor, 2079·2
Kilovit, 2079·2
Kilpane, 2079·2
Kimafan, 2079·2
Kiminto, 2079·2
Kin, 2079·2
KIN-493, 366·3
Kin Soff, 2079·2
Kinabide, 2079·2
Kinasten, 2079·3
Kincare, 2079·3
Kinciclina, 2079·3
Kindaren, 2079·3
Kindcalcio, 2079·3
Kindcetin, 2079·3
Kindelmin, 2079·3
Kinder Em-eukal Hustensaft, 2079·3
Kinder Erkaltungsbalsam, 2079·3
Kinder Finimal, 2079·3
Kinder Luuf, 2079·3
Kindercal, 2079·3
Kindergen, 2079·3
Kinderval, 2079·3
Kindomet, 2079·3
Kindpasm, 2079·3
Kinedak, 2079·3
Kinerase, 2079·3
Kineret, 2079·3
Kinestase, 2079·3
Kinet, 2079·3
Kinetizine, 2079·3
Kineto, 2079·3
Kinetone, 2079·3
Kinevac, 2079·3
Kinex, 2079·3
Kinfil, 2079·3
King's Cureall, 1686·3
Kinidin, 2079·3
Kinidin Durules, 2079·4
Kinidine, 2079·4
Kiniduron, 2079·4
Kinin, 2079·4
Kininogen, High Molecular Weight, 735·3
Kinkeliba, 1703·3
Kinline, 2079·4
Kinnab, 1666·1
Kinogen, 2079·4
Kinolymphat, 2079·4
Kinot, 2079·4
Kinson, 2079·4
Kintavit, 2079·4
Kinupril, 2079·4
Kinurea H, 2079·4
Kionex, 2079·4
Kiper, 2079·4
Kipress, 2079·4
Kir Richter, 2079·4
Kira, 2079·4
Kiri, 2079·4
Kirim, 2079·4
Kirim Gyn, 2079·4
Kirin, 2079·4
Kiro Rub, 2079·4
Kirsan, 2079·4
Kisolv, 2079·4
Kitacne, 2079·4
Kitacne AR, 2079·4
Kitacne PB, 2079·4
Kitadol Preparations, 2079·4
Kitapen, 2080·1
Kitasamicina, 225·3
Kitasamycin, 225·3
Kitasamycin $A_4$, 225·3
Kitasamycin $A_5$, 225·3
Kitasamycin Tartrate, 225·3
Kit-kat, 1302·3
Kitnos, 2080·1
Kiton, 2080·1
Kit-Syrup, 2080·1
Kivat, 2080·1
KL-255, 878·1
Klacid, 2080·1
Klacid— *see* Klacid HP 7, 2080·1
Klacid— *see* Losec Hp 7, 2105·4
Klacid— *see* Losec 20 Triple, 2106·1
Klacid— *see* Pylorid-KA, 2247·2
Klacid HP 7, 2080·1
Klaciped, 2080·1
Klafotaxim, 2080·1
Klamacin, 2080·1
Klari, Linimento— *see* Linimento Klari, 2097·4
Klaricid, 2080·1
Klaricid— *see* Heliclear, 2038·1
Klaricid— *see* HeliMet, 2038·1
Klariderm, 2080·1
Klaridex, 2080·1
Klarivitina, 2080·1
Klaron, 2080·1
Klaryl, 2080·1
Klatschrose, 1058·1
KLB6, 2080·1
KLB6 Fruit Diet, 2080·1
Klean-Prep, 2080·1
K-Lease, 2080·1
Klebsiella Pneumoniae Glycoprotein, 1703·3
Kleen-Handz, 2080·1
Kleenocid, 2080·1
Kleenosept, 2080·2
Kleer, 2080·2
Kleer Cream, 2080·2
Kleie, 1253·2
Klenac, 2080·2
Kleotrat, 2080·2
Klerist-D, 2080·2
Klestran, 2080·2
Klevasin, 2080·2
Klevistamin, 2080·2
Klexane, 2080·2
KLGH 3, 2080·2
Kliacef, 2080·2
Klifem, 2080·2
Klimadynon, 2080·2
Klimaktoplant, 2080·2
Klimaktoplant H, 2080·2
Klimaktosin, 2080·2
Klimalet, 2080·2
Klimapur, 2080·2
Klimareduct, 2080·2
Klimasyx, 2080·2
Klimax-Gastreu S R10, 2080·2
Klimaxil, 2080·2
Klimicin, 2080·2
Klimofol, 2080·2
Klimonorm, 2080·2
Klinefelter's Syndrome— *see* Hypogonadism, 1316·1
Klinna, 2080·2
Klinoc, 2080·2
Klinomycin, 2080·2
Klinotab, 2080·2
Klinoxid, 2080·3
Kliofem, 2080·3
Kliogest, 2080·3
Kliogest N, 2080·3
Klion, 2080·3
Kliovance, 2080·3
Klipal, 2080·3
Klipal Codeine, 2080·3
Klismacort, 2080·3
Klispel, 2080·3
Klistier, 2080·3
Klizin, 2080·3
KLN, 2080·3
Kloclor, 2080·3
Klodin, 2080·3
Klodipin, 2080·3
Klomazole, 2080·3
Klomeprax, 2080·3
Klomicina, 2080·3
Klonacid, 2080·3
Klonadroxil, 2080·3
Klonadryl, 2080·3
Klonadryl Antitusivo, 2080·3
Klonafenac, 2080·3
Klonalfenicol, 2080·3
Klonalmox, 2080·3
Klonalol, 2080·3
Klonam, 2080·3
Klonametacina, 2080·3
Klonamicin, 2080·4
Klonatropina, 2080·4
Klonazol, 2080·4
Klonocarpina, 2080·4
Klonopin, 2080·4
Klont, 2080·4
Klopoxid, 2080·4
K-Lor, 2080·4
Kloraetyl, 2080·4
Kloramfenikol, 185·1
Klor-Con, 2080·4
Klor-Con/EF, 2080·4
Klor-De, 2080·4
Kloref, 2080·4
Kloren, 2080·4
Klorhexol, 2080·4
Klor-Kleen, 2080·4
Klorokin, 2080·4
Kloroplatinasyra, 1670·2
Klorpo, 2080·4
Klorproman, 2080·4
Klorsept, 2080·4
Klorvess, 2080·4
Klosartan, 2080·4
Klosidol, 2080·4
Klosidol B1 B6 B12, 2080·4
Klosterfrau Aktiv, 2080·4
Klosterfrau Franzbranntwein, 2081·1
Klosterfrau Franzbranntwein Latschenkiefer, 2081·1
Klosterfrau Melissengeist, 2081·1
Klosterfrau-Beruhigungskapseln, 2081·1
Klotricid, 2081·1
Klotriptyl, 2081·1
Klotrix, 2081·1
$KL_4$-surfactant, 1736·2
Klyndaken, 2081·1
Klysma Salinisch, 2081·1
Klysma Sorbit, 2081·1
Klysmol, 2081·1
K-Lyte, 2081·1
K-Lyte DS, 2081·1
K-Lyte/Cl, 2081·1
Klyx, 2081·1
Klyx Magnum, 2081·1
KM-65, 1115·3
KMA, 2081·1
K-Mag, 2081·1
K-Med, 2081·1
KMG Plus, 2081·1
KMH, 2081·1
K-Mizol, 2081·1
KN Solution, 2081·1
Kneipp Preparations, 2081·1
Kneipplax N, 2081·4
Knob Root, 1749·3
Knoblauch, 1691·1
Knoblauch Dragees N, Kneipp— *see* Kneipp Knoblauch Dragees N, 2081·3
Knoblauch-Pflanzensaft, Kneipp— *see* Kneipp Knoblauch-Pflanzensaft, 2081·3
Knoblauch-Vital, 2081·4
Knochenzement, 2081·4
Kno-Paine, 2081·4
K-Norm, 2081·4
Knotted Wrack, 1742·3
Knowful, 2081·4
Kö-1173, 958·1
Ko-1366, 878·1
Koal, 2081·4
Koate, 2081·4
Koate-DVI, 2081·4
Koate-HP, 2081·4
Koate-HS, 2081·4
Ko-Cap, 2081·4
Kochsalz mit Glucose, 2081·4
Kodakon, 2081·4
Kodamid, 2081·4
Kodan Tinktur Forte, 2081·4
Kodimagnyl, 2081·4
Kodipar, 2082·1
Kofarest, 2082·1
Kof-Eze, 2082·1
Koffazon, 2082·1
Koffex, 2082·1
Koffex DM, 2082·1
Koffex DM-D, 2082·1
Koffex DM-D-E, 2082·1
Koffex DM+Decongestant— *see* Koffex DM-D, 2082·1
Koffex DM+Decongestant+Expectorant— *see* Koffex DM-D-E, 2082·1
Koffex DM-E, 2082·1

Koffex DM+Expectorant— see Koffex DM-E, 2082·1
Koffex Expectorant, 2082·1
Koffisal, 2082·1
Kofron, 2082·1
Kogenate, 2082·1
Kohle-Compretten, 2082·1
Kohle-Hevert, 2082·1
Kohlensaurebad Bastian, 2082·1
Kohle-Pulvis, 2082·1
Kohle-Tabletten, 2082·1
Kohrsolin, 2082·1
Kohrsolin FF, 2082·1
Kohrsolin ID, 2082·1
Kojic Acid, 1151·2
Koki Ment Tiro, Pastillas— see Pastillas Koki Ment Tiro, 2207·4
Ko-Kure, 2082·1
Kola, 1765·3
Kola Astier, 2082·1
Kola Fosfatada Soel, 2082·1
Kola, Gota, 1144·3
Kola, Gotu, 1144·3
Kola Nuts, 1765·3
Kola-Dallmann, 2082·1
Kola-Dallmann mit Lecithin, 2082·1
Koladex, 2082·1
Kolampept, 2082·1
Kolanticon, 2082·2
Kolantyl, 2082·2
Kolantyl DMP, 2082·2
Kolemed, 2082·2
Kolephrin, 2082·2
Kolephrin GG/DM, 2082·2
Kolephrin/DM, 2082·2
Kolestop, 2082·2
Kolibel, 2082·2
Kolkin, 2082·2
Kollagenase, 2082·2
Kollagenase com Cloranfenicol, 2082·2
Kollaps-Gastreu N R67, 2082·2
Kollateral, 2082·2
Kollateral A + E, 2082·2
Kollodiumwolle, 1156·2
Koloquinthen, 1260·3
Kolplex, 2082·2
Kolpovent, 2082·2
Kolsan, 2082·2
Kolsuspension, 2082·2
Kolton Bronchiale Erkaltungssaft, 2082·2
Kolton Grippale N, 2082·2
Komasin, 2082·2
Kombé Strophanthin, 1009·1
Kombetin, 2082·2
Komb-H-Insulin, 2082·2
Kombicrom, 2082·2
Kombinax, 2082·3
Komb-Insulin, 2082·3
Komb-Insulin S, 2082·3
Kombi-Stulln N, 2082·3
Komil, 2082·3
Kompensan, 2082·3
Kompensan Dimeticon, 2082·3
Kompensan-S, 2082·3
Kona, 2082·3
Konaderm, 2082·3
Konakion, 2082·3
Konakion MM, 2082·3
Konakion Novum, 2082·3
Konaturil, 2082·3
Konazil, 2082·3
Konazol, 2082·3
Konazol Shampoo, Hexal— see Hexal Konazol Shampoo, 2043·3
Kondon's Nasal, 2082·3
Kondremul, 2082·3
Konicortil, 2082·3
Koniderm, 2082·3
Konifungil, 2082·3
Konirub, 2082·3
Konjac Flour, 1693·3
Konjac Mannan, 1693·3
Konjax, 2082·3
Konjunktival, 2082·3
Konjunktival Thilo, 2082·4
Konlax, 2082·4
Konor, 2082·4
Konorderm, 2082·4
Konovid, 2082·4
Konstitutin, 2082·4
Konsyl, 2082·4
Konsyl-D, 2082·4
Kontagripp Mono, 2082·4
Kontakto Derm, 2082·4
Kontal, 2082·4
Kontexin, 2082·4
Kontic, 2082·4
Konyne, 2082·4
Konyne 80, 2082·4
Kop Alerge Vacina, 2082·4
Kop Hepar, 2082·4
Kopen, 2082·4
Kophane Cough and Cold Formula, 2082·4
Korandil, 2082·4
Kordinol Compuesto, 2082·4
Koreberon, 2082·4
Korec, 2082·4
Koretic, 2082·4
Korifen, 2082·4
Koro, 2082·4
Korodin, 2082·4
Koromex, 2082·4
Koro-Nyhadin, 2083·1
Korsakoff's Syndrome— see Wernicke-Korsakoff Syndrome, 1455·3
Korseng, 2083·1
Korsolex Preparations, 2083·1
Korticoid, 2083·1
Korticoid Polyvalent, 2083·1
Kortikoid-ratiopharm, 2083·1
Korynase, 2083·1
Korzen, 2083·1
Kos, 2083·1
Kosteo, 2083·1
Kovan, 2083·1
Kovilen, 2083·1
Kovinal, 2083·1
Kovitonic, 2083·1
KP, 2083·1
KP-363, 395·2
K-Pek, 2083·1
K-Pek II, 2083·1
K-Phos MF, 2083·1
K-Phos Neutral, 2083·1
K-Phos No.2, 2083·1
K-Phos Original, 2083·1
Kpl, 2083·1
KPN, 2083·1
KPP, 2083·1
K-Profen, 2083·2
Kraftol, 2083·2
Krallendorn, 2083·2
Krama, 2083·2
Krameria, 1738·1
Krameria Root, 1738·1
*Krameria triandra*, 1738·1
Kranit Nova, 2083·2
Kratalgin, 2083·2
Kratium, 2083·2
Kratofin Simplex, 2083·2
Krauter Hustensaft, 2083·2
Krauter Hustensaft N Kneipp Tannolsaft, Kneipp— see Kneipp Krauter Hustensaft N Kneipp Tannolsaft, 2081·3
Krauter Taschenkur Nerven und Schlaf N, Kneipp— see Kneipp Krauter Taschenkur Nerven und Schlaf N, 2081·3
Krauterdoktor Preparations, 2083·2
Krauterelixier, 2083·2
Krautergeist S, 2083·2
Krauterhaus Mag Kottas Preparations, 2083·3
Krauterlax A, 2083·3
Krauterlax-S, 2083·3
Krauterpfarrer Weidinger Tee Preparations, 2083·3
Krautertee Preparations— see Neuners Krautertee Preparations, 2162·4
Krebiozen, 1703·3
Krebsilasi, 2083·4
Kredex, 2083·4
Kreislauf Katovit, 2083·4
Kreislaufja, 2083·4
Kreislauftropen, 2083·4
Kremil, 2083·4
Kremil-S, 2083·4
Krenosin, 2083·4
Krenosine, 2084·1
Kreon, 2084·1
Kresolum Venale, 1177·3
Kresse, 2084·1
Krestin, 1733·2
Kreuzdorn, 1254·1
Kreuzlinger Klosterliniment, 2084·1
Kriadex, 2084·1
Kriolen, 2084·1
Kriptiser, 2084·1
Kripton, 2084·1
Kriptonal, 2084·1
Krisovin, 2084·1
Kristallviolett, 1186·1
Kristalose, 2084·1
Kritel, 2084·1
Krol, 2084·1
Kronel, 2084·1
Kronofed-A, 2084·1
Krophan N, 2084·1
Krucef, 2084·1
Kruschels, 2084·1
Kruses Fluid Magnesia, 2084·1
KRX-101, 1009·2
Kryobulin, 2084·1
Kryobulin TIM 3, 2084·1
Kryobulin TIM 3-I, 2084·1
Kryobuline S-TIM 3, 2084·1
Kryptocur, 2084·1
Krypton-81m, 1525·1
Kryptoxanthine, 1422·3
KSR, 2084·1
K-SR, 2084·1
KT-611, 964·1
KT-3777, 228·1
K-Tab, 2084·1
K-Thrombin, 2084·1
Kudona, 2084·2
Kudrox Double Strength, 2084·2
Kuhlprednon, 2084·2
Kümmel, 1667·2
Kümmelöl, 1667·3
Kupa, 2084·2
Kupfersulfat, 1426·1
Kuracid, 2084·2
Kurapel, 2084·2
Kürbissamen, 1677·3
Kurgan, 2084·2
Kurom, 2084·2
Kurrol's Salt, Potassium, 1734·3
Kuson, 2084·2
Kutapressin, 2084·2
Kutesan, 2084·2
Kutrase, 2084·2
Ku-Zyme, 2084·2
Ku-Zyme HP, 2084·2
Kveim Antigen, 1703·3
Kvilla, 2084·2
KVX-478, 628·2
KW, 1730·3, 2084·2
KW-110, 1248·1
KW-1062, 231·3
KW-1070, 158·3
KW-3049, 868·1
KW-4679, 438·1
Kwai, 2084·2
Kwan Loong Oil, 2084·2
KWD-2019, 797·2
KWD-2183, 781·2
Kwelcof, 2084·2
Kwell, 2084·2
Kwellada, 2084·2
Kwellada-P, 2084·2
Kwells, 2084·2
Kwicap, 2084·2
Kwikprep, 2084·2
Kwim, 2084·2
K-Y, 2084·2
K-Y Personal Lubricant— see K-Y Plus Spermicidal Lubricant, 2084·3
K-Y Plus Spermicidal Lubricant, 2084·3
Kyasamur Forest Fever— see Haemorrhagic Fevers, 618·2
Kyaugutt, 2084·3
Kybernin, 2084·3
Kybernin P, 2084·3
Kymazol, 2084·3
Kyolarte, 2084·3
Kyolic Preparations, 2084·3
Kytinon, 2084·3
Kytinon ABC, 2084·3
Kytril, 2084·3
Kytta Preparations, 2084·3
Kyypakkaus, 2084·4

**L**

L, 1439·1
L1, 1033·1
L-8, 1342·3
L 25, 2084·4
L 28, 2084·4
L 52, 2084·4
L-67, 1382·3
L 72, 2084·4
L-105, 254·1
L 114, 2084·4
L-542, 1185·3
L-554, 443·3
L-627, 165·3
L-743, 632·2
L-846, 727·3
L-1573, 1712·1
L-1633, 1130·2
L-1718, 1725·1
L-2214, 414·3
L-2329, 415·1
L-3428, 859·2
L-5103, 250·2
L-5458, 1096·2
L-6257, 470·2
L-11473, 253·3
L-12507, 264·3
L-154803, 949·1
L-154826, 946·3
L-588357-0, 956·1
L-620388, 177·2
L-642957, 188·1
L-643341, 1265·2
L-644128-000U, 997·1
L-670452, 765·3
L-671152, 908·3
L-700462, 1013·3
L-706631, 788·3
L-735524, 638·2
L-743726, 632·2
L-743873, 395·3
L-749345, 207·3
L-791456, 38·2
LA-III, 690·1
LA-12, 2084·4
LA-391, 1289·3
LA-956, 1591·2
LA-1221, 878·2
LA-6023, 342·3
LA 40221, 463·1
LA Morph, 2084·4
La Rocha, 698·3
LAAM, 54·1
Lab/A, 2084·4
Labarraque's Solution, 1192·2
L'Abbe Chaupitre Preparations— see Formule de l'Abbe Chaupitre Preparations, 2007·3
Labdiazina, 2084·4
Label, 2084·4
Labello Active, 2084·4
Labello UV, 2084·4
Labelphen, 2084·4
Labenda, 2084·4
Labentrol, 2084·4
Labetalol, Hidrocloruro de, 943·3
Labetalol Hydrochloride, 943·3
Labetaloli Hydrochloridum, 943·3
Labfcilina, 2084·4
Labigeron, 2084·4
Labile Factor, 735·3
Labileno, 2084·4

Labilex, 2084·4
Labiline— *see* Vitafissan N, 2380·4
Labimion, 2084·4
Labiosan, 2084·4
Labirin, 2084·4
Labisan, 2084·4
Labistatin, 2084·4
Labiton, 2084·4
Labitrix, 2084·4
Labocaina, 2084·4
Labocane, 2084·4
Labocne, 2085·1
Labocton, 2085·1
Labopal, 2085·1
Labosalic, 2085·1
Labosept, 2085·1
Labosona, 2085·1
Labosona G, 2085·1
Labosona N, 2085·1
Labotensil, 2085·1
Laboterol, 2085·1
Labour Augmentation— *see* Labour Induction and Augmentation, 1511·1
Labour Induction— *see* Labour Induction and Augmentation, 1511·1
Labour, Management of— *see* Labour Induction and Augmentation, 1511·1
Labour Pain, 6·2
Labour, Premature, Infections in— *see* Premature Labour, 143·2
Labour, Premature— *see* Premature Labour, 794·1
Labour, Third Stage— *see* Postpartum Haemorrhage, 1684·3
Laboxantryl, 2085·1
Labrocol, 2085·1
Labstix, 2085·1
Labstix SG, 2085·1
Laburide, 2085·1
Laburnum, 1703·3
*Laburnum anagyroides*, 1703·3
*Laburnum vulgare*, 1703·3
Labycarbol, 2085·1
Labydon, 2085·1
Labymetacyn, 2085·1
Labypurol, 2085·1
Labysal, 2085·1
LAC-43, 1371·1
Lac 4 N, 2085·1
Lacalut, 2085·1
Lacbon, 2085·1
Lacca, 1743·3
Lacca in Tabulis, 1743·3
*Laccifer lacca*, 1743·3
Laccoderme a l'huile de Cade, 2085·1
Lacdigest, 2085·1
Lac-Dol, 2085·1
Laceran, 2085·1
Laceran Piel Seca, 2085·1
Lacerdermol, 2085·1
Lacerdermol Complex, 2085·1
Lacermucin, 2085·1
Lacerol, 2085·2
Lacgel, 2085·2
Lachemistol, 2085·2
Lachess, 2085·2
Lachydrin, 2085·2
Lac-Hydrin, 2085·2
Lacidipine, 944·2
Lacidipino, 944·2
Laciken, 2085·2
Lacimen, 2085·2
Lacin, 2085·2
Lacipil, 2085·2
Lacirex, 2085·2
Laclorene, 2085·2
Laclorhex, 2085·2
LAC-Lotion, 2085·2
Lacoerdin Mg Plus, 2085·2
Lacoerdin-N, 2085·2
Lac-Oph, 2085·2
Lacophtal, 2085·2
Lacovin, 2085·2
Lacribase, 2085·2
Lacrifluid, 2085·2
Lacrigel, 2085·2
Lacri-Gel, 2085·2
Lacrigel A, 2085·2
Lacril, 2085·2
Lacrilube, 2085·2
Lacri-Lube, 2085·2
Lacrilux, 2085·3
Lacrim, Neo— *see* Neo Lacrim, 2156·3
Lacrima, 2085·3
Lacrima Plus, 2085·3
Lacrimal, 2085·3
Lacrimal OK, 2085·3
Lacrimalfa, 2085·3
Lacrimart, 2085·3
Lacrime, 2085·3
Lacrimill, 2085·3
Lacrimol, 2085·3
Lacrinorm, 2085·3
Lacripharma, 2085·3
Lacrisert, 2085·3
Lacrisic, 2085·3
Lacrisifi, 2085·3
Lacrisol, 2085·3
Lacri-Stulln, 2085·3
Lacri-Tears, 2085·3
Lacromycin, 2085·3
Lacrycon, 2085·3
Lacrypos, 2085·3
Lacrystat, 2085·3
Lacrytube, 2085·3
Lacryvisc, 2085·3
Lacson, 2085·3
Lactacyd, 2085·4
Lactacyd Antibatterico, 2085·4
Lactacyd Derma, 2085·4
Lactacyd Femina, 2085·4
Lactacyd Intimo, 2085·4
Lactagel, 2085·4
Lacta-Gynecogel, 2085·4
Lactaid, 2085·4
Lactal, 2085·4
Lactamax, 2085·4
Lactar, 2085·4
Lac-Tas, 2085·4
Lactase, 1756·2
Lactase Deficiency— *see* Lactose Intolerance, 1439·1
Lactation Induction— *see* Lactation Inhibition and Induction, 1317·1
Lactation Inhibition— *see* Lactation Inhibition and Induction, 1317·1
Lactato de Amonio, 1142·3
Lactato de Amrinona, 862·3
Lactato de Biperideno, 479·3
Lactato de Ciclizina, 429·3
Lactato de Ciprofloxacino, 188·3
Lactato de Etacridina, 1165·3
Lactato de Etilo, 1147·1
Lactato de Milrinona, 959·2
Lactato de Pentazocina, 79·3
Lactato de Prenilamina, 1735·1
Lactato de Sodio, 1223·2
Lact-Easy, 2085·4
Lactec, 2085·4
Lactec D, 2085·4
Lactec G, 2085·4
Lactel, 2085·4
Lacteol, 2085·4
Lacteol Fort, 2085·4
Lacteol Forte, 2085·4
Lactess, 2085·4
Lactic Acid, 1704·1
(*S*)-Lactic Acid, 1704·1
Lactic Acid Lactate, 1704·1
Lactic Acidosis— *see* Metabolic Acidosis, 1217·2
Lactic-acid-producing Organisms, 1704·2
Lacticare, 2085·4
Lacticare-HC, 2085·4
Láctico, Ácido, 1704·1
Láctico, Organismos Productores de Ácido, 1704·2
Lacticum, Acidum, 1704·1
Lactiderm, 2085·4
Lactiderm HC, 2085·4
Lactidorm, 2085·4
Lactifero, 2085·4
Lactigriet, 2086·1
Lactinex, 2086·1
Lactinol, 2086·1
Lactinol-E, 2086·1
Lactipan, 2086·1
Lactisan, 2086·1
Lactisol, 2086·1
Lactisona, 2086·1
Lactisporin, 2086·1
Lactisyn, 2086·1
Lactit, 1269·1
Lactitol, 1269·1
Lactitol Monohydrate, 1269·1
Lactitolum, 1269·1
Lactivis, 2086·1
Lacto Calamine, 2086·1
Lacto Pregomine, 2086·1
Lacto Vagin, 2086·1
Lactoacridine, 1165·3
Lactobac, 2086·1
*Lactobacillus acidophilus*, 1642·1, 1704·2
*Lactobacillus bulgaricus*, 1704·2
Lactobionato de Eritromicina, 208·2
Lactobiosit, 1269·1
Lactocal-F, 2086·1
Lacto-Cev Zn, 2086·1
Lactocol, 2086·1
Lactocol Expectorante, 2086·1
Lactocrem, 2086·1
Lactocrem Bebe, 2086·1
Lactocreosote, 1117·2
Lactocur, 2086·1
Lactofalk, 2086·1
Lactoferment, 2086·1
Lactoferrina, 2086·2
Lactofilus, 2086·2
Lactofit, 2086·2
Lactoflavin, 1456·1
Lactofree, 2086·2
Lactogen, 1337·3
Lactogenic Hormone, 1337·3
Lactoger, 2086·2
Lactogermine, 2086·2
Lacto-Gin, 2086·2
Lactolas, 2086·2
Lactolavol, 2086·2
Lactolife, 2086·2
Lactoliofil, 2086·2
Lactomannan, 2086·2
Lactomina, 2086·2
1.13-3.4-Lactone, 204·2
Lactonico, 2086·2
Lactonorm, 2086·2
Lactopectin, 2086·2
Lactophilus, 2086·2
Lactopregomine, 2086·2
Lacto-Purga, 2086·2
Lactopurum, 2086·2
Lactored, 2086·2
Lactosa, 1438·3
Lactose, 1438·3
Lactose, Anhydrous, 1438·3
Lactose Breath Test, 1269·2
Lactose Intolerance, 1439·1
Lactose Monohydrate, 1438·3
Lactosec, 2086·2
Lactositol, 1269·1
Lactosum, 1438·3
Lactotropin, 1337·3
Lactovit, 2086·2
Lactoyl-lactic Acid, 1704·1
17β-(*S*)-Lactoyl-17-methylestra-4,9-dien-3-one, 1573·3
Lactrase, 2086·2
Lactrex, 2086·2
*Lactuca virosa*, 1765·2
Lactucarium, 1765·2
Lactucol, 2086·2
Lactuflor, 2086·2
Lactugal, 2086·3
Lactul, 2086·3
Lactulax, 2086·3
Lactulon, 2086·3
Lactulona, 2086·3
Lactulosa, 1269·1
Lactulose, 1269·1
Lactulose Concentrate, 1269·1
Lactulose, Liquid, 1269·1
Lactulose Solution, 1269·1
Lactulosum, 1269·1
Lactumed, 2086·3
Lactuverlan, 2086·3
Lactyl, 2086·3
Ladakamycin, 529·2
Ladazol, 2086·3
Ladinin, 2086·3
Ladip, 2086·3
Ladiwin, 2086·3
Ladocort, 2086·3
Ladogal, 2086·3
Ladose, 2086·3
Ladropen, 2086·3
Lady, 1373·3
Lady-35, 2086·3
Lady Fittig, 2086·3
Ladylen, 2086·3
Ladylen Duo, 2086·3
Ladymega, 2086·3
Lady-Ten 35, 2086·3
Ladytone, 2086·3
Ladyvital, 2086·3
Laetrile, 1704·3
Laevadosin, 2086·3
Laev-Amin, 2086·3
Laevilac S, 2086·3
Laevodex, 2086·4
Laevo-dopa, 1205·2
Laevofusin Isoton, 2086·4
Laevofusin-Starter, 2086·4
Laevolac, 2086·4
Laevomycetinum, 185·1
Laevoral, 2086·4
Laevosan, 2086·4
Laevostrophan, 2086·4
Laevostrophan Compositum, 2086·4
Laevovit $D_3$, 2086·4
Laevulose, 1431·3
Laevulosum, 1431·3
Lafarclor, 2086·4
Lafarin, 2086·4
Lafedam, 2086·4
Lafena, 2086·4
Lafigesic, 2086·4
Lafigin, 2086·4
Lafol, 2086·4
Lafurex, 2086·4
Lafutidine, 1269·3
Lagarmicin, 2086·4
Lagatrim, 2086·4
Lagenbach, 2086·4
Lagin, 2086·4
Lagricel, 2086·4
Lagricel Ofteno, 2086·4
Lagrifilm Plus, 2086·4
Lagrima Artificial, 2086·4
Lagrima Humectante, 2086·4
Lagrimas, Alcon— *see* Alcon Lagrimas, 1783·3
Lagrimas Artificiales, 2086·4
Lagrimas de Santa Lucia, 2086·4
Lagun, 2086·4
Lagur, 2086·4
Lagylan, 2086·4
Laidor, 2087·1
Laif, 2087·1
Laikan 100, 2087·1
Laiken, 2087·1
Lait Auto-Bronzant, 2087·1
Lait Bronzage, 2087·1
Lait Ecran Total, 2087·1
Lait Hydratant Bronzage, 2087·1
Lait Protecteur, 2087·1
Lait Solaire Ecran Total, 2087·1
Lait Solaire Haute Protection, 2087·1
Laitan, 2087·1
LAK, 563·3
Lake, 2087·1
Lakrima, 2087·1
Lakriment Neu, 2087·1
Laktipex, 2087·1
Lalax, 2087·1
LAM, 54·1

Lama, 2087·1
Lamaline, 2087·1
Lambda, 2087·1
Lambda-cyhalothrin, 1502·3
Lambert-Eaton Myasthenic Syndrome— *see* Eaton-Lambert Myasthenic Syndrome, 1485·1
Lamblit, 2087·1
Lambutol, 2087·1
Lamcoin, 2087·1
Lametec, 2087·1
Lamictal, 2087·1
Lamictin, 2087·2
Lamidac, 2087·2
Lamiden, 2087·2
Lamiderm, 2087·2
Lamifiban, 944·3
Lamilea, 2087·2
Laminaria, 1704·3
*Laminaria digitata*, 1704·3
*Laminaria japonica*, 1704·3
Laminariae, Stipites, 1704·3
Laminariae, Styli, 1704·3
Lamisil, 2087·2
Lamivudina, 648·2
Lamivudine, 648·2
Lamnotyl, 2087·2
Lamoryl, 2087·2
Lamotrigina, 363·3
Lamotrigine, 363·3
Lampicin, 2087·2
Lampocef, 2087·2
Lampocillina, 2087·2
Lampoflex, 2087·2
Lampomandol, 2087·2
Lampren, 2087·2
Lamprene, 2087·2
Lamra, 2087·2
Lamuna, 2087·2
Lamuran, 2087·2
Lamuzid, 2087·2
Lanabiotic, 2087·2
Lanacaina, 2087·2
Lanacane, 2087·2
Lanacane Medicated Cream, 2087·3
Lanacane Medicated Powder, 2087·3
Lanacef, 2087·3
Lanacine, 2087·3
Lanacordin, 2087·3
Lanacort, 2087·3
Lanacrist, 2087·3
Lanalcolum, 1482·3
Lanalget, 2087·3
Lanamont, 2087·3
Lanaphilic, 2087·3
Lanate, 2087·3
Lanatilin, 2087·3
Lanatin, 2087·3
Lanatoside A, 894·2
Lanatoside C, 945·1
Lanatosides A, B, and C, 945·1
Lanatósido C, 945·1
Lanatosidum C, 945·1
Lancome Preparations, 2087·3
Lander Dandruff Control, 2087·3
Landiolol Hydrochloride, 945·1
Lanex, 2087·3
Lanexat, 2087·3
Lanfast, 2087·3
Langerhans-cell Histiocytosis— *see* Histiocytic Syndromes, 505·2
Langoran, 2087·3
Laniazid, 2087·3
Lanicor, 2087·3
Lanirapid, 2087·3
Lanitop, 2087·3
Lanoc, 2087·4
Lanoclav, 2087·4
Lanoconazol, 405·2
Lanoconazole, 405·2
Lanofene, 2087·4
Lanogastro, 2087·4
Lanohex, 2087·4
Lanol, 2087·4
Lanolate, Isopropyl, 1483·3
Lanoléine, 1483·1
Lanolept, 2087·4
Lanolin, 1483·1
Lanolin Alcohols, 1482·3
Lanolin, Anhydrous, 1483·1
Lanolin, Ethoxylated, 1483·3
Lanolin, Hydrous, 1483·2
Lanolin, Modified, 1483·2
Lanolin Oil, 1483·3
Lanolin, Poloxyl, 1483·3
Lanolin, Purified, 1483·1
Lanolin Wax, 1483·3
Lanolina, 1483·1
Lanolina Anhidra, 1483·1
Lanolor, 2087·4
Lanomycin, 2087·4
Lanorinal, 2087·4
Lanoteplasa, 945·1
Lanoteplase, 945·1
Lanoxicaps, 2087·4
Lanoxin, 2087·4
Lanreotida, Acetato de, 1330·3
Lanreotide Acetate, 1330·3
Lanseka, 2087·4
Lansinoh, 2087·4
Lanso— *see* Lanfast, 2087·3
Lansoprazol, 1269·3
Lansoprazole, 1269·3
Lansoprazole Sulfone, 1270·1
Lansox, 2087·4
Lansoyl, 2087·4
Lantadin, 2087·4
Lantanon, 2087·4
Lantarel, 2087·4
Lanthanum Carbonate, 1219·1
Lantigen B, 2087·4
Lantogent, 2087·4
Lantus, 2087·4
Lanuretic, 2087·4
Lanvis, 2087·4
Lanz, 2087·4
Lanzo, 2088·1
Lanzo— *see* Helipak A, 2038·2
Lanzo— *see* Helipak K, 2038·2
Lanzo— *see* Helipak T, 2038·2
Lanzogastro, 2088·1
Lanzol, 2088·1
Lanzopral, 2088·1
Lanzor, 2088·1
Lao-Dal, 2088·1
LAPDAP, 452·1
Lapenax, 2088·1
Lapices Epiderm Metadier, 2088·1
Lapidar, 2088·1
Lapidar 10, 2088·1
Lapis Pumicis, 1140·1
Lappa, 1704·3
Lappa Root, 1704·3
Lappaconitine Hydrobromide, 945·1
Laprazol, 2088·1
Lapril, 2088·1
Laprilen, 2088·1
Lapsus, 2088·1
Laracit, 2088·1
Laractone, 2088·1
Larafen, 2088·1
Laraflex, 2088·1
Laragon, 2088·1
Laranja, Essência de, 1724·1
Laranjeira, Essência de Flor de, 1719·2
Larapam, 2088·1
Laratrim, 2088·1
Larch Resin Comp., 2088·1
Larcooral, 2088·1
Largactil, 2088·1
Largal Ultra, 2088·1
Largatrex, 2088·1
Largitor, 2088·2
Largon, 2088·2
Lariago, 2088·2
Lariam, 2088·2
Lariamar, 2088·2
Laridal, 2088·2
Laridox, 2088·2
Larifikehl, 2088·2
Larilon, 2088·2
Larimicina, 2088·2
Laringex, 2088·2
Larintil, 2088·2
Larither, 2088·2
Larjancaina, 2088·2
Larjanfilina, 2088·2
Larmabak, 2088·2
Larmadex, 2088·2
Larmax, 2088·2
Larmecran, 2088·2
Larmes Artificielles, 2088·2
Larodopa, 2088·2
Laroferon, 2088·2
Laronidase, 1705·1
Laron-type Dwarfism— *see* Growth Retardation, 1314·2
Laroscorbine, 2088·2
Larotabe, 2088·2
Laroxyl, 2088·2
Larpose, 2088·3
*Larrea tridentata*, 566·1, 1670·1
Larry, 2088·3
Lars, 2088·3
Larsen, 2088·3
Larsimal, 2088·3
Larva Migrans, Cutaneous— *see* Cutaneous Larva Migrans, 98·1
Larva Migrans, Ocular— *see* Toxocariasis, 101·1
Larva Migrans, Visceral— *see* Toxocariasis, 101·1
Larvas, 1151·3
LarvE, 2088·3
Larvitan, 2088·3
Larydol, 2088·3
Larylin Preparations, 2088·3
Laryngarsol, 2088·3
Laryngeal Carcinoma— *see* Malignant Neoplasms of the Head and Neck, 517·3
Laryng-O-Jet, 2088·3
Laryngomedin N, 2088·3
Laryngotracheobronchitis— *see* Croup, 1079·1
Laryngsan, 2088·3
Lary-Phary, 2088·3
LAS-3876, 1248·2
LAS-9273, 1260·3
LAS-31416, 465·2
Lasa, 2088·3
Lasa Antiasmatico, 2088·3
Lasa con Codeina, 2088·3
Lasain, 2088·3
Lasalar-Y, 2088·3
Lasalar-Y Simple, 2088·3
Lasalocid, 606·1
Lasalocid Sódico, 606·1
Lasalocid Sodium, 606·1
Lasar, 2088·3
Laser, 2088·3
Laservis, 2088·3
Lasikal, 2088·4
Lasilacton, 2088·4
Lasilactona, 2088·4
Lasilactone, 2088·4
Lasiletten, 2088·4
Lasilix, 2088·4
Lasiride, 2088·4
Lasitace, 2088·4
Lasitone, 2088·4
Lasix, 2088·4
Lasma, 2088·4
Lasonil, 2088·4
Lasonil H, 2088·4
Lasonil N, 2088·4
Lasoproct, 2088·4
Lasoreuma, 2088·4
Lasoride, 2088·4
Lasoven, 2088·4
L-Asp, 2088·4
Laspar, 2088·4
Lassa Fever— *see* Haemorrhagic Fevers, 618·2, 652·3
Lassadermil, 2088·4
Lassarmex, 2088·4
Lassatina, 2088·4
Lassativi Vetegali, 2088·4
Lassifar, 2089·1
Lasten/Barn, 2089·1
Lastet, 2089·1
Lasticom, 2089·1
Lastin, 2089·1
Lastrim, 2089·1
Lastuss, 2089·1
LAS-W-090, 433·1
Latamoxef Disódico, 225·3
Latamoxef Disodium, 225·3
Latanoprost, 1519·1
Latensin, 2089·1
Latesil, 2089·1
Latesyl, 2089·1
Latex, 1741·1
Latiazem Hydrochloride, 900·1
Laticort, 2089·1
Latimit, 2089·1
Latoconazole, 405·2
Latof, 2089·1
Latof-T, 2089·1
Latonid, 2089·1
Latonina, 2089·1
Latoren, 2089·1
Latotryd, 2089·1
*Latrodectus mactans* Antiserum, 1640·1
*Latrodectus mactans* Antivenin, 1640·1
*Latrodectus mactans* Antivenom, 1640·1
Latschenöl, 1737·1
Lattosio, 1438·3
Lattubio, 2089·1
Lattulac, 2089·1
Latycin, 2089·1
Latycyn, 2089·1
Laubeel, 2089·1
Laudamonium, 2089·1
Laudanosine, 1402·1
Laudefen, 2089·1
Laudil, 2089·1
Laughing Gas, 1304·3
Launol, 2089·1
Laur, 2089·1
Laurak, 2089·1
Lauralkonium Bromide, 1170·2
Lauralkonium Chloride, 1170·2
Laurato de Nandrolona, 1561·2
Laurato de Sorbitán, 1416·1
Laurel Dulce, Aceite Esencial de, 1659·1
Laurel Leaf Oil, 1659·1
Laureth 4, 1412·3
Laureth 9, 1412·3
Laureth Compounds, 1412·3
Lauricin, 2089·1
Laurilsulfato de Sodio, 1574·2
Laurimic, 2089·2
Laurimicina, 2089·2
Laurina, 2089·2
Laurinol Plus, 2089·2
Lauritran, 2089·2
Laurocapram, 1481·2
Lauroderme, 2089·2
Lauroderme Po, 2089·2
Lauromacrogol 400, 1412·3
Lauromacrogols, 1412·3
Lauromentol, 2089·2
Lauromicina, 2089·2
*Laurus nobilis*, 1659·1
Lauryl Gallate, 1168·1
Lauryldimethylbenzylammonium Bromide, 1170·2
Laurylum Gallicum, 1168·1
Lavaflac, 2089·2
Lavagin, 2089·2
Lavanda, Aceite Esencial de, 1705·2
Lavanda Sofar, 2089·2
Lavande, Huile Essentielle de, 1705·2
*Lavandula angustifolia*, 1705·1, 1705·2
*Lavandula latifolia*, 1749·2
*Lavandula officinalis*, 1705·1, 1705·2
*Lavandula spica*, 1749·2
Lavandulae Aetheroleum, 1705·2
Lavandulae Flos, 1705·1
Lavandulae, Oleum, 1705·2
Lavandulae Spicatae, Oleum, 1749·2
Lavasept, 2089·2
Lavement Au Phosphate, 2089·2
Lavendelblüten, 1705·1
Lavendelöl, 1705·2

Lavender, 1705·1
Lavender Flower, 1705·1
Lavender Flower Oil, 1705·2
Lavender Oil, 1705·2
Lavender Oil, English, 1705·2
Lavender Oil, Foreign, 1705·2
Lavender Oil, Spike, 1749·2
Laver, 2089·2
Laveran, 2089·2
Lavichthol, 2089·2
Laviest, 2089·2
Lavisa, 2089·2
Lavolen, 2089·2
Lavolho, 2089·2
Lawefluor N, 2089·2
Lawsone, 1705·2
Lawsonia, 1696·3, 1705·2
*Lawsonia*, 1705·2
*Lawsonia alba*, 1696·3
*Lawsonia inermis*, 1696·3
Lax Pills, 2089·2
Laxa, 2089·2
Laxabon, 2089·2
Laxaco, 2089·2
Laxadin, 2089·2
Laxadoron, 2089·2
Laxagel, 2089·3
Laxagetten, 2089·3
Laxal, 2089·3
Laxalpin, 2089·3
Laxamalt, 2089·3
Laxamin, 2089·3
Laxamucil, 2089·3
Laxan, 2089·3
Laxanin N, 2089·3
Laxans, 2089·3
Laxans-ratiopharm, 2089·3
Laxans-ratiopharm Pico, 2089·3
Laxante Bescansa, 2089·3
Laxante Bescansa Aloico, 2089·3
Laxante Bescansa Normal, 2089·3
Laxante Derly, 2089·3
Laxante Olan, 2089·3
Laxante Salud, 2089·3
Laxante Sanatorium, 2089·3
Laxantil, 2089·3
Laxarine, 2089·3
Laxarol, 2089·3
Laxaron, 2089·3
Laxasan, 2089·3
Laxative, 2089·4
Laxative Comp, 2089·4
Laxative Pills, 2089·4
Laxative & Stool Softener, 2089·4
Laxative Tablets, 2089·4
Laxatives, 1239·3
Laxativum Nouvelle Formule, 2089·4
Laxatol, 2089·4
Laxavit, 2089·4
Laxbene, 2089·4
Laxcodyl, 2089·4
Laxen, 2089·4
Laxen Busto, 2089·4
Laxette, 2089·4
Laxettes, 2089·4
Laxicaps P, 2089·4
Laxicon, 2089·4
Laxicona, 2089·4
Laxikal Forte, 2089·4
Laxilose, 2089·4
Laxiplant, 2089·4
Laxiplant cum Senna, 2089·4
Laxiplant Soft, 2089·4
Laxisoft, 2089·4
Laxitab, 2089·4
Laxo Vian, 2089·4
Laxoberal, 2089·4
Laxoberal Bisa, 2090·1
Laxoberon, 2090·1
Laxocodyl, 2090·1
Laxodal, 2090·1
Laxofalk, 2090·1
Laxogeno, 2090·1
Laxol, 2090·1
Laxolen, 2090·1
Laxolind, 2090·1
Laxolyne, 2090·1
Laxomax, 2090·1
Laxomild, 2090·1
Laxomundin, 2090·1
Laxonol, 2090·1
Laxopol, 2090·1
Laxose, 2090·1
Laxsol, 2090·1
Laxtam, 2090·1
Laxuave Enteral, 2090·1
Laxucil, 2090·1
Laxvital, 2090·1
Laxyl, 2090·1
Laxysat Burger, 2090·1
Laxysat Mono, 2090·1
Layor Carang, 1576·3
Lazabemida, 1205·2
Lazabemide, 1205·2
Lazercreme, 2090·1
Lazerformaldehyde, 2090·1
LazerSporin-C, 2090·1
L-75-1362B, 1674·3
LB-46, 983·2
LB-502, 919·3
LB-20304, 216·3
LB-20304a, 216·3
LB Jabon con Purcelin, 2090·1
LC-33, 1706·3
LC-44, 699·1
LC-65, 2090·1
L-Carn, 2090·1
LCB-29, 1394·3
L-Cimexyl, 2090·2
L-Combur-5-Test, 2090·2
LCP, 2090·2
LDP-341, 532·1
29060-LE, 591·2
Le 100 B, 2090·2
Le 500 D, 2090·2
Le Face Protection, 2090·2
Le Fibre, 2090·2
Le Pont Tratamiento Ungueal Formula 405, 2090·2
Le Stick a Levres, 2090·2
Le Tan Preparations, 2090·2
Le Thermogene, 2090·2
Le Trim-BM, 2090·2
Lead, 1705·3
Lead Acetate, 1706·1
Lead Carbonate, 1706·1
Lead Monoxide, 1706·1
Lead Oleate, 1706·1
Lead Plaster-mass, 1706·1
Lead Subacetate, 1706·1
Leaf, 1373·3
Lealgin, 2090·2
LEAN Formula w/ Advantra, 2090·3
Leanor, 2090·3
Leaton fur Erwachsene, 2090·3
Leaton fur Kinder, 2090·3
Lebensenergie-Kapseln, 2090·3
Leber- und Gallentee, Tiroler Adler— *see* Tiroler Adler Leber- und Gallentee, 2333·4
Leberetic, 2090·3
Leber-Galle-Tropfen 83, 2090·3
Leber-Galletropfen SN, 2090·3
Leberinfusion, 2090·3
Leber's Optic Atrophy, 1459·1
Lebersal, 2090·3
Leberschutz, 2090·3
Lebertran, 1425·2
Lebic, 2090·3
Lebilon, 2090·3
Lebocar, 2090·3
Lebopride, 2090·3
Lebriton N, 2090·3
Lebrocetin, 2090·3
Lecarge, 2090·3
Leche Autobronceadora, 2090·3
Leche Autobronceadora Cara y Cuerpo, 2090·3
Leche de Magnesia Phillips, 2090·3
Leche de Proteccion Total, 2090·3
Lechuga Silvestre, 1765·2
Lecia, 2090·3
Lecibral, 2090·3
Lecicarbon, 2090·3
Leciderm, 2090·3
Lecifar-K, 2090·3
Lecikur, 2090·3
Lecimar, 2090·4
Lecinova, 2090·4
Leciplus, 2090·4
Lecithin, 1706·1
Lecithin ACE, 2090·4
Lecithin AE, 2090·4
Lecitina, 1706·1
Lecitone, 2090·4
Lecivital, 2090·4
Leclor A, 2090·4
Leclyte, 2090·4
Lecrolyn, 2090·4
Lectil, 2090·4
Lectopam, 2090·4
Lectrum, 2090·4
Ledclair, 2090·4
Ledercillin VK, 2090·4
Ledercort, 2090·4
Ledercort con Neomicina, 2090·4
Ledercort-N, 2090·4
Lederderm, 2090·4
Lederfen, 2090·4
Lederfolat, 2090·4
Lederfolin, 2090·4
Lederfoline, 2090·4
Lederlind, 2090·4
Lederlon, 2090·4
Ledermicina, 2090·4
Ledermix, 2091·1
Ledermycin, 2091·1
Lederpaediat, 2091·1
Lederpax, 2091·1
Lederplatin, 2091·1
Lederscon, 2091·1
Lederspan, 2091·1
Ledertam, 2091·1
Ledertepa, 2091·1
Ledertrexate, 2091·1
Ledervorin, 2091·1
Ledion, 2091·1
Ledolid, 2091·1
Ledoren, 2091·1
Ledovit C, 2091·1
Ledox, 2091·1
Ledoxid Acne, 2091·1
Ledoxina, 2091·1
Ledum Med Complex, 2091·1
Leech, 945·1
Lefaenteril, 2091·1
Lefax, 2091·1
Lefaxin, 2091·1
Lefcar, 2091·1
Leferdivin, 2091·2
Lefetamina, Hidrocloruro de, 53·1
Lefetamine Hydrochloride, 53·1
Lefkacid, 2091·2
Lefkaflam, 2091·2
Lefkur, 2091·2
Leflunomida, 53·2
Leflunomide, 53·2
Lefrine, 2091·2
Left Ventricular Dysfunction— *see* Heart Failure, 820·3
Leftose, 2091·2
Leg Cramps, Hylands— *see* Hylands Leg Cramps, 2052·3
Leg Cramps with Quinine, 2091·2
Legalon, 2091·2
Legalon SIL, 2091·2
Legapas, 2091·2
Legapas Comp, 2091·2
Legapas Mono— *see* Legapas, 2091·2
Legapas N— *see* Legapas comp, 2091·2
Legatrin PM, 2091·2
Legatrin Rub, 2091·2
Leg-Care, Extralife— *see* Extralife Leg-Care, 1986·3
Legederm, 2091·2
Legendal, 2091·2
Legifol CS, 2091·2
Legil, 2091·2
Legionella Pneumonia— *see* Legionnaires' Disease, 133·1
Legionellosis— *see* Legionnaires' Disease, 133·1
Legionnaires' Disease, 133·1
Legofer, 2091·2
Legrand, Colirio— *see* Colirio Legrand, 1899·4
Lehydan, 2091·2
Leiba, 2091·2
Leicester Retard, 2091·2
Leiguar, 2091·2
Leinöl, 1707·2
Leinsamen, 1707·2
Leioderm, 2091·2
Leioderm P, 2091·2
Leiomyomas— *see* Fibroids, 1326·1
Leios, 2091·2
Leishmaniasis, 597·2
Leishmaniasis Vaccines, 1622·1
Leishmanin, 1706·2
Leishmanina, 1706·2
Leite de Magnesia, 2091·3
Leite de Magnesia de Phillips, 2091·3
Lejguar, 2091·3
Lektinol, 2091·3
Lelco Preparations, 2091·3
Lelong Contusions, 2091·3
Lelong Irritations, 2091·3
Lema C, 2091·3
Lemakalim, 890·3
Lemazol, 2091·3
Lemblastine, 2091·3
Lembrol, 2091·3
Lemdopa, 2091·3
L-Emental, 2091·3
Lemeron, 2091·3
Lemesil, 2091·3
Lemgrip, 2091·3
Lemivit, 2091·3
Lemlax, 2091·3
Lemnis Fatty Cream, 2091·3
Lemnis Fatty Cream HC, 2091·3
Lemocin, 2091·3
Lemocin CX, 2091·4
Lemocin Flexibels, 2091·4
Lemon, 1706·2
Lemon Balm, 1711·1
Lemon Balm Oil, 1711·2
Lemon Grass Oil, 1706·3
Lemon Oil, 1706·2
Lemon Oil, California-type, 1706·2
Lemon Oil, Italian-type, 1706·2
Lemon Oil, Terpeneless, 1706·3
Lemon Peel, Dried, 1706·2
Lemon Time, 2091·4
Lemon Verbena, 1706·3
Lemongrass, Aceite de, 1706·3
Lemongrass Oil, 1706·3
Lemonvit, 2091·4
Lemophar, 2091·4
Lemotussin-DM, 2091·4
Lemoxin, 2091·4
Lemoxol, 2091·4
Lem-Plus, 2091·4
Lemsip Preparations, 2091·4
Lemtosid, 2092·1
Lemuval, 2092·1
Lemyflox, 2092·1
Lemytriol, 2092·1
Len V.K., 2092·1
Lenactin, 2092·1
Lenadol, 2092·1
Lenafen, 2092·1
Lenamet, 2092·1
Lenapain, 2092·2
Lenar, 2092·2
Lenasone, 2092·2
Lenazine, 2092·2
Lenazine Forte, 2092·2
Lendianon, 2092·2
Lenditro, 2092·2
Lendorm, 2092·2
Lendormin, 2092·2
Lendormine, 2092·2
Lendrex, 2092·2

Lenen, 2092·2
Lengua de Vaca, 1766·1
Leniartril, 2092·2
Lenicalm, 2092·2
Lenicet, 2092·2
Lenident, 2092·2
Leniderm, 2092·2
Lenidermyl, 2092·2
Lenide-T, 2092·2
Lenidolor, 2092·2
Lenidor, 2092·2
Lenifren, 2092·2
Lenil, 2092·2
Leniline, 2092·2
Lenipasta, 2092·2
Lenirit, 2092·2
Lenirose, 2092·2
Lenisan, 2092·2
Lenisolone, 2092·2
Lenistar, 2092·3
Lenitil, 2092·3
Lenitin, 2092·3
Lenitral, 2092·3
Lenium, 2092·3
Lenixil, 2092·3
Lennox-Gastaut Syndrome— *see* Epilepsy, 349·1
Leño de Cuasia, 1737·2
Lenocef, 2092·3
Lenocin, 2092·3
Lenograstim, 755·3
Lenolax, 2092·3
Lenoltec Preparations, 2092·3
Lenovate, 2092·3
Lenovor, 2092·3
Lenoxin, 2092·3
Lenpryl, 2092·3
Lens Fresh, 2092·3
Lens Lubricant, 2092·3
Lens Plus, 2092·3
Lens Plus Buffered Saline Solution, 2092·3
Lens Plus Rewetting Drops, 2092·3
Lens Tears, 2092·3
Lens Wet, 2092·3
Lensan A, 2092·3
Lensan B, 2092·3
Lensept, 2092·3
Lensrins NT, 2092·3
Lenta, 2092·3
Lentard, 2092·3
Lentard MC, 2092·3
Lentare, 2092·3
Lentaron, 2092·3
Lente, 2092·4
Lente Iletin I, 2092·4
Lente Iletin II, 2092·4
Lente, Insulin, 334·2
Lente L, 2092·4
Lente MC, 2092·4
Lentinan, 1706·3
Lentinano, 1706·3
*Lentinus edodes*, 1706·3
Lentisol, 2092·4
Lentizol, 2092·4
Lento C, 2092·4
Lentocilin-S, 2092·4
Lentogesic, 2092·4
Lentogest, 2092·4
Lento-Kalium, 2092·4
Lentolith, 2092·4
Lentopenil, 2092·4
Lentoquine, 2092·4
Lentorem, 2092·4
Lentorsil, 2092·4
Lentusin, 2092·4
Leo-114, 1565·3
Leo-400, 2092·4
Leo-640, 305·3
Leo-1031, 581·2
Leo-Doce, 2092·4
Leodrin, 2092·4
Leogumil, 2092·4
Leonal, 2092·4
Leonitren, 2092·4
Leonuri Cardiacae Herba, 1717·1
Leonurus, 1717·1
*Leonurus cardiaca*, 1717·1
Leopard's Bane, 1656·3
Leopin, 2092·4
Leotrim, 2092·4
Leovinezal, 2092·4
Leparan, 2092·4
Lepargylic Acid, 1142·3
Lepheton, 2092·4
Lephin, 2092·4
Lepicortinolo, 2092·4
Lepinal, 2093·1
Lepinaletten, 2093·1
Lepirudin, 945·2
Lepirudina, 945·2
Lepisor, 2093·1
Lepobron, 2093·1
Leponex, 2093·1
Lepra Reactions— *see* Leprosy, 133·1
Leprolin, 1707·1
Lepromin, 1706·3
Lepromin A, 1706·3
Lepromin H, 1706·3
Lepromina, 1706·3
Leprosin A, 1707·1
Leprosy, 133·1
Leprosy Vaccines, 1622·1
Leptanal, 2093·1
Leptazol, 1592·1
Lepticur, 2093·1
Leptilan, 2093·1
Leptilanil, 2093·1
Leptin, 1707·1
Leptina, 1707·1
Leptofen, 2093·1
Leptoprol, 2093·1
Leptopsique, 2093·1
*Leptospermum scoparium*, 1709·3
*Leptospira interrogans*, 1622·2
Leptospira Vaccines, 1622·2
Leptospirosis, 133·3
Leptospirosis Vaccines, 1622·2
Lepur, 2093·1
Lercadip, 2093·1
Lercan, 2093·1
Lercanidipine Hydrochloride, 946·1
Lercanidipino, Hidrocloruro de, 946·1
Lerdelimumab, 1707·1
Lerdip, 2093·1
Lergigan, 2093·1
Lergigan Comp, 2093·1
Lergocil, 2093·1
Lerin, 2093·1
Leritine, 2093·1
Lerivon, 2093·1
Lermex, 2093·1
Lerogin, 2093·1
Leroid, 2093·1
Lertamine, 2093·1
Lertamine D, 2093·2
Lertamine Extra, 2093·2
Lertus, 2093·2
Lertus Biotic, 2093·2
Leruze, 2093·2
Lervipan, 2093·2
Lerzam, 2093·2
Les Yeux 1, 2093·2
Les Yeux 2, 2093·2
Lesch-Nyhan Syndrome, 682·2
Lescol, 2093·2
Leshcutan, 2093·2
Lesil, 2093·2
Lesoxyephedrine, 1124·1
Lespenefril, 2093·2
Lespenephryl, 2093·2
Lesser Celandine, 1732·1
Lessina, 2093·2
Lessmusec, 2093·2
Lesspain, 2093·2
Lesterol, 2093·2
Lestid, 2093·2
Lestric, 2093·2
Lestrin, 2093·2
Letansil, 2093·2
Letequatro, 2093·2
Lethyl, 2093·2
Letigen, 2093·3
Letofort, 2093·3
Letondal, 2093·3
Letoprol, 2093·3
Letosteína, 1123·3
Letosteine, 1123·3
Letrazuril, 606·1
Letrazurilo, 606·1
Letrozol, 565·1
Letrozole, 565·1
Letter, 2093·3
Letterer-Siwe Syndrome— *see* Histiocytic Syndromes, 505·2
Lettuce Opium, 1765·2
Lettuce, Wild, 1765·2
Letus, 2093·3
Letynol, 2093·3
Leu, 1439·1
Leucina, 1439·1
LeucinAde, 2093·3
Leucine, 1439·1
L-Leucine, 1439·1
[2-Leucine,7-isoleucine]vasopressin, 1336·1
1-L-Leucine-2-L-threonine-63-desulfohirudin, 945·2
Leucinum, 1439·1
Leuco-4, 2093·3
Leuco Hubber, 2093·3
Leucobasal, 2093·3
Leucocalcin, 2093·3
Leucocianidol, 1688·2
Leucocida, 2093·3
Leucocitim, 2093·3
Leucocitos, 756·1
Leucocyanidin, 1688·2
Leucocyanidol, 1688·2
Leucocyte Endogenous Mediator, 1701·3
Leucocyte Interferon, 640·3
Leucocytes, 756·1
Leucocytoclastic Vasculitis— *see* Hypersensitivity Vasculitis, 1081·3
Leucodin, 2093·3
Leucodinine B, 2093·3
Leucodinin-M, 2093·3
Leucogen, 2093·3
Leucomax, 2093·3
Leucomethylene Blue, 1043·1
Leucomycin, 225·3
Leucomycin $A_3$, 224·3
Leucomycin V $3^B$, 9-Diacetate $3,4^B$-Dipropanoate, 231·3
*Leuconostoc mesenteroides*, 745·2, 745·3, 746·1, 746·2, 747·1
Leucoplakia, 531·3
Leucorsan, 2093·3
Leucotrofina, 2093·3
Leucovorin, 1431·1
Leucovorin Calcium, 1431·1
Leu-enkephalin, 73·3
Leukaemia, Acute Myelogenous— *see* Acute Myeloid Leukaemias, 506·3
Leukaemia, Acute Myeloid— *see* Acute Myeloid Leukaemias, 506·3
Leukaemia, Acute Non-lymphoblastic— *see* Acute Myeloid Leukaemias, 506·3
Leukaemia, Acute Promyelocytic— *see* Acute Myeloid Leukaemias, 506·3
Leukaemia, Burkitt Cell— *see* Acute Lymphoblastic Leukaemia, 506·1
Leukaemia, Chronic Granulocytic— *see* Chronic Myeloid Leukaemia, 507·3
Leukaemia, Chronic Lymphocytic— *see* Chronic Lymphocytic Leukaemia, 507·2
Leukaemia, Chronic Myelogenous— *see* Chronic Myeloid Leukaemia, 507·3
Leukaemia, Chronic Myeloid— *see* Chronic Myeloid Leukaemia, 507·3
Leukaemia, Hairy-cell— *see* Hairy-cell Leukaemia, 508·2
Leukaemia, Smouldering— *see* Myelodysplastic Syndromes, 508·2
Leukaemias, Acute, 505·3
Leukaemias, Chronic, 507·2
Leukase, 2093·3
Leukase N, 2093·3
Leukase-Kegel, 2093·3
Leukeran, 2093·3
Leukichtan, 2093·4
Leukine, 2093·4
Leuko Fungex Antifungal— *see* Eulactol Antifungal, 1982·2
Leukoencephalopathy, Progressive Multifocal— *see* Infections in Immunocompromised Patients, 624·2
Leukominerase, 2093·4
Leukona Preparations, 2093·4
LeukoNorm, 2093·4
LeukoScan, 2093·4
Leukotriene Antagonists, 777·1
Leukotriene Inhibitors, 777·1
Leukotrienes, 1511·1
Leumostin, 2093·4
Leunase, 2093·4
Leuplin, 2093·4
Leuprogel One-Month Depot— *see* Eligard, 1965·3
Leuprolide, 1331·1
Leuprolide Acetate, 1331·1
Leuprorelin, 1331·1
Leuprorelin Acetate, 1331·1
Leuprorelina, Acetato de, 1331·1
Leuprorelinum, 1331·1
Leurocristine Sulphate, 592·2
Leustat, 2093·4
Leustatin, 2093·4
Leustatine, 2094·1
Leutrol, 2094·1
Levacecarnine Hydrochloride, 1646·1
Levacetilmetadol, 54·1
Levacetylmethadol, 54·1
Levacetylmethadol Hydrochloride, 54·1
Levadin, 2094·1
Levadol, 2094·1
Levadura Desecada, 1469·1
Levaknel, 2094·1
Levalbuterol Hydrochloride, 788·2
Levaliver, 2094·1
Levall, 2094·1
Levamfetamine, 1584·3
Levamin, 2094·1
Levamisol, Hidrocloruro de, 107·2
Levamisole, 107·1
Levamisole Hydrochloride, 107·2
Levamisole for Veterinary Use, 107·1
Levamisoli Hydrochloridum, 107·2
Levamizol, Cloridrato de, 107·2
Levant Storax, 1749·3
Levantol Procaina, 2094·1
Levanxol, 2094·1
Levaquin, 2094·1
Levarterenol Acid Tartrate, 974·3
Levarterenol Bitartrate, 974·3
Levarterenoli Bitartras, 974·3
Levate, 2094·1
Levatol, 2094·1
Levaxin, 2094·1
Levbid, 2094·1
Levcromakalim, 890·3
Levdropropizine, 1119·3
Levedad, 2094·1
Levedura Sêca, 1469·1
Leveglutan, 2094·1
Level Up, 2094·1
Levelina, 2094·1
Levetiracetam, 366·1
Leviax, 2094·1
Levicor, 2094·1
Leviden, 2094·1
Levifusa, 2094·1
Levistici Radix, 1708·1
Levístico, 1708·1
*Levisticum officinale*, 1708·1
Levitra, 2094·1
Levium, 2094·1
Levlen, 2094·1
Levlen ED, 2094·1
Levlite, 2094·2
Levmetamfetamine, 1124·1
Levobens, 2094·2
Levobeta C, 2094·2
Levobetaxolol, Hidrocloruro de, 946·1
Levobetaxolol Hydrochloride, 946·1
Levobren, 2094·2

Levobunolol, Hidrocloruro de, 946·2
Levobunolol Hydrochloride, 946·2
Levobupivacaína, 1377·1
Levobupivacaína, Hidrocloruro de, 1377·1
Levobupivacaine, 1377·1
Levobupivacaine Hydrochloride, 1377·1
Levo-C, 2094·2
Levocabastina, Hidrocloruro de, 435·2
Levocabastine Hydrochloride, 435·2
Levocabastini Hydrochloridum, 435·2
Levocarb, 2094·2
Levocarnil, 2094·2
Levocarnin, 2094·2
Levocarnitina, 1423·3
Levocarnitine, 1423·3
Levocarnitinum, 1423·3
Levocarvit, 2094·2
Levocetirizina, 435·3
Levocetirizine, 435·3
Levocetirizine Hydrochloride, 435·3
Levocina, 2094·2
Levocomp, 2094·2
Levodex, 2094·2
Levodexan, 2094·2
Levodop, 2094·2
Levodopa, 1205·2
Levodopa Comp, 2094·2
Levodopa Comp B, 2094·2
Levodopa Comp C, 2094·2
Levodopa-Carbi, 2094·2
Levodopum, 1205·2
Levo-Dromoran, 2094·2
Levodropropizina, 1119·3
Levodropropizine, 1119·3
Levodropropizinum, 1119·3
Levofamil, 2094·2
Levofenil, 2094·2
Levofloxacin, 225·3
Levofloxacino, 225·3
Levofolene, 2094·2
Levofolinate, 1431·1
Levofolinato de Calcio, 1431·1
Levoglutamida, 1433·2
Levoglutamide, 1433·2
Levoglutil Vitaminado, 2094·2
Levograf, 2094·2
Levolac, 2094·2
Levoleucovorin Calcium, 1431·1
Levomed, 2094·2
Levomenol, 1707·1
Levomenthol, 1711·3
Levomepromazina, 703·2
Levomepromazina, Hidrocloruro de, 703·2
Levomepromazina, Maleato de, 703·2
Levomepromazine, 703·2
Levomepromazine Embonate, 703·3
Levomepromazine Hydrochloride, 703·2
Levomepromazine Maleate, 703·2
Levomepromazine Sulfoxide, 703·2
Levomepromazini Hydrochloridum, 703·2
Levomepromazini Maleas, 703·2
Levomet, 2094·2
Levometadona, Hidrocloruro de, 54·1
Levometanfetamina, 1124·1
Levomethadone Hydrochloride, 54·1
Levomethadoni Hydrochloridum, 54·1
Levomethadyl Acetate, 54·1
Levomethadyl Acetate Hydrochloride, 54·1
Levomycetin, 2094·2
Levonelle, 2094·3
Levonordefrin, 1675·3
Levonorgestrel, 1563·2
Levonorgestrelum, 1563·2
Levonova, 2094·3
Levopa, 2094·3
Levopa-C, 2094·3
Levopar, 2094·3
Levopar Plus, 2094·3
Levopenbutolol Sulfate, 979·1
Levophed, 2094·3
Levophta, 2094·3
Levoplus, 2094·3
Levopraid, 2094·3
Levoprome, 2094·3
Levopront, 2094·3
Levopropoxifeno, Napsilato de, 1124·1
Levopropoxyphene Dibudinate, 1124·1
Levopropoxyphene Napsilate, 1124·1
Levopropoxyphene Napsylate, 1124·1
Levopropylhexedrine, 353·3
Levopropylhexedrine Hydrochloride, 1593·1
Levoptin, 2094·3
Levora, 2094·3
Levordiol, 2094·3
Levorenin, 852·2
Levorfanol, Tartrato de, 54·1
Levorin, 2094·3
Levormeloxifene, 1564·3
Levorphan Tartrate, 54·1
Levorphanol Bitartrate, 54·1
Levorphanol Tartrate, 54·1
Levosalbutamol, Hidrocloruro de, 788·2
Levosalbutamol Hydrochloride, 788·2
Levosimendan, 946·2
Levostab, 2094·3
Levosulpiride, 722·2, 722·3
Levosulpride, 722·2
Levo-T, 2094·3
Levotec, 2094·3
Levothroid, 2094·3
Levothym, 2094·3
Levothyrox, 2094·3
Levothyroxine Sodium, 1600·1
Levothyroxinnatrium, 1600·1
Levothyroxinum Natricum, 1600·1
Levotiroxina, 2094·3
Levotiroxina Sódica, 1600·1
Levotonine, 2094·3
Levotrin, 2094·3
Levotuss, 2094·4
Levovist, 2094·4
Levoxacin, 2094·4
Levoxine— *see* Levoxyl, 2094·4
Levoxyl, 2094·4
Levozin, 2094·4
Levozine, 2094·4
Levsin, 2094·4
Levsinex, 2094·4
Levucal, 2094·4
Levucal D, 2094·4
Levudin, 2094·4
Levugen, 2094·4
Levulan Kerastick, 2094·4
Lévulinate Calcique, 1225·3
Levulosado, 2094·4
Levulosado Vitulia, Suero— *see* Suero Levulosado Vitulia, 2310·4
Levulosalino Isot, 2094·4
Levulose, 1431·3
Levunolol, 2094·4
Levuplex, 2094·4
Levure de Bière, 1469·1
Levure Or, 2094·4
Levurinetten, 2094·4
Levurinetten N, 2094·4
Levusalino, 2094·4
Levviax, 2094·4
Lewy-body Dementia— *see* Dementia, 1484·1
Lexapro, 2094·4
Lexat, 2094·4
Lexatin, 2094·4
Lexavite, 2094·4
Lexemin, 2094·4
Lexfor, 2095·1
Lexibiotico, 2095·1
Lexidronam, Samarium ($^{153}$Sm), 1525·2
Lexiflox, 2095·1
Lexil, 2095·1
Lexilium, 2095·1
Lexin, 2095·1
Lexincef, 2095·1
Lexinor, 2095·1
Lexipafant, 1707·2
Lexis, 2095·1
Lexiva, 2095·1
Lexobene, 2095·1
Lexomil, 2095·1
Lexostad, 2095·1
Lexotan, 2095·1
Lexotanil, 2095·1
Lexpec, 2095·1
Lexpec with Iron, 2095·1
Lexpec with Iron-M, 2095·1
Lextarol, 2095·1
Lextrasa, 2095·1
Lexxel, 2095·1
Lexxema, 2095·1
Leza, 2095·1
Lezidim, 2095·1
Lezole, 2095·1
LF-178, 915·2
LF-17895, 952·2
LFA-3/1gG$_1$ Fusion Protein, Recombinant Human, 1141·2
LFA3TIP, 1141·2
LG-11457, 914·1
LG-30158, 1740·1
LG-100057, 526·2
LG-100069, 529·3
L-G Vita, 2095·1
LGD-1057, 526·2
LGD-1069, 529·3
L-Gel, 2095·1
LH, 1332·1
LH Predict, 2095·1
LH/FSH-RF, 1325·1
LH/FSH-RH, 1325·1
LH-RF, 1325·1
LH-RH, 1325·1
Li 450, 2095·1
Liaderyl, 2095·1
Liamba, 1666·1
Liamycin, 2095·2
Lianda, 1666·1
Liatriz, 2095·2
Libeeda, 2095·2
Libenar, 2095·2
Liberal, 2095·2
Liberalgium, 2095·2
Liberan, 2095·2
Liberanas, 2095·2
Liberate, 2095·2
Liberbil, 2095·2
Liberen, 2095·2
Liberim T, 2095·2
Liberol Preparations, 2095·2
Liberprost, 2095·2
Libertin, 2095·2
Libertrim, 2095·2
Liberty Cap, 1736·1
Libexin, 2095·2
Libexin Mucolitico, 2095·2
Libexine, 2095·2
Libexine Compositum, 2095·2
Libiam, 2095·2
Libidomega, 2095·2
Libiocid, 2095·3
Libiplus, 2095·3
Liblan, 2095·3
Libradin, 2095·3
Librax, 2095·3
Libraxin, 2095·3
Libritabs, 2095·3
Librium, 2095·3
Librofem, 2095·3
Libronchin, 2095·3
Libronchin Prikkelhoest, 2095·3
Licab, 2095·3
Licain, 2095·3
Licarb, 2095·3
Licarbium, 2095·3
Licarpin, 2095·3
Lice— *see* Pediculosis, 1499·1
Lice Blaster, 2095·3
Lice Rid, 2095·3
Licetrol, 2095·3
Lichen Planus, 1136·2
Lichtena, 2095·3
Licide, 2095·3
Licilon, 2095·3
Liconar, 2095·3
Licor Amoniacal, 2095·3
Licor de Cacau, 2095·3
Licor de Tayuya, 2095·3
Licorice, 1270·2, 1270·3
Licostrata, 2095·4
Licovit, 2095·4
Licrease, 2095·4
Licuamon, 2095·4
Lidaflan, 2095·4
Lidaltrin, 2095·4
Lidaltrin Diu, 2095·4
LidaMantle, 2095·4
LidaMantle HC, 2095·4
Lidamidina, Hidrocloruro de, 1270·2
Lidamidine Hydrochloride, 1270·2
Lidaprim, 2095·4
Lidazon, 2095·4
Lid-Care, 2095·4
Lidemol, 2095·4
Lidene, 2095·4
Lidenix, 2095·4
Lident Adrenalina, 2095·4
Lident Andrenor, 2095·4
Liderclox, 2095·4
Liderflex, 2095·4
Liderma, 2095·4
Liderman, 2095·4
Liderplus, 2095·4
Lidesthesin, 2095·4
Lidex, 2095·4
LIDFLN, 1377·3, 1689·1
Lidial, 2095·4
Lidifen, 2095·4
Lidinal, 2096·1
Lidixin, 2096·1
Lidl, 2096·1
Lido Spray, 2096·1
Lido Tea, 2096·1
Lidobama Complex, 2096·1
Lidocabbott, 2096·1
Lidocadren, 2096·1
Lidocaína, 1377·3
Lidocaína, Hidrocloruro de, 1377·3
Lidocaine, 1377·3
Lidocaine, Carbonated, 1369·2, 1379·2
Lidocaine Hydrochloride, 1377·3
Lidocaine Hydrochloride, Anhydrous, 1377·3
Lidocaine Sodium, 1379·2
Lidocaini Hydrochloridum, 1377·3
Lidocainum, 1377·3
Lidocalm, 2096·1
Lidocard, 2096·1
Lidocation, 2096·1
Lidocaton, 2096·1
Lidocord, 2096·1
Lidocorit, 2096·1
Lidodan, 2096·1
Lidoderm, 2096·1
Lidofenin, Technetium ($^{99m}$Tc), 1526·1
Lidoflazina, 946·3
Lidoflazine, 946·3
Lidogel, 2096·1
Lidogeyer, 2096·1
Lidohex, 2096·1
Lido-Hyal, 2096·1
Lidoject, 2096·1
Lidojet, 2096·1
Lidomol, 2096·1
Lidomyxin, 2096·1
Lidonostrum, 2096·1
LidoPen, 2096·2
LidoPosterine, 2096·2
Lidosen, 2096·2
Lidosporin, 2096·2
Lidospray, 2096·2
Lidoston, 2096·2
Lidoxin, 2096·2
Lid-Pack, 2096·2
Lidrian, 2096·2
Lidrone, 2096·2
Lierre Terrestre, 1696·1
Lievistar, 2096·2
Lievitosohn, 2096·2
Lievitovit, 2096·2
Lievitovit 300, 2096·2
Lifar, 2096·2
Lifaton B12, 2096·2
Life Brand Baby Sunblock, 2096·2
Life Brand Cough Lozenges, 2096·2

Life Brand Kids Sunblock— *see* Life Brand Baby Sunblock and Kids Sunblock, 2096·2
Life Brand Natural Source, 2096·2
Life Brand Sport Sunblock, 2096·2
Life Brand Sunblock, 2096·2
Life Drops, 2096·2
Life Support, Advanced Cardiac— *see* Advanced Cardiac Life Support, 812·2
Life Support, Basic— *see* Advanced Cardiac Life Support, 812·2
Lifechange Circulation Aid, 2096·2
Lifechange Menopause Formula, 2096·2
Lifechange Mens Complex with Saw Palmetto, 2096·2
Lifechange Multi Plus Antioxidant, 2096·3
Lifedrops, 2096·3
Lifenac, 2096·3
Lifermycin, 2096·3
Liferoot, 1743·1
Liferost, 2096·3
Liferxina, 2096·3
Liferzit, 2096·3
Lifespan Antioxidant, Natures Way— *see* Natures Way Lifespan Antioxidant, 2153·3
Lifestyle, 2096·3
Lifestyles, 2096·3
Lifesystem Preparations, 2096·3
Lifibrol, 946·3
Lifo-Scrub, 2096·3
Lifril, 2096·3
Lifurom, 2096·4
Lifurox, 2096·4
Liga, 2096·4
Light Ammonium Bituminosulfonate, 1148·2
Light Kaolin, 1268·3
Light Kaolin (Natural), 1268·3
Light Liquid Paraffin, 1479·1
Light Liquid Petrolatum, 1479·1
Light Mineral Oil, 1479·1
Light Mineral Oil, Topical, 1479·1
Light Petroleum, 1476·3
Light Sodium Bituminosulphonate, 1148·3
Light White Mineral Oil, 1479·1
Lightening, 2096·4
Lightning Cough Remedy, 2096·4
Lignaform, 2096·4
Lignoc. Hydrochlor., 1377·3
Lignocaine, 1377·3
Lignocaine, Carbonated— *see* Xylocaine, 2389·2
Lignocaine Hydrochloride, 1377·3
Lignospan, 2096·4
Lignospan Special, 2096·4
Lignosporin, 2096·4
Lignostab— *see* Xylocaine 2% Plain, 2389·2
Lignostab-A, 2096·4
Lignum Vitae, 1696·2
Ligofragmin, 2096·4
Ligramex, 2096·4
*Ligusticum chuanxiong*, 1750·2
Ligvites, Gerard House— *see* Gerard House Ligvites, 2022·1
Li-iL Rheuma-Bad, 2096·4
Likacin, 2096·4
Likenil, 2096·4
Likuden M, 2096·4
Lilacillin, 2096·4
Liliam, 2096·4
Li-Liquid, 2096·4
Lilium Med Complex, 2096·4
Lilly-53858, 39·2
Lilly-61169, 39·2
Lilly-67314, 611·1
Lilly-69323, 39·2
Lilly-79891, 611·1
Lilly-109514, 1277·1
Lillypen Profil, 2096·4
Lillypen Protamine Isophane, 2096·4
Lillypen Rapide, 2096·4
Lily of the Valley, 1675·3
Liman, 2096·4
Limao Bravo, 2096·4
Limao Bravo com Vitamina C, 2097·1
Limao Bravo, Xarope de— *see* Xarope de Limao Bravo, 2387·3
Limão, Essência de, 1706·2
Limaprost, 1519·2
Limaprost Alfadex, 1519·2
Limarin, 2097·1
Limbao, 2097·1
Limbatril, 2097·1
Limbial, 2097·1
Limbitrol, 2097·1
Limbitryl, 2097·1
Limcee, 2097·1
Limclair, 2097·1
Lime, 1664·3
Lime, Chloride of, 1175·3
Lime, Chlorinated, 1175·3
Lime Flower, 1756·2
Lime Solution, Sulfurated, 1158·2
Lime, Sulfurated, 1158·2
Lime, Sulphate of, 1665·1
Lime, Sulphurated, 1158·2
Lime Water, 1664·3
Limeciclina, 228·2
Limectant, 2097·1
Limed, 2097·1
Lime-flower Tea, 1756·2
Lime-sulphur, 1158·3
Limethason, 2097·1
Limexx, 2097·1
Limican, 2097·1
Limifen, 2097·1
Liminate, 2097·1
Liminos, 2097·1
Limit-X, 2097·1
Limón, Aceite Esencial de, 1706·2
Limón, Acido del, 1673·1
Limón Exento de Terpeno, Aceite Esencial de, 1706·3
Limonal, 2097·1
Limone, 2097·1
Limonene, 1283·2, 1673·2, 1706·2, 1710·2, 1724·1, 1740·2, 1760·1
Limonis Aetheroleum, 1706·2
Limonis Deterpenatum, Oleum, 1706·3
Limonis, Oleum, 1706·2
Limovan, 2097·1
Limoxin, 2097·1
Limpacid, 2097·1
Limpele, 2097·1
Limpidex, 2097·1
Limptar, 2097·1
Limptar N, 2097·2
Lin, 1707·2
LIN-1418, 723·1
Lin, Huile de, 1707·2
Linadin, 2097·2
Linalol, 1655·2, 1676·1, 1724·1
(+)-Linalol, 1724·2
Linalyl Acetate, 1660·1
Linamin Plus, 2097·2
Lin-Amox, 2097·2
Linapen, 2097·2
Linaris, 2097·2
Linatil, 2097·2
Linatil Comp, 2097·2
Linaza, 1707·2
Linaza, Aceite de, 1707·2
Linazine, 2097·2
Lincaina, 2097·2
Lincil, 2097·2
Linco, 2097·2
Lincocin, 2097·2
Lincocina, 2097·2
Lincocine, 2097·2
Lincoflan, 2097·2
Lincogin, 2097·2
Lincolan, 2097·2
Lincomicina, Hidrocloruro de, 226·2
Lincomiral, 2097·2
Lincomy, 2097·2
Lincomycin, 226·2
Lincomycin Hydrochloride, 226·2
Lincomycin Hydrochloride Monohydrate, 226·2
Lincomycini Hydrochloridum, 226·2
Lincomyn, 2097·2
Lincono, 2097·2
Linco-Ped, 2097·2
Lincoplax, 2097·2
Linco-Plus, 2097·2
Lincorex, 2097·2
Lincosamides, 118·1
Lincotax, 2097·2
Linctifed, 2097·3
Linctodyl, 2097·3
Linctosan, 2097·3
Linctus Tussi Infans, 2097·3
Lindane, 1506·3
Lindano, 1506·3
Lindanoxil, 2097·3
Lindanum, 1506·3
Lindasol, 2097·3
Lindemil, 2097·3
Linden, 1756·2
Lindigoa S, 2097·3
Lindilane, 2097·3
Lindiol, 2097·3
Lindisc, 2097·3
Lindisc Duo, 2097·3
Lindofluid N, 2097·3
Lindormin, 2097·3
Lindotab, 2097·3
Lindoxyl, 2097·3
Linea, 2097·3
Linea F, 2097·3
Lineafarm, 2097·3
Linervidol, 2097·3
Linestrenol, 1557·1
Linezolid, 226·3
Linfocilin, 2097·3
Linfogex, 2097·3
Linfoglobulina, 2097·3
Linfol, 2097·3
Linfolysin, 2097·3
Lingo, 2097·3
Lingopen, 2097·3
Lingraine, 2097·4
Linho, 1707·2
Lini Oleum, 1707·2
Lini Semen, 1707·2
Lini Semina, 1707·2
Lini-Bombe— *see* Linibon, 2097·4
Linibon, 2097·4
Liniderm, 2097·4
Liniment Balm, 2097·4
Linimento de Sloan, 2097·4
Linimento Klari, 2097·4
Linimento Naion, 2097·4
Linimento Sloan, 2097·4
Liniplant, 2097·4
Linisol, 2097·4
Linitul, 2097·4
Linitul Antibiotico, 2097·4
Link, 2097·4
Links-Glaukosan, 2097·4
Linmycin, 2097·4
Linna-Oil, 2097·4
Linobion Preparations, 2097·4
Linoforce, 2097·4
Linola, 2097·4
Linola Gamma, 2097·4
Linola Gras, 2098·1
Linola Mi-gras, 2098·1
Linola Urea, 2098·1
Linoladiol, 2098·1
Linoladiol N, 2098·1
Linoladiol-H N, 2098·1
Linola-Fett, 2098·1
Linola-Fett 2000, 2098·1
Linola-Fett-N Olbad, 2098·1
Linola-H N, 2098·1
Linola-H-compositum N, 2098·1
Linola-H-Fett N, 2098·1
Linola-sept, 2098·1
Linoleic Acid, 1690·2
Linoleic Acid Glyceride, 1656·1
Linoleico, Ácido, 1690·2
γ-Linolenic Acid, 1690·2
Linolic Acid, 1690·2
Linomide, 583·2
Linopril, 2098·1
Linoril, 2098·1
Linosun, 2098·1
Linotar, 2098·1
Linox, 2098·1
Linsal, 2098·1
Linseed, 1707·2
Linseed, Crushed, 1707·2
Linseed Oil, 1707·2
Linseed Oil, Boiled, 1707·2
Linseed Oil Soap, 1575·2
Linseed Oil, Virgin, 1707·2
Linsidomina, Hidrocloruro de, 946·3
Linsidomine Hydrochloride, 946·3
L-Insulin, 2098·1
L-Insulin SNC, 2098·1
Lintia, 2098·1
Linum, 1707·2
*Linum usitatissimum*, 1707·2
Linurin, 2098·1
Linusit Creola, 2098·1
Linusit Darmaktiv Leinsamen, 2098·1
Linusit Gold, 2098·1
Linvas, 2098·1
Linvite, 2098·1
Liobifar, 2098·1
Liocarpina, 2098·1
Liofindol, 2098·2
Liogynon, 2098·2
Lio-Levedura, 2098·2
Liomagen, 2098·2
Liometacen, 2098·2
Lio-Morbillo, 2098·2
Lion, 2098·2
Lion Cleansing Herbs, 2098·2
Lioram, 2098·2
Lioresal, 2098·2
Lioresyl, 2098·2
Liosiero, 2098·2
Liotec, 2098·2
Liothyronine Hydrochloride, 1602·3
Liothyronine Sodium, 1602·2
Liothyroninum Natricum, 1602·2
Liotironina Sódica, 1602·2
Lioton, 2098·2
Liotrex, 2098·2
Liotrix, 1600·1, 1602·2
Liotropina, 2098·2
Liozim, 2098·2
Lip Block Sunscreen, 2098·2
Lip Medex, 2098·2
Lip Tone, 2098·2
Lip Treatment, 2098·2
Lipactin, 2098·2
Lipanon, 2098·2
Lipanor, 2098·2
Lipanthyl, 2098·2
Lipantil, 2098·3
Liparison, 2098·3
Liparol, 2098·3
Lipaten, 2098·3
Lipaxan, 2098·3
Lipaz, 2098·3
Lipazil, 2098·3
Lipazym, 2098·3
Lipbalm with Sunscreen, 2098·3
Lipcor, 2098·3
Lipcut, 2098·3
Lipdaune, 2098·3
Lipei, 2098·3
Lipemol, 2098·3
Lipenan, 2098·3
Liperol, 2098·3
Lipex, 2098·3
Lip-Eze, 2098·3
Lipibec, 2098·3
Lipicard, 2098·3
Lipid Complex— *see* Abelcet, 1768·2
Lipidal, 2098·3
Lipidavit, 2098·3
Lipidax, 2098·3
Lipidem, 2098·3
Lipiderm, 2098·3
Lipidil, 2098·3
Lipidless, 2098·3
Lipidos, 2098·3
Lipidys, 2098·4
Lipifen, 2098·4

Lipikar, 2098·4
Lipilim, 2098·4
Lipiodol, 2098·4
Lipirex, 2098·4
Lipiscor, 2098·4
Lipison, 2098·4
Lipisorb, 2098·4
Lipistorol, 2098·4
Lipitor, 2098·4
Lipitrol, 2098·4
Lipivas, 2098·4
Liplat, 2098·4
Liple, 2098·4
Lipmagik, 2098·4
Lipo Cordes, 2098·4
Lipo Sol, 2098·4
Lipoabsorver, 2098·4
Lipobalsamo, 2098·4
Lipobase, 2098·4
Lipobay, 2098·4
Lipocal, 2098·4
Lipocambi, 2098·4
Lipochol, 2098·4
Lipociden, 2099·1
Lipocin, 2099·1
Lipoclar, 2099·1
Lipoclin, 2099·1
Lipocol, 2099·1
Lipodel, 2099·1
Lipoenergy, 2099·1
Lipofacton, 2099·1
Lipofen, 2099·1
Lipofene, 2099·1
Lipoflavonoid, 2099·1
Lipofor, 2099·1
Lipoforte, 2099·1
Lipofren, 2099·1
Lipofundin Preparations, 2099·1
Lipofundina MCT/LCT, 2099·1
Lipogen, 2099·1
Lipogis, 2099·1
Lipograsil, 2099·1
Lipoic Acid, 1754·3
Lipoicin, 2099·2
Lipoite, 2099·2
Lipolan, 2099·2
Lipolest, 2099·2
Lipoleum, 2099·2
Lipolo, 2099·2
Lipolotion, 2099·2
Lipomax, 2099·2
Lipomega, 2099·2
Lipo-Merz, 2099·2
Lipomul, 2099·2
Liponet, 2099·2
α-Liponic Acid, 1754·3
Liponol, 2099·2
Liponorm, 2099·2
Lipopharm, 2099·2
Lipoplasmin, 2099·2
Liporex, 2099·2
Liporon, 2099·2
Liposcler, 2099·2
Liposel, 2099·2
Liposic, 2099·2
Liposit, 2099·2
Liposom, 2099·2
Liposperse, 2099·2
Lipostabil, 2099·2
Lipostat, 2099·3
Liposterol, 2099·3
Lipostop, 2099·3
Liposyn, 2099·3
Liposyn II, 2099·3
Liposyn III, 2099·3
Lipotalon, 2099·3
Lipoton, 2099·3
Lipotop, 2099·3
Lipotrend Cholesterol, 2099·3
Lipotriad, 2099·3
Lipotril, 2099·3
β-Lipotrophin, 1332·2
Lipotropic, 2099·3
Lipotropic Factors, 2099·3
Lipovastinklonal, 2099·3
Lipoven, 2099·3
Lipovenoes, 2099·3
Lipovenoes MCT, 2099·3
Lipovenos, 2099·3
Lipovenos MCT, 2099·3
Lipovit, 2099·3
Lipovitan, 2099·3
Lipovitasi-Or, 2099·3
Lipox, 2099·3
5-Lipoxygenase Inhibitors, 777·1
Lipozid, 2099·3
Lipozil, 2099·4
*Lippia citriodora*, 1706·3
Liprace, 2099·4
Lipraken, 2099·4
Lipram, 2099·4
Lipreren, 2099·4
Lipresina, 1342·3
Lipressina, 1342·3
Liprevil, 2099·4
Lipril, 2099·4
Liprocil, 2099·4
Lip-Sed, 2099·4
Lipshield Lipbalm, 2099·4
Lipsin, 2099·4
Lipsorex, 2099·4
Lipur, 2099·4
Lipus, 2099·4
Liq. Hydrog. Perox., 1182·2
Liqiprin, 2099·4
Liquefied Phenol, 1188·1
Liquemin, 2099·4
Liquemin N, 2099·4
Liquemine, 2099·4
Liquemine, Low— *see* Low Liquemine, 2106·3
Liqufruta Garlic Cough Medicine, 2099·4
LiquiBand, 2099·4
Liquibid, 2099·4
Liquibid-D, 2099·4
Liquibid-PD, 2099·4
Liquicard, 2099·4
Liqui-Char, 2099·4
Liquid X, 1308·3
Liquid Antacid, 2099·4
Liquid Antacid Plus Simethicon, 2099·4
Liquid B Complex, 2099·4
Liquid Ecstasy, 1308·3
Liquid Glucose, 1432·2
Liquid Maltitol, 1439·3
Liquid Nitrogen, 1236·3
Liquid Oxygen, 1237·2
Liquid Paraffin, 1479·1
Liquid Paraffin, Light, 1479·1
Liquid Petrolatum, 1479·1
Liquid Petrolatum, Heavy, 1479·1
Liquid Petrolatum, Light, 1479·1
Liquid Pred, 2099·4
Liquid Soap Pre-Op, 2099·4
Liquid Storax, 1749·3
Liquida, Pix, 1159·3
*Liquidambar orientalis*, 1749·3
*Liquidambar styraciflua*, 1749·3
Liquidepur, 2100·1
Liquido de Dakin, 2100·1
Liquidorm N, 2100·1
Liqui-Doss, 2100·1
Liquifer, 2100·1
Liquified Phenol, 1188·1
Liquifilm, 2100·1
Liquifilm Lagrimas, 2100·1
Liquifilm OK, 2100·1
Liquifilm Tears, 2100·1
Liquifilm Wetting, 2100·1
Liquifresh, 2100·1
Liquigel, 2100·1
Liquigen, 2100·1
Liquigesic Co, 2100·1
Liqui-Histine DM, 2100·1
Liquilax, Adco- — *see* Adco-Liquilax, 1775·3
Liquimat, 2100·1
Liquipake, 2100·1
Liquipom Dexa Antib, 2100·1
Liquipom Dexa Const, 2100·1
Liquipom Dexamida, 2100·1
Liquipom Medrisone, 2100·1
Liquiprin, 2100·1
Liquirit N, 2100·1
Liquiritiae Radix, 1270·2
Liquisorbon MCT, 2100·1
Liquisorbon MCT— *see* Nutrison MCT, 2181·3
LiquiVent, 2100·1
Liquivisc, 2100·1
Liquor Ammoniae, 1653·3
Liquor Ammoniae Dilutus, 1653·3
Liquor Ammoniae Fortis, 1653·3
Liquor Carbonis Detergens, 1159·2
Liquor Hydrogenii Peroxidi, 1182·2
Liquor Picis Carbonis, 1159·2
Liquorice, 1270·2
Liquorice, Deglycyrrhizinised, 1270·3
Liquorice, Indian, 1645·1
Liquorice Root, 1270·2
Liracol, 2100·2
Liroken, 2100·2
Lironex, 2100·2
Lirugen, 2100·2
Lis, 2100·2
Lisa, 2100·2
Lisac, 2100·2
Lisacef, 2100·2
Lisacne, 2100·2
Lisacol, 2100·2
Lisadimate, 1151·2
Lisadimato, 1151·2
Lisador, 2100·2
Lisaglucon, 2100·2
Lisaler, 2100·2
Lisaler Beta, 2100·2
Lisalgil, 2100·2
Lisalgil Compuesto, 2100·2
Lisan, 2100·2
Lisanirc, 2100·2
Lisapres, 2100·2
Lisaspin, 2100·2
Lisba, 2100·2
Lisbak, 2100·2
Lisedema, 2100·2
Lisenteral, 2100·2
Liserdol, 2100·2
Lisergida, 1708·2
Liseta, 2100·2
Lisi, 2100·2
Lisi Lich, 2100·2
Lisibeta, 2100·2
Lisiflen, 2100·3
Lisigamma, 2100·3
Lisigon, 2100·3
Lisihexal, 2100·3
Lisiken, 2100·3
Lisil, 2100·3
Lisin Sorb, 2100·3
Lisina, 1439·1
Lisina, Acetato de, 1439·2
Lisina, Hidrocloruro de, 1439·2
Lisinal, 2100·3
Lisinfos, 2100·3
Lisino, 2100·3
Lisinopril, 946·3
Lisinopril Dihydrate, 946·3
Lisinoprilum, 946·3
Lisinospes, 2100·3
Lisinotyrol, 2100·3
Lisinvitan, 2100·3
Lisiofer, 2100·3
Lisipril, 2100·3
Lisipril Comp, 2100·3
Lisi-Puren, 2100·3
Liskantin, 2100·3
Liskonum, 2100·3
Lismol, 2100·3
Lisoder, 2100·3
Lisoderma, 2100·3
Lisodren, 2100·3
Lisodur, 2100·3
Lisodura, 2100·3
Lisofenicol, 2100·3
Lisoflu, 2100·3
Lisolac, 2100·3
Lisolip, 2100·3
Lisomuc, 2100·3
Lisomucil, 2100·3
Lisomucil Gola, 2100·3
Lisomucil Tosse Sedativo, 2100·4
Lisomucin, 2100·4
Lisoneurin B12, 2100·4
Lisonotec, 2100·4
Lisopress, 2100·4
Lisopride, 2100·4
Lisopulm, 2100·4
Lisoquinol, 2100·4
Lisorane, 2100·4
Lisoril, 2100·4
Lisoril-5HT, 2100·4
Lisosmalen, 2100·4
Lisotox, 2100·4
Lisotran, 2100·4
Lisotrex, 2100·4
Lisovyr, 2100·4
Lispor, 2100·4
Lispril, 2100·4
Lispro, Insulin, 334·3, 340·2
Lissamine Green, 1057·3
Listaflex, 2100·4
Listerfluor, 2100·4
Listerine Preparations, 2100·4
Listeriosis, 134·1
Listermint, 2101·1
Listermint Arctic Mint Mouthwash, 2101·1
Listermint con Fluor, 2101·1
Listermint with Fluoride, 2101·1
Listran, 2101·1
Lisurida, Maleato de, 1210·3
Lisuride Maleate, 1210·3
Lisvifar, 2101·1
Lit-300, 2101·1
Litak, 2101·1
Litalgin, 2101·1
Litalir, 2101·1
Litarek, 2101·1
Litarex, 2101·1
Lithane, 2101·1
Lithanthracis, Oleum, 1159·2
Lithanthracis, Pix, 1159·2
Lithanthracis, Pyroleum, 1159·2
Litheum, 2101·1
Lithiagel, 2101·1
Lithias-cyl N Ho-Len-Complex, 2101·1
Lithicarb, 2101·1
Lithii Carbonas, 301·1
Lithii Citras, 301·1
Lithimole, 2101·1
Lithioderm, 2101·1
Lithiofor, 2101·1
Lithionit, 2101·1
Lithium Acetate, 305·2
Lithium Benzoate, 1707·2
Lithium Carb., 301·1
Lithium Carbonate, 301·1
Lithium Citrate, 301·1
Lithium Gamolenate, 1690·3
Lithium Gluconate, 305·2
Lithium Glutamate, 305·2
Lithium Hydroxide, 301·1
Lithium Orotate, 1724·3
Lithium Salicylate, 54·2
Lithium Succinate, 1151·2
Lithium Sulfate, 305·2
Lithiumeel, 2101·1
Lithiun, 2101·1
Lithizine, 2101·1
Lithobid, 2101·1
Lithocholic Acid, 1660·3, 1670·1, 1761·1
Lithofalk, 2101·1
Lithol Rubine BK, 1057·3
Litholrubine BK, 1057·3
Lithonate, 2101·1
Lithostat, 2101·2
Lithosun, 2101·2
Lithurex S, 2101·2
Litiax, 2101·2
Litican, 2101·2
Litio, Benzoato de, 1707·2
Litio, Carbonato de, 301·1
Litio, Citrato de, 301·1
Litiocar, 2101·2
Litiofarm, 2101·2

Lito, 2101·2
Litobile, 2101·2
Litocit, 2101·2
Litoff, 2101·2
Litolrubina BK, 1057·3
Litosmil, 2101·2
Litoxol, 2101·2
Litrison, 2101·2
Litursol, 2101·2
Liv 52, 2101·2
Liva-Care, Extralife— *see* Extralife Liva-Care, 1986·3
Livadex, 2101·2
Livamine, 2101·2
Liv-Detox, 2101·2
Live (Oral) Poliomyelitis Vaccines, 1633·3
Liver Abscess— *see* Abscess, Liver, 120·3
Liver Cancer— *see* Malignant Neoplasms of the Liver, 518·3
Liver Fluke Infections, 99·3
Liver of Sulphur, 1158·3
Liver Tonic Capsules, 2101·2
Liver Tonic Herbal Formula 6, 2101·2
Liver Transplantation, 1346·3
Liverall, 2101·2
Liverasi, 2101·2
Livercrom, 2101·2
Liver-Vite, Bioglan— *see* Bioglan Liver-Vite, 1844·1
Livesan, 2101·2
Livial, 2101·2
Liviane Compuesto, 2101·3
Liviel, 2101·3
Liviella, 2101·3
Livifem, 2101·3
Liviton, 2101·3
Livitrinsic-f, 2101·3
Livo Luk, 2101·3
Livocab, 2101·3
Livogen, 2101·3
Livolon, 2101·3
Livomarin, 2101·3
Livomedrox, 2101·3
Livomonil, 2101·3
Livostin, 2101·3
Livten, 2101·3
Lixacol, 2101·3
Lixamide, 2101·3
Lixidol, 2101·3
Lixir, 2101·3
Lixogan, 2101·3
Lizarona, 2101·3
Lizepat, 2101·3
Lizipaina, 2101·3
Lizovag, 2101·3
Lizul, 2101·3
LJ-206, 1116·2
LJC-10141, 39·1
LJC-10627, 165·3
LJC-10846, 727·3
LJP-394, 1348·2
LL-1530, 963·3
LL-1558, 1011·2
LL-1656, 877·2
Llantén, 1733·1
Llantusil, 2101·3
Llorentecaina Noradrenal, 2101·3
Lloyd's Cream, 2101·3
Lluvia de Oro, 1703·3
LM6, 2101·4
LM-91, 1501·3
LM-94, 1700·1
LM-123, 918·2
LM-192, 1764·3
LM-208, 316·3
LM-209, 437·2
LM-427, 249·1
LM-550, 1013·2
LM-2717, 358·2
LMB-2, 508·2
LMD, 745·3
LMTH, 1337·3
LMW Heparins, 949·2
LMWD, 745·3
LMW-DS, 892·2
L-M-X4, 2101·4
L-NMMA, 1752·1
LO-44, 873·2
Lo-Acid, 2101·4
Loads, 701·2
Lobac, 2101·4
Lobacin, 2101·4
Lobak, 2101·4
Lobamine-Cysteine, 2101·4
Lobana, 2101·4
Lobana Body, 2101·4
Lobana Derm-Aide, 2101·4
Lobana Peri-Garde, 2101·4
Lobaplatin, 565·1
Lobaplatino, 565·1
Lobate, 2101·4
Lobate-G, 2101·4
Lobate-GM, 2101·4
Lobate-M, 2101·4
Lobelia, 1589·1
Lobelia Composta, 2101·4
Lobelia Composto, Xarope de— *see* Xarope de Lobelia Composto, 2387·3
Lobelia Compound, 2101·4
*Lobelia inflata*, 1589·1
Lobelia Med Complex, 2101·4
Lobelina, Hidrocloruro de, 1589·1
Lobelina, Sulfato de, 1589·1
Lobeline, 1589·1
Lobeline Hydrochloride, 1589·1
Lobeline Sulfate, 1589·1
Lobeline Sulphate, 1589·1
Lobelini Hydrochloridum, 1589·1
Lobenzarit Disódico, 1707·2
Lobenzarit Sódico, 1707·2
Lobenzarit Sodium, 1707·2
Lobesol, 2101·4
Lobeta, 2101·4
Lobevat, 2101·4
Lobione, 2101·4
Lobivon, 2101·4
Lobu, 2101·4
Lobucavir, 649·3
Locabase, 2101·4
Locabiosol, 2101·4
Locabiotal, 2101·4
Locacid, 2102·1
Locacorten Preparations, 2102·1
Locacortene, 2102·1
Locacortene Tar, 2102·1
Locacortene Vioforme, 2102·1
Local Anaesthesia, 1369·1
Local Anaesthetics, 1367·1
Local Anaesthetics, Amide Type, 1367·1
Local Anaesthetics, Ester Type, 1367·1
Localin, 2102·1
Localisation-related Seizures— *see* Epilepsy, 349·1
Localone, 2102·1
Localyn, 2102·1
Localyn SV, 2102·1
Localyn-Neomicina, 2102·1
Locao Mancha Branca, 2102·1
Locapred, 2102·1
Locasalen, 2102·1
Locasalene, 2102·1
Locaseptil-Neo, 2102·1
Locasil, 2102·1
Locasol, 2102·2
Locasol New Formula, 2102·2
Locason, 2102·2
Locasyn, 2102·2
Locatop, 2102·2
Locemix, 2102·2
Loceptin, 2102·2
Loceryl, 2102·2
Locetar, 2102·2
Lochol, 2102·2
Locholes, 2102·2
Locholest, 2102·2
Lociherp, 2102·2
Locilan, 2102·2
Locion Axel, 2102·2
Locion Corporal Suavizante AHA Formula 405, 2102·2
Locion Limpiadora AHA Formula 405, 2102·2
Lockesol, 2102·2
Lockets, 2102·2
Lockets Medicated Linctus, 2102·2
Lockjaw— *see* Tetanus, 149·2
Locko, 2102·2
Lockolys, 2102·2
Lockolys— *see* CAPD/DPCA, 1867·4
Locobase, 2102·2
Locoid, 2102·2
Locoid C, 2102·3
Locoid Crelo, 2102·3
Locoide N, 2102·3
Locoidol, 2102·3
Locoidon, 2102·3
LOCOL, 2102·3
Locomin, 2102·3
Locomucil, 2102·3
Locorten Preparations, 2102·3
Locortene, 2102·3
Locortene Vioformo, 2102·3
Locose, 2102·3
Locrim, 2102·3
Loctenk, 2102·3
Locula, 2102·3
Locust Bean Gum, 1579·1
Locust Bean Tree, 1579·1
Lodales, 2102·3
Loderix, 2102·3
Loderm, 2102·3
Loderm Retinoico, 2102·3
Lodiarid, 2102·3
Lodimol, 2102·3
Lodine, 2102·3
Lodipen, 2102·3
Lodipres, 2102·3
Lodis, 2102·4
Lodixal, 2102·4
Lodoc, 2102·4
Lodopin, 2102·4
Lodosyn, 2102·4
Lodot, 2102·4
Lodoxamida Trometamol, 1707·3
Lodoxamide Ethyl, 1707·3
Lodoxamide Trometamol, 1707·3
Lodoxamide Tromethamine, 1707·3
Lodoz, 2102·4
Lodrane, 2102·4
Lodrane 12, 2102·4
Lodrane Allergy— *see* Lodrane 12, 2102·4
Lodrane 12D, 2102·4
Lodronat, 2102·4
Lodyfen, 2102·4
Loesfer, 2102·4
Loesfer + Acide Folique, 2102·4
Loestrin, 2102·4
Loestrin 1.5/30, 2102·4
Loestrin Fe, 2102·4
Loette, 2102·4
Loexom, 2102·4
Lofacol, 2102·4
Lofenac, 2102·4
Lofenalac, 2102·4
Lofenalac— *see* Phenyl-Free, 2217·2
Lofenoxal, 2102·4
Lofensaid, 2102·4
Lofepramina, Hidrocloruro de, 305·3
Lofepramine Hydrochloride, 305·3
Lofexidina, Hidrocloruro de, 1041·2
Lofexidine Hydrochloride, 1041·2
Lofibra, 2102·4
Loflazepato de Etilo, 698·1
Lofoxin, 2103·1
Loftan, 2103·1
Lofton, 2103·1
Loftyl, 2103·1
Logacron, 2103·1
Logan, 2103·1
Logascid, 2103·1
Logastin, 2103·1
Logastric, 2103·1
Logat, 2103·1
Logecine, 2103·1
Logen, 2103·1
Logesic, 2103·1
Logical, 2103·1
Logican, 2103·1
Logicin Preparations, 2103·1
Logiflox, 2103·2
Logimat, 2103·2
Logimax, 2103·2
Logiparin, 2103·2
Logirene, 2103·2
Logoderm, 2103·2
Logradin, 2103·2
Logrosal, 2103·2
Logroton, 2103·2
Logryx, 2103·2
Logynon, 2103·2
Logynon ED, 2103·2
Lohp, 2103·2
Loiasis, 99·3
Loisan, 2103·2
Loisan-D, 2103·2
Loitin, 2103·2
Lokalicid, 2103·2
Lokalison-antimikrobiell Creme N, 2103·2
LoKara, 2103·3
Lokilan, 2103·3
Lokilan Nasal, 2103·3
Lomabronchin N, 2103·3
Lomac, 2103·3
Lomacin, 2103·3
Lomadryl, 2103·3
Lomaherpan, 2103·3
Lomahypericum, 2103·3
Lomal, 2103·3
Lomar, 2103·3
Lomarheumin N, 2103·3
Lomarin, 2103·3
Lomasatin M, 2103·3
Lomasleep, 2103·3
Lomatol, 2103·3
Lomatuell H, 2103·3
Lomax, 2103·3
Lomazell Forte N, 2103·3
Lombalgina, 2103·3
Lombriareu, 2103·3
Lombrimade, 2103·3
Lomef, 2103·3
Lomeflon, 2103·3
Lomefloxacin Hydrochloride, 227·2
Lomefloxacin Mesilate, 227·2
Lomefloxacin Mesylate, 227·2
Lomefloxacino, Hidrocloruro de, 227·2
Lomepral, 2103·3
Lomesone, 2103·3
Lomex, 2103·3
Lomexin, 2103·3
Lomfer, 2103·3
Lomflox, 2103·4
Lomide, 2103·4
Lomine, 2103·4
Lomir, 2103·4
Lomofen, 2103·4
Lomont, 2103·4
Lomoparan, 891·2
Lomotil, 2103·4
Lomper, 2103·4
Lomprax, 2103·4
Lomudal, 2103·4
Lomupren, 2103·4
Lomupren Compositum, 2103·4
Lomusol, 2103·4
Lomusol Plus Xylometazoline, 2103·4
Lomusol-X, 2103·4
Lomuspray, 2103·4
Lomustina, 565·2
Lomustine, 565·2
Lomustinum, 565·2
Lomy, 2103·4
LON-798, 927·2
Lonactene, 2103·4
Lonaflam, 2103·4
Lonalac, 2103·4
Lonalgal, 2103·4
Lonarid, 2103·4
Lonarid Aplo, 2103·4
Lonarid Mono, 2103·4
Lonarid N, 2103·4
Lonarid-N, 2104·1
Lonavar, 2104·1
Lonazolac Calcium, 54·2

Lonazolaco Cálcico, 54·2
Lonchocarpus, 1510·1
*Lonchocarpus utilis*, 1510·1
Loncord, 2104·1
Londerm-N, 2104·1
London Drugs Preparations, 2104·1
London Paste, 1665·1, 1748·1
Lonestin, 2104·1
Long Buchu, 1663·1
Long Lasting Nasal Mist, 2104·1
Longachin, 2104·1
Longacilin, 2104·1
Longacor, 2104·1
Longactil, 2104·1
Longalgic, 2104·1
Longastatina, 2104·1
Longasteril 40, 2104·1
Longasteril 70, 2104·1
Longatren, 2104·1
Longazem, 2104·1
Longbalsem, 2104·1
Longevit, 2104·1
Longevit Plus, 2104·1
Longevital, 2104·1
Longifene, 2104·2
Longifolene, 1760·1
Longimin, 2104·2
Longivol, 2104·2
Longtussin Duplex Tag und Nacht N, 2104·2
Longum, 2104·2
Lonidamina, 565·3
Lonidamine, 565·3
Lonikan, 2104·2
Lonine, 2104·2
Loniten, 2104·2
Lonnoten, 2104·2
Lonol, 2104·2
Lonol Sport, 2104·2
Lonolox, 2104·2
Lonoten, 2104·2
Lonox, 2104·2
Lonseren, 2104·2
Lontadex, 2104·2
Lontadex D, 2104·2
Lonza, 2104·2
Loop Diuretics, 811·2
Loortan, 2104·2
Loortan Plus, 2104·2
Lo/Ovral, 2104·2
Lopalind, 2104·2
Lopamide, 2104·2
Lopamine, 2104·2
Lo-P-Caps, 2104·3
Lop-Dia, 2104·3
Lopediar, 2104·3
Lopedium, 2104·3
Lopela, 2104·3
Lopelin, 2104·3
Lopemid, 2104·3
Lopepham, 2104·3
Loperacap, 2104·3
LoperaGen, 2104·3
Loperamerck, 2104·3
Loperamida, Hidrocloruro de, 1271·1
Loperamide Hydrochloride, 1271·1
Loperamide Oxide, 1271·1
Loperamide Oxide Monohydrate, 1271·1
Loperamidi Hydrochloridum, 1271·1
Loperamidi Oxidum Monohydricum, 1271·1
Loperamil, 2104·3
Loperan, 2104·3
Loperastat, 2104·3
Loperax, 2104·3
Lopercin, 2104·3
Loperdium, 2104·3
Loperhoe, 2104·3
Loperia, 2104·3
Loperid, 2104·3
Loperidol, 2104·3
Loperium, 2104·3
Loperkey, 2104·3
Lopermide, 2104·3
Loperyl, 2104·3
Lopetrans, 2104·3
Lopex, 2104·3
Lophakomp Preparations, 2104·3
Lophakomp-Hypericum— *see* Lomahypericum, 2103·3
*Lophophora williamsii*, 1713·3
Lopid, 2104·4
Lopiden, 2104·4
Lopimed, 2104·4
Lopinavir, 649·3
Lopiretic, 2104·4
Lopirin, 2104·4
Lopitrex, 2104·4
Loporic, 2104·4
Lopramine Hydrochloride, 305·3
Loprazol, 2104·4
Loprazolam Mesilate, 704·1
Loprazolam, Mesilato de, 704·1
Loprazolam Mesylate, 704·1
Loprazolam Methanesulphonate, 704·1
Lopremone, 1337·3
Lopresor, 2104·4
Lopresor, Slow- — *see* Slow-Lopresor, 2295·1
Lopress, 2104·4
Lopressor, 2104·4
Lopressor HCT, 2104·4
Lopril, 2104·4
Loproc, 2104·4
Loprofin, 2104·4
Loprox, 2104·4
Loptomit, 2104·4
Lopurax, 2104·4
Lora, 2104·4
Lorabenz, 2104·4
Lorabid, 2105·1
Loracarbef, 228·1
Loraclar, 2105·1
Loradine, 2105·1
Loradur, 2105·1
Lorafem, 2105·1
Loraga, 2105·1
Loragalen, 2105·1
Loragamma, 2105·1
Loralerg, 2105·1
Loralerg-D, 2105·1
Lora-Lich, 2105·1
Loramed, 2105·1
Loramet, 2105·1
Loramide, 2105·1
Loranil, 2105·1
Loranil D, 2105·1
Lorano, 2105·1
Loranox, 2105·1
Lorans, 2105·1
Lorapam, 2105·1
Lora-Puren, 2105·1
Lorasifar, 2105·1
Lorastine, 2105·1
Lorastyne, 2105·1
Loratab, 2105·1
Lora-Tabs, 2105·1
Loratadina, 436·1
Loratadine, 436·1
Loratadura, 2105·1
Loratamed, 2105·2
Loratin, 2105·2
Loratyn, 2105·2
Loratyne, 2105·2
Lorax, 2105·2
Lorazene, 2105·2
Lorazep, 2105·2
Lorazepam, 704·1
Lorazepam Pivalate, 705·1
Lorazepamum, 704·1
Lorazepan, 2105·2
Lorbef, 2105·2
Lorbi, 2105·2
Lorcainida, Hidrocloruro de, 947·2
Lorcainide Hydrochloride, 947·2
Lorcet 10/650, 2105·2
Lorcet Plus, 2105·2
Lorcet-HD, 2105·2
Loremex, 2105·2
Loremix, 2105·2
Loremix D, 2105·2
Lorenin, 2105·2
Lorentin, 2105·2
Lorenzo, Aceite de, 1707·3
Lorenzo's Oil, 1707·3, 2105·2
Loretam, 2105·2
Loretic, 2105·2
Lorexen, 2105·2
Lorfast, 2105·2
Lorfenil, 2105·2
Loricin, 2105·2
Loride, 2105·2
Loridem, 2105·2
Loriderm, 2105·2
Loridin, 2105·2
Loridin-D, 2105·2
Lorien, 2105·3
Lorinden T, 2105·3
Lorita, 2105·3
Loriter, 2105·3
Lorityne, 2105·3
Lorium, 2105·3
Lorivan, 2105·3
Lormetazepam, 705·2
Lormine, 2105·3
Lornazol, 2105·3
Lornox, 2105·3
Lornoxicam, 54·2
Loron, 2105·3
Lorophyn, 2105·3
Loroxide, 2105·3
Lorpa, 2105·3
Lorsacor, 2105·3
Lorsedal, 2105·3
Lorsedin, 2105·3
Lortaan, 2105·3
Lortaan Plus, 2105·3
Lortab, 2105·3
Lortab ASA, 2105·3
Lortadine, 2105·3
Lortuss DM, 2105·3
Lortuss HC, 2105·3
Lorvas, 2105·3
Lorzaar, 2105·3
Lorzaar Plus, 2105·3
Lorzem, 2105·3
Losacar, 2105·4
Losacar-H, 2105·4
Losacor, 2105·4
Losacor D, 2105·4
Losalen, 2105·4
Losamel, 2105·4
Losan Fe, 2105·4
Losapan, 2105·4
Losapres, 2105·4
Losapres-D, 2105·4
Losaprex, 2105·4
Losaprol, 2105·4
Losar, 2105·4
Losartán Potásico, 947·2
Losartan Potassium, 947·2
Losartec, 2105·4
Losatal, 2105·4
Losazid, 2105·4
Loscalcon, 2105·4
Loscon, 2105·4
Losec Preparations, 2105·4
Losec— *see* Klacid HP 7, 2080·1
Lose.Lax, 2106·1
Losferron, 2106·1
Losferron-Fol, 2106·1
Losigamona, 366·2
Losigamone, 366·2
Losna, 1645·1
Losnesium, 2106·1
Losopil, 2106·1
Lostapres, 2106·1
Lostatin, 2106·1
Lostradyl, 2106·1
Lotadine, 2106·1
Lotem, 2106·1
Lotemax, 2106·1
Lotemp, 2106·1
Loten, 2106·1
Lo-Ten, 2106·1
Lotensin, 2106·1
Lotensin H, 2106·1
Lotensin HCT, 2106·1
Loteprednol Etabonate, 1105·3
Loteprednol, Etabonato de, 1105·3
Loteprednol Ethyl Carbonate, 1105·3
Loteprol, 2106·1
Lotesoft, 2106·1
Lotharin, 2106·1
Lotil, 2106·1
Lotin, 2106·1
Lotio Decapans, 2106·1
Lotio Plumbi, 1706·1
Lotio Zinc, 2106·1
Lotio Zinci, 2106·1
Lotioblanc, 2106·1
Lotion Ecran Solaire Extreme, 2106·2
Lotion Pour Feux Sauvages, 2106·2
Lotoquis, 2106·2
Lotoquis Simple, 2106·2
Lotrel, 2106·2
Lotremin, 2106·2
Lotremine, 2106·2
Lotrial, 2106·2
Lotrial D, 2106·2
Lotricomb, 2106·2
Lotriderm, 2106·2
Lotrimin, 2106·2
Lotrimin AF, 2106·2
Lotrimin Ultra, 2106·2
Lotrisone, 2106·2
Lotrix, 2106·2
Lotronex, 2106·2
Lotusix, 2106·2
Lotussin, 2106·2
Lotussin Expectorant, 2106·2
Lou Gehrig's Disease— *see* Motor Neurone Disease, 1739·1
Louisiana Long Pepper, 1667·1
Louisiana Sport Pepper, 1667·1
Louse Infections— *see* Pediculosis, 1499·1
Louse-borne Typhus— *see* Typhus, 152·3
Louten, 2106·2
Lovacol, 2106·2
Lovacor, 2106·2
Lovage Root, 1708·1
Lovalip, 2106·3
Lovamine, 2106·3
Lovan, 2106·3
Lovarin, 2106·3
Lovarin P, 2106·3
Lovasc, 2106·3
Lovast, 2106·3
Lovastatin, 949·1
Lovastatina, 949·1
Lovastatinum, 949·1
Lovastin, 2106·3
Lovatex, 2106·3
Lovaton, 2106·3
Lovatop, 2106·3
Love Drug, 1593·3
Love Pill, 1593·3
Lovelle, 2106·3
Lovenox, 2106·3
Loveral, 2106·3
Lovilia, 2106·3
Lovina, 2106·3
Lovir, 2106·3
Lovire, 2106·3
Loviscol, 2106·3
Lovrak, 2106·3
Low Back Pain, 7·1
Low Back Pain, Hylands— *see* Hylands Low Back Pain, 2052·3
Low Centyl K, 2106·3
Low Liquemine, 2106·3
Lowadina, 2106·3
Lowasa, 2106·3
Lowden, 2106·3
Lowe-Komplex Preparations, 2106·3
Lowenzahn-Pflanzensaft, Kneipp— *see* Kneipp Lowenzahn-Pflanzensaft, 2081·3
Löwenzahnwurzel, 1751·3
Lowfin, 2106·3
Lowila Cake, 2106·3
Lowin, 2106·3
Lowlipid, 2106·3
Low-molecular-mass Heparins, 949·2
Low-molecular-weight Dextran, 745·3

Low-molecular-weight Heparins, 949·2
Lowpre, 2106·4
Lowpress, 2106·4
Lowsium Plus, 2106·4
Low-Substituted Carboxymethylcellulose Sodium, 1578·1
Low-Substituted Hydroxypropyl Cellulose, 1579·3
Loxam, 2106·4
Loxapac, 2106·4
Loxapin, 2106·4
Loxapina, 705·2
Loxapina, Hidrocloruro de, 705·2
Loxapina, Succinato de, 705·2
Loxapine, 705·2
Loxapine Hydrochloride, 705·2
Loxapine Succinate, 705·2
Loxapine-*N*-oxide, 705·3
Loxavit, 2106·4
Loxazol, 2106·4
Loxen, 2106·4
Loxetine, 2106·4
Loxibest, 2106·4
Loxifen, 2106·4
Loxiflan, 2106·4
Loxiglumida, 1271·3
Loxiglumide, 1271·3
Loxin, 2106·4
Loxina, 2106·4
Loxitan, 2106·4
Loxitane, 2106·4
Loxitenk, 2106·4
Loxonin, 2106·4
Loxoprofen Sodium, 54·3
Loxoprofeno Sódico, 54·3
Loxyn, 2106·4
Lozan, 2106·4
Lozap, 2106·4
Lozapin, 2106·4
Lozapine, 2106·4
Lozaprin, 2106·4
Lozide, 2106·4
Lozione Same AS, 2106·4
Lozione Same Urto, 2106·4
Lozione Vittoria, 2106·4
Lozitan, 2106·4
Lozol, 2106·4
Lozopin, 2107·1
LP Drink, 2107·1
LP Mix, 2107·1
β-LPH, 1332·2
L-Polamidon, 2107·1
LP-Truw Mono, 2107·1
LPV, 2107·1
LRCL-3794, 21·1
LRX-15, 1521·2
LS-121, 964·1
LS-519, 488·1
LS-2616, 583·2
LS-519-Cl2, 488·1
LSD, 1708·2
LSD-25, 1708·2
LSP, 2107·1
LT-31-200, 875·3
LTH, 1337·3
Lu-10-171, 289·1
Lu-10-171B, 289·1
Lu-23-174, 721·3
Lu-26-054/0, 292·1
LU-200134, 12·1
Luan, 2107·1
Luar-G, 2107·1
Luar-G Compositum, 2107·1
Luarprofeno, 2107·1
Luase, 2107·1
Lubafax, 2107·1
Lubalix, 2107·1
Lubarol, 2107·1
Lubeluzol, 950·2
Lubeluzole, 950·2
Lubentyl, 2107·1
Lubentyl a la Magnesie, 2107·1
Lubex, 2107·1
Lubexyl, 2107·1
Lubical, 2107·1
Lubo, 2107·1
Lubogliss, 2107·1
Luborant, 2107·1
LubraSol, 2107·1
Lubricans, 2107·1
Lubriderm, 2107·1
Lubriderm AHA, 2107·1
Lubriderm Daily UV, 2107·1
Lubriderm UV 15, 2107·2
Lubrificante Anestesico, 2107·2
Lubrifilm, 2107·2
Lubrigel, 2107·2
Lubrik, 2107·2
Lubrikano, 2107·2
Lubrilax, 2107·2
Lubrilent, 2107·2
Lubrilin, 2107·2
Lubrin, 2107·2
Lubrirhin, 2107·2
Lubrisec, 2107·2
Lubri-Tears, 2107·2
LubriTears, 2107·2
Lubritina Franklin, 2107·2
Lubrizal, 2107·2
Lucebanol, 2107·2
Lucen, 2107·2
Lucenfal, 2107·2
Lucerne, 1649·1
Luci, 2107·2
Lucibran, 2107·2
Lucidex, 2107·2
Lucidril, 2107·2
*Lucilia sericata*, 1151·3
Lucilium, 2107·2
Lucinactant, 1736·2
Lucisan, 2107·2
Lucitan, 2107·2
Luckyhepa, 2107·2
Luco-Oph, 2107·2
Lucopenin, 2107·3
Lucosil, 2107·3
Lucretin, 2107·3
Lucrin, 2107·3
Luctor, 2107·3
Ludeal, 2107·3
Ludilat, 2107·3
Ludiomil, 2107·3
Luditec, 2107·3
Lufenuron, 1507·1
Luffa Preparations, 2107·3
Luffa-loges, 2107·3
Luffasan, 2107·3
Luffeel Comp, 2107·3
Luforan, 2107·3
Luftal, 2107·3
Luftgaz, 2107·3
Lufyllin, 2107·3
Lufyllin-EPG, 2107·3
Lufyllin-GG, 2107·3
Lugesteron, 2107·3
Lugol's Solution, 1598·3
LüH6, 1046·3
Luiflex, 2107·3
Luitase, 2107·3
Luivac, 2107·3
Luizym, 2107·4
Lukadin, 2107·4
Lukair, 2107·4
Lukasm, 2107·4
Luliberin, 1325·1
Lullan, 2107·4
Lumaren, 2107·4
Lumat, 2107·4
Lumbago— *see* Low Back Pain, 7·1
Lumbago-Gastreu S R11, 2107·4
Lumbalgine, 2107·4
Lumbicid, 2107·4
Lumbinon, 2107·4
Lumbriquil, 2107·4
Lumefantrina, 453·3
Lumefantrine, 453·3
Lumiactiv, 2107·4
Lumiclar, 2107·4
Lumidrops, 2107·4
Lumifurex, 2107·4
Lumigan, 2107·4
Lumin, 2107·4
Luminal, 2107·4
Luminale, 2107·4
Luminaletas, 2107·4
Luminalette, 2107·4
Luminaletten, 2107·4
Luminalettes, 2107·4
Luminovag, 2107·4
Lumiracoxib, 54·3
Lumirelax, 2107·4
Lumirem, 2107·4
Lumitens, 2108·1
Lumix, 2108·1
Lumox, 2108·1
Lunadon, 2108·1
Lunch Money Drug, 698·3
Lundiran, 2108·1
Lunelax, 2108·1
Lunelax Comp, 2108·1
Lunelle, 2108·1
Lunerin, 2108·1
Lung Abscess— *see* Pneumonia, 141·3
Lung Cancer— *see* Malignant Neoplasms of the Lung, 519·2
Lung Disease, Chronic— *see* Bronchopulmonary Dysplasia, 1077·2
Lung Disease, Chronic Obstructive— *see* Chronic Obstructive Pulmonary Disease, 779·2
Lung Disease, Diffuse Parenchymal— *see* Diffuse Parenchymal Lung Disease, 1079·3
Lung Disease, Interstitial— *see* Diffuse Parenchymal Lung Disease, 1079·3
Lung Fluke Infections, 99·3
Lung Injury, Acute— *see* Acute Respiratory Distress Syndrome, 1075·2
Lung Transplantation, 1347·2
Lunibron, 2108·1
Lunis, 2108·1
Luparen, 2108·1
Lupectrim, 2108·1
Lupectrim Balsamico, 2108·1
Lu-Peracina, 2108·1
Lupercaina, 2108·1
Luperzol, 2108·1
Lupidon, 2108·1
Lupidon G, 2108·1
Lupidon H, 2108·1
Lupidon H+G, 2108·1
Lupihist, 2108·1
Lupizyme, 2108·1
Lupovalin, 2108·1
Luprac, 2108·1
Lupride, 2108·1
Lupron, 2108·1
Lupron— *see* Procren, 2237·1
Luprostiol, 1519·2
Lupuli Flos, 1708·1
Lupuli Strobulus, 1708·1
Lúpulo, 1708·1
Lupulus, 1708·1
Lupus Erythematosus, Systemic— *see* Systemic Lupus Erythematosus, 1088·3
Lupus Nephritis— *see* Systemic Lupus Erythematosus, 1088·3
Lupus Pernio— *see* Sarcoidosis, 1087·2
Lurdex, 2108·1
Luret, 2108·2
Luride, 2108·2
Lurline PMS, 2108·2
Lurselle, 2108·2
Lusap, 2108·2
Lusemin, 2108·2
Lustra, 2108·2
Lustra-AF, 2108·2
Lustral, 2108·2
Lustys Herbalene, 2108·2
Lutalmin, 2108·2
Lutamidal, 2108·2
Luteal Hormone, 1566·2
Lutebiol, 2108·2
Lutein, 1056·1, 1423·1
Luteine, 1566·2
Luteinising Hormone, 1330·1, 1332·1
Luteinising Hormone-releasing Factor, 1325·1
Lutene, 2108·2
Lutenil, 2108·2
Lutenyl, 2108·2
Luteohormone, 1566·2
Luteoliberina, 2108·2
Luteomammotropic Hormone, 1337·3
Luteotrophic Hormone, 1337·3
Luteotropin, 1337·3
Luteran, 2108·2
Lutionex, 2108·2
Lutogin, 2108·2
Lutoginestryl F, 2108·2
Lutogynestryl, 2108·2
Lutometrodiol, 2108·2
Lutopolar, 2108·2
Lutoral, 2108·2
Lutoral E, 2108·2
Lutrax, 2108·2
Lutrelef, 2108·3
Lutrepulse, 2108·3
Lutropin, 1332·1
Lutropin Alfa, 1332·1
Lutropina, 1332·1
Lutropina Alfa, 1332·1
Luuf Preparations, 2108·3
Luva Invisivel, 2108·3
Luvased, 2108·3
Luvased-Tropfen N, 2108·3
Luveris, 2108·3
Luvier, 2108·3
Luvion, 2108·3
Luvos Heilerde, 2108·3
Luvox, 2108·3
Luxazone, 2108·3
Luxazone Eparina, 2108·3
Luxiq, 2108·3
Luxiva, 2108·3
Luxiva Changing, 2108·3
Luxivia— *see* Luxiva, 2108·3
Luxivia Ultra, 2108·3
Luxoben, 2108·3
Luxofort, 2108·3
Luxomicina, 2108·4
Luzolona Simple, 2108·4
Luzolona Y, 2108·4
Luzone, 2108·4
LVD, 745·3
L-Vist, 2108·4
LVP, 1342·3
LY-048740, 159·1
LY-061188, 168·1
LY-097964, 172·3
LY-099094, 593·3
LY-110140, 292·1
LY-127809, 1211·2
LY-127935, 225·3
LY-135252, 1585·1
LY-137998, 1327·2
LY-139037, 1277·2
LY-139381, 180·2
LY-139481, 1568·3
LY-139602, 1585·1
LY-139603, 1585·1
LY-146032, 204·2
LY-156758, 1568·3
LY-163892, 228·1
LY-170053, 710·3
LY-174008, 905·3
LY-177370, 271·2
LY-188011, 558·1
LY-188695, 433·2
LY-198561, 866·3
LY-203638, 759·2
LY-231514, 579·1
LY-237216, 206·1
LY-246708, 1498·3
LY-246736, 1250·2
LY-248686, 291·3
LY-253351, 1009·2
LY-303366, 395·1
LY-307640, 1285·1
LY-326869, 962·3
LY-333328, 240·2
LY-333334, 775·2
LY-335348, 546·3
LY-544349, 1746·3
Lyapolate Sodium, 1000·2

Lyasin, 2108·4
Lyban, 2108·4
Lybovit, 2108·4
Lycazid, 2108·4
Lyceft, 2108·4
Lycia Luminique, 2108·4
Lycine, 1660·1
Lycitrope, 2108·4
Lyclear, 2108·4
Lycoaktin, 2108·4
Lycoaktin M, 2108·4
Lycobiol, 2108·4
Lycopene, 1056·1
*Lycopodium serratum*, 1703·1
Lycovowen-N, 2108·4
Lyderm, 2108·4
Lydonide, 2108·4
Lydroxil, 2108·4
Lyell's Syndrome— *see* Drug-induced Skin Reactions, 1134·3
Lyell's Syndrome— *see* Toxic Epidermal Necrolysis, 1138·3
Lyflex, 2108·4
Lyforan, 2108·4
Lygal Preparations, 2108·4
Lyman, 2108·4
Lyme Borreliosis— *see* Lyme Disease, 134·1
Lyme Disease, 134·1
Lyme Disease Vaccines, 1622·2
Lymecycline, 228·2
LYMErix, 2108·4
Lymetel, 2108·4
Lymphaden N, 2108·4
Lymphaden PE, 2109·1
Lymphadenomtropfen N, 2109·1
Lymphatic Filariasis, 100·1
Lymphazurin, 2109·1
Lymphdiaral, 2109·1
Lymphdiaral Aktiv, 2109·1
Lymphex, 2109·1
Lymphoblastic Leukaemia, Acute— *see* Acute Lymphoblastic Leukaemia, 506·1
Lymphoblastoid Interferon, 640·3
Lymphocyte Activating Factor, 1701·3
Lymphocyte Immune Globulin, 1348·3
Lymphocytic Antiserum, 1348·3
Lymphocytic Leukaemia, Acute— *see* Acute Lymphoblastic Leukaemia, 506·1
Lymphocytic Leukaemia, Chronic— *see* Chronic Lymphocytic Leukaemia, 507·2
Lymphoglobulin, 2109·1
Lymphoglobuline, 2109·1
Lymphogranuloma Venereum, 134·2
Lymphokines, 1701·3
Lymphoma, Burkitt's, 511·1
Lymphoma, Diffuse Large Cell— *see* Non-Hodgkin's Lymphomas, 510·1
Lymphoma, Follicular— *see* Non-Hodgkin's Lymphomas, 510·1
Lymphoma, Lymphoblastic— *see* Non-Hodgkin's Lymphomas, 510·1
Lymphoma, Lymphoplasmacytic, 511·3
Lymphoma, MALT, 511·1
Lymphoma, Ocular— *see* Malignant Neoplasms of the Eye, 516·1
Lymphoma, Primary CNS, 510·3
Lymphomas, 509·1
Lymphomas, AIDS-related, 510·3
Lymphomas, Cutaneous T-cell, 511·2
Lymphomas, Non-Hodgkin's— *see* Non-Hodgkin's Lymphomas, 510·1
Lymphomas, Primary Effusion, 510·3
Lymphomyosot, 2109·1
Lymphoplasmacytic Lymphoma, 511·3
Lymphotoxin, 590·2
Lymphozil, 2109·1
Lymphtropfen S, 2109·1
Lyndak, 2109·1
Lyndiol, 2109·1
Lyndiol, Neo— *see* Neo Lyndiol, 2156·3
Lyndiolett, 2109·1
Lynenol, 1557·1
Lynestrenol, 1557·1
Lynestrenolum, 1557·1
Lynoestrenol, 1557·1
Lynoral, 2109·1
Lyn-ratiopharm, 2109·1
Lyn-ratiopharm-Sequenz, 2109·1
Lynx, 2109·1
Lyobalsam, 2109·1
Lyo-Bifidus, 2109·1
Lyofoam, 2109·1
Lyofoam C, 2109·1
Lyogen, 2109·1
Lyomer, 2109·1
Lyorodin, 2109·1
Lyostypt, 2109·1
Lyovac Cosmegen, 2109·1
Lyphocin, 2109·1
Lypholyte, 2109·1
Lypressin, 1342·3
Lyprinol, 2109·2
Lypsyl Cold Sore Gel, 2109·2
Lyrica, 2109·2
Lyrinel XL, 2109·2
Lys, 1439·1
Lys Acetate, 1439·2
Lys Hydrochloride, 1439·2
Lysalgo, 2109·2
Lysantin, 2109·2
Lysanxia, 2109·2
Lysbex, 2109·2
Lysedem, 2109·2
Lysedil, 2109·2
Lysedil Compositum, 2109·2
Lyseen, 2109·2
D-Lysergic Acid Amide, 1723·2
Lysergic Acid Diethylamide, 1708·2
Lysergide, 1708·2
Lysergol, 1723·2
Lysetol FF, 2109·2
Lysetol Med, 2109·2
Lysetol V, 2109·2
Lysine, 1439·1
L-Lysine, 1439·1
Lysine Acetate, 1439·2
Lysine Acetylsalicylate, 54·3
DL-Lysine Acetylsalicylate, 54·3
Lysine Amidotrizoate, 1061·1
Lysine Aspirin, 54·3
Lysine Hydrochloride, 1439·2
L-Lysine Monoacetate, 1439·2
Lysine Monohydrate, 1439·1
L-Lysine Monohydrochloride, 1439·2
Lysine Orotate, 1724·3
L-Lysine-(1-benzyl-1*H*-indazol-3-yloxy)acetic Acid, 20·3
[8-Lysine]vasopressin, 1342·3
Lysini Acetas, 1439·2
Lysini Hydrochloridum, 1439·2
Lysinotol, 2109·2
Lysinuric Protein Intolerance— *see* Hyperammonaemia, 1425·2
Lysivit $B_{12}$ a l'inositol, 2109·2
Lyso-6, 2109·2
Lysocalm, 2109·2
Lysocline, 2109·2
Lysodren, 2109·2
Lysodrop, 2109·2
Lysofon, 2109·2
Lysoform, 2109·2
Lysoform Killavon, 2109·2
Lysoformin, 2109·2
Lysoformin 3000, 2109·2
Lysoformin Spezial, 2109·3
Lysol, 1178·1
Lysomucil, 2109·3
Lysopaine, 2109·3
Lysoprin, 2109·3
Lysosomal α-Glucosidase, 1646·2
Lysosomal Storage Disease— *see* Gaucher Disease, 1649·2
Lysosomal Storage Disorder— *see* Fabry Disease, 1651·2
Lysovir, 2109·3
Lysox, 2109·3
Lysozyme Hydrochloride, 1717·2
Lyssavac N, 2109·3
Lyssuman, 2109·3
Lysthenon, 2109·3
Lystin, 2109·3
Lysuride Maleate, 1210·3
Lysuron, 2109·3
Lyteers, 2109·3
Lyteprep, 2109·3
Lytos, 2109·3
Lytren, 2109·3
Lytren RHS, 2109·3
Lytta, 1666·3
*Lytta vesicatoria*, 1667·1
Lyzyme, 2109·3

M

M, 1042·1
M-14, 253·2
M-99, 38·3
M-141, 255·2
683-M, 1126·1
M-811, 1741·3
M-1028, 401·2
M5050, 1037·3
M-5943, 452·1
M & M, 2109·3
Ma Ma Sustagen, 2109·3
Maalox Preparations, 2109·3
Maalox Antacid/Anti-Gas, Extra Strength— *see* Extra Strength Maalox Antacid/Anti-Gas, 1986·2
Maaloxan, 2109·4
Maaloxan Ca, 2109·4
Mab, 2109·4
MAb-B43.13, 577·1
MabCampath, 2109·4
Mabicrol, 2109·4
Mabis, 2109·4
Mabogastrol, 2109·4
Mabosil, 2109·4
Maboterpen, 2109·4
Mabron, 2110·1
Mabthera, 2110·1
Mabuprofen, 47·1
Mac, 2110·1
Mac Dual Action, 2110·1
Mac Extra— *see* Mac Dual Action, 2110·1
MAC Infections— *see* Opportunistic Mycobacterial Infections, 137·2
Mac Sugar Free, 2110·1
Macaine, 2110·1
Macalvit, 2110·1
Macbirs, 2110·1
Macbirs Minoxidil, 2110·1
Mace, 1670·1, 1708·2
Mace Oil, 1708·2
Macgel, 2110·1
Mach-2, 2110·1
Machlor, 2110·1
Machto, 2110·1
Macis, Aceite de, 1708·2
Mackenzies Menthoids, 2110·1
Mackenzies Smelling Salts, 2110·1
Macladin, 2110·1
Maclar, 2110·1
Maclean Indigestion Tablets, 2110·1
Macleans Mouthguard, 2110·1
Macleans Sensitive, 2110·1
Maclov, 2110·2
Macmiror, 2110·2
Macmiror Complex, 2110·2
Macmiror Complex V, 2110·2
Macobal, 2110·2
Macoderm, 2110·2
Macodin, 2110·2
Maconha, 1666·1
Maconia, 1666·1
Macorel, 2110·2
Macosil, 2110·2
Macril, 2110·2
Macro Antioxidant, 2110·2
Macro Anti-Stress, 2110·2
Macro B, 2110·2
Macro C, 2110·2
Macro E, 2110·2
Macro Garlic, 2110·2
Macro Maxepa, 2110·2
Macro Multi M, 2110·2
Macro Natural Vitamin E Cream, 2110·2
Macroadenoma— *see* Hyperprolactinaemia, 1315·2
Macrobid, 2110·2
Macrocilin, 2110·2
Macrocin, 274·3
Macrodantin, 2110·2
Macrodantina, 2110·2
Macrodex, 2110·2
Macrodexin, 2110·2
Macrofurin, 2110·2
Macroglobulinaemia, Waldenström's, 511·3
Macrogol Cetostearyl Ethers, 1412·2
Macrogol Esters, 1411·1
Macrogol Ethers, 1411·2
Macrogol 15 Hydroxystearate, 1412·3
Macrogol Lauril Ethers, 1412·3
Macrogol Lauryl Ethers, 1412·3
Macrogol Monomethyl Ethers, 1413·1
Macrogol Nonylphenyl Ethers, 1413·2
Macrogol Oleyl Ethers, 1413·1
Macrogol Ricinoleate, 1414·3
Macrogol Stearate, 1413·2
Macrogol 8 Stearate, 1413·2
Macrogol 40 Stearate, 1413·2
Macrogol Stearate 400, 1413·2
Macrogol Stearate 2000, 1413·2
Macrogol Stearates, 1413·2
Macrogol Tetramethylbutylphenyl Ethers, 1414·1
Macrogol Trihydroxystearate, 1414·3
Macrogola, 1708·2
Macrogoles, 1708·2
Macrogolglycerol Hydroxystearate, 1414·3
Macrogolglycerol Ricinoleate, 1414·3
Macrogolglyceroli Hydroxystearas, 1414·3
Macrogolglyceroli Ricinoleas, 1414·3
Macrogoli Aether Cetostearylicus, 1412·2
Macrogoli Aether Laurilicum, 1412·3
Macrogoli Aether Oleicum, 1413·1
Macrogoli 15 Hydroxystearas, 1412·3
Macrogoli Stearas, 1413·2
Macrogols, 1708·2
Macrolax, 2110·3
Macrolides, 118·2
Macrolin, 2110·3
Macromax, 2110·3
Macromicina, 2110·3
Macromin, 2110·3
Macro-P, 2110·3
Macropen, 2110·3
Macrophage Colony-stimulating Factors, 756·3
Macrophage-targeted β-Glucocerebrosidase, 1649·1
Macroral, 2110·3
Macrosalb ($^{99m}$Tc), 1525·3
Macrosan, 2110·3
Macrosil, 2110·3
Macroten, 2110·3
Macsoralen, 2110·3
Mactam, 2110·3
Mactex, 2110·3
Macular Oedema, Cystoid— *see* Postoperative Inflammatory Ocular Disorders, 70·3
Madagascar Vanilla, 1762·3
Madar, 2110·3
Made B12, 2110·3
Madecassic Acid, 1144·3
Madecassol Preparations, 2110·3
Maderan, 2110·3
Maderil, 2110·3
Madi, 1666·1
Madicure, 2110·3
Madiplot, 2110·3
Madiprazole, 2110·3
Maditez, 2110·3
Madol, 2110·3
Madola, 2110·4
Madomine, 2110·4
Madonna, 2110·4
Madopar, 2110·4
Madopark, 2110·4
Madoxy, 2110·4
Madura Foot— *see* Mycetoma, 136·2, 388·3
Maduramicin, 606·1
Maduramicin Ammonium, 606·1

Maduramicina, 606·1
Madurase, 2110·4
Mafel, 2110·4
Mafen, 2110·4
Mafena, 2110·4
Mafenida, Acetato de, 228·2
Mafenide, 228·2
Mafenide Acetate, 228·2
Mafenide Hydrochloride, 228·3
Mafenide Propionate, 228·3
Maflurell, 2110·4
Maformin, 2110·4
Mafosfamida, 565·3
Mafosfamide, 565·3
Mafu, 2110·4
Mag-200, 2110·4
Mag 2, 2110·4
Mag 50, 2110·4
Mag 77, 2110·4
Mag Cit Prep, 2110·4
Mag Doskar's Preparations, 2110·4
Mag Kottas Preparations, 2110·4
Magagel, 2111·2
Magaininas, 228·3
Magainins, 228·3
Magalba, 2111·2
Magaldrate, 1271·3
Magaldrato, 1271·3
Magaldratum, 1271·3
Magalite, 2111·2
Magalphil, 2111·2
Magan, 2111·2
Magasan, 2111·2
Magastron, 2111·2
Mag-Cal Mega, 2111·2
Magcal Plus, Celloid Compounds— *see* Celloid Compounds Magcal Plus, 1877·2
Mag-Carb, 2111·2
Magcol, 2111·2
Magel, 2111·2
Magen-700, 2111·2
Magen-Darmtropfen S, 2111·2
Magenpulver Hafter, 2111·2
Magenta, 1185·1
Magenta, Acid, 1646·3
Magenta, Basic, 1185·1
Magenta Paint, 1185·2
Magenta, Trisulfonic Acid, Diammonium Salt, 1646·3
Magenta, Trisulfonic Acid, Disodium Salt, 1646·3
Magentabletten Hafter, 2111·2
Magentee, 2111·2
Magentee EF-EM-ES, 2111·2
Magen-Tee, Kneipp— *see* Kneipp Magen-Tee, 2081·3
Magentee Solu-Vetan, Heumann— *see* Heumann Magentee Solu-Vetan, 2042·4
Magen-Tee Stada N, 2111·2
Magentropen N Legastol, 2111·3
Magesto, 2111·3
Mag-G, 2111·3
Maggots, 1151·3
Magic Methyl, 1714·1
Magic Mix, 2111·3
Magic Mushroom, 1736·1
Magicul, 2111·3
Magion, 2111·3
Magisbile, 2111·3
Magistery of Bismuth, 1252·2
Magium, 2111·3
Magium E, 2111·3
Magium K, 2111·3
Magiyam, 1666·1
Maglid, 2111·3
Maglucate, 2111·3
Magluphen, 2111·3
Maglut, 2111·3
Magmed, 2111·3
Magmin, 2111·3
Mag-Min, 2111·3
Magnacal, 2111·3
Magnalox, 2111·3
Magnalum, 2111·3
Magnamycin, 2111·3
Magnapen, 2111·3
Magnaprin, 2111·3
Magnaspart, 2111·4
Magnaspor, 2111·4
Magnatil, 2111·4
Magnatil Calcico, 2111·4
Magne-$B_6$, 2111·4
Magnebe, 2111·4
MagneBind, 2111·4
Magnecyl, 2111·4
Magnecyl-koffein, 2111·4
Magneforte, 2111·4
Magnefusin, 2111·4
Magnerot, 2111·4
Magnerot A, 2111·4
Magnerot Classic, 2111·4
Magnerot N, 2111·4
Magnesia, 2111·4
Magnesia Bisurada, 2111·4
Magnesia Bisurata, 2111·4
Magnesia Bisurata Aromatic, 2111·4
Magnesia Bisurata Aromatic Plus, 2111·4
Magnesia Effervescente Sella, 2111·4
Magnesia Fluida, 2111·4
Magnesia Pasteur, 2111·4
Magnesia Phosphorica I Oligoplex, 2111·4
Magnesia S Pellegrino, 2111·4
Magnesia San Pellegrino, 2111·4
Magnesia Volta, 2111·4
Magnesiamaito, 2112·1
Magnesie Plus, 2112·1
Magnesie S Pellegrino, 2112·1
Magnesii Acetas Tetrahydricus, 1227·3
Magnesii Aspartas Dihydricus, 1227·3
Magnesii Chloridum Hexahydricum, 1228·1
Magnesii Chloridum 4.5-Hydricum, 1228·1
Magnesii Glycerophosphas, 1228·1
Magnesii Hydroxidum, 1272·2
Magnesii Oxidum, 1272·3
Magnesii Oxidum Leve, 1272·3
Magnesii Oxidum Ponderosum, 1272·3
Magnesii Peroxidum, 1185·2
Magnesii Pidolas, 1228·2
Magnesii Stearas, 1574·2
Magnesii Subcarbonas, 1272·1
Magnesii Subcarbonas Levis, 1272·1
Magnesii Subcarbonas Ponderosus, 1272·1
Magnesii Sulfas Heptahydricus, 1228·2
Magnesii Trisilicas, 1272·3
Magnesin, 2112·1
Magnesio, 1227·3
Magnesio, Acetato de, 1227·3
Magnesio, Ascorbato de, 1227·3
Magnesio, Aspartato de, 1227·3
Magnesio, Carbonato de, 1272·1
Magnesio, Citrato de, 1272·1
Magnésio, Cloreto de, 1228·1
Magnesio, Cloruro de, 1228·1
Magnesio + C/Mag-CE, 2112·1
Magnesio, Fosfato de, 1228·1
Magnesio, Glicerofosfato de, 1228·1
Magnesio, Glucoheptonato de, 1228·1
Magnesio, Gluconato de, 1228·1
Magnesio, Hidróxido de, 1272·2
Magnesio, Lactato de, 1228·1
Magnesio, Óxido de, 1272·3
Magnesio, Pidolato de, 1228·2
Magnesio, Sulfato de, 1228·2
Magnesio, Trisilicato de, 1272·3
Magnesioboi, 2112·1
Magnesiocard, 2112·1
Magnesiol, 2112·1
Magnesiomix, 2112·1
Magnesit, 2112·1
Magnesium, 1227·3
Magnesium Acetate, 1227·3
Magnesium Acetate Tetrahydrate, 1227·3
Magnesium Alginate, 1577·1
Magnesium Aluminium Silicate, 1577·1
Magnesium Aluminometasilicate, 1577·2
Magnesium Aluminosilicate, 1577·2
Magnesium Aluminosilicate Hydrate, 1248·2
Magnesium Aluminum Silicate, 1577·1
Magnesium Aluminum Silicate Hydrate, 1248·2
Magnesium α-Aminoglutarate Hydrobromide, 1709·2
Magnesium Aminosuccinate Dihydrate, 1227·3
Magnesium Ascorbate, 1227·3
Magnesium Aspartate, 1227·3
Magnesium Aspartate Dihydrate, 1227·3
Magnesium Aspartate Hydrobromide, 706·1
Magnesium L-Aspartate Hydrobromide Trihydrate, 706·1
Magnesium Aspartate Hydrochloride, 1229·1
Magnesium Biomed, 2112·1
Magnesium Bromoglutamate, 1709·2
Magnesium Carbonate, 1272·1
Magnesium Carbonate, Heavy, 1272·1
Magnesium Carbonate, Light, 1272·1
Magnesium Chloratum, 1228·1
Magnesium Chloride, 1228·1
Magnesium Chloride Hexahydrate, 1228·1
Magnesium Chloride 4.5-Hydrate, 1228·1
Magnesium Chloride, Partially Hydrated, 1228·1
Magnesium Citrate, 1272·1
Magnesium Clofibrate, 885·1
Magnesium Complexe, 2112·1
Magnesium Compositum, 2112·1
Magnésium Cristallisé, Chlorure de, 1228·1
Magnesium Deoxyribonucleate, 1679·2
Magnesium Di[(*S*)-2-aminohydrogenobutane-1,4-dioate], 1227·3
Magnesium Diasporal, 2112·1
Magnesium (*R,S*)-2,3-Dihydroxypropyl Phosphate, 1228·1
Magnesium Fosforylcholine, 1690·1
Magnesium Gluceptate, 1228·1
Magnesium Glucoheptonate, 1228·1
Magnesium Gluconate, 1228·1
Magnesium D-Gluconate Hydrate, 1228·1
Magnesium Glutamate Hydrobromide, 1709·2
Magnesium Glycerinophosphate, 1228·1
Magnesium Glycerophosphate, 1228·1
Magnesium Glycocolle Lafarge, 2112·1
Magnesium Hydrate, 1272·2
Magnesium Hydrogen Phosphate Trihydrate, 1228·1
Magnesium Hydroxide, 1272·2
Magnesium 2-Hydroxy-1-(hydroxymethyl)ethyl Phosphate, 1228·1
Magnesium 2-Hydroxypropionate, 1228·1
Magnesium Isospaglumate, 1702·2
Magnesium Lactate, 1228·1
Magnesium Laurilsulfate, 1574·3
Magnesium Levulinate, 1229·1
Magnesium Metrizoate, 1067·2
Magnesium Orotate, 1229·1, 1724·3
Magnesium Oxide, 1272·3
Magnesium Oxide, Heavy, 1272·3
Magnesium Oxide, Light, 1272·3
Magnesium 5-Oxopyrrolidine-2-carboxylate, 1228·2
Magnesium Palmitate, 1574·2
Magnesium Pemoline, 1592·1
Magnesium Perhydrolum, 1185·2
Magnesium Peroxide, 1185·2
Magnesium Phosphate, 1228·1
Magnesium Phosphate, Tribasic, 1228·1
Magnesium Phosphate Trihydrate, Dibasic, 1228·1
Magnesium Pidolate, 1228·2
Magnesium Plus, 2112·1
Magnesium Polystyrene Sulfonate, 1053·3
Magnesium Pyre, 2112·1
Magnesium Pyroglutamate, 1228·2
Magnesium Salicylate, 55·1
Magnesium Silicate, 1159·1, 1580·2
Magnesium Silicate, Hydrated, 1272·3
Magnesium Silicofluoride, 1446·3
Magnesium Stearate, 1574·2
Magnesium Sulfate, 1228·2
Magnesium Sulphate, 1228·2
Magnesium Sulphate, Dried, 1228·2
Magnesium Sulphate Heptahydrate, 1228·2
Magnesium Thiosulfate, 1054·1
Magnesium Tonil, 2112·1
Magnesium Tonil N, 2112·1
Magnesium Tonil Vitamin E, 2112·1
Magnesium Trisilicate, 1272·3
Magnesium Valproate, 382·2
Magnesium Verla, 2112·1
Magnesium Vital, 2112·1
Magnesium-B, 2112·1
Magnesium-Eufidol, 2112·1
Magnesium-OK, 2112·1
Magnesium-Plus-Hevert, 2112·1
Magnesoide, 2112·2
Magnesona, 2112·2
Magnesorot, 2112·2
Magnespasmil, 2112·2
Magnespasmyl, 2112·2
Magnesplus, 2112·2
Magnetic Resonance Imaging, 1059·1
Magnetop, 2112·2
Magnetrans Forte, 2112·2
Magnevist, 2112·2
Magnevistan, 2112·2
Magnezie, 2112·2
Magnezyme, 2112·2
Magnidol-Plus, 2112·2
Magnihexal, 2112·2
Magnil, 2112·2
Magniton-R, 2112·2
Magno Sanol, 2112·2
Magnodor, 2112·2
Magnofit, 2112·2
Magnogen, 2112·2
Magnogene, 2112·2
Magnograf, 2112·2
Magnol, 2112·2
Magnolat, 2112·2
Magnolax, 2112·2
Magnolex, 2112·2
Magnonorm, 2112·2
Magnoplasm, 2112·3
Magnopyrol, 2112·3
Magnoral, 2112·3
Magnorbin, 2112·3
Magnorell, 2112·3
Magnorol, 2112·3
Magnoscorbol, 2112·3
Magnosol, 2112·3
Magnosolv, 2112·3
Magnostase, 2112·3
Magnoston, 2112·3
Magnotab, 2112·3
Magnovit, 2112·3
Magnox, 2112·3
Magnurol, 2112·3
Magnus, 2112·3
Magnyl, 2112·3
Magocean, 2112·3
Magonate, 2112·3
Magopsor, 2112·3
Magoral, 2112·3
Mag-Oro, 2112·3
Mag-Ox, 2112·3
Magralibi, 2112·3
Magrilan, 2112·3
Magrinex, 2112·3
Magroton, 2112·3
Magsal, 2112·3
Magsil, 2112·4
Magsons, 2112·4
Mag-SR, 2112·4
Mag-SR Plus Calcium, 2112·4
Mag-Tab, 2112·4
Mag-Tab SR, 2112·4
Magto, 2112·4
Magtrate, 2112·4
Magvital, 2112·4
Mahiou, 2112·4
Ma-huang, 1119·3
Maiblume, 1675·3
Maidenhair Tree, 1692·3
Maiglöckchenkraut, 1675·3
Mainnox, 2112·4
Maintain, 2112·4
Maintane, 2112·4
Maiorad, 2112·4
Maïs, Huile de, 1439·2
Maíz, Barba Del, 1676·1

Maizar, 2112·4
Maize, 1676·1
Maize Oil, 1439·2
Maize Oil, Refined, 1439·2
Maize Starch, 1449·1
Majeptil, 2112·4
Majocarmin Forte, 2112·4
Majocarmin Mite, 2112·4
Majocarmin-Tee, 2112·4
Majolat, 2112·4
Major Antithrombin, 735·3, 742·2
Major Tranquillisers, 663·1
Major-Con, 2112·4
Major-gesic, 2112·4
Majorpen, 2112·4
Makatussin Preparations, 2112·4
Makhlif, 1666·1
Makovan, 2113·1
Makrocilin, 2113·1
Malachite Green, 1185·2
Malachite Green G, 1171·1
Maladin, 2113·1
Malafene, 2113·1
Malak, 1666·1
Malandil, 2113·1
Malarex, 2113·1
Malaria, 444·1
Malaria Vaccines, 1622·2
Malaridine Phosphate, 460·1
Malarone, 2113·1
Malastop, 2113·1
Malathion, 1507·1
Malathionum, 1507·1
Malatión, 1507·1
Malato de Almotriptán, 465·2
Malato de Cleboprida, 1260·3
Malato de Pizotifeno, 470·3
Malato de Tietilperazina, 442·1
Malaviron, 2113·1
Malayan Filariasis— *see* Lymphatic Filariasis, 100·1
Malayan Pit-viper, 863·2
Maldison— *see* Cleensheen, 1892·2
Maldison— *see* Lice Rid, 2095·3
Male +, 2113·1
Male Breast Cancer— *see* Malignant Neoplasms of the Male Breast, 515·2
Male Contraception— *see* Contraception, 1535·3
Male Fern, 108·2
Male Formula Herbal Plus Formula 2, 2113·1
Maleapril, 2113·1
Maleato de Acepromazina, 668·3
Maleato de Azatadina, 425·1
Maleato de Bromfeniramina, 426·1
Maleato de Carbinoxamina, 426·3
Maleato de Cinepazet, 884·2
Maleato de Cinepazida, 884·2
Maleato de Clorfenamina, 427·3
Maleato de Dexbromfeniramina, 426·1
Maleato de Dexclorfeniramina, 427·3
Maleato de Dimetindeno, 431·2
Maleato de Dizocilpina, 1683·1
Maleato de Domperidona, 1263·2
Maleato de Enalapril, 909·2
Maleato de Ergometrina, 1684·1
Maleato de Ergonovina, 1684·1
Maleato de Feniramina, 438·3
Maleato de Flupirtina, 43·3
Maleato de Fluvoxamina, 298·2
Maleato de Irsogladina, 1267·3
Maleato de Levomepromazina, 703·2
Maleato de Lisurida, 1210·3
Maleato de Mepiramina, 437·1
Maleato de Metilergometrina, 1714·2
Maleato de Metisergida, 469·3
Maleato de Midazolam, 707·2
Maleato de Perhexilina, 980·2
Maleato de Proclorperazina, 716·3
Maleato de Proglumetacina, 85·2
Maleato de Propiomazina, 440·3
Maleato de Rosiglitazona, 345·2
Maleato de Tegaserod, 1293·2
Maleato de Tietilperazina, 442·1
Maleato de Timolol, 1012·2
Maleato de Trimebutina, 1758·1
Maleato de Trimipramina, 320·2
Maleic Acid, 1709·2
Maleico, Ácido, 1709·2
Malen, 2113·1
Male-pattern Baldness— *see* Alopecia, 1134·1
Malexin, 2113·1
Malfin, 2113·1
Maliasin, 2113·1
Malic Acid, 1709·2
Málico, Ácido, 1709·2
Malidens, 2113·1
Malignancies, HIV-associated— *see* HIV-associated Malignancies, 623·1
Malignancy, Hypercalcaemia of— *see* Hypercalcaemia of Malignancy, 1218·1
Malignant Ascites— *see* Ascites, 815·1
Malignant Effusions, 512·2
Malignant Hyperpyrexia— *see* Malignant Hyperthermia, 1394·2
Malignant Hypertension— *see* Hypertension, 825·1
Malignant Hyperthermia, 1394·2
Malignant Melanoma— *see* Melanoma, 522·3
Malignant Neoplasms of the Aerodigestive Tract— *see* Malignant Neoplasms of the Head and Neck, 517·3
Malignant Neoplasms of the Bladder, 512·3
Malignant Neoplasms of the Bone, 513·1
Malignant Neoplasms of the Brain, 513·2
Malignant Neoplasms of the Breast, 514·1
Malignant Neoplasms of the Breast, Prophylaxis— *see* Prophylaxis of Breast Cancer, 515·1
Malignant Neoplasms of the Cervix, 515·3
Malignant Neoplasms of the Colon— *see* Malignant Neoplasms of the Gastrointestinal Tract, 516·2
Malignant Neoplasms of the Endometrium, 516·1
Malignant Neoplasms of the Eye, 516·1
Malignant Neoplasms of the Gastrointestinal Tract, 516·2
Malignant Neoplasms of the Head and Neck, 517·3
Malignant Neoplasms of the Kidney, 518·1
Malignant Neoplasms of the Liver, 518·3
Malignant Neoplasms of the Lung, 519·2
Malignant Neoplasms of the Male Breast, 515·2
Malignant Neoplasms of the Mouth— *see* Malignant Neoplasms of the Head and Neck, 517·3
Malignant Neoplasms of the Oesophagus— *see* Malignant Neoplasms of the Gastrointestinal Tract, 516·2
Malignant Neoplasms of the Ovary, 520·2
Malignant Neoplasms of the Pancreas, 521·1
Malignant Neoplasms of the Prostate, 521·2
Malignant Neoplasms of the Rectum— *see* Malignant Neoplasms of the Gastrointestinal Tract, 516·2
Malignant Neoplasms of the Skin, 522·2
Malignant Neoplasms of the Skin, Prophylaxis— *see* Malignant Neoplasms of the Skin, 522·2
Malignant Neoplasms of the Stomach— *see* Malignant Neoplasms of the Gastrointestinal Tract, 516·2
Malignant Neoplasms of the Testis, 523·1
Malignant Neoplasms of the Thymus, 523·3
Malignant Neoplasms of the Thyroid, 523·3
Malignant Osteopetrosis, Infantile— *see* Osteopetrosis, 1085·2
Malignant Pericardial Effusions— *see* Malignant Effusions, 512·2
Malignant Pleural Effusions— *see* Malignant Effusions, 512·2
Malignant Thyroid Nodule— *see* Malignant Neoplasms of the Thyroid, 523·3
Malimed, 2113·2
Malinert, 2113·2
Malipuran, 2113·2
Malirid, 2113·2
Malival, 2113·2
Malival Compuesto, 2113·2
Malix, 2113·2
Mallamint, 2113·2
Mallazine, 2113·2
Mallebrin, 2113·2
Mallebrin Konzentrat, 2113·2
Mallebrinetten— *see* Mallebrin, 2113·2
Mallorol, 2113·2
Mallow, 1709·3
Mallow Flower, 1709·3
Mallow Leaf, 1709·3
Malocide, 2113·2
Malocin, 2113·2
Malogen Aqueous, 2113·2
Malogen in Oil, 2113·2
Malogex, 2113·2
Malonato de Bopindolol, 875·3
Maloprim, 2113·2
Malortil, 2113·2
Malotilate, 1709·3
Malotilato, 1709·3
Malt Extract, 1439·2
MALT Lymphoma, 511·1
Malt Soup Extract, 1439·2
Maltase, Acid, 1646·2
Malted Grain of Barley, 1439·2
Malted Grain of Wheat, 1439·2
Maltitol, 1439·3
D-Maltitol, 1439·3
Maltitol, Jarabe de, 1439·3
Maltitol, Liquid, 1439·3
Maltitol Solution, 1439·3
Maltitol Syrup, 1439·3
Maltitolum, 1439·3
Maltitolum Liquidum, 1439·3
Maltlevol, 2113·2
Maltlevol-M, 2113·2
Maltodextrin, 1439·3
Maltodextrina, 1439·3
Maltodextrinum, 1439·3
Maltofer, 2113·2
Maltofer Fol, 2113·2
Maltofer Vitaminado, 2113·2
Maltogen, 2113·2
Malton E, 2113·2
Malto-oligosaccharides, 1417·1
Maltosa, 1440·1
Maltose, 1440·1
Maltose, Hydrogenated, 1439·3
Maltose-glucose Syrup, High, Hydrogenated, 1439·3
Maltovis, 2113·2
Maltsupex, 2113·2
Maltyl, 2113·2
Maludil, 2113·2
Malugel, 2113·3
Malva, 1666·1
Malva Composta, 2113·3
*Malva neglecta*, 1709·3
*Malva sylvestris*, 1709·3
Malvae Folium, 1709·3
Malvae Sylvestris Flos, 1709·3
Malvaliz, 2113·3
Malvasen, Natusor— *see* Natusor Malvasen, 2154·1
Malvatricin, 2113·3
Malvavisco, 1651·3
Malvedrin, 2113·3
Malvenblätter, 1709·3
Malvenblüten, 1709·3
Malveol, 2113·3
Malvitona, 2113·3
Malvodon, 2113·3
Malvol, 2113·3
Malvona, 2113·3
Malvosulfam, 2113·3
Mamellin, 2113·3
Mamíferos, Extractos Tisulares, 1709·3
Mammalian Tissue Extracts, 1709·3
Mammol, 2113·3
Mammotropin, 1337·3
Mamofen, 2113·3
Mamograf, 2113·3
Man Formula, 2113·3
Maná, 1273·1
Manaderm, 2113·3
Manceau, 2113·3
Mancef, 2113·3
Mandafen, 2113·3
Mandal 425, 2113·3
Mandalyn Expectorant, 2113·3
Mandalyn Paediatric, 2113·3
Mandanol, 2113·3
Mandarine, 2113·3
(7*R*)-7-D-Mandelamido-3-(1-methyl-1*H*-tetrazol-5-ylthiomethyl)-3-cephem-4-carboxylic Acid, 169·3
7-[(*R*)-Mandelamido]-3-(1-sulphomethyl-1*H*-tetrazol-5-ylthiomethyl)-3-cephem-4-carboxylic Acid, Disodium Salt, 174·2
Mandelamine, 2113·3
Mandelan, 2113·3
Mandelato de Metenamina, 230·2
Mandelic Acid, 228·3
Mandelic Acid, Racemic, 228·3
Mandélico, Ácido, 228·3
Mandelip, 2113·3
Mandelo-katt, 2113·4
Mandelöl, 1651·1
(+)-Mandelonitrile Glucoside, 1765·2
(1*R*,3*r*,5*S*)-3-[(±)-Mandeloyloxy]-8-methyltropanium Bromide, 483·2
Mandepiril, 2113·4
Mandokef, 2113·4
Mandol, 2113·4
Mandolgin, 2113·4
Mandolsan, 2113·4
Mandorla, Olio di, 1651·1
Mandragora Comp, 2113·4
Mandragora Med Complex, 2113·4
Mandrake, American, 1155·2
Mandrogripp, 2113·4
Mandrolax, 2113·4
Mandrolax Lactu, 2113·4
Mandrolax Pico, 2113·4
Mandros Diarstop, 2113·4
Mandros Reise, 2113·4
Maneon, 2113·4
Manerix, 2113·4
Manevac, 2113·4
Mangafodipir Trisódico, 1067·1
Mangafodipir Trisodium, 1067·1
Manganese, 1440·1
Manganese Amino Acid Chelate, 1440·2
Manganese Chloride, 1440·1
Manganese Dioxide, 1440·2
Manganese Gluconate, 1440·1
Manganese D-Gluconate, 1440·1
Manganese Hydrogen Citrate, 1440·2
Manganese Sulfate, 1440·1
Manganese Sulphate, 1440·1
Manganese Sulphate Monohydrate, 1440·1
Manganese (II) Sulphate Monohydrate, 1440·1
Manganeso, 1440·1
Manganeso, Cloruro de, 1440·1
Manganeso, Gluconato de, 1440·1
Manganeso, Sulfato de, 1440·1
Mangani Sulfas Monohydricum, 1440·1
Mangaplexe, 2113·4
Mania— *see* Bipolar Disorder, 278·2
Manibee Complejo, 2113·4
Manibee-C, 2113·4
Manic, 2113·4
Manic Depression— *see* Bipolar Disorder, 278·2
Manicol, 2113·4
Manidipine Hydrochloride, 950·2
Manidipino, Hidrocloruro de, 950·2
Manidon, 2113·4
*Manihot utilissima*, 1449·1
Manimon, 2113·4
Maninil, 2113·4
Maniprex, 2113·4
Manita, 950·2
Manitol, 950·2
Maniton, 2113·4
Manivasc, 2113·4
Manmox, 2113·4
Mann, 2113·4
Manna, 1273·1

Manna Sugar, 950·2
Manne en Larmes, 1273·1
Mannex, 2113·4
Mannistol, 2114·1
Mannite, 950·2, 2114·1
Mannit-Losung, 2114·1
Mannitol, 950·2
D-Mannitol, 950·2
Mannitolum, 950·2
Mannose, 950·2
D-Mannuronic Acid, 1576·3
Mano, 2114·1
Manobrozil, 2114·1
Manodepo, 2114·1
Manoflox, 2114·1
Manoglucon, 2114·1
Manoketo, 2114·1
Manolio, 2114·1
Manolone, 2114·1
Manomet, 2114·1
Manon, 2114·1
Manorfen, 2114·1
Manorifcin, 2114·1
Manoron, 2114·1
Manotran, 2114·1
Manovon, 2114·1
Mansal, 2114·1
Mansil, 2114·1
Mansonella Infections, 100·1
Mantadan, 2114·1
Mantadix, 2114·1
Mantai, 2114·1
Manteca de Cacao, 1482·3
Manteca de Karité, 1482·1
Manteiga de Cacau, 1482·3
Mantidan, 2114·1
Mantoux Test, 1759·1
Mantus, 2114·1
Manugel, 2114·1
Manuka, 1709·3
Manusept, 2114·1
Manusept HD, 2114·1
Manzan, 2114·1
Manzan Plus, 2114·2
Manzanilla, 1669·3
Manzanilla Ordinaria, 1669·3
Manzanilla Romana, 1669·3
Manzul, 1666·1
MAOIs, 278·2, 316·1
Maolate, 2114·2
Maoni, 2114·2
Maosig, 2114·2
MAOtil, 2114·2
Maox, 2114·2
Map An, 2114·2
Mapap, 2114·2
Mapap, Childrens— *see* Childrens Mapap, 1882·4
Mapap Cold Formula, 2114·2
Mapezine, 2114·2
Mapin, 2114·2
Maple Melts, 2114·2
Mapluxin, 2114·2
Mapox, 2114·2
Mappine, 1663·2
Mapro-GRY, 2114·2
Maprolu, 2114·2
Maprotilina, Hidrocloruro de, 306·1
Maprotiline, 306·1
Maprotiline Hydrochloride, 306·1
Maprotiline Mesilate, 306·2
Maprotiline Resinate, 306·2
Maprotiline-*N*-oxide, 306·2
Maprotilini Hydrochloridum, 306·1
Mapurit, 2114·2
Maquil, 2114·2
Maqui-Libre, 2114·2
Mar, 2114·2
Mar Plus, 2114·2
Maracugina, 2114·2
Maracuja Composto, Elixir de— *see* Elixir de Maracuja Composto, 1965·4
Maraguango, 1666·1
Marajuana, 1666·1
Marament Balsam W, 2114·2
Marament-N, 2114·2
Maranon H, 2114·2
Maranox, 2114·2
Maranox— *see* Double-Action Toothache Kit, 1952·2
Maranta, 1422·1
*Maranta arundinacea*, 1422·1
Marathon, 2114·2
Marathon Antioxidante, 2114·2
Marax, 2114·2
Marben, 2114·3
Marblen, 2114·3
Marbofloxacin, 228·3
Marbofloxacino, 228·3
Marcain, 2114·3
Marcain with Fentanyl, 2114·3
Marcain with Pethidine, 2114·3
Marcaina, 2114·3
Marcaine, 2114·3
Marcelle Moisture Eye Cream, 2114·3
Marcelle Multi-Defense, 2114·3
Marcelle Protective Block, 2114·3
Marcelle Sunblock, 2114·3
Marcen, 2114·3
Marcillin, 2114·3
Marclorhex, 2114·3
Marco Rub Camphorated, 2114·3
Marco Sweet Light, 2114·3
Marco Sweett, 2114·3
Marcocid, 2114·3
Marcodine, 2114·3
Marcof, 2114·3
Marcoumar, 2114·3
Marcumar, 2114·3
Marcuphen, 2114·4
Marduk, 2114·4
Mareamin, 2114·4
Mareen, 2114·4
Marespin, 2114·4
Marevan, 2114·4
Marevit, 2114·4
Marezine, 2114·4
Maregesic, 2114·4
Margesic H, 2114·4
Margosa, 1658·2
Margosa Oil, 1658·2
Marianon, 2114·4
Mariazeller, 2114·4
Marienbader Pillen N, 2114·4
Mariendistel Curarina, 2114·4
Marigold, 1665·2
Marigongo, 1666·1
Marihuana, 1666·1
Marijuana, 1666·1
Maril, 2114·4
Marimastat, 565·3
Marimer, 2114·4
Marine, 2114·4
Marine Lipid Concentrate, 2114·4
Marinepa, 2114·4
MarinEx, 2114·4
Marinheiro, Elixir de— *see* Elixir de Marinheiro, 1965·4
Marinol, 2114·4
Mariquita, 1666·1
Mariston, 2114·4
Markalakt, 2114·4
Marks-Losung, 2114·4
Marlidan, 2114·4
Marlin Salt System, 2115·1
Marlyn Formula 50, 2115·1
Marly-Skin, 2115·1
Marnatal-F, 2115·1
Marolderm, 2115·1
Maronil, 2115·1
Marovil, 2115·1
Marovilina, 2115·1
Marplan, 2115·1
Marpres, 2115·1
Marron d'Inde, 1648·2
Marrón FK, 1056·2
Marrón HT, 1056·3
Marrubene Codethyline, 2115·1
Marrubio, 1124·1
Marrubium, 1124·1
*Marrubium vulgare*, 1124·1
*Marsdenia condurango*, 1675·3
Marsh Trefoil, 1712·1
Marshmallow, 1651·3
Marshmallow Leaf, 1651·3
Marshmallow Root, 1651·3
Marsil, 2115·1
Marsilid, 2115·1
Marsonil, 2115·1
Marten-Tab, 2115·1
Marthritic, 2115·1
Martigene, 2115·1
Martimil, 2115·1
Martindale Methadone Mixture DTF, 2115·1
Martispasmol, 2115·1
Martos-10, 2115·1
Maruamba, 1666·1
Mar-V, 2115·1
Marvelon, 2115·1
Marvil, 2115·1
Marviol, 2115·1
Marybud, 1665·2
Marzine, 2115·1
Marzolam, 2115·1
Masa Balm, 2115·2
Masaga, 2115·2
Masagil, 2115·2
Masarax, 2115·2
Masaren, 2115·2
Masarol, 2115·2
Masaworm, 2115·2
Masaworm-1, 2115·2
Masculine Herbal Complex, 2115·2
Masdil, 2115·2
Masdil, Uni— *see* Uni Masdil, 2358·2
Masern-Impfstoff Merieux, 2115·2
Masern-Lebend-Impfstoff, 2115·2
Masern-Vaccinol, 2115·2
Masern-Virus-Impfstoff, 2115·2
Masferol, 2115·2
Masflex, 2115·2
Masigel K, 2115·2
Masivol, 2115·2
Masivol Urea, 2115·2
Maskam Krauter-Tee, 2115·2
Masnidipine Hydrochloride, 946·1
Masnoderm, 2115·2
Masoprocol, 566·1
Masor, 2115·2
Massa Estearínica, 1481·1
Massage Balm with Calendula, 2115·2
Massageol, 2115·2
Massagim, 2115·2
Masse, 2115·2
Masse Cream, 2115·3
Massengill, 2115·3
Massengill Disposable, 2115·3
Massengill Feminine Cleansing Wash, 2115·3
Massengill Medicated, 2115·3
Massorax, 2115·3
Massubal, 2115·3
Mast Cell Stabilisers, 777·1
Mastaflu, 2115·3
Mastalgia, 1546·3
Master-Aid, 2115·3
Masterelax, 2115·3
Master-Gel, 2115·3
Mastia, 2115·3
Mastic, 1710·1
Mastic Paint, Compound, 1710·1
Mastical, 2115·3
Mastiche, 1710·1
Mastika, 2115·3
Mastiol, 2115·3
Mastix, 1710·1
Mastocytosis, 797·1
Mastodanatrol, 2115·3
Mastodynon, 2115·3
Mastu S, 2115·3
Masvitalin Ginseng, 2115·3
Maswin, 2115·3
Matai, 2115·3
Matcine, 2115·3
Maté, 1765·3
Matekwane, 1666·1
Matenol, 2115·3
Mater Test, 2115·3
Matergam, 2115·4
Matergam-P, 2115·4
Materlac, 2115·4
Materna, 2115·4
Materna Nova, 2115·4
Materna Tsimchit, 2115·4
MaternAid, 2115·4
Maternity One, 2115·4
Matersupre, 2115·4
Matervit, 2115·4
Mathieu Cough Syrup, 2115·4
Mathoine, 2115·4
Matico Compuesto, 2115·4
Matidan, 2115·4
Matiga, 2115·4
Matikomp, 2115·4
Matmille, 2115·4
Mato, 2115·4
Matrabec, 2115·4
Matricaria, 469·1
Matricaria C/Vit AED2 Composta, 2115·4
Matricaria Flower, 1669·3
Matricaria Flowers, 1669·3
Matricaria Oil, 1669·3
*Matricaria recutita*, 1669·3
Matricaria Vitam AED, 2115·4
Matricariae Flos, 1669·3
Matrifolin, 2115·4
Matrix, 2115·4
Matulane, 2115·4
Maturation, Delayed— *see* Delayed Puberty, 1314·1
Mature Balance, 2115·4
Maturity Test, 2115·4
Mauve des Bois, 1709·3
Maux de Gorge, 2115·4
Maveral, 2115·4
Mavid, 2115·4
Mavigen Sebo, 2115·4
Mavik, 2115·4
Mavipiu, 2116·1
Mavitalon, 2116·1
Mavixan, 2116·1
Maw Oil, 1733·3
Max, 2116·1
Max Uric, 2116·1
Maxacalcitol, 1462·1
Maxadol, 2116·1
Maxadol Forte, 2116·1
Maxadol-P, 2116·1
Maxair, 2116·1
Maxalt, 2116·1
Maxamaid Preparations 2116·1
Maxamaid MSUD— *see also* MSUD Maxamaid, 2142·2
Maxamaid, RVHB— *see* also RVHB Maxamaid, 2272·4; XMET Maxamaid, 2388·3
Maxamaid XLys Low Try— *see also* XLys Low Try Maxamaid, 2388·3
Maxamaid XMET— *see also* XMET Maxamaid, 2388·3
Maxamaid XMET, THRE, VAL, ISOLEU— *see* XMTVI Maxamaid, 2388·3
Maxamaid, XMTVI— *see also* XMTVI Maxamaid, 2388·3
Maxamaid XP— *see also* XP Maxamaid, 2388·4
Maxamaid XPhen, Tyr— *see* XPhen, Tyr Maxamaid, 2388·4
Maxamin Forte, 2116·1
Maxamox, 2116·1
Maxamum Preparations, 2116·1
Maxamum, MSUD— *see also* MSUD Maxamum, 2142·2
Maxamum, XMET— *see also* XMET Maxamum, 2388·3
Maxamum, XMTVI— *see also* XMTVI Maxamum, 2388·3
Maxamum, XP— *see also* XP Maxamum, 2388·4
Maxamum, XPhen, Tyr— *see also* XPhen, Tyr Maxamum, 2388·4
Maxaquin, 2116·1
Maxcef, 2116·2
Maxcil, 2116·2
Maxenal, 2116·2

Maxepa, 2116·2
Maxepa, Bioglan— *see* Bioglan Maxepa, 1844·1
Maxepa & EPO, 2116·2
Maxepa, Natures Own— *see* Natures Own Maxepa, 2153·3
Maxepa Plus, 2116·2
Maxeran, 2116·2
Maxeron, 2116·2
Maxi-6, 2116·2
Maxi-10, 2116·2
Maxi B, Natures Own— *see* Natures Own Maxi B, 2153·3
Maxi Force Energy Cocktail, 2116·2
Maxi-B, 2116·2
Maxibol, 2116·2
Maxibone, 2116·2
Maxicaine, 2116·2
Maxi-calc, 2116·2
Maxi-Calsor, 2116·2
Maxicardil, 2116·2
Maxicilina, 2116·2
Maxicrom, 2116·2
Maxid, 2116·2
Maxidauno, 2116·2
Maxidex, 2116·2
Maxidon, 2116·2
Maxidone, 2116·2
Maxidraine, 2116·2
Maxidrol, 2116·3
Maxifed, 2116·3
Maxifed DM, 2116·3
Maxifed DMX, 2116·3
Maxifed G, 2116·3
Maxifem, 2116·3
Maxiflor, 2116·3
Maxijul, 2116·3
Maxi-Kalz, 2116·3
Maxi-Kalz Vit D3, 2116·3
Maxilase, 2116·3
Maxilase-Bacitracine, 2116·3
Maxilief, 2116·3
Maxiliv, 2116·3
Maxilube, 2116·3
Maxim Hp, 2116·3
Maximiton, 2116·3
Maximum Blue Label, 2116·3
Maximum Green Label, 2116·3
Maximum Once A Day, 2116·3
Maximum Potential for Men, 2116·3
Maximum Red Label, 2116·3
Maximum Relief Ex-Lax, 2116·3
Maximum Strength Allergy Drops, 2116·3
Maximum Strength Anbesol, 2116·3
Maximum Strength Aqua-Ban, 2116·3
Maximum Strength Arthriten, 2116·3
Maximum Strength Desenex Antifungal, 2116·3
Maximum Strength Dristan Cold, 2116·4
Maximum Strength Dynafed— *see* Dynafed Plus, 1960·1
Maximum Strength Flexall 454, 2116·4
Maximum Strength Ornex, 2116·4
Maximum Strength Sine-Aid, 2116·4
Maximum Strength Sinutab Without Drowsiness, 2116·4
Maximum Strength Sleepinal, 2116·4
Maximum Strength Sudogest Sinus, 2116·4
Maximum Strength TheraFlu Non-Drowsy, 2116·4
Maximum Strength Tylenol Allergy Sinus, 2116·4
Maximum Strength Tylenol Allergy Sinus NightTime, 2116·4
Maximum Strength Tylenol Cough— *see* Multi-Symptom Tylenol Cough, 2145·1
Maximum Strength Tylenol Cough with Decongestant— *see* Multi-Symptom Tylenol Cough with Decongestant, 2145·1
Maximum Strength Tylenol Sinus, 2116·4
Maximum Strength Unisom SleepGels, 2116·4
Maxiphen DM, 2116·4
Maxipime, 2116·4
Maxipro, 2116·4
Maxipro HBV, 2116·4
Maxipro HBV, Super Soluble— *see* Super Soluble Maxipro HBV, 2313·3
Maxiquin, 2116·4
Maxisalic, 2116·4
Maxisona, 2116·4
Maxisorb, 2116·4
Maxisporin, 2116·4
Maxitone, 2116·4
Maxitratobes, 2116·4
Maxitrol, 2116·4
Maxi-Tuss HCG, 2117·1
Maxi-Tuss HCX, 2117·1
Maxius, 2117·1
Maxivalet, 2117·1
Maxivate, 2117·1
Maxivent, 2117·1
Maxivision, 2117·1
Maxivit, 2117·1
Maxi-Vite, 2117·1
Maxolon, 2117·1
Maxomat, 2117·1
Maxor, 2117·1
Maxoral, 2117·1
Maxovite, 2117·1
Max-Pax, 2117·1
Maxsoten, 2117·1
Maxsulid, 2117·1
Maxtral, 2117·1
Maxtrex, 2117·1
Maxtrim, 2117·1
Maxudin, 2117·1
Maxum Multi-vite, 2117·1
Maxus, 2117·1
Maxzide, 2117·1
May Apple Root, 1155·2
May Lily, 1675·3
Maycor, 2117·1
May-Cur-Tee, Mag Kottas— *see* Mag Kottas May-Cur-Tee, 2111·2
Maydis Amylum, 1449·1
Maydis, Oleum, 1439·2
Maydis Oleum Raffinatum, 1439·2
Mayfung, 2117·1
Maygace, 2117·1
Maylox, 2117·1
Maylyt, 2117·2
Maynar, 2117·2
Mayogel, 2117·2
Mayopirina, 2117·2
May-pop, 1729·1
May-Vita, 2117·2
Mazanor, 2117·2
Mazetol, 2117·2
Mazicon— *see* Romazicon, 2269·3
Mazindol, 1589·1
Mazipredone, 1105·3
Mazipredone Hydrochloride, 1105·3
Mazitrom, 2117·2
Mazon Medicated Cream, 2117·2
Mazon Medicated Shampoo, 2117·2
Mazon Medicated Soap, 2117·2
M&B-760, 264·1
M&B-782, 1191·2
M&B-800, 613·2
M&B-15497, 603·2
M&B-39831, 587·1
M&B Cough Syrup, 2117·2
M&B-17803A, 848·1
Mbanje, 1666·1
MB-530B, 949·1
MB-46030, 1505·3
M-Bentabs, 2117·2
M-beta, 2117·2
MC-903, 1144·1
MC Modulo Calorico, 2117·2
M-Caps, 2117·2
McArdle's Disease— *see* Glycogen Storage Disease Type V, 1450·2
McCune-Albright Syndrome— *see* Precocious Puberty, 1318·2
MCE, 1211·2
MCI-186, 909·2
MCI-2016, 1660·2
MCI-9038, 864·3
MCI-9042, 996·3
McN-1025, 1507·3
McN-2559, 94·2
McN-2559-21-98, 94·2
McN-4853, 378·3
McN-A-2673-11, 292·1
McN-A-2833, 980·2
McN-A-2833-109, 980·2
McN-JR-1625, 701·2
McN-JR-2498, 727·1
McN-JR-3345, 716·1
McN-JR-4263-49, 40·1
McN-JR-4584, 671·2
McN-JR-4749, 697·2
McN-JR-6218, 701·1
McN-JR-6238, 715·1
McN-JR-7904, 946·3
McN-JR-8299-11, 114·1
McN-JR-15403-11, 1261·2
McN-JR-16341, 713·2
McN-R-726-47, 488·2
McN-R-1967, 553·1
McN-X-181, 727·2
MCNU, 582·2
MCP, 2117·2
MCPham, 2117·2
MCR, 2117·2
MCR-50, 2117·2
MCT, 2117·2
MCT Duocal, 2117·2
MCT Oil, 2117·2
MCT Oljy, 2117·2
MCT Pepdite, 2117·2
MCT Peptide, 2117·2
Mct Psycho Dragees N, 2117·2
M-D, 2117·3
MD-60, 2117·3
MD-76, 2117·3
MD-141, 749·3
516-MD, 428·3
MD-805, 864·3
MD-2028, 698·2
MD-67350, 884·2
MD Complejo, 2117·3
MDA, 1593·3
MDE, 1593·3
MDEA, 1593·3
MD-Gastroview, 2117·3
MDi-193, 891·1
Mdiltiwas, 2117·3
MDL-458, 1096·2
MDL-473, 253·3
MDL-507, 264·3
MDL-832, 1121·3
MDL-9918, 441·1
MDL-14042, 1041·2
MDL-14042A, 1041·2
MDL-16455A, 433·3
MDL-17043, 911·1
MDL-19438, 911·1
MDL-62198, 249·1
MDL-71754, 383·2
MDL-71782, 604·2
MDL-71782A, 604·2
MDL-73147EF, 1262·3
MDL 74,156, 1263·1
MDM, 1589·3
MDMA, 1589·3
M-Dolor, 2117·3
MDP, 773·2
MDR Fitness Tabs, 2117·3
MDS Quick, 2117·3
ME-1206, 172·1
ME-1207, 172·1
ME-3737, 776·1
MEA, 1712·1
Meadow Anemone, 1737·1
Meadow Clover, 1737·3
Meadow Saffron, 416·3
Meadowsweet, 1710·1
Mealin, 2117·3
Measlegam, 2117·3
Measles, 624·3
Measles Immunoglobulin, Human, 1623·1
Measles Immunoglobulins, 1623·1
Measles, Mumps and Rubella Vaccine (Live), 1625·1
Measles, Mumps, and Rubella Vaccines, 1625·1
Measles, Mumps, Rubella, and Varicella-Zoster Vaccines, 1626·1
Measles, Mumps, and Rubella Virus Vaccine Live, 1625·1
Measles and Mumps Vaccines, 1624·3
Measles and Rubella Vaccines, 1624·3
Measles and Rubella Virus Vaccine Live, 1624·3
Measles Vaccine (Live), 1623·1
Measles Vaccines, 1623·1
Measles Virus Vaccine Live, 1623·1
Meas/Vac(Live), 1623·1
Meaverin, 2117·3
Meaverin "A" mit Adrenalin, 2117·3
Meaverin Hyperbar, 2117·3
Meaverin "N" mit Noradrenaline, 2117·3
MEB-6401, 396·2
Meba, 2117·3
Meballymal, 721·2
Meballymalnatrium, 721·2
Meban, 2117·3
Mebandozer, 2117·3
Mebaral, 2117·3
Mebaxin, 2117·3
Mebaxol, 2117·3
Mebeciclol, 2117·3
Mebelmin, 2117·3
Mebemerck, 2117·3
Meben, 2117·3
Mebendan, 2117·3
Mebenda-P, 2117·3
Mebendazol, 108·2
Mebendazole, 108·2
Mebendazolum, 108·2
Mebendazotil, 2117·3
Mebendil, 2117·3
Mebenix, 2117·3
Mebenlax, 2117·4
Mebensole, 2117·4
Mebental, 2117·4
Mebentiasis, 2117·4
Mebentine, 2117·4
Mebentral, 2117·4
Mebetin, 2117·4
Mebeverina, Hidrocloruro de, 1273·1
Mebeverine Embonate, 1273·1
Mebeverine Hydrochloride, 1273·1
Mebex, 2117·4
Mebhidrolina, 436·3
Mebhidrolina, Napadisilato de, 436·3
Mebhydrolin, 436·3
Mebhydrolin Napadisilate, 436·3
Mebhydrolin Napadisylate, 436·3
Mebhydrolin Naphthalenedisulphonate, 436·3
Mebhydrolin Naphthalene-1,5-disulphonate, 436·3
Mebo, 2117·4
Mebocaina, 2117·4
Mebonat, 2117·4
Meb-Overoid, 2117·4
Mebran, 2117·4
Mebrofenin, Technetium ($^{99m}$Tc), 1526·1
Mebron, 2117·4
Mebrophenhydramine Hydrochloride, 433·2
Mebrophenhydraminium Chloratum, 433·2
Mebryl, 2117·4
Mebubarbital, 713·2
Mebucaine, 2117·4
Mebucalets F, 2117·4
Mebucasol F, 2117·4
Mebumal, 713·2
Mebumalnatrium, 713·3
Mebutamate, 951·2
Mebutamato, 951·2
Mebutan, 2117·4
Mebutar, 2117·4
Mebutar Compuesto, 2117·4
Mebutizida, 951·2
Mebutizide, 951·2
Mebutol, 2117·4
Mebzol, 2117·4
Mecain, 2117·4
Mecamilamina, Hidrocloruro de, 951·3

Mecamine Hydrochloride, 951·3
Mecamylamine Hydrochloride, 951·3
Mecanyl, 2117·4
Mecasermin, 1338·3
Mecasermina, 1338·3
Mecca, 2117·4
Mecetronio, Etilsulfato de, 1185·2
Mecetronium Ethylsulfate, 1185·2
Mecetronium Ethylsulphate, 1185·2
Mecetronium Etilsulfate, 1185·2
Mechanical Ventilation— *see* Intensive Care, 1398·1
Mechlorethamine Hydrochloride, 537·1
Mecholyl, 2117·4
Mechovit, 2117·4
Mecilinam, 228·3
Mecillinam, 228·3
Mecillinam, Pivaloyloxymethyl Ester, 244·3
Mecisteína, Hidrocloruro de, 1124·1
Meclan, 2117·4
Meclastine Fumarate, 429·1
Meclifar, 2117·4
Meclizine Hydrochloride, 436·3
Meclizinium Chloride, 436·3
Meclociclina, Sulfosalicilato de, 229·1
Meclocycline, 229·1
Meclocycline Sulfosalicylate, 229·1
Meclocycline Sulphosalicylate, 229·1
Meclocycline 5-Sulphosalicylate, 229·1
Mecloderm, 2117·4
Mecloderm Antiacne, 2117·4
Mecloderm F, 2118·1
Mecloderm Ovuli, 2118·1
Mecloderm Polvere Aspersoria, 2118·1
Meclodol, 2118·1
Meclofenamate Sodium, 55·1
Meclofenamato Sódico, 55·1
Meclofenamic Acid, 55·1
Meclofenámico, Ácido, 55·1
Meclofenoxane Hydrochloride, 1710·1
Meclofenoxate Hydrochloride, 1710·1
Meclofenoxato, Hidrocloruro de, 1710·1
Meclomen, 2118·1
Meclomid, 2118·1
Meclon, 2118·1
Mecloprodine Fumarate, 429·1
Meclosil, 2118·1
Meclosorb, 2118·1
Mecloxamina, Citrato de, 485·3
Mecloxamine Citrate, 485·3
Meclozina, Hidrocloruro de, 436·3
Meclozine, 437·1
Meclozine Hydrochloride, 436·3
Meclozini Hydrochloridum, 436·3
Meclutin, 2118·1
Meclutin Semplice, 2118·1
Mecobalamin, 1459·1
Mecolin, 2118·1
Meconha, 1666·1
Mecoten, 2118·1
Mecrilate, 1678·1
Mecrylate, 1678·1
Mectizan, 2118·1
Mecysteine Hydrochloride, 1124·1
MED-15, 14·3
Meda, 2118·1
Medacaps N, 2118·1
Medacter, 2118·1
Med-Actigen, 2118·1
Medalgin, 2118·1
Medalginan, 2118·1
Medamet, 2118·1
Medamol Co, 2118·1
Medamor, 2118·1
Med-Anspasmic, 2118·1
Medapur, 2118·1
Medaren, 2118·1
Medarex, 2118·1
Medaspor, 2118·1
Medazepam, 706·1
Medazepam Hydrochloride, 706·1
Medazine, 2118·2
Medazol, 2118·2
Medazol Gel, 2118·2
Medazole, 2118·2
Medazyl, 2118·2
Med-Broncodil, 2118·2
Med-Broncodil Expectorant, 2118·2
Med-Circuron, 2118·2
Medebar, 2118·2
Medebiotin, 2118·2
Medecitral, 2118·2
Medefizz, 2118·2
Medefoam, 2118·2
Medefungin, 2118·2
Medemycin, 2118·2
Medenorex, 2118·2
Medent-DM, 2118·2
Mede-Prep, 2118·2
Mederebro, 2118·2
Mederebro Compuesto, 2118·2
Mederma, 2118·2
Mederreumol, 2118·2
Medescan, 2118·2
Medeserpine Co, 2118·2
Medesup, 2118·2
Medetomidina, Hidrocloruro de, 706·1
Medetomidine Hydrochloride, 706·1
Medeton, 2118·2
Medevac, 2118·2
Medex Rub, 2118·2
Med-Gastramet, 2118·3
Medgesic, 2118·3
Med-Glionil, 2118·3
Med-Guaiphan, 2118·3
Medi Creme, 2118·3
Medi Pulv, 2118·3
Mediabet, 2118·3
Medialipide, 2118·3
Mediamik, 2118·3
Mediamox, 2118·3
Medianox, 2118·3
Medianut, 2118·3
Mediatensyl, 2118·3
Mediator, 2118·3
Mediaven, 2118·3
Mediaxal, 2118·3
Medibronc, 2118·3
Medic, 2118·3
Medica, 2118·3
*Medicago sativa*, 1649·1
Medicaid, 2118·3
Medicaina, 2118·3
Medical Air, 1236·3
Medical Pic, 2118·3
Medicament Sinus, 2118·3
Medicap, 2118·3
Medicated Analgesic Cream, 2118·3
Medicated Chest Rub, 2118·3
Medicated Extract of Rosemary, 2118·3
Medicated Pain Relief Plaster, Boots— *see* Boots Medicated Pain Relief Plaster, 1851·1
Medichrom, 2118·3
Medicillin, 2118·4
Medicinal Air, 1236·3
Medicinal Air, Synthetic, 1236·3
Medicinal Gargle, 2118·4
Mediclear, 2118·4
Medicoal, 2118·4
Medicone, 2118·4
Medicone Derma, 2118·4
Medicone Rectal, 2118·4
Medicreme, 2118·4
Medicyclomine, 2118·4
Medi-Dan, 2118·4
Medident, 2118·4
Medifed, 2118·4
Medifen, 2118·4
Medifer, 2118·4
Medi-First Sinus Decongestant, 2118·4
Mediflex, 2118·4
Mediflor Preparations, 2118·4
Medifolin, 2119·1
Medifome, 2119·1
Medifon, 2119·1
Medifungol, 2119·1
Medigel, 2119·1
Medigesic, 2119·1
Medigoxin, 955·2
Medihaler, 2119·1
Medihaler-Epi, 2119·1
Medihaler-Iso, 2119·1
Medijel, 2119·1
Medi-Kain, 2119·1
Medi-Keel A, 2119·1
Medikem, 2119·1
Mediker, 2119·1
Mediklin, 2119·1
Medikol, 2119·2
Medi-Kord, 2119·2
Medil, 2119·2
Medilar, 2119·2
Medilax, 2119·2
Medilaxan, 2119·2
Medilet, 2119·2
Medilium, 2119·2
Medilyn, 2119·2
Medimegen, 2119·2
Medin G, 2119·2
Medinait, Vicks— *see* Vicks Medinait, 2375·3
Medinat Esten, 2119·2
Medinat PMT-Eze, 2119·2
Medinol, 2119·2
Mediocin, 2119·2
Mediolax, 2119·2
Medipam, 2119·2
Medipax, 2119·2
Medipe, 2119·2
Medipekt, 2119·2
Medipina, 2119·2
Medipirol, 2119·2
Mediplant, 2119·2
Mediplant Inhalations, 2119·2
Mediplant Krauter, 2119·2
Mediplast, 2119·2
Mediplaster, 2119·2
Mediplex, 2119·2
Mediplus, 2119·3
Medipo, 2119·3
Medi-Prep, 2119·3
Mediprim, 2119·3
Medipulv, 2119·3
Medi-Quik, 2119·3
Medised, 2119·3
Medised Infant, 2119·3
Medisense, 2119·3
Medisense G2, 2119·3
MediSense Sof-Tact, 2119·3
Medisept, 2119·3
Medisepta, 2119·3
Medismon, 2119·3
Medi-Sol, 2119·3
Medisport Athlete's Foot, 2119·3
Medi-Swab, 2119·3
Medi-Swab H, 2119·3
Meditapp, 2119·3
Meditapp Expectorant, 2119·3
Meditar, 2119·3
Mediterranean Fever, Familial— *see* Familial Mediterranean Fever, 416·2
Mediterranean Spotted Fever— *see* Spotted Fevers, 147·1
Medi-Test Tests, 2119·3
Medithane, 2119·4
Medi-Tissue, 2119·4
Meditoina, 2119·4
Meditonsin, 2119·4
Medituss, 2119·4
Medium-chain Triglycerides, 1440·3
Medium-Chain Triglycerides, 1440·3
Mediuresix, 2119·4
Mediveine, 2119·4
Medivitan N, 2119·4
Medivitan N Neuro, 2119·4
Medi-Wipe, 2119·4
Medixel, 2119·4
Medixil, 2119·4
Medixin, 2119·4
Medizinalbad, Biokosma— *see* Biokosma Medizinalbad, 1844·3
Medizol, 2119·4
Medizyme, 2119·4
Med-Kafuzone, 2119·4
Medkofen, 2119·4
Med-Mucolo, 2119·4
Med-Myolax, 2119·4
Mednil, 2119·4
Medobeta, 2119·4
Medobiotin, 2119·4
Medocalum, 2120·1
Medocarnitin, 2120·1
Medocef, 2120·1
Medociprin, 2120·1
Medoclazide, 2120·1
Medoclor, 2120·1
Medocodene, 2120·1
Medocor, 2120·1
Medocriptine, 2120·1
Medocycline, 2120·1
Medodermone, 2120·1
Medoenzym, 2120·1
Medofloxine, 2120·1
Medofulvin, 2120·1
Medoglycin, 2120·1
Medolexin, 2120·1
Medolin, 2120·1
Medomet, 2120·1
Medomycin, 2120·1
Medonol, 2120·1
Medopa, 2120·1
Medopal, 2120·1
Medopam, 2120·1
Medopate, 2120·1
Medophyll, 2120·1
Medopren, 2120·1
Medoric, 2120·1
Medostatin, 2120·2
Medotar, 2120·2
Medotifen, 2120·2
Medovascin, 2120·2
Medovent, 2120·2
Medovir, 2120·2
Medoxem, 2120·2
Medoxim, 2120·2
Medoxin, 2120·2
Medozem, 2120·2
Medozide, 2120·2
Medozine, 2120·2
Medphalan, 566·1
Medphlem, 2120·2
Med-Phylline, 2120·2
Medpramol, 2120·2
Medral, 2120·2
Medralone, 2120·2
Medramil, 2120·2
Medramine Retard, 2120·2
Medramine-$B_6$ Rectocaps, 2120·2
Medrate, 2120·2
Medricol, 2120·2
Medrisocil, 2120·2
Medrisona, 1106·1
Medrivas, 2120·2
Medrivas Antib, 2120·2
Medrivas Antibiotico, 2120·2
Medrocil, 2120·2
Medrocis, 2120·2
Medrogestona, 1557·1
Medrogestone, 1557·1
Medrol, 2120·3
Medrol Acne Lotion, 2120·3
Medrol, Depo- — *see* Depo-Medrol, 1925·3
Medrol Lozione Antiacne, 2120·3
Medrol, Solu— *see* Solu-Medrol, 2298·2
Medrol Topical— *see* Medrol Veriderm, 2120·3
Medrol Veriderm, 2120·3
Medronate, 2120·3
Medronate Disodium, 773·2
Medronate, Technetium ($^{99m}$Tc), 1526·1
Medronato Disódico, 773·2
Medrone, 2120·3
Medronic Acid, 773·2
Medrónico, Ácido, 773·2
Medrosterona, 2120·3
Medroxiprogesterona, Acetato de, 1557·2
Medroxitest, 2120·3
Medroxyhexal, 2120·3
Medroxyprogesterone Acetate, 1557·2
Medroxyprogesteroni Acetas, 1557·2
Medroxyurea, 2120·3

MED-Rx, 2120·3
MED-Rx DM, 2120·3
Medrysone, 1106·1
Medsara, 2120·3
Medsatrexate, 2120·3
Medsavorina, 2120·3
Med-Spastic, 2120·3
Med-Sultrim, 2120·3
Med-Tricocide, 2120·3
Med-Tussin, 2120·3
Medulloblastoma— *see* Malignant Neoplasms of the Brain, 513·2
Medusit, 2120·3
Med-Xyzarax, 2120·3
Medyn, 2120·3
Meerzwiebel, 1130·3
ME-F, 2120·3
Mefa, 2120·3
Mefac, 2120·3
Mefacap, 2120·3
Mefamic, 2120·4
Mefazil, 2120·4
Mefe-basan, 2120·4
Mefedra-N, 2120·4
Mefen, 2120·4
Mefenacide, 2120·4
Mefenamic Acid, 55·2
Mefenámico, Ácido, 55·2
Mefenamicum, Acidum, 55·2
Mefenan, 2120·4
Mefenesina, 1394·3
Mefenidramium Metilsulfate, 432·2
Mefenitoína, 366·2
Mefenix, 2120·4
Mefenix Relax, 2120·4
Mefenorex, Hidrocloruro de, 1589·2
Mefenorex Hydrochloride, 1589·2
Mefentermina, Sulfato de, 952·1
Mefic, 2120·4
Mefiron, 2120·4
Mefliam, 2120·4
Mefloquina, Hidrocloruro de, 453·3
Mefloquine Hydrochloride, 453·3
Mefloquini Hydrochloridum, 453·3
Meflotas, 2120·4
Meflox, 2120·4
Meformed, 2120·4
Mefoxil, 2120·4
Mefoxin, 2120·4
Mefoxitin, 2120·4
Mefpa, 2120·4
Mefren Incolore, 2120·4
Mefren Pastilles, 2120·4
Mefrusida, 951·3
Mefruside, 951·3
Mega 65, 2120·4
Mega Acidophilus, 2120·4
Mega AO, 2120·4
Mega B, 2120·4
Mega B Extra Strength, 2121·1
Mega B, Natures Way— *see* Natures Way Mega B, 2153·3
Mega B Slow Release, 2121·1
Mega Balance, 2121·1
Mega C, Bioglan— *see* Bioglan Mega C, 1844·1
Mega C, Slow Release— *see* Slow Release Mega C, 2295·1
Mega Cal Calcium, 2121·1
Mega Capsule, 2121·1
Mega E, 2121·1
Mega Men, 2121·1
Mega Multi, 2121·1
Mega Multi, Natures Way— *see* Natures Way Mega Multi, 2153·3
Mega Multi, Slow Release— *see* Slow Release Mega Multi, 2295·1
Mega Stress Vitamins, 2121·1
Mega Swiss One, 2121·1
Mega Vim, 2121·1
Mega VM, 2121·1
Mega-Antioxidant, 2121·1
Mega-B + L-Tryptophan, Natures Own— *see* Natures Own Mega-B + L-Tryptophan, 2153·3
Megabrain, 2121·1
Megabron, 2121·1
Megabyl, 2121·1
Mega-Cal, 2121·1
Mega-Cal with Vit D, 2121·1
Mega-Calcium, 2121·1
Mega-calcium Sandoz, 2121·1
Megace, 2121·1
Megacillin, 2121·1
Megacillin Oral, 2121·1
Megacilline, 2121·1
Megacina, 2121·1
Megacistin, 2121·1
Megacistin G, 2121·1
Megacort, 2121·1
Megadin, 2121·2
Megadophilus, Ultra Strength— *see* Ultra Strength Megadophilus, 2356·2
Megadose, 2121·2
Megadoxa, 2121·2
Megafer, 2121·2
Megaflox, 2121·2
Megafol, 2121·2
Megagrisevit, 2121·2
Megal Simple, 2121·2
Megalac, 2121·2
Megalat, 2121·2
Megalax, 2121·2
Megalex, 2121·2
Megaloblastic Anaemia, 734·1
Megalocin, 2121·2
Megalotect, 2121·2
Megamag, 2121·2
Megamilbedoce, 2121·2
Megamox, 2121·2
Megamylase, 2121·2
Meganest, 2121·2
Megapen, 2121·2
Megapenil, 2121·2
Megapenil Forte, 2121·2
Megaplatin, 2121·2
Megaplus, 2121·2
Megapress, 2121·2
Mega-Prim, 2121·2
Megapyn, 2121·2
Megareal, 2121·3
Megasin, 2121·3
Megastene, 2121·3
Megastrol, 2121·3
Megatears, 2121·3
Megaton, 2121·3
Megaval, 2121·3
Megavir, 2121·3
Megavis, 2121·3
Megavit, 2121·3
Megavit Natal, 2121·3
Megavites, 2121·3
Megavix, 2121·3
Megaxin, 2121·3
Megefren, 2121·3
Megestat, 2121·3
Megestil, 2121·3
Megestin, 2121·3
Megestran, 2121·3
Megestrol Acetate, 1558·2
Megestrol, Acetato de, 1558·2
Megestroli Acetas, 1558·2
Meggezones, 2121·3
Meglucon, 2121·3
Meglum, 2121·3
Meglumina, 1710·1
Meglumine, 1710·1, 1710·2
Meglumine Adipiodone, 1060·1
Meglumine Amidotrizoate, 1060·2
Meglumine Antimonate, 600·3
Meglumine Antimoniate, 600·3
Meglumine Diatrizoate, 1060·2
Meglumine Gadobenate, 1062·1
Meglumine Gadopentetate, 1062·2
Meglumine Gadoterate, 1062·3
Meglumine Indometacin, 49·1
Meglumine Iodamide, 1063·2
Meglumine Iodipamide, 1060·1
Meglumine Iodoxamate, 1064·1
Meglumine Ioglicate, 1064·1
Meglumine Iotalamate, 1065·3
Meglumine Iothalamate, 1065·3
Meglumine Iotroxate, 1066·1
Meglumine Iotroxinate, 1066·1
Meglumine Ioxaglate, 1066·2
Meglumine Ioxitalamate, 1066·3
Meglumine Metrizoate, 1067·2
Megluminum, 1710·1
Meglutol, 952·1
Megostat, 2121·3
Megral, 2121·3
Meiact, 2121·3
Meibi, 2121·3
Meicelin, 2121·3
Meiceral, 2121·3
Meiclox, 2121·3
Meige Syndrome— *see* Blepharospasm, 1390·1
Meilax, 2121·3
Meimendro, 485·2
Meinfusona, 2121·4
Meinvenil Fisiologico, 2121·4
Meinvenil Glucosalina, 2121·4
Meixil, 2121·4
Mejoral, 2121·4
Mejoral Cafeina, 2121·4
Mejoralito, 2121·4
Mejorultra, 2121·4
MEK, 1476·2
Mekan, 2121·4
Mel B, 606·1
Mel de Jatahy, 2121·4
Mel Depuratum, 1434·2
Mel Despumatum, 1434·2
Melablock, 2121·4
Melabon, 2121·4
Melabon Infantil, 2121·4
Melabon K, 2121·4
Melabon N, 2121·4
Melabon Plus C, 2121·4
Melac, 2121·4
Melacine, 2121·4
Melacler, 2121·4
Melactone, 2121·4
Meladinina, 2121·4
Meladinine, 2121·4
Melagatran, 952·1
Melagel, 2121·4
Melagesic PM, 2121·4
Melagriao, 2121·4
Melaleuca, Aceite de, 1710·2
*Melaleuca alternifolia*, 1710·2
*Melaleuca cajuputi*, 1664·1
*Melaleuca dissitiflora*, 1710·2
*Melaleuca leucadendron*, 1664·1
*Melaleuca linariifolia*, 1710·2
Melaleuca Oil, 1710·2
*Melaleuca quinquenervia*, 1719·3
*Melaleuca viridiflora*, 1719·3
Melaleucae Aetheroleum, 1710·2
Melaleucae, Oleum, 1710·2
Melanasa, 2121·4
Melanex, 2122·1
Melanex Duo, 2122·1
Melanocyl, 2122·1
Melanocyte-stimulating Hormone, 1332·2
Melanocyte-stimulating-hormone-release-inhibiting Factor, 1332·3
Melanocyte-stimulating-hormone-releasing Factor, 1332·2
Melanoma, Cutaneous— *see* Melanoma, 522·3
Melanoma, Ocular— *see* Malignant Neoplasms of the Eye, 516·1
Melanostatin, 1332·3
Melanostatina, 1332·3
Melanotropin, 1332·2
Melanotropin Release-inhibiting Factor, 1332·3
Melanox, 2122·1
Melaoline, 2122·1
Melaprugna, 2122·1
Melapure, 2122·1
Melarsen Oxide-BAL, 606·1
Melarsomina, 109·2
Melarsomine, 109·2
Melarsonyl Potassium, 606·3
Melarsoprol, 606·1
Melasma— *see* Pigmentation Disorders, 1137·2
Melasmax, 2122·1
Melasoft, 2122·1
Melatol, 2122·1
Melatonin, 1710·2
Melatonina, 1710·2
Melatouch, 2122·1
Melavir, 2122·1
Melaxose, 2122·1
Melbetese, 2122·1
Melbin, 2122·1
Mel-C, 2122·1
Meldopa, 2122·1
Meleril, 2122·1
Melfalán, 566·1
Melfen, 2122·1
Melfiat, 2122·1
Melgar, 2122·1
Melgisorb, 2122·1
Mel-H, 2122·1
Melhoral, 2122·1
Melhoral C, 2122·1
Melhoral Infantil, 2122·1
Meli Rephastasan, 2122·1
*Melia azadirachta*, 1658·2
Meliane, 2122·1
Melic, 2122·2
Melicat, 2122·2
Melicron, 2122·2
Melioidosis, 134·3
Melipass, 2122·2
Melipramine, 2122·2
Melisa, 1711·1
Meliseptol, 2122·2
Meliseptol Rapid, 2122·2
Melisol, 2122·2
Melissa, 1711·1
Melissa Comp., 2122·2
Melissa Leaf, 1711·1
*Melissa officinalis*, 1711·1
Melissa Oil, 1711·2
Melissa Oil, Indian, 1706·3
Melissa (Specie Composta), 2122·2
Melissa Tonic, 2122·2
Melissae Folium, 1711·1
Melisse Pflanzensaft, Kneipp— *see* Kneipp Melisse Pflanzensaft, 2081·3
Melissenblatt, 1711·1
Melissengeist, 2122·2
Melissin, 2122·2
Melitase, 2122·2
Melitoxin, 894·2
Melitracen Hydrochloride, 306·3
Melitraceno, Hidrocloruro de, 306·3
Melitrast, 2122·2
Melittin, 1655·3
Melival, 2122·2
Melix, 2122·2
Melizid, 2122·2
Melizide, 2122·2
Mellaril, 2122·2
Mellerette, 2122·2
Melleretten, 2122·2
Mellerettes, 2122·2
Melleril, 2122·2
Mellin, 2122·3
Mellin AR, 2122·3
Mellin HA, 2122·3
Mellin Polilat, 2122·3
Mellitron, 2122·3
Mellow Drug of America, 1593·3
Melneurin, 2122·3
Melocin, 2122·3
Melocotón, Aceite de, 1730·2
Mel-OD, 2122·3
Meloden, 2122·3
Melodene, 2122·3
Melodene 15, 2122·3
Melodia, 2122·3
Melodil, 2122·3
Melodol, 2122·3
Melograno, 112·1
Méloides, 1666·3
Meloids, 2122·3
Meloka, 2122·3
Melol, 2122·3
Melon Pumpkin Seeds, 1677·3

Melopat, 2122·3
Melosteral, 2122·3
Melotec, 2122·3
Melox Plus, 2122·3
Meloxat, 2122·3
Meloxicam, 56·1
Meloxigran, 2122·3
Meloxil, 2122·3
Melpax, 2122·3
Melpaz, 2122·3
Melperomerck, 2122·3
Melperona, Hidrocloruro de, 706·1
Melperone Hydrochloride, 706·1
Melphalan, 566·1
Mel-Puren, 2122·3
Melrose, 2122·4
Melrosum, 2122·4
Melrosum Codein Hustensirup, 2122·4
Melrosum Extra Sterk, 2122·4
Melrosum Hustensirup, 2122·4
Melrosum Hustensirup N, 2122·4
Melrosum Medizinalbad, 2122·4
Melsept, 2122·4
Melsept SF, 2122·4
Melsept Spray, 2122·4
Melsitt, 2122·4
Meltonar, 2122·4
Meltus Preparations, 2122·4
Meltus for Chesty Coughs & Catarrh, Adult— *see* Adult Meltus for Chesty Coughs & Catarrh, 1777·3
Melubrin, 2122·4
Melubrina, Neo— *see* Neo Melubrina, 2156·3
Melur, 2122·4
Melvit, 2122·4
Melxi, 2122·4
Melzine, 2122·4
Memac, 2122·4
Memantina, Hidrocloruro de, 1711·2
Memantine Hydrochloride, 1711·2
Membracel, 2122·4
MembraneBlue, 2122·4
Membrane-stabilising Drugs, 809·3
Membranoproliferative Glomerulonephritis— *see* Glomerular Kidney Disease, 1080·2
Membranous Glomerulonephritis— *see* Glomerular Kidney Disease, 1080·2
Membranous Nephropathy— *see* Glomerular Kidney Disease, 1080·2
Memento, 2122·4
Memento NF, 2123·1
Memfit, 2123·1
Memoactive, 2123·1
Memocap, 2123·1
Memoloba, 2123·1
Memonol, 2123·1
Memo-Puren, 2123·1
Memoq, 2123·1
Memorandum, 2123·1
Memorex, 2123·1
Memorex Compuesto, 2123·1
Memorfix, 2123·1
Memoria, 2123·1
Memoril, 2123·1
Memorino, 2123·1
Memorioglutan, 2123·1
Memoriol B6, 2123·1
Memorisan, 2123·1
Memorit, 2123·1
Memory Booster, 2123·1
Memory Plus, 2123·1
Memoserina S, 2123·1
Memosprint, 2123·1
Memovigor, 2123·1
Memovisus, 2123·1
Memovit B12, 2123·1
Memphil— *see* Mempil, 2123·1
Mempil, 2123·1
Memzotil, 2123·1
Men Hormone, 2123·1
Menabil Complex, 2123·1
Menabol, 2123·2
Menaderm, 2123·2
Menaderm Clio, 2123·2
Menaderm Neomicina, 2123·2
Menaderm Otologico, 2123·2
Menaderm, Recto— *see* Recto Menaderm, 2253·2
Menaderm Simple, 2123·2
Menaderm Simplex, 2123·2
Menadiol Diacetate, 1466·3
Menadiol Dibutyrate, 1468·1
Menadiol, Fosfato Sódico de, 1466·3
Menadiol Potassium Sulfate, 1466·3
Menadiol Sodium Diphosphate, 1466·3
Menadiol Sodium Phosphate, 1466·3
Menadiol Sodium Sulfate, 1466·3
Menadiolum Solubile, 1466·3
Menadiona, 1466·3
Menadiona, Bisulfito Sódico de, 1466·3
Menadione, 1466·3
Menadione Sodium Bisulfite, 1466·3
Menadione Sodium Bisulphite, 1466·3
Menadionum, 1466·3
Menadol, 2123·2
Menalation, 2123·2
Menalcol, 2123·2
Menalgil B6, 2123·2
Menalgon, 2123·2
Menalgon B6, 2123·2
Menalmina, 2123·2
Menamin, 2123·2
Menaph., 1466·3
Menaph. Sod. Bisulphite, 1466·3
Menaphthene, 1466·3
Menaphthone, 1466·3
Menaphthone Sodium Bisulphite, 1466·3
Menaquinone-4, 1467·1
Menaquinone 4, 1467·1
Menaquinone K4, 1467·1
Menaquinones, 1467·3
Menarini-Metforal, 2123·2
Menatetren, 1467·1
Menatetrenona, 1467·1
Menatetrenone, 1467·1
Menatetrenonum, 1467·1
Menaven, 2123·2
Menbutona, 1711·3
Menbutone, 1711·3
Mencalisvit, 2123·2
Mencevax, 2123·2
Mencevax AC, 2123·2
Mencevax ACWY, 2123·2
Mencirax, 2123·2
Mencogrin, 2123·2
Mencogrin AP, 2123·2
Mendelson's Syndrome— *see* Aspiration Syndromes, 1240·1
Menegradil, 2123·3
Meneparol, 2123·3
Menest, 2123·3
Menfazona, 2123·3
Menfegol, 1413·2
Mengivac (A+C), 2123·3
Menglitato, 1124·2
Menglytate, 1124·2
Meni-D, 2123·3
Ménière's Disease, 422·1
Meniero, 2123·3
Meniex, 2123·3
Menifazepam, 710·1
Meningitec, 2123·3
Meningitis, Bacterial— *see* Meningitis, 134·3
Meningitis, Cryptococcal— *see* Cryptococcosis, 387·3
Meningitis, Fungal— *see* Meningitis, 388·3
Meningo A+C, 2123·3
Meningococcal A+C, 2123·3
Meningococcal Group C Conjugate Vaccine, 1626·1
Meningococcal Infections, 135·3
Meningococcal Meningitis— *see* Meningitis, 134·3
Meningococcal Polysaccharide Vaccine, 1626·1
Meningococcal Vaccines, 1626·1
Meningocoele— *see* Neural Tube Defects, 1430·1
Meningoencephalitis, Amoebic, Primary— *see* Primary Amoebic Meningoencephalitis, 595·3
Meningokokken-Impfstoff A + C, 2123·3
Meningomyelocoele— *see* Neural Tube Defects, 1430·1
Meningovax A+C, 2123·3
Meninvact, 2123·3
Menisole, 2123·3
Menjugate, 2123·3
Menkes' Disease— *see* Deficiency States, 1426·2
Menobarb, 2123·3
Menobiol, 2123·3
Menocal, 2123·3
Meno-Care, Extralife— *see* Extralife Meno-Care, 1986·3
Menoconfort, 2123·3
Meno-cyl Ho-Len-Complex, 2123·3
Menodoron, 2123·3
Menofem, 2123·3
Menoflavon, 2123·3
Menoflush, 2123·3
Menoflush + $\frac{1}{4}$, 2123·3
Menoflush-Menogloed +$\frac{1}{4}$— *see* Menoflush + $\frac{1}{4}$, 2123·3
Menogen, 2123·4
Menogon, 2123·4
Menograine, 2123·4
Meno-Implant, 2123·4
Menolistica, 2123·4
Meno-MPA, 2123·4
Menomune, 2123·4
Menomune ACYW, 2123·4
Meno-Net, 2123·4
Menopace, 2123·4
Meno-Patch, 2123·4
Menopausal Disorders, 1540·2
Menopausal Gonadotrophins, Human, 1330·1
Menopause, 2123·4
Menopause L122, 2123·4
Menopause, Modern Herbals— *see* Modern Herbals Menopause, 2138·2
Menopause Test, 2123·4
Menopax, 2123·4
Menophase, 2123·4
Menoplex, 2123·4
Menoprem, 2123·4
Menopur, 2123·4
Menorest, 2123·4
Menoring, 2123·4
Menorrhagia, 1567·3
Menosan, 2123·4
Menosedan, 2123·4
Menosedan Ciclo, 2123·4
Menosedan Fase, 2123·4
Menosedan MPA, 2124·1
Menoselect, 2124·1
Menosor, 2124·1
Menostress, 2124·1
Menotensil, 2124·1
Menotime, 2124·1
Menotrophin, 1330·1
Menotropina, 1330·1
Menotropins, 1330·1
Menotropinum, 1330·1
Menovis, 2124·1
Menoxicor, 2124·1
Menphegol, 1413·2
Menpovax 4, 2124·1
Menpovax A+C, 2124·1
Menpros, 2124·1
Mens Super Soy/Clover, Bioglan— *see* Bioglan Mens Super Soy/Clover, 1844·1
Mensalgin, 2124·1
Mensana, 2124·1
Mensifem, 2124·1
Mensiso, 2124·1
Mensoma, 2124·1
Mensoton, 2124·1
Menstrogen, 2124·1
Menstrual Bleeding, Excessive— *see* Menorrhagia, 1567·3
Menstrual Cramps, Hylands— *see* Hylands Menstrual Cramps, 2052·3
Menstruasan, 2124·1
Menstruation, Absence of— *see* Amenorrhoea, 1313·1
Menstruation, Painful— *see* Dysmenorrhoea, 6·1
Menstrunat, 2124·1
MENT, 1536·1
Ment Vital, 2124·1
Menta, 1749·1
Menta, Aceite Esencial de, 1749·1
Menta, Aceite Esencial Desmentolado de, 1715·2
Menta, Hoja de, 1283·2
Menta Piperita, Aceite Esencial de, 1283·2
Menta Piperita, Hoja de, 1283·2
Mentacur, 2124·1
Mental Alertness, 2124·1
Mentalgina, 2124·1
Mentalol, 2124·1
Mentamida, 2124·1
Mentania, 2124·1
Mentax, 2124·1
Menth. Pip., 1283·2
*Mentha*, 1711·3
*Mentha arvensis*, 1715·2
*Mentha canadensis*, 1715·2
*Mentha cardiaca*, 1749·1
Mentha Oil, 1715·2
*Mentha* × *piperita*, 1283·2
Mentha Piperita, 1283·2
*Mentha pulegium*, 1736·1
*Mentha spicata*, 1749·1
Mentha Viridis, 1749·1
*Mentha viridis*, 1749·1
Menthacin, 2124·1
Menthae Arvensis Aetheroleum Partim Mentholi Privum, 1715·2
Menthae Crispae Folium, 1749·1
Menthae Crispae, Oleum, 1749·1
Menthae Piperitae Aetheroleum, 1283·2
Menthae Piperitae Folium, 1283·2
Menthae Piperitae, Oleum, 1283·2
Menthae Viridis, Oleum, 1749·1
*p*-Menthane-1,8-diol Monohydrate, 1131·1
*p*-Menthan-3-ol, 1711·3
Menthe Crépue, Huile Essentielle de, 1749·1
Menthe Poivrée, 1283·2
Menthe Poivrée, Essence de, 1283·2
*p*-Menth-6-ene-2,8-diol, 1130·2
Menthodex, 2124·1
Menthofuran, 1283·2
Menthol, 1283·2, 1711·3
Menthol Cough Drops, Vicks— *see* Vicks Menthol Cough Drops, 2375·3
Menthol Ethylglycolate, 1124·2
Menthol, Racemic, 1711·3
Mentholatum Preparations, 2124·2
Mentholease, 2124·2
Mentholon Original N, 2124·2
Mentholum, 1711·3
Mentholyptus, Halls— *see* Halls Mentholyptus, 2035·3
Menthone, 1283·2
Menthoneurin, 2124·2
Menthoneurin-Salbe, 2124·2
Menthoneurin-Vollbad N, 2124·2
MenthoRub, 2124·2
Menthose, 2124·2
Menthyl Acetate, 1283·2
Menthyl *O*-Aminobenzoate, 1151·3
Menthyl Anthranilate, 1151·3
*p*-Menth-3-yl Ethoxyacetate, 1124·2
α-[*p*-(*p*-Menthyl)phenyl]-ω-hydroxypoly(oxyethylene), 1413·2
Menthymin Mono, 2124·3
Mentis, 2124·3
Mentium, 2124·3
Mentobox, 2124·3
Mentobox Antitusivo, 2124·3
Mentocaina R, 2124·3
Mentodrin, 2124·3
Mentofenol, 2124·3
Mentol, 1711·3
Mentolatun, 2124·3
Mento-O-Cap, 2124·3
Mentopin Preparations, 2124·3
Mentor, 2124·3

Mentoval, 2124·3
Mentozil, 2124·3
Menutil, 2124·3
Menyanthes, 1712·1
*Menyanthes trifoliata*, 1712·1
Menyanthidis Trifoliatae Folium, 1712·1
Menzotil, 2124·3
Meocil, 2124·3
282 Mep, 2124·3
Mepacrina, Hidrocloruro de, 606·3
Mepacrine Hydrochloride, 606·3
Mepacrine Mesilate, 607·1
Mepacrini Hydrochloridum, 606·3
Mepagyl, 2124·3
Mepalax, 2124·3
Meparfynol, 707·1
Mepartricin, 405·2
Mepartricin Sodium Laurilsulfate, 405·2
Mepartricina, 405·2
Mepastat, 2124·4
Mepenzolate Bromide, 485·3
Mepenzolate Methylbromide, 485·3
Mepenzolato, Bromuro de, 485·3
Mepenzolone Bromide, 485·3
Mepergan, 2124·4
Meperidine Hydrochloride, 80·2
Meperidinic Acid, 81·2
Meperol, 2124·4
15-Me-$PGF_{2\alpha}$, 1514·2
Mephadolor, 2124·4
Mephamesone, 2124·4
Mephanol, 2124·4
Mephaquin, 2124·4
Mephaquine, 2124·4
Mephathiol, 2124·4
Mephatussine, 2124·4
Mephatussine Compositum, 2124·4
Mephaxine, 2124·4
Mephaxine Compositum, 2124·4
Mephenamine Citrate, 486·1
Mephenamine Hydrochloride, 486·1
Mephenesin, 1394·3
Mephenetoin, 366·2
Mephenoxalone, 1395·1
Mephentermine Sulfate, 952·1
Mephentermine Sulphate, 952·1
Mephentermini Sulfas, 952·1
Mephentine, 2124·4
Mephenytoin, 366·2
Mephetedrine Sulphate, 952·1
Mephobarbital, 366·3
Mephyton, 2124·4
Mepibil, 2124·4
Mepicain, 2124·4
Mepicaton, 2124·4
Mepident, 2124·4
Mepiforan, 2124·4
Mepiform, 2124·4
Mepihexal, 2124·4
Mepi-Mynol, 2124·4
Mepinaest, 2124·4
Mepindolol Sulfate, 952·2
Mepindolol, Sulfato de, 952·2
Mepindolol Sulphate, 952·2
Mepiramina, Hidrocloruro de, 437·1
Mepiramina, Maleato de, 437·1
Mepirizole, 36·3
Mepirodipine Hydrochloride, 866·3
Mepisolver, 2124·4
Mepitel, 2124·4
Mepitiostane, 1559·1
Mepitiostano, 1559·1
Mepivacaína, Hidrocloruro de, 1381·2
Mepivacaine Hydrochloride, 1381·2
Mepivacaini Chloridum, 1381·2
Mepivacaini Hydrochloridum, 1381·2
Mepivamol, 2124·4
Mepivastesin, 2125·1
Mepivirgi, 2125·1
Mepotin, 2125·1
Mepral, 2125·1
Meprate, 2125·1
Mepraz, 2125·1
Meprazan, 2125·1
Meprednisona, 1106·1
Meprednisone, 1106·1
Meprednisone Acetate, 1106·1
Meprednisone Sodium Hemisuccinate, 1106·1
Mepril, 2125·1
Meprizina, 2125·1
Mepro, 2125·1
Meprobamate, 706·2
Meprobamato, 706·2
Meprobamatum, 706·2
Meprodil, 2125·1
Meprofen, 2125·1
Meprogesic, 2125·1
Meprogest, 2125·1
Meprolol, 2125·1
Meprolol Comp, 2125·1
Mepromol, 2125·1
Mepron, 2125·1
Mepronet, 2125·1
Mepronizine, 2125·1
Meprosona-F, 2125·1
Meprotanum, 706·2
Meptazinol, Hidrocloruro de, 56·3
Meptazinol Hydrochloride, 56·3
Meptid, 2125·1
Meptidol, 2125·1
Meptin, 2125·1
Mepyl, 2125·1
Mepyraderm, 2125·2
Mepyramine Acefyllinate, 437·1
Mepyramine Hydrochloride, 437·1
Mepyramine Hydrogen Maleate, 437·1
Mepyramine Maleate, 437·1
Mepyramine Tannate, 437·1
Mepyramini Maleas, 437·1
Mepyrimal, 2125·2
Mequin, 2125·2
Mequinol, 1151·3
Mequitazina, 437·2
Mequitazine, 437·2
Mequiverine Hydrochloride, 1764·3
MER-41, 1542·2
Meracilina, 2125·2
Meracote, 2125·2
Meractinomycin, 545·1
Meradimate, 1151·3
Meradimato, 1151·3
Meralluride, 952·2
Meralop, 2125·2
Meralops, 2125·2
Meramide, 2125·2
Merankol Pastiglie, 2125·2
Merapiran, 2125·2
Merapril, 2125·2
Merasyn, 2125·2
Merbenloc, 2125·2
Merbentyl, 2125·2
Merbromin, 1185·3
Merbromina, 1185·3
Mercalm, 2125·2
Mercamine, 1712·1
Mercap, 2125·2
Mercaptamina, 1712·1
Mercaptamina, Bitartrato de, 1712·1
Mercaptamina, Hidrocloruro de, 1712·2
Mercaptamine, 1712·1
Mercaptamine Bitartrate, 1712·1
Mercaptamine Hydrochloride, 1712·2
Mercaptina, 2125·2
Mercaptizol, 2125·2
Mercaptoacetic Acid, 1160·3
Mercaptomerin Sodium, 952·2
(±)-*N*-[α-(Mercaptomethyl)hydrocinnamoyl]glycine Benzyl Ester Acetate, 1285·2
*N*-(2-Mercapto-2-methylpropionyl)-L-cysteine, 1663·2
1-[(2*S*)-3-Mercapto-2-methylpropionyl]-L-proline, 879·2
*N*-{1-[(*S*)-3-Mercapto-2-methylpropionyl]-L-prolyl}-3-phenyl-L-alanine Acetate, 856·2
2-Mercapto-6-methylpyrimidin-4-ol, 1602·3
3-Mercaptopropane-1,2-diol, 1186·3
1-(3-Mercaptopropionic Acid)-8-D-arginine-vasopressin, 1322·3
1-(3-Mercaptopropionic Acid)-oxytocin, 1322·3
*N*-(2-Mercaptopropionyl)glycine, 1054·3
*N*-(2-Mercaptopropionyl)glycine 2-Thiophenecarboxylate, 1130·3
2-Mercapto-6-propylpyrimidin-4-ol, 1603·1
Mercaptopurina, 567·2
Mercaptopurine, 567·2
6-Mercaptopurine Monohydrate, 567·2
Mercaptopurine Riboside, 568·1
Mercaptopurine Sodium, 568·1
Mercaptopurinum, 567·2
D-3-Mercaptovaline, 1046·3
Mercaptyl, 2125·2
Mercazolylum, 1603·3
Merced, 2125·2
Mercilon, 2125·2
Mercina, 2125·2
Merck-Cough Linctus, 2125·2
Merckenzyme, 2125·2
Merck-Expectorant, 2125·2
Merck-Fed, 2125·2
Merck-Flu, 2125·3
Merck-Gesic, 2125·3
Mercodol with Decapryn, 2125·3
Mercromina, 2125·3
Mercrotona, 2125·3
Mercryl, 2125·3
Mercryl Lauryle, 2125·3
Mercryl Plus, 2125·3
Mercuchrom, 2125·3
Mercural, 2125·3
Mercure, 1713·1
Mercurescéine Sodique, 1185·3
Mercureux (Chlorure), 1712·3
Mercuric Ammonium Chloride, 1152·1
Mercuric Chlor., 1712·3
Mercuric Chloride, 1712·3
Mercuric Cyanide, 1506·2
Mercuric Oxide, Yellow, 1712·3
Mercúrico Amarillo, Óxido, 1712·3
Mercúrico, Cloruro, 1712·3
Mercurin, 2125·3
Mercurio, 1713·1
Mercurio Amoniacal, 1152·1
Mercurio, Bicloruro de, 1712·3
Mercurio Cromo, 2125·3
Mercurio, Oxido Amarillo de, 1712·3
Mercurio, Protocloruro de, 1712·3
Mercurioso, Cloruro, 1712·3
Mercurique (Chlorure), 1712·3
Mercurique (Oxyde) Jaune, 1712·3
Mercurius Dulcis, 1712·3
Mercurobromo, 2125·3
Mercurobutol, 1185·3
Mercurochrome, 1185·3
Mercurodibromofluorescein, 1185·3
Mercurophylline Sodium, 952·2
Mercurothiolate, 1194·1
Mercurothiolate Sodique, 1194·1
Mercurous Chloride, 1712·3
Mercurous Chloride, Mild, 1712·3
Mercurous Chloride, Precipitated, 1712·3
Mercury, 1713·1
Mercury Amide Chloride, 1152·1
Mercury Aminochloride, 1152·1
Mercury, Ammoniated, 1152·1
Mercury Bichloride, 1712·3
Mercury Monochloride, 1712·3
Mercury Perchloride, 1712·3
Mercury Subchloride, 1712·3
Mercutina Brota, 2125·3
Mercuval, 2125·3
Merebral, 2125·3
Meredazol, 2125·3
Mereprine, 2125·3
Meresa, 2125·3
Meretek UBT, 2125·3
Merethoxylline Procaine, 952·2
Merex, 2125·3
Merfen, 2125·3
Merfene, 2125·3
Merfluan Sali Dentali, 2125·3
Mericomb, 2125·3
Meridia, 2125·3
Meridol, 2125·4
Meridol-D, 2125·4
Meriestra, 2125·4
Merigest, 2125·4
Merigest Combi— *see* Merigest Sequi, 2125·4
Merigest Sequi, 2125·4
Merimono, 2125·4
Merional, 2125·4
Merional-HMG, 2125·4
Merislon, 2125·4
Meristel, 2125·4
Meritene, 2125·4
Meritene, Resource— *see* Resource Meritene, 2259·2
Merlin, 2125·4
Merlit, 2125·4
Merluzzo, Olio di Fegato di, 1425·2
Mermid, 2125·4
Merocaine, 2125·4
Merocets, 2125·4
Merocets Plus, 2125·4
Meroken New, 2125·4
Merol, 2125·4
Meromycin, 2125·4
Meronem, 2125·4
Meropen, 2125·4
Meropenem, 229·1
Merothol— *see* Merocets Plus, 2125·4
Merozen, 2125·4
Merpal, 2125·4
Merphalan, 566·1
Merphen, 2125·4
Merrem, 2126·1
Mersal. Acid, 952·2
Mersálico, Ácido, 952·2
Mersalilo, 952·2
Mersalyl, 952·2
Mersalyl Acid, 952·2
Mersalyl Sodium, 952·2
Mersalylum Acidum, 952·2
MerSol, 2126·1
Mersol, 2126·1
Mersyndol, 2126·1
Mersyndol with Codeine, 2126·1
Mersyndol Daystrength, 2126·1
Merthiolate, 2126·1
Mertiatide, Technetium ($^{99m}Tc$), 1526·1
Meruvax, 2126·1
Meruvax II, 2126·1
Merxil, 2126·1
Merz Spezial, 2126·1
Merz Spezial Dragees N, 2126·1
Merzbiotin, 2126·1
Mesacol, 2126·1
Mesactol, 2126·1
Mesaflor, 2126·1
Mesagin, 2126·1
Mesalamine, 1273·2
Mesalazina, 1273·2
Mesalazine, 1273·2
Mesalazinum, 1273·2
Mesangiocapillary Glomerulonephritis— *see* Glomerular Kidney Disease, 1080·2
Mesantoin, 2126·1
Mesasal, 2126·1
Mesatil, 2126·1
Mesatonum, 1126·3
Mescal Buttons, 1713·3
Mescalina, 1713·3
Mescaline, 1713·3
Mescolor, 2126·1
Mescorit, 2126·1
Mesid, 2126·1
Mesigyna, 2126·1
Mesiken, 2126·1
Mesilato de Alatrofloxacino, 154·1
Mesilato de Amidefrina, 1115·1
Mesilato de Antazolina, 424·2
Mesilato de Benzatropina, 479·2
Mesilato de Betahistina, 1660·1
Mesilato de Bitolterol, 781·3
Mesilato de Bromocriptina, 1200·3
Mesilato de Camostat, 1665·2
Mesilato de Clorprotixeno, 682·3
Mesilato de Crisnatol, 540·2
Mesilato de Dalfopristina, 248·1
Mesilato de Danofloxacino, 202·2
Mesilato de Deferoxamina, 1033·1

Mesilato de Delavirdina, 630·2
Mesilato de Dihidroergotamina, 465·3
Mesilato de Dimetotiazina, 431·3
Mesilato de Dolasetrón, 1262·3
Mesilato de Doxazosina, 908·3
Mesilato de Endralazina, 910·3
Mesilato de Eprosartán, 912·1
Mesilato de Fenoldopam, 915·3
Mesilato de Fentolamina, 982·1
Mesilato de Gabexato, 1690·1
Mesilato de Gemifloxacino, 216·3
Mesilato de Hicantona, 105·3
Mesilato de Imatinib, 562·1
Mesilato de Isoetarina, 788·1
Mesilato de Loprazolam, 704·1
Mesilato de Nelfinavir, 650·1
Mesilato de Pefloxacino, 241·3
Mesilato de Pentamidina, 613·2
Mesilato de Pergolida, 1211·2
Mesilato de Pridinol, 1395·2
Mesilato de Proclorperazina, 716·3
Mesilato de Quinupristina, 248·2
Mesilato de Reboxetina, 316·3
Mesilato de Saquinavir, 653·3
Mesilato de Tioproperazina, 724·1
Mesilato de Tirilazad, 1013·2
Mesilato de Trovafloxacino, 274·3
Mesin, 2126·1
Mesitol, 2126·2
M-Eslon, 2126·2
Mesmerin, 2126·2
Mesna, 1041·2
Mesna Disulfide, 1041·3
Mesnex, 2126·2
Mesnil, 2126·2
Mesnum, 1041·2
Mesocaine, 2126·2
Mesocarb, 1589·2
Mesodal, 2126·2
Mesoglicano Sódico, 1714·1
Mesoglycan Sodium, 1714·1
Mesolex, 2126·2
Mesolona, 2126·2
Mesonex, 2126·2
Mesonordihydroguaiaretic Acid, 566·1
Mesopran, 2126·2
Mesorfan, 2126·2
Mesoridazina, Besilato de, 706·3
Mesoridazine, 706·3, 724·3
Mesoridazine Benzenesulphonate, 706·3
Mesoridazine Besilate, 706·3
Mesoridazine Besylate, 706·3
Mesotina, 2126·2
Mesoxalonitrile (−)-{*p*-[(*R*)-1,4,5,6-Tetrahydro-4-methyl-6-oxo-3-pyridazinyl]phenyl}hydrazone, 946·2
Mespafin, 2126·2
Mespiperone ($^{11}$C), 1523·1
Mesporan, 2126·2
Mesporin, 2126·2
Mesren, 2126·2
Mestacine, 2126·2
Mesterolona, 1559·1
Mesterolone, 1559·1
Mesterolonum, 1559·1
Mestian, 2126·2
Mestil-Ka, 2126·2
Mestinon, 2126·2
Mesto-Of, 2126·2
Mestoranum, 2126·2
Mestranol, 1559·2
Mestranolum, 1559·2
Mestrel, 2126·2
Mesulfen, 1152·1
Mesulfeno, 1152·1
Mesulid, 2126·2
Mesulphen, 1152·1
Mesupon, 2126·2
Mesura, 2126·3
Mesuridazine, 706·3
Mesuridazine Benzenesulphonate, 706·3
Mesuximida, 366·2
Mesuximide, 366·2
Met, 2126·3
Meta, 1507·2
Meta Framan, 2126·3
Metabiarex, 2126·3
Metabisulfito Potásico, 1193·1
Metabisulfito Sódico, 1193·1
Metabol, 2126·3
Metabolic Acidosis, 1217·2
Metabolic Alkalosis, 1217·3
Metabolic Bone Disease of Prematurity— *see* Rickets of Prematurity, 1232·1
Metabolic Disorders, Amino Acid— *see* Amino Acid Metabolic Disorders, 1417·2
Metabolic Mineral Mixture, 2126·3
Metabolic Syndrome— *see* Cardiovascular Risk Reduction, 819·1
Metabolicum, 2126·3
Metabolite-A, 2126·3
Metabromsalan, 1171·2
Metabyn, 2126·3
Metacaf, 2126·3
Metacaine Mesylate, 1385·3
Metacard, 2126·3
Metacen, 2126·3
Metaciclina, Hidrocloruro de, 230·1
Metacidil, 2126·3
Metacolina, Cloruro de, 1492·1
Metacortandracin, 1109·3
Metacortandralone, 1108·1
Metacresol, 1178·1
Metacresolsulfonic Acid-Formaldehyde, 756·1
Metacresolsulphonic Acid-Formaldehyde, 756·1
Metacresolum, 1178·1
Metacrilato de Metilo, 1714·3
Metacualona, 707·1
Metacuprol, 2126·3
Metacycline, 230·1
Metacycline Hydrochloride, 230·1
Metacyclini Chloridum, 230·1
Metadate, 2126·3
Metadec, 2126·3
Metadol, 2126·3
Metadon, 2126·3
Metadona, Hidrocloruro de, 57·2
Metadoxil, 2126·3
Metadoxine, 1456·3
Metadyne, 2126·3
Metafar, 2126·3
Metaflex, 2126·3
Metaflex NF, 2126·3
Metaflex Plus, 2126·3
Metaflex Plus NF, 2126·3
Metagin, 1183·3
Metaginkgo, 2126·3
Metaglip, 2126·3
Metagliz, 2126·3
Metagliz Bismutico, 2126·3
Metagonimiasis— *see* Intestinal Fluke Infections, 99·2
Metagyl, 2126·3
Metahydrin, 2126·4
Meta-K, 2126·4
Metakaveron, 2126·4
Metakelfin, 2126·4
Metakes, 2126·4
Metal Fume Fever, 1469·3, 1713·1
Metalax, 2126·4
Metalcaptase, 2126·4
Metaldehído, 1507·1
Metaldehyde, 1507·1
Metalgin, 2126·4
Metalkonium Chloride, 1185·3
Metallic Soaps, 1574·1
Metalon, 2126·4
Metalpha, 2126·4
Metals, Heavy, Poisoning, 1050·1
Metals, Radioactive, Poisoning, 1050·1
Metalyse, 2126·4
Metamagnesol, 2126·4
Metamelfalan, 576·2
Metamfepramone Hydrochloride, 1714·1
Metamfepyramone Hydrochloride, 1714·1
Metamfetamine Hydrochloride, 1589·2
Metamide, 2126·4
Metamidol, 2126·4
Metamizol Sódico, 35·3
Metamizole Calcium, 36·1
Metamizole Magnesium, 36·1
Metamizole Sodium, 35·3, 36·1
Metamizolum Natricum, 35·3
Metampicilina Sódica, 229·3
Metampicillin Sodium, 229·3
Metamucil, 2126·4
Metandienona, 1559·3
Metandienone, 1559·3
Metandren, 2126·4
Metanephrine, 854·1
Metanfepramona, Hidrocloruro de, 1714·1
Metanfetamina, Hidrocloruro de, 1589·2
Metaniazida, 230·1
Metanium, 2126·4
Metanol, 1475·2
Metanopirone Citrate, 723·2
Metanor, 2126·4
Metantelinio, Bromuro de, 485·3
Metaossylen, 2126·4
Metaoxedrini Chloridum, 1126·3
Metaphyllin, 780·2
Metapio, 2126·4
Metapirona, 2126·4
Metaplatin, 2126·4
Metaplex, 2126·4
Metaplexan, 2126·4
Metaproterenol Sulfate, 790·2
Metaproterenol Sulphate, 790·2
Metaradrine Bitartrate, 952·2
Metaraminol Acid Tartrate, 952·2
Metaraminol Bitartrate, 952·2
Metaraminol Tartrate, 952·2
Metaraminol, Tartrato de, 952·2
Metargen Pediatrico, 2126·4
Metasal, 2126·4
Metasedin, 2126·4
Metasin, 2127·1
Metasolidago S, 2127·1
Metasolvens, 2127·1
Metason, 2127·1
Metaspirine, 2127·1
Metaspray, 2127·1
Metastatic Bone Disease— *see* Malignant Neoplasms of the Bone, 513·1
Metastatic Brain Tumours— *see* Malignant Neoplasms of the Brain, 513·2
Metastatic Breast Cancer— *see* Malignant Neoplasms of the Breast, 514·1
Metastatic Liver Disease— *see* Malignant Neoplasms of the Liver, 518·3
Metastatic Lung Disease— *see* Malignant Neoplasms of the Lung, 519·2
Metastron, 2127·1
Metasulfobenzoato Sódico de Dexametasona, 1097·2
Metasulfobenzoato Sódico de Prednisolona, 1108·1
Metatartaric Acid, 1752·1
Metatensin, 2127·1
Metatone, 2127·1
Metavirulent, 2127·1
Metax, 2127·1
Metaxalona, 1395·1
Metaxalone, 1395·1
Metaxol, 2127·1
Metazem, 2127·1
Metazepium Iodide, 480·2
Metazin, 2127·1
Metazinc, 2127·1
Metazol, 2127·1
Metazolamida, 953·1
Metbay, 2127·1
Metblock, 2127·1
Metcon, 2127·1
Metcort, 2127·1
Meted, 2127·1
Metenamina, 230·1
Metenamina, Hipurato de, 230·2
Metenamina, Mandelato de, 230·2
Metenammina, 230·1
Metenan, 2127·1
Meteneprost, 1519·2
Metenix 5, 2127·1
Met-enkephalin, 73·3
Metenolona, Acetato de, 1559·2
Metenolona, Enantato de, 1559·3
Metenolone Acetate, 1559·2
Metenolone Enantate, 1559·3
Meteophyt Forte, 2127·1
Meteophyt N, 2127·1
Meteophyt S, 2127·1
Meteoril, 2127·1
Meteosan, 2127·2
Meteosim, 2127·2
Meteospasmyl, 2127·2
Meteoxane, 2127·2
Meteozym, 2127·2
Meterfolic, 2127·2
Metergolina, 1211·2
Metergoline, 1211·2
Metescufylline, 1714·1
Metesculetol Sódico, 1714·1
Metesculetol Sodium, 1714·1
Meteverine Hydrochloride, 1717·2
Metex, 2127·2
Metfin, 2127·2
Metfirex, 2127·2
Metfogamma, 2127·2
Metfor, 2127·2
Metfor-500, 2127·2
Metforal, 2127·2
Metforal, Menarini— *see* Menarini-Metforal, 2123·2
Metforem, 2127·2
Metfori, 2127·2
Metform, 2127·2
Metformax, 2127·2
Metformin Chlorophenoxyacetate, 342·3
Metformin Embonate, 342·3
Metformin Hydrochloride, 342·3
Metformina, Hidrocloruro de, 342·3
Metformini Hydrochloridum, 342·3
Metfron, 2127·2
Meth, 1589·2
Methachalonum, 707·1
Methacholine Chloride, 1492·1
Methacholinium Chloratum, 1492·1
Methacin, 2127·2
Methacrylate Copolymer, Basic Butylated, 1714·3
Methacrylate Copolymer (Type A), Ammonio, 1714·3
Methacrylate Copolymer (Type B), Ammonio, 1714·3
Methacrylic Acid, 1733·2
Methacrylic Acid Copolymer, 1714·3
Methacrylic Acid-Ethyl Acrylate Copolymer (1:1), 1714·3
Methacrylic Acid-Ethyl Acrylate Copolymer (1:1) Dispersion 30 Per Cent, 1714·3
Methacrylic Acid-Methyl Methacrylate Copolymer (1:1), 1714·3
Methacrylic Acid-Methyl Methacrylate Copolymer (1:2), 1714·3
Methacycline, 230·1
Methacycline Hydrochloride, 230·1
Methaddict, 2127·2
Methadol, 58·2
Methadone Hydrochloride, 57·2
(−)-Methadone Hydrochloride, 54·1
(±)-Methadone Hydrochloride, 57·2
Methadone Mixture DTF, Martindale— *see* Martindale Methadone Mixture DTF, 2115·1
Methadoni Hydrochloridum, 57·2
Methadose, 2127·2
*l*-Methadyl Acetate, 54·1
Methaemoglobinaemia, 1043·1
Methagual, 2127·2
Methalamic Acid, 1065·3
Methalgen, 2127·2
Methaminodiazepoxide, 674·2
Methaminodiazepoxide Hydrochloride, 674·2
*l*-Methamphetamine, 1124·1
Methamphetamine Hydrochloride, 1589·2, 1589·3
Methamphetamini Hydrochloridum, 1589·2
Methampyrone, 35·3
Methanamide, 1474·3
Methandienone, 1559·3
Methandrostenolone, 1559·3

β-[(*p*-Methanesulfonamidophenethyl)methylamino]methanesulfono-*p*-phenetidide, 906·3
Methaniazide, 230·1
Methaniazide Calcium, 230·1
Methaniazide Sodium, 230·1
Methanol, 1475·2
Methanolquinoline Antimalarials, 444·1
Methantheline Bromide, 485·3
Methanthelinium Bromide, 485·3
Methantoin, 366·2
Methaqualone, 707·1
Methaqualonum, 707·1
Metharmon-F, 2127·2
β-Methasone, 1093·1
Methatabs, 2127·2
Methatropic, 2127·2
Methazil, 2127·2
Methazolamide, 953·1
Methdilazine, 437·2
Methdilazine Hydrochloride, 437·2
Methenamine, 230·1, 230·2
Methenamine Calcium Thiocyanate, 230·3
Methenamine Hippurate, 230·2
Methenamine Mandelate, 230·2
Methenaminum, 230·1
Methenolone Acetate, 1559·2
Methenolone Enanthate, 1559·3
Methenolone Oenanthate, 1559·3
Methergin, 2127·2
Methergine, 2127·2
Methergoline, 1211·2
Methex, 2127·3
Methexenyl, 703·1
Met-HGH, 1327·2
Methicillin Sodium, 230·3
Methimazole, 1603·3
Methionine, 1042·1
DL-Methionine, 1042·1
L-Methionine, 1042·1
L-Methionine ($^{11}$C), 1523·1
*S*-Methionine, 1042·1
245-L-Methionine Plasminogen Activator, 909·2
Methioninum, 1042·1
DL-Methioninum, 1042·1
Methioninyl Adenylate, 1647·2
Methionyl Bovine Growth Hormone, 1327·2
Methionyl Human Growth Hormone, 1327·2
Methionyl Porcine Growth Hormone, 1327·2
Méthioplégium, 1017·3
Methiosulfonium Chloride, 1714·1
Methiotrans, 2127·3
Methisoprinol, 640·2
Methixene Hydrochloride, 485·3
Methixene Hydrochloride Monohydrate, 485·3
Methnine, 2127·3
Methoblastin, 2127·3
Methoblastine, 2127·3
Methocaps, 2127·3
Methocarbamol, 1395·1
Methocel, 2127·3
Methochalcone, 1714·3
Method M, 2127·3
Methohexital, 1303·2
Methohexital Sodium, 1303·2
Methohexital Sodium for Injection, 1303·2
Methohexitone, 1303·2
Methohexitone Sodium, 1303·2
Methoin, 366·2
Methomyl, 1507·2
Methoprene, 1507·2
Methopt, 2127·3
α-Methopterin, 568·2
Methorcon, 2127·3
Methorphinan Tartrate, 54·1
Methotrexate, 568·2
Methotrexate Disodium, 568·3
Methotrexate Sodium, 568·3
Methotrexatum, 568·2
Methotrimeprazine, 703·2
Methotrimeprazine Hydrochloride, 703·2
Methotrimeprazine Hydrogen Maleate, 703·2
Methotrimeprazine Maleate, 703·2
Methoxacet, 2127·3
Methoxacet-C, 2127·3
Methoxadone, 1395·1
Methoxamedrine Hydrochloride, 953·1
Methoxamine Hydrochloride, 953·1
Methoxiphenadrin Hydrochloride, 1124·2
Methoxisal, 2127·3
Methoxisal-C, 2127·3
Methoxsalen, 1152·1
Methoxyamfetamine, 1593·3
4-Methoxyamfetamine, 1593·3
*p*-Methoxyamfetamine, 1593·3
1-(4-Methoxybenzoyl)-2-pyrrolidinone, 1655·1
α-(α-Methoxybenzyl)-4-(β-methoxyphenethyl)-1-piperazineethanol Dihydrochloride, 1132·3
4-Methoxy-*N*,*N'*-bis(3-pyridinylmethyl)-1,3-benzenedicarboxamide Monohydrate, 982·3
2-{3-Methoxycarbonyl-2-[2-nitro-5-(propylthio)phenyl]guanidino}ethanesulphonic Acid, 110·1
(1*R*,2*R*,3*S*,5*S*)-2-Methoxycarbonyltropan-3-yl Benzoate, 1373·3
Methoxychlor, 1507·2
(8*R*,9*S*)-6'-Methoxycinchonan-9-ol, 991·3
(8*S*,9*R*)-6'-Methoxycinchonan-9-ol, 460·1
17β-(1-Methoxycyclopentyloxy)-2α,3α-epithio-5α-androstane, 1559·1
Methoxy-DDT, 1507·2
10α-Methoxy-1,6-dimethylergolin-8β-ylmethyl 5-Bromonicotinate, 1719·3
2-Methoxy-*N*α-dimethylphenethylamine Hydrochloride, 1124·2
2-Methoxyethanol, 1475·2
*N*-[5-(2-Methoxyethoxy)pyrimidin-2-yl]benzenesulphonamide Sodium, 333·2
Methoxyflurane, 1304·1
9-Methoxy-7*H*-furo[3,2-*g*][1]benzopyran-7-one, 1152·1
4-Methoxy-7*H*-furo[3,2-*g*]chromen-7-one, 1154·1
9-Methoxyfuro[3,2-*g*]chromen-7-one, 1152·1
12-Methoxyibogamine, 1700·2
*N*-[2-(5-Methoxyindol-3-yl)ethyl]acetamide, 1710·2
1-{[(5-Methoxyindol-3-yl)methylene]amino}-3-pentylguanidine Maleate, 1293·2
Methoxymethane, 1236·1
5-Methoxy-2-{(*S*)-[(4-methoxy-3,5-dimethyl-2-pyridyl)methyl]sulfinyl}benzimidazole Magnesium (2:1) Trihydrate, 1265·1
(*RS*)-5-Methoxy-2-(4-methoxy-3,5-dimethyl-2-pyridylmethylsulphinyl)benzimidazole, 1278·2
4-Methoxy-2-(5-methoxy-3-methylpyrazol-1-yl)-6-methylpyrimidine, 36·3
(+)-3-Methoxy-9a-methylmorphinan, 1117·3
2-Methoxy-2-methylpropane, 1475·3
7-Methoxy-1-methyl-9*H*-pyrido[3,4-*b*]indole, 1696·3
*N*-{4-(Methoxymethyl)-1-[2-(2-thienyl)ethyl]-4-piperidyl}propionanilide, 90·2
*N*-{4-(Methoxymethyl)-1-[2-(2-thienyl)ethyl]-4-piperidyl}propionanilide Citrate, 90·2
(*R*)-5-(Methoxymethyl)-3-{*p*-[(*R*)-4,4,4-trifluoro-3-hydroxybutoxy]phenyl}-2-oxazolidinone, 287·1
6-Methoxy-2-naphthylacetic Acid, 64·1
4-(6-Methoxy-2-naphthyl)butan-2-one, 63·3
4-(4-Methoxy-1-naphthyl)-4-oxobutyric Acid, 1711·3
(+)-2-(6-Methoxy-2-naphthyl)propionic Acid, 65·1
3-Methoxy-19-nor-17α-pregna-1,3,5(10)-trien-20-yn-17β-ol, 1559·2
Methoxyphenamine Hydrochloride, 1124·2
3-[4-(β-Methoxyphenethyl)piperazin-1-yl]-1-phenylpropan-1-ol Dihydrochloride, 1121·1
2-Methoxyphenol, 1122·1
4-Methoxyphenol, 1151·3
3-(2-Methoxyphenothiazin-10-yl)-2-methylpropyldimethylamine, 703·2
(±)-2-(*o*-Methoxyphenoxy)-2-methyl-1,3-benzodioxan-4-one, 1122·2
5-(2-Methoxyphenoxymethyl)oxazolidin-2-one, 1395·1
(*RS*)-3-(2-Methoxyphenoxy)propane-1,2-diol, 1122·1
*o*-Methoxyphenyl Salicylate Acetate, 1121·3
5-(4-Methoxyphenyl)-3*H*-1,2-dithiole-3-thione, 1655·1
2-(4-Methoxyphenyl)indan-1,3-dione, 863·3
(±)-4-(*o*-Methoxyphenyl)-α-[(1-naphthyloxy)methyl]-1-piperazineethanol, 964·1
6-[3-(4-*o*-Methoxyphenylpiperazin-1-yl)propylamino]-1,3-dimethyluracil, 1018·1
(*E*)-1-Methoxy-4-(prop-1-enyl)benzene, 1654·3
17β-Methoxy-3-propoxyestra-1,3,5(10)-triene, 1568·2
2-({[4-(3-Methoxypropoxy)-3-methyl-2-pyridyl]methyl}sulfinyl)-1*H*-benzimidazole Sodium, 1285·1
5-Methoxypsoralen, 1154·1
8-Methoxypsoralen, 1152·1
$N^1$-(3-Methoxypyrazin-2-yl)sulphanilamide, 263·1
$N^1$-(6-Methoxypyridazin-3-yl)sulphanilamide, 263·1
$N^1$-(6-Methoxypyrimidin-4-yl)sulphanilamide Monohydrate, 263·2
1-(6-Methoxy-4-quinolyl)-3-(3-vinyl-4-piperidyl)propan-1-one Hydrochloride, 1764·3
(α*R*)-α-(6-Methoxy-4-quinolyl)-α-[(2*S*,4*S*,5*R*)-(5-vinylquinuclidin-2-yl)]methanol, 460·1
(+)-(α*S*)-α-(6-Methoxy-4-quinolyl)-α-[(2*R*,4*S*,5*R*)-(5-vinylquinuclidin-2-yl)]methanol, 991·3
$N^1$-(4-Methoxy-1,2,5-thiadiazol-3-yl)sulphanilamide, 263·2
(*E*)-5-Methoxy-4'-trifluoromethylvalerophenone *O*-2-Aminoethyloxime Maleate, 298·2
(2*E*,4*E*,6*E*,8*E*)-9-(4-Methoxy-2,3,6-trimethylphenyl)-3,7-dimethylnona-2,4,6,8-tetraenoic Acid, 1140·2
(*all-trans*)-9-(4-Methoxy-2,3,6-trimethylphenyl)-3,7-dimethyl-2,4,6,8-nonatetraenoic Acid, 1140·2
Methoxyverapamil Hydrochloride, 922·3
Methozane, 2127·3
Methscopolamine Bromide, 483·3
Methscopolamine Nitrate, 483·3
Methsuximide, 366·2
Methyclothiazide, 953·2
Methycobal, 2127·3
Methyl 4-Acetamido-2-ethoxybenzoate, 605·1
Methyl Alcohol, 1475·2
Methyl 2-Aminobenzoate, 1154·1
Methyl 6-Amino-7-chloro-6,7,8-trideoxy-*N*-[(2*S*,4*R*)-1-methyl-4-propylprolyl]-1-thio-L-*threo*-D-*galacto*-octopyranoside, 194·2
Methyl 6-Amino-6,8-dideoxy-*N*-[(2*S*,4*R*)-1-methyl-4-propylprolyl]-1-thio-α-D-*erythro*-D-*galacto*-octopyranoside, 226·2
Methyl Aminolaevulinate Hydrochloride, 527·2
Methyl Aminolevulinate Hydrochloride, 527·2
Methyl L-2-Amino-3-mercaptopropionate Hydrochloride, 1124·1
Methyl 5-Amino-4-oxopentanoate Hydrochloride, 527·2
Methyl Anthranilate, 1154·1
Methyl *N*-L-α-Aspartyl-L-phenylalaninate, 1422·1
Methyl Benzoquate, 607·2
Methyl 5-Benzoyl-1*H*-benzimidazol-2-ylcarbamate, 108·2
Methyl Benzoylecgonine, 1373·3
Methyl Benzylidene Camphor, 1147·1
Methyl 7-Benzyloxy-6-butyl-1,4-dihydro-4-oxoquinoline-3-carboxylate, 607·2
Methyl Bromide, 1507·2
Methyl Butetisalicylate, 59·2
Methyl *tert*-Butyl Ether, 1475·3
Methyl Butyl Ketone, 1476·1
Methyl *n*-Butyl Ketone, 1476·1
Methyl 1-(Butylcarbamoyl)benzimidazol-2-ylcarbamate, 1500·2
Methyl Catechol, 1122·1
Methyl Chloride, 1476·2
Methyl 6-[3-(2-Chloroethyl)-3-nitrosoureido]-6-deoxy-α-D-glucopyranoside, 582·2
Methyl (+)-(*S*)-α-(*o*-Chlorophenyl)-6,7-dihydrothieno[3,2-*c*]pyridine-5(4*H*)-acetate Sulphate, 888·3
Methyl (*S*)-2-Chlorophenyl(4,5,6,7-tetrahydrothieno[3,2-*c*]pyridin-5-yl)acetate Bisulphate, 888·3
Methyl 7-Chloro-6,7,8-trideoxy-6-(*cis*-4-ethyl-L-pipecolamido)-1-thio-L-*threo*-α-D-*galacto*-octopyranoside Monohydrochloride Monohydrate, 244·1
Methyl Cyanide, 1471·1
Methyl 2-Cyanoacrylate, 1678·1
Methyl (*Z*)-7-{(1*R*,2*S*,3*R*,5*S*)-2-[(3*S*)-5-Cyclohexyl-3-hydroxypent-1-ynyl]-3,5-dihydroxycyclopentyl}hept-5-enoate, 1512·3
Methyl Cysteine Hydrochloride, 1124·1
Methyl Dacisteine, 1124·2
Methyl 11-Demethoxy-*O*-(3,4,5-trimethoxybenzoyl)reserpate, 892·3
Methyl Diacetylcysteinate, 1124·2
Methyl *N*,*S*-Diacetyl-L-cysteinate, 1124·2
Methyl 16,17-Didehydro-19α-methyl-18-oxayohimban-16-carboxylate, 994·3
Methyl (1*R*,2*R*,4*S*)-4-(*O*-{2,6-Dideoxy-4-*O*-[(2*R*,6*S*)-tetrahydro-6-methyl-5-oxopyran-2-yl]-α-L-*lyxo*-hexopyranosyl}-(1→4)-2,3,6-trideoxy-3-dimethylamino-L-*lyxo*-hexopyranosyloxy)-2-ethyl-1,2,3,4,6,11-hexahydro-2,5,7-trihydroxy-6,11-dioxonaphthacene-1-carboxylate, 525·2
Methyl Diethylacetylsalicylate, 59·2
Methyl 2-(2-Diethylaminoacetamido)-*m*-toluate Hydrochloride, 1385·3
β-Methyl Digoxin, 955·2
Methyl (3α,16α)-14,15-Dihydro-14β-hydroxyeburnamenine-14-carboxylate, 1764·2
Methyl (2*E*,13*E*)-(8*R*,11*R*,12*R*,15*R*)-11,15-Dihydroxy-16,16-dimethyl-9-oxoprosta-2,13-dienoate, 1518·1
(±)-Methyl (13*E*)-11,16-Dihydroxy-16-methyl-9-oxoprost-13-enoate, 1519·2
Methyl 11,17α-Dimethoxy-18β-(3,4,5-trimethoxybenzoyloxy)-3β,20α-yohimbane-16β-carboxylate, 995·1
Methyl Ethyl Ketone, 1476·2
Methyl *O*-(2-Ethylbutyryl)salicylate, 59·2
Methyl Flavone Carboxylic Acid, 482·2
Methyl 5-(4-Fluorobenzoyl)-1*H*-benzimidazol-2-ylcarbamate, 105·2
Methyl Fluorosulfate, 1714·1
Methyl Fluorosulphate, 1714·1
Methyl Fluorosulphonate, 1714·1
Methyl Gentisate, 59·2
Methyl Hexyl Ether, 1476·1
Methyl Hydroxybenzoate, 1183·3
Methyl 2-Hydroxybenzoate, 59·3
Methyl 4-Hydroxybenzoate, 1183·3
Methyl Hydroxybenzoate, Sodium, 1183·3
Methyl Hydroxybenzoate, Soluble, 1183·3
Methyl (*E*)-7-{(1*R*,2*R*,3*R*)-3-Hydroxy-2-[(*E*)-(3*R*)-3-hydroxy-4,4-dimethyloct-1-enyl]-5-oxocyclopentyl}hept-2-enoate, 1518·1
Methyl (−)-(1*R*,2*R*,3*R*)-3-Hydroxy-2-[(*E*)-(3*S*,5*S*)-3-hydroxy-5-methyl-1-nonenyl]-ε,5-dioxocyclopentaneheptanoate, 1520·3
(±)-Methyl 7-{(1*R*,2*R*,3*R*)-3-Hydroxy-2-[(*E*)-(4*RS*)-4-hydroxy-4-methyloct-1-enyl]-5-oxocyclopentyl}heptanoate, 1519·2
Methyl 3-[4-(2-Hydroxy-3-isopropylaminopropoxy)phenyl]propionate Hydrochloride, 913·1
Methyl Hydroxypropyl Cellulose, 1579·3
Methyl 17α-Hydroxy-yohimban-16α-carboxylate Hydrochloride, 1766·2
Methyl Isobutyl Ketone, 1476·2
Methyl Lomustine, 583·2
Methyl 2-Methylacrylate, 1714·3

*S*-Methyl *N*-(Methylcarbamoyloxy)thioacetimidate, 1507·2
*O*-Methyl [2-(2-Methyl-5-nitroimidazol-1-yl)ethyl]thiocarbamate, 603·1
Methyl 2-Methylpropenoate, 1714·3
Methyl 4-Methyl-3-(2-propylaminopropionamido)thiophene-2-carboxylate Hydrochloride, 1370·3
Methyl Mitomycin, 581·1
Methyl Nicotinate, 59·2
Methyl Parahydroxybenzoate, 1183·3
Methyl Parahydroxybenzoate, Sodium, 1183·3
Methyl 1-Phenethyl-4-(*N*-phenylpropionamido)isonipecotate Citrate, 25·1
Methyl Phenidate Hydrochloride, 1590·2
Methyl (2*R*)-Phenyl[(2*R*)-piperidin-2-yl]acetate Hydrochloride, 1587·1
Methyl α-Phenyl-2-piperidylacetate Hydrochloride, 1590·2
Methyl 5-Phenylsulphinyl-1*H*-benzimidazol-2-ylcarbamate, 111·1
Methyl 5-Phenylthio-1*H*-benzimidazol-2-ylcarbamate, 105·2
Methyl Phthalate, 1504·1
Methyl 2-[4-(2-Piperidinoethoxy)benzoyl]benzoate Hydrochloride, 1732·3
Methyl Polysiloxane, 1482·1
Methyl 5-Propoxy-1*H*-benzimidazol-2-ylcarbamate, 111·2
Methyl (8*R*,10*R*)-6-Propylergolin-8-ylmethyl Sulphide Methanesulphonate, 1211·2
Methyl 5-Propylthio-1*H*-benzimidazol-2-ylcarbamate, 101·2
Methyl Pyridine-3-carboxylate, 59·2
Methyl 3-Quinoxalin-2-ylmethylenecarbazate 1,4-Dioxide, 166·1
Methyl Sal., 59·3
Methyl Salicylate, 59·3
Methyl Salicylate Compound Liniment, 2127·3
Methyl Salicylate Ointment Compound, 2127·3
Methyl Sulphoxide, 1473·2
Methyl Terbutyl Ether, 1475·3
Methyl Tertiary Butyl Ether, 1475·3
Methyl *O*-(3,4,5-Trimethoxybenzoyl)reserpate, 995·1
Methyl Undecenoate, 411·1
Methyl Violet, 1186·2
Methylacetopyronone, 1178·1
Methylacetoxyprogesterone, 1557·2
α-Methyl-1-adamantanemethylamine Hydrochloride, 653·1
Methylal, 1680·3
4-[(2-Methylallyl)amino]hydratropic Acid, 14·1
4-Methyl-amino-antipyrine, 36·1
1-Methylamino-1-deoxy-D-glucitol, 1710·1
4-(2-Methylaminoethyl)-*o*-phenylene Diisobutyrate, 937·3
4-[2-(1-Methylamino-2-nitrovinylamino)ethylthiomethyl]thiazol-2-ylmethyl(dimethyl)amine, 1277·2
(+)-(1*S*,2*S*)-2-Methylamino-1-phenylpropan-1-ol, 1129·2
(1*R*,2*S*)-2-Methylamino-1-phenylpropan-1-ol, 1120·1
4-(2-Methylaminopropyl)phenol Sulfate, 982·3
*l*-Methylamphetamine, 1124·1
Methylamphetamine Hydrochloride, 1589·2
17α-Methyl-2′*H*-5α-androst-2-eno[3,2-*c*]pyrazol-17β-ol, 1569·2
$N^{\omega}$-Methyl-L-arginine, 1752·1
*N*-Methyl-D-aspartate, 1683·1
Methylated Spirits, 1185·3
Methylated Spirits, Industrial, 1185·3
Methylated Spirits, Mineralised, 1185·3
Methylatropine Bromide, 476·3, 477·1
Methylatropine Nitrate, 477·1
Methylatropini Bromidum, 476·3
Methylatropini Nitras, 477·1
Methylatropinium Bromatum, 476·3
Methylbenactyzium Bromide, 485·3
Methylbenzene, 1477·1
Methylbenzethonium Chloride, 1186·1
Methylbenzoic Acid, 1478·3
α-Methyl-5*H*-[1]-benzopyrano[2,3-*b*]pyridine-7-acetic Acid, 85·2
2-(2-Methylbenzo[*b*]thienylmethyl)-2-imidazoline Hydrochloride, 1124·3
$N^1$-{3-[(*S*)-(α-Methylbenzyl)amino]propyl}bleomycinamide Sulphate, 579·3
3-(4-Methylbenzylidene)bornan-2-one, 1147·1
3-(4-Methylbenzylidene)camphor, 1147·1
2-Methylbutan-2-ol, 1471·2
Methylbutanol Nitrite Esters, 1032·1
Methylbutanol Nitrites, 1032·1
4-(3-Methylbut-2-enyl)-1,2-diphenylpyrazolidine-3,5-dione, 43·1
2-Methylbutyl 4-Dimethylaminobenzoate, 1155·1
3-Methylbutyl 2-Hydroxybenzoate, 14·3
5-(1-Methylbutyl)-5-vinylbarbituric Acid, 727·2
Methyl-CCNU, 583·2
Methylcellulose, 1580·2
Methylcellulose Propylene Glycol Ether, 1579·3
Methylcellulosum, 1580·2
Methylcephaëline Hydrochloride, 604·3
Methylchloroform, 1477·3
Methylchloroisothiazolinone, 1185·1
5-[(*Z*,*E*)-β-Methylcinnamylidene]-4-oxo-2-thioxo-3-thiazolidineacetic Acid, 331·1
Methylcloxazolam, 707·1
Methylcobalamin, 1459·1
6α-Methylcompactin, 949·1
Methyl-cyclohexenylmethyl-barbitursäure, 703·1
Methylcysteine Hydrochloride, 1124·1
4-(*N*-Methyl-2,2-dichloroacetamido)phenyl 2-Furoate, 604·1
β-Methyldigoxin, 955·2
*o*-Methyldihydroartemisinin, 447·2
Methyl-2,5-dimethoxyamfetamine, 1593·3
Methyldinitrobenzamide, 604·2
Methyldinoprost, 1514·2
4-Methyl-1,3-dioxolan-2-one, 1476·3
11β-Methyl-3,20-dioxo-19-norpregn-4-en-17α-yl Acetate, 1563·2
6-Methyl-3,20-dioxopregna-4,6-dien-17α-yl Acetate, 1558·2
6α-Methyl-3,20-dioxopregn-4-en-17α-yl Acetate, 1557·2
2-Methyl-1,2-di(3-pyridyl)propan-1-one, 1715·1
3-*O*-Methyldobutamine, 906·1
Methyldopa, 953·2
α-Methyldopa, 956·1
3-*O*-Methyldopa, 1208·3
α-Methyldopa Hydrazine, 1204·3
α-Methyldopamine, 956·1
Methyldopate Hydrochloride, 953·2
Methyldopum, 953·2
Methyldopum Hydratum, 953·2
Methylene Blue, 1042·2
Methylene Chloride, 1473·1
16-Methylene-17-alpha-acetoxy-19 Norprogesterone, 1549·3
6-Methyleneandrosta-1,4-diene-3,17-dione, 552·3
2,2′-Methylenebis[6-bromo-4-chlorophenol], 1171·1
2,2′-Methylenebis(4-chlorophenol), 104·1
2,2′-Methylenebis(6-chlorothymole), 1171·1
3,3′-Methylenebis(4-hydroxycoumarin), 894·2
*N*,*N*″-Methylenebis{*N*′-[3-(hydroxymethyl)-2,5-dioxo-4-imidazolidinyl]urea}, 1184·2
Methylenebis(hydroxytoluenesulphonic Acid) Polymer, 756·1
4,4′-Methylenebis(perhydro-1,2,4-thiadiazine 1,1-Dioxide), 264·2
Methylenebis(phosphonic Acid), 773·2
2,2′-Methylenebis(3,4,6-trichlorophenol), 1181·2
Méthylènecycline Chlorhydrate, 230·1
Methylenedioxyamphetamine, 1593·3
3,4-Methylenedioxyamphetamine, 1593·3
3,4-Methylenedioxyethamfetamine, 1593·3
3,4-Methylenedioxy-*N*-hydroxyamfetamine, 1593·3
Methylenedioxymethamfetamine, 1589·3
Methylenedioxymethamphetamine, 1589·3
3,4-Methylenedioxymethamphetamine, 1589·3
6-Methyleneoxytetracycline Hydrochloride, 230·1
16-Methyleneprednisolone, 1109·3
Methylenesulfathiazole, 214·2
Methyleni Chloridum, 1473·1
Methylenii Caeruleum, 1042·2
Methylephedrine Hydrochloride, 1124·2
Methylergobasine Maleate, 1714·2
Methylergobrevin, 2127·3
Methylergol Carbamide Maleate, 1210·3
Methylergometrine Maleate, 1714·2
Methylergonovine Maleate, 1714·2
6-*O*-Methylerythromycin, 192·2
1,1′-[(Methylethanediylidene)dinitrilo]diguanidine Dihydrochloride, 573·3
*N*-Methyl-9,10-ethanoanthracene-9(10*H*)-propylamine, 306·1
1-[4-(1-Methylethyl)phenyl]-3-phenyl-1,3-propanedione, 1148·3
3-Methylfentanyl, 40·3
Methylflurether, 1298·1
Methyl-GAG, 573·3
6′*N*-Methylgentamicin $C_{1A}$ Sulphate, 231·3
*N*-Methylglucamine, 1710·1
*N*-Methylglucamine 3,5-Diacetamido-2,4,6-tri-iodobenzoate, 1060·2
Methylglucamine Diatrizoate, 1060·2
[1-(*N*-Methylglycine)-5-L-valine-8-L-alanine]-angiotensin II Acetate Hydrate, 996·3
Methylglyoxal Bisguanylhydrazone, 573·3
Methylhexabarbital, 703·1
Methylhippuric Acid, 1478·3
Methylhomatropinium Bromatum, 483·2
Methylhomatropinium Bromide, 483·2
Methylhydrazine, 1717·3
Methylhydrocupreine Hydrobromide, 1699·3
Methylhydroxyethylcellulose, 1579·2
Methylhydroxyethylcellulosum, 1579·2
α-Methyl-ω-hydroxypoly(oxyethylene), 1413·1
Methylhydroxypropylcellulose, 1579·3
Methylhydroxypropylcellulose Phthalate, 1579·3
Methylhydroxypropylcellulosi Phthalas, 1579·3
Methylhydroxypropylcellulosum, 1579·3
Methylhydroxyquinoline Methylsulphate, 1714·2
Methylhydroxyquinoline Metilsulfate, 1714·2
1-Methyl-8-hydroxyquinolinium Methyl Sulphate, 1714·2
Methylhyoscini Nitras, 483·3
(Methylidynetrithio)triacetic Acid, 1191·3
2-Methylimidazole Polymer with 1-Chloro-2,3-epoxypropane, 889·2
1-Methylimidazole-2-thiol, 1603·3
2,2′-Methyliminobis(diethyldimethylammonium) Dibromide, 866·2
*N*,*N*′-[(Methylimino)dimethylidyne]di-2,4-xylidine, 1500·2
Methylin, 2127·3
(−)-(*R*)-1-Methylindol-3-yl 4,5,6,7-Tetrahydro-5-benzimidazolyl Ketone Hydrochloride, 1285·2
Methylis Oxybenzoas, 1183·3
Methylis Parahydroxybenzoas, 1183·3
Methylis Parahydroxybenzoas Natricum, 1183·3
Methylis Paraoxibenzoas, 1183·3
Methylis Salicylas, 59·3
Methylisothiazolinone, 1185·1
2-Methyl-4-isothiazolin-3-one, 1185·1
2-Methyl-3(2*H*)-isothiazolone, 1185·1
3-{4-[3-(3-Methyl-5-isoxazolyl)propoxy]-3,5-xylyl}-5-(trifluoromethyl)-1,2,4-oxadizole, 651·3
$N^1$-(5-Methylisoxazol-3-yl)sulphanilamide, 261·1
1-Methyl-D-lysergic Acid Butanolamide, 469·3
Methylmelubrin, 35·3
Methylmercadone, 611·2
Methylmercaptoimidazole, 1603·3
Methylmercury, 1713·1
Methylmethacrylate, 1714·3
Methylmethionine Sulfonium Chloride, 1714·1
1-Methyl-*N*-(9-methyl-9-azabicyclo[3.3.1]non-3-yl)-1*H*-indazole-3-carboxamide Hydrochloride, 1267·1
4′-{[4-Methyl-6-(1-methyl-2-benzimidazolyl)-2-propyl-1-benzimidazolyl]methyl}-2-biphenylcarboxylic Acid, 1010·1
(2*S*,3*R*)-5-Methyl-3-{[(α*S*)-α-(methylcarbamoyl)phenethyl]carbamoyl}-2-[(2-thienylthio)methyl]hexanohydroxamic Acid, 529·2
(−)-6-Methyl-2-(4-methyl-3-cyclohexen-1-yl)-5-hepten-2-ol, 1707·1
α-Methyl-3,4-methylenedioxyphenethylamine, 1593·3
5-Methyl-2-(1-methylethyl)-cyclohexyl 2-Aminobenzoate, 1151·3
1-Methyl-5-(1-methyl-2-pentynyl)-5-(2-propenyl)-2,4,6(1*H*,3*H*,5*H*)-pyrimidinetrione, 1303·2
(*R*)-Methyl(α-methylphenethyl)prop-2-ynylamine Hydrochloride, 1214·1
(−)-*N*-Methyl-γ-(2-methylphenoxy)-benzenepropanamine Hydrochloride, 1585·1
2-Methyl-4-(4-methyl-1-piperazinyl)-10*H*-thieno[2,3-*b*][1,5]benzodiazepine, 710·3
*N*-Methyl-3-(1-methyl-4-piperidyl)indole-5-ethanesulfonamide Hydrochloride, 470·1
4-Methyl-5-[4-(methylthio)benzoyl]-4-imidazolin-2-one, 911·1
17-Methyl-9α,13α,14α-morphinan-3-ol, 1679·3
(−)-9a-Methylmorphinan-3-ol Hydrogen Tartrate Dihydrate, 54·1
Methylmorphine, 27·1
Methylmorphine Phosphate, 27·1
(+)-1-(3-Methyl-4-morpholino-2,2-diphenylbutyryl)pyrrolidine, 28·2
1-Methyl-3-morpholinopropyl Perhydro-4-phenylpyran-4-carboxylate, 1121·2
Methylnaltrexone, 1045·3
2-Methylnaphthalene-1,4-diyl Bis(disodium Phosphate) Hexahydrate, 1466·3
3-Methylnaphthalene-1,2,4-triol 2-(4-Aminobenzoate), 741·3
Methylnaphthochinonum, 1466·3
Methylnaphthochinonumnatrium Bisulfurosum, 1466·3
2-Methyl-1,4-naphthoquinone, 1466·3
2-Methyl-1,4-naphthylene Diacetate, 1466·3
(+)-(*S*)-*N*-Methyl-γ-(1-naphthyloxy)-2-thiophenepropylamine Hydrochloride, 291·3
*N*-Methylnicotinamide, 1441·3
3-*O*-Methyl-6-*O*-nicotinoylmorphine, 1125·2
4-Methyl-4′-(*p*-nitroanilino)thio-1-piperazinecarboxanilide, 102·3
2-Methyl-5-nitroimidazole-1-acetic Acid, 609·2
2-Methyl-5-nitroimidazole-1-propanol, 616·3
2-(2-Methyl-5-nitroimidazol-1-yl)ethanol, 607·2
2-(2-Methyl-5-nitroimidazol-1-yl)ethyl Benzoate, 607·2
(1-Methyl-5-nitroimidazol-2-yl)methyl Carbamate, 615·2
1-(2-Methyl-5-nitroimidazol-1-yl)propan-2-ol, 615·3
6-(1-Methyl-4-nitroimidazol-5-ylthio)purine, 1349·1
4-[(*E*)-2-(1-Methyl-5-nitroimidazol-2-yl)vinyl]pyrimidin-2-ylamine, 602·3
5-Methyl-2-nitro-7-oxa-8-mercurabicyclo[4.2.0]octa-1,3,5-triene, 1186·3
1-Methyl-4-nitro-5-thioimidazole, 1349·3
α-Methylnoradrenaline, 956·1
7α-Methylnorethynodrel, 1572·3
17α-Methyl-19-norpregna-4,9-diene-3,20-dione, 1547·2
7-α-Methyl-19-nortestosterone, 1536·1
6-Methyl-1,2,3-oxathiazin-4(3*H*)-one 2,2-Dioxide Potassium, 1420·3
3-Methyl-1-(5-oxohexyl)-7-propylxanthine, 989·3
(1-Methyl-4-oxo-2-imidazolidinylidene)phosphoramidic Acid, 1689·3

(2*S*-{2α(*E*),3β,4β,5α[$2R^*$,$3R^*$($1R^*$,$2R^*$)]})-9-{[3-Methyl-1-oxo-4-(tetrahydro-3,4-dihydroxy-5-{[3-(2-hydroxy-1-methyl-propyl)oxiranyl]methyl}-2*H*-pyran-2-yl)-2-butenyl]oxy}nonanoic Acid, 233·1
Methylparaben, 1183·3
Methylparaben Sodium, 1183·3
Methylparafynol, 707·1
Methylpartricin, 405·2
2-Methyl-2,4-pentanediol, 1697·1
4-Methylpentan-2-one, 1476·2
5-Methyl-2-pentylphenol, 1168·2
Methylpentynol, 707·1
3-Methylpent-1-yn-3-ol, 707·1
Methylperidol Hydrochloride, 710·1
Methylperone Hydrochloride, 706·1
(*R,S*)-α-Methylphenethylamine, 1584·3
(*R,S*)-α-Methylphenethylamine Sulphate, 1584·3
(+)-α-Methylphenethylamine Sulphate, 1585·3
7-[2-(α-Methylphenethylamino)ethyl]theophylline Hydrochloride, 1588·2
α-(α-Methylphenethylamino)-α-phenylacetonitrile, 1584·3
(±)-3-(α-Methylphenethylamino)propionitrile Hydrochloride, 1588·3
(*S*)-α-Methylphenethylammonium Sulphate, 1585·3
3-(α-Methylphenethyl)-*N*-(phenylcarbamoyl)syndnone Imine, 1589·2
*d-threo*-Methylphenidate, 1587·1
Methylphenidate Hydrochloride, 1590·2
Methylphenobarbital, 366·3
Methylphenobarbitalum, 366·3
Methylphenobarbitone, 366·3
Methylphenol, 1177·3
2-(2-{4-[2-Methyl-3-(phenothiazin-10-yl)propyl]piperazin-1-yl}ethoxy)ethanol, 697·2
2-[1-Methyl-2-(4-phenoxyphenoxy)ethoxy]pyridine, 1509·3
2-Methyl-1,4-phenylenediamine, 1728·3
(7*R*)-3-Methyl-7-(α-D-phenylglycylamino)-3-cephem-4-carboxylic Acid Monohydrate, 168·1
*p*-(5-Methyl-3-phenyl-4-isoxazolyl)benzenesulfonamide, 96·1
(5-Methyl-3-phenyl-4-isoxazolyl)penicillin Sodium, 240·2
*N*-{[*p*-(5-Methyl-3-phenyl-4-isoxazolyl)phenyl]sulfonyl}propionamide Sodium, 79·2
(±)-*trans*-3-Methyl-2-phenylmorpholine Hydrochloride, 1592·2
α-{1-[Methyl(3-phenyl-2-propenyl)amino]ethyl}benzenemethanol Hydrochloride, 1672·2
1-Methyl-4-phenyl-4-propionoxypiperidine, 81·1
3-Methyl-1-phenyl-2-pyrazolin-5-one, 909·2
5-Methyl-1-phenyl-2(1*H*)-pyridone, 1732·3
*N*-Methyl-2-phenylsuccinimide, 370·1
1-Methyl-4-phenyl-1,2,3,6-tetrahydropyridine, 81·1
*N*-Methyl-4-[(α-phenyl-*o*-tolyl)oxy]butylamine, 1660·2
(±)-*N*-Methyl-3-phenyl-3-(α,α,α-trifluoro-*p*-tolyloxy)propylamine Hydrochloride, 292·1
Methylphosphonothioic Acid S-{2-[bis(1-methylethyl)amino]ethyl} *O*-Ethyl Ester, 1719·2
Methylphytylnaphthochinonum, 1467·1
3-(4-Methylpiperazin-1-yliminomethyl)rifamycin SV, 250·2
10-[3-(4-Methylpiperazin-1-yl)propyl]phenothiazine Dimalonate, 713·3
10-[3-(4-Methylpiperazin-1-yl)propyl]-2-trifluoromethylphenothiazine Dihydrochloride, 726·3
α-(4-Methyl-1-piperazinyl)-3′-{[4-(3-pyridyl)-2-pyrimidinyl]amino}-*p*-tolu-*p*-toluidide Methanesulfonate, 562·1
4-(1-Methylpiperidin-4-ylidene)-4*H*-benzo[4,5]cyclohepta-[1,2-*b*]thiophen-10(9*H*)-one Hydrogen Fumarate, 788·1
1-Methyl-4-piperidyl Diphenylpropoxyacetate Hydrochloride, 489·1
(±)-2′-[2-(1-Methyl-2-piperidyl)ethyl]-*p*-anisanilide Hydrochloride, 910·3
10-[2-(1-Methyl-2-piperidyl)ethyl]-2-(methylsulphinyl)phenothiazine, 706·3
10-[2-(1-Methyl-2-piperidyl)ethyl]-2-methylthiophenothiazine, 724·2
(1-Methyl-2-piperidyl)formo-2′,6′-xylidide Hydrochloride, 1381·2
9-(1-Methyl-4-piperidylidene)thioxanthene, 439·1
(*RS*)-9-(1-Methyl-3-piperidylmethyl)thioxanthene Hydrochloride Monohydrate, 485·3
Methylprednisolone, 1106·1
6α-Methylprednisolone, 1106·1
Methylprednisolone Aceponate, 1106·3
Methylprednisolone Acetate, 1106·1
Methylprednisolone 21-Acetate, 1106·1
Methylprednisolone Cipionate, 1107·1
Methylprednisolone Hemisuccinate, 1106·1, 1106·2
Methylprednisolone Hydrogen Succinate, 1106·1
Methylprednisolone 21-(Hydrogen Succinate), 1106·1
Methylprednisolone Sodium Hemisuccinate, 1106·2
Methylprednisolone Sodium Succinate, 1106·2
Methylprednisolone 21-(Sodium Succinate), 1106·2
Methylprednisolone Suleptanate, 1107·1
Methylprednisoloni Acetas, 1106·1
Methylprednisoloni Hydrogenosuccinas, 1106·1
Methylprednisolonum, 1106·1
16β-Methylprednisone, 1106·1
2-Methylpropane, 1236·2
17α-Methyl-17-propionylestra-4,9-dien-3-one, 1568·1
2-Methyl-2-propyltrimethylene Carbamate Isopropylcarbamate, 1392·1
2-Methyl-2-propyltrimethylene Dicarbamate, 706·2
(1*R*,3*r*,5*S*)-8-Methyl-3-(2-propylvaleryloxy)tropanium Bromide, 486·1
*N*-Methyl-*N*-2-propynylbenzylamine Hydrochloride, 978·3
(15*S*)-15-Methylprostaglandin $F_{2\alpha}$, 1514·2
5-Methylpyrazine-2-carboxylic Acid 4-Oxide, 851·1
4-Methylpyrazole, 1039·2
4-Methyl-1*H*-pyrazole, 1039·2
(±)-5-{*p*-[2-(Methyl-2-pyridylamino)ethoxy]benzyl}-2,4-thiazolidinedione Maleate (1:1), 345·2
*N*-Methyl-2-(2-pyridyl)ethylamine, 1660·1
*N*-Methyl-2-(2-pyridyl)ethylamine Bismethanesulphonate, 1660·1
*N*-Methyl-2-(2-pyridyl)ethylamine Dihydrochloride, 1660·1
5-Methyl-3-(2-pyridyl)-2*H*,5*H*-1,3-oxazino[5,6-*c*]-[1,2]benzothiazine-2,4(3*H*)-dione 6,6-Dioxide, 36·2
$N^1$-(4-Methylpyrimidin-2-yl)sulphanilamide, 260·3
10-(1-Methylpyrrolidin-3-ylmethyl)phenothiazine, 437·2
3-{[(*R*)-1-Methyl-2-pyrrolidinyl]methyl}-5-[2-(phenylsulfonyl)ethyl]indole Hydrobromide, 467·1
(*S*)-3-(1-Methylpyrrolidin-2-yl)pyridine, 1720·1
(±)-1-{1-[(4-Methyl-4*H*,6*H*-pyrrolo[1,2-*a*][4,1]benzoxazepin-4-yl)methyl]-4-piperidyl}-2-benzimidazolinone, 1294·3
5-Methylquinolin-8-ol, 617·1
Methylrosaniline Chloride, 1186·1
Methylrosanilinii Chloridum, 1186·1
Methylrosanilinium Chloride, 1186·1
Methylscopolamini Nitras, 483·3
β-Methylserine, 1451·1
6β-[(Methyl[$^{75}$Se]seleno)methyl]-19-norcholest-5(10)-en-3β-ol, 1525·2
(±)-*cis*-2-Methylspiro[1,3-oxathiolane-5,3′-quinuclidine] Hydrochloride Hemihydrate, 1488·3
Methylstanazole, 1569·2
Methylsulfathiazole, 263·1
6-[*N*-(3-Methylsulfonyl-2-oxoimidazolidin-1-ylcarbonyl)-D-phenylglycylamino]penicillanic Acid, 231·1
4-[*p*-(Methylsulfonyl)phenyl]-3-phenyl-2(5*H*)-furanone, 86·3
*N*-(4-Methyl-2-sulphamoyl-$\Delta^2$-1,3,4-thiadiazolin-5-ylidene)acetamide, 953·1
1-[3-(2-Methylsulphonylphenothiazin-10-yl)propyl]piperidine-4-carboxamide, 1276·3
Methylsynephrine Hydrochloride, 977·3
Methyltestosterone, 1559·3
Methyltestosteronum, 1559·3
4-Methyl-1-tetradecylpyridinium Chloride, 1186·3
5-Methyltetrahydrofolate, 1429·2
(2*R*,4*R*)-4-Methyl-1-[(*S*)-$N^2$-{[(*RS*)-1,2,3,4-tetrahydro-3-methyl-8-quinolyl]sulfonyl}arginyl]pipecolic Acid, 864·3
2-Methyl-3-(3,7,11,15-tetramethyl-2,6,10,14-hexadeca-tetraenyl)-1,4-naphthoquinone, 1467·1
2-Methyl-3-[3,7,11,15-tetramethylhexadec-2-enyl] Naphthalene-1,4-dione, 1467·1
Methyltheobromine, 782·1
7-Methyltheophylline, 782·1
$N^1$-(5-Methyl-1,3,4-thiadiazol-2-yl)sulphanilamide, 260·3
3-[(5-Methyl-1,3,4-thiadiazol-2-yl)thiomethyl]-7-(tetrazol-1-ylacetamido)-3-cephem-4-carboxylic Acid, 170·3
6-Methylthiochroman-7-sulphonamide 1,1-Dioxide, 955·2
3-Methylthiofentanyl, 40·3
3-Methyl-2-thiohydantoin, 1597·2
5-Methylthiomethyl-3-(5-nitrofurfurylideneamino)-2-oxazolidone, 611·2
8β-Methylthiomethyl-6-propylergoline Methanesulphonate, 1211·2
Methylthioninii Chloridum, 1042·2
Methylthioninium Chloride, 1042·2
Methylthioninium Chloride, Commercial, 1042·2
(*E*)-1-{2-(Methylthio)-1-[*o*-(pentyloxy)phenyl]vinyl}imidazole Hydrochloride, 406·3
Methylthiouracil, 1602·3
6-Methyl-2-thiouracil, 1602·3
3-*O*-Methyltolcapone, 1216·2
*N*-[(1-Methyl-5-*p*-toluoylpyrrol-2-yl)acetyl]glycine, 14·3
2-Methyl-3-*o*-tolylquinazolin-4-(3*H*)-one, 707·1
5-(3-Methyl-1-triazeno)imidazole-4-carboxamide, 544·3, 587·1
2-({3-Methyl-4-(2,2,2-trifluoroethoxy)-2-pyridyl)methyl} Sulphinylbenzimidazole, 1269·3
2-[α-Methyl-3-(trifluoromethyl)phenethylamino]ethyl Benzoate Hydrochloride, 868·1
2-{[2-Methyl-3-(trifluoromethyl)phenyl]amino}-3-pyridinecarboxylic Acid Compounded with 1-Deoxy-1-(methylamino)-D-glucitol (1:1), 43·3
1-Methyl-3-(4-{*p*-[(trifluoromethyl)thio]phenoxy}-*m*-tolyl)-*s*-triazine-2,4,6-(1*H*,3*H*,5*H*)-trione, 617·3
5-Methyl-6-(3,4,5-trimethoxyanilinomethyl)quinazolin-2,4-diyldiamine Mono-D-glucuronate, 410·2
Methyl-*O*-(3,4,5-trimethoxycinnamoyl)reserpate, 994·3
*N*-Methyl-2,3,3-trimethylbicyclo[2.2.1]hept-2-ylamine Hydrochloride, 951·3
(1*R*,3*r*,5*S*)-8-Methyl-3-[(±)-tropoyloxy]tropanium Bromide, 476·3
(1*R*,3*r*,5*S*)-8-Methyl-3-[(±)-tropoyloxy]tropanium Nitrate, 477·1
α-Methyltyramine, 956·1
α-Methyltyrosine, 956·1
α-Methyl-*p*-tyrosine, 956·1
(−)-α-Methyl-L-tyrosine, 956·1
(±)-α-Methyl-DL-tyrosine, 956·1
Methyluric Acid, 783·1
1-Methyluric Acid, 804·1
(*E*)-8-Methyl-*N*-vanillylnon-6-enamide, 24·2
Methylxanthine, 783·1
1-Methylxanthine, 804·1
3-Methylxanthine, 804·1
1-Methyl-2-(2,6-xylyloxy)ethylamine Hydrochloride, 958·1
Methyment, 2127·3
Methypranolol, 955·3
Methysergide, 469·3
Methysergide Maleate, 469·3
Methysticin, 1703·2
Metibasol, 2127·3
Meticel, 2127·3
Meticil, 2127·3
Meticilina Sódica, 230·3
Meticillin Sodium, 230·3
Meticillinum Natricum, 230·3
Meticlorpindol, 603·1
Meticlotiazida, 953·2
Meticortelone, 2127·4
Meticorten, 2127·4
Meticrane, 955·2
Meticrano, 955·2
Metifarma, 2127·4
Metifarma Mucolit, 2127·4
Metifex, 2127·4
Metifex-L, 2127·4
Metiguanide, 2127·4
Metil Carboprost, 1514·2
Metilarsinato de Sodio, 1748·1
Metilbenactio, Bromuro de, 485·3
Metilbencetonio, Cloruro de, 1186·1
Metilbetasone Solubile, 2127·4
Metilbromuro de Homatropina, 483·2
Metilbromuro de Octatropina, 486·1
Metilbutilcetona, 1476·1
Metilcelulosa, 1580·2
Metilcloroisotiazolinona, 1185·1
Metilcord, 2127·4
Metildigoxin, 955·2
Metildigoxina, 955·2
Metildopa, 953·2
Metildopato, Cloridrato de, 953·2
Metildopato, Hidrocloruro de, 953·2
Metilefedrina, Hidrocloruro de, 1124·2
Metilendioximetanfetamina, 1589·3
Metilene, Blu di, 1042·2
Metileno, Azul de, 1042·2
Metilergometrina, Maleato de, 1714·2
Metiletilcetona, 1476·2
Metilfenidato, Hidrocloruro de, 1590·2
Metilfenobarbital, 366·3
Metilhidroxiquinolina, Metilsulfato de, 1714·2
Metilisobutilcetona, 1476·2
Metilisotiazolinona, 1185·1
Metilmorfina, 27·1
Metilnitrato de Atropina, 477·1
Metilon, 2127·4
Metilparabeno, 1183·3
Metilparabeno Sódico, 1183·3
Metilpentinol, 707·1
Metilpirimifós, 1509·2
Metilprednisolona, 1106·1
Metilprednisolona, Acetato de, 1106·1
Metilprednisolona, Hidrogenosuccinato de, 1106·1
Metilprednisolona, Succinato Sódico de, 1106·2
Metilpren, 2127·4
Metilrosanilina, Cloruro de, 1186·1
Metilsedor, 2127·4
Metilsulfato de Amezinio, 858·2
Metilsulfato de Difemanilo, 481·3
Metilsulfato de Poldina, 488·2
Metilsulfato de Toloconio, 1194·3
Metiltestosterona, 1559·3
Metiltioninio, Cloruro de, 1042·2
Metiltiouracilo, 1602·3
Metimyd, 2127·4
Metina, 2127·4
Metinal-Idantoina, 2127·4
Metinal-Idantoina L, 2127·4
Metindo, 2127·4
Metinet, 2127·4
Metiocolin B12, 2127·4
Metiocolin Composto, 2127·4
Metioduro de Buzepida, 480·2
Metionina, 1042·1, 2127·4
DL-Metionina, 1042·1

Metionina Composta, 2127·4
Metiosulfonio, Cloruro de, 1714·1
Metipranolol, 955·3
Metipregnone, 1557·2
Metirapona, 1715·1
Metirel, 2127·4
Metirosina, 956·1
Metirosine, 956·1
Metisergida, Maleato de, 469·3
Metison, 2127·4
Metisona, 2127·4
Metisoprinol, 640·2
Metivirol, 2127·4
Metixen, 2127·4
Metixene Hydrochloride, 485·3
Metixeni Hydrochloridum, 485·3
Metixeno, Hidrocloruro de, 485·3
Metizolina, Hidrocloruro de, 1124·3
Metizoline Hydrochloride, 1124·3
Meto, 2127·4
Meto Comp, 2127·4
Metobeta, 2128·1
Metobeta Comp, 2128·1
Metoblock, 2128·1
Metoc, 2128·1
Metocal, 2128·1
Metocal Vitamina D, 2128·1
Metocalcium, 2128·1
Metocalcona, 1714·3
Metocar, 2128·1
Metocarbamol, 1395·1
Metochalcone, 1714·3
Metocinium Iodide, 486·1
Metoclan, 2128·1
Metoclopramida, Hidrocloruro de, 1274·3
Metoclopramide, 1274·3
Metoclopramide Dihydrochloride, 1276·2
Metoclopramide Glycyrrhizinate, 1276·2
Metoclopramide Hydrochloride, 1274·3
Metoclopramidi Hydrochloridum, 1274·3
Metoclopramidum, 1274·3
Metoclor, 2128·1
Metoclosan, 2128·1
Meto-comp, 2128·1
Metocontin, 2128·1
Metocor, 2128·1
Metocurine Iodide, 1403·3
Metocyl, 2128·1
Metodilazina, 437·2
Metodilazina, Hidrocloruro de, 437·2
Metodine, 2128·1
Metodoc, 2128·1
Metodura, 2128·1
Metodura Comp, 2128·1
Metofen Compound, 2128·1
Metofen Forte, 2128·1
Metogastron, 2128·1
Metohexal, 2128·1
Metohexal Comp, 2128·1
Metohexital, 1303·2
Metohexital Sódico, 1303·2
Metolar, 2128·1
Metolazona, 956·2
Metolazone, 956·2
Metole, 2128·1
Metolol, 2128·1
Metolol Compositum, 2128·1
Metolon, 2128·2
MetoMed, 2128·2
Metomerck, 2128·2
Metomide, 2128·2
Metomilo, 1507·2
Metomin, 2128·2
Metomit, 2128·2
Metono, 2128·2
Metop, 2128·2
Metopal, 2128·2
Metopimazina, 1276·3
Metopimazine, 1276·3
Metopiron, 2128·2
Metopirone, 2128·2
Metoplex, 2128·2
Metopram, 2128·2
Metopreno, 1507·2
Metopresol, 2128·2
Metopress, 2128·2
Metoprin, 2128·2
Metoprin Balsamico, 2128·2
Metoprogamma, 2128·2
Metoprolin, 2128·2
Metoprolol, 956·3
Metoprolol Fumarate, 956·3
Metoprolol Succinate, 957·1
Metoprolol Tartrate, 957·1
Metoprolol, Tartrato de, 957·1
Metoprololi Succinas, 957·1
Metoprololi Tartras, 957·1
Metoral, 2128·2
Metorene, 2128·2
Metorfan, 2128·2
Metoros, 2128·2
Metosan, 2128·2
Metosix, 2128·2
Metostad Comp, 2128·2
Metosyn, 2128·2
Meto-Tablinen, 2128·3
Meto-thiazid, 2128·3
Metotrexate Sodium, 568·3
Metotrexato, 568·2
Metotrexato Sódico, 568·3
Metotyrol, 2128·3
Metovit, 2128·3
Metoxaleno, 1152·1
Metoxamina, Hidrocloruro de, 953·1
2-Metoxietanol, 1475·2
Metoxifenamina, Hidrocloruro de, 1124·2
Metoxiflurano, 1304·1
Metoxiprim, 2128·3
5-Metoxipsoraleno, 1154·1
4-Metoxypyridoxine, 1692·3
Metozoc, 2128·3
Metozzard, 2128·3
Metral, 2128·3
Metram, 2128·3
Metran, 2128·3
Metrazole, 2128·3
Metrazone, 2128·3
Metrecina, 2128·3
Metrergina, 2128·3
Metreton, 2128·3
Metrexato, 2128·3
Metricom, 2128·3
Metrifonate, 109·2
Metrifonato, 109·2
Metrifonatum, 109·2
Metrigen Fuerte, 2128·3
Metrim, 2128·3
Metrine, 2128·3
Metriphonate, 109·2
Metrizamida, 1067·1
Metrizamide, 1067·1
Metrizoate Meglumine, 1067·2
Metrizoate Sodium, 1067·2
Metrizoato de Meglumina, 1067·2
Metrizoato de Sodio, 1067·2
Metrizoic Acid, 1067·1
Metrizoico, Ácido, 1067·1
Metrizol, 2128·3
Metro, 2128·3
Metrocide, 2128·3
Metrocream, 2128·3
Metrodax, 2128·3
Metroderme, 2128·3
Metrodin, 2128·3
Metrodine, 2128·3
Metrodiyod, 2128·3
Metrofur, 2128·4
Metrogel, 2128·4
Metrogel Vaginal, 2128·4
Metrogestone, 1557·1
Metrogyl, 2128·4
Metrogyl-F, 2128·4
Metrolex, 2128·4
Metrolyl, 2128·4
Metronib, 2128·4
Metronidazol, 607·2
Metronidazol, Benzoato de, 607·2
Metronidazol, Hidrocloruro de, 607·2
Metronidazole, 607·2
Metronidazole Benzoate, 607·2
Metronidazole Hydrochloride, 607·2
Metronidazoli Benzoas, 607·2
Metronidazolum, 607·2
Metronide, 2128·4
Metronid-Puren, 2128·4
Metronil, 2128·4
Metronimerck, 2128·4
Metronix, 2128·4
Metronour, 2128·4
Metront, 2128·4
Metropast, 2128·4
Metrosa, 2128·4
Metroson, 2128·4
Metrostat, 2128·4
Metrotex, 2128·4
Metrotop, 2128·4
Metroval, 2128·4
Metrozine, 2128·4
Metrozol, 2128·4
Metrozole, 2128·4
Met-Rx, 2128·4
Metsal Preparations, 2128·4
Metsec, 2129·1
Met-Sil, 2129·1
Metubine, 2129·1
Metussa, 2129·1
Metussan, 2129·1
Metvix, 2129·1
Metxaprim, 2129·1
Metypred, 2129·1
Metypresol, 2129·1
Metyrapol, 1715·1
Metyrapone, 1715·1
Metyrapone Tartrate, 1715·1
Metyrosine, 956·1
Metysolon, 2129·1
Metyzoline Hydrochloride, 1124·3
Mevacor, 2129·1
Mevalon, 2129·1
Mevalotin, 2129·1
Mevamox, 2129·1
Mevaren, 2129·1
Mevastatin, 958·1
Mevastatina, 958·1
Mevasterol, 2129·1
Mevastin, 2129·1
Mevedal, 2129·1
Mevilin-L, 2129·1
Mevinacor, 2129·1
Mevinol, 2129·1
Mevinolin, 949·1
Mevlor, 2129·1
Mex, 2129·1
Mexalen, 2129·1
Mexan, 2129·1
Mexasone, 2129·2
Mexa-Vit C, 2129·2
Mexazolam, 707·1
Mexcyn, 2129·2
Mexe N, 2129·2
Mexenona, 1154·2
Mexenone, 1154·2
Mexican Aspirin, 36·1
Mexican Scammony Resin, 1267·3
Mexican Scammony Root, 1267·3
Mexican Valium, 698·3
Mexican Vanilla, 1762·3
Mexilen, 2129·2
Mexiletina, Hidrocloruro de, 958·1
Mexiletine Hydrochloride, 958·1
Mexiletini Hydrochloridum, 958·1
Mexitil, 2129·2
Mexitilen, 2129·2
Mexona, 2129·2
Mexoryl SX, 1146·3
Mexsana, 2129·2
Mexyphamine Hydrochloride, 1124·2
Meylon, 2129·2
Mezabox, 2129·2
Mezclas de Hidrocloruros de Alcaloides del Opio, 74·3
Mezen, 2129·2
Mezenol, 2129·2
Mezinc, 2129·2
Meziv, 2129·2
Mezlin, 2129·2
Mezlocilina Sódica, 231·1
Mezlocillin, 231·1
Mezlocillin Sodium, 231·1
Mezolitan, 2129·2
Mezym F, 2129·2
MF 110, 2129·2
MF-465a, 984·2
MF-701, 892·2
MF-934, 254·3
MFP Sodium, 1446·2
MFT, 1593·3
MFV-Ject, 2129·2
Mg 5-Granoral, 2129·2
Mg 5-Granulat, 2129·2
Mg 5-Longoral, 2129·2
Mg 5-Oraleff, 2129·2
Mg 5-Sulfat, 2129·3
MG 50, 2129·2
MG217 Medicated, 2129·2
MG217 Medicated Tar-Free, 2129·2
MG217 Sal-Acid, 2129·3
MG400, 2129·2
Mg-4833, 1687·1
MG-13054, 916·2
MG-13608, 1119·1
MG Cold Sore Formula, 2129·2
MGBG, 573·3
Mg-nor, 2129·3
MH-532, 715·1
MHP-A, 2129·3
M-I-36, 914·1
Mi85, 20·1
MI-216, 1065·3
MI-217, 1490·2
Miabene, 2129·3
Miacalcic, 2129·3
Miacalcin, 2129·3
Mi-Acid, 2129·3
Mi-Acid Gelcaps, 2129·3
Miadenil, 2129·3
Mialgex, 2129·3
Mialin, 2129·3
Miambutol, 2129·3
Mianeurin, 2129·3
Mianin, 1194·3
Mianserin Hydrochloride, 306·3
Mianserina, Hidrocloruro de, 306·3
Mianserini Hydrochloridum, 306·3
Miantor, 2129·3
Miantrex, 2129·3
Miaxan, 2129·3
Miazide, 2129·3
Miazide B6, 2129·3
Mibazol, 2129·3
Mibefradil Dihydrochloride, 959·1
Mibefradil, Hidrocloruro de, 959·1
Mibefradil Hydrochloride, 959·1
MIBK, 1476·2
Mibolerona, 1560·1
Mibolerone, 1560·1
Mibrox, 2129·3
Miburell, 2129·3
Miburell— *see* Dularell Classic, 1956·3
Mica, 2129·3
Micafungin Sodium, 405·2
Mical, 2129·3
Micalpha, 2129·3
Micane, 2129·3
Micanol, 2129·3
Micar, 2129·4
Micardis Preparations, 2129·4
Micarzin, 2129·4
Micatin, 2129·4
Micaveen, 2129·4
Micazin, 2129·4
Miccil, 2129·4
Micebrina, 2129·4
Micelle A Plus E, Bioglan— *see* Bioglan Micelle A plus E, 1844·1
Micelle E, 2129·4
Micelle E, Bioglan— *see* Bioglan Micelle E, 1844·1
Micerfin, 2129·4
Micetal, 2129·4
Micetinoftalmina, 2129·4
Miciclin, 2129·4
Micifrona, 2129·4
Mickey Finn, 684·3

Miclast, 2129·4
Miclobet, 2129·4
Miclonazol, 2129·4
Micoban, 2129·4
Micocert, 2129·4
Micocid, 2129·4
Micocide, 2130·1
Micoderm, 2130·1
Micoespec, 2130·1
Micofenolato de Mofetilo, 1361·2
Micoffen, 2130·1
Micofim, 2130·1
Micofin, 2130·1
Micofitex, 2130·1
Micofoot, 2130·1
Micofulvin, 2130·1
Micogal, 2130·1
Micogel, 2130·1
Micogen, 2130·1
Micogin, 2130·1
Micogyn, 2130·1
Micoisdin, 2130·1
Micoless, 2130·1
Micolette, 2130·1
Micolis, 2130·1
Micolis Novo, 2130·1
Micoliv, 2130·1
Micomax, 2130·1
Micomazol, 2130·1
Micomazol B, 2130·1
Micomazol Deo, 2130·1
Micomicen, 2130·1
Micomisan, 2130·1
Miconacina, 2130·1
Miconal, 2130·1
Miconan, 2130·1
Miconax, 2130·1
Miconazol, 405·2
Miconazol, Nitrato de, 405·3
Miconazole, 405·2
Miconazole Nitrate, 405·3
Miconazoli Nitras, 405·3
Miconazolum, 405·2
Miconol, 2130·1
Micopirox, 2130·2
Micoplex, 2130·2
Micoral, 2130·2
Micoren, 2130·2
Micos, 2130·2
Micosan, 2130·2
Micoser, 2130·2
Micoset, 2130·2
Micosid, 2130·2
Micosil, 2130·2
Micosol, 2130·2
Micosona, 2130·2
Micostatin, 2130·2
Micosten, 2130·2
Micostop, 2130·2
Micostyl, 2130·2
Micotar, 2130·2
Micotarin, 2130·2
Micotef, 2130·2
Micotenk, 2130·2
Micotiazol, 2130·2
Micoticum, 2130·2
Micotissim, 2130·2
Micotopic, 2130·2
Micotox, 2130·2
Micotral, 2130·2
Micotrat, 2130·2
Micotrim, 2130·2
Micotrim P, 2130·2
Micotrim S, 2130·2
Micotrizol, 2130·2
Micoxolamina, 2130·2
Micoz, 2130·3
Micozen, 2130·3
Micozol Compuesto, 2130·3
Micozole, 2130·3
Micrainin, 2130·3
Micral Test, 2130·3
Micral Test II, 2130·3
Micral Test S, 2130·3
Micralax, 2130·3
Micraleve, 2130·3
Micraltest II, 2130·3
Micranet, 2130·3
Micranil, 2130·3
Micreme, 2130·3
Micreme H, 2130·3
MICRhoGAM, 2130·3
Micristin, 2130·3
Micro +, 2130·3
Micro I, 2130·3
Micro Cr, 2130·3
Micro Cu, 2130·3
Micro Mn, 2130·3
Micro Se, 2130·3
Micro Zn, 2130·3
Microadenoma— *see* Hyperprolactinaemia, 1315·2
Microalbustix, 2130·3
Microangiopathies, Thrombotic— *see* Thrombotic Microangiopathies, 758·1
Microbactim, 2130·3
Microbamat, 2130·3
Microbar-Colon, 2130·3
Microbar-HD (E-Z-HD), 2130·3
Microbiogen, 2130·3
Microbumintest, 2130·3
Microcasen, 2130·4
Microcid, 2130·4
Microcidal, 2130·4
Microcide, 1694·2
Microclisma Evacuante AD-BB, 2130·4
Microclismi Marco Viti, 2130·4
Microclismi Sella, 2130·4
Microcrystalline Cellulose, 1578·3
Microcrystalline Cellulose and Carboxymethylcellulose Sodium, 1578·3
Microcrystalline Wax, 1481·3
Microdiol, 2130·4
Microdit, 2130·4
Microdoine, 2130·4
Microfemin, 2130·4
Microfer, 2130·4
Microgel, 2130·4
Microgen, 2130·4
Microgest, 2130·4
Microgeste, 2130·4
Microginon, 2130·4
Microgyn, 2130·4
Microgynon, 2130·4
Microgynon 30, 2130·4
Micro-K, 2130·4
Microka, 2130·4
Micro-Kalium, 2130·4
Microklist, 2130·4
Microlax, 2130·4
Microlet, 2131·1
Microlev, 2131·1
Microlevlen ED, 2131·1
Microlipid, 2131·1
Microlite, 2131·1
Microlut, 2131·1
Microluton, 2131·1
Micromex, 2131·1
*Micromonospora*, 116·1, 158·3
*Micromonospora inyoensis*, 255·1
Micromycin, 2131·1
Micronase, 2131·1
MicroNefrin, 2131·1
Micronema, 2131·1
Micronoan, 2131·1
Micronomicin Sulfate, 231·3
Micronomicin Sulphate, 231·3
Micronomicina, Sulfato de, 231·3
Micronor, 2131·1
Micronor, Evorel— *see* Evorel Micronor, 1984·3
Micronor HRT, 2131·1
Micronor, Ortho— *see* Ortho Micronor, 2193·3
Micronovum, 2131·1
Micronutrients, 1419·1
Micropaque, 2131·1
Microphta, 2131·1
Microphyllin, 2131·1
Micropil, 2131·1
Micropirin, 2131·1
Micropur, 2131·1
Micropyrin, 2131·1
Microrgan, 2131·1
Microsan N, 2131·1
Microscopic Polyangiitis— *see* Polyarteritis Nodosa and Microscopic Polyangiitis, 1085·3
Microser, 2131·1
Microshield Preparations, 2131·1
Microsol, 2131·2
Microsona, 2131·2
Microsona C, 2131·2
Microsona Otica, 2131·2
Microsporidiosis, 598·2
Microstix-3, 2131·2
Microstix Candida, 2131·2
Microsulf, 2131·2
Microterol, 2131·2
Microtid, 2131·2
Microtrast, 2131·2
Microtrim, 2131·2
Microvacin, 2131·2
Microval, 2131·2
Microvibrate, 2131·2
Microvita, 2131·2
Microvlar, 2131·2
Microx— *see* Mykrox, 2147·4
Microxin, 2131·2
Microzepam, 2131·2
Microzide, 2131·2
Mictarin, 2131·2
Mictasol, 2131·2
Mictasol Azul, 2131·3
Mictasol Bleu, 2131·3
Mictasol com Sulfa, 2131·3
Mictasone, 2131·3
Mictonetten, 2131·3
Mictonorm, 2131·3
Mictral, 2131·3
Mictrex, 2131·3
Mictrin, 2131·3
Micturition Disorders, 475·3
Micturol Sedante, 2131·3
Micutrin, 2131·3
Micutrin Beta, 2131·3
Midacina, 2131·3
Midaglizol, 343·2
Midaglizole, 343·2
Midalcipran Hydrochloride, 307·3
Midalet, 2131·3
Midalgan, 2131·3
Midalgan, Balsamo— *see* Balsamo Midalgan, 1827·3
Midamor, 2131·3
Midarine, 2131·3
Midaselect, 2131·3
Midatenk, 2131·3
Midax, 2131·3
Midazol, 2131·4
Midazolam, 707·1
Midazolam, Hidrocloruro de, 707·2
Midazolam Hydrochloride, 707·2
Midazolam Maleate, 707·2
Midazolam, Maleato de, 707·2
Midazolamum, 707·1
Midchlor, 2131·4
Midecamicina, 231·3
Midecamin, 2131·4
Midecamycin, 231·3
Midecamycin $A_1$, 231·3
Midecamycin Acetate, 231·3
Midecamycin Diacetate, 231·3
Midecin, 2131·4
Midelin, 2131·4
Miderm, 2131·4
Midermus, 2131·4
Midetol, 2131·4
Midium, 2131·4
Midodrina, Hidrocloruro de, 959·2
Midodrine Hydrochloride, 959·2
Midol Preparations, 2131·4
Midolam, 2131·4
Midolen, 2131·4
Midon, 2131·4
Midoride, 2131·4
Midotens, 2131·4
Midrat, 2132·1
Midriati, 2132·1
Midriaticum, 2132·1
Midrid, 2132·1
Midrin, 2132·1
Midriodavi, 2132·1
Midro, 2132·1
Midro Abfuhr, 2132·1
Midro Pico, 2132·1
Midro Tee, 2132·1
Midro-Tea, 2132·1
Miduret, 2132·1
Midy Vitamine C, 2132·1
Midysalb, 2132·1
Miegel, 2132·1
Miel Blanc, 1434·2
Miel Purificada, 1434·2
Mielocol, 2132·1
Mielogen, 2132·1
Mielomade, 2132·1
Mielucin, 2132·1
MIF, 1332·3
Mifegest, 2132·1
Mifegyne, 2132·1
Mifeprex, 2132·1
Mifepristona, 1560·2
Mifepristone, 1560·2
Miferen, 2132·1
Miflasona, 2132·2
Miflasone, 2132·2
Miflonide, 2132·2
Miformin, 2132·2
Migard, 2132·2
Migea, 2132·2
Migent, 2132·2
Miglitol, 343·2
Miglucan, 2132·2
Miglustat, 1715·2
Migpriv, 2132·2
Migra Dioxadol, 2132·2
Migra Dorixina, 2132·2
Migracin, 2132·2
Migradol, Ordov— *see* Ordov Migradol, 2192·1
Migradon, 2132·2
Migraeflux MCP, 2132·2
Migraeflux N, 2132·2
Migraeflux Orange N, 2132·2
Migrafen, 2132·2
Migrafin, 2132·2
Migragesic, 2132·2
Migrai-Care, Extralife— *see* Extralife Migrai-Care, 1986·3
Migraine, 464·2
Migraine, Abdominal— *see* Abdominal Migraine, 470·3
Migraine Ice, 2132·2
Migraine-Kranit, 2132·2
Migraine-Kranit Nova, 2132·2
Migrainous Neuralgia— *see* Cluster Headache, 464·1
Migral, 2132·2
Migral II, 2132·2
Migral Compositum, 2132·2
Migralave N, 2132·3
Migraleve, 2132·3
Migralgine, 2132·3
Migraliv, 2132·3
Migramax, 2132·3
Migranal, 2132·3
Migranat, 2132·3
Migrane, 2132·3
Migra-Nefersil, 2132·3
Migrane-Gastreu R16, 2132·3
Migrane-Kranit Duo, 2132·3
Migrane-Kranit Kombi, 2132·3
Migrane-Kranit Mono, 2132·3
Migrane-Kranit N, 2132·3
Migrane-Neuridal, 2132·3
Migranerton, 2132·3
Migranil, 2132·3
Migranin, 2132·3
Migranin Ibuprofen, 2132·3
Migranol, 2132·3
Migraprim, 2132·3
Migraspirina, 2132·3
Migrastick, 2132·3

Migratam, 2132·3
Migratan S, 2132·3
Migratapsin, 2132·4
Migratine, 2132·4
Migravess, 2132·4
Migrax, 2132·4
Migrenin, 82·3
Migretil, 2132·4
Migrexa, 2132·4
Migril, 2132·4
Migristene, 2132·4
Migwell, 2132·4
Mihexine, 2132·4
Mijal, 2132·4
Mijex, 2132·4
Mijex Extra, 2132·4
Mikacin, 2132·4
Mikan, 2132·4
Mikanil, 2132·4
Mikavir, 2132·4
Mikazul, 2132·4
Mikelan, 2132·4
Mikesan, 2132·4
Mi-Ke-Sons, 2132·4
Miketos, 2132·4
Mikium, 2132·4
Miklogen, 2132·4
Mikostat, 2132·4
Mikostat Baby Ointment, 2132·4
Mikozal, 2133·1
Mikozal, Gyno-— *see* Gyno-Mikozal, 2034·1
Mikro-30, 2133·1
Mikrobac, 2133·1
Mikrozid, 2133·1
Mikutan N, 2133·1
Mil Cobalin Nueva Formula, 2133·1
Mila-Asma, 2133·1
Mila-Cono, 2133·1
Milafed, 2133·1
Milagin, 2133·1
Milamet, 2133·1
Milamox, 2133·1
Milanidazole, 2133·1
Milanolone, 2133·1
Mila-Tercon, 2133·1
Milavir, 2133·1
Milax, 2133·1
Milbedoce Anabolico, 2133·1
Milbemicina Oxima, 110·1
Milbemycin Oxime, 110·1
Milbeta, 2133·1
Milbron, 2133·1
Milchsäure, 1704·1
Milco, 2133·1
Milcopen, 2133·1
Mild Mercurous Chloride, 1712·3
Mild Silver Protein, 1746·2
Mildison, 2133·1
Miles Nervine, 2133·1
Milfarin, 2133·1
Milfoil, 1646·2
Milgamma, 2133·1
Milgamma Mono, 2133·1
Milgamma N, 2133·1
Milgamma-NA, 2133·1
Milgex, 2133·2
Milical, 2133·2
Milice, 2133·2
Milid, 2133·2
Milidon, 2133·2
Milidon CF, 2133·2
Milidon Compound, 2133·2
Miliken Mucol Med Retard, 2133·2
Miliken Mucol Retard, 2133·2
Miliken Mucolitico, 2133·2
Milithin, 2133·2
Milk of Magnesia, 2133·2
Milk of Magnesia, Phillips'— *see* Phillips' Milk of Magnesia, 2217·2
Milk Sugar, 1438·3
Milk of Sulfur, 1158·2
Milk Thistle, 1043·3, 2133·2
Milk Thistle Formula, 2133·2
Milk-Alkali Syndrome— *see* Metabolic Alkalosis, 1217·3
Milkinol, 2133·2
Milk-Thistle Fruit, 1043·3
Milla, 2133·2
Millefolii Herba, 1646·2
Millepertuis, 299·1
Millerspas, 2133·2
Milli Anovlar, 2133·2
Millibar, 2133·2
Millicortene, 2133·2
Millicortenol, 2133·2
Millicorten-Vioform, 2133·2
Milligynon, 2133·2
Millisrol, 2133·2
Millypar, 2133·2
Milnaciprán, Hidrocloruro de, 307·3
Milnacipran Hydrochloride, 307·3
Milneuron NA, 2133·3
Milneuron Plus, 2133·3
Miloderme, 2133·3
Milodistim, 755·3
Milorex, 2133·3
Miloride, 2133·3
Milpar, 2133·3
Mil-Par, 2133·3
Milrila, 2133·3
Milrinona, 959·2
Milrinona, Lactato de, 959·2
Milrinone, 959·2
Milrinone Lactate, 959·2
Milrosina, 2133·3
Milrosina Nistatina, 2133·3
Milsan, 2133·3
Milsana, 2133·3
Miltaun, 2133·3
Miltefosina, 573·2
Miltefosine, 573·2
Miltex, 2133·3
Miltina HA, 2133·3
Miltina IPO, 2133·3
Milton, 2133·3
Milton Anti-Bacterial, 2133·3
Miltown, 2133·3
Milumel AR, 2133·3
Milumel HA, 2133·3
Milumil, 2133·3
Milupa Preparations, 2133·3
Milupan, Aptamil HA Con— *see* Aptamil HA con LCP Milupan, 1809·3
Milurit, 2133·4
Milvane, 2133·4
Milyzer, 2133·4
Milzine, 2133·4
Mimedran, 2133·4
Mimixin, 2133·4
Min Huil, 2133·4
Min O, 2133·4
Minac 50, 2133·4
Minachlor, 2133·4
Minadex, 2133·4
Minadex Mix, 2133·4
Minadex Mix Ginseng, 2133·4
Minakne, 2133·4
Minalfene, 2134·1
Minalgin, 2134·1
Minalka, 2134·1
Minamino, 2134·1
Minaphlex, 2134·1
Min-A-Pon, 2134·1
Minard's Liniment, 2134·1
Minax, 2134·1
Minaxen, 2134·1
Minaza, 2134·1
Minazol, 2134·1
Mincifit, 2134·1
Mindac, 2134·1
Mindiab, 2134·1
Mindol, 2134·1
Mindol-Merck, 2134·1
Mindosan V, 2134·1
Minegyl, 2134·1
Minegyl C/Nistatina, 2134·1
Mineral, 2134·1
Mineral Oil, 1479·1
Mineral Oil, Light, 1479·2
Mineral Oil, Light, Topical, 1479·2
Mineral Oil, Light, White, 1479·1
Mineral Oil, Topical Light, 1479·2
Mineral Oil, White, 1479·1
Mineral Soap, 1577·2
Mineralis, Pix, 1159·2
Mineralised Methylated Spirits, 1185·3
Mineralocorticoids, 1068·1
Minerals, 1417·1
Minerasol, 2134·1
Minerell, 2134·1
Minerva, 2134·1
Minervicomplex, 2134·1
Minervit, 2134·1
Minervit Plus, 2134·1
Minesol, 2134·1
Minesse, 2134·1
Minestril, 2134·2
Minestrin, 2134·2
Minfaden, 2134·2
Minha, 2134·2
28 Mini, 2134·2
Mini New Gen, 2134·2
Mini Ovulo Lanzas, 2134·2
Mini Pregnon, 2134·2
Mini Pseudo, 2134·2
Mini Thin Asthma Relief— *see* Mini Two-Way Action, 2134·2
Mini Thin Pseudo— *see* Mini Pseudo, 2134·2
Mini Two-Way Action, 2134·2
Minian, 2134·2
Minias, 2134·2
Miniasal, 2134·2
Minibit, 2134·2
Miniblock, 2134·2
Minidalton, 2134·2
Miniderm, 2134·2
Minidex, 2134·2
Minidiab, 2134·2
Minidine, 2134·2
Minidol, 2134·2
Minidril, 2134·2
Minidyne, 2134·2
Minifom, 2134·2
Mini-Gamulin Rh, 2134·2
Minigeste, 2134·2
Mini-Glynase, 2134·2
Mini-Gravigard, 2134·2
Minihep, 2134·3
Minilax, 2134·3
Minima, 2134·3
Minimal Brain Dysfunction— *see* Hyperactivity, 1583·1
Minimal Change Disease— *see* Glomerular Kidney Disease, 1080·2
Minimal Change Nephropathy— *see* Glomerular Kidney Disease, 1080·2
Minims Artificial Tears, 2134·3
Mini-Pe, 2134·3
Miniphase, 2134·3
Minipil, 2134·3
Mini-Pill, 2134·3
Minipres, 2134·3
Minipress, 2134·3
Minirin, 2134·3
Minirin/DDAVP, 2134·3
Miniscap, 2134·3
Mini-sintrom, 2134·3
Minisiston, 2134·3
Minisol, 2134·3
Minison, 2134·3
Ministat, 2134·3
Miniten, 2134·3
Minitran, 2134·3
MinitranS, 2134·3
Minit-Rub, 2134·3
Minizide, 2134·3
Mino-50, 2134·4
Mino T, 2134·4
Minobese, 2134·4
Minocalve, 2134·4
Minociclina, Hidrocloruro de, 231·3
Minocin, 2134·4
Minoclin, 2134·4
Minoclir, 2134·4
Minocycline, 231·3
Minocycline Hydrochloride, 231·3
Minocyclini Hydrochloridum, 231·3
Minoderm, 2134·4
Minodiab, 2134·4
Minofen, 2134·4
Minogal, 2134·4
Minogalen, 2134·4
Minolis, 2134·4
Minomax, 2134·4
Minomex, 2134·4
Minomycin, 2134·4
Minona, 2134·4
Minoplus, 2134·4
Minopres, 2134·4
Minor, 2134·4
Minor Tranquillisers, 663·1
Minoral, 2134·4
Minorplex, 2134·4
Minostad, 2134·4
Minot, 2134·4
Minotab, 2134·4
Minotabs, 2134·4
Minoton, 2134·4
Minotrex, 2134·4
Minotyrol, 2134·4
Minovag, 2134·4
Minovital, 2135·1
Min-Ovral, 2135·1
Mino-Wolff, 2135·1
Minox, 2135·1
Minoxi, 2135·1
Minoxidil, 960·1
Minoxidilum, 960·1
Minoxidine, 2135·1
Minoxigaine, 2135·1
Minoximen, 2135·1
Minoxitrim, 2135·1
Minozinan, 2135·1
Minprog, 2135·1
Minprostin, 2135·1
Minprostin $E_2$, 2135·1
Minprostin $F_{2}\alpha$, 2135·1
Minra, 2135·1
Minrin, 2135·1
Mint, 1749·1
Mint, Black, 1283·2
Mint Oil, 1715·2
Mint Oil, Dementholised, 1715·2
Mint Oil, Partly Dementholised, 1715·2
Mint Weed, 1730·3
Mint, White, 1283·2
Mintaglos, 2135·1
Mintamox, 2135·1
Mintavit-C, 2135·1
Mintec, 2135·1
Mintetten Truw, 2135·1
Mintezol, 2135·1
Mint-Lysoform, 2135·1
Mintox, 2135·1
Mintox Plus, 2135·1
Mintox Plus, Extra Strength— *see* Extra Strength Mintox Plus, 1986·2
Minulet, 2135·1
Minulette, 2135·2
Minuric, 2135·2
Minurin, 2135·2
Minus Fat, 2135·2
Minus Fat Extra, 2135·2
Minuslip, 2135·2
Minusorb, 2135·2
Minute-Gel, 2135·2
Minutil, 2135·2
MinVitin, 2135·2
Minzol Trost Tropfen, Kneipp— *see* Kneipp Minzol Trost Tropfen, 2081·3
Mio Aldoron, 2135·2
Mio Relax, 2135·2
Miocacin, 2135·2
Miocalven, 2135·2
Miocalven D, 2135·2
Miocamen, 2135·2
Miocamycin, 231·3, 2135·2
Miocardin, 2135·2
Miocarpine, 2135·2
Miochol, 2135·2
Miochol-E, 2135·2
Miochole, 2135·2

Miociclin, 2135·2
Mio-Citalgan, 2135·2
Miocor, 2135·2
Miocoron, 2135·2
Miocrin, 2135·2
Miocuril, 2135·3
Miodarid, 2135·3
Miodaron, 2135·3
Miodene, 2135·3
Miodom, 2135·3
Miodrina, 2135·3
Miodrone, 2135·3
Mioflex, 2135·3
Miogesil, 2135·3
Miokacin, 2135·3
Miokalium, 2135·3
Miokamycin, 231·3
Miol, 2135·3
Miolastan, 2135·3
Miolene, 2135·3
Mionevrasi, 2135·3
Mionevrix, 2135·3
Miopat, 2135·3
Miopropan, 2135·3
Miopropan Proctologico, 2135·3
Miopropan-T, 2135·3
Miorel, 2135·3
Miorrelax, 2135·3
Mios, 2135·3
Miosal, 2135·3
Miosan, 2135·3
Miosen, 2135·3
Miostat, 2135·3
Miostenil, 2135·4
Miosys, 2135·4
Miotenk, 2135·4
Miotens, 2135·4
Miotic Double, 2135·4
Mioticol, 2135·4
Miotin, 2135·4
Miotonachol, 2135·4
Miotonal, 2135·4
Miotyn, 2135·4
Mio-Virobron, 2135·4
Miovisin, 2135·4
Miowas G, 2135·4
Miozac, 2135·4
Miozets, 2135·4
Miphar, 2135·4
Mi-Pilo, 2135·4
Mipramid, 2135·4
Mipraz, 2135·4
MIR, 2135·4
Mira Klonal, 2135·4
Miraa, 1585·2
Mirabel, 2135·4
Mirabol, 2135·4
Miracef, 2135·4
Miracid, 2135·4
Miraclar, 2135·4
Miracle Fruit, 1715·2
Miraclid, 2135·4
Miraclin, 2135·4
Miracorten, 2135·4
Miraculin, 1715·2
Miradol, 2135·4
Miradon, 2135·4
Miraflow, 2135·4
Mirafur, 2135·4
Miral, 2136·1
MiraLax, 2136·1
Miralis, 2136·1
Miraluma, 2136·1
Miramycin, 2136·1
Miranax, 2136·1
Miranova, 2136·1
Mirantal, 2136·1
Mirapex, 2136·1
Mirapexin, 2136·1
Mirapront N, 2136·1
Mirasan, 2136·1
MiraSept, 2136·1
Miraton, 2136·1
Mirax, 2136·1
Miraxid, 2136·1
Miraxx, 2136·1
Mirazul, 2136·1
Mirbane, Oil of, 1722·2
Mircette, 2136·1
Mircol, 2136·1
Mirelle, 2136·1
Mirena, 2136·1
Miretic, 2136·2
Mireze, 2136·2
Mirfat, 2136·2
Mirfudorm, 2136·2
Mirfulan, 2136·2
Mirfulan Spray N, 2136·2
Mirfusot, 2136·2
Mirimostim, 756·3
Mirion, 2136·2
Miripirio, Cloruro de, 1186·3
Miripirium Chloride, 1186·3
Miristalconio, Cloruro de, 1186·3
Miristalkonium Chloride, 1186·3
Miristato de Isopropilo, 1481·2
Mirococept, 1675·2
Mirorroidin, 2136·2
Miroton, 2136·2
Miroton N, 2136·2
Mirpan, 2136·2
Mirquin, 2136·2
Mirra, 1718·3
Mirsol, 2136·2
Mirtaz, 2136·2
Mirtazapina, 307·3
Mirtazapine, 307·3
Mirtazon, 2136·2
Mirtecaína, 1381·3
Mirtex P, 2136·2
Mirtilene, 2136·2
Mirtilene Forte, 2136·2
Mirtilo, 1718·3
Mirtilus, 2136·2
Mirtilvedo C, 2136·2
Mirtiros, 2136·2
Mirtivit, 2136·2
Mirus, 2136·2
Mirus-S, 2136·2
Misari, 1666·1
Miscidon, 2136·2
Misodex, 2136·2
Misodomin, 2136·2
Misofenac, 2136·2
Misone, 2136·3
Misoprostol, 1519·2
Misoprostol Acid, 1519·3
Misordil, 2136·3
Misostol, 2136·3
Misotrol, 2136·3
Misovan, 2136·3
Mission Prenatal, 2136·3
Mission Surgical Supplement, 2136·3
Mist, 1730·3
Mist Expect Stim, 2136·3
Mistabron, 2136·3
Mistabronco, 2136·3
Mistalin, 2136·3
Mistaline, 2136·3
Mistamin, 2136·3
Mistamine, 2136·3
Mistel Curarina, 2136·3
Mistel, Kneipp Pflanzen-Dragees— *see* Kneipp Pflanzen-Dragees Mistel, 2081·3
Mistelkraut, 1715·3
Mistel-Krautertabletten, 2136·3
Mistelol-Kapseln, 2136·3
Mistel-Pflanzensaft, Kneipp— *see* Kneipp Mistel-Pflanzensaft, 2081·3
Misteltropfen, 2136·3
Misteltropfen Hofmanns, 2136·3
Mistick Verde, 2136·3
Mistletoe, 1715·3
Mistletoe, European, 1715·3
Mistral, 2136·3
Misubar, 2136·3
Misulban, 2136·3
Misultina, 2136·3
Misura, 2136·3
Misurid, 2136·3
Misurid Plus, 2136·3
MIT, 1594·1
Mita-c, 2136·3
Mitan, 2136·3
Mitchell Expel Anti Lice Spray, 2136·4
Miten, 2136·4
Miten Plus, 2136·4
Mite-X, 2136·4
Mitex, 2136·4
Mitexan, 2136·4
Mithen, 2136·4
Mithracin, 2136·4
Mithracine, 2136·4
Mithramycin, 580·2
Miticocan, 2136·4
Mitiderma, 2136·4
Mitil, 2136·4
Mitilase, 2136·4
Mitituss, 2136·4
Mitobronitol, 573·2
Mitocin, 2136·4
Mitocin-C, 2136·4
Mitocor, 2136·4
Mitocortyl, 2136·4
Mitocyna, 2136·4
Mitog, 2136·4
Mitoguazona, Dihidrocloruro de, 573·3
Mitoguazone Acetate, 573·3
Mitoguazone Dihydrochloride, 573·3
Mitokebir, 2136·4
Mitokor, 2136·4
Mitolactol, 573·3
Mitolem, 2136·4
Mito-medac, 2136·4
Mitomicina, 573·3
Mitomycin, 573·3
Mitomycin C, 573·3
Mitomycine C, 573·3
Mitomycinum, 573·3
Mitonovag, 2136·4
Mitostat, 2136·4
Mitosyl, 2136·4
Mitotane, 575·1
Mitotano, 575·1
Mitotic Inhibitors, 492·1
Mitotie, 2136·4
Mitoxal, 2136·4
Mitoxana, 2137·1
Mitoxantrona, Hidrocloruro de, 575·2
Mitoxantrone Hydrochloride, 575·2
Mitoxantroni Hydrochloridum, 575·2
Mitoxgen, 2137·1
Mitoxmar, 2137·1
Mitozantrone Hydrochloride, 575·2
Mitozytrex, 2137·1
Mitran, 2137·1
Mitranax, 2137·1
Mitroken, 2137·1
Mitrolan, 2137·1
Mitrotan, 2137·1
Mitrotil, 2137·1
Mitroxone, 2137·1
Mit's Linctus Codeinae Co, 2137·1
Mittavin, 2137·1
Mittoval, 2137·1
Mivacron, 2137·1
Mivacurio, Cloruro de, 1403·3
Mivacurium Chloride, 1403·3
Mivalen, 2137·1
Mivazerol, 961·2
Mivitase 2000, 2137·1
Mixandex, 2137·1
Mixavit, 2137·1
Mixavit, New— *see* New Mixavit, 2165·4
Mixavit-M, 2137·1
Mixed Botulinum Antitoxin, 1610·3
Mixed Vegetable Tablets, 2137·1
Mixer, 2137·1
Mixgen, 2137·1
Mixobar, 2137·1
Mixogen, 2137·1
Mixotone, 2137·1
Mixtard Preparations, 2137·2
Mixtard, Human— *see* Human Mixtard, 2049·2
Mixtard 30/70— *see also* Pork Mixtard 30, 2228·3
Mixtard, Pork— *see* Pork Mixtard 30, 2228·3
Mixtus, 2137·2
Miya-BM, 2137·2
Mizar, 2137·2
Mizolastina, 437·3
Mizolastine, 437·3
Mizolen, 2137·2
Mizollen, 2137·2
Mizolmex, 2137·2
Mizoltec, 2137·3
Mizonase, 2137·3
Mizoribina, 1360·3
Mizoribine, 1360·3
Mizoron, 2137·3
Mizosin, 2137·3
MJ-1999, 1001·3
MJ-4309-1, 486·3
MJ-5190, 1115·1
MJ-9022-1, 672·2
MJ-9067-1, 910·3
MJ-10061, 414·3
MJ-13105-1, 877·1
MJ-13754-1, 309·2
MJ-13805-1, 701·1
MJD-30, 424·2
MJF-9325, 561·1
MJF-10938, 1029·2
MJF-11567-3, 167·2
MJF-12264, 586·2
MK4, 1467·1
MK-130, 1393·1
MK-135, 889·3
MK-188, 1573·3
MK-191, 244·1
MK-208, 1265·2
MK-0217, 765·3
MK-217, 765·3
MK-231, 91·2
MK-240, 316·2
MK-306, 177·2
MK-341, 806·3
MK-351, 953·2
MK-360, 114·2
MK-366, 238·3
MK-383, 1013·3
MK-0383, 1013·3
MK-397, 105·2
MK-401, 103·3
MK-421, 909·2
MK-422, 909·3
MK-462, 471·1
MK-0462, 471·1
MK-476, 788·3
MK-485, 1204·3
MK-486, 1204·3
MK-507, 908·3
MK-0507, 908·3
MK-521, 946·3
MK-595, 913·2
MK-639, 638·2
MK-0639, 638·2
MK-647, 34·1
MK-650, 1096·2
MK-0663, 38·2
MK-0681, 1055·2
MK-733, 997·1
MK-745, 1274·3
MK-781, 956·1
MK-787, 221·1
MK-0787, 221·1
MK-790-, 54·1
MK-791, 188·1
MK-793, 900·1
MK-801, 1683·1
MK-803, 949·1
MK-826, 207·3
MK-0826, 207·3
MK-0869, 1250·3
MK-870, 858·2
MK-905, 103·3
MK-0906, 1554·2
MK-906, 1554·2
MK-0936, 101·2
MK-950, 1012·2
MK-0954, 947·2

MK-955, 214·2
MK-965, 528·3
MK-0966, 86·3
MK-990, 114·1
MK-0991, 395·3
ML 20, 2137·3
ML-236B, 958·1
ML-1024, 914·2
ML-1129, 1514·1
ML-1229, 1514·1
ML Cu 250, 2137·3
ML Cu 375, 2137·3
M-long, 2137·3
M&M, 1589·3
MM-14151, 193·3
MM Diplovax, 2137·3
MM Expectorante, 2137·3
M-M Vax, 2137·3
MMH, 1717·3
MMR, 2137·3
MMR II, 2137·3
MMR Triplovax, 2137·3
MMR Vax, 2137·3
MMR/Vac(Live), 1625·1
MN-1695, 1267·3
MND, 2137·3
MnDPDP, 1067·1
Mnesis, 2137·3
MN-Fusin, 2137·3
Mnoana, 1666·1
MO-911, 978·3
Moban, 2137·3
Mobec, 2137·3
Mobemide, 2137·3
Moben, 2137·3
Mobex, 2137·3
Mobic, 2137·3
Mobicox, 2137·4
Mobidin, 2137·4
Mobiflex, 2137·4
Mobiforton, 2137·4
Mobigesic, 2137·4
Mobilat Preparations, 2137·4
Mobilis, 2137·4
Mobilisin, 2137·4
Mobilisin Composto, 2137·4
Mobilisin Plus, 2137·4
Mobilyzer, 2137·4
Mobisyl, 2137·4
Mobloc, 2137·4
Moclamine, 2137·4
Moclix, 2138·1
Moclo A, 2138·1
Moclobemida, 308·2
Moclobemide, 308·2
Moclodura, 2138·1
Moctanin, 2138·1
Mocydone, 2138·1
Mod, 2138·1
Modafinil, 1591·1
Modafinil, Acid, 1591·1
Modafinilo, 1591·1
Modal, 2138·1
Modalim, 2138·1
Modalina, 2138·1
Modamide, 2138·1
Modane, 2138·1
Modane Bulk, 2138·1
Modane Soft, 2138·1
Modantis, 2138·1
Modasomil, 2138·1
Modaton, 2138·1
Modaton NI, 2138·1
Modavigil, 2138·1
Modecate, 2138·1
Modecate Acutum, 2138·1
Modekal, 2138·1
Modellsweet, 2138·1
Modenol, 2138·1
Moderil, 2138·1
Moderin Acne, 2138·2
Moderin, Neo— *see* Neo Moderin, 2156·4
Moderine, 2138·2
Moderlax, 2138·2
Modern Herbals Preparations, 2138·2
Modernel, 2138·2
Modicef, 2138·2
Modicon, 2138·2
Modiem, 2138·2
Modifast, 2138·2
Modifenac, 2138·2
Modifical, 2138·2
Modified Black Fluids, 1193·3
Modified Cellulose Gum, 1578·1
Modified Lanolin, 1483·2
Modified White Fluids, 1193·3
Modil, 2138·2
Modilac AR, 2138·2
Modilac HA, 2138·2
Modilac Sans Lactose, 2138·2
ModimMunal, 2138·2
Modina, 2138·3
Modiodal, 2138·3
Modip, 2138·3
Modisal, 2138·3
Modiscop, 2138·3
Moditen, 2138·3
Moditen Depot, 2138·3
Modium, 2138·3
Modival, 2138·3
Modivid, 2138·3
Modizide, 2138·3
Modomed, 2138·3
Modopar, 2138·3
Modrasone, 2138·3
Modrenal, 2138·3
MODS— *see* Septicaemia, 144·3
Moducal, 2138·3
Moducren, 2138·3
Moducrin, 2138·3
Modula, 2138·3
Modul'Aid, 2138·3
Modulamin, 2138·3
Modulan, 2138·3
Modulanzime, 2138·3
Modulator, 2138·3
Modulen IBD, 2138·3
Modulo Calorico, 2138·4
Modulon, 2138·4
Modu-Puren, 2138·4
Moduret, 2138·4
Moduretic, 2138·4
Moduretic Mite, 2138·4
Moduretik, 2138·4
Modus, 2138·4
Modustatina, 2138·4
Modustatine, 2138·4
Modutrol, 2138·4
Moenomycin A, 162·2
Moenomycin C, 162·2
Moex, 2138·4
Moexipril, Hidrocloruro de, 961·2
Moexipril Hydrochloride, 961·2
Moexiprilat, 961·2
Mofebutazona, 60·1
Mofebutazone, 60·1
Mofebutazone Sodium, 60·1
Mofesal, 2138·4
Mofesal N, 2138·4
Mofetilo, Micofenolato de, 1361·2
Mofezolac, 60·1
Mofezolaco, 60·1
Mogadan, 2138·4
Mogadon, 2138·4
Mogasinte, 2138·4
Mogetic, 2138·4
Mohave Yucca, 1766·2
Mohexal, 2138·4
Mohnfrucht, 1129·1
Mohrus, 2138·4
Moisol, 2138·4
Moist Again, 2138·4
Moi-Stir, 2138·4
Moi-Stir— *see* Entertainer's Secret, 1971·3
Moisture Drops, 2139·1
Moisture Eyes, 2139·1
Moisture Lift Protective, 2139·1
Moisture Shield, 2139·1
Moisture Therapy, 2139·1
Moisturel, 2139·1
Molagar, 2139·1
Molax, 2139·1
Molca, 2139·1
Molcain, 2139·1
Molcer, 2139·1
Moldina, 2139·1
Mole, Invasive— *see* Gestational Trophoblastic Tumours, 505·1
Molelant, 2139·1
Molevac, 2139·1
Molfenac, 2139·1
Molgramostim, 756·1
Molgramostim Concentrated Solution, 756·1
Molgramostimi Solutio Concentrata, 756·1
Molibdato de Amonio, 1440·3
Molibdato de Sodio, 1440·3
Molibdeno, 1440·3
Molindona, Hidrocloruro de, 709·3
Molindone Hydrochloride, 709·3
Molipaxin, 2139·1
Molival, 2139·1
Mollifene, 2139·1
Mollipect, 2139·1
Molluscicides, 1499·1
Molnia, 2139·1
Molsi-Azu, 2139·1
Molsicor, 2139·1
Molsidain, 2139·1
Molsidaine, 2139·1
Molsidirex, 2139·1
Molsidolat, 2139·1
Molsidomina, 961·3
Molsidomine, 961·3
Molsihexal, 2139·1
Molsiket, 2139·2
Molsi-Puren, 2139·2
Molybdene Injectable, 2139·2
Molybdenum, 1440·3
Molybdenum-99, 1525·3
Molypen, 2139·2
Molzyme, 2139·2
MOM, 231·3
Mom Preparations, 2139·2
Momea, 1666·1
Momeka, 1666·1
Momendol, 2139·2
Moment, 2139·2
Momentol, 2139·2
Momentum, 2139·2
Momentum Analgetikum, 2139·2
Momentum Muscular Backache Formula, 2139·2
Mometasona, Furoato de, 1107·2
Mometasone Furoate, 1107·2
Mometasoni Furoas, 1107·2
Momicine, 2139·2
Monacolin K, 949·1
Monafed, 2139·2
Monafed DM, 2139·2
Mona-Lisa, 2139·2
Monapax, 2139·2
Monarc-M, 2139·2
Monarit, 2139·2
Monaspor, 2139·2
Monaxin, 2139·2
Monazol, 2139·2
Monazole, 2139·2
Mönchspfeffer, 1649·1
Mondrian, 2139·3
Mondus, 2139·3
Monensin, 611·1
Monensin Sodium, 611·1
Monensina Sódica, 611·1
Moneva, 2139·3
Moni, 2139·3
Monic Acid, 233·2
Monicil, 2139·3
Monicor, 2139·3
Monilac, 2139·3
Monilen, 2139·3
Monipax, 2139·3
Monistat, 2139·3
Monit, 2139·3
Monitan, 2139·3
Monit-Puren, 2139·3
Monizole, 2139·3
Monkey B Virus Infection— *see* Herpesvirus Simiae Infections, 621·1
Monkey Dust, 1730·3
Monkey Gland, 1730·3
Monkshood Root, 1646·3
Mono Acis, 2139·3
Mono Corax, 2139·3
Mono Demetrin, 2139·3
Mono- and Di-glycerides, 1413·2
Mono- and Diglycerides of Food Fatty Acids, Self-emulsifying, 1412·2
Mono & Disaccharide Free Diet Powder (Product 3232A), 2139·3
Mono Mack, 2139·3
Mono Maycor, 2139·3
Mono Praecimed, 2139·3
Mono Wolff, 2139·3
Mono y Diglicéridos, 1413·2
Mono-A, 2139·3
Monoacetyldapsone, 204·1
Monoacetylhydrazine, 224·1
6-*O*-Monoacetylmorphine, 31·1
Monoacylglycerols, 1412·1
Monoamine Oxidase Inhibitors, 278·2, 316·1
Monoamine Oxidase Type A Inhibitors, Reversible, 278·2, 316·1
Monobac, 2139·3
Monobactams, 117·3
Monobasic Ammonium Phosphate, 1654·2
Monobasic Calcium Phosphate, 1664·2
Monobasic Potassium Phosphate, 1230·3
Monobasic Sodium Phosphate, 1230·3
Monobenzona, 1154·2
Monobenzone, 1154·2
Monobeta, 2139·3
Monobios, 2139·3
Monobiotic, 2139·3
Monobromomethane, 1507·2
Monobutazone, 60·1
Monocal, 2139·3
Monocalcium Phosphate, 1664·2
Monocaps, 2139·3
Mono-Cedocard, 2139·4
Monocef, 2139·4
Monocetin, 2139·4
Monochlorethane, 1376·2
Monochlorimipramine Hydrochloride, 289·3
Monochloroacetic Acid, 1154·2
Monochloromethane, 1476·2
Monochlorothymol, 1177·2
Monocid, 2139·4
Monocide, 2139·4
Monocinque, 2139·4
Monoclair, 2139·4
Monoclate-P, 2139·4
Monocline, 2139·4
Monoclonal Antibodies, 492·1
Monoclonal Antibody 17-1A, 550·2
Monoclonal Antibody, Endotoxin, 1615·2
Monoclonal CD4 Antibodies, 1668·3
Monoclox, 2139·4
Monocomponent Insulins, 334·2
Monocontin, 2139·4
Monocor, 2139·4
Monocord, 2139·4
Monocordil, 2139·4
Monoctanoin, 1715·3
Monoctanoína, 1715·3
Monodesethylchloroquine, 450·2
*N*-Monodesethyltiapride, 725·1
*N*-2-Monodesmethylnizatidine, 1277·3
*N*-Monodesmethyl-rizatriptan, 471·1
Monodox, 2139·4
Monodoxin, 2139·4
Monodur, 2139·4
Mono-Embolex, 2139·4
Monoestearato de Aluminio, 1574·1
Monoestearato de Glicerilo, 1412·1
Monoestearato de Glicerilo Autoemulsionable, 1412·2
Monoetanolamina, Oleato de, 1716·1
Monoethanolamine, 1716·1, 1758·2
Monoethanolamine Ioxitalamate, 1066·3
Monoethanolamine Laurilsulfate, 1574·3
Monoethanolamine Oleate, 1716·1

Monoethyl Fumarate, 1147·3
Monoethylglycinexylidide, 1379·1
Monofed, 2139·4
Monofeme, 2139·4
Monoferro, 2139·4
Monofix, 2139·4
Monofix-VF, 2139·4
Monoflam, 2139·4
Monoflocet, 2139·4
Monofluorofosfato Sódico, 1446·2
Monofoscin, 2140·1
Monogen, 2140·1
Mono-Gesic, 2140·1
Monogestin, 2140·1
Monoginal, 2140·1
Monoglicéridos Diacetilados, 1411·2
Monoglycerides, Diacetylated, 1411·2
Monoglycerides of Food Fatty Acids, Self-emulsifying, 1412·2
Monoglycerylphosphoric Acid, 1695·2
Monohidrocloruro de Flurazepam, 700·3
Monohydrated Selenium Dioxide, 1444·1
Monohydroxyethylrutoside, 1688·2
Monohydroxyethylrutosides, 1688·2
L-Mono-iodotyrosine, 1594·1
Mono-Jod, 2140·1
Monoket, 2140·1
Mono-Latex, 2140·1
Monolein, 1412·1
Monolin, 2140·1
Monolin NPH, 2140·1
Monolin Regular, 2140·1
Monolinolein, 1412·1
Monolitum, 2140·1
Monolong, 2140·1
Monomax, 2140·1
Monomethoxypolyethylene Glycol Succinimidyl L-Asparaginase, 528·3
Monomethylarsonic Acid, 1657·3
Monomethylhydrazine, 1717·3
Monomycin, 2140·1
Monomycin A Sulphate, 612·3
Monomycine, 2140·1
Mononine, 2140·1
Mononit, 2140·1
Mononitrat, 2140·1
Mononitrato de Isosorbida, 942·1
Mononitril, 2140·1
Mononitrogen Monoxide, 973·3
Monooctanoin, 1715·3
Mono-octanoin, 1715·3
Monooleato de Glicerilo, 1412·1
Monopalmitoestearato de Etilenglicol, 1411·3
Monopalmitoestearato de Propilenglicol, 1415·3
Monoparin, 2140·1
Monophenylbutazone, 60·1
Monophosadénine, 1647·3
Monophosphothiamine, 1455·3
Monopina, 2140·1
Monoplus, 2140·1
Monopotassium Carbonate, 1223·1
Monopotassium Phosphate, 1230·3
Monopress, 2140·1
Monopril, 2140·1
Monopril Comp, 2140·1
Monopril-HCT, 2140·2
Monoprim, 2140·2
Monopront, 2140·2
Monopur, 2140·2
Monoquin, 2140·2
Monores, 2140·2
Monorythm, 2140·2
Monos, 2140·2
Monosaccharides, 1417·1
Monosodium Alendronate, 765·3
Monosodium 4-Aminosalicylate Dihydrate, 155·1
Monosodium L-Ascorbate, 1460·2
Monosodium Carbonate, 1223·2
Monosodium (6*R*)-6-[2-Carboxy-2-(3-thienyl)acetamido]penicillanate Monohydrate, 270·2
Monosodium D-Gluconate, 1747·3
Monosodium Glutamate, 1441·1
Monosodium Risedronate, 774·3
Monosodium Tartrate, 1290·1
Monosol, 2140·2
Monosorb— *see* Trangina, 2340·3
Monosorbitrate, 2140·2
Monosordil, 2140·2
Monostearin, 1412·1
Monostearin Emulsificans, 1412·2
Monostearin, Self-emulsifying, 1412·2
Monostearoylglycerol, 1412·1
Monostenase, 2140·2
MonoStep, 2140·2
Monostop, 2140·2
Monosulfato de Guanetidina, 926·3
Monosulfiram, 1510·1
Monotard, 2140·2
Monotard HM, 2140·2
Monotard, Human— *see* Human Monotard, 2049·2
Monotard MC, 2140·2
Monotest, 2140·2
Monothioglycerol, 1186·3
α-Monothioglycerol, 1186·3
Mono-Tildiem, 2140·2
Monotioglicerol, 1186·3
Monotrate, 2140·2
Monotrean, 2140·2
Monotrean B6, 2140·2
Mono-Tridin, 2140·2
Monotrim, 2140·2
Monotrin, 2140·2
Monotussin, 2140·3
Mono-Vacc Test (O.T.), 2140·3
Monovacc-Test, 2140·3
Monovax, 2140·3
Monovent, 2140·3
Monoxerutin, 1688·2
Monoxerutina, 1688·2
Monóxido de Carbono, 1235·2
Monoxychlorosene, 1187·2
Monozide, 2140·3
Monozol, 2140·3
Monphytol, 2140·3
Monsel's Solution, 1428·3
Montair, 2140·3
Montalen, 2140·3
Montamed, 2140·3
Montana, 2140·3
Montana N, 2140·3
Montavon, 2140·3
Montegen, 2140·3
Montelukast Sódico, 788·3
Montelukast Sodium, 788·3
Montenegro Test, 1706·2
Monteplasa, 961·3
Monteplase, 961·3
Monticina, 2140·3
Montmorillonite, 1039·3, 1577·2
Montricin, 2140·3
Monuril, 2140·3
Monurol, 2140·3
Monydrin, 2140·3
MoodLift, 2140·3
Moorbad-Saar N, 2140·3
Moorland, 2140·3
Moorlauge Bastian, 2140·4
Mopen, 2140·4
Moperidona, 2140·4
Moperidona AF, 2140·4
Moperidona Enzimatica, 2140·4
Moperona, Hidrocloruro de, 710·1
Moperone Hydrochloride, 710·1
Mopral, 2140·4
Mopsoralen, 2140·4
Moracizina, Hidrocloruro de, 962·1
Moracizine, 961·3
Moracizine Hydrochloride, 962·1
Moradorm, 2140·4
Moradorm S, 2140·4
*d*-Moramid, 28·2
Morantel Citrate, 110·1
Morantel, Citrato de, 110·1
Morantel Hydrogen Tartrate for Veterinary Use, 110·1
Morantel Tartrate, 110·1
Morantel, Tartrato de, 110·1
Moranteli Hydrogenotartras, 110·1
Morapid, 2140·4
Moraten, 2140·4
Moraxen, 2140·4
Morbil, 2140·4
Morbilvax, 2140·4
Morcap, 2140·4
Morclofona, 1124·3
Morclofone, 1124·3
Morclofone Hydrochloride, 1124·3
Morclophon, 1124·3
Morcontin, 2140·4
Morde X, 2140·4
MoreDophilus, 2140·4
Morelin, 2140·4
Morelle Noire, 1661·2
Morera Compuesta, 2140·4
Morfex, 2140·4
Morfina, 60·1
Morfina, Hidrocloruro de, 60·1
Morfina, Sulfato de, 60·2
Morfina, Tartrato de, 60·3
Morgenxil, 2140·4
Morhulin, 2140·4
Moriamin, 2140·4
Moricizine, 961·3
Moricizine Hydrochloride, 962·1
Morinamida, 233·1
Morinamide, 233·1
Morinamide Hydrochloride, 233·1
Morlan FB 25, 2140·4
Morniflu, 2140·4
Morniflumate, 60·1
Morniflumato, 60·1
Morning Glory, 1723·2
Morning Sickness— *see* Nausea and Vomiting, 1245·2
Moroccan Type Rosemary Oil, 1740·2
Moroctic Acid, 976·2
Moroctocog Alfa, 751·2
Moronal, 2140·4
Moronal V, 2140·4
Moroxidina, Hidrocloruro de, 649·3
Moroxydine Hydrochloride, 649·3
Morphalgin, 2140·4
Morphazinamide, 233·1
Morphea— *see* Scleroderma, 1348·1
Morphethylbutyne, 1129·2
Morphex, 2140·4
Morphgesic, 2141·1
Morphine, 27·3, 60·1
Morphine Hydrochloride, 60·1
Morphine Methyl Ether, 27·1
Morphine Sulfate, 60·2
Morphine Sulphate, 60·2
Morphine Tartrate, 60·3
Morphine-3-glucuronide, 61·2
Morphine-6-glucuronide, 61·2
Morphini Hydrochloridum, 60·1
Morphini Sulfas, 60·2
Morphinii Chloridum, 60·1
Morphinum Chloratum, 60·1
Morphitec, 2141·1
Morpholine Salicylate, 63·3
2-Morpholinoethyl (*E*)-6-(4-Hydroxy-6-methoxy-7-methyl-3-oxo-5-phthalanyl)-4-methyl-4-hexenoate, 1361·2
2-Morpholinoethyl 2-Methyl-2-phenoxypropionate, 1129·2
2-Morpholinoethyl 2-(α,α,α-Trifluoro-*m*-toluidino)nicotinate, 60·1
3-*O*-(2-Morpholinoethyl)morphine Monohydrate, 1128·3
1-(Morpholinoformimidoyl)guanidine Hydrochloride, 649·3
(±)-5-Morpholinomethyl-3-(5-nitrofurfurylideneamino)oxazolidin-2-one Hydrochloride, 215·2
*N*-Morpholinomethylpyrazine-2-carboxamide, 233·1
3-Morpholinosydnonimine Hydrochloride, 946·3
Morrhuae, Oleum, 1425·2
Morrhuate Sodium, 1748·1
Morrhulan, 2141·1
Morruato de Sodio, 1748·1
Morruetil, 2141·1
Morrugripe, 2141·1
Morstel, 2141·1
Morsydomine, 961·3
Morton Salt Substitute, 2141·1
Morubel, 2141·1
Morue, Huile de Foie de, 1425·2
Moruman, 2141·1
Morupar, 2141·1
MoRu-Viraten, 2141·1
MOS, 2141·1
Mosalan, 2141·1
Mosapramina, 710·1
Mosapramine, 710·1
Mosaprida, Citrato de, 1276·3
Mosapride Citrate, 1276·3
Mosar, 2141·1
Mosc., 1718·2
Moscada, Essência de, 1722·3
Moschus, 1718·2
*Moschus moschiferus*, 1718·2
Mosco, 2141·1
Moscontin, 2141·1
Mosegor, 2141·1
Moselar, 2141·1
Mosil, 2141·1
Moskizol, 2141·1
Mostarda Preta, 1718·2
Mostardina, 2141·1
Mostaza, Aceite Esencial de, 1718·2
Mostaza Blanca, 1718·2
Mostaza Negra, 1718·2
Mostaza, Semilla de, 1718·2
Mostrelan, 2141·1
Mota, 1666·1
Motens, 2141·1
Mother and Child Vitamin Drops, 2141·1
Motherwort, 1717·1
Motherwort Compound, Gerard House— *see* Gerard House Motherwort Compound, 2022·1
Motherwort Herb, 1717·1
Motiax, 2141·1
Moticlod, 2141·1
Moticon, 2141·1
Motidine, 2141·2
Motidom, 2141·2
Motifene, 2141·2
Motilex, 2141·2
Motilidone, 2141·2
Motilium, 2141·2
Motilyo, 2141·2
Motion Sickness, Hylands— *see* Hylands Motion Sickness, 2052·3
Motion Sickness— *see* Nausea and Vomiting, 1245·2
Motional, 2141·2
Motipress, 2141·2
Motitrel, 2141·2
Motival, 2141·2
Motivan, 2141·2
Motiven, 2141·2
Motivone, 2141·2
Motofen, 2141·2
Motoneuron Disease— *see* Motor Neurone Disease, 1739·1
Motor Neurone Disease, 1739·1
Motosol, 2141·2
Motozina, 2141·2
Motrax, 2141·2
Motretinida, 1154·2
Motretinide, 1154·2
Motrim, 2141·2
Motrin, 2141·2
Motrin Cold, Childrens— *see* Childrens Motrin Cold, 1882·4
Motrin IB Sinus, 2141·2
Mountain Balm, 1121·2
Mountain Sickness, Acute— *see* High-altitude Disorders, 822·2
Mountain Tobacco, 1656·3
Moura Brasil, Colirio— *see* Colirio Moura Brasil, 1899·4
Moutarde Jonciforme, 1718·2
Moutarde Noire, Graine de, 1718·2
Mouth Cancer— *see* Malignant Neoplasms of the Head and Neck, 517·3
Mouth Infections, Bacterial— *see* Mouth Infections, 136·1

Mouth Kote, 2141·2
Mouth Ulceration, 1245·1
MouthKote, 2141·2
MouthKote F/R, 2141·3
MouthKote O/R, 2141·3
MouthKote P/R, 2141·3
Mouthrinse, 2141·3
Mouthwash, 2141·3
Mouthwash Antiseptic & Gargle, 2141·3
Mouthwash & Gargle, 2141·3
Mouthwash Mint/Peppermint, 2141·3
Mova Nitrat, 2141·3
Movacox, 2141·3
Movalis, 2141·3
Movana, 2141·3
Movatec, 2141·3
Movelat, 2141·3
Movelium, 2141·3
Movens, 2141·3
Movent, 2141·3
Mover, 2141·3
Movergan, 2141·3
Movergan— *see* Antiparkin, 1805·1
Movex, 2141·3
Movicard, 2141·3
Movicol, 2141·3
Movicolon, 2141·3
Movicox, 2141·3
Movidone, 2141·3
Moviflex, 2141·4
Movilat, 2141·4
Movilisin, 2141·4
Movin, 2141·4
Movina, 2141·4
Movistal, 2141·4
Movithiol, 2141·4
Movon, 2141·4
Movone, 2141·4
Movox, 2141·4
Movoxicam, 2141·4
Mowineuron, 2141·4
Mowivit, 2141·4
Mox, 2141·4
Moxacef, 2141·4
Moxacil, 2141·4
Moxacin, 2141·4
Moxadent, 2141·4
Moxal, 2141·4
Moxal II, 2141·4
Moxal Plus, 2141·4
Moxalactam Disodium, 225·3
Moxaline, 2141·4
Moxan, 2141·4
Moxan— *see* Losec 20 Triple, 2106·1
Moxapen, 2141·4
Moxaverina, Hidrocloruro de, 1717·2
Moxaverine, 1717·2
Moxaverine Hydrochloride, 1717·2
Moxcil, 2141·4
Moxcin, 2141·4
Moxicam, 2141·4
Moxicel, 2141·4
Moxiclav, 2142·1
Moxidectin, 110·1
Moxidectina, 110·1
Moxif, 2142·1
Moxifloxacin Hydrochloride, 233·1
Moxifloxacino, Hidrocloruro de, 233·1
Moxilcap, 2142·1
Moxilen, 2142·1
Moxilin, 2142·1
Moximed, 2142·1
Moxina, 2142·1
Moxipan, 2142·1
Moxipen, 2142·1
Moxiplus, 2142·1
Moxiral, 2142·1
Moxiren, 2142·1
Moxisilita Clorhidrato, 962·2
Moxisilita, Hidrocloruro de, 962·2
Moxisylyte Hydrochloride, 962·2
Moxitral, 2142·1
Moxlin, 2142·1
Moxon, 2142·1
Moxonidina, 962·3
Moxonidine, 962·3
Moxonidinum, 962·3
Moxycarb, 2142·1
Moxyclav, 2142·1
Moxydar, 2142·1
Moxymax, 2142·1
Moxypen, 2142·1
Moxyvit, 2142·1
Moz-Bite, 2142·1
Mozzie Patch, 2142·1
4-MP, 1039·2
6MP, 567·2
MP-302, 1066·2
MP-328, 1066·2
MP-620, 1063·2
MP-1177, 1063·1
MPA, 1362·1, 2142·1
MPA Gyn, 2142·1
MPA-beta, 2142·1
MPA-Noury, 2142·1
MPC-1304, 864·2
MPI-5010, 539·2
MPP, 418·2
MPPP, 81·1, 1196·2
MPR, 955·3
M-Prednisol, 2142·1
α-MPT, 956·1
MPTP, 81·1, 1196·2
MPV-785, 706·1
MPV-1248, 1032·3
MPV-1440, 689·3
MPV-253-AII, 689·3
M-19-Q, 254·1
MR-654, 1307·3
Mr. Multy, 2142·1
Mr Nits, 2142·1
MRA, 1757·1
MRF, 1332·2
MRL-41, 1542·2
Mrs Cullen's Powders, 2142·2
MRSA Infections— *see* Staphylococcal Infections, 147·2
M-R-Vax II, 2142·2
MRX, 2142·2
MRX-115, 1067·2
MS-551, 972·2
MS Contin, 2142·2
MS Direct, 2142·2
MS Mono, 2142·2
MSD-803, 949·1
MSG, 1441·1
MSH, 1332·2
α-MSH, 1332·2
β-MSH, 1332·2
γ-MSH, 1332·2
MSI, 2142·2
MSI-78, 228·3
MSI-93, 228·3
MSI-94, 228·3
MSIR, 2142·2
MS-Long, 2142·2
MSP, 2142·2
MSP-1, 1622·3
MSP-2, 1622·3
MSP-3, 1622·3
MSP-Blu, 2142·2
MSPD, 2142·2
MSP/RESA, 1622·3
MSR, 2142·2
MST, 2142·2
MST-16, 583·3
MST Continus, 2142·2
MST Unicontinus, 2142·2
MSTA, 2142·2
M-Stada, 2142·2
MSUD, 2142·2
MSUD 1, 2142·2
MSUD 2, 2142·2
MSUD III, 2142·2
MSUD Aid, 2142·2
MSUD Analog, 2142·2
MSUD, Analog— *see* Analog MSUD, 1798·3
MSUD Diet, 2142·2
MSUD Maxamaid, 2142·2
MSUD, Maxamaid— *see* Maxamaid MSUD, 2116·1
MSUD Maxamum, 2142·2
MSUD, Maxamum— *see* Maxamum MSUD, 2116·1
α-MT, 956·1
MT-141, 174·1
MTA, 579·1
MTB-51, 485·3
MTBE, 1475·3
MTC-DOX, 549·3
MTE, 2142·2
MTHPC, 586·3
MTIC, 544·3, 587·1
M-Trim, 2142·2
MTX, 568·2, 2142·3
Mu Tong, 1656·3
Mucabrox, 2142·3
Mucaderma S, 2142·3
Mucaine, 2142·3
Mucaine 2 in 1, 2142·3
Mucal, 2142·3
Mucalan, 2142·3
Mucantil, 2142·3
Mucasept-A, 2142·3
Mucato de Isometepteno, 1702·1
Mucedokehl, 2142·3
Muchan, 2142·3
Mucibron, 2142·3
Muciclar, 2142·3
Mucil, 2142·3
Mucilar, 2142·3
Mucilar Avena, 2142·3
Mucilax, 2142·3
Mucilin, 2142·3
Mucilloid, 2142·3
Mucin, Gastric, 1579·1
Mucina Gástrica, 1579·1
Mucine, 2142·3
Mucinex, 2142·3
Mucinol, 2142·3
Mucinum, 2142·4
Mucinum a l'Extrait de Cascara, 2142·4
Mucinum Cascara, 2142·4
Muciplasma, 2142·4
Mucipulgite, 2142·4
Mucisol, 2142·4
Muciteran, 2142·4
Mucitux, 2142·4
Mucivital, 2142·4
Muclox, 2142·4
Muco4, 2142·4
Muco Cortos, 2142·4
Muco Dosodos, 2142·4
Muco Dosodos Biotic, 2142·4
Muco Panoral, 2142·4
Muco Rhinathiol, 2142·4
Muco Sanigen, 2142·4
Muco-Anestyl, 2142·4
Muco-Aspecton, 2142·4
Mucobase, 2142·4
Mucobene, 2142·4
Mucobrol, 2142·4
Mucobron, 2142·4
Mucobronchyl, 2143·1
Mucobroxol, 2143·1
Mucocaps, 2143·1
Mucocedyl, 2143·1
Mucocef, 2143·1
Mucocil, 2143·1
Mucocis, 2143·1
Mucocistein, 2143·1
Mucoclean, 2143·1
Mucocutaneous Lymph Node Syndrome of Childhood— *see* Kawasaki Disease, 1629·3
Muco-cyl Ho-Len-Complex, 2143·1
Muco-Dest, 2143·1
Mucodestrol, 2143·1
Mucodex, 2143·1
Mucodic, 2143·1
Mucodil, 2143·1
Mucodox, 2143·1
Mucodrenol, 2143·1
Mucodyne, 2143·1
Mucofalk, 2143·1
Mucofan, 2143·1
Muco-Fen, 2143·1
Muco-Fen DM, 2143·1
Muco-Fen-LA, 2143·1
Mucofial, 2143·1
Muco-Fips, 2143·1
Mucoflem, 2143·1
Mucofluid, 2143·1
Mucoflux, 2143·2
Mucofor, 2143·2
Mucogel, 2143·2
Mucogen, 2143·2
Mucogeran, 2143·2
Mucogyne, 2143·2
Mucojet, 2143·2
Mucokehl, 2143·2
Mucola, 2143·2
Mucolair, 2143·2
Mucolan, 2143·2
Mucolase, 2143·2
Mucolator, 2143·2
Mucolavi, 2143·2
Mucolene, 2143·2
Mucoless, 2143·2
Mucolex, 2143·2
Mucolexin, 2143·2
Mucolid, 2143·2
Mucolin, 2143·2
Mucolin A, 2143·2
Mucolinc, 2143·2
Mucolinct, 2143·2
Mucolisil, 2143·2
Mucolit, 2143·2
Mucolitic, 2143·3
Mucolitic Antitusivo, 2143·3
Mucolitico, 2143·3
Mucolitico Maggioni, 2143·3
Mucolix, 2143·3
Mucolysin, 2143·3
Mucolyt, 2143·3
Mucolyte, 2143·3
Mucolytics, 1112·1
Mucomax, 2143·3
Mucomed, 2143·3
Muco-Mepha, 2143·3
Mucomex, 2143·3
Mucomix, 2143·3
Mucomyst, 2143·3
Muconorm, 2143·3
Mucopec, 2143·3
Mucophlogat, 2143·3
Mucopolysaccharides, Sulfated, 810·2
Mucoporetta, 2143·3
Mucoprednibron, 2143·3
Mucopront, 2143·3
Mucoral— *see* Mucorhinathiol Mucoral, 2143·4
Mucoral, Mucorhinathiol— *see* Mucorhinathiol Mucoral, 2143·4
Mucorama, 2143·3
Mucorama TS, 2143·4
Mucorem, 2143·4
Mucorex, 2143·4
Mucorex Ampicilina, 2143·4
Mucorex Ciclin, 2143·4
Mucorhinathiol Mucoral, 2143·4
Mucorhinyl, 2143·4
Mucormycosis, 388·3
Mucosa Compositum, 2143·4
Mucosal Protectants, 1240·1
Mucosan, 2143·4
Muco-Sana, 2143·4
Mucoseptal, 2143·4
Mucosil, 2143·4
Mucosirop, 2143·4
Mucosol, 2143·4
Mucosolvan, 2143·4
Mucosolvan Compositum, 2143·4
Mucosolvon, 2143·4
Mucosolvon Compositum, 2143·4
Mucospas, 2143·4
Mucospect, 2143·4
Mucospire, 2143·4
Mucosta, 2143·4
Mucostar, 2143·4
Mucosteine, 2144·1
Mucostop, 2144·1
Mucosyt, 2144·1

Mucotablin, 2144·1
Muco-Tablinen, 2144·1
Mucotectan, 2144·1
Mucothera, 2144·1
Mucotherm, 2144·1
Mucothiol, 2144·1
Mucotic, 2144·1
Mucotoss, 2144·1
Mucotreis, 2144·1
Muco-Trin, 2144·1
Mucotrophir, 2144·1
Mucotuss, Chemists Own— *see* Chemists Own Chesty Cough, 1881·4
Mucovibrol, 2144·1
Mucovibrol C, 2144·1
Mucovibrol T, 2144·1
Mucovin, 2144·1
Mucovital, 2144·1
Mucoxan, 2144·1
Mucoxin, 2144·1
Mucoxine-F, 2144·1
Mucoxol, 2144·1
Mucoxolan, 2144·1
Mucoza, 2144·1
Mucozan, 2144·1
Mucozym, 2144·2
Mucret, 2144·2
Mu-Cron, 2144·2
Mu-Cron, Otrivine— *see* Otrivine Mu-Cron, 2197·2
Muc-Sabona, 2144·2
*Mucuna pruriens*, 1680·3
Mudagrip, 2144·2
Mudantil, 2144·2
Mudantos H, 2144·2
Mudapenil, 2144·2
Mudd Acne, 2144·2
Mudrane, 2144·2
Mudrane GG, 2144·2
Mudrane GG-2, 2144·2
Muelita, 2144·2
Muérdago, 1715·3
Muérdago, Tallo de, 1715·3
Muflex, 2144·2
Muforan, 2144·2
Mugo, Olio di, 1737·1
Muguet, 1675·3
Mulatinha, 1666·1
Mulcatel, 2144·2
Mulimen, 2144·2
Mulkine, 2144·2
Mullein, 1764·1
Mullein Flower, 1764·1
Mulmicor, 2144·2
Mulsal A Megadosis, 2144·2
Mulsal N, 2144·2
Mul-Tab, 2144·2
Multene, 2144·2
Multe-Pak, 2144·2
Multi-12, 2144·2
Multi II, 2144·2
Multi II IV VI, 2144·2
Multi 75, 2144·2
Multi 1000, 2144·2
Multi B, 2144·2
Multi B Complex, 2144·2
Multi Cal-Mag, 2144·2
Multi Formula for Men 50+, 2144·2
Multi Forte 29, 2144·3
Multi Hance, 2144·3
Multi Up, 2144·3
Multi Vit Drops with Iron, 2144·3
Multi for Women, 2144·3
Multi-Action Actifed Preparations, 2144·3
Multialchilpeptide, 576·2
Multialquilpéptido, 576·2
Multi-B Forte, 2144·3
Multi-B Strong, 2144·3
Multibay, 2144·3
Multibionta Preparations, 2144·3
Multicap, 2144·3
Multicebrina Efevit, 2144·3
Multicentrum, 2144·3
Multichew, 2144·3
Multicrom, 2144·3
Multi-Day, 2144·3
Multiderm, 2144·3
Multielmin, 2144·3
Multifebrin, 2144·3
Multiferon, 2144·3
Multifluorid, 2144·3
Multiformil, 2144·3
Multifung, 2144·3
Multifungin, 2144·4
Multifungin H, 2144·4
Multigen AL, 2144·4
Multigesic, 2144·4
Multi-gesic, 2144·4
Multiglyco, 2144·4
Multigotas, 2144·4
Multi-Gyn, 2144·4
MultiHance, 2144·4
Multi-12/K1, 2144·4
Multilase, 2144·4
Multilens Solution, 2144·4
Multilex, 2144·4
Multilim, 2144·4
Multilim RG, 2144·4
Multilind, 2144·4
Multiload, 2144·4
Multilyte, 2144·4
Multi-Mam Compressas, 2144·4
Multi-Mam Lanolina, 2144·4
Multi-Mega, 2144·4
Multi-Min, 2144·4
Multi-Min Electro, 2144·4
MultiMineral, 2144·4
Multi-Mins, 2144·4
Multi-Mulsin N, 2144·4
Multin, 2145·1
Multiparin, 2145·1
Multipax, 2145·1
Multi-Phyto, 2145·1
Multiple Myeloma, 511·3
Multiple Organ Dysfunction Syndrome— *see* Septicaemia, 144·3
Multiple Sclerosis, 646·2
Multiple Sclerosis Vaccines, 1626·3
Multipore, 2145·1
Multi-Pro, 2145·1
Multi-Purpose Lens Drops, 2145·1
Multiron, 2145·1
Multi-Sanasol, 2145·1
Multi-Sanostol, 2145·1
Multi-Sanosvit mit Eisen, 2145·1
Multisedil, 2145·1
Multiselect 29, 2145·1
Multisoy, 2145·1
Multistix Tests, 2145·1
Multi-Symptom PMS Relief, Extra Strength— *see* Extra Strength Multi-Symptom PMS Relief, 1986·2
Multi-Symptom Tylenol Preparations, 2145·1
Multi-Tabs Neo, 2145·2
Multi-Tar, 2145·2
Multi-Tar Plus, 2145·2
Multi-targeted Antifolate, 579·1
Multitest, 2145·2
Multitest CMI, 2145·2
Multitest IMC, 2145·2
Multiton, 2145·2
Multivac VR, 2145·2
Multi-Vi-Min, 2145·2
Multivit, 2145·2
Multi-Vit, 2145·2
Multivit Biovital, 2145·2
Multi-Vitamin Day & Night, 2145·2
Multivitamin Phytopharma V, 2145·2
Multivitamin-Aufbau-Kapseln, 2145·2
Multivitamin-Dragees-Pascoe, 2145·2
Multivitamines, 2145·2
Multivitaminico, Perfus— *see* Perfus Multivitaminico, 2213·2
Multivitaplex, 2145·2
Multivit-B, 2145·2
Multi-Vite, 2145·2
Multivite Six, 2145·2
Multivitol, 2145·2
Multodrin, 2145·2
Multojod-Gastreu N R12, 2145·2
Multosin, 2145·2
Multovitan, 2145·2
Multum, 2145·2
Mulungu, 1717·2
Mulvidren-F Softab, 2145·2
Mulvitin, 2145·3
Mumaten, 2145·3
Mumps Immunoglobulins, 1626·3
Mumps and Measles Vaccines, 1624·3
Mumps, Rubella, and Measles Vaccines, 1625·1
Mumps and Rubella Vaccine (Live), Measles, 1625·1
Mumps and Rubella Vaccines, 1638·2
Mumps, and Rubella Virus Vaccine Live, Measles, 1625·1
Mumps Skin Test Antigen, 1717·2
Mumps Vaccine (Live), 1626·3
Mumps Vaccines, 1626·3
Mumps Virus Vaccine Live, 1627·1
Mumps Virus Vaccine Live, Rubella and, 1638·2
Mumpsvax, 2145·3
Mump/Vac(Live), 1627·1
Mundidol, 2145·3
Mundil, 2145·3
Mundiphyllin, 2145·3
Mundisal, 2145·3
Mundisept, 2145·3
Mundra, 2145·3
Mundyadi Vatika, 1666·1
Municaps, 2145·3
Munit-E, 2145·3
Munitren H, 2145·3
Munleit, 2145·3
Munobal, 2145·3
Munolan, 2145·3
Munostin, 2145·3
Munti-Vim, 2145·3
Mupaten, 2145·3
Mupax, 2145·3
Muphoran, 2145·3
Mupiderm, 2145·3
Mupirocin, 233·1, 233·2
Mupirocin Calcium, 233·2
Mupirocina, 233·1
Mupirocinum, 233·1
Mupirocinum Calcicum, 233·2
Mupirox, 2145·3
Muporin, 2145·3
Muraligne, 2145·3
Muramidasa, Hidrocloruro de, 1717·2
Muramidase Hydrochloride, 1717·2
Muramyl, 2145·3
Murazyme, 2145·3
Murelax, 2145·3
Muriate of Ammonia, 1115·2
Muriatic Acid, 1699·1
Muriaticum Acidum, 1699·2
Muricalm, 2145·3
Murine Preparations, 2145·4
Murine Typhus— *see* Typhus, 152·3
Muro 128, 2145·4
Murocel, 2145·4
Murocoll-2, 2145·4
Murode, 2145·4
Murodermina, 1294·2
Muromonab-CD3, 1360·3
Muroptic, 2145·4
Murri Antidolorifico, 2145·4
Mus, 2145·4
Musapam, 2145·4
Musaril, 2145·4
Musashi, 2145·4
Musashi Barras Growling Dog, 2145·4
Musashi Creatina, 2145·4
Muscade, 1722·2
Muscade, Essence de, 1722·3
Muscadol, 2145·4
Muscalax, 2145·4
Muscaran, 2145·4
Muscarine, 1717·3
Muscarsan, 2145·4
Muscelax, 2145·4
Muscimol, 1717·3
Muscinil, 2146·1
Muscle Adenylic Acid, 1647·3
Muscle & Back Pain Relief, 2146·1
Muscle & Back Pain Relief-8, 2146·1
Muscle Relaxant and Analgesic, 2146·1
Muscle Relaxants, 1386·1
Muscle Rub, 2146·1
Muscle Spasm, 1386·1
Muscoflex, 2146·1
Muscol, 2146·1
Muscoril, 2146·1
Musco-ril, 2146·1
Muscular Dystrophies, 1083·3
Muscular Pain, Modern Herbals— *see* Modern Herbals Muscular Pain, 2138·2
Muscular Rheumatism— *see* Soft-tissue Rheumatism, 11·1
Musculoskeletal and Joint Disorders— *see* Soft-tissue Rheumatism, 11·1
Muscunor, 2146·1
Muse, 2146·1
Mushroom, Fool's, 1717·3
Mushroom, Magic, 1736·1
Mushrooms, 1717·3
Musk, 1718·2
Musk Ambrette, 1718·2
Musk, Deer, 1718·2
Muskatöl, Átherisches, 1722·3
Muskelat, 2146·1
Muskol, 2146·1
Muslax, 2146·1
Musocalm, 2146·1
Musocan, 2146·1
Mussel, Green-lipped, 1696·1
Musside, 2146·1
Mustard, Black, 1718·2
Mustard, Essence of, 1718·2
Mustard Gas, 1679·3
Mustard Oil, Expressed, 1718·2
Mustard Oil, Volatile, 1718·2
Mustard, White, 1718·2
Mustargen, 2146·1
Musterole, 2146·1
Musterole Extra, 2146·1
Mustine Hydrochloride, 537·1
Mustoforan, 2146·1
Musxan, 2146·1
Mutabase, 2146·1
Mutabon, 2146·1
Mutabon D, 2146·1
Mutacol, 2146·1
Mutaflor, 2146·2
Mutagrip, 2146·2
Mutamycin, 2146·2
Mutamycine, 2146·2
Mutan, 2146·2
Mutellon, 2146·2
Mutesa, 2146·2
Muthesa, 2146·2
Muthesa N, 2146·2
Mutum, 2146·2
Muvial, 2146·2
Muvidina, 2146·2
Muxol, 2146·2
M-Vac, 2146·2
MVI, 2146·2
MVI-12, 2146·2
MVI Paediatric, 2146·2
MVI-Ped, 2146·2
MVM, 2146·2
MXL, 2146·2
MY-5116, 791·2
Myacyne, 2146·2
Myadec, 2146·2
Myalgesic, 2146·2
Myalgol N, 2146·2
Myambutol, 2146·3
Myambutol-INH, 2146·3
Myasthenia, Congenital— *see* Congenital Myasthenia, 1489·1
Myasthenia Gravis, 1486·2
Myasthenia, Hereditary— *see* Congenital Myasthenia, 1489·1
Myasthenic Syndrome, Eaton-Lambert— *see* Eaton-Lambert Myasthenic Syndrome, 1485·1
Mybacin, 2146·3
Mybacin Dermic, 2146·3
Mybulen, 2146·3

Mycardol, 2146·3
Mycatox, 2146·3
Mycel, 2146·3
Mycelex Preparations, 2146·3
Mycella, 2146·3
Mycetin, 2146·3
Mycetoma, Bacterial— *see* Mycetoma, 136·2
Mycetoma, Fungal— *see* Mycetoma, 388·3
Myciclid, 2146·3
Mycidal, 2146·3
Mycidex, 2146·3
Mycifradin, 2146·3
Myciguent, 2146·3
Mycil, 2146·3
Mycil Gold, 2146·3
Mycil Healthy Feet, 2146·3
Mycinette, 2146·4
Mycinettes, 2146·4
Mycinopred, 2146·4
Myci-Spray, 2146·4
Mycitracin, 2146·4
Mycitracin Plus, 2146·4
Myclo-Derm, 2146·4
Myclo-Gyne, 2146·4
Myco-Aid, 2146·4
Mycoapaisyl, 2146·4
Mycobacter, 2146·4
Mycobacterial Infections, Atypical— *see* Opportunistic Mycobacterial Infections, 137·2
Mycobacterial Infections, Opportunistic— *see* Opportunistic Mycobacterial Infections, 137·2
Mycobacterium Avium Complex Infections— *see* Opportunistic Mycobacterial Infections, 137·2
*Mycobacterium bovis*, 1609·2, 1759·1
*Mycobacterium leprae*, 1622·1, 1706·3
*Mycobacterium tuberculosis*, 1609·2, 1759·1
*Mycobacterium vaccae*, 151·1, 1627·2
Mycobacterium Vaccae Vaccines, 1627·2
*Mycobacterium w*, 1622·1
Mycoban, 2146·4
Myco-Biotic II, 2146·4
Mycobutin, 2146·4
Mycobutol, 2146·4
Mycochlorin, 2146·4
Mycocid, 2146·4
Mycocide NS, 2146·4
Mycodecyl, 2146·4
Mycoderm, 2146·4
Mycoderm-C, 2146·4
Mycodermil, 2146·4
Mycodib, 2146·4
Mycofebrin, 2146·4
Mycofen, 2147·1
Myco-flusemidon, 2147·1
Mycofug, 2147·1
Mycogel, 2147·1
Mycogen II, 2147·1
Mycohaug C, 2147·1
Myco-Hermal, 2147·1
Mycohexal, 2147·1
Mycol, 2147·1
Mycolog, 2147·1
Mycolog-II, 2147·1
Myconel, 2147·1
Myconex, 2147·1
Myconil, 2147·1
Myconip, 2147·1
Mycophenolate Mofetil, 1361·2
Mycophenolate Morpholinoethyl, 1361·2
Mycophenolate Sodium, 1362·2
Mycophenolic Acid, 1362·1
Mycopol, 2147·1
Mycoral, 2147·1
Mycoril, 2147·1
Mycosamthong, 2147·1
Mycosin, 2147·1
Mycosis Fungoides, 511·2
Mycospor, 2147·1
Mycospor Carbamid, 2147·1
Mycospor Nagelset, 2147·1
Mycospor Onicoset, 2147·1
Mycosporan, 2147·1
Mycosporan Karbamid, 2147·2
Mycosporan Onycoset, 2147·2
Mycosquam, 2147·2
Mycostatin, 2147·2
Mycostatin V, 2147·2
Mycostatine, 2147·2
Mycostatin-Zinkoxid, 2147·2
Mycoster, 2147·2
Myco-Synalar, 2147·2
Mycota, 2147·2
Mycotel, 2147·2
Myco-Triacet II, 2147·2
Mycotricide, 2147·2
Myco-Ultralan, 2147·2
Mycozole, 2147·2
Mycurium, 2147·2
Mydecamycin, 231·3
Mydfrin, 2147·2
Mydocalm, 2147·2
Mydocalm-A, 2147·2
Mydosone, 2147·2
Mydral, 2147·2
Mydramide, 2147·2
Mydriacil, 2147·3
Mydriacyl, 2147·3
Mydrial— *see* Neo-Mydrial, 2159·2
Mydrial-Atropin, 2147·3
Mydrian, 2147·3
Mydriasert, 2147·3
Mydriasine, 476·3
Mydriasis— *see* Mydriasis and Cycloplegia, 476·2
Mydriasis, Reversal of— *see* Reversal of Mydriasis, 1487·1
Mydriaticum, 2147·3
Mydriatin, 1127·3
Mydril, 2147·3
Mydrilate, 2147·3
Mydrin-P, 2147·3
Mydriolytics, 1487·1
Mydrum, 2147·3
Myelinolysis, Central Pontine— *see* Hyponatraemia, 1220·3
Myelobromol, 2147·3
Myelodysplasia— *see* Myelodysplastic Syndromes, 508·2
Myelogenous Leukaemia, Acute— *see* Acute Myeloid Leukaemias, 506·3
Myelogenous Leukaemia, Chronic— *see* Chronic Myeloid Leukaemia, 507·3
Myeloid Leukaemia, Chronic— *see* Chronic Myeloid Leukaemia, 507·3
Myeloma, 511·3
Myelomatosis, 511·3
Myelosan, 532·2
Myelostim, 2147·3
Myfortic, 2147·3
Myfungar, 2147·3
Mygale Compositum, 2147·3
Mygdalon, 2147·3
Mygel, 2147·3
Mygesal, 2147·3
Myk, 2147·3
Myk-1, 2147·3
Myko Cordes, 2147·3
Myko Cordes Plus, 2147·3
Mykoderm Heilsalbe, 2147·3
Mykoderm Mund-Gel, 2147·3
Mykofungin, 2147·3
Mykohaug, 2147·3
Mykontral, 2147·3
MykoPosterine N, 2147·4
Mykoproct Sine, 2147·4
Mykosert, 2147·4
Mykotin, 2147·4
Mykrox, 2147·4
Mykundex, 2147·4
Mykundex Heilsalbe, 2147·4
Mykundex Mono, 2147·4
Mylabris, 1667·1
*Mylabrus cichorii*, 1667·1
*Mylabrus phalerata*, 1667·1
*Mylabrus pustulator*, 1667·1
*Mylabrus sidae*, 1667·1
Mylagen, 2147·4
Mylanta Preparations, 2147·4
Mylepsinum, 2148·1
Myleran, 2148·1
Myleuca, 2148·1
Mylicon, 2148·1
Mylocel, 2148·1
Mylocort, 2148·1
Mylol, 2148·1
Mylom, 2148·1
Mylotarg, 2148·1
Mylproin, 2148·1
Mymin C, 2148·1
Myminic Expectorant, 2148·1
Myminic Syrup, 2148·1
Myminicol, 2148·1
Mynah, 2148·1
Mynatal, 2148·1
Mynate 90 Plus, 2148·1
Mynocine, 2148·1
Myo Hermes, 2148·1
Myobid, 2148·1
Myobloc, 2148·1
Myocardial Infarction, 828·2
Myocardial Infarction, Non-Q Wave— *see* Angina Pectoris, 813·1
Myocardial Infarction, Non-ST Elevation— *see* Angina Pectoris, 813·1
Myocardial Infarction Pain, 7·1
Myocardial Ischaemia, Asymptomatic Transient— *see* Angina Pectoris, 813·1
Myocardial Ischaemia, Silent— *see* Angina Pectoris, 813·1
Myocardon, 2148·2
Myocardon Mono, 2148·2
Myocardon N, 2148·2
Myocet, 2148·2
Myocholine, 2148·2
Myochrysine, 2148·2
Myocin, 2148·2
Myoclonic Seizures— *see* Epilepsy, 349·1
Myoclonic Seizures— *see* Myoclonus, 353·1
Myoclonus, 353·1
Myocord, 2148·2
Myocrisin, 2148·2
Myodipine, 2148·2
Myodrine, 2148·2
Myodura, 2148·2
Myo-Echinacin, 2148·2
Myofascial Pain— *see* Soft-tissue Rheumatism, 11·1
Myofedrin, 2148·2
Myoflex, 2148·2
Myoflex Ice, 2148·2
Myoflex Ice Plus, 2148·2
Myogard, 2148·2
Myogeloticum N, 2148·2
Myogit, 2148·2
Myolastan, 2148·2
Myolax, 2148·2
Myolosyx, 2148·2
Myomethol, 2148·2
Myonac, 2148·3
Myonal, 2148·3
Myoneuronal Blockers, 1397·1
Myonil, 2148·3
Myonit, 2148·3
Myopar, 2148·3
Myopax, 2148·3
Myophen, 2148·3
Myoplege, 2148·3
Myoplegine, 2148·3
Myoprin, 2148·3
Myoquin, 2148·3
Myoscain, 2148·3
Myoscint, 2148·3
Myosic, 2148·3
Myositis Ossificans Progressiva— *see* Ectopic Ossification, 762·2
Myositis— *see* Polymyositis and Dermatomyositis, 1086·2
Myoson, 2148·3
Myospasmal, 2148·3
Myospaz, 2148·3
Myospaz Forte, 2148·3
Myotenlis, 2148·3
Myotonachol, 2148·3
Myotonia Congenita— *see* Myotonia, 376·1
Myotonine, 2148·3
Myovek, 2148·3
Myoview, 2148·3
Myovin, 2148·3
Myoviton, 2148·3
Myoxam, 2148·3
Myoxan, 2148·3
Mypaid, 2148·3
Myphetane DC, 2148·3
Myphetane DX, 2148·4
Myprodol, 2148·4
Myproflam, 2148·4
Myra 300-E, 2148·4
Myralact, 1186·3
β-Myrcene, 1724·1, 1740·2, 1760·1
Myrcia Oil, 1659·1
Myrciae, Oleum, 1659·1
Myriacyl, 2148·4
Myrica, 1659·2
*Myrica cerifera*, 1659·2
Myrin, 2148·4
Myrin Plus, 2148·4
Myrin-P, 2148·4
Myristica, 1722·2
*Myristica fragrans*, 1708·2, 1722·2, 1722·3
Myristica Oil, 1722·3
Myristicae Fragrantis Aetheroleum, 1722·3
Myristicae, Oleum, 1722·3
Myristicin, 1722·3
Myristoll, 2148·4
Myristyl Alcohol, 1718·3
Myristylbenzalkonium Chloride, 1186·3
Myristyl-gamma-picolinium Chloride, 1186·3
Myrol, 2148·4
*Myroxylon balsamum*, 1131·3, 1730·2
Myrrh, 1718·3
Myrrha, 1718·3
Myrrhinil-Intest, 2148·4
Myrtaven, 2148·4
Myrtecaine, 1381·3
Myrtecaine Laurilsulfate, 1381·3
Myrtilen, 2148·4
Myrtilli, Baccae, 1718·3
Myrtilli Fructus, 1718·3
Myrtillus, 1718·3
Myrtle, Tropical, 1673·2
Myser, 2148·4
Mysial, 2148·4
Myslee, 2148·4
Mysocort, 2148·4
Mysoline, 2148·4
Mysolone-N, 2148·4
Mysoven, 2148·4
Mysteclin, 2148·4
Mysteclin-V, 2148·4
Mytancid, 2148·4
Mytelase, 2148·4
Mytex, 2148·4
Mytic 810, 2149·1
Mytobrin, 2149·1
Mytrex, 2149·1
Mytussin Preparations, 2149·1
My-Vitalife, 2149·1
Myvlar, 2149·1
Myxina, 2149·1
Myxoedema— *see* Hypothyroidism, 1595·3
Myxoedema Coma— *see* Hypothyroidism, 1595·3
Myxofat, 2149·1
MZM, 2149·1
M-Zole, 2149·1


## N


N, 1422·1
N-5′, 806·3
N-22, 60·1
N-0252, 1481·2
N-399, 491·3
N-553, 1396·3
N-714, 682·3
N-746, 730·3
N7001, 306·3
N-7009, 699·1
51087N, 859·2
N32 Collutorio, 2149·1

N D Clear, 2149·1
NA-97, 1404·3
NA-274, 1115·3
NA-872, 1114·3
Naabak, 2149·1
Naaprep, 2149·1
Naaxia, 2149·1
NAB-365, 784·2
Nabicortin, 2149·1
Nabi-HB, 2149·1
Nabilona, 1277·1
Nabilone, 1277·1
Nabone, 2149·1
Nabonet, 2149·1
NABQI, 76·3
Nabuco, 2149·1
Nabucox, 2149·1
Nabumetona, 63·3
Nabumetone, 63·3
Nabumetonum, 63·3
Nabuser, 2149·1
Nabutil, 2149·2
Nabuton, 2149·2
NAC, 2149·2
Nac, 2149·2
Nacgel, 2149·2
Nacha, 2149·2
Naclof, 2149·2
Naclon, 2149·2
Nacom, 2149·2
Nacor, 2149·2
Nacozil, 2149·2
Nacro, 2149·2
Nactol, 2149·2
Nad, 2149·2
NAD, 1719·1
Nadamen, 2149·2
Nadelholzteer, 1159·3
Nadem, 2149·2
Nadem Forte, 2149·2
Nadetos, 2149·2
Nadex, 2149·2
β-NADH, 1719·1
Nadib, 2149·2
Nadida, 1719·1
Nadide, 1719·1
Nadifloxacin, 233·3
Nadifloxacino, 233·3
Nadinola, 2149·2
Nadione, 2149·2
Nadipinia, 2149·2
Naditone, 2149·2
Nadiwil, 2149·2
Nadixa, 2149·2
Nadolol, 963·1
Nadololum, 963·1
Nadona, 2149·2
Nadopen-V, 2149·2
Nadostine, 2149·3
Nadoxolol, Hidrocloruro de, 963·3
Nadoxolol Hydrochloride, 963·3
NADP, 1442·1
NADPH, 1719·1
Nadrifor, 2149·3
Nadroparin Calcium, 963·3
Nadroparina Cálcica, 963·3
Nadroparinum Calcicum, 963·3
Naegleria Infections— *see* Primary Amoebic Meningoencephalitis, 595·3
Naetene, 2149·3
Naf Buches, 2149·3
Nafacil, 2149·3
Nafamostat Mesilate, 1719·1
Nafamostat Mesylate, 1719·1
Nafarelin Acetate, 1332·3
Nafarelina, Acetato de, 1332·3
Nafasol, 2149·3
Nafato de Cefamandol, 169·3
Nafazair, 2149·3
Nafazair A, 2149·3
Nafazolina, 1124·3
Nafazolina, Hidrocloruro de, 1124·3
Nafazolina, Nitrato de, 1124·3
Nafcilina Sódica, 233·3
Nafcillin Sodium, 233·3
Nafcillinum Natricum, 233·3
Nafcon A, 2149·3
Naferon, 2149·3
Naflapen, 2149·3
Naflex, 2149·3
Nafloxin, 2149·3
Nafluor, 2149·3
Nafluryl, 2149·3
Nafluvent, 2149·3
Nafordyl, 2149·3
NaFril, 2149·3
Nafrine, 2149·3
Nafronyl Oxalate, 964·1
Naftaleno, 1507·3
Naftalofos, 110·1
Naftazolina, 2149·3
Naftazona, 757·1
Naftazone, 757·1
Naftenato de Cobre, 397·1
Nafti, 2149·3
Naftidrofurilo, Oxalato de, 964·1
Naftidrofuryl Hydrogen Oxalate, 964·1
Naftidrofuryl Oxalate, 964·1
Naftidrofuryli Hydrogenooxalas, 964·1
Naftifina, Hidrocloruro de, 406·2
Naftifine Hydrochloride, 406·2
Naftifungin Hydrochloride, 406·2
Naftilacético, Ácido, 1719·1
Naftilong, 2149·3
Naftilux, 2149·3
Naftin, 2149·3
Naftoclizine, 427·3, 1130·3
Naftodril, 2149·3
β-Naftol, 103·2
Naftopidil, 964·1
Naganinum, 615·3
Naganol, 615·3
Nagel Batrafen, 2149·3
Nagun, 2149·3
Nahora, 2149·3
Nail Infections, Fungal— *see* Skin Infections, 390·1
Nail Nutrition, 2149·3
4 Nails, 2149·3
NailVit, 2149·3
Naion, Linimento— *see* Linimento Naion, 2097·4
Nakadipine Hydrochloride, 868·1
Nalador, 2149·3
Nalapres, 2149·4
Nalapril, 2149·4
Nalaprix, 2149·4
Nalbu, 2149·4
Nalbufina, Hidrocloruro de, 64·2
Nalbufine Hydrochloride, 64·2
Nalbuphine Hydrochloride, 64·2
Nalcrom, 2149·4
Nalcron, 2149·4
Nalcryn, 2149·4
Naldecol NF, 2149·4
Naldecol-D, 2149·4
Naldecon Preparations, 2149·4
Naldelate DX Adult, 2149·4
Naled, 1507·3
Nalerona, 2149·4
Nalex, 2149·4
Nalex DH, 2149·4
Nalex-A, 2149·4
Nalfan, 2149·4
Nalfon, 2149·4
Nalgesic, 2149·4
Nalgest, 2150·1
Nalidin, 2150·1
Nalidix, 2150·1
Nalidixan, 2150·1
Nalidixic Acid, 234·1
Nalidíxico, Ácido, 234·1
Nalidixin, 2150·1
Nalidixinic Acid, 234·1
Nalidoid, 2150·1
Naligram, 2150·1
Naline, 2150·1
Nalion, 2150·1
Nalissina, 2150·1
Nalix, 2150·1
Nalixone, 2150·1
Nallpen, 2150·1
Nalmefene, 1044·1
Nalmefene Hydrochloride, 1044·1
Nalmefeno, Hidrocloruro de, 1044·1
Nalmetrene, 1044·1
Nalmetrene Hydrochloride, 1044·1
Nalone, 2150·1
Nalopril, 2150·1
Nalorex, 2150·1
Nalorfina, 1044·2
Nalorfina, Hidrobromuro de, 1044·2
Nalorfina, Hidrocloruro de, 1044·2
Nalorphine, 1044·2
Nalorphine Hydrobromide, 1044·2
Nalorphine Hydrochloride, 1044·2
Nalorphini Hydrochloridum, 1044·2
Nalorphinium Chloride, 1044·2
Nalox, 2150·1
Naloxona, Cloridrato de, 1044·3
Naloxona, Hidrocloruro de, 1044·3
Naloxone Hydrochloride, 1044·3
Naloxone Hydrochloride Dihydrate, 1044·3
Naloxoni Hydrochloridum, 1044·3
6-β-Naltrexol, 1046·1
Naltrexona, Hidrocloruro de, 1046·1
Naltrexone, 1046·1
Naltrexone Hydrochloride, 1046·1
Naltrox, 2150·1
Naluril, 2150·1
Nalvir, 2150·1
Namba, 1666·1
Namenda, 2150·1
Nametone, 2150·1
Namic, 2150·1
Namifen, 2150·1
Namir, 2150·1
Nan, 2150·1
Nan AR, 2150·1
Nan HA, 2150·1
Nan HA/AR, 2150·1
Nan Sin Lactosa, 2150·1
Nan Soya, 2150·1
Nanafed, 2150·2
Nanalan, 2150·2
Nanalan Plus, 2150·2
Nanbacine, 2150·2
Nandain, 2150·2
Nandrol, 2150·2
Nandrolona, 1561·2
Nandrolona, Ciclohexilpropionato de, 1561·2
Nandrolona, Decanoato de, 1561·2
Nandrolona, Fenilpropionato de, 1561·3
Nandrolona, Laurato de, 1561·2
Nandrolona, Sulfato Sódico de, 1561·3
Nandrolona, Undecilato de, 1561·3
Nandrolone, 1561·2
Nandrolone Cyclohexanepropionate, 1561·2
Nandrolone Cyclohexylpropionate, 1561·2
Nandrolone Decanoate, 1561·2
Nandrolone Dodecanoate, 1561·2
Nandrolone Hexyloxyphenylpropionate, 1561·3
Nandrolone Hydrocinnamate, 1561·3
Nandrolone Laurate, 1561·2
Nandrolone Phenpropionate, 1561·3
Nandrolone Phenylpropionate, 1561·3
Nandrolone Propionate, 1561·3
Nandrolone Sodium Sulfate, 1561·3
Nandrolone Sodium Sulphate, 1561·3
Nandrolone Undecanoate, 1561·3
Nandrolone Undecylate, 1561·3
Nandrosande, 2150·2
Nani Pre Dental, 2150·2
Nanocoll, 2150·2
Nanophyetiasis— *see* Intestinal Fluke Infections, 99·2
Nanotiv, 2150·2
Nansius, 2150·2
Naox, 2150·2
Napa, 2150·2
NAPA, 848·3
Napacod, 2150·2
Napadisilato de Mebhidrolina, 436·3
Napamide, 2150·2
Napamol, 2150·2
Napan, 2150·2
NaPCA, 1158·1
Napflam, 2150·2
Napha Forte, 2150·2
Naphacel, 2150·2
Naphasal, 2150·2
Naphazoline, 1124·3
Naphazoline Acetate, 1125·1
Naphazoline Hydrochloride, 1124·3
Naphazoline Nitrate, 1124·3
Naphazoline Plus, 2150·2
Naphazolini Hydrochloridum, 1124·3
Naphazolini Nitras, 1124·3
Naphazolinium Nitricum, 1124·3
Naphcon, 2150·2
Naphcon Forte, 2150·2
Naphcon-A, 2150·2
Naphensyl, 2150·2
Naphoptic-A, 2150·2
Naphtears, 2150·2
Naphthalene, 1507·3
1-Naphthaleneacetic Acid, 1719·1
*N*-[(1*R*)-1-(Naphthalen-1-yl)ethyl]-3-[3-(trifluoromethyl)phenyl]propan-1-amine Hydrochloride, 770·2
Naphthalin, 1507·3
Naphthalophos, 110·1
Naphthammonum, 103·2
Naphthizinum, 1124·3
Naphthol, 103·2
Naphth-2-ol, 103·2
1,2-Naphthoquinone 2-Semicarbazone, 757·1
*O*-2-Naphthyl *m*,*N*-Dimethylthiocarbanilate, 410·1
1-Naphthyl Methylcarbamate, 1501·2
Naphthylacetic Acid, 1719·1
1-Naphthylacetic Acid, 1719·1
β-Naphthylamine, 1471·3
2-(1-Naphthylmethyl)-2-imidazoline, 1124·3
α-Naphthylthiourea, 1500·2
1-(1-Naphthyl)-2-thiourea, 1500·2
Naphthyridine Antimalarials, 444·1
Napilene, 2150·3
Napiro, 2150·3
Naplin, 2150·3
Napmel, 2150·3
Nappy Rash Powder, 2150·3
Nappy Rash Relief Cream, 2150·3
Nappy-Hippo, 2150·3
Nappy-Mate, 2150·3
Napratec, 2150·3
Napreben, 2150·3
Naprel, 2150·3
Naprelan, 2150·3
Napren, 2150·3
Naprex, 2150·3
Naprilene, 2150·3
Naprina, 2150·3
Naprius, 2150·3
Naprix, 2150·3
Naprix D, 2150·3
Naprizide, 2150·3
Naprobene, 2150·3
Naprocet, 2150·3
Naprocoat, 2150·3
Naprodil, 2150·3
Naprodol, 2150·3
Napro-Dorsch, 2150·3
Naprofidex, 2150·4
Naprogen, 2150·4
Naprogesic, 2150·4
Naprokes, 2150·4
Naprometin, 2150·4
Napromex, 2150·4
Napronet, 2150·4
Naprontag, 2150·4
Naprontag Flex, 2150·4
Naprorex, 2150·4
Naproscript, 2150·4
Naprosian, 2150·4
Naproso, 2150·4
Naprosyn, 2150·4
Naprosyne, 2150·4
Naproval, 2150·4

Naprovite, 2150·4
Naprox, 2150·4
Naproxen, 65·1
Naproxen Aminobutanol, 65·3
Naproxen Cetrimonium, 65·3
Naproxen Lysine, 65·3
Naproxen Piperazine, 65·3
Naproxen Sodium, 65·1
Naproxeno, 65·1
Naproxeno Sódico, 65·1
Naproxenum, 65·1
Naproxi, 2150·4
Naprux, 2150·4
Napsen, 2150·4
Napsilato de Dextropropoxifeno, 28·3
Napsilato de Levopropoxifeno, 1124·1
Napxen, 2150·4
Naqua, 2150·4
Naquinto, 2150·4
Naragran, 2150·4
Naramig, 2151·1
Naranja, 1724·1
Naranja, Aceite Esencial de, 1724·1
Naranja Amarga, 1723·3
Naranja Amarga, Corteza de, 1723·3
Naranja de Acridina, 1647·1
Naranja Sin Terpeno, Aceite Esencial de, 1724·2
Naranocor, 2151·1
Naranocut H, 2151·1
Naranofem, 2151·1
Naranopect P, 2151·1
Naranotox, 2151·1
Naranotox Plus, 2151·1
Narapril, 2151·1
Narasin, 611·1
Narasin Granular, 611·1
Narasina, 611·1
Naratriptán, Hidrocloruro de, 470·1
Naratriptan Hydrochloride, 470·1
Narcan, 2151·1
Narcanti, 2151·1
Narcaricin, 2151·1
Narcaricina, 2151·1
Narcolepsy— *see* Narcoleptic Syndrome, 1583·2
Narcoleptic Syndrome, 1583·2
Narcoral, 2151·1
Narcotan, 2151·1
Narcotic Analgesics, 1·3
Narcotine, 1125·3
L-α-Narcotine, 1125·3
Narcotine Hydrochloride, 1125·3
Narcotuss, 2151·1
Narcozep, 2151·1
Nard, Wild, 1658·1
Nardelzine, 2151·1
Nardil, 2151·1
Nardyl, 2151·1
Narfen, 2151·1
Narial, 2151·1
Naribel, 2151·1
Naricin, 2151·1
Naride, 2151·1
Naridex, 2151·1
Naridrin, 2151·1
Narifont, 2151·1
Narifresh, 2151·2
Narigen, 2151·2
Narilet, 2151·2
Narine, 2151·2
Naringin, 1723·3
Narisoro, 2151·2
Naristar, 2151·2
Naritec, 2151·2
Narium, 2151·2
Narix, 2151·2
Narixan, 2151·2
Narizima, 2151·2
Narizima Adulto, 2151·2
Narizima Pediatrico, 2151·2
Narizine, 2151·2
Narlisim, 2151·2
Narobic, 2151·2
Narocin, 2151·2
Narol, 2151·2
Narop, 2151·2
Naropeine, 2151·2
Naropin, 2151·2
Naropin with Fentanyl, 2151·2
Naropina, 2151·2
Narphen, 2151·2
Nartap, 2151·2
Nartograstim, 757·1
Narvizol, 2151·3
Narzen, 2151·3
Nasa-12, 2151·3
Nasa Rhinathiol, 2151·3
Nasabid, 2151·3
Nasacor, 2151·3
Nasacort, 2151·3
Nasacort AQ, 2151·3
NaSal, 2151·3
Nasal Congestion, 1112·3
Nasal Decongestant, 2151·3
Nasal Decongestants, 1112·1
Nasal Inhaler, 2151·3
Nasal Jelly, 2151·3
Nasal Moist, 2151·3
Nasal Relief, 2151·3
Nasal & Sinus Cold Formula, 2151·3
Nasal & Sinus Relief, 2151·3
Nasal Spray, 2151·3
Nasal Spray for Hayfever, 2151·3
Nasalate, 2151·3
Nasal-Bec, 2151·3
Nasalcrom, 2151·3
Nasal-Ease, 2151·3
Nasalemed, 2151·3
Nasaleze, 2151·3
Nasalflu, 2151·3
Nasalgen, 2151·3
Nasalide, 2151·3
Nasamine, 2151·4
Nasan, 2151·4
Nasanal, 2151·4
Nasapert, 2151·4
Nasarel, 2151·4
Nasarox, 2151·4
Nasaruplasa, 964·2
Nasaruplase, 964·2
Nasaruplase Beta, 964·2
Nasasinutab, 2151·4
Nasatab LA, 2151·4
Nasben, 2151·4
Nasben Soft, 2151·4
Nasciodine, 2151·4
Nascobal, 2151·4
Nasdro, 2151·4
Nasea, 2151·4
Nasengel, 2151·4
Nasengel AL, 2151·4
Nasenspray AL, 2151·4
Nasenspray E, 2151·4
Nasenspray K, 2151·4
Nasentropfen AL, 2151·4
Nasentropfen E, 2151·4
Nasentropfen K, 2151·4
Nasentropfen-ratiopharm, 2151·4
Naseptin, 2151·4
Nasex, 2151·4
Nasic, 2152·1
Nasicortin, 2152·1
Nasicur, 2152·1
Nasil, 2152·1
Nasilex, 2152·1
Nasimild, 2152·1
Nasin, 2152·1
Nasivin Preparations, 2152·1
Nasivine, 2152·1
Nasivinetten Gegen Schnupfen, 2152·1
Nasivinetten— *see* Nasivinettes, 2152·1
Nasivinettes, 2152·1
Nasivion, 2152·1
Nasmer, 2152·1
Naso Instil, 2152·1
Naso Pekamin, 2152·1
Nasobec, 2152·1
Nasobol, 2152·1
Naso-Calma, 2152·1
Nasocan, 2152·1
Nasoclean, 2152·1
Nasocort, 2152·1
Nasoferm, 2152·1
Nasoflux, 2152·1
Nasogrip, 2152·1
Nasojol, 2152·2
Nasolac, 2152·2
Nasolin, 2152·2
Nasolina, 2152·2
Nasomet, 2152·2
Nasomicina, 2152·2
Nasomicina Salina, 2152·2
Nasomin, 2152·2
Nasomixin, 2152·2
Nasonex, 2152·2
Nasopan, 2152·2
Nasopharyngeal Carcinoma— *see* Malignant Neoplasms of the Head and Neck, 517·3
Nasopomada, 2152·2
Naso-Prieulina, 2152·2
Nasorest, 2152·2
Nasosil, 2152·2
Nasotic Oto, 2152·2
Nasovalda, 2152·2
Naspor, 2152·2
Nasterid, 2152·2
Nasteril, 2152·2
Nastifrin, 2152·2
Nastifrin Compuesto, 2152·3
Nastifrin DN Compuesto, 2152·3
Nastil, 2152·3
Nastizol Preparations, 2152·3
Nastizol-L, 2152·3
Nastop, 2152·3
Nastoren, 2152·3
Nastul, 2152·3
Nastul Compuesto, 2152·3
*Nasturtium armoracia*, 1697·3
Nasulind, 2152·3
NAT-333, 786·1
Nat. Mur., 1234·3
Natabec, 2152·3
Natabec F, 2152·3
NataChew, 2152·3
Natacyn, 2152·3
Natafort, 2152·3
Natafucin, 2152·3
Natal, 2152·3
Natal Extra, 2152·3
NatalCare, 2152·3
Natalin, 2152·3
Natalins, 2152·3
Natalins Com Fluor, 2152·3
Natalins Folico, 2152·4
Natalins Rx, Enfamil— *see* Enfamil Natalins Rx, 1970·3
Natalizumab, 1719·1
Natamicina, 406·2
Natamycin, 406·2
Nataral, 2152·4
Natarex Prenatal, 2152·4
NataTab, 2152·4
Natavite, 2152·4
Natead, 2152·4
Natecal, 2152·4
Natecal D, 2152·4
Nateglin, 2152·4
Nateglinida, 343·3
Nateglinide, 343·3
Nateplase, 964·2
Nathergen, 2152·4
Naticardina, 2152·4
Natigesta, 2152·4
Nati-K, 2152·4
Natiken, 2152·4
Natil, 2152·4
Natinate, 2152·4
Natisedina, 2152·4
Natisedine, 2152·4
Natispray, 2152·4
Nativa HA, 2152·4
Nativit, 2152·4
Nativit Fluor, 2152·4
Na-To-Caps, 2152·4
Natopherol, 2152·4
Natopherol Dermal-Day, 2152·4
Natoss, 2152·4
Natovit, 2152·4
Natracalm, 2152·4
NatraFlex, 2153·1
Natraleze, 2153·1
Natrapel, 2153·1
Natrasleep, 2153·1
Natrecor, 2153·1
Natri Sulfis Anhydricus, 1193·1
Natriclo, 2153·1
Natrii Acetas Trihydricus, 1223·1
Natrii Alendronas, 765·3
Natrii Alginas, 1577·1
Natrii Amidotrizoas, 1060·2
Natrii Aminosalicylas Dihydricus, 155·1
Natrii Ascorbas, 1460·2
Natrii Benzoas, 1169·3
Natrii Bicarbonas, 1223·2
Natrii Calcii Edetas, 1051·3
Natrii Caprylas, 1723·1
Natrii Carbonas, 1747·2
Natrii Carbonas Anhydricus, 1747·1
Natrii Carbonas Decahydricus, 1747·2
Natrii Carbonas Monohydricus, 1747·2
Natrii Cetylo- et Stearylosulfas, 1574·2
Natrii Chloridum, 1233·3
Natrii Citras, 1223·2
Natrii Cromoglicas, 795·3
Natrii Cyclamas, 1426·2
Natrii Dihydrogenophosphas, 1230·3
Natrii Dihydrogenophosphas Dihydricus, 1230·3
Natrii Disulfis, 1193·1
Natrii Docusas, 1262·2
Natrii Edetas, 1037·3
Natrii Ferrigluconas, 1444·3
Natrii Fluoridum, 1444·3
Natrii Fusidas, 215·2
Natrii Gentisas, 90·1
Natrii Glutamas, 1441·1
Natrii Glycerophosphas, 1695·2
Natrii Hyaluronas, 1697·3
Natrii Hydrogenocarbonas, 1223·2
Natrii Hydroxidum, 1747·3
Natrii Iodetum, 1598·1
Natrii Iodidum, 1598·1
Natrii Jodidum, 1598·1
Natrii Laurilsulfas, 1574·2
Natrii Metabisulfis, 1193·1
Natrii Molybdas Dihydricus, 1440·3
Natrii Monofluorophosphas, 1446·2
Natrii Nitras, 1192·2
Natrii Nitris, 1052·3
Natrii Nitroprussias, 1000·2
Natrii Para-aminosalicylas, 155·1
Natrii Perboras, 1192·2
Natrii Phosphas, 1231·1
Natrii Picosulfas, 1289·3
Natrii Polystyrenesulfonas, 1053·1
Natrii Propionas, 408·1
Natrii Salicylas, 90·1
Natrii Selenis Pentahydricus, 1444·1
Natrii Stearas, 1574·3
Natrii Stearylis Fumaras, 1575·1
Natrii Sulfas Anhydricus, 1290·1
Natrii Sulfas Decahydricus, 1290·1
Natrii Sulfis Anhydricus, 1193·1
Natrii Sulfis Heptahydricus, 1193·1
Natrii Sulfis Siccatus, 1193·1
Natrii Sulphas, 1290·1
Natrii Sulphis, 1193·1
Natrii Tetraboras, 1661·3
Natrii Thiosulfas, 1053·3
Natrii Valproas, 380·1
Natrilix, 2153·1
Natrioxen, 2153·1
Natrium Aceticum, 1223·1
Natrium Arsenicicum, 1747·1
Natrium Benzoicum, 1169·3
Natrium Boricum, 1661·3
Natrium Carbonicum Calcinatum, 1747·1
Natrium Carbonicum Crystallisatum, 1747·2
Natrium Carbonicum Siccatum, 1747·1
Natrium Cetylosulphuricum, 1574·2
Natrium Cetylstearylosulphuricum, 1574·2

Natrium Chloricum, 1747·2
Natrium Citricum Acidum, 1223·2
Natrium Fluoratum, 1444·3
Natrium Glycerophosphoricum, 1695·2
Natrium Hydricum, 1747·3
Natrium Hydroxydatum, 1747·3
Natrium Iodatum, 1598·1
Natrium Isopentylaethylthiobarbituricum (cum Natrio Carbonico), 1309·1
Natrium Lauryl Sulphuricum, 1574·2
Natrium Methylarsonicum, 1748·1
Natrium Muriaticum, 1234·3
Natrium Nitricum, 1192·2
Natrium Nitrosum, 1052·3
Natrium Novaminsulfonicum, 35·3
Natrium Phosphoricum Monobasicum, 1230·3
Natrium Sulfaminochloratum, 1194·3
Natrium Sulfobituminosum Decoloratum, 1148·3
Natrium Sulfuricum Crystallisatum, 1290·1
Natrium Sulfuricum Siccatum, 1290·1
Natrium Thiosulfuricum, 1053·3
Natrium-Homaccord, 2153·1
Natriumseleniat, 1444·1
Natriuretic Peptides, 964·2
Natrocitral, 2153·1
Natropas, 2153·1
Natrosteril, 2153·1
Natsurf, 2153·1
Natucor, 2153·1
Natuderm, 2153·1
Natudolor, 2153·1
Natudophilus, 2153·1
Natudor, 2153·1
Natu-fem, 2153·1
Natulan, 2153·1
Natulanar, 2153·1
Natulax, 2153·1
Natura Preparations, 2153·1
Naturaform Fruchtewurfel Mit Manna, 2153·2
Natural Camphor, 1665·3
Natural Defense, 2153·2
Natural Diet, 2153·2
Natural E, Bioglan— *see* Bioglan Natural E, 1844·1
Natural Fibre, 2153·2
Natural Herb Tablets, 2153·2
Natural Horizons Solar Block Extreme, 2153·2
Natural Horizons Solar Block Lotion, 2153·2
Natural Horizons Solar Block Toddler, 2153·2
Natural Ice Extreme, 2153·2
Natural Ice Lipbalm, 2153·2
Natural Laxative with Softener, Chemists Own— *see* Chemists Own Natural Laxative with Softener, 1882·1
Natural Source Laxative, 2153·2
Natural Vitamin A Ester Concentrate, 1451·3
Natural Wealth Beta, 2153·2
Natural Zanzy, 2153·2
Naturalag, 2153·2
Naturalass, 2153·2
Naturalist, 2153·2
Naturalyte, 2153·2
Naturcil, 2153·2
Nature Throid, 2153·2
Nature's Choice, 2153·2
Natures Own Preparations, 2153·2
Natures Remedy, 2153·3
Nature's Tears, 2153·3
Natures Way Preparations, 2153·3
Naturest, 2153·3
Naturetin, 2153·3
Naturetti, 2153·3
Naturgen Terre Silice, 2153·3
Naturgen Terre Volcanique, 2153·3
Naturine, 2153·4
Naturland Preparations, 2153·4
Naturlax, 2153·4
Naturogest, 2153·4
Naturvite, 2153·4
Natus Gerin, 2153·4
Natusan, 2153·4
Natuscap Retard, 2153·4
Natuscilin, 2153·4
Natusgel, 2153·4
Natusor Preparations, 2153·4
Natuvit, 2154·1
Natuzilium, 2154·1
Natyl, 2154·1
Naudicelle Preparations, 2154·1
Naudivite, 2154·1
Naupathon, 2154·1
Nausamine, 2154·1
Nausea Relief, 2154·1
Nausea and Vomiting, 1245·2
Nauseatol, 2154·1
Nausedron, 2154·1
Nausefe, 2154·1
Nausetum, 2154·1
Nausex, 2154·2
Nausicalm, 2154·2
Nausigon, 2154·2
Nausil, 2154·2
Nausilen, 2154·2
Nausilon B6, 2154·2
Nausyn, 2154·2
Nautamine, 2154·2
Nautigo, 2154·2
Nautisol, 2154·2
Nautrol, 2154·2
Nauzelin, 2154·2
Nauzine, 2154·2
Navamed, 2154·2
Navamin, 2154·2
Navane, 2154·2
Navasprin, 2154·2
Navelbine, 2154·2
Navicalm, 2154·2
Navidoxine, 2154·2
Navidrex, 2154·2
Naviga, 2154·2
Navispare, 2154·3
Navixen, 2154·3
Navoban, 2154·3
Naxan, 2154·3
Naxen, 2154·3
Naxidine, 2154·3
Naxil, 2154·3
Naxilan-Plus, 2154·3
Naxo, 2154·3
Naxo C, 2154·3
Naxo TV, 2154·3
Naxocina, 2154·3
Naxoclinda, 2154·3
Naxodol, 2154·3
Naxogil, 2154·3
Naxogin, 2154·3
Naxogin Compositum, 2154·3
Naxogin Composto, 2154·3
Naxogin Dos, 2154·3
Naxogyn, 2154·3
Naxolan, 2154·3
Naxopren, 2154·3
Naxpa, 2154·3
Naxy, 2154·3
Naxyn, 2154·3
Nazalet, 2154·3
Nazalin, 2154·3
Nazamit, 2154·4
Nazasetron Hydrochloride, 1251·1
Nazene, 2154·4
Nazicol, 2154·4
Nazobel, 2154·4
Nazobio, 2154·4
Nazodin, 2154·4
Nazolfarm, 2154·4
Nazolin, 2154·4
Nazophyl, 2154·4
Nazosoro, 2154·4
Nazotiran, 2154·4
9-NC, 583·2
NC-14, 864·1
NC-123, 706·3
NC-150, 83·1
NC-1264, 1757·2
NC-1400, 873·2
N-Combur Test, 2154·4
NDC-0082-4155, 545·3
2′-NDG, 635·3
NDGA, 1187·1
*meso*-NDGA, 566·1
ND-Gesic, 2154·4
NDR-5998A, 786·1
NE-10064, 866·3
NE-58095, 774·3
Nealorin, 2154·4
Neamine, 235·1
Neat Effect, 2154·4
Neat Feat, 2154·4
Neat One, 2154·4
Neat Touch, 2154·4
Neatenol, 2154·4
Neatenol Diu, 2154·4
Neatenol Diuvas, 2154·4
Nebacetin, 2154·4
Nebacetin N, 2154·4
Nebacetina, 2154·4
Nebacina, 2154·4
Nebacitrin, 2154·4
Nebacumab, 1615·2
Nebal, 2154·4
Nebalon, 2154·4
Nebapol B, 2154·4
Nebapul, 2154·4
Nebasulf, 2155·1
Nebcin, 2155·1
Nebcina, 2155·1
Nebcine, 2155·1
Nebicina, 2155·1
Nebilet, 2155·1
Nebilox, 2155·1
Nebiotin, 2155·1
Nebivolol, 964·3
Nebivolol, Hidrocloruro de, 964·3
Nebivolol Hydrochloride, 964·3
Neblic, 2155·1
Neblik, 2155·1
Nebracetam, 1719·2
Nebramycin Factor 2, 158·2
Nebramycin Factor 6, 271·2
Nebril, 2155·1
Nebris, 2155·1
Nebufur, 2155·1
Nebulasma, 2155·1
Nebulcort, 2155·1
Nebulcrom, 2155·1
Nebulicina, 2155·1
NebuPent, 2155·1
NEC, 2155·1
Necamin, 2155·1
Necatoriasis— *see* Hookworm Infections, 99·2
Necid, 2155·1
Neck Cancer— *see* Malignant Neoplasms of the Head and Neck, 517·3
Necloral, 2155·1
Neclovir, 2155·1
Necon, 2155·1
Necon 1/50, 2155·1
Necon 10/11, 2155·1
Necopen, 2155·1
Necro B-6, 2155·2
Necrohepat, 2155·2
Necroplex, 2155·2
Necrotising Enteritis— *see* Necrotising Enterocolitis, 129·2
Necrotising Enterocolitis, 129·2
Necrotising Fasciitis, 136·2
Necrotising Ulcerative Gingivitis, Acute— *see* Mouth Infections, 136·1
Necrotising Vasculitis— *see* Vasculitic Syndromes, 1090·1
Necrotising Vasculitis, Systemic— *see* Polyarteritis Nodosa and Microscopic Polyangiitis, 1085·3
Necta C, 2155·2
Necyrane, 2155·2
Neda Fruchtewurfel, 2155·2
Neda Lactiv Importal, 2155·2
Nedaplatin, 576·2
Nedaplatino, 576·2
Nedax, 2155·2
Nedax Plus, 2155·2
Nedeltran, 2155·2
Nedios, 2155·2
Nedis, 2155·2
Nedocromil Calcium, 789·3
Nedocromil Sodium, 789·3
Nedocromilo Sódico, 789·3
Nedolon P, 2155·2
NEE 1/35, 2155·2
Neem, 1658·2
Neem Oil, 1658·2
Nefadar, 2155·2
Nefadol, 2155·2
Nefam, 2155·2
Nefazan, 2155·2
Nefazodona, Hidrocloruro de, 309·2
Nefazodone Hydrochloride, 309·2
Nefazol, 2155·2
Nefelid, 2155·2
Nefersil, 2155·2
Nefersil B, 2155·2
Nefiracetam, 1719·2
Nefirel, 2155·2
Nefluan, 2155·2
Nefoben, 2155·2
Nefopam, Hidrocloruro de, 66·2
Nefopam Hydrochloride, 66·2
Nefrin, 2155·2
Nefro Diet, 2155·2
Nefroamino, 2155·2
Nefrocarnit, 2155·3
Nefrodial, 2155·3
Nefrolactona, 2155·3
Nefroplasmal, 2155·3
Nefrosol, 2155·3
Nefro-Zinc, 2155·3
Nefryl, 2155·3
Negaban, 2155·3
Negacef, 2155·3
Negacne, 2155·3
Negadix, 2155·3
Negalerg, 2155·3
Negalerg L, 2155·3
Negaporosis, 2155·3
Negatol, 2155·3
Negatol Dental, 2155·3
Negazole, 2155·3
NegGram, 2155·3
Negram, 2155·3
Negro PN, 1056·2
Nehydrin, 2155·3
Nehydrin N, 2155·3
Neimen/Vac, 1626·1
*Neisseria gonorrhoeae*, 1616·1
*Neisseria meningitidis*, 1626·1
NeisVac, 2155·3
NeisVac-C, 2155·3
Nekacin, 2155·3
Nelapine, 2155·3
Nelbinex, 2155·3
Nelconil, 2155·3
Nelex, 2155·4
Nelfilea, 2155·4
Nelfinavir Mesilate, 650·1
Nelfinavir, Mesilato de, 650·1
Nelfinavir Mesylate, 650·1
Nelfir, 2155·4
Nelin, 2155·4
Nelkenöl, 1673·3
Nelova Preparations, 2155·4
Nelsons Clikpak Series, 2155·4
Neltenexina, 1125·2
Neltenexine, 1125·2
Neltenexine Hydrochloride, 1125·2
Nemactil, 2155·4
Nemapres, 2155·4
Nemasol, 2155·4
Nemasole, 2155·4
Nematode Infections, 97·1
Nembutal, 2155·4
Nemdyn, 2155·4
Nemegel, 2155·4
Nemesil, 2155·4
Nemestran, 2155·4
Nemexin, 2155·4
Nemicina, 2155·4
Nemocebral, 2155·4
Nemocid, 2155·4

Nemodine, 2155·4
Nemonaprida, 710·1
Nemonapride, 710·1
Nemozole, 2155·4
Nene Dent, 2155·4
Nene Dent N, 2155·4
Nene-Lax, 2155·4
NEO, 235·1
Neo Analsona, 2156·1
Neo Aritmina, 2156·1
Neo Artrol, 2156·1
Neo Atromid, 2156·1
Neo A-V, 2156·1
Neo Axedil, 2156·1
Neo Baby Cream, 2156·1
Neo Bace, 2156·1
Neo Bacitrin, 2156·1
Neo Bacitrin Hidrocortis, 2156·1
Neo Bendazol, 2156·1
Neo Benzil, 2156·1
Neo Borocillina, 2156·1
Neo Borocillina Balsamica, 2156·1
Neo Borocillina C, 2156·1
Neo Borocillina Collutorio, 2156·1
Neo Borocillina Spray, 2156·1
Neo Borocillina Tosse Compresse, 2156·1
Neo Borocillina Tosse Sciroppo, 2156·1
Neo Butartrol, 2156·1
Neo Butazol, 2156·1
Neo Cal, 2156·1
Neo Cal D, 2156·1
Neo Carbone Belloc, 2156·1
Neo Cardiol, 2156·1
Neo Cebetil, 2156·1
Neo Cefadril, 2156·1
Neo Cefix, 2156·1
Neo Ceflex, 2156·1
Neo Cepacol Collutorio, 2156·2
Neo Cepacol Pastiglie, 2156·2
Neo Citran, 2156·2
Neo Citran A, 2156·2
Neo Citran Calorie Reduced, 2156·2
Neo Citran Chest Congestion & Cough, 2156·2
Neo Citran Cough Cold & Flu, 2156·2
Neo Citran Daycaps, 2156·2
Neo Citran DM, 2156·2
Neo Citran Extra Strength, 2156·2
Neo Citran Grippe/refroidissement, 2156·2
Neo Citran Nutrasweet— *see* Neo Citran Calorie Reduced, 2156·2
Neo Citran Sinus, 2156·2
Neo Citran Sore Throat & Cough, 2156·2
Neo Clodil, 2156·2
Neo Clotrimazyl, 2156·2
Neo Coltirot, 2156·2
Neo Coricidin, 2156·2
Neo Coricidin Gola, 2156·2
Neo Cortofen, 2156·2
Neo Decabutin, 2156·2
Neo Decapeptyl, 2156·2
Neo Dohyfral, 2156·2
Neo Dulceril, 2156·2
Neo Duplofer, 2156·2
Neo Eblimon, 2156·2
Neo Elixifilin, 2156·2
Neo Emocicatrol, 2156·3
Neo Emoform, 2156·3
Neo Esoformolo, 2156·3
Neo Expectan, 2156·3
Neo Fedipina, 2156·3
Neo Fenicol, 2156·3
Neo Fertinorm, 2156·3
Neo Fluostomygen, 2156·3
Neo Folico, 2156·3
Neo Formitrol, 2156·3
Neo Fulvigal, 2156·3
Neo Furasil, 2156·3
Neo Gastrausil, 2156·3
Neo Genyl, 2156·3
Neo Gripe Mixture, 2156·3
Neo H2, 2156·3
Neo Hidroclor, 2156·3
Neo Hubber, 2156·3
Neo Iloticina, 2156·3
Neo Isocaden, 2156·3
Neo Itrax, 2156·3
Neo Kef, 2156·3
Neo Kodan, 2156·3
Neo Lacrim, 2156·3
Neo Lactoflorene, 2156·3
Neo Linco, 2156·3
Neo Loratadin, 2156·3
Neo Lyndiol, 2156·3
Neo Makatussin N, 2156·3
Neo Mebend, 2156·3
Neo Melubrina, 2156·3
Neo Metrodazol, 2156·3
Neo Mistatin, 2156·4
Neo Moderin, 2156·4
Neo Moldava, 2156·4
Neo Mom, 2156·4
Neo Moxicilin, 2156·4
Neo Nifalium, 2156·4
Neo Nisidina C-Fher, 2156·4
Neo Nisidina-Fher, 2156·4
Neo OPT, 2156·4
Neo Pelvicillin, 2156·4
Neo Perginol, 2156·4
Neo POM, 2156·4
Neo Propranol, 2156·4
Neo Quimica Colirio, 2156·4
Neo Rhinovit, 2156·4
Neo Rinactive, 2156·4
Neo Rinoleina, 2156·4
Neo Sampoon, 2156·4
Neo Sativan, 2156·4
Neo Silvikrin, 2156·4
Neo Soluzione Sulfo Balsamica, 2156·4
Neo Stress, Bioglan— *see* Bioglan Neo Stress, 1844·1
Neo Sulfazina, 2156·4
Neo Tionazol, 2156·4
Neo Tomizol, 2156·4
Neo Topico Giusto, 2156·4
Neo Uniplus, 2156·4
Neo Uniplus C, 2156·4
Neo Urgenin, 2156·4
Neo Vastrictol, 2157·1
Neo Verpamil, 2157·1
Neo Visage, 2157·1
Neo Vitalisan, 2157·1
Neo Zeta-Foot, 2157·1
Neo-Acarina, 2157·1
Neo-adlibamin, 2157·1
Neo-Alcos-Anal, 2157·1
Neo-Ampiplus, 2157·1
Neo-Angin Preparations, 2157·1
Neo-antiperstam, 2157·1
Neo-Audiocort, 2157·1
Neobac, 2157·1
Neobacigrin, 2157·1
Neobacina, 2157·1
Neobacipan, 2157·1
Neobacitracina, 2157·1
Neobacitracine, 2157·1
Neo-Ballistol, 2157·2
Neobar, 2157·2
Neobes, 2157·2
Neo-Bex, 2157·2
Neo-Bex Forte, 2157·2
Neo-Biphyllin, 2157·2
Neobitiol Compuesto, 2157·2
Neobloc, 2157·2
Neo-Boldolaxine, 2157·2
Neobonsen, 2157·2
Neo-botacreme, 2157·2
Neobradoral, 2157·2
Neobron, 2157·2
Neo-Bronchol, 2157·2
Neobrontyl, 2157·2
NeoBros, 2157·2
NeoBros 10, 2157·2
NeoBros C, 2157·2
Neobrufen, 2157·2
Neo-Bucosin, 2157·2
Neo-C, 2157·2
Neocaina, 2157·2
Neocalcit, 2157·2
Neo-Calglucon, 2157·2
Neocalmans, 2157·2
Neocapil, 2157·2
Neocarbo, 2157·3
Neocarbon, 2157·3
Neocardon, 2157·3
Neocarzinostatin, 594·3
Neocate, 2157·3
Neocate One +, 2157·3
Neocef, 2157·3
Neocefal, 2157·3
Neoceflex, 2157·3
Neoceftriona, 2157·3
Neocel, 2157·3
Neocepacilina, 2157·3
Neoceptin-R, 2157·3
Neocetrin, 2157·3
Neoceuticals Preparations, 2157·3
Neochinosol, 2157·3
Neocibalena, 2157·3
Neo-Cibalgin, 2157·3
Neo-Cibalgina, 2157·3
Neociclina, 2157·3
Neociclina Vitaminada, 2157·3
Neo-Cimexon, 2157·3
Neo-Cimexon G, 2157·3
Neocin, 2157·4
Neocina, 2157·4
Neocinolon, 2157·4
Neocitec, 2157·4
NeoCitran, 2157·4
Neocitran, 2157·4
NeoCitran Antitussif, 2157·4
NeoCitran Expectorant, 2157·4
Neoclaritine, 2157·4
Neoclarityn, 2157·4
Neo-Cleanse, 2157·4
Neoclym, 2157·4
Neo-Cobefrin— *see* Carbocaine with Neo-Cobefrin, 1869·3
Neo-Codion, 2157·4
Neo-Codion N, 2157·4
Neo-Codion NN, 2157·4
Neocof, 2157·4
Neocoflan, 2157·4
Neocolan, 2157·4
Neocon, 2157·4
Neocones, 2157·4
Neocontrast, 2158·1
Neocopan, 2158·1
Neo-Cortef, 2158·1
Neocortin, 2158·1
Neocortizul, 2158·1
Neo-Cratylen, 2158·1
Neocristin, 2158·1
Neo-Cromaton Bicomplesso, 2158·1
Neo-Currino, 2158·1
Neo-Cutigenol, 2158·1
Neocutis, 2158·1
Neo-Cystine, 2158·1
Neo-Cytamen, 2158·1
Neo-Dagracycline, 2158·1
Neo-Davisolona, 2158·1
Neodazol, 2158·1
Neo-Debiol AD3, 2158·1
Neo-Deca, 2158·1
NeoDecadron, 2158·1
Neo-Decongestine, 2158·1
Neo-Delphicort, 2158·1
Neo-Dentocain, 2158·1
Neoderm, 2158·1
Neoderm Ginecologico, 2158·2
Neodesfila, 2158·2
Neo-Desogen, 2158·2
Neo-Destomygen, 2158·2
Neodetoxergon, 2158·2
Neodex, 2158·2
Neo-Dex (Improved), 2158·2
Neodexa, 2158·2
Neodexa Plus, 2158·2
Neo-Dexameth, 2158·2
Neodexasone, 2158·2
Neodexon, 2158·2
Neodextril 40, 2158·2
Neodextril 70, 2158·2
Neo-Diaral, 2158·2
Neodicumarinum, 914·1
Neo-Diophen, 2158·2
Neo-Disterin, 2158·2
Neodol, 2158·2
Neodolito, 2158·2
Neodolpasse, 2158·2
Neodone, 2158·2
Neodox, 2158·2
Neo-DP, 2158·2
Neodrea, 2158·3
Neoduplamox, 2158·3
Neo-Durabolic, 2158·3
Neodyn, 2158·3
Neoefodil, 2158·3
Neo-egmol, 2158·3
Neo-Emedyl, 2158·3
Neoendorphins, 73·3
Neo-endusix, 2158·3
Neo-enteroseptol, 2158·3
Neo-Eparbiol, 2158·3
Neo-Eunomin, 2158·3
Neo-Eunomine, 2158·3
Neofam, 2158·3
Neofarmotox, 2158·3
Neofazol, 2158·3
Neofed, 2158·3
Neofenox, 2158·3
Neo-Fepramol, 2158·3
Neo-Fer, 2158·3
Neo-Fer, Nycoplus— *see* Nycoplus Neo-Fer, 2182·2
Neoflogin, 2158·3
Neofloxin, 2158·3
Neofolin, 2158·3
Neofomiral, 2158·3
Neo-fradin, 2158·3
Neofrin, 2158·3
Neoftalm, 2158·3
Neoftalm Dexa, 2158·3
Neofulvin, 2158·4
Neo-Furadantin, 2158·4
Neofyllin, 2158·4
Neogadine, 2158·4
Neogadine SG, 2158·4
Neogama, 2158·4
Neogama D Novo, 2158·4
Neogasol, 2158·4
Neogecim, 2158·4
Neogel, 2158·4
Neogentrol, 2158·4
Neogest, 2158·4
Neo-Geynevral, 2158·4
Neo-Gilurythmal, 2158·4
Neo-Gilurytmal, 2158·4
Neogluconin, 2158·4
Neogobion, 2158·4
Neo-Golaseptine, 2158·4
Neogram, 2158·4
Neogrip, 2158·4
Neogynon, 2158·4
Neogynona, 2158·4
Neo-Healar, 2158·4
Neo-Heparbil, 2158·4
Neo-Hesna, 2158·4
Neohexal, 2158·4
Neo-Hydro, 2158·4
Neo-Hytisone, 2158·4
Neo-Intol, 2159·1
Neoiodarsolo, 2159·1
Neo-Ipertas, 2159·1
Neo-Kap, 2159·1
Neokratin, 2159·1
Neo-Lapitrypsin, 2159·1
Neolapril, 2159·1
Neo-Laryngobis, 2159·1
Neolasil, 2159·1
Neolette, 2159·1
Neo-Lidocaton, 2159·1
Neolidona, 2159·1
Neolipid, 2159·1
Neoloid, 2159·1
Neolon-D, 2159·1
Neo-Lotan, 2159·1
Neo-Lotan Plus, 2159·1
Neomas, 2159·1
Neomas L, 2159·1
Neomed, 2159·1
Neomedil, 2159·1
Neo-Medrol, 2159·1

Neo-Medrol Acne, 2159·1
Neo-Medrol Comp, 2159·1
Neo-Medrol Veriderm, 2159·2
Neo-Medrone, 2159·2
Neomelin, 2159·2
Neo-Melubrina, 2159·2
Neo-Mercazole, 2159·2
Neomercurocromo, 2159·2
Neomeritine, 2159·2
Neo-Meton, 2159·2
Neomicina, 235·1
Neomicina Composta, 2159·2
Neomicina, Sulfato de, 235·1
Neomicina, Undecilenato de, 235·2
Neomicol, 2159·2
Neomigran, 2159·2
Neo-Mindol, 2159·2
Neomite, 2159·2
Neomixen, 2159·2
Neomixin, 2159·2
Neomonovar, 2159·2
Neo-Mudapenil, 2159·2
Neo-Mune, 2159·2
Neomycin, 235·1
Neomycin A, 235·1
Neomycin B, 235·1
Neomycin B Sulphate, 215·1
Neomycin C, 235·1
Neomycin E Sulphate, 612·3
Neomycin Hydrochloride, 236·1
Neomycin Sulfate, 235·1
Neomycin Sulphate, 235·1
Neomycin Undecenoate, 235·2
Neomycin Undecylenate, 235·2
Neomycini Sulfas, 235·1
Neo-mycodermol, 2159·2
Neo-Mydrial, 2159·2
Neomyrt Plus, 2159·2
Neo-NaClex, 2159·2
Neo-NaClex-K, 2159·2
Neonatal Apnoea, 806·1
Neonatal Conjunctivitis, 136·3
Neonatal Intraventricular Haemorrhage, 740·1
Neonatal Myasthenia— *see* Myasthenia Gravis, 1486·2
Neonatal Opioid Dependence— *see* Neonatal Abstinence Syndrome, 72·1
Neonatal Opioid Withdrawal Syndrome— *see* Neonatal Abstinence Syndrome, 72·1
Neonatal Respiratory Distress Syndrome, 1084·2
Neonatal Seizures, 353·2
Neonatal Sepsis— *see* Septicaemia, 144·3
Neonates, Pain in— *see* Choice of Analgesics in Children, 3·2
Neonaxil, 2159·2
Neo-Nevral, 2159·2
Neoniagar, 2159·2
Neo-omnipen, 2159·2
Neo-Optal, 2159·3
Neo-Optalidon, 2159·3
NeoOstrogynal, 2159·3
Neopam, 2159·3
Neopan, 2159·3
Neopankreoflat, 2159·3
Neo-Panlacticos, 2159·3
Neo-Panlacticos Plus, 2159·3
Neoparyl Framycetine, 2159·3
Neopect, 2159·3
Neopelle, 2159·3
Neo-Penotran, 2159·3
Neopenyl, 2159·3
Neopeptine, 2159·3
Neoperazona, 2159·3
Neo-Pergonal, 2159·3
Neopermease, 2159·3
Neophedan, 2159·3
Neo-Phlogicid, 2159·3
Neophyllin, 2159·3
Neopiridin, 2159·3
Neo-Planotest, 2159·3
Neoplasms, Malignant, 499·1
Neoplastic Fever— *see* Fever and Hyperthermia, 8·2
Neoplatin, 2159·3
Neoplaxol, 2159·3
Neoplex, 2159·3
Neoplex B, 2159·3
Neoplex B+C, 2159·3
Neo-Plex Concentrate— *see* Neo-C, 2157·2
Neoplus, 2159·3
Neopolydex, 2159·4
Neoprazol, 2159·4
Neopred, 2159·4
Neo-Preocil, 2159·4
Neopress, 2159·4
Neoprex, 2159·4
Neo-Primovlar, 2159·4
Neoproct, 2159·4
Neo-Prunex, 2159·4
Neopulmonier, 2159·4
Neo-Pyodron, 2159·4
Neo-Pyrazol, 2159·4
Neo-Pyrazon, 2159·4
Neopyrin, 2159·4
Neoquassin, 1737·2
Neoquin, 2159·4
Neoquin Forte, 2159·4
Neoral, 2159·4
Neoral-Sandimmun, 2159·4
NeoRecormon, 2159·4
Neorinol, 2159·4
Neorlest, 2159·4
Neo-Rowachol, 2159·4
Neo-Rowatinex, 2159·4
Neorutin, 2159·4
Neorythmin, 2159·4
Neos Nitro OPT, 2159·4
Neo-Sabenyl, 2159·4
Neosac, 2159·4
Neosaldina, 2160·1
Neosar, 2160·1
Neosayomol, 2160·1
Neosec, 2160·1
Neosed, 2160·1
Neosemid, 2160·1
Neoseptil, 2160·1
Neosidantoina, 2160·1
Neo-Sinedol, 2160·1
Neo-Sinefrina, 2160·1
Neo-Sintrom, 2156·4
Neosol, 2160·1
Neosolets, 2160·1
Neosona, 2160·1
Neosoralen, 2160·1
Neosorexa, 1504·1
Neosoro, 2160·1
Neo-Soyal, 2160·1
Neospect, 2160·1
Neosporin Preparations, 2160·1
Neossolvan, 2160·2
Neostatin, 2160·2
Neo-Stediril, 2160·2
Neostesin, 2160·2
Neostig. Brom., 1492·2
Neostig. Methylsulph., 1492·2
Neostigmina, 1492·2
Neostigmina, Bromuro de, 1492·2
Neostigmina, Metilsulfato de, 1492·2
Neostigmine, 1492·2
Neostigmine Bromide, 1492·2
Neostigmine Methylsulfate, 1492·2
Neostigmine Methylsulphate, 1492·2
Neostigmine Metilsulfate, 1492·2
Neostigmine Min-I-Mix, 2160·2
Neostigmini Bromidum, 1492·2
Neostigmini Metilsulfas, 1492·2
Neostigminii Bromidum, 1492·2
Neostigminum Bromatum, 1492·2
Neostig-Reu, 2160·2
Neostil, 2160·2
Neostix-N, 2160·2
Neo-Stomygen, 2160·2
Neostrata Preparations, 2160·2
Neosulf, 2160·3
Neosulida, 2160·3
Neosulin Lenta, 2160·3
Neosulin NPH, 2160·3
Neosulin Regular, 2160·3
Neo-Suxigal, 2160·3
Neo-Synalar, 2160·3
Neosynephrine, 2160·3
Neo-Synephrine, 2160·3
Neo-Synephrine 12 Hour, 2160·3
Neosynephrin-POS, 2160·3
Neo-Synodorm, 2160·3
Neotaflan, 2160·3
Neotalem, 2160·3
Neotame, 1441·1
Neotaren, 2160·3
NeoTect, 2160·3
Neotenol, 2160·3
Neotensin, 2160·3
Neotensin Diu, 2160·3
Neotest, 2160·3
Neotetranase, 2160·3
Neo-Thyreostat, 2160·3
Neotica, 2160·3
Neotigason, 2160·3
Neo-Tinic, 2160·3
Neo-Tiroimade, 2160·3
Neo-Tizide, 2160·4
Neotomic, 2160·4
Neoton, 2160·4
Neotonico, 2160·4
Neotop, 2160·4
Neotopic, 2160·4
Neo-Tosel, 2160·4
Neotoss, 2160·4
Neotrace, 2160·4
Neotracin, 2160·4
Neotretin, 2160·4
Neotrexate, 2160·4
Neotri, 2160·4
Neotricin, 2160·4
Neotricin HC, 2160·4
Neo-Trim Fibre, 2160·4
Neo-Trim Meal Replacement, 2160·4
Neotrin, 2160·4
Neotrin Balsamico, 2160·4
Neotroparin, 2160·4
Neo-Tuss, 2160·4
NeoTussan, 2160·4
Neotyf, 2160·4
Neo-Ulcoid, 2160·4
Neo-Uridixico, 2160·4
Neo-Ustiol, 2160·4
Neovastat, 525·3
Neovermin, 2160·4
Neovis, 2160·4
NeoVisc, 2161·1
Neovita, 2161·1
Neo-Vites, 2161·1
Neo-Vivactil, 2161·1
Neovlar, 2161·1
Neovletta, 2161·1
Neoxane, 2161·1
Neoxene, 2161·1
Neoxidil, 2161·1
Neoxil, 2161·1
Neoxinal, 2161·1
Neo-Xylestesin Preparations, 2161·1
Neoyod, 2161·1
Neozep, 2161·1
Neozimina, 2161·1
Neozine, 2161·1
Neo-Zol, 2161·1
Neozolone, 2161·1
Nepenic, 2161·1
Neper, 2161·1
*Nepeta hederacea*, 1696·2
NephPlex RX, 2161·1
Nephral, 2161·1
Nephramine, 2161·2
Nephrex, 2161·2
Nephril, 2161·2
Nephrisan P, 2161·2
Nephrisol Mono, 2161·2
Nephritin, 2161·2
Nephritis, Anti-GBM— *see* Glomerular Kidney Disease, 1080·2
Nephritis, Immune-complex— *see* Glomerular Kidney Disease, 1080·2
Nephritis, Lupus— *see* Systemic Lupus Erythematosus, 1088·3
Nephritis Syndrome, Acute— *see* Glomerular Kidney Disease, 1080·2
Nephroblastoma— *see* Wilms' Tumour, 518·2
Nephro-Calci, 2161·2
Nephrocaps, 2161·2
Nephrocare, 2161·2
Nephro-Fer, 2161·2
Nephro-Fer Rx, 2161·2
Nephrogenic Diabetes Insipidus— *see* Diabetes Insipidus, 1314·1
Nephrogesic, 2161·2
Nephrolith Mono, 2161·2
Nephrolithol N, 2161·2
Nephro-loges, 2161·2
Nephron, 2161·2
Nephron FA, 2161·2
Nephronorm Med, 2161·2
Nephro-Pasc, 2161·2
Nephropathy, Diabetic— *see* Diabetic Complications, 326·2
Nephropathy, IgA— *see* Glomerular Kidney Disease, 1080·2
Nephropathy, Membranous— *see* Glomerular Kidney Disease, 1080·2
Nephropathy, Minimal Change— *see* Glomerular Kidney Disease, 1080·2
Nephroplasmal N, 2161·2
Nephropur Tri, 2161·2
Nephroselect M, 2161·2
Nephrosolid, 2161·2
Nephrosteril, 2161·2
Nephrotect, 2161·2
Nephrotic Syndrome— *see* Glomerular Kidney Disease, 1080·2
Nephrotrans, 2161·2
Nephro-Vite, 2161·2
Nephro-Vite +Fe, 2161·3
Nephrox, 2161·3
Nephrubin-N, 2161·3
Nephur 4, 2161·3
Nephur 6, 2161·3
Nephur 7, 2161·3
Nephur-Test + Leucocytes, 2161·3
Nepinalona, 1125·2
Nepinalone, 1125·2
Nepinalone Hydrochloride, 1125·2
Nepituss, 2161·3
Nepresol, 2161·3
Nepressol, 2161·3
Nepro, 2161·3
Neptal, 2161·3
Neptazane, 2161·3
Nequinate, 607·2
Nequinato, 607·2
Neral, 1673·2, 1706·2, 1724·1
Nerapin, 2161·3
Nerdipina, 2161·3
Nerdipine, 2161·3
Nereflun, 2161·3
Nerelid, 2161·3
Nerex, 2161·3
Nergadan, 2161·3
Neribas, 2161·3
Neribase, 2161·3
Neribax, 2161·3
Nericur, 2161·3
Neriderm, 2161·3
Neridronate Sodium, 773·2
Neridronic Acid, 773·2
Neridrónico, Ácido, 773·2
Neriforte, 2161·3
Neriquinol, 2161·4
Nerisalic, 2161·4
Nerisona, 2161·4
Nerisona C, 2161·4
Nerisone, 2161·4
Nerisone C, 2161·4
*Nerium oleander*, 1723·1
Nerixia, 2161·4
Nerizina, 2161·4
Nero, 2161·4
Nerofen— *see* Nurofen, 2180·2
Neroli Oil, 1719·2
Neroli, Oleum, 1719·2
Nerolid, 2161·4
Nerpemide, 2161·4
Nerprun, 1254·1
Nervade, 2161·4

Nervan, 2161·4
Nervatona, 2161·4
Nervatona Plus, 2161·4
Nervaxon, 2161·4
Nerve Agents, 1719·2
Nerve Block, Central— *see* Central Nerve Block, 1370·1
Nerve Block, Peripheral— *see* Peripheral Nerve Block, 1370·2
Nerve Block, Regional— *see* Regional Nerve Block, 1370·1
Nerve Block, Sympathetic— *see* Sympathetic Nerve Block, 1370·2
Nerve Blocks, 1369·1, 1369·3
Nerve Gases, 1719·2
Nerve Growth Factor, 1679·1
Nerve Tonic, 2161·4
Nervei, 2161·4
Nerven und Schlaf N, Kneipp Krauter Taschenkur— *see* Kneipp Krauter Taschenkur Nerven und Schlaf N, 2081·3
Nerven- und Schlaf-Tee N, Kneipp— *see* Kneipp Nerven- und Schlaf-Tee N, 2081·3
Nervencreme S, 2161·4
Nerven-Dragees, 2161·4
Nervendragees, 2161·4
Nervenja, 2161·4
Nervenruh, 2161·4
Nerventee EF-EM-ES, 2162·1
Nerven-Tee Stada N, 2162·1
Nervfluid S, 2162·1
Nervifene, 2162·1
Nervifloran, 2162·1
Nervigenol Magnesio, 2162·1
Nervikan, 2162·1
Nervine, 2162·1
Nervine, Miles— *see* Miles Nervine, 2133·1
Nervinetten, 2162·1
Nervinfant N, 2162·1
Nervipan, 2162·1
Nervistop L, 2162·1
Nervita, 2162·1
Nervitone, 2162·1
Nervium, 2162·1
Nervo OPT N, 2162·1
Nervobion, 2162·1
Nervobion Fuerte, 2162·1
Nervocaine, 2162·1
Nervocalm, 2162·1
Nervocur, 2162·1
Nervoforcan, 2162·1
Nervogastrol N, 2162·1
Nervoheel, 2162·1
Nervoject N, 2162·1
Nervolta, 2162·1
Nervomax TB12, 2162·1
Nervonocton N, 2162·1
Nervopax, 2162·1
Nervoregin Forte, 2162·2
Nervoregin H, 2162·2
Nervosal, 2162·2
Nervosana, 2162·2
Nervostal, 2162·2
Nervpin N, 2162·2
Nervuton N, 2162·2
Neryl Acetate, 1706·2
Nesacain, 2162·2
Nesacaine, 2162·2
Nesdonal, 2162·2
Nesentials, Vitelle— *see* Vitelle Nesentials, 2382·2
Nesfare, 2162·2
Nesfare Antibiotico— *see* Nesfare, 2162·2
Nesiritide Citrate, 964·3
Nesivine, 2162·2
Nesol, 2162·2
Nesoro, 2162·2
NESP, 745·2
Nespo, 2162·2
Nestabs, 2162·2
Nestabs, Vitelle— *see* Vitelle Nestabs, 2382·2
Nestargel, 2162·2
Nesthakchen, 2162·2
Nestic, 2162·2
Nestle VHC, 2162·2
Nestosyl, 2162·2
Nestrex, Vitelle— *see* Vitelle Nestrex, 2382·2
Nestum, 2162·2
Nesvital, 2162·2
Netaf, 2162·2
Nethaprin Dospan, 2162·2
Nethaprin Expectorant, 2162·3
Neticin, 2162·3
Neticonazol, Hidrocloruro de, 406·3
Neticonazole Hydrochloride, 406·3
Netillin, 2162·3
Netilmicin Sulfate, 236·3
Netilmicin Sulphate, 236·3
Netilmicina, Sulfato de, 236·3
Netilmicini Sulfas, 236·3
Netilyn, 2162·3
Netira, 2162·3
Netobimin, 110·1
Netobimina, 110·1
Netocur, 2162·3
Netocur Balsamico, 2162·3
Netra, 2162·3
Netrocin, 2162·3
Netromicina, 2162·3
Netromicine, 2162·3
Netromycin, 2162·3
Netromycine, 2162·3
Nettacin, 2162·3
Nettinerv S, 2162·3
Nettle, Dwarf, 1762·1
Nettle Rash L88, 2162·3
Nettle, Stinging, 1762·1
Nettlerash— *see* Urticaria and Angioedema, 1138·3
Netunal, 2162·3
Netux, 2162·3
Neu Viplex, 2162·3
Neuart, 2162·3
Neubee, 2162·3
Neucare, 2162·3
Neucor, 2162·3
Neuer, 2162·3
Neufil, 2162·3
Neuflo, 2162·3
Neugal, 2162·3
Neugen, 2162·3
Neugeron, 2162·3
Neugra N, 2162·3
Neulactil, 2162·3
Neulasta, 2162·4
Neuleptil, 2162·4
Neumak, 2162·4
Neumega, 2162·4
Neumobacticel, 2162·4
Neumopectolina, 2162·4
Neumoral, 2162·4
Neumoterol, 2162·4
Neumotex, 2162·4
Neuners Krautertee Preparations, 2162·4
Neupax, 2163·2
Neupogen, 2163·2
Neupram, 2163·2
Neupramir, 2163·2
Neuquinon, 2163·2
Neuraben, 2163·2
Neurabol, 2163·2
Neuractin, 2163·2
Neuractiv, 2163·2
Neuragon, 2163·2
Neural Tube Defects, 1430·1
Neuralgia, Migrainous— *see* Cluster Headache, 464·1
Neuralgia, Postherpetic— *see* Postherpetic Neuralgia, 7·3
Neuralgia, Trigeminal— *see* Trigeminal Neuralgia, 8·2
Neuralgietabletten N, 2163·2
Neuralgietropfen CM, 2163·2
Neuralgin, 2163·2
Neuralgin ASS, 2163·2
Neuralin, 2163·2
Neuralprona, 2163·2
Neuralysan S, 2163·2
Neuramag P, 2163·2
Neuramate, 2163·2
Neuramide Sherman, 2163·2
Neuramin, 2163·3
Neuramizone, 2163·3
Neur-Amyl, 2163·3
Neuranidal, 2163·3
Neuranidal Duo, 2163·3
Neurapas, 2163·3
Neurax, 2163·3
NeuRecover, 2163·3
Neurex, 2163·3
Neuri B6, 2163·3
Neuriberi, 2163·3
Neuriclor, 2163·3
Neuriclor Vascular, 2163·3
Neuri-cyl N Ho-Len-Complex, 2163·3
Neuridon, 2163·3
Neuridon Forte, 2163·3
Neuril, 2163·3
Neurilan, 2163·3
Neurinase, 2163·3
Neuriplege, 2163·3
Neurium, 2163·3
Neuro, 2163·3
Neuro B, 2163·3
Neuro B1-6-12, 2163·3
Neuro Calme, 2163·3
Neuro Nutrients, 2163·3
Neuro Uno, 2163·3
Neuroactil, 2163·4
Neuro-AS N, 2163·4
Neuro-B Forte, 2163·4
Neurobex, 2163·4
Neurobiol, 2163·4
Neurobion, 2163·4
Neurobion N, 2163·4
Neurobionta, 2163·4
Neuroblastoma, 524·1
NeuroBloc, 2163·4
Neurobrucellosis— *see* Brucellosis, 122·3
Neurocalcium, 2163·4
Neurocam, 2163·4
Neurocardiogenic Syncope— *see* Hypotension, 828·1
Neurocardol, 2163·4
Neurocatavin Dexa, 2163·4
Neurochol C, 2163·4
Neurocil, 2163·4
Neurocine, 2163·4
Neurocysticercosis— *see* Cysticercosis, 98·1
Neurodavur, 2163·4
Neurodavur Plus, 2163·4
Neurodep, 2163·4
Neurodex, 2163·4
Neurodif, 2164·1
Neuro-Do, 2164·1
Neurodol Tissugel, 2164·1
Neuro-Effekton B, 2164·1
Neurofenac, 2164·1
Neurofitol, 2164·1
Neuroflax, 2164·1
Neuroflorine, 2164·1
Neurofor, 2164·1
Neuroforte, 2164·1
Neuroftal, 2164·1
Neurogamma, 2164·1
Neurogen-E, 2164·1
Neurogenic Pain, 2·1
Neurogeron, 2164·1
Neuroglutamin, 2164·1
Neurogrisevit N, 2164·1
Neurokinin-1 Receptor Antagonists, 1239·2
Neurol, 2164·1
Neurolea, 2164·1
Neurolep, 2164·1
Neurolepsin, 2164·1
Neuroleptanaesthesia— *see* Anaesthetic Techniques, 1296·2
Neuroleptanalgesia— *see* Anaesthetic Techniques, 1296·2
Neuroleptic, 663·1
Neuroleptic Malignant Syndrome, 677·3
Neuro-Lichtenstein, 2164·1
Neuro-Lichtenstein N, 2164·1
Neurolil, 2164·1
Neurolite, 2164·1
Neurolithium, 2164·2
Neuromade, 2164·2
Neuromax, 2164·2
Neuromerck, 2164·2
Neuromet, 2164·2
Neuromethyn, 2164·2
Neuromins, 2164·2
Neuromultivit, 2164·2
Neuromuscular Blockers, 1397·1
Neuronal Vascular, 2164·2
Neuronika, 2164·2
Neurontin, 2164·2
Neuropathic Pain, 2·1
Neuropathy, Acute Idiopathic Demyelinating— *see* Guillain-Barré Syndrome, 1630·2
Neuropathy, Diabetic— *see* Diabetic Complications, 326·2
Neuropax, 2164·2
Neurophosphates, 2164·2
Neuroplant, 2164·2
Neuroplus, 2164·2
Neuroprotectants, 836·3
Neuro-ratiopharm, 2164·2
Neuro-ratiopharm N, 2164·2
Neurorestol, 2164·2
Neurorubin, 2164·2
Neurorubine, 2164·2
Neurosande, 2164·2
Neurosedol, 2164·2
Neuroselect, 2164·2
Neurosine, 2164·2
NeuroSlim, 2164·2
Neurosthenol, 2164·3
Neurostil, 2164·3
Neurostop, 2164·3
Neurostop Complex, 2164·3
Neurosyphilis— *see* Syphilis, 148·2
Neurotab, Vida— *see* Vida Neurotab, 2376·2
Neurotensyl, 2164·3
Neurothioct, 2164·3
Neurotic Depression, 278·1
Neurotioct, 2164·3
Neurotisan, 2164·3
Neurotol, 2164·3
Neuroton, 2164·3
Neurotonico, 2164·3
Neurotop, 2164·3
Neurotrat, 2164·3
Neurotrat $B_{12}$, 2164·3
Neurotrat S, 2164·3
Neurotropan, 2164·3
Neurovegetalin, 2164·3
Neuro-Vibolex, 2164·3
Neurovit, 2164·3
Neurovitan, 2164·3
Neuro-Wied, 2164·3
Neurozan, 2164·4
Neurozepam, 2164·4
Neuryl, 2164·4
Neusinol, 2164·4
Neut, 2164·4
Neutracido, 2164·4
Neutracol, 2164·4
Neutrafluor, 2164·4
Neutraforte, 2164·4
NeutraGard Advanced, 2164·4
Neutragel, 2164·4
Neutral Acriflavine, 1165·3
Neutral Endopeptidase Inhibitors, 964·2
Neutral Insulin, 334·2
Neutral Metalloendopeptidase Inhibitors, 964·2
Neutral Proflavine Sulphate, 1165·3
Neutral Quinine Hydrochloride, 460·1
Neutral Quinine Sulphate, 460·1
Neutral Red, 1719·3
Neutral Red Chloride, 1719·3
Neutralca-S, 2164·4
Neutralfett, 1481·1
Neutralice, 2164·4
Neutramine, 2164·4

Neutran, 2164·4
Neutra-Phos, 2164·4
Neutra-Phos-K, 2164·4
Neutrexin, 2164·4
Neutro Bar, 2164·4
Neutrodor, 2164·4
Neutrofer, 2164·4
Neutrofer Folico, 2164·4
Neutroflavin, 1165·3
Neutrogen TGel, 2164·4
Neutrogena Preparations, 2164·4
Neutrogerm, 2165·2
Neutrogin, 2165·2
Neutrolac, 2165·2
Neutromax, 2165·3
Neutromed, 2165·3
Neutronorm, 2165·3
Neutropenia, 740·2
Neutropenic Patients, Fever in— *see* Infections in Immunocompromised Patients, 131·2
Neutrose S Pellegrino, 2165·3
Neutroses, 2165·3
Neuvita, 2165·3
Neuzym, 2165·3
Neuzyme, 2165·3
Nevacort, 2165·3
Nevimune, 2165·3
Neviralea, 2165·3
Neviran, 2165·3
Nevirapina, 650·2
Nevirapine, 650·2
Nevralgex, 2165·3
Nevralgina, 2165·3
Nevramin, 2165·3
Nevril, 2165·3
Nevril Crono, 2165·3
Nevrine Codeine, 2165·3
Nevrol, 2165·3
Nevrosthenine Glycocolle Freyssinge, 2165·3
New B-Cool, 2165·4
New Daigaku, 2165·4
New Decongestant Pediatric, 2165·4
New Diatabs— *see* Diatabs, 1935·4
New Era Preparations, 2165·4
New Eye Lotion, 2165·4
New Gen, 2165·4
New Hands, 2165·4
New Mixavit, 2165·4
New Patecs A, 2165·4
New Zealand Tea Tree, 1709·3
NewAce, 2165·4
Newderm, 2165·4
Newrelax, 2165·4
New-Skin, 2165·4
NEX-002, 683·1
Nexadron, 2165·4
Nexadron Compuesto, 2165·4
Nexen, 2165·4
Nexiam, 2165·4
Nexit, 2165·4
Nexium, 2165·4
Nexium Hp, 2165·4
Nexvep, 2165·4
Nexxair, 2165·4
NeyArthros (Revitorgan-Dilutionen Nr 43), 2165·4
NeyArthros-Liposome (Revitorgan Lp Nr 83), 2165·4
NeyCalm (Revitorgan-Dilutionen Nr 98, Revitorgan-Lingual Nr 98), 2166·1
NeyChondrin (Revitorgan-Dilutionen Nr 68), 2166·1
NeyChondrin (Revitorgan-Lingual Nr. 68), 2166·1
NeyChondrin N (Revitorgan-Dilutionen N Nr 68), 2166·1
NeyCorenar (Revitorgan-Dilutionen Nr 6), 2166·1
NeyDesib (Revitorgan-Dilutionen Nr 78), 2166·1
Neydin-F, 2166·1
Neydin-M, 2166·1
NeyDop (Revitorgan-Dilutionen Nr 97), 2166·1
NeyDop (Revitorgan-Lingual Nr. 97), 2166·1
NeyDop N (Revitorgan-Dilutionen N Nr 97), 2166·1
NeyFaexan (Revitorgan-Dilutionen Nr 55), 2166·1
NeyFegan (Revitorgan-Dilutionen Nr 26), 2166·1
NeyGeront (Revitorgan-Dilutionen Nr 64), 2166·1
NeyGeront (Revitorgan-Lingual Nr 64), 2166·1
NeyGeront N (Revitorgan-Dilutionen N Nr 64), 2166·1
NeyGeront-Vitalkapseln, 2166·1
NeyImmun (Revitorgan-Dilutionen Nr 73), 2166·1
NeyNormin (Revitorgan-Dilutionen Nr 65), 2166·1
NeyNormin (Revitorgan-Lingual Nr 65), 2166·2
NeyNormin N (Revitorgan-Dilutionen N Nr 65), 2166·1
NeyParadent-Liposome, 2166·2
NeyPsorin (Revitorgan-Dilutionen Nr 5), 2166·2
NeyPulpin (Revitorgan-Dilutionen Nr 10), 2166·2
NeyPulpin N (Revitorgan-Dilutionen N Nr 10), 2166·2
Neythymun, 2166·2
NeyTroph (Revitorgan-Dilutionen Nr 96), 2166·2
NeyTroph (Revitorgan-Lingual Nr 96), 2166·2
NeyTumorin (Revitorgan-Dilutionen Nr 66), 2166·2
NeyTumorin (Revitorgan-Lingual Nr 66), 2166·2
NeyTumorin N (Revitorgan-Dilutionen N Nr 66), 2166·2
Nezeril, 2166·2
NF Cough Syrup with Codeine, 2166·2
NGT, 2166·2
Nia, 2166·2
Niacel, 2166·2
Niacex, 2166·2
Niacin, 1441·1
Niacinamide, 1441·2
Niacor, 2166·2
Nialamida, 310·2
Nialamide, 310·2
Nialen, 2166·2
Niaouli, Essence de, 1719·3
Niaouli Oil, 1719·3
Niaprazina, 438·1
Niaprazine, 438·1
Niar, 2166·2
Niaspan, 2166·2
NiaStase, 2166·3
Niberan, 2166·3
Nibiol, 2166·3
Nibocin, 2166·3
Nibren, 2166·3
Nicabate, 2166·3
Nicam, 2166·3
Nican, 2166·3
Nican, Gotas— *see* Gotas Nican, 2030·2
Nicangin, 2166·3
Nicant, 2166·3
Nicaphlogyl, 2166·3
Nicapress, 2166·3
Nicaraven, 1719·3
Nicarbazin, 611·2
Nicarbazina, 611·2
Nicardal, 2166·3
Nicardia, 2166·3
Nicardipine Hydrochloride, 965·1
Nicardipino, Hidrocloruro de, 965·1
Nicardium, 2166·3
Nicarpin, 2166·3
Nicaven, 2166·3
N'ice, 2166·3
N'ice 'N Clear, 2166·3
N'ice Vitamin C, 2166·3
Nicef, 2166·3
Nicene, 2166·3
Nicene N, 2166·3
Nicer, 2166·3
Nicergobeta, 2166·3
Nicergolent, 2166·3
Nicergolina, 1719·3
Nicergoline, 1719·3
Nicergoline Tartrate, 1720·1
Nicergolinum, 1719·3
Niceritrol, 965·3
Nicerium, 2166·3
Nicethamidum, 1591·2
Nicetile, 2166·3
Nicholin, 2166·3
Nicizina, 2166·3
Niclosamida, 110·1
Niclosamida Anidra, 110·1
Niclosamida Mono-hidratada, 110·2
Niclosamida Monohidrato, 110·2
Niclosamide, 110·1
Niclosamide, Anhydrous, 110·1
Niclosamide Monohydrate, 110·2
Niclosamidum Anhydricum, 110·1
Niclosamidum Monohydricum, 110·2
Niclosan, 2166·3
Nico Hepatocyn, 2166·4
Nicobid, 2166·4
Nicobio, 2166·4
Nicobion, 2166·4
NicoBloc, 2166·4
Nicoboxil, 66·3
Nicoboxilo, 66·3
Nicobrevin, 2166·4
Nicocodina, 1125·2
Nicocodine, 1125·2
Nicocodine Hydrochloride, 1125·2
Nicodan, 2166·4
Nicodan N, 2166·4
Nicoderm, 2166·4
Nicodisc, 2166·4
Nicofibrate Hydrochloride, 965·3
Nicofibrato, Hidrocloruro de, 965·3
Nicogelat— *see* Bronchostop, 1855·3
Nicogum, 2166·4
Nicojuvel, 2166·4
Nicol, 2166·4
Nicolan, 2166·4
Nicolip, 2166·4
Nicolmycetin, 2166·4
Nicolsint, 2166·4
Nicomax, 2166·4
Nicomide, 2166·4
Nicomorfina, Hidrocloruro de, 66·3
Nicomorphine Hydrochloride, 66·3
Niconil, 2166·4
Nicopatch, 2166·4
Nicopaverina, 2166·4
Nicopaverina B6, 2166·4
Nicoprive, 2166·4
Nicorandil, 965·3
Nicord, 2166·4
Nicorette, 2166·4
Nicostop TTS, 2167·1
Nicosyn, 2167·1
Nicotabs, 2167·1
Nicotears, 2167·1
*Nicotiana tabacum*, 1720·1
Nicotibine, 2167·1
Nicotina, 1720·1
Nicotinamida, 1441·2
Nicotinamide, 1441·2
Nicotinamide Adenine Dinucleotide, 1442·1, 1719·1
Nicotinamide Adenine Dinucleotide Phosphate, 1442·1
Nicotinamidum, 1441·2
Nicotinate-fibrate Derivatives, 811·3
Nicotinates, 811·3
Nicotinato de Bencilo, 21·2
Nicotinato de Etilo, 37·2
Nicotinato de Hexilo, 45·1
Nicotinato de Inositol, 939·3
Nicotinato de Metilo, 59·2
Nicotinato de Propilo, 85·3
Nicotinato de Xantinol, 1029·1
Nicotine, 1720·1
Nicotine Bitartrate, 1720·1
Nicotine Citrate, 1720·1
Nicotine Malate, 1720·1
Nicotine Polacrilex, 1720·1
Nicotine Resinate, 1720·1
Nicotine Tartrate, 1720·1
Nicotinell, 2167·1
Nicotinell TTS, 2167·1
Nicotine-*N*-oxide, 1721·1
Nicotinex, 2167·1
Nicotinic Acid, 1441·1
Nicotinic Acid Amide, 1441·2
Nicotinic Acid Diethylamide, 1591·2
Nicotinic Alcohol, 966·1
Nicotínico, Ácido, 1441·1
Nicotinicum, Acidum, 1441·1
Nicotinílico, Alcohol, 966·1
Nicotinoid, 2167·1
6-Nicotinoylcodeine, 1125·2
Nicotinoyldiaethylamidum, 1591·2
2-Nicotinoyloxyethyl 2-(4-Chlorophenoxy)-2-methylpropionate, 914·2
Nicotinum, 1720·1
Nicotinuric Acid, 1441·3
Nicotinyl Alcohol, 966·1
Nicotinyl Alcohol Tartrate, 966·2
Nicotinyl Tartrate, 966·2
Nicotinylmethylamide, 1700·1
Nicotrans, 2167·1
Nicotrol, 2167·1
Nicotylamide, 1441·2
Nicoumalone, 848·3
Nicovitol, 2167·1
Nicozid, 2167·1
Nicozinc, 2167·1
NidaGel, 2167·1
Nidal, 2167·1
Nidal AR, 2167·1
Nidal HA, 2167·1
Nidazolem, 2167·1
Nidazolin, 2167·1
NIDDM— *see* Diabetes Mellitus, 324·1
Nide, 2167·1
Nidem, 2167·1
Nidex, 2167·1
Nidina Confort, 2167·1
Nidina HA, 2167·1
Nidina Probiotico, 2167·1
Nidol, 2167·1
Nidralon, 2167·2
Nidran, 2167·2
Nidrel, 2167·2
Nidrozol, 2167·2
Nieral, 2167·2
Nierano HM, 2167·2
Nieren-Elixier ST, 2167·2
Nierentee 2000, 2167·2
Nierentee EF-EM-ES, 2167·2
Nieron Blasen- und Nieren-Tee VI, 2167·2
Nieron S, 2167·2
Nieron-Tee N, 2167·2
Nieroxin N, 2167·2
Nifadil, 2167·2
Nifal, 2167·2
Nifalin, 2167·2
Nifangin, 2167·2
Nif-Atenil, 2167·2
Nifatenol, 2167·2
Nifdemin, 2167·2
Nife, 2167·2
Nife Uno, 2167·2
Nife-basan, 2167·2
Nifebene, 2167·2
Nifecard, 2167·2
Nifeclair, 2167·2
Nifecodan, 2167·2
Nifecor, 2167·2
Nifed, 2167·2
Nifed Sol, 2167·2
Nifedalat, 2167·3
Nifedate, 2167·3
Nifedax, 2167·3
Nifedel, 2167·3
Nifediac, 2167·3
Nifedical, 2167·3
Nifedicor, 2167·3
Nifedicron, 2167·3
Nifedi-Denk, 2167·3

Nifedigel, 2167·3
Nifedin, 2167·3
Nifedine, 2167·3
Nifedipat, 2167·3
Nifedipina, 966·2
Nifedipine, 966·2
Nifedipino, 966·2
Nifedipinum, 966·2
Nifedipres, 2167·3
Nifedipress, 2167·3
Nifehexal, 2167·3
Nifehexal Sali, 2167·3
Nifekalant, Hidrocloruro de, 972·2
Nifekalant Hydrochloride, 972·2
Nifelat, 2167·3
Nifelease, 2167·3
Nifenazona, 66·3
Nifenazone, 66·3
Niferex, 2167·3
Niferex Forte, 2167·3
Niferex Prenatal, 2167·3
Niferex-PN, 2167·3
Nifesal, 2167·3
Nifetex, 2167·3
Nifetolol, 2167·3
Nifezzard, 2167·3
Nifical, 2167·3
Nificard, 2167·3
Nifint, 2167·4
Nifiran, 2167·4
Niflactol, 2167·4
Niflam, 2167·4
Niflamol, 2167·4
Niflan, 2167·4
Niflucan, 2167·4
Niflugel, 2167·4
Niflumic Acid, 67·1
Niflumic Acid Glycinamide, 67·1
Niflúmico, Ácido, 67·1
Nifluril, 2167·4
Niflux, 2167·4
Nifopress, 2167·4
Nifostin, 2167·4
Nifreal, 2167·4
Nif-Ten, 2167·4
Nifucin, 2167·4
Nifur, 2167·4
Nifuran, 2167·4
Nifurantin, 2167·4
Nifurantin B 6, 2167·4
Nifurat, 2167·4
Nifuratel, 611·2
Nifurazolidonum, 605·2
Nifuretten, 2167·4
Nifurol, 2167·4
Nifuroxazida, 237·2
Nifuroxazide, 237·2
Nifuroxazidum, 237·2
Nifuroxima, 406·3
Nifuroxime, 406·3
Nifursol, 611·2
Nifurtimox, 611·2
Nifurtoinol, 237·2
Nifurtox, 2167·4
Nifurzida, 237·2
Nifurzide, 237·2
Nigalax, 2168·1
Nigersan, 2168·1
Night Cold Comfort, 2168·1
Night Cough Pastilles— *see* Potters Day & Night Cough Pastilles, 2229·3
Night Cramp— *see* Muscle Spasm, 1386·1
Night Nurse, 2168·1
Night Terrors— *see* Parasomnias, 667·3
Night Time, 2168·1
Night Time Cold/Flu Relief, 2168·1
Night Time Liquigels, 2168·1
Night-blooming Cereus, 1669·2
Nightcalm, 2168·1
Night-Care, 2168·1
Nightmares— *see* Parasomnias, 667·3
Nightpeel, 2168·1
Nightshade, Black, 1661·2
Nightshade, Deadly, 479·1
Nightshade, Woody, 1683·1
Night-Time, 2168·1
Night-Time Effervescent Cold, 2168·1
Nighttime Cold & Flu, 2168·1
Nighttime Pamprin, 2168·1
NightTime Theraflu, 2168·1
Niglinar, 2168·1
Nigrantyl, 2168·1
Nigroids, 2168·1
NIH-7958, 79·3
NIH-8805, 21·3
NIH-10567, 1700·2
Nij-Terol, 2168·1
Nikableomicina, 2168·1
Nikarin, 2168·1
Nikethamide, 1591·2
Nikethamide Calcium Thiocyanate, 1591·2
Nikethylamide, 1591·2
Nikion, 2168·1
Nikkho Vac, 2168·1
Niklod, 2168·1
Nikofrenon, 2168·1
Nikorazol, 2168·1
Nikoril, 2168·1
Nikotinsäure, 1441·1
Nikotugg, 2168·1
Nilandron, 2168·2
Nilcid, 2168·2
Nilcid-MPS, 2168·2
Nilevar, 2168·2
Nilflux, 2168·2
Nilgrip, 2168·2
Nilken, 2168·2
NilnOcen, 2168·2
Nilodor, 2168·2
Nilperidol, 2168·2
Nilstat, 2168·2
Nilutamida, 576·2
Nilutamide, 576·2
Nilvadipine, 972·2
Nilvadipino, 972·2
Nim, 2168·2
Nimadorm, 2168·2
Nimalgex, 2168·2
Nimaz, 2168·2
Nimbex, 2168·2
Nimbisan, 2168·2
Nimbium, 2168·2
Nimbus, 2168·2
Nimed, 2168·2
Nimedex, 2168·2
Nimeflan, 2168·2
Nimegen, 2168·2
Nimelide, 2168·2
Nimenol, 2168·2
Nimepast, 2168·2
Nimesil, 2168·2
Nimesilam, 2168·2
Nimesul, 2168·2
Nimesulene, 2168·2
Nimesulida, 67·1
Nimesulide, 67·1
Nimesulide Betacyclodextrin Complex, 67·1
Nimesulide Betadex, 67·1
Nimesulidum, 67·1
Nimesulin, 2168·3
Nimesulix, 2168·3
Nimesulon, 2168·3
Nimesyl, 2168·3
Nimesyl Gel, 2168·3
Nimetazepam, 710·1
Nimex, 2168·3
Nimexan, 2168·3
Nimfast, 2168·3
Nimicon, 2168·3
Nimicor, 2168·3
Nimodil, 2168·3
Nimodilat, 2168·3
Nimodilat Plus, 2168·3
Nimodipine, 972·3
Nimodipino, 972·3
Nimodipinum, 972·3
Nimodrel, 2168·3
Nimopect, 2168·3
Nimorazol, 611·3
Nimorazole, 611·3
Nimoreagin, 2168·3
Nimotop, 2168·3
Nimovas, 2168·3
Nims, 2168·3
Nimulid, 2168·3
Nimulid Nugel, 2168·3
Nimus, 2168·3
Nimustina, Hidrocloruro de, 576·3
Nimustine Hydrochloride, 576·3
Nimusyp, 2168·3
Nimutab, 2168·3
Nina, 2168·3
Nina cum Diphenhydramino, 2168·3
Ninazol, 2168·3
Nindaxa, 2168·3
Ninderm, 2168·3
Nine Rubbing Oils, 2168·4
Ninjin, 1693·1
Ninjin-yoei-to, Kanebo— *see* Kanebo Ninjin-yoei-to, 2074·2
Ninlium, 2168·4
Ni-No-Fluid N, 2168·4
Niocitran, 2168·4
Niofen, 2168·4
Niofen Flu, 2168·4
Niong Retard, 2168·4
Niopam, 2168·4
Niotal, 2168·4
Nipactrin, 2168·4
Nipaxon, 2168·4
Nipent, 2168·4
Niperotidina, Hidrocloruro de, 1277·2
Niperotidine Hydrochloride, 1277·2
Nipin, 2168·4
Nipiol, 2168·4
Nipodur, 2168·4
Nipogalin, 2168·4
Nipolept, 2168·4
Nipradilol, 973·2
Nipradolol, 973·2
Nipress, 2168·4
Nipride, 2168·4
Niprina, 2168·4
Niprus, 2168·4
Niprusodio, 2168·4
Nipruss, 2168·4
Niquetamida, 1591·2
NiQuitin, 2168·4
Niraben, 2168·4
Nirapel, 2168·4
Nirason N, 2168·4
Nirolex Preparations, 2168·4
Nirox, 2169·1
Nirulid, 2169·1
Nirvanol, 366·2
Nirvaxal, 2169·1
Nisaid, 2169·1
Nisal, 2169·1
Nisalgen, 2169·1
Nisapulvol, 2169·1
Nisaseptol, 2169·1
Nisasol, 2169·1
Nise, 2169·1
Nisicur, 2169·1
Nisin, 237·2
Nisina, 237·2
Nisis, 2169·1
Nisisco, 2169·1
Nisita, 2169·1
Nisodipen, 2169·1
Nisoldipine, 973·2
Nisoldipino, 973·2
Nisolid, 2169·1
Nisolone, Depo- — *see* Depo-Nisolone, 1925·4
Nistaglos, 2169·1
Nistagrand, 2169·1
Nistagyn, 2169·1
Nistaken, 2169·2
Nistan, 2169·2
Nistanil, 2169·2
Nistaquim, 2169·2
Nistat, 2169·2
Nistatina, 406·3
Nistaval, 2169·2
Nistax, 2169·2
Nistazol, 2169·2
Nistoral, 2169·2
Nisuflex, 2169·2
Nisulid, 2169·2
Nisural, 2169·2
Nisvastatin, 984·1
Nisylen, 2169·2
Nit. Acid, 1722·1
Nitagon, 2169·2
Nitalapram Hydrobromide, 289·1
Nitan, 2169·2
Nitavan, 2169·2
Nitazoxanida, 612·1
Nitazoxanide, 612·1
Nite Time Cold Formula, 2169·2
Nite Time Diet, 2169·2
Nitecall, 2169·2
Niten, 2169·2
Niten D, 2169·2
Nitens, 2169·2
Nitepax, 2169·2
Niterey, 2169·2
Nitesco Smagliature, 2169·2
Nitised, 2169·2
Nitisinona, 1722·1
Nitisinone, 1722·1
Nitlotion, 2169·2
Nitoman, 2169·2
Nitopro, 2169·2
Nitorol, 2169·3
Nitossil, 2169·3
Nitradisc, 2169·3
Nitrados, 2169·3
Nitramin, 2169·3
Nitrangin, 2169·3
Nitrangin Compositum, 2169·3
Nitrangin Forte, 2169·3
Nitrapamil, 2169·3
Nitrapan, 2169·3
Nitrates, 811·3, 1190·1
Nitrato de Bismutilo, 1252·2
Nitrato de Butoconazol, 395·2
Nitrato de Cerio, 1144·3
Nitrato de Econazol, 397·2
Nitrato de Estricnina, 1750·1
Nitrato de Fenticonazol, 397·3
Nitrato de Isoconazol, 401·3
Nitrato de Miconazol, 405·3
Nitrato de Nafazolina, 1124·3
Nitrato de Omoconazol, 407·2
Nitrato de Oxiconazol, 407·3
Nitrato de Plata, 1746·1
Nitrato de Prata, 1746·1
Nitrato de Sertaconazol, 408·1
Nitrato de Sulconazol, 408·2
Nitrato de Tiamina, 1455·1
Nitrato Potásico, 1190·1
Nitrato Sódico, 1192·2
Nitratophenylmercury, 1189·2
Nitravet, 2169·3
Nitrazadon, 2169·3
Nitrazep, 2169·3
Nitrazepam, 710·1
Nitrazepamum, 710·1
Nitrazepan, 2169·3
Nitrazepol, 2169·3
Nitrazine Paper, 2169·3
Nitre, 1190·1, 2169·3
Nitregamma, 2169·3
Nitrek, 2169·3
Nitren, 2169·3
Nitren Lich, 2169·3
Nitrencord, 2169·3
Nitrendepat, 2169·3
Nitrendicor, 2169·3
Nitrendidoc, 2169·3
Nitrendil, 2169·3
Nitrendimerck, 2169·3
Nitrendipine, 973·3
Nitrendipino, 973·3
Nitrendipinum, 973·3
Nitrenpress, 2169·3
Nitrensal, 2169·3
Nitrepress, 2169·3
Nitre-Puren, 2169·3
Nitrex, 2169·4
Nitriate, 2169·4

Nitric Acid, 1722·1
Nitric Oxide, 973·3
Nitric Oxide Synthase Inhibitors, 145·2
Nítrico, Ácido, 1722·1
Nitridazol, 2169·4
Nitriderm TTS, 2169·4
Nitrilan, 2169·4
Nitrileno, 2169·4
2,2′,2″-Nitrilotriethanol, 1758·2
Nitrimidazine, 611·3
Nitrito de Amilo, 1032·1
Nitrito de Butilo, 1663·3
Nitrito Sódico, 1052·3
Nitro, 2169·4
Nitro Mack, 2169·4
Nitro Pohl, 2169·4
Nitro Solvay, 2169·4
Nitrobenceno, 1722·2
Nitrobenzene, 1722·2
Nitrobenzol, 1722·2
Nitro-Bid, 2169·4
Nitrobid, 2169·4
9-Nitrocamptothecin, 583·2
9-Nitro-20(*S*)-camptothecin, 583·2
Nitrochloroform, 1502·1
Nitrocine, 2169·4
Nitrocit, 2169·4
Nitrocod, 2169·4
Nitrocontin, 2169·4
Nitrocor, 2169·4
Nitro-Crataegutt, 2169·4
Nitro-cum, 2169·4
Nitroder, 2169·4
Nitro-Derm, 2169·4
Nitroderm, 2169·4
Nitroderm TTS, 2169·4
Nitrodex, 2169·4
Nitrodisc, 2169·4
Nitro-Dur, 2169·4
Nitrodyl, 2170·1
Nitroerythrite, 913·1
Nitroerythrol, 913·1
Nitroflu, 2170·1
Nitrofural, 238·2
5-Nitro-2-furaldehyde Oxime, 406·3
5-Nitro-2-furaldehyde Semicarbazone, 238·2
Nitrofuralum, 238·2
Nitrofurantoin, 237·2, 237·3
Nitrofurantoína, 237·2
Nitrofurantoinum, 237·2
Nitrofurazone, 238·2
Nitrofur-C, 2170·1
1-(5-Nitrofurfurylideneamino)hydantoin, 237·2
1-(5-Nitrofurfurylideneamino)imidazolidine-2,4-dione, 237·2
3-(5-Nitrofurfurylideneamino)-2-oxazolidone, 605·2
2′-(5-Nitrofurfurylidene)-4-hydroxybenzohydrazide, 237·2
1-{[3-(5-Nitro-2-furyl)allylidene]amino}hydantoin, 215·2
Nitrogard, 2170·1
Nitrogen, 1236·3
Nitrogen-13, 1525·1
Nitrogen, Liquid, 1236·3
Nitrogen, Low-oxygen, 1236·3
Nitrogen Monoxide, 973·3, 1304·3
Nitrogen Mustard, 537·1
Nitrogen Mustards, 492·1
Nitrogen Oxide, 1304·3
Nitrogen 97 Percent, 1236·3
Nitrogenii Monoxidum, 1304·3
Nitrogenii Oxidum, 973·3, 1304·3
Nitrogenium, 1236·3
Nitrogenium Oxydulatum, 1304·3
Nitrógeno, 1236·3
Nitrógeno 13, 1525·1
Nitrogesic, 2170·1
Nitroglicerina, 923·2
Nitroglycerin, 923·2
Nitroglycerol, 923·2
Nitroglyn, 2170·1
Nitrogray, 2170·1
4-[2-(5-Nitroimidazol-1-yl)ethyl]morpholine, 611·3
Nitroina, 2170·1
Nitroject, 2170·1
Nitrokapseln-ratiopharm, 2170·1
Nitrokor, 2170·1
Nitrol, 2170·1
Nitrolan— *see* Nitro-pro, 2170·2
Nitrolerg, 2170·1
Nitrolingual, 2170·1
Nitromed, 2170·1
Nitromersol, 1186·3
Nitromex, 2170·1
Nitromidager, 2170·1
Nitromin, 2170·1
Nitromint, 2170·1
Nitronal, 2170·1
Nitronasal, 2170·1
Nitrong, 2170·1
Nitro-Obsidan, 2170·1
Nitropacin, 2170·2
Nitropentaerythrol, 979·1
Nitropenthrite, 979·1
Nitro-Pflaster-ratiopharm TL, 2170·2
4′-Nitro-2′-phenoxymethanesulphonanilide, 67·1
4-(4-Nitrophenoxy)phenyl Isothiocyanate, 110·2
Nitroplast, 2170·2
Nitro-Praecordin N, 2170·2
Nitropresabbott, 2170·2
Nitropress, 2170·2
Nitro-pro, 2170·2
Nitroprus, 2170·2
Nitroprusiato Sódico, 1000·2
Nitroprussiat, 2170·2
Nitroprusside Reagent Tablets— *see* Acetest, 1770·2
Nitropulse, 2170·2
NitroQuick, 2170·2
5-Nitroquinolin-8-ol, 238·3
Nitroretard-Faran, 2170·2
Nitrosamines, 1052·3
Nitroscanate, 110·2
Nitroscanato, 110·2
Nitrosid, 2170·2
*S*-Nitroso-*N*-acetylpenicillamine, 597·3
1-Nitroso-3,5-dimethyl-adamantane, 1711·2
Nitrosofenfluramine, 1588·3
Nitrosorbide, 2170·2
Nitrosorbon, 2170·2
Nitrosoureas, 492·1
Nitrostat, 2170·2
Nitrosum, Oxydum, 1304·3
Nitrosylon, 2170·2
NitroTab, 2170·2
Nitro-Tablinen, 2170·2
Nitrotard, 2170·2
*N*-(5-Nitro-2-thiazolyl)salicylamide Acetate, 612·1
*N*-(5-Nitrothiazol-2-yl)thiophene-2-carboxamide, 616·3
5-Nitro-2-thiophenecarboxylic Acid [3-(5-Nitro-2-furyl)allylidene]hydrazide, 237·2
Nitro-Time, 2170·2
Nitrourean, 2170·2
Nitrous Oxide, 1304·3
Nitrovasodilators, 811·3
Nitroven, 2170·2
Nitrovis, 2170·2
Nitroxinil, 110·3
Nitroxinilo, 110·3
Nitroxolina, 238·3
Nitroxoline, 238·3
*N*-[2-(Nitroxy)ethyl]-3-pyridinecarboxamide, 965·3
Nitroxynil, 110·3
Nitrumon, 2170·2
Nitux, 2170·2
Nivabetol, 2170·2
Nivadil, 2170·2
Nivadipine, 972·2
Nivador, 2170·2
Nivagin, 2170·3
Nivalin, 2170·3
Nivaquine, 2170·3
Nivaquine-P, 2170·3
Nivas, 2170·3
Nivas Plus, 2170·3
Nivea, 2170·3
Nivea Sun, 2170·3
Nivea Visage, 2170·3
Nivelan, 2170·3
Nivelipol, 2170·3
Nivelon, 2170·3
Nivemycin, 2170·3
Niven, 2170·3
Niver, 2170·3
Nivoflox, 2170·3
Nix, 2170·3
Nixal, 2170·3
Nixin, 2170·3
Nixoderm, 2170·3
Nixyn, 2170·3
Niyaplat, 2170·3
Nizacol, 2170·3
Nizale, 2170·4
Nizatidina, 1277·2
Nizatidine, 1277·2
Nizatidine *N*-2-Oxide, 1277·3
Nizatidine *S*-Oxide, 1277·3
Nizatidinum, 1277·2
Nizax, 2170·4
Nizaxid, 2170·4
Nizcreme, 2170·4
Nizofenona, 1722·2
Nizofenone, 1722·2
Nizole, 2170·4
Nizoral, 2170·4
Nizorelle, 2170·4
Nizoretic, 2170·4
Nizovules, 2170·4
Nizshampoo, 2170·4
NK-104, 984·1
NK341, 92·3
NK-421, 590·3
NK-631, 579·3
NK-1006, 162·2
NKK-105, 1709·3
NKT-01, 1360·2
N-Labstix, 2170·4
NM-441, 246·3
N-Multistix, 2170·4
N-Multistix SG, 2170·4
NN-304, 340·3
NNC-05-0328, 378·1
NND-318, 405·2
NO-05-0328, 378·1
No 440, 2170·4
No Doz, 2170·4
No Doz Plus, 2170·4
No Drowsiness Sinarest, 2170·4
No Gas, 2170·4
No Grip, 2170·4
No Grip C, 2170·4
No Name Cough Lozenge, 2170·4
No Pain-HP, 2170·4
Noacid, 2170·4
No-Acid, 2170·4
NO-AD Preparations, 2170·4
Noalgil, 2171·1
Noalgos, 2171·1
Noameba-DS, 2171·1
Noan, 2171·1
Nobactam, 2171·1
Nobactam Bronquial, 2171·1
Nobacter, 2171·1
Nobec, 2171·1
Nobecutan, 2171·1
Nobecutane, 2171·1
Nobese, 2171·1
Nobese No. 1, 2171·1
No-Bite, 2171·1
Nobiten, 2171·1
Nobligan, 2171·1
Nobliten, 2171·1
Nobritol, 2171·1
Noc, 2171·1
*Nocardia orientalis*, 275·2
Nocardiosis, 137·1
Noce Vomica, 1722·3
Noceptin, 2171·1
Nocertone, 2171·1
Nociceptive Pain, 2·1
Nociclin, 2171·1
Nocid, 2171·1
Nocloprost, 1520·3
Nocpaz, 2171·1
Noctal, 2171·1
Noctamid, 2171·1
Noctamide, 2171·2
Noctazepam, 2171·2
Noctilan, 2171·2
Noctiplon, 2171·2
Noctirex, 2171·2
Noctis, 2171·2
Noctisan, 2171·2
Noctium, 2171·2
Nocton, 2171·2
Noctor, 2171·2
Noctran, 2171·2
Noctura, 2171·2
Nocturnal Enuresis, 475·3
Nocturne, 2171·2
Nocturno, 2171·2
Noctyl, 2171·2
Nocutil, 2171·2
Nocvalene, 2171·2
Node DS, 2171·2
Node G, 2171·2
Node P, 2171·2
Node Tar, 2171·2
Nodepe, 2171·2
Nodex, 2171·2
Nodict, 2171·2
Nodipir, 2171·2
Nodoff, 2171·2
Nodolex, 2171·2
Nodolfen, 2171·2
Nodor, 2171·2
NoDoz, 2171·3
No-Drowsiness Allerest, 2171·3
Nodryl, 2171·3
Noducil, 2171·3
Noemin N, 2171·3
Noesude, Chemists Own— *see* Chemists Own Chesty Mucus Cough, 1881·4
Nofagus, 2171·3
Nofebrin, 2171·3
Nofedol, 2171·3
Nofetumomab Merpentan, Technetium ($^{99m}$Tc), 1526·1
Noflam, 2171·3
Noflam-N, 2171·3
No-Flu, 2171·3
Noflux, 2171·3
No-Gas, 2171·3
Nogastra, 2171·3
No-Gravid, 2171·3
No-Hist, 2171·3
Noiafren, 2171·3
Noir Brillant BN, 1056·2
Noivy, 2171·3
Noix d'Arec, 1656·2
Noix de Galle, 1690·2
Noix Vomique, 1722·3
Nok, 2171·3
Nokatar, 2171·3
Nokid, 2171·3
Noklot, 2171·3
Noktone, 2171·3
Nolac, 2171·3
Nolahist, 2171·3
Nolamine, 2171·3
Nolarac, 2171·3
Nolatrexed, 576·3
Nolder, 2171·3
Noleptan, 2171·4
Nolgen, 2171·4
Nolil, 2171·4
Nolipax, 2171·4
Nolipid, 2171·4
Nolol, 2171·4
Nolotil, 2171·4
Nolotil Compositum, 2171·4
Nolvadex, 2171·4
Nomafen, 2171·4
Nomapam, 2171·4
Nomegestrol Acetate, 1562·1
Nomegestrol, Acetato de, 1562·1
Nomegestroli Acetas, 1562·1

Nomigrain, 2171·4
Nominfone, 2171·4
Nomon Mono, 2171·4
Nomopain, 2171·4
Nomotec, 2171·4
Non Acid, 2171·4
Nonacog Alfa, 752·3
Nonafluoro-2-(trifluoromethyl)butane, 1067·2
Nonak, 2171·4
No-Name Dandruff Treatment, 2171·4
Nonan, 2171·4
Nonanedioic Acid, 1142·3
3,6,9,12,15,18,21,24,27-Nonaoxaoctacosyl 4-Butylaminobenzoate, 1115·3
Nonathymulin, 1756·1
Nonavit, 2171·4
Non-brewed Condiment, 1645·3
Non-depolarising Muscle Relaxants, 1397·1
Non-depolarising Neuromuscular Blockers, 1397·1
Non-Drowsy Sinutab, 2171·4
Non-Drowsy Sudafed Preparations, 2171·4
No-Nerviol, 2172·1
Nongonococcal Urethritis— *see* Urethritis, 152·3
Non-Hodgkin's Lymphomas, 510·1
Non-insulin-dependent Diabetes Mellitus— *see* Diabetes Mellitus, 324·1
Nonionic Surfactants, 1411·1
Nonivamida, 67·2
Nonivamide, 67·2
Nonketotic Hyperglycinaemia, 1750·2
Non-lymphoblastic Leukaemia, Acute— *see* Acute Myeloid Leukaemias, 506·3
Non-Ovlon, 2172·1
Nonoxinol, 1413·2
Nonoxinol 9, 1413·3
Nonoxinol 10, 1413·3
Nonoxinol 11, 1413·3
Nonoxinoles, 1413·2
Nonoxinols, 1413·2
Nonoxinolum 9, 1413·3
Nonoxynol 4, 1413·2
Nonoxynol 9, 1413·3
Nonoxynol 10, 1413·3
Nonoxynol 11, 1413·3
Nonoxynol 15, 1413·2
Nonoxynol 30, 1413·2
Nonoxynols, 1413·2
Non-Q Wave Myocardial Infarction— *see* Angina Pectoris, 813·1
Nonseminomatous Testicular Cancer— *see* Malignant Neoplasms of the Testis, 523·1
Non-small Cell Lung Cancer— *see* Malignant Neoplasms of the Lung, 519·2
Nonspecific Interstitial Pneumonia— *see* Diffuse Parenchymal Lung Disease, 1079·3
Nonspecific Urethritis— *see* Urethritis, 152·3
Nonspecific Vaginitis— *see* Bacterial Vaginosis, 121·2
Non-ST Elevation Myocardial Infarction— *see* Angina Pectoris, 813·1
Non-starch Polysaccharides, 1253·3, 1417·1
Nonsteroidal Anti-inflammatory Drugs, 67·3
Non-ulcer Dyspepsia— *see* Dyspepsia, 1242·1
α-(4-Nonylphenyl)-ω-hydroxydeca(oxyethylene), 1413·3
α-(4-Nonylphenyl)-ω-hydroxynona(oxyethylene), 1413·3
α-(4-Nonylphenyl)-ω-hydroxypoly(oxyethylene), 1413·2
α-(4-Nonylphenyl)-ω-hydroxyundeca(oxyethylene), 1413·3
Nonylvanillamide, 67·2
Noocetam, 2172·1
Noodipina, 2172·1
Noodis, 2172·1
Noostan, 2172·1
Nootrofic, 2172·1
Nootron, 2172·1
Nootrop, 2172·1
Nootropil, 2172·1
Nootropyl, 2172·1
Nopain, 2172·1
Nopan, 2172·1
Nopar, 2172·1
Nopika— *see* Prulit, 2244·2
Nopil, 2172·1
Noplak, 2172·1
Nopoxamine, 1381·3
Nopres, 2172·1
Nopriken, 2172·1
Nopron, 2172·2
Noprop, 2172·2
Nopucid, 2172·2
Nopucid Composto, 2172·2
Nopucid Compuesto, 2172·2
Nopucid MC, 2172·2
Nopyn, 2172·2
Noquerat, 2172·2
Nor 2, 2172·2
Nora, 2172·2
Norabromol N, 2172·2
Norace, 2172·2
Noracin, 2172·2
Noradran, 2172·2
Noradrenaline, 974·3
Noradrenaline Acid Tartrate, 974·3
Noradrenaline Bitartrate, 975·1
Noradrenaline Hydrochloride, 975·1
Noradrenaline Reuptake Inhibitors, Serotonin and, 278·2
Noradrenaline Tartrate, 975·1
Noradrenaline Theophylline Hydrochloride, 1754·3
Noradrenalini Hydrochloridum, 975·1
Noradrenalini Tartras, 975·1
Norakin N, 2172·2
Noralget, 2172·2
Noralone, 2172·2
Noramidazophenum, 35·3
Noraminophenazonum, 36·1
Nor-Anaesthol, 2172·2
Noranat, 2172·2
19-Norandrostenolone Phenylpropionate, 1561·3
5′-Nor-anhydrovinblastine Tartrate, 594·1
Norapomorphine, 1199·3
Nora-ratiopharm, 2172·2
Norastemizole, 424·2
Noravid, 2172·2
Noraxin, 2172·2
Norbactin, 2172·2
Norbal, 2172·2
Norbiline, 2172·2
Norbixin, 1056·1
Norboral, 2172·2
Norbormida, 1507·3
Norbormide, 1507·3
Norbuprenorphine, 22·3
Norcalcin, 2172·2
Norcholesterol, Iodinated ($^{131}$I), 1524·3
Norciden, 2172·2
Norcin, 2172·3
Norcisapride, 1260·2
Norclozapine, 688·2
Norco, 2172·3
Norcocaine, 1375·3
Norcodeine, 27·3
Norcolut, 2172·3
Norcuron, 2172·3
Norcyclizine, 430·1
Nordapanin N, 2172·3
Nordathricin N, 2172·3
Nordaz, 2172·3
Nordazepam, 710·3
*l*-Nordefrin, 1675·3
Norden, 2172·3
2′-Nor-2′-deoxyguanosine, 635·3
Nordet, 2172·3
Nordette, 2172·3
Nordextropropoxyphene, 29·3
Nordhausen, 1750·3
Nordiate, 2172·3
Nordiazepam, 710·3
Nordicort, 2172·3
Nordihidroguayarético, Ácido, 1187·1
Nordihydrocodeine, 35·2
Nordihydroguaiaretic Acid, 1187·1
Nordimmun, 2172·3
Nordiol, 2172·3
Nordiol-21, 2172·3
Norditropin, 2172·3
Norditropine, 2172·3
Nordolce, 2172·3
Nordonil, 2172·3
Nordotol, 2172·3
Nordox, 2172·3
Nordyl, 2172·3
Norebox, 2172·4
Norecil, 2172·4
No-Ref, 2172·4
Norel, 2172·4
Norel DM, 2172·4
Norel Plus, 2172·4
Norel SD, 2172·4
Norelbin, 2172·4
Norelgestromin, 1562·1
*d,l*-Norephedrine, 1128·1
(±)-Norephedrine, 1127·3, 1128·1
Norepine, 2172·4
Norepinefrina, 974·3
Norepinefrina, Bitartrato de, 974·3
Norepinefrina, Hidrocloruro de, 975·1
Norepinephrine, 974·3
Norepinephrine Acid Tartrate, 975·1
Norepinephrine Bitartrate, 974·3
*l*-Norepinephrine Bitartrate, 975·1
Norepinephrine Hydrochloride, 975·1
Norepirenamine, 974·3
Noreskin, 2172·4
Norestin, 2172·4
Noretandrolona, 1562·2
Norethandrolone, 1562·2
Norethin 1/35E, 2172·4
Norethin 1/50M, 2172·4
Norethindrone, 1562·2
Norethindrone Acetate, 1562·2
Norethindrone Enanthate, 1562·2
Norethisterone, 1562·2
Norethisterone Acetate, 1562·2
Norethisterone Enantate, 1562·2
Norethisterone Enanthate, 1562·2
Norethisterone Heptanoate, 1562·2
Norethisteroni Acetas, 1562·2
Norethisteronum, 1562·2
Norethynodrel, 1563·1
Noretinodrel, 1563·1
Noretisterona, 1562·2
Noretisterona, Acetato de, 1562·2
Noretisterona, Enantato de, 1562·2
Noretisterone, 1562·2
Noretynodrel, 1563·1
Norfcin, 2172·4
Norfemac, 2172·4
Norfenazin, 2172·4
Norfenefrina, Hidrocloruro de, 975·3
Norfenefrine Hydrochloride, 975·3
Norfenon, 2172·4
Norfisar, 2172·4
Norflam T, 2172·4
Norflamin, 2172·4
Norflex, 2172·4
Norflex Co, 2172·4
Norflex Plus, 2172·4
Norflo, 2172·4
Norflocin, 2172·4
Norflocine, 2172·4
Norflohexal, 2172·4
Norflok, 2172·4
Norflol, 2172·4
Norflosal, 2173·1
Norflox, 2173·1
Norfloxacin, 238·3
Norfloxacin Pivoxil, 239·1
Norfloxacino, 238·3
Norfloxacinum, 238·3
Norfloxasan, 2173·1
Norflox-Azu, 2173·1
Norfloxbeta, 2173·1
Norfloxin, 2173·1
Norfloxinor, 2173·1
Norflox-Puren, 2173·1
Norfluoxetine, 296·2
Norflurane, 1236·2
Norflurano, 1236·2
Norforms, 2173·1
Norgagil, 2173·1
Norgalax, 2173·1
Norgalax Miniklistier, 2173·1
Norgeal, 2173·1
Norgesic, 2173·1
Norgesic N, 2173·1
Norgestimate, 1563·2
Norgestimato, 1563·2
Norgestomet, 1563·2
Norgeston, 2173·1
Norgestrel, 1563·2
D-Norgestrel, 1563·2
DL-Norgestrel, 1563·2
*dl*-Norgestrel, 1563·2
Norgestrel Max, 2173·1
Norgestrel Plus, 2173·1
Norgestrelum, 1563·2
Norgestrienona, 1564·3
Norgestrienone, 1564·3
Norgic, 2173·1
Norglicem, 2173·1
Norgotin, 2173·1
Norica, 2173·1
Noricaven, 2173·1
Noricaven Novo, 2173·1
Noriclan, 2173·1
Noriday, 2173·2
Noriderm, 2173·2
Norifortan, 2173·2
Norimin, 2173·2
Norimode, 2173·2
Norincol, 2173·2
Norinyl Preparations, 2173·2
Noripam, 2173·2
Noripurum, 2173·2
Noripurum Folico, 2173·2
Noripurum Vitaminado, 2173·2
Norisodrine with Calcium Iodide, 2173·2
Noristerat, 2173·2
Norit, 2173·2
Noritate, 2173·2
Norit-Carbomix, 2173·2
Noritet, 2173·2
Noritren, 2173·2
Norivite, 2173·2
Norivite-12, 2173·2
Norizal, 2173·2
Norizine, 2173·2
Norketamine, 1302·3
Norkotral Tema, 2173·3
Norlevo, 2173·3
Norline, 2173·3
Norlip, 2173·3
Norlutate, 2173·3
Norluten, 2173·3
Normabenzil, 2173·3
Normabrain, 2173·3
Normacidine, 2173·3
Normacol Preparations, 2173·3
Normafenac, 2173·3
Normafibe, 2173·3
Normaflu, 2173·3
Normaform, 2173·3
Normagit, 2173·3
Normagrin, 2173·3
Normal Immunoglobulin, Human, 1627·2
Normal Immunoglobulin for Intravenous Administration, Human, 1627·2
Normal Immunoglobulins, 1627·2
Normal Propyl Alcohol, 1191·2
Normalac, 2173·3
Normalax, 2173·3
Normalene, 2173·3
NormaLine, 2173·4
Normaline, 2173·4
Normalip, 2173·4
Normalip Pro, 2173·4
Normalite, 2173·4
Normaloe, 2173·4
Normalol, 2173·4
Normamor, 2173·4
Normapril, 2173·4

Normase, 2173·4
Normasol, 2173·4
Normastigmin, 2173·4
Normastigmin mit Pilocarpin, 2173·4
Normaten, 2173·4
Normaten Plus, 2173·4
Normatens, 2173·4
Normatensil, 2173·4
Normatol, 2173·4
Normavom, 2173·4
Normax, 2173·4
Normaxin, 2173·4
Normell, 2173·4
Normensan, 2173·4
Normeperidine, 81·3
Normeperidinic Acid, 81·3
Normetadona, Hidrocloruro de, 1125·2
Normethadol, 58·2
Normethadone Hydrochloride, 1125·2
Normex, 2173·4
Normhydral, 2174·1
Normicina, 2174·1
Normiflo, 2174·1
Normin, 2174·1
Normison, 2174·1
Normiten, 2174·1
Normitrol, 2174·1
Normix, 2174·1
Normlgel, 2174·1
Normo Gastryl, 2174·1
Normo Nar, 2174·1
Normobren, 2174·1
Normoc, 2174·1
Normochromic Anaemia, 732·1
Normocir, 2174·1
Normocytic-normochromic Anaemia, 734·2
Normodiar, 2174·1
Normodyne, 2174·1
Normofenicol, 2174·1
Normofer, 2174·1
Normoflex, 2174·1
Normofundin Preparations, 2174·1
Normofusin, 2174·1
Normogam, 2174·1
Normogamma, 2174·1
Normogastryl, 2174·1
Normogin, 2174·2
Normoglaucon, 2174·2
Normoglucon, 2174·2
Normolaxil, 2174·2
Normolip, 2174·2
Normo-Loges, 2174·2
Normolose, 2174·2
Normolyt, 2174·2
Normolytoral, 2174·2
Normomensil, 2174·2
Normonal, 2174·2
Normoparin, 2174·2
Normophasic, 2174·2
Normopres, 2174·2
Normopresan, 2174·2
Normopresil, 2174·2
Normopress, 2174·2
Normopride Enzimatico, 2174·2
Normoprost, 2174·2
Normoprost Compuesto, 2174·2
Normoprost Plus, 2174·2
Normo-real, 2174·2
Normorix, 2174·2
Normorphine, 27·3, 61·2
Normorytmin, 2174·2
Normosang, 2174·2
Normoskin, 2174·2
Normosol Preparations, 2174·2
Normospor, 2174·3
Normosteril, 2174·3
Normotensin, 2174·3
Normotensor, 2174·3
Normothen, 2174·3
Normotherin, 2174·3
Normotil, 2174·3
Normotin V1, 2174·3
Normotin-R, 2174·3
Normovite Antianemico, 2174·3
Normovlar ED, 2174·3
Normoxidil, 2174·3
Normoxin, 2174·3
Normpress, 2174·3
Normulen, 2174·3
Normum, 2174·3
Norocin, 2174·3
Norogil, 2174·3
No-Roma, 2174·3
Noronal, 2174·3
Noroxin, 2174·3
Noroxine, 2174·3
Noroxycodone, 75·2
Nor-Pa, 2174·3
Norpace, 2174·3
Norpethidine, 81·3
Norpethidinic Acid, 81·3
Norphen, 2174·3
Norphenazone, 82·3, 909·2
Norphenylephrine Hydrochloride, 975·3
Norphin, 2174·4
Norphyllin, 2174·4
Norpid, 2174·4
Norpilen, 2174·4
2-[2-(10-Norpin-2-en-2-yl)ethoxy]triethylamine, 1381·3
Norplant, 2174·4
Norpramin, 2174·4
19-Nor-17α-pregna-1,3,5(10)-trien-20-yne-3,17β-diol, 1553·2
Norpregneninolone, 1562·2
19-Nor-17α-pregn-4-en-17β-ol, 1554·1
19-Nor-17α-pregn-4-en-20-yne-3β,17β-diol Diacetate, 1554·2
19-Nor-17α-pregn-4-en-20-yn-17β-ol, 1557·1
Norpress, 2174·4
Norpril, 2174·4
Norprolac, 2174·4
Norpropoxyphene, 29·3
*d*-Norpseudoephedrine, 1128·1
(+)-Norpseudoephedrine, 1585·2
Nor-QD, 2174·4
Norrbotten Disease— *see* Gaucher Disease, 1649·2
Norsa, 2174·4
(7*E*,22*E*)-19-Nor-9,10-secoergosta-5,7,22-triene-1α,3β,25-triol, 1462·1
Norselegiline, 1214·3
Norsertindole, 722·1
Norset, 2174·4
Norsic, 2174·4
Norsol, 2174·4
Norspor, 2174·4
Norsulfazole, 264·1
*m*-Norsynephrine Hydrochloride, 975·3
Nortase, 2174·4
Nortec, 2174·4
Nortem, 2174·4
Norterol, 2174·4
19-Nortestosterone, 1561·2
Nortestosterone Cyclohexylpropionate, 1561·2
Nortestosterone Decanoate, 1561·2
Nortestosterone Decylate, 1561·2
Nortestosterone Laurate, 1561·2
Nortestosterone Phenylpropionate, 1561·3
Nortestosterone Sodium Sulphate, 1561·3
Nortestosterone Undecanoate, 1561·3
Northiaden, 291·1
Northiron, 2174·4
Nortilidate, 94·1
Nortilidine, 94·1
Nortimil, 2174·4
Nortolan, 2174·4
Norton, 2174·4
Nortrel, 2174·4
Nortrilen, 2174·4
Nortriptilina, Hidrocloruro de, 310·2
Nortriptyline Hydrochloride, 310·2
Nortriptylini Hydrochloridum, 310·2
Nortrix, 2174·4
Nortron, 2174·4
Nortuss, 2174·4
Nortussine, 2175·1
Nortussine Mono, 2175·1
Nortylin, 2175·1
Nortyline, 2175·1
Norum, 2175·1
Noruxol, 2175·1
Norvancomycin Hydrochloride, 239·2
Norvas, 2175·1
Norvasc, 2175·1
Norvectan, 2175·1
Norvedan, 2175·1
Norventyl, 2175·1
Norverapamil, 1020·3
Norvetal, 2175·1
Norvic, 2175·1
Norvil, 2175·1
Norvir, 2175·1
Norwegian Scabies— *see* Scabies, 1499·1
Norwich Extra Strength, 2175·1
Norxacin, 2175·1
Norxia, 2175·1
Norxin, 2175·1
Norzac, 2175·1
Norzetam, 2175·1
Norzol, 2175·1
Norzotepine, 730·3
Nos, 2175·1
Nosatel, 2175·1
Noscaflex, 2175·1
Noscal, 2175·2
Nosca-Mereprine, 2175·2
Noscapina, 1125·3
Noscapina, Camsilato de, 1125·3
Noscapina, Hidrocloruro de, 1125·3
Noscapine, 1125·3
Noscapine Ascorbate, 1125·3
Noscapine Camphor-10-sulphonate, 1125·3
Noscapine Camsilate, 1125·3
Noscapine Camsylate, 1125·3
Noscapine Embonate, 1125·3
Noscapine Hydrochloride, 1125·3
Noscapini Hydrochloridum, 1125·3
Noscapinium Chloride, 1125·3
Noscapinum, 1125·3
Noscorex, 2175·2
Nose Candy, 1373·3
Nose Fresh, 2175·2
Nosebo, 2175·2
NoseEase, 2175·2
Nosenil, 2175·2
Nosipren, 2175·2
Nositrol, 2175·2
No-Sor Nose Balm, 2175·2
No-Sor Vapour Rub, 2175·2
No-Spa, 2175·2
Nospan, 2175·2
Nospasmin, 2175·2
Nospasmin Compuesto, 2175·2
Nossacin, 2175·2
Nostaden, 2175·2
Nostimex, 2175·2
Nostress, 2175·2
Nostril, 2175·2
Nostrilet, 2175·2
Nostrilla, 2175·2
Nostroline, 2175·2
Nosweat, 2175·2
Notacilin, 2175·2
Notagol, 2175·2
Notakehl, 2175·2
Notatin, 1694·2
Notem, 2175·2
Noten, 2175·3
Notensyl, 2175·3
Notezine, 2175·3
Nothav, 2175·3
Notoginseng, Radix, 1693·1
Notorium, 2175·3
No-Tos Preparations, 2175·3
Notosil, 2175·3
Notoxid, 2175·3
Notoxin, 2175·3
Notozen, 2175·3
Notrab, 2175·3
Notta, 2175·3
Nottem, 2175·3
Notul, 2175·3
Notuss, 2175·3
Notuss PD, 2175·3
Nourilax, 2175·3
Nourishake, 2175·3
Noury Hoofdlotion, 2175·3
Nourymag, 2175·3
Nourytam, 2175·3
Nova Derm, 2175·3
Nova Paratopina, 2175·3
Nova Paratropina Compositum, 2175·3
Nova Perfecting Lotion, 2175·4
Nova Rectal, 2175·4
Nova Vizol, 2175·4
Novaban, 2175·4
Novaboin, 2175·4
Novabritine, 2175·4
Novabupi, 2175·4
NovaCare, 2175·4
Novacef, 2175·4
Novacefrex, 2175·4
Novacet, 2175·4
Novacetol, 2175·4
Novacil, 2175·4
Novacilina, 2175·4
Novacler, 2175·4
Novaclox, 2175·4
Novacloxab, 2175·4
Novacnyl, 2175·4
Novacort, 2175·4
Novacrium, 2175·4
Nova-Dec, 2175·4
Novaderm, 2175·4
Novadex, 2175·4
Novador, 2175·4
Novadral, 2175·4
Novadrel, 2175·4
Novafac, 2176·1
Novafac 30, 2176·1
Novafac CC, 2176·1
Novafed A, 2176·1
Novafem, 2176·1
Novafix, 2176·1
Novafix Extra Fuerte, 2176·1
Novafur, 2176·1
Novag Grip, 2176·1
Novagcilina, 2176·1
Novagest Expectorant with Codeine, 2176·1
Novagon, 2176·1
Novahaler, 2176·1
Novahistex Preparations, 2176·1
Novahistine Preparations, 2176·1
Novain, 2176·2
Novalac Preparations, 2176·2
Novalan, 2176·2
Novalexin, 2176·2
Novalgin, 2176·2
Novalgina, 2176·2
Novalgine, 2176·2
Novalgrip, 2176·2
Novalm, 2176·2
Novalona, 2176·2
Novalox, 2176·2
Novalucol, 2176·2
Novaluzid, 2176·2
Novamet, 2176·2
Novamidazofen, 35·3
Novamilor, 2176·2
Novamin, 2176·2
Novamina, 2176·2
Novamine, 2176·2
Novaminsulfon, 36·1, 2176·3
Novaminsulfone Sodium, 35·3
Novamir, 2176·3
Novamix, 2176·3
Novamox, 2176·3
Novamoxin, 2176·3
Novanaest, 2176·3
Novaneurina B12, 2176·3
Novanox, 2176·3
Novantron, 2176·3
Novantrone, 2176·3
Novapam, 2176·3
Novapamyl, 2176·3
Novapen, 2176·3
Novaphylline, 2176·3
Novapirina, 2176·3
Novapres, 2176·3
Novaprin, 2176·3
Novapsyl, 2176·3

Novarel, 2176·3
Novarnela, 2176·3
Novarok, 2176·3
Novarrutina, 2176·3
Novartril, 2176·3
Novasal, 2176·3
Novasen, 2176·3
Novasone, 2176·4
Novasource Preparations, 2176·4
Novastan, 2176·4
Novasten, 2176·4
NovaStep, 2176·4
Novasulfon, 2176·4
Nova-T, 2176·4
Novatec, 2176·4
Novativ, 2176·4
Novatox, 2176·4
Novatrex, 2176·4
Novatrim, 2176·4
Novatropina, 2176·4
Novavir, 2176·4
Novaxen, 2176·4
Novazam, 2176·4
Novazepam, 2176·4
Novazyd, 2176·4
Novegam, 2176·4
Novel, 2176·4
Novel 1000, 2176·4
Novel Erythropoiesis Stimulating Protein, 745·2
Novel Ginkgo, 2176·4
Novel Jelly, 2177·1
Novelciclina, 2177·1
Noveldexis, 2177·1
Novelian, 2177·1
Novelmin, 2177·1
Novelon, 2177·1
Novemina, 2177·1
Noveril, 2177·1
Novesin, 2177·1
Novesina, 2177·1
Novesine, 2177·1
Novhepar, 2177·1
Novial, 2177·1
Novicarbon, 2177·1
Novid, 2177·1
Novidat, 2177·1
Novidol, 2177·1
Novidrine, 2177·1
Novidroxin, 2177·1
Noviform, 2177·1
Noviforme-Blache, 2177·1
Novifort, 2177·1
Novilax, 2177·1
Novim, 2177·1
Novimax, 2177·1
Novipec, 2177·1
Novirasin, 2177·1
Novirell B, 2177·1
Novirell B Duo, 2177·1
Novirell B Mono, 2177·2
Novital, 2177·2
Novitan, 2177·2
Novitropan, 2177·2
Novo AC and C, 2177·2
Novo Aerofil Sedante, 2177·2
Novo B, 2177·2
Novo Bacticort, 2177·2
Novo Bacticort Complex, 2177·2
Novo Dermoquinona, 2177·2
Novo E, 2177·2
Novo Mandrogallan N, 2177·2
Novo Melanidina, 2177·2
Novo Paramicon, 2177·2
Novo Petrin, 2177·2
Novo Rino, 2177·2
Novo Rino-S, 2177·2
Novo Vagran, 2177·2
Novo Vagran D, 2177·2
Novo Vegestabil, 2177·2
Novo V-K, 2177·2
Novo Wilpan, 2177·2
Novo-Alprazol, 2177·2
Novo-Atenol, 2177·2
Novo-AZT, 2177·2
Novobedouze, 2177·2
Novobiocin, 239·2
Novobiocin Calcium, 239·2
Novobiocin Sodium, 239·2
Novobiocina, 239·2
Novobiocina Cálcica, 239·2
Novobiocina Sódica, 239·2
Novobiocinum Calcium, 239·2
Novobiocinum Natricum, 239·2
Novobiocyl, 2177·2
Novobroncol, 2177·2
Novo-Butamide, 2177·2
Novo-Butazone, 2177·3
Novocain, 2177·3
Novocain, Ravocaine and— *see* Ravocaine and Novocain, 2252·3
Novocainamidum, 987·1
Novocainum, 1383·2
Novocalm, 2177·3
Novo-Captoril, 2177·3
Novo-Carbamaz, 2177·3
Novocephal, 2177·3
Novo-Cerusol, 2177·3
Novocetam, 2177·3
Novo-Chlorocap, 2177·3
Novo-Cholamine, 2177·3
Novocholin, 2177·3
Novocilin, 2177·3
Novocilin Balsamico, 2177·3
Novocillin, 2177·3
Novo-Cimetine, 2177·3
Novo-Clopamine, 2177·3
Novo-Clopate, 2177·3
Novo-Cloxin, 2177·3
Novocortal, 2177·3
Novo-Cromolyn, 2177·3
Novo-Cycloprine, 2177·3
Novodentin, 2177·3
Novo-Difenac, 2177·3
Novodig, 2177·3
Novodigal, 2177·3
Novodil, 2177·3
Novo-Diltazem, 2177·3
Novo-Dimenate, 2177·3
Novo-Dipam, 2177·3
Novo-Dipiradol, 2177·3
Novo-Doparil, 2177·4
Novo-Doxylin, 2177·4
Novofarma Champu, 2177·4
Novofem, 2177·4
Novofemme, 2177·4
Novofen, 2177·4
Novofer, 2177·4
Novo-Ferrogluc, 2177·4
Novo-Ferrosulfate, 2177·4
Novo-Fibrate, 2177·4
Novo-Fibre, 2177·4
Novofilin, 2177·4
Novo-Flupam, 2177·4
Novo-Flurazine, 2177·4
Novo-Flurprofen, 2177·4
Novo-Folacid, 2177·4
Novo-Fumar, 2177·4
Novo-Furantoin, 2177·4
Novogel, 2177·4
Novogent, 2177·4
Novo-Gesic, 2177·4
Novo-Gesic C, 2177·4
Novogyn, 2177·4
Novo-Helisen, 2177·4
Novo-Herklin 2000, 2177·4
Novo-Hexidyl, 2177·4
Novo-Hydrazide, 2177·4
Novo-Hydrocort, 2177·4
Novo-Hylazin, 2177·4
Novo-Ipramide, 2178·1
Novo-Keto, 2178·1
Novolax, 2178·1
NovoLet Preparations, 2178·1
Novo-Lexin, 2178·1
Novolin Preparations, 2178·1
NovoLog, 2178·1
NovoLog Mix 70/30, 2178·1
Novo-Lorazem, 2178·1
Novo-Medopa, 2178·1
Novo-Medrone, 2178·1
Novo-Meprazine, 2178·2
Novo-Mepro, 2178·2
Novomet, 2178·2
Novo-Methacin, 2178·2
Novo-Metoprol, 2178·2
Novomin, 2178·2
Novomint N, 2178·2
Novomit, 2178·2
No-Vomit, 2178·2
NovoMix 30, 2178·2
Novo-Mucilax, 2178·2
Novomyxine, 2178·2
Novo-Naprox, 2178·2
Novo-Nastizol, 2178·2
Novonausin, 2178·2
Novo-Nidazol, 2178·2
Novo-Nifedin, 2178·2
NovoNorm, 2178·2
Novopac, 2178·2
Novopasmil Compuesto, 2178·2
Novopen, 2178·2
Novo-Pen-G, 2178·2
Novo-Pen-VK, 2178·2
Novo-Peridol, 2178·2
Novo-Pheniram, 2178·2
Novopin MIG, 2178·2
Novo-Pindol, 2178·2
Novo-Pirocam, 2178·2
Novoplat, 2178·2
Novoplatinum, 2178·2
Novo-Plus, 2178·3
Novo-Poxide, 2178·3
Novo-Pramine, 2178·3
Novo-Pranol, 2178·3
Novo-Prazin, 2178·3
Novo-Profen, 2178·3
Novo-Propamide, 2178·3
Novo-Propoxyn, 2178·3
Novoprotect, 2178·3
Novoptine, 2178·3
Novopulmon, 2178·3
Novo-Purol, 2178·3
Novo-Pyrazone, 2178·3
Novoquin, 2178·3
Novo-Ranidine, 2178·3
NovoRapid, 2178·3
Novo-Renal, 2178·3
Novo-Ridazine, 2178·3
Novorutin, 2178·3
Novo-Rythro, 2178·3
Novosal, 2178·3
Novo-Salmol, 2178·3
Novo-Semide, 2178·3
NovoSeven, 2178·3
Novo-Sorbide, 2178·3
Novo-Soxazole, 2178·3
Novo-Spiroton, 2178·3
Novo-Spirozine, 2178·3
Novospray, 2178·3
Novostrep, 2178·4
Novo-Sucralate, 2178·4
Novo-Sundac, 2178·4
Novo-Tears, 2178·4
Novoter, 2178·4
Novoter Gentamicin, 2178·4
Novoter Gentamicina, 2178·4
Novo-Tetra, 2178·4
Novo-Thalidone, 2178·4
Novo-Theophyl, 2178·4
Novothyral, 2178·4
Novothyrox, 2178·4
Novo-Timol, 2178·4
Novotiral, 2178·4
Novotossil, 2178·4
Novo-Triamzide, 2178·4
Novo-Trimel, 2178·4
Novo-Triolam, 2178·4
Novo-Triphyl, 2178·4
Novo-Tripramine, 2178·4
Novo-Triptyn, 2178·4
Novotussan, 2178·4
Novo-Veramil, 2178·4
Novo-Vites, 2178·4
Novoxapam, 2178·4
Novoxil, 2178·4
Novozitron, 2178·4
Novo-Zolamide, 2178·4
Novral, 2178·4
Nov/Ser, 1615·3
Novutrax, 2178·4
Novuxol, 2178·4
Novynette, 2179·1
Nowax, 2179·1
Noxacorn, 2179·1
Noxalide, 2179·1
Noxema 2-In-1, 2179·1
Noxenur, 2179·1
Noxenur S, 2179·1
Noxidil, 2179·1
Noxiflex, 2179·1
Noxigram, 2179·1
Noxigur, 2179·1
Noxine, 2179·1
Noxinor, 2179·1
Noxitiolina, 1187·1
Noxobran, 2179·1
Noxom S, 2179·1
Noxotab, 2179·1
Nox-Pain, 2179·1
Noxraxin, 2179·1
Noxworm, 2179·1
Noxyflex, 2179·1
Noxyflex S, 2179·1
Noxythiolin, 1187·1
Noxytiolin, 1187·1
Noyaux, Huile de, 1651·1
Noz Moscada, 1722·2
Nozid, 2179·1
Nozinan, 2179·1
Nozolon, 2179·1
NP-113, 640·2
NPAB, 984·3
NPH Iletin I, 2179·1
NPH Iletin II, 2179·1
NPH Insulin, 334·2
NPT-10381, 640·2
N'rama, 1666·1
NRDC-149, 1502·3
NRDC-161, 1503·1
NS-718, 394·2
NS-75A, 1320·2
NSAID-associated Ulcer— *see* Peptic Ulcer Disease, 1246·3
NSAIDs, 67·3
NSC-675, 1143·2
NSC-740, 568·2
NSC-750, 532·2
NSC-752, 588·2
NSC-755, 567·2
NSC-758, 1694·1
NSC-762, 537·1
NSC-763, 1473·2
NSC-1390, 412·2
NSC-1771, 1755·1
NSC-1879, 83·1
NSC-2101, 1740·3
NSC-3053, 545·1
NSC-3070, 1548·1
NSC-3088, 536·1
NSC-3590, 1431·1
NSC-3951, 1170·2
NSC-4112, 397·3
NSC-5366, 1125·3
NSC-5648, 1757·2
NSC-6091, 202·2
NSC-6365, 1758·2
NSC-6396, 588·1
NSC-6738, 1503·2
NSC-7571, 1165·3
NSC-7760, 1050·1
NSC-8549, 1718·3
NSC-8806, 566·1
NSC-9120, 1108·1
NSC-9166, 1570·1
NSC-9324, 668·3
NSC-9564, 1562·2
NSC-9566, 1550·1
NSC-9701, 1559·3
NSC-9704, 1566·2
NSC-9894, 1556·3
NSC-9895, 1550·1
NSC-10023, 1109·3
NSC-10108, 1542·1

NSC-10483, 1103·3
NSC-10973, 1553·2
NSC-12165, 1555·3
NSC-13875, 526·2
NSC-14210, 566·1
NSC-15200, 772·2
NSC-15432, 1563·1
NSC-16895, 301·1
NSC-17590, 1550·2
NSC-17591, 1570·1
NSC-17592, 1556·3
NSC-18268, 545·1
NSC-19043, 75·2
NSC-19893, 554·2
NSC-19987, 1106·1
NSC-20264, 1647·3
NSC-20272, 1719·1
NSC-20293, 1550·1
NSC-20526, 1171·2
NSC-20527, 1171·2
NSC-21548, 1755·3
NSC-21626, 1191·2
NSC-23162, 1561·3
NSC-23759, 587·3
NSC-24559, 580·2
NSC-25141, 426·3
NSC-25154, 580·1
NSC-25159, 1591·2
NSC-25855, 1756·2
NSC-26154, 741·3
NSC-26271, 540·2
NSC-26386, 1557·2
NSC-26492, 1604·2
NSC-26980, 573·3
NSC-27640, 553·1
NSC-29863, 926·3
NSC-32065, 559·1
NSC-32363, 727·2
NSC-32942, 1172·1
NSC-32946, 573·3
NSC-34249, 1050·1
NSC-34632, 228·2
NSC-34652, 366·2
NSC-35051, 566·1
NSC-35770, 1542·2
NSC-37725, 1557·1
NSC-38297, 532·2
NSC-38721, 575·1
NSC-39069, 590·2
NSC-39084, 1349·1
NSC-39415, 1179·1
NSC-39470, 1093·1
NSC-39661, 637·3
NSC-39690, 1735·2
NSC-40725, 941·1
NSC-40902, 1730·3
NSC-42722, 1559·3
NSC-43193, 1569·2
NSC-43798, 978·3
NSC-45388, 544·2
NSC-47439, 1102·3
NSC-49171, 88·1
NSC-49506, 939·3
NSC-49842, 591·2
NSC-50364, 607·2
NSC-55926, 255·3
NSC-56410, 581·1
NSC-56769, 1145·3
NSC-58775, 710·1
NSC-59687, 1282·3
NSC-59989, 1177·3
NSC-60584, 1158·3
NSC-61815, 1060·2
NSC-63278, 1106·1
NSC-63878, 543·1
NSC-64013, 360·1
NSC-64087, 730·3
NSC-64198, 893·2
NSC-64393, 255·3
NSC-64967, 1559·3
NSC-65411, 1555·2
NSC-66847, 1752·3
NSC-67068, 1565·1
NSC-67574, 592·2
NSC-68982, 926·2
NSC-69200, 882·3
NSC-69856, 594·3
NSC-70731, 226·2
NSC-70762, 348·1
NSC-71047, 1162·2
NSC-71423, 1558·2
NSC-72005, 1195·1
NSC-72260, 1560·1
NSC-73205, 35·3
NSC-73713, 1585·3
NSC-74226, 1559·2
NSC-75054, 1559·1
NSC-75520, 655·3
NSC-77213, 581·2
NSC-77370, 1687·2
NSC-77518, 690·1
NSC-77625, 1016·2
NSC-78194, 485·3
NSC-78502, 229·1
NSC-78559, 700·3
NSC-79037, 565·2
NSC-79389, 884·3
NSC-80998, 1096·2
NSC-81430, 1544·1
NSC-82151, 545·3
NSC-82174, 234·1
NSC-82261, 217·1
NSC-82699, 43·2
NSC-83653, 1197·2
NSC-84054, 1556·2
NSC-84223, 1308·3
NSC-85791, 913·2
NSC-85998, 584·1
NSC-89199, 551·1
NSC-91523, 989·3
NSC-92336, 1549·2
NSC-92338, 1542·1
NSC-92339, 1101·2
NSC-94100, 573·2
NSC-94219, 395·3
NSC-95072, 240·2
NSC-95441, 583·2
NSC-100071, 401·2
NSC-101791, 1101·3
NSC-102816, 529·2
NSC-102824, 20·1
NSC-104800, 573·3
NSC-106563, 872·3
NSC-106566, 913·1
NSC-106568, 272·2
NSC-106962, 1065·2
NSC-107079, 1671·1
NSC-107430, 79·3
NSC-107431, 1067·2
NSC-107433, 616·3
NSC-107434, 1067·3
NSC-107654, 408·1
NSC-107677, 431·2
NSC-107678, 863·3
NSC-107679, 890·3
NSC-107680, 1101·1
NSC-108160, 291·2
NSC-108161, 984·2
NSC-108164, 911·3
NSC-108165, 725·2
NSC-108166, 274·1
NSC-109229, 528·3
NSC-109723, 590·2
NSC-109724, 561·1
NSC-110364, 240·3
NSC-110430, 880·2
NSC-110431, 953·2
NSC-110432, 1304·1
NSC-110433, 263·1
NSC-111071, 166·2
NSC-111180, 1112·3
NSC-113926, 250·2
NSC-114649, 482·2
NSC-114650, 1587·2
NSC-114901, 290·2
NSC-115748, 674·2
NSC-115944, 1298·1
NSC-119875, 538·1
NSC-122758, 1161·1
NSC-122819, 587·2
NSC-123018, 1557·1
NSC-123127, 547·3
NSC-125973, 577·3
NSC-127716, 546·2
NSC-129224, 1648·1
NSC-129943, 582·2
NSC-130044, 442·1
NSC-134087, 581·2
NSC-134434, 105·3
NSC-134454, 1264·2
NSC-141046, 197·1
NSC-141540, 551·3
NSC-141633, 558·3
NSC-148958, 586·2
NSC-157365, 594·3
NSC-157658, 1679·2
NSC-164011, 594·3
NSC-169780, 1036·1
NTSC-177023, 107·2
NSC-178248, 538·1
NSC-182986, 546·3
NSC-208734, 525·2
NSC-218321, 579·2
NSC-220537, 540·2
NSC-226080, 1363·1
NSC-239336, 550·2
NSC-241240, 533·3
NSC-245382, 576·3
NSC-245467, 593·3
NSC-246131, 590·3
NSC-249008, 410·2
NSC-249992, 527·3
NSC-256439, 560·2
NSC-262168, 1060·1
NSC-265489, 590·3
NSC-266046, 577·1
NSC-0270516, 582·2
NSC-296961, 1031·3
NSC-301467, 551·2
NSC-301739, 575·2
NSC-312887, 553·2
NSC-325319, 546·3
NSC-337766, 530·2
NSC-351521, 580·1
NSC-352122, 410·2
NSC-356894, 1360·2
NSC-362856, 587·1
NSC-368390, 1351·2
NSC-406087, 1588·1
NSC-406239, 1416·1
NSC-408735, 603·2
NSC-409962, 535·1
NSC-515776, 903·1
NSC-526046, 966·1
NSC-526280, 1171·2
NSC-527579, 1106·1
NSC-527604, 1033·1
NSC-528986, 157·1
NSC-606170, 657·1
NSC-612049, 630·3
NSC-628503, 547·1
NSC-648766, 589·3
NSC-659772, 526·2
NSC 378348, 1444·1
NSC 620261, 528·2
NSC 648539, 528·2
N-Statin, 2179·1
NTA-194, 94·1
NTBC, 1722·1
NTG, 923·2
NTR, 2179·2
Ntsangu, 1666·1
NTZ Long Acting Nasal, 2179·2
NU-445, 260·1
NU-903, 718·1
NU-2121, 966·1
Nu-Alpraz, 2179·2
Nu-Amilzide, 2179·2
Nu-Amoxi, 2179·2
Nu-Ampi, 2179·2
Nuardin, 2179·2
Nu-Atenol, 2179·2
Nu-Baclo, 2179·2
Nubain, 2179·2
Nubaina, 2179·2
Nubak, 2179·2
Nubevital BB, 2179·2
Nubevital P, 2179·2
Nubevital Sunblock Ultra, 2179·2
Nubral Preparations, 2179·2
Nu-Cal, 2179·2
Nu-Capto, 2179·2
Nu-Cephalex, 2179·2
Nu-Cidex, 1187·3, 2179·2
Nu-Cimet, 2179·2
Nuclav, 2179·2
Nuclear Fast Red, 1719·3
Nucleic Acid, 1722·2
Nucleic Acid, Animal, 1679·2
Nucleic Acid, Plant, 1738·2
Nucleic Acid, Ribose, 1738·2
Nucleic Acid, Thymus, 1679·2
Nucleic Acid, Yeast, 1738·2
Nucleico, Ácido, 1722·2
Nucleicum, Acidum, 1722·2
Nucleinic Acid, 1722·2
Nucleo CMP, 2179·2
Nucleodoxina, 2179·3
Nucleserina, 2179·3
Nuclevit $B_{12}$, 2179·3
Nuclosina, 2179·3
Nu-Cloxi, 2179·3
Nucoa, 2179·3
Nucobrox, 2179·3
Nucofed, 2179·3
Nucofed Expectorant, 2179·3
Nucolox, 2179·3
Nucosef, 2179·3
Nucosef DM, 2179·3
Nu-Cotrimox, 2179·3
Nucotuss Expectorant, 2179·3
Nuctalon, 2179·3
Nuctane, 2179·3
Nu-Diclo, 2179·3
Nu-Diltiaz, 2179·3
Nudopa, 2179·3
Nuelin, 2179·3
Nuevapina, 2179·3
Nueve Lunas, 2179·3
Nuez Moscada, 1722·2
Nuez Moscada, Aceite Esencial de, 1722·3
Nuez Moscada, Esencia de, 1722·3
Nuez Vómica, 1722·3
Nueza, 1663·1
Nufarol, 2179·3
Nufex, 2179·3
Nu-Gel, 2179·3
Nuhair, 2179·4
Nuhist, 2179·4
Nu-Hydral, 2179·4
Nuicalm, 2179·4
Nuidor, 2179·4
Nu-Indo, 2179·4
Nu-Iron, 2179·4
Nu-Iron V, 2179·4
Nu-Iron Plus, 2179·4
Nujol, 2179·4
Nulacin, 2179·4
Nulacin Fermentos, 2179·4
Nulagrip C, 2179·4
Nularef, 2179·4
Nularef Cort, 2179·4
Nularef-D, 2179·4
Nulastres, 2179·4
Nulceran, 2179·4
Nulcerin, 2179·4
Nuleron, 2179·4
NuLev, 2179·4
Nu-Levocarb, 2179·4
Nulip, 2179·4
Nullatuss, 2179·4
Nulobes, 2179·4
Nu-Loraz, 2179·4
Nu-Lotan, 2179·4
NuLytely, 2179·4
Numalin, 2180·1
Numark, 2180·1
Numatol, 2180·1
Numbon, 2180·1
Nu-Medopa, 2180·1
Numencial, 2180·1
Nu-Metop, 2180·1
Numidan, 2180·1
Numonyl, 2180·1

Numonyl C, 2180·1
Numonyl D, 2180·1
Numonyl T, 2180·1
Numonyl Tex, 2180·1
Numorphan, 2180·1
Numosol, 2180·1
Numzident, 2180·1
Numzit, 2180·1
Num-Zit, 2180·1
Nu-Naprox, 2180·1
Nu-Nifed, 2180·1
Nuomin, 2180·1
Nu-Oxybutyn, 2180·1
Nu-Pen-VK, 2180·1
Nupercainal, 2180·1
Nupercaine Heavy, 2180·2
Nu-Pindol, 2180·2
Nu-Pirox, 2180·2
Nupra, 2180·2
Nuprafen, 2180·2
Nu-Prazo, 2180·2
Nuprilan, 2180·2
Nuprin, 2180·2
Nuprin Backache, 2180·2
Nu-Prochlor, 2180·2
Nur 1 Tropfen Chlorhexidin, 2180·2
Nur 1 Tropfen Medizinisches Mundwasser, 2180·2
Nu-Ranit, 2180·2
Nurasic, 2180·2
Nureflex, 2180·2
Nuriban, 2180·2
Nuriban A, 2180·2
Nuri-Kapseln, 2180·2
Nuril, 2180·2
Nuriphasic, 2180·2
Nur-Isterate, 2180·2
Nurocain, 2180·2
Nurocain with Sympathin, 2180·2
Nurofen Preparations, 2180·2
Nurogrip, 2180·3
Nurolasts, 2180·3
Nuromax, 2180·3
Nurse Harvey's Gripe Mixture, 2180·3
Nurse Sykes Balsam, 2180·3
Nurse Sykes Powders, 2180·3
Nursoy, 2180·3
Nurture Nourishing, 2180·3
Nu-Salt, 2180·3
Nu-Seals, 2180·3
Nussidex, 2180·3
Nustasium, 2180·3
Nut Oil, 1656·1
Nuta, 2180·3
Nutacough, 2180·3
Nutamol, 2180·3
Nutcracker Oesophagus— *see* Oesophageal Motility Disorders, 1246·3
Nu-Tears, 2180·3
Nu-Tears II, 2180·3
Nutegen A, 2180·3
Nutegen G, 2180·3
Nutegen H, 2180·4
Nu-Tetra, 2180·4
Nutgall, 1690·2
Nutilis, 2180·4
Nutmeg, 1722·2
Nutmeg Oil, 1722·3
Nutra Fibra, 2180·4
Nutra Nutrabain, 2180·4
Nutra Nutraderme, 2180·4
Nutrabase, 2180·4
Nutrabeaute, 2180·4
Nutrabiotique, 2180·4
Nutracel, 2180·4
Nutracort, 2180·4
Nutra-D, 2180·4
Nutraderm, 2180·4
Nutraderme, 2180·4
Nutradex, 2180·4
Nutrafilm, 2180·4
Nutraflow, 2180·4
Nutraforme, 2180·4
Nutraisdin, 2180·4
Nutralcon, 2180·4
Nutralona, 2180·4
Nutraloric, 2180·4
Nutrament, 2180·4
Nutramigen, 2180·4
Nutramigen, Enfalac— *see* Enfalac Nutramigen, 1970·2
Nutramince, 2181·1
Nutra'Mix, 2181·1
NutraMX, 2181·1
Nutraplus, 2181·1
Nutrapurete, 2181·1
Nutrarepos, 2181·1
Nutra-Soothe, 2181·1
Nutrasoothe, 2181·1
Nutrasorb, 2181·1
Nutrasweet, 2181·1
Nutravit Light, 2181·1
Nutren, 2181·1
Nutren IBD, 2181·1
Nutr-E-Sol, 2181·1
Nutrex, 2181·1
Nutri Concentrated, 2181·1
Nutri 2000 (Nutrinaut), 2181·1
Nutri Twin, 2181·1
Nutri Yin-Nutri Yang, 2181·1
Nu-Triazide, 2181·1
Nutribraun, 2181·1
Nutrical, 2181·1
Nutricalcio, 2181·1
Nutricap, 2181·2
Nutricomp, 2181·2
Nutricon, 2181·2
Nutricremal, 2181·2
Nutrideen, 2181·2
Nutridoral, 2181·2
Nutridrink, 2181·2
Nutrifac, 2181·2
Nutriflex, 2181·2
Nutriflex Lipid, 2181·2
Nutriflex Lipid N, 2181·2
Nutriflex Lipide, 2181·2
NutriFocus, 2181·2
Nutrifol, 2181·2
Nutrigel, 2181·2
Nutrigene, 2181·2
Nutrigil, 2181·2
NutriHeal, 2181·2
Nutri-Junior, 2181·2
Nutrilac, 2181·2
Nutrilamine, 2181·2
Nutrilan, 2181·2
Nutrilife Pro, 2181·2
Nutrilin, 2181·2
Nutrilon AR, 2181·2
Nutrilon Lactomin, 2181·2
Nutrilon L-K, 2181·2
Nutrilon Pepti, 2181·2
Nutrilon Soja, 2181·3
Nutrilon Soya, 2181·3
Nutrilon Soya— *see* Infasoy, 2061·2
Nutrilyte, 2181·3
Nutrimaiz SM, 2181·3
Nutrimed, 2181·3
Nutri-Mega, 2181·3
Nutri-Min, 2181·3
Nutrinaut— *see* Nutri 2000 (Nutrinaut), 2181·1
Nutrineal Preparations, 2181·3
Nutrini, 2181·3
Nutri-Ped, 2181·3
Nutriperi Lipid, 2181·3
Nutriplasmal, 2181·3
NutriPlus, 2181·3
Nutriplus Lipid, 2181·3
Nutrisan, 2181·3
NutriScience, 2181·3
Nutri-Soija, 2181·3
Nutrisol, 2181·3
Nutrisol-S, 2181·3
Nutrison, 2181·3
Nutrison MCT, 2181·3
Nutrison Pepti, 2181·3
Nutrisource, 2181·3
Nutrispecial Lipid, 2181·3
Nutrisun Lait Solaire Insectifuge 16, 2181·3
Nutrisun Lait Solaire Insectifuge 30, 2181·4
Nutrisun Lotion Solaire Insectifuge 8, 2181·4
Nutritional Agents and Vitamins, 1417·1
Nutritrace, 2181·4
NutriTwin G, 2181·4
Nutrivisc, 2181·4
Nutrivit, 2181·4
Nutrizim, 2181·4
Nutrizima, 2181·4
Nutrizym, 2181·4
Nutrizym N, 2181·4
Nutrocal, 2181·4
Nutrocal DM, 2181·4
Nutrodrip, 2181·4
Nutrodrip— *see* Isosource (Nutrodrip), 2068·4
Nutrol Preparations, 2181·4
Nutrolin-B, 2181·4
Nutropin, 2181·4
Nutroplex, 2181·4
Nutroplex with Iron & Lysine, 2181·4
Nutroplex Lysine, 2181·4
Nutrosa, 2182·1
Nutrox, 2182·1
Nuvacthen Depot, 2182·1
Nuvapen, 2182·1
NuvaRing, 2182·1
Nuvelle, 2182·1
Nuvelle Continuous, 2182·1
Nuvelle TS, 2182·1
Nu-Verap, 2182·1
Nuvir, 2182·1
Nuvit, 2182·1
Nuvorell, 2182·1
Nux ISO, 2182·1
Nux Med Complex, 2182·1
Nux Moschata, 1722·2
Nux Vom., 1722·3
Nux Vomica, 1722·3
Nux Vomica Oligoplex, 2182·1
Nux Vomica-Homaccord, 2182·1
Nux Vomica-Injeel, 2182·1
Nuxil, 2182·1
Nuzak, 2182·1
Nwonkaka, 1666·1
NY-198, 227·2
Nyaderm, 2182·1
Nyal Preparations, 2182·1
Nycodol, 2182·2
Nycoflox, 2182·2
Nycoheparin, 2182·2
Nycopin, 2182·2
Nycoplus Neo-Fer, 2182·2
Nycopren, 2182·2
Nycovir, 2182·2
Nydrazid, 2182·2
Nyefax, 2182·2
Nylax with Senna, 2182·2
Nylex, 2182·2
Nylidrin Hydrochloride, 1663·2
Nylidrinium Chloride, 1663·2
Nylipark, 2182·2
Nymix Mucolytikum, 2182·2
Nyogel, 2182·2
Nyolol, 2182·2
NyQuil, 2182·2
NyQuil Allergy/Head Cold, Vicks Children's— *see* Vicks Children's NyQuil Allergy/Head Cold, 2375·2
Nyquil, Childrens— *see* Childrens Nyquil, 1882·4
NyQuil Hot Therapy, 2182·2
NyQuil LiquiCaps, Vicks— *see* Vicks NyQuil LiquiCaps, 2375·3
Nyquil Night-time Cold/Cough Liquid, Vicks Children's— *see* Vicks Children's NyQuil Night-time Cold/Cough Liquid, 2375·2
NyQuil Nighttime Cold/Flu, 2182·2
Nyrene, 2182·3
Nyrin, 2182·3
Nysconitrine, 2182·3
Nyspes, 2182·3
Nystacid, 2182·3
Nystacortone, 2182·3
Nystaderm, 2182·3
Nystaderm Comp, 2182·3
Nystadermal, 2182·3
Nystaform, 2182·3
Nystaform-HC, 2182·3
Nystalocal, 2182·3
Nystamont, 2182·3
Nystan, 2182·3
Nystasan, 2182·3
Nystatin, 406·3
Nystatin $A_1$, 406·3
Nystatin-Dome, 2182·3
Nystatinum, 406·3
Nystex, 2182·3
Nystin, 2182·3
Nystop, 2182·3
Nytamel, 2182·3
Nytcold Medicine, 2182·3
Nytol, 2182·3
Nytol Herbal, 2182·3
Nytol Natural Source, 2182·3
NYU-CS, 1622·3
NYVAC-Pf7, 1622·3
NZ-105, 909·2


## O


O A R, 2182·3
O-4 Cycline, 2182·3
Oak Bark, 1722·3
Oak, Common, 1722·3
Oak, Durmast, 1722·3
Oasil, 2182·3
Oasil Simes, 2182·4
Oasis, Canesten— *see* Canesten Oasis, 1867·2
Oat Milk Treatment Cream, 2182·4
Oatmeal, 1658·2
Oatmeal, Colloidal, 1658·2
Oats, 1658·2
Oaxen, 2182·4
Obaron, 2182·4
Obbekjaers, 2182·4
Obducti Laxativi Vegetabiles S— *see* PhytoLaxin, 2219·1
Obecirol, 2182·4
Obeflorine, 2182·4
Obegyn Prenatal, 2182·4
Obelin, 2182·4
Obe-Nix, 2182·4
Obesan-X, 2182·4
Obesidex, 2182·4
Obesifran, 2182·4
Obesity, 1583·3
Obestat, 2182·4
Obetine, 2182·4
Obetrol— *see* Adderall, 1775·3
Obex-LA, 2182·4
Ob-gene, 1584·1
Obidoxima, Cloruro de, 1046·3
Obidoxime Chloride, 1046·3
Obifen, 2182·4
Obimin, 2182·4
Obimin-AF, 2182·4
Obimin-AZ, 2182·4
Obimol, 2182·4
Obinese, 2182·4
O-Biol, 2182·4
O-Biol P, 2182·4
Obiron Extra, 2182·4
Obisin, 2182·4
Obituin, 1689·1
Oblax A-1-1, 2182·4
Obleas Chinas, 2182·4
Oblimersen Sodium, 577·1
Oblioser, 2182·4
Obliterol, 2182·4
Oboliz, 2182·4
Obracin, 2182·4
Obry, 2183·1
Obrydex, 2183·1
Obrypre, 2183·1
Obsessive-compulsive Disorder, 663·2
Obsidan, 2183·1
Obsidan Comp, 2183·1
Obsilazin N, 2183·1
Obstar, 2183·1
Obstetrix, 2183·1

Obstilax, 2183·1
Obstinol M, 2183·1
Obstructive Airways Disease, Chronic— *see* Chronic Obstructive Pulmonary Disease, 779·2
Obstructive Pulmonary Disease, Chronic— *see* Chronic Obstructive Pulmonary Disease, 779·2
Obtrex, 2183·1
Obus Form Therapeutic Heat, 2183·1
Obus Form Therapeutic Ice, 2183·1
Obusforme, 2183·1
Obusonid, 2183·1
Ocacin, 2183·1
Ocadrik, 2183·1
O-Cal, 2183·1
O-Cal Prenatal, 2183·1
Occhivit, 2183·1
Occidal, 2183·1
Occipital Epilepsy— *see* Epilepsy, 349·1
Occlucort, 2183·1
Occlusal, 2183·1
Occlusion, Arterial, Acute— *see* Peripheral Arterial Thromboembolism, 830·3
Occlusive Arterial Disease— *see* Peripheral Vascular Disease, 831·2
Occodem, 2183·1
Occu System, 2183·1
Ocean, 2183·1
Oceantone, 2183·1
Ocefax, 2183·1
Oceral, 2183·1
Oceral GB, 2183·2
Ochozim, 2183·2
Ocid, 2183·2
OCL, 2183·2
Oclovir, 2183·2
OCM, 2183·2
*Ocotea*, 1742·1
Ocrilate, 1678·1
Ocrylate, 1678·1
Ocsaar, 2183·2
Ocsaar Plus, 2183·2
OCT, 1462·1
Octacaína, Hidrocloruro de, 1382·1
Octacaine Hydrochloride, 1382·1
1,2,4,5,6,7,8,8-Octachloro-2,3,3a,4,7,7a-hexahydro-4,7-methanoindene, 1501·3
Octacosanol, 984·2, 2183·2
(*Z*,*Z*)-Octadeca-9,12-dienoic Acid, 1690·2
Octadecafluorooctane, 1730·2
Octadecanoic Acid, 1749·2
1-Octadecanol, 1482·3
(*Z*,*Z*,*Z*)-Octadeca-6,9,12-trienoic Acid, 1690·2
(*Z*)-Octadec-9-enoic Acid, 1481·3
Octadec-9-enol, 1481·3
9-Octadecenylamine Hydrofluoride, 1427·1
Octadecyl Alcohol, 1482·3
Octadon P, 2183·2
Octafluoropropane, 1067·2
Octafonio, Cloruro de, 1187·1
Octafonium Chloride, 1187·1
Octagam, 2183·2
1,1′,2,2′,3,3′,4,4′-Octahydro-6,6′,7,7′,8,8′-hexamethoxy-2,2′-dimethyl-1,1′-bis(3,4,5-trimethoxybenzyl)-2,2′-[butanedioylbis(oxytrimethylene)]di-isoquinolinium Dichloride, 1403·1
(4*S*,7*S*,10a*S*)-Octahydro-4-[(*S*)-α-mercaptohydrocinnamamido]-5-oxo-7*H*-pyrido[2,1-*b*][1,3]thiazepine-7-carboxylic Acid, 976·1
(*E*)-1,1′,2,2′,3,3′,4,4′-Octahydro-6,6′,7,7′-tetramethoxy-2,2′-dimethyl-1,1′-bis(3,4,5-trimethoxybenzyl)-2,2′-[oct-4-enedioylbis(oxytrimethylene)]di-isoquinolinium Dichloride, 1403·3
(3*R*,5a*S*,6*R*,8a*S*,9*R*,12*S*,12a*R*)-Octahydro-3,6,9-trimethyl-3,12-epoxy-12*H*-pyrano[4,3-*j*]-1,2-benzodioxepin-10(3*H*)-one, 447·2
Octamide, 2183·2
Octanal, 1724·1
Octanate, 2183·2
Octane-1,8-dicarboxylic Acid, 1157·3
Octanine, 2183·2
Octanoato Sódico, 1723·1
Octanoic Acid, 1723·1
Octanoic Acid ($^{13}$C), 1723·1
Octanoico, Ácido, 1723·1
Octanyl, 2183·2
Octanyne, 2183·2
Octanyne— *see* Octanine, 2183·2
Octaphonium Chloride, 1187·1
Octaplas, 2183·2
Octapressin— *see* Citanest Octapressin, 1889·2
Octapressin— *see* Citanest con Octapressin, 1889·1
Octapressin— *see* Citanest with Octapressin, 1889·2
Octapressin— *see* Xylonest-Octapressin, 2389·2
Octapressine, Citanest— *see* Citanest Octapressine, 1889·2
Octastatin, 1342·2
Octatron, 2183·2
Octatropina, Metilbromuro de, 486·1
Octatropine Methylbromide, 486·1
Octavi, 2183·2
Octegra, 2183·2
Octelmin, 2183·2
Octenidina, Hidrocloruro de, 1187·2
Octenidine Hydrochloride, 1187·2
Octenisept, 2183·2
Octex, 2183·2
Octiban, 2183·2
Octicair, 2183·2
Octil, 2183·2
Octil 2-Cyanoacrylate, 1678·1
Octil Gallate, 1168·1
Octil Hydrogen Fumarate, 1147·3
Octil Triazone, 1154·3
7-(2-Octilcyclopentyl)heptanoic Acid, 1511·1
Octildodecanol, 1476·3
Octilia, 2183·2
Octim, 2183·3
Octinoxate, 1154·3
Octinoxato, 1154·3
Octinum, 2183·3
Octinum-D, 2183·3
Octisalate, 1154·3
Octisalato, 1154·3
Octiveran, 2183·3
Octocaine, 2183·3
Octocog Alfa, 751·2
Octocrilene, 1154·3
Octocrileno, 1154·3
Octocrylene, 1154·3
Octodrina, 975·3
Octodrine, 975·3
Octodrine Camsilate, 975·3
Octodrine Phosphate, 975·3
Octofene, 2183·3
Octonativ-M, 2183·3
Octonox, 2183·3
*m*-Octopamine, 975·3
*p*-Octopamine, 975·3
Octopil, 2183·3
Octorax, 2183·3
Octostim, 2183·3
Octotensina, 2183·3
Octotiamina, 1455·1
Octotiamine, 1455·1
Octovit, 2183·3
Octoxinol, 1414·1
Octoxinol 9, 1414·1
Octoxinol 10, 1414·1
Octoxinoles, 1414·1
Octoxinols, 1414·1
Octoxynol 9, 1414·1
Octoxynols, 1414·1
Octreoscan, 2183·3
Octreotida, Acetato de, 1333·1
Octreotide Acetate, 1333·1
Octyl Dimethyl PABA, 1155·1
Octyl Gallate, 1168·1
Octyl Methoxycinnamate, 1154·3
Octyl Salicylate, 1154·3
Octyl Triazone, 1154·3
Octyl 3,4,5-Trihydroxybenzoate, 1168·1
Octyldodecanol, 1476·3
(*RS*)-2-Octyldodecan-1-ol, 1476·3
Octyldodecanolum, 1476·3
Octylis Gallas, 1168·1
Octylonium Bromide, 1725·1
Octylphenoxy Polyethoxyethanol, 1414·1
Ocubrax, 2183·3
Ocu-Caine, 2183·3
OcuCaps, 2183·3
Ocu-Carpine, 2183·3
Ocuclear, 2183·3
Ocucoat, 2183·3
Ocudiafan, 2183·3
Ocufen, 2183·3
Ocuflox, 2183·3
Ocuflur, 2183·4
Ocufort, 2183·4
Ocufri, 2183·4
Ocugel, 2183·4
Ocugram, 2183·4
Ocuhist, 2183·4
Oculac, 2183·4
Ocular Cicatricial Pemphigoid— *see* Pemphigus and Pemphigoid, 1085·2
Ocular Hypertension— *see* Glaucoma and Ocular Hypertension, 1485·1
Ocular Inflammatory Disorders, Postoperative— *see* Postoperative Inflammatory Ocular Disorders, 70·3
Ocular Larva Migrans— *see* Toxocariasis, 101·1
Ocular Melanoma— *see* Malignant Neoplasms of the Eye, 516·1
Ocular Myasthenia— *see* Myasthenia Gravis, 1486·2
Oculastin, 2183·4
Oculoforte, 2183·4
Oculoheel, 2183·4
Oculosan, 2183·4
Oculosan Forte, 2183·4
Oculosan N, 2183·4
Oculotec, 2183·4
Oculotect, 2183·4
Oculotect Fluid, 2183·4
Oculotect Sine, 2183·4
Oculube, 2183·4
Ocu-Lube, 2183·4
Ocu-Mycin, 2183·4
Ocu-Pentolate, 2183·4
Ocu-Phrin, 2183·4
Ocupol, 2183·4
Ocupol-D, 2183·4
Ocupres, 2183·4
Ocupress, 2184·1
Ocuprost, 2184·1
Ocurest, 2184·1
Ocurest-AH, 2184·1
Ocurest-Z, 2184·1
Ocusert, 2184·1
Ocusoft Pads, 2184·1
Ocusoft VMS, 2184·1
Ocusol, 2184·1
Ocu-Spor-B, 2184·1
Ocu-Spor-G, 2184·1
Ocustil, 2184·1
Ocustress, 2184·1
Ocusulf-10, 2184·1
Ocu-Tears, 2184·1
Ocutears, 2184·1
Ocuton, 2184·1
Ocutricin, 2184·1
Ocutrien, 2184·1
Ocu-Trol, 2184·1
Ocu-Tropic, 2184·1
Ocu-Tropine, 2184·1
Ocutrulan, 2184·1
Ocuvite, 2184·1
ODA-914, 1322·3
Odaban, 2184·1
Odala Wern, 2184·2
Odamesol, 2184·2
Odamida, 2184·2
Odanet, 2184·2
Odanex, 2184·2
Odasol, 2184·2
Oddibil, 2184·2
Oddispasmol, 2184·2
Odemase, 2184·2
Odemin, 2184·2
Odenil Unas, 2184·2
Odermennigkraut, 1649·1
Odiron-C, 2184·2
Odisor, 2184·2
Odo-fre, 2184·2
Odol Control Sarro, 2184·2
Odol Med Antiplaca, 2184·2
Odol Med Dental, 2184·2
Odol Tratamiento de Encias, 2184·2
Odongi, 2184·2
Odon-Pyr, 2184·2
Odontalg, 2184·2
Odontalgiche (Dentali), 2184·2
Odontalgico Dr. Knapp con Vit. B1, 2184·2
Odontocromil C Sulfamida, 2184·2
Odonton-Echtroplex, 2184·2
Odontovac, 2184·2
Odontoxina, 2184·3
Odor Eze, 2184·3
Odourless Garlic, 2184·3
Odoxil, 2184·3
Odranal, 2184·3
Odric, 2184·3
Odrik, 2184·3
O-Due, 2184·3
Odupril, 2184·3
Oecotrim, 2184·3
Oecozol, 2184·3
Oedema, Pulmonary— *see* Shock, 835·1
Oedemex, 2184·3
Oeillette, Huile d', 1733·3
OeKolp, 2184·3
Oemine, 2184·3
Oenobiol, 2184·3
*Oenothera biennis*, 1686·3
Oesclim, 2184·3
Oesophageal Cancer— *see* Malignant Neoplasms of the Gastrointestinal Tract, 516·2
Oesophageal Candidiasis— *see* Candidiasis, 386·3
Oesophageal Disorders— *see* Oesophageal Motility Disorders, 1246·3
Oesophageal Impaction— *see* Oesophageal Motility Disorders, 1246·3
Oesophageal Spasm— *see* Oesophageal Motility Disorders, 1246·3
Oesophageal Varices— *see* Variceal Haemorrhage, 1716·1
Oesophagitis, Reflux— *see* Gastro-oesophageal Reflux Disease, 1242·3
Oesophagus, Nutcracker— *see* Oesophageal Motility Disorders, 1246·3
Oest...— *see also under* Est...
Oesto-Mins, 2184·3
Oestraclin, 2184·3
Oestradiol, 1550·1
Oestradiol Benzoate, 1550·1
Oestradiol Cyclopentylpropionate, 1550·1
Oestradiol Cypionate, 1550·1
Oestradiol Dipropionate, 1550·1
Oestradiol Enanthate, 1550·1
Oestradiol 17-Heptanoate, 1550·1
Oestradiol Hexahydrobenzoate, 1550·1
Oestradiol 17-Nicotinate 3-Propionate, 1552·3
Oestradiol Phenylpropionate, 1550·2
Oestradiol Valerate, 1550·2
Oestrifen, 2184·3
Oestrilin, 2184·3
Oestring, 2184·3
Oestriol, 1552·3
Oestriol 3-Cyclopentyl Ether, 1568·2
Oestriol Sodium Succinate, 1552·3
Oestriol Succinate, 1552·3
Oestrodienolum, 1547·3
Oestrodose, 2184·3
Oestro-Feminal, 2184·3
Oestrofeminal, 2184·3
Oestrogel, 2184·3
Oestrogen Replacement Therapy, 1536·3
Oestrogens, 1527·1
Oestrogens, A, Synthetic Conjugated, 1543·3
Oestrogens, B, Synthetic Conjugated, 1543·3

Oestrogens, Conjugated, 1543·2
Oestrogens, Esterified, 1549·3
Oestro-Gynaedron M, 2184·3
Oestro-Gynaedron Nouveau, 2184·3
Oestrone, 1553·1
OestroTabs Plus Cyclic, 2184·4
Oestrugol N, 2184·4
Ofal, 2184·4
Ofal P, 2184·4
Ofcin, 2184·4
Off Skintastic, 2184·4
Offeno, 2184·4
Offentina, 2184·4
Off-Ezy, 2184·4
Ofil, 2184·4
Ofisolona, 2184·4
O-Flam, 2184·4
Oflin, 2184·4
Oflocee, 2184·4
Oflocet, 2184·4
Oflocin, 2184·4
Oflodex, 2184·4
Oflodura, 2184·4
Oflohexal, 2184·4
Oflono, 2184·4
Oflovir, 2184·4
Oflox, 2184·4
O-Flox, 2184·4
Ofloxa, 2184·4
Ofloxacin, 239·3
*S*-(−)-Ofloxacin, 225·3
Ofloxacin Hydrochloride, 240·1
Ofloxacino, 239·3
Ofloxacinum, 239·3
Ofloxan, 2184·4
Ofloxcin, 2184·4
Ofloxin, 2184·4
O-fluor, 2184·4
Ofnifenil, 2184·4
Ofnimarex, 2184·4
O-folin, 2184·4
Ofoxin, 2185·1
Oframax, 2185·1
Oftabiotico, 2185·1
Oftacilox, 2185·1
Oftaciprox, 2185·1
Oftacon, 2185·1
Oftadil, 2185·1
Oftagel, 2185·1
Oftagen, 2185·1
Oftagen Compuesto, 2185·1
Oftal, 2185·1
Oftalar, 2185·1
Oftalbrax, 2185·1
Oftaler, 2185·1
Oftalirio, 2185·1
Oftalmet, 2185·1
Oftalmil, 2185·1
Oftalmo, 2185·1
Oftalmocaina, 2185·1
Oftalmoflogol, 2185·1
Oftalmol Dexa, 2185·1
Oftalmol Ocular, 2185·1
Oftalmolets, 2185·1
Oftalmolosa Cusi de Icol, 2185·1
Oftalmolosa Cusi Virucida, 2185·1
Oftalmotonil, 2185·2
Oftalmotrim, 2185·2
Oftalmotrim Dexa, 2185·2
Oftalmowell, 2185·2
Oftalzina, 2185·2
Oftamolol, 2185·2
Oftan Preparations, 2185·2
Oftapinex, 2185·2
Oftaquin, 2185·2
Oftaquix, 2185·2
Oftasona N, 2185·2
Oftasona P, 2185·2
Oftasteril, 2185·2
Oftavir, 2185·2
Oftazil, 2185·2
Oftazul, 2185·2
Oftcor, 2185·3
Oftic, 2185·3
Ofticlin, 2185·3
Oftimolo, 2185·3
Oftinal, 2185·3
Oftrim, 2185·3
Oftyll Desoxydrop, 2185·3
Ogamma, 2185·3
Ogast, 2185·3
Ogasto, 2185·3
Ogastro, 2185·3
Ogen, 2185·3
Ogenest, 2185·3
Ogestane, 2185·3
Oglos, 2185·3
OGT-918, 1715·2
Ogyline, 2185·3
OH B12, 2185·3
OH B12 B1, 2185·3
4-OHA, 557·1
4-OHAD, 557·1
1α-OH-$D_2$, 1462·1
1α-$OHD_3$, 1461·2
1α,25$(OH)_2D_3$, 1461·2
25-$(OH)D_3$, 1461·2
Ohexine, 2185·3
OHM-11771, 973·3
*l*-OHP, 577·1
OIF, 2185·3
Oil of American Wormseed, 103·3
Oil, Boiled, 1707·2
Oil of Mirbane, 1722·2
Oil of Olay, 2185·3
Oil of Vitriol, 1750·3
Oil of Wintergreen, 59·3
Oilalfo, 2185·3
Oilatum Preparations, 2185·3
Oil-Free Acne Wash, 2185·4
Oil-Free Active Sunscreen, 2185·4
Oil-Free Sunblock, 2185·4
Oil-Free Sunscreen, 2185·4
Oil-Free Sunspray, 2186·1
Oils, Sulfated, 1574·1
Ojensalve Neutral, 2186·1
Ojosbel, 2186·1
Ojosbel Azul, 2186·1
OK-432, 1731·3
Okacin, 2186·1
Okacyn, 2186·1
Okal, 2186·1
Okalcin, 2186·1
Okavax, 2186·1
Oki, 2186·1
Oklaricid, 2186·1
Okokit II, 2186·1
Okoubarell, 2186·1
Okoubasan, 2186·1
Oksibutin, 2186·1
OKT3, 1360·3
Okuzell, 2186·1
OKY-046, 1725·2
OL-27-400, 1351·2
OL-110, 1160·3
O-Lac, 2186·1
Oladin, 2186·1
Olaflur, 1442·3
Olam, 2186·1
Olamin, 2186·1
Olamin P, 2186·1
Ol-Amine, 2186·1
Olamyc, 2186·1
Olan-Gin, 2186·1
Olanzapina, 710·3
Olanzapine, 710·3
Olaquindox, 1723·1
Olbad Cordes, 2186·1
Olbad Cordes Comp, 2186·1
Olbad Cordes F, 2186·1
Olbas, 2186·2
Olbas for Children, 2186·2
Olbemox, 2186·2
Olbenorm, 2186·2
Olbetam, 2186·2
Ol-Bi, 2186·2
Olbiacor, 2186·2
Olcadil, 2186·2
Olcam, 2186·2
Old Louisiana Sport Capsicum, 1667·1
Old Tuberculin, 1759·1
Oldamin, 2186·2
Oldan, 2186·2
*Olea europaea*, 1723·2
Olea Herbaria, 1763·3
Oleander, 1723·1
Oleanderblätter, 1723·1
Oleandomicina, Fosfato de, 240·2
Oleandomycin Phosphate, 240·2
Oleandomycin, Triacetyl Ester, 274·1
Oleandri Folium, 1723·1
Oleandrin, 1723·1
Oleato de Etilo, 1685·2
Oleato de Monoetanolamina, 1716·1
Oleato de Sodio, 1574·3
Oleato de Sorbitán, 1416·1
Oleatum, 2186·2
Oleatum Bar, 2186·2
Oleatum Emollient, 2186·2
Oleatum Gel, 2186·2
Oleic Acid, 1481·3, 1707·3
Oleic Acid Glyceride, 1656·1
Oleico, Ácido, 1481·3
Oleicum, Acidum, 1481·3
Oleo Calcarea, 2186·2
Oléo de Algodoeiro, 1676·1
Oleo de Amêndoas, 1651·1
Óleo de Amendoim, 1656·1
Óleo de Bacalhau, 1425·2
Oleo de Primula, 2186·2
Oleo Dermosina Simples, 2186·2
Oleo Eletrico, 2186·3
Oleobal, 2186·3
Oleoban, 2186·3
Oleoban Composto, 2186·3
Oleoban Gel, 2186·3
Oleocal, 2186·3
Oleoderm, 2186·3
Oleoderm Plus, 2186·3
Oleo-Lax, 2186·3
Oleomycetin, 2186·3
Oleomycetin-Prednison, 2186·3
Oleosint, 2186·3
Oleosorbate, 2186·3
Oleovit, 2186·3
Oleovit A, 2186·3
Oleovit A + D, 2186·3
Oleovit A + $D_3$, 2186·3
Oleovit $D_3$, 2186·3
Oleovitamin A, 1451·2
2-Oleoyl-1-palmitoyl-*sn*-glycero(3)phospho(1)-*sn*-glycerol, 1736·2
Olestra, 1451·1
Olethytan 20, 1415·2
Oleum, 1750·3
Oleum Anethi, 1680·2
Oleum Anisi, 1655·2
Oleum Arachis, 1656·1
Oleum Aurantii Deterpenatum, 1724·2
Oleum Bergamottae, 1659·3
Oleum Betulae Albae, 1159·2
Oleum Betulae Empyreumaticum, 1159·2
Oleum Betulae Pyroligneum, 1159·2
Oleum Cacao, 1482·3
Oleum Cadinum, 1159·2
Oleum Cajuputi, 1664·1
Oleum Cari, 1667·3
Oleum Carui, 1667·3
Oleum Carvi, 1667·3
Oleum Caryophylli, 1673·3
Oleum Cassiae, 1668·2
Oleum Cinnamomi, 1668·2, 1672·2
Oleum Cinnamomi Cassiae, 1668·2
Oleum Citri, 1706·2
Oleum Citronellae, 1673·2
Oleum Cocois, 1481·1
Oleum Cocos Raffinatum, 1481·1
Oleum Cocosis, 1481·1
Oleum Coriandri, 1676·1
Oleum Crotonis, 28·2
Oleum Eucalypti, 1686·2
Oleum Foeniculi, 1687·3
Oleum Geranii, 1692·2
Oleum Gossypii Seminis, 1676·1
Oleum Graminis Citrati, 1706·3
Oleum Helianthi, 1451·1
Oleum Hippoglossi, 1434·1
Oleum Jecoris Aselli, 1425·2
Oleum Jecoris Hippoglossi, 1434·1
Oleum Juniperi, 1703·1
Oleum Juniperi Empyreumaticum, 1159·2
Oleum Lavandulae, 1705·2
Oleum Lavandulae Spicatae, 1749·2
Oleum Limonis, 1706·2
Oleum Limonis Deterpenatum, 1706·3
Oleum Lini, 1707·2
Oleum Lithanthracis, 1159·2
Oleum Maydis, 1439·2
Oleum Melaleucae, 1710·2
Oleum Menthae Crispae, 1749·1
Oleum Menthae Piperitae, 1283·2
Oleum Menthae Viridis, 1749·1
Oleum Morrhuae, 1425·2
Oleum Myrciae, 1659·1
Oleum Myristicae, 1722·3
Oleum Neroli, 1719·2
Oleum, Olivae, 1723·2
Oleum Papaveris, 1733·3
Oleum Papaveris Seminis, 1733·3
Oleum Persicorum, 1730·2
Oleum Petrolei, 1479·1
Oleum Pini Pumilionis, 1737·1
Oleum Rapae, 1737·3
Oleum Rhinale, 2186·3
Oleum Ricini, 1668·2
Oleum Ricini Sulphatum, 1575·3
Oleum Roris Marini, 1740·2
Oleum Rosae, 1740·2
Oleum Rosmarini, 1740·2
Oleum Rusci, 1159·2
Oleum Rutae, 1741·1
Oleum Sassafras, 1742·1
Oleum Sesami, 1743·3
Oleum Sinapis Volatile, 1718·2
Oleum Terebinthinae, 1760·1
Oleum Terebinthinae Depuratum, 1760·1
Oleum Theobromatis, 1482·3
Oleum Thymi, 1755·3
Oleum Tiglii, 28·2
Oleum Tropaeoli, 1659·3
Oleum Vaselini, 1479·1
Olexa, 2186·3
Olexin, 2186·3
Oleyl Acetate, 1481·3
Oleyl Alcohol, 1481·3
Olf, 2186·3
Olfen, 2186·3
Olfex, 2186·3
Olfosonide, 2186·3
Olibanum, 1690·1
Olibanum RA, 2186·3
Olicard, 2186·3
Olicardin, 2186·4
Olicide, 2186·4
Oliclinomel, 2186·4
Olidermil, 2186·4
Oligobs, 2186·4
Oligocean, 2186·4
Oligocean Minceur, 2186·4
Oligocean Xtra, 2186·4
Oligocomplesso, 2186·4
Oligocure, 2186·4
Oligoderm, 2186·4
Oligoelementos, 2186·4
Oligo-elements Aguettant, 2186·4
Oligo-Essentials, 2186·4
Oligofer, 2186·4
Oligoforme, 2186·4
Oligogranul, 2186·4
Oligomenorrhoea— *see* Amenorrhoea, 1313·1
Oligophytum, 2186·4
Oligoplex, 2186·4
Oligorhine, 2186·4
Oligosaccharides, 1417·1
Oligosol, 2186·4
Oligossac, 2186·4
Oligostim, 2186·4
Oligo-Yang, 2186·4
Olimag, 2186·4
Olio di Fegato di Merluzzo, 1425·2
Olio di Mandorla, 1651·1
Olio di Mugo, 1737·1
OlioClinomel, 2186·4

Olivae Oleum, 1723·2
Olivae Oleum Raffinatum, 1723·2
Olivae Oleum Virginale, 1723·2
Olive Leaf, 1723·2
Olive Oil, 1723·2
Olive Oil, Refined, 1723·2
Olive Oil, Virgin, 1723·2
Oliveira Junior, Xarope Grindelia de— *see* Xarope Grindelia de Oliveira Junior, 2387·4
Oliviase, 2186·4
Olivysat, 2186·4
Olmesartan Medoxomil, 975·3
Olmetec, 2186·4
Olmifon, 2186·4
Olmo Resbaladizo, 1747·1
Olmoran, 2186·4
Olocynan, 2187·1
Ologyn, 2187·1
Olohepat, 2187·1
Ololiuqui, 1723·2
Olopatadina, Hidrocloruro de, 438·1
Olopatadine Hydrochloride, 438·1
Oloprim, 2187·1
Olprinona, Hidrocloruro de, 976·1
Olprinone Hydrochloride, 976·1
Olren N, 2187·1
Olsalazina Sódica, 1278·1
Olsalazine Sodium, 1278·1
Olsalazinum Natricum, 1278·1
Ölsäure, 1481·3
Oltens, 2187·1
Olter, 2187·1
Olux, 2187·1
Olympic Balm, 2187·1
Olynth, 2187·1
Olynth Erkaltungsbalsam, 2187·1
Olynth Kombi, 2187·1
Olynth Salin, 2187·1
Olyspal, 2187·1
Olyster, 2187·1
OM-518, 1395·1
Omacor, 2187·1
Omadine, 2187·1
Omaflaxina, 2187·1
Omalizumab, 790·1
Omapatrilat, 964·2, 976·1
Omapatrilato, 976·1
Omapren, 2187·1
Omatropina Bromidrato, 483·2
Ombolan, 2187·1
Ombravist, 2187·1
Ombrelle Preparations, 2187·1
Omca, 2187·2
Omcilon A, 2187·2
Omcilon A M, 2187·2
Omcilon A Orabase, 2187·2
Om-Dicynone, 2187·2
OMDS, 1146·1
Omebeta, 2187·2
Omega, 2187·2
Omega-3, 2187·2
Omega-3 Acid Ethyl Esters, 976·2
Omega-3 Acidorum Esteri Ethylici, 976·2
Omega-3 Acidorum Triglycerida, 976·2
Omega-3 Marine Triglycerides, 976·2
Omega-3 Triglycerides, 976·1
Omega-3-acid Ethyl Esters, 976·2
Omega-3-Acid Ethyl Esters 60, 976·2
Omega-3-Acid Ethyl Esters 90, 976·2
Omega-3-Acid Triglycerides, 976·2
Omega-3-Acids, Fish Oil, Rich in, 976·2
Omega 3+, 2187·2
Omega 7, 2187·2
Omega 100, 2187·2
Omega 100 Bronquial, 2187·2
Omega 100 L, 2187·2
Omegacoeur, 2187·2
Omega-H3, 2187·2
Omegaline, 2187·2
Omegaven, 2187·2
Omelind, 2187·2
Ome-nerton, 2187·2
Omep, 2187·2
Omepra, 2187·2
Omepradex, 2187·2
Omepral, 2187·2
Omeprasec, 2187·3
Omeprax, 2187·3
Omeprazen, 2187·3
Omeprazin, 2187·3
Omeprazol, 1278·2
Omeprazol Magnésico, 1278·2
Omeprazol Sódico, 1278·2
Omeprazole, 1278·2
Omeprazole Magnesium, 1278·2
Omeprazole Sodium, 1278·2
Omeprazole Sulfone, 1280·1
Omeprazolum, 1278·2
Omeprazolum Natricum, 1278·2
Omeprol, 2187·3
Omeprotec, 2187·3
Ome-Puren, 2187·3
Omerol, 2187·3
Omesan, 2187·3
Omesec, 2187·3
Ometon, 2187·3
Omez, 2187·3
Omezol, 2187·3
Omezolan, 2187·3
Omezole, 2187·3
Omic, 2187·3
Omicite, 2187·3
Omida Gel Antirhumatismal, 2187·3
Omida Granules Relaxants, 2187·3
Omida Spray Nasal, 2187·3
Omifin, 2187·3
Omilcal, 2187·3
Omilipis, 2187·3
Ominol, 2187·3
Omix, 2187·3
Ommunal, 2187·3
Omnalio, 2187·3
Omnatax, 2187·3
Omneo, 2187·4
Omnia, 2187·4
Omnia T, 2187·4
Omniadol, 2187·4
Omniapharm, 2187·4
Omnibionta, 2187·4
Omnibionta Integral, 2187·4
Omnic, 2187·4
Omnic— *see* Flomax, 2000·2
Omnicare, 2187·4
Omnicare Daily Cleaner, 2187·4
Omnicare 1 Step, 2187·4
Omnicef, 2187·4
Omniderm, 2187·4
Omniflora, 2187·4
Omniflora Akut, 2187·4
Omniflora N, 2187·4
Omnigeriat, 2187·4
Omnigraf, 2187·4
OmniHIB, 2187·4
Omnihist LA, 2187·4
Omnipaque, 2187·4
Omnipen, 2187·4
Omnipen-N, 2187·4
Omniplex, 2187·4
Omniscan, 2187·4
Omnisept, 2188·1
Omnitest, 2188·1
Omnitrace, 2188·1
Omnitrast, 2188·1
Omni-Tuss, 2188·1
Omnival, 2188·1
Omnopon, 2188·1
Omnoponum, 74·3
Omoconazol, Nitrato de, 407·2
Omoconazole Nitrate, 407·2
OMP, 2188·1
Ompranyt, 2188·1
Omr-IgG, 2188·1
Omri-Hep-B, 2188·1
Omrixate, 2188·1
OMS-1, 1507·1
OMS-14, 1503·2
OMS-29, 1501·2
OMS-658, 1501·1
OMS-1825, 1500·2
OMS-2000, 1505·2
OMS-3047, 1505·3
OMS Concentrate, 2188·1
Omsk Haemorrhagic Fever— *see* Haemorrhagic Fevers, 618·2
Omycet, 2188·1
Onagra, Aceite de, 1686·3
Onagre, 2188·1
Onaka, 2188·1
Onapan, 2188·1
Oncaspar, 2188·1
Once A Day, Improved— *see* Improved Once A Day, 2058·4
Once A Day, Super— *see* Super Once A Day, 2313·3
Once-a-Day, 2188·1
Oncet, 2188·1
Onchocerciasis, 100·2
Onciplus, 2188·1
Onclast, 2188·1
Onco Tiotepa, 2188·1
Oncocarb, 2188·1
Onco-Carbide, 2188·1
Oncocarbil, 2188·1
Onco-Cloramin, 2188·1
Oncofu, 2188·1
Oncosal, 2188·1
OncoScint, 2188·1
OncoScint CR 103, 2188·1
OncoScint CR/OV, 2188·2
OncoSeeds, 2188·2
Oncotam, 2188·2
Oncotaxina, 2188·2
OncoTICE, 2188·2
Oncotron, 2188·2
Oncovin, 2188·2
Oncovite, 2188·2
Onctose, 2188·2
Onctose a l'Hydrocortisone, 2188·2
Onctose Hydrocortisone, 2188·2
Ondansetron, 1281·1
Ondansetrón, Hidrocloruro de, 1281·1
Ondansetron Hydrochloride, 1281·1
Ondansetron Hydrochloride Dihydrate, 1281·1
Ondansetroni Hydrochloridum, 1281·1
Ondax, 2188·2
Ondolen, 2188·2
Ondroly-A, 2188·2
Ondrox, 2188·2
One, 2188·2
One A Day, 2188·2
One Step, 2188·2
One Touch, 2188·2
One-a-Day Antihistamine— *see* Boots Hayfever Relief Antihistamine, 1851·1
Onealfa, 2188·2
One-Alpha, 2188·2
Onefin, 2188·2
Onelacne, 2188·2
Onemer, 2188·2
One-Tablet-Daily, 2188·2
Onfor, 2188·2
Onglinex, 2188·3
Onguent Hemorrhoidal, 2188·3
Onguent Nasal Ruedi, 2188·3
Onico Fitex, 2188·3
Onion, 1723·2
Onixol, 2188·3
Oniz, 2188·3
Onkocristin, 2188·3
Onkofluor, 2188·3
Onkomorphin, 2188·3
Onkoposid, 2188·3
Onkotrone, 2188·3
Onkovertin, 2188·3
Onkovertin N, 2188·3
Only One, 2188·3
ONO-802, 1518·1
ONO-1078, 791·1
ONO-1101, 945·1
ONO-1206, 1519·2
ONO-2235, 331·1
ONO-5046, 1746·3
Onoact, 2188·3
Onofin-K, 2188·3
Onon, 2188·3
Ononidis Radix, 1723·3
Ononis, 1723·3
*Ononis spinosa*, 1723·3
Onopordon Comp B, 2188·3
Onoprose, 2188·3
Onoton, 2188·3
Onrectal, 2188·3
Onsia, 2188·3
Onsudil, 2188·3
Onsukil, 2188·3
Ontak, 2188·3
Ontop, 2188·3
Ontosein, 2188·3
Ontrax, 2188·3
Onxol, 2188·3
Onycho Phytex, 2188·4
Onychomal, 2188·4
Onychomycoses— *see* Skin Infections, 390·1
Ony-Clear, 2188·4
OP-1, 768·2
OP-21-23, 978·3
OP-370, 892·2
OP-1206, 1519·2
Opacist ER, 2188·4
Opacite, 2188·4
Opalgyne, 2188·4
Opalia, 2188·4
Opalino, 2188·4
Opalmon, 2188·4
Opam, 2188·4
Opamox, 2188·4
Oparsan con Lisina y L-Glutamina, 2188·4
Opas, 2188·4
Opatanol, 2188·4
Opazimes, 2188·4
OPC-21, 884·1
OPC-31, 671·1
OPC-1085, 880·3
OPC-2009, 791·1
OPC-7251, 233·3
OPC-8212, 1022·1
OPC-13013, 884·1
OPC-14597, 671·1
OPC-17116, 220·3
Opcon-A, 2188·4
Opebacan, 1658·3
Operand, 2188·4
Operium, 2188·4
Ophan, 2188·4
Ophcillin N, 2188·4
Ophdilvas N, 2188·4
Ophidus, 2188·4
Ophtacalm, 2188·4
Ophtadil, 2188·4
Ophtagram, 2188·4
Ophtaguttal, 2188·4
Ophtal, 2189·1
Ophtalin, 2189·1
Ophtalmin, 2189·1
Ophtalmin N, 2189·1
Ophtalmine, 2189·1
Ophtalmotrim, 2189·1
Ophtamedine, 2189·1
Ophtasiloxane, 2189·1
Ophtasone, 2189·1
Ophtaxia, 2189·1
Ophthalgan, 2189·1
Ophthalin, 2189·1
Ophthalmia Neonatorum— *see* Neonatal Conjunctivitis, 136·3
Ophthalmopathy, Graves'— *see* Hyperthyroidism, 1594·3
Ophthetic, 2189·1
Ophthifluor, 2189·1
Ophtho-Bunolol, 2189·1
Ophtho-Chloram, 2189·1
Ophthocort, 2189·1
Ophtho-Sulf, 2189·1
Ophtho-Tate, 2189·1
Ophtilan, 2189·1
Ophtim, 2189·1
Ophtocain N, 2189·1
Ophtol-A, 2189·1
Ophtopur-N, 2189·1
Ophtopur-Z, 2189·1
Ophtosan, 2189·1

Ophtrivin-A, 2189·1
Opialum, 74·3
Opiate Analgesics, 1·3
Opidina, 2189·1
Opidol, 2189·1
Opii, Extractum Concentratum, 74·3
Opii Hydrochloridum, Alkaloidorum, 74·3
Opii Pulvis Normatus, 74·2
Opilet, 2189·2
Opilon, 2189·2
Opino, 2189·2
Opino N, 2189·2
Opino N Spezial, 2189·2
Opio, 74·2
Opioid Analgesics, 1·3, 71·2
Opioid Dependence— *see* Treatment of Opioid Dependence, 71·2
Opioid Dependence, Neonatal— *see* Neonatal Abstinence Syndrome, 72·1
Opioid Detoxification.— *see* Treatment of Opioid Dependence, 71·2
Opioid Peptides, 73·2
Opioid Receptors, 73·3
Opioid Withdrawal Syndrome— *see* Treatment of Opioid Dependence, 71·2
Opioid Withdrawal Syndrome, Neonatal— *see* Neonatal Abstinence Syndrome, 72·1
Opipramol, Hidrocloruro de, 311·1
Opipramol Hydrochloride, 311·1
Opiren, 2189·2
Opisthorchiasis— *see* Liver Fluke Infections, 99·3
Opium, 74·2, 74·3
Opium Alkaloids, Mixed, Hydrochlorides of, 74·3
Opium Concentratum, 74·3
Opium Crudum, 74·2
Opium, Gum, 74·2
Opium, Powdered, 74·3
Opium, Prepared, 74·2
Opium, Raw, 74·2
O-Plat, 2189·2
Opliphon, 2189·2
Opnol, 2189·2
Opobyl, 2189·2
Opobyl-phyto, 2189·2
Opocarbon, 2189·2
Opocler, 2189·2
Opoenterol, 2189·2
Oponaf, 2189·2
Opoplex, 2189·2
Opo-Veinogene, 2189·2
Opovital B12, 2189·2
Opplin, 2189·2
Opportunistic Mycobacterial Infections, 137·2
Oprad, 2189·2
Opragen, 2189·2
Oprazole, 2189·2
Oprazon, 2189·2
Opredsone, 2189·2
Oprelvekin, 757·1
Oprelvekina, 757·1
Opren, 21·1
Opridan, 2189·2
Oprimol, 2189·3
O'Prin, 2189·3
Oprisine, 2189·3
Opsacin, 2189·3
Opsa-His, 2189·3
Opsar, 2189·3
Opsaram, 2189·3
Opsardex, 2189·3
Opsil, 2189·3
Opsil Tears, 2189·3
Opsil-A, 2189·3
Opsite, 2189·3
Opsonat, 2189·3
Optacilin, 2189·3
Optacilin Balsamico, 2189·3
Optafen, 2189·3
Optaflan, 2189·3
Optal, 2189·3
Optalgin, 2189·3
Optalia, 2189·3
Optalidon, 2189·3
Optalidon a la Noramidopyrine, 2189·3
Optalidon N, 2189·3
Optalidon Special NOC, 2189·3
Optamid, 2189·3
Optamide, 2189·3
Optamine, 2189·4
Optamox, 2189·4
Optasid, 2189·4
Optavite, 2189·4
Optazine, 2189·4
Optazine Fresh, 2189·4
Optazol, 2189·4
Opteron, 2189·4
Opthaflox, 2189·4
Opthavir, 2189·4
Optibiol, 2189·4
Optic Atrophy, Leber's, 1459·1
Optical, 2189·4
Optical mit Eisen, 2189·4
Opticare PMS, 2189·4
Opticef, 2189·4
Opticide, 2189·4
Opti-Clean, 2189·4
Opti-Clean II, 2189·4
Opticrom, 2189·4
Opticron, 2189·4
Opticyl, 2189·4
Optidase, 1668·3
Optiderm, 2189·4
Optiderme, 2189·4
Optidorm, 2189·4
Optifast VLCD, 2189·4
Optifen, 2190·1
Optifluor, 2190·1
Opti-Free Preparations, 2190·1
Optigen, 2190·1
Optigene, 2190·1
Optigene 3, 2190·1
Opti-Genta, 2190·1
Optiject, 2190·1
Optil, 2190·1
Optilac, 2190·1
Optilast, 2190·1
Optilax, 2190·1
Optilets, 2190·1
Optilets-M, 2190·1
Optilube, 2190·1
Optilube PVA, 2190·1
Optima, 2190·1
Optima 50 Plus, 2190·1
Opti-Mag, 2190·1
Optimal, 2190·1
Optimark, 2190·1
Optimax, 2190·1
Optimin, 2190·2
Optimina + Ginseng Con Vit, 2190·2
Optimina Plus, 2190·2
Optimine, 2190·2
Optimoist, 2190·2
Optimol, 2190·2
Optimyxin, 2190·2
Optimyxin Plus, 2190·2
Optinate, 2190·2
Optinem, 2190·2
Optineuron, 2190·2
Optipect, 2190·2
Optipect Kodein, 2190·2
Optipect N, 2190·2
Optipect Neo, 2190·2
Opti-Plus, 2190·2
OptiPranolol, 2190·2
Optipres, 2190·2
Optipyrin, 2190·2
Optiray, 2190·2
Optisedine, 2190·2
Optisen, 2190·2
Opti-Soak, 2190·2
Opti-Soft, 2190·3
Optisol, 2190·3
Optison, 2190·3
Opti-Tears, 2190·3
Optium, 2190·3
Opti-Up, 2190·3
Optivar, 2190·3
Optivit, 2190·3
Optivite PMT, 2190·3
Optizoline, 2190·3
Optizor, 2190·3
Opti-Zyme, 2190·3
Optobet, 2190·3
Optocain, 2190·3
Optochinidin Retard, 2190·3
Optocillin, 2190·3
Optocor, 2190·3
Optomicin, 2190·3
Optovit, 2190·3
Optovit E, 2190·3
Optovite B12, 2190·3
Optrelam, 2190·3
Optrex Preparations, 2190·3
Optrex Eye Dew— *see* Eye Dew, 1986·4
Optrol, 2190·4
Optruma, 2190·4
Optryl, 2190·4
Opturem, 2190·4
OPV, 1634·1, 2190·4
OPV-Merieux, 2190·4
OR-611, 1205·1
(−)-OR-1259, 946·2
Ora, 2190·4
ORA5, 2190·4
Orabase Preparations, 2190·4
Orabet, 2190·4
Orabiot UD, 2190·4
Oracef, 2190·4
Oracefal, 2190·4
Oracilin, 2190·4
Oracilline, 2190·4
Oracit, 2190·4
Oracort, 2190·4
Oracort E, 2190·4
Oracyclin, 2190·4
Oraday, 2190·4
Oradex, 2190·4
Oradexon, 2190·4
Oradroxil, 2191·1
Oradyne-Z, 2191·1
Orafen, 2191·1
Orafer Comp, 2191·1
Oragalin Espasmolitico, 2191·1
Ora-Gallin, 2191·1
Ora-Gallin Compositum, 2191·1
Ora-Gallin Purum, 2191·1
Oragallin S, 2191·1
Oragard, 2191·1
Oragard Baby, 2191·1
Oragesic, 2191·1
Orageston, 2191·1
Oragrafin, 2191·1
Orahesive, 2191·1
Oraica, 2191·1
Orajel Preparations, 2191·1
Orajel, Baby— *see* Baby Orajel, 1824·2
Orajel Tooth and Gum Cleanser, Baby— *see* Baby Orajel Tooth and Gum Cleanser, 1824·2
Orakef, 2191·1
Orakit, 2191·2
Oral Cancer— *see* Malignant Neoplasms of the Head and Neck, 517·3
Oral Contraceptives, 1527·3
Oral Impact, 2191·2
Oral Plan, 2191·2
Oral Rehidr Sal Farmasur, 2191·2
Oral Rehydration Solutions, 1222·2
Oral Rehydration Therapy, 1222·3
Oral Spray, 2191·2
Oral Ulceration— *see* Mouth Ulceration, 1245·1
Oral-Aid, 2191·2
Oralav, 2191·2
Oral-B Preparations, 2191·2
Oralbalance, 2191·2
Oralbiotico, 2191·2
Oralcef, 2191·2
Oralcer, 2191·2
Oralcon, 2191·2
Oralcrom, 2191·2
Oraldene, 2191·2
Oraldine, 2191·2
Oralesper, 2191·2
Oralfene, 2191·2
Oralgan, 2191·2
Oralgan Codeine— *see* Klipal Codeine, 2080·3
Oralgar, 2191·2
Oralgen, 2191·2
Oralgene, 2191·3
Oralife Peppermint, 2191·3
Oralipin, 2191·3
Oral-K, 2191·3
Oralmox, 2191·3
Oralmuv, 2191·3
Oralone Dental, 2191·3
Oralovite, 2191·3
Oralpadon, 2191·3
Oralsan, 2191·3
Oralsone, 2191·3
Oralsone B C— *see* Aftasone B C, 1779·3
Oralsone C, 2191·3
Oralsone Topic, 2191·3
Oralspray, 2191·3
Oral-T, 2191·3
Oralten Troche, 2191·3
Oralube, 2191·3
Oralvac, 2191·3
Oral-Virelon, 2191·3
Oramec— *see* Mectizan, 2118·1
Oramedy, 2191·3
Oramet, 2191·3
Oramil, 2191·3
Oraminax, 2191·3
Oraminic II, 2191·3
Oramorph, 2191·3
Oramox, 2191·3
Orange Crush, 530·2
Orange, Essence of, 1724·1
Orange Flower Oil, 1719·2
Orange Flower Oil, Bitter, 1719·2
Orange Mullein, 1764·1
Orange Oil, 1724·1
Orange Oil, California-type, 1724·1
Orange Oil, Florida-type, 1724·1
Orange Oil, Sweet, 1724·1
Orange Oil, Terpeneless, 1724·2
Orange Peel, Sweet, 1724·1
Orangé S, Jaune, 1058·2
Orange Shellac, 1743·3
Orange, Sweet, 1724·1
Orange Yellow S, 1058·2
Orange-flower Oil, 1719·2
Orangel, 2191·3
Oranol, 2191·4
Oranor, 2191·4
Orap, 2191·4
Oraphen-PD, 2191·4
Orapred, 2191·4
Orascan, 2191·4
Ora-Sed, 2191·4
Ora-Sed Jel, 2191·4
Orasept, 2191·4
Oraseptate, Scope with— *see* Scope, 2280·1
Oraseptic, 2191·4
Oraseptic Gola, 2191·4
Orasol, 2191·4
Orasorbil, 2191·4
Orastel, 2191·4
Orasthin, 2191·4
Orastina, 2191·4
Oratane, 2191·4
Oratol, 2191·4
Oratol F, 2191·4
Oratrol, 2191·4
Oravil, 2191·4
Oravir, 2191·4
Oraxim, 2191·4
Orazamida, 1724·2
Orazamide, 1724·2
Orazinc, 2191·4
Orbenil, 2192·1
Orbenin, 2192·1
Orbenine, 2192·1
Orbifen, 2192·1
Orbifloxacin, 240·2
Orbifloxacino, 240·2
Orbofiban Acetate, 977·2
Orbofibrán, Acetato de, 977·2
Orcel, 2192·1

Orchibion, 2192·1
Orcilone, 2192·1
Orcinol, 2192·1
Orciprenalina, Sulfato de, 790·2
Orciprenaline Sulfate, 790·2
Orciprenaline Sulphate, 790·2
Orciprenalini Sulfas, 790·2
Orcl, 2192·1
Orclor, 2192·1
Ordeal Bean, 1494·1
Ordiflazine, 946·3
Ordinal Forte, 2192·1
Ordine, 2192·1
Ordov Preparations, 2192·1
Ordrine AT Extended-Release, 2192·1
Oreda, 2192·1
Oregovomab, 577·1
Orellanine, 1717·3
Orelox, 2192·1
Oretic, 2192·1
Oreton Methyl, 2192·1
Orexin, 2192·1
ORF-10131, 1563·2
ORF-11676, 1044·1
ORF-15817, 632·1
ORF-17070, 1329·3
ORF-22164, 1319·1
Orfarin, 2192·1
Orfen, 2192·2
Orfenace, 2192·2
Orfenadrina, Citrato de, 486·1
Orfenadrina, Hidrocloruro de, 486·1
Orfenal, 2192·2
Orfidal, 2192·2
Orfidora, 2192·2
Orfilept— *see* Orfiril, 2192·2
Orfiril, 2192·2
Orflex, 2192·2
Org-538, 1570·1
Org-2766, 538·3
Org-2969, 1547·2
Org-3236, 1554·1
Org-3770, 307·3
Org-5730, 868·1
Org-6216, 1110·1
Org-9426, 1405·2
Org-9487, 1405·2
Org-10172, 891·2
Org-31338, 1330·1
Org-31540, 918·3
Org-32489, 1324·2
Org-37462, 1325·1
Org 33062, 701·1
Orgalutran, 2192·2
Orgametril, 2192·2
Organ and Tissue Transplantation, 1344·2
Organex, 2192·2
Organic Mineral, Bioglan— *see* Bioglan Organic Mineral, 1844·1
Organic Solvents, 1471·1
Organidin NR, 2192·2
Organochlorine Insecticides, 1501·3
Organoneuro Cerebral, 2192·2
Organoneuro Optico, 2192·2
Organophosphate Insecticides, 1507·3
Organophosphorus Insecticides, 1507·3
Orgaplasma, 2192·2
Orgaran, 2192·2
Orgasuline 30/70, 2192·2
Orgasuline NPH, 2192·2
Orgasuline Rapide, 2192·2
Orgestriol, 2192·2
Org-GB-94, 306·3
Org-NA-97, 1404·3
Org-NC-45, 1409·3
Org-OD-14, 1572·3
Orgotein, 92·2
Orgoteína, 92·2
Orgran, 2192·2
Oribiox, 2192·2
Oributol, 2192·2
Oricant, 2192·2
Oricitral, 2192·2
Oriconazole, 401·3
Oricyclin, 2192·2
Oricyclin— *see* Helipak T, 2038·2
Oriens, 2192·2
Oriental Spotted Fever— *see* Spotted Fevers, 147·1
Orifer F, 2192·3
Orifungal, 2192·3
Original, 2192·3
Original Alka-Seltzer Effervescent Tablets, 2192·3
Original Cabdrivers Expectorant, 2192·3
Original Schneckensirup, 2192·3
Original Sensodyne, 2192·3
Original-Tinktur N Truw, 2192·3
Origlucon, 2192·3
Orimeten, 2192·3
Orimetene, 2192·3
Orimune, 2192·3
Orinase, 2192·3
Orinase Diagnostic, 2192·3
Oriprim, 2192·3
Oris, 2192·3
Oritavancin, 240·2
Oritavancin Phosphate, 240·2
Oritaxim, 2192·3
Oritaxime, 2192·3
Orivan, 2192·3
Orivir, 2192·3
Orizaba Jalap Root, 1267·3
Orizanol, 1725·1
OrLAAM, 2192·3
Orlamix, 2192·3
Orla-Wax, 2192·3
Orlaxyl, 2192·3
Orlept, 2192·3
Orlipastat, 1724·2
Orlistat, 1724·2
Orlobin, 2192·3
Orloc, 2192·3
Orlon, 2192·3
Ormeloxifene, 1564·3
Ormeloxifeno, 1564·3
Ormetein, 92·2
Ormetoprim, 240·2
Ormetoprima, 240·2
Ormigrein, 2192·3
Ormir, 2192·4
Ormobyl CM, 2192·4
Ormodon, 2192·4
Ormox, 2192·4
Ornade, 2192·4
Ornade Expectorant, 2192·4
Ornade-DM, 2192·4
Ornatrol, 2192·4
Ornex, 2192·4
Ornex, Maximum Strength— *see* Maximum Strength Ornex, 2116·4
Ornicetil, 2192·4
Ornicetil S, 2192·4
Ornidazol, 612·2
Ornidazole, 612·2
Ornidyl, 2192·4
Ornihepat, 2192·4
Ornil, 2192·4
Ornil KGF, 2192·4
Ornipresina, 1335·3
Ornipressin, 1335·3
Ornitaine, 2192·4
Ornitargin, 2192·4
Ornithine, 1442·3
L-Ornithine, 1442·3
Ornithine Aspartate, 1442·3
Ornithine Hydrochloride, 1442·3
Ornithine Ketoglutarate, 1442·3
Ornithine Oxoglurate, 1442·3
Ornithine-α-ketoglutarate, 1433·3
[8-Ornithine]-vasopressin, 1335·3
Ornithosis— *see* Psittacosis, 143·2
Ornitina, 1442·3
Ornoprostil, 1520·3
Ornoprostilo, 1520·3
Oro, 1695·3
Oro 198, 1523·3
Oro B12, 2192·4
Oroacid, 2192·4
Orobicin, 2192·4
Orobiotic, 2192·4
Orocaine, 2192·4
Orocal, 2193·1
Orocal $D_3$, 2193·1
Orochlor, 2193·1
Orochol, 2193·1
Orocholin, 2193·1
Orocil, 2193·1
Oro-Clense, 2193·1
Or-O-Derm, 2193·1
Orodina, 2193·1
Orofacial Pain, 7·2
Orofar, 2193·1
Orofar Lidocaine, 2193·1
Orofen, 2193·1
Orofluor, 2193·1
Orofungin, 2193·1
Oroken, 2193·1
Oromag, 2193·1
Oromedine, 2193·1
Oromone, 2193·1
Oro-NaF, 2193·1
Oropharyngeal Candidiasis— *see* Candidiasis, 386·3
Oropharyngeal Carcinoma— *see* Malignant Neoplasms of the Head and Neck, 517·3
Oro-Pivalone, 2193·1
Oropivalone Bacitracine, 2193·1
Oropur, 2193·1
Ororhinathiol, 2193·1
Orosanyl, 2193·1
Orosept, 2193·1
Oroseptol Lysozyme, 2193·2
Orostat, 2193·2
Orostick, 2193·2
Orotic Acid, 1724·3
Orótico, Ácido, 1724·3
Orotre, 2193·2
Orotrix, 2193·2
Orovite, 2193·2
Orovite '7', 2193·2
Orovite Comploment $B_6$, 2193·2
Oroxadin, 2193·2
Oroxamide, 1724·2
Oroxine, 2193·2
Orozuz, 1270·2
Orpar, 2193·2
Orpec, 2193·2
Orphenadin Citrate, 486·1
Orphenadin Hydrochloride, 486·1
Orphenadol, 2193·2
Orphenadrine Citrate, 486·1
Orphenadrine Hydrochloride, 486·1
Orphenadrini Citras, 486·1
Orphenadrini Hydrochloridum, 486·1
Orphengesic, 2193·2
Orphipal, 2193·2
Orphol, 2193·2
Orpidix, 2193·2
Orravina, 2193·2
Orrepaste, 2193·2
ORS Bicarbonate, 2193·2
Orsanil, 2193·2
Orset, 2193·2
Orsinon, 2193·2
Orstanorm, 2193·2
Ortenal, 2193·2
Ortensan, 2193·2
Orthangin N, 2193·2
Orthangin Novo, 2193·2
Ortho, 2193·3
Ortho 0.5/35, 2193·3
Ortho 1/35, 2193·3
Ortho 7/7/7, 2193·3
Ortho 10/11, 2193·3
Ortho Cyclen, 2193·3
Ortho Evra, 2193·3
Ortho Gynest Depot, 2193·3
Ortho Gyne-T, 2193·3
Ortho Micronor, 2193·3
Ortho Shields, 2193·3
Ortho Tri-Cyclen, 2193·3
Orthoboric Acid, 1662·1
Orthocardon-N, 2193·3
Ortho-Cept, 2193·3
Orthoclone OKT3, 2193·3
Ortho-Creme, 2193·3
Orthodichlorobenzene, 1724·3
Ortho-Dienestrol, 2193·3
Ortho-Dienoestrol, 2193·3
Ortho-Est, 2193·3
Orthoforms, 2193·3
Ortho-Gel, 2193·3
Ortho-Gynest, 2193·3
Ortho-Gynol, 2193·3
Ortho-Gynol II, 2193·3
Ortholan mit Salicylester, 2193·3
Ortho-Maren Retard, 2193·4
Orthon, 2193·4
Orthonett Novum, 2193·4
Ortho-Novin, 2193·4
Ortho-Novum Preparations, 2193·4
Orthophenylphenol, 1187·2
Orthophosphoric Acid, 1731·2
Orthoplex SAD, 2193·4
Ortho-Prefest— *see* Prefest, 2231·4
*Orthosiphon aristatus*, 1702·3
*Orthosiphon spicatus*, 1702·3
*Orthosiphon stamineus*, 1702·3
Orthosiphonblätter, 1702·3
Orthosiphonblatter Indischer Nierentee, 2193·4
Orthosiphonis Folium, 1702·3
Orthostatic Hypotension, 1100·2
Orthovisc, 2193·4
OrthoWash, 2193·4
Orthoxicol Preparations, 2193·4
Orti B, 2194·1
Ortic C, 2194·1
Ortiga, 1762·1
Ortisan, 2194·1
Ortitruw, 2194·1
Orti-Vite, Super— *see* Super Orti-Vite, 2313·3
Orto Dermo P, 2194·1
Orto Nasal, 2194·1
Ortociclina, 2194·1
Ortocilin, 2194·1
Ortodermina, 2194·1
Ortodiclorobenceno, 1724·3
Ortofenilfenol, 1187·2
Ortoflan, 2194·1
Ortopsique, 2194·1
Ortoserpina, 2194·1
Ortosifón, 1702·3
Ortosol P, 2194·1
Ortoton, 2194·1
Ortoton Plus, 2194·1
Ortovermin, 2194·1
Ortóxibenzoico, Acido, 1157·1
Ortoxine, 2194·1
Ortran, 2194·1
Ortrip, 2194·1
Ortrizol, 2194·1
Or-Tyl, 2194·1
Orucote, 2194·1
Orudis, 2194·1
Orugesic, 2194·1
Oruject, 2194·1
Orulop, 2194·1
Oruvail, 2194·1
*Oryza sativa*, 1449·1
Oryzae Amylum, 1449·1
Oryzanol, 1725·1
γ-Oryzanol, 1725·1
Os, Aar— *see* Aar Os, 1767·3
Osa, 2194·2
Osa Gel de Dentition aux Plantes, 2194·2
Osaline, 2194·2
Osalmid, 1725·1
Osalmida, 1725·1
Osangin, 2194·2
Osanit, 2194·2
Osarsolum, 600·2
Osaten, 2194·2
Os-Cal, 2194·2
Oscal, 2194·2
Os-Cal D, 2194·2
Oscal D, 2194·2
Os-Cal + D, 2194·2
Os-Cal Forte, 2194·2
Os-Cal Fortified, 2194·2
Os-Cal Plus, 2194·2

Oscalcio, 2194·2
Oscevitin-A, 2194·2
Oscillococcinum, 2194·2
Oscorel, 2194·2
Osdron, 2194·2
Oseille, 1749·1
Oseltamivir Carboxylate, 651·1
Oseltamivir, Fosfato de, 651·1
Oseltamivir Phosphate, 651·1
Osemin, 2194·2
Oseotal, 2194·2
Oseototal, 2194·2
Oseum, 2194·2
Osfolate, 2194·2
Osfolato, 2194·2
O-Sid, 2194·2
Osigraft, 2194·2
Osiren, 2194·2
Osmil, 2194·3
Osmitrol, 2194·3
Osmo, 2194·3
Osmo-Adalat, 2194·3
Osmofundin 10%, 2194·3
Osmofundin 20%, 2194·3
Osmofundin 15% N, 2194·3
Osmofundina, 2194·3
Osmofundina Concentrada, 2194·3
Osmogel, 2194·3
Osmogenol, 2194·3
Osmoglyn, 2194·3
Osmohes, 2194·3
Osmolac, 2194·3
Osmoleine, 2194·3
Osmolite, 2194·3
Osmolite HN, 2194·3
Osmopak-Plus, 2194·3
Osmoran, 2194·3
Osmorich, 2194·3
Osmorol, 2194·3
Osmosal, 2194·3
Osmosteril 10%, 2194·4
Osmosteril 20%, 2194·4
Osmotan G, 2194·4
Osmotic Demyelination— *see* Hyponatraemia, 1220·3
Osmotic Diuretics, 811·2
Osmotic Laxatives, 1239·3
Osmotil, 2194·4
Osmotol, 2194·4
Osmovist, 2194·4
Osnervan, 2194·4
Ospamox, 2194·4
Ospamox— *see* Klacid HP 7, 2080·1
Ospen, 2194·4
Ospen KV, 2194·4
Ospexin, 2194·4
Ospocard, 2194·4
Ospolot, 2194·4
Ospor, 2194·4
Osporin, 2194·4
Ospronim, 2194·4
Ospur Ca, 2194·4
Ospur $D_3$, 2194·4
Ospur F, 2194·4
Osra, 2194·4
Osseans D3, 2194·4
Osseocalcina, 2194·4
Ossidal, 2194·4
Ossification, Ectopic— *see* Ectopic Ossification, 762·2
Ossigeno, 1236·3
Ossin, 2194·4
Ossiplex, 2194·4
Ossiten, 2194·4
Ossivite, 2194·4
Ossocal-D, 2195·1
Ossofluor, 2195·1
Ossofortin, 2195·1
Ossofortin Forte, 2195·1
Ossomax, 2195·1
Ossopan, 2195·1
Osspulvit S, 2195·1
Osspulvit S Forte, 2195·1
Oss-regen, 2195·1
OST Vit, 2195·1
Ostac, 2195·1
Ostaren, 2195·1
Ostatac, 2195·1
Ostedron, 2195·1
Osteitis Deformans— *see* Paget's Disease of Bone, 764·2
Osteitis Fibrosa— *see* Renal Osteodystrophy, 764·3
Ostelin, 2195·1
Osten, 2195·1
Ostenan, 2195·1
Ostenil, 2195·1
Osteo, 2195·1
Osteo Bi-Flex, 2195·1
Osteo Complex, 2195·1
Osteo D, 2195·1
Osteo Support, 2195·1
Osteoapatite with Boron, 2195·1
Osteoarthritis, 9·2
Osteoarthrosis— *see* Osteoarthritis, 9·2
Osteobion, 2195·1
Osteocal, 2195·1
Osteocal D3, 2195·1
Osteocalcic, 2195·2
Osteocalcil, 2195·2
Osteocalcin, 2195·2
Osteocalmine, 2195·2
Osteocare, 2195·2
Osteochondrin S, 2195·2
Osteocis, 2195·2
Osteoclastoma— *see* Bone Sarcoma, 524·3
Osteocur, 2195·2
Osteocynesine, 2195·2
Osteodidronel, 2195·2
Osteodystrophy, Renal— *see* Renal Osteodystrophy, 764·3
OsteoEze Bone & Joint Care, 2195·2
Osteofem, 2195·2
Osteofix, 2195·2
Osteoflam-MR, 2195·2
Osteofluor, 2195·2
Osteoform, 2195·2
Osteofos D3, 2195·2
Osteogen, 2195·2
Osteogenesis Imperfecta, 762·3
Osteogenic Protein-1, 768·2
Osteogenic Sarcoma— *see* Bone Sarcoma, 524·3
Osteogenin, 768·2
Osteogenon, 2195·2
Osteomalacia, 762·3
Osteomar, 2195·2
Osteomerck, 2195·2
Osteomin, 2195·2
Osteomyelitis— *see* Bone and Joint Infections, 122·1
Osteopetrosis, 1085·2
Osteopetrosis, Juvenile— *see* Osteopetrosis, 1085·2
Osteoplex, 2195·2
Osteo-Plus, 2195·2
Osteoplus, 2195·2
Osteopor, 2195·2
Osteoporosis, 763·1
Osteoporosis Mineral Plus Formula 9, 2195·3
Osteoporosis, Post-traumatic— *see* Complex Regional Pain Syndrome, 5·3
Osteopro, 2195·3
Osteoral, 2195·3
Osteos, 2195·3
Osteosan, 2195·3
Osteosarcoma— *see* Bone Sarcoma, 524·3
Osteosil, 2195·3
Osteostab, 2195·3
Osteostabil, 2195·3
Osteoton, 2195·3
Osteotonina, 2195·3
Osteotop, 2195·3
Osteotrat, 2195·3
Osteotriol, 2195·3
Osteovis, 2195·3
Osteovit, 2195·3
Ostepam, 2195·3
Osteral, 2195·3
Osteum, 2195·3
Osteus, 2195·3
Osticalcin, 2195·3
Ostiderm, 2195·3
Ostidil-D3, 2195·3
Ostifix, 2195·3
Ostine, 2195·3
Ostobon, 2195·3
Ostocalcium, 2195·3
Ostocalcium B-12, 2195·4
Ostochont, 2195·4
Ostofen, 2195·4
Ostoforte, 2195·4
Ostogene, 2195·4
Ostone-B12, 2195·4
Ostopor, 2195·4
Ostosalm, 2195·4
Ostostabil, 2195·4
Ostram, 2195·4
Ostram $D_3$, 2195·4
Ostram D3, 2195·4
Ostram Vitamine $D_3$, 2195·4
Ostram-Vit $D_3$, 2195·4
Ostranorm, 2195·4
Ostron, 2195·4
Ostronara, 2195·4
Ostro-Primolut, 2195·4
Osvical, 2195·4
Osvical D, 2195·4
Osyrol, 2195·4
Osyrol Lasix, 2195·4
Otalex G, 2195·4
Otalgan, 2195·4
Otalgicin, 2196·1
Otandrol, 2196·1
Otarex, 2196·1
Otastat, 586·3
Otauril, 2196·1
Otazol, 2196·1
Otek-AC, 2196·1
O-Tet, 2196·1
Otex, 2196·1
Otex HC, 2196·1
Otiborin, 2196·1
Otic Domeboro, 2196·1
Otic-Care, 2196·1
Oticerim, 2196·1
Oticum, 2196·1
Otidin, 2196·1
Otidrops, 2196·1
Otigent, 2196·1
Otilin, 2196·1
Otilonio, Bromuro de, 1725·1
Otilonium Bromide, 1725·1
Oti-Med, 2196·1
Otipax, 2196·1
Otised, 2196·1
Otitex, 2196·1
Otitis Externa, 138·1
Otitis Media, 138·1
OtiTricin, 2196·1
Otix, 2196·1
Oto Betnovate, 2196·1
Oto Biotaer, 2196·2
Oto Difusor, 2196·2
Oto Neomicin Calm, 2196·2
Oto Vitna, 2196·2
Oto Xilodase, 2196·2
Otobacid N, 2196·2
Otobel, 2196·2
Otobiotic, 2196·2
Oto-Biotic, 2196·2
Otobrain, 2196·2
Otocain, 2196·2
Otocalm, 2196·2
Otocalma, 2196·2
Otocalmia, 2196·2
Otocalmine, 2196·2
Oto-Cer, 2196·2
Otoceril, 2196·2
Otocerum, 2196·2
Otocipro, 2196·2
Otoclean Gotas Oticas, 2196·2
Otoclean Solucion de Limpieza, 2196·2
Otocomb Otic, 2196·2
Otocort, 2196·2
Otocuril, 2196·3
Oto-cyl Ho-Len-Complex, 2196·3
Otodex, 2196·3
Otodol, 2196·3
Otodolor, 2196·3
Otofa, 2196·3
Otofenicol-D, 2196·3
Oto-Flexiole N, 2196·3
Otoflogin, 2196·3
Otoflour, 2196·3
Otoflox, 2196·3
Otofluor, 2196·3
Otogen Calmante, 2196·3
Otogesic, 2196·3
Otoial, 2196·3
Otolin, 2196·3
Otolisan, 2196·3
Otolitan N Farblos, 2196·3
Otolitan N mit Rivanol, 2196·3
Otoloide, 2196·3
Otolone, 2196·3
Otolys, 2196·3
Otolysine, 2196·3
Otomar-HC, 2196·3
Otomicetina, 2196·3
Otomicina, 2196·3
Otomide, 2196·4
Otomidone, 2196·4
Otomidrin, 2196·4
Otomixyn, 2196·4
Otomize, 2196·4
Otomycin, 2196·4
Otomycin-HPN, 2196·4
Otonal, 2196·4
Otonasal, 2196·4
Otonax, 2196·4
Otonina, 2196·4
Otonorthia, 2196·4
Otopax, 2196·4
Oto-Ped, 2196·4
Otopen, 2196·4
Oto-Phen, 2196·4
Oto-Phen Forte, 2196·4
Otoralgyl, 2196·4
Otoralgyl a la Phenylephrine, 2196·4
Otoralgyl Sulfamide, 2196·4
Otorinazol, 2196·4
Oto-Rinil, 2196·4
Otosal, 2196·4
Otosamthong, 2196·4
Otosan, 2197·1
Otosan Natural Ear Drops, 2197·1
Otosedol, 2197·1
Otosedol Biotico, 2197·1
Otoseptil, 2197·1
Otosil, 2197·1
Otosporin, 2197·1
Otosporin L, 2197·1
Otospray, 2197·1
Otosulf, 2197·1
Otosynalar, 2197·1
Oto-Synalar N, 2197·1
Otothricinol, 2197·1
Otovix, 2197·1
Otovowen, 2197·1
Otowaxol, 2197·1
Otradrops, 2197·1
Otrasel, 2197·1
Otraspray, 2197·1
Otreon, 2197·1
O-trexat, 2197·1
Otriflu, 2197·1
Otrinol, 2197·1
Otrisal, 2197·2
Otrisalin, 2197·2
Otriven, 2197·2
Otriven gegen Schnupfen, 2197·2
Otriven H, 2197·2
Otriven mit Dexpanthenol, 2197·2
Otrivin, 2197·2
Otrivin Menthol, 2197·2
Otrivina, 2197·2
Otrivine, 2197·2
Otrivine Preparations, 2197·2
Otrivine-Antistin, 2197·2
Otrivini, 2197·2
Otrozol, 2197·2
Otsuka MV, 2197·2
Otto of Rose, 1740·2

Ottocid, 2197·2
Ottoclor, 2197·2
Ottovis, 2197·2
Oturga, 2197·2
Otylol, 2197·2
138OU, 162·2
OU-1308, 1520·3
Ouabain, 977·3
Ouabaína, 977·3
Ouabainum, 977·3
Ouate Hemostatique, 2197·2
Out of Africa, 2197·2
Outgro, 2197·2
Outlook, 2197·2
Out-of-Sorts, 2197·3
Ouvidonal, 2197·3
Ova, 2197·3
Oval Buchu, 1663·1
Ova-Mit, 2197·3
Ovanon, 2197·3
Ovarell, 2197·3
Ovarian Cancer— *see* Malignant Neoplasms of the Ovary, 520·2
Ovarian Dysfunction, 1317·2
Ovarian Extracts, 1565·1
Ovariusedan, 2197·3
Ovariuteran, 2197·3
Ovary Extracts, 1565·1
Ovary, Polycystic— *see* Polycystic Ovary Syndrome, 1317·2
Ovastat, 2197·3
Ovcon 35, 2197·3
Ovcon 50, 2197·3
Overal, 2197·3
Overoid, 2197·3
Overpon, 2197·3
Ovesterin, 2197·3
Ovestin, 2197·3
Ovestinon, 2197·3
Ovestrion, 2197·3
Ovex, 2197·3
Ovide, 2197·3
Ovidol, 2197·3
Ovidrel, 2197·3
Ovidrelle, 2197·3
Ovidrelle— *see* Ovitrelle, 2197·4
Ovinol, 2197·3
Ovinum, 2197·3
Oviol, 2197·3
Ovipreg, 2197·3
*Ovis aries*, 1483·1
Ovis Neu, 2197·3
Ovitrelle, 2197·4
Ovofar, 2197·4
Ovol, 2197·4
Ovoplex, 2197·4
Ovoresta, 2197·4
Ovoresta M, 2197·4
Ovosiston, 2197·4
Ovostat, 2197·4
Ovo-Vinces, 2197·4
Ovral, 2197·4
Ovran, 2197·4
Ovran 30, 2197·4
Ovranet, 2197·4
Ovranette, 2197·4
Ovrette, 2197·4
OvuGen, 2197·4
Ovukalen, 2197·4
Ovukit, 2197·4
Ovules Sedo-Hemostatiques du Docteur Jouve, 2197·4
Ovuplan, 2197·4
Ovuquick, 2197·4
Ovutest, 2197·4
Ovysmen, 2197·4
Owbridges for Chesty Coughs, 2197·4
Owencet, 2197·4
Owentar— *see* Psorigel, 2245·1
Owentar II— *see* Ionil-T Plus, 2065·3
OX-373, 683·1
Ox Bile, 1660·3
Oxa, 2197·4
Oxa B12, 2198·1
Oxa Forte, 2198·1
Oxa Sport, 2198·1
Oxabenal, 2198·1
Oxabenz, 2198·1
Oxabolona, Cipionato de, 1565·1
Oxabolone Cipionate, 1565·1
Oxabolone Cypionate, 1565·1
22-Oxacalcitriol, 1462·1
Oxacant N, 2198·1
Oxacant-forte N, 2198·1
Oxacant-Khella N, 2198·1
Oxacant-mono, 2198·1
Oxacant-sedativ, 2198·1
Oxacatin, 2198·1
Oxacephalosporins, 117·3
Oxaceprol, 1725·1
Oxacil, 2198·1
Oxacilina Sódica, 240·2
Oxacillin Sodium, 240·2
Oxacillinum Natricum, 240·2
Oxacillinum Natrium, 240·2
Oxacycle-P, 2198·1
Oxadilene, 2198·1
Oxadisten, 2198·1
Oxadol, 2198·1
Oxagesic, 2198·1
Oxahexal, 2198·1
OXAIDS, 1715·2
Oxaine-M, 2198·1
Oxalaldehyde, 1181·1
Oxalato de Cerio, 1255·2
Oxalato de Naftidrofurilo, 964·1
Oxalgin, 2198·1
Oxalgin-DP, 2198·1
Oxalic Acid, 1304·2, 1725·1
Oxálico, Ácido, 1725·1
Oxaliplatin, 577·1
Oxaliplatino, 577·1
Oxaliplatinum, 577·1
Oxaltie, 2198·1
*N,N′*-Oxalylbis(*N*-2-aminoethyl-*N*-2-chlorobenzyldiethylammonium) Dichloride, 1487·3
Oxalyt, 2198·1
Oxamin, 2198·1
Oxaminozoline Phosphate, 996·1
Oxamniquina, 110·3
Oxamniquine, 110·3
Oxamphetamine Hydrobromide, 1699·3
Oxandrin, 2198·2
Oxandrolona, 1565·1
Oxandrolone, 1565·1
Oxanest, 2198·2
Oxantel Embonate, 111·1
Oxantel, Embonato de, 111·1
Oxantel Pamoate, 111·1
Oxapam, 2198·2
Oxapax, 2198·2
Oxapen, 2198·2
Oxaphenamide, 1725·1
Oxaprost, 2198·2
Oxaprozin, 75·1
Oxaprozina, 75·1
Oxarol, 2198·2
Oxascand, 2198·2
Oxathos, 2198·2
Oxatokey, 2198·2
Oxatomida, 438·1
Oxatomide, 438·1
Oxazacort, 1096·2
Oxazepam, 712·2
Oxazepam Hemisuccinate, 712·3
Oxazepamum, 712·2
Oxazimédrine, 1592·2
Oxazolam, 712·3
Oxazolazepam, 712·3
Oxazolidinone Antibacterials, 120·2
Oxbarukain, 2198·2
OxBipp, 2198·2
Oxcarbazepina, 366·3
Oxcarbazepine, 366·3
Oxcazen, 2198·2
Oxcord, 2198·2
Oxedrine, 977·3
Oxedrine Hydrochloride, 977·3
Oxedrine Tartrate, 977·3
Oxedrini Tartras, 977·3
Oxeladin Citrate, 1126·1
Oxeladin Hydrogen Citrate, 1126·1
Oxeladina, Hidrocloruro de, 1126·1
Oxeladini Hydrogenocitras, 1126·1
Oxelio, 2198·2
Oxema Improved, 2198·2
Oxendolone, 1565·2
Oxeno, 2198·2
Oxeol, 2198·2
Oxepa, 2198·2
Oxepam, 2198·2
Oxeprax, 2198·2
Oxeron, 2198·2
Oxerutinas, 1688·2
Oxerutins, 1688·2
Oxetacaína, 1382·1
Oxetacaine, 1382·1
Oxetacaine Hydrochloride, 1382·1
2-Oxetanone, 1191·2
Oxethazaine, 1382·1
Oxetine, 2198·2
Oxetorona, Fumarato de, 470·2
Oxetorone Fumarate, 470·2
Oxez, 2198·2
Oxeze, 2198·2
Oxfendazol, 111·1
Oxfendazole, 111·1
Oxfendazole for Veterinary Use, 111·1
Oxfendazolum, 111·1
Oxibato Sódico, 1308·3
Oxibendazol, 111·2
Oxibendazole, 111·2
Oxibenzona, 1154·3
Oxibran, 2198·2
Oxibron, 2198·2
Oxibron NF, 2198·2
Oxibuprocaína, Hidrocloruro de, 1382·1
Oxibut, 2198·2
Oxibutinina, Hidrocloruro de, 486·3
Oxicam, 2198·2
Oxicanol, 2198·3
Oxichinolini Sulfas, 1700·1
Oxichlorochin Sulphate, 452·3
Oxicloroseno, 1187·2
Oxiclozanida, 111·2
Oxicodal, 2198·3
Oxicodona, Hidrocloruro de, 75·2
Oxicodona, Tereftalato de, 75·2
Oxiconazol, Nitrato de, 407·3
Oxiconazole Nitrate, 407·3
Oxiderma, 2198·3
Oxidermiol Antihist, 2198·3
Oxidermiol Enzima, 2198·3
Oxidermiol Fuerte, 2198·3
Oxidermiol Lassar, 2198·3
Oxidine, 2198·3
Oxidised Cellulose, 757·1
Oxidized Cellulose, 757·1, 757·2
Oxidized Regenerated Cellulose, 757·2
Oxido Amari, 2198·3
Oxido Amarillo de Mercurio, 1712·3
Óxido de Aluminio, 1140·1
Óxido de Bismuto, 1252·1
Óxido de Calcio, 1664·3
Óxido de Etileno, 1179·1
Óxido de Hierro, 1057·3
Óxido de Polietileno, 1581·1
Óxido Nítrico, 973·3
Óxido Nitroso, 1304·3
Oxidronate Disodium, 773·3
Oxidronate Sodium, 773·3
Oxidronate, Technetium ($^{99m}$Tc), 1526·1
Oxidronato Disódico, 773·3
Oxidronic Acid, 773·3
Oxidrónico, Ácido, 773·3
Oxifedrina, Hidrocloruro de, 978·2
Oxifedrini Chloridum, 978·2
Oxifenbutazona, 76·1
Oxifenciclimina, Hidrocloruro de, 487·2
Oxifenisatina, 1282·3
Oxifenisatina, Acetato de, 1282·3
Oxifenonio, Bromuro de, 487·2
Oxi-Freeda, 2198·3
Oxifungol, 2198·3
Oxigen, 2198·3
Oxígeno, 1236·3
Oxígeno 15, 1525·1
Oxiken, 2198·3
Oxiklorin, 2198·3
Oxilan, 2198·3
Oxilapine, 705·2
Oxilin, 2198·3
Oxilium, 2198·3
Oxilofrina, Hidrocloruro de, 977·3
Oxilofrine Hydrochloride, 977·3
Oximar, 2198·3
Oximar Respiratorio, 2198·3
Oximen, 2198·3
Oximetazolina, Hidrocloruro de, 1126·1
Oximetolona, 1565·2
Oximorfona, Hidrocloruro de, 76·1
Oximorphone Hydrochloride, 76·1
5-Oxin, 2198·3
Oxine Sulphate, 1700·1
Oxinovag, 2198·3
Oxinovag Complex, 2198·3
Oxipertina, 713·1
Oxipoligelatina, 757·2
Oxipor, 2198·3
Oxipor VHC, 2198·3
Oxipurinol, 413·2
Oxiquinol Potásico, 1734·2
Oxiracetam, 1725·2
Oxirane, 1179·1
Oxis, 2198·3
Oxisept, 2198·3
Oxistat, 2198·4
Oxi-T, 2198·4
Oxi-Tabs C+E, 2198·4
Oxitetraciclina, 241·1
Oxitetraciclina Cálcica, 241·1
Oxitetraciclina, Hidrocloruro de, 241·1
Oxitina, 2198·4
Oxitocina, 1336·1
Oxiton, 2198·4
Oxitopisa, 2198·4
Oxitover, 2198·4
Oxitraklin, 2198·4
Oxitrat, 2198·4
Oxitriptan, 311·1
DL-Oxitriptan, 311·1
Oxitropio, Bromuro de, 790·3
Oxitropium Bromide, 790·3
Oxiurazina, 2198·4
Oxivel, 2198·4
Oxivent, 2198·4
Oxivite, 2198·4
Oxizole, 2198·4
Oxlip, 1735·1
3-Oxoandrost-4-en-17β-yl 3-Cyclopentylpropionate, 1569·3
3-Oxoandrost-4-en-17β-yl Decanoate, 1570·1
3-Oxoandrost-4-en-17β-yl Heptanoate, 1570·1
3-Oxoandrost-4-en-17β-yl 4-Methylpentanoate, 1570·1
3-Oxoandrost-4-en-17β-yl 3-Phenylpropionate, 1570·1
3-Oxoandrost-4-en-17β-yl Propionate, 1570·1
3-Oxoandrost-4-en-17β-yl Undecanoate, 1570·1
Oxobenzopyrancarboxylic Acid, Diethylamine Salt, 1670·3
3-Oxo-2′,5′-bis(trifluoromethyl)-4-aza-5α-androst-1-ene-17β-carboxanilide, 1549·2
Oxobron, 2198·4
4-(3-Oxobutyl)-1,2-diphenylpyrazolidine-3,5-dione, 51·1
Oxociprofloxacin, 191·1
Oxodal, 2198·4
5-Oxo-desethylzaleplon, 727·3
4-Oxo-1,4-dihydroquinoline, 119·1
3-Oxo-enoxacin, 207·2
1-Oxoestazolam, 697·3
3-Oxoestr-4-en-17β-yl, 1561·2
3-Oxoestr-4-en-17β-yl 3-Cyclohexylpropionate, 1561·2
3-Oxoestr-4-en-17β-yl Decanoate, 1561·2
3-Oxoestr-4-en-17β-yl Dodecanoate, 1561·2
3-Oxoestr-4-en-17β-yl 3-Phenylpropionate, 1561·3

3-Oxoestr-4-en-17β-yl Sodium Sulphate, 1561·3
3-Oxoestr-4-en-17β-yl Undecanoate, 1561·3
Oxoferin, 2198·4
3-Oxo-L-gulofuranolactone, 1460·2
3-Oxo-L-gulofuranolactone 6-Palmitate, 1168·2
3-Oxo-L-gulofuranolactone Sodium Enolate, 1460·2
6-[*N*-(2-Oxoimidazolidin-1-ylcarbonyl)-D-phenylglycylamino]penicillanic Acid, 160·2
Oxoinex, 2198·4
(±)-2-[4-(1-Oxo-isoindolin-2-yl)phenyl]butyric Acid, 939·1
4-Oxo-isotretinoin, 1150·3
Oxolam, 2198·4
Oxolamina, 1126·1
Oxolamina, Citrato de, 1126·1
Oxolamina, Fosfato de, 1126·1
Oxolamine, 1126·1
Oxolamine Citrate, 1126·1
Oxolamine Phosphate, 1126·1
Oxolamine Tannate, 1126·1
Oxolinic Acid, 240·3
Oxolínico, Ácido, 240·3
Oxolinicum, Acidum, 240·3
Oxomar, 2198·4
Oxomemazina, 438·2
Oxomemazina, Hidrocloruro de, 438·2
Oxomemazine, 438·2
Oxomemazine Hydrochloride, 438·2
Oxomifer, 2198·4
Oxonic Acid, 586·3
3-Oxo-19-nor-17α-pregn-4-en-20-yn-17β-yl Acetate, 1562·2
(6*R*,8*r*,9a*S*)-3-Oxoperhydro-2*H*-2,6-methanoquinolizin-8-yl Indole-3-carboxylate Methanesulphonate, 1262·3
2-Oxo-4-phenyl-1-pyrrolidineacetamide, 1731·1
1-[*N*-(5-Oxo-L-prolyl)-L-histidyl]-L-prolinamide, 1337·3
(*R*)-3-[(*S*)-5-Oxoprolyl]-4-thiazolidinecarboxylic Acid, 1731·3
6-Oxo-prostaglandin $F_{1\alpha}$, 1517·2
Oxopurin, 2198·4
2-Oxo-1-pyrrolidineaceto-2′,6′-xylidide, 1719·2
2-(2-Oxopyrrolidin-1-yl)acetamide, 1732·1
(*S*)-2-(2-Oxopyrrolidin-1-yl)butanamide, 366·1
2-Oxoquazepam, 718·2
Oxoquin, 2198·4
4-Oxo-*cis*-retinoic Acid, 1161·2
4-Oxo-*trans*-retinoic Acid, 1161·2
Oxosint, 2198·4
*N*-[4-Oxo-2-(1*H*-tetrazol-5-yl)-4*H*-1-benzopyran-8-yl]-*p*-(4-phenylbutoxy)benzamide, 791·1
Oxo-Val, 2198·4
22-Oxovincaleukoblastine Sulphate, 592·2
Oxoway, 2198·4
5-Oxo-zaleplon, 727·3
Ox-Pam, 2198·4
Oxpentifylline, 979·3
Oxphenonii Bromidum, 487·2
Oxprenolol, Hidrocloruro de, 978·1
Oxprenolol Hydrochloride, 978·1
Oxprenololi Hydrochloridum, 978·1
Oxrate, 2198·4
Oxsac, 2198·4
Oxsoralen, 2198·4
Oxsoralon, 2199·1
Oxtolyltropine Hydrobromide, 483·2
Oxtriphylline, 784·2
Oxy Preparations, 2199·1
Oxyb, 2199·1
Oxybase, 2199·2
Oxybenzone, 1154·3
β,β′-Oxybis(aceto-*p*-phenetidide), 104·1
4,4′-Oxybis(butan-2-ol), 1680·2
Oxybismethane, 1236·1
1,1′-[Oxybis(methylene)]bis[4-(hydroxyimino)methyl]pyridinium Dichloride, 1046·3
Oxyboldine, 2199·2
Oxybubene, 2199·2
Oxybugamma, 2199·2
Oxybuprocaine Hydrochloride, 1382·1
Oxybuprocaini Hydrochloridum, 1382·1
Oxybutin, 2199·2
Oxybuton, 2199·2
Oxybutyn, 2199·2
Oxybutynin Chloride, 486·3
Oxybutynin Hydrochloride, 486·3
Oxybutynini Hydrochloridum, 486·3
Oxy-Care, 2199·2
Oxycedri, Pix, 1159·2
Oxycedri, Pyroleum, 1159·2
Oxycel, 2199·2
Oxychlorosene, 1187·2
Oxychlorosene Sodium, 1187·2
Oxycline, 2199·2
Oxyclozanide, 111·2
Oxycocet, 2199·2
Oxycod, 2199·2
Oxycodan, 2199·2
Oxycodone Hydrochloride, 75·2
Oxycodone Pectinate, 75·3
Oxycodone Terephthalate, 75·2
Oxycone Hydrochloride, 75·2
Oxycontin, 2199·2
Oxyde de Fer Sucré, 1438·2
Oxyde Nitreux, 1304·3
Oxyderm, 2199·2
Oxydermine, 2199·2
Oxydol, 1182·2
Oxydum Nitrosum, 1304·3
Oxyephedrine Hydrochloride, 977·3
Oxyetophylline, 785·1
Oxyfast, 2199·2
Oxyfedrine Hydrochloride, 978·2
Oxyflux, 2199·2
Oxygen, 1236·3
Oxygen-15, 1525·1
Oxygen 93 Percent, 1237·1
Oxygen, Hyperbaric, 1237·2
Oxygen, Liquid, 1237·2
Oxygenium, 1236·3
Oxygeron, 2199·2
Oxygesic, 2199·2
Oxygirex, 2199·2
OxyIR, 2199·2
Oxylim, 2199·2
Oxylin, 2199·2
Oxymedin, 2199·2
Oxymet, 2199·2
Oxymetazoline Hydrochloride, 1126·1
Oxymetazolini Hydrochloridum, 1126·1
Oxymetholone, 1565·2
Oxymethurea, 1187·2
Oxymorphone Hydrochloride, 76·1
Oxymycin, 2199·2
Oxyno, 2199·2
Oxynorm, 2199·3
Oxypan, 2199·3
Oxypangam, 2199·3
Oxyperol, 2199·3
Oxypertine, 713·1
Oxyphenbutazone, 76·1
Oxyphenbutazone Piperazine, 76·1
Oxyphenbutazonum, 76·1
Oxyphencyclimine Hydrochloride, 487·2
Oxyphenisatin, 1282·3
Oxyphenisatin Acetate, 1282·3
Oxyphenisatin Diacetate, 1282·3
Oxyphenisatine, 1282·3
Oxyphenisatine Acetate, 1282·3
Oxyphenisatine Diacetate, 1282·3
Oxyphenonium Bromatum, 487·2
Oxyphenonium Bromide, 487·2
Oxyphenylmethylaminoethanol Tartrate, 977·3
Oxyplastine, 2199·3
Oxypolygelatin, 757·2
Oxyprenolol Hydrochloride, 978·1
Oxyquinol, 1700·1
Oxyquinol Potassium, 1734·2
Oxyquinoline Sulfate, 1700·1
Oxysept, 2199·3
Oxysept Comfort, 2199·3
Oxyspas, 2199·3
Oxytel, 2199·3
Oxytetracycline, 241·1
Oxytetracycline Calcium, 241·1
Oxytetracycline Dihydrate, 241·1
Oxytetracycline Hydrochloride, 241·1
Oxytetracyclini Hydrochloridum, 241·1
Oxytetracyclinum, 241·1
Oxytetral, 2199·3
Oxytetramix, 2199·3
Oxythyol, 2199·3
Oxytocin, 1336·1
Oxytocin Bulk Solution, 1336·1
Oxytocin Citrate, 1337·1
Oxytocinum, 1336·1
Oxytrol, 2199·3
Oxyurin, 2199·3
Oxyzal, 2199·3
Oyo, 2199·3
Oysco, 2199·3
Oysco D, 2199·3
Oyst-Cal, 2199·3
Oyst-Cal-D, 2199·3
Oyster Calcium, 2199·3
Oyster Calcium with Vitamin D, 2199·3
Oyster Shell Calcium, 2199·4
Oyster Shell Calcium with Vitamin D, 2199·4
Oystercal, 2199·4
Oystercal-D, 2199·4
Oz, 2199·4
γ-OZ, 1725·1
Ozagrel, 1725·2
Ozagrel Hydrochloride, 1725·2
Ozagrel Sodium, 1725·2
Ozex, 2199·4
Ozidia, 2199·4
Ozogamicin, Gemtuzumab, 558·3
Ozoken, 2199·4
Ozolinone, 914·2
Ozonol, 2199·4
Ozonol Antibiotic Plus, 2199·4
Ozonosol, 2199·4
Ozonyl, 2199·4
Ozonyl Aquoso, 2199·4
Ozonyl Expectorante, 2199·4
Ozopulmin, 2199·4
Ozopulmin G, 2199·4
Ozothin, 2199·4
Ozothine, 2199·4
Ozothine a la Diprophylline, 2199·4
Ozovit, 2199·4
Ozym, 2199·4

## P

P, 1443·2
3P, 2199·4
P-12, 240·2
P-25, 198·2
P-30 Protein, 582·2
P-50, 157·1
P-071, 427·1
P-113, 996·3
P-286, 1066·2
P-725, 713·3
P-1011, 205·2
P-1134, 983·1
P-1202, 527·2
P-1393, 868·1
P-1496, 1573·3
P-1779, 858·1
P-1888, 1750·3
P-2105, 911·3
P-2525, 984·2
P-3693A, 291·2
P-4125, 1750·3
P-5604, 1105·3
P & S, 2200·1
P & S Plus, 2200·1
P. Veinos, 2200·1
PA-93, 239·2
PA-105, 240·2
PA-109, 1569·1
PA-144, 580·2
Paan, 1656·2
PAB, 1142·2
PABA, 1142·2
Pabacidum, 1142·2
Pabafilm, 2200·1
Pabalat, 2200·1
Pabalate, 2200·1
Pabanox, 2200·1
Pabasol, 2200·1
Pabasun, 2200·1
Pabrinex, 2200·1
P-A-C, 2200·1
Pac Merieux, 2200·1
Pacaps, 2200·1
Paceco, 2200·1
Paceflex, 2200·1
Pacemol, 2200·1
Pacerone, 2200·1
Pacetal, 2200·1
Paceum, 2200·1
Pacifen, 2200·1
Pacifene, 2200·1
Pacifenity, 2200·1
Pacimol, 2200·1
Pacinax, 2200·1
Pacinol, 2200·1
Pacinone, 2200·1
Pacis, 2200·2
Pacisyn, 2200·2
Pacitane, 2200·2
Pacium, 2200·2
Paclikebir, 2200·2
Paclitax, 2200·2
Paclitaxel, 577·3
Pacliteva, 2200·2
Pacofen, 2200·2
Pacopan, 2200·2
Pactens, 2200·2
Pacyl, 2200·2
Padamin, 2200·2
Paderyl, 2200·2
Padet, 2200·2
Padiacrom, 2200·2
Padiafusin, 2200·2
Padiafusin OP, 2200·2
Padiamol, 2200·2
Padiamuc, 2200·2
Padiatifen, 2200·2
Padiken, 2200·2
Padimate, 1155·1
Padimate A, 1155·1
Padimate O, 1155·1
Padimato, 1155·1
Padimato O, 1155·1
Padma 28, 2200·2
Padma-Lax, 2200·2
Padmed Circosan, 2200·3
Padrin, 2200·3
Padutin, 2200·3
Paedamin, 2200·3
Paedialgon, 2200·3
Paediasure, 2200·3
Paediathrocin, 2200·3
Paediatric Seravit, 2200·3
Paedisup, 2200·3
Paf, 2200·3
Paferxin, 2200·3
Paftec, 2200·3
Paget's Disease of Bone, 764·2
PAHA, 1653·2
Pahtlisan, 2200·3
Paididont, 2200·3
Paidocin, 2200·3
Paidoflor, 2200·3
Paidolax, 2200·3
Paidomal, 2200·3
Paidorinovit, 2200·3
Paidoterin Descongestivo NF, 2200·3
Paidovit, 2200·3
Paidozim, 2200·3
Paigastrol, 2200·3
Pain, 2·1
Pain Aid, 2200·3
Pain Aid Free, 2200·3
Pain, Bone— *see* Cancer Pain, 5·1
Pain, Breast— *see* Mastalgia, 1546·3
Pain Buster, 2200·3
Pain Bust-R II, 2200·3
Pain, Cancer— *see* Cancer Pain, 5·1

Pain, Central— *see* Central Post-stroke Pain, 5·3
Pain, Central Post-stroke.— *see* Central Post-stroke Pain, 5·3
Pain, Chemists Own— *see* Chemists Own Pain, 1882·1
Pain in Children— *see* Choice of Analgesics in Children, 3·2
Pain, Colic— *see* Biliary and Renal Colic, 4·3
Pain of Diabetic Neuropathy— *see* Diabetic Neuropathy, 6·1
Pain Doctor, 2200·4
Pain, Facial— *see* Orofacial Pain, 7·2
Pain & Fever, Chemists Own— *see* Chemists Own Pain & Fever, 1882·1
Pain And Fever Relief, 2200·4
Pain, Labour— *see* Labour Pain, 6·2
Pain, Low Back— *see* Low Back Pain, 7·1
Pain, Menstrual— *see* Dysmenorrhoea, 6·1
Pain, Myocardial Infarction— *see* Myocardial Infarction Pain, 7·1
Pain, Myofascial— *see* Soft-tissue Rheumatism, 11·1
Pain, Neurogenic, 2·1
Pain, Neuropathic, 2·1
Pain, Nociceptive, 2·1
Pain, Orofacial— *see* Orofacial Pain, 7·2
Pain, Pancreatic— *see* Pancreatic Pain, 7·3
Pain, Phantom Limb— *see* Phantom Limb Pain, 7·3
Pain, Postoperative— *see* Postoperative Analgesia, 4·1
Pain Relief Syrup for Children, 2200·4
Pain Reliever, 2200·4
Pain Reliever, Extra Power— *see* Extra Power Pain Reliever, 1986·1
Pain Relieving Ointment, 2200·4
Pain, Sickle-cell Crisis— *see* Sickle-cell Crisis, 8·1
Pain, Somatic, 2·1
Pain Syndromes, Sympathetic— *see* Complex Regional Pain Syndrome, 5·3
Pain, Visceral, 2·1
Painagon, 2200·4
Painaid, 2200·4
Painaid BRF Back Relief Formula, 2200·4
Painaid ESF Extra-Strength Formula, 2200·4
Painaid PMF Premenstrual Formula, 2200·4
Painamol, 2200·4
Painamol Plus, 2200·4
Paincod, 2200·4
Paindol, 2200·4
Painex, 2200·4
Painil, 2200·4
Painnox, 2200·4
Painrite, 2200·4
Painrite SA, 2200·4
Pains-of, 2200·4
Painstop, 2200·4
Painza, 2200·4
Pakinase, 2200·4
Paklitaxfil, 2200·4
Pakurat, 2200·4
Palacos Preparations, 2200·4
Palacril, 2201·1
Paladac, 2201·1
Palafer, 2201·1
Palafer CF, 2201·1
Palamed, 2201·1
Palamed G, 2201·1
Palan, 2201·1
Palane, 2201·1
Palaprin, 2201·1
*Palaquium gutta*, 1696·2
Palatinit, 1438·3
Palatol, 2201·1
Palatol N, 2201·2
Palatrobil, 2201·2
Palcid, 2201·2
Palcol, 2201·2
Paldar, 2201·2
Paldesic, 2201·2
Paleodina, 2201·2
Palfium, 2201·2
Palgic DS, 2201·2
Palgic-D, 2201·2
Paliatil, 2201·2
Palindromic Rheumatism— *see* Rheumatoid Arthritis, 9·3
Palistop, 2201·2
Paliuryl, 2201·2
Palivizumab, 1637·2
Palladon, 2201·2
Palladone, 2201·2
Pallia, 2201·2
Palliative Care, Nausea and Vomiting in— *see* Nausea and Vomiting, 1245·2
Pallidone, 2201·2
Palm, American Dwarf, 1569·1
Palm Kernel Oil, 1481·3
Palm Kernel Oil, Fractionated, 1481·3
Palmer's Cocoa Butter Formula, 2201·2
Palmer's Cocoa Butter Formula Nappy Rash, 2201·2
Palmer's Cocoa Butter Formula Nursing, 2201·2
Palmetto Plus, 2201·2
Palmiclor, 2201·2
Palmicol, 2201·2
Palmidrol, 1725·3
Palmiffer, 2201·2
Palmil, 2201·2
Palmisan, 2201·2
Palmisol, 2201·2
Palmitan, 2201·2
Palmitate-A, 2201·2
Palmitato de Cloranfenicol, 185·1
Palmitato de Colfoscerilo, 1736·2
Palmitato de Isopropilo, 1481·2
Palmitato de Pipotiazina, 716·1
Palmitato de Sorbitán, 1416·2
Palmitato de Xantofila, 1765·3
Palmitic Acid ($^{11}$C), 1523·1
Palmitic Acid Triglyceride, 1763·3
Palmitylchloramphenicol, 185·1
Palon, 2201·2
Palonosetron Hydrochloride, 1282·3
Palpipax, 2201·3
Palpitations— *see* Cardiac Arrhythmias, 816·1
Pals, 2201·3
Palsy, Bell's— *see* Bell's Palsy, 1076·3
Paltomiel, 2201·3
Paltomiel Plus, 2201·3
Paludil, 2201·3
Paludrin, 2201·3
Paludrine, 2201·3
Paluken, 2201·3
Palukin, 2201·3
Paluquina, 2201·3
Paluther, 2201·3
Palux, 2201·3
Palygorskite, 1251·1
Pam, 2201·3
PAM, 566·1
2-PAM, 1050·1
2-PAM Chloride, 1050·1
2-PAM Iodide, 1050·1
Pamabrom, 978·2
Pamabromo, 978·2
Pamba, 2201·3
PAMBA, 742·1
2-PAMCl, 1050·1
Pamecil, 2201·3
Pamedox, 2201·3
Pamelor, 2201·3
Pamergan, 2201·3
Pamergan P100, 2201·3
2-PAMI, 1050·1
Pamid, 2201·3
Pamidran, 2201·3
Pamidronate Disodium, 773·3
Pamidronato Disódico, 773·3
Pamidronic Acid, 773·3
Pamidrónico, Ácido, 773·3
Pamine, 2201·3
Pamisol, 2201·3
Pamiteplase, 978·3
2-PAMM, 1050·1
Pamocil, 2201·3
Pamol, 2201·3
Pamoxan, 2201·4
Pamoxet, 2201·4
Pampe, 2201·4
Pamprin, 2201·4
Pamprin, Nighttime— *see* Nighttime Pamprin, 2168·1
Pan C, 2201·4
Pan Limpiador AL, 2201·4
Panac, 2201·4
Panac K, 2201·4
Panacef, 2201·4
Panacet, 2201·4
Panacod, 2201·4
Panacrearell, 2201·4
Panadeine, 2201·4
Panadeine Plus, 2201·4
Panado, 2201·4
Panado-Co, 2201·4
Panadol Preparations, 2201·4
*see also* Childrens Panadol Preparations, 1883·1
*Panaeolus*, 1717·3
Panafcort, 2202·1
Panafcortelone, 2202·1
Panafen, 2202·1
Panafil, 2202·1
Panafil-White, 2202·1
Panaflu, 2202·1
Panaflu Plus, 2202·1
Panagesic, 2202·1
Panagesic con Cafeina, 2202·1
Panalba, 2202·1
Panaleve, 2202·1
Panalgesic, 2202·1
Panalgesic Gold, 2202·1
Panaline, 2202·2
Panama Wood, 1416·1
Panamax, 2202·2
Panamax Co, 2202·2
Panamic, 2202·2
Pan-Amin, 2202·2
Panamor, 2202·2
Panasal, 2202·2
Panasol-S, 2202·2
Panasorbe, 2202·2
Panataxel, 2202·2
Panax, 1693·1, 2202·2
Panax Complex, 2202·2
*Panax ginseng*, 1693·1
*Panax japonicus*, 1693·1
Panax N, 2202·2
*Panax notoginseng*, 1693·1
*Panax pseudoginseng*, 1693·1
*Panax quinquefolius*, 1693·1
*Panax schinseng*, 1693·1
Panaxid, 2202·2
Panaxosides, 1693·1
Panazyme, Bioglan— *see* Bioglan Panazyme, 1844·1
Panbesy, 2202·2
Pancardiol, 2202·2
Pancebrin, 2202·2
Pancenz, 2202·2
Panchelidon N, 2202·2
Pancholtruw N, 2202·2
Pancillin, 2202·2
Panclasa, 2202·2
Panclor, 2202·2
Pancof, 2202·2
Pancof PD, 2202·2
Pancof XP, 2202·2
Pancof-EXP, 2202·2
Pancof-HC, 2202·2
Pancof-XL, 2202·3
Panconium, 2202·3
Pancoran, 2202·3
Pancreal Kirchner, 2202·3
Pancreas Powder, 1725·3
Pancreas Transplantation— *see* Pancreatic Transplantation, 1347·3
Pancrease, 2202·3
Pancrease HL, 2202·3
Pancreatic Adenocarcinoma— *see* Malignant Neoplasms of the Pancreas, 521·1
Pancreatic Cancer— *see* Malignant Neoplasms of the Pancreas, 521·1
Pancreatic Cholera, 505·1
Pancreatic Endocrine Tumours— *see* Carcinoid Tumours and Other Secretory Neoplasms, 504·1
Pancreatic Enzymes, 1725·3
Pancreatic Extract, 1725·3
Pancreatic Pain, 7·3
Pancreatin, 1725·3
Pancreatina, 1725·3
Pancreatinum, 1725·3
Pancreatis Pulvis, 1725·3
Pancreatitis, 1726·3
Pancrecura, 2202·3
Pancrelase, 2202·3
Pancrelipasa, 1725·3
Pancrelipase, 1725·3
Pancreocimina, 1727·2
Pancreoflat, 2202·3
Pancreolauryl, 2202·3
Pancreolauryl-Test, 2202·3
Pancreolauryl-Test N, 2202·3
Pancreon, 2202·3
Pancreon Compositum, 2202·3
Pancreozymin, 1727·2
Pancresil, 2202·3
Pancrex, 2202·3
Pancrezyme 4X, 2202·3
Pancrin, 2202·3
Pancrit, 2202·3
Pancrotanon, 2202·3
Pancuron, 2202·3
Pancuronii Bromidum, 1404·3
Pancuronio, Bromuro de, 1404·3
Pancuronium Bromide, 1404·3
Pancurox, 2202·3
Pancutan, 2202·3
Pancutan Base, 2202·3
Panda Baby Cream, 2202·3
Pandel, 2202·3
Panderm, 2202·3
Pandermil, 2202·4
Pandigal, 2202·4
Panectyl, 2202·4
Pan-Emecort, 2202·4
Panencephalitis, Subacute Sclerosing— *see* Measles, 624·3
Pan-Enteral, 2202·4
Panfil G, 2202·4
Panflavin, 2202·4
Panflogin, 2202·4
Panfugan, 2202·4
Pan-Fungex, 2202·4
Panfungol, 2202·4
Panfurex, 2202·4
Pangamic Acid, 1727·2
Pangámico, Ácido, 1727·2
Pangamox, 2202·4
Pangastren, 2202·4
Pangavit Hypak, 2202·4
Pangavit Pediatrico, 2202·4
Pangel, 2202·4
Pangen, 2202·4
Pangest, 2202·4
Panglobulin, 2202·4
Pangon, 2202·4
Pangrol, 2202·4
Panhematin, 2202·4
Panic Attacks, 663·3
Panimun Bioral, 2202·4
Panimycin, 2202·4
Paniodal, 2202·4
Paniodine, 2202·4
Panipenem, 241·3
Panitol, 2202·4
Panitone, 2203·1
Panix, 2203·1
Pankreaden, 2203·1
Pankreaplex Neu, 2203·1
Pankreas M Comp, 2203·1
Pankreas S Comp, 2203·1
Pankrease, 2203·1
Pankreatan, 2203·1
Pankreaticum, 2203·1
Pankreaticum N, 2203·1
Pankreoflat, 2203·1
Pankreoflat Sedante, 2203·1

Pankreon, 2203·1
Pankreon Compositum, 2203·1
Pankreon Compuesto, 2203·1
Pankreon Forte, 2203·1
Pankreon Total, 2203·1
Pankreozym, 2203·1
Pankrevowen, 2203·1
Panlem, 2203·1
Panlor DC, 2203·1
Pan-masala, 1656·2
Panmicol, 2203·1
Panmist JR, 2203·1
Panmist LA, 2203·1
PanMist-DM, 2203·1
Panmist-S, 2203·1
Panmycin, 2203·1
Pannag, 1693·1
Pannaz, 2203·1
Pannocort, 2203·2
Pannogel, 2203·2
Panocaine, 2203·2
Panocod, 2203·2
Panodil, 2203·2
Panolase, 2203·2
Pan-Ophtal, 2203·2
Panoptic, 2203·2
Panoral, 2203·2
Panorex, 2203·2
Panos, 2203·2
Panotil, 2203·2
Panotile, 2203·2
Panotile N, 2203·2
Panotos, 2203·2
Panotos NF, 2203·2
Panoxi, 2203·2
PanOxyl, 2203·2
PanOxyl Clear Acne, 2203·2
Panpeptal N, 2203·2
Panpur, 2203·2
Panpurol, 2203·2
Panquil, 2203·2
Panretin, 2203·3
Pansan, 2203·3
Panscol, 2203·3
Pansebase, 2203·3
Pansebase Composto, 2203·3
Pansebase Solido, 2203·3
Pansements Coricides, 2203·3
Panseptil, 2203·3
Pansoral, 2203·3
Pansporin, 2203·3
Pansteryl, 2203·3
Pan-Streptomycin, 2203·3
Pansulfox, 2203·3
Pan-Sun, 2203·3
Pantacid, 2203·3
Pantaflux, 2203·3
Pantasol, 2203·3
Pantec, 2203·3
Pantecta, 2203·3
Pantederm, 2203·3
Pantelmin, 2203·3
Pantenil, 2203·3
Panteston, 2203·3
Pantestone, 2203·3
Pantethine, 978·3
Pantetina, 978·3, 2203·3
Pantevit, 2203·3
Panthenol, 1727·2, 2203·4
*dl*-Panthenol, 1727·2
Panther Cap, 1717·3
Panthisone, 2203·4
Panthoderm, 2203·4
Panthoderm-A, 2203·4
Panthogenat, 2203·4
Pantiban, 2203·4
Pantinol, 2203·4
Panto, 2203·4
Panto Liquid, 2203·4
Pantobamin, 2203·4
Pantobionta, 2203·4
Pantobron, 2203·4
Pantoc, 2203·4
Pantocal, 2203·4
Pantocarm, 2203·4
Pantocide, 1181·2
Pantocrinale, 2203·4
Pantocycline, 2203·4
Pantodac, 2203·4
Pantodrin, 2203·4
Pantogar, 2203·4
Pantok, 2203·4
Pantolax, 2203·4
Pantoloc, 2203·4
Pantometil, 2203·4
Pantomicina, 2203·4
Pantomin, 2203·4
Pantomucol, 2204·1
Pantonate, 2204·1
Pantop, 2204·1
PantoPAC, 2204·1
Pantopan, 2204·1
Pantopaz, 2204·1
Pantopept, 2204·1
Pantoprazol, 1283·1
Pantoprazole, 1283·1
Pantoprazole Sodium, 1283·1
Pantoprazole Sodium Sesquihydrate, 1283·1
Pantorc, 2204·1
Pantosin, 2204·1
Pantostin, 2204·1
Pantotenato de Calcio, 1442·3
Pantoténico, Ácido, 1442·3
Pantothen, 2204·1
Pantothenic Acid, 1442·3
D-Pantothenic Acid, 1727·3
Pantothenol, 1727·2
±-Pantothenyl Alcohol, 1727·2
Pantovigar N, 2204·1
Pantovit, 2204·1
Pantovit Vital, 2204·1
Pantozol, 2204·1
Pantozol-Rifun, 2204·1
Pantricine, 2204·1
Pantrop, 2204·1
Pantus, 2204·1
Pantyson, 2204·1
Panverm, 2204·1
Panvermin, 2204·1
Panvit, 2204·1
Panvitan-M, 2204·1
Panvitina BC, 2204·1
Panvitrop, 2204·1
Panwarfin, 2204·1
Panxeol, 2204·2
Panzid, 2204·2
Panzimine, 2204·2
Panzynorm, 2204·2
Panzynorm Forte-N, 2204·2
Panzynorm-N, 2204·2
Panzytrat, 2204·2
Papain, 1727·3
Papaína, 1727·3
Papaine, 2204·2
Papase, 2204·2
Papasine, 2204·2
Papatropin, 2204·2
*Papaver rhoeas*, 1058·1
*Papaver somniferum*, 74·3, 1129·1, 1733·3
Papaveretum, 74·3
Papaverina, 1728·1
Papaverina, Hidrocloruro de, 1728·1
Papaverine, 1728·1
Papaverine Codecarboxylase Derivative, 1728·2
Papaverine Cromesilate, 1728·2
Papaverine Hydrobromide, 1728·2
Papaverine Hydrochloride, 1728·1
Papaverine Monophosadenine, 1728·2
Papaverine Nicotinate, 1728·2
Papaverine Sulfate, 1728·2
Papaverine Teprosilate, 1728·2
Papaverini Hydrochloridum, 1728·1
Papaverinii Chloridum, 1728·1
Papaverinium Chloride, 1728·1
Papaveris Capsula, 1129·1
Papaveris, Oleum, 1733·3
Papaveris Rhoeados Flos, 1058·1
Papaveris Seminis, Oleum, 1733·3
Papaya, 1671·1
Papaya Enzyme, 2204·2
Papaya Plus, 2204·2
Papayasanit-N, 2204·2
Papayotin, 1727·3
Papenzima, 2204·2
Papilo Lisin, 2204·2
Papoose Root, 1661·2
Paprika, 1056·1, 1667·1
Paps, 2204·2
Papulex, 2204·2
Papytazyme, 2204·2
Par, 2204·2
Par Glycerol, 2204·2
Para, 1728·3, 2204·2
Para Lentes, 2204·2
Para Piojicida, 2204·2
Para Plus, 2204·2
Para Repulsif, 2204·2
Para Special Poux, 2204·2
Para Z Mol, 2204·2
Para-aminobenzoic Acid, 1142·2
Para-aminohippuric Acid, 1653·2
Para-aminosalicylic Acid, 154·3
Parabenos, 1183·2
Parabens, 1183·2
Parabowl, 2204·3
Parabromdylamine Maleate, 426·1
Paracalcin, 1462·1
Paracap, 2204·3
Paracare, 2204·3
Paracefan, 2204·3
Paracet, 2204·3
Paracet Comp, 2204·3
Paracetacod, 2204·3
Paracetaldehyde, 713·1
Paracetamol, 76·2
Paracetamol Comp, 2204·3
Paracetamol Plus, 2204·3
Paracetamol-aspirin Ester, 20·3
Paracetamolum, 76·2
Paracetophenetidin, 82·2
Paracets, 2204·3
Paracets Cold Relief, 2204·3
Paracets Plus, 2204·3
Parachloramine Hydrochloride, 436·3
Parachlorometacresol, 1177·1
Parachlorometaxylenol, 1177·2
Parachlorophenol, 1187·3
Parachlorophenol, Camphorated, 1187·3
Parachlorophenylalanine, 1687·2
Parachoc, 2204·3
Paracin, 2204·3
Paraclear, 2204·3
Paraclim, 2204·3
Paraclorofenol, 1187·3
Paracne, 2204·3
Paracoccidioidomycosis, 389·1
Paracod, 2204·3
Paracodin, 2204·3
Paracodin N, 2204·3
Paracodin Retard, 2204·3
Paracodina, 2204·3
Paracodine, 2204·4
Paracodol, 2204·4
Paractol, 2204·4
Paradenton, 2204·4
Paraderm, 2204·4
Paraderm Plus, 2204·4
Paradex, 2204·4
Paradichlorobenzene, 1728·3
Paradiclorobenceno, 1728·3
Parador, 2204·4
Paradote, 2204·4
Paradrine, 2204·4
Paradroxil, 2204·4
Paradryl med Efedrin, 2204·4
Parafenilendiamina, 1728·3
Paraff. Dur., 1479·1
Paraff. Liq. Lev., 1479·1
Paraff. Moll. Alb., 1479·3
Paraff. Moll. Flav., 1479·3
Paraffin, 1475·1, 1479·1
Paraffin, Dickflüssiges, 1479·1
Paraffin, Dünnflüssiges, 1479·1
Paraffin, Hard, 1479·1
Paraffin, Light Liquid, 1479·2
Paraffin, Liquid, 1479·1
Paraffin, Liquid, Light, 1479·1
Paraffin, Spray, 1479·1
Paraffin, Synthetic, 1479·1
Paraffin Wax, 1479·1
Paraffin, White Soft, 1479·3
Paraffin, Yellow Soft, 1479·3
Paraffins and Similar Bases, 1479·1
Paraffinum Durum, 1479·1
Paraffinum Liquidum, 1479·1
Paraffinum Liquidum Leve, 1479·1
Paraffinum Liquidum Tenue, 1479·1
Paraffinum Molle Album, 1479·3
Paraffinum Molle Flavum, 1479·3
Paraffinum Perliquidum, 1479·1
Paraffinum Solidum, 1479·1
Paraffinum Subliquidum, 1479·1
Parafina Líquida, 1479·1
Parafina Sólida, 1479·1
Paraflex, 2204·4
Paraflex AN, 2204·4
Paraflex Comp, 2204·4
Paraflex Crema, 2204·4
Paraflex Plus, 2204·4
Para-fluorofentanyl, 40·3
Parafon, 2204·4
Parafon DSC, 2204·4
Parafon Forte, 2204·4
Parafon Forte C8, 2204·4
Parafon Forte DSC, 2204·4
Paraform, 1187·3
Paraformaldehído, 1187·3
Paraformaldehyde, 1187·3
Paraformic Aldehyde, 1187·3
Paragar, 2204·4
Paragard T380A, 2205·1
Paragel, 2205·1
Paraghurt, 2205·1
Paragip, 2205·1
Paragol N, 2205·1
Paragonimiasis— *see* Lung Fluke Infections, 99·3
Paragrippe, 2205·1
Paraguay Tea, 1765·3
Parahexal, 2205·1
Parahidroxibenzoato de Bencilo, 1183·2
Para-Hist HD, 2205·1
Parahydroxybenzoate Phenoxyethanol, 1195·3
Parahypon, 2205·1
Parakapton, 2205·1
Parake, 2205·1
Paral, 2205·1
Paraldehído, 713·1
Paraldehyde, 713·1
Paraldehydum, 713·1
Paralergin, 2205·1
Paralgen, 2205·1
Paralgesic, 2205·1
Paralgin, 2205·1
Paralice, 2205·1
Paralief, 2205·1
Paralink, 2205·1
Paralon, 2205·1
Paralymphine, 2205·1
Paralyoc, 2205·1
Paralysis Agitans— *see* Parkinsonism, 1196·1
Paralysis, Hyperkalaemic Periodic— *see* Hyperkalaemic Periodic Paralysis, 1219·3
Paralysis, Hypokalaemic Periodic— *see* Hypokalaemic Periodic Paralysis, 1220·1
Paralysis, Hysterical— *see* Conversion and Dissociative Disorders, 696·2
Paralysis, Sleep— *see* Narcoleptic Syndrome, 1583·2
Paralytic Ileus— *see* Decreased Gastrointestinal Motility, 1241·1
Paramax, 2205·1
Paramet, 2205·1
Parametasona, Acetato de, 1107·3
Paramethasone Acetate, 1107·3
Paramethasone Disodium Phosphate, 1107·3
Paramettes, 2205·1
Paramin, 2205·1
Paraminan, 2205·1

Paramine, 2205·1
Paraminol, 2205·1
Paramol, 2205·2
Paramol Forte, 2205·2
Paramol TP, 2205·2
Paramolan, 2205·2
Paramolan C, 2205·2
*Paramyxovirus parotitidis*, 1626·3
Paranal, 2205·2
Paranal-L, 2205·2
Paranorm, 2205·2
Paranthil, 2205·2
Paranzol, 2205·2
Paraoxon, 1494·1
Parapaed, 2205·2
Parapenzolate Bromide, 487·2
Paraphenylenediamine, 1728·3
Paraphilias— *see* Disturbed Behaviour, 665·1
Para-Pio, 2205·2
Paraplatin, 2205·2
Paraplatine, 2205·2
Para-plus, 2205·2
Parapres, 2205·2
Parapres Plus, 2205·2
Parapsyllium, 2205·2
Paraquat, 1508·1
Paraquat Dichloride, 1508·1
Paraqueimol, 2205·2
Pararosaniline Hydrochloride, 1185·1
Parartrin, 2205·2
Paras, 2205·2
Parasidose, 2205·2
Parasimed, 2205·2
Parasin, 2205·2
Parasomnias, 667·3
Parasone, 2205·2
Para-Speciaal, 2205·2
Para-Suppo, 2205·3
Parasympatholytics, 475·1
Parasympathomimetics, 1484·1
Parat, 2205·3
Paratabs, 2205·3
Para-Tabs, 2205·3
Parathion, 1508·2
Parathormone, 774·3
1-34 Parathormone (Human), 775·2
Parathyrin, 774·3
Parathyroid Hormone, 774·3
Parathyroid Hormone (1-34), Human, 775·2
Parathyroid Hormone Peptide (1-34), 775·2
Paratión, 1508·2
Paratirina, 774·3
Paratol, 2205·3
Paratoluendiamina, 1728·3
Paratoluenediamine, 1728·3
Paratosse, 2205·3
Paratral, 2205·3
Paratropina, 2205·3
Paratropina Compuesta, 2205·3
Paratulle, 2205·3
Paratyphoid Fever— *see* Typhoid and Paratyphoid Fever, 152·2
Paraverm, 2205·3
Paravertebral LWS, 2205·3
Paraxanthine, 783·1
Paraxin, 2205·3
Paraxin Ear, 2205·3
Parcaine, 2205·3
Parcel, 2205·3
Parche Leon Fortificante, 2205·3
Parconazol, Hidrocloruro de, 407·3
Parconazole Hydrochloride, 407·3
Parcono, 2205·3
Pardelprin, 2205·3
Pa-Real, 2205·3
Parecid, 2205·3
Parecoxib Sódico, 79·2
Parecoxib Sodium, 79·2
Paredrine, 2205·3
Paregorico, Elixir— *see* Elixir Paregorico, 1965·4
Paregorique, 2205·3
Parelmin, 2205·3
Paremyd, 2205·3
Parenchymal Lung Disease, Diffuse— *see* Diffuse Parenchymal Lung Disease, 1079·3
Parencias, 2205·3
Parenciclina, 2205·3
Parengesico, 2205·3
Parentamin Preparations, 2205·3
Parenteral, 2205·4
Parenteral BG, 2205·4
Parenteral BX, 2205·4
Parenteral EK Cal GX, 2205·4
Parenteral EK G, 2205·4
Parenteral EK X, 2205·4
Parenteral G, 2205·4
Parenteral HG, 2205·4
Parenteral HX, 2205·4
Parenteral K10, 2205·4
Parenteral NS, 2205·4
Parenteral Nutrition, 1418·2
Parenteral OP, 2205·4
Parenteral X, 2205·4
Parenterin, 2205·4
Parentrovite, 1455·2
Parenzyme, 2205·4
Parenzyme Ampicilina, 2205·4
Parenzyme Analgesico, 2205·4
Parenzyme Tetraciclina, 2205·4
Parethoxycaine Hydrochloride, 1382·2
Paretoxicaína, Hidrocloruro de, 1382·2
Parexel, 2205·4
Par-F, 2205·4
Parfenac, 2205·4
Parfenac Basisbad, 2205·4
Parfenal, 2205·4
Par-Gamma, 2205·4
Pargeverine Hydrochloride, 487·3
Pargilina, Hidrocloruro de, 978·3
Pargin, 2205·4
Pargine, 2206·1
Pargitan, 2206·1
Pargo, 2206·1
Pargyline Hydrochloride, 978·3
Paricalcitol, 1462·1
Pariet, 2206·1
Parilac, 2206·1
Parinix, 2206·1
Paritrel, 2206·1
Parizac, 2206·1
Parkadina, 2206·1
Parkelase, 2206·1
Parkelase Chloromycetin, 2206·1
Parkemed, 2206·1
Parkexin, 2206·1
Parkinane, 2206·1
Parkinsan, 2206·1
Parkinsol, 2206·1
Parkinsonism, 1196·1
Parkinson's Disease— *see* Parkinsonism, 1196·1
Parkipan, 2206·1
Parkopan, 2206·1
Parkotil, 2206·1
Parks, 2206·1
Parlax, 2206·1
Parlib, 2206·1
Parlide, 2206·1
Parlodel, 2206·1
Parmecal, 2206·2
Parmentier, 2206·2
Parmid, 2206·2
Parmodalin, 2206·2
Parmol, 2206·2
Parnaparin Sodium, 978·3
Parnaparina Sódica, 978·3
Parnaparinum Natricum, 978·3
Par-Natal Plus 1 Improved, 2206·2
Parnate, 2206·2
Parnoxil, 2206·2
Paro, 2206·2
Parocin, 2206·2
Parodium, 2206·2
Parodontal, 2206·2
Parodontal F5 Med, 2206·2
Parodontax, 2206·2
Paroex, 2206·2
Parogencyl, 2206·2
Parogencyl Anti-age Gencives, 2206·2
Parogencyl Bi-Actif, 2206·2
Parogencyl Gencives Fragilisees, 2206·2
Parogencyl Sensibilite Gencives, 2206·2
Parol, 2206·2
Paromomicina, Sulfato de, 612·3
Paromomycin Sulfate, 612·3
Paromomycin Sulphate, 612·3
Paronal, 2206·3
Paroplak, 2206·3
Parotiditis, Prueba Cutánea Contra El Antígeno de la, 1717·2
Paroven, 2206·3
Parox, 2206·3
Parox Meltab, 2206·3
Paroxat, 2206·3
Paroxedura, 2206·3
Paroxetina, Hidrocloruro de, 311·2
Paroxetine, 311·2
Paroxetine Hydrochloride, 311·2
Paroxetine Hydrochloride Hemihydrate, 311·2
Paroxetine Mesilate, 311·2
Paroxetine Mesylate, 311·2
Paroxetini Hydrochloridum Hemihydricum, 311·2
Paroxysmal Atrial Tachycardia— *see* Cardiac Arrhythmias, 816·1
Paroxysmal Hemicrania, Chronic— *see* Cluster Headache, 464·1
Paroxysmal Polyserositis— *see* Familial Mediterranean Fever, 416·2
Paroxysmal Supraventricular Tachycardia— *see* Cardiac Arrhythmias, 816·1
Parsal, 2206·3
Parsel, 2206·3
Parsilid, 2206·3
Parsimonil, 2206·3
Parsistene, 2206·3
Parsitan, 2206·3
Parsley, 1728·3
Parsley Piert, 1729·1
Parsol 1789, 1142·3
Parsol MCX, 1154·3
Parstelin, 2206·3
Partamol, 2206·3
Partane, 2206·3
Parthenolide, 469·2
Partial Seizures— *see* Epilepsy, 349·1
Partial Status Epilepticus— *see* Status Epilepticus, 352·1
Partially Hydrated Magnesium Chloride, 1228·1
Partoben, 2206·3
Partobulin, 2206·3
Partocon, 2206·3
Partogamma, 2206·3
Parto-Gamma, 2206·3
Partogamma-T, 2206·3
Partusisten, 2206·3
Partuss LA, 2206·3
Parulon, 2206·3
Paruman, 2206·3
Parvisedil, 2206·3
Parvlex, 2206·4
Parvodex, 2206·4
Parvolex, 2206·4
Parvon, 2206·4
Parvon Forte, 2206·4
Parvon-N, 2206·4
Parvon-Spas, 2206·4
PAS, 154·3
Pas Hain, 2206·4
Pasaden, 2206·4
Pasalen, 2206·4
Pasalicylum, 154·3
Pasalicylum Solubile, 155·1
Pasalix, 2206·4
Pascalium, 2206·4
Pascallerg, 2206·4
Pascobilin Novo, 2206·4
Pascodolor Tropfen, 2206·4
Pascofemin, 2206·4
Pascohepan Novo, 2206·4
Pascoletten N, 2206·4
Pascoleucyn, 2206·4
Pascolibrin, 2206·4
Pascomag, 2206·4
Pascomucil, 2206·4
Pasconal Forte Nerventropfen, 2206·4
Pasconal Nerventropfen, 2206·4
Pasconeural-Injektopas, 2206·4
Pascopankreat, 2206·4
Pascopankreat Novo, 2206·4
Pascopankreat S, 2207·1
Pascorenal, 2207·1
Pascosabal, 2207·1
Pascosedon, 2207·1
Pascotox, 2207·1
Pascotox Forte-Injektopas, 2207·1
Pascotox Mono, 2207·1
Pascovegeton, 2207·1
Pascovenol Novo, 2207·1
Pasedon, 2207·1
Pasem, 2207·1
Paser, 2207·1
Pas-Fatol N, 2207·1
Pasgensin, 2207·1
Pasifen, 2207·1
Pasiflora, 1729·1
Pasil, 2207·1
Pasiniazid, 224·2
Pasionari, 1729·1
Pasisana, 2207·1
Pasivital H, 2207·1
Pasmalgin, 2207·1
Pasminox, 2207·1
Pasminox Somatico, 2207·1
Pasmocalm, 2207·1
Pasmodil, 2207·1
Pasmodina, 2207·1
Pasmolit, 2207·1
Pasmosedan, 2207·1
Pasmosedan Compuesto, 2207·1
Pasmovit, 2207·1
Paspat, 2207·1
Paspat Oral, 2207·2
Paspertase, 2207·2
Paspertin, 2207·2
Pasque Flower, 1737·1
Pasrin, 2207·2
Passacanthine, 2207·2
Passagen, 2207·2
Passaja, 2207·2
Passaneuro, 2207·2
Passedan, 2207·2
Passedyl, 2207·2
Passelyt, 2207·2
Passi Catha, 2207·2
Passicalm, 2207·2
Passicarbone, 2207·2
Passiflora, 1729·1, 2207·2
Passiflora Complex, 2207·2
Passiflora Compose, 2207·2
Passiflora Composta, 2207·2
Passiflora Compound, 2207·2
Passiflora Curarina, 2207·2
Passiflora GHL, 2207·2
Passiflorae Herba, 1729·1
Passiflorin, 2207·2
Passiflorine, 2207·3
Passifuril, 2207·3
Passilex, 2207·3
Passilin, 2207·3
Passin, 2207·3
Passinevryl, 2207·3
Passion Flower, 1729·1
Passionflower Plus, 2207·3
Passiorin N, 2207·3
Passive Immunisation, 1605·1
Past Ail, 2207·3
Pasta, 1373·3
Pasta Arsenicale, 2207·3
Pasta Boli, 2207·3
Pasta Cool, 2207·3
Pasta d'Agua, 2207·3
Pasta de Lassar, 2207·3
Pasta Dermic, 2207·3
Pasta Devitalizzante, 2207·3
Pasta Dicofarm, 2207·3
Pasta Lactisol, 2207·3
Pasta Lassar, 2207·3

Pasta Lassar Imba, 2207·3
Pasta Lassar Orravan, 2207·3
Pasta Rubra Salicylata, 2207·3
Pastiglie Valda, 2207·3
Pastilhas Valda, 2207·3
Pastillas Antisep Garg L, 2207·3
Pastillas Antisep Garg M, 2207·3
Pastillas Dr Andreu, 2207·3
Pastillas Juanola, 2207·4
Pastillas Koki Ment Tiro, 2207·4
Pastillas Lorbi, 2207·4
Pastillas Medex, 2207·4
Pastillas Pectoral Kely, 2207·4
Pastilles d'Ems, 2207·4
Pastilles Medicinales Vicks, 2207·4
Pastilles Monleon, 2207·4
Pastilles Pectorales Demo N, 2207·4
Pastilles Pectorales Formule 541, 2207·4
Pastilles pour la Gorge No 535, 2207·4
Pastilles Valda, 2207·4
Pastimmun, 2207·4
Pasuma-Dragees, 2207·4
Patanol, 2207·4
Pat-Chobet, 2207·4
Pate a l'Eau Roche-Posay, 2207·4
Pate d'Unna, 2207·4
Pate Iodoforme du Prof Dr Walkhoff, 2207·4
Patecs A, New— *see* New Patecs A, 2165·4
Patector, 2207·4
Patent Blue V, 1729·1, 1750·3
Patent Blue AC, 1056·2
Patent Ductus Arteriosus, 49·2
Patentex, 2207·4
Patentex Oval, 2207·4
Patentex Oval N, 2207·4
Pates Pectorales, 2207·4
Pathilon, 2207·4
Pathocil, 2208·1
Patient-controlled Analgesia, 3·3
Patriot, 2208·1
Patropin, 2208·1
Patsolin, 2208·1
Patuxan, 2208·1
Patxen, 2208·1
Paucimycin Sulphate, 612·3
*Paullinia cupana*, 1765·3
Pausafren T, 2208·1
Pausanol, 2208·1
Pausedal, 2208·1
Pausene, 2208·1
Pausigin, 2208·1
*Pausinystalia yohimbe*, 1766·2
PAVA, 67·2
Pavabid, 2208·1
Pa-Vaccinol, 2208·1
Pavacol-D, 2208·1
Pavedal, 2208·1
Paveriwern, 2208·1
Pavertrin, 2208·1
Paverysat Forte N, 2208·1
Pavitron, 2208·1
Pavot, Fruit du, 1129·1
Pavulon, 2208·1
Pawa-Rutan, 2208·1
Pax, 2208·1
Paxadorm, 2208·1
Paxam, 2208·1
Paxapride, 2208·1
Paxarel, 2208·1
Paxate, 2208·1
Paxel, 2208·1
Paxeladine, 2208·1
Paxeladine Noctee, 2208·1
Paxene, 2208·2
Paxetil, 2208·2
Paxical, 2208·2
Paxidal, 2208·2
Paxidorm, 2208·2
Paxil, 2208·2
Paxilfar, 2208·2
Paxipam, 2208·2
Paxium, 2208·2
Paxon, 2208·2
Paxon-D, 2208·2
Paxtibi, 2208·2
Paxtine, 2208·2
Paxum, 2208·2
Paxxet, 2208·2
Paxyl, 2208·2
Payasanit Gastro, 2208·2
*Payena*, 1696·2
Pazbronquial, 2208·2
Pazo, 2208·2
Pazolam, 2208·2
Pazolini, 2208·2
Pazucross, 2208·2
Pazufloxacin Mesilate, 241·3
PB-005, 1566·1
PB-89, 1121·3
P-4657B, 725·2
PB Gel, 2208·2
PBB, 1501·3
PBZ, 2208·2
PC 30 N, 2208·3
PC 30 V, 2208·3
PC-1020, 1156·1
PC-1421, 716·1
PC Arthri-Spray, 2208·3
PC Regulax, 2208·3
PC Rei-shi, 2208·3
PCB, 1501·3
PCC, 1730·3
PC-Cap, 2208·3
PCDDs, 1681·1
PCDFs, 1681·1
PCE, 1730·3, 2208·3
PCF N, 2208·3
PCL, 2208·3
PCM, 2208·3
PCMC, 1177·1
PCMX, 1177·2
PCP, 1508·3, 1730·3
PCP— *see* Pneumocystis Carinii Pneumonia, 389·1
PCR-4099, 888·3
PC-SPES, 522·1
PD-93, 244·1
PD-81565, 579·2
PD-107779, 207·2
PD-110843, 384·3
PD-127391, 194·2
PD Cough, 2208·3
PDB, 488·2
PD-135711-15B, 361·3
PDDB, 1179·1
PDF, 2208·3
PDP Liquid Protein, 2208·3
Peace, 2208·3
Peace Pills, 1730·3
Peace Weed, 1730·3
Peacef, 2208·3
Peacetime, 2208·3
Peach Kernel Oil, 1730·2
Peanut Oil, 1656·1
Pebegal, 2208·3
PEC, 2208·3
Pecasolin, 2208·3
Pe-Ce, 2208·3
Pe-Ce Ven N, 2208·3
Pect Hustenloser, 2208·3
Pectal, 2208·3
Pectalin, 2208·3
Pectamol, 2208·3
Pectapas, 2208·3
Pectikon— *see* Betapect, 1838·3
Pectimax, 2208·3
Pectin, 1580·3
Pectina, 1580·3
Pectin-K, 2208·3
Pecto-Baby, 2208·4
Pectobal Dextro, 2208·4
Pectobron, 2208·4
Pectocalmine, 2208·4
Pectocalmine Junior N, 2208·4
Pectocor N, 2208·4
Pectoderme, 2208·4
Pectodrill, 2208·4
Pectoids, 2208·4
Pectojuvene, 2208·4
Pectomucil, 2208·4
Pectoral, 2208·4
Pectoral Brum, 2208·4
Pectoral Edulcor— *see* Codedrill, 1896·4
Pectoral Funk Antitus, 2208·4
Pectoral Hebert, 2208·4
Pectoral Kely, Pastillas— *see* Pastillas Pectoral Kely, 2207·4
Pectoral N, 2208·4
Pectoral Pagliano, 2208·4
Pectoral Pasteur, 2208·4
Pectorina, 2208·4
Pectosan Preparations, 2208·4
Pectoserum, 2208·4
Pectosorin, 2209·1
Pectoss, 2209·1
Pectothymin, 2209·1
Pectotussyl, 2209·1
Pectover, 2209·1
Pectox, 2209·1
Pectox Ampicilina, 2209·1
Pectramin, 2209·1
Pectrolyte, 2209·1
Pectyl, 2209·1
Pedameth, 2209·1
Ped-El, 2209·1
Ped-Element, 2209·1
PediaCare Preparations, 2209·1
Pediacel, 2209·1
Pediacof, 2209·1
Pedia-Col, 2209·1
Pediacon DX, 2209·1
Pediacon EX, 2209·1
Pediaderm, 2209·1
Pediaflor, 2209·2
Pedialyte, 2209·2
Pediamino PLM, 2209·2
PediaPatch, Trans-Ver-Sal— *see* Trans-Ver-Sal PediaPatch, 2341·2
Pediapirin, 2209·2
Pediapred, 2209·2
Pediaprofen, 2209·2
Pediaprofen— *see* Motrin, 2141·2
Pediarix, 2209·2
PediaSure, 2209·2
Pediatex, 2209·2
Pediatex-D, 2209·2
Pediatex-DM, 2209·2
Pedia-Tric, 2209·2
Pediatric, 2209·2
Pediatric Cough Syrup, 2209·2
Pediatric Electrolyte, 2209·2
Pediatric Formula, 2209·2
Pediatrivite, 2209·2
Pediatrix, 2209·2
Pediazole, 2209·2
Pedi-Bath, 2209·2
Pedi-Boro Soak Paks, 2209·2
Pedic, 2209·2
Pedi-Cort V, 2209·2
Pedicrem, 2209·2
Pediculosis, 1499·1
Pedi-Dent, 2209·2
Pedi-Dri, 2209·2
Pedifan, 2209·2
Pedigesic, 2209·2
Pedikurol, 2209·3
Pedil, 2209·3
Pediletan, 2209·3
Pedimed, 2209·3
Pediotic, 2209·3
Pediox, 2209·3
Pedi-Pro, 2209·3
Pediron, 2209·3
Pedisafe, 2209·3
Pedisol, 2209·3
Peditrace, 2209·3
Peditral, 2209·3
Pedituss Cough, 2209·3
Pedi-Vit-A, 2209·3
Pedoc, 2209·3
Pedopur, 2209·3
Pedoz, 2209·3
Pedpain, 2209·3
Pedriachol, 2209·3
PedTE-PAK, 2209·3
Pedtrace, 2209·3
PedvaxHIB, 2209·3
Pedvitin, 2209·3
PeeHoo, 2209·3
Peerless Composition Essence, 2209·4
Peetalix, Chemists Own— *see* Chemists Own Peetalix, 1882·1
Pefamic, 2209·4
Pefbid, 2209·4
Peflacin, 2209·4
Peflacina, 2209·4
Peflacine, 2209·4
Peflox, 2209·4
Pefloxacin Mesilate, 241·3
Pefloxacin Mesilate Dihydrate, 241·3
Pefloxacin Mesylate, 241·3
Pefloxacini Mesilas Dihydricus, 241·3
Pefloxacino, Mesilato de, 241·3
Pefloxidina, 2209·4
Pefrakehl, 2209·4
Pega, 2209·4
Pegacaristim, 760·2
PEG-ADA, 1729·2
Pegademasa, 1729·2
Pegademase, 1729·2
PEG-Adenosine Deaminase, 1729·2
Pegaldesleukin, 563·3
Peganix, 2209·4
Peganone, 2209·4
Peganum, 1696·3
*Peganum harmala*, 1696·3
PEG-L-asparaginase, 528·3
Pegaspargasa, 528·3
Pegaspargase, 528·3
Pegasys, 2209·4
Pegatron, 2209·4
Pegfilgrastim, 753·3
PEG-IL2, 563·3
Pegina, 2209·4
Peginterferon Alfa-2a, 640·3
Peginterferon Alfa-2b, 640·3
PegIntron, 2209·4
PEG-Intron— *see* Pegatron, 2209·4
Peglyte, 2209·4
PEG-megakaryocyte Growth and Development Factor, 760·2
PEG-MGDF, 760·2
Pegorgotein, 92·3
Pegorgoteína, 92·3
PEGs, 1708·2
PEG-SOD, 92·3
Pegvisomant, 1337·2
Pegylation, 1709·1
Peinfort, 2209·4
Peinka, 1666·1
Peitel, 2209·4
Peitoral Angico Pelotense, 2209·4
Pekamin, 2209·4
Peking Ginseng Royal Jelly N, 2209·4
Peking Royal Jelly N, 2209·4
Pekiron, 2209·4
Pel Cupron, 2209·4
Pelargon, 2209·4
Pelargonii, Aetheroleum, 1692·2
*Pelargonium*, 1692·2
Pelargonium Oil, 1692·2
Pelargonyl Vanillylamide, 67·2
Peldesina, 579·1
Peldesine, 579·1
Peledox, 2210·1
Pelicrep, 2210·1
Pelin, 1645·1
Pelina, 2210·1
Peliphane, 2210·1
Pellagra, 1442·1
Pellexeme, 2210·1
Pellidol, 1178·2
Pellit, 2210·1
Pellit Dermal Wund- und Heilsalbe, 2210·1
Pellit Insektenstich, 2210·1
Pellit Sonnenallergie— *see* Pellit Insektenstich, Pellit Sonnenallergie, 2210·1
Pellit Sonnenbrand, 2210·1
Pelmec, 2210·1
Pelmec Duo, 2210·1
Pelmic, 2210·1

Pelo Libre, 2210·1
Pelox, 2210·1
Pelsana Med, 2210·1
Pelsano, 2210·1
Pelsano— *see* Pelsana Med, 2210·1
Pelson, 2210·1
Peltazon, 2210·1
Pelvic Inflammatory Disease, 139·2
Pelvichthol, 2210·1
Pelvichthol N, 2210·1
Pelvo Magnesium, 2210·1
PemADD, 2210·1
Pemar, 2210·1
Pemazine Dimalonate, 713·3
Pemetrexed Disódico, 579·1
Pemetrexed Disodium, 579·1
Pemine, 2210·1
Pemirolast Potásico, 790·3
Pemirolast Potassium, 790·3
Pemix, 2210·2
PE-Mix, 2210·2
Pemol, 2210·2
Pemolina, 1591·2
Pemoline, 1591·2
Pemoline, Magnesium, 1592·1
Pemphigoid— *see* Pemphigus and Pemphigoid, 1137·1
Pemphigoid, Ocular Cicatricial— *see* Pemphigus and Pemphigoid, 1085·2
Pemphigus— *see* Pemphigus and Pemphigoid, 1137·1
Pemtumomab, 579·2
Pen, 2210·2
Pen Di Ben, 2210·2
Pen Mega, 2210·2
Pen Oral, 2210·2
Penaderm, 2210·2
Penadur, 2210·2
Penadur 6.3.3, 2210·2
Penagrand, 2210·2
Penalta, 2210·2
Penamox, 2210·2
Penamox M, 2210·2
Penanyst, 2210·2
Penaten, 2210·2
Penaten Crema Disinfettante, Johnson's— *see* Johnson's Penaten Crema Disinfettante, 2071·3
Penatoel, 2210·2
Penbaccin, 2210·2
Pen-BASF, 2210·2
Penbene, 2210·2
Penbeta, 2210·2
Penbritin, 2210·2
Penbutolol Hemisulfate, 979·1
Penbutolol Sulfate, 979·1
Penbutolol, Sulfato de, 979·1
Penbutolol Sulphate, 979·1
Penbutololi Sulfas, 979·1
Penciclovir, 651·2
Penclox, 2210·2
Pencom, 2210·2
Pencor, 2210·2
Pencotrex, 2210·2
Pendiben Compuesto, 2210·2
Pendine, 2210·2
Pendium, 2210·3
Pendramine, 2210·3
Pendysin, 2210·3
Penecare, 2210·3
Penecort, 2210·3
Penederm, 2210·3
Penedil, 2210·3
Penegra, 2210·3
Penek, 1666·1
Pener, 2210·3
Penetamato, Hidroioduro de, 242·1
Penethamate Hydriodide, 242·1
Penetran, 2210·3
Penetrating Rub, 2210·3
Penetrex, 2210·3
Penetro, 2210·3
Penfantil, 2210·3
Penfill Preparations, 2210·3
Penfluridol, 713·2
Pengesic, 2210·3
Pengesod, 2210·3
Penglobe, 2210·3
Penhexal, 2210·3
Penhexal VK, 2210·3
Penibiot, 2210·3
Penibiot Lidocaina, 2210·3
Penibrin, 2210·3
Penicigran, 2210·3
Penicil, 2210·3
Penicil Dermol, 2210·4
Penicilamina, 1046·3
Penicilina-benetamina, 162·3
Penicillamine, 1046·3
D-Penicillamine, 1046·3
Penicillaminum, 1046·3
Penicillanic Acid 1,1-Dioxide, 257·2
Penicillanoyloxymethyl (6*R*)-6-(D-2-Phenylglycylamino)penicillanate *S'*,*S'*-Dioxide, 264·2
Penicillat, 2210·4
Penicillenic Acid, 163·3
Penicillin, 163·2
Penicillin 356, 198·1
Penicillin B, 242·1
Penicillin F, 118·3
Penicillin Fortified, 2210·4
Penicillin G, 163·2
Penicillin G Benzathine, 162·3
Penicillin G Clemizole, 194·1
Penicillin G Potassium, 163·2
Penicillin G Procaine, 246·1
Penicillin G Sodium, 163·2
Penicillin K, 118·3
Penicillin, Phenoxymethyl, 242·1
Penicillin V, 242·1
Penicillin V Benzathine, 163·2
Penicillin V Calcium, 242·1
Penicillin V Potassium, 242·1
Penicillin X, 118·3
Penicillinase, 118·3
Penicillinase-resistant Penicillins, 118·3
Penicillins, 118·3
Penicillins, Natural, 118·3
Penicillins, Penicillinase-resistant, 118·3
Penicillins, Semisynthetic, 118·3
*Penicillium chrysogenum*, 118·3
*Penicillium citrinum*, 958·1
*Penicillium griseofulvum*, 400·3
*Penicillium notatum*, 118·3, 163·2, 242·1
*Penicillium stoloniferum*, 1362·2
Penicilloic Acid, 163·3
Penicilloyl-polylysine, 1729·2
Peniciloil Polilisina, 1729·2
Penicina, 2210·4
Penidural, 2210·4
Penidural D/F, 2210·4
Penidure, 2210·4
Penilan, 2210·4
Penilente Forte, 2210·4
Penilente LA, 2210·4
Penilevel, 2210·4
Penilevel Retard, 2210·4
Penilfedrin P, 2210·4
Penillic Acid, 163·3
Penimox, 2210·4
Peni-Oral, 2210·4
Penipot, 2210·4
Peniroger, 2210·4
Penisintex Bronquial, 2210·4
Penisodina, 2210·4
Penisol, 2210·4
Penka, 1666·1
Penkaron, 2210·4
Pen-Kera, 2210·4
Penlac, 2210·4
Penles, 2210·4
Penlol, 2210·4
PenMix, 2210·4
Penmox, 2210·4
Pennsaid, 2211·1
Pennsylvanian Sumach, 1738·1
Penntuss, 2211·1
Pennyroyal, 1736·1
Pennyroyal Oil, 1736·1
Pennywort, Indian, 1144·3
Pen-Os, 2211·1
Penotran, 2211·1
Penoxil V, 2211·1
Penprocilina, 2211·1
Penrazol, 2211·1
Penrazole, 2211·1
Penrite, 2211·1
Pensodital, 2211·1
Penstad, 2211·1
Penstapho, 2211·1
Penstaphon, 2211·1
Pensulan, 2211·1
Pensulvit, 2211·1
Penta, 1508·3
Penta 500, 2211·1
Penta-3B, 2211·1
Penta-3B + C, 2211·1
Penta-3B Plus, 2211·1
Pentabil, 2211·1
Pentacard, 2211·1
Pentacarinat, 2211·1
Pentacel, 2211·1
3,3',5,5',6-Pentachloro-2'-hydroxysalicylanilide, 111·2
Pentachlorophenol, 1508·3
Pentachlorophenol Sodium, 1508·3
Pentacine, 2211·1
Pentacis, 2211·1
Pentaclorofenol, 1508·3
Pentacol, 2211·1
Pentacoq, 2211·1
Pentacort, 2211·2
Pentacrom, 2211·2
Pentact, 2211·2
Pentact-HIB, 2211·2
Pentadecan, 2211·2
Pentadent, 2211·2
Pentaderm, 2211·2
Pentaerithrityl Tetranitrate, 979·1
Pentaerithrityl Tetranitrate, Diluted, 979·2
Pentaerithrityl Trinitrate, 979·2
Pentaerithrityli Tetranitras, 979·1
Pentaeritritilo, Tetranitrato de, 979·1
Pentaeritritol, 1283·2
Pentaerythritol, 1283·2
Pentaerythritol Tetranicotinate, 965·3
Pentaerythritol Tetranitrate, 979·1
Pentaerythritolum Tetranitricum, 979·1
Pentafluoroisopropenyl Fluoromethyl Ether, 1308·1
Pentafluoromethoxy Isopropyl Fluoromethyl Ether, 1308·1
7α-[9-(4,4,5,5,5-Pentafluoropentylsulfinyl)nonyl]estra-1,3,5(10)-triene-3,17β-diol, 557·3
Pentafresh, 2211·2
Pentafuside, 633·1
Pentagastrin, 1729·3
Pentagastrina, 1729·3
Pentagin, 2211·2
Pentaglobin, 2211·2
Pentaglucano, 2211·2
3,3',4',5,7-Pentahydroxyflavone, 1688·2
(2*S*,16*Z*,18*E*,20*S*,21*S*,22*R*,23*R*,24*R*,25*S*,26*S*,27*S*,28*E*)-5,6,21,23,25-Pentahydroxy-27-methoxy-2,4,11,16,20,22,24,26-octamethyl-2,7-(epoxypentadeca[1,11,13]trienimino)benzofuro[4,5-*e*]pyrido[1,2-*a*]benzimidazole-1,15(2*H*)-dione 25-Acetate, 254·1
Pentakis ($N^2$-Acetyl-L-glutaminato)tetrahydroxytrialuminium, 1248·1
3,3',4',5,7-Pentakis(benzyloxy)flavone, 1688·2
Pental Forte, 2211·2
Pentalgina, 2211·2
Pentalmicina, 2211·2
Pentalong, 2211·2
Pentam, 2211·2
Pentamethazene Bromide, 866·2
Pentamethazol, 1592·1
4,4'-(Pentamethylenedioxy)dibenzamidine Bis(2-hydroxyethanesulphonate), 613·2
1,5-Pentamethylenetetrazole, 1592·1
Pentamethylmelamine, 526·3
Pentamethylpararosaniline Hydrochloride, 1186·2
Pentamicina, 407·3
Pentamidina, Isetionato de, 613·2
Pentamidina, Mesilato de, 613·2
Pentamidine Diisetionate, 613·2
Pentamidine Dimethanesulphonate, 613·2
Pentamidine Dimethylsulphonate, 613·2
Pentamidine Isethionate, 613·2
Pentamidine Isetionate, 613·2
Pentamidine Mesilate, 613·2
Pentamidine Mesylate, 613·2
Pentamidine Methanesulphonate, 613·2
Pentamidini Diisetionas, 613·2
Pentamidini Isethionas, 613·2
Pentamina, 2211·2
Pentaminum, 866·2
Pentamol, 2211·2
Pentamycetin, 2211·2
Pentamycetin-HC, 2211·2
Pentamycin, 407·3
Pentanedial, 1180·3
Pentane-1,5-dial, 1180·3
Pentanitrol, 979·1
Pentanolis Nitris, 1032·1
*N*-Pentanoyl-*N*-[2'-(1*H*-tetrazol-5-yl)biphenyl-4-ylmethyl]-L-valine, 1018·3
Pentasa, 2211·2
Pentasodium Colistinmethanesulfonate, 199·1
Pentaspan, 2211·2
Pentastarch, 750·1
Penta-Thion, 2211·2
Pentatop, 2211·2
Pentavac, 2211·2
Pentavalent Antimony Compounds, 600·3
Pentavite, 2211·3
Penta-Vite Chewable Multi Vitamins with Minerals, 2211·3
Penta-Vite Childrens Vitamins with Iron, 2211·3
Penta-Vite Infant Vitamins, 2211·3
Pentavitol, 2211·3
Pentawin, 2211·3
Pentazine VC with Codeine, 2211·3
Pentazocina, 79·3
Pentazocina, Hidrocloruro de, 79·3
Pentazocina, Lactato de, 79·3
Pentazocine, 79·3
Pentazocine Hydrochloride, 79·3
Pentazocine Lactate, 79·3
Pentazocini Hydrochloridum, 79·3
Pentazocinum, 79·3
Pentazol, 1592·1
Pentazole, 2211·3
Pentcillin, 2211·3
Pentetate, Calcium, 1050·1
Pentetate Calcium Trisodium, 1050·1
Pentetate, Technetium ($^{99m}$Tc), 1526·1
Pentetato Cálcico Trisódico, 1050·1
Pentetic Acid, 1050·1
Pentetrazol, 1592·1
Pentetrazolum, 1592·1
Pentetreotide, 1334·2
Pentetreotide, Indium ($^{111}$In), 1524·1
Pent-HIBest, 2211·3
Penthiobarbital Sodique, 1309·1
Penthotal, 2211·3
Penthrox, 2211·3
Pentibrom, 2211·3
Pentibroxil, 2211·3
Penticlox, 2211·3
Penticort, 2211·3
Penticort Neomycine, 2211·3
Pentidix, 2211·3
Pentids, 2211·3
Pentifilina, 979·2
Pentifylline, 979·2
Pentilzeno, 2211·3
Pentiver, 2211·3
Pento, 2211·3
Pentobarbital, 713·2, 1309·3
Pentobarbital Cálcico, 713·3
Pentobarbital Calcium, 713·3
Pentobarbital Sódico, 713·3
Pentobarbital Sodium, 713·3
Pentobarbitalum, 713·2
Pentobarbitalum Natricum, 713·3
Pentobarbitone, 713·2
Pentobarbitone Calcium, 713·3

Pentobarbitone Sodium, 713·3
Pentobarbitone, Soluble, 713·3
Pentoclave, 2211·3
Pentoflux, 2211·3
Pentohexal, 2211·3
Pentolab, 2211·3
Pentolair, 2211·3
Pentolate, Bell— *see* Bell Pentolate, 1832·3
Pentomer, 2211·3
Pento-Puren, 2211·3
Pentorel, 2211·3
Pentosan Polysulfate Sodium, 979·2
Pentosan Polysulphate Sodium, 979·2
Pentosano Polisulfato de Sodio, 979·2
Pentostam, 2211·3
Pentostatin, 579·2
Pentostatina, 579·2
Pentothal, 2211·4
Pentovena, 2211·4
Pentox, 2211·4
Pentoxi, 2211·4
Pentoxifilina, 979·3
Pentoxifylline, 979·3
Pentoxifyllinum, 979·3
Pentoximed, 2211·4
Pentoxin, 2211·4
Pentoxiverina, 1126·2
Pentoxiverina, Citrato de, 1126·2
Pentoxiverina, Hidrocloruro de, 1126·3
Pentoxy, 2211·4
Pentoxyverine, 1126·2
Pentoxyverine Citrate, 1126·2
Pentoxyverine Hydrochloride, 1126·3
Pentoxyverine Hydrogen Citrate, 1126·2
Pentoxyverine Tannate, 1126·3
Pentoxyverini Hydrogenocitras, 1126·2
Pentrax, 2211·4
Pentrax Gold, 2211·4
Pentrexyl, 2211·4
Pentrexyl Expec, 2211·4
Pentrinitrol, 979·2
Pentyl 1-(5-Deoxy-β-D-ribofuranosyl)-5-fluoro-1,2-dihydro-2-oxo-4-pyrimidinecarbamate, 533·2
Pentyl 4-Dimethylaminobenzoate, 1155·1
Pentyl Ether, 1476·1
6-Pentyl-*m*-cresol, 1168·2
Pentylenetetrazol, 1592·1
Pentymalnatrium, 670·1
Pentymalum, 670·1
Pen-V, 2211·4
Pen-V-basan, 2211·4
Pen-Vee, 2211·4
Pen-Vee K, 2211·4
Penveno, 2211·4
Pen-Ve-Oral, 2211·4
Penvicilin, 2211·4
Pen-Vi-K, 2211·4
Penvir, 2211·4
Pen-V-Merck, 2211·4
Penzaethinum G, 162·3
PEP, 2211·4
PEPAP, 81·1
Pepcid, 2211·4
Pepcid Complete, 2212·1
Pepcid Duo, 2212·1
Pepcidac, 2212·1
Pepciddual, 2212·1
Pepcidduo, 2212·1
Pepcidin, 2212·1
Pepcidina, 2212·1
Pepcidine, 2212·1
Pepcidtwo, 2212·1
Pepcine, 2212·1
Pepdenal, 2212·1
Pepdine, 2212·1
Pepdite, 2212·1
Pepdual, 2212·1
Pepdul, 2212·1
Pepevit, 2212·1
Pepfamin, 2212·1
Pepleomycin Sulphate, 579·3
Peplomicina, Sulfato de, 579·3
Peplomycin Sulfate, 579·3
Peplomycin Sulphate, 579·3
Pepo, 1677·3
Pepp, 2212·1
Pepper, Cayenne, 1667·1
Pepper, Louisiana Long, 1667·1
Pepper, Louisiana Sport, 1667·1
Pepper Sprays, 67·2, 1667·1
Pepper, Tabasco, 1667·1
Peppermint, 1283·2
Peppermint Leaf, 1283·2
Peppermint Oil, 1283·2
Pep-Rani, 2212·1
Peprazol, 2212·1
Pepsaletten N, 2212·1
Pepsamar, 2212·1
Pepsamar Plus, 2212·1
Pepsane, 2212·1
Pepsicaps, 2212·2
Pepsidol, 2212·2
Pepsin, 1729·3
Pepsin Powder, 1729·3
Pepsin, Saccharated, 1729·3
Pepsina, 1729·3
Pepsini Pulvis, 1729·3
Pepsitase, 2212·2
Pepsiton, 2212·2
Pepsivit, 2212·2
Pepsogel, 2212·2
Pepsytoin, 2212·2
Peptab, 2212·2
Peptac, 2212·2
Peptamen, 2212·2
Peptan, 2212·2
Peptavlon, 2212·2
Peptazol, 2212·2
Peptgel, 2212·2
Pepti-2000, 2212·2
Pepti-2000 LF, 2212·2
Peptic Guard, 2212·2
Peptic Relief, 2212·2
Peptic Ulcer— *see* Peptic Ulcer Disease, 1246·3
Peptic Ulcer, Bleeding— *see* Peptic Ulcer Disease, 1246·3
Peptica, 2212·2
Pepticaine, 2212·2
Peptical, 2212·2
Peptichemio, 2212·2
Pepticum, 2212·2
Pepticus, 2212·2
Peptide T, 651·3
Peptides, Opioid, 73·2
Peptiditutteli, 2212·2
Péptido Relacionado con el Gen de la Calcitonina, 878·3
Péptido T, 651·3
Péptido Vasoactivo Intestinal, 1763·2
Péptidos Natriuréticos, 964·2
Peptifar, 2212·2
Pepti-Junior, 2212·2
Pepti-Junior, Cow & Gate— *see* Cow & Gate Pepti-Junior, 1910·3
Peptimax, 2212·3
Peptinal, 2212·3
Peptinal Forte, 2212·3
Peptinaut, 2212·3
Peptinex, 2212·3
Peptireal, 2212·3
Peptison, 2212·3
Peptisorb, 2212·3
Peptizole, 2212·3
Pepto Diarrhea Control, 2212·3
Pepto-Bismol, 2212·3
Peptoci, 2212·3
Peptol, 2212·3
Peptomet, 2212·3
Peptonorm, 2212·3
Peptonum, 2212·3
Peptopancreasi, 2212·3
Pepto-Pancreasi, 2212·3
Peptophen— *see* Thermalife, 2329·2
Peptulan, 2212·3
Pepzan, 2212·3
Pepzitrat, 2212·3
Pepzol, 2212·3
Peracel, 2212·3
Peracetic Acid, 1187·3
Peracético, Ácido, 1187·3
Peracil, 2212·3
Peracon, 2212·3
Peracon Expectorant, 2212·4
Peragit, 2212·4
Peralgin, 2212·4
Peran, 2212·4
Perasian, 2212·4
Perasthman N, 2212·4
Perative, 2212·4
Peratsin, 2212·4
Perazina, Dimalonato de, 713·3
Perazine Dimaleate, 714·1
Perazine Dimalonate, 713·3
Perbel, 2212·4
Perbilen, 2212·4
Perborato Sódico, 1192·2
Percaine, 1373·2
Percainum, 1373·2
Percapyl, 2212·4
Percas, 2212·4
Perchloracap, 2212·4
Perchloroethylene, 1477·1
Perclar, 2212·4
Perclorato Potásico, 1602·3
Perclorato Sódico, 1603·3
Perclusone, 2212·4
Percocet, 2212·4
Percodan, 2212·4
Percoffedrinol N, 2212·4
Percogesic, 2212·4
Percolone, 2212·4
Percorina, 2212·4
Percut. BCG Vaccine, 1609·2
Percutafeine, 2212·4
Percutalgine, 2212·4
Percutalin, 2212·4
Percutaneous Bacillus Calmette-Guérin Vaccine, 1609·2
Percutaneous Transluminal Angioplasty— *see* Reperfusion and Revascularisation Procedures, 834·1
Percutase N, 2213·1
Percutol, 2213·1
Perderm, 2213·1
Perdiem, 2213·1
Perdiem Fiber, 2213·1
Perdiphen, 2213·1
Perdiphen Phyto, 2213·1
Perdipina, 2213·1
Perdipine, 2213·1
Perdix, 2213·1
Perdogrip, 2213·1
Perdolan, 2213·1
Perdolan Codeine, 2213·1
Perdolan Compositum, 2213·1
Perdolan Duo— *see* Perdolan Codeine, 2213·1
Perdolan Mono— *see* Perdolan, 2213·1
Perdolan Mono C, 2213·1
Perduretas Codeina, 2213·1
Perebron, 2213·1
Pereflat, 2213·1
Perejil, 1728·3
Peremesin, 2213·1
Peremesin N, 2213·1
Peremin, 2213·1
Perenal, 2213·1
Perenan, 2213·1
Perennia, 2213·1
Perental, 2213·1
Perenterol, 2213·1
Perenteryl, 2213·2
Peresal, 2213·2
Perfadex, 2213·2
Perfalgan, 2213·2
Perfan, 2213·2
Perfane, 2213·2
Perfarin, 2213·2
Perfect Climate, 2213·2
Perfectil, 2213·2
Perfenazina, 714·2
Perfenazina, Decanoato de, 714·2
Perfenazina, Enantato de, 714·2
Perflenapent, 1067·2
Perflexane, 1067·2
Perflisopent, 1067·2
Perfluamine, 1730·1
Perflubron, 1730·1
Perflunafene, 1730·1
Perfluoroalkylpolyether, 1733·2
Perfluorocarbon Blood Substitutes, 1730·1
Perfluorocarbons, 1730·1
Perfluorodecahydronaphthalene, 1730·1
Perfluorodecalin, 1730·1
Perfluoron, 2213·2
Perfluoro-n-octane, 1730·2
Perfluoro-octa, 1730·2
Perfluorooctane, 1730·2
Perfluorooctylbromide, 1730·1
Perfluoropropane, 1067·2
Perfluorotripropylamine, 1730·1
Perflutren, 1067·2
Perflux, 2213·2
Perfocyn, 2213·2
Perfolate, 2213·2
Perfolin, 2213·2
Perform, 2213·2
Performer, 2213·2
Perf/Ser, 1615·3
Perfudal, 2213·2
Perfudan, 2213·2
Perfungol, 2213·2
Perfus Multivitaminico, 2213·2
Perfusion de PAS, 2213·2
Perfusion Mixte, 2213·2
Pergalen, 2213·2
Pergamid, 2213·2
Perganit, 2213·2
Pergastric, 2213·2
Pergidal, 2213·2
Perginol, 2213·3
Pergogreen, 2213·3
Pergolida, Mesilato de, 1211·2
Pergolide Mesilate, 1211·2
Pergolide Mesylate, 1211·2
Pergolidi Mesilas, 1211·2
Pergonal, 2213·3
Pergotime, 2213·3
Perhexilina, Maleato de, 980·2
Perhexiline Maleate, 980·2
2-(Perhydroazepin-1-yl)ethyl α-Cyclohexyl-α-(3-thienyl)acetate Dihydrogen Citrate Monohydrate, 882·1
(6*R*)-6-(Perhydroazepin-1-ylmethyleneamino)penicillanic Acid, 228·3
1-(Perhydroazepin-1-yl)-3-{4-[2-(5-methylisoxazole-3-carboxamido)ethyl]benzenesulphonyl}urea, 333·1
1-(Perhydroazepin-1-yl)-3-*p*-tolylsulphonylurea, 348·1
1-(Perhydroazepin-1-yl)-3-tosylurea, 348·1
1-[2-(Perhydroazocin-1-yl)ethyl]guanidine Monosulphate, 926·3
Perhydro-1,4-diazepin-1,4-diylbis(trimethylene 3,4,5-Trimethoxybenzoate) Dihydrochloride, 900·1
*N*-(Perhydro-2-oxo-3-thienyl)acetamide, 1672·3
Perhydrosqualène, 1482·2
Perhydro-4a,7,9-trihydroxy-2-methyl-6,8-bis(methylamino)pyrano[2,3-*b*][1,4]benzodioxin-4-one, 255·2
Periactin, 2213·3
Periactine, 2213·3
Periamin, 2213·3
Periamin X, 2213·3
Periamin G, 2213·3
Periatin, 2213·3
Periatin BC, 2213·3
Periavita, 2213·3
Peribilan, 2213·3
Periblastine, 2213·3
Pericaina, 2213·3
Perical, 2213·3
Pericam, 2213·3
Pericardial Effusions, Malignant— *see* Malignant Effusions, 512·2
Pericarditis, 416·2
Pericate, 2213·3
Pericel, 2213·3
Pericephal, 2213·3
Periciazina, 714·1

Periciazine, 714·1
Peri-Colace, 2213·3
Pericristine, 2213·3
Pericyazine, 714·1
Pericyazine Mesilate, 714·1
Pericyazine Tartrate, 714·1
Perida, 2213·3
Peridal, 2213·3
Peridane, 2213·3
Perident, 2213·4
Peridex, 2213·4
Peridil, 2213·4
Peridin-C, 2213·4
Peridol, 2213·4
Peridon, 2213·4
Peridor, 2213·4
Peri-Dos Softgels, 2213·4
Peridys, 2213·4
Perifazo, 2213·4
Perifem, 2213·4
Perifer H1, 2213·4
Periflex, 2213·4
Perifusin, 2213·4
Perikabiven, 2213·4
Perikan, 2213·4
Perikliman, 2213·4
Perikursal, 2213·4
Perilax, 2213·4
Perilox, 2213·4
Perinal, 2213·4
Perinatal Streptococcal Infections, 139·3
Perindopril, 980·2
Perindopril *tert*-Butylamine, 980·2
Perindopril, Erbrumina de, 980·2
Perindopril Erbumine, 980·2
Perindoprilat, 980·3
Perindoprilum, *tert*-Butylamini, 980·2
Perinorm, 2213·4
Perio-Aid, 2213·4
Perio-Aid C Cloruro de Cetilpiridinio, 2213·4
Periobacter, 2213·4
Periochip, 2213·4
Periochip, Blend-a-Med— *see* Blend-a-Med Periochip, 1848·4
Periocline, 2213·4
Period Pain Relief, 2213·4
Periodent, 2213·4
Periodentix, 2214·1
Periodentyl, 2214·1
Periodic Disease— *see* Familial Mediterranean Fever, 416·2
Periodic Limb Movements in Sleep— *see* Parasomnias, 667·3
Periodine Anti-Malarico, 2214·1
Periodontal Disease— *see* Mouth Infections, 136·1
Periodontil, 2214·1
Periodontitis— *see* Mouth Infections, 136·1
Periofem Ciclico, 2214·1
Periofem Continuo, 2214·1
Periogard, 2214·1
Periogard Chlorohex, 2214·1
Periogard Plus, 2214·1
PerioMed, 2214·1
Periostat, 2214·1
Perioxidin, 2214·1
Peripan, 2214·1
Peripheral Arterial Disease— *see* Peripheral Vascular Disease, 831·2
Peripheral Arterial Embolism— *see* Peripheral Arterial Thromboembolism, 830·3
Peripheral Arterial Thromboembolism, 830·3
Peripheral Arterial Thrombosis— *see* Peripheral Arterial Thromboembolism, 830·3
Peripheral Blood Stem Cell Transplantation— *see* Haematopoietic Stem Cell Transplantation, 1344·3
Peripheral Nerve Block, 1370·2
Peripheral Vascular Disease, 831·2
Periphramine, 2214·1
Periplasmal, 2214·1
Periplasmal G, 2214·1
Periplasmal XE, 2214·1
*Periploca sepium*, 1744·1
Periplum, 2214·1
Peripress, 2214·1
Peristaltine, 2214·1
Peritoflex, 2214·2
Peritofundin, 2214·2
Peritofundinas, 2214·2
Peritol, 2214·2
Peritone, 2214·2
Peritoneal Dialysis, 1221·3
Peritonitis, Bacterial— *see* Peritonitis, 140·1
Peritonitis, Fungal— *see* Peritonitis, 389·1
Peritrast, 2214·2
Peritrast Comp, 2214·2
Peritrast-Infusio 160/32%, 2214·2
Peritrast-Infusio 180/31%, 2214·2
Peritrast-Oral CT, 2214·2
Peritrast-Oral-GI, 2214·2
Peritrast-RE, 2214·2
Peritrate, 2214·2
Perivar, 2214·2
Perivar Rosskaven, 2214·2
Perivar Venensalbe, 2214·2
Periventricular Haemorrhage— *see* Neonatal Intraventricular Haemorrhage, 740·1
Perkamillon, 2214·2
Perketan, 2214·2
Perkod, 2214·2
Perlas de PMMA con Gentamicina, 2214·2
Perlatos, 2214·2
Perlax, 2214·2
Perlea, 2214·2
Perles d'huile de Foie de Morue du Dr Geistlich, 2214·2
Perlice, 2214·2
Perlinganit, 2214·2
Perlinsol Cutaneo, 2214·3
Perlol, 2214·3
Perludil, 2214·3
Perlutal, 2214·3
Perlutan, 2214·3
Perlutex, 2214·3
Permadoze, 2214·3
Permanganato Potásico, 1190·2
Permapen, 2214·3
Permax, 2214·3
Permease, 2214·3
Permecil, 2214·3
Permetel, 2214·3
Permethrin, 1508·3
Permethylpolysiloxane, 1482·1
Permetrina, 1508·3
Permetrix, 2214·3
Permicaps, 2214·3
Permitabs, 2214·3
Permitil, 2214·3
Permixon, 2214·3
*Perna canaliculus*, 1696·1
Pernaemyl, 2214·3
Pernamed, 2214·3
Pernazene, 2214·3
Pernazine, 2214·3
Pernexin, 2214·3
Pernicious Anaemia— *see* Megaloblastic Anaemia, 734·1
Pernionin, 2214·3
Pernionin N, 2214·3
Pernionin Teil-Bad, 2214·3
Pernionin Voll-Bad N, 2214·3
Perniosis— *see* Raynaud's Syndrome, 833·3
Pernox, 2214·3
Pernutrin, 2214·4
Pernyzol, 2214·4
Pero, 2214·4
Perocef, 2214·4
Perocur, 2214·4
Perofen, 2214·4
Perospirone Hydrochloride, 714·1
Perossido d'Idrogeno Soluzione, 1182·3
Peroxacne, 2214·4
Peroxiben, 2214·4
Peroxiben Plus, 2214·4
Peróxido de Benzoilo, 1143·2
Peróxido de Hidrógeno, 1182·2
Peróxido de Hidrógeno, Solución al 3%, 1182·2
Peróxido de Hidrógeno, Solución al 6%, 1182·2
Peróxido de Hidrógeno, Solución al 27%, 1182·3
Peróxido de Hidrógeno, Solución al 30%, 1182·3
Peróxido de Hidrógeno y Urea, 1195·3
Peróxido de Magnesio, 1185·2
Peróxido de Zinc, 1195·3
Peroximicina, 2214·4
Peroxin, 2214·4
Peroxyacetic Acid, 1187·3
Peroxyl, 2214·4
Perozon Erkaltungsbad, 2214·4
Perozon Heublumen, 2214·4
Perozon Rosmarin-Olbad Mono, 2214·4
Perpector, 2214·4
Perphenan, 2214·4
Perphenazine, 714·2
Perphenazine Decanoate, 714·2
Perphenazine Enantate, 714·2
Perphenazine Enanthate, 714·2
Perphenazine Heptanoate, 714·2
Perphenazine Maleate, 714·2
Perphenazinum, 714·2
Perphyllon, 2214·4
Perprazole, 1265·1
Persa-Gel, 2214·4
Persantin, 2214·4
Persantin Plus, 2214·4
Persantin S, 2214·4
Persantine, 2214·4
Persian Liquorice, 1270·2
Persic Oil, 1730·2
Persicae Semen, 1730·2
Persicorum, Oleum, 1730·2
Persil, 1728·3
Persistent Fetal Circulation— *see* Pulmonary Hypertension, 832·1
Persistent Pulmonary Hypertension of the Newborn— *see* Pulmonary Hypertension, 832·1
Persivate, 2214·4
Perskindol, 2214·4
Persol, 2215·1
Persol Forte, 2215·1
Persolv Richter, 2215·1
Personnel, 2215·1
Personnelle Contre le Rhume, 2215·1
Personnelle DM, 2215·1
Persumbrax, 2215·1
Pert Plus, 2215·1
Pertacel, 2215·1
Pertacilon, 2215·1
Pertamin, 2215·1
Pertaxol, 2215·1
Pertechnetate ($^{99m}$Tc) Sodium, 1525·3
Pertensal, 2215·1
Pertenso, 2215·1
Pertenso N, 2215·1
Pertil, 2215·1
Pertiroid, 2215·1
Pertix Preparations, 2215·1
Pertofran, 2215·1
Pertoglobulin, 2215·1
Pertranquil, 2215·1
Pertrim, 2215·1
Pertriptyl, 2215·1
Pertrombon, 2215·1
Pertudoron, 2215·1
Pertudoron 1, 2215·1
Pertudoron 2, 2215·1
Pertusan, 2215·1
Pertus-Gamma, 2215·2
Pertussex Compositum, 2215·2
Pertussin, 2215·2
Pertussis, 140·2
Pertussis (Acellular, Component) and Haemophilus Type B Conjugate Vaccine (Adsorbed), Diphtheria, Tetanus, 1614·2
Pertussis (Acellular, Component), Hepatitis B (rDNA), Poliomyelitis (Inactivated) and Haemophilus Type B Conjugate Vaccine (Adsorbed), Diphtheria, Tetanus, 1614·3
Pertussis (Acellular, Component) and Hepatitis B (rDNA) Vaccine (Adsorbed), Diphtheria, Tetanus, 1614·3
Pertussis (Acellular, Component), Poliomyelitis (Inactivated) and Haemophilus Type B Conjugate Vaccine (Adsorbed), Diphtheria, Tetanus, 1615·1
Pertussis (Acellular, Component) and Poliomyelitis (Inactivated) Vaccine (Adsorbed), Diphtheria, Tetanus, 1615·1
Pertussis (Acellular, Component) Vaccine (Adsorbed), Diphtheria, Tetanus and, 1613·3
Pertussis, Diphtheria, and Tetanus Vaccines, 1613·3
Pertussis, Haemophilus Influenzae, Diphtheria, and Tetanus Vaccines, 1614·2
Pertussis Immune Globulin, 1631·2
Pertussis Immunoglobulins, 1631·2
Pertussis, Poliomyelitis, Diphtheria, and Tetanus Vaccines, 1615·1
Pertussis, Poliomyelitis, Haemophilus Influenzae, Diphtheria, and Tetanus Vaccines, 1615·1
Pertussis, Poliomyelitis (Inactivated) and Haemophilus Type B Conjugate Vaccine (Adsorbed), Diphtheria, Tetanus, 1615·1
Pertussis and Poliomyelitis (Inactivated) Vaccine (Adsorbed), Diphtheria, Tetanus, 1615·1
Pertussis Vaccine, 1631·2
Pertussis Vaccine (Acellular, Component, Adsorbed), 1631·2
Pertussis Vaccine (Acellular, Co-purified, Adsorbed), 1631·3
Pertussis Vaccine (Adsorbed), 1631·2
Pertussis Vaccine (Adsorbed), Diphtheria, Tetanus and, 1613·3
Pertussis Vaccines, 1631·2
Pertuvac, 2215·2
Peru Balsam, 1730·2
Perubare, 2215·2
Perubore, 2215·2
Perudent, 2215·2
Peru-Lenicet, 2215·2
Perusliuos-K, 2215·2
Peruvian Bark, 1671·3
Peruvian Leaf, 1373·3
Peruvian Rhatany, 1738·1
Per/Vac, 1631·2
Per/Vac/Ads, 1631·2
Pervasum, 2215·2
Perviam, 2215·2
Pervinox, 2215·2
Pervinox D, 2215·2
Pervioral, 2215·2
Pervita, 2215·2
Pervivo, 2215·2
Pervone, 2215·2
Perycit, 2215·2
Perzine, 2215·2
Pesendorfer, 2215·2
Pesex-R, 2215·2
Pespir, 2215·2
Pessarios Profilaticos Rendell, 2215·2
Pest Control— *see* Vector Control, 1500·1
Pestarin, 2215·2
Pesticides and Repellents, 1499·1
Petadolex, 2215·2
Petadolor, 2215·2
Petaforce V, 2215·2
Pétalos de Amapola, 1058·1
Pétalos de Rosa, 1058·1
Pe-Tam, 2215·3
*Petasites hybridus*, 1663·3
*Petasites officinalis*, 1663·3
Peteha, 2215·3
Petercillin, 2215·3
Peterkaien, 2215·3
Peterphyllin, 2215·3
Peter's Sirop, 2215·3
Petersilie N, Kneipp— *see* Kneipp Petersilie N, 2081·3
Pethidine Hydrochloride, 80·2

Pethidini Hydrochloridum, 80·2
Pethidinic Acid, 81·2
Petibelle, 2215·3
Petidina, Hidrocloruro de, 80·2
Petidion, 2215·3
Petiflog, 2215·3
Petina Compound, 2215·3
Petinimid, 2215·3
Petinutin, 2215·3
Petit Mal— *see* Epilepsy, 349·1
Petite Centaurée, 1669·2
Petites Pilules Carters, 2215·3
PETN, 965·3, 979·1
Petnidan, 2215·3
Petogen, 2215·3
Petrasch-Anthozym N, 2215·3
Petrol, 1476·3
Petrolagar No. 2, 2215·3
Petrolagar with Phenolphthalein, 2215·3
Petrolatum, 1479·3
Petrolatum, Liquid, 1479·1
Petrolatum, Liquid, Heavy, 1479·1
Petrolatum, Liquid, Light, 1479·1
Petrolatum, White, 1479·3
Petrolatum, Yellow, 1479·3
Petrolei, Oleum, 1479·1
Petroleum Benzin, 1476·3
Petroleum Ether, 1476·3
Petroleum Jelly, 1479·3
Petroleum Jelly, White, 1479·3
Petroleum Jelly, Yellow, 1479·3
Petroleum, Light, 1476·3
Petroleum Med Complex, 2215·3
Petroleum Spirit, 1476·3
Petroselinum, 1728·3
*Petroselinum crispum*, 1728·3
Petylyl, 2215·3
Peumus, 1661·2
*Peumus boldus*, 1661·2
Pevalip, 2215·3
Pevaryl, 2215·3
Pevaryl TC, 2215·3
Pevidine, 2215·3
Pevison, 2215·3
Pevisone, 2215·4
Pexan E, 2215·4
Pexelizumab, 1675·2
Pexeva, 2215·4
Pexid, 2215·4
Pexid— *see* Pexsig, 2215·4
Pexiganan Acetate, 228·3
Pexola, 2215·4
Pexsig, 2215·4
Peyote, 1713·3
Peyotl, 1713·3
Peyrone's Salt, 538·1
P-FAD, 1694·2
*Pfaffia paniculata*, 1693·1
Pfeffer, Spanischer, 1667·1
Pfefferminzblätter, 1283·2
Pfefferminzöl, 1283·2
Pfeiffer's Cold Sore, 2215·4
Pfeil, 2215·4
P-Fen, 2215·4
Pfizerpen, 2215·4
Pflanzen-Dragees Brennessel, Kneipp— *see* Kneipp Pflanzen-Dragees Brennessel, 2081·3
Pflanzen-Dragees Mistel, Kneipp— *see* Kneipp Pflanzen-Dragees Mistel, 2081·3
Pflanzen-Dragees Weissdorn, Kneipp— *see* Kneipp Pflanzen-Dragees Weissdorn, 2081·3
PFOB, 1730·1
PFT, 1659·2, 2215·4
PG 53, 2215·4
PG/53, 2215·4
PGA, 1429·1
$PGA_2$, 1511·1
$PGB_2$, 1511·1
$PGC_2$, 1511·1
$PGE_1$, 1512·3
$PGE_1$ α-CD, 1512·3
$PGE_2$, 1515·1
$PGF_{2\alpha}$, 1514·3
$PGF_{2\alpha}$ THAM, 1514·3
$PGG_2$, 1511·1
$PGH_2$, 1511·1
$PGI_2$, 1516·3
PGX, 1516·3
pH4, 2215·4
PH 4 Plus, 2215·4
pH5-Eucerin, 2217·2
pH5-Eucerin Solar, 2217·2
Ph-549, 397·3
pH 550, 2215·4
PH-5776, 612·1
PH Maxi, 2215·4
Phacobiotic, 2215·4
Phacocef, 2215·4
Phacotrex, 2215·4
Phaeochromocytoma, 831·3
Phaeophytins, 1057·1
Phaeva, 2215·4
Phakan, 2215·4
Phakolen, 2215·4
Phalloidin, 1717·3
Phallolysin, 1717·3
Phallotoxins, 1717·3
Phaloin, 1717·3
Phamopril, 2215·4
Phamoprofen, 2216·1
Phamoranit, 2216·1
Phamoxi, 2216·1
Phamuc, 2216·1
Phanadex Cough, 2216·1
Phanalgin, 2216·1
Phanate, 2216·1
Phanatuss Cough, 2216·1
Phantogeusia— *see* Taste Disorders, 682·2
Phantom Limb Pain, 7·3
Phapax, 2216·1
Pharcina, 2216·1
Phardol Mono, 2216·1
Phardol Rheuma, 2216·1
Pharken, 2216·1
Pharma Plus, 2216·1
Pharma Plus Oil Free, 2216·1
Pharma Plus Sport, 2216·1
Pharmacare Aspec, 2216·1
Pharmacen, 2216·1
Pharmacetin, 2216·1
Pharmaceutix, 2216·1
Pharmacilline, 2216·1
Pharmacists Creme, 2216·1
Pharmacists Lotion, 2216·1
Pharmacol DM, 2216·1
Pharma-Col Junior, 2216·1
Pharmacycare Preparations, 2216·1
Pharma-Dentix, 2216·2
Pharmadol, 2216·2
Pharmadose Alcool, 2216·2
Pharmadose Mercuresceine, 2216·2
Pharmadose Teinture d'Arnica, 2216·2
Pharmaethyl, 2216·2
Pharmaflex, 2216·2
Pharmaflur, 2216·2
Pharmafort, 2216·2
Pharmagrip, 2216·2
Pharmalgen, 2216·2
Pharmapress, 2216·2
Pharmapress Co, 2216·2
Pharmatex, 2216·2
Pharmaton, 2216·2
Pharmaton Complex, 2216·2
Pharmaton, Geriatric— *see* Geriatric Pharmaton, 2022·2
Pharmaton Kiddi, 2216·2
Pharmaton, Kiddi— *see* Kiddi Pharmaton, 2079·1
Pharmaton SA, 2216·2
Pharmatovit, 2216·2
Pharmetapp, 2216·2
Pharmilin-DM, 2216·3
Pharminicol DM, 2216·3
Pharminil DM, 2216·3
Pharmitussin DM, 2216·3
Pharmorubicin, 2216·3
Pharmotidine, 2216·3
Pharnax, 2216·3
Pharo-Tus, 2216·3
Pharyngine a la Vitamine C, 2216·3
Pharyngitis, 140·3
Pharyngor, 2216·3
Pharynx, 2216·3
Pharysyx N, 2216·3
Phase O, 2216·3
Phased Oral Contraceptives, 1535·1
Phatropine, 2216·3
Phazyme, 2216·3
Phe, 1443·1
Pheasant's Eye, Vernal, 1648·1
Phelypressine, 1324·2
Phemitone, 366·3
Phen...— *see also under* Fen...
Phenacemide, 367·3
Phenacetin, 82·2
Phenacetinum, 82·2
Phenacyl Chloride, 1670·1
Phenadone, 57·2
Phenadoz, 2216·3
Phenaemal, 2216·3
Phenaemaletten, 2216·3
Phenahist-TR, 2216·3
Phenamacide Hydrochloride, 487·3
Phenamazide Hydrochloride, 487·3
Phenameth DM, 2216·3
Phenamin, 2216·3
Phenaminum, 1584·3
9-Phenanthrenemethanol Antimalarials, 444·1
Phenantoin, 366·2
Phenantoinum, 370·2
Phenapap, 2216·3
Phenapap Sinus Headache & Congestion, 2216·3
Phenaphen with Codeine, 2216·3
Phenasale, 110·1
Phenaseptic, 2216·3
Phenate, 2216·3
PhenaVent, 2216·4
Phenazepam, 715·1
Phenazin, 2216·4
Phenazine, 2216·4
Phenazo, 2216·4
Phenazocine Hydrobromide, 82·2
Phenazolinum, 424·2
Phenazone, 82·3
Phenazone and Caffeine Citrate, 82·3
Phenazone Salicylate, 82·3
Phenazonum, 82·3
Phenazopyridine Hydrochloride, 83·1
Phenchlor SHA, 2216·4
Phencodin, 2216·4
Phencyclidine Hydrochloride, 1730·3
Phendex, 2216·4
Phendimetrazine Acid Tartrate, 1592·1
Phendimetrazine Bitartrate, 1592·1
Phendimetrazine Hydrochloride, 1592·1
Phendimetrazine Tartrate, 1592·1
Phendiridine, 2216·4
Phenedrine, 2216·4
Phenelzine Sulfate, 312·1
Phenelzine Sulphate, 312·1
Phenemalnatrium, 367·3
Phenemalum, 367·3
Phenerbel-S, 2216·4
Phenergan Preparations, 2216·4
Phenethanolum, 1188·1
Phenethicillin Potassium, 242·1
Phenethyl Alcohol, 1188·1
4-{2-[6-(Phenethylamino)hexylamino]ethyl}pyrocatechol Dihydrochloride, 908·2
1-Phenethylbiguanide Hydrochloride, 344·1
Phenethylhydrazine Hydrogen Sulphate, 312·1
1-(2-Phenethyl)-4-*N*-(*N*-hydroxypropionylanilino) Piperidine, 41·1
8-Phenethyl-1-oxa-3,8-diazaspiro[4.5]decan-2-one Hydrochloride, 786·1
*N*-(1-Phenethyl-4-piperidyl) Propionanilide, 40·1
*N*-(1-Phenethyl-4-piperidyl)propionanilide Dihydrogen Citrate, 40·1
Pheneticillin Potassium, 242·1
Pheneticillin Sodium, 242·1
Pheneticillinum Kalicum, 242·1
Pheneturide, 367·3
Phenex, 2216·4
Phenexpect, 2217·1
Phenexpect CD, 2217·1
Phenformin Hydrochloride, 344·1
Phenhalal, 2217·1
Phenhist DH with Codeine, 2217·1
Phenhist Expectorant, 2217·1
Phenhydan, 2217·1
Phenic Acid, 1188·1
Phenicarbazide, 83·2
Phenicol, 2217·1
Phenimixin, 2217·1
Phenindamine Acid Tartrate, 438·2
Phenindamine Tartrate, 438·2
Phenindamini Tartras, 438·2
Phenindaminium Tartrate, 438·2
Phenindione, 981·1
Pheniramine, 438·3
Pheniramine 4-Amino-2-hydroxybenzoate, 438·3
Pheniramine Aminosalicylate, 438·3
Pheniramine *p*-Aminosalicylate, 438·3
Pheniramine 4-Aminosalicylate, 438·3
Pheniramine Hydrochloride, 438·3
Pheniramine Hydrogen Maleate, 438·3
Pheniramine Maleate, 438·3
Pheniramine Para-aminosalicylate, 438·3
Pheniramine Tannate, 438·3
Pheniramini Maleas, 438·3
Pheniraminium Maleate, 438·3
Phenlaxine, 1282·3
Phenmetrazine, 1592·1
Phenmetrazine Hydrochloride, 1592·2
Phenobarb, 2217·1
Phenobarbital, 367·3
Phenobarbital Diethylamine, 369·3
Phenobarbital Magnesium, 369·3
Phenobarbital Sodium, 367·3
Phenobarbitalum, 367·3
Phenobarbitalum Natricum, 367·3
Phenobarbitone, 367·3
Phenobarbitone Sodium, 367·3
Phenobarbitone, Soluble, 367·3
Phenocillin, 2217·1
Phenoctide, 1187·1
Phenododecinium Bromide, 1179·1
Phenol, 1188·1
Phenol, Liquified, 1188·1
Phenol Red, 1730·3
Phenolphtaleinum, 1284·1
Phenolphthalein, 1284·1
Phenolphthalein, Yellow, 1284·1
Phenolphthaleinum, 1284·1
Phenolsulfonphthalein, 1730·3
Phenolsulfonphthaleinum, 1730·3
Phenolsulphonphthalein, 1730·3
Phenolum, 1188·1
Phenomerborum, 1189·2
Phénomycilline, 242·1
Phenonip— *see* Tantol Skin Cleanser, 2319·4
Phenoperidine Hydrochloride, 83·2
Phenoptic, 2217·1
Phenoris, 2217·1
Phenoro, 2217·1
Phenotal, 2217·1
Phenothrin, 1509·1
Phenoxazole, 1591·2
Phenoxine, 2217·1
(6*R*)-6-(2-Phenoxyacetamido)penicillanic Acid, 242·1
Phenoxyaethanol, 1189·1
Phenoxybenzamine Hydrochloride, 981·2
3-Phenoxybenzyl (1*RS*,3*RS*)-(1*RS*,3*SR*)-3-(2,2-Dichlorovinyl)-2,2-dimethylcyclopropanecarboxylate, 1508·3
3-Phenoxybenzyl (1*RS*,3*RS*)-(1*RS*,3*SR*)-2,2-Dimethyl-3-(2-methylprop-1-enyl)cyclopropanecarboxylate, 1509·1
Phenoxyethanol, 1189·1
2-Phenoxyethanol, 1189·1
Phenoxyethanolum, 1189·1
β-Phenoxyethyl Alcohol, 1189·1
2-Phenoxyethyl *p*-Hydroxybenzoate, 1195·3
Phenoxyisopropanol, 1189·2
Phenoxyisopropyl Alcohol, 1189·2

Phenoxyisopropylnorsuprifen, 1702·2
Phenoxymethyl Penicillin, 242·1
Phenoxymethylpenicillin, 242·1
Phenoxymethylpenicillin Calcium, 242·1
Phenoxymethylpenicillin Potassium, 242·1, 242·2
Phenoxymethylpenicillini Dibenzylaethylendiaminum, 163·2
Phenoxymethylpenicillinum, 242·1
Phenoxymethylpenicillinum Calcicum, 242·1
Phenoxymethylpenicillinum Kalicum, 242·1
Phenoxypenicillins, 118·3
Phenoxypropanol, 1189·1
1-Phenoxypropan-2-ol, 1189·2
4-Phenoxy-3-(pyrrolidin-1-yl)-5-sulphamoylbenzoic Acid, 983·3
16-Phenoxy-ω-17,18,19,20-tetranor-prostaglandin $E_2$-methylsulfonylamide, 1520·3
4-[3-(α-Phenoxy-*p*-tolyl)propyl]morpholine Hydrochloride, 1376·3
Phenpro, 2217·1
Phenprobamate, 715·1
Phenprocoumon, 981·3
Phenpropamine Citrate, 1250·2
Phensedyl, 2217·1
Phensedyl Dry Family Cough, 2217·1
Phensedyl Plus, 2217·1
Phensic, 2217·1
Phensic Dual Action, 2217·1
Phensic Ibuprofen, 2217·1
Phensuximide, 370·1
Phentanyl Citrate, 40·1
Phentermine, 1592·2
Phentermine Hydrochloride, 1592·2
Phentolamine Hydrochloride, 982·1
Phentolamine Mesilate, 982·1
Phentolamine Mesylate, 982·1
Phentolamine Methanesulphonate, 982·1
Phentolamini Mesilas, 982·1
Phenyl Hydrate, 1188·1
Phenyl Hydride, 1471·3
Phenyl Salicylate, 88·1
Phenyl Sulfate, 1188·3
*N*-Phenylacetamide, 11·3
(6*R*)-6-(2-Phenylacetamido)penicillanic Acid, 163·2
Phenylacetic Acid, 528·2
Phenylacetic Acid Mustard, 536·2
3-Phenylacetylamino-2,6-piperidinedione, 528·2
Phenylacetylglutamine, 528·2
(Phenylacetyl)urea, 367·3
Phenylade, 2217·1
Phenylalanine, 1443·1
L-Phenylalanine, 1443·1
Phenylalanine Mustard, 566·1
Phenylalanine Nitrogen Mustard, 566·1
[2-Phenylalanine,8-lysine]vasopressin, 1324·2
Phenylalaninum, 1443·1
Phenylamine, 1471·2
Phenylaminopropanum Racemicum Sulfuricum, 1584·3
4-Phenylazobenzene-1,3-diamine Hydrochloride Citrate, 1670·3
3-Phenylazopyridine-2,6-diyldiamine Hydrochloride, 83·1
Phenylbenzene, 1681·2
Phenylbenzimidazole Sulphonic Acid, 1147·1
2-Phenyl-1*H*-benzimidazole-5-sulphonic Acid, 1147·1
2-Phenyl-1,2-benzisoselenazolin-3-one, 1683·2
8-(*p*-Phenylbenzyl)atropinium Bromide, 491·3
Phenylbutazone, 83·2
Phenylbutazone Calcium, 84·1
Phenylbutazone Megallate, 84·1
Phenylbutazone Piperazine, 84·1
Phenylbutazone Sodium, 84·1
Phenylbutazonum, 83·2
(2-Phenylbutyryl)urea, 367·3
Phenylcarbinol, 1170·2
1-(1-Phenylcyclohexyl)piperidine Hydrochloride, 1730·3
1-(1-Phenylcyclohexyl)pyrrolidine, 1730·3
(±)-*trans*-2-Phenylcyclopropylamine Sulphate, 318·3
Phenyldimazone Hydrochloride, 1125·2
Phenyldimethylpyrazolone, 82·3
Phenyldrine, 2217·2
4,4′-*o*-Phenylenebis(ethyl 3-Thioallophanate), 114·2
4,4′-[*p*-Phenylenebis(methyleneamino)]bis(isoxazolidin-3-one), 266·2
*NN*′-*p*-Phenylenedimethylenebis[2,2-dichloro-*N*-(2-ethoxyethyl)acetamide], 616·3
(±)-(3*E*,3′*E*)-3,3′-(*p*-Phenylenedimethylidyne)bis[2-oxo-10-bornanesulfonic Acid], 1146·3
Phenylephrine, 1126·3
Phenylephrine Acid Tartrate, 1126·3
Phenylephrine Bitartrate, 1126·3
Phenylephrine Hydrochloride, 1126·3
Phenylephrine Tannate, 1127·3
Phenylephrine Tartrate, 1126·3
Phenylephrini Hydrochloridum, 1126·3
Phenylephrinum, 1126·3
2-Phenylethanol, 1188·1
Phenylethyl Alcohol, 1188·1
Phenylethylbarbituric Acid, 367·3
16α,17α-(1-Phenylethylidenedioxy)pregn-4-ene-3,20-dione, 1541·3
Phenylethylmalonamide, 377·1
Phenylethylmalonylurea, 367·3
1-Phenylethyl-4-phenyl-4-acetoxypiperidine, 81·1
Phenylfenesin LA, 2217·2
Phenyl-Free, 2217·2
Phenylgesic, 2217·2
Phenylglucuronide, 1188·3
Phenylglycolic Acid, 228·3
(6*R*)-6-(α-D-Phenylglycylamino)penicillanic Acid, 157·1
Phenylhydrargyri Acetas, 1189·2
Phenylhydrargyri Boras, 1189·2
Phenylhydrargyri Nitras, 1189·2
Phenylic Acid, 1188·1
2-Phenylindan-1,3-dione, 981·1
Phenylindanedione, 981·1
Phenylinium, 981·1
Phenylisohydantoin, 1591·2
Phenylketonuria— *see* Amino Acid Metabolic Disorders, 1417·2
Phenylmercuric Acetate, 1189·2
Phenylmercuric Borate, 1189·2
Phenylmercuric Dinaphthylmethanedisulfonate, 1182·2
Phenylmercuric Hydroxide, 1189·2
Phenylmercuric Nitrate, 1189·2
Phenylmercuric Orthoborate, 1189·2
Phenylmercuric Salts, 1189·2
Phenylmercury Nitrate, Basic, 1189·2
Phenylmethane, 1477·1
Phenylmethanol, 1170·2
Phenylmethylaminopropane Hydrochloride, 1589·2
1-Phenylpentan-1-ol, 1687·2
*N*-(4-Phenylphenacyl)-1-hyoscyaminium Bromide, 482·2
(−)-(1*R*,3*r*,5*S*)-8-(4-Phenylphenacyl)-3-[(*S*)-tropoyloxy]tropanium Bromide, 482·2
(*S*)-3-Phenyl-1′-(phenylmethyl)-(3,4′-bipiperidine)-2,6-dione, 481·1
3-(4-Phenylpiperazin-1-yl)propane-1,2-diol, 1119·3
2-Phenyl-2-piperidyl Acetic Acid, 1590·3
Phenylpiperone Hydrochloride, 35·3
4-Phenylpiracetam, 1731·1
Phenylprenazone, 43·1
2-Phenyl-1,3-propanediol Dicarbamate, 361·1
Phenylpropanol, 1731·1
1-Phenylpropan-1-ol, 1731·1
Phenylpropanolamine, 1127·3
Phenylpropanolamine Bitartrate, 1127·3, 1128·3
Phenylpropanolamine Hydrochloride, 1127·3
Phenylpropanolamine Polistirex, 1128·3
Phenylpropanolamine Sulfate, 1128·3
Phenylpropanolamini Hydrochloridum, 1127·3
*trans*-3-Phenylpropenoic Acid, 1177·3
3-Phenylpropyl Carbamate, 715·1
Phenylpropylhydroxycoumarin, 981·3
Phenylpseudohydantoin, 1591·2
6-Phenylpteridine-2,4,7-triamine, 1016·2
Phenylsemicarbazide, 83·2
1-Phenylsemicarbazide, 83·2
Phenylsulphoacetamidopenicillanic Acid, Disodium Salt, 257·2
5-Phenylthiazole-2,4-diamine Hydrochloride, 1584·3
Phenyltoloxamine Citrate, 439·1
Phenyltoloxamine Polistirex, 439·1
Phenyltolyloxamine Citrate, 439·1
2-[(α-Phenyl-*p*-tolyl)oxy]triethylamine Hydrochloride, 587·3
Phenyphrine-Azol, 2217·2
Phenytek, 2217·2
Phenytoin, 370·2
Phenytoin Sodium, 370·2
Phenytoin, Soluble, 370·2
Phenytoinum, 370·2
Phenytoinum Natricum, 370·2
Phenzone and Caffeine Citrate, 82·3
Pheramin N, 2217·2
Pherarutin, 2217·2
Pherazine with Codeine, 2217·2
Pherazine DM, 2217·2
Pherazine VC, 2217·2
Pherazine VC with Codeine, 2217·2
Phescode, Chemists Own— *see* Chemists Own Phescode, 1882·1
Phexin, 2217·2
Phicon, 2217·2
Phicon-F, 2217·2
Philinal, 2217·2
Philinet, 2217·2
Phillips' Chewable, 2217·2
Phillips Gelcaps, 2217·2
Phillips' Milk of Magnesia, 2217·2
Phillips P.T.Y. Yeast Tablets— *see* Tonic Yeast, 2336·4
pHisoDerm, 2217·2
pHisoHex, 2217·2
pHisoHex Face Wash, 2217·3
pHisoHex Reformulated, 2217·3
Phisomain, 2217·3
pHiso-MED, 2217·3
Phlebocreme, 2217·3
Phlebodril, 2217·3
Phlebodril Mono, 2217·3
Phlebodril N, 2217·3
Phlebogel, 2217·3
Phlebosedol, 2217·3
Phlebostasin, 2217·3
Phlebostasin Compositum, 2217·3
Phlebosup, 2217·3
Phlexy, 2217·3
Phlexy Vits, 2217·3
Phlexyvits, 2217·3
Phlogenzym, 2217·3
Phlogidermil, 2217·3
Phlogont, 2217·3
Phlogont Rheuma, 2217·3
Phlogont-Thermal, 2217·3
Phloroglucin, 1731·1
Phloroglucinol, 1731·1
Phloropropiophenone, 1689·1
PHNCYC, 480·3, 1126·3
PHNL, 1126·3
Phobias— *see* Phobic Disorders, 663·3
Phobic Disorders, 663·3
Phocytan, 2217·3
Pholcodine, 1128·3
Pholcodine Citrate, 1128·3
Pholcodine Polistirex, 1128·3
Pholcodinum, 1128·3
Pholcodyl, 2217·4
Pholcolin, 2217·4
Pholcolinct, 2217·4
Pholco-Mereprine, 2217·4
Pholcones, 2217·4
Pholcones Bismuth, 2217·4
Pholedrine Sulfate, 982·3
Pholedrine Sulphate, 982·3
Pholtex, 2217·4
Pholtrate, 2217·4
Phol-Tussil, 2217·4
Phol-Tux, 2217·4
Phonal, 2217·4
Phonix Preparations, 2217·4
Phono Arnica Comp, 2217·4
Phono Chol, 2217·4
Phono Gripp, 2217·4
Phono Uren, 2217·4
Phono Ven, 2217·4
Phor Pain, 2217·4
*Phoradendron flavescens*, 1715·3
Phorpain, 2217·4
Phos Kola, 2217·4
PhosChol, 2217·4
Phoscortil, 2217·4
Phosetamin, 2217·4
Phos-Ex, 2218·1
Phos-Flur, 2218·1
Phosfo Enema, 2218·1
Phosfomin, 2218·1
Phosfomin Iron, 2218·1
Phosfonema, 2218·1
Phosforid, 2218·1
Phosgene, 1731·1
Phoslo, 2218·1
PhosLo, 2218·1
Phosmet, 1509·1
Phos-NaK, 2218·1
Phosoforme, 2218·1
Phosph. Acid, 1731·2
Phosphalugel, 2218·1
Phosphate, 1230·3
Phosphate Tertiaire de Calcium, 1225·3
Phosphate-Novartis, 2218·1
Phosphates, 2218·1
Phosphate-Sandoz, 2218·1
Phosphate-Sandoz— *see* Phosphate-Novartis, 2218·1
Phosphatides, 1706·1
Phosphatidyl Choline, 1706·1, 1731·1
Phosphatidyl Glycerol, 1736·2
Phosphatidyl Inositol, 1706·1
Phosphatidyl Olamine, 1706·1
Phosphatidyl Serine, 1706·1, 1731·2
Phosphatidylcholine, 1731·1
Phosphatidylserine, 1731·2
Phosphine, 1500·1
Phosphinic Acid, 1700·2
Phosphocalcina Iodada, 2218·1
Phosphocholine, 2218·1
Phosphocol, 2218·1
Phosphocreatine, 1677·2
Phosphocreatinine, 1689·3
Phosphocysteamine, 1712·2
Phosphodiesterase Inhibitors, 811·1
Phosphoestrolum, 1555·3
Phospho-Lax, 2218·1
Phospholine Iodide, 2218·1
Phosphomycin, 214·2
Phosphonatoformate Trisodium, 634·2
Phosphoneuros, 2218·1
Phosphonic Acid Antibacterials, 120·2
Phosphonoformate Trisodium, 634·2
9-[2-(Phosphonomethoxy)ethyl]adenine, 628·1
9-[(*R*)-2-(Phosphonomethoxy)propyl]adenine Monohydrate, 655·1
*N*-(Phosphonomethyl)glycine, 1505·3
*cis*-4-(Phosphonomethyl)pipecolic Acid, 1743·1
Phosphonomycin, 214·2
2-Phosphono-oxybenzoic Acid, 44·2
Phosphonorm, 2218·1
Phosphoprep, 2218·1
Phosphoral, 2218·1
Phosphoramide Mustard, 541·3
Phosphore-Medifa, 2218·2
Phosphor-Homaccord, 2218·2
Phosphoric Acid, 1731·2
Phosphoric Acid, Concentrated, 1731·2
Phosphoric Acid, Dilute, 1731·2
Phosphoric Acid, Diluted, 1731·2
Phosphoric Acid Tributyl Ester, 1477·3

Phosphorothioic Tri(ethyleneamide), 588·1
Phosphorsäure, 1731·2
Phosphorus, 1731·2
Phosphorus-32, 1525·1
Phosphorus Med Complex, 2218·2
Phosphorus White, 1731·2
Phosphorus, Yellow, 1731·2
Phosphorylcholine, 1690·1
4-Phosphoryloxy-*NN*-dimethyltryptamine, 1736·1
Phospho-Soda, Fleet— *see* Fleet Phospho-Soda, 1998·4
Phostal, 2218·2
Phostarac, 2218·2
Photoallergy— *see* Light-induced Skin Reactions, 1136·3
Photochemotherapy, 1153·1
Photochemotherapy, Extracorporeal, 1153·2
Photoderm, 2218·2
Photoderm Latte, 2218·2
Photoderm Max, 2218·2
Photoderm Mineral, 2218·2
Photoderm Special, 2218·2
Photodynamic Therapy, 581·1
Photofrin, 2218·2
Photopheresis, 1153·2
Photoplex, 2218·2
Photoscreen, 2218·2
Photosensitivity— *see* Light-induced Skin Reactions, 1136·3
Phototoxicity— *see* Light-induced Skin Reactions, 1136·3
Phoxim, 1509·1
PHP, 1730·3
Phrenilin, 2218·2
Phrenotropin, 718·1
*o*-Phthalaldehyde, 1189·3
Phthalazine-1,4-diyldihydrazine Sulphate Hemipentahydrate, 899·3
Phthalazolum, 242·3
*o*-Phthaldialdehyde, 1189·3
2-Phthalimidoglutarimide, 1752·3
Phthalophos, 110·1
Phthalylsulfathiazole, 242·3
Phthalylsulfathiazolum, 242·3
Phthalylsulphathiazole, 242·3
Phthiriasis Palpebrarum— *see* Pediculosis, 1499·1
Phthivazid, 215·2
Phthivazidum, 215·2
Phthorothanum, 1299·3
PhXA-41, 1519·1
Phycocyane, 2218·2
Phylarm, 2218·2
Phyllocontin, 2218·2
Phylloquinone, 1467·1
Phyllotemp, 2218·2
Phylobid, 2218·2
Phyloday, 2218·2
Phylorinol, 2218·2
Phymet DTF, 2218·2
Phymorax, 2218·2
Phy-O, 2218·2
Phyone, 1327·2
Physalis, 1731·3
*Physalis alkekengi*, 1731·3
*Physalis peruviana*, 1731·3
Physeptone, 2218·2
Physex, 2218·3
Physiodose, 2218·3
Physiogel, 2218·3
Physiogesic, 2218·3
Physiogine, 2218·3
Physiolax, 2218·3
Physiologic, 2218·3
Physiologica, 2218·3
Physiological Saline, 1233·3
Physiolyte, 2218·3
Physiomenthol, 2218·3
Physiomer, 2218·3
Physiomint, 2218·3
Physiomycine, 2218·3
Physioneal, 2218·3
Physioneal Glucosa, 2218·3
Physiorhine, 2218·3
Physio-Rub, 2218·3
Physiosoin, 2218·3
PhysioSol, 2218·3
Physiostat, 2218·3
Physiotens, 2218·3
Physiotherm, 2218·3
Physiotulle, 2218·3
Physium, 2218·3
Physostig. Sal., 1494·1
Physostig. Sulph., 1494·2
*Physostigma venenosum*, 1494·1
Physostigmine, 1494·1
Physostigmine Aminoxide Salicylate, 1491·2
Physostigmine Monosalicylate, 1494·1
Physostigmine *N*-Oxide Salicylate, 1491·2
Physostigmine Salicylate, 1494·1
Physostigmine Sulfate, 1494·2
Physostigmine Sulphate, 1494·2
Physostigmini Salicylas, 1494·1
Physostigmini Sulfas, 1494·2
Phytat, 2218·4
Phytate Sodium, 1052·3
Phytemag, 2218·4
Phytentielles, 2218·4
Phytex, 2218·4
Phytic Acid, 2218·4
Phyto Corrective Gel, 2218·4
Phytoberidin, 2218·4
Phytobronchin, 2218·4
Phytobronchin— *see* Phytohustil, 2218·4
Phytocalm, 2218·4
Phyto-Care, 2218·4
Phytocean, 2218·4
Phytocold, 2218·4
Phytocortal, 2218·4
Phytoderm Compositum, 2218·4
Phytodiet, 2218·4
Phytodolor, 2218·4
Phytodorma, 2218·4
Phyto-Embryonnaire, 2218·4
Phytoestrin, 2218·4
Phytoestrol N, 2218·4
Phytofibre, 2218·4
Phytogran, 2218·4
Phytohepar, 2218·4
Phytohustil, 2218·4
Phyto-Hypophyson C, 2219·1
Phyto-Hypophyson L, 2219·1
*Phytolacca americana*, 1733·1
*Phytolacca decandra*, 1733·1
*Phytolacca dodecandra*, 1504·3, 1733·1
Phytolax, 2219·1
Phyto-Laxia, 2219·1
PhytoLaxin, 2219·1
Phytolife, 2219·1
Phytolife Plus, 2219·1
Phytolithe, 2219·1
Phytomed Preparations, 2219·1
Phytomelis, 2219·1
Phytomenad., 1467·1
Phytomenadione, 1467·1
Phytomenadionum, 1467·1
Phytonadione, 1467·1
Phytonoctu, 2219·1
Phytonoxon N, 2219·1
Phytophanere, 2219·1
Phytopure, 2219·1
Phytorelax, 2219·1
Phytoslim, 2219·1
Phytosterol, 982·3
Phytosterolum, 982·3
Phytosyl Plus, 2219·1
Phytotherapie Boribel No 8, 2219·1
Phytotherapie Boribel No 9, 2219·1
Phytotherapie Titree, 2219·1
Phytotux, 2219·2
Phytotux H, 2219·2
Phytovim, 2219·2
PI Antiseptic Ointment, 2219·2
Piascledine, 2219·2
Piat, 2219·2
Piazofolina, 2219·2
Picalm, 2219·2
Picapan, 2219·2
Picariz, 2219·2
Picibanil, 1731·3, 2219·2
Picillin, 2219·2
Picis Carbonis, Liquor, 1159·2
Pickles Preparations, 2219·2
Picktooth Fruit, 1653·3
Picloxydine Dihydrochloride, 1190·1
Picolamine Salicylate, 84·1
Picolax, 2219·2
Picolax— *see* Colonprep, 1900·3
Picolaxine, 2219·2
Picolite, 2219·2
Picolon, 2219·2
Picoprep, 2219·2
PicoPrep— *see* Prep Kit-C, 2233·1
Pico-Salax, 2219·2
Picosulfato de Sodio, 1289·3
Picosulphol, 1289·3
Picosyl, 2219·2
Picot, 2219·2
Picot Sans Gluten, 2219·2
Picot Sans Lactose, 2219·2
Picotamida, 982·3
Picotamide, 982·3
Picotamide Monohydrate, 982·3
Picotamidum Monohydricum, 982·3
*Picraena excelsa*, 1737·2
*Picrasma excelsa*, 1737·2
Picric Acid, 1758·1
Picrinic Acid, 1758·1
Picrocrocine, 1058·2
Picroprep, 2219·2
Pidilat, 2219·3
Pidocal, 2219·3
Pidolato de Calcio, 1226·1
Pidolato de Magnesio, 1228·2
Pidolato Sódico, 1158·1
Pidomag, 2219·3
Pidorubicin Hydrochloride, 550·2
Pidotimod, 1731·3
Piecidex, 2219·3
Piedra Pómez, 1140·1
Piel Vital, 2219·3
Pielograf, 2219·3
Pierami, 2219·3
Pierre Ponce Granulée, 1140·1
PIF, 1196·1
Pifatidine Hydrochloride, 1288·1
PIFE, 1308·1
Pifrol, 2219·3
Pigbel— *see* Necrotising Enterocolitis, 129·2
Pigbel Vaccines, 1632·3
Pigenil, 2219·3
Pigitil, 2219·3
Pigmal, 2219·3
Pigmanorm, 2219·3
Pigment Hormone, 1332·2
Pigment Rubine, 1057·3
Pigmentasa, 2219·3
Pigmentation Disorders, 1137·2
Pigmented Purpuric Dermatosis— *see* Non-infective Skin Disorders, 401·2
Piketofen, 2219·3
Piketoprofen, 84·1
Piketoprofen Hydrochloride, 84·1
Piketoprofeno, 84·1
Pik-Gel, 2219·3
PIL, 1495·1
Pilagan, 2219·3
Pilax, 2219·3
Pilder, 2219·3
Pildoras Ferrug Sanatori, 2219·3
Pildoras Zeninas, 2219·3
Pileabs, 2219·3
Pilem, 2219·3
Pilensar, 2219·3
Piles— *see* Haemorrhoids, 1243·1
Piletabs, 2219·3
Pilewort, 1732·1
Pilewort Compound, 2219·3
Pil-Food, 2219·3
Pilfood, 2219·4
Pilfor P, 2219·4
Pil-G Uso, 2219·4
Pilison, 2219·4
Pilka, 2219·4
Pilka F, 2219·4
Pilka Forte, 2219·4
Pill-bearing Spurge, 1686·3
Pillole Fattori, 2219·4
Pilmolite, 2219·4
Pilo, 2219·4
Pilobloc, 2219·4
Pilocar, 2219·4
Pilocarcil, 2219·4
Pilocarp. Hydrochlor., 1495·1
Pilocarp. Nit., 1495·1
Pilocarpic Acid, 1495·3
Pilocarpina, 1494·3
Pilocarpina, Borato de, 1495·1
Pilocarpina, Hidrocloruro de, 1495·1
Pilocarpina, Nitrato de, 1495·1
Pilocarpine, 1494·3
Pilocarpine Borate, 1495·1
Pilocarpine Hydrochloride, 1495·1
Pilocarpine Monohydrochloride, 1495·1
Pilocarpine Mononitrate, 1495·1
Pilocarpine Nitrate, 1495·1
Pilocarpini Chloridum, 1495·1
Pilocarpini Hydrochloridum, 1495·1
Pilocarpini Nitras, 1495·1
Pilocarpinii Nitras, 1495·1
Pilocarpinium Chloratum, 1495·1
Pilocarpinium Nitricum, 1495·1
Pilocarpol, 2219·4
*Pilocarpus microphyllus*, 1494·3
Pilocollyre, 2219·4
Pilodren, 2219·4
Pilo-Eserin, 2219·4
Pilof Nicolich, 2219·4
Piloftal, 2219·4
Pilogel, 2219·4
Pilogel HS, 2219·4
Pilomann, 2219·4
Pilomann-Ol, 2219·4
Pilomed, 2220·1
Pilopine HS, 2220·1
Piloplex, 2220·1
Pilopos, 2220·1
Pilopt, 2220·1
Piloptic, 2220·1
Pilopto-Carpine, 2220·1
Pilostat, 2220·1
Pilostigmin Puroptal, 2220·1
Pilo-Stulln, 2220·1
Pilosuryl, 2220·1
Pilotim, 2220·1
Pilotina, 2220·1
Pilotonina, 2220·1
Pilovital, 2220·1
Piloxil, 2220·1
Pilriteiro, 1677·1
Pilsicainida, Hidrocloruro de, 983·1
Pilsicainide Hydrochloride, 983·1
Pilulas De Witt's, 2220·1
Pilulas Ross, 2220·1
Pilules de Vichy, 2220·1
Pilzcin, 2220·1
Pima, 2220·1
Pima Biciron N, 2220·1
Pimafucin, 2220·1
Pimafucort, 2220·1
Pimagedina, 344·1
Pimagedine, 344·1
Pimaricin, 406·2
Pimecrolimus, 1155·1
Piment Rouge, 1667·1
*Pimenta racemosa*, 1659·1
Pimentão , 1667·1
Pimethixene, 439·1
Pimetixene, 439·1
Pimetixeno, 439·1
Pimiken, 2220·1
Pimobendan, 983·1
Pimozida, 715·1
Pimozide, 715·1
Pimozidum, 715·1
Pimpinela Mayor, 1663·2
*Pimpinella anisum*, 1655·2
Pimustine Hydrochloride, 576·3
Pin de Montagne, Essence de, 1737·1
Pinacidil, 983·1
Pinaclav, 2220·1
Pinaclor, 2220·1

Pinacolyl Methylphosphonofluoridate, 1719·2
Pinadone DTF, 2220·2
Pinadrina, 2220·2
Pinal N, 2220·2
Pinal S, 2220·2
Pin-Alcol, 2220·2
Pinalgesic, 2220·2
Pinamet, 2220·2
Pinamox, 2220·2
Pinaverio, Bromuro de, 1732·1
Pinaverium Bromide, 1732·1
Pinazepam, 715·3
Pinazone, 43·2
Pindac, 2220·2
Pinden, 2220·2
Pindione, 2220·2
Pindocor, 2220·2
Pindol, 2220·2
Pindolol, 983·2
Pindololum, 983·2
Pindoptan, 2220·2
Pindoreal, 2220·2
Pine Needle Oil, Dwarf, 1737·1
Pine Oil, Pumilio, 1737·1
Pine OPC, 2220·2
Pine Tar, 1159·3
Pineal, 2220·2
Pinealoblastoma— *see* Retinoblastoma, 524·2
Pineapple, 1662·3
Pinedrin, 2220·2
α-Pinene, 1710·2, 1724·1, 1740·2, 1760·1
β-Pinene, 1706·2, 1724·1, 1740·2, 1760·1
Pinetarsol, 2220·2
Pinex Preparations, 2220·2
Pingus, 698·3
Pini, Pix, 1159·3
Pini Pumilionis, Oleum, 1737·1
Pini, Pyroleum, 1159·3
Pini, Resina, 1675·1
Pinifed, 2220·2
Pinikehl, 2220·2
Piniment, 2220·2
Pinimenthol Preparations, 2220·3
Piniol, 2220·3
Piniol Erkaltungsbalsam, 2220·3
Piniol Nasensalbe, 2220·3
Piniol Nasenspray, 2220·3
Pink Bismuth Rose, 2220·3
Pinklot, 2220·3
Pinloc, 2220·3
Pino Mugo, Aceite Esencial de, 1737·1
Pino-Cort, 2220·3
Pinorhinol, 2220·3
Pinosil, 2220·3
Pin-Rid, 2220·3
Pinselina Knapp, 2220·3
Pinsken, 2220·3
Pinta— *see* Syphilis, 148·2
Pintacrom, 2220·3
Pintal, 2220·3
*Pinus*, 1675·1
*Pinus mugo*, 1737·1
*Pinus pinaster*, 1760·1
Pinworm Infections— *see* Enterobiasis, 99·1
Pin-X, 2220·3
Piodermina, 2220·4
Piodrex, 2220·4
Pioglit, 2220·4
Pioglitazona, Hidrocloruro de, 344·1
Pioglitazone Hydrochloride, 344·1
Pioletal, 2220·4
Piolhol, 2220·4
Piolhol Plus, 2220·4
Piolin, 2220·4
Pionax, 2220·4
Pioral Pasta, 2220·4
Piorlis, 2220·4
Piosan, 2220·4
Piosol, 2220·4
Piostop, 2220·4
Pipacid, 2220·4
Pipamperona, Hidrocloruro de, 716·1
Pipamperone, 716·1
Pipamperone Hydrochloride, 716·1
Pipazetate, 1129·1
Pipazetate Hydrochloride, 1129·1
Pipazetato, Hidrocloruro de, 1129·1
Pipazethate, 1129·1
Pipazethate Hydrochloride, 1129·1
Pipcil, 2220·4
Pipeacid, 2220·4
2′,6′-Pipecoloxylidide, 1381·2
Pipecurium Bromide, 1405·2
Pipecuronio, Bromuro de, 1405·2
Pipecuronium Bromide, 1405·2
Pipedac, 2220·4
Pipedic, 2220·4
Pipefort, 2220·4
Pipemed, 2220·4
Pipemid, 2220·4
Pipemidic Acid, 243·1
Pipemidic Acid Trihydrate, 243·1
Pipemídico, Ácido, 243·1
Pipemidicum Trihydricum, Acidum, 243·1
Pipemidol, 2220·4
Pipenzolate Bromide, 487·3
Pipenzolate Methylbromide, 487·3
Pipenzolato, Bromuro de, 487·3
*Piper betle*, 1656·2
*Piper methysticum*, 1703·2
Pipera, 2220·4
Piperac, 2220·4
Piperacetazina, 716·1
Piperacetazine, 716·1
Piperacilina, 243·1
Piperacilina Sódica, 243·1
Piperacillin, 243·1
Piperacillin Sodium, 243·1
Piperacillinum, 243·1
Piperacillinum Natricum, 243·1
Piperamic Acid, 243·1
Piperaquina, Fosfato de, 456·1
Piperaquine Phosphate, 456·1
Piperaquini Phosphas, 456·1
Piperawitt DS, 2220·4
Piperaz. Adip., 111·2
Piperazil, 2220·4
Piperazina, 111·2
Piperazina, Adipato de, 111·2
Piperazina, Citrato de, 111·2
Piperazina, Fosfato de, 111·2
Piperazina Hexahidrato, 111·2
Piperazine, 111·2
Piperazine Adipate, 111·2
Piperazine Bis(theophyllin-7-ylacetate) (1:1), 780·1
Piperazine Citrate, 111·2
Piperazine Estrone Sulfate, 1553·1
Piperazine Hexahydrate, 111·2
Piperazine Hydrate, 111·2
Piperazine Oestrone Sulphate, 1553·1
Piperazine 17-Oxoestra-1,3,5-(10)-trien-3-yl Hydrogen Sulphate, 1553·1
Piperazine Phosphate, 111·2, 111·3
Piperazine Theophylline Ethanoate, 780·1
1,1′-[Piperazine-1,4-diylbis(formimidoyl)]bis[3-(4-chlorophenyl)guanidine] Dihydrochloride, 1190·1
Piperazini Adipas, 111·2
Piperazini Citras, 111·2
Piperazini Hydras, 111·2
Piperazini Phosphas, 111·2
4-Piperazinoquinoline Antimalarials, 444·1
Piperazinum Adipicum, 111·2
Piperazinum Hydricum, 111·2
Pipercream, 2220·4
Piperestazine Hydrochloride, 1129·1
Piperidic Acid, 1690·2
*p*-Piperidinoacetilaminobenzoato de Etilo, 1376·3
1-Piperidinocyclohexanecarbonitrile, 1730·3
2-(2-Piperidinoethoxy)ethyl Pyrido[3,2-*b*][1,4]benzothiazine-10-carboxylate, 1129·1
2-Piperidinoethyl Bicyclohexyl-1-carboxylate Hydrochloride, 481·3
2-Piperidinoethyl 3-Methyl-4-oxo-2-phenyl-4*H*-chromene-8-carboxylate Hydrochloride, 482·2
3-Piperidino-4′-propoxypropiophenone, 1383·3
3-Piperidinopropylene Bis(phenylcarbamate) Hydrochloride, 1376·2
*N*-{3-[(α-Piperidino-*m*-tolyl)oxy]propyl}glycolamide Acetate Monohydrochloride, 1288·1
4-[(1-Piperidinylacetyl)amino]benzoic Acid Ethyl Ester, 1376·3
Piperidolate Hydrochloride, 487·3
Piperidolato, Hidrocloruro de, 487·3
Piperidyl Methadone Hydrochloride, 35·3
Piperidylamidone Hydrochloride, 35·3
α-2-Piperidylbenzhydrol Hydrochloride, 1592·3
*N*-(2-Piperidylmethyl)-2,5-bis(2,2,2-trifluoroethoxy)benzamide Acetate, 916·2
Piperilate Ethobromide, 487·3
Piperilline, 2220·4
Piperital, 2220·4
Pipermed, 2220·4
Pipermel, 2220·4
Piperonal, 1509·1
Piperonil, 2220·4
Piperonyl Butoxide, 1509·2
Piperonyl Ranitidine Hydrochloride, 1277·2
Piperonylaldehyde, 1509·1
10-[(4-Piperonyl-1-piperazinyl)acetyl]phenothiazine, 1687·3
2-(4-Piperonylpiperazin-1-yl)pyrimidine, 1212·2
Pipersal, 2220·4
Pipertex, 2221·1
Pipertox, 2221·1
Pipervermin, 2221·1
Pipetanato, Etobromuro de, 487·3
Pipetecan, 2221·1
Pipetexina, 2221·1
Pipethanate Ethobromide, 487·3
Pipiol, 2221·1
Piplex, 2221·1
Pipobroman, 580·1
Piportil, 2221·1
Piportil L4, 2221·1
Piportyl, 2221·1
Piportyl L4, 2221·1
Pipothiazine, 716·1
Pipothiazine Palmitate, 716·1
Pipotiazina, 716·1
Pipotiazina, Palmitato de, 716·1
Pipotiazine, 716·1
Pipotiazine Palmitate, 716·1
Pipoxolan, 1732·1
Pipoxolan Hydrochloride, 1732·1
Pippen, 2221·1
Pipracil, 2221·1
Pipracin, 2221·1
Pipradrol, Hidrocloruro de, 1592·3
Pipradrol Hydrochloride, 1592·3
Pipralen, 2221·1
Pipram, 2221·1
Pipratecol, 983·3
Pipril, 2221·1
Piprine, 2221·1
Piprinhidrinato, 439·1
Piprinhydrinate, 439·1
Piprol, 2221·1
Piproxen, 2221·1
*Piptadenia macrocarpa*, 1663·2
*Piptadenia peregrina*, 1663·2, 1680·3
Piptalake P, 2221·1
Pipurin, 2221·1
Pipurol, 2221·1
Pira, 2221·1
Pirabene, 2221·1
Piracalamina, 2221·1
Piracebral, 2221·1
Piracetam, 1732·1
Piracetam Complex, 2221·2
Piracetamum, 1732·1
Piracetrop, 2221·2
Piraclofós, 1509·2
Pirafoid, 2221·2
Pirafrin, 2221·2
Piraldin, 2221·2
Piraldina, 2221·2
Piralgina, 2221·2
Piralone, 2221·2
Piram, 2221·2
Piramagno, 2221·2
Piram-D, 2221·2
Piramin, 2221·2
Pirandall, 2221·2
Pirantel, Embonato de, 113·2
Pirantel Pamoate, 113·2
Pirantrim, 2221·2
Pirarubicin, 580·1
Pirarubicin Hydrochloride, 580·1
Pirarubicina, 580·1
Piraside, 2221·2
Piratam, 2221·2
Pirawil, 2221·2
Pirax, 2221·2
Pirazer, 2221·2
Pirazinamida, 246·3
Pirazinon, 2221·2
Pirbuterol Acetate, 790·3
Pirbuterol, Acetato de, 790·3
Pirbuterol, Hidrocloruro de, 790·3
Pirbuterol Hydrochloride, 790·3
Pirehexal, 2221·2
Piren-basan, 2221·2
Pirenoxina Sódica, 1732·2
Pirenoxine Sodium, 1732·2
Pirenzepina, Hidrocloruro de, 488·1
Pirenzepine Dihydrochloride Monohydrate, 488·1
Pirenzepine Hydrochloride, 488·1
Pirenzepini Dihydrochloridum Monohydricum, 488·1
Piretanida, 983·3
Piretanide, 983·3
Piretanide Sodium, 983·3
Piretanidum, 983·3
Piretanyl, 2221·2
Piretro, 1509·3
Pireuma, 2221·2
Pirexyl, 2221·2
Pirfalin, 2221·2
Pirfenidona, 1732·3
Pirfenidone, 1732·3
Pirfenoxone Sodium, 1732·2
Pirglutargine, 1732·3
Piribedil, 1212·2
Piribedil Mesilate, 1212·2
Piricarbato, 1737·1
Piridasmin, 2221·2
Piridofilina, 791·2
Piridossina Cloridrato, 1456·3
Piridostigmina, Bromuro de, 1496·1
Piridoxilate, 1732·3
Piridoxilato, 1732·3
Piridoxina, Hidrocloruro de, 1456·3
Pirifedrina, 2221·2
Pirifibrate, 984·1
Pirifibrato, 984·1
Pirifur, 2221·3
Piriject, 2221·3
Pirilene, 2221·3
Pirimat, 2221·3
Pirimetamina, 458·1
Pirimetan, 2221·3
Pirimiphos-Methyl, 1509·2
Pirimir, 2221·3
Pirinace, 2221·3
Pirinasol, 2221·3
Pirinitramide, 84·1
Pirinovag, 2221·3
Piriproxifeno, 1509·3
Pirisudanol, Dimaleato de, 1732·3
Pirisudanol Maleate, 1732·3
Piriteze, 2221·3
Piritildiona, 718·1
Piritinol, Hidrocloruro de, 1737·2
Piritiona Cíncica, 1156·2
Piriton, 2221·3
Piriton Expectorant, 2221·3
Piritosse, 2221·3
Piritramida, 84·1
Piritramide, 84·1
Piritramide Tartrate, 84·1
Piritrexim Isethionate, 580·1

Piritrexim Isetionate, 580·1
Piritrexima, Isetionato de, 580·1
Pirium, 2221·3
Pirkam, 2221·3
Pirlimicina, Hidrocloruro de, 244·1
Pirlimycin Hydrochloride, 244·1
Pirlindol, 316·2
Pirlindole, 316·2
Pirmenol, Hidrocloruro de, 984·1
Pirmenol Hydrochloride, 984·1
Piro, 2221·3
Piro KD, 2221·3
Piroalgin, 2221·3
Pirobac, 2221·3
Pirobeta, 2221·3
Pirobutil, 2221·3
Pirocal, 2221·3
Pirocam, 2221·3
Piroctona Olamina, 1155·2
Piroctone Olamine, 1155·2
Pirodax, 2221·3
Pirofix, 2221·3
Piroflam, 2221·3
Piroflex, 2221·3
Piroftal, 2221·3
Pirogálico, Ácido, 1156·2
Pirogina, 2221·4
Pirohexal-D, 2221·4
Piroli-N, 2221·4
Pirom, 2221·4
Piromav, 2221·4
Piromebrina, 2221·4
Piromidic Acid, 244·1
Piromídico, Ácido, 244·1
Pironal, 2221·4
Pironaridina, Fosfato de, 460·1
Pironet, 2221·4
Pirongil, 2221·4
Pirophen, 2221·4
Piro-Phlogont, 2221·4
Piroplasmosis— *see* Babesiosis, 595·3
Piro-Puren, 2221·4
Pirorheum, 2221·4
PirorheumA, 2221·4
Pirosol, 2221·4
Pirox, 2221·4
Piroxal, 2221·4
Piroxam, 2221·4
Piroxan, 2221·4
Pirox-basan, 2221·4
Piroxcin, 2221·4
Piroxen, 2221·4
Piroxene, 2221·4
Piroxgel, 2221·4
Piroxicam, 84·2
Piroxicam Beta Cyclodextrin, 84·2
Piroxicam Beta Cyclodextrin Complex, 84·2
Piroxicam Betadex, 84·2
Piroxicam Choline, 85·1
Piroxicam Cinnamate, 85·1
Piroxicam Pivalate, 85·1
Piroxicamum, 84·2
Piroxifen, 2221·4
Piroxiflam, 2222·1
Piroxigea, 2222·1
Piroxil, 2222·1
Piroxilina, 1156·2
Piroximerck, 2222·1
Piroxin, 2222·1
Piroxiplus, 2222·1
Piroxistad, 2222·1
Piroxityrol, 2222·1
Piroxsil, 2222·1
Pirox-Spondyril, 2222·1
Piroxy, 2222·1
Pirozadil, 984·1
Pirozip, 2222·1
Pirrolfungin, 2222·1
Pirrolnitrina, 408·1
Piruvato de Sodio, 1748·2
Pirvinio, Embonato de, 113·3
Pirxane, 2222·1
Pirzinol, 2222·1
Pisacaina, 2222·1
Pisatrina, 2222·1
Piscidia, 1702·3
*Piscidia erythrina*, 1702·3
*Piscidia piscipula*, 1702·3
Piscis Oleum Omega-3 Acidis Abundams, 976·2
Pissenlit, 1751·3
*Pistacia lentiscus*, 1710·1
Pistofil, 2222·1
Pitavastatin, 984·1
Pitavastatin Calcium, 984·1
Pitcher Plant, 88·2
Pitiriax, 2222·1
Pitkin's Menstruum, 755·2
Pito, 1666·1
Pitocin, 2222·1
Pitofenona, Hidrocloruro de, 1732·3
Pitofenone Hydrochloride, 1732·3
Pitressin, 2222·1
Pitrex, 2222·1
Pitrion, 2222·1
Pitrisan, 2222·1
Pituitarium Posterius Pulveratum, 1337·3
Pituitary, 1337·3
Pituitary Diabetes Insipidus— *see* Diabetes Insipidus, 1314·1
Pituitary Hormones, 1312·1
Pituitary, Posterior, 1337·3
Pituitary (Posterior Lobe), Powdered, 1337·3
Pit-viper, Malayan, 863·2
Pityker, 2222·1
Pityriasis Capitis— *see* Seborrhoeic Dermatitis, 1138·3
Pityriasis Versicolor— *see* Skin Infections, 390·1
Pityval, 2222·1
Pivalato de Clocortolona, 1096·1
Pivalato de Desoxicortona, 1097·1
Pivalato de Flumetasona, 1101·1
Pivalato de Fluocortolona, 1102·1
Pivalato de Prednisolona, 1108·1
Pivalato de Tixocortol, 1110·1
Pivalic Acid, 244·2, 244·3
Pivalone, 2222·2
Pivalone Compositum, 2222·2
Pivalone Neomycin, 2222·2
Pivalone Neomycine, 2222·2
Pivaloxicam, 2222·2
Pivaloyloxymethyl (+)-(6*R*,7*R*)-7-[2-(2-Amino-4-thiazolyl)glyoxylamido]-3-[(*Z*)-2-(4-methyl-5-thiazolyl)vinyl]-8-oxo-5-thia-1-azabicyclo[4.2.0]oct-2-ene-2-carboxylic Acid $7^2$-(*Z*)-(*O*-Methyloxime), 172·1
Pivaloyloxymethyl (*Z*)-7-[2-(2-Aminothiazol-4-yl)-2-methoxyiminoacetamido]-3-(5-methyl-2*H*-tetrazol-2-ylmethyl)-3-cephem-4-carboxylic Acid, 181·3
Pivaloyloxymethyl (+)-(6*R*,7*R*)-7-[(*Z*)-2-(2-Amino-4-thiazolyl)-2-pentenamido]-3-(hydroxymethyl)-8-oxo-5-thia-1-azabicyclo[4.2.0]oct-2-ene-2-carboxylic Acid Carbamate Monohydrochloride Monohydrate, 171·3
Pivaloyloxymethyl (6*R*)-6-(Perhydroazepin-1-ylmethyleneamino)penicillanate, 244·2
Pivaloyloxymethyl (6*R*)-6-(α-D-Phenylglycylamino)penicillanate, 244·1
Pivamdinocillin, 244·2
Pivamiser, 2222·2
Pivampicilina, 244·1
Pivampicilina, Hidrocloruro de, 244·2
Pivampicillin, 244·1, 244·2
Pivampicillin Hydrochloride, 244·2
Pivampicillinum, 244·1
Pivanozolo, 2222·2
Pivmecilinam, 244·2
Pivmecilinam, Hidrocloruro de, 244·2
Pivmecillinam, 244·2
Pivmecillinam Hydrochloride, 244·2
Pivmecillinami Hydrochloridum, 244·2
Piv2PMEA, 628·1
Pix Abietinarum, 1159·3
Pix Betulae, 1159·2
Pix Cadi, 1159·2
Pix Carbon., 1159·2
Pix Carbonis, 1159·2
Pix Juniperi, 1159·2
Pix Liquida, 1159·3
Pix Lithanthracis, 1159·2
Pix Mineralis, 1159·2
Pix Oxycedri, 1159·2
Pix Pini, 1159·3
Pixfix, 2222·2
Pixicam, 2222·2
Pixidin, 2222·2
Pixor Stick Anti-acne N, 2222·2
PIXY-321, 755·3
Piz Buin, 2222·2
Pizide, 2222·2
Pizomed, 2222·2
Pizotifen, 470·3
Pizotifen Hydrochloride, 470·3
Pizotifen Hydrogen Malate, 470·3
Pizotifen Malate, 470·3
Pizotifeno, 470·3
Pizotifeno, Malato de, 470·3
Pizotyline, 470·3
Pizotyline Malate, 470·3
PK-10169, 910·3
PK-26124, 1738·3
PK Aid, 2222·2
PK-Levo, 2222·2
PK-Merz, 2222·2
PKU Preparations, 2222·2
Plac Out, 2222·2
Placatus, 2222·2
Placentex, 2222·2
Placentina, 2222·2
Placentrex, 2222·2
Placidox, 2222·2
Placidyl, 2222·2
Placil, 2222·3
Placinoral, 2222·3
Placis, 2222·3
Plactidil, 2222·3
Plactosse, 2222·3
Plafonyl, 2222·3
Plagex, 2222·3
Plagon, 2222·3
Plague, 141·2
Plague Vaccines, 1633·1
Plain Caramel, 1057·1
Plak, 2222·3
Plak Out, 2222·3
Plaket, 2222·3
Plamet, 2222·3
Plamidasil, 2222·3
Plamin, 2222·3
Plamivon, 2222·3
Plan B, 2222·3
Plander, 2222·3
Plander R, 2222·3
Planitrix, 2222·3
Planizol, 2222·3
Planocid, 2222·3
Planor, 2222·3
Planphylline, 2222·3
Plant Nucleic Acid, 1738·2
Plant Protease Concentrate, 1662·2
Plant Spray, 2222·3
Planta Genista, 1742·2
Planta Lax, 2222·3
Plantaben, 2222·3
Plantacard N, 2222·3
Plantactiv, 2222·3
Plantaginis Lanceolatae, 1738·2
Plantaginis Lanceolatae Folium, 1738·2
Plantaginis Ovatae Semen, 1268·1
Plantaginis Ovatae Seminis Tegumentum, 1268·1
*Plantago afra*, 1268·1
*Plantago arenaria*, 1268·1
*Plantago depressa*, 1733·1
*Plantago indica*, 1268·1
*Plantago ispaghula*, 1268·1
*Plantago lanceolata*, 1738·2
*Plantago major*, 1733·1
*Plantago ovata*, 1268·1
*Plantago psyllium*, 1268·1
Plantago Seed, 1268·1
Plantaguar, 2222·3
Plantain, 1733·1
Plantain Herb, 1738·2
Plantain, Ribwort, 1738·2
PlantarPatch, Trans-Ver-Sal— *see* Trans-Ver-Sal PlantarPatch, 2341·2
Plantax, 2222·3
Planten, 2222·4
Plantiodine Plus, 2222·4
Plantival, 2222·4
Plantival Novo, 2222·4
Plantmobil, 2222·4
Plantocur, 2222·4
Planum, 2222·4
Plaqacide, 2222·4
Plaquenil, 2222·4
Plaquetal, 2222·4
Plaquetas, 758·3
Plaquetil, 2222·4
Plaquinol, 2222·4
Plas-Amino, 2222·4
Plasbumin, 2222·4
Plasil, 2222·4
Plasil Enzimatico, 2222·4
Plasimine, 2222·4
Plaskine Neomicina, 2222·4
Plasma, 757·3
Plasma Cell Neoplasms, 511·3
Plasma, Cryoprecipitate Depleted, 757·3
Plasma du Dr Quinton, 2222·4
Plasma Expanders, 732·1, 835·2
Plasma for Fractionation, Human, 757·3
Plasma Humanum ad Separationem, 757·3
Plasma Humanum Collectum Deinde Conditum ad Viros Exstinguendos, 757·3
Plasma Marin Hypertonique, 2222·4
Plasma (Pooled and Treated for Virus Inactivation), Human, 757·3
Plasma Protein Fraction, 758·2
Plasma Thromboplastin Antecedent, 735·3
Plasma Thromboplastin Component, 735·3, 752·2
Plasmacair, 2222·4
Plasmaclar, 2223·1
Plasmafusin, 2223·1
Plasmagel, 2223·1
Plasma-Lyte, 2223·1
Plasma-Lyte IV, 2223·1
Plasma-Lyte O, 2223·1
Plasmanate, 2223·1
Plasma-Plex, 2223·1
Plasmarine, 2223·1
Plasmasteril, 2223·1
Plasmatein, 2223·1
Plasmaviral, 2223·1
Plasmin, 916·2
Plasminogen, 735·3, 984·1
Plasminogen Activator, 245-L-Methionine, 909·2
Plasminogen Activator, Recombinant Human Single-chain Urokinase-type, 996·3
Plasminogen Activator, Recombinant Tissue-type, 857·1
Plasminogen Activator, Tissue, 735·3
Plasminogen Streptokinase Activator Complex, Anisoylated, 863·3
Plasminógeno, 984·1
Plasminokinase, 1005·2
Plasmion, 2223·1
Plasmocolit, 2223·1
Plasmodex, 2223·1
*Plasmodium falciparum*, 1622·2
Plasmonsoy, 2223·1
Plasmoquine, 2223·1
Plasmotrim, 2223·1
Plasonil, 2223·1
Plast Apyr Fisio Irrigac, 2223·1
Plast Apyr Fisiologico, 2223·1
Plast Apyr Glucosado, 2223·1
Plast Apyr Glucosalino, 2223·1
Plastenan, 2223·1
Plastenan con Neomicina, 2223·1
Plastenan Neomicina, 2223·1
Plaster of Paris, 1665·1
Plastesol, 2223·1
Plásticos, 1733·1
Plastics, 1733·1
Plastistil, 2223·1
Plastranit, 2223·2
Plastufer, 2223·2

Plastulen N, 2223·2
Plastules, 2223·2
Plasvit, 2223·2
Plata, 1746·1
Plata, Acetato de, 1746·1
Plata, Nitrato de, 1746·1
Plata, Proteína de, 1746·2
Plata, Proteinato de, 1746·2
Plata, Vitelinato de, 1746·2
Platamine, 2223·2
Platelet Concentrate, 758·3
Platelet-derived Growth Factor, 1679·1
Platelets, 758·3
Platenk, 2223·2
Platiblastin, 2223·2
Platiblastin-S, 2223·2
Platicarb, 2223·2
Platin, 2223·2
Platinex, 2223·2
Platinic Chloride, 1670·2, 1699·1
Platino II, 2223·2
Platinol, 2223·2
Platinostyl, 2223·2
Platinum Diamminodichloride, 538·1
Platinum Years, 2223·2
Platinwas, 2223·2
Platiran, 2223·2
Platistil, 2223·2
Platistin, 2223·2
Platistine, 2223·2
Platium, 2223·2
Plato, 2223·2
Platocillina, 2223·2
Platosin, 2223·2
Plâtre Cuit, 1665·1
Platsul A, 2223·2
Platsul-A, 2223·2
Platyphylline Acid Tartrate, 488·2
Platyphylline Bitartrate, 488·2
Platyphyllini Hydrotartras, 488·2
Plau-noi, 1284·2
Plaunotol, 1284·1
Plausital, 2223·3
Plausitin, 2223·3
Plavix, 2223·3
Plax, 2223·3
Plax, Advanced Formula— *see* Advanced Formula Plax, 1777·3
Plazolit, 2223·3
Ple-1053, 866·3
Plebe, 2223·3
Pleconaril, 651·3
Pleconarilo, 651·3
Plecor, 2223·3
*Plectranthus barbatus*, 1674·3
Plegicil, 2223·3
Plegine, 2223·3
Plegisol, 2223·3
Plegivex, 2223·3
Pleiadon, 2223·3
Pleiamide, 2223·3
Plenacor, 2223·3
Plenacor D, 2223·3
Plenactol, 2223·3
Plenaer, 2223·3
Plenax, 2223·3
Plenaxis, 2223·3
Plendil, 2223·3
Plendur, 2223·3
Plenidon, 2223·4
Plenifem, 2223·4
Plenigraf, 2223·4
Plenish-K, 2223·4
Plenitude Excell A-3, 2223·4
Plenocedan, 2223·4
Plenogripe, 2223·4
Plenolyt, 2223·4
Plenomicina, 2223·4
Plenosol N, 2223·4
Plenovit, 2223·4
Plentiva, 2223·4
Plentiva Cycle 5, 2223·4
Plenty, 2223·4
Plenum, 2223·4
Plenur, 2223·4
Plenyl, 2223·4
Pleo Vitamin, 2223·4
Pleocortex, 2223·4
Pleocortex B6, 2223·4
Pleomix-Alpha, 2223·4
Pleomix-B, 2223·4
Pleon, 2223·4
Pleon RA, 2223·4
Plesmet, 2223·4
Pletaal, 2223·4
Pletal, 2223·4
Pletil, 2223·4
Pleural Effusions, Malignant— *see* Malignant Effusions, 512·2
Pleurisy Root, 1733·1
Plex B, 2224·1
Plex Ton, 2224·1
Plexion, 2224·1
Plexium, 2224·1
Plexivita, 2224·1
Plexo Enterin, 2224·1
Plexoton B12, 2224·1
Plexus, 2224·1
Pliagel, 2224·1
Plicamicina, 580·2
Plicamycin, 580·2
Plidan, 2224·1
Plidan Compuesto, 2224·1
Plidex, 2224·1
Plinzene, 2224·1
Plissamur, 2224·1
Plitican, 2224·1
Plokon, 2224·1
Plomo, 1705·3
Plomurol, 2224·1
Plorinoc, 2224·1
Plostim, 2224·1
Plovacal, 2224·1
Plumarol, 2224·1
Plumger, 2224·1
Pluravit, 2224·1
Pluravit Super B, 2224·1
Plurexid, 2224·1
Pluribios, 2224·1
Pluricefo, 2224·1
Pluriderm, 2224·1
Pluridoxina, 2224·1
Plurifactor, 2224·2
Plurilac, 2224·2
Plurimen, 2224·2
Plurimineral, 2224·2
Plurisalina, 2224·2
Plurisan, 2224·2
Plurisemina, 2224·2
Pluriverm, 2224·2
Plurivermil, 2224·2
Pluriviron Mono, 2224·2
Plurivitamin, 2224·2
30 Plus, 2224·2
30 Plus Sunblock, 2224·2
45 Plus, 2224·2
50 Plus, 2224·2
Plus Kalium Retard, 2224·2
Plus & Plus, 2224·2
Plus Sinus, 2224·2
Plus & White, 2224·2
Plusapetit, 2224·2
Pluscal, 2224·2
Pluscloran, 2224·2
Plusderm, 2224·2
Plusderm ATB, 2224·2
Plusgel, 2224·2
Plusgin, 2224·2
Plusplatin, 2224·3
Plustaxano, 2224·3
Plusvent, 2224·3
Plusvit, 2224·3
Pluviton, 2224·3
Pluviton B, 2224·3
PLV2, 1324·2
PM, 2224·3
PM-150, 96·3
PM-396, 366·2
PM-671, 360·1
PM-185184, 615·3
PMA, 1189·2, 1593·3
PMEA, 628·1
P-Mega-Tablinen, 2224·3
PMFE, 1308·1
PML Crono, 2224·3
PMMA, 1714·3
PMN, 1189·2
PMPA, 655·1
(*R*)-PMPA, 655·1
PMQ-INGA, 2224·3
PMS, 2224·3
PMS— *see* Premenstrual Syndrome, 1551·3
PMS, Hylands— *see* Hylands PMS, 2052·3
PMS L21, 2224·3
PMS Support, 2224·3
PMS-Artificial Tears, 2224·3
PMS-Artificial Tears Extra, 2224·3
PMS-Baximycin, 2224·3
PMS-Care, Extralife— *see* Extralife PMS-Care, 1986·3
PMS-Dicitrate, 2224·3
PMS-Egozinc, 2224·3
PMS-Egozinc-HC, 2224·3
PMS-Enemol, 2224·3
PMS-Levazine, 2224·3
PMS-Phosphates, 2224·3
PMS-Polytrimethoprim, 2224·3
PMT, 254·1
PMT— *see* Premenstrual Syndrome, 1551·3
PMT Complex, 2224·3
PMT Formula, 2224·3
PMT Oral Spray, 2224·3
PMT-Eze, Bioglan— *see* Bioglan PMT-Eze, 1844·1
PN-200-110, 942·2
Pneucid, 2224·4
Pneumaseptic, 2224·4
Pneumo 23, 2224·4
Pneumo 23 Imovax, 2224·4
Pneumoclar, 2224·4
Pneumococcal Meningitis— *see* Meningitis, 134·3
Pneumococcal Polysaccharide Vaccine, 1633·1
Pneumococcal Vaccines, 1633·1
Pneumoconiosis— *see* Diffuse Parenchymal Lung Disease, 1079·3
Pneumocystis Carinii Pneumonia, 389·1
*Pneumocystis jiroveci*, 389·1
Pneumodoron Preparations, 2224·4
Pneumogeine, 2224·4
Pneumogenol, 2224·4
Pneumolat, 2224·4
Pneumolat Expectorante, 2224·4
Pneumomist, 2224·4
Pneumonia, 141·3
Pneumonia, Aspiration— *see* Pneumonia, 141·3
Pneumonia, Legionella— *see* Legionnaires' Disease, 133·1
Pneumonia, Pneumocystis Carinii— *see* Pneumocystis Carinii Pneumonia, 389·1
Pneumonia, Q Fever— *see* Q Fever, 143·3
Pneumonitis— *see* Pneumonia, 141·3
Pneumopan, 2224·4
Pneumopect, 2224·4
Pneumopent, 2224·4
Pneumoplasme, 2224·4
Pneumoplasme a l'Histamine, 2224·4
Pneumopur, 2224·4
Pneumorel, 2224·4
Pneumotussin, 2224·4
Pneumo/Vac, 1633·1
Pneumovax, 2224·4
Pneumovax II, 2224·4
Pneumovax 23, 2224·4
Pneumune, 2224·4
PNU-98528-E, 1212·2
PNU-100766, 226·3
PNU-140690, 655·3
PNU-142300, 227·2
PNU-142586, 227·2
PNU-155950E, 316·3
PNU-180638E, 465·2
PNU-200583E, 489·3
Pnu-Imune, 2224·4
Pnu-Imune 23, 2225·1
Pnu-Inmune, 2225·1
P.O. 12, 2225·1
Po Antisseptico, 2225·1
Pobrax, 2225·1
Pocin, 2225·1
Pocin G, 2225·1
Pocin H, 2225·1
Pocket Energy, Fon Wan— *see* Fon Wan Pocket Energy, 2006·2
PocketScan, 2225·1
Pockinal, 2225·1
Poconeol Preparations, 2225·1
Pocophage, 2225·1
Pocyl, 2225·1
Podactin, 2225·1
Podase, 2225·1
Pod-Ben-25, 2225·1
Podertonic, 2225·1
Podine, 2225·1
Podium, 2225·1
Podocon, 2225·1
Podofilia, 2225·1
Podofilino, 1155·2
Podofilm, 2225·1
Podófilo, 1155·2
Podófilo Indio, 1155·2
Podofilotoxina, 1155·3
Podofilox, 1155·3, 2225·1
Podofin, 2225·1
Podomexef, 2225·1
Podoph., 1155·2
Podoph. Resin, 1155·2
Podophylli Resina, 1155·2
Podophyllin, 1155·2
Podophyllotoxin, 1155·3
Podophyllum, 1155·2
*Podophyllum emodi*, 1155·2
*Podophyllum hexandrum*, 1155·2
Podophyllum, Indian, 1155·2
*Podophyllum peltatum*, 1155·2
Podophyllum Resin, 1155·2
Podophyllum Rhizome, 1155·2
Podophyllum Rhizome, Indian, 1155·2
Podoxin, 2225·1
Poen Efrina, 2225·1
Poenbioptal, 2225·1
Poenbiotico, 2225·1
Poen-Caina NF, 2225·1
Poenfenicol, 2225·2
Poenflox, 2225·2
Poenglaucol, 2225·2
Poenglausil, 2225·2
Poenkerat, 2225·2
Poentimol, 2225·2
Poentobral Plus, 2225·2
Pofol, 2225·2
Poikicholan, 2225·2
Poikigastran N, 2225·2
Poikigeron, 2225·2
Poikilocard Mono, 2225·2
Poikiven T, 2225·2
Poinoxilina, 1190·1
Point, 2225·2
Point-Two, 2225·2
Poison Antidote Kit, 2225·2
Poison Ivy, 1738·1
Poison Ivy/Oak, 2225·2
Poison Oak, 1738·1
Poisoning, Acute— *see* Acute Poisoning, 1030·1
Poisoning, Aluminium— *see* Aluminium Overload, 1035·1
Poisoning, Amanita, 1043·3
Poisoning, Anticholinesterases, 1050·2
Poisoning, Bromate— *see* Bromate Poisoning, 1054·1
Poisoning, Ciguatera— *see* Ciguatera Poisoning, 951·1
Poisoning, Cyanide, 1052·3, 1054·1
Poisoning, Food— *see* Gastro-enteritis, 127·3
Poisoning, Heavy Metals, 1050·1
Poisoning, Heparin, 1051·1
Poisoning, Iron— *see* Iron Poisoning, 1035·3
Poisoning, Mushroom, 1043·3

Poisoning, Nerve Gas— *see* Nerve Gas Poisoning, 1496·3
Poisoning, Opioids, 1045·1
Poisoning, Organophosphorus Insecticides, 1050·2
Poisoning, Paracetamol— *see* Overdosage, 76·2
Poisoning, Radioactive Metals, 1050·1
Poisoning, Tetrodotoxin— *see* Tetrodotoxin Poisoning, 1491·1
Poisoning, Thallium, 1051·2
Poisonous Mushrooms or Toadstools, 1717·3
Poke Root, 1733·1
Pokeroot, 1733·1
Polacrilin Potassium, 1733·1
Polacrilina Potásica, 1733·1
Polacrilinum Kalii, 1733·1
Polagen, 2225·2
Polamin, 2225·2
Polamine, 2225·2
Polaprezinc, 1284·2
Polar Ice, 2225·2
Polaramin, 2225·2
Polaramin Espettorante, 2225·2
Polaramine Preparations, 2225·2
Polaratyne, 2225·3
Polaratyne D, 2225·3
Polaronil, 2225·3
Polase, 2225·3
Polcortolon TC, 2225·3
Poldina, Metilsulfato de, 488·2
Poldine Methosulphate, 488·2
Poldine Methylsulfate, 488·2
Poldine Methylsulphate, 488·2
Poldine Metilsulfate, 488·2
Poledin, 2225·3
Polenat, 2225·3
Polendiamina, 2225·3
Poleo, Aceite Esencial de, 1736·1
Polery, 2225·3
Poli...— *see also under* Poly...
POLI-67, 93·2
Poli (A). Poli (U), 1733·2
Poli ABE, 2225·3
Poli B Fuerte, 2225·3
Poli (I). Poli (C), 1733·2
Poli Miner Vit, 2225·3
Poliacel, 2225·3
Poliacel-Act-Hib, 2225·3
Polial, 2225·3
Poliantib, 2225·3
Polibac, 2225·3
Polibar Preparations, 2225·3
Polibatrin, 2225·3
Poliben, 2225·3
Polibeta B12, 2225·3
Polibimbi, 2225·4
Polibiotic, 2225·4
Polibroxol, 2225·4
Polibutin, 2225·4
Policarbofilo, 1284·2
Policarbofilo Cálcico, 1284·2
Poli-Cifloxin, 2225·4
Policol, 2225·4
Policold, 2225·4
Policolinosil, 2225·4
Policosanol, 984·2
Policresolsulfonato, 756·1
Policresulen, 1190·1
Poli-Cycline, 2225·4
Polidasa, 2225·4
Polideltaxin, 2225·4
Poliderms, 2225·4
Polides, 2225·4
Polidocanol, 1412·3
Polienzim, 2225·4
Poliésteres de la Sacarosa, 1450·3
Poliestirenosulfonato Cálcico, 1032·3
Poliestirenosulfonato Potásico, 1050·1
Poliestirenosulfonato Sódico, 1053·1
Poliestradiol, Fosfato de, 1565·3
Poliestriol, Fosfato de, 1565·3
Poli-Fibrozil, 2225·4
Polifloroglucinol, Fosfato de, 1156·1
Polifluidil, 2225·4
Poli-Flunarin, 2225·4
Poli-Formin, 2225·4
Polifosfato Potásico, 1734·3
Polígala Raíz, 1130·2
Poligelina, 759·1
Poliginax, 2225·4
Poliglicol Anti Acne, 2225·4
Poligot, 2225·4
Poligot-CF, 2225·4
Poligram, 2225·4
Polihexanida, 1190·1
Polihexanide, 1190·1
Polijodurato, 2225·4
Polilevo, 2225·4
Polilevo N, 2225·4
Polimerosa, 2225·4
Polimetafosfato de Sodio, 1748·2
Polimixina B Composto, 2225·4
Polimixina B, Sulfato de, 245·1
Polimod, 2226·1
Polimoxil, 2226·1
Polimucil, 2226·1
Polinazolo, 2226·1
Polineural, 2226·1
Polinorm, 2226·1
Polinoxilina, 1190·1
Polio Sabin, 2226·1
Polio Vaccines, 1633·3
Poliodine, 2226·1
Polioftal, 2226·1
PolioHib, 2226·1
Poliomyelan, 2226·1
Poliomyelitis, Diphtheria, Tetanus, and Pertussis Vaccines, 1615·1
Poliomyelitis, Diphtheria, and Tetanus Vaccines, 1615·2
Poliomyelitis, Haemophilus Influenzae, Diphtheria, Tetanus, and Pertussis Vaccines, 1615·1
Poliomyelitis (Inactivated) and Haemophilus Type B Conjugate Vaccine (Adsorbed), Diphtheria, Tetanus, Pertussis, 1615·1
Poliomyelitis (Inactivated) and Haemophilus Type B Conjugate Vaccine (Adsorbed), Diphtheria, Tetanus, Pertussis (Acellular, Component), 1615·1
Poliomyelitis (Inactivated) and Haemophilus Type B Conjugate Vaccine (Adsorbed), Diphtheria, Tetanus, Pertussis (Acellular, Component), Hepatitis B (rDNA), 1614·3
Poliomyelitis (Inactivated) Vaccine (Adsorbed), Diphtheria, Tetanus, Pertussis and, 1615·1
Poliomyelitis (Inactivated) Vaccine (Adsorbed), Diphtheria, Tetanus, Pertussis (Acellular, Component) and, 1615·1
Poliomyelitis and Tetanus Vaccines, 1641·3
Poliomyelitis Vaccine (Inactivated), 1633·3
Poliomyelitis Vaccine, Live (Oral), 1634·1
Poliomyelitis Vaccine (Oral), 1634·1
Poliomyelitis Vaccines, 1633·3
Polioral, 2226·1
Polio-Vaccinol, 2226·1
Poliovax-IN, 2226·1
Poliovirus Vaccine Inactivated, 1634·1
Poliovirus Vaccines, 1633·3
Polipectol, 2226·1
Polipirox, 2226·1
Poliplex, 2226·1
Poli(I)$^2$poli($C_{12}$U), 651·3
Polipred, 2226·1
Poliprenoico, Ácido, 1156·1
Poliptal, 2226·1
Poli-Relaxane, 2226·1
Polireumin, 2226·1
Poliroxin, 2226·1
Polirreumin, 2226·1
Polisacárido-K, 1733·2
Polisan, 2226·1
Polised, 2226·1
Poliseng, 2226·1
Polisep, 2226·1
Polisilan Gel, 2226·1
Polisilon, 2226·2
Polisorbato 20, 1415·1
Polisorbato 40, 1415·1
Polisorbato 60, 1415·1
Polisorbato 80, 1415·2
Polisorbato 85, 1415·2
Polisorbatos, 1415·1
Polistin Pad, 2226·2
Polistin T-Caps, 2226·2
Polistirex, Codeine, 28·1
Polistirex, Dihydrocodeine, 35·2
Polistirex, Hydrocodone, 45·1
Polisulfade, 2226·2
Politef, 1733·2
Politefo, 1733·2
Politelmin, 2226·2
Politiazida, 984·2
Politifen, 2226·2
Politosse, 2226·2
Poli-Uretic, 2226·2
Polivitaminico, 2226·2
Poliwit, 2226·2
Polixan, 2226·2
Polixima, 2226·2
Polixin, 2226·2
Polizep, 2226·2
Polizine, 2226·2
Pollcapsan M, 2226·2
Pollen Royal, 2226·2
Pollenase Allergy, 2226·2
Pollenase Antihistamine, 2226·2
Pollenase Hayfever— *see* Pollenase Nasal, 2226·2
Pollenase Nasal, 2226·2
Pollen-B, 2226·2
Pollenna, 2226·2
Pollergon, 2226·2
Pollinex, 2226·2
Pollinex Quattro, 2226·2
Pollinex-R, 2226·2
Pollingel, 2226·2
Pollingel Con Ginkgo Biloba, 2226·2
Pollingel Ginseng, 2226·2
Pollinil, 2226·2
Pollinosan, 2226·2
Pollinose S, 2226·2
Pollstimol, 2226·2
Pollyferm, 2226·3
Polmonin, 2226·3
Polocaine, 2226·3
Polopiryna, 15·1
Poloral, 2226·3
Poloren, 2226·3
Poloris, 2226·3
Poloxalene, 1414·2
Poloxaleno, 1414·2
Poloxalkol, 1414·2
Poloxamer, 1414·1
Poloxamer 124, 1414·1
Poloxamer 182D, 1414·1
Poloxamer 182LF, 1414·1
Poloxamer 188, 1414·2
Poloxamer 188LF, 1414·1
Poloxamer 237, 1414·1
Poloxamer 331, 1414·1
Poloxamer 338, 1414·1
Poloxamer 407, 1414·2
Poloxamera, 1414·1
Poloxámero 188, 1414·2
Poloxámero 407, 1414·2
Poloxámeros, 1414·1
Poloxamers, 1414·1
Poloxyl Lanolin, 1483·3
Polper B12, 2226·3
Polper Calcio-Magnesio, 2226·3
Polper Vascular, 2226·3
Polvac, 2226·3
Pol/Vac(Inact), 1633·3
Pol/Vac(Oral), 1634·1
Polviderm NF, 2226·3
Polvilho Antisseptico, 2226·3
Polvo Roge, 2226·3
Polvos Alcalinos, 2226·3
Polvos Antibioticos, 2226·3
Polvos Wilfe, 2226·3
Poly...— *see also under* Poli...
Poly A.poly U, 1733·2
Poly C, 2226·3
Poly Gel, 2226·3
Poly I.poly C, 1733·2
Poly I.poly C12U, 651·3
Poly (2-Oxopyrrolidin-1-ylethylene), 1581·2
Poly Pred, 2226·3
Poly Visc, 2226·3
Polyacrylate Dispersion 30 Per Cent, 1714·3
Polyacrylic Acid, 1284·2, 1577·2
Polyadenylic and Polyuridylic Acids, 1733·2
Polyadenylic-polyuridylic Acid, 1733·2
Poly(alcohol Vinylicus), 1581·1
Polyangiitis, Microscopic— *see* Polyarteritis Nodosa and Microscopic Polyangiitis, 1085·3
Polyanhydroglucuronic Acid, 757·1
Polyanion, 2226·3
Polyarteritis Nodosa— *see* Polyarteritis Nodosa and Microscopic Polyangiitis, 1085·3
Polyäthylenglykol-Sorbitanoleat, 1415·2
Poly-B con Vitamina C, 2226·3
Polybactrin, 2226·3
Polybamycin, 2226·3
Polybee, 2226·3
Poly[benzene-1,3,5-triol Mono(dihydrogen Phosphate)], 1156·1
Polybion, 2226·3
Polybion Forte, 2226·3
Polybion N, 2226·3
Poly{[bis(hydroxymethyl)ureylene]methylene}, 1190·1
Polybrominated Biphenyl Compounds, 1501·3
Polycal, 2226·4
Polycarbophil, 1284·2
Polycarbophil Calcium, 1284·2
Polycarbophilum Calcii, 1284·2
Polycare, 2226·4
Polychlorinated Biphenyl Compounds, 1501·3
Polychlorinated Dibenzo-*p*-dioxins, 1681·1
Polychlorinated Dibenzofurans, 1681·1
Polychlorinated Terphenyl Compounds, 1501·3
Polychondritis, 1086·1
Polycidin, 2226·4
Polycin, 2226·4
Polycin-B, 2226·4
Polycitra, 2226·4
Polycitra-K, 2226·4
Polycitra-LC, 2226·4
Polyclean, 2226·4
Polyclens, 2226·4
Polyclox, 2226·4
Polycolvit, 2226·4
Polycose, 2226·4
Polycresolsulfonate, 756·1
Polycrol, 2226·4
Polycutan, 2226·4
Polycystic Ovary Syndrome, 1317·2
Polycythaemia Rubra Vera— *see* Polycythaemia Vera, 508·3
Polycythaemia, Secondary— *see* Erythrocytosis, 806·1
Polycythaemia Vera, 508·3
Polycytidylic Acids, Polyinosinic and, 1733·2
Polyderm, 2226·4
Polydex, 2226·4
Poly-Dex, 2226·4
Polydexa, 2226·4
Polydexa a la Phenylephrine, 2226·4
Polydiet, 2226·4
Poly(dimethylsiloxane), 1482·1
Polydine, 2226·4
Polydipsia— *see* Hyponatraemia, 1220·3
Polydol, 2227·1
Polydona, 2227·1
Polyenzyme-I, 2227·1
Polyenzyme-N, 2227·1
Polyerga, 2227·1
Polyestradiol Phosphate, 1565·3
Polyestriol Phosphate, 1565·3
Polyethoxylated Castor Oils, 1414·3
Polyethylene Glycol, 1708·3

Polyethylene Glycol 1000 Monocetyl Ether, 1412·2
Polyethylene Glycol Monomethyl Ether, 1413·1
Polyethylene Glycol Monomethyl Ethers, 1413·1
Polyethylene Glycol Mono-oleyl Ether, 1413·1
Polyethylene Glycols, 1708·2
Polyethylene Granules, 1140·1
Polyethylene Oxide, 1581·1
Polyethylene-polypropylene Glycol, 1414·1
Polyfax, 2227·1
Polyfra, 2227·1
Polyfructosan, 1702·1
*Polygala chinensis*, 1703·1
*Polygala senega*, 1130·2
Polygalae Radix, 1130·2
Polygalic Acid, 1130·2
Polygam, 2227·1
Polygeline, 759·1
Polygelinum, 759·1
Polyglobin, 2227·1
Polyglucin, 746·2
Poly[3→-(*O*-β-D-glucopyranosyl-(1→3)-*O*-[β-D-glucopyranosyl-(1→6)]-*O*-β-D-glucopyranosyl-(1→3)-*O*-β-D-glucopyranosyl)→1], 583·3
Polygot, 2227·1
Polygynax, 2227·1
Polygynax Virgo, 2227·1
Polyhadol, 2227·1
Polyhexamethylene Biguanide Hydrochloride, 1190·1
Poly(1-hexamethylenebiguanide Hydrochloride), 1190·1
Polyhexanide, 1190·1
Poly-Histine, 2227·1
Poly-Histine CS, 2227·1
Poly-Histine D, 2227·1
Poly-Histine DM, 2227·1
Polyhydramnios, 49·3
Poly(ICLC), 1733·2
Polyinosinic and Polycytidylic Acids, 1733·2
Polyinosinic-polycytidylic Acid, 1733·2
Polyionique, 2227·1
Poly(I):poly($C_{12}$,U), 651·3
Poly-Iron, 2227·1
Poly-Iron Forte, 2227·1
Poly-Joule, 2227·1
Poly-Karaya, 2227·1
Polylactic Acids, 1704·1
Polymannuronic Acid, 1576·3
Polymanoacetate, 1645·2
Polymeric Diet, 1417·3
Polymerised Formaldehyde, 1187·3
Polymethylmethacrylate, 1714·3
Polymorphic Light Eruption— *see* Light-induced Skin Reactions, 1136·3
Polymox, 2227·1
Polymyalgia Rheumatica, 1086·2
Polymycin, 2227·2
Polymyositis— *see* Polymyositis and Dermatomyositis, 1086·2
Polymyxin B Sulfate, 245·1
Polymyxin B Sulphate, 245·1
Polymyxin E Sulphate, 198·3
Polymyxini B Sulfas, 245·1
Polymyxins, 120·2
Polynase, 2227·2
Polyneuropathy, Acute Idiopathic Inflammatory— *see* Guillain-Barré Syndrome, 1630·2
Polyneuropathy, Acute Infectious— *see* Guillain-Barré Syndrome, 1630·2
Polyneuropathy, Sensory— *see* Diabetic Neuropathy, 6·1
Polynoxylin, 1190·1
Polyoestradiol Phosphate, 1565·3
Polyoestriol Phosphate, 1565·3
Polyols, 1417·1
Polyoph, 2227·2
Polyoxyethylene Castor Oils, 1414·3
Polyoxyethylene Glycol 1000 Monocetyl Ether, 1412·2
Polyoxyethylene Glycol Stearates, 1413·2
Polyoxyethylene Glycols, 1708·2
Polyoxyethylene 20 Sorbitan Monolaurate, 1415·1
Polyoxyethylene 20 Sorbitan Mono-oleate, 1415·2
Polyoxyethylene 20 Sorbitan Monopalmitate, 1415·1
Polyoxyethylene 20 Sorbitan Monostearate, 1415·1
Polyoxyethylene 20 Sorbitan Trioleate, 1415·2
Polyoxyethylene Stearates, 1413·2
Polyoxyethyleneamine, 1506·1
Polyoxyl Castor Oil, 1414·3
Polyoxyl 35 Castor Oil, 1414·3
Polyoxyl Castor Oils, 1414·3
Polyoxyl 20 Cetostearyl Ether, 1412·2
Polyoxyl 40 Hydrogenated Castor Oil, 1414·3
Polyoxyl Hydrogenated Castor Oils, 1414·3
Polyoxyl Lauryl Ether, 1412·3
Polyoxyl Lauryl Ethers, 1412·3
Polyoxyl 10 Oleyl Ether, 1413·1
Polyoxyl 8 Stearate, 1413·2
Polyoxyl 40 Stearate, 1413·2
Polyoxyl Stearates, 1413·2
Polyoxymethylene, 1187·3
Polypeptide Antibacterials, 120·2
Polyphed, 2227·2
Polyphloroglucin Phosphate, 1156·1
Polyphloroglucinol Phosphate, 1156·1
Polypirine, 2227·2
Polyplasdone XL, 1581·2
Polypred, 2227·2
Poly-Pred, 2227·2
Polyprenic Acid, 1156·1
Polyprenoic Acid, 1156·1
Polypress, 2227·2
Polyquin, 2227·2
Polyrhinium, 2227·2
Polyrinse, 2227·2
Polyrinse Desinfektionssystem, 2227·2
Polyrinse-Aufnahmelosung, 2227·2
Polyrinse-Augenelement, 2227·2
Poly-Rivitin, 2227·2
Polysaccharide B 1459, 1582·3
Polysaccharide-Iron Complex, 1443·2
Polysaccharide-K, 1733·2
Polysaccharides, 1417·1
Polysaccharides, Non-starch, 1253·3, 1417·1
Polysept, 2227·2
Polyseptol, 2227·2
Polyserositis, Paroxysmal— *see* Familial Mediterranean Fever, 416·2
Polyserositis, Recurrent— *see* Familial Mediterranean Fever, 416·2
Polysilane, 2227·2
Polysilane Delalande, 2227·2
Polysilane Joullie, 2227·2
Polysilic III, 2227·2
Polysilon, 2227·3
Poly(sodium Ethylenesulphonate), 1000·2
Polysorb, 2227·3
Polysorbate 20, 1415·1
Polysorbate 40, 1415·1
Polysorbate 60, 1415·1
Polysorbate 80, 1415·2
Polysorbate 85, 1415·2
Polysorbates, 1415·1
Polysorbatum 20, 1415·1
Polysorbatum 40, 1415·1
Polysorbatum 60, 1415·1
Polysorbatum 80, 1415·2
Polysorbitanum 80 Oleinatum, 1415·2
Polyspectran, 2227·3
Polyspectran HC, 2227·3
Polysporin, 2227·3
Polysporin Burn Formula— *see* Polysporin Plus Pain Relief, 2227·3
Polysporin Plus Pain Relief, 2227·3
Polysporin Triple Antibiotic, 2227·3
Polysporina, 2227·3
Polytab, 2227·3
Polytabs-F, 2227·3
Polytamin, 2227·3
Polytanol, 2227·3
Polytar, 2227·3
Polytar— *see* Dan-Tar Plus, 1918·3
Polytar AF, 2227·3
Polytar Emollient, 2227·3
Polytar Liquid, 2227·4
Polytar Plus, 2227·4
Poly-Tears, 2227·4
Polytef, 1733·2
Poly(tetrafluoroethylene), 1733·2
Polythiazide, 984·2
Polytonyl, 2227·4
Polytopic, 2227·4
Polytracin, 2227·4
Polytrim, 2227·4
Poly-Tussin, 2227·4
Polyuridylic Acids, Polyadenylic and, 1733·2
Polyvalent Snake Antivenom, 2227·4
Polyvidone, 1581·2
Polyvidone-Iodine, 1190·3
Polyvidonum, 1581·2
Poly-Vi-Flor, 2227·4
Poly-Vi-Fluor, 2227·4
Polyvinyl Acetate Phthalate, 1581·1
Polyvinyl Alcohol, 1581·1
Poly(Vinyl Alcohol), 1581·1
Polyvinylpyrrolidone, 1581·2
Polyvinylpyrrolidone-Iodine Complex, 1190·3
Poly-Visc, 2227·4
Poly-Vi-Sol, 2227·4
Polyvit, 2227·4
Polyvit 30 Plus, 2227·4
Polyvita, 2227·4
Poly-Vitamin Plus, 2227·4
Polyxan-Blau N, 2227·4
Polyxan-Blau N Comp, 2227·4
Polyxan-Gelb N, 2227·4
Polyxan-Gelb N Comp, 2227·4
Polyxan-Grun N, 2227·4
Polyxan-Grun N Comp, 2227·4
Polyxen, 2227·4
Polyxicam, 2227·4
Polyxit, 2228·1
Polyzalip, 2228·1
*catena*-Poly{zinc-μ-[β-alanyl-L-histidinato(2-)-*N*,$N^N$,*O*:$N^τ$ ]}, 1284·2
Polyzym, 2228·1
Pomada Antibiotica, 2228·1
Pomada Antihemorroidal, 2228·1
Pomada Balsamica, 2228·1
Pomada Blumen, 2228·1
Pomada Heridas, 2228·1
Pomada Infantil Vera, 2228·1
Pomada Martel, 2228·1
Pomada Minancora, 2228·1
Pomada Revulsiva, 2228·1
Pomada Vitaminica, 2228·1
Pomada Wilfe, 2228·1
Pomaderme, 2228·1
Pomadom, 2228·1
Pomaglos, 2228·1
Pomaglos Pomada, 2228·1
Pomalgex, 2228·1
Pomata Midy HC, 2228·1
Pomegranate, 112·1
Pomegranate Bark, 112·1
Pomegranate Root Bark, 112·1
Pomeranze, 1723·3
Pommade au The des Bois, 2228·1
Pommade Lelong, 2228·1
Pommade Maurice, 2228·1
Pommade Midy, 2228·1
Pommade Mo Cochon, 2228·1
Pommade Nasale Ruedi, 2228·1
Pommade Po-Ho N A Vogel, 2228·2
Pompe Disease, 1646·2
*Bis*(POM)PMEA, 628·1
Ponac, 2228·2
Ponalar, 2228·2
Ponalgic, 2228·2
Ponaris, 2228·2
Ponce, Pierre Granulée, 1140·1
Ponceau 4R, 1057·3
Ponceau 4RC, Brilliant, 1057·3
Pondactil, 2228·2
Pondactone, 2228·2
Pondarmett, 2228·2
Pondera, 2228·2
Ponderax Pacaps, 1588·3
Pondicilina, 2228·2
Pondnacef, 2228·2
Pondnadysmen, 2228·2
Pondnoxcill, 2228·2
Pondocillin, 2228·2
Pondperdone, 2228·2
Ponds Prevent, 2228·2
Pondtroxin, 2228·2
Pondusvitam, 2228·2
Pongesic, 2228·2
Ponmel, 2228·2
Ponnac, 2228·2
Ponnesia, 2228·2
Ponoxylan, 2228·2
Ponsinomycin, 231·3
Ponsolit, 2228·2
Ponstan, 2228·2
Ponstel, 2228·2
Ponstil, 2228·2
Ponstil Mujer, 2228·3
Ponstin, 2228·3
Ponstyl, 2228·3
Pontacid, 2228·3
Pontalon, 2228·3
Pontefix, 2228·3
Pontiac Fever— *see* Legionnaires' Disease, 133·1
Pontin, 2228·3
Pontine Myelinolysis, Central— *see* Hyponatraemia, 1220·3
Pontiride, 2228·3
Pontocaine, 2228·3
Pontuc, 2228·3
Pontyl, 2228·3
Pool 8, 2228·3
Poplar Buds, 1733·3
PO-PLL, 1729·2
Po-Pon-S, 2228·3
Poppers, 1032·2
Poppy Capsule, 1129·1
Poppy Heads, 1129·1
Poppy Straw, 62·2
Poppy-seed Oil, 1063·2, 1733·3
*Populus balsamifera*, 1733·3
*Populus candicans*, 1733·3
*Populus gileadensis*, 1733·3
*Populus nigra*, 1733·3
*Populus tacamahacca*, 1733·3
POR 8, 2228·3
Poractant Alfa, 1736·2
Porazine, 2228·3
Porcelana— *see* Porcelana Nighttime Formula, 2228·3
Porcelana Daytime Formula, 2228·3
Porcelana Nighttime Formula, 2228·3
Porcelana with Sunscreen— *see* Porcelana Daytime Formula, 2228·3
Porcine Growth Hormone, Methionyl, 1327·2
Porcine Insulin, 333·3, 334·1
Porcine Skin, 1158·1
Porcoll, 2228·3
Poremax-C, 2228·3
Porfimer Sodium, 580·3
Porfímero Sódico, 580·3
Porfirin 12, 2228·3
Porfiromicina, 581·1
Porfiromycin, 581·1
*Poria cocos*, 1750·2
Pork Actrapid, 2228·3
Pork Calcitonin, 768·2
Pork Insulatard, 2228·3
Pork Mixtard 30, 2228·3
Pork Tapeworm Infections— *see* Taeniasis, 101·1
Poro, 2228·3
Porosis D, 2228·3
Porostenina, 2228·3
Porphin, 2228·3
Porphyria, Convulsions in— *see* Porphyria, 353·2
Porphyrias, 1040·3
Porphyrocin, 2228·3

Porriver, 2228·3
Portagen, 2228·4
Portal Systemic Encephalopathy— *see* Hepatic Encephalopathy, 1243·2
Portamin, 2228·4
Portia, 2228·4
Portolac, 2228·4
Portugal, Essence of, 1724·1
Posaconazole, 407·3
Posalfilin, 2228·4
Posanin, 2228·4
Posatirelin, 1337·2
Posatirelina, 1337·2
Posdrink, 2228·4
Pose-Bac, 2228·4
Pose-CM, 2228·4
Posecus, 2228·4
Posedene, 2228·4
Pose-Dex, 2228·4
Poselium, 2228·4
Posene, 2228·4
Posicycline, 2228·4
Posidol, 2228·4
Posifenicol, 2228·4
Posifenicol C, 2228·4
Posiformin, 2228·4
Posiject, 2228·4
Posilent, 2228·4
Posine, 2228·4
Posipen, 2228·4
Positivum, 2228·4
Positon, 2228·4
Positron-emitters, 1522·2
Posivil, 2228·4
Posivyl, 2228·4
Posmox, 2229·1
Posnac, 2229·1
Posorutin, 2229·1
Postacne, 2229·1
Postadoxin N, 2229·1
Postadoxine, 2229·1
Postafen, 2229·1
Postafene, 2229·1
Postafeno, 2229·1
Postanaesthetic Tremor, Spontaneous— *see* Shivering and its Treatment, 1295·2
Postap, 2229·1
Postap Expectorant, 2229·1
Postarax, 2229·1
Postavit-B, 2229·1
Postcoital Contraception— *see* Emergency Contraception, 1536·1
Postcoital Contraceptives, 1527·3
Post-dural Puncture Headache, 1368·1
Posterine, 2229·1
Posterine Corte, 2229·1
Posterior Pituitary, 1337·3
Posterior Pituitary Hormones, 1312·1
Posterisan, 2229·1
Posterisan Forte, 2229·1
Postherpetic Neuralgia, 7·3
Posti N, 2229·1
Post-immunisation Fever— *see* Fever and Hyperthermia, 8·2
Post-infectious Glomerulonephritis— *see* Glomerular Kidney Disease, 1080·2
Postinor, 2229·1
Postinor-2, 2229·1
PostMI, 2229·1
Postoperative Inflammatory Ocular Disorders, 70·3
Postoperative Nausea and Vomiting— *see* Nausea and Vomiting, 1245·2
Postoperative Ocular Inflammation— *see* Postoperative Inflammatory Ocular Disorders, 70·3
Postoperative Pain— *see* Postoperative Analgesia, 4·1
Postoperative Shivering— *see* Shivering and its Treatment, 1295·2
Postopyl, 2229·1
Postoval, 2229·1
Postpartum Haemorrhage, 1684·3
Post-stroke Pain, Central— *see* Central Post-stroke Pain, 5·3
Post-traumatic Osteoporosis— *see* Complex Regional Pain Syndrome, 5·3
Post-traumatic Seizures, 376·1
Post-traumatic Stress Disorder, 664·1
Postural Hypotension— *see* Orthostatic Hypotension, 1100·2
Posture, 2229·1
Posture D, 2229·2
Posture-D, 2229·2
Pot, 1666·1
Pot. Iod., 1598·1
Pot Marigold, 1665·2
Pot. Permang., 1190·2
Potaba, 2229·2
Potabex, 2229·2
Potable Aqua, 2229·2
Potacol-R, 2229·2
Potasa Sulfurada, 1158·3
Potasalan, 2229·2
Potash Alum, 1652·1
Potash, Caustic, 1734·2
Potash Lye, 1734·2
Potash Soap, 1575·2
Potasi, 2229·2
Potasio, 1232·1
Potasio, Acetato de, 1232·1
Potasio C, 2229·2
Potasio, Cloruro de, 1232·2
Potasio, Gluconato de, 1232·2
Potasio, Sulfato de, 1232·2
Potasio, Tartrato de, 1232·2
Potasion, 2229·2
Potasion Solucion, 2229·2
Potasoral, 2229·2
Potassa Sulphurata, 1158·3
Potassii Chloras, 1734·2
Potassii Hydroxyquinolini Sulphas, 1734·2
Potassii Iodidum, 1598·1
Potassii Sulphas, 1232·2
Potássio, Cloreto de, 1232·2
Potassion, 2229·2
Potassium, 1232·1
Potassium Acetate, 1232·1
Potassium Acid Phosphate, 1230·3
Potassium Acid Tartrate, 1284·3
Potassium Alginate, 1577·1
Potassium Alum, 1652·1
Potassium Aluminium Sulphate Dodecahydrate, 1652·1
Potassium Aminobenzoate, 1733·3
Potassium 4-Aminobenzoate, 1733·3
Potassium Antimonyltartrate, 103·1
Potassium Ascorbate, 1233·1, 1461·1
Potassium Aspartate, 1233·1
Potassium Benzoate, 1233·1
Potassium Bicarbonate, 1223·1
Potassium Biphosphate, 1230·3
Potassium 1,4-Bis(2-ethylhexyl) Sulphosuccinate, 1262·1
Potassium Bisulfite, 1193·1
Potassium Bisulphite, 1193·1
Potassium Bitartrate, 1284·3
Potassium Borotartrate, 1734·1
Potassium Bromate, 1734·1
Potassium Bromide, 1662·3
Potassium Canrenoate, 984·2
Potassium Chlorate, 1734·2
Potassium Chloride, 1232·2
Potassium 7-Chloro-2,3-dihydro-2-oxo-5-phenyl-1*H*-1,4-benzodiazepine-3-carboxylate, 685·1
Potassium Citrate, 1223·1
Potassium Clavulanate, 193·3
Potassium Clavulanate, Diluted, 193·3
Potassium Clorazepate, 685·1
Potassium Cyanide, 1506·2
Potassium [*o*-(2,6-Dichloroanilino)phenyl]acetate, 32·1
Potassium Dichloroisocyanurate, 1191·3
Potassium (6*R*)-6-[2-(3,4-Dichlorophenyl)-2-methoxyacetamido]penicillanate, 198·1
Potassium Dichromate, 1670·3
Potassium Dihydrogen Orthophosphate, 1230·3
Potassium Dihydrogen Phosphate, 1230·3
Potassium Ferricyanide, 1506·2
Potassium Fluoride, 1446·1
Potassium Gluceptate, 1233·1
Potassium Gluconate, 1232·2
Potassium D-Gluconate, 1232·2
Potassium Guaiacolsulfonate, 1131·1
Potassium Guaiacolsulphonate, 1131·1
Potassium (*E,E*)-Hexa-2,4-dienoate, 1192·3
Potassium Hydrogen Carbonate, 1223·1
Potassium Hydrogen Sulphite, 1193·1
Potassium Hydrogen Tartrate, 1284·3
Potassium Hydroxide, 1734·2
Potassium Hydroxymethoxybenzenesulphonate Hemihydrate, 1131·1
Potassium 17-Hydroxy-3-oxo-17α-pregna-4,6-diene-21-carboxylate, 984·2
Potassium Hydroxyquinoline Sulfate, 1734·2
Potassium Hydroxyquinoline Sulphate, 1734·2
Potassium Hypochlorite, 1192·2
Potassium Iodate, 1598·1
Potassium Iodide, 1598·1
Potassium Iodide and Stramonium Compound, 2229·2
Potassium (Iodure de), 1598·1
Potassium Kurrol's Salt, 1734·3
Potassium Menaphthosulfate, 1466·3
Potassium Metabisulfite, 1193·1
Potassium Metabisulphite, 1193·1
Potassium Metaphosphate, 1734·3
Potassium 9-Methyl-3-(1*H*-tetrazol-5-yl)-4*H*-pyrido[1,2-*a*]pyrimidin-4-one, 790·3
Potassium MG, 2229·2
Potassium Monofluorophosphate, 1446·3
Potassium Nitrate, 1190·1
Potassium Nitrite, 1053·1
Potassium Oleate, 1574·3
Potassium Orotate, 1724·3
Potassium Oxyquinoline Sulphate, 1734·2
Potassium Perchlorate, 1602·3
Potassium Permanganate, 1190·2
Potassium (6*R*)-6-(2-Phenoxybutyramido)penicillanate, 246·3
Potassium α-Phenoxyethylpenicillin, 242·1
Potassium (6*R*)-6-(2-Phenoxypropionamido)penicillanate, 242·1
Potassium α-Phenoxypropylpenicillin, 246·3
Potassium Phosphate, 1230·3
Potassium Phosphate, Dibasic, 1230·3
Potassium Phosphate, Monobasic, 1230·3
Potassium Polymetaphosphate, 1734·3
Potassium Polystyrene Sulfonate, 1050·1
Potassium Polystyrene Sulphonate, 1050·1
Potassium Polysulfides, 1158·3
Potassium Propionate, 408·1
Potassium Pyrosulphite, 1193·1
Potassium Selenate, 1444·1
Potassium Silicofluoride, 1446·3
Potassium Soap, 1575·2
Potassium Sodium Borotartrate, 1734·1
Potassium Sodium Cyanide, 1506·2
Potassium Sodium Tartrate, 1284·3
Potassium Sodium Tartrate Tetrahydrate, 1284·3
Potassium Sorbate, 1192·3
Potassium Sulfate, 1232·2
Potassium Sulphate, 1232·2
Potassium Sulphate for Homoeopathic Use, 1232·2
Potassium Tartrate, 1232·2
Potassium Tetraborate, 1662·1
Potassium Troclosene, 1191·3
Potassium-channel Activators, 812·1
Potassium-channel Openers, 812·1
Potassium-Rougier, 2229·2
Potassium-sparing Diuretics, 811·2
Potassride, 2229·2
Potato Starch, 1449·1
Pota-Vi-Kin, 2229·2
Potcit, 2229·2
Potekam, 2229·2
Potenciator, 2229·2
Potencil, 2229·2
Potencort, 2229·2
Potendal, 2229·2
Potensone, 2229·2
*Potentilla erecta*, 1757·2
*Potentilla tormentilla*, 1757·2
Potentol, 2229·2
Potenzia, 2229·2
*Poterium officinalis*, 1663·2
Potional, 2229·2
Potklor, 2229·2
Po-Trim, 2229·3
Potsilo N, 2229·3
Potter's Preparations, 2229·3
Povadine, 2229·3
Povanyl, 2229·3
Povi Complex, 2229·3
Povibac, 2229·3
Povicler, 2229·3
Poviderm, 2229·3
Povid-Derme, 2229·3
Povidine, 2229·3
Povidona, 1581·2
Povidona Yodada, 1190·3
Povidone, 1581·2
Povidone, Iodinated, 1190·3
Povidone-Iodine, 1190·3
Povidonum, 1581·2
Povidonum Iodinatum, 1190·3
Povin, 2229·3
Poviral, 2229·3
Powdered C, 2229·3
Powdered Cellulose, 1578·3
Powdered Garlic, 1691·2
Powdered Ipecac, 1123·1
Powdered Opium, 74·3
Powdered Pituitary (Posterior Lobe), 1337·3
Powdered Talc, 1159·1
Power Orot, 2229·3
Power Rub, 2229·3
Powercef, 2229·3
Powergel, 2229·3
PowerLean, 2229·3
PowerMate, 2229·3
PowerSleep, 2229·4
PowerVites, 2229·4
Poxider, 2229·4
Pozapam, 2229·4
Pozato, 2229·4
Pozhexol, 2229·4
PP-563, 1502·3
PPD Tine Test, 2229·4
PPG, 2229·4
PPG-5, 2229·4
PPI-149, 1319·1
PPL, 1729·2
PPoma— *see* Carcinoid Tumours and Other Secretory Neoplasms, 504·1
PPS, 2229·4
PPSB Konzentrat S-TIM, 2229·4
PR 100, 2229·4
PR 100-Cloressidina, 2229·4
PR-934-423, 377·2
PR-934-423A, 377·2
PR-934423, 377·2
PR Freeze Spray, 2229·4
PR Heat Spray, 2229·4
Prabioquim, 2229·4
Pra-Brexidol, 2229·4
Pracap, 2229·4
Pracem, 2229·4
Pracne, 2229·4
Practazin, 2229·4
Practil, 2229·4
Practin, 2229·4
Practiser, 2229·4
Practizol, 2229·4
Practo-Clyss, 2229·4
Practomil, 2229·4
Practon, 2229·4
Pradente, 2229·4
Prader-Willi Syndrome, 1584·1
Pradif, 2229·4
Pradinolol, 2229·4
Praecicor, 2230·1
Praeciglucon, 2230·1
Praecineural, 2230·1
Praecipitatum Album, 1712·3
Praecordin S, 2230·1
Praedex, 2230·1
Praefeminon Plus, 2230·1
Praesidin, 2230·1

Pragman, 2230·1
Pragmatar, 2230·1
Pragmaten, 2230·1
Prairie Gold, 2230·1
Prajmaline Bitartrate, 984·3
Prajmalio, Bitartrato de, 984·3
Prajmalium Bitartrate, 984·3
Pralenal, 2230·1
Pralidoxima, 1050·1
Pralidoxima, Cloruro de, 1050·1
Pralidoxima, Ioduro de, 1050·1
Pralidoxima, Mesilato de, 1050·1
Pralidoxima, Metilsulfato de, 1050·2
Pralidoxime, 1050·1
Pralidoxime Chloride, 1050·1
Pralidoxime Iodide, 1050·1
Pralidoxime Mesilate, 1050·1
Pralidoxime Mesylate, 1050·1
Pralidoxime Methanesulphonate, 1050·1
Pralidoxime Methylsulphate, 1050·2
Pralidoxime Metilsulfate, 1050·2
Pralifan, 2230·1
Pralmorelin, 1314·3
Pralol, 2230·1
Pramace, 2230·1
PrameGel, 2230·1
Pramet, 2230·1
Pramet FA, 2230·1
Pramidal, 2230·1
Pramide, 2230·1
Pramidin, 2230·1
Pramigel, 2230·1
Pramilem, 2230·1
Pramilet FA, 2230·1
Pramin, 2230·1
Praminan, 2230·1
Pramino, 2230·1
Pramipexol, Hidrocloruro de, 1212·2
Pramipexole Dihydrochloride, 1212·2
Pramipexole Hydrochloride, 1212·2
Pramiracetam Sulfate, 1734·3
Pramiracetam, Sulfato de, 1734·3
Pramiracetam Sulphate, 1734·3
Pramistar, 2230·2
Pramiverina, Hidrocloruro de, 1734·3
Pramiverine Hydrochloride, 1734·3
Pramlintida, 344·3
Pramlintide, 344·3
Pramocaína, Hidrocloruro de, 1382·2
Pramocaine Hydrochloride, 1382·2
Pramosone, 2230·2
PramOtic, 2230·2
Pramotil, 2230·2
Pramox, 2230·2
Pramox HC, 2230·2
Pramoxine Hydrochloride, 1382·2
Pramoxinium Chloride, 1382·2
Pranactin— *see* Meretek UBT, 2125·3
Pranadox, 2230·2
Prandase, 2230·2
Prandin, 2230·2
Prandin $E_2$, 2230·2
Pranlukast, 791·1
Pranlukast Hydrate, 791·1
Pranoflog, 2230·2
Pranolol, 2230·2
Pranoprofen, 85·2
Pranoprofeno, 85·2
Pranosine, 2230·2
Pranox, 2230·2
Pranoxen, 2230·2
Prantal, 2230·2
Pranzo, 2230·2
Praparation H, Sperti— *see* Sperti Praparation H, 2303·2
Praquantel, 2230·2
Prareduct, 2230·2
Prascolend, 2230·2
Prasepine, 2230·2
Prasig, 2230·2
Prasikon, 2230·2
Prasterol, 2230·2
Prasterona, 1565·3
Prasterona, Enantato de, 1565·3
Prasterona, Sulfato Sódico de, 1566·1
Prasterone, 1565·3
Prasterone Enantate, 1565·3
Prasterone Enanthate, 1565·3
Prasterone Sodium Sulfate, 1566·1
Prasterone Sodium Sulphate, 1566·1
Prata, Nitrato de, 1746·1
Prata, Proteinato de, 1746·2
Prata, Vitelinato de, 1746·2
Pratazine, 2230·2
Praticef, 2230·2
Pratsiol, 2230·2
Prava, 2230·2
Pravachol, 2230·3
Pravacilin, 2230·3
Pravacol, 2230·3
Pravaselect, 2230·3
Pravasin, 2230·3
Pravasine, 2230·3
Pravastatin Sodium, 984·3
Pravastatina Sódica, 984·3
Pravastatinum Natricum, 984·3
Pravator, 2230·3
Pravidel, 2230·3
Pravigard PAC, 2230·3
Prax, 2230·3
Praxel, 2230·3
Praxilene, 2230·3
Praxinor, 2230·3
Praxis, 2230·3
Praxiten, 2230·3
Prayanol, 2230·3
Prayer Beads, 1645·1
Prazac, 2230·3
Prazam, 2230·3
Prazen, 2230·3
Prazene, 2230·3
Prazentol, 2230·3
Prazepam, 716·2
Prazepamum, 716·2
Prazicuantel, 112·2
Prazidec, 2230·3
Prazine, 2230·3
Prazinil, 2230·3
Praziquantel, 112·2
Praziquantelum, 112·2
Prazite, 2230·3
Prazocor, 2230·3
Prazohexal, 2230·4
Prazoken, 2230·4
Prazol, 2230·4
Prazolene, 2230·4
Prazolit, 2230·4
Prazolo, 2230·4
Prazonil, 2230·4
Prazosin Hydrochloride, 985·1
Prazosina, Hidrocloruro de, 985·1
Prazosini Hydrochloridum, 985·1
Pre Clean Mom, 2230·4
Pre Clor, 2230·4
Pre Natal, 2230·4
Pre Nutrison, 2230·4
Preastig, 2230·4
Pre-Attain, 2230·4
PreCare, 2230·4
Precedex, 2230·4
Precef, 2230·4
Precidona, 2230·4
Precifen, 2230·4
Precifenac, 2230·4
Precileucin, 2230·4
Precipitated Sulfur, 1158·2
Precision, 2230·4
Precision Plus, 2230·4
Precitene, 2230·4
Precitene MCT 50, 2230·4
Pre-Clar, 2230·4
Precocious Puberty, 1318·2
Preconceive, 2230·4
Precopen, 2230·4
Precopen Mucolitico, 2230·4
Precortalon Aquosum, 2230·4
Precortil, 2230·4
Precortisyl, 2230·4
Precosa, 2230·4
Precose, 2230·4
Precosol, 2231·1
Prectal, 2231·1
Precurgen, 2231·1
Precyclan, 2231·1
Pred, 2231·1
PRED, 1108·2
Pred Fort, 2231·1
Pred Forte, 2231·1
Pred G, 2231·1
Pred Mild, 2231·1
Pred Oph, 2231·1
Predalgic, 2231·1
Predalon, 2231·1
Predalone, 2231·1
Pred-Clysma, 2231·1
Predcor, 2231·1
Predeltin, 2231·1
Predenema, 2231·1
Predermid, 2231·1
Predesic, 2231·1
Predex, 2231·1
Predfoam, 2231·1
Predicor, 2231·1
Predicorten, 2231·1
Predictor, 2231·1
Predigested Diets, 1417·3
Predigested Elemental Diet, 1417·3
Predisole, 2231·1
Predmetil, 2231·1
Predmicin, 2231·1
Predmix, 2231·2
Predmycin, 2231·2
Predmycin P, 2231·2
Predmycin-P, 2231·2
Prednabene, 2231·2
Prednacinolone Acetonide, 1096·3
Prednazolina, 1129·1
Prednazoline, 1129·1
Prednefrin, 2231·2
Prednefrin SF, 2231·2
Prednersone, 2231·2
Prednesol, 2231·2
Predni, 2231·2
Predni Azuleno, 2231·2
Predni H, 2231·2
Predni M, 2231·2
Predni Tablinen, 2231·2
Prednicarbate, 1107·3
Prednicarbato, 1107·3
Prednicarbatum, 1107·3
Prednicort, 2231·2
Prednicortelone, 2231·2
Predniderma, 2231·2
Prednidib, 2231·2
Prednifarma, 2231·2
Predni-F-Tablinen, 2231·2
Predniftalmina, 2231·2
Prednigalen, 2231·2
Predni-Helvacort, 2231·2
Prednihexal, 2231·2
Prednilem, 2231·2
Prednilideno, 1109·3
Predniment, 2231·2
Prednimustina, 581·2
Prednimustine, 581·2
Predniocil, 2231·2
Predni-Ophtal, 2231·2
Prednipirine, 2231·2
Predni-POS, 2231·3
Prednis Neomic, 2231·3
Prednisil, 2231·3
Prednisil-N, 2231·3
Prednisol, 2231·3
Prednisolona, 1108·1
Prednisolona, Acetato de, 1108·1
Prednisolona, Caproato de, 1108·1
Prednisolona, Esteaglato de, 1108·2
Prednisolona, Fosfato Sódico de, 1108·1
Prednisolona, Hidrogenosuccinato de, 1108·1
Prednisolona, Metasulfobenzoato Sódico de, 1108·1
Prednisolona, Pivalato de, 1108·1
Prednisolona, Succinato Sódico de, 1108·2
Prednisolona, Tebutato de, 1108·2
Prednisolone, 1108·1
Prednisolone Acetate, 1108·1
Prednisolone 21-Acetate, 1108·1
Prednisolone Butylacetate, 1108·2
Prednisolone 21-*tert*-Butylacetate, 1108·2
Prednisolone Caproate, 1108·1
Prednisolone 21-(3,3-Dimethylbutyrate), 1108·2
Prednisolone 21-(Disodium Orthophosphate), 1108·1
Prednisolone Farnesil, 1109·2
Prednisolone Hemisuccinate, 1108·1
Prednisolone Hexanoate, 1108·1
Prednisolone 21-Hexanoate, 1108·1
Prednisolone Hydrogen Succinate, 1108·1
Prednisolone 21-(Hydrogen Succinate), 1108·1
Prednisolone Metasulfobenzoate Sodium, 1108·1
Prednisolone Metasulphobenzoate Sodium, 1108·1
Prednisolone Palmitate, 1109·2
Prednisolone Phosphate, 1109·1
Prednisolone Pivalate, 1108·1
Prednisolone 21-Pivalate, 1108·1
Prednisolone Sesquihydrate, 1108·1
Prednisolone Sodium Hemisuccinate, 1108·2
Prednisolone Sodium Metasulphobenzoate, 1108·1
Prednisolone Sodium Phosphate, 1108·1
Prednisolone Sodium Succinate, 1108·2
Prednisolone Sodium Succinate for Injection, 1108·2
Prednisolone 21-(Sodium *m*-Sulphobenzoate), 1108·1
Prednisolone Sodium Tetrahydrophthalate, 1109·2
Prednisolone Steaglate, 1108·2
Prednisolone 21-Stearoylglycolate, 1108·2
Prednisolone Tebutate, 1108·2
Prednisolone Tertiary-butylacetate, 1108·2
Prednisolone Trimethylacetate, 1108·1
Prednisolone-Fenoxazoline Compound, 1129·1
Prednisoloni Acetas, 1108·1
Prednisoloni Natrii Phosphas, 1108·1
Prednisoloni Pivalas, 1108·1
Prednisolonum, 1108·1
Prednisolut, 2231·3
Prednisona, 1109·3
Prednisona, Acetato de, 1109·3
Prednisone, 1109·3
Prednisone Acetate, 1109·3
Prednisone 21-Acetate, 1109·3
Prednisone Monohydrate, 1109·3
Prednisonum, 1109·3
Prednistyle, 2231·3
Prednitone, 2231·3
Prednitop, 2231·3
Prednitracin, 2231·3
Prednylidene, 1109·3
Prednylidene Diethylaminoacetate Hydrochloride, 1109·3
Predonium, 2231·3
Pred-Phosphate, 2231·3
Predsim, 2231·3
Predsol, 2231·3
Predsol-N, 2231·3
Predsolets, 2231·3
Predual, 2231·3
Predual Descongestivo, 2231·3
Predual DI, 2231·3
Predualito, 2231·3
Predval, 2231·3
Pre-eclampsia— *see* Eclampsia and Pre-eclampsia, 352·3
Pre-eclampsia— *see* Hypertension, 825·1
Pre-emptive Analgesia— *see* Postoperative Analgesia, 4·1
Prefagyl, 2231·3
Prefamone, 2231·3
Prefem, 2231·3
Prefemine, 2231·4
Preferid, 2231·4
Preferred Remedies Preparations, 2231·4
Prefest, 2231·4
Prefesta, 2231·4
Prefin, 2231·4
Prefine, 2231·4
Preflex Daily Cleaner, 2231·4

Prefolic, 2231·4
Preforms, 2231·4
Prefrin, 2231·4
Prefrin A, 2231·4
Prefrin Z, 2231·4
Pregabalin, 376·2
Pregabalina, 376·2
Pregaday, 2231·4
Pregamal, 2231·4
Pregelatinised Starch, 1449·1
Pregelatinized Starch, 1449·2
Pregestimil, 2231·4
Pregestimil, Enfalac— *see* Enfalac Pregestimil, 1970·3
Preglandin, 2231·4
Pregnacare, 2231·4
Pregna-Cert, 2231·4
9β,10α-Pregna-4,6-diene-3,20-dione, 1549·2
17α-Pregna-2,4-dien-20-yno[2,3-*d*]isoxazol-17β-ol, 1545·2
Pregnafort, 2231·4
Pregnancy, Ectopic— *see* Ectopic Pregnancy, 572·2
Pregnancy and Fertility Tests, 1734·3
Pregnancy Formula, 2231·4
Pregnancy, Hypertension in— *see* Hypertension, 825·1
Pregnancy, Nausea and Vomiting in— *see* Nausea and Vomiting, 1245·2
Pregnancy, Termination of— *see* Termination of Pregnancy, 1512·2
Pregnancy, Tubal— *see* Ectopic Pregnancy, 572·2
Pregnancy-urine Hormone, 1320·3
Pregnanediol, 1567·1
Pregna-Sure HCG, 2231·4
Pregnatal, 2231·4
Pregnavit, 2231·4
Pregnavit F, 2231·4
Pregnavite Forte F, 2231·4
Pregnazon, 2231·4
Pregnenedione, 1566·2
Pregn-4-ene-3,20-dione, 1566·2
Pregnesin, 2232·1
Pregnidoxin, 2232·1
Pregnifer, 2232·1
Pregnon L, 2232·1
Pregnon, Mini— *see* Mini Pregnon, 2134·2
Pregnorm, 2232·1
Pregnosis, 2232·1
Pregnospia Duoclon, 2232·1
Pregnosticon, 2232·1
Pregnyl, 2232·1
Pregomin, 2232·1
Pregomine, 2232·1
Prehist, 2232·1
Prehist D, 2232·1
Prejomin, 2232·1
Prekallikrein, 735·3
Prelac, 2232·1
Prelafel, 2232·1
Prêle, 1684·1
Prelectal, 2232·1
Prelertan, 2232·1
Preleukaemia— *see* Myelodysplastic Syndromes, 508·2
Prelis, 2232·1
Prelis Comp, 2232·1
Prelisin, 2232·1
Prelloran, 2232·1
Prelone, 2232·1
Prelu-2, 2232·1
Prelude, 2232·1
Prelus, 2232·1
Premagnol, 2232·1
Premandol, 2232·2
Premaril, 2232·2
Premaril MP, 2232·2
Premaril Plus MP, 2232·2
Premarin Preparations, 2232·2
Premarin— *see* Menoprem, 2123·4
Premarin— *see* Premplus, 2232·4
Premarin— *see* Provelle, 2243·3
Premarina, 2232·2
Premature Labour, 794·1
Premature Labour, Infections in— *see* Premature Labour, 143·2
Prematurity, Metabolic Bone Disease of— *see* Rickets of Prematurity, 1232·1
Prematurity, Retinopathy of— *see* Retinopathy of Prematurity, 1466·1
Prematurity, Rickets of— *see* Rickets of Prematurity, 1232·1
Premdoc, 2232·2
Preme, 2232·2
Premedication— *see* Anaesthesia, 1296·1
Premedication in Endoscopy— *see* Endoscopy, 666·2
Premella, 2232·2
Premelle Preparations, 2232·2
Premence, 2232·3
PreMens, 2232·3
Premenstrual Dysphoric Disorder— *see* Premenstrual Syndrome, 1551·3
Premenstrual Syndrome, 1551·3
Premenstrual Tension— *see* Premenstrual Syndrome, 1551·3
Prementaid, 2232·3
PremesisRx, 2232·3
Premia, 2232·3
Premia Continuous, 2232·3
Premia Low, 2232·3
Premicia, 2232·3
Premid, 2232·3
Premique, 2232·3
Premique Cycle, 2232·3
Premium, 2232·3
Premjact, 2232·3
Premofil M, 2232·3
Premosan, 2232·3
Premox, 2232·3
Prempac Sekvens— *see* Premelle Sekvens, 2232·3
Prempak, 2232·3
Prempak-C, 2232·4
Prempak N, 2232·4
Premphase, 2232·4
Premplus, 2232·4
Prempro, 2232·4
Prempro Bifasico, 2232·4
Prempro Monofasico, 2232·4
Premsyn PMS, 2232·4
Premular, 2232·4
Prenacid, 2232·4
Prenadona, 2232·4
Prenafort, 2232·4
Prenalex, 2232·4
Prenalon, 2232·4
Prenalterol, Hidrocloruro de, 986·3
Prenalterol Hydrochloride, 986·3
Prenatabs, 2232·4
Prenatal, 2232·4
Prenatal with Folic Acid, 2232·4
Prenatal Nutrients, 2232·4
Prenatal PC, 2232·4
Prenatal Plus, 2232·4
Prenatal Plus Iron, 2232·4
Prenatal Plus-Improved, 2232·4
Prenatal-S, 2232·4
Prenate, 2233·1
Prenatex, 2233·1
Prenatol, 2233·1
Prenavit, 2233·1
Prenavite, 2233·1
Prenazone, 43·1
Prenefrin, 2233·1
Prenilamina, Lactato de, 1735·1
Prenilone, 2233·1
Prenisonal, 2233·1
Prenolol, 2233·1
Prenomod, 2233·1
Prenoretic, 2233·1
Prenormine, 2233·1
Prenoxan au Phenobarbital, 2233·1
Prenoxdiazin Hydrochloride, 1129·1
Prenoxdiazina, Hidrocloruro de, 1129·1
Prenoxdiazine Hibenzate, 1129·1
Prenoxdiazine Hydrochloride, 1129·1
Prent, 2233·1
Pre-Nutrison, 2233·1
Prenylamine, 1735·1
Prenylamine Lactate, 1735·1
Prenylaminii Lactas, 1735·1
Pre-Op, 2233·1
Prep Kit-C, 2233·1
Prepacol, 2233·1
Prepacort H, 2233·1
Prepadine, 2233·1
Pre-Par, 2233·1
Preparacion H, 2233·1
Preparado H, 2233·1
Preparation H Preparations, 2233·1
Preparazione Antiemorroidaria, 2233·2
Preparazione H, 2233·2
Prepared Belladonna Herb, 479·1
Prepared Opium, 74·2
Prepcare, 2233·2
Prepcat, 2233·2
Pre-Pen, 2233·2
Prephen, 2233·2
Prepidil, 2233·2
Preptin, 2233·2
Prepulsid, 2233·2
Prepurex, 2233·2
Preran, 2233·2
Pres, 2233·2
Pres Plus, 2233·2
Presabet, 2233·2
Prescaina, 2233·2
Prescal, 2233·2
Presco, 2233·2
Prescol, 2233·2
Pre-senile Dementia— *see* Dementia, 1484·1
Presept, 2233·2
Preservatives, 1164·1
Preservex, 2233·2
Presi Regul, 2233·2
Presi Regul D, 2233·2
President's Choice Preparations, 2233·3
Presilam, 2233·3
Presinex, 2233·3
Presinol, 2233·3
Presistin, 2233·3
Preslow, 2233·3
Presocor, 2233·3
Presoken, 2233·3
Presokin, 2233·3
Presol, 2233·3
Presolar, 2233·3
Presolol, 2233·3
Presomen, 2233·3
Presomen Compositum, 2233·3
Presoquim, 2233·3
Prespir, 2233·3
Press-12, 2233·3
Pressalolo, 2233·3
Pressalolo Diuretico, 2233·3
Pressamina, 2233·3
Pressat, 2233·3
Pressel, 2233·3
Presselin Preparations, 2233·3
Pressimed, 2233·4
Pressimedin, 2233·4
Pressin, 2233·4
Pressitan, 2233·4
Pressitan Plus, 2233·4
Pressodipin, 2233·4
Pressolat, 2233·4
Pressomax, 2233·4
Pressotec, 2233·4
Pressunic Compositum, 2233·4
Pressural, 2234·1
Pressuril, 2234·1
Pressyn, 2234·1
Prestim, 2234·1
Prestodol, 2234·1
Prestole, 2234·1
Presun Preparations, 2234·1
Presyc, 2234·1
Pretcamida, 1592·3
Preterax, 2234·1
Preterm Labour— *see* Premature Labour, 794·1
Prethcamide, 1592·3
Pretinha, 1666·1
Pretts Diet Aid, 2234·1
Pretuval, 2234·1
Pretuval C, 2234·2
Pretz, 2234·2
Pretz-D, 2234·2
Prevacid, 2234·2
Prevacid— *see* Hp-Pac, 2048·4
Prevacid— *see* Prevpac, 2234·3
Prevacid NapraPAC, 2234·2
Prevagin-Premaril, 2234·2
Prevalin, 2234·2
Prevalina, 2234·2
Prevalite, 2234·2
Prevalon, 2234·2
Prevax, 2234·2
Prevecilina, 2234·2
Prevegyne, 2234·2
Preven, 2234·2
Prevenar, 2234·2
Prevencal Preparations, 2234·2
Prevencor, 2234·2
Prevent, 2234·2
Preventan, 2234·2
Preventol BP— *see* Hygienist, 2052·2
Preventol CMK— *see* Hygienist, 2052·2
Preventol Extra— *see* Hygienist, 2052·2
Prevepen, 2234·2
Prevepen Forte, 2234·2
Prevex Preparations, 2234·2
Prevident, 2234·3
Previfem, 2234·3
Previgrip, 2234·3
Previnfec, 2234·3
Previscan, 2234·3
Previum, 2234·3
Prevnar, 2234·3
Prevolac, 2234·3
Prevpac, 2234·3
Prewash, 2234·3
Prexan, 2234·3
Prexene, 2234·3
Prexidine, 2234·3
Prezal, 2234·3
Prezatida Cúprica, Acetato de, 1156·1
Prezatide Copper Acetate, 1156·1
Prezatim, 2234·3
Prezolon, 2234·3
Priadel, 2234·3
Priamide, 2234·3
Priapism, 952·3, 1513·1
Priaxim, 2234·3
Pricam, 2234·3
Priciasol, 2234·3
Pricillin, 2234·3
Prickly Ash Berries, 1766·3
Prickly Heat Powder, 2234·4
Pridam, 2234·4
Pridana, 2234·4
Pridecil, 2234·4
Pri-De-Sid, 2234·4
Pridinol, 2234·4
Pridinol Hydrochloride, 1395·2
Pridinol Mesilate, 1395·2
Pridinol, Mesilato de, 1395·2
Pridinol Mesylate, 1395·2
Pridio, 2234·4
PRIF, 1196·1
Prifinio, Bromuro de, 488·2
Prifinium Bromide, 488·2
Priftin, 2234·4
Prigost, 2234·4
Prilace, 2234·4
Prilagin, 2234·4
Prilan, 2234·4
Priliximab, 1668·3
Prilocaína, Hidrocloruro de, 1382·3
Prilocaine, 1382·3
Prilocaine, Carbonated, 1369·2
Prilocaine Hydrochloride, 1382·3
Prilocaini Hydrochloridum, 1382·3
Prilocainum, 1382·3
Prilosec, 2234·4
Prilovase, 2234·4
Prilpressin, 2234·4
Priltam, 2234·4
Priltenk, 2234·4
Primacaine, 2234·4
Prima-Cal, 2234·4

Prima-Cal Plus Vit D, 2234·4
Primacard, 2234·4
Primachina Fosfato, 456·2
Primachini Phosphas, 456·2
Primacin, 2234·4
Primacine, 2234·4
Primaclone, 376·3
Primacor, 2234·4
Primacton, 2234·4
Primacy C+AHA, 2234·4
Primacy Phyto +, 2234·4
Primaderm, 2234·4
Primafen, 2234·4
Primafluor, 2235·1
Primahex, 2235·1
Primakinder, 2235·1
Primalan, 2235·1
Primamed, 2235·1
Primanol, 2235·1
Primanol-Borage, 2235·1
Primaquin, 2235·1
Primaquin MP, 2235·1
Primaquin MP Continuo, 2235·1
Primaquina, Fosfato de, 456·2
Primaquine Diphosphate, 456·2
Primaquine Phosphate, 456·2
Primaquini Diphosphas, 456·2
Primaquinum Phosphoricum, 456·2
Primary Biliary Cirrhosis, 1761·2
Primary CNS Lymphoma, 510·3
Primary Effusion Lymphoma, 510·3
Primary Propyl Alcohol, 1191·2
Primary Thrombocythaemia, 509·1
Primasept Med, 2235·1
Primasone, 2235·1
Primaspan, 2235·1
Primastick, 2235·1
Primatene Preparations, 2235·1
Primatenol, 2235·1
Primatenol Plus, 2235·1
Primatime, 2235·1
Primatour, 2235·1
Primatuss Cough Mixture 4, 2235·1
Primatuss Cough Mixture 4D, 2235·1
Primavax, 2235·1
Primavera-N, 2235·1
Primaxin, 2235·1
Primbactam, 2235·1
Primcillin, 2235·1
Prime Time, 2235·1
Primelwurzel, 1735·1
Primene, 2235·1
Primera, 2235·2
Primeral, 2235·2
Primeran, 2235·2
Primesin, 2235·2
Primevére, Racine de, 1735·1
Primidona, 376·3
Primidone, 376·3
Primidonum, 376·3
Primil, 2235·2
Primiprost, 2235·2
Primobolan, 2235·2
Primobolan Depot, 2235·2
Primobolan S, 2235·2
Primocef, 2235·2
Primodian Depot, 2235·2
Primodium, 2235·2
Primofenac, 2235·2
Primofol Depot, 2235·2
Primogonyl, 2235·2
Primogyn, 2235·2
Primogyn Depot, 2235·2
Primogyna, 2235·2
Primolut Depot, 2235·2
Primolut Depot— *see* Proluton Depot, 2239·3
Primolut N, 2235·2
Primolut-Nor, 2235·2
Primoniat Depot, 2235·2
Primonil, 2235·3
Primoris, 2235·3
Primosiston, 2235·3
Primostat, 2235·3
Primoteston Depot, 2235·3
Primotussan, 2235·3
Primover, 2235·3
Primovist, 2235·3
Primovlar, 2235·3
Primoxil, 2235·3
Primperan, 2235·3
Primperan Complex, 2235·3
Primperil, 2235·3
Primperoxane, 2235·3
Primpesasy, 2235·3
Primrose Micelle, Bioglan— *see* Bioglan Primrose Micelle, 1844·1
Primrose Root, 1735·1
Primrose-E, Bioglan— *see* Bioglan Primrose-E, 1844·1
Primsol, 2235·3
Prímula, 1735·1
*Primula elatior*, 1735·1
*Primula officinalis*, 1735·1
Primula Root, 1735·1
*Primula veris*, 1735·1
*Primula vulgaris*, 1735·1
Primulae Radix, 1735·1
Primum, 2235·3
Primyxine, 2235·3
Prinachol, 2235·3
Prinactizide, 2235·3
Princi B1 + B6, 2235·3
Princi-B, 2235·3
Princi-B Fort, 2235·4
Principen, 2235·4
Princol, 2235·4
Prindex, 2235·4
Prindolol, 983·2
Prinil, 2235·4
Prinivil, 2235·4
Prinivil Plus, 2235·4
Prinodolol, 983·2
Prinol Plus, 2235·4
Prinox, 2235·4
Prinsyl, 2235·4
Printan, 2235·4
Printania, 2235·4
Printol, 2235·4
Prinzide, 2235·4
Prinzmetal's Angina— *see* Angina Pectoris, 813·1
Prioderm, 2235·4
Priorin, 2235·4
Priorin Biotin, 2235·4
Priorin N, 2235·4
Priorix, 2235·4
Priovit 12, 2235·4
Priper, 2235·4
Priper Plus, 2235·4
Pripsen, 2235·4
Priscol, 2236·1
Priscoline, 2236·1
Prisdal, 2236·1
Prisma, 2236·1
Prisoventril, 2236·1
Pristinamicina, 246·1
Pristinamycin, 246·1
Pristinamycin I, 246·1
Pristinamycin II, 246·1
Pristine, 2236·1
Pristinex, 2236·1
Pritor, 2236·1
Pritor Plus, 2236·1
Pritoral, 2236·1
PritorPlus, 2236·1
Privacom, 2236·1
Privin, 2236·1
Privin, Antistin— *see* Antistin-Privin, 1805·3
Privina, 2236·1
Privine, 2236·1
Privituss, 2236·1
Prixar, 2236·1
Prixin, 2236·1
Prizem, 2236·1
Prizma, 2236·1
PRN, 439·1
Pro, 1443·2
Pro Dorm, 2236·1
Pro Lertus, 2236·1
Pro Ulco, 2236·1
Proaccelerin, 735·3
Pro-Actidil, 2236·1
Proadifen Hydrochloride, 1735·2
Proadifeno, Hidrocloruro de, 1735·2
Proaf, 2236·2
Proagil, 2236·2
Proaller, 2236·2
ProAmatine, 2236·2
Proampi, 2236·2
Proartinal, 2236·2
Proasma-T, 2236·2
Proazamine Chloride, 439·1
Proazulenes, 1646·2
Pro-Banthine, 2236·2
Probase 3, 2236·2
Probax, 2236·2
Probec, 2236·2
Probecid, 2236·2
Probecilin, 2236·2
Probec-T, 2236·2
Probeks, 2236·2
Proben, 2236·2
Probenecid, 416·3
Probenecidum, 416·3
Probenxil, 2236·2
Probenzima, 2236·2
Probenzima Ampicilina, 2236·2
Probenzima Analgesico, 2236·2
Probeta, 2236·2
Probi-Albumin, 2236·2
Probigol, 2236·2
Pro-Bionate, 2236·2
Probiophyt V, 2236·2
Probiotics, 1704·2
Probiox, 2236·2
Probi-Rho D, 2236·2
Probi-Tet, 2236·2
Probitor, 2236·2
Probofex, 2236·3
Probucol, 986·3
Probufen, 2236·3
Pro-C, 2236·3
Pro-30C, 2236·3
Procadax, 2236·3
Procadil, 2236·3
Procaína, Hidrocloruro de, 1383·2
Procaína Penicilina, 246·1
Procainamida, Hidrocloruro de, 987·1
Procainamide Hydrochloride, 987·1
Procainamidi Chloridum, 987·1
Procainamidi Hydrochloridum, 987·1
Procaine Ascorbate, 1383·3
Procaine Benzylpenicillin, 246·1
Procaine Hydrochloride, 1383·2
Procaine Penicillin G, 246·1
Procaine-*N*-glucoside Hydrochloride, 1383·3
Procaini Benzylpenicillinum, 246·1
Procaini Hydrochloridum, 1383·2
Procainii Chloridum, 1383·2
Procainium Chloride, 1383·2
Pro-Cal, 2236·3
Procal, 2236·3
ProcalAmine, 2236·3
Procal-D, 2236·3
Pro-Cal-Sof, 2236·3
Procamide, 2236·3
Procan, 2236·3
Procan SR— *see* Procanbid, 2236·3
Procanbid, 2236·3
Procanest, 2236·3
Procaneural, 2236·3
Procaptan, 2236·3
Procarbazina, Hidrocloruro de, 581·2
Procarbazine Hydrochloride, 581·2
Procardia, 2236·3
Procardin, 2236·3
Procardol, 2236·3
Pro-Cas, 2236·3
Procaterol, Hidrocloruro de, 791·1
Procaterol Hydrochloride, 791·1
Procaterol Hydrochloride Hemihydrate, 791·1
Procavit, 2236·3
Proceane Hypertonique, 2236·3
Proceane Isotonique, 2236·3
Procef, 2236·3
Procelac, 2236·4
Procephal, 2236·4
Proceptin, 2236·4
Procetofene, 915·2
Procetoken, 2236·4
Prochieve, 2236·4
Prochlor, 2236·4
Prochlorpemazine, 716·2
Prochlorpemazine Edisylate, 716·2
Prochlorpemazine Maleate, 716·3
Prochlorpemazine Mesylate, 716·3
Prochlorperazine, 716·2
Prochlorperazine Dihydrogen Maleate, 716·3
Prochlorperazine Dimaleate, 716·3
Prochlorperazine Dimethanesulphonate, 716·3
Prochlorperazine Edisilate, 716·2
Prochlorperazine Edisylate, 716·2
Prochlorperazine Ethanedisulphonate, 716·2
Prochlorperazine Ethane-1,2-disulphonate, 716·2
Prochlorperazine Maleate, 716·3
Prochlorperazine Mesilate, 716·3
Prochlorperazine Mesylate, 716·3
Prochlorperazine Methanesulphonate, 716·3
Prochlorperazini Maleas, 716·3
Prochlorperazini Mesylas, 716·3
Prochol, 2236·4
Prochor, 2236·4
Prociclide, 2236·4
Prociclidina, Hidrocloruro de, 488·2
Pro-Cid, 2236·4
Procilin, 2236·4
Procillin, 2236·4
Procimeti, 2236·4
Procin, 2236·4
Procinonida, 1110·1
Procinonide, 1110·1
Procion, 2236·4
Procirex, 2236·4
Proclim, 2236·4
Proclimine, 2236·4
Proclor, 2236·4
Procloril, 2236·4
Proclorperazina, 716·2
Proclorperazina, Edisilato de, 716·2
Proclorperazina, Maleato de, 716·3
Proclorperazina, Mesilato de, 716·3
Proclozine, 2236·4
Procodazol, 1735·2
Procodazole, 1735·2
Procodazole Ethyl Ester, 1735·2
Procodazole Sodium, 1735·2
Procodin, 2236·4
Procodine, 2236·4
Procof, 2236·4
Procofen, 2236·4
Procold, 2236·4
Pro-Coll, 2236·4
Procomfrin, 2236·4
Procomvax, 2236·4
Proconfial, 2237·1
Proconvertin, 735·3, 750·3
Procor, 2237·1
Procor S, 2237·1
Procordal, 2237·1
Procordal Gold, 2237·1
Procort, 2237·1
Procorum, 2237·1
Procosamine, 2237·1
Procoutol, 2237·1
Procren, 2237·1
Procrin, 2237·1
Procrit, 2237·1
Proctalgen, 2237·1
Proctase-P, 2237·1
Proctena, 2237·1
Proctidol, 2237·1
Proctil, 2237·1
Proctitis— *see* Inflammatory Bowel Disease, 1243·3
Proctitis, Infective— *see* Proctitis, 143·2

Proctium, 2237·1
Procto, 2237·1
Procto Synalar, 2237·1
Proctoacid, 2237·1
Proctocolitis— *see* Inflammatory Bowel Disease, 1243·3
Proctocort, 2237·1
Proctocream HC, 2237·1
Proctocream HC 2.5%, 2237·1
Proctodan-HC, 2237·1
Proctofoam, 2237·2
Proctofoam-HC, 2237·2
Proctogel, 2237·2
Procto-Glyvenol, 2237·2
Procto-Ikatral, 2237·2
Procto-Jellin, 2237·2
Procto-Kaban, 2237·2
Proctolog, 2237·2
Proctolyn, 2237·2
Proctomyxin, 2237·2
Proctonet, 2237·2
Proctonostrum, 2237·2
Proctoparf, 2237·2
Proctoplex, 2237·2
Proctopure, 2237·2
Proctor's Pinelyptus, 2237·2
Proctosan, 2237·2
Proctosedyl, 2237·2
Proctosoll, 2237·3
Proctosone, 2237·3
Proctosor, 2237·3
Proctospre, 2237·3
Proctosteroid, 2237·3
Procto-Synalar, 2237·3
Procto-Synalar N, 2237·3
Proctozorin-N, 2237·3
Proctyl, 2237·3
Procuazona, 86·1
Proculin, 2237·3
Procur, 2237·3
Pro-Cure, 2237·3
Procuta, 2237·3
Procutan, 2237·3
Pro-Cute, 2237·3
Procyclid, 2237·3
Procyclidine Hydrochloride, 488·2
Procyclidini Hydrochloridum, 488·2
Procyclo, 2237·3
Procythol, 2237·3
Procytox, 2237·3
Pro-Dafalgan, 2237·3
Prodafem, 2237·4
Prodamox, 2237·4
Prodasone, 2237·4
Prodazol, 2237·4
Prodeine, 2237·4
Prodel, 2237·4
Prodel B, 2237·4
Prodep, 2237·4
Proderm, 2237·4
Proderma, 2237·4
Prodessal, 2237·4
Pro-Diaban, 2237·4
Prodicard, 2237·4
Prodiem Plain, 2237·4
Prodiem Plus, 2237·4
Prodifer, 2237·4
Prodigrip, 2237·4
Prodil, 2237·4
Prodilantin, 2237·4
Prodis, 2237·4
Prodium, 2237·4
Prodiuret, 2237·4
Prodolina, 2237·4
Prodon, 2237·4
Prodop, 2237·4
Prodopa, 2237·4
Prodorol, 2237·4
Prodoxidil, 2237·4
Prodoxil, 2238·1
Prodoxin, 2238·1
Prodren, 2238·1
Product 3232A— *see* Mono & Disaccharide Free Diet Powder (Product 3232A), 2139·3
Product 80056— *see* Protein Free Diet (Product 80056), 2242·4
Product Code 889, 2238·1
Produvir, 2238·1
Prodynorphin, 73·3
Pro-Efferalgan, 2238·1
Proendotel, 2238·1
Pro-enkephalin, 73·3
Proepa, 2238·1
Pro-Epanutin, 2238·1
Proesten, 2238·1
Proetzonide, 2238·1
Proetztotal, 2238·1
Prof, 2238·1
Profact, 2238·1
Profamid, 2238·1
Profar, 2238·1
Profargil, 2238·1
Profasi, 2238·1
Profasi HP, 2238·1
Profed, 2238·1
Profelina, 2238·1
Profelixir, 2238·1
Profemina, 2238·1
Profemina CC, 2238·1
Profemina MP, 2238·1
Profen, 2238·2
Profen II, 2238·2
Profen II DM, 2238·2
Profen Forte DM, 2238·2
Profena, 2238·2
Profenal, 2238·2
Profenamina, Hidrocloruro de, 488·3
Profenamine Hydrochloride, 488·3
Profenamini Hydrochloridum, 488·3
Profenda, 2238·2
Profenid, 2238·2
Profenil, 2238·2
Profeno, 2238·2
Profenzol, 2238·2
Profer, 2238·2
Profergan, 2238·2
Profex, 2238·2
Profiber, 2238·2
Profibra, 2238·2
Profil, 2238·2
Profilasmim-Ped, 2238·2
Profilate, 2238·2
Profilnine, 2238·2
Profinal, 2238·2
Profisin, 2238·2
Profiten, 2238·2
Profium, 2238·2
Proflag, 2238·2
Proflam, 2238·2
Proflavanol, 2238·2
Proflavanol C, 2238·3
Proflavina, Hemisulfato de, 1165·3
Proflavine Hemisulfate, 1165·3
Proflavine Hemisulphate, 1165·3
Proflavine Sulphate, Neutral, 1165·3
Proflax, 2238·3
Proflex, 2238·3
Proflo, 2238·3
Proflox, 2238·3
Profloxin, 2238·3
Profluid, 2238·3
Profol, 2238·3
Profolen, 2238·3
Proformiphen, 715·1
Profort, 2238·3
ProFree, 2238·3
Profrin-A, 2238·3
Profungal, 2238·3
Profylac, 2238·3
Progabida, 377·2
Progabide, 377·2
Progandol, 2238·3
Progastrit, 2238·3
Progediol, 2238·3
Progeffik, 2238·3
Progemox, 2238·3
Progenar, 2238·3
Progendo, 2238·3
Proger-F, 2238·3
Progeril, 2238·3
Progesic, 2238·3
Progest, 2238·4
Progestagens, 1527·2
Progestan, 2238·4
Progestasert, 2238·4
Progesterona, 1566·2
Progesteron-Depot, 2238·4
Progesterone, 1566·2
Progesterone-retard Pharlon, 2238·4
Progesteronum, 1566·2
Progestins, 1527·2
Progestogel, 2238·4
Progestogen-only Oral Contraceptives, 1527·3
Progestogen-releasing Intra-uterine Devices, 1527·3
Progestogens, 1527·1
Progestol, 2238·4
Progestosol, 2238·4
Progestrol, 2238·4
Progevera, 2238·4
Progevera 250, 2238·4
Progezzard, 2238·4
Proginkgo, 2238·4
Proglan, 2238·4
Proglicem, 2238·4
Proglumetacin Maleate, 85·2
Proglumetacina, Maleato de, 85·2
Proglumida, 1284·3
Proglumide, 1284·3
Proglycem, 2238·4
Pro-Gola, 2238·4
Progona, 2238·4
Progor, 2238·4
Progout, 2238·4
Prograf, 2238·4
Graft, 2238·4
PRO'gram, 2238·4
Progras, 2238·4
Progray, 2238·4
Progress, 2239·1
Progresse, 2239·1
Proguanide Hydrochloride, 457·1
Proguanil, Hidrocloruro de, 457·1
Proguanil Hydrochloride, 457·1
Proguanili Hydrochloridum, 457·1
Pro-Guard, Bioglan— *see* Bioglan Pro-Guard, 1844·1
Proguval, 2239·1
Progyluton, 2239·1
Progynon, 2239·1
Progynon C, 2239·1
Progynon Depot, 2239·1
Progynon Depot 10, 2239·1
Progynova, 2239·1
Prohair, 2239·1
Prohance, 2239·1
Pro-HDL, 2239·1
Prohelmin, 2239·1
Prohep, 2239·1
Proheparum, 2239·1
Proheptatriene Hydrochloride, 1393·1
Prohexal, 2239·1
ProHIBiT, 2239·1
Prohist, 2239·1
Proinsulin, 334·1, 340·3
Projuvex, 2239·1
Proken M, 2239·1
Prokids, 2239·1
Prokinate, 2239·1
Prokinetic Drugs, 1240·1
Prokinyl, 2239·1
Prol, 2239·2
Prolacam, 2239·2
Prolactin, 1337·3
Prolactina, 1337·3
Prolactinoma— *see* Hyperprolactinaemia, 1315·2
Prolactin-release Inhibiting Factor, 1196·1
Proladone, 2239·2
Prolair, 2239·2
Prolaken, 2239·2
Prolamine, 1694·2
Prolan, 2239·2
Prolapsed Disc— *see* Low Back Pain, 7·1
Prolastin, 2239·2
Prolastina, 2239·2
Prolax, 2239·2
Pro-Lax, 2239·2
Prolert, 2239·2
Proleukin, 2239·2
Prolidon, 2239·2
Prolief, 2239·2
Prolifen, 2239·2
Prolift, 2239·2
Proligestona, 1568·1
Proligestone, 1568·1
Prolina, 1443·2
Proline, 1443·2
L-Proline, 1443·2
Prolintane Hydrochloride, 1592·3
Prolintano, Hidrocloruro de, 1592·3
Prolinum, 1443·2
Prolipase, 2239·2
Prolisina E2, 2239·2
Prolisina VR, 2239·2
Prolitrol, 2239·2
Prolixan, 2239·2
Prolixana, 2239·2
Prolixin, 2239·2
Prolmon, 2239·2
Proloid S, 2239·2
Prolol, 2239·2
Prolong, 2239·3
Prolonium Iodide, 1603·1
Prolopa, 2239·3
Proloprim, 2239·3
Proluton, 2239·3
Proluton Depot, 2239·3
Promac, 2239·3
Promacet, 2239·3
Promal, 2239·3
Promani, 2239·3
Promanum N, 2239·3
Promatussin DM, 2239·3
Promaxol, 2239·3
Promazina, Embonato de, 717·3
Promazina, Hidrocloruro de, 717·3
Promazine Embonate, 717·3
Promazine Hydrochloride, 717·3
Promazine Pamoate, 717·3
Promazini Hydrochloridum, 717·3
Promeal, 2239·3
Promecilina, 2239·3
Promedolum, 95·3
Promedyl, 2239·3
Promega, 2239·3
Promegestona, 1568·1
Promegestone, 1568·1
Promelasa, 1735·2
Promelase, 1735·2
Promelatonin, 2239·3
Promensil, 2239·3
Promestriene, 1568·2
Promestrieno, 1568·2
Prometax, 2239·3
Prometazina, 439·1
Prometazina, Hidrocloruro de, 439·1
Prometazina, Teoclato de, 439·2
Prometh with Dextromethorphan, 2239·3
Prometh VC Plain, 2239·3
Promethawern, 2239·3
Promethazine, 439·1
Promethazine Compound Linctus, 2239·3
Promethazine Dioxide Hydrochloride, 440·1
Promethazine Embonate, 440·1
Promethazine Expectorants, 2239·3
Promethazine Hydrochloride, 439·1, 439·2
Promethazine Maleate, 440·1
Promethazine Sulfoxide, 439·3
Promethazine Teoclate, 439·2
Promethazine Theoclate, 439·2
Promethazine VC with Codeine, 2239·3
Promethazini Hydrochloridum, 439·1
Promethazinium Chloride, 439·1
Prometidine, 2239·4
Prometrium, 2239·4
Promibasol, 2239·4
Promibasol-Plus, 2239·4
Promiced, 2239·4
Promictuline, 2239·4

Promidan, 2239·4
Promifen, 2239·4
Prominal, 2239·4
Promincil, 2239·4
Prominol, 2239·4
Promise, 2239·4
Promit, 2239·4
Promiten, 2239·4
Promix, 2239·4
Promix 3, 2239·4
Promixin, 2239·4
Promocard, 2239·4
ProMod, 2239·4
Promogran, 2239·4
Promolan, 2239·4
Promolate, 1129·2
Promote, 2239·4
Promoxil, 2239·4
Prompt, 2239·4
Promune, 2239·4
Promyelocytic Leukaemia, Acute— *see* Acute Myeloid Leukaemias, 506·3
Promyrtil, 2239·4
Pronaestin, 2239·4
Pronasteron, 2240·1
Pronat, 2240·1
Pro-Nat, 2240·1
Pronaxen, 2240·1
Pronaxil, 2240·1
Pronax-P, 2240·1
Pronazol, 2240·1
Pronemia Hematinic, 2240·1
Pronerv, 2240·1
Pronervon Phyto, 2240·1
Pronervon T, 2240·1
Pronest, 2240·1
Pronestyl, 2240·1
Proneurin, 2240·1
Proneurit, 2240·1
Pronicol, 2240·1
Pronitol, 2240·1
Pronivel, 2240·1
Pronoctan, 2240·1
Pronose, 2240·1
Pronosil, 2240·1
Pronovan, 2240·1
Pronoxen, 2240·1
Prontalgin, 2240·1
Prontalgine, 2240·1
Prontamid, 2240·1
Prontinal, 2240·1
Pronto, 2240·2
Pronto Emoform, 2240·2
Pronto Platamine, 2240·2
Prontoalivio, 2240·2
Prontobario, 2240·2
Prontocid N, 2240·2
Prontodex, 2240·2
Prontoferro, 2240·2
Prontofort, 2240·2
Prontogest, 2240·2
Prontokef, 2240·2
Prontoket, 2240·2
Prontol, 2240·2
Prontolax, 2240·2
Prontomixin, 2240·2
Prontomucil, 2240·2
Prontopyrin Plus, 2240·2
Prontosil, 119·2
Prontovent, 2240·2
Proof Spirit, 1166·1
Pro-opiomelanocortin, 73·3, 1332·2
Propa, 2240·2
Propa PH, 2240·2
Propabloc, 2240·2
Propac, 2240·2
Propace, 2240·2
Propacet, 2240·2
Propacetamol, Hidrocloruro de, 85·3
Propacetamol Hydrochloride, 85·3
Propacetamoli Hydrochloridum, 85·3
Propacil, 2240·2
Propacor, 2240·2
Propaderm, 2240·2
Propafen, 2240·2
Propafenona, Hidrocloruro de, 988·3
Propafenone Hydrochloride, 988·3
Propagermanio, 652·1
Propagermanium, 652·1
Propagest, 2240·3
Propagin, 1183·3
Propain, 2240·3
Propain Forte, 2240·3
Propain Plus, 2240·3
Propal, 2240·3
Propalem, 2240·3
Propalen, 2240·3
Propalgin, 2240·3
Propalgina Plus, 2240·3
Propalgina PS Hot Lemon, 2240·3
Propalong, 2240·3
Propam, 2240·3
Propamerck, 2240·3
Propamide, 2240·3
Propamidina, Isetionato de, 1191·2
Propamidine Isethionate, 1191·2
Propamidine Isetionate, 1191·2
Propan, 2240·3
Propan Gel-S, 2240·3
Propane, 1238·2
(±)-Propane-1,2-diol, 1735·2
Propane-1,2-diol Alginate, 1576·3
Propanediol Diacetate, 1415·3
Propane-1,2,3-triol, 1694·3
1,2,3-Propanetriol Triacetate, 410·2
Propane-1,2,3-triol Trinitrate, 923·2
Propanidid, 1305·3
Propano, 1238·2
Propanocaína, Hidrocloruro de, 1383·3
Propanocaine Hydrochloride, 1383·3
Propanoic Acid, 407·3
Propanoico, Ácido, 407·3
Propanol, 1191·2, 2240·3
Propan-1-ol, 1191·2
2-Propanol, 1184·3
Propan-2-ol, 1184·3
Propanolide, 1191·2
Propanolum, 1191·2
2-Propanone, 1471·1
Propantel, 2240·3
Propantelina, Bromuro de, 489·1
Propanthel, 2240·3
Propantheline Bromide, 489·1
Propanthelini Bromidum, 489·1
PropapH, 2240·3
Propaphenin, 2240·3
Proparacaine Hydrochloride, 1384·1
Proparakain-POS, 2240·3
Propargile, 2240·3
Proparin, 2240·3
Propass, 2240·4
Propast, 2240·4
Propastad, 2240·4
Propatilnitrato, 989·3
Propatyl Nitrate, 989·3
Propatylnitrate, 989·3
Propavan, 2240·4
Propavent, 2240·4
Propavente, 2240·4
Propaxoline Citrate, 1735·3
Propayerst, 2240·4
Propayerst Plus, 2240·4
Propazinum, 717·3
Propazol, 1735·2
Propazole, 1735·2
Propecia, 2240·4
Propedil, 2240·4
Propellant 11, 1236·1
Propellant 12, 1236·1
Propellant 22, 1236·1
Propellant 114, 1235·3
Propellant 134A, 1236·2
Propellant 142B, 1236·1
Propellant 152A, 1236·2
Propellants, Aerosol, 1235·1
Prop-2-enal, 1647·1
Propenamide, 1647·1
Propentofilina, 989·3
Propentofylline, 989·3
*p*-Propenylanisole, 1654·3
Propericiazine, 714·1
Properil, 2240·4
Propeshia, 2240·4
Propess, 2240·4
Propetamfós, 1509·2
Propetamphos, 1509·2
Prophage, 2240·4
Prophedin, 2240·4
Prophenamini Chloridum, 488·3
Prophenpyridamine, 438·3
Prophenpyridamine Maleate, 438·3
Pro-Phree, 2240·4
Prophthal, 2240·4
Prophyllin, 2240·4
Prophylux, 2240·4
Propibay, 2240·4
Propicilina Potásica, 246·3
Propicillin Potassium, 246·3
Propicillinum Kalicum, 246·3
Propiden, 2240·4
Propifenazona, 85·3
Propil, 2240·4
Propilenglicol, 1735·2
Propilenoglicol, 1735·2
Propilhexedrina, 1592·3
Propilhexedrina, Hidrocloruro de, 1592·3
Propiliodona, 1067·3
Propilparabeno, 1183·3
Propilparabeno Sódico, 1183·3
Propilracil, 2240·4
Propiltiouracilo, 1603·1
Propimex, 2240·4
Propine, 2240·4
Propinox Hydrochloride, 487·3
Propiochrone, 2241·1
Propiocine, 2241·1
Propioform, 2241·1
Propiolactona, 1191·2
Propiolactone, 1191·2
β-Propiolactone, 1191·2
Propiomazina, Hidrocloruro de, 440·3
Propiomazina, Maleato de, 440·3
Propiomazine, 440·3
Propiomazine Hydrochloride, 440·3
Propiomazine Hydrogen Maleate, 440·3
Propiomazine Maleate, 440·3
Propionat, 2241·1
Propionato de Clobetasol, 1095·2
Propionato de Eritromicina, 208·2
Propionato de Fluticasona, 1102·3
Propionato de Josamicina, 224·3
Propionato de Sodio, 408·1
Propionato de Testosterona, 1570·1
Propionato de Ulobetasol, 1111·3
*Propionibacterium acnes*, 540·2
Propionic Acid, 407·3
Propionilpromazina, 718·1
Propiono-3-lactone, 1191·2
Propionyl Erythromycin Mercaptosuccinate, 211·1
4-*N*-(*N*-Propionylanilino) Piperidine, 41·1
Propionylerythromycin, 208·2
Propionylerythromycin Lauryl Sulphate, 208·1
3″-Propionyl-leucomycin $A_5$, 254·1
Propionylpromazine, 718·1
Propiopromazine, 718·1
Propiosalic, 2241·1
Propiosol, 2241·1
Propipocaína, 1383·3
Propipocaine, 1383·3
Propiral, 2241·1
Propitocaine Hydrochloride, 1382·3
Propiverina, Hidrocloruro de, 489·1
Propiverine Hydrochloride, 489·1
Proplax, 2241·1
Proplex, 2241·1
Proplex T, 2241·1
Pro-Plus, 2241·1
Propoabbott, 2241·1
Propocam, 2241·1
Propofan, 2241·1
Propofol, 1305·3
Propofolum, 1305·3
Propol, 2241·1
Propolcream, 2241·1
Propóleo, 1735·2
Propoleos, 2241·1
Propolis, 1735·2
Propolisept Urtinktur, 2241·1
Propolisept-Salbe, 2241·1
Propomill, 2241·1
Proponol, 2241·1
Propoten, 2241·1
Propovan, 2241·1
Propoxicaína, Hidrocloruro de, 1384·1
Propoxur, 1509·2
Propoxycaine Hydrochloride, 1384·1
Propoxycainium Chloride, 1384·1
Propoxyphene, 28·3
Propoxyphene Hydrochloride, 28·3
Propoxyphene Napsylate, 28·3
Propoxypiperocaine, 1383·3
Propra, 2241·1
Propra Comp, 2241·1
Proprahexal, 2241·1
Propral, 2241·1
Propranet, 2241·1
Propranolol, Hidrocloruro de, 989·3
Propranolol Hydrochloride, 989·3
Propranololi Hydrochloridum, 989·3
Propranur, 2241·1
Propra-ratiopharm, 2241·1
Pro-PS, 2241·2
Propulm, 2241·2
Propulsid, 2241·2
Propulsin, 2241·2
Propycil, 2241·2
Propyderm, 2241·2
Propyl, 2241·2
Propyl Alcohol, 1191·2
Propyl Alcohol, Normal, 1191·2
Propyl Alcohol, Primary, 1191·2
Propyl 4-Diethylcarbamoylmethoxy-3-methoxyphenylacetate, 1305·3
Propyl 1,4-Dihydro-3,5-di-iodo-4-oxo-1-pyridylacetate, 1067·3
Propyl Gallate, 1168·1
Propyl Hydride, 1238·2
Propyl Hydroxybenzoate, 1183·3
Propyl 4-Hydroxybenzoate, 1183·3
Propyl Hydroxybenzoate, Sodium, 1183·3
Propyl Hydroxybenzoate, Soluble, 1183·3
Propyl Nicotinate, 85·3
Propyl Parahydroxybenzoate, 1183·3
Propyl Parahydroxybenzoate, Sodium, 1183·3
Propyl Salicylate, 1157·2
Propyl 3,4,5-Trihydroxybenzoate, 1168·1
Propyl Undecenoate, 411·1
Propy-Lacticare, 2241·2
Propyladiphenine Hydrochloride, 1735·2
*N*-Propylajmalinium Hydrogen Tartrate, 984·3
2-Propylaminopropiono-*o*-toluidide, 1382·3
Propylene Carbonate, 1476·3
Propylene Dichloride, 1473·1
Propylene Dilaurate, 1415·3
Propylene Glycol, 1735·2
Propylene Glycol Alginate, 1576·3
Propylene Glycol Diacetate, 1415·3
Propylene Glycol Dilaurate, 1415·3
Propylene Glycol Laurate, 1415·3
Propylene Glycol Monolaurate, 1415·3
Propylene Glycol Monopalmitate, 1415·3
Propylene Glycol Monopalmitostearate, 1415·3
Propylene Glycol Monostearate, 1415·3
Propylene Glycol Stearate, 1415·3
(±)-*N*,*N*′-Propylenebis[nicotinamide], 1719·3
(±)-4,4′-Propylenebis(piperazine-2,6-dione), 582·2
(+)-(*S*)-4,4′-Propylenebis(piperazine-2,6-dione), 1036·1
Propylèneglycol (Stéarate de), 1415·3
Propylenglycoli Dilauras, 1415·3
Propylenglycoli Monolauras, 1415·3
Propylenglycoli Monopalmitostearas, 1415·3
Propylenglycoli Monostearas, 1415·3
Propylenglycolum, 1735·2
Propyless, 2241·2
Propylhexed, 1592·3
Propylhexedrine, 1592·3

Propylhexedrine Hydrochloride, 1592·3
14a,17α-Propylidene Dioxypregn-4-ene-3,20-dione, 1568·1
Propyliodone, 1067·3
Propyliodonum, 1067·3
Propylis Gallas, 1168·1
Propylis Oxybenzoas, 1183·3
Propylis Parahydroxybenzoas, 1183·3
Propylis Parahydroxybenzoas Natricum, 1183·3
Propylis Paraoxibenzoas, 1183·3
19-Propylorvinol Hydrochloride, 38·3
Propylparaben, 1183·3
Propylparaben Sodium, 1183·3, 1184·1
2-Propylpentanoic Acid, 380·1
1-(α-Propylphenethyl)pyrrolidine Hydrochloride, 1592·3
2-Propylpyridine-4-carbothioamide, 246·3
Propylthiocil, 2241·2
Propylthiouracil, 1603·1
6-Propyl-2-thiouracil, 1603·1
Propylthiouracilum, 1603·1
Propyl-Thyracil, 2241·2
Propylum Gallicum, 1168·1
2-Propylvaleramide, 380·1
2-Propylvaleric Acid, 380·1
2-Propylvaleric Acid—Sodium 2-Propylvalerate (1:1), 380·1
Propyphenazone, 85·3
Propyphenazonum, 85·3
Propyre T, 2241·2
Pro-Q, 2241·2
Proquazone, 86·1
Proquin, 2241·2
P-Roquine, 2241·2
Prorhinel, 2241·2
Proroxan, 990·3
Prorynorm, 2241·2
Pro-Sabona Uno, 2241·2
Prosatietil, 2241·2
Proscar, 2241·2
Proscar, Chibro-— *see* Chibro-Proscar, 1882·3
Proscilaridina, 990·3
Proscillaridin, 990·3
Proscillaridin A, 990·3
Proscope, 2241·2
Prosedar, 2241·2
Prosed/DS, 2241·2
Prosed-X, 2241·2
Proser, 2241·2
Proserinum, 1492·2
Prosgutt, 2241·2
Pro-Shape, 2241·3
Prosicca, 2241·3
ProSight Lutein, 2241·3
Prosiston, 2241·3
Proskin, 2241·3
Proslender, 2241·3
Proslim-Lipid, 2241·3
Prosmin, 2241·3
Prosobee, 2241·3
Prosom, 2241·3
Pro-Sope, 2241·3
Prosoyal, 2241·3
Prospan, 2241·3
Prospec, 2241·3
Prost-1, 2241·3
Prosta, 2241·3
Prosta Fink Forte, 2241·3
Prosta Fink N, 2241·3
Prosta Urgenin Uno, 2241·3
Prostabiol, 2241·3
Prosta-Caps Chassot N, 2241·3
Prosta-Caps Fink, 2241·3
Prostacur, 2241·3
Prostacyclin, 1516·3
Prostadilat, 2241·3
Prostadirex, 2241·4
Prostaflor, 2241·4
Prostafort, 2241·4
Prostaforton, 2241·4
Prostagalen, 2241·4
Prostaglandin $A_2$, 1511·1
Prostaglandin $B_2$, 1511·1
Prostaglandin $C_2$, 1511·1
Prostaglandin $D_2$, 1511·1
Prostaglandin $E_1$, 1512·3
Prostaglandin $E_1$ α-Cyclodextrin Clathrate Compound, 1512·3
Prostaglandin $E_2$, 1515·1
Prostaglandin $F_{2\alpha}$, 1514·3
Prostaglandin $F_{2\alpha}$ Trometamol, 1514·3
Prostaglandin $G_2$, 1511·1
Prostaglandin $H_2$, 1511·1
Prostaglandin $I_2$, 1516·3
Prostaglandin X, 1516·3
Prostaglandins, 1511·1
Prostagutt, 2241·4
Prostagutt Forte, 2241·4
Prostagutt Mono, 2241·4
Prostagutt Uno, 2241·4
Prostagutt-F, 2241·4
Prostaherb Cucurbitae— *see* Vesiherb, 2374·1
Prostaherb N, 2241·4
Prostakan, 2241·4
Prostal, 2241·4
Prostalium, 2241·4
Prostall, 2241·4
Prostalog, 2241·4
Prostamal, 2241·4
Prostamed, 2241·4
Prostamed Urtica, 2241·4
Prostamid, 2241·4
Prostamustin, 2241·4
Prostan, 2241·4
Prostandin, 2241·4
Prostaneurin, 2241·4
Prostanoic Acid, 1511·1
Prostanoids, 1511·1
Prostanovag, 2241·4
Prostap, 2241·4
Prostaphlin-A, 2241·4
Prostarell, 2241·4
Prostasal, 2241·4
Prostasan, 2241·4
Prostascint Kit, 2241·4
Prostaselect, 2242·1
Prostaserene, 2242·1
Prostasyx, 2242·1
Prostata, 2242·1
Prostata-Gastreu N R25, 2242·1
Prostata-Komplex N Ho-Fu-Complex, 2242·1
Prostata-Kurbis S, 2242·1
Prostatal, 2242·1
Prostate Cancer— *see* Malignant Neoplasms of the Prostate, 521·2
Prostate Support, 2242·1
Prostatic Cancer— *see* Malignant Neoplasms of the Prostate, 521·2
Prostatic Hyperplasia, Benign— *see* Benign Prostatic Hyperplasia, 1555·1
Prostatin F, 2242·1
Prostatitis, Bacterial— *see* Urinary-tract Infections, 153·1
Prostatonin, 2242·1
Prosta-Urgenin, 2242·1
Prosta-Urgenine, 2242·1
Prostavasin, 2242·1
Prostawern, 2242·1
Prostazosina, 2242·1
Prostearin, 1415·3
Prostease, 2242·1
Prostec, 2242·1
Prostem, 2242·1
Prostem Plus, 2242·1
Prostene, 2242·1
Prosteo, 2242·1
Prostep, 2242·1
Prosteren, 2242·1
Prostess, 2242·1
Prostetin, 2242·1
Prostex, 2242·1
ProstGard, 2242·1
Prosthetic Heart Valves— *see* Valvular Heart Disease, 838·2
Prostica, 2242·1
Prostide, 2242·1
Prostigmin, 2242·1
Prostigmina, 2242·2
Prostigmine, 2242·2
Prostin, 2242·2
Prostin E2, 2242·2
Prostin F2, 2242·2
Prostin F2 Alpha, 2242·2
Prostin/15M, 2242·2
Prostin Pediatrico, 2242·2
Prostin VR, 2242·2
Prostine $E_2$, 2242·2
Prostine $F_2$ Alpha, 2242·2
Prostine VR, 2242·2
Prostinfenem, 2242·2
Prostivas, 2242·2
Prostodin, 2242·2
Prostogenat, 2242·2
Prosturol, 2242·2
Prost-X, 2242·2
Prosulf, 2242·2
Prosultiamina, 1455·1
Prosultiamine, 1455·1
Prosure, 2242·2
Prosymbioflor, 2242·2
Pro-Symbioflor, 2242·2
Prota, 2242·2
Protacine Maleate, 85·2
Protact, 2242·3
Protactyl, 2242·3
Protagent, 2242·3
Protalgia, 2242·3
Protamide, 2242·3
Protamina, 1050·3
Protamina, Cloridrato de, 1050·3
Protamina, Hidrocloruro de, 1050·3
Protamina, Sulfato de, 1050·3
Protamine, 1050·3
Protamine Hydrochloride, 1050·3
Protamine Insulin, Isophane, 334·2
Protamine Sulfate, 1050·3
Protamine Sulphate, 1050·3
Protamine Zinc Insulin, 334·2
Protamini Hydrochloridum, 1050·3
Protamini Sulfas, 1050·3
Protan, 2242·3
Protangix, 2242·3
Protanol, 2242·3
Protaphan, 2242·3
Protaphane, 2242·3
Protaphane HM, 2242·3
Protaphane HM— *see* Insulatard HM, 2063·3
Protaphane MC, 2242·3
Protargin, Mild, 1746·2
Protargin, Strong, 1746·2
Protargolum, 1746·2
Protarin, 2242·3
Protasol, 2242·3
Protat, 2242·3
Protaxil, 2242·3
Protaxol, 2242·3
Protaxon, 2242·3
Protease, 2242·3
Protease Concentrate, Plant, 1662·2
Proteazone, 2242·3
Protec, 2242·3
Pro-Tec Sport, 2242·3
Protec T, 2242·3
Proteccion Ultra, 2242·3
ProTech, 2242·3
Protecor, 2242·3
Protectaid, 2242·3
Protecteur Levres, 2242·4
Protectina, 2242·4
Protecto, 2242·4
Protecto-Derm, 2242·4
Protectol, 2242·4
Protector, 2242·4
Protegra Antioxid, 2242·4
Proteigeno, 2242·4
Proteika, 2242·4
Protein C, 735·3, 759·2
Protein C Deficiency— *see* Thromboembolic Disorders, 837·3
Protein Free Diet (Product 80056), 2242·4
Protein Plus, 2242·4
Protein S, 735·3
Protein S Deficiency— *see* Thromboembolic Disorders, 837·3
Proteína Bactericida Incrementadora de la Permeabilidad, 1658·3
Proteína C, 759·2
Protein-A Immuno-adsorption Column, 758·2
Proteínas Morfogenéticamente Óseas, 768·1
Proteinato de Plata, 1746·2
Proteinato de Prata, 1746·2
Protein-Free, 2242·4
Proteins, 1417·1
Proteinsteril Hepa, 2242·4
Proteinsteril KE, 2242·4
Proteita, 2242·4
Protemp, 2242·4
Proten Plus, 2242·4
Protenac, 2242·4
Protenate, 2242·4
Protensin-M, 2242·4
Proteoferrina, 2242·4
Proteozym, 2242·4
Proterenal, 2242·4
Proteval, 2242·4
Protevis, 2242·4
Protexel, 2242·4
Prothanon, 2242·4
Prothanon Cromo, 2242·4
Prothazin, 2242·4
Prothazine, 2242·4
Prothiaden, 2242·4
Prothiazide, 2243·1
Prothiazine, 2243·1
Prothiazine Expectorant, 2243·1
Prothicid, 2243·1
Prothil, 2243·1
Prothionamide, 246·3
Prothipendyl Hydrochloride, 718·1
Prothiucil, 2243·1
Prothrombin, 735·3
Prothrombin Complex Concentrate, Activated, 752·2
Prothrombin Complex, Dried, 752·2
Prothrombin Time, 735·3
Prothrombinex, 2243·1
Prothrombinkomplex BaWu, 2243·1
Prothrombinum Multiplex Humanum, 752·2
Prothromplex Preparations, 2243·1
Prothuril, 2243·1
Prothyrid, 2243·1
Prothyrysat, 2243·1
Proti 5, 2243·1
Protiaden, 2243·1
Protiadene, 2243·1
Protical, 2243·1
Protid, 2243·1
Protideal, 2243·1
Protiderm, 2243·1
Protidiet, 2243·1
Protifar, 2243·1
Protifar Plus, 2243·1
Protifortf, 2243·1
Protifortifiant, 2243·1
Protil, 2243·1
Protilase, 2243·1
Protina G, 2243·1
Protina Torre MP, 2243·1
Protinex, 2243·1
Protinin, 2243·1
Protinules, 2243·2
Protinutril, 2243·2
Protionamida, 246·3
Protionamide, 246·3
Protionamide Hydrochloride, 246·3
Protipendilo, Hidrocloruro de, 718·1
Protipharm, 2243·2
Protireal, 2243·2
Protirelin, 1337·3
Protirelin Tartrate, 1338·2
Protirelina, 1337·3
Protirelinum, 1337·3
Protium, 2243·2
Protobex, 2243·2
Proto-Boric, 2243·2
Protocide, 2243·2
Protocloruro de Mercurio, 1712·3

Protogyl, 2243·2
Protol, 2243·2
Proton, 2243·2
Proton Pump Inhibitors, 1239·3
Protonix, 2243·2
Protopam, 2243·2
Protopic, 2243·2
Protoporfirina IX Disódica, 1735·3
Protoporfirina-Estaño, 1756·3
Protoporphyrin Disodium, 1735·3
Protoporphyrin IX Disodium, 1735·3
Protosin, 2243·2
Protosol, 2243·2
Protossido, Azoto, 1304·3
Protostat, 2243·2
Protostib, 600·3
Protothecosis, 390·1
Protoveratrine A, 1764·1
Protoveratrine B, 1764·1
Protovit, 2243·2
Protovit N, 2243·2
Protoxyde d'Azote, 1304·3
Protozoal Gastro-enteritis— *see* Gastro-enteritis, 596·3
Protozoal Infections in Immunocompromised Patients— *see* Infections in Immunocompromised Patients, 597·1
Protozone, 2243·2
Protriptilina, Hidrocloruro de, 316·2
Protriptyline Hydrochloride, 316·2
Protromplex, 2243·2
Protromplex TIM 3, 2243·2
Protropin, 2243·2
Protuss, 2243·2
Protussa, 2243·2
Protuss-D, 2243·2
Protuss-DM, 2243·2
Pro-Uro, 2243·3
Prourokinase, 735·3
Prourokinase, Glycosylated, 964·2
Prourokinase, Non-glycosylated, 996·3
Provacsin Nasal, 2243·3
Provail, 2243·3
Provames, 2243·3
Provamicina, 2243·3
Provas, 2243·3
Provas Comp, 2243·3
Provascul, 2243·3
Provatine, 2243·3
Provax, 2243·3
Provegol, 2243·3
Provelle, 2243·3
Provenal, 2243·3
Provenen, 2243·3
Proveno N, 2243·3
Pro-Vent, 2243·3
Proventil, 2243·3
Provera, 2243·3
Provera— *see* Estrapak, 1979·3
Provera— *see* Menoprem, 2123·4
Provera— *see* Provelle, 2243·3
Provera, Depo- — *see* Depo-Provera, 1925·4
Provertin-UM TIM 3, 2243·3
Provetal, 2243·3
Provette Continuous, 2243·3
Provette Sequential, 2243·3
Provical, 2243·3
Provictol, 2243·3
Provide, 2243·3
Providex, 2243·3
ProvideXtra, 2243·3
Provigil, 2243·4
Provimin, 2243·4
Proviodine, 2243·4
Proviron, 2243·4
Provironum, 2243·4
Provisc, 2243·4
Provisc— *see* Duovisc, 1957·4
Provisual, 2243·4
Provisual Compuesto, 2243·4
Provita, 2243·4
Provitamin A, 1422·3
Provitamin A + D + E, 2243·4
Provitamin A-E, 2243·4
Proviton, 2243·4
Provive, 2243·4
Provixen-N, 2243·4
Provocholine, 2243·4
Provokit, 2243·4
Provotest, 2243·4
Prowess, 2243·4
Prowess Plain, 2243·4
Pro-Whey, 2243·4
ProWohl, 2243·4
PROX, 1384·1
Proxacin, 2243·4
Proxalin, 2243·4
Proxalin-Plus, 2243·4
Proxalyoc, 2243·4
Proxazol, Citrato de, 1735·3
Proxazole Citrate, 1735·3
Proxen, 2243·4
PROXFLN, 1384·1, 1689·1
Proxibarbal, 718·1
Proxibarbital, 718·1
Proxidin, 2244·1
Proxifilina, 791·2
Proxigel, 2244·1
Proxil, 2244·1
Proximetacaína, Hidrocloruro de, 1384·1
Proxin, 2244·1
Proxine, 2244·1
Proxinor, 2244·1
Proxitec, 2244·1
Proxol, 2244·1
Proxymetacaine Hydrochloride, 1384·1
Proxyphylline, 791·2
Proxyphyllinum, 791·2
Proxytab, 2244·1
Proxyvon, 2244·1
Proyeast, 2244·1
Prozac, 2244·1
Prozamel, 2244·1
Prozapina, Hidrocloruro de, 1736·1
Prozapine Hydrochloride, 1736·1
Prozatan, 2244·1
Prozef, 2244·1
Prozen, 2244·1
Proziere, 2244·1
Prozin, 2244·1
Prozina, 2244·1
Prozine, 2244·1
Prozit, 2244·1
Prozitel, 2244·1
Prozolin, 2244·1
ProZone Preparations, 2244·1
Prozyme, 2244·2
Prozyn, 2244·2
PRP-D, 1616·2
PRP-OMP, 1616·2
PRP-OMPC, 1616·2
PRP-T, 1616·2
Prudencial, 2244·2
Pruderm, 2244·2
Prueba de Schick, 1742·2
Pruebas de Embarazo Y de Fertilidad, 1734·3
Prueboi, 2244·2
Pruina, 2244·2
Prulifloxacin, 246·3
Prulifloxacino, 246·3
Prulit, 2244·2
Prunasin, 1765·2
Prunasine, 2244·2
Prune, 1285·1
Prune, African, 1568·2
Prune Bark, Virginian, 1765·2
Prune, Virginian, 1765·2
Prunetol, 1692·1
Pruni Africanae, 1568·2
Prunier d'Afrique, 1568·2
Prunodiet, 2244·2
Prunogil, 2244·2
Prunus, 1285·1
*Prunus africana*, 1568·2
*Prunus amygdalus*, 1651·1
*Prunus armeniaca*, 1730·2
*Prunus avium*, 1058·1
*Prunus cerasus*, 1058·1
*Prunus domestica*, 1285·1
*Prunus dulcis*, 1651·1
*Prunus persica*, 1730·2
*Prunus serotina*, 1765·2
Prunus-Bad, 2244·2
Prurex, 2244·2
Pruriced, 2244·2
Pruridermase, 2244·2
Pruridol, 2244·2
Prurigel, 2244·2
Pruri-med, 2244·2
Prurimix, 2244·2
Pruripelen, 2244·2
Prurisedan, 2244·2
Prurisedan Antimicotico, 2244·2
Prurisedan Biotic, 2244·2
Pruritrat, 2244·2
Pruritus, 1137·3
Prurix, 2244·2
Prurizin, 2244·2
Prussian Blue, 1051·2
Prussic Acid, 1506·1
Pryleugan, 2244·3
Pryndette, 2244·3
Prysma, 2244·3
Prysoline, 2244·3
P2S, 1050·1
PS-341, 532·1
PSC-801, 990·3
PSC-833, 591·1
PSE CPM, 2244·3
PSE MSC, 2244·3
Pselac, 2244·3
Pserhofer's, 2244·3
Pseudo, 2244·3
Pseudocapsaicin, 67·2
Pseudo-Car DM, 2244·3
Pseudocef, 2244·3
Pseudo-Chlor, 2244·3
Pseudoefedrina, 1129·2
Pseudoefedrina, Hidrocloruro de, 1129·2
Pseudoefedrina, Sulfato de, 1129·2
Pseudoephedrine, 1129·2
Pseudoephedrine Hydrochloride, 1129·2
Pseudoephedrine Polistirex, 1130·1
Pseudoephedrine Sulfate, 1129·2
Pseudoephedrine Sulphate, 1129·2
Pseudoephedrine Tannate, 1130·1
Pseudoephedrini Hydrochloridum, 1129·2
Pseudofrin, 2244·3
Pseudo-Gest, 2244·3
Pseudo-Gest Plus, 2244·3
Pseudohypericin, 299·2
Pseudohypoparathyroidism— *see* Hypoparathyroidism, 765·2
Pseudoisoeugenyl 2-Methylbutyrate, 1655·2
Pseudomembranous Colitis— *see* Antibiotic-associated Colitis, 128·1
Pseudomonal Meningitis— *see* Meningitis, 134·3
*Pseudomonas fluorescens*, 233·3
Pseudomonas Immunoglobulins, 1635·2
*Pseudomonas pyrrocinia*, 408·1
Pseudomonas Vaccines, 1635·2
Pseudomonic Acid, 233·1
Pseudono, 2244·3
Pseudo-obstruction— *see* Decreased Gastrointestinal Motility, 1241·1
Pseudophage, 2244·3
Pseudotumour Cerebri— *see* Raised Intracranial Pressure, 833·1
Psico Blocan, 2244·3
Psicoasten, 2244·3
Psicocen, 2244·3
Psicofar, 2244·3
Psicoglut, 2244·3
D-Psicose, 1432·1
Psicosedin, 2244·3
Psicosoma Solucion, 2244·3
Psilo-Balsam N, 2244·3
Psilocibina, 1736·1
Psilocin, 1736·1
Psilocina, 1736·1
*Psilocybe*, 1717·3
*Psilocybe mexicana*, 1736·1
*Psilocybe semilanceata*, 1736·1
Psilocybin, 1736·1
Psilocybine, 1736·1
Psilocyn, 1736·1
Psilumax, 2244·3
Psipax, 2244·3
Psiquial, 2244·3
Psittacosis, 143·2
Psiu, 2244·4
PSK, 1733·2
PS-K, 1733·2
Psocortene, 2244·4
Psodermil, 2244·4
Pso-Rad, 2244·4
Psoraderm 5, 2244·4
Psoradexan, 2244·4
Psoradrate, 2244·4
Psoralen, 1153·2
Psoralon MT, 2244·4
Psorantral, 2244·4
Psor-a-set, 2244·4
Psor-Asist, 2244·4
Psorasolv, 2244·4
Psorcon, 2244·4
Psorcutan, 2244·4
Psorex, 2244·4
Psoriacen, 2244·4
Psoriacreme, 2244·4
Psoriasdin, 2244·4
Psoriasis, 1137·3
Psoriasis-Bad, 2244·4
Psoriasis-Salbe M, 2244·4
Psoriasis-Salbe S, 2244·4
Psoriasis-Solution, 2244·4
Psoriasis-Sulfur L12, 2244·4
Psoriasis-Tabletten, 2244·4
Psoriasol, 2244·4
Psoriatec, 2244·4
Psoriatic Arthritis— *see* Spondyloarthropathies, 11·1
Psoriatic Arthropathy— *see* Spondyloarthropathies, 11·1
Psoricreme, 2244·4
Psoriderm, 2244·4
Psorigel, 2245·1
Psorigerb N, 2245·1
Psorimed, 2245·1
Psorin, 2245·1
Psorinase, 2245·1
PSP, 1730·3
Psychobald, 2245·1
Psychogenic Polydipsia— *see* Hyponatraemia, 1220·3
Psychomotor Epilepsy— *see* Epilepsy, 349·1
Psychoneuroticum (Rowo-578), 2245·1
Psychopax, 2245·1
Psychoses, 665·1
Psychoses, Hypochondriacal— *see* Hypochondriasis, 664·3
Psychotic Disorders— *see* Psychoses, 665·1
Psychotonin, 2245·1
Psychotonin M, 2245·1
Psychotonin-sed, 2245·1
Psycoton, 2245·1
Psylia, 2245·1
Psyllii Semen, 1268·1
Psylli-Mucil Plus, Bioglan— *see* Bioglan Psylli-Mucil Plus, 1844·1
Psyllium Husk, 1268·1
Psyllium Seed, 1268·1
Psymion, 2245·1
Psyquil, 2245·1
Psyrazine, 2245·1
PSY-stabil, 2245·1
PT-9, 1660·1
PTA, 735·3, 2245·1
P-Tanna, 2245·1
Ptarmiganberry Leaves, 1659·2
PTC, 735·3, 752·2
PTE, 2245·1
Pteroylglutamic Acid, 1429·1
Pteroylmonoglutamic Acid, 1429·1
Pterygium, 574·3
PTFE, 1733·2
PTH, 774·3
PTH 1-34, 774·3

Pthiriasis Palpebrarum— *see* Pediculosis, 1499·1
Ptinolin, 2245·1
Ptyalin, 1654·2
PU, 1320·3
Puamin, 2245·1
Pubergen, 2245·1
Puberty, Delayed— *see* Delayed Puberty, 1314·1
Puberty, Precocious— *see* Precocious Puberty, 1318·2
Pubic Lice— *see* Pediculosis, 1499·1
Pudan-Lebertran-Zinksalbe, 2245·1
Puernol, 2245·1
Puersan, 2245·1
Puerzym, 2245·2
Pufolic— *see* Elageno OS, 1964·4
Pulbil, 2245·2
Pulbronc, 2245·2
Pulbronc Simple, 2245·2
Pulegium Oil, 1736·1
Pulegone, 1283·2, 1736·1
Pulibex, 2245·2
Pulin, 2245·2
Pulkrin, 2245·2
Pulmadil, 2245·2
Pulmagol, 2245·2
Pulmarin, 2245·2
Pulmax, 2245·2
Pulmaxan, 2245·2
Pulmeno, 2245·2
Pulmex, 2245·2
Pulmex Baby, 2245·2
Pulmiben, 2245·2
Pulmicort, 2245·2
Pulmicret, 2245·2
Pulmictan, 2245·2
Pulmidur, 2245·2
Pulmilide, 2245·3
Pulminflamatoria, 2245·3
Pulmison, 2245·3
Pulmist, 2245·3
Pulmo Preparations, 2245·3
Pulmocare, 2245·3
Pulmocilin, 2245·3
Pulmocis, 2245·3
Pulmoclase, 2245·3
Pulmocler, 2245·3
Pulmocod, 2245·3
Pulmo-Cod, 2245·3
Pulmo-Cod (C & G), 2245·3
Pulmocordio Forte, 2245·3
Pulmocordio Mite SL, 2245·3
Pulmo-cyl Ho-Len-Complex, 2245·3
Pulmodexane, 2245·3
Pulmodex-C, 2245·3
Pulmofasa, 2245·3
Pulmofasa Antihist, 2245·4
Pulmofluide Simple, 2245·4
Pulmoflux, 2245·4
Pulmofor, 2245·4
Pulmoformil, 2245·4
Pulmoforte, 2245·4
Pulmogripe, 2245·4
Pulmoiodo, 2245·4
Pulmolite, 2245·4
Pulmoll, 2245·4
Pulmoll au Menthol et a l'Eucalyptus, 2245·4
Pulmonar, 2245·4
Pulmonary Disease, Chronic Obstructive— *see* Chronic Obstructive Pulmonary Disease, 779·2
Pulmonary Embolism— *see* Venous Thromboembolism, 839·1
Pulmonary Fibrosis, Idiopathic— *see* Diffuse Parenchymal Lung Disease, 1079·3
Pulmonary Hypertension, 832·1
Pulmonary Hypertension of the Newborn, Persistent— *see* Pulmonary Hypertension, 832·1
Pulmonary Oedema— *see* Heart Failure, 820·3
Pulmonary Oedema, High-altitude— *see* High-altitude Disorders, 822·2
Pulmonary Oedema— *see* Shock, 835·1
Pulmonary Surfactants, 1736·1
Pulmonase, 2245·4
Pulmonilo Synergium, 2245·4
Pulmonium N, 2245·4
Pulmonix, 2245·4
Pulmophyllin, 2245·4
Pulmophylline, 2245·4
Pulmoquin, 2245·4
Pulmorell, 2245·4
Pulmo-Rest, 2245·4
Pulmo-Rest Expectorant, 2245·4
Pulmorex DM, 2245·4
Pulmorien, 2245·4
Pulmorphan, 2246·1
Pulmorphan Pediatrique, 2246·1
Pulmosan, 2246·1
Pulmo-San, 2246·1
Pulmoserum, 2246·1
Pulmosin, 2246·1
Pulmosina, 2246·1
Pulmosodyl, 2246·1
Pulmospin, 2246·1
Pulmosterin Duo, 2246·1
Pulmosterin Retard, 2246·1
Pulmotide, 2246·1
Pulmo-Timelets, 2246·1
Pulmotin, 2246·1
Pulmotosse, 2246·1
Pulmotropic, 2246·1
Pulmovax, 2246·1
Pulmovent, 2246·1
Pulmoverina, 2246·1
Pulmovital, 2246·1
Pulmozyme, 2246·1
Pulpa de Caña Fístula, 1255·2
Pulpomixine, 2246·1
Pulsalux, 2246·1
Pulsar, 2246·1
Pulsar Enzimatico, 2246·2
Pulsar Plus, 2246·2
Pulsatilla, 1737·1
Pulsatilla Med Complex, 2246·2
*Pulsatilla pratensis*, 1737·1
*Pulsatilla vulgaris*, 1737·1
Pulseless Electrical Activity— *see* Advanced Cardiac Life Support, 812·2
Pulsit, 2246·2
Pulsitil, 2246·2
Pulsol, 2246·2
Pulsor, 2246·2
Pulsoton, 2246·2
Pulverizador Nasal, 2246·2
Pulvhydrops Mono, 2246·2
Pulvicin, 2246·2
Pulvinal Beclometasone Dipropionate, 2246·2
Pulvinal Salbutamol, 2246·2
Pulvis-3, 2246·2
Pulvispray, 2246·2
Pulvo Preparations, 2246·2
Pumactant, 1736·2
Pumex, 1140·1
Pumex Granulatus, 1140·1
Pumice, 1140·1
Pumice Flour, 1140·1
Pumice Stone, 1140·1
Pumicis, Lapis, 1140·1
Pumilene Vapo, 2246·2
Pumilen-N, 2246·2
Pumilio Pine Oil, 1737·1
Pumilsan, 2246·2
Pumonal Eco Natura, 2246·2
Pumpan, 2246·2
Pump-Hep, 2246·2
Punarnaba, 1737·1
Punarnava, 1737·1
Punarnavine, 1737·1
Puncto E, 2246·2
Pungino, 2246·2
*Punica granatum*, 112·1
Punktyl, 2246·2
Puntol, 2246·2
Puntual, 2246·2
Puntualex, 2246·3
Pupiletto, 2246·3
Pupilla, 2246·3
Pupilla Antistaminico, 2246·3
Pupilla Light, 2246·3
Puraloe, 2246·3
Puralube, 2246·3
Puran T4, 2246·3
Purata, 2246·3
Purbac, 2246·3
Pur-Bloka, 2246·3
Pure Health, 2246·3
Pure Omega, 2246·3
Pure Plan, 2246·3
Pureduct, 2246·3
Puregon, 2246·3
Pureness Blemish Control, 2246·3
Puresis, 2246·3
Puretam, 2246·3
Purethal, 2246·3
Purfalox, 2246·3
Purfilx, 2246·3
Purganol, 2246·3
Purgante, 2246·3
Purgatives, 1239·3
Purgazen, 2246·3
Purge, 2246·3
Purgoleite, 2246·4
Purgo-Pil, 2246·4
Purgoxin, 2246·4
Puricin, 2246·4
Puricos, 2246·4
Purid, 2246·4
Puride, 2246·4
Purified Bentonite, 1577·2
Purified Honey, 1434·2
Purified Insulins, 334·2
Purified Siliceous Earth, 1581·3
Purified Stearic Acid, 1749·2
Purified Talc, 1159·1
Purified Water, 1764·3
Purigoa, 2246·4
Purilon, 2246·4
Purinethiol, 567·2
Purine-6-thiol Monohydrate, 567·2
Puri-Nethol, 2246·4
Purinol, 2246·4
Puriphyl, 2246·4
Purisole, 2246·4
Puritabs, 2246·4
Puritenk, 2246·4
Purmolax, 2246·4
Purmycin, 2246·4
Purochin, 2246·4
Purofilina, 2246·4
Purol, 2246·4
Puromylon, 2246·4
Purple Clover, 1737·3
Purple Medick, 1649·1
Purporent, 2246·4
Purpose, 2246·4
Purpose Alpha Hydroxy, 2246·4
Purpose Dual, 2246·4
Purpura, Autoimmune Thrombocytopenic— *see* Idiopathic Thrombocytopenic Purpura, 1082·1
Purpura, Henoch-Schönlein— *see* Hypersensitivity Vasculitis, 1081·3
Purpura, Idiopathic Thrombocytopenic— *see* Idiopathic Thrombocytopenic Purpura, 1082·1
Purpura, Thrombotic Thrombocytopenic— *see* Thrombotic Microangiopathies, 758·1
Purpuralin, 2246·4
Purpuric Dermatosis, Pigmented— *see* Non-infective Skin Disorders, 401·2
Pur-Rutin, 2246·4
Pursana, 2246·4
Pursenid, 2247·1
Pursennid, 2247·1
Pursennid Complex, 2247·1
Pursennid Fibra, 2247·1
Pursennide, 2247·1
Pursennid-In, 2247·1
Pursept A, 2247·1
Puru-C, 2247·1
Pusiran, 2247·1
Putaren, 2247·1
Putatone, 2247·1
PUVA, 1153·1
Puvadin, 2247·1
Puvasoralen, 2247·1
PV Carpine, 2247·1
PVA, 2247·1
P-vate, 2247·1
PVF, 2247·1
PVFK, 2247·1
P-Vidine, 2247·1
PVK, 2247·1
PVP, 1581·2
PVPI, 2247·1
PVP-Iodine, 1190·3
P-V-Tussin, 2247·1
Pyal, 2247·1
Pycnogenol Plus, 2247·1
Pydrin, 1505·2
Pyelodion, 2247·1
Pyelonephritis— *see* Urinary-tract Infections, 153·1
Pygeum Africanum, 1568·2
*Pygeum africanum*, 1568·2
Pygeum Africanum Bark, 1568·2
Pygeum Bark, 1568·2
Pygmal, 2247·1
Pygno-Vite, Bioglan— *see* Bioglan Pygno-Vite, 1844·1
Pygosal, 2247·1
Pykaryl T, 2247·2
Pykno, 2247·2
Pylobactel, 2247·2
Pylobactell, 2247·2
Pylori 13, 2247·2
Pylori Chek, 2247·2
Pylorid, 2247·2
Pylorid-KA, 2247·2
Pyloripac, 2247·2
Pyloriset, 2247·2
Pylorisin, 2247·2
Pynamic, 2247·2
Pynclear, 2247·2
Pynmed, 2247·2
Pynstop, 2247·2
Pyocefal, 2247·2
Pyocoline, 2247·2
Pyoctaninum Caeruleum, 1186·1
Pyoderma Gangrenosum, 1138·2
Pyoderma, Superficial Granulomatous— *see* Pyoderma Gangrenosum, 1138·2
Pyodontyl, 2247·2
Pyolysin, 2247·2
Pyoralene, 2247·2
Pyoredol, 2247·2
Pyorex, 2247·2
Pyostacine, 2247·2
Pyraclofos, 1509·2
Pyracon, 2247·2
Pyradol, 2247·2
Pyrafat, 2247·2
Pyralfin, 2247·2
Pyralin, 2247·3
Pyralvex, 2247·3
Pyranisamine Hydrochloride, 437·1
Pyranisamine Maleate, 437·1
Pyranol, 2247·3
Pyrantel Embonate, 113·2
Pyrantel Pamoate, 113·2
Pyranteli Embonas, 113·2
Pyrantin, 2247·3
Pyrantrin, 2247·3
Pyrapam, 2247·3
Pyratab, 2247·3
Pyrazide, 2247·3
Pyrazinamide, 246·3
Pyrazinamidum, 246·3
Pyrazine-2-carboxamide, 246·3
Pyrazinoic Acid, 247·3
Pyrazinoic Acid Amide, 246·3
1*H*-Pyrazolo[3,4-*d*]pyrimidine-4-thiol, 418·2
1*H*-Pyrazolo[3,4-*d*]pyrimidin-4-ol, 412·2
Pyrbuterol Acetate, 790·3
Pyrbuterol Hydrochloride, 790·3
Pyrcon, 2247·3
Pyreazid, 2247·3
Pyrecol, 2247·3
Pyreflor, 2247·3

Pyretal, 2247·3
Pyrethri Flos, 1509·3
Pyrethric Acid, 1509·3
Pyrethrins, 1509·3
Pyrethroid Insecticides, 1509·3
Pyrethrum Extract, 1509·3
Pyrethrum Flower, 1509·3
Pyrethrum Spray, 2247·3
Pyrexia— *see* Fever and Hyperthermia, 8·2
Pyrexon, 2247·3
Pyribenzamine, 2247·3
Pyricarbate, 1737·1
Pyricontin, 2247·3
Pyridiate, 2247·3
4-Pyridinamine, 1491·2
2-Pyridine Aldoxime Methochloride, 1050·1
Pyridine-3-carboxamide, 1441·2
Pyridine-3-carboxylic Acid, 1441·1
2,6-Pyridinediyldimethylene Bis(methylcarbamate), 1737·1
2,6-Pyridinediyldimethylene Bis(3,4,5-trimethoxybenzoate), 984·1
3-Pyridinemethanol, 966·1
(7*R*)-3-(1-Pyridiniomethyl)-7-[(2-thienyl)acetamido]-3-cephem-4-carboxylate, 168·3
Pyridinolcarbamate, 1737·1
Pyridium, 2247·3
Pyridium Plus, 2247·3
Pyridofylline, 791·2
Pyridophylline, 791·2
Pyridostig. Brom., 1496·1
Pyridostigmine Bromide, 1496·1
Pyridostigmini Bromidum, 1496·1
Pyridoxal Phosphate, 1456·3
Pyridoxal 5-Phosphate, 1456·3
Pyridoxamine Dihydrochloride, 1456·3
Pyridoxamine Hydrochloride, 1456·3
4-Pyridoxic Acid, 1457·1
Pyridoxine Citrate, 1457·2
Pyridoxine $\alpha_5$-Hemiacetal Glyoxylate, 1732·3
Pyridoxine Hydrochloride, 1456·3
Pyridoxine Oxoglurate, 1457·2
Pyridoxine L-5-Oxopyrrolidine-2-carboxylate, 1456·3
Pyridoxine Phosphate, 1457·2
Pyridoxine Phosphoserinate, 1457·2
Pyridoxine Pidolate, 1456·3, 1457·2
Pyridoxine *O*-(Theophyllin-7-ylethyl)sulphate, 791·2
Pyridoxini Hydrochloridum, 1456·3
Pyridoxinii Chloridum, 1456·3
Pyridoxinium Chloride, 1456·3
Pyridoxol Hydrochloride, 1456·3
Pyridoxylate, 1732·3
β-Pyridylcarbinol, 966·1
3-Pyridylmethanol, 966·1
3-Pyridylmethanol Hydrogen (2*R*,3*R*)-Tartrate, 966·2
3-Pyridylmethyl 2-(4-Chlorophenoxy)-2-methylpropionate Hydrochloride, 965·3
4,4′-(2-Pyridylmethylene)di(phenyl Acetate), 1251·3
$N^1$-(2-Pyridyl)sulphanilamide, 263·3
Pyrifin, 2247·3
Pyrifoam, 2247·3
Pyrigesic, 2247·3
Pyril, 2247·3
Pyrilamine Hydrochloride, 437·1
Pyrilamine Maleate, 437·1
Pyrilax, 2247·3
Pyrimel, 2247·3
Pyrimethamine, 458·1
Pyrimethaminum, 458·1
1-(2-Pyrimidinyl)-piperazine, 673·1
8-[4-(4-Pyrimidin-2-ylpiperazin-1-yl)butyl]-8-azaspiro[4.5]decane-7,9-dione Hydrochloride, 672·2
2-[4-(4-Pyrimidin-2-ylpiperazin-1-yl)butyl]-1,2-benzothiazol-3(2*H*)-one 1,1-Dioxide Hydrochloride, 703·1
(1R*,2S*,3R*,4S*)-*N*-{4-[4-(2-Pyrimidinyl)-1-piperazinyl]butyl}-2,3-norbornanedicarboximide Citrate, 723·2
$N^1$-(Pyrimidin-2-yl)sulphanilamide, 258·2
Pyrimon, 2247·3
Pyrinex, 2247·3
Pyrinyl II, 2247·3
Pyrinyl Plus, 2247·4
Pyriped, 2247·4
Pyriproxyfen, 1509·3
Pyrisept, 2247·4
Pyrisuccideanol Maleate, 1732·3
Pyrithione Magnesium, 1156·2
Pyrithione Zinc, 1156·2
Pyrithioxine Hydrochloride, 1737·2
Pyrithyldione, 718·1
Pyritil, 2247·4
Pyritinol Hydrochloride, 1737·2
Pyrocaps, 2247·4
Pyrodifenium Bromide, 488·2
Pyrogallic, 2247·4
Pyrogallic Acid, 1156·2
Pyrogallol, 1156·2
Pyrogastrone, 2247·4
Pyrogenium, 2247·4
L-Pyroglutamyl-L-histidyl-L-prolinamide, 1337·3
Pyroleum Betulae, 1159·2
Pyroleum Juniperi, 1159·2
Pyroleum Lithanthracis, 1159·2
Pyroleum Oxycedri, 1159·2
Pyroleum Pini, 1159·3
Pyromed, 2247·4
Pyron, 2247·4
Pyronaridine Phosphate, 460·1
Pyrophosphate, Technetium ($^{99m}$Tc), 1526·1
Pyroxin, 2247·4
Pyroxy, 2247·4
Pyroxylin, 1156·2
Pyroxylinum, 1156·2
Pyr-Pam, 2247·4
Pyrrolamidol, 28·2
L-Pyrrolidine-2-carboxylic Acid, 1443·2
Pyrrolidine-2,5-dione, 1750·2
Pyrrolidinomethyltetracycline, 254·1
1-(Pyrrolidin-1-ylcarbonylmethyl)-4-(3,4,5-trimethoxycinnamoyl)piperazine Hydrogen Maleate, 884·2
$N^2$-(Pyrrolidin-1-ylmethyl)tetracycline, 254·1
(*E*)-2-[3-(Pyrrolidin-1-yl)-1-*p*-tolylprop-1-enyl]pyridine Hydrochloride Monohydrate, 442·3
(*E*)-3-{6-[(*E*)-3-Pyrrolidin-1-yl-1-*p*-tolylprop-1-enyl]-2-pyridyl}acrylic Acid, 423·3
Pyrrolidone Acetamide, 1732·1
Pyrrolizidine Alkaloids, 1743·1
Pyrrolnitrin, 408·1
Pyrroxate, Extra Strength— *see* Extra Strength Pyrroxate, 1986·2
Pyrvin, 2247·4
Pyrvinium Embonate, 113·3
Pyrvinium Pamoate, 113·3
Pytazen, 2247·4
Pytest, 2247·4
Pyverm, 2247·4
Pyzin, 2247·4
PZ-51, 1683·2
PZ-68, 979·2
PZ-1511, 674·2
PZ-17105, 1735·3
PZA, 2247·4
PZA-Ciba, 2247·4
P-Zide, 2247·4


## Q


Q, 1433·2
Q 10, 2247·4
Q-35, 162·2
Q200, 2247·4
Q300, 2247·4
Q Fever, 143·3
Q Fever Vaccines, 1635·3
Q-Age, 2247·4
Qari, 2247·4
Qat, 1585·2
QDALL, 2247·4
QED, 2247·4
QED A-150, 2247·4
Qiftrin, 2248·1
Qinghaosu, 447·2
Qinolon, 2248·1
QM-6008, 671·3
QM Integratore, 2248·1
QT, 2248·1
Q-Tech, 2248·1
QTest, 2248·1
QTest Ovulation, 2248·1
Quackgrass, 1676·2
Quadblock, 2248·1
Quadezyme, 2248·1
Quadion, 2248·1
Quadracel, 2248·1
Quadracel— *see* Pentacel, 2211·1
Quadra-Hist D, 2248·1
Quadramet, 2248·1
Quadrasa, 2248·1
Quadratic Acid Dibutylester, 1158·1
Quadrax, 2248·1
Quadriderm, 2248·1
Quadriderm CD, 2248·1
Quadriderm NF, 2248·1
Quadriderme, 2248·1
Quadrikin, 2248·1
Quadrilon, 2248·1
Quadrinal, 2248·1
Quadriplus, 2248·1
Quadronal ASS Comp, 2248·1
Quadronal Comp, 2248·1
Quadropril, 2248·1
Quagu-Test, 2248·1
Quait, 2248·2
Qual, 2248·2
Qualecon, 2248·2
Qualiton, 2248·2
Quam, 2248·2
Quamatel, 2248·2
Quanil, 2248·2
Quantaffirm, 2248·2
Quantalan, 2248·2
Quantor, 2248·2
Quardin, 2248·2
Quarelin, 2248·2
Quark, 2248·2
Quartamon Med, 2248·2
Quarzan, 2248·2
Quasar, 2248·2
Quassia, 1737·2
*Quassia amara*, 1737·2
Quassia, Jamaica, 1737·2
Quassia, Surinam, 1737·2
Quassia Wood, 1737·2
Quassiae Lignum, 1737·2
Quassiaholz, 1737·2
Quassin, 1737·2
Quaternary Ammonium Compounds, 1172·3
Quaternium-15, 1176·3
Quaternium 18-Bentonite, 1143·1
Quatohex, 2248·2
Quatro-Soda, 2248·2
Quatro-Virelon, 2248·2
Quazepam, 718·2
Quazium, 2248·2
Québrachine, Chlorhydrate de, 1766·2
Quecksilber, 1713·1
Quecksilberchlorid, 1712·3
Quecksilberchlorür, 1712·3
Quecksilberoxyd, Gelbes, 1712·3
Queen Anne's Lace, 1765·1
Queen Bee Jelly, 1740·3
Queen of the Meadow, 1695·3
Queen of the Meadows, 1710·1
Quefeno, 2248·2
Quelacid, 2248·2
Quelicin, 2248·2
Quelidrine, 2248·2
Quellada Preparations, 2248·2
Quelodin, 2248·3
Quelodin F, 2248·3
Quem Plus, 2248·3
Quemicetina, 2248·3
Quemicetina con Hidrocortisona, 2248·3
Quemox, 2248·3
Quenobilan, 2248·3
Quenocol, 2248·3
Quenodeoxicólico, Ácido, 1670·1
Quenopodio Vermifuga, Esencia de, 103·3
Quensyl, 2248·3
Quentakehl, 2248·3
Queratil, 2248·3
Queratinasa, 1703·3
Quercetin, 1688·2
Quercetina, 1688·2
Quercetol Hemostatico, 2248·3
Quercetol K, 2248·3
Quercitannic Acid, 1723·1
Quercus, 1722·3
Quercus Cortex, 1722·3
*Quercus infectoria*, 1690·2, 1751·2
*Quercus petraea*, 1723·1
*Quercus pubescens*, 1723·1
*Quercus robur*, 1723·1
Queroseno, 1475·1
Querto, 2248·3
Query Fever— *see* Q Fever, 143·3
Quest Gamma Oil, 2248·3
Questran, 2248·3
Quetiapina, Fumarato de, 718·2
Quetiapine Fumarate, 718·2
Quetidin, 2248·3
Quetzal, 2248·3
Qugyl, 2248·3
Quiacort, 2248·3
Quiacort G, 2248·3
Quiacort G Plus, 2248·3
Quibron, 2248·4
Quibron-T, 2248·4
Quick N Easy, 2248·4
Quick Pep, 2248·4
Quickcal, 2248·4
QuickCal, 2248·4
QuickCare, 2248·4
Quicklime, 1664·3
Quicksilver, 1713·1
QuickVue, 2248·4
Quiedorm, 2248·4
Quiens, 2248·4
Quies, 2248·4
Quiet Days, 2248·4
Quiet Life, 2248·4
Quiet Night, Heath & Heather— *see* Heath & Heather Quiet Night, 2037·3
Quiet Nite, 2248·4
Quiet Tyme, 2248·4
Quietan, 2248·4
Quietiline, 2248·4
Quietude, 2248·4
Quifenadine Hydrochloride, 440·3
Quiflox, 2248·4
Quifloxona, 2248·4
Quik, 2248·4
Quilagen, 2248·4
Qui-Lea, 2248·4
Quilla Simplex, 2248·4
Quillaia, 1416·1
Quillaia Bark, 1416·1
Quillaiae Cortex, 1416·1
Quillaiasapotoxin, 1416·1
Quillaic Acid, 1416·1
*Quillaja saponaria*, 1416·1
Quillay, 1416·1
Quilonorm, 2248·4
Quilonum, 2248·4
Quimalan, 2248·4
Quimefuran, 2248·4
Quimio-Ped, 2248·4
Quimio-Ped Balsamico, 2249·1
Quimobrom, 2249·1
Quimocyclar, 2249·1
Quimodril, 2249·1
Quimolactona, 2249·1
Quimolauril, 2249·1
Quimopapaina, 1671·1
Quimosporina, 2249·1
Quimotrase, 2249·1
Quimotrip, 2249·1
Quimotripsina, 1671·2
Quimpe Amida, 2249·1
Quimpe Antibiotico, 2249·1
Quimpe Vitamin, 2249·1
Quimpedor, 2249·1

Quina, 1671·3
Quina Vermelha, 1671·3
Quinaband, 2249·1
Quinacrine Hydrochloride, 606·3
Quinaglute, 2249·1
Quinagolida, Hidrocloruro de, 1213·1
Quinagolide Hydrochloride, 1213·1
Quinalan, 2249·1
Quinalbarbitone, 721·2
Quinalbarbitone Sodium, 721·2
Quinalbital, 937·3
Quinapril, Hidrocloruro de, 991·1
Quinapril Hydrochloride, 991·1
Quinaprilat, 991·1
Quinate, 2249·1
Quinax, 2249·1
Quinazide, 2249·1
Quinazil, 2249·1
Quinbisul, 2249·1
Quindoleina, 2249·1
Quinestradiol, 1568·2
Quinestradol, 1568·2
Quinestrol, 1568·2
Quinetazona, 991·2
Quinethazone, 991·2
Quineuron, 2249·1
Quinfamex, 2249·1
Quinfamide, 615·2
Quingamine, 448·2
Quini, 2249·1
Quinicardina, 2249·1
Quinicardine, 2249·1
Quinicine Hydrochloride, 1764·3
Quinidex, 2249·1
Quinidina, 991·3
Quinidina, Bisulfato de, 991·3
Quinidina, Gluconato de, 991·3
Quinidina, Poligalacturonato de, 991·3
Quinidina, Sulfato de, 991·3
Quinidine, 991·3
Quinidine Bisulfate, 991·3
Quinidine Bisulphate, 991·3
Quinidine Gluconate, 991·3
Quinidine Polygalacturonate, 991·3
Quinidine Poly(D-galacturonate) Hydrate, 991·3
Quinidine Sulfate, 991·3
Quinidine Sulphate, 991·3
Quinidini Sulfas, 991·3
Quinidinium Gluconate, 991·3
Quiniduran, 2249·1
Quinidurule, 2249·1
Quinimax, 2249·2
Quinina, 460·1
Quinina, Ascorbato de, 1737·2
Quinina, Bisulfato de, 460·1
Quinina, Dihidrocloruro de, 460·1
Quinina, Etilcarbonato de, 460·1
Quinina, Hidrobromuro de, 460·2
Quinina, Hidrocloruro de, 460·2
Quinina, Sulfato de, 460·2
Quinina y Urea, Hidrocloruro de, 1737·2
Quinine, 460·1
Quinine Acid Hydrochloride, 460·1
Quinine Acid Sulphate, 460·1
Quinine, Anhydrous, 460·1
Quinine Ascorbate, 1737·2
Quinine Benzoate, 462·3
Quinine Biascorbate, 1737·2
Quinine Bisulfate, 460·1
Quinine Bisulphate, 460·1
Quinine Camsilate, 462·2
Quinine Dihydrochloride, 460·1
Quinine Dihydrochloride, Carbamidated, 1737·2
Quinine Etabonate, 460·1
Quinine Ethyl Carbonate, 460·1
Quinine Formate, 462·2
Quinine Gluconate, 462·2
Quinine Hydrobromide, 460·2
Quinine Hydrobromide, Basic, 460·2
Quinine Hydrochloride, 460·2
Quinine Hydrochloride, Basic, 460·2
Quinine Hydrochloride, Neutral, 460·1
Quinine Monohydrobromide, 460·2
Quinine Monohydrochloride, 460·2
Quinine Sulfate, 460·2
Quinine Sulphate, 460·2
Quinine Sulphate, Basic, 460·2
Quinine Sulphate, Neutral, 460·1
Quinine and Urea Hydrochloride, 1737·2
Quininga, 2249·2
Quinini Bisulfas, 460·1
Quinini Dihydrochloridum, 460·1
Quinini Hydrochloridum, 460·2
Quinini Sulfas, 460·2
Quiniodochlor, 196·3
Quinisedine, 2249·2
Quinisocaína, Hidrocloruro de, 1384·2
Quinisocaine Hydrochloride, 1384·2
Quinivax-in, 2249·2
Quino, Corteza del, 1671·3
Quinobact, 2249·2
Quinobarb, 2249·2
Quinobiot, 2249·2
Quinoc, 2249·2
Quinocarbine, 2249·2
Quinocort, 2249·2
Quinoctal, 2249·2
Quinoderm, 2249·2
Quinoderm Antibacterial Face Wash, 2249·2
Quinoderm-H, 2249·2
Quinodermil, 2249·2
Quinodermil-AS, 2249·2
Quinodis, 2249·2
Quinoflex, 2249·2
Quinoflox, 2249·2
Quinoform, 2249·2
Quinoforme, 2249·2
Quinol, 1148·1
Quinoline Yellow, 1057·3
8-Quinolinol Benzoate (Ester), 1170·2
Quinolin-8-ol Sulfate, 1734·2
8-Quinolinol Sulphate, 1700·1
Quinolin-8-ol Sulphate, 1700·1
Quinolonecarboxylic Acids, 119·1
Quinolones, 119·1
4-Quinolones, 119·1
Quinolylindanedione Sulfonic Acid, Sodium Salt, 1057·3
Quinomed, 2249·2
Quinoped, 2249·2
Quinophthalone Sulfonic Acid, Sodium Salt, 1057·3
Quinora, 2249·2
Quinoret, 2249·2
Quinortar, 2249·2
Quinox, 2249·3
$N^1$-(Quinoxalin-2-yl)sulphanilamide, 263·3
Quinoxan, 2249·3
Quinquina, 1671·3
Quinquina Rouge, 1671·3
Quinradon, 2249·3
Quinradon-N, 2249·3
Quinsana Plus, 2249·3
Quinsul, 2249·3
Quintabs, 2249·3
Quintasa, 2249·3
Quintelmin, 2249·3
Quintex, 2249·3
Quintex Pediatrique, 2249·3
Quintonine, 2249·3
Quintopan, 2249·3
Quintopan Enfant, 2249·3
3-Quinuclidinyl Acetate Hydrochloride, 1487·1
10-(Quinuclidin-3-ylmethyl)phenothiazine, 437·2
Quinupramina, 316·3
Quinupramine, 316·3
Quinupristin, 248·1
Quinupristin Mesilate, 248·2
Quinupristin Mesylate, 248·2
Quinupristina, Mesilato de, 248·2
Quinupristina/dalfopristina, 248·1
Quinupristin/Dalfopristin, 248·1
Quipro, 2249·3
Quiralam, 2249·3
Quirgel, 2249·3
Quiss, 2249·3
Quit, 2249·3
Quitadrill, 2249·3
Quitaxon, 2249·3
Quitoso, 2249·3
QuitX, 2249·3
Quixil, 2249·3
Quixin, 2249·3
Quocel, 2249·3
Quocin, 2249·3
Quoderm, 2249·3
Quomem, 2249·3
Quool, 2249·4
Quosten, 2249·4
Quotal NF, 2249·4
Quotane, 2249·4
Quotivit O.E., 2249·4
Qura, 2249·4
QV, 2249·4
QV Flare Up, 2249·4
QV Lip Balm, 2249·4
Qvar, 2249·4
Q-Vax, 2249·4
QZ-2, 707·1

## R

R, 1421·1
R-2, 698·3
R-13-615, 1557·1
R-54, 573·2
R-75, 946·1
R-100, 1653·2
R-148, 707·1
R-516, 428·3
R-661, 480·2
R-720-11, 1588·2
R-738, 66·2
R-798, 791·3
R-802, 214·2
R-805, 67·1
R-812, 1108·1
R-818, 916·2
R-837, 638·1
R-848, 652·1
R-1132, 1261·3
R-1406, 83·2
R-1569, 1757·1
R-1575, 428·3
R-1625, 701·2
R-1658, 710·1
R-1929, 671·2
R-2028, 698·2
R-2113, 1096·3
R-2167, 698·2
R-2323, 1556·2
R-2453, 1547·2
R-2498, 727·1
R-3345, 716·1
R-3365, 84·1
R-3763, 178·3
R-3827, 1319·1
R-4263, 40·1
R-4318, 43·2
R-4584, 671·2
R-4749, 697·2
R-4845, 21·2
R-5020, 1568·1
R-6218, 701·1
R-6238, 715·1
R-7904, 946·3
R-8299, 114·1
R-11333, 672·1
R-12564, 107·2
R-13423, 205·2
R-13672, 701·3
R-14827, 397·2
R-14889, 405·3
R-14950, 434·1
R-15403, 1261·2
R-15454, 401·3
R-15889, 947·2
R-16341, 713·2
R-16470, 481·1
R-16659, 1299·1
R-17635, 108·2
R-17889, 105·2
R-18134, 405·2
R-18553, 1271·1
R-23979, 397·3
R-25061, 93·1
R-25831, 603·1
R-26490, 1299·1
R-28096, 603·1
R-30730, 90·2
R-31520, 104·1
R-33799, 25·1
R-33800, 90·2
R-33812, 1263·2
R-34828, 104·1
R-35443, 438·1
R-39209, 12·2
R-39500, 407·3
R-41400, 403·3
R-41468, 943·1
R-42470, 409·3
R-43512, 424·2
R-46541, 672·1
R-49945, 943·1
R-50547, 435·2
R-51211, 401·3
R-51619, 1259·2
R-55667, 721·1
R-58425, 1271·1
R-58735, 1741·2
R-62690, 603·1
R-64433, 603·2
R-64766, 719·2
R-65824, 964·3
R-66905, 408·1
R-67555, 964·3
R-83842, 594·3
R-87926, 950·2
R & C, 2249·4
R Calm, 2249·4
R Calm + B6, 2249·4
RA-8, 903·1
RA Lotion, 2249·4
RA Morph, 2249·4
Rábano Rusticano, 1697·3
Rabarbaro, 1287·3
Rabarbaroni, 2249·4
RabAvert, 2249·4
Rabec, 2249·4
Rabeloc, 2249·4
Rabeprazol Sódico, 1285·1
Rabeprazole Sodium, 1285·1
Rabies, 1636·2
Rabies Antisera, 1635·3
Rabies Gamma, 2249·4
Rabies Immune Globulin, 1635·3
Rabies Immunoglobulin, Human, 1635·3
Rabies Immunoglobulins, 1635·3
Rabies Vaccine, 1635·3, 1636·1
Rabies Vaccine for Human Use Prepared in Cell Cultures, 1635·3
Rabies Vaccines, 1635·3
Rabies-Imovax, 2249·4
Rabigam, 2249·4
Rabipor, 2249·4
Rabipur, 2249·4
Rabivac, 2249·4
Rablas, 2249·4
Raboldo, 2249·4
Rabro, 2250·1
Rabro N, 2250·1
Rabugen, 2250·1
Rabuman, 2250·1
Rab/Vac, 1636·1
Racecadotril, 1285·2
Racecadotrilo, 1285·2
Racementhol, 1711·3
Racemethionine, 1042·1
Racemetirosine, 956·1
Racemic Adrenaline, 854·2
Racemic Calcium Pantothenate, 1443·1
Racephedrine Hydrochloride, 1120·1, 1120·3
Racephenicol, 269·2
Racepinefrine, 852·2, 854·2
Racepinefrine Hydrochloride, 852·2, 854·2
Racepinephrine, 852·2
Racepinephrine Hydrochloride, 852·2
Racestyptin, 2250·1
Racestyptine, 2250·1

Racetam, 2250·1
Racine de Bugrane, 1723·3
Racine de Primevére, 1735·1
Ra-Cliss, 2250·1
Raclioprida, 719·2
Raclopride, 719·2
Raclopride ($^{11}$C), 1523·1
Racovel, 2250·1
RAD-001, 1360·1
Radacef, 2250·1
Radalgin, 2250·1
Radan, 2250·1
Radanil, 2250·1
Radecol, 2250·1
Radedorm, 2250·1
Radenarcon, 2250·1
Radepur, 2250·1
RadiaGel, 2250·1
Radialar 280, 2250·1
Radian, 2250·1
Radian-B, 2250·1
Radian-B Ibuprofen, 2250·1
Radian-B Red Oils, 2250·2
Radiation Protection, 1599·3
*Radicula armoracia*, 1697·3
Radicura, 2250·2
Radicut, 2250·2
Radigen, 2250·2
Radikal, 2250·2
Radilem, 2250·2
Radin, 2250·2
Radina, 2250·2
Radina Dex, 2250·2
Radine, 2250·2
Radio Salil, 2250·2
Radioactive Metals, Poisoning, 1050·1
Radioced, 2250·2
Radiogardase, 2250·2
Radiogardase-Cs, 2250·2
Radiological Terms, 1522·3
Radiomiron, 2250·2
Radionuclide Generators, 1522·2
Radionuclides, 1522·1
Radiopaque, 2250·2
Radiopharmaceuticals, 1522·1
Radioselectan, 2250·2
Radiotherapy-induced Nausea and Vomiting— *see* Nausea and Vomiting, 1245·2
Radix Aconiti, 1646·3
Radix Notoginseng, 1693·1
Radix Ononidis, 1723·3
Radix Scutellariae, 1746·3
Radol, 2250·2
Rado-Salil, 2250·2
Rado-Spray, 2250·2
Raductil, 2250·2
Radyn, 2250·2
Rafacalcin, 2250·2
Rafapen V-K, 2250·2
Rafapen Mega, 2250·2
Rafassal, 2250·2
Rafathricin, 2250·2
Rafathricin with Benzocaine, 2250·2
Rafazocine, 2250·2
Rafazocine X, 2250·3
Rafe, 1666·1
Rafen, 2250·3
Raffo-Ca, 2250·3
Raffolutil, 2250·3
Raffonin, 2250·3
Raffreddoremed, 2250·3
Rafi, 1666·1
Rafo, 1666·1
Rafocilina, 2250·3
Rafoxanida, 114·1
Rafoxanide, 114·1
Raftace, 2250·3
Raft-Eze, 2250·3
Rafton, 2250·3
Rafuzone, 2250·3
Ragaden, 2250·3
Rage— *see* Disturbed Behaviour, 665·1
Ragonil, 2250·3
Ragwort, 1743·1
Raikocef, 2250·3
Raised Intracranial Pressure, 833·1
Raíz de Eupatorio, 1695·3
Raiz de Genciana, 1692·2
Raíz de Harpagofito, 28·2
Raíz de Polígala, 1130·2
Raiz de Regaliz, 1270·2
Ralcidin, 2250·3
Ralgex Preparations, 2250·3
Ralgex, Ibutop— *see* Ibutop Ralgex, 2055·1
Ralicid, 2250·3
Ralinet, 2250·3
Ralodantin, 2250·3
Ralofekt, 2250·3
Ralogaine, 2250·3
Ralopar, 2250·3
Ralovera, 2250·3
Ralovera, Depo- — *see* Depo-Ralovera, 1925·4
Raloxifene Hydrochloride, 1568·3
Raloxifeno, Hidrocloruro de, 1568·3
Ralozam, 2250·3
Ralsifen-X, 2250·3
Raltitrexed, 582·1
Ralur, 2250·4
Ramace, 2250·4
Ramavit, 2250·4
Ramend, 2250·4
Ramend Krauter, 2250·4
Ramet Cade, 2250·4
Ramet Dalibour, 2250·4
Ramet Pain, 2250·4
Ramfin, 2250·4
Rami Slijmoplossende, 2250·4
Rami-Dextromethorphan, 2250·4
Ramidox, 2250·4
Ramifenazona, 86·1
Ramifenazone, 86·1
Ramifenazone Hydrochloride, 86·1
Ramifenazone Salicylate, 86·1
Ramipres, 2250·4
Ramipril, 994·1
Ramiprilat, 994·1
Ramiprilum, 994·1
Ramistos, 2250·4
Ramivan, 2250·4
Ramno Fix, 2250·4
Ramno-Flor, 2250·4
Ramnosa, 1738·1
Ramol, 2250·4
Ramoplanin, 249·1
Ramoplanina, 249·1
Ramosetrón, Hidrocloruro de, 1285·2
Ramosetron Hydrochloride, 1285·2
Ramp, 2250·4
Rampicin, 2250·4
Ramses, 2250·4
Ramulus Uncariae Cum Uncis, 1668·3
Ramysis, 2250·4
Ran, 2250·4
Ran H2, 2250·4
Ran Lich, 2250·4
Ranacid, 2250·4
Ranamp, 2250·4
Ranceph, 2250·4
Rancil, 2250·4
Ranclav, 2251·1
Ranclosil, 2251·1
Randex, 2251·1
Randoclin, 2251·1
Randum, 2251·1
Ranepal, 2251·1
Ranfen, 2251·1
Ranfradin, 2251·1
Rani, 2251·1
Rani 2, 2251·1
Raniben, 2251·1
Raniberl, 2251·1
Ranibeta, 2251·1
Ranibloc, 2251·1
Ranic, 2251·1
Ranicel, 2251·1
Ranicid, 2251·1
Raniclon, 2251·1
Ranicodan, 2251·1
Ranicur, 2251·1
Ranicux, 2251·1
Ranidil, 2251·1
Ranidin, 2251·1
Ranidina, 2251·1
Ranidine, 2251·2
Ranidura T, 2251·2
Ranifarma, 2251·2
Raniflex, 2251·2
Ranifur, 2251·2
Ranigyl, 2251·2
Ranihexal, 2251·2
Ranikur, 2251·2
Ranil, 2251·2
Ranilonga, 2251·2
Ranimed, 2251·2
Ranimerck, 2251·2
Ranimex, 2251·2
Ranimustina, 582·2
Ranimustine, 582·2
Rani-nerton, 2251·2
Raniplex, 2251·2
Raniprotect, 2251·2
Rani-Q, 2251·2
Ranisen, 2251·2
Ranisifar, 2251·2
Ranitak, 2251·2
Ranitax, 2251·2
Ranitic, 2251·2
Ranitidi GNO, 2251·2
Ranitidina, Hidrocloruro de, 1285·2
Ranitidine, 1285·2
Ranitidine Bismuth Citrate, 1287·2
Ranitidine Bismutrex, 1287·2
Ranitidine Hydrochloride, 1285·2, 1285·3
Ranitidini Hydrochloridum, 1285·2
Ranitidoc, 2251·2
Ranitil, 2251·2
Ranitine, 2251·3
Ranitinol, 2251·3
Ranition, 2251·3
Ranitral, 2251·3
Ranitrat, 2251·3
Ranitul, 2251·3
Ranityrol, 2251·3
Ranivel, 2251·3
Ranix, 2251·3
Ranixal, 2251·3
Ranmoxy, 2251·3
Ranolazina, Hidrocloruro de, 994·2
Ranolazine Hydrochloride, 994·2
Ranolta, 2251·3
Ranomustine, 582·2
Ranopine, 2251·3
Ranoprin, 2251·3
Ranoxyl, 2251·3
Ranozol, 2251·3
Ranpirnasa, 582·2
Ranpirnase, 582·2
Ranpuric, 2251·3
Rantac, 2251·3
Rantag, 2251·3
Rantec, 2251·3
Ranteen, 2251·3
Ranthrocin, 2251·3
Rantudal, 2251·3
Rantudil, 2251·3
Ranuber, 2251·3
Ranulin, 2251·4
*Ranunculus ficaria*, 1732·1
Ranvil, 2251·4
Ranvir, 2251·4
Ranxas, 2251·4
Ranzac, 2251·4
Ranzil, 2251·4
Ranzol, 2251·4
Rap, Creme— *see* Creme Rap, 1911·3
Rapacuronio, Bromuro de, 1405·2
Rapacuronium Bromide, 1405·2
Rapae, Oleum, 1737·3
Rapaid Preparations, 2251·4
Rapako Comp, 2251·4
Rapako Xylo, 2251·4
Rapamic, 2251·4
Rapamune, 2251·4
Rapamycin, 1363·1
Rape Oil, 1737·3
Rapeseed Oil, 1737·3
Rapeseed Oil, Refined, 1737·3
Rap-eze, 2251·4
Raphanus S Potier, 2251·4
Rapicort, 2251·4
Rapid Gel, 2251·4
Rapid Strand, 2251·4
Rapid-acting Insulins, 339·3
Rapidal, 2251·4
Rapidica, 2251·4
Rapidocaine, 2251·4
Rapidol, 2251·4
RapidVue, 2251·4
Rapifen, 2251·4
Rapignost Basic Screen Plus, 2251·4
Rapignost Diabetes Profile, 2251·4
Rapignost Total Screen LSG, 2252·1
Rapilax, 2252·1
Rapilax Fibras, 2252·1
Rapilin, 2252·1
Rapilysin, 2252·1
Rapimix, 2252·1
Rapi-snooze, 2252·1
Rapitard MC, 2252·1
Rapitil, 2252·1
Rapitux, 2252·1
Rapivir, 2252·1
Raplon, 2252·1
Rapolyte, 2252·1
Rappell, 2252·1
Raptiva, 2252·1
Rapura, 2252·1
Raquiferol, 2252·1
Rarical, 2252·1
Raricap, 2252·1
Raricap L, 2252·1
Rariplex, 2252·1
RAS, 2252·1
Rasal, 2252·1
Rasburicasa, 418·3
Rasburicase, 418·3
Raset, 2252·1
Rashfree, 2252·1
Rasilvax, 2252·1
Raspberry, 1057·3
Raspberry Leaf, 1737·3
Raspberry Tea, 1737·3
Rastinon, 2252·1
Ratacand, 2252·1
Ratacand Plus, 2252·2
Ratanhiae Radix, 1738·1
Ratania, Raíz de, 1738·1
Rat-bite Fever— *see* Bites and Stings, 121·3
Rati Salil Preparations, 2252·2
Ratic, 2252·2
Ratica, 2252·2
Raticina, 2252·2
RatioAllerg, 2252·2
RatioDolor, 2252·2
RatioGast, 2252·2
RatioGrippal + C, 2252·2
RatioHepar, 2252·2
RatioMobil, 2252·2
Rationale, 2252·2
Rationasal, 2252·2
Ratiopyrin, 2252·2
RatioSept, 2252·2
Rattlesnake Root, 1130·2
Raubasina, 994·3
Raubasine, 994·3
Raudil, 2252·2
Raudopen, 2252·2
Raufuncton N, 2252·2
Raunormine, 892·3
Rauserpin, 2252·2
Rauvolfia, 994·3
Rauwiplus, Diu— *see* Diu Rauwiplus, 1946·1
Rauwolfia, 994·3
*Rauwolfia canescens*, 892·3
Rauwolfia Serpentina, 994·3
*Rauwolfia serpentina*, 994·3, 995·2
Rauwolfia Vomitoria, 994·3
*Rauwolfia vomitoria*, 995·2
Rauwolfiae Radix, 994·3
RauwolfiaViscomp, 2252·2

Rauwolfiawurzel, 994·3
Rauwolfine, 856·1, 994·3
Rauwolfinine, 994·3
Rauwolsan H, 2252·2
Rauwoplant, 2252·2
Rauzide, 2252·3
Ravalgen, 2252·3
Ravalton, 2252·3
Ravamil, 2252·3
Ravenol, 2252·3
Raveron, 2252·3
Ravigona, 2252·3
Ravocaine and Novocain, 2252·3
Ravotril, 2252·3
Raw Opium, 74·2
Raw Prostate, 2252·3
Raxamida, 2252·3
Raxedin, 2252·3
Raxeto, 2252·3
Ray Block, 2252·3
Raycept, 2252·3
Rayepen, 2252·3
Rayetetra, 2252·3
Raynaud's Disease— *see* Raynaud's Syndrome, 833·3
Raynaud's Phenomenon— *see* Raynaud's Syndrome, 833·3
Raynaud's Syndrome, 833·3
Rayne, 2252·3
Rayvist, 2252·3
Rayvist 180, 2252·3
Razagleda Plus, 2252·3
Razene, 2252·3
Razoxane, 582·2
Razoxano, 582·2
1489-RB, 243·1
RB-1509, 565·2
1532-RB, 231·3
1589-RB, 241·3
1609RB, 580·1
RBC, 2252·3
RBPI-21, 1658·3
RC-61-91, 938·1
RC-160, 1342·2
RC-172, 1141·2
RC-173, 1141·2
R-Cetate, 2252·3
RCF, 2252·3
R-Cin, 2252·3
R-Cinex, 2252·3
R-Cinex Z, 2252·3
RD-13621, 45·3
RD-20000, 1096·3
R-Den, 2252·4
Reabilan, 2252·4
Reacel-A, 2252·4
Reach Junior Fluoride, 2252·4
Reactine, 2252·4
Reactine Plus, 2252·4
Reactivan, 2252·4
Reactive Arthritis— *see* Bone and Joint Infections, 122·1
Reactive Arthritis— *see* Spondyloarthropathies, 11·1
Reactive Depression, 278·1
Reafix, 2252·4
Reagin, 2252·4
Reagin Vascular, 2252·4
Real Lemon Cold Powders, 2252·4
Realderm, 2252·4
Realdiet, 2252·4
Realdrax, 2252·4
Real-Vit, 2252·4
Reanima, 2252·4
Reapam, 2252·4
Reasec, 2252·4
Re-Azo, 2252·4
Rebacil, 2252·4
ReBalance, 2252·4
Rebamipida, 1287·3
Rebamipide, 1287·3
Rebaten, 2252·4
Rebaudin, 1449·3
Rebaudioside A, 1449·3
Rebetol, 2252·4
Rebetol— *see* Intron A/Rebetol, 2064·3
Rebetol— *see* Pegatron, 2209·4
Rebetol— *see* Rebetron, 2252·4
Rebetron, 2252·4
Rebif, 2252·4
Rebladerm, 2252·4
Rebone, 2253·1
Re-BONE, 2253·1
Rebound Headache— *see* Analgesic-induced Headache, 464·1
Reboxetina, Mesilato de, 316·3
Reboxetine Mesilate, 316·3
Reboxetine Mesylate, 316·3
Rec-7-0040, 482·2
Rec-7/0267, 1587·2
Rec-15/0691, 1756·2
Rec-15/1476, 397·3
Rec-15-2375, 946·1
Reca, 2253·1
Recaflex, 2253·1
Recal, 2253·1
Recalfe, 2253·1
Recalplex, 2253·1
Recamicina, 2253·1
Recanescine, 892·3
Recarcin, 2253·1
Recatol Algin, 2253·1
Recatol Mono, 2253·1
Recatol N, 2253·1
Receant, 2253·1
Recef, 2253·1
Receptozine, 2253·1
Recessan, 2253·1
RechLH, 1332·2
Recilugo, 2253·1
Recipect, 2253·1
Recital, 2253·1
Reclomide, 2253·1
Reclor, 2253·1
Rececef, 2253·1
Recofen, 2253·1
Recofen-D, 2253·1
Recofol, 2253·1
Recombinant H-B Vax II, 2253·1
Recombinant Human Single-Chain Urokinase-type Plasminogen Activator, 996·3
Recombinant Interleukin-2, 562·3
Recombinant Macrophage-targeted β-Glucocerebrosidase, 1649·2
Recombinant Tissue-type Plasminogen Activator, 857·1
Recombinate, 2253·1
Recombivax HB, 2253·1
Recomvax B, 2253·2
Reconvan, 2253·2
Recormon, 2253·2
Recormon— *see* NeoRecormon, 2159·4
Recort Plus, 2253·2
Recoveron, 2253·2
Recoveron N, 2253·2
Recoveron NC, 2253·2
Recovery Food, 2253·2
Recozil, 2253·2
Recrea, 2253·2
Rectacaine, 2253·2
Rectagene Medicated Balm, 2253·2
Rectagene Medicated Rectal Balm, 2253·2
Rectal Cancer— *see* Malignant Neoplasms of the Gastrointestinal Tract, 516·2
Rectalad, 2253·2
Rectamigdol, 2253·2
Rectanus, 2253·2
Rectified Spirit, 1166·1
Rectified Turpentine Oil, 1760·1
Rectinol, 2253·2
Rectinol HC, 2253·2
Rectiole, 2253·2
Recto Bronco Tosse, 2253·2
Recto Menaderm, 2253·2
Recto Menaderm NF, 2253·2
Rectocort, 2253·2
Rectodelt, 2253·2
Rectogel, 2253·2
Rectogel HC, 2253·2
Rectogesic, 2253·2
Rectolax Kits— *see* X-Prep Bowel Evacuant Kits, 2388·4
Rectopanbiline, 2253·2
Rectophedrol, 2253·3
Rectoplexil, 2253·3
Rectopred, 2253·3
Rectopulmo Adultos, 2253·3
Rectopulmo Infantil, 2253·3
Rectoquintyl, 2253·3
Rectoquintyl-Promethazine, 2253·3
Rectoquotane, 2253·3
Recto-Reparil, 2253·3
Rectosan, 2253·3
Rectosellan, 2253·3
Rectosellan H, 2253·3
Rectoseptal-Neo Preparations, 2253·3
Rectovalone, 2253·3
Rectovasol, 2253·3
Rectozorin, 2253·3
Recugel, 2253·3
Recupex, 2253·3
Recurrent Polyserositis— *see* Familial Mediterranean Fever, 416·2
Recvalysat, 2253·3
Recycline, 2253·3
Red A, Cochineal, 1057·3
Red AC, Allura, 1056·1
Red 1, Acid, 1058·1
Red Aniline, 1185·1
Red Away, 2253·3
Red 10B, 1058·1
Red Blood Cells, 759·3
Red Cherry, 1058·1
Red Chloride, Neutral, 1719·3
Red Cinchona Bark, 1671·3
Red Clover, 1737·3
Red, Congo, 1675·3
Red Cross Toothache, 2253·3
Red Flower Oil, 59·3
Red 2G, 1058·1
Red Ginseng, 1693·1
Red Kooga Preparations, 2253·4
Red, Neutral, 1719·3
Red, Nuclear Fast, 1719·3
Red Off, 2253·4
Red Off Plus, 2253·4
Red Oil, 2253·4
Red, Phenol, 1730·3
Red Point-Massagecreme, Biokosma— *see* Biokosma Red Point-Massagecreme, 1844·3
Red Poppy Petals, 1058·1
Red Puccoon, 1741·3
Red Rose Petals, 1058·1
Red, Scarlet, 1191·3
Red Seal Liquid Calcium, 2253·4
Red Seaweeds, 1578·2
Red Squill, 1509·3
Red, Toluylene, 1719·3
Red Whortleberry, 1676·3
Redac, 2253·4
Redacid, 2253·4
Redactiv, 2253·4
Redaflam, 2253·4
Redalip, 2253·4
Redap, 2253·4
Redaxa Fit, 2253·4
Redaxa Lax, 2253·4
Redentil, 2253·4
Redeptin, 2253·4
Redergin, 2253·4
Redergot, 2253·4
Rediarin, 2253·4
Redicres Rapido, 2253·4
Redimune, 2253·4
Redipred, 2253·4
Redisol, 2253·4
Redken Solve Acid Balance, 2253·4
Redol, 2253·4
Redol Comp, 2253·4
Redolet, 2253·4
Redomex, 2253·4
ReDormin, 2254·1
Redotex NF, 2254·1
Redotrin, 2254·1
Redox-Injektopas, 2254·1
Redoxon Preparations, 2254·1
Red-Poppy Petal, 1058·1
Redrate, 2254·1
Redrocin, 2254·1
Red-Rose Petal, 1058·1
Reducap, 2254·1
Reducealin, 2254·1
Reduced DPN, 1719·1
Reduced Haloperidol, 702·1
Reducelle, 2254·1
Reducin, 2254·1
Reducin-A, 2254·1
Reducing Agents, 1164·2
Reducol, 2254·1
Reductel, 2254·1
Reducterol, 2254·1
Reductil, 2254·1
Reducto, 2254·2
Reducto-special, 2254·2
Reducto-spezial, 2254·2
Redudiet, 2254·2
Redufen, 2254·2
Redulip, 2254·2
Redupon, 2254·2
Redupres, 2254·2
Redupress, 2254·2
Reduprost, 2254·2
Redurate, 2254·2
Redusa, 2254·2
Redusan, 2254·2
Redusan Plus, 2254·2
Reduscar, 2254·2
Redusterol, 2254·2
Redutemp, 2254·2
Reduten, 2254·2
Redutensil, 2254·2
Reduterm, 2254·2
Redutona, 2254·2
Reduvit, 2254·2
Re-Dux, 2254·2
Reduxade, 2254·2
Reduxpain, 2254·2
Redvit, 2254·2
Reedvit, 2254·2
Reef Preparations, 2254·2
Reemplazante Gastri Mein, 2254·3
Reemplazante Intesti, 2254·3
Reese's Pinworm, 2254·3
ReFacto, 2254·3
Refenax Preparations, 2254·3
Refenesen, 2254·3
Refenesen Plus, 2254·3
Refesan T, 2254·3
Refex, 2254·3
Refined Arachis Oil, 1656·1
Refined Oil, 1763·3
Refined Olive Oil, 1723·2
Refined Sesame Oil, 1743·3
Refined Sugar, 1450·1
Refined Wool Fat, 1483·1
Reflax, 2254·3
Reflex, 2254·3
Reflex Anoxic Seizures— *see* Anoxic Seizures, 478·2
Reflex Sympathetic Dystrophy— *see* Complex Regional Pain Syndrome, 5·3
Reflexan, 2254·3
Reflexgel, 2254·3
Reflexspray, 2254·3
Reflin, 2254·3
Reflocheck, 2254·3
Reflor, 2254·3
Reflotron, 2254·3
Refludan, 2254·3
Refludin, 2254·4
Reflux, 2254·4
Reflux Oesophagitis— *see* Gastro-oesophageal Reflux Disease, 1242·3
Refluxin, 2254·4
Refluxine, 2254·4
Refobacin, 2254·4
Refobacin-Palacos R, 2254·4
Refolinon, 2254·4
Reforce, 2254·4
Reforgan, 2254·4
Refortrix, 2254·4
Refotax, 2254·4
Refrane Bronce, 2254·4

Refrane Gel, 2254·4
Refresh Preparations, 2254·4
Refrianex, 2254·4
Refrianex Compuesto, 2254·4
Refrigerant 11, 1236·1
Refrigerant 12, 1236·1
Refrigerant 22, 1236·1
Refrigerant 114, 1235·3
Refrigerant 134A, 1236·2
Refrigerant 152A, 1236·2
Refrigerant 142B, 1236·1
Refrigerants, 1235·1
Reftax, 2254·4
Refulgin, 2255·1
Refusal, 2255·1
Regadrin B, 2255·1
Regain, 2255·1
Regaine, 2255·1
Regaine— *see* Rogaine, 2269·1
Regal, 2255·1
Regalil, 2255·1
Regalisa, 2255·1
Regaliz, 1270·2
Regaliz Americano, 1645·1
Regaliz, Raiz de, 1270·2
Regamint, 2255·1
Regard, 2255·1
Regasinum Preparations 2255·1
Regavasal N, 2255·1
Regelan, 2255·1
Regelan N, 2255·1
Regena-Haut G, 2255·1
Regena-Haut W, 2255·1
Regenaplex Preparations, 2255·1
Regender, 2255·1
Regeneresen, 2255·1
Regenerin, 2255·1
Regenesis, 2255·1
Regenom, 2255·1
Regenon, 2255·1
Regental, 2255·1
Regepar, 2255·1
Regepithel, 2255·1
Regibloc, 2255·2
Regina Royal Concorde, 2255·2
Regina Royal Five, 2255·2
Regina Royal One Hundred, 2255·2
Regiocaina, 2255·2
Regional Nerve Block, 1370·1
Regitin, 2255·2
Regitina, 2255·2
Regitine, 2255·2
Regla PH, 2255·2
Regla PH Forte, 2255·2
Reglan, 2255·2
ReglaPh, 2255·2
Reglosedyl, 2255·2
Reglovar, 2255·2
Reglumax, 2255·2
Reglusan, 2255·2
Regolact Plus, 2255·2
Regolpause, 2255·2
Regomed, 2255·2
Regonol, 2255·2
Regran, 2255·2
Regranex, 2255·2
Regro, 2255·2
Regroton, 2255·3
Regrowth, 2255·3
Regubil, 2255·3
Regucal, 2255·3
Regucal D, 2255·3
Regucel, 2255·3
Regudig, 2255·3
Regufer, 2255·3
Regulacid, 2255·3
Regulacor-POS, 2255·3
Regulact, 2255·3
Regulador Blumen, 2255·3
Regulador Gesteira, 2255·3
Regulador Xavier N-1, 2255·3
Regulador Xavier N-2, 2255·3
Regulan, 2255·3
Regulane, 2255·3
Regulane AF, 2255·3
Regular Iletin I, 2255·3
Regular Iletin II, 2255·3
Regular Insulin, 334·2
Regular Strength Bayer, 2255·3
Regular Strength Cold Daytime Relief, 2255·3
Regular Strength Cold Nighttime Relief, 2255·3
Regular Strength Sinus, 2255·3
Regulaten, 2255·3
Regulax, 2255·3
Regulax N, 2255·3
Regulax Picosulfat, 2255·3
Regulax SS, 2255·3
Reguletts, 2255·3
Regulex, 2255·3
Regulex-D, 2255·4
Regulim, 2255·4
Regulin, 2255·4
Regulip, 2255·4
Reguloid, 2255·4
Regulose, 2255·4
Regulton, 2255·4
Regunon, 2255·4
Regurin, 2255·4
Rehalyt, 2255·4
Rehidrat, 2255·4
Rehsal, 2255·4
Rehydralyte, 2255·4
Rehydration Therapy, Oral, 1222·3
Rehydrex Med Glucos, 2255·4
Rehydrex Med Glucose, 2255·4
Reidramax, 2255·4
Reidrax, 2255·4
Reina de los Prados, 1710·1
Reine des Prés, 1710·1
Reise Superpep-K, 2255·4
Reisedragee Eu Rho, 2255·4
Reisegold, 2255·4
Reisetabletten, 2255·4
Reisevit, 2255·4
Reiter's Syndrome— *see* Bone and Joint Infections, 122·1
Reiter's Syndrome— *see* Spondyloarthropathies, 11·1
Rejuva, 2255·4
Rejuva-A, 2256·1
Rejuvesol, 2256·1
Rekamide, 2256·1
Rekasitin, 2256·1
Rekawan, 2256·1
Rekiv, 2256·1
Rekod, 2256·1
Rekont, 2256·1
Rekord B12, 2256·1
Rekord Ferro, 2256·1
Relacon-DM, 2256·1
Relacon-HC, 2256·1
Relact, 2256·1
Relafen, 2256·1
Relaflex, 2256·1
Relampago, 2256·1
Relapamil, 2256·1
Relapsing Fever, 143·3
Relapsing Polychondritis— *see* Polychondritis, 1086·1
Relar, 2256·1
Relasan, 2256·1
Relaten, 2256·1
Relatene, 2256·1
Relatrac, 2256·1
Relavit Fosforo, 2256·1
Relax, 2256·1
Relax B$^{+}$, 2256·1
Relax and Sleep, 2256·1
Relaxan, 2256·1
Relaxaplex, 2256·1
Relaxar, 2256·1
Relaxa-Tabs, 2256·2
Relaxedans, 2256·2
Relaxibys, 2256·2
Relaxil, 2256·2
Relaxin, 1737·3
Relaxina, 1737·3
Relaxine, 2256·2
Relaxin-P, 2256·2
Relaxit, 2256·2
Relaxoddi, 2256·2
Relaxophen, 2256·2
Relaxyl, 2256·2
Relaxyl Plus, 2256·2
Relazepam, 2256·2
Relcofen, 2256·2
Releaf for PMS, 2256·2
Release, 2256·2
Relefact, 2256·2
Relefact LH-RH, 2256·2
Relefact TRH, 2256·2
Relefact TRH— *see* Thyrel-TRH, 2330·4
Relenza, 2256·2
Relepax, 2256·2
Relert, 2256·2
Reless, 2256·2
Relestat, 2256·3
Relexic, 2256·3
Relexil, 2256·3
Reliberan, 2256·3
Relief, 2256·3
Relief Rub, 2256·3
Relief-Coff, 2256·3
Reliev, 2256·3
Reliev 76%, 2256·3
Relievol Allergy Sinus, 2256·3
Relievol PMS, 2256·3
Relievol Sinus, 2256·3
Relif, 2256·3
Relifen, 2256·3
Relifex, 2256·3
Relisan, 2256·3
Reliser, 2256·3
Relisorm, 2256·3
Relisorm L, 2256·3
Relitone, 2256·3
Reliv, 2256·3
Reliveran, 2256·3
Relivora Komplex, 2256·3
Relmus, 2256·3
Relmus Compositum, 2256·3
Relomycin, 274·3
Reloxyl, 2256·3
Reloxyl Mucolitico, 2256·4
Relpax, 2256·4
Relvene, 2256·4
Relyomycin, 2256·4
Relyovix, 2256·4
Rem, 2256·4
Remacemida, Hidrocloruro de, 377·2
Remacemide Hydrochloride, 377·2
Remafen, 2256·4
Remdue, 2256·4
Remedacen, 2256·4
Remedeine, 2256·4
Remederm, 2256·4
Remederm HC, 2256·4
Remedium Nervinum N EKF, 2256·4
Remedium Sinutale N EKF, 2256·4
Remedol, 2256·4
Remeflin, 2256·4
Remegel, 2256·4
Remegel Wind Relief, 2256·4
Remen, 2256·4
Remena, 2256·4
Remens, 2256·4
Remergil, 2256·4
Remergon, 2256·4
Remeron, 2256·4
Remestan, 2256·4
Remethan, 2256·4
Remexal, 2256·4
Remicade, 2256·4
Remicaine, 2257·1
Remicard, 2257·1
Remid, 2257·1
Remiderm, 2257·1
Remidol, 2257·1
Remifemin, 2257·1
Remifemin Plus, 2257·1
Remifentanil Hydrochloride, 86·1
Remifentanilo, Hidrocloruro de, 86·1
*Remijia pedunculata*, 991·3
Remikin, 2257·1
Remikiren, 994·3
Remikireno, 994·3
Reminyl, 2257·1
Remiprostan Uno, 2257·1
Remisan, 2257·1
Remisan Mucolitico, 2257·1
Remisol, 2257·1
Remisol-PLS, 2257·1
Remitex, 2257·1
Remitex D, 2257·1
Remnant Hyperlipoproteinaemia— *see* Hyperlipidaemias, 823·1
Remnant Particle Disease— *see* Hyperlipidaemias, 823·1
Remnos, 2257·1
Remodil, 2257·1
Remodulin, 2257·1
Remontal, 2257·1
Remoplexe, 2257·1
Remotil, 2257·1
Remotiv, 2257·1
Remotive, 2257·1
Remotrox, 2257·1
Remov, 2257·1
Remove, 2257·2
Remular-S, 2257·2
Remy, 2257·2
Remycin, 2257·2
Remydrial, 2257·2
Ren Hematocis, 2257·2
Rena, 2257·2
Renacalcio, 2257·2
Renacidin, 2257·2
Renacor, 2257·2
Renagel, 2257·2
Renal Calculi, 936·2
Renal Cancer— *see* Malignant Neoplasms of the Kidney, 518·1
Renal Caps, 2257·2
Renal Care, 2257·2
Renal Colic— *see* Biliary and Renal Colic, 4·3
Renal Disease, End-stage— *see* Chronic Renal Failure, 1222·1
Renal Disease, Hypertension in— *see* Hypertension, 825·1
Renal Failure, Acute— *see* Acute Renal Failure, 1221·3
Renal Failure, Chronic— *see* Chronic Renal Failure, 1222·1
Renal Failure, Chronic, Dietary Modification in— *see* Renal Failure, 1418·1
Renal, Natusor— *see* Natusor Renal, 2154·1
Renal Osteodystrophy, 764·3
Renalapril, 2257·2
Renal-cell Carcinoma— *see* Malignant Neoplasms of the Kidney, 518·1
Renalin, 1183·1
Renal-Vit, 2257·2
Renamel, 2257·2
RenAmin, 2257·2
Renapur, 2257·2
Renase, 2257·2
Renaton, 2257·2
Rena-Vite, 2257·2
Renax, 2257·2
Renbiocid, 2257·2
Rencef, 2257·2
Rendell, Pessarios Profilaticos— *see* Pessarios Profilaticos Rendell, 2215·2
Rendells, 2257·2
Rendells Plus, 2257·2
Renedil, 2257·2
Re/Neph, 2257·2
Renese, 2257·3
Renese R, 2257·3
Reneuron, 2257·3
Reneuu Invisible Glove, 2257·3
RenewTrient, 1308·3
Renezide, 2257·3
Renidur, 2257·3
Renilon, 2257·3
Renio 186, 1525·1
Renipress, 2257·3
Renipril, 2257·3
Renipril Plus, 2257·3
Renistad, 2257·3
Renitec, 2257·3

Renitec Comp, 2257·3
Renitec Plus, 2257·3
Renitecmax, 2257·3
Reniten, 2257·3
Reniten Plus, 2257·3
Rennie Preparations, 2257·3
Rennie, Antacidum— *see* Antacidum Rennie, 1802·3
Rennie, Digestif— *see also* Digestif Rennie, 1939·1
Rennie, Digestive— *see* Digestive Rennie, 1939·1
Rennie, Digestivo— *see* Digestivo Rennie, 1939·1
Renob Blasen- und Nierentee, 2257·4
Renocil, 2257·4
Renocis, 2257·4
Renoclear, 2257·4
Renofundina, 2257·4
Renografin, 2257·4
Renolip, 2257·4
Reno-M, 2257·4
Renopen, 2257·4
Renorell, 2257·4
Renormax, 2257·4
Renotol, 2257·4
Renova, 2257·4
Renovascular Hypertension— *see* Hypertension, 825·1
Renovator, 2257·4
Renpress, 2257·4
Renshen, 1693·1
Rentamine Pediatric, 2257·4
Rentibloc, 2257·4
Rentylin, 2257·4
Renu, 2257·4
ReNu, Bausch & Lomb— *see* Bausch & Lomb ReNu, 1829·3
Renu Enzymatic Cleaner, 2257·4
Renu Multiplus, 2257·4
Renu Plus, 2257·4
Ren-Ur, 2257·4
Renusor, 2257·4
Renutrin, 2257·4
Renutryl, 2257·4
Renutryl 500, 2258·1
Renzaprida, 1287·3
Renzapride, 1287·3
Reocol, 2258·1
Reodyn, 2258·1
Reoferol, 2258·1
Reoflus, 2258·1
Reolase, 2258·1
Reomax, 2258·1
Reomucil, 2258·1
ReoPro, 2258·1
Reotan, 2258·1
Repaglinida, 344·3
Repaglinide, 344·3
Repalyte, 2258·1
Repan, 2258·1
Repan CF, 2258·1
Reparcillin, 2258·1
Reparex, 2258·1
Reparil, 2258·1
Reparil N, 2258·1
Reparil-Gel N, 2258·1
Repariven, 2258·1
Repasma, 2258·1
RepaVen, 2258·1
Rep-Cartil, 2258·1
Repelente Rep, 2258·1
Repelex, 2258·2
Repellents, Insect, 1499·1
Repeltin, 2258·2
Repentil, 2258·2
Reperfusion and Revascularisation Procedures, 834·1
Repertaxin L-Lysine, 1363·1
Repervit, 2258·2
Repevax, 2258·2
Repha Orphon, 2258·2
Rephacimin, 2258·2
Rephacratin, 2258·2
Rephahyval, 2258·2
Rephalgin, 2258·2
Rephalysin C, 2258·2
Repha-Os, 2258·2
Rephaprossan, 2258·2
Rephastasan, 2258·2
Rephastasan, Meli— *see* Meli Rephastasan, 2122·1
Rephenyl, 2258·2
Repilysin, 2258·2
Repirinast, 791·2
Repisan, 2258·2
Repivate, 2258·2
Replagal, 2258·2
Replasyn, 2258·2
Replavit, 2258·2
Replavite, 2258·2
Replena, 2258·2
Replena— *see* Suplena, 2313·4
Replenate, 2258·2
Replenine, 2258·2
Replenine VF, 2258·2
Replens, 2258·2
Replete, 2258·2
Replicare, 2258·2
Repligen, 2258·2
Repogen, 2258·2
Repogen Ciclo, 2258·3
Repogen Conti, 2258·3
Reposans, 2258·3
Reposo-Mono, 2258·3
Reposton, 2258·3
Repotin, 2258·3
Repovit, 2258·3
Repowine Mono, 2258·3
Repowinon, 2258·3
Repriadol, 2258·3
Repronex, 2258·3
Reprost, 2258·3
Reproterol, Hidrocloruro de, 791·2
Reproterol Hydrochloride, 791·2
Reproven N, 2258·3
Reptilase, 2258·3
Repursan, 2258·3
Repursan M, 2258·3
Repursan ST, 2258·3
Requiesan, 2258·3
Requip, 2258·3
Res Vin, 2258·3
Resaid, 2258·3
Resakal, 2258·3
Resalt, 2258·3
Resaltex, 2258·3
Resan Mucolitico, 2258·3
Resan Retard, 2258·3
Resata, 2258·3
Rescaps-D SR, 2258·4
Rescinamina, 994·3
Rescinnamine, 994·3
Rescold, 2258·4
Rescon Preparations, 2258·4
Rescriptor, 2258·4
RescueFlow, 2258·4
Rescuesol, 2258·4
Rescula, 2258·4
Rescuvolin, 2258·4
Resdan, 2258·4
Resectal, 2258·4
Resectisol, 2258·4
Reser, 2258·4
Reseril, 2258·4
Reserpic Acid, 994·3
Reserpina, 995·1, 2258·4
Reserpine, 994·3, 995·1
Reserpinum, 995·1
Reset, 2258·4
Resfenol, 2258·4
Resfin, 2258·4
Resfolin, 2258·4
Resfrialgina, 2258·4
Resfry, 2259·1
Resfry Infantil, 2259·1
Resical, 2259·1
Residex P55, 2259·1
Resilar, 2259·1
Resimatil, 2259·1
Resin, 1675·1
Resina Carbolica Dentilin, 2259·1
Resina de Guayaco, 1696·2
Resina de Ipomoea, 1267·3
Resina de Jalapa, 1268·3
Resina Pini, 1675·1
Resina Terebinthinae, 1675·1
Resincalcio, 2259·1
Resincolestiramina, 2259·1
Resinol, 2259·1
Resinsodio, 2259·1
Resiquimod, 652·1
Resistan, 2259·1
Resisten Retard, 2259·1
Resivit, 2259·1
Resma, 2259·1
Resmethrin, 1509·3
Resmetrina, 1509·3
Resnedal, 2259·1
Resochin, 2259·1
Resochina, 2259·1
Resochine, 2259·1
Resodermil, 2259·1
Resoferon, 2259·1
Resol, 2259·1
Resolution, 2259·1
Resolutivo Regium, 2259·1
Resolve, 2259·2
Resolve Extra, 2259·2
Resolve Plus, 2259·2
Resolve Thrush, 2259·2
Resolve/GP, 2259·2
Resonium, 2259·2
Resonium A, 2259·2
Resonium Calcium, 2259·2
Resorbane, 2259·2
Resorborina, 2259·2
Resorcin, 1156·3
Resorcin Acetate, 1156·3
Resorcinol, 1156·3
Resorcinol Monoacetate, 1156·3
Resorcinol, Monoacetato de, 1156·3
Resorcinolphthalein Sodium, 1689·1
Resorcinolum, 1156·3
Resostyl, 2259·2
Resource Preparations, 2259·2
Resovist, 2259·2
Respa-1st, 2259·3
Respa-ARM, 2259·2
Respacal, 2259·2
Respa-DM, 2259·3
Respa-GF, 2259·3
Respahist, 2259·3
Respaire, 2259·3
Respalis, 2259·3
Respalor, 2259·3
Respatona Decongestant Formula, 2259·3
Respatona Plus Bronchial Cough Relief, 2259·3
Respax, 2259·3
Respbid, 2259·3
Respexil, 2259·3
Respibien, 2259·3
Respibron, 2259·3
Respicilin, 2259·3
Respicort, 2259·3
Respicur, 2259·3
RespiGam, 2259·3
Respilene, 2259·3
Respimex, 2259·3
Respimox, 2259·3
Respinol, 2259·3
Respinol Compound, 2259·3
Respir, 2259·3
Respir Balsamico, 2259·4
Respiral, 2259·4
Respiratory Distress Syndrome, Acute— *see* Acute Respiratory Distress Syndrome, 1075·2
Respiratory Distress Syndrome, Neonatal— *see* Neonatal Respiratory Distress Syndrome, 1084·2
Respiratory Failure, 1237·3
Respiratory Syncytial Virus Immunoglobulins, 1637·2
Respiratory Syncytial Virus Infection, 625·1
Respiratory Syncytial Virus Vaccines, 1637·2
Respiratory-tract Infections, Bacterial— *see* Respiratory-tract Infections, 144·1
Respiratory-tract Infections, Fungal— *see* Respiratory-tract Infections, 390·1
Respiret, 2259·4
Respiro, 2259·4
Respirol, 2259·4
Respiroma, 2259·4
Respisniffers, 2259·4
Respitol, 2259·4
Resplant, 2259·4
Respocort, 2259·4
Respolin, 2259·4
Responsar, 2259·4
Respontin, 2259·4
Resprax, 2259·4
Respreve, 2259·4
Resprim, 2259·4
Resprin, 2259·4
Restal, 2259·4
Restameth-SR, 2259·4
Restandol, 2259·4
Restasis, 2259·4
Restaslim, 2259·4
Restaurene, 2259·4
Restavit, 2259·4
Resteclin, 2259·4
Restenil, 2259·4
Restex, 2260·1
Restful, 2260·1
Restharrow Root, 1723·3
Restin, 2260·1
Restless Legs Syndrome— *see* Parasomnias, 667·3
Restlessness— *see* Disturbed Behaviour, 665·1
Restol, 2260·1
Restopon, 2260·1
Restorativ Glucosamine Muscle and Joint, 2260·1
Restore, 2260·1
Restoril, 2260·1
Restovar, 2260·1
Restrical, 2260·1
Restructa Forte ST, 2260·1
Restwel, 2260·1
Restylane, 2260·1
Resulax, 2260·1
Resulin, 2260·1
Resurmide, 2260·1
Resuscitation, Cardiopulmonary— *see* Advanced Cardiac Life Support, 812·2
Resvelife, 2260·1
Resyl, 2260·1
Resyl DM, 2260·1
Resyl mit Codein, 2260·1
Resyl Plus, 2260·1
Retabolin Forte, 2260·1
Retacillin Compositum, 2260·1
Retacnyl, 2260·1
Re-82-TAD-15, 528·3
Retafer, 2260·1
Retafyllin, 2260·1
Retalzem, 2260·1
Retama Negra, 1742·2
Retan, 2260·1
Ret-A-Pres, 2260·2
Retardent, 2260·2
Retardex, 2260·2
Retardin, 2260·2
Retarpen, 2260·2
Retarpen Balsamico, 2260·2
Retarpen Compositum, 2260·2
Retarpen Mucolitico, 2260·2
Retavase, 2260·2
Retavit, 2260·2
Retcin, 2260·2
Retebem, 2260·2
Retef, 2260·2
Retemic, 2260·2
Retens, 2260·2
Reteplasa, 995·2
Reteplase, 995·2
Reticulogen, 2260·2
Reticulogen Fortificado, 2260·2
Reticus, 2260·2

Retimax, 2260·2
Retin-A, 2260·2
Retinar, 2260·2
Retinitis Pigmentosa, 1454·2
Retinoblastoma, 524·2
Retinoic Acid, 1161·1
*all-trans*-Retinoic Acid, 1161·1
9-*cis*-Retinoic Acid, 526·2
13-*cis*-Retinoic Acid, 1148·3
Retinol, 1451·2, 2260·2
Retinol Acetate, 1451·2
Retinol Concentrate (Oily Form), Synthetic, 1451·3
Retinol Concentrate (Powder Form), Synthetic, 1451·3
Retinol Concentrate, Solubilisate/Emulsion, Synthetic, 1451·3
Retinol Palmitate, 1451·2
Retinol Propionate, 1451·2
Retinol-A, 2260·2
Retinopathy, Diabetic— *see* Diabetic Complications, 326·2
Retinopathy of Prematurity, 1466·1
Retinova, 2260·2
Retinovit, 2260·2
Retinyl Acetate, 1451·2
Retinyl Palmitate, 1451·2
Retinyl Propionate, 1451·2
Retirides, 2260·2
Retisdin, 2260·3
Retisol-A, 2260·3
Retitop, 2260·3
Retodol Compositum, 2260·3
Retofar, 2260·3
Retolen, 2260·3
Retoxil, 2260·3
ReTrieve, 2260·3
Retrocollis— *see* Spasmodic Torticollis, 1391·1
Retrolental Fibroplasia— *see* Retinopathy of Prematurity, 1466·1
Retrovir, 2260·3
Retrovir/3TC Post-HIV Exposure, 2260·3
Rettavate, 2260·3
Retterspitz Preparations, 2260·3
Reucam, 2260·3
Reudene, 2260·3
Reufel, 2260·3
Reufirron, 2260·3
Reuflodol, 2260·3
Reugast, 2260·3
Reugot, 2260·3
Reukamicin, 2260·3
Reumacid, 2260·3
Reumacort, 2260·3
Reumadil, 2260·4
Reumagel, 2260·4
Reumagil, 2260·4
Reumaless, 2260·4
Reumalex, Gerard House— *see* Gerard House Reumalex, 2022·1
Reumaren, 2260·4
Reumat, 2260·4
Reumatosil, 2260·4
Reumazine, 2260·4
Reumilase Plus, 2260·4
Reumin, 2260·4
Reumine, 2260·4
Reumix, 2260·4
Reumo, 2260·4
Reumol, 2260·4
Reumon, 2260·4
Reumophan, 2260·4
Reumoquin, 2260·4
Reumoxican, 2260·4
Reupax, 2260·4
Reuplex, 2260·4
Reuprofen, 2260·4
Reusan, 2260·4
Reusin, 2260·4
Reutaren, 2260·4
Reutenox, 2260·4
Reutricam, 2260·4
Reuxen, 2260·4
REV-6000A, 892·2
Revalid, 2260·4
Revange, 2261·1
Revanil, 2261·1
Revapol, 2261·1
Revasc, 2261·1
Revascularisation Procedures— *see* Reperfusion and Revascularisation Procedures, 834·1
Revastin, 2261·1
Revaton, 2261·1
Revaxis, 2261·1
Reve, 2261·1
Reveal, 2261·1
Revectina, 2261·1
Revelatest, 2261·1
Revellex, 2261·1
Revelplac, 2261·1
Revelplac 2001, 2261·1
Revenil, 2261·1
Revenil Dospan, 2261·1
Revenil Expectorante, 2261·1
Revenox, 2261·1
Reverin, 2261·1
Reversa, 2261·1
Reversa AHA HQ, 2261·1
Reversa UV, 2261·1
Reverse $T_3$, 1594·1
Reverse Tri-iodothyronine, 1594·1
Reversible Inhibitors of Monoamine Oxidase Type A, 278·2, 316·1
Reversol, 2261·1
Revex, 2261·1
Rev-Eyes, 2261·1
Revez, 2261·1
Revia, 2261·1
Revic, 2261·2
Revicain, 2261·2
Revicain Comp, 2261·2
Revicain Comp Plus, 2261·2
Revicon, 2261·2
Revil, 2261·2
Revimine, 2261·2
Revion, 2261·2
Reviparin Sodium, 995·3
Reviparina Sódica, 995·3
Revirax, 2261·2
Revit, 2261·2
Revital, 2261·2
Revitaleyes, 2261·2
Revitalizing, 2261·2
Revitalose, 2261·2
Revitalose C, 2261·2
Revitam, 2261·2
Revitan, 2261·2
Revitex, 2261·2
Revitonil, 2261·2
Revitonus C, 2261·2
Revitorgan Lp Nr 83— *see* NeyArthros-Liposome, 2165·4
Revitorgan-Dilutionen Nr 5— *see* NeyPsorin, 2166·2
Revitorgan-Dilutionen Nr 6— *see* NeyCorenar, 2166·1
Revitorgan-Dilutionen Nr 10— *see* NeyPulpin, 2166·2
Revitorgan-Dilutionen Nr 26— *see* NeyFegan, 2166·1
Revitorgan-Dilutionen Nr 43— *see* NeyArthros, 2165·4
Revitorgan-Dilutionen Nr 55— *see* NeyFaexan, 2166·1
Revitorgan-Dilutionen Nr 64— *see* NeyGeront, 2166·1
Revitorgan-Dilutionen Nr 65— *see* NeyNormin, 2166·1
Revitorgan-Dilutionen Nr 66— *see* NeyTumorin, 2166·2
Revitorgan-Dilutionen Nr 68— *see* NeyChondrin, 2166·1
Revitorgan-Dilutionen Nr 73— *see* NeyImmun, 2166·1
Revitorgan-Dilutionen Nr 78— *see* NeyDesib, 2166·1
Revitorgan-Dilutionen Nr 96— *see* NeyTroph, 2166·2
Revitorgan-Dilutionen Nr 97— *see* NeyDop, 2166·1
Revitorgan-Dilutionen Nr 98— *see* NeyCalm, 2166·1
Revitorgan-Dilutionen N Nr 10— *see* NeyPulpin N, 2166·2
Revitorgan-Dilutionen N Nr 64— *see* NeyGeront N, 2166·1
Revitorgan-Dilutionen N Nr 65— *see* NeyNormin N, 2166·1
Revitorgan-Dilutionen N Nr 66— *see* NeyTumorin N, 2166·2
Revitorgan-Dilutionen N Nr 68— *see* NeyChondrin N, 2166·1
Revitorgan-Dilutionen N Nr 97— *see* NeyDop N, 2166·1
Revitorgan-Lingual Nr 64— *see* NeyGeront, 2166·1
Revitorgan-Lingual Nr 65— *see* NeyNormin, 2166·2
Revitorgan-Lingual Nr 66— *see* NeyTumorin, 2166·2
Revitorgan-Lingual Nr 68— *see* NeyChondrin, 2166·1
Revitorgan-Lingual Nr 96— *see* NeyTroph, 2166·2
Revitorgan-Lingual Nr 97— *see* NeyDop, 2166·1
Revitorgan-Lingual Nr 98— *see* NeyCalm, 2166·1
Revivan, 2261·2
Revive, 2261·2
Revivon, 38·3
Revivona, 2261·2
Revixil, 2261·3
Revocon, 2261·3
Revolyt, 2261·3
Revulsan, 2261·3
Rewodina, 2261·3
Rex, 2261·3
Rexachlor, 2261·3
Rexacin, 2261·3
Rexalgan, 2261·3
Rexall Preparations, 2261·3
Rexamat, 2261·3
Rexan, 2261·3
Rexer, 2261·3
Rexgenta, 2261·3
Rexichlor, 2261·3
Rexigen Forte, 2261·3
Rexilen, 2261·3
Rexiluven S, 2261·3
Reximide, 2261·3
Rexitene, 2261·3
Rexitol, 2261·3
Rexivin, 2261·3
Rexolate, 2261·3
Rexophtal N, 2261·3
Rexort, 2261·3
Rexorubia, 2261·4
Reyataz, 2261·4
Reye's Syndrome, 16·2
Reynolds, 698·3
Rezamid, 2261·4
Rezamid D, 2261·4
Rezamid F— *see* Rezamid D, Rezamid F, Rezamid M, 2261·4
Rezamid M— *see* Rezamid D, Rezamid F, Rezamid M, 2261·4
Rezulin, 2261·4
Rezult, 2261·4
RFG-Kit, 2261·4
RFS-2000, 583·2
R-GCR, 1649·2
RG-CSF, 755·3
R-Gel, 2261·4
R-Gen, 2261·4
R-Gene, 2261·4
RGH-1106, 1405·2
RGH-2202, 1337·2
RGH-4405, 1764·2
RH-2267, 1541·3
$Rh_o$ (D) Immune Globulin, 1608·1
Rhabarber, 1287·3
Rhabarex B, 2261·4
Rhabdomyosarcoma— *see* Soft-tissue Sarcoma, 525·2
Rhamni Frangulae Cortex, 1266·3
Rhamni Purshianae Cortex, 1255·1
Rhamni Purshiani Cortex, 1255·1
3β-(α-L-Rhamnopyranosyloxy)-1β,5,11α,14,19-pentahydroxy-5β,14β-card-20(22)-enolide Octahydrate, 977·3
Rhamnose, 1738·1
L-Rhamnose, 1738·1
*Rhamnus cathartica*, 1254·1
*Rhamnus frangula*, 1266·3
*Rhamnus purshianus*, 1255·1
Rhapontic Rhubarb, 1287·3
Rhapontica, Chinese, 1287·3
Rhatany, Peruvian, 1738·1
Rhatany Root, 1738·1
RhBMP-2, 768·1
RhDNase, 1119·1
Rheaban Maximum Strength, 2261·4
Rhefluin, 2261·4
Rhei Radix, 1287·3
Rhei Rhizoma, 1287·3
Rheila Medicated Cough Drops, 2261·4
Rheila Stringiet N, 2261·4
Rhein, 30·2, 1288·1
Rhein Diacetate, 30·1
Rhem, 2261·4
Rhemofenax, 2261·4
Rhenium-186, 1525·1
Rhenium ($^{186}$Re) Etidronate, 1525·1
Rhenium Sulfide, Colloidal, Technetium ($^{99m}$Tc), 1525·3
Rhenus Med, 2261·4
Rheobral, 2261·4
Rheoflux, 2261·4
Rheofusin, 2261·4
Rheogen, 2261·4
Rheohes, 2261·4
Rheomacrodex, 2261·4
Rheotromb, 2261·4
Rhesogam, 2261·4
Rhesogamma, 2261·4
Rhesogamma P, 2262·1
Rhesonativ, 2262·1
Rhesugam, 2262·1
Rhesuman, 2262·1
Rhesus (D) Incompatibility— *see* Haemolytic Disease of the Newborn, 1608·2
Rheu, 2262·1
Rheubalmin Preparations, 2262·1
Rheucastin, 2262·1
Rheucostan M, 2262·1
Rheufenac, 2262·1
Rheuferm Phyto, 2262·1
Rheugesal, 2262·1
Rheugesic, 2262·1
Rheum, 1287·3, 1288·1
*Rheum coreanum*, 1288·1
*Rheum emodi*, 1287·3
*Rheum officinale*, 1288·1
*Rheum palmatum*, 1288·1
*Rheum rhaponticum*, 1287·3
*Rheum tanguticum*, 1288·1
*Rheum webbianum*, 1287·3
Rheuma, 2262·1
Rheuma Lindofluid, 2262·1
Rheuma Salbe, Kneipp— *see* Kneipp Rheuma Salbe, 2081·3
Rheuma V + T Bad N, 2262·1
RheumaASS, 2262·1
Rheuma-Bad, 2262·1
Rheuma-Bad, Kneipp— *see* Kneipp Rheuma-Bad, 2081·3
Rheumabene, 2262·1
Rheumacin, 2262·1
Rheumadoron, 2262·1
Rheumadyn PMD, 2262·2
Rheuma-Gastreu R46, 2262·2
Rheuma-Gel, 2262·2
Rheuma-Hek, 2262·2
Rheuma-Hevert, 2262·2
Rheumajecta, 2262·2
Rheumakaps, 2262·2
Rheumalan, 2262·2
Rheumaliment N, 2262·2
Rheuma-Liquidum, 2262·2
Rheuma-loges, 2262·2
Rheumamed AC, Gothaplast— *see* Gothaplast Rheumamed AC, 2030·2
Rheumanox, 2262·2
Rheuma-Pasc, 2262·2

Rheuma-Pasc N, 2262·2
Rheuma-Plantina, 2262·2
Rheumaplast N, 2262·2
Rheumasalbe, 2262·2
Rheuma-Salbe, 2262·2
Rheuma-Salbe N, 2262·2
Rheumasan, 2262·2
Rheumasan Moor-Bad S, 2262·2
Rheumasan N, 2262·2
Rheumaselect, 2262·2
Rheuma-Sern, 2262·2
Rheumasit, 2262·2
Rheumasol, 2262·2
Rheumatab Salicis, 2262·2
Rheumatabletten N, 2262·3
Rheumatac, 2262·3
Rheuma-Teufelskralle HarpagoMega, 2262·3
Rheumatex, 2262·3
Rheumatic Carditis— see Rheumatic Fever, 144·2
Rheumatic Diseases— see Soft-tissue Rheumatism, 11·1
Rheumatic Fever, 144·2
Rheumatic Heart Disease— see Rheumatic Fever, 144·2
Rheumatic Pain, 2262·3
Rheumatic Pain, Modern Herbals— see Modern Herbals Rheumatic Pain, 2138·2
Rheumatic Pain Relief, 2262·3
Rheumatic Pain Remedy, 2262·3
Rheumatic Pain Tablets, 2262·3
Rheumatica, 2262·3
Rheumatism, Desert— see Coccidioidomycosis, 387·3
Rheumatism, Muscular— see Soft-tissue Rheumatism, 11·1
Rheumatism, Palindromic— see Rheumatoid Arthritis, 9·3
Rheumatism Rhus Tox, 2262·3
Rheumatism, Soft-tissue— see Soft-tissue Rheumatism, 11·1
Rheumatisme— see Rhumatisme, 2263·4
Rheumatoid Arthritis, 9·3
Rheumatoid Arthritis Vaccine, 10·2
Rheumaton, 2262·3
Rheumatrex, 2262·3
Rheumatropfen N, 2262·3
Rheumavek, 2262·3
Rheumax, 2262·3
Rheumed, 2262·3
Rheumeda, 2262·3
Rheumesser, 2262·3
Rheumex, 2262·3
Rheumichthol Bad, 2262·3
Rheumitin, 2262·3
Rheumodoron 1, 2262·3
Rheumodoron 2, 2262·3
Rheumodoron 102 A, 2262·3
Rheumon, 2262·3
Rheumox, 2262·3
Rheunervol N, 2262·3
Rheutrop, 2262·3
Rhewlin, 2262·3
RhIGF-1, 1338·3
RhIGF-I/rhIGFBP-3, 1339·1
RhIL-1ra, 14·3
Rhinaaxia, 2262·4
Rhinadine, 2262·4
Rhinadvil, 2262·4
Rhinal, 2262·4
Rhinalar, 2262·4
Rhinall, 2262·4
Rhinallergy, 2262·4
Rhinamide, 2262·4
Rhinar, 2262·4
Rhinaris, 2262·4
Rhinaris Saline, 2262·4
Rhinatate, 2262·4
Rhinatate-NF, 2262·4
Rhinathiol Preparations, 2262·4
Rhinathiol Antitussivum— see Tusso Rhinathiol, 2353·1
Rhinathiol, Muco— see Muco Rhinathiol, 2142·4
Rhinathiol Mucolyticum— see Muco Rhinathiol, 2142·4
Rhinathiol, Tusso— see Tusso Rhinathiol, 2353·1
RhinATP, 2262·4
Rhinedrine, 2262·4
Rhinedrine Lubricant, 2262·4
Rhinedrine Moisturizing, 2262·4
Rhinex, 2262·4
Rhinidine, 2263·1
Rhinipan, 2263·1
Rhiniramine, 2263·1
Rhinirex, 2263·1
Rhinisan, 2263·1
Rhinitis, 422·3
Rhinitisan, 2263·1
Rhinivict, 2263·1
Rhinobeta, 2263·1
Rhinobiotal, 2263·1
Rhinocap, 2263·1
Rhinocaps, 2263·1
Rhinocillin B, 2263·1
Rhinoclir, 2263·1
Rhinocort, 2263·1
Rhinocortol, 2263·1
Rhinocure, 2263·1
Rhinocure Simplex, 2263·1
Rhinodex, 2263·1
Rhinodoron, 2263·1
Rhinodrin, 2263·1
Rhinofeb, 2263·1
Rhinofebral, 2263·2
Rhinofebryl, 2263·2
Rhinofluimucil, 2263·2
Rhino-Gastreu N R49, 2263·2
Rhinogen, 2263·2
Rhinoguttae Argenti Diacetylotannici Proteinici, 2263·2
Rhinoguttae Dexamethasoni cum Naphazolino, 2263·2
Rhinoguttae Pro Infantibus N, 2263·2
Rhinohist, 2263·2
Rhino-Lacteol, 2263·2
Rhinolar-EX, 2263·2
Rhinolast, 2263·2
Rhinolex, 2263·2
Rhinomer, 2263·2
Rhino-Mex, 2263·2
Rhino-Mex-N, 2263·2
Rhinon, 2263·2
Rhinoperd, 2263·2
Rhinoperd Comp, 2263·2
Rhinophen-C, 2263·2
Rhinophyma— see Rosacea, 1138·2
Rhinopront, 2263·2
Rhinopront Top, 2263·2
Rhinopten, 2263·3
Rhinosept, 2263·3
Rhinoside, 2263·3
Rhinosinusitis— see Sinusitis, 146·1
Rhinosol, 2263·3
Rhinosovil, 2263·3
Rhinospray, 2263·3
Rhinospray Antialergico, 2263·3
Rhinospray Atlantik, 2263·3
Rhinospray Plus, 2263·3
Rhino-stas, 2263·3
Rhinostop, 2263·3
Rhino-Sulfuryl, 2263·3
Rhinosyn, 2263·3
Rhinosyn-DM, 2263·3
Rhinosyn-DMX, 2263·3
Rhinosyn-X, 2263·3
Rhinothricinol, 2263·3
Rhinoton Plus, 2263·3
Rhinotrophyl, 2263·3
Rhinotussal, 2263·3
Rhinovac, 2263·3
Rhinovalon, 2263·3
Rhinovalon Neomycine, 2263·3
Rhinovent, 2263·3
Rhinovis, 2263·4
Rhinox, 2263·4
Rhinureflex, 2263·4
Rhinyl, 2263·4
Rhizoma Filicis Maris, 108·2
Rhizoma Panacis Japonica, 1693·1
Rhizoma Panacis Majoris, 1693·1
Rhodacine, 2263·4
Rhodamer, 2263·4
Rhodiaprox, 2263·4
Rhodine, 2263·4
Rhodis, 2263·4
Rhodogil, 2263·4
Rhodophyceae, 1578·2
Rhoead. Pet., 1058·1
Rhoeados Petalum, 1058·1
RhoGAM, 2263·4
Rhoival, 2263·4
Rho-kinase, 914·3
Rhonal, 2263·4
Rhonuracil, 2263·4
Rhophylac, 2263·4
Rhotral, 2263·4
Rhotrimine, 2263·4
Rhovail, 2263·4
Rhovane, 2263·4
RhTSH, 1341·1
Rhu GM-CSF, 760·1
Rhuaka, 2263·4
Rhubarb, 1287·3, 1288·1
Rhubarb, Chinese, 1287·3
Rhubarb, Garden, 1288·1
Rhubarb, Himalayan, 1287·3
Rhubarb, Indian, 1287·3
Rhubarb, Rhapontic, 1287·3
Rhubarb Rhizome, 1287·3
RhuIL-4R, 778·3
Rhuli Gel, 2263·4
Rhuli Spray, 2263·4
Rhum Creosotado, 2263·4
RhuMAb HER2, 589·3
RhuMab-E25, 790·1
Rhumagrip, 2263·4
Rhumalgan, 2263·4
Rhumanol, 2263·4
Rhumantin, 2263·4
Rhumatisme, 2263·4
Rhume, 2263·4
Rhus, 1738·1
*Rhus*, 1751·2
*Rhus aromatica*, 1738·1
*Rhus coriaria*, 1738·1
*Rhus glabra*, 1738·1
Rhus Med Complex, 2263·4
Rhus Opodeldoc, 2264·1
*Rhus radicans*, 1738·1
*Rhus toxicodendron*, 1738·1
Rhus Toxicodendron Oligoplex, 2264·1
Rhus-Rheuma-Gel N, 2264·1
Rhu-TNFR:Fc, 36·3
Rhythmocor, 2264·1
Rhythmy, 2264·1
Riabal, 2264·1
Riacen, 2264·1
Riamba, 1666·1
Riamet, 2264·1
Rib, 698·3
Rib. Nig., 1661·1
Ribastamin, 2264·1
Ribatra, 2264·1
Ribatran, 2264·1
Ribav, 2264·1
Ribavin, 2264·1
Ribavirin, 652·1
Ribavirina, 652·1
Ribavirinum, 652·1
Ribaviron C, 2264·1
Ribelfan, 2264·1
Ribes Nigrum, 1661·1
*Ribes nigrum*, 1661·1
Ribex, 2264·1
Ribex Flu, 2264·1
Ribex Nasale, 2264·1
Ribex Tosse, 2264·1
Ribexen con Espettorante, 2264·1
Ribocarbo, 2264·1
Ribociclina, 2264·1
Ribodoxo-L, 2264·1
Riboflavin, 1456·1
Riboflavin 5′-Phosphate Sodium, 1456·1
Riboflavin Sodium Phosphate, 1456·1
Riboflavin Tetrabutyrate, 1456·3
Riboflavina, 1456·1
Riboflavina, Fosfato Sódico de, 1456·1
Riboflavine, 1456·1
Riboflavine Phosphate, 1456·1
Riboflavine Phosphate, Sodium Salt, 1456·1
Riboflavine Sodium Phosphate, 1456·1
Riboflavini Natrii Phosphas, 1456·1
Riboflavinum, 1456·1
Ribofluor, 2264·1
Ribofolin, 2264·1
*N*-(9-β-D-Ribofuranosyl-9*H*-purin-6-yl)butyramide Cyclic 3′,5′-(Hydrogen Phosphate) 2′-Butyrate Sodium, 1663·2
1-β-D-Ribofuranosylpyrimidine-2,4(1*H*,3*H*)-dione, 1760·3
1-β-D-Ribofuranosyl-1*H*-1,2,4-triazole-3-carboxamide, 652·1
1-β-D-Ribofuranosyluracil, 1760·3
Ribolac, 2264·1
Ribomicin, 2264·1
Ribomunyl, 2264·1
Ribomustin, 2264·1
Ribon, 2264·1
Ribonucleasa, 1738·1
Ribonuclease, 1738·1
Ribonucleic Acid, 1738·2
Ribonucleico, Ácido, 1738·2
Riboposid, 2264·2
Ribose Nucleic Acid, 1738·2
Ribostat, 2264·2
Ribotrex, 2264·2
Ribotripsin, 2264·2
Ribovac, 2264·2
Ribovir, 2264·2
Ribo-Wied, 2264·2
Ribozym, 2264·2
Ribozymes, 498·2
Ribrain, 2264·2
Ribufen, 2264·2
Ribujet, 2264·2
Ribusol, 2264·2
Ribwort Plantain, 1738·2
RIC Calcio, 2264·2
Rical, 2264·2
Riccomycine, 2264·2
Riccovitan, 2264·2
Rice Bran Oil, 1725·1
Rice Embryo Bud Oil, 1725·1
Rice Starch, 1449·1
Ricelyt, 2264·2
Ricelyte— see Infalyte, 2060·4
Ricerca System, 2264·2
Ricerca System Anagen, 2264·2
Ricerca System Elios, 2264·2
Ricerca System Hidra, 2264·2
Ricerca System Iposeb, 2264·2
*Richardella dulcifica*, 1715·2
Richmond Antiseptic Cream, 2264·2
Ricilin, 2264·2
Ricilina, 2264·2
Ricin, 1738·2, 2264·2
Ricin, Huile de, 1668·2
Ricini Oleum Hydrogenatum, 1668·2
Ricini Oleum Virginale, 1668·2
Ricini Sulphatum, Oleum, 1575·3
Ricinis, 2264·2
Ricino, 1738·2
Ricino, Aceite de, 1668·2
Ricino Koki, 2264·2
Ricinoleic Acid, 1738·3
Ricinoleico, Ácido, 1738·3
*Ricinus communis*, 1668·2, 1738·2
Rickamicin Sulphate, 254·3
Rickets— see Osteomalacia, 762·3
Rickets of Prematurity, 1232·1
Rickettsial Infections, 144·3
Rickettsialpox— see Spotted Fevers, 147·1
Ricola, 2264·2
Riconazol, 2264·3
Ricridene, 2264·3
Ricura, 2264·3
RID, 2264·3
Ridamin, 2264·3
Rid-a-Pain, 2264·3
Rid-a-Pain HP, 2264·3

Ridaq, 2264·3
Ridasa, 2264·3
Ridaura, 2264·3
Ridauran, 2264·3
Ridazin, 2264·3
Ridazine, 2264·3
Ridene, 2264·3
Ridenol, 2264·3
Rideril, 2264·3
Ridersweet, 2264·3
Ridinox, 2264·3
Ridiodent, 2264·3
Ri-Donna, 2264·3
Riduton Ergo, 2264·3
Ridutox, 2264·3
Riduvir, 2264·3
Rielex, 2264·3
Rifa, 2264·3
Rifa E, 2264·3
Rifabutin, 249·1
Rifabutina, 249·1
Rifabutine, 249·1
Rifabutinum, 249·1
Rifacilin, 2264·3
Rifacol, 2264·4
Rifacom E-Z, 2264·4
Rifadecina, 2264·4
Rifadin, 2264·4
Rifadine, 2264·4
Rifafour, 2264·4
Rifagen, 2264·4
Rifaldazine, 250·2
Rifaldin, 2264·4
Rifam, 2264·4
Rifamate, 2264·4
Rifamcilin, 2264·4
Rifamcin, 2264·4
Rifamicina Sódica, 253·2
Rifamiso, 2264·4
Rifam-P, 2264·4
Rifamp, 2264·4
Rifampicin, 250·2
Rifampicin Sodium, 252·3
Rifampicina, 250·2
Rifampicinum, 250·2
Rifampin, 250·2
Rifampyzid, 2264·4
Rifamycin, 2264·4
Rifamycin AMP, 250·2
Rifamycin B, 253·2
Rifamycin Sodium, 253·2
Rifamycin SV, 253·2
Rifamycin SV Sodium, 253·2
Rifamycins, 117·1
Rifamycinum Natricum, 253·2
Rifan, 2264·4
Rifanicozid, 2264·4
Rifano, 2264·4
Rifapentina, 253·3
Rifapentine, 253·3
Rifapiam, 2264·4
Rifaprim, 2264·4
Rifasynt, 2264·4
Rifater, 2264·4
Rifaxidin, 254·1
Rifaximin, 254·1
Rifaximina, 254·1
Rifaximine, 254·1
Rifazida, 2264·4
Rifedot, 2264·4
Rifex, 2264·4
Rifinah, 2265·1
Rifocin, 2265·1
Rifocina, 2265·1
Rifocine, 2265·1
Rifocort, 2265·1
Rifocyna, 2265·1
Rifoldin, 2265·1
Rifoldin INH, 2265·1
Rifomycins, 117·1
Rift Valley Fever— *see* Haemorrhagic Fevers, 618·2
Rift Valley Fever Vaccines, 1637·2
Rifun, 2265·1
Riganpil, 2265·1
Rigentex, 2265·1
Riget, 2265·1
Rigevidon, 2265·1
Rigidur, 2265·1
Rigidur Duo, 2265·1
Rigix, 2265·1
Rigmoz, 2265·1
Rigoletten, 2265·1
Rigoran, 2265·1
Rigotax, 2265·1
Rikamycin, 254·1
Riker-594, 377·3
Riker 52G, 742·3
Riklinak, 2265·1
Rikodeine, 2265·1
Rikoderm, 2265·1
Rikospray, 2265·1
RIL-2, 562·2
Rilamir, 2265·2
Rilan, 2265·2
Rilaprost, 2265·2
Rilaquin, 2265·2
Rilastil, 2265·2
Rilastil Anti-Oxidante, 2265·2
Rilastil Dermo Solar, 2265·2
Rilaten, 2265·2
Rilatine, 2265·2
Rilcapton, 2265·2
Rilex, 2265·2
Rilfit, 2265·2
Rilmenidina, Fosfato de, 996·1
Rilmenidine Acid Phosphate, 996·1
Rilmenidine Dihydrogen Phosphate, 996·1
Rilmenidine Hydrogen Phosphate, 996·1
Rilmenidine Phosphate, 996·1
Rilmenidini Dihydrogenophosphas, 996·1
Rilutek, 2265·2
Riluzol, 1738·3
Riluzole, 1738·3
Rimacid, 2265·2
Rimacillin, 2265·2
Rimactan, 2265·2
Rimactan + INH, 2265·2
Rimactane, 2265·2
Rimactazid, 2265·2
Rimactazid + Z, 2265·2
Rimactazide, 2265·2
Rimactazide + Z, 2265·2
Rimafen, 2265·2
Rimafungol, 2265·2
Rimagrip, 2265·2
Rimantadina, Hidrocloruro de, 653·1
Rimantadine Hydrochloride, 653·1
Rimapam, 2265·2
Rimapen, 2265·3
Rimapurinol, 2265·3
Rimarex, 2265·3
Rimarin, 2265·3
RIMAs, 278·2, 316·1
Rimasal, 2265·3
Rimastine, 2265·3
Rimbol, 2265·3
Rimcure, 2265·3
Rimcure 3-FDC, 2265·3
Rimevax, 2265·3
Rimexel, 2265·3
Rimexolona, 1110·1
Rimexolone, 1110·1
Rimidol, 2265·3
Rimifon, 2265·3
Rimiterol, Hidrobromuro de, 791·3
Rimiterol Hydrobromide, 791·3
Rimodar, 2265·3
Rimopride Citrate, 1276·3
Rimoxallin, 2265·3
Rimoxol, 2265·3
Rimoxyn, 2265·3
Rimpazid, 2265·3
Rimsalin, 2265·3
Rimso, 2265·3
Rimycin, 2265·3
Rin Up, 2265·3
Rinactive, Neo— *see* Neo Rinactive, 2156·4
Rinade BID, 2265·3
Rinadine, 2265·3
Rinafed, 2265·3
Rinafort, 2265·3
Rinalix, 2265·3
Rinantipiol, 2265·3
Rinatec, 2265·4
Rinatrol, 2265·4
Rinaze, 2265·4
Rinazina, 2265·4
Rince Bouche Antiseptique, 2265·4
Rinedrone, 2265·4
Rinelon, 2265·4
Rinerge, 2265·4
Rinex, 2265·4
Rinexin, 2265·4
Ring N, 2265·4
Ringer Lactato Vitulia, Suero— *see* Suero Ringer Lactato Vitulia, 2310·4
Ringersteril, 2265·4
Ringworm— *see* Skin Infections, 390·1
Ringworm Ointment, 2265·4
Rinil, 2265·4
Rinilyn, 2265·4
Rinisone, 2265·4
Rinnova, 2265·4
Rino Calyptol, 2265·4
Rino Clenil, 2265·4
Rino Dexa, 2265·4
Rino Ebastel, 2265·4
Rino Naftazolina, 2265·4
Rino Resfenol, 2265·4
Rino Spray, 2265·4
Rino-Azetin, 2265·4
Rino-B, 2265·4
Rinobactil, 2265·4
Rinobalsamiche, 2265·4
Rinobanedif, 2266·1
Rinoben, 2266·1
Rinoblanco, 2266·1
Rinoblanco Dexa Antibio, 2266·1
Rinocidina, 2266·1
Rinocorin, 2266·1
Rinocron, 2266·1
Rinocusi Vitaminico, 2266·1
Rinodan, 2266·1
Rinodif, 2266·1
Rinofen, 2266·1
Rinofilax AG M, 2266·1
Rinofluimucil, 2266·1
Rinofluimucil-S, 2266·1
Rinoflumil, 2266·1
Rinoflux, 2266·1
Rinofomentil, 2266·1
Rinofren, 2266·1
Rinofren Pediatrico, 2266·1
Rinofrenal, 2266·1
Rinofrenal Plus, 2266·1
Rinofrim, 2266·1
Rinogan, 2266·1
Rinogel, 2266·2
Rinogerol, 2266·2
Rinoglin, 2266·2
Rinogutt Antiallergico Spray, 2266·2
Rinogutt Eucalipto-Fher, 2266·2
Rinogutt Spray-Fher, 2266·2
Rinojet, 2266·2
Rinojet SF, 2266·2
Rinoklin, 2266·2
Rinolan, 2266·2
Rino-Lastin, 2266·2
Rinolergan, 2266·2
Rinomar, 2266·2
Rinomax, 2266·2
Rinomex, 2266·2
Rinomicine, 2266·2
Rinomicine Activada, 2266·2
Rinopaidolo, 2266·2
Rinopanteina, 2266·2
Rinoparin, 2266·2
Rino-Ped, 2266·2
Rinoretard, 2266·2
Rinorix, 2266·2
Rinos, 2266·2
Rinos-A, 2266·2
Rinosbon, 2266·2
Rinosedin, 2266·3
Rinosil, 2266·3
Rinosite, 2266·3
Rinosol, 2266·3
Rinosone, 2266·3
Rinosoro, 2266·3
Rinospray, 2266·3
Rinostat, 2266·3
Rinostil, 2266·3
Rinotil, 2266·3
Rinotricina, 2266·3
Rinovagos, 2266·3
Rinoval, 2266·3
Rinovel, 2266·3
Rinoven, 2266·3
Rinoven Compuesto, 2266·3
Rinovit, 2266·3
Rinovit Nube, 2266·3
Rinowash, 2266·3
Rinox Adulto, 2266·3
Rinox Pediatrico, 2266·3
Rinozin, 2266·3
Rinsoderm, 2266·3
Rinstead, 2266·3
Rinstead Teething Gel, 2266·3
Rintac, 2266·3
Rinurel, 2266·4
Rinutan, 2266·4
Riodine, 2266·4
Rio-Josipyrin N, 2266·4
Riomet, 2266·4
Riomitsin, 241·1
Riopan, 2266·4
Riopan Plus, 2266·4
Riopone, 2266·4
Riostatin, 2266·4
Riotane, 2266·4
Riotapen, 2266·4
Rioven, 2266·4
Ripason, 2266·4
Riphenidate, 2266·4
Ripix, 2266·4
Ripol, 2266·4
Riposon, 2266·4
Risatarun, 2266·4
Riscalon, 2266·4
Rischiaril, 2266·4
Risedronate Sodium, 774·3
Risedronato Sódico, 774·3
Risedronic Acid, 774·3
Risedrónico, Ácido, 774·3
Risek, 2266·4
Riselle, 2266·4
Risicordin, 2266·4
Risidon, 2266·4
Risinetten, 2266·4
Risocalm, 2266·4
Risolid, 2266·4
Risoltuss, 2267·1
Risoniac, 2267·1
Risordan, 2267·1
Risperdal, 2267·1
Risperidona, 719·2
Risperidone, 719·2
Risperidonum, 719·2
Risperin, 2267·1
Rispid, 2267·1
Ristalen, 2267·1
Risthal, 2267·1
Risto, 2267·1
Ristolzit, 2267·1
Ritalin, 2267·1
Ritalina, 2267·1
Ritaline, 2267·1
Ritalinic Acid, 1590·3
Ritalmex, 2267·1
Ritamine, 2267·1
Ritanserin, 721·1
Ritanserina, 721·1
Ritaphen, 2267·1
Riteban, 2267·1
Rite-Diet, 2267·1
Ritiometan, 1191·3
Ritiometan Magnesium, 1191·3
Rition, 2267·1
Ritmocardyl, 2267·1
Ritmocit, 2267·1
Ritmocor, 2267·1
Ritmodan, 2267·2

Ritmoforine, 2267·2
Ritmogel, 2267·2
Ritmolol, 2267·2
Ritmoneuran, 2267·2
Ritmonorm, 2267·2
Ritodrina, Hidrocloruro de, 1739·2
Ritodrine Hydrochloride, 1739·2
Ritonavir, 653·2
Ritopar, 2267·2
Ritro, 2267·2
Ritrocel, 2267·2
Ritromine, 2267·2
Ritroprim, 2267·2
Rituxan, 2267·2
Rituximab, 582·3
Ritvir, 2267·2
Rityne, 2267·2
Rivacefin, 2267·2
Rivanase, 2267·2
Rivanol, 2267·2
Rivanol, Anaesthesin-— *see* Anaesthesin-Rivanol, 1797·4
Rivasa, 2267·2
Rivasol, 2267·2
Rivasol HC, 2267·2
Rivasone, 2267·2
Rivastigmina, Hidrogenotartrato de, 1497·1
Rivastigmine, 1497·1
Rivastigmine Bitartrate, 1497·1
Rivastigmine Hydrogen Tartrate, 1497·1
Rivastigmine Tartrate, 1497·1
Rivatril, 2267·2
*Rivea corymbosa*, 1723·2
Rivecrum, 2267·2
Rivela, 2267·2
Riveparin, 2267·2
River Blindness— *see* Onchocerciasis, 100·2
Rivervan, 2267·2
Rivescal Tar, 2267·2
Rivescal ZPT, 2267·2
Rivial, 2267·2
Rividose, 2267·2
Rivistel, 2267·2
Rivitin BC, 2267·2
Rivodarone, 2267·2
Rivodol, 2267·3
Rivoltan, 2267·3
Rivopen-V, 2267·3
Rivostatin, 2267·3
Rivotril, 2267·3
Rivovit, 2267·3
Rivoxicillin, 2267·3
Rivozol, 2267·3
Riwa Franzbranntwein, 2267·3
α-Rix, 2267·3
Rixapen, 2267·3
Rizaben, 2267·3
Rizalief, 2267·3
Rizaliv, 2267·3
Rizalt, 2267·3
Rizatriptan Benzoate, 471·1
Rizatriptán, Benzoato de, 471·1
Rize, 2267·3
Rizen, 2267·3
Rizinusöl, 1668·2
R-Loc, 2267·3
RM-1601, 1505·3
R-metHuG-CSF, 753·3
R-metHuSCF, 742·2
RMI-9384A, 290·2
RMI-9918, 441·1
RMI-10482A, 1124·3
RMI-14042A, 1041·2
RMI-17043, 911·1
RMI-71754, 383·2
RMI-71782, 604·2
RMS, 2267·3
RN13 Regeneresen, 2267·3
RNA, 1738·2
RNA Interference, 1738·2
RNase, 1738·1
RNH-6270, 975·3
Ro-01-6794/706, 1679·3
Ro-1-5155, 966·1
Ro-1-7683, 491·1
Ro-1-9334, 603·2
Ro-1-9569, 1752·2
Ro-02-2985, 606·1
Ro-2-3248, 866·2
Ro-2-3773, 480·2
Ro-2-9757, 554·2
Ro-2-9915, 399·3
Ro-4-0403, 682·3
Ro-4-1544/6, 103·1
Ro-4-1557, 1393·1
Ro-4-2130, 261·1
Ro-4-3476, 263·2
Ro-4-3780, 1148·3
Ro-4-3816, 1398·3
Ro-4-4393, 259·3
Ro-4-4602, 1200·2
Ro-4-5282, 1589·2
Ro-4-5360, 710·1
Ro-4-6467/1, 581·2
Ro-5-0690, 674·2
Ro-5-2180, 710·3
Ro-5-2807, 690·1
Ro-5-3059, 710·1
Ro-5-3307/1, 891·3
Ro-5-3350, 671·3
Ro-5-4023, 359·1
Ro-5-4200, 698·2
Ro-5-4556, 706·1
Ro-5-5345, 723·2
Ro-5-6901, 700·3
Ro-5-9754, 240·2
Ro-6-4563, 331·3
Ro-7-0207, 612·2
Ro-7-1051, 602·3
Ro-07-5965, 806·3
Ro-09-1978/000, 533·2
Ro-10-1670, 1140·2
Ro-10-1670/000, 1140·2
Ro-10-6338, 877·2
Ro-10-9070, 228·3
Ro-10-9071, 244·2
Ro-10-9359, 1147·1
Ro-11-1163, 308·2
Ro-11-1163/000, 308·2
Ro-11-1430, 1154·2
Ro-11-2933, 498·3
Ro-11-7891, 1659·2
Ro-12-0068, 93·1
Ro-12-0068/000, 93·1
Ro-12-8095, 308·3
Ro-13-5057, 1655·1
Ro-13-8996, 407·3
Ro-13-8996/000, 407·3
Ro-13-8996/001, 407·3
Ro-13-9297, 54·2
Ro-13-9904, 182·3
Ro-13-9904/000, 182·3
Ro-14-4767/000, 391·1
Ro-14-4767/002, 391·1
Ro-15-1788, 1038·3
Ro-15-1788/000, 1038·3
Ro-15-8074, 172·3
Ro-15-8075, 172·3
Ro-17-2301, 166·3
Ro-17-2301/006, 166·3
Ro-18-0647, 1724·2
Ro-18-0647/002, 1724·2
Ro-19-6327, 1205·2
Ro-19-6327/000, 1205·2
Ro-20-5720/000, 25·1
Ro-21-3971, 707·1
Ro-21-3981/001, 707·2
Ro-21-3981/003, 707·2
Ro-21-5104, 455·2
Ro-21-5535, 1461·2
Ro-21-5998, 453·3
Ro-21-5998/001, 453·3
Ro-21-8837/001, 551·1
Ro-21-9738, 547·3
Ro-22-2296/000, 551·1
Ro-22-7796, 883·1
Ro-22-7796/001, 883·1
Ro-22-8181, 640·3
Ro-22-9000, 1512·3
Ro 23-4194, 1462·1
Ro-23-6240, 213·2
Ro-23-6240/000, 213·2
Ro-24-2027, 657·1
Ro-24-2027/000, 657·1
Ro-24-7375, 1359·3
Ro-24-7472/000, 1701·3
Ro-31-2848, 883·3
Ro-31-2848/006, 883·3
Ro-31-8959, 653·3
Ro-31-8959/003, 653·3
Ro-40-5967, 959·1
Ro-40-5967/001, 959·1
Ro-40-7592, 1216·1
Ro-42-5892, 994·3
Ro-44-9883, 944·3
Ro-44-9883/000, 944·3
Ro-47-0203/029, 875·3
Ro-48-3657/001, 996·3
Ro-63-8695, 567·1
Ro-64-0796/002, 651·1
Ro-107-9070/194, 656·3
Ro-0783/B, 311·1
Ro-50831, 300·3
Roaccutan, 2267·3
Roaccutane, 2267·3
Roach-2, 698·3
Roacnetan, 2267·3
Roacutan, 2267·3
Roapies, 698·3
Ro-A-Vit, 2267·3
Robafen AC Cough, 2267·3
Robafen CF, 2267·3
Robafen DAC, 2267·4
Robafen DM, 2267·4
Robanul, 2267·4
Robatar, 2267·4
RoBathol, 2267·4
Robaxacet, 2267·4
Robaxacet-8, 2267·4
Robaxifen, 2267·4
Robaxin, 2267·4
Robaxisal Preparations, 2267·4
Robaz, 2267·4
Robenidina, Hidrocloruro de, 615·2
Robenidine Hydrochloride, 615·2
Robenzidene Hydrochloride, 615·2
Roberfarin, 2267·4
Robervital, 2267·4
Robidone, 2267·4
Robidrine, 2267·4
Robiflam, 2267·4
Robi-Flu, 2267·4
Robigesic, 2267·4
Robimycin Robitabs, 2267·4
Robinax, 2267·4
Robinaxol, 2267·4
Robinaz, 2267·4
Robinia Med Complex, 2267·4
Robinia Ro-Plex (Rowo-99), 2267·4
Robinul, 2267·4
Robinul-Neostigmin, 2267·4
Robinul-Neostigmine, 2268·1
Robitussin Preparations, 2268·1
Robovites, 2268·3
Robovites Multivitamin, 2268·3
Roburis, 2268·3
Roburvit, 2268·3
Robusta Coffee, 1765·3
Robutal, 698·3
Robuvalen, 2268·3
RoC Sunscreen Stick, 2268·3
RoC Total Sunblock, 2268·3
Rocal, 2268·3
Rocaltrol, 2268·3
Rocanal Imediat, 2268·3
Rocanal Permanent Gangrene, 2268·3
Rocanal Permanent Vital, 2268·3
Roccal, 2268·3
Roccaxin, 2268·3
Rocefalin, 2268·3
Rocefin, 2268·3
Rocephalin, 2268·3
Rocephin, 2268·3
Rocephine, 2268·3
Roceron, 2268·3
Roceron-A, 2268·3
Roceron-A— *see* Roferon-A, 2269·1
Rocgel, 2268·4
Rochagan, 2268·4
Roche, 2268·4
Rochelle Salt, 1284·3
Rochevit, 2268·4
Rociclyn, 2268·4
Rocid, 2268·4
Rocilin, 2268·4
Rociverina, 1740·1
Rociverine, 1740·1
Rock, 1373·3
Rocket Fuel, 1730·3
Rocky Mountain Spotted Fever— *see* Spotted Fevers, 147·1
Rocmaline, 2268·4
Rocodin, 2268·4
Rocof, 2268·4
Rocornal, 2268·4
Roctylan, 2268·4
Rocuronio, Bromuro de, 1405·2
Rocuronium Bromide, 1405·2
Rodakin, 2268·4
Rodase, 2268·4
Rodavan, 2268·4
Rodazol, 2268·4
Rodenal, 2268·4
Rodenticides, 1499·1
Rodepan, 2268·4
Rodermil, 2268·4
Rodinac, 2268·4
Rodinac Biotic, 2268·4
Rodinac Flex, 2268·4
Rodinac Gesic, 2268·4
Rodogyl, 2268·4
Rodopsin Plus, 2268·4
Rodovit, 2268·4
RO-Dry Eyes, 2268·4
RO-Eye Drops, 2268·4
RO-Eyewash, 2268·4
Rofact, 2268·4
Rofatuss, 2268·4
Rofecoxib, 86·3
Rofenid, 2269·1
Rofepain, 2269·1
Roferon-A, 2269·1
Rofetab, 2269·1
Rofex, 2269·1
Rofiz, 2269·1
Roflatol Phyto (Rowo-146), 2269·1
Roflumilast, 791·3
Rofoxin, 2269·1
Rogaan, 2269·1
Rogadermis, 2269·1
Rogaine, 2269·1
Rogal, 2269·1
Rogasti, 2269·1
Rogastril, 2269·1
Roge, 2269·1
Rogelina, 2269·1
Rogitine, 2269·1
Roha-Fenchel-Tee, 2269·1
Rohasal, 2269·1
Rohasal N, 2269·1
Rohipnol, 2269·1
Rohto Zi, 2269·1
Rohto Zi Contact, 2269·1
Rohto Zi Fresh, 2269·1
Rohypnol, 2269·1
Roical, 2269·2
Roidhemo, 2269·2
Roiplon, 2269·2
Roipnol, 2269·2
Rojema, 2269·2
Rojo Allura AC, 1056·1
Rojo Cereza, 1058·1
Rojo Congo, 1675·3
Rojo de Cochinilla A, 1057·3
Rojo de Remolacha, 1056·2
Rojo Escarlata, 1191·3
Rojo 2G, 1058·1
Rojo Neutro, 1719·3
Rojobacter, 2269·2
Rokacet, 2269·2
Rokacet Plus, 2269·2
Rokadin, 2269·2
Rokal, 2269·2

Rokal Plus, 2269·2
Rokamol, 2269·2
Rokamol Plus Codeine, 2269·2
Rokan, 2269·2
Rokanite, 2269·2
Rokital, 2269·2
Rokitamicina, 254·1
Rokitamycin, 254·1
Rokumi-ga, Tsumura— *see* Tsumura Rokumi-gan, 2351·1
Rolac Plus, 2269·2
Rolaids, 2269·2
Rolaket, 2269·2
Rolandic Epilepsy— *see* Epilepsy, 349·1
Rolap, 2269·2
Rolar, 2269·2
Rolatuss Expectorant, 2269·2
Rolatuss with Hydrocodone, 2269·2
Rolatuss Plain, 2269·2
Roleca Wacholder, 2269·2
Roleca-S, 2269·2
Rolene, 2269·2
Rolicyclidine, 1730·3
Rolip, 2269·3
Rolitetraciclina, 254·1
Rolitetracycline, 254·1
Roliwol, 2269·3
Roliwol B, 2269·3
Roliwol S, 2269·3
Roll-bene, 2269·3
Roll-On, 2269·3
Roloken, 2269·3
Rolsical, 2269·3
Romadin, 2269·3
Roman Chamomile Flower, 1669·3
Romarene, 2269·3
Romarin, Essence de, 1740·2
Romarinex, 2269·3
Romarinex-Choline, 2269·3
Romazicon, 2269·3
Rombay, 2269·3
Rombellin, 2269·3
Rombox, 2269·3
Romeira, 112·1
Romero, Aceite Esencial de, 1740·2
Romero, Esencia de, 1740·2
Romesa, 2269·3
Romesec, 2269·3
Romet, 2269·3
Romicin, 2269·3
Romidon, 2269·3
Romifidina, 721·2
Romifidine, 721·2
Romigal, 2269·3
Romilar Preparations, 2269·3
Rominafort, 2269·4
Romir, 2269·4
Romiver, 2269·4
Rommix, 2269·4
Romulin, 2269·4
Ronabin, 2269·4
Ronal, 2269·4
Roname, 2269·4
RO-Naphz, 2269·4
Rondamine-DM, 2269·4
Rondec, 2269·4
Rondec Compositum, 2269·4
Rondec-DM, 2269·4
Rondimen, 2269·4
Ronemox, 2269·4
Ronexine, 2269·4
Ronfase, 2269·4
Ronfnyl, 2269·4
Rongony, 1666·1
Ronic, 2269·4
Ronidazol, 615·2
Ronidazole, 615·2
Ronifibrate, 996·1
Ronifibrato, 996·1
Ronmix, 2269·4
Ronpirin APCQ, 2269·4
Ronpirin Cold Remedy, 2269·4
Rontafor, 2269·4
Rontagel, 2270·1
Rontilona, 2270·1
Ronvan, 2270·1
Ronvir, 2270·1
Roofies, 698·3
Rope, 698·3
Ropect, 2270·1
Rophelin, 2270·1
Rophies, 698·3
Ropinirol, Hidrocloruro de, 1213·3
Ropinirole Hydrochloride, 1213·3
Ropion, 2270·1
Ropivacaína, Hidrocloruro de, 1384·2
Ropivacaine Hydrochloride, 1384·2
Ropril, 2270·1
Roquinimex, 583·2
R.O.R., 2270·1
Rora, 1666·1
Rorela, 1683·1
Rorellae, Herba, 1683·1
Roris Marini, 1740·2
Roris Marini, Oleum, 1740·2
ROS, 1740·1
Ros. Pet., 1058·1
Ros Solis, 1683·1
Rosa, Aceite Esencial de, 1740·2
*Rosa alba*, 1740·2
*Rosa canina*, 1740·1
*Rosa centifolia*, 1740·2
*Rosa damascena*, 1740·2
Rosa de Bengala Sódico, 1740·1
Rosa, Esencia de, 1740·2
*Rosa gallica*, 1058·1, 1740·2
Rosa Maria, 1666·1
*Rosa pendulina*, 1740·1
Rosac, 2270·1
Rosacea, 1138·2
Rosae Fructus, 1740·1
Rosae Gallicae Petala, 1058·1
Rosae, Oleum, 1740·2
Rosae Petalum, 1058·1
Rosae Pseudo-fructus, 1740·1
Rosagenus, 2270·1
Rosalgin, 2270·1
Rosalox, 2270·1
Rosanil, 2270·1
Rosaniline Hydrochloride, 1185·1
Rosarthron, 2270·1
Rosarthron Forte, 2270·1
Rosary Beans, 1645·1
Rosased, 2270·1
Rosatil BB, 2270·1
Roscillin, 2270·1
Rose, Attar of, 1740·2
Rose Bay, 1723·1
Rose Bengal, 1740·1
Rose Bengal Sodium, 1740·1
Rose Bengal Sodium ($^{131}$I), 1524·3
Rose Bengale, 1740·1
Rose, Fleur de, 1058·1
Rose Fruit, 1740·1
Rose Geranium Oil, 1692·2
Rose Hips, 1740·1
Rose Oil, 1740·2
Rose, Otto of, 1740·2
Rose Rouge, 1058·1
Roseine, Acid, 1646·3
Roseliane Creme, 2270·1
Roseliane Lait, 2270·1
Rosemary, 1740·2
Rosemary Leaf, 1740·2
Rosemary Oil, 1740·2
Rosemary Oil, Moroccan Type, 1740·2
Rosemary Oil, Spanish Type, 1740·2
Rosemary Oil, Tunisian Type, 1740·2
Rosenblüte, 1058·1
Rosets, 2270·1
Rosiced, 2270·1
Rosiden, 2270·1
Rosig, 2270·1
Rosiglitazona, Maleato de, 345·2
Rosiglitazone Maleate, 345·2
Rosilan, 2270·1
Rosils, 2270·1
Rosin, 1675·1
Rosital, 2270·1
Rosken Skin Repair, 2270·1
Rosmarini Aetheroleum, 1740·2
Rosmarini Folium, 1740·2
Rosmarini, Oleum, 1740·2
Rosmarinic Acid, 1711·1, 1740·2
Rosmarinöl, 1740·2
*Rosmarinus officinalis*, 1740·2
Rosol-Gamma, 2270·2
Rosone, 2270·2
Rosovax, 2270·2
Rosoxacin, 254·1
Rosoxacino, 254·1
Ross, Pilulas— *see* Pilulas Ross, 2220·1
Rossepar, 2270·2
Rossitrol, 2270·2
Rosskastaniensamen, 1648·2
Rossofolin, 2270·2
Ro-Strumal NEU (Rowo-221), 2270·2
Rosula, 2270·2
Rosuvastatin Calcium, 996·2
Rotane, 2270·2
Rotavirus Vaccines, 1637·2
Rotenona, 1510·1
Rotenone, 1510·1
Rotenonum, 1510·1
Roter, 2270·2
Roter Complex, 2270·2
Rotersept, 2270·2
Rotesan, 2270·2
Rothacin, 2270·2
Rothera's Tablets— *see* Acetest, 1770·2
Rothonal, 2270·2
Rothricin, 2270·2
Roth's RKT Tropfen, 2270·2
Roth's Ropulmin N, 2270·2
Roth's Rotacard, 2270·2
Rotilen, 2270·2
Rotol, 2270·2
Rotram, 2270·2
Rotramin, 2270·2
Rotuss, 2270·2
Roubac, 2270·2
Rouge Cochenille A, 1057·3
Roug-mycin, 2270·2
Rouhex-G, 2270·2
Round Buchu, 1663·1
Roundup, 1506·1
Roundworm Infections, 97·1
Rounox, 2270·2
Rouphylline, 2270·2
Rouvax, 2270·2
Rouvax Merieux, 2270·3
Rovacor, 2270·3
Rovalcyte, 2270·3
Rovamicina, 2270·3
Rovamycin, 2270·3
Rovamycine, 2270·3
Rovericlin, 2270·3
Roveril, 2270·3
Rovigon, 2270·3
Rovigon G, 2270·3
Rovit, 2270·3
Rovit C, 2270·3
Rowachol, 2270·3
Rowachol Comp, 2270·3
Rowachol, Neo- — *see* Neo-Rowachol, 2159·4
Rowachol-Digestiv, 2270·3
Rowaclimax, 2270·3
Rowadermat, 2270·3
Rowalind, 2270·3
Rowanefrin, 2270·3
Rowapraxin, 2270·3
Rowarolan, 2270·4
Rowasa, 2270·4
Rowatanal, 2270·4
Rowatinex, 2270·4
Rowatinex, Neo- — *see* Neo-Rowatinex, 2159·4
Rowo-15— *see* Cardiotonicum, 1871·1
Rowo-52, 2270·4
Rowo-99— *see* Robinia Ro-Plex, 2267·4
Rowo-100— *see* Antinicoticum sine, 1804·4
Rowo-138— *see* Rowo-Sedaphin 138, 2270·4
Rowo-146— *see* Roflatol Phyto, 2269·1
Rowo-210— *see* Asthmalyticum-Ampullen N, 1817·3
Rowo-216, 2270·4
Rowo-221— *see* Ro-Strumal NEU, 2270·2
Rowo-298, 2270·4
Rowo-415— *see* Echinacea Ro-Plex, 1961·3
Rowo-576— *see* Rowo-Rytesthin, 2270·4
Rowo-578— *see* Psychoneuroticum, 2245·1
Rowo-629, 2270·4
Rowo-633— *see* Antineuralgicum, 1804·4
Rowo-776— *see* Symphytum Ro-Plex, 2316·1
Rowo-849 Echinacea Ro-Plex (Rowo-849), 2270·4
Rowo-Rytesthin (Rowo-576), 2270·4
Rowo Rytesthin Ro-Plex (Rowo-318), 2270·4
Rowo-778 Symphytum Ro-Plex T (Rowo-778), 2270·4
Rowo-Sedaphin 138 (Rowo-138), 2270·4
Row-shay, 698·3
Roxacilin, 2270·4
Roxadimate, 1157·1
Roxadimato, 1157·1
Roxalia, 2270·4
Roxane, 2270·4
Roxanol, 2270·4
Roxarsona, 1740·3
Roxarsone, 1740·3
Roxatidina, Hidrocloruro de Acetato de, 1288·1
Roxatidine Acetate Hydrochloride, 1288·1
Roxatine, 2270·4
Roxazin, 2270·4
Roxcin, 2270·4
Roxen, 2270·4
Roxene, 2270·4
Roxenil, 2270·4
Roxeptin, 2270·4
Roxflan, 2270·4
Roxi, 2271·1
Roxibion, 2271·1
Roxicam, 2271·1
Roxicet, 2271·1
Roxicilline, 2271·1
Roxicin, 2271·1
Roxicodone, 2271·1
Roxid, 2271·1
Roxiden, 2271·1
Roxidura, 2271·1
Roxifen, 2271·1
Roxigrun, 2271·1
Roxiklinge, 2271·1
Roxilan, 2271·1
Roxillin, 2271·1
Roxilox, 2271·1
Roximin, 2271·1
Roximin-Galenica, 2271·1
Roxin, 2271·1
Roxina, 2271·1
Roxine, 2271·1
Roxinox, 2271·1
Roxiprin, 2271·1
Roxi-Puren, 2271·1
Roxit, 2271·1
Roxitan, 2271·1
Roxithro-Lich, 2271·1
Roxithromycin, 254·2
Roxithromycinum, 254·2
Roxithrostad, 2271·1
Roxithroxyl, 2271·1
Roxitin, 2271·1
Roxitran, 2271·1
Roxitricina, 2271·1
Roxitrol, 2271·2
Roxitrom, 2271·2
Roxitromicina, 254·2
Roxitromin, 2271·2
Roxium, 2271·2
Roxiwas, 2271·2
Roxlecon, 2271·2
Roxo, 2271·2
Roxomycin, 2271·2
Roxorin, 2271·2
Roxthomed, 2271·2
Roxthrin, 2271·2
Roxto, 2271·2

Roxtrocin, 2271·2
Roxy, 2271·2
Roxycam, 2271·2
Roxyn, 2271·2
Roxyrol, 2271·2
Roxyspes, 2271·2
Royal E, 2271·2
Royal Galanol, 2271·2
Royal Jelly, 1740·3
Royal Life, 2271·2
Royalin, 2271·2
Roycefax, 2271·2
Roychlor, 2271·2
Royen, 2271·2
Royflex, 2271·2
Royl 6, 2271·2
Roytrin, 2271·2
Royvac Kit, 2271·2
Rozacreme, 2271·2
Rozagel, 2271·2
Rozex, 2271·2
Rozicel, 2271·3
Rozovin, 2271·3
RP-2090, 264·1
RP-2168, 600·3
RP-2512, 613·2
RP-2632, 260·3
RP-2831, 1697·1
RP-2987, 481·3
RP-3359, 457·1
RP-3377, 448·2
RP-3799, 104·1
RP-3854, 606·1
RP-4753, 458·1
RP-4909, 675·1
RP-5171, 1735·2
RP-5337, 255·3
RP-6847, 438·2
RP-7044, 703·2
7162-RP, 320·2
RP-7204, 689·2
RP-7293, 246·1
RP-7542, 1646·1
RP-7843, 724·1
RP-7891, 333·1
8599-RP, 431·3
RP-8823, 607·2
RP-8909, 714·1
RP-9712, 607·2
RP-9715, 1393·1
RP-9778, 246·3
RP-9921, 742·3
RP-9965, 1276·3
RP-13057, 545·3
13228-RP, 456·1
RP-13907, 1689·1
14539-RP, 615·3
RP-14539, 615·3
RP-19366, 716·1
RP-19552, 716·1
RP-19583, 51·2
RP-20605, 107·2
RP-22050, 594·3
RP-22410, 333·1
27267-RP, 729·3
41982-RP, 241·3
RP-54274, 1738·3
RP-54476, 248·1
RP-54563, 910·3
RP-54780, 577·1
RP-56976, 547·1
RP-57669, 248·2
RP-59500, 248·1
RPA, 995·2
RP-Pose, 2271·3
RPR-251526, 1095·2
R-Rax, 2271·3
RRV, 1637·3
RRV-TV, 1637·2
RS-1301, 1547·2
RS-1320, 1101·1
RS-2252, 1100·1
RS-2362, 1110·1
RS-2386, 1095·2
RS-3540, 65·1
RS-3650, 65·1
RS-3999, 1101·1
RS-4691, 1096·1
RS-8858, 111·1
RS-10085-197, 961·2
RS-21592, 635·3
RS-25259-197, 1282·3
RS-26306, 1325·1
RS-35887, 395·2
RS-35887-00-10-3, 395·2
RS-37619-00-31-3, 52·1
RS-43285, 994·2
RS-44872, 408·2
RS-44872-00-10-3, 408·2
RS-61443, 1361·2
RS-61443-190, 1361·2
RS-69216, 965·1
RS-69216-XX-07-0, 965·1
RS-079070-194, 656·3
RS-94991298, 1332·3
$RT_3$, 1594·1
R-Tanna, 2271·3
R-Tanna S Pediatric, 2271·3
R-Tannamine, 2271·3
R-Tannate, 2271·3
R-Tannic-S, 2271·3
RTH, 2271·3
Rt-PA, 857·1
RTS,S, 1622·2
RTS,S/AS02, 1622·3
R-Tyflam, 2271·3
RU-43-715-n, 86·1
RU-486, 1560·2
RU-965, 254·2
RU-1697, 1573·2
RU-2267, 1541·3
RU-2323, 1556·2
RU-15060, 93·3
RU-15750, 43·2
RU-19110, 605·3
RU-23908, 576·2
RU-24756, 175·3
RU-27987, 1573·3
RU-28965, 254·2
RU-31158, 704·1
RU-38486, 1560·2
RU-41740, 1703·3
RU-44570, 1016·1
RU-66647, 265·2
Ru Xiang, 1690·1
Rubacina, 2271·3
Rubber, 1741·1
Rubeaten, 2271·3
Rubefacients, 4·3
Rubella, Diphtheria, and Tetanus Vaccines, 1615·2
Rubella Immunoglobulin, Human, 1637·3
Rubella Immunoglobulins, 1637·3
Rubella, Measles, and Mumps Vaccines, 1625·1
Rubella and Measles Vaccines, 1624·3
Rubella and Mumps Vaccines, 1638·2
Rubella and Mumps Virus Vaccine Live, 1638·2
Rubella Vaccine (Live), 1637·3
Rubella Vaccine (Live), Measles, Mumps and, 1625·1
Rubella Vaccines, 1637·3
Rubella Virus Vaccine Live, 1638·1
Rubella Virus Vaccine Live, Measles and, 1624·3
Rubella Virus Vaccine Live, Measles, Mumps, and, 1625·1
Rubellovac, 2271·3
Rubesal, 2271·3
Rubeuman, 2271·3
Rubex, 2271·3
Rubi Idaei Folium, 1737·3
Rubia Paver, 2271·3
Rubicalm, 2271·3
Rubicolan F, 2271·3
Rubi-Dex, 2271·3
Rubidio 82, 1525·2
Rubidio, Ioduro de, 1741·1
Rubidiosin Composto, 2271·3
Rubidium-81, 1525·1
Rubidium-82, 1525·2
Rubidium Chloride ($^{82}$Rb), 1525·2
Rubidium Iodide, 1741·1
Rubidomycin Hydrochloride, 545·3
Rubidox, 2271·3
RubieDorm, 2271·3
RubieFol, 2271·4
RubieMag + E, 2271·4
RubieMen, 2271·4
RubieMol, 2271·4
RubieNex Mono, 2271·4
RubieNex Spezial, 2271·4
RubieSed, 2271·4
Rubifarm, 2271·4
Rubifen, 2271·4
Rubifort, 2271·4
Rubilax, 2271·4
Rubilem, 2271·4
Rubilin, 2271·4
Rubina, 2271·4
Rubine, Acid, 1646·3
Rubio N, 2271·4
Rubion, 2271·4
Rubiron, 2271·4
Rubiron B12, 2271·4
Rubisan, 2271·4
Rubistenol, 2271·4
Rubitecan, 583·2
Rubiten, 2271·4
Rubiulcer, 2271·4
Rubizon-Rheumagel, 2271·4
Rubizuel, 2271·4
Rubjovit, 2271·4
Rublex D, 2271·4
Rublex Massage Cream, 2271·4
Rubocord, 2272·1
Ruboderm, 2272·1
Ruboril, 2272·1
Rubozinc, 2272·1
Rubracobal, 2272·1
Rubralong, 2272·1
Rubramin, 2272·1
Rubranova, 2272·1
Rubraplex, 2272·1
Rubrargil, 2272·1
Rubreserine, 1494·2
Rubriment, 2272·1
Rubriment-N, 2272·1
Rubrina, 2272·1
Rubrobion, 2272·1
Rubrocalcium, 2272·1
Rubrociclina, 2272·1
Rubrocortin, 2272·1
Rubroferrina, 2272·1
Rubrum Congoensis, 1675·3
Rubrum Scarlatinum, 1191·3
Rubus Complex, 2272·1
Rubus Idaeus, 1057·3
*Rubus idaeus*, 1057·3, 1737·3
Rub/Vac(Live), 1638·1
Rucaina, 2272·1
Rucaten Forte, 2272·1
Rucaten Prednisolona, 2272·1
Rucin, 2272·1
Ruda, Aceite Esencial de, 1741·1
Rudbeckia, 1683·2
Rudd-U, 2272·1
Rudesol, 2272·1
Rudi-Rouvax, 2272·2
Rudistrol, 2272·2
Rudivax, 2272·2
Rudocaine, 2272·2
Rudocycline, 2272·2
Rudolac, 2272·2
Rudotel, 2272·2
Rue, 1741·1
Rue Oil, 1741·1
Ru-Ef-Tb, 2272·2
RUF-331, 377·3
Ruffles, 698·3
Rufinamida, 377·3
Rufinamide, 377·3
Ruflox, 2272·2
Rufloxacin Hydrochloride, 254·3
Rufol, 2272·2
Ruibarbo, 1287·3
Ru-lets, 2272·2
Rulicalcin, 2272·2
Rulid, 2272·2
Rulide, 2272·2
Rulivan, 2272·2
Rulofer G, 2272·2
Rulofer N, 2272·2
RuLox, 2272·2
RuLox Plus, 2272·2
Rulun, 2272·2
Rumadene, 2272·2
Rumalon, 2272·2
Rumasian, 2272·2
Rumatab, 2272·2
Rumatifen, 2272·2
Rumatifen-Plus, 2272·2
*Rumex acetosa*, 1749·1
*Rumex crispus*, 1766·1
Rumicine, 2272·2
Rumisedan, 2272·3
Rumisedan Fuerte, 2272·3
Rumitex, 2272·3
Rum-K, 2272·3
Runde, 2272·3
Rupan, 2272·3
Rupatadine, 440·3
Rupatadine Fumarate, 440·3
Rupecef, 2272·3
Rupediz, 2272·3
Rupegen, 2272·3
Rupe-N, 2272·3
Rupe-N Compuesto, 2272·3
Rupton, 2272·3
Rupton Chronules, 2272·3
Rupture-wort, 1697·1
Rusci, Oleum, 1159·2
Ruscimel, 2272·3
Ruscogenin, 1741·1
Ruscogenina, 1741·1
Ruscorectal, 2272·3
Ruscoroid, 2272·3
Ruscovarin, 2272·3
Ruscus, 2272·3
*Ruscus aculeatus*, 1741·1
Rusedal, 2272·3
Russedyl, 2272·3
Russian Flies, 1666·3
Russian Ginseng, 1693·1, 1744·1
Russian Liquorice, 1270·2
Russian Red, 1156·3
Rusyde, 2272·3
Ruta Grav., 1741·1
*Ruta graveolens*, 1741·1
Rutae, Oleum, 1741·1
Ruta-Gastreu N R55, 2272·3
Ruticalzon, 2272·3
Ruticalzon VC, 2272·3
Rutice Fuerte, 2272·3
Rutin, 1688·2
Rutinice Fortissimo, 2272·3
Rutinion, 2272·3
Rutisan CE, 2272·3
Rutiscorbin, 2272·3
Rutisept Extra, 2272·3
Rutiviscal, 2272·4
Rutoside, 1688·2
Rutoside Trihydrate, 1688·2
Rutósido, 1688·2
Rutosidum, 1688·2
Ru-Tuss Preparations, 2272·4
Ruvamed, 2272·4
Ruvominox, 2272·4
Ruxicolan, 2272·4
RV-12424, 43·3
RV Paque, 2272·4
R-Vac, 2272·4
RVHB Maxamaid, 2272·4
RWJ-10131, 1563·2
RWJ-10553, 1562·1
RWJ-15817, 632·1
RWJ-17021, 378·3
RWJ-17070, 1329·3
RWJ-22164, 1319·1
RWJ-25213, 225·3
RWJ-26251, 539·3
RWJ-26251-000, 539·3
RWJ-60235, 1143·1

RX-6029-M, 21·3
RX-781094, 1700·2
Ryccard, 2272·4
Rydene, 2272·4
Rye, 2272·4
Rylosol, 2272·4
Rymed, 2272·4
Rymed-TR, 2272·4
Ryna, 2272·4
Ryna-12, 2272·4
Ryna-C, 2272·4
Rynacrom Preparations, 2272·4
Ryna-CX, 2273·1
Rynatan, 2273·1
Rynatanic, 2273·1
Rynatus, 2273·1
Rynatuss, 2273·1
Ryol, 2273·1
Ryped, 2273·1
Rythmex, 2273·1
Rythmical, 2273·1
Rythmodan, 2273·1
Rythmodul, 2273·1
Rythmogastryl, 2273·1
Rythmol, 2273·1
Rythmonopm, 2273·1
Rythocin, 2273·1
Rytmobeta, 2273·1
Rytmogenat, 2273·1
Rytmonorm, 2273·1
Rytmonorma, 2273·1
Rytmopasc, 2273·1
Rytmo-Puren, 2273·1
Ry-Tuss, 2273·1

## S

S, 1444·3
S-1, 586·3
S-2, 2273·1
S-7, 397·3
S.8, 2273·1
S-26 AR, 2273·2
S-26 HA, 2273·2
S-26 LF, 2273·2
S-26 Sem Lactose, 2273·2
S-041, 1062·1
S-46, 367·3
S73-4118, 983·3
S74-6766, 1319·2
S-77-0777, 1107·3
S-095, 1067·1
S-222, 905·3
S-596, 865·1
S-752, 1505·2
S-768, 1588·2
883-S, 1669·2
S-940, 110·1
S-1320, 1094·2
S-1530, 710·1
S-1694, 280·3
S-2395, 1011·1
S-2539, 1509·1
S-2620, 1584·2
S-3341-3, 996·1
S-4522, 996·2
S-5602, 1505·2
S-5614, 1586·3
6059-S, 225·3
6315-S, 213·2
7432-S, 182·1
S-8527, 884·3
S-9318, 1509·3
S-9490, 980·2
S-9490-3, 980·2
S-10036, 557·2
S-10364, 1559·1
S-12911, 775·2
S-26308, 638·1
S-28463, 652·1
S-31183, 1509·3
710674-S, 397·1
S-771221B, 174·1
S Amet, 2273·1
SA-7, 1376·3
SA14-14-2, 1621·3
SA-79, 988·3
SA-96, 1663·2
SA-504, 489·3
Saak, 2273·2
SAB, 2273·2
SAB Simplex, 2273·2
Saba, 2273·2
Sabacur Uno, 2273·2
Sabadilla, 1763·3
Sabadilla Med Complex, 2273·2
Sabal, 1569·1, 2273·2
*Sabal serrulata*, 1569·1
Sabal Uno, 2273·2
Sabalia, 2273·2
Sabalin, 2273·2
Sabalis Serrulatae, 1569·1
Sabalvit, 2273·2
Sabanotropico, 2273·2
Sabão Mole, 1575·2
Sabatif, 2273·2
Sabax Fosenema, 2273·2
Sabax Gentamix, 2273·2
SabCaps, 2273·2
Sabeluzol, 1741·2
Sabeluzole, 1741·2
Sabima, 2273·2
Sabin, 2273·2
Sabin Vaccine, 1633·3
Sabinene, 1706·2, 1710·2, 1724·1
Sabofen, 2273·2
Sabonal Uno, 2273·2
Sabonete Sulfuroso, 2273·2
Sabril, 2273·2
Sabrilan, 2273·3
Sabrilex, 2273·3
Sabro, 2273·3
Sabsi, 1666·1
Sabugueiro, 1741·3
Saburgen-N, 2273·3
Sabutol, 2273·3
Sacarato Cálcico, 1665·1
Sacarina, 1443·2
Sacarina Cálcica, 1443·3
Sacarina Sódica, 1443·3
Sacarosa, 1450·1
Sacarosa, Octaacetato de, 1750·2
Saccarina, 1443·2
Sacch. Ust., 1056·3
Saccharated Iron Oxide, 1438·2
Saccharated Pepsin, 1729·3
Saccharin, 1443·2
Saccharin Calcium, 1443·3
Saccharin Sod., 1443·3
Saccharin Sodium, 1443·3
Saccharinnatrium, 1443·3
Saccharinum, 1443·2
Saccharinum Natricum, 1443·3
Saccharoidum Natricum, 1443·3
*Saccharomyces boulardii*, 1704·2
*Saccharomyces carlsbergensis*, 1469·1
*Saccharomyces cerevisiae*, 1469·1
*Saccharomyces monacensis*, 1469·1
Saccharomyces Siccum, 1469·1
Saccharose, 1450·1
Saccharum, 1450·1
Saccharum Lactis, 1438·3
*Saccharum officinarum*, 1450·1
Saccharum Ustum, 1056·3
Sacietyl, 2273·3
Sacin, 2273·3
Sacnel, 2273·3
Sacolene, 2273·3
Sacred Bark, 1255·1
Sacrosidasa, 1741·2
Sacrosidase, 1741·2
Sacsol, 2273·3
Sacsol NF, 2273·3
Sactabs, 2273·3
Sadda, 1666·1
Sadefen, 2273·3
Sadeltan F, 2273·3
Sadol, 2273·3
SAE, 2273·3
Saetil, 2273·3
Safarol, 2273·3
Saf-Clens, 2273·3
Safe Tussin 30, 2273·3
Safeway Cough Lozenges, 2273·3
Safeway Nasal, 2273·3
Safflower, 1443·3
Safflower Oil, 1443·3
Safflower Oil, Refined, 1443·3
Saffron, 1058·2
Saffron, Bastard, 1444·1
Saffron, False, 1444·1
Saffron for Homoeopathic Preparations, 1058·2
Saffron, Indian, 1058·3
Saffron, Meadow, 416·3
Saforelle, 2273·3
Safran, 1058·2
Safrole, 1742·1
Safyr Bleu Antihistamine, 2273·3
Sagadreps, 2273·3
Sagamicin, 2273·3
Sagamicin Sulphate, 231·3
Sagamicina, 2273·3
Sage, 1741·2
Sage Leaf Oil, 1741·2
Sage Leaf (Salvia Officinalis), 1741·2
Sage Leaf, Three-lobed, 1741·2
Sage Oil, 1741·2
Sagitta Kamillbad, 2273·3
Sagittacin N, 2273·3
Sagittacortin, 2273·3
Sagittamuc, 2273·4
Sagittaproct, 2273·4
Sagittaproct S, 2273·4
Sagrada-Lax, 2273·4
Sagrosept, 2273·4
SaH-42548, 1589·1
Saintbois, 2273·4
Sairei-to, Kanebo— *see* Kanebo Sairei-to, 2074·2
Sairei-to, Tsumura— *see* Tsumura Sairei-to, 2351·1
Sais Andrews, 2273·4
Sais de Frutos, 2273·4
Sais Zitos, 2273·4
Saizen, 2273·4
Sal Amarum, 1228·2
Sal Ammoniac, 1115·2
Sal de Andrews, 2273·4
Sal de Fruta Eno, 2273·4
Sal de Vichy, 1223·2
Sal De Yasta, 2273·4
Sal Dietetica, 2273·4
Sal Lite, 2273·4
Sal Liviana En Sodio, 2273·4
Sal Sedativa de Homberg, 1662·1
Salac, 2273·4
Sal-Acid, 2273·4
Salact, 2273·4
Salactic Film, 2273·4
Salactol, 2273·4
Salagen, 2274·1
Salagesic, 2274·1
Salamidacetic Acid, 87·3
Salamidacético, Ácido, 87·3
Salamol, 2274·1
Salamol, Steri-Neb— *see* Steri-Neb Salamol, 2306·4
Salapin, 2274·1
Salatac, 2274·1
Salatac Gel, 2274·1
Salazine, 2274·1
Salazopirina, 2274·1
Salazoprin, 2274·1
Salazopyrin, 2274·1
Salazopyrina, 2274·1
Salazopyrine, 2274·1
Salazosulfapyridine, 1291·1
Salbei Curarina, 2274·1
Salbeiblätter, 1741·2
Salbei-Halspastillen, 2274·1
Salbetol, 2274·1
Salbu, 2274·1
Salbudan, 2274·1
Salbufax, 2274·1
Salbuhexal, 2274·1
Salbulair, 2274·1
Salbulin, 2274·1
Salbulind, 2274·1
Salbumol, 2274·1
Salbunova, 2274·1
Salbupp, 2274·1
Salburin, 2274·1
Salbusian, 2274·1
Salbutac, 2274·1
Salbutalan, 2274·1
Salbutalin, 2274·2
Salbutam, 2274·2
Salbutamax, 2274·2
Salbutamol, 791·3
Salbutamol Hemisulphate, 791·3
Salbutamol Sulfate, 791·3
Salbutamol, Sulfato de, 791·3
Salbutamol Sulphate, 791·3
Salbutamoli Sulfas, 791·3
Salbutamolum, 791·3
Salbutard, 2274·2
Salbuterol, 2274·2
Salbutib, 2274·2
Salbutol, 2274·2
Salbutol Beclo, 2274·2
Salbuvent, 2274·2
Salcacam, 2274·2
Salcal, 2274·2
Salcat, 2274·2
Salcatonin, 768·2
Salcedogen, 2274·2
Salcedol, 2274·2
Salcemetic, 2274·2
Salceryl, 2274·2
Salco, 2274·2
Salcoat, 2274·2
Salcotan, 2274·2
Saldac, 2274·2
Salder S, 2274·2
Saldeva, 2274·2
Salena, 2274·2
Sales de Frutas P G, 2274·2
Sales Fruta Mag Viviar, 2274·2
Saleto, 2274·2
Saleto-200, 2274·3
Saleto-D, 2274·3
Salflex, 2274·3
Salf-Pas, 2274·3
Salguer, 2274·3
Salgydal a la Noramidopyrine, 2274·3
Salhumin Preparations, 2274·3
Sali d'Achille, 2274·3
Sali di Salsomaggiore, 2274·3
Sali Iodati di Montecatini, 2274·3
Sali Lassativi di Chianciano, 2274·3
Sali Tamerici di Montecatini, 2274·3
Sali-Adalat, 2274·3
Sali-Aldopur, 2274·3
Salibra, 2274·3
Salic, 2274·3
Salicairine, 2274·3
Salicalcium, 2274·3
SaliCept, 2274·3
Salicil, 2274·3
Salicilamida, 87·3
Salicilato de Amonio, 14·2
Salicilato de Bismuto, 1252·1
Salicilato de Bismuto Composto, 2274·4
Salicilato de Bornilo, 21·2
Salicilato de Colina, 26·2
Salicilato de Dietilamina, 34·1
Salicilato de Eseridina, 1491·2
Salicilato de Etilo, 37·3
Salicilato de Fenilo, 88·1
Salicilato de Glicol, 44·3
Salicilato de Imidazol, 47·2
Salicilato de Isoamilo, 14·3
Salicilato de Litio, 54·2
Salicilato de Metilo, 59·3
Salicilato de Morfolinio, 63·3
Salicilato de Picolamina, 84·1
Salicilato de Trietanolamina, 95·3
Salicilato de Turfilo, 93·3
Salicilato Magnésico, 55·1
Salicilato Sódico, 90·1
Salicflico, Ácido, 1157·1
Salicin, 87·3
Salicina, 2274·4
Salicin-C, 2274·4

Salicis Cortex, 87·3
Salicort, 2274·4
Salicort-R, 2274·4
Salicrem, 2274·4
Salicrem K, 2274·4
Salicrem Miconazol, 2274·4
Salicyl, 2274·4
Salicyl Phenolic Glucuronide, 17·3
Salicyl Salicylate, 88·1
Salicylamide, 87·3
Salicylamide *O*-Acetic Acid, 87·3
Salicylanilides, Brominated, 1171·2
Salicylazosulfapyridine, 1291·1
Salicylcafeina, 2274·4
Salicylic Acid, 1157·1
Salicylic Acid Acetate, 15·1
Salicylic Acyl Glucuronide, 17·3
Salicylicum, Acidum, 1157·1
Salicylosalicylic Acid, 88·1
Salicylsalicylic Acid, 88·1
Salicylsyrevaselin— *see* Salsyvase, 2275·2
Salicyluric Acid, 17·3
Sali-Decoderm, 2274·4
Salidex, 2274·4
Salidur, 2274·4
Saliject, 2274·4
Salikaren, 2274·4
Saliker, 2274·4
Salilax, 2274·4
Salimar-Bad L, 2274·4
Saliment, 2274·4
Salimetin, 2274·4
Salimidin, 2274·4
Salimont, 2274·4
Salinal, 2274·4
SALINE, 1233·3
Saline Laxatives, 1239·3
Saline, Physiological, 1233·3
Salinex, 2274·4
Salinol, 2274·4
Salinomicina Sódica, 615·2
Salinomycin Sodium, 615·2
Salipads, 2274·4
Salipax, 2275·1
Salipran, 2275·1
Sali-Prent, 2275·1
Sali-Puren, 2275·1
Salipyrin, 82·3
Salirub, Vida— *see* Vida Salirub, 2376·2
*Salisburia adiantifolia*, 1692·3
Salisoap, 2275·1
Salisol, 2275·1
Sali-Spiroctan, 2275·1
Salisteril, 2275·1
Salistoperm, 2275·1
Salitanol Estreptomicina, 2275·1
Saliton, 2275·1
Saliva Medac, 2275·1
Saliva Orthana, 2275·1
Salivace, 2275·1
Salivan, 2275·1
Salivart, 2275·1
Saliveze, 2275·1
Salivix, 2275·1
Salix, 87·3, 2275·1
*Salix daphnoides*, 87·3
*Salix fragilis*, 87·3
*Salix purpurea*, 87·3
Salizylsäure, 1157·1
Salk Vaccine, 1633·3
Sallowthorn, 1742·2
Salmagne, 2275·1
Salmaplon, 2275·1
Salmaterol Xinafoate, 795·1
Salmax, 2275·1
Salmetedur, 2275·1
Salmeter, 2275·1
Salmeterol 1-Hydroxy-2-naphthoate, 795·1
Salmeterol Xinafoate, 795·1
Salmeterol, Xinafoato de, 795·1
Salmiak, 2275·1
Salmocalcin, 2275·1
Salmocide, 2275·1
Salmofar, 2275·1
Salmol, 2275·1
Salmol Expectorant, 2275·2
Salmon Calcitonin, 768·2
Salmon Oil, Farmed, 976·3
Salmonella Enteritis, 129·3
*Salmonella typhi*, 1642·2
Salmonellosis— *see* Salmonella Enteritis, 129·3
Salmonis Domestici Oleum, 976·3
Salmoten, 2275·2
Salmundin, 2275·2
Salnacedin, 1157·2
Salodiur, 2275·2
Salofalk, 2275·2
Sal-Oil-T, 2275·2
Salol, 88·1
Salomethyl, 2275·2
Salomol, 2275·2
Salonair, 2275·2
Salongo, 2275·2
Salonpas, 2275·2
Salopyrine, 2275·2
Salospir, 2275·2
Salpad, 2275·2
Salpetersäure, 1722·1
Salpingitis— *see* Pelvic Inflammatory Disease, 139·2
Sal-Plant, 2275·2
Salsalate, 88·1
Salsalato, 88·1
Salsaparilha, 1742·1
Salseb, 2275·2
Salsepareille, 1742·1
Salsitab, 2275·2
Salsol, 2275·2
Salsyvase, 2275·2
Salt, 1233·3
Salt Substitute, Morton— *see* Morton Salt Substitute, 2141·1
Saltadol, 2275·2
Saltamol, 2275·2
Saltermox, 2275·3
Salterpyn, 2275·3
Saltos, 2275·3
Saltpetre, 1190·1
Saltpetre, Chile, 1192·2
Saltrates, 2275·3
Saltrates Rodell, 2275·3
Sal-Tropine, 2275·3
Saltucin, 2275·3
Salubion, 2275·3
Salucur, 2275·3
Saludopin, 2275·3
Salugliben, 2275·3
Saluket-H1, 2275·3
Salures, 2275·3
Salures-K, 2275·3
Saluretin, 2275·3
Saluric, 2275·3
Salurin, 2275·3
Saluron, 2275·3
Salus Preparations, 2275·3
Salusa, 2275·4
Salusan, 2275·4
Salutaris, 2275·4
Salutensin, 2275·4
Salutina, 2275·4
Salva Infantes, 2275·4
Salvacam, 2275·4
Salvacolina NF, 2275·4
Salvacolon, 2275·4
Salvado, 1253·2
Salvalerg, 2275·4
Salvalion, 2275·4
Salvapen, 2275·4
Salvapen Mucolitico, 2275·4
Salvara, 2275·4
Salvarina, 2275·4
Salvatrim, 2275·4
Salvaxil, 2275·4
Salvent, 2275·4
Salverina, Hidrocloruro de, 1741·3
Salverine Hydrochloride, 1741·3
Salvesept, 2275·4
Salvi CAL E-G, 2275·4
Salvi CAL GX, 2275·4
Salvia, 1741·2
*Salvia fructicosa*, 1741·2
*Salvia officinalis*, 1741·2
*Salvia triloba*, 1741·2
Salviae Officinalis Folium, 1741·2
Salviae Trilobae Folium, 1741·2
Salviamin G-E, 2276·1
Salviamin GX-E, 2276·1
Salviamin Hepar, 2276·1
Salviamin X-E, 2276·1
Salviathymol N, 2276·1
Salvibest, 2276·1
Salvicutan, 2276·1
Salviette H, 2276·1
Salvilipid, 2276·1
Salvit M, 2276·1
Salvital, 2276·1
Salvitass, 2276·1
Salvstrumpa— *see* Zipzoc Salvstrumpa, 2394·2
Salvstrumpa, Zipzoc— *see* Zipzoc Salvstrumpa, 2394·2
Salvyl, 2276·1
Salvysat, 2276·1
Salycilina, 2276·1
Salysal, 88·1
Salzone, 2276·1
Salzsäure, 1699·1
Samarin, 2276·1
Samario 153, 1525·2
Samarium-153, 1525·2
Samarium ($^{153}$Sm) EDTMP, 1525·2
Samarium ($^{153}$Sm) Lexidronam, 1525·2
Sambil, 2276·1
Sambuc., 1741·3
Sambuci Flos, 1741·3
Sambuco (Specie Composta), 2276·1
Sambucol, 2276·1
Sambucus, 1741·3
Sambucus Complex, 2276·1
*Sambucus nigra*, 1741·3
SAMe, 1647·2
Same Plast, 2276·1
Samertan, 2276·1
Same-Seb, 2276·1
Same-Seb Beta, 2276·1
Samilstin, 2276·1
Samonil, 2276·1
Samonter, 2276·1
Samox, 2276·1
Samoxin, 2276·2
Samyr, 2276·2
Sanabronchiol, 2276·2
Sanaco, 2276·2
Sanacol, 2276·2
Sanacorte, 2276·2
Sanaden Reforzado, 2276·2
Sanaderm, 2276·2
Sanadermil, 2276·2
Sanadiar, 2276·2
Sanador, 2276·2
Sanadorn, 2276·2
Sanafen, 2276·2
Sanaform, 2276·2
Sanagas, 2276·2
Sanalepsi N, 2276·2
Sanaler, 2276·2
Sanaler-D, 2276·2
Sanalgin, 2276·2
Sanalgin N, 2276·2
Sanamidol, 2276·2
Sanaprav, 2276·2
Sana-Scrub, 2276·2
Sanasepton, 2276·2
Sana-Sol, 2276·2
Sanasthmax, 2276·2
Sanasthmyl, 2276·2
Sanatison Mono, 2276·3
Sanatogen, 2276·3
Sanato-Rhev, 2276·3
Sanaven, 2276·3
Sanaven Venentabletten, 2276·3
Sanavir, 2276·3
Sanavitan S, 2276·3
Sanaxin, 2276·3
Sanblex, 2276·3
Sancago, 2276·3
Sancap, 2276·3
Sancipro, 2276·3
Sancor Biosalud, 2276·3
Sanctura, 2276·3
Sanderson's Throat Specific, 2276·3
Sandimmun, 2276·3
Sandimmun Neoral, 2276·3
Sandimmune, 2276·3
Sandival, 2276·3
Sandival Desleible, 2276·3
Sandival NF, 2276·3
Sandocal, 2276·3
Sandocal-D, 2276·3
Sandoglobulin, 2276·4
Sandoglobulina, 2276·4
Sandoglobuline, 2276·4
Sando-K, 2276·4
Sandolanid, 2276·4
Sandomigran, 2276·4
Sandomigrin, 2276·4
Sandonorm, 2276·4
Sandoparin, 2276·4
Sandoparine, 2276·4
Sandopart, 2276·4
Sandoretic, 2276·4
Sandosource, 2276·4
Sandosource GI Control— *see* Novasource GI Control, 2176·4
Sandosource Peptide, 2276·4
Sandostatin, 2276·4
Sandostatina, 2276·4
Sandostatine, 2276·4
Sandovac, 2276·4
Sandoven, 2276·4
Sandoz Ca-D, 2276·4
Sandoz Calcium, 2276·4
Sandoz Calcium + Vitamine C, 2277·1
Sandoz Calcium-C, 2277·1
Sandrena, 2277·1
Sanein, 2277·1
Sanelor, 2277·1
Sanepa Forte, 2277·1
Sanerva, 2277·1
Sangcya, 2277·1
Sangen, 2277·1
Sangen Casa, 2277·1
Sangen Sapone Disinfettante, 2277·1
Sangenor, 2277·1
Sangerol, 2277·1
Sangobion, 2277·1
Sangotone, 2277·1
Sangre, 743·3
Sangsue, 945·1
Sanguessugas, 945·1
Sanguijuela, 945·1
Sanguinaria, 1741·3
Sanguinaria Canadensis, 1741·3
*Sanguinaria canadensis*, 1741·3
Sanguinarine, 1741·3
Sanguinarine Canadensis, 1741·3
Sanguinaris Canadensis, 1741·3
Sanguisan N, 2277·1
Sanguisorba, 1663·2
*Sanguisorba officinalis*, 1663·2
Sanguisorbis N, 2277·1
Sanguisuga, 945·1
Sangur-Test, 2277·1
Sanhelios Preparations, 2277·1
Sanicel, 2277·1
Sanicolax, 2277·1
Sanicopyrine, 2277·2
SaniDrox, 2277·2
Sanieb, 2277·2
Sanifer, 2277·2
Saniflor Collutorio, 2277·2
Saniflor Vena, 2277·2
Sanifolin, 2277·2
Sanifug, 2277·2
Sanigermin, 2277·2
Sanil Menta Bucal, 2277·2
Sanilin, 2277·2
Sanipresin, 2277·2
Sanipresin-D, 2277·2
Saniprostol, 2277·2
Saniquiet, 2277·2
SaniSteril Deterferri, 2277·2
SaniSteril Sterilferri, 2277·2

SaniSteril Strumenti Alcolico, 2277·2
Sani-Supp, 2277·2
Saniter Compuesto, 2277·2
Sanitos, 2277·2
Sanivit, 2277·2
Sanjin Royal Jelly, 2277·2
Sankombi, 2277·2
Sanmigran, 2277·2
Sano Tuss, 2277·2
Sanobamat, 2277·2
Sanoclorofila, 2277·2
Sanoderm, 2277·2
Sanodin, 2277·2
Sanoformine, 2277·2
Sanogyl, 2277·3
Sanogyl Bianco, 2277·3
Sanogyl Fluo, 2277·3
Sanogyl Junior, 2277·3
Sanoma, 2277·3
Sanomigran, 2277·3
Sanopinwern, 2277·3
Sanopinwern T, 2277·3
Sanor, 2277·3
Sanoral, 2277·3
Sanorex, 2277·3
Sanorvil, 2277·3
Sanostol, 2277·3
Sanovit, 2277·3
Sanoxit, 2277·3
Sanoyodo, 2277·3
Sanpronol, 2277·3
Sans Soleil Skin Ceuticals, 2277·3
Sansacne, 2277·3
Sans-Acne, 2277·3
Sansanal, 2277·3
Sansert, 2277·3
Sansudor, 2277·3
Santa Flora S, 2277·3
Santaherba, 2277·3
Santalyt, 2277·3
Santamex-Expectorant, 2277·3
Santane $A_4$, 2277·3
Santane $C_6$, 2277·4
Santane $D_5$, 2277·4
Santane $F_{10}$, 2277·4
Santane $H_7$, 2277·4
Santane $N_9$, 2277·4
Santane $O_1$, 2277·4
Santane $R_8$, 2277·4
Santane $V_3$, 2277·4
Santasal N, 2277·4
Santasapina V, 2277·4
Santasapina Nouvelle Formule, 2277·4
Santax S, 2277·4
Santenol, 2277·4
Santevini, 2277·4
Santheose, 798·2
Santin, 2277·4
Santonica, 114·1
Santonin, 114·1
Santonina, 114·1
Santoninum, 114·1
Santus, 2277·4
Santussal, 2277·4
Santyl, 2277·4
Sanukehl, 2277·4
Sanutri Osseo, 2277·4
Sanuvis, 2277·4
Sanvapress, 2277·4
Sanvar, 1342·2
Sanvita Bronchial, 2277·4
Sanvita Enerlecit, 2278·1
Sanvita Leber-Galle, 2278·1
Sanvita Magen, 2278·1
Sanxon, 2278·1
Sanyrene, 2278·1
Sanytol, 2278·1
Sanzur, 2278·1
Sanzyme-DS, 2278·1
Sanzyme-S, 2278·1
Sao Joao, Xarope— *see* Xarope Sao Joao, 2387·4
Sapec, 2278·1
Saperconazol, 408·1
Saperconazole, 408·1
Sapo Mollis, 1575·2
Sapoderm, 2278·1
Saponite, 1577·1
Sapresta, 2278·1
Sapriken, 2278·1
Sapropterin Hydrochloride, 1742·1
Sapropterina, Hidrocloruro de, 1742·1
Sapucai, 2278·1
Saquat, 2278·1
Saquinavir, 653·3
Saquinavir Mesilate, 653·3
Saquinavir, Mesilato de, 653·3
Saquinavir Mesylate, 653·3
Saquinavir Methanesulfonate, 653·3
Sara, 2278·1
Sarafem, 2278·1
Sarafloxacin Hydrochloride, 254·3
Sarafloxacino, Hidrocloruro de, 254·3
Saralasin Acetate, 996·3
Saralasina, Acetato de, 996·3
Sarapin, 2278·1
Saratoga, 2278·1
Sarcoderma, 2278·1
Sarcoidosis, 1087·2
Sarcolysine, 566·1
L-Sarcolysine, 566·1
Sarcoma of Bone— *see* Bone Sarcoma, 524·3
Sarcoma, Ewing's— *see* Bone Sarcoma, 524·3
Sarcoma, Kaposi's— *see* Kaposi's Sarcoma, 524·3
Sarcoma, Osteogenic— *see* Bone Sarcoma, 524·3
Sarcoma, Soft-tissue— *see* Soft-tissue Sarcoma, 525·2
Sarcomas, 524·3
Sarcop, 2278·1
Sarcoton, 2278·1
Sarf, 2278·1
Sargenor, 2278·1
Sargenor a la Vitamine C, 2278·1
Sargepirine, 2278·1
Sargramostim, 760·1
Saridine, 2278·1
Saridon, 2278·1
Saridon N, 2278·2
Saridon Neu— *see* Saridon, 2278·1
Sarilen, 2278·2
Sarin, 1719·2
Sarna Preparations, 2278·2
Sarnapen, 2278·2
Sarnaton, 2278·2
Sarnigal, 2278·2
Sarnisan, 2278·2
Sarnodex, 2278·2
Sarnol, 2278·2
Sarolin, 2278·2
Saromet, 2278·2
Saroten, 2278·2
Sarotena, 2278·2
Sarotex, 2278·2
*Sarothamnus scoparius*, 1742·2
Sarpagandha, 994·3
Sarpagine, 994·3
Sarpiol, 2278·2
Sarpogrelate Hydrochloride, 996·3
Sarpogrelato, Hidrocloruro de, 996·3
Sarpul, 2278·2
Sarracenia Purpurea, 88·2
SARS, 625·1
Sarsa, 1742·1
Sarsaparilla, 1742·1
Sarsaparilla Root, 1742·1
Sarsaparol Uro, 2278·2
Sarsapsor, 2278·2
Sartol, 2278·2
Sartuzin, 2278·2
Saruplasa, 996·3
Saruplase, 996·3
SAS, 2278·2
Sasafrás, Aceite Esencial de, 1742·1
Sasapyrine, 88·1
Saspryl, 2278·2
*Sassafras albidum*, 1742·1
Sassafras Oil, 1742·1
Sassafras, Oleum, 1742·1
Sastid, 2278·2
Sastid Anti-Fungal, 2278·3
Sastid Jabon, 2278·3
Sasulen, 2278·3
Satedon, 2278·3
Satigene, 2278·3
Satinique Anti-Dandruff, 2278·3
Sativol, 2278·3
Saton, 2278·3
Satraplatin, 583·2
Satraplatino, 583·2
Satumomab Pendetide, Indium ($^{111}$In), 1524·1
Saturnil, 2278·3
Saúco, 1741·3
Sauerstoff, 1236·3
Sauge, Feuilles de, 1741·2
Saugella, 2278·3
Saugella Gel, 2278·3
Saugella Idrocrema, 2278·3
Saugella Intilac, 2278·3
Saugella Salviettine, 2278·3
Saugella Uomo, 2278·3
Sauran, 2278·3
Saurat, 2278·3
Savacol Mouth and Throat Rinse, 2278·3
Savarine, 2278·3
Savecal, 2278·3
Saventrine, 2278·3
Savex Preparations, 2278·3
Savilen, 2278·3
Savior, 2278·3
Savlodil, 2278·3
Savlodil— *see* Hibicet verdunning, 2044·2
Savlon Preparations, 2278·3
Savlon— *see* Hibicet concentraat, 2044·2
Savlon Hospital Concentrate— *see* Hibicet, 2044·2
Savoral, 2278·4
Savorix T, 2278·4
Saw Palmetto, 1569·1
Saw Palmetto Formula, 2278·4
Saw Palmetto Fruit, 1569·1
Sawmetto Vivo-Livo, 2278·4
Saxitoxin, 1742·1
Saxitoxina, 1742·1
Sayomol, 2278·4
Sazo, 2278·4
SB-1, 912·2
Sb-58, 103·1
SB-75, 1320·2
SB-075, 1320·2
SB-5833, 674·1
SB-7505, 937·3
SB-265805, 216·3
SB-209509AX, 469·2
SB-265805S, 216·3
SBOB, 2278·4
SBP, 1750·3
SBPA Analgesic/Calmative, 2278·4
SC-300, 2278·4
SC-0735, 1722·1
SC-1749, 1711·3
SC-2910, 485·3
SC-4642, 1563·1
SC-7031, 903·3
SC-9376, 879·1
SC-9420, 1003·1
SC-9880, 1555·2
SC-10295, 607·2
SC-10363, 1558·2
SC-11585, 1565·1
SC-11800, 1554·2
SC-13957, 903·3
SC-14266, 984·2
SC-18862, 1422·1
SC-21009, 1563·2
SC-29333, 1519·2
SC-30695, 1519·3
SC-32642, 607·2
SC-37681, 1518·1
SC-47111, 227·2
SC-47111A, 227·2
SC-47111B, 227·2
SC-48334, 1715·2
SC-49088, 202·1
SC-54684A, 1029·2
SC-57099-B, 977·2
SC-58635, 25·2
SC-65872, 96·1
SC-66110, 911·3
SC-69124A, 79·2
Scabecid, 2278·4
Scabene, 2278·4
Scabenzil, 2278·4
Scabexyl, 2278·4
Scabicin, 2278·4
Scabies, 1499·1
Scabiex, 2278·4
Scabine, 2278·4
Scabioderm, 2279·1
Scabioid, 2279·1
Scabisan, 2279·1
Scabisan Plus, 2279·1
Scadan, 2279·1
Scaflam, 2279·1
Scalded Skin Syndrome— *see* Drug-induced Skin Reactions, 1134·3
Scalded Skin Syndrome— *see* Toxic Epidermal Necrolysis, 1138·3
Scalded Skin Syndrome, Staphylococcal— *see* Skin Infections, 146·2
Scalid, 2279·1
Scalpicin, 2279·1
Scalpicin Anti-Dandruff Anti-Itch, 2279·1
Scalpicin Capilar, 2279·1
Scalpin, 2279·1
Scalpvit, 2279·1
Scammony Resin, 1267·3
Scammony Root, 1267·3
Scandicain, 2279·1
Scandicaine, 2279·1
Scandine, 2279·1
Scandinibsa, 2279·1
Scandinor, 2279·1
Scandishake, 2279·1
Scandonest, 2279·1
Scanlux, 2279·1
Scannotrast, 2279·1
Scarfade, 2279·1
Scarlet, Brilliant, 1057·3
Scarlet Fever, Staphylococcal— *see* Skin Infections, 146·2
Scarlet GN, 545·3
Scarlet Red, 1191·3
Scavenger, 2279·1
SCE-129, 180·2
SCE-963, 177·2
SCE-1365, 173·2
SCF, 742·2
Sch-1000, 787·1
Sch-1000-Br-monohydrate, 787·1
Sch-3444, 487·2
Sch-4358, 1106·1
Sch-4831, 1093·1
Sch-4855, 1129·2
Sch-6783, 893·2
Sch-9384, 1126·1
Sch-9724, 217·1
Sch-10144, 410·1
Sch-10159, 726·2
Sch-10304, 26·3
Sch-10649, 425·1
Sch-11460, 1093·1
Sch-12041, 701·2
Sch-13475, 254·3
Sch-13521, 556·2
Sch-13949W, 791·3
Sch-14714, 43·3
Sch-15719W, 943·3
Sch-16134, 718·2
Sch-18020W, 1091·1
Sch-20569, 236·3
Sch-21420, 222·2
Sch-22219, 1090·3
Sch-25298, 213·3
Sch-28316Z, 939·1
Sch-29851, 436·1
Sch-30500, 640·3
Sch-32088, 1107·2
Sch-32481, 110·1
Sch-33844, 1003·1

Sch-34117, 431·1
Sch-39300, 756·1
Sch-39304, 400·3
Sch-39720, 182·1
Sch-52000, 1700·3
Sch-52365, 587·1
Sch-56592, 407·3
Sch-58235, 914·2
Sch-60936, 912·2
Sch-209579, 1462·1
Schachtelhalmkraut, 1684·1
Schafgarbe, 1646·2
Schamill, 2279·2
Scharlachrot, 1191·3
Scheinpharm Artificial Tears, 2279·2
Scheinpharm Artificial Tears Plus, 2279·2
Scheinpharm Testone-Cyp, 2279·2
Scheinpharm Triamcine-A, 2279·2
Schellack, 1743·3
Scheribar, 2279·2
Scheribase, 2279·2
Schericur, 2279·2
Scheriderm, 2279·2
Schering Base, 2279·2
Schering PC4, 2279·2
Scheriproct, 2279·2
Scheriproct N, 2279·2
Scheriproct Neo, 2279·2
Scherisorb— *see* Intrasite, 2064·2
Scherogel, 2279·2
Schias-Amaro Medicinale, 2279·2
Schick Control, 1742·2
Schick Test, 1742·2
Schick Test Control, 1742·2
Schick Test Toxin, 1742·2
Schiff Reagent, 1185·2
Schiller's Iodine, 1599·1
Schinsent, 1693·1
Schistosomiasis, 100·3
Schistosomiasis Vaccines, 1638·2
Schiwalys Hemofiltration, 2279·2
Schizophrenia, 665·3
Schizophyllan, 583·3
*Schizophyllum commune*, 583·3
Schizopol, 2279·2
Schlaf- und Nerventee, 2279·2
SchlafTabs, 2279·2
Schlehepar N, 2279·2
Schleimhaut-Komplex Ho-Fu-Complex, 2279·2
Schlüsselblumenwurzel, 1735·1
Schmerz-Dolgit, 2279·2
Schneckensaft N, 2279·2
Schneckensirup, 2279·2
Schneckensirup, Original— *see* Original Schneckensirup, 2192·3
Schnupfen Endrine, 2279·2
*Schoenocaulon officinale*, 1763·3
Scholl Preparations, 2279·2
Schöllkraut, 1695·3
Schoolife, 2279·3
Schoum, 2279·3
Schrundensalbe Dermi-cyl, 2279·3
Schufen, 2279·3
Schultz No. 1038, 1042·2
Schupps Preparations, 2279·3
Schwarzer Senfsame, 1718·2
Schwarze-Salbe, 2279·3
Schwarzwalder Heublumen-Extrakt, 2279·3
Schwedenbitter, Tiroler Adler— *see* Tiroler Adler Schwedenbitter, 2333·4
Schweden-Mixtur H Nouvelle Formulation, 2279·4
Schwedentrunk, 2279·4
Schwedentrunk Elixier, 2279·4
Schwedentrunk mit Ginseng, 2279·4
Schwefel, 1158·2
Schwefelbad Dr Klopfer, 2279·4
Schwefelbad-Saar, 2279·4
Schwefel-Diasporal, 2279·4
Schwefelkohlenstoff, 1472·1
Schwefelleber, 1158·3
Schwohepan S, 2279·4
Schwoneural, 2279·4
Schworalgan, 2279·4
Schworocard, 2279·4
Schworocor, 2279·4
Schworosin, 2279·4
Schworotox, 2279·4
Schworotox N, 2279·4
Sciargo, 2279·4
Sciatica— *see* Low Back Pain, 7·1
SCID, 1729·2
Scilla, 1130·3
Scillacor, 2279·4
Scillae Bulbus, 1130·3
Scillase N, 2279·4
Scille, 1130·3
Scilliroside, 1509·3
Scintadren, 2279·4
Sciomir, 2279·4
Sciroppo Berta, 2279·4
Sciroppo Fenoglio, 2279·4
Sciroppo Merck all'Efetonina, 2279·4
Scitropin, 2279·4
Sclane, 2279·4
Scleramin, 2279·4
Scleremo, 2280·1
Scleril, 2280·1
Scleritis, 1088·1
Sclerobion, 2280·1
Sclerocalcine, 2280·1
Scleroderma, 1348·1
Sclerodex, 2280·1
Sclerodine, 2280·1
Sclerofin, 2280·1
Scleromate, 2280·1
Sclerosis, Systemic— *see* Scleroderma, 1348·1
Sclerosol, 2280·1
Sclerovein, 2280·1
SCMC, 1577·3, 2280·1
SCMC Promethazine, 2280·1
S-Coaltar, 2280·1
Scoburen, 2280·1
Scoline, 2280·1
Scolybil, 2280·1
Scopace, 2280·1
Scopanil, 2280·1
Scoparii Cacumina, 1742·2
Scoparium, 1742·2
Scopas, 2280·1
Scope, 2280·1
Scope with Oraseptate— *see* Scope, 2280·1
Scopex, 2280·1
Scopex Co, 2280·1
Scopinal, 2280·1
Scopoderm, 2280·1
Scopoderm TTS, 2280·1
Scopolamine, 483·3
Scopolamine Bromhydrate, 483·3
Scopolamine *N*-Butyl Bromide, 483·3
Scopolamine Butylbromide, 483·3
Scopolamine Hydrobromide, 483·3
Scopolamine Methobromide, 483·3
Scopolamine Methonitrate, 483·3
Scopolamine Methylbromide, 483·3
Scopolamine Methylnitrate, 483·3
Scopolamini Hydrobromidum, 483·3
Scopoletin, 1762·1
Scopolomini Butylbromidum, 483·3
Scorbex, 2280·1
Scordal, 2280·1
Scorotox, 2280·2
Scorpion Antivenins, 1638·3
Scorpion Antivenoms, 1638·3
Scorpion Stings, 1638·3
Scorpion Venom Antisera, 1638·3
Scotch Spearmint, 1749·1
Scott Dandruff Shampoo, 2280·2
Scott, Emulsao— *see* Emulsao Scott, 1968·3
Scottopect, 2280·2
Scott's Cod Liver, 2280·2
Scott's Emulsion, 2280·2
Scott's Emulsion Orange, 2280·2
Scott's Emulsion Original, 2280·2
Scot-Tussin Preparations, 2280·2
SCR, 2280·2
SCR1, 1675·2
SCR1-3, 1675·2
Scriptolyte, 2280·2
Scripto-Metic, 2280·2
Scrub Typhus— *see* Typhus, 152·3
SCT-1, 768·2
Scuffle, 1730·3
Scullcap, 1746·3
Scullcap & Gentian Tablets, 2280·2
ScuPA, 996·3
Scurvy, 1461·1
Scutellaria, 1746·3
*Scutellaria*, 1746·3
*Scutellaria baicalensis*, 1746·3
*Scutellaria barbata*, 1746·3
*Scutellaria lateriflora*, 1746·3
SD-271-12, 1585·3
SD-1248-17, 491·1
SD-1750, 1503·2
SD-8447, 1510·2
SD-17102, 955·2
SD-43775, 1505·2
SD2-CV-205-502, 1213·1
SD-Hermal, 2280·2
SDL, 2280·2
SDV, 2280·2
SDZ-212-713, 1497·1
SDZ-ASM-981, 1155·1
SDZ-CHI-621, 1351·1
SDZ-DJN-608, 343·3
SDZ-ENA-713, 1497·1
SDZ-HTF-919, 1293·2
SDZ-PSC-833, 591·1
711-SE, 983·3
SE-780, 868·1
SE-1520, 938·2
SE-1702, 332·1
SE-2395, 1011·1
Sea Breeze, 2280·2
Sea Buckthorn, 1742·2
Sea Buckthorn Oil, 1742·3
Sea Sickness— *see* Nausea and Vomiting, 1245·2
Sea Squirt, 546·3
Sea Wasp Antivenin, 1621·3
Sea Wasp Sting— *see* Box Jellyfish Sting, 1621·3
Seabell, 2280·2
Sea-buckthorn, 1742·2
Sea-Cal, 2280·2
Seacor, 2280·2
Seal On, 2280·2
Seal Finger— *see* Bites and Stings, 121·3
Sealdin, 2280·2
Sea-Legs, 2280·2
Seale's Lotion, 2280·3
Seal-On, 2280·3
SeaMist, 2280·3
Sea-Omega, 2280·3
Seaprose S, 1735·2
Seasonal Affective Disorder, 278·1
Seasonale, 2280·3
Seasorb Soft, 2280·3
Seatone, 2280·3
Seaweeds, Kelps, and Wracks, 1742·3
Sebacato de Dibutilo, 1679·3
Sebacic Acid, 1157·3
Sebácico, Ácido, 1157·3
Sebacnol, 2280·3
Sebaklen, 2280·3
Sebamed, 2280·3
Sebamed, Baby— *see* Baby Sebamed, 1824·2
Sebamed Suncream 20, 2280·3
Sebamed Suncream 28, 2280·3
Sebamed Sunlotion, 2280·3
Seba-Nil, 2280·3
Sebaquin, 2280·3
Sebasorb, 2280·3
Sebaveen, 2280·3
Sebcur, 2280·3
Sebcur/T, 2280·3
Sebercim, 2280·3
Sebex, 2280·3
Sebexol, 2280·3
Sebexol cum Urea, 2280·3
Sebex-T, 2280·3
Sebiprox, 2280·3
Sebirinse, 2280·3
Sebitar, 2280·3
Sebium K2, 2280·3
Sebizole, 2280·4
Sebizon, 2280·4
Sebo, 2280·4
Sebo Concept D/A, 2280·4
Sebo Creme, 2280·4
Sebo Shampooing, 2280·4
Sebolic, 2280·4
Sebolith, 2280·4
Sebomin, 2280·4
Sebophane, 2280·4
Sebo-Psor, 2280·4
Seborrhoeic Dermatitis, 1138·3
Seborrhoeic Folliculitis— *see* Seborrhoeic Dermatitis, 1138·3
Seborrol, 2280·4
Sebosel, 2280·4
Sebo-Soufrol, 2280·4
Sebosquam, 2280·4
Sebrane, 2280·4
Sebrane Rhume, 2280·4
Sebryl, 2280·4
Sebryl Plus, 2280·4
Sebucare, 2280·4
Sebulex, 2280·4
Sebulon, 2280·4
Sebumselen, 2280·4
Sebutone, 2280·4
Secabiol, 2280·4
Secadine, 2280·4
Secadrex, 2281·1
Secalan, 2281·1
Secalbum, 2281·1
Secale, 2281·1
*Secale cereale*, 1685·1
Secale Cornutum, 1685·1
Secale Med Complex, 2281·1
Secalip, 2281·1
Secalosan N, 2281·1
Secalysat, 2281·1
Secalysat EM, 2281·1
Secamin, 2281·1
Secand, 2281·1
Secaris, 2281·1
Secbutabarbital, 721·2
Secbutabarbital Sódico, 721·2
Secbutabarbital Sodium, 721·2
Secbutobarbital, 721·2
Secbutobarbital Sodium, 721·2
Secbutobarbitone, 721·2
Secbutobarbitone Sodium, 721·2
Seclodin, 2281·1
Secnid, 2281·1
Secnidal, 2281·1
Secnidalin, 2281·1
Secnidazol, 615·3
Secnidazole, 615·3
Secnil, 2281·1
Secni-Plus, 2281·1
Secnizol, 2281·1
Secnol, 2281·1
Seco, 2281·1
Secobarbital, 721·2
Secobarbital Sódico, 721·2
Secobarbital Sodium, 721·2
Secobarbitalum, 721·2
Secobarbitalum Natricum, 721·2
Secobarbitone, 721·2
Secobarbitone Sodium, 721·2
(5*Z*,7*E*)-9,10-Secocholesta-5,7,10(19)-triene-1α,3β-diol, 1461·2
(5*Z*,7*E*)-9,10-Secocholesta-5,7,10(19)-triene-3β,25-diol Monohydrate, 1461·2
(5*Z*,7*E*)-9,10-Secocholesta-5,7,10(19)-triene-1α,3β,25-triol, 1461·2
(+)-(5*Z*,7*E*,24*R*)-9,10-Secocholesta-5,7,10(19)-triene-1α,3β,24-triol Monohydrate, 1158·3
(5*Z*,7*E*)-9,10-Secocholesta-5,7,10(19)-trien-3β-ol, 1461·3
(5*Z*,7*E*,22*E*)-9,10-Secoergosta-5,7,10(19),22-tetraene-1α,3β-diol, 1462·1
(5*Z*,7*E*,22*E*)-9,10-Secoergosta-5,7,10(19),22-tetraen-3β-ol, 1462·1

(*5E,7E,22E*)-10α-9,10-Secoergosta-5,7,22-trien-3β-ol, 1461·3
Secokapton, 2281·1
Seconal, 2281·1
Secondary Propyl Alcohol, 1184·3
Secotex, 2281·1
Secpel, 2281·1
Secpel Composto, 2281·1
Secran, 2281·1
SecreFlo, 2281·1
Secrelux, 2281·1
Secrepat, 2281·1
Secrepina, 2281·2
Secresol, 2281·2
Secret 28, 2281·2
Secretil, 2281·2
Secretin, 1742·3
Secretina, 1742·3
Secretory Neoplasms— *see* Carcinoid Tumours and Other Secretory Neoplasms, 504·1
Sectam, 2281·2
Sectral, 2281·2
Sectrazide, 2281·2
Secubar, 2281·2
Secubar Diu, 2281·2
Secuentex-21, 2281·2
Secumalnatrium, 721·2
Se-Cure, 2281·2
Securgin, 2281·2
Securo, 2281·2
Securon, 2281·2
Securon, Half— *see* Half Securon, 2035·2
Securopen, 2281·2
Securpres, 2281·2
Seczol, 2281·2
Seda Kneipp N, 2281·2
Sedabarb, 2281·2
Sedabel, 2281·2
Sedaben, 2281·2
Sedacalman, 2281·2
Sedacollyre, 2281·2
Sedacoron, 2281·2
Sedacris, 2281·2
Sedactrim, 2281·2
Sedactrim Balsamico, 2281·2
Sedacur, 2281·2
Seda-Do, 2281·2
Sedadom, 2281·3
Seda-Gel, 2281·3
Sedagin, 2281·3
Seda-Grandelat, 2281·3
Sedagripe, 2281·3
Sedagul, 2281·3
Sedakatt, 2281·3
Sedalen Cort, 2281·3
Sedalene, 2281·3
Sedalex, 2281·3
Sedalgina, 2281·3
Sedalin, 2281·3
Sedalint Baldrian, 2281·3
Sedalint Kava, 2281·3
Sedalipid, 2281·3
Sedalito, 2281·3
Sedalmerck, 2281·3
Sedalmerck TH, 2281·3
Sedalozia, 2281·3
Sedalpan, 2281·3
Sedanium-R, 2281·3
Sedans, 2281·3
Sedante Arceli, 2281·3
Sedante Dia, 2281·3
Sedante Nativa, 2281·4
Sedante Noche, 2281·4
Sedantol, 2281·4
Sedanxol— *see* Ciatyl-Z, 1885·2
Sedapain, 2281·4
Sedapap, 2281·4
Sedaplaie, 2281·4
Seda-Plantina, 2281·4
Sedaplus, 2281·4
Seda-Rash, 2281·4
Sedarene, 2281·4
Sedariston, 2281·4
Sedariston Konzentrat, 2281·4
Sedartryl, 2281·4
Sedaselect, 2281·4
Sedaselect D, 2281·4
Sedasept, 2281·4
Sedasol eco natura, 2281·4
Sedasor, 2281·4
Sedaspir, 2281·4
Sedastip, 2281·4
Sedasyx, 2281·4
Sedatif PC, 2281·4
Sedatif Tiber, 2281·4
Sedation, 666·2
Sedation, Dental— *see* Dental Sedation, 666·2
Sedation in Endoscopy— *see* Endoscopy, 666·2
Sedation in Intensive Care— *see* Intensive Care, 666·3
Sedatival, 2281·4
Sedativum-Hevert, 2282·1
Sedatol, 2282·1
Sedatonyl, 2282·1
Sedatoss, 2282·1
Sedatruw S, 2282·1
Sedatus, 2282·1
Sedatuss, 2282·1
Sedatuss DM, 2282·1
Sedatux, 2282·1
Sedauric, 2282·1
Sedazin, 2282·1
Sedergine, 2282·1
Sedergine C, 2282·1
Sedermyl, 2282·1
Sedesterol, 2282·1
Sedevil, 2282·1
Sedex, 2282·1
Sediat, 2282·1
Sedibaine, 2282·1
Sedicepan, 2282·1
Sediclon, 2282·1
Sediel, 2282·1
Sedilax, 2282·1
Sedilene Procto, 2282·1
Sedilit, 2282·1
Sedilix, 2282·1
Sedilix DM, 2282·2
Sedilor, 2282·2
Sedinal, 2282·2
Sedinfant N, 2282·2
Sedinol, 2282·2
Sedioton, 2282·2
Sedisan, 2282·2
Sediten, 2282·2
Sediver, 2282·2
Sedizepan, 2282·2
Sedlitz, Sel de, 1228·2
Sedo, 2282·2
Sedobex, 2282·2
Sedobion, 2282·2
Sedobrina, 2282·2
Sedocalcio, 2282·2
Sedocardin, 2282·2
Sedodermil, 2282·2
Sedofan, 2282·2
Sedofan II, 2282·2
Sedofan DM, 2282·2
Sedofan P, 2282·2
Sedofan T, 2282·2
Sedofantil, 2282·2
Sedofarin, 2282·2
Sedofit, 2282·2
Sedogastrol, 2282·2
Sedogelat, 2282·2
Sedogelat Forte, 2282·2
Sedol, 2282·3
Sedonat, 2282·3
Sedonium, 2282·3
Sedopal, 2282·3
Sedopect, 2282·3
Sedophon, 2282·3
Sedopretten, 2282·3
Sedopuer F, 2282·3
Sedoran, 2282·3
Sedorrhoide, 2282·3
Sedosan N, 2282·3
Sedosil, 2282·3
Sedosolvin, 2282·3
Sedotensil, 2282·3
Sedotime, 2282·3
Sedotus, 2282·3
Sedotusse, 2282·3
Sedotussin Preparations, 2282·3
Sedovegan, 2282·4
Sedovegan Novo, 2282·4
Sedovent, 2282·4
Sedoxil, 2282·4
Sedural, 2282·4
Seduspar, 2282·4
Sefal, 2282·4
Sefaretic, 2282·4
Sefasin, 2282·4
Sefdene, 2282·4
Sefdin, 2282·4
Seferin, 2282·4
Sefloc, 2282·4
Sefmal, 2282·4
Sefmex, 2282·4
Sefmic, 2282·4
Sefnor, 2282·4
Seforman, 2282·4
Seftem, 2282·4
Seftil, 2282·4
Sefulken, 2282·4
Segel, 2282·4
Seglor, 2282·4
Segurex, 2282·4
Seguril, 2282·4
$^{75}$SeHCAT, 1525·2
Seide, 2282·4
Seifenrinde, 1416·1
Seignette Salt, 1284·3
Seikivita, 2282·4
Seis-B, 2282·4
Seizures, Alcohol Withdrawal— *see* Alcohol Withdrawal and Abstinence, 1166·2
Seizures, Anoxic— *see* Anoxic Seizures, 478·2
Seizures, Eclamptic— *see* Eclampsia and Pre-eclampsia, 352·3
Seizures, Epileptic— *see* Epilepsy, 349·1
Seizures, Febrile— *see* Febrile Convulsions, 353·1
Seizures, Neonatal— *see* Neonatal Seizures, 353·2
Seizures, Post-traumatic— *see* Post-traumatic Seizures, 376·1
Sejungin B, 2282·4
Sekalax, 2282·4
Seki, 2283·1
Sekin, 2283·1
Sekisan, 2283·1
Sekitol, 2283·1
Sekretolin, 2283·1
Sekretovit, 2283·1
Sekretovit Amoxi, 2283·1
Sekretovit Ex, 2283·1
Sekucid, 2283·1
Sekucid Konz, 2283·1
Sekudrill, 2283·1
Sekugerm, 2283·1
Sekumatic, 2283·1
Sekumatic FD, 2283·1
Sekumatic FDR, 2283·1
Sekusept Preparations, 2283·1
Sel Anglais, 1228·2
Sel D, 2283·1
Sel de Sedlitz, 1228·2
Sel d'Ems, 2283·1
Seladin, 2283·1
Selamectin, 114·1
Selamectina, 114·1
Selan, 2283·1
Selanac, 2283·1
Selanir, 2283·1
Selax, 2283·2
Selaxa, 2283·2
Selbex, 2283·2
Sel'bis, 2283·2
Seldane, 2283·2
Selebound, 2283·2
Selecid, 2283·2
Selecim, 2283·2
Selecom, 2283·2
Select 1/35, 2283·2
Selectadoce, 2283·2
Selectadril, 2283·2
Selectafer N, 2283·2
Selectan, 2283·2
Selecten, 2283·2
Selectin, 2283·2
Selective Alpha$_1$ Blockers, 809·2
Selective Digestive Tract Decontamination— *see* Intensive Care, 132·2
Selective Serotonin Reuptake Inhibitors, 278·2, 296·3
Selecto, 2283·2
Selectocalcio, 2283·2
Selecto-D, 2283·2
Selectofen, 2283·2
Selectofur, 2283·2
Selectografin, 2283·2
Selectol, 2283·2
Selectomycin, 2283·2
Selectovit, 2283·2
Selectrim, 2283·2
Selecturon, 2283·2
Selectus, 2283·2
Selectus FN, 2283·3
Seledat, 2283·3
Seledie, 2283·3
Selefusin, 2283·3
Selegam, 2283·3
Selegel, 2283·3
Selegil, 2283·3
Selegilina, Hidrocloruro de, 1214·1
Selegiline Hydrochloride, 1214·1
Selegilini Hydrochloridum, 1214·1
Selegos, 2283·3
Selektine, 2283·3
Selemax, 2283·3
Selemerck, 2283·3
Selemite-B, 2283·3
Selemite B Tablets, Vitaglow— *see* Vitaglow Selemite B, 2381·1
Selemix, 2283·3
Selemun, 2283·3
Selemycin, 2283·3
Selen, 2283·3
Selenarell, 2283·3
Selenase, 2283·3
Selenato Potásico, 1444·1
Selene, 2283·3
*Selenicereus grandiflorus*, 1669·2
Selenii Disulfidum, 1157·3
Selenio, 1444·1
Selenio 75, 1525·2
Selenio Composto, 2283·3
Selenion, 2283·3
Selenioso Ácido, 1444·1
Selenious Acid, 1444·1
Selenito Sódico, 1444·1
Selenium, 1444·1
Selenium-75, 1525·2
Selenium Bonus, 2283·3
Selenium Dioxide, Monohydrated, 1444·1
Selenium Disulphide, 1157·3
Selenium E, 2283·3
Selenium Med Complex, 2283·3
Selenium Plus, 2283·3
Selenium Sulfide, 1157·3
Selenium Sulphide, 1157·3
Selenium-ACE, 2283·3
Selenix, 2283·3
Seleno-6, 2283·3
Selenocysteine, 1444·1
Selenokehl, 2283·3
Selenol, 2283·3
Selenomethionine, 1444·1
Selenonorcholestenol ($^{75}$Se), 1525·2
Selen-Wied, 2283·3
Sele-Pak, 2283·4
Seleparina, 2283·4
Selepark, 2283·4
Selepen, 2283·4
Seleplus, 2283·4
Seler, 2283·4
Seles Beta, 2283·4
Selexid, 2283·4
Selexid N, 2283·4

Selezen, 2283·4
Self-emulsifying Diglycerides of Food Fatty Acids, 1412·2
Self-emulsifying Glyceryl Monostearate, 1412·2
Self-emulsifying Mono- and Diglycerides of Food Fatty Acids, 1412·2
Self-emulsifying Monoglycerides of Food Fatty Acids, 1412·2
Self-emulsifying Monostearin, 1412·2
Selfotel, 1743·1
Selg, 2283·4
Selgene, 2283·4
Selg-Esse, 2283·4
Selgimed, 2283·4
Selgin, 2283·4
Selgina, 2283·4
Selgine, 2283·4
Selimax, 2283·4
Seline, 2283·4
Selinol, 2283·4
Selipran, 2283·4
Selit, 2283·4
Selm, 2283·4
Selobloc, 2283·4
Selocomp ZOC, 2283·4
Selokeen, 2283·4
Seloken, 2283·4
Seloken Retard Plus, 2283·4
Seloken ZOC, 2283·4
Seloken ZOC/ASA, 2284·1
Selokomb, 2284·1
Selon, 2284·1
Selopral, 2284·1
Selopres, 2284·1
Selopresin, 2284·1
Selopress, 2284·1
Selozide, 2284·1
Selo-Zok, 2284·1
Selpar, 2284·1
Selpiran, 2284·1
Selpiran-S, 2284·1
Sels Calcaires Nutritifs, 2284·1
Selso, 2284·1
Selsun, 2284·1
Selsun Blu, 2284·1
Selsun Plus, 2284·1
Selsun with Provitamin $B_5$, 2284·1
Selsun-R, 2284·1
Seltoc, 2284·1
Seltomylon, 2284·1
Seltouch, 2284·1
Seltrans, 2284·1
Selukos, 2284·1
Selva N, 2284·1
Selvigon, 2284·1
Selvigon Hustensaft, 2284·2
Selvjgon, 2284·2
Semap, 2284·2
Semax, 2284·2
Semble, 2284·2
Sembrina, 2284·2
Semduramicin, 615·3
Semduramicina, 615·3
Semen Foenugraeci, 1688·1
Semen Sinapis, 1718·2
Semen Trigonellae, 1688·1
Semence de Courge, 1677·3
Semeth, 2284·2
Semibiocin, 2284·2
Semicid, 2284·2
Semi-Daonil, 2284·2
Semi-Euglucon, 2284·2
Semi-Euglucon N, 2284·2
Semiglen, 2284·2
Semi-Gliben-Puren N, 2284·2
Semilente, 2284·2
Semilente, Insulin, 334·2
Semilente MC, 2284·2
Semilla de Lino, 1707·2
Semilla de Mostaza, 1718·2
Semilla de Psilio, 1268·1
Seminoma— *see* Malignant Neoplasms of the Testis, 523·1
Semipenil, 2284·2
Semisodium Valproate, 380·1
Semper, 2284·2
Sempera, 2284·2
Semprex, 2284·2
Semprex-D, 2284·2
Semuele, 2284·2
Semustina, 583·2
Semustine, 583·2
Sen, 1288·2
Senagar, 2284·2
Senaglinide, 343·3
Senalsor, 2284·2
Sendoxan, 2284·2
Sene Composta, 2284·3
Seneca Snakeroot, 1130·2
Senecio, 1743·1
*Senecio aureus*, 1743·1
*Senecio jacobaea*, 1743·1
Senecion, 2284·3
Senefor, 2284·3
Senega, 1130·2
Senega and Ammonia, 2284·3
Senega Root, 1130·2
Seneuval, 2284·3
Senexon, 2284·3
Senexon E, 2284·3
Senexon Plus, 2284·3
Senfsame, Schwarzer, 1718·2
Senicor, 2284·3
Senikolp, 2284·3
Senilezol, 2284·3
Senior, 2284·3
Senior Formula, 2284·3
Senior Multi-One, 2284·3
Senioral, 2284·3
Seniospray, 2284·3
Seniovita Aktiv, 2284·3
Senlax, 2284·3
Senlizumab, 1743·2
Senna, 1288·2
Senna, Alexandrian, 1288·2
Senna Fruit, 1288·2
Senna, Khartoum, 1288·2
Senna Leaf, 1288·2
Senna Pods, Alexandrian, 1288·2
Senna Pods, Tinnevelly, 1288·2
Senna, Tinnevelly, 1288·2
Sennae Folium, 1288·2
Sennae Fructus Acutifoliae, 1288·2
Sennae Fructus Angustifoliae, 1288·2
Senna-Gen, 2284·3
SennaPlus, 2284·3
Sennapur, 2284·3
Senna-Specie Composta, 2284·3
Sennesoft, 2284·3
Sennetabs, 2284·3
Sennetsu Fever— *see* Ehrlichiosis, 125·1
Sennocol, 2284·3
Sennoside B, 1288·2
Sennosides, 1288·2
Senociclin, 2284·3
Senodin-AN, 2284·3
Senokot, 2284·3
Senokot Direct Relief, 2284·4
Senokot-S, 2284·4
Senokot-S— *see* X-Prep Bowel Evacuant Kit-1, 2388·4
Senokotxtra, 2284·4
Senol, 2284·4
Senolax, 2284·4
Senophile, 2284·4
Senorm, 2284·4
Senosan, 2284·4
Senro, 2284·4
Sensaid con Fluor, 2284·4
Sensaval, 2284·4
Senselle— *see* Durex Sensilube, 1959·2
Sensibit, 2284·4
Sensibit D, 2284·4
Sensicutan, 2284·4
Sensiderme, 2284·4
Sensifluid, 2284·4
Sensigard, 2284·4
Sensigel, 2284·4
Sensilacer, 2284·4
Sensilube, 2284·4
Sensilube, Durex— *see* Durex Sensilube, 1959·2
Sensinerv Forte, 2284·4
Sensiotin, 2284·4
Sensipar, 2284·4
Sensiquell, 2284·4
Sensit, 2285·1
Sensitex, 2285·1
Sensit-F, 2285·1
Sensitiner, 2285·1
Sensitive Care, 2285·1
Sensitive Eyes, 2285·1
Sensitivity Protection Crest, 2285·1
Sensitram, 2285·1
Sensival, 2285·1
Sensivision au Plantain, 2285·1
Sensodent, 2285·1
Sensodyne Preparations, 2285·1
Sensodyne, Original— *see* also Original Sensodyne, 2192·3
SensoGARD, 2285·1
Sensorcaine, 2285·1
Sensoricaine, 2285·1
Sensory Polyneuropathy— *see* Diabetic Neuropathy, 6·1
Sens-Out, 2285·1
Sentidol, 2285·1
Sentril, 2285·2
Seocalcitol, 583·3
Sepan, 2285·2
Sepatren, 2285·2
Sepazon, 2285·2
Sepcen, 2285·2
Sepdine, 2285·2
Sepex, 2285·2
Sepexin, 2285·2
Sepfadine, 2285·2
Sephros, 2285·2
Sepia, 1743·2
Sepmax, 2285·2
Se-Power, 2285·2
Seprafilm, 2285·2
Sepram, 2285·2
Sep/Ser, 1615·3
Sepsilem, 2285·2
Sepsis— *see* Septicaemia, 144·3
Sepsis Syndrome— *see* Septicaemia, 144·3
Sepso J, 2285·2
Sepsol, 2285·2
Septa, 2285·2
Septacare, 2285·2
Septacef, 2285·2
Septacin, 2285·2
Septacin Amoxi, 2285·2
Septacin Ex, 2285·2
Septacord, 2285·2
Septadine, 2285·2
Septadine Scrub, 2285·2
Septal, 2285·3
Septalibour, 2285·3
Septalone, 2285·3
Septanest, 2285·3
Septeal, 2285·3
Septi-Aid, 2285·3
Septic Arthritis— *see* Bone and Joint Infections, 122·1
Septic Shock— *see* Septicaemia, 144·3
Septic Shock— *see* Shock, 835·1
Septicaemia, 144·3
Septicide, 2285·3
Septicol, 2285·3
Septicon, 2285·3
Septicortin, 2285·3
Septidiaryl, 2285·3
Septidine, 2285·3
Septidron, 2285·3
Septil, 2285·3
Septilisin, 2285·3
Septiolan, 2285·3
Septiolan Balsamico, 2285·3
Septiphene, 1177·3
Septirose, 2285·3
Septisan, 2285·3
Septisept, 2285·3
Septi-Soft, 2285·3
Septisol, 2285·3
Septison, 2285·3
Septisooth, 2285·3
Septivon, 2285·4
Septivon N, 2285·4
Septobore, 2285·4
Septocaine, 2285·4
Septocipro, 2285·4
Septocoll, 2285·4
Septol, 2285·4
Septolit, 2285·4
Septomandolo, 2285·4
Septomixine, 2285·4
Septone, 2285·4
Septonsil, 2285·4
Septopal, 2285·4
Septoprin, 2285·4
Septoral, 2285·4
Septosan, 2285·4
Septosol, 2285·4
Septra, 2285·4
Septran, 2285·4
Septrin, 2285·4
Sepurin, 2285·4
Sequals G, 2285·4
Sequax, 2285·4
Sequennia, 2286·1
Sequential Oral Contraceptives, 1535·1
Sequilar, 2286·1
Sequilar ED, 2286·1
Sequinan, 2286·1
Sequostat, 2286·1
Ser, 1444·3
Seracalm, 2286·1
Seraccel, 2286·1
Seracin, 2286·1
Seractil, 2286·1
Seractiv, 2286·1
Serad, 2286·1
Serag-HAES, 2286·1
Seraim, 2286·1
Seralbuman, 2286·1
Seralbumin, 2286·1
Seramed, 2286·1
Seranex Sans Codeine, 2286·1
Ser-Ap-Es, 2286·1
Serasa, 2286·1
Seratrodast, 795·3
Seravit, 2286·1
Seravit, Paediatric— *see* Paediatric Seravit, 2200·3
Serax, 2286·1
Serazide Hydrochloride, 1200·2
Serc, 2286·1
Sercerin, 2286·1
Sercim, 2286·1
Serdolect, 2286·1
Serebon, 2286·1
Serecid, 2286·1
Serecor, 2286·1
Seredyn, 2286·1
Serefodipine Hydrochloride, 909·2
Serefrex, 2286·2
Sereine, 2286·2
Sere-Mit, 2286·2
Serenace, 2286·2
Serenade, 2286·2
Serenal, 2286·2
Serenase, 2286·2
Serene, 2286·2
Serenelfi, 2286·2
Serenex, 2286·2
Serengrav, 2286·2
Serenight, 2286·2
Serenil, 2286·2
Serenity, Gerard House— *see* Gerard House Serenity, 2022·1
Serenity, Tranquillity and Peace, 1593·3
Serenoa Complex, 2286·2
*Serenoa repens*, 1569·1
*Serenoa serrulatum*, 1569·1
Serenoa-C, 2286·2
Serenol, 2286·2
Serentil, 2286·2
Serenus, 2286·2
Serepax, 2286·2
Serepress, 2286·2

Sereprid, 2286·2
Sereprile, 2286·2
Sereprostat, 2286·2
Seresis, 2286·2
Seresta, 2286·2
Seretaide, 2286·3
Seretide, 2286·3
Seretran, 2286·3
Sereupin, 2286·3
Serevent, 2286·3
Serezac, 2286·3
Serfabiotic, 2286·3
Serfinato, 2286·3
Serformin, 2286·3
Serfoxide, 2286·3
Sergast, 2286·3
Serianon, 2286·3
Seriglutan B12, 2286·3
Serimol, 2286·3
Serina, 1444·3
Serine, 1444·3
L-Serine, 1444·3
DL-Serine 2-(2,3,4-Trihydroxybenzyl)hydrazide, 1200·2
125-L-Serine-2–133-interleukin 2 (Human Reduced), 562·3
Serinum, 1444·3
Serivo, 2286·3
Serlain, 2286·3
Serless, 2286·3
Sermaka, 2286·3
Sermetrol, 2286·3
Sermion, 2286·3
Sermonil, 2286·3
Sermorelin Acetate, 1339·2
Sermorelina, Acetato de, 1339·2
Serobid, 2286·3
Serobif, 2286·3
Serocalcin, 2286·3
Serocryptin, 2286·4
Serocytol, 2286·4
Serodox, 2286·4
Serofene, 2286·4
Seroflo, 2286·4
Serofusine, 2286·4
Seroglubin, 2286·4
Seromex, 2286·4
Seromida, 2286·4
Seromycin, 2286·4
Seronegative Arthritides— *see* Spondyloarthropathies, 11·1
Seronex, 2286·4
Seronil, 2286·4
Serophene, 2286·4
Serophy, 2286·4
Seroplatin, 2286·4
Seroposide, 2286·4
Seropram, 2286·4
Seroquel, 2286·4
Seroscand, 2286·4
Serostim, 2286·4
Serotabir, 2286·4
Sero-Tet, 2286·4
Serotone, 2286·4
Serotonin, 1743·2
Serotonin and Noradrenaline Reuptake Inhibitors, 278·2
Serotonin Reuptake Inhibitors, Selective, 278·2, 296·3
Serotonin Syndrome, 313·1
Serotonina, 1743·2
Serotron, 2286·4
Serotulle, 2287·1
Serovidina, 2287·1
Serovin, 2287·1
Seroxat, 2287·1
Serozinc, 2287·1
Serpafar, 2287·1
Serpax, 2287·1
Serpens, 2287·1
Serpentaria, 1656·3
Serpentary, 1656·3
Serpentine, 994·3
Serpentines, 1658·1
Serradase, 2287·1
Serranit, 2287·1
Serrano, 2287·1
Serrao, 2287·1
Serrapep, 2287·1
Serrapeptasa, 1743·2
Serrapeptase, 1743·2
Serrason, 2287·1
*Serratia*, 1743·2
Serratia Extracellular Proteinase, 1743·2
Serratiopeptidase, 1743·2
Serratol, 2287·1
Serrazyme, 2287·1
Serrin, 2287·1
Serta, 2287·1
Sertaconazol, Nitrato de, 408·1
Sertaconazole Nitrate, 408·1
Sertaconazoli Nitras, 408·1
Sertacream, 2287·1
Sertadie, 2287·1
Sertagyn, 2287·1
Sertal, 2287·1
Sertal Compuesto, 2287·1
Sertalia, 2287·1
Sertenef, 590·2
Serterol, 2287·1
Sertidine, 2287·1
Sertinal, 2287·1
Sertindol, 721·3
Sertindole, 721·3
Sertopic, 2287·1
Sertralina, Hidrocloruro de, 317·2
Sertraline Hydrochloride, 317·2
Sertrixen, 2287·1
Serum, 744·3
Serum Sickness— *see* Drug-induced Skin Reactions, 1134·3
Serum Thymic Factor, 1756·1
Serutan, 2287·1
Servambutol, 2287·2
Servamox, 2287·2
Servamox CLV, 2287·2
Servamox-F, 2287·2
Servanolol, 2287·2
Servatrin, 2287·2
Servazolin, 2287·2
Servetinal, 2287·2
Servicef, 2287·2
Servicillin, 2287·2
Servicimet, 2287·2
Serviclazide, 2287·2
Serviclor, 2287·2
Serviclox, 2287·2
Servicol, 2287·2
Servicyclin, 2287·2
Servidapsone, 2287·2
Servidiclox, 2287·2
Servidipine, 2287·2
Servidopa, 2287·2
Servidoxyne, 2287·2
Servidrat, 2287·2
Servidrat Low Sodium, 2287·2
Serviflox, 2287·2
Servigenta, 2287·2
Servin, 2287·2
Servinadine, 2287·2
Servinaprox, 2287·3
Servindomet, 2287·3
Servipen-V, 2287·3
Servipep, 2287·3
Serviprofen, 2287·3
Serviproxan, 2287·3
Serviradine, 2287·3
Servispor, 2287·3
Servitamol, 2287·3
Servitenol, 2287·3
Servitet, 2287·3
Servithiazid, 2287·3
Servitifen, 2287·3
Servitrim, 2287·3
Servitrocin, 2287·3
Servium, 2287·3
Servizol, 2287·3
Serzone, 2287·3
Serzonil, 2287·3
Sesal, 2287·3
Sesalgin, 2287·3
Sesame Oil, 1743·3
Sesame Oil, Refined, 1743·3
Sesame Street, 2287·3
Sesami, Oleum, 1743·3
Sesami Oleum Raffinatum, 1743·3
Sésamo, Aceite de, 1743·3
*Sesamum indicum*, 1743·3
Sesden, 2287·3
Sesquioleato de Sorbitán, 1416·2
Sesquiterpene Lactone Antimalarials, 444·1
Sessoforte, 2287·3
Sestamibi, Technetium ($^{99m}$Tc), 1526·1
Sestrine, 2287·3
Setacol, 2287·3
Setamol, 2287·3
Setarin, 2287·4
Setarin H, 2287·4
Setas Venenosas, 1717·3
Setastina, Hidrocloruro de, 441·1
Setastine Hydrochloride, 441·1
Setcillin, 2287·4
Sethro, 2287·4
Setin, 2287·4
Setlers Preparations, 2287·4
Setlers Wind-Eze— *see* Wind-Eze, 2386·2
Setlinctus, 2287·4
Setmenate, 2287·4
Setmotil, 2287·4
Setmoxil, 2287·4
Setprodine, 2287·4
Setrilan, 2287·4
Setromol, 2287·4
Setron, 2287·4
Setronges, 2287·4
Setronil, 2287·4
Setrosone, 2287·4
Setrozole, 2287·4
Setsolone, 2287·4
Setux, 2287·4
Setux Expectorante, 2287·4
Seudotabs, 2287·4
Sevelamer Hydrochloride, 1051·2
Sevelámero, Hidrocloruro de, 1051·2
Seven Barks, 1698·3
Seven Seas, 2287·4
Sevenal, 2287·4
Sevenaleta, 2287·4
Severe Acute Respiratory Syndrome— *see* SARS, 625·1
Severin, 2287·4
Severon, 2288·1
Seville Orange, 1723·3
Sevinol, 2288·1
Sevirumab, 1612·1
Sevium, 2288·1
Sevocris, 2288·1
Sevoflurane, 1307·3
Sevoflurano, 1307·3
Sevorane, 2288·1
Sevorex, 2288·1
Sevredol, 2288·1
Sevre-Long, 2288·1
Sevrium, 2288·1
Sex Hormones, 1527·1
Sexadien, 2288·1
Sexormom, 2288·1
Sexual Behaviour, Deviant— *see* Disturbed Behaviour, 665·1
Sexually Transmitted Diseases, 145·3
Sézary Syndrome, 511·2
SF-86-327, 408·2
SF-277, 30·1
SF-86327, 408·2
SF Gel, 2288·1
SFC Lotion, 2288·1
SF-R11, 1736·2
SG-75, 965·3
SGD-301-76, 407·3
S/Gel, 2288·1
Sguardi, 2288·1
SH-206, 2288·1
SH-213AB, 1066·1
SH-261, 1731·1
SH-567, 1559·2
SH-582, 1556·2
SH-601, 1559·3
SH-714, 1544·1
SH-717, 333·2
SH-723, 1559·1
SH-742, 1102·1
SH-770, 1102·1
SH-863, 1096·1
SH-881, 1544·1
SH-926, 1063·2
SH-968, 1099·3
Shade, 2288·1
Shade UVAGuard, 2288·1
Shak Iso, 2288·1
Shaklee Dandruff Control, 2288·1
Shaklee Lip Protection Stick, 2288·1
Shaklee Sunscreen, 2288·2
Shamday Antiforfora, 2288·2
Shampoo SDE Tar, 2288·2
Shampoo SDE Zinc, 2288·2
Shampoo Tersa-Tar, 2288·2
Shampooing Anti-Pelliculaire, 2288·2
Shampooing Extra-doux, 2288·2
Shampooing Traitant Antipelliculaire, 2288·2
Shampoux, 2288·2
Shampoux Repel, 2288·2
Shanvac-B, 2288·2
Shark Cartilage Extract, 525·3
Shark-liver Oil, 1243·2
Sharkoferrol, 2288·2
Sharkomalt, 2288·2
Sharkovit, 2288·2
SHB-286, 1520·3
SH-B-331, 1556·1
She, 1373·3
SHE-222, 952·2
Shea Butter, 1482·1
Sheepdips, 1508·1
Sheets, 1730·3
Sheik, 2288·2
Sheik Elite, 2288·2
Sheko, 2288·2
Shellac, 1743·3
Shellac, Purified, 1743·3
Shellgel, 2288·2
Shemol, 2288·2
Shepard's, 2288·2
Shepherds Burse Herb, 1744·1
Shepherd's Purse, 1744·1
SH-H-200-AB, 1064·1
Shield, 2288·2
Shields, 2288·2
Shigella Enteritis— *see* Shigellosis, 130·1
Shigella Vaccines, 1638·3
Shigellosis, 130·1
Shigellosis Vaccines, 1638·3
Shii-ta-ker, 2288·2
Shin-Biofermin S, 2288·2
Shinbit, 2288·2
Shincef, 2288·2
Shincort, 2288·2
Shinfomycin, 2288·2
Shingles— *see* Varicella-zoster Infections, 621·1
Shingles Pain Relief, 2288·2
Shinoxol, 2288·2
Shintamet, 2288·2
Shiomarin, 2288·2
Shiseido Preparations, 2288·3
Shivering, Postoperative— *see* Shivering and Its Treatment, 1295·2
Shiwalax, 2288·3
SH-K-203, 1102·1
SH-L-451-A, 1062·2
Shock, 835·1
Shock, Anaphylactic— *see* Anaphylactic Shock, 855·2
Shock, Cardiogenic— *see* Shock, 835·1
Shock, Hypovolaemic— *see* Shock, 835·1
Shock, Septic— *see* Septicaemia, 144·3
Shock, Septic— *see* Shock, 835·1
Shock, Toxic, Syndrome— *see* Toxic Shock Syndrome, 149·2
Shop Vervain Wort, 1764·1
Short Buchu, 1663·1
Short Stature— *see* Growth Retardation, 1314·2

Sho-saiko-to, Kanebo— see Kanebo Sho-saiko-to, 2074·2
Sho-saiko-to, Tsumura— see Tsumura Sho-saiko-to, 2351·1
Sho-seiryu-to, Tsumura— see Tsumura Sho-seiryu-to, 2351·1
Shoulder-hand Syndrome— see Complex Regional Pain Syndrome, 5·3
Shur-Seal, 2288·3
SH-Y-579A, 645·3
SI-88, 1291·1
Si o No, 2288·3
SIADH— see Syndrome of Inappropriate ADH Secretion, 1318·3
Siadocin, 2288·3
Siagoside, 1691·1
Sialexin, 2288·3
Sialin, 2288·3
Sialor, 2288·3
Siam Benzoin, 1744·1
Siamdopa, 2288·3
Siamformet, 2288·3
Siamidine, 2288·3
Siamik, 2288·3
Sia-Mox, 2288·3
Siampicil, 2288·3
Siampraxol, 2288·3
Siarizine, 2288·3
Siaten, 2288·3
Sibelium, 2288·3
Sibelium Plus, 2288·4
Siberian Ginseng, 1693·1, 1744·1
Sibicort, 2288·4
Sibrafiban, 996·3
Sibudan, 2288·4
Sibu-Estirol, 2288·4
Sibutral, 2288·4
Sibutramina, Hidrocloruro de, 1593·1
Sibutramine Hydrochloride, 1593·1
Sicadentol Plus, 2288·4
Sicadol, 2288·4
Sical, 2288·4
Sicaril, 2288·4
Sicatem, 2288·4
Sicazine, 2288·4
Siccafluid, 2288·4
Siccagent, 2288·4
Siccalix, 2288·4
Siccapos, 2288·4
Siccaprotect, 2288·4
Sicca-Stulln, 2288·4
Sicco, 2288·4
Siccoral, 2288·4
Sicef, 2288·4
Sickle-cell Crisis— see Sickle-cell Disease, 734·3
Sickle-cell Crisis Pain— see Sickle-cell Crisis, 8·1
Sickle-cell Disease, 734·3
Sickle-cell Disease, Infection Prophylaxis— see Spleen Disorders, 146·3
Sickle-cell Trait— see Sickle-cell Disease, 734·3
Si-Cliss, 2288·4
Sico Relax, 2288·4
Sicobal, 2288·4
Sicombyl, 2288·4
Sic-Ophtal, 2288·4
Sicoplus, 2288·4
Sicorten, 2288·4
Sicorten Plus, 2289·1
Sicriptin, 2289·1
Sicrit, 2289·1
Siddhi, 1666·1
Sidenar, 2289·1
Sideralce, 2289·1
Siderblut, 2289·1
Siderfol, 2289·1
Sideril, 2289·1
Sideroblastic Anaemia, 734·2
Sideroglobina, 2289·1
Sidervim, 2289·1
Sidroga Preparations, 2289·1
Siduol, 2289·1
Siduro, 2289·1
Siepex, 2289·1
Sieral, 2289·1
Siero Antiofidico, 2289·1
Sies, 2289·1
Siesta-1, 2289·1
Siete Mares Higado Bacal, 2289·2
Sifaclor, 2289·2
Sifamic, 2289·2
Sificetina, 2289·2
Sificrom, 2289·2
Sifiviral, 2289·2
Siframin, 2289·2
Sifrol, 2289·2
Sigabloc, 2289·2
Sigabroxol, 2289·2
Sigacalm, 2289·2
Sigacap Cor, 2289·2
Sigacefal, 2289·2
Sigacimet, 2289·2
Sigacora, 2289·2
Sigadoc, 2289·2
Sigadoxin, 2289·2
Sigafam, 2289·2
Sigafenac, 2289·2
Sigamopen, 2289·2
Sigamuc, 2289·2
Sigamucil, 2289·2
Sigaperidol, 2289·2
Sigaprim, 2289·2
Sigaprolol, 2289·2
Sigapurol, 2289·2
Sigas, 2289·2
Sigasalur, 2289·2
Sigatricin, 2289·3
Sighirma, 1666·1
Sigma Liquid Antacid, 2289·3
Sigma Relief, 2289·3
Sigma Relief Chest Rub, 2289·3
Sigma Relief Junior, 2289·3
Sigmacort, 2289·3
Sigmafon, 2289·3
Sigmalin $B_6$, 2289·3
Sigmalin $B_6$ Forte, 2289·3
Sigmalin $B_6$ ohne Coffein, 2289·3
Sigman-Haustropfen, 2289·3
Sigmart, 2289·3
Sigmasporin, 2289·3
Sigmatriol, 2289·3
Sigmaxin, 2289·3
Sigmetadine, 2289·3
Signal, 2289·3
Sigtab-M, 2289·3
Siguent Hycor, 2289·3
Siguent Neomycin, 2289·3
SIL-1000, 2289·3
SIL-5000— see SIL-1000, -5000, 2289·3
Silace, 2289·3
Silace-C, 2289·3
Silact, 2289·3
Siladryl, 2289·3
Silafed, 2289·4
Silain, 2289·4
Silaminic Cold, 2289·4
Silaminic Expectorant, 2289·4
Sil-A-Mox, 2289·4
Silan, 2289·4
Silapap, 2289·4
Silarine, 2289·4
Silartrin, 2289·4
Silastic, 2289·4
Silaxa, 2289·4
Silaxon, 2289·4
Silbecor, 2289·4
Silbephylline, 2289·4
Silberne, 2289·4
Silcon, 2289·4
Silcor, 2289·4
Sildec-DM, 2289·4
Sildefil, 2289·4
Sildenafil Citrate, 1744·2
Sildenafilo, Citrato de, 1744·2
Sildicon-E, 2289·4
Silencium, 2289·4
Silent Myocardial Ischaemia— see Angina Pectoris, 813·1
Silentan, 2289·4
Silepar, 2289·4
Sileton, 2289·4
Silettum, 2289·4
Silfedrine, 2289·4
Silflam, 2289·4
Silfox, 2290·1
Silgel, 2290·1
Silibene, 2290·1
Silibinin, 1043·3
Silibinin Dihemisuccinate, Disodium, 1043·3
Silibinina, 1043·3
Silic, 2290·1
Silic 15, 2290·1
Silica, Anhydrous, Colloidal, 1581·3
Silica, Colloidal Anhydrous, 1582·1
Silica, Colloidal Hydrated, 1581·3
Silica Colloidalis Anhydrica, 1581·3
Silica Colloidalis Hydrica, 1581·3
Silica, Dental Type, 1581·3
Silica, Dental-Type, 1581·3
Silica Gel, 1581·3
Silica, Hydrated, Colloidal, 1581·3
Silica L11, 2290·1
Silica, Precipitated, 1581·3
Silica-OK, 2290·1
Silicare, 2290·1
Silicas, 1581·3
Silicato de Magnesio, 1580·2
Silicato de Sodio, 1748·3
Silicato de Sodio y de Aluminio, 1250·2
Silica-Vite, Bioglan— see Bioglan Silica-Vite, 1844·1
Sílice, 1581·3
Silicea, 1582·1
Silicea Purificada Terra, 1581·3
Siliceous Earth, Purified, 1581·3
Silicic Complex, 2290·1
Silicin, 2290·1
Silicol, 2290·1
Silicon Dioxide, 1581·3
Silicon Dioxide, Colloidal, 1581·3
Siliconas, 1482·1
Silicone, Huile de, 1482·1
Silicone Oil, 1482·1
Silicones, 1482·1
Siliconum Liquidum, 1482·1
Silicosis— see Diffuse Parenchymal Lung Disease, 1079·3
Silicristin, 1043·3
Silicristina, 1043·3
Silicur, 2290·1
Silidermil, 2290·1
Silidianin, 1043·3
Silidianina, 1043·3
Silidral, 2290·1
Silidron, 2290·1
Siligaz, 2290·1
Siligel, 2290·1
Silimag, 2290·1
Silimalon, 2290·1
Silimarin, 2290·1
Silimarina, 1043·3
Silimarit, 2290·1
Silimazu, 2290·1
Sili-Met-San, 2290·1
Siliprele, 2290·1
Silirex, 2290·1
Silisan, 2290·1
Siliver, 2290·1
Silkis, 2290·1
Silliver, 2290·2
Sillix, 2290·2
Sillix C, 2290·2
Sillix Donna, 2290·2
Silmar, 2290·2
Silmycetin, 2290·2
Sil-Norboral, 2290·2
Siloderm, 2290·2
Silomat, 2290·2
Silomat Compositum, 2290·2
Silomat DA, 2290·2
Silomat Plus, 2290·2
Silomat-Fher, 2290·2
Silon, 2290·2
Silostar, 2290·2
Silox-50, 2290·2
Siloxan, 2290·2
Siloxogene, 2290·2
Silphen, 2290·2
Silphen DM, 2290·2
Silpin, 2290·2
Silrelax, 2290·2
Siltapp, 2290·2
Sil-Tex, 2290·2
Siltussin, 2290·2
Siltussin DM, 2290·3
Siltussin-CF, 2290·3
Silubin, 2290·3
Siludrox, 2290·3
Silvadene, 2290·3
Silvadiazin, 2290·3
Silvana, 2290·3
Silvaysan, 2290·3
Silvazine, 2290·3
Silvederma, 2290·3
Silvedine, 2290·3
Silver, 1746·1
Silver Acetate, 1746·1
Silver Allantoinate, 1746·1
Silver Birch Leaf, 1660·3
Silver Borate, 1746·1
Silver Carbonate, 1746·1
Silver Chloride, 1746·1
Silver Chromate, 1746·1
Silver Clove Medicated Balm, 2290·3
Silver Glycerolate, 1746·1
Silver Iodide, Colloidal, 1746·1
Silver Lactate, 1746·1
Silver Manganite, 1746·1
Silver Nitrate, 1746·1
Silver Nucleinate, 1746·2
Silver Protein, 1746·2
Silver Proteinate, 1746·2
Silver Sulfadiazine, 259·1
Silver Sulphadiazine, 259·1
Silver Vitellin, 1746·2
Silver Zinc Allantoinate, 1746·1
Silvercef, 2290·3
Silverex, 2290·3
Silver-nylon, 1746·1
Silverol, 2290·3
Silvertone, 2290·3
Silybin, 1043·3
Silybon, 2290·3
Silybum Complex, 2290·3
Silybum Marianum, 1043·3
*Silybum marianum*, 1043·3
Silybum Substance $E_6$, 1043·3
Silychristin, 1043·3
Silydianin, 1043·3
Silyhexal, 2290·3
Silymarin, 1043·3
Silymarin Phytosome, 2290·3
Sily-Sabona, 2290·3
Silzolin, 2290·3
Simaal Gel 2, 2290·3
Simacort, 2290·3
Simagel, 2290·4
Simaglen, 2290·4
Simaphil, 2290·4
Simar, 2290·4
Simatin, 2290·4
Simbion, 2290·4
Simcone, 2290·4
Simdax, 2290·4
Simeco, 2290·4
Simeco Plus, 2290·4
Simecon, 2290·4
Simecon Antiacido, 2290·4
Simegel, 2290·4
Simepar, 2290·4
Simetac, 2290·4
Simet-AF, 2290·4
Simethicone, 1289·2
Simeticona, 1289·2
Simeticone, 1289·2
Simeticonum, 1289·2
Simetyl, 2290·4
Simex, 2290·4
Simfibrate, 997·1
Simfibrato, 997·1
Simic, 2290·4
Simicol, 2290·4

Similac Preparations, 2290·4
Similasan 1, 2291·1
Similia, 2291·1
Similibus, 2291·1
Simoph Tears, 2291·1
Simovil, 2291·1
Simoxil, 2291·1
Simoyiam, 2291·1
Simp, 2291·1
Simperten, 2291·1
Simperten-D, 2291·1
Simplamox, 2291·1
Simple, 2291·1
Simple Cleaner, 2291·1
Simplene, 2291·1
Simplet, 2291·1
Simplex, 2291·1
Simplex-Fieberblasen, 2291·1
Simplicity, 2291·1
Simplotan, 2291·1
Simply Cough, 2291·1
Simply Sleep, 2291·1
Simply Stuffy, 2291·1
Simpottantacinque, 2291·1
Simprox, 2291·1
Simpsons, 2291·1
Simron Plus, 2291·1
Simrose, 2291·1
Simtec, 2291·1
Simulcium G3, 2291·2
Simulect, 2291·2
Simultan, 2291·2
Simusol, 2291·2
Simvacol, 2291·2
Simvacor, 2291·2
Simvador, 2291·2
Simvast, 2291·2
Simvastatin, 997·1
Simvastatina, 997·1
Simvastatinum, 997·1
Simvasten, 2291·2
Simvor, 2291·2
Simvotin, 2291·2
SIN-10, 961·3
Sin Mareo X 4, 2291·2
Sin-A Crud, 2291·2
Sinacarb, 2291·2
Sinacid, 2291·2
Si-Nade, 2291·2
Sinadrin Plus, 2291·2
Sinadrin, Super Strength— *see* Super Strength Sinadrin, 2313·3
Sinaf, 2291·2
Sin-A-Gen, 2291·2
Sinaler, 2291·2
Sinaler B, 2291·2
Sinalfa, 2291·2
Sinalgia, 2291·2
Sinalgico, 2291·2
Sin-Algin, 2291·2
Sinamida Cicatrizante, 2291·2
Sinamida Econazol, 2291·2
Sinamida Pies, 2291·3
Sinamida-D, 2291·3
Sinapause, 2291·3
Sinapet, 2291·3
Sinapils, 2291·3
Sinapis Alba, 1718·2
Sinapis Nigra, 1718·2
Sinapis, Semen, 1718·2
Sinapis Volatile, Oleum, 1718·2
Sinapisme Rigollot, 2291·3
Sinaplin, 2291·3
Sinapsan, 2291·3
Sinapultide, 1736·2
Sinaqua, 2291·3
Sinarest, 2291·3
Sinarest Linctus, 2291·3
Sinarest, No Drowsiness— *see* No Drowsiness Sinarest, 2170·4
Sinarest Vapocaps, 2291·3
Sinarest-PD, 2291·3
Sinarona, 2291·3
Sinartrol, 2291·3
Sinaryl, 2291·3
Sinase, 2291·3
Sinasmal, 2291·3
Sinaspril-Paracetamol, 2291·3
Sinaxial, 2291·3
Sincalida, 1746·2
Sincalide, 1746·2
Sincerck, 2291·3
Sincerum, 2291·3
Sincerum Biotic, 2291·3
Sincerum Biotic L, 2291·3
Sincon, 2291·4
Sincosan, 2291·4
Sincrivit, 2291·4
Sindol, 2291·4
Sindopa, 2291·4
Sindrat, 2291·4
Sindrolen, 2291·4
Sindrolen Vitaminado, 2291·4
Sine-Aid IB, 2291·4
Sine-Aid Maximum Strength, 2291·4
Sine-Aid, Maximum Strength— *see* Maximum Strength Sine-Aid, 2116·4
Sinease, 2291·4
Sinecod, 2291·4
Sinecod Bocca, 2291·4
Sinecod Tosse Fluidificante, 2291·4
Sinecod Tosse Sedativo, 2291·4
Sinedal, 2291·4
Sinedol, 2291·4
Sinedopa, 2291·4
Sinedyston, 2291·4
Sinefricol, 2291·4
Sinefrina, 977·3
Sinefrina, Hidrocloruro de, 977·3
Sinefrina Tartrato, 977·3
Sinefrina, Tartrato de, 977·3
Sinegastrin, 2291·4
Sinemet, 2291·4
Sinemet, Half— *see* Half Sinemet, 2035·2
Sine-Off Preparations, 2291·4
Sinequan, 2292·1
Sinerbe, 2292·1
Sinergen, 2292·1
Sinergina, 2292·1
Sinertec, 2292·1
Sinesalin, 2292·1
Sinestic, 2292·1
Sinestron, 2292·1
Sinevrile, 2292·1
Sinex, 2292·1
Sinex, Vicks— *see* Vicks Sinex, 2375·4
Sinex, Wick— *see* Wick Sinex, 2386·1
Sinezan, 2292·1
Sinfrontal, 2292·1
Singastril, 2292·1
Singlauc, 2292·1
Single-peak Insulins, 334·2
Singlet, 2292·1
Singril, 2292·1
Singrilen, 2292·1
Singulair, 2292·1
Sinhcloran, 2292·2
Siniphen, 2292·2
Sinistrin— *see* Inutest, 2064·3
Sinketol, 2292·2
Sinkron, 2292·2
Sinlergia, 2292·2
Sinmaren, 2292·2
Sinmol, 2292·2
Sinobid, 2292·2
Sinogan, 2292·2
Sinografin, 2292·2
Sinolax-Milder, 2292·2
Sinomarin, 2292·2
Sinop, 2292·2
Sinophenin, 2292·2
Sinopil, 2292·2
Sinoral, 2292·2
Sinorphan, 964·2, 1285·2
Sinotar, 2292·2
Sinovula, 2292·2
Sinoxis, 2292·2
Sinozol, 2292·2
Sinozzard, 2292·2
Sinpasmon, 2292·2
Sinpet, 2292·2
Sinpor, 2292·2
Sinpro N, 2292·2
Sinquan, 2292·2
Sinquane, 2292·2
Sinsia, 2292·3
Sinsurrene, 2292·3
Sintalgin, 2292·3
Sintamin, 2292·3
Sintebron, 2292·3
Sintegran, 2292·3
Sintemicina, 2292·3
Sintenyl, 2292·3
Sintepul, 2292·3
Sinteroid, 2292·3
Sinthrome, 2292·3
Sintisone, 2292·3
Sintobil, 2292·3
Sintocalcin, 2292·3
Sintocef, 2292·3
Sintoclar, 2292·3
Sintodian, 2292·3
Sintofenac, 2292·3
Sintoftona, 2292·3
Sintolatt, 2292·3
Sintomicetina, 2292·3
Sintomodulina, 2292·3
Sintonal, 2292·3
Sintopen, 2292·3
Sintoplus, 2292·3
Sintotrat, 2292·3
Sintozima, 2292·3
Sintrocid, 2292·3
Sintrogel, 2292·3
Sintrom, 2292·3
Sintrom Mitis, 2292·4
Sinuberase, 2292·4
Sinuc, 2292·4
Sinuclear, 2292·4
Sinuclear P, 2292·4
Sinucon, 2292·4
Sinudec, Ordov— *see* Ordov Sinudec, 2192·1
Sinufed Preparations, 2292·4
Sinuforce, 2292·4
Sinuforton, 2292·4
Sinugesic, 2292·4
Sinugex, 2292·4
Sinulan, Natusor— *see* Natusor Sinulan, 2154·1
Sinulen, 2292·4
Sinulin, 2292·4
Sinumax Preparations, 2292·4
Sinumed, 2292·4
Sinumine, 2292·4
Sinumist-SR, 2292·4
Sinupan, 2293·1
Sinupas N, 2293·1
Sinupret, 2293·1
Sinurit, 2293·1
Sinus, 2293·1
Sinus & Congestion Relief, 2293·1
Sinus Excedrin, 2293·1
Sinus and Hayfever, 2293·1
Sinus, Hylands— *see* Hylands Sinus, 2052·3
Sinus Inhalaciones, 2293·1
Sinus Medication, 2293·1
Sinus Pain & Nasal Congestion Relief, 2293·1
Sinus Relief, 2293·1
Sinus Relief with Antihistamine, Nyal Plus+ — *see* Nyal Plus+ Sinus Relief with Antihistamine, 2182·2
Sinus Relief, Chemists Own— *see* Chemists Own Sinus Relief, 1882·1
Sinus Relief, Nyal— *see* Nyal Sinus Relief, 2182·2
Sinus Relief, Nyal Plus+ Day Night— *see* Nyal Plus+ Day Night Sinus Relief, 2182·2
Sinusaid, 2293·1
Sinusal, 2293·1
Sinusalia, 2293·1
Sinuselect, 2293·1
Sinusitis, 146·1
Sinusitis Hevert N, 2293·1
Sinusitis PMD, 2293·1
Sinusitis-Komplex N, 2293·1
Sinusitis-Weliplex, 2293·1
Sinusol, 2293·1
Sinusol-Schleimlosender Tee, 2293·1
Sinus-Pain Relief, Chemists Own— *see* Chemists Own Sinus-Pain Relief, 1882·1
Sinuspax, 2293·1
Sinus-Relief, 2293·1
Sinustat, 2293·1
Sinustop Pro, 2293·1
Sinustrat, 2293·1
Sinustrat Solucao Natural, 2293·1
Sinustrat Vasoconstritor, 2293·1
Sinusyx, 2293·2
Sinutab Preparations, 2293·2
Sinutab, Non-Drowsy— *see* Non-Drowsy Sinutab, 2171·4
Sinutab Without Drowsiness, Maximum Strength— *see* Maximum Strength Sinutab Without Drowsiness, 2116·4
SINUtuss DM, 2293·3
SINUvent, 2293·3
Sinuvent PE, 2293·3
Sinuzin, 2293·3
Sinuzin-D, 2293·3
Sinvacor, 2293·3
Sinvascor, 2293·3
Sinvastacor, 2293·3
Sinvastil, 2293·3
Sinvatrox, 2293·3
Siochrome, 2293·3
Siofor, 2293·3
Siokof-P, 2293·3
Sioneuron, 2293·3
Siopel, 2293·3
Sioplex, 2293·3
Sioplex Lysine, 2293·3
Sioplex-Z, 2293·3
Sioril, 2293·3
Siosol, 2293·3
Siozwo, 2293·3
Siozwo N, 2293·3
Sipam, 2293·3
Sipcar, 2293·3
Sipental, 2293·3
Siphene, 2293·4
Sipirac, 2293·4
Siprofen, 2293·4
Siqualine, 2293·4
Squalone, 2293·4
Siquial, 2293·4
Siquil, 2293·4
Siran, 2293·4
Sirani, 2293·4
Sirben, 2293·4
Sirdalud, 2293·4
Sirepar, 2293·4
Siridone, 2293·4
Sirigen, 2293·4
Sirmia Abfuhrkapseln, 2293·4
Sirmia Artischockenelixier N, 2293·4
Sirmia Knoblauchsaft N, 2293·4
Sirmione, Acqua di— *see* Acqua di Sirmione, 1772·3
Sirmiosta Nervenelixier N, 2293·4
Sirodina, 2293·4
Sirolax, 2293·4
Sirolimus, 1363·1
Sirop Antitussif Wyss a Base de Codeine, 2293·4
Sirop Boin, 2293·4
Sirop Cocillana Codeine, 2293·4
Sirop contre la Toux Nouvelle Formule, 2293·4
Sirop Dentition, 2293·4
Sirop des Vosges Expectorant, 2293·4
Sirop des Vosges Toux Seche, 2293·4
Sirop DM, 2294·1
Sirop Expectorant, 2294·1
Sirop Passi-Par, 2294·1
Sirop Pectoral Preparations, 2294·1
Sirop pour le Sommeil, 2294·1
Sirop S contre la Toux et la Bronchite, 2294·1
Sirop Teyssedre, 2294·1
Sirop Toux du Larynx, 2294·1
Sirop Wyss contre la Toux, 2294·1
Siros, 2294·1

Sirotamicin BG, 2294·1
Sirotamicin HC, 2294·1
Siroxyl, 2294·1
SIRS— *see* Septicaemia, 144·3
Sirtal, 2294·1
Sisare, 2294·1
Sisare Mono, 2294·1
Sisomicin Sulfate, 254·3
Sisomicin Sulphate, 254·3
Sisomicina, Sulfato de, 254·3
Sisomina, 2294·1
Sisoptin, 2294·1
Sissomicin Sulphate, 254·3
Sistalgina, 2294·1
Sita, 2294·1
Sitem, 2294·1
Siterone, 2294·1
Siticox, 2294·2
Siticox-INH, 2294·2
Sito-Lande, 2294·2
β-Sitosterin, 982·3
Sitosterol, 982·3, 1762·1
β-Sitosterol, 982·3
Sitrac, 2294·2
Sitriol, 2294·2
Sitzmarks, 2294·2
Sivastin, 2294·2
Sivelestat, 1746·3
Sivelestat Sodium, 1746·3
Sivlor, 2294·2
Sizofiran, 583·3
Sizopin, 2294·2
SJ-1977, 485·3
SJ Liniment, 2294·2
Sjögren's Syndrome— *see* Dry Eye, 1576·1
Sjögren's Syndrome— *see* Dry Mouth, 1576·2
SK7, 979·2
SK-331A, 1029·1
Skaelud, 2294·2
Skakuyaku-kanzo-to, Tsumura— *see* Tsumura Shakuyaku-kanzo-to, 2351·1
Skeeter Stik, 2294·2
Skelan, 2294·2
Skelan IB, 2294·2
Skelaxin, 2294·2
Skelid, 2294·2
Skema, 2294·2
Skenan, 2294·2
Skezide, 2294·2
SKF-5, 1593·3
SKF-51, 975·3
SKF-385, 318·3
SKF-478, 1261·1
SKF-478-A, 1261·1
SKF-478-J, 1261·1
SKF-525-A, 1735·2
SKF-525A, 1735·2
SKF-688A, 981·2
SKF-1717, 1655·1
SKF-2208, 1434·2
SKF-5116, 703·2
SKF-5883, 724·1
SKF-7988, 277·3
SKF-8542, 1016·2
SKF-9976, 1126·1
SKF-14287, 637·3
SKF-18667, 1414·2
SKF-20716, 714·1
SKF-30310, 111·2
SKF-33134-A, 859·2
SKF-38094, 1427·1
SKF-38095, 1442·3
SKF-39162, 19·1
SKF-41558, 170·3
SKF-60771, 170·3
SKF-62698, 1012·2
SKF-62979, 101·2
SKF-70230-A, 1129·1
SKF-82526-j, 915·3
SKF-83088, 173·3
SKF-88373-Z, 182·2
SKF-92334, 1255·3
SKF-96022, 1283·1
SKF-100168, 937·3
SKF-101468, 1213·3
SKF-0101468-A, 1213·3
SKF-102362, 972·2
SKF-104864A, 589·1
SKF-108566-J, 912·1
SK-F, BIC-F, 2294·2
SKF-D-39162, 19·1
SKF-D-39304, 179·3
SKF-D-75073-Z, 174·2
SKF-D-75073-$Z_2$, 174·2
SKFS-104864-A, 589·1
Skiacol, 2294·2
Skiatropine, 2294·2
Skid, 2294·2
Skid E, 2294·2
Skilax, 2294·2
Skin Bond Cement, 2294·2
Skin, Bovine, 1158·1
Skin C, 2294·2
Skin Cancer— *see* Malignant Neoplasms of the Skin, 522·2
Skin Cancer, Prophylaxis— *see* Malignant Neoplasms of the Skin, 522·2
Skin Cap, 2294·2
Skin Care Nutrients, 2294·2
Skin Cleanser & Deodorizer, 2294·3
Skin Cleansing, 2294·3
Skin Clear, 2294·3
Skin Conditioner & Bath Oil, 2294·3
Skin Cure, 2294·3
Skin Dry, 2294·3
Skin Equivalent, Bioengineered Human, 1158·1
Skin Eruptions Mixture, 2294·3
Skin Hair & Nails, 2294·3
Skin Healing Cream, 2294·3
Skin Infections, Bacterial— *see* Skin Infections, 146·2
Skin Infections, Fungal— *see* Skin Infections, 390·1
Skin, Porcine, 1158·1
Skin Prep, 2294·3
Skin Repair, 2294·3
Skin Repair Daily Care, 2294·3
Skin Shield, 2294·3
Skin So Soft Antibacterial, 2294·3
Skin Sol P, 2294·3
Skin Sol T, 2294·3
Skin Substitutes, 1158·1
Skin Ulceration, Infections in— *see* Skin Infections, 146·2
Skinat, 2294·3
Skincalm, 2294·3
Skin-Cap, 2294·3
Skinderm A, 2294·3
Skindure, 2294·3
Skinfect, 2294·3
Skinicles, 2294·3
Skinman Intensiv, 2294·3
Skinman Soft, 2294·3
Skinocyclin, 2294·3
Skinoderm, 2294·3
Skinola-Fett, 2294·3
Skinoren, 2294·3
Skinsept, 2294·4
Skinsept F, 2294·4
Skinsept G, 2294·4
Skinsept Mucosa, 2294·4
Skintex, 2294·4
SkinVit, 2294·4
Skleremo, 2294·4
Sklerofibrat, 2294·4
Sklerosol N, 2294·4
Sklerovenol N, 2294·4
Sklerovitol, 2294·4
Skudal, 2294·4
Skullcap, 1746·3
Skunk, 1666·2
Skunk Cabbage, 1746·3
Skunkweed, 1746·3
SL-76-002, 377·2
SL-80.0750, 728·3
SL-80.0750-23N, 728·3
SL-85.0324-00, 437·3
SL-501, 1117·1
SL-75212-10, 873·1
SL-77499, 856·2
SL-77499-10, 856·2
Slaked Lime, 1664·3
Slap, 2294·4
Sleep Aid, 2294·4
Sleep Aid, Modern Herbals— *see* Modern Herbals Sleep Aid, 2138·2
Sleep Disorders, 667·1
Sleep Paralysis— *see* Narcoleptic Syndrome, 1583·2
Sleep Walking— *see* Parasomnias, 667·3
Sleep-Care, Extralife— *see* Extralife Sleep-Care, 1986·3
Sleepeaze, 2294·4
Sleep-Ettes D, 2294·4
Sleep-eze 3, 2294·4
Sleep-Eze D, 2294·4
Sleep-Eze V Natural, 2294·4
Sleepeze PM, 2294·4
Sleepia, 2294·4
Sleepinal, Maximum Strength— *see* Maximum Strength Sleepinal, 2116·4
Sleeping Sickness— *see* African Trypanosomiasis, 599·3
Sleeplessness & Insomnia Relief, 2294·4
Sleepwell 2-Nite, 2294·4
Slepan, 2294·4
Slim Caps, 2294·4
Slim Mint, 2294·4
Slim 'n Trim, 2294·4
Slimase, 2294·4
SlimLinea, 2294·4
Slimmer, 2294·4
Slimomin, 2295·1
Slimum, 2295·1
Slippery Elm, 1747·1
Slippery Elm Bark, 1747·1
Slippery Elm Stomach Tablets, 2295·1
Sloan, 2295·1
Sloan Baume, 2295·1
Sloan Liniment, 2295·1
Sloan, Linimento— *see* Linimento Sloan, 2097·4
Sloan's Balsem, 2295·1
Slo-Bid, 2295·1
Slofedipine, 2295·1
Slofenac, 2295·1
Slo-Indo, 2295·1
Slo-Morph, 2295·1
Slo-Niacin, 2295·1
Slo-Phyllin, 2295·1
Slo-Phyllin GG, 2295·1
Slo-Salt-K, 2295·1
Slo-Theo, 2295·1
Slow Deralin, 2295·1
Slow Fe with Folic Acid, 2295·1
Slow K, 2295·1
Slow Release Mega C, 2295·1
Slow Release Mega Multi, 2295·1
Slow-channel Blockers, 810·3
Slow-Fe, 2295·1
Slow-Fe Folic, 2295·1
Slow-K, 2295·1
Slow-Lopresor, 2295·1
Slow-Mag, 2295·2
Slow-Sodium, 2295·2
Slow-Trasicor, 2295·2
Slow-Trasitensine, 2295·2
Slozem, 2295·2
SLT, 2295·2
Slumber, 2295·2
SM-33, 2295·2
SM-33 Adult Formula, 2295·2
SM-224, 447·2
SM-227, 447·2
SM-804, 447·2
SM-1652, 178·2
SM-3997, 723·2
SM-5887, 527·3
SM-7338, 229·1
SM-8668, 400·3
SM-9018, 714·1
SM-9527, 909·2
8SM— *see* Replenate, 2258·2
SMA AR, 2295·2
SMA High Energy, 2295·2
SMA LF, 2295·2
SMA Sin Lactosa, 2295·2
Small Airways Disease— *see* Chronic Obstructive Pulmonary Disease, 779·2
Small Cell Lung Cancer— *see* Malignant Neoplasms of the Lung, 519·2
Smallpox Vaccine, 1639·1
Smallpox Vaccines, 1639·1
SMANCS, 594·3
Smaril, 2295·2
Smart Fizz, 2295·2
Smecta, 2295·2
Smelling Salts, 1654·1
Smilacis Rhizoma, 1742·1
*Smilax*, 1742·1
Smilitene, 2295·2
Smok Quits, 2295·2
Smoke-Eze, 2295·2
Smokeless, 2295·2
Smokerette, 2295·2
Smoking Cessation, 1721·2
Smoking Withdrawal Support, 2295·2
Smooth Hydrangea, 1698·3
Smooth Sumach, 1738·1
SMS-201-995, 1333·1
SMZ-TMP, 2295·2
SN-38, 564·3
SN-105-843, 406·2
SN-307, 1281·1
SN-654, 405·2
SN-7618, 448·2
SN-12,837, 457·1
SN-13,272, 456·2
Snake Antivenins, 1639·1
Snake Antivenoms, 1639·1
Snake Bite, 2295·2
Snake Bites, 1639·2
Snake Venom Antisera, 1639·1
Snake Venom Antiserum, 1639·1
Snake Weed, 1686·3
Snakeroot, 1656·3
SNAP, 597·3
Snap Skin Cleanser Normal, 2295·2
Snap Skin Cleanser Sensitive, 2295·2
Snaplets-DM, 2295·2
Snaplets-EX, 2295·2
Snaplets-Multi, 2295·2
SND-5008, 1488·3
SND-919-CL-2Y, 1212·2
Snell Cell, 2295·3
Snell'it, 2295·3
SNI-2011, 1488·3
Snif, 2295·3
Snip, 2295·3
SNK-508, 1488·3
Sno Phenicol, 2295·3
Sno Pro, 2295·3
Sno Strips, 2295·3
Sno Tears, 2295·3
Snoffocin, 2295·3
Snooze Fast, 2295·3
Sno-Pro, 2295·3
Snor-Away, 2295·3
Snore Calm, 2295·3
Snore Eze, 2295·3
Snore No More, 2295·3
Snore Stop, 2295·3
Snoreeze, 2295·3
Snore-No-More, 2295·3
Snorenz, 2295·3
Snow, 1373·3
Snowdrop, Caucasian, 1491·2
Snowdrop, Voronov's, 1491·2
Snowfire, 2295·3
SNP, 2295·3
(Sn)-protoporphyrin, 1756·3
SNRIs, 278·2
Snufflebabe, 2295·3
Snufflebabe Cradle Cap, 2295·3
Snup, 2295·3
SNX-111, 96·3
Soaclens, 2295·3
Soam, 2295·3
Soap Bark, 1416·1
Soap, Castile, 1575·2
Soap Clay, 1577·2

Soap, Curd, 1575·2
Soap, Green, 1575·2
Soap, Hard, 1575·2
Soap, Linseed Oil, 1575·2
Soap, Potash, 1575·2
Soap, Potassium, 1575·2
Soap, Soft, 1575·2
Soapex, 2295·3
Soaps, 1574·1
Soaps, Alkali-metal, 1574·1
Soaps, Amine, 1574·1
Soaps, Ammonium, 1574·1
Soaps, Metallic, 1574·1
Soaps and Other Anionic Surfactants, 1574·1
Sobelin, 2295·4
Sobrepin, 2295·4
Sobrepina, 2295·4
Sobrerol, 1130·2
Sobrerolo, 1130·2
Sobrial, 2295·4
Sobril, 2295·4
Sobrius, 2295·4
Sobuzoxane, 583·3
Sobuzoxano, 583·3
Socainide Hydrochloride, 947·2
Social Anxiety Disorder— *see* Phobic Disorders, 663·3
Social Phobia— *see* Phobic Disorders, 663·3
Socian, 2295·4
Socloxin, 2295·4
Socosep, 2295·4
SOD, 92·2
Sod. Cyclam., 1426·2
Sod. Iod., 1598·1
Sod. Perbor., 1192·2
Sod. Stibogluc., 600·3
Soda Ash, 1747·1
Soda, Baking, 1223·2
Soda, Cenizas de, 1747·1
Soda Lime, 1747·1
Soda Lye, 1747·3
Soda, Washing, 1747·2
Sodemethin, 2295·4
Soden, 2295·4
Soderm, 2295·4
Soderm Plus, 2295·4
Sodexx, 2295·4
Sodibic, 2295·4
Sodical Plus, Celloid Compounds— *see* Celloid Compounds Sodical Plus, 1877·2
Sodiclo, 2295·4
Sodii Benzoas, 1169·3
Sodii Chloras, 1747·2
Sodii et Potassii Tartras, 1284·3
Sodii Iodidum, 1598·1
Sodilen, 2295·4
Sodilin, 2295·4
Sodio, 1233·3
Sódio, Cloreto de, 1233·3
Sodio, Cloruro de, 1233·3
Sodiofolin, 2295·4
Sodiopen, 2295·4
Sodioral con Inulina, 2295·4
Sodiparin, 2295·4
Sodipen, 2295·4
Sodipental, 2295·4
Sodip-phylline, 2295·4
Sodipryl Retard, 2295·4
Sodium, 1233·3
Sodium Acetate, 1223·1
Sodium Acetate, Theobromine and, 798·2
Sodium Acetate, Theophylline and, 805·2
Sodium Acetate Trihydrate, 1223·1
Sodium Acetazolamide, 849·1
Sodium (12*Z*,14*E*,24*E*)-(2*S*,16*S*,17*S*,18*R*,19*R*,20*R*,21*S*,22*R*,23*S*)-21-Acetoxy-1,2-dihydro-6,9,17,19-tetrahydroxy-23-methoxy-2,4,12,16,18,20,22-heptamethyl-1,11-dioxo-2,7-(epoxypentadeca-1,11,13-trienimino)-naphtho[2,1-*b*]furan-5-olate, 253·2
Sodium (7*R*)-3-Acetoxymethyl-7-[(*Z*)-2-(2-aminothiazol-4-yl)-2-(methoxyimino)acetamido]-3-cephem-4-carboxylate, 175·3
Sodium (7*R*)-3-Acetoxymethyl-7-[2-(4-pyridylthio)acetamido]-3-cephem-4-carboxylate, 170·2
Sodium (7*R*)-3-Acetoxymethyl-7-[2-(2-thienyl)acetamido]-3-cephem-4-carboxylate, 168·3
Sodium Acexamate, 1646·2
Sodium Acid Carbonate, 1223·2
Sodium Acid Citrate, 1223·2
Sodium Acid Phosphate, 1230·3
Sodium Aescin Polysulfate, 1648·2
Sodium Aescinate, 1648·2
Sodium Alendronate, 765·3
Sodium Alginate, 1577·1
Sodium Alkyl Sulfates, 1574·2
Sodium Alkyl Sulfoacetates, 1574·3
Sodium 5-Allyl-5-(1-methylbutyl)barbiturate, 721·2
Sodium 5-Allyl-5-(1-methylbutyl)-2-thiobarbiturate, 1309·1
Sodium Aluminium Silicate, 1250·2
Sodium Aluminosilicate, 1250·2
Sodium Amidotrizoate, 1060·2
Sodium Aminarsonate, 158·3
Sodium Aminoacetate, Theophylline, 805·2
Sodium Aminobenzoate, 1747·1
Sodium 4-Aminobenzoate, 1747·1
Sodium [2-Amino-3-(*p*-bromobenzoyl)phenyl]acetate Sesquihydrate, 21·3
Sodium 7-{2-[(*S*)-2-Amino-2-carboxyethyl]thioacetamido}-7-methoxy-3-(1-methyl-1*H*-tetrazol-5-ylthiomethyl)-3-cephem-4-carboxylate, 174·1
Sodium Aminohippurate, 1653·2
Sodium 4-Amino-2-hydroxybenzoate Dihydrate, 155·1
Sodium 4-Aminophenylarsonate, 158·3
Sodium Aminosalicylate, 155·1
Sodium Aminosalicylate Dihydrate, 155·1
Sodium (7*R*)-7-[(*Z*)-2-(2-Aminothiazol-4-yl)-2-(methoxyimino)acetamido]cephalosporanate, 175·3
Sodium (*Z*)-7-[2-(2-Aminothiazol-4-yl)-2-methoxyiminoacetamido]-3-cephem-4-carboxylate, 182·2
Sodium Amobarbital, 670·1
Sodium Anilarsonate, 158·3
Sodium Antimony Gluconate, 600·3
Sodium Antimonyltartrate, 103·1
Sodium Apolate, 1000·2
Sodium Arsanilate, 158·3
Sodium Arsenate, 1747·1
Sodium Arseniate, 1747·1
Sodium Artelinate, 448·1
Sodium Artesunate, 447·2
Sodium Ascorbate, 1460·2
Sodium Aspirin, 18·1
Sodium 3-Aurothio-2-hydroxypropane-1-sulphonate, 20·1
Sodium Aurothiomalate, 88·2
Sodium Aurothiosuccinate, 88·2
Sodium Aurothiosulphate, 90·1
Sodium Aurotiosulfate, 90·1
Sodium Azide, 1191·3
Sodium (6*R*)-6-(D-2-Azido-2-phenylacetamido)penicillanate, 159·1
Sodium Azodisalicylate, 1278·1
Sodium Benzoate, 1169·3
Sodium Benzoate, Caffeine and, 783·2
Sodium Benzosulphimide, 1443·3
Sodium Biborate, 1661·3
Sodium Bicarbonate, 1223·2
Sodium Biphosphate, 1230·3
Sodium 1,4-Bis(2-ethylhexyl) Sulphosuccinate, 1262·2
Sodium Bisulfite, 1193·1
Sodium Bisulphite, 1193·1
Sodium Bituminosulfonate, 1148·3
Sodium Bituminosulphonate, Light, 1148·3
Sodium Borate, 1661·3
Sodium Bromide, 1662·3
Sodium Butabarbital, 721·2
Sodium Butyl Hydroxybenzoate, 1183·3
Sodium Butyl Parahydroxybenzoate, 1183·3
Sodium 5-*sec*-Butyl-5-ethylbarbiturate, 721·2
Sodium Butylparaben, 1183·3
Sodium 2-(3-Butyramido-2,4,6-tri-iodobenzyl)butyrate, 1067·3
Sodium Calcium Edetate, 1051·3
Sodium Calciumedetate, 1051·3
Sodium Caprylate, 1723·1
Sodium 3-Carbamoyloxymethyl-7-methoxy-7-[2-(2-thienyl)acetamido]-3-cephem-4-carboxylate, 177·2
Sodium 3-(4-Carbamoylpyridiniomethyl)-7-[(2*R*)-2-phenyl-2-sulphoacetamido]-3-cephem-4-carboxylate, 180·2
Sodium Carbonate, 1747·2
Sodium Carbonate Anhydrous, 1747·1
Sodium Carbonate, Anhydrous, 1747·2
Sodium Carbonate Decahydrate, 1747·2
Sodium Carbonate, Exsiccated, 1747·1
Sodium Carbonate Monohydrate, 1747·2
Sodium Carbonate Peroxide, 1192·3
Sodium (Carbonato)dihydroxyaluminate(1-), 1261·2
Sodium Carboxymethyl Starch, 1582·1
Sodium Carboxymethylcellulose, 1577·3
Sodium (4*R*,5*S*,6*S*)-3-({(3*S*,5*S*)-5-[(*m*-Carboxyphenyl)carbamoyl]-3-pyrrolidinyl}thio)-6-[(1*R*)-1-hydroxyethyl]-4-methyl-7-oxo-1-azabicyclo[3.2.0]hept-2-ene-2-carboxylate, 207·3
Sodium (2-Carboxyphenylthio)ethylmercury, 1194·1
Sodium Cellulose Glycollate, 1577·3
Sodium Cellulose Phosphate, 1052·1
Sodium Cephalothin, 168·3
Sodium Cetostearyl Sulfate, 1574·2
Sodium Cetostearyl Sulphate, 1574·2
Sodium Cetyl Sulfate, 1574·2
Sodium Chlorate, 1747·2
Sodium Chloride, 1233·3
Sodium *N*-Chlorobenzenesulphonimidate Sesquihydrate, 1195·1
Sodium 1-(4-Chlorobenzoyl)-5-methoxy-2-methylindole-3-acetate, Trihydrate, 47·3
Sodium (±)-(*Z*)-7-{(1*R*,2*R*,3*R*,5*S*)-2-[(*E*)-(3*R*)-4-(3-Chlorophenoxy)-3-hydroxybut-1-enyl]-3,5-dihydroxycyclopentyl}hept-5-enoate, 1514·3
Sodium 1-[({(*R*)-*m*-[(*E*)-2-(7-Chloro-2-quinolyl)-vinyl]-α-[*o*-(1-hydroxy-1-methylethyl)phenethyl]-benzyl}thio)methyl] Cyclopropaneacetate, 788·3
Sodium Chlorothiazide, 882·2
Sodium *N*-Chlorotoluene-*p*-sulphonimidate Trihydrate, 1194·3
Sodium, Chlorure de, 1233·3
Sodium Chondroitin Sulfate, 1670·2
Sodium Chromate ($^{51}$Cr), 1523·2
Sodium Citrate, 1223·2
Sodium Clodronate, 770·2
Sodium Colistimethate, 199·1
Sodium Colistinmethanesulphonate, 199·1
Sodium Cromoglicate, 795·3
Sodium Cromoglycate, 795·3
Sodium Cyanide, 1506·2
Sodium Cyclamate, 1426·2
Sodium Cyclohexanehexyl(hexaphosphate), 1052·3
Sodium Cyclohexanesulphamate, 1426·2
Sodium 5-(Cyclohex-1-enyl)-1,5-dimethylbarbiturate, 703·1
Sodium *N*-Cyclohexylsulphamate, 1426·2
Sodium Dehydroacetate, 1178·1
Sodium Deoxyribonucleate, 1679·2
Sodium Dexamethasone Phosphate, 1097·2
Sodium Dextrothyroxine, 893·2
Sodium 3,5-Diacetamido-2,4,6-tri-iodobenzoate, 1060·2
Sodium Diacetate, 1191·3
Sodium 2′,4′-Diaminoazobenzene-4-sulphonate, 1056·2
Sodium 2′,4′-Diamino-5′-methylazobenzene-4-sulphonate, 1056·2
Sodium Diaphenylsulphonacetate, 153·3
Sodium Diatrizoate, 1060·2
Sodium Dibunate, 1130·2
Sodium 2,6-Di-*tert*-butylnaphthalene-1-sulphonate, 1130·2
Sodium Dichloroacetate, 1747·2
Sodium [2-(2,6-Dichloroanilino)phenyl]acetate, 32·1
Sodium Dichloroisocyanurate, 1191·3
Sodium Dichloro-*s*-triazinetrione, 1191·3
Sodium Dichromate, 1670·3
Sodium Dicloxacillin Monohydrate, 205·2
Sodium α-(4-Diethylaminophenyl)-α-(4-diethyliminiocyclo-hexa-2,5-dienylidene)toluene-2,4-disulfonate, 1750·3
Sodium α-(4-Diethylaminophenyl)-α-(4-diethyliminiocyclo-hexa-2,5-dienylidene)toluene-2,5-disulfonate, 1750·3
Sodium 5,5-Diethylbarbiturate, 671·2
Sodium Diethyldithiocarbamate, 1038·2
Sodium 17α-Dihydroequilin Sulfate, 1543·2
Sodium 17β-Dihydroequilin Sulfate, 1543·2
Sodium Dihydrogen Orthophosphate, 1230·3
Sodium Dihydrogen Phosphate, 1230·3
Sodium Dihydrogen Phosphate, Anhydrous, 1230·3
Sodium Dihydrogen Phosphate Dihydrate, 1230·3
Sodium Dihydrogen Phosphate Monohydrate, 1230·3
Sodium 2,5-Dihydroxybenzoate Dihydrate, 90·1
Sodium 2,3-Dimercaptopropanesulfonate, 1055·3
Sodium (6*R*)-6-(2,6-Dimethoxybenzamido)penicillanate Monohydrate, 230·3
Sodium 1-[4-Dimethylamino-α-(4-dimethyliminiocyclohexa-2,5-dienylidene)benzyl]-2-hydroxynaphthalene-3,6-disulphonate, 1057·3
Sodium 3-(3-Dimethylaminomethyleneamino-2,4,6-tri-iodophenyl)propionate, 1065·2
Sodium *N*-(2,3-Dimethyl-5-oxo-1-phenyl-3-pyrazolin-4-yl)-*N*-methylaminomethanesulphonate Monohydrate, 35·3
Sodium 2-{7-[1,1-Dimethyl-3-(4-sulphobutyl)benz[*e*]indolin-2-ylidene]hepta-1,3,5-trienyl}-1,1-dimethyl-1*H*-benz[*e*]indolio-3-(butyl-4-sulphonate), 1701·1
Sodium Dioctyl Sulphosuccinate, 1262·2
Sodium Disulphite, 1193·1
Sodium Dithionite, 1747·3
Sodium Dithiosulfatoaurate, 90·1
Sodium Dodecyl Sulphate, 1574·2
Sodium Edetate, 1037·3
Sodium Equilin Sulfate, 1543·2, 1549·3
Sodium 17α-Estradiol Sulfate, 1543·2
Sodium Estrone Sulfate, 1543·2, 1549·3
Sodium Etacrynate, 913·3
Sodium Ethacrynate, 913·3
Sodium (6*R*)-6-(2-Ethoxy-1-naphthamido)penicillanate Monohydrate, 233·3
Sodium 8-Ethoxy-5-quinolinesulfonate, 1647·2
Sodium Ethyl Hydroxybenzoate, 1183·3
Sodium Ethyl Mercurithiosalicylate, 1194·1
Sodium (7*R*)-7-[(*R*)-2-(4-Ethyl-2,3-dioxopiperazin-1-ylcarboxamido)-2-(4-hydroxyphenyl)acetamido]-3-[(1-methyl-1*H*-tetrazol-5-yl)thiomethyl]-3-cephem-4-carboxylate, 174·3
Sodium 4-Ethyl-1-isobutyloctyl Sulfate, 1575·1
Sodium 5-Ethyl-5-isopentylbarbiturate, 670·1
Sodium 5-Ethyl-5-(1-methylbutyl)barbiturate, 713·3
Sodium 5-Ethyl-5-(1-methylbutyl)-2-thiobarbiturate, 1309·1
Sodium 5-Ethyl-5-phenylbarbiturate, 367·3
Sodium (2*R*)-2-{(2*R*,5*S*,6*R*)-6-[(1*S*,2*S*,3*S*,5*R*)-5-{(2*S*,5*S*,7*R*,9*S*,10*S*,12*R*,15*R*)-2-[(2*R*,5*R*,6*S*)-5-Ethyltetrahydro-5-hydroxy-6-methylpyran-2-yl]-15-hydroxy-2,10,12-trimethyl-1,6,8-trioxadispiro[4.1.5.3]pentadec-13-en-9-yl}-2-hydroxy-1,3-dimethyl-4-oxoheptyl]tetrahydro-5-methylpyran-2-yl}butyrate, 615·2
Sodium Etidronate, 771·2
Sodium Etoquinol, 1647·2
Sodium Feredetate, 1444·3
Sodium Ferric Gluconate, 1444·3
Sodium Ferric Gluconate Complex, 1444·3
Sodium Ferrigluconate, 1444·3
Sodium Fluorescein, 1689·1

Sodium Fluoride, 1444·3
Sodium Fluoride ($^{18}$F), 1523·3
Sodium Fluoroacetate, 1510·1
Sodium (±)-2-(2-Fluoro-4-biphenylyl)propionate Dihydrate, 44·1
Sodium 6-Fluoro-2-(2′-fluoro-4-biphenylyl)-3-methyl-4-quinolinecarboxylate, 1351·2
Sodium (±)-(3*R*$^*$,5*S*$^*$,6*E*)-7-[3-(*p*-Fluorophenyl)-1-isopropylindol-2-yl]-3,5-dihydroxy-6-heptenoate, 918·2
Sodium {*S*-[*R*$^*$,*S*$^*$-(*E*)]}-7-[4-(4-Fluorophenyl)-5-(methoxymethyl)-2,6-bis(1-methylethyl)-3-pyridinyl]-3,5-dihydroxy-6-heptenoate, 881·3
Sodium Fluorophosphate, 1446·2
Sodium Fluorosilicate, 1446·3
Sodium Fluosilicate, 1446·3
Sodium Folate, 1429·3
Sodium Folinate, 1431·3
Sodium Formaldehyde Sulfoxylate, 1192·1
Sodium Formaldehyde Sulphoxylate, 1192·1
Sodium Formate, 1689·3
Sodium (7*R*)-7-[(2*R*)-2-Formyloxy-2-phenylacetamido]-3-(1-methyl-1*H*-tetrazol-5-ylthiomethyl)-3-cephem-4-carboxylate, 169·3
Sodium Fumarate, 1147·3
Sodium Fusidate, 215·2
Sodium Fytate, 1052·3
Sodium Gamma-hydroxybutyrate, 1308·3
Sodium Gentisate, 90·1
Sodium Gluconate, 1747·3
Sodium Glutamate, 1441·1
Sodium Glycerophosphate, 1695·2
Sodium Glycerylphosphate, 1695·2
Sodium Glycinate, Theophylline, 805·2
Sodium Guaiacolglycolate, 1122·1
Sodium Gualenate, 1658·3
Sodium 5′-Guanylate, 1681·3
Sodium Heparin, 928·1
Sodium Heparitin Sulphate, 1009·1
Sodium Hexafluorosilicate, 1446·3
Sodium (3*R*,5*R*)-7-{(1*S*,2*S*,6*S*,8*S*,8a*R*)-1,2,6,7,8,8a-Hexahydro-6-hydroxy-2-methyl-8-[(*S*)-2-methylbutyryloxy]-1-naphthyl}-3,5-dihydroxyheptanoate, 984·3
Sodium Hexametaphosphate, 1748·2
Sodium Hexobarbital, 703·1
Sodium Hyaluronate, 1697·3
Sodium Hydrogen L-(+)-2-Aminoglutarate Monohydrate, 1441·1
Sodium Hydrogen Bis(2-propylvalerate) Oligomer, 380·1
Sodium Hydrogen 4-(Carbamoylmethylamino)phenylarsonate Hemihydrate, 617·3
Sodium Hydrogen Carbonate, 1223·2
Sodium Hydrogen Diacetate, 1191·3
Sodium Hydrogen Sulphite, 1193·1
Sodium Hydrosulfite, 1747·3
Sodium Hydrosulphite, 1747·3
Sodium Hydroxide, 1747·3
Sodium 2-Hydroxybenzoate, 90·1
Sodium 4-Hydroxybutyrate, 1308·3
Sodium 2-(1-Hydroxycyclohexyl)butyrate, 1678·2
Sodium 4-*O*-(4-Hydroxy-3,5-di-iodophenyl)-3,5-di-iodo-D-tyrosinate Hydrate, 893·2
Sodium 4-*O*-(4-Hydroxy-3,5-di-iodophenyl)-3,5-di-iodo-L-tyrosine Hydrate, 1600·1
Sodium (+)-(5*R*,6*S*)-6-[(1*R*)-1-Hydroxyethyl]-7-oxo-3-[(2*R*)-tetrahydro-2-furyl]-4-thia-1-azabicyclo[3.2.0]hept-2-ene-2-carboxylate, 213·1
Sodium 4-*O*-(4-Hydroxy-3-iodophenyl)-3,5-di-iodo-L-tyrosine, 1602·2
Sodium Hydroxymethanesulphinate Dihydrate, 1192·1
Sodium 1-Hydroxy-5-oxo-5*H*-pyrido[3,2-*a*]phenoxazine-3-carboxylate, 1732·2
Sodium 2-Hydroxypropionate, 1223·2
Sodium Hydroxyquinoline Sulfate, 1700·1
Sodium Hypochlorite, 1192·1
Sodium Hypochlorite Solution, 1192·1
Sodium Hypochlorite Solution, Dilute, 1192·1
Sodium Hypochlorite Solution, Strong, 1192·1
Sodium Hypochlorite Topical Solution, 1192·1
Sodium Hyposulphite, 1053·3
Sodium Ibandronate, 772·3
Sodium (6*R*)-6-[2-(Indan-5-yloxycarbonyl)-2-phenylacetamido]penicillanate, 166·3
Sodium Indigotindisulphonate, 1700·3
Sodium 5′-Inosinate, 1681·3
Sodium Iodamide, 1063·2
Sodium Iodide, 1598·1
Sodium Iodide ($^{123}$I), 1524·1
Sodium Iodide ($^{125}$I), 1524·2
Sodium Iodide ($^{131}$I), 1524·3
Sodium Iodide, Caffeine and, 783·2
Sodium Iodoheparinate, 1748·1
Sodium Iodohippurate ($^{123}$I), 1524·1
Sodium Iodohippurate ($^{125}$I), 1524·2
Sodium Iodohippurate ($^{131}$I), 1524·3
Sodium (Iodure de), 1598·1
Sodium Ioglicate, 1064·2
Sodium Iopodate, 1065·2
Sodium Iotalamate, 1065·3
Sodium Iotalamate ($^{125}$I), 1524·2
Sodium Iothalamate, 1065·3
Sodium Ioxaglate, 1066·2
Sodium Ioxitalamate, 1066·3
Sodium Ipodate, 1065·2
Sodium Ironedetate, 1444·3
Sodium 2-(4-Isobutylphenyl)butyrate, 23·3
Sodium Isospaglumate, 1702·2
Sodium α-Ketopropionate, 1748·2
Sodium Lactate, 1223·2
Sodium Lactate Solution, 1223·2
Sodium Lauril Ether Sulfate, 1574·3
Sodium Lauril Sulfoacetate, 1574·3
Sodium Laurilsulfate, 1574·2
Sodium Lauryl Sulfate, 1574·2
Sodium Lauryl Sulphate, 1574·2
Sodium Liothyronine, 1602·2
Sodium Lyapolate, 1000·2
Sodium 2-Mercaptoethanesulphonate, 1041·2
Sodium (6*R*)-6-[D-2-(3-Mesyl-2-oxoimidazolidine-1-carboxamido)-2-phenylacetamido]penicillanate Monohydrate, 231·1
Sodium Metabisulfite, 1193·1
Sodium Metabisulphite, 1193·1
Sodium Metharsinite, 1748·1
Sodium α-{*p*-[(6-Methoxy-3-pyridazinyl)sulfamoyl]anilino}-2,3-dimethyl-5-oxo-1-phenyl-3-pyrazoline-4-methanesulphonate, 260·3
Sodium Methyl Hydroxybenzoate, 1183·3
Sodium Methyl Parahydroxybenzoate, 1183·3
Sodium Methylarsinate, 1748·1
Sodium (6*R*)-6-(D-2-Methyleneamino-2-phenylacetamido)penicillanate, 229·3
Sodium (2*S*,3*S*,5*R*)-3-Methyl-7-oxo-3-(1*H*-1,2,3-triazol-1-ylmethyl)-4-thia-1-azabicyclo[3.2.0]-heptane-2-carboxylate 4,4-Dioxide, 264·3
Sodium Methylparaben, 1183·3
Sodium (6*R*)-6-(5-Methyl-3-phenylisoxazole-4-carboxamido)penicillanate Monohydrate, 240·2
Sodium (1-Methyl-5-*p*-toluoylpyrrol-2-yl)acetate Dihydrate, 94·2
Sodium Metrizoate, 1067·2
Sodium Molybdate, 1440·3
Sodium Molybdate Dihydrate, 1440·3
Sodium Monofluoroacetate, 1510·1
Sodium Monofluorophosphate, 1446·2
Sodium Morrhuate, 1748·1
Sodium Nitrate, 1192·2
Sodium Nitrite, 1052·3
Sodium Nitroferricyanide Dihydrate, 1000·2
Sodium Nitroprussiate, 1000·2
Sodium Nitroprusside, 1000·2
Sodium Nitrosylpentacyanoferrate(III) Dihydrate, 1000·2
Sodium Noramidopyrine Methanesulphonate, 35·3
Sodium Novobiocin, 239·2
Sodium Octanoate, 1723·1
Sodium Oleate, 1574·3
Sodium Oxidronate, 773·3
Sodium (±)-*p*-[(2-Oxocyclopentyl)methyl]hydratropate Dihydrate, 54·3
Sodium (6*R*)-6-[D-2-(2-Oxoimidazolidine-1-carboxamido)-2-phenylacetamido]penicillanate, 160·2
Sodium 2-Oxo-3-[(1*RS*)-3-oxo-1-phenylbutyl]-2*H*-1-benzopyran-4-olate, 1022·2
Sodium 2-Oxopropanoate, 1748·2
Sodium 5-Oxopyrrolidine-2-carboxylate, 1158·1
Sodium Oxybate, 1308·3
Sodium Oxybutyrate, 1308·3
Sodium Oxychlorosene, 1187·2
Sodium Palmitate, 1574·3
Sodium Pangamate, 1727·2
Sodium Pantothenate, 1443·1
Sodium Para-aminosalicylate, 155·1
Sodium Pariprazole, 1285·1
Sodium PAS, 155·1
Sodium Pentachlorophenate, 1508·3
Sodium Pentobarbital, 713·3
Sodium Pentosan Polysulphate, 979·2
Sodium Perborate, 1192·2
Sodium Perborate, Hydrated, 1192·2
Sodium Perborate Monohydrate, 1192·3
Sodium Percarbonate, 1192·3
Sodium Perchlorate, 1603·3
Sodium Pertechnetate ($^{99m}$Tc), 1525·3
Sodium (6*R*)-6-(2-Phenoxycarbonyl-2-phenylacetamido)penicillanate, 166·3
Sodium Phenylacetate, 1748·2
Sodium Phenylbutyrate, 1748·2
Sodium 4-Phenylbutyrate, 1748·2
Sodium Phenylethylbarbiturate, 367·3
Sodium Phosphate, 1231·1
Sodium Phosphate ($^{32}$P), 1525·1
Sodium Phosphate, Dibasic, 1231·1
Sodium Phosphate Dihydrate, 1231·1
Sodium Phosphate, Monobasic, 1230·3
Sodium Phosphate, Tribasic, 1231·1
Sodium Phytate, 1052·3
Sodium Picosulfate, 1289·3
Sodium Picosulphate, 1289·3
Sodium Pidolate, 1158·1
Sodium Poly(hydroxyaluminium) Carbonate-hexitol Complex, 1248·1
Sodium Polymannuronate, 1577·1
Sodium Polymetaphosphate, 1748·2
Sodium Polystyrene Sulfonate, 1053·1
Sodium Polystyrene Sulphonate, 1053·1
Sodium Potassium Tartrate, 1284·3
Sodium Propanoate, 408·1
Sodium Propionate, 408·1
Sodium Propyl Hydroxybenzoate, 1183·3, 1184·1
Sodium Propyl Parahydroxybenzoate, 1183·3, 1184·1
Sodium Propylparaben, 1183·3
Sodium 2-Propylpentanoate, 380·1
Sodium 2-Propylvalerate, 380·1
Sodium (7*R*)-7-[2-(4-Pyridylthio)acetamido]cephalosporanate, 170·2
Sodium Pyroborate, 1661·3
Sodium Pyroglutamate, 1158·1
Sodium Pyrosulphite, 1193·1
Sodium Pyrrolidone Carboxylate, 1158·1
Sodium Pyruvate, 1748·2
Sodium 5′-Ribonucleotide, 1681·3
Sodium Ricinoleate, 1575·3
Sodium Risedronate, 774·3
Sodium Rose Bengal, 1740·1
Sodium Saccharin, 1443·3
Sodium Salamidacetate, 87·3
Sodium Salicylate, 90·1
Sodium Salicylate, Caffeine and, 783·2
Sodium Salicylate, Theobromine and, 798·2
Sodium Selenate, 1444·1
Sodium Selenite, 1444·1
Sodium Selenite Pentahydrate, 1444·1
Sodium Selenium Oxide, 1444·1
Sodium Silicate, 1581·3, 1748·3
Sodium Silicoaluminate, 1250·2
Sodium Silicofluoride, 1446·3
Sodium Starch Glycolate, 1582·1
Sodium Starch Glycolate (Type A), 1582·1
Sodium Starch Glycolate (Type B), 1582·1
Sodium Starch Glycolate (Type C), 1582·2
Sodium Starch Glycollate, 1582·1
Sodium Stearate, 1574·3
Sodium Stearyl Fumarate, 1575·1
Sodium Stearyl Sulfate, 1574·2
Sodium Stibocaptate, 103·1
Sodium Stibogluconate, 600·3
Sodium Succinate, 1748·3
Sodium Sulamyd, 2295·4
Sodium Sulfadiazine, 258·2
Sodium Sulfate, 1290·1
Sodium Sulfite, 1193·1
Sodium Sulfobromophthalein, 1750·3
Sodium Sulfosuccinated Undecenoic Acid Monoethanolamide, 411·1
Sodium Sulphate, 1290·1
Sodium Sulphate, Anhydrous, 1290·1
Sodium Sulphate Decahydrate, 1290·1
Sodium Sulphate, Dried, 1290·1
Sodium Sulphate, Exsiccated, 1290·1
Sodium Sulphite, 1193·1
Sodium Sulphite, Anhydrous, 1193·1
Sodium Sulphite, Exsiccated, 1193·1
Sodium Sulphite Heptahydrate, 1193·1
Sodium Sulphoxylate, 1747·3
Sodium Tartrate, 1290·1
Sodium Tequinol, 1647·2
Sodium Tetraborate, 1661·3
Sodium Tetradecyl Sulfate, 1575·1
Sodium Tetradecyl Sulphate, 1575·1
Sodium Tetradecyl Sulphate Concentrate, 1575·1
Sodium (±)-(1*R*,2*R*,3a*S*,8b*S*)-2,3,3a,8b-Tetrahydro-2-hydroxy-1-[(*E*)-(3*S*,4*RS*)-3-hydroxy-4-methyl-1-octen-6-ynyl]-1*H*-cyclopenta[*b*]benzofuran-5-butyrate, 1514·1
Sodium 1,2,3,4-Tetrahydro-2-methyl-1,4-dioxonaphthalene-2-sulphonate Trihydrate, 1466·3
Sodium 2-{2-[2-(*p*-1,3,3-Tetramethylbutylphenoxy)ethoxy]ethoxy}ethanesulfonate, 1683·3
Sodium (7*R*)-7-[2-(1*H*-Tetrazol-1-yl)acetamido]-3-(1,3,4-thiadiazol-2-ylthiomethyl)-3-cephem-4-carboxylate, 182·1
Sodium (7*R*)-7-[2-(2-Thienyl)acetamido]cephalosporanate, 168·3
Sodium Thioctate, 1754·3
Sodium Thiosalicylate, 90·2
Sodium Thiosulfate, 1053·3
Sodium Thiosulphate, 1053·3
Sodium 2,2,2-Trichloroethyl Hydrogen Orthophosphate, 726·2
Sodium Triclofos, 726·2
Sodium Trihydrogen (4-Amino-1-hydroxybutylidene)diphosphonate Trihydrate, 765·3
Sodium Trihydrogen [1-Hydroxy-2-(3-pyridyl)ethylidene]diphosphonate, 774·3
Sodium Troclosene, 1191·3
Sodium Tyropanoate, 1067·3
Sodium Valproate, 380·1
Sodium Versenate, 1037·3
Sodium Warfarin, 1022·2
Sodium Xylanpolysulphate, 979·2
Sodium-free Condiments, 1233·2
Sodium-Iron(III) Gluconate Complex, 1444·3
Sodium-*o*-phenylphenol, 1187·2
Sodixen, 2295·4
Sodol Compound, 2296·1
Sodolac, 2296·1
Sodorant, 2296·1
Sofarcid, 2296·1
Sofargen, 2296·1
Sofasin, 2296·1
Sofenol, 2296·1
Soffodex, 2296·1
Soficlor, 2296·1
Sofidrox, 2296·1
Sofilex, 2296·1
Soflax, 2296·1
Soflax EX, 2296·1
Sofloran, 2296·1
Sof/Pro Clean, 2296·1

Sofracort, 2296·1
Sofradex, 2296·1
Sofradex-F, 2296·1
Sofraline, 2296·1
Soframycin, 2296·1
Soframycine, 2296·2
Soframycine Hydrocortisone, 2296·2
Soframycine Naphazoline, 2296·2
Sofrasolone, 2296·2
Sofra-Tull, 2296·2
Sofra-Tulle, 2296·2
Sof-Sof, 2296·2
Sof-T, 2296·2
Soft Kilnits, 2296·2
Soft Lips, 2296·2
Soft Lips Crystal Ice, 2296·2
Soft Lips French Vanilla, 2296·2
Soft Lips Sparkle, 2296·2
Soft Lips Ultra, 2296·2
Soft Mate, 2296·2
Soft Mate Consept, 2296·2
Soft Mate Consept 1, 2296·2
Soft Mate Consept 2, 2296·2
Soft Mate Enzyme Plus Cleaner, 2296·2
Soft Paraffin, White, 1479·3
Soft Paraffin, Yellow, 1479·3
Soft Soap, 1575·2
Softa Man, 2296·2
Softab, 2296·2
Sof-Tact, MediSense— *see* MediSense Sof-Tact, 2119·3
Softasept N, 2296·2
Soft-drink Caramel, 1057·1
Softene, 2296·2
Softin, 2296·2
Softixol, 2296·2
Softon, 2296·2
Softon Plus, 2296·3
Soft-tissue Rheumatism, 11·1
Softwash, 2296·3
Softwear, 2296·3
Sogilen, 2296·3
Sogoon, 2296·3
Soiae Oleum Hydrogenatum, 1447·2
Soiae Oleum Raffinatum, 1447·2
Soijatutteli, 2296·3
Soin Autobronzant, 2296·3
Soja Bean, 1447·2
Soja Bean Oil, 1447·2
Sojae Oleum, 1447·2
Sojar Men, 2296·3
Sojar Plus-Calcio, 2296·3
Sojar Pro, 2296·3
Sojarlech, 2296·3
Soklinal, 2296·3
Sol Bronce Vital, 2296·3
Solacap, 2296·3
Solacid, 2296·3
Solacy, 2296·3
Solage, 2296·3
Solamin, 2296·3
Solani Amylum, 1449·1
Solanine, 1661·2
Solan-M, 2296·3
Solantal, 2296·3
*Solanum dulcamara*, 1683·1
*Solanum incanum*, 1260·3
*Solanum nigrum*, 1661·2
*Solanum tuberosum*, 1449·1
Solapsor, 2296·3
Solaquin, 2296·3
Solaquin Forte, 2296·3
Solar Block, 2296·4
Solar Block Baby, 2296·4
Solar Block Surf/Sport, 2296·4
Solar Keratosis— *see* Basal Cell and Squamous Cell Carcinoma, 522·3
Solaraze, 2296·4
Solarcaine Preparations, 2296·4
Solardril Composto, 2296·4
Solart, 2296·4
Solatran, 2296·4
Solaurit, 2296·4
Solavert, 2296·4
Solaxin, 2296·4
SolBar, 2296·4
SolBar Plus, 2296·4
Solblastin, 2296·4
Solciclina, 2296·4
Solclin, 2296·4
Solcode, 2297·1
Solcoderm, 2297·1
Solco-Derman, 2297·1
Solcogyn, 2297·1
Solcoseryl, 2297·1
Solcoseryl Comp— *see* Solcoseryl Dental, 2297·1
Solcoseryl Dental, 2297·1
Solcosplen, 2297·1
Solco-Trichovac, 2297·1
Soldactone, 2297·1
Soldermil Ecran Total, 2297·1
Soldermil Protector Solar, 2297·1
Soldesam, 2297·1
Soldesanil, 2297·1
Soldrin, 2297·1
Solecin, 2297·1
Soledum Preparations, 2297·1
Soleil Ecran, 2297·1
Soleil, Jaune, 1058·2
Solemar, 2297·1
Solemil, 2297·1
Solevita, 2297·1
Solex A15, 2297·2
Solexa, 2297·2
Soleze, 2297·2
Solf...— *see also under* Sulf... *and* Sulph...
Solfa, 2297·2
Solfac, 2297·2
Solfadiazina, 258·2
Solfadimetossina, 259·2
Solfadimetossipirimidina, 259·2
Solfaguanidina, 260·3
Solfamerazina, 260·3
Solfametazina, 259·2
Solfametopirazina, 263·1
Solfametossipirazina, 263·1
Solfametossipiridazina, 263·1
Solfammide, 263·2
Solfapirimidina, 258·2
Solfatiazolo, 264·1
Solfen, 2297·2
Solfidin, 2297·2
Solfomucil, 2297·2
Solfoton, 2297·2
Solfranicol, 2297·2
Solfurol, 2297·2
Solganal, 2297·2
Solgeretik, 2297·2
Solgol, 2297·2
Solian, 2297·2
Solibay, 2297·2
Solicam, 2297·2
Solid Carbon Dioxide, 1235·2
Solid Green, 1171·1
Solidage, 1748·3
Solidaginis Herba, 1748·3
Solidaginis Virgaureae Herba, 1748·3
Solidago, 1748·3
*Solidago canadensis*, 1748·3
*Solidago gigantea*, 1748·3
Solidago M, 2297·2
Solidago Virga Aurea, 1748·3
*Solidago virgaurea*, 1748·3
Solidagoren N, 2297·2
Solidagosan N, 2297·2
Solidon, 2297·2
Solifenacin Succinate, 489·2
Solin, 2297·2
Solinase, 2297·2
Solinitrina, 2297·2
Solipid, 2297·2
Solisan, 2297·2
Solitab, 2297·2
Solivito N, 2297·2
Sol-Jod, 2297·2
Solkan, 2297·3
Sollival, 2297·3
Solmag, 2297·3
Solmucaine, 2297·3
Solmucalm, 2297·3
Solmucol, 2297·3
Solmux, 2297·3
Soloc, 2297·3
Solocalm, 2297·3
Solocalm Plus, 2297·3
Solocalm-B, 2297·3
Solocalm-Flex, 2297·3
Solocare, 2297·3
Solo-care, 2297·3
Solo-care Hard, 2297·3
Solo-care Soft, 2297·3
Solomet, 2297·3
Solomet C Bupivacain Hydrochlorid, 2297·3
Solone, 2297·3
Solosa, 2297·3
Solosin, 2297·3
SoloSite, 2297·3
Solosprin, 2297·3
Solotrim, 2297·3
Solotron, 2297·3
Solovite, 2297·3
Solpadeine, 2297·3
Solpadeine Max, 2297·3
Solpadeine Plus, 2297·4
Solpadol, 2297·4
Solpaflex, 2297·4
Solpat, 2297·4
Solphyllex, 2297·4
Solphyllin, 2297·4
Solpic, 2297·4
Solplex 40, 2297·4
Solplex 70, 2297·4
Solprene, 2297·4
Solprin, 2297·4
Solsavit, 2297·4
Solsolona, 2297·4
Soltamox, 2297·4
Soltice, 2297·4
Soltric, 2297·4
Soltrictor con Lagrifilm, 2297·4
Soltrim, 2297·4
Soltrimox, 2297·4
Solubacter, 2297·4
Solubeol, 2297·4
Solubilising Agents, 1411·1
Solu-Biloptin, 2297·4
Solubitrat, 2297·4
Soluble Amylobarbitone, 670·1
Soluble Barbitone, 671·2
Soluble Fluorescein, 1689·1
Soluble Glass, 1748·3
Soluble Gluside, 1443·3
Soluble Guncotton, 1156·2
Soluble Heparin, 928·1
Soluble Hexobarbitone, 703·1
Soluble Insulin, 334·2
Soluble Methyl Hydroxybenzoate, 1183·3
Soluble Pentobarbitone, 713·3
Soluble Phenobarbitone, 367·3
Soluble Phenytoin, 370·2
Soluble Propyl Hydroxybenzoate, 1183·3
Soluble Saccharin, 1443·3
Soluble Sulphacetamide, 257·3
Soluble Sulphadiazine, 258·2
Soluble Sulphadimidine, 259·2
Soluble Sulphamerazine, 260·3
Soluble Sulphathiazole, 264·1
Soluble Thiopentone, 1309·1
Solucalcine, 2297·4
Solucamphre, 2298·1
Solucao ABC, 2298·1
Solucao Aminon, 2298·1
Solucao Aminorin, 2298·1
Solucao Anticoagulante, 2298·1
Solucao Nasal de Nafazolina, 2298·1
Solucao Stago, 2298·1
Solucaps, 2298·1
Solucel, 2298·1
Solu-Celestan, 2298·1
Solucer, 2298·1
Soluchrom, 2298·1
Solución de Bióxido de Hidrogeno, 1182·2
Solucion De Lugol, 2298·1
Solucion Detergente, 2298·1
Solucion DP, 2298·1
Solucion Fisio, 2298·1
Solucion Schoum, 2298·1
Soluciones de Rehidratación Oral, 1222·2
Soluciones para Diálisis, 1221·1
Solucionic, 2298·1
Solucis, 2298·1
Solucol, 2298·1
Solucort, 2298·1
Solu-Cortef, 2298·1
Solu-Cortef— *see* Emergent-Ez, 1967·2
Solu-Crom, 2298·1
Soludacortin, 2298·1
Solu-Dacortin, 2298·1
Solu-Dacortin H, 2298·1
Solu-Dacortina, 2298·1
Solu-Dacortine, 2298·2
Soludactone, 2298·2
Soludecadron, 2298·2
Solu-Decortin-H, 2298·2
Soluderme, 2298·2
Soludial, 2298·2
Soludor, 2298·2
Solufen, 2298·2
Solufena, 2298·2
Solufilina, 2298·2
Solufilina Sedante, 2298·2
Solufilina Simple, 2298·2
Solu-Flur, 2298·2
Solufos, 2298·2
Solugastril, 2298·2
Solugel, 2298·2
Solukapton, 2298·2
Solulexin, 2298·2
Solulip, 2298·2
Solumag, 2298·2
Solu-Medrol, 2298·2
Solu-Medrone, 2298·2
Solumerin, 2298·3
Solumidazol, 2298·3
Solu-Moderin, 2298·3
Solumol, 2298·3
Soluna, 2298·3
Solunac, 2298·3
Solupen, 2298·3
Solupen Enzimatico, 2298·3
Solupen N, 2298·3
Solupen-D, 2298·3
Solupred, 2298·3
Soluprick SQ, 2298·3
Solupsa, 2298·3
Solupsan, 2298·3
Solurex, 2298·3
Soluric, 2298·3
Solurin, 2298·3
Solurrinol, 2298·3
Solurutine Papaverine F. Retard, 2298·3
Solus, 2298·3
Solusprin, 2298·3
Solusteril, 2298·3
Soluston, 2298·3
Solustrep, 2298·3
Solustres, 2298·3
Soluté Officinal d'Eau Oxygénée, 1182·2
Solutina, 2298·3
Solutio Cordes, 2298·3
Solutio Cordes Dexa N, 2298·3
Solutio Hydrogenii Peroxydati, 1182·3
Solution Antiseptique, 2298·3
Solution ChKM du Prof Dr Walkhoff, 2298·3
Solution Stago Diluee, 2298·4
Solutrast, 2298·4
Solutrat, 2298·4
Solutricine, 2298·4
Solutricine Expectorant, 2298·4
Solutricine Maux de Gorge, 2298·4
Solutricine Tetracaine, 2298·4
Solutricine Vitamine C, 2298·4
Soluver, 2298·4
Soluver Plus, 2298·4
Soluvit, 2298·4
Soluvit N, 2298·4
Soluvit Neu, 2298·4
Soluvite, 2298·4
Solu-Volon A, 2298·4

Soluzione Composta Alcoolica Saponosa di Coaltar, 2298·4
Soluzione Darrow, 2298·4
Soluzione Schoum, 2298·4
Soluzyme, 2298·4
Solvanol, 2298·4
Solvazinc, 2298·4
Solve Dandruff, 2298·4
Solvent Ether, 1474·2
Solvent Hexane, 1476·3
Solvente Indoloro, 2298·4
Solvents, 1471·1
Solvetan, 2298·4
Solvex, 2298·4
Solvex Liquido Fungicida, 2298·4
Solvezink, 2299·1
Solviflu, 2299·1
Solvin, 2299·1
Solving, 2299·1
Solvipect, 2299·1
Solvipect Comp, 2299·1
Solvisol, 2299·1
Solvium, 2299·1
Solvobil, 2299·1
Solvolin, 2299·1
Solvomed, 2299·1
Solvopret, 2299·1
Solvopret TP, 2299·1
Solyptol, 2299·1
Som, 2299·1
Soma, 2299·1
Soma Balsamico, 2299·1
Soma Complex, 2299·1
Soma Compound, 2299·1
Soma Compound with Codeine, 2299·1
Somabion, 2299·1
Somac, 2299·1
Somacid, 2299·2
Somac-MA, 2299·2
Somadril, 2299·2
Somadril Comp, 2299·2
Somaflam, 2299·2
Somaflex, 2299·2
Somagerol, 2299·2
Somalgen, 2299·2
Somalgesic, 2299·2
Somalgin, 2299·2
Somalium, 2299·2
Soman, 1719·2
Somanol, 2299·2
Somanol + Ethanol, 2299·2
Somapam, 2299·2
Somaplus, 2299·2
Somarexin, 2299·2
Somarexin & C, 2299·2
Somasedin, 2299·2
Somastin, 2299·2
Somatarax, 2299·2
Somatic Pain, 2·1
Somatin, 2299·2
Somatofalk, 2299·2
Somatolan, 2299·2
Somatoliberin, 1339·2
Somatoline, 2299·2
Somatomax PM, 1308·3
Somatomedin C, 1338·3
Somatomedinas, 1338·3
Somatomedins, 1338·3
Somatorelin, 1339·2
Somatorelina, 1339·2
Somatosan, 2299·2
Somatostatin, 1339·3
Somatostatin Acetate, 1340·1
Somatostatina, 1339·3
Somatostatinoma— *see* Carcinoid Tumours and Other Secretory Neoplasms, 504·1
Somatostatinum, 1339·3
Somatotrophin, 1327·2
Somatotrophin, Bovine, 1329·3
Somatotrophin-release-inhibiting Factor, 1339·3
Somatotropin, 1327·2
Somatotropin, Bovine, 1329·3
Somatotropina, 1327·2
Somatran, 2299·2
Somatrel, 2299·2
Somatrem, 1327·2
Somatron, 2299·3
Somatrop, 2299·3
Somatropil, 2299·3
Somatropin, 1327·2
Somatropin Bulk Solution, 1327·2
Somatropina, 1327·2
Somatropinoma— *see* Acromegaly and Gigantism, 1312·1
Somatropinum, 1327·2
Somatulin, 2299·3
Somatulina, 2299·3
Somatuline, 2299·3
Somatyl, 2299·3
Somavert, 2299·3
Somazina, 2299·3
Somese, 2299·3
Sometribove, 1327·2
Sometripor, 1327·2
Somiaton, 2299·3
Somidobove, 1327·2
Somin, 2299·3
Sominex, 2299·3
Sominex Pain Relief, 2299·3
Somit, 2299·3
Somnal, 2299·3
Somnambulism— *see* Parasomnias, 667·3
Somnatrol, 2299·3
Somnil, 2299·3
Somnipax, 2299·3
Somnipron, 2299·3
Somnisedan, Natusor— *see* Natusor Somnisedan, 2154·1
Somnite, 2299·3
Somnium, 2299·3
Somno, 2299·3
Somnol, 2299·4
Somnosan, 2299·4
Somnovit, 2299·4
Somnubene, 2299·4
Somnus, Gerard House— *see* Gerard House Somnus, 2022·1
Somnuvis S, 2299·4
Somoblon, 2299·4
Somol, 2299·4
Somonal, 2299·4
Sompraz, 2299·4
Somsanit, 2299·4
Son, 1253·2
Sonacide, 2299·4
Soñadora, 1666·1
Sonadryl, 2299·4
Sonalent, 2299·4
Sonata, 2299·4
Sondalis, 2299·4
Sone, 2299·4
Sonebon, 2299·4
Soneriper, 2299·4
Sonermin, 590·2
Soneryl, 2299·4
Songar, 2299·4
Songha, 2299·4
Songha Day, 2299·4
Songha Night, 2299·4
Sonhare, 2299·4
Sonicur, 2299·4
Sonidal, 2299·4
Sonidar, 2299·4
Sonide, 2299·4
Sonifilan, 2299·4
Sonin, 2299·4
Soni-Slo, 2300·1
Sonnenbrandspray, 2300·1
Sonnenbraun, 2300·1
Sonnenhutkraut, 1683·2
Sonodor, 2300·1
Sonofit, 2300·1
Sonoripan, 2300·1
SonoRx, 2300·1
Sonotabs, 2300·1
Sonotrat, 2300·1
Sonotryl, 2300·1
SonoVue, 2300·1
Sonrisal, 2300·1
Sons Piral, 2300·1
Sontedril, 2300·1
Soolan, 2300·1
Soor-Gel, 2300·1
Soorphenesin, 2300·1
Sootha, 2300·1
Soothaderm, 2300·1
Soothake Toothache Gel, 2300·1
Soothake Toothache Tincture, 2300·1
Soothe Aid, 2300·1
Soothelip, 2300·1
Soothe'n Heal, 2300·1
Soothene— *see* Kleer Cream, 2080·2
Soothex, 2300·1
Soothing Ice Rub, 2300·1
Soothol, 2300·1
Soov Bite, 2300·1
Soov Burn, 2300·1
Soov Cream, 2300·1
Soov Prickly Heat, 2300·2
Sopa-K, 2300·2
Sopalamin 3B, 2300·2
Sopalamine 3B, 2300·2
Sopalamine 3B Plus, 2300·2
Sopalamine 3B Plus C, 2300·2
Sopax, 2300·2
Sophidone, 2300·2
Sophipren, 2300·2
Sophixin, 2300·2
*Sophora japonica*, 1688·2
Sophtal, 2300·2
Sophtal-POS N, 2300·2
Soporin, 2300·2
Soprol, 2300·2
Soproxen, 2300·2
Sopulmin, 2300·2
Soquette, 2300·2
Soraderm, 2300·2
Soral, 2300·2
Soramin, 2300·2
Sorbalgon, 2300·2
Sorbangil, 2300·2
Sorbates, 1192·3
Sorbato Potásico, 1192·3
Sorbatos, 1192·3
Sorbecal, 2300·2
Sorbenor, 2300·2
Sorbic Acid, 1192·3
Sorbicet, 2300·2
Sorbichew, 2300·2
Sorbiclis, 2300·2
Sórbico, Ácido, 1192·3
Sorbid, 2300·2
Sorbide Nitrate, 941·1
Sorbidilat, 2300·2
Sorbidin, 2300·3
Sorbidon Hydrate, 2300·3
Sorbifer, 2300·3
Sorbilax, 2300·3
Sorbiline, 2300·3
Sorbimacrogol Laurate 300, 1415·1
Sorbimacrogol Oleate 300, 1415·2
Sorbimacrogol Palmitate 300, 1415·1
Sorbimacrogol Stearate 300, 1415·1
Sorbimacrogol Trioleate 300, 1415·2
Sorbimon, 2300·3
Sorbinil, 345·3
Sorbinilo, 345·3
Sorbisal, 2300·3
Sorbisterit, 2300·3
Sorbitan Derivatives, 1411·2
Sorbitan Esters, 1416·1
Sorbitan Laurate, 1416·1
Sorbitan Monolaurate, 1416·1
Sorbitan Monooleate, 1416·1
Sorbitan Mono-oleate, 1416·1
Sorbitan Monopalmitate, 1416·2
Sorbitan Monostearate, 1416·2
Sorbitan Oleate, 1416·1
Sorbitan Palmitate, 1416·2
Sorbitan Sesquioleate, 1416·2
Sorbitan Stearate, 1416·2
Sorbitan Trioleate, 1416·2
Sorbitan Tristearate, 1416·3
Sorbitani Lauras, 1416·1
Sorbitani Oleas, 1416·1
Sorbitani Palmitas, 1416·2
Sorbitani Sesquioleas, 1416·2
Sorbitani Stearas, 1416·2
Sorbitani Trioleas, 1416·2
Sorbitol, 1446·3
D-Sorbitol, 1446·3
Sorbitolum, 1446·3
Sorbitrate, 2300·3
Sorbitur, 2300·3
Sorbon, 2300·3
Sorboxaethenum Laurinicum, 1415·1
Sorboxaethenum Oleinicum, 1415·2
Sorboxaethenum Stearinicum, 1415·1
Sorbsan, 2300·3
Sorcal, 2300·3
Sorciclina, 2300·3
Sore Eyes, Murine— *see* Murine Sore Eyes, 2145·4
Sore Mouth Gel, 2300·3
Sore Throat Chewing Gum, 2300·3
Sore Throat, Hylands— *see* Hylands Sore Throat, 2052·3
Sore Throat L39, 2300·3
Sore Throat Lozenges, 2300·3
Sore Throat Relief, 2300·3
Sorebral, 2300·3
Soredine, 2300·3
Soren, 2300·3
Sorethytan 20 Mono-oleate, 1415·2
Sorgoa, 2300·3
Sorgoran, 2300·3
Soriacur, 2300·3
Sorial, 2300·3
Soriatane, 2300·3
Soridermal, 2300·3
Sorine Adulto, 2300·4
Sorine Infantil, 2300·4
Sorivudina, 654·2
Sorivudine, 654·2
Sormodren, 2300·4
Sormon, 2300·4
Sornil, 2300·4
Soro de Manutencao H, 2300·4
Soro Nasal, 2300·4
Soroliv, 2300·4
Soronal, 2300·4
Soroneo, 2300·4
Soropon, 2300·4
Sorot, 2300·4
Sorquetan, 2300·4
Sorrel, 1749·1
Sorrel Dock, 1749·1
Sorsis, 2300·4
Sorsis Beta, 2300·4
Sortis, 2300·4
Sosegon, 2300·4
Sosenol, 2300·4
Sostac, 2300·4
Sostatin, 2300·4
Sostenon, 2300·4
Sostilar, 2300·4
Sostril, 2300·4
Sota, 2300·4
Sota Lich, 2300·4
Sotab, 2300·4
Sotabet, 2300·4
Sotabeta, 2301·1
Sotacor, 2301·1
Sotagamma, 2301·1
Sota-Gry, 2301·1
Sotahexal, 2301·1
Sotalex, 2301·1
Sotalin, 2301·1
Sotalodoc, 2301·1
(+)-Sotalol, 1002·2
*d*-Sotalol, 1002·2
Sotalol, Hidrocloruro de, 1001·3
Sotalol Hydrochloride, 1001·3
*d,l*-Sotalol Hydrochloride, 1001·3
Sotaloli Hydrochloridum, 1001·3
Sotamed, 2301·1
Sotamol, 2301·1
Sotanorm, 2301·1
Sotaper, 2301·1
Sotapor, 2301·1
Sota-Puren, 2301·1
Sotaryt, 2301·1
Sota-saar, 2301·1

Sotastad, 2301·1
Sotatyrol, 2301·1
Sotaziden N, 2301·1
Sotilen, 2301·1
Sotoger, 2301·1
Sotolone, 1688·1
Sotomycin, 2301·1
Sotradecol, 2301·1
Sotret, 2301·1
Souci, 1665·2
Soufrane, 2301·1
Soufre, 1158·2
Soufre, Foie de, 1158·3
Soufrol, 2301·1
Soufrol TP, 2301·1
Soufrol ZNP, 2301·1
Sour Cherry, 1058·1
Sour Dock, 1749·1, 1766·1
Soussi, 1666·1
South American Blastomycosis— *see* Paracoccidioidomycosis, 389·1
Sovcainum, 1373·2
Sovel, 2301·1
Soventol, 2301·2
Soventol HC, 2301·2
Soviclor, 2301·2
Soviet Gramicidin, 220·3
Sovipan, 2301·2
Soy Forte with Block Cohosh, 2301·2
Soy Power Plus, Bioglan— *see* Bioglan Soy Power Plus, 1844·1
Soya Bean, 1447·2
Soya Diet, 2301·2
Soya Oil, 1447·2
Soya Protein, 1447·2
Soyabean, 1447·2
Soyabean Oil, 1447·2
Soya-bean Oil, 1447·2
Soya-bean Oil, Hydrogenated, 1447·2
Soya-bean Oil, Refined, 1447·2
Soyac, 2301·2
Soyacal, 2301·2
Soyal, 2301·2
Soyalac, 2301·2
Soyaloid, 2301·2
Soyaven, 2301·2
Soybean, 1447·2
Soybean Oil, 1447·2
Soybean Oil, Hydrogenated, 1447·2
Soydex, 2301·2
Soymen, 2301·2
SoyPlus, 2301·2
SP, 2301·2
SP54, 2301·2
SP-54, 979·2
SP-63, 1725·1
SP95, 2301·2
Sp-281, 1764·2
S-640P, 170·3
SP-732, 1592·3
SP Betaisodona, 2301·2
SP Cream, 2301·2
SP Troches, 2301·2
Spablock, 2301·2
Space Dust, 1373·3
Spaciclina, 2301·2
Spagall, 2301·2
Spagulax, 2301·2
Spagulax au Citrate de Potassium, 2301·2
Spagulax au Sorbitol, 2301·2
Spagulax Mucilage, 2301·2
Spagymun, 2301·3
Spagyrom, 2301·3
Spai, 2301·3
Spalgin, 2301·3
Spalt, 2301·3
Spalt N, 2301·3
Spalt Schmerz-Gel, 2301·3
Spalt Schmerztabletten, 2301·3
Spamus, 2301·3
Span C, 2301·3
Spanidin, 2301·3
Spanischer Pfeffer, 1667·1
Spanish Fly, 1666·3
Spanish Liquorice, 1270·2
Spanish Psyllium, 1268·1
Spanish Tummy Mixture, 2301·3
Spanish Type Rosemary Oil, 1740·2
Span-K, 2301·3
Spanor, 2301·3
Spanplex, 2301·3
Spara, 2301·3
Sparaplaie, 2301·3
Spardac, 2301·3
Sparfloxacin, 255·1
Sparine, 2301·3
Sparkal, 2301·3
Sparkles, 2301·3
Sparkling White Eye Drops, 2301·3
Sparksol, 2301·3
Spart. Sulph., 1749·1
Sparteine Sulfate, 1749·1
Sparteine Sulphate, 1749·1
(−)-Sparteine Sulphate, 1749·1
*l*-Sparteine Sulphate, 1749·1
Sparteinum Sulfuricum, 1749·1
Spartiol, 2301·3
Spartocine, 2301·4
Spartocine N, 2301·4
Sparx, 2301·4
SPA-S-160, 405·2
Spascopan, 2301·4
Spasdic, 2301·4
Spasen, 2301·4
Spasen Somatico, 2301·4
Spasfon, 2301·4
Spasfon-Lyoc, 2301·4
Spasgone, 2301·4
Spasgone-H, 2301·4
Spasm, Gastrointestinal— *see* Gastrointestinal Spasm, 1242·2
Spasm, Muscle— *see* Muscle Spasm, 1386·1
Spasm, Oesophageal— *see* Oesophageal Motility Disorders, 1246·3
Spasma, 2301·4
Spasmag, 2301·4
Spasmalgan, 2301·4
Spasmalgin, 2301·4
Spasman, 2301·4
Spasman Scop, 2301·4
Spasmaverine, 2301·4
Spasmend, 2301·4
Spasmeridan, 2301·4
Spasmex, 2301·4
Spasmhalt, 2301·4
Spasmhalt-ASA, 2301·4
Spasmidenal, 2301·4
Spasmine, 2301·4
Spasmium, 2302·1
Spasmium Comp, 2302·1
Spasmo Claim, 2302·1
Spasmo Gallo Sanol, 2302·1
Spasmo Gallo Sanol Mint, 2302·1
Spasmo Inalgon Neu, 2302·1
Spasmo Nil, 2302·1
Spasmo-Barbamin, 2302·1
Spasmo-Barbamine Compositum, 2302·1
Spasmo-Bomaleb, 2302·1
Spasmo-Canulase, 2302·1
Spasmo-Cibalgin, 2302·1
Spasmo-Cibalgin Comp, 2302·1
Spasmo-Cibalgin Compositum S, 2302·1
Spasmo-Cibalgin S, 2302·1
Spasmo-Cibalgina, 2302·1
Spasmo-Cibalgine, 2302·1
Spasmocor, 2302·1
Spasmoctyl, 2302·1
Spasmocyclon, 2302·1
Spasmodene, 2302·1
Spasmodex, 2302·1
Spasmodic Torticollis, 1391·1
Spasmodil, 2302·1
Spasmofen, 2302·1
Spasmofides S, 2302·1
Spasmogel, 2302·1
Spasmo-Granobil-Krampf- und Reizhusten, 2302·2
Spasmoliv, 2302·2
Spasmolyt, 2302·2
Spasmo-Lyt, 2302·2
Spasmolytine, 1648·1
Spasmomen, 2302·2
Spasmomen Somatico, 2302·2
Spasmo-Mucosolvan, 2302·2
Spasmonal, 2302·2
Spasmonal Fibre, 2302·2
Spasmo-Nervogastrol, 2302·2
Spasmo-Oxepam, 2302·2
Spasmoplex, 2302·2
Spasmoplus, 2302·2
Spasmopriv, 2302·2
Spasmo-Proxyvon, 2302·2
Spasmo-Proxyvon Forte, 2302·2
Spasmo-Rhoival TC, 2302·2
Spasmosarto, 2302·2
Spasmosedine, 2302·2
Spasmosol, 2302·2
Spasmo-Solugastril, 2302·2
Spasmosyx F, 2302·2
Spasmotropin, 2302·3
Spasmo-Urgenin, 2302·3
Spasmo-Urgenin TC, 2302·3
Spasmo-Urgenine Neo, 2302·3
Spasmowern, 2302·3
Spasmoxyl, 2302·3
Spasms, Infantile— *see* Epilepsy, 349·1
Spassirex, 2302·3
Spasticity, 1386·2
Spastrex, 2302·3
Spasuret, 2302·3
Spasuri, 2302·3
Spasyt, 2302·3
Spatab, 2302·3
Spatix, 2302·3
Spaziron, 2302·3
Spazol, 2302·3
SPCA, 735·3, 750·3
Spearmint, 1749·1
Spearmint, Common, 1749·1
Spearmint Oil, 1749·1
Spearmint, Scotch, 1749·1
Speciafoldine, 2302·3
Special Defense Sun Block, 2302·3
Special K, 1302·3
Specicef-N, 2302·3
Speci-Chol, 2302·3
Species Carvi Comp, 2302·3
Species Nervinae, 2302·3
Specifthir, 2302·3
Specilid, 2302·3
Specinor, 2302·3
Spec-T, 2302·3
Spec-T Sore Throat/Decongestant, 2302·3
Spectazole, 2302·3
Spectinomycin, 255·2
Spectinomycin Dihydrochloride Pentahydrate, 255·2
Spectinomycin Hydrochloride, 255·2
Spectinomycini Hydrochloridum, 255·2
Spectra, 2302·3
Spectraban, 2302·4
Spectraban 55, 2302·4
Spectraban T, 2302·4
Spectraban Ultra, 2302·4
Spectracef, 2302·4
Spectracil, 2302·4
Spectramedryn, 2302·4
Spectramox, 2302·4
Spectrapain, 2302·4
Spectrapain Forte, 2302·4
Spectrasone, 2302·4
Spectratet, 2302·4
Spectrim, 2302·4
Spectro Derm, 2302·4
Spectro Gluvs, 2302·4
Spectro Gram, 2302·4
Spectro Jel, 2302·4
Spectro Tar, 2302·4
Spectrobid, 2302·4
Spectrocef, 2302·4
Spectrocin, 2302·4
Spectrocin Plus, 2303·1
Spectro-Jel, 2303·1
Spectroxyl, 2303·1
Spectrum, 2303·1
Specyton Cartilage-parathyroide, 2303·1
Spedifen, 2303·1
Spedralgin sans Codeine, 2303·1
Spedro, 2303·1
Speed, 1589·2
Spektramox, 2303·1
Spel, 2303·1
Spencer's Bronchitis, 2303·1
Spenglersan, 2303·1
Spenglersan Kolloid, 2303·1
Spermaceti, 1480·3
Spermaceti, Synthetic, 1480·3
Spersacarbachol, 2303·1
Spersacarpin, 2303·1
Spersacarpine, 2303·1
Spersacet, 2303·1
Spersacet C, 2303·1
Spersadex, 2303·1
Spersadex Comp, 2303·1
Spersadex Med Kloramfenikol, 2303·1
Spersadexolin, 2303·1
Spersadexoline, 2303·1
Spersallerg, 2303·2
Spersamide, 2303·2
Spersanicol, 2303·2
Spersapolymyxin, 2303·2
Spersatear, 2303·2
Sperti Plus Preparacion H, 2303·2
Sperti Praparation H, 2303·2
Sperti Preparacao H, 2303·2
Sperti Preparacion H, 2303·2
Sperti (Preparacion H) Clear Gel, 2303·2
Sperti Preparation H, 2303·2
Sperti (Preparation H), 2303·2
Spesicor, 2303·2
Speton, 2303·2
Spevin, 2303·2
SPf66, 1622·3
SPF 15 For Body, 2303·2
Spherex, 2303·2
Spherocytosis— *see* Haemolytic Anaemia, 733·1
Spherulin, 2303·2
Sphingogel, 2303·2
S.P.H.P., 2303·2
Spicae Aetheroleum, 1749·2
Spicline, 2303·2
Spider Antivenins, 1640·1
Spider Antivenoms, 1640·1
Spider Bites, 1640·1
Spider Venom Antisera, 1640·1
Spidifen, 2303·2
Spidox, 2303·2
Spidufen, 2303·3
Spigelon, 2303·3
Spike Lavender, 1749·2
Spike Lavender Oil, 1749·2
Spike Oil, 1749·2
Spilacnet, 2303·3
Spilan, 2303·3
Spina Bifida— *see* Neural Tube Defects, 1430·1
Spinacane, 1482·2
Spinal Block— *see* Central Nerve Block, 1370·1
Spinal Cord Injury, 1088·2
Spindle Tree Bark, 1265·2
Spiny Restharrow, 1723·3
Spir, 2303·3
Spiracin, 2303·3
Spiractin, 2303·3
*Spiraea ulmaria*, 1710·1
Spiraeae Herba, 1710·1
Spiralgin, 2303·3
Spiramycin, 255·3
Spiramycin I, 255·3
Spiramycin Adipate, 256·1
Spiramycinum, 255·3
Spiraphan, 2303·3
Spirapril Hydrochloride, 1003·1
Spirapril Hydrochloride Monohydrate, 1003·1
Spiraprilat, 1003·1
Spiraprili Hydrochloridum, 1003·1
Spiravet, 2303·3
Spirbon, 2303·3
Spiresis, 2303·3
Spiretic, 2303·3

Spirial, 2303·3
Spiricort, 2303·3
Spiridazide, 2303·3
Spiridon, 2303·3
Spirillon, 2303·3
Spirit Caramel, 1057·1
Spirit, Proof, 1166·1
Spirit, Rectified, 1166·1
Spirit Salicyl, 2303·3
Spirit, White, 1478·1
Spirit Whitfield, 2303·3
Spirits of Salt, 1699·1
Spirits of Turpentine, 1760·1
Spiriva, 2303·3
Spirix, 2303·3
Spiro, 2303·3
Spiro Comp, 2303·3
Spirobene, 2303·3
Spirobeta, 2303·3
Spiro-Co, 2303·3
Spirocort, 2303·3
Spiroctan, 2303·4
Spiroctazine, 2303·4
Spiro-D, 2303·4
Spiroderm, 2303·4
Spirofur, 2303·4
Spirogamma, 2303·4
Spirogel, 2303·4
Spirohexal, 2303·4
Spirolactone, 1003·1
Spirolair, 2303·4
Spirolang, 2303·4
Spirolept, 2303·4
Spirometon, 2303·4
Spiromide, 2303·4
Spiromix, 2303·4
Spiron, 2303·4
Spironex, 2303·4
Spirono, 2303·4
Spirono Comp, 2303·4
Spironol, 2303·4
Spironolacton Plus, 2303·4
Spironolactone, 1003·1
Spironolactonum, 1003·1
Spironone, 2303·4
Spironothiazid, 2303·4
Spiropal, 2303·4
Spiropent, 2303·4
Spiroscand, 2303·4
Spirosine, 2303·4
Spirospare, 2303·4
Spirostada Comp, 2304·1
(25*R*)-Spirost-5-ene-1β,3β-diol, 1741·1
Spiro-Tablinen, 2304·1
Spirotone, 2304·1
Spirox, 2304·1
Spirsa, 2304·1
Spirulina, 1749·2
Spitacid, 2304·1
Spitaderm, 2304·1
Spitalen, 2304·1
Spitzwegerich, 1738·2
Spitzwegerich, Kneipp Hustensaft— *see* Kneipp Hustensaft Spitzwegerich, 2081·3
Spitzwegerichkraut, 1738·2
Spizef, 2304·1
SPL, 2304·1
Spleen Disorders, Infection Prophylaxis— *see* Spleen Disorders, 146·3
Splendil, 2304·1
Splenectomy, Infection Prophylaxis— *see* Spleen Disorders, 146·3
Splenocarbine, 2304·1
Splenofigon, 2304·1
Splenomegaly Syndrome, Hyperreactive Malarial— *see* Malaria, 444·1
Splenomegaly Syndrome, Tropical— *see* Malaria, 444·1
Splen-Uvocal, 2304·1
Splinting— *see* Muscle Spasm, 1386·1
SPM-925, 961·2
Spm-OK, 2304·1
Spolera, 2304·1
Spondylitis, Ankylosing— *see* Spondyloarthropathies, 11·1
Spondyloarthropathies, 11·1
Spondylon, 2304·1
Spondylonal, 2304·1
Spondyvit, 2304·1
Spongostan, 2304·1
Sponsin, 2304·1
Sponwiga, 2304·1
Sporacid, 2304·1
Sporahexal, 2304·1
Sporal, 2304·1
Sporanox, 2304·1
Sporasec, 2304·2
Sporcid, 2304·2
Sporex, 2304·2
Sporicef, 2304·2
Sporicidin, 2304·2
Sporidex, 2304·2
Sporidox Plus, 2304·2
Sporiline, 2304·2
Sporinex, 2304·2
Sporlab, 2304·2
Sporlac, 2304·2
Spornar, 2304·2
Sporostatin, 2304·2
Sporotrichosis, 391·1
Sporoxyl, 2304·2
Sport Sunblock, 2304·2
Sportenine, 2304·2
Sportino, 2304·2
Sportino Akut, 2304·2
Sportium, 2304·2
Sports Eze Bruising Relief, 2304·2
Sports Eze Joint & Muscle, 2304·2
Sports Multi, 2304·2
Sportscreme, 2304·2
Sportscreme Ice, 2304·2
Sportsman Rub, 2304·2
Sportsmega, 2304·2
Sportupac M, 2304·2
Sportusal, 2304·2
Sportusal Spray Sine Heparino, 2304·3
Sportz Sunscreen, 2304·3
Spotof, 2304·3
Spotoway, 2304·3
Spotted Fevers, 147·1
Spozal, 2304·3
Spozol, 2304·3
Sprains— *see* Soft-tissue Rheumatism, 11·1
Spray Anti-Septico, 2304·3
Spray Auto-Bronzant, 2304·3
Spray de Proteccion Total, 2304·3
Spray Paraffin, 1479·1
Spray Solaire Bronzage Rapide, 2304·3
Spray Solaire Bronzage Securite, 2304·3
Spraychrome, 2304·3
Spray-on Bande, 2304·3
Spray-Pax, 2304·3
Spray-Tish, 2304·3
Spray-U-Thin, 2304·3
Sprediol, 2304·3
Spregal, 2304·3
Spren, 2304·3
Spreor, 2304·3
Sprilon, 2304·3
Sprinsol, 2304·3
Sprintec, 2304·3
Sprue, Tropical— *see* Gastro-enteritis, 127·3
SPS, 2304·3
SPZ, 2304·3
SQ-1089, 559·1
SQ-1489, 1755·1
SQ-9343, 1052·3
SQ-9453, 1473·2
SQ-9538, 587·3
SQ-11436, 179·3
SQ-11725, 963·1
SQ 13050, 397·1
SQ-13050, 397·2
SQ-13396, 1064·3
SQ-14055, 270·2
SQ-14225, 879·2
SQ-15101, 1541·3
SQ-15659, 254·1
SQ-15874, 1129·1
SQ-16123, 230·3
SQ-16150, 1550·1
SQ-16360, 215·2
SQ-16374, 1559·3
SQ-16401, 220·3
SQ-16423, 240·2
SQ-16496, 1559·2
SQ-16603, 215·2
SQ-18566, 1103·2
SQ-19844, 1746·2
SQ-20881, 1010·3
SQ-21982, 1064·1
SQ-22022, 179·3
SQ-22947, 270·2
SQ-26333, 1029·3
SQ-26776, 160·3
SQ-26991, 1029·3
SQ-26992, 161·1
SQ-28555, 919·1
SQ-31000, 984·3
SQ-32692, 1062·3
SQ-32756, 654·2
SQ-34514, 649·3
Squad, 2304·3
Squalane, 1482·2
Squalanum, 1482·2
Squalene, 1482·2
Squam, 2304·3
Squamasol, 2304·4
Squa-med, 2304·4
Squamous Cell Carcinoma of the Skin— *see* Basal Cell and Squamous Cell Carcinoma, 522·3
Squaphane, 2304·4
Squaric Acid Dibutylester, 1158·1
Squaw Root, 1661·2
Squaw Weed, 1743·1
Squibb-HC, 2304·4
Squill, 1130·3
Squill, Indian, 1130·3
Squill, Red, 1509·3
Squill, White, 1130·3
Squint— *see* Strabismus, 1487·1
SR-720-22, 956·2
SR-2508, 551·2
SR-4233, 588·3
SR-25990C, 888·3
SR-29142, 418·3
SR-41319, 776·1
SR-41319B, 776·1
SR-47436, 940·1
SR-90107A, 918·3
SR-96225, 851·2
SR-96669, 577·1
SRC Expectorant, 2304·4
SRG-95213, 893·2
Srilane, 2304·4
SRL172, 1627·2
SRM-Rhotard, 2304·4
SRO, 2304·4
SS-320A, 1121·3
SS-717, 406·3
SSD, 2304·4
SSKI, 2304·4
SSRIs, 278·2, 296·3
SST, 2304·4
SSZ, 2304·4
ST 37, 2304·4
ST-52, 2304·4
ST-155, 885·2
ST-198, 1423·3
ST-200, 1646·1
ST 630, 1462·1
ST-679, 14·3
ST-813, 407·3
ST-1059, 959·2
ST-1085, 959·2
ST-1191, 292·1
ST-1435, 1549·3
ST-1512, 786·3
ST-7090, 931·2
ST-9067, 1658·3
S-T Cort, 2304·4
S-T Forte, 2304·4
S-T Forte 2, 2304·4
St Bonifatius-Tee, 2304·4
St. Jakobs-Balsam Mono, 2304·4
St James Balm, 2304·4
St. John's Wort, 299·1
St Johnswort Compound, 2304·4
St. Joseph Adult Chewable, 2304·4
St. Joseph Cold Tablets For Children, 2304·4
St. Joseph Cough Suppressant, 2304·4
St Luke's Oil, 2304·4
St Luke's Sports Oil, 2305·1
St Mary's Thistle Plus, 2305·1
St. Peter-224, 959·2
St Radegunder Preparations, 2305·1
St Vitus' Dance— *see* Chorea, 664·2
Stabicilline, 2305·2
Stabilanol, 2305·2
Stabilisers, 1411·1
Stabilising and Suspending Agents, 1576·1
Stable Factor, 735·3, 750·3
Stablon, 2305·2
Stacer, 2305·2
Stacho-Zym N, 2305·2
Stacin, 2305·2
Stacort-A, 2305·2
Stadaglicin, 2305·2
Stadalax, 2305·2
Stadelant, 2305·2
Stadol, 2305·2
Stadovir, 2305·2
Stadyl, 2305·2
Staficilin N, 2305·2
Staficyn, 2305·2
Stafilon, 2305·2
Staflocil, 2305·2
Stafoxil, 2305·2
Stagesic, 2305·2
Stagid, 2305·2
Stago, 2305·2
Stahist, 2305·2
Stalcin, 2305·2
Stalene, 2305·2
Stalevo, 2305·2
Stallergenes MRV, 2305·2
Staloral, 2305·3
Staltor, 2305·3
Stamar, 2305·3
Stamaril, 2305·3
Stamina, 2305·3
Stammering— *see* Stuttering, 702·3
Stamoist E, 2305·3
Stamoist LA, 2305·3
Stamoneyrol, 2305·3
Stancare, 2305·3
Standacillin, 2305·3
Standard III, 2305·3
Stangyl, 2305·3
Stanhexidine, 2305·3
Stanilo, 2305·3
Stanno-Bardane, 2305·3
Stannosi Fluoridum, 1448·3
Stannous Fluoride, 1448·3
Stanol, 2305·3
Stanol Esters, 1448·3
Stanolone, 1541·3
Stanozolol, 1569·2
Stanozololum, 1569·2
Stantar— *see* Clinitar, 1893·3
Stantar— *see* Cosmetar-S, 1909·2
Stantar— *see* Meditar, 2119·3
Stapenor, 2305·3
Staphlex, 2305·3
Staphycid, 2305·3
Staphyclox, 2305·3
Staphylase, 2305·3
Staphylex, 2305·3
Staphylococcal Infections, 147·2
Staphylococcal Scalded Skin Syndrome— *see* Skin Infections, 146·2
Staphylococcal Scarlet Fever— *see* Skin Infections, 146·2
Staphylococcal Vaccines, 1640·2
Staphylokinase, 1005·2
Staphypan, 2305·3
Staporos, 2305·3
Star Anise, 1655·2
Star Anise Fruit, 1655·2
Star Anise Oil, 1655·2

Starcef, 2305·3
Starch, 1449·1
Starch, Alant, 1702·1
Starch, Cassava, 1449·2
Starch, Corn, 1449·1
Starch Gum, 1427·1
Starch, Maize, 1449·1
Starch, Potato, 1449·1
Starch, Pregelatinised, 1449·1
Starch, Pregelatinized, 1449·2
Starch, Rice, 1449·1
Starch Sodium Glycolate, 1582·1
Starch, Tapioca, 1449·1
Starch, Topical, 1449·1
Starch, Wheat, 1449·1
Starem, 2305·3
Starflower Oil, 1661·3
Staril, 2305·4
Stärke, 1449·1
Starkungs- Und Kraftigungstee, Bioreform— *see* Bioreform-Starkungs- und Kraftigungstee, 1845·3
Starlep, 2305·4
Starlix, 2305·4
Starnoc, 2305·4
Starogyn, 2305·4
Star-Otic, 2305·4
Starox, 2305·4
Star-Pen, 2305·4
Start NP, 2305·4
Startle Disease, Familial— *see* Stiff-man Syndrome, 696·3
Startonyl, 2305·4
Starwort, 1696·3
Stas Preparations, 2305·4
Stat-Crit, 2305·4
Statex, 2305·4
Staticin, 2305·4
Staticine, 2305·4
Staticum, 2305·4
Statiflex G, 2305·4
Statinclyne, 2305·4
Statins, 811·3
Stativa, 2305·4
Statrol, 2305·4
Status Asthmaticus— *see* Asthma, 777·2
Status Epilepticus, 352·1
Status Migrainosus— *see* Migraine, 464·2
Statuss Expectorant, 2306·1
Statuss Green, 2306·1
Staurodorm, 2306·1
Staurodorm Neu, 2306·1
Stavacin, 2306·1
Stavir, 2306·1
Stavudine, 654·2
Stay Alert, 2306·1
Stay-Wet 3, 2306·1
Stay-Wet 4, 2306·1
ST-155-BS, 885·2
STD, 2306·1
Stearic Acid, 1749·2
Stearic Acid 50, 1749·2
Stearic Acid 70, 1749·2
Stearic Acid 95, 1749·2
Stearic Acid Triglyceride, 1763·3
Stearine, 1749·2
Stearinsäure, 1749·2
Stearyl Alcohol, 1482·3
STEC, 129·2
Stechapfel, 489·2
Stecort-NM, 2306·1
Stediril, 2306·1
Stediril 30, 2306·1
Stediril D, 2306·1
Stedon, 2306·1
Stefolant, 2306·1
Steicardin N, 2306·1
Steicorton, 2306·1
Steigal, 2306·1
Steinaclox, 2306·1
Steinkohlenteer, 1159·2
Steiprostat, 2306·1
Steirocall N, 2306·1
Steiroplex, 2306·1
Steitonit, 2306·1
Stelabid, 2306·1
Stelapar, 2306·1
Stelazine, 2306·1
Stelea, 2306·2
Stelium, 2306·2
Stella, 2306·2
Stellamicina, 2306·2
Stellatropine, 2306·2
Stellisept, 2306·2
Stellorphinad, 2306·2
Stellorphine, 2306·2
Stem Cell Factor, 742·2
Stemetil, 2306·2
Stemgen, 2306·2
Stemiz, 2306·2
Stemzine, 2306·2
Sten, 2306·2
Stenobronchial, 2306·2
Stenocrat, 2306·2
Steno-loges N, 2306·2
Stenoptin, 2306·2
Stenosara, 2306·2
Stenox, 2306·2
Stenting— *see* Reperfusion and Revascularisation Procedures, 834·1
Steocalcin, 2306·2
Steocar, 2306·2
Steocin, 2306·2
Steovit D3, 2306·2
Step 2, 2306·2
Stephadilat-S, 2306·2
Stepronin, 1130·3
Stepronin Lysinate, 1130·3
Stepronin Sodium, 1130·3
Sterac, 2306·2
Steradent, 2306·3
Sterades, 2306·3
Steramin, 2306·3
Steramina G, 2306·3
Steranabol Ritardo, 2306·3
Steranios, 2306·3
Sterapred, 2306·3
Sterax, 2306·3
Sterculia, 1290·2
Sterculia Gum, 1290·2
*Sterculia urens*, 1290·2
Ster-Dex, 2306·3
Sterets, 2306·3
Sterets H, 2306·3
Sterets Unisept, 2306·3
Sterex, 2306·3
Sterexidine, 2306·3
Stericlens, 2306·3
Stericol Hospital Disinfectant, 1193·3
Steridine, 2306·3
Steridol, 2306·3
Steridrolo, 2306·3
Steridrolo a Rapida Idrolisi, 2306·3
Sterigel, 2306·3
Sterigin, 2306·3
Sterigynon, 2306·3
Steril Zeta, 2306·3
Sterile Erythromycin Gluceptate, 208·2
Sterile Erythromycin Lactobionate, 208·2
Sterile Larvae, 1151·3
Sterilene, 2306·3
Sterilent, 2306·3
Sterilite, 2306·3
Sterillium, 2306·3
Sterillium Virugard, 2306·3
Sterilon, 2306·4
Sterimar, 2306·4
Sterimar Cu, 2306·4
Sterimycine, 2306·4
Steri-Neb Cromogen, 2306·4
Steri-Neb Salamol, 2306·4
Sterinet, 2306·4
Sterinor, 2306·4
Sterinova, 2306·4
Steripaste, 2306·4
Steripod, 2306·4
Steripod Chlorhexidine Gluconate, 2306·4
Steripod Chlorhexidine Gluconate with Cetrimide, 2306·4
Steripod Pink— *see* Steripod Chlorhexidine Gluconate, 2306·4
Steripod Yellow— *see* Steripod Chlorhexidine Gluconate with Cetrimide, 2306·4
Sterisol, 2306·4
Steri/Sol, 2306·4
Steriwipe, 2306·4
Sterk Hostesirup, 2306·4
Sterlane, 2306·4
Stern Biene Fenchelhonig, 2306·4
Stern Biene Fenchelsirup, 2306·4
Sternanis, 1655·2
Sterocort, 2306·4
Sterodelta, 2306·4
Sterodex, 2306·4
Sterofrin, 2306·4
Sterofundin Preparations, 2306·4
Sterogyl, 2307·1
Steroids, Anabolic, 1527·2
Sterolone, 2307·1
Steromien, 2307·1
Steron, 2307·1
Steronase Aq, 2307·1
Steronide, 2307·1
Steropotassium, 2307·1
Steroprim, 2307·1
Sterosan, 2307·1
Steros-Anal, 2307·1
Sterosone, 2307·1
Sterostatine, 2307·1
Ster-Zac, 2307·1
Stesiron, 2307·1
Stesolid, 2307·1
Stetic, 2307·1
Stevencillin, 2307·1
Stevens-Johnson Syndrome— *see* Drug-induced Skin Reactions, 1134·3
Stevens-Johnson Syndrome— *see* Erythema Multiforme, 1135·3
Stevia Dulri, 2307·1
*Stevia rebaudiana*, 1449·3
Stevin, 1449·3
Stevioside, 1449·3
Steviosin, 1449·3
STH, 1327·2
STH-2130, 721·2
Sthenorex, 2307·1
STI-571, 562·1
Stibii et Kalii Tartras, 103·1
Stibium Natrium Tartaricum, 103·1
Stibocaptate, 103·1
Stibogluconate, Sodium, 600·3
Stibophen, 103·1
Stibophenum, 103·1
Stick Ecran Solaire, 2307·1
Stick Ecran Total, 2307·1
Stick Labial de Proteccion Total, 2307·2
Stick Solaire Haute Protection, 2307·2
Stickoxydul, 1304·3
Stiebenyl, 2307·2
Stiedex, 2307·2
Stiedex LP, 2307·2
Stiefcortil, 2307·2
Stiefderm, 2307·2
Stiefotrex, 2307·2
Stiemycin, 2307·2
Stiemycine, 2307·2
Stieprox, 2307·2
Stieva-A, 2307·2
Stievamycin, 2307·2
Stiff-man Syndrome, 696·3
Stigma Maydis, 1676·1
Stigmast-5-en-3β-ol, 982·3
Stigmicarpin, 2307·2
Stilamin, 2307·2
Stilaze, 2307·2
Stilbestrol, 1548·1
Stilboestrol, 1548·1
Stilboestrol Diphosphate, 1555·3
Stilboestrol Dipropionate, 1548·1
Stilene, 2307·2
Stilex, 2307·2
Stilgrip, 2307·2
Still, 2307·2
Stilla, 2307·2
Stilla Decongestionante, 2307·2
Stilla Delicato, 2307·2
Stillacor, 2307·3
Stillargol, 2307·3
Still's Disease, 11·2
Stilnoct, 2307·3
Stilnox, 2307·3
Stilomagic, 2307·3
Stilpane, 2307·3
Stilphostrol, 2307·3
Stimate, 2307·3
Stimilfar, 2307·3
Stimlor, 2307·3
Stimol, 2307·3
Stimolfit, 2307·3
Stimtes, 2307·3
Stimu-ACTH, 2307·3
Stimubral, 2307·3
Stimu-GH, 2307·3
Stimul, 2307·3
Stimulance, 2307·3
Stimulants and Anorectics, 1583·1
Stimulants, Central, 1583·1
Stimulex, 2307·3
Stimu-LH, 2307·3
Stimulnerv, 2307·3
Stimunal, 2307·3
Stimuplexe, 2307·3
Stimu-TSH, 2307·3
Stimuzim, 2307·3
Stimycine, 2307·4
Stin, 2307·4
Sting-Eze, 2307·4
Stinging Nettle, 1762·1
Stinging Nettle for Homoeopathic Preparations, Common, 1762·1
Sting-Kill, 2307·4
Stingose, 2307·4
Stings, Box Jellyfish— *see* Box Jellyfish Sting, 1621·3
Stings, *Chironex fleckeri*— *see* Box Jellyfish Sting, 1621·3
Stings, Infections in— *see* Bites and Stings, 121·3
Stings, Jellyfish— *see* Jellyfish Sting, 1645·3
Stings, Scorpion— *see* Scorpion Stings, 1638·3
Stings, Sea Wasp— *see* Box Jellyfish Sting, 1621·3
Stioxyl, 2307·4
Stipites Laminariae, 1704·3
Stipo, 2307·4
Stiprox, 2307·4
Stiproxal, 2307·4
Stiripentol, 377·3
Stivane, 2307·4
Stivate, 2307·4
Stobcon, 2307·4
Stockholm Tar, 1159·3
Stocof, 2307·4
Stocrin, 2307·4
Stodal, 2307·4
Stodal for Children, 2307·4
Stoddard Solvent, 1478·1
Stofilan, 2307·4
Stogar, 2307·4
STOI-X, 2307·4
Stolina, 2307·4
Stoma Anestesia Dental, 2307·4
Stomaax, 2307·4
Stomaax Plus, 2307·4
Stomac, 2308·1
Stomach Calm, 2308·1
Stomach Cancer— *see* Malignant Neoplasms of the Gastrointestinal Tract, 516·2
Stomach Mixture, 2308·1
Stomachicon N, 2308·1
Stomachysat N, 2308·1
Stomacine, 2308·1
Stoma-Gastreu S R5, 2308·1
Stomagel N, 2308·1
Stomahesive, 2308·1
Stomakon, 2308·1
Stomasal Med, 2308·1
Stomatitis, Aphthous— *see* Mouth Ulceration, 1245·1
Stomec, 2308·1
Stomedine, 2308·1

Stomet, 2308·1
Stomidros, 2308·1
Stomigen, 2308·1
Stomosan, 2308·1
Stomygen, 2308·1
Stone, Blue, 1426·1
Stone Fish Antivenins, 1640·2
Stone Fish Antivenoms, 1640·2
Stone Fish Venom Antisera, 1640·2
Stone Root, 1749·3
Stongel, 2308·1
Stop, 2308·1
Stop Espinilla Normaderm, 2308·1
Stop Hemo, 2308·1
Stop Itch, 2308·1
Stopain, 2308·2
Stopaler, 2308·2
Stop-Allerg, 2308·2
Stoparen, 2308·2
Stopayne, 2308·2
Stopcold, 2308·2
Stopen, 2308·2
Stopex, 2308·2
Stopit, 2308·2
Stopitch, 2308·2
Stoppers, 2308·2
Stoptoss, 2308·2
Storax, 1749·3
Storax, American, 1749·3
Storax, Levant, 1749·3
Storax, Liquid, 1749·3
Storax, Prepared, 1749·3
Storax, Purified, 1749·3
Stosstherapie, 1464·1
Stovalid N, 2308·2
Stoxil, 2308·2
STP, 1593·3
Strabismus, 1487·1
Strafortin, 2308·2
Strains Cream, 2308·2
Strains— *see* Soft-tissue Rheumatism, 11·1
Stramoine, 489·2
Stramonii Folium, 489·2
Stramonii Pulvis Normatus, 489·2
Stramonium, 489·2
Stramonium Leaf, 489·2
Stramonium Leaf, Powdered, 489·2
Stramonium, Prepared, 489·2
Stranoval, 2308·2
Stratene, 2308·2
Strattera, 2308·2
Strawberry Tomato, 1731·3
Strefen, 2308·2
Streflam, 2308·2
Strength, 2308·2
Strepfen, 2308·2
Strepsils Preparations, 2308·2
Strepsils Pain Relief Spray— *see* Dequaspray, 1926·3
Strepsilspray Lidocaine, 2308·4
Streptase, 2308·4
Strepto, 2308·4
Streptocidum, 263·2
Streptococcal Deoxyribonuclease, 1749·3
Streptococcal Infections, Group B, Perinatal— *see* Perinatal Streptococcal Infections, 139·3
*Streptococcus*, 1005·2
Streptococcus Group B Vaccines, 1640·2
*Streptococcus haemolyticus*, 1749·3
*Streptococcus lactis*, 237·2
*Streptococcus mutans*, 1612·2
*Streptococcus pneumoniae*, 1633·1
*Streptococcus thermophilus*, 1704·2
Streptocol, 2308·4
Streptodornase, 1749·3
Strepto-Erbazide, 2308·4
Strepto-Fatol, 2308·4
Streptogramins, 118·3
Strepto-Hefa, 2308·4
Streptokinase, 1005·2
Streptokinase Bulk Solution, 1005·2
Streptokinasi Solutio ad Praeparationem, 1005·2
Streptokinasum, 1005·2
Streptomagma, 2308·4
*Streptomyces*, 116·1, 117·3, 118·2, 119·3
*Streptomyces albus*, 615·3
*Streptomyces ambofaciens*, 255·3
*Streptomyces antibioticus*, 240·2, 657·1
*Streptomyces argillaceus*, 580·2
*Streptomyces aureofaciens*, 187·3, 204·3, 405·2, 611·1
*Streptomyces avermitilis*, 106·2
*Streptomyces azureus*, 270·2
*Streptomyces bambergiensis*, 162·2
*Streptomyces caespitosus*, 573·3
*Streptomyces candidus*, 159·1
*Streptomyces capreolus*, 166·1
*Streptomyces carzinostaticus*, 594·3
*Streptomyces cattleya*, 221·1
*Streptomyces chrysomallus*, 545·1
*Streptomyces cinnamonensis*, 611·1
*Streptomyces clavuligerus*, 193·3
*Streptomyces coeruleorubidus*, 545·3, 547·3
*Streptomyces decaris*, 215·1
*Streptomyces erythreus*, 208·1
*Streptomyces fradiae*, 214·2, 215·1, 235·1, 274·3, 1703·3
*Streptomyces galilaeus*, 525·2
*Streptomyces garyphalus*, 202·1
*Streptomyces griseus*, 256·1, 395·3, 1502·1
*Streptomyces hygroscopicus*, 1363·2
*Streptomyces kanamyceticus*, 225·1
*Streptomyces kitasatoensis*, 225·3
*Streptomyces lasaliensis*, 606·1
*Streptomyces lincolnensis*, 118·1, 226·2
*Streptomyces mycarofaciens*, 231·3
*Streptomyces narbonensis*, 224·3
*Streptomyces natalensis*, 406·3
*Streptomyces niveus*, 239·2
*Streptomyces nodosus*, 391·2
*Streptomyces noursei*, 406·3
*Streptomyces orchidaceus*, 202·1
*Streptomyces orientalis*, 275·2
*Streptomyces parvulus*, 545·1
*Streptomyces pentaticus*, 407·3
*Streptomyces peucetius*, 545·3, 547·3
*Streptomyces plicatus*, 580·2
*Streptomyces pristina spiralis*, 246·1
*Streptomyces rimosus*, 241·1, 612·3
*Streptomyces spectabilis*, 255·2
*Streptomyces spheroides*, 239·2
*Streptomyces tanashiensis*, 580·2
*Streptomyces tenebrarius*, 158·2, 271·2
*Streptomyces tsukubaensis*, 1365·2
*Streptomyces venezuelae*, 117·3, 185·1
*Streptomyces verticillus*, 530·2
*Streptomyces virginiae*, 277·3
Streptomycin, 256·1
Streptomycin Calcium Chloride, 257·1
Streptomycin Hydrochloride, 256·1
Streptomycin Pantothenate, 257·1
Streptomycin Sesquisulphate, 256·2
Streptomycin Sulfate, 256·2
Streptomycin Sulphate, 256·2
Streptomycini Sulfas, 256·2
Streptonase, 2308·4
Streptonivicin, 239·2
Strepto-Plus, 2308·4
Streptosil con Neomicina-Fher, 2308·4
Streptosil L PMC, 2308·4
Streptozocin, 584·1
Streptozotocin, 584·1
Streptozyme, 2308·4
Streptuss, 2308·4
Stresam, 2308·4
Stress, 2308·4
Stress 600, 2308·4
Stress B Complex, 2308·4
Stress Disorder, Acute— *see* Anxiety Disorders, 663·1
Stress Disorder, Post-traumatic— *see* Post-traumatic Stress Disorder, 664·1
Stress Formula, 2308·4
Stress Formula B Compound Plus Vitamin C, 2308·4
Stress Formula C/Zinc, 2308·4
Stress, Modern Herbals— *see* Modern Herbals Stress, 2138·2
Stress Plex C, 2308·4
Stress Relief, 2309·1
Stress Tab, 2309·1
Stress Tab with Iron, 2309·1
Stress Tab with Zinc, 2309·1
Stress Tablets, 2309·1
Stress Ulceration— *see* Peptic Ulcer Disease, 1246·3
Stressan, 2309·1
Stresscaps, 2309·1
Stressease, 2309·1
Stressen, 2309·1
StressForm "605" with Iron, 2309·1
Stressigal, 2309·1
Stressless, 2309·1
Stresson, 2309·1
Stresson Multifibra, 2309·1
Stress-Relax, Bioglan— *see* Bioglan Stress-Relax, 1844·2
Stresstabs, 2309·1
Stresstabs with Zinc, 2309·1
Stresstein, 2309·1
Strialisin, 2309·1
Striant, 2309·1
Striaton, 2309·1
Striatridin, 2309·1
Strictus, 2309·1
Stri-Dex Antibacterial Cleansing, 2309·1
Stri-Dex Clear, 2309·1
Stri-Dex Face Wash, 2309·1
Stri-Dex Pads, 2309·1
Stringan, 2309·1
Strobili Lupuli, 1708·1
Strocain, 2309·1
Strodival, 2309·1
Strogen, 2309·1
Stroke, 836·1
Stromba, 2309·1
Strombaject, 2309·1
Stromectol, 2309·2
Stromic, 2309·2
217 Strong, 2309·2
Strong Ammonia Solution, 1653·3
Strong Cetrimide Solution, 1172·2
Strong Glutaraldehyde Solution, 1180·3
Strong Sodium Hypochlorite Solution, 1192·1
StrongStart, 2309·2
Strongus, 2309·2
Strongyloidiasis, 100·3
Strontium-89, 1525·2
Strontium Acetate, 1749·3
Strontium Chloride, 1749·3
Strontium Chloride ($^{89}$Sr), 1525·2
Strontium Ranelate, 775·2
Strophantab, 2309·2
Strophanthin, 1009·1
Strophanthin-G, 977·3
Strophanthin-Herztabletten Compositum, 2309·2
Strophanthin-K, 1009·1
Strophanthinum, 977·3
Strophanthoside-G, 977·3
Strophanthoside-K, 1009·1
Strophanthus, 1009·1, 2309·2
*Strophanthus gratus*, 977·3
*Strophanthus kombe*, 1009·1
*Stropharia*, 1717·3
*Stropharia cubensis*, 1736·1
Stropheupas-forte, 2309·2
Strotan, 2309·2
Strovite, 2309·2
Strox, 2309·2
Strubelin, 2309·2
Structolipid, 2309·2
Structolipide, 2309·2
Structum, 2309·2
Strumazol, 2309·2
Strumedical 400, 2309·2
Strumex, 2309·2
Strych. Hydrochlor., 1750·1
Strychni Semen, 1722·3
Strychnidin-10-one, 1750·1
Strychnina, 1750·1
Strychninae Hydrochloridum, 1750·1
Strychninae Nitras, 1750·1
Strychninae Sulphas, 1750·1
Strychnine, 1750·1
Strychnine Hydrochloride, 1750·1
Strychnine Nitrate, 1750·1
Strychnine Sulfate, 1750·1
Strychnine Sulphate, 1750·1
Strychninum Nitricum, 1750·1
Strychninum Sulfuricum, 1750·1
*Strychnos ignatii*, 1722·3
*Strychnos nux-vomica*, 1722·3
Stryphnasal, 2309·2
Stryphnon, 2309·2
Stryphonasal— *see* Stryphnasal, 2309·2
STS-557, 1548·1
St-Tissues, 2309·2
Stuart Factor, 735·3
Stuart Formula, 2309·2
Stuart Prenatal, 2309·2
Stuartnatal 1+1, 2309·2
Stuartnatal Plus, 2309·2
Stuart-Prower Factor, 735·3
Stud, 2309·2
Stud 100, 2309·2
Stugerina, 2309·2
Stugeron, 2309·2
Stullmaton, 2309·3
Stunarone, 2309·3
Stuno, 2309·3
Stutgeron, 2309·3
Stuttering, 702·3
STV, 2309·3
Stye, 2309·3
Styli Laminariae, 1704·3
Stylo Sport, 2309·3
Stypro, 2309·3
Styptanon, 2309·3
Styptin, 2309·3
Stypto-Caine, 2309·3
Styptocid, 2309·3
Styptysat, 2309·3
Styrax, 1749·3
*Styrax benzoin*, 1751·1
*Styrax paralleloneurus*, 1751·1
*Styrax tonkinensis*, 1744·1
Styrene Copolymer with Divinylbenzene, Sulfonated, Sodium Salt, 1053·2
Styrene Polymer, Sulfonated, Calcium Salt, 1032·3
Styrene Polymer, Sulfonated, Potassium Salt, 1050·1
SU-101, 53·2
Su-4885, 1715·1
Su-5864, 926·3
Su-6518, 431·2
Su-8341, 890·3
Suadian, 2309·3
Sual, 2309·3
Sualim, 2309·3
Sualyn, 2309·3
Suamoxil, 2309·3
Suanzaoren, 1750·2
Suanzaorentang, 1750·2
Suarda, 1483·1
Suavene, 2309·3
Suavigel, 2309·3
Suavisan, 2309·3
Suavisan N, 2309·3
Suavisol, 2309·3
Suavit Calcio, 2309·3
Suaviter, 2309·3
Suavithiol, 2309·3
Suavuret, 2309·4
Sub Tensin, 2309·4
Subacute Sclerosing Panencephalitis— *see* Measles, 624·3
Subamycin, 2309·4
Subarachnoid Haemorrhage— *see* Stroke, 836·1
Subazotato de Bismuto, 1252·2
Subcarbonato de Bismuto, 1252·1
Subcutin N, 2309·4
Subcuvia, 2309·4
Subdue, 2309·4
Subgalato de Bismuto, 1252·2
Subitan, 2309·4
Subji, 1666·1
Sublimaze, 2309·4

Sublimed Sulfur, 1158·2
Sublivac, 2309·4
Sublivac B.E.S.T., 2309·4
Subnitrato de Bismuto, 1252·2
Suboffen, 2309·4
Suboxone, 2309·4
Subreum, 2309·4
Substi, 2309·4
Substitol, 2309·4
Subsyde, 2309·4
Subutex, 2309·4
Sucadermil, 2309·4
Sucari, 2309·4
Sucaryl, 2309·4
Successia, 2309·4
Succi, 2309·4
Succi Pharmacetin, 2309·4
Succicaptal, 2309·4
Succicuran, 2309·4
Succicurarium Chloride, 1406·2
Succilate, 2309·4
Succimer, 1054·2
Succimer, Technetium ($^{99m}$Tc), 1526·1
Succímero, 1054·2
Succin, 2310·1
Succinato de Abacavir, 625·2
Succinato de Doxilamina, 432·3
Succinato de Estriol, 1552·3
Succinato de Litio, 1151·2
Succinato de Loxapina, 705·2
Succinato de Sodio, 1748·3
Succinato de Sumatriptán, 471·2
Succinato Sódico de Cloranfenicol, 185·1
Succinato Sódico de Estriol, 1552·3
Succinato Sódico de Hidrocortisona, 1104·1
Succinato Sódico de Metilprednisolona, 1106·2
Succinato Sódico de Prednisolona, 1108·2
Succinic Dialdehyde, 1180·2
Succinilsolfatiazolo, 257·1
Succinilsulfatiazol, 257·1
Succinimida, 1750·2
Succinimide, 1750·2
Succinolin, 2310·1
Succinyl, 2310·1
Succinylated Gelatin, 755·2
Succinylcholine Chloride, 1406·2
2,2′-Succinyldioxybis(ethyltrimethylammonium) Dichloride Dihydrate, 1406·2
Succinylmonocholine, 1408·3
Succinylsulfathiazole, 257·1
Succinylsulfathiazolum, 257·1
Succinylsulphathiazole, 257·1
Succosa, 2310·1
Succus Cineraria Maritima, 2310·1
Sucedal, 2310·1
Sucee, 2310·1
Sucontral, 2310·1
Sucrabest, 2310·1
Sucrafen, 2310·1
Sucrafilm, 2310·1
Sucrager, 2310·1
Sucraid, 2310·1
Sucral, 2310·1
Sucralan, 2310·1
Sucralbene, 2310·1
Sucralfate, 1290·2
Sucralfato, 1290·2
Sucralfin, 2310·1
Sucralmax, 2310·1
Sucralosa, 1450·1
Sucralose, 1450·1, 2310·1
Sucralstad, 2310·1
Sucralum, 2310·1
Sucramal, 2310·1
Sucramed, 2310·1
Sucraphil, 2310·1
Sucrate, 2310·1
Sucrato, 2310·1
Sucratyrol, 2310·1
Sucre, 1450·1
Sucre de Gélatine, 1433·3
Sucredulcor, 2310·1
Sucret, 2310·1
Sucrets Preparations, 2310·1
Sucrets, Childrens Cherry— *see* Childrens Cherry Sucrets, 1882·4
Sucrets, Cough Control— *see also* Cough Control Sucrets, 1909·4
Sucrin, 2310·2
Sucro, Bioglan— *see* Bioglan Sucro, 1844·2
Sucroril, 2310·2
Sucrose, 1450·1
Sucrose Esters, 1416·3
Sucrose Hydrogen Sulphate Basic Aluminium Salt, 1290·2
Sucrose, Iron, 1438·2
Sucrose Octaacetate, 1750·2
Sucrose Octa-acetate, 1750·2
Sucrose Octakis(hydrogen Sulphate) Aluminium Complex, 1290·2
Sucrose Octasulfate, 1290·2
Sucrose Polyesters, 1450·3
Sucrosum, 1450·1
Suczulen Mono, 2310·2
Sudafed Preparations, 2310·2
Sudafed Co— *see* Non-Drowsy Sudafed Congestion Cold & Flu, 2171·4
Sudafed Cold & Cough, Childrens— *see* Childrens Sudafed Cold & Cough, 1883·1
Sudafed Congestion Cold & Flu, Non-Drowsy— *see* Non-Drowsy Sudafed Congestion Cold & Flu, 2171·4
Sudafed Decongestant Nasal Spray, Non-Drowsy— *see* Non-Drowsy Sudafed Decongestant Nasal Spray, 2172·1
Sudafed Decongestant, Non-Drowsy— *see* Non-Drowsy Sudafed Decongestant, 2171·4
Sudafed Dual Relief Max, Non-Drowsy— *see* Non-Drowsy Sudafed Dual Relief Max, 2172·1
Sudafed Dual Relief, Non-Drowsy— *see* Non-Drowsy Sudafed Dual Relief, 2172·1
Sudafed Expectorant, Non-Drowsy— *see* Non-Drowsy Sudafed Expectorant, 2172·1
Sudafed Linctus, Non-Drowsy— *see* Non-Drowsy Sudafed Linctus, 2172·1
Sudafed Nasal Decongestant, Childrens— *see* Childrens Sudafed Nasal Decongestant, 1883·1
Sudagesic, 2310·3
Sudal, 2310·3
Sudan IV, 1191·3
Suda-Tussin, 2310·3
Sudeck's Atrophy— *see* Complex Regional Pain Syndrome, 5·3
Sudevil Vita, 2310·3
Sudhinol, 2310·3
Sudis, 2310·3
Sudismasa, 92·3
Sudismase, 92·3
Sudocrem, 2310·3
Sudodrin, 2310·3
Sudogest Sinus, Maximum Strength— *see* Maximum Strength Sudogest Sinus, 2116·4
Sudol, 2310·3
Sudomyl, 2310·3
Sudonol, 2310·3
Sudosian, 2310·3
Sudosin, 2310·3
SUD-919Y, 1212·2
Suero Antiofidico Polivalente, 2310·3
Suero Fisiologico, 2310·3
Suero Fisiologico Vitulia, 2310·3
Suero Glucosado Vitulia, 2310·3
Suero Glucosalino Vitulia, 2310·4
Suero Levulosado Vitulia, 2310·4
Suero Potassico Bieffe ME, 2310·4
Suero Ringer Braun, 2310·4
Suero Ringer Lactato Vitulia, 2310·4
Sueroral, 2310·4
Suevitine, 2310·4
Sufenta, 2310·4
Sufentanil, 90·2
Sufentanil Citrate, 90·2
Sufentanili Citras, 90·2
Sufentanilo, Citrato de, 90·2
Sufentanilum, 90·2
Suffisance, 2310·4
Sufil, 2310·4
Sufisal, 2310·4
Sufortan, 2310·4
Sufortanon, 2310·4
Sufralem, 2310·4
Sufrexal, 2310·4
Suganril, 2310·4
Sugar, 2310·4
Sugar Absorption Test, 1269·2
Sugar Alcohols, 1417·1
Sugar Bloc, 2310·4
Sugar, Burnt, 1056·3
Sugar, Cane, 1450·1
Sugar, Compressible, 1450·1
Sugar, Confectioner's, 1450·1
Sugar, Invert, 1434·3
Sugar, Manna, 950·2
Sugar, Refined, 1450·1
Sugar Spheres, 1450·1
Sugar, Wood, 1766·1
Sugar-beet, 1450·1
Sugarbil, 2310·4
Sugar-cane, 1450·1
Sugarceton, 2310·4
Sugarless C, 2310·4
Sugast, 2310·4
Sugiran, 2310·4
Sugril, 2310·4
Suguan, 2310·4
Suguan M, 2310·4
Suifac, 2310·4
Suiflox, 2311·1
Suimel, 2311·1
Suint Purifiée, Graisse de, 1483·1
Suipen, 2311·1
Sukar-Sin, 2311·1
Sukcee, 2311·1
Sukepar, 2311·1
Sukir, 2311·1
Sukolin, 2311·1
Sul 10, 2311·1
Sulamid, 2311·1
Sulamyd, Sodium— *see* Sodium Sulamyd, 2295·4
Sular, 2311·1
Sulartrene, 2311·1
Sulazine, 2311·1
Sulbacin, 2311·1
Sulbacta, 2311·1
Sulbactam, 257·2
Sulbactam Sódico, 257·2
Sulbactam Sodium, 257·2
Sulbamox, 2311·1
Sulbenicilina Sódica, 257·2
Sulbenicillin Sodium, 257·2
Sulbutiamina, 1455·1
Sulbutiamine, 1455·1
Sulcain, 2311·1
Sulcephalosporin Sodium, 180·2
Sulcoline, 2311·1
Sulconazol, Nitrato de, 408·2
Sulconazole Nitrate, 408·2
Sulcran, 2311·1
Sulcrate, 2311·1
Suldiamin, 2311·1
Sulen, 2311·1
Suleo-M, 2311·1
Suleparoid, 1009·1
Suleparoid Sodium, 1009·1
Suleparoide, 1009·1
Sulesomab, Technetium ($^{99m}$Tc), 1526·1
Sulf...— *see also under* Solf... *and* Sulph...
SULF, 257·3
Sulf-10, 2311·1
Sulfa 10, 2311·1
Sulfa Cloran, 2311·1
Sulfa Hidro, 2311·1
Sulfabenzamida, 257·3
Sulfabenzamide, 257·3
Sulfabenzpyrazine, 263·3
Sulfac, 2311·1
Sulfacarbamida, 257·3
Sulfacarbamide, 257·3
Sulfacet, 2311·2
Sulfacetam, 2311·2
Sulfacetamida, 257·3
Sulfacetamida Sódica, 257·3
Sulfacetamide, 257·3
Sulfacetamide Sodium, 257·3
Sulfacetamidum Natricum, 257·3
Sulfacet-R, 2311·2
Sulfachloramphenicol, 2311·2
Sulfachlorpyridazine, 258·1
Sulfachrysoidine, 258·1
Sulfacid, 2311·2
Sulfaclorpiridazina, 258·1
Sulfaclozina, 258·1
Sulfaclozine, 258·1
Sulfacollyre, 2311·2
Sulfacrisoidina, 258·1
Sulfacylum, 257·3
Sulfaderm, 2311·2
Sulfadiazina, 258·2
Sulfadiazina Argéntica, 259·1
Sulfadiazina de Plata, 2311·2
Sulfadiazina Sódica, 258·2
Sulfadiazinac, 2311·2
Sulfadiazine, 258·2
Sulfadiazine Silver, 259·1
Sulfadiazine Sodium, 258·2
Sulfadiazinum, 258·2
Sulfadiazinum Argentum, 259·1
Sulfadiazinum Natricum, 258·2
Sulfadicramida, 259·2
Sulfadicramide, 259·2
Sulfadimerazine, 259·2
Sulfadimethoxine, 259·2
Sulfadimethylpyrimidine, 264·1
Sulfadimetoxina, 259·2
Sulfadimezinum, 259·2
Sulfadimidina, 259·2
Sulfadimidina Sódica, 259·2
Sulfadimidine, 259·2
Sulfadimidine Sodium, 259·2
Sulfadimidinum, 259·2
Sulfadoxina, 259·3
Sulfadoxine, 259·3
Sulfadoxinum, 259·3
Sulfafer, 2311·2
Sulfafurazol, 260·1
Sulfafurazol Diolamina, 260·1
Sulfafurazole, 260·1
Sulfafurazole, Acetyl, 260·1
Sulfafurazole Diolamine, 260·1
Sulfafurazolum, 260·1
Sulfagine, 2311·2
Sulfagrand, 2311·2
Sulfaguanidina, 260·3
Sulfaguanidine, 260·3
Sulfaguanidinum, 260·3
Sulfa-isodimérazine, 264·1
Sulfaisodimidine, 264·1
Sulfalene, 263·1
Sulfaleno, 263·1
Sulfamazone Sodium, 260·3
Sulfamerazina, 260·3
Sulfamerazina Sódica, 260·3
Sulfamerazine, 260·3
Sulfamerazine Sodium, 260·3
Sulfamerazinum, 260·3
Sulfamerazinum Natricum, 260·3
Sulfamethazine, 259·2
Sulfamethazine Sodium, 259·2
Sulfamethizole, 260·3
Sulfamethizole Monoethanolamine, 261·1
Sulfamethizolum, 260·3
Sulfamethoxazole, 261·1
Sulfamethoxazole Lysine, 262·3
Sulfamethoxazolum, 261·1
Sulfamethoxypyrazine, 263·1
Sulfamethoxypyridazine, 263·1
Sulfamethoxypyridazine Sodium, 263·1
Sulfamethoxypyridazine for Veterinary Use, 263·1
Sulfamethoxypyridazinum, 263·1
Sulfamethyldiazine, 260·3
Sulfamethylpyrimidine, 260·3
Sulfamethylthiazole, 263·1
Sulfametiltiazol, 263·1
Sulfametizol, 260·3

Sulfametopyrazine, 263·1
Sulfametoxazol, 261·1
Sulfametoxipiridazina, 263·1
Sulfametrol, 263·2
Sulfametrole, 263·2
Sulfamide, 2311·2
Sulfamidinum, 260·3
Sulfaminum, 263·2
Sulfamonomethoxine, 263·2
Sulfamonometoxina, 263·2
Sulfamoxol, 263·2
Sulfamoxole, 263·2
2-Sulfamoylacetylphenol, 385·2
Sulfamylon, 2311·2
Sulfan Blue, 1750·3
Sulfanicole, 2311·2
Sulfanil, 2311·2
Sulfanilamida, 263·2
Sulfanilamide, 263·2
Sulfanilamide Camsilate, 263·3
Sulfanilamide Sodium, 263·3
Sulfanilamide Sodium Mesilate, 263·3
Sulfanilamidothiazolum, 264·1
Sulfanilamidum, 263·2
Sulfanilcarbamide, 257·3
Sulfanoral T, 2311·2
Sulfaphtalylthiazol, 242·3
Sulfapirazinmetossina, 263·1
Sulfapiridina, 263·3
Sulfaplat, 2311·2
Sulfapyrazin Methoxyne, 263·1
Sulfapyridine, 263·3, 1292·2
Sulfaquinoxalina, 263·3
Sulfaquinoxaline, 263·3
Sulfaquinoxaline Sodium, 263·3
Sulfarlem, 2311·2
Sulfarlem Choline, 2311·2
Sulfarlem S 25, 2311·2
Sulfaryl, 2311·2
Sulfasalazina, 1291·1
Sulfasalazine, 1291·1
Sulfasalazinum, 1291·1
Sulfasomidine, 264·1
Sulfasuccinamida, 264·1
Sulfasuccinamide, 264·1
Sulfasuccinamide Sodium, 264·1
Sulfate d'Orthoxyquinoléine, 1700·1
Sulfated Castor Oil, 1575·3
Sulfated Fatty Alcohols, 1574·1
Sulfated Glucosaminoglycans, 810·2, 931·1
Sulfated Hydrogenated Castor Oil, 1575·3
Sulfated Insulin, 334·2
Sulfated Mucopolysaccharides, 810·2, 931·1
Sulfated Oils, 1574·1
Sulfathiazole, 264·1
Sulfathiazole Sodium, 264·1
Sulfathiazolum, 264·1
Sulfathiazolum Natricum, 264·1
Sulfatiazol, 264·1
Sulfatiazol Sódico, 264·1
Sulfatina, 2311·2
Sulfato Cálcico, 1665·1
Sulfato Cálcico Anhidro, 1665·1
Sulfato de Abacavir, 625·2
Sulfato de Amikacina, 154·1
Sulfato de Anfetamina, 1584·3
Sulfato de Antazolina, 424·2
Sulfato de Apramicina, 158·2
Sulfato de Arbekacina, 158·3
Sulfato de Astromicina, 158·3
Sulfato de Bametán, 866·3
Sulfato de Bario, 1061·1
Sulfato de Bekanamicina, 162·2
Sulfato de Betanidina, 872·3
Sulfato de Bleomicina, 530·2
Sulfato de Butacaína, 1372·3
Sulfato de Capreomicina, 166·1
Sulfato de Cefpiroma, 178·2
Sulfato de Cloroquina, 448·2
Sulfato de Cobre, 1426·1
Sulfato de Colistina, 198·3
Sulfato de Debrisoquina, 891·3
Sulfato de Dexanfetamina, 1585·3
Sulfato de Dibekacina, 205·2
Sulfato de Dihidralazina, 899·3
Sulfato de Dihidroestreptomicina, 205·3
Sulfato de Esparteína, 1749·1
Sulfato de Estreptomicina, 256·2
Sulfato de Estricnina, 1750·1
Sulfato de Fenelzina, 312·1
Sulfato de Foledrina, 982·3
Sulfato de Framicetina, 215·1
Sulfato de Gentamicina, 217·1
Sulfato de Guanadrel, 926·3
Sulfato de Guanoxano, 927·3
Sulfato de Hexoprenalina, 786·3
Sulfato de Hidroxicloroquina, 452·3
Sulfato de Indinavir, 638·2
Sulfato de Isepamicina, 222·2
Sulfato de Isoprenalina, 940·2
Sulfato de Kanamicina, 225·1
Sulfato de Lobelina, 1589·1
Sulfato de Mefentermina, 952·1
Sulfato de Mepindolol, 952·2
Sulfato de Micronomicina, 231·3
Sulfato de Neomicina, 235·1
Sulfato de Netilmicina, 236·3
Sulfato de Orciprenalina, 790·2
Sulfato de Paromomicina, 612·3
Sulfato de Penbutolol, 979·1
Sulfato de Peplomicina, 579·3
Sulfato de Polimixina B, 245·1
Sulfato de Pramiracetam, 1734·3
Sulfato de Protamina, 1050·3
Sulfato de Pseudoefedrina, 1129·2
Sulfato de Salbutamol, 791·3
Sulfato de Sisomicina, 254·3
Sulfato de Terbutalina, 797·2
Sulfato de Tobramicina, 271·3
Sulfato de Tranilcipromina, 318·3
Sulfato de Trospectomicina, 274·2
Sulfato de Tuaminoheptano, 1132·1
Sulfato de Vimblastina, 591·2
Sulfato de Vinblastina, 591·2
Sulfato de Vincristina, 592·2
Sulfato de Vindesina, 593·3
Sulfato Ferroso Composto, 2311·2
Sulfato Sódico, 1290·1
Sulfato Sódico Anhidro, 1290·1
Sulfato Sódico de Nandrolona, 1561·3
Sulfato Sódico de Prasterona, 1566·1
Sulfatofer, 2311·2
Sulfatral, 2311·2
Sulfatral-Cerio, 2311·2
Sulfatrex, 2311·2
Sulfatril, 2311·2
Sulfatrim, 2311·3
Sulfa+Trim, 2311·3
Sulfatroxazol, 264·1
Sulfatroxazole, 264·1
Sulfaurea, 257·3
Sulfawal, 2311·3
Sulfenazone, 260·3
Sulfer Plus, 2311·3
Sulferro, 2311·3
Sulferrol, 2311·3
Sulfestrep, 2311·3
Sulfex, 2311·3
Sulfile, 2311·3
Sulfinona, 2311·3
Sulfinpirazona, 417·3
Sulfinpyrazone, 417·3
Sulfinpyrazonum, 417·3
Sulfintestin Neom, 2311·3
Sulfintestin Neomicina, 2311·3
Sulfiram, 1510·1
Sulfiramum, 1510·1
Sulfiselen, 2311·3
Sulfisomezole, 261·1
Sulfisomidina, 264·1
Sulfisomidine, 264·1, 264·2
Sulfisomidine Sodium, 264·2
Sulfisomidinum, 264·1
Sulfisoxazole, 260·1
Sulfisoxazole Acetyl, 260·1
Sulfisoxazole Diolamine, 260·1
Sulfite Ammonia Caramel, 1057·1
Sulfites and Sulfur Dioxide, 1193·1
Sulfito Sódico, 1193·1
Sulfitos y Dióxido de Azufre, 1193·1
Sulfitrat, 2311·3
Sulfix, 2311·3
Sulfizax, 2311·3
Sulfoam, 2311·3
*o*-Sulfobenzimide, 1443·2
α-Sulfobenzylpenicillin Sodium, 257·2
Sulfobromoftaleína Sódica, 1750·3
Sulfobromophthalein Sodium, 1750·3
Sulfocillin Sodium, 257·2
Sulfociprofloxacin, 191·1
Sulfogaiacol, 1131·1
Sulfoguayacol, 1131·1
Sulfoid Trimetho, 2311·3
Sulfoil, 2311·3
Sulfometh, 2311·3
Sulfona, 2311·3
Sulfonamides, 119·2
Sulfonated Castor Oil, 1575·3
Sulfonated Diethenylbenzene-ethenylbenzene Copolymer Complex, Codeine and, 28·1
Sulfonated Diethenylbenzene-ethenylbenzene Copolymer Complex, Hydrocodone and, 45·1
Sulfonated Styrene Copolymer with Divinylbenzene, Sodium Salt, 1053·2
Sulfonated Styrene Polymer, Calcium Salt, 1032·3
Sulfonated Styrene Polymer, Potassium Salt, 1050·1
Sulfonazolum, 264·1
Sulfones, 117·1
4,4′-Sulfonylbis-benzenamine, 202·2
Sulfonylurea Antidiabetics, 346·1
Sulfo-Olbad Cordes, 2311·3
Sulfopino, 2311·3
Sulforcin, 2311·3
Sulforidazine, 724·3
Sulformethoxine, 259·3
Sulfort, 2311·3
Sulforthomidine, 259·3
Sulfo-Salicyl, 2311·3
Sulfo-Schwefelbad, 2311·3
Sulfo-Selenium, 2311·3
Sulfotrim, 2311·3
Sulfoxyl, 2311·3
Sulfredox, 2311·4
Sulf+Trim, 2311·4
Sulfur, 1158·2
Sulfur, Colloidal, 1158·2
Sulfur Dioxide, 1193·2
Sulfur, Flowers of, 1158·2
Sulfur Hexafluoride, 1067·3
Sulfur Med Complex, 2311·4
Sulfur, Milk of, 1158·2
Sulfur Mustard, 1679·3
Sulfur, Precipitated, 1158·2
Sulfur, Sublimed, 1158·2
Sulfurated Lime, 1158·2
Sulfurated Potash, 1158·3
Sulfurell, 2311·4
Sulfuretten, 2311·4
Sulfuric Acid, 1750·3
Sulfuric Acid, Fuming, 1750·3
Sulfúrico, Ácido, 1750·3
Sulfuro de Hidrógeno, 1236·2
Sulfuro de Selenio, 1157·3
Sulfurous Acid, 1193·2
Sulfuryl, 2311·4
Sulgan 99, 2311·4
Sulgan— *see* F 99 Sulgan N, 1987·1
Sulgan N, 2311·4
Sulginum, 260·3
Sulglicotida, 1293·2
Sulglicotide, 1293·2
Sulglycotide, 1293·2
Sulidamor, 2311·4
Sulide, 2311·4
Sulimed, 2311·4
Sulindac, 91·2
Sulindac Sodium, 92·1
Sulindac Sulfone, 552·3
Sulindaco, 91·2
Sulindacum, 91·2
Sulindal, 2311·4
Sulindor, 2311·4
Sulinol, 2311·4
Sulisobenzona, 1158·3
Sulisobenzone, 1158·3
Sulkine, 2311·4
Sulmasque, 2311·4
Sulmetin, 2311·4
Sulmetin Papaver, 2311·4
Sulmetin Papaverina, 2311·4
Sulmycin, 2311·4
Sulmycin Mit Celestan-V, 2312·1
Sulmyn, 2312·1
Sulnil, 2312·1
Sulobil, 2312·1
Sulocten, 2312·1
Sulodexida, 1009·2
Sulodexide, 1009·2
Sulorane, 2312·1
Sulotil, 2312·1
Suloves, 2312·1
Sulp, 2312·1
Sulpan, 2312·1
Sulparex, 2312·1
Sulperazon, 2312·1
Sulph...— *see also under* Solf... *and* Sulf...
Sulphacarbamide, 257·3
Sulphacetamide, 257·3
Sulphacetamide Sodium, 257·3
Sulphacetamide, Soluble, 257·3
Sulphacetamidum Sodium, 257·3
Sulphachlorpyridazine, 258·1
Sulphadiazine, 258·2
Sulphadiazine Silver, 259·1
Sulphadiazine Sodium, 258·2
Sulphadiazine, Soluble, 258·2
Sulphadimethoxine, 259·2
Sulphadimethyloxazole, 263·2
Sulphadimethylpyrimidine, 259·2
Sulphadimidine, 259·2
Sulphadimidine Sodium, 259·2
Sulphadimidine, Soluble, 259·2
Sulphafuraz, 260·1
Sulphafurazole, 260·1
Sulphafurazole, Acetyl, 260·1
Sulphafurazole Diethanolamine, 260·1
Sulphafurazole Diolamine, 260·1
Sulphafurazole, Iminobisethanol Salt, 260·1
Sulphaguanidine, 260·3
Sulphalene, 263·1
Sulphamerazine, 260·3
Sulphamerazine Sodium, 260·3
Sulphamethazine, 259·2
Sulphamethizole, 260·3
Sulphamethoxazole, 261·1
Sulphamethoxypyridazine, 263·1
Sulphamide, 2312·1
*p*-Sulphamidoaniline, 263·2
Sulphamoxole, 263·2
*p*-Sulphamoylbenzoic Acid, 1668·2
4′-Sulphamoylsuccinanilic Acid, 264·1
*N*-(5-Sulphamoyl-1,3,4-thiadiazol-2-yl)acetamide, 849·1
Sulphan Blue, 1750·3
Sulphanilamide, 263·2
*N*-Sulphaniloylacetamide, 257·3
*N*-Sulphanilylbenzamide, 257·3
1-Sulphanilylguanidine, 260·3
*N*-*p*-Sulphanilylphenylglycine Sodium, 153·3
Sulphanilylurea, 257·3
Sulphanilylurea Monohydrate, 257·3
Sulphanum Caeruleum, 1750·3
Sulphapyridine, 263·3
Sulphaquinoxalina, 263·3
Sulphaquinoxaline, 263·3
Sulphasalazine, 1291·1
Sulphasomidine, 264·1
Sulphate of Lime, 1665·1
Sulphated Castor Oil, 1575·3
Sulphathiazole, 264·1
Sulphathiazole Sodium, 264·1
Sulphation Factors, 1338·3
Sulphaurea, 257·3
Sulphenazone, 260·3
Sulphinpyrazone, 417·3
Sulphinylbismethane, 1473·2
Sulphobromophthalein Sodium, 1750·3

12-Sulphodehydroabietic Acid, Monosodium Salt, 1264·3
Sulpho-Lac, 2312·1
Sulphonyldianiline, 202·2
Sulphonylurea Antidiabetics, 346·1
Sulphormethoxine, 259·3
Sulphorthodimethoxine, 259·3
Sulphoxyphenylpyrazolidine, 417·3
Sulphur, 1158·2
Sulphur Dioxide, 1193·2
Sulphur for External Use, 1158·2
Sulphur Fluoride, 1067·3
Sulphur Hexafluoride, 1067·3
Sulphur, Liver of, 1158·3
Sulphurated Lime, 1158·2
Sulphurated Potash, 1158·3
Sulphuretted Hydrogen, 1236·2
Sulphuric Acid, 1750·3
Sulpilan, 2312·1
Sulpiren, 2312·1
Sulpirida, 722·2
Sulpiride, 722·2
L-Sulpiride, 722·2
Sulpiridum, 722·2
Sulpitil, 2312·1
Sulpivert, 2312·1
Sulpor, 2312·1
Sulpril, 2312·1
Sulprim, 2312·1
Sulprostona, 1520·3
Sulprostone, 1520·3
Sulpyrin, 2312·1
Sulpyrine, 35·3
Sulquibron, 2312·1
Sulquipen, 2312·1
Sultamicilina, 264·2
Sultamicillin, 264·2
Sultamicillin Toluene-4-sulphonate, 264·2
Sultamicillin Tosilate, 264·2
Sultamicillin Tosylate, 264·2
Sultanol, 2312·1
Sulterline, 2312·1
Sulthiame, 377·3
Sultiame, 377·3
Sultiamo, 377·3
Sultiprim, 2312·1
Sulton, 2312·1
Sultoprida, Hidrocloruro de, 723·1
Sultopride Hydrochloride, 723·1
Sultrin, 2312·1
Sultrona, 2312·2
Sultroquin, 2312·2
Sulvi, Colirio— *see* Colirio Sulvi, 1899·4
SUM-3170, 705·2
Sumac, 1751·2
Sumacal, 2312·2
Sumach Berries, 1738·1
Sumaclina, 2312·2
Sumal, 2312·2
Sumapen, 2312·2
Sumatra Benzoin, 1751·1
Sumatriptan Succinate, 471·2
Sumatriptán, Succinato de, 471·2
Sumatriptani Succinas, 471·2
Sumax, 2312·2
Sumedium, 2312·2
Sumenan, 2312·2
Sumial, 2312·2
Sumidin, 2312·2
Sumiferon, 2312·2
Sumigrene, 2312·2
Suminat, 2312·2
Sumir, 2312·2
Summavac, 2312·2
Summavit, 2312·2
Summavit ME, 2312·2
Summers Eve Preparations, 2312·2
Summitates Cannabis, 1666·1
Sumo, 2312·3
Sumycin, 2312·3
SUN-0588, 1742·1
SUN-1165, 983·1
SUN-5555, 213·1
Sun-9216, 945·1
Sun Block, E45— *see* E45 Sun Block, 1960·4
Sun Buffer, 2312·3
Sun Defense Preparations, 2312·3
Sun, E45— *see* E45 Sun, 1960·4
Sun High Protection Kids Sunblock, 2312·3
Sun Lip Balm, 2312·3
Sun Management Preparations, 2312·3
Sun Pacer Preparations, 2312·3
Sun Tanning, 2312·3
Sun-Benz, 2312·3
Sunblock, 2312·3
Sunblock for Face, 2312·3
Sunblock Lotion, 2312·3
Sunburn— *see* Light-induced Skin Reactions, 1136·3
Suncodin, 2312·3
Sundays Maximum Protection, 2312·3
Sundew, 1683·1
Sundown Preparations, 2312·3
SuNerven, 2312·4
Sunfilter, 2312·4
Sunflower Oil, 1451·1
Sunflower Oil, Refined, 1451·1
Sunflowerseed Oil, 1451·1
Sun-Glizide, 2312·4
Suniderma, 2312·4
Sunkist, 2312·4
SunKist Multivitamins Complete, Children's— *see* Children's SunKist Multivitamins Complete, 1883·1
SunKist Multivitamins + Extra C, Children's— *see* Children's SunKist Multivitamins + Extra C, 1883·1
SunKist Multivitamins + Iron, Children's— *see* Children's SunKist Multivitamins + Iron, 1883·1
Sunmax 30, 2312·4
Sunmax 60, 2312·4
Sunnie, 2312·4
Sunolut, 2312·4
Sunprox, 2312·4
Sunrythm, 2312·4
Sunsan-Heillotion, 2312·4
Sunscreen Lotion, 2313·1
Sunscreen Lotion Ecran, 2313·1
Sunscreens, 1133·2
Sunseekers, 2313·1
Sunsense Preparations, 2313·1, 2313·2
Sunset Yellow FCF, 1058·2
Sunsmackers, 2313·2
Sunspot, 2313·2
Supa C, 2313·2
Supa-Boost, 2313·2
Supac, 2313·2
Supacef, 2313·2
Supadol, 2313·2
Supartz, 2313·2
Super Acid, 1302·3
Super Active Multi, 2313·2
Super Antioxidant Plus, 2313·2
Super Anti-Oxydant Formula, 2313·2
Super AO Formula, 2313·2
Super B, 2313·2
Super B Complex, 2313·2
Super B Complex, Natures Own— *see* Natures Own Super B Complex, 2153·3
Super B Plus, 2313·2
Super B Plus Liver Tonic, 2313·2
Super B Stress, 2313·2
Super Banish, 2313·2
Super C, 2313·2
Super Cal C, Bioglan— *see* Bioglan Super Cal C, 1844·2
Super Cal-C Bio, 2313·2
Super Cal-Mag, 2313·2
Super Cold Tabs, 2313·2
Super Cough, 2313·2
Super Cromer Orto, 2313·2
Super D Perles, 2313·2
Super Daily, 2313·2
Super Energex Plus, 2313·3
Super 28 Formula, 2313·3
Super Galanol, 2313·3
Super Gamma Oil with Vitamin E, 2313·3
Super GammaOil Marine, 2313·3
Super GLA, 2313·3
Super Hi Potency, 2313·3
Super Ivy Dry, 2313·3
Super K, 1302·3
Super Kids, 2313·3
Super Mega B+C, 2313·3
Super Once A Day, 2313·3
Super Orti-Vite, 2313·3
Super Plenamins, 2313·3
Super Quints, 2313·3
Super Soluble Maxipro HBV, 2313·3
Super Strength Sinadrin, 2313·3
Super Stress Mega B Plus Vitamin C, 2313·3
Super Vikaps, 2313·3
Super Vita Vim, 2313·3
Super Vitalex, 2313·3
Super Wate-On, 2313·3
Super Weed, 1730·3
Superan, 2313·3
Superantioxidante, 2313·3
Supercarotene C&E, Bioglan— *see* Bioglan Supercarotene C&E, 1844·2
Superdophilus, 2313·3
Superdophilus, Bioglan— *see* Bioglan Superdophilus, 1844·2
SuperEPA, 2313·3
Superfade, 2313·3
Supergan, 2313·3
Superglue, 1678·1
Superhist, 2313·3
Superinone, 1416·3
Superlipid, 2313·3
Supermin, 2313·3
Supero, 2313·3
Superol, 2313·3
Superoxide Dismutase, 92·2
Superoxide Dismutase, Bovine, 92·2
Superoxidised Water, 1164·3
Superóxido Dismutasa, 92·2
Superpeni, 2313·4
Superpep, 2313·4
Superplex-T, 2313·4
Supersan, 2313·4
SuperSkin, 2313·4
Supertar, 2313·4
Supertendin 2000 N, 2313·4
Supertendin-Depot, 2313·4
Superthiol, 2313·4
Supertonic, 2313·4
Supervit, 2313·4
Supeudol, 2313·4
Suplac, 2313·4
Suplan, 2313·4
Suplasyn, 2313·4
Suplatast Tosilate, 797·2
Suplatast, Tosilato de, 797·2
Suplatast Tosylate, 797·2
Suplatastum Tosilas, 797·2
Supledin, 2313·4
Suplena, 2313·4
Suplevit, 2313·4
Supligol, 2313·4
Supo Gliz, 2313·4
Supo Kristal, 2313·4
Supofen, 2313·4
Supositorio Hamamelis Composto, 2313·4
Supositorios Senosiain, 2313·4
Supotron, 2313·4
Supoviol, 2313·4
Supplamins F, 2313·4
Supplemaman, 2313·4
Supplementary Drugs and Other Substances, 1645·1
Suppletive, 2313·4
Supplex, 2313·4
Suppomaline, 2314·1
Supportan, 2314·1
Supprelin, 2314·1
Suppress, 2314·1
Supra, 2314·1
Supraalox, 2314·1
Supracaine, 2314·1
Supracam, 2314·1
Supracef, 2314·1
Supracid, 2314·1
Supracombin, 2314·1
Supracortin 3, 2314·1
Supracream, 2314·1
Supracyclin, 2314·1
Supracycline, 2314·1
Supradol, 2314·1
Supradyn, 2314·1
Supradyn Ginseng, 2314·1
Supradyn N, 2314·1
Supradyn Vital 50+, 2314·1
Supradyne, 2314·1
Supradynvital, 2314·1
Supragesic, 2314·1
Supralan, 2314·1
Supralan-N, 2314·1
Supralef, 2314·1
Supralip, 2314·2
Supralox, 2314·2
Supramol, 2314·2
Supramox, 2314·2
Supramycin, 2314·2
Supran, 2314·2
Suprane, 2314·2
Supranitrin, 2314·2
Suprapen, 2314·2
Supraproct-S, 2314·2
Suprarenal Cortex, 1110·1
Suprarenin, 852·2, 2314·2
Suprasec, 2314·2
Suprasten, 2314·2
Suprastin, 2314·2
Supratonin, 2314·2
Supraventricular Arrhythmias— *see* Cardiac Arrhythmias, 816·1
Supraventricular Tachycardia, Paroxysmal— *see* Cardiac Arrhythmias, 816·1
Supra-Vir, 2314·2
Supraviran, 2314·2
Supravite, 2314·2
Supravite C, 2314·2
Suprax, 2314·2
Suprecur, 2314·2
Suprefact, 2314·2
Suprema, 2314·2
Supremase, 2314·3
Suprenoat, 2314·3
Supres, 2314·3
Supresol, 2314·3
Supressin, 2314·3
Suprexon, 2314·3
Sup-Rhinite, 2314·3
Suprim, 2314·3
Suprimal, 2314·3
Suprimox, 2314·3
Supristol, 2314·3
Suprium, 2314·3
Suprofen, 93·1
Suprofeno, 93·1
Suprotide, 2314·3
Suracton, 2314·3
Suralgan, 2314·3
Suramin Hexasodium, 615·3
Suramin Sodium, 615·3
Suramina Sódica, 615·3
Surazem, 2314·3
Surbex, 2314·3
Surbex with C, 2314·3
Surbex C, 2314·3
Surbex Plus Iron, 2314·3
Surbex Plus Zinc, 2314·3
Surbex T, 2314·3
Surbex with Zinc, 2314·3
Surbronc, 2314·3
Surbu-Gen-T, 2314·3
Surdolin, 2314·3
Sureau, Fleurs de, 1741·3
SureLac, 2314·3
Sure-Lax, 2314·4
Sure-Lax (Herbal), 2314·4
Surelen, 2314·4
Surem, 2314·4
Sureptil, 2314·4
Sureskin, 2314·4
Suretin, 2314·4
Surfa-Base, 2314·4
Surface Anaesthesia, 1370·2
Surfactal, 2314·4
Surfactant TA, 1736·2

Surfactante B, 2314·4
Surfactants, Ampholytic, 1574·1
Surfactants, Amphoteric, 1574·1
Surfactants, Anionic, 1574·1
Surfactants, Nonionic, 1411·1
Surfacten, 2314·4
Surfactil, 2314·4
Surfak, 2314·4
Surfaz, 2314·4
Surfaz-SN, 2314·4
Surfer, 1730·3
Surfexo Neonatal, 2314·4
Surfol, 2314·4
Surfolase, 2314·4
Surfont, 2314·4
Surfortan, 2314·4
Surgam, 2314·4
Surgamic, 2314·4
Surgamyl, 2314·4
Surgel, 2314·4
Surgestone, 2315·1
Surgibone, 1751·1
Surgical Infection, 147·3
Surgical Spirit, 1186·1
Surgical Wax, Aseptic, 1480·2
Surgical Wax, Bone, 1480·2
Surgicel, 2315·1
Surgicoll, 2315·1
Surgident, 2315·1
Surgi-Gel, 2315·1
Surgras Physiologique, 2315·1
Surifarm, 2315·1
Suril, 2315·1
Surinam Quassia, 1737·2
Sur-Lax, 2315·1
Surlid, 2315·1
Surmenalit, 2315·1
Surmontil, 2315·1
Surmoruine, 2315·1
Surnox, 2315·1
Suronit, 2315·1
Surpass, 2315·1
Surplex, 2315·1
Surquina, 2315·1
Sursum, 2315·1
Suruma, 1666·1
Survanta, 2315·1
Survanta-Vent, 2315·1
Survector, 2315·1
Survimed, 2315·1
Survitine, 2315·1
Susano, 2315·1
Suscard, 2315·2
Suspectim, 2315·2
Suspending Agents, 1576·1
Sus-Phrine, 2315·2
Suss, 2315·2
Suss Balsamico, 2315·2
Süssholzwurzel, 1270·2
Sustac, 2315·2
Sustacal, 2315·2
Sustagen, 2315·2
Sustain, 2315·2
Sustained Release Buffered C, 2315·2
Sustained Release Executive B Plus Herbs, 2315·2
Sustaire, 2315·2
Sustanon, 2315·2
Sustanon 100, 2315·2
Sustanon 250, 2315·2
Sustemial, 2315·2
Sustenan, 2315·2
Sustenan 250, 2315·2
Sustenium, 2315·2
Sustenon 250, 2315·2
Sustitutos de la Piel, 1158·1
Sustiva, 2315·2
Sustrate, 2315·3
Sustress Plus, 2315·3
Sutac, 2315·3
Sutif, 2315·3
Sutilaína, 1751·1
Sutilains, 1751·1
Sutin, 2315·3
Sutoprofen, 93·1
Sutrico, 2315·3
Sutrico Tar, 2315·3
Sutril, 2315·3
Su-Tuss DM, 2315·3
Su-Tuss HD, 2315·3
Suvalan, 2315·3
Suvipen, 2315·3
Suxamethonii Chloridum, 1406·2
Suxamethonium Bromide, 1409·1
Suxamethonium Chloride, 1406·2
Suxamethonium Iodide, 1409·1
Suxametonio, Cloruro de, 1406·2
Suxametonklorid, 1406·2
Suxar, 2315·3
Suxibuzona, 93·1
Suxibuzone, 93·1
Suxibuzonum, 93·1
Suxidina, 2315·3
Suxilep, 2315·3
Suxinutin, 2315·3
Svedocain sin Vasoconstr, 2315·3
Sviroxit, 2315·3
Svitalark, 2315·3
SVR 50B, 2315·3
SVR Creme Antimoustique, 2315·3
Swarm, 2315·3
Sweating, Excessive— *see* Hyperhidrosis, 1136·1
Sweatosan N, 2315·3
Swecon, 2315·3
Sween— *see* Coloplast OAD (Sween), 1900·3
Sween Cream, 2315·3
Sweet Almond Oil, 1651·1
Sweet Birch Oil, 59·3
Sweet Cherry, 1058·1
Sweet Fennel, 1687·2
Sweet Flag, 1664·1
Sweet Flag Root, 1664·1
Sweet Gale, 1661·2
Sweet Orange, 1724·1
Sweet Orange Oil, 1724·1
Sweet Touch, 2315·3
Sweetabb, 2315·3
Sweetex, 2315·3
Swiff, 2315·3
Swim-Ear, 2315·3
Swimming Pool Granuloma— *see* Opportunistic Mycobacterial Infections, 137·2
Swiss Herb Cough Drops, 2315·3
Swiss One, 2315·4
Swiss-Kal Eff, 2315·4
Swiss-Kal SR, 2315·4
SX Carduus, 2315·4
SX Mentha, 2315·4
SX Sabal, 2315·4
SX Valeriana Comp, 2315·4
SY-5555, 213·1
Sycold, 2315·4
Sycot, 2315·4
Sydenham's Chorea— *see* Chorea, 664·2
Sydolil, 2315·4
Sygen, 2315·4
Sykofen, 2315·4
Sylador, 2315·4
Syllact, 2315·4
Syllamalt, 2315·4
Symadal M, 2315·4
Symax, 2315·4
Symbial, 2315·4
Symbicort, 2315·4
Symbiocort, 2315·4
Symbioflor 1, 2315·4
Symbioflor I, 2315·4
Symbioflor 2, 2315·4
Symbioflor II, 2315·4
Symbioflor-Antigen, 2315·4
Symbyax, 2315·4
Symclosene, 1191·3
Symfona N, 2315·4
Symmetrel, 2315·4
Symoron, 2316·1
Symoxyl, 2316·1
Sympaethaminum, 977·3
Sympal, 2316·1
Sympalept, 2316·1
Sympaneurol, 2316·1
Sympathetic Dystrophy, Reflex— *see* Complex Regional Pain Syndrome, 5·3
Sympathetic Nerve Block, 1370·2
Sympathetic Pain Syndromes— *see* Complex Regional Pain Syndrome, 5·3
Sympathin, Nurocain with— *see* Nurocain with Sympathin, 2180·2
Sympathomimetics, 812·1
Sympathyl, 2316·1
Sympatol, 2316·1
Sympavagol, 2316·1
Symphocal, 2316·1
Symphytum, 1675·2
*Symphytum officinale*, 1675·2
Symphytum Ro-Plex (Rowo-776), 2316·1
Symphytum-Komplex, 2316·1
*Symplocarpus foetidus*, 1746·3
Sympropaminum, 982·3
Symptofed, 2316·1
Syn MD, 2316·1
Synacol CF, 2316·1
Synacort, 2316·1
Synacthen, 2316·1
Synacthen Depot, 2316·1
Synacthen Retard, 2316·1
Synacthene, 2316·1
Syn-A-Gen, 2316·1
Synagis, 2316·1
Synalar Preparations, 2316·1
Synalar, Neo- — *see* Neo-Synalar, 2160·3
Synaleve, 2316·2
Synalgo, 2316·2
Synalgos-DC, 2316·2
*Synanceja trachynis* Antiserum, 1640·2
*Synanceja trachynis* Antivenin, 1640·2
*Synanceja trachynis* Antivenom, 1640·2
Synap, 2316·2
Synapausa, 2316·2
Synapause, 2316·2
Synapause E, 2316·2
Synapause-$E_3$, 2316·2
Synarel, 2316·3
Synarela, 2316·3
Synarome, 2316·3
Synastone, 2316·3
Synbetamine, 2316·3
Synbrozil, 2316·3
Syncaine, 1383·2
Syncarpin-N, 2316·3
Synchlolim, 2316·3
Synchrocell, 2316·3
Synchro-Levels, 2316·3
Synchrorose, 2316·3
Synchrovit, 2316·3
Syncillin, 2316·3
Synclovir, 2316·3
Synco-CFN, 2316·3
Syncoforte, 2316·3
Syncomet, 2316·3
Syncope— *see* Hypotension, 828·1
Syncoquin, 2316·3
Syncortyl, 2316·3
Syncro, 2316·3
Syndette, 2316·3
Syndol, 2316·3
Syndopa, 2316·3
Syndrome of Inappropriate ADH Secretion, 1318·3
Synedil, 2316·3
Synemol, 2316·3
Synephrine, 977·3
*m*-Synephrine, 1126·3
*p*-Synephrine, 977·3
Synephrine Tartrate, 977·3
Synerbiol, 2316·4
Synercid, 2316·4
Synerga, 2316·4
Synergistic Manganese, 2316·4
Synergistic Selenium, 2316·4
Synergomycin, 2316·4
Synergon, 2316·4
Synergy B, Bioglan— *see* Bioglan Synergy B, 1844·2
Synergyl, 2316·4
Synermox, 2316·4
Synerpril, 2316·4
Synestrol, 1556·3
Syneudon, 2316·4
Synfase, 2316·4
Synflex, 2316·4
Syngamosis, 101·1
Syngel, 2316·4
Syngynon, 2316·4
Synitidine, 2316·4
Synizoral, 2316·4
Synkapton, 2316·4
Synkavit, 2316·4
Synobel, 2316·4
Synoestrol, 1556·3
Synogin, 2316·4
Synoxicam, 2316·4
Synpharma Preparations, 2316·4
Synphase, 2317·1
Synphasec, 2317·1
Synphasic, 2317·1
Synrelin, 2317·1
Synrelina, 2317·1
Syn-Rx, 2317·1
Syn-Rx DM, 2317·1
*Synsepalum dulcificum*, 1715·2
Synstigminium Bromatum, 1492·2
Syntaris, 2317·1
Syntestan, 2317·1
Synthamin, 2317·1
Synthetic Air, 1236·3
Synthetic Conjugated Oestrogens, A, 1543·3
Synthetic Conjugated Oestrogens, B, 1543·3
Synthetic Paraffin, 1479·1
Synthetic Retinol Concentrate (Oily Form), 1451·3
Synthetic Retinol Concentrate (Powder Form), 1451·3
Synthetic Retinol Concentrate, Solubilisate/Emulsion, 1451·3
Synthocilin, 2317·1
Synthol, 2317·1
Synthomanet, 2317·1
Synthomycine, 2317·1
Synthroid, 2317·1
Synti, 2317·1
Syntocinon, 2317·1
Syntoclox, 2317·1
Syntofene, 2317·1
Syntometrin, 2317·1
Syntometrine, 2317·2
Syntonol, 2317·2
Syntopressin, 2317·2
Synum C, 2317·2
Synuretic, 2317·2
Synureticum, 2317·2
Synvinolin, 997·1
Synvisc, 2317·2
Synvomin, 2317·2
Syphilis, 148·2
Syprine, 2317·2
Syprol, 2317·2
Syracol CF, 2317·2
Syraprim, 2317·2
Syrea, 2317·2
Syrup DM, 2317·2
Syrup DM-D, 2317·2
Syrup DM-D-E, 2317·2
Syrup DM-E, 2317·2
Syrvite, 2317·2
Syscan, 2317·2
Syscor, 2317·2
Systaflam, 2317·2
Systemic Capillary Leak Syndrome, 798·2
Systemic Inflammatory Response Syndrome— *see* Septicaemia, 144·3
Systemic Lupus Erythematosus, 1088·3
Systemic Necrotising Vasculitis— *see* Po yarteritis Nodosa and Microscopic Po angiitis, 1085·3
Systemic Sclerosis— *see* Sclerod 1348·1
Systen, 2317·2
Systen Conti, 2317·2
Systen Sequi, 2317·2
Systepin, 2317·2
Systodin, 2317·2

Systral, 2317·3
Systral C, 2317·3
Systral Hydrocort, 2317·3
Systrason, 2317·3
Sytron, 2317·3
Syu, 2317·3
Syviman N, 2317·3
Syxal, 2317·3
Syxyl-Vitamin-Comb, 2317·3
*Syzygium aromaticum*, 1673·2
Szillosan Forte, 2317·3

**T**

T, 1451·1, 1730·3
2,4,5-T, 1510·3
$T_3$, 1602·2
$T_3$, Reverse, 1594·1
T3, 2317·3
$T_4$, 1600·1
T4, 2317·3
T5, 2317·3
T-20, 633·1
T-1220, 243·1
T-1551, 174·3
T-1824, 1658·3
T-1982, 171·2
T-2588, 181·3
T-3761, 241·3
T-3762, 241·3
T. Polio, 2317·3
T & T Antioxidant, 2317·3
TA-058, 158·3
TA-064, 892·2
TA-870, 906·3
TA-0910, 1340·1
TA-2711, 1264·3
TA-6366, 938·2
TA Baume, 2317·3
TA Graser, 2317·3
TA MIX, 2317·3
Tab Vaccine, 2317·3
Tabalon, 2317·3
Tabarell, 2317·3
Tabasco Pepper, 1667·1
Tab-A-Vite, 2317·3
Tabcin, 2317·3
Tabcin Antigripal, 2317·3
Tabcin Compuesto, 2317·3
Tabcin Expectorante, 2317·3
Taben 450, 2317·3
*Tabernanthe iboga*, 1700·2
Tabine, 2317·3
Tabletas Antiacidas, 2317·3
Tabletas Phillips, 2317·4
Tabletas Quimpe, 2317·4
Tabletes Valda, 2317·4
Tabloid, 2317·4
Taborcil, 2317·4
Tabotamp, 2317·4
Tabrin, 2317·4
Tabritis, 2317·4
Tabun, 1719·2
Tac, 2317·4
TAC Esofago, 2317·4
Tacalcitol, 1158·3
Tacardia, 2317·4
Tacef, 2317·4
Tacex, 2317·4
Tachidol, 2317·4
Tachiflu, 2317·4
Tachifludec, 2317·4
Tachipirina, 2317·4
Tachmalcor, 2317·4
...chmalin, 2317·4
...mb, 2317·4
...317·4
...·4
... see Cardiac Arrhyth-
... Cardiac Arrhyth-
...ular, Paroxys-
...nias, 816·1
...Cardiac Ar-
...less— *see*
...ort, 812·2
Tachycardia, Ventricular, Pulseless— *see* Cardiac Arrhythmias, 816·1
Tachydaron, 2317·4
Tachyfenon, 2317·4
Tachynerg Campher Herzsalbe, 2317·4
Tachynerg N, 2317·4
Tachystin, 2317·4
Tachytalol, 2317·4
Tacid-4, 2318·1
Tacidina, 2318·1
Tacinol, 2318·1
Taclipaxol, 2318·1
Tacrina, Hidrocloruro de, 1497·2
Tacrinal, 2318·1
Tacrine Hydrochloride, 1497·2
Tacrolimus, 1363·3
Tacron, 2318·1
Tacryl, 2318·1
Tactu-nerval, 2318·1
TAD, 2318·1
TAD+, 2318·1
Tadalafil, 1751·1
Tadalafilo, 1751·1
Tadenan, 2318·1
Tadenom, 2318·1
Tadex, 2318·1
Taeniasis, 101·1
Tafenil, 2318·1
Tafenoquina, 463·3
Tafenoquine, 463·3
Tafenoquine Succinate, 463·3
Tafil, 2318·1
Tafirol, 2318·1
Tafloc, 2318·1
Taflox, 2318·1
Tagadine, 2318·1
Tagagel, 2318·1
Tagal, 2318·1
Tagaliv, 2318·1
Tagamet, 2318·1
Tagatose, 1269·1
TAGG, 2318·2
Tagonis, 2318·2
Tagozzard, 2318·2
Taguinol, 2318·2
Taharmayim, 2318·2
Taharsept, 2318·2
Tahartaf, 2318·2
Tahgalim, 1666·1
Tahitian Vanilla, 1762·3
Tahor, 2318·2
Tai Ginseng N, 2318·2
Taido, 2318·2
Taigalor, 2318·2
Taingel, 2318·2
Tairal, 2318·2
Takadol, 2318·2
Takata, 2318·2
Takayasu's Arteritis, 1089·3
Takecef, 2318·2
Takepron, 2318·2
Takesulin, 2318·2
Taketiam, 2318·2
Takil, 2318·2
Takrouri, 1666·1
Taks, 2318·2
Takus, 2318·2
Talacen, 2318·2
Talam, 2318·2
Talasa NF, 2318·2
Talavir, 2318·2
Talc, 1159·1
Talc, Powdered, 1159·1
Talc, Purified, 1159·1
Talcid, 2318·2
Talco Alivio, 2318·3
Talco Antihistam Calber, 2318·3
Talco Purificado, 1159·1
Talcum, 1159·1
Talcum Purificatum, 1159·1
Talerc, 2318·3
Talflex, 2318·3
Talidat, 2318·3
Talidomida, 1752·3
Talinolol, 1009·2
Talio 201, 1526·2
Talio, Acetato de, 1754·2
Talion, 2318·3
Talipexol, Hidrocloruro de, 1215·3
Talipexole Hydrochloride, 1215·3
Talizer, 2318·3
Talkosona, 2318·3
Tallo de Muérdago, 1715·3
Talofen, 2318·3
Talofilina, 2318·3
Talohexal, 2318·3
Taloken, 2318·3
Talol, 2318·3
Talowin, 2318·3
Taloxa, 2318·3
Taloxoral— *see* Taloxa, 2318·3
Talpramin, 2318·3
Talquis Cusi, 2318·3
Talquissar, 2318·3
Talquistina, 2318·3
Talseclin, 2318·3
Talso, 2318·3
Talsutin, 2318·3
Taltirelin, 1340·1
Taltirelina, 1340·1
Taludon, 2318·3
Talusin, 2318·3
Taluvian, 2318·3
Talval, 2318·3
Talvosilen, 2318·4
Talwin, 2318·4
Talwin— *see* Emergent-Ez, 1967·2
Talwin Compound, 2318·4
Talwin NX, 2318·4
Tam, 2318·4
Tamagon, 2318·4
Tamanybonsan, 2318·4
Tamaril, 2318·4
Tamarind, 1293·2
Tamarindo, 1293·2
*Tamarindus indica*, 1293·2
Tamarine, 2318·4
Tamarix, 2318·4
Tamax, 2318·4
Tamaxin, 2318·4
Tambocor, 2318·4
Tambocur, 2318·4
Tambutec, 2318·4
Tamec, 2318·4
Tameran, 2318·4
Tametin, 2318·4
Tamexin, 2318·4
Tamibarotene, 507·1
Tamifen, 2318·4
Tamiflu, 2318·4
Tamigen, 2318·4
Tamik, 2319·1
Tamilan, 2319·1
Tamin, 2319·1
Tamine SR, 2319·1
Tamisa, 2319·1
Tamizam, 2319·1
Tamobeta, 2319·1
Tamofen, 2319·1
Tamofene, 2319·1
Tamokadin, 2319·1
Tamolan, 2319·1
Tamolem, 2319·1
Tamone, 2319·1
Tamooex, 2319·1
Tamopham, 2319·1
Tamophar, 2319·1
Tamoplex, 2319·1
Tamosin, 2319·1
Tamox, 2319·1
Tamoxan, 2319·1
Tamoxasta, 2319·1
Tamoxen, 2319·1
Tamoxene, 2319·1
Tamoxi, 2319·1
Tamoxifen Citrate, 584·1
Tamoxifeni Citras, 584·1
Tamoxifeno, Citrato de, 584·1
Tamoxigenat, 2319·1
Tamoximerck, 2319·1
Tamoxin, 2319·1
Tamoxis, 2319·1
Tamoxistad, 2319·1
Tamper, 2319·2
Tampo, 2319·2
Tamposit N, 2319·2
Tampositorien H, 2319·2
Tampositorien mit Belladonna, 2319·2
Tampovagan, 2319·2
Tampovagan c Acid Lact, 2319·2
Tamsulosin Hydrochloride, 1009·2
Tamsulosina, Hidrocloruro de, 1009·2
Tamyl, 2319·2
Tan Express, 2319·2
Tanac, 2319·2
Tanac Dual Core, 2319·2
Tanacet, 2319·2
Tanaceti Parthenii Herba, 469·1
Tanaceto, 1751·3
*Tanacetum parthenium*, 469·1
*Tanacetum vulgare*, 1751·3
Tanadopa, 2319·2
Tanafed, 2319·2
Tanafed DM, 2319·2
Tanafed DMX, 2319·2
Tanafed DP, 2319·2
Tanagel, 2319·2
Tanagel Papeles, 2319·2
Tanakan, 2319·2
Tanakene, 2319·2
Tanalbina, 2319·2
Tanalone, 2319·2
Tanasid, 2319·2
Tanatril, 2319·2
Tanavat, 2319·3
Tancilina, 2319·3
Tandax, 2319·3
Tandem Icon, 2319·3
Tandene, 2319·3
Tanderalgin, 2319·3
Tanderil, 2319·3
Tanderon, 2319·3
Tandial, 2319·3
Tandiur, 2319·3
Tandix, 2319·3
Tandorene, 2319·3
Tandospirona, Citrato de, 723·2
Tandospirone Citrate, 723·2
Tandrex, 2319·3
Tandrex A, 2319·3
Tandrexin, 2319·3
Tandriflan, 2319·3
Tandrilax, 2319·3
Tanezox, 2319·3
Tanganil, 2319·3
Tangenol, 2319·3
Tánico, Ácido, 1751·2
Tanidina, 2319·3
Tanin, 1751·2
Tanizona, 2319·3
Tann. Acid, 1751·2
Tannacomp, 2319·3
Tannalbin, 2319·3
Tannic-12, 2319·3
Tannic Acid, 1751·2
Tannidin Plus, 2319·3
Tannin, 1751·2
Tannin Albuminate, 1248·1
Tanninum, 1751·2
Tannisol, 2319·3
Tannolact, 2319·3
Tannolil, 2319·4
Tannolsaft, Kneipp Krauter Hustensaft N Kneipp— *see* Kneipp Krauter Hustensaft N Kneipp Tannolsaft, 2081·3
Tannopon, 2319·4
Tannosynt, 2319·4
Tanoral, 2319·4
Tanrix, 2319·4
Tanser, 2319·4
Tanston, 2319·4
Tansy, 1751·3
Tansy Oil, 1751·3
Tantacol DM, 2319·4
Tantafed, 2319·4
Tantalum, 1059·1
Tantaphen, 2319·4
Tantapp, 2319·4

Tantol Skin Cleanser, 2319·4
Tantol Skin Lotion, 2319·4
Tantum, 2319·4
Tantum Ciclina, 2319·4
Tantum Rosa, 2319·4
Tantum Verde, 2319·4
Tantumar, 2319·4
Tanvimil, 2319·4
Tanyl, 2319·4
Tanzal, 2319·4
TAO, 2319·4
TAP-144, 1331·1
Tapal-2, 2320·1
Tapanol, 2320·1
Tapazol, 2320·1
Tapazole, 2320·1
Tapeworm Infections, Beef— *see* Taeniasis, 101·1
Tapeworm Infections, Dwarf— *see* Hymenolepiasis, 99·2
Tapeworm Infections, Fish— *see* Diphyllobothriasis, 98·1
Tapeworm Infections, Pork— *see* Taeniasis, 101·1
Tapioca Starch, 1449·1, 1449·2
Taponoto, 2320·1
Taporin, 2320·1
Taprodex, 2320·1
Tapsin Analgesico, 2320·1
Tapsin 2 Analgesico, 2320·1
Tapsin Compuesto, 2320·1
Tapsin Compuesto con Clorfenamina, 2320·1
Tapsin Compuesto Dia/Noche Plus, 2320·1
Tapsin Periodo Menstrual, 2320·1
Tapsin sin Cafeina, 2320·1
Tapzol, 2320·1
Tapzol con Neomicina, 2320·1
Taquicord, 2320·1
Tar, 1159·3
Tar Acids, 1193·3
Tar, Coal, 1159·2
Tar Doak, 2320·1
Tar Isdin Champu, 2320·1
Tar Isdin Plus, 2320·1
Tar, Juniper, 1159·2
Tar Oil, Birch, 1159·2
Tar Oil, Juniper, 1159·2
Tar Oils, Tars and, 1159·2
Tar, Pine, 1159·3
Tar, Prepared, 1159·2
Tar, Stockholm, 1159·3
Tar Weed, 1696·1
Tar, Wood, 1159·3
Tara, 1751·2, 2320·1
Tara Abfuhrsirup, 2320·1
Taradyl, 2320·1
Taraleon, 2320·1
Taraphilic, 2320·1
Tara-Plus, 2320·1
Tarassaco (Specie Composta), 2320·1
Taraten, 2320·1
Taraxacum, 1751·3
Taraxacum Compuesto, 2320·1
Taraxacum Herb, 1751·3
Taraxacum Med Complex, 2320·2
*Taraxacum officinale*, 1751·3
Taraxacum Root, 1751·3
Taraxin, 2320·2
Tarband, 2320·2
Tardan, 2320·2
Tardigal, 2320·2
Tardive Dyskinesia— *see* Extrapyramidal Disorders, 677·1
Tardocillin, 2320·2
Tardotol, 2320·2
Tardyferon, 2320·2
Tardyferon $B_9$, 2320·2
Tardyferon-Fol, 2320·2
Tareg, 2320·2
Tareg-D, 2320·2
Tarflex, 2320·2
Targel, 2320·2
Targel SA, 2320·2
Target, 2320·2
Targifor, 2320·2
Targifor C, 2320·2
Targinina, 1752·1
Targinine, 1752·1
Targocid, 2320·2
Targosid, 2320·3
Targretin, 2320·3
Targus, 2320·3
Tariquidar, 499·1
Tarisdin, 2320·3
Taritux, 2320·3
Tarivid, 2320·3
Tarjen, 2320·3
Tarjena, 2320·3
Tarka, 2320·3
Tarlene, 2320·3
Tarmed, 2320·3
Taro Gel, 2320·3
Tarocidin, 2320·3
Tarocidin D, 2320·3
Taroctyl, 2320·3
Tarocyn, 2320·3
Tarodent, 2320·3
Tarodex, 2320·3
Tarophed, 2320·3
Tarophenicol, 2320·3
Taro-Sone, 2320·3
Tars and Tar Oils, 1159·2
Tarseb, 2320·3
Tarsum, 2320·3
Tart. Acid, 1752·1
Tartar Control Listerine, 2320·3
Tartar Emetic, 103·1
Tartar, Purified Cream of, 1284·3
Tartar, Soluble Cream of, 1734·1
Tartaric Acid, 1752·1
(+)-L-Tartaric Acid, 1752·1
Tartárico, Ácido, 1752·1
Tartaricum, Acidum, 1752·1
Tartarus Depuratus, 1284·3
Tartarus Natronatus, 1284·3
Tartarus Stibiatus, 103·1
Tartarus Vitriolatus, 1232·2
Tartephedreel, 2320·3
Tartrato Ácido de Potasio, 1284·3
Tartrato de Alimemazina, 423·3
Tartrato de Brimonidina, 876·3
Tartrato de Butorfanol, 23·3
Tartrato de Ciclizina, 429·3
Tartrato de Dextromoramida, 28·2
Tartrato de Dihidrocodeína, 34·3
Tartrato de Dihidroergotamina, 466·1
Tartrato de Ergotamina, 467·2
Tartrato de Fendimetrazina, 1592·1
Tartrato de Fenindamina, 438·2
Tartrato de Gepefrina, 923·2
Tartrato de Ifenprodil, 938·1
Tartrato de Ketanserina, 943·1
Tartrato de Levorfanol, 54·1
Tartrato de Metaraminol, 952·2
Tartrato de Metoprolol, 957·1
Tartrato de Morantel, 110·1
Tartrato de Potasio Y de Sodio, 1284·3
Tartrato de Tilosina, 275·1
Tartrato de Tolterodina, 489·3
Tartrato de Vinorelbina, 594·1
Tartrato de Zolpidem, 728·3
Tartrato Sódico, 1290·1
Tartrazin., 1058·2
Tartrazina, 1058·2
Tartrazine, 1058·2
Tartrazol Yellow, 1058·2
Tartrina, 2320·3
Tartrique (Acide), 1752·1
Tartrique, Jaune, 1058·2
Tarvexol, 2320·4
Tarytar, 2320·4
Tasakal, 2320·4
Tasedan, 2320·4
Tasep, 2320·4
Tasmaderm, 2320·4
Tasmar, 2320·4
Tasonermin, 590·2
Tasonermina, 590·2
Tasosartan, 1009·3
Taste Disorders, 682·2
Tasty C, 2320·4
TATBA, 1110·2
TATD, 1455·1
Tatig, 2320·4
Tationil, 2320·4
TAU-284, 425·3
Tau Kit, 2320·4
Taucor, 2320·4
Tauglicolo, 2320·4
Tauliz, 2320·4
Tauma, 2320·4
Taumatina, 1451·1
Taural, 2320·4
Taurargin, 2320·4
Tauredon, 2320·4
Taurina, 1752·1
Taurine, 1752·1
Tauro, 2320·4
Taurobetina, 2320·4
Taurochenodeoxycholic Acid, 1660·3
Taurocholic Acid, 1660·3
Taurolidina, 264·2
Taurolidine, 264·2
Taurolin, 2320·4
Tauroselcholic Acid ($^{75}$Se), 1525·2
Tauroursodeoxycholic Acid, 1761·1
Taurovit, 2320·4
Taurultam, 264·2
Tausendgüldenkraut, 1669·2
Tautoss, 2320·4
Tauval, 2320·4
Tauxolo, 2320·4
Tavanic, 2320·4
Tavan-SP 54, 2321·1
Tavegil, 2321·1
Tavegyl, 2321·1
Taver, 2321·1
Tavidan, 2321·1
Tavinex, 2321·1
Tavinex Expectorante, 2321·1
Tavinex Expectotabs, 2321·1
Tavipec, 2321·1
Tavist, 2321·1
Tavist Allergy, 2321·1
Tavist ND, 2321·1
Tavist-1— *see* Tavist Allergy, 2321·1
Tavist-D, 2321·1
Tavolax, 2321·1
Tavolax Nouvelle Formule, 2321·1
Tavonin, 2321·1
Tavor, 2321·1
Taxagon, 2321·1
Taxfeno, 2321·1
Taxifur, 2321·1
Taxilan, 2321·1
Taxocris, 2321·1
Taxodiol, 2321·1
Taxofen, 2321·1
Taxol, 577·3, 2321·1
Taxol A, 577·3
Taxotere, 2321·2
Taxus, 2321·2
*Taxus baccata*, 547·2, 578·2
*Taxus brevifolia*, 578·2
Taxyl, 2321·2
Taycovit, 2321·2
Tayuya, Licor de— *see* Licor de Tayuya, 2095·3
Tazac, 2321·2
Tazarotene, 1160·2
Tazarotenic Acid, 1160·2
Tazaroteno, 1160·2
Tazepin, 2321·2
Tazicef, 2321·2
Tazidem, 2321·2
Tazidime, 2321·2
Taziken, 2321·2
Tazobac, 2321·2
Tazobactam Sódico, 264·3
Tazobactam Sodium, 264·3
Tazocel, 2321·2
Tazocilline, 2321·2
Tazocin, 2321·2
Tazonam, 2321·2
Tazorac, 2321·2
Taztia, 2321·2
Tazusin, 2321·2
TBHQ, 1193·3
TBI/698, 269·3
T-BMP, 2321·2
TBS, 1171·2
TBTO, 1756·3
TBV, 2321·2
3TC, 648·2, 2321·2
3TC/AZT, 2321·3
3TC Complex, 2321·3
3TC/Epivir, 2321·3
TC-109, 616·3
TCC, 1195·1
TCDD, 1681·1
TCDO, 1752·3
T-cell Growth Factor, 562·2
TCK-1 Hematocis, 2321·3
TCK 6, 2321·3
TCK 7 Angiocis, 2321·3
TCK-17 Nanocis, 2321·3
TCK 18, 2321·3
TCK-21, 2321·3
TCO, 2321·3
TCP, 1730·3, 2321·3
TCV-116, 878·3
TD, 2321·3
TD Spray Iso Mack, 2321·3
T/Derm, Neutrogena— *see* Neutrogena T/Derm, 2165·2
Td-Impfstoff, 2321·3
Td-Polio, 2321·3
Td-pur, 2321·3
Td-Rix, 2321·3
Td-Vaccinol, 2321·3
Td-Virelon, 2321·3
TE-031, 192·2
TE-114, 489·3
Te Anatoxal, 2321·3
Tea, 1765·3
Tea, Abyssinian, 1585·2
Tea, African, 1585·2
Tea, Arabian, 1585·2
Tea, Paraguay, 1765·3
Tea Test, 2321·3
Tea Tree, New Zealand, 1709·3
Tea Tree Oil, 1710·2
Tea Tree & Witch Hazel Cream, 2321·3
Tealep, 2321·3
Tealine, 2321·3
Tear Gas, 1676·3, 1677·3
Teardrops, 2321·3
TearGard, 2321·3
Tear-Gel, 2321·4
Teargel, 2321·4
Teargen, 2321·4
Tearisol, 2321·4
Tears Again, 2321·4
Tears Again MC, 2321·4
Tears Encore, 2321·4
Tears Gel— *see* Tears Lubricante, 2321·4
Tears Humectante, 2321·4
Tears Lubricante, 2321·4
Tears Natural, 2321·4
Tears Naturale, 2321·4
Tears Night & Day, 2321·4
Tears Plus, 2321·4
Tears Renewed, 2321·4
Teatrois, 2321·4
Tebacón, Hidrocloruro de, 1131·2
Tebamide, 2321·4
Tebasedan, 2321·4
Tebege-Tannin, 2321·4
Tebertin, 2321·4
Tebesium, 2321·4
Tebesium-s, 2321·4
Tebetane Composto, 2321·4
Tebetane Compuesto, 2321·4
Tebezide, 2321·4
Tebezonum, 269·3
Tebloc, 2321·4
Tebofortan, 2322·1
Tebofortin, 2322·1
Tebokan, 2322·1
Tebonin, 2322·1
Teboroxime, Technetium (9
Teboven, 2322·1
Te-Br, 2322·1

Tebraxin, 2322·1
Tebrazid, 2322·1
Tebutato de Prednisolona, 1108·2
Tecastemizole, 424·2
Teceeme, 2322·1
Tecelac, 2322·1
Teceleukin, 562·3
Tecfazolina, 2322·1
Tecfoline, 2322·1
TechneScan DMSA, 2322·1
TechneScan DTPA, 2322·1
TechneScan Enxofre, 2322·1
TechneScan HDP, 2322·1
TechneScan MAA, 2322·1
TechneScan MAG3, 2322·1
TechneScan MDB, 2322·1
TechneScan PYP, 2322·1
TechneScan Q12, 2322·1
Technetium ($^{99m}$Tc) Albumin, 1525·3
Technetium ($^{99m}$Tc) Apcitide, 1525·3
Technetium ($^{99m}$Tc) Arcitumomab, 1526·1
Technetium ($^{99m}$Tc) Betiatide, 1526·1
Technetium ($^{99m}$Tc) Bicisate, 1526·1
Technetium ($^{99m}$Tc) Colloidal Rhenium Sulfide, 1525·3
Technetium ($^{99m}$Tc) Depreotide, 1526·1
Technetium ($^{99m}$Tc) Disofenin, 1526·1
Technetium ($^{99m}$Tc) Etifenin, 1526·1
Technetium ($^{99m}$Tc) Exametazime, 1526·1
Technetium ($^{99m}$Tc) Gluceptate, 1526·1
Technetium ($^{99m}$Tc) Gluconate, 1526·1
Technetium ($^{99m}$Tc) Lidofenin, 1526·1
Technetium ($^{99m}$Tc) Mebrofenin, 1526·1
Technetium ($^{99m}$Tc) Medronate, 1526·1
Technetium ($^{99m}$Tc) Mertiatide, 1526·1
Technetium ($^{99m}$Tc) Nofetumomab Merpentan, 1526·1
Technetium ($^{99m}$Tc) Oxidronate, 1526·1
Technetium ($^{99m}$Tc) Pentetate, 1526·1
Technetium ($^{99m}$Tc) Pyrophosphate, 1526·1
Technetium ($^{99m}$Tc) Sestamibi, 1526·1
Technetium ($^{99m}$Tc) Succimer, 1526·1
Technetium ($^{99m}$Tc) Sulesomab, 1526·1
Technetium ($^{99m}$Tc) Teboroxime, 1526·1
Technetium ($^{99m}$Tc) Tetrofosmin, 1526·1
Technetium-99m, 1525·2
Techniques Anti-Dandruff, 2322·1
Teclind, 2322·1
Teclothiazide Potassium, 1010·1
Teclotiazida Potásica, 1010·1
Teclozan, 616·3
Tecnal, 2322·1
Tecnal C, 2322·1
Tecnecio 99M, 1525·2
Tecnemab K1, 2322·1
Tecnid, 2322·1
Tecnocarb, 2322·1
Tecnocris, 2322·1
Tecnofen, 2322·1
Tecnoflut, 2322·2
Tecnolip, 2322·2
Tecnomicina, 2322·2
Tecnoplatin, 2322·2
Tecnosal, 2322·2
Tecnotax, 2322·2
Tecnotecan, 2322·2
Tecnovorin, 2322·2
Teconam, 2322·2
Tecyn, 2322·2
Teczem, 2322·2
Teczol, 2322·2
Teddy-C, 2322·2
Tedec Profer, 2322·2
rin Sodium, 891·1
322·2

Teekanne Preparations, 2322·2
Teel Oil, 1743·3
Teen Derm, 2322·3
Teen Formula, 2322·3
Teen Vitamins, 2322·3
Teenstick, 2322·3
Teer-Linola-Fett, 2322·3
Teerol, 2322·3
Teerol-H, 2322·3
Teeth Tough, 2322·3
Teetha, 2322·3
Teething, 2322·3
Teething Granules— *see* Teetha, 2322·3
Teething Relief, 2322·3
Tefaclor, 2322·3
Tefamin, 2322·3
Tefavinca, 2322·3
Tefilin, 2322·3
Tefizox, 2322·3
Teflan, 2322·3
Teflon, 1733·2
Tegafur, 586·2
Tegagen, 2322·3
Tegaserod Maleate, 1293·2
Tegaserod, Maleato de, 1293·2
Tegasorb, 2322·3
Tegeline, 2322·3
Tegens, 2322·3
Tegisec, 2322·3
Tegison, 2322·3
Tegopen, 2322·3
Tegra, 2322·3
Tegreen, 2322·3
Tegretal, 2322·3
Tegretard, 2322·4
Tegretol, 2322·4
Tegrex, 2322·4
Tegrezin, 2322·4
Tegrin, 2322·4
Tegrin, Advanced Formula— *see* Advanced Formula Tegrin, 1777·3
Tegrin Medicated, 2322·4
Tegrin-HC, 2322·4
Tegrin-LT, 2322·4
Tegrital, 2322·4
Tegunal, 2322·4
Teguphen, 2322·4
Teguran, 2322·4
Teichomycin $A_2$, 264·3
Teicomid, 2322·4
Teicoplanin, 264·3
Teicoplanina, 264·3
Teicox, 2322·4
Teiklonal, 2322·4
Tejel, 2322·4
Tejuntivo, 2322·4
Tekaval, 2322·4
Tekfema, 2322·4
Teladar, 2322·4
Telament, 2322·4
Telarix, 2322·4
Telaroid, 2322·4
Telbibur N, 2322·4
Telbon, 2322·4
Teldafen, 2322·4
Teldane, 2322·4
Teldane D, 2323·1
Teldanex, 2323·1
Teldrin, 2323·1
Telebar, 2323·1
Telebrix Preparations, 2323·1
Telen, 2323·1
Telepaque, 2323·1
Telepathine, 1696·3
Telergon 1, Apiserum con— *see* Apiserum con Telergon 1, 1807·3
Telergon II, 2323·1
Telesol, 2323·1
Tele-Stulln, 2323·1
Telfast, 2323·1
Telfast Decongestant, 2323·2
Telfast-D, 2323·2
Telithromycin, 265·2
Telitromicina, 265·2
Telmesteína, 1131·1
Telmesteine, 1131·1

Telmisartan, 1010·1
Telmitin, 2323·2
Telo Cypro, 2323·2
Teloeut, 1666·1
Telos, 2323·2
Telset, 2323·2
Teltonal, 2323·2
Telugren, 2323·2
Telugren Plus, 2323·2
Teluron, 2323·2
Telus, 2323·2
Telvodin, 2323·2
Temaco, 2323·2
Temador, 2323·2
Temafloxacin, 266·1
Temafloxacin Hydrochloride, 266·1
Temafloxacino, 266·1
Temaze, 2323·2
Temazep, 2323·2
Temazepam, 723·2
Temazepamum, 723·2
Temazin Cold, 2323·2
Temazine, 2323·2
Temefos, 1510·2
Temephos, 1510·2
Temesta, 2323·2
Temetex, 2323·2
Temgesic, 2323·2
Temgesic-nX, 2323·2
Temic, 2323·2
Temigran, 2323·2
Temocapril, Hidrocloruro de, 1010·2
Temocapril Hydrochloride, 1010·2
Temocaprilat, 1010·2
Temocilina Sódica, 266·1
Temocillin, 266·1
Temocillin Disodium, 266·1
Temocillin Sodium, 266·1
Temodal, 2323·2
Temodar, 2323·3
Temolan, 2323·3
Temoporfin, 586·3
Temoporfina, 586·3
Temovate, 2323·3
Temoxol, 2323·3
Temozolomida, 587·1
Temozolomide, 587·1
Temperal, 2323·3
Temperax, 2323·3
Tempil, 2323·3
Tempil N, 2323·3
Tempire, 2323·3
Templadol, 2323·3
Tempo, 2323·3
Tempofin, 2323·3
Tempolax, 2323·3
Temporal Arteritis— *see* Giant Cell Arteritis, 1080·1
Temporal Lobe Epilepsy— *see* Epilepsy, 349·1
Tempo-Rinolo, 2323·3
Temporol, 2323·3
Temposil, 2323·3
Tempra, 2323·3
Tempra CD, 2323·3
Tempra MF, 2323·3
Temprin, 2323·3
Temserin, 2323·3
Temtabs, 2323·3
Temzzard, 2323·3
Tenacid, 2323·3
Tenadin, 2323·3
Tenadren, 2323·4
Tenadrin, 2323·4
Tenag, 2323·4
Tenalgin, 2323·4
Tenalif, 2323·4
Tenamfetamine, 1593·3
Tenanfetamina, 1593·3
Tenaron, 2323·4
Tenat, 2323·4
Tenax, 2323·4
Tenben, 2323·4
Ten-Bloka, 2323·4
Tencef, 2323·4
Tencet, 2323·4

Tenchlor, 2323·4
Tencilan, 2323·4
Tencon, 2323·4
Tender Age, 2323·4
TenderWet, 2323·4
Tendinitis— *see* Soft-tissue Rheumatism, 11·1
Tendolon, 2323·4
Tendrin, 2323·4
Tenectéplasa, 1010·2
Tenecteplase, 1010·2
Tenelid, 2323·4
Teneretic, 2323·4
Tenex, 2323·4
Tenibex, 2323·4
Tenidon, 2323·4
Tenif, 2323·4
Teniken, 2323·4
Tenildiamina, Hidrocloruro de, 442·1
Teniposide, 587·2
Tenipósido, 587·2
Tenitramina, 1010·3
Tenitramine, 1010·3
Tenitran, 2323·4
Teniverme, 2323·4
Ten-K, 2323·4
Tenkafruse, 2323·4
Tenkdol, 2323·4
Tenliv, 2324·1
Tenlol, 2324·1
Tennis Elbow— *see* Soft-tissue Rheumatism, 11·1
Teno, 2324·1
Tenoblock, 2324·1
Tenocam, 2324·1
Tenocard, 2324·1
Tenoclor, 2324·1
Tenocor, 2324·1
Tenofed, 2324·1
Tenofovir, 655·1
Tenofovir Disoproxil Fumarate, 655·1
Tenofovir, Fumarato del Disoproxilo de, 655·1
Tenoic Acid, 269·2
Tenoico, Ácido, 269·2
Tenolin, 2324·1
Tenolol, 2324·1
Tenolone, 2324·1
Tenomax, 2324·1
Tenon, 2324·1
Tenonitrozol, 616·3
Tenonitrozole, 616·3
Tenopres, 2324·1
Tenopres D, 2324·1
Tenoprin, 2324·1
Tenopt, 2324·1
Tenordate, 2324·1
Tenoret, 2324·1
Tenoretic, 2324·1
Tenoric, 2324·1
Tenormin, 2324·1
Tenormine, 2324·1
Ten-O-Six, 2324·2
Tenosynovitis— *see* Soft-tissue Rheumatism, 11·1
Tenotec, 2324·2
Tenovate, 2324·2
Tenovate G, 2324·2
Tenovate M, 2324·2
Tenox, 2324·2
Tenoxen, 2324·2
Tenoxicam, 93·1
Tenoxicamum, 93·1
Tenoxil, 2324·2
Tenoxol, 2324·2
Tenpril, 2324·2
Ten-Quat, 2324·2
Tens, 2324·2
Tensadiur, 2324·2
Tensaldin, 2324·2
Tensaliv, 2324·2
Tensamon, 2324·2
Tensan, 2324·2
Tensanil, 2324·2
Tensazol, 2324·2
Tensiben, 2324·2

Tensidol, 2324·2
Tensig, 2324·2
Tensikey, 2324·2
Tensikey Compl
Tensil, 2324·2
Tensilon, 2324·2
Tensimin, 2324·2
Tensioactivos Pu
Tensiocap, 2324·
Tensiocomplet, 2
Tensiomax, 2324
Tensiomin, 2324·
Tensiomin-Cor, 2
Tension Headac— *see* Boots Tension 51·1
Tensionorme, 232
Tension-type Hea
Tensioval, 2324·3
Tensipine, 2324·3
Tensiplex, 2324·3
Tensispes, 2324·3
Tensitruw, 2324·3
Tensium, 2324·3
Tenso Stop, 2324·
Tenso Stop Plus,
Tensobon, 2324·3
Tensobon Comp, 2
Tensocardil, 2324·
Tensoderm, 2324·3
Tensodin, 2324·3
Tensodox, 2324·3
Tensofar, 2324·3
Tensoflux, 2324·3
Tensogard, 2324·3
Tensogradal, 2324·
Tensoliv, 2324·3
Tensolve, 2324·3
Tensoprel, 2324·3
Tensopril, 2324·3
Tensopril D, 2324·3
Tensopyn, 2324·4
Tensostad, 2324·4
Tensotin, 2324·4
Tensozide, 2324·4
Tenstaten, 2324·4
Tenston, 2324·4
Tensulan, 2324·4
Tensuril, 2324·4
Tentrini, 2324·4
Tenualax, 2324·4
Tenuate, 2324·4
Tenuate Dospan, 232
Tenuate Retard, 2324
Tenuatina, 2324·4
Tenutex, 2324·4
Tenvatil, 2324·4
Tenzone, 2324·4
Teobid, 2324·4
Teobroma, 1754·3
Teobromina, 798·2
Teoclato de Prometaz
Teoden, 2324·4
Teodosis, 2324·4
Teodrenalina, Hidrocl
Teodrin, 2324·4
Teofilina, 798·3
Teofilina Hidrato, 798
Teofilinato de Colina,
Teofillina, 798·3
Teofylamin, 2324·4
Teogrand, 2324·4
Teolixir, 2324·4
Teolixir Compositum,
Teolong, 2324·4
Teonanácatl, 1736·1
Teonibsa, 2324·4
Teonim, 2324·4
Teonova, 2325·1
Teophyl, 2325·1
Teoptic, 2325·1
Teoremac, 2325·1
Teoremin, 2325·1
Teosona, 2325·1
Teosona Sol, 2325·1
Teoston, 2325·1
Teovent, 2325·1

Teovit, 2325·1
TEPA, 588·1
Tepam, 2325·1
Tepanil, 2325·1
Tepavil, 2325·1
Tepazepan, 2325·1
Tepilta, 2325·1
Tepirubicin, 580·1
Tepox Cal, 2325·1
Teprenona, 1293·3
Teprenone, 1293·3
Teprotide, 1010·3
Teprótido, 1010·3
Tequin, 2325·1
Teraciton, 2325·1
Teraclox, 2325·1
Teradyl, 2325·1
Terafluss, 2325·1
Teragran, 2325·1
Teragran Junior, 2325·1
Teragran M, 2325·1
Terak, 2325·1
Teralithe, 2325·1
Teramic, 2325·2
Teranic, 2325·2
Terapéutica Génica, 1691·3
Terapova, 2325·2
Teraprost, 2325·2
Terasep, 2325·2
Teraumon, 2325·2
Terazol, 2325·2
Terazosin Hydrochloride, 1010·3
Terazosina, Hidrocloruro de, 1010·3
Terbac, 2325·2
Terbasmin, 2325·2
Terbasmin Expectorante, 2325·2
Terbinafina, Hidrocloruro de, 408·2
Terbinafine, 408·2
Terbinafine Hydrochloride, 408·2
Terbolan, 2325·2
Terbosil, 2325·2
Terbron, 2325·2
Terbron Expectorant, 2325·2
Terbuken, 2325·2
Terbul, 2325·2
Terbulin, 2325·2
Terbulin Expectorant, 2325·2
Terbuno, 2325·2
Terbutalina, Sulfato de, 797·2
Terbutaline Sulfate, 797·2
Terbutaline Sulphate, 797·2
Terbutalini Sulfas, 797·2
Terbutastad, 2325·2
Terbuturmant, 2325·2
Tercian, 2325·2
Terco-C, 2325·2
Terco-D, 2325·2
Terconazol, 409·3
Terconazole, 409·3
Terconazolum, 409·3
Terden, 2325·2
Terdine, 2325·2
Térébenthine, Essence de, 1760·1
Terebinthinae, Aetheroleum, 1760·1
Terebinthinae Depuratum, Oleum, 1760·1
Terebinthinae, Oleum, 1760·1
Terebinthinae, Resina, 1675·1
Terebinthini Aetheroleum ab Pinum Pinastrum, 1760·1
Terekol, 2325·2
Terelit, 2325·2
Terephthalylidene-3,3′-dicamphor-10,10′-disulfonic Acid, 1146·3
Terfadine, 2325·2
Terfedura, 2325·3
Terfegen, 2325·3
Terfemax, 2325·3
Terfemundin, 2325·3
Terfen, 2325·3
Terfenadina, 441·1
Terfenadina DG, 2325·3
Terfenadine, 441·1
Terfenadine Carboxylate Hydrochloride, 433·3
Terfenadinum, 441·1
Terfenor, 2325·3

Terfenor Antihistamine, 2325·3
Terfex, 2325·3
Terfin, 2325·3
Terfium, 2325·3
Terfluzine, 2325·3
Tergil, 2325·3
Tergil-T, 2325·3
Tergurida, 1216·1
Terguride, 1216·1
Tergynan, 2325·3
Teriaki, 1666·1
Tericin AT, 2325·3
Teriflunomide, 53·3
Teril, 2325·3
Teriparatida, 775·2
Teriparatida, Acetato de, 775·2
Teriparatide, 775·2
Teriparatide Acetate, 775·2
Teriparatidum, 775·2
Terivalidin, 2325·3
Terizidona, 266·2
Terizidone, 266·2
Terlane, 2325·3
Terlipresina, 1340·1
Terlipressin, 1340·1
Terlipressin Acetate, 1340·1
Terlipressin Diacetate, 1340·1
Terloc, 2325·3
Terloc Duo, 2325·3
Terlomexin, 2325·3
Termalgin, 2325·3
Termalgin Codeina, 2325·3
Termination of Pregnancy, 1512·2
Termizol, 2325·3
Termofren, 2325·3
Termogripe C, 2325·3
Termol, 2325·4
Termonal, 2325·4
Termonil, 2325·4
Termo-Ped, 2325·4
Termoprin, 2325·4
Termopriona, 2325·4
Termosan, 2325·4
Termotrin, 2325·4
Ternadin, 2325·4
Ternalin, 2325·4
Ternalin-D, 2325·4
Ternel, 2325·4
Terneurine, 2325·4
Ternidazol, 616·3
Ternidazole, 616·3
Ternolol, 2325·4
Terocaps, 2325·4
Terodul, 2325·4
Terol, 2325·4
Terolut, 2325·4
Teromol, 2325·4
Teronac, 2325·4
Terost, 2325·4
Terostrant, 2325·4
Terpalate, 2325·4
Terpect, 2325·4
Terpene Hydrate, 1131·1
Terpeneless Lemon Oil, 1706·3
Terpeneless Orange Oil, 1724·2
Terpestrol H, 2325·4
Terphylin, 2325·4
Terpin Hydrate, 1131·1
Terpin Hydrochloride, 1131·1
Terpina, Hidrato de, 1131·1
Terpine des Monts-Dore, 2325·4
Terpine Gonnon, 2325·4
α-Terpinene, 1710·2
γ-Terpinene, 1706·2, 1710·2
Terpinen-4-ol, 1710·2
Terpineol, 1752·2
α-Terpineol, 1655·2, 1706·2, 1710·2, 1740·2, 1752·2
(+)-Terpineol, 1724·2
Terpinol, 1131·1
Terpinolene, 1710·2
Terpoin, 2326·1
Terpone, 2326·1
Terponil, 2326·1
Terposen, 2326·1
Terra Fullonica, 1039·3

Terra Silicea Purificada, 1581·3
Terra-Cortil, 2326·1
Terra-Cortril Preparations, 2326·1
Terradermina, 2326·1
Terrados, 2326·1
Terrafor, 2326·1
Terrafungine, 241·1
Terrakal, 2326·1
Terralin, 2326·1
Terramicina Preparations, 2326·2
Terramycin Preparations, 2326·2
Terramycine, 2326·2
Terramycine Solu-Retard, 2326·2
Terranilo, 2326·2
Terranumonyl, 2326·2
Terrasil, 2326·2
Terricil, 2326·2
Tersac, 2326·2
Tersaseptic, 2326·2
Tersatar, 2326·2
Tersa-Tar, 2326·2
Tersif, 2326·3
Tersigat, 2326·3
Tersoderm Anticaspa, 2326·3
Tersoderm Cabellos Grasos, 2326·3
Tersoderm Plus, 2326·3
Tertatolol, Hidrocloruro de, 1011·1
Tertatolol Hydrochloride, 1011·1
Tertensif, 2326·3
Tertiary Amyl Alcohol, 1471·2
Tertiary Butylhydroquinone, 1193·3
Tertroxin, 2326·3
Tervalon, 2326·3
Terveson, 2326·3
Terzine, 2326·3
Terzolin, 2326·3
Tesacof, 2326·3
Tesalon, 2326·3
Tesamone, 2326·3
Tesical, 2326·3
Teslac, 2326·3
Teslascan, 2326·3
Tesmilifene Hydrochloride, 587·3
Tesopalmed Forte cum Yohimbine, 2326·3
Tesopen, 2326·3
Tesoprel, 2326·3
Tesor-C, 2326·3
Tesos, 2326·3
TESPA, 588·1
Tess, 2326·3
Tessalon, 2326·3
Tessifol, 2326·3
Tessofort, 2326·3
Test Pack Plus, 2326·3
Testac, 2326·3
Testanon 25, 2326·3
Testanon 50, 2326·3
Tes-Tape, 2326·4
Testasa E, 2326·4
Testerell, 2326·4
Test-Estro, 2326·4
Testex, 2326·4
Testicular Cancer— *see* Malignant Neoplasms of the Testis, 523·1
Testicular Extracts, 1569·3
Testicular Maldescent— *see* Cryptorchidism, 1313·1
Testiculi, 2326·4
Testim, 2326·4
Testinfex, 2326·4
Testiormina, 2326·4
Testis Extracts, 1569·3
Testisan, 2326·4
Testo, 2326·4
Testoderm, 2326·4
Testo-Enant, 2326·4
Testofran, 2326·4
Testogel, 2326·4
Testolactona, 587·3
Testolactone, 587·3
Testonus, 2326·4
Testopel, 2326·4
Testosterona, 1569·3
Testosterona, Cipionato de, 1569·3
Testosterona, Decanoato de, 1570·1
Testosterona, Enantato de, 1570·1

Testosterona, Fenilpropionato de, 1570·1
Testosterona, Isocaproato de, 1570·1
Testosterona, Propionato de, 1570·1
Testosterona, Undecilato de, 1570·1
Testosterone, 1569·3
Testosterone Cipionate, 1569·3
Testosterone Cyclopentylpropionate, 1569·3
Testosterone Cypionate, 1569·3
Testosterone Decanoate, 1570·1
Testosterone Enantate, 1570·1
Testosterone Enanthate, 1570·1
Testosterone Hemisuccinate, 1571·3
Testosterone Heptanoate, 1570·1
Testosterone Hexahydrobenzoate, 1571·3
Testosterone Hexahydrobenzylcarbonate, 1571·3
Testosterone Implants, 2326·4
Testosterone Isocaproate, 1570·1
Testosterone Isohexanoate, 1570·1
Testosterone Phenylpropionate, 1570·1
Testosterone Propionate, 1570·1
Testosterone Undecanoate, 1570·1
Testosterone Undecylate, 1570·1
Testosteroni Enantas, 1570·1
Testosteroni Propionas, 1570·1
Testosteronum, 1569·3
Testotard, 2326·4
Testotonic B, 2326·4
Testotoxicosis, Familial— *see* Precocious Puberty, 1318·2
Testoviron Preparations, 2326·4
Testovis, 2327·1
Testozzard, 2327·1
Testpack HCG-Urine, 2327·1
TestPack Plus HCG-Urine, 2327·1
Testred, 2327·1
Tesurene, 2327·1
TET, 1385·1
Teta Extra, 2327·1
Tetabulin, 2327·1
Tetabuline, 2327·1
Tetacid, 2327·1
Tetagam, 2327·1
Tetagam N, 2327·1
Tetagamma, 2327·1
Tetagamma P, 2327·1
Tetagam-P, 2327·1
Tetaglobulina, 2327·1
Tetaglobuline, 2327·1
Tetagrip, 2327·1
Tetamer, 2327·1
Tetamun SSW, 2327·1
Tetamyn, 2327·1
Tetanobulin, 2327·1
Tetanogamma, 2327·1
Tetanol, 2327·1
Tetanosimultan, 2327·1
Tetanospasmin, 1398·2
Tetanus, 149·2, 1398·2
Tetanus Antitoxin for Human Use, 1640·2
Tetanus Antitoxins, 1640·2
Tetanus and Diphtheria Toxoids Adsorbed for Adult Use, 1613·1
Tetanus and Diphtheria Vaccines, 1613·1
Tetanus Formol Toxoid, 1641·1
Tetanus, Haemophilus Influenzae, and Diphtheria Vaccines, 1613·3
Tetanus, and Hepatitis B (rDNA) Vaccine (Adsorbed), Diphtheria, 1613·3
Tetanus Immune Globulin, 1640·3
Tetanus Immunoglobulin, Human, 1640·3
Tetanus Immunoglobulins, 1640·3
Tetanus and Influenza Vaccines, 1641·3
Tetanus, Pertussis (Acellular, Component) and Haemophilus Type B Conjugate Vaccine (Adsorbed), Diphtheria, 1614·2
Tetanus, Pertussis (Acellular, Component), Hepatitis B (rDNA), Poliomyelitis (Inactivated) and Haemophilus Type B Conjugate Vaccine (Adsorbed), Diphtheria, 1614·3
Tetanus, Pertussis (Acellular Component) and Hepatitis B (rDNA) Vaccine (Adsorbed), Diphtheria, 1614·3
Tetanus, Pertussis (Acellular, Component), Poliomyelitis (Inactivated) and Haemophilus Type B Conjugate Vaccine (Adsorbed), Diphtheria, 1615·1
Tetanus, Pertussis (Acellular, Component) and Poliomyelitis (Inactivated) Vaccine (Adsorbed), Diphtheria, 1615·1
Tetanus and Pertussis (Acellular, Component) Vaccine (Adsorbed), Diphtheria, 1613·3
Tetanus, Pertussis, and Diphtheria Vaccines, 1613·3
Tetanus, Pertussis, Haemophilus Influenzae, and Diphtheria Vaccines, 1614·2
Tetanus, Pertussis, Poliomyelitis, and Diphtheria Vaccines, 1615·1
Tetanus, Pertussis, Poliomyelitis, Haemophilus Influenzae, and Diphtheria Vaccines, 1615·1
Tetanus, Pertussis, Poliomyelitis (Inactivated) and Haemophilus Type B Conjugate Vaccine (Adsorbed), Diphtheria, 1615·1
Tetanus, Pertussis and Poliomyelitis (Inactivated) Vaccine (Adsorbed), Diphtheria, 1615·1
Tetanus and Pertussis Vaccine (Adsorbed), Diphtheria, 1613·3
Tetanus, Poliomyelitis, and Diphtheria Vaccines, 1615·2
Tetanus and Poliomyelitis Vaccines, 1641·3
Tetanus, Rubella, and Diphtheria Vaccines, 1615·2
Tetanus Toxoid, 1641·1
Tetanus Toxoid Adsorbed, 1641·1
Tetanus and Typhoid Vaccines, 1643·1
Tetanus Vaccine, 1641·1
Tetanus Vaccine (Adsorbed), 1640·3
Tetanus Vaccine (Adsorbed) for Adults and Adolescents, Diphtheria and, 1613·1
Tetanus Vaccine (Adsorbed), Diphtheria and, 1613·1
Tetanus Vaccines, 1640·3
Tetanus-Gamma, 2327·1
Teta-S, 2327·2
Tetasorbat SSW, 2327·2
Tetatox, 2327·2
Tetavax, 2327·2
Tetaven, 2327·2
Tetavenin, 2327·2
Tetefit Vitamin E, 2327·2
Tetesept, 2327·2
Tetesept Calcium, 2327·2
Tetesept Magnesium, 2327·2
Tetesept Vitamin C, 2327·2
Tethexal, 2327·2
Tetinox, 2327·2
Tetmosol, 2327·2
Tetra, 2327·2
Tetra Caplets, 2327·2
Tetra Central, 2327·2
Tetra Hubber, 2327·2
Tetra Tripsin, 2327·2
1,3,5,7-Tetraazatricyclo[3.3.1.1$^{3,7}$]decane, 230·1
Tetrabamate, 698·2
Tetrabenazina, 1752·2
Tetrabenazine, 1752·2
Tetrabioptal, 2327·2
3,3′,5,5′-Tetrabromo-2,2′-biphenyldiolmono(dihydrogen Phosphate), 103·3
Tetrabromocresol, 1193·3
3,4,5,6-Tetrabromo-*o*-cresol, 1193·3
Tetrabromofluorescein, Disodium Salt, 1057·2
4,5,6,7-Tetrabromo-2-hydroxy-1,3,2-benzodioxabismole, 1660·2
Tetrabromopyrocatechol Bismuth, 1660·2
Tetrabronco, 2327·2
Tetrac, 1601·3
Tetracaína, 1385·1
Tetracaína, Hidrocloruro de, 1385·1
Tetracaine, 1385·1
Tetracaine Hydrochloride, 1385·1
Tetracaini Hydrochloridum, 1385·1
Tetracainii Chloridum, 1385·1
Tetracap, 2327·2
Tetracem, 2327·2
Tetracemate, Disodium, 1037·3
Tetracemic Acid, 1038·2
Tetrachlormethiazide Potassium, 1010·1
Tetrachlorodecaoxide, 1752·3
Tetrachlorodecaoxygen Anion Complex, 1752·3
2,3,7,8-Tetrachlorodibenzo-*p*-dioxin, 1681·1
Tetrachloroethane, 1477·1
1,1,2,2-Tetrachloroethane, 1477·1
Tetrachloroethene, 1477·1
Tetrachloroethylene, 1477·1
Tetrachloroethylenum, 1477·1
Tetrachloromethane, 1472·2
Tetrachlorotetraiodofluorescein, Disodium Salt, 1740·1
Tetrachlorvinphos, 1510·2
Tetraciclina, 266·2
Tetraciclina, Complejo con Fosfato, 266·2
Tetraciclina, Hidrocloruro de, 266·2
Tetracina, 2327·2
Tetraclin, 2327·2
Tetraclorodecaóxido, 1752·3
Tetracloroetano, 1477·1
Tetracloroetileno, 1477·1
Tetracloruro de Carbono, 1472·2
Tetraclorvinfós, 1510·2
Tetracoq, 2327·2
Tetracoq— *see* Pentacoq, 2211·1
Tetracosactida, 1340·2
Tetracosactide, 1340·2
Tetracosactide Acetate, 1340·3
Tetracosactido, 1340·2
Tetracosactidum, 1340·2
Tetracosactrin, 1340·2
Tetract-HIB, 2327·3
Tetracycline, 266·2
Tetracycline Hydrochloride, 266·2
Tetracycline Phosphate Complex, 266·2
Tetracyclinemethylene Lysine, 228·2
Tetracyclines, 119·3
Tetracyclini Hydrochloridum, 266·2
Tetracyclinum, 266·2
Tetracyn, 2327·3
Tetradecafluorohexane, 1067·2
Tetradecanoic Acid 1-Methylethyl Ester, 1481·2
1-Tetradecanol, 1718·3
Tetradecilsulfato de Sodio, 1575·1
Tetraderm, 2327·3
Tetradin, 2327·3
Tetradox, 2327·3
*O,O,O′,O′*-Tetraethyl *S,S′*-Methylenediphosphorodithioate, 1505·1
Tetraethylthiuram Disulphide, 1681·3
Tetraethylthiuram Monosulphide, 1510·1
Tetrafluor, 2327·3
Tetrafluorodichloroethane, 1235·3
1,1,1,2-Tetrafluoroethane, 1236·2
Tetrafosammina, 2327·3
Tetra-Gelomyrtol, 2327·3
Tetraglycine Hydroperiodide, 1194·1
Tetragynon, 2327·3
Tetrahelmin, 2327·3
1,2,3,4-Tetrahydroacridin-9-ylamine Hydrochloride, 1497·2
Tetrahydroaminoacridine Hydrochloride, 1497·2
Tetrahydrobiopterin, 1742·1
(6*R*)-5,6,7,8-Tetrahydrobiopterin Hydrochloride, 1742·1
Tetrahydrocannabinol, 1666·1
$\Delta^9$-Tetrahydrocannabinol, 1264·2
Tetrahydrocannabinolic Acid, 1666·1
Tetrahydrocortisol, 1104·2
Tetrahydrocortisone, 1104·2
(2*R*,3*S*,4*S*,5*R*,6*S*)-Tetrahydro-2,4-dihydroxy-6-{(*R*)-1-[(2*S*,5*R*,7*S*,8*R*,9*S*)-9-hydroxy-2,8-dimethyl-2-{(2*S*,2′*R*,3′*S*,5′*R*)-octahydro-2-methyl-5′-[(2*S*,3*S*,5*R*,6*S*)-tetrahydro-6-hydroxy-3,5,6-trimethyl-2*H*-pyran-2-yl]-3′-[(2*S*,5*S*,6*R*)-tetrahydro-5-methoxy-6-methyl-2*H*-pyran-2-yloxy]-2,2′-bifuran-5-yl}-1,6-dioxaspiro[4.5]dec-7-yl]ethyl}-5-methoxy-3-methyl-2*H*-pyran-2-ylacetic Acid, 615·3
1,1′,4,4′-Tetrahydro-*N,N′*-dioctyl-1,1′-decamethylenedi-(4-pyridylideneamine) Dihydrochloride, 1187·2
1,2,3,6-Tetrahydcine-4-carboxylic Ac
Tetrahydrofolate
α-(Tetrahydrofuly(oxyethylene), 14
Tetrahydrofurfuhylene Glycol Ether,
Tetrahydrofurfui
(3*S*)-Tetrahydro)-1-hydroxy-2-(*N*ilamido)ethyl]phen3·2
(3*S*)-Tetrahydro)-1-hydroxy-2-(*N*ilamido)ethyl]pheralcium Phosphate (1:
(5*S*,5a*R*,8a*S*,9*R*ro-5-(4-hydroxy-3,5-c(4,6-*O*-thenylidene-pxy)isobenzofuro[5,e6(5a*H*)-one, 587·2
(+)-2,3α,3aα,7ydroxy-8(*R**)-(4-hydenyl)-4-(3α,5,7-trihyomanyl)-3,6-methan*H*)-one, 1043·3
(α*S*)-Tetrahydr*S*)-2-hydroxy-4-pherxy)acetamido]butyl]ropyl-2-oxo-1(2*H*)-py649·3
(±)-*p*-(5,6,7,8-1,5-*a*]pyridin-5-yl)beydrochloride, 553·1
1,2,3,4-Tetrahminomethyl-7-nitro-( 110·3
1,2,3,4-Tetrah-carboxamidine Sulp
Tetrahydrolips
7,8,9,10-Tetranoazepino[4,5-*g*]qui
*O*-(1,2,3,4-Teno-6-naphthyl) *m,N*-Date, 410·1
(6*R*)-5,6,7,8-Taminocarbazole-3-car
(6a*R*)-5,6,6aethyl-4*H*-dibenzo[*de*,liol Hydrochloride He
(−)-(*R*)-5,6,9,[(2-methylimidazol-1-rido[3,2,1-*jk*]carbazol-3
4,5,6,7-Tetramethylamino)-2*H*-inda
(±)-1,2,3,9-T-3-(2-methylimidazolazol-4(9*H*)-one, 1281·1
2,3,4,5-Tetra[(5-methylimidazol-4pyrido[4,3-*b*]indol-1-o 1248·3
(*E*)-1,4,5,6-hyl-2-[2-(3-methyl-2-tmidine Citrate Monol
Tetrahydro-ofurfurylideneamino)-ioxide, 611·2
1,2,3,4-Tetr-9-phenyl-2-azafluorenete, 438·2
3,4,5,6-Tetr-1-phenyl-1*H*-2,5-benzoxloride, 66·2
2,3,4,9-Tetr9-phenyl-1*H*-indeno[2,ydrogen Tartrate, 438·
1,4,5,6-Tetryrimidin-2-yl-methyl αelate Hydrochloride,
(*E*)-3-[2-(1,-1-methylpyrimidin-2-y4′-Methylenebis(3-hydro 111·1
1,4,5,6-Tetl-2-[(*E*)-2-(2-thienyl)v 4,4′-Methylenebis(3-hoate), 113·2
2-(5,6,7,8-Thylamino)-2-imidazoli Monohydrate, 1131·3
2-(1,2,3,4-hthyl)-2-imidazoline Hy1·2
1-(1,2,3,4-o-6-quinolyl)-4-veratroyl1
(±)-({[(Te-3-thienyl)carbamoyl]m Acid, 1121·1
L-Tetrahydr3·1
*p*-[1-(5,6,75,5,8,8-pentamethyl-2-nbenzoic Acid, 529·3
(*S*)-2,3,5,6-phenylimidazo[2,1-*b*]07·1

(±)-2,3,5,6-Tetrahydro-6-phenylimidazo[2,1-*b*]thiazole Hydrochloride, 114·1
Tetrahydro-1*H*-pyrrolizine-7a(5*H*)-aceto-2′,6′-xylidide Hydrochloride, 983·1
(*S*)-*N*-(5,6,7,9-Tetrahydro-1,2,3,10-tetramethoxy-9-oxobenzo[α]heptalen-7-yl)acetamide, 415·1
6,7,8,9-Tetrahydro-5*H*-tetrazoloazepine, 1592·1
4-(Tetrahydro-2*H*-1,2-thiazin-2-yl)benzenesulphonamide *S,S*-Dioxide, 377·3
5,6,7,8-Tetrahydro-3-[2-(4-*o*-tolyl-1-piperazinyl)ethyl]-*s*-triazolo[4,3-*a*]pyridine Monohydrochloride, 1679·1
(−)-1,2,3,4-Tetrahydro-1-(3,4,5-trimethoxybenzyl)isoquinoline-6,7-diol Hydrochloride Monohydrate, 806·3
(3*S*,3a*S*,5a*S*,9b*S*)-3a,5,5a,9b-Tetrahydro-3,5a,9-trimethylnaphtho[1,2-*b*]furan-2,8(3*H*,4*H*)-dione, 114·1
(6a*R*,10a*R*)-6a,7,8,10a-Tetrahydro-6,6,9-trimethyl-3-pentyl-6*H*-dibenzo[*b,d*]pyran-1-ol, 1264·2
Tetrahydroxyethylrutoside, 1688·2
(9*S*,12*E*,14*S*,15*R*,16*S*,17*R*,18*R*,19*R*,20*S*,21*S*,22*E*,24*Z*)-6,16,18,20-Tetrahydroxy-1′-isobutyl-14-methoxy-7,9,15,17,19,21,25-heptamethylspiro[9,4-(epoxypentadeca[1,11,13]trienimino)-2*H*-furo-[2′,3′:7,8]naphth[1,2-*d*]imidazole-2,4′-piperidine]-5,10,26-(3*H*,9*H*)-trione-16-acetate, 249·1
*meso*-Tetrahydroxyphenylchlorin, 586·3
*meta*-Tetrahydroxyphenylchlorin, 586·3
(*R*)-11β,16α,17,21-Tetrahydroxypregna-1,4-diene-3,20-dione Cyclic 16,17-Acetal, 1095·2
Tetrahydrozoline Hydrochloride, 1131·2
Tetraiodofluorescein, Disodium Salt, Monohydrate, 1057·2
3,5,3′,5′-Tetraiodo-D-thyronine Sodium, 893·2
3,5,3′,5′-Tetra-iodo-L-thyronine Sodium, 1600·1
*N,N′,N″,N‴*-Tetrakis(2,3-dihydroxy-1-hydroxymethylpropyl)-2,2′,4,4′,6,6′-hexaiodo-5,5′-(*N,N′*-dimethylmalonyldiimino)di-isophthalamide, 1066·1
*NNN′N′*-Tetrakis(2-hydroxyethyl)ethylenediamine Tetranitrate, 1010·3
Tetralgin, 2327·3
Tetralgin Novo, 2327·3
Tetralim, 2327·3
Tetralisal, 2327·3
Tetrallobarbital, 673·3
Tetralution, 2327·3
Tetralysal, 2327·3
Tetram, 2327·3
Tetra-Mag, 2327·3
Tetramax, 2327·3
Tetramdura, 2327·3
Tetramel, 2327·3
DL-1,2,9,10-Tetramethoxyaporphine, 1121·3
6′,7′,10,11-Tetramethoxyemetan Dihydrochloride Heptahydrate, 604·3
(+)-6,6′,7′,12′-Tetramethoxy-2,2,2′,2′-tetramethyltubocuraranium Di-iodide, 1403·3
Tetramethrin, 1510·2
Tetramethylammonium Iodide, 1752·3
4-(1,1,3,3-Tetramethylbutyl)phenol, 1416·3
α-[4-(1,1,3,3-Tetramethylbutyl)phenyl]-ω-hydroxypoly(oxyethylene), 1414·1
1,1,1′,1′-Tetramethyl-4,4′-(3α,17β-diacetoxy-5α-androstan-2β,16β-diyl)dipiperazinium Dibromide, 1405·2
Tetramethylene Di(methanesulphonate), 532·2
(*all-E*)-3,7,11,15-Tetramethyl-2,4,6,10,14-hexadecapentaenoic Acid, 1156·1
Tetramethylmelamine, 526·3
6,10,14,18-Tetramethyl-5,9,13,17-nonadecatetraen-2-one, 1293·3
(*all-E*)-1,1′-(3,7,12,16-Tetramethyl-1,3,5,7,9,11,13,15,17-octadecanonaene-1,18-diyl)bis[2,6,6-trimethylcyclohexene], 1422·3
Tetramethylolmethane, 1283·2
Tetramethylpararosaniline Hydrochloride, 1186·2
1,2,2,6-Tetramethyl-4-piperidyl Mandelate Hydrochloride, 482·1
Tetramethylthionine Chloride Trihydrate, 1042·2
Tetramethylthiuram Disulphide, 1755·1
α,α,α′,α′-Tetramethyl-5-(1*H*-1,2,4-triazol-1-ylmethyl)-*m*-benzenediacetonitrile, 528·1
(±)-2,5,7,8-Tetramethyl-2-(4,8,12-trimethyltridecyl)chroman-6-ol, 1464·3
(+)-2,5,7,8-Tetramethyl-2-(4,8,12-trimethyltridecyl)chroman-6-ol, 1464·3
2,5,7,8-Tetramethyl-2-(4,8,12-trimethyltridecyl)-6-chromanyl 2-(4-Chlorophenoxy)-2-methylpropionate, 1015·1
Tetrametilamonio, Ioduro de, 1752·3
Tetrametrina, 1510·2
Tetramicin, 2327·3
Tetramil, 2327·3
Tetramisol, Hidrocloruro de, 114·1
Tetramisole Hydrochloride, 114·1
*l*-Tetramisole Hydrochloride, 107·2
Tetramizol Composto, 2327·3
Tetramizotil, 2327·3
Tetramune, 2327·3
Tetrana, 2327·4
Tetranase, 2327·4
Tetranitrato de Eritritilo, 913·1
Tetranitrato de Pentaeritritilo, 979·1
Tetranitrol, 913·1
Tetrano, 2327·4
Tetranovax, 2327·4
3,3′-(4,7,10,13-Tetraoxahexadecanedioyldiamino)bis(2,4,6-tri-iodobenzoic Acid), 1064·1
Tetrapres, 2327·4
Tetraprocyn, 2327·4
Tetrapulmo, 2327·4
Tetra-saar, 2327·4
Tetrasan, 2327·4
Tetrasine, 2327·4
Tetrasine Extra, 2327·4
Tetrasodium 4-Acetamido-5-hydroxy-6-[7-sulphonato-4-(4-sulphonatophenylazo)-1-naphthylazo]naphthalene-1,7-disulphonate, 1056·2
Tetrasodium 1,1′-Diamino-8,8′-dihydroxy-7,7′-(2,2′-dimethylbiphenyl-4,4′-diylbisdiazo)di-(naphthalene-2,4-disulphonate), 1658·3
Tetrasodium 3,3′-[(3,3′-Dimethylbiphenyl-4,4′-diyl)bisazo]bis[5-amino-4-hydroxynaphthalene-2,7-disulphonate], 1758·3
Tetrasodium 6,6′-[3,3′-Dimethylbiphenyl-4,4′-diylbis(azo)]bis[4-amino-5-hydroxynaphthalene-1,3-disulphonate], 1658·3
Tetra-Tablinen, 2327·4
Tetratiomolibdato de Amonio, 1032·1
TetraTITER, 2327·4
Tetratoss, 2327·4
Tetravac, 2327·4
Tetraxil, 2327·4
Tetrazep, 2327·4
Tetrazepam, 724·1
Tetrazepamum, 724·1
Tetrazil, 2327·4
*N*-[*p*-(*o*-1*H*-Tetrazol-5-ylphenyl)benzyl]-*N*-valeryl-L-valine, 1018·3
Tetrerba, 2327·4
Tetrex, 2327·4
Tetrex-F, 2327·4
Tetrib, 2327·4
Tetridamina, 93·2
Tetridamine, 93·2
Tetridamine Maleate, 93·2
Tetrilin, 2327·4
Tetrim, 2327·4
Tetrisal, 2327·4
Tetrizolina, Hidrocloruro de, 1131·2
Tetrodotoxin Poisoning, 1491·1
Tetrofosmin, Technetium ($^{99m}$Tc), 1526·1
Tetroid, 2327·4
Tetroxoprim, 269·2
Tetroxoprim Embonate, 269·2
Tetroxoprima, 269·2
Tetroxoprima y Sulfadiazina, 199·3
Tetrydamine, 93·2
Tetryzoline Hydrochloride, 1131·2
Tetryzoline Nitrate, 1131·2
Tetryzoline Phosphate, 1131·2
Tetryzoline Sulfate, 1131·2
Tet/Ser, 1640·2
Tetterwort, 1695·3
Tet-Tox, 2327·4
Tetuman, 2328·1
Tet/Vac/Ads, 1641·1
Tet/Vac/FT, 1641·1
Teufelskralle, 2328·1
Teufelskrallenwurzel, 28·2
Teutocilin, 2328·1
Teutoformin, 2328·1
Teutolax, 2328·1
Teutomicina, 2328·1
Teutonico, 2328·1
Teutoss, 2328·1
Teutrin, 2328·1
Teutrin Balsamico, 2328·1
Tevacaine, 2328·1
Tevacor, 2328·1
Tevacutan, 2328·1
Tevacycline, 2328·1
Tevapirin, 2328·1
Tevax, 2328·1
Teveten, 2328·1
Teveten HCT, 2328·1
Teveten Plus, 2328·1
Tevetens, 2328·1
Tevetenz, 2328·1
Tevoril, 2328·1
Tev-Tropin, 2328·1
Texacort, 2328·1
Texan Snakeroot, 1656·3
Texate, 2328·1
Texicam, 2328·1
Texodil, 2328·1
Texot, 2328·1
Texoven, 2328·1
Texx, 2328·1
Teylor, 2328·2
Tezosentan, 1011·1
TFE, 2328·2
TFT, 2328·2
TFT Ophtiole, 2328·2
6-TG, 588·2
T/Gel, 2328·2
T/Gel, Neutrogena— *see* Neutrogena T/Gel, 2165·2
T-Gen, 2328·2
T-Gesic, 2328·2
TGF-β2 Antisense Oligonucleotide, 528·2
TGS, 1450·1
Th-152, 790·2
TH-1165a, 785·2
1314-TH, 212·3
TH-1321, 246·3
TH-2180, 1305·3
THA, 1497·2, 2328·2
Thacapzol, 2328·2
Thaden, 2328·2
Thais, 2328·2
Thalamic Syndrome— *see* Central Post-stroke Pain, 5·3
Thalamonal, 2328·2
Thalaris, 2328·2
β-Thalassaemia, 735·2
Thalidomide, 1752·3
Thalitone, 2328·2
Thallium-201, 1526·2
Thallium Acetate, 1754·2
Thallous Acetate, 1754·2
Thallous Chloride ($^{201}$Tl), 1526·2
Thallus Eckloniae, 1704·3
Thallus Laminariae, 1704·3
Thalomid, 2328·2
THAM, 1758·2
Tham, 2328·2
Thamacetat, 2328·2
Thamesol, 2328·2
Thaumatin, 1451·1
Thaumatin I, 1451·1
Thaumatin II, 1451·1
*Thaumatococcus daniellii*, 1451·1
T/h-basan, 2328·2
$\Delta^9$-THC, 1264·2
Thé, 1765·3
The Blue One, Bioglan— *see* Bioglan The Blue One, 1843·4
The Brioni, 2328·2
The Chambard-Tee, 2328·2
The Franklin, 2328·2
The Ginseng King, 2328·2
The Laxatif Solubilax, 2328·2
Thea, 1765·3
Thebacon Hydrochloride, 1131·2
Thecodine, 75·2
Thedox, 2328·2
Theelol, 1552·3
Théine, 782·1
Theinol, 2328·2
Thelban, 2328·3
Thelmox, 2328·3
Themibutol, 2328·3
Themisalum, 798·2
Thenitrazole, 616·3
Thenoate Lithium, 269·2
Thenoate Monoethanolamine, 269·2
Thenoate Sodium, 269·2
Thenoic Acid, 269·2
2-[4-(2-Thenoyl)phenyl]propionic Acid, 93·1
2-(α-Thenoylthio)-propionylglycine, 1130·3
Thenyldiamine Hydrochloride, 442·1
Thenyldiaminium Chloride, 442·1
Theo, 2328·3
Theo-24, 2328·3
Theo Max, 2328·3
Theo PA, 2328·3
Theo-Asthalin, 2328·3
Theobid Duracaps, 2328·3
Theobric, 2328·3
Theobrom., 1754·3
Theobroma, 1754·3
*Theobroma cacao*, 1482·3, 1754·3
Theobroma Oil, 1482·3
Theobromatis, Oleum, 1482·3
Theobromine, 798·2
Theobromine and Calcium Salicylate, 798·2
Theobromine and Sodium Acetate, 798·2
Theobromine and Sodium Salicylate, 798·2
Theobrominum, 798·2
Theobromsal, 798·2
Theo-Bronc, 2328·3
Theo-Bros, 2328·3
Theochron, 2328·3
Theocol, 2328·3
Theodrenaline Hydrochloride, 1754·3
Theodrine, 2328·3
Theo-Dur, 2328·3
Theofibrate, 914·2
Theofol, 2328·3
Theofol Comp, 2328·3
Theogel, 2328·3
Theohexal, 2328·3
Theolair, 2328·3
Theolan, 2328·3
Theolin, 2328·3
Theolong, 2328·3
Theomax DF, 2328·3
Theophar, 2328·3
Theophen, 2328·3
Theophen Comp, 2328·3
Theophyllaminum, 780·2, 2328·4
Theophyllard, 2328·4
Theophylline, 798·3
Theophylline, Anhydrous, 798·3
Theophylline Calcium Glycinate, 805·2
Theophylline Calcium Salicylate, 805·2
Theophylline Cholinate, 784·2
Theophylline Ethanoate, Heptaminol, 786·3
Theophylline and Ethylenediamine, 780·2
Theophylline Ethylenediamine Compound, 780·2
Theophylline Glycinate, 805·2
Theophylline Hydrate, 798·3
Theophylline Monoethanolamine, 805·2
Theophylline Monohydrate, 798·3
Theophylline Olamine, 805·2
Theophylline Sodium Acetate, 805·2
Theophylline and Sodium Acetate, 805·2
Theophylline Sodium Aminoacetate, 805·2
Theophylline Sodium Glycinate, 805·2
Theophylline-aminoisobutanol, 781·3
Theophylline-ethylenediamine, 780·2
Theophylline-ethylenediamine Hydrate, 780·2
Theophyllinum, 798·3
Theophyllinum et Ethylenediaminum, 780·2
Theophyllinum Monohydricum, 798·3
Theophyllinylacetic Acid, Aminomethylheptanol, 786·3

2-(Theophyllin-7-yl)ethyl 2-(4-Chlorophenoxy)-2-methylpropionate, 914·2
Theopirina, 2328·4
Theoplus, 2328·4
Theosal, 2328·4
Theosalicin, 798·2
Theospan-SR, 2328·4
Theospirex, 2328·4
Theo-SR, 2328·4
Theostat, 2328·4
Theo-Talusin, 2328·4
Theotard, 2328·4
Theotex, 2328·4
Theotrim, 2328·4
Theovent, 2328·4
Theo-X, 2328·4
Thephorin, 2328·4
Theprubicine, 2328·4
Thera Hematinic, 2328·4
Thera Tears, 2328·4
Therabid, 2328·4
Therac, 2328·4
Theracap, 2328·4
Theracaps, 2328·4
Theraclox, 2328·4
Theracne, 2328·4
Theracof Plus, 2328·4
Theracort, 2328·4
TheraCys, 2328·4
Theradol, 2328·4
TheraFlu, 2328·4
TheraFlu Flu and Cold, 2329·1
TheraFlu Flu, Cold & Cough, 2329·1
Theraflu, NightTime— *see* NightTime Theraflu, 2168·1
TheraFlu Non-Drowsy, Maximum Strength— *see* Maximum Strength TheraFlu Non-Drowsy, 2116·4
TheraFlu Vapor Stick, 2329·1
Thera-Flur, 2329·1
Theragen, 2329·1
Theragenerix, 2329·1
Theragenerix-H, 2329·1
Thera-gesic, 2329·1
Theragran, 2329·1
Theragran AntiOxidant, 2329·1
Theragran Hematinic, 2329·1
Theragran-M, 2329·1
Thera-Hist, 2329·1
Theralen, 2329·1
Theralene, 2329·1
Theralene Pectoral, 2329·1
Theralene Pectoral Nourrisson, 2329·1
Thera-M, 2329·1
Theramycin Z, 2329·1
Theranal, 2329·1
Theranyl, 2329·1
TheraPatch Cold Sore, 2329·1
Therapeutic Bath, 2329·1
Therapeutic Bath Oil, 2329·1
Therapeutic Mineral Ice, 2329·1
Therapeutic Skin Lotion, 2329·1
Therapeutic Skin Lotion— *see* Therapeutic Bath Oil, 2329·1
Therapeutic Soothing Ice, 2329·1
Theraplex T, 2329·1
Theraplex Z, 2329·1
Therapsor, 2329·2
Therapy Bayer— *see* Regular Strength Bayer, 2255·3
Therasa, 2329·2
Therasona, 2329·2
Theratar, 2329·2
Theravee, 2329·2
Theravee Hematinic, 2329·2
Theravim, 2329·2
Theravite, 2329·2
Therems, 2329·2
Therevac Plus, 2329·2
Therevac SB, 2329·2
Therma Ayoral, 2329·2
Thermal, 2329·2
Thermalife, 2329·2
Thermalife C, 2329·2
Thermazene, 2329·2
Thermo Burger, 2329·2
Thermo Mobilisin, 2329·2
Thermo Rub, 2329·2
Thermocream, 2329·2
Thermocutan, 2329·2
Thermodent, 2329·2
Thermo-Gel, 2329·2
Thermogene, 2329·2
Thermo-loges, 2329·2
Thermo-Menthoneurin, 2329·2
Thermo-Menthoneurin Bad, 2329·2
Thermo-Rheumon, 2329·2
Thermo-Rub, 2329·3
Thermorub, 2329·3
Thermosenex, 2329·3
Thesit, 2329·3
Thesit P, 2329·3
*Thevetia peruviana*, 1723·1
Thevier, 2329·3
Thex Forte, 2329·3
THF, 1756·1
THFES (HM), 1573·3
Thiaben, 2329·3
Thiabena, 2329·3
Thiabendazole, 114·2
Thiabet, 2329·3
Thiabutazide, 878·2
Thiacetarsamide, 114·1
Thiacetazone, 269·3
Thiacomin, 2329·3
Thiamazole, 1603·3
Thiamazolum, 1603·3
Thiamcin, 2329·3
Thiamfenicol, 269·2
Thiamin Hydrochloride, 1455·1
Thiamine Chloride, 1455·1
Thiamine Dicamsylate, 1455·3
Thiamine Disulfide, 1455·3
Thiamine Hydrobromide, 1455·1
Thiamine Hydrochloride, 1455·1
Thiamine Mononitrate, 1455·1
Thiamine Monophosphate, 1455·3
Thiamine Nitrate, 1455·1
Thiamine Propyl Disulphide, 1455·1
Thiamine Pyrophosphate, 1455·2
Thiamine Tetrahydrofurfuryl Disulphide, 1454·3
Thiamini Hydrochloridum, 1455·1
Thiamini Nitras, 1455·1
Thiaminii Chloridum, 1455·1
Thiaminose, 2329·3
Thiamphenicol, 269·2
Thiamphenicol Aminoacetate Hydrochloride, 269·2
Thiamphenicol Glycinate Hydrochloride, 269·2
Thiamphenicol Glycine Acetylcysteinate, 269·3
Thiamphenicol Palmitate, 269·3
Thiamphenicol Sodium Glycinate Isophthalolate, 269·3
Thiamphenicolum, 269·2
Thiamylal Sodium, 1309·1
Thianax, 2329·3
Thianthol, 1152·1
Thiavit, 2329·3
Thiazid-comp, 2329·3
Thiazide Diuretics, 811·2
Thiazolidine-4-carboxylic Acid, 1756·2
Thiazolidinedione Antidiabetics, 345·3
2-(Thiazol-4-yl)-1*H*-benzimidazole, 114·2
5-Thiazolylmethyl {(α*S*)-α-[(1*S*,3*S*)-1-Hydroxy-3-((2*S*)-2-{3-[(2-isopropyl-4-thiazolyl)methyl]-3-methylureido}-3-methylbutyramido)-4-phenylbutyl]phenethyl}carbamate, 653·2
4′-(1,3-Thiazol-2-ylsulphamoyl)phthalanilic Acid, 242·3
4′-(1,3-Thiazol-2-ylsulphamoyl)succinanilic Acid Monohydrate, 257·1
$N^1$-(1,3-Thiazol-2-yl)sulphanilamide, 264·1
Thick & Easy, 2329·3
Thickened Juice, 2329·3
Thienamycin, 221·1
Thienopyridines, 810·3
1-[1-(2-Thienyl)cyclohexyl]piperidine, 1730·3
Thierry, 2329·3
Thiethylperazine, 442·1
Thiethylperazine Dimaleate, 442·1
Thiethylperazine Malate, 442·1
Thiethylperazine Maleate, 442·1
Thilo Tears, 2329·3
Thilo Wet, 2329·3
Thiloadren, 2329·3
Thiloadren N, 2329·3
Thilocanfol, 2329·3
Thilocanfol C, 2329·3
Thilocof, 2329·3
Thilocombin, 2329·3
Thilodexine, 2329·4
Thilodigon, 2329·4
Thilodrin, 2329·4
Thilogel, 2329·4
Thilol, 2329·4
Thilo-micine, 2329·4
Thilomide, 2329·4
Thilorbin, 2329·4
Thilo-Tears, 2329·4
Thilotim, 2329·4
Thiloxedine, 2329·4
Thimerosal, 1194·1
Thinz, 2329·4
Thioacetazone, 269·3
Thiobarbital, 1309·1
2,2′-Thiobis(4-chlorophenol), 397·3
2,2′-Thiobis(4,6-dichlorophenol), 103·3
Thiobitum, 2329·4
Thiocarbamazine, 102·3
Thiocolchicoside, 1395·2
Thioctacid, 2329·4
Thioctamide, 1754·3
Thioctic Acid, 1754·3
Thioctic Acid Amide, 1754·3
Thioctothiamine, 1455·1
Thiodantol, 2329·4
Thiodeol, 2329·4
Thioderon, 2329·4
*O,O*′-(Thiodi-*p*-phenylene) *O,O,O*′,*O*′-Tetramethyl Bis(phosphorothioate), 1510·2
Thiofentanyl, 40·3
Thiogamma, 2329·4
(1-Thio-D-glucopyranosato)gold, 19·3
(1-Thio-β-D-glucopyranosato)(triethylphosphine)gold 2,3,4,6-Tetra-acetate, 19·1
Thioglycerol, 1186·3
Thioglycollic Acid, 1160·3
Thioguanine, 588·2
6-Thioguanine, 588·2
Thioguanylic Acid, 588·3
Thioinosine, 568·1
Thiola, 2329·4
Thiomebumalnatrium cum Natrii Carbonate, 1309·1
Thiomed, 2329·4
Thiomersal, 1194·1
Thiomersalate, 1194·1
Thiomersalum, 1194·1
7α-Thiomethylspirolactone, 1004·1
Thiomucase, 1755·1, 2329·4
Thionembutal, 2329·4
Thiopental Sodium, 1309·1
Thiopental Sodium and Sodium Carbonate, 1309·1
Thiopentalum Natricum, 1309·1
Thiopentalum Natricum et Natrii Carbonas, 1309·1
Thiopentax, 2329·4
Thiopentobarbitalum Solubile, 1309·1
Thiopentone Sodium, 1309·1
Thiophanate, 114·2
Thiophene-2-carboxylic Acid, 269·2
2-Thiophenic Acid, 269·2
Thiophenicol, 269·2, 2329·4
Thiophosphamide, 588·1
Thioplex, 2329·4
Thiopon, 2329·4
Thiopon Balsamique, 2329·4
Thiopon Pantothenique, 2329·4
Thioprine, 2329·4
Thioproline, 1756·2
Thiopronine, 1054·3
Thioproperazine Dimethanesulphonate, 724·1
Thioproperazine Mesilate, 724·1
Thioproperazine Mesylate, 724·1
Thioproperazine Methanesulphonate, 724·1
Thiopurine Methyltransferase, 1350·1
Thioridazine, 724·2
Thioridazine Hydrochloride, 724·2
Thioridazini Hydrochloridum, 724·2
Thioridazinum, 724·2
Thioril, 2330·1
Thiorubrol, 2330·1
Thiosan, 2330·1
Thiosedal, 2330·1
Thiosept, 2330·1
Thiosia, 2330·1
Thiosol, 2330·1
Thiospot, 2330·1
Thiostrepton, 270·2
Thiosulfil Forte, 2330·1
Thiotepa, 588·1
Thiothixene, 725·2
Thiothixene Hydrochloride, 725·2
Thiouric Acid, 568·1, 588·3
6-Thiouric Acid, 1349·3
Thiovalone, 2330·1
Thioxanthine, 588·3
Thioxene, 2330·1
Thioxolone, 1160·3
Thiozine, 2330·1
Thiprasolan, 2330·1
Thiram, 1755·1
Thirial, 2330·1
Thixit, 2330·1
*Thlaspi bursa-pastoris*, 1744·1
Thohelur I, 2330·1
Thohelur II, 2330·1
Thomaeamin Hepar, 2330·1
Thomaeamin N, 2330·1
Thomaeamin X E, 2330·1
Thomaedex 40, 2330·1
Thomaedex 60, 2330·1
Thomaegelin, 2330·1
Thomaejonin, 2330·1
Thomaemannit, 2330·1
Thomapyrin, 2330·1
Thomapyrin Akut, 2330·1
Thomapyrin C, 2330·1
Thomapyrin mit Vitamin C, 2330·1
Thomapyrine, 2330·2
Thomasin, 2330·2
Thombran, 2330·2
Thonzonium Bromide, 1757·2
Thonzylamine Hydrochloride, 442·2
Thorazine, 2330·2
Thorium Dioxide, 1059·1, 1755·1
Thorium Oxide, 1755·1
Thornapple, 489·2
Thoroughwort, 1661·3
THP-ADM, 580·1
THP-doxorubicin, 580·1
THR, 1688·3, 2330·2
Thr, 1451·1
THR-221, 174·1
Threadworm Infections— *see* Enterobiasis, 99·1
Threadworm Infections— *see* Strongyloidiasis, 100·3
Threamine DM, 2330·2
Threchop, 2330·2
L-Threitol 1,4-Dimethanesulphonate, 590·2
Threohydrobupropion, 288·2
Threolone, 2330·2
Threonine, 1451·1
L-Threonine, 1451·1
Threoninum, 1451·1
$N^2$-[1-($N^2$-L-Threonyl-L-lysyl)-L-prolyl]-L-arginine, 1759·3
Threptin Micromix, 2330·2
Thriazol, 2330·2
Thrioniren, 2330·2
Thriostaxil, 2330·2
Thriusedon, 2330·2
Throat, 2330·2
Throat Discs, 2330·2
Throat Lozenges, 2330·2
Throaties Anti-Bacterial Pastilles, 2330·2
Throaties Pastilles, 2330·2
Thrombace, 2330·2
Thrombace Neo, 2330·2
Thrombareduct, 2330·2
Thrombate, 2330·2
Thrombate III, 2330·2
Thrombhibin, 2330·2
Thrombin, 760·1
Thrombin Clotting Time, 735·3
Thrombinar, 2330·2
Thrombo AS, 2330·2
Thrombo ASS, 2330·2

Thromboangiitis Obliterans— *see* Peripheral Vascular Disease, 831·2
Thrombocid, 2330·2
Thrombocoll, 2330·3
Thrombocythaemia— *see* Primary Thrombocythaemia, 509·1
Thrombocytopenia— *see* Haemorrhagic Disorders, 737·3
Thrombocytopenic Purpura, Autoimmune— *see* Idiopathic Thrombocytopenic Purpura, 1082·1
Thrombocytopenic Purpura, Idiopathic— *see* Idiopathic Thrombocytopenic Purpura, 1082·1
Thrombocytopenic Purpura, Thrombotic— *see* Thrombotic Microangiopathies, 758·1
Thrombocytosis— *see* Primary Thrombocythaemia, 509·1
Thrombodine, 2330·3
Thromboembolic Disorders, 837·3
Thromboembolism, Peripheral Arterial— *see* Peripheral Arterial Thromboembolism, 830·3
Thromboembolism— *see* Thromboembolic Disorders, 837·3
Thromboembolism, Venous— *see* Venous Thromboembolism, 839·1
Thrombogen, 2330·3
Thrombohexal, 2330·3
Thrombokinase, 760·2
Thrombolytics, 812·1
Thrombophilias— *see* Thromboembolic Disorders, 837·3
Thrombophob, 2330·3
Thrombophob-S, 2330·3
Thromboplastin, 760·2
Thromboplastin Antecedent, Plasma, 735·3
Thromboplastin Component, Plasma, 735·3
Thromboplastin, Tissue, 735·3
Thrombopoietin, 760·2
Thrombosantin, 2330·3
Thrombosis, Arterial— *see* Thromboembolic Disorders, 837·3
Thrombosis, Deep-vein— *see* Venous Thromboembolism, 839·1
Thrombosis, Peripheral Arterial— *see* Peripheral Arterial Thromboembolism, 830·3
Thrombosis— *see* Thromboembolic Disorders, 837·3
Thrombosis, Venous— *see* Thromboembolic Disorders, 837·3
Thrombosis, Venous— *see* Venous Thromboembolism, 839·1
Thrombostat, 2330·3
Thrombotic Microangiopathies, 758·1
Thrombotic Thrombocytopenic Purpura— *see* Thrombotic Microangiopathies, 758·1
Thrombotrol, 2330·3
Thrombotrol-VF, 2330·3
Thromboxane $A_2$, 1511·1
Thromboxane $B_2$, 1511·1
Thromboxanes, 1511·1
Thrush— *see* Candidiasis, 386·3
Thuja, 1755·1
Thuja Med Complex, 2330·3
*Thuja occidentalis*, 1755·1
Thuja Oligoplex, 2330·3
Thujaderm, 2330·3
Thujone, 1645·1, 1741·2
Thunas Preparations, 2330·3
Thurfyl Salicylate, 93·3
THY, 962·2
Thybon, 2330·3
Thycapzol, 2330·3
Thymalfasin, 1755·2
Thyme, 1755·2
Thyme, Common, 1755·2
Thyme, French, 1755·2
Thyme, Garden, 1755·2
Thyme Oil, 1755·3
Thyme, Rubbed, 1755·2
Thymi Aetheroleum, 1755·3
Thymi Herba, 1755·2
Thymi, Oleum, 1755·3
Thymi Syrup, 2330·3
Thymian Erkaltungs-Bad, 2330·3
Thymic Humoral Factor, 1756·1
Thymidine, 1755·3
Thymi-Fips, 2330·4
Thymine 2-Desoxyriboside, 1755·3
Thymipin N, 2330·4
Thymitaq, 577·1
Thymitic Antiserum, 1348·3
Thymiverlan, 2330·4
Thymodrosin, 2330·4
Thymodrosin N, 2330·4
Thymogene A, 1756·1
Thymo-Glanduretten, 2330·4
Thymoglobulin, 2330·4
Thymoglobuline, 2330·4
Thymoject, 2330·4
Thymol, 1194·2
Thymol Iodide, 1194·3
Thymol Mouthwash Red, 2330·4
Thymolum, 1194·2
Thymoma— *see* Malignant Neoplasms of the Thymus, 523·3
Thymomodulin, 1756·1
Thymopentin, 1756·1
Thymophysin, 2330·4
Thymopoietin, 1756·1
Thymopoietin Pentapeptide, 1756·1
Thymorell, 2330·4
Thymoseptine, 2330·4
Thymosin α1, 1755·2
Thymosin Fraction 5, 1756·1
Thymostimulin, 1756·1
Thymoval, 2330·4
Thymowied, 2330·4
Thymoxamine Hydrochloride, 962·2
Thymulin, 1756·1
Thymunes, 2330·4
Thymus Cancer— *see* Malignant Neoplasms of the Thymus, 523·3
Thymus Extracts, 1756·1
Thymus Hormones, 1756·1
Thymus Nucleic Acid, 1679·2
*Thymus vulgaris*, 1755·2, 1755·3
*Thymus zygis*, 1755·2, 1755·3
Thym-Uvocal, 2330·4
2-Thymyloxymethyl-2-imidazoline Hydrochloride, 1132·1
Thypinone, 2330·4
Thyradin-S, 2330·4
Thyrar, 2330·4
Thyrax, 2330·4
Thyrefact, 2330·4
Thyrel-TRH, 2330·4
Thyreocomb N, 2330·4
Thyreogutt, 2330·4
Thyreogutt Mono, 2330·4
Thyreoidin, 1604·2
Thyreo-loges Comp, 2330·4
Thyreo-loges N, 2330·4
Thyreo-Pasc N, 2331·1
Thyreostat II, 2331·1
Thyreotom, 2331·1
Thyrex, 2331·1
Thyro-4, 2331·1
Thyro-Block, 2331·1
Thyrocalcitonin, 768·2
Thyrogen, 2331·1
Thyroglobulin, 1604·1
Thyrohormone, 2331·1
Thyroid, 1604·2
Thyroid and Antithyroid Drugs, 1594·1
Thyroid Cancer— *see* Malignant Neoplasms of the Thyroid, 523·3
Thyroid, Dry, 1604·2
Thyroid Extract, 1604·2
Thyroid Gland, 1604·2
Thyroid Nodule, Malignant— *see* Malignant Neoplasms of the Thyroid, 523·3
Thyroid Nodules, Non-malignant— *see* Goitre and Thyroid Nodules, 1594·1
Thyroidea, 1604·2
Thyroideum Siccum, 1604·2
Thyroiditis, Atrophic— *see* Hypothyroidism, 1595·3
Thyroiditis, Hashimoto's— *see* Hypothyroidism, 1595·3
Thyroid-stimulating Hormone, 1341·1
Thyrolar, 2331·1
Thyroliberin, 2331·1
Thyroliberin TRH, 2331·1
Thyronajod, 2331·1
Thyrosit, 2331·1
Thyrostat, 2331·1
Thyrotardin N, 2331·1
Thyrotoxicosis— *see* Hyperthyroidism, 1594·3
Thyrotrophic Hormone, 1341·1
Thyrotrophin, 1341·1
Thyrotrophin-releasing Hormone, 1337·3
Thyrotropin, 1341·1
Thyrotropin Alfa, 1341·1
Thyrotropin-releasing Hormone, 1337·3
Thyroxine Sodium, 1600·1
D-Thyroxine Sodium, 893·2
L-Thyroxine Sodium, 1600·1
Thyroxinum Natricum, 1600·1
Thyrozol, 2331·1
Thytropar, 2331·1
TI-211-950, 1003·1
TI Baby Natural, 2331·1
TI Lite, 2331·1
TI Screen, 2331·1
TI Screen Natural, 2331·1
TI Screen Sunless, 2331·1
Tiabendazol, 114·2
Tiabendazole, 114·2
Tiabendazolum, 114·2
Tiabenzol, 2331·1
Tiabexol, 2331·1
Tiabiose, 2331·1
Tiabrenolo, 2331·1
Tiacetarsamida, 114·1
Tiacid, 2331·1
Tiaden, 2331·1
Tiadenol, 1011·2
Tiadil, 2331·2
Tiadilon, 2331·2
Tiadipona, 2331·2
Tiadyl, 2331·2
Tiadyl Plus, 2331·2
Tiagabina, Hidrocloruro de, 378·1
Tiagabine Hydrochloride, 378·1
Tiakem, 2331·2
Tial, 2331·2
Tiamate, 2331·2
Tiamazol, 1603·3
Tiamfenicolo, 269·2
Tiamfenicolo Glicinato Cloridrato, 269·2
Tiamidexal, 2331·2
Tiamilal Sódico, 1309·1
Tiamin, 2331·2
Tiamina, Hidrocloruro de, 1455·1
Tiamina, Nitrato de, 1455·1
Tiaminal $B_{12}$, 2331·2
Tiaminal $B_{12}$ Trivalente, 2331·2
Tiamol, 2331·2
Tiamon Mono, 2331·2
Tiamulin Fumarate, 270·2
Tiamulin Hydrogen Fumarate for Veterinary Use, 270·2
Tiamulina, Fumarato de, 270·2
Tiamulini Hydrogenofumaras, 270·2
Tianeptina Sódica, 318·2
Tianeptine Sodium, 318·2
Tianeptinum Natricum, 318·2
Tianfenicol, 269·2
Tianfenicol, Hidrocloruro del Glicinato de, 269·2
Tiaperamide Hydrochloride, 94·1
Tiaplex, 2331·2
Tiaprida, Hidrocloruro de, 725·1
Tiapridal, 2331·2
Tiapride Hydrochloride, 725·1
Tiapridex, 2331·2
Tiapridi Hydrochloridum, 725·1
Tiaprizal, 2331·2
Tiaprofen, 2331·2
Tiaprofenic Acid, 93·3
Tiaprofenic Acid, Trometamol Salt, 94·1
Tiaprofénico, Ácido, 93·3
Tiaprofenicum, Acidum, 93·3
Tiaprorex, 2331·2
Tiaprost Trometamol, 1521·1
Tiaramida, Hidrocloruro de, 94·1
Tiaramide Hydrochloride, 94·1
Tiatral 100 SR, 2331·2
Tiaven, 2331·2
Tiazac, 2331·2
Tiazen, 2331·2
Tiazida, Urocaudal— *see* Urocaudal Tiazida, 2361·4
Tiazolidin, 2331·2
Tiba, 2331·2
Tiberal, 2331·2
Tibezonio, Ioduro de, 1756·2
Tibezonium Iodide, 1756·2
Tibifor, 2331·2
Tibinide, 2331·2
Tibirim, 2331·3
Tibirim INH, 2331·3
Tibitol, 2331·3
Tibofem, 2331·3
Tibolona, 1572·3
Tibolone, 1572·3
Tiburon, 2331·3
Tic Douloureux— *see* Trigeminal Neuralgia, 8·2
Ticalma, 2331·3
Ticar, 2331·3
Ticarcilina Sódica, 270·2
Ticarcillin Disodium, 270·2
Ticarcillin Monosodium, 270·2
Ticarcillin Sodium, 270·2
Ticarcillinum Natricum, 270·2
Ticarpen, 2331·3
Ticdine, 2331·3
Tice, 2331·3
Tick Antivenins, 1641·3
Tick Antivenoms, 1641·3
Tick Typhus— *see* Spotted Fevers, 147·1
Tick Venom Antisera, 1641·3
Tick-borne Encephalitis Immunoglobulins, 1642·1
Tick-borne Encephalitis Vaccine (Inactivated), 1642·1
Tick-borne Encephalitis Vaccines, 1642·1
Tickly Cough & Sore Throat Relief, 2331·3
Ticlid, 2331·3
Ticlidil, 2331·3
Ticlobal, 2331·3
Ticlodix, 2331·3
Ticlodone, 2331·3
Ticlogi, 2331·3
Ticlomed, 2331·3
Ticlop, 2331·3
Ticlopat, 2331·3
Ticlopidina, Hidrocloruro de, 1011·2
Ticlopidine Hydrochloride, 1011·2
Ticlopidini Hydrochloridum, 1011·2
Ticloproge, 2331·3
Ticoflex, 2331·3
Ticolcin, 2331·3
Ticon, 2331·3
Ticovac, 2331·3
Ticrynafen, 1012·2
Tics, 664·2
Tidact, 2331·3
Tiddy, 2331·3
Tidigesic, 2331·3
Tielle, 2331·4
Tiemonio, Ioduro de, 489·3
Tiemonio, Metilsulfato de, 489·3
Tiemonium Iodide, 489·3
Tiemonium Methylsulphate, 489·3
Tiemonium Metilsulfate, 489·3
Tiempe, 2331·4
Tienam, 2331·4
Tienilic Acid, 1012·2
Tienílico, Ácido, 1012·2
Tienor, 2331·4
Tierlite, 2331·4
Tierra de Diatomeas, 1581·3
Tierra de Fuller, 1039·3
Tietilperazina, 442·1
Tietilperazina, Malato de, 442·1
Tietilperazina, Maleato de, 442·1
Tietze's Syndrome— *see* Mastalgia, 1546·3
Tietze's Syndrome— *see* Soft-tissue Rheumatism, 11·1
Tifacogin, 145·3
Tifell, 2331·4
Tifen, 2331·4
Tifenso, 2331·4
Tiffy, 2331·4
Tiffy Fu, 2331·4
Tiffyrub, 2331·4
Tifox, 2331·4
Tigan, 2331·4

Tigan— *see* Emergent-Ez, 1967·2
Tigason, 2331·4
Tigel IRM, 2331·4
Tiger Balm Preparations, 2331·4
Tiger Balsam Rot, 2332·1
Tiger Liniment, 2332·1
Tiger Snake, 2332·1
Tiglii, Oleum, 28·2
Tiglio (Specie Composta), 2332·1
Tigridol, 2332·1
Tikacillin, 2332·1
Tikl, 2332·1
Tikleen, 2332·1
Tiklid, 2332·1
Tiklyd, 2332·1
Tikosyn, 2332·1
TIL, 563·3
Tilactasa, 1756·2
Tilactase, 1756·2
Tilad, 2332·1
Tilade, 2332·1
Tilaire, 2332·1
Tilarginine, 1752·1
Tilarin, 2332·1
Tilatil, 2332·1
Tilavist, 2332·1
Tilazem, 2332·1
Tilbroquinol, 617·1
Tilcitin, 2332·1
Tilcotil, 2332·1
Tildiem, 2332·1
Tilekin, 2332·1
Tilene, 2332·1
Tiletamina, Hidrocloruro de, 1310·2
Tiletamine Hydrochloride, 1310·2
Tilexim, 2332·1
Tilfilin, 2332·2
Tili, 2332·2
Tili Comp, 2332·2
Tilia, 1756·2
*Tilia cordata*, 1756·2
*Tilia platyphyllos*, 1756·2
Tiliae Flos, 1756·2
*Tilia × vulgaris*, 1756·2
Tilicomp, 2332·2
Tilidalor, 2332·2
Tilidate Hydrochloride, 94·1
Tilidin Comp, 2332·2
Tilidin N, 2332·2
Tilidin Plus, 2332·2
Tilidina, Hidrocloruro de, 94·1
Tilidine Hydrochloride, 94·1
Tilidine Hydrochloride Hemihydrate, 94·1
Tilidine Phosphate, 94·2
Tilidini Hydrochloridum Hemihydricum, 94·1
Tilidin-saar, 2332·2
Tilidura, 2332·2
Tiligetic, 2332·2
Tilimerck, 2332·2
Tili-Puren, 2332·2
Tiliquinol, 617·1
Tilitrate, 2332·2
Tilker, 2332·2
Till, 2332·2
Tilleul, 1756·2
Tilmicosin, 271·2
Tilmicosin Phosphate, 271·2
Tilmicosina, 271·2
Tilnalox, 2332·2
Tilo, 1756·2
Tilodene, 2332·2
Tiloptic, 2332·2
Tiloryth, 2332·2
Tilosin, 2332·2
Tilosina, 274·3
Tilosina, Tartrato de, 275·1
Tiloxapol, 1416·3
Tiloxican, 2332·2
Tilstigmin, 2332·2
Tiltab, 2332·2
Tiltis, 2332·2
Ti-Lub, 2332·3
Tiludronate Disodium, 776·1
Tiludronate Sodium, 776·1
Tiludronato Sódico, 776·1
Tiludronic Acid, 776·1
Tiludrónico, Ácido, 776·1
Tilur, 2332·3
TIM, 1012·2, 2332·3
Timabak, 2332·3
Timacar, 2332·3
Timacor, 2332·3
Tim-Ak, 2332·3
Timalfasina, 1755·2
Timarol, 2332·3
Timasen, 2332·3
Timax, 2332·3
Timazolina, Hidrocloruro de, 1132·1
Timbo, 1510·1
Time Action B Complex with C, 2332·3
Time Released Balanced B, 2332·3
Timecef, 2332·3
Timed, 2332·3
Timed Action Balanced B, 2332·3
Timed D, 2332·3
Timed Release C, 2332·3
Timed Release Ester C, 2332·3
Timed Release Mega Men, 2332·3
Timed Release Swiss One, 2332·3
Timed Release Ultra Mega, 2332·3
Timed Release Vita-Vim, 2332·3
Timed Release Womens Ultra Mega, 2332·3
Timelit, 2332·3
Timenten, 2332·3
Timentin, 2332·3
Timepidio, Bromuro de, 489·3
Timepidium Bromide, 489·3
Timezol, 2332·3
Timi, 2332·3
Timico, Acido, 1194·2
Timicolid, 2332·3
Timicon, 2332·3
Timidina, 1755·3
Timiperona, 725·2
Timiperone, 725·2
Timisol, 2332·3
T-Immun, 2332·4
Timnodonic Acid, 976·2
Timo, 1755·2
Timo, Hormonas del, 1756·1
Timo (Specie Composta), 2332·4
Timo-COMOD, 2332·4
Timocomod, 2332·4
Timodine, 2332·4
Timodrop, 2332·4
TimoEDO, 2332·4
Timoferol, 2332·4
Timoftal, 2332·4
Timoftol, 2332·4
Timogel, 2332·4
Timoglau, 2332·4
Timoglau Plus, 2332·4
Timoglobulina, 2332·4
Timohexal, 2332·4
Timol, 1194·2
Timolabak, 2332·4
Timolen, 2332·4
Timoler, 2332·4
Timolide, 2332·4
Timolo, 2332·4
Timolol Hemihydrate, 1012·3
Timolol Maleate, 1012·2
Timolol, Maleato de, 1012·2
Timololi Maleas, 1012·2
Timolux, 2332·4
Timomann, 2332·4
Timonacic, 1756·2
Timonacic Methyl Hydrochloride, 1756·3
Timonácico, 1756·2
Timonil, 2332·4
Timo-Optal, 2332·4
Timop, 2332·4
Tim-Ophtal, 2332·4
Timoptic, 2332·4
Timoptol, 2332·4
Timoptol-XE, 2333·1
Timosan, 2333·1
Timosil, 2333·1
Timosin, 2333·1
Timosine, 2333·1
Timosoft, 2333·1
Timo-Stulln, 2333·1
Timox, 2333·1
Timozzard, 2333·1
Timpanol, 2333·1
Timpilo, 2333·1
Timpron, 2333·1
Timsopt, 2333·1
Timunox, 2333·1
Tin, 1756·3
Tin-113, 1524·1
Tin Fluoride, 1448·3
Tin Oxide, 1756·3
Tina, 2333·1
Tinacef, 2333·1
Tinactin, 2333·1
Tinaderm, 2333·1
Tinaderm Extra, 2333·1
Tinaderme, 2333·1
Tinaderm-M, 2333·1
Tinagel, 2333·1
Tinaroc Preparations, 2333·1
Tinasol, 2333·1
Tinasolve, 2333·2
Tinatox, 2333·2
Tinax, 2333·2
Tinazol, 2333·2
Tinazole, 2333·2
TinBen, 2333·2
TinCoBen, 2333·2
Tinctura Justi, 2333·2
Tine Test, 1759·1
Tine Test PPD, 2333·2
Tinea— *see* Skin Infections, 390·1
Tinea Versicolor— *see* Skin Infections, 390·1
Tineafax, 2333·2
Tinerol, 2333·2
Ting, 2333·2
Tingosan, 2333·2
Tini, 2333·2
Tiniazol, 2333·2
Tinidafyl, 2333·2
Tinidafyl Plus, 2333·2
Tinidazol, 617·1
Tinidazole, 617·1
Tinidazolum, 617·1
Tin-mesoporphyrin, 1756·3
Tinnevelly Senna, 1288·2
Tinnevelly Senna Fruit, 1288·2
Tinnitin, 2333·2
Tinnitus, 1381·1
Tinok AF, 2333·2
Tinoral, 2333·2
Tinox, 2333·2
Tin-protoporphyrin, 1756·3
Tinsenol, 2333·2
Tinset, 2333·2
Tintorine, 2333·2
Tintu. Mertiolato Asens, 2333·2
Tintura Benjui, 2333·2
Tintura de Salsa Caroba e Manaca, 2333·2
Tintus, 2333·2
Tinver, 2333·2
Tinzaparin Sodium, 1013·1
Tinzaparina Sódica, 1013·1
Tinzaparinum Natricum, 1013·1
Tioacetazona, 269·3
Tiobarbital, 2333·2
Tiobec, 2333·2
Tiobutarit, 1663·2
Tiocalmina, 2333·2
Tioclomarol, 1013·2
Tiocolchicósido, 1395·2
Tioconax, 2333·3
Tioconazol, 409·3
Tioconazole, 409·3
Tioconazolum, 409·3
Tiocosol, 2333·3
Tioctan, 2333·3
Tioctan-S, 2333·3
Tióctico, Ácido, 1754·3
Tiof, 2333·3
Tiofacic, 1130·3
Tiofanato, 114·2
Tiofeniclin, 2333·3
Tioglicolato Cálcico, 1160·3
Tioglicólico, Ácido, 1160·3
Tioguaialina, 2333·3
Tioguanina, 588·2, 2333·3
Tioguanine, 588·2
Tioguanine Nucleotide, 1349·2
Tioguanine Sodium, 588·3
Tiomersal, 1194·1
Tiomicol, 2333·3
Tiomucasa, 1755·1
Tionamil, 2333·3
Tionazen, 2333·3
Tioner, 2333·3
Tiopental Sódico, 1309·1
Tiopronin, 1054·3
Tiopronin Sodium, 1055·1
Tiopronina, 1054·3
Tioproperazina, Mesilato de, 724·1
Tiorfan, 2333·3
Tioridazina, 724·2
Tioridazina, Hidrocloruro de, 724·2
Tiorilene, 2333·3
Tiosalicilato Sódico, 90·2
Tiosalis, 2333·3
Tiosalprin, 2333·3
Tioscina, 2333·3
Tioside, 2333·3
Tiosol, 2333·3
Tiostreptón, 270·2
Tiosulfato Sódico, 1053·3
Tiotau, 2333·3
Tioten, 2333·3
Tiotepa, 588·1
Tiotil, 2333·3
Tiotixene, 725·2
Tiotixene Hydrochloride, 725·2
Tiotixeno, 725·2
Tiotixeno, Hidrocloruro de, 725·2
Tiotropio, Bromuro de, 806·2
Tiotropium Bromide, 806·2
Tiotropium Bromide Monohydrate, 806·2
Tiovalone, 2333·3
Tioxal, 2333·3
Tioxolona, 1160·3
Tioxolone, 1160·3
TIP, 2333·3
Tipac, 2333·3
Tiparol, 2333·3
Tipepidina, Hibenzato de, 1131·3
Tipepidine Hibenzate, 1131·3
Tipepidine Hybenzate, 1131·3
Tiperal, 2333·3
Tipidin, 2333·3
Tipidine, 2333·3
Tipkin, 2333·3
Tiplac, 2333·4
Tipodex, 2333·4
Tipotaf, 2333·4
Tipranavir, 655·3
Tiprocin, 2333·4
Tiptipot, Afalpi— *see* Afalpi Tiptipot, 1778·4
Tipuric, 2333·4
Tiq'Aouta, 2333·4
Tiquizio, Bromuro de, 1757·1
Tiquizium Bromide, 1757·1
Tirabicin, 2333·4
Tiracaspa, 2333·4
Tiracrin, 2333·4
Tiradine, 2333·4
Tirakallos, 2333·4
Tiralcol, 2333·4
Tiram, 1755·1
Tiramina, Hidrocloruro de, 1760·1
Tirapazamina, 588·3
Tirapazamine, 588·3
Tiratosse, 2333·4
Tiratricol, 1602·2, 1604·3
Tirgon, 2333·4
Tirilazad Mesilate, 1013·2
Tirilazad, Mesilato de, 1013·2
Tirilazad Mesylate, 1013·2
Tirlor, 2333·4
Tirocal, 2333·4
Tirocular, 2333·4
Tirodril, 2333·4
Tirofibán, Hidrocloruro de, 1013·3
Tirofiban Hydrochloride, 1013·3
Tiroglobulina, 1604·1
Tiroide Amsa, 2333·4
Tiroide Secca, 1604·2
Tiroide Vister, 2333·4
Tiroides, 1604·2
Tiroidine, 2333·4

Tirolaxo, 2333·4
Tiroler Adler Leber- und Gallentee, 2333·4
Tiroler Adler Schwedenbitter, 2333·4
Tiroler Steinol, 2333·4
Tiropanoato de Sodio, 1067·3
Tiropramida, Hidrocloruro de, 1757·1
Tiropramide Hydrochloride, 1757·1
Tirosina, 1451·1
Tirosint, 2333·4
Tirossina, 1600·1
Tirotax, 2333·4
Tirotricina, 275·1
Tirotrofina, 1341·1
Tirotropina Alfa, 1341·1
Tirovel, 2333·4
Tiroxina Sodica, 1600·1
Tirozol 5/10, 2333·4
Tirs, 2334·1
Tisamid, 2334·1
Tisana Arnaldi, 2334·1
Tisana Cisbey, 2334·1
Tisana Kelemata, 2334·1
Tisane Antibiliaire et Stomachique, 2334·1
Tisane Antiflatulente pour Nourissons et Enfants, 2334·1
Tisane Antirhumatismale, 2334·1
Tisane Calmante pour les Enfants, 2334·1
Tisane Clairo, 2334·1
Tisane contre la Tension, 2334·1
Tisane contre les Refroidissements, 2334·1
Tisane Depurative "les 12 Plantes", 2334·1
Tisane des Familles, 2334·1
Tisane Digestive Weleda, 2334·1
Tisane Diuretique, 2334·1
Tisane Favorisant l'Allaitement, 2334·1
Tisane Grande Chartreuse, 2334·1
Tisane Hepatique de Hoerdt, 2334·2
Tisane Hepatique et Biliaire, 2334·2
Tisane Laxative, 2334·2
Tisane Laxative H Nouvelle Formulation, 2334·2
Tisane Laxative Natterman No 13, 2334·2
Tisane Laxative Natterman No 13 Instant, 2334·2
Tisane Mexicaine, 2334·2
Tisane Orientale Soker, 2334·2
Tisane Pectorale, 2334·2
Tisane Pectorale et Antitussive, 2334·2
Tisane Pectorale pour les Enfants, 2334·2
Tisane pour Dormir, 2334·2
Tisane pour le Coeur et la Circulation, 2334·2
Tisane pour le Foie, 2334·2
Tisane pour le Sommeil et les Nerfs, 2334·2
Tisane pour les Enfants, 2334·2
Tisane pour les Reins et la Vessie, 2334·2
Tisane pour l'Estomac, 2334·2
Tisane Provencale No1, 2334·2
Tisane Purgative, 2334·2
Tisane Relaxante N, 2334·3
Tisane Sedative Weleda, 2334·3
Tisane Touraine, 2334·3
Tisanes de l'Abbe Hamon Preparations, 2334·3
Tisatin, 2334·3
Tisept, 2334·3
Tisercin, 2334·3
Tisit, 2334·3
Tisobrif, 2334·3
Tisogen, 2334·3
TiSol— *see* Oragesic, 2191·1
Tisopurina, 418·2
Tisopurine, 418·2
Tisorek, 2334·3
Tisplal, 2334·3
Tispol Ibu-DD, 2334·3
Tispol S, 2334·3
Tisseel, 2334·3
Tisseel Duo, 2334·3
Tisseel Duo Quick, 2334·3
Tissucol Preparations, 2334·4
TissuCone, 2334·4
Tissue Factor, 735·3, 760·2
Tissue Factor Pathway Inhibitor, 145·3
Tissue Plasminogen Activator, 735·3, 857·1
Tissue Thromboplastin, 735·3
Tissue-type Plasminogen Activator, Recombinant, 857·1
TissuFleece, 2334·4
TissuFoil, 2334·4
TissuVlies, 2334·4
Tisuderma, 2334·4
Tis-U-Sol, 2334·4
Titan, 2334·4
Titanii Dioxidum, 1160·3
Titanio, 1757·1
Titanium, 1757·1
Titanium Dioxide, 1160·3
Titanium Oxide, 1160·3
Titanium Peroxide, 1160·3
Titanium Salicylate, 1160·3
Titanorein, 2334·4
Titanoreine, 2334·4
Titanoreine Lidocaine, 2334·4
Titanox, 2334·4
Tition, 2334·4
Titmus Losung 1, 2334·4
Titmus Losung 2, 2335·1
Titralac, 2335·1
Titralac Extra Strength, 2335·1
Titralac Plus, 2335·1
Titralac-Sil, 2335·1
Titralgan, 2335·1
Titrane, 2335·1
Ti-Tre, 2335·1
Ti-tree Oil, 1710·2
Titretta, 2335·1
Titus, 2335·1
Ti-U-Lac, 2335·1
Ti-U-Lac HC, 2335·1
Ti-UVA-B, 2335·1
TIVA— *see* Anaesthetic Techniques, 1296·2
Tivision, 2335·1
Tivitis, 2335·1
Tixair, 2335·1
Tixobar, 2335·1
Tixocortol Pivalate, 1110·1
Tixocortol, Pivalato de, 1110·1
Tixycolds Preparations, 2335·1
Tixylix Preparations, 2335·1
Tixylix Inhalant— *see* Tixycolds Cold and Hayfever, 2335·1
Tixymol, 2335·2
Tixyplus, 2335·2
Tizanidina, Hidrocloruro de, 1395·3
Tizanidine Hydrochloride, 1395·3
Tizoxim, 2335·2
TJN-318, 405·2
TKC, 2335·2
T-KI, 2335·2
T-Koff, 2335·2
T-LI, 2335·2
TLM, 2335·2
T-LU, 2335·2
T-MA, 2335·2
TMA, 1593·3
TMA-2, 1593·3
TMB-4, 1050·3
T-Medevax, 2335·2
TMG Folic, 2335·2
TMP, 2335·2
TMS, 2335·2
TMS-19Q, 254·1
TMT, 1755·1
TMTD, 1755·1
TNF, 590·2
TNFα, 590·2
TNFβ, 590·2
TNFα-1a, 590·2
TNKase, 2335·2
TNK-tPA, 1010·2
Toa, 2335·2
Toads, 1663·2
Toadstools, 1717·3
Toallet Benzal, 2335·2
Tobacco Amblyopia, 1459·1
Tobacco, Indian, 1589·1
Tobacin, 2335·2
Tobazon, 2335·2
Tobe, 2335·2
Tobedoce, 2335·2
Tobi, 2335·2
Tobitil, 2335·2
Tobra, 2335·2
Tobra Gobens, 2335·2
Tobrabact, 2335·2
Tobra-cell, 2335·2
Tobracil, 2335·3
Tobracort, 2335·3
Tobradex, 2335·3
Tobradistin, 2335·3
Tobrafen, 2335·3
Tobragan, 2335·3
Tobral, 2335·3
Tobralex, 2335·3
Tobra-M, 2335·3
Tobramaxin, 2335·3
Tobramicina, 271·2
Tobramicina, Sulfato de, 271·3
Tobramina, 2335·3
Tobramycin, 271·2
Tobramycin Sulfate, 271·3
Tobramycin Sulphate, 271·3
Tobramycinum, 271·2
Tobraneg, 2335·3
Tobranom, 2335·3
Tobrasix, 2335·3
Tobrasol, 2335·3
Tobrasone, 2335·3
Tobrex, 2335·3
Tobridavi, 2335·3
Tobrin, 2335·3
Tobrin-D, 2335·3
Tobutol, 2335·3
Tocainida, Hidrocloruro de, 1014·1
Tocainide, 1014·1
Tocainide Hydrochloride, 1014·1
Tocalfa, 2335·3
Tocalm, 2335·3
Tocid, 2335·3
Tocilizumab, 1757·1
Toclapekt, 2335·3
Toclase, 2335·3
Toclase Expectorant, 2335·4
Toclase Toux Seche, 2335·4
Toco, 2335·4
Tocodrine, 2335·4
Tocoferil Nicotinate, 1015·1
Tocoferil Palmitate, *dl*-Alpha, 1465·3
*d*-α-Tocoferilo, Acetato de, 1465·1
*dl*-α-Tocoferilo, Acetato de, 1465·1
Tocoferilo, Nicotinato de, 1015·1
*d*-α-Tocoferilo, Succinato Ácido, 1465·1
*dl*-α-Tocoferilo, Succinato Ácido, 1465·1
*d*-α-Tocoferol, 1464·3
*dl*-α-Tocoferol, 1464·3
Tocofersolan, 1465·3
Tocofibrate, 1015·1
Tocofibrato, 1015·1
Tocogen, 2335·4
Tocogestan, 2335·4
Tocolion, 2335·4
Tocolysis— *see* Premature Labour, 794·1
Tocomine, 2335·4
Tocomizol, 2335·4
Toconal, 2335·4
Tocopa, 2335·4
Tocophan— *see* Tocopa, 2335·4
α-Tocopherol, 1464·3
*d*-α-Tocopherol, 1464·3
*dl*-α-Tocopherol, 1464·3
*RRR*-α-Tocopherol, 1464·3
α-Tocopherol Acetate, 1465·1
(±)-α-Tocopherol Acetate, 1465·1
(+)-α-Tocopherol Acetate, 1465·1
α-Tocopherol Acetate Concentrate (Powder Form), 1465·1
Tocopherol, Alpha, 1464·3
Tocopherol, *d*-Alpha, 1464·3
Tocopherol, *dl*-Alpha, 1464·3
(±)-α-Tocopherol Hydrogen Succinate, 1465·1
(+)-α-Tocopherol Hydrogen Succinate, 1465·1
α-Tocopherol, Natural, 1464·3
(±)-α-Tocopherol Nicotinate, 1015·1
α-Tocopherol, Synthetic, 1464·3
α-Tocopheroli Acetas, 1465·1
*RRR*-α-Tocopheroli Acetas, 1465·1
α-Tocopheroli Acetatis Pulvis, 1465·1
DL-α-Tocopheroli Hydrogenosuccinas, 1465·1
*RRR*-α-Tocopheroli Hydrogenosuccinas, 1465·1
Tocopherols, 1464·3
α-Tocopherolum, 1464·3
*RRR*-α-Tocopherolum, 1464·3
Tocopheronic Acid, 1465·2
Tocophersolan, 1465·3
*RRR*-α-Tocopheryl Acetate, 1465·1
*d*-α-Tocopheryl Acetate, 1465·1
*dl*-α-Tocopheryl Acetate, 1465·1
Tocopheryl Acetate, Alpha, 1465·1
Tocopheryl Acetate, *d*-Alpha, 1465·1
Tocopheryl Acetate, *dl*-Alpha, 1465·1
*d*-α-Tocopheryl Acid Succinate, 1465·1
*dl*-α-Tocopheryl Acid Succinate, 1465·1
Tocopheryl Acid Succinate, *d*-Alpha, 1465·1
Tocopheryl Acid Succinate, *dl*-Alpha, 1465·1
DL-α-Tocopheryl Hydrogen Succinate, 1465·1
*RRR*-α-Tocopheryl Hydrogen Succinate, 1465·1
Tocopheryl Hydrogen Succinate, Alpha, 1465·1
Tocopheryl Nicotinate, 1015·1
Tocorell, 2335·4
Tocotrienols, 1464·3
Tocovenos, 2335·4
Tocovid, 2335·4
Tocovid Suprabio, 2335·4
Tocovital, 2335·4
Tocrat, 2335·4
Todalgil, 2335·4
Today, 2335·4
Today Ovulation Test, 2335·4
Todexona, 2335·4
Todolac, 2335·4
Todralazina, Hidrocloruro de, 1015·1
Todralazine Hydrochloride, 1015·1
Toepedo, 2335·4
Tofen, 2335·4
Tofisopam, 725·3
Tofizopam, 725·3
Toflamixina, 2335·4
Toflamixina Plus, 2335·4
Toflex, 2335·4
Tofranil, 2335·4
Tofranil-PM, 2336·1
Togal Preparations, 2336·1
Togamycin, 2336·1
Togasan, 2336·1
Togine, 2336·1
Togrel, 2336·1
Togrisol, 2336·1
Toilax, 2336·1
Tokelau— *see* Skin Infections, 390·1
Toki-shakuyaku-san, Tsumura— *see* Tsumura Toki-shakuyaku-san, 2351·1
Tokovitan, 2336·1
Tol, 2336·1
Tol 12, 2336·1
Tol Total, 2336·1
Tolan, 2336·1
Tolanase, 2336·1
Tolazamida, 348·1
Tolazamide, 348·1
Tolazol. Hydrochlor., 1015·1
Tolazolina, Hidrocloruro de, 1015·1
Tolazoline Hydrochloride, 1015·1
Tolazolinium Chloratum, 1015·1
Tolbetol, 2336·1
Tolbin, 2336·1
Tolbutamida, 348·1
Tolbutamide, 348·1
Tolbutamide Sodium, 348·1
Tolbutamidum, 348·1
Tolcapona, 1216·1
Tolcapone, 1216·1
Tolchicine, 2336·1
Tolciclate, 410·1
Tolciclato, 410·1
Tolcyclamide, 333·1
Toldex, 2336·1
Toldimfos, 1231·3
Tolecen, 2336·1
Tolectin, 2336·1
Tolep, 2336·2
Tolerance Extreme, 2336·2

Tolerane, 2336·2
Tolerex, 2336·2
Toleriane, 2336·2
Tolestan, 2336·2
Tolexine, 2336·2
Tolfamic, 2336·2
Tolfenamic Acid, 94·2
Tolfenámico, Ácido, 94·2
Tolfenamicum, Acidum, 94·2
Tolfrinic, 2336·2
Tolgin, 2336·2
Tolglybutamide, 348·1
Tolicaína, Hidrocloruro de, 1385·3
Tolid, 2336·2
Toliken, 2336·2
Toliman, 2336·2
Tolimed, 2336·2
Tolinase, 2336·2
Tolindol, 2336·2
Tolinol, 1680·3
Tollkirschen, 479·1
Tollwutglobulin, 2336·2
Tollwut-Impfstoff (HDC), 2336·2
Tolmetin, 94·3
Tolmetin Sodium, 94·2
Tolmetina Sódica, 94·2
Tolmicen, 2336·2
Tolmicil, 2336·2
Tolmicol, 2336·2
Tolmin, 2336·2
Tolnaderm, 2336·2
Tolnaftate, 410·1
Tolnaftato, 410·1
Tolnaftatum, 410·1
Toloconio, Metilsulfato de, 1194·3
Toloconium Methylsulphate, 1194·3
Toloconium Metilsulfate, 1194·3
Tolodina, 2336·2
Tolonio, Cloruro de, 1757·1
Tolonium Chloride, 1757·1
Toloran, 2336·2
Toloxane, 2336·2
Toloxatona, 318·2
Toloxatone, 318·2
Toloxim, 2336·2
Toloxin, 2336·3
Tolperisona, Hidrocloruro de, 1396·3
Tolperisone Hydrochloride, 1396·3
Tolpropamina, Hidrocloruro de, 442·2
Tolpropamine Hydrochloride, 442·2
Tolrest, 2336·3
Tolrestat, 327·1
Toltem, 2336·3
Tolterodina, Tartrato de, 489·3
Tolterodine Tartrate, 489·3
Tolterodine L-Tartrate, 489·3
Toltrazuril, 617·3
Toltrazurilo, 617·3
Tolu Balsam, 1131·3
Tolu, Baume de, 1131·3
Toluene, 1477·1
Tolueno, 1477·1
Toluic Acid, 1478·3
Toluidinblau, 2336·3
*o*-Toluidine, 1383·1
Toluidine Blue O, 1757·1
Toluol, 1477·1
Toluole, 1477·1
Toluric Acid, 1478·3
Tolu-Sed DM, 2336·3
Tolusil, 2336·3
Tolutanum, Balsamum, 1131·3
Toluylene Red, 1719·3
Tolvin, 2336·3
Tolvon, 2336·3
Tolycaine Hydrochloride, 1385·3
1-[4-(*o*-Tolylazo)-*o*-tolylazo]naphth-2-ol, 1191·3
1-(*p*-Tolyl)ethanol, 1680·3
*p*-Tolylmethylcarbinol, 1680·3
3-(*o*-Tolyloxy)propane-1,2-diol, 1394·3
*p*-[5-*p*-Tolyl-3-(trifluoromethyl)pyrazol-1-yl]benzenesulfonamide, 25·2
Tolynol, 1394·3, 1680·3
Tolynolum, 1680·3
*Tolypocladium inflatum*, 1351·2
Tolyprin, 2336·3
Tomabef, 2336·3
Tomag, 2336·3
Tomanil, 2336·3
Tomato, Strawberry, 1731·3
Tomcin, 2336·3
Tomevis, 2336·3
Tomevit, 2336·3
Tomid, 2336·3
Tomilho, Essência de, 1755·3
Tomillo, 1755·2
Tomillo, Aceite Esencial de, 1755·3
Tomillo, Esencia de, 1755·3
Tomiporan, 2336·3
Tomiron, 2336·3
Tomizol, Neo— *see* Neo Tomizol, 2156·4
Tomocat, 2336·3
Tomoray, 2336·3
Tomoxetina, Hidrocloruro de, 1585·1
Tomoxetine Hydrochloride, 1585·1
Tomudex, 2336·3
Tomycin, 2336·3
Tomycine, 2336·3
Ton Was, 2336·3
Tonactil, 2336·3
Tonactiv, 2336·4
Tonalgen, 2336·4
Tonamil, 2336·4
Tonaril, 2336·4
Tonaton, 2336·4
Tonavir, 2336·4
Tonavital, 2336·4
Toncard-Do, 2336·4
Toncils, 2336·4
Tondex, 2336·4
Tondinel H, 2336·4
Tonekin, 2336·4
Tonekin Plus, 2336·4
Toneon, 2336·4
Toness, 2336·4
Tonex, 2336·4
Tonexis, 2336·4
Tonexis HP, 2336·4
Tongill, 2336·4
Tonginal, 2336·4
Toniazol, 2336·4
Tonible, 2336·4
Tonibral, 2336·4
Tonibral Adulte, 2336·4
Tonic Seizures— *see* Epilepsy, 349·1
Tonic Yeast, 2336·4
Tonicalcium, 2336·4
Tonic-clonic Seizures— *see* Epilepsy, 349·1
Tonic-clonic Status Epilepticus— *see* Status Epilepticus, 352·1
Tonice, 2336·4
Tonico Blumen, 2336·4
Tonico Juventus, 2336·4
Tonico No 1, 2336·4
Tonico Pasteur, 2336·4
Tonico Prata, 2337·1
Tonicol & ADC, 2337·1
Tonicum, 2337·1
Tonid, 2337·1
Tonilax, 2337·1
Tonimax, 2337·1
Tonimed, 2337·1
Tonimer, 2337·1
Tonimol, 2337·1
Tonipan, 2337·1
Tonique D Nouvelle Formule, 2337·1
Tonique Vegetal, 2337·1
Tonisan, 2337·1
Tonizin, 2337·1
Tonka Bean, 1676·2
Tonka Bean Camphor, 1676·2
Tonka Seed, 1676·2
Tono, 2337·1
Tonobexol, 2337·1
Tonocalcin, 2337·1
Tonocaltin, 2337·1
Tonocard, 2337·1
Tono-Cis, 2337·1
Tonoferon, 2337·1
Tonofit, 2337·1
Tonoflex, 2337·1
Tonofolin, 2337·1
Tonoftal, 2337·1
Tonogen, 2337·1
Tonogen S, 2337·1
Tonoglutal, 2337·1
Tonoklen, 2337·2
Tonopan, 2337·2
Tonopaque, 2337·2
Tonoplantin Mono, 2337·2
Tonoplus, 2337·2
Tonopres, 2337·2
Tonopron ACD, 2337·2
Tonopron Fuerte con Vit. B12, 2337·2
Tonoprotect, 2337·2
Tonosai, 2337·2
Tonosol, 2337·2
Tonotensil, 2337·2
Tonotensil D, 2337·2
Tonovin, 2337·2
Tonovital Antioxidante, 2337·2
Tonovital E, 2337·2
Tonovital Plus Antioxidante, 2337·2
Tonovix, 2337·2
Tonox, 2337·2
Tonquin Bean, 1676·2
Tonsan Akut, 2337·2
Tonsan Chronisch, 2337·2
Tonsan-K, 2337·2
Tonsicur, 2337·2
Tonsildrops, 2337·2
Tonsilgon, 2337·2
Tonsillitis— *see* Pharyngitis, 140·3
Tonsillitis PMD, 2337·2
Tonsillol, 2337·2
Tonsillopas, 2337·2
Tonsillosyx, 2337·2
Tonsiotren, 2337·2
Tonsiotren H, 2337·2
Tonterin, 2337·2
Tonum, 2337·2
Tonus, 2337·3
Tonus-forte-Tablinen, 2337·3
Tonval, 2337·3
Tonzilamina, Hidrocloruro de, 442·2
Tonzonio, Bromuro de, 1757·2
Tonzonium Bromide, 1757·2
Toose, 2337·3
Toot, 1373·3
Toothache Bark, 1766·3
Toothache Drops, 2337·3
Toothache Drops, Nyal— *see* Nyal Toothache Drops, 2182·2
Toothache Gel, 2337·3
Toothed Wrack, 1742·3
Top C, 2337·3
Top Calcium, 2337·3
Top Dent Fluor, 2337·3
Top Flog, 2337·3
Top Life Preparations, 2337·3
Top Marks, 2337·3
Topaal, 2337·3
Topaben-N, 2337·3
Topace, 2337·3
Topadol, 2337·3
Topal, 2337·3
Topalgic, 2337·3
Topamac, 2337·3
Topamax, 2337·3
Toparal, 2337·3
Topase, 2337·3
Topasel, 2337·3
Topcal D3, 2337·3
Top-Cat, 2337·4
Top-Dal, 2337·4
Toperit, 2337·4
Topestin, 2337·4
Topfans, 2337·4
Topfena, 2337·4
Topher-E, 2337·4
Tophi— *see* Gout and Hyperuricaemia, 412·1
Topialyse, 2337·4
Topic, 2337·4
Topicaina, 2337·4
Topicaine, 2337·4
Topical, 2337·4
Topical Anaesthesia— *see* Surface Anaesthesia, 1370·2
Topical Analgesics, 4·3
Topicasone, 2337·4
Topicasone with Neomycin, 2337·4
Topicil, 2337·4
Topico Denticion Vera, 2337·4
Topicort, 2337·4
Topicorte, 2337·4
Topicorten V, 2337·4
Topicorten-Tar, 2337·4
Topicrem, 2337·4
Topicycline, 2337·4
Topidexa, 2337·4
Topifort, 2337·4
Topifram, 2338·1
Topiglos, 2338·1
Topilact 12, 2338·1
Topilene, 2338·1
Topilone, 2338·1
Topimax, 2338·1
Topionic, 2338·1
Topiramate, 378·3
Topiramato, 378·3
Topisalen, 2338·1
Topisolon, 2338·1
Topisolon mit Salicylsaure, 2338·1
Topisone, 2338·1
Topivate, 2338·1
Toplexil, 2338·1
Top-Mag, 2338·1
Top-Nitro, 2338·1
Topo Worth, 2338·1
Topoderm N, 2338·1
Topoisomerase Inhibitors, 492·1
Topokebir, 2338·1
Toposar, 2338·1
Topotag, 2338·1
Topotecán, Hidrocloruro de, 589·1
Topotecan Hydrochloride, 589·1
Topotel, 2338·1
Toppyc, 2338·1
Topramine, 2338·1
Toprec, 2338·1
Toprek, 2338·1
Toprel, 2338·1
Toprilem, 2338·2
Toprim, 2338·2
Toprol, 2338·2
Toprol XL, 2338·2
Topromel, 2338·2
Topron, 2338·2
Top-Sabona, 2338·2
Topsiton, 2338·2
Topster, 2338·2
Topsym, 2338·2
Topsym Polyvalent, 2338·2
Topsymin, 2338·2
Topsymin F, 2338·2
Topsyn, 2338·2
Topsyne, 2338·2
Topsyne Neomycine, 2338·2
Topsyn-Y, 2338·2
Toptabs, 2338·2
Toquilone Compositum, 2338·2
Toradiur, 2338·2
Toradol, 2338·2
Tora-Dol, 2338·2
Toral, 2338·2
Torasemida, 1015·3
Torasemide, 1015·3
Toraseptol, 2338·2
Torbetol, 2338·2
Torecan, 2338·2
Torem, 2338·3
Toremifene Citrate, 589·2
Torental, 2338·3
Torfan, 2338·3
Torfan H, 2338·3
Torgyn, 2338·3
Toriac, 2338·3
Torio, Dióxido de, 1755·1
Toriol, 2338·3
Torlanbulina Antitenani, 2338·3
Torlasporin, 2338·3
Tormentil, 1757·2
Tormentilla, 1757·2
Tormentillae Rhizoma, 1757·2
Tornalate, 2338·3
Tornix, 2338·3
Torolac, 2338·3
Torrat, 2338·3
Torrem, 2338·3
Torsade de Pointes— *see* Cardiac Arrhythmias, 816·1
Torsemide, 1015·3

Torsilax, 2338·3
Torticollis— *see* Spasmodic Torticollis, 1391·1
Torvast, 2338·3
Torymycin, 2338·3
Toryxil, 2338·3
T-OS, 2338·3
Tos Mai, 2338·3
Tosactide, 1322·2
Toscacalm, 2338·3
Toscal, 2338·3
Toscal Compuesto, 2338·3
Toscalmin, 2338·3
Toscamycin-R, 2338·3
Tosdetan, 2338·3
Tosdiazina, 2338·3
Tosdrope, 2338·4
Toseina NF, 2338·4
Tosfriol, 2338·4
Tosicalcin, 2338·4
Tosidrin, 2338·4
Tosifar, 2338·4
Tosilab, 2338·4
Tosilato de Bretilio, 876·2
Tosilato de Suplatast, 797·2
Tosilato de Tosufloxacino, 272·2
Tosilcloramida Sódica, 1194·3
Tositumomab, 589·3
Tosrhimatiol, 2338·4
Tossamine, 2338·4
Tossamine Plus, 2338·4
Tossanil, 2338·4
Tossarel, 2338·4
Tossbel, 2338·4
Tossec, 2338·4
Tossedrin, 2338·4
Tossefedrin, 2338·4
Tossefin, 2338·4
Tossefluid, 2338·4
Tosseina, 2338·4
Tossemed, 2338·4
Tosseque, 2338·4
Tossestop, 2338·4
Tossex, 2338·4
Tossex-S, 2338·4
Tossilerg, 2338·4
Tossimel, 2338·4
Tossin, 2338·4
Tossivitan, 2338·4
Tossoral, 2339·1
Tosufloxacin, 272·2
Tosufloxacin Toluene-4-sulphonate Monohydrate, 272·2
Tosufloxacin Tosilate, 272·2
Tosufloxacin Tosylate, 272·2
Tosufloxacino, Tosilato de, 272·2
Tosuman, 2339·1
Tosylchloramide Sodium, 1194·3
Tosylchloramide Sodium B, 1195·1
Tosylchloramidum Natricum, 1194·3
Totacef, 2339·1
Totacide, 2339·1
Totacillin, 2339·1
Totaforte, 2339·1
Total, 2339·1
Total Care, 2339·1
Total Cover Sunblock, 2339·1
Total Eclipse, 2339·1
Total Eclipse Moisturizing, 2339·1
Total Formula, 2339·1
Total Magnesiano, 2339·1
Total Magnesiano Antioxidante, 2339·1
Total Magnesiano con Vit C, 2339·1
Total Magnesiano E, 2339·1
Total Magnesiano Energizante, 2339·1
Total Magnesiano Fem, 2339·1
Total Magnesiano Limon, 2339·1
Total Magnesiano Sport, 2339·1
Total Magnesiano Stress, 2339·1
Total Parenteral Nutrition, 1418·2
Total Vitamins, 2339·1
Total Woman, 2339·1
Total Zinc, Natures Way— *see* Natures Way Total Zinc, 2153·3
Totalbloc Maximum Protection, 2339·1
TotalCare, 2339·1
Totalens, 2339·1
Totalflora, 2339·2
Totalip, 2339·2
Totalos Plus, 2339·2
Totam, 2339·2
Totamine, 2339·2
Totapen, 2339·2
Totaquine, 1672·1
Totaretic, 2339·2
Totasedan, 2339·2
Totasex, 2339·2
Totatrom, 2339·2
Totelle, 2339·2
Totelle Cyclo, 2339·2
Totelle Sekvens, 2339·2
Totelmin, 2339·2
Totephan, 2339·2
Tot'Hema, 2339·2
Totipen, 2339·2
Totocortin, 2339·2
Totonik, 2339·2
Toularynx, 2339·2
Toulumad, 2339·2
Tourette's Syndrome— *see* Tics, 664·2
Touristil, 2339·2
Tournesol, Huile de, 1451·1
Touro Preparations, 2339·2
Touxium, 2339·3
Tovene, 2339·3
Toverine, 2339·3
T.O.Vir, 2339·3
Toxal, 2339·3
Toxanal, 2339·3
Toxepasi, 2339·3
Toxex, 2339·3
Toxic Epidermal Necrolysis, 1138·3
Toxic Epidermal Necrolysis— *see* Drug-induced Skin Reactions, 1134·3
Toxic Nodular Goitre— *see* Hyperthyroidism, 1594·3
Toxic Shock Syndrome, 149·2
Toxicarb, 2339·3
Toxicerna, 2339·3
Toxicol, 2339·3
Toxi-L 90 N, 2339·3
Toxilic Acid, 1709·2
Toxi-loges, 2339·3
Toxi-loges N, 2339·3
Toximer, 2339·3
Toximer C, 2339·3
Toxina Botulínica A, 1388·3
Toxina Botulínica B, 1388·3
Toxinas Botulínicas, 1388·3
Toxinas de Fusión de Interleucina 2, 1701·3
Toxinum Botulinicum Typum A ad Iniectabile, 1388·3
Toxiselect, 2339·3
Toxocariasis, 101·1
Toxogonin, 2339·3
Toxogonine, 2339·3
Toxoplasmosis, 598·3
TP-1, 1756·1, 2339·3
TP-5, 1756·1
TP-10, 1675·2
TP-21, 724·2
T-PA, 857·1
TPA, 735·3
T-PA, 2339·3
TPE 1800 GX, 2339·3
TPH, 2339·3
T-Phyl, 2339·3
TPMT, 1350·1
TPN, 1418·2
TPN Additive, 2339·3
TP-Ophtal, 2339·3
TPS-23, 706·3
TPT, 2339·4
TR-495, 707·1
Trabar, 2339·4
Trabectedin, 589·3
Trabilin, 2339·4
Trabit, 2339·4
Trablok, 2339·4
Trabona, 2339·4
Trac Tabs 2X, 2339·4
Tracefusin, 2339·4
Tracel, 2339·4
Tracelyte, 2339·4
Tracer Glucose, 2339·4
Tracheo Fresh, 2339·4
Trachiform, 2339·4
Trachisan, 2339·4
Trachisan N, 2339·4
Trachitol, 2339·4
Trachoma, 149·3
Trachyl, 2339·4
Tracilarin, 2339·4
Tracin, 2339·4
Tracine, 2339·4
Tracitrans Plus, 2340·1
Tracleer, 2340·1
Traconal, 2340·1
Tracozon, 2340·1
Tracrium, 2340·1
Tractocile, 2340·1
Tractoven, 2340·1
Tractur, 2340·1
Tracur, 2340·1
Tracurix, 2340·1
Tracuron, 2340·1
Tracutil, 2340·1
Tracyne, 2340·1
Tradelia, 2340·1
Tradexol, 2340·1
Tradil, 2340·1
Tradol, 2340·1
Tradolan, 2340·1
Tradolgesic, 2340·1
Tradon, 2340·1
Tradonal, 2340·1
Tradox, 2340·1
Trafermin, 1160·3
Trafloxal, 2340·1
Trafuril, 2340·1
Trag., 1582·2
Tragacanth, 1582·2
Tragacanth, Gum, 1582·2
Tragacanth, Indian, 1290·2
Tragacantha, 1582·2
Tragacanto, 1582·2
Tragant, 1582·2
Tralen, 2340·1
Tralgiol, 2340·2
Trali, 2340·2
Tralic, 2340·2
Trama, 2340·2
Tramabene, 2340·2
Tramabeta, 2340·2
Tramacet, 2340·2
Tramadex, 2340·2
Tramadin, 2340·2
Tramadoc, 2340·2
Tramadol, Hidrocloruro de, 94·3
Tramadol Hydrochloride, 94·3
Tramadol-Dolgit, 2340·2
Tramadoli Hydrochloridum, 94·3
Tramadolor, 2340·2
Tramadon, 2340·2
Trama-Dorsch, 2340·2
Tramadura, 2340·2
Tramagetic, 2340·2
Tramagit, 2340·2
Tramahexal, 2340·2
Tramake, 2340·2
Trama-Klosidol, 2340·2
Tramal, 2340·2
Tramalan, 2340·2
Tramamed, 2340·2
Tramamerck, 2340·2
Tramapine, 2340·2
Tramastad, 2340·2
Tramatyrol, 2340·2
Tramax, 2340·2
Tramazac, 2340·2
Tramazolina, Hidrocloruro de, 1131·3
Tramazoline Hydrochloride, 1131·3
Tramazoline Hydrochloride Monohydrate, 1132·1
Tramazolini Hydrochloridum, 1131·3
Trambo, 2340·2
Tramedphano, 2340·3
Tramex, 2340·3
Tramic, 2340·3
Tramil, 2340·3
Tramisal, 2340·3
Tramo, 2340·3
Tramoda, 2340·3
Tramsilione, 2340·3
Tramundal, 2340·3
Tramundin, 2340·3
Tranavan, 2340·3
Tranazol, 2340·3
Trancap, 2340·3
Tranclor, 2340·3
Trancolon, 2340·3
Trancolon P, 2340·3
Trancon, 2340·3
Trancopal Dolo, 2340·3
Trandate, 2340·3
Trandiur, 2340·3
Trandolapril, 1016·1
Trandolaprilat, 1016·1
Trandor, 2340·3
Trandrozine, 2340·3
Trane, 2340·3
Tranex, 2340·3
Tranexamic Acid, 760·3
Tranexámico, Ácido, 760·3
Trangina, 2340·3
Trangorex, 2340·3
Tranilast, 806·3
Tranilcipromina, Sulfato de, 318·3
Tranimet, 2340·3
Trankilium, 2340·3
Trankimazin, 2340·3
Tranqipam, 2340·3
Tranquase, 2340·4
Tranquil, 2340·4
Tranquillisers, 663·1
Tranquilyn, 2340·4
Tranquinal, 2340·4
Tranquinal Soma, 2340·4
Tranquirit, 2340·4
Tranquital, 2340·4
Tranquo, 2340·4
Trans Act$_{LAT}$ — *see* Transact, 2340·4
Transacalm, 2340·4
Transact, 2340·4
Transact Lat, 2340·4
Transamin, 2340·4
Transamine Sulphate, 318·3
Transannon, 2340·4
Transbil, 2340·4
Transbilix, 2340·4
Transbronchin, 2340·4
Transbronquina, 2340·4
Transbronquina Rectal, 2340·4
Transcop, 2340·4
Transcortin, 1073·2
TransCyte, 2340·4
Transderm Scop, 2340·4
Transderma B, 2340·4
Transderma H, 2340·4
Transdermal Contraceptives, 1527·3
Transdermal-NTG, 2340·4
Transderm-Nitro, 2340·4
Transderm-V, 2340·4
Transdiol, 2340·4
Transene, 2340·4
Transfer Factor, 1757·2
Transferal, 2340·4
Transferencia, Factor de, 1757·2
Transfert, 2340·4
Transformal, 2340·4
Transforming Growth Factor, 1679·1
Transforming Growth Factor Antibodies, 1757·2
Transforming Growth Factor-β2-specific Phosphorothioate Antisense Oligodeoxynucleotide, 528·2
Transiderm-Nitro, 2341·1
Transient Ischaemic Attack— *see* Stroke, 836·1
Transilane, 2341·1
Transimune, 2341·1
Transipeg, 2341·1
Transipen, 2341·1
Transitol, 2341·1
Transix, 2341·1
Translet, 2341·1
Translet Plus One, 2341·1
Translet Plus Two, 2341·1
Translight, 2341·1
Transmer, 2341·1
Transmetil, 2341·1
Transoak, 2341·1
Transoddi, 2341·1
Transol, 2341·1

Transoxyl, 2341·1
Trans-Plantar, 2341·1
Trans-Plantar— *see* Trans-Ver-Sal Plantar-Patch, 2341·2
Transplantation, Bone Marrow— *see* Haematopoietic Stem Cell Transplantation, 1344·3
Transplantation, Heart— *see* Heart Transplantation, 1345·2
Transplantation, Intestinal— *see* Intestinal Transplantation, 1346·1
Transplantation, Islet-cell— *see* Pancreatic Transplantation, 1347·3
Transplantation, Kidney— *see* Kidney Transplantation, 1346·2
Transplantation, Liver— *see* Liver Transplantation, 1346·3
Transplantation, Lung— *see* Lung Transplantation, 1347·2
Transplantation, Organ and Tissue— *see* Organ and Tissue Transplantation, 1344·2
Transplantation, Pancreas— *see* Pancreatic Transplantation, 1347·3
Transplantation, Peripheral Blood Stem Cell— *see* Haematopoietic Stem Cell Transplantation, 1344·3
Transpulmin Preparations, 2341·1
Transpulmina, 2341·1
Transpulmina Gola, 2341·1
Transpulmina Tosse, 2341·1
Transtec, 2341·2
Transulose, 2341·2
Transvane, 2341·2
Transvasin Preparations, 2341·2
Transvercid, 2341·2
Trans-Ver-Sal Preparations, 2341·2
Transvital, 2341·2
Transzone, 2341·2
Trantalol, 2341·2
Trantil, 2341·2
Tranvagal, 2341·2
Tranxal, 2341·2
Tranxen, 2341·2
Tranxene, 2341·2
Tranxilene, 2341·2
Tranxilium, 2341·2
Tranxilium N, 2341·2
Tranylcypromine Sulfate, 318·3
Tranylcypromine Sulphate, 318·3
Tranzicalm, 2341·2
Trapanal, 2341·2
Trapax, 2341·2
Trapidil, 1016·2
Trapidilum, 1016·2
Trapped Wind & Indigestion, Modern Herbals— *see* Modern Herbals Trapped Wind & Indigestion, 2138·2
Traqueobron, 2341·2
Traquivan, 2341·3
Trasedal, 2341·3
Trasicor, 2341·3
Trasicor, Slow-— *see* Slow-Trasicor, 2295·2
Trasidrex, 2341·3
Trasitensin, 2341·3
Trasitensine, 2341·3
Trasitensine, Slow-— *see* Slow-Trasitensine, 2295·2
Trastocir, 2341·3
Trastuzumab, 589·3
Trasylol, 2341·3
Tratacne, 2341·3
Tratamiento Hormonal Sustitutivo, 1536·2
Tratenamin, 2341·3
Tratobes, 2341·3
Tratocoli, 2341·3
Tratoderm, 2341·3
Tratul, 2341·3
Trauma Relief, 2341·3
Traumac, 2341·3
TraumaCal, 2341·3
Traumacel P, 2341·3
Trauma-cyl, 2341·3
Trauma-cyl N Complex, 2341·3
Trauma-Dolgit, 2341·3
Traumadyn, 2341·3
Traumafusin, 2341·3
Traumagel, 2341·3
Traumal, 2341·3
Traumalgyl, 2341·4
Traumalitan, 2341·4
Traumalix, 2341·4
Traumanase, 2341·4
Traumaparil, 2341·4
Traumaplant, 2341·4
Trauma-Puren, 2341·4
Traumasalbe, 2341·4
Trauma-Salbe Kuhlend, 2341·4
Trauma-Salbe Rodler 301 N, 2341·4
Trauma-Salbe Rodler 302 N, 2341·4
Trauma-Salbe Warmend, 2341·4
Traumasenex, 2341·4
Traumasept, 2341·4
Traumasive, 2341·4
Traumasport, 2341·4
Traumasteril Kohlenhydratfrei, 2341·4
Traumatociclina, 2341·4
Traumazol, 2341·4
Traumed, 2341·4
Traumeel, 2341·4
Traumeel S, 2341·4
Traumicid, 2341·4
Traumon, 2341·4
Traumox, 2341·4
Trausan, 2341·4
Trautil, 2342·1
Travacalm, 2342·1
Travacalm HO, 2342·1
Travacalm Natural, 2342·1
Travad, 2342·1
Travahex, 2342·1
Travamin, 2342·1
Travamine, 2342·1
Travasept, 2342·1
Travasol, 2342·1
Travasorb, 2342·1
Travatan, 2342·1
Travel Aid, 2342·1
Travel Calm, 2342·1
Travel Sickness, 2342·1
Travel Sickness Cocculus, 2342·1
Travel Sickness— *see* Nausea and Vomiting, 1245·2
Travel Tabs, 2342·1
Travel Well, 2342·1
Travelaide, 2342·1
Travelbac, 2342·1
Travel-Caps, 2342·1
Traveleeze, 2342·1
Travelgum, 2342·1
Travel-Gum, 2342·1
Travella, 2342·1
Travellers, 2342·1
Travellers' Diarrhoea— *see* Gastro-enteritis, 127·3
Travello, 2342·1
Travelmate, 2342·1
Traveltabs, 2342·1
Travert, 2342·2
Travex, 2342·2
Traviata, 2342·2
Travilan, 2342·2
Travisco, 2342·2
Travocort, 2342·2
Travogen, 2342·2
Travogyn, 2342·2
Travoprost, 1521·1
Trawell, 2342·2
Traxam, 2342·2
Traxamic, 2342·2
Traxaton, 2342·2
Tray-Te, 2342·2
Trazidex, 2342·2
Trazil, 2342·2
Trazinac, 2342·2
Trazodil, 2342·2
Trazodona, Hidrocloruro de, 319·1
Trazodone Hydrochloride, 319·1
Trazograf, 2342·2
Trazolan, 2342·2
Trazone, 2342·2
Trazorel, 2342·2
Trazoteva, 2342·2
Trazyl, 2342·2
TRCS-Verorab, 2342·2
TRD-Contin, 2342·2
Trébol de Agua, 1712·1
Trébol Rojo, 1737·3
Trebon, 2342·2
Trebon-N, 2342·2
Trecalmo, 2342·2
Trecator, 2342·3
Trecloran, 2342·3
Treda, 2342·3
Tredalat, 2342·3
Tredemine, 2342·3
Tredol, 2342·3
Trèfle d'Eau, 1712·1
Trefoil, 1737·3
Trefoil, Marsh, 1712·1
Trefovital, 2342·3
Tregor, 2342·3
Trelibec, 2342·3
Treloc, 2342·3
Trelstar, 2342·3
Tremacamra, 655·3
Tremafarm, 2342·3
Tremaril, 2342·3
Tremarit, 2342·3
Trematode Infections, 97·1
Tremblex, 2342·3
Trementina, 1478·1
Trementina, Aceite Esencial de, 1760·1
Trementina, Esencia de, 1760·1
Tremexal, 2342·3
Tremix, 2342·3
Tremoforat, 2342·3
Tremopar, 2342·3
Tremoquil, 2342·3
Tremor, 872·3
Tremor, Postural— *see* Tremor, 872·3
Tremor, Spontaneous Postanaesthetic— *see* Shivering and Its Treatment, 1295·2
Tremorex, 2342·3
Tren, 2342·3
Trenantone, 2342·3
Trenbolona, Acetato de, 1573·2
Trenbolone Acetate, 1573·2
Trenbolone Hexahydrobenzylcarbonate, 1573·2
Trench Fever, 150·1
Trench Mouth— *see* Mouth Infections, 136·1
Trendar PMS, 2342·3
Trendinol, 2342·3
Trenelone, 2342·3
Trenlin, 2342·3
Trentadil, 2342·3
Trental, 2342·3
Treo, 2342·4
Treo Comp, 2342·4
Treomycin, 2342·4
Treonina, 1451·1
Treosulfan, 590·2
Treosulfano, 590·2
Treparin, 2342·4
Trepibutona, 1757·2
Trepibutone, 1757·2
Trepidan, 2342·4
Trepiline, 2342·4
Trepionate, 1757·2
Trepol, 2342·4
Treponematosis— *see* Syphilis, 148·2
Trepress, 2342·4
Treprostinil, 1521·2
Treprostinil Sodium, 1521·2
Treprostinol, 1521·2
Tres Orix Forte, 2342·4
Tresal, 2342·4
Tresite F, 2342·4
Tresium, 2342·4
Tresivac, 2342·4
Tresleen, 2342·4
Tresos B, 2342·4
Trestolone, 1536·1
Tretamine, 526·3
Tretin, 2342·4
Tretinoderm, 2342·4
Tretinoin, 1161·1
Tretinoína, 1161·1
Tretinoine, 2342·4
Tretinoine Kefrane, 2342·4
Tretinoinum, 1161·1
Tretinon, 2342·4
Tretoquinol, Hidrocloruro de, 806·3
Tretoquinol Hydrochloride, 806·3
Treupel Comp, 2342·4
Treupel Mono, 2342·4
Treupel N, 2342·4
Treupel sans Codeine, 2342·4
Treupel Simplex, 2342·4
Treuphadol, 2342·4
Treuphadol Plus, 2342·4
Trevilor, 2343·1
Trevina, 2343·1
Trevis, 2343·1
Trewilor, 2343·1
Trex, 2343·1
Trexall, 2343·1
Trexan, 2343·1
Trexan— *see* Revia, 2261·1
Trexen, 2343·1
Trexeron, 2343·1
Trexirol NF, 2343·1
Trexofin, 2343·1
Trexol, 2343·1
Trexydin, 2343·1
Trexyl, 2343·1
Trezor, 2343·1
TRF, 1337·3
TRH, 1337·3, 2343·1
TRH-221, 174·1
TRH Prem, 2343·1
TRH, Synthetic, 1337·3
Trhelea, 2343·1
Tri Hachemina, 2343·1
Tri Vit with Fluoride, 2343·1
Triac, 1604·3, 2343·1
Triacana, 2343·1
Triacel, 2343·1
Triacelluvax, 2343·1
Triacet, 2343·1
Triacetin, 410·2
Triacetina, 410·2
Triacetinum, 410·2
Triacetyloleandomycin, 274·1
Triacilline, 2343·1
Triacomb, 2343·1
Triaconazole, 409·3
Triacontanyl 3-(4-Hydroxy-3-methoxyphenyl)prop-2-enoate, 1725·1
Triactin, 2343·2
Triacylglycerols, 1412·1
Triad, 2343·2
Triada, 2343·2
Triadapin, 2343·2
Tri-Adcortyl, 2343·2
Triadene, 2343·2
Triaderm, 2343·2
Triafed with Codeine, 2343·2
Triaformo, 2343·2
Triagin, 2343·2
Triagynon, 2343·2
Triaken, 2343·2
Trial AG, 2343·2
Trial Antacid, 2343·2
Trial Combi, 2343·2
Trial Gel, 2343·2
Trial Gest, 2343·2
Trial Pack, 2343·2
Trial Sat, 2343·2
Trialix, 2343·2
Trialmin, 2343·2
Trialona, 2343·2
Trialone, 2343·2
Trialyn DM, 2343·2
Triam, 2343·2
Triam-A, 2343·3
Triama, 2343·2
Triamaxco, 2343·3
Triamcinolona, 1110·2
Triamcinolona, Acetónido de, 1110·2
Triamcinolona, Diacetato de, 1110·2
Triamcinolona, Hexacetónido de, 1110·2
Triamcinolone, 1110·2
Triamcinolone Acetonide, 1110·2
Triamcinolone Acetonide Acetate, 1110·2
Triamcinolone Acetonide 21-(3,3-Dimethylbutyrate), 1110·2
Triamcinolone Acetonide Dipotassium Phosphate, 1111·1
Triamcinolone Acetonide 21-Disodium Phosphate, 1110·2
Triamcinolone Acetonide Hemisuccinate, 1111·1
Triamcinolone Acetonide Metembonate, 1111·1

Triamcinolone Acetonide Sodium Phosphate, 1110·2
Triamcinolone Aminobenzal Benzamidoisobutyrate, 1111·1
Triamcinolone Benetonide, 1111·1
Triamcinolone Diacetate, 1110·2
Triamcinolone 16α,21-Diacetate, 1110·2
Triamcinolone Hexacetonide, 1110·2
Triamcinoloni Acetonidum, 1110·2
Triamcinoloni Hexacetonidum, 1110·2
Triamcinolonum, 1110·2
Triamciterap, 2343·3
Triamco, 2343·3
Triam-Co, 2343·3
Triamcort, 2343·3
TriamCreme, 2343·3
Triamer, 2343·3
Triamgalen, 2343·3
Trianhexal, 2343·3
Trianid, 2343·3
Trianinic Preparations, 2343·3
Triarinicflu, 2344·1
Trianinicin, 2344·1
Triaminicin Cold, Allergy, Sinus, 2344·1
Triamnicol DM, 2344·1
Triamnicol Multi-Symptom Cough and Col 2344·1
Triamicol Multi-Symptom Relief, 2344·1
Triamodil— *see* Aminotril, 1794·2
2,4,7-Tiamino-6-phenylpteridine, 1016·2
Triamide, 2344·1
Triamonium Aurintricarboxylate, 1757·3
Triamonium Citrate, 1654·1
Triamcide, 2344·1
Triampen, 2344·1
Triamp Compositum, 2344·1
TriamSbe, 2344·1
Triamsirt, 2344·1
Triamten Comp, 2344·2
Triamtene, 1016·2, 1016·3
Triamten-H, 2344·2
Triamten/HCT, 2344·2
Triamteno, 1016·2
Triamterum, 1016·2
Triam-Tiida R, 2344·2
Triamvir, 2344·2
Trianal, 44·2
Trianal C2344·2
Triancil, 44·2
Tri-Anem, 2344·2
2,4,6-Trialino-*p*-(carbo-2′-ethylhexyl-1′-oxy)-1,3-triazine, 1154·3
Tri-*p*-anishloroethylene, 1542·1
Trianteren 1016·2
Triapin, 24·2
Triapten, 14·2
Triarese, 24·2
Triasox, 21·2
Triaspar, 24·2
Triasporin,44·2
Triastad H 2344·2
Triastonal, 44·2
Triatec Preations, 2344·2
Triativ, 234
Triatop, 232
Triaval, 234
Triavil, 234
Tri-A-Vite 1344·3
Triax, 1604·
Triaxin, 234
Triaxone, 233
Triaxton, 233
Triaz, 2344·
Triazid, 2344
Triazine, 234
Triazol, 2344
Triazolam, 7
Triazole Antigals, 386·1
4,4′-(1*H*-1-Triazol-1-ylmethylene)dibenzile, 565·1
Tribakin, 234
Triban, 2344·
Tribasic CalciPhosphate, 1226·1
Tribasic Magum Phosphate, 1228·1
Tribasic SodiPhosphate, 1231·1
Tribavirin, 65
Tribdoze, 234
Tribe 12, 234
Tribedex, 234
Tribedoxyl, 2344·3
Tribemin, 2344·3
Tribenoside, 1757·3
Tribenósido, 1757·3
Tribenosidum, 1757·3
Tribesian, 2344·3
Tribesona, 2344·3
Tribeton, 2344·3
Tribiot, 2344·3
Tribiotic Plus, 2344·3
Tri-Biozene, 2344·3
Tribonat, 2344·3
3,4′,5-Tribromosalicylanilide, 1171·2
Tribromsalan, 1171·2
Tri-Buffered ASA, 2344·3
Tributyl Acetylcitrate, 1757·3
Tributyl 2-(Acetyloxy)propane-1,2,3-tricarboxylate, 1757·3
Tributyl Phosphate, 1477·3
Tri-*n*-butyl Phosphate, 1477·3
Tributylis Acetylcitras, 1757·3
Tri-*n*-butylis Phosphas, 1477·3
Tri(*n*-butyl)phosphate, 1477·3
Tributyltin Oxide, 1756·3
Tricaína, Mesilato de, 1385·3
Tricaine Mesilate, 1385·3
Tricaine Mesylate, 1385·3
Tricaine-MPS, 2344·4
Tri-Cal, 2344·4
Tricalcico, Fosfato, 1225·3
Tricalcii Phosphas, 1225·3
Tricalcio Com Fluor, 2344·4
Tricalcium Citrate, 1225·1
Tricalcium Diorthophosphate, 1226·1
Tricalcium 2-Hydroxypropane-1,2,3-tricarboxylate Tetrahydrate, 1225·1
Tricalcium Phosphate, 1225·3
Trical-D, 2344·4
Tricalma Retard, 2344·4
Tricalvit, 2344·4
Trican, 2344·4
Tricandil, 2344·4
Tricangine, 2344·4
Tricarbaurinio, 1757·3
Tricarbaurinium, 1757·3
Tricef, 2344·4
Tricefin, 2344·4
Tricen, 2344·4
Tricephin, 2344·4
Tricept, 2344·4
Tricerol, 2344·4
Trichazole, 2344·4
Trichex, 2344·4
Trichinellosis— *see* Trichinosis, 101·1
Trichinosis, 101·1
Tri-Chlor, 2344·4
Trichloracetic Acid, 1162·1
Trichloraceticum, Acidum, 1162·1
Trichlorbutanolum, 1176·3
Trichloressigsäure, 1162·1
Trichlorethylene, 1310·3
Trichlorethylenum, 1310·3
Trichlorfon, 109·2
Trichlorisobutylicus, Alcohol, 1176·3
Trichlormethiazide, 1017·2
Trichlormethiazidum, 1017·2
Trichloroacetic Acid, 684·3, 1162·1, 1311·1, 1477·1, 1477·3
1,1,1-Trichloro-2,2-bis(4-chlorophenyl)ethane, 1502·1
1,1,1-Trichloro-2-2-bis(*p*-methoxyphenyl)-ethane, 1507·2
3,4,4′-Trichlorocarbanilide, 1195·1
Trichloroethane, 1477·3
α-Trichloroethane, 1477·3
1,1,1-Trichloroethane, 1477·3
2,2,2-Trichloroethane-1,1-diol, 684·1
Trichloroethanol, 684·3, 726·3, 1311·1, 1477·3
Trichloroethene, 1310·3
Trichloroethylene, 1310·3
Trichloroethylenum, 1310·3
(*R*)-1,2-*O*-(2,2,2-Trichloroethylidene)-α-D-glucofuranose, 1501·2
Trichlorofluoromethane, 1236·1
Trichlorogalactosucrose, 1450·1
2,4,4′-Trichloro-2′-hydroxydiphenyl Ether, 1195·2
Trichloroisocyanuric Acid, 1191·3
Trichlorol, 2344·4
Trichloromethane, 1296·3
1,1,1-Trichloro-2-methylpropan-2-ol, 1176·3
Trichloromonofluoromethane, 1236·1
Trichloronitromethane, 1502·1
Trichlorophenoxyacetic Acid, 1510·3
2,4,5-Trichlorophenoxyacetic Acid, 1510·3
Trichlorphon, 109·2
Trichobiol, 2344·4
Trichomoniasis, 599·3
Trichomoniasis Vaccines, 1642·1
Trichonas, 2344·4
*Trichosanthes kirilowii*, 655·3
Trichosanthin, 655·3
Trichostrongyliasis, 101·2
Trichotine, 2344·4
Trichozole, 2344·4
Trichuriasis, 101·2
Tri-Ciclomex, 2344·4
Triciclor, 2344·4
Triciderm, 2344·4
Tricidine, 2344·4
Tricidine Dequalinium, 2344·4
Tricifa, 2344·4
TriCilest, 2345·1
Tricilon, 2345·1
Tricin, 2345·1
Tricivir, 2345·1
Triclabendazol, 115·2
Triclabendazole, 115·2
Triclin, 2345·1
Triclocarban, 1195·1
Tricloderm, 2345·1
Triclofós Sódico, 726·2
Triclofos Sodium, 726·2
Triclonam, 2345·1
Triclormetiazida, 1017·2
Tricloroacético, Ácido, 1162·1
Tricloroetano, 1477·3
Tricloroetileno, 1310·3
Triclorofenoxiacético, Ácido, 1510·3
Triclorofluorometano, 1236·1
Tricloryl, 2345·1
Triclosan, 1195·2
Triclose, 2345·1
Tri-Co, 2345·1
Tricobalt Tetroxide, 1674·1
Tricocel, 2345·1
Tricocet, 2345·1
Tricodein, 2345·1
Tricodene Preparations, 2345·1
Tricoderm F, 2345·1
Tricodex, 2345·1
Tricofarma, 2345·1
Tricofin, 2345·1
Tricogyn, 2345·1
Tricolam, 2345·1
Tricold, 2345·1
Tri-Cold, 2345·1
Tricolocion, 2345·2
Tricolpex, 2345·2
Tricomed, 2345·2
Tricomox, 2345·2
Triconal, 2345·2
Triconidazol, 2345·2
Tricoplus, 2345·2
Tricoplus Conef, 2345·2
Tricor, 2345·2
Tricorex, 2345·2
Tricortin, 2345·2
Tricosantina, 655·3
Tricosten, 2345·2
Tricovivax, 2345·2
Tricowas B, 2345·2
Tricox, 2345·2
Tricoxane, 2345·2
Tricoxidil, 2345·2
Tricozone, 2345·2
Tricresol, 1177·3
Tri-Cyclen, 2345·2
Tricyclic Antidepressants, 278·2, 285·2
Tricyclo[3.3.1.1$^{3,7}$]dec-1-ylamine Hydrochloride, 1197·2
Tridelta, 2345·2
Trident, 2345·2
Triderm, 2345·2
Triderm 5, 2345·2
Triderm Zeta, 2345·2
Tridermal, 2345·2
Triderm-C, 2345·3
Tridesilon, 2345·3
Tridesonit, 2345·3
Tridestan N, 2345·3
Tridestra, 2345·3
Tridette, 2345·3
*Tridídemnum*, 546·3
Tridigestivo Soubeiran, 2345·3
Tridihexethyl Chloride, 490·2
Tridihexetilo, Cloruro de, 490·2
Tridil, 2345·3
Tridin, 2345·3
Tridin Forte, 2345·3
Triditol-G, 2345·3
Tridocemine, 2345·3
Tridomose, 2345·3
Tridyl, 2345·3
Triefect, 2345·3
Triella, 2345·3
Tri-Emcortina, 2345·3
Trien Hydrochloride, 1055·2
Trienbolone Acetate, 1573·2
Triene, 2345·3
Trientina, Dihidrocloruro de, 1055·2
Trientine Dihydrochloride, 1055·2
Trientine Hydrochloride, 1055·2
Triestearato de Sorbitán, 1416·3
Trietanolamina, Salicilato de, 95·3
Triethanolamine, 1758·2
Triethanolamine Salicylate, 95·3
3-(2,4,5-Triethoxybenzoyl)propionic Acid, 1757·2
Triethoxymethane, 1121·2
Triethyl Citrate, 1757·3
Triethyl Orthoformate, 1121·2
Triethylenemelamine, 526·3
Triethylenephosphoramide, 588·1
Triethylenetetramine Dihydrochloride, 1055·2
Triethylenethiophosphoramide, 588·1
Triethylis Citras, 1757·3
Trietilo, Citrato de, 1757·3
Trietioduro de Galamina, 1403·2
Trietoximetano, 1121·2
Triette, 2345·3
Triexidyl, 2345·3
Triexifenidila, Cloridrato de, 490·2
Trifacilina, 2345·3
Trifacta, 2345·3
Trifamox, 2345·3
Trifamox Bronquial, 2345·4
Trifamox Duo, 2345·4
Trifamox IBL, 2345·4
Trifas, 2345·4
Trifed, 2345·4
Trifed-C Cough, 2345·4
Trifedrin, 2345·4
Trifeme, 2345·4
Tri-Femoden, 2345·4
Trifen, 2345·4
Trifene, 2345·4
Triferon, 2345·4
Trifibra Mix, 2345·4
Tri-Filena, 2345·4
Triflucan, 2345·4
Trifluid, 2345·4
Triflumann, 2345·4
Triflumed, 2345·4
Triflumuron, 1510·3
Trifluoperazina, Hidrocloruro de, 726·3
Trifluoperazine Hydrochloride, 726·3
Trifluoperazini Hydrochloridum, 726·3
Trifluoroacetic Acid, 1300·3
*N*-Trifluoroacetyladriamycin-14-valerate, 590·3
*N*-Trifluoroacetyldoxorubicin-14-valerate, 590·3
6-Trifluoromethoxy-1,3-benzothiazol-2-ylamine, 1738·3
Trifluoromethylhydrothiazide, 937·2
α,α,α-Trifluoro-5-methyl-4-isoxazolecarboxy-*p*-toluidide, 53·2
α,α,α-Trifluoro-2-methyl-4′-nitro-*m*-propionotoluidide, 556·2
2-{4-[3-(2-Trifluoromethylphenothiazin-10-yl)propyl]piperazin-1-yl}ethanol, 699·3
2-{4-[3-(2-Trifluoromethylthioxanthen-9-ylidene)propyl]piperazin-1-yl}ethanol Dihydrochloride, 699·1

(*Z*)-2-{4-[3-(2-Trifluoromethylthioxanthen-9-ylidene)propyl]piperazin-1-yl}ethyl Decanoate, 699·1
α′,α′,α′-Trifluoro-4′-nitroisobutyro-*m*-toluidide, 556·2
2-(α,α,α-Trifluoro-2-nitro-*p*-toluoyl)-1,3-cyclohexanedione, 1722·1
Trifluorothymidine, 655·3
ααα-Trifluorothymidine, 655·3
2-(ααα-Trifluoro-*m*-toluidino)nicotinic Acid, 67·1
*N*-(ααα-Trifluoro-*m*-tolyl)anthranilic Acid, 43·2
2-($\alpha^3$,$\alpha^3$,$\alpha^3$-Trifluoro-2,3,-xylidino)nicotinic Acid compounded with 1-Deoxy-1-(methylamino)-D-glucitol (1:1), 43·3
Trifluperidol, 727·1
Trifluperidol, Hidrocloruro de, 727·1
Trifluperidol Hydrochloride, 727·1
Triflupromazina, 727·1
Triflupromazina, Hidrocloruro de, 727·1
Triflupromazine, 727·1
Triflupromazine Hydrochloride, 727·1
Trifluridina, 655·3
Trifluridine, 655·3
Trifluron, 1510·3
Triflusal, 1017·3
Triflusalum, 1017·3
Triflux, 2345·4
Trifolium Complex, 2345·4
*Trifolium pratense*, 1737·3
Trifosfaneurina, 2345·4
Trifosfaneurina B6, 2345·4
Trifosfaneurina B2 B12, 2345·4
Trifyba, 2346·1
Trigastril, 2346·1
Tri-Gel, 2346·1
Trigeminal Neuralgia, 8·2
Trigen, 2346·1
Trigesico, 2346·1
Triglicen, 2346·1
Triglicéridos de Cadena Media, 1440·3
Triglicéridos Marinos Omega 3, 976·2
Trigliceril CM, 2346·1
Triglobe, 2346·1
Triglycerida Saturata Media, 1440·3
Triglycerides, Medium-chain, 1440·3
Triglycyl-lysine-vasopressin, 1340·1
Trigoa, 2346·1
Trigogine, 2346·1
Trigon Depot, 2346·1
Trigon Rectal, 2346·1
Trigon Topico, 2346·1
*Trigonella foenum-graecum*, 1688·1
Trigonellae, Semen, 1688·1
Trigyn, 2346·1
Trigynera, 2346·1
Tri-Gynera, 2346·1
Trigynon, 2346·1
Trigynovin, 2346·1
TriHEMIC, 2346·1
Triherpine, 2346·1
Trihexifenidilo, Hidrocloruro de, 490·2
Trihexy, 2346·1
Trihexyphenidyl Hydrochloride, 490·2
Trihexyphenidyli Hydrochloridum, 490·2
Trihexyphenidylium Chloratum, 490·2
TriHIBit, 2346·1
Trihistalex, 2346·1
Trihistan, 2346·1
Trihist-CS, 2346·1
Trihist-D, 2346·2
Trihist-DM, 2346·2
(5*Z*,7*E*,22*E*,24*E*)-24a,26a,27a-Trihomo-9,10-secocholesta-5,7,10(19),22,24-pentaene-1α,3β,25-triol, 583·3
Tri-Hydroserpine, 2346·2
Trihydroxybenzylhydrazine, 1200·2
(1′*R*,6*R*,6a*R*,7*R*,13*S*,14*S*,16*R*)-6′,8,14-Trihydroxy-7′,9-dimethoxy-4,10,23-trimethyl-19-oxo-3′,4′,6,7,12,13,14,16-octahydrospiro[6,16-(epithiopropanoxymethano)-7,13-imino-6a*H*-1,3-dioxolo[7,8]isoquino[3,2-*b*][3]benzazocine-20,1′(2′*H*)-isoquinolin]-5-yl Acetate, 589·3
11β,17α,21-Trihydroxy-6,16α-dimethyl-2′-phenyl-2′*H*-pregna-2,4,6-trieno[3,2-*c*]pyrazol-20-one 21-Acetate, 1096·2
Trihydroxyethylrutoside, 1688·3
3,5,7-Trihydroxy-2-[3-(4-hydroxy-3-methoxyphenyl)-2-(hydroxymethyl)-1,4-benzodioxan-6-yl]-4-chromanone, 1043·3
4′,5,7-Trihydroxyisoflavone, 1692·1
3′,5,7-Trihydroxy-4′-methoxyflavone 7-[6-*O*-(6-Deoxy-α-L-mannopyranosyl)-β-D-glucopyranoside], 1688·2
Trihydroxymethylaminomethane, 1758·2
11β,17α,21-Trihydroxy-16-methylenepregna-1,4-diene-3,20-dione, 1109·3
11β,17α,21-Trihydroxy-6α-methylpregna-1,4-diene-3,20-dione, 1106·1
(5*Z*,13*E*)-(8*R*,9*S*,11*R*,12*R*,15*S*)-9,11,15-Trihydroxy-15-methylprosta-5,13-dienoic Acid, 1514·2
7-[2-(3,4,β-Trihydroxyphenethylamino)ethyl]theophylline Hydrochloride, 1754·3
7-{3-[(3,5,β-Trihydroxyphenethyl)amino]propyl}theophylline Hydrochloride, 791·2
11β,17α,21-Trihydroxypregna-1,4-diene-3,20-dione, 1108·1
11β,17,21-Trihydroxypregna-1,4-diene-3,20-dione 21-(4-{4-[Bis(2-chloroethyl)amino]phenyl}butyrate), 581·2
11β,17α,21-Trihydroxypregna-1,4-diene-3,20-dione 21-(Dihydrogen Phosphate) Compound with 2-(2-Isopropylphenoxymethyl)-2-imidazoline, 1129·1
11β,17,21-Trihydroxypregna-1,4-diene-3,20-dione 17-(Ethyl Carbonate) 21-Propionate, 1107·3
11β,17α,21-Trihydroxypregna-1,4-diene-3,20-dione 21-(Sodium Succinate), 1108·2
11β,17α,21-Trihydroxypregn-4-ene-3,20-dione, 1103·3
11β,17α,21-Trihydroxypregn-4-ene-3,20-dione 21-Diethylaminoacetate Hydrochloride, 1103·3
2′,4′,6′-Trihydroxypropiophenone, 1689·1
(5*Z*,13*E*)-(8*R*,9*S*,11*R*,12*R*,15*S*)-9,11,15-Trihydroxyprosta-5,13-dienoic Acid, 1514·3
Trihydroxystearate Ester of Ethoxylated Glycerol, 1414·3
Tri-Immunol, 2346·2
Tri-iodomethane, 1184·2
Triiodothyroacetic Acid, 1604·3
Triiodothyronine Injection, 2346·2
Triiodothyronine, Reverse, 1594·1
L-Tri-iodothyronine Sodium, 1602·2
3,5,3′-Tri-iodo-L-thyronine Sodium, 1602·2
Tri-K, 2346·2
Trikacide, 2346·2
Triketocholanic Acid, 1679·2
Trikof-D, 2346·2
Tri-Kort, 2346·2
Trikozol, 2346·2
Trikozol— *see* Helipak A, 2038·2
Trikozol— *see* Helipak T, 2038·2
Trikresolum, 1177·3
Trikvilar, 2346·2
Trilafon, 2346·2
Trilam, 2346·2
Trilax, 2346·2
Trileptal, 2346·2
Trileptin, 2346·2
Tri-Levlen, 2346·2
Trilifan, 2346·2
Trilisate, 2346·2
Trillium Complex, 2346·2
Triloc, 2346·2
Trilog, 2346·2
Trilombrin, 2346·2
Trilon, 2346·2
Trilone, 2346·2
Trilophosphamide, 590·2
Trilor, 2346·3
Trilosil, 2346·3
Trilosil N, 2346·3
Trilostane, 1757·3
Trilostano, 1757·3
Triloxane, 2346·3
Triludan, 2346·3
Trilufen, 2346·3
Tri-Luma, 2346·3
Trim, 2346·3
Tri-Mactex, 2346·3
Trimadiaz Antrima, 2346·3
Trimag, 2346·3
Trimagnesium Phosphate, 1228·1
Trimasone, 2346·3
Trimate-Ace, 2346·3
Trimaze, 2346·3
Trimazide, 2346·3
Trimazol, 2346·3
Trimebutina, Maleato de, 1758·1
Trimebutine, 1758·1
Trimebutine Maleate, 1758·1
Trimecaína, Hidrocloruro de, 1385·3
Trimecaine Hydrochloride, 1385·3
Trimecainium Chloratum, 1385·3
Trimedal, 2346·3
Trimedat, 2346·3
Trimedil, 2346·3
Trimedoxime Bromide, 1050·3
Trimegestona, 1573·3
Trimegestone, 1573·3
Trimel, 2346·3
Trim-Elim, 2346·3
Trimepaz, 2346·3
Trimeperidine Hydrochloride, 95·3
Trimeprazine *SS*-Dioxide, 438·2
Trimeprazine Tartrate, 423·3
Trimeprimine, 320·2
Trimesul, 2346·3
Trimesuxol, 2346·3
Trimetabol, 2346·3
Trimetadiona, 379·3
Trimetafán, Cansilato de, 1017·3
Trimetaphan Camphorsulphonate, 1017·3
Trimetaphan Camsilate, 1017·3
Trimetaphan Camsylate, 1017·3
Trimetaphani Camsylas, 1017·3
Trimetazidina, Hidrocloruro de, 1018·1
Trimetazidine Dihydrochloride, 1018·1
Trimetazidine Hydrochloride, 1018·1
Trimetazidini Dihydrochloridum, 1018·1
Trimetazine Hydrochloride, 1018·1
Trimethadione, 379·3
Trimethadionum, 379·3
Trimethaphan Camsylate, 1017·3
Trimethinum, 379·3
Trimetho Comp, 2346·4
Trimethobenzamide Hydrochloride, 442·2
Trimethoprim, 272·2
Trimethoprim Hydrochloride, 272·2, 273·3
Trimethoprim Lactate, 273·3
Trimethoprim Sulfate, 272·2, 273·3
Trimethoprim Sulphate, 272·2
Trimethoprimum, 272·2
Trimethoquinol Hydrochloride, 806·3
Trimethox, 2346·4
2,4,5-Trimethoxyamfetamine, 1593·3
1-(2,3,4-Trimethoxybenzyl)piperazine Dihydrochloride, 1018·1
5-(3,4,5-Trimethoxybenzyl)pyrimidine-2,4-diamine, 272·2
Trimethoxychalcone, 1714·3
2′,4,4′-Trimethoxychalcone, 1714·3
3,4,5-Trimethoxyphenethylamine, 1713·3
(±)-3,4,5-Trimethoxy-*N*-3-piperidylbenzamide, 1294·2
Trimethoxyprim, 272·2
2′,4′,6′-Trimethoxy-4-(pyrrolidin-1-yl)butyrophenone Hydrochloride, 877·2
Trimethylamine, 1423·3
Trimethylamine-*N*-oxide, 1423·3
Trimethylaminuria— *see* Fish Odour Syndrome, 1417·3
[2-(Trimethylammonio)ethyl][hexadecyloxyphosphonate], 573·2
1,7,7-Trimethylbicyclo[2.2.1]heptan-2-ol Acetate, 1662·2
1,7,7-Trimethylbicyclo[2.2.1]heptan-2-one, 1665·3
3,3,5-Trimethylcyclohexyl Mandelate, 890·3
3,3,5-Trimethylcyclohexyl Salicylate, 1148·1
(±)-2,4,5-Trimethyl-3,6-dioxo-ζ-phenyl-1,4-cyclohexadiene-1-heptanoic Acid, 795·3
Trimethylene, 1297·1
Trimethylene Bis[2-(4-chlorophenoxy)-2-methylpropionate], 997·1
4,4′-Trimethylenedioxydibenzamidine Bis(2-hydroxyethanesulphonate), 1191·2
2,5,9-Trimethyl-7*H*-furo[3,2-*g*][1]benzopyran-7-one, 1162·2
Trimethylglycine, 1660·1
Trimethylglycine Hydrochloride, 1660·2
1,5,*N*-Trimethylhex-4-enylamine Hydrochloride, 1702·1
1,7,7-Trimethyl-3-[(4-methylphenyl)methylene]bicyclo[2.2.1]heptan-2-one, 1147·1
1,3,3-Trimethyl-2-oxabicyclo[2.2.2]octane, 1672·1
3,5,5-Trimethyl-1,3-oxazolidine-2,4-dione, 379·3
*N*,α,α-Trimethylphenethylamine Sulphate Dihydrate, 952·1
1,2,5-Trimethyl-4-phenyl-4-piperidyl Propionate Hydrochloride, 95·3
Trimethylphloroglucinol, 1731·1
4,5′,8-Trimethylpsoralen, 1162·2
1,3,7-Trimethylpurine-2,6(3*H*,1*H*)-dione, 782·1
Trimethyltetradecylammonium Bromide, 1172·2
Trimethyl[1-(*p*-tolyl)dodecyl]ammonium Methylsulphate, 1194·3
2,4,6-Trimethyl-1,3,5-trioxane, 713·1
Trimethyltubocurarine Iodide, 1403·3
1,3,7-Trimethylxanthine, 782·1
Trimetin, 2346·4
Trimetin Duplo, 2346·4
Trimetobenzamida, Hidrocloruro de, 442·2
Trimetoger, 2346·4
Trimeton, 2346·4
Trimetoprim Balsamico, 2346·4
Trimetoprima, 272·2
Trimetoprima y Sulfadiazina, 199·3
Trimetoprim-Sulfa, 2346·4
Trimetoquinol Hydrochloride, 806·3
Trimetox, 2346·4
Trimetrexate Glucuronate, 410·2
Trimetrexato, Glucuronato de, 410·
Trimetrox, 2346·4
Trimex, 2346·4
Trimexazol, 2346·4
Trimexazol Balsamico, 2346·4
Trimexazole, 2346·4
Trimexine, 2346·4
Trimexole, 2346·4
Trimexole Compositum, 2346·4
Trimexolone, 1110·1
Trimezole, 2346·4
Trim-Fit, 2346·4
Trimicon, 2346·4
Tri-Micon, 2346·4
Trimicro, 2346·4
Trimidura, 2346·4
Trimin Sulfa, 2346·4
Trimineurin, 2346·4
Triminol Cough, 2346·4
Tri-Minulet, 2346·4
Trimipramim, 2347·1
Trimipramina, 320·2
Trimipramina, Maleato de, 320
Trimipramine, 320·2
Trimipramine Hydrochloride, 3 3
Trimipramine Hydrogen Malea 320·2
Trimipramine Maleate, 320·2
Trimipramine Mesilate, 320·3
Trimipramini Maleas, 320·2
Trimiron, 2347·1
TriMix, 2347·1
Trimogal, 2347·1
Trimoks, 2347·1
Trimol, 2347·1
Trimol-A, 2347·1
Trimonase, 2347·1
Trimonil, 2347·1
Trimono, 2347·1
Trimopan, 2347·1
Trimo-San, 2347·1
Trimovate, 2347·1
Trimovax, 2347·1
Trimox, 2347·1
Trimox— *see* Prevpac, 223
Trimoxazole, 2347·1
Trimoxol, 2347·1
Trimoxzol, 2347·1
Trimpex, 2347·1
Trimstat, 2347·1
Trim-Vit, 2347·1
Trimzol, 2347·1
Trinaderm, 2347·1
Trinagesic, 2347·1
Trinalgen, 2347·1

Trinalin, 2347·2
Trinalion, 2347·2
Tri-Nasal, 2347·2
Trinate, 2347·2
Trinavet, 2347·2
Tri-Nefrin Extra Strength, 2347·2
Trinelax, 2347·2
Trinergic, 2347·2
Trinergot, 2347·2
TriNessa, 2347·2
Trinestril, 2347·2
Trinettriol, 989·3
Trineurin, 2347·2
Trinevral, 2347·2
Trinevrina B6, 2347·2
Triniagar, 2347·2
Trinicalm, 2347·2
Trinicalm Forte, 2347·2
Trinicalm Plus, 2347·2
Trinidex, 2347·2
Triniol, 2347·2
Trinipatch, 2347·2
Triniplas, 2347·2
Triniscon, 2347·2
Trinispray, 2347·2
Triniton, 2347·2
Trinitrin, 923·2
Trinitrina, 2347·2
Trinitrine, 2347·2
Trinitrine Simple Laleuf, 2347·3
Trinitrofenol, 1758·1
Trinitroglycerin, 923·2
Trinitron, 2347·3
Trinitrophenol, 1758·1
2,4,6-Trinitrophenol, 1758·1
Trinitrosan, 2347·3
Trinizol, 2347·3
Trinizol M, 2347·3
Trinolone, 2347·3
Trinordiol, 2347·3
Tri-Norinyl, 2347·3
Trinorm, 2347·3
TRI-Normin, 2347·3
Trinotecan, 2347·3
Trinotrex, 2347·3
Trinovum, 2347·3
Trinsicon, 2347·3
Trintek, 2347·3
Trio D, 2347·3
Trio S, 2347·3
Trio Val, 2347·3
Trio Val Dia y Noche, 2347·3
TrioBe, 2347·3
Triocalcio, 2347·3
Triocaps, 2347·4
Triocetin, 2347·4
Trio-D, 2347·4
Triodanin, 2347·4
Triodeen, 2347·4
Trioden, 2347·4
Triodena, 2347·4
Triodene, 2347·4
Triofan, 2347·4
Triofed, 2347·4
Triogene, 2347·4
Triogesic, 2347·4
Triogestena, 2347·4
Triogestin, 2347·4
Triolax, 2347·4
Trioleato de Sorbitán, 1416·2
Triolip, 2347·4
TRI-OM, 2347·4
Triomar, 2347·4
Triomer, 2347·4
Triomin, 2347·4
Triominic, 2347·4
Trionetta, 2347·4
Trioral/HCT, 2347·4
Triospan, 2347·4
Triostat, 2347·4
Triotann, 2347·4
Tri-Otic, 2347·4
Triotonico, 2347·4
Triovit, 2348·1
Triox NF, 2348·1
3,3′-(3,6,9-Trioxaundecanedioyldi-imino)bis(2,4,6-tri-iodobenzoic Acid), 1066·1
Trioxina, 2348·1
Trioxisaleno, 1162·2
3,7,12-Trioxo-5β-cholan-24-oic Acid, 1679·2
Trioxsalen, 1162·2
Trioxyethylrutin, 1688·3
Trioxyméthylène, 1187·3
Trioxysalen, 1162·2
Tri-P, 2348·1
Tripac-Cyano, 2348·1
Tripacel, 2348·1
Tripalmitin, 1736·2
Tripamida, 1018·1
Tripamide, 1018·1
Triparen, 2348·1
Triparsamida, 617·3
Triparsean, 2348·1
Tripe P, 2348·1
Tripedia, 2348·1
Tripelenamina, Citrato de, 442·3
Tripelenamina, Hidrocloruro de, 442·3
Tripelennamine Citrate, 442·3
Tripelennamine Hydrochloride, 442·3
Tripelennaminium Chloride, 442·3
Tripelennaminium Citrate, 442·3
Triperidol, 2348·1
Triphacycline, 2348·1
Triphasil, 2348·1
Tri-Phen-Chlor TR, 2348·1
Triphenyl, 2348·1
Triphenyl Expectorant, 2348·1
Triphidus, 2348·1
Triphosadénine, 1648·1
Triphosmag, 2348·1
Triphthazinum, 726·3
Tripiperazine Dicitrate, Hydrous, 111·2
Triple Antibiotic, 2348·1
Triple Antigen, 2348·1
Triple Care Cleanser, 2348·1
Triple Care Cream, 2348·1
Triple Paste, 2348·1
Triple Protection, 2348·1
Triple Sulfa, 2348·1
Triple X, 2348·1
Tri-Plen, 2348·2
Triplex, 2348·2
Tripo, 2348·2
Tripondil, 2348·2
Triposed, 2348·2
Tripotassium Citrate, 1223·1
Tripotassium Dicitratobismuthate, 1252·2
Tripotassium 2-Hydroxypropane-1,2,3-tricarboxylate Monohydrate, 1223·1
Tripress, 2348·2
Triprim, 2348·2
Tripro-amylin, 344·3
Triprodrine, 2348·2
Triprofed, 2348·2
Tri-Profen, 2348·2
Tri-Profen Cold & Flu, 2348·2
Triprolidina, Hidrocloruro de, 442·3
Triprolidine Hydrochloride, 442·3
Tripsina, 1758·3
Tripsol, 2348·2
Tripsor, 2348·2
Tripsyline, 2348·2
Tripta, 2348·2
Triptafen, 2348·2
Triptil, 2348·2
Triptizol, 2348·2
Triptófano, 320·3
Tript-OH, 2348·2
Triptone, 2348·2
Triptorelin, 1341·2
Triptorelin Acetate, 1341·2
Triptorelin Diacetate, 1341·2
Triptorelin Embonate, 1341·2
Triptorelin Pamoate, 1341·2
Triptorelina, 1341·2
Triptoreline, 1341·2
Triptyl, 2348·2
Triptyline, 2348·2
Tripulmin, 2348·2
Tripulmin Balsamico, 2348·3
Tripvac, 2348·3
Triquilar, 2348·3
Tri-Regol, 2348·3
Triricinoleate Ester of Ethoxylated Glycerol, 1414·3
Tririnol, 2348·3
Trirubin, 2348·3
Trirutin, 2348·3
Trirutin N, 2348·3
TRIS, 1758·2
Tris, 2348·3
Trisalgina, 2348·3
Trisalicilato de Colina y Magnesio, 26·2
Trisan, 2348·3
Tris(aziridin-1-yl)phosphine Sulphide, 588·1
Trisdazol, 2348·3
2,4,6-Tris(dimethylamino)-1,3,5-triazine, 526·2
Trisekvens, 2348·3
Trisel, 2348·3
Trisenox, 2348·3
Triseptil, 2348·3
Trisequens, 2348·3
3′,4′,7-Tris[*O*-(2-hydroxyethyl)]rutin, 1688·3
Tris(hydroxymethyl)aminomethane, 1758·2
Tri-Sinerge, 2348·3
Trisiston, 2348·3
Tris(lactato)aluminium, 1653·1
Trisodium Calcium Diethylenetriaminepentaacetate, 1050·1
Trisodium Citrate, 1223·2
Trisodium 4,4′,4″-(2,4-Diaminobenzene-1,3,5-triazo)tribenzenesulphonate, 1056·3
Trisodium Edetate, 1037·3
Trisodium Hydrogen Ethylenediaminetetraacetate, 1037·3
Trisodium Hydrogen (1-Hydroxy-2-imidazol-1-ylethylidene)diphosphonate Hydrate (5:2), 776·2
Trisodium 2-Hydroxypropane-1,2,3-tricarboxylate Dihydrate, 1223·2
Trisodium 3-Hydroxy-4-(4-sulphonato-1-naphthylazo)naphthalene-2,7-disulphonate, 1056·1
Trisodium 7-Hydroxy-8-(4-sulphonato-1-naphthylazo)naphthalene-1,3-disulphonate, 1057·3
Trisodium 5-Hydroxy-1-(4-sulphonatophenyl)-4-(4-sulphonatophenylazo)pyrazole-3-carboxylate, 1058·2
Trisodium Orthophosphate, 1231·1
Trisodium Phosphate, 1231·1
Trisodium Phosphonatoformate Hexahydrate, 634·2
Trisodium Trihydrogen (*OC*-6-13)-*N*,*N*′-Ethane-1,2-diylbis{N-[2-methyl-3-oxido-κ*O*-5-(phosphonatooxymethyl)-4-pyridylmethyl]glycinato(*O*,*N*)}manganate(II), 1067·1
Trisodium Trihydrogen (*OC*-6-13)-{[*N*,*N*-′-Ethylenebis(*N*-{[3-hydroxy-5-(hydroxymethyl)-2-methyl-4-pyridyl]methyl}glycine) 5,5′-Bis(phosphato)](8-)}Manganate(6-), 1067·1
Trisodium Uridine Triphosphate, 1760·3
Trisofort, 2348·3
Trisolvit, 2348·4
Trisoralen, 2348·4
Trisorcin, 2348·4
Trisporal, 2348·4
Tri-Sprintec, 2348·4
Trissil, 2348·4
Tri-Statin II, 2348·4
TriStep, 2348·4
Tristina, 2348·4
Tristoject, 2348·4
Trisufin, 2348·4
Trisul, 2348·4
Trisulfaminic, 2348·4
Trisulfose, 2348·4
Trisulprim, 2348·4
Trisyn, 2348·4
Tritab, 2348·4
Tritace, 2348·4
Tritace Comp, 2348·4
Tritace-HCT, 2348·4
Tritan, 2348·4
Tri-Tannate, 2348·4
Tri-Tannate Plus Pediatric, 2348·4
Tritanrix, 2348·4
Tritanrix HB, 2348·4
Tritanrix HB-HIB, 2349·1
Tritanrix HB/Hiberix, 2349·1
Tritazide, 2349·1
Tritec, 2349·1
Tritenk, 2349·1
Tritet, 2349·1
Tri-Thiazid, 2349·1
Tri-Thiazid Reserpin, 2349·1
Trithioparamethoxyphenylpropene, 1655·1
Tritiated Water, 1526·2
Tritici Amylum, 1449·1
Triticin, 1676·2
Triticum, 1676·2, 2349·1
*Triticum aestivum*, 1253·2, 1439·2, 1449·1
*Triticum compactum*, 1253·2
*Triticum durum*, 1253·2
*Triticum turgidum*, 1439·2
*Triticum vulgare*, 1449·1
Tritio, 1526·2
Tritium, 1526·2
Tritocualina, 443·3
Tritopan, 2349·1
Tritoqualine, 443·3
Tri-Torrat, 2349·1
Trittico, 2349·1
Triv, 2349·1
Trivacuna, 2349·1
Trivagel N, 2349·1
Trivalent Antimony Compounds, 103·1
Trivanex, 2349·1
Trivastal, 2349·1
Trivastan, 2349·1
Trivax, 2349·1
Trivax-AD, 2349·1
Trivax-Hib, 2349·1
Trive, 2349·1
Trivemil, 2349·1
Trivermon, 2349·1
Tri-Vi-Flor, 2349·1
Tri-Vi-Fluor, 2349·2
Triviken, 2349·2
Trivina, 2349·2
Triviraten, 2349·2
Trivisol, 2349·2
Tri-Vi-Sol Preparations, 2349·2
Tri-Vitamin, 2349·2
Trivitamin Fluoride Drops, 2349·2
Trivitan, 2349·2
Trivitana DM, 2349·2
Trivitana Q10, 2349·2
Trivit-B, 2349·2
Trivitol, 2349·2
Trivon, 2349·2
Trivora, 2349·2
Tri-Wycillina, 2349·2
Trixidine, 2349·2
Trixilan, 2349·2
Trixilem, 2349·2
Trixne, 2349·2
Trixol, 2349·2
Trixone, 2349·2
Trixotene, 2349·2
Trixzol, 2349·2
Triyodisan, 2349·2
Triyosom, 2349·2
Triyotex, 2349·3
Triz, 2349·3
Trizele, 2349·3
Trizid, 2349·3
Trizina, 2349·3
Trizivir, 2349·3
Trizol Balsamico, 2349·3
Trizolin, 2349·3
TRK-100, 1514·1
TRO, 491·1
Trobicin, 2349·3
Trobicine, 2349·3
Troca Cationi, 2349·3
Troca Flu, 2349·3
Troca Flu Spray Nasale, 2349·3
Trocacin, 2349·3
Trocaine, 2349·3
Trocal, 2349·3
Trochain, 2349·3
Trocium, 2349·3
Trockenhefe, 1469·1
Troclosene Potassium, 1191·3
Troclosene, Sodium, 1191·3
Trodrine, 2349·3
Trofalgon, 2349·3
Trofen, 2349·3
Trofentyl, 2349·3

Troferit, 2349·3
Trofesil, 2349·3
Trofi Milina, 2349·3
Troficardil, 2349·3
Trofinan, 2349·3
Trofinerv, 2349·4
Trofinerv Antiox, 2349·4
Trofo 5, 2349·4
Trofocalcium, 2349·4
Trofocard, 2349·4
Trofodermin, 2349·4
Trofodermin Neomicina, 2349·4
Trofodermin-S, 2349·4
Trofogin, 2349·4
Trofomed, 2349·4
Troforex Pepsico, 2349·4
Trofoseptine, 2349·4
Trofosfamida, 590·2
Trofosfamide, 590·2
Troglitazona, 348·2
Troglitazone, 348·2
Trois Fleurs d'Orient, Creme des— *see* Creme des 3 Fleurs d'Orient, 1911·2
Trojan, 2349·4
Trolamina, 1758·2
Trolamine, 1758·2
Trolamine Laurilsulfate, 1574·3
Trolamine Polypeptide Oleate-Condensate, 1758·2
Trolamine Salicylate, 95·3
Trolaminum, 1758·2
Troleandomicina, 274·1
Troleandomycin, 274·1
Troliber, 2349·4
Trolip, 2349·4
Trolit, 2349·4
Trolovol, 2349·4
Tromadil, 2349·4
Tromagesic, 2349·4
Tromalyt, 2349·4
Tromantadina, Hidrocloruro de, 656·1
Tromantadine Hydrochloride, 656·1
Tromasin, 2349·4
Tromasin con Aspirina, 2349·4
Trombenal, 2349·4
Trombenox, 2349·4
Trombina, 760·1
Trombofob, 2349·4
Trombolisin, 2349·4
Trombolysin, 2349·4
Tromboparin, 2350·1
Trombopat, 2350·1
Tromboplastina, 760·2
Trombopoyetina, 760·2
Trombosol, 2350·1
Trombovar, 2350·1
Tromboxanil, 2350·1
Trombyl, 2350·1
Tromcardin, 2350·1
Tromderm, 2350·1
Tromedal, 2350·1
Trometamol, 1758·2
Trometamol Acefyllinate, 1758·3
Trometamol Citrate, 1758·3
Trometamol Thioctate, 1754·3
Trometamolum, 1758·2
Tromethamine, 1758·2
Tromicol, 2350·1
Tromigal, 2350·1
Tromir, 2350·1
Tromlipon, 2350·1
Trommcardin, 2350·1
Trommgallol, 2350·1
Trompersantin, 2350·1
Tromphyllin, 2350·1
Tronadora, 1666·1
Tronan, 2350·1
Troneo, 2350·1
Tronex, 2350·1
Tronolane, 2350·1
Tronotene, 2350·1
Tronothane, 2350·1
Tronoxal, 2350·1
Tropaeoli, Oleum, 1659·3
*Tropaeolum majus*, 1659·3
$1\alpha H,5\alpha H$-Tropan-$3\alpha$-yl Indole-3-carboxylate, 1293·3
($1R,3r,5S$)-Tropan-3-yl ($RS$)-Mandelate, 483·2
(−)-($1R,3r,5S$)-Tropan-3-yl ($S$)-Tropate, 485·1
($1R,3r,5S,8r$)-Tropan-3-yl ($RS$)-Tropate, 476·3
Tropargal, 2350·1
Troparin, 2350·1
Troparin Compositum, 2350·1
Tropatepina, Hidrocloruro de, 491·1
Tropatepine Hydrochloride, 491·1
Tropergen, 2350·1
Tropex, 2350·2
Tropfen gegen Venenbeschwerden, 2350·2
Trophamine, 2350·2
Trophicard, 2350·2
Trophicreme, 2350·2
Trophiderm, 2350·2
Trophigil, 2350·2
Trophires, 2350·2
Trophires Compose, 2350·2
Trophoblastic Tumours, Gestational— *see* Gestational Trophoblastic Tumours, 505·1
Trophoseptine, 2350·2
Trophosphamide, 590·2
Trophox, 2350·2
Trophysan, 2350·2
Tropicacyl, 2350·2
Tropical Blend, 2350·2
Tropical Blend Dark Tanning, 2350·2
Tropical Blend Dry Oil, 2350·2
Tropical Blend Tan Magnifier, 2350·2
Tropical Gold Dark Tanning, 2350·2
Tropical Gold Sunblock, 2350·2
Tropical Gold Sunscreen, 2350·2
Tropical Myrtle, 1673·2
Tropical Pulmonary Eosinophilia— *see* Lymphatic Filariasis, 100·1
Tropical Sprue— *see* Gastro-enteritis, 127·3
Tropicamida, 491·1
Tropicamide, 491·1
Tropicamidum, 491·1
Tropicil Top, 2350·2
Tropico, 2350·2
Tropicol, 2350·3
Tropicur, 2350·3
Tropimil, 2350·3
Tropinal, 2350·3
Tropinom, 2350·3
Tropiovent, 2350·3
Tropisetron, 1293·3
Tropisetrón, Hidrocloruro de, 1293·3
Tropisetron Hydrochloride, 1293·3
Tropisol, 2350·3
Tropium, 2350·3
Tropivag, 2350·3
Tropivag Plus, 2350·3
Tropixal, 2350·3
Tropoderm, 2350·3
Tropyl Mandelate Hydrobromide, 483·2
Tropyn, 2350·3
Trorix, 2350·3
Trosderm, 2350·3
Trosic, 2350·3
Trosid, 2350·3
Trospectomicina, Sulfato de, 274·2
Trospectomycin Sulfate, 274·2
Trospectomycin Sulphate, 274·2
Trospi, 2350·3
Trospio, Cloruro de, 491·2
Trospium Chloride, 491·2
Trosycort, 2350·3
Trosyd, 2350·3
Trosyl, 2350·3
Trova, 2350·3
Trovafloxacin Mesilate, 274·3
Trovafloxacin Mesylate, 274·3
Trovafloxacino, Mesilato de, 274·3
Trovan, 2350·3
Troxerutin, 1688·3
Troxerutina, 1688·3
Troxeven, 2350·3
Troxidone, 379·3
Troxipida, 1294·2
Troxipide, 1294·2
Troxxil, 2350·3
Troxyderm, 2350·3
Trozocina, 2350·4
Trozolet, 2350·4
Trozolite, 2350·4
Trozyman, 2350·4
D-Trp$^{6}$-LHRH, 1341·2
Tru, 2350·4
Tru Compuesto, 2350·4
True Illusion, 2350·4
True Test, 2350·4
Trufree, 2350·4
Trumsal, 2350·4
Truoxin, 2350·4
Truphylline, 2350·4
Truquil, 2350·4
Trusopt, 2350·4
Truxa, 2350·4
Truxa R, 2350·4
Truxal, 2350·4
Truxaletten, 2350·4
α-Truxilline, 1373·3
Truxillo Leaf, 1373·3
Try, 2350·4
Tryasol, 2350·4
Trycam, 2350·4
Trymo, 2350·4
Trypan Blue, 1758·3
Trypanosomiasis, African— *see* African Trypanosomiasis, 599·3
Trypanosomiasis, American— *see* American Trypanosomiasis, 600·1
Trypanum Caeruleum, 1758·3
Tryparsam., 617·3
Tryparsamide, 617·3
Tryparsone, 617·3
Trypsin, 1758·3
Trypsin, Crystallized, 1758·3
Trypsinum, 1758·3
Tryptal, 2351·1
Tryptan, 2351·1
Tryptanol, 2351·1
Tryptil, 2351·1
Tryptine, 2351·1
Tryptizol, 2351·1
Tryptoferm, 2351·1
Tryptomer, 2351·1
Tryptophan, 320·3
DL-Tryptophan, 321·2
L-Tryptophan, 320·3
[6-D-Tryptophan] Luteinising Hormone-releasing Factor, 1341·2
2-L-Tryptophan-3-de-L-leucine-4-de-L-proline-8-L-glutaminebradykinin Potentiator B, 1010·3
Tryptophanum, 320·3
Trysul, 2351·1
TS-1, 586·3
TS-222, 1385·3
TS-408, 1104·1
T's and Blues, 79·3, 442·3
TSAA-291, 1565·2
T/Sal, Neutrogena— *see* Neutrogena T/Sal, 2165·2
T/Scalp, Neutrogena— *see* Neutrogena T/Scalp, 2165·2
TSH, 1341·1
TSPA, 588·1
TSST-1, 149·2
T-Stat, 2351·1
Tsumura Preparations, 2351·1
TTC, 2351·2
TTD, 1681·3
TTD-$B_3$-$B_4$, 2351·2
TTFD, 1454·3
Tuaminoheptane Carbonate, 1132·1
Tuaminoheptane Sulfate, 1132·1
Tuaminoheptane Sulphate, 1132·1
Tuaminoheptano, Sulfato de, 1132·1
Tuaplex, 2351·2
Tuba Root, 1510·1
Tubal Pregnancy— *see* Ectopic Pregnancy, 572·2
Tubarine, 2351·2
Tubazid, 222·2
Tuberculin, 1759·1
Tuberculin for Human Use, Old, 1759·1
Tuberculin, Old, 1759·1
Tuberculin Purified Protein Derivative for Human Use, 1759·1
Tuberculinas, 1759·1
Tuberculins, 1759·1
Tuberculosis, 150·1
Tuberen, 2351·2
Tubergen-Test, 2351·2
Tubersol, 2351·2
Tubersol PPD, 2351·2
Tubertest, 2351·2
Tubetam, 2351·2
Tubial 50B, 2351·2
Tubilux, 2351·2
Tubilysin, 2351·2
Tubocurarina, Cloruro de, 1409·2
Tubocurarine Chloride, 1409·2
*d*-Tubocurarine Chloride, 1409·2
(+)-Tubocurarine Chloride Hydrochloride Pentahydrate, 1409·2
Tubocurarini Chloridum, 1409·2
Tub/Vac/BCG, Dried, 1609·2
Tub/Vac/BCG (Perc), 1609·2
Tucaresol, 1759·3
Tucks, 2351·2
Tuclase, 2351·2
Tudcabil, 2351·2
Tueor, 2351·2
Tuftsin, 1759·3
Tuftsin Acetate, 1759·3
Tuinal, 2351·2
Tukol, 2351·2
Tukson, 2351·2
Tularaemia, 152·1
Tularaemia Vaccines, 1642·1
Tulgrasum Antibiotico, 2351·2
Tulgrasum Cicatrizante, 2351·2
Tulip, 2351·2
Tulipe-R, 2351·2
Tulle Gras Lumiere, 2351·2
Tulle Vaseline, 2351·2
Tulobuterol, Hidrocloruro de, 806·3
Tulobuterol Hydrochloride, 806·3
Tulotract, 2351·2
Tulox, 2351·2
Tumarol, 2351·3
Tumarol Kinderbalsam, 2351·3
Tumarol-N, 2351·3
Tumax, 2351·3
Tumdi, 2351·3
Tumenol Ammonium, 1148·2
Tumour Necrosis Factor, 590·2
Tumour Necrosis Factor Receptor, 145·2
Tumour Necrosis Factor Receptor Fusion Protein, 10·2
1-235 Tumour Necrosis Factor Receptor (Human) Fusion Protein with 236-467-Immunoglobulin G1 (Human γ1-Chain Fc Fragment), 36·3
Tumours, Fungating— *see* Skin Infections, 146·2
Tums, 2351·3
Tums Plus, 2351·3
Tundra, 2351·3
Tundrax, 2351·3
Tuneluz, 2351·3
Tunik, 2351·3
Tunik B12, 2351·3
Tunisian Type Rosemary Oil, 1740·2
Tunitol-BX, 2351·3
Tuosomin, 2351·3
Tupast, 2351·3
Turbatherm, 2351·3
Turbaund, 2351·3
Turbinal, 2351·3
Turbocalcin, 2351·3
Turbogesic, 2351·3
Turbovit, 2351·3
Turexan Preparations, 2351·3
Turfa, 2351·4
Turgoral, 2351·4
Turicard, 2351·4
Turifarm, 2351·4
Turimonit, 2351·4
Turimycin, 2351·4
Turinal, 2351·4
Turineurin, 2351·4
Turiplex, 2351·4
Turisan, 2351·4
Turisteron, 2351·4
Turixin, 2351·4
Turkish Opium, 74·3
Turmeric, 1058·3

Turmeric, Javanese, 1759·3
Turmeric Oleoresin, 1058·3
Turmerik, 2351·4
Turnera, 1679·1
*Turnera diffusa*, 1679·1
Turner's Syndrome, 1317·3
Turoptin, 2351·4
Turpentine Oil, 1760·1
Turpentine Oil, Pinus Pinaster Type, 1760·1
Turpentine Oil, Rectified, 1760·1
Turpentine, Spirits of, 1760·1
Turpentine White Liniment, 2351·4
Turresis, 2351·4
Tusabron, 2351·4
Tusant, 2351·4
Tusben, 2351·4
Tuscalman, 2351·4
Tusco, 2351·4
Tuscolgen, 2351·4
Tusehli, 2351·4
Tuselin Descongestivo, 2351·4
Tuselin Expectorante, 2351·4
Tuseran, 2352·1
Tusibron, 2352·1
Tusibron-DM, 2352·1
Tusical, 2352·1
Tusigen, 2352·1
Tusilen, 2352·1
Tusilen Pediatrico, 2352·1
Tusitato, 2352·1
Tusitinas, 2352·1
Tusminal, 2352·1
Tusno, 2352·1
Tusofren, 2352·1
Tusol, 2352·1
Tusolven, 2352·1
Tusorama, 2352·1
Tuspel, 2352·1
Tuspel Plus, 2352·1
Tuspress, 2352·1
Tusquelin, 2352·1
Tusquit, 2352·1
Tuss, 2352·1
Tuss Hustenstiller, 2352·1
Tussa, 2352·1
Tussafed, 2352·1
Tussafed HC, 2352·2
Tussafed-LA, 2352·2
Tussafin Expectorant, 2352·2
Tussafug, 2352·2
Tuss-Allergine Modified TD, 2352·2
Tussamag Preparations, 2352·2
Tussamed, 2352·2
Tussaminic C, 2352·2
Tussaminic DH, 2352·2
Tussanil Compositum, 2352·2
Tussanil DH, 2352·2
Tussanil N, 2352·2
Tussanil Plain, 2352·2
Tussantiol, 2352·2
Tussanyl, 2352·2
Tussar-2, 2352·2
Tussar DM, 2352·2
Tussar SF, 2352·2
Tusscodin, 2352·3
Tuss-DM, 2352·3
Tussed, 2352·3
Tussefar, 2352·3
Tussend, 2352·3
Tussi-12, 2352·3
Tussi-12 D, 2352·3
Tussi-12D S, 2352·3
Tussibron, 2352·3
Tussicare, 2352·3
Tussicon, 2352·3
Tussidane, 2352·3
Tussidermil N, 2352·3
Tussidex, 2352·3
Tussidoron, 2352·3
Tussidrill, 2352·3
Tussidyl, 2352·3
Tussifed, 2352·3
Tussifen, 2352·3
Tussiflex, 2352·3
Tussiflex D, 2352·3
Tussiflorin Forte, 2352·3
Tussiflorin Hustensaft, 2352·3
Tussiflorin Hustenstiller, 2352·3
Tussiflorin Hustentropfen, 2352·3
Tussiflorin N, 2352·3
Tussigon, 2352·3
Tussilage, 1117·2
*Tussilago farfara*, 1117·2
Tussilene, 2352·3
Tussilinct, 2352·4
Tussiliv, 2352·4
Tussils, 2352·4
Tussimag Codein, 2352·4
Tussimont, 2352·4
Tussin Antitussive, 2352·4
Tussin Antitussive, Expectorant, Decongestant, 2352·4
Tussin Children's DM, 2352·4
Tussin, Diabetic— *see* Diabetic Tussin, 1934·1
Tussin DM, Diabetic— *see* Diabetic Tussin DM, 1934·1
Tussin EX, Diabetic— *see* Diabetic Tussin EX, 1934·1
Tussin Expectorant, 2352·4
TUSSinfant N, 2352·4
Tussinol Preparations, 2352·4
Tussin-Pinho, 2352·4
Tussionex, 2352·4
Tussionex Pennkinetic, 2352·4
Tussi-Organidin DM NR, 2352·4
Tussi-Organidin NR, 2352·4
Tussipax, 2352·4
Tussipax a l'Euquinine, 2352·4
Tussipect, 2352·4
Tussiphane, 2353·1
Tussiplex, 2353·1
Tussirex, 2353·1
Tussis, 2353·1
Tussisana N, 2353·1
Tussisedal, 2353·1
Tussistin, 2353·1
Tussistin N, 2353·1
Tussitot, 2353·1
Tussiverlan, 2353·1
Tussivit, 2353·1
Tussizone, 2353·1
Tuss-LA, 2353·1
Tusso, 2353·1
Tusso Rhinathiol, 2353·1
Tussocal, 2353·1
Tussodan DM, 2353·1
Tussodina, 2353·1
Tussogest Extended-Release, 2353·1
Tussol, 2353·1
Tussolvina, 2353·1
Tussophedrine, 2353·1
Tussoret, 2353·1
Tussoretard SN— *see* Tussoret, 2353·1
Tussoretardin, 2353·1
Tussosedan, 2353·2
Tuss-Tan, 2353·2
Tusstat, 2353·2
Tussucalman, 2353·2
Tussycalm, 2353·2
Tutiverm, 2353·2
Tutofusin Preparations, 2353·2
Tutoplast Dura, 2353·2
Tutoplast Fascia Lata, 2353·2
Tutoseral, 2353·2
Tuttozem N, 2353·2
Tuvirumab, 1617·3
Tux, 2353·2
Tuxi, 2353·2
Tuxidrin, 2353·2
Tuxium, 2353·2
Tuya, 1755·1
Tuzanil, 2353·2
Tuzo, 2353·2
Tuzzil, 2353·3
TV-485, 38·1
T-Vites, 2353·3
TVX-485, 38·1
TVX-1322, 11·3
TVX-Q-7821, 703·1
Twice-A-Day, 2353·3
Twilite, 2353·3
Twina, 2353·3
Twin-K, 2353·3
Twinrix, 2353·3
Twitch, 1676·2
Two Cal HN, 2353·3
TwoCal, 2353·3
TwoCal HN, 2353·3
TWSb/6, 103·1
$TXA_2$, 1511·1
Tybikin, 2353·3
Tycoytycoy, 2353·3
Tydamine, 2353·3
Tyklid, 2353·3
Tylenol Preparations, 2353·3
Tylenol Preparations, Children's— *see* Children's Tylenol Preparations, 1883·1
Tylenol Preparations, Extra Strength— *see* Extra Strength Tylenol Preparations, 1986·2
Tylenol Preparations, Infant's— *see* Infant's Tylenol, 2061·1
Tylenol Preparations, Junior— *see* Junior Strength Tylenol, 2072·2
Tylenol Preparations, Maximum Strength— *see* Maximum Strength Tylenol Preparations, 2116·4
Tylenol Preparations, Multi-Symptom— *see* Multi-Symptom Tylenol Preparations, 2145·1
Tylephen, 2354·1
Tylex, 2354·1
Tylex CD, 2354·1
Tylex Flu, 2354·1
Tylidol, 2354·1
Tyll, 2354·1
Tylosin, 274·3
Tylosin A, 274·3
Tylosin B, 274·3
Tylosin C, 274·3
Tylosin D, 274·3
Tylosin Phosphate, 275·1
Tylosin Tartrate, 275·1
Tylosin Tartrate for Veterinary Use, 275·1
Tylosin for Veterinary Use, 274·3
Tylosinum, 274·3
Tylox, 2354·1
Tyloxapol, 1416·3
Tymazoline Hydrochloride, 1132·1
Tymelyt, 2354·1
Tymol, 2354·1
Tympagesic, 2354·1
Tympalgine, 2354·1
Type 2 Breath Holding Attacks— *see* Anoxic Seizures, 478·2
Typherix, 2354·1
Typhim Vi, 2354·2
Typhoid Fever— *see* Typhoid and Paratyphoid Fever, 152·2
Typhoid Polysaccharide Vaccine, 1642·2
Typhoid and Tetanus Vaccines, 1643·1
Typhoid Vaccine, 1642·2
Typhoid Vaccine, Freeze-dried, 1642·2
Typhoid Vaccine (Live, Oral, Strain Ty 21a), 1642·2
Typhoid Vaccines, 1642·2
Typhoid/Vac, 1642·2
Typhoid/Vac, Dried, 1642·2
Typhoid/Vac(Oral), 1642·2
Typhoid/Vi/Vac, 1642·2
Typhoral, 2354·2
Typhoral L, 2354·2
Typhovax, 2354·2
Typhus Fevers— *see* Typhus, 152·3
Typhus, Tick— *see* Spotted Fevers, 147·1
Typhus Vaccines, 1643·1
Typh-Vax, 2354·2
Tyr, 1451·1
Tyramine Hydrochloride, 1760·1
*p*-Tyramine Hydrochloride, 1760·1
Tyrazol, 2354·2
Tyrcine, 2354·2
Tyrenol, 2354·2
Tyrex, 2354·2
Tyrocaine, 2354·2
Tyrocidine, 275·1
Tyrocombine, 2354·2
Tyrodone, 2354·2
Tyro-Drops, 2354·2
Tyromex, 2354·2
Tyroneomicin, 2354·2
Tyropanoate Sodium, 1067·3
Tyroplus, 2354·2
Tyroqualine, 2354·2
Tyrosamine Hydrochloride, 1760·1
Tyroseng, 2354·2
Tyrosidon, XPT— *see* XPT Tyrosidon, 2388·4
Tyrosidon, XPTM— *see* XPTM Tyrosidon, 2388·4
Tyrosin TU, 2354·2
Tyrosine, 1451·1
L-Tyrosine, 1451·1
Tyrosinum, 1451·1
Tyrosolvetten, 2354·2
Tyrosolvetten-C, 2354·2
Tyrosum, 2354·2
Tyrosur, 2354·2
Tyrothricin, 220·2, 275·1, 2354·3
Tyrothricin Co, 2354·3
Tyrothricin Comp, 2354·3
Tyrothricin Compositum, 2354·3
Tyrothricine + Gramicidine, 2354·3
Tyrothricine Lafran, 2354·3
Tyrothricinum, 275·1
Tyrozets, 2354·3
Tytin, 2354·3
Tyzine, 2354·3
T-ZA, 2354·3
Tzoali, 2354·3
TZU-0460, 1288·1


## U


256U87, 656·1
1592U89, 625·2
U-4527, 1502·1
U-6013, 1105·3
U-6591, 239·2
U-6987, 330·3
U-7800, 1102·3
U-8471, 1106·1
U-9889, 584·1
U-10136, 1512·3
U-10149, 226·2
U-10858, 960·1
U-10997, 1560·1
U-12062, 1515·1
U-14583, 1514·3
U-14583E, 1514·3
U-14624, 1038·2
U-14743, 581·1
U-17323, 1102·2
U-17835, 348·1
U-18409AE, 255·2
U-18496, 529·2
U-18573, 45·3
U-19646, 1392·2
U-19920, 543·1
U-19920A, 543·1
U-21251, 194·2
U-24973A, 306·3
U-25179E, 194·2
U-26225A, 94·3
U-26452, 331·2
U-26597A, 889·2
U-27182, 43·3
U-28288D, 926·3
U-28508, 194·2
U-28774, 703·1
U-31889, 668·3
U-32070E, 1461·2
U-32921, 1514·2
U-32921E, 1514·2
U-33030, 725·3
U-34865, 1099·3
U-36059, 1500·2
U-36384, 1514·2
U-42585, 1707·3
U-42585E, 1707·3
U-42718, 1707·3
U-46785, 1519·2
U-53217, 1516·3
U-53217A, 1516·3
U-54461, 532·2
U-54461S, 532·2
U-57930E, 244·1
U-62840, 1521·2
U-63366, 274·2
U-63366F, 274·2
U-64279A, 182·2
U-64279E, 182·2
U-70226E, 938·1
U-72107A, 344·1
U-72107E, 344·1

U-72791, 173·3
U-72791A, 173·3
U-74006F, 1013·2
U-76252, 178·3
U-76253, 178·3
U-87201, 629·1
U-87201E, 629·1
U-90152S, 630·2
U-100766, 226·3
U-101440E, 564·1
U-140690, 655·3
U Lactin, 2354·3
UAA, 2354·3
Uabaina, 977·3
UAD-Otic, 2354·3
Ubaína, 977·3
Ubenimex, 590·3
Ubenzima, 2354·3
Ubicarden, 2354·3
Ubicardio, 2354·3
Ubicondrial, 2354·3
Ubicor, 2354·3
Ubidecarenona, 1760·2
Ubidecarenone, 1760·2
Ubidecarenonum, 1760·2
Ubidenone, 2354·3
Ubidex, 2354·3
Ubifactor, 2354·3
Ubimaior, 2354·3
Ubiquinone-10, 1760·2
Ubisint, 2354·3
Ubistesin, 2354·3
Ubiten, 2354·3
Ubivis, 2354·4
Ubizol, 2354·4
Ublosid, 2354·4
Ubretid, 2354·4
Ubtest, 2354·4
UCB-1967, 1119·3
UCB-2543, 1126·2
UCB-3412, 697·2
UCB-3928, 1121·2
UCB-3983, 1041·2
UCB-4445, 426·3
UCB-5033, 671·3
UCB-6215, 1732·1
UCB-22059, 366·1
UCB-22073, 961·2
UCB-L059, 366·1
UCB-P071, 427·1
Ucecal, 2354·4
Ucee D, 2354·4
Ucemine PP, 2354·4
Ucephan, 2354·4
Ucerax, 2354·4
UCG-Slide, 2354·4
Ucholine, 2354·4
Ucine, 2354·4
Ucort, 2354·4
UDC, 2354·4
UDCA, 1760·3, 2354·4
UDCG-115, 983·1
Udesospray, 2354·4
Udicil, 2354·4
Udiliv, 2354·4
Udima, 2354·4
Udima Ery, 2354·4
UDPG, 1674·3
Udramil, 2354·4
Udrik, 2354·4
UF-021, 1521·3
Ufarin, 2354·4
Ufexil, 2354·4
Ufocard, 2354·4
Ufonitren, 2354·4
Ufor, 2354·4
UFT, 586·3, 2354·4
Uftoral, 2355·1
Ugal, 2355·1
Ugrilon, 2355·1
Ugurol, 2355·1
UH-AC-62, 56·1
UH-AC-62XX, 56·1
Ujostabil, 2355·1
UK-2964-18, 110·1
UK-4271, 110·3
UK-14304-18, 876·3
UK-20349, 409·3
UK-33274-27, 908·3
UK-48340-11, 862·1
UK-48340-26, 862·1
UK-49858, 398·1
UK-61689, 615·3
UK-61689-2, 615·3
UK-67994, 105·1
UK-68798, 906·3
UK-69578, 879·1
UK-76654-2, 491·3
UK-79300, 879·1
UK-88525, 481·1
UK-92480-10, 1744·2
UK-109496, 411·2
UK-116044-04, 467·1
UK-124114, 114·1
Ukidan, 2355·1
UL 250, 2355·1
U-Lactin Foot Cream, 2355·1
U-Lactin Forte, 2355·1
Ularitide, 964·2
Ulcaid, 2355·1
Ulcar, 2355·1
Ulcecur, 2355·1
Ulcedin, 2355·1
Ulcedine, 2355·1
Ulcedor, 2355·1
Ulcefate, 2355·1
Ulcefor, 2355·1
Ulcegel, 2355·1
Ulcekon, 2355·1
Ulcelac, 2355·1
Ulcemet, 2355·1
Ulcemex, 2355·2
Ulcenon, 2355·2
Ulcepin, 2355·2
Ulcer— *see* Wounds and Ulcers, 1139·2
Ulcer, Aphthous— *see* Mouth Ulceration, 1245·1
Ulcer, Duodenal— *see* Peptic Ulcer Disease, 1246·3
Ulcer, Gastric— *see* Peptic Ulcer Disease, 1246·3
Ulcer, NSAID-associated— *see* Peptic Ulcer Disease, 1246·3
Ulcer, Peptic— *see* Peptic Ulcer Disease, 1246·3
Ulcerac, 2355·2
Ulceracid, 2355·2
Ulceral, 2355·2
Ulceran, 2355·2
Ulcerase, 2355·2
Ulceration, Mouth— *see* Mouth Ulceration, 1245·1
Ulceration, Oral— *see* Mouth Ulceration, 1245·1
Ulceration, Skin, Infections in— *see* Skin Infections, 146·2
Ulcerative Colitis— *see* Inflammatory Bowel Disease, 1243·3
Ulcerease, 2355·2
Ulcerfen, 2355·2
Ulceridine, 2355·2
Ulcerim, 2355·2
Ulcerit, 2355·2
Ulcerlmin, 2355·2
Ulcermin, 2355·2
Ulcerocin, 2355·2
Ulcerol, 2355·2
Ulcerone, 2355·2
Ulcerosol, 2355·2
Ulcertec, 2355·2
Ulcesep, 2355·2
Ulcesium, 2355·2
Ulcestop, 2355·2
Ulcetrax, 2355·2
Ulcevarin, 2355·2
Ulcex, 2355·2
Ulcidine, 2355·3
Ulcim, 2355·3
Ulcimet, 2355·3
Ulcin, 2355·3
Ulcinax, 2355·3
Ulcirex, 2355·3
Ulcitag, 2355·3
Ulcitrat, 2355·3
Ulco-cyl Ho-Len-Complex, 2355·3
Ulcoderma, 2355·3
Ulcodina, 2355·3
Ulcofam, 2355·3
Ulcogant, 2355·3
Ulcoid, 2355·3
Ulcoid-Zol, 2355·3
Ulcolind Amoxi, 2355·3
Ulcolind $H_2$, 2355·3
Ulcolind Metro, 2355·3
Ulcolind Rani, 2355·3
Ulcolind Wismut, 2355·3
Ulcomedina, 2355·3
Ulcomet, 2355·3
Ulcometin, 2355·3
Ulcometion, 2355·3
Ulconar, 2355·3
Ulcopir, 2355·4
Ulcoprotect, 2355·4
Ulcoren, 2355·4
Ulcosafe, 2355·4
Ulcosal, 2355·4
Ulcostad, 2355·4
Ulcotenal, 2355·4
Ulcotenk, 2355·4
Ulcotruw N, 2355·4
Ulcourona, 2355·4
Ulc-Out, 2355·4
Ulcozol, 2355·4
Ulcrafate, 2355·4
Ulcrast, 2355·4
Ulcrux, 2355·4
Ulcubloc, 2355·4
Ulcufato, 2355·4
Ulcu-Pasc, 2355·4
Ulcurilen, 2355·4
Ulcurilen N, 2355·4
Ulcusan, 2355·4
Ulcyte, 2355·4
Uldadin, 2355·4
Uldapril, 2355·4
Ulfamet, 2355·4
Ulfon, 2355·4
Ulgarine, 2355·4
Ulgastrin, 2355·4
Ulgastrin Bis, 2356·1
Ulgastrin Neu, 2356·1
Ulgel, 2356·1
Ulgescum, 2356·1
Ulgut, 2356·1
Ulinastatin, 1760·2
Ulinastatina, 1760·2
Ulis, 2356·1
Ulkodin, 2356·1
Ulkowis, 2356·1
Ullus Preparations, 2356·1
Ulmaria, 1710·1
Ulmus, 1747·1
Ulmus Fulva, 1747·1
*Ulmus fulva*, 1747·1
*Ulmus rubra*, 1747·1
Ulobetasol Propionate, 1111·3
Ulobetasol, Propionato de, 1111·3
Ulogen, 2356·1
Ulone, 2356·1
Ulpax, 2356·1
Ulprazole, 2356·1
ULR-LA, 2356·1
Ulsal, 2356·1
Ulsanic, 2356·1
Ulsaven, 2356·1
Ulsen, 2356·1
Ulserch, 2356·1
Ulserral, 2356·1
Ultacit, 2356·1
Ultacite, 2356·1
Ultak, 2356·1
Ultane, 2356·1
Ultec, 2356·2
Ultexiv, 2356·2
Ulticadex, 2356·2
Ultidin, 2356·2
Ultilac N, 2356·2
Ultimag, 2356·2
Ultiva, 2356·2
Ultra, 2356·2
Ultra Adsorb, 2356·2
Ultra Augenschutz, 2356·2
Ultra Chloraseptic, 2356·2
Ultra, Clearasil— *see* Clearasil Ultra, 1892·1
Ultra Derm, 2356·2
Ultra Energizer, 2356·2
Ultra Heartburn Relief, 2356·2
Ultra Mide, 2356·2
Ultra Strength Megadophilus, 2356·2
Ultra Tears, 2356·2
Ultra Vita Time, 2356·2
Ultra Vita-Min, 2356·2
Ultrabas, 2356·2
Ultrabase, 2356·2
Ultrabeta, 2356·2
Ultrabion, 2356·2
Ultrabion Balsamico, 2356·2
Ultrabiotic, 2356·2
ULTRAbrom, 2356·2
Ultrac, 2356·2
Ultrac E, 2356·3
Ultrac Q10, 2356·3
Ultracain Preparations, 2356·3
Ultracaine D-S, 2356·3
Ultracal, 2356·3
Ultracalcium, 2356·3
Ultracarbon, 2356·3
Ultracare, 2356·3
UltraCare, 2356·3
UltraCare Daily Cleaner, 2356·3
Ultracef, 2356·3
Ultracet, 2356·3
Ultracillin, 2356·3
Ultra-Clear-A-Med, 2356·3
Ultracorten H, 2356·4
Ultracortene-H, 2356·4
Ultracortenol, 2356·4
Ultracortin, 2356·4
Ultracur S, 2356·4
Ultra-Demoplas, 2356·4
Ultraderm, 2356·4
Ultraderme, 2356·4
Ultradermis, 2356·4
Ultradina, 2356·4
Ultradol, 2356·4
Ultrafen, 2356·4
Ultraflu, 2356·4
Ultrafort, 2356·4
Ultra-Freeda, 2356·4
Ultragin, 2356·4
Ultra-K, 2356·4
Ultralan, 2356·4
Ultralan M, 2356·4
Ultralan-crinale, 2356·4
Ultralanum Plain, 2356·4
Ultralente, 2356·4
Ultralente, Insulin, 334·2
Ultralente MC, 2357·1
Ultra-Levura, 2357·1
Ultra-Levure, 2357·1
Ultram, 2357·1
Ultra-Mag, 2357·1
Ultra-Mg, 2357·1
Ultramicina, 2357·1
Ultramicina Plus, 2357·1
Ultramidol, 2357·1
Ultramol, 2357·1
Ultramop, 2357·1
Ultramox, 2357·1
Ultran, 2357·1
Ultra-Natal, 2357·1
Ultrapenil, 2357·1
Ultraplex 31, 2357·1
Ultraproct, 2357·1
Ultraquin, 2357·1
Ultraquin Plain, 2357·1
Ultra-R, 2357·1
Ultra-Rich, 2357·1
Ultrase, 2357·2
Ultrasep, 2357·2
Ultrasept, 2357·2
Ultrasine, 2357·2
Ultrasol-F, 2357·2
Ultrasol-S, 2357·2
Ultrassol, 2357·2
Ultratard, 2357·2
Ultratard HM, 2357·2
Ultrathon, 2357·2
Ultravate, 2357·2
Ultra-Vinca, 2357·2
Ultraviolet Light, 1136·3
Ultraviral, 2357·2

Ultraviral Duo, 2357·2
Ultraviro C, 2357·2
Ultravisin, 2357·2
Ultravist, 2357·2
Ultravite, 2357·2
Ultravite with Minerals— *see* Ultravite, 2357·2
Ultrazon N, 2357·2
Ultrazyme, 2357·2
Ultren, 2357·2
Ultreon, 2357·2
Ultrex, 2357·2
Ultrimin, 2357·2
Ulxit, 2357·2
Ulzec, 2357·3
Ulzol, 2357·3
UM-952, 21·3
UM Instante, 2357·3
Um Minuto, 2357·3
Um Segundo, 2357·3
Uman Preparations, 2357·3
Umasam, 2357·3
Umatrope, 2357·3
Umbradol, 2357·3
Umbrium, 2357·3
Umckaloabo, 2357·3
Umine, 2357·3
Umizan, 2357·3
Umoder, 2357·3
Umolit, 2357·3
Umoril, 2357·3
Umprel, 2357·3
Umuline Preparations, 2357·3
Umya, 1666·1
Uña de Gato, 2357·4
Unacid, 2357·4
Unacid PD, 2357·4
Unacil, 2357·4
Unacim, 2357·4
Unakalm, 2357·4
Un-Alfa, 2357·4
Unalmes, 2357·4
Unamine, 2357·4
Unamol, 2357·4
UN-Aspirin, 2357·4
Unasyn, 2357·4
Unasyna, 2357·4
Unasyn-S, 2357·4
Unat, 2357·4
Unathen, 2357·4
Unatol, 2357·4
Unava, 2357·4
Uncadol, 2357·4
*Uncaria gambier*, 1668·3
Uncariae Uncis cum Ramulus, 1668·3
Undebenzophene, 1195·3
Undecenoic Acid, 410·3
Undec-10-enoic Acid, 410·3
Undecenoic Acid Monoethanolamide, 411·1
Undecilato de Nandrolona, 1561·3
Undecilato de Testosterona, 1570·1
Undecilenato de Calcio, 410·3
Undecilenato de Neomicina, 235·2
Undecilenato de Zinc, 411·1
Undecilénico, Ácido, 410·3
Undecilinato de Zinco, 411·1
Undecyl, 2357·4
Undecylenic Acid, 410·3
Undecylenicum, Acidum, 410·3
Undelenic, 2357·4
Underan, 2358·1
Undestor, 2358·1
Undex, 2358·1
Undulant Fever— *see* Brucellosis, 122·3
Unergol, 2358·1
Unex Amarum, 2358·1
Unexym MD S, 2358·1
Unexym Mono, 2358·1
Ung Vernleigh, 2358·1
Ungel, 2358·1
Unguentacid, 2358·1
Unguentine, 2358·1
Unguentine Plus, 2358·1
Unguento Callicida Naion, 2358·1
Unguento Dermico Antibiotico, 2358·1
Unguento Leon, 2358·1
Unguento Morry, 2358·1
Unguentolan, 2358·1
Unguentum Bossi, 2358·1
Unguentum Cardiacum Kneipp, Kneipp Herzsalbe— *see* Kneipp Herzsalbe Unguentum Cardiacum Kneipp, 2081·2
Unguentum Lactisol, 2358·1
Unguentum Lymphaticum, 2358·1
Unguentum M, 2358·1
Unguentum Truw, 2358·1
Ungvita, 2358·1
Uni Amox, 2358·1
Uni B Complex Poliv, 2358·1
Uni Bromazepax, 2358·1
Uni Carbamaz, 2358·2
Uni Cetotifen, 2358·2
Uni Dexametason, 2358·2
Uni Diazepax, 2358·2
Uni Doxiciclin, 2358·2
Uni Gliben, 2358·2
Uni Haloper, 2358·2
Uni Hioscin, 2358·2
Uni Masdil, 2358·2
Uni Mist, 2358·2
Uni Propralol, 2358·2
Uni Salve, 2358·2
Uni Vir, 2358·2
Uni-Ace, 2358·2
Unibac, 2358·2
Unibar, 2358·2
Unibaryt, 2358·2
Unibaryt— *see* Barilux, 1828·4
Unibaryt-R, 2358·2
Unibase, 2358·2
Uni-Bent Cough, 2358·2
Unibios Simple, 2358·2
Unicaine, 2358·2
Unical, 2358·2
Unicalm, 2358·2
Unicap, 2358·2
Unicap M, 2358·2
Unicarbazan, 2358·2
Unicef, 2358·2
Uni-Check, 2358·2
Unichew, 2358·2
Unichol, 2358·2
Unicid, 2358·2
Unicide, 2358·3
Unicilin, 2358·3
Unicilina, 2358·3
Uniclar, 2358·3
Uniclor, 2358·3
Uni-Colex, 2358·3
Unicomplex-T & M, 2358·3
Unicontin, 2358·3
Unicordium, 2358·3
Unidasa, 2358·3
Uni-Decon, 2358·3
Uniderm, 2358·3
Unidermo, 2358·3
Unidie, 2358·3
Unidixina, 2358·3
Unidor, 2358·3
Unidose, 2358·3
Unidox, 2358·3
Unidrol, 2358·3
Uni-Dur, 2358·3
Unienzyme C MPS, 2358·3
Unif, 2358·3
Uni-Febrin, 2358·3
Uni-Fedra Compound, 2358·3
Unifenobarb, 2358·3
Unifer, 2358·3
Unifiber, 2358·4
Unifibre, 2358·4
Unifilin, 2358·4
Uniflex, 2358·4
Uniflex-N, 2358·4
Uniflox, 2358·4
Uniflu & Gregovite C, 2358·4
Uniflu with Gregovite C, 2358·4
Unifluid, 2358·4
Unifyl, 2358·4
Unigamol, 2358·4
Unigan, 2358·4
Unigo, 2358·4
Uni-Gold HCG, 2358·4
Unigrip, 2358·4
Unigyn, 2358·4
Unihep, 2358·4
Uni-Kaotin, 2358·4
Uniket, 2358·4
Unik-Zoru, 2358·4
Unilair, 2358·4
Unilan, 2358·4
Unilarm, 2358·4
Uniloc, 2358·4
Unilong, 2358·4
Unilux, 2358·4
Uni-Ma, 2358·4
Unimaalox, 2359·1
Unimax, 2359·1
Unimazole, 2359·1
Unimer, 2359·1
Unimest, 2359·1
Unimezol, 2359·1
Unimicebrina, 2359·1
Unimol, 2359·1
Unimox, 2359·1
Uniparin, 2359·1
Unipen, 2359·1
Unipexil, 2359·1
Uni-Phen, 2359·1
Uni-Pholco, 2359·1
Uniphyl, 2359·1
Uniphyllin, 2359·1
Uniphyllin Continus, 2359·1
Unipine XL, 2359·1
Uniplant, 1562·1
Uniplex, 2359·1
Uniplus, 2359·1
Unipolar Disorder, 278·1
Uniprazol, 2359·1
Unipred, 2359·1
Unipril, 2359·1
Unipridiur, 2359·1
Uniprofen, 2359·1
Unique PH, 2359·1
Unique Plus, 2359·1
Uniquin, 2359·2
Uni-Ramine, 2359·2
Uni-Ramine CE, 2359·2
Uni-Ramine Expectorant, 2359·2
Uniren, 2359·2
Uniretic, 2359·2
Unirhinol, 2359·2
Uniroid-HC, 2359·2
Unisal, 2359·2
Uniscrub, 2359·2
Unisedil, 2359·2
Unisedyl, 2359·2
Unisept, 2359·2
Unisept, Sterets— *see* Sterets Unisept, 2306·3
Unisoil, 2359·2
Unisol, 2359·2
Unisolve, 2359·2
Unisom Preparations, 2359·2
Unisom SleepGels, Maximum Strength— *see* Maximum Strength Unisom SleepGels, 2116·4
Unisom-C, 2359·2
Unison Enema, 2359·2
Unison Ointment, 2359·2
Unistep HCG, 2359·2
Unistin, 2359·2
Unitable, 2359·3
Unithiol, 1055·3
Unithroid, 2359·3
Unitifed, 2359·3
Unitimoftol, 2359·3
Unitinase, 2359·3
Unitiol, 1055·3
Unitone, 2359·3
Uni-Tranxene, 2359·3
Unitrexate, 2359·3
Unitril, 2359·3
Unitrim, 2359·3
Unitrol, 2359·3
Unitul Complex, 2359·3
Unitulle, 2359·3
Unituss, 2359·3
Unituss HC, 2359·3
Uni-tussin, 2359·3
Uni-tussin DM, 2359·3
Unival, 2359·3
Univasc, 2359·3
Uni-Vasin, 2359·3
Univate, 2359·3
Univer, 2359·3
Universal Antidote, 1030·3, 1751·3
Universal Concentration Tablets, 2359·3
Universal Earache Drops, 2359·3
Universal Eye Drops, 2359·3
Universal Nasal Drops, 2359·4
Universal Throat Lollies, 2359·4
University of Wisconsin Solution, 414·2, 851·3
Univol, 2359·4
Uniwarfin, 2359·4
Uniwash, 2359·4
UniXan, 2359·4
Unixime, 2359·4
Unizen, 2359·4
Unizink, 2359·4
Unizitro, 2359·4
Unizol, 2359·4
Unizuric, 2359·4
Unizyme, 2359·4
Unkei-to, Tsumura— *see* Tsumura Unkei-to, 2351·2
Unmodified Insulin, 334·2
UnoCardil, 2359·4
Uno-Ciclo, 2359·4
Uno-Enantone, 2359·4
Uno-Lin, 2359·4
Unoplex, 2359·4
Unoprost, 2359·4
Unoprostona de Isopropilo, 1521·3
Unoprostone Isopropyl, 1521·3
Unorox, 2359·4
Unotex N Feminin, 2359·4
Unotex N Masculin, 2359·4
Uno-Vit, 2359·4
Unprozy, 2359·4
Unsayna, 2359·4
Untano, 2359·4
Untigex, 2359·4
Unwind Herbal Nytol, 2359·4
UO, 2359·4
Uonin, 2359·4
UP-57, 481·3
UP-83, 67·1
UP-164, 60·1
UP-339-01, 883·1
Up Mep, 2360·1
U-Pasta, 2360·1
Upderm, 2360·1
Upelva, 2360·1
Upfen, 2360·1
Upha C, 2360·1
Upha Dextrophan, 2360·1
Upha Lozenges, 2360·1
Uphacol, 2360·1
Uphadeq, 2360·1
Uphadyl CD, 2360·1
Uphadyl Forte, 2360·1
Uphageron, 2360·1
Uphalexin, 2360·1
Uphalyte, 2360·1
Uphamol, 2360·1
Uphanormin, 2360·1
Uphastatin, 2360·1
Uphavit Plus, 2360·1
Uphaxicam, 2360·1
Uphazhexol, 2360·1
Uprima, 2360·1
U-Proxyn, 2360·1
Upsa C, 2360·1
Upsa Plus, 2360·1
Upsadex, 2360·1
Upsalgin C, 2360·1
Upsalgina, 2360·1
Upsalgine, 2360·1
Upsalgin-N, 2360·2
Upsavit C, 2360·2
Upset Stomach, 2360·2
Upset Stomach, Hylands— *see* Hylands Upset Stomach, 2052·3
UR-112, 885·1
UR-1501, 1017·3
UR-1521, 44·2
UR-4056, 400·3
UR-12592, 440·3
Uracid, 2360·2
Uracil, 637·3, 2360·2
Uracil Arabinoside, 543·3
Uracil Riboside, 1760·3
Uracil-6-carboxylic Acid, 1724·3

Uractazide, 2360·2
Uractone, 2360·2
Uractonum, 2360·2
Uracyst-S, 2360·2
Uracyst-S Test Kit, 2360·2
Ural, 2360·2
Uralgin, 2360·2
Uralyt, 2360·2
Uralyt Urato, 2360·2
Uralyt-U, 2360·2
Uramilon, 2360·2
Uramox, 2360·2
Uranin, 1689·1
Urantin, 2360·2
Urantoin, 2360·2
Urapidil, 1018·1
Urapidil Fumarate, 1018·2
Urapidil, Hidrocloruro de, 1018·1
Urapidil Hydrochloride, 1018·1
Uraplex, 2360·2
Urapro, 2360·2
Urarthone, 2360·2
Urasal, 2360·2
Urasin, 2360·2
Urate Overproduction— *see* Gout and Hyperuricaemia, 412·1
Urate Oxidase, 418·3
Urate Underexcretion— *see* Gout and Hyperuricaemia, 412·1
Urazamide, 1760·3
Urazol, 2360·2
Urbadan, 2360·2
Urbal, 2360·2
Urbanil, 2360·3
Urbanol, 2360·3
Urbanyl, 2360·3
Urbason, 2360·3
Urdes, 2360·3
Urdox, 2360·3
Urdrim, 2360·3
Urea, 1162·2
Urea Cycle Disorders— *see* Hyperammonaemia, 1421·2
Urea Hydrochloride, Quinine and, 1737·2
Urea Hydrogen Peroxide, 1195·3
Urea Peroxide, 1195·3
Ureacin, 2360·3
Ureadin Preparations, 2360·3
Ureaphil, 2360·3
Urea-Quinine, 1737·2
Ureata S, 2360·3
Urecare, 2360·3
Urecholine, 2360·3
Urecrem, 2360·3
Urecrem Hidro, 2360·3
Urederm, 2360·3
Uree, 2360·3
Uregyt, 2360·3
Ureia, 1162·2
5-Ureidohydantoin, 1141·3
5-Ureidoimidazolidine-2,4-dione, 1141·3
Ureidopenicillins, 119·1
Ureina, 2360·3
Urekolin, 2360·3
Urelief Plus, 2360·3
Urelium Neu, 2360·4
Urelle, 2360·4
Urem, 2360·4
Uremiase, 2360·4
Uremide, 2360·4
Uremol, 2360·4
Uremol-HC, 2360·4
Uren, 2360·4
Ureotop, 2360·4
Ureotop + VAS, 2360·4
Urequin, 2360·4
Ureteral Colic— *see* Biliary and Renal Colic, 4·3
Urethral Syndrome— *see* Urinary-tract Infections, 153·1
Urethritis, 152·3
Uretil, 2360·4
Uretren Comp, 2360·4
Uretron, 2360·4
Ureum, 1162·2
Urex, 2360·4
Urfadyn PL, 2360·4
Urfadyne, 2360·4
Urfamycin, 2360·4
Urfamycine, 2360·4
Urgendol, 2360·4
Urgenin, 2360·4
Urgenin Cucurbitae Oleum, 2360·4
Urgenin, Neo— *see* Neo Urgenin, 2156·4
Urgenine, 2360·4
Urginea, 1130·3
*Urginea maritima*, 1509·3
Urginol, 2360·4
Urgis, 2360·4
Urgo Activ Huhneraugenpflaster, 2361·1
Urgocall, 2361·1
Urgofroid, 2361·1
Urgomed, 2361·1
Urgosorb, 2361·1
Urgotul, 2361·1
Uriage Preparations, 2361·1
Uri-Alk, 2361·1
Uribac, 2361·1
Uriben, 2361·1
Uribenz, 2361·1
Uricad, 2361·1
Uricalm, 2361·1
Uri-Care, Extralife— *see* Extralife Uri-Care, 1986·3
Uricasa, 418·3
Uricase, 418·3
Uricemil, 2361·1
Uricodue, 2361·1
Uriconorme, 2361·1
Uricont, 2361·1
Uricosal, 2361·2
Uricovac, 2361·2
Uricozyme, 2361·2
Uridactone, 2361·2
Urideal, 2361·2
Uridina, 1760·3
Uridina Trifosfato, 1760·3
Uridine, 1760·3
Uridine 5′-(Tetrahydrogen Triphosphate), 1760·3
Uridine Triphosphate, 1760·3
Uridine Triphosphoric Acid, 1760·3
Uridine-5′-diphosphoglucose Sodium, 1674·3
Uridon Modified, 2361·2
Uridoz, 2361·2
Uriduct, 2361·2
Uriflex Preparations, 2361·2
Uri-Flor, 2361·2
Urifron, 2361·2
Uriginex Urtica, 2361·2
Urigon, 2361·2
Urigram, 2361·2
Urihesive, 2361·2
Urikal, 2361·2
Uriken, 2361·2
Urilin, 2361·2
Urimar-T, 2361·2
Urimax, 2361·2
Urinary Incontinence— *see* Urinary Incontinence and Retention, 476·1
Urinary Retention— *see* Urinary Incontinence and Retention, 476·1
Urinary-tract Infections, 153·1
Urinase, 2361·2
Urinastatin, 1760·2
Urination Disorders— *see* Micturition Disorders, 475·3
Urinefrol, 2361·2
Urinex, 2361·2
Urinorm, 2361·2
Urinox, 2361·2
Urion, 2361·3
Uripiser, 2361·3
Uri-Plus Rubia, 2361·3
Uriprim, 2361·3
Uripurinol, 2361·3
Urirex-K, 2361·3
Urisan, 2361·3
Uriscreen, 2361·3
Urisec, 2361·3
Urised, 2361·3
Urisept NF, 2361·3
Uriseptic, 2361·3
Urisor, 2361·3
Urispadol, 2361·3
Urispas, 2361·3
Uristix, 2361·3
Uristix 2, 2361·3
Uristix 4, 2361·3
Uritab, 2361·3
Uritact, 2361·3
Uritest, 2361·3
Uritest 2, 2361·3
Uritracin, 2361·3
Uritrat, 2361·3
Uritrate, 2361·3
Urival, 2361·3
Urizal, 2361·3
Urizine, 2361·3
Urizone, 2361·3
Urlix, 2361·3
Urmidin, 2361·3
Uro 3000, 2361·4
Uro Angiografin, 2361·4
Uro Bac Septin, 2361·4
Uro Bactrim, 2361·4
Uro Batrox, 2361·4
Uro Blue, 2361·4
Uro Duoctrim, 2361·4
Uro Fink, 2361·4
Uro Furan, 2361·4
Uro Heractrim, 2361·4
Uro Septoprin, 2361·4
Uroalquine, 2361·4
Uroanthelone, 1294·2
Urobac, 2361·4
Urobacid, 2361·4
Urobactam, 2361·4
Uro-Bacteracin, 2361·4
Urobactrex, 2361·4
Uro-Bactrim, 2361·4
Uro-Baxapril, 2361·4
Urobine, 2361·4
Urobioctrin, 2361·4
Urobiotic, 2361·4
Urobiotic-250, 2361·4
Uroc, 2361·4
Urocalun, 2361·4
Urocarb, 2361·4
Urocarf, 2361·4
Urocaudal, 2361·4
Urocaudal Tiazida, 2361·4
Uro-Cephoral, 2361·4
Urochinasi, 2361·4
Urochloralic Acid, 684·3
Urocit-K, 2361·4
Urocrasina, 2362·1
Urocridin, 2362·1
Uroctal, 2362·1
Uroctrin, 2362·1
Urodene, 2362·1
Urodie, 2362·1
Urodil Blasen-Nieren Arzneitee, 2362·1
Urodil Phyto, 2362·1
Urodilatin, 964·2
Urodin, 2362·1
Urodonal, 2362·1
Urodyn, 2362·1
Uroenterone, 1294·2
Urofar, 2362·1
Urofen, 2362·1
Uroflan, 2362·1
Uroflo, 2362·1
Uroflox, 2362·1
Urofolitropina, 1342·1
Urofollitrophin, 1342·1
Urofollitropin, 1342·1
Urofollitropinum, 1342·1
Urofos, 2362·1
Urofossat, 2362·1
Urogal, 2362·1
Urogastrone, 1294·2
Urogem, 2362·1
Urogesic, 2362·1
Urogesic Blue, 2362·1
Urogliss, 2362·1
Urogliss-S, 2362·1
Urogonadotrophin, 1330·1
Urogotan A, 2362·1
Urografin, 2362·1
Urografin Meglumin, 2362·2
Urografina, 2362·2
Urografine, 2362·2
Urogram, 2362·2
Urogutt, 2362·2
Urokinase, 1018·2
Urokinasum, 1018·2
Urokit, 2362·2
Uroknop, 2362·2
Uro-KP-Neutral, 2362·2
Urol Mono, 2362·2
Uro-L 90 N, 2362·2
Urolene Blue, 2362·2
Uro-Leotrim, 2362·2
Uro-Linfol, 2362·2
Urolithico, 2362·2
Urologicum PMD, 2362·2
Urologicum-Echtroplex, 2362·2
Urologin, 2362·2
Urolosin, 2362·2
Urolux Retro, 2362·2
Uro-Mag, 2362·2
Uromethin, 2362·2
Uro-Micinovo, 2362·2
Uromil, 2362·2
Uromiro Preparations, 2362·2
Uromiron, 2362·2
Uromitexan, 2362·2
Uromix, 2362·3
Uromont, 2362·3
Uro-Munal, 2362·3
Uromykol, 2362·3
Uronalin, 2362·3
Uro-Nebacetin N, 2362·3
Uronefrex, 2362·3
Uroneotrim, 2362·3
Uronid, 2362·3
Uronor, 2362·3
Uronorm, 2362·3
Uronovag, 2362·3
Uropac, 2362·3
Uro-Pasc, 2362·3
Uro-Phosphate, 2362·3
Urophytum, 2362·3
Uropielon, 2362·3
Uropimid, 2362·3
Uropimide, 2362·3
Uropipedil, 2362·3
Uropipemid, 2362·3
Uropirite, 2362·3
Uroplant, 2362·3
Uroplex, 2362·3
Uropol, 2362·3
Uro-POS, 2362·3
Uro-Pract, 2362·3
Uro-Pract N, 2362·3
Uroprot, 2362·4
Uropurat, 2362·4
Uropyrine, 2362·4
Uroqid-Acid, 2362·4
Uroquidan, 2362·4
Uroquina, 2362·4
Uroquinasa, 1018·2
Urorenal, 2362·4
Uro-Ripirin, 2362·4
Urosalin, 2362·4
Urosan, 2362·4
Uroselect, 2362·4
Uroseptal, 2362·4
Uroseptin, 2362·4
Uro-Septiolan, 2362·4
Uroseptol, 2362·4
Urosetic, 2362·4
Urosin, 2362·4
Urosiphon, 2362·4
Urospasmon, 2362·4
Urospasmon Sine, 2362·4
Urostei, 2362·4
Uro-Stilloson, 2362·4
Urostix, 2362·4
Urosulphanum, 257·3
Uro-Tablinen, 2362·4
Uro-Tainer Preparations, 2362·4
Urotal, 2363·1
Uro-Tarivid, 2363·1
Urotem, 2363·1
Uro-Teutrim, 2363·1
Urothelial Cancer— *see* Malignant Neoplasms of the Bladder, 512·3
Urotonine, 2363·1
Urotoxicity, Cytotoxic, 1041·3
Urotractan, 2363·1
Urotractin, 2363·1

Urotrate, 2363·1
Urotricef, 2363·1
Urotril, 2363·1
Urotrol, 2363·1
Urotropine, 230·1
Urotruw S, 2363·1
Uroval, 2363·1
Uro-Vaxom, 2363·1
Urovec, 2363·1
Urovison, 2363·1
Urovisona, 2363·1
Uroxacin, 2363·1
Uroxate, 2363·1
UroXatral, 2363·1
Uroxazol, 2363·1
Uroxazol-N, 2363·1
Uroxin, 2363·1
Uroxina, 2363·1
Urozyl-SR, 2363·1
Ursacol, 2363·2
Ursilon, 2363·2
Ursinus Inlay-Tabs, 2363·2
Urso, 2363·2
Urso Mix, 2363·2
Ursobil, 2363·2
Ursobilane, 2363·2
Ursochol, 2363·2
Ursodamor, 2363·2
Ursodeoxicólico, Ácido, 1760·3
Ursodeoxycholic Acid, 1660·3, 1760·3
Ursodesoxycholic Acid, 1760·3
Ursodexil, 2363·2
Ursodiol, 1760·3, 2363·2
Ursofalk, 2363·2
Ursofalk + Chenofalk, 2363·2
Ursoflor, 2363·2
Ursogal, 2363·2
Ursolac, 2363·2
Ursolin, 2363·2
Ursolisin, 2363·2
Ursolit, 2363·2
Ursolite, 2363·2
Ursolvan, 2363·2
Urson, 2363·2
Ursoproge, 2363·2
Ursosan, 2363·2
Ursotan, 2363·2
Urtias, 2363·2
Urtica, 1762·1
*Urtica dioica*, 1762·1
Urtica Plus, 2363·2
Urtica Plus N, 2363·2
*Urtica urens*, 1762·1
Urticalcin, 2363·2
Urticaprostat Uno, 2363·3
Urticaria— *see* Urticaria and Angioedema, 1138·3
Urticur, 2363·3
Urtigen, 2363·3
Urtikalma, 2363·3
Urtipret, 2363·3
Urtivac, 2363·3
Urtivit, 2363·3
Urumogi, 1666·1
Urupan, 2363·3
Urushiol, 1738·1
Urzac, 2363·3
Usanimals, 2363·3
Usar Fibras, 2363·3
Usedent, 2363·3
Useton, 2363·3
Usix, 2363·3
Uskan, 2363·3
Usnea Barbata, 1762·1
*Usnea barbata*, 1762·1
Usneabasan, 2363·3
Usnic Acid, 1762·1
Usnicon, 2363·3
U-Spa, 2363·3
Ustilakehl, 2363·3
Ustimon, 2363·3
Ustiosan, 2363·3
UT-15, 1521·2
UT 380, 2363·3
Utabon, 2363·3
Utefos, 2363·3
Uteplex, 2363·3
Utergin, 2363·3
Uterine, 2363·3
Uterine Bleeding, Dysfunctional— *see* Menorrhagia, 1567·3
Uterine Fibroids— *see* Fibroids, 1326·1
Uterovarol, 2363·3
Uticox, 2363·3
Utidol, 2363·3
Utilin, 2363·3
Utilin H, 2363·4
Utilin N, 2363·4
Utilin S, 2363·4
Utin, 2363·4
Utinor, 2363·4
Utira, 2363·4
Utisept, 2363·4
Utk, 2363·4
Utolid, 2363·4
Utolincomycin, 2363·4
Utoral, 2363·4
Utovlan, 2363·4
UTP, 1760·3
Utrim, 2363·4
Utrogest, 2363·4
Utrogestan, 2363·4
UV Light, 1136·3
UV Protectant, 2363·4
UV Sport Gel, 2363·4
UV Triplegard Preparations, 2363·4
UV Ultrablock, 2364·1
Uvacin, 2364·1
Uvadex, 2364·1
Uvae Ursi Folium, 1659·2
Uvalysat, 2364·1
Uvamin, 2364·1
Uvamine Retard, 2364·1
Uvanox, 2364·1
Uvasal, 2364·1
Uva-Ursi, 1659·2
Uva-Ursi Complex, 2364·1
Uva-Ursi Plus, 2364·1
Uvavit, 2364·1
Uveal Melanoma— *see* Malignant Neoplasms of the Eye, 516·1
Uvedose, 2364·1
Uvega, 2364·1
Uveitis, 1090·1
Uveline, 2364·1
Uvestat, 2364·1
Uvesterol, 2364·1
Uvesterol D, 2364·1
Uvicin, 2364·1
Uvicol, 2364·1
Uvimag $B_6$, 2364·1
Uvirgan Mono, 2364·1
Uvirgan N, 2364·1
Uvistat Preparations, 2364·1
UV-Luar, 2364·2
UW Solution, 414·2, 851·3
Uxalun, 2364·2
Uxen, 2364·2
Uxicolin, 2364·2
Uzara, 2364·2
Uzix, 2364·2

## V

V, 1451·2
3V, 2364·2
V Day Preparations, 2364·2
V Infusionslosung, 2364·2
Vaben, 2364·2
Vabeta, 2364·2
Vabicin, 2364·2
Vabon, 2364·2
Vac Antigrip Frac, 2364·2
Vac Antimeningococic A+C, 2364·2
Vac Antiparotiditis, 2364·2
Vac Antipolio Or, 2364·2
Vac Antipolio Oral, 2364·2
Vac Antirrabica, 2364·2
Vac Antirrubeola, 2364·2
Vac Antitetanica, 2364·2
Vac Antitifica Or, 2364·2
Vac Polio Sabin, 2364·2
Vac Poliomielitica, 2364·2
Vac Triple MSD, 2364·2
Vacanyl, 2364·2
Vaccin DTCP, 2364·2
Vaccin DTP, 2364·2
Vaccin Meningococcique Merieux, 2364·3
Vaccin Rubeole Merieux, 2364·3
Vaccin Tab, 2364·3
Vaccin TP, 2364·3
Vaccination, 1605·1
Vaccine Antipoliomyelitique/Merieux, 2364·3
Vaccines, 1605·3
Vaccines Immunoglobulins and Antisera, 1605·1
Vaccinia Immune Globulin, 1643·1
Vaccinia Immunoglobulins, 1643·1
*Vaccinium macrocarpon*, 1676·3
*Vaccinium myrtillus*, 1718·3
*Vaccinium oxycoccos*, 1676·3
*Vaccinium vitis-idaea*, 1676·3
Vaccino Antipiogeno, 2364·3
Vaccino Antipneumocatarrale, 2364·3
Vaccino Difto Tetano, 2364·3
Vaccino DPT, 2364·3
Vaccino Tab Te, 2364·3
Vaccinum Cholerae, 1611·2
Vaccinum Cholerae Cryodesiccatum, 1611·2
Vaccinum Diphtheriae Adsorbatum, 1612·3
Vaccinum Diphtheriae Adulti et Adulescentis Adsorbatum, 1612·3
Vaccinum Diphtheriae et Tetani Adsorbatum, 1613·1
Vaccinum Diphtheriae et Tetani Adulti et Adulescentis Adsorbatum, 1613·1
Vaccinum Diphtheriae, Tetani et Hepatitidis B (ADNr) Adsorbatum, 1613·3
Vaccinum Diphtheriae, Tetani et Pertussis Adsorbatum, 1613·3
Vaccinum Diphtheriae, Tetani et Pertussis sine Cellulis ex Elementis Praeparatum Adsorbatum, 1613·3
Vaccinum Diphtheriae, Tetani, Pertussis et Poliomyelitidis Inactivatum Adsorbatum, 1615·1
Vaccinum Diphtheriae, Tetani, Pertussis, Poliomyelitidis Inactivatum et Haemophili Stirpe B Conjugatum Adsorbatum, 1615·1
Vaccinum Diphtheriae, Tetani, Pertussis sine Cellulis ex Elementis Praeparatum et Haemophili Stirpe B Conjugatum Adsorbatum, 1614·2
Vaccinum Diphtheriae, Tetani, Pertussis sine Cellulis ex Elementis Praeparatum et Hepatitidis B (ADNr) Adsorbatum, 1614·3
Vaccinum Diphtheriae, Tetani, Pertussis sine Cellulis ex Elementis Praeparatum et Poliomyelitidis Inactivatum Adsorbatum, 1615·1
Vaccinum Diphtheriae, Tetani, Pertussis sine Cellulis ex Elementis Praeparatum, Hepatitidis B (ADNr), Poliomyelitidis Inactivatum et Haemophili Stirpe B Conjugatum Adsorbatum, 1614·3
Vaccinum Diphtheriae, Tetani, Pertussis sine Cellulis ex Elementis Praeparatum Poliomyelitidis Inactivatum et Haemophili Stirpe B Conjugatum Adsorbatum, 1615·1
Vaccinum Encephalitidis Ixodibus Advectae Inactivatum, 1642·1
Vaccinum Febris Flavae Vivum, 1644·2
Vaccinum Febris Typhoidi, 1642·2
Vaccinum Febris Typhoidi Cryodesiccatum, 1642·2
Vaccinum Febris Typhoidis Polysaccharidicum, 1642·2
Vaccinum Febris Typhoidis Vivum Perorale (Stirpe Ty 21a), 1642·2
Vaccinum Haemophili Stirpe B Conjugatum, 1616·1
Vaccinum Haemorrhagia Febris Cum Renis Sindronum, 1617·1
Vaccinum Hepatitidis A Inactivatum Adsorbatum, 1617·1
Vaccinum Hepatitidis A Inactivatum et Hepatitidis B (ADNr) Adsorbatum, 1620·1
Vaccinum Hepatitidis A Inactivatum Virosomale, 1617·1
Vaccinum Hepatitidis B (ADNr), 1618·1
Vaccinum Influenzae Inactivatum ex Corticis Antigeniis Praeparatum, 1620·2
Vaccinum Influenzae Inactivatum ex Corticis Antigeniis Praeparatum Virosomale, 1620·2
Vaccinum Influenzae Inactivatum ex Viris Integris Praeparatum, 1620·2
Vaccinum Influenzae Inactivatum ex Virorum Fragmentis Praeparatum, 1620·2
Vaccinum Meningitidis Cerebrospinalis, 1626·1
Vaccinum Meningococcale Classis C Coniugatum, 1626·1
Vaccinum Morbillorum, Parotitidis et Rubellae Vivum, 1625·1
Vaccinum Morbillorum Vivum, 1623·1
Vaccinum Parotitidis Vivum, 1626·3
Vaccinum Pertussis, 1631·2
Vaccinum Pertussis Adsorbatum, 1631·2
Vaccinum Pertussis sine Cellulis Copurificatum Adsorbatum, 1631·3
Vaccinum Pertussis sine Cellulis ex Elementis Praeparatum Adsorbatum, 1631·2
Vaccinum Pneumococcale Polysaccharidum, 1633·1
Vaccinum Poliomyelitidis Inactivatum, 1633·3
Vaccinum Poliomyelitidis Perorale, 1634·1
Vaccinum Rabiei ex Cellulis ad Usum Humanum, 1635·3
Vaccinum Rubellae Vivum, 1637·3
Vaccinum Tetani Adsorbatum, 1640·3
Vaccinum Tuberculosis (BCG) Cryodesiccatum, 1609·2
Vaccinum Varicellae Vivum, 1643·2
Vacillin, 2364·3
Vacina Antipiogenica, 2364·3
Vacina Antipneumocatarral, 2364·3
Vacina Catarral, 2364·3
Vacina Dupla DT, 2364·3
Vacina Meningococica A+C, 2364·3
Vacina Meningococica Conjugada Grupo C, 2364·3
Vacina Pneumococica Conjugada 7-Valate, 2364·3
Vacina Poliomielitica, 2364·3
Vacina Triplice DPT, 2364·3
Vacinolone, 2364·3
Vaclox, 2364·3
Vacolax, 2364·3
Vacontil, 2364·3
Vacopan, 2364·3
Vacrax, 2364·3
Vacromil, 2364·3
Vactyph, 2364·4
Vacudol, 2364·4
Vacudol Forte, 2364·4
Vaculin, 2364·4
Vacuna Antigripal, 2364·4
Vacuna Antipiogena, 2364·4
Vacuna Doble, 2364·4
Vacuna Haptenica, 2364·4
Vacuna Triple, 2364·4
Vacunas, 1605·3
Vacunas Anticonceptivas, 1611·3
Vacunas BCG, 1609·2
Vacunas contra el Campylobacter Jejuni, 1611·1
Vacunas contra el Cáncer, 1611·2
Vacunas contra el Citomegalovirus, 1612·1
Vacunas contra Estreptococos del Grupo B, 1640·2
Vacunas contra Shigella, 1638·3
Vacunas de Escherichia Coli, 1615·3
Vacunas de Haemophilus Influenzae, 1616·1
Vacunas de Haemophilus Influenzae y la Hepatitis B, 1616·3
Vacunas de Helicobacter Pylori, 1617·1
Vacunas de la Brucelosis, 1611·1
Vacunas de la Caries Dental, 1612·2
Vacunas de la Difteria, 1612·3
Vacunas de la Difteria, el Tétanos, la Tos Ferina, la Poliomielitis y Haemophilus Influenzae, 1615·1
Vacunas de la Difteria, el Tétanos, la Tos Ferina y Haemophilus Influenzae, 1614·2
Vacunas de la Difteria, el Tétanos, la Tos Ferina y la Hepatitis B, 1614·3
Vacunas de la Difteria, el Tétanos, la Tos Ferina y la Poliomielitis, 1615·1
Vacunas de la Difteria, el Tétanos y Haemophilus Influenzae, 1613·3
Vacunas de la Difteria, el Tétanos y la Poliomielitis, 1615·2

Vacunas de la Difteria, el Tétanos y la Rubéola, 1615·2
Vacunas de la Difteria, el Tétanos y la Tos Ferina, 1613·3
Vacunas de la Difteria y el Tétanos, 1613·1
Vacunas de la Encefalitis Japonesa, 1621·2
Vacunas de la Encefalitis Transmitida por Garrapatas, 1642·1
Vacunas de la Enfermedad de Lyme, 1622·2
Vacunas de la Enteritis Necrotizante, 1632·3
Vacunas de la Esclerosis Múltiple, 1626·3
Vacunas de la Esquistosomiasis, 1638·2
Vacunas de la Fiebre Amarilla, 1644·2
Vacunas de la Fiebre del Valle del Rift, 1637·2
Vacunas de la Fiebre Hemorrágica Argentina, 1609·2
Vacunas de la Fiebre Q, 1635·3
Vacunas de la Fiebre Renal Epidémica, 1617·1
Vacunas de la Fiebre Tifoidea, 1642·2
Vacunas de la Fiebre Tifoidea y del Tétanos, 1643·1
Vacunas de la Gonorrea, 1616·1
Vacunas de la Gripe, 1620·2
Vacunas de la Hepatitis A, 1617·1
Vacunas de la Hepatitis A y Fiebre Tifoidea, 1620·1
Vacunas de la Hepatitis B, 1618·1
Vacunas de la Leishmaniasis, 1622·1
Vacunas de la Lepra, 1622·1
Vacunas de la Leptospirosis, 1622·2
Vacunas de la Parotiditis, 1626·3
Vacunas de la Peste, 1633·1
Vacunas de la Poliomielitis, 1633·3
Vacunas de la Rabia, 1635·3
Vacunas de la Rickettsiosis Típica, 1643·1
Vacunas de la Rubéola, 1637·3
Vacunas de la Rubéola y la Parotiditis, 1638·2
Vacunas de la Tos Ferina, 1631·2
Vacunas de la Tricomoniasis, 1642·1
Vacunas de la Tularemia, 1642·1
Vacunas de la Varicela Zóster, 1643·2
Vacunas de la Viruela, 1639·1
Vacunas de las Hepatitis A y B, 1620·1
Vacunas de Mycobacterium Vaccae, 1627·2
Vacunas de Polisacáridos Meningocócicos, 1626·1
Vacunas de Pseudomonas, 1635·2
Vacunas de Rotavirus, 1637·2
Vacunas del Carbunco, 1608·1
Vacunas del Cólera, 1611·2
Vacunas del Dengue, 1612·2
Vacunas del Herpes Simple, 1620·1
Vacunas del Paludismo, 1622·2
Vacunas del Sarampión, 1623·1
Vacunas del Sarampión, la Parotiditis y la Rubéola, 1625·1
Vacunas del Sarampión y la Parotiditis, 1624·3
Vacunas del Sarampión y la Rubéola, 1624·3
Vacunas del SIDA, 1607·3
Vacunas del Tétanos, 1640·3
Vacunas del Tétanos y la Gripe, 1641·3
Vacunas del Tétanos y la Poliomielitis, 1641·3
Vacunas del Virus de Epstein-Barr, 1615·3
Vacunas del Virus del Papiloma Humano, 1620·2
Vacunas del Virus Sincitial Respiratorio, 1637·2
Vacunas Estafilocócicas, 1640·2
Vacunas Neumocócicas, 1633·1
Vacuobil, 2364·4
Vacuobil Plus, 2364·4
Vadarex, 2364·4
Vademin-Z, 2364·4
Vadicate, 2364·4
Vadilex, 2364·4
Vadinar, 2364·4
Vadiral, 2364·4
Vaditon, 2364·4
Vadol, 2364·4
Vadolax, 2364·4
Vadosilan, 2364·4
Vafluson, 2364·4
Vag Oral, 2364·4
Vagaka, 2364·4
Vagantin, 2364·4
Vagarne, 2364·4
Vagarsol, 2364·4
Vagi Biotic, 2365·1
Vagi-C, 2365·1
Vagicillin, 2365·1
Vagicin, 2365·1
Vagicural, 2365·1
Vagicural Plus, 2365·1
Vagifem, 2365·1
Vagiflor, 2365·1
Vagi-Gard Medicated Cream, 2365·1
Vagi-Gard Medicated Disposable Douche, 2365·1
Vagi-Gard Personal Lubricating Gel, 2365·1
Vagi-Hex, 2365·1
Vagiklin, 2365·1
Vagil, 2365·1
Vagilen, 2365·1
Vagimax, 2365·1
Vagimid, 2365·1
Vaginal Contraceptives, 1527·3
Vaginex, 2365·1
Vaginitis— *see* Bacterial Vaginosis, 121·2
Vaginitis, Atrophic— *see* Menopausal Disorders, 1540·2
Vaginitis, Hylands— *see* Hylands Vaginitis, 2052·3
Vaginosis— *see* Bacterial Vaginosis, 121·2
Vaginyl, 2365·1
Vagisan, 2365·1
Vagisan Compuesto, 2365·1
Vagisil, 2365·1
Vagistat, 2365·1
Vagi-Sulfa, 2365·2
Vagitrene, 2365·2
Vagitrin-N, 2365·2
Vagitrol-V, 2365·2
Vagmicor, 2365·2
Vagmycin, 2365·2
Vagoclyss, 2365·2
Vagolisal, 2365·2
Vagomine, 2365·2
Vagopax, 2365·2
Vagophemanil Methylsulphate, 481·3
Vagoplex, 2365·2
Vagostabyl, 2365·2
Vagostal, 2365·2
Vagostesyl, 2365·2
Vagotrope-S, 2365·2
Vagran, 2365·2
Vagran Descongestivo, 2365·2
Vagyl, 2365·2
Vainilla, 1762·3
Vainillina, 1763·1
Val, 1451·2
VAL-13081, 1254·1
Valaciclovir, Hidrocloruro de, 656·1
Valaciclovir Hydrochloride, 656·1
Valacyclovir Hydrochloride, 656·1
Valamin 12, 2365·2
Valatux, 2365·2
Valavir, 2365·2
Valaxona, 2365·2
Valbet, 2365·2
Valbet-N, 2365·2
Valbil, 2365·2
Valcaps, 2365·2
Valcatil, 2365·2
Valclair, 2365·2
Valcote, 2365·2
Valcyte, 2365·3
Valda, 2365·3
Valda F3, 2365·3
Valda Septol, 2365·3
Valda, Tabletes— *see* Tabletes Valda, 2317·4
Valda, Xarope— *see* Xarope Valda, 2387·4
Valdatos, 2365·3
Valdecoxib, 96·1
Valdefer, 2365·3
Valderma, 2365·3
Valdig-N Burger, 2365·3
Valdispert, 2365·3
Valdispert Comp, 2365·3
Valdispert Complex, 2365·3
Valdorm, 2365·3
Valeans, 2365·3
Valecid, 2365·3
Valederm, 2365·3
Valena N, 2365·3
Valencene, 1724·1
Valenium, 2365·3
Valepotriates, 1762·2
Valepotriatos, 1762·2
Valer, 1762·2
Valerato de Betametasona, 1093·2
Valerato de Diflucortolona, 1099·3
Valerato de Estradiol, 1550·2
Valerato de Hidrocortisona, 1104·2
Valerbe, 2365·3
Valerbet, 2365·3
Valerecen, 2365·3
Valergen, 2365·3
Valerial, 2365·3
Valerian, 1762·2, 2365·3
Valerian Compound, Gerard House— *see* Gerard House Valerian Compound, 2022·1
Valerian, Japanese, 1762·2
Valerian Passiflora and Hops, 2365·3
Valerian Plus Herbal Plus Formula 12, 2365·4
Valerian Rhizome, 1762·2
Valerian Root, 1762·2
Valeriana, 1762·2
Valeriana Comp Novum, 2365·4
*Valeriana fauriei*, 1762·2
Valeriana Forte N, 2365·4
Valeriana Mild, 2365·4
*Valeriana officinalis*, 1762·2
Valeriana Oligoplex, 2365·4
Valeriana Orto, 2365·4
Valeriana (Specie Composta), 2365·4
Valerianae Radix, 1762·2
Valerianaheel, 2365·4
Valeric, 2365·4
Valerin, 2365·4
Valerina Day Time, 2365·4
Valerina Night-Time, 2365·4
Valerix, 2365·4
Valerocalma, 2365·4
Valertest, 2365·4
Valesono, 2365·4
Valetamato, Bromuro de, 491·3
Valethamate Bromide, 491·3
Valeton, 2365·4
Valette, 2365·4
Valezen, 2365·4
Valfam, 2365·4
Valfiran, 2365·4
Valflex, 2365·4
Valganciclovir, Hidrocloruro de, 656·3
Valganciclovir Hydrochloride, 656·3
Valherpes, 2365·4
Valifol, 2365·4
Valin Baldrian, 2365·4
Valina, 1451·2
Valine, 1451·2
L-Valine, 1451·2
Valinor, 2365·4
Valinum, 1451·2
Valiquid, 2365·4
Valirem, 2365·4
Valisone, 2366·1
Valisone-G, 2366·1
Valium, 2366·1
Valium— *see* Emergent-Ez, 1967·2
Valix, 2366·1
Valken, 2366·1
Vallergan, 2366·1
Valley Fever— *see* Coccidioidomycosis, 387·3
Valmane, 2366·1
Valmarin Bad N, 2366·1
Valmicin, 2366·1
Valnar, 2366·1
Valnemulin, 275·1
Valnemulin Hydrochloride, 275·2
Valnemulina, 275·1
Valnémuline, 275·1
Valnoctamida, 727·2
Valnoctamide, 727·2
Valocordin-Diazepam, 2366·1
Valoid, 2366·1
Valonorm, 2366·1
Valontan, 2366·1
Valopin, 2366·1
Valopride, 2366·1
Valoran, 2366·1
Valorel, 2366·1
Valoron, 2366·1
Valoron N, 2366·1
Valpakine, 2366·1
Valpam, 2366·1
Valpar, 2366·1
Valparin, 2366·1
Valpax, 2366·1
Valpeda, 2366·2
Valpex, 2366·2
Valpiform, 2366·2
Valpin, 2366·2
Valpinax, 2366·2
Val-Plus, 2366·2
Valporal, 2366·2
Valprene, 2366·2
Valpression, 2366·2
Valpridol, 2366·2
Valpro, 2366·2
Valpro Beta, 2366·2
Valproate, 380·1
Valproate Pivoxil, 380·1
Valproate Semisodium, 380·1
Valproate Sodium, 380·1
Valproato, 380·1
Valproato de Pivoxilo, 380·1
Valproato Semisódico, 380·1
Valproato Sódico, 380·1
Valprodura, 2366·2
Valproflux, 2366·2
Valproic Acid, 380·1
Valproico, Ácido, 380·1
Valprolept, 2366·2
Valpromida, 380·1
Valpromide, 380·1
ValproNa, 2366·2
Valprosid, 2366·2
Valrian, 2366·2
Valrubicin, 590·3
Valrubicina, 590·3
Vals, 2366·2
Valsartan, 1018·3
Valsartan/HCTZ, 2366·2
Valsera, 2366·2
Valspodar, 591·1
Valstar, 2366·2
Valsweet, 2366·2
Valtaxin, 2366·2
Valtran, 2366·2
Valtrate, 1762·2
Valtrax, 2366·2
Valtrex, 2366·2
Val-Uno, 2366·2
Valupass, 2366·2
Valus, 2366·2
Valverde Preparations, 2366·3
Valvular Heart Disease, 838·2
Vamazole, 2366·3
Va-Mengoc-BC, 2366·3
Vamin Preparations, 2366·3
Vamina, 2366·4
Vamina Glucose, 2366·4
Vamine Glucose, 2366·4
Vaminolac, 2366·4
Vaminolact, 2366·4
Vanadiol, 2366·4
Vanadyl Sulfate, 325·1
Vanafen, 2366·4
Vanafen-S, 2366·4
Vanamide, 2366·4
Vanaurus, 2366·4
Vancam, 2366·4
Vancenase, 2366·4
Vanceril, 2366·4
Vanclomin, 2366·4
Vanco, 2366·4
Vancoabbott, 2366·4
Vancocid, 2366·4
Vancocin, 2366·4
Vancocina, 2366·4
Vancocine, 2366·4
Vancolan, 2366·4

Vancoled, 2367·1
Vancomax, 2367·1
Vancomicina, Hidrocloruro de, 275·2
Vancomycin, 275·2
Vancomycin Hydrochloride, 275·2
Vancomycini Hydrochloridum, 275·2
Vancoplus, 2367·1
Vanco-saar, 2367·1
Vancoscand, 2367·1
Vancoson, 2367·1
Vancotenk, 2367·1
Vanco-Teva, 2367·1
Vancox, 2367·1
Vanderbumin, 2367·1
Vanderm, 2367·1
Vandisul, 2367·1
Vandol, 2367·1
Vandral, 2367·1
Vanesten, 2367·1
Vanex Expectorant, 2367·1
Vanex Forte, 2367·1
Vanex Forte-R, 2367·1
Vanex-HD, 2367·1
Vanicream, 2367·1
Vanidene, 2367·1
Vanilla, 1762·3
Vanilla Beans, 1762·3
Vanilla, Bourbon, 1762·3
Vanilla, Madagascar, 1762·3
Vanilla, Mexican, 1762·3
*Vanilla planifolia*, 1762·3
Vanilla Pods, 1762·3
*Vanilla tahitensis*, 1762·3
Vanilla, Tahitian, 1762·3
Vanillic Acid Diethylamide, 1588·1
Vanillic Aldehyde, 1763·1
Vanillic Diethylamide, 1588·1
Vanillin, 1763·1
Vanillinum, 1763·1
2′-Vanillylideneisonicotinohydrazide Monohydrate, 215·2
Vanillylmandelic Acid, 854·1
*N*-Vanillylnonamide, 67·2
Vanilone, 2367·1
Vaniqa, 2367·1
Vanmicina, 2367·1
Vanmycetin, 2367·1
Vanocin, 2367·1
Vanoxide, 2367·1
Vanoxide-HC, 2367·1
Vanquin, 2367·1
Vanquish, 2367·1
Vansil, 2367·2
Vantaggio, 2367·2
Vantal, 2367·2
Vanticon, 2367·2
Vantin, 2367·2
Vantux, 2367·2
Vanzor, 2367·2
Vaopin N, 2367·2
Vap Air, 2367·2
Vapex, 2367·2
Vapin, 2367·2
Vapin Complex, 2367·2
Vapio, 2367·2
Vapo Syrup, Wick— *see* Wick Vapo Syrup, 2386·1
Vapodrops with Butter and Menthol, Vicks— *see* Vicks Vapodrops with Butter and Menthol, 2375·4
Vapodrops, Vicks— *see* Vicks Vapodrops, 2375·4
Vapoflu, 2367·2
Vapolatum Inhalador, 2367·2
Vapolatum Labial, 2367·2
Vapolatum Unguento, 2367·2
Vapo-Myrtol, 2367·2
Vaponefrin, 2367·2
Vapor Flay, 2367·2
Vapor Rub, Mentholatum— *see* Mentholatum Vapour Rub, 2124·2
Vapores Pyt, 2367·2
Vaporil, 2367·2
Vaporisateur Medicamente, 2367·2
Vaporisateur Nasal Decongestionnant, 2367·2
Vaporiser Fluid, Gold Cross— *see* Gold Cross Vaporiser Fluid, 2029·3
Vaporizing Chest Rub, 2367·2
Vaporizing Colds Rub, 2367·3
Vaporizing Ointment, 2367·3
Vaporub, Vick— *see* Vick Vaporub, 2375·1
Vaporub, Vicks— *see* Vicks Vaporub, 2375·4
Vaporub, Wick— *see* Wick Vaporub, 2386·1
Vapour Rub, 2367·3
Vapreotida, 1342·2
Vapreotide, 1342·2
Vapresan, 2367·3
Vapresan Diur, 2367·3
VAQTA, 2367·3
Vardenafil, 1763·1
Vardenafil Dihydrochloride, 1763·1
Vardenafil Hydrochloride, 1763·1
Vardenafil Hydrochloride Trihydrate, 1763·2
Vardenafil Monohydrochloride, 1763·1
Varedet, 2367·3
Varemoid, 2367·3
Varenicline, 1763·2
Varenicline Tartrate, 1763·2
Varfine, 2367·3
Variargil, 2367·3
Varibiotic, 2367·3
Varicare, 2367·3
Variceal Haemorrhage, 1716·1
Varicela Biken, 2367·3
Varicell, 2367·3
Varicella, 2367·3
Varicella— *see* Varicella-zoster Infections, 621·1
Varicella Immunoglobulin, Human, 1643·1
Varicella Immunoglobulin for Intravenous Administration, Human, 1643·1
Varicella Immunoglobulins, 1643·1
Varicella Vaccine (Live), 1643·2
Varicella Vaccines, 1643·2
Varicella-Zoster Immune Globulin, 1643·2
Varicella-Zoster Immunoglobulins, 1643·1
Varicella-zoster Infections, 621·1
Varicella-Zoster Vaccines, 1643·2
Varicellon, 2367·3
Varices, Bleeding— *see* Variceal Haemorrhage, 1716·1
Varicex, 2367·3
Varicofit, 2367·3
Varicogel, 2367·3
Varicose Ointment, 2367·3
Varicose Veins, 1717·1
Varicylum, 2367·3
Varicylum N, 2367·3
Varicylum-S, 2367·3
Varidasa, 2367·3
Varidase, 2367·3
Varidoid, 2367·3
Varigerm, 2367·4
Varigestrol, 2367·4
Varigloban, 2367·4
Variglobin, 2367·4
Varihes, 2367·4
Varihesive, 2367·4
Varihesive Hydroactive, 2367·4
Varikromo, 2367·4
Varilise, 2367·4
Varilisin, 2367·4
Varilrix, 2367·4
Varimer, 2367·4
Varimesna, 2367·4
Varimine, 2367·4
Variplant, 2367·4
Variplastic, 2367·4
Variplex, 2367·4
Varison, 2367·4
Varitan N, 2367·4
Varitect, 2367·4
Variton, 2367·4
Varivax, 2367·4
Varizin, 2367·4
Varizol, 2367·4
Varlane, 2367·4
Varnoline, 2367·4
Varson, 2367·4
Vartalan, 2368·1
Vartalan D, 2368·1
Vartalon, 2368·1
Vartalon Complemento, 2368·1
Var/Vac(Live), 1643·2
Var-Zeta, 2368·1
Vas, 2368·1
V-AS, 2368·1
VAS, Carbamid + — *see* Carbamid + VAS, 1869·1
Vasactife, 2368·1
Vasactin, 2368·1
Vasa-Gastreu N R63, 2368·1
Vascace, 2368·1
Vascace Plus, 2368·1
Vascal, 2368·1
Vascalpha, 2368·1
Vascard, 2368·1
Vascase, 2368·1
Vascase Plus, 2368·1
Vascer, 2368·1
Vasclin, 2368·1
Vascocitrol, 2368·1
Vascoman, 2368·1
Vascopan, 2368·1
Vascor, 2368·1
Vascoray, 2368·1
Vascoten, 2368·1
Vascular Dementia— *see* Dementia, 1484·1
Vascular Disease, Peripheral— *see* Peripheral Vascular Disease, 831·2
Vascular Endothelial Growth Factor, 1763·2
Vasculat, 2368·1
Vasculene, 2368·2
Vasculin, 2368·2
Vasculine, 2368·2
Vasculitic Syndromes, 1090·1
Vasculitis, Granulomatous— *see* Vasculitic Syndromes, 1090·1
Vasculitis, Hypersensitivity— *see* Hypersensitivity Vasculitis, 1081·3
Vasculitis, Leucocytoclastic— *see* Hypersensitivity Vasculitis, 1081·3
Vasculitis, Necrotising— *see* Vasculitic Syndromes, 1090·1
Vasculitis, Necrotising, Systemic— *see* Polyarteritis Nodosa and Microscopic Polyangiitis, 1085·3
Vasculoflex, 2368·2
Vascunormyl, 2368·2
Vasdalat, 2368·2
Vasdilat, 2368·2
Vaselastic, 2368·2
Vaselatum, 2368·2
Vaselina, 2368·2
Vaselina Amarela, 1479·3
Vaselina Amarilla, 1479·3
Vaselina Boricada, 2368·2
Vaselina Branca, 1479·3
Vaselina Filante, 1479·3
Vaselina Líquida, 1479·1
Vaselina Mentolada, 2368·2
Vaseline, 1479·3, 2368·2
Vaseline Épaisse, Huile de, 1479·1
Vaseline Fluide, Huile de, 1479·1
Vaseline Preparations, 2368·2
Vaseline Officinale, 1479·3
Vaselini, Oleum, 1479·1
Vaselinöl, 1479·1
Vaselinum Album, 1479·3
Vaselinum Flavum, 1479·3
Vaselinum Liquidum, 1479·1
Vaselitulle, 2368·2
Vaselpin, 2368·2
Vaseretic, 2368·2
Vasesana-Vasoregulans, 2368·3
Vasian, 2368·3
Vasican, 2368·3
Vasil, 2368·3
Vasilium, 2368·3
Vaslip, 2368·3
Vasoactive Intestinal Octacosapeptide (Swine), 1763·2
Vasoactive Intestinal Peptide, 1763·2
Vasobrain, 2368·3
Vasobral, 2368·3
Vasobrix, 2368·3
Vasocardol, 2368·3
Vasocedine, 2368·3
Vasocedine Pseudoephedrine, 2368·3
Vasocidin, 2368·3
Vasocine, 2368·3
VasoClear, 2368·3
VasoClear A, 2368·3
Vasocon, 2368·3
Vasocon Ant, 2368·3
Vasocon-A, 2368·3
Vasoconstr, 2368·3
Vasoconstrictor Pensa, 2368·3
Vasocor, 2368·3
Vasodepressor Syncope— *see* Hypotension, 828·1
Vasodexa, 2368·3
Vasodil, 2368·3
Vasodilan, 2368·4
Vaso-Dilatan, 2368·4
Vasodilators, 812·2
Vasodin, 2368·4
Vasodip, 2368·4
Vasodipina, 2368·4
Vasodual, 2368·4
Vaso-E-Bion, 2368·4
Vasofed, 2368·4
Vasofen, 2368·4
Vasoflex, 2368·4
Vasofluina, 2368·4
Vasoforte N, 2368·4
Vasofrinic, 2368·4
Vasofrinic Plus, 2368·4
Vasofyl, 2368·4
Vasogen, 2368·4
Vasojet, 2368·4
Vasolan, 2368·4
Vasolastine, 2368·4
Vasolat, 2368·4
Vasolipid, 2368·4
Vasomax, 2368·4
Vasomed, 2368·4
Vasomil, 2368·4
Vasomine, 2368·4
Vasomotal, 2368·4
Vasonase, 2368·4
Vasonett, 2368·4
Vasonit, 2369·1
Vasonorm, 2369·1
Vasopos N, 2369·1
Vasopresina, 1342·2
Vasopressin, 1342·2, 2369·1
Vasopressin Deficiency— *see* Diabetes Insipidus, 1314·1
Vasopressin Resistance— *see* Diabetes Insipidus, 1314·1
Vasopressin Tannate, 1343·2
Vasopressin $V_2$ Receptor Antagonists, 1319·1
Vasopril, 2369·1
Vasopril Plus, 2369·1
Vasoprost, 2369·1
Vasopt, 2369·1
Vasopten, 2369·1
Vasorbate, 2369·1
Vasorema, 2369·1
Vasoretic, 2369·1
Vasorinil, 2369·1
Vasosan, 2369·1
Vasospastic Arterial Disease— *see* Raynaud's Syndrome, 833·3
Vasosterone, 2369·1
Vasosterone Antibiotico, 2369·1
Vasosterone Collirio, 2369·1
Vasosterone Oto, 2369·1
Vasosulf, 2369·1
Vasosuprina Ilfi, 2369·1
Vasotec, 2369·1
Vasotenal, 2369·1
Vasoton, 2369·1
Vasotonal, 2369·1
Vasotonin, 2369·1
Vasotonin Forte, 2369·1
Vasotop, 2369·2
Vasovagal Syncope— *see* Hypotension, 828·1
Vasovitol, 2369·2
Vasoxine, 2369·2
Vasoxyl, 2369·2
Vasperdil, 2369·2
Vaspit, 2369·2
Vastarel, 2369·2
Vasten, 2369·2
Vastensium, 2369·2
Vastin, 2369·2

Vastina, 2369·2
Vastinol, 2369·2
Vastribil, 2369·2
Vastrictol, 2369·2
Vastripine, 2369·2
Vastus, 2369·2
Vasurix Polividona, 2369·2
Vasurix-Polyvidone— *see* Telebrix Polyvidone, 2323·1
Vasylox, 2369·2
Vatran, 2369·2
Vatrasin, 2369·2
Vatrem, 2369·2
Vatrix-S, 2369·2
Vavifor, 2369·2
Vaxem Hib, 2369·2
Vaxicoq, 2369·2
Vaxicum NA, 2369·2
Vaxidina, 2369·2
Vaxigrip, 2369·2
Vaxim HIB, 2369·3
Vaxipar, 2369·3
Vaxitiol, 2369·3
Vazigam, 2369·3
Vazosin, 2369·3
Vcanalare, 2369·3
VCF, 2369·3
V-Cil-K, 2369·3
V-Cillin K, 2369·3
VCM, 1764·3
V-Crima, 2369·3
V-Dec-M, 2369·3
Ve, 2369·3
Veafer, 2369·3
V-Echinocandin, 395·1
Veclam, 2369·3
Vecredil, 2369·3
Vectarion, 2369·3
Vectavir, 2369·3
Vectidan, 2369·3
Vector Control, 1500·1
Vectrin, 2369·3
Vectrine, 2369·3
Vecural, 2369·3
Vecuron, 2369·3
Vecuronio, Bromuro de, 1409·3
Vecuronium Bromide, 1409·3
Vedaprofen, 96·3
Vedaprofeno, 96·3
Vedrin, 2369·3
Veemycin, 2369·3
Veenac, 2369·3
Veetids, 2369·3
Vefed, 2369·3
Vefluxan, 2369·4
Vefren, 2369·4
Vegadeine, 2369·4
Vegal, 2369·4
Veganin, 2369·4
Veganin 3, 2369·4
Veganine, 2369·4
Vege Swiss One, 2369·4
Vegebaby, 2369·4
Vegebom, 2369·4
Vegebyl, 2369·4
Vegelact, 2369·4
Vegelax, 2369·4
Vegelose, 2369·4
Vegesan, 2369·4
Vegestabil, 2369·4
Vegestabil Digest, 2369·4
Vegetable Black, 1058·3
Vegetable Carbon, 1058·3
Vegetable Charcoal, 1031·1
Vegetable Cough Remover, 2369·4
Vegetable Fatty Oils, 1763·3
Vegetable Oil, Hydrogenated, 1763·3
Vegetable Oil, Thin, 1481·1
Vegetal Tonic, 2369·4
Vegetalin, 2369·4
Vegetallumina, 2369·4
Vegetarian Protein Supplement, 2369·4
Vegetex, 2369·4
Vegetoserum, 2369·4
Vegicap Vegetarian, 2370·1
Vegital, 2370·1
Vehem, 2370·1
Veil, 2370·1
Veinamitol, 2370·1
Veineva, 2370·1
Veinobiase, 2370·1
Veinoconfort, 2370·1
Veinoglobuline, 2370·1
Veino-Gouttes-N, 2370·1
Veinophytum, 2370·1
Veinopress A3, 2370·1
Veinopress A4— *see* Veinopress A3 and A4, 2370·1
Veinosane, 2370·1
Veinosclerol— *see* Aetoxisclerol, 1778·4
Veinostase, 2370·1
Veinotonyl, 2370·1
Vekfazolin, 2370·1
Velamox, 2370·1
Velaned, 2370·1
Velastatin, 997·1
Velasulin, 2370·1
Velasulin Human, 2370·1
Velasulin MC, 2370·1
Velaten, 2370·1
Velbacil, 2370·1
Velban, 2370·1
Velbe, 2370·1
Velcade, 2370·1
Veldrol, 2370·1
Velexina, 2370·2
Veliten, 2370·2
Vellutan, 2370·2
Velmonit, 2370·2
Velnacrine, 1498·1
Velocef, 2370·2
Velodan, 2370·2
Velonarcon, 2370·2
Velopural, 2370·2
Velorin, 2370·2
Velosalic, 2370·2
Velosef, 2370·2
Velosulin Preparations, 2370·2
Velosuline Humanum, 2370·2
Veloudiet, 2370·2
Velpro, 2370·2
Velsay, 2370·2
Veltex, 2370·2
Velutrix, 2370·2
Velvachol, 2370·2
Velvelan, 2370·2
Vemizol, 2370·2
Vemol, 2370·2
Venacol, 2370·2
Venactive, 2370·2
Venacton, 2370·3
Venactone, 2370·3
Venalisin, 2370·3
Venalitan, 2370·3
Venalot Preparations, 2370·3
Venartel, 2370·3
Venastat, 2370·3
Venbig, 2370·3
Vencipon N, 2370·3
Vendal, 2370·3
Venderol, 2370·3
Ven-Detrex, 2370·3
Vendrex, 2370·3
Venelbin, 2370·3
Venelbin N, 2370·3
Venelbin Ruscus, 2370·3
Venen-Dragees, 2370·3
Venen-Fluid, 2370·3
Venengel, 2370·3
Venen-Salbe, 2370·3
Venen-Salbe N, 2370·3
Venen-Tabletten, 2370·3
Venentabs, 2370·3
Venen-Tropfen, 2370·3
Venen-Tropfen N, 2370·3
Venereal Diseases— *see* Sexually Transmitted Diseases, 145·3
Venex, 2370·4
Vengesic, 2370·4
Venimmun, 2370·4
Venimmun N, 2370·4
Venimmuna, 2370·4
Venirene, 2370·4
Veniten, 2370·4
Venitrin, 2370·4
Venium, 2370·4
Venlafaxina, Hidrocloruro de, 321·3
Venlafaxine Hydrochloride, 321·3
Venlax, 2370·4
Venlor, 2370·4
Veno, 2370·4
Veno SL, 2370·4
Venobene, 2370·4
Venobiase, 2370·4
Venobiase Mono, 2370·4
Veno-biomo, 2370·4
Venocaina, 2370·4
Venocur Triplex, 2370·4
Venodin, 2370·4
Venodura, 2370·4
Venofer, 2370·4
Venoferrum, 2370·4
Venofit, 2370·4
Venofortan, 2370·4
Venoful, 2370·4
Venogal, 2370·4
Venogamma, 2371·1
Venogamma Anti-Rho (D), 2371·1
Venogamma Polivalente, 2371·1
Venoglobulin, 2371·1
Venoglobulin-H, 2371·1
Venoglobulin-S, 2371·1
Venogyl, 2371·1
Veno-Hexanicit, 2371·1
Veno-Kattwiga N, 2371·1
Veno-L 90 N, 2371·1
Venolen, 2371·1
Venolep, 2371·1
Venomenhal, 2371·1
Venomhal, 2371·1
Venomil, 2371·1
Venoparil, 2371·1
Venoplant Preparations, 2371·1
Venoplus, 2371·1
Venopril, 2371·1
Venopyronum, 2371·1
Venopyronum N, 2371·2
Venorell, 2371·2
Venoruton, 2371·2
Venoruton Emulgel, 2371·2
Venoruton Heparin, 2371·2
Venos Cough Mixture, 2371·2
Venos Expectorant, 2371·2
Venos Honey & Lemon, 2371·2
Venos for Kids, 2371·2
Venosan, 2371·2
Venoselect N, 2371·2
Venoserin, 2371·2
Venosin, 2371·2
Venosmil, 2371·2
Venosmine, 2371·2
Venostasin, 2371·2
Venostasin Composto, 2371·2
Veno-Tebonin N, 2371·2
Venotop, 2371·2
Venotrauma, 2371·2
Venotrulan, 2371·2
Venotrulan N, 2371·3
Venous Thromboembolism, 839·1
Venous Thrombosis— *see* Thromboembolic Disorders, 837·3
Veno-V, 2371·3
Venovit, 2371·3
Vensa, 2371·3
Vent Retard, 2371·3
Ventadur, 2371·3
Ventamol, 2371·3
Ventamol Expectorant, 2371·3
Ventavis, 2371·3
Venter, 2371·3
Venterol, 2371·3
Ventexxair, 2371·3
Venteze, 2371·3
Ventide, 2371·3
Ventilan, 2371·3
Ventilastin, 2371·3
Ventilat, 2371·3
Ventilation, Mechanical— *see* Intensive Care, 1398·1
Ventimax, 2371·3
Ventisol, 2371·3
Ventmax, 2371·3
Ventnaze, 2371·3
Ventodisk, 2371·3
Ventodisks, 2371·3
Ventoflu, 2371·3
Ventolair, 2371·3
Ventolase, 2371·3
Ventoliber, 2371·3
Ventolin Preparations, 2371·4
Ventoline, 2371·4
Ventomol, 2371·4
Ventor, 2371·4
Ventorlin, 2371·4
Ventox, 2371·4
Ventracid N, 2371·4
Ventre Livre, 2371·4
Ventricon N, 2371·4
Ventricor, 2371·4
Ventricular Arrhythmias— *see* Cardiac Arrhythmias, 816·1
Ventricular Fibrillation— *see* Advanced Cardiac Life Support, 812·2
Ventricular Fibrillation— *see* Cardiac Arrhythmias, 816·1
Ventricular Tachycardia— *see* Cardiac Arrhythmias, 816·1
Ventricular Tachycardia, Pulseless— *see* Advanced Cardiac Life Support, 812·2
Ventricular Tachycardia, Pulseless— *see* Cardiac Arrhythmias, 816·1
Ventrigutt N, 2371·4
Ventri-loges N, 2371·4
Ventrimarin Novo, 2371·4
Ventrux, 2371·4
Ventzone, 2371·4
Venucreme, 2371·4
Venugel, 2371·4
Venusmin, 2371·4
Venustas Antiforfora, 2371·4
Venustas Lozione Caduta, 2371·4
Venustas Shampoo per Capelli con Forfora e/o Grassi, 2371·4
Venutabs, 2371·4
Venyl, 2371·4
Vepan, 2372·1
Vepar, 2372·1
Vepen, 2372·1
Vepesid, 2372·1
Vepeside, 2372·1
Vepicombin, 2372·1
Vera, 2372·1
Vera Cruz Jalap, 1268·3
Verabeta, 2372·1
Veracaps, 2372·1
Veracapt, 2372·1
Veracef, 2372·1
Veracim, 2372·1
Veracol, 2372·1
Veracolate, 2372·1
Veracor, 2372·1
Veracoron, 2372·1
Veractil— *see* Nozinan, 2179·1
Veracur, 2372·1
Veracuril, 2372·1
Veraday, 2372·1
Veradin, 2372·1
Veradol, 2372·1
Veragamma, 2372·1
Veragel, 2372·1
Veragel DMS, 2372·1
Verahexal, 2372·2
Verakard, 2372·2
Veraken, 2372·2
Veral, 2372·2
Veralan, 2372·2
Veraldid, 2372·2
Vera-Lich, 2372·2
Veraligral, 2372·2
Veralipral, 2372·2
Veralipral T, 2372·2
Veraliprida, 727·2
Veralipride, 727·2
Veralipril, 2372·2
Veraloc, 2372·2
Veralox, 2372·2
Veramex, 2372·2
Veramil, 2372·2
Veramina, 2372·2
Veramon, 2372·2
Veranorm, 2372·2
Veranzol, 2372·2
Verap, 2372·2
Verapabene, 2372·2
Verapal, 2372·2

Verapam, 2372·2
Verapamil Hydrochloride, 1019·1
Verapamili Hydrochloridum, 1019·1
Verapamilo, Hidrocloruro de, 1019·1
Verapin, 2372·2
Veraplex, 2372·2
Verapress, 2372·2
Veraptin, 2372·2
Verasal, 2372·3
Verasifar, 2372·3
Veraskin, 2372·3
Veraspir, 2372·3
Verastad, 2372·3
Veratensin, 2372·3
Veratide, 2372·3
Veratran, 2372·3
Veratric Acid, 1273·1
Veratrina, 1763·3
Veratrine, 1763·3
Veratro Verde, 1764·1
Veratropan Composto, 2372·3
Veratrum Album, 1764·1
*Veratrum album*, 1764·1
Veratrum, American, 1764·1
Veratrum, Green, 1764·1
Veratrum Med Complex, 2372·3
Veratrum Viride, 1764·1
*Veratrum viride*, 1764·1
Veratrum, White, 1764·1
5-Veratrylpyrimidine-2,4-diyldiamine, 603·2
Veratyrol, 2372·3
Veraval, 2372·3
Veravorin, 2372·3
Verax, 2372·3
Verazinc, 2372·3
Verbalem, 2372·3
Verbasci Flos, 1764·1
Verbascum, 1764·1
Verbascum Complex, 2372·3
*Verbascum densiflorum*, 1764·1
*Verbascum phlomoides*, 1764·1
*Verbascum thapsus*, 1764·1
Verbena, 1764·1
*Verbena officinalis*, 1764·1
Verbena Oil, Indian, 1706·3
*Verbena triphylla*, 1706·3
Verbenone, 1740·2
Verbesol, 2372·3
Verbex, 2372·3
Verbital, 2372·3
Verboril, 2372·3
Vercef, 2372·3
Vercite, 2372·3
Vercol, 2372·3
Vercyte, 2372·3
Verdal, 2372·3
Verdauungs-Tee N, Kneipp— *see* Kneipp Verdauungs-Tee N, 2081·4
Verde Brillante, 1171·1
Verde de Indocianina, 1701·1
Verde de Malaquita, 1185·2
Verde S, 1057·3
Verdünnte Schwefelsäure, 1750·3
Verecolene CM, 2372·3
Verel, 2372·4
Verelait, 2372·4
Verelan, 2372·4
Verexamil, 2372·4
Verfid, 2372·4
Vergentan, 2372·4
Vergeturine, 2372·4
Vergo, 2372·4
Vergon, 2372·4
Vericaps, 2372·4
Vericardine, 2372·4
Vericordin, 2372·4
Vericordin Compuesto, 2372·4
Vericort, 2372·4
Veriderm, 2372·4
Veriga, 2372·4
Verilax, 2372·4
Verimex, 2372·4
Verintex, 2372·4
Verintex N, 2372·4
Verisan, 2372·4
Veriscal D, 2372·4
Verisop, 2372·4
Verladyn, 2372·4
Verla-Lipon, 2372·4
Verlim 3, 2372·4
Verlin, 2372·4
Verlost, 2372·4
Vermepen, 2372·4
Vermex, 2372·4
Vermi, 2372·4
Vermiclase, 2372·4
Vermicol, 2373·1
Vermidil, 2373·1
Vermifran, 2373·1
Vermifuge, 2373·1
Vermilan, 2373·1
Vermilen, 2373·1
Vermilen Composto, 2373·1
Vermin, 2373·1
Vermin-Dazol, 2373·1
Vermine, 2373·1
Verminon, 2373·1
Vermin-Plus, 2373·1
Vermirax, 2373·1
Vermis, 2373·1
Vermisen, 2373·1
Vermisol, 2373·1
Vermital, 2373·1
Vermixide, 2373·1
Vermizol, 2373·1
Vermizym, 2373·1
Vermol, 2373·1
Vermonon, 2373·1
Vermoplex, 2373·1
Vermoral, 2373·1
Vermox, 2373·1
Vernal Pheasant's Eye, 1648·1
Vernarin, 2373·1
Vernausin, 2373·1
Vernelan, 2373·1
Vernies, 2373·1
Vernleigh Baby Cream, 2373·2
Verolax, 2373·2
Veroptinstada, 2373·2
Verorab, 2373·2
Verospiron, 2373·2
Verotina, 2373·2
Verotonil, 2373·2
Veroven, 2373·2
Veroxil, 2373·2
Verpacor, 2373·2
Verpamil, 2373·2
Verpir, 2373·2
Verra-med, 2373·2
Verruca Removal, Scholl— *see* Scholl Verucca Removal, 2279·3
Verrucare, 2373·2
Verrucas— *see* Warts, 1139·2
Verrucid, 2373·2
Verruclean, 2373·2
Verrucosal, 2373·2
Verrufilm, 2373·2
Verrugon, 2373·2
Verrulia, 2373·2
Verrulyse-Methionine, 2373·2
Verrumal, 2373·2
Verrupan, 2373·3
Verrupatch, 2373·3
Verruplan, 2373·3
Verrupor, 2373·3
Verrutopic, 2373·3
Verrutopic AS, 2373·3
Verrutrix, 2373·3
Verrux, 2373·3
Verruxane, 2373·3
Versacaps, 2373·3
Versal, 2373·3
Versal, Improved— *see* Improved Versal, 2058·4
Versamiv, 2373·3
Versan, 2373·3
Versatic, 2373·3
Versed, 2373·3
Versel, 2373·3
Versiclear, 2373·3
Versigen, 2373·3
Versiva, 2373·3
Versol, 2373·3
Verstadol, 2373·3
Versus, 2373·3
Vertab, 2373·3
Vertebralon N, 2373·3
Vertel, 2373·3
Verteporfin, 591·1
Verteporfina, 591·1
Vertex, 2373·3
Vertiginkgo, 2373·3
Vertigirex, 2373·3
Vertigo, 423·2
Vertigoheel, 2373·3
Vertigo-Hevert, 2373·3
Vertigo-Meresa, 2373·4
Vertigon, 2373·4
Vertigo-neogama, 2373·4
Vertigopas, 2373·4
Vertigo-Vomex, 2373·4
Vertin, 2373·4
Vertipam, 2373·4
Vertirosan, 2373·4
Vertirosan Vitamin $B_6$, 2373·4
Vertisal, 2373·4
Vertiserc, 2373·4
Vertix, 2373·4
Vertizine D, 2373·4
Vertizole, 2373·4
Verucasep, 2373·4
Verucca Removal System, 2373·4
Verucid, 2373·4
Verufil, 2373·4
Verunec, 2373·4
Verutal, 2373·4
Verutex, 2373·4
Vervain, 1764·1
Verveine Odorante, 1706·3
Very Low Calorie Diets, 1418·1
Very-Test, 2373·4
Verytracin, 2373·4
Very-Vit, 2373·4
Verzol, 2373·4
Verzum, 2373·4
Vesadol, 2373·4
Vesagex, 2373·4
Vesagex Heelbalm, 2373·4
Vesalion Preparations, 2374·1
Vesalium, 2374·1
Vesanoid, 2374·1
Vesdil, 2374·1
Vesdil Plus, 2374·1
Vesibil, 2374·1
Vesiherb, 2374·1
Vesilax, 2374·1
Vesirig, 2374·1
Vesix, 2374·1
Vesnarinona, 1022·1
Vesnarinone, 1022·1
Vesparax, 2374·1
Vesprin, 2374·1
Vessel, 2374·1
Vessel Due F, 2374·1
Vesselvite, 2374·1
Vessiflex, 2374·1
Vestaclav, 2374·1
Vesyca, 2374·1
Vetamol, 2374·1
Vetedol, 2374·1
Vethisel, 2374·1
Vethoine, 2374·1
Vetio, 2374·1
Vetiprost, 2374·1
Vetrabutina, Hidrocloruro de, 1764·2
Vetrabutine Hydrochloride, 1764·2
Vetren, 2374·2
Vetuss HC, 2374·2
Vexol, 2374·2
Vexolon, 2374·2
Vexurat, 2374·2
Veybirol-Tyrothyricine, 2374·2
Vfend, 2374·2
Via Mal, 2374·2
Via Mal Traumagel, 2374·2
Viabom, 2374·2
Viacin, 2374·2
Viactiv, 2374·2
Viadent, 2374·2
Viaderm-KC, 2374·2
Viadetres, 2374·2
Viadil, 2374·2
Viadil Compuesto, 2374·2
Viadur, 2374·2
Viafen, 2374·2
Viafurox, 2374·2
Viaggio, 2374·2
Viagra, 2374·2
Vial's Tonischer Wein, 2374·2
Viamon, 2374·2
Viani, 2374·3
Viapres, 2374·3
Viarex, 2374·3
Viarox, 2374·3
Viartril, 2374·3
Viartril S, 2374·3
Viaspan, 2374·3
ViATIM, 2374·3
Viatine, 2374·3
Viatol, 2374·3
Viavent, 2374·3
Viaxol, 2374·3
Viazem, 2374·3
Vibalgan, 2374·3
Vi-Balsabron, 2374·3
Vibazine, 2374·3
Vibeden, 2374·3
Vibee, 2374·3
Viberol Tirotricina, 2374·3
Vibetrat, 2374·3
Vibetrat Dexa, 2374·3
Vibion, 2374·3
Vibolex E, 2374·3
Vibracina, 2374·4
Vibradox, 2374·4
Vibragel, 2374·4
Vibral, 2374·4
Vibramicina, 2374·4
Vibramycin, 2374·4
Vibramycine, 2374·4
Vibramycine N, 2374·4
Vibra-S, 2374·4
Vibratab, 2374·4
Vibra-Tabs, 2374·4
Vibraveineuse, 2374·4
Vibravenos, 2374·4
Vibravenosa, 2374·4
*Vibrio cholerae*, 1611·2
Vibrio Infections— *see* Cholera and Other Vibrio Infections, 128·3
Vibrocil, 2374·4
Vibrocil NF, 2374·4
Vibrocil-S, 2374·4
Vibrumin, 2374·4
Vibtil, 2374·4
Viburcol, 2374·4
Viburcol N, 2374·4
Viburnum Complex, 2374·4
Vi-C, 2374·4
Vicam, 2374·4
Vicapan N, 2375·1
Vi-Caps, 2375·1
Vicard, 2375·1
Viccillin, 2375·1
Viccillin-S, 2375·1
Vi-Ce, 2375·1
Vicedent, 2375·1
Vicefeno, 2375·1
Vicemex, 2375·1
Vicenrik, 2375·1
ViCetamol, 2375·1
Vichy, Sal de, 1223·2
Vichy-Autobronzant, 2375·1
Vichy-Creme Ecran Total, 2375·1
Vichy-Lait Ecran Enfants, 2375·1
Vichy-Lait Ecran Extreme, 2375·1
Vichy-Lait Protecteur, 2375·1
Vici, 2375·1
Vicilan, 2375·1
Vicitina, 2375·1
Vick Preparations, 2375·1
Vick, Inalador— *see* Inalador Vick, 2059·1
Vick, Xarope— *see* Xarope Vick, 2387·4
Vicks Preparations, 2375·2
Vicks Cough Drops, Extra Strength— *see* Extra Strength Vicks Cough Drops, 1986·2
Vicks, Pastilles Medicinales— *see* Pastilles Medicinales Vicks, 2207·4
Vicks, Sirop Pectoral— *see* Sirop Pectoral Vicks, 2294·1
Vi-Claro, 2376·1
Viclor, 2376·1
Viclor Grip, 2376·1

Vicmafen, 2376·1
Vicnas, 2376·1
Vicodin, 2376·1
Vicodin Tuss, 2376·1
Vicoferell, 2376·1
Vicombil, 2376·1
Vicomin A C, 2376·1
Vicon, 2376·1
Vicoprofen, 2376·1
Vicortin, 2376·1
Vicrom, 2376·1
Victan, 2376·1
Victoril, 2376·1
Victors Dual Action Cough Drops, Vicks— *see* Vicks Victors Dual Action Cough Drops, 2376·1
Victrix, 2376·1
Vida Preparations, 2376·1
Vida-Butaline, 2376·2
Vidaclofen-Plus, 2376·2
Vidaclovir, 2376·2
Vi-Dailin, 2376·2
Vidalat, 2376·2
Vidalidine, 2376·2
Vidan, 2376·2
Vidang, 105·1
Vidaperamide, 2376·2
Vidapirocam, 2376·2
Vidapril, 2376·2
Vidarabina, 657·1
Vidarabina, Fosfato de, 657·1
Vidarabine, 657·1
Vidarabine 5′-Monophosphate, 657·1
Vidarabine Phosphate, 657·1
Vidarabine Sodium Phosphate, 657·1
Vidaspan, 2376·2
Vidatapp, 2376·2
Vidatifen, 2376·2
Vidavit, 2376·2
Vidaylin, 2376·2
Vi-Daylin, 2376·2
Vi-Daylin Plus Iron, 2376·2
Vi-Daylin/F, 2376·2
Vidaza, 2376·2
Vidcalm, 2376·2
Vi-De$_3$, 2376·2
Videne, 2376·2
Video, 2376·2
Video Capsule con Mirtillo, 2376·2
Video-Light, 2376·3
Video-Mill, 2376·3
Video-Net, 2376·3
Videorelax, 2376·3
Viderm, 2376·3
Vidermina, 2376·3
Videx, 2376·3
Vidilac, 2376·3
Vidirakt S, 2376·3
Vidisept, 2376·3
Vidisept EDO, 2376·3
Vidisept N, 2376·3
Vidiseptal EDO Sine, 2376·3
Vidisic, 2376·3
Vidora, 2376·3
Vidox, 2376·3
Vidyn, 2376·3
Vie Ca Rad, 2376·3
Vienna Paste, 1664·3, 1734·2
Vieta, 2376·3
Viewgam, 2376·3
Vifarcap, 2376·3
Vifazolin, 2376·3
Vifenac, 2376·3
Vi-Ferrin, 2376·3
Vifolyt, 2376·3
Vifortol, 2376·3
Vig, 2376·3
Vig Recovery, 2376·4
Vigabatrin, 383·2
Vigabatrina, 383·2
Vigam, 2376·4
Vigamox, 2376·4
Vigam-S, 2376·4
Vigantol, 2376·4
Vigantoletten, 2376·4
Vigarol, 2376·4
Vigem, 2376·4
Vigencial, 2376·4
Vigicer, 2376·4
Vigil, 2376·4
Vigilia, 2376·4
Vigilon, 2376·4
Vigiten, 2376·4
Vigodana, 2376·4
Vigodana N, 2376·4
Vigofortal, 2376·4
Vigogel, 2376·4
Vigomar Forte, 2376·4
Vigonal, 2376·4
Vigoplus, 2376·4
Vigor Plus, 2376·4
Vigor-Ace, 2376·4
Vigoran, 2376·4
Vigorsan, 2376·4
Vigortol, 2376·4
Vigortonic, 2376·4
Vigour S, 2376·4
Vigranon B, 2377·1
Vikaman, 2377·1
Vikasolum, 1466·3
Vikatron, 2377·1
Vikela, 2377·1
Viken, 2377·1
Vilam, 2377·1
Vilan, 2377·1
Vilbine, 2377·1
Vilerm, 2377·1
Vilne, 2377·1
Vilona, 2377·1
Viloxazina, Hidrocloruro de, 323·3
Viloxazine Hydrochloride, 323·3
Viltar, 2377·1
Vilterm, 2377·1
Vima, Colirio— *see* Colirio Vima, 1899·4
Vi-Magna, 2377·1
Vimax, 2377·1
Vimblastina, Sulfato de, 591·2
Vimepan, 2377·1
Vimeral, 2377·1
Viminate, 2377·1
Vimineral, 2377·1
Viminfort, 2377·1
Viminol, Hidroxibenzoato de, 96·3
Viminol Hydroxybenzoate, 96·3
Vimoli, 2377·1
Vimotadine, 2377·1
Vimultisa, 2377·1
Vin Tonique de Vial, 2377·1
Vinagrera, 1749·1
Vinarine, 2377·1
Vinatal, 2377·1
Vinate GT, 2377·1
Vinblastina, Sulfato de, 591·2
Vinblastine Sulfate, 591·2
Vinblastine Sulphate, 591·2
Vinblastini Sulfas, 591·2
Vinburnina, 1764·2
Vinburnine, 1764·2
Vinburnine Phosphate, 1764·2
Vinca, 2377·1
*Vinca minor*, 1764·2
*Vinca rosea*, 591·2, 592·2
Vincacen, 2377·1
Vincadar, 2377·1
Vincafolina, 2377·1
Vincafor, 2377·2
Vincagil, 2377·2
Vincaleukoblastine Sulphate, 591·2
Vincamina, 1764·2
Vincamine, 1764·2
Vincamine Hydrochloride, 1764·2
Vincamine Hydrogen Tartrate, 1764·2
Vincamine Oxoglurate, 1764·2
Vincamine Teprosilate, 1764·2
Vincaminol, 2377·2
Vincamone, 1764·2
Vincapan, 2377·2
Vincapront, 2377·2
Vinca-Ri, 2377·2
Vincarutine, 2377·2
Vincasar, 2377·2
Vincasar PFS, 2377·2
Vinca-Tablinen, 2377·2
Vinca-Treis, 2377·2
Vincent's Infection— *see* Mouth Infections, 136·1
Vincent's Powders, 2377·2
Vinces, 2377·2
Vincetron, 2377·2
Vincidol, 2377·2
Vincigrip, 2377·2
Vincigrip Balsamico, 2377·2
Vincimax, 2377·2
Vinciseptil Otico, 2377·2
Vincitos, 2377·2
Vincizina, 2377·2
Vinco Forte, 2377·2
Vinco-Abfuhr-Perlen, 2377·2
Vincosedan, 2377·2
Vincrin, 2377·2
Vincristex, 2377·2
Vincristina, Sulfato de, 592·2
Vincristine Sulfate, 592·2
Vincristine Sulphate, 592·2
Vincristini Sulfas, 592·2
Vincrisul, 2377·2
Vindesina, Sulfato de, 593·3
Vindesine Sulfate, 593·3
Vindesine Sulphate, 593·3
Vindesini Sulfas, 593·3
Vinecort, 2377·2
Vinegar, 1645·3
Vinegar, Artificial, 1645·3
Vinelbine, 2377·2
Vingel, 2377·3
Vingional, 2377·3
Vinho Ferruginoso, 2377·3
Vinho Reconstituinte, 2377·3
Vinho Tonificante, 2377·3
Vinilbital, 727·2
Vinilo, Cloruro de, 1764·3
Vinkhum, 2377·3
Vinocard Q10, 2377·3
Vinone, 2377·3
Vinopepsin, 2377·3
Vinorelbina, Tartrato de, 594·1
Vinorelbine Ditartrate, 594·1
Vinorelbine Tartrate, 594·1
Vinorelbini Tartras, 594·1
Vinorgen, 2377·3
Vinpocetina, 1764·2
Vinpocetine, 1764·2
Vinracine, 2377·3
Vinsal, 2377·3
Vinsen, 2377·3
Vintec, 2377·3
Vintene, 2377·3
γ-Vinyl Aminobutyric Acid, 383·2
Vinyl Chloride, 1764·3
Vinyl Chloride Monomer, 1764·3
Vinylbital, 727·2
Vinylbitone, 727·2
γ-Vinyl-GABA, 383·2
Vinylpyrrolidinone Polymer, 1581·2
Vinymalum, 727·2
Vinzam, 2377·3
Viobeta, 2377·3
Viocidina, 2377·3
Viocort, 2377·3
Viodenum, 2377·3
Viodine, 2377·3
Viodor, 2377·3
Vioform, 2377·3
Vioform-Hydrocortisone, 2377·3
Vioformio-Hidrocortisona, 2377·3
Vioformo, 2377·3
Vioformo-Cort, 2377·3
Viogen-C, 2377·3
Viokase, 2377·3
Viola, 2377·4
Viola Crystallina, 1186·1
Violent Behaviour— *see* Disturbed Behaviour, 665·1
Violet, Crystal, 1186·1
Violet, Gentian, 1186·1
Violet, Methyl, 1186·2
Violgen, 2377·4
Violin, 2377·4
Vioneurin, 2377·4
Vioridon, 2377·4
Viosterol, 1462·1
Viotisone, 2377·4
Vioxx, 2377·4
Vioxxalt, 2377·4
VIP, 1763·2
Viper Venom Antiserum, European, 1639·1
Viperfav, 2377·4
Vipirim, 2377·4
Viplex, 2377·4
Viplura, 2377·4
Viplus, 2377·4
Vipocem, 2377·4
Vipodo, 2377·4
Vipoma— *see* Carcinoid Tumours and Other Secretory Neoplasms, 504·1
Vipral, 2377·4
Vipratox, 2377·4
Vipres, 2377·4
Viprinex, 2377·4
Vipro, 2377·4
Viprofen, 2377·4
Viprynium Embonate, 113·3
Viprynium Pamoate, 113·3
Vipsogal, 2377·4
Viquidil, Hidrocloruro de, 1764·3
Viquidil Hydrochloride, 1764·3
Viquin Forte, 2377·4
Vir, Aar— *see* Aar Vir, 1767·3
Vira-A, 2377·4
Viraban, 2377·4
Virac, 2377·4
Viracept, 2378·1
Viracillina, 2378·1
Virafer, 2378·1
Viraferon, 2378·1
ViraferonPeg, 2378·1
Viral Diarrhoea— *see* Gastro-enteritis, 618·2
Viral Encephalitis— *see* Encephalitis, 618·2
Viral Gastro-enteritis— *see* Gastro-enteritis, 618·2
Viral Haemorrhagic Fevers— *see* Haemorrhagic Fevers, 618·2
Viral Hepatitis— *see* Hepatitis, 618·3
Viral Infections in Immunocompromised Patients— *see* Infections in Immunocompromised Patients, 624·2
Viralief, 2378·1
Viralin, 2378·1
Viramid, 2378·1
Vira-MP, 2378·1
Viramune, 2378·1
Viranet, 2378·1
Virasolve, 2378·1
Virasorb, 2378·1
Viratin, 2378·1
Viravan, 2378·1
Viravan-DM, 2378·1
Virax, 2378·1
Viraxy, 2378·1
Virazid, 2378·1
Virazid— *see* Virazole, 2378·1
Virazide, 2378·1
Virazole, 2378·1
Virazone, 2378·1
Virbelte, 2378·1
Virdex, 2378·1
Viread, 2378·2
Viregyt, 2378·2
Virelon C, 2378·2
Virest, 2378·2
Virexen, 2378·2
Virfen, 2378·2
Virflutam, 2378·2
Virgamelis, 2378·2
Virgan, 2378·2
Virgilocard, 2378·2
Virgimycin, 277·3
Virgin Castor Oil, 1668·2
Virgin Linseed Oil, 1707·2
Virgin Oil, 1763·3
Virgin Olive Oil, 1723·2
Virginiamicina, 277·3
Virginiamycin, 277·3
Virginiamycin $M_1$, 277·3
Virginiamycin $S_1$, 277·3
Virginian Prune, 1765·2
Virginian Prune Bark, 1765·2
Virginian Snakeroot, 1656·3
Virginiana Gocce Verdi, 2378·2
Virherpes, 2378·2
Viridal, 2378·2
Viride Malachitum, 1185·2

Viride Nitens, 1171·1
Viridin, 2378·2
Virigen, 2378·2
Virilis-Gastreu S R41, 2378·2
Virilisterona, 2378·2
Virilit, 2378·2
Virilon, 2378·2
Virin, 2378·2
Virivac, 2378·2
Virless, 2378·2
Virlix, 2378·2
Virlix-D, 2378·2
Virman Plus, 2378·2
Virmax, 2378·2
Virmen, 2378·2
Virobin, 2378·2
Virobis, 2378·3
Virobron, 2378·3
Virobron B12 NF, 2378·3
Viro-Do, 2378·3
Virofral, 2378·3
Virogon, 2378·3
Virohep-A, 2378·3
Virolan, 2378·3
ViroMed, 2378·3
Viromed, 2378·3
Viromidin, 2378·3
Viron Wart Lotion, 2378·3
Vironida, 2378·3
Vironox, 2378·3
Viropect, 2378·3
Virophta, 2378·3
Viropox, 2378·3
Viroptic, 2378·3
Virormone, 2378·3
Virosol, 2378·3
Virostat, 2378·3
Virovir, 2378·3
Viroxy, 2378·3
Virozid, 2378·3
Virtamox, 2378·3
Virubact, 2378·3
Virucalm, 2378·3
Virucid, 2378·3
Viruderm, 2378·3
Virudermin, 2378·3
Virudin, 2378·4
Virulex, 2378·4
Virulex Forte, 2378·4
Viru-Merz, 2378·4
Viru-Merz Serol, 2378·4
Virunguent, 2378·4
Virunguent P, 2378·4
Virupos, 2378·4
Viru-Salvysat, 2378·4
Virusan, 2378·4
Viruseen, 2378·4
Viruserol, 2378·4
Viru-Serol, 2378·4
Virustat, 2378·4
Virusteril, 2378·4
Virustop, 2378·4
Viruxan, 2378·4
Virval, 2378·4
Virzin, 2378·4
VISA Infections— *see* Staphylococcal Infections, 147·2
Visacare, 2378·4
Visadron, 2378·4
Visage, Neo— *see* Neo Visage, 2157·1
Visaline, 2378·4
Visalmin, 2378·4
Visamin, 2378·4
Visammin, 1653·3
Visano N, 2378·4
VisanoCor— *see* VisanoCor N, 2379·1
VisanoCor N, 2379·1
Visano-mini N, 2379·1
Viscaplus, 2379·1
Viscard, 2379·1
Viscasan, 2379·1
Visceral Larva Migrans— *see* Toxocariasis, 101·1
Visceralgine, 2379·1
Visceralgine Compositum, 2379·1
Visceralgine Forte, 2379·1
Visci Caulis, 1715·3
Visclair, 2379·1
Viscoat, 2379·1
Viscoat— *see* Duovisc, 1957·4
Viscocort, 2379·1
Viscofresh, 2379·1
Viscolex, 2379·1
Viscolyt, 2379·1
Viscomucil, 2379·1
Visconisan N, 2379·1
Viscopaste, 2379·1
Viscopaste PB7, 2379·1
Visc-Ophtal, 2379·1
Viscophyll, 2379·1
Viscorapas Duo, 2379·1
Viscoseal, 2379·1
Viscotears, 2379·1
Viscoteina, 2379·1
Viscoter, 2379·1
Viscotiol, 2379·2
Viscotirs, 2379·2
Viscotoxins, 1715·3
Viscotraan, 2379·2
Viscozyme, 2379·2
Viscum, 1715·3
Viscum Album, 1715·3
*Viscum album*, 1715·3
Viscum Album H, 2379·2
Viscysat, 2379·2
Visderm, 2379·2
Visergil, 2379·2
Vi-Siblin, 2379·2
Vi-Siblin S, 2379·2
Visicol, 2379·2
Visidic, 2379·2
Visinal, 2379·2
Visine Preparations, 2379·2
Visine, Advanced Relief— *see also* Advanced Relief Visine, 1777·3
Visiodose, 2379·3
Visiolyre, 2379·3
Visio-Max, 2379·3
Vision Care Enzymatic Cleaner, 2379·3
Visionace, 2379·3
Visional Gotas, 2379·3
VisionBlue, 2379·3
Vision-Eze, Bioglan— *see* Bioglan Vision-Eze, 1844·2
Visionom, 2379·3
Visipaque, 2379·3
Visiplex, 2379·3
Viskaldix, 2379·3
Viskazide, 2379·3
Viskeen, 2379·3
Visken, 2379·3
Viskene, 2379·3
Viskenit, 2379·3
Viskoferm, 2379·3
Viskose Ojendraber, 2379·3
Vislin, 2379·3
Vislube, 2379·3
Vislube— *see* Vismed, 2379·3
Vismed, 2379·3
Visnadina, 1653·3
Visnadine, 1653·3
Visnaga, 1653·3
Visodin, 2379·3
Visogenol, 2379·4
Visolon, 2379·4
Visolux, 2379·4
Visonest, 2379·4
Visopt, 2379·4
Visotone, 2379·4
Visoy, 2379·4
Vispring, 2379·4
Vistabel, 2379·4
Vistacarpin, 2379·4
Vista-Cetamide, 2379·4
Vistacloran, 2379·4
Vistacrom, 2379·4
Vistacrom— *see* Stop-Allerg, 2308·2
Vistafrin, 2379·4
Vistagan, 2379·4
Vistalbalon, 2379·4
Vista-Methasone, 2379·4
Vista-Methasone N, 2379·4
Vista-Phenicol, 2379·4
Vistaril, 2379·4
Vistazine, 2379·4
Vistide, 2379·4
Vistimon, 2379·4
Vistofilm, 2379·4
Vistosan, 2379·4
Vistoxyn, 2380·1
Visu Q10, 2380·1
Visual, 2380·1
Visual-Eyes, 2380·1
Visublefarite, 2380·1
Visubril, 2380·1
Visucloben, 2380·1
Visucloben Antibiotico, 2380·1
Visucloben Decongestionante, 2380·1
Visudyne, 2380·1
Visuglican, 2380·1
Visumetazone Preparations, 2380·1
Visumicina, 2380·1
Visumidriatic, 2380·1
Visumidriatic Antiflogistico, 2380·1
Visumidriatic Fenilefrina, 2380·1
Visustrin, 2380·1
Visutensil, 2380·1
Vi-Syneral, 2380·1
Vi-Syneral GE, 2380·1
Vi-Syneral Plus, 2380·1
Vit Eparin, 2380·1
Vita, 2380·1
Vita 3, 2380·2
Vita 3B, 2380·2
Vita B6, 2380·2
Vita B Compound 100, 2380·2
Vita B Plus C, 2380·2
Vita 3B Plus C, 2380·2
Vita Bee, 2380·2
Vita Buer-G-plus, 2380·2
Vita Buerlecithin, 2380·2
Vita C, 2380·2
Vita Calmag Zn, 2380·2
Vita Cris, 2380·2
Vita Day, 2380·2
Vita Dino Buddies, 2380·2
Vita E, 2380·2
Vita Ferin C, 2380·2
Vita Gerine, 2380·2
Vita Grip, 2380·2
Vita Menal, 2380·2
Vita Multicap, 2380·2
Vita Senior, 2380·2
Vita Stress, 2380·2
Vita Truw, 2380·2
Vita Vim, 2380·2
Vita Vim, Super— *see* Super Vita Vim, 2313·3
Vita-B, 2380·2
Vita-B1, 2380·2
Vita-B2, 2380·2
Vita-B6, 2380·2
Vitabact, 2380·2
Vitabase, 2380·2
Vitabase Complexo Vitaminico C/Minerais, 2380·2
Vitabase Vitamina C, 2380·2
Vitabe, 2380·3
Vita-Bel, 2380·3
Vitaber A E, 2380·3
Vitaber PP + E, 2380·3
Vitableu, 2380·3
Vita-Bob, 2380·3
Vita-Brachont, 2380·3
Vitac, 2380·3
Vita-C, 2380·3
Vita-C R15, 2380·3
Vitacal, 2380·3
Vita-Cal Mag with Zinc and Vitamin D, 2380·3
Vita-Cal Plus, 2380·3
Vitacap, 2380·3
VitaCarn, 2380·3
Vitace, 2380·3
Vita-Ce, 2380·3
Vitacelsia Plus, 2380·3
Vitacic, 2380·3
Vitacid, 2380·3
Vitacimin, 2380·3
Vitacimin Sweetlet, 2380·3
Vitacitrus, 2380·3
Vitacolor, 2380·3
Vitacortil, 2380·3
Vitacrecil, 2380·3
Vitacrecil— *see* Crecil, 1911·1
Vitactiv E, 2380·3
Vitadece, 2380·3
Vita-Dermacide, 2380·3
Vitaderme, 2380·3
Vitadesan, 2380·4
Vita-D-Grin, 2380·4
Vita-Diem, 2380·4
Vitadol-C, 2380·4
Vitadral, 2380·4
Vit-A-drops— *see* Viva-Drops, 2383·1
Vitadye, 2380·4
Vita-E, 2380·4
Vita-E Plus Selenium, 2380·4
Vitaendil C K P, 2380·4
VitaEPA, 2380·4
VitaEPA Plus, 2380·4
Vitafardi C B12, 2380·4
Vitafem, 2380·4
Vitaferro, 2380·4
Vitafissan N, 2380·4
Vitafluid, 2380·4
Vitaflur, 2380·4
Vitafol, 2380·4
Vitaforte, 2380·4
Vitafran, 2380·4
Vitagama Fluor, 2380·4
Vitagama Fluor Complex, 2380·4
Vita-Gard, 2380·4
Vitagel, 2380·4
Vitagenol, 2380·4
Vitagenol Plus, 2380·4
Vitageran, 2380·4
Vita-Gerin, 2380·4
Vita-Gerin N, 2380·4
Vitageyer B, 2381·1
Vitageyer C, 2381·1
Vitaglow Selemite B, 2381·1
Vitaglumil, 2381·1
Vitagripe, 2381·1
Vitagutt Knoblauch, 2381·1
Vitagutt Vitamin E, 2381·1
Vita-Hexin, 2381·1
Vitaject, 2381·1
Vitakid, 2381·1
Vita-Kid, 2381·1
Vital, 2381·1
Vital Eyes, 2381·1
Vital Floramin, 2381·1
Vital High Nitrogen, 2381·1
Vital HN, 2381·1
Vitalaif, 2381·1
Vitalax, 2381·1
Vita-Lea, 2381·1
Vitalen C, 2381·1
Vitaleph, 2381·1
Vitaler, 2381·1
Vitalets, 2381·1
Vitaleyes, 2381·1
Vitalgine, 2381·1
Vitalin, 2381·1
Vitaline, 2381·1
Vitalipid, 2381·1
Vitalipid N, 2381·1
Vitalipid Neu, 2381·2
Vitalipide, 2381·2
Vitalisin, 2381·2
Vitalitan, 2381·2
Vitalium, 2381·2
Vitalize, 2381·2
Vital-Kapseln, 2381·2
Vitalle, 2381·2
Vitalmin Nutraenergy, 2381·2
Vitalmix Complex, 2381·2
Vitalmix Fos, 2381·2
Vitalmix Junior, 2381·2
Vita-Logos, 2381·2
Vitalorange, 2381·2
Vitalpen, 2381·2
Vitalux, 2381·2
Vitalux Plus, 2381·2
Vitalyn, 2381·2
Vitam Doce, 2381·2
Vitamag, 2381·2
Vita-Max, 2381·2
Vitamedin, 2381·2
Vita-Mefren, 2381·2
Vitamen, 2381·2
Vita-Merfen, 2381·2
Vita-Merfen NF, 2381·2

Vita-Merfen Soins Dermatologiques, 2381·2
Vitamfenicolo, 2381·3
Vitamidyne A and D, 2381·3
Vitamil, 2381·3
Vitamin A, 1451·2, 1451·3
Vitamin A Acetate, 1451·2
Vitamin A Acid, 1161·1, 2381·3
Vitamin A Alcohol, 1451·2
Vitamin A Concentrate (Oily Form), Synthetic, 1451·3
Vitamin A Concentrate (Powder Form), Synthetic, 1451·3
Vitamin A Concentrate (Solubilisate/Emulsion), Synthetic, 1451·3
Vitamin A Ester Concentrate, Natural, 1451·3
Vitamin A Palmitate, 1451·2
Vitamin A Propionate, 1451·2
Vitamin, Antixerophthalmic, 1451·2
Vitamin $B_1$, 1455·1
Vitamin $B_1$ Mononitrate, 1455·1
Vitamin $B_1$ Substances, 1454·3
Vitamin $B_2$, 1456·1
Vitamin $B_2$ Phosphate, 1456·1
Vitamin $B_2$ Substances, 1456·1
Vitamin $B_3$, 1441·2
Vitamin $B_4$, 1647·3
Vitamin $B_5$, 1442·3
Vitamin $B_6$, 1456·3
Vitamin $B_6$ Substances, 1456·3
Vitamin $B_9$, 1429·1
Vitamin $B_{11}$, 1429·1
Vitamin $B_{12}$, 1458·2
Vitamin $B_{12}$ Substances, 1458·2
Vitamin $B_{12}$-deficiency Anaemia— *see* Megaloblastic Anaemia, 734·1
Vitamin $B_{15}$, 1727·2
Vitamin $B_{17}$, 1704·3
Vitamin B Duo, 2381·3
Vitamin B Substances, 1454·3
Vitamin $B_T$, 1423·3
Vitamin C, 1460·2
Vitamin C Palmitate, 1168·2
Vitamin C Substances, 1460·2
Vitamin C-Calcium, 2381·3
Vitamin $D_2$, 1462·1
Vitamin $D_3$, 1461·3
Vitamin D Substances, 1461·2
Vitamin D Tablets, Calcium and— *see* Calcium and Ergocalciferol Tablets, 1863·3
Vitamin D-dependent Rickets— *see* Osteomalacia, 762·3
Vitamin D-pseudodeficiency Rickets— *see* Osteomalacia, 762·3
Vitamin E, 1464·3, 1465·1
Vitamin E Nicotinate, 1015·1
Vitamin E Polyethylene Glycol Succinate, 1465·1
Vitamin E Substances, 1464·3
Vitamin F, 2381·3
Vitamin for the Hair, 2381·3
Vitamin G, 1456·1
Vitamin H, 1423·2
Vitamin H′, 1142·2
Vitamin K, 1302·3
Vitamin K Deficiency Bleeding, 1468·2
Vitamin K Substances, 1466·3
Vitamin $K_1$, 1467·1
Vitamin $K_2$, 1467·3
Vitamin $K_{2(20)}$, 1467·1
Vitamin $K_3$, 1466·3
Vitamin $K_3$ Sodium Bisulphite, 1466·3
Vitamin $K_4$ Diacetate, 1466·3
Vitamin $K_4$ Sodium Phosphate, 1466·3
Vitamin MK 4, 1467·1
Vitamin P Substances, 1688·2
Vitamin PP, 1441·2
Vitamin U, 1714·1
Vitamina A, 1451·2
Vitamina C-Complex, 2381·3
Vitamina F99 Topica, 2381·3
Vitaminas B, 1454·3
Vitaminas $B_1$, 1454·3
Vitaminas $B_2$, 1456·1
Vitaminas $B_6$, 1456·3
Vitaminas $B_{12}$, 1458·2
Vitaminas C, 1460·2
Vitaminas D, 1461·2
Vitaminas E, 1464·3
Vitaminas K, 1466·3
Vitaminas Lorenzini, 2381·3
Vitamine 15, 2381·3
Vitamine F99, 2381·3
Vitaminer S, 2381·3
Vitamineral, 2381·3
Vitaminex, 2381·3
Vitaminic A-D, 2381·3
Vita-Minis Cold & Flu, 2381·3
Vita-Minis Vitamin C Plus, 2381·3
Vitaminoftalmina, 2381·3
Vitaminol, 2381·3
Vitaminorum, 2381·3
Vitamins, Nutritional Agents and, 1417·1
Vitamins Only, 2381·3
Vitaminum A, 1451·2
Vitaminum A in Aqua Dispergibile, 1451·3
Vitaminum A Densatum Oleosum, 1451·3
Vitaminum A Pulvis, 1451·3
Vitamischka, 2381·3
Vitamon K, 2381·3
Vitamorrhuine, 2381·3
Vitamult, 2381·3
Vitamuruine, 2381·3
Vitamycetin, 2381·3
Vitan, 2381·3
Vit-A-N, 2381·3
Vitana-EZ, 2381·3
Vita-Nat, 2381·3
Vitanatur, 2381·4
Vitaneed, 2381·4
Vitaneuron, 2381·4
Vitanol, 2381·4
Vitanol-A, 2381·4
Vitanor, 2381·4
Vitanovit, 2381·4
Vitapan, 2381·4
Vitapantol, 2381·4
Vita-Ped, 2381·4
Vitapelen, 2381·4
Vitapen, 2381·4
Vitaphakol, 2381·4
Vitaplex, 2381·4
Vitaplex Comp, 2381·4
Vitaplex Mineral, 2381·4
Vita-Plus, 2381·4
Vitaplus B, 2381·4
Vitaplus B Plus, 2381·4
Vitaplus C Plus, 2381·4
Vita-Plus E, 2381·4
Vita-PMS, 2381·4
Vitapore, 2381·4
Vita-Preg, 2381·4
Vitaquick, 2381·4
Vitaral, 2381·4
Vitarex, 2381·4
Vitargenol, 2381·4
Vitarical, 2381·4
Vitarnin, 2381·4
Vitarubin, 2381·4
Vitarutine, 2381·4
Vitasana, 2382·1
Vitasana-Lebenstropfen, 2382·1
Vitasavoury, 2382·1
Vitasay, 2382·1
Vitascarbol, 2382·1
Vita-Schlanktropfen, 2382·1
Vitascorb, 2382·1
Vitascorbol, 2382·1
Vitasedine, 2382·1
Vitaseptine, 2382·1
Vitaseptol, 2382·1
Vitaseve, 2382·1
Vitasic, 2382·1
Vitasma, 2382·1
VitaSohn, 2382·1
Vitasprint, 2382·1
Vitasprint $B_{12}$, 2382·1
Vitasprint Complex, 2382·1
Vita-Squares, 2382·1
Vitasten, 2382·1
Vita-Suple, 2382·1
Vitathion, 2382·1
Vita-Thion, 2382·1
Vitathion-ATP, 2382·1
Vitaton, 2382·1
Vitatona, 2382·1
Vitatonin, 2382·2
Vitatonus Dexa, 2382·2
Vitatron, 2382·2
Vitaveran Folico, 2382·2
Vitavir, 2382·2
Vitavitin, 2382·2
Vitavox Pastillas, 2382·2
Vita-Worth B Complex, 2382·2
Vitawund, 2382·2
Vitawund Baby, 2382·2
Vitax, 2382·2
Vitax Derm, 2382·2
Vitaxicam, 2382·2
Vitayde C, 2382·2
Vitazell E, 2382·2
Vitazinc, 2382·2
Vitazyme, 2382·2
Vitcaroten, 2382·2
Vit-C-Lutsch, 2382·2
Vitec, 2382·2
Vitecaf, 2382·2
Vitef, 2382·2
Vitelinato de Plata, 1746·2
Vitelinato de Prata, 1746·2
Vitelle Nesentials, 2382·2
Vitelle Nestabs, 2382·2
Vitelle Nestrex, 2382·2
Vitelsix, 2382·2
Vitenur, 2382·2
Viteral, 2382·2
Vitergan Master, 2382·2
Vitergan Pre-natal, 2382·3
Vitergan Zinco, 2382·3
Viternum, 2382·3
Viternum Vitaminado, 2382·3
Viterra, 2382·3
Vitestable, 2382·3
Vitex, 2382·3
*Vitex agnus-castus*, 1649·1
Vitexid, 2382·3
Vitexin, 1677·1, 1729·1
Vitialgin, 2382·3
Viticromin, 2382·3
Vitiligo— *see* Pigmentation Disorders, 1137·2
Vitinoin, 2382·3
Vitintra, 2382·3
Vitiral, 2382·3
Vitiron, 2382·3
Vitiveine, 2382·3
ViTiX, 2382·3
Vitlipid N, 2382·3
Vitneurin, 2382·3
Vito Bronches, 2382·3
Vitobasan N, 2382·3
Vitobel, 2382·3
Vitogen, 2382·3
Vitogen Spectrum, 2382·3
Vitol, 2382·3
Vit-o-Mar, 2382·3
Vitonic, 2382·3
Vitonico, 2382·3
Vitonil, 2382·3
Vitoral, 2382·3
Vitosal, 2382·4
Vitotal, 2382·4
Vit-Porphyrin, 2382·4
Vitrace, 2382·4
Vitraday, 2382·4
Vitrafem, 2382·4
Vitrasert, 2382·4
Vitravene, 2382·4
Vitrax, 2382·4
Vitreoclar, 2382·4
Vitreolent, 2382·4
Vitreolent Plus, 2382·4
Vitreolux, 2382·4
Vitreosan, 2382·4
Vitrical, 2382·4
Vitrimix, 2382·4
Vitrimix KV, 2382·4
Vitriol, Blue, 1426·1
Vitriol, Brown Oil of, 1750·3
Vitriol, Concentrated Oil of, 1750·3
Vitriol, Green, 1428·2
Vitriol, Oil of, 1750·3
Vitriol, White, 1469·3
Vitrite, 2382·4
Vitron, 2382·4
Vitron-C, 2382·4
Vitrosups, 2382·4
Vits, 2382·4
Vitulpas, 2382·4
Vit-u-pept, 2382·4
Vitussin, 2382·4
Vivabec, 2383·1
Vivacor, 2383·1
Vivactil, 2383·1
Vivadone, 2383·1
Viva-Drops, 2383·1
Vival, 2383·1
Vivalan, 2383·1
Vivalessence, 2383·1
Vivamag, 2383·1
Vivamyne, 2383·1
Vivance, 2383·1
Vivapryl, 2383·1
Vivarin, 2383·1
Vivarint, 2383·1
Vivatak, 2383·1
Vivatec, 2383·1
Vivatec Comp, 2383·1
Vivaxim, 2383·1
Vivaxine, 2383·1
Vivazid, 2383·1
Vivelle, 2383·1
Vivelle— *see* Estalis Sequi, 1978·4
Vivena AR, 2383·1
Vivena HA, 2383·1
Vivene, 2383·1
Viverdal, 2383·1
Vivicrom, 2383·1
Vividrin Preparations, 2383·1
Vividyl, 2383·2
Vivimed, 2383·2
Vivin C, 2383·2
Vivinox, 2383·2
Vivinox N, 2383·2
Vivinox Stark, 2383·2
Vivinox-Schlafdragees, 2383·2
Vivioptal, 2383·2
Viviplus, 2383·2
Vivir, 2383·2
ViviRhin S, 2383·2
Vivisun, 2383·2
Vivol, 2383·2
Vivolan, 2383·2
Vivonex, 2383·2
Vivotif, 2383·2
Vivradoxil, 2383·2
Vivural, 2383·2
Vix Plex, 2383·2
Vixcef, 2383·2
Vixiderm E, 2383·2
Vixidone, 2383·2
Vixidone T, 2383·2
Vixin, 2383·3
Vixmicina, 2383·3
Vixorfit, 2383·3
Vi-Zac, 2383·3
Vizax, 2383·3
Vizerul, 2383·3
Vizole, 2383·3
Viz-On, 2383·3
Vizoptal, 2383·3
Vizylac, 2383·3
VLB, 591·2
Vleminckx's Solution, 1158·2
VM 26, 2383·3
VM-26, 587·2
VM-2000, 2383·3
VM Drosan, 2383·3
VMA, 854·1
VML-251, 469·2
VML-600, 652·1
Vobaderm, 2383·3
Vobamyk, 2383·3
Vocadys, 2383·3
Vocalzone, 2383·3
Vocara, 2383·3
Vodol, 2383·3
Vofenal, 2383·3
Vogalene, 2383·3
Vogalib, 2383·3
Voglibosa, 348·3

Voglibose, 348·3
Voglisan, 2383·3
Voir, 2383·3
Voker, 2383·3
Volamin, 2383·3
Volatile Bitter Almond Oil, 1659·3
Volatile Mustard Oil, 1718·2
Volatile Oils, 1763·3
Volcidol-S, 2383·3
Volcolon, 2383·3
Voldal, 2383·3
Volfenac, 2383·3
Vollmers Praparierter Gruner N, 2383·3
Volmac, 2383·4
Volmax, 2383·4
Volnac, 2383·4
Vologen, 2383·4
Volon Preparations, 2383·4
Volon, Solu— *see* Solu-Volon A, 2298·4
Volonimat, 2383·4
Volonimat N, 2383·4
Volonimat Plus N, 2383·4
Volonten, 2383·4
Volplex, 2383·4
Volraman, 2383·4
Volsaid, 2383·4
Volta, 2383·4
Voltaflan, 2383·4
Voltaflex, 2383·4
Voltamicin, 2383·4
Voltamicine, 2383·4
Voltanac, 2383·4
Voltaren Preparations, 2383·4
Voltarene, 2384·1
Voltarene Rapide, 2384·1
Voltarol, 2384·1
Voltarol Ophtha, 2384·1
Voltax, 2384·1
Voltfast, 2384·1
Voltil, 2384·1
Voltric, 2384·1
Voltrix, 2384·1
Volumax D 40, 2384·1
Volumax D 70, 2384·1
Volutine, 2384·1
Volutol, 2384·1
Voluven, 2384·1
Volverac, 2384·2
Vomacur, 2384·2
Vomex A, 2384·2
Vomidon, 2384·2
Vomidrine, 2384·2
Vomifene, 2384·2
Vominar, 2384·2
Vominil, 2384·2
Vomisin, 2384·2
Vomistop, 2384·2
Vomiting— *see* Nausea and Vomiting, 1245·2
Vomitron, 2384·2
Vomitusheel, 2384·2
Vomix, 2384·2
Von Willebrand Factor, 735·3
Von Willebrand's Disease— *see* Haemorrhagic Disorders, 737·3
Voncon, 2384·2
Vonifin, 2384·2
Vonil, 2384·2
Vonil Enzimatico, 2384·2
Vontrol, 2384·2
Vonum, 2384·2
Vopar, 2384·2
Vopax, 2384·2
V-Optic, 2384·2
Voraclor, 2384·2
Vorange, 2384·2
Vo-Remi, 2384·2
Voren, 2384·2
Voren Plus, 2384·2
Voriconazol, 411·2
Voriconazole, 411·2
Vorigeno, 2384·2
VoriNa, 2384·2
Voronov's Snowdrop, 1491·2
Vorozol, 594·3
Vorozole, 594·3
Vorst, 2384·2
VoSoL, 2384·3
VoSoL HC, 2384·3
VoSpire, 2384·3
Vostar, 2384·3
Votag, 2384·3
Votamed, 2384·3
Voveran, 2384·3
Voxpax, 2384·3
Voxsuprine, 2384·3
VP-16, 551·3
VP-16-213, 551·3
VP-63843, 651·3
V-Pen, 2384·3
VP-Gen, 2384·3
VP-Tec, 2384·3
VR, 2384·3
Vraap, 2384·3
Vridol, 2384·3
VRSA Infections— *see* Staphylococcal Infections, 147·2
V-Tablopen, 2384·3
V-Talgin, 2384·3
V-Tears, 2384·3
VTEC, 129·2
VUAB-6453 (SPOFA), 955·3
Vuclodir, 2384·3
Vudirax, 2384·3
Vueffe, 2384·3
VUFB-6453, 955·3
Vulbegal, 2384·3
Vulcase, 2384·3
Vulcasid, 2384·3
Vulgix, 2384·3
Vulnofilin Compuesto, 2384·3
Vulnopur, 2384·3
Vulnostimulin, 2384·4
Vulpuran, 2384·4
Vulvovaginal Candidiasis— *see* Candidiasis, 386·3
Vumon, 2384·4
Vunsu, 2384·4
Vurdon, 2384·4
VVS, 2384·4
VWf, 735·3
VX, 1719·2
VX-478, 628·2
Vykmin, 2384·4
Vypen, 2384·4
Vysorel, 2384·4
Vytinal, 2384·4
Vytone, 2384·4
Vytral, 2384·4
V-Zoline, 2384·4

## W

W, 320·3
W5, 2384·4
W-37, 330·3
51W89, 1399·1
W-090, 433·1
141W94, 628·2
W-554, 361·1
W-583, 951·2
W-1655, 83·1
W-1929, 199·1
W-2900A, 914·2
W-2946M, 791·2
W-2964M, 43·3
W-2979M, 425·2
W-3566, 1568·2
W-4020, 716·2
W-4565, 240·3
W-5219, 1284·3
W-5759A, 94·1
W-5975, 1093·1
W-6309, 1100·1
W-7000A, 946·2
W-19053, 1376·3
W-36095, 1014·1
Wacholderbeeren, 1703·1
Wacholderöl, 1703·1
Wacholderteer, 1159·2
Wachs, Gebleichtes, 1480·1
Wachs, Gelbes, 1480·2
Wahoo Bark, 1265·2
Wakamoto, 2384·4
Wake-Up Tablets, 2384·4
Walacort, 2384·4
Walagesic, 2384·4
Walamycin, 2384·4
Walaphage, 2384·4
Walavin, 2384·4
WAL-801-Cl, 433·3
Waldenström's Macroglobulinaemia, 511·3
Walekof, 2384·4
Walesolone, 2384·4
Walix, 2384·4
Wallerox, 2384·4
Walsedyl, 2384·4
Walyte, 2384·4
Wampole Bronchial Cough Syrup, 2385·1
Wampole Vitamin Syrup, 2385·1
Wandonorm, 2385·1
Wanmycin, 2385·1
Wanse, 2385·1
War Lin, 2385·1
Waran, 2385·1
Warca, 2385·1
Warfant, 2385·1
Warfarin Potassium, 1022·2
Warfarin Sodium, 1022·2
Warfarin Sodium Clathrate, 1022·2
Warfarina Sódica, 1022·2
Warfarina Sódica, Clatrato de, 1022·2
Warfarin-deanol, 1028·1
Warfarinum Natricum, 1022·2
Warfarinum Natricum Clathratum, 1022·2
Warfilone, 2385·1
WariActiv, 2385·1
Wari-Diclowal, 2385·1
Waridipin, 2385·1
Warimazol, 2385·1
Wari-Procomil, 2385·1
Wariviron, 2385·1
Warix, 2385·1
Warme-Gel, 2385·1
Warm-Up, 2385·1
Wart Remover, 2385·1
Wart Remover, Scholl— *see* Scholl Wart Remover, 2279·3
Wartec, 2385·1
Wartex, 2385·1
Warticon, 2385·1
Wartner, 2385·1
Wart-Off, 2385·1
Warts, 1139·2
Waruzol, 2385·1
Warz-ab Extor, 2385·1
Warzen-Alldahin, 2385·2
Warzenmittel, 2385·2
Warzin, 2385·2
WAS-2160, 397·1
Wash E45, 2385·2
Washing Soda, 1747·2
Wasp-Eze, 2385·2
Wasser, 1764·3
Wasser für Injektionszwecke, 1765·1
Wasserhaltiges Aluminiumoxid, 1249·2
Wasserstoffsuperoxydlösung, 1182·2
Wassertrat, 2385·2
Water, 1764·3
Water ($^{15}$O), 1525·1
Water Babies, 2385·2
Water Babies Little Licks, 2385·2
Water Babies UVGuard, 2385·2
Water Balance, HRI— *see* HRI Water Balance, 2048·4
Water, Disinfection of— *see* Disinfection of Water, 1165·1
Water Glass, 1748·3
Water, Highly Purified, 1764·3
Water for Injection, 1765·1
Water for Injections, 1765·1
Water Intoxication— *see* Hyponatraemia, 1220·3
Water Naturtabs, 2385·2
Water Pill c Potasio, 2385·2
Water, Purified, 1764·3
Water Relief Tablets, Heath & Heather— *see* Heath & Heather Water Relief Tablets, 2037·3
Water Retention, Modern Herbals— *see* Modern Herbals Water Retention, 2138·2
Water Soluble E, Bioglan— *see* Bioglan Water Soluble E, 1844·2
Water, Tritiated, 1526·2
Water-insoluble Fibre, 1253·2
Waterlex, Gerard House— *see* Gerard House Waterlex, 2022·2
Watershed, 2385·2
Water-soluble Fibre, 1253·2
Waucosin, 2385·2
Wax Alcohols, Wool, 1482·3
Wax, Aseptic Surgical, 1480·2
Wax, Bone, Sterile Surgical, 1480·2
Wax, Candelilla, 1480·2
Wax, Caranda, 1668·1
Wax, Carnauba, 1668·1
Wax, Cetyl Esters, 1480·3
Wax, Emulsifying, 1481·1
Wax, Emulsifying, Anionic, 1481·1
Wax, Horsley's, 1480·2
Wax, Microcrystalline, 1481·3
Wax Myrtle Bark, 1659·2
Wax, Paraffin, 1479·1
Wax, White, 1480·2
Wax, Yellow, 1480·2
Waxolve, 2385·2
Waxsol, 2385·2
Waxsol NF, 2385·2
Waxwane, 2385·2
4-Way Fast Acting, 2385·2
4-Way Long Lasting, 2385·2
WAY-ANA-756, 1009·3
Waycital, 2385·2
WAY-CMA-676, 558·3
Wayfrato, 2385·2
Waynazol, 2385·2
Waysen, 2385·2
Waysul, 2385·2
Waytifeno, 2385·3
Waytrax, 2385·3
WBA-8119, 1500·3
WCS Dusting Powder, 2385·3
We-941, 672·1
We-941-BS, 672·1
WEB-1881, 1719·2
WEB-2086, 781·1
WEB-2086-BS, 781·1
Wechseltee EF-EM-ES, 2385·3
Wee, 1666·1
Wegener's Granulomatosis, 1090·2
Weiche Zinkpaste, 2385·3
Weifapenin, 2385·3
Weight Control, 2385·3
Weight Loss Aid, 2385·3
Weight Loss Kit, 2385·3
Weight Watchers Punto, 2385·3
Weil's Disease— *see* Leptospirosis, 133·3
Weimerquin, 2385·3
Weinsäure, 1752·1
Weinstein, 1284·3
Weiscal, 2385·3
Weiscalina, 2385·3
Weisen-U, 2385·3
Weissdorn, 1677·1
Weissdorn, Kneipp Pflanzen-Dragees— *see* Kneipp Pflanzen-Dragees Weissdorn, 2081·3
Weissdorn-Planzensaft Sebastianeum, Kneipp— *see* Kneipp Weissdorn-Pflanzensaft Sebastianeum, 2081·4
Weissdorn-Tee, Kneipp— *see* Kneipp Weissdorn-Tee, 2081·4
Weisser Ton, 1268·3
Welchol, 2385·3
Weleda Hamorrhoidalzapfchen, 2385·3
Weleda-Rheumasalbe M, 2385·3
Wellbutrin, 2385·3
Wellcid, 2385·3
Wellconal, 2385·3
Wellcoprim, 2385·3
Wellcovorin, 2385·3
Welldorm, 2385·3
Wellferon, 2385·3
Wellman, 2385·3
Wellvone, 2385·3
Wellwoman, 2385·4
Welticilina, 2385·4
Welt-Sulfazol, 2385·4
Wemid, 2385·4
Wepox, 2385·4
Weraplex Plain, 2385·4
Wermutkraut, 1645·1
Wernicke-Korsakoff Syndrome, 1455·3
Wernicke's Encephalopathy— *see* Wernicke-Korsakoff Syndrome, 1455·3
West Indian Tamarind, 1293·2

Westcan Century Plus MV & Mineral, 2385·4
Westcort, 2385·4
Westphal Variant Chorea— *see* Chorea, 664·2
West's Syndrome— *see* Epilepsy, 349·1
Wet, 2385·4
Wetol, 2385·4
Wetting Agents, 1411·1
Wetting Solutions, 1164·2
Wewe, 1666·1
WF-10, 1752·3
WG-253, 791·3
WH-5668, 1305·3
Wheat Bran, 1253·2
Wheat, Malted Grain of, 1439·2
Wheat Starch, 1449·1
Wheat-germ Oil, 1465·3
Whey Factor, 1724·3
Whippit, 1305·1
Whipple's Disease, 153·3
Whipworm Infections— *see* Trichuriasis, 101·2
White Arsenic, 1657·1
White Asbestos, 1658·1
White Beeswax, 1480·1
White Bismuth, 1252·2
White Breath Holding Attacks— *see* Anoxic Seizures, 478·2
White Cloverine, 2385·4
White Copperas, 1469·3
White Destroying Angel, 1717·3
White Fluids, 1193·3
White Girl, 1373·3
White Hellebore, 1764·1
White Hellebore Rhizome, 1764·1
White Horehound, 1124·1
White Lady, 1373·3
White Mineral Oil, 1479·1
White Mineral Oil, Light, 1479·1
White Mint, 1283·2
White Mustard, 1718·2
White Petrolatum, 1479·3
White Petroleum Jelly, 1479·3
White Precipitate, 1152·1, 1712·3
White Shellac, 1743·3
White Shellac (Bleached), 1743·3
White Soft Paraffin, 1479·3
White Spirit, 1478·1
White Squill, 1130·3
White Veratrum, 1764·1
White Vitriol, 1469·3
White Wax, 1480·1, 1480·2
Whiteheads— *see* Acne, 1133·3
Whitethorn, 1677·1
Whitfield, 2385·4
Whitfield Plus, 2385·4
Whitfields (Benzoic Acid Compound) Ointment, 2385·4
Whitfields Ointment— *see* Whitfields (Benzoic Acid Compound) Ointment, 2385·4
*Whitmania acranulata*, 945·1
*Whitmania pigra*, 945·1
Whole Blood, 743·3
Whole Blood, ACD, 744·1
Whole Blood, CPD, 744·1
Whole Blood, CPDA-1, 744·1
Whole Blood, Heparin, 744·1
Whooping Cough— *see* Pertussis, 140·2
Whooping-cough Vaccine, 1631·2
Whortleberry, 1718·3
Whortleberry, Red, 1676·3
WHR-5020, 38·1
WHR-1142A, 1270·2
WHR-2908A, 305·3
Wibi, 2385·4
Wibophorin, 2385·4
Wibotin H, 2385·4
Wicaran, 2385·4
Wicarba, 2385·4
Wick Preparations, 2385·4
Wicne, 2386·1
Wicnecarb, 2386·1
Wicnelact, 2386·1
Wicnevit, 2386·1
Wiedimmun, 2386·1
Wiesensauerampfer, 1749·1
Wifibrin, 2386·1
Wigraine, 2386·1
Wild Black Cherry Bark, 1765·2
Wild Carrot, 1765·1
Wild Cherry, 1765·2
Wild Cherry Bark, 1765·2
Wild Hydrangea, 1698·3
Wild Lettuce, 1765·2
Wilkinite, 1577·2
Willlong, 2386·1
Willospon, 2386·1
Willospon Forte, 2386·1
Willow Bark, 87·3
Willowbark Plus Herbal Formula 11, 2386·2
Wilms' Tumour, 518·2
Wilpan, 2386·2
Wilpan C, 2386·2
Wilprafen, 2386·2
Wilson's Disease, 1049·3
Wilyfenicol, 2386·2
Win-1258-2, 452·3
Win-3406, 787·3
Win-5063, 269·2
Win-5063-2, 269·2
Win-8077, 1487·3
Win-8851-2, 1067·3
Win-9154, 939·3
Win-9317, 989·3
Win-11318, 1371·1
Win-11450, 20·3
Win-13146, 616·3
Win-14833, 1569·2
Win-17757, 1545·2
Win-18320, 234·1
Win-18501-2, 713·1
Win-20228, 79·3
Win-22118, 92·3
Win-24540, 1757·3
Win-24933, 105·3
Win-32729, 1683·3
Win-32784, 781·3
Win-35213, 254·1
Win-35833, 884·2
Win-39103, 1067·1
Win-39424, 1064·2
Win-40014, 615·2
Win-40350, 1699·3
Win-40680, 862·3
Win-41464, 1187·2
Win-41464-2, 1187·2
Win-41464-6, 1187·2
Win-47203-2, 959·2
Win-59010, 1067·1
Win-59010-2, 1067·1
Win-59075, 588·3
Win-63843, 651·3
Win-90000, 883·2
Winar, 2386·2
Winasma, 2386·2
Winasorb, 2386·2
Winasorb Flex, 2386·2
Wincef, 2386·2
Wincoram, 2386·2
Wind & Dyspepsia Relief, 2386·2
Windcheaters, Asilone— *see* Asilone Windcheaters, 1815·3
Wind-Eze, 2386·2
Windol, 2386·2
Windol Basisbad, 2386·2
Windtreibender Tee, Bioreform— *see* Bioreform-Windtreibender Tee, 1845·3
Wingel, 2386·2
Wink, 2386·2
40 Winks, 2386·2
Winlomylon, 2386·2
Winobanin, 2386·2
Winofit, 2386·2
Winol, 2386·2
Winpac, 2386·2
Winpain, 2386·2
Winpred, 2386·2
WinRho, 2386·2
Winstrol, 2386·3
Winter AP, 2386·3
Winter Cherry, 1731·3
Wintergreen, 59·3
Wintergreen Oil, 59·3
Wintogeno, 2386·3
Wintomilon, 2386·3
Wintomylon, 2386·3
Winton, 2386·3
Wintonin, 2386·3
Wisamt, 2386·3
Wisamt N, 2386·3
Wismut Comp, 2386·3
Wismutgallat, Basisches, 1252·2
Wismutkarbonat, Basisches, 1252·1
Wismutnitrat, Basisches, 1252·2
Witch Doctor, 2386·3
Witch Hazel, 1696·3
Witch Sunsore, 2386·3
Withdrawal Syndrome, Alcohol— *see* Alcohol Withdrawal and Abstinence, 1166·2
Withdrawal Syndrome, Barbiturate— *see* Dependence and Withdrawal, 670·2
Withdrawal Syndrome, Benzodiazepine— *see* Benzodiazepine Withdrawal Syndrome, 690·2
Withdrawal Syndrome, Cocaine— *see* Withdrawal, 1375·2
Withdrawal Syndrome, Ergotamine— *see* Dependence, 468·1
Withdrawal Syndrome, Opioid— *see* Treatment of Opioid Dependence, 71·2
Withdrawal Syndrome, Opioid, Neonatal— *see* Neonatal Abstinence Syndrome, 72·1
Witromin, 2386·3
Witte Kruis, 2386·3
Witty, 2386·3
WI-140, 1284·2
WL-43775, 1505·2
Wobe-Mugos, 2386·3
Wobe-Mugos E, 2386·3
Wobe-Mugos Th, 2386·3
Wobenzimal, 2386·3
Wobenzym, 2386·3
Wobenzym N, 2386·3
Woerisetten S, 2386·3
Wokadine, 2386·3
Wokex-2, 2386·3
Wokex-3, 2386·4
Wokex-4, 2386·4
Wolff Basis, 2386·4
Wolff-Parkinson-White Syndrome— *see* Cardiac Arrhythmias, 816·1
Wolfies, 698·3
Wolf's Bane, 1656·3
Wolfsbane, 1656·3
Wolfsbane Root, 1646·3
Wollblumen, 1764·1
Wollfett, 1483·1
Wollwachs, 1483·1
Wollwachsalkohole, 1482·3
Woloderma, 2386·4
Woman Formula, 2386·4
Woman Kind, 2386·4
Womens All-in-One, Natures Way— *see* Natures Way Womens All-in-One, 2153·3
Womens Change Formula, 2386·4
Womens Exclusive Formula, 2386·4
Women's Formula Herbal Formula 3, 2386·4
Womens Support, 2386·4
Women's Timed Release Ultra Mega Without Iron, 2386·4
Womens Tylenol Multi-Symptom Menstrual Relief, 2386·4
Womosol Solar, 2386·4
Wonder Ice, 2386·4
Wondergel, 2386·4
Wondra, 2386·4
Wood Charcoal, 1031·1
Wood Creosote, 1117·2
Wood Naphtha, 1475·3
Wood Sugar, 1766·1
Wood Tar, 1159·3
Woodwards Preparations, 2386·4
Woody Nightshade, 1683·1
Wool Alcohols, 1482·3
Wool Alcohols, Acetylated, 1483·1
Wool Alcohols, Ethoxylated, 1483·1
Wool Fat, 1483·1
Wool Fat, Hydrogenated, 1483·2
Wool Fat, Hydrous, 1483·2
Wool Fat, Refined, 1483·1
Wool Green B, 1057·3
Wool Wax Alcohols, 1482·3
Woolly Foxglove Leaf, 894·2
Worisetten S, Kneipp— *see* Kneipp Worisetten S, 2081·4
Worm, 2386·4
Wormex, 2386·4
Wormgo, 2386·4
Wormin, 2386·4
Wormseed, Oil of American, 103·3
Wormstop, 2386·4
Wormwood, 114·1, 1645·1
Wotinex, 2386·4
Wound Disinfection, 1165·2
Wound-A-Sept, 2386·4
Wounds— *see* Wounds and Ulcers, 1139·2
WR-1065, 1031·3
WR-1141, 588·2
WR-2721, 1031·3
WR-2785, 567·2
WR-13045, 575·1
WR-19039, 568·2
WR-19508, 532·2
WR-19813, 566·1
WR-28453, 543·1
WR-45312, 588·1
WR-69596, 554·2
WR-83799, 559·1
WR-95704, 526·2
WR-135675, 772·2
WR-138719, 540·2
WR-138720, 553·1
WR-138743, 573·3
WR-139007, 544·2
WR-139013, 536·1
WR-139017, 565·2
WR-139021, 535·1
WR-142490, 453·3
WR-147650, 537·1
WR-171669, 452·2
WR-220057, 573·2
WR-220066, 586·2
WR-220076, 583·2
WR-238605, 463·3
Wright's Vaporizing Fluid, 2386·4
Wrinkle Defence, 2387·1
Writer's Cramp— *see* Dystonias, 1209·3
WSM-3978G, 980·2
W-Tropfen, 2387·1
Wund- und Brand-Gel Eu Rho, 2387·1
Wund- und Heilsalbe N, 2387·1
Wundesin, 2387·1
Wurmsamenöl, 103·3
WV-569, 975·3
Wy-401, 37·2
Wy-806, 1382·1
Wy-1359, 440·3
Wy-3277, 233·3
Wy-3467, 690·1
Wy-3478, 1308·3
Wy-3498, 712·2
Wy-3707, 1563·2
Wy-3917, 723·2
Wy-4036, 704·1
Wy-4082, 705·2
Wy-4508, 188·1
Wy-5104, 1563·2
Wy-8138, 1253·2
Wy-8678, 926·2
Wy-16225, 30·1
Wy-21743, 75·1
Wy-21894, 43·1
Wy-21901, 939·2
Wy-22811, 56·3
Wy-44635, 178·2
Wy-45030, 321·3
Wy-49605, 213·1
Wy-090217, 1363·1
Wy-90493-RD, 864·3
Wyamine, 2387·1
Wyamine— *see* Emergent-Ez, 1967·2
Wyanoids Relief Factor, 2387·1
Wycillin, 2387·1
Wycillin R, 2387·1
Wycillina, 2387·1
Wycort, 2387·1
Wycort c Neomycin, 2387·1
Wydase, 2387·1
Wydora, 2387·1
Wygesic, 2387·1

Wylaxine, 2387·1
Wymesone, 2387·1
Wymox, 2387·1
Wypresin, 2387·1
Wysolone, 2387·1
Wysoy, 2387·1
Wytens, 2387·1
Wytensin, 2387·1
WZ-884642, 988·3
WZ-884643, 988·3

X

X-2, 2387·1
X-1497, 230·3
XA-41, 1519·1
Xacin, 2387·1
X-Adene, 2387·1
Xagrid, 2387·1
Xaken, 2387·1
Xal, 2387·1
Xalacom, 2387·2
Xalatan, 2387·2
Xalazin, 2387·2
Xalcom, 2387·2
Xaliplat, 2387·2
Xalyn-Or, 2387·2
Xamamina, 2387·2
Xamoterol Fumarate, 1029·1
Xamoterol, Fumarato de, 1029·1
Xanacine, 2387·2
Xanagis, 2387·2
Xanalin, 2387·2
Xanax, 2387·2
Xanbon, 2387·2
Xanef, 2387·2
Xanidine, 2387·2
Xanol, 2387·2
Xanolam, 2387·2
Xanomel, 2387·2
Xanomelina, 1498·3
Xanomeline, 1498·3
Xanomeline Tartrate, 1498·3
Xanor, 2387·2
Xantervit, 2387·2
Xantervit Antibiotico, 2387·2
Xantervit Eparina, 2387·2
Xantham Gum, 1582·3
Xanthan Gum, 1582·3
Xanthani Gummi, 1582·3
Xanthine Oxidase Inhibitor, 413·3
Xanthine-containing Beverages, 1765·2
Xanthines, 777·2
Xanthinol Niacinate, 1029·1
Xanthinol Nicotinate, 1029·1
Xanthium, 2387·3
Xanthomax, 2387·3
*Xanthomonas campestris*, 1582·3
Xanthophyl Dipalmitate, 1765·3
Xanthophylls, 1056·1
Xanthotoxin, 1152·1
Xanthoxylum, 1766·3
*Xanthoxylum piperitum*, 1766·3
Xantina B12, 2387·3
Xantina, Bebidas con, 1765·2
Xantinol Nicotinate, 1029·1
Xantinol, Nicotinato de, 1029·1
Xantinon B12, 2387·3
Xantinon Complex, 2387·3
Xantium, 2387·3
Xantivent, 2387·3
Xantofila, Palmitato de, 1765·3
Xantofyl Palmitate, 1765·3
Xantox, 2387·3
Xantromid, 2387·3
Xanturenasi, 2387·3
Xao Pil, 2387·3
Xao T, 2387·3
Xao-Dex, 2387·3
Xapro, 2387·3
Xarator, 2387·3
Xarope Antigripal, 2387·3
Xarope Comp Mel E Agriao, 2387·3
Xarope das Criancas, 2387·3
Xarope de Caraguata, 2387·3
Xarope de Eucalipto, 2387·3
Xarope de Iodeto de Potassio, 2387·3
Xarope de Iodeto de Potassio Composto, 2387·3
Xarope de Limao Bravo, 2387·3
Xarope de Lobelia Composto, 2387·3
Xarope de Macas Rainetas, 2387·3
Xarope 44E, 2387·4
Xarope Grindelia de Oliveira Junior, 2387·4
Xarope Iodo-Suma, 2387·4
Xarope Neo, 2387·4
Xarope Peitoral de Ameixa Composto, 2387·4
Xarope Sao Joao, 2387·4
Xarope Valda, 2387·4
Xarope Vick, 2387·4
Xasmun, 2387·4
Xaten, 2387·4
Xatral, 2387·4
Xebramol, 2387·4
Xedenol, 2387·4
Xedenol B12, 2387·4
Xedenol Flex, 2387·4
Xefo, 2387·4
Xeloda, 2387·4
Xeltic, 2387·4
Xemilofibán, Hidrocloruro de, 1029·2
Xemilofiban Hydrochloride, 1029·2
Xemos, 2387·4
Xenalon, 2387·4
Xenar, 2387·4
Xenazine, 2387·4
Xenetix, 2387·4
Xenical, 2388·1
Xenid, 2388·1
Xenisalato, Hidrocloruro de, 1163·1
Xenitropio, Bromuro de, 491·3
Xenobid, 2388·1
Xenon, 1311·2
Xenon-127, 1526·3
Xenon-133, 1526·3
Xenotransplantation— *see* Organ and Tissue Transplantation, 1344·2
Xenovate, 2388·1
Xenysalate Hydrochloride, 1163·1
Xenytropium Bromide, 491·3
Xepagan, 2388·1
Xepamet, 2388·1
Xepanicol, 2388·1
Xepasone, 2388·1
Xepin, 2388·1
Xerac AC, 2388·1
Xeracil, 2388·1
Xeragel, 2388·1
Xeramax, 2388·1
Xeramel, 2388·1
Xerand, 2388·1
Xeraspor, 2388·1
Xerazole, 2388·1
Xerenal, 2388·1
Xerial, 2388·1
Xerodent, 2388·1
Xeroderm, 2388·1
Xerogesic, 2388·1
Xeroil, 2388·1
Xerophthalmia, 1454·1
Xeroprim, 2388·1
Xerostomia— *see* Dry Mouth, 1576·2
Xerotens, 2388·1
Xerumenex, 2388·2
Xet, 2388·2
Xflu, 2388·2
XI-921, 1438·2
Xibornol, 277·3
Xibornol Prodes, 2388·2
Xicam, 2388·2
Xicane, 2388·2
Xicil, 2388·2
Xiclav, 2388·2
Xiclovir, 2388·2
Xidanef, 2388·2
Xiemed, 2388·2
Xigris, 2388·2
Xilazina, 1765·3
Xilazina, Hidrocloruro de, 1766·1
Xileno, 1478·2
Xilinum, 2388·2
Xilitol, 1469·1
Xilodase, 2388·2
Xilometazolina, Hidrocloruro de, 1132·2
Xilo-Mynol, 2388·2
Xilonibsa, 2388·2
Xilopar, 2388·2
Xilosa, 1766·1
Ximaken, 2388·2
Ximelagatran, 952·1
Ximovan, 2388·2
Xinafoato de Salmeterol, 795·1
Xinder, 2388·2
Xinia, 2388·2
Xintoprost, 2388·2
Xipamid, 2388·2
Xipamida, 1029·2
Xipamide, 1029·2
Xipral, 2388·3
Xiprine, 2388·3
Xiprocan, 2388·3
Xiral, 2388·3
Xiratuss, 2388·3
Xismox, 2388·3
Xiten, 2388·3
Xitix, 2388·3
Xitocin, 2388·3
XLEU, Analog— *see* Analog XLEU, 1798·3
XLEU, Maxamaid— *see* Maxamaid XLEU, 2116·1
XLYS, Analog— *see* Analog XLYS, 1798·3
XLYS Low Try, Analog— *see* Analog XLYS Low Try, 1798·3
XLys Low Try Maxamaid, 2388·3
XLYS Low Try, Maxamaid— *see* Maxamaid XLYS, Low Try, 2116·1
XLYS Low Try, Maxamum— *see* Maxamum XLYS, Low Try, 2116·1
XMET Analog, 2388·3
XMET, Analog— *see* Analog XMET, 1798·3
XMET Cys, Analog— *see* Analog XMET, Cys, 1798·3
XMET Cys, Maxamaid— *see* Maxamaid XMET, Cys, 2116·1
XMET Maxamaid, 2388·3
XMET, Maxamaid— *see* Maxamaid XMET, 2116·1
XMET Maxamum, 2388·3
XMET, Maxamum— *see* Maxamum XMET, 2116·1
XMET Maximum, 2388·3
XMet, Thre, Val, Isoleu Maxamum— *see* XMTVI Maxamum, 2388·3
XMTVI Analog, 2388·3
XMTVI, Analog— *see* Analog XMTVI, 1798·3
XMTVI Asadon, 2388·3
XMTVI Maxamaid, 2388·3
XMTVI, Maxamaid— *see* Maxamaid XMTVI, 2116·1
XMTVI Maxamum, 2388·3
XMTVI, Maxamum— *see* Maxamum XMTVI, 2116·1
Xolaam, 2388·3
Xolair, 2388·3
Xolof, 2388·3
Xolof D, 2388·3
Xonatil, 2388·3
Xopenex, 2388·3
Xorox, 2388·3
Xorpic, 2388·3
Xotic— *see* Zoto-HC, 2395·4
Xozacil, 2388·3
XP-03, 703·2
XP Analog, 2388·4
XP Analog— *see* Analog XP, 1798·3
XP Analog LCP, 2388·4
XP Maxamaid, 2388·4
XP Maxamum, 2388·4
Xpe SPC, 2388·4
XPhen, Tyr Analog, 2388·4
Xphen, Tyr, Analog— *see* Analog Xphen, Tyr, 1798·3
XPhen, Tyr Maxamaid, 2388·4
XPhen, Tyr Maxamum, 2388·4
XPHEN Tyr, Maxamum— *see* Maxamum XPhen, Tyr, 2116·1
X-Praep, 2388·4
X-Prep, 2388·4
X-Prep Bowel Evacuant Kit-1, 2388·4
X-Prep Bowel Evacuant Kit-2, 2388·4
XPT Tyrosidon, 2388·4
XPTM, Analog— *see* Analog XPTM, 1798·3
XPTM, Maxamaid— *see* Maxamaid XPTM, 2116·1
XPTM Tyrosidon, 2388·4
X-Seb, 2388·4
X-Seb Plus, 2388·4
X-Seb T, 2388·4
X-Seb T Plus, 2388·4
XSP-Bena, 2388·4
X'tac, 2388·4
X-Tar, 2388·4
XTC, 1589·3
XU-62-320, 918·2
Xuprin, 2388·4
Xusal, 2388·4
Xycam, 2388·4
Xylamide, 1284·3
Xylanaest, 2389·1
Xylazine, 1765·3
Xylazine Hydrochloride, 1766·1
Xylazine Hydrochloride for Veterinary Use, 1766·1
Xylene, 1478·2
Xylenol, 1478·3
Xylenols, 1193·3
Xylesine, 2389·1
Xylestesin Preparations, 2389·1
Xylestin-A, 2389·1
Xylit, 1469·1, 2389·1
Xylitol, 1469·1
*meso*-Xylitol, 1469·1
Xylitolum, 1469·1
Xylo, 2389·1
Xylo Siozwo, 2389·1
Xylocain Preparations, 2389·1
Xylocaina, 2389·1
Xylocaine Preparations, 2389·2
Xylocard, 2389·2
Xylocitin, 2389·2
Xylocitin Cor, 2389·2
Xylo-COMOD, 2389·2
Xylol, 1478·2
Xylole, 1478·2
Xylolin, 2389·2
Xyloma, 2389·2
Xylomed— *see* Xylose-BMS, 2389·3
Xylometazoline Hydrochloride, 1132·2
Xylometazolini Hydrochloridum, 1132·2
Xylonest, 2389·2
Xylonest-Octapressin, 2389·2
Xyloneural, 2389·2
Xylonibsa, 2389·2
Xylonor, 2389·2
Xylonor Especial, 2389·3
Xylonor 2% sin Vasoconst, 2389·3
Xylo-Pfan, 2389·3
Xyloproct, 2389·3
Xyloprocto, 2389·3
α-D-Xylopyranose, 1766·1
Xylose, 1766·1
D-Xylose, 1766·1
Xylose-BMS, 2389·3
Xylosum, 1766·1
Xylotocan, 2389·3
Xylotox, 2389·3
Xylovit, 2389·3
*N*-(2,3-Xylyl)anthranilic Acid, 55·2
(*S*)-4-[1-(2,3-Xylyl)ethyl]imidazole Hydrochloride, 689·3
(±)-4-[1-(2,3-Xylyl)ethyl]imidazole Monohydrochloride, 706·1
5-(3,5-Xylyloxymethyl)oxazolidin-2-one, 1395·1
Xymel, 2389·3
Xymiazole, 1502·3
Xyrem, 2389·3
Xyzal, 2389·3
Xyzall, 2389·3
XZ-450, 159·1

Y

Y, 1451·1
129Y83, 1736·2
Y-516, 710·1
Y-4153, 683·1
Y-6047, 685·2
Y-7131, 698·1
Y-9179, 1722·2
Y-25130, 1251·1
Yacutin, 2389·3
Yadalan, 2389·3

Yadegal Compuesto, 2389·3
Yagé, 1696·3
Yakona N, 2389·3
Yal, 2389·3
Yamalen, 2389·3
Yamatetan, 2389·3
Yamba, 1666·1
Yamcon, 2389·3
Yanal, 2389·4
Yangonin, 1703·2
Yanurax, 2389·4
Yapamicin, 2389·4
Yariba, 2389·4
Yarrow, 1646·2
Yasmin, 2389·4
Yasta, 2389·4
Yatropan, 2389·4
Yatrox, 2389·4
Yatushan Plus, 2389·4
Yavit, 2389·4
Yaws— *see* Syphilis, 148·2
YB-2, 939·1
YC-93, 965·1
Ydroquinidine Cooper, 2389·4
Yeast, Brewers', 1469·1
Yeast Clear, 2389·4
Yeast, Dried, 1469·1
Yeast Nucleic Acid, 1738·2
Yeast Vite, 2389·4
Yeast-Gard, 2389·4
Yeast-X, 2389·4
Yectafer, 2389·4
Yectafer Complex, 2389·4
Yectames, 2389·4
Yectamicina, 2389·4
Yectamid, 2389·4
Yectofer, 2389·4
Yedoc, 2389·4
Yeiamin-2, 2389·4
Yelets, 2389·4
Yellow Beeswax, 1480·2
Yellow Canary, 1057·3
Yellow Cross Liquid, 1679·3
Yellow Dock, 1766·1
Yellow FCF, Sunset, 1058·2
Yellow Fever— *see* Haemorrhagic Fevers, 618·2
Yellow Fever Vaccine, 1644·2
Yellow Fever Vaccine (Live), 1644·2
Yellow Fever Vaccines, 1644·2
Yellow 2G, 1058·3
Yellow 2G, Acid Light, 1058·3
Yellow Jasmine Root, 1691·3
Yellow Mercuric Oxide, 1712·3
Yellow Oleander, 1723·1
Yellow Petrolatum, 1479·3
Yellow Petroleum Jelly, 1479·3
Yellow Phenolphthalein, 1284·1
Yellow Precipitate, 1712·3
Yellow, Quinoline, 1057·3
Yellow Root, 1698·3
Yellow S, Orange, 1058·2
Yellow Soft Paraffin, 1479·3
Yellow, Tartrazol, 1058·2
Yellow Wax, 1480·2
Yelnac, 2389·4
Yel/Vac, 1644·2
Yendol, 2389·4
Yerba Dulce, 1449·3
Yerba Santa, 1121·2
Yermonil, 2389·4
Yersinia Enteritis, 130·2
Yersiniosis— *see* Yersinia Enteritis, 130·2
Yesan, 2389·4
Yeso Blanco, 1665·1
Yestamin, 2389·4
Yewtaxan, 2390·1
YF-Vax, 2390·1
Yirala, 2390·1
Ylox, 2390·1
YM-026, 343·3
YM-044, 213·1
YM-060, 1285·2
YM-175, 773·1
YM-617, 1009·2
YM-730, 866·3
YM-866, 978·3
YM-905, 489·2
YM-08316, 786·1
YM-09151-2, 710·1
YM-09330, 177·1
YM-09538, 862·3
YM-09730-5, 866·3
YM-11170, 1265·2
*R*-(−)-YM-12617, 1009·2
YM-12617-1, 1009·2
YM-67905, 489·2
YMDL-17043, 911·1
YN-72, 654·2
Yocon, 2390·1
Yocoral, 2390·1
Yodacua, 2390·1
Yodine, 2390·1
Yodo, 1598·1
Yodo Tio Calci, 2390·1
Yodofrixon Salicilado, 2390·1
Yodolactina, 2390·1
Yodolin, 2390·1
Yodon, 2390·1
Yodoxin, 2390·1
Yodozona, 2390·1
Yogurt, 1704·2
Yohimbina, Hidrocloruro de, 1766·2
δ-Yohimbine, 994·3
Yohimbine Hydrochloride, 1766·2
Yohimex, 2390·1
Yohydrol, 2390·1
Yokel, 2390·1
Yomax, 2390·1
Yomesan, 2390·1
Yonka, 2390·1
Yopin, 2390·1
Yoquin, 2390·1
Yoruba, 1666·1
Youngflex Massage 168, 2390·1
Your Choice, 2390·1
Yovis, 2390·1
Yovita, 2390·1
Yperite, 1679·3
Ypsiloheel N, 2390·1
Yrelan, 2390·2
YSE, 2390·2
YSE Glutamique, 2390·2
Ysol 206, 2390·2
YS-20P, 224·3
Ystheal, 2390·2
YTR-830, 264·3
YTR-830H, 264·3
Ytracis, 2390·2
Yttrium-90, 1526·3
Yttrium Citrate ($^{90}$Y), 1526·3
Yttrium ($^{90}$Y) Ibritumomab Tiuxetan, 1526·3
Yttrium Silicate ($^{90}$Y), 1526·3
Yuca, 1766·2
Yucca, 1766·2
*Yucca arborescens*, 1766·2
*Yucca brevifolia*, 1766·2
*Yucca filamentosa*, 1766·2
*Yucca mohavensis*, 1766·2
*Yucca schidigera*, 1766·2
Yucomy, 2390·2
Yurelax, 2390·2
Yuremetil D, 2390·2
Yuremid, 2390·2
Yusin, 2390·2
Yutopar, 2390·2
Yuyo, 2390·2
Yuzpe Regimen, 1536·2
Yxin, 2390·2
Yxin Tears, 2390·2

## Z

Z-103, 1284·2
Z 300, 2390·2
Z-326, 482·2
Z-424, 96·3
Z-1282, 214·3
Z-4828, 590·2
Z-4942, 561·1
Z Frin, 2390·2
Z Span, 2390·2
Zaart-H, 2390·2
Zaba, 2390·2
Zabysept, 2390·2
Zacam, 2390·2
Zacate Chino, 1666·1
Zacetin, 2390·2
Zacin, 2390·2
Zacnan, 2390·2
Z-Acne, 2390·2
ZacPac, 2390·2
Zactin, 2390·2
Zactos, 2390·2
Zadaxin, 2390·2
Zaden, 2390·2
Zad-G, 2390·3
Zadine, 2390·3
Zadino, 2390·3
Zadipina, 2390·3
Zaditen, 2390·3
Zaditor, 2390·3
Zadolina, 2390·3
Zadorin, 2390·3
Zadstat, 2390·3
Zadyl, 2390·3
Zaedoc, 2390·3
Zafarismal, 2390·3
Zafen, 2390·3
Zafibral, 2390·3
Zafimida, 2390·3
Zafirlukast, 807·1
Zafirst, 2390·3
Zafluox, 2390·3
Zafor, 2390·3
Zagam, 2390·3
Zagastrol, 2390·3
Zagreb Antivenom, 1639·2
Zagyl, 2390·3
Zaharina, 1443·2
Zahnerol N, 2390·3
Zahnungstropfen Escatitona, 2390·3
Zainexpect, 2390·3
Zainexpect C & F, 2390·4
Zainexpect CD, 2390·4
ZAL-846, 727·3
Zalain, 2390·4
Zalcitabina, 657·1
Zalcitabine, 657·1, 657·2
Zaldarida, 1294·3
Zaldaride, 1294·3
Zaldaride Maleate, 1294·3
Zaldiar, 2390·4
Zaleplon, 727·3
Zalig, 2390·4
Zaltoprofen, 96·3
Zaltoprofeno, 96·3
Zalvor, 2390·4
Zamacort, 2390·4
Zamadol, 2390·4
Zamanon, 2390·4
Zambesil, 2390·4
Zam-Buk, 2390·4
Zamene, 2390·4
Zamifenacin, 491·3
Zamifenacina, 491·3
Zamocilline, 2390·4
Zamudol, 2390·4
Zanaflex, 2390·4
Zanahoria Silvestre, 1765·1
Zanamet, 2390·4
Zanamivir, 658·1
Zandine, 2390·4
Zanedip, 2390·4
Zanfel, 2390·4
Zanicor, 2390·4
Zanidex, 2390·4
Zanidin, 2390·4
Zanidip, 2390·4
Zanizal, 2390·4
Zanoc, 2390·4
Zanocin, 2391·1
Zanosar, 2391·1
Zanprol, 2391·1
Zantab, 2391·1
Zantac, 2391·1
Zantarac, 2391·1
Zanthoxylum, 1766·3
*Zanthoxylum americanum*, 1766·3
*Zanthoxylum clavaherculis*, 1766·3
Zanthoxylum Fruit, 1766·3
Zanthoxylum, Fruto de, 1766·3
*Zanthoxylum piperitum*, 1766·3
Zantic, 2391·1
Zantidon, 2391·1
Zantipres, 2391·1
Zantril, 2391·1
Zantryl, 2391·1
Zanzipik, 2391·1
Zapain, 2391·1
Zapazole, Chemists Own— *see* Chemists Own Zapazole, 1882·1
Zaperin, 2391·1
Zaplon, 2391·1
Zappelin, 2391·1
Zaprin, 2391·1
Zapto, 2391·1
Zapto Co, 2391·1
Zaramol, 2391·1
Zarator, 2391·1
Zarcop, 2391·1
Zarent, 2391·1
Zarex, 2391·1
Zargus, 2391·1
Zaricort, 2391·1
Zarin, 2391·2
Zariviz, 2391·2
Zarocs, 2391·2
Zarondan, 2391·2
Zarontin, 2391·2
Zaroxolyn, 2391·2
Zaroxolyne, 2391·2
Zarzaparrilla, 1742·1
Zasten, 2391·2
Zatinol, 2391·2
Zatofug, 2391·2
Zatrol, 2391·2
Zatur, 2391·2
Zavedos, 2391·2
Zavesca, 2391·2
Zayasel, 2391·2
Zaymaz, Chemists Own— *see* Chemists Own Cold & Allergy, 1881·4
Z-Bec, 2391·2
ZBM, 2391·2
ZBT, 2391·2
ZC-102, 96·3
Z-Cof, 2391·2
Z-Cof HC, 2391·2
ZD-1033, 528·1
ZD-1694, 582·1
ZD-1839, 557·3
ZD-4433, 207·3
ZD-4522, 996·2
ZD-5077, 718·2
ZD-9238, 557·3
Z-Dorm, 2391·2
Ze Caps, 2391·2
Zea, 1676·1
*Zea mays*, 1439·2, 1449·1, 1676·1
Zeadema, 2391·2
Zearalanol, 1573·3
ZeaSorb, 2391·2
ZeaSorb AF, 2391·3
Zeaxanthin, 1423·1
Zeben, 2391·3
Zebeta, 2391·3
Zebrak, 2391·3
Zebu, 2391·3
Zeclar, 2391·3
Zeclar— *see* Helipak K, 2038·2
Zeclaren OD, 2391·3
Zecnil, 2391·3
Zedax, 2391·3
Zedex, 2391·3
Zedex-P, 2391·3
Zeefra, 2391·3
Zeel, 2391·3
Zeel Comp, 2391·3
Zeel P, 2391·3
Zeel Plus, 2391·3
Zeel T, 2391·3
Zeelulean with Escin, Bioglan— *see* Bioglan Zellulean with Escin, 1844·2
Zee-Seltzer, 2391·3
Zeet Expectorant, 2391·3
Zeet Linctus, 2391·3
Zefa, 2391·3
Zefaxone, 2391·4
Zefazone, 2391·4
Zeffix, 2391·4
Zefirol, 2391·4
Zeftam, 2391·4
Zefxon, 2391·4

Zehu-Ze, 2391·4
Zein, 1766·3
Zeína, 1766·3
Zeisin, 2391·4
Zelapar, 2391·4
Zelderme, 2391
Zeldox, 2391·4
Zelfin, 2391·4
Zelicrema, 2391
Zeliderm, 2391·
Zelis, 2391·4
Zelitrex, 2391·4
Zelium, 2391·4
Zelix, 2391·4
Zellaforte, 2391
Zellaforte N Pl 2391·4
Zellaforte Plus, 391·4
Zeller-Augenwar, 2391·4
Zellox-II, 2391
Zelmac, 2391·4
Zelmar, 2391·4
Zelnorm, 2391·
Zemaira, 2391·
Zemalex, 2392
Zemide, 2392·
Zemplar, 2392·
Zemtard, 2392
Zemuron, 2392
Zen, 2392·1
Zenalb, 2392·1
Zenapax, 2392
Zenas, 2392·1
Zenate, Advsed Formula— *see* Advanced Form Zenate, 1777·3
Zenavan, 2392
Zenaxin, 2392
Zenda, 2392·1
Zendhin, 2392
Zendol, 2392·
Zengac, 2392·
Zeniac, 2392·1
Zeniac LP, 2391
Zeniac LP Fo 2392·1
Zenicide, 2392
Zenium, 2392·
Zenmolin, 239
Zenodian, 239
Zenoxone, 239
Zenpro, 2392·
Zensil, 2392·1
Zentavion, 239
Zentel, 2392·1
Zentius, 2392·
Zentralin, 239
Zentramin Basn N, 2392·2
Zentropil, 239
Zenusin, 2392
Zenzera, 2392
Zepac, 2392·2
Zepan, 2392·2
Zepelan, 2392
Zepelin, 2392·
Zepelindue, 22·2
Zephiran, 239
Zephirol, 239
Zepholin, 239
Zephrex, 2392
Zepiken, 2392
Zepilen, 2392·
Zeplex, 2392·
Zepobrax, 2392
Zeprat, 2392·
Zera, 2392·2
Zerandin, 2392
Zeranol, 1573
Zerella, 2392·
Zerene, 2392·
Zerfenazin, 22·2
Zerinetta, 2392
Zerinetta-Fher 2392·2
Zerinoflu, 2393
Zerinol-Fher, 92·3
Zerit, 2392·3
Zeritavir, 2393
Zermed, 2392
Zeroac, 2392·
Zerobase, 2393
Zeroflog, 2393
Zeropenem, 2392·3
Zeropyn, 2392·3
Zerosorin SN, 2392·3
Zerospam, 2392·3
Zerouali, 1666·1
Zertine, 2392·3
Zesger, 2392·3
Zestan, 2392·3
Zestomax, 2392·3
Zestoretic, 2392·3
Zestril, 2392·3
Zeta N, 2392·3
Zetacet, 2392·3
Zeta-cypermethrin, 1502·3
Zetagal, 2392·3
Zetalax, 2392·3
Zetalerg, 2392·3
Zetamicin, 2392·3
Zetar, 2392·4
Zetarina, 2392·4
Zetavir, 2392·4
Zetavit, 2392·4
Zetavudin, 2392·4
Zetaxim, 2392·4
Zetia, 2392·4
Zetir, 2392·4
Zetir-D, 2392·4
Zetitec, 2392·4
Zetix, 2392·4
Zeto, 2392·4
Zetofen, 2392·4
Zetomax, 2392·4
Zetoridal, 2392·4
Zetran, 2392·4
Zetron, 2392·4
Zetrotax, 2392·4
Zevalin, 2392·4
Zevin, 2392·4
Z-gen, 2392·4
Zhi Qiao, 1723·3
Zhi Shi, 1723·3
Zhimu, 1750·2
Zi, Rohto— *see* Rohto Zi, 2269·1
Ziac, 2392·4
Ziagen, 2392·4
Ziagenavir, 2392·4
Ziak, 2392·4
Zibelant, 2392·4
Zibil, 2392·4
Zibor, 2392·4
Zibren, 2393·1
Ziclin, 2393·1
Ziconal, 2393·1
Ziconotida, 96·3
Ziconotide, 96·3
Zidac, 2393·1
Zideron, 2393·1
Zidicef, 2393·1
Zidis, 2393·1
Zidix, 2393·1
Zidolam, 2393·1
Zidonil, 2393·1
Zidoval, 2393·1
Zidovimm, 2393·1
Zidovir, 2393·1
Zidovudina, 658·2
Zidovudine, 658·2
Zidovudinum, 658·2
Zidovusan, 2393·1
Ziele konopi indyjskich, 1666·1
Zienam, 2393·1
Zifartel, 2393·1
Zig C, 2393·1
Ziga-Gel, 2393·1
Ziken, 2393·1
Ziks, 2393·1
Zil, 2393·1
Zilaben, 2393·1
Zilactin Preparations, 2393·1
Zilak, 2393·2
Zildem, 2393·2
Zilden, 2393·2
Zileuton, 807·3
Zileze, 2393·2
Zilisten, 2393·2
Zilium, 2393·2
Ziloxican, 2393·2
Zilutrol, 2393·2
Zimadoce, 2393·2
Zimaina, 2393·2
Zimalgin, 2393·2
Zimanel, 2393·2
Zimaquin, 2393·2
Zimbacol, 2393·2
Zimbro, 1703·1
Zimerol, 2393·2
Zimicina, 2393·2
Zimmex, 2393·2
Zimocel, 2393·2
Zimoclone, 2393·2
Zimor, 2393·2
Zimovane, 2393·2
Zimox, 2393·2
Zimt, 1672·2
Zimtöl, 1672·2
Zinabol, 2393·2
Zinacef, 2393·2
Zinaderm, 2393·2
Zinadiur, 2393·2
Zinadol, 2393·2
Zinadril, 2393·2
Zinaf, 2393·3
Zinalerg, 2393·3
Zinamide, 2393·3
Zinasen, 2393·3
Zinat, 2393·3
Zinaxin, 2393·3
Zinaxin Plus, 2393·3
Zinc, 1469·2
Zinc Acetate, 1469·2
Zinc Acetate Dihydrate, 1469·2
Zinc, Acetato de, 1469·2
Zinc Acexamate, 1646·2
Zinc for Acne, 2393·3
Zinc B, E & C, 2393·3
Zinc Bacitracin, 161·3
Zinc, Blanc de, 1163·2
Zinc Borate, 1662·1
Zinc + C250, 2393·3
Zinc C Plus, 2393·3
Zinc Carbonate, 1163·2
Zinc Carbonate, Basic, 1144·1
Zinc Carbonate, Hydrated, 1163·2
Zinc Carbonate Hydroxide, 1163·2
Zinc, Carbonato Básico de, 1163·2
Zinc, Carbonato de, 1163·2
Zinc Chelate, Bioglan— *see* Bioglan Zinc Chelate, 1844·2
Zinc Chloride, 1469·2
Zinc, Cloruro de, 1469·2
Zinc Cream White, 2393·3
Zinc Defence, 2393·3
Zinc Di(undec-10-enoate), 411·1
Zinc, Fenosulfonato de, 1163·3
Zinc, Flores de, 1163·2
Zinc Gluconate, 1469·2
Zinc, Gluconato de, 1469·2
Zinc Hyaluronate, 1697·3
Zinc 4-Hydroxybenzenesulphonate, 1163·3
Zinc *p*-Hydroxybenzenesulphonate, 1163·3
Zinc Lotion, 2393·3
Zinc Menthol, 2393·3
Zinc Oleate, 1574·3, 1575·3
Zinc Orotate, 1724·3
Zinc Oxide, 1144·1, 1163·2
Zinc, Óxido de, 1163·2
Zinc Palmitate, 1575·3
Zinc Peroxide, 1195·3
Zinc Phenolsulfonate, 1163·3
Zinc Phenolsulphonate, 1163·3
Zinc Phosphate, 1163·3
Zinc Phosphide, 1500·1
Zinc Plus, 2393·3
Zinc 2-Pyridinethiol 1-Oxide, 1156·2
Zinc Pyridinethione, 1156·2
Zinc Salicylate, 1157·2
Zinc Stearate, 1575·3
Zinc Subcarbonate, 1163·2
Zinc Sulfate, 1469·3
Zinc Sulfate Heptahydrate, 1469·3
Zinc Sulfate Hexahydrate, 1469·3
Zinc Sulfate Monohydrate, 1469·3
Zinc, Sulfato de, 1469·3
Zinc Sulphate, 1469·3
Zinc Sulphate Heptahydrate, 1469·3
Zinc Sulphate Hexahydrate, 1469·3
Zinc Supplement, 2393·3
Zinc Undecenoate, 411·1
Zinc Undecylenate, 411·1
Zinc White, 1163·2
Zinc Zenith, 2393·3
Zincaband, 2393·3
Zinc-ACE, 2393·3
Zinca-Pak, 2393·3
Zincaps, 2393·3
Zincate, 2393·3
Zincation, 2393·3
Zincation Plus, 2393·3
Zincfrin, 2393·3
Zincfrin Antihistaminicum, 2393·3
Zincfrin-A, 2393·4
Zincfrin-A— *see* Zincfrin Antihistaminicum, 2393·3
Zinci Acetas Dihydricus, 1469·2
Zinci Chloridum, 1469·2
Zinci Oxidum, 1163·2
Zinci Oxydum, 1163·2
Zinci Stearas, 1575·3
Zinci Sulfas, 1469·3
Zinci Sulfas Heptahydricus, 1469·3
Zinci Sulfas Hexahydricus, 1469·3
Zinci Undecylenas, 411·1
Zinc-Ichtyol, 2393·4
Zinc-Imizol, 2393·4
Zinco all' Acqua, 2393·4
Zinco Sulpha, 2393·4
Zincod, 2393·4
Zincoderm, 2393·4
Zincoderma, 2393·4
Zincofax, 2393·4
Zincol, 2393·4
Zincolok, 2393·4
Zincometil, 2393·4
Zincon, 2393·4
Zincopan, 2393·4
Zincoral, 2393·4
Zincosol, 2393·4
Zincotape, 2393·4
Zincotex, 2393·4
Zincovit, 2393·4
Zincoxid, 2393·4
Zincream, 2393·4
Zincstic, 2393·4
Zinctab, 2393·4
Zincum Chloratum, 1469·2
Zincum Oxydatum, 1163·2
Zincum Sulfuricum, 1469·3
Zincum Valerianicum-Hevert, 2393·4
Zincvit, 2393·4
Zindaclin, 2393·4
Zindacline, 2393·4
Zinecard, 2393·4
Zineli, 2393·4
Zineryt, 2393·4
Zinetac, 2394·1
Zinetrin, 2394·1
Zinga, 2394·1
Zingib., 1267·1
Zingiber, 1267·1
*Zingiber officinale*, 1267·1
Zingiberis Rhizoma, 1267·1
Zink Beta, 2394·1
Zink Verla, 2394·1
Zinkamin, 2394·1
Zinkbrause, 2394·1
Zink-Calmitol, 2394·1
Zink-D Longoral, 2394·1
Zinkit, 2394·1
Zink'N'Swim, 2394·1
Zinkokehl, 2394·1
Zinkolie, 2394·1
Zinkorell, 2394·1
Zinkorot, 2394·1
Zinkosalb, 2394·1
Zinkotase, 2394·1
Zinkpaste, 2394·1
Zink-Ratiopharm, 2394·1
Zinksalbe, 2394·1
Zinksalbe Dialon, 2394·1
Zink-Sandoz, 2394·1
Zinkzalf, 2394·1
Zinnat, 2394·1
Zinnkraut-Tropfen, 2394·1
Zinocep, 2394·1

Zinopril, 2394·1
Zinostatin, 594·3
Zinostatin Stimalamer, 594·3
Zinostatina, 594·3
Zintona, 2394·1
Zinulin, 2394·1
Zinvit, 2394·2
Zinvit C, 2394·2
Zinvit G, 2394·2
Zipeprol, Hidrocloruro de, 1132·3
Zipeprol Hydrochloride, 1132·3
Zipos, 2394·2
Zipra, 2394·2
Ziprasidona, 728·1
Ziprasidone, 728·1
Ziprasidone Hydrochloride, 728·1
Ziprasidone Mesilate, 728·1
Ziprasidone Mesylate, 728·1
Ziprol, 2394·2
Zipzoc, 2394·2
Zipzoc Salvstrumpa, 2394·2
Ziradryl, 2394·2
Zirconio, 1766·3
Zirconium, 1766·3
Zirconium Dioxide, 1766·3
Zirconium Lactate, 1766·3
Zirconium Oxychloride, 1766·3
Ziremex, 2394·2
Zirkulin Beruhigungs-Tee, 2394·2
Zirpine, 2394·2
Zirtec, 2394·2
Zirtek, 2394·2
Zirvit, 2394·2
Zirvit Beta, 2394·2
Zirvit E, 2394·2
Zispin, 2394·2
Zita, 2394·2
Zitazonium, 2394·2
Zithromax, 2394·2
Zitos, Sais— *see* Sais Zitos, 2273·4
Zitrix, 2394·2
Zitromax, 2394·2
Zitroneo, 2394·2
Zitumex, 2394·2
Ziverone, 2394·2
Zix, 2394·2
Ziz, 2394·2
Ziziphus Soup, 1750·2
*Zizyphus spinosus*, 1750·2
ZK-30595, 1549·1
ZK-35760, 1065·2
ZK-36374, 1518·2
ZK-39482, 1066·1
ZK-43649, 1050·1
ZK-57671, 1520·3
ZK-62498, 1142·3
ZK-00091106, 770·2
ZK-94006, 1145·1
ZK-112004, 1062·3
ZK-112119, 668·1
ZK-132281, 1061·3
Z-Kraft, 2394·3
ZL-101, 1277·2
Zleep, 2394·3
ZM-204636, 718·2
Z-Max, 2394·3
ZN 220, 2394·3
ZN Xampu, 2394·3
Zn-A-C, Bioglan— *see* Bioglan Zn-A-C, 1844·2
Zn-Fusin, 2394·3
ZNP, 2394·3
Znupril, 2394·3
Zobacide, 2394·3
Zoben, 2394·3
Zocor, 2394·3
Zocord, 2394·3
Zocord/ASA, 2394·3
Zocovin, 2394·3
Zodeac, 2394·3
Zodol, 2394·3
Zodorm, 2394·3
Zodormdura, 2394·3
Zodurat, 2394·3
Zofen, 2394·3
Zofenil, 2394·3
Zofenopril Cálcico, 1029·3
Zofenopril Calcium, 1029·3
Zofenoprilat, 1029·3
Zoff, 2394·3
Zoflut, 2394·3
Zoflux, 2394·3
Zofora, 2394·3
Zofran, 2394·3
Zofron, 2394·4
Zogamicin, Gemtuzumab, 558·3
Zoiral, 2394·4
Zok-Zid, 2394·4
Zolac, 2394·4
Zoladex, 2394·4
Zolam, 2394·4
Zolamid, 2394·4
Zolamox, 2394·4
Zolanix, 2394·4
Zolapin, 2394·4
Zolaten, 2394·4
Zolazepam, Hidrocloruro de, 728·3
Zolazepam Hydrochloride, 728·3
Zolben, 2394·4
Zolben C, 2394·4
Zoldan-A, 2394·4
Zoldicam, 2394·4
Zole, 2394·4
Zoledronate Disodium, 776·2
Zoledronate Trisodium, 776·2
Zoledronato Disódico, 776·2
Zoledronato Trisódico, 776·2
Zoledronic Acid, 776·2
Zoledrónico, Ácido, 776·2
Zole-F, 2394·4
Zoleprim, 2394·4
Zoleptil, 2394·4
Zoles, 2394·4
Zolicef, 2394·4
Zolidan, 2394·4
Zoliden, 2395·1
Zoliderm, 2395·1
Zolidime, 2395·1
Zolidin, 2395·1
Zolief, 2395·1
Zolim, 2395·1
Zolimomab Aritox, 1738·3
Zolin, 2395·1
Zolina, 2395·1
Zoliparin, 2395·1
Zolisint, 2395·1
Zolistam, 2395·1
Zolistan, 2395·1
Zolival, 2395·1
Zolken, 2395·1
Zollinger-Ellison Syndrome, 1247·3
Zolmic, 2395·1
Zolmitriptan, 473·3
Zolnod, 2395·1
Zoloft, 2395·1
Zolpidem Hemitartrate, 728·3
Zolpidem Tartrate, 728·3
Zolpidem, Tartrato de, 728·3
Zolpidemi Tartras, 728·3
Zolpi-Lich, 2395·1
Zolpinox, 2395·1
Zolpramex, 2395·1
Zolstatin, 2395·1
Zoltec, 2395·1
Zoltenk, 2395·1
Zolterol, 2395·1
Zoltren, 2395·1
Zol-Triq, 2395·1
Zoltum, 2395·2
Zolvera, 2395·2
Zomacton, 2395·2
Zomepral, 2395·2
Zomera, 2395·2
Zometa, 2395·2
Zometic, 2395·2
Zomig, 2395·2
Zomigon, 2395·2
Zomigoro, 2395·2
Zomni, 2395·2
Zomorph, 2395·2
Zon, 2395·2
Zonal, 2395·2
Zonalon, 2395·2
Zonap, 2395·2
Zoncef, 2395·2
Zondar, 2395·2
Zone-A, 2395·2
Zonegran, 2395·2
Zonisamida, 384·3
Zonisamide, 384·3
Zonite, 2395·2
Zonivent, 2395·2
Zoo Chews, 2395·2
Zoo Chews with Iron, 2395·2
Zoodermina Cream, 2395·2
Zop, 2395·2
Zopam, 2395·3
Zopax, 2395·3
Zophren, 2395·3
Zopicalm, 2395·3
Zopicalma, 2395·3
Zopiclodura, 2395·3
Zopiclona, 729·3
Zopiclone, 729·3
Zopiclone *N*-Oxide, 730·1
Zopiclonum, 729·3
Zopimed, 2395·3
Zopinox, 2395·3
Zopi-Puren, 2395·3
Zopitan, 2395·3
Zopranol, 2395·3
Zorac, 2395·3
Zorail, 2395·3
Zorak, 2395·3
Zoral, 2395·3
Zoran, 2395·3
Zorax, 2395·3
Zorbtive, 2395·3
Zorclone, 2395·3
Zordyl, 2395·3
Zoref, 2395·3
Zorinax, 2395·3
Zoroxin, 2395·3
ZORprin, 2395·3
Zoru, 2395·3
Zorubicin Hydrochloride, 594·3
Zorubicina, Hidrocloruro de, 594·3
Zost, 2395·3
Zoster— *see* Varicella-zoster Infections, 621·1
Zostex, 2395·3
Zostrix, 2395·3
Zostrum, 2395·3
Zosvir, 2395·4
Zosyn, 2395·4
Zo-Tab, 2395·4
Zotepina, 730·2
Zotepine, 730·2
Zotinar, 2395·4
Zotinar-N, 2395·4
Zoto-HC, 2395·4
Zoton, 2395·4
Zoton— *see* Heliclear, 2038·1
Zoton— *see* HeliMet, 2038·1
Zotran, 2395·4
Zotrim, 2395·4
Zov800, 2395·4
Zovia, 2395·4
Zoviplus, 2395·4
Zovir, 2395·4
Zovirax, 2395·4
Zoxan, 2395·4
Zoxil, 2395·4
Zoylex, 2395·4
ZP 11, 2395·4
ZP Dermil, 2395·4
Z-Pak, 2395·4
Z-Pam, 2395·4
Z-Plus, 2395·4
ZR-515, 1507·2
ZR-3210, 1505·3
ZSC, 2395·4
ZSU, 1469·3
Zubes, 2395·4
Zucker, 1450·1
Zuclomifene, 1542·2
Zuclopenthixol, 730·3
Zuclopenthixol Acetate, 730·3
Zuclopenthixol Decanoate, 730·3
Zuclopenthixol Dihydrochloride, 730·3
Zuclopenthixol Hydrochloride, 730·3
Zuclopenthixoli Decanoas, 730·3
Zuclopentixol, 730·3
Zuclopentixol, Acetato de, 730·3
Zuclopentixol, Decanoato de, 730·3
Zuclopentixol, Hidrocloruro de, 730·3
Zuflax, 2395·4
Zuk Rheuma— *see* Zuk Schmerzgel, Zuk Schmerzsalbe, 2395·4
Zuk Schmerzgel, 2395·4
Zuk Thermo, 2396·1
Zuledine, 2396·1
Zuleptan, 2396·1
Zulex, 2396·1
Zumalgic, 2396·1
Zumaque, 1738·1
Zumba, 2396·1
Zumenon, 2396·1
Zumetil, 2396·1
Zunden, 2396·1
Zundic, 2396·1
Zurcal, 2396·1
Zurcale, 2396·1
Zurcazol, 2396·1
Zurfix, 2396·1
Zurim, 2396·1
Zurinel, 2396·1
Zuvair, 2396·1
Zwitsalax/N, 2396·1
Zwitsanal, 2396·1
Zwitsavit-D, 2396·1
Z-Xtra, 2396·1
Zyban, 2396·1
Zycalcit, 2396·2
Zycel, 2396·2
Zyclir, 2396·2
Zyderm, 2396·2
Zydol, 2396·2
Zydone, 2396·2
Zydowin, 2396·2
Zyflo, 2396·2
Zygomycosis— *see* Mucorcosis, 388·3
Zykinase, 2396·2
Zykolat-EDO, 2396·2
Zylapour, 2396·2
Zylium, 2396·2
Zyllergy, 2396·2
Zylol, 2396·2
Zyloprim, 2396·2
Zyloric, 2396·2
Zymacap, 2396·2
Zyma-D2, 2396·2
Zymaduo, 2396·2
Zymafluor, 2396·2
Zymafluor D, 2396·3
Zymamed, 2396·3
Zymar, 2396·3
Zymase, 2396·3
Zymelin, 2396·3
Zymerol, 2396·3
Zymine, 2396·3
Zymizinc, 2396·3
Zymonucléique, Acide, 172[illegible]
Zymoplex, 2396·3
Zynace, 2396·3
Zynal, 2396·3
Zynicor, 2396·3
Zynor, 2396·3
Zynox, 2396·3
Zyntabac, 2396·3
Zyomet, 2396·3
Zyplast, 2396·3
Zyplo, 2396·3
Zyprexa, 2396·3
Zyquin, 2396·4
Zyrantol, 2396·4
Zyrazine, 2396·4
Zyrcon, 2396·4
Zyrex, 2396·4
Zyrlex, 2396·4
Zyrtec Preparations, 2396·4
Zyrzine, 2396·4
Zytaz, 2396·4
Zytee, 2396·4
Zytine, 2396·4
Zytofen, 2396·4
Zytram, 2396·4
Zytrim, 2396·4
Zyvox, 2396·4
Zyvoxam, 2396·4
Zyvoxid, 2396·4